This book is due for return on or before the last date shown below.

PEDIATRIC
INFECTIOUS
DISEASES

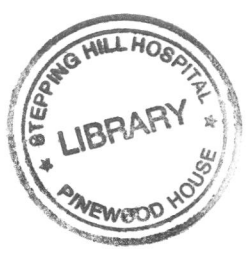

PRINCIPLES AND PRACTICE OF

PEDIATRIC
INFECTIOUS
DISEASES

FOURTH EDITION

Editor

Sarah S. Long, MD
Professor of Pediatrics
Drexel University College of Medicine
Chief, Section of Infectious Diseases
St. Christopher's Hospital for Children
Philadelphia, PA, USA

Associate Editors

Larry K. Pickering, MD
Senior Advisor to the Director
National Center for Immunization and Respiratory Diseases
Executive Secretary
Advisory Committee on Immunization Practices
Centers for Disease Control and Prevention
Professor of Pediatrics, Emory University School of Medicine
Atlanta, GA, USA

Charles G. Prober, MD
Professor of Pediatrics, Microbiology and Immunology
Senior Associate Dean, Medical Education
Stanford School of Medicine
Stanford, CA, USA

For additional online content visit expertconsult.com

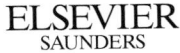

ELSEVIER
SAUNDERS

Edinburgh London New York Oxford Philadelphia St Louis Sydney Toronto

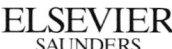

First edition 1997, Churchill Livingstone
Second edition 2003, Churchill Livingstone, an imprint of Elsevier Science
Third edition 2008, Churchill Livingstone

Chapters
1, 3, 6, 52, 54, 57, 58, 61, 91, 113, 158, 159, 169, 170, 174, 175, 178, 179, 213, 214, 215, 216, 217, 218, 219, 220, 229, 237, 239, 240, 241, 265, 271, 274, 278, 279, 281, 283 and 284 are in the public domain and may be used and reprinted without special permission; citation of the source, however, is appreciated.

Cover figure: Transmission electron micrograph of parainfluenza virus

British Library Cataloguing in Publication Data

Principles and practice of pediatric infectious diseases. –
4th ed.
1. Communicable diseases in children.
I. Long, Sarah S. II. Pickering, Larry K. III. Prober,
Charles G., 1949–
618.9'29-dc22

ISBN-13: 9781437727029

E-book ISBN: 9781437720594

Content Strategist: Belinda Kuhn
Content Development Specialist: Rachael Harrison
Content Coordinators: Alexandra Jones & Trinity Hutton
Project Managers: Joannah Duncan & Lucy Boon
Design: Charles Gray
Illustration Manager: Bruce Hogarth
Illustrator: Graeme Chambers
Marketing Managers (UK/USA): Gaynor Jones & Carla Holloway

Working together to grow
libraries in developing countries

www.elsevier.com | www.bookaid.org | www.sabre.org

ELSEVIER   BOOK AID International   Sabre Foundation

Printed in China
Last digit is the print number: 9 8 7 6 5 4 3 2 1

Preface

The field of infectious diseases is ever changing – with emerging pathogens, globalization, escalating antimicrobial resistance, novel diagnostic methods, expanding therapeutic options, and continuous development of vaccines and strategies for implementation. The landscape is increasingly complex – with deepening recognition of the role of infectious agents and the host in a damage–response framework of disease.

Our goal is to provide a comprehensive, reliable, up-to-date reference focused on evidence-based, practical information that is required to care for neonates, infants, children, and adolescents with any infectious disease. Entries always address the four imperatives of pediatric infectious diseases: understand the problem, diagnose the etiology, manage the patient to optimize outcome, and prevent a recurrence or first occurrence. The scope also includes epidemiology, control, and prevention of infectious diseases with guidance for establishing policy as well as managing individual patients. Features permeating the fourth edition include web-based resources, important contact information, and electronic links to primary literature to aid easy access to expanded, current information as well as to obtain restricted therapeutic agents or access to experts for management of rare diseases. New tables, figures, illustrated cases, scan- and slide-ready graphics and algorithms, and "Key Points" boxes of concise summaries have been added. New patient images and radiologic images have been added.

We have engaged subject-specific experts as authors and have edited all chapters to reflect a prescribed, predictable, and focused format that will reward the reader with answers to "What should I do next?" With a substantial number of authors from the Centers for Disease Control and Prevention, the American Academy of Pediatrics' Committee on Infectious Diseases and the Section on Infectious Diseases, the Pediatric Infectious Diseases Society and infection prevention advisory groups, we have attempted to present consistent recommendations and to build a compendium of best practices. Examples of new content are highlighted here, within the context of the four major sections of the book.

Part I. Understanding, Controlling, and Preventing Infectious Diseases: expanded primer in biostatistics; expanded use of immunoglobulin products; latest vaccines, schedule of immunizations, adverse event reporting; listings of resources in electronic, telephone, and paper media; newest recommendations for infection prevention for hospitals and offices; special considerations for children who have out-of-home care, are exposed to pets and exotic animals, are traveling, or are immigrating.

Part II. Clinical Syndromes and Cardinal Features of Infectious Diseases: Approach to Diagnosis and Initial Management: new content on conditions that mimic infectious diseases (such as hemophagocytic lymphohistiocytosis and macrophage activation syndrome); developmental stages of innate and adaptive immunity; mechanisms, clinical manifestations, and management strategies for systemic inflammatory response syndrome; recognizing and managing infections and risks due to congenital or acquired immunocompromising conditions in uniquely susceptible hosts; expanded content on central nervous system infectious and parainfectious conditions; new morbidities and evidence-based approaches to preventing healthcare-associated infections.

Part III. Etiologic Agents of Infectious Diseases: significant new entries related to antimicrobial resistance and therapies for bacterial infections, especially infections due to staphylococci, enterococci, pneumococci, gonococci, mycobacteria, and gram-negative bacilli; recently discovered viruses, new antiviral therapies, and new vaccines; evidence and guidance where evidence is incomplete for treatment of fungal infections; comprehensive and latest guidance for management of protozoal infections, including toxoplasmosis and malaria.

Part IV. Laboratory Diagnosis and Therapy of Infectious Diseases: through the burgeoning world of molecular diagnostics, the *best tests* for laboratory identification of infectious agents; *differentiating features* of commonly used laboratory tests to measure the inflammatory response and predict the cause; *new insights* into principles of use of anti-infective therapies; *expanded primer* on the pharmacodynamic basis of optimal use of antimicrobial agents; mechanisms and *best laboratory techniques* to detect newly emerging antimicrobial resistance; *new antimicrobial agents* for treating bacterial, fungal, viral, and parasitic infections.

The primary audience for our textbook is the subspecialist in infectious diseases who provides care for or advises on policy regarding infants, children, and adolescents. We hope that our book also will serve as a daily "consultant" for pediatricians and family physicians and a valuable resource for surgeons, clinical microbiologists, experts in infection control, health policy makers, and other health professionals who care for children.

Sarah S. Long
Larry K. Pickering
Charles G. Prober

Dedication and Acknowledgments

*With our families and other loved ones,
whose patience and endurance are our inspiration,*

We share the achievement of this book

*To our mentors and colleagues, who share
knowledge and stimulate learning,*

We give credit for the book's value

*To those who practice medicine as an art based on science,
and for the children whom they will serve,*

We offer the book's lessons

*To Bill and Melinda Gates
for their unprecedented contributions
to child health through eradication of infectious diseases worldwide*

We dedicate this book

With special contributions by James H. Brien, DO, Department of Pediatrics, Texas A & M University College of Medicine, Scott & White Memorial Hospital, Temple, Texas; and Eric N. Faerber, MD, Department of Radiology, Drexel University College of Medicine, St. Christopher's Hospital for Children, Philadelphia, Pennsylvania.

Contributors

Elisabeth E. Adderson, MD
Associate Professor of Pediatrics and
Molecular Sciences, University of
Tennessee Health Sciences Center;
Associate Member, Department of
Infectious Diseases, St. Jude Children's
Research Hospital, Memphis, Tennessee
*Infectious Complications of Antibody
Deficiency*

Aarti Agarwal, MD
Epidemic Intelligence Service Officer,
Malaria Branch, Division of Parasitic
Diseases and Malaria, Center for Global
Health, Centers for Disease Control and
Prevention, Atlanta, Georgia
Plasmodium *Species (Malaria)*

Grace M. Aldrovandi, MD, CM
Professor of Pediatrics, Pathology,
Molecular Microbiology & Immunology,
Departments of Pediatrics and Pathology,
Keck School of Medicine, Saban Research
Institute, University of Southern
California, Los Angeles, California
Immunopathogenesis of HIV-1 Infection

**Upton D. Allen, MBBS, MSc, FRCPC,
FRCP (UK)**
Professor of Pediatrics, Senior Associate
Scientist, Research Institute; Chief,
Division of Infectious Diseases,
Department of Pediatrics, Hospital for
Sick Children, University of Toronto,
Ontario, Canada
Adenoviruses

Manuel R. Amieva, MD, PhD
Assistant Professor of Pediatrics,
Microbiology & Immunology, Stanford
University School of Medicine; Attending
Physician, Division of Infectious Diseases,
Lucile Packard Children's Hospital,
Stanford, California
Campylobacter jejuni *and*
Campylobacter coli; *Other* Campylobacter
Species

Krow Ampofo, MB, ChB
Associate Professor, Department of
Pediatrics, University of Utah School of
Medicine; Attending Physician, Infectious
Diseases, Primary Children's Hospital,
Salt Lake City, Utah
Streptococcus pneumoniae

Alicia D. Anderson, DVM, MPH
Veterinary Epidemiologist, Rickettsial
Zoonoses Branch, Division of Vector-
Borne Diseases, National Center for
Emerging and Zoonotic Diseases, Centers
for Disease Control and Prevention,
Atlanta, Georgia
Coxiella burnetii *(Q fever)*

Margot Anderson, MD
Fellow, Section of Pediatric Infectious
Diseases, Department of Pediatrics,
Tulane University Medical Center,
New Orleans, Louisiana
Filoviruses and Arenaviruses

Paul M. Arguin, MD
Domestic Unit Chief, Malaria Branch,
Division of Parasitic Diseases and
Malaria, Center for Global Health,
Centers for Disease Control and
Prevention, Atlanta, Georgia
Plasmodium *Species (Malaria)*

John C. Arnold, MD
Staff, Pediatrics and Infectious Diseases,
Department of Pediatrics, Naval Medical
Center, San Diego, California
Pharyngitis; Streptococcus pyogenes
(Group A Streptococcus)

Ann M. Arvin, MD
Lucile Packard Professor of Pediatrics,
Professor of Microbiology and
Immunology, Stanford School of
Medicine; Chief, Division of Infectious
Diseases, Lucile Packard Children's
Hospital, Stanford, California
Varicella-Zoster Virus

Shai Ashkenazi, MD, MSc
The Pickel Chair for Pediatric Research,
Professor of Pediatrics, Sackler Faculty of
Medicine, Tel Aviv, Israel; Chairman,
Pediatrics, Schneider Children's Medical
Center, Petach Tikva, Israel
Plesiomonas shigelloides; Shigella *Species*

Carol J. Baker, MD
Professor of Pediatrics, Molecular
Virology and Microbiology, Baylor
College of Medicine; Attending Physician,
Infectious Diseases, Texas Children's
Hospital; Medical Director of Infection
Control, Woman's Hospital of Texas,
Houston, Texas
Bacterial Infections in the Neonate;
Streptococcus agalactiae *(Group B
Streptococcus)*

William J. Barson, MD
Professor of Pediatrics, The Ohio State
University College of Medicine and
Public Health; Attending Physician,
Section of Infectious Diseases,
Nationwide Children's Hospital,
Columbus, Ohio
Klebsiella *and* Raoultella *Species;* Proteus,
Providencia, *and* Morganella *Species*

Daniel G. Bausch, MD, MPH&TM
Associate Professor, Department of
Tropical Medicine, Tulane School of
Public Health and Tropical Medicine;
Clinical Associate Professor, Department
of Internal Medicine, Section of Adult
Infectious Diseases, Tulane University
Medical Center, New Orleans, Louisiana
Filoviruses and Arenaviruses

Kirsten Bechtel, MD
Associate Professor of Pediatrics
(Emergency Medicine), Yale University
School of Medicine, New Haven,
Connecticut
Infectious Diseases in Child Abuse

Daniel K. Benjamin, Jr, MD, PhD
Professor of Pediatrics, Duke University
School of Medicine; Faculty Associate
Director, Duke Clinical Research Institute,
Durham, North Carolina
*Necrotizing Enterocolitis; Clinical Approach
to the Infected Neonate*

Frank E. Berkowitz, MBBCh, MPH
Professor of Pediatrics, Emory University
School of Medicine, Atlanta, Georgia
Balantidium coli; Blastocystis *Species;*
Endolimax nana; Leishmania *Species
(Leishmaniasis);* Sarcocystis *Species;*
Trypanosoma *Species (Trypanosomiasis)*

Margaret J. Blythe, MD
Professor of Pediatrics, Adjunct Professor
of Gynecology, Indiana University School
of Medicine; Medical Director of the Teen
Care and Wellness Program, Wishard
Hospital Health Care Services,
Indianapolis, Indiana
Sexually Transmitted Infection Syndromes

Joseph A. Bocchini, Jr, MD
Professor, Chairman, Department of
Pediatrics, Louisiana State University
Health Science Center–Shreveport;
Medical Director, Children's Hospital,
Shreveport, Louisiana
Infections Related to Pets and Exotic Animals

Michael Boeckh, MD
Associate Professor of Medicine,
University of Washington School of
Medicine; Associate Member, Division of
Infectious Diseases, Fred Hutchinson
Cancer Research Center, Seattle,
Washington
BK, JC, and Other Human Polyomaviruses

Anna Bowen, MD, MPH
Medical Epidemiologist, Waterborne
Disease Prevention Branch, Division of
Foodborne, Waterborne, and
Environmental Diseases, National Center
for Emerging and Zoonotic Infectious
Diseases, Centers for Disease Control and
Prevention, Atlanta, Georgia
*Enteric Diseases Transmitted through Food,
Water, and Zoonotic Exposures*

William R. Bowie, MD, FRCPC
Professor of Medicine, Division of
Infectious Diseases, Department of
Medicine, University of British Columbia,
Vancouver, British Columbia
Epididymitis, Orchitis, and Prostatitis

Thomas G. Boyce, MD, MPH
Associate Professor of Pediatrics,
Department of Pediatric and Adolescent
Medicine, Division of Infectious Diseases,
Mayo Clinic, Rochester, Minnesota
*Otitis Externa and Necrotizing Otitis
Externa*

John S. Bradley, MD
Professor, Chief, Division of Infectious
Diseases, Department of Pediatrics,
University of California School of
Medicine; Director, Division of Infectious
Diseases, Rady Children's Hospital San
Diego, San Diego, California
*Chemoprophylaxis; Principles of Anti-
Infective Therapy; Antimicrobial Agents*

Michael T. Brady, MD
Professor and Chair, Department of
Pediatrics, The Ohio State University
College of Medicine; Physician-In-Chief,
Nationwide Children's Hospital,
Columbus, Ohio
*Less Commonly Encountered Nonenteric
Gram-Negative Bacilli; Eikenella,
Pasteurella, and Chromobacterium Species*

Denise F. Bratcher, DO
Professor of Pediatrics, University of
Missouri–Kansas City School of
Medicine; Attending Physician, Section of
Infectious Diseases; Pediatrics Residency
Program Director, Children's Mercy
Hospitals and Clinics, Kansas City,
Missouri
*Archanobacterium haemolyticum;
Bacillus Species (Anthrax); Other
Corynebacteria; Other Gram-Positive Bacilli*

Paula K. Braverman, MD
Professor of Clinical Pediatrics, University
of Cincinnati College of Medicine;
Attending Physician, Division of
Adolescent Medicine, Cincinnati
Children's Hospital Medical Center,
Cincinnati, Ohio
Urethritis, Vulvovaginitis, and Cervicitis

Caroline Breese Hall, MD
Professor of Pediatrics and Medicine,
University of Rochester School of
Medicine and Dentistry; Attending
Physician, Divisions of Infectious
Diseases in Pediatrics and Medicine,
University of Rochester Medical Center,
Rochester, New York
*Human Herpesviruses 6 and 7 (Roseola,
Exanthem Subitum); Human Herpesvirus 8
(Kaposi Sarcoma-Associated Herpesvirus)*

Joseph S. Bresee, MD
Chief, Epidemiology and Prevention
Branch, Influenza Division, National
Center for Immunizations and
Respiratory Diseases, Centers for Disease
Control and Prevention, Atlanta, Georgia
Viral Gastroenteritis; Astroviruses

Itzhak Brook, MD, MSc
Professor of Pediatrics, Georgetown
University School of Medicine; Attending
Physician, Georgetown University
Hospital, Washington, DC
*Anaerobic Bacteria: Classification, Normal
Flora, and Clinical Concepts; Clostridium
tetani (Tetanus); Other Clostridium
Species; Bacteroides and Prevotella Species
and Other Gram-Negative Bacilli*

Kristina Bryant, MD
Associate Professor, Department of
Pediatrics, University of Louisville School
of Medicine; Division of Infectious
Diseases, Kosair Children's Hospital,
Louisville, Kentucky
Tickborne Infections

E. Stephen Buescher, MD
Professor of Pediatrics, Eastern Virginia
Medical School; Attending Physician,
Division of Infectious Diseases,
Children's Hospital of The King's
Daughters, Norfolk, Virginia
*Evaluation of the Child with Suspected
Immunodeficiency; Infectious Complications
of Dysfunction or Deficiency of
Polymorphonuclear and Mononuclear
Phagocytes*

Jane L. Burns, MD
Professor of Pediatrics, University of
Washington School of Medicine;
Attending Physician, Division of
Infectious Diseases, Seattle Children's
Hospital, Seattle, Washington
*Infectious Complications in Special Hosts;
Pseudomonas Species and Related
Organisms; Burkholderia cepacia Complex
and Other Burkholderia Species;
Stenotrophomonas maltophilia*

Gale R. Burstein, MD, MPH
Associate Professor of Clinical Pediatrics,
University at Buffalo, The State University
of New York; Division of Adolescent
Medicine, Women and Children's
Hospital, Buffalo, New York
Sexually Transmitted Infection Syndromes

Carrie L. Byington, MD
H.A. and Edna Benning Presidential
Professor of Pediatrics, Vice Chair
Research Enterprise, Department of
Pediatrics, University of Utah School of
Medicine; Section of Infectious Diseases,
Primary Children's Hospital, Salt Lake
City, Utah
Streptococcus pneumoniae

Kathy K. Byrd, MD, MPH
Medical Epidemiologist, Prevention
Branch, Division of Viral Hepatitis,
National Center for HIV/AIDS, Viral
Hepatitis, STD, and TB Prevention,
Centers for Disease Control and
Prevention, Atlanta, Georgia
Hepatitis B and Hepatitis D Viruses

Michael Cappello, MD
Professor of Pediatrics, Microbial
Pathogenesis, and Public Health;
Director, Yale Program in International
Child Health, Yale University School of
Medicine, New Haven, Connecticut
*Intestinal Nematodes; Taenia solium,
Taenia asiatica, and Taenia saginata
(Taeniasis and Cysticercosis); Taenia
(Multiceps) multiceps and Taenia serialis
(Coenurosis)*

Bryan D. Carter, PhD
Professor of Child and Adolescent
Psychiatry, Associate Professor of
Pediatrics, University of Louisville School
of Medicine; Director, Pediatric
Consultation–Liaison Service, Kosair
Children's Hospital, Louisville, Kentucky
Chronic Fatigue Syndrome

Emily J. Cartwright, MD
Epidemic Intelligence Service Officer,
Division of Foodborne, Waterborne and
Environmental Diseases, National Center
for Emerging and Zoonotic Infectious
Diseases, Centers for Disease Control and
Prevention, Atlanta, Georgia
Other Vibrio Species

Mary T. Caserta, MD
Professor of Pediatrics, University of
Rochester School of Medicine and
Dentistry; Attending Physician, Division
of Pediatric Infectious Diseases,
University of Rochester Medical Center,
Rochester, New York
*Human Herpesviruses 6 and 7 (Roseola,
Exanthem Subitum); Human Herpesvirus 8
(Kaposi Sarcoma-Associated Herpesvirus)*

Chiara Cerini, MD
Fellow in Pediatrics, Luigi Sacco Hospital,
University of Milan School of Medicine,
Milan, Italy
Immunopathogenesis of HIV-1 Infection

Ellen Gould Chadwick, MD
Professor of Pediatrics, Feinberg School
of Medicine, Northwestern University;
Associate Director, Section of Pediatric
and Maternal HIV Infection, Division of
Infectious Diseases, Children's Memorial
Hospital, Chicago, Illinois
Nocardia Species

Beth Cheesebrough, MD
Specialist Registrar in Paediatrics, Ealing Hospital, Middlesex, United Kingdom
The Systemic Inflammatory Response Syndrome (SIRS), Sepsis, and Septic Shock

P. Joan Chesney, MD, CM
Professor of Pediatrics, University of Tennessee Health Sciences Center; Staff Physician, Pediatric Infectious Disease Section, Le Bonheur Children's Medical Center; Vice-President, Director, Office of Clinical Education and Training; Member, Department of Pediatric Infectious Diseases, St. Jude Children's Research Hospital, Memphis, Tennessee
Lymphatic System and Generalized Lymphadenopathy; Mediastinal and Hilar Lymphadenopathy

John C. Christenson, MD
Professor of Clinical Pediatrics, Indiana University School of Medicine; Director, Ryan White Center for Pediatric Infectious Disease; Director, Pediatric Travel Medicine Clinic, Riley Hospital for Children, Indianapolis, Indiana
Laboratory Diagnosis of Infection Due to Bacteria, Fungi, Parasites, and Rickettsiae

Thomas G. Cleary, MD
Professor, Center for Infectious Diseases, Division of Epidemiology, University of Texas School of Public Health, Houston, Texas
Shigella Species

Susan E. Coffin, MD, MPH
Associate Professor of Pediatrics, Division of Infectious Diseases, University of Pennsylvania School of Medicine; Hospital Epidemiologist and Medical Director, Infection Prevention and Control, Children's Hospital of Philadelphia, Philadelphia, Pennsylvania
Healthcare-Associated Infections

Laura M. Conklin, MD
Medical Officer, Division of Bacterial Diseases, Division of Emerging Infections and Surveillance Services, National Center for Preparedness, Detection and Control of Infectious Diseases, Centers for Disease Control and Prevention, Atlanta, Georgia
Chlamydophila (Chlamydia) psittaci (Psittacosis)

Laurie S. Conklin, MD
Assistant Professor of Pediatrics, George Washington University School of Medicine; Attending, Department of Gastroenterology, Hepatology, and Nutrition, Children's National Medical Center, Washington, DC
Acute Hepatitis

Beverly L. Connelly, MD
Professor of Pediatrics, University of Cincinnati College of Medicine; Director, Infection Control Program; Director, Infectious Diseases Training Program, Division of Infectious Diseases, Cincinnati Children's Hospital Medical Center, Cincinnati, Ohio
Granulomatous Hepatitis; Acute Pancreatitis; Cholecystitis and Cholangitis

Despina Contopoulos-Ioannidis, MD
Clinical Associate Professor, Division of Infectious Diseases and Geographic Medicine, Department of Medicine, Stanford University School of Medicine, Stanford, California
Toxoplasma gondii (Toxoplasmosis)

James H. Conway, MD, FAAP
Associate Professor of Pediatrics, University of Wisconsin School of Medicine & Public Health; Division of Pediatric Infectious Diseases, American Family Children's Hospital, Madison, Wisconsin
Mastoiditis

Margaret M. Cortese, MD
Captain, United States Public Health Service; Medical Epidemiologist, Division of Viral Diseases, National Center for Immunization and Respiratory Diseases, Centers for Disease Control and Prevention, Atlanta, Georgia
Rotaviruses

C. Michael Cotten, MD
Associate Professor of Pediatrics, Duke University School of Medicine; Director, Neonatology Clinical Research, Duke University Medical Center, Durham, North Carolina
Necrotizing Enterocolitis

Elaine Cox, MD
Assistant Clinical Professor of Pediatrics, Indiana University School of Medicine; Attending Physician, Section of Infectious Diseases, James Whitcomb Riley Hospital for Children, Indianapolis, Indiana
Agents of Eumycotic Mycetoma: Pseudallescheria boydii (Anamorph Scedosporium apiospermum)

Maryanne E. Crockett, MD, MPH, FRCPC, DTM&H
Assistant Professor, Pediatrics and Child Health, Medical Microbiology, University of Manitoba; Pediatric Infectious Diseases Consultant, Pediatrics and Child Health, Winnipeg Children's Hospital, Winnipeg, Canada
Protection of Travelers

James E. Crowe, Jr, MD
Ingram Professor of Cancer Research, Professor of Pediatrics, Microbiology and Immunology, and the Vanderbilt Vaccine Center, Vanderbilt University Medical Center, Nashville, Tennessee
Human Metapneumovirus

Nigel Curtis, FRCPH, PhD
Professor, Department of Paediatrics, The University of Melbourne; Head, Infectious Diseases Unit, Department of General Medicine, Murdoch Children's Research Institute, Royal Children's Hospital Melbourne, Parkville, Australia
Infections Related to the Upper and Middle Airways; Mycobacterium Species Non-tuberculosis

Dennis J. Cunningham, MD
Associate Professor of Pediatrics, The Ohio State University College of Medicine; Medical Director, Epidemiology; Attending Physician, Section of Infectious Diseases, Nationwide Children's Hospital, Columbus, Ohio
Enterobacter, Cronobacter, and Pantoea Species

Linda Marie Dairiki Shortliffe, MD
Stanley McCormick Memorial Professor, Department of Urology, Lucile Packard Children's Hospital, Stanford University School of Medicine, Stanford, California
Urinary Tract Infections; Renal Abscess and Other Complex Renal Infections

Toni Darville, MD
Carol Ann Craumer Professor of Pediatrics and Immunology, University of Pittsburgh School of Medicine; Chief of Infectious Diseases, Children's Hospital of Pittsburgh of UPMC, Pittsburgh, Pennsylvania
Chlamydia trachomatis

Gregory A. Dasch, PhD
Rickettsial Team Leader, Rickettsial Zoonoses Branch, Division of Vector-Borne Diseases, National Center for Emerging and Zoonotic Infectious Diseases, Centers for Disease Control and Prevention, Atlanta, Georgia
Other Rickettsia Species

Irini Daskalaki, MD
Assistant Professor of Pediatrics, Drexel University College of Medicine; Attending Physician, St. Christopher's Hospital for Children, Philadelphia, Pennsylvania
Corynebacterium diphtheriae

Robert S. Daum, MD
Professor of Pediatrics, Microbiology and Molecular Medicine, University of Chicago; Attending Physician, Department of Pediatrics, University of Chicago Comer Children's Hospital, Chicago, Illinois
Staphylococcus aureus

Fatimah S. Dawood, MD
Medical Officer, Influenza Division, National Center for Immunization and Respiratory Diseases, Centers for Disease Control and Prevention, Atlanta, Georgia
Influenza Viruses

Gail J. Demmler, MD
Professor of Pediatrics, Baylor College of Medicine; Attending Physician, Division of Infectious Diseases; Director of Diagnostic Virology Laboratory, Texas Children's Hospital, Houston, Texas
Adenoviruses

Dickson D. Despommier, PhD
Emeritus Professor of Public Health and Microbiology, Columbia University, New York, New York
Tissue Nematodes

Karen A. Diefenbach, MD
Assistant Professor of Surgery, Yale University School of Medicine; Attending Physician, Division of Pediatric Surgery, Children's Hospital at Yale-New Haven, New Haven, Connecticut
Intra-Abdominal, Visceral, and Retroperitoneal Abscesses

Christopher C. Dvorak, MD
Assistant Professor of Clinical Pediatrics, University of California, San Francisco School of Medicine; Attending Physician, Division of Pediatric Blood and Marrow Transplantation, UCSF Benioff Children's Hospital, San Francisco, California
Antifungal Agents

Kathryn M. Edwards, MD
Sarah H. Sell and Cornelius Vanderbilt Chair in Pediatrics, Department of Pediatrics, Vanderbilt University; Attending Physician, Division of Infectious Diseases, Vanderbilt Children's Hospital, Nashville, Tennessee
Prolonged, Recurrent and Periodic Fever Syndromes; Bordetella pertussis *(Pertussis) and Other* Bordetella *Species*

Morven S. Edwards, MD
Professor of Pediatrics, Baylor College of Medicine; Attending Physician, Infectious Diseases, Texas Children's Hospital, Houston, Texas
Bacterial Infections in the Neonate; Streptococcus agalactiae *(Group B Streptococcus)*

Lawrence F. Eichenfield, MD
Professor of Clinical Pediatrics and Medicine (Dermatology), University of California San Diego School of Medicine; Chief, Pediatric & Adolescent Dermatology; Medical Director of Research, Children's Hospital, San Diego, California
Purpura

Dirk M. Elston, MD, FAAD
Director, Department of Dermatology, Geisinger Medical Center, Danville, Pennsylvania
Ectoparasites (Lice and Scabies)

Janet A. Englund, MD
Professor, Department of Pediatrics, University of Washington School of Medicine; Attending Physician, Seattle Children's Hospital; Clinical Associate, Fred Hutchinson Cancer Research Center, Seattle, Washington
Infectious Complications in Special Hosts

Veronique Erard, MD, MSc
Clinic of Medicine, Infectious Diseases, Hôpital Cantonal Fribourg, Fribourg, Switzerland
BK, JC, and Other Human Polyomaviruses

Marina E. Eremeeva, MD, PhD, ScD
Senior Service Fellow, Rickettsial Zoonoses Branch, Division of Vector-Borne Diseases, National Center for Emerging and Zoonotic Infectious Diseases, Centers for Disease Control and Prevention, Atlanta, Georgia
Other Rickettsia *Species*

Anat R. Feingold, MD
Assistant Professor of Clinical Pediatrics, UMDNJ-Robert Wood Johnson Medical School at Camden; Chief, Division of Pediatric Infectious Diseases, Cooper University Hospital, Camden, New Jersey
Anaerobic Cocci; Anaerobic Gram-Positive, Nonsporulating Bacilli (including Actinomycosis)

Adam Finn, MA, BM, BCh, PhD, FRCP, FRCPCH
David Baum Professor of Paediatrics, Schools of Clinical Sciences & Cellular & Molecular Medicine, University of Bristol; Honorary Consultant Paediatrician, Bristol Royal Hospital for Children, Bristol, United Kingdom
Neisseria meningitidis

Anthony E. Fiore, MD, MPH
Associate Director for Science, Division of Parasitic Diseases and Malaria, Center for Global Health, Centers for Disease Control and Prevention, Atlanta, Georgia
Influenza Viruses

Marc Fischer, MD, MPH
Medical Epidemiologist, Arboviral Diseases Branch, Division of Vector-Borne Diseases, National Center for Emerging and Zoonotic Infectious Diseases, Centers for Disease Control and Prevention, Fort Collins, Colorado
Coltivirus (Colorado Tick Fever); Flaviviruses

Sarah J. Fitch, MD
Attending Physician, Department of Radiology, Virginia Commonwealth University; Main Hospital of the Medical College of Virginia, Richmond, Virginia
Mediastinal and Hilar Lymphadenopathy

Patricia M. Flynn, MD, MS
Professor of Pediatrics and Preventive Medicine, University of Tennessee Health Science Center; Member, Department of Infectious Diseases, St. Jude Children's Research Hospital, Memphis, Tennessee
Cryptosporidium *Species; Cystoisospora (Isospora) and Cyclospora Species; Microsporidia*

LeAnne M. Fox, MD, MPH, DTM&H
Division of Parasitic Diseases and Malaria, Center for Global Health, Centers for Disease Control and Prevention, Atlanta, Georgia
Blood and Tissue Nematodes (Filarial Worms); Intestinal Trematodes

Michael M. Frank, MD
Samuel L. Katz Professor of Pediatrics, Professor of Medicine and Immunology, Duke University Medical Center, Durham, North Carolina
Infectious Complications of Complement Deficiencies

Douglas R. Fredrick, MD
Clinical Professor of Ophthalmology and Pediatrics, Stanford University School of Medicine, Stanford, California
Conjunctivitis in the Neonatal Period (Ophthalmia Neonatorum); Conjunctivitis beyond the Neonatal Period; Infective Keratitis; Uveitis, Retinitis, and Chorioretinitis; Endophthalmitis

Sheila Fallon Friedlander, MD
Professor of Clinical Pediatrics and Medicine, University of California School of Medicine; Chief, Section of Dermatology, Rady Children's Hospital, San Diego, California
Subcutaneous Tissue Infections and Abscesses; Dermatophytes and Other Superficial Fungi

Hayley A. Gans, MD
Assistant Professor of Pediatrics, Stanford University School of Medicine; Attending Physician, Division of Infectious Diseases, Lucile Packard Children's Hospital, Stanford, California
Hemophagocytic Lymphohistiocytosis and Macrophage Activation Syndrome

Carla G. Garcia, MD
Assistant Professor of Pediatrics, University of Texas Southwestern Medical Center at Dallas; Attending Physician, Division of Pediatric Infectious Diseases, Children's Medical Center at Dallas, Dallas, Texas
Acute Bacterial Meningitis beyond the Neonatal Period

Maria C. Garzon, MD
Professor of Clinical Dermatology and Clinical Pediatrics, Columbia University; Director, Division of Dermatology, The University Hospital of Columbia and Cornell, New York, New York
Papules, Nodules, and Ulcers

Jeffrey S. Gerber, MD, PhD, MSCE
Attending Physician, Division of
Infectious Diseases, The Children's
Hospital of Philadelphia, Philadelphia,
Pennsylvania
*Clinical Syndromes of Device-Associated
Infections*

Michael D. Geschwind, MD, PhD
Associate Professor of Neurology,
University of California San Francisco;
Michael J. Homer Chair in Neurology,
University of California San Francisco;
Department of Neurology, Memory &
Aging Center, San Francisco, California
Prion Diseases

Laura B. Gieraltowski, PhD, MPH
Lieutenant, U.S. Public Health Service;
Epidemic Intelligence Service Officer,
Enteric Diseases Epidemiology Branch,
Division of Foodborne, Waterborne, and
Environmental Diseases, National Center
for Emerging and Zoonotic Infectious
Diseases, Centers for Disease Control and
Prevention, Atlanta, Georgia
*Enteric Diseases Transmitted through Food,
Water, and Zoonotic Exposures*

Francis Gigliotti, MD
Professor of Pediatrics, Microbiology and
Immunology, Associate Chair of
Pediatrics for Academic Affairs,
University of Rochester School of
Medicine and Dentistry; Chief, Division
of Infectious Diseases, Golisano
Children's Hospital at Strong, Rochester,
New York
Pneumocystis jirovecii

Peter H. Gilligan, PhD
Professor of Microbiology, Immunology
and Pathology, Laboratory Medicine,
University of North Carolina School of
Medicine; Director, Clinical
Microbiology-Immunology Laboratories,
University of North Carolina Hospitals,
Chapel Hill, North Carolina
*Mechanisms and Detection of Antimicrobial
Resistance*

Carol Glaser, DVM, MD
Chief, Encephalitis and Special
Investigations Section, Division of
Communicable Disease Control,
California Department of Public Health;
Associate Clinical Professor of Pediatrics,
Infectious Disease, Department of
Pediatrics, University of California, San
Francisco, California
*Encephalitis; Para- and Postinfectious
Neurologic Syndromes*

Benjamin D. Gold, MD
Children's Center for Digestive
Healthcare, LLC Pediatric
Gastroenterology; Hepatology and
Nutrition, Children's Healthcare of
Atlanta; Guest Research Scientist,
Helicobacter Laboratory, Centers for
Disease Control and Prevention, Atlanta,
Georgia
*Helicobacter pylori; Other Gastric and
Enterohepatic Helicobacter Species*

Brahm Goldstein, MD, MCR
Senior Medical Director, Clinical
Research, Ikaria, Inc., Hampton, New
Jersey
*The Systemic Inflammatory Response
Syndrome (SIRS), Sepsis, and Septic Shock*

Jane M. Gould, MD
Assistant Professor of Pediatrics, Drexel
University College of Medicine; Attending
Physician, Section of Infectious Diseases,
St. Christopher's Hospital for Children,
Philadelphia, Pennsylvania
*Infection following Burns; Topical
Antimicrobial Agents*

Michael Green, MD, MPH
Professor of Pediatrics, Surgery, Clinical
and Translational Science, University of
Pittsburgh School of Medicine; Attending
Physician, Division of Infectious Diseases,
Children's Hospital of Pittsburgh,
Pittsburgh, Pennsylvania
*Infections in Solid Organ Transplant
Recipients*

David Greenberg, MD
Associate Professor of Pediatrics and
Infectious Diseases, Soroka University
Medical Center; Faculty of Health
Sciences, Ben-Gurion University of the
Negev, Beer-Sheva, Israel
*Moraxella and Psychrobacter Species;
Kingella Species*

Patricia M. Griffin, MD
Chief, Enteric Diseases Epidemiology
Branch, Division of Foodborne,
Waterborne, and Environmental Diseases,
National Center for Emerging and
Zoonotic Infectious Diseases, Centers for
Disease Control and Prevention, Atlanta,
Georgia
Other Vibrio Species

Alexei A. Grom, MD
Associate Professor of Pediatrics,
University of Cincinnati College of
Medicine; Attending Physician, Division
of Rheumatology, Cincinnati Children's
Hospital Medical Center, Cincinnati,
Ohio
Fever and the Inflammatory Response

Kathleen Gutierrez, MD
Associate Professor of Pediatrics, Stanford
School of Medicine; Attending Physician,
Division of Infectious Diseases, Lucile
Packard Children's Hospital, Stanford,
California
*Musculoskeletal Symptom Complexes;
Osteomyelitis; Infectious and Inflammatory
Arthritis; Diskitis; Transient Synovitis;
Mumps Virus*

Judith A. Guzman-Cottrill, DO
Assistant Professor of Pediatrics, Oregon
Health and Science University; Attending
Physician, Division of Infectious Diseases,
Doernbecher Children's Hospital,
Portland, Oregon
*The Systemic Inflammatory Response
Syndrome (SIRS), Sepsis, and Septic Shock*

Aron J. Hall, DVM, MSPH, DACVPM
Epidemiologist, Division of Viral
Diseases, National Center for
Immunization and Respiratory Diseases,
Centers for Disease Control and
Prevention, Atlanta, Georgia
*Enteric Diseases Transmitted through Food,
Water, and Zoonotic Exposures; Caliciviruses*

Marvin B. Harper, MD
Associate Professor of Pediatrics, Harvard
Medical School; Senior Associate in
Medicine, Division of Infectious Diseases
and Division of Emergency Medicine,
Children's Hospital Boston, Boston,
Massachusetts
*Pneumonia in the Immunocompromised
Host; Infection following Bites*

Christopher J. Harrison, MD
Professor of Pediatrics, University of
Missouri – Kansas City; Director of
Infectious Diseases Laboratory, Children's
Mercy Hospitals and Clinics, Kansas City,
Missouri
*Chronic Meningitis; Recurrent Meningitis;
Focal Suppurative Infections of the Nervous
System*

David B. Haslam, MD
Associate Professor of Pediatrics and
Molecular Microbiology, Washington
University School of Medicine; Attending
Physician, Division of Infectious Diseases,
St. Louis Children's Hospital, St. Louis,
Missouri
*Classification of Streptococci; Enterococcus
Species; Viridans Streptococci, Abiotrophia
and Granulicatella Species, and
Streptococcus bovis; Groups C and G
Streptococci; Other Gram-Positive, Catalase-
Negative Cocci*

Sarah J. Hawkes, MBBS, PhD
Reader in Global Health, Institute of
Global Health, University College
London, London, United Kingdom
Treponema pallidum (Syphilis)

Edward B. Hayes, MD
Research Professor, Barcelona Centre for
International Health Research, Barcelona,
Spain
Togaviridae: Alphaviruses; Flaviviruses

Rohan Hazra, MD
Medical Officer, Pediatric Adolescent
Maternal AIDS (PAMA) Branch, Eunice
Kennedy Shriver National Institute of
Child Health and Human Development,
National Institutes of Health, Bethesda,
Maryland
Management of HIV Infection

Sara Jane Heilig, MD
Resident in Dermatology, Department of
Dermatology, Penn State/M.S. Hershey
Medical Center, Hershey, Pennsylvania
Erythematous Macules and Papules

J. Owen Hendley, MD
Professor of Pediatrics, University of
Virginia School of Medicine; Attending
Physician, Division of Pediatric Infectious
Disease, University of Virginia Health
System, Charlottesville, Virginia
The Common Cold; Rhinoviruses

Marion C.W. Henry, MD, MPH
Fellow, Department of Pediatric Surgery,
Children's National Medical Center,
Washington DC
Appendicitis

Joseph A. Hilinski, MD
Assistant Professor of Pediatrics, Emory
University School of Medicine, Children's
Healthcare of Atlanta; Division of
Pediatric Infectious Diseases,
Epidemiology, and Immunology, Emory
Children's Center, Atlanta, Georgia
Myocarditis; Pericarditis

Scott D. Holmberg, MD, MPH
Chief, Epidemiology & Surveillance
Branch, Division of Viral Hepatitis,
National Center for HIV/AIDS, Viral
Hepatitis, STD, and TB Prevention,
Centers for Disease Control and
Prevention, Atlanta, Georgia
Hepatitis C Virus

Deborah Holtzman, PhD
Associate Director for Science, Division of
Viral Hepatitis, National Center for HIV/
AIDS, Viral Hepatitis, STD, and TB
Prevention, Centers for Disease Control
and Prevention, Atlanta, Georgia
Hepatitis C Virus

Peter J. Hotez, MD, PhD
Dean, National School of Tropical
Medicine, Baylor College of Medicine;
Professor, Pediatrics and Molecular &
Virology and Microbiology, Endowed
Chair of Tropical Pediatrics; Head,
Section of Pediatric Tropical Medicine,
Texas Children's Hospital; Director,
Center for Vaccine Development;
President, Sabin Vaccine Institute;
President, American Society of Tropical
Medicine & Hygiene; Co-Editor-in-Chief,
PLoS Neglected Tropical Diseases, Feigin
Center, Houston, Texas
*Classification of Parasites; Intestinal
Nematodes; Tissue Nematodes*

Katherine K. Hsu, MD, MPH
Assistant Professor of Pediatrics, Boston
University Medical Center; Medical
Director, Division of STD Prevention &
HIV/AIDS Surveillance, Massachusetts
Department of Public Health, Boston,
Massachusetts
*Neisseria gonorrhoeae; Other Neisseria
Species*

Dale J. Hu, MD, MPH
Epidemiology Research Team Leader,
Division of Viral Hepatitis, National
Center for HIV/AIDS, Viral Hepatitis,
STD, and TB Prevention, Centers for
Disease Control and Prevention, Atlanta,
Georgia
Hepatitis B and Hepatitis D Viruses

Loris Y. Hwang, MD
Assistant Professor of Pediatrics and
Adolescent Medicine, University of
California San Francisco School of
Medicine, San Francisco, California
Human Papillomaviruses

David Y. Hyun, MD
Assistant Professor of Pediatrics, George
Washington University School of
Medicine; Attending Physician,
Children's National Medical Center,
Washington, DC
Clostridium difficile

Mary Anne Jackson, MD
Professor of Pediatrics, University of
Missouri, Kansas City School of
Medicine; Chief, Section of Infectious
Diseases, Children's Mercy Hospitals and
Clinics, Kansas City, Missouri
*Lymphatic System and Generalized
Lymphadenopathy; Mediastinal and Hilar
Lymphadenopathy; Abdominal and
Retroperitoneal Lymphadenopathy; Localized
Lymphadenitis, Lymphadenopathy, and
Lymphangitis*

Richard F. Jacobs, MD
Robert H. Fiser, Jr, M.D. Endowed Chair
in Pediatrics, Professor and Chairman,
Department of Pediatrics, University of
Arkansas for Medical Sciences; President,
Arkansas Children's Hospital Research
Institute; Attending Physician, Pediatric
Infectious Diseases, Arkansas Children's
Hospital, Little Rock, Arkansas
Bartonella Species (Cat-Scratch Disease)

Jeffrey L. Jones, MD, MPH
Medical Epidemiologist, Division of
Parasitic Diseases and Malaria, Center for
Global Health, Centers for Disease
Control and Prevention, Atlanta, Georgia
*Clonorchis, Opisthorchis, Fasciola, and
Paragonimus Species*

Saleem Kamili, PhD
Chief, Assay Development and Diagnostic
Reference Laboratory, Division of Viral
Hepatitis, National Center for HIV/AIDS,
Viral Hepatitis, STD, and TB Prevention,
Centers for Disease Control and
Prevention, Atlanta, Georgia
Hepatitis E Virus

M. Gary Karlowicz, MD
Professor of Pediatrics, Eastern Virginia
Medical School; Attending Physician,
Division of Neonatal-Perinatal Medicine,
Children's Hospital of The King's
Daughters, Norfolk, Virginia
Hospital-Associated Infections in the Neonate

Ben Z. Katz, MD
Professor of Pediatrics, Northwestern
University Feinberg School of Medicine;
Attending Physician, Division of
Infectious Diseases, Children's Memorial
Hospital, Chicago, Illinois
*Epstein–Barr Virus (Mononucleosis and
Lymphoproliferative Disorders)*

Gilbert J. Kersh, PhD
Senior Service Fellow, Rickettsial
Zoonoses Branch, Division of Vector-
Borne Diseases, National Center for
Emerging and Zoonotic Infectious
Diseases, Centers for Disease Control and
Prevention, Atlanta, Georgia
Coxiella burnetii (Q fever)

Laura M. Kester, MD
Fellow in Adolescent Medicine,
Department of Pediatrics, Indiana
University School of Medicine, James
Whitcomb Riley Hospital, Indianapolis,
Indiana
Sexually Transmitted Infection Syndromes

**Jay S. Keystone, MD, MSc(CTM),
FRCPC(C)**
Professor of Medicine, University of
Toronto; Staff Physician, Tropical Disease
Unit, Department of Medicine, Division
of Infectious Disease, Toronto General
Hospital, University Health Network,
Toronto, Ontario, Canada
Protection of Travelers

David W. Kimberlin, MD
Professor of Pediatrics, University of
Alabama at Birmingham; Division of
Pediatric Infectious Diseases, Children's
Hospital, Birmingham, Alabama
Antiviral Agents

Martin B. Kleiman, MD
Ryan White Professor of Pediatrics
(emeritus), Indiana University School of
Medicine; Director, Infection Control,
James Whitcomb Riley Hospital for
Children, Indianapolis, Indiana
*Classification of Fungi; Histoplasma
capsulatum (Histoplasmosis); Blastomyces
dermatitidis (Blastomycosis); Coccidioides
immitis and Coccidioides posadasii
(Coccidiomycosis); Agents of Eumycotic
Mycetoma: Pseudallescheria boydii
(Anamorph Scedosporium apiospermum)*

Mark W. Kline, MD
J.S. Abercrombie Professor and
Chairman, Department of Pediatrics,
Baylor College of Medicine; Physician-in-
Chief, Texas Children's Hospital,
Houston, Texas
*Diagnosis and Clinical Manifestations of
HIV Infection; Infectious Complications of
HIV Infection*

Andrew Y. Koh, MD
Assistant Professor, Department of Pediatrics (Hematology/Oncology and Infectious Diseases) and Microbiology, University of Texas Southwestern Medical Center; Director of Pediatric Hematopoietic Stem Cell Transplantation, Children's Medical Center Dallas, Dallas, Texas
Fever and Granulocytopenia; Infections in Children with Cancer

Andreas Konstantopoulos, MD
Professor of Pediatrics, University of Athens; President of European Pediatric Association (EPA); President-elect of International Pediatric Association (IPA), Athens, Greece
Giardia intestinalis *(Giardiasis)*

Katalin I. Koranyi, MD
Professor of Clinical Pediatrics, The Ohio State University College of Medicine and Public Health; Attending Physician, Section of Infectious Diseases, Nationwide Children's Hospital, Columbus, Ohio
Less Commonly Encountered Enterobacteriaceae

E. Kent Korgenski, MS, MT
Microbiology Technical Supervisor, Microbiology Laboratory, Primary Children's Medical Center, Salt Lake City, Utah
Laboratory Diagnosis of Infection Due to Bacteria, Fungi, Parasites, and Rickettsiae

Andrew T. Kroger, MD, MPH
Medical Officer, National Center for Immunization and Respiratory Diseases, Centers for Disease Control and Prevention, Atlanta, Georgia
Active Immunization

Paul Krogstad, MD
Professor, Departments of Pediatrics and Molecular and Medical Pharmacology, David Geffen School of Medicine at UCLA Los Angeles, California
Diagnosis and Clinical Manifestations of HIV Infection

Christine T. Lauren, MD
Assistant Professor of Clinical Dermatology and Clinical Pediatrics, Columbia University Medical Center, New York, New York
Papules, Nodules, and Ulcers

Hillary S. Lawrence, MD
Department of Dermatology, University of Kansas Medical Center, Kansas City, Kansas
Superficial Bacterial Skin Infections and Cellulitis

Eugene Leibovitz, MD
Pediatric Infectious Diseases Unit, Soroka University Medical Center; Department of Pediatrics, Ben-Gurion University of the Negev, Beer-Sheva, Israel
Moraxella *and* Psychrobacter *Species*

Stéphanie Levasseur, MD
Assistant Professor of Clinical Pediatrics; Division of Pediatric Cardiology, Columbia University Medical Center, New York, New York
Endocarditis and Other Intravascular Infections

David B. Lewis, MD
Professor of Pediatrics, Stanford University School of Medicine; Attending Physician in Immunology and Infectious Diseases, Lucile Packard Children's Hospital; Institute for Immunity, Transplantation, and Infectious Disease; Interdepartmental Program in Immunology, Stanford University, Stanford, California
Hemophagocytic Lymphohistiocytosis and Macrophage Activation Syndrome; Infectious Complications of Cell-Mediated Immune Deficiency Other than AIDS: Primary Immunodeficiencies

Jay M. Lieberman, MD
Medical Director, Infectious Diseases, Focus and Quest Diagnostics, Nichols Institute, Cypress, California
Neisseria gonorrhoeae; *Other* Neisseria *Species*

Jen-Jane Liu, MD
Chief Resident in Urology, Lucile Packard Children's Hospital, Stanford University School of Medicine, Stanford, California
Urinary Tract Infections; Renal Abscess and Other Complex Renal Infections

Robyn A. Livingston, MD
Assistant Professor of Pediatrics, University of Missouri at Kansas City; Director of Infection Prevention and Control, Attending Physician in Pediatric Infectious Diseases, Children's Mercy Hospital and Clinics, Kansas City, Missouri
Recurrent Meningitis

Eloisa Llata, MD, MPH
Medical Epidemiologist, Epidemiology and Surveillance Branch, Division of STD Prevention, National Center for HIV/AIDS, Viral Hepatitis, STD, and TB Prevention, Centers for Disease Control and Prevention, Atlanta, Georgia
Pelvic Inflammatory Disease

Anagha R. Loharikar, MD
Epidemic Intelligence Service Officer, Division of Foodborne, Waterborne and Environmental Diseases, National Center for Emerging and Zoonotic Infectious Diseases, Centers for Disease Control and Prevention, Atlanta, Georgia
Vibrio cholerae *(Cholera)*

Sarah S. Long, MD
Professor of Pediatrics, Drexel University College of Medicine; Chief, Section of Infectious Diseases, St. Christopher's Hospital for Children, Philadelphia, Pennsylvania
Mucocutaneous Symptom Complexes; Prolonged, Recurrent and Periodic Fever Syndromes; Respiratory Tract Symptom Complexes; Encephalitis; Bordetella pertussis *(Pertussis) and Other* Bordetella *Species; Anaerobic Bacteria: Classification, Normal Flora, and Clinical Concepts;* Clostridium botulinum *(Botulism); Laboratory Manifestations of Infectious Diseases; Principles of Anti-Infective Therapy*

Ben A. Lopman, MSc, PhD
Epidemiology Branch, Division of Viral Diseases, National Center for Immunizations and Respiratory Diseases, Centers for Disease Control and Prevention, Atlanta, Georgia
Viral Gastroenteritis

Bennett Lorber, MD, DSc(hon)
Thomas M. Durant Professor of Medicine, Temple University School of Medicine; Attending Physician, Infectious Diseases; Temple University Hospital, Philadelphia, Pennsylvania
Listeria monocytogenes

Donald E. Low, MD, FRCPC
Professor, Department of Laboratory Medicine and Pathobiology, Department of Medicine, University of Toronto; Microbiologist-in-Chief, University Health Network/Mount Sinai Hospital, Toronto, Ontario, Canada
Myositis, Pyomyositis, and Necrotizing Fasciitis

Yalda C. Lucero, MD, PhD
Assistant Professor of Pediatrics, Faculty of Medicine, University of Chile, Santiago, Chile
Aeromonas *Species*

Jorge Luján-Zilbermann, MD
Associate Professor of Pediatrics, University of South Florida College of Medicine; Attending Physician, Division of Infectious Diseases, All Children's Hospital, St. Petersburg; Attending Physician, Tampa General Hospital; Attending Physician, St. Joseph's Children's Hospital, Tampa, Florida
Infections in Hematopoietic Stem Cell Transplant Recipients

Katherine Luzuriaga, MD
Professor of Pediatrics, Division of Immunology and Infectious Diseases, University of Massachusetts Medical School, Worcester, Massachusetts
Introduction to Retroviridae; Human T-Cell Lymphotropic Viruses; Human Immunodeficiency Viruses

Noni E. MacDonald, MD, MSc, FRCPC
Professor of Pediatrics, Dalhousie University; Attending Physician, Division of Infectious Diseases, Department of Pediatrics, IWK Health Centre; Head, Health and Policy and Translation Group, Canadian Centre for Vaccinology, Halifax, Canada
Epididymitis, Orchitis, and Prostatitis

Adam MacNeil, PhD, MPH
Epidemiologist, Viral Special Pathogens Branch, Division of High-Consequence Pathogens and Pathology, National Center for Emerging and Zoonotic Infectious Diseases, Centers for Disease Control and Prevention, Atlanta, Georgia
Bunyaviruses

Yvonne A. Maldonado, MD
Professor, Department of Pediatrics, Stanford School of Medicine; Chief, Division of Infectious Diseases, Lucille Packard Children's Hospital; Professor, Health Research and Policy, Stanford School of Medicine, Stanford, California
Rubella Virus; Rubeola Virus (Measles and Subacute Sclerosing Panencephalitis); Polioviruses

Chitra S. Mani, MBBS, DCH
Associate Professor of Pediatrics, Medical College of Georgia; Attending Physician, Division of Infectious Diseases, Associate Hospital Epidemiologist, Children's Medical Center, Augusta, Georgia
Acute Pneumonia and Its Complications; Persistent and Recurrent Pneumonia

Mario J. Marcon, PhD
Clinical Associate Professor of Pathology and Pediatrics, The Ohio State University College of Medicine and Public Health; Director, Clinical/Molecular Microbiology and Immunodiagnostics, Department of Laboratory Medicine, Nationwide Children's Hospital, Columbus, Ohio
Klebsiella and Raoultella Species; Enterobacter, Cronobacter, and Pantoea Species; Citrobacter Species; Less Commonly Encountered Enterobacteriaceae; Proteus, Providencia, and Morganella Species; Serratia Species; Acinetobacter Species; Less Commonly Encountered Nonenteric Gram-Negative Bacilli; Eikenella, Pasteurella, and Chromobacterium Species

Gary S. Marshall, MD
Professor of Pediatrics, University of Louisville School of Medicine; Chief, Division of Pediatric Infectious Diseases, Kosair Children's Hospital, Louisville, Kentucky
Chronic Fatigue Syndrome

Stacey W. Martin, MSc
Epidemiologist and Statistician, Meningitis and Vaccine Preventable Diseases Branch, Division of Bacterial Diseases, National Center for Immunization and Respiratory Diseases, Centers for Disease Control and Prevention, Atlanta, Georgia
Principles of Epidemiology and Public Health

Catalina Matiz, MD
Resident in Dermatology, University of California San Diego School of Medicine, San Diego, California
Subcutaneous Tissue Infections and Abscesses

Alison C. Mawle, PhD
Associate Director for Laboratory Science, National Center for Immunization and Respiratory Diseases, Centers for Disease Control and Prevention, Atlanta, Georgia
Active Immunization

Tony Mazzulli, MD, FRCPC, FACP
Professor, Department of Laboratory Medicine and Pathobiology, University of Toronto; Deputy Chief Microbiologist, Mount Sinai Hospital and University Health Network, Toronto, Ontario, Canada
Laboratory Diagnosis of Infection Due to Viruses, Chlamydia, Chlamydophila, *and* Mycoplasma

George H. McCracken, Jr, MD
Professor of Pediatrics, GlaxoSmithKline Distinguished Professor of Pediatric Infectious Disease, Department of Pediatrics, University of Texas Southwestern Medical Center at Dallas; Attending Physician, Children's Medical Center of Dallas, Dallas, Texas
Acute Bacterial Meningitis beyond the Neonatal Period

Matthew B. McDonald, III, MD
Assistant Professor of Pediatrics, Drexel University College of Medicine; Attending Physician in Pediatrics, St. Christopher's Hospital for Children, Philadelphia, Pennsylvania
Abdominal Symptom Complexes

Robert S. McGregor, MD
Professor of Pediatrics, Interim Chair, Department of Pediatrics, Drexel University College of Medicine; Residency Program Director, Attending Physician in Pediatrics, St. Christopher's Hospital for Children, Philadelphia, Pennsylvania
Abdominal Symptom Complexes

Kenneth McIntosh, MD
Professor of Pediatrics, Department of Pediatrics, Harvard Medical School; Emeritus Chief, Division of Infectious Diseases, Children's Hospital Boston, Boston, Massachusetts
Pneumonia in the Immunocompromised Host

Meredith McMorrow, MD, MPH
Malaria Branch, Division of Parasitic Diseases and Malaria, Center for Global Health, Centers for Disease Control and Prevention, Atlanta, Georgia *Plasmodium Species (Malaria)*

Candice McNeil, MD, MPH
Postdoctoral Fellow, Division of Infectious Diseases and Geographic Medicine, Department of Medicine, Stanford School of Medicine, Stanford, California; Attending Physician, Division of AIDS Medicine, Santa Clara Valley Medical Center, San Jose, California
Entamoeba histolytica *(Amebiasis); Other* Entamoeba, *Amebas, and Intestinal Flagellates;* Naegleria fowleri; Acanthamoeba *Species*

Jennifer H. McQuiston, DVM, MS
Epidemiology Activity Chief, Rickettsial Zoonoses Branch, Division of Vector-Borne Diseases, National Center for Emerging and Zoonotic Infectious Diseases, Centers for Disease Control and Prevention, Atlanta, Georgia
Rickettsia rickettsii *(Rocky Mountain Spotted Fever)*

Debrah Meislich, MD
Assistant Professor of Clinical Pediatrics, UMDNJ-Robert Wood Johnson Medical School at Camden; Attending Physician, Pediatric Infectious Diseases, Cooper University Hospital, Camden, New Jersey
Anaerobic Cocci; Anaerobic Gram-Positive, Nonsporulating Bacilli (including Actinomycosis)

H. Cody Meissner, MD
Professor of Pediatrics, Tufts University School of Medicine; Chief, Pediatric Infectious Disease, Tufts Medical Center, Boston, Massachusetts
Passive Immunization; Bronchiolitis; Respiratory Syncytial Virus

Asunción Mejías, MD, PhD
Assistant Professor of Pediatrics, The Ohio State University College of Medicine; Division of Pediatric Infectious Diseases, The Research Institute at Nationwide Children's Hospital, Columbus, Ohio
Parainfluenza Viruses

Manoj P. Menon, MD, MPH
Medical Officer, Enteric Diseases Epidemiology Branch, Division of Foodborne, Waterborne, and Environmental Diseases, National Center for Emerging and Zoonotic Infectious Diseases, Centers for Disease Control and Prevention, Atlanta, Georgia
Vibrio cholerae *(Cholera)*

Jussi Mertsola, MD
Professor in Pediatrics, Turku University Hospital, Turku, Finland
Bordetella pertussis *(Pertussis) and Other* Bordetella *Species*

Marian G. Michaels, MD, MPH
Professor of Pediatrics and Surgery, University of Pittsburgh School of Medicine; Attending Physician, Division of Infectious Diseases, Children's Hospital of Pittsburgh of UPMC, Pittsburgh, Pennsylvania
Eosinophilic Meningitis; Infections in Solid Organ Transplant Recipients

Melissa B. Miller, PhD
Associate Professor, Department of Pathology and Laboratory Medicine, University of North Carolina School of Medicine; Director, Clinical Molecular Microbiology Laboratory; Associate Director, Clinical Microbiology-Immunology Laboratories, University of North Carolina Hospitals, Chapel Hill, North Carolina
Mechanisms and Detection of Antimicrobial Resistance

Eric D. Mintz, MD, MPH
Team Lead, Global Water, Sanitation and Hygiene Epidemiology Team, Waterborne Disease Prevention Branch, Division of Foodborne, Waterborne, and Environmental Diseases, National Center for Emerging and Zoonotic Infectious Diseases, Centers for Disease Control and Prevention, Atlanta, Georgia
Vibrio cholerae (Cholera)

John F. Modlin, MD
Professor of Pediatrics and Medicine, Chair Department of Pediatrics, Senior Associate Dean for Clinical Affairs, Dartmouth Medical School, Dartmouth-Hitchcock Medical Center, Lebanon, New Hampshire
Introduction to Picornaviridae; Enteroviruses and Parechoviruses

Parvathi Mohan, MD
Programs Director, Hepatology Program, Neurophysiology Program, Children's National Medical Center, Washington, DC
Chronic Hepatitis

Susan P. Montgomery, DVM, MPH
Epidemiology Team Lead, Parasitic Diseases Branch, Division of Parasitic Diseases and Malaria, Center for Global Health, Centers for Disease Control and Prevention, Atlanta, Georgia
Diphyllobothrium, Dipylidium, and Hymenolepis Species

Jose G. Montoya, MD
Associate Professor of Medicine, Division of Infectious Diseases, Stanford School of Medicine, Stanford, California
Toxoplasma gondii (Toxoplasmosis)

Zack S. Moore, MD, MPH
Medical Epidemiologist, Communicable Disease Branch, North Carolina Department of Health and Human Services, Raleigh, North Carolina
Poxviridae

Maite de la Morena, MD
Associate Professor of Pediatrics and Internal Medicine, University of Texas Southwestern Medical Center in Dallas; Division of Allergy and Immunology, Children's Medical Center Dallas, Dallas, Texas
Immunologic Development and Susceptibility to Infection

Pedro L. Moro, MD, MPH
Epidemiologist, Immunization Safety Office, Division of Healthcare Quality Promotion, National Center for Emerging and Zoonotic Infectious Diseases, Centers for Disease Control and Prevention, Atlanta, Georgia
Echinococcus Species (Agents of Cystic, Alveolar, and Polycystic Echinococcosis)

Anna-Barbara Moscicki, MD
Professor of Pediatrics and Adolescent Medicine, Department of Pediatrics, University of California San Francisco School of Medicine, San Francisco, California
Human Papillomaviruses

R. Lawrence Moss, MD
E. Thomas Boles Jr Professor of Surgery, The Ohio State University College of Medicine; Surgeon-in-Chief, Nationwide Children's Hospital, Columbus, Ohio
Peritonitis; Appendicitis; Intra-Abdominal, Visceral, and Retroperitoneal Abscesses

Trudy V. Murphy, MD
Chief, Vaccine Unit, Division of Viral Hepatitis, National Center for HIV/AIDS, Viral Hepatitis, STD, and TB Prevention, Centers for Disease Control and Prevention, Atlanta, Georgia
Hepatitis B and Hepatitis D Viruses

Dennis L. Murray, MD
Professor of Pediatrics, Georgia Health Sciences University; Chief, Pediatric Infectious Diseases, Associate Medical Director, Children's Medical Center, Augusta, Georgia
Acute Pneumonia and Its Complications; Persistent and Recurrent Pneumonia

Angela L. Myers, MD, MPH
Assistant Professor of Pediatrics, University of Missouri, Kansas City School of Medicine; Pediatric Infectious Diseases Fellowship Program Director, Children's Mercy Hospitals and Clinics, Kansas City, Missouri
Abdominal and Retroperitoneal Lymphadenopathy; Localized Lymphadenitis, Lymphadenopathy, and Lymphangitis

Simon Nadel, FRCP
Consultant in Paediatric Intensive Care, Department of Paediatrics, Imperial College London; Department of Paediatrics, St. Mary's Hospital, London, United Kingdom
The Systemic Inflammatory Response Syndrome (SIRS), Sepsis, and Septic Shock

James P. Nataro, MD, PhD, MBA
Benjamin Armistead Shepherd Professor and Chair, Department of Pediatrics, University of Virginia School of Medicine, Charlottesville, Virginia
Inflammatory Enteritis; Escherichia coli

Michael N. Neely, MD
Assistant Professor of Pediatrics, Keck School of Medicine, University of Southern California; Pediatric Infectious Diseases and Clinical Pharmacology, Los Angeles County and University of Southern California Medical Center and Children's Hospital Los Angeles, Los Angeles, California
Pharmacokinetic–Pharmacodynamic Basis of Optimal Antibiotic Therapy

William L. Nicholson, PhD
Activity Chief, Disease Assessment, Rickettsial Zoonoses Branch, Division of Vector-Borne Diseases, National Center for Emerging and Zoonotic Infectious Diseases, Centers for Disease Control and Prevention, Atlanta, Georgia
Ehrlichia and Anaplasma Species (Ehrlichiosis and Anaplasmosis)

Victor Nizet, MD
Professor of Pediatrics and Pharmacy, School of Medicine and Skaggs School of Pharmacy and Pharmaceutical Sciences, University of California San Diego; Chief, Division of Pediatric Pharmacology and Drug Discovery, Rady Children's Hospital San Diego, San Diego, California
Pharyngitis; Streptococcus pyogenes (Group A Streptococcus)

Amy Jo Nopper, MD
Attending Physician, Division of Dermatology, Children's Mercy Hospital, Kansas City, Missouri
Superficial Bacterial Skin Infections and Cellulitis

Anna Norrby-Teglund, PhD
Professor, Department of Medicine, Karolinska Institute, Stockholm, Sweden
Myositis, Pyomyositis, and Necrotizing Fasciitis

Theresa J. Ochoa, MD
Assistant Professor of Pediatrics, Universidad Peruana Cayetano Heredia, Lima, Peru; Assistant Professor of Epidemiology, University of Texas School of Public Health, Houston, Texas
Yersinia Species

Miguel O'Ryan, MD
Full Professor, Vice President for Research and Development, University of Chile, Santiago, Chile
Yersinia Species; Aeromonas Species

Walter A. Orenstein, MD
Professor of Medicine and Pediatrics, Division of Infectious Diseases, Emory University School of Medicine; Associate Director, Emory Vaccine Center, Atlanta, Georgia
Active Immunization

Christopher D. Paddock, MD, MPHTM
Staff Pathologist and Research Medical Officer, Infectious Diseases Pathology Branch, Division of High Consequence Pathogens and Pathology, National Center for Emerging and Zoonotic Infectious Diseases, Centers for Disease Control and Prevention, Atlanta, Georgia
Rickettsia rickettsii *(Rocky Mountain Spotted Fever)*

Diane E. Pappas, MD, JD
Professor of Clinical Pediatrics, University of Virginia School of Medicine; University of Virginia Health System, Charlottesville, Virginia
The Common Cold; Rhinoviruses

Robert F. Pass, MD
Professor of Pediatrics and Microbiology, University of Alabama Birmingham School of Medicine, Division of Infectious Diseases, Children's Hospital of Alabama, Birmingham, Alabama
Viral Infections in the Fetus and Neonate; Cytomegalovirus

Thomas F. Patterson, MD
Professor of Medicine; Chief, Division of Infectious Diseases Fellowship; Director, San Antonio Center for Medical Mycology; Attending Physician, Division of Infectious Diseases, University of Texas Health Science Center at San Antonio, and the South Texas Veterans Health Care System, San Antonio, Texas
Agents of Hyalohyphomycosis and Phaeohyphomycosis; Agents of Mucormycosis (Zygomycosis); Malassezia species; Sporothrix schenckii (Sporotrichosis); Cryptococcus Species

Stephen I. Pelton, MD
Professor of Pediatrics and Epidemiology, Boston University Schools of Medicine and Public Health; Chief, Section of Pediatric Infectious Diseases, Boston Medical Center, Boston, Massachusetts
Otitis Media

Larry K. Pickering, MD
Senior Advisor to the Director, National Center for Immunization and Respiratory Diseases; Executive Secretary, Advisory Committee on Immunization Practices, Centers for Disease Control and Prevention; Professor of Pediatrics, Emory University School of Medicine, Atlanta, Georgia
Infections Associated with Group Childcare; Active Immunization; Approach to the Diagnosis and Management of Gastrointestinal Tract Infections; Infections Related to Pets and Exotic Animals; Giardia intestinalis *(Giardiasis)*

Caroline Diane Sarah Piggott, MD
Clinical Fellow in Pediatric Dermatology, University of California San Diego School of Medicine, San Diego, California
Dermatophytes and Other Superficial Fungi

Philip A. Pizzo, MD
Dean, The Carl and Elizabeth Naumann Professor of Pediatrics, Microbiology and Immunology, Stanford School of Medicine
Fever and Granulocytopenia; Infections in Children with Cancer

Andrew J. Pollard, FRCPCH, PhD
Professor of Paediatric Infection and Immunity, Director of the Oxford Vaccine Group, University of Oxford; Honorary Consultant Paediatrician, Children's Hospital, Oxford, United Kingdom
Neisseria meningitidis

Klara M. Posfay-Barbe, MD, MS
Head of Pediatric Infectious Diseases, Department of Pediatrics, University Hospitals of Geneva, University of Geneva School of Medicine, Geneva, Switzerland
Eosinophilic Meningitis

Susan M. Poutanen, MD, MPH, FRCPC
Assistant Professor, Departments of Laboratory Medicine and Pathobiology and Medicine, University of Toronto; Medical Microbiologist and Infectious Disease Consultant, University Health Network and Mount Sinai Hospital, Toronto, Canada
Human Coronaviruses

Dwight A. Powell, MD
Professor of Pediatrics, The Ohio State University College of Medicine and Public Health; Chief, Section of Infectious Diseases, Nationwide Children's Hospital, Columbus, Ohio
Citrobacter *Species;* Serratia *Species;* Acinetobacter *Species*

Alice S. Prince, MD
Professor of Pediatrics, Columbia University College of Physicians and Surgeons; Attending Physician, Infectious Diseases, Morgan Stanley Children's Hospital of New York, New York, New York
Pseudomonas aeruginosa

Charles G. Prober, MD
Professor of Pediatrics, Microbiology & Immunology, Senior Associate Dean, Medical Education, Stanford School of Medicine, Stanford, California
Introduction to Herpesviridae; Herpes Simplex Virus

Octavio Ramilo, MD
Henry G. Cramblett Chair in Infectious Diseases, Professor of Pediatrics, Ohio State University; Chief, Infectious Diseases, Nationwide Children's Hospital, Columbus, Ohio
Parainfluenza Viruses

Shawn J. Rangel, MD, MSCE
Instructor, Pediatric Surgery, Harvard Medical School; Staff Surgeon, Children's Hospital Boston, Boston, Massachusetts
Peritonitis

Sarah A. Rawstron, MB, BS
Associate Professor of Clinical Pediatrics, Weill Medical College of Cornell University; Director, Pediatric Residency Program, The Brooklyn Hospital Center, Brooklyn, New York
Treponema pallidum *(Syphilis); Other* Treponema *Species*

Jennifer S. Read, MD, MS, MPH, DTM&H
National Vaccine Program Office, Office of the Assistant Secretary for Health, Department of Health and Human Services, Washington, DC
Epidemiology and Prevention of HIV Infection in Children and Adolescents

Michael D. Reed, PharmD, FCCP, FCP
Professor of Pediatrics, Northeast Ohio Medical University College of Medicine; Director, Rebecca D. Considine Research Institute, Clinical Pharmacology and Toxicology Associate Chair, Department of Pediatrics, Akron Children's Hospital, Rootstown, Ohio
Pharmacokinetic–Pharmacodynamic Basis of Optimal Antibiotic Therapy

Joanna J. Regan, MD, MPH
Medical Epidemiologist, Rickettsial Zoonoses Branch, Division of Vector-Borne Diseases, National Center for Emerging and Zoonotic Infectious Diseases, Centers for Disease Control and Prevention, Atlanta, Georgia
Ehrlichia *and* Anaplasma *Species (Ehrlichiosis and Anaplasmosis);* Rickettsia rickettsii *(Rocky Mountain Spotted Fever)*

Megan E. Reller, MDCM, MPH, DTM&H
Assistant Professor of Pathology, Division of Medical Microbiology, Department of Pathology, Johns Hopkins University School of Medicine, Baltimore, Maryland
Salmonella *Species*

Melissa A. Reyes, MD
Clinical Fellow, Department of Dermatology, Rady Children's Hospital, San Diego, California
Purpura

Peter A. Rice, MD
Professor, Infectious Diseases and Immunology, University of Massachusetts School of Medicine, North Worcester, Massachusetts
Neisseria gonorrhoeae

Samuel E. Rice-Townsend, MD
Post Doctor Fellow, Pediatric Surgery and Critical Care, Harvard Medical School; Post Doctor Fellow, Pediatric Surgery and Critical Care Children's Hospital, Boston, Massachusetts
Peritonitis

Frank O. Richards, Jr, MD
Director, Malaria, River Blindness, Lymphatic Filariasis, Schistosomiasis, The Carter Center, Atlanta, Georgia; Assistant Adjunct Professor of Pediatrics, Associate Adjunct Professor of Global Health, Emory University; Professional Staff, Children's Health Care Atlanta, Atlanta, Georgia
Diphyllobothrium, Dipylidium, and Hymenolepis Species; Blood Trematodes (Schistosomiasis)

Gail L. Rodgers, MD
Senior Director, Scientific Affairs, Vaccines, Pfizer, Collegeville, Pennsylvania
Infection following Burns; Topical Antimicrobial Agents

Pierre E. Rollin, MD
Deputy Branch Chief, Viral Special Pathogens Branch, Division of High-Consequence Pathogens and Pathology, National Center for Emerging and Zoonotic Infectious Diseases, Centers for Disease Control and Prevention, Atlanta, Georgia
Bunyaviruses

José R. Romero, MD
Professor of Pediatrics, University of Arkansas for Medical Sciences; Section of Infectious Diseases, Arkansas Children's Hospital, Little Rock, Arkansas
Aseptic and Viral Meningitis

G. Ingrid J.G. Rours, MD, PhD
Associate Professor of Pediatrics, Department of Pediatric Infectious Diseases and Immunology, Erasmus Medical Centre, Rotterdam, Netherlands
Chlamydia trachomatis

Anne H. Rowley, MD
Professor of Pediatrics, Microbiology/Immunology, Northwestern University Feinberg School of Medicine; Attending Physician, Division of Infectious Diseases, The Children's Memorial Hospital, Chicago, Illinois
Kawasaki Disease

Sharon L. Roy, MD
Medical Epidemiologist, Waterborne Disease Prevention Branch, Division of Foodborne, Waterborne, and Environmental Diseases, National Center for Emerging and Zoonotic Infectious Diseases, Centers for Disease Control and Prevention, Atlanta, Georgia
Enteric Diseases Transmitted through Food, Water, and Zoonotic Exposures

Lorry G. Rubin, MD
Professor of Pediatrics, Hofstra North Shore-LIJ School of Medicine, Hempstead; Professor of Pediatrics, Albert Einstein College of Medicine; Chief, Division of Infectious Diseases, Steven and Alexandra Cohen Children's Medical Center of the North Shore-LIJ Health System, New Hyde Park, New York
Capnocytophaga Species; Francisella tularensis (Tularemia); Legionella Species; Streptobacillus moniliformis (Rat-Bite Fever); Other Gram-Negative Coccobacilli

Guillermo M. Ruiz-Palacios, MD
Professor of Internal Medicine, Chair of the Department of Infectious Diseases of the National Institute of Medical Sciences and Nutrition, Mexico City, Mexico
Other Campylobacter Species

Lisa Saiman, MD, MPH
Professor of Clinical Pediatrics, Columbia University College of Physicians & Surgeons; Attending Physician, Section of Infectious Diseases, Morgan Stanley Children's Hospital of New York, New York-Presbyterian Hospital; Hospital Epidemiologist, Department of Infection Prevention and Control, New York-Presbyterian Hospital, New York, New York
Endocarditis and Other Intravascular Infections

Laura Sass, MD
Assistant Professor of Pediatrics, Eastern Virginia Medical School; Attending Physician, Division of Pediatric Infectious Disease; Attending Physician, Cystic Fibrosis Center, Children's Hospital of the King's Daughters, Norfolk, Virginia
Hospital-Associated Infections in the Neonate

Jason B. Sauberan, PharmD
Assistant Clinical Professor, University of California San Diego Skaggs School of Pharmacy and Pharmaceutical Sciences; Department of Pharmacy, University of California San Diego Medical Center, San Diego, California
Antimicrobial Agents

Peter M. Schantz, VMD, PhD
Adjunct Professor, Department of Global Health, Rollins School of Public Health, Emory University, Atlanta, Georgia
Taenia solium, Taenia asiatica, and Taenia saginata (Taeniasis and Cysticercosis); Echinococcus Species (Agents of Cystic, Alveolar, and Polycystic Echinococcosis); Taenia (Multiceps) multiceps and Taenia serialis (Coenurosis)

Eileen Schneider, MD
Medical Epidemiologist, Division of Viral Diseases, National Center for Immunization and Respiratory Diseases, Centers for Disease Control and Prevention, Atlanta, Georgia
Human Parvoviruses

Gordon E. Schutze, MD
Professor of Pediatrics, Vice Chairman for Educational Affairs, Department of Pediatrics, Baylor College of Medicine; Vice President, International Medical Services, Baylor College of Medicine International Pediatric AIDS Initiative at Texas Children's Hospital, Houston, Texas
Bartonella Species (Cat-Scratch Disease)

Benjamin Schwartz, MD
Senior Science Advisor, National Vaccine Program Office, U.S. Department of Health and Human Services, Washington, DC
Principles of Epidemiology and Public Health

Heidi Schwarzwald, MD, MPH
Associate Professor of Pediatrics, Baylor College of Medicine; Section Head and Service Chief, Retrovirology and Global Health Department of Pediatrics, Texas Children's Hospital, Houston, Texas
Diagnosis and Clinical Manifestations of HIV Infection

Kara N. Shah, MD, PhD
Associate Professor of Pediatrics and Dermatology, University of Cincinnati College of Medicine; Chief of Dermatology, Cincinnati Children's Hospital, Cincinnati, Ohio
Urticaria and Erythema Multiforme

Samir S. Shah, MD, MSCE
Associate Professor of Pediatrics, University of Cincinnati College of Medicine; Attending Physician, Division of Infectious Diseases and Hospital Medicine, Cincinnati Children's Hospital Medical Center, Cincinnati, Ohio
Chlamydophila (Chlamydia) pneumoniae; Mycoplasma pneumoniae; Other Mycoplasma Species; Ureaplasma urealyticum

Andi L. Shane, MD, MPH, MSc
Assistant Professor, Department of Pediatrics, Emory University School of Medicine; Division of Infectious Diseases, Emory Children's Center, Atlanta, Georgia
Infections Associated with Group Childcare; Approach to the Diagnosis and Management of Gastrointestinal Tract Infections

Craig A. Shapiro, MD
Fellow, Emory University School of Medicine and Children's Healthcare of Atlanta; Division of Pediatric Infectious Diseases, Epidemiology, and Immunology, Emory Children's Center, Atlanta, Georgia
Myocarditis; Pericarditis

Eugene D. Shapiro, MD
Professor of Pediatrics, Epidemiology and Investigative Medicine, Yale University School of Medicine; Attending Physician, Pediatrics, Children's Hospital at Yale-New Haven, New Haven, Connecticut
Fever without Localizing Signs; Leptospira Species (Leptospirosis); Borrelia burgdorferi (Lyme Disease); Other Borrelia Species and Spirillum minus

Umid M. Sharapov, MD, MSc
Medical Epidemiologist, Division of Viral Hepatitis, National Center for HIV/AIDS, Viral Hepatitis, STD, and TB Prevention, Centers for Disease Control and Prevention, Atlanta, Georgia
Hepatitis A Virus

Jana Shaw, MD, MPH
Assistant Professor of Pediatrics, Pediatric Infectious Diseases, SUNY Upstate Medical University; Division of Infectious Diseases, Upstate Golisano Children's Hospital, Syracuse, New York
Infections of the Oral Cavity

George Kelly Siberry, MD, MPH
Medical Officer, Pediatric, Adolescent, and Maternal AIDS (PAMA) Branch, Eunice Kennedy Shriver National Institute of Child Health and Human Development, National Institutes of Health, Bethesda, Maryland
Management of HIV Infection

Jane D. Siegel, MD
Professor of Pediatrics, University of Texas Southwestern Medical Center at Dallas; Attending Physician in Infectious Diseases, Medical Director, Infection Prevention and Control, Children's Medical Center of Dallas; Attending Physician, Parkland Health and Hospital System, Dallas, Texas
Pediatric Infection Prevention and Control

Robert David Siegel, MD, PhD
Associate Professor (Teaching), Department of Microbiology and Immunology, Program in Human Biology, and Center for African Studies, Stanford University, Stanford, California
Classification of Human Viruses

Nalini Singh, MD, MPH
Professor of Pediatrics, Epidemiology, and Global Health, George Washington University Schools of Medicine and Public Health; Chief, Division Infectious Diseases, Children's National Medical Center, Washington DC
Clostridium difficile

Upinder Singh, MD
Associate Professor, Departments of Internal Medicine and Microbiology and Immunology, Stanford University School of Medicine; Chief, Division of Infectious Diseases and Geographic Medicine, Stanford University Medical Center, Stanford, California
Entamoeba histolytica (Amebiasis); Other Entamoeba, Amebas, and Intestinal Flagellates; Naegleria fowleri; Acanthamoeba Species

P. Brian Smith, MD, MPH, MHS
Associate Professor of Pediatrics, Duke University Medical Center, Duke Clinical Research Institute, Durham, North Carolina
Clinical Approach to the Infected Neonate; Candida Species

John D. Snyder, MD
Professor of Pediatrics, George Washington University School of Medicine, Washington, DC
Acute Hepatitis; Chronic Hepatitis

David E. Soper, MD
J. Marion Sims Professor of Obstetrics and Gynecology, Professor of Medicine, Division of Infectious Diseases, Medical University of South Carolina, Charleston, South Carolina
Pelvic Inflammatory Disease

Mary Allen Staat, MD, MPH
Professor of Pediatrics, University of Cincinnati College of Medicine; Director, International Adoption Center, Department of Pediatrics, Division of Infectious Diseases, Cincinnati Children's Hospital Medical Center, Cincinnati, Ohio
Infectious Diseases in Refugee and Internationally Adopted Children

J. Erin Staples, MD, PhD
Medical Epidemiologist, Arboviral Diseases Branch, Division of Vector-Borne Diseases, National Center for Emerging and Zoonotic Infectious Diseases, Centers for Disease Control and Prevention, Fort Collins, Colorado
Coltivirus (Colorado Tick Fever); Togaviridae: Alphaviruses

Jeffrey R. Starke, MD
Professor of Pediatrics, Baylor College of Medicine; Infection Control Officer, Texas Children's Hospital, Houston, Texas
Mycobacterium tuberculosis

William J. Steinbach, MD
Associate Professor of Pediatrics, Molecular Genetics & Microbiology, Duke University School of Medicine; Division of Pediatric Infectious Diseases, Duke University Medical Center, Durham, North Carolina
Candida Species; Aspergillus Species; Antifungal Agents

Ina Stephens, MD
Pediatric Residency Program Director, Sinai Hospital of Baltimore, Baltimore, Maryland
Inflammatory Enteritis

Joseph W. St. Geme, III, MD
Professor of Pediatrics and Molecular Genetics and Microbiology, Chairman of the Department of Pediatrics, Duke University Medical Center; Chief Medical Officer and Attending Physician, Duke Children's Hospital, Durham, North Carolina
Classification of Bacteria; Classification of Streptococci; Enterococcus Species; Viridans Streptococci, Abiotrophia and Granulicatella Species, and Streptococcus bovis; Groups C and G Streptococci; Other Gram-Positive, Catalase-Negative Cocci; Haemophilus influenzae

Bradley P. Stoner, MD, PhD
Associate Professor of Medicine and Anthropology, Washington University in St. Louis, St. Louis, Missouri
Klebsiella (Calymmatobacterium) granulomatis (Granuloma Inguinale)

Jonathan B. Strober, MD
Associate Clinical Professor, Neurology & Pediatrics, University of California San Francisco; Director, Pediatric Muscular Dystrophy Clinic; Director of Ambulatory Services, Safety and Compliance, Division of Child Neurology, UCSF Benioff Children's Hospital, San Francisco, California
Para- and Postinfectious Neurologic Syndromes

Kanta Subbarao, MBBS, MPH
Senior Investigator, Laboratory of Infectious Diseases, National Institutes of Allergy and Infectious Diseases, National Institutes of Health, Bethesda, Maryland
Influenza Viruses

Deanna A. Sutton, PhD
Associate Professor/Research, Department of Pathology, University of Texas Health Science Center at San Antonio, San Antonio, Texas
Agents of Hyalohyphomycosis and Phaeohyphomycosis; Agents of Mucormycosis (Zygomycosis); Malassezia species; Sporothrix schenckii (Sporotrichosis)

Douglas Swanson, MD
Associate Professor of Pediatrics, University of Missouri – Kansas City School of Medicine; Attending Physician, Section of Infectious Diseases, Children's Mercy Hospitals and Clinics, Kansas City, Missouri
Chronic Meningitis

Leonel T. Takada, MD
PhD student, Neurology, Hospital das Clinicas, University of Sao Paulo Medical School, Sao Paulo, Brazil; Visiting Scholar, Memory and Aging Center, Neurology Department, University of California, San Francisco, California
Prion Diseases

Jacqueline E. Tate, PhD
Epidemiologist, Division of Viral Diseases, National Center for Immunization and Respiratory Diseases, Centers for Disease Control and Prevention, Atlanta, Georgia
Astroviruses

Robert V. Tauxe, MD, MPH
Deputy Director, Division of Foodborne, Bacterial and Mycotic Diseases, National Center for Zoonotic, Vector-Borne and Enteric Diseases, Centers for Disease Control and Prevention, Atlanta, Georgia
Vibrio cholerae (Cholera)

Marc Tebruegge, DTM&H, DLSHTM, MRCPCH, MSc, MD
Postgraduate Scholar, Department of Paediatrics, The University of Melbourne; Honorary Clinical Research Fellow, Infectious Diseases Unit, Department of General Medicine; Postgraduate Scholar, Murdoch Children's Research Institute, Royal Children's Hospital Melbourne, Parkville, Australia
Infections Related to the Upper and Middle Airways; Mycobacterium *Species Non-tuberculosis*

Eyasu H. Teshale, MD
Epidemiologist, Division of Viral Hepatitis, National Center for HIV/AIDS, Viral Hepatitis, STD, and TB Prevention, Centers for Disease Control and Prevention, Atlanta, Georgia
Hepatitis E Virus

George R. Thompson, III, MD
Assistant Professor of Medicine, University of California Davis School of Medicine; Assistant Director, Coccidioidomycosis Serology Laboratory, Department of Medical Microbiology and Immunology, Davis, California
Cryptococcus *Species*

Herbert A. Thompson, PhD
Chief, Viral and Rickettsial Zoonoses Branch, Division of Viral and Rickettsial Diseases, National Center for Infectious Diseases, Centers for Disease Control and Prevention, Atlanta, Georgia
Coxiella burnetii *(Q Fever)*

Richard B. Thomson, Jr, PhD
Medical Microbiologist and Director, Microbiology Laboratories, Department of Pathology and Laboratory Medicine, NorthShore University HealthSystem, Illinois; Clinical Professor of Pathology, The University of Chicago Pritzker School of Medicine, Chicago, Illinois
Nocardia *Species*

Emily A. Thorell, MD
Assistant Professor of Pediatrics, University of Utah School of Medicine; Director, Antimicrobial Stewardship Program, Associate Hospital Epidemiologist, Primary Children's Medical Center, Salt Lake City, Utah
Cervical Lymphadenitis and Neck Infections

Rania A. Tohme, MD, MPH
Epidemiology & Surveillance Branch, Division of Viral Hepatitis, National Center for HIV/AIDS, Viral Hepatitis, STD, and TB Prevention, Centers for Disease Control and Prevention, Atlanta, Georgia
Hepatitis C Virus

Robert W. Tolan, Jr, MD
Clinical Associate Professor of Pediatrics, Drexel University College of Medicine, Philadelphia, Pennsylvania; Chief, Division of Allergy, Immunology and Infectious Diseases, The Children's Hospital at Saint Peter's University Hospital, New Brunswick, New Jersey
Fusobacterium *Species;* Babesia *Species (Babesiosis)*

Philip Toltzis, MD
Professor of Pediatrics, Case Western Reserve University School of Medicine; Attending Physician, Divisions of Pharmacology and Critical Care, Rainbow Babies and Children's Hospital, Cleveland, Ohio
Staphylococcus epidermidis *and Other Coagulase-Negative Staphylococci*

James Treat, MD
Assistant Professor of Pediatrics and Dermatology, University of Pennsylvania School of Medicine; Fellowship Director, Pediatric Dermatology, Education Director, Pediatric Dermatology, Children's Hospital of Philadelphia, Philadelphia, Pennsylvania
Vesicles and Bullae

Stephanie B. Troy, MD
Assistant Professor, Division of Infectious Diseases, Department of Medicine, Eastern Virginia Medical School, Norfolk, Virginia
Polioviruses

Russell B. Van Dyke, MD
Professor of Pediatrics, Section of Pediatrics Infectious Diseases, Pediatrics, Tulane University Health Sciences Center, New Orleans, Louisiana
Infectious Complications of HIV Infection

Jorge J. Velarde, MD
Division of Infectious Diseases, Children's Hospital Boston, Boston, Massachusetts
Escherichia coli

Jennifer Vodzak, MD
Instructor of Pediatrics, Drexel University College of Medicine; Fellow, Section of Infectious Diseases, St. Christopher's Hospital for Children, Philadelphia, Pennsylvania
Other Hemophilus *Species*

Ellen R. Wald, MD
Alfred Dorrance Daniels Professor and Chair, Department of Pediatrics, University of Wisconsin School of Medicine and Public Health; Physician-in-Chief, American Family Children's Hospital, Madison, Wisconsin
Mastoiditis; Sinusitis; Periorbital and Orbital Infections

Geoffrey A. Weinberg, MD
Professor of Pediatrics, Department of Pediatrics, University of Rochester School of Medicine and Dentistry; Director, Pediatric HIV Program, Golisano Children's Hospital, University of Rochester Medical Center, Rochester, New York
Neurologic Symptom Complexes

A. Clinton White, Jr, MD
The Paul R. Stalnaker, MD Distinguished Professor of Internal Medicine; Director, Infectious Disease Division, Department of Internal Medicine, University of Texas Medical Branch, Galveston, Texas
Taenia solium, Taenia asiatica, *and* Taenia saginata *(Taeniasis and Cysticercosis);* Taenia (Multiceps) multiceps *and* Taenia serialis *(Coenurosis)*

Marc-Alain Widdowson, MA, MSc, VetMB
Medical Epidemiologist, National Center for Immunization and Respiratory Diseases, Centers for Disease Control and Prevention, Atlanta, Georgia
Caliciviruses

Harold C. Wiesenfeld, MD, CM
Associate Professor of Obstetrics, Gynecology and Reproductive Sciences and Medicine, University of Pittsburgh School of Medicine; Director, Division of Reproductive Infectious Diseases and Immunology, University of Pittsburgh Medical Center, Pittsburgh, Pennsylvania
Pelvic Inflammatory Disease

John V. Williams, MD
Assistant Professor of Pediatrics, Division of Pediatric Infectious Diseases, Vanderbilt University Medical Center, Nashville, Tennessee
Human Metapneumovirus

Roxanne E. Williams, MD, MPH
Division of Viral Hepatitis, National Center for HIV/AIDS, Viral Hepatitis, STD, and TB Prevention, Centers for Disease Control and Prevention, Atlanta, Georgia
Hepatitis A Virus

Rodney E. Willoughby, Jr, MD
Professor of Pediatrics, Medical College of Wisconsin; Attending Physician, Division of Infectious Diseases, Children's Hospital of Wisconsin, Milwaukee, Wisconsin
Rabies Virus

Craig M. Wilson, MD
Professor of Epidemiology, Pediatrics and Microbiology; Director, UAB Sparkman Center for Global Health, University of Alabama at Birmingham, Birmingham, Alabama
Antiparasitic Agents

Sarah L. Wingerter, MD
Instructor of Pediatrics, Harvard Medical School; Division of Pediatric Emergency Medicine, Children's Hospital, Boston, Massachusetts
Infection following Trauma

Jerry A. Winkelstein, MD
Emeritis Professor of Pediatrics, Johns Hopkins University School of Medicine, Baltimore, Maryland
Infectious Complications of Complement Deficiencies

Kimberly A. Workowski, MD
Professor of Medicine, Division of Infectious Diseases, Emory University School of Medicine; Team Lead, Guidelines Unit, Division of STD Prevention, National Center for HIV/AIDS, Viral Hepatitis, STD, and TB Prevention, Centers for Disease Control and Prevention, Atlanta, Georgia
Skin and Mucous Membrane Infections and Inguinal Lymphadenopathy; Trichomonas vaginalis

Terry W. Wright, PhD
Associate Professor of Pediatrics, Microbiology and Immunology, University of Rochester School of Medicine and Dentistry; Golisano Children's Hospital at Strong, Rochester, New York
Pneumocystis jirovecii

Pablo Yagupsky, MD
Professor of Pediatrics and Clinical Microbiology, Ben-Gurion University of the Negev, Beer-Sheva, Israel
Kingella *Species*

Nada Yazigi, MD
Assistant Professor of Clinical Pediatrics, University of Cincinnati School of Medicine; Attending Physician, Division of Gastroenterology, Hepatology and Nutrition, Cincinnati Children's Hospital Medical Center, Cincinnati, Ohio
Granulomatous Hepatitis; Acute Pancreatitis; Cholecystitis and Cholangitis

Catherine Yen, MD, MPH
Epidemic Intelligence Service Officer, Division of Viral Diseases, National Center for Immunization and Respiratory Diseases, Centers for Disease Control and Prevention, Atlanta, Georgia
Rotaviruses

Edward J. Young, MD
Professor of Medicine and Molecular Virology and Microbiology, Baylor College of Medicine; Attending Physician, Michael E. DeBakey Veterans Affairs Medical Center, Houston, Texas
Brucella *Species (Brucellosis)*

Andrea L. Zaenglein, MD
Associate Professor of Dermatology and Pediatrics, Penn State/Milton S. Hershey Medical Center, Hershey, Pennsylvania
Erythematous Macules and Papules

Theoklis E. Zaoutis, MD, MSCE
Associate Professor of Pediatrics and Epidemiology, University of Pennsylvania School of Medicine; Associate Chief, Division of Infectious Diseases, The Children's Hospital of Philadelphia, Philadelphia, Pennsylvania
Healthcare-Associated Infections; Clinical Syndromes of Device-Associated Infections

Contents

Part I: Understanding, Controlling, and Preventing Infectious Diseases

A. Epidemiology and Control of Infectious Diseases

1   Principles of Epidemiology and Public Health *1*
    Benjamin Schwartz and Stacey W. Martin

2   Pediatric Infection Prevention and Control *9*
    Jane D. Siegel

3   Infections Associated with Group Childcare *24*
    Andi L. Shane and Larry K. Pickering

4   Infectious Diseases in Refugee and Internationally Adopted Children *32*
    Mary Allen Staat

B. Prevention of Infectious Diseases

5   Passive Immunization *37*
    H. Cody Meissner

6   Active Immunization *44*
    Andrew T. Kroger, Alison C. Mawle, Larry K. Pickering, and Walter A. Orenstein

7   Chemoprophylaxis *68*
    John S. Bradley

8   Protection of Travelers *76*
    Maryanne E. Crockett and Jay S. Keystone

C. Host Defenses against Infectious Diseases

9   Immunologic Development and Susceptibility to Infection *83*
    Maite de la Morena

10 Fever and the Inflammatory Response *91*
    Alexei A. Grom

Part II: Clinical Syndromes and Cardinal Features of Infectious Diseases: Approach to Diagnosis and Initial Management

A. Septicemia, Toxin- and Inflammation-Mediated Syndromes

11 The Systemic Inflammatory Response Syndrome (SIRS), Sepsis, and Septic Shock *97*
    Judith A. Guzman-Cottrill, Beth Cheesebrough, Simon Nadel, and Brahm Goldstein

12 Hemophagocytic Lymphohistiocytosis and Macrophage Activation Syndrome *103*
    Hayley A. Gans and David B. Lewis

B. Cardinal Symptom Complexes

13 Mucocutaneous Symptom Complexes *108*
    Sarah S. Long

14 Fever without Localizing Signs *114*
    Eugene D. Shapiro

15 Prolonged, Recurrent and Periodic Fever Syndromes *117*
    Sarah S. Long and Kathryn M. Edwards

16 Lymphatic System and Generalized Lymphadenopathy *127*
    Mary Anne Jackson and P. Joan Chesney

17 Cervical Lymphadenitis and Neck Infections *135*
    Emily A. Thorell

18 Mediastinal and Hilar Lymphadenopathy *148*
    Mary Anne Jackson, P. Joan Chesney, and Sarah J. Fitch

19 Abdominal and Retroperitoneal Lymphadenopathy *155*
    Angela L. Myers and Mary Anne Jackson

Contents

20 Localized Lymphadenitis, Lymphadenopathy, and Lymphangitis 157
Angela L. Myers and Mary Anne Jackson

21 Respiratory Tract Symptom Complexes 162
Sarah S. Long

22 Abdominal Symptom Complexes 171
Matthew B. McDonald, III and Robert S. McGregor

23 Neurologic Symptom Complexes 176
Geoffrey A. Weinberg

24 Musculoskeletal Symptom Complexes 182
Kathleen Gutierrez

C. Oral Infections and Upper and Middle Respiratory Tract Infections

25 Infections of the Oral Cavity 190
Jana Shaw

26 The Common Cold 196
Diane E. Pappas and J. Owen Hendley

27 Pharyngitis 199
John C. Arnold and Victor Nizet

28 Infections Related to the Upper and Middle Airways 205
Marc Tebruegge and Nigel Curtis

29 Otitis Media 213
Stephen I. Pelton

30 Otitis Externa and Necrotizing Otitis Externa 220
Thomas G. Boyce

31 Mastoiditis 222
Ellen R. Wald and James H. Conway

32 Sinusitis 227
Ellen R. Wald

D. Lower Respiratory Tract Infections

33 Bronchiolitis 231
H. Cody Meissner

34 Acute Pneumonia and Its Complications 235
Chitra S. Mani and Dennis L. Murray

35 Persistent and Recurrent Pneumonia 245
Dennis L. Murray and Chitra S. Man

36 Pneumonia in the Immunocompromised Host 252
Kenneth McIntosh and Marvin B. Harper

E. Cardiac and Vascular Infections

37 Endocarditis and Other Intravascular Infections 256
Stéphanie Levasseur and Lisa Saiman

38 Myocarditis 265
Craig A. Shapiro and Joseph A. Hilinski

39 Pericarditis 268
Craig A. Shapiro and Joseph A. Hilinski

F. Central Nervous System Infections

40 Acute Bacterial Meningitis beyond the Neonatal Period 272
Carla G. Garcia and George H. McCracken, Jr

41 Chronic Meningitis 279
Douglas Swanson and Christopher J. Harrison

42 Recurrent Meningitis 287
Robyn A. Livingston and Christopher J. Harrison

43 Aseptic and Viral Meningitis 292
José R. Romero

44 Encephalitis 297
Carol Glaser and Sarah S. Long

45 Para- and Postinfectious Neurologic Syndromes 314
Carol Glaser and Jonathan B. Strober

46 Focal Suppurative Infections of the Nervous System 319
Christopher J. Harrison

47 Eosinophilic Meningitis 330
Marian G. Michaels and Klara M. Posfay-Barbe

48 Prion Diseases 333
Leonel T. Takada and Michael D. Geschwind

G. Genitourinary Tract Infections

49 Urinary Tract Infections 339
Jen-Jane Liu and Linda Marie Dairiki Shortliffe

50 Renal Abscess and Other Complex Renal Infections 343
Jen-Jane Liu and Linda Marie Dairiki Shortliffe

51 Sexually Transmitted Infection Syndromes 345
Laura M. Kester, Gale R. Burstein, and Margaret J. Blythe

52 Skin and Mucous Membrane Infections and Inguinal Lymphadenopathy 349
Kimberly A. Workowski

53 Urethritis, Vulvovaginitis, and Cervicitis 353
Paula K. Braverman

54 Pelvic Inflammatory Disease 363
Eloisa Llata, Harold C. Wiesenfeld, and David E. Soper

55 Epididymitis, Orchitis, and Prostatitis 367
Noni E. MacDonald and William R. Bowie

56 Infectious Diseases in Child Abuse 370
Kirsten Bechtel

H. Gastrointestinal Tract Infections and Intoxications

57 Approach to the Diagnosis and Management of Gastrointestinal Tract Infections 372
Larry K. Pickering and Andi L. Shane

58 Viral Gastroenteritis 377
Ben A. Lopman and Joseph S. Bresee

59 Inflammatory Enteritis *382*
Ina Stephens and James P. Nataro

60 Necrotizing Enterocolitis *388*
C. Michael Cotten and Daniel K. Benjamin, Jr

61 Enteric Diseases Transmitted through Food, Water, and Zoonotic Exposures *392*
Laura B. Gieraltowski, Sharon L. Roy, Aron J. Hall, and Anna Bowen

I. Intra-Abdominal Infections

62 Acute Hepatitis *400*
Laurie S. Conklin and John D. Snyder

63 Chronic Hepatitis *404*
Parvathi Mohan and John D. Snyder

64 Granulomatous Hepatitis *407*
Nada Yazigi and Beverly L. Connelly

65 Acute Pancreatitis *410*
Nada Yazigi and Beverly L. Connelly

66 Cholecystitis and Cholangitis *412*
Nada Yazigi and Beverly L. Connelly

67 Peritonitis *414*
Samuel E. Rice-Townsend, R. Lawrence Moss, and Shawn J. Rangel

68 Appendicitis *420*
Marion C.W. Henry and R. Lawrence Moss

69 Intra-Abdominal, Visceral, and Retroperitoneal Abscesses *423*
Karen A. Diefenbach and R. Lawrence Moss

J. Skin and Soft-Tissue Infections

70 Superficial Bacterial Skin Infections and Cellulitis *427*
Hillary S. Lawrence and Amy Jo Nopper

71 Erythematous Macules and Papules *435*
Sara Jane Heilig and Andrea L. Zaenglein

72 Vesicles and Bullae *438*
James Treat

73 Purpura *441*
Melissa A. Reyes and Lawrence F. Eichenfield

74 Urticaria and Erythema Multiforme *445*
Kara N. Shah

75 Papules, Nodules, and Ulcers *449*
Christine T. Lauren and Maria C. Garzon

76 Subcutaneous Tissue Infections and Abscesses *454*
Catalina Matiz and Sheila Fallon Friedlander

77 Myositis, Pyomyositis, and Necrotizing Fasciitis *462*
Donald E. Low and Anna Norrby-Teglund

K. Bone and Joint Infections

78 Osteomyelitis *469*
Kathleen Gutierrez

79 Infectious and Inflammatory Arthritis *477*
Kathleen Gutierrez

80 Diskitis *483*
Kathleen Gutierrez

81 Transient Synovitis *485*
Kathleen Gutierrez

L. Eye Infections

82 Conjunctivitis in the Neonatal Period (Ophthalmia Neonatorum) *487*
Douglas R. Fredrick

83 Conjunctivitis beyond the Neonatal Period *490*
Douglas R. Fredrick

84 Infective Keratitis *494*
Douglas R. Fredrick

85 Uveitis, Retinitis, and Chorioretinitis *498*
Douglas R. Fredrick

86 Endophthalmitis *503*
Douglas R. Fredrick

87 Periorbital and Orbital Infections *506*
Ellen R. Wald

M. Infections Related to Trauma

88 Infection following Trauma *512*
Sarah L. Wingerter

89 Infection following Burns *516*
Jane M. Gould and Gail L. Rodgers

90 Infection following Bites *521*
Marvin B. Harper

91 Infections Related to Pets and Exotic Animals *526*
Joseph A. Bocchini, Jr and Larry K. Pickering

92 Tickborne Infections *531*
Kristina Bryant

N. Infections of the Fetus and Newborn

93 Clinical Approach to the Infected Neonate *536*
P. Brian Smith and Daniel K. Benjamin, Jr

94 Bacterial Infections in the Neonate *538*
Morven S. Edwards and Carol J. Baker

95 Viral Infections in the Fetus and Neonate *544*
Robert F. Pass

96 Hospital-Associated Infections in the Neonate *548*
M. Gary Karlowicz and Laura Sass

O. Infections and Transplantation

97 Infections in Solid Organ Transplant Recipients *555*
Michael Green and Marian G. Michaels

98 Infections in Hematopoietic Stem Cell Transplant Recipients *562*
Jorge Luján-Zilbermann

P. Infections and Cancer

99 Fever and Granulocytopenia 567
Andrew Y. Koh and Philip A. Pizzo

100 Infections in Children with Cancer 573
Andrew Y. Koh and Philip A. Pizzo

Q. Infections Associated with Hospitalization and Medical Devices

101 Healthcare-Associated Infections 579
Susan E. Coffin and Theoklis E. Zaoutis

102 Clinical Syndromes of Device-Associated Infections 588
Jeffrey S. Gerber and Theoklis E. Zaoutis

R. Infections in Patients with Deficient Defenses

103 Evaluation of the Child with Suspected Immunodeficiency 600
E. Stephen Buescher

104 Infectious Complications of Antibody Deficiency 609
Elisabeth E. Adderson

105 Infectious Complications of Complement Deficiencies 615
Michael M. Frank and Jerry A. Winkelstein

106 Infectious Complications of Dysfunction or Deficiency of Polymorphonuclear and Mononuclear Phagocytes 619
E. Stephen Buescher

107 Infectious Complications of Cell-Mediated Immunity Other Than AIDS: Primary Immunodeficiencies 626
David B. Lewis

108 Infectious Complications in Special Hosts 633
Janet A. Englund and Jane L. Burns

S. Human Immunodeficiency Virus and the Acquired Immunodeficiency Syndrome

109 Epidemiology and Prevention of HIV Infection in Children and Adolescents 641
Jennifer S. Read

110 Immunopathogenesis of HIV-1 Infection 648
Grace M. Aldrovandi and Chiara Cerini

111 Diagnosis and Clinical Manifestations of HIV Infection 650
Paul Krogstad, Heidi Schwarzwald, and Mark W. Kline

112 Infectious Complications of HIV Infection 657
Russell B. Van Dyke and Mark W. Kline

113 Management of HIV Infection 664
George Kelly Siberry and Rohan Hazra

Part III: Etiologic Agents of Infectious Diseases

A. Bacteria

114 Classification of Bacteria 673
Joseph W. St. Geme, III

Gram-Positive Cocci

115 Staphylococcus aureus 675
Robert S. Daum

116 Staphylococcus epidermidis and Other Coagulase-Negative Staphylococci 689
Philip Toltzis

117 Classification of Streptococci 695
David B. Haslam and Joseph W. St. Geme, III

118 Streptococcus pyogenes (Group A Streptococcus) 698
Victor Nizet and John C. Arnold

119 Streptococcus agalactiae (Group B Streptococcus) 707
Morven S. Edwards and Carol J. Baker

120 Enterococcus Species 712
David B. Haslam and Joseph W. St. Geme, III

121 Viridans Streptococci, Abiotrophia and Granulicatella Species, and Streptococcus bovis 716
David B. Haslam and Joseph W. St. Geme, III

122 Groups C and G Streptococci 719
David B. Haslam and Joseph W. St. Geme, III

123 Streptococcus pneumoniae 721
Krow Ampofo and Carrie L. Byington

124 Other Gram-Positive, Catalase-Negative Cocci 729
David B. Haslam and Joseph W. St. Geme, III

Gram-Negative Cocci

125 Neisseria meningitidis 730
Andrew J. Pollard and Adam Finn

126 Neisseria gonorrhoeae 741
Katherine K. Hsu, Peter A. Rice, and Jay M. Lieberman

127 Other Neisseria Species 748
Katherine K. Hsu and Jay M. Lieberman

Gram-Positive Bacilli

128 Archanobacterium haemolyticum 750
Denise F. Bratcher

129 Bacillus Species (Anthrax) 751
Denise F. Bratcher

130 Corynebacterium diphtheriae 754
Irini Daskalaki

131 Other Corynebacteria 759
Denise F. Bratcher

132 *Listeria monocytogenes* 762
Bennett Lorber

133 Other Gram-Positive Bacilli 767
Denise F. Bratcher

134 *Mycobacterium tuberculosis* 771
Jeffrey R. Starke

135 *Mycobacterium* Species Non-*tuberculosis* 786
Marc Tebruegge and Nigel Curtis

136 *Nocardia* Species 792
Ellen Gould Chadwick and Richard B. Thomson, Jr

Enterobacteriaceae: Gram-Negative Bacilli

137 *Escherichia coli* 796
James P. Nataro and Jorge J. Velarde

138 *Klebsiella* and *Raoultella* Species 799
William J. Barson and Mario J. Marcon

139 *Klebsiella (Calymmatobacterium) granulomatis*
(Granuloma Inguinale) 802
Bradley P. Stoner

140 *Enterobacter, Cronobacter,* and *Pantoea*
Species 804
Dennis J. Cunningham and Mario J. Marcon

141 *Citrobacter* Species 806
Dwight A. Powell and Mario J. Marcon

142 Less Commonly Encountered
Enterobacteriaceae 808
Katalin I. Koranyi and Mario J. Marcon

143 *Plesiomonas shigelloides* 810
Shai Ashkenazi

144 *Proteus, Providencia,* and *Morganella* Species 811
William J. Barson and Mario J. Marcon

145 *Serratia* Species 813
Dwight A. Powell and Mario J. Marcon

146 *Salmonella* Species 814
Megan E. Reller

147 *Shigella* Species 819
Shai Ashkenazi and Thomas G. Cleary

148 *Yersinia* Species 823
Theresa J. Ochoa and Miguel O'Ryan

**Nonenterobacteriaceae:
Gram-Negative Bacilli**

149 *Acinetobacter* Species 828
Dwight A. Powell and Mario J. Marcon

150 *Aeromonas* Species 830
Miguel O'Ryan and Yalda C. Lucero Alvarez

151 Less Commonly Encountered Nonenteric
Gram-Negative Bacilli 832
Michael T. Brady and Mario J. Marcon

152 *Eikenella, Pasteurella,* and *Chromobacterium*
Species 835
Michael T. Brady and Mario J. Marcon

153 *Moraxella* and *Psychrobacter* Species 839
Eugene Leibovitz and David Greenberg

154 *Pseudomonas* Species and Related
Organisms 841
Jane L. Burns

155 *Pseudomonas aeruginosa* 842
Alice S. Prince

156 *Burkholderia cepacia* Complex and Other
Burkholderia Species 846
Jane L. Burns

157 *Stenotrophomonas maltophilia* 849
Jane L. Burns

158 *Vibrio cholerae* (Cholera) 849
Anagha R. Loharikar, Manoj P. Menon,
Robert V. Tauxe, and Eric D. Mintz

159 Other *Vibrio* Species 854
Emily J. Cartwright and Patricia M. Griffin

Gram-Negative Coccobacilli

160 *Bartonella* Species (Cat-Scratch Disease) 856
Gordon E. Schutze and Richard F. Jacobs

161 *Brucella* Species (Brucellosis) 861
Edward J. Young

162 *Bordetella pertussis* (Pertussis) and Other
Bordetella Species 865
Sarah S. Long, Kathryn M. Edwards and
Jussi Mertsola

163 *Campylobacter jejuni* and *Campylobacter coli* 873
Manuel R. Amieva

164 Other *Campylobacter* Species 878
Manuel R. Amieva and Guillermo M. Ruiz-Palacios

165 *Capnocytophaga* Species 880
Lorry G. Rubin

166 *Chlamydophila (Chlamydia) pneumoniae* 881
Samir S. Shah

167 *Chlamydia trachomatis* 883
Toni Darville and G. Ingrid J.G. Rours

168 *Chlamydophila (Chlamydia) psittaci*
(Psittacosis) 889
Laura M. Conklin

169 *Coxiella burnetii* (Q fever) 891
Gilbert J. Kersh, Alicia D. Anderson, and
Herbert A. Thompson

170 *Ehrlichia* and *Anaplasma* Species (Ehrlichiosis
and Anaplasmosis) 893
Joanna J. Regan and William L. Nicholson

171 *Francisella tularensis* (Tularemia) 897
Lorry G. Rubin

172 *Haemophilus influenzae* 899
Joseph W. St. Geme, III

173 Other *Haemophilus* Species 906
Jennifer Vodzak

174 *Helicobacter pylori* 908
Benjamin D. Gold

175 Other Gastric and Enterohepatic
Helicobacter Species 916
Benjamin D. Gold

176 *Kingella* Species 919
Pablo Yagupsky and David Greenberg

177 *Legionella* Species 922
Lorry G. Rubin

178 *Rickettsia rickettsii* (Rocky Mountain
Spotted Fever) 926
Jennifer H. McQuiston, Joanna J. Regan, and
Christopher D. Paddock

179 Other *Rickettsia* Species 930
Marina E. Eremeeva and Gregory A. Dasch

180 *Streptobacillus moniliformis*
(Rat-Bite Fever) 938
Lorry G. Rubin

181 Other Gram-Negative Coccobacilli 939
Lorry G. Rubin

Treponemataceae (Spiral Organisms)

182 *Treponema pallidum* (Syphilis) 941
Sarah A. Rawstron and Sarah J. Hawkes

183 Other *Treponema* Species 948
Sarah A. Rawstron

184 *Leptospira* Species (Leptospirosis) 949
Eugene D. Shapiro

185 *Borrelia burgdorferi* (Lyme Disease) 952
Eugene D. Shapiro

186 Other *Borrelia* Species and *Spirillum*
minus 957
Eugene D. Shapiro

Anaerobic Bacteria

187 Anaerobic Bacteria: Classification, Normal
Flora, and Clinical Concepts 958
Itzhak Brook and Sarah S. Long

188 *Clostridium tetani* (Tetanus) 966
Itzhak Brook

189 *Clostridium botulinum* (Botulism) 970
Sarah S. Long

190 *Clostridium difficile* 977
Nalini Singh and David Y. Hyun

191 Other *Clostridium* Species 979
Itzhak Brook

192 *Bacteroides* and *Prevotella* Species and Other
Gram-Negative Bacilli 982
Itzhak Brook

193 *Fusobacterium* Species 985
Robert W. Tolan, Jr

194 Anaerobic Cocci 988
Debrah Meislich and Anat R. Feingold

195 Anaerobic Gram-Positive,
Nonsporulating Bacilli
(including Actinomycosis) 990
Anat R. Feingold and Debrah Meislich

Mycoplasma

196 *Mycoplasma pneumoniae* 993
Samir S. Shah

197 Other *Mycoplasma* Species 998
Samir S. Shah

198 *Ureaplasma urealyticum* 1000
Samir S. Shah

Diseases of Possible Infectious or Unknown Etiology

199 Kawasaki Disease 1002
Anne H. Rowley

200 Chronic Fatigue Syndrome 1007
Gary S. Marshall and Bryan D. Carter

B. Viruses

201 Classification of Human Viruses 1015
Robert David Siegel

DNA Viruses: Poxviridae

202 Poxviridae 1020
Zack S. Moore

DNA Viruses: Herpesviridae

203 Introduction to Herpesviridae 1025
Charles G. Prober

204 Herpes Simplex Virus 1026
Charles G. Prober

205 Varicella-Zoster Virus 1035
Ann M. Arvin

206 Cytomegalovirus 1044
Robert F. Pass

207 Human Herpesviruses 6 and 7 (Roseola,
Exanthem Subitum) 1052
Caroline Breese Hall and Mary T. Caserta

208 Epstein–Barr Virus (Mononucleosis and
Lymphoproliferative Disorders) 1059
Ben Z. Katz

209 Human Herpesvirus 8 (Kaposi Sarcoma-
Associated Herpesvirus) 1066
Caroline Breese Hall and Mary T. Caserta

DNA Viruses: Adenoviridae

210 Adenoviruses 1067
Upton D. Allen and Gail J. Demmler

DNA Viruses: Papovaviridae

211 Human Papillomaviruses *1071*
Loris Y. Hwang and Anna-Barbara Moscicki

212 BK, JC, and Other Human
Polyomaviruses *1075*
Veronique Erard and Michael Boeckh

DNA Viruses: Hepadnaviridae

213 Hepatitis B and Hepatitis D Viruses *1077*
*Kathy K. Byrd, Trudy V. Murphy, and
Dale J. Hu*

DNA Viruses: Parvoviridae

214 Human Parvoviruses *1087*
Eileen Schneider

RNA Viruses: Reoviridae

215 Coltivirus (Colorado Tick Fever) *1092*
Marc Fischer and J. Erin Staples

216 Rotaviruses *1094*
Catherine Yen and Margaret M. Cortese

RNA Viruses: Togaviridae, Flaviviridae, and Bunyaviridae

217 Togaviridae: Alphaviruses *1097*
Edward B. Hayes and J. Erin Staples

218 Flaviviruses *1099*
Edward B. Hayes and Marc Fischer

219 Bunyaviruses *1102*
Adam MacNeil and Pierre E. Rollin

220 Hepatitis C Virus *1105*
*Rania A. Tohme, Deborah Holtzman, and
Scott D. Holmberg*

221 Rubella Virus *1112*
Yvonne A. Maldonado

RNA Viruses: Coronaviridae

222 Human Coronaviruses *1117*
Susan M. Poutanen

RNA Viruses: Paramyxoviridae

223 Parainfluenza Viruses *1121*
Asunción Mejías and Octavio Ramilo

224 Mumps Virus *1125*
Kathleen Gutierrez

225 Respiratory Syncytial Virus *1130*
H. Cody Meissner

226 Human Metapneumovirus *1134*
John V. Williams and James E. Crowe, Jr

227 Rubeola Virus (Measles and Subacute
Sclerosing Panencephalitis) *1137*
Yvonne A. Maldonado

RNA Viruses: Rhabdoviridae

228 Rabies Virus *1145*
Rodney E. Willoughby, Jr

RNA Viruses: Orthomyxoviridae

229 Influenza Viruses *1149*
*Fatimah S. Dawood, Kanta Subbarao, and
Anthony E. Fiore*

RNA Viruses: Arenaviridae and Filoviridae

230 Filoviruses and Arenaviruses *1159*
Margot Anderson and Daniel G. Bausch

RNA Viruses: Retroviridae

231 Introduction to Retroviridae *1164*
Katherine Luzuriaga

232 Human T-Cell Lymphotropic Viruses *1165*
Katherine Luzuriaga

233 Human Immunodeficiency Viruses *1166*
Katherine Luzuriaga

RNA Viruses: Picornaviridae

234 Introduction to Picornaviridae *1167*
John F. Modlin

235 Polioviruses *1168*
Stephanie B. Troy and Yvonne A. Maldonado

236 Enteroviruses and Parechoviruses *1172*
John F. Modlin

237 Hepatitis A Virus *1180*
Roxanne E. Williams and Umid M. Sharapov

238 Rhinoviruses *1186*
Diane E. Pappas and J. Owen Hendley

RNA Viruses: Caliciviridae

239 Caliciviruses *1187*
Aron J. Hall and Marc-Alain Widdowson

240 Astroviruses *1190*
Jacqueline E. Tate and Joseph S. Bresee

241 Hepatitis E Virus *1191*
Eyasu H. Teshale and Saleem Kamili

C. Fungi

242 Classification of Fungi *1194*
Martin B. Kleiman

243 *Candida* Species *1196*
P. Brian Smith and William J. Steinbach

244 *Aspergillus* Species *1203*
William J. Steinbach

245 Agents of Hyalohyphomycosis and
Phaeohyphomycosis *1209*
Thomas F. Patterson and Deanna A. Sutton

246 Agents of Mucormycosis
(Zygomycosis) *1212*
Thomas F. Patterson and Deanna A. Sutton

Contents

247 *Malassezia* Species *1215*
Deanna A. Sutton and Thomas F. Patterson

248 *Sporothrix schenckii* (Sporotrichosis) *1218*
Thomas F. Patterson and Deanna A. Sutton

249 *Cryptococcus* Species *1220*
George R. Thompson, III and Thomas F. Patterson

250 *Histoplasma capsulatum* (Histoplasmosis) *1224*
Martin B. Kleiman

251 *Pneumocystis jirovecii 1230*
Francis Gigliotti and Terry W. Wright

252 *Blastomyces dermatitidis* (Blastomycosis) *1234*
Martin B. Kleiman

253 *Coccidioides immitis* and *Coccidioides posadasii* (Coccidiomycosis) *1239*
Martin B. Kleiman

254 Dermatophytes and Other Superficial Fungi *1246*
Caroline Diane Sarah Piggott and Sheila Fallon Friedlander

255 Agents of Eumycotic Mycetoma: *Pseudallescheria boydii* (Anamorph *Scedosporium apiospermum*) *1250*
Martin B. Kleiman and Elaine Cox

D. Human Parasites and Vectors

256 Classification of Parasites *1254*
Peter J. Hotez

257 Ectoparasites (Lice and Scabies) *1257*
Dirk M. Elston

Protozoa

258 *Babesia* Species (Babesiosis) *1261*
Robert W. Tolan, Jr

259 *Balantidium coli 1266*
Frank E. Berkowitz

260 *Blastocystis* Species *1268*
Frank E. Berkowitz

261 *Cryptosporidium* Species *1269*
Patricia M. Flynn

262 *Endolimax nana 1271*
Frank E. Berkowitz

263 *Entamoeba histolytica* (Amebiasis) *1273*
Candice McNeil and Upinder Singh

264 Other *Entamoeba*, Amebas, and Intestinal Flagellates *1278*
Candice McNeil and Upinder Singh

265 *Giardia intestinalis* (Giardiasis) *1279*
Larry K. Pickering and Andreas Konstantopoulos

266 *Cystoisospora* (*Isospora*) and *Cyclospora* Species *1283*
Patricia M. Flynn

267 *Leishmania* Species (Leishmaniasis) *1285*
Frank E. Berkowitz

268 Microsporidia *1291*
Patricia M. Flynn

269 *Naegleria fowleri 1293*
Candice McNeil and Upinder Singh

270 *Acanthamoeba* Species *1295*
Candice McNeil and Upinder Singh

271 *Plasmodium* Species (Malaria) *1298*
Aarti Agarwal, Meredith McMorrow and Paul M. Arguin

272 *Sarcocystis* Species *1306*
Frank E. Berkowitz

273 *Toxoplasma gondii* (Toxoplasmosis) *1308*
Despina Contopoulos-Ioannidis and Jose G. Montoya

274 *Trichomonas vaginalis 1317*
Kimberly A. Workowski

275 *Trypanosoma* Species (Trypanosomiasis) *1319*
Frank E. Berkowitz

Nematodes

276 Intestinal Nematodes *1326*
Michael Cappello and Peter J. Hotez

277 Tissue Nematodes *1334*
Dickson D. Despommier and Peter J. Hotez

278 Blood and Tissue Nematodes (Filarial Worms) *1342*
LeAnne M. Fox

Cestodes

279 *Diphyllobothrium, Dipylidium,* and *Hymenolepis* Species *1347*
Frank O. Richards, Jr and Susan P. Montgomery

280 *Taenia solium, Taenia asiatica,* and *Taenia saginata* (Taeniasis and Cysticercosis) *1350*
Michael Cappello, Peter M. Schantz, and A. Clinton White, Jr

281 *Echinococcus* Species (Agents of Cystic, Alveolar, and Polycystic Echinococcosis) *1356*
Pedro L. Moro and Peter M. Schantz

282 *Taenia* (*Multiceps*) *multiceps* and *Taenia serialis* (Coenurosis) *1362*
Michael Cappello, Peter M. Schantz, and A. Clinton White, Jr

Trematodes

283 Intestinal Trematodes *1363*
LeAnne M. Fox

284 *Clonorchis, Opisthorchis, Fasciola,* and *Paragonimus* Species *1365*
Jeffrey L. Jones

285 **Blood Trematodes (Schistosomiasis)** *1368*
Frank O. Richards, Jr

Part IV: Laboratory Diagnosis and Therapy of Infectious Diseases

A. The Clinician and the Laboratory

286 **Laboratory Diagnosis of Infection Due to Bacteria, Fungi, Parasites, and Rickettsiae** *1373*
John C. Christenson and E. Kent Korgenski

287 **Laboratory Diagnosis of Infection Due to Viruses, *Chlamydia*, *Chlamydophila*, and *Mycoplasma* 1384**
Tony Mazzulli

288 **Laboratory Manifestations of Infectious Diseases** *1400*
Sarah S. Long

B. Anti-Infective Therapy

289 **Principles of Anti-Infective Therapy** *1412*
John S. Bradley and Sarah S. Long

290 **Mechanisms and Detection of Antimicrobial Resistance** *1421*
Melissa B. Miller and Peter H. Gilligan

291 **Pharmacokinetic–Pharmacodynamic Basis of Optimal Antibiotic Therapy** *1433*
Michael N. Neely and Michael D. Reed

292 **Antimicrobial Agents** *1453*
John S. Bradley and Jason B. Sauberan

293 **Antifungal Agents** *1484*
William J. Steinbach and Christopher C. Dvorak

294 **Topical Antimicrobial Agents** *1493*
Jane M. Gould and Gail L. Rodgers

295 **Antiviral Agents** *1502*
David W. Kimberlin

296 **Antiparasitic Agents** *1518*
Craig M. Wilson

Index *1547*

All references are available online at www.expertconsult.com

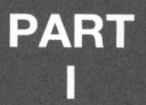

1 Principles of Epidemiology and Public Health

Benjamin Schwartz and Stacey W. Martin

Epidemiology is the study of the distribution and determinants of disease or other health-related states or events in specified populations and the application of this study to control of health problems.[1] The key component of this definition is the link between epidemiology and populations, which distinguishes it from clinical case studies that focus on individuals.

Health events can be characterized by their distribution (descriptive epidemiology) and by factors that influence their occurrence (analytic epidemiology). In both descriptive and analytic epidemiology, health-related questions are addressed using quantitative methods to identify patterns or associations from which inferences can be drawn and interventions developed, applied, and assessed.

DESCRIPTIVE EPIDEMIOLOGY

Surveillance

The goals of descriptive epidemiology are to define the frequency of health-related events and their distribution by person, place, and time. The foundation of descriptive epidemiology is surveillance, or case detection. Retrospective surveillance identifies health events from existing data, such as clinical or laboratory records, hospital discharge data, and death certificates. Prospective surveillance identifies and collects information about cases as they occur, for example, through ongoing laboratory-based reporting.

With *passive surveillance*, case reports are supplied voluntarily by clinicians, laboratories, health departments, or other sources. The completeness and accuracy of passive reporting are affected by whether reporting is legally mandated, whether a definitive diagnosis can be established, illness severity, interest of the public and the medical community in a condition, and whether a report will elicit a public health response. Because more severe illness is more likely to be diagnosed and reported, the severity and clinical spectrum of passively reported cases are likely to differ from that of all cases of an illness. Passively collected reports of nationally notifiable diseases are tabulated in the *Morbidity and Mortality Weekly Report* (http://www.cdc.gov/mmwr/).

In *active surveillance*, effort is made to ascertain all cases of a condition occurring in a defined population. Active case finding can be prospective (involving routine contacts with reporting sources), retrospective (through record audit) or both. Population-based active surveillance, in which all cases in a defined geographic area are identified and reported, provides the most complete and unbiased ascertainment of disease and is optimal for describing the rate of a disease and its clinical spectrum. By contrast, active surveillance conducted at only one or several participating facilities can yield biased information on disease frequency or spectrum based on the representativeness of the patient population and the size of the sample obtained.

Case Definition

Establishing a standard case definition is an important first step for surveillance and description of the epidemiology of a disease or health event.[2] Formulation of a case definition is important particularly where laboratory diagnostic testing is not definitive. More restrictive case definitions minimize misclassification but may exclude true cases and are most useful when investigating a newly recognized condition, in which the ability to determine etiology, pathogenesis, or risk factors is decreased by inclusion of noncases in the study population. A more inclusive definition might be important in an outbreak setting when cases are being detected for further investigation or when preventive interventions can be applied. Multiple research or public health objectives can be addressed by developing a tiered case definition that incorporates varying degrees of diagnostic certainty for definite and probable cases.

Sensitivity, Specificity, and Predictive Value

Sensitivity, specificity, and predictive values can be used to quantify the performance of a case definition or the results of a diagnostic test or algorithm (Table 1-1). Unlike sensitivity and specificity, predictive values vary with the prevalence of a condition within a population. Even with a highly specific diagnostic test, if a disease is uncommon among those tested, a large proportion of positive test results will be false positives, and the positive predictive value will be low (Table 1-2). If the test is applied more selectively, where the proportion of people tested who truly have disease is greater, the test's predictive value will be improved. Thus, sensitivity and specificity are characteristics of the test, whereas predictive values depend on the disease prevalence in the population in which the test is applied. Often, the sensitivity and specificity of a test are inversely related. Selecting the optimal balance of sensitivity and specificity depends on the purpose for which the test is used. Generally, a screening test should be highly sensitive, whereas a follow-up confirmatory test should be highly specific.

Incidence and Prevalence

Characterizing disease frequency is one of the most important aspects of descriptive epidemiology. Frequency measures typically include a count of new or existing cases of disease as the numerator and a quantification of the population at risk as the denominator. *Cumulative incidence* is expressed as a proportion and describes the number of new cases of an illness occurring in a fixed at-risk population over a specified period of time, generally 1 year, unless otherwise stated. *Incidence density* is defined as the rate of new cases of disease in a dynamic at-risk population; for this measure the denominator typically is expressed as the population-time at-risk (e.g., person-time). Because the occurrence of many infections varies with season, extrapolating annual incidence from cases detected during a short observation period can be inaccurate. In describing the risk of acquiring illness during a disease outbreak, the *attack rate*, defined as the number of new cases of disease occurring in a specified population and time period, is a useful measure.

Prevalence refers to the proportion of the population having a condition at a specific point in time. As such, it is a better measure

TABLE 1-1. Definitions and Formulae for the Calculation of Important Epidemiologic Parameters

Measures of test accuracy	*Sensitivity:* Proportion of true positives (diseased) with a positive test	$A/(A + C)$	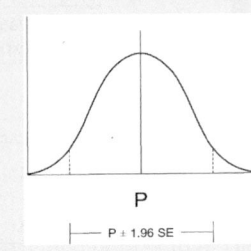
	Specificity: Proportion of true negatives (nondiseased) with a negative test	$D/(B + D)$	
	Positive predictive value (PPV): Proportion of positive tests that are true positives	$A/(A + B)$	
	Negative predictive value (NPV): Proportion of negative tests that are true negatives	$D/(C + D)$	
Measures of data dispersion and precision	*Variance:* Statistic describing variability of individuals in a population	$[1/(n-1)][(x_1 - \bar{x})^2 + (x_2 - \bar{x})^2 + \ldots + (x_n - \bar{x})^2]$	
	Standard error: Statistic describing the variability of sample-based point estimates (*Po*) around the true population value being estimated	$\sqrt{\text{Variance}}$	
	Confidence interval: A range of values that is believed to contain the true value within a defined level of certainty (usually 95%, as shown)		
Absolute measures of association and risk	*Absolute risk reduction* (ARR), *excess risk* or *attributable risk:* Difference in the incidence of the outcome between exposed and unexposed	$(A/(A + B)) - (C/(C + D))$	
	Number needed to treat (NNT): Number of individuals that must receive an intervention (or exposure) to prevent one negative outcome	$1/\text{ARR}$	
Relative measures of association and risk	*Relative risk* or *risk ratio* (RR): Risk (probability) of a health event in those with a given exposure divided by the risk in those without the exposure	$\dfrac{A/(A + B)}{C/(C + D)}$	
	Odds ratio (OR): Odds of a given exposure among those with a health event divided by odds of exposure among those without the health event	AD/BC	
Measure of impact	*Population attributable fraction:* The proportion of disease in a population due to the specific exposure	$[P_e\,(\text{RR} - 1)]/[1 + P_e\,(\text{RR} - 1)]$ (Proportion exposed, P_e = $(A + B)/(A + B + C + D)$)	

TABLE 1-2. Positive and Negative Predictive Values for a Hypothetical Diagnostic Test Having a Sensitivity of 90% and Specificity of 90%

Proportion with Condition	Positive Predictive Value	Negative Predictive Value
1%	8%	>99%
10%	50%	99%
20%	69%	97%
50%	90%	90%

of disease burden for chronic conditions than is incidence or attack rate, which identify only new (incident) cases. Prevalent cases of disease can be ascertained in a cross-sectional survey, whereas determining incidence requires longitudinal surveillance. When disease prevalence is low and incidence and duration are stable, prevalence is a function of disease incidence multiplied by its average duration.

Describing Illness by Person, Place, and Time

Characterizing disease by person, place, and time is often useful. Demographic variables, including age, sex, socioeconomic status, and race or ethnicity are often associated with the risk of disease. Describing a disease by place can help define risk groups; for example, when an illness is caused by an environmental exposure or is vector-borne, or in an outbreak with a point source exposure. Time, also, is a useful descriptor of disease occurrence. Evaluating

long-term (secular) trends provides information that can be used by policymakers or clinicians to identify emerging health problems or to assess the impact of prevention programs. The timing of illness in outbreaks can be displayed in an epidemic curve and can be useful in defining the mode of transmission of an infection or its incubation period and in assessing the effectiveness of control measures.

ANALYTIC EPIDEMIOLOGY

Study Design

The goal of analytic studies is to identify predictors of an outcome. This goal can be addressed in experimental or epidemiologic (observational) studies. Ecological or trend studies also can be used to assess predictors when the frequency or distribution of an outcome has changed over time or differs between populations. In contrast to experimental or observational studies that analyze information about individuals, ecological studies draw inferences from data on a population level. Inferences from ecological studies must be made with caution because populations differ in multiple ways and because relationships observed for groups do not necessarily apply to individuals (known as the "ecological fallacy"). Because of these drawbacks, ecological studies are suited best to generating hypotheses that can be tested using other study methods.

In *experimental studies,* hypotheses are tested by systematically allocating an exposure of interest to subjects in separate groups to achieve the desired comparison. Such studies include randomized, controlled, double-blinded treatment trials, and laboratory experiments. By carefully controlling study variables, investigators can

TABLE 1-3. Types of Observational Studies and Their Advantages and Disadvantages

Type of Study	Design, Characteristics	Advantages	Disadvantages
Cohort	Prospective or retrospective	Ideal for outbreak investigations in defined populations	Unsuited for rare diseases or those with long latency
	Select study group	Prospective design ensures that exposure preceded disease	Expensive
	Observe for exposures and disease	Selection of study group is unbiased by knowledge of disease status	May require long follow-up periods
	Calculate relative risk (RR) or hazard ratio (HR) of disease given exposure	RR and HR accurately describe risk given exposure	Difficult to investigate multiple exposures
Cross-sectional	Nondirectional	Rapid, easy to perform, and inexpensive	Timing of exposure and disease may be difficult to determine
	Select study group	Ideal to determine knowledge, attitudes, and behaviors	Biases may affect recall of past exposures
	Determine exposure and disease status		
	Calculate RR for disease given exposure		
Case-control	Retrospective	Rapid, easy to perform, and inexpensive	Timing of exposure and disease may be difficult to determine
	Identify cases with disease	Ideal for studying rare diseases, those with long latency, new diseases	Biases can occur in selecting cases and controls and determining exposures
	Identify controls without disease		OR only provides an estimate of the RR if disease is rare
	Determine exposures in cases and controls		
	Calculate odds ratio (OR) for an exposure given disease		

restrict differences among groups, thereby increasing the likelihood that the observed differences are a consequence of the specific factor being studied. Because experiments are prospective, the temporal sequence of exposure and outcome can be clearly established, making it easy to define cause and effect.

By contrast, *epidemiologic studies* test hypotheses using observational methods to assess exposures and outcomes among individuals in populations and identifying statistical associations from which inferences regarding causation are drawn. Although observational studies cannot be controlled to the same degree as experiments, they are practical in circumstances in which exposures or behaviors cannot be assigned. Moreover, the results are more generalizable to a real population having a wide range of attributes. The three basic types of observational studies are cohort studies, cross-sectional studies, and case-control studies (Table 1-3). Hybrid study designs, incorporating components of these three, have also been developed.[3] In planning observational studies care must be taken in the selection of participants to minimize the possibility of bias. Selection bias results when study subjects have differing probabilities of being selected that are related to the risk factors or outcomes under evaluation.

Cohort Studies

In a *cohort study*, subjects are categorized based on their exposure to a suspected risk factor and are observed for the development of disease. Associations between exposure and disease are expressed by the relative risk of disease in exposed and unexposed groups (see Table 1-1). Cohort studies typically are prospective, with exposure being defined before disease occurs. In retrospective cohort studies, in which the cohort is selected after the outcome has occurred, exposures are determined from existing records that preceded the outcome, and, thus, the directionality of the exposure–disease relationship is still forward. By characterizing exposures before development of disease, selection bias is minimized and inference of cause and effect is easier. A major disadvantage of cohort studies is that they are impractical for studying rare diseases or conditions with a long latent period between

exposure and the onset of clinical illness. Moreover, whereas cohort studies can assess multiple potential outcomes resulting from an exposure, it is difficult to investigate multiple exposures as risk factors for a single outcome. In general, cohort studies are unsuited for investigating risk factors for new or rare diseases or for generating new hypotheses about possible exposure–disease relationships.

Cohort studies provide data not only on whether an outcome occurs but, for those experiencing the outcome, on when it occurs. Analysis of time-to-event data for outcomes such as death or illness is a powerful approach to assess or compare the impacts of preventive or therapeutic interventions. The probability of remaining event-free over time can be expressed in a *Kaplan–Meier survival curve* where, initially, the event-free probability is 1 and declines in a step-function as the outcomes of interest occur (Figure 1-1A). Time-to-event data can also be displayed as the *cumulative hazard* of an event occurring among members of a cohort, increasing from 0 at enrollment (Figure 1-1B). These two approaches are related in that the hazard reflects the incident event rate while survival reflects the cumulative nonoccurrence of that outcome.[4,5] With time-to-event analysis, the association between exposure and disease is often expressed as a hazard ratio. Like a relative risk, the hazard ratio is a comparative measure of risk between exposed and unexposed groups, the primary difference being the hazard ratio compares event experience over the entire time period, whereas the relative risk compares event occurrence only at the study endpoint.[6]

Cross-Sectional Studies

In a *cross-sectional study*, or survey, a sample is selected and at a single point in time exposures and outcome are determined. Outcomes may include disease status or behaviors and beliefs. Unlike cohort studies, multiple exposures can be evaluated as explanations for the outcome. Associations are characterized by the *prevalence ratio* similar to the relative ratio in cohort studies. Because neither exposures nor outcomes are used in selection of the study group, their prevalence is an estimate of that in the

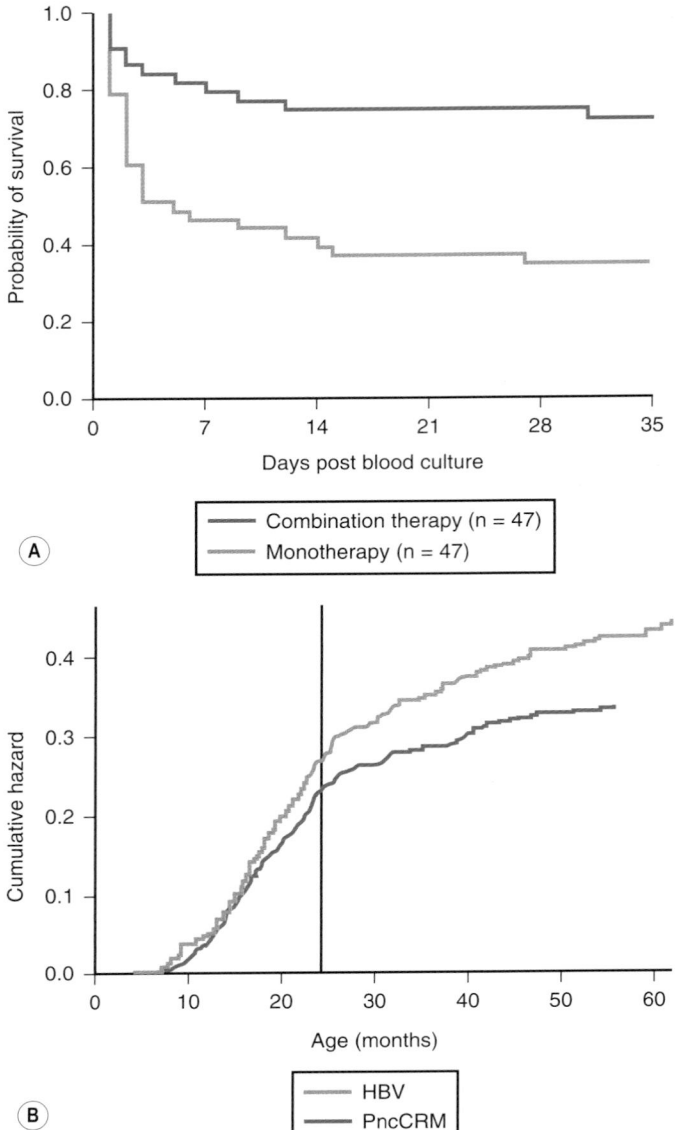

Figure 1-1. Example of Kaplan–Meier and cumulative hazard curves. **(A)** Survival plot for critically ill patients with *Streptococcus pneumoniae* bacteremia treated with monotherapy or combination therapy. (Redrawn from Baddour LM, Yu VL, Klugman KP, et al. Combination antibiotic therapy lowers mortality among severely ill patients with pneumococcal bacteremia. Am J Respir Crit Care Med 2004;170:440–444.) **(B)** Cumulative hazard of tympanostomy tube placement from 2 months until 4–5 years of age in children who received pneumococcal conjugate vaccine (PncCRM) or a control vaccine (HBV). (Redrawn from Palmu AAI, Verho J, Jokinen J, et al. The seven-valent pneumococcal conjugate vaccine reduced tympanostomy tube placement in children. Pediatr Infect Dis J 2004;23:732–738.)

overall population from which the sample was drawn. National survey data characterizing health status, behaviors, and medical care are available from the National Center for Health Statistics (http://www.cdc.gov/nchs/index.htm).

Case-Control Studies

In a *case-control study,* the investigator identifies a group of people with a disease or outcome of interest (cases) and compares their exposures with those in a selected group of people who do not have disease (controls). Differences between the groups are expressed by an *odds ratio,* which compares the odds of an exposure in case and control groups (see Table 1-1). Case-control studies are retrospective in that disease status is known and serves as the basis for selecting the two comparison groups; exposures are then determined by reviewing available records or by interview.

A major advantage of case-control studies is their efficiency in studying uncommon diseases or those with a long latency. Case-control studies also can evaluate multiple exposures that may contribute to a single outcome. They tend to be less costly and more time-efficient than cohort studies because study subjects can be identified from existing sources (such as hospital or laboratory records, disease registries, or surveillance reports) and, after identification of suitable control subjects, data on prior exposures can be collected rapidly. Case-control studies also have several drawbacks: bias can be introduced during selection of cases and controls and in retrospectively determining exposures, and inferring causation from statistically significant associations can be complicated by difficulty in determining the temporal sequence of exposure and disease in a retrospective study.

Causal Inference and the Impact of Bias

Care must be taken in the design of all analytic studies, whether experimental or observational; however, concerns about validity and the impact of potential biases are particularly important for observational studies.

The *validity* of a study is the degree to which inferences drawn from a study are warranted. Internal validity refers to the correctness of study conclusions for the population from which the study sample was drawn, whereas external validity refers to the extent to which the study results can be generalized beyond the population sampled. The validity of a study can be affected by bias, or *systematic error,* in selecting the study participants (sampling), in ascertaining their exposures, or in analyzing and interpreting study data. For errors to result in bias, they must be systematic, or directional. *Nonsystematic error* (random misclassification) decreases the ability of a study to identify a true association but does not result in detection of a spurious association.

Several sources of bias can occur in selection of study participants (Box 1-1). *Diagnosis bias* results when persons with a given exposure are more likely to be diagnosed as having disease than are people without the exposure; this can occur because diagnostic testing is more likely to be done or because the interpretation of a test may be affected by knowledge of exposure status. For hospital-based studies, differential referral also can bias selection of a study sample. This bias would occur if, for example, the frequency of an exposure varied with socioeconomic status and a hospital predominantly admitted persons from either a high- or low-income group. Bias also can occur when eligible subjects refuse to participate in a study as cases or controls. However, nonresponse, even at high rates, does not result in bias if responders and nonresponders are similar with respect to the exposures of interest.

Determining exposures can be affected by several types of bias. Recall of exposures may be different for persons who have had an illness compared with people who were well. This bias occurs in either direction: cases may be more likely to remember an exposure that they associate with their illness (e.g., what was eaten before an episode of diarrhea) or less likely to recall an exposure if a severe illness affected memory. Interviewers can introduce bias by questioning cases and controls differently about their exposures. Misclassification of exposures can result from errors in measurement such as might occur with the use of an inaccurate laboratory test; these errors often are random rather than systematic.

Even a carefully designed study that minimizes potential biases can make erroneous causal inferences. An exposure can appear falsely to be associated with disease because it is closely linked to the true, but undetermined, risk factor. Race is often found to be associated with the risk of a disease, whereas the true risk factor may be an unmeasured variable that is linked to race, such as socioeconomic status. The risk of making incorrect inferences can be minimized by considering certain general criteria for

BOX 1-1. Potential Sources of Bias in Observational Studies[a]

BIAS IN CASE ASCERTAINMENT AND CASE/CONTROL SELECTION

Surveillance bias: differential surveillance or reporting for exposed and unexposed

Diagnosis bias: differential use of diagnostic tests in exposed and unexposed

Referral bias: differential admission to hospital based on an exposure or a variable associated with exposure

Selection bias: differential sampling of cases based on an exposure or a variable associated with exposure

Nonresponse bias: differential outcome or exposures of responders and nonresponders

Survival bias: differential exposures between those who survive to be included in a study and those who die following an illness

Misclassification bias: systematic error in classification of disease status

BIAS IN ESTIMATION OF EXPOSURE

Recall bias: differential recall of exposures based on disease status

Interviewer bias: differential ascertainment of exposures based on disease status

Misclassification bias: systematic errors in measurement or classification of exposure

[a]A more complete listing is provided by Sackett.[7]

establishing causation. These include the strength of an association, the presence of a dose–response effect, a clear temporal sequence of exposure to disease, the consistency of findings with those of other studies, and the biologic plausibility of the hypothesis.[8]

Statistical Analysis

Characteristics of Populations and Samples

Whereas epidemiologic analysis seeks to make valid conclusions about populations, the entire population rarely is included in a study. An assumption underlying statistical analysis is that the sample evaluated was selected randomly from the population. Often, this criterion is not met and calls into question the appropriateness and interpretation of statistical analyses.

The mean, median, and mode describe a central value for samples and populations. The arithmetic *mean* is the average, determined by summing individual values and dividing by the sample size. When data are not normally distributed (skewed), calculation of a geometric mean can limit the impact of outlying values. The geometric mean is calculated by taking the *n*th root of the *product* of all the individual values, where *n* is the total number of individual values. For example, immunogenicity of vaccines is usually expressed by the geometric mean titer. The *median*, or middle value, is another way to describe nonnormally distributed data. The *mode*, or most commonly occurring value in a sample, is rarely used.

Several measures can be used to describe the variability in a sample. The *range* describes the difference between the highest and lowest value, whereas the *interquartile range* defines the difference between the 25th and 75th percentiles. Variation among individuals is most often characterized by the variance or standard deviation. The *variance* is defined as the mean of the squared deviation of each observation from the sample's mean. The *standard deviation* is the square root of the variance (see Table 1-1). For a normally distributed population, 68% of values fall within 1 standard deviation of the mean and 95% of values within 1.96 standard deviations. The *standard error* represents a type

of standard deviation and is used to describe the standard deviation of an estimate (e.g., mean, odds ratio, relative risk).

When analyzing a sample, the mean or other statistics describing the sample represent a *point estimate* of that parameter for the entire population. If another random sample were drawn from the same population, the point estimate for the parameter of interest would likely be different, depending on the variability in the population and the sample size selected. A *confidence interval* defines a range of values that includes the true population value, within a defined level of certainty. Most often, the 95% confidence interval is presented (see Table 1-1).

Absolute and Relative Measures of Association

Measures of association are used by investigators to assess the strength of an association between an exposure and an outcome. In a cohort study, the *absolute risk reduction* (also known as *excess risk, attributable risk,* or *risk difference*) is the difference in the incidence of the outcome between exposed and unexposed. The *number needed to treat* is a measure of the number of individuals that must receive a treatment to prevent one negative outcome and is calculated as the reciprocal of the *absolute risk reduction*. In addition to absolute measures, relative measures also are useful for describing the strength of an association. In a cohort study or survey, the relative risk or risk ratio compares the risk of disease for those with versus those without an exposure (see Table 1-1). In case-control studies, association is assessed by the odds ratio, which compares the odds of exposure among those with and without a disease or health outcome; when disease is uncommon (<10%) in both exposed and unexposed groups, the odds ratio approximates the relative risk. For time-to-event analyses, the comparative risk is expressed as the *hazard ratio*. Odds ratios, relative risks, and hazard ratios greater than 1 signify increased risk given exposure and values less than 1 suggest that exposure decreases the risk of an outcome. Because observational studies generally do not include all members of a population, these measures of association represent an estimate of the true value within the entire population. Statistical analyses can help guide investigators in making causal inferences based on a point estimate of these measures of association.

Statistical Significance

Statistical tests are applied to assess the likelihood that the study results were obtained by chance alone rather than representing a true difference within the population. Most investigators consider a P value <0.05 as being *statistically significant*, indicating a less than 5% risk that the observed association is the result of chance alone (designated a *type I error*, the probability of which is the *alpha level*). Although use of this cutoff for significance testing has become conventional, ignoring higher P values can lead to missing a real and important association, whereas blind faith in the significance of lower P values can lead to erroneous conclusions. Statistical testing should contribute to, but not replace, criteria for evaluating possible causation. Statistical significance can also be defined based on 95% confidence intervals, which approximately correspond to a P value of 0.05. An odds ratio, relative risk, or hazard ratio is considered statistically significant if the 95% confidence interval does not include 1. An advantage of using confidence intervals to define statistical significance is that they provide information on whether a finding is statistically significant and on the possible range of values for the point estimate in the population, with 95% certainty.

Another pitfall in interpreting statistical significance is ignoring the *magnitude* of an effect in favor of its "significance." A very large study can identify small, perhaps trivial, differences between study groups as significant. Some epidemiologists have proposed that, despite statistical significance, odds ratios less than 2 or 3 in an observational study should not be interpreted because unidentified bias or confounding could have accounted for a difference of this magnitude.[9] Conversely, the relative risk or odds ratio associating an exposure and outcome may be large but, if the exposure is uncommon in both groups, will not explain most cases of illness. The public health importance of an exposure can be described by the *population-attributable fraction*, or the proportion of the disease in a population that is related to the exposure of interest.

Sample Size

One reason that a study may fail to identify a true risk factor as statistically significant is that the sample size was too small (designated a *type II error*, the probability of which is the *beta level*). Statistical power is defined as $1 - \beta$ and is the complement of type II error, that is, the probability of correctly identifying a difference of specified size between groups, if such a difference truly exists. The problem of inadequate sample size in clinical studies was highlighted in an analysis of "negative" randomized controlled trials reported in three leading medical journals between 1975 and 1990. Of 70 reports, only 16% and 36% had sufficient statistical power (80%) to detect a true 25% or 50% relative difference, respectively, between treatment groups.[10]

In calculating sample sizes for testing hypotheses, investigators must select type I and type II errors and define the magnitude of the difference that is deemed clinically important. Often, the type II error is set at 0.2, indicating acceptance of a 20% likelihood that a true difference exists but would not be identified by the study. Sample size calculations can be performed using a range of computer software. The program Epi-Info can be used to perform sample size calculations as well as other statistical functions and is available at no charge from the Centers for Disease Control and Prevention (www.cdc.gov/epiinfo/).

Ensuring an adequate sample size is particularly important for studies attempting to prove *equivalence* or *noninferiority* of a new treatment compared with standard therapy. Food and Drug Administration guidance recommends that noninferiority trials adopt a null hypothesis that a difference exists between treatments; this hypothesis is rejected if the lower 95% confidence limit for the new treatment is within a specified margin of the point estimate for standard therapy. Because the null hypotheses can never be proven or accepted, the failure to reject a null hypothesis of no difference between treatments or exposure does not prove equivalence. The importance of this distinction is illustrated by an analysis of 25 studies claiming equivalence of therapies for pediatric bacterial meningitis. Twenty-three studies claimed equivalence based on a failure to detect a significant difference between treatment groups. However, only 3 of these trials could exclude a 10% difference in mortality, potentially missing a clinically significant difference.[11]

In some situations, an investigator would want to detect a significant difference among study groups as soon as possible, for example, when a therapeutic or preventive intervention could be applied once a risk group is identified or when there are concerns about the safety of a drug or vaccine. One approach to this situation is to include in the study design an *interim analysis* after a specified number of subjects are evaluated. Because the likelihood of identifying chance differences as significant increases with the number of analyses, it is recommended that the threshold for defining statistical significance should become more stringent as the number of planned analyses increases.[12] If each interim analysis can lead to stopping the trial, this study design is considered a group sequential method.[13] Another example of a group sequential design is when concordance or discordance in outcome is tabulated for each matched set exposed to alternate treatments. Results for each set are plotted on a graph and data collection continues until a preset threshold for a significant difference between study groups is crossed or no significant difference is detected at a given power.[12]

Statistical Inference

Statistical testing is used to determine the significance of differences between study groups, and, thus, it provides guidance on whether to accept or reject the null hypothesis. Although providing details of specific statistical tests is outside the scope of this chapter, Table 1-4 provides examples of statistical tests that can be applied in analyzing different types of exposure and outcome variables.

Using appropriate analytic and statistical methods is important in identifying significant predictors of an outcome (i.e., risk factors) correctly. *Confounding variables* are associated with the disease of interest and with other exposure variables that are associated with the disease and are not part of the causal pathway (Figure 1-2). For example, in a study evaluating the link between childcare attendance and pharyngeal carriage of penicillin-resistant pneumococci, recent antimicrobial use would be a confounding variable because it is associated with both childcare attendance and carriage of resistant pneumococci. Failure to adjust for recent antimicrobial use as a confounding variable would result in overestimating the relationship between childcare and resistant pneumococcal carriage. *Effect modifiers* interact with risk factors to affect their impact on outcome but may or may not themselves affect outcome. Frequently, age is an effect modifier, with an exposure associated significantly with an outcome in one age group but not in another.

There are several approaches to control for confounding variables and effect modifiers. In study design, an extraneous variable can be controlled for by randomization, restricting sampling to one category of the variable or by *frequency matching* to obtain similar proportions of cases and controls in each stratum. A more extreme form of matching is to select control subjects who are similar to individual cases for extraneous variables (e.g., age, sex, underlying disease) and to analyze whether exposures are concordant or discordant within matched sets. A newer approach to study design is the *case-crossover*[14] or *case series*[15] analysis. In this method, exposures occurring in a defined risk period before the outcome are compared with exposures occurring outside the risk window. This approach has been adapted to the study of adverse events after vaccination. If the vaccine causes the event, the rate of the event would be greater within a defined risk window than would be predicted by chance alone based on the expected distribution of the event.[16] The strength of this approach is

TABLE 1-4. Types of Statistical Tests Used to Evaluate the Significance of Associations among Categorical and Continuous Variables

Independent Variable (Exposure, Risk Factor)	Dependent Variable (Disease, Outcome)	
	Categorical and Dichotomous	Continuous
CATEGORICAL		
Dichotomous	Chi-square test	Student-test (parametric)
	Fisher exact test	Wilcoxon rank sum test (nonparametric)
>2 categories	Chi-square test	Analysis of variance (parametric)
		Kruskal–Wallis test (nonparametric)
CONTINUOUS	Logistic regression	Linear regression
		Correlation (Pearson: parametric; Spearman: nonparametric)

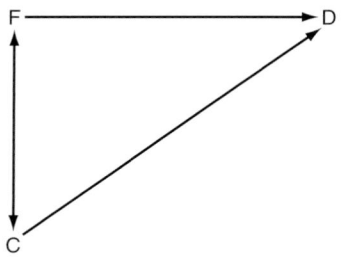

Figure 1-2. Path diagram illustrating association between a confounding variable (*C*), another risk factor (*F*), and the disease outcome (*D*).

that each case serves as his or her own control, decreasing confounding.

At the analysis stage, the impact of confounding variables and effect modifiers can be limited by performing a stratified analysis or using a multivariable model. In a *stratified analysis*, the possible association between a risk factor and an outcome is determined separately within different categories, or strata, of the extraneous variable. Stratum-specific estimates can be combined into a single estimate using an appropriate statistical test (e.g., a *Mantel–Haentzel odds ratio*). If a stratification variable is an effect modifier, the relative risk or odds ratio will differ substantially between the strata; for example, an exposure may be a strong risk factor in one age group but not another. In this setting, a summary statistic should not be presented and results for each stratum should be presented separately. When the extraneous variable is confounding, an unstratified analysis can identify an exposure as a significant risk factor; when the analysis is stratified by the confounding variable, however, the apparent association with outcome is abolished in each stratum, indicating that the exposure is not an independent risk factor for disease.

Because stratified analyses rapidly become confusing as the number of strata increases, techniques of *mathematical modeling* have been developed that permit the simultaneous control of multiple variables. Significant risk factors determined in a *multivariable model* are interpreted as each contributing independently and significantly to the outcome, thus controlling for confounding. Effect modification can be taken into account by including terms expressing the interaction between a risk factor and effect modifier in the model. Various multivariable models are appropriate for discrete, continuous, and time-dependent outcomes. A limitation of multivariable modeling is *multicollinearity*, which occurs when two or more explanatory variables of interest are highly correlated, and can result in inaccurate measures of association and decreased statistical power. The risk of multicollinearity can be reduced by assessing correlations between potential risk factors and selecting which variables to include in the model. Various methods to identify and minimize multicollinearity have been developed.[17]

VACCINE EFFICACY STUDIES

With advances in vaccine development and the licensure of new vaccines, the ability to interpret results of vaccine efficacy studies becomes increasingly important. Most prelicensure efficacy studies are experimental randomized, double-blind, controlled trials in which *vaccine efficacy* (VE) is calculated by comparing the attack rates (AR) for disease in the vaccinated and unvaccinated groups (VE (%) = ((AR unvaccinated − AR vaccinated)/AR unvaccinated) × 100; or (1 − RR) × 100).

After licensure, conducting controlled studies, which requires withholding vaccine from a control group, is no longer ethical. Therefore, further studies of efficacy must be observational rather than experimental, comparing persons who have chosen to be immunized with those who have not. In *case-control efficacy studies*, vaccination status of persons with disease is compared with vaccination status of healthy controls. The number of vaccinated and unvaccinated cases and controls is included in a two-by-two table, and vaccine efficacy is calculated as 1 minus the odds ratio (VE (%) = (1 − OR) × 100). When the proportion of cases who have been vaccinated is less than the proportion of vaccinated controls, the odds ratio is <1 and the point estimate for efficacy indicates that immunization is protective. The precision of the estimate is expressed by the 95% confidence interval. A lower 95% confidence limit that is greater than 0% indicates statistically significant protection; often investigators set power of vaccine efficacy studies so that the lower confidence limit is much greater than zero and consistent with meaningful levels of protection. The most important component of a case-control efficacy study is selecting controls who have the same opportunity for immunization as do cases. If cases had less opportunity to be immunized, results will be biased toward showing protection. Factors such as low socioeconomic status, which may increase the risk of disease and

decrease the chance of being immunized, are potential confounding variables and can be controlled for by matching controls to cases for those factors.

Cohort studies also can be used to determine vaccine efficacy after licensure. A study design called the *indirect-cohort method* was developed by researchers at the Centers for Disease Control and Prevention to evaluate the efficacy of the pneumococcal polysaccharide vaccine using data collected by disease surveillance.[18] The study cohort included persons identified with invasive pneumococcal infections. The study hypothesis was that, if vaccine was protective, the proportion of vaccinated persons infected with pneumococcal serotypes that are included in the vaccine formulation would be less than the proportion of unvaccinated persons infected with vaccine-type strains. Vaccine efficacy was calculated from the relative serotype distributions overall and for each individual serotype. In a study of pneumococcal polysaccharide vaccine efficacy that utilized this approach, the point estimate of efficacy for preventing invasive infection was 57% (95% confidence interval, 45% to 66%);[19] this estimate is similar to that obtained in a case-control efficacy study.[20]

DISEASE CONTROL AND PUBLIC HEALTH POLICY
Outbreak Investigations

Outbreak investigations require knowledge of disease transmission and use of descriptive and analytic epidemiologic tools. Possible outbreaks can be identified from surveillance data showing an increased rate of an infection or an unusual clustering in person, place, and time. Comparing the incidence rate of disease with a baseline rate from a previous period is helpful in validating the occurrence of an outbreak. Other explanations for changes in the apparent rate of disease occurrence, such as diagnostic error, seasonal variations, and changes in reporting, must be considered. Using sensitive molecular methods to assess similarity between isolates from cases may be helpful in documenting that an apparent cluster of cases represents an outbreak, because most outbreaks are caused by a single strain.

After establishing the presence of an outbreak, the next steps of an investigation are to develop a case definition, identify cases, and characterize the descriptive epidemiology. An *epidemic curve* depicts number of cases over time and can provide information on possible transmission. In an outbreak with a *point source exposure*, an index case may be identified, with other cases occurring after an incubation period or at multiples of an incubation period (Figures 1-3 and 1-4). Plotting the location of cases on a spot map may be helpful in determining possible exposures. Describing host characteristics can be important in identifying at-risk populations for further investigation or targeting control measures, and for developing hypotheses that can be investigated in an analytic study.

Cohort studies are optimal for investigating outbreaks that occur in small, well-defined populations. These include outbreaks in school or childcare, social gatherings, and hospitals. In populations that are not well defined, a case-control study is the most feasible approach. It is important to select controls who had an opportunity equal to that of cases for exposure to potential risk factors and developing disease. Neighbors of cases or patients from the same medical-provider practice or hospital as the case are commonly selected as controls. Friends of cases have been used as controls in some investigations, but concerns have been raised about possible "overmatching," because friends may be more likely than others to have similar exposures. When the number of cases is relatively small, enrolling multiple controls per case increases the power of the study to find significant risk factors. After a standard questionnaire is administered, significant risk factors are determined by comparing exposures of cases and controls. The results of analyses may lead to inferences of causation and development of prevention and control strategies or to further hypotheses that can be evaluated later. The impact of intervention can be determined by ongoing surveillance and continuing to plot additional cases on the epidemic curve (Figure 1-4).

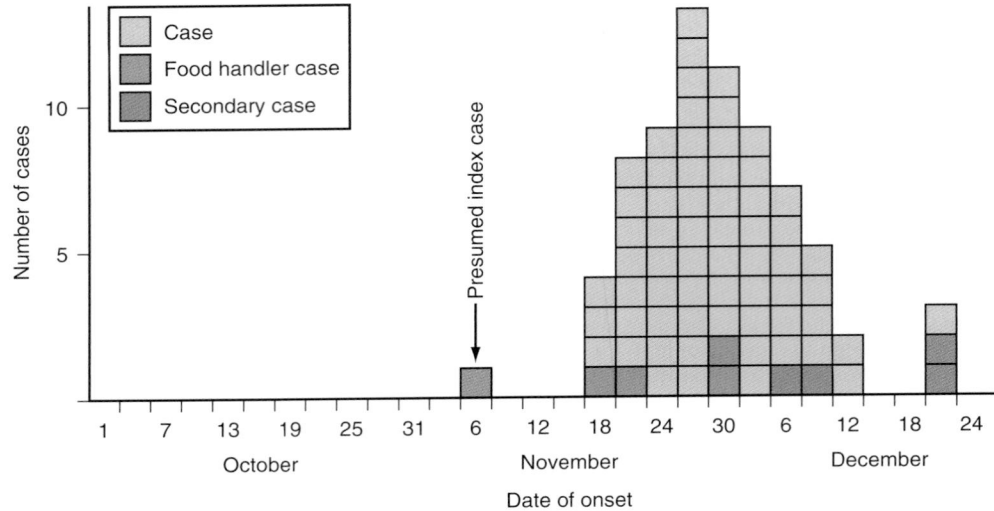

Figure 1-3. Example of an epidemic curve for a common source outbreak with continuous exposure. Cases of hepatitis A by date of onset, Fayetteville, Arkansas, November to December 1979. (Centers for Disease Control and Prevention, unpublished data.)

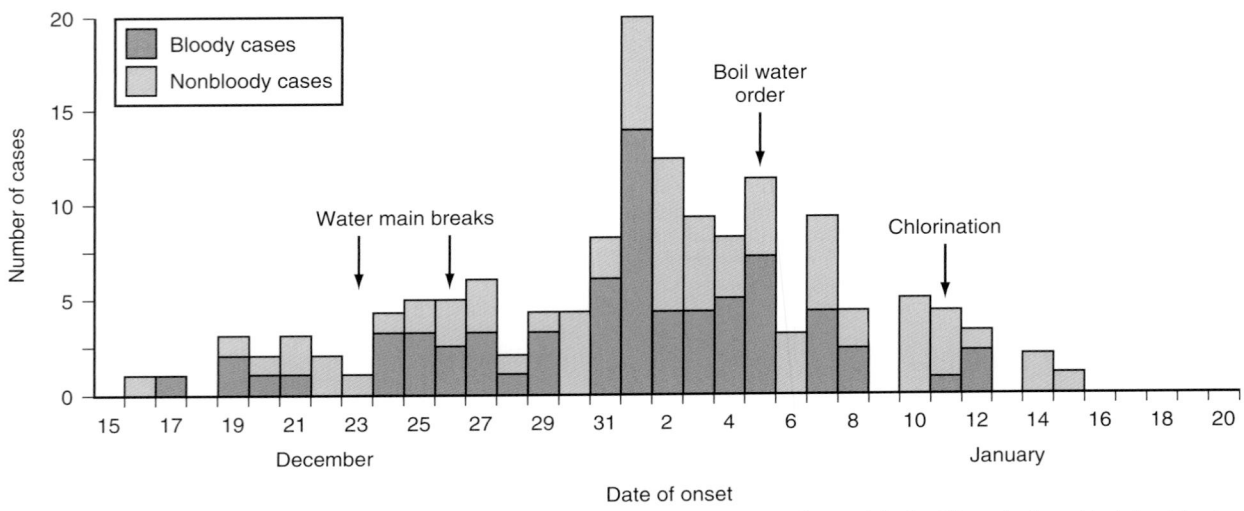

Figure 1-4. Example of an epidemic curve for a common source outbreak with continuous exposure. Cases of diarrheal illness in city residents by date of onset and character of stool, Cabool, Missouri, December 1989 to January 1990. (Centers for Disease Control and Prevention, unpublished data.)

Impact and Economic Analysis of Disease Prevention

Assessing health and economic impacts of public health interventions is important in developing or supporting policy decisions. Health impacts can be expressed directly as cases of disease, deaths, and sequelae prevented. Vaccine efficacy is a specific example of the *prevented fraction* (PF), where PF=$P(1-RR)$, with P representing the proportion exposed to an intervention. Secondary measures of health impact include *years of potential life lost (YPLLs)* or *quality-adjusted life-years (QALYs)* lost, which quantify the impact of death, or death and disability, respectively, based on the age at which these events occur.[21] A measure of the efficiency of an intervention is the *number needed to treat* (NNT), which describes how many persons must be exposed to an intervention to avoid one case of adverse health outcome; for example, the number of persons who would need to be immunized to prevent a case or a death, or to be given antibiotic prophylaxis to prevent one case of infection.

Because public health resources are limited, it is becoming increasingly important to calculate impact in economic as well as in health terms and to compare an intervention with other potential uses of available resources. *Cost-effectiveness* analyses determine the cost per health outcome achieved, such as the cost per death or complication averted. In a cost-effectiveness formula, costs appear in the numerator and health benefits appear in the denominator. The numerator includes expenditures for the prevention program from which cost savings occurring with disease prevention are subtracted. In addition to direct costs averted (e.g., savings from decreased medical care), indirect costs savings occur from increased productivity of people who do not become ill or miss time from work while receiving care or caring for ill family members. *Cost–utility* calculations are similar to cost-effectiveness but assess cost per QALY saved or YPLL averted.

Cost–benefit analyses differ from cost-effectiveness analyses in that the calculation is made entirely in economic terms. Health benefits are assigned an economic value and expenditures are compared with savings. One problem with this approach lies in the difficulty assigning an economic value to a health effect. For example, the value of a life saved may be quantified as the estimated value of a person's earnings over his or her lifetime, forgone earnings due to premature death, or by a standard amount; both economic and ethical issues may be raised by the choice of approach. Because the parameters used in economic analyses often are uncertain or based on limited data, and because choices made by the investigator (e.g., regarding the value of life) may be influential to the analysis, *sensitivity analyses* often are performed where parameters are varied across a range of potential values. In addition to defining a range of possible economic outcomes, sensitivity analyses can identify the factors that most influence the results, elucidating where further studies may be important.

EVALUATING THE MEDICAL LITERATURE

Basic epidemiologic knowledge is important in evaluating studies reported in the medical literature. Steps in reviewing published medical research are shown in Box 1-2. The ability to assess published studies carefully often is limited by the information presented in the report. To improve reporting of randomized controlled trials, a group of investigators and editors developed a Consolidated Standards of Reporting Trials (CONSORT)[23] (http://www.consort-statement.org/) and later extended these recommendations to reporting of noninferiority and equivalence randomized trials.[24] Although these standards have been adopted by many journals and editorial groups, reporting often does not adhere to the quality standards proposed.[25,26] Although the guidelines refer to experimental rather than observational studies, most criteria still apply.

Assessing the *research hypothesis* allows readers to determine the relevance of the study to their practice and to judge whether the analyses were done to test the hypothesis or to identify other interesting associations. The ability to make causal inferences from a confirmatory study that tests a single hypothesis is greater than from an exploratory study in which multiple exposures are considered as potential explanations for an outcome.

Several components of *study design* are important to consider. Details should be presented regarding the criteria for selecting a cohort or cases and controls. *Exposure* and *outcome variables* should be clearly defined, and the potential for misclassification and its impact should be considered. Quantifying exposure may be important to establish a dose–response relationship. Finally, *sample size estimates* should be presented, making clear the magnitude of difference between study groups considered clinically meaningful and the type I and type II error levels.

In the *analysis*, it is important that outcomes for all study subjects are reported, even if that outcome is "lost to follow-up." *Intent-to-treat* analyses consider outcomes for all enrolled subjects, whether or not they completed the therapy (e.g., those who were nonadherent with therapy or who received only part of a vaccination series). The appropriateness of the statistical tests should be assessed; for example, if data are not normally distributed, they can be transformed to a scale that is more normally distributed (e.g., geometric mean titers) or nonparametric statistical tests should be used. In assessing a multivariable model, the reader

> **BOX 1-2.** Steps in the Critical Evaluation of Epidemiologic Literature[22]
>
> 1. Consider the research hypothesis
> 2. Consider the study design
>   - Type of study
>   - Selection of study participants
>   - Selection and definition of outcome variables
>   - Selection and definition of exposure (predictor) variables
>   - Sample size and power
> 3. Consider the analysis
>   - Complete accounting of study subjects and outcomes
>   - Appropriateness of statistical tests
>   - Potential sources and impact of bias
>   - Potential impact of confounding and effect modification
> 4. Consider the interpretation of results
>   - Magnitude and importance of associations
>   - Study limitations
>   - Ability to make causal inferences

should critically evaluate the type of model chosen, the variables included, and whether interaction terms were considered. Missing data pose a particular problem in modeling, in that study subjects can only be included if data are available for each variable in the model; thus, the power of a multivariate model may be much less than that predicted in a sample size calculation.

Bias can have an important impact on study results and must be carefully considered. Approaches to minimize bias should be clearly described. The direction and potential magnitude of remaining bias should be estimated and its impact on results considered. Potential confounding, the presence of important unmeasured variables, and possible effect modification can have a major impact on the results. Investigators should openly discuss the potential limitations of the investigation and describe the strategies they applied to overcome those limitations.

Finally, *interpretation* of study results includes assessing the magnitude of the associations, their relevance to practice, and the likelihood that the relationships observed are causal. The importance of an exposure in explaining an outcome can be expressed by the attributable proportion. The *external validity* of the results, however, and the potential impact on one's own patient population must still be assessed.

Acknowledgment

Thanks to Paul M. Gargiullo, PhD, for assistance.

---

2 Pediatric Infection Prevention and Control

Jane D. Siegel

During the past decade, there has been a surge in interest to reduce healthcare-associated infection (HAI) as an integral part of patient safety. Involvement of new stakeholders for improving patient safety and outcomes related to HAI (e.g., Child Health Corporation of America (CHCA), National Association of Children's Hospitals and Related Institutions (NACHRI), individual states' mandatory HAI public reporting programs, the Centers for Medicare and Medicaid Services (CMS), the Joint Commission) has broadened the arena for HAI prevention efforts. Of note, 5 of

the 15 Joint Commission National Patient Safety Goals for 2011 target prevention of HAIs (www.jointcommission.org/hap_2011_npsgs/). Additionally, the National Healthcare Safety Network (NHSN) (previously National Nosocomial Infection Surveillance (NNIS) System) now is reporting more pediatric-specific rates of device-associated infections.[1] An understanding of the complexities of prevention and control of HAIs in children is critical to many different leaders of healthcare facilities caring for children.

Infection Prevention and Control (IPC) for the pediatric population is a unique science that requires understanding of various host factors, sources of infection, routes of transmission, behaviors associated with care of infants and children, pathogens and their virulence factors, treatments, preventive therapies, and behavioral theory. Although the term *nosocomial* still applies to infections that are acquired in acute care hospitals, a more general term, *healthcare-associated infections* (HAIs), now is used since much care of high-risk patients, including those with medical devices (e.g., central venous catheters (CVCs), ventilators, ventricular shunts, peritoneal dialysis catheters), has shifted to ambulatory settings, rehabilitation or chronic care facilities, and to the home; thus, the geographic location of acquisition of the infection often cannot be determined. A true *nosocomial* infection is defined as an infection that was not incubating or present at the time of hospital admission, and that develops ≥48 hours after hospital admission or ≤48 hours after hospital discharge. A *surgical site infection* is classified as an HAI (www.cdc.gov/nhsn) if it develops within ≤30 days of the procedure or within one year after a permanently placed nonhuman-derived implant. In neonates, a transplacental infection is not considered a nosocomial infection. An infection is nosocomial, however, if a mother is not infected at the time of admission but delivers an infected infant ≥48 hours after her admission. The principles of transmission of infectious agents in healthcare settings and recommendations for prevention are reviewed in the Guideline for Isolation Precautions: Preventing Transmission of Infectious Agents in Healthcare Settings, 2007.[2]

Historically, HAI rates between 2% and 13% of admissions or discharges from pediatric intensive care units have been reported.[3,4] Rates of all HAIs as high as 7% to 25% are reported in neonatal intensive care units (NICUs) and are inversely proportional to birthweight.[1,5,6] NICU outbreaks are unique and often involve large numbers of patients due to the traditional design of housing large numbers of high-risk infants in close proximity.[7] However, infection rates have decreased substantially in recent years with consistent adherence to bundled practices for insertion and maintenance of CVCs,[8,9] care of patients on ventilators,[10] and high-risk surgical procedures.[11] Children who have complex underlying diseases are at greatest risk for prolonged hospitalization, complications, and mortality associated with acquisition of new infections in the hospital.[4,6,12,13] Severely immunosuppressed patients (e.g., allogeneic hematopoietic stem cell transplant (HSCT) recipients, children with leukemia undergoing intensive chemotherapy, solid-organ transplant recipients during the periods of most intense immunosuppression) also are at increased risk for invasive aspergillosis and other environmental fungal infections, especially during periods of facility renovation, construction, and water leaks.[14,15]

RISK FACTORS FOR HAIs IN CHILDREN

Unique aspects of HAIs in children have been reviewed in detail[4,16,17] and are summarized below. Specific risks and pathogens are addressed in multiple other chapters in this textbook.

Host or Intrinsic Factors

Intensive care units, oncology services, and gastroenterology services caring for patients with short gut syndrome who are dependent on total parenteral nutrition (TPN and lipids) have the highest rates of bacterial and fungal infection associated with CVCs. HAIs can result in the serious morbidity and mortality such as occur in adults and in lifetime physical, neurologic, and developmental disabilities. Host, or intrinsic, factors that make children particularly vulnerable to infection are immaturity of the immune system, congenital abnormalities, and congenital or acquired immunodeficiencies. Innate deficiencies of the immune system in prematurely born infants, who may be hospitalized for prolonged periods of time and exposed to intensive monitoring, supportive therapies, and invasive procedures, contribute to the high rates of infection in the NICU. All components of the immune system are compromised in neonates and the degree of deficiency is proportional inversely to the gestational age (see Chapter 9,

Immunologic Development and Susceptibility to Infection). Additionally, the underdeveloped skin of the very-low-birthweight (VLBW, <1000 g) infant provides another mode of entry for pathogens. Populations of immunosuppressed children have expanded with the advent of more intense immunosuppressive therapeutic regimens used for oncologic conditions, HSCTs, solid-organ transplantation, and rheumatologic conditions and inflammatory bowel disease for which immunosuppressive agents and tumor necrosis factor-α inhibitors (infliximab (Remicade)) and other immune modulators are used.

Children with congenital anomalies have a high risk of HAI because their unusual anatomy may predispose to contamination of normally sterile sites with body fluids. Also, they require prolonged and repeated hospitalizations, undergo many complex surgical procedures, and have extended exposure to invasive supportive and monitoring equipment. For example, at the University of Virginia Medical Center, children with myelomeningocele have had an average of 9 hospitalizations (range, 3 to 50) and 6 surgical procedures (range, 2 to 30) by 15 years of age (personal communication, Leigh Grossman).

Fortunately, the population of children with perinatally acquired human immunodeficiency virus (HIV) infection and acquired immunodeficiency syndrome (AIDS) has decreased dramatically since 1994, but new cases of sexually transmitted HIV infection continue to be diagnosed in teens who are cared for in children's hospitals. Finally, young infants who have not yet been immunized, or immunosuppressed children who do not respond to vaccines or lose their antibody during treatment (e.g., patients with nephrotic syndrome), have increased susceptibility to infections that would be prevented by vaccines.

Sources or Extrinsic Factors

The source of many HAIs is the endogenous flora of the patient.[2,18,19] An asymptomatic colonizing pathogen can invade a patient's bloodstream or be transmitted on the hands of healthcare personnel (HCP) to other patients. Other important sources of HAIs in infants and children include the mother; invasive monitoring and supportive equipment, blood products, total parenteral nutrition fluids, lipids; infant formula and human milk; HCP, and other contacts, including adult and sibling visitors. Maternal infection with *Neisseria gonorrhoeae*, *Treponema pallidum*, HIV, hepatitis B virus, parvovirus B19, *Mycobacterium tuberculosis*, herpes simplex virus, group B streptococcus, or colonization with multidrug-resistant organisms, pose substantial threats to the neonate. During perinatal care, procedures such as fetal monitoring using scalp electrodes, fetal transfusion and surgery, umbilical cannulation, and circumcision are risk factors for infection. Intrinsically contaminated powdered formulas and infant formulas prepared in contaminated blenders or improperly stored or handled, or both, have resulted in sporadic and epidemic infections in the nursery (e.g., *Cronobacter* (formerly *Enterobacter*) *sakazakii*).[20] Human milk that has been contaminated by maternal flora or by organisms transmitted through breast pumps has caused isolated serious infections and epidemics. The risks of neonatal hepatitis, cytomegalovirus (CMV) infection, and HIV infection from human milk warrant further caution for handling.

Devices. Rates of central line associated bloodstream infections (CLABSIs) in the pediatric intensive care units (PICUs) and high-risk nurseries (HRNs) in the NNIS system, now the NHSN, from January 2002 to June 2004 were among the highest for all reporting ICUs, with a mean of 6.6 CLABSIs per 1000 catheter-days in the PICUs; this rate was surpassed only in trauma and burn units, with a mean of 7.4 and 7.0 CLABSIs per 1000 catheter-days, respectively[21] (Table 2-1). Rates of umbilical catheter- and CVC-associated BSIs varied by birthweight (BW) from 3.5 per 1000 catheter-days in those >2500 g BW, to 9.1 per 1000 catheter-days in those <1000 g BW (Table 2-2). Medical device-related infections (e.g., CLABSIs, ventilator-associated pneumonia (VAP), and surgical site infections (SSIs)) can be prevented by implementing 3 to 5 sets or "bundles" of evidence-based practices, as defined in the Institute for Healthcare Improvement (IHI) 100,000 Lives

TABLE 2-1. Comparison of Laboratory-Confirmed Central Line-Associated Bloodstream Infection (CLABSI) Rates in ICUs from National Nosocomial Infection Surveillance (NNIS) 2002–2004[5] with National Healthcare Safety Network (NHSN) 2009[1]

	No. ICUs Reporting		Rate/1000 Catheter-Days[a]: Pooled Mean (Median, Range 10–90%) Mean Device Utilization Ratio[b]	
ICU Type	2002–2004	2009	2002–2004	2009
Trauma	22	74	7.4 (5.2, 1.9–11.9) 0.61	2.6 (2.0, 0–6.7) 0.59
Burn	14	33	7.0 (NA[c]) 0.56	5.3 (3.8, 0.2–12.4) 0.50
Pediatric	54	–	6.6 (5.2, 0.9–11.2) 0.46	–[d] –
Cardiothoracic	–	21	– –	2.5 (2.7, 0.4–4.0) 0.70
Medical	–	13	– –	2.6 (NA) 0.40
Medical/Surgical	–	135	– –	2.2 (1.7, 0–4.5) 0.50
Medical	94	–	5.0 (3.9, 0.5–8.8) 0.52	– –
Major teaching facility	–	134	– –	2.2 (1.7, 0.2–4.7) 0.62
All other facilities	–	183	– –	1.6 (0–4.1) 0.43
Respiratory	6	9	4.8 (NA) 0.47	2.1 (NA) 0.58
Surgical	99	223	4.6 (3.4, 0–8.7) 0.61	1.8 (1.2, 0–4.2) 0.60
Neurosurgical	30	79	4.6 (3.1, 0–10.6) 0.48	1.5 (1.2, 0–3.6) 0.46
Coronary (medical cardiac)	60	252	3.5 (3.2, 1.0–9.0) 0.38	1.7 (1.1, 0–4.2) 0.40
Medical-surgical				
Major teaching facility	100	192	4.0 (3.4, 1.7–7.6) 0.57	1.7 (1.3, 0–3.8) 0.58
All other facilities	109	–	3.2 (3.1, 0.8–6.1) 0.50	– –
≤15 beds	–	771	– –	1.4 (0, 0–3.8) 0.39
>15 beds	–	323	– –	1.3 (0.9, 0–3.0) 0.48
Surgical cardiothoracic	48	219	2.7 (1.8, 0–4.9) 0.79	1.2 (0.8, 0–2.5) 0.71

[a]Number of CLABSIs/number of central line days × 1000.

[b]Number of central line days/number of patient days.

[c]Not available.

[d]Not reported.

Campaign (www.ihi.org/IHI/Programs/Campaign), the NACHRI collaboratives (www.childrenshospitals.net),[9] and single center studies. This effect is evident in the NHSN data summary for 2009.[1] Although the highest rates of CLABSI (5.3 per 1000 catheter-days) in ICUs occurred in burn ICUs, and in smallest infants in NICUs (3.4 per 1000 catheter-days at ≤750 g) rates fell in all units/groups measured (Tables 2-1 and 2-2). In the NHSN reports for 2006–2008[22] and for 2009,[1] data are presented for CLABSI in pediatric hematology-oncology units: permanent-line CLABSI rates per 1000 catheter-days were 2.3 and 3.0, respectively, and temporary-line CLABSI rates were 4.6 and 4.8, respectively. Use of more specialized life-saving technologies, such as extracorporeal membrane oxygenation (ECMO), hemodialysis/hemofiltration, pacemakers, and implantable ventricular assist devices (VADs), further increases the risk of infection in the sickest children who require the most intense, prolonged, and invasive support. However, these infections are not included in the NHSN device-associated module and no benchmarking data are available.

Many standard infection prevention and control procedures for prevention of device-related infections in adults cannot be followed routinely for children. In adults, for example, peripheral intravascular catheters are changed routinely every 3 to 4 days to reduce the risk of catheter colonization and subsequent BSI. Infants, however, may have such limited vascular access that catheters remain in place until they become unnecessary, nonfunctional, or contaminated. Additionally, the specific indications for

TABLE 2-2. Comparison of Laboratory-Confirmed Central Line-Associated Bloodstream Infection (CLABSI) Rates in Level III Neonatal Intensive Care Units (NICUs) from the National Nosocomial Infection Surveillance (NNIS) 1992-2004[5] with National Healthcare Safety Network (NHSN) 2009[1,a]

Birthweight Group Category	No. NICUs Reporting		Rate/1000 Catheter-Days[b]: Pooled Mean (Median, Range 10–90%) Mean Device Utilization Ratio[c]	
	1992–2004	2009	1992–2004	2009
≤750 grams	–[d]	150	–	3.4 (2.7, 0–8.6) 0.37
751–1000 grams	–	159	–	2.7 (1.4, 0–8.8) 0.31
≤1000 grams	104	–	9.1 (8.5, 1.6–16.1) 0.42	– –
1001–1500 grams	98	156	5.4 (4.0, 0–12.2) 0.30	1.9 (0, 0–5.8) 0.23
1501–2500 grams	97	134	4.1 (3.2, 0–8.9) 0.21	1.5 (0,0–4.7) 0.16
>2500 grams	94	106	3.5 (1.9, 0–7.4) 0.29	1.3 (0,0–3.5) 0.19

[a]Inborn NICUs with very-low-birthweight infants are combined with outborn NICUs with larger-birthweight infants usually requiring surgical procedures.

[b]Number of CLABSIs/number of central line days × 1000.

[c]Number of central line/number of patient days.

[d]Not reported.

prophylaxis against deep-vein thrombosis and peptic ulcers have not been defined for children requiring mechanical ventilator support; some evidence suggests that prophylaxis against peptic ulcers is associated with an increased risk of necrotizing enterocolitis and candidemia in LBW (<1500 g) infants.[23]

Practices. Several practices must be evaluated with respect to the associated risk of infection. A significant association between reduced levels of nurse staffing and appropriately trained nurses has been demonstrated to increase risk in many studies in both children and adults.[24] There are theoretical concerns that infection risk also will increase in association with the innovative practices of co-bedding and kangaroo care in the NICU because of increased opportunity for skin-to-skin exposure of multiple-gestation infants to each other and to their mothers, respectively. Overall, the infection risk is reduced with kangaroo care,[25] but transmission of tuberculosis[26] and RSV[27] has occurred in kangaroo mother care units in South Africa. Neither the benefits nor the safety of co-bedding multiple-birth infants in the hospital setting have been demonstrated in studies reviewed by the American Academy of Pediatrics in 2007. With increasing numbers of procedures being performed by pediatric interventional radiologists, an understanding of appropriate aseptic technique and recommended regimens for antimicrobial prophylaxis is important.[28]

Antimicrobial selective pressure. Exposure to vancomycin and to third-generation cephalosporins contributes substantially to the increase in infections caused by vancomycin-resistant enterococcus (VRE)[29] and multidrug-resistant gram-negative bacilli, including extended-spectrum β-lactamase (ESBL)-producing organisms,[30] respectively. Exposure to third-generation cephalosporins also is a risk factor for the development of invasive candidiasis in LBW infants in the NICU.[31] Trends in resistance of certain organisms to certain antibiotics as tracked by NHSN show increasing resistance of *Pseudomonas aeruginosa*, *Klebsiella pneumoniae*, and *Escherichia coli*.

Transmission

Modes

The principal modes of transmission of infectious agents are direct and indirect contact, droplet, and airborne. Most infectious agents are transmitted by the contact route via hands of HCP, but many pathogens can be transmitted by more than one route. Viruses, bacteria, and *Candida* spp. can be transmitted horizontally. Although the source of most *Candida* HAIs is the patient's endogenous flora, horizontal transmission, most likely via HCP's hands, has been demonstrated in studies using DNA fingerprinting in the NICU and in a pediatric oncology unit.[32] Transmission of infectious agents by the droplet route requires exposure of mucous membranes to large respiratory droplets (>5 μm) within 1 to 2 meters (3 to 6 feet) of the infected individual, who may be coughing or sneezing. Large respiratory droplets do not remain suspended in the air. Adenovirus, influenza virus, and rhinovirus are transmitted primarily by the droplet route whereas other respiratory viruses (e.g., RSV, parainfluenza) are transmitted primarily by the contact route. Although influenza virus can be transmitted via the airborne route under unusual conditions of reduced air circulation or relative humidity, there is ample evidence that transmission of influenza is prevented by droplet precautions and, in the care of infants, the addition of contact precautions.[33]

Some agents (e.g., severe acute respiratory syndrome–coronavirus (SARS-CoV)) can be transmitted as small-particle aerosols under special circumstances of aerosol-producing procedures (e.g., endotracheal intubation, bronchoscopy); therefore, an N95 or higher respirator is indicated for those in the same airspace when these procedures are performed, but an airborne infection isolation room (AIIR) may not always be required. Roy and Milton proposed a new classification for aerosol transmission when evaluating routes of SARS transmission:[34] (1) *obligate*: under natural conditions, disease occurs following transmission of the agent only through small-particle aerosols (e.g., tuberculosis); (2) *preferential*: natural infection results from transmission through multiple routes, but small-particle aerosols are the predominant route (e.g., measles, varicella); and (3) *opportunistic*: agents naturally cause disease through other routes, but under certain environmental conditions can be transmitted via fine-particle aerosols. This conceptual framework may explain rare occurrences of airborne transmission of agents that are transmitted most frequently by other routes (e.g., smallpox, SARS, influenza, noroviruses). Concern about airborne transmission of influenza arose again during the 2009 influenza A (H1N1) pandemic. However, the conclusion from all published experiences during the 2009 pandemic is that droplet transmission is the usual route of transmission and that surgical masks were non-inferior to N95 respirators in preventing laboratory-confirmed influenza, including 2009 H1N1, among HCP.[35,36] Concerns about unknown or possible routes of transmission of agents that can cause severe disease and have no known treatment often result in more extreme prevention strategies than may be necessary; therefore, recommended precautions could change as the epidemiology of emerging agents is defined and these controversial issues are resolved. Although transmission of *M. tuberculosis* can occur rarely from an infant or young child with active tuberculosis, the more frequent source is the adult visitor who has not been diagnosed with active pulmonary tuberculosis; thus screening of visiting family members is an important component for control of tuberculosis in pediatric healthcare facilities.[37]

Transmission of microbes among children and between children and HCP is a frequent risk due to the very close contact that occurs during care of infants and young children. Traditionally, multi-bed rooms are crowded with children, parents, and HCP. However, with the increasing evidence that single-patient rooms provide improved environments for patients, which include reduced risk of transmission of infectious agents and reduced medical errors, the American Institute of Architects' 2006 Guidelines for Design and Construction of Health Care Facilities recommends single-patient rooms for acute medical/surgical and postpartum patients as the standard for all new construction (www.aia.org/aah_gd_hospcons). Although there are insufficient data at this time to support a definitive recommendation for single-patient rooms in NICUs, there is increasing experience that suggests a benefit to reduce the risk of infection and to improve neurosensory development.[38] Toddlers often share waiting rooms, playrooms, toys, books, and other items and therefore have the potential of transmitting pathogens directly and indirectly to one another. Contaminated bath toys were implicated in an outbreak of multidrug-resistant *P. aeruginosa* in a pediatric oncology unit.[39]

Before effective preventive measures[40] were established, 17% of preschool children hospitalized for >1 week had a nosocomial viral respiratory tract illness.[41] Infection of pediatric HCP also was common. Since routine care of infants and younger children involves holding, cuddling, wiping noses, feeding, and changing diapers, it is easy to see how RSV and other respiratory tract viral agents can be transmitted in secretions that are then inoculated onto mucous membranes of HCP. RSV infections were more likely to develop in healthy volunteers who held or cuddled infants with RSV infection (cuddlers, 70%) or in those who handled items that the infants had touched, but did not touch the infant (touchers, 41%); infection did not develop in those who sat in the patients' rooms (sitters) but had no direct contact with the patient, items, or surfaces.[42] HCP with mild symptoms of infection also can unknowingly become intermediary hosts and transmit organisms to susceptible children.

Healthcare Personnel

Transmission of infectious agents is facilitated by overcrowding, understaffing, and too few appropriately trained nurses. Several studies have established the association of understaffing and overcrowding with increased rates of HAIs in NICUs, PICUs, and general pediatrics units.[24,43] The 2007 Guideline for Isolation Precautions recommends that healthcare facilities consider staffing levels and composition as important components of an effective infection control program.[2] HCP rarely are the *source* of outbreaks of HAIs caused by bacteria and fungi, but when they are, there usually are factors present that increase their risk of transmission (e.g., sinusitis, draining otitis externa, respiratory tract infections, dermatitis, onychomycosis, wearing of artificial nails).[44] Individuals with direct patient contact who were wearing artificial nails have been implicated in outbreaks of *P. aeruginosa* and ESBL-producing *K. pneumoniae* in NICUs;[45,46] therefore, the use of artificial nails or extenders is prohibited in individuals who have direct contact with high-risk patients.[2,47] Several published studies

have shown that infected pediatric HCP, including resident physicians, transmitted *Bordetella pertussis* to other patients.[48] HCP also have been implicated as the source of outbreaks of rotavirus[49] and influenza.[50]

Environment

The role of environmental surfaces in transmission of a variety of pathogens during outbreaks (e.g., *Clostridium difficile*, norovirus, methicillin-resistant *Staphylococcus aureus* (MRSA), VRE, MDR/gram-negative bacilli (GNB)) has been defined in recent years.[51] Therefore, heightened attention is directed appropriately toward cleaning and monitoring the effectiveness of cleaning by training, observation, and feedback[52] and by using various markers (e.g., an invisible fluorescein powder[53] and adenosine triphosphate (ATP) bioluminescence[54]).

PATHOGENS

While there is no agreed-upon definition for what constitutes an "epidemiologically important organism," the following characteristics apply and are presented for guidance to infection control staff in the 2007 Healthcare Infection Control Practice Advisory Committee of the Centers for Disease Control and Prevention (HICPAC/CDC) Guideline for Isolation Precautions in Healthcare Settings:[2]

1. A propensity for transmission within healthcare facilities based on published reports and the occurrence of temporal or geographic clusters of infection in >2 patients (e.g., VRE, MRSA, and methicillin-susceptible *S. aureus* (MSSA), *C. difficile*, norovirus, RSV, influenza, rotavirus, *Enterobacter* spp., *Serratia* spp., group A streptococcus). A single case of HA invasive disease caused by certain pathogens (e.g., group A streptococcus postoperatively or in burn units; *Legionella* sp.; *Aspergillus* sp.) should trigger an investigation.
2. Antimicrobial resistance (e.g., MRSA, VRE, ESBL-producing GNB, *Burkholderia cepacia*, *Ralstonia* spp., *Stenotrophomonas maltophilia*, and *Acinetobacter* species. Many of the intrinsically resistant GNB also suggest possible contamination of water or medication.
3. Association with serious clinical disease, increased morbidity and mortality (e.g., MRSA and MSSA, group A streptococcus).
4. A newly discovered or re-emerging pathogen (e.g., vancomycin-insensitive or -resistant *S. aureus* (VISA, VRSA), *C. difficile*).

Pathogens associated with HAIs in children differ from those in adults. The importance of HA respiratory viral infections in pediatrics was first recognized in 1984.[3] The viruses most frequently associated with transmission in a pediatric healthcare facility are RSV, rotavirus, and influenza. With the dramatic reduction in rotavirus infections following introduction of the vaccine, rotavirus now is a rare cause of HAI. However, other respiratory viruses (e.g., parainfluenza, adenovirus, human metapnuemovirus) have been implicated in outbreaks in high-risk units. As more respiratory viruses are identified by using highly sensitive molecular methods, epidemiologic studies will be required to define further the risk of transmission in healthcare facilities.[55] HA outbreaks of varicella and measles now are rare events due to consistent uptake during the past decade of vaccines in children and HCP. Clinical manifestations of certain pathogens (e.g., RSV and *Bordetella pertussis*) can be life-threatening in infants and young children, especially those with underlying conditions. Excessive burden of disease and mortality also is associated with influenza in infants and young children.[56,57] Children <18 years of age accounted for approximately 35% (20 million) of cases, 32% (87,000) of hospitalizations, and 10% (1,280) of deaths during the 2009 influenza A(H1N1) pandemic.[58]

The emergence of community-associated (CA)-MRSA isolates characterized by the unique Scc *mec* type IV element was first observed among infants and children. As rates of colonization with CA-MRSA at the time of hospital admission increased, so did transmission of community strains, most often USA 300, within

TABLE 2-3. Trends in Resistance of Selected Pathogens and Drugs in the National Nosocomial Infection Surveillance System (NNIS) 1998–2003 and the National Healthcare Safety Network (NHSN) 2006–2007

Pathogen Antimicrobial Agent	1998–2002[5] All ICU Isolates	2003[5] All Isolates	2006–2007[a] All CLABSI Isolates
Staphylococcus aureus			
Oxacillin R	51.3%	59.5%	56.8%
Enterococcus spp.			
Vancomycin R	12.8%	28.5%	36.4%
			78.9% for *E. faecium*
Klebsiella pneumoniae			
3rd-geneneration cephalosporin R	6.1%	20.6%	27.1%
Carbapenem R	_[b]	–	10.8%
E. coli			
3rd-geneneration cephalosporin R	1.2%	5.8%	8.1%
Fluoroquinolone R	5.8%	–	30.8%
Enterobacter spp.			
3rd-geneneration cephalosporin R	26.3%	31.1%	–
Pseudomonas aeruginosa			
Cefipime R	–	–	12.6%
Carbapenem R	19.6%	21.1%	23.0%
Fluoroquinolone R	36.3%	29.5%	30.5%
Acinetobacter baumannii			
Carbapenem R	–	–	29.2%

R, resistant.

[a]Hidron AI, Edwards JR, Patel J, et al. Infect Control Hosp Epidemiol 2008;29:996–1011.

[b]Not reported.

the hospital and especially within the NICU,[59] making prevention especially challenging. Other multidrug-resistant organisms, e.g., VRE, ESBLs, and carbapenemase-producing gram-negative bacilli (carbapenem-resistant Enterobacteriaceae, *K. pneumoniae* carbapenemase), have emerged as the most challenging HA pathogens in both pediatric and adult settings, and otherwise healthy children in the community can be asymptomatically colonized with these multidrug-resistant organisms.[60–62] GNB, including ESBL and other multidrug-resistant isolates, are more frequent than MRSA and VRE in many PICUs and NICUs. Patients who are transferred from chronic care facilities can be colonized with MDR-GNB at the time of admission to the PICU.[18] Trends in targeted MDR organisms (MDROs) as tracked in the NNIS/NHSN ICUs are summarized in Table 2-3. Continued increases in MRSA, VRE, and certain resistant GNB are a "call to action" for all healthcare facilities. The CDC campaign to prevent antimicrobial resistance by judicious use of antimicrobial agents (GET SMART, www.cdc.gov/getsmart/) and the Guideline for Management of MDROs in Healthcare Settings, 2006[63] provide more epidemiologic information. Of note, in 2004, rates of HA-MRSA and VRE plateaued, but the incidence of *K. pneumoniae* resistant to third-generation cephalosporins in ICUs reporting to NHSN increased (www.cdc.gov/ncidod/dhqp/ar_mrsa_data.html). HAIs caused by MDROs are associated with increased length of stay, increased morbidity and mortality, and increased cost, in part due to the delay in initiating effective antimicrobial therapy.[64] While there is lower prevalence of specific MDROs in pediatric institutions, the same principles of target identification and interventions to control MDROs apply in all settings.

The incidence of *Candida* infections increased in incidence in most PICUs and NICUs during the 1990s, but decreased 2000–2004. There is considerable center-to-center variability in both the incidence of invasive candidiasis and the proportion of *Candida* infections caused by *Candida* non-*albicans* sp., most of which are resistant to fluconazole. Risk factors for *Candida* infections include prolonged length of stay in an ICU, use of CVCs, intralipids, H2-blocking agents, and exposure to third-generation cephalosporins. GNB and *Candida* sp. are especially important pathogens for HAIs

in patients with short gut who are receiving TPN and can cause repeated episodes of sepsis.[23,65] There is now evidence that fluconazole prophylaxis in a subset of very high-risk low-birthweight infants is safe and effective in preventing invasive candidiasis;[65] however, the staff of each NICU first must optimize infection practices and then must assess the remaining local risk of *Candida* infections. Finally, environmental fungi (e.g., *Aspergillus, Fusarium, Scedosporium, Bipolaris,* Zygomycetes), are important sources of infection for severely immunocompromised patients, demanding meticulous attention to the conditions of the internal environment of any facility that provides care for severely immunocompromised patients and prevention of possible exposure to construction dust in and around healthcare facilities.[66] With the advent of more effective and less toxic antifungal agents, it is important to identify the infecting agent by obtaining tissue samples and to determine susceptibility to candidate antifungal agents.[15]

PREVENTION

Prevention remains the mainstay of infection control and requires special considerations in children. The goals of infection prevention and control (IPC) are to prevent the transmission of infectious agents among individual patients or groups of patients, visitors, and HCP who care for them. If prevention cannot always be achieved, the strategy of early diagnosis, treatment, and containment is critical. This chapter focuses on the unique principles and practice of infection control for the care of children. Specific pathogens and diseases are discussed in detail in chapters dedicated to those topics. Recommended isolation precautions by infectious agent can be found in the *Red Book Report of the Committee on Infectious Diseases* of the American Academy of Pediatrics (AAP) and in the Guideline for Isolation Precautions: Preventing Transmission of Infectious Agents in Healthcare Settings, 2007.[2]

A series of IPC guidelines have been developed and updated by HICPAC/CDC and others to provide evidence-based/rated recommendations for practices that are associated with reduced rates of

BOX 2-1. Resources for Infection Prevention and Control Recommendations

CENTERS FOR DISEASE CONTROL AND PREVENTION/ HEALTHCARE INFECTION CONTROL PRACTICES COMMITTEE (HICPAC)

www.cdc.gov/hicpac/pubs.html

General

- Guideline for Disinfection and Sterilization in Health-Care Facilities, 2008
- Guideline for Isolation Precautions: Preventing Transmission of Infectious Agents in Healthcare Settings, 2007
- Management of Multi-Drug Resistant Organisms (MDROs) in Healthcare Settings, 2006
- Guidelines for Environmental Infection Control in Health-Care Facilities, 2003
- Guidelines for Hand Hygiene in Healthcare Settings, 2002

Device-/Procedure-Related

- Guidelines for the Prevention of Intravascular Catheter-Related Infections, 2011
- Guideline for Prevention of Catheter-Associated Urinary Tract Infections, 2009
- Guideline for Preventing Healthcare-Associated Pneumonia, 2003
- Guideline for the Prevention of Surgical Site Infection, 1999

Other

- Guideline for the Prevention and Control of Norovirus Gastroenteritis Outbreaks in Healthcare Settings, 2011

AMERICAN ACADEMY OF PEDIATRICS

- Committee on Infectious Diseases. 2009 Report of the Committee on Infectious Diseases. In: Pickering LK, Baker CJ, Kimberlin DW, Long SS (eds) Red Book, 28th ed. Illinois, American Academy of Pediatrics, 2009 (update 2012)
- Pickering LK, Marano N, Bocchini JA, Angulo FJ and the Committee on Infectious Diseases. Exposure to nontraditional pets at home and to animals in public settings: risk to children. Pediatrics 2008;122:876–886

- Committee on Infectious Diseases, American Academy of Pediatrics
- Infection prevention and control in pediatric ambulatory settings. Pediatrics 2007;120:650–665

OTHER

- Petersen BT, Chennat J, Cohen J, et al. Multisociety guideline on reprocessing flexible GI endoscopes: 2011. Infect Control Hosp Epidemiol 2011;32:527–537
- Talbot TR, Babcock H, Caplan AL, et al. Revised SHEA Position Paper: Influenza vaccination of healthcare personnel. Infect Control Hosp Epidemiol 2010;31:987–995
- Cohen SH, Gerding DN, Johnson S, et al. Clinical practice guidelines for *Clostridium difficile* infection in adults: 2010 Update by the Society for Healthcare Epidemiology of America (SHEA) and the Infectious Diseases Society of America (IDSA). Infect Control Hosp Epidemiol 2010;31:431–455
- Henderson DK, Dembry L, Fishman NO, et al. SHEA guideline for management of healthcare workers who are infected with hepatitis B virus, hepatitis C virus, and/or human immunodeficiency virus. Infect Control Hosp Epidemiol 2010;31:203–231
- Yokoe D, Casper C, Dubberke E, et al. Infection prevention and control in health-care facilities in which hematopoietic cell transplant recipients are treated. Bone Marrow Transplant 2009;44:495–507
- Yokoe D, Casper C, Dubberke E, et al. Safe living after hematopoietic cell transplantation. Bone Marrow Transplant 2009;44:509–519
- Saiman L, Siegel JD, and the Cystic Fibrosis Foundation Consensus Conference on Infection Control Participants. Infection control recommendations for patients with cystic fibrosis: microbiology, important pathogens, and infection control practices to prevent patient-to-patient transmission. Infect Control Hosp Epidemiol 2003;24(5 Suppl):S6–52 (update in progress)

HAIs, especially those associated with the use of medical devices and surgical procedures (Box 2-1). Bundled practices are groups of 3 to 5 evidence-based "best practices" with respect to a disease process that individually improve care, but when applied together result in substantially greater reduction in infection rates. Adherence to the individual measures within a bundle is readily measured. Bundles for the reduction of CLABSIs,[9] SSIs,[11] VAP[12] established for adults have been adapted to pediatrics (www.ihi.org/IHI/Programs/Campaign). Detailed information on advances in prevention strategies for pediatrics have been reviewed.[16,17]

Administrative Factors

The importance of certain administrative measures for a successful IPC program has been demonstrated. There is evidence to designate IPC as one component of the institutional culture of safety and to obtain support from senior leadership of healthcare organizations to provide necessary fiscal and human resources for a proactive, successful IPC program. Critical elements requiring administrative support include: (1) access to appropriately trained healthcare epidemiology and IPC personnel; (2) access to clinical microbiology laboratory services needed to support infection control outbreak investigations, including ability to perform molecular testing; (3) access to data-mining programs and information technology specialists; (4) multidisciplinary programs to assure judicious use of antimicrobial agents and control of resistance; (5) delivery of effective educational information to HCP, patients, families, and visitors; and (6) provision of adequate

numbers of well-trained infection preventionists and bedside nursing staff.[2,24]

The IPC Team

An effective IPC program should improve safety of patients and HCP, and decrease short- and long-term morbidity, mortality, and healthcare costs.[67] The IPC Committee establishes policies and procedures to prevent or reduce the incidence and costs associated with HAIs. This committee should be one of the strongest and most accessible committees in the hospital; committee composition should be considered carefully and limited to active, authoritative participants who have well-defined committee responsibilities and who represent major groups within the hospital. The chairperson should be a good communicator with expertise in IPC issues, healthcare epidemiology, and clinical pediatric infectious diseases. An important function of the IPC committee is the regular review of IPC policies and the development of new policies as needed. Annual review of all policies is required by the Joint Commission and can be accomplished optimally by careful review of a few policies each month. With the advent of unannounced inspections, a constant state of readiness is required.

The hospital epidemiologist or medical director of the IPC division usually is a physician with training in pediatric infectious diseases and dedicated expertise in healthcare epidemiology. In multidisciplinary medical centers, pediatric infectious disease experts should be consulted for management of pediatric IPC and report to the broader IPC leadership. Infection preventionists (IPs) are specialized professionals with advanced training, and preferably certification, in IPC. Although the majority of IPs are registered nurses, others, including microbiologists, medical technologists, pharmacists, and epidemiologists, are successful in this position. Pediatric patients should have IP services provided by someone with expertise and training in the care of children. In a large, general hospital, at least one IP should be dedicated to IPC services for children. The responsibilities of IPs have expanded greatly in the last decade and include the following: (1) surveillance and IPC in facilities affiliated with primary acute care hospitals (e.g., ambulatory clinics, day-surgery centers, long-term care facilities, rehabilitation centers, home care) in addition to the primary hospital; (2) oversight of occupational health services related to IPC, (e.g., assessment of risk and administration of recommended prophylaxis following exposure to infectious agents, tuberculosis screening, influenza and pertussis vaccination, respiratory protection fit testing, administration of other vaccines as indicated during infectious disease crises such as pre-exposure smallpox vaccine in 2003 and pandemic influenza A(H1N1) vaccine in 2009); (3) preparedness planning for annual influenza outbreaks, pandemic influenza, SARS, bioweapons attacks; (4) adherence monitoring for selected IPC practices; (5) oversight of risk assessment and implementation of prevention measures associated with construction, renovation, and other environmental conditions associated with increased infection risk; 6) participation in antimicrobial stewardship programs, focusing on prevention of transmission of MDROs; (7) evaluation of new products that could be associated with increased infection risk (e.g., intravenous infusion materials) and for introduction and assessment of performance after implementation; (8) mandatory public reporting of HAI rates in states according to enacted legislation; (9) increased communication with the public and with local public health departments concerning infection control-related issues; and (10) participation in local and multicenter research projects. IPC programs must be adequately staffed to perform all of these activities. Thus, the ratio of 1 IP per 250 beds that was associated with a 30% reduction in the rates of nosocomial infection in the Study on Efficacy of Nosocomial Infection Control (SENIC) study performed in the 1970s is no longer sufficient, as the complexity of patient populations and responsibilities have increased. Many experts recommend that a ratio of 1 IP per 100 beds is more appropriate for the current workload, but no study has been performed to confirm the effectiveness of that ratio. There is no information on the number of individuals required outside acute care, but it is clear that individuals well trained in IPC must be available for all sites where healthcare is delivered.[2]

Surveillance

Surveillance for HAIs consists of a systematic method of determining the incidence and distribution of infections acquired by hospitalized patients. The CDC recommends the following: (1) prospective surveillance on a regular basis by trained IPs, using standardized definitions; (2) analysis of infection rates using established epidemiologic and statistical methods (e.g., calculation of rates using appropriate denominators that reflect duration of exposure; use of statistical process control charts for trending rates); (3) regular use of data in decision-making; and (4) employment of an effective and trained healthcare epidemiologist who develops IPC strategies and policies and serves as a liaison with the medical community and administration.[68-71] The CDC has established a set of standard definitions of HAIs that have been validated and accepted widely with updates posted on the CDC NHSN website or published in HICPAC/CDC guidelines. Standardization of surveillance methodology has become especially important with the advent of state legislation for mandatory reporting of HAI infection rates to the public.[72]

Although various surveillance methods are used, the basic goals and elements are similar and include using standardized definitions of infection, finding and collecting cases of HAIs, tabulating data, using appropriate denominators that reflect duration

---

> **BOX 2-2.** Sources of Data for Surveillance
>
> - Clinical rounds with physicians and/or nurses
> - Review of:
>   Patient orders
>   Radiology reports/databases
>   Pharmacy reports/databases
>   Operating room diagnoses and procedures
>   Microbiology: bacteriology, virology, mycology, acid-fast bacilli, serology reports autopsy reports, data-mining reports
> - Postdischarge surveillance, especially for surgical site infections
> - Public health surveillance
> - Review of:
>   Employee health reports
>   Admission diagnoses
>   Outpatient diagnoses
>   Administrative databases, but should not be used as sole source due to inaccurate coding of healthcare-associated infections

---

of risk, analyzing and interpreting the data, reporting important deviations from endemic rates (epidemic, outbreaks) to the bedside care providers and to the facility administrators, implementing appropriate control measures, auditing adherence rates for recommended measures, and assessing efficacy of the control measures. Medical centers can utilize different methods of surveillance, as outlined in Box 2-2. Most experts agree that a combination of methods enhances surveillance and reliability of data, and that some combination of clinical chart review and database retrieval is important.[68-71] Administrative databases created for the purposes of billing should not be used as the sole source to identify HAIs because of both the overestimates and underestimates that result from inaccurate coding of HAIs.[72] Use of software designed specifically for IPC data entry and analysis facilitates real-time tracking of trends and timely intervention when clusters are identified. The IPC team should participate in the development and update of electronic medical record systems for a healthcare organization, to be sure that the surveillance needs will be met.

In the past decade, there has been much controversy over the importance of obtaining active surveillance cultures from all patients admitted to an acute care hospital, especially to an ICU, to detect asymptomatic colonization with MRSA. With the implementation of bundled practices to prevent device-related and surgical site infections, emergence of new MDROs, and evidence from well-designed studies, it is clear that active surveillance cultures should be obtained in a targeted fashion in units where there is an indication of ongoing transmission of MRSA or other MDROs, according to 2006 guidelines.[63]

The microbiology laboratory can provide online culture information about individual patients, outbreaks of infection, antibiotic susceptibility patterns of pathogens in periodic antibiotic susceptibility summary reports, and employee infection data. This laboratory also can assist with surveillance cultures and facilitation of molecular typing of isolates during outbreak investigations. Rapid diagnostic testing of clinical specimens for identification of respiratory and gastrointestinal tract viruses and *B. pertussis* is especially important for pediatric facilities. The IPC division and the microbiology laboratory must communicate daily, because even *requests* for cultures from physicians (e.g., *M. tuberculosis, Neisseria meningitidis, C. difficile*) can be an early marker for identifying patients who are infected, are at high risk of infection, or require isolation. If microbiology laboratory work is outsourced, it is important to assure that the services needed to support an effective infection control program will be available, as described in a policy statement of the Infectious Diseases Society of America.[73]

The pharmacy is an important collaborative member of any multidisciplinary team working on strategies to prevent antimicrobial resistance. Antimicrobial utilization in the hospital should be assessed for appropriateness, efficacy, cost, and association with emergence of resistant organisms. For surveillance purposes, use of specific antimicrobial agents can alert the IP to potentially infected patients (e.g., tuberculosis). The need to restrict use of antimicrobial agents is a collaborative decision based on review of all data. Restriction of new, potent broad-spectrum antimicrobial agents is advised to prevent emergence of resistance that occurs with increased exposure to most antimicrobial agents (e.g., extended-spectrum cephalosporins, quinolones, linezolid, daptomycin).[30,74-76]

Control of unusual infections or outbreaks in the community generally is the responsibility of the local or state public health department; however, the individual facility must be responsible for preventing transmission within that facility. Public health agencies can be helpful particularly in alerting hospitals of community outbreaks so that outpatient and inpatient diagnosis, treatment, necessary isolation, and other preventive measures are implemented promptly to avoid further spread. Conversely, designated individuals in the hospital must notify public health department personnel of reportable infections so as to facilitate early diagnosis, treatment, and infection control in the community. Benefits of community or regional collaboratives of individual healthcare facilities and local public health departments for prevention of HAIs, especially those caused by MDROs, have been demonstrated and should be encouraged.[2]

ISOLATION PRECAUTIONS

Isolation of patients with potentially transmissible infectious diseases is a proven strategy for reducing transmission of infectious agents in healthcare settings. During the past decade, many published studies, including those performed in pediatric settings, have provided a strong evidence base for most recommendations for isolation precautions. However, controversies still exist concerning the most clinically and cost-effective measures for preventing certain HAIs, especially those associated with MDROs. Since 1970, the guidelines for isolation developed by CDC have responded to the needs of the evolving healthcare systems in the United States. For example, universal precautions became a required standard in response to the HIV epidemic and the need to prevent transmission of bloodborne pathogens (e.g., HIV, hepatitis B and C viruses (HBV and HCV), rapidly fatal infections such as the viral hemorrhagic fevers). The Occupational Safety and Health Administration (OSHA) published specific requirements[77] in 1991 for universal precautions (now, Standard Precautions) for HCP who, as a result of their required duties, are at increased risk for skin, eye, mucous membrane, or parenteral contact with blood or other potentially infectious materials. Although all requirements may not have been proven to be clinically or cost-effective, healthcare facilities must enforce these measures. The federal Needlestick Safety and Prevention Act, signed into law in November, 2000, authorized OSHA's revision of its Bloodborne Pathogens Standard more explicitly to require the use of safety-engineered sharp devices (www.osha.gov/SLTC/bloodbornepathogens/index.html).

The most recent Guideline for Isolation Precautions published in 2007[2] affirms *Standard Precautions*, a combination of universal precautions and body substance isolation, as the foundation of transmission prevention measures, and *Transmission-based Precautions* for certain suspected pathogens. HCP must recognize the importance of body fluids, excretions, and secretions in the transmission of infectious pathogens and take appropriate protective precautions by using personal protective equipment (PPE) (e.g., masks, gowns, gloves, face shields, or goggles) and safety devices even if an infection is not suspected or known. In addition, these updated guidelines provide recommendations for all settings in which healthcare is delivered (acute care hospitals, ambulatory surgical and medical centers, long-term care facilities, and home health agencies). Evidence and recommendations are provided for the prevention of transmission of MDROs such as MRSA, VRE, VISA, VRSA, and GNB.[63] The components of a protective environment for prevention of environmental fungal infections in HSCT

recipients are summarized. Finally, evidence-based, rated recommendations for administrative measures that are necessary for effective prevention of infection in healthcare settings are provided.

Standard Precautions

The term *Standard Precautions* replaced Universal Precautions and Body Substance Isolation in 1996. Standard Precautions should be used when there is likely to be exposure to: (1) blood; (2) all other body fluids, secretions, and excretions, whether or not they contain visible blood, except sweat; (3) nonintact skin; or (4) mucous membranes. Standard Precautions strategy is designed to reduce the risk of transmission of microorganisms from both identified and unidentified sources of infection. The components of Standard Precautions are summarized in Table 2-4. In the updated isolation guideline, safe injection practices are included as a component of Standard Precautions, because recent outbreaks of HBV and HCV in ambulatory care settings as a result of failure to follow recommended practices indicate a need to reiterate the established effective practices.[78] There were two additions to Standard Precautions in 2007: (1) *Respiratory hygiene/cough etiquette* for source containment by people with signs and symptoms of respiratory tract infection; and (2) *Use of a mask* by the individual inserting an epidural anesthesia needle or performing a myelogram when prolonged exposure of the puncture site is likely. Both components have a strong evidence base.

Implementation of Standard Precautions requires critical thinking from all HCP and the availability of PPE in proximity to all patient care areas. HCP with exudative lesions or weeping dermatitis must avoid direct patient care and handling of patient care equipment. Individuals having direct patient contact should be able to anticipate an exposure to blood or other potentially infectious material and to take proper protective precautions. Individuals also should know what steps to take if high-risk exposure occurs. Exposures of concern are exposures to blood or other potentially infectious material defined as an injury with a contaminated sharp object (e.g., needlestick, scalpel cut); a spill or splash of blood or other potentially infectious material onto nonintact skin (e.g., cuts, hangnails, dermatitis, abrasions, chapped skin) or onto a mucous membrane (e.g., mouth, nose, eye); or a blood exposure covering a large area of normal skin. Handling food trays or furniture, pushing wheelchairs or stretchers, using restrooms or phones, having personal contact with patients (e.g., giving information, touching intact skin, bathing, giving a back rub, shaking hands), or doing clerical or administrative duties for a patient do not constitute high-risk exposures. If hands or other skin surfaces are exposed to blood or other potentially infectious material, the area should be washed immediately with soap and water for at least 10 seconds and rinsed with running water for at least 10 seconds. If an eye, the nose, or mouth is splashed with blood or body fluids, the area should be irrigated immediately with a large volume of water. If a skin cut, puncture, or lesion is exposed to blood or other potentially infectious material, the area should be washed immediately with soap and water for at least 10 seconds and rinsed with 70% isopropyl alcohol. Any exposure incident should be reported immediately to the occupational health department and a determination must be made if blood samples are required from the source patient and the exposed individual and if immediate prophylaxis is indicated.

All HCP should know where to find the exposure control plan that is specific to each place of employment, whom to contact, where to go, and what to do if inadvertently exposed to blood or body fluids. Important resources include the occupational health department, the emergency department, and the infection control/hospital epidemiology division. The most important recommendation in any accidental exposure is to seek advice and intervention immediately, because the efficacy of recommended prophylactic regimens is improved with shorter intervals after exposure, such as for hepatitis B immune globulin administration after exposure to HBV or for antiretroviral therapy after percutaneous exposure to HIV. Chemoprophylaxis following exposure to

TABLE 2-4. Recommendations for Application of Standard Precautions for the Care of all Patients in all Healthcare Settings[2]

Component	Recommendations for Performance
Hand hygiene	After touching blood, body fluids, secretions, excretions, contaminated items; immediately after removing gloves; between patient contacts. Alcohol-containing antiseptic handrubs preferred except when hands are visibly soiled with blood or other proteinaceous materials or if exposure to spores (e.g., *Clostridium difficile, Bacillus anthracis*) is likely to have occurred
Gloves	For touching blood, body fluids, secretions, excretions, contaminated items; for touching mucous membranes and nonintact skin
Gown	During procedures and patient care activities when contact of clothing/exposed skin with blood/body fluids, secretions, and excretions is anticipated
Mask,[a] eye protection (goggles), face shield	During procedures and patient care activities likely to generate splashes or sprays of blood, body fluids, secretions, especially suctioning, endotracheal intubation to protect healthcare personnel. For patient protection, use of a mask by the individual inserting an epidural anesthesia needle or performing myelograms when prolonged exposure of the puncture site is likely to occur
Soiled patient-care equipment	Handle in a manner that prevents transfer of microorganisms to others and to the environment; wear gloves if visibly contaminated; perform hand hygiene
Environmental control	Develop procedures for routine care, cleaning, and disinfection of environmental surfaces, especially frequently touched surfaces in patient care areas
Textiles and laundry	Handle in a manner that prevents transfer of microorganisms to others and to the environment
Injection practices (use of needles and other sharps)	Do not recap, bend, break, or hand-manipulate used needles; if recapping is required, use a one-handed scoop technique only; use needle-free safety devices when available; place used sharps in a puncture-resistant container. Use a sterile, single-use, disposable needle and syringe for each injection given. Single-dose medication vials are preferred when medications are administered to >1 patient
Patient resuscitation	Use mouthpiece, resuscitation bag, or other ventilation devices to prevent contact with mouth and oral secretions
Patient placement	Prioritize for single-patient room if the patient is at increased risk of transmission, is likely to contaminate the environment, does not maintain appropriate hygiene, or is at increased risk of acquiring infection or developing adverse outcome following infection
Respiratory hygiene/cough etiquette[b]	Instruct symptomatic persons to cover mouth/nose when sneezing/coughing; use tissues and dispose in no-touch receptacle; observe hand hygiene after soiling of hands with respiratory secretions; wear surgical mask if tolerated or maintain spatial separation, >1–2 meters (3–6 feet) if possible

[a]During aerosol-generating procedures on patients with suspected or proven infections transmitted by aerosols (e.g., severe acute respiratory syndrome), wear a fit-tested N95 or higher respirator in addition to gloves, gown, and face/eye protection.

[b]Source containment of infectious respiratory secretions in symptomatic patients, beginning at initial point of encounter (e.g., triage and reception areas in emergency departments and physician offices).

HIV-infected material is most effective if initiated within 4 hours of exposure.[79] Updates are posted on the CDC website. Reporting a work-related exposure is required for subsequent medical care and workers' compensation.

Transmission-Based Precautions

Transmission-based Precautions are designed for patients with documented or suspected infection with pathogens for which additional precautions beyond Standard Precautions are needed to prevent transmission. The three categories of Transmission-based Precautions are: *Contact Precautions, Droplet Precautions,* and *Airborne Precautions,* and are based on the likely routes of transmission of specific infectious agents. They may be combined for infectious agents that have more than one route of transmission. Whether used singly or in combination, they are always used in addition to Standard Precautions. Transmission-based Precautions are applied at the time of initial contact, based on the clinical presentation and the most likely pathogens – so-called *Empiric* or *Syndromic Precautions.* This approach is useful especially for emerging agents (e.g., SARS-CoV, avian influenza, pandemic influenza), for which information concerning routes of transmission is still evolving. The categories of clinical presentation are as follows: diarrhea, central nervous system, generalized rash/exanthem, respiratory, skin or wound infection. Single-patient rooms are always preferred for children needing Transmission-based Precautions. If unavailable, cohorting of patients, and preferably of staff, according to clinical diagnosis is recommended.

Table 2-5 lists the three categories of isolation based on routes of transmission and the necessary components. Table 2-6 lists

precautions by syndromes, to be used when a patient has an infectious disease and the agent is not yet identified. It should be noted that for infectious agents that are more likely to be transmitted by the droplet route (e.g., pandemic influenza), droplet precautions (with use of surgical mask) is appropriate; however, during an aerosol-producing procedure, N95 or higher respirators are indicated (www.pandemicflu.gov/plan/healthcare/maskguidancehc.html).

ENVIRONMENTAL MEASURES

Contaminated environmental surfaces and noncritical medical items have been implicated in transmission of several HAIs, including VRE, *C. difficile, Acinetobacter* sp., MRSA, and RSV.[1,51,52] Pathogens on surfaces are transferred to the hands of HCP and then transferred to patients or items. Most often, the failure to follow recommended procedures for cleaning and disinfection contributes more than the specific pathogen to the environmental reservoir during outbreaks. Education of environmental services personnel combined with observations of cleaning procedures and feedback has been associated with a persistent decrease in the acquisition of VRE in a medical ICU;[52] monitoring for adherence to recommended environmental cleaning practices is an important determinant of success. Certain infectious agents (e.g., rotavirus, noroviruses, *C. difficile*) can be resistant to some routinely used hospital disinfectants; thus, when there is ongoing transmission and cleaning procedures have been observed to be appropriate, a 1:10 dilution of 5.25% sodium hypochlorite (household bleach) or other special disinfectants may be indicated.[80] Pediatric facilities should use disinfectants active against rotavirus.

TABLE 2-5. Transmission-Based Precautions[2,a]

Component	Contact	Droplet	Airborne
Hand hygiene	Per Standard Precautions. 5 moments of hand hygiene,[47] and **upon entry** into room. Soap and water preferred over alcohol handrub for *Clostridium difficile, Bacillus anthracis* spores	Per Standard Precautions. 5 moments of hand hygiene, and **upon entry** into room	Per Standard Precautions. 5 moments of hand hygiene, and **upon entry** into room
Gown	Yes. Don before or **upon entry** into room	Per Standard Precautions. Add to droplet precautions for infants, young children, and/or presence of diarrhea	Per Standard Precautions and, if infectious, draining skin lesions present
Gloves	Yes. Don before or **upon entry** into room	Per Standard Precautions. Add for infants, young children and/or presence of diarrhea	Per Standard Precautions. Add for infants, young children and/or presence of diarrhea
Mask	Per Standard Precautions	Yes. Don before or **upon entry** into room	Don N95 particulate respirator or higher **before entry** into room
Goggles/face shield	Per Standard Precautions	Per Standard Precautions. Always for SARS, avian influenza	Per Standard Precautions. Always for SARS, avian influenza
N95 or higher respirator Always don **before entry** into room	When aerosol-producing procedures performed for influenza, SARS[b], VHF[c]	When aerosol-producing procedures performed for influenza, SARS, VHF	Yes. Don before entry into room
Room placement	Single-patient room preferred. Cohort like-infections if single-patient rooms unavailable	Single-patient room preferred. Cohort like-infections if single-patient rooms unavailable	Single-patient room. Negative air pressure; 12 air changes/hour for new construction, 6 air changes/hour for existing rooms
Environmental measures	Increased frequency, especially in the presence of diarrhea, transmission of *Clostridium difficile*, norovirus. Bleach for VRE, *C.difficilie*, norovirus	Routine	Routine
Transport	Mask patient if coughing. Cover infectious skin lesions. PPE not routinely required for transporter	Mask patient	Mask patient. Cover infectious skin lesions

[a]*An addition to Standard precautions, use Transmission-based Precautions, use Transmission-based Precautions for patients with highly transmisible or epidemiologically important pathogens for which additional precautions are needed.*

[b]*SARS, severe acute respiratory syndrome.*

[c]*VHF, viral hemorrhagic fever.*

VISITATION POLICIES

Since acquisition of a seemingly innocuous viral infection in neonates and in children with underlying diseases can result in unnecessary evaluations and empiric therapies for suspected septicemia as well as serious life-threatening disease, special visitation policies are required in pediatric units, especially the high-risk units. All visitors with signs or symptoms of respiratory or gastrointestinal tract infection should be restricted from visiting patients in healthcare facilities. During the influenza season, it is preferred for all visitors to have received influenza vaccine. Increased restrictions may be required during a community outbreak (e.g., SARS, pandemic influenza). For patients requiring Contact Precautions, the use of PPE by visitors is determined by the nature of the interaction with the patient and the likelihood that the visitor will frequent common areas on the patient unit or interact with other patients and their families.

Although most pediatricians encourage visits by siblings in inpatient areas, the medical risk must not outweigh the psychosocial benefit. Studies demonstrate that parents favorably regard sibling visitation[81] and that bacterial colonization[82,83] or subsequent infection[84] does not increase in the neonate or older child who has been visited by siblings, but these studies are limited by small numbers. Strict guidelines for sibling visitation should be established and enforced in an effort to maximize visitation opportunities and minimize risks of transmission of infectious agents. The following recommendations regarding visitation may guide policy development:

1. Sibling visitation is encouraged in the well-child nursery and NICU, as well as in areas for care of older children.

2. Before visitation, parents should be interviewed by a trained staff nurse concerning the current health status of the sibling. Siblings should not be allowed to visit if they are delinquent in recommended vaccines, have fever or symptoms of an acute illness, or are within the incubation period following exposure to a known infectious disease. After the interview, the physician or nurse should place a written consent for sibling visitation in the permanent patient record and a name tag indicating that the sibling has been approved for visitation for that day.

3. Asymptomatic siblings who recently were exposed to varicella but who previously were immunized can be assumed to be immune.

4. The visiting sibling should visit only his or her sibling and not be allowed in playrooms with groups of patients.

5. Visitation should be limited to periods of time that ensure adequate screening, observation, and monitoring of visitors by medical and nursing staff members.

6. Children should observe hand hygiene before and after contact with the patient.

7. During the entire visit, sibling activity should be supervised by parents or another responsible adult.

PETS

Pets can be of substantial clinical benefit to the child hospitalized for prolonged periods of time; therefore it is important for healthcare facilities to provide guidance for safe visitation. Many zoonoses and infections are attributable to animal exposure (see Chapter 91, Infections Related to Pets and Exotic Animals). Most infections result from inoculation of animal flora through a bite

TABLE 2-6. Clinical Syndromes or Conditions Warranting Empiric Transmission-Based Precautions in Addition to Standard Precautions Pending Confirmation of Diagnosis[a]

Clinical Syndrome or Condition[b]	Potential Pathogens[c]	Empiric Precautions (Always Includes Standard Precautions)
DIARRHEA		
Acute diarrhea with a likely infectious cause in an incontinent or diapered patient	Enteric pathogens[d]	Contact Precautions (pediatrics and adult)
MENINGITIS	Neisseria meningitidis	Droplet Precautions for first 24 hours of antimicrobial therapy; mask and face protection for intubation
	Enteroviruses	Contact Precautions for infants and children
	Mycobacterium tuberculosis	Airborne Precautions if pulmonary infiltrate.
		Airborne Precautions plus Contact Precautions if potentially infectious draining body fluid present
RASH OR EXANTHEMS, GENERALIZED, ETIOLOGY UNKNOWN		
Petechial/ecchymotic with fever (general)	Neisseria meningitidis	Droplet Precautions for first 24 hours of antimicrobial therapy
If traveled in an area with an ongoing outbreak of VHF in the 10 days before onset of fever	Ebola, Lassa, Marburg viruses	Droplet Precautions plus Contact Precautions, with face/eye protection, emphasizing safety sharps and barrier precautions when blood exposure likely. Use N95 or higher respiratory protection when aerosol-generating procedure performed
Vesicular	Varicella-zoster, herpes simplex, variola (smallpox), vaccinia viruses	Airborne plus Contact Precautions. Contact Precautions only if herpes simplex, localized zoster in an immunocompetent host, or vaccinia viruses most likely
Maculopapular with cough, coryza, and fever	Rubeola (measles) virus	Airborne Precautions
RESPIRATORY INFECTIONS		
Cough/fever/upper-lobe pulmonary infiltrate in an HIV-negative patient or a patient at low risk for HIV infection	Mycobacterium tuberculosis, respiratory viruses, Streptococcus pneumoniae, Staphylococcus aureus (MSSA or MRSA)	Airborne Precautions plus Contact Precautions until M. tuberculosis ruled out; Droplet if respiratory viruses most likely
Cough/fever/pulmonary infiltrate in any lung location in an HIV-infected patient or a patient at high risk for HIV infection	Mycobacterium tuberculosis, respiratory viruses, Streptococcus pneumoniae, Staphylococcus aureus (MSSA or MRSA)	Airborne Precautions plus Contact Precautions. Use eye/face protection if aerosol-generating procedure performed or contact with respiratory secretions anticipated. If tuberculosis is unlikely and there are no AIIRs and/or respirators available, use Droplet Precautions instead of airborne precautions. Tuberculosis more likely in HIV-infected than in HIV-negative individuals
Cough/fever/pulmonary infiltrate in any lung location in a patient with a history of recent travel (10–21 days) to country with outbreak of SARS, avian influenza	Mycobacterium tuberculosis, severe acute respiratory syndrome virus–coronavirus (SARS-CoV), avian influenza	Airborne plus Contact Precautions plus eye protection. If SARS and tuberculosis unlikely, use Droplet Precautions instead of Airborne Precautions
Respiratory infections, particularly bronchiolitis and pneumonia, in infants and young children	Respiratory syncytial virus, parainfluenza virus, adenovirus, influenza virus, human metapneumovirus	Contact Precautions plus Droplet Precautions; Droplet Precautions may be discontinued when adenovirus and influenza have been ruled out
SKIN OR WOUND INFECTION		
Abscess or draining wound that cannot be covered	Staphylococcus aureus (MSSA or MRSA), group A streptococcus	Contact Precautions. Add droplet precautions for the first 24 hours of appropriate antimicrobial therapy if invasive group A streptococcal disease is suspected

AIIR, airborne infection isolation room; HIV, human immunodeficiency virus; MRSA, methicillin-resistant Staphylococcus aureus; *MSSA, methicillin-susceptible* Staphylococcus aureus; *VHF, viral hemorrhagic fever.*

[a]*Infection control professionals should modify or adapt this table according to local conditions. To ensure that appropriate empiric precautions are always implemented, hospitals must have systems in place to evaluate patients routinely according to these criteria as part of their preadmission and admission care.*

[b]*Patients with the syndromes or conditions listed may have atypical signs or symptoms (e.g., neonates and adults with pertussis may not have paroxysmal or severe cough). The clinician's index of suspicion should be guided by the prevalence of specific conditions in the community, as well as clinical judgment.*

[c]*The organisms listed under the column "Potential Pathogens" are not intended to represent the complete, or even most likely, diagnoses, but rather possible etiologic agents that require additional precautions beyond standard precautions until they can be ruled out.*

[d]*These pathogens include enterohemorrhagic* Escherichia coli *O157:H7,* Shigella *spp., hepatitis A virus, noroviruses, rotavirus,* Clostridium difficile.

or scratch or self-inoculation after contact with the animal, the animal's secretions or excretions, or contaminated environment. Although there are few data to support a true evidence-based guideline for pet visitation in healthcare facilities, recommendations are provided in the Guidelines for Environmental Infection Control in Health-Care Facilities[80] to guide institutional policies.

Additionally, a guideline has been developed by the Association for Professionals in Infection Control and Epidemiology (APIC) that provides rationale, evidence-based recommendations (when possible), and consensus opinion.[85]

Prudent visitation policies should limit visitation to animals who: (1) are domesticated; (2) do not require a water environment; (3) do not bite or scratch; (4) can be brought to the hospital in a carrier or easily walked on a leash; (5) are trained to defecate and urinate outside or in appropriate litter boxes; (6) can be bathed before visitation; and (7) are known to be free of respiratory, dermatologic, and gastrointestinal tract disease. Despite the established risk of salmonellosis associated with reptiles (e.g., turtles, iguanas), there continue to be many reports of outbreaks of invasive disease associated with reptiles; reptiles should be excluded from pet visitation programs and families should be advised not to have pet reptiles in the home with young infants or immunocompromised individuals.[86,87] Exotic animals that are imported should be excluded because of unpredictable behavior and the potential for transmission of unusual pathogens (e.g., monkey-pox in the U.S. in 2003).[88] Visitation should be limited to short periods of time and confined to designated areas. Visiting pets need to have a certificate of immunization from a licensed veterinarian. Children should observe hand hygiene after contact with pets. Most pediatric facilities restrict pet interaction with severely immunosuppressed patients and those in ICUs.

DISINFECTION, STERILIZATION, AND REMOVAL OF INFECTIOUS WASTE

Disinfection and sterilization as they relate to infection prevention and control have been reviewed[89] and comprehensive guidelines were made by the CDC in 2008.[90] *Cleaning* is the removal of all foreign material from surfaces and objects. This process is accomplished using soap and enzymatic products. Failure to remove all organic material from items before disinfection and sterilization reduces the effectiveness of these processes. *Disinfection* is a process that eliminates all forms of microbial life except the endospore. Disinfection usually requires liquid chemicals. Disinfection of an inanimate surface or object is affected adversely by the presence of organic matter; a high level of microbial contamination; use of too dilute germicide; inadequate disinfection time; an object that can harbor microbes in protected cracks, crevices, and hinges; and pH and temperature.

Sterilization is the eradication of all forms of microbial life, including fungal and bacterial spores. Sterilization is achieved by physical and chemical processes such as steam under pressure, dry heat, ethylene oxide, and liquid chemicals. The Spaulding classification of patient care equipment as *critical, semicritical,* and *noncritical* items with regard to sterilization and disinfection is used by the CDC.[90] *Critical items* require sterilization because they enter sterile body tissues and carry a high risk of causing infection if contaminated; *semicritical items* require disinfection because they may contact mucous membranes and nonintact skin; and *noncritical items* require routine cleaning because they only come in contact with intact skin. If noncritical items used on patients requiring Transmission-based Precautions, especially Contact Precautions, must be shared, these items should be disinfected between uses. Guidelines for specific objects and specific disinfectants are published and updated by the CDC. Multiple published reports and manufacturers similarly recommend the use and reuse of objects with appropriate sterilization, disinfection, or cleaning recommendations. Recommendations in guidelines for reprocessing endoscopes focus on training of personnel, meticulous manual cleaning, high-level disinfection followed by rinsing, air-drying, and proper storage to avoid contamination.[91] Medical devices that are designed for single use (e.g., specialized catheters, electrodes, biopsy needles) must be reprocessed by third parties or hospitals according to the guidance issued by the Food and Drug Administration (FDA) in August, 2000 with amendments in September, 2006; such reprocessors are considered and regulated as "manufacturers." Available data show that single-use devices reprocessed according to the FDA regulatory requirements are as safe and effective as new devices (www.fda.gov/cdrh/reprocessing).

Deficiencies in disinfection and sterilization leading to infection have resulted either from failure to adhere to scientifically based guidelines or failures in the disinfection or sterilization processes. When such failures are discovered, an investigation

must be completed including notification of patients and, in some cases, testing for infectious agents. Rutala and Weber[92] have published an excellent guidance document for risk assessment and communication to patients in such situations.

Healthcare facility waste is all biologic or nonbiologic waste that is discarded and not intended for further use. *Medical waste* is material generated as a result of use with a patient, such as for diagnosis, immunization, or treatment, and includes soiled dressings and intravenous tubing. *Infectious waste* is that portion of medical waste that could potentially transmit an infectious disease. Microbiologic waste, pathologic waste, contaminated animal carcasses, blood, and sharps are all examples of infectious waste. Methods of effective disposal of infectious waste include incineration, steam sterilization, drainage to a sanitary sewer, mechanical disinfection, chemical disinfection, and microwave. State regulations guide the treatment and disposal of regulated medical waste. Recommendations for developing and maintaining a program within a facility for safe management of medical waste are available.[80]

OCCUPATIONAL HEALTH

Occupational health (OH) and student health collaboration with the IPC Department of a healthcare facility is required by OSHA[77] and is essential for a successful program. The OH program is of paramount importance in hospitals caring for children because HCP are at increased risk of infection because: (1) children have a high incidence of infectious diseases; (2) personnel may be susceptible to many pediatric pathogens; (3) pediatric care requires close contact; (4) children lack good personal hygiene; (5) infected children can be asymptomatic; and (6) HCP are exposed to multiple family members who also can be infected.

The OH Department is an educational resource for information on infectious pathogens in the healthcare workplace. In concert with the IPC service, OH provides pre-employment education and respirator fit testing; annual retraining for all employees regarding routine health maintenance, available recommended and required vaccines, standard precautions and isolation categories, and exposure plans. Screening for tuberculosis at regular intervals, as determined by the facility's risk assessment, may use either tuberculin skin testing (TST) or interferon-γ release assays (IGRAs).[93] With new pathogens being isolated, new diseases and their transmission described, and new prophylactic regimens and treatment available, it is mandatory that personnel have an up-to-date working knowledge of IPC and know where and what services, equipment, and therapies are available for HCP.

All HCP should be screened by history or serologic testing, or both, to document their immune status to specific agents, and immunization should be provided for the following for all employees who are nonimmune and who do not have contraindications to receiving the vaccine: diphtheria toxoid, HBV, influenza (yearly), mumps, poliomyelitis, rubella, rubeola, varicella, adult pertussis vaccine (Tdap). The 2006 Advisory Committee on Immunization Practices (ACIP) recommendation to provide HCP with a single dose of Tdap vaccine was amended in 2011 to have no restriction based on age or on the time since the last Td dose. Providing vaccines at no cost to HCP increases acceptance.

The failure to increase influenza vaccine coverage above an average of 60% using novel strategies and signed declination forms led to the recommendation by many professional societies to implement a mandatory influenza vaccine program for all employees who work in a facility where healthcare is delivered.[94,95] Publications from several large institutions, including children's hospitals, indicate that mandatory programs with only medical and religious exemptions are well received with only rare employees being terminated for failure to be vaccinated.[96,97]

Special Concerns of Healthcare Personnel

HCP who have common underlying medical conditions should be able to obtain general information on wellness and screening when needed from the OH service. HCP with direct patient contact who have infants <1 year of age at home are concerned about acquiring infectious agents from patients and transmitting them to their susceptible children. An immune healthcare worker who is exposed to varicella-zoster virus (VZV) does not become a silent "carrier" of VZV. However, pathogens to which the healthcare worker is partially immune or nonimmune can cause a severe, mild, or asymptomatic infection in the employee that can be transmitted to family members. Examples include influenza, pertussis, RSV and other respiratory viruses, rotavirus, and tuberculosis. Important preventive procedures for HCP with infants at home are: (1) consistent observance of Standard Precautions, Transmission-based Precautions, and hand hygiene according to published recommendations;[2,47] (2) annual influenza and one-time Tdap immunization; (3) routine tuberculosis screening; (4) assurance of immunity or immunization against poliomyelitis, measles, mumps, hepatitis B, and rubella; (5) early medical evaluation for infectious illnesses; (6) routine, on-time immunization of infants; and (7) prompt initiation of prophylaxis/therapy following exposure/development of certain infections.

HCP who are, could be, or anticipate becoming pregnant should feel comfortable working in the healthcare workplace. In fact, with Standard Precautions and appropriate adherence to environmental cleaning and isolation precautions, vigilant HCP can be at less risk than a preschool teacher, childcare provider, or mother of children with many playmates in the home. Pathogens of potential concern to pregnant HCP include cytomegalovirus, HBV, influenza, measles, mumps, parvovirus B19, rubella, VZV, and *M. tuberculosis*. Important preventive procedures include documentation of immunity or immunization before pregnancy for rubella, mumps, measles, poliomyelitis, and HBV; annual influenza vaccine; routine tuberculosis screening; early medical evaluation for infectious illnesses; and prompt prophylaxis or therapy if exposed to or infected with certain pathogens. It is important to note that pregnancy is an *indication* for influenza vaccine to prevent the increased risk of serious disease and hospitalization that occurs in second- and third-trimester women who develop influenza infection. In 2011, the CDC recommended universal immunization with Tdap (if previously not immunized with Tdap) for pregnant women after 20 weeks of gestation.[98] Pregnant workers should assume that all patients are potentially infected with cytomegalovirus and other "silent" pathogens and should use gloves (followed by hand hygiene) when handling body fluids, secretions, and excretions. Table 2-7 summarizes the

TABLE 2-7. The Pregnant Healthcare Worker: Guide to Management of Occupational Exposure to Selected Infectious Agents[a]

Agent	In-Hospital Source	Potential Effect on the Fetus	Rate of Perinatal Transmission	Maternal Screening	Prevention
Bioweapons Agents Category A Smallpox (vaccinia)	Respiratory secretions, contents of pustulovesicular lesions	Fetal vaccinia, premature delivery, spontaneous abortion, and perinatal death	Limited data	History of successful vaccination with "take" within previous 5 years	Pre-event vaccination contraindicated during pregnancy. Vaccine and vaccinia-immune globulin (VIG) after exposure; pre-exposure vaccine only if smallpox present in the community and exposure to patients with smallpox likely. Airborne plus Contact Precautions
Cytomegalovirus (CMV)	Urine, blood, semen, vaginal secretion, immunosuppressed, transplant, dialysis, day care	Classic disease[b] (5–10%); hearing loss (10–15%)	Primary infection (25–50%); recurrent infection (52%); symptomatic (<5–15%)	Routine screening not recommended; antibody is incompletely protective	Efficacy of CMV immune globulin not established. No vaccine available. Standard Precautions. Restriction from care of known CMV patient not required
Hepatitis A (HAV)	Feces (most common), blood (rare)	No fetal transmission described; transmission can occur at the time of delivery if mother still in the infectious phase and can cause hepatitis in the infant	Unknown	Routine screening not recommended	Vaccine is a killed viral vaccine and can safely be used in pregnancy. Contact Precautions during acute phase
Hepatitis B (HBV)	Blood, bodily fluids, vaginal secretions, semen	Hepatitis, early-onset hepatocellular carcinoma	HBeAg⁻ and HBsAg⁺ (10%) HBeAg⁺ and HbsAg⁺ (90%)	Routine HBsAg testing advised during pregnancy and at delivery	HBV vaccine during pregnancy if indications exist. Neonate: HBIG plus vaccine at birth. Standard Precautions
Hepatitis C (HCV)	Blood, vaginal secretions, semen	Hepatitis	5% (0–25%)	Routine screening not recommended	No vaccine or immune globulin available; postexposure treatment with antiviral agents investigational. Standard Precautions
Herpes simplex virus (HSV)	Vesicular fluid, oropharyngeal and vaginal secretions	Sepsis, encephalitis, meningitis, mucocutaneous lesions, congenital malformation (rare)	Primary genital (33–50%) Recurrent genital (1–2%)	Antibody testing minimally useful. Genital inspection for lesions if in labor	Chemoprophylaxis at 36 weeks decreases shedding. Standard precautions. Contact Precautions for patients with mucocutaneous lesions

Continued

Agent	In-Hospital Source	Potential Effect on the Fetus	Rate of Perinatal Transmission	Maternal Screening	Prevention
Human immunodeficiency virus (HIV)	Blood, bodily fluids, vaginal secretions, semen	No congenital syndrome. If fetus infected, AIDS in 2–4 years	Depends on HIV viral load and use of antiretroviral agents during pregnancy, labor and postnatally in the infant. If viral load <1000 (rate 2%). If viral load >10000 (rate up to 25%)	Routine maternal screening advised. If exposed, testing every 3 months	Antiretroviral chemoprophylaxis for exposures; intrapartum postnatal chemoprophylaxis for HIV+ mothers and post partum for their infants indicated to prevent perienatal transmission. Standard Precautions
Influenza	Sneezing and coughing, respiratory tract secretions	No congenital syndrome (influenza in mother could cause hypoxia in fetus). Severe disease in pregnant women, especially with 2009 influenza A (H1N1)	Rare	None	Trivalent inactivated vaccine (TIV) for all pregnant women during influenza season to decrease risk of hospitalizations for cardiopulmonary complications in mother. No risk if exposed to individuals who received live attenuated influenza vaccine (LAIV). Droplet Precautions. Add Contact Precautions for young infants
Parvovirus B19	Respiratory secretion, blood, immunocompromised patients	Fetal hydrops, stillbirth; no congenital syndrome	Approximately 25%; fetal death <10%	No routine screening. B19 DNA can be detected in serum, leukocytes, respiratory secretions, urine, tissue specimens	No vaccine. Defer care of immunocompromised patients with chronic anemia when possible. Droplet Precautions
Rubella	Respiratory secretions	Congenital syndrome	90% in first trimester; 40–50% overall	Routine rubella IgG testing in pregnancy. Preconceptional screening recommended	Vacccine. No congenital rubella syndrome described for vaccine. Droplet Precautions. Contact Precautions for patients with congenital rubella
Syphilis	Blood, lesion, fluid, amniotic fluid	Congenital syndrome	Variable 10–90%; depends upon stage of maternal disease and trimester of the infection	VDRL, RPR. FTA-ABS	Postexposure prophylaxis with penicillin. Standard Precautions; wear gloves when handling infant or caring for patients with primary syphilis with mucocutaneous lesions until completion of 24 hours of treatment
Tuberculosis	Sputum, skin lesions	Neonatal tuberculosis; liver most frequently infected	Rare	Skin test: PPD. Chest radiograph	Varies with PPD reaction size and chest radiograph result; therapy for active disease during pregnancy. Airborne Precautions. Contact Precautions if draining skin lesions
Varicella-zoster virus	Respiratory secretion, vesicle fluid	Malformations, skin, limb, central nervous system, eye. Disseminated or localized disease	Congenital syndrome (2%)	Varicella IgG serology; history 90% correct	Vaccine[c]; VariZIG within 96 hours of exposure if susceptible.[d] Airborne plus Contact Precautions

AIDS, acquired immunodeficiency syndrome; FTA-ABS, fluorescent treponemal antigen-antibody test; HBeAg, hepatitis B e antigen; HBIG, hepatitis B immune globulin; HBsAg, hepatitis B surface antigen; IgG, immunoglobulin G; PPD, purified protein derivative; RPR, rapid plasma reagin test; VDRL, Venereal Disease Research Laboratory test.

[a]Employment, prepregnancy screening/vaccination is primary prevention for certain agents. Annual immunization for influenza is primary prevention.

[b]Congenital syndrome: varying combinations of jaundice, hepatosplenomegaly, microcephaly, thrombocytopenia, anemia, retinopathy, skin, and bone lesions.

[c]Live virus vaccine given before or after pregnancy.

[d]See Chapter 205, Varicella-Zoster Virus.

information about infectious agents that are relevant to the pregnant woman, and a comprehensive review has been published.[99]

INFECTION PREVENTION AND CONTROL IN THE AMBULATORY SETTING

The risk of HAIs in ambulatory settings has been reviewed,[100,101] is substantial, and is associated with lack of adherence to routine IPC practices and procedures, especially recommended safe injection practices, disinfection and sterilization, and hand hygiene.[78,102] Respiratory viral agents and *M. tuberculosis* are noteworthy infectious agents transmitted in ambulatory settings. Transmission of RSV in an HSCT outpatient clinic has been demonstrated using molecular techniques.[103] Crowded waiting rooms, toys, furniture, lack of isolation of children, unwell children, contaminated hands, contaminated secretions, and susceptible HCP are only some of the factors that result in sporadic and epidemic illness in outpatient settings. The association of CA-MRSA in HCP working in an outpatient HIV clinic with environmental CA-MRSA contamination of that clinic indicates the potential for transmission in this setting.[104] Patient-to-patient transmission of *Burkholderia* species and *P. aeruginosa* in outpatient clinics for people with cystic fibrosis has been confirmed and prevented by implementing recommended IPC methods.[105,106] IPC guidelines and policies for pediatric outpatient settings have been published.[101] Prevention strategies include definition of policies, education, and strict adherence to guidelines. In pediatrics, one of the most important interventions is segregation of children with respiratory tract illnesses and consistent implementation of respiratory etiquette/cough hygiene. A guideline for infection prevention and control for outpatient settings with a checklist was posted on the CDC website in July, 2011: www.cdc.gov/HAI/pdfs/guidelines/standatds-of-ambulatory-care-7-2011.pdf.

3 Infections Associated with Group Childcare

Andi L. Shane and Larry K. Pickering

In 2007, 325,289 licensed childcare facilities in the United States provided care for 9.5 million children, employing 1.2 million providers (http://www.naccrra.org). Aggregation of young children potentiates transmission of organisms that can produce disease in other children, adult care providers, parents, and community contacts. Group childcare settings can increase the frequency of certain diseases and amplify outbreaks of illness (Table 3-1). An increase in antibiotic use to facilitate earlier return to care enhances the potential for emergence of resistant organisms, resulting in an increased economic burden to individuals and society.[1-3] Children newly entered into group childcare are at especially high risk of enteric and respiratory tract infections.[4-9] As a consequence of these infections, attendees may be protected against respiratory tract viral infections and reactive airway diseases during subsequent years.[10] An 8-year prospective cohort study conducted from 1998 to 2006 in Quebec comparing children enrolled in home care with those in small or large group childcare observed an increase in infections at initiation of large group care. Enrollment in group childcare before 2.5 years of age resulted in decreased maternal reporting of respiratory and gastrointestinal tract infections and otitis media during elementary school years.[11] Frequent infections early in life, resulting from sibling and group childcare exposure, may be protective against atopic disease in later childhood.[12] A prospective evaluation of a birth cohort of almost 4000 children in the Netherlands demonstrated that children who were enrolled in group childcare between birth and 2 years of age had more parental reported episodes of airway symptoms in the first 4 years of life but fewer reported symptoms from 4 to 8 years of age. A longitudinal repeated-event analysis did not reveal protection from early childcare enrollment with respect to asthma symptoms, hyperresponsiveness, or allergic sensitization at the age of 8 years.[13]

CHILDCARE ARRANGEMENTS

Quantifying the types of childcare arrangements and the number of children participating in each is challenging because of different ascertainment methods used in several data sources. The U.S. Census Bureau conducts the Survey of Income and Program participation (SIPP), which collects information about childcare arrangements for children <15 years of age. A primary care arrangement is defined as the arrangement used the most hours per week. In 2006, 47% of children <15 years of age were cared for by a relative; 24% attended an organized care facility including group childcare, nursery or preschool or Head Start; 16% were in non-relative provided care, the majority of which was outside the child's primary residence; 11% were in an unspecified arrangement; and 2% were not enrolled in a regular arrangement[14] (www.census.gov/population/www/socdemo/2006_detailedtables.html). Types of facilities can be classified by size of enrollment, age of enrollees, and environmental characteristics of the facility. Grouping of children by age varies by setting but in organized care facilities children usually are separated into: infants (6 weeks through 12 months), toddlers (13 through 35 months), preschool (36 months through 59 months), and school-aged children (5 through 12 years), which has relevance to infectious disease epidemiology with regard to regulation and monitoring. Most non-relative care provided in an organized care facility is subject to state licensing and regulation, whereas care by a relative in a child's or provider's home may not be subject to state regulations and monitoring.

EPIDEMIOLOGY AND ETIOLOGY OF INFECTIONS

Although most infectious diseases have the propensity to propagate in childcare settings, diseases shown in Table 3-1 commonly are associated with outbreaks.

Enteric Infections

Outbreaks of diarrhea occur at a rate of approximately 3 per year per childcare center and are associated most frequently with organisms that cause infection after ingestion of a low inoculum. These organisms generally are transmitted from person to person[15,16] and include: rotavirus, sapovirus, norovirus, astrovirus, enteric adenovirus, *Giardia intestinalis*, *Cryptosporidium*, *Shigella*, *Escherichia coli* O157:H7 and other Shiga-toxin producing *E. coli* (STEC), *E. coli* O114, enteropathogenic *E. coli*, and *Clostridium difficile*.[15,17-29] These fecal coliforms[30,31] and enteric viruses contaminate the environment;[32] contamination rates are highest during outbreaks of diarrhea. Attack rates and frequency of asymptomatic excretion of these organisms in children attending group childcare are shown

TABLE 3-1. Association of Infectious Diseases with Group Childcare Settings

Disease or Infection	Risk Factors and Association with Outbreaks
Enteric	Close person-to-person contact, fecal-oral contact, suboptimal hand hygiene, and food preparation practices
Viral	
Rotaviruses, enteric adenoviruses, astroviruses, noroviruses, hepatitis A virus (HAV)	Commonly associated with outbreaks HAV and rotavirus are vaccine preventable
Bacterial	
Shigella, Escherichia coli O157:H7	Commonly associated with outbreaks
Campylobacter spp., *Salmonella* spp., *Clostridium difficile*	Less commonly associated with outbreaks
Parasitic	
Giardia intestinalis *Cryptosporidium parvum*	Commonly associated with outbreaks
Respiratory tract (acute upper and lower respiratory tract infections and invasive disease)	Aerosolization and respiratory droplets, person-to-person contact, suboptimal hand hygiene
Bacterial	
Haemophilus influenzae type b (Hib)	Few outbreaks; Hib is vaccine preventable
Streptococcus pneumoniae	Few outbreaks; vaccine preventable invasive *S. pneumoniae* caused by serotypes not in vaccine
Group A streptococcus	Few outbreaks and low risk of secondary cases
Neisseria meningitidis	Few outbreaks; some serogroups vaccine preventable; *N. meningitidis* caused by serogroups not in vaccine in people ≥2 years of age
Bordetella pertussis	Increasingly associated with outbreaks in childcare centers and schools; vaccine preventable
Mycobacterium tuberculosis	Occasional outbreaks, usually as a result of contact with an infectious adult care provider
Kingella kingae	Outbreaks rare; oropharynx usual habitat; usually manifest as arthritis and osteomyelitis
Viral	
Rhinoviruses, parainfluenza, influenza, respiratory vaccinesyncytial virus (RSV), respiratory adenoviruses, influenza, metapneumoviruses, bocavirus	Disease usually caused by same organisms circulating in the community; influenza is vaccine preventable in children ≥6 months of age
Multiple organ systems	
Cytomegalovirus	Prevalent asymptomatic excretion with transmission from children to providers
Parvovirus B19	Outbreaks reported; risk to susceptible pregnant women and immunocompromised
Varicella-zoster virus (VZV)	Outbreaks in childcare centers occur. VZV is vaccine preventable in children ≥12 months of age. Zoster lesions present low risk of infection
Herpes simplex virus (HSV)	Low risk of transmission from active lesions and oral secretions
Hepatitis B virus	Rarely occurs in childcare centers; vaccine preventable
Hepatitis C virus	No documented cases of transmission in the childcare setting
Human immunodeficiency virus (HIV)	No documented cases of transmission in the childcare setting
Skin	Close person-to-person contact
Staphylococcal and streptococcal impetigo	Transmission increased by close person-to-person contact with lesions; outbreaks less likely with decreased incidence of varicella infections; methicillin-resistant *Staphylococcus aureus* (MRSA) infection common
Scabies	Outbreaks in group childcare reported
Pediculosis	Common in children attending group childcare
Ringworm	*Tinea corporis* and *T. capitis* outbreaks associated with childcare
Conjunctiva	Outbreaks in group childcare reported with both bacterial and viral etiologies

in Table 3-2. Reported attack rates depend on several factors, including methods used for organism detection.[23,24]

Enteric viruses are the predominant etiology of diarrheal syndromes among children in group care.[33] Environmental swabs corroborated stool virus detection in 45% of outbreaks.[34] With the marked decline in rotavirus disease due to the success of the rotavirus immunization program, norovirus may be the most common viral enteric pathogen in childcare centers.

Organisms generally associated with foodborne outbreaks, including *Salmonella* and *Campylobacter jejuni*, infrequently are associated with diarrhea in the childcare setting. Report of an outbreak of diarrhea in 14 of 67 (21%) exposed children and adult care providers associated with ingestion of fried rice contaminated with *Bacillus cereus*,[35] however, highlights the fact that foodborne outbreaks can occur in the childcare setting, especially when food is prepared and served at the center.

Bacterial pathogens that have the potential to cause severe systemic infections, including *E. coli* O157:H7 and other STEC,[28] have been associated with fecal-oral transmission in group childcare settings. An outbreak of *E. coli* O157:H7 occurred in a childcare center in Alberta, Canada in 2002 likely after introduction by a

3-year-old enrollee who developed hemolytic–uremic syndrome following farm animal contact. The diarrheal attack rate was 23% among enrollees, which is comparable with attack rates reported during previous childcare-associated outbreaks of *E. coli* O157:H7. Prolonged asymptomatic shedding and subclinical cases in concert with poor hygiene and toileting practices likely contributed to propagation of the outbreak.[36]

Shigella sonnei causes periodic multicommunity outbreaks in group childcare. Childcare attendance and age <60 months were associated with illness in a dispersed community outbreak of molecularly related strains of *S. sonnei* among traditionally observant Jewish children in New York City in 2000.[37] Multiple illnesses in a single household were determined to be due to intrahousehold secondary transmission. A multicommunity outbreak of over 1600 culture-confirmed cases in the greater metropolitan area of Cincinnati, Ohio from May to September, 2001 had an overall mean attack rate of 10% among childcare center enrollees. Highest attack rates occurred among newly or incompletely toilet-trained enrollees and lowest attack rates among diapered children. The attack rate was 6% among staff. Secondary transmission was facilitated by poor hygiene practices, including inaccessible

TABLE 3-2. Outbreaks of Diarrhea by Organism

Organism	Attack Rate (Enrollees) (%)	Secondary Attack Rate (Family Members) (%)	Asymptomatic Excretion (Enrollees)
Rotavirus	50	15–80	Common
Enteric adenovirus	40	Unknown	Common
Astrovirus	50–90	Unknown	Common
Calicivirus	50	Unknown	Common
Giardia intestinalis	17–54	15–50	Common
Cryptosporidium	33–74	25–60	Common
Shigella	33–73	25–50	Uncommon
Escherichia coli			
O157:H7	29, 34	Unknown	Uncommon
O114:NM	67	Unknown	Uncommon
O111:K58	56, 94	Unknown	Uncommon
Clostridium difficile	32	Unknown	Common

handwashing supplies and incomplete diaper disposal practices, as well as recreational activities involving water.[38] A prolonged multistate increase of shigellosis due to organisms with similar biochemical and genetic profiles occurred in the south and mid-Atlantic areas from June 2001 to March 2003. A substantial proportion of cases were associated with group childcare.[39] From May to October of 2005, 639 cases of multidrug-resistant *S. sonnei* were reported in northwest Missouri. A case-control investigation of 39 licensed childcare centers demonstrated that centers with ≥1 sink or a diapering station in each room were less likely to have cases, showing the essential importance of these practices to reduce the propagation of shigellosis in childcare centers.[40] Investigators in North Carolina demonstrated that proper diapering and hand hygiene practices, and food-preparation equipment decreased the incidence of diarrheal illness among children and staff in out-of-home childcare centers.[41]

Spread of diarrhea pathogens from index cases in the childcare setting into families has been reported for many enteropathogens (see Table 3-2), with secondary attack rates ranging from 15% to 80%. A retrospective evaluation of transmission of infectious gastroenteritis (80% due to rotavirus) in 936 households in northern California revealed a secondary household attack rate of 9%. Older children in the households had a 2- to 8-fold greater risk of secondary infection than adults.[42] During outbreaks of diarrhea in childcare centers, asymptomatic excretion of enteropathogens is frequent[15,23,24,43–46] (see Table 3-2). During outbreaks associated with enteric viruses and *G. intestinalis* in children <3 years of age, asymptomatic infection occurs in up to 50% of infected children. In one longitudinal study of diarrhea in 82 children <2 years of age in a childcare center, more than 2700 stool specimens were collected on a weekly basis.[45] Using enzyme immunoassays, 21 of 27 (78%) children infected with *G. intestinalis* were asymptomatic and 19 of 37 (51%) children with rotavirus were asymptomatic. A point-prevalence evaluation of 230 asymptomatic preschool children attending childcare in southwest Wales and inner London demonstrated a 1.3% fecal colonization rate with both *Cryptosporidium* and *Giardia* spp.[47] The role that asymptomatic excretion of enteropathogens plays in spread of disease is unknown.

Acute infectious diarrhea is two to three times more common in children in childcare than in age-matched children cared for in their homes.[4,48,49] Approximately 20% of clinic visits for acute diarrheal illness among children younger than 3 years of age are attributable to childcare attendance [4]. In addition, the incidence of diarrheal illness is 3-fold higher among children in their first month in out-of-home childcare than in children cared for at home.[4,5]

Diarrhea occurs 17 times more frequently in diapered children than in children not wearing diapers.[50] Children who are diapered are more likely to be younger than children who are not; therefore, higher attack rates merely may represent exposure of a younger, nonimmune cohort. In a multicommunity group childcare outbreak of *S. sonnei*, the highest attack rates were noted in rooms where both toilet-trained and diapered children were co-mingled (14%) compared with rooms with toilet-trained children only (9%) and rooms with diapered children only (5%), despite comparable availability of sinks and toilets.[38]

Rotavirus

Rotaviruses are the most common etiology of significant symptomatic diarrhea in children <2 years of age, although rates of diarrhea have decreased since implementation of rotavirus immunization.[51] Infections are transmitted primarily from person to person by the fecal-oral route. Rotavirus can be isolated from human stools for approximately 21 days after illness onset and rotavirus RNA has been detected on toys and surfaces in childcare centers.[32] The highest attack rates for rotavirus infections have occurred in infants and children enrolled in group childcare.

Primary prevention of rotavirus in all settings has been accomplished with administration of one of two licensed rotavirus vaccines. Before introduction of rotavirus vaccines in the U.S. in 2006, rotavirus caused an estimated 20 to 60 deaths, 55,000 to 70,000 hospitalizations, 205,000 to 272,000 emergency department visits, and 400,000 outpatient visits annually among children less than 5 years of age. The 2007–08 and 2008–09 rotavirus seasons were notable for their decreased duration, later onset, and fewer positive tests, compared with median data for 2000–2006 from a national network of sentinel laboratories.[52,53]

Hepatitis A Virus

Hepatitis A virus (HAV) infections usually are mild or asymptomatic in children. Less than 5% of children <3 years of age and <10% of children between 4 and 6 years of age with HAV infection develop jaundice. The first outbreak of HAV in a childcare center was reported in 1973 in North Carolina;[54] outbreaks subsequently were recognized throughout the U.S.[55] Peak viral titers in stool and greatest infectivity occur during the 2 weeks before onset of symptoms. Outbreaks in childcare centers generally are not recognized until illness becomes apparent in older children or adults.[55] Prior to routine use of hepatitis A vaccine in children in the U.S., approximately 15% of episodes of HAV infection were estimated to be associated with childcare centers. HAV infections are transmitted in the childcare setting by the fecal-oral route and occur more frequently in settings that include diapered children. Large size and long hours of operation also are risk factors for outbreaks of HAV infection.[56]

The mainstays for prevention of HAV infection include maintenance of personal hygiene, hand hygiene, and disinfecting procedures. Universal administration of hepatitis A vaccine to toddlers in Israel in 1999 resulted in a notable absence of outbreaks of HAV in childcare and elementary school settings from 2000 through 2006.[57] Universal administration of 2 doses of hepatitis A vaccine to all children, beginning at 1 year (12 through 23 months) of age, with the 2 doses administered at least 6 months apart is recommended in the U.S.[58] Administration of hepatitis A vaccine or immune globulin to unimmunized, immunocompetent people 12 months through 40 years of age for postexposure prophylaxis also is recommended.[59,60] A case-control study to evaluate the effectiveness of an HAV vaccination program targeted at childcare attendees between 2 and 5 years of age found that people with direct contact with a childcare center were protected against disease. Furthermore, the 6-fold greater risk of HAV infection that occurred in people who had contact with a childcare center prior to implementation of the hepatitis A immunization program in Maricopa County, Arizona was not found in the postvaccination case-control study.[61] Enhanced population-based surveillance conducted by health departments among six U.S. sites from 2005 to 2007 was notable for 1156 cases among 29.8 million people. Being an employee or child in a childcare center accounted for 8% of cases, while international travel and contact with a case were more frequent risk factors associated with 46% and 15% of hepatitis A cases. Despite the decline in the incidence of HAV, continued education, training, and monitoring of staff regarding appropriate hygienic practices are essential components of any preventive plan.

Respiratory Tract Infections

Children <2 years of age attending childcare centers have an increased number of upper and lower respiratory tract illnesses compared with age-matched children cared for at home.[4,6,62,63] Approximately 10% to 17% of respiratory tract illnesses in U.S. children <5 years of age are attributable to childcare attendance.[64,65] A prospective cohort study found that 89% of disease episodes among children attending a childcare center are respiratory tract infections (RTIs).[66] Another prospective cohort study following 119 children through 24 months of age from 2006 to 2008 demonstrated a mean annual incidence of RTI of 4.2 per child during the first year and 1.2 during the second year of the study. One or more viruses were detected by real-time reverse transcriptase polymerase chain reaction (rRT-PCR) from two-thirds of the episodes.[67] Infections with human metapneumovirus (HMPV) and human bocavirus (HBoV) also have been reported in childcare enrollees.[67-69]

In a retrospective cohort study of 2568 children from 1 to 7 years of age, 1-year-old children cared for in childcare centers, when compared to those cared for at home, had an increased risk of the common cold (relative risk (RR), 1.7; 95% CI, 1.4 to 2.0), otitis media (RR, 2.0; 95% CI, 1.6 to 2.5), and pneumonia (RR, 9.7; 95% CI, 2.3 to 40.6).[62] In a prospective cohort study in France, the risk of upper respiratory tract illnesses (URTIs) was higher for those cared for in small centers (odds ratio (OR), 2.2; 95% CI, 1.4–3.4) and large centers (OR, 1.2; 95% CI, 0.8–1.8) compared with those in family childcare homes. The intermediate risk for those in large childcare centers may have resulted from segregation in those centers into small classrooms. A national registry-based study of Danish children from birth to 5 years of age revealed that for children under 1 year of age, the first 6 months of enrollment in group childcare were associated with a 69% higher incidence of hospitalizations for acute respiratory tract infections compared with children in home care. The incidence of hospitalization decreased after 6 months of group childcare enrollment and was comparable with children in home care after >12 months of enrollment.[70]

Respiratory tract infections that have been studied in the childcare setting include pharyngitis, sinusitis, otitis media, common cold, bronchiolitis, and pneumonia.[6,62,63,65,71] Organisms responsible for illness in children in childcare settings are similar to organisms that circulate in the community and include respiratory syncytial virus, parainfluenza viruses, adenovirus, rhinovirus, coronavirus, influenza viruses, parvovirus B19, and *Streptococcus pneumoniae*. Infections due to *Bordetella pertussis* in the U.S. have increased, with 8296 cases of pertussis reported in 2002 and 25,827 cases reported in 2004.[72-74] In 2010 over 6000 cases of pertussis were reported in California including 10 deaths in infants <3 months of age.[75] Incompletely immunized infants under 12 months of age often experience severe clinical disease. In many group childcare arrangements, adolescents and adults experiencing mild to moderate illnesses may be the source cases of pertussis. An outbreak of pertussis, occurring in a childcare center in northern Israel with 88% immunization coverage, resulted in infection among all of the unvaccinated children and only 7% of the vaccinated children.[76] In 2005, the American Academy of Pediatrics (AAP) and Advisory Committee on Immunization Practices (ACIP) recommended universal use of one of the licensed Tdap vaccines for those aged 10 through 64 years.[73,74] Childcare providers of any age with routine contact with infants <12 months of age also should receive a single dose of Tdap.[77]

An adult or adolescent also can be the index case for *Mycobacterium tuberculosis* infections in a group childcare setting; child-to-child transmission occurs infrequently.[78,79] An outbreak of tuberculosis (TB) associated with a private-home childcare facility

in San Francisco, California occurred between 2002 and 2004.[80] Of 11 outbreak cases, 9 (82%) occurred in children <7 years of age; all had extensive contact with the private-home childcare facility, where the adult index patient spent considerable time. Isolates from 4 of the pediatric patients and 2 of the adult patients had identical molecular patterns. Thirty-six additional children and adult contacts had latent TB infections.[80] In a Swedish outbreak of TB following prolonged contact with a provider with cavitary disease in a childcare center, 17 children had radiographic evidence of pulmonary disease; 1 child had miliary disease and 17 had latent tuberculosis infection. The tuberculin skin test was effective in identifying infected children.[81] These outbreaks demonstrate that detection and contact investigation are paramount in reducing tuberculosis infection. High transmissibility of TB among residents of adult daycare centers also has been demonstrated.[82]

Person-to-person transmission of *Chlamydophila pneumoniae* among children in the childcare setting has been reported without occurrence of disease.[83] *Kingella kingae* colonizes the oropharynx and respiratory tracts of young children and has been associated with invasive disease.[84] The first reported outbreak of invasive *K. kingae* osteomyelitis/pyogenic arthritis occurred in a childcare center in 2003; 15 (13%) children older than 16 months of age were found to be colonized, with 9 children (45%) in the same class as the 2 children with invasive disease. Matching pulse field gel electrophoresis (PFGE) patterns supported child-to-child transmission.[85] Successive cases of *K. kingae* endocarditis and osteomyelitis occurred in two children attending a North Carolina childcare center in 2007 with a child enrollment of 14 children and 5 staff. Interaction with children from a co-owned childcare facility with 19 children >21 months of age and 5 staff resulted in an epidemiologic investigation of the attendees at both. A high rate of invasive disease, but a low rate of colonization (4%) was noted.[86]

Outbreaks of group A streptococcal (GAS) infection among children and adult staff in the childcare setting have been reported.[87-89] In a study of prevalence of GAS conducted in a childcare center after a fatal case of invasive disease, 25% of 258 children and 8% of 25 providers had GAS isolated from throat cultures.[87] Risk of carriage was increased in children who shared the room of the index case (OR, 2.7; 95% CI, 0.8 to 9.4). Perianal GAS infection and infection associated with varicella also have been reported.[88,90] A clone of GAS (emm type 4) was responsible for a community outbreak of streptococcal toxic shock syndrome among children attending a childcare center in northern Spain. The outbreak-associated strains were not isolated from pharyngotonsillar swabs of staff, childcare or household contacts of the colonized and infected children.[91]

The risk of acute otitis media (AOM) is increased in children in childcare, especially in children <2 years of age.[65,66,92,93] In one study, the incidence rate ratio for AOM was 1.5 in children in childcare compared with that in children in home care.[65] AOM is responsible for most antibiotic use in children <3 years of age in the childcare setting. Childcare attendance also has been associated with risk of developing recurrent AOM (>6 episodes in 1 year), as well as chronic otitis media with effusion persisting for more than 6 months.[94] The size of the childcare center was an important variable in the occurrence of frequent AOM in children younger than 12 months of age, varying from 16% in small care groups to 36% in large care groups.[93] Genotypically similar strains of nontypable *Haemophilus influenzae* and pneumococci were isolated from nasopharyngeal cultures from children attending childcare centers.[95,96]

Handwashing decreases the frequency of acute respiratory tract diseases in childcare.[97,98] A cluster, randomized, controlled trial of an infection control intervention including training of childcare staff regarding handwashing, transmission modes of infection, and aseptic techniques related to nose-wiping demonstrated a significant reduction in URTI among enrollees <24 months of age over 311 child-years of surveillance.[97] Because most infectious agents are communicable for a few days before and after clinical illness, exclusion from childcare of children with symptoms of upper respiratory tract infections probably will not decrease spread.

Influenza

Rates of virus infection are highest among children <2 years of age and elderly people, and rates of complications are greatest among children of all ages with predisposing or underlying medical conditions. Among preschool-aged children with influenza infections, hospitalization rates range from 100 to 500/100,000 children, with highest hospitalization rates among children from birth to 1 year of age.[99] Influenza viruses are spread from person to person primarily through large respiratory tract droplets, either directly or by secondary contact with objects that are contaminated with infectious droplets. Children shed virus for several days prior to onset of clinical symptoms and are contagious for >10 days following symptom onset. Transmission of infections may be increased by close contact among children who are not able to contain their secretions.

Annual vaccination against influenza is the primary method for preventing influenza infection. Influenza vaccine is recommended annually for all people 6 months of age and older.[99] A single-blind randomized controlled trial conducted during the 1996 to 1997 influenza season in 10 childcare centers in San Diego, California revealed that vaccinating children against influenza reduced influenza-related illness among their household contacts.[100-102] In addition to preventing respiratory tract illness, several studies have shown the effectiveness of influenza vaccine in preventing AOM among children in childcare.[97,98,103] In one study of children 6 to 30 months of age in childcare centers, OR for AOM was 0.69 and the 95% CI was 0.49 to 0.98 for children who received influenza immunization.[104]

Routine use of intranasal influenza vaccine among healthy children may be cost effective and can be maximized by using group-based vaccination approaches. A prospective 2-year efficacy trial of intranasal influenza vaccine in healthy children 15 through 71 months of age demonstrated clinical as well as economic efficacy associated with focusing vaccination efforts on children in group settings.[105] Vaccinating children has been associated with protection of older people as well.[105-107]

Children with signs and symptoms of URTI should be cohorted. Ill childcare providers should be discouraged from providing care or having contact with children in group childcare. Vaccination of both child attendees and adult providers annually is recommended and both children and providers should receive frequent reminders regarding hand hygiene and respiratory etiquette to reduce influenza infections in group childcare settings. Frequently touched surfaces, toys, and commonly shared items should be cleaned at least daily and when visibly soiled as these items can serve as fomites in the transmission of viruses.[108]

The issue of childcare center closure as a strategy to prevent community spread of influenza was raised by the 2009 novel H1N1 influenza pandemic. A survey of 58% of families of 402 students in Perth, Australia who were affected by pandemic-related school closures revealed a substantial disruption of daily schedules. Almost half of the parents had work absences and 35% made alternative childcare arrangements. Children impacted by the school closures were more likely to report out-of-home activities during the closure period. Less than half (47%) of the parent respondents felt that the school closures were an effective response.[109] Childcare center and elementary school absences were two components of a surveillance system used for monitoring influenza activity in a U.S.–Mexico border community during the 2009 novel H1N1 influenza pandemic.[110]

Invasive Bacterial Infection

Studies conducted before routine use of *Haemophilus influenzae* type b (Hib) vaccine in the U.S. showed that the risk of developing primary invasive Hib infection was higher among children attending childcare centers than in children cared for at home, independent of other possible risk factors.[107,111] Incorporation of conjugated Hib vaccines into the routine immunization schedule of children in the U.S. has reduced dramatically the frequency of invasive Hib disease.[112]

Risk of disease due to *Neisseria meningitidis* may be increased in children in group childcare. Using space–time cluster analysis of invasive infections during 9 years of surveillance, from 1993 to 2001, in the Netherlands, researchers noted that clustering beyond chance occurred at a rate of 3% and concluded that this rate was likely the result of direct transmission. Childcare center attendance was reported as the likely exposure for 8 of 40 (20%) clusters, accounting for 13 of 82 (16%) cases of invasive disease with multiple serosubtypes.[113] For children from 2 through 10 years of age, routine immunization with meningococcal conjugate vaccine is recommended only for children at continued increased risk of invasive disease.[114]

The risks of developing primary invasive disease due to *S. pneumoniae*, nasopharyngeal carriage of *S. pneumoniae*, and carriage of antibiotic-resistant strains are increased for children in childcare centers[115-123] and childcare homes.[117] In Finland, an increased risk of invasive pneumococcal disease in children <2 years of age was associated with childcare attendance (OR, 36; 95% CI, 5.7 to 233) and family childcare (OR, 4.4; 95% CI, 1.7 to 112).[117] Secondary spread of *S. pneumoniae* in the childcare setting has been reported, but the exact risks are not known.[110,122,124-126] Colonization with *S. pneumoniae* in one childcare center was 59% for children 2 to 24 months of age; 75% of the strains were penicillin-nonsusceptible.[118] In an evaluation of the childcare cohort of an 11-month enrollee with multidrug-resistant *S. pneumoniae* infection in southwest Georgia, *S. pneumoniae* was isolated from 19 of 21 (90%) nasopharyngeal cultures; 10 (53%) matched the serotype[14] and susceptibility pattern of the strain from the index child; 4 of the 10 children with index-strain carriage had shared a childcare room with the index child, suggesting person-to-person transmission.[127]

Incorporation of heptavalent pneumococcal conjugate vaccine (PCV7) into the routine childhood immunization schedule in the U.S. in August 2000 has resulted in a dramatic reduction in the frequency of invasive pneumococcal disease (IPD).[128] The impact of vaccination on AOM and reduction of penicillin-nonsusceptible pneumococcal infection is less dramatic and more variable, with evidence of increasing nasopharyngeal colonization and respiratory tract infections caused by nonvaccine serotypes and nontypable strains of pneumococcus.[128-131] Serotype 19A, not included in PCV7, has been associated with IPD in many communities[132] and in childcare.[133] A 13-valent pneumococcal conjugate vaccine (PCV13) was licensed by the Food and Drug Administration (FDA) in 2010 to replace PCV7.[134,135] The impact of broader serotype coverage, including serotype 19A, with PCV13 on epidemiology will be important to monitor as PCV13 is administered to a notable proportion of enrollees in group childcare.

Viral Infections

Echovirus

During an outbreak of echovirus 30 infection in children and care providers in a childcare center, and in exposed parents, infection occurred in 75% of children and 60% of adults; aseptic meningitis was more frequent in infected adults (12 in 65, 18%) than in children (2 in 79, 3%).[139] A retrospective cohort study of four childcare centers, attendees, employees, and household contacts in Germany revealed that 42% of childcare attendees, 13% of their household contacts, 5% of childcare center employees, and 2% of their household contacts were ill over a 31-day period. Thirteen percent (12 of 92) of childcare attendees had meningitis. This outbreak likely began among children enrolled in group childcare, with secondary cases occurring among their household contacts.[140] An association with childcare also was noted in an outbreak of echovirus 18 meningitis in a rural Missouri community with an attack rate of 1 per 1000 people; contact with childcare was noted as the most common risk factor among ill people.[141]

Parvovirus B19

Parvovirus B19, the agent of erythema infectiosum (fifth disease), can cause arthropathy, transient aplastic crisis, persistent anemia in immunocompromised hosts, and nonimmune fetal hydrops. Serologic evidence of past infection has been reported to be 30% to 60% in adults, 15% to 60% in school-aged children, and 2% to 15% in preschool children.[178] The virus is endemic among young children and has caused outbreaks of disease in the childcare setting.[179,180] Parvovirus B19 spreads by the respiratory route or through contact with oropharyngeal secretions. In an outbreak during which more than 571 school and childcare personnel were tested serologically, the overall attack rate among susceptible individuals was 19%, with the highest rate (31%) occurring in childcare personnel.[179] A cross-sectional study of 477 childcare staff revealed a seroprevalence for parvovirus B19 IgG antibodies of 70%. Seropositivity was associated with age, and among staff less than 40 years of age, with length of group childcare contact.[181] The greatest concern is that an infected pregnant woman could transmit the virus transplacentally, leading to fetal hydrops; neonatal illness and congenital malformations have not been linked to prenatal parvovirus B19 infection. Estimates of the risk of fetal loss when a pregnant woman of unknown antibody status is exposed are 3% for fetal death after household exposure and 2% after occupational exposure in a school.[182]

Cytomegalovirus

Young childcare attendees shed cytomegalovirus (CMV) chronically after acquisition and often transmit virus to other children and adults with whom they have close daily contact.[142–145] Transmission is thought to occur through direct person-to-person contact and from contaminated toys, hands of childcare providers, or classroom surfaces.[146] Prevalence studies have shown that 10% to 70% of children <3 years of age (peak, 13 through 24 months) in childcare settings have CMV detected in urine or saliva.[142,144,147] CMV-infected children can transmit the virus to women, with rates from 8% to 20% in their childcare providers and 20% in their mothers per year[148–150] compared with rates of 1% to 3% per year in women whose toddlers are not infected.

Bloodborne Viral Pathogens

There is concern about the potential for spread of bloodborne organisms in the childcare setting: hepatitis B virus (HBV), hepatitis C virus (HCV), and human immunodeficiency virus (HIV).[151–154] The highest concentrations of HBV in infected people are found in blood and blood-containing body fluids. The most common and efficient routes of transmission are percutaneous blood exposure, sexual exposure, and, perinatally, from mothers to offspring at the time of delivery. Other recognized but less efficient modes of transmission include bites and mucous membrane exposure to blood or other body fluids.[155,156] Two case reports and a larger study have demonstrated possible transmission of HBV among children in the childcare setting.[156–158] Investigators in Denmark and the Netherlands demonstrated high levels of HBV DNA in saliva of 46 HBeAg-positive children, suggesting that exposure to saliva could be a means of horizontal transmission of hepatitis B infection.[159] Other investigators have failed to demonstrate transmission in childcare, despite long-term exposure to children positive for hepatitis B surface antigen (HBsAg).[160] Because of the small number of studies, the risk of HBV transmission in childcare cannot be quantified precisely. With implementation of universal immunization of infants with HBV vaccine beginning in 1991, the potential for horizontal HBV transmission in the childcare setting has been reduced to negligible. If a known HBsAg carrier bites and breaks the skin of an unimmunized child, hepatitis B immune globulin and the HBV vaccine series should be administered.[152] The transmission risk of HCV infection in childcare settings is unknown. The general risk of HCV infection from percutaneous exposure to infected blood is estimated to be 10 times greater than HIV but less than HBV.

No cases of HIV infection are known to have resulted from transmission of the virus in out-of-home childcare. Children with

HIV infection in the childcare setting should be monitored for exposure to infectious diseases, and their health and immune status should be evaluated frequently. The risk of transmission of HIV by percutaneous body fluid exposure, such as biting, is low. Complete evaluation of the source and extent of exposure should be undertaken to assess the possible risk of HIV transmission and benefits of postexposure prophylaxis.[152]

Precautions for prevention of HBV, HCV, and HIV infection should be directed toward preventing transfer of blood or secretions from person to person. Childcare providers should be educated about modes of transmission of bloodborne diseases and their prevention, and each center should have written policies for managing illnesses and common injuries[161] such as bite wounds.[162] Standard precautions for handling blood and blood-containing body fluids should be practiced in all childcare settings.[152] Children infected with HIV or HCV or children who are HBsAg carriers should be included in childcare activities. Decisions regarding attendance at childcare and the optimal childcare environment should be made by parents and the child's physician after considering the possible risks and benefits.

Skin Infection and Infestation

The magnitude of skin infections or infestations and the rates of occurrence in children in group childcare compared with rates in age-matched children not in group childcare are not known. The most frequently recognized nonvaccine-preventable conditions are impetigo or cellulitis (due to *S. aureus* or GAS), pediculosis, and scabies.[88,98,163] Other conditions with skin manifestations that occur in children in childcare include herpes simplex virus (HSV) infection, varicella, ringworm, and molluscum contagiosum.[88,164–166]

Varicella Zoster

Unimmunized children in childcare facilities are susceptible to varicella infection; most reported cases occur in children <10 years of age.[88,165] An outbreak of varicella was reported when a child with zoster attended a childcare center.[164] Although the lesions were covered, the child continually scratched and showed others the lesions, indicating the potential difficulties with enforcement of preventive policies. Universal immunization with varicella vaccine has reduced cases of chickenpox among children in group childcare.[58,167] However, several outbreaks of varicella have been reported among childcare attendees in the post-licensure era.[89,168,169] A varicella outbreak occurring among elementary school attendees in Maine in December to January 2003 was due to failure to vaccinate. The vaccination rates were notable for a decrease from 90% of kindergarten attendees to 60% of third-grade enrollees. Vaccine effectiveness in this cohort of 296 students was 89% against all varicella disease and 96% against moderate to severe disease. This outbreak illustrates the importance of vaccination of susceptible older children and adolescents to decrease the incidence of severe disease in unvaccinated children.[167] In June 2005 and June 2006, ACIP recommended the implementation of a routine 2-dose varicella vaccination program for children, with the first dose administered at 12 through 15 months and the second dose at 4 through 6 years of age.[167] An outbreak among elementary school student recipients of 1-dose and 2-dose varicella immunizations with a pre-outbreak coverage rate of 97% resulted in 84 reported infections (most cases with <50 lesions). Of these, 25 (30%) of children had received 2 doses and 53 (63%) had received one dose of varicella vaccine. The severity of disease and vaccine effectiveness of 1 and 2 doses were comparable.[170] An outbreak in an elementary school in Philadelphia in 2006 demonstrated that second-dose varicella vaccination for outbreak control was an effective intervention to reduce varicella incidence among classroom contacts of a case.[171–173] This strategy may be employed as a control measure among age-eligible childcare attendees who have not received the 2-dose varicella series in an outbreak setting.

TABLE 3-3. Vaccine-Preventable Infections

Organism	Immunization Indicated	
	Childcare Attendee	**Childcare Provider**
Diphtheria, pertussis, tetanus	As part of the 5-dose DTaP series	Tdap booster as adolescent and one time dose of Tdap to adults who have not received Tdap then Td every 10 years
Haemophilus influenzae type b (Hib)	As part of the 3–4-dose series, depending on vaccine used	Not indicated
Hepatitis A	2-dose series beginning at 1 year (12 through 23 months) of age	2-dose series recommended for adults at high risk for hepatitis A virus infection; not routinely recommended for childcare providers
Hepatitis B	3-dose series beginning at birth	3-dose series recommended for hepatitis B virus infection; not routinely recommended for childcare providers
Influenza A and B	Annual immunization for all children 6 months of age and older; 2 doses if first influenza immunization and ≤8 years of age	Annual immunization with trivalent inactivated or live attenuated influenza vaccine
Measles, mumps, rubella	2-dose series starting at 12 months of age	Booster immunization if only one dose received
Meningococcal disease	Conjujate vaccine for children 2 through 10 years of age in high-risk groups and routinely at 11 through 18 years of age for all children and adolescents	Conjugate vaccine recommended for adults 19 through 55 years of age or polysaccharide vaccine for adults ≥56 years of age at increased risk
Pneumococcal disease	4 doses of 13-valent conjugate vaccine (PCV13) for all children 2 through 23 months of age; 1 dose of PCV13 for certain children 24 through 59 months of age. Polysaccharide vaccine in addition to conjugate vaccine for certain high-risk groups 2 through 18 years of age	Pneumococcal polysaccharide vaccine for adults with chronic conditions and for high-risk groups 19 through 64 years of age and all adults at ≥65 years of age
Poliomyelitis	4-dose series; final dose administered at or after the fourth birthday	Most adults are immune; inactivated poliovirus vaccine may be indicated in select populations
Rotavirus	2 or 3-dose series beginning at 2 months of age and completed by 8 months of age	Not indicated
Varicella	2 doses, one at 12 through 15 months of age and the second at 4 through 6 years of age	2 doses for susceptible people ≥13 years of age
Human papillomavirus	3 doses for females and males 9 years through 26 years of age	3 doses for females through 26 years of age

Herpes Simplex

Clusters of primary HSV infections occur in children in childcare, most frequently manifesting as gingivostomatitis.[166] In one study, restriction endonuclease analysis of DNA of isolated HSV revealed that a single strain of HSV-1 had been transmitted among children.[174] Molluscum contagiosum is a benign, usually asymptomatic viral infection of the skin; humans are the only source. Virus is spread by direct contact or by fomites. Infectivity is low, but outbreaks have been reported. The frequency of occurrence in the childcare setting is unknown. The incidence of pediculosis capitis (head lice) among children in childcare facilities in Seattle was 0.02 per 100 child-weeks[175] and 0.03 per child-year in San Diego.[176] Because head lice are transmitted by direct head-to-head contact, childcare centers with shared sleeping areas may facilitate transmission. Treatment of infested children and their contacts with pediculicides may be considered as control measures.[177]

Methicillin-Resistant *Staphylococcus aureus*

Infections due to methicillin-resistant *Staphylococcus aureus* (MRSA) were reported infrequently in the group childcare setting before 2000.[136,137] However, with the emergence of community-acquired (CA)-MRSA and its predisposition for affecting people in crowded conditions where sharing of fomites and skin-to-skin contact occurs, and where hygiene is compromised, children in group care are at risk. A molecular epidemiologic study of MRSA prevalence among 104 children, 32 employees, and 17 household contacts of attendees affiliated with a university medical center childcare facility in Texas noted an overall 7% colonization rate with MRSA. MRSA was isolated from one employee (3%), 6 (35%) family members and 4 (2%) environmental samples. Molecular typing revealed closely related, mostly community-associated

isolates. The use of macrolide antibiotics and asthma medications were associated with MRSA colonization.[138] MRSA colonization of a child in a childcare setting is not a reason for exclusion from the setting.

VACCINE-PREVENTABLE DISEASES

In the United States, there are 16 diseases against which children should be immunized, unless there are medical contraindications: diphtheria, tetanus, pertussis, Hib, measles, mumps, rubella, poliomyelitis, HBV, varicella, *S. pneumoniae*, HAV, influenza, rotavirus, human papillomavirus, and meningococcal disease.[58] Immunization of children and their care providers should be high priority (Table 3-3) and immunization especially is likely to benefit children in childcare settings.[183] High levels of immunization exist among children in licensed childcare facilities, partially because laws requiring age-appropriate immunizations of children attending licensed childcare programs exist in almost all states. Vaccine mandates for HBV are active in 47 (94%) states as of June 2010, hepatitis A in 17 (34%) states as of October 2010, pneumococcus in 31 (62%) of states as of October 2010, and varicella in 49 (98%) states as of December 2010 (http://www.immunize.org/laws/#inf). In a study of exemptions to immunizations, children of childcare age (3 through 5 years) with exemptions to immunizations were 66 times more likely to acquire measles and 17 times more likely to acquire pertussis than were age-matched immunized children.[184]

INFECTIONS ASSOCIATED WITH ANIMALS

Animal exposure has been associated with sporadic zoonotic infections as well as outbreaks, injuries, and allergies, most notably in children <5 years of age. The increased prevalence of infections in this age group is likely due to compromised hand hygiene resulting in transmission of pathogens from animal to child. Animal interaction can occur in locations where childcare is provided, with a resident pet or visiting animal display, or in public venues where children visit, including petting zoos, aquariums, county fairs, parks, carnivals, circuses, or farms. Guidelines to reduce opportunities for transmission and infection have been developed to prevent disease transmission in many of these settings.[185,186] Inadequate hand hygiene, suboptimal supervision of children's activities following animal contact, and hand-to-mouth activities following animal contact are risk factors for infection. Infections that have been associated with close contact with animals include those caused by *Escherichia coli* O157:H7, *Salmonella enterica* serotype Typhimurium, *Cryptosporidium parvum*, *Campylobacter jejuni*, Shiga toxin-producing *E. coli* (STEC), and *Giardia intestinalis*.[187–190] In addition to enteric infections, animal exposure can result in transmission of ecto- and endoparasites, *Mycobacterium tuberculosis* in certain settings, and local or systemic infections as a consequence of bites, scratches, stings, and other injuries.

Contact with animals within the childcare environment should occur where controls are established to reduce the risk of injuries and disease. Specific recommendations for group childcare settings include close supervision of children during animal contact, strict hand hygiene after direct animal contact or contact with animal products or environment, designation of areas for animal contact that are separate from areas in which food or drink are consumed, disinfection and cleaning of all animal areas with supervision of children >5 years of age who may be participating in this task. Amphibians, reptiles, and weasels (ferrets and mink) should be housed in a cage and not handled by children. Wild or exotic animals, nonhuman primates, mammals with a high risk of transmitting rabies, wolf-dog hybrids, aggressive wild or domestic animals, stray animals, venomous or toxin-producing spiders, and insects should not be permitted in the group childcare setting,[190] (http://www.cdc.gov/healthypets/).

ANTIBIOTIC USE AND RESISTANCE PATTERNS

During an 8-week period of observation of 270 children, antimicrobial agents were used by 36% of children in childcare centers compared with 7% and 8% of children in childcare homes or in home care, respectively (P<0.001). The mean duration of antibiotic therapy prescribed for children in childcare centers (20 days) differed significantly (P<0.001) from children in childcare homes (4 days) and children in home care (5 days).[128] The estimated annual rates of antibiotic treatment ranged from 2.4 to 3.6 times higher for children in group care compared with children in home care.[191,192] A prospective, population-based survey of 818 families with one or more 18-month-old children from 2002 to 2003 in rural and central Sweden revealed that a high concern about infectious illness was associated with more frequent physician consultations and more prescriptions for antibiotics. Concern for infection was more common in children enrolled in group childcare than children not enrolled in group childcare. Concern about infectious illness was an important determining factor for physician consultation and antibiotic prescriptions. Directed consultations in which providers address parental concerns may result in less antibiotic prescribing with preserved parental satisfaction.[193]

Multiple studies have documented an association of childcare center attendance and colonization or infection due to resistant bacteria, including outbreaks of illness due to resistant *S. pneumoniae*[115,117,119–121,126,194,195] and *S. sonnei*,[22,39,40] as well as colonization due to resistant *H. influenzae*,[196] *E. coli*,[197,198] and MRSA.[137]

INFECTIOUS DISEASES IN ADULTS

Parents of children who attend a childcare facility and people who provide care to these children have increased risk of acquiring infections such as CMV,[143,144,146,147,199–201] parvovirus B19,[179,180] HAV,[202,203] and diarrhea.[44,50] Childcare providers have annual rates of CMV seroconversion ranging between 8% and 20%, compared with hospital employees whose seroconversion rate is about 2%.[143,144,147,201] During community outbreaks of erythema infectiosum, childcare providers were found to be among the most affected occupational groups, with seroconversion rates ranging from 9% to 31%.[179,180] In a prevalence study of HAV antibodies among childcare providers employed in 37 randomly selected childcare centers in Israel during 1997, 90% (402 of 446) of the childcare providers had HAV antibodies; the authors postulated a 2-fold increased risk of acquiring HAV among providers.[203] During outbreaks of diarrhea in childcare centers, 40% of care providers developed diarrhea.[50] During a multicommunity outbreak of shigellosis, the overall median attack rate among employed staff of childcare centers was 6%, with a range of 0% to 17%.[38] In outbreaks of GAS and echovirus 30 infection[139] in childcare centers, adult providers and parents were affected. Similar prevalence rates of pneumococcal colonization (5% among adult employees of childcare centers with child contact and 5% among nonclinical employees at a tertiary care center) were noted in a study performed in 2003 in Galveston, Texas; these data suggest that childcare providers are not at an increased risk for pneumococcal colonization in the universal pneumococcal conjugate vaccine era.[204] Compared with nonproviders childcare providers have a significantly higher annual risk of at least one infectious disease and loss of work days due to infectious diseases.[205] Childcare providers should receive all immunizations routinely recommended for adults, as shown on the adult immunization schedule (see Table 3-3) (www.cdc.gov/vaccines).

ECONOMIC IMPACT OF GROUP CHILDCARE ILLNESS

The economic burden of illness associated with group childcare was estimated at $1.5 billion annually adjusted to 2005 U.S. dollars.[206] Precise mechanisms for estimating illness burden and for evaluating effectiveness of infection control interventions are rare due to multiple challenges associated with performing such assessments.[207] Attributing an outbreak to group childcare is challenging, because although these settings may promote transmission of infection, childcare attendees and staff interact with household contacts external to the childcare arrangement, thus facilitating secondary spread. A prospective evaluation of 208 families with at least one childcare enrollee, conducted from November 2000 to May 2001 in the Boston area, documented 2072 viral illnesses over 105,352 person-days. Among the 834 subjects, 1683 URTIs and 389 gastrointestinal tract (GI) illnesses were reported during the study period, with a total mean cost of $49 per URTI and $56 per GI episode. Decreased parental productivity during missed days of work to care for a child who had to be withdrawn from childcare accounted for a significant proportion of the nonmedical cost.[206]

PREVENTION

Specific standards should be established for personal hygiene, especially hand hygiene, maintenance of current immunization records of children and providers, exclusion policies, targeting frequently contaminated areas for environmental cleaning, and appropriate handling of food and medication. In studies in which improved infection control measures were implemented and monitored, both upper respiratory tract illness and diarrhea were reduced in intervention centers.[97,208] In addition, in children at intervention centers, 24% children were given fewer antibiotic prescriptions and parents had fewer absences from work.[98]

Educational sessions on health topics by healthcare professionals were found to be the most efficacious means of promoting health education in simultaneous surveys of licensed childcare center directors, parents, and health providers in Boston.[209] A prospective observational study of a convenience sample of 134 childcare centers in Pennsylvania noted that sites that were located in suburban, non-profit, parent-funded centers had improved health and safety practices compared with sites that were located in urban areas, received their funding through state subsidies, or were designated as for profit.[210] However, the translation of knowledge into continued practice beyond the education and focus on the intervention remains a challenge. A cross-sectional survey conducted in 2000 childcare providers, parents, and pediatricians in Baltimore revealed deficits of knowledge among all groups. Compared with national guidelines on exclusion for 12 symptoms, childcare providers and parents were over exclusive and pediatricians were under exclusive. More childcare providers and parents than pediatricians felt that exclusion would reduce transmission of disease.[211]

As asymptomatic excretion and potential for transmission precede the onset of clinical symptoms in many childcare-associated infectious diseases, strategies that involve prevention would be most efficacious. In addition to traditional handwashing, the use of alcohol-based hand-sanitizing products in healthcare and other settings is an efficacious means of achieving hand hygiene.[212] Ethanol hand sanitizers are more effective than handwashing with soap and water in removing detectable rhinovirus from hands of adult volunteers. An additional evaluation of the effectiveness of adding organic acids to hand sanitizers was notable for residual rhinovirus virucidal activity of up to 4 hours.[213] In support of this preventive strategy, a cluster-randomized, controlled trial was conducted in the homes of 292 families with children who were enrolled in out-of-home childcare centers. A multifactorial intervention emphasizing alcohol-based hand sanitizer use in the home reduced transmission of GI illnesses within families. The effect on reduction of respiratory tract illness transmission in this evaluation was less pronounced and may relate to use of hand-sanitizing gel following toilet use but not following sneezing, coughing, or blowing/wiping of nasal secretions.[214] A follow-up study that added surface disinfection to a hand sanitizer intervention in a school-based cluster-randomized controlled trial demonstrated a greater decrease in adjusted absenteeism rates due to GI compared with respiratory tract illness. Norovirus was the only virus isolated more frequently from classroom surfaces in the control group.[215] A comparative evaluation of antibacterial liquid soap and alcohol-based hand sanitizer for inactivation of norovirus on human finger pads demonstrated a greater virucidal effectiveness with the antibacterial soap compared to the ethanol-based hand sanitizer. Despite utility of alcohol-based sanitizers for control of enteric and respiratory tract pathogen transmission, they may be relatively ineffective against norovirus.[216] Molecular techniques, including DNA probes, could be used as surrogate markers to study transmission of enteric pathogens in childcare centers and from centers to children's homes.[217] Further evaluations of molecular techniques during outbreak investigations, hand hygiene strategies, and educational interventions could assist with allocation of resources to the most effective prevention regimens.

Written policies should be available for the following areas: managing child and employee illness, including exclusion policies; maintaining health, including immunizations; diaper-changing procedures; hand hygiene; personal hygiene policies for staff and children; environmental sanitation policies and procedures; handling, serving, and preparation of food; dissemination of information about illness; and handling of animals. Local health authorities should be notified about cases of communicable diseases involving children or care providers in the childcare setting. The AAP and the American Public Health Association jointly published the National Health and Safety Performance Standards: Guidelines for Out-of-Home Childcare Programs, available at http://nrckids.org. This comprehensive manual provides guidelines regarding infectious diseases and other health-related matters pertinent to out-of-home childcare. Additional resources include information about group childcare infection rates[218] and guidance for preparation of childcare programs for pandemic response (http://www.aap.org/disasters/).

Future investigation of outbreaks of illness associated with group childcare will need to utilize newly developed computerized models and paradigms to assess the economic impact of outbreaks. In an era of limited funding, an understanding of expenses and allocation of resources will be important information to justify utility of interventions.

4 Infectious Diseases in Refugee and Internationally Adopted Children

Mary Allen Staat

Each year thousands of immigrant children come to the United States to begin a new life. In this chapter, the infectious disease issues of two groups of immigrants will be discussed: refugees and internationally adopted children. Refugees are noncitizen immigrants who are unable or unwilling to return to their country of origin because of persecution or a fear of persecution.[1] Internationally adopted children are immigrants who are classified as orphans; most are not truly orphaned, but have been abandoned by or separated from both parents.

In 2009, 74,602 refugees arrived in the U.S.[1] Of these, 34% were <18 years of age. Nearly 80% of refugees came from just five countries: Iraq (25%), Burma (24%), Bhutan (18%), Iran (7%), and Cuba (6%).[1]

Since 1999, more than 200,000 children have been internationally adopted in the U.S. with a peak in 2004 with 22,990 children adopted.[2] However, from 2004 to 2010 there was a decline in the number of children adopted to 11,059 with a shift in the source countries. In 2004, 83% of children came from five countries: China (31%), Russia (26%), Guatemala (14%), South Korea (8%), and Kazakhstan (4%), while in 2010, the same percentage came from eight countries: China (31%), Ethiopia (23%), Russia (10%), South Korea (8%), the Ukraine (4%), Taiwan (3%), India (2%), and Colombia (2%).[2]

Because refugees and internationally adopted children come from resource-poor countries, healthcare providers should be cognizant of the global prevalence of infectious diseases that are seen less commonly in native-born North Americans. Both groups are at increased risk for common infectious diseases such as tuberculosis, intestinal parasites, dermatologic infections, and infestations. In addition, infection due to hepatitis B virus (HBV), hepatitis C virus (HCV), human immunodeficiency virus (HIV), and *Treponema pallidum* (syphilis) are far more prevalent in the countries of immigrants where there are few resources for screening and prevention compared to the U.S.

Refugee children and internationally adopted children differ in terms of the general medical screening they receive before arrival in the U.S.[3-8] Most refugees are subjected to organized screening evaluations including a physical examination, before emigration visas are issued. For children >15 years of age, pre-departure screening includes serologic testing for HIV and syphilis and a chest radiograph to assess for evidence of tuberculosis. In contrast, only adoptees from certain countries with high rates of tuberculosis, such as China and Ethiopia, have been required to undergo this organized screening procedure for tuberculosis.[5,7] Second, because medical screening for refugees usually is sponsored by responsible medical organizations, results of such testing are typically accurate. In international adoptees, HIV, syphilis, and HBV serology typically are provided with the referral information; in recent years, testing generally has proven to be accurate when repeated in the U.S. Third, preventive measures such as immunizations, vitamin supplementation, and dental care are undertaken in most refugees; in adoptees, preventive care is inconsistent. Last, differences in the types of infectious diseases may also distinguish refugees from adopted children. Although both populations are susceptible to a variety of infectious agents, because the countries of origin and the living conditions differ, refugee children are more likely to have been exposed to infections such as typhoid fever, malaria, filariasis, flukes, or schistosomiasis, which occur less commonly in internationally adopted children from countries outside of Africa.

GUIDELINES FOR EVALUATION

Because of the predominance of infectious diseases in developing nations, recommendations for screening tests are weighted toward infectious disease processes, but aspects of general health, including vision, hearing, dental, and developmental examinations, also should be included.[3–8] Despite the healthy appearance of many immigrant children, children should be evaluated by a healthcare professional within 2 weeks after arrival to assure that they are screened properly and receive preventive healthcare services. Table 4-1 outlines the recommended infectious disease screening for refugees and internationally adopted children. The reader also is referred to pathogen-specific chapters.

Hepatitis A

Virtually all inhabitants of resource-poor countries have contracted hepatitis A virus (HAV) by early adulthood and will have HAV immunoglobulin (Ig) G antibodies. Now that HAV vaccine is recommended for all children ≥12 months of age,[9] IgG anti-HAV testing in children >1 year of age should be considered for all immigrants to determine which children should be immunized.[10] Screening for IgM anti-HAV can be useful for determining whether the child has acute HAV infection so that secondary prevention through HAV vaccine can be provided to unvaccinated family members and close contacts. Since HAV infection is anicteric in young children[9] and most young children are asymptomatic, the only way to identify children who may shed HAV for months is by screening with an IgM anti-HAV test. Symptoms of HAV infection should prompt evaluation for viral hepatitis in recently arrived immigrants or adoptees, even in the absence of jaundice.[9]

Hepatitis B

Routine screening for HBV infection is recommended for all refugees and internationally adopted children.[4–8] Early identification of HBV infection is important so that appropriate management can be initiated and household contacts and caregivers can be vaccinated. The prevalence of chronic HBV infection varies by region and the rates in refugee and internationally adopted children mirror the rates of infection in their country. Children typically acquire HBV by vertical transmission, although blood-borne infection and horizontal transmission also have been implicated.[11–28] In international adoptees, the prevalence of chronic HBV infection was 20% in Romanian adoptees from the early 1990s;[14–16] however, more recent studies have consistently shown a prevalence of 1% to 5%.[17–25]

HBV screening tests, including the HBV surface antigen (HBsAg) and antibodies to surface (anti-HBs) and core (anti-HBc) antigens, are recommended in the medical evaluation of internationally

TABLE 4-1. Recommended Tests for Refugee and Internationally Adopted Children

Test	Refugee Children	Internationally Adopted Children
Tuberculin skin test (TST)	All	All[a]
HEPATITIS B VIRUS SEROLOGIC TESTING	All	All[a]
Hepatitis B surface antigen (HBsAg)		
Hepatitis B surface antibody (anti-HBs)		
Hepatitis B core antibody (anti-HBc)		
Hepatitis C virus serologic testing	Some	Some[a]
Human immunodeficiency virus 1 and 2 serologic testing	≥15 years of age	All[a]
SYPHILIS SEROLOGIC TESTING		
Nontreponemal test (RPR, VDRL, or ART)	≥15 years of age	All
Treponemal test (TPPA, MHA-TP, or FTA-ABS)	Not recommended	All
STOOL EXAMINATION		
Microscopic evaluation for ova and parasites (3 specimens)	All[b]	All
Giardia intestinalis and *Cryptosporidium* antigen (1 specimen)	All[b]	All
Complete blood count	All	All
Urinalysis	All	Not recommended

*ART, automated reagin test; FTA-ABS, fluorescent treponemal antibody absorption; MHA-TP, microhemagglutination-*Treponema pallidum*; RPR, rapid plasma reagin; TPPA, *Treponema pallidum *particle agglutination; VDRL, Venereal Disease Research Laboratory.*

[a]*Consider reassessing 6 months after arrival.*

[b]*All should be screened if there was no presumptive treatment prior to arrival to the U.S. See text for CDC website.*

adopted children and refugees.[4–8] All three tests should be performed to determine whether the child is immune due to immunization, recovered from infection, or has acute or chronic hepatitis B. Common patterns of hepatitis B serology profile are shown in Chapter 213, Hepatitis B and Hepatitis D Viruses. In a child who is found to be HBsAg-positive, repeat testing should be done 6 months later; if HBsAg persists for ≥6 months, the child has chronic hepatitis B infection. If the child no longer has HBsAg and has developed anti-HBs, the child had acute infection and has recovered and is no longer able to transmit the virus to others. Children with acute or chronic HBV (positive HBsAg) can transmit HBV to others and should have additional testing done, including testing for HBeAg, HBeAb, and serum hepatic enzyme levels. HBsAg-positive children should be followed by a hepatologist for management. For children with negative tests initially, some experts recommend repeat testing for HBV approximately 6 months after arrival to insure that the child was not infected just prior to arrival to the U.S.[8,25] In addition, children with acute or chronic HBV also should have serologic testing for HAV to determine the need for HAV vaccination, and HCV for overall management and treatment considerations.

Vaccination of household contacts of children with acute or chronic HBV (HBsAg-positive) must occur promptly. Epidemiologic studies have demonstrated that up to 20% of unvaccinated household contacts of HBV cases become HBsAg-positive within ≥5 years of exposure within the home[26,27] and transmission of

HBV from newly adopted children to their parents has been documented.[26–28]

Hepatitis C

Until more is known regarding the incidence and prevalence of HCV in refugee and internationally adopted children, screening for this virus is not recommended routinely.[4–8] However, if there is a history of specific risk factors such as current or former injection drug use, receipt of blood products, or residence in settings with a documented high prevalence of HCV, testing should be performed.[29] These risk factors often are difficult to ascertain in either group of children. In one study, the prevalence of HCV antibody in internationally adopted children was <1%.[21] Antibody testing is performed initially and if the antibody is positive, polymerase chain reaction (PCR) is performed to confirm infection. Children found to have HCV infection should be immunized for HAV and HBV and should be referred to a hepatologist for further management.

Human Immunodeficiency Virus-1 and Human Immunodeficiency Virus-2 Infection

Refugees ≥15 years of age are tested routinely for HIV prior to coming to the U.S.[5] Children <15 years of age are not tested unless they are in a high-risk situation. Otherwise, for children not tested abroad, routine testing is not recommended for refugees unless indicated clinically. In contrast, most internationally adopted children have been tested for antibodies to HIV-1 by enzyme immunoassay (EIA) in their birth country. While reports of HIV infection in internationally adopted children are rare,[16,21] routine screening by EIA is recommended for all internationally adopted children upon arrival to the U.S.[7,8] Positive or indeterminate results should be resolved with use of HIV DNA PCR. If there is a clinical suspicion of HIV infection, HIV DNA PCR testing should be considered if the antibody testing by EIA is negative. Retesting ≥6 months after arrival to the U.S. should be considered.[8] Families are now permitted to adopt children with HIV infection. Thus, clinicians should be prepared to provide care and resources for children arriving to the U.S. with HIV infection.

Preadoptive testing for HIV-2 infection is not performed routinely. HIV-2 infection is prevalent in some African nations and is now recognized on several other continents; perinatal transmission appears to be limited. Symptoms suggestive of HIV infection with negative EIA results for HIV-1 should prompt testing for HIV-2.

Tuberculosis

Tuberculosis is highly prevalent in the countries of origin for both refugees and internationally adopted children; therefore, screening upon arrival to the U.S. is recommended for both groups.[4–8] In 2010, 60% of all tuberculosis cases in the U.S. were among foreign-born people, with significantly higher rates in foreign-born (18.1/100,000) compared to U.S.-born persons (1.6/100,000).[30] In addition, 89% of multidrug-resistant tuberculosis cases in the U.S. were in foreign-born persons.[30] In children, 22% of all tuberculosis cases were foreign-born, with tuberculosis rates in foreign-born 12-fold higher than in U.S.-born children.[31] Both refugees and internationally adopted children are at increased risk for *Mycobacterium tuberculosis* infection. A high proportion of immigrants and refugees are found to have latent tuberculosis infection (LTBI) ranging from 20% to 76%.[32–36] One study found that 7% of immigrants had active pulmonary tuberculosis.[36] LTBI is lower in internationally adopted children compared with refugees, ranging from 14% to 21%,[37–39] and tuberculosis disease rarely has been reported.[40,41] With the increased numbers of children coming from Ethiopia, a country with high rates of tuberculosis, the rates of LTBI and tuberculosis in internationally adopted children is likely to increase. Retesting children at least 3 months after arrival to the U.S. has been supported by

data from two studies, in which children with initially negative tuberculin skin test (TST) had repeat TST >3 months later with 13% to 20% of the TSTs positive.[38,39]

In the past, refugees ≥15 years of age and children <15 years of age with concern about tuberculosis exposure or disease were screened with a chest radiograph prior to arriving in the U.S. If the chest radiograph was abnormal, microscopic evaluation of sputum or gastric aspirate for acid-fast bacilli was performed. Sputum-positive people are banned from entry until sputum smears are negative. The overseas screening requirements for tuberculosis for immigrants and refugees bound for the U.S. underwent a major revision in 2007, including tuberculosis screening for all people.[42] These requirements are still in the process of being implemented. International adoptees from certain countries with high rates of tuberculosis (China and Ethiopia) now fall under the same requirements as other immigrants and refugees.[42] For other adoptees, screening in the country of origin is inconsistently done and generally is documented only in older children.

For both refugees and internationally adopted children, screening for tuberculosis should be performed at the initial assessment by placement of a TST (5 TU purified protein derivative).[5–8,43] The test should be read 48 to 72 hours later by a healthcare professional. A reading of ≥10 mm of induration is considered positive for both refugees and internationally adopted children. A reading of ≥5 mm is considered positive if there is a known contact with a person with active tuberculosis, an abnormal chest radiograph, signs or symptoms suggestive of tuberculosis, or evidence of immunosuppression. Children with a positive TST should have a thorough physical examination and chest radiograph performed to assess for *M. tuberculosis* disease. If the chest radiograph and physical examination are normal and the skin test is ≥10 mm, the diagnosis of LTBI is made and treatment with a 9-month course of isoniazid is begun. Similarly, a child with TST induration of 5 mm to 9 mm who has known exposure to someone with active tuberculosis or who is receiving immunosuppressive therapy or has an immunosuppressive condition, including HIV, with no evidence of disease, should receive isoniazid therapy. Retesting of skin test-negative children ≥6 months after arrival should be considered for all children given the high rate of false-negative TSTs shortly after arrival to the U.S.[38,39]

Interferon-gamma release assays (IGRAs), such as QuantiFERON Gold and T-SPOT.TB are available, but are not currently recommended for use in children <5 years of age.[43] For tuberculosis disease, their sensitivity is comparable with the TST. For tuberculosis infection, their specificity is higher compared with TST but the sensitivity is not known. Samples must be tested within 8 to 12 hours of being drawn to ensure viability of cells. For immune-competent children ≥5 years of age, IGRAs can be used in place of a TST to confirm cases of active or latent tuberculosis. Similar to children with a positive TST result, a child with a positive result from an IGRA should be considered infected with *M. tuberculosis* complex; however, a negative result from an IGRA cannot definitively rule out tuberculosis infection.

While most refugees and internationally adopted children with *M. tuberculosis* infection have LTBI, disease should be considered in children with pneumonia or nonspecific symptoms such as fever, malaise, growth delay, weight loss, cough, night sweats, and chills. Pulmonary tuberculosis is the most common site of infection in children, accounting for 77% of cases, followed by lymphatic tuberculosis in 16% of children.[31] Chest radiographs can reveal hilar or mediastinal lymphadenopathy, segmental or lobar infiltrates, or pleural effusion. Cavitary lesions and miliary disease are less common. Extrapulmonary manifestations in the central nervous system, middle ear and mastoids, lymph nodes, bone, joints, and skin can be seen. Recovery of the responsible organism is paramount, because many children arrive from countries in which drug-resistant *M. tuberculosis* is common. Gastric aspirates or bronchoscopy, or both, can be useful adjuncts in a child too young or too ill to expectorate sputum.[43]

Vaccination with BCG is common in most resource-poor countries, but is not a contraindication to the placement of a TST.[8,43]

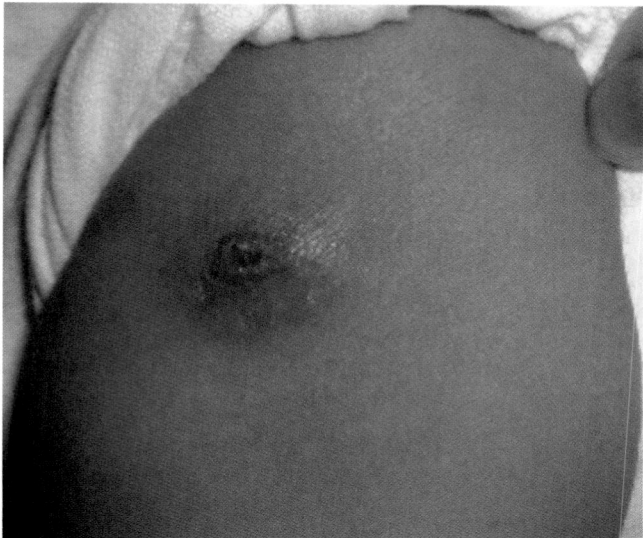

Figure 4-1. Child with granuloma due to *Mycobacterium bovis* at site of BCG vaccination.

Previous studies have demonstrated that TST after BCG vaccination does not elicit induration of ≥10 mm, and thus a history of BCG does not affect the interpretation of the TST.[44,45]

BCG vaccination can be recognized by a 2- to 4-mm scarification, typically on the left deltoid. Occasional complications include enlargement of the regional lymph nodes or nodularity or ulceration at the vaccination site. The granuloma typically is located in the deltoid region and may or may not be draining and can be associated with regional or distant sites of infection (Figure 4-1). Culture of the drainage yields *Mycobacterium bovis*. There is no consensus regarding the management of this condition. Some lesions resolve without treatment, whereas other lesions require excision or treatment with isoniazid, erythromycin, or clarithromycin.[43,46,47]

Enteric Infections

Intestinal parasites are common in both refugee and internationally adopted children; infection rates vary by age and country of origin.[12-14,17-24,48-52] While most children will not have had testing prior to coming to the U.S., presumptive treatment of refugees from certain regions of the world is recommended prior to departure to the U.S.[53] All refugees from the Middle East, South and Southeast Asia are recommended to receive albendazole for round worm infestation and ivermectin for *Strongyloides stercoralis*. African refugees also should receive presumptive treatment for *Strongyloides* and for those originating from areas endemic for schistosomiasis, treatment with praziquantel should be given. In African countries where microfilarial *Loa loa* infection is endemic, ivermectin should not be given for *Strongyloides* since treatment with ivermectin in the presence of *Loa loa* has been associated with encephalopathy; instead, a 7-day course of albendazole is given. Additional details of country-specific recommendations, timing, dosing and duration of treatment can be found in Centers for Disease Control and Prevention (CDC) guidelines for refugee and immigrant care and are available on the CDC website (http://www.cdc.gov/immigrantrefugeehealth/guidelines/domestic/intestinal-parasites-domestic.html).[53]

A wide variety of parasites, both pathogenic and nonpathogenic (Table 4-2), can be seen in both groups of immigrants. Refugees are more likely to have nematodes and trematodes compared with internationally adopted children. In adoptees, the prevalence of intestinal parasites varies from 9% to 51%, depending on the child's age and country of origin; older children and children originating from countries other than Korea have higher rates.[17-24,52] In one study in internationally adopted children, the

TABLE 4-2. Pathogenic and Nonpathogenic Intestinal Parasites

Parasite Type	Pathogens	Nonpathogens
Protozoa	Giardia intestinalis	Endolimax nana
	Entamoeba histolytica	Entamoeba coli
	Dientamoeba fragilis[a]	Entamoeba gingivalis
	Balantidium coli	Entamoeba hartmanni
	Blastocystis hominis[a]	Entamoeba polecki
	Cystoisopora belli	Iodamoeba butschlii
	Cryptosporidium parvum	Chilomastix mesnili
	Cyclospora cayentensis	Enteromonas hominis
	Microsporidium species	Retortamonas intestinalis
		Trichomonas hominis
		Trichomonas tenax
HELMINTHS		
Nematodes (roundworms)	Ascaris lumbricoides (roundworm)	
	Trichuris trichiura (whipworm)	
	Strongyloides stercoralis (threadworm)	
	Enterobius vermicularis (pinworm)	
	Necator americanus (hookworm)	
	Ancyclostoma duodenale (hookworm)	
Cestodes (tapeworms)	Hymenolepis species	
	Taenia saginata (beef tapeworm)	
	Taenia solium (pork tapeworm)	
	Schistosoma species	

[a]Controversy exists regarding the pathogenicity of this organism.

overall prevalence of intestinal parasites was 29%; 19% had *Giardia intestinalis* and <1% had helminths.[52] A higher prevalence was found in older children but there was no increased risk with the presence of malnutrition or gastrointestinal symptoms.[52,53] In contrast, in refugees, 17% of children had *Giardia*, while 19% had helminths.[51]

Both refugees (who cannot be presumed to have been treated) and adoptees should be screened for intestinal parasites upon arrival to the U.S.[5-8] The diagnosis is made by examination of preserved stool for ova and parasite testing; testing multiple specimens increases the sensitivity,[52,54,55] with a yield of 79% for 1 specimen, 92% for 2 specimens, and an additional 8% for a 3rd specimen.[52] One stool specimen should also be evaluated for *G. intestinalis* and *Cryptosporidium parvum* using antigen testing.[8] Repeat stool samples are essential to assess the effectiveness of treatment for the identified parasite and to determine the presence of new (or newly found) pathogens. If the child remains persistently symptomatic, additional stool examinations are warranted and testing for other parasites such as *Cyclospora* and *S. stercoralis* should be considered. In adoptees, screening for parasitosis with eosinophil counts is not indicated because most infections are due to protozoa *(G. intestinalis)* and nonmigrating nematodes (pinworms) which do not elicit peripheral blood eosinophilia.[8] However, for either group, for children with negative stool ova and parasite examinations and eosinophilia (absolute eosinophil count exceeding 450 cells/mm³), additional serologic testing should be done.[4,5,8] In this case, serologic testing for *S. stercoralis* should be performed, regardless of country of origin. Also, for children with eosinophilia who are from sub-Saharan Africa, Southeast Asia, or areas of Latin America where schistosomiasis is endemic should have serologic testing for *Schistosoma* species. Similarly, testing for filariasis should be performed in children with eosinophilia who come from areas where filariasis is endemic. Since a variety of parasites can cause filariasis (see Chapter 278, Blood and Tissue Nematodes (Filiarial Worms)), if testing is positive, consultation with an infectious disease specialist with expertise in this disease is recommended to ensure that correct treatment is given.

Bacterial enteric pathogens appear to be less common than intestinal parasites in immigrants and adoptees; however, most studies have not assessed systematically for bacterial causes. Children with bloody diarrhea or diarrhea associated with high fever should have stool examined for bacterial enteropathogens (e.g., *Salmonella, Shigella, Yersinia, Campylobacter*) as part of the initial evaluation.[8]

Chagas Disease (American Trypanosomiasis)

Chagas disease, caused by *Trypanosoma cruzi*, is endemic throughout much of Mexico, Central and South America. The risk of Chagas disease varies by region within endemic countries. While the prevalence of Chagas disease in refugees or internationally adopted children is unknown, screening is warranted since treatment of infected children is highly effective compared with treatment in adults.[8] Serologic testing should only be performed in children ≥12 months of age because of the potential presence of maternal antibody.

Syphilis

Refugees ≥15 years of age routinely are screened for syphilis before resettlement.[5] Although refugees are not screened routinely upon arrival in the U.S., refugees of any age should be tested if there is clinical suspicion for syphilis or there is evidence or concern for sexual exposure.

Most internationally adopted children have documentation of syphilis screening in their birth country; syphilis rarely has been reported after arrival in the U.S.[17-24] In children with a history of syphilis, it is often difficult to obtain the details of the birth mother's history, treatment, and management. In addition, in children with suspected *T. pallidum* exposure, details of the evaluation and prescribed treatment regimens often are incomplete or uninterpretable. For internationally adopted children, screening with both a nontreponemal and treponemal test is recommended.[8] A positive treponemal test result warrants a complete and thorough evaluation to document the extent of the disease and to provide optimal treatment.

Other Testing

A complete blood count is recommended for refugees and internationally adopted children.[5-8] The hemoglobin and red blood cell indices can identify children with anemia, iron deficiency, hemoglobinopathies, or malaria. Low white blood cell count and lymphopenia can indicate HIV infection or malnutrition. Eosinophilia is common among refugees and suggests parasitic infection.[4-8,53] For refugees, a urinalysis is recommended to assess for hematuria and pyuria.[4,53] Hematuria may indicate schistosomiasis and pyuria may reflect a urinary tract infection or renal tuberculosis. Routine screening for malaria is not recommended, but malaria should always be considered in children with fever who come from endemic areas.[5]

Elevated blood lead levels have been reported in internationally adopted children and lead testing is recommended for all international adoptees.[56] There is no formal recommendation for refugees; however, it is likely that they could benefit from this screening as well.

Other Infections

Dermatologic Infections

Lice, scabies, tinea, and molluscum contagiosum are common in both refugees and internationally adopted children. The incidence of these conditions has not been well documented. The physical examination should include careful evaluation for these entities so that appropriate treatment is given.

Upper Respiratory Tract Infections

Upper respiratory tract infections, occur in a large percentage of adopted children within the first month of arrival.[57] Since the past history of otitis media often is unknown and since many children have language delays, referral to an otolaryngologist for hearing test evaluation should be considered for children with otitis media and language delays.

Other Less Common Infections

Clinicians should be aware of other potential diseases and clinical manifestations that can be seen in refugees and internationally adopted children. These diseases are less prevalent than those discussed and do not have readily available screening tests. In addition, some diseases may have long incubation periods, as long as several years, such as neurocysticercosis. In most cases, however, the longer the interval from arrival to the U.S. and development of a clinical syndrome, the less likely the syndrome will be attributed to a pathogen acquired in the country of origin.

PREVENTIVE MEASURES

Immunizations

Most refugees arrive in the U.S. without immunization records, while most adoptees have some documentation of receipt of immunizations. The recommended approach to optimize immunization for these two groups of immigrants differs.

The Immigration and Nationality Act (INA) of 1996 requires immigrant visa applicants to provide proof of vaccination with receipt of at least the first dose of the ACIP-recommended vaccines before entry into the U.S.[5,6] These regulations apply to most immigrant children entering the U.S.; however, internationally adopted children who are ≤10 years of age can obtain an exemption from these requirements; adoptive parents are required to sign a waiver indicating their intention to comply with the ACIP immunization requirements within 30 days after the child's arrival in the U.S. Refugees are not required to meet immunization requirements of the INA at the time of entry into the U.S. but must show proof of immunization when they apply for permanent residency, typically 1 year after arrival.

Refugee children. For refugees, if immunization documents exist, they should be reviewed and may be accepted as valid if the immunizations were provided at ages and intervals acceptable to U.S. standards.[5-8,58,59] The clinical diagnosis of vaccine-preventable diseases may not be reliable, especially for rubella and mumps; vaccine should be given. In addition, a history of varicella infection may be unavailable or unreliable in these populations; therefore, children should be immunized for varicella or have antibody testing performed.

Refugees who have no records or have incomplete immunizations should receive vaccines at their first visit. Guidelines for routine and catch-up immunizations should be followed.[6,58,59] There are few data on verifying immunization status by antibody testing in refugees; however, one study found screening for varicella was more cost-effective than providing immediate vaccine for people >5 years of age.[60]

International adoptees. Several studies have used antibody testing to verify the immunization status of internationally adopted children.[20-24,61-69] Results differ, with some studies showing inadequate protection while others found good protection. Differences in study design, laboratory methods, and definitions of protection likely account for the differences. With a lack of consensus, currently there are two acceptable approaches recommended to insure that internationally adopted children are protected against vaccine-preventable diseases.[8,58,59] The

TABLE 4-3. Serologic Testing Available for Verifying Immunization Status

Children ≥5 Months of Age	Children ≥12 Months of Age
Diphtheria IgG EIA	Diphtheria IgG EIA
Tetanus IgG EIA	Tetanus IgG EIA
Poliovirus serotypes 1–3 neutralizing antibody	Poliovirus serotypes 1–3 neutralizing antibody
Hepatitis B surface antibody	Hepatitis B surface antibody
	Rubeola (measles) antibody
	Mumps antibody
	Rubella antibody
	Varicella antibody
	Hepatitis A antibody

EIA, enzyme immunoassay; IgG, immunoglobulin G.

first approach is to reinitiate immunizations regardless of documentation; the second approach is to use serologic testing to determine which immunizations are needed. Because antibody testing for one vaccine-preventable disease may not be predictive for others, a combination of reimmunization and antibody testing could be utilized. Serologic testing is available for most vaccine antigens (Table 4-3). For children ≥5 months of age, testing for diphtheria, tetanus, polio, and hepatitis B can be performed. Testing for measles, mumps, rubella, varicella, and HAV antibodies could be considered only in children ≥12 months of age because of the possible presence of maternal antibody. For varicella, testing is performed to verify whether the child had previous infection since varicella immunization is not available in most countries from which children are adopted.

Providing care for new immigrants can be rewarding. Application of directed screening tests upon arrival yields incalculable dividends for prevention and for the welfare of adoptees, refugees, and their families.

SECTION B: Prevention of Infectious Diseases

5 Passive Immunization

H. Cody Meissner

Passive immunization provides individuals with preformed antibodies that can prevent or treat infectious diseases. Over a century ago, hyperimmune animal sera were produced to treat specific infections. After human plasma fractionation was developed (during World War II), immune globulin (human) (IG) became available for passive immunization. Although this was an enormous breakthrough, intravenous (IV) infusion of the product was found to evoke a variety of severe adverse reactions. Therefore, the IV route of administration was precluded, and IG largely was limited to intramuscular (IM) injection. For some indications, this was not a disadvantage. However, for treatment of primary immunodeficiency, it became clear that the volume (and hence the amount of immunoglobulin G (IgG)) that could be administered by the intramuscular route was suboptimal. In 1981, the first United States-licensed (human) IGIV was approved by the Food and Drug Administration (FDA). This changed immunoglobulin therapy dramatically. IGIV enabled clinicians to administer large doses of IgG with minimal discomfort and to produce an immediate rise in both total plasma IgG and titers of specific antibodies.

The products available for passive immunization can be grouped as follows: (1) standard immune globulin (IG) for intramuscular administration (hepatitis A, measles, rubella); (2) hyperimmune globulins that can be administered intramuscularly (hepatitis B immune globulin, rabies immune globulin, tetanus immune globulin, varicella immune globulin) or intravenously (cytomegalovirus, vaccinia, botulism immune globulins); (3) IGIV; and (4) monoclonal antibodies (Table 5-1). In addition, two antitoxins of animal origin still are available for limited distribution.

Passive immunization can be used for a variety of clinical indications, including: (1) treatment of primary and, in certain cases, secondary immunodeficiency or its sequelae; and (2) prophylaxis against infections due to specific organisms. In general, treatment of established infections has been less successful, even when the specific organism or toxin can be identified. However, the use of IGIV for the treatment of various conditions that involve immune dysregulation, such as immune thrombocytopenic purpura (ITP) and Kawasaki disease, has become routine and has stimulated much investigation of immunomodulation.

In the following sections, the various products and their uses are discussed. Pathogen- and disease-specific chapters also should be consulted. An effort has been made to use nonproprietary product names as they appear in the labeling, but for brevity, there is liberal use of abbreviations. Emphasis is placed on FDA approved indications (i.e., those that appear in the product package inserts). In the case of IGIV, not all products have been approved or studied for all indications (Table 5-2). Moreover, in contrast to IGs for IM administration, IGIV products undergo a variety of manufacturing processes, utilize a number of different stabilizers and excipients, are formulated in various concentrations or physical states, and can differ in subtle ways (e.g., IgA content). Furthermore, licensed manufacturers constantly are studying processes to improve products, and additional manufacturers have products undergoing clinical trials in the hope of bringing them to market. The clinician

TABLE 5-1. Immune Globulins Prepared from Human Plasma

Nonproprietary Name	Abbreviation
FOR INTRAMUSCULAR ADMINISTRATION	
Standard immune globulin (human)	IG
Hepatitis B immune globulin (human)	HBIG
Rabies immune globulin (human)[a]	RIG
Tetanus immune globulin (human)	TIG
Varicella-zoster immune globulin (human)[b]	VariZIG
FOR INTRAVENOUS ADMINISTRATION	
Immune globulin intravenous (human)	IGIV
Cytomegalovirus immune globulin intravenous (human)	CMV-IGIV
Botulism immune globulin intravenous (human)	BIG-IGIV
Vaccinia immune globulin intravenous (human)	VIG-IGIV

[a]*As much of the dose as possible should be instilled around the wound.*
[b]*See text.*

TABLE 5-2. Available Immune Globulin Intravenous Products in the United States

Product Registered Name	Manufacturer	FDA-Approved Indication
Carimune NF	ZLB Behring	ITP, PID
Vivaglobulin	ZLB Behring (subcutaneous)	PID
Privigen	CSL Behring	PID, chronic ITP
Gammar-P IV	ZLB Behring	PID
Venoglobulin S	Griflos U.S.A	PID, ITP, KS
Flebogamma S	Griflos U.S.A	PID
Gammagard Liquid	Baxter	PID
Gammagard S/D	Baxter	CLL, ITP, KD, PID
Polygam	Baxter	PID, ITP
Iveegam EN	Baxter	KD, PID
Gamimune N	Talecris Biotherapeutics	PID, ITP, HIV, bone marrow transplantation
Gamunex	Talecris Biotherapeutics	ITP, PID
Octagam	Octapharma U.S.A	PID
WinRho SDF	Baxter	Chronic or acute ITP and HIV-immune related conditions

CLL, chronic lymphocytic leukemia; FDA, Food and Drug Administration; HIV, human immunodeficiency virus; ITP, immune thrombocytopenia purpura; KD, Kawasaki disease; PID, primary immunodeficiency.

should consult the current package insert for the specific IGIV product being used.

IMMUNE GLOBULIN (HUMAN)

IG is prepared by cold alcohol fractionation of pooled human plasma. It is formulated as a 16.5% protein solution. At least 96% of the total protein is IgG; small quantities of IgM and IgA are present. Each lot of product must represent the pooled plasma of at least 1000 donors so as to provide a wide diversity of antibodies. In practice, however, each lot represents many more donors (up to 60,000). Individual donations of the plasma, like those used as the source for all human plasma derivatives, are screened for markers of a variety of viruses (hepatitis B, hepatitis C, human immunodeficiency) to minimize the potential for transmission of infections. Other steps taken to minimize such transmission are noted at the end of this chapter.

Hepatitis A

A major use of standard IG is for postexposure prophylaxis of hepatitis A virus (HAV) in susceptible persons.[1] When injected deep into a large muscle mass within 14 days of exposure, IG is 80% to 90% effective in preventing clinical hepatitis. IG is most effective when administered early in the incubation period. When administered later in the incubation period, IG may only attenuate the severity of HAV disease expression. The usual dose is 0.02 mL/kg, given as soon as possible after exposure. For persons 12 months through 40 years of age, HAV vaccine is preferred over IG for postexposure prophylaxis. IG is preferred for people >40 years of age, for children <12 months of age, for immunocompromised people and for people with chronic liver disease.[2]

IG also is effective for pre-exposure prophylaxis of hepatitis A in travelers to areas where hepatitis A is prevalent. However, for travelers who are at least 1 year old and whose departure is not imminent, hepatitis A vaccine largely has replaced IG. If IG is to

be used, the dose depends on the circumstances. For a child younger than 1 year, the dose is 0.02 mL/kg if the anticipated stay is 3 months or less and 0.06 mL/kg if it is longer. In older persons whose departure is imminent, the dose of IG is 0.02 mL/kg, concomitant with the vaccine, for a stay of up to 5 months; and 0.06 mL/kg, concomitant with vaccine, for a longer stay.

For people ≥12 months of age for whom IG is given for pre-exposure or postexposure prophylaxis, hepatitis A vaccine is given simultaneously, at a separate site and using a separate syringe.[3]

Measles

Vaccination is, by far, the major strategy for achieving protection against measles. More than 99% of persons who receive 2 doses of measles vaccine (with the first dose administered no earlier than first birthday) develop serologic evidence of immunity.[4] Nonetheless, prophylaxis for measles remains an important indication for IG in children <12 months of age, in older children who have not been vaccinated, and in immunocompromised children who are not receiving routine immunoglobulin replacement therapy. Prophylaxis is indicated for susceptible household or hospital contacts of a case. A single dose of 0.25 mL/kg administered within 6 days of exposure may prevent or modify disease and provide temporary protection. Immunocompromised children should receive 0.50 mL/kg. (In either case, no more than 15 mL should be injected, and small children should be given no more than 3 mL at any single site.) A child who is receiving routine IgG replacement therapy is already protected, and no further dosage is indicated. If the child is ≥12 months of age, live measles vaccine should be administered about 5 months later if there is no underlying disease contraindicating use. For children 6 through 11 months of age traveling to areas where measles is endemic, MMR vaccine (rather than IG) should be given; this dose is not counted in the required two-dose series at ≥12 months of age.

Rubella

IG can be considered for prophylaxis of rubella-susceptible women exposed to rubella early in pregnancy. As many as 85% of infants infected in the first trimester of pregnancy will have signs of congenital rubella syndrome. This option is only recommended for women if termination of pregnancy is declined. Limited data indicate that intramuscular IG in a dose of 0.55 mL/kg may decrease clinically apparent infection, viral shedding and rates of viremia in infected susceptible people. Theoretically, the reduction in viral replication may decrease the likelihood of fetal infection. The absence of clinical signs in a woman who has received IG does not guarantee that fetal infection has been prevented. Infants with congenital rubella have been born to mothers who were given IG shortly after exposure.

SPECIFIC IMMUNE GLOBULINS FOR INTRAMUSCULAR ADMINISTRATION

Specific IGs for IM use are IgG preparations produced from plasma that is selected by screening donations or collected from donors who have been deliberately immunized or given immune booster therapy. Either approach can ensure the presence of high levels of antibody directed against one or more specific antigens. The manufacturing process is essentially the same as that used to prepare IG. The protein concentration differs for individual products; this can be found in the "Description" section of the package insert. Specific products available for IM administration are listed in Table 5-1. They are used to prevent hepatitis B, rabies, tetanus, and varicella-zoster virus (VZV).

Hepatitis B Immune Globulin (HBIG)

All pregnant women should be tested for circulating hepatitis B surface antigen (HBsAg). Infants born to women who are HBsAg-positive (either acutely or chronically infected with HBV) are at high risk of acute and chronic HBV infection. HBV vaccination and one dose of HBIG administered within 24 hours of birth are 85% to 95% effective in preventing both acute HBV infection and chronic infection. HBIG (0.5 mL) should be administered IM, preferably within 12 hours of birth. The first of 3 doses of HBV vaccine should be given at the same time as HBIG but at a different site.

In general, HBIG is not recommended if the mother's HBsAg status is not known, but HBV vaccination series should begin at once. Ideally, in such a case, the mother should be tested for HBsAg as soon as possible after delivery. If the test result is positive, the infant should receive 0.5 mL of HBIG as soon as possible and within 7 days of birth, and the vaccination series should be completed according to schedule. Preterm infants (<2 kg) constitute a special class. If the mother's HBsAg status is unknown and cannot be determined rapidly, the child should be given 0.5 mL of HBIG as well as vaccine, because the premature infant may respond suboptimally to HBV vaccine.

After a percutaneous (needlestick, laceration or bite) or mucosal exposure that contains or might contain HBV, blood should be obtained from the person who was the source of the exposure (if possible) to deteremine their HBsAg status. Management of the exposed person depends on the HBsAg status of the source and the vaccination and anti-HBs response status of the exposed person. Recommended postexposure prophylaxis for different scenarios is described.[5]

Human Rabies Immune Globulin (HRIG)

Rabies IG (human) (RIG) is always used in association with rabies vaccine.[6] HRIG is administered to previously unvaccinated persons to provide rabies virus neutralizing antibody until the patient responds to vaccination by actively producing virus-neutralizing antibodies. HRIG is administered once at the same time postexposure prophylaxis is initiated with the human rabies vaccine.[7,8]

The dose of HRIG is 20 IU/kg. If anatomically feasible, the full dose should be infiltrated around the wound and any remaining dose should be administered intramuscularly at an anatomic site distant from the vaccine administration. HRIG is supplied in 2 mL (300 IU) and 10 mL (1500 IU) vials with an average potency of 150 IU/mL. Thus, the contents of a 2 mL vial can be used to treat a child of up to 15 kg; for larger children, additional vials are required. A 10 mL vial is sufficient to treat a 75 kg adult, making it less suitable for pediatric use. However, if the smaller vials are not available, an appropriate portion can be withdrawn to treat a child. The product contains no preservative; once a vial has been entered, the contents should be administered promptly, and the remainder discarded.

Tetanus Immune Globulin (TIG)

TIG is the oldest of the specific IGs. TIG still is recommended for the treatment of tetanus and for prophylaxis in certain circumstances. Tetanus is so rare in persons whose immunization history includes at least 3 doses of tetanus toxoid that TIG is not recommended for such individuals. The need for active immunization with or without passive immunization depends on the condition of the wound and the patient's immunization history. Specific guidance is provided.[9] Persons with wounds that are neither clean nor minor and who have had 0–2 prior doses of tetanus toxoid or have an uncertain history of prior doses should receive TIG as well as DT, Td, DTaP or Tdap (depending on age and other needed vaccines). TIG can only remove unbound tetanus toxin. It cannot affect toxin bound to nerve endings. A single IM dose of 3000 to 5000 units TIG is generally recommended for children and adults, with part of the dose infiltrated around the wound. IGIV contains tetanus antitoxin and can be used if TIG is not available.

Varicella-Zoster Immune Globulin (VariZIG)

Postexposure prophylaxis should be targeted toward patients without evidence of immunity to varicella who are at high risk for severe disease and complications and who have been exposed to varicella. Such individuals include: (1) immunocompromised people; (2) nonimmune pregnant women; (3) neonates whose mothers have signs and symptoms of varicella within 5 days before delivery to 48 hours after delivery; (4) premature infants born at 28 weeks of gestation or later who are exposed in the neonatal period and whose mothers do not have evidence of immunity; (5) premature infants born before 28 weeks of gestation or who weigh <1000 g at birth and are exposed during the neonatal period regardless of maternal history of varicella disease or vaccination (because transfer of maternal antibody may not have occurred). Significant exposure can occur through residence in the same household, close contact with a playmate, proximity to a contagious patient, or contact with a contagious visitor or hospital staff member.

In the past, varicella-zoster IG (human) (VZIG) was used routinely for postexposure prophylaxis. The only manufacturer of VZIG discontinued production in 2004 and supplies were depleted by 2006. Physicians should access http://www.cdc.gov/MMWRpreview/MMWRhtml/mm5508a5.htm for relevant recommendations. In February 2006, an investigational VZIG product, VariZIG (Cangene Corporation, Winnipeg, Canada) became available under an investigational new drug application to the FDA.[10] Similar to VZIG, VariZIG is a purified human IG preparation made from plasma containing high levels of varicella IgG antibodies. This product is lyophilized, and after reconstitution is administered IM within 96 hours of exposure. The dose is 125 U (1 vial)/10 kg body weight up to a maximum of 625 U (5 vials). The minimum dose is 125 U. VariZIG is distributed by FFF Enterprises (Temecula, California: 24-hour telephone, 800-843-7477) under expanded access protocol. Pharmacists and healthcare providers who expect to need VariZIG can participate in a program that permits acquisition of an inventory in advance.

If VariZIG cannot be obtained within 96 hours after exposure, IGIV can be given at a dose of 400 mg/kg. Although licensed IGIV preparations are known to contain varicella antibody, the titer in any specific lot is uncertain. An alternative to postexposure prophylaxis with IGIV is administration of oral acyclovir, which should be started 7 to 10 days after exposure and continued for a total of 7 days. This approach can be considered in immunocompetent, seronegative adults with significant exposure. The dose for adults is 800 mg given 4 times a day. If a child requires acyclovir preemptively, the dose is 40 to 80 mg/kg per day, divided into 4 doses. As an alternative, exposed immunocompetent children can be given varicella vaccine within 96 hours of exposure if they have not previously received vaccine and have no contraindication.

IMMUNE GLOBULIN INTRAVENOUS (HUMAN) (IGIV)

IGIV, like IG, is prepared from large pools of plasma derived from as many as 60,000 donors. The early steps in its manufacture are similar to those used for preparing IG. Further processing of individual products is performed by a variety of techniques, including steps such as polyethylene glycol precipitation, ion exchange chromatography, and exposure to low pH. This variation reflects, in part, the lack of consensus on the optimal procedure for preparing IGIV on a commercial scale in a form that is safe for IV administration. Final formulations are diverse, e.g., freeze-dried or in solution, different protein concentrations of the latter, different pH, and various stabilizers and other excipients that can be used in a number of different combinations. This variety and the dynamic state of the industry render any compilation of manufacturing methods or formulations rapidly obsolete. The clinician who intends to use a particular product should consult the "Description" section of the product package insert for a brief synopsis of the product's preparation and properties.

Although each lot of IGIV must contain at least minimal levels of antibodies to certain infectious organisms or toxoids (measles, poliovirus, and diphtheria), these levels were established to ensure lot-to-lot consistency rather than to match the clinical indications for individual products. Even though the use of large plasma pools enhances consistency, IGIV products differ in sources of plasma as well as in processing methods. As a result, antibody titers to other bacterial and viral pathogens can vary significantly among preparations and lots.[10-12] In addition, processing steps can alter functional capabilities of IgG or change the relative distribution of immunoglobulin subclasses. These changes may or may not be reflected in antibody titers measured by routine laboratory tests. Moreover, most individual products have undergone clinical trials for only a certain subset of indications. In addition, even when many IGIV products carry the same indication, direct comparisons of the efficacy of multiple products in a single clinical trial are rare. For all of these reasons, IGIV cannot be considered a uniform generic product. Available products in the U.S. (2011) are shown in Table 5-2. Certain physiologic properties intrinsic to IGIV preparations (and variable among products) should be considered in all individuals for whom administration is considered and especially in those who have underlying conditions. Such considerations include high volume load, sodium content and osmolality, especially in neonates and young children as well as those with cardiac disease, renal impairment, or thromboembolic risk; 2% to 10% carbohydrate content, in those with diabetes or renal impairment; low pH in neonates; and average IgA content (<2 to 720 µg/mL) in those with anti-IgA antibodies.

Approved Indications

There are currently 6 FDA-approved indications for IGIV: (1) replacement therapy for primary immunodeficiency disorders associated with defects in humoral immunity; (2) treatment of idiopathic thrombocytopenic purpura to induce a rapid rise in platelet count when needed to prevent or control bleeding; (3) prevention of infection and graft-versus-host disease (GvHD) in adult bone marrow transplant recipients; (4) prevention of coronary artery aneurysms associated with Kawasaki disease; (5) prevention of infection in children with HIV; and (6) prevention of bacterial infections in patients with hypogammaglobulinemia associated with B-cell chronic lymphocytic leukemia (Table 5-3).

Primary Immune Deficiencies

During the past 20 years, IGIV has become the drug of choice for replacement therapy in primary immunodeficiency and all IGIV products carry this indication.[13,14] Although most subjects enrolled in IGIV efficacy trials have had the more common primary immunodeficiencies, clinical experience with IGIV in a wide variety of these conditions has been favorable. Patients with the following primary immunodeficiencies have associated hypogammaglobulinemia and may benefit from replacement IGIV therapy: X-linked agammaglobulinemia, common variable immunodeficiency, severe combined immunodeficiency, hyper-IgM syndrome, congenital agammaglobulinemia, and Wiskott–Aldrich syndrome.

As clinical experience has grown, physicians have learned to tailor dosage to the individual patient. The objective is to determine the dose and regimen that will achieve and maintain freedom from serious infections. Monitoring the trough levels of IgG in parallel with the patient's clinical course has been helpful in accomplishing this objective. A range of effective doses, dosing schedules, and trough levels has been observed. However, the usual schedule for IGIV infusion is once every 3 or 4 weeks, and typical dose is approximately 400 mg/kg (range 300 to 800 mg/kg). Trough concentrations of IgG should be maintained in the range of 400 to 500 mg/dL.[12] In 2006, the FDA approved IG subcutaneous (Vivaglobulin, ZLB Behring) for people with primary immunodeficiency. It is the first subcutaneous IG approved that can be self-administered weekly (158 mg/kg) using a portable pump.

Secondary Immune Deficiencies

Chronic lymphocytic leukemia (CLL) and the immune suppression that occurs in patients undergoing bone marrow transplantation (BMT) result in quantitative and/or qualitative humoral immunodeficiency. Although IGIV reduces infections in these conditions, unresolved issues are selection of patients most likely to benefit, optimal timing and duration of administration, and the relative effectiveness of IGIV and other anti-infective therapies.

Infection with human immunodeficiency virus (HIV) causes dysregulation of humoral immunity with impaired functional antibody activity. Some HIV-infected children have been shown to experience fewer bacterial infections while receiving IGIV; hence, IGIV may benefit selected patients.[15,16] In these studies, a benefit was observed for children with CD4+ lymphocyte counts >200/mm³. Antimicrobial prophylaxis (e.g., trimethoprim-sulfamethoxazole) is an alternative approach to IGIV for preventing bacterial infections and is effective in preventing *Pneumocystis jirovecii* pneumonia.[17]

Immunomodulation

Mechanism of immunomodulation by IGIV and its use in treatment of inflammatory and autoimmune diseases have been reviewed recently.[18] Potential anti-inflammatory mechanisms include: neutralization of pathologic autoantibodies, enhanced clearance of autoantibodies, inhibition of phagocytosis by effector cells, altered complement deposition, altered cytokine expression, neutralization of superantigens, and modulation of lymphocyte function.[19] Because "immunomodulation" does not appear as a separate category in the labeling of IGIV, the labeled indications in this category are considered individually in this discussion.

Immune thrombocytopenic purpura. ITP can follow viral infections. Antibodies that are specific for or that cross-react with platelet surface antigens coat the cell surface and promote greater clearance of platelets by the spleen. In patients with ITP, IGIV can affect a rapid increase in platelet counts (often within 24 hours of infusion) and thereby can avert life-threatening bleeding. The prevailing hypothesis is that IgG in IGIV interacts with phagocytic Fc receptors, blocking clearance of platelets and allowing them to enter or remain in the circulation.[20] However, the mechanism may be more complex, involving induction of receptor expression.[21]

Many different IGIV products have been shown to be effective for treatment of ITP, although few direct comparisons of effectiveness have been made. Compounding the lack of data is the fact that no laboratory tests can predict efficacy in ITP, either of individual products or for individual patients. IGIV has been studied in acute and chronic ITP in both adults and children. Not all cases respond; however, in general, children show a response more frequently than do adults, and the increase in platelet count is

---

TABLE 5-3. Approved Indications for Immune Globulin Intravenous Therapy

Indications	Dosage	Comments
REPLACEMENT THERAPY		
Primary immunodeficiency	~400 mg/kg q4 weeks (average dose)	Adjust dose according to individual response
Chronic lymphocytic leukemia	400 mg/kg q3–4 weeks	Cost-effectiveness questioned
Bone marrow transplantation	500 mg/kg q1 week	Other anti-infective therapies also effective
Human immunodeficiency virus infection in children	400 mg/kg q2–4 weeks	Useful in selected symptomatic patients
IMMUNE MODULATION		
Idiopathic thrombocytopenic purpura (ITP)	400 mg/kg daily for 5 days, *or* 1 g/kg single dose	Useful in acute and chronic immune thrombocytopenia purpura
Kawasaki disease	2 g/kg single dose	10–20% of patients may need a second dose

more prolonged in children treated for acute ITP. (A B-lymphocyte-suppressive effect may account for prolonged decrease in antiplatelet antibodies.) Because acute ITP can resolve spontaneously, especially in young children, it is important to obtain the consultation of an experienced hematologist during the planning of the therapeutic approach.[22]

Initially, the dosage of IGIV employed for treatment of ITP was 400 mg/kg daily for 5 consecutive days.[20] This regimen is still in use, but monitoring of the platelet count may indicate that dosage can be stopped after the second, third, or fourth day. On the other hand, some IGIV products have been shown to raise the platelet count adequately when a single dose of 1 g/kg is infused. If the rise is insufficient, this dose can be repeated the next day or on alternate days, depending on the product used. In all cases, it is important: (1) not to exceed the rate of administration recommended in the package insert for the particular IGIV product; and (2) to avoid the higher dose in patients with expanded fluid volume.

Kawasaki disease. Immune dysregulation may play a role in diseases for which a specific etiology has not been identified. Kawasaki disease is an acute inflammatory condition with multisystem vasculitis that can result in arterial aneurysms, particularly of the coronary vessels. Several IGIV preparations have been studied for the treatment of this condition. IGIV administered concurrently with oral aspirin rapidly downregulates the inflammatory response. IGIV plus aspirin reduces the incidence of coronary artery aneurysms from 20% to 25% to <5%.[23,24] Treatment with IGIV should be administered within the first 10 days of illness and within 7 days of onset of symptoms if possible; a single dose of 2 g/kg infused over 10 to 12 hours is recommended (http://aappolicy.aappublications.org/). Patients with Kawasaki disease who are diagnosed after 10 days of fever also should receive aspirin and IGIV promptly although benefit has not been studied in this setting.

The initial dose of aspirin usually is 80 to 100 mg/kg per day divided into 4 equal doses.[25,26] When fever has resolved, a once daily 3 to 5 mg/kg dose of aspirin is recommended. Children who have persistent or recrudescent symptoms may be treated with a second IGIV dose of 2 g/kg. Inasmuch as the etiology of Kawasaki disease is unknown, it is possible that not all IGIV preparations (or all lots) are equally effective, even among products that carry this indication. Some clinicians recommend oral prednisolone for retreatment when the response to IGIV is inadequate.[27]

Bone marrow transplantation. IGIV can reduce the risk of infection in recipients of bone marrow transplants. In addition, several studies have reported IGIV to lower the incidence of acute GvHD, but in one of the studies this result was only observed in patients who were older than 20 years.[28,29]

Other Uses

The number of clinical conditions for which IGIV has been tried greatly exceeds that of its approved indications. The reasons for this are many. The simplest is the obvious fact that clinical research necessarily precedes the compilation of data by the manufacturer, submission of the data to regulatory authorities, and review and approval by the latter. Thus, in principle, a manufacturer simply might choose not to request approval of a particular indication if it offers no market advantage. Other reasons are more complex. A well-received, concisely written paper published in the medical literature might present positive results but might not include all of the less common adverse effects or might not address statistical nuances or subtleties of trial design that raise concerns. Alternatively, widespread use (indeed, commonly accepted treatment) for a particular condition can be generated by the enthusiastic endorsement of a respected clinician. In practice, such use may or may not be confirmed by appropriately controlled and adequately powered studies. In addition, placebo-controlled randomized trials for treatment of an uncommon disease may be difficult to conduct in a reasonable time frame because of slow accrual of eligible patients. The growing off-label use of IGIV has been implicated in shortages of IGIV (see below). This section includes some

of the better-known off-label uses of IGIV, but no attempt has been made to include all or even most of them.

Toxic shock syndrome. IGIV has been used an adjuvant for the treatment of toxic shock syndrome associated with staphylococci and invasive streptococcal disease. IGIV typically contains antibodies against superantigen toxins (including toxic shock syndrome toxin-1, staphylococcal enterotoxins and streptococcal exotoxins) produced by both of these organisms. Furthermore, the anti-inflammatory properties of IGIV may help ameliorate the exaggerated cytokine response induced by superantigens. Both animal studies and case reports suggest the utility of IGIV as adjuvant therapy for the treatment of toxic shock syndrome secondary to staphylococcal toxin and streptococcal infection.[30,31] The efficacy of IGIV as adjunctive therapy in streptococcal toxin shock syndrome was studied in a double-blind, placebo-controlled trial but the trial was ended early because of poor patient accrual. Although statistical significance was not reached, results suggested a 3.6-fold higher mortality rate in placebo recipients. Because most patients respond rapidly to fluids, vasopressor therapy and antimicrobials, some experts would reserve IGIV for those patients who do not respond to initial therapy. Typical dose of IGIV for this purpose is 1 g/kg, although a range of doses has been used.

Neonates. Because of the high morbidity and mortality rates in preterm infants, the effects of IGIV in this population have been studied extensively.[32] Despite enthusiasm and the apparent logic of replacing missing antibodies, many studies have shown minimal benefit.[32-34] One prospective, randomized trial was conducted with preterm (gestational age <33 weeks) infants whose IgG levels at birth were <400 mg/dL. Those who received IGIV had no fewer infectious episodes and no lower mortality rate than those who received an albumin placebo.[35]

Parvovirus B19. Most parvovirus B19 infections are mild and do not require treatment. However, illness can be prolonged in patients with a variety of immunodeficiencies, including: primary immunodeficiencies, HIV infection, sickle-cell disease, organ transplantation, and cytotoxic therapies. In such patients, parvovirus B19 causes chronic, severe anemia. IGIV (400 mg/kg daily for 5 days) has been reported to reduce the viral load and to restore erythropoiesis in selected patients.[36,37] Anemia, hydrops, and persistent neonatal infection also can occur with intrauterine infection. In conjunction with intrauterine transfusions of red blood cells, IGIV may be helpful in ameliorating anemia associated with congenital parvovirus B19 infection.[38]

Immune-mediated cytopenias. Patients with a variety of immune-mediated cytopenias, including anemia and neutropenia, have been treated with IGIV, with some success.[39] Published reports support the use of IGIV in HIV-infected individuals with ITP, although none of the licensed IGIV products carries this specific indication.[40,41]

Guillain–Barré syndrome (GBS). GBS is an acute immune-mediated inflammatory polyneuropathy. IGIV or plasma exchange represent the main methods of treatment. Large, randomized controlled trials of IGIV in children with GBS are not available. Results from small trials in children with GBS are consistent with data from larger randomized trials in adults suggesting that IGIV therapy can shorten the time to recovery. The mechanism of IGIV in this illness is uncertain.[42,43]

SPECIFIC IMMUNE GLOBULINS FOR INTRAVENOUS ADMINISTRATION

Currently four specific, plasma-derived hyperimmune polyclonal products for IV administration are approved for prophylaxis or therapy of infectious disease (see Table 5-1).

Cytomegalovirus Immune Globulin (CMV-IGIV)

Cytomegalovirus (CMV) IGIV (human) is indicated for the prophylaxis of CMV disease associated with stem cell or solid-organ transplantation.[44-46] The use of CMV-IGIV for prophylaxis of CMV disease varies among transplant centers. Factors that influence the susceptibility of transplant recipients to CMV disease include: organ type, immunosuppressive regimen, and donor/recipient CMV status. CMV-negative transplant recipients who receive an organ from a CMV-positive donor are at highest risk for CMV disease and typically receive some form of CMV prophylaxis. This can include ganciclovir (using a prophylactic or pre-emptive strategy) alone, CMV-IGIV alone, or CMV-IGIV in combination with ganciclovir therapy. CMV-IGIV for in utero CMV infection is not recommended routinely but has been used in selected instances with confirmed infection.

Botulism Immune Globulin (BIG-IV)

Botulism IGIV (human) was approved by the FDA in 2003 under the orphan drug program. It is indicated in infants <12 months of age for treatment of botulism suspected to be caused by either toxin type A or B. Produced by immunization of healthy adult donor, BIG-IV is available under the trade name BabyBIG, only through the California Department of Health Services (510-231-7600, all days/hours). A 5-year randomized, placebo-controlled treatment trial demonstrated the safety and efficacy of BIG-IV in reducing the mean hospital stay per case from approximately 5.5 weeks to 2.5 weeks as well as a reduced mean hospitalization cost per case by about $90,000. Treatment with BIG-IV should be initiated as soon as possible to neutralize toxin and should not be delayed for laboratory confirmation of a suspected case.[47] BabyBIG is not indicated for foodborne or wound botulism. In 2010, an investigational heptavalent equine botulism antitoxin (HBAT) containing antitoxin to types A, B, C, D, E, F, and G replaced previous A, B, and E products as the only product available in the U.S. for naturally occurring non-infant botulism and is available only through the Centers for Disease Control and Prevention (CDC) (770-488-7100 all hours/days).[48]

Vaccinia Immune Globulin (VIG-IV)

Vaccinia IG (human) (VIG) was developed in the 1960s for ameliorating side effects associated with smallpox (vaccinia) immunization, including eczema vaccinatum, generalized, and progressive vaccinia.[49] The original preparation contained a high proportion of protein aggregates and thus was administered IM and is no longer available. Vaccinia immune globulin intravenous (VIG-IV) is the only product currently available for treatment of complications of vaccinia vaccination. The use of VIG-IV has become extremely limited since the eradication of smallpox. It is considered valuable "insurance," to be held in reserve if a patient is receiving an experimental vaccine that involves a vaccinia carrier virus, or to prevent or manage complications of smallpox vaccination should such be required for a bioterrorism threat. Supplies of VIG-IV are stored in the Strategic National Stockpile. Release of VIG-IV from the stockpile must be approved by the CDC.

MONOCLONAL ANTIBODIES

The development of hybridoma technology in the 1970s permitted the production of essentially unlimited supplies of any monoclonal antibody (mAb). Monoclonal antibodies are being explored as antimicrobial and immunomodulating agents. Monoclonal antibodies have been studied in an attempt to modify septic shock syndrome either by blocking bacterial components that induce septic shock or by modifying the proinflammatory cytokines that mediate septic shock. Early attempts to utilize mAb against endotoxin in the treatment of gram-negative bacillary septicemia were not successful.[50,51] The advantages of mAb include the avoidance of a requirement for a large IV infusion over several hours, predictable supply of a highly standardized product, elimination of concern for adventitious agents, and avoidance of unwanted antibody in a polyclonal product that might interfere with a live virus vaccine.[52]

Palivizumab is a humanized murine mAb directed against the surface fusion glycoprotein of respiratory syncytial virus (RSV). Monthly intramuscular administration of palivizumab demon-

strated a reduction in the risk of RSV hospitalization among high-risk infants by approximately 50%.[53]

In June 1998, the FDA licensed this monoclonal antibody, establishing palivizumab as the first monoclonal antibody introduced into clinical practice for prevention of an infectious disease. Recommendations for use of palivizumab have been made and revised by the American Academy of Pediatrics.[54,55]

IMMUNOGLOBULIN PRODUCTS PREPARED FROM ANIMAL PLASMA

In the past, there existed an array of approved animal-derived immunoglobulin products specific for various infectious agents or their toxins. Few are in use currently, most having been supplanted by analogues of human origin (e.g., RIG, TIG) or by other therapeutic modalities. (There are approved animal-derived products for the treatment of venomous bites and digoxin intoxication and for prevention of organ rejection; these are beyond the scope of this chapter.) The only available products in this category are botulism antitoxin and diphtheria antitoxin. They can be obtained from the CDC for emergency use in the treatment of foodborne botulism and diphtheria, respectively. These equine immunoglobulin products are only provided when specifically indicated. Because immediate anaphylaxis and delayed serum sickness are possible adverse reactions, these products should only be used when their life-saving potential clearly outweighs the risk. Procedures for skin testing and desensitization are readily available and the physician should always be prepared to treat any adverse event.[56]

ADVERSE REACTIONS TO IMMUNE GLOBULINS PREPARED FROM HUMAN PLASMA

The most common adverse reaction to IM-administered IGs is pain at the injection site. Local or facial flushing can occur, as can headache, chills, or nausea, but these symptoms are less common. Severe systemic reactions are rare.

Infusion-Related Reactions

Reactions such as fever, headache, myalgia, chills, nausea, and vomiting often are related to the rate of IGIV infusion and usually are mild to moderate and self-limited (Box 5-1). These reactions may result from formation of IgG aggregates during manufacture or storage. There may be product-to-product variations in adverse effects among individual patients. Isoimmune hemolytic reaction

---

BOX 5-1. Adverse Effects of Immune Globulin Intravenous Therapy

MINOR SYSTEMIC REACTIONS
Headache, back or hip pain, fever, dizziness or lightheadedness, nausea, flushing

PYROGENIC REACTIONS
High fever and systemic symptoms

VASOMOTOR/CARDIOVASCULAR MANIFESTATIONS
Changes in blood pressure and heart rate

INFREQUENT, SERIOUS REACTIONS
Aseptic meningitis[a]
Acute renal failure
Hypersensitivity reactions[b]
Anaphylaxis

[a]Aseptic meningitis may be more common in adults or children with specific underlying conditions.
[b]Reaction reports are more common for products that contain sucrose.

is described rarely, especially if large doses of IGIV are infused. Less common but severe reactions include hypersensitivity and anaphylactoid reactions marked by flushing, changes in blood pressure, and tachycardia; thromboembolic events; aseptic meningitis; and renal insufficiency and failure. The causes of these reactions are unknown. Adverse events often can be decreased by following the package insert for the individual product carefully with regard to rate of administration. Aseptic meningitis associated with pleocytosis can occur, especially among patients receiving high doses of IGIV (2 g/kg).[57–60] Acute renal failure has been reported rarely following IGIV infusions, particularly among patients with pre-existing renal disease who receive IGIV products containing sucrose.

Anaphylactic reactions induced by anti-IgA can occur in patients with primary antibody deficiency who have a total absence of circulating IgA and develop IgG antibodies to IgA.[61] These reactions are rare in patients with panhypogammaglobulinemia and potentially are more common in patients with selective IgA deficiency and subclass IgG deficiencies. In rare instances in which reactions related to anti-IgA antibodies have occurred, use of IgA-depleted IGIV preparations may decrease the likelihood of further reactions. Because of the extreme rarity of these reactions, however, screening for IgA deficiency and anti-IgA antibodies is not recommended routinely.

Interference with Active Immunization

Antibodies present in IGs can interfere with the immune response to the corresponding live virus vaccines. This is rarely a problem when the vaccine is a substance such as a toxoid, a polysaccharide, or a killed virus preparation, even when the vaccine is given simultaneously with the IG, provided that the two products are administered with separate syringes at different sites. However, antibodies in IG can interfere with viral replication after administration of live-virus vaccines and, thus, prevent successful immunization. The effect on the immune response to measles immunization has been demonstrated, but in principle, similar interference could occur with any live-virus vaccine. Measles, mumps, rubella or varicella vaccine should not be given in the 2 weeks before or 3 months after an individual receives any IgG preparation or whole or fractionated blood. Because high doses of IGIV can inhibit the response to measles vaccine for extended periods, longer intervals are required as the IGIV dose is increased (up to 11 months after 2 g/kg IGIV as for Kawasaki disease) to provide sufficient time for passively acquired antibodies to wane.

Transmission of Infectious Agents

Although IGs prepared from human plasma are biologic products and, hence, must always be considered to carry a theoretical risk for transmission of viruses, they have a remarkable record of safety. Even IGIV, which is administered directly into the bloodstream, often in large quantities, has been extremely safe. The many investigations conducted have revealed no documented case of transmission of hepatitis by U.S. licensed IGs for IM use. Similarly, there is no evidence of transmission of HIV by U.S.-licensed IGs for either IM or IV administration.[62]

Several cases of non-A, non-B hepatitis were associated with IGIV administration between 1983 and 1987.[63,64] These cases involved sources of IGIV that were not commercial lots available in the U.S. In February 1994, however, a worldwide recall of U.S. licensed IGIV products manufactured by Baxter Healthcare Corporation was initiated because of hepatitis C virus (HCV) transmissions.[65] Cases of hepatitis C occurred in several countries, including the U.S., among individuals who received these products between April 1, 1993, and February 23, 1994 (when they were removed from the market).[66,67]

The reason for these transmissions of hepatitis illustrates the complex relationships that underlie the production of IGs and all human plasma derivatives. These products had initially been licensed in February 1986 and, like other U.S. licensed IGIV products, had an impeccable safety record. In 1990, the first test for

antibody to HCV – a single-antigen anti-HCV test – became available commercially. In 1992, a more sensitive test (a multi-antigen anti-HCV test) came into use. Although using these tests to screen donors of blood and blood components (e.g., red blood cells, platelets) was of obvious benefit, application of the more sensitive test for screening of donors of plasma for fractionation had a paradoxical effect; that is, although withholding units of plasma that gave a positive test result meant that fewer infectious donors were represented in the plasma pools, these pools also were depleted with respect to beneficial anti-HCV antibodies that had co-circulated with the antibodies detected by the test. These beneficial antibodies had served two functions: (1) neutralization of viruses; and (2) complexing with viruses so as to partition them away from the protein fraction that became the final product.

As a consequence, many lots of IGIV manufactured by Baxter Healthcare Corporation from plasma collected from donors who had been tested by the more sensitive test contained infectious (i.e., non-neutralized, noncomplexed) virus.[66,67] By contrast, IGIV made by other manufacturers from plasma collected from donors who had undergone the same type of testing did not transmit hepatitis C.[65–67] This finding showed that the margin of safety had differed among individual IGIV products.

Concerns about the potential transmission of prion disease by IG products have been raised. These concerns are highlighted by the lack of serologic assays to screen blood products for prions. The findings of several studies suggest that the likelihood of prion transmission via plasma products is exceedingly small. This includes the observations that very low levels of prions are found in the plasma of affected individuals and that the processing of plasma for the production of IGs typically inactivates prions.[68–71] To date, no case of prion disease has been linked to IG therapy.

Studies performed on a laboratory scale have shown that many manufacturing steps that are intrinsic to the process for preparing IgG greatly lower viral and prion burden. For example, alcohol fractionation of plasma partitions virus and prions away from the IgG fraction.[72] If the alcohol concentration at a particular manufacturing step is sufficiently high and the virus is sufficiently labile (e.g., HIV), alcohol is viricidal.[72] Other precipitating agents, such as polyethylene glycol, can achieve similar partitioning of viruses. Incubation at low pH, either in the presence or in the absence of enzymes, has a strong antiviral effect.[73,74]

Solvent-detergent treatment is one step that has been deliberately introduced to achieve viral inactivation in various IGs. This treatment destroys enveloped viruses such as HBV, HCV, and HIV.[75] It is used in the manufacturing of numerous IGs for IM and IV use (including current IGIV products made by Baxter Healthcare Corporation). Another deliberate viral inactivation used for some products is heat treatment, which can be performed in the presence of stabilizers to prevent denaturation of the IgG.[76] The process for making some IG products now includes so-called nanofiltration, that is, filtration of the product through membranes with pore dimensions that permit the passage of proteins but not viruses. Brief summaries of these procedures as well as of the experiments demonstrating inactivation and removal of specific viruses are generally provided in the "Description" sections of the package inserts for the individual products.

PRODUCT SHORTAGES

There have been periodic shortages of certain IG products. The reasons for this are multiple. In some cases, there have been specific production problems. In others, increased demand is a major factor. For example, use of IGIV in the U.S. has increased steadily by approximately 10% each year, and production has not always kept pace. Off-label use of IGIV contributes importantly to shortage. A study of 12 academic health centers revealed that 52% of IGIV prescribed was used for off-label indications.[77] In response to these shortages, some hospitals have developed committees to review and restrict usage of IGIV. It is incumbent on clinicians to employ IGs appropriately so that products will be available for use in conditions for which they have proven benefit.

THE FUTURE

In the immediate future, we may anticipate additional IG products for IV administration. Some of these are likely to be specific IGs directed against known infectious agents. In the future, additional specific mAb products will become available. Furthermore, advances in molecular biology have made possible the humanization of murine mAb, whereby the murine sequences are limited to the variable region of the antibody. This process leads to decreased antigenicity, improved pharmacokinetics, and presumably results in fewer side effects. In the past 10 years, a number of mAbs have been licensed for use, including those for: (1) organ transplantation (via inhibition of cytokine activity or depletion of lymphocyte subsets); (2) treatment of malignancies (i.e., lymphoma, colon and breast cancer); and (3) immunologic modulation (i.e., asthma and Crohn disease). A variety of mAbs for the treatment and prevention of infectious diseases are in clinical development related to the following pathogens: *Cryptococcus neoformans, Staphylococcus aureus,* HIV, and *Candida albicans.* The advantages provided by mAbs have led some to hope that these reagents will be helpful in dealing with the problems of drug-resistant pathogens and potential bioterrorism attacks.

In parallel with continuing product development, it is reasonable to expect improvements in the design and conduct of clinical trials. One example might be streamlining the design of trials involving well-known products (e.g., IGIV) used to treat well-understood conditions such as primary immunodeficiency. Another, one hopes, is the conduct of trials that are sufficiently powered to permit major "off-label" uses to be either approved or abandoned.

6 Active Immunization

Andrew T. Kroger, Alison C. Mawle, Larry K. Pickering, and Walter A. Orenstein

Vaccines are among the most effective means of preventing disease, disability, and death. The use of vaccines, initiated by Jenner in 1796 with demonstration that inoculation of material from cowpox lesions could prevent smallpox, predates the germ theory of disease. Use of conventional viral and bacterial culture techniques led to development of vaccines to prevent 7 diseases in 1985. Subsequently, advances in understanding the immunologic basis of immunity and new molecular biologic techniques, including genome sequencing, have facilitated definition of the precise composition and structure of antigens, development and extensive use of new vaccines, and an expansion of their potential uses beyond prevention of childhood diseases.

The profound impact of vaccines on disease incidence is a result not only of availability of safe and effective vaccines but also of strategies for disease control and programs to deliver vaccines to target groups. Eradication of smallpox in 1977 is among the greatest public health achievements and was based on competent disease surveillance and containment of spread of disease with a highly effective vaccine.[1] Global efforts under way to eradicate poliomyelitis and to certify eradication of polio involve more comprehensive disease control strategies. National and multi-country mass vaccination campaigns, intensive surveillance for wild poliovirus, and house-to-house vaccination programs have succeeded in terminating transmission of wild poliovirus in the Americas, the Western Pacific, and Europe, and gains are being made in the remaining endemic countries in the Indian subcontinent and Africa (www.polioeradication.org).[2-4] Efforts to reduce or even eliminate measles and neonatal tetanus, two of the major causes of child fatality worldwide, also are progressing, although cases of measles continue to occur worldwide.[5,6] The Global Alliance for Vaccines and Immunization, an alliance between organizations in the public and private sectors, provides support for introduction of vaccines in countries that previously could not support their use. (www.gavialliance.org).

Benefits of successful vaccines include not only reductions in disease incidence, disability, pain, and suffering, but also savings in healthcare costs in both the economically developed and developing world. Studies in the United States have reaffirmed benefits of childhood immunization.[7-9] A cost–benefit analysis covering vaccine-preventable diseases of childhood, including diphtheria, tetanus, pertussis, polio, hepatitis B, *Haemophilus influenzae* type b (Hib), measles, mumps, rubella, and varicella (MMRV), estimated that for every dollar spent on childhood immunization in 2011, there were $2.37 dollars saved in direct costs and $11.69 saved by society.[9]

IMMUNIZATION AND VACCINES

Immunization is the process of artificially inducing immunity or providing protection from disease. *Active immunization* is the process of stimulating the body to produce antibody and other immune responses (e.g., cell-mediated immunity) through administration of a vaccine or toxoid. *Passive immunization* is provision of temporary immunity by administration of preformed antibodies derived from humans or animals (see Chapter 5, Passive Immunization).

Vaccine Content

Biologic agents used to induce active immunization include vaccines and toxoids. Traditionally, a *vaccine* is defined as a suspension of live (usually attenuated) or inactivated microorganisms, or fractions thereof, which is administered to induce immunity and prevent infectious disease or its sequelae; efforts to develop vaccines to increase immune response to cancers or to treat diseases like diabetes mellitus necessitate rethinking of this definition. *Live-attenuated* vaccines traditionally have been developed by means of serial passage (in culture or animals) of an initially pathogenic bacteria or virus strain with selection for strains that are less pathogenic for humans but which induce protective immunity (e.g., MMR). Live-attenuated vaccines also can be developed with use of reassortants of attenuated animal or human virus strains with virus coat antigens from pathogenic strains (e.g., cold-adapted influenza, rotavirus). *Inactivated* vaccines can consist of: (1) whole organisms inactivated by heat, formalin, or other agents (polio, hepatitis A, rabies); (2) purified protein (acellular pertussis and influenza) or polysaccharide antigens (pneumococcal, meningococcal, and intramuscular typhoid) from whole organisms; (3) purified antigens produced by genetically altered organisms (e.g., hepatitis B and human papillomavirus (HPV) vaccines produced by yeast); or (4) chemically modified antigens, such as polysaccharides conjugated to carrier proteins to increase immune response (e.g., conjugated Hib, pneumococcal and meningococcal vaccines (PCV and MCV)). *Toxoids* are bacterial toxins produced in bacterial culture that have been rendered nontoxic but retain the ability to stimulate formation of antitoxin.

Vaccine and toxoid preparations also contain other constituents intended to enhance immunogenicity and stability but that also can be responsible for adverse reactions.[10] Such constituents include: (1) suspending fluid, which can be saline or complex fluids containing constituents derived from the biologic system or medium in which the vaccine is produced (e.g., egg or serum proteins); (2) preservatives, stabilizers, and antimicrobial agents, which are used to inhibit bacterial growth in viral cultures or the final product or to stabilize antigens (e.g., mercurials, phenols, albumin, glycine, neomycin); and (3) adjuvants, which enhance response to inactivated antigens (e.g., aluminum phosphate or hydroxide (alone or combined with monophosphoryl lipid A, ASO_4)). Concern about the possibility of adverse effects from cumulative exposure to mercury in the environment has led to removal of thimerosal as a preservative from U.S. vaccines recommended for infants.[11] The only vaccines administered to infants that contain thimerosal as a preservative are influenza vaccine and DT vaccine (that should only be administered in rare circumstances). Physicians should be knowledgeable about the constituents of each vaccine, which are described in vaccine information package inserts.

TYPES OF VACCINES

Immunologic Basis of Response to Vaccines

The two major approaches to active immunization are use of: (1) live-attenuated vaccines and (2) inactivated or detoxified agents or their purified components. For some diseases, such as poliomyelitis and influenza, both approaches have been used.

Live-attenuated vaccines have the advantage of producing a complex immunologic response simulating natural infection. Because replication of the organism and processing of antigens mimic those of the natural pathogen, both humoral and cell-mediated responses can be generated to a variety of antigens. Generally, immunity induced by one dose of a live-attenuated vaccine is long-lasting, possibly lifelong. However, the strength of response, particularly the humoral response, usually is less robust than the response following natural infection, and detectable antibodies can wane with time, resulting in some loss of protection. Induction of immunity by live vaccines can be inhibited by passive antibody, whether from transplacental acquisition from the mother or receipt of immunoglobulin-containing blood products; thus, optimal response depends on ensuring that this level of passive antibody has declined (e.g., primary measles vaccination at 12 months of age instead of earlier, delay of measles vaccination after administration of blood products). In addition, because response may be only 90% to 95% after a single dose, a two-dose or multiple-dose regimen may be necessary to induce higher levels of protection in the community and prevent spread of disease if the population is exposed (herd protection).

Inactivated or purified antigen vaccines induce response only to components present in the vaccine. Generally, multiple doses, usually three or more, are necessary to induce satisfactory antibody levels that persist for long periods of time; booster doses at longer intervals (e.g., 10 or more years for tetanus and diphtheria toxoids (Td)) sometimes are required to ensure lasting protection. The nature of vaccine responses depends on antigen type. Protein (and glycoprotein) antigens usually induce both humoral immunity and memory (response through T-helper lymphocytes) after multiple doses, evidenced as more rapid, broad and intense (anamnestic) response to successive doses. Polysaccharide antigens by themselves induce only humoral antibody without T-lymphocyte stimulation and fail to induce an anamnestic response with repeated antigenic challenge. This limitation can be overcome by conjugation of polysaccharides to protein carriers (e.g., Hib polysaccharide conjugated to whole or modified diphtheria or tetanus toxoids or to outer-membrane protein (OMP) complex of *Neisseria meningitidis*) to induce both a stronger immune response in younger children and immunologic memory.

Immune Response to Active Immunization

The general mechanism by which a long-term protective memory immune response is induced requires activation of T lymphocytes by antigen presenting cells (APCs), which then provide help to B lymphocytes to develop into antibody-producing plasma cells (T-lymphocyte dependent response).[12,13] Polysaccharide antigens bypass T-lymphocyte help (T-lymphocyte independent response) and induce B-lymphocyte differentiation directly. However, T-lymphocyte independent responses do not induce immunologic memory. Initiation of a T-lymphocyte dependent antibody response occurs by activation of naïve $CD4^+$ T-helper lymphocytes in response to presentation of antigen by APCs, generally dendritic cells (DCs). This interaction occurs through recognition of the major histocompatibility complex (MHC)/peptide complex on the APC by the T-lymphocyte receptor, and secretion of cytokines that are necessary for maturation of naïve T-helper $CD4^+$ lymphocytes to differentiate toward a Th1 or Th2 response.[14] Th1 responses are predominantly cell-mediated, whereas Th2 responses are predominantly humoral. In the presence of interleukin (IL)-12, Th1 response is differentiated, and is associated with secretion of IL-2 and interferon (IFN)-γ. In the presence of IL-4, Th2 response is differentiated, and is associated with secretion of IL-4 and IL-5. These 2 cytokines are essential for differentiation and maturation of B lymphocytes into antibody-secreting plasma cells. A small subset of $CD4^+$ lymphocytes do not differentiate into effector cells, but mature to become long-lived memory cells, which form the nucleus of the secondary immune response upon re-exposure to antigen. The overall response is regulated by a further class of $CD4^+$ T lymphocytes (Treg).

In a primary response, naïve B lymphocytes recognize a specific antigenic epitope on native antigen through the immunoglobulin receptor on their surface, and differentiate into antibody-secreting cells in response to help from $CD4^+$ Th2 lymphocytes. A given B lymphocyte is activated by a T lymphocyte responding to the same antigen. B-lymphocyte proliferation and maturation then occurs in a clonal manner, and during this process, immunoglobulin class switching (from IgM to IgG and IgA) and affinity maturation occur. Antigen-specific plasma cells develop and secrete large amounts of clonal antibody. The polyclonal response to a given immunogen reflects the sum of the multiple individual clonal B lymphocyte responses that make up an antibody response. A minority of activated B lymphocytes mature into long-lived memory B lymphocytes, which form the basis of the rapid secondary response upon the next encounter with antigen. The mechanism of maintenance of these lymphocytes is an area of active research, since the ability to mount a strong secondary response after many years is a critical component of the adaptive immune response.

Initiation of the specific immune response to a pathogen is dependent upon the innate immune response, which is rapid, does not exhibit memory, and historically has been considered nonspecific. However, discovery of germ-line encoded pattern recognition receptors (PRRs) has led to an understanding that specific molecular structures are recognized by pathogen-associated molecular patterns (PAMPs). These specific structures include toll-like receptors (TLRs), which are membrane associated, and NOD-like receptors (NLRs), which are found in the cytoplasm and include the NALP family of receptors and others, all of which contribute to immune activation by inducing proinflammatory cytokines, which in turn modulates the adaptive immune response. TLRs and NLRs are found on APCs and recognize a wide variety of molecules commonly found in pathogens. TLR4 binds lipopolysaccharide, and TLR5 binds flagellin, both common bacterial components. The NALP3 inflammasome is activated by aluminum and has been shown to be the pathway through which aluminum adjuvants enhance immunogenicity.

Antibodies produced in response to immunization can mediate protection by a variety of extracellular mechanisms including: (1) direct neutralization of bacterial toxin; (2) facilitation of intracellular digestion of bacteria by phagocytes (opsonization); (3) initiation of or combination with the complement pathway to cause lysis; or (4) sensitization of macrophages to promote phagocytosis. Antibodies cannot readily reach the intracellular space, which is the site of viral and some bacterial replication. However, antibodies are effective against many viral diseases by interacting with a virus before initial intracellular penetration occurs (neutralization), and preventing locally replicating virus from disseminating from the site of entry to an important target organ, as in spread of poliovirus from the gut to the central nervous system or of rabies from a puncture wound to peripheral neural tissue. Antigen-specific cytotoxic T-lymphocyte-mediated responses are an important component of the response to viral infections.

The cell-mediated immune response also has an innate and memory effector arm. Natural killer (NK) cells recognize virally infected cells in a nonspecific manner, without generation of memory. Activated NK cells secrete a variety of soluble mediators, including IFNs that kill virally infected cells, and ILs that modulate differentiation and response of CD4+ T-helper lymphocytes. Cytotoxic CD8+ T lymphocytes require help of CD4+ cells (generally Th1), in order to differentiate and mature. CD8+ cytotoxic T lymphocytes are an important part of the immune response to intracellular bacteria and viruses. As viruses replicate in a cell, viral proteins are processed and presented on the cell surface as an MHC class I/peptide complex. The complex is recognized by cytotoxic T lymphocytes. As with CD4+ T lymphocytes, a small subset develops into long-lived memory CD8+ T lymphocytes, capable of rapid reactivation as part of a secondary immune response.

Rarely, vaccination can result in immune responses that alter the course of natural infection detrimentally. For example, killed measles vaccine, a formalin-inactivated vaccine administered to some children in the U.S. between 1963 and 1967, sensitized some vaccine recipients so that when exposed to wild virus they developed an atypical infection with enhanced severity of disease. The prevailing theory has been that failure of formalin-inactivated vaccine to produce response to the measles virus fusion protein led to altered immune response and atypical disease upon subsequent challenge. More recent theories suggest that killed measles virus failed to induce high-avidity antibody, and immune-complex deposition was the major determinant of atypical measles.[15]

Following primary immunization with inactivated antigens, antibody response develops in 2 to 6 weeks but may be incomplete even after two doses; after effective priming, booster responses occur within 4 to 14 days. The initial response usually is immunoglobulin M (IgM) antibodies, followed within weeks by IgG antibodies. Response to live vaccines requires one incubation period, followed by several weeks to months for development of a strong immune response. Response to measles vaccination usually is maximal by 6 weeks, but in younger children, antibody levels can continue to rise for several months. However, protection against measles begins much earlier and some evidence suggests that disease can be prevented even when vaccine is administered within 72 hours of exposure.

Determinants of Response

Vaccine immunogenicity and response is determined by characteristics of the vaccine and the host. Vaccine dose, presence of an adjuvant, route and site of administration, timing of doses, and vaccine handling can affect response. Vaccine doses are adjusted before licensure to ensure a high level of response (generally >90% of subjects); adjuvants permit a better response with a lower dose of inactivated antigen. The routes of administration (e.g., intradermal, subcutaneous, intramuscular, and mucosal) can determine the strength and nature of the immune response. Mucosal administration (intranasal or oral) stimulates higher levels of mucosal IgA antibodies that can inhibit disease transmission with greater effectiveness than parenteral administration, which induces limited or no mucosal response.[16] Intradermal vaccination with lower antigen doses can induce antibody responses similar to responses induced by intramuscular or subcutaneous administration of recommended doses, but intradermal vaccine is more difficult to deliver precisely and, in practice, achieves less predictable responses.

Sites of Administration

Intramuscular injections should be given in the anterior thigh (infants and toddlers) or deltoid muscle (children and adults); injection into the buttocks may produce lower antibody response, which has been documented for hepatitis B and rabies vaccines in adults, probably owing to delivery of vaccine into adipose tissue.[17,18] Vaccines with adjuvants should be given in deep muscle, because subcutaneous or intradermal injection can induce local inflammation, granuloma formation, or necrosis.[19] Timing of doses of killed vaccines is important; a minimal interval of 1 month between primary doses is usual,[8] as is delay of a fourth or reinforcing dose for 10 months or longer after the first dose to enhance response and duration of antibody persistence. The recommended routes and sites of administration and timing of doses are devised to ensure optimal effectiveness in disease prevention and should be used.

Host Factors

Intrinsic factors in the host that affect immune response include genetic factors,[20,21] age, nutritional or disease status, primary or secondary immunodeficiency, sex, pregnancy, and smoking. Although genetic factors such as MHC polymorphism are known to affect both cellular and humoral immune response at a molecular level for some vaccines, the precise mechanisms for these genetic influences often are unknown.[20-22] Age is an important factor in response to immunization. With killed vaccines, neonates generally do not develop as brisk a response as older infants or children (i.e., hepatitis B), and with certain vaccines, too early immunization can result in poor response or development of tolerance or interference (DTaP, inactivated poliovirus vaccine (IPV), Hib conjugates). For live (and some killed) vaccines, inhibition of response by maternal antibodies determines the optimal timing for vaccination in early childhood (measles, hepatitis A). Generally, response to all vaccines is excellent in young children, adolescents, and young adults but diminishes with increasing age. In adults, pregnancy and male sex have minor dampening effects on antibody response, with limited significance; smoking decreases response to many antigens and may raise risk of nonresponse to vaccination when other negative factors are present.[17,19] Extreme debilitation, primary or secondary immunodeficiency disorders (including diseases or treatments that cause immunosuppression) and some chronic diseases (renal disease, diabetes mellitus) can diminish immune response. For people with such conditions, inactivated vaccines may be recommended although higher or more frequent doses may be required; live vaccines often are contraindicated because of the risk of disseminated disease and possible death due to the vaccine organism.[19,23]

Measurement of Response

Ideally, reliable laboratory tests should be available to measure the presence and strength of each of the major effectors of protection against the disease for which the vaccination is administered. In routine practice, a wide variety of tests are available to assess presence, absence, and level of antibodies. These include enzyme immunoassay (EIA), complement fixation, and immunofluorescent techniques. Assays for functional antibody, such as neutralization or opsonophagocytosis, generally are performed in reference or research laboratories, as are tests for T-lymphocyte function. CD4+ Th1 and Th2 lymphocytes and CD8+ lymphocytes generally are characterized by their cytokine profiles using assays such as ELISpot or intracellular cytoplasmic staining.

For certain diseases, such as hepatitis B, poliovirus, rubella, and measles, reliable tests exist and antibody levels that correlate with protection are known. For some diseases, such as pertussis, no serologic correlate of protection has been defined. Development of improved laboratory methods to measure protection and to permit rapid diagnosis of acute disease continues to be a priority of vaccine-preventable disease control programs.

Vaccine Licensure and Approval

Before U.S. Food and Drug Administration (FDA) licensure, a new vaccine generally requires 10 to 15 years of preclinical testing and clinical trials. Prior to testing a vaccine in humans, a manufacturer files an investigational new drug (IND) application with the FDA, followed by three phases of clinical trials that are performed to study vaccine safety, immunogenicity, and efficacy.[24,25] Following completion of the prelicensure clinical trials, the following steps are required: the manufacturer must apply for a Biologics Licensure Application (BLA) with the FDA; the FDA must license the vaccine; the Advisory Committee on Immunization Practices (ACIP) of the Centers for Disease Control and Prevention (CDC), the American Academy of Family Physicians (AAFP), and the Committee on Infectious Diseases (COID) of the American Academy of Pediatrics (AAP) must recommend the vaccine for use in children and adolescents; and financing for the vaccine must be secured for people in the public and private sectors (Figure 6-1). The ACIP, AAFP, the American College of Obstetricians and Gynecologists (ACOG), the American College of Nurse-Midwives the American College of Physicians make recommendations for and use of vaccines in the adult schedule.

Following FDA licensure of a new vaccine, information about the vaccine is reviewed by the ACIP. The ACIP is comprised of 15 voting members appointed by the Secretary of the Department of Health and Human Services. In addition, many professional medical and public health societies and organizations and industry representatives participate in ACIP discussions. To formulate recommendations, the ACIP establishes subject-specific work groups to review and synthesize data months to years before presentation to the ACIP where votes are taken on vaccine use. ACIP recommendations are subject to the approval of the director of the CDC (www.cdc.gov/vaccines/recs/acip/charter.htm). The COID of the AAP also develops recommendations for vaccine use in children and adolescents, which are approved by the Board of Directors of the AAP. The AAP recommendations usually are the same as, or similar to, recommendations of the ACIP.

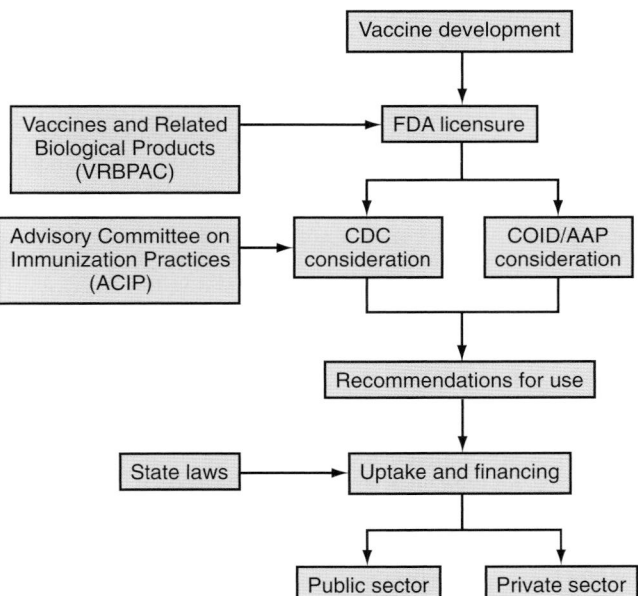

Figure 6-1. Development of pediatric vaccine recommendations and policies. FDA, Food and Drug Administration; CDC, Centers for Disease Control and Prevention; COID, Committee on Infectious Diseases; AAP, American Academy of Pediatrics, Board of Directors. (Redrawn from Pickering LK, Orenstein WA. Development of pediatric vaccine recommendations and policies. Semin Pediatr Infect Dis 2002;13:148–154, with permission.)

Following vaccine licensure, monitoring for rare adverse events continues for some vaccines through formal phase IV trials conducted by the manufacturer, which often are required and monitored by the FDA. In addition, postmarketing surveillance for adverse events is performed and permits detection of new or unanticipated adverse events. Reporting of adverse events observed after vaccine administration is required by the National Childhood Vaccine Injury Act for vaccines covered under the Vaccine Injury Compensation Program (VICP).[26] The importance of postmarketing surveillance was demonstrated following licensure and wide use of tetravalent rhesus rotavirus vaccine (RRV) in the U.S. for infants in 1999. Surveillance of adverse events detected cases of intussusception within 1 week after receipt of the first or second doses of RRV. Follow-up studies determined that risk of intussusception was 1 case per 10,000 doses of vaccine administered.[27] Subsequently, the vaccine was withdrawn from distribution, and recommendation for universal use in infants in the U.S. was withdrawn.[28]

PRINCIPLES OF IMMUNIZATION PROGRAMS

Disease Reduction

Childhood immunization programs have reduced substantially the occurrence of vaccine-preventable diseases in the U.S. from the representative annual morbidity during the 20th century (Table 6-1).[29-31] Declines exceed 95% for all diseases for which universal vaccination has been well implemented, with the exception of hepatitis B, which remains a common clinical disease in adults not reached by universal vaccine programs,[32] and pertussis.[33] Smallpox has been eradicated, poliomyelitis due to indigenous wild poliovirus has not occurred since 1979 in the U.S., and endemic rubella has been declared eliminated in the U.S.[34,35] Fewer than 10 cases each of diphtheria and tetanus in children are now reported each year, and indigenous transmission of measles has been interrupted. Wide use of Hib conjugate vaccines has reduced Hib disease by >98% in the U.S. and in some European countries.[36,37] Use of PCV has led to marked reductions in invasive pneumococcal disease among vaccinated children as well as unvaccinated young infants, adolescents, and adults.[38-41] Building on the success of the program to date, the U.S. Public Health Service established 2010 goals to eliminate indigenous transmission of measles, rubella and congenital rubella syndrome, mumps, diphtheria, poliomyelitis, Hib disease in children <5 years of age, and tetanus in people <35 years of age, and to reduce hepatitis B in people 2 through 18 years of age by 90%.[42] These goals were achieved for measles, rubella, congenital rubella, poliomyelitis, and hepatitis B. The new Healthy People 2020 objectives include specific goals for the vaccination of adolescents, including 1 dose of Tdap, and ≥2 doses of varicella vaccine (excluding persons who have had varicella disease) (http://www.healthypeople.gov/hp2020/objectives/topicarea.aspx?id=30&topicarea=immunization+and+infectious+diseases).

Immunization Coverage

Immunization coverage among preschool children has increased steadily after the measles resurgence that began in 1989 and stimulated unprecedented efforts to improve delivery of immunization. In 2010, coverage with three doses of DTaP, polio, and hepatitis B virus (HBV) vaccines, and one dose of MMR vaccine among children 19 through 35 months of age each reached or exceeded 92%, whereas coverage with ≥1 dose of varicella vaccine was 90%.[43] Among school-aged children as well as attendees of childcare centers and Head Start programs, coverage with recommended vaccines has exceeded 95% since the early 1980s, as a result of enforcement of comprehensive state immunization laws requiring receipt of specified vaccines for school attendance. School laws now are being expanded to include newly recommended vaccines.[44] In 2010, 69% of adolescents received one dose of Tdap vaccine, 63% received one dose of MCV4 vaccine, and 32% of females received three doses of HPV vaccine.[45]

TABLE 6-1. Reported Morbidity of Selected Vaccine-Preventable Diseases and Vaccine Coverage Levels – United States, 20th Century and 2010

Disease	United States, 20th-Century Annual Morbidity[a]	United States, 2010 Morbidity[b]	Vaccine Coverage Levels, 2009 %[c]	Healthy People 2010 Coverage Level Goals	Reduction in Morbidity
Diphtheria	175,885	0	84% (≥4 doses)	90%	100%
Tetanus	1314	8	84% (≥4 doses)	90%	99.4%
Pertussis	147,271	21,291	84% (≥4 doses)	90%	86%
Poliomyelitis (paralytic)	16,316	0	93%[d] (≥3 doses)	90%	100%
Measles	503,282	61	90% (≥1 dose)	90%	99.9%
Mumps	152,209	2528	90% (≥1 dose)	90%	98.4%
Congenital rubella	823	0	90% (≥1 dose)	90%	100%
Acquired rubella	47,745	6	90% (≥1 dose)	90%	90%
Haemophilus influenzae type b and unknown; <5 years of age	20,000	270	92% (≥2 or 3 doses, depending on brand)	90%	
Varicella	Unknown	16,207	90% (≥1 dose)	90%	

[a]MMWR 2004;53:687–696, number of reported cases.

[b]CDC. MMWR January 7, 2011;59(52):1704–1716, (provisional MMWR week 52 data).

[c]National Immunization Survey, 2009. Accessed 02/07/11 at www.cdc.gov/vaccines/stats-surv/nis/data/tables_2009.htm

[d]Inactivated poliovirus vaccine.

Vaccine Administration

Vaccine Schedules

The CDC, the AAFP, and AAP annually publish harmonized childhood and adolescent immunization schedules. The ACIP, AAFP, and ACP also publish an annual adult immunization schedule (www.cdc.gov/vaccines).[45a] The ACIP, with input from many liaison organizations, periodically reviews the schedules to ensure consistency with new vaccine developments and policies. The first harmonized childhood immunization schedule was published in 1995 and recommended 6 vaccines containing antigens against 9 infectious diseases:[46] diphtheria and tetanus toxoids and whole-cell pertussis vaccine (DTP); Td; MMR; Hib; oral poliovirus vaccine (OPV); and HBV vaccine. Since November 2010, vaccines have been recommended universally in the childhood and adolescent immunization schedule to protect against 16 infectious diseases (Figures 6-2, 6-3 and 6-4). The harmonized schedule specifies both timing and the acceptable range of timing recommended for each dose of universally recommended vaccine and for vaccines recommended for children and adolescents in selected high-risk populations.

Since inception, the major focus of the U.S. immunization program has been immunization of infants and young children. In 1996, following growing concern about morbidity associated with vaccine-preventable diseases in the hard-to-reach adolescent population, the ACIP recommended expanding efforts to immunize adolescents (11 through 18 years of age) by establishing a routine vaccination visit at 11 to 12 years of age.[47] In addition to providing Td and previously missed vaccinations, the report emphasized that this visit should be used to provide other important preventive health services. The addition of several new vaccines for adolescents (tetravalent MCV (MCV4), tetanus toxoid and reduced-content diphtheria toxoid and acellular pertussis vaccine (Tdap) and HPV) to the recommended schedule has stimulated a reappraisal of approaches that will most effectively and efficiently increase the proportion of adolescents who receive newly recommended vaccines and develop ways to integrate these approaches into other adolescent health, education, and development programs.[48]

Vaccine Spacing

Minimal spacing of vaccine doses generally is 1 month for the initial doses of killed vaccines; longer intervals are needed for booster doses to provide optimal responses.[8] For children with delayed initiation of immunization (after 6 months of age), an accelerated schedule is recommended (Figure 6-2).[8,49] To optimize adherence to the schedule in this circumstance, visits should be scheduled at 1-month intervals, and all recommended vaccines should be given at each visit. There is no need to restart any of the vaccine series among people with long delays between doses. The minimal spacing for MMR-containing vaccines is 28 days.

Simultaneous Administration

All childhood vaccines can be administered simultaneously. This practice is based on extrapolation of data from multiple studies showing that most vaccines can be administered at the same time without compromising safety or immunogenicity.[50] Thus, DTaP, Hib, IPV, HBV, PCV, MMR, varicella, and rotavirus vaccines (RV) can be administered simultaneously, and for inactivated vaccines within any interval of one another when otherwise indicated.[8,49] It is possible that Menactra's MCV4 vaccine interferes with the immune response to PCV13. Interference between live virus vaccines other than OPV and rotavirus (e.g., MMR and varicella) theoretically can occur if they are given within a short interval; live virus vaccines should be given either simultaneously or at least 1 month apart. Vaccines should not be mixed in the same syringe unless specifically licensed for such use. Interference has been found between certain vaccines (cholera and yellow fever).

Spacing of Antibody-Containing Products and Vaccines

Immunoglobulins or blood products containing immunoglobulins inhibit response to certain live-virus vaccines (MMR and possibly varicella). The duration of inhibition of response is related to the dose of immunoglobulin delivered, and algorithms for calculating appropriate delays of MMR after receipt of such products are available.[19,49,51] In general, MMR vaccines should be delayed 3 months or longer after administration of usual doses of immunoglobulin (e.g., to prevent hepatitis A) or blood products, and for longer periods of time after higher doses (e.g., ≥10 months after 2 g/kg immune globulin intravenous administered for treatment of Kawasaki disease).

Interchangeability of Vaccines

Available data support interchangeability of most vaccines produced by different manufacturers to prevent the same disease

Vaccine ▼　　　　Age ►	Birth	1 month	2 months	4 months	6 months	9 months	12 months	15 months	18 months	19–23 months	2–3 years	4–6 years	
Hepatitis B[1]	Hep B	HepB					HepB						Range of recommended ages for all children
Rotavirus[2]			RV	RV	RV[2]								
Diphtheria, tetanus, pertussis[3]			DTaP	DTaP	DTaP		see footnote[3]	DTaP				DTaP	
Haemophilus influenzae type b[4]			Hib	Hib	Hib[4]		Hib						
Pneumococcal[5]			PCV	PCV	PCV		PCV				PPSV		Range of recommended ages for certain high-risk groups
Inactivated poliovirus[6]			IPV	IPV	IPV							IPV	
Influenza[7]					Influenza (Yearly)								
Measles, mumps, rubella[8]							MMR		see footnote[8]			MMR	Range of recommended ages for all children and certain high-risk groups
Varicella[9]							Varicella		see footnote[9]			Varicella	
Hepatitis A[10]							Dose 1[10]				HepA Series		
Meningococcal[11]							MCV4 — see footnote[11]						

This schedule includes recommendations in effect as of December 23, 2011. Any dose not administered at the recommended age should be administered at a subsequent visit, when indicated and feasible. The use of a combination vaccine generally is preferred over separate injections of its equivalent component vaccines. Vaccination providers should consult the relevant Advisory Committee on Immunization Practices (ACIP) statement for detailed recommendations, available online at http://www.cdc.gov/vaccines/pubs/acip-list.htm. Clinically significant adverse events that follow vaccination should be reported to the Vaccine Adverse Event Reporting System (VAERS) online (http://www.vaers.hhs.gov) or by telephone (800-822-7967).

1. **Hepatitis B (HepB) vaccine.** (Minimum age: birth)
   At birth:
   • Administer monovalent HepB vaccine to all newborns before hospital discharge.
   • For infants born to hepatitis B surface antigen (HBsAg)–positive mothers, administer HepB vaccine and 0.5 mL of hepatitis B immune globulin (HBIG) within 12 hours of birth. These infants should be tested for HBsAg and antibody to HBsAg (anti-HBs) 1 to 2 months after completion of at least 3 doses of the HepB series, at age 9 through 18 months (generally at the next well-child visit).
   • If mother's HBsAg status is unknown, within 12 hours of birth administer HepB vaccine for infants weighing ≥2,000 grams, and HepB vaccine plus HBIG for infants weighing <2,000 grams. Determine mother's HBsAg status as soon as possible and, if she is HBsAg-positive, administer HBIG for infants weighing ≥2,000 grams (no later than age 1 week).
   Doses after the birth dose:
   • The second dose should be administered at age 1 to 2 months. Monovalent HepB vaccine should be used for doses administered before age 6 weeks.
   • Administration of a total of 4 doses of HepB vaccine is permissible when a combination vaccine containing HepB is administered after the birth dose.
   • Infants who did not receive a birth dose should receive 3 doses of a HepB-containing vaccine starting as soon as feasible (Figure 3).
   • The minimum interval between dose 1 and dose 2 is 4 weeks, and between dose 2 and 3 is 8 weeks. The final (third or fourth) dose in the HepB vaccine series should be administered no earlier than age 24 weeks and at least 16 weeks after the first dose.
2. **Rotavirus (RV) vaccines.** (Minimum age: 6 weeks for both RV-1 [Rotarix] and RV-5 [Rota Teq])
   • The maximum age for the first dose in the series is 14 weeks, 6 days; and 8 months, 0 days for the final dose in the series. Vaccination should not be initiated for infants aged 15 weeks, 0 days or older.
   • If RV-1 (Rotarix) is administered at ages 2 and 4 months, a dose at 6 months is not indicated.
3. **Diphtheria and tetanus toxoids and acellular pertussis (DTaP) vaccine.** (Minimum age: 6 weeks)
   • The fourth dose may be administered as early as age 12 months, provided at least 6 months have elapsed since the third dose.
4. **Haemophilus influenzae type b (Hib) conjugate vaccine.** (Minimum age: 6 weeks)
   • If PRP-OMP (PedvaxHIB or Comvax [HepB-Hib]) is administered at ages 2 and 4 months, a dose at age 6 months is not indicated.
   • Hiberix should only be used for the booster (final) dose in children aged 12 months through 4 years.
5. **Pneumococcal vaccines.** (Minimum age: 6 weeks for pneumococcal conjugate vaccine [PCV]; 2 years for pneumococcal polysaccharide vaccine [PPSV])
   • Administer 1 dose of PCV to all healthy children aged 24 through 59 months who are not completely vaccinated for their age.
   • For children who have received an age-appropriate series of 7-valent PCV (PCV7), a single supplemental dose of 13-valent PCV (PCV13) is recommended for:
     — All children 14 through 59 months
     — Children aged 60 through 71 months with underlying medical conditions.
   • Administer PPSV at least 8 weeks after last dose of PCV to children aged 2 years or older with underlying medical conditions, including a cochlear implant. See MMWR 2010:59(No. RR-11), available at http://www.cdc.gov/mmwr/pdf/rr/rr5911.pdf.
6. **Inactivated poliovirus vaccine (IPV).** (Minimum age: 6 weeks)
   • If 4 or more doses are administered before age 4 years, an additional dose should be administered at age 4 through 6 years.
   • The final dose in the series should be administered on or after the fourth birthday and at least 6 months after the previous dose.

7. **Influenza vaccines.** (Minimum age: 6 months for trivalent inactivated influenza vaccine [TIV]; 2 years for live, attenuated influenza vaccine [LAIV])
   • For most healthy children aged 2 years and older, either LAIV or TIV may be used. However, LAIV should not be administered to some children, including 1) children with asthma, 2) children 2 through 4 years who had wheezing in the past 12 months, or 3) children who have any other underlying medical conditions that predispose them to influenza complications. For all other contraindications to use of LAIV, see MMWR 2010;59(No. RR-8), available at http://www.cdc.gov/mmwr/pdf/rr/rr5908.pdf.
   • For children aged 6 months through 8 years:
     — For the 2011–12 season, administer 2 doses (separated by at least 4 weeks) to those who did not receive at least 1 dose of the 2010–11 vaccine. Those who received at least 1 dose of the 2010–11 vaccine require 1 dose for the 2011–12 season.
     — For the 2012–13 season, follow dosing guidelines in the 2012 ACIP influenza vaccine recommendations.
8. **Measles, mumps, and rubella (MMR) vaccine.** (Minimum age: 12 months)
   • The second dose may be administered before age 4 years, provided at least 4 weeks have elapsed since the first dose.
   • Administer MMR vaccine to infants aged 6 through 11 months who are traveling internationally. These children should be revaccinated with 2 doses of MMR vaccine, the first at ages 12 through 15 months and at least 4 weeks after the previous dose, and the second at ages 4 through 6 years.
9. **Varicella (VAR) vaccine.** (Minimum age: 12 months)
   • The second dose may be administered before age 4 years, provided at least 3 months have elapsed since the first dose.
   • For children aged 12 months through 12 years, the recommended minimum interval between doses is 3 months. However, if the second dose was administered at least 4 weeks after the first dose, it can be accepted as valid.
10. **Hepatitis A (HepA) vaccine.** (Minimum age: 12 months)
    • Administer the second (final) dose 6 to18 months after the first.
    • Unvaccinated children 24 months and older at high risk should be vaccinated. See MMWR 2006;55(No. RR-7), available at http://www.cdc.gov/mmwr/pdf/rr/rr5507.pdf.
    • A 2-dose HepA vaccine series is recommended for anyone aged 24 months and older, previously unvaccinated, for whom immunity against hepatitis A virus infection is desired.
11. **Meningococcal conjugate vaccines, quadrivalent (MCV4).** (Minimum age: 9 months for Menactra [MCV4-D], 2 years for Menveo [MCV4-CRM])
    • For children aged 9 through 23 months 1) with persistent complement component deficiency; 2) who are residents of or travelers to countries with hyperendemic or epidemic disease; or 3) who are present during outbreaks caused by a vaccine serogroup, administer 2 primary doses of MCV4-D, ideally at ages 9 months and 12 months or at least 8 weeks apart.
    • For children aged 24 months and older with 1) persistent complement component deficiency who have not been previously vaccinated; or 2) anatomic/functional asplenia, administer 2 primary doses of either MCV4 at least 8 weeks apart.
    • For children with anatomic/functional asplenia, if MCV4-D (Menactra) is used, administer at a minimum age of 2 years and at least 4 weeks after completion of all PCV doses.
    • See MMWR 2011;60:72–6, available at http://www.cdc.gov/mmwr/pdf/wk/mm6003. pdf, and Vaccines for Children Program resolution No. 6/11-1, available at http://www. cdc.gov/vaccines/programs/vfc/downloads/resolutions/06-11mening-mcv.pdf, and MMWR 2011;60:1391–2, available at http://www.cdc.gov/mmwr/pdf/wk/mm6040. pdf, for further guidance, including revaccination guidelines.

This schedule is approved by the Advisory Committee on Immunization Practices (http://www.cdc.gov/vaccines/recs/acip), the American Academy of Pediatrics (http://www.aap.org), and the American Academy of Family Physicians (http://www.aafp.org). Department of Health and Human Services • Centers for Disease Control and Prevention Recommended immunization schedules for persons aged 0–18 years – United States, 2012. MMWR 2012;61(5):1-2

Figure 6-2. Recommended immunization schedule for persons aged 0 through 6 years – United States, 2012 (for those who fall behind or start late, see the catch-up schedule [Figure 6-4]).

Vaccine ▼ Age ▶	7–10 years	11–12 years	13–18 years	
Tetanus, diphtheria, pertussis[1]	1 dose (if indicated)	1 dose	1 dose (if indicated)	Range of recommended ages for all children
Human papillomavirus[2]	See footnote[2]	3 doses	Complete 3-dose series	
Meningococcal[3]	See footnote[3]	Dose 1	Booster at age 16 years	
Influenza[4]	Influenza (yearly)			Range of recomended ages for catch-up immunization
Pneumococcal[5]	See footnote[5]			
Hepatitis A[6]	Complete 2-dose series			
Hepatitis B[7]	Complete 3-dose series			
Inactivated poliovirus[8]	Complete 3-dose series			Range of recommended ages for certain high-risk groups
Measles, mumps, rubella[9]	Complete 2-dose series			
Varicella[10]	Complete 2-dose series			

This schedule includes recommendations in effect as of December 23, 2011. Any dose not administered at the recommended age should be administered at a subsequent visit, when indicated and feasible. The use of a combination vaccine generally is preferred over separate injections of its equivalent component vaccines. Vaccination providers should consult the relevant Advisory Committee on Immunization Practices (ACIP) statement for detailed recommendations, available online at http://www.cdc.gov/vaccines/pubs/acip-list.htm. Clinically significant adverse events that follow vaccination should be reported to the Vaccine Adverse Event Reporting System (VAERS) online (http://www.vaers.hhs.gov) or by telephone (800-822-7967).

1. **Tetanus and diphtheria toxoids and acellular pertussis (Tdap) vaccine.** (Minimum age: 10 years for Boostrix and 11 years for Adacel)
   - Persons aged 11 through 18 years who have not received Tdap vaccine should receive a dose followed by tetanus and diphtheria toxoids (Td) booster doses every 10 years thereafter.
   - Tdap vaccine should be substituted for a single dose of Td in the catch-up series for children aged 7 through 10 years. Refer to the catch-up schedule if additional doses of tetanus and diphtheria toxoid–containing vaccine are needed.
   - Tdap vaccine can be administered regardless of the interval since the last tetanus and diphtheria toxoid–containing vaccine.
2. **Human papillomavirus (HPV) vaccines (HPV4 [Gardasil] and HPV2 [Cervarix]).** (Minimum age: 9 years)
   - Either HPV4 or HPV2 is recommended in a 3-dose series for females aged 11 or 12 years. HPV4 is recommended in a 3-dose series for males aged 11 or 12 years.
   - The vaccine series can be started beginning at age 9 years.
   - Administer the second dose 1 to 2 months after the first dose and the third dose 6 months after the first dose (at least 24 weeks after the first dose).
   - See *MMWR* 2010;59:626–32, available at http://www.cdc.gov/mmwr/pdf/wk/mm5920.pdf.
3. **Meningococcal conjugate vaccines, quadrivalent (MCV4).**
   - Administer MCV4 at age 11 through 12 years with a booster dose at age 16 years.
   - Administer MCV4 at age 13 through 18 years if patient is not previously vaccinated.
   - If the first dose is administered at age 13 through 15 years, a booster dose should be administered at age 16 through 18 years with a minimum interval of at least 8 weeks after the preceding dose.
   - If the first dose is administered at age 16 years or older, a booster dose is not needed.
   - Administer 2 primary doses at least 8 weeks apart to previously unvaccinated persons with persistent complement component deficiency or anatomic/functional asplenia, and 1 dose every 5 years thereafter.
   - Adolescents aged 11 through 18 years with human immunodeficiency virus (HIV) infection should receive a 2-dose primary series of MCV4, at least 8 weeks apart.
   - See *MMWR* 2011;60:72–76, available at http://www.cdc.gov/mmwr/pdf/wk/mm6003.pdf, and Vaccines for Children Program resolution No. 6/11-1, available at http://www.cdc.gov/vaccines/programs/vfc/downloads/resolutions/06-11mening-mcv.pdf, for further guidelines.
4. **Influenza vaccines (trivalent inactivated influenza vaccine [TIV] and live, attenuated influenza vaccine [LAIV].**
   - For most healthy, nonpregnant persons, either LAIV or TIV may be used, except LAIV should not be used for some persons, including those with asthma or any other underlying medical conditions that predispose them to influenza complications. For all other contraindications to use of LAIV, see *MMWR* 2010;59(No.RR-8), available at http://www.cdc.gov/mmwr/pdf/rr/rr5908.pdf.
   - Administer 1 dose to persons aged 9 years and older.
   - For children aged 6 months through 8 years:
     — For the 2011–12 season, administer 2 doses (separated by at least 4 weeks) to those who did not receive at least 1 dose of the 2010–11 vaccine. Those who received at least 1 dose of the 2010–11 vaccine require 1 dose for the 2011–12 season.
     — For the 2012–13 season, follow dosing guidelines in the 2012 ACIP influenza vaccine recommendations.

5. **Pneumococcal vaccines (pneumococcal conjugate vaccine [PCV] and pneumococcal polysaccharide vaccine [PPSV]).**
   - A single dose of PCV may be administered to children aged 6 through 18 years who have anatomic/functional asplenia, HIV infection or other immunocompromising condition, cochlear implant, or cerebral spinal fluid leak. See *MMWR* 2010:59(No. RR-11), available at http://www.cdc.gov/mmwr/pdf/rr/rr5911.pdf.
   - Administer PPSV at least 8 weeks after the last dose of PCV to children aged 2 years or older with certain underlying medical conditions, including a cochlear implant. A single revaccination should be administered after 5 years to children with anatomic/functional asplenia or an immunocompromising condition.
6. **Hepatitis A (HepA) vaccine.**
   - HepA vaccine is recommended for children older than 23 months who live in areas where vaccination programs target older children, who are at increased risk for infection, or for whom immunity against hepatitis A virus infection is desired. See *MMWR* 2006;55(No. RR-7), available at http://www.cdc.gov/mmwr/pdf/rr/rr5507.pdf.
   - Administer 2 doses at least 6 months apart to unvaccinated persons.
7. **Hepatitis B (HepB) vaccine.**
   - Administer the 3-dose series to those not previously vaccinated.
   - For those with incomplete vaccination, follow the catch-up recommendations (Figure 3).
   - A 2-dose series (doses separated by at least 4 months) of adult formulation Recombivax HB is licensed for use in children aged 11 through 15 years.
8. **Inactivated poliovirus vaccine (IPV).**
   - The final dose in the series should be administered at least 6 months after the previous dose.
   - If both OPV and IPV were administered as part of a series, a total of 4 doses should be administered, regardless of the child's current age.
   - IPV is not routinely recommended for U.S. residents aged 18 years or older.
9. **Measles, mumps, and rubella (MMR) vaccine.**
   - The minimum interval between the 2 doses of MMR vaccine is 4 weeks.
10. **Varicella (VAR) vaccine.**
   - For persons without evidence of immunity (see *MMWR* 2007;56[No. RR-4], available at http://www.cdc.gov/mmwr/pdf/rr/rr5604.pdf), administer 2 doses if not previously vaccinated or the second dose if only 1 dose has been administered.
   - For persons aged 7 through 12 years, the recommended minimum interval between doses is 3 months. However, if the second dose was administered at least 4 weeks after the first dose, it can be accepted as valid.
   - For persons aged 13 years and older, the minimum interval between doses is 4 weeks.

This schedule is approved by the Advisory Committee on Immunization Practices (http://www.cdc.gov/vaccines/recs/acip),
the American Academy of Pediatrics (http://www.aap.org), and the American Academy of Family Physicians (http://www.aafp.org).
Centers for Disease Control and Prevention. Recommended immunization schedules for persons aged 0–18 years – United States, 2012. MMWR 2012; 61(5):3

Figure 6-3. Recommended immunization schedule for persons aged 7 through 18 years – United States, 2012 (for those who fall behind or start late, see the schedule below and the catch-up schedule [Figure 6-4]).

Vaccine	Minimum Age for Dose 1	Minimum Interval Between Doses			
		Dose 1 to dose 2	Dose 2 to dose 3	Dose 3 to dose 4	Dose 4 to dose 5
Persons aged 4 months through 6 years					
Hepatitis B	Birth	4 weeks	8 weeks and at least 16 weeks after first dose; minimum age for the final dose is 24 weeks		
Rotavirus[1]	6 weeks	4 weeks	4 weeks[1]		
Diphtheria, tetanus, pertussis[2]	6 weeks	4 weeks	4 weeks	6 months	6 months[2]
Haemophilus influenzae type b[3]	6 weeks	4 weeks if first dose administered at younger than age 12 months / 8 weeks (as final dose) if first dose administered at age 12–14 months / No further doses needed if first dose administered at 15 months or older	4 weeks[3] if current age is younger than 12 months / 8 weeks (as final dose)[3] if current age is 12 months or older and first dose administered at younger than age 12 months and second dose administered at younger than 15 months / No further doses needed if previous dose administered at age 15 months or older	8 weeks (as final dose) This dose only necessary for children aged 12 months through 59 months who received 3 doses before 12 months	
Pneumococcal[4]	6 weeks	4 weeks if first dose administered at younger than age 12 months / 8 weeks (as final dose for healthy children) if first dose administered at age 12 months or older or current age 24 through 59 months / No further doses needed for healthy children if first dose administered at age 24 months or older	4 weeks if current age is younger than 12 months / 8 weeks (as final dose for healthy children) if current age is 12 months or older / No further doses needed for healthy children if previous dose administered at age 24 months or older	8 weeks (as final dose) This dose only necessary for children aged 12 months through 59 months who received 3 doses before age 12 months or for children at high risk who received 3 doses at any age	
Inactivated poliovirus[5]	6 weeks	4 weeks	4 weeks	6 months[5] minimum age 4 years for final dose	
Meningococcal[6]	9 months	8 weeks[6]			
Measles, mumps, rubella[7]	12 months	4 weeks			
Varicella[8]	12 months	3 months			
Hepatitis A	12 months	6 months			
Persons aged 7 through 18 years					
Tetanus, diphtheria/ tetanus, diphtheria, pertussis[9]	7 years[9]	4 weeks	4 weeks if first dose administered at younger than age 12 months / 6 months if first dose administered at 12 months or older	6 months if first dose administered at younger than age 12 months	
Human papillomavirus[10]	9 years	Routine dosing intervals are recommended[10]			
Hepatitis A	12 months	6 months			
Hepatitis B	Birth	4 weeks	8 weeks (and at least 16 weeks after first dose)		
Inactivated poliovirus[5]	6 weeks	4 weeks	4 weeks[5]	6 months[5]	
Meningococcal[6]	9 months	8 weeks[6]			
Measles, mumps, rubella[7]	12 months	4 weeks			
Varicella[8]	12 months	3 months if person is younger than age 13 years / 4 weeks if person is aged 13 years or older			

1. **Rotavirus (RV) vaccines (RV-1 [Rotarix] and RV-5 [Rota Teq]).**
   - The maximum age for the first dose in the series is 14 weeks, 6 days; and 8 months, 0 days for the final dose in the series. Vaccination should not be initiated for infants aged 15 weeks, 0 days or older.
   - If RV-1 was administered for the first and second doses, a third dose is not indicated.
2. **Diphtheria and tetanus toxoids and acellular pertussis (DTaP) vaccine.**
   - The fifth dose is not necessary if the fourth dose was administered at age 4 years or older.
3. ***Haemophilus influenzae* type b (Hib) conjugate vaccine.**
   - Hib vaccine should be considered for unvaccinated persons aged 5 years or older who have sickle cell disease, leukemia, human immunodeficiency virus (HIV) infection, or anatomic/functional asplenia.
   - If the first 2 doses were PRP-OMP (PedvaxHIB or Comvax) and were administered at age 11 months or younger, the third (and final) dose should be administered at age 12 through 15 months and at least 8 weeks after the second dose.
   - If the first dose was administered at age 7 through 11 months, administer the second dose at least 4 weeks later and a final dose at age 12 through 15 months.
4. **Pneumococcal vaccines.** (Minimum age: 6 weeks for pneumococcal conjugate vaccine [PCV]; 2 years for pneumococcal polysaccharide vaccine [PPSV])
   - For children aged 24 through 71 months with underlying medical conditions, administer 1 dose of PCV if 3 doses of PCV were received previously, or administer 2 doses of PCV at least 8 weeks apart if fewer than 3 doses of PCV were received previously.
   - A single dose of PCV may be administered to certain children aged 6 through 18 years with underlying medical conditions. See age-specific schedules for details.
   - Administer PPSV to children aged 2 years or older with certain underlying medical conditions. See *MMWR* 2010:59(No. RR-11), available at http://www.cdc.gov/mmwr/pdf/rr/rr5911.pdf.

5. **Inactivated poliovirus vaccine (IPV).**
   - A fourth dose is not necessary if the third dose was administered at age 4 years or older and at least 6 months after the previous dose.
   - In the first 6 months of life, minimum age and minimum intervals are only recommended if the person is at risk for imminent exposure to circulating poliovirus (i.e., travel to a polio-endemic region or during an outbreak).
   - IPV is not routinely recommended for U.S. residents aged 18 years or older.
6. **Meningococcal conjugate vaccines, quadrivalent (MCV4).** (Minimum age: 9 months for Menactra [MCV4-D]; 2 years for Menveo [MCV4-CRM])
   - See Figure 1 ("Recommended immunization schedule for persons aged 0 through 6 years") and Figure 2 ("Recommended immunization schedule for persons aged 7 through 18 years") for further guidance.
7. **Measles, mumps, and rubella (MMR) vaccine.**
   - Administer the second dose routinely at age 4 through 6 years.
8. **Varicella (VAR) vaccine.**
   - Administer the second dose routinely at age 4 through 6 years. If the second dose was administered at least 4 weeks after the first dose, it can be accepted as valid.
9. **Tetanus and diphtheria toxoids (Td) and tetanus and diphtheria toxoids and acellular pertussis (Tdap) vaccines.**
   - For children aged 7 through 10 years who are not fully immunized with the childhood DTaP vaccine series, Tdap vaccine should be substituted for a single dose of Td vaccine in the catch-up series; if additional doses are needed, use Td vaccine. For these children, an adolescent Tdap vaccine dose should not be given.
   - An inadvertent dose of DTaP vaccine administered to children aged 7 through 10 years can count as part of the catch-up series. This dose can count as the adolescent Tdap dose, or the child can later receive a Tdap booster dose at age 11–12 years.
10. **Human papillomavirus (HPV) vaccines (HPV4 [Gardasil] and HPV2 [Cervarix]).**
    - Administer the vaccine series to females (either HPV2 or HPV4) and males (HPV4) at age 13 through 18 years if patient is not previously vaccinated.
    - Use recommended routine dosing intervals for vaccine series catch-up; see Figure 2 ("Recommended immunization schedule for persons aged 7 through 18 years").

Clinically significant adverse events that follow vaccination should be reported to the Vaccine Adverse Event Reporting System (VAERS) online (http://www.vaers.hhs.gov) or by telephone (800-822-7967). Suspected cases of vaccine-preventable diseases should be reported to the state or local health department. Additional information, including precautions and contraindications for vaccination, is available from CDC online (http://www.cdc.gov/vaccines) or by telephone (800-CDC-INFO [800-232-4636]). Centers for Disease Control and Prevention. Recommended immunization schedules for persons aged 0–18 years – United States, 2012. MMWR 2012;61(5):4

Figure 6-4. Catch-up immunization schedule for persons aged 4 months through 18 years who start late or who are more than 1 month behind – United States, 2012. The figure below provides catch-up schedules and minimum intervals between doses for children whose vaccinations have been delayed. A vaccine series does not need to be restarted, regardless of the time that has elapsed between doses. Use the section appropriate for the child's age. Always use this table in conjunction with the accompanying childhood and adolescent immunization schedules [Figures 6-2 and 6-3] and their respective footnotes.

(tetanus, diphtheria, hepatitis B, and hepatitis A). Studies indicate that response to a 3-dose series using different Hib conjugate vaccines equals or exceeds that when the same vaccine is used for all doses.[52] The ACIP and AAP recommend that, when feasible, the same vaccine should be used for the primary series but that three doses of any vaccine are sufficient.[8,49] Data are limited regarding safety, immunogenicity, and efficacy of using acellular pertussis (as DTaP) vaccines from different manufacturers for successive doses of the pertussis series. Data suggest that two of the current DTaP preparations can be used interchangeably for the first 3 doses of the DTaP series without affecting safety or immunogenicity.[53] When the specific product is not known or available, any DTaP vaccine should be used to continue or complete the series.

Vaccine Safety and Compensation for Vaccine Injury

In 1986, the National Childhood Vaccine Injury Act (NCVIA) was passed, creating a compensation program for families affected by childhood vaccine-associated adverse events. Several other government programs and committees to ensure safety of the vaccine supply also were created by this Act (Table 6-2).

Studies of Vaccine Safety

As many vaccine-preventable diseases approach or reach elimination in the U.S., continuing to balance the risks and benefits of each vaccine becomes increasingly important.[54] For example, OPV, formerly recommended for routine use in the U.S., was associated with vaccine-associated paralytic poliomyelitis (VAPP in 1 case among 2.5 million vaccine doses distributed). This rare adverse event was no longer considered acceptable following elimination of polio in the U.S. and in 2000, the ACIP recommended using IPV for all doses of polio vaccine.[55] Public perceptions of vaccine safety are a challenge to the continued success of the vaccination program. New parents and younger physicians grew up without

TABLE 6-2. National Childhood Vaccine Injury Act, 1986

National Vaccine Injury Compensation Program	• Limits manufacturer liability • Provides payments to families of children who sustain documented injuries following routine immunization
National Vaccine Program	• Develops and coordinates a comprehensive national vaccine plan
Advisory Commission on Childhood Vaccines	• Advises Secretary of Health and Human Services on injury compensation program
National Vaccine Advisory Committee	• Advises Secretary of Health and Human Services on national vaccine policy
Federal Excise Tax on Childhood Vaccines	• 1987 amendment to Compensation Act • Proceeds used to finance payments to families of children affected by a vaccine-associated adverse event

Data from Schwartz B, Orenstein WA. Vaccination policies and programs: the federal government's role in making the system work. Prim Care 2001;28:697–711.

appreciating the morbidity and mortality of several vaccine-preventable diseases. Therefore risk, or perception of risk, for adverse events becomes an important concern.

In the early 1990s, the Institute of Medicine (IOM) reviewed available information regarding the possible causality of serious adverse events after each of the then licensed childhood vaccines.[56–58] For many events, information was considered insufficient to determine causality. For some events, however, the investigating panels classified events more definitively, as follows: (1) evidence establishes definitively that vaccine plays a causal role; (2) evidence supports a causal role for the vaccine; and (3) evidence indicates that the vaccine definitely does not play a causal role. These events are summarized in Table 6-3. These investigations represented a comprehensive compilation of data on

TABLE 6-3. Summary of Institute of Medicine (IOM) Findings on the Relationship of Adverse Events to Individual Vaccines

Vaccine	Established Causation	Favoring Causation	Favoring Rejection of Causation
DT/Td/TT	Anaphylaxis	Guillain–Barré syndrome[a] Brachial neuritis	Encephalopathy Infantile spasms Death from SIDS
Pertussis (whole-cell) (DTP)	Anaphylaxis; protracted, inconsolable crying	Acute encephalopathy Shock and unusual shocklike state (hypotonic-hyporesponsive episode) Chronic encephalopathy (after acute encephalopathy)	Infantile spasms Hypoarrhythmia Reye syndrome SIDS
Measles	Death from measles vaccine strain in primarily immunocompromised individuals	Anaphylaxis	–
MMR	Anaphylaxis Thrombocytopenia	–	Autistic spectrum disorders
Mumps (see MMR)	–	–	–
OPV	Poliomyelitis Death from polio vaccine strain, mainly in immunocompromised people	Guillain–Barré syndrome[a]	–
IPV	–	–	–
Hepatitis B	Anaphylaxis	–	–
Hib (conjugate)	–	–	Early-onset *Haemophilus influenzae* b disease
Rubella[b] (see MMR)	Acute arthritis	Chronic arthritis	–

DT, diphtheria and tetanus toxoid; DTP, diphtheria and tetanus toxoid and pertussis (whole-cell) vaccine; Hib, Haemophilus influenzae type b conjugate vaccine; IPV, inactivated poliovirus vaccine; MMR, measles, mumps, and rubella vaccine; OPV, live oral poliovirus vaccine; SIDS, sudden infant death syndrome; T, tetanus toxoid; Td, tetanus and diphtheria toxoids.

[a]*The Advisory Committee on Immunization Practice of the United States Public Health Service disagreed with these IOM findings (see reference 33).*

[b]*Data were reviewed by an earlier IOM committee. Initial report categories corresponding to those table headings were "Evidence indicates a causal relationship, Evidence is consistent with a causal relationship," and "Evidence does not indicate a causal relationship."*

vaccine safety, although controversy persists regarding certain events. Reanalysis of available data on the occurrence of Guillain–Barré syndrome (GBS) after OPV suggests that evidence does not support causation.[59]

Two prominent public vaccine safety concerns are the perceived causal association of MMR with autism and thimerosal-containing vaccines with autism. As a result of continued concerns about vaccine safety, in 2000, the CDC and National Institutes of Health commissioned the National Academy of Science IOM to convene an Immunization Safety Review Committee.[60] Between 2001 and 2004, this independent expert committee published eight reports related to various immunization safety concerns. The committee has made recommendations in the areas of public health response, policy review, research, and communications for each of the eight subjects reviewed (Box 6-1). With respect to autism, the IOM concluded that the body of epidemiologic evidence favors rejection of a causal relationship between the MMR vaccine and autism. The committee also concluded that there is no relationship between thimerosal-containing vaccines and autism.[60] None of the eight IOM reports recommended a policy review of the current vaccine recommendations or change in the immunization schedule.

Monitoring of Vaccine Safety

To help ensure safety of vaccines, a robust infrastructure consisting of several systems has been established to monitor vaccine safety following vaccine licensure. The Vaccine Adverse Event Reporting System (VAERS), operated jointly by the CDC and FDA, is a national passive surveillance system used to detect early warning signals and generate hypotheses about possible new vaccine adverse events or changes in frequency of recognized events.[61] Intussusception associated with receipt of rotavirus vaccine, leading to withdrawal of the vaccine from the market in 1999, was an adverse event detected by VAERS.[27,28] A second system is the Vaccine Safety Datalink (VSD), which consists of large linked databases from health maintenance organizations.[54,62] Associations between serious medical events and immunizations can be evaluated through the VSD. A third system is the Clinical Immunization Safety Assessment centers network, which consists of selected clinical academic medical centers in partnership with CDC to study the pathophysiology of vaccine reactions and develop clinical management protocols for affected patients. These systems are crucial to the vitality and strength of the U.S. immunization program.

Reporting System for Adverse Events after Immunization

In addition to mandating review of causality of adverse events and creating a unified reporting system for adverse events after vaccination, the 1986 NCVIA established a program to provide compensation to people who experience permanent injury after vaccination.[26] A table of injuries eliciting automatic compensation was developed and has been revised on the basis of the findings of the IOM studies; in addition, any person who shows medical evidence of causality may be compensated. This program is funded by a special excise tax on each dose of vaccine ($0.75 per antigen) to which the program applies (at present, vaccines to prevent diphtheria, tetanus, pertussis, *Haemophilus influenza* type b infection, polio, measles, mumps, rubella, hepatitis A, hepatitis B, invasive pneumococcal disease, varicella, rotavirus, meningococcal disease, human papillomavirus infection, and influenza). People who believe they have been injured by vaccines should call 800-338-2382 or go to www.hrsa.gov/osp/vicp to obtain information or to file a claim.

Physicians should be aware of contraindications to and precautions for each vaccine as defined in package inserts and by the ACIP and AAP. To view the NCVIA Reporting and Compensation table and for qualifications and aids to interpretation of the table, go to www.hrsa.gov/vaccinecompensation/table.htm. Parents should be questioned about the presence of such conditions before any vaccine is administered to their children.

Vaccination in Special Situations

Infants Who Weigh Less Than 2000 Grams

Studies show that infants with birthweight <2000 grams may have a diminished response after administration of HBV vaccine at birth.[63] However, by 1 month chronologic age, all preterm infants, regardless of gestational age or weight at birth, are as likely to respond as older and larger infants.[19,49] Preterm infants born to hepatitis B surface antigen (HBsAg)-positive mothers and mothers with unknown HBsAg status should receive immunoprophylaxis with HBV vaccine and hepatitis B immunoglobulin (HBIG) within 12 hours of birth. If these infants weigh <2000 grams at birth, the initial vaccine dose should not be counted towards completion of the HBV vaccine series, and 3 additional doses of vaccine should be administered, beginning when the infant is 1 month of age. Preterm infants weighing <2000 grams and born to HBsAg-negative mothers should receive the first dose of the HBV vaccine series at 1 month of postnatal age (if medically stable) or at hospital discharge if the infant is younger than one month at discharge.

Pregnant Women

Risk of vaccination during pregnancy is largely theoretical. The benefit of vaccinating a pregnant woman may outweigh the risk when the risk for disease exposure is high; infection may harm the mother or infant, and the vaccine is unlikely to cause harm. Td or Tdap and influenza vaccines are indicated for susceptible pregnant women. Women's healthcare providers should implement a material Tdap vaccination program for women who have not previously received Tdap. Healthcare personnel (HCP) should administer Tdap preferably during the third or late trimester (after 20 weeks' gestation).[64] Alternatively administer Tdap immediately postpartum as part of the cocoon strategy (http://www.cdc.gov/vaccines/recs/acip/). Hepatitis B, hepatitis A, meningococcal and pneumococcal polysaccharide vaccines can be given to pregnant women at high risk for these diseases (see adult immunization schedule at www.cdc.gov/vaccines). The greatest concerns have been raised about live vaccines. MMR vaccine is contraindicated in pregnant women on theoretical grounds; however, because no case of congenital rubella syndrome has been reported after MMR vaccination among susceptible women exposed to rubella virus through MMR vaccine, inadvertent vaccination is not a reason to interrupt pregnancy. Varicella-containing vaccines also are contraindicated in pregnant women because of the theoretical risk that they may cause birth defects. Reporting of inadvertent immunization with a varicella-containing vaccine during pregnancy is encouraged (1-800-986-8999). Pregnancy in a household member is not a reason to postpone vaccination of other family members. In fact, vaccination of family members may be the best way to protect a pregnant mother from being exposed to natural infection. Breastfeeding does not adversely affect the responses to live or killed vaccines; breastfed infants should be vaccinated according to the recommended childhood and adolescent immunization schedule.[8]

Immunocompromised People

People with altered immunocompetence require special considerations for vaccination[19,23,49,65,66] since they may be at increased risk for serious adverse consequences of disease, at risk for serious consequences of vaccination, or at risk for poor response to vaccination. The safety and efficacy of vaccines in people with immune deficiencies are determined by the nature and degree of immune suppression. Immunodeficiency conditions can be grouped into primary and secondary (acquired) disorders. Primary disorders of the immune system generally are inherited as single-gene disorders, may involve any part of the immune system, and share the common feature of susceptibility to infection with various organisms, depending on the specific deficiency. Categories of immunocompromised people with acquired immune deficiency disorders include people with human immunodeficiency virus (HIV) infection; hematopoietic or solid-organ transplants; malignancies; immunosuppression due to administration of chemotherapy, systemic corticosteroids, radiation, monoclonal antibodies, or other drugs with significant side effects; and with other chronic conditions, including splenectomy. People in these categories can be vaccinated safely with killed vaccines, which usually are recommended in the same doses and on the same schedules as for immunocompetent people. Response to both killed and live vaccines may be suboptimal, and higher doses or additional doses may be needed to ensure protection. Live vaccines generally are not recommended for any of these groups because of known or theoretical risks of disseminated infection due to the vaccine. Exceptions are MMR and varicella vaccines, which are either recommended or can be considered for susceptible people with HIV infection with CD4+ T-lymphocyte counts ≥15% that are expected for age and no or mild symptoms of disease.[19,49,65,66] Table 6-4 shows recommendations for immunization of children and adolescents with primary and secondary immune deficiencies.

International Travelers

International travelers frequently have increased risk of exposure to vaccine-preventable diseases, even in economically developed countries. Parents and physicians of children and adolescents planning international travel should ensure that all routine childhood and adolescent immunizations are up-to-date and that adults are up-to-date on their immunizations. Infants ≥6 months of age should be given MMR vaccine. The need for other vaccines should be determined through consultation with specific guidelines for travelers.[67] Additional information for international travelers can be found on the CDC website at www.cdc.gov/travel or the World Health Organization website at www.who.int/ith/en.

Immigrants

The immunization status of all children immigrating from other countries should be reviewed upon their entry into the U.S., and necessary vaccinations administered. Since 1996, the Immigration and Naturalization Act has required that people seeking permanent U.S. residency show proof of having received the recommended vaccines as established by the ACIP. Most vaccines given in other countries meet high standards of potency, and immunizations that are documented on an immunization record generally can be presumed to have been effective. Doses that are consistent in initial timing and intervals with U.S. recommendations can be considered acceptable, and only doses needed to comply with U.S. recommendations for age need be given.[8] If a child has no immunization record, the immunization series should be initiated; the most significant risk of serious reaction may be to the tetanus component of DTP or DTaP, for which immunization in the presence of high levels of antibody due to prior undocumented immunization can cause serious local Arthus-type reactions.

International Adoptees

Studies have shown that immunization records for international adoptees from some areas (e.g., eastern Europe, the former Soviet Union, and China), especially children from orphanages, may not accurately reflect protection because of inaccurate or unreliable records, lack of vaccine potency, poor nutritional status, or other problems. For any international adoptee, if there is a question as to whether vaccines were administered or were immunogenic, the best course is to administer all vaccines recommended by age. If there is desire to avoid unnecessary injections, the judicious use of serologic testing may help to determine which injections can be avoided (see Chapter 4, Infectious Diseases in Refugee and Internationally Adopted Children).

Other Programmatic Issues

Responsibility for ensuring that children and adolescents are immunized adequately lies with parents and primary care providers. For children and adolescents without primary healthcare providers, public and hospital-based clinics provide immunizations through federal- and state-funded programs. Each child's immunization status should be assessed every time the child is seen for healthcare, whether for preventive or curative treatment. Physicians should ensure that each child has an immunization record and that the record is updated each time an immunization is given.[68] Parents should be encouraged to bring the immunization record for each healthcare visit. Immunization information systems (i.e., immunization registries) are intended to compile and make available to all providers the immunization records of all children in a city or state. These registries will provide a system whereby reminders about impending or missed immunizations can be generated and providers can gain access to a reliable record for mobile children.[69]

TABLE 6-4. Vaccination of Persons with Primary and Secondary Immunodeficiencies

	Specific Immunodeficiency	Contraindicated Vaccines[a]	Risk-Specific Recommended Vaccines[a]	Effectiveness and Comments
PRIMARY				
B-lymphocyte (humoral)	Severe antibody deficiencies (e.g., X-linked agammaglobulinemia and common variable immunodeficiency)	OPV[b] Smallpox LAIV BCG Ty21a (live typhoid) Yellow fever	Pneumococcal Consider measles and varicella vaccination	The effectiveness of any vaccine is uncertain if it depends only on the humoral response (e.g., PPSV or MPSV4) IGIV interferes with the immune response to measles vaccine and possibly varicella vaccine

Continued

TABLE 6-4. Vaccination of Persons with Primary and Secondary Immunodeficiencies—cont'd

	Specific Immunodeficiency	Contraindicated Vaccines[a]	Risk-Specific Recommended Vaccines[a]	Effectiveness and Comments
	Less severe antibody deficiencies (e.g., selective IgA deficiency and IgG subclass deficiency)	OPV[b] BCG Yellow fever Other live vaccines appear to be safe	Pneumococcal	All vaccines likely effective; immune response might be attenuated
T-lymphocyte (cell-mediated and humoral)	Complete defects (e.g., severe combined immunodeficiency [SCID] disease, complete DiGeorge syndrome)	All live vaccines[c,d,e]	Pneumococcal	Vaccines might be ineffective
	Partial defects (e.g., most patients with DiGeorge syndrome, Wiskott-Aldrich syndrome, ataxia-telangiectasia)	All live vaccines[c,d,e]	Pneumococcal Meningococcal Hib (if not administered in infancy)	Effectiveness of any vaccine depends on degree of immune suppression
Complement	Persistent complement, properdin, or factor B deficiency	None	Pneumococcal Meningococcal	All routine vaccines likely effective
Phagocytic function	Chronic granulomatous disease, leukocyte adhesion defect, and myeloperoxidase deficiency	Live bacterial vaccines[c]	Pneumococcal[f]	All inactivated vaccines safe and likely effective Live viral vaccines likely safe and effective
SECONDARY				
	HIV/AIDS	OPV[b] Smallpox BCG LAIV Withhold MMR and varicella in severely immunocompromised persons Yellow fever vaccine might have a contraindication or a precaution depending on clinical parameters of immune function[i]	Pneumococcal Consider Hib (if not administered in infancy) and meningococcal vaccination	MMR, varicella, rotavirus, and all inactivated vaccines, including inactivated influenza, might be effective[g]
	Malignant neoplasm, transplantation, immunosuppressive or radiation therapy	Live viral and bacterial, depending on immune status[c,d]	Pneumococcal	Effectiveness of any vaccine depends on degree of immune suppression
	Asplenia	None	Pneumococcal Meningococcal Hib (if not administered in infancy)	All routine vaccines likely effective
	Chronic renal disease	LAIV	Pneumococcal Hepatitis B[h]	All routine vaccines likely effective

AIDS, acquired immunodeficiency syndrome; BCG, bacille Calmette-Guérin; Hib, Haemophilus influenzae type b; HIV, human immunodeficiency virus; IG, immunoglobulin; IGIV, immune globulin intravenous; LAIV, live, attenuated influenza vaccine; MMR, measles, mumps, and rubella; MPSV4, quadrivalent meningococcal polysaccharide vaccine; OPV, oral poliovirus vaccine (live); PPSV, pneumococcal polysaccharide vaccine; TIV, trivalent inactivated influenza vaccine.

[a]Other vaccines that are universally or routinely recommended should be given if not contraindicated.

[b]OPV is no longer available in the United States.

[c]Live bacterial vaccines: BCG and oral Ty21a Salmonella Typhi vaccine.

[d]Live viral vaccines: MMR, MMRV, OPV, LAIV, yellow fever, zoster, rotavirus, varicella, and vaccinia (smallpox). Smallpox vaccine is not recommended for children or the general public.

[e]Regarding T-lymphocyte immunodeficiency as a contraindication for rotavirus vaccine, data exist only for severe combined immunodeficiency.

[f]Pneumococcal vaccine is not indicated for children with chronic granulomatous disease beyond age-based universal recommendations for PCV. Children with chronic granulomatous disease are not at increased risk for pneumococcal disease.

[g]HIV-infected children should receive IG after exposure to measles and may receive varicella and measles vaccine if CD4+ T-lymphocyte count is ≥15%.

[h]Indicated based on the risk from dialysis-based bloodborne transmission.

[i]Symptomatic HIV infection or CD4+ T-lymphocyte count of <200/mm³ or <15% of total lymphocytes for children aged <6 years is a contraindication to yellow fever vaccine administration. Asymptomatic HIV infection with CD4+ T-lymphocyte count of 200–499/mm³ for persons aged ≥6 years or 15%–24% of total lymphocytes for children aged <6 years is a precaution for yellow fever vaccine administration. Details of yellow fever vaccine recommendations are available from CDC. (CDC. Yellow fever vaccine: recommendations of the Advisory Committee on Immunization Practices [ACIP]. MMWR 2010;59[No. RR-7].)

From Centers for Disease Control and Prevention; General Recommendations on Immunization: Recommendations of the Advisory Committee on Immunization Practices (ACIP). MMWR 2011;60:2

Clinical Practice Guidelines for Child and Adolescent Immunization

The Infectious Diseases Society of America (IDSA) has developed specific guidelines for child and adolescent immunization practices to help providers maintain practices that optimize the immunization status of children and adults.[68] These are guidelines for appropriate clinic practices, including identification of appropriate contraindications to immunization (www.cdc.gov/vaccines/recs/vac-admin/contraindications-vacc.htm), use of tracking systems, and avoidance of missed opportunities. The Task Force for Community Preventive Services has reviewed extensively the scientific literature regarding best practices to improve immunization of young children.[70,71] The most effective and most strongly recommended interventions are divided into: (1) interventions that increase community demand for vaccines (client reminder-recall systems, multicomponent interventions that include education, and vaccination requirements for school, childcare, and college attendance); (2) interventions that enhance access to vaccination services (reducing out-of-pocket costs for vaccination, expanding access in medical or public health settings, including the Women, Infants, and Children program); and (3) interventions that utilize provider-based interventions (reminder-recall and assessment and feedback for vaccine providers). Conducting audits of patient immunization records in both public clinics and private provider offices is recommended to educate providers about the immunization status of patients as well as to identify practices that can be changed to improve immunization coverage. Routine use of audits in public clinics has reduced missed opportunities for immunization and markedly improved immunization coverage. Self-assessment methods are available from the CDC and AAP.

Education of parents regarding the importance of immunization as well as informed consent are critical features of successful immunization programs. The NCVIA mandated that parents should be provided with written materials for vaccines covered by NVICP that describe the diseases that vaccines are intended to prevent, the risks and benefits of the vaccines, and the procedure for reporting adverse events and seeking compensation for vaccine-related injury.[26] Vaccine information statements, including some not covered by NVICP, are available at www.cdc.gov/vaccines/pubs/vis/default.htm.

Vaccine Shortages

In addition to the rising cost of vaccines, an unparalleled number of vaccine shortages in the U.S. have had a substantial impact on vaccine delivery. From 2000 through 2010, vaccine shortages, vaccine supply issues, and changes in routine recommendations occurred for almost all vaccines in the childhood and adolescent immunization schedule.[72-79] The shortages affected millions of children and their healthcare providers, even triggering suspension of school entry requirements for vaccines.[79-81] Three vaccine shortages (PCV7, Td, and Hib (PRP-OMP)) lasted nearly 2 years, one (PCV7) occurred twice, and one (inactivated influenza vaccine, 2004/2005 season) halved the nation's influenza vaccine supply virtually overnight.[77]

The causes of these widespread vaccine shortages are multifactorial. One important long-term factor is the decrease in the number of vaccine manufacturers of childhood vaccines routinely recommended in the U.S. In 1993, six manufacturers produced the six vaccines. Over a decade later, although several vaccines (PCV7, varicella, influenza, Tdap, rotavirus, MMRV, herpes zoster, MCV and HPV) have been added to the recommended schedules, the number of manufacturers has only increased to seven. In addition, there are single manufacturers for many of the childhood and adolescent vaccines (MMR, MMRV, varicella, and PCV13). In response to concerns over the fragility of the U.S. vaccine supply, the General Accounting Office and National Vaccine Advisory Committee both conducted indepth reviews of the vaccine shortages and concluded that future disruptions in vaccine supply are likely to continue, and they proposed solutions.[72,82] The current status of vaccine shortages in the U.S. can be found at http://www.cdc.gov/vaccines/vac-gen/shortages/default.htm.

Handling and Storage of Vaccines

Vaccines are perishable products that require specific care in handling and storage; ensuring that a vaccine maintains potency and safety is a responsibility shared by the manufacturer and all people handling the vaccine. Live-attenuated vaccines are more susceptible to degradation when exposed to temperature extremes, and inactivated vaccines (particularly those containing adjuvants) and toxoids must be protected from freezing to ensure potency.[19] Vaccines that are exposed to damaging environmental conditions can suffer loss of potency without a change in appearance. A vaccine quality control program should be established in each clinical practice and should focus on education of personnel, maintenance of equipment, and adherence to established daily monitoring of vaccines.

Vaccine Financing

Ensuring that all children and adolescents, regardless of health insurance status or income level, have access to recommended vaccines requires a complex system of financing which includes private and public funding mechanisms (Table 6-5). In 2009, 53% of U.S. children received vaccines purchased through the public sector, and 47% received vaccines purchased through the private sector. Most of the public-purchase vaccines are financed through the Vaccines for Children (VFC) program, an entitlement program

Table 6-5. Major Financing Programs for Childhood Immunization

Variable	Vaccines for Children Program	Section 317	State/Local Government	Private Insurance
Financing source	Entitlement funded through Medicaid trust fund	Annual discretionary appropriation by Congress	Appropriations through state or local legislatures	Employer-based insurance
Eligibility	Age <19 years and membership in ≥1 of the following categories: Medicaid-eligible; uninsured; Alaska Native or American Indian; or underinsured at a federally qualified health center or rural health clinic	No federal eligibility restrictions	Varies by state or local area	Individuals covered by private insurance, including Employee Retirement Income Security Act (ERISA) plans
Financing of new vaccines and recommendations	Vote of ACIP and establishment of a federal contract; funds are approved by the Office of Management and Budget	Funding appropriated by Congress annually	Funding must be sought from state legislatures	ACIP recommended vaccines must be covered with no copay or deductible
Proportion of childhood vaccine market purchased	46%	4%	3%	47%

ACIP, Advisory Committee on Immunization Practices.

TABLE 6-6. Composition of Selected Vaccines with Tetanus Toxoid, Diphtheria Toxoid, and Acellular Pertussis Components Licensed in the United States, 2008

Vaccines for children <7 years of age	Trade name	PT	FHA	PRN	FIM	Recommended Use
DTaP	Infanrix	25	25	8	–	All 5 doses
DTaP–IPV–HepB	Pediarix	25	25	8	–	First 3 doses
DTaP	Daptacel	10	5	3	5	All 5 doses
DTaP–IPV/Hib	Pentacel	20	20	3	5	First 4 doses
DTaP	Tripedia	23.4	23.4	–	–	All 5 doses
DTaP–IPV	Kinrix	25	25	8	–	Fifth dose only
DT	No trade name	–	–	–	–	Use instead of DTaP if pertussis contraindicated
Vaccines for people ≥7 years of age						
Tdap	Boostrix	8	8	2.5	–	Single dose indicated for people 10 years of age and older
Tdap	Adacel	2.5	5	3	5	Single dose indicated for people 11 through 64 years of age
Td	Several	–	–	–	–	Every 10 years

DT, diphtheria and tetanus toxoid; DTaP, diphtheria and tetanus toxoids, and acellular pertussis for use <7 years of age; FHA, filamentous hemagglutinin antigen; FIM, fimbriae; HepB, hepatitis B; IPV, inactivated poliovirus vaccine; PRN, pertactin; PT, pertussis toxoid, Td, tetanus and reduced-content diphtheria toxoid for use ≥7 years of age; Tdap, tetanus toxoid and reduced-content diphtheria toxoid and acellular pertussis vaccine for use in adolescents.

established in 1994 as part of the Social Security Act.[24,25] Other government funding mechanisms include Section 317 of the Public Health Service Act of 1962, a federal grant program, and state and local government funding. These programs support states to provide immunizations to children who do not qualify for the VFC program but who are not covered by private insurance. Several states use a combination of federal and state funding to purchase and distribute vaccines recommended for children to all immunization providers in private and public sectors. Insurance programs provide vaccines for children in the private sector.

Surveillance for Vaccine-Preventable Diseases and Adverse Events

Surveillance for vaccine-preventable diseases is mandated by each state, and data are compiled in the National Notifiable Disease Surveillance System at the CDC.[83] Results are no longer published weekly in MMWR but are available at www.cdc.gov/mmwr. These data are monitored to assess effectiveness of vaccines and of the vaccination program. For each reported case of disease, confirmation of disease by laboratory testing and documentation of the patient's vaccination status are critical to determining whether continued occurrence of disease is due to failure to deliver vaccine or failure of vaccine. As programs approach elimination of indigenous transmission, determination of chains of disease transmission as well as whether the case is indigenous or imported, and rapid implementation of control measures also become critical. All physicians are urged to report all suspected cases of vaccine-preventable diseases promptly to their local and state health departments.

Monitoring for adverse events after vaccination is the joint responsibility of the FDA and CDC.[26,54] Physicians are required to report certain events that occur after vaccination and should report all suspected adverse reactions after vaccination to VAERS. VAERS forms are available through state health departments, physicians, and from VAERS at 800-822-7967; forms also can be obtained and submitted electronically through a secure website at http://vaers.hhs.gov.

ROUTINE CHILDHOOD AND ADOLESCENT VACCINES

Diphtheria and Tetanus Toxoids, and Pertussis Vaccines

In 1980 cutaneous diphtheria was no longer a nationally notifiable disease in the U.S. Between 1990 and 2009, 28 cases of respiratory tract diphtheria were reported. From 2000 through 2009,

284 cases of tetanus were reported in the U.S., with a peak of 41 cases in 2006.[30] In 2004 the number of reported cases of pertussis increased for the third consecutive year, with 25,827 cases reported, the highest since 1959.[30] In 2009 the number of cases was 16,858 and in 2010 over 21,000 cases were reported, resulting in changes in pertussis vaccine recommendations.[8] Although infants have the highest morbidity associated with pertussis, adolescents and adults account for the majority of reported cases.[84]

Immunization of children and adolescents to prevent diphtheria, tetanus, and pertussis usually is completed with a vaccine composed of diphtheria and tetanus toxoids combined with an acellular pertussis component.[33,64,85–87] Diphtheria and tetanus toxoids are purified preparations of formalin-inactivated diphtheria and tetanus toxins, respectively. Table 6-6 shows the composition and recommended use of vaccines with tetanus toxoid, diphtheria toxoid, and acellular pertussis components licensed in the U.S. for children <7 years of age and people ≥7 years of age. Whole-cell DTP was the only pertussis vaccine available from 1948 through 1992; because of its relatively high rate of adverse reactions compared with the newer acellular pertussis vaccines, DTP is no longer used in the U.S.[86] Whole-cell DTP continues to be the most frequently used pertussis-containing vaccine worldwide.

Recommendations for DTaP Immunization for Children <7 Years of Age

Immunization with DTaP vaccine is recommended for all children <7 years of age. Primary vaccination consists of 3 doses of DTaP vaccine given at 2, 4, and 6 months of age; the minimal age for initiating vaccination is 6 weeks, and the minimal interval between doses is 4 weeks (see Figure 6-2).[8,85,86] To ensure protection, a reinforcing dose of DTaP is given at 15 to 18 months of age, and a booster dose at school entry (4 through 6 years of age). Diphtheria and tetanus (DT) toxoids are used in children for whom pertussis vaccination is contraindicated. If the schedule is interrupted, there is no need to restart the series.

The vaccination advisory bodies consider data insufficient to support expression of a preference among the different acellular pertussis vaccines.[85] Whenever feasible, the same brand of DTaP vaccine should be used for all doses of the primary vaccination series, although data suggest that two of the available preparations can be used interchangeably for the first 3 doses of the series.[53] If the provider does not know or does not have available the type of DTaP vaccine previously administered, any of the DTaP vaccines can be used to complete the series. DTaP vaccines can be given simultaneously with other recommended childhood vaccines (HBV, Hib, IPV or OPV, PCV13, rotavirus) at 2, 4, and 6 months of age, and can be given with these vaccines as well as with MMR, varicella, and HAV vaccines at 15 through 18 months of age. DTaP is not licensed for use in adults or in children ≥7 years of age. Vaccination to prevent diphtheria and tetanus is recommended for previously unvaccinated children (≥7 years of age and in whom pertussis vaccine is contraindicated) and adults. Children 7 through 10 years of age who are not fully immunized with DTaP against pertussis should receive a single dose of Tdap.[7,88]

Use of tetanus toxoid-containing preparations, with or without tetanus immunoglobulin, can be indicated after penetrating or other types of injuries in people who are not adequately vaccinated.[87] For any such person who has not previously received the 3-dose primary series, initiation or continuation of the primary vaccination appropriate for age (DTaP, Tdap, DT, or Td) is recommended after any wound. Vaccination is not necessary in people who have received 3 prior doses of tetanus vaccine, unless: (1) the last vaccination occurred more than 10 years previously (5 years for wounds other than clean and minor wounds); or (2) only 3 doses of fluid (nonadjuvant) tetanus toxoid were received, in which case one dose of Td vaccine should be given (see Chapter 188, *Clostridium tetani* (Tetanus)).

Precautions and Contraindications

Vaccination with any pertussis-containing vaccine is contraindicated in any child who has had an anaphylactic reaction to any component of the vaccine or has experienced acute encephalopathy within 7 days of administration of a previous dose.[85] The following events are considered precautions to pertussis immunization: (1) temperature ≥40.5°C within 48 hours of a prior dose not attributed to another cause; (2) collapse or shocklike state (hypotonic-hyporesponsive episode) within 48 hours of DTP or DTaP administration; (3) persistent inconsolable crying (≥3 hours) within 48 hours of administration of DTP or DTaP; and (4) convulsions with or without fever within 3 days of immunization. When these events occur, the physician may elect to continue vaccination if the benefits are judged to outweigh the risks, as when a pertussis outbreak is occurring in the community. DTaP immunization should be deferred in children with evolving neurologic disorders until the situation is clarified; when stable, the child should be given DTaP vaccine. Decisions about pertussis vaccination of such children should be made before the first birthday. If pertussis vaccine is not used, pediatric DT should be administered.

Recommendations for Tdap Immunization for Adolescents 11 through 18 Years of Age

Adolescents 11 through 18 years of age should receive a single dose of Tdap instead of Td for booster immunization against tetanus, diphtheria, and pertussis if they have completed the recommended childhood DTP/DTaP vaccination series[8] and have not received Tdap. The preferred age for Tdap vaccination is 11 to 12 years of age (Figure 6-3).

Adolescents 11 through 18 years of age who received Td, but not Tdap, are encouraged to receive a single dose of Tdap to provide protection against pertussis if they have completed the recommended childhood DTP/DTaP vaccination series.[8,33,64,88] If more doses of tetanus and diphtheria toxoids are needed to complete the primary series in such older children, Td should be used. Tdap has not been licensed for more than a single dose.

Contraindications, Precautions, and Reasons to Defer Tdap or Td among Adolescents 11 through 18 Years of Age

Contraindications to Tdap include a history of serious allergic reaction (i.e., anaphylaxis) to vaccine components or encephalopathy (e.g., coma or prolonged seizures) not attributable to an identifiable cause within 7 days of administration of a vaccine with pertussis components. This is a contraindication for the pertussis components; Td can be used.

Precautions and reasons to defer Tdap include: GBS less than 6 weeks after a previous dose of a tetanus toxoid-containing vaccine; progressive neurologic disorder, including progressive encephalopathy, or uncontrolled epilepsy, until the condition has stabilized (these conditions are precautions for the pertussis components; Td can be used); moderate or severe acute illness; and history of an Arthus reaction after a tetanus toxoid-containing and/or diphtheria toxoid-containing vaccine administered <10 years previously.

Special Situations for Tdap (Single-Dose) and Td Use among Adolescents 11 through 18 Years of Age

If simultaneous vaccination is not feasible, inactivated vaccines can be administered at any time before or after a different inactivated or live vaccine. ACIP recommends that Tdap (or Td) and MCV4 vaccines (which all contain diphtheria toxoid) can be administered using any sequence and timing.

The following situations for administration of Tdap should be considered:[8,33,88]

- Use of Td when Tdap is not available. When Tdap is indicated but not available, vaccine providers should administer Td if the last pediatric DTP/DTaP/DT or Td dose was >10 years earlier to provide protection against tetanus and diphtheria.
- Tetanus prophylaxis in wound management. Adolescents who require a tetanus toxoid-containing vaccine as part of wound management should receive a single dose of Tdap instead of Td if they previously have not received Tdap; if Tdap is not available or previously was administered, adolescents who need a tetanus toxoid-containing vaccine should receive Td.
- History of pertussis. Adolescents who have a history of pertussis generally should receive Tdap according to the routine recommendations.
- No history of pertussis vaccination. Adolescents who have not received vaccines with pertussis components but completed the recommended tetanus and diphtheria vaccination series with pediatric DT or Td should generally receive Tdap according to the routine recommendations if they do not have a contraindication to the pertussis components.
- No history of pediatric DTP/DTaP or Td/Tdap vaccination. Adolescents who have never received tetanus-diphtheria-pertussis vaccination should receive a series of three vaccinations. The preferred schedule is a single Tdap dose, followed by a dose of Td ≥4 weeks after the Tdap dose and a second dose of Td 6 to 12 months after the earlier Td dose. Tdap can be substituted for any one of the three Td doses in the series.
- Use of Td and Tdap in pregnant women. See "Pregnant Women" section.[33,64,89]
- Providers who administer Tdap to pregnant women are encouraged to report Tdap administrations to the appropriate manufacturer's pregnancy registry: for Boostrix to GlaxoSmithKline Biologicals at 1-888-825-5249, or for Adacel to Sanofi Pasteur at 1-800-822-2463 (1-800-vaccine).

Haemophilus influenzae Type b Conjugate Vaccines

Before introduction of conjugated Hib vaccines in 1987, the incidence of invasive Hib diseases among children <5 years of age was estimated to be 100 cases/100,000. In 2009, the incidence of invasive Hib disease from all serotypes and all age groups was 1.01 cases per 100,000. In 2010, there were 270 cases of invasive disease due to *H. influenzae* reported in children <5 years of age, of which 6% were type b and 94% were of unknown serotype.[90]

Hib conjugate vaccines, first licensed for 18-month-old children in 1987 and for infants 2 months of age and older in 1990, have replaced the polysaccharide vaccines available from 1985 to 1989.[91] Hib conjugate vaccines contain Hib polysaccharide covalently linked with a protein carrier, which induces a T-lymphocyte-dependent immune response and immune memory not induced by polysaccharide (polyribosylribitol phosphate (PRP)) vaccine alone. The carrier protein for a vaccine licensed for infants is OMP of *Neisseria meningitidis* (PRP-OMP). Another tetanus-toxoid conjugate (PRP-T, Hiberix) vaccine is licensed for children 15 months through 4 years of age. Two combination vaccines containing either PRP-OMP or PRP-T are available.

When given as a 2-dose (PRP-OMP) or 3-dose (PRP-T) primary series to infants, Hib vaccine induces a high level of antibody to Hib polysaccharide, which wanes over the next 6 through 15 months, necessitating a booster dose at 12 through 18 months of age. PRP-OMP induces a substantial response after a single dose and may be preferred for populations at highest risk of infant infection (Native Americans, including Alaska Natives); the other vaccines require 3 doses for optimal response in infants.[91] Controlled trials showed 93% efficacy for PRP-OMP in infants in the U.S.; licensing of PRP-T was based on comparable immunogenicity and efficacy data from a British trial, and ecologic data from Finland. Several studies have shown that giving different Hib vaccines during the primary series induces a response similar to that induced by a primary series with the same vaccine and that booster doses with different vaccines induce strong responses.[52,91]

Recommendations for Immunization

Hib vaccination is recommended for all infants starting at 6 weeks to 2 months of age (Figure 6-2).[8,49,65,91] For PRP-T, 3 primary doses are given at 2-month intervals (1 month is acceptable), with a booster dose at 12 through 15 months of age. For PRP-OMP, 2 doses are given at 2-month intervals followed by a booster at 12 through 15 months of age. When primary immunization is delayed, the number of doses is reduced; for children vaccinated beginning at 6 through 11 months of age, 2 or 3 primary doses are recommended for each of the 3 vaccines, followed by a booster at >12 months of age. If vaccination is initiated at 12 through 14 months of age, 2 doses with a 2-month interval are indicated. For initiation of vaccination in children 15 through 59 months of age, a single dose of any of the licensed vaccines is recommended. Although the primary series ideally should be completed with the same vaccine, 3 doses of any vaccine are sufficient if the initial vaccine is not available or is unknown. Booster doses can consist of any of the licensed vaccines. Hib vaccines can be given simultaneously with all other childhood vaccines, including DTaP, IPV or OPV, hepatitis B, PCV13, MMR, varicella, hepatitis A, and rotavirus vaccines.

Vaccination of children >59 months of age can be considered for certain high-risk groups, including children with sickle-cell disease, splenectomy, leukemia, or HIV infection.[19,49,65,91] For these children, one dose of vaccine is indicated but may not be as highly immunogenic as in healthy children. Immunization is indicated in children with prior Hib disease during the first 2 years of life, in whom adequate immunity may not develop after infection, but is not necessary in older children who have had Hib disease.

Contraindications and Precautions

The only known common adverse events following administration of Hib vaccines are fever and local reactions, observed in <4% of recipients. The only contraindication to Hib vaccine is an anaphylactic reaction to a previous dose of the same vaccine.

Hepatitis B Vaccine

During 1990 to 2008, the number of acute HBV cases reported annually declined 83%.[32,92] This steady decline coincides with implementation of a national strategy to achieve elimination of HBV. The primary elements of this strategy are: (1) screening of all pregnant women for HBV infection with the provision of postexposure prophylaxis to infants born to infected women; (2) routine vaccination of all infants and children <19 years of age; and (3) vaccination of others at increased risk for hepatitis B (e.g., HCP, men who have sex with men (MSM), injection drug users (IDUs), household and sexual contacts of people with chronic HBV infection) and adults with diabetes.[32,93]

In 2004, the incidence of HBV among children <12 years of age was 0.36 per 100,000 population, representing a 94% decline for that age group from 1990 to 2004. During that time, the disparity between the population with the highest (Asian Pacific Islanders) and the lowest (whites) incidence has been reduced by >90%. From 1990 to 2004 rates among adolescents 12 through 19 years of age declined 54% but the 2004 rate (2.8 per 100,000 population) remains substantially higher than the rate for children <12 years of age.[93]

During 1990 to 1999, HBV rates among adults declined 63%, but through 2009 rates have remained essentially unchanged. Among adults, a high proportion of cases occur among people in identified risk groups (i.e., IDUs, MSM, and people with multiple sex partners), indicating a need to strengthen efforts to reach these populations with vaccine.[32]

Recommendations for Immunization

HBV vaccine consists of purified HBsAg particles produced through recombinant DNA technology in yeast. Table 6-7 shows vaccine products that contain hepatitis B antigen licensed in the U.S. Vaccine usually is given as a 3-dose series; doses 2 and 3 are administered 1 and 6 months, respectively, after the first dose. Alternative schedules include 0, 1, 4 months; 0, 2, 4 months; and a schedule that includes 4 doses, with doses 2, 3, and 4 given at 1, 2, and 12 months, respectively, after the first. Schedules that vary the timing of the second and third doses to permit integration into the recommended childhood and adolescent immunization schedule have resulted in high immunogenicity. The final (third or fourth) dose in the hepatitis B series should be administered no earlier than 24 weeks after the first. A two-dose schedule (second dose given 4 to 6 months after the first) has been approved for adolescents 11 through 15 years of age for one HBV vaccine. Dosages vary by age, vaccine, and whether the child is born to an HBsAg-positive mother; dosages for infants and children are half of those required for adults. Minimal intervals between doses should be 1 month between the first two doses, and 2 months, but preferably 4 to 6 months or more, between the second and third doses; lapsed immunization does not necessitate restarting the vaccine series.[8] Three products that combine HBV vaccine with other vaccine antigens are licensed for use at various ages (Table 6-7).

Response to a 3-dose series is excellent in all age groups, producing anti-HBV antibodies (anti-HBs) in 85% to 99% of recipients; response is highest in children 2 through 18 years of age.[32,93] People with immunocompromising conditions, such as renal failure, have poorer response, and higher dosages are recommended. Vaccine efficacy measured in placebo-controlled trials in both high-risk children (infants of HBsAg-positive mothers) and adults has shown a short-term efficacy of 80% to 95%. Long-term follow-up of children and adults has demonstrated protection against serious consequences of infection (chronic carriage and chronic liver disease) in almost all people who show response to the initial series (anti-HBs level of ≥10 mIU/mL), but continued

TABLE 6-7. Hepatitis B-Containing Vaccines Licensed in the United States

Vaccine	Antigen Content	Recommended Age Group
Recombivax HB	Hepatitis B	All age groups
Engerix-B	Hepatitis B	All age groups
Comvax	Hepatitis B and Hib conjugate	6 weeks through 71 months of age
Pediarix	Hepatitis B + DTaP + IPV	6 weeks through 6 years of age
Twinrix	Hepatitis B + hepatitis A	≥18 years of age

DTaP, diphtheria and tetanus toxoids and acellular pertussis; Hib, Haemophilus influenzae, type b; IPV, inactivated poliovirus vaccine.

studies are needed. Booster doses of hepatitis B vaccine are not recommended for any age group; however, the need for booster continues to be evaluated. HBV vaccine can be given simultaneously with all other childhood vaccines.

Contraindications and Precautions

HBV vaccination is contraindicated for people with a history of hypersensitivity to yeast or to any HBV vaccine component. Despite a theoretical risk for allergic reaction to vaccination in people with allergy to *Saccharomyces cerevisiae* (baker's yeast), no evidence exists for adverse reactions after vaccination of people with a history of yeast allergy.

People with a history of serious adverse events (e.g., anaphylaxis) after receipt of HBV vaccine should not receive additional doses. As with other vaccines, immunization of people with moderate or severe acute illness, with or without fever, should be deferred until the acute phase of the illness resolves. Immunization is not contraindicated in people with a history of multiple sclerosis, Guillain–Barré syndrome, autoimmune disease (e.g., systemic lupus erythematosus or rheumatoid arthritis), or other chronic diseases.[59,60] Pregnancy is not a contraindication to vaccination. Limited data indicate no apparent risk for adverse events to developing fetuses when HBV vaccine is administered to pregnant women.

Measles, Mumps, and Rubella Vaccine

Vaccination programs have reduced the incidence of disease due to measles, mumps, and rubella in the U.S.[30] Implementation of these strategies has resulted in interruption of measles transmission in the U.S. and an all-time low number of 37 measles cases reported in 2004, 27 of which were imported and resulted in 6 secondary cases. A large outbreak of 34 cases of measles occurred in the U.S. in 2005.[94] In 2008, multiple outbreaks of measles occurred in the U.S., totaling 140 cases, the highest number since 1996. These cases occurred as a result of importation or re-importation into community clusters with large proportions of unvaccinated persons. In 2011, outbreak data show that the total number of measles cases exceeded cases in 2008 with the majority of cases associated with importation from other countries.[95]

On October 29, 2004, a nine-person independent panel unanimously agreed that rubella is no longer endemic in the U.S.[34] In 2006 there was one case of congenital rubella reported in the U.S. The incidence of reported cases of mumps in the U.S. had been decreasing until 2006 when an outbreak involving several thousand people occurred.[96] On average, around 1100 cases of mumps have occurred annually from 2007 through 2009. Protection against measles, mumps, and rubella is provided by the combined MMR and MMRV vaccines.[8,97,98] Measles vaccine is a live-attenuated virus vaccine produced from the Moraten strain of measles virus, which was derived from the Edmonston B strain. Mumps vaccine is a live-attenuated vaccine derived from the Jeryl Lynn strain of mumps virus. Rubella vaccine is a live-attenuated vaccine derived from the RA27/3 strain of rubella virus that was grown on human diploid cells. Other rubella strains, with slightly different safety and efficacy profiles, were used in the U.S. before 1979. These vaccines also are available in monovalent and bivalent preparations, use of which is limited for outbreak control.

Recommendations for Immunization

A single dose of measles vaccine given to children ≥12 months of age induces antibody and produces protection in 95% to 98% of recipients; protection is long-lasting, and waning of immunity, although documented in several studies, appears to be uncommon and plays a minimal role in measles outbreaks,[97,99] which occur in the U.S. because of importation and spread to unimmunized people.[94,95] Nevertheless, because infrequent vaccine failure with one dose led to frequent measles outbreaks among schoolchildren, a second dose of MMR vaccine is now recommended for all children. In most studies, the second dose increases measles

antibody response to >99%, whether it is given within 3 months of the initial dose or years later upon a child's entry to primary or middle school. Additionally the booster dose can induce antibody increases in people with low levels of antibody, but the increases appear to be short-lived.

A single dose of mumps vaccine given at 12 through 15 months of age induces detectable antibodies in 80% to 85% of recipients. Immunity is long-lasting, possibly lifelong, but waning immunity (or possibly primary vaccine failure) has been suggested as a contributing cause in some mumps outbreaks in highly vaccinated school populations. A large mumps outbreak that began in Iowa in December 2005 and spread to several other states prompted a change in recommendations for use of mumps-containing vaccines.[96] In addition to routine immunization, the CDC recommends MMR vaccine for people born after 1957 who do not have a history of physician-diagnosed mumps infection, laboratory evidence of immunity, or immunity through vaccine, which the ACIP has redefined as 1 dose of mumps vaccine for preschool children and adults not at high risk, and 2 doses for children in grades K through 12 and adults at high risk (HCP, international travelers, and post high-school students).

During an outbreak, a second dose should be considered for all adults and children 1 to 4 years of age who have not received 2 doses; the second dose is given at least 28 days after the first dose. The CDC suggests that unvaccinated HCP born before 1957 who do not have other evidence of immunity also should receive 2 doses of the vaccine during an outbreak.

Rubella vaccine induces a primary response in 95% to 98% of children vaccinated at 12 months of age or older; protection is long-lasting, with >90% of recipients protected against clinical disease and viremia for >15 years.

Vaccination to prevent measles, mumps, and rubella is recommended for all children and adolescents.[8,97] Measles vaccination and now mumps vaccine are recommended in a 2-dose series, given as MMR or MMRV, for all susceptible people. MMRV vaccine is indicated for simultaneous immunization against measles, mumps, rubella, and varicella among children 12 months through 12 years of age; MMRV is not licensed for people outside this age group.[98] For infants and young children, the first dose should be given at 12 through 15 months of age, and the second at 4 through 6 years of age.[97] The timing of the first dose is based on the likelihood that maternal antibody does not persist during the second year of life; in the past, persistence of maternal antibody accounted for lower efficacy when vaccine was given at 12 through 14 months of age. Later studies have shown that younger mothers, who have acquired antibody through vaccination, may transfer less measles antibody to their infants (because vaccine induces lower titers than natural measles infection), who then become susceptible at a younger age.[100] During outbreaks that affect children <1 year of age (and for international travel to areas where measles is endemic), the age of measles vaccination should be lowered to 6 months; children vaccinated before 12 months of age still should be vaccinated with 2 doses of MMR or MMRV at the recommended ages.[101]

For dose 1 of the 2-dose MMR series, there is an increased risk of febrile seizures in children who received MMRV compared with children who received simultaneous but separate MMR and varicella vaccines. For first dose at ages 12 through 47 months, either MMR and varicella vaccines or MMRV vaccine can be used. However, unless the parent prefers MMRV as a single injection, CDC recommends that MMR and varicella vaccines should be given separately for the first dose. There is no evidence for increased risk of febrile seizures with MMRV when used for dose 2 of the 2-dose series; MMRV is preferred over separate MMR and varicella vaccines for dose 2.

Recommendations for timing of the second dose of MMR are based on: (1) the major benefit of the second MMR in reducing the proportion of children who remain susceptible to measles because of failure of the primary vaccine; and (2) the ease of implementation by using the preschool immunization visit. All children should be given the second dose of MMR vaccine at school entry if it was not given previously. The ACIP recommends that states implement requirements that all children entering school have received 2 doses of MMR after the first birthday.[97] Receipt of 2 doses of MMR vaccine also is recommended for all people entering or enrolled in college; many states now implement prematriculation requirements, which have been shown to reduce the risk of measles outbreaks in these populations.

Rubella vaccination is recommended for all susceptible adults.[97] Adolescents and adults should be considered susceptible to rubella and should be vaccinated unless they have a history of ≥1 dose of vaccine or have serologic evidence of immunity. Ensuring rubella immunity is especially important in women of childbearing age. A clinical history of rubella is not sufficiently reliable. Delivery of rubella vaccine to adults is more successful in programs that do not use prevaccination screening, because screening requires a second visit for susceptible people to be vaccinated.

Programs to ensure immunity to measles, mumps, and rubella are recommended for all HCP and for international travelers, who may be exposed to these diseases in countries with less effective control programs.[97] Among people born after 1956, measles immunity should be based on receipt of 2 doses of measles vaccine, serologic evidence of immunity, or a prior physician-diagnosed case of measles. Acceptable presumptive evidence of immunity to mumps includes one of the following: (1) documentation of adequate vaccination; (2) laboratory evidence of immunity; (3) birth before 1957; or (4) documentation of physician-diagnosed mumps. Evidence of immunity through documentation of adequate vaccination is now defined as 1 dose of a live mumps virus vaccine for preschool-aged children and adults not at high risk and 2 doses for school-aged children (i.e., grades K through 12) and for adults at high risk (i.e., HCP, international travelers, and students at post high-school educational institutions).

Contraindications and Precautions

Measles, MMR, and MMRV vaccines produce minor reactions, including fever ≥39.4°C in 5% to 15% and transient rash in 15% of recipients. Fever and rash occur between 4 and 14 days after vaccination and last for several days. More serious reactions include febrile convulsion, in 1 per 2000-to-3000 recipients 1 to 2 years of age; risk is higher in people with a personal or family history of convulsions.[59,98,102] Thrombocytopenia, which usually is transient, can occur in 1 per 30,000 recipients of MMR vaccine, and anaphylaxis, more rarely.[97] Cases of encephalitis have been reported, with an onset of about 10 days after vaccination, after <1 per 1 million vaccine doses, but a causal role of measles vaccination has not been established. Available data do not support a relationship between measles-containing vaccine and subacute sclerosing panencephalitis (SSPE); in fact, widespread use of measles vaccines virtually has eliminated SSPE; no case of SSPE confirmed to be caused by vaccine virus has been reported.[58,97,103] The IOM rejected a hypothesized causal relationship between MMR vaccine and autism spectrum disorders.[59] Uncommon adverse events after mumps vaccines include aseptic meningitis, parotitis, orchitis, and low-grade fever. Reactions are expected to be less frequent among recipients of the second dose.

Adverse events after rubella vaccination include fever and mild rash in 5% to 10% of recipients, and joint pain, generally without arthritis. The frequency of arthritis increases with age of vaccination, particularly for recipients >15 years of age, and can reach 40% in older adult women.[97] The rate of acute arthritis is lower than that observed for natural rubella in the same age group.[56,59] In one study, the IOM concluded that rubella vaccination may cause chronic arthritis in adult women at rates as high as 5%.[59] However, other studies have found no evidence for a risk of onset of chronic arthropathy after rubella vaccination, and a randomized trial found only a small risk of persistent joint pains.[104,105] The RA 27/3 rubella vaccine has not been linked to radiculoneuritis or neuropathy.

Vaccination with MMR or any component vaccine is contraindicated in pregnant women, people with anaphylaxis to neomycin or gelatin, and in people who are immunocompromised because of the following: (1) congenital or acquired immune disorders, such as leukemia, lymphoma, and HIV infection with

severe immunocompromise; (2) long-term systemic corticosteroid treatment; or (3) chemotherapy.[97] Rarely, disseminated infection and death due to measles encephalitis have been reported in immunocompromised people who were inadvertently given measles vaccine.[57] Measles (and MMR) vaccination is indicated for people with asymptomatic HIV infection, because measles disease can be severe in such people and vaccine can induce immunity; vaccination should be considered for symptomatic HIV-infected people if they do not have evidence of severe immunocompromise and they lack measles immunity.[23,65] Data show that even people with severe egg allergy can be vaccinated. Most anaphylactic reactions appear to be related to other vaccine components (e.g., gelatin).[106]

Rubella vaccine virus is able to cross the placenta and cause fetal infection; however, no case of congenital rubella syndrome due to vaccine virus has been reported in infants of 680 susceptible women who received rubella vaccine within 3 months of conception and who carried their pregnancies to term.[107] The ACIP recommends that rubella vaccination not be considered a reason to interrupt pregnancy, but also that rubella vaccine not be given knowingly to a pregnant woman. A reasonable approach is to ask women whether they are pregnant now or may become pregnant within the next 28 days after immunization and to vaccinate only women who answer negatively.

Pneumococcal Conjugate and Polysaccharide Vaccines

Before use of PCV7, *Streptococcus pneumoniae* was the most common bacterial cause of acute otitis media and invasive bacterial infections in children, with >17,000 cases of invasive disease in the U.S. in children <5 years of age. After introduction of routine PCV7 immunization, the incidence of invasive pneumococcal disease (IPD) declined dramatically, especially in children <2 years of age.[108–110] U.S. population-based active surveillance data show that within 2 years of PCV7 licensure the rate of IPD in children <2 years of age declined by 69%.[111] In tandem with the decrease in IPV, data suggest that the incidence of pneumococcal noninvasive disease, including otitis media, also decreased.[112–114] In addition to decreasing the burden of pediatric pneumococcal disease, PCV7 may have an impact on reducing pediatric antibiotic prescriptions and procedures such as blood cultures in young febrile children and decrease in disease due to *S. pneumoniae* in adults.[38–41]

In February 2010, a 13-valent pneumococcal polysaccharide-protein conjugate vaccine (PCV13) was licensed. PCV13 contains the 7 serotypes included in the previously licensed PCV7 (4, 6B, 9V, 14, 18C, 19F, and 23F) plus 6 additional serotypes (1, 3, 5, 6A, 7F, and 19A) each conjugated to cross-reactive material (CRM) 197, a nontoxic variant of diphtheria toxin. By 2008, 8 years after licensure of PCV7, 3 serotypes contained in PCV13 (3, 7F, and 19A) accounted for >90% of IPD cases caused by the 6 additional serotypes.[108] PCVs induce a T-lymphocyte-dependent response that includes a primary response in infants and an anamnestic response to booster doses. Three doses of vaccine in infants induce significant increases in serum antibody concentrations to all 13 serotypes.

Pneumococcal polysaccharide vaccine (PPSV23) consists of purified capsular polysaccharides of 23 serotypes of *S. pneumoniae*, which represent 85% of strains isolated from cases of invasive pneumococcal disease in the U.S. in people of all ages.[115] PPSV23 vaccine induces increases in antibodies to pneumococcal polysaccharides in 80% to 95% of healthy recipients after a single dose. Initial studies showed high efficacy in young healthy adults (South African miners and military recruits); subsequent studies have shown about 60% efficacy against IPD in adults at risk for disease but lower effectiveness in adults who are immunocompromised, who have cirrhosis or renal failure, or who are older.[116] Efficacy in children has not been measured, and immunogenicity in children <2 years of age is limited. PPSV23 does not induce immunologic memory.

Recommendations for Immunization

Pneumococcal vaccination with PCV13 is recommended for all children <2 years of age.[26,108] The vaccine is given to infants as a 4-dose series at 2, 4, 6, and 12 through 15 months of age. Catch-up immunization is recommended for all children through 59 months of age, using fewer doses depending on age. For high-risk children, catch-up is recommended through 71 months of age. PCV13 should be used to complete a series that has begun with PCV7. For children who have received a complete series of PCV7, a supplemental dose of PCV13 is recommended through 59 months of age (71 months of age if high risk). Providers may give a dose of PCV13 to children at extremely high risk of invasive disease (functional or anatomic asplenia, immunosuppression, or renal disease), between the ages of 6 years and 18 years if they have not previously received PCV13.[8]

PPSV23 is given in a single dose to high-risk children ≥2 years of age and to adults.[115] PPSV23 is recommended for children at increased risk of pneumococcal disease irrespective of PCV receipt, because PPSV23 provides protection against additional serotypes. One-time revaccination is recommended for people who are at highest risk of invasive disease (asplenia, immunosuppression, nephrotic syndrome), if 5 years have elapsed since the last dose. No more than 2 doses of PPSV23 are recommended. Children with high-risk conditions should first receive PCV13 followed by PPSV23 ≥2 months later (see Chapter 123, *Streptococcus pneumoniae*).

Contraindications and Precautions

Adverse events after PCV13 administration are minor; examples are injection site erythema, swelling, and soreness, which occur in 35% to 49% of recipients, low-grade fever, in about 40%, and higher fever (>39°C) in 5%.[108] No serious adverse events have been associated with use of PCV13. Use of PCV13 is contraindicated in people who have had prior anaphylactic reactions to a previous dose or to a vaccine component. Safety during pregnancy has not been evaluated. Systemic reactions to PPSV23 are uncommon, but mild local reactions occur in about one-half of recipients and may be worse in people revaccinated within 5 years of initial vaccination.[115] PPSV23 vaccine is contraindicated in people who have had prior anaphylactic reactions to the vaccine or to vaccine components.

Poliovirus Vaccines

Through use of OPV, the last case of indigenously transmitted poliomyelitis in the U.S. occurred in 1979. In 2005 in the U.S., poliovirus infections occurred in 4 children who were not vaccinated due to religious reasons.[117] All 4 children were asymptomatic and were infected with a poliovirus derived from viruses found in attenuated OPVs used in much of the world. In another report, an unimmunized 22-year-old woman acquired VAPP from a child immunized with OPV in Central America.[118] This was the first case of paralytic polio identified in the U.S. since 1999 and the first imported VAPP case ever documented in the U.S. In December 2008, a 44-year-old immunosuppressed woman due to common variable immunodeficiency acquired VAPP and died from complications of her chronic illness, including neurologic sequelae.[119] These reports raise concerns about transmission of both vaccine-derived and wild polioviruses and the risk of a polio outbreak occurring in the U.S. Worldwide, polio remains endemic in only 4 countries (Afghanistan, India, Nigeria, and Pakistan).[4]

Enhanced IPV is the only poliovirus vaccine now available in the U.S.[120] IPV is derived from 3 wild strains of poliovirus, types 1, 2, and 3, which are inactivated by formalin. Until 2000, when recommendations were made for exclusive use of IPV for routine immunization, live-attenuated OPV was available in the U.S. OPV is still the most commonly used poliovirus vaccine in the world. OPV is constituted from 3 Sabin strains of polioviruses, types 1, 2, and 3, in concentrations of 1,000,000, 100,000, and 600,000 infective units ($TCID_{50}$) per dose, respectively. Both IPV and OPV,

when given as 3-dose primary series, induce protective antibody to each type of poliovirus in 95% to 99% of recipients. Antibody levels decline gradually, and booster doses of each vaccine are recommended at school entry. OPV induces higher levels of intestinal immunity than IPV and, thus, provides greater protection against infection because OPV better prevents replication and shedding of wild-type poliovirus in the intestine. In developing countries, OPV has lower per-dose effectiveness than in industrialized countries. Therefore, more doses are needed to reach the immunity thresholds in the community that are needed to terminate transmission than would be needed in developed countries.

Vaccination against poliovirus is recommended for all children. With the progress in global polio eradication and the continued risk of VAPP after OPV vaccination (approximately 8 cases per year from 1980 to 1994), the U.S. vaccination policy was modified, first to a sequential schedule of two doses of IPV followed by two doses of OPV in 1997, and subsequently to a schedule of all IPV in the year 2000.[120–122]

Recommendations for Immunization

IPV is recommended to be given at 2, 4, and 6 through 18 months of age, simultaneously with other childhood vaccines. Vaccination can start at 6 weeks of age, and 4-week minimal intervals are acceptable for the interval between dose 1 and 2 and dose 2 and 3.[120] The interval between the next-to-last and last dose should be 6 months, and this booster dose is recommended at school entry and must be after the fourth birthday.[121] There is no need to restart the series if interrupted. OPV may be used in the same schedule, but OPV is no longer being produced in the U.S. and, for practical purposes, is no longer available. OPV continues to be the preferred vaccine in countries where poliomyelitis is or recently was endemic, and it is the only vaccine suitable for eradication of the disease.[2,120]

Contraindications and Precautions

IPV is only contraindicated in children who have experienced a severe allergic reaction to a previous dose of IPV or to streptomycin, polymyxin B, or neomycin. OPV is contraindicated in children who have immunosuppressive conditions due to congenital immunodeficiency (agammaglobulinemia or hypogammaglobulinemia), cancer (leukemia or lymphoma), immunosuppressive chemotherapy, or acquired immunodeficiency syndrome (AIDS).[23,120] OPV also is contraindicated for family and other close contacts of immunocompromised people because of the risk of transmission of OPV to the affected person. Vaccination in pregnancy should be avoided on theoretical grounds, but, if necessary, IPV can be given.

No significant adverse reactions have been observed after administration of IPV. The major adverse reaction to OPV is VAPP, which develops at a rate of 1 per 2.5 million vaccine doses.[123] Before the policy change in the U.S., healthy vaccine recipients represented about 40% of cases, contacts of recipients represented about 40% of cases, and immunosuppressed people represented 20%. Highest risk is associated with receipt of the first vaccine dose (1 per 700,000 recipients) and is 10-fold lower for subsequent doses. Risk in people with congenital immunodeficiency is about 2000-fold higher than in healthy recipients. The risk of VAPP appears to be raised by receipt of multiple doses of injectable antibiotics 1 to 30 days after immunization.[124] OPV rarely can cause disseminated infection and death in immunocompromised people.[57]

Varicella Vaccine

Live-attenuated varicella-zoster vaccine was licensed for use in U.S. children and adults in March 1995, and by 2009, 90% of 19- through 35-month-old children were immunized.[30] Varicella vaccine, developed in Japan from the Oka strain of varicella virus, is >95% effective in protecting against severe disease and 70% to 90% effective against mild to moderate illness for children 1 to 2 years of age, for at least 7 to 9 years after vaccination.[125–128] Children and adults who experience breakthrough infection with wild varicella-zoster virus usually demonstrate mild disease, with an average of <50 lesions (compared with >250 lesions observed in typical varicella).

Recommendations for Immunization

In 2005 and 2006, the ACIP made policy changes for use of live, attenuated varicella-containing vaccines for prevention of varicella.[128] A routine 2-dose schedule of varicella vaccination of children is now recommended along with a second-dose catch-up varicella vaccination for children, adolescents, and adults who previously had received only 1 dose. The basis for these changes was: (1) the recognition that vaccine failures occur after a first dose; (2) outbreaks of varicella had been reported in populations with high coverage with 1 dose of vaccine; (3) emergency revaccination during outbreaks, which had previously been recommended, was difficult and costly; and (4) evidence showed that a second dose could decrease vaccine failure rates. The ACIP also expanded recommendations for varicella-containing vaccines to promote wider use of the vaccine for adolescents, adults, and HIV-infected children and approved new criteria for evidence of immunity to varicella. Specific recommendations are as follows:

- All children <13 years of age routinely should receive 2 doses of varicella-containing vaccine, with the first dose administered at 12 through 15 months of age and the second dose at 4 through 6 years of age (i.e., before a child enters kindergarten or first grade). The second dose can be administered at an earlier age provided the interval between doses 1 and 2 is at least 3 months. However, if the second dose is administered at least 28 days following the first dose, the second dose does not need to be repeated.[8]
- A second catch-up dose of varicella vaccination is recommended for children, adolescents, and adults who previously have received 1 dose, to improve individual protection against varicella and for more rapid impact on school outbreaks. Catch-up vaccination can be implemented during routine health provision visits and through school and college entry requirements. Catch-up second dose can be administered at any interval ≥3 months after the first dose (Figures 6-2, 6-3 and 6-4). The minimum 3-month interval is the package insert allowance based on studies of the second dose. Future research is likely to evaluate intervals as short as 1 month. The 2-dose varicella vaccination schedule is similar to the MMR vaccination schedule. MMRV vaccine is licensed and indicated for simultaneous vaccination against measles, mumps, rubella, and varicella among children 12 months through 12 years of age. MMRV is associated with an increased risk of febrile seizures following the first dose in people 12 through 47 months of age. Unless a parent prefers MMRV, separate simultaneous administration of MMR and varicella vaccines is preferred to the combination vaccine for the first dose if the dose is given at 12 through 47 months of age. For second doses or doses administered at 48 months of age or older, the combination product generally is preferred, but providers need to consider the number of injections, the availability of vaccines, the timeliness of series completion, the likelihood of patient return, storage/cost considerations, patient choice, and the likelihood of adverse events. Students at all grade levels (including college) and children in childcare facilities should be protected against varicella.

HIV-infected children >12 months of age with CD4+ T-lymphocyte counts of >15% of expected for age and without evidence of varicella immunity may receive 2 doses of single antigen varicella vaccine at a minimum interval of 3 months. Because data are not available on safety, immunogenicity, or efficacy of MMRV vaccine in HIV-infected children, MMRV vaccine should not be administered as a substitute for the component vaccines when vaccinating HIV-infected children.

Women should be assessed prenatally for evidence of varicella immunity. Upon completion or termination of their pregnancies, women who do not have evidence of varicella immunity should receive the first dose of varicella vaccine before discharge from the healthcare facility. The second dose should be administered 4 to 8 weeks later (at the postpartum or other healthcare visit). To ensure administration of varicella vaccine, standing orders are recommended for healthcare settings where completion or termination of pregnancy occurs.

Varicella vaccine previously was recommended for people ≥13 years of age without evidence of immunity who: (1) have close contact with people at high risk for severe disease (HCP and family contacts of immunocompromised people); or (2) are at high risk for exposure or transmission. The ACIP now recommends that all people 13 years of age and older without evidence of immunity be vaccinated with 2 doses of varicella vaccine at an interval of 4 to 8 weeks. The vaccine may be offered during routine healthcare visits.

During a varicella outbreak, people who have received 1 dose of varicella vaccine should receive a second dose, provided the appropriate vaccination interval has elapsed since the first dose (3 months for people 12 months through 12 years of age, and at least 4 weeks for people ≥13 years of age).

Revised criteria for evidence of immunity to varicella include any of the following: (1) documentation of age-appropriate vaccination (preschool-aged children ≥12 months of age: 1 dose; school-aged children, adolescents, and adults: 2 doses); (2) laboratory evidence of immunity or laboratory confirmation of disease; (3) birth in the U.S. before 1980 (although for HCP and pregnant women, birth before 1980 should not be considered evidence of immunity); (4) a healthcare provider diagnosis of varicella or healthcare provider verification of history of varicella disease; and (5) history of herpes zoster based on healthcare provider diagnosis.[128]

Varicella vaccine can be given simultaneously with all other childhood vaccines. The vaccine also is recommended for postexposure prophylaxis of susceptible people exposed to varicella, and it can be used for control of outbreaks.

Contraindications and Precautions

Varicella vaccine induces mild varicelliform rash and fever in 5% to 10% of recipients.[125] Vaccine virus rarely can be transmitted from healthy people who experience rash. More serious adverse events (e.g., encephalitis, ataxia) have been reported rarely, at rates lower than expected after natural varicella and lower than background rates in the community. Varicella vaccine is contraindicated in people who have a blood dyscrasia, in people with primary or acquired immunodeficiency (including immunodeficiency due to HIV infection), in pregnant women, and in people who have had an anaphylactic reaction to varicella vaccine or any component, including gelatin. However, vaccine can be given to people with humoral immunodeficiency and can be considered for people with asymptomatic or mildly symptomatic HIV infection with age-specific CD4+ T-lymphocyte counts >15%, after the risks and benefits have been weighed.[126–128] As with measles-containing vaccines, vaccination should be delayed for ≥3 months after receipt of immunoglobulin or blood products, because response to vaccine administered within this interval is unknown. Although varicella vaccine virus rarely has been isolated from patients with herpes zoster, the risk of clinical herpes zoster after varicella vaccination appears to be substantially lower than risk after natural varicella infection.

Hepatitis A Vaccine

Since routine childhood vaccination was recommended in 1999 in states where hepatitis A rates consistently were elevated, the overall hepatitis A rate has declined dramatically. In 2009, the rate (0.66 per 100,000 population) was the lowest recorded, with 1987 cases reported.[92] Declines have been greater among age groups and regions where routine vaccination of children is recommended, likely reflecting the result of the current vaccination strategy. To maintain and further reduce the current low rates, the strategy was expanded in October 2005 to include routine vaccination nationwide of children 12 through 23 months of age.[129,130]

Recommendations for Immunization

HAV vaccines are produced in tissue culture and purified and inactivated with formalin; two vaccines have been licensed for use in the U.S. since 1995.[130] These vaccines are highly immunogenic and are >95% effective in preventing HAV infection when given as a 2-dose series to children or adults.[130,131] HAV vaccine also can provide protection after exposure and can be useful in controlling hepatitis A outbreaks in well-defined populations. HAV vaccine is licensed for use in children ≥12 months of age.[130] A combination product consisting of HAV and HBV vaccine given on a 0-, 1-, and 6-month schedule is licensed for people ≥18 years of age.

HAV vaccine is given as a 2-dose series, with doses separated by 6 to 18 months.[130] Recommendations for use of hepatitis A vaccine in children are as follows:

- All children should receive HAV vaccine at 1 year of age (i.e., 12 through 23 months). Vaccination should be completed according to the licensed schedules and integrated into the recommended childhood immunization schedule. Children who are not vaccinated by 2 years of age can be vaccinated at subsequent visits.
- States, counties, and communities with existing HAV vaccination programs for children 2 through 18 years of age are encouraged to maintain these programs. In these areas, new efforts focused on routine vaccination of children 1 year of age should enhance, not replace, ongoing programs directed at a broader population of children.
- In areas without existing HAV vaccination programs, catch-up vaccination of unvaccinated children 2 through 18 years of age can be considered. Such programs might be warranted, especially in the context of increasing incidence or ongoing outbreaks among children or adolescents.

In addition, high-risk groups recommended to receive HAV vaccine include MSM, users of illicit drugs, people with cirrhosis or clotting factor disorders, and people traveling to or working in countries where hepatitis A is highly endemic.

Contraindications and Precautions

Adverse reactions to HAV vaccine appear to be limited to pain at the injection site. The only contraindication to the vaccine is a severe reaction to a previous dose of the vaccine or to one of its components (alum or phenoxyethanol). Because HAV vaccine is inactivated, no special precautions need to be taken when immunizing immunocompromised people.

Influenza Vaccines

Since the worldwide influenza pandemic of 1918 that caused an estimated 25 to 50 million deaths, the control of influenza circulation has been a major challenge to clinicians and public health experts. During 1976–2007, annual estimates of influenza-associated deaths from respiratory and circulatory causes ranged from 3349 (in 1986–1987) to 48,614 (in 2003–2004). During seasons when influenza A (H3N2) circulating strains were prominent, 2.7 times more deaths occurred compared with seasons when A (H3N2) was not prominent.[132] The 2009 H1N1 influenza pandemic, which caused an estimated 12,000 deaths, has renewed awareness of influenza. Additionally, influenza causes >200,000 hospitalizations annually.[133] Because of the frequent antigenic changes in influenza viruses, the antigenic content of influenza vaccine is changed annually to optimize protection against influenza type A and B strains expected to circulate during the following winter and spring. Influenza viruses of type A (H1N1 and H3N2) and B are selected on the basis of immunologic match with circulating strains; viruses are grown in chicken embryos and combined into a single vaccine containing components of all these strains. The efficacy of vaccine is related to the degree of match between the vaccine and circulating influenza viruses. Major antigenic drift in the circulating strain(s) is associated with seasonal epidemics because the vaccine's effectiveness may be reduced substantially. Annual vaccination is necessary to ensure protection against each year's influenza strains.[134,135]

Recommendations for Immunization

Two types of influenza vaccines are licensed for use in the U.S., a trivalent inactivated vaccine (TIV) that is purified, split with a detergent, and inactivated with formalin; and a cold-adapted, live, nasally administered vaccine (live-attenuated influenza vaccine or LAIV) licensed for healthy people 2 through 49 years of age, including close contacts of high-risk people. In 2010, the ACIP and AAP recommended expansion of annual influenza vaccination to all people 6 months of age and older. TIV can be used for all people without contraindications. LAIV can be used for people 2 through 49 years of age. A quadrivalent nasally administered LAIV was licensed in 2012 by the FDA and is expected to be available for the 2013–2014 influenza season.

For previously unvaccinated children 6 months through 8 years of age, or children who did not receive 2010–2011 seasonal influenza vaccine, 2 doses of vaccine, given at 4-week intervals, are recommended. This 2-dose recommendation also includes children 6 months through 8 years of age who were vaccinated for the very first time in the previous season (exactly one season prior) and received only 1 dose. For other groups, only a single dose is necessary.

Contraindications and Precautions

Inactivated influenza vaccine should not be administered to people known to have anaphylactic hypersensitivity to eggs or to other components of the influenza vaccine without first consulting a physician. People with egg allergy who may have experienced a mild reaction to eggs (e.g., hives) can receive influenza vaccine (TIV) with in-office observation for 30 minutes and availability of appropriate resuscitative equipment.[136] People with anaphylaxis or a severe reaction should be referred to an allergist for evaluation. Chemoprophylactic use of antiviral agents is an option for preventing influenza among such people.[137] However, people who have a history of anaphylactic hypersensitivity to vaccine components but who are also at high risk for complications from influenza can benefit from vaccine after appropriate allergy evaluation and desensitization. The list of children/adolescents with high-risk conditions includes:

- Children 6 months through 4 years of age.
- People who have chronic pulmonary (including asthma), cardiovascular (except hypertension), renal, hepatic, neurologic, hematologic, or metabolic disorders (including diabetes mellitus).
- People who are immunosuppressed (including immunosuppression caused by medications or by human immunodeficiency virus).
- People who are or will be pregnant during the influenza season.
- People who are aged 6 months through 18 years and receiving long-term aspirin therapy and who therefore might be at risk for experiencing Reye syndrome after influenza virus infection.
- Residents of nursing homes and other chronic-care facilities.
- American Indians/Alaska Natives.
- People who are morbidly obese (body-mass index ≥40).

People with moderate-to-severe acute febrile illness usually should not be immunized until their symptoms have resolved. However, minor illnesses with or without fever do not contraindicate use of influenza vaccine, particularly among children with mild upper respiratory tract infection or allergic rhinitis.

About 3% to 5% of recipients experience local tenderness or fever after vaccination. The occurrence of GBS within 6 weeks of influenza vaccination was observed in adults after the swine influenza vaccine program campaign (1976) but was not observed subsequently until 1990, when a case-control study suggested a slightly elevated risk in persons 18 through 64 years of age but not in people >65 years of age.[134] Given the substantial benefits of influenza vaccination among the target populations, the risk of GBS, if any, is exceeded by the benefits. LAIV should not be used in people of the following ages/with the following conditions: age <2 years or ≥50 years; asthma, reactive airways disease, or other chronic disorders of the pulmonary or cardiovascular systems; other underlying medical conditions, including metabolic diseases such as diabetes mellitus, renal dysfunction, and hemoglobinopathies; known or suspected immunodeficiency diseases or receipt of immunosuppressive therapies; receipt of aspirin or other salicylates (because of the association of Reye syndrome with wild-type influenza virus infection); history of GBS within 6 weeks of a dose of influenza vaccine; pregnancy; or history of hypersensitivity, including anaphylaxis, to any of the components of LAIV or to eggs.

Meningococcal Vaccines

From 2000 to 2004, approximately 2400 to 3000 cases of invasive meningococcal disease occurred annually in the U.S. In 2009, there were 980 reported cases.[92] The case-fatality ratio for meningococcal disease is approximately 10%, and severe sequelae (e.g., neurologic disability, limb loss) occur in approximately 10% of survivors.[138,139] Infants <1 year of age have the highest rates of meningococcal disease. During the 1990s, incidence rates of meningococcal disease increased among adolescents and young adults.[138] Evidence also showed that college freshmen living in dormitories have a modestly increased risk of meningococcal disease (4.6 cases per 100,000) compared with other people of the same age.[139]

Recommendations for Immunization

A meningococcal polysaccharide (MPSV4) vaccine, containing antigens of serogroups A, C, Y, and W135, has been used in the U.S. since licensure in 1981. This vaccine protects against the serogroups that cause approximately two-thirds of meningococcal disease in people 18 to 23 years of age in the U.S. More than half of the cases in infants are due to serogroup B, for which a licensed vaccine does not exist in the U.S.[139] Similar to other polysaccharide vaccines, MPSV4 induces a T-lymphocyte-independent immune response resulting in poor long-term immunity and inconsistent immunogenicity in children <2 years of age. An additional shortcoming is that MPSV4 does not reduce nasopharyngeal carriage or induce herd protection.[139] Before February 2005, MPSV4 vaccine was recommended for people at high risk for meningococcal disease and for outbreak control. Educating college freshmen about the potential for the MPSV4 vaccine to prevent severe infection also was recommended.

Employing the same technology used to develop PCV7, a meningococcal serogroup C conjugate vaccine was licensed in the United Kingdom in 1999. The vaccine was introduced into the routine infant schedule, with catch-up vaccination for older children and adolescents. In the 2 years after introduction of infant MCV, the incidence of serogroup C meningococcal disease declined by 87% in vaccinated people.[140,141] Substantial reductions in disease also occurred in unvaccinated populations as a result of herd immunity.

In the U.S., two quadrivalent MCVs (serogroups A, C, Y, and W-135) (MCV4) are licensed for use in people 2 through 55 years of age. MCV4 D (Menactra) is licensed for use down to the age of 9 months, and is recommended at that age only for children with persistent terminal complement component deficiency and infants in certain settings (see Fig 6-2). Each of the polysaccharides is linked to either a diphtheria toxoid or CRM 197. During prelicensure clinical trials, antibody levels postvaccination to MCV4 were at least as high among adolescents and adults as responses to MPSV4, the prior licensed product. Because MCV4 induces T-lymphocyte-mediated immunity and higher-quality immune responses, the duration of protection is thought to be longer than immunity produced by MPSV4.[139]

The latest recommendations for the use of MCV4 were published by CDC in 2011[142] (Figure 6-2). For people 11 through 18 years of age, a routine revaccination dose is recommended. The age for routine recommendation for dose 1 is 11 to 12 years. A dose of MCV4 (or MPSV4) administered at 10 years of age can be counted as the 11- to 12-year dose. Doses administered before age 10 are not counted as part of the routine adolescent MCV4 series.

People vaccinated at 11 through 15 years of age should have a revaccination dose at 16 through 18 years of age. The maximum age for the first routine dose is 18 years unless the person is going to college, in which case it is 21 years of age. If the first dose is not received before the 16th birthday only one dose is recommended routinely. The maximum age for the routine booster dose is 21 years (before the 22nd birthday) including people who receive the first dose at 11 through 15 years of age. Children who received the first dose at 11 through 15 years of age and did not receive the booster dose on schedule (age 16 through 18 years) may receive the booster dose upon entry to college. The minimum interval between doses is 8 weeks. Children who received the first dose at 11 through 15 years and did not receive the booster dose on schedule, and who are not entering college may receive the booster dose at age 19 through 21 years at the clinician's discretion.

For people 11 through 18 years with HIV, a primary series should be given, with 2 doses separated by 2 months. Recommendations for a booster dose are similar to people without HIV. HIV infection is not an indication per se for immunization of persons 2 through 10 years or ≥19 years of age, but the vaccine should be administered in a 2-dose schedule if it is administered (such as for international travel). People 19 through 21 years of age attending college also should be vaccinated.

For people 2 through 55 years with persistent complement component deficiency and asplenia (functional and anatomic) a primary series should be given. Two doses of MCV4 are separated by 2 months. A routine booster dose should be given thereafter. The interval to the first booster is 3 years if the primary series is completed by the seventh birthday, otherwise it is 5 years, with continued boosters every 5 years thereafter. For infants and children 9 through 23 months of age the MCV4 vaccine licensed for this age group should be given as a 2-dose series 3 months apart to those at high risk for meningococcal disease (complement deficiency, travel to high-risk area or during an epidemic.)

For people without HIV, without persistent complement component deficiency, and without asplenia (functional and anatomic), who may have received a first dose of MCV4 at 2 through 10 years of age (e.g., for international travel), subsequent doses should be administered at the following intervals, if the child remains at risk: after 3 years if the first dose was given at 2 through 6 years, or 5 years if the first dose was given at 7 years of age or older.[143]

Serogroup B capsular polysaccharide is poorly immunogenic in humans, so the focus in vaccine development has been on common proteins. OMP vaccines to prevent group B meningococcal disease have been shown to be safe and effective in older children and adults but not among infants and young children, in whom rates of serogroup B diseases are highest. In addition the variability in OMP strains causing endemic disease will likely limit their usefulness in the U.S. since individual vaccines might need to be made for each strain.

Precautions and Contraindications

Vaccination should be deferred for people with moderate or severe acute illness until the person's condition improves. Vaccination with MCV4 or MPSV4 is contraindicated among people known to have a severe allergic reaction to any component of the vaccine, including diphtheria toxoid (for MCV4), or to dry natural rubber latex. Because both MCV4 and MPSV4 are inactivated vaccines, they can be administered to people who are immunosuppressed as a result of disease or medications; however, response to the vaccine might be less than optimal.

Studies of vaccination with MPSV4 during pregnancy have not documented adverse effects among either pregnant women or newborns. On the basis of these data, pregnancy should not preclude vaccination with MPSV4 if indicated. MCV4 is safe and immunogenic among nonpregnant people 11 through 55 years of age, but data are not available on the safety of MCV4 during pregnancy. Women of childbearing age who become aware that they were pregnant at the time of MCV4 vaccination should contact their healthcare provider or the vaccine manufacturer.

Rotavirus Vaccine

Rotavirus is the most common cause of severe gastroenteritis in infants and young children worldwide. In developing countries, rotavirus gastroenteritis is a major cause of childhood death and is responsible for more than half a million deaths per year in children <5 years of age.[144,145] Prior to routine use of rotavirus vaccines, rotavirus gastroenteritis resulted in relatively few childhood deaths in the U.S. (approximately 20 to 70 per year). However, nearly every child in the U.S. was infected with rotavirus by 5 years of age and most developed gastroenteritis, leading to >400,000 physician visits, >200,000 emergency department visits, 55,000 to 70,000 hospitalizations each year, and direct and indirect costs of approximately $1 billion.[145]

A live-attenuated tetravalent rotavirus vaccine prepared from rhesus rotavirus type 3 and human-rhesus reassortant types 1, 2, and 4 was licensed in 1999 for use in infants in the U.S. In precensure controlled trials, this vaccine, was shown to be safe and highly effective, preventing >90% of hospitalizations for rotavirus diarrhea.[146] After licensure, the vaccine was recommended in early March 1999 by the ACIP, AAP, and AAFP. In early June 1999, reports of adverse events suggested that cases of intussusception might follow rotavirus vaccination. Subsequent studies demonstrated that children given this rotavirus vaccine had a relative risk of intussusception of 24.8 during 3 to 7 days after the first dose, with an estimated risk of 1 case per 10,000 vaccinated infants.[27] On the basis of these data, the ACIP and the AAP rescinded the recommendation for routine use of rotavirus vaccine in the U.S., and the manufacturer withdrew the vaccine from distribution.[28]

The next generation of rotavirus vaccines thus far has resulted in two products. The ACIP states no preference between the two products. The first vaccine is a pentavalent reassortant vaccine (RV5, or Rotateq, Merck) that was licensed in the U.S. by the FDA in February 2006. This vaccine is a live oral vaccine that contains 5 reassortant rotaviruses (G1, G2, G3, G4, and P1A) developed from human and bovine parent rotavirus strains.[147] Data from prelicensure trials showed immunogenicity of 93% to 100%, and efficacy of 74% against rotavirus gastroenteritis of any severity, and 98% against severe gastroenteritis.[148] The incidence of serious adverse events, intussusception, fever, and irritability was similar among RV5 and placebo recipients.[145,149] The second is a monovalent rotavirus vaccine based on an attenuated human rotavirus strain of P1A[8]G1 specificity, RIX 4414 (RV1, or Rotarix, GlaxoSmithKline Biologicals) which was licensed in 2008. This orally administered vaccine, given in 2 doses, has shown good clinical efficacy[150] and in a trial of more than 60,000 infants, no increase in intussusception was noted among recipients of the vaccine versus placebo.[151] In postlicensure studies in Mexico and Brazil, RV1 prevented approximately 80,000 hospitalizations and 1300 deaths annually and was associated with a short-term risk of intussusception in approximately 1 per 51,000–68,000 vaccinated infants.[152]

Introduction of RV5 and RV1 has been associated with a dramatic reduction in rotavirus-associated hospitalizations, office visits, and overall burden of disease due to rotavirus in the U.S.[153–157]

In 2010, a virus or parts of a virus called porcine circovirus was found in both rotavirus vaccines. This virus does not cause disease in humans and is not thought to be a safety or efficacy concern.[158,159]

Recommendations for Immunization

All infants should be immunized routinely with 3 doses of RV5 administered orally at 2, 4, and 6 months of age, or 2 doses of RV1 administered orally at 2 and 4 months of age. The first dose should be administered between 6 weeks and 14 weeks 6 days of age. Subsequent doses should be administered at 4- to 10-week intervals, and all doses of vaccine should be administered by 8 months 0 days of age. RV can be administered together with other childhood vaccines indicated at the same visits.

Premature infants (i.e., infants born at <37 weeks' gestation) can be immunized if they are at least 6 weeks of age, are being or have been discharged from the hospital nursery, and clinically are stable. Infants living in households with people who have or are suspected of having an immunodeficiency disorder or impaired immune status can be vaccinated, including infants living in households with pregnant women.

Readministration of a dose of RV to an infant who regurgitates, spits out, or vomits during or after administration of vaccine is not recommended. The infant should receive the remaining recommended doses of RV at appropriate intervals. If a recently vaccinated child is hospitalized for any reason, no measure other than routine universal precautions need be taken to prevent the spread of vaccine virus in the hospital setting.

Contraindications and Precautions

Contraindications for use of RV: history of severe hypersensitivity to any component of the vaccine; history of serious allergic reaction to a previous dose of vaccine; history of intussusception; or history of severe combined immunodeficiency (SCID). SCID is a contraindication because 5 cases of SCID have been diagnosed in infants who received RV vaccine with evidence of gastrointestinal tract symptoms presumably caused by vaccine virus.[160,161]

Human Papillomavirus Vaccine

More than 100 types of papillomaviruses have been recognized on the basis of DNA sequence analyses,[162] over 40 of which infect the genital area. HPV is associated with a variety of clinical conditions that range from benign skin and mucous membrane lesions to cancer. Clinical manifestations with the most frequently associated HPV types include skin warts (types 1, 2, 3, and 10), recurrent respiratory papillomatosis (types 6 and 11), condyloma acuminata (types 6 and 11), and cervical cancer (types 16, 18, 31, 33, and 45). HPV is one of the most common causes of sexually transmitted infections in the U.S. and worldwide, causing almost all of the morbidity and mortality associated with cervical cancer.[162] Based on the association of HPV with cervical cancer and precursor lesions, HPVs can be grouped into low-risk and high-risk HPV types. In the U.S. and Europe, HPV-16 accounts for approximately 50% of cases of cervical cancer, with types 18, 31, and 45 accounting for an additional 25% to 30% of cases.[163]

Vaccination against high-risk HPV types could substantially reduce the incidence of cervical cancer. Administration of HPV-16 vaccine has been shown to reduce the incidence of HPV-16 infection and HPV-related cervical intraepithelial neoplasia.[164] In addition, a bivalent HPV vaccine was efficacious in preventing persistent cervical infections with HPV-16 and HPV-18 and associated cytologic abnormalities and lesions.[165] Two HPV vaccines are licensed: a quadrivalent vaccine containing virus-like particles of serotypes 6, 11, 16, and 18; and a bivalent vaccine containing virus-like particles of serotypes 16 and 18.[166–168]

Recommendations for Immunization

HPV vaccination is recommended for females, and there is no preference for use of quadrivalent or bivalent vaccines (HPV4 and HPV2) for prevention of cervical cancer. Recommendations for use of HPV vaccine include routine vaccination of females 11 to 12 years of age[166,167] (Figure 6-3). Vaccination can be started in females as young as 9 years of age. Vaccination also is recommended for females 13 through 26 years of age who previously have not been vaccinated or who have not completed the full vaccine series. HPV vaccine is administered intramuscularly in a 3-dose schedule. Doses should be administered at times 0, 1–2 months, and 6 months. HPV vaccine can be administered at the same visit as other age-appropriate vaccines, such as Tdap, Td, and MCV4. Cervical cancer screening recommendations have not changed for females who receive HPV vaccine because approximately 30% of cervical cancers are caused by types not in the vaccine.[166]

HPV vaccine is not recommended for use in pregnancy. The vaccine has not been associated causally with adverse outcomes of pregnancy or adverse events to the developing fetus. However, data on vaccination in pregnancy are limited. Any exposure to vaccine in pregnancy should be reported to the vaccine pregnancy registry (Merck: 800-986-8999, GlaxoSmithKline: 888-452-9622).

HPV4 vaccine is licensed for males 9 through 26 years of age[168] and has been shown to be effective for prevention of genital warts.[169] HPV4 has been licensed by the FDA for prevention of anal cancer, and is recommended for males 11 through 21 years of age and for males 22 through 26 years of age who are immunosuppressed, have HIV infection, or are men who have sex with men. HPV4 may be given to males 9 through 10 years and 22 through 26 years of age at the provider's discretion.

Contraindications and Precautions

HPV vaccine is contraindicated for people with a history of immediate hypersensitivity to any vaccine component. Quadrivalent HPV vaccine is produced in yeast cells. Bivalent HPV vaccine is produced using a baculovirus-infected insect cell line. HPV vaccine can be administered to people with minor acute illnesses (e.g., diarrhea or mild upper respiratory tract infections, with or without fever). Vaccination of people with moderate or severe acute illnesses should be deferred until after the illness improves.

SELECTED OTHER VACCINES THAT MAY BE USED IN CHILDREN AND ADOLESCENTS

Calmette-Guérin Bacillus Vaccine

A live-attenuated vaccine prepared from the Calmette-Guérin bacillus (formerly bacille Calmette-Guérin, BCG) strain of *Mycobacterium bovis*, BCG vaccine is intended to prevent serious *M. tuberculosis* disease.[167] The vaccine is used routinely throughout most of the developing world but only in restricted situations in the U.S. Data regarding the efficacy of BCG are highly variable and conflicting. Meta-analyses suggest that a single dose of BCG vaccine given at or soon after birth is about 50% effective in preventing the most severe outcomes of *M. tuberculosis* infection (disseminated or miliary tuberculosis).[170,171] Vaccine efficacy data in adults, such as HCP, are inconclusive. BCG vaccine can cause reactivity of the tuberculin skin test, and thus reduce its utility for monitoring for *M. tuberculosis* infection and aiding in the decision whether preventive antimicrobial therapy is indicated.

In the U.S., BCG vaccine should only be considered for tuberculin-negative infants and children who continually are exposed and cannot be separated from adults who have active tuberculosis and are untreated, are treated inadequately, or have strains resistant to rifampin and isoniazid.[170–172] Information about BCG vaccine can be found at www.cdc.gov/tb/publications/factsheets/prevention/BCG.htm/.

Vaccines for Travelers

Cholera Vaccine

Cholera vaccine is not available in the U.S. The previously available vaccine prepared from killed whole *Vibrio cholerae* organisms was approximately 50% effective for 6 months after vaccination, but use was not recommended routinely except to satisfy requirements for entry into certain countries. An oral cholera vaccine (DuKoral) is available in some European countries and in Canada but it is not recommended for travelers. Other vaccines are under development.[173]

Japanese Encephalitis (JE) Vaccine

JE virus (JEV), a mosquito-borne flavivirus, is the most common vaccine-preventable cause of encephalitis in Asia. Among an estimated 35,000 to 50,000 annual cases, 20% to 30% of patients die, and 30% to 50% of survivors have neurologic or psychiatric sequelae. No treatment exists. For most travelers to Asia, the risk for JE is very low but varies on the basis of destination, duration, season, and activities.

JEV vaccine is recommended for travelers who plan to spend a month or longer in endemic areas during the JEV transmission season and for laboratory workers with a potential for exposure to infectious JEV. Vaccine should be considered for: (1) short-term (<1 month) travelers to endemic areas during the JEV transmission season if they plan to travel outside of an urban area and will have an increased risk for JEV exposure; (2) travelers to an area with an ongoing JEV outbreak; and (3) travelers to endemic areas who are uncertain of specific destinations, activities, or duration of travel. JEV vaccine is not recommended for short-term travelers whose visit will be restricted to urban areas or times outside of a well-defined JEV transmission season.

Two JEV vaccines are licensed in the U.S. An inactivated mouse brain-derived JEV vaccine (JE-VAX (JE-MB)) has been licensed since 1992 to prevent JE in people ≥1 year of age traveling to JE-endemic countries. Supplies of this vaccine are limited because production has ceased. In March 2009, an inactivated Vero cell culture-derived vaccine (IXIARO (JE-VC)) was licensed for use in people aged ≥17 years of age. All remaining doses of JE-MB expired in May 2011. Current options for U.S. providers to protect children younger than 17 years include enrolling the child in a clinical trial, administering JE-VC off-label, or advising the patient to receive JE vaccine at an international health travelers clinic in Asia.[174]

Typhoid Fever Vaccine

Two typhoid vaccines are available in the U.S. for travelers: a purified capsular polysaccharide parenteral vaccine prepared from the typhoid Vi antigen, and an oral live-attenuated vaccine (*Salmonella* Typhi Ty21a strain).[175] The inactivated Vi vaccine is given as a single dose, with booster doses at 2-year intervals if exposure continues. The oral vaccine is given as a 4-dose series of enterically coated capsules at 2-day intervals, taken before meals; the need for booster doses after this vaccine is uncertain. Both vaccines have efficacy of 50% to 80%. The minimal recommended ages for use of these vaccines are 2 years for the inactivated Vi vaccine and 6 years for the oral vaccine.

Typhoid vaccination is indicated for people who potentially will be exposed to contaminated food and water while traveling to areas in which typhoid is endemic, for laboratory workers exposed to the organism, and for people exposed to typhoid carriers in the household. Inactivated Vi vaccine produces local reactions (swelling, induration) in 7% and fever or headache in fewer than 3% of recipients. Oral typhoid vaccine produces only minor adverse events, including nausea, vomiting, and abdominal discomfort. Oral typhoid vaccine should not be given to immunocompromised people (including people with HIV infection).

Yellow Fever

Yellow fever (YF) is a vector-borne disease transmitted to a human from the bite of an infected mosquito. YF is endemic to sub-Saharan Africa and tropical South America and is estimated to cause 200,000 cases of clinical disease and 30,000 deaths annually. Infection in humans is capable of producing hemorrhagic fever and is fatal in 20% to 50% of people with severe disease.[176] No treatment exists for YF disease. A traveler's risk for acquiring YF virus is determined by multiple factors, including immunization status, location of travel, season, duration of exposure, occupational and recreational activities while traveling, and local rate of virus transmission at the time of travel.

All travelers to countries in which YF is endemic should be advised of the risks for contracting the disease and available methods to prevent it, including use of personal protective measures and receipt of vaccine. Administration of YF vaccine is recommended for people ≥9 months of age who are traveling to or living in areas of South America and Africa where a risk exists for YF virus transmission. Because serious adverse events can occur following YF vaccine administration, HCP should vaccinate only people who are at risk for exposure or who require proof of vaccination for country entry. To minimize the risk for serious adverse events, HCP should observe the contraindications, consider the precautions to vaccination before administering vaccine, and issue a medical waiver if indicated.[177,178] The YF vaccine is only available in the U.S. from providers certified by state health departments (wwwnc.cdc.gov/travel/yellow-fever-vaccination-clinics/search.htm).

YF vaccine should not be given to pregnant women; however, if a pregnant woman is traveling to an endemic area and cannot avoid potential exposure, she may be given the vaccine. The vaccine is contraindicated in people who have anaphylactic allergy to eggs and people who are immunocompromised. There is evidence that vaccine virus can be transferred from breastfeeding mothers to infants in human milk, as a breastfeeding infant has developed encephalitis following vaccination. Breastfeeding should be considered a precaution for YF vaccine.[178]

SOURCES OF INFORMATION ON VACCINES

Important sources for information about vaccines are as follows:
Official package information insert. Manufacturers provide product-specific information for each vaccine; some of these are reproduced in their entirety in *Physicians' Desk Reference* (PDR) and are dated.
Centers for Disease Control and Prevention. Specific information on immunization and vaccine-preventable diseases is available from the following sources: (1) National Center for Immunization and Respiratory Diseases, Centers for Disease Control and Prevention, Atlanta GA 30333; (2) CDC Information Center: voice, 1-800-232-INFO (CDC-INFO); and (3) the CDC website at www.cdc.gov/vaccines/
Morbidity and Mortality Weekly Report. This report, published weekly by the CDC, contains vaccine recommendations, reports of specific disease activity, policy statements, and regular and special recommendations of the ACIP. Subscription information is available from the following sources: MMWR Morb Mort Wkly Rep, Superintendent of Documents, United States Government Printing Office, Washington, DC 20402-9235 (202-783-3238); and online at www.cdc.gov/mmwr/.
Health Information for International Travel. CDC publishes this booklet as a guide to the requirements and recommendations for specific immunizations and health practices for travel to various countries. The booklet can be obtained from the Superintendent of Documents, United States Government Printing Office, Washington, DC 20402-9235. Travelers' health information can also be obtained through the CDC internet site, at www.cdc.gov/travel, or through the CDC information center (1-800-232-4636).
AAP Red Book: Report of the Committee on Infectious Diseases. The full report containing recommendations on all licensed vaccines, published by the AAP, is updated every 3 years. The most recent *Red Book* was published in 2012 and can be ordered from American Academy of Pediatrics, 141 Northwest Point Blvd, PO Box 927, Elk Grove Village, IL 60009-0927, or from the AAP website, at www.aap.org/bookstore/, or 888-227-1770.
Control of Communicable Diseases in Man. The American Public Health Association publishes this manual at approximately 5-year intervals. The 18th edition (2004) is available. The manual contains valuable information concerning infectious diseases; their occurrence worldwide; immunization, diagnostic, and therapeutic information; and up-to-date recommendations on isolation and other control measures for each disease presented. The manual can be ordered from the American Public Health Association, 1015 15th St NW, Washington, DC 20005.
Health departments. Most state and many local health departments provide routine immunizations, immunization cards, and schedules to patients. They also send out routine reports of disease incidence. Many states have print information online to be downloaded.
World Health Organization. Additional information about the World Health Organization and international vaccine programs may be found online at www.who.int/vaccines/.
Global Alliance for Vaccines and Immunization. Information on the Global Alliance for Vaccines and Immunization may be found at the website www.vaccinealliance.org/.
Additional useful sources of information. The Immunization Action Coalition, online at www.immunize.org/; the National Network for Immunization Information, online at www.idsociety.org/; the Vaccine Education Center, online at www.chop.edu/service/vaccine-education-center/home.html; the Institute for Vaccine Safety, online at www.vaccinesafety.edu.

7 Chemoprophylaxis

John S. Bradley

Chemoprophylaxis is prevention of disease by administration of a drug. An antimicrobial agent is given to an individual who is at risk of developing an infection because of exposure. The term "prophylaxis" as used in this chapter does not apply to those situations in which infection is already established; however, for some children who are already infected, the term has been used in situations to denote the prevention of "disease" rather than infection. Immunoprophylaxis (see Chapter 5, Passive Immunization; Chapter 6, Active Immunization), barrier prophylaxis (e.g., use of condoms; see Chapter 53, Urethritis, Vulvovaginitis, and Cervicitis; Chapter 54, Pelvic Inflammatory Disease), and chemical repellents for arthropod vectors are discussed elsewhere. Specific discussions of the prevention of travelers' diarrhea (see Chapter 8, Protection of Travelers), neonatal conjunctivitis (see Chapter 82, Conjunctivitis in the Neonatal Period (Ophthalmia Neonatorum)), malaria (see Chapter 271, *Plasmodium* Species (Malaria)), and human immunodeficiency virus (HIV) infection (see Chapter 109, Epidemiology and Prevention of HIV Infection in Children

and Adolescents) can also be found elsewhere. Similarly, immune or chemoprophylaxis for immunocompromised hosts, such as solid organ or bone marrow transplant subjects, or those subjects being treated for cancer, are not discussed specifically in this chapter.

Ideally, recommendations for antimicrobial prophylaxis should be based on data documenting efficacy in prospective, randomized, controlled studies. This standard is met uncommonly because of the infrequency and highly variable rate of infection after a given exposure, which necessitates studies with very large sample sizes. Most prophylactic regimens are presumed to be efficacious on the basis of small clinical trials, supporting pharmacology and biologic plausibility. Also, prophylaxis may be justified solely by the severe consequences of possible infection (e.g., infection of implanted neurosurgical or cardiac foreign material).

Chemoprophylaxis of infection in children can be classified as general or specific. Chemoprophylaxis is *general* when all children, regardless of underlying disease or other factors, are at substantial risk of infection following exposure to a pathogen and administration of an antimicrobial agent may prevent disease (e.g., *Neisseria meningitidis* in households). *Specific* chemoprophylaxis is administered to certain children who are deemed at special risk for infection due to the presence of an immunodefective state or anatomic structural anomalies. Chemoprophylaxis should be administered during the entire interval of documented increased risk of infection. The duration of general or specific chemoprophylaxis vary. Prophylaxis can be short term, following a specific exposure (e.g., *Neisseria meningitidis*), more prolonged with ongoing exposure (e.g., malaria) or over several years (e.g., rheumatic fever prophylaxis).

The benefits of chemoprophylaxis strategies to decrease morbidity and mortality and their attendant costs to the healthcare system should be weighed against potential risks, including drug toxicities, costs, and the development and spread of antimicrobial resistance. Every effort should be made to limit the duration of prophylaxis or to find alternative methods to prevent infection (e.g., clean intermittent catheterization of the urinary bladder to prevent urinary tract infections). Recommendations change periodically on the basis of evolving knowledge, changing pathogens, and the susceptibility to antimicrobial agents. Updated guidelines are published periodically by the Centers for Disease Control and Prevention (CDC) in *Morbidity and Mortality Weekly Report*, the American Academy of Pediatrics (AAP) in the *Red Book*, Report of the Committee on Infectious Diseases[1] in the *Medical Letter on Drugs and Therapeutics*[2] by the American Heart Association (AHA),[3] and in peer-reviewed journals.

GENERAL PRINCIPLES

For chemoprophylaxis to be effective, four criteria should be met:

1. The antimicrobial drug(s) used must have activity against the likely infectious agent or must disrupt pathogenesis (e.g., prevent toxin production).
2. The host should have a well-defined increased risk of disease. Other important factors considered in assessing the need for prophylaxis are the likelihood of development of infection following exposure, the severity of infection, and communicability to others.
3. The safety of a chemoprophylactic agent must be such that complications of its administration do not outweigh the risks of infection (i.e., an acceptable risk-to-benefit ratio).
4. The chemoprophylactic agent must have adequate tissue concentrations present at the time of exposure to the infectious agent.

CHEMOPROPHYLAXIS IN HEALTHY CHILDREN

Chemoprophylaxis is recommended to prevent surgical and trauma-related infections (Table 7-1) or to prevent disease associated with significant morbidity and mortality caused by bacterial, viral, fungal, mycobacterial, and parasitic agents (Table 7-2).

Specific Pathogens with a Defined Point of Exposure

Neisseria meningitidis

For meningococcal disease, the reported secondary attack rates among household contacts of index cases range from 0.25% in adults to 10% for infants younger than 1 year. Prophylaxis is reviewed in Chapter 125, *Neisseria meningitidis*, and doses of primary and alternative agents are listed in Table 7-2. Regimens using rifampin, ciprofloxacin, and ceftriaxone are effective in eliminating nasopharyngeal carriage of *N. meningitidis*.[4] Use of rifampin has the largest experience in children. Prophylaxis should be instituted as soon as possible (preferably within 24 hours) for contacts in households and childcare centers, and sometimes for

TABLE 7-1. Classification of Operative Wounds and Risk of Infection

Classification	Criteria	Risk (%)
Clean	Elective, not emergency, nontraumatic; primarily closed; no acute inflammation; no break in technique; respiratory, GI, biliary, and GU tracts not entered	<2
Clean-contaminated	Urgent or emergent, otherwise clean; elective opening of respiratory, GI, biliary, or GU tract with minimal spill and not infected urine or bile; minor technique break	<10
Contaminated	Nonpurulent inflammation; gross spill from GI tract; entry into biliary or GU tract in the presence of infection; major break in technique; penetrating trauma <4 hours' duration; chronic open wounds to be grafted or covered	~20
Dirty	Purulent inflammation (e.g., abscess); preoperative perforation of respiratory GI or GU tract; penetrating trauma >4 hours' duration	~40

GI, gastrointestinal; GU, genitourinary.

school contacts as well as for persons who have had contact with infected oral secretions. Rifampin is excreted into body fluids, causing red discoloration of urine and tears in 80% of individuals. Rifampin alters the metabolism of some drugs, including oral contraceptives, phenytoin, phenobarbital, carbamazepine, warfarin compounds, and other agents utilizing the hepatic cytochrome P450 enzyme system. Safety of rifampin in pregnancy has not been established. Alternative agents include ceftriaxone and ciprofloxaxin.[4] Ceftriaxone requires injections, but compliance and antimicrobial exposure is assured. Ciprofloxacin has been evaluated in adults and demonstrated to eradicate carriage; fluoroquinolone agents are relatively contraindicated in pregnant women, and prepubertal children due to concerns for possible arthropathy. However, arthropathy is unlikely to occur with a single fluoroquinolone dose administered for prophylaxis and may assure compliance compared with the 2-day, 4-dose regimen required with rifampin.

Haemophilus influenzae type b

Prophylaxis of *Haemophilus influenzae* infections is discussed in Chapter 172, *Haemophilus influenzae*, and Chapter 173, Other *Haemophilus* Species. Doses of primary and alternative agents for prophylaxis are listed in Table 7-2. Rifampin is approximately 95% effective in the eradication of nasopharyngeal carriage of *Haemophilus influenzae* type b (Hib) in children, but studies have fallen short of clearly documenting its efficacy in prevention of disease.[5,6] Prophylaxis is indicated if an incompletely immunized child younger than 4 years has close exposure to a case of invasive *Haemophilus* disease. The efficacy of prophylaxis for invasive strains of *H. influenzae* other than type b (e.g., types a, f, and others) has not been evaluated. Recommendations for initiation of prophylaxis in childcare or school settings vary; local public health authorities should be consulted.

In general, prophylaxis is recommended in childcare settings when: (1) 2 or more cases of Hib disease have occurred within a 60-day period; or (2) incompletely immunized children younger than 4 years have been exposed. Similar prophylactic regimens should be considered when exposure to other invasive *H. influenzae* infection occurs, including exposure to encapsulated serotypes such as types a and f, although there are no data supporting the efficacy of rifampin prophylaxis against serotypes other than Hib.

TABLE 7-2. Chemoprophylaxis for Healthy Children Exposed to Specific Pathogens[a]

Pathogen	Prophylactic Agent	Dose/Day	Maximum Dose/Day	Divided Doses	Duration
Bordetella pertussis[b]	Erythromycin	40–50 mg/kg	2.0 g	4	14 days
	Azithromycin	10 mg/kg	500 mg	1	5 days
	or				
	Clarithromycin	15 mg/kg	1.0 g	2	7 days
Haemophilus influenzae type b	Rifampin	20 mg/kg	600 mg	1	4 days
Corynebacterium diphtheriae	Erythromycin	40–50 mg/kg	20 g	4	7 days
	or				
	Benzathine penicillin	600,000 units (IM) if <30 kg 1.2 million units (IM) if ≥30 kg			Once
Neisseria meningitidis	Rifampin	20 mg/kg	1.2 g *or* 600 mg	2 / 1	2 days / 4 days
	or				
	Ceftriaxone	125 mg (IM) if <12 years 250 mg (IM) if ≥12 years			Once
	or				
	Ciprofloxacin	500 mg if ≥18 years			Once
Yersinia pestis (pneumonic)	Sulfonamide	40 mg/kg if <9 years		2	7 days
	or				
	TMP-SMX	8 mg/kg TMP		2	7 days
	Tetracycline	15 mg/kg if ≥9 years	1.0 g	4	7 days
Vibrio cholerae[c]					
<9 years	TMP-SMX	8 mg/kg TMP		2	3 days
9 through 17 years	Tetracycline	50 mg/kg	2.0 g	4	3 days
≥18 years	Ciprofloxacin	15 mg/kg	1.0 g	2	3 days
Streptococcus agalactiae	Ampicillin (maternal intrapartum)		2.0 g; then 1.0 g (IV) q4 h		Until delivery
	or				
	Penicillin G (maternal intrapartum)		5 million units; then 2.5 to 3 million q4h		Until delivery
Mycobacterium leprae (borderline or lepromatous)	Dapsone	1 mg/kg	100 mg	1	3 years
Herpes simplex virus[d]	Acyclovir (neonate; see text)	15 mg/kg (IV)		3	7–10 days
	Acyclovir (suppression of oral, genital or ocular infection)	10–20 mg/kg	800	2–4	Up to 12 months or longer
Influenza A[e]	Amantadine, rimantadine	5 mg/kg	150 mg if 1–9 years 200 mg if ≥10 years	1–2	See text
	Oseltamivir	30 mg if 1–2 years; 45 mg if 3–5 years 60 mg if 6–12 years	75 mg if ≥13 years	1	See text
	Zanamivir inhaled (for prophylaxis for children 5 years of age and older)	2 inhalations (5 mg per inhalation, 10 mg total per dose)	2 inhalations total	1	See text
Scabies	5% permethrin	Topically			Once
Neisseria gonorrhoeae					
Ophthalmia neonatorum	0.5% erythromycin	Topically			Once
Sexual exposure					
<45 kg	Ceftriaxone	125 mg (IM)			Once
45 kg and ≥9 years	Ceftriaxone	250 mg (IM)			Once
	or				
	Cefixime	400 mg			Once
Chlamydia trachomatis					
<9 years	Erythromycin	50 mg/kg	2.0 g	4	7 days
≥9 years	Doxycycline	4 mg/kg	200 mg	2	7 days
	or				
	Azithromycin	1.0 g			Once

Continued

TABLE 7-2. Chemoprophylaxis for Healthy Children Exposed to Specific Pathogens—cont'd

Pathogen	Prophylactic Agent	Dose/Day	Maximum Dose/Day	Divided Doses	Duration
Treponema pallidum	Benzathine penicillin G alt	50,000 units/kg (IM)	2.4 million units (IM)	2	Once[a]
	Doxycycline if ≥9 years alt	4 mg/kg	200 mg		14 days
	Azithromycin	2 g			Once
Klebsiella granulomatis	Doxycycline if ≥9 years or	4 mg/kg	200 mg	2	3 weeks
	TMP-SMX	8 mg/kg TMP	320 mg TMP	2	3 week

alt, alternative; IM, intramuscularly; IV, intravenously; SMX, sulfamethoxazole; TMP, trimethoprim.

[a]Alternative drugs used only if other(s) cannot be used; listings are not exhaustive. Some regimens are not of proven benefit. Administration is oral except as noted.

[b]See Chapter 162, Bordetella pertussis (Pertussis) and Other Bordetella Species, for doses by age.

[c]Resistance of isolate requires revision of chemoprophylactic regimen.

[d]Agents listed only as guidelines to possible dosing; data evolving.

[e]Agents not approved for use in children younger than 1 year.

Group B Streptococcus

Early-onset disease due to group B streptococcus (*Streptococcus agalactiae*) can be prevented by intrapartum administration of ampicillin or penicillin to women[7] (see Chapter 119, *Streptococcus agalactiae* (Group B Streptococcus)). Intrapartum administration of antibiotics does not prevent disease in infants who were infected before starting therapy, or prevent late-onset GBS infections.

Human Immunodeficiency Virus (HIV)

Perinatal or intrauterine transmission of HIV is diminished by the administration of zidovudine and other anti-HIV retroviral therapy to the mother during pregnancy, with continued treatment of the infant for various periods of time after delivery, depending on the regimen used. An area of active investigation, the most current information on treatment and prophylaxis is posted on the website of the NIH (AIDSinfo: http://aidsinfo.nih.gov/). Specific 2010 recommendations on regimens to prevent neonatal HIV infection can be found at: http://aidsinfo.nih.gov/ContentFiles/PerinatalGL.pdf. Current HIV maternal/neonatal prophylactic regimens with zidovudine and other agents or cesarean delivery have reduced the rate of transmission in worldwide studies to <2% (see Chapter 109, Epidemiology and Prevention of HIV Infection in Children and Adolescents).[8] For recommendations for health-care worker exposure[9] or sexual/injection-drug nonoccupational HIV exposure,[10] detailed antiviral drug recommendations, based on risks of transmission balanced by risks of antiviral drug toxicity with chemoprophylaxis, also are provided at the NIH's AIDSinfo website. The risk of HIV infection may be decreased post exposure, particularly if antiviral prophylaxis is provided within 12 to 24 hours of exposure (see Chapter 109, Epidemiology and Prevention of HIV Infection in Children and Adolescents).

Herpes Simplex Virus

Neonatal herpes simplex virus (HSV) infection usually results from transmission at the time of labor and delivery. Prophylaxis for both pregnant women and the exposed neonate is not well defined.[11] With vaginal delivery during maternal primary genital infection, transmission of HSV to the infant may exceed 50%, whereas delivery during maternal reactivation disease carries a risk of less than 5%. It may be difficult to determine whether an active HSV infection is primary or recurrent, because primary genital infection often is asymptomatic. Diagnostic tests for maternal HSV infection, including specific tests for HSV-1 and HSV-2, and rapid PCR testing for HSV DNA from mucosal surfaces, will aid in defining risk of infection to the neonate. For pregnant women, data on

the efficacy of preventing infection using antiviral prophylaxis with acyclovir or valacyclovir has prompted recommendations for the use of antiviral agents during the last month of pregnancy to prevent recurrent infection at the time of delivery, although the impact of prophylaxis on preventing neonatal infection has not yet been demonstrated.[11,12]

For the neonate potentially exposed to a mother with recurrent HSV-2 at the time of delivery, many experts recommend cultures (e.g., cultures of the umbilicus, conjunctiva, mouth, and nasopharynx) at 12–24 hours of age in all infants who are asymptomatic without antiviral therapy, while others consider that documented exposure to virus at the time of vaginal delivery constitutes sufficient risk to the infant to begin intravenous acyclovir therapy to prevent symptomatic infection. Positive results from culture specimens taken 24 hours or more after delivery are more likely to indicate infection, with a higher risk of developing symptomatic disease; many experts recommend intravenous acyclovir therapy to prevent symptomatic infection.[13]

For neonates with documented central nervous system HSV-2 infection, oral acyclovir prophylaxis for the first 6 months of life has been associated with a modest benefit in improved cognitive development at 5 years of age, compared with those who did not receive prophylaxis.[14]

Acyclovir and valacyclovir prophylaxis to prevent recurrent symptomatic disease has been used to reduce the number of recurrent genital and oral-cutaneous HSV infections in adolescents and adults with frequent recurrences.[15] In addition, acyclovir has been used prophylactically in children younger than 3 years who were exposed to HSV infections in childcare center outbreaks (30 to 60 mg/kg per day in 3 to 5 divided doses).[16] Some experts also recommend acyclovir prophylaxis for ocular HSV infections (recurrent HSV keratitis or recurrent infection of skin adjacent to the eye), to prevent corneal ulcerations and scarring, although no data exist on the safety and efficacy of prophylaxis for children in this situation[17] (see Chapter 295, Antiviral Agents).

Respiratory Tract Bacterial and Viral Pathogens

Mycobacterium tuberculosis. Isoniazid is effective in preventing symptomatic tuberculosis disease in latently infected asymptomatic children, and is believed to be effective in preventing acquisition of *Mycobacterium tuberculosis* infection in uninfected children following close exposure.[18,19] Treatment of latent tuberculosis infection is actually therapy rather than prophylaxis, because isoniazid administration eradicates inapparent, ongoing latent infection and prevents the progression to symptomatic disease (see Chapter 134, *Mycobacterium tuberculosis*).

Bordetella pertussis. Macrolide agents are felt to be effective in preventing the transmission of *Bordetella pertussis* and in halting the development of clinical pertussis in household contacts before symptoms occur.[20-22] Both 5 days of azithromycin and 7 days of clarithromycin administration in older children and adults are likely to be as effective as 14 days of erythromycin administration in preventing disease following exposure. Of the effective macrolides, azithromycin is the best tolerated and therefore the preferred agent. Given the association of idiopathic hypertrophic pyloric stenosis (IHPS) with administration of erythromycin to neonates, azithromycin also is the preferred agent for newborns; however, the safety profile of this agent in the newborn is not well defined and cases of IHPS following azithromycin have been reported. Risk for severe or fatal pertussis following exposure in neonates warrants administration of azithromycin, with close observation.

Influenza virus. Protection against influenza in high-risk patients, such as those with underlying cardiac or pulmonary disease, is best achieved by annual immunization. However, when this is not possible or is delayed, antiviral prophylaxis to prevent infection until immunization can be completed is an appropriate strategy.[23,24] Prophylaxis also should be considered for immune-compromised children for whom active immunization may not be protective. Neuraminidase inhibitors (zanamivir and oseltamivir) are effective for treatment and prophylaxis of both influenza A and influenza B virus infections. Although oseltamivir is not FDA-approved for infants less than 12 months of age, uncontrolled data on the safety and efficacy for treatment in this age group have been published, and use for treatment and prophylaxis is recommended down to 3 months of age.[25] Insufficient data exist for infants less than 3 months of age; prophylaxis is not recommended routinely.[23,26] Since 2005–2006, influenza A viruses have demonstrated widespread resistance to both amantadine and rimantadine, and influenza B virus is intrinsically resistant to these agents. However, for adamantane-susceptible strains of influenza A virus, these agents are also effective as prophylaxis. Healthcare providers should follow annual recommendations by the CDC and AAP for optimal prophylaxis strategies, particularly for winter seasons in which vaccine strains of influenza are not well matched with circulating strains.

Unusual Agents

Prophylaxis is recommended for a number of infrequent infections (see Table 7-2), including diphtheria, plague, cholera, and leprosy. Consultation with public health or infectious disease experts is recommended for dealing with these unusual infections in the United States.

Sexually Transmitted Agents

Prophylaxis is recommended after exposure to certain sexually transmitted agents. Despite the lack of evidence, prophylaxis is justified because: (1) transmission rates of disease after exposure are high; and (2) the diagnosis of infection may be difficult until active disease develops. Additionally, identification and treatment of index cases and contacts are critical to decreasing transmission in the community. Therefore, for certain infections that may be asymptomatic and for which transmission rates exceed 50%, such as gonorrhea, *Chlamydia trachomatis* infection, and syphilis, it is reasonable to provide therapy on an empiric basis, as outlined by the CDC[27] (see Table 7-2). There are also guidelines for evaluation and treatment of sexually abused children and adolescents.[27] (Chapter 56, Infectious Diseases in Child Abuse). Infants born to mothers who have untreated gonorrhea are at high risk of infection and should be given ceftriaxone 25–50 mg/kg IV or IM once, not to exceed 125 mg.[27]

CHEMOPROPHYLAXIS FOR SURGICAL PROCEDURES AND TRAUMA

Surgical procedures (see Chapter 102, Clinical Syndromes of Device-Associated Infections) and traumatic injuries (see Chapter 88, Infection Following Trauma) are associated with a variable risk for infection. Studies documenting the efficacy of systemic prophylaxis of surgical wound infections have been performed primarily in adults, but the pathogenesis of such infections is assumed to be similar in children. Risk of infection can be estimated by categorizing the type of surgical procedure as clean, clean-contaminated, contaminated, or dirty, yielding risk of infection from less than 2% up to approximately 40% (see Table 7-1).[28] Further assessment of risk is based on patient type.[29] Antibiotic prophylaxis is warranted in all procedures that are clean-contaminated, contaminated, or dirty (see Chapter 67, Peritonitis; Chapter 68, Appendicitis; Chapter 88, Infection Following Trauma; Chapter 102, Clinical Syndromes of Device-Associated Infections).

Principles

During surgical procedures, the time of maximum risk of infection is relatively finite, and, therefore, chemoprophylactic regimens should be limited in duration. A single dose of antimicrobial agent given 60 minutes or less before the initial incision usually provides adequate tissue concentrations throughout operations of less than 4 hours' duration.[30-33] When surgery is prolonged, major blood loss occurs, or the agent used has a short half-life (e.g., 1–2 hours) a second dose is advisable during the procedure.[32]

Surgical prophylaxis should be reserved for use in situations in which: (1) the risks of infection outweigh the risks of toxicity of antibiotic therapy or the development of antibiotic resistance; and (2) infection would have major consequence (e.g., when foreign material such as a ventriculoperitoneal shunt is implanted). The choice of antibiotic is based on spectrum of activity against the most likely pathogens and the penetration at the site of interest. Periodic consensus recommendations for prophylaxis during surgical procedures are published in the *Medical Letter on Drugs and Therapeutics.*[2] Quality standards for prophylaxis in surgical procedures have been proposed.[34] With rising rates of infection caused by community-associated methicillin-resistant *Staphylococcus aureus* (MRSA), the use of surgical prophylaxis with an agent with activity against MRSA, such as vancomycin, is now recommended for certain procedures in settings with a high rate of postsurgical infections caused by MRSA. In addition, anti-MRSA prophylaxis is used for selected patients known to be colonized with MRSA who are to undergo extensive surgery, particularly involving the placement of foreign material.[2]

Surgical Procedures

Neurosurgery. Placement of a ventriculoperitoneal shunt is classified as a clean procedure. However, the morbidity associated with infection of ventriculoperitoneal shunts is high. A favorable role has been demonstrated for prophylactic antibiotic therapy.[35,36]

Head and neck surgery. For clean-contaminated surgery involving the head and neck, prospective studies of adults with cancer suggest that more prolonged therapy beyond 24 hours is not associated with lower infection rates.[37] A meta-analysis of studies investigating antimicrobial prophylaxis for tonsillectomy demonstrated decreased fever, but no decrease in rates of secondary hemorrhage or pain.[38]

Noncardiac thoracic surgery. Few studies document the efficacy of prophylactic antibiotics in thoracic surgery, but antibiotics nearly always are given. Studies in adults undergoing chest procedures for trauma generally have shown that antibiotic administration reduces rates of infection and that therapy through the time of use of a chest tube has variable effects on the incidence of pneumonia and empyema.[39] No prospective studies have been performed in children.

Cardiac surgery. In cardiovascular surgery, antibiotic prophylaxis almost always is given. Even with a small risk of perioperative infection, the high morbidity of infection has justified its use as currently proposed in surgical infection guidelines.[2,40-42] Treatment for 24 hours is likely to provide maximum benefit with acceptable risks; treatment greater than 48 hours is not likely to provide additional benefit. For surgeries that last longer than 400 minutes, patients who were given a second dose of cefazolin demonstrated a statistically significant decrease in infections compared with those who were not (7.7% versus 16%).[42]

Evaluation of risk factors for pacemaker infections suggested an increased risk of infection in the absence of antimicrobial prophylaxis.[43] Subsequent prospective study of antimicrobial prophylaxis during implantation of pacemakers in adults has demonstrated a significant reduction in the incidence of infection with the use of prophylaxis.[44] Routine antimicrobial prophylaxis is recommended for cardiovascular implantable electronic devices in the 2010 Guidelines by the AHA.[45]

Abdominal surgery. A large number of studies performed in adults document efficacy of antimicrobial prophylaxis in abdominal surgical procedures, particularly for colorectal procedures and appendectomy when perforation has occurred.[29] Prophylactic agents should have activity against common flora of the gastrointestinal tract, especially gram-negative enteric and anaerobic bacteria. For an appendectomy for acute appendicitis, a Cochrane meta-analysis demonstrated that prophylaxis compared with placebo provides improved outcomes.[46] However, for nonperforated appendicitis, a single preoperative antibiotic dose was as effective as either 24 hours or 5 days of prophylaxis.[47]

Orthopedic surgery. Prophylactic antibiotics (particularly antistaphylococcal agents) reduce the incidence of infection after several orthopedic procedures when a foreign body (such as an artificial joint or internal fixation device) is implanted. Efficacy of prophylaxis has been demonstrated most strikingly in joint replacement procedures in adults.[48] Current regimens most commonly employ single-dose or short-course (24 hours or less) cefazolin or a similar agent with good antistaphylococcal activity, with a caution to screen for MRSA colonization, and, if the patient is already known to be colonized or infected by MRSA, to use vancomycin prophylaxis.[2,49]

Genitourinary surgery. Prophylactic antibiotics are not routinely required for cystoscopy in a patient who does not have an indwelling catheter, and the urine is documented to be sterile. If the urine is not sterile, or is not known to be sterile (e.g., a culture has not been performed), a single dose of prophylactic antibiotic is recommended prior to the procedure. If the procedure is more invasive and involves ureteroscopy, or the implantation of prosthetic material, prophylaxis is recommended.[2]

Trauma

Traumatic injury has, understandably, a higher risk for infection than controlled surgical procedures, but the risk varies by type and location of injury (see Chapter 88, Infection Following Trauma; Chapter 90, Infection Following Bites). Trials of prophylactic antibiotics after significant trauma have inconsistently demonstrated a benefit in preventing infection, but may not always adequately identify the population most likely to benefit. One prospective, randomized, double-blind trial of intravenous cefonicid for patients requiring thoracostomy with chest tube placement after chest trauma found significantly fewer infections in those receiving antibiotic prophylaxis (1.6% in treated patients versus 10.7% in untreated patients).[50]

Mammalian Bite Wounds

Prophylaxis or early treatment of animal bite wound injuries is controversial (see Chapter 90, Infection Following Bites). A meta-analysis of 8 studies of antibiotic prophylaxis of mammalian bite wounds suggested a benefit for antibiotics when the bites were caused by humans, and when the mammalian bites occurred on the hand.[51] Amoxicillin-clavulanate (20 to 40 mg/kg per day of the amoxicillin component in 3 divided doses for 5 to 7 days) provides the best spectrum of activity for both animal and human bites, considering the most frequently responsible pathogens: *Pasteurella multocida* (in cat and dog bites), *Eikenella corrodens* (in human bites), anaerobic bacteria, streptococci, and *Staphylococcus aureus*.

CHEMOPROPHYLAXIS IN SPECIAL SITUATIONS AND IN CHILDREN WITH CONDITIONS PREDISPOSING TO INFECTION

Children predisposed to development of infection by virtue of underlying conditions, defined immunodeficient state, or underlying anatomic defect may benefit from chemoprophylaxis (see Table 7-3). Prophylaxis is required over a prolonged period of risk, and strict compliance with regimens is critical to preventing "breakthrough" infections.

Prior Rheumatic Fever

Patients who have a well-documented history of acute rheumatic fever (ARF) (including disease manifested by carditis, arthritis, or chorea) should receive continuous antibiotic prophylaxis to prevent recurrent attacks associated with either symptomatic or asymptomatic group A streptococcal infection. Prophylaxis should be initiated as soon as the diagnosis of acute rheumatic fever is made. The preferred prophylaxis agent is penicillin. To ensure adherence, monthly administration of benzathine penicillin (1.2 million units IM for children weighing more than 27 kg (60 lb); 600,000 units for those weighing less than 27 kg) is recommended, but for those believed to be adherent to oral therapy, continuous prophylaxis with penicillin V (phenoxymethyl penicillin), 250 mg twice daily, should be effective at preventing a streptococcal infection if an exposure occurs. For those receiving monthly intramuscular injections, adequate serum antibiotic levels may not persist beyond 3 weeks in some, and, in high-exposure situations, recurrences are less likely if IM therapy is provided every 3 weeks rather than every 4 weeks.[52]

The appropriate duration of chemoprophylaxis for rheumatic fever is not known; some studies suggest that treatment can be discontinued in young adults who are at low risk for recurrent episodes of group A streptococcal infection.[53,54] Current recommendations for minimum duration are 5 years (or until age 21 years) for those *without* carditis, and 10 years (or until age 21 years, whichever is longer) for those *with* carditis, without residual heart disease. For those with carditis *and* residual heart disease, prophylaxis should continue at least 10 years or until age 40 years (whichever is longer), with consideration given to lifelong prophylaxis[55] (Table 7-3).

Recommendations for other infections associated with *Streptococcus pyogenes* are less certain. Most experts recommend prophylaxis for children with poststreptococcal Sydenham chorea, similar to that for rheumatic fever. Some experts recommend prophylaxis for one year in children who have had an episode of poststreptococcal reactive arthritis (PSRA) but have no evidence of rheumatic fever, based on concerns that PSRA is an incomplete manifestation of ARF. If no evidence of rheumatic fever is present after 12 months of prophylaxis, therapy can be discontinued, but the child with PSRA should continue to be followed long term for new evidence of cardiac involvement.[56-58] The cost–benefit, safety, and efficacy of prophylaxis of pediatric autoimmune neuropsychiatric disorders associated with streptococcal infection (PANDAS) have not been established; currently, routine prophylaxis is not recommended.

For persons exposed to cases of severe invasive group A streptococcal disease, including toxic shock syndrome and necrotizing fasciitis, the theoretical small increased risk of infection is not sufficient to recommend prophylaxis routinely, and studies have not been conducted to establish the efficacy of such prophylactic treatment.

Asplenia

Children with functional or anatomic asplenic states, particularly sickle-cell anemia, have been shown to benefit from continuous penicillin prophylaxis to prevent pneumococcal and other bacterial infections (see Chapter 108, Infectious Complications in Special Hosts). A single prospective controlled study showed an

TABLE 7-3. Chemoprophylaxis in Special Situations (see text for references)

Disorder	Prophylactic Agents	Dosing	Duration
Prior rheumatic fever	Benzathine penicillin G	1.2 million units every 4 weeks (every 3 weeks if high-risk)	RF without carditis: 5 years after episode, or 21 years of age, whichever is longer
	or		
	Penicillin V	250 mg twice daily	RF with carditis, without regurgitation (clinical or echocardiograph): 10 years after episode, or well into adulthood, whichever is longer
	or		
	Sulfisoxazole	500 mg if ≤27 kg (60 lb); 1 g if >27 kg; once daily	
	or		
	Erythromycin	250 mg twice daily	RF with carditis, with regurgitation: 10 years after episode, or at least 40 years of age, sometimes lifelong
Asplenic states[a] [47,49]	Penicillin V	125 mg twice daily if <5 years 250 mg twice daily if ≤5 years	At least until 5 years of age or 5 years after surgical removal, whichever is longer; see text
Recurrent otitis media	Sulfisoxazole	50 mg/kg at bedtime	3–6 months
	or		
	Amoxicillin	20 mg/kg at bedtime	3–6 months
	or		
	Amoxicillin	40 mg/kg per day divided q8 hours at onset of upper respiratory tract infection	3–5 days
Recurrent urinary tract infection	TMP-SMX	2 mg/kg TMP once daily	Variable
	or		
	Nitrofurantoin	1–2 mg/kg once daily	
Endocarditis Dental, oral, or upper respiratory tract procedures	Standard Amoxicillin (PO)	50 mg/kg (maximum 2 g) procedure; then 25 mg/kg 6 hours after initial dose	Once 30 to 60 minutes before the procedure
	Standard (penicillin-allergic) Clindamycin (PO)	20 mg/kg (maximum 600 mg)	
	or		
	Oral medication impossible Ampicillin (IM or IV)	50 mg/kg (maximum 2 g)	
	or		
	Azithromycin	15 mg/kg (maximum 500 mg)	Once 30 to 60 minutes before the procedure
	or		
	Clarithomycin		
	Cefazolin	50 mg/kg (maximum 1 g)	Once 30 to 60 minutes before the procedure
	or		
	Ceftriaxone		
	Gentamicin (IM or IV)		2 mg/kg (maximum 80 mg) before procedure; can be repeated 8 hours after initial dose

IM, intramuscularly; IV, intravenously; PO, by mouth; RF, rheumatic fever; SMX, sulfamethoxazole; TMP, trimethoprim.

[a]*Asplenic states include congenital and surgical asplenia, and splenic dysfunction associated with hemoglobinopathies; also considered for individuals with complement disorders. Vaccinations are also very important.*

84% reduction in rate of infection in children younger than 3 years of age who received daily oral penicillin V (125 mg twice daily for children <5 years; 250 mg twice daily for children ≥5 years) compared with those receiving placebo.[59] A follow-up placebo-controlled trial of penicillin prophylaxis beyond 5 years of age in children receiving comprehensive care for sickle-cell disease showed a low incidence of infection and no significant benefit for prophylaxis in preventing pneumococcal bacteremia or meningitis (2% in penicillin group versus 1% in placebo group).[60] It is recommended that prophylaxis be discontinued in children older than 5 years, provided that they have not previously had invasive pneumococcal infection and are appropriately immunized for age.

Asplenia from other causes (congenital, surgical, functional) also is associated with increased risk of fulminant septicemia. Compared with the incidence in healthy children, the incidence of mortality from septicemia is 50-fold higher after splenectomy for trauma (compared with >350-fold higher in children with sickle-cell disease). Although the risk is higher in younger children

and in the first 5 years after splenectomy, fulminant septicemia has been reported in adults more than 25 years after splenectomy.[61,62] There is general consensus that asplenic children with malignancy, thalassemia, congenital anomalies, or other diseases with high risk of fulminant infection should receive daily chemoprophylaxis.[61] There is less certainty about the need for prophylaxis in otherwise healthy children who undergo splenectomy for trauma. In general, prophylaxis (in addition to appropriate immunization) should be strongly considered for asplenic children younger than 5 years and should be considered for older children. Asplenic children should receive conjugate pneumococcal, meningococcal, and Hib vaccines as recommended in Chapter 6, Active Immunization.

Underlying Immunocompromising Conditions

The prevention of bacterial, viral, fungal, and mycobacterial infections in immune-compromised hosts is an area of active research. As new regimens for treatment of disease evolve, collaborative guidelines are published by professional organizations to aid the practitioner in decisions regarding prophylaxis for various high-risk populations, including children undergoing cancer chemotherapy,[63] stem cell transplantation,[64] solid organ transplantation,[65,66] and therapy of HIV.[67]

Similarly, as primary immunodeficiency disorders are identified increasingly and better characterized, a systematic approach to antimicrobial prophylaxis for each entity is considered, based on the expected pathogens and risks of infection.[68] For example, individuals lacking terminal components of complement, properdin deficiency, or other abnormalities of complement pathways are at risk of recurrent meningococcal infections and may benefit from penicillin prophylaxis. Immunization with a protein-conjugate vaccine is likely to be more protective than antibiotic prophylaxis for those immune deficiencies in which the child can mount an appropriate, protective response to immunization (see Chapter 105, Infectious Complications of Complement Deficiencies).[69]

Other Underlying Conditions

Recurrent Otitis Media

The widespread use of conjugate pneumococcal vaccines has been associated with a decrease in the incidence of acute and recurrent otitis media. The numbers of children who require antimicrobial prophylaxis for recurrent otitis media has decreased. In the past, sulfisoxazole, amoxicillin, and TMP-SMX have been shown effective for prophylaxis in otitis-prone children, although not all placebo-controlled investigations have documented benefit.[70–75] Children may be considered as candidates for prophylaxis if they have experienced 3 episodes of acute otitis media within the previous 6 months or 4 episodes within the previous 12 months. The development of colonization with antibiotic resistant organisms, as well as transmission to contacts (both adults and children) should be considered. Most experts recommend a trial of prophylactic antimicrobial therapy before consideration of placement of tympanostomy tubes.[76]

Urinary Tract Infection

Antibiotic prophylaxis is effective in preventing recurrent urinary tract infection and is indicated in children with underlying anatomic or neurologic lesions leading to a higher risk of infection, especially those with obstructive lesions or high-grade vesicoureteral reflex (grades III–V).[77–79] Prophylaxis is primarily designed to prevent incremental renal damage with each episode of pyelonephritis that may ultimately lead to renal failure later in life. In the past, children without the identifiable increased risk factors listed above who suffered recurrent infections also were believed to benefit from prophylaxis. In this group, documentation of 3 or more urinary tract infections within a 1-year period was considered a reasonable indication for prophylaxis. The benefit of prophylaxis in this group is limited to decreasing pain and discomfort that accompany UTIs, rather than in prevention of pyelonephritis and renal scarring, although even this benefit has been questioned in some well-controlled studies, which also document increased antimicrobial resistance associated with prophylaxis.[80–84]

Current American Urology Association guidelines suggest that more high-quality data are required before recommendations regarding antimicrobial prophylaxis can be made, particularly for specific high-risk groups that may benefit most from prevention of recurrent infections.[85]

Nitrofurantoin (1 to 2 mg/kg per day), and TMP-SMX (1 to 2 mg/kg per day of TMP component) are the best-studied regimens in children for prophylaxis.

Cardiac Abnormalities

The AHA periodically publishes guidelines for endocarditis prophylaxis. In 2007, major changes were made based on the Committee's conclusions that (1) extremely small numbers of cases of infective endocarditis might be prevented by antibiotic prophylaxis for dental procedures, even if prophylaxis were 100% protective; (2) prophylaxis should not be recommended solely on the basis of an increased lifetime risk of acquisition of endocarditis; (3) infective endocarditis prophylaxis for dental procedures should be recommended only for people with underlying conditions associated with the highest risk of adverse outcome from infective endocarditis; (4) for patients with these underlying conditions, prophylaxis should be given for all dental procedures that involve manipulation of gingival tissue or the periapical region of teeth or perforation of the oral mucosa.[3] Recommendations also focus emphasis on good oral hygiene, access to routine dental care, and eradication of dental disease to minimize the frequency of bacteremia that may be associated with daily brushing and flossing. Cardiac conditions associated with the highest risk of adverse outcome from endocarditis for which prophylaxis with dental procedures is still recommended are shown in Box 7-1. Antibiotic prophylaxis is no longer recommended for any other form of congenital heart disease, including mitral valve prolapse with regurgitation, acquired valvulopathy, hypertrophic cardiomyopathy, or presence of cardiac pacemakers or implanted defibrillators, unless there is a history of previous endocarditis or placement of a prosthetic valve. Antibiotic prophylaxis is not recommended for shedding of deciduous teeth or bleeding from trauma to the lips or oral mucosa.

BOX 7-1. Prophylaxis for Infective Endocarditis According to Cardiac Conditions and Dental Procedures[3]

Cardiac conditions associated with highest risk of adverse outcome from endocarditis for which prophylaxis with dental procedures is recommended

- Prosthetic cardiac valve
- Previous infective endocarditis
- Congenital heart disease (CHD)[a]
  - Unrepaired cyanotic CHD including palliative shunts and conduits
  - Completely repaired congenital heart defect with prosthetic material or device, whether placed by surgery or by catheter intervention, during the first 6 months after the procedure[b]
  - Repaired CHD with residual defects at the site or adjacent to the site of a prosthetic patch or prosthetic device (which inhibit endothelialization)
- Cardiac transplantation in which cardiac valvulopathy has developed

Dental procedures for which endocarditis prophylaxis *is* recommended for patients above

- All dental procedures that involve manipulation of gingival tissue or the periapical region of teeth or perforation of the oral mucosa
  - Professional cleaning with gingival probing, biopsies, suture removal, placement of orthodontic bands

Dental procedures for which endocarditis prophylaxis *is not* recommended even for patients above

- Routine anesthetic injections through noninfected tissue
- Taking of dental radiographs
- Drilling of carious teeth
- Orthodontic/prosthodontic procedures
  - placement or removal of appliances
  - placement of orthodontic brackets
  - adjustment of orthodontic appliances

[a]Except for conditions listed, antibiotic prophylaxis is no longer recommended for any other form of CHD.
[b]Prophylaxis is recommended because endothelialization of prosthetic material occurs within 6 months after the procedure.

Antibiotics recommended when prophylaxis is appropriate according to Box 7-1 are shown in Table 7-3. A single dose of antibiotic should be administered before the procedure. If the dose was inadvertently omitted, it can be administered up to 2 hours after the procedure.

Antibiotic prophylaxis is no longer recommended for routine respiratory tract procedures (e.g., intubation, extubation, bronchoscopy).[3] Antibiotic prophylaxis may be considered for patients listed in Box 7-1 who undergo an invasive procedure that involves incision or biopsy of the respiratory tract mucosa (e.g., tonsillectomy, adenoidectomy, bronchoscopy with incision of the respiratory mucosa) or when performed to treat an established infection (e.g., to drain an abscess or empyema). Antibiotic regimens should always include an agent active against oral (viridans) streptococci, but additional suspected pathogens from an abscess being drained may dictate broader spectrum prophylaxis.

Antibiotic prophylaxis is no longer recommended solely to prevent endocarditis in patients who undergo genitourinary (GU) or gastrointestinal (GI) tract procedures, including diagnostic esophagogastro-duodenoscopy or colonoscopy.[3] For patients listed in Box 7-1 who have an established GU or GI tract infection or for those who receive antibiotic therapy to prevent wound infection or septicemia associated with a GU or GI procedure, it is reasonable to include an agent active against *Enterococcus* species.[3] For patients listed in Box 7-1 scheduled for elective cystoscopy or other urinary tract manipulation who have enterococcal urinary tract infection or colonization, antibiotic therapy to eradicate/suppress enterococci in the urine before the procedure may be reasonable. If the procedure is not elective, it may be reasonable that the empiric or specific antimicrobial regimen administered include an agent active against enterococci.[3]

Antibiotic prophylaxis is recommended for procedures on infected skin, skin structures, or musculoskeletal tissue only for patients listed in Box 7-1. In 2007, the AHA reaffirmed previous recommendations of settings for which endocarditis prophylaxis is *not* indicated (including cardiac catheterization and cesarean delivery) and added the following procedures: ear and body piercing, tattooing, vaginal delivery, and hysterectomy.[3]

---

8 Protection of Travelers

Maryanne E. Crockett and Jay S. Keystone

Close to 900 million people travel internationally each year and estimates suggest that up to 7% of travelers are children.[1-3] Consequently, upwards of 60 million children may travel internationally each year. Annually up to 8% of travelers to the developing regions of the world are ill enough to seek medical healthcare while abroad or upon returning home.[4,5] Although travel can expose children to some risks, the benefits are many. Therefore, a careful pretravel evaluation to provide appropriate guidance and preparation is critical to protect pediatric travelers and their families and allow them to enjoy their time abroad.

PREPARATION FOR TRAVEL

General Advice

A pretravel evaluation should be performed at least 6 to 10 weeks prior to travel. The entire itinerary for the trip should be reviewed, including destinations, time and duration of travel, types of accommodation, activities, and potential exposure to insects and animals. The evaluation also should review the medical and particularly the immunization history of the child in order to ensure that appropriate advice is given regarding preventive measures, including necessary vaccines. This evaluation can be accomplished by providing a form for parents to complete and bring to the initial pretravel assessment visit. Particular attention should be given to children of immigrants who are returning to their home countries to visit friends and relatives because these children have been shown to be at increased risk of many infectious diseases and may be less likely to seek pretravel advice.[6-8] Many excellent resources, the majority of which are accessible online, provide pretravel advice for pediatricians (Box 8-1).

Travel health guidance should be provided regarding safety issues and infectious diseases.[9-12] Motor vehicle crashes are the most common cause of death among travelers; therefore, particular attention must be given to use of seat belts and car seats as recommended according to the age and size of the child. Car seats may not be available readily at the destination and therefore should accompany the family. Other injury concerns for children include drowning, falls from unprotected balconies or windows, and electrical injuries from unprotected outlets. Children and adolescents who participate in extreme sports and outdoor activities while traveling also should be informed of the potential risks. A parent traveling alone with children should have notarized documentation authorizing him or her to travel with the children.

Advice regarding food and water precautions and insect avoidance should be reviewed thoroughly. Skin protection is an important topic and includes both risk of serious sunburn and avoidance of infectious diseases. For sunblock, 30 is the minimum sun protection factor (SPF) recommended for children. Sunblock should be applied 30 minutes before exposure and always before insect repellent is applied where both are needed. Adolescent travelers should be counseled regarding safer sex practices and risks of body piercing and tattooing in less developed countries. Fresh water exposure of any kind should be avoided in areas that are endemic for schistosomiasis or where *Leptospira* organisms can contaminate the water. Exposure to infected stool of animals or humans can result in several types of parasitic infection either directly (e.g., hookworm) or through fecal–oral exposure (e.g., *Toxocara* spp.). Shoes provide more protection than sandals for children exposed to contaminated environments. Animal bites can result in injury, bacterial infection at the site, or rabies; therefore, children should be cautioned to avoid unknown animals, particularly dogs, while traveling. Since disposable diapers may not be available in some countries, parents should be aware that cloth diapers must be ironed after washing to kill eggs and larvae deposited on clothing by the tumbu fly, the vector of myiasis, in parts of Africa.

A travel medical kit should be assembled prior to travel and carried with the family at all times (Box 8-2). As at home, medications should be stored in childproof containers out of reach of children. A discussion of travel health insurance and what to do in the event of illness should be included in the evaluation. Written material summarizing the pretravel advice also may be helpful for families.

Immunizations

Although immunization rates have been increasing in the United States, there remain a significant number of children who are

BOX 8-1. Resources and Additional Information for Travelers

- *International Travel and Health,* print version updated biannually, online version updated regularly by the World Health Organization (WHO). Available online at www.who.int/ith/
- WHO vaccine summaries: www.who.int/vaccines/globalsummary/immunization/countryprofileselect.cfm
- Centers for Disease Control and Prevention (CDC) *Health Information for International Travel,* updated approximately every 2 years by the CDC, Atlanta, USA: U.S. Department of Health and Human Services (*The Yellow Book*). Available online at http://wwwnc.cdc.gov/travel/content/yellowbook/home-2010.aspx
- CDC travel information section: www.cdc.gov/travel/
- CDC *Morbidity and Mortality Weekly Report* (MMWR): http://www.cdc.gov/mmwr/
- CDC *Emerging Infectious Diseases Journal:* http://www.cdc.gov/ncidod/EID/index.htm
- CDC Malaria Hotline: 770-488-7788
- CDC Travelers' Health Automated Information Line (toll-free): 1-877-FYI-TRIP
- GIDEON (Global Infectious Diseases and EpidemiOlogy Network), available online at www.gideononline.com/
- Pickering LK, Baker CJ, Kimberlin DW, Long SS, (eds) *Red Book: 2009 Report of the Committee on Infectious Diseases,* 28th ed. Elk Grove Village, IL, American Academy of Pediatrics, 2009 (1-888-227-1770 Publications) – a new edition is published every 3 years
- The Pan American Health Organization, the regional office of the WHO: www.paho.org/
- Immunization Action Coalition: www.immunize.org/izpractices/p5120.pdf
- United States State Department Hotline for American Travelers (202-647-5225)
- United States State Department: http://travel.state.gov/
- International Association for Medical Assistance to Travellers: www.iamat.org
- Program for Monitoring Emerging Diseases (Pro-MED-mail): www.promedmail.org
- Committee to Advise on Tropical Medicine and Travel (CATMAT): http://www.phac-aspc.gc.ca/tmp-pmv/catmat-ccmtmv/index-eng.php
- Travax: www.travax.scot.nhs.uk/
- United States: American Society for Tropical Medicine and Hygiene travel health: www.astmh.org
- The International Society for Travel Medicine: www.istm.org
- United Kingdom: www.travelhealth.co.uk/diseases/travelclinics.htm
- Canada: www.travelhealth.gc.ca
- University of Minnesota Travel Handouts (in 20 languages): http://www.tropical.umn.edu/TTM/VFR/index.htm

BOX 8-2. Pediatric Travel Medical Kit

NONPRESCRIPTION ITEMS

- Personal information card: name, birth date, chronic medical conditions, regular medications, allergies, blood type, vaccination record, emergency contact information
- First-aid supplies: bandages, adhesive tape, gauze, antiseptic cleaning solution, commercial suture/syringe kit (with letter from physician)
- Thermometer
- Analgesics/antipyretics: acetaminophen, ibuprofen
- Skin care products: sunscreen (≥SPF 30), barrier ointment/cream, topical corticosteroid cream, disinfectant solution (e.g., chlorhexidine)
- Antihistamine (e.g., diphenhydramine)
- Insect repellent (diethyltoluamide: DEET), insecticide (permethrin)
- Water purification system
- Oral rehydration packets
- Antimotility agent (e.g., loperamide) if older child (≥2 years)
- Extra pair of prescription glasses

PRESCRIPTION ITEMS

- Currently prescribed medications
- Antimalarial prophylaxis
- Antibiotic for severe travelers' diarrhea (see text)
- Topical antibacterial ointment/cream
- Topical antifungal ointment/cream
- Topical ophthalmic/otic antibiotic solution

be required for entry into or travel from endemic countries. Vaccination against meningococcus, influenza, and polio are required for travelers to the Hajj in Saudi Arabia.[16] *Recommended* travel vaccines include vaccines that should be considered according to the risk of infection during travel.

During the pretravel evaluation, some children may need to receive vaccines in the recommended childhood and adolescent immunization schedule administered in an accelerated manner to complete their primary series, catch-up with routine vaccinations, or complete the recommended pretravel vaccine series prior to departure[16–19] (Table 8-1). The routine or catch-up schedule for immunizations should be continued when the child returns.

If administered simultaneously, ≥2 inactivated vaccines, as well as inactivated and live vaccines can be given. There is no required interval between different inactivated vaccines. Two parenterally administered live vaccines, if not given at the same time, should be administered at least 28 days apart.[20] Caution must be used when scheduling live vaccine administration following immune globulin (IG) administration because decreased immunogenicity of the vaccines can result.[18] This is particularly true of measles and varicella vaccines. Measles and varicella-containing vaccines should be deferred from 3 to 11 months after IG administration depending on the indication and dose of IG required (see Chapter 5, Passive Immunization). Although the effect of IG administration on the immunogenicity of varicella vaccine is unknown, the current recommendation is to use the same guidelines for varicella vaccine and IG as are used for measles-containing vaccines.[21] IG administration does not interfere with the immune response to yellow fever, oral polio virus (OPV), rotavirus vaccines, or any inactivated vaccines. IG should not be given <14 days after administration of a live vaccine.

Routine Immunizations

Most North American vaccine-preventable diseases are endemic globally; therefore, a child's routine vaccination schedule should be brought up to date prior to travel.[19] In particular, the primary series of vaccines, including at least 3 doses of the diphtheria and

underimmunized.[13] Many countries with low immunization rates have ongoing transmission of vaccine-preventable illnesses that rarely are seen in North America. Consequently, children who travel must have up-to-date immunization coverage to minimize their risk of contracting vaccine-preventable diseases if they travel to countries where these diseases are prevalent. Country-specific vaccine-preventable disease statistics and immunization schedules can be found on the World Health Organization (WHO) website and a listing of international vaccine names also is available online.[14,15]

Travel vaccines are divided into the categories of routine, required, and recommended. *Required* travel vaccines are needed by travelers to cross international borders, according to health regulations at destination. Proof of yellow fever vaccination may

TABLE 8-1. Acceleration of Routine Vaccine Schedule for Travel

Vaccine	Earliest Age for First Dose	Minimum Interval Between Doses
Combined hepatitis A and B[a]	1 year	1 week, 2 weeks between 2nd and 3rd doses (booster after 1 year)
Hepatitis A	1 year	6 months[b]
DTaP	6 weeks	4 weeks, 6 months between 3rd and 4th doses
IPV	6 weeks	4 weeks
OPV	Birth	4 weeks
Hib (conjugate)	6 weeks	4 weeks (booster after 12 months of age)
Hepatitis B	Birth	4 weeks, 8 weeks between 2nd and 3rd doses (3rd dose should be given ≥16 weeks after 1st dose)
PCV13	6 weeks	4 weeks, 8 weeks between 3rd and 4th doses (after 12 months of age)
Measles	6 months followed by MMR at 12 months and at 4 to 6 years of age	4 weeks
MMR	12 months	4 weeks
Rotavirus[c]	6 weeks	4 weeks
Varicella	12 months	4 weeks if ≥13 years of age 3 months if <13 years of age

DTaP, diphtheria, tetanus, acellular pertussis; Hib, Haemophilus influenzae *b; IPV, inactivated polio virus; MMR, measles, mumps, rubella; OPV, oral polio virus; PCV13, pneumococcal conjugate. Regular immunization schedule should be reinstituted upon return from the endemic area.*

[a]*Combined hepatitis A and B accelerated schedule is an off-label use for children.*

[b]*Hepatitis A booster does not need to be given as an accelerated schedule as seroconversion rate following the first dose is high. The second dose can be given any time after 6 months to induce long-lasting immunity.*

[c]*For rotavirus vaccine, the maximum age for the first dose is 14 weeks and 6 days, and the maximum age for the last dose is 8 months and 0 days.*

tetanus toxoid or the acellular pertussis (DTaP) vaccine, should be administered by standard or accelerated schedules (see Table 8-1). The Tdap adolescent preparation with acellular pertussis vaccine should be used as the adolescent booster beginning at 11 years of age.[22,23] People 7 through 10 years of age who are not fully immunized against pertussis should receive a single dose of Tdap. Tdap can be administered regardless of the interval since the last tetanus and diphtheria-containing vaccine. Underimmunized children <6 years of age also should receive the conjugate *Haemophilus influenzae* type b (Hib) vaccine prior to travel.

Although global polio eradication had been targeted for 2005, polio remains endemic in several countries in Asia and Africa (an up-to-date listing of polio cases can be found at www.polioeradication.org). OPV, although widely used in the WHO Expanded Programme on Immunization – Plus (EPI-PLUS), is not available in the U.S. An accelerated schedule for inactivated poliovirus vaccine (IPV) should be initiated if required, with the first dose given at 6 weeks of age and subsequent doses given at least 4 weeks apart.[19] If a child is traveling in the first few weeks of life and OPV is available, vaccination with OPV can be initiated at birth, with subsequent doses at 4-week intervals.[16] A booster dose of IPV should be given at 4 to 6 years of age and at least 6 months following the previous dose.

More than half a million children die of measles annually, with children <1 year of age having the highest risk of severe disease.

Also, the risk of subacute sclerosing panencephalitis is related to acquisition of measles virus at a young age. Maternal antibodies generally protect infants for <6 months. Children between 6 and 12 months of age who are traveling to countries where measles is endemic (including all countries where measles vaccination is not universal) should receive one dose of measles, mumps, rubella (MMR) vaccine prior to travel. Only doses given at or after 12 months of age count as part of the routine U.S. immunization schedule. Children >12 months of age should receive two doses of MMR given at least 28 days apart prior to travel.

Hepatitis B is part of the routine immunization schedule in the U.S.[24] Children who have not completed their routine hepatitis B series should receive hepatitis B vaccine prior to travel to highly endemic areas. The hepatitis B series can be accelerated with doses given at 0, 1, and 2 months, followed by a fourth dose at 12 months. A hyper-accelerated schedule of 0, 7, and 21 days with a fourth dose at 12 months can be used if necessary. Although this schedule is not licensed by the U.S. Food and Drug Administration, it is used widely in travel clinics. A 2-dose schedule of adult Recombivax HB at 0 and 4 to 6 months is licensed in the U.S. for adolescents 11 through 15 years of age.[24]

Hepatitis A vaccine is recommended universally for children in the U.S. and should be given as a 2-dose schedule beginning at 12 to 24 months of age with the second dose 6 months later.[25] Children who have not received the hepatitis A vaccine series should be vaccinated prior to travel to developing countries. The majority of hepatitis A cases imported into the U.S. by travelers are related to travel to Mexico and Central America.[25] Although hepatitis A generally causes asymptomatic or mild infection in young children, such children can shed virus for prolonged periods. Consequently, vaccination of young travelers is recommended to protect both the recipient and any contacts. Children from birth to <12 months of age who are at high risk of exposure to hepatitis A can be given 0.02 mL/kg of IG intramuscularly as passive hepatitis A prophylaxis.[25] For travel lasting longer than 3 months, a larger dose of 0.06 mL/kg should be used.

Twinrix (GlaxoSmithKline) is a combined hepatitis A and B vaccine that is licensed for people ≥18 years of age.[16,24] Twinrix-Junior is not licensed in the U.S. but is available in Europe and Canada for children 1 through 15 years of age. These vaccines are given in a 3-dose schedule at 0, 1, and 6 months. For last-minute travel they can be accelerated in a schedule of 0, 7, and 21 days with a booster given at 1 year.[26,27] In Canada and parts of Europe, two *adult* doses of the vaccine 6 months apart have been approved for children 1 through 15 years of age.[28,29]

Varicella vaccine is recommended for all susceptible children and is given in the U.S. as 2 doses to children from 12 months through 12 years of age. For children <13 years of age, the second dose should be given 3 months after the first. For adolescents 13 years of age and older, 2 doses are required with an interval of at least 4 weeks between doses.[19]

Conjugate pneumococcal vaccine (PCV13) is part of the routine childhood immunization schedule and should be given as a 4-dose series at 2, 4, 6, and 12 through 15 months of age, although PCV also can be accelerated as needed (see Chapter 123, *Streptococcus pneumoniae*).

Two quadrivalent conjugate meningococcal vaccines for serogroups A/C/Y/W-135 (MCV) are licensed in the U.S. for children. Both are recommended for people 2 through 54 years of age who are at increased risk of meningococcal disease, including travelers to countries with hyperendemic or epidemic meningococcal disease. MPSV4 is preferred for at-risk people ≥55 years of age. Also, MCV is recommended routinely for use in all children 11 to 12 years of age with a booster dose at 16 years of age.[30] Administer one dose at 13 through 18 years of age if not previously vaccinated (see Chapter 125, *Neisseria meningitidis*).[31,32]

Influenza vaccine is recommended for all people without medical contraindications 6 months of age and older.[33] It is noteworthy that the influenza season occurs from April to September in the southern hemisphere and year-round in the tropics.[2] Influenza outbreaks have occurred on cruise ships and on organized group tours in any latitude and season.[33]

Rotavirus vaccine is recommended for all children in the U.S. starting at 2 months of age in a 2- or 3-dose schedule depending on which of the 2 licensed vaccines is used.[34] Rotavirus vaccine can be given in an accelerated dosing schedule if needed (see Table 8-1).

Two human papillomavirus (HPV) vaccines are licensed in the U.S. and Canada and are recommended for use in all females at 11 to 12 years of age.[35,36] HPV4 vaccine is recommended for males and females at 11 to 12 years of age. HPV vaccines are administered in a 3-dose schedule, the second and third dose 2 and 6 months after the first dose. The first dose can be given as early as 9 years of age.

Required and Recommended Vaccines for Travel

Table 8-2 provides details regarding travel vaccines recommended for children.

Cholera Vaccine

The risk of cholera is low for travelers. Cholera vaccines are not available in the U.S. Cholera vaccines are licensed in some countries: WC/rBS (Dukoral) and two closely related bivalent cholera vaccines Shanchol and mORCVAX.[37] Dukoral is licensed for children ≥2 years of age. Cholera vaccine is not required for entry into any country. The WHO recommends use of cholera vaccine only for travelers at high risk such as emergency or relief workers who plan to work in refugee camps or as healthcare personnel in endemic areas.[38]

Typhoid Vaccine

Typhoid vaccine is recommended for pediatric travelers to the Indian subcontinent and other developing countries in Central and South America, the Caribbean, Africa, and Asia.[39] Children are particularly at risk of developing typhoid disease and of becoming chronic carriers. Two vaccines are available for prevention of typhoid: a live attenuated oral vaccine (Ty21a), which can be used in children ≥6 years of age, and a purified Vi capsular polysaccharide vaccine that is delivered intramuscularly to children ≥2 years of age. The efficacy of both vaccines is approximately 50% to 70%; receipt of the vaccine does not eliminate the need

for food and water precautions.[40–42] If exposure continues, revaccination is recommended every 2 years for the polysaccharide vaccine and every 5 years for the oral Ty21a vaccine.

The Ty21a vaccine only is available in capsules in the U.S., which limits usefulness in younger children. The Ty21a vaccine must be refrigerated and taken with cool liquids approximately 1 hour before eating. The Ty21a vaccine should not be taken concurrently with the antimalarial proguanil, and antibiotics should not be used from the day before the first capsule until 7 days after completing the vaccine course. Clinical trials of a Vi conjugate vaccine demonstrating safety, efficacy, and immunogenicity in children ≥2 years of age are ongoing.[43,44]

Yellow Fever Vaccine

Yellow fever vaccine is a live attenuated vaccine that may be required or recommended for travel to central South America and sub-Saharan Africa. Some countries in Africa require an international certificate of vaccination (or physician waiver letter) against yellow fever for all entering travelers; other countries may require evidence of vaccination for travelers coming from or traveling through endemic or infected areas. The vaccine is recommended for all children ≥9 months of age traveling to endemic areas. Yellow fever vaccine is effective 10 days after administration of the first dose and a booster is required every 10 years for travelers at ongoing risk. Risks and benefits of yellow fever vaccination and likelihood of infection must be considered carefully in pregnant women and people who are immunocompromised.[45] Yellow fever vaccine contains egg protein; therefore, people with previous anaphylaxis to eggs should not receive the vaccine. The vaccine is only available in the U.S. from providers certified by state health departments.[46]

A yellow fever vaccine-associated encephalitis syndrome has been reported in young infants at a rate of 0.5 to 4 per 1000 infants vaccinated.[16] Neurologic symptoms occur 7 to 21 days after immunization; disease is related to reversion of vaccine virus to wild-type neurotropic virus. Consequently, the vaccine is contraindicated in infants <6 months of age. For infants 6 to 9 months of age who cannot avoid travel to a yellow fever-endemic area, consultation with an expert in the field is recommended. Yellow fever vaccine-associated viscerotropic disease, a severe systemic illness that can result in fatal organ failure, rarely has been reported.

TABLE 8-2. Schedule and Dosing for Travel Vaccines

Vaccine	Schedule	Minimum Age	Dose (mL)	Route	Booster Dose
BCG (live attenuated)	1 dose	Birth	<30 days: 0.3 mL (dilute to half concentration) >30 days: 0.3 mL	Intradermal preferred but subcutaneous acceptable	None
Hepatitis A/B, combined (inactivated/recombinant)	3 doses: 0, 1, and 6 months	1 year	0.5 mL	Intramuscular	None
Meningococcal – A/C/Y/W-135 (polysaccharide)	1 dose	3 months (see text)	0.5 mL	Subcutaneous	<4 years: 2–3 years ≥4 years: 3–5 years
Meningococcal – A/C/Y/W-135 (conjugated polysaccharide)	1 dose	2 years	0.5 mL	Intramuscular	<7 years: 3 years ≥7 years: 5 years
Rabies (inactivated cell culture)	3 doses: 0, 7, 21 or 28 days	Birth	1.0 mL	Intramuscular	Consider at 2 years if high-risk
Typhoid, Ty21a (live attenuated)	4 doses: alternate days	6 years	1 capsule	Oral	5 years
Typhoid, Vi (capsular polysaccharide)	1 dose	2 years	0.5 mL	Intramuscular	2 years
Yellow fever (live attenuated)	1 dose	9 months	0.5 mL	Subcutaneous	10 years
Japanese encephalitis (IXIARO)	2 doses: 0 and 28 days	17 years	0.5 mL	Intramuscular	1 year

BCG, bacille Calmette-Guérin

Rabies Vaccine

Rabies is highly endemic in Africa, Asia (particularly India, China, and Indonesia), and in parts of Latin America, but the risk to travelers is low. Pre-exposure rabies immunization is recommended for travelers with an occupational risk of exposure, for people planning extended stays in endemic areas where medical care is limited, and for outdoor travelers.[47] Given that children are more likely to interact with animals and not report an animal bite, rabies pre-exposure vaccination should be considered for children traveling to endemic countries for at least 1 month. The pre-exposure vaccine is 3 doses of 1.0 mL each given intramuscularly at 0, 7, and 21 or 28 days.[47] The series can be administered using either of the two licensed vaccines in the U.S.: human diploid cell vaccine (HDCV), or purified chick embryo cell vaccine (PCECV). If a vaccinated child is bitten or sustains a skin-penetrating scratch by a potentially rabid animal, the wound must be washed thoroughly and 2 additional doses must be completed as soon as possible (given 3 days apart); rabies IG is not required.[48] Without pre-exposure immunization, rabies IG and 4 doses of an approved vaccine (given over 14 days) are required in the U.S. Current WHO recommendations are for 5 intramuscular or intradermal doses of vaccine.[49] (Note: rabies IG is often not available in many developing countries.)

Japanese Encephalitis Virus Vaccine

Japanese encephalitis, an arboviral infection transmitted by night-biting *Culex* mosquitoes, is endemic in rural areas of Asia although occasional epidemics occur in periurban areas. In temperate regions, transmission occurs from April to November, but disease occurs year-round in tropical and subtropical areas. The disease is uncommon in travelers.[50] Although the majority of cases are subclinical, half of patients with clinical disease have persistent neurologic abnormalities and the case fatality rate is close to 25%.[51] Vaccine is recommended for all travelers >12 months of age who are traveling in rural endemic areas for at least 1 month. Currently there is only one Japanese encephalitis vaccine (IXIARO/JE-VC), which is licensed in the U.S. for people ≥17 years of age.[51a] An inactivated mouse-brain-derived vaccine (JE-VAX/JE-MB) was previously licensed in the U.S. for children I through 16 years of age but is no longer available. Ongoing clinical trials of JE-VC are underway in children between 2 months and 17 years. Current options for JE vaccination for travelers <17 years include enrolling children in the ongoing clinical trials, administering JE-VC off-label, or obtaining JE vaccine in Asia at an international travel health clinic. A recent study found that half an adult dose of JE-VC was safe and immunogenic in children ages 1–3 years.[51b] Therefore, off-label use of JE-VC may be considered with an adult dose of the vaccine above 3 years and half a dose from 1 to 3 years. Two doses of JE-VC are given 1 month apart with the series being completed at least 1 week prior to travel. The duration of immunity is unknown. A booster dose of JE-VC may be given one year after the two dose primary series.

Meningococcal Vaccine

Five serogroups of *Neisseria meningitidis* (A, B, C, Y, and W135) are responsible for the vast majority of meningococcal disease. The epidemiology of serogroups responsible for disease is changing worldwide; B, C, and Y are most prevalent in the U.S., whereas A, C, and W135 (more recently) cause the majority of epidemic disease in sub-Saharan Africa where the incidence of meningococcal disease can be as high as 30 cases per 100,000 annually.[31,32]

Meningococcal vaccine is required for travelers to the Hajj and also is recommended for people traveling to the "meningitis belt" in equatorial Africa during the dry season from December to June. The quadrivalent conjugate vaccines for serogroups A/C/Y/W-135 (MCV4) can be given to children beginning at 2 years of age. Although there is little response to polysaccharide vaccines in children less than 2 years of age, some short-term protection to serogroup A may be provided by two doses of the vaccine given 3 months apart; consequently, this is advised for infants from 3 to 24 months of age who are traveling to high-risk areas. Children who received the conjugate or polysaccharide meningococcal vaccine before 7 years of age should be revaccinated within 3 years if they remain at risk.[32,51]

Conjugate vaccines for serogroups A, C, and A/C are available in a number of countries other than the U.S. for use in infants and older children.[52] A new 4-component vaccine for group B meningococcus has shown strong immunogenicity and good tolerance.[53]

Tickborne Encephalitis Virus Vaccine

Tickborne encephalitis is transmitted by *Ixodes ricinus* ticks in the forests of central and eastern Europe during the summer months.[54] Two vaccines are licensed in Europe for use in children ≥1 year of age (FSME-IMMUN and Encepur), and FSME-IMMUN is licensed in Canada, for use in people ≥16 years of age; however, neither is available in the U.S.[3,42]

BCG

Bacille Calmette-Guérin (BCG) vaccine is part of the routine vaccination schedule in many developing countries where tuberculosis (TB) is highly endemic. BCG does not prevent TB infection but has been shown to decrease the incidence of severe TB disease such as miliary TB and TB meningitis. Vaccination with BCG can be considered for a young human immunodeficiency virus (HIV)-negative traveler (<5 years of age) who will be spending a substantial period of time in a country that is highly endemic for TB when contact with people with active TB is likely.[16,55] In addition, children who do not receive BCG and who have traveled to a country with a high TB burden should have a tuberculin skin test prior to and 3 months after returning from travel.[2]

MALARIA

Prophylaxis

Malaria is caused by infection with *Plasmodium* species, most commonly through the bite of an infected female *Anopheles* mosquito. Malaria is one of the leading causes of death among children <5 years of age worldwide, causing more than half a billion infections and 1 million deaths each year. Young children, pregnant women, and people who previously or recently have not been exposed to malaria have the highest risk of severe disease. Although malaria is endemic throughout the tropics, the highest risk for malaria infection in travelers occurs in sub-Saharan Africa, Papua New Guinea, the Solomon Islands, and Vanuatu.[56] There is no vaccine available for prevention of malaria infection in travelers; therefore, families traveling with children must be provided with advice regarding personal protective measures and malaria chemoprophylaxis if they are traveling to endemic areas.

Chemoprophylaxis

The type of chemoprophylaxis recommended depends on the likelihood of drug resistance, potential adverse reactions, cost, and convenience. In addition, characteristics of the individual traveler, including age, ability to swallow tablets, and any specific contraindications, are relevant.[57] Breastfeeding infants require prophylaxis since antimalarial drugs do not reach high enough levels in human milk. Several medications are recommended for prevention of malaria in children: chloroquine, mefloquine, doxycycline, atovaquone/proguanil (AP, Malarone).[57,58] Primaquine is recommended as a primary agent in high *P. vivax* areas such as Central America, except for Honduras, and as a second-line agent in other areas when other antimalarial drugs cannot be used (see Chapter 271, *Plasmodium* Species (Malaria)).[59] Chloroquine and mefloquine should be initiated 1 to 2 weeks prior to travel although doxycycline, AP, and primaquine may be started 1 day before exposure. All chemoprophylactic agents must be continued for 4 weeks after departure from malaria-endemic areas, except for AP

BOX 8-3. Precautions for Use of Diethyltoluamide (DEET)

- Use repellents containing ≥30% DEET only
- Apply sparingly to exposed skin
- Apply only to intact skin
- Apply to face by wiping; avoid eyes and mouth; do not spray directly on face
- Wash off with soap and water when coming indoors
- Do not inhale or ingest repellent
- Do not apply on hands or other areas that are likely to come in contact with the eyes or mouth
- Do not allow children under 10 years of age to apply DEET themselves. Apply to your own hands then apply to the child
- Do not use on children less than 2 months of age

and primaquine which need be continued for only 1 week after exposure. Updated guidelines from national organizations such as the Centers for Disease Control and Prevention (CDC) and the Committee to Advise on Tropical Medicine and Travel (CATMAT) can be found online (see Box 8-1).

Protective Measures

Because no malaria chemoprophylaxis is 100% effective, personal protective measures, such as barrier and chemical protection and exposure avoidance, should be used to minimize risk of contact with mosquitoes. These protective measures also can decrease risk of other insectborne diseases, such as dengue and other arboviruses.

Since *Anopheles* mosquitoes that transmit malaria bite from dusk to dawn, children must have adequate protection during these hours. The *Aedes* mosquito that transmits yellow fever, chikungunya, and dengue virus bites primarily in the early morning and late afternoon. The vector of Japanese encephalitis, the *Culex* mosquito, bites between dusk and dawn. When thereis a risk of insect exposure, children should be dressed in light-colored clothing that covers their arms and legs. Other measures to avoid insect bites include staying in air-conditioned or well-screened accommodation or using insecticide-treated bed nets.

Chemical protection provides additional defense against insect-borne diseases. The safest and best studied is *N,N*-diethyl-meta-toluamide (DEET).[57] Although adverse reactions, such as encephalopathy and rashes, have been described with excessive or prolonged use of high concentrations of DEET in children, this compound is considered safe when used appropriately according to product label instructions[56,60] (Box 8-3). The concentration of DEET correlates with duration of protection; therefore, products with lower concentrations need to be reapplied. DEET is approved by the Environmental Protection Agency and the American Academy of Pediatrics in a concentration of 30% for children of ages down to 2 months; in standard preparations, this concentration will provide 4 to 6 hours of protection.[61] Non-DEET-containing repellents such as picaridin and oil of lemon eucalyptus appear to be safe and well tolerated but need to be reapplied more frequently.[59] Oil of lemon eucalyptus is not recommended in children <3 years of age.

Permethrin (a safe chrysanthemum derivative) is a contact insecticide that may be used for treatment of bed nets and clothing.[62] Permethrin-treated fabric has a duration of efficacy between 2 weeks and 6 months depending on the method of treatment. The best chemical protection against mosquito bites is use of a combination of permethrin-treated clothing and an effective insecticide on exposed skin.

TRAVELERS' DIARRHEA

Risk

Travelers' diarrhea is one of the most common illnesses among travelers, affecting 9% to 40% of children who travel.[62] Both the

incidence and severity of travelers' diarrhea are age-dependent, with the highest rates, longest duration, and greatest severity occurring in infants and children under 3 years of age.[63,64] Children's stools may normally can be quite variable; consequently, travelers' diarrhea is defined as ≥2-fold increase in the frequency of unformed stools, lasting at least 2 to 3 days. The infectious causes of travelers' diarrhea in children and adults predominantly are bacterial and include enterotoxigenic *Escherichia coli* (ETEC), which is the most common cause, enteroaggregative *Escherichia coli* (EAEC), *Salmonella, Campylobacter, Shigella,* enteropathogenic *Escherichia coli* (EPEC), and, rarely, shigatoxin-producing *Escherichia coli* (STE). Viral and parasitic infections are less common causes of pediatric travelers' diarrhea, although rotavirus, norovirus, *Cryptosporidium parvum, Giardia lamblia,* and *Entamoeba histolytica* also account for a small proportion of diarrhea in young travelers.

The risk of developing travelers' diarrhea depends on the travel destination, with rates as high as 73% among children traveling to North Africa and 61% among children visiting India.[63] Travel to Southeast Asia, Latin America, and other African countries has been associated with rates of approximately 40%.

Although travelers' diarrhea generally is a self-limited infection, it can cause significant morbidity, particularly if it results in moderate to severe dehydration. Parents must be counseled regarding the symptoms and signs of dehydration as well as the approach to oral rehydration and when to seek medical attention.

Preventive Measures

Because there are no vaccines licensed in the U.S. for prevention of travelers' diarrhea in children, counseling regarding food and water precautions is the most important preventive measure. Vaccines are in development in preclinical and clinical phases against ETEC, *Shigella* spp., and *Campylobacter jejuni;* a cholera vaccine that cross-protects against ETEC is licensed in Canada and Europe for children ≥2 years of age.[65]

General rules regarding food and water precautions when traveling apply to both children and adults; however, young children are more likely to explore the environment with their hands and mouths, thus creating opportunities for infection. Frequent handwashing with soap and water is critical, particularly before eating, although alcohol-based handwashes may be used when water is not available.

Children must be reminded to use safe water sources for all drinking, tooth brushing, and food preparation. Safe water sources include bottled water from a trusted source or water that has been boiled, chemically treated, or filtered. Combination chemical and filter pumps may provide the best protection as filters vary in the size of microbes which are removed.[66] Water should be boiled for at least 1 minute at altitudes <2000 meters and 3 minutes at >2000 meters.[2] Carbonated drinks also are considered safe for drinking, but water used to make ice may be contaminated. For infants, breastfeeding is the safest form of nutrition. In addition to its many health benefits, breastfeeding does not require a source of clean water, unlike the use of formula, both in its preparation and the cleaning of bottles.

The selection and preparation of foods are important during travel to minimize the risk of travelers' diarrhea. Although the advice to "boil it, cook it, peel it, or forget it" frequently is given, this often is not practical to follow. If possible, only steaming-hot freshly made food should be consumed. Families traveling with children should have a ready supply of snacks and avoid buying food from street vendors (Box 8-4).

Additional food and water precautions can decrease risk of other infectious diseases while traveling. These include avoidance of unpasteurized dairy products to eliminate risk of brucellosis and other bacterial infections. Raw or undercooked meat and fish should not be consumed due to risk of parasitic infections. Avoiding undercooked seafood can decrease risk of hepatitis A. In developing countries, raw vegetables and fruit that cannot be self-peeled should be avoided.

Chemoprophylaxis for travelers' diarrhea generally is not advised in children.[63] However, short-term prophylaxis (<3 weeks)

BOX 8-4. Prevention of Travelers' Diarrhea in Children

DO

- Eat only thoroughly cooked food served hot
- Peel fruit
- Drink only bottled, carbonated, boiled, chemically treated, or filtered water
- Prepare all beverages and ice cubes with boiled or bottled water
- Wash hands before eating or preparing foods
- Continue breastfeeding throughout travel period

DON'T

- Eat raw vegetables or unpeeled fruit
- Eat raw seafood or shellfish or undercooked meat
- Eat food from street vendors
- Drink tap water
- Consume milk or dairy products unless labeled as pasteurized or irradiated

---

could be considered for children with increased susceptibility to travelers' diarrhea, such as children with achlorhydria, or children in whom travelers' diarrhea might have significant medical consequences (e.g., children with chronic renal failure, congestive heart failure, diabetes mellitus, or inflammatory bowel disease).[67]

Treatment

Treatment of travelers' diarrhea in children must include close attention to hydration status, and parents should be counseled regarding early signs of dehydration. Oral rehydration therapy (ORT) using a homemade or commercially prepared oral rehydration solution (ORS) can be used to prevent dehydration associated with diarrheal disease. Commercial ORS should be used to treat mild to moderate dehydration; severe dehydration may require intravenous fluid resuscitation.[68,69] ORS packets should be part of a family's travel medical kit. Locally made preparations can be used early in therapy, although they differ in composition from the reduced-osmolarity ORS recommended by WHO (Table 8-3).[68,69] Breastfeeding should be continued in infants, and solid food intake should be maintained along with rehydration with ORT throughout the diarrheal episode, although foods high in simple sugars should be avoided because the increased osmotic load may worsen fluid losses.

Loperamide generally is used in combination with antibiotics for treatment of travelers' diarrhea in adults; however, the role of loperamide in pediatric travelers' diarrhea remains controversial, despite being licensed for use in children ≥2 years of age. Although loperamide has been shown to decrease duration and severity of acute diarrhea in children, this drug has been associated with significant side effects in children and is not recommended for children <3 years of age.[68,70,71] Zinc supplementation has been associated with improved outcomes in diarrheal disease in children in developing countries, but zinc supplementation is not recommended in treatment of travelers' diarrhea.[68]

Empiric treatment with antimicrobial agents can be considered in pediatric travelers' diarrhea.[3] Azithromycin often is used as the first choice for treatment of pediatric travelers' diarrhea, especially in areas with a high prevalence of fluoroquinolone-resistant *Campylobacter* species such as India and Thailand because it is given once a day and has a known safety profile in children. A dose of 10 mg/kg once daily for 3 days (maximum dose of 500 mg) is appropriate.[63] In adults a single dose of antibiotic has been shown to be as effective as 3 days' treatment; therefore, in children a full 3-day course may not be necessary.[72,73]

Fluoroquinolones for 1 to 3 days are the drug of choice for adults with travelers' diarrhea that is moderate to severe, persistent (>3 days), or associated with fever or bloody stools. Although there are concerns regarding the potential for development of arthropathy and antimicrobial resistance with fluoroquinolone use in children, the U.S. FDA has approved ciprofloxacin for anthrax and as a second-line agent for the treatment of urinary tract infections in children from 1 through 17 years of age.[74,75] Therefore, fluoroquinolones could be considered safe in children for the short course required for travelers' diarrhea. A 1- to 3-day course of ciprofloxacin at a dose of 20 to 30 mg/kg per day divided twice daily with a maximum dose of 500 mg bid is recommended for children with moderate to severe or bloody diarrhea.[63]

Rifaximin (Xifaxan), a nonabsorbed rifamycin derivative, has been approved in the U.S. for treatment and prevention of travelers' diarrhea for people ≥12 years of age.[76] A liquid preparation is available in some countries for pediatric use. The drug is indicated for the management of non-invasive diarrheas such as ETEC, cholera, or EAEC when fever and bloody diarrhea are absent.

If travelers' diarrhea does not respond to a course of antimicrobial therapy, medical attention should be sought to investigate other possible causes of the diarrhea.

EMERGING INFECTIOUS DISEASES

Over the past decade, several infectious agents, such as severe acute respiratory syndrome (SARS) coronavirus, the H5N1 strain of avian influenza, and the pandemic (H1N1) 2009 influenza virus have emerged as potentially widespread health threats. Given the constantly changing epidemiology of infectious diseases, pediatricians who advise families regarding travel health must keep informed of the current status of emerging infectious diseases that may pose a threat to the traveler. Several websites provide up-to-date information regarding such infections, including that of the WHO and the CDC (see Box 8-1).

THE IMMUNOCOMPROMISED TRAVELER

Children with immunodeficiencies require special consideration at their pretravel evaluation because of increased risk of travel-related illness.[77] Most patients with an altered immune system, particularly people with decreased T-lymphocyte immunity, should not receive live vaccines because of risk of developing clinical illness from the vaccine strain.[78] IPV should be given instead of OPV to all members in the family of an immunocompromised person, and Vi typhoid vaccine should be administered instead of the Ty21a vaccine to an immunocompromised child, although there is no risk to the patient if family members receive the live oral vaccine.[18,79] However, MMR, varicella, and yellow fever vaccines should be considered for HIV-seropositive children who are not severely immunocompromised (see Chapter 227, Rubeola Virus (Measles and Subacute Sclerosing Panencephalitis); Chapter 205, Varicella-Zoster Virus). Killed or subunit vaccines may be administered to children with altered immunity, although responses to the vaccines can be diminished.[78] Asplenic patients may respond poorly to polysaccharide vaccines in particular. Patients with certain B-lymphocyte deficiencies, such as X-linked and common variable agammaglobulinemia, should avoid OPV, vaccinia, and live bacterial vaccines, although other patients with

---

TABLE 8-3. Formulation of Oral Rehydration Solution (ORS)

World Health Organization	Home Formula
• Sodium chloride 2.6 g/L (75 mmol/L sodium)	• 3.5 g NaCl (¾-teaspoon table salt)
• Potassium chloride 1.5 g/L (20 mmol/L potassium)	• 1.5 g KCl (1 cup orange juice)
• Trisodium citrate, dihydrate 2.9 g/L (10 mmol/L citrate)	• 2.5 g NaHCO₃ (1 teaspoon baking soda)
• Glucose, anhydrous 13.5 g/L (75 mmol/L glucose)	• 20 g glucose (4 tablespoons sugar)
	• Water to final volume of 1 L (33 oz)

humoral deficiencies, including selective immunoglobulin A (IgA) and IgG subclass deficiency, need only avoid OPV; other live vaccines can be considered.

Some travel-associated illnesses can be more severe in immunocompromised travelers. Asplenic travelers are at greater risk of severe babesiosis and malaria, and organ and stem cell transplant recipients are more likely to develop bacteremia associated with gastroenteritis due to *Salmonella* or *Campylobacter* spp.[80] HIV-seropositive travelers with low CD4+ lymphocyte counts must be particularly conscious of risk factors associated with opportunistic infections such as *Toxoplasma gondii, Cystoisospora* (previously *Isospora*) *belli, Salmonella* spp. and *Cryptosporidium parvum*,[80] and, therefore, must be particularly cautious regarding food, water, and animal exposures. In addition, because of the risk of disseminated strongyloidiasis in immunocompromised hosts, closed footwear should be encouraged strongly in such travelers.

RETURN FROM TRAVEL

Routine posttravel screening generally is not required for asymptomatic, short-term travelers, although screening may be considered for long-term travelers, expatriates, adventure travelers, and people who have experienced significant illness while traveling.[5,81]

If post-travel screening is indicated, the tests required should be determined by the potential exposures associated with the travel itinerary and any symptoms, if present.

Children who develop fever after travel should seek immediate medical attention, and parents must inform the physicians caring for them of their travel itinerary. This is particularly critical if the itinerary has included a malaria-endemic area, since chemoprophylaxis cannot prevent all cases of malaria. Because malaria can manifest with nonspecific symptoms in children, any symptoms of fever, rigors, headache, malaise, abdominal pain, vomiting, diarrhea, poor feeding, or cough following travel to an endemic country should be evaluated promptly by a physician.[82,83]

Travel-related illness has been shown to be highly dependent on itinerary. In a report of disease and relationship to place of exposure among ill returned travelers, significant regional differences in proportionate morbidity were reported.[5] Typhoid fever was seen most frequently in travelers returning from South Asia. Malaria was the most frequent cause of febrile illness among travelers returning from sub-Saharan Africa, whereas dengue was a more frequent cause of fever in most other areas. Rickettsial infections, primarily tickborne spotted fever, occur more frequently than malaria or dengue among travelers returning from southern Africa.[5]

SECTION C: Host Defenses against Infectious Diseases

Immunologic Development and Susceptibility to Infection

Maite de la Morena

The human immune system has evolved to protect the individual from infectious microbes. It does this by utilizing a complex interactive network of cells, proteins, and organs. Experiments of nature in humans, such as those recognized as the inherited disorders of immune function,[1,2] have taught us that despite the apparent redundancy of the system, quantitative and qualitative defects in individual components and/or pathways result in abnormal function and susceptibility to particular infections.

This chapter provides a general overview of the development of innate and adaptive immune responses, addresses some immunologic developmental characteristics unique to the fetus and newborn, and addresses pathogen susceptibility in general terms.

THE INNATE IMMUNE RESPONSE

The innate immune system represents the first line of host defense against infection and includes: (a) antimicrobial products and physical barriers such as skin and mucosal surfaces; (b) receptors for pathogens (toll-like receptors (TLRs), C-type lectin receptors, nucleotide-binding oligoimerization domain (NOD), leucine-rich-repeat containing receptors (NLRs), and retinoic acid-inducible gene I protein (RIG-I) helicase receptors) that allow for the recruitment of immune cells to site of infection (for review see Netea and van den Meer[3]); (c) phagocytic cells such as neutrophils and macrophages; (d) dendritic cells; (e) complement proteins; and (f) natural killer cells.

Antimicrobial Products, the Skin and Mucosal Barriers

In mammals, epithelial cells are capable of secreting antimicrobial peptides such as defensins and cathelicidins. Defensins contribute to host defense by disrupting the cytoplasmic membranes of microbes. α-Defensins are produced by neutrophils, monocytes and Paneth cells of the gut while β-defensins are produced by

epithelial cells. hCap18/LL-37, a human cathelicidin, has been found in epithelial cells, mast cells, monocytes, and lymphocytes and has neutralizing capability against lipopolysaccharide (LPS), stimulates angiogenesis, and acts as a chemoattractant for neutrophils, monocytes, and T lymphocytes.[4–7]

The skin's tight junctions between epithelial cells, thickness, and dry environment offer a shield against microbes. Loss of skin integrity as seen in wounds, burns, and inflammation allows the entry of pathogens through this barrier. Both psoriasis and atopic dermatitis (AD) are known inflammatory skin conditions associated with skin disruption. While infection rarely is associated with psoriasis, patients with AD are commonly infected with *Staphylococcus aureus*. Human β-defensin 2 (HBD2) and the cathelicidin LL-37 appear to be strongly expressed in psoriasis and not in eczematous skin. Interleukin (IL)-13, produced under atopic conditions, suppresses the induction of these antimicrobial peptides.[8]

During the third trimester of pregnancy, the fetus becomes covered by the vernix caseosa that contains antimicrobial peptides including α-defensins, LL-37, and psoriasin, a calcium binding protein upregulated in psoriasis. Vernix extracts have antibacterial activity against gram-negative bacteria and antifungal properties against *Candida albicans,* whereas amniotic fluid derived proteins/peptides show only the former activity.[9]

Experimental models of mucocutaneous candidiasis have unraveled the role that Th17 cells plays at the mucosal/epithelial interface in the control of *Candida*. Chemoattractants for neutrophils and synthesis of defensins by keratinocytes locally contribute to such control. In addition, these models have shed light on the pathogenesis of *Candida* infections in patients with hyper-IgE, the autoimmune polyendocrinopathy syndrome, in patients with ectodermal dysplasia (APECED), and in patients with defects in the caspase recruitment domain (CARD)-9 protein.[10–15]

The more common entry pathway for pathogens is through the mucosal barrier. Mucosal epithelial cells secrete mucus which contains antimicrobial peptides. Mucus coats pathogens, allowing antimicrobial peptides to exert their action, and provides a vehicle for particles and pathogens to be cleared by the action of cilia. Within the respiratory tract, cilia move the mucus towards the upper airways where it is either expelled though the cough mechanism or swallowed. Ineffective clearance as seen in patients with immotile cilia syndrome or cystic fibrosis and after lung transplantation favors pathogen colonization. Potential therapeutic approaches utilizing novel antimicrobial peptides show promise.[16] Human defensin β2 (HDB2) and LL37 appear to be elevated consistently in states of infection and may contribute to pathogen clearance as knock-out β-defensin mice cannot clear *H. Influenzae.*[17]

Surfactant-associated proteins, specifically surfactant protein A (SP-A) and surfactant protein D (Sp-D), contribute to the innate immune responses in the lung. Produced by type II pneumocytes and nonciliated respiratory epithelial cells, they belong to the family of proteins called collectins. SP-A and SP-D can interact with microorganisms, modulate local inflammatory responses, modulate neutrophil responses in vitro, and participate in clearance of pollens and other complex organic antigens.[18] Lysozyme, lactoferrin, and phospholipase A2 in tears and saliva, and histatins in saliva, are potent antibacterial enzymes as well.[19,20] The gastrointestinal tract is protected by digestive enzymes, bile salts, fatty acids, and lysolipids. Paneth cells in the human gut secrete α-defensins and influence the virulence of orally ingested bacteria. Thus, children and adults with infections due to *Shigella* or virulent *Salmonella* strains have demonstrated decreased synthesis by colonic enterocyte of HBD1 and cathelicidin LL-37. HBD2 expression also is reduced in enterocytes of patients with Crohn disease, and gastric mucosa derived β-defensins are seen in *Helicobacter pylori* infections. Interestingly, in vitro, this microbe is susceptible to HBD2.

Commensal bacteria are resistant to endogenous antimicrobial peptides but induce epithelial defensins. *Porphyromonas gingivalis* does not induce HBD2 and behaves as a silent invader (see Zasloff[21]).

Pathogen Receptors and Toll-like Receptors

Pathogen-associated molecular patterns (PAMPs) represent pathogen-specific sugars/lipoproteins or nucleic acids expressed as part of their life cycle (i.e., bacterial DNA as unmethylated repeats of dinucleotide CpG, double-stranded (ds) or single-stranded (ss) RNA). Host proteins capable of recognizing such specific microbial patterns are called pathogen recognition receptors (PRRs). An example is mannose-binding lectin (MBL), a circulating soluble protein that binds mannose or fucose residues on microbes, permitting their phagocytosis. Macrophages carry a C-type lectin, called macrophage mannose receptor (MMR), which not only binds sugar moieties found on the surface of bacteria but also can recognize viruses such as the human immunodeficiency virus (HIV).[22]

Toll-like receptors are a type of PRR capable of linking the innate and adaptive immune systems (see Chapter 10, Fever and the Inflammatory Response). These proteins are present on many cells including airway and gut epithelial cells, antigen presenting cells (B lymphocytes, macrophages, dendritic cells, monocytes), hematopoietic stem cells, mast cells, regulatory T lymphocytes, NK cells, and endothelial cells.[23] A total of 10 different TLRs have been identified in humans: TLR1, TLR2, TLR4, TLR5, TLR6, and TLR10 are found on cell surfaces, while TLR3, TLR7, TLR8, and TLR9 are localized within the endosomes. TLR2 is involved in responses to gram-positive bacteria (peptidoglycans and lipoproteins) and yeast.[24] TLR4 mediates the interaction of gram-negative bacteria by transducing signals derived from LPS. A mouse model for TLR4 mutations renders the animal resistant to endotoxin but highly susceptible to gram-negative infection.[25] All TLRs are capable of interacting with different ligands (see Table 10-1). RSV F protein, lipopolysaccharide (LPS), and *Pseudomonas* exoenzyme S have been shown to interact with TLR4 while flagellin is recognized by TLR5.[26] TLR2 recognizes envelope proteins of HSV while TLR9 identifies CpG motifs within the viral genome.[27]

TLR recognition of microbial products triggers the activation of downstream signaling pathways where myeloid differentiation factor 88 (MyD88) and/or toll-IL-1 receptor domain containing adaptor inducing IFN-β (TRIF) lead to activation of NF-κB and subsequent transcription of proinflammatory cytokines: tumor necrosis factor (TNF)-α, IL-1, and IL-6. MyD88 recruits the IL-1R-associated kinase (IRAK) family of proteins: IRAK1 and IRAK4. Humans and mice with IRAK4 deficiency have severe impairment of IL-1 and TLR downstream signaling and are susceptible to recurrent bacterial infections.[28,29] TRIF signaling results in the activation of interferon regulatory factor (IRF)-3 and induction of type 1 interferon (IFN) genes such as IFN-α and IFN-β,[30] helpful for viral clearance.

TLR polymorphism may be linked to diseases such as asthma[31] and atherosclerosis,[23] TLR-2 has been linked to different responses to ischemia/reperfusion injury after solid-organ transplantation,[32] and a deletion of the signaling domain of TLR5 has been found to increase susceptibility to Legionnaire disease.[33] Finally toll signaling pathways have been implicated in the pathogenesis of sepsis and shock.[34-36] Defects in TLR3 have identified inherited susceptibility to HSV encephalitis.[37-41] The stage of human development in which toll receptors appear is not clearly established. However, there is evidence that TLR2 is developmentally expressed during fetal life from early pseudoglandular to canalicular stages of human lung development.[42] (See Chapter 11, The Systemic Inflammatory Response Syndrome (SIRS), Sepsis, and Septic Shock, for review.)

Phagocytes

The major phagocytic cells are neutrophils and macrophages. In humans, myeloid precursors are found in the yolk sac by day 19 of development, 2 days before the onset of blood circulation. Hematopoiesis then shifts to the fetal liver and finally to the bone marrow. In the bone marrow phagocyte development is under the control of multiple growth factors, including interleukin 3 (IL-3), granulocyte-macrophage colony-stimulating factor (GM-CSF), granulocyte colony-stimulating factor (G-CSF), and macrophage colony-stimulating factor (M-CSF). The marrow pool of neutrophils in adults is 20 times the number of neutrophils in circulation. The mechanisms responsible for the release of neutrophils from the marrow are complex. In familial neutropenias associated with maturational arrest, genes such as *CSF3R, ELA2,* and *WAS* have been identified as essential for neutrophil development.[43-46] Chemokines such as CXCR2 and CXCR4 also appear to play key roles in both the release and return of neutrophils to the bone marrow.[47,48] Once in the circulation neutrophils circulate for a few hours and then move into the tissues where they are active for 2 to 6 days.

At term, the neonatal peripheral neutrophil count is higher than that of adults, but there appears to be little reserved capacity to respond with an outpouring of phagocytic cells, which often are immature, during infection. Newborn infants with septicemia often have severe neutropenia and depletion of phagocytic storage pools, a finding associated with a high mortality rate.[49,50] The cause of depletion remains unknown; it often occurs in the presence of increased numbers of neutrophil precursors and elevated levels of CSFs in blood.[51] Perhaps a decreased number of neutrophils at the site of infection contribute to the susceptibility of neonates to pneumonia and skin infection and to the development of multiple sites of infection after bacteremia or fungemia.[52] This lack of adequate numbers of cells at the site of infection may cause or result in functional deficiencies.

Monocytes also move from the circulation to tissue spaces, where they develop into macrophages and live for 2 to 3 months, assuming specialized characteristics most determined by their location (e.g., lung, liver, or spleen). Circulating monocytes also have chemotactic and phagocytic activities and have receptors for immunoglobulin G (IgG) Fc domains (FcR), complement, and TLRs 2 to 9 along with CD14, an important molecule that mediates TLR4 activation by LPS.[53,54]

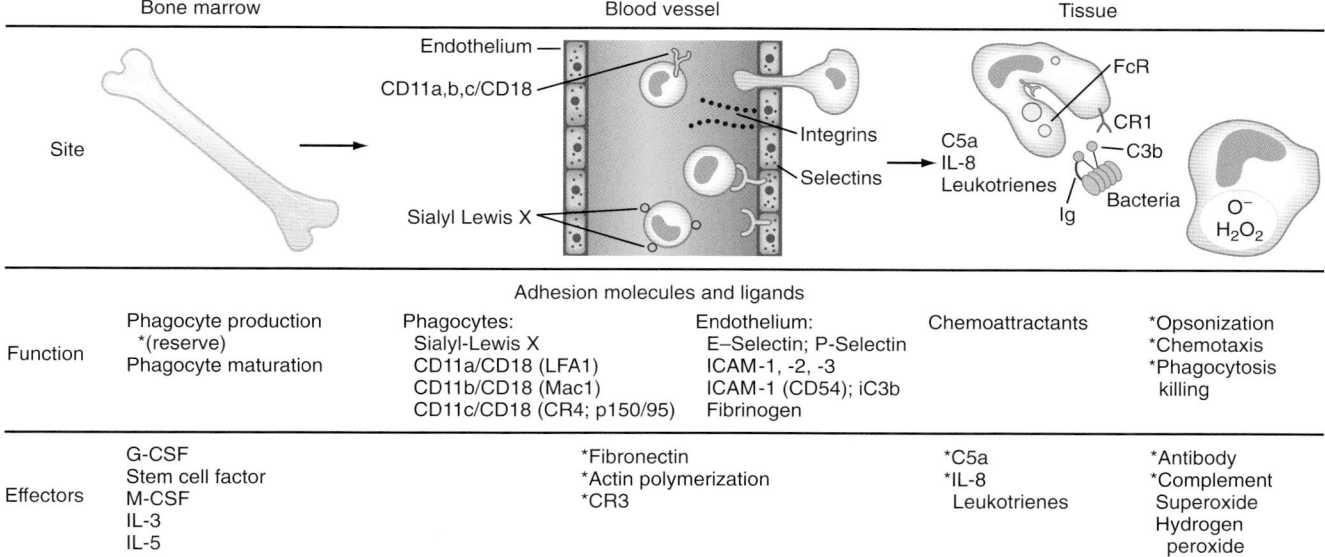

Figure 9-1. Aspects of immunologic function. *Indicates aspects that are immature or defective in the neonatal period. C, complement; CD, cluster of differentiation; CR, complement receptor; G-CSF, granulocyte colony-stimulating factor; Ig, immunoglobulin; IL, interleukin; M-CSF, macrophage colony-stimulating factor.

The function of phagocytes (which are particularly important in defense against bacteria and fungi) requires not only sufficient numbers of cells but adequate ability to sense and migrate toward the site of infection (chemotaxis) and to ingest and kill (phagocytosis) microorganisms. These processes are mediated by the expression of adhesion molecules, opsonins (complement and antibodies), and release of toxic substances (Figure 9-1).

Chemotaxis is the process by which phagocytes reach the site of infection. As a result of a local inflammatory response, endothelial cells within the local vessels express adhesion molecules called selectins (CD62E, CD62P). These molecules reversibly bind to ligands on neutrophils (sialyl-Lewis X and PSGL1) and consequently make the neutrophil slow down and "roll" along the endothelium. Subsequently, another group of adhesion molecules, called integrins, are upregulated on the surface of neutrophils. Integrins are composed of one of three different α chains: CD11a, CD11b (CR3), or CD11c (CR4); they are noncovalently linked to a β chain, CD18, thus forming CD11a/CD18 or LFX1, CD11b/CD18 or MAC-1, and CD11c/CD18 or p150,95 integrin complex. Integrin molecules "stop" the neutrophil, which then undergoes skeletal changes and migrates through the vascular lumen into the extravascular space by adhering to intracellular adhesion molecules (ICAMs). Interestingly, the sialic constituent of the group B streptococcus (GBS) capsular polysaccharide mimics the human Lewis X antigen, making this a poor immunogen, and perhaps renders the neonate more susceptible to this organism.[55] Defects in the expression of adhesion molecules have been described in humans: leukocyte adhesion defect (LAD) type I, II, and III. Lack of integrin expression causes LAD I, lack of sialyl-Lewis X expression causes LAD II, and defects of integrin activation cause LAD III. Patients present with persistent leukocytosis, delayed separation of the cord, skin ulcers, periodontitis, and delayed wound healing.[56] L-selectin (CD62L) levels on fetal and immature infant neutrophils are comparable with those of adults. However, their expression is downregulated in the term neonate and is further diminished during acute bacterial infection in vivo.[57] Other defects in chemotaxis have been described.[56,58–61] In the newborn, defects in chemotaxis have been linked to decreased expression of Rac2, a signaling molecule, on to cord blood neutrophils.[52]

Phagocytosis is an active process by which a previously bound pathogen is engulfed by a phagocyte in a membrane-bound vesicle called a phagosome. Both macrophages and neutrophils contain lysosomes, which are membrane-bound acidic organelles containing proteolytic enzymes and are capable of producing toxic products: nitric oxide (NO), superoxide anion (O_2^-), and hydrogen peroxide (H_2O_2). Fusion of the lysosome and phagosome membranes is necessary for killing of the organism. Within azurophilic granules, a bactericidal/permeability-increasing protein (BPI) binds to bacterial lipopolysaccharide and kills gram-negative bacteria. BPI has been implicated in both neonatal sepsis[62] and chronic *Pseudomonas* infection in cystic fibrosis patients.[63]

Superoxide and H_2O_2 production is dependent on the NADPH oxidase enzyme complex (see Chapter 106, Infectious Complications of Dysfunction or Deficiency of Polymorphonuclear and Mononuclear Phagocytes). Defects in the different components of this enzyme result in the immunodeficiency chronic granulomatous disease. Affected patients are susceptible to infections with catalase-positive organisms, *Aspergillus* and *Nocardia* species. Because phagocytes are unable to kill the microbes, the host tries to contain the infection by calling in more macrophages and lymphocytes, resulting in granuloma formation. Once bacteria are killed, neutrophils die whereas macrophages are capable of generating new lysosomes.

There are no well-described phagocytic defects in the developing human embryo. The capability of the newborn for non-opsonic adherence to organisms and phagocytosis is nearly equal to that of adult cells. However, deficiencies in chemotaxis and superoxide production have been described.[55,64–66] Bacterial killing of cord blood phagocytes is effective against *Escherichia coli* and *Streptococcus pyogenes* and is similar to adults, but appears abrogated against GBS.[67] Abnormalities in chemoattractants (IL8, complement fragment C5a, fibronectin)[68,69] and defective expression of complement receptors, such as C5a receptor, caused by C5a-mediated exocytosis of myeloperoxidase[70] also have been described. Membrane fluidity defects and cytoskeletal changes may contribute to neutrophil motility defects as well.[71] Intrapartum administration of magnesium sulfate results in an alteration in neutrophil motility and phagocytosis of cord blood neutrophils as measured by chemotaxis, random motility, and chemiluminescence.[72]

Dendritic Cells

Dendritic cells (DCs) are the prototypic antigen presenting cell. In humans, CD34+ hematopoietic stem cells (HSCs) capable of generating dendritic cells are detected in the fetal liver at 20 weeks' gestation, after which they are found mainly in the bone marrow. After birth 1% to 3% of cord blood cells express CD34. During differentiation these CD34+ cells lose CD34 expression and express CD4, CD45RA, IL-3R, and major histocompatibility complex (MHC) class II antigens.[73,74] A class of dendritic cells called Langerhans cells (LCs) were first described in 1868. It is difficult to identify lineage ontogeny of dendritic cells in humans. Bone marrow differentiation studies of dendritic cells suggest a dual origin of dendritic cells: myeloid and lymphoid.[75,76] LCs can derive from blood dendritic cells.[77] While lineage specific markers are still being defined, three transcription factors have been shown to regulate their development: PU.1, RelB, and Ikaros. PU.1 is important for myeloid-derived DCs,[78] RelB is associated with DC activation,[79] and Ikaros proteins are transcriptional activators and influence chromatin remodeling and histone deacetylation.[80]

DCs are capable of regulating both innate and adaptive immune responses. With unique morphologic characteristics when activated, several pathogen receptors have been identified: TLRs that appear to be involved in DC maturation, and scavenger receptors that mediate bacterial internalization. MAC-1 (CD11b/CD18) or the CR3 complement receptor is demonstrated for phagocytosis of complement-coated bacteria.[81]

In the skin, LCs are localized to the basal and suprabasal layers of the epidermis, in the murine gut, DCs are found in the Peyer patches, and in the human lungs they can be found within the airway epithelium, alveolar septa, visceral pleura, and vascular walls.[82-84]

While surveying the tissue environment, DCs can be recognized by an "immature" phenotype (CD11b^{bright}, CD11c^{mod}, CD86^{low}, ClassII^{low}, CD4$^-$). Upon uptake of antigen/microbial products by different mechanisms of phagocytosis, they migrate via the afferent lymphatics to the regional lymph node where they arrive as mature nonphagocytic DCs (CD40^{high}). These DCs can produce inflammatory cytokines and chemokines. Bacterial uptake of *Mycobacterium tuberculosis*, BCG, *Saccharomyces cerevisiae*, *Corynebacterium parvum*, *Staphylococcus aureus*, *Leishmania* spp., and *Borrelia burgdorferi* has been demonstrated in vitro[85-88] (also for review see Granucci et al.[81]).

Complement

The complement system comprises a series of serum proteins that function in host defense as an enzymatic cascade (see Chapter 105, Infectious Complications of Complement Deficiencies). When microorganisms invade the host, activation of complement occurs locally by one of three pathways that converge at the stage of the formation of an enzyme called C3 convertase. This enzyme cleaves complement component C3 into C3b and C3a. C3b, the major effector molecule of the complement system, binds to the bacterial cell membrane. This important molecule functions as an opsonin (to facilitate phagocytosis) and also helps cleave C5 into C5a and C5b. C5a is a potent chemoattractant, and C5b is an integral part of the membrane-attack complex along with other terminal components: C6, C7, and C9. One pathway (classical) is activated by antibody–antigen complexes and,

thus, depends on and enhances specific humoral immunity. A second pathway (alternative) can be activated by direct binding to the surface of some microorganisms and, thus, functions to provide innate (nonspecific) immunity. A third pathway (MBL pathway) is initiated by the binding of MBL on mannose- and fucose-containing surfaces of bacteria and viruses, favoring their phagocytosis.

Until 18 months of age, the concentration of most complement proteins is lower than that of adults, with the exception of C7. Between 28 and 33 weeks of gestation, there appears to be little development of the complement system. Levels of C8 and C9 are the most markedly reduced at all gestational ages. Levels correlate with gestational age, but not with birthweight, type of delivery, or sex.[89] Deficiencies of complement activation in both classical and alternative pathways have been described.[90,91] Low levels of total hemolytic complement activity are a significant predictor of mortality in neonates with septicemia.[91]

The molecular basis for defects in complement function in neonates and the details of the consequences are only partially understood. For example, a possible defect has been described in formation of a reactive thioester bond on C3 that is essential for opsonic and covalent binding of C3b to bacteria.[92] Inefficient killing of *E. coli* by neonatal sera appears to correlate with low concentrations of C9.[93] and can be overcome by adding C9 to ampicillin-treated serum from neonates in vitro.[94] Finally, deficient formation of C5a may also increase the newborn infant's risk of infection. Although levels of C5 are similar in adult and neonatal sera, neonatal sera form significantly less C5a on exposure to type III group B streptococcus.[95] This deficiency was apparent in newborn sera with antibody levels similar to those of adults and could be corrected by in vitro addition of C3.

Hemolytic uremic syndrome (HUS) occurs in childhood and frequently is preceded by a diarrheal illness caused by *E. coli* O157:H7. Plasma protein factor H and plasma serine protease I, regulatory proteins of the alternative complement pathway, have been associated with the nondiarrheal form of HUS.[96,97] A study of 120 patients with nondiarrheal HUS found that 10% of patients had mutations in the membrane cofactor protein (MCP; CD46). The onset typically was in early childhood, most did not develop end-stage renal failure.[98]

Natural Killer Cells

Natural killer (NK) cells are a subgroup of lymphocytes that exhibit cytolytic activity against tumor cells or cells infected with viruses (Table 9-1). In humans, NK cells are similar to T lymphocytes in their effector function, but lack the T-lymphocyte receptor/CD3 complex and express the low affinity Fc receptor for IgG (CD16, FcγRIII). They comprise up to 10% of peripheral blood lymphocytes (PBLs) in adults.

NK cells appear in substantial numbers by 6 to 9 weeks of gestation in the embryonic liver and later in the fetal liver, thymus, and spleen. After birth, NK cells develop primarily from HSCs in the marrow and are driven to maturity by cytokines, in particular IL-15. IL-15 has the same intracellular signaling molecule, the

TABLE 9-1. Comparison of Natural Killer Cells and Cytolytic T Lymphocytes

Characteristic	Natural Killer Cell	Cytolytic T Lymphocyte
Identification of target for kill	Nonspecific killing of virus-infected cells *or* Binding to antibody-coated cells via CD16 (ADCC)	TCR specifically identifies viral peptide complexed with MHC class I molecule on surface of infected cell
Surface markers	CD16 and/or CD56	CD3/CD8
Signal(s) for activation	IFN-α, IFN-β, IL-12	IL-2 and antigen (on surface of antigen-presenting cell)
Onset of function	1–6 days after infection	5–10 days after infection
Mechanism of killing	Granule exocytosis and secretion of toxin	Granule exocytosis and secretion of toxin

ADCC, antibody-dependent cell-mediated cytotoxicity; IFN, interferon; IL, interleukin; TCR, T-cell receptor.

common γ chain (γC), as other cytokines (IL-2, IL-4, IL-7, IL9, and IL-21). Mutations in γC are responsible for a form of severe combined immunodeficiency (SCID) that lacks both T and NK cells.

Unlike cytotoxic T lymphocytes (CTLs), NK cells do not require MHC class I antigens to recognize their targets, do not recognize particular viral antigens,[99] and can be activated by cytokines without previous exposure to the antigen, making this cell an important contributor to innate responses. However, NK cells can function with some degree of antigenic specificity because they can lyse cells that have been previously coated with specific antibody molecules. This process is called antibody-dependent cell-mediated cytotoxicity (ADCC). Both NK cells and CTLs mediate cytolysis in a similar manner because these two cell populations contain granules composed of cytolytic proteins called perforin and enzymes called granzymes. Perforin polymerizes when in contact with the target cell plasma membrane creating pores; granzyme introduced through these pores induces target cell apoptosis.[100] Defects in the vesicle membrane fusion, perforin and granzyme have been described in patients with hemophagocytic lymphohistiocytosis syndromes (see Chapter 12, Hemophagocytic Lymphohistiocytosis and Macrophage Activation Syndrome).

NK cell activity in cord blood from infants born between 32 and 36 weeks of gestation is low compared with activity in infants born after 36 weeks. Interestingly, antenatal glucocorticoid therapy for preterm labor can accelerate maturation of NK cells.[101] Compared with adult NK cells, neonatal NK cells have decreased cytotoxic activity and diminished ADCC until at least 6 months of age.[102] On the other hand when interferons (IFNs), IL-2, IL-12, and IL-15 are added to cultured neonatal NK cells, they are capable of responding like adult cells.[99]

Neonatal herpes simplex virus (HSV) infection and severe recurrent herpesvirus infections in adults provide evidence of the importance of NK cells in host defense.[103,104] Human umbilical cord blood cells demonstrate defective NK cell cytotoxicity and ADCC against HSV-infected targets,[105–107] and evidence for the relevance of ADCC in protecting the infant from HSV is provided by the association of high levels of maternal- or neonatal-specific ADCC to HSV or high levels of neonatal HSV-neutralizing antibodies with absence of disseminated HSV infection in infants.[108] The higher risk of preterm infants developing HSV encephalitis or disseminated disease is not clearly understood and underscores the role of decreased maternal transfer of neutralizing antibodies in the preterm child.[109]

Term infants infected perinatally with HIV are deficient in ADCC, while preterm infants are deficient in both NK cell cytotoxicity and ADCC against HIV-infected targets. These observations may relate to an increased risk of HIV transmission in preterm neonates. Low NK cell cytotoxicity and ADCC of newborn lymphocytes to HIV-infected cells may further explain the newborn's inability to reduce plasma levels of HIV after acute infection.[110] NK defects have been recognized as either part of a broad immunodeficiency syndrome or as isolated defects within the NK populations.[111]

THE ADAPTIVE IMMUNE RESPONSE

The adaptive immune response is essential for host defense as shown by the primary immunodeficiency syndromes. Specificity and immunologic memory are the two most important consequences of adaptive immunity. Specificity is determined by the vast range of molecular diversity of the antigen receptor. Immunologic memory is the ability to respond rapidly and effectively to pathogens previously encountered. The effector cells of the adaptive immune response are T and B lymphocytes. These cells derive from a common HSC (Figure 9-2). Lymphopoiesis is a tightly regulated sequence of events that leads to the expression of a functional antigen receptor on the surface of the lymphocyte. For the B lymphocytes it is the immunoglobulin molecule and for the T lymphocyte, the T cell receptor (TCR) complex. Cellular microenvironment, growth factors, cytokines, and chemokines along with silencing or activation of certain genes at different stages of lineage commitment are some of the multiple factors contributing to a successful and mature lymphocyte (for review see Blom and Spits[112]).

B Lymphocytes

B lymphocytes play a critical role in pathogen-specific immunity by producing antibodies. B lymphocytes recognize soluble antigens via immunoglobulins anchored on their surface and differentiate into antibody-producing cells, called plasma cells, capable of secreting immunoglobulins. These proteins function alone (neutralization) or with complement or phagocytes to inactivate microorganisms.

The B-lymphocyte system is fully developed at birth. The origin of the human B lymphocyte is not well defined but fetal B lymphocytes can be recognized in the yolk sac, omentum, and fetal liver.[113] After birth B-lymphocyte development takes place in the bone marrow. The ordered steps of B-lymphocyte development are marked by rearrangement of the immunoglobulin genes (see Figure 9-2). Recombinase-activating gene (RAG) 1 and 2, transcription factors, and signaling molecules are required for normal B-lymphocyte development, defects of which result in the classic X-linked mutations in Bruton's tyrosine kinase or autosomal recessive forms of agammaglobulinemia. A mature B lymphocyte can be identified by the cells surface molecules: CD19, CD20, CD21 (the EBV receptor) and CD40 (ligand for CD154, defective in hyper-IgM syndrome) amongst others. All of these B surface molecules are lost when the cell reaches the plasma cell state. Thus the monoclonal antibody anti-CD20, used for management of B-cell CD20[+] lymphomas and autoimmune conditions, will not deplete the plasma cell pool.

Passively Acquired Antibodies

Neonates have a limited serum antibody repertoire (at least 10[11]) of actively formed (self-produced) antibodies as they have not had the opportunity of encountering pathogens. This is alleviated by transplacental transfer of maternal antibody, which occurs by a selective, active process, that can occur as early as 20 to 24 weeks but more consistently after 35 weeks of gestation.[114] Only immunoglobulin G (IgG) antibodies appear in umbilical cord blood, and some IgG subclasses are transferred better than others.[115,116] This mechanism may be related to differential binding of FcRII isoforms in the placenta.[117,118] At birth, full-term infants have serum IgG levels that are equal to or exceed maternal level by 5% to 10%.[119] Because most antibody transfer occurs during the third trimester of pregnancy, preterm infants may have very low levels. For example, most infants born at 32 weeks of gestation or earlier have serum IgG levels below 400 mg/dL.[120] Transplacentally acquired antibody disappears rapidly after birth, reaching a nadir at 3 months (Table 9-2). Average concentrations at this time are 60 mg/dL for infants born at 25 to 28 weeks of gestation, 104 mg/dL for infants born at 29 to 32 weeks, and 430 mg/dL for infants born at term.[121,122] However, these low levels of maternal IgG antibody appear to be associated with less risk of infection than might be expected. A longitudinal study of the ability of preterm infants to form specific antibodies provides a partial explanation for this low risk.[123] By about 9 months of age, infants have formed specific IgG antibodies in response to immunization with diphtheria, tetanus toxoids, and pertussis vaccine. Also by about this age, their antibodies have functional opsonic activity against *E. coli* and coagulase-negative staphylococci.

The maternal repertoire of specific antibodies is critical for protection of the newborn infant from commonly encountered pathogens.[124] Baker and Kasper[125] demonstrated that a concentration of 2 μg/mL or less of serum antibody to type III group B streptococcus in cord blood correlated with susceptibility to invasive disease. Evidence of the protective effect of maternal antibodies against HSV[108,126] and varicella-zoster virus infection is well established.[127] Many gram-negative organisms require IgM antibodies and complement for efficient opsonization.[128,129] Since IgM does not cross the placenta, neonatal sera opsonize these organisms poorly.[123]

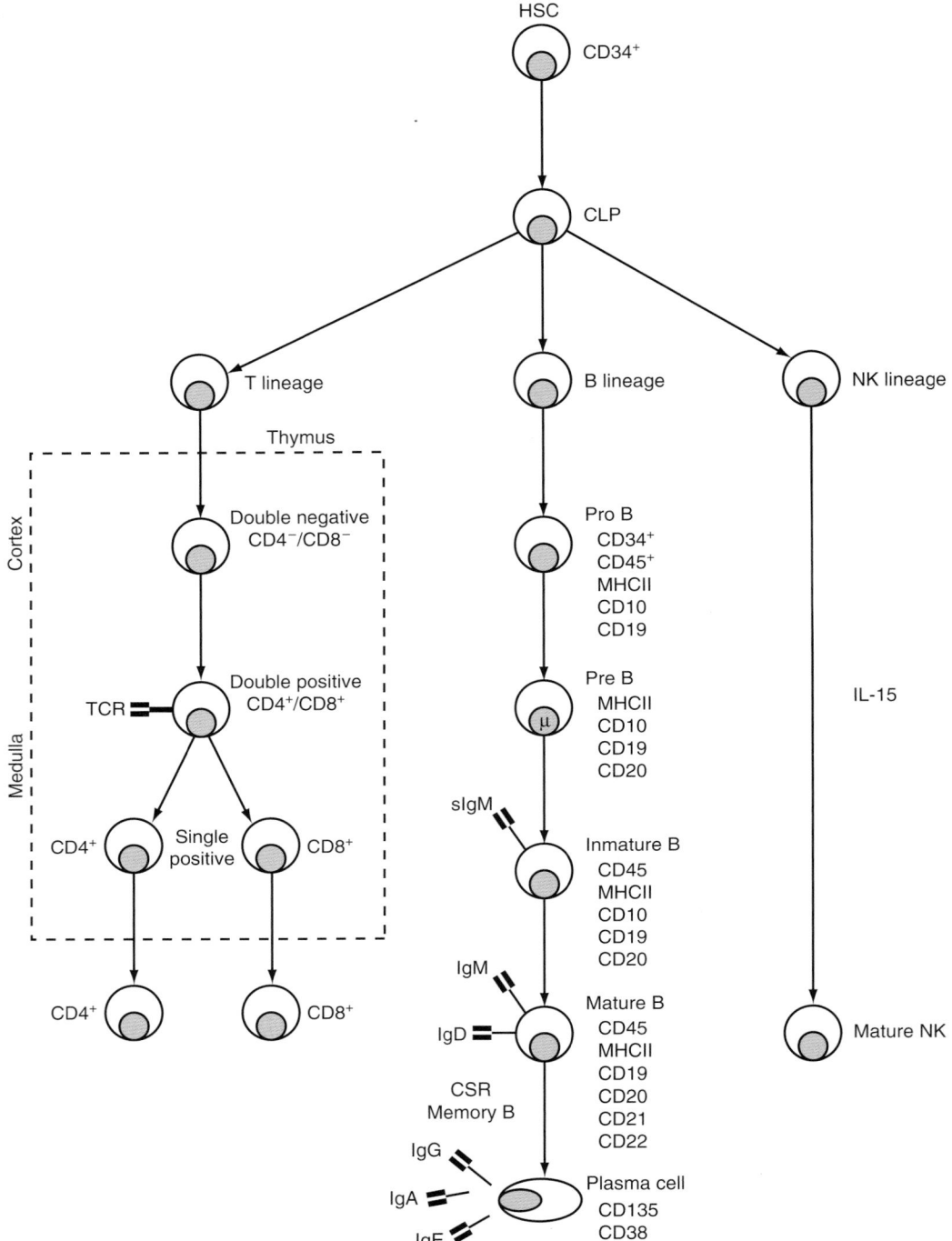

Figure 9-2. Developmental stages of T, B, and natural killer (NK) lymphocytes. B, B lymphocyte; CD, cluster of differentiation; CLP, common lymphoid precursor; CSR, class switch recombination; HSC, hematopoietic stem cell; IG, immunoglobulin; MHC, major histocompatibility complex; T, T lymphocyte.

TABLE 9-2. Concentration of Serum IgG in Term and Premature Infants

Postnatal Age	Gestational Age: Mean Serum IgG (mg/dL)		
	25–28 weeks[a]	29–32 weeks[a]	Term[b]
1 week	251	368	1031
3 months	60	104	430
6 months	159	179	427

[a]Data for premature infants based on samples at 1 week, 3 months, and 6 months of age.[121]

[b]Data for term infants based on cord blood and samples at 1–3 months and 4–6 months of age.[122]

The apparent protective role of transplacental IgG antibodies against group B streptococcus infection has led to extensive attempts to prevent or treat such infection with passively administered antibody, in which variable efficacy underscores confounding mechanisms necessary for the newborn to clear pathogens[130,131] or by immunization of women with group B streptococcal vaccines.[132]

Active Production of Antibodies

The ability of newborn infants to produce an active antibody response to antigenic stimulation develops in an orderly fashion. An adult pattern of antibody responses is not acquired until 4 to 5 years of age. Analysis of the factors responsible for this developmental pattern is complex because production of antibody depends not only on B-lymphocyte maturity but also on interactions with other cells that mature at different rates (Table 9-3).

After birth, active production of IgG slowly increases, with differences among IgG subclasses; IgG1 and IgG3 production matures before IgG2 and IgG4.[115] The last isotype to achieve adult concentrations is IgA.[133–135]

Postmortem studies of fetuses suggest that secretory IgA (sIgA)-containing epithelial cells appear at 20 to 21 weeks of gestation and their number increases from 2.5 cells per 10,000 μm at 23 to 26 weeks, to 8 cells per 10,000 μm at 36 to 40 weeks. In fetuses with pneumonia or sepsis, the number of sIgA-containing epithelial cells in the trachea, bronchi, and intrahepatic duct decreases and, at times, completely disappears. This suggests that sIgA is an important component of mucosal immunity at as early as 20 weeks of gestation.[135,136]

Fetuses can produce IgM antibodies predominantly in response to intrauterine infection.[137] Preterm infants respond nearly as well as term infants to immunization beginning at 2 months with DTP,

TABLE 9-3. Developmental Milestones of Humoral Immunity Event

Event	Age
Surface-positive B lymphocytes of all isotypes present in liver	16 weeks of gestation
Surface-positive B lymphocytes of all isotypes present in bone marrow	22 weeks of gestation
Stimulated B lymphocytes secrete primarily IgM	Fetus–newborn
Production of antibody in response to protein antigens	Fetus–newborn
Serum IgG reaches 60% of adult levels	1 year
Production of antibody in response to polysaccharide antigens	2–3 years
Stimulated B lymphocytes secrete all isotypes	2–5 years
Serum IgA reaches 60% of adult levels	6–8 years

DTaP, poliovirus, and hepatitis B vaccines.[138–140] Term infants immunized or infected during the first few days of life usually produce protective antibody responses, although at somewhat lower levels than adults.[141–143] The presence of fetal bone marrow B-lymphocyte pools similar in size to those of adults and with comparable isotype diversity suggests that their functional deficits may reflect a developing memory repertoire with increased specificity to antigen (and thus can have interference of antigens) or the need to generate T lymphocytes capable of producing strong B-lymphocyte signals, rather than inherent B-lymphocyte immaturity as a sole factor. Studies of B-lymphocyte activation have revealed much about the complexities of B-lymphocyte signaling[144] and suggest possible mechanisms for deficits of B-lymphocyte function that can be examined in healthy neonates.[145]

In contrast to the early development of antibody responses to most protein antigens, responses to thymus (T)-independent antigens, such as polysaccharides, develop much later. The basis for this remains unclear.[146,147] Cord blood B lymphocytes are capable of activation in vitro with T-independent activators. This suggests that signal transduction pathways within the B lymphocyte are normal.[148] However, the mechanism of B-lymphocyte activation by polysaccharides differs from protein antigens in that it involves costimulation through a B-lymphocyte surface molecule called CD21 and may be influenced by the expression of yet another B-cell surface molecule: CD22.[146] Both CD21 and CD22 were noted to be reduced on neonatal B lymphocytes upon stimulation, suggesting a unique role for these molecules in antibody production to polysaccharide antigens.[146,149]

Although the extent to which neonatal deficiencies of neutrophil function, complement, or antibody contribute to the increased risk of infection is unknown, these factors are important in vitro to the opsonophagocytic killing of E. coli, group B streptococcus, and Candida species. Thus the combined effect of these deficiencies no doubt contributes to the increased risk of serious infection with these pathogens in this group of children.[124]

T Lymphocytes

T lymphocytes play a central role in regulation of antigen-specific immune responses, modulating the function of antigen presenting cells, B and other T lymphocytes, both through contact with (receptor binding) and secretion of cytokines.[144] T lymphocytes are effector cells of cell-mediated immune response and function as cytotoxic cells (CTLs), able to kill target cells that express foreign antigens.

Most mature T lymphocytes (95%) recognize antigen through a T-cell receptor (TCR). Contrary to B lymphocytes, T lymphocytes can only recognize antigens that are displayed on cell surfaces. These antigens can be derived from pathogens that replicate within the cell such as viruses or intracellular bacteria or products internalized from the extracellular space. The reason T lymphocytes can recognize intracellular pathogens is that these infected cells display on their surface fragments/peptides derived from the pathogens' proteins. The molecules responsible for holding these peptides within their groove are the MHC molecules. Two classes of MHC molecules are recognized: class I, which include human leukocyte antigen (HLA)-A, HLA-B and HLA-C, and class II: HLA-DR, HLA -DQ and HLA -DP. MHC class I are present on all nucleated cells, whereas MCH class II are present on antigen presenting cells and other specialized cells. Peptide:MCH class I complexes (MHC I) present antigen to cytotoxic T cells (CD8) and peptide:MHC-class II complexes (MHC II) present to helper T cells (Th1/CD4).

Cytosolic peptides derived from vaccinia virus, influenza virus, rabies, and Listeria are coupled to MHC I molecules on the surface of the infected cell. These peptide:MHC I complexes can then be recognized by cytotoxic CD8+ cells that kill the targeted infected cell. Mycobacterium tuberculosis, Mycobacterium leprae, Leishmania donovani, and Pneumocystis jirovecii are localized within macrophage vesicles and their derived peptides are coupled to MHC II molecules on their surface. Peptide:MHC II are recognized by CD4 (Th1) cells. These activated T cells then produce IFN-γ which recruit more macrophages, a granuloma is formed and the activated macrophage kills its intracellular pathogen by releasing the antimicrobial products within its vesicles. *Clostridium tetani*, *Staphylococcus aureus*, *Streptococcus pneumoniae*, Polioviruses, *P. jirovecii*, and *Trichinella spiralis* require both humoral and cellular immune response for effective killing.[22] It is therefore understandable that defects in antigen processing, presentation and both T- and B-effector functions make the individual susceptible to those pathogens that require a particular pathway for clearance.

Sir Peter Medawar first recognized that antigen presentation in fetal life leads to a form of immunologic tolerance which was different than in adult life.[150] This mechanism was postulated to be due to a state of immunologic naiveté of the fetus. However, an alternative hypothesis suggests perhaps that certain adaptive immune responses may be actively suppressed in the developing fetus, which are mediated by an important population of T lymphocytes called regulatory T cells.[151] This theory is favored by the fact that that fetuses are capable of generating specific adaptive responses after transplacental spread of infectious agents.[152-154]

HSC progenitors migrate to the thymus where, similar to B cells, T cells rearrange their TCR genes by somatic recombination. In contrast to BCRs, TCRs do not diversify their variable (V) region genes through somatic hypermutation. Also, unlike the B cells, T cells must develop into two populations: αβ-T cells (the most abundant, 95% of the circulating pool) or γδ T cells (approximately 5% of the circulating pool). Maturing T lymphocytes move within the thymus in a directed manner from the cortex to the medulla (see Figure 9-2) The expression of surface molecules identifies their state of maturity. Thus T cells start as double negative (CD4−/CD8−)stage → double positive (CD4+/CD8+) → single positive CD4+ or CD8+ just before being released to the periphery. During maturation in the thymus, T cells are selected to proceed to the next developmental stage thanks to the interactions of a successfully assembled TCR with self-MHC:self-peptide complexes. As with B lymphocytes, *RAG1/2* genes and their products are identified during early stages of development and the expression of transcription factors and signaling events drive clonal commitment.[155-158]

The ontogeny of T-lymphocyte immunity in the neonate has been reviewed (Table 9-4).[159,160] Cord blood has an increased absolute number of T lymphocytes compared with the peripheral blood of older children and adults. The mean T-lymphocyte counts in newborn infants, children, and adults are 3100 cells/mm³, 2500 cells/mm³, and 1400 cells/mm³, respectively. The ratio of CD4+ to CD8+ cells in cord blood is the same as that in adults (1.2), but it is increased to 1.9 from birth through 11 months of life.[161,162] Although the absolute number of T lymphocytes decreases beyond the neonatal period, the percentage of T lymphocytes among the total lymphocyte population increases.

Proliferative Responses

Neonatal T lymphocytes proliferate normally in response to phytohemagglutinin (PHA) and allogeneic cell stimulation but have a limited ability to develop immunologic memory.[163-165] Cord blood cell populations have been shown to contain large numbers of naive T lymphocytes (CD45RA+) versus memory T lymphocytes (CD45RO+).[166,167] This proportion declines slowly to 61% by 7 years of age, as naive lymphocytes are replaced by memory lymphocytes, which probably represents an intrinsic maturation of T lymphocytes as a consequence of antigenic stimulation.[159,168]

Cytokine Production

The predominant naive phenotype of newborn T lymphocytes may further account for differences in cytokine production. Neonatal T lymphocytes produce less INF-γ, IL-2, IL-4, IL-10, and TNF-α than adult T lymphocytes in response to various stimuli. Modest reduction of GM-CSF and decreased G-CSF and IL-3 production and gene expression have also been described.[168-172] Dysregulation of various immunoregulatory and cytokine genes in cord blood mononuclear cells could explain the apparent immaturity of neonatal cell mediated immunity.[173]

A group of soluble polypeptide mediators, called chemokines, also are important in immune surveillance. Chemokines regulate leukocyte chemotaxis, inflammation, antitumor activity, and HIV infection in humans. Placental cord blood mononuclear cells in comparison to adult peripheral blood mononuclear cells, produce smaller amounts of the chemokine called RANTES (regulated upon activation, T lymphocyte expressed). Since RANTES is a known ligand for CCR5, it suggests a role of this chemokine in HIV pathogenesis.[174,175]

T lymphocytes influence the functional activity of many other cell types responsible for both natural and specific immunity. Decreased T-lymphocyte function in neonates is likely to increase their susceptibility to infection by many pathogens. For example, decreased T-lymphocyte help for antibody production and isotype switching via CD40L–CD40 interaction,[176] along with decreased phagocytic function, probably contribute to increased susceptibility to bacterial infection. Susceptibility to viral infection and other intracellular pathogens, such as *Toxoplasma gondii* and *Listeria*, probably results from decreased cytolytic activity of T lymphocytes and decreased IFN-γ.[168] The specific role of T-lymphocyte immaturity in severe clinical HSV infection in neonates is suggested by the observation that neonates infected with HSV showed decreased antigen-specific cellular responses (decreased proliferation and IFN-γ production) compared with adults who had primary HSV infection.[177] Finally NK cell cytotoxicity and ADCC, along with defective chemokine production, may be contributors to perinatally acquired HIV infection.

INTERRELATIONSHIPS AND THE FUTURE

Humans resist infection in several ways. The innate defense mechanisms act first and may be capable of eliminating the pathogen completely. If not, adaptive responses are initiated and put in place, releasing clonally expanded effector T and B lymphocytes to the sites of infection. The mechanisms that regulate the final clearance are dependent on the pathogen itself. For certain pathogens, an effective adaptive immune response leads to a state of protective immunity. However, many pathogens evolve mechanisms that permit evasion from an effective immune response. Since Edward Jenner's studies of cowpox 200 years ago, vaccination has become a successful application of our interpretation of nature's experiments. Furthermore, the study of patients with primary immunodeficiency has provided not only a better understanding of biologic systems as they relate to humans but has in turn offered therapeutic options not only for this group of patients but for others as well. Only through the understanding of the basic intrinsic mechanisms that regulate immunity will further pathogenic mechanism be elucidated and therapies develop.

TABLE 9-4. Comparison of Newborn and Adult T Lymphocytes

Characteristics	Newborn	Adult
Repertoire of TCR binding specificity	Unknown	Broad
Mean T-lymphocyte count	3100/mm³	1400/mm³
CD4+/CD8+ (ratio)	1.2	1.2
Proliferation (mitogen-stimulated)	Good	Good
Proliferation (antigen-stimulated)	Poor	Good
Ability to provide help to B lymphocytes	Poor	Good
CD45RA+ (naive CD4+ T lymphocytes)	90%	48%
Production of cytokines	Decreased IFN-γ, IL-4, G-CSF, GM-CSF, IL-3	Multiple

10 Fever and the Inflammatory Response

Alexei A. Grom

FEVER

Pathogenesis

Fever is defined as a centrally mediated rise of body temperature above the normal daily variation in response to many different pathologic insults.[1] The rise in the body temperature is a regulated process triggered by the elevation of the set point in the thermoregulatory center located in the hypothalamus. This elevation can be elicited by exogenous or endogenous pyrogenic substances. A variety of microbial products, including endotoxins and exotoxins, are exogenous pyrogens. Although these molecules can act directly to induce fever, evidence indicates that they stimulate host cells to secrete mediators known as endogenous pyrogens. The pivotal endogenous pyrogens are cytokines produced during the inflammatory response, most notably, tumor necrosis factor-α (TNF-α), interleukin-1 (IL-1), IL-6, and to a lesser degree, the interferons (IFNs).[2–4] Fever is more likely to be caused by infection, but any inflammatory, neoplastic, immunologic, or traumatic event also can generate fever.

Once these pyrogenic cytokines are produced, they enter the systemic circulation and stimulate the rich vascular network surrounding the preoptic area of the hypothalamus (thermoregulatory center). Here they activate phospholipase A_2, liberating plasma membrane arachidonic acid as a substrate for the cyclooxygenase pathway.[5,6] Some cytokines can increase cyclooxygenase expression directly, causing liberation of the arachidonate metabolite prostaglandin (PG) E_2. Because this small lipid molecule diffuses easily across the blood–brain barrier, some believe it to be the local mediator that activates thermoregulatory neurons, which in turn raise the thermostat set point (Figure 10-1). Although the blood–brain barrier prevents migration of large proteins such as circulating cytokines, the presence of the pyrogenic substances has been demonstrated at certain sites known as circumventricular organs, which lack a blood–brain barrier.[6]

As a result, activation of peripheral mechanisms that stimulate the sympathetic chain and terminal adrenergic efferent nerves leads to vasoconstriction (heat conservation) and muscle contraction (heat production), which generate fever. Autonomic (decreased sweating) and endocrine (decreased vasopressin secretion to reduce amount of body fluid to be heated) pathways contribute to thermoregulation.[6] Conservation and production of heat continue until the temperature of the blood bathing the hypothalamic neurons matches the new elevated setting. When cytokine stimulation ceases, the hypothalamic set point is reset downward and the processes of heat loss through vasodilatation and sweating are initiated. In addition to these thermoregulatory mechanisms, certain areas in the cerebral cortex are stimulated to promote behavioral changes designed to help control temperature. Thus, a child who desires extra blankets during a shaking chill is manifesting a heat-saving effector behavior, and a child who removes clothing is exhibiting a heat-loss behavioral mechanism.

Fever must be distinguished from hyperthermia, which is an uncontrolled increase in the body temperature. Hyperthermia typically develops when exogenous heat exposure or endogenous heat production exceeds the body's ability to lose heat. This occurs despite a normal hypothalamic set point.

Clinical Aspects

Body temperature varies with age, physical activity, and at various times of the day, fluctuating from values less than 37°C in the early morning to values near 38°C in the late afternoon. Normal diurnal fluctuation also is exhibited in febrile patients. In general, values higher than 37.8°C are considered to be fever, although single elevations do not always imply a pathologic process. Very young infants tend to have blunted fever rises more often than older infants and children do in response to the same antigenic stimulus. In clinical practice, core temperature is measured best by use of a rectal thermometer; oral temperatures can be influenced by prior ingestion of hot or cold foods and are reduced in the presence of open-mouth breathing in patients with tachypnea. Axillary readings are less reliable and typically are 0.5°C lower than oral values and 1°C lower than rectal readings. In theory, the tympanic membrane is an ideal site for measuring core body temperature because it is perfused by a tributary artery supplying the body's thermoregulatory center. Unfortunately, numerous studies of many different tympanic membrane thermometers have shown that although convenient, such instruments tend to give highly variable readings that correlate poorly with simultaneously obtained oral or rectal readings.[7,8]

Antipyretic Therapy

Substantial evidence suggests that fever is more beneficial than harmful for the host.[9] High temperatures interfere with the replication and virulence of certain pathogens and may speed the recovery of infected patients. In addition, some immunologic responses (e.g., leukocyte migration and phagocytosis, as well as interferon production) are enhanced by temperature elevation.

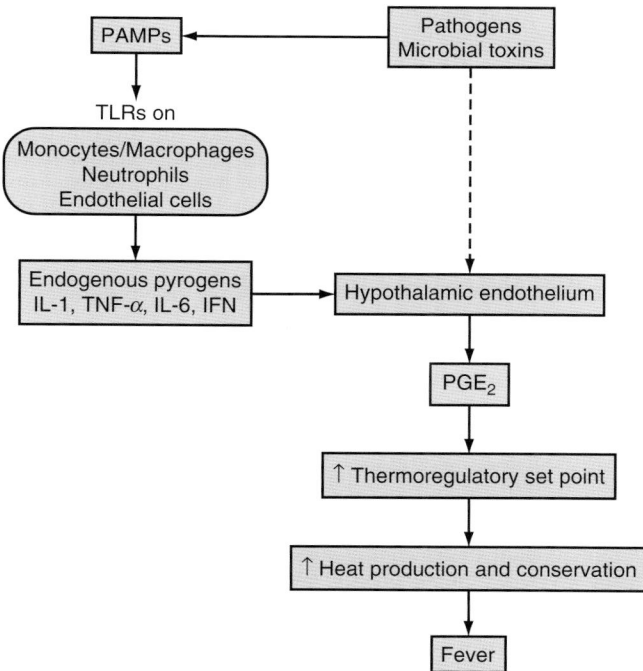

Figure 10-1. Induction of fever. Central and peripheral mechanisms. IFN, interferon; IL-1, interleukin-1; PAMPs, pathogen-associated molecular patterns; PGE_2, prostaglandin E_2; TLRs, toll-like receptors; TNF-α, tumor necrosis factor-α.

Moreover, fever is likely to represent a regulatory mechanism to reduce cytokine activation of the acute inflammatory response through a negative biofeedback process. Finally, nonspecific suppression of fever may eliminate an important clue for the need for further diagnostic investigations or for changes in therapy. Short courses of approved doses of standard antipyretic drugs carry a low risk of toxicity, and most of these drugs have analgesic properties as well. Their use may reduce the intensity of the symptoms of an illness, but also can prolong an illness or diminish a vaccine response.

Antipyretic Agents

Because fever is generated after local hypothalamic stimulation by PGs, inhibitors of the cyclooxygenase enzyme system are potent antipyretics. Although acetaminophen is a poor cyclooxygenase inhibitor in peripheral tissue, this agent is oxidized in the brain, and the resulting compound inhibits cyclooxygenase activity. Aspirin inhibits PG synthetase in a wide variety of tissues, and its antipyretic effect is equivalent to that of acetaminophen. Because these drugs are broad cyclooxygenase inhibitors, they can cause many side effects. The potential association between aspirin therapy in children with influenza or varicella and the development of Reye syndrome precludes its use in children with these conditions.

Several nonsteroidal anti-inflammatory drugs (e.g., ibuprofen, naproxen) have antipyretic effects similar to those of aspirin and acetaminophen. Because these agents are associated with more adverse effects than is acetaminophen, their use for treatment of simple fever is ill-advised as its anti-inflammatory effect could have adverse effect on clinical course of infection. Thus they should be restricted to those conditions requiring an anti-inflammatory agent.

Corticosteroids are among the most potent antipyretic drugs because not only do they inhibit the activity of phospholipase A_2, thereby interfering with arachidonic acid metabolism and PG synthesis, and also block the production of pyrogenic cytokines (i.e., TNF, IL-1, and IL-6) at a proximal step in the genesis of a febrile response. Although corticosteroids are excellent anti-inflammatory agents, they should not be used in management of simple febrile episodes or infectious diseases without specific indications.

The use of a cooling blanket or water-alcohol bathing an attempt to accelerate peripheral heat losses is uncomfortable, and the latter can lead to alcohol toxicity. Peripheral cooling, in the absence of pharmacologic downregulation of the hypothalamic set point, can be counterproductive because cold receptors in the skin send signals to the spinal cord and brain for reactive vasoconstriction and shivering, thus increasing heat conservation, and eliciting oxygen consumption and heat production.

THE INFLAMMATORY RESPONSE

The body has a sentinel system that maintains immunologic surveillance to avoid pathogen-induced derangements of homeostasis. Once this background activity is circumvented, a host inflammatory response ensues. The inflammatory response is a complex reaction that involves the migration of elements of the immune system into sites of tissue injury or microbial invasion.[10] In most clinical situations, the inflammatory response, with or without the aid of antimicrobial therapy, is effective in resolving the infection and contributes to tissue remodeling. If the infection is not brought under control, however, the infectious stimulus gains access to the circulation and stimulates the release of a cascade of systemic and local effector molecules. This host reaction, called the systemic inflammatory response syndrome, can be caused by a variety of immunologic, traumatic, surgical, or drug-induced insults; most often, however, an infectious agent is the trigger (see Chapter 11, The Systemic Inflammatory Response Syndrome (SIRS), Sepsis, and Septic Shock). The sum of the balance of microbial damage–host response framework can result in host damage due to the microbe, the host, or both.

The Innate and Adaptive Immune Systems

The immune response to infection and cellular injury can be broadly divided into two categories: innate and adaptive immunity.[11] The immediate response, associated with the production of the pyrogenic cytokines IL-1, IL-6, and TNF-α, is mounted by the innate immune system that involves neutrophils, monocyte/macrophage, dendritic cells, and natural killer (NK) cells. The main receptors of the innate immune system recognize broad patterns of conserved and often integral structural components of microbes that are not present in human cells. These highly conserved microbial structural components are often called pathogen-associated molecular patterns or PAMPs, while the host receptors are called pattern recognition receptors or PRRs. The binding of PAMPs to PRRs results in rapid changes in expression of genes including those encoding pyrogenic cytokines. In addition to inflammatory cytokines, many other pathways are activated including synthesis of degradative enzymes and enzymes responsible for production of small molecule mediators of inflammation such as arachidonic acid derivatives (Figure 10-2).

The contribution of the adaptive immune system becomes important at later stages of the immune response. The adaptive immune response is mediated by T and B lymphocytes and is characterized by high specificity and long-lasting memory. The adaptive immunity is influenced by the generation of helper T-lymphocyte subsets (Th) and the subsequent production of "effector" cytokines by these cells. Thus, naïve T lymphocytes that recognize the antigen presented by antigen-presenting cells (APCs), undergo activation and expansion. At this stage, they can differentiate into two subsets: Th1 or Th2, determined by the cytokine milieu at this step. The IFNs and IL-12 drive Th1 differentiation, whereas IL-4 induces Th2 differentiation.[12] Th1 cells secrete IFN-γ and promote mainly cellular immunity, whereas Th2 cells produce IL-4, IL-5, IL-10, and IL-13 and primarily promote humoral immunity. Infection of intracellular pathogens induces primarily a Th1-dominated response that protects against the majority of microorganisms, while some parasitic infections induce a Th2 response that is associated with resistance to helminths.

In addition to instructive cytokines, APCs use several costimulatory molecules, including CD80 and CD86, to signal T cells and to induce clonal expansion of antigen-specific T cells. Antigen presentation in the absence of costimulatory molecules leads to cell anergy. Since the engagement of the innate receptors on APCs leads to upregulation of expression of the costimulatory molecules and enhances antigen presentation, the interaction between the innate and adaptive systems at this step becomes very important.[11]

Receptors of the Innate System

The PRRs that initiate recognition of infectious agents respond to PAMPs, which are shared by large groups of microorganisms but are not present in mammalian cells.[11] Probably the best-known example of PAMPs are lipopolysacharides. Lipopolysacharides (LPS) are the mixture of fragments of the outer membrane of gram-negative bacteria. LPS administration induces local and systemic inflammation and tissue damage that is similar to that observed in infection caused by gram-negative bacteria. For this reason, the LPS-induced response has been used for several decades as a model of inflammation. In 1998, the principal component of the human receptor system recognizing LPS was identified as toll-like receptor (TLR) 4. The term is based on structural similarities with the *Drosophila* protein "toll" which is required for the normal development of the flies and protection against the fungus *Aspergillus*.[13,14] Over the last several years, at least nine other human TLRs have been identified. Each appears to recognize a distinct set of PAMPs (see Table 10-1). It is becoming clear that, collectively, TLRs can detect most (if not all) microbes[11,15–17] including protozoa, bacteria, viruses, and fungi. Evidence exists to suggest that some TLRs also may recognize endogenous ligands

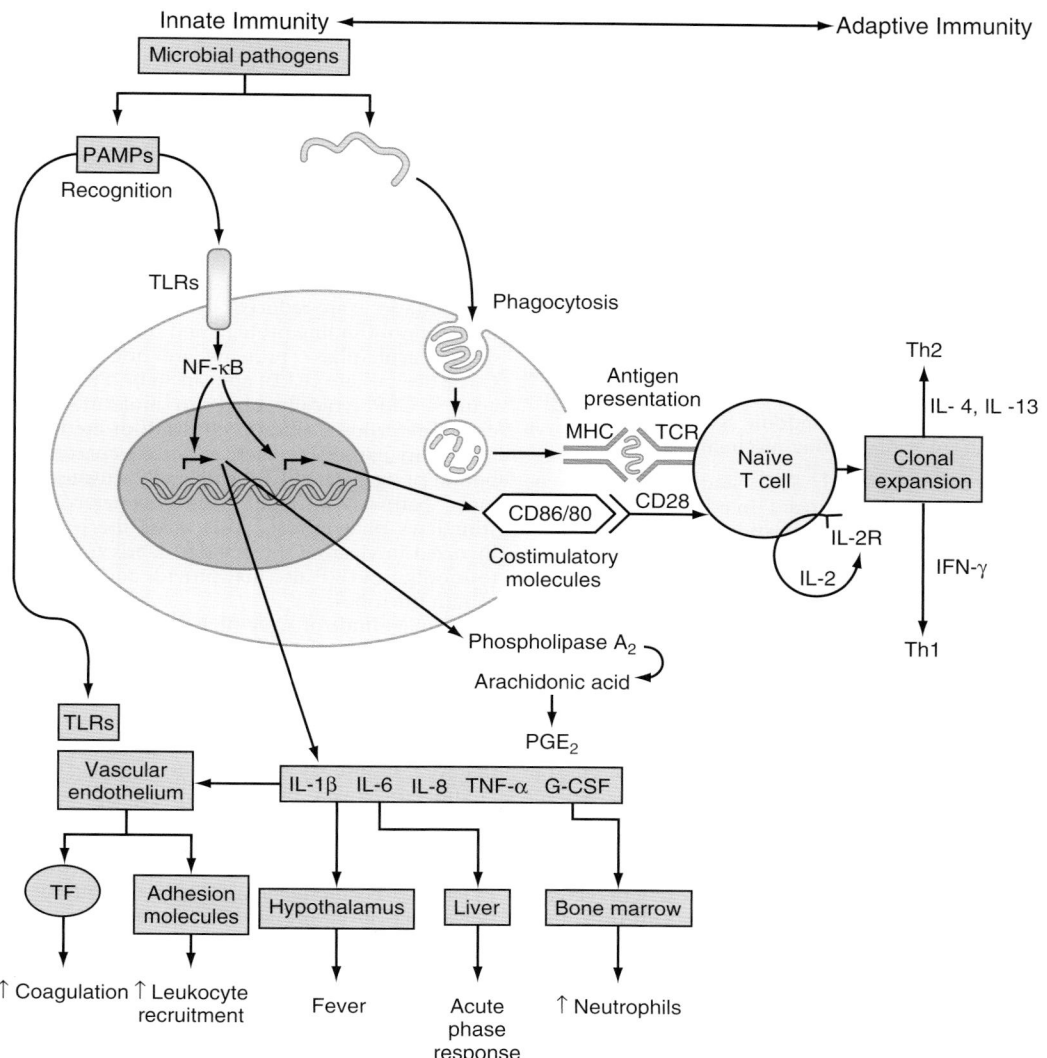

Figure 10-2. Induction of the innate and adaptive immune responses. The recognition of pathogen-associated molecular patterns (PAMPs) by toll-like receptors (TLRs) results in the activation of intracellular signaling pathways leading to the activation of the transcription factor NF-κB. The translocation of NF-κB into the nucleus leads to upregulation of expression of genes encoding proinflammatory cytokines interleukin-1 (IL-1), interleukin-6 (IL-6), tumor necrosis factor-α (TNF-α), and colony-stimulating factors (CSFs). It also leads to increased expression of costimulatory molecules involved in antigen presentation and induction of the adaptive immune responses. The cytokines IL-1, IL-6, TNF, and granulocyte CSF (G-CSF), through their effects on hypothalamus, bone marrow, liver, and vascular endothelial cells, initiate the inflammatory cascade. IFN, interferon; MHC, major histocompatibility complex; TCR, T-cell receptor; TF, tissue factor.

TABLE 10-1. Toll-like Receptors (TLRs) and Their Microbial Ligands

TLR	Ligand	Microbial Source
TLR2	Lipoproteins	Bacteria
	Peptidoglycan	Gram-positive bacteria
	Lipopolysaccharide	*Leptospira*
	Zymosan	Yeast
TLR3	Double-stranded RNA	Viruses
TLR4	Lipopolysaccharide	Gram-negative bacteria
TLR5	Flagellin	Various bacteria
TLR7/8	Single-stranded RNA	Viruses
TLR9	CpG DNA	Bacteria, protozoa

such as degradation products of various extracellular matrix components released as a result of tissue damage. The term damage-associated molecular patterns (DAMPs) collectively describes these endogenous TLR ligands. The recognition of DAMPs by TLRs may contribute to the development of inflammation, and in some infections, may lead to a greatly exaggerated inflammatory response. For instance, TLR4 increases severity of the inflammatory response to H5N1 influenza virus infection by recognizing a DAMP rather then the virus itself. More specifically, acute lung injury caused by H5N1 virus produces endogenous oxidized phospholipids, which stimulate TLR4.[18]

TLRs are expressed in different and important cells of the innate immune system including monocyte/macrophages, dendritic cells, neutrophils, vascular endothelial cells, and epithelial cells lining mucosal surfaces. While some TLRs (such as TLR1, 2, 4, 5, and 6) are expressed on the cell surface, others (TLR3, 7, and 9) are found almost exclusively in intracellular compartments such as endosomes.[17] Pathogens that have evaded cell surface or endosomal TLRs and have gained access to the cytosol are recognized by another group of PRRs called NOD-like receptors (NLRs). The activation of at least some of the NLRs induces activation of caspase 1, which catalyzes the proteolytic processing of pro-IL-1β to into mature active IL-1β.

The binding of microbial molecules to TLRs leads to the activation of intracellular signaling pathways. The predominant pathway used by TLRs leads to the activation of NF-κB, a nuclear transcription factor that initiates rapid changes in expression of several groups of genes (Figure 10-2). Most important are those encoding:

- cytokines and chemokines (including the pyrogenic cytokines TNF-α, IL-1, IL-6 as well as IL-8, colony-stimulating factors, platelet-activating factor among others)
- enzymes involved in the degradation of extracellular matrix proteins
- enzymes responsible for the production of small molecule mediators of inflammation such as arachidonic acid derivatives
- proteins involved in microbial killing mechanisms.

A subset of TLRs comprising TLR3, TLR7, and TLR9 recognize nucleic acids derived mainly from viruses. In addition to production of proinflammatory cytokines, activation of these TLRs also leads to the production of type I interferons that have the ability to induce proteins that interfere with viral replication.[17]

The engagement and activation of TLRs expressed on vascular endothelial cells also leads to increased expression of chemokines and adhesion molecules (selectins and integrin ligands).[19,20] Combined with the simultaneous upregulation of selectin ligands and integrins on leukocytes (also stimulated by TLR engagement), the result is increased adhesion of leukocytes to the vascular endothelium. Once these cells are firmly attached, they begin transmigration across endothelial surfaces (i.e., extravasation) to the sites of microbial invasion and tissue damage. During extravasation, degranulation of neutrophils can occur. Such degranulation is associated with the release of several proteolytic enzymes and toxic oxygen radicals that contribute to increased vascular permeability. Furthermore, activation of the complement system (classic and alternate pathways) and coagulation cascades (intrinsic and extrinsic pathways) occurs concurrently with cytokine stimulation. Release of the anaphylatoxins C3a and C5a promotes vascular abnormalities and neutrophil activation.

The cytokines and chemokines whose production is stimulated by TLR engagement in turn produce multiple effects that further amplify the inflammatory response:

- the cytokines IL-1, TNF-α, and IL-6 stimulate metabolism of arachidonic acid to form leukotrienes, thromboxane A_2, and prostaglandins (especially PGE_2 and PGI_2)
- IL-1, TNF-α, and IL-6 increase PGE_2 synthesis in the vascular and perivascular cells of hypothalamus leading to generation of fever[2-4]
- Granulocyte colony-stimulating factor (G-CSF) increases production and release of neutrophils from the bone marrow to replace those consumed by inflammation, often leading to an increase in absolute neutrophil counts
- IL-1 and TNF-α stimulate endothelial cells to synthesize secondary factors that contribute to the inflammatory process, including endothelial-cell adhesion molecules, chemokines (IL-8, MIP-1α), hemostatic tissue factor (TF), as well as IL-1, PGI_2, and granulocyte-macrophage colony-stimulating factor (GM-CSF).

The release of the hemostatic TF by endothelial cells and macrophages appears to be pivotal in the activation of the coagulation cascade, which activation in turn can trigger activation of the complement system. Together, activation of these pathways can lead to disseminated intravascular coagulation often seen in severe systemic inflammatory responses.[21] Platelets are primed to interact with endothelium and to aggregate in dense masses that interfere with blood supply to tissues. This generalized endothelial cell activation is critical in the pathogenesis of vascular injury and capillary permeability associated with acute inflammation that can progress to shock and multiorgan dysfunction in some patients.[21]

Acute-Phase Response

In response to mainly IL-1 and IL-6, a structurally and functionally heterogeneous group of proteins change their concentration in peripheral blood. These proteins are known as acute-phase response proteins.[1,22] Some of these are known as *positive acute-phase proteins* because they increase in concentration after antigenic stimuli. These proteins are synthesized mainly by the liver, the most important examples being C-reactive protein, serum amyloid A, $α_1$-acid glycoprotein, $α_1$-antitrypsin, haptoglobin, ceruloplasmin, and fibrinogen. Other acute-phase proteins are referred to as *negative acute-phase proteins* because their plasma concentrations are reduced. Examples include albumin, prealbumin, retinol-binding protein, and transferrin. The exact functions of the acute-phase proteins are not completely understood. C-reactive protein (CRP) appears to be a pattern recognition molecule.[23] CRP typically binds to molecular configurations that either are exposed during cell death or are found on the surface of certain pathogens such as *Streptococcus pneumoniae*. Ligand-bound or aggregated CRP efficiently activates the classic complement pathway through a direct interaction with C1q, and stimulates phagocytosis. This raises the possibility that CRP is involved in clearing the cellular debris from necrotic and apoptotic cells, but CRP also may provide additional protection against certain microbes.

The magnitude of acute-phase responses provides a guide to the intensity of the inflammation or the extent of tissue involvement. For instance, the rise in fibrinogen causes erythrocytes to form stacks (rouleaux) that sediment more rapidly than do individual erythrocytes. This is the basis for measuring erythrocyte sedimentation rate as a simple test for the magnitude of systemic inflammatory response regardless of the initiating stimuli.

Mineral changes are uniformly present during the acute-phase host response. The best-documented alterations are decreased serum concentrations of iron and zinc caused by the uptake in hepatocytes and phagocytes. Conversely, serum copper levels are elevated as a consequence of increased synthesis of ceruloplasmin, the copper carrier protein. Because of hypoferremia, reduction of red blood cell synthesis, and decreased red blood cell lifespan, mild but reversible anemia usually accompanies a significant acute inflammatory response.

Profound alterations in utilization of carbohydrates, proteins, and lipids occur during acute inflammatory responses.[1,24,25] The hypermetabolic state typically seen in patients with sepsis requires massive use of carbohydrate and lipid stores to meet energy needs. In addition, amino acids from muscle tissue are used by the liver to produce glucose (gluconeogenesis). These changes are presumably provoked by cytokine-induced production of cortisol, insulin, glucagon, and growth hormone. Clinically, these abnormalities manifest as reactive hyperglycemia, substantial fluctuation in plasma concentrations of free fatty acids, hypertriglyceridemia, and negative nitrogen balance resulting from catabolism of amino acids. Many of these effects are mediated by TNF-α.

The Regulatory Anti-Inflammatory Pathways

The overproduction of proinflammatory substances can lead to extensive tissue damage and vascular injury, disseminated intravascular coagulation, and shock. To attenuate potential damage to the host, the inflammatory cascade stimulates modulating pathways that involve anti-inflammatory cytokines such as transforming growth factor-β (TGF-β), IL-4, and IL-10. TGF-β also has the ability to stimulate production of extracellular matrix proteins and, thus, contribute to tissue remodeling after the resolution of inflammation. Natural inhibitors of inflammatory cytokines also exist.[26] For instance, many inflammatory cells including neutrophils and macrophages have the ability to shed their TNF receptors. These soluble TNF receptors bind free TNF and neutralize its proinflammatory activity. Also, the IL-1 system has unique pathways of negative regulation that involve natural IL-1 receptor antagonists and the type II decoy receptor. Interestingly, some anti-inflammatory cytokines (e.g., IL-4, IL-10) can simultaneously inhibit the production of IL-1 and stimulate production of receptor antagonists and the decoy receptor. Thus, an intricate network of positive and negative biofeedback loops operates during the course of a systemic inflammatory response and the net balance determines clinical expression and severity of disease.

Interaction of Innate and Adaptive Immune Responses

In summary, the *immediate* inflammatory response to microbial invasion or tissue injury is controlled mainly by the innate immune system. This innate response is triggered by the binding of PAMPs to the pattern recognition receptors (i.e., TLRs and NLRs) expressed in host cells. The subsequent intracellular signaling in host cells leads to increased expression of several groups of genes including those encoding pyrogenic and proinflammatory cytokines TNF-α, IL-1, and IL-6. TLR activation also leads to upregulation of expression of the costimulatory molecules involved in antigen presentation (i.e., CD80/CD86). This leads to the enhancement of adaptive immunity that becomes more important in *the later stages* of the inflammatory response. Anti-inflammatory pathways are activated simultaneously, and the net balance between proinflammatory and anti-inflammatory stimuli determines the magnitude and the outcome of the inflammatory response. Basic mechanisms of the inflammatory response remain regardless whether the response is systemic or local. For instance, in bacterial meningitis, local production of cytokines within the subarachnoidal space in response to presence of bacteria, or their cell wall components, induces the disruption of the blood–brain barrier, increased vascular permeability, and chemotactic attraction of neutrophils to the meningeal site of microbial invasion.[27]

The effective coordination of the adaptive and innate immunity eventually leads to the elimination of the invading microbes. The absence of microbial stimulation leads to the cessation of the proinflammatory stimuli and resolution of inflammation. At this stage, several cytokines and growth factors (including TGF-β) contribute to the repair of the damaged tissues. This allows the host to return to and maintain a relative state of homeostasis until the next microbial challenge.

11 The Systemic Inflammatory Response Syndrome (SIRS), Sepsis, and Septic Shock

Judith A. Guzman-Cottrill, Beth Cheesebrough, Simon Nadel, and Brahm Goldstein

Sepsis remains a major cause of morbidity and mortality among children.[1-4] Sepsis-associated mortality in children has decreased from 97% in 1966[5] to 9% among infants in the early 1990s.[6] A recent population-based study of United States children with severe septicemia (bacterial or fungal infection with at least one acute organ dysfunction) reported a mortality rate of 10.3%.[7] Although this represents a significant improvement over past decades, severe sepsis remains one of the leading causes of death in children, with over 4300 deaths annually (7% of all deaths among children) and estimated annual total costs of $1.97 billion.[8]

In a seminal study, Watson et al.[8] analyzed the impact of age, sex, birthweight, underlying disease, and microbiologic etiology on the incidence, mortality, and hospital costs of children who develop septicemia using 1995 hospital discharge and population data from seven states. Table 11-1 shows the annual incidence, case fatality, and national estimates of severe sepsis by age. The incidence is highest in infants (5.16 per 1000), falls significantly in older children (0.20 per 1000 in 10- to 14-year-olds), and also exhibits a sex difference, being 15% higher in boys than in girls (0.60 versus 0.52 per 1000, P < 0.001).[8] Overall hospital mortality was 10.3%, or 4383 deaths nationally (6.2 per 100,000 population).[8] Of interest, about 50% of the cases had an underlying disease and over 20% were low-birthweight neonates. The most common infections were respiratory tract (37%) and primary bloodstream infections (BSIs) (25%).[8] The mean length of hospital stay was 31 days, and the cost was $40,600 per admission.[8]

DEFINITIONS

An international panel of experts in the fields of adult and pediatric septicemia and clinical research proposed the first set of specific definitions and criteria for the components of the sepsis continuum that can be applied consistently in the pediatric population in 2005.[6] These definitions were used again in the international guidelines for management of sepsis and septic shock.[9] The consensus definitions for systemic inflammatory response syndrome (SIRS), infection, sepsis, severe sepsis, septic shock, and multiple organ dysfunction syndrome in children are listed in Box 11-1. It is important to recognize that these definitions were meant for use in the design, conduct, and analysis of large, multicenter, international therapeutic trials rather than as a clinical tool at the bedside. It is clear that, given the intra- and inter-individual differences in the time course of disease progression, these definitions often have limited clinical utility.

The diagnosis and thus the definition of septic shock in children can be challenging. Children often maintain blood pressure until severely ill;[10] while there is no requirement for systemic hypotension in order to make the diagnosis of septic shock as there is in adults, a recent expert review committee recommends early recognition of septic shock in premature neonates, infants, and children using clinical examination, not biochemical tests.[11] Shock can occur long before hypotension occurs in children. Thus, shock can be diagnosed clinically before hypotension occurs by clinical signs, which include hypothermia or hyperthermia, altered mental status, and peripheral vasodilation (warm shock) or vasoconstriction with capillary refill >2 seconds (cold shock).[11] Hypotension is a sign of late and decompensated shock in children and is confirmatory of shock state if present in a child with suspected or proven infection.[12] Although there are distinct clinical presentations and classifications of shock in children (e.g., warm and cold shock; fluid-refractory and catecholamine-resistant shock), septic shock is defined as septicemia in the presence of cardiovascular dysfunction (i.e., severe sepsis with cardiovascular dysfunction).[6]

ETIOLOGY

Several factors influence the potential pathogens causing septicemia in children, including age, host immune status, and geographic location at the time of infection. In addition, organisms causing community-onset infections differ from those acquired in the hospital setting. During the neonatal period, common bacterial causes include group B streptococci and enteric bacilli, such as *Escherichia coli*. Other less common pathogens include enterococci, *Listeria monocytogenes*, *Staphylococcus*

TABLE 11-1. Annual Incidence, Case Fatality, and National Estimates of Severe Sepsis by Age

Age	Incidence (Per 1000 Population)	National Estimate of Cases	Case Fatality (%)	National Estimate of Deaths
<1 year[a]	5.16	20,145	10.6	2135
0–28 days[b]	3.60	14,049	10.3	1361
29–364 days[b]	1.56	6,096	13.5	774
1–4 years[a]	0.49	7,583	10.4	786
5–9 years[a]	0.22	4,168	9.9	413
10–14 years[a]	0.20	3,836	9.6	368
15–19 years[a]	0.37	6,633	9.7	644
All children	0.56	42,364	10.3	4383

[a]National estimates are generated from the seven-state cohort using state and national age- and sex-specific population estimates from the National Center for Health Statistics and the United States Census.

[b]Results for these ages are based on data from the five states (MA, MD, NJ, NY, and VA) in which neonates could be identified (n = 6349 or 66% of the entire seven-state cohort).

From Watson RS, Carcillo JA, Linde-Zwirble WT, et al. The epidemiology of severe sepsis in children in the United States. Am J Respir Crit Care Med 2003;167:695–701.

PART II Clinical Syndromes and Cardinal Features of Infectious Diseases: Approach to Diagnosis and Initial Management

SECTION A Septicemia, Toxin- and Inflammation-Mediated Syndromes

BOX 11-1. Definitions of Systemic Inflammatory Response Syndrome, Infection, Sepsis, Severe Sepsis, and Septic Shock

SYSTEMIC INFLAMMATORY RESPONSE SYNDROME (SIRS)

The presence of two or more of the following criteria, one of which must be abnormal temperature or leukocyte count:

- Core[a] temperature of >38.5°C *or* <36°C
- Tachycardia, defined as a mean heart rate >2 SD above normal for age in the absence of external stimulus, chronic drugs, or painful stimuli; or otherwise unexplained persistent elevation over a 0.5- to 4-hour time period *or* for children <1 year old: Bradycardia, defined as a mean heart rate <10th percentile for age in the absence of external vagal stimulus, beta-blocker drugs, or congenital heart disease; or otherwise unexplained persistent depression over a 0.5-hour time period
- Mean respiratory rate >2 SD above normal for age or mechanical ventilation for an acute process not related to underlying neuromuscular disease or the receipt of general anesthesia
- Leukocyte count elevated or depressed for age (not secondary to chemotherapy-induced leukopenia) or >10% immature neutrophils

INFECTION

A suspected or proven (by positive culture, tissue stain, or polymerase chain reaction test) infection caused by any pathogen *or* a clinical syndrome associated with a high probability of infection. Evidence of infection includes positive findings on clinical exam, imaging, or laboratory tests (e.g., white blood cells in a normally sterile body fluid, perforated viscus, chest X-ray consistent with pneumonia, petechial or purpuric rash, or purpura fulminans)

SEPSIS

SIRS in the presence of or as a result of suspected or proven infection

SEVERE SEPSIS

Sepsis plus the following: cardiovascular organ dysfunction, acute respiratory distress syndrome (ARDS), or two or more other organ dysfunctions

SEPTIC SHOCK

Sepsis and cardiovascular organ dysfunction

[a]Core temperature must be measured by rectal, oral, or central catheter probe.

From Goldstein B, Giroir B, Randolph A. International pediatric sepsis consensus conference: definitions for sepsis and organ dysfunction in pediatrics. Pediatr Crit Care Med 2005;6:2–8.

aureus (including methicillin-resistant *Staphylococcus aureus*) and *Streptococcus pneumoniae*. Advances in neonatology and survival of extremely- and very-low-birthweight infants affect the epidemiology of hospital-associated neonatal sepsis. The use of central venous catheters (CVCs) and other foreign bodies further predispose these already compromised neonates to pathogens such as coagulase-negative staphylococci, *S. aureus*, less common gram-negative bacilli, and *Candida* spp. Viral neonatal sepsis may be indistinguishable clinically from bacterial infection. Viral pathogens include herpes simplex virus, enteroviruses, respiratory syncytial virus, and influenza virus.

Beyond the neonatal period, *S. pneumoniae* and *Neisseria meningitidis* are common causes of sepsis in otherwise healthy children. *Haemophilus influenzae* type b (Hib) should be considered in the incompletely vaccinated child. In 2005, only 9 cases of invasive Hib disease in children <5 years of age were reported in the U.S.[13] In 2008, this increased to 30 cases.[14] Since the routine administration of the heptavalent pneumococcal conjugate vaccine in 2000, the overall incidence of invasive pneumococcal disease in children <5 years of age has declined by 76%.[15] Other organisms include *S. aureus* and *Streptococcus pyogenes* (also causing toxic shock syndrome), *Salmonella* spp., and rickettsia in certain geographic regions (Rocky Mountain spotted fever and ehrlichiosis). In hospitalized infants and children with indwelling CVCs, coagulase-negative staphylococci, *S. aureus*, gram-negative bacilli, and *Candida* spp. are important causes of sepsis due to central line associated bloodstream infection (CLABSI).

Children with underlying immunodeficiency states can develop septicemia due to the same pathogens as healthy children; however, some conditions predispose to additional organisms. Neutropenic cancer patients with mucositis are at risk of sepsis due to the Enterobacteriaceae, other gram-negative bacilli such as *Pseudomonas aeruginosa*, and alpha-hemolytic (viridans) streptococci. The last are associated with acute respiratory distress syndrome (ARDS) and can cause meningitis.[16,17] As most oncology patients have indwelling CVCs, they also remain at risk for the typical CLABSI pathogens. Other conditions increase risk of sepsis due to certain pathogens, e.g., acquired immunodeficiency virus (AIDS) for *S. pneumoniae*, *P. aeruginosa*, *S. aureus*, and Hib; anatomic or functional asplenia (including sickle-cell disease) for encapsulated organisms such as *S. pneumoniae*, *Salmonella* spp., Hib, and *N. meningitidis*; and cyclic neutropenia for *Clostridium* species.

PATHOPHYSIOLOGY

If a microbe gains access to the intravascular compartment, the host activates defensive mechanisms. Transient bacteremia without significant clinical consequences occurs commonly in healthy children. In others, probably depending on the age and immunocompetence of the patient, the virulence and number of pathogens in the blood, and the timing and nature of a therapeutic intervention, the host's systemic inflammatory response ensues and can progress independently, despite successful eradication of the microbe. Although infection is a major cause of the systemic inflammatory response syndrome (SIRS), a number of other entities, including trauma, ARDS, neoplasm, burn injury, pancreatitis, and dysfunctional macrophage activation, are also recognized causes.

Most pathophysiologic consequences of the sepsis syndrome result from an imbalance between pro- and anti-inflammatory mediators in combination with microbial toxins.[18] In children, severe sepsis arises from coordinated activation of the innate immune response.[19] This response, triggered by diverse pathogens, is multifaceted.[18–20] Once triggered, the response leads to secretion of pro- and anti-inflammatory cytokines, activation and mobilization of leukocytes, activation of coagulation and inhibition of fibrinolysis,[21,22] and increased apoptosis.[23] As a result of coagulation activation, thrombin generated promotes fibrin deposition in the microvasculature and also exacerbates ongoing inflammation by direct and indirect mechanisms.[18] Although evolutionarily designed to limit microbial dissemination, overexuberant innate inflammatory processes may be detrimental, resulting in cardiac dysfunction, vasodilation, capillary injury, and micro- and macrovascular thromboses. Despite antimicrobial therapy and intensive supportive care, these processes frequently lead to organ dysfunction, thrombotic complications, long-term neurologic morbidity, or death (Table 11-1).[1,24]

The clinical manifestations of sepsis are the result of systemic inflammation and include abnormal temperature regulation, flushed warm skin, widened pulse pressure, tachycardia, tachypnea, metabolic acidosis (elevated serum lactate, decreased base excess), renal and/or hepatic dysfunction, thrombocytosis, and leukocytosis. As the syndrome progresses, multiorgan failure, including acute respiratory failure, hypotension, myocardial failure, decreased neurologic function, oliguric or anuric renal failure, hepatic failure, leukopenia, anemia, and thrombocytopenia, can ensue and can lead to death.

CLINICAL AND LABORATORY FINDINGS

Fever, tachycardia, and tachypnea are the most common physiologic abnormalities associated with sepsis, even though they are insensitive and nonspecific. Other clinical signs include decreased tone, diminished activity, pale or grey skin color, prolonged capillary refill time, and poor feeding or sucking.[25] Biochemical markers of inflammation may one day prove to be more objective and reliable than physiologic findings; however, no biochemical marker has been confirmed to be robust enough to use for the definitive diagnosis of sepsis or for tracking response to therapy and disease progression. Early recognition of septic shock depends on clinical recognition, as there are no reliable biochemical tests available to date.[11] Early treatment with antibiotics and fluid resuscitation has been demonstrated clearly to reduce both morbidity and mortality.[11,12,26]

Clinical Signs

The earliest clinical sign of clinical infection is age-dependent changes in body temperature.[27] In immune-competent children the earliest sign is fever. In immune-compromised children and premature infants the earliest sign can be hypothermia or fever.[27] Fever in association with changes in a child's behavior, such as an infant's loss of smiling or playfulness (especially after fever has been controlled with antipyretic therapy), are signs of serious infection, which may benefit from antibacterial, antiviral, or antifungal therapy.[28-30]

Tachycardia is a useful sign of sepsis in the neonate born at term,[31] as is tachycardia and/or tachypnea in older children.[27] Fever can account for some tachycardia, as each 1°C increase can result in an increase in heart rate of 10%; however, the heart rate and respiratory rate should become normal for age when fever is controlled with antipyretic therapy or falls spontaneously.[27] Heart rate >150 beats/minute in children and >160 beats/minute in infants, and respiratory rates >50 breaths/minute in children and >60 breaths/minute in infants are associated with increased mortality risk and commonly presage the development of septic shock.[6] A minimum mean arterial pressure of >30 mmHg is considered absolutely the lowest tolerable blood pressure in the extremely premature infant.[11,32] Specific hemodynamic abnormalities at the time of coming to medical attention have been associated with increasing mortality: eucardia (1%), tachycardia/bradycardia (3%), hypotension with capillary refill <3 seconds (5%), normotension with capillary refill >3 seconds (7%), hypotension with capillary refill >3 seconds (33%).[11]

Laboratory Findings

Numerous biologic markers of sepsis in children have been studied; however, none has independent high positive or negative predictive value for decision making in clinical practice based on evidence of prospective clinical trials.[27,33] Biomarkers that are commonly used clinically include: the total peripheral white blood cell (WBC) count,[34,35] platelet count, erythrocyte sedimentation rate (ESR), base excess/base deficit, lactate,[36,37] procalcitonin (PCT),[38-41] C-reactive protein (CRP),[42-45] and interleukin-6 (IL-6).[41,46,47] Many tests and biologic markers currently under study and development are promising and include specific rapid antigen assays,[48] polymerase chain reaction tests,[49-51] genomic testing (for guiding therapy and determining host response),[52,53] and proteomic testing (for identification of differentially expressed proteins and peptides).[54-58] Use of combinations of tests may improve independent predictive values.[59]

MANAGEMENT

Antimicrobial Therapy

Empiric antimicrobial therapy for severe sepsis should be administered urgently, targeting likely causative pathogens (Table 11-2). Important considerations when selecting a regimen include: the

TABLE 11-2. Suggested Initial Antimicrobial Choices for Empiric Therapy in Infants and Children with Suspected Sepsis[a]

Age or Clinical Situation	Antimicrobial Agent(s)
Neonate (community-onset)	Ampicillin + gentamicin
Neonate (hospital-onset)	Vancomycin + gentamicin or cefotaxime[b]
Child (community-onset)	Cefotaxime or ceftriaxone + vancomycin
Child (hospital-onset)	Vancomycin + anti-pseudomonal penicillin or ceftazidime or carbapenem[b]
Skin or soft-tissue involvement	Vancomycin or semi-synthetic penicillin + clindamycin
Toxic shock syndrome	Vancomycin or semi-synthetic penicillin + clindamycin
Neonatal HSV[c]	Acyclovir
Rocky Mountain spotted fever Ehrlichiosis	Doxycycline

[a]Antimicrobials should be modified as laboratory data is available and based on clinical course.

[b]Antimicrobial should be based on patient-specific risk factors and local antimicrobial susceptibility trends (see text).

[c]HSV, herpes simplex virus.

child's age, community versus hospital acquisition, host immune status, and penetration into affected or at-risk tissues and compartments (such as central nervous system). In U.S. cities, as many as 76% of invasive, community-associated *S. aureus* isolates can be methicillin resistant.[60] Vancomycin should be included in the empiric regimen if *S. aureus* is suspected. Once the causative organism is isolated and antibiotic susceptibilities are available, antimicrobial therapy is adjusted appropriately. When possible, broad-spectrum agents (such as vancomycin, third-generation cephalosporins and carbapenems) should be discontinued to minimize the emergence of multidrug-resistant organisms in the patient and spread in the patient's environment. If *Escherichia coli* or *Klebsiella* spp. (or other gram-negative bacilli in certain hospital settings) are isolated, the organism is tested for extended-spectrum β-lactamase (ESBL) production. Carbapenems are the treatment of choice for serious infections with ESBL-producing organisms.[61]

Supportive Care

Effective treatment of sepsis and septic shock is dependent on prompt recognition and initiation of supportive as well as specific therapy. The basic principles of initial critical care include ensuring adequate circulation, airway patency, and gas exchange. The interventions required to achieve these goals depend on the specific physiologic state of the patient at the time of presentation. Shock that occurs during sepsis results from decreased intravascular volume, maldistribution of intravascular volume, and/or impaired myocardial function, all of which can occur at different times during the course of septic shock.[62] Children with sepsis who receive early aggressive fluid resuscitation (>40 mL/kg in the first hour with isotonic intravenous fluids) demonstrate improved survival without increased risk of noncardiogenic pulmonary edema or ARDS.[63,64]

Determination of when, what type, and how much pharmacologic support is needed in a patient with septic shock requires careful consideration of many factors. These factors include the patient's clinical state (e.g., capillary refill time, urine output, peripheral versus core temperature gradient), information obtained from monitoring devices (heart rate, blood pressure, central venous pressure, pulmonary artery pressure, cardiac output, stroke volume, and systemic vascular resistance), and knowledge of basic drug effects (including dopamine, norepinephrine, epinephrine, and phenylephrine) in the setting of septic shock.

Septic shock causes multisystem organ dysfunction, and it is important to evaluate and treat abnormalities in other organ systems, including the kidney and gastrointestinal tract. Patients with acute renal failure may require renal replacement therapy. The gastrointestinal tract is vulnerable to disturbances such as hemorrhage, ileus, brush border atrophy, and translocation of enteric organisms into the blood. Additionally, early institution of nutritional support, particularly enteral feeding, may ameliorate gastrointestinal atrophy, bacterial translocation, and improve multiorgan function.[65]

Maintaining tight control of serum glucose has been shown to be beneficial in some studies in critically ill adult patients and is currently being evaluated in children.[66]

Endotoxin Physiology and Antiendotoxin Therapy

Endotoxin is one of the most important bacterial components contributing to the inflammatory process. Levels of endotoxin correlate directly with severity of meningococcal disease and other forms of sepsis, and with elaboration and release of inflammatory mediators. Endotoxin upregulates TNF-α, IL-1 and IL-6, complement and coagulation pathways. Endotoxin also can be found in the presence of critical illness, not related to gram-negative sepsis,[67,68] where its presence appears to be related to severity of disease and outcome. It is postulated that the presence of endotoxin in the blood in these circumstances is related to altered gut permeability.

The assumption that the inflammatory process is related to the presence of endotoxin in the bloodstream is based on the finding that the pathophysiology of gram-negative sepsis can be reproduced by administration of purified endotoxin or a variety of endotoxin-free inflammatory mediators, which are upregulated by endotoxin.

A variety of antiendotoxin strategies have been proposed in the management of severe sepsis, including agents that bind to and neutralize endotoxin, enhance endotoxin clearance, or inhibit the interaction of endotoxin with its receptors (see Table 11-3).

Cytokine Physiology and Anticytokine Therapy

Cytokines have a central role in the pathogenesis of bacterial infection and sepsis. Cytokines coordinate a wide variety of inflammatory reactions at the tissue level. The cytokine network can be divided roughly into a proinflammatory arm and an anti-inflammatory arm. Prominent proinflammatory cytokines are TNF-α and IL-1. Anti-inflammatory cytokines, of which IL-10 is a well-studied example, inhibit the synthesis of proinflammatory cytokines and exert several direct anti-inflammatory effects on different cell types. The action of proinflammatory cytokines can be further inhibited by naturally occurring soluble inhibitors, such as soluble TNF receptors type I and type II which inhibit TNF activity, soluble IL-1 receptor type II, and IL-1ra, which both inhibit IL-1 activity.

The plasma concentrations of cytokines are rapidly dynamic and vary greatly in patients with sepsis. Some patients who fulfill the clinical criteria for SIRS may not have detectable levels of proinflammatory cytokines in their circulation because they are studied late in the septic process.[69] This may explain why the cytokines TNF-α, IL-1β, IL-12, and IFN-β, which according to animal models play a central role in the pathogenesis of septic shock, are not consistently correlated with disease severity or outcome in patients with septic shock.

Infection models that use an initially localized source of infection such as pneumonia and peritonitis have suggested that proinflammatory cytokines have a crucial role in host defense against bacterial infection. Neutralization of endogenous TNF-α during murine pneumonia caused by either gram-positive or gram-negative bacteria resulted in an accelerated course of the infection, and was associated with greater outgrowth of bacteria in the lungs, and decreased survival.[70] Conversely, the elimination of IL-10 improved survival of murine pneumonia and reduced the bacterial load within the pulmonary compartment.[71] Evidence for anticytokine therapies is summarized in Table 11-3.

Immunoparalysis

Induction of anti-inflammatory pathways to inhibit excessive proinflammatory activity can be demonstrated in most patients with sepsis. This has led to the concept of "compensatory anti-inflammatory response," following SIRS in time course.[72] In addition, shortly after the onset of a septic event, a refractory state develops that is characterized by a relative inability of host inflammatory cells to respond to usual proinflammatory stimuli (such as endotoxin challenge).[73] The diminished responsiveness involves monocytes, granulocytes, and lymphocytes. Although the mechanisms that underlie immunoparalysis have not been explained completely, it is conceivable that anti-inflammatory cytokines, particularly IL-10 and transforming growth factor-β (TGF-β) are involved.

It has been proposed that immunoparalysis could contribute to the increased susceptibility to nosocomial infection and late mortality of patients who survive the acute sepsis. As a result, strategies aiming to restore immune function have been developed and evaluated partially in patients with sepsis. Cytokines are able to reverse monocyte deactivation in vitro and in animals; IFN-γ and granulocyte-macrophage colony-stimulating factor (GM-CSF) have been studied with the results summarized in Table 11-3.[74-76]

Arachidonic Acid Metabolism and Inhibitor Therapy

Products of the cyclooxygenase (COX) and lipooxygenase pathways of arachidonic acid metabolism include leukotrienes, prostaglandins, and thromboxane. These products appear to play a major role in diminishing systemic vascular resistance and causing platelet aggregation, membrane lysis, and increased capillary permeability, which are the hallmarks of SIRS and shock. Drugs that interfere with these pathways have been tested as treatments for sepsis and are summarized in Table 11-3.

Immune Globulin Intravenous (IGIV) Therapy

Immune globulin intravenous (IGIV), like IFN-γ and GM-CSF, can be regarded as a treatment method aimed to improve host defense. Although plasma immune globulin concentration may be reduced in patients with sepsis, the use of IGIV therapy is not supported by randomized clinical trials. Indeed, no individual well-designed trial has been undertaken in adults with sepsis. A small non-blinded study in 21 patients with streptococcal toxic shock syndrome showed a reduced mortality (6% versus 34%, P = 0.02), suggesting possible benefit in pyrogenic exotoxin-mediated shock.[77] Results of the International Neonatal Immunotherapy Study (INIS trial), which enrolled 3493 infants, are expected to be published in the near future.[78]

Corticosteroids

Since the 1960s, investigators have attempted to modulate the inflammatory response to sepsis with corticosteroids, given at doses much higher than normal physiologic concentrations. These studies failed to show a beneficial effect of glucocorticoids in patients with sepsis.[79,80] However, more recent investigations indicate that glucocorticoids in much lower doses (supposedly inducing less immunosuppressive effects) could be of benefit to patients with septic shock.

Adrenal failure is common in critical illness, particularly in vasopressor-dependent septic shock. High baseline total serum cortisol together with a low response to a corticotropin stimulation test is correlated with a poor outcome in sepsis.[81] Several studies in children and adults with septic shock have demonstrated abnormalities of control of adrenal corticosteroid secretion over the course of illness.[82,83]

Various randomized controlled trials comparing hydrocortisone to placebo have been performed in septic shock. There is general

TABLE 11-3. Evidence for Potential Therapies for Severe Sepsis and Shock

Agent	Mechanism of Action	Studies
ANTIENDOTOXIN THERAPIES		
E5	Murine monoclonal antibody against core elements of endotoxin	915 adults with confirmed gram-negative sepsis in a multicenter placebo-controlled trial; no statistical difference in mortality[96]
HA-1A	Humanized monoclonal antibody against lipid A moiety of endotoxin	621 adults with presumed gram-negative bacillary shock in placebo-controlled trial; significantly higher mortality in those treated[97,98]
		269 children with meningococcal septicemia in a placebo-controlled trial; reduced mortality by 33% (nonsignificant)[99]
rBPI21	Bactericidal-permeability inducing factor (neutrophil granule protein that can neutralize endotoxin)	393 children with meningococcal septicemia in placebo-controlled trial; no statistical difference in mortality; fewer treated patients required multiple amputations (3.2% vs. 7.4%)[100]
Statin therapy[101]	Elevates HDL levels (HDL binds to and neutralizes endotoxin); modifies T-lymphocyte activity; enhances expression of endothelial nitric oxide; modulates inflammatory cell signaling and release of cytokines; has antioxidant effects	69,168 Canadian adults in matched cohort study; reduced incidence of sepsis in treated overall and in high-risk groups, i.e., those receiving corticosteroids, patients with diabetes mellitus and malignancy[102]
Plasmapheresis or exchange transfusion	Removes endotoxin and other inflammatory mediators	Anecdotal reports of good outcomes[103–110]
Polymyxin B hemoperfusion	Binds and neutralizes endotoxin	64 adults with intra-abdominal infection in randomized 2-session hemoperfusion vs. conventional therapy; reduced vasopressor requirements and reduced 28-day mortality (32% vs. 53%)[111]
ANTICYTOKINE THERAPIES		
Monoclonal antibody against TNF-α	Removes TNF-α	Pooled data from clinical trials; reduced mortality 3.5%[112]
Soluble TNF-α receptor constructs	Mops up TNF-α	Most studies failed to demonstrate an effect. One adult placebo-controlled trial showed increased mortality in patients receiving high-dose dimeric type II TNF-α receptors[113]
Afelimomab	F(ab') 2 fragment of murine monoclonal antibody binds to TNF-α	Adults with severe infection and high IL-6 levels in multicenter trial; relative risk of death reduced 11.9% and more rapid improvement in organ dysfunction scores[114]
Recombinant IL-1ra	Inhibits IL-1 activity	Administered in continuous infusion; no reduction in mortality[115,116]
ARACHIDONIC ACID METABOLISM THERAPIES		
Ibuprofen	Inhibits cyclooxygenase pathway	455 adults with sepsis in randomized study; reduced prostaglandin I₂, thromboxane levels, and lactic acidosis; no reduction in acute respiratory distress syndrome or mortality[117]
		Adults with sepsis and hypothermia; reduced 30-day mortality[118]
Pentoxifylline	Inhibits phosphodiestaerase resulting in suppression of TNF-α, IL-1, and IL-10; prevents endothelial cell dysfunction; stimulates release of tissue plasminogen activator; attenuates thromboxane release	51 adults; improved scores of organ dysfunction[119]
		Neonatal studies; reduced all-cause mortality[120,121]
ANTICOAGULANT THERAPIES		
Recombinant tissue factor pathway inhibitor (TFPI)	Inhibits factor Xa and possibly exerts other effects on inflammatory mediators distinct from its effect on coagulation	Improved outcome in septic animals[122]
		Adult phase II study; trend toward reduced mortality and no increase in adverse effects[123]
		1754 adults with severe sepsis in phase III multicenter study, no effect on 28-day mortality; possible benefit in subset with severe community-acquired pneumonia[124]
		2100 adults with severe community-acquired pneumonia in a prospective randomized study (CAPTIVATE) to assess 28-day mortality; results pending
Antithrombin	Inhibits thrombin, factors IXa and Xa; binds to endothelial cells modulating the inflammatory response	Continuous infusion in adults with sepsis; reduced IL-6 levels and diminished CRP[125]
		2314 adults with severe sepsis in randomized trial; absolute reduction in 90-day mortality of 7.6%; difference was negated in those receiving concomitant heparin for prophylaxis of deep vein thrombosis[126]
Activated protein C (aPC)	Inactivates factors Va and VIIIa	1690 adults with severe sepsis in multicenter trial; reduced 28-day mortality[127]
		477 children with severe sepsis in a randomized, placebo-controlled trial; halted early for failure to demonstrate benefit in any endpoints and appearance of increased risk of hemorrhagic complications in children <60 days of age[128]

Continued

PART II Clinical Syndromes and Cardinal Features of Infectious Diseases: Approach to Diagnosis and Initial Management

SECTION A Septicemia, Toxin- and Inflammation-Mediated Syndromes

TABLE 11-3. Evidence for Potential Therapies for Severe Sepsis and Shock—cont'd

Agent	Mechanism of Action	Studies
Tissue plasminogen activator (tPA)	Inhibits intravascular thrombosis by catalyzing conversion of plasminogen to plasmin	Rescue therapy in children with meningococcal septicemia; unacceptable level of adverse events, including fatal intracranial haemorrhage[129]
THERAPIES TARGETING THE ENDOTHELIUM		
BB-882	Antagonizes platelet-activating factor (PAF activates endothelial cells and amplifies the release of inflammatory mediators)	100 adults with severe infection; no reduction in mortality and no improvement in hemodynamic or respiratory scores[130]
TCV-309	Antagonizes PAF	98 adults; reduced organ dysfunction; no effect on mortality[131]
BN52021	Antagonizes PAF	609 adults with severe sepsis; statistically insignificant reduction in mortality[132]
Platelet-activating factor acetyl-hydrolase (PAF-AH)	A secreted plasma protein that inactivates PAF and other oxidized phospholipids	127 adults with severe sepsis; reduced all-cause mortality[133] 1261 adults with severe sepsis in a multicenter, international trial; halted early for failure to demonstrate improved 28-day mortality or secondary endpoints[134]

agreement that hydrocortisone supplementation improves the hemodynamic condition of vasopressor-dependent septic shock.[84] What remains more controversial is the definition of adrenal insufficiency, the optimal dose and timing of corticosteroid supplementation, whether this should then be tapered slowly, and the impact of corticosteroid supplementation on outcome. A multicenter, randomized, placebo-controlled trial of 499 patients with septic shock[85] found that hydrocortisone did not improve overall survival or in the subgroup of patients who did not have a response to corticotropin, although shock was reversed more quickly in the hydrocortisone-treated group than in the placebo group.

Although no study has evaluated the efficacy of corticosteroids in children with sepsis, several well-designed trials conducted in children with bacterial meningitis, most of whom had bacteremia when enrolled, have shown that early administration of dexamethasone was associated with significant reduction in hemodynamic instability in the 6 hours after initiation of antibiotic therapy.[86]

Anticoagulant Therapies

Virtually all patients with sepsis have coagulation abnormalities. These abnormalities can vary from subclinical alterations in clotting times, to full-blown disseminated intravascular coagulation (DIC). Because of the recognized interactions between inflammation and coagulation, manipulation of the coagulation cascade would appear to be an attractive target for new therapies (see Table 11-3).

Therapies Targeting the Endothelium

Endothelial dysfunction appears to be pivotal as the primary pathologic feature of severe sepsis. Restoration of endothelial function by interventions to reduce endothelial cell injury and dysfunction are being developed (see Table 11-3).

Nitric Oxide Balance

Activation of the inflammatory response results in elaboration of a number of mediators with direct effects on vasomotor tone. Nitric oxide (NO), bradykinin, histamine, and prostaglandin I_2 (PGI_2) can all decrease vascular tone and cause hypotension. NO is a highly diffusible compound that activates soluble guanylate cyclase in smooth-muscle cells. This converts guanosine triphosphate (GTP) to cyclic guanosine monophosphate (cGMP), which relaxes the smooth-muscle cell via a protein kinase, by promoting calcium entry into the sarcoplasmic reticulum.[87]

The inflammatory response in sepsis, including increased NO production, can result in endothelial cell dysfunction affecting vascular smooth muscle. The resulting effects on organ perfusion may be instrumental in the pathogenesis of the multiple organ dysfunction syndrome seen in septic shock, which is associated with increased morbidity and mortality. The implication of NO in the vascular hyporesponsiveness and cardiac depression of sepsis supports the hypothesis that blockage or reduction of NO production may produce clinical benefit in patients with sepsis (see Table 11-3).

However, there are many animal models of sepsis in which various inhibitors of NO production have demonstrated potentially harmful effects as well as potential benefit. It has become clear, however, that nonspecific NO inhibitors cause detrimental effects secondary to reduced organ perfusion, elevation of pulmonary artery pressures, and increased renal vascular resistance[88,89] as well as increased capillary permeability, increased lactic acidosis, and hepatic toxicity.[90] This is likely to be due to inhibition of baseline NO production which is essential for control of organ perfusion under normal circumstances.

Innate Immune Responses and Toll-Like Receptors (TLRs)

The most exciting new development in sepsis research in the past years is the discovery of TLRs as signal-transducing elements of multiple antigens and the rapidly unfolding picture of TLRs as essential in the innate immune response to infection.[91]

Upon first encounter with a microorganism, the innate immune system can distinguish between different classes of pathogenic bacteria, viruses, and fungi. The innate immune system can recognize conserved motifs on pathogens that are not seen on higher eukaryotes. These motifs have been referred to as "pathogen-associated molecular patterns" or PAMPs, whereas their binding partners on immunocompetent cells have been termed "pattern recognition receptors."

Endotoxin, for example, interacts with cells via the pattern recognition receptor CD14. Spontaneous binding of endotoxin to CD14 occurs at very slow rates. Lipopolysaccharide (LPS) CD14-binding is greatly accelerated in the presence of an acute-phase reactant mainly derived from the liver, lipopolysaccharide-binding protein (LBP). CD14 does not have an intracellular domain; cells respond to endotoxin via signaling through TLR4, which requires the presence of a secreted protein, MD-2. TLR2 in turn is essential for signaling the proinflammatory effects of the bacterial lipoproteins, peptidoglycan and zymosan, whereas TLR5 mediates cellular effects induced by bacterial flagellin, and TLR9 mediates effects induced by unmethylated CpG-containing oligonucleotides present in bacterial (but not eukaryotic) DNA. Different members of the TLR family can act together in activating cells in response to pathogens; e.g., TLR2 and TLR6 cooperate in detecting certain bacterial components, including peptidoglycan.[92] The in vivo relevance of induction of an effective innate immune response to infection has been shown with specific-TLR-deficient mice. TLR2 knockout mice are highly susceptible to infection due to gram-positive organisms, whereas TLR4 knockout mice have reduced resistance to gram-negative infection.[93]

Designing methods to neutralize microbial products or block their interaction with specific receptor on immune cells is an attractive concept. Monoclonal antibodies (IC14) against CD14 have been evaluated in phase I studies.[94,95] IC14 was shown to attenuate LPS-induced clinical symptoms and strongly inhibited LPS-induced proinflammatory cytokine release, while delaying the release of the anti-inflammatory cytokines. The results suggest that CD14 blockade with IC14 warrants further clinical investigation to determine its ability to attenuate the proinflammatory response due to infection.

FUTURE CONSIDERATIONS

The publication of the human genome will lead to advances in genomics and proteomics in the coming decade. The possibilities for individualized drug treatment of patients with sepsis, related to their genotype, may become reality. New technology may allow bedside testing of patients' genotypes or determination of protein or peptide biomarkers associated with poor outcome, to allow targeted therapy of even the sickest patients.

It is probable that many new agents will be developed based on the unraveling of the host–pathogen interaction. However, until this time we must utilize currently available therapies to the best of our knowledge. Despite huge advances, treatment of sepsis is still dependent upon administration of appropriate antibiotics, intravenous fluid support, and relatively crude methods of organ support. We can only improve upon current treatment of pediatric sepsis *after* there is agreement that properly conducted multicenter clinical trials can and must be carried out in critically ill children in order to test new therapies. To reach this goal, we should model pediatric sepsis trials after the successful clinical trial programs such as those that have so greatly improved survival from childhood cancer.

There have only been three large properly controlled phase III studies in children with sepsis, none of which has recruited adequate numbers to definitively determine efficacy. Although these and all the many adult studies except one have failed to demonstrate a significant survival advantage, there is much that can be learned from these unsuccessful studies that is relevant to the design of future sepsis trials. Children with severe sepsis and shock should be enrolled in double-blind, placebo-controlled studies to evaluate new treatments. These studies should be large enough to minimize random error and avoid type II error. Definitions for the target population should be explicit, reproducible, and include illness severity scores. Protocols for both the use of the investigational agent and conventional treatment should be standardized. Outcomes should be clinically relevant and predefined, and should include measures of both benefit and harm. In addition, the analysis of results should be carried out, both on evaluable patients and on the intent-to-treat population. Finally, a health economic evaluation of the implications of the introduction of ever-increasingly expensive therapies should be mandatory. Only in this way will we be likely to influence the unacceptably high mortality rate of severe sepsis in children, with the added advantage of limiting the widespread use of extremely expensive new therapies that have been insufficiently evaluated.

12 Hemophagocytic Lymphohistiocytosis and Macrophage Activation Syndrome

Hayley A. Gans and David B. Lewis

HEMOPHAGOCYTIC LYMPHOHISTIOCYTOSIS

Hemophagocytic lymphohistiocytosis (HLH) is characterized by the accumulation of activated T lymphocytes and well-differentiated macrophages (histiocytes) in the bone marrow, lymph nodes, liver, spleen, and, often, the central nervous system (CNS). HLH is typified by fever, hepatosplenomagaly, peripheral blood cytopenias, and, most characteristically, hemophagocytosis, i.e., the presence of intact red blood cells, leukocytes, platelets, or their precursors within infiltrating macrophages of the liver, spleen, bone marrow, and the CNS.[1,2] Most cases of HLH appear to be due to lymphocyte hyperactivation, particularly CD8+ T lymphocytes,[3] with cytokine hypersecretion resulting in systemic mononuclear phagocyte activation, inflammation, coagulopathy, and, potentially, multiorgan failure.

HLH is divided into primary and secondary forms.[4] In the primary form, HLH is the predominant presenting feature of a small group of genetic disorders, including familial hemophagocytic lymphohistiocytosis (FHL).[3] Systemic infections are a precipitant of the hemophagocytic syndrome in many, but not all primary cases.[1,5] Secondary HLH encompasses all other causes and also most often is triggered by systemic infections, especially in immunocompromised hosts,[6–8] or by untreated hematologic malignancies.[4] The macrophage activation syndrome (MAS), which occurs in rheumatologic autoinflammatory/autoimmune disorders, has some pathologic similarities to HLH,[9] but is treated differently and discussed at the end of this chapter.

ETIOLOGY AND INCIDENCE

Primary HLH

Classic FHL, which was first reported in 1952,[10] accounts for approximately 25% of all HLH cases worldwide. FHL is estimated to affect 1 in 50,000 live births in northern Europe,[1] and likely occurs at a higher frequency in countries in which consanguinity is common.[11] There are four genetically defined autosomal recessive (AR) causes of FHL[3,12] due to mutations in the genes (indicated in italics) encoding perforin (*PRF1*; FHL2), Munc13-4 (*UNC13D*; FHL3), syntaxin 11 (*STX11*; FHL4), and syntaxin-binding protein 2 (*STXB2*; FHL5) (Table 12-1), all of which play critical roles in cell-mediated cytotoxicity. The AR genetic defect for FHL1 is unknown.[12] In FHL, HLH typically is fulminant and develops in the first few months of life or even in utero.[13] HLH rarely can be manifest first in adulthood, especially in cases where hypomorphic FHL mutations preserve some protein function.[12] In addition to HLH, FHL5 can manifest with hypogammaglobulinemia, bleeding, or colitis.[14]

X-linked lymphoproliferative (XLP) disease (SAP/*SH2D1A* deficiency) only affects males and usually presents in association

PART II Clinical Syndromes and Cardinal Features of Infectious Diseases: Approach to Diagnosis and Initial Management

SECTION A Septicemia, Toxin- and Inflammation-Mediated Syndromes

TABLE 12-1. Classification of Pediatric Hemophagocytic Lymphohistiocytosis

Primary HLH		
Familial HLH	**Chromosome**	**Protein/Gene**
FHL1	9q21.3-22	Unknown
FHL2	10q22	Perforin IPRF1
FHL3	17q25.1	MUNC13-4/UNC13D
FHL4	6q24	Syntaxin-11/STX11
FHL5	19p13.3-p13.2	MUNC18-2/STXBP2
IMMUNODEFICIENCY DISEASE		
CHS-1	1q42.1-q42.2	LYST
XLP disease	Xq25	SAP/SH2D1A
XFLH disease	Xq25	XIAP/BIRC4
GS type 2	15q21	RAB27A

Secondary HLH	
Infections	**Frequent Inciting Agents**
Viral	Adenovirus, enteroviruses, herpesviruses (EBV, CMV, HSV, HHV-6, HHV-8, VZV), HIV (including acute infection), influenza (including H5N1), measles, parvovirus B19
Bacterial	*Mycobacterium tuberculosis, Brucella, Coxiella,* rickettsioses, gram-negative or gram-positive bacteremia
Parasitic	*Plasmodium* spp., *Leishmania* spp.
Fungal	*Histoplasma capsulatum, Penicillium* sp., *Fusarium* sp.

Non-infectious Categories	
Therapy	HAART, phenytoin, other anticonvulsants, BMT, solid organ transplant, chemotherapy
Oncologic (as presenting feature)	Lymphomas, pre-B-cell ALL
Rheumatologic	JIA, SLE, Kawasaki disease

ALL, acute lymphoblastic leukemia; BMT, bone marrow transplantation; CHS, Chédiak–Higashi syndrome; CMV, cytomegalovirus; EBV, Epstein–Barr virus; EEE, eastern equine encephalitis virus; FHL, familial hemophagocytic lymphohistiocytosis; GS, Griscelli syndrome; HAART, highly active antiretroviral therapy; HIV, human immunodeficiency virus; HHV-6, human herpesvirus 6; HHV-8, human herpesvirus 8; HLH, hemophagocytic lymphohistiocytosis; HSV, herpes simplex virus; JIA, juvenile idiopathic arthritis; SLE, systemic lupus erythematosus; XLH, X-linked hemophagocytic syndrome; XLP, X-linked lymphoproliferative syndrome; VZV, varicella-zoster virus.

Adapted from Janka G, Zur Stadt U. Familial and acquired hemophagocytic lymphohistiocytosis. Hematol (Am Soc Hematol Educ Program) 2005;82–88; and Janka G, Imashuku S, Elinder G, et al. Infection- and malignancy-associated hemophagocytic syndromes. Secondary hemophagocytic lymphohistiocytosis. Hematol Oncol Clin North Am 1998;12:435–444.

with primary Epstein–Barr virus (EBV) infection, with about 60% of cases developing fulminant HLH.[15] In contrast to FHL, hypogammaglobulinemia, often prior to EBV infection,[15] is frequent, as is the rapid development of EBV-related lymphoproliferative disease and/or lymphomas.

X-linked familial hemophagocytic lymphohistiocytosis (XFHL) disease (XIAP/BIRC4 deficiency),[16,17] only affects males and can present similarly to FHL. XFHL also can have a more delayed, mild, and/or recurrent course, with recovery without cytotoxic chemotherapy.[17] In contrast to XLP disease, EBV-related lymphoproliferative disease or lymphoma is infrequent, and it is not clear whether hypogammaglobulinemia frequently occurs prior to the onset of HLH.[16,17]

Griscelli syndrome (GS) type II (AR *RAB27A* gene deficiency) typically manifests as early-onset HLH in manner indistinguishable from FHL.[18] Melanosome transport also is defective, resulting in partial albinism and the hair having a characteristic silvery sheen.[3]

In Chediak–Higashi syndrome (CHS) (AR *LYST* gene deficiency), HLH frequently develops during infancy or childhood.[19] CHS is readily distinguished from other forms of primary HLH by oculocutaneous albinism, dysfunctional neutrophils with giant inclusions, and platelet dysfunction.[20]

Secondary HLH

Secondary HLH most often is triggered by severe and/or prolonged infections in immunocompromised patients (see Table 12-1), particularly those with severe acquired immunodeficiencies,[21] e.g., due to human immunodeficiency virus (HIV) infection/AIDS,[22] cancer chemotherapy[23] or potent immunosuppression. Secondary HLH also can be a complication of severe infection in patients with primary immunodeficiencies other than those that are causes of primary HLH, including chronic granulomatous disease,[24,25] severe combined immunodeficiency (SCID),[26,27] DiGeorge syndrome (22q11.2 deletion),[28] Wiskott–Aldrich syndrome,[29] and X-linked agammaglobulinemia.[30] Although secondary HLH originally was considered to be mainly a complication of primary EBV infection in previously healthy older children, HLH can occur in all ages in association with severe infections with a wide variety of pathogens (see Table 12-1).[7,8,31] Common non-EBV viral triggers include infections with other herpesviruses (e.g., cytomegalovirus (CMV), HHV-6, HHV-8), adenovirus, dengue, enterovirus, influenza A,[32] and parvovirus B19. There are case reports of many other types of viral infection that also have been associated with HLH, suggesting that HLH potentially can complicate any severe systemic viral infection. Severe bacterial infections, particularly those involving the reticuloendothelial system, e.g., typhoid fever, rickettsial diseases, brucellosis, and disseminated *Mycobacterium tuberculosis*,[8] are frequent precipitants of HLH, and systemic fungal infections, e.g., *Histoplasma* and *Penicillium* infection, are recognized causes. Visceral leishmaniasis, which has been misdiagnosed as FHL,[33] and malaria are frequent protozoal triggers.[8]

Rarer non-infectious conditions associated with secondary HLH in children (see Table 12-1) include lymphoid malignancies,[34,35] highly active antiretroviral therapy for HIV, anti-epileptic drug therapy, acute allograft rejection, graft-versus-host disease (GvHD), including by maternal T lymphocyte engraftment in infants with severe combined immunodeficiency,[27] hemolytic anemia, and certain inherited metabolic disorders, e.g., lysinuric protein intolerance.

PATHOGENESIS

In primary HLH, most of the identified genetic defects compromise the ability of T lymphocytes and natural killer (NK) cells to kill target cells by the secretion of perforin and granzymes from intracellular cytotoxic granules. Antigenically naïve CD8+ T lymphocytes acquire their cytotoxic granules after activation and differentiation into effector cells, whereas newly produced NK cells emerge from the bone marrow containing these granules. Cytotoxic granules are released by CD8+ T lymphocytes after their surface αβ-T-cell receptors are engaged by antigenic peptide/MHC complexes on the infected target cell, whereas NK-cell granule release occurs when the NK cells encounters infected target cells that lack MHC class I expression. Cell-mediated cytotoxicity requires the concerted activity of the LYST, Rab27a, MUNC13-4, syntaxin 11, and MUNC18-2 proteins for the intracellular maturation, trafficking, pre-release priming, and exocytosis of cytotoxic granules; genetic mutations encoding these proteins result in CHS, GS type II, FHL3, FHL4, and FHL5, respectively.[3] The release of perforin, which is defective in FHL2, perforates the target cell membrane, allowing the cytoplasmic entry of granzymes that trigger target cell apoptosis.[3] It is not yet known how XIAP deficiency promotes HLH.

Activated CD8[+] T lymphocytes and NK cells also release large amounts of interferon-gamma (IFN-γ) and tumor necrosis factor-alpha (TNF-α), which potently activate macrophages and dendritic cells. A plausible scenario for primary HLH occurring in association with viral infection is that T cells and NK cells are activated by severe infection to secrete cytotoxins and cytokines, but that cytotoxicity is ineffective in killing and eliminating the viral antigenic stimulus. This results in prolonged and persistent lymphocyte activation and cytokine secretion which, in turn, persistently activates macrophages and dendritic cells leading them to become hemophagocytic[4,21,36] and to secrete additional proinflammatory cytokines. This combined lymphocyte and mononuclear phagocyte "cytokine storm" appears to be a common final pathway for HLH pathogenesis,[4,37] accounting for fever, hyperlipidemia, endothelial activation, coagulopathy, tissue infiltration of T cells and macrophages, CNS vasculitis and demyelination, marrow hyperplasia or aplasia, and multiorgan dysfunction and failure. In XLP disease, SAP deficiency selectively impairs recognition and killing of EBV-infected B lymphocytes by CD8[+] T lymphocytes and NK cells,[38,39] resulting in a high EBV viral load; other forms of activation and cytokine secretion by CD8 T cells and NK cells are intact and driven by the persistent viral load. However, cases of HLH can occur in FHL without apparent associated infections, and these observations, along with animal model studies suggest that perforin-dependent cell-mediated cytotoxicity, in addition to its antimicrobial role, also directly regulates lymphocyte activation and homeostasis.[3]

Secondary HLH most commonly occurs when overwhelming infection in an immunocompromised host triggers marked and/or prolonged T-lymphocyte and NK-cell activation and hypercytokinemia. Lymphocyte and mononuclear phagocyte-derived hypercytokinemia also is likely the cause of HLH in untreated leukemia/lymphoma, GvHD, or HLH following chemotherapy.

More enigmatic is the basis for HLH and hypercytokinemia following primary EBV infection (EBV-HLH) in previously healthy children, as only a minority of cases are accounted for by primary HLH genetic disorders.[40] In EBV-HLH and EBV infection complicating primary HLH there often are high levels of EBV genomes in circulating T lymphocytes,[41,42] but the importance of this T-lymphocyte tropism by EBV for HLH pathogenesis remains unclear.

CLINICAL AND RADIOLOGIC FEATURES

Primary and secondary HLH cannot be distinguished reliably on the basis of clinical, laboratory, or histopathologic features. Prolonged high fever, hepatosplenomegaly, and cytopenias generally are hallmarks of HLH. Rash, lymphadenopathy, respiratory tract and gastrointestinal symptoms, failure to thrive, and irritability are frequent (Table 12-2).[43] Clinical and laboratory abnormalities often peak at days 6 to 10 of illness, although there is substantial variability.[43]

Systemic Manifestations

Fever, often prolonged, is present in all patients. HLH is an important diagnostic consideration in fever of unknown origin.[43] Organomegaly, often pronounced and progressive, is found in more than 90% of cases. A diffuse erythematous maculopapular or petechial rash may transiently appear with high fevers.[43] Respiratory tract symptoms are frequent and can vary from mild cough to acute respiratory distress syndrome requiring ventilatory support.[43] Cardiovascular collapse and renal failure can occur.[43] Lymphadenopathy, often prominent, is frequent (50% to 70% of patients).[43] Gastrointestinal symptoms, including vomiting, diarrhea, and abdominal pain, occur in about 40% of patients.

CNS Manifestations

The majority of HLH patients have neurologic symptoms and/or cerebrospinal fluid (CSF) abnormalities (mononuclear pleocytosis and/or elevated protein) at the time of diagnosis.[48] Rarely, hemophagocytosis of white blood cells of the CSF can be observed,[2] a finding that is specific for HLH. Neurologic symptoms can be the presenting feature, precede clinical HLH by 2 or more years,[49] or can develop only later in the course.[2] Seizures, meningismus, and irritability are present commonly.[50] Cranial nerve palsies, ataxia, nystagmus, disturbances of gait and vision, hemiplegia or tetraplegia, delayed psychomotor development, and increased intracranial pressure have been reported. Frequent findings on magnetic resonance imaging or computed tomography include multiple nodular or ring-enhancing parenchymal lesions in the cerebrum and cerebellum, leptomeningeal enhancement, confluent parenchymal lesions with or without hemorrhage, and ventriculomegaly, which can be due to cerebral atrophy or hydrocephalus.[48,51] Demyelination can occur and mimic acute disseminated encephaloymyelitis.[52] Definitive diagnosis of CNS disease may require biopsy of the meninges and white matter.[53]

HLH in the Fetus and Neonate

HLH manifesting with liver failure[54,55] is more common in the fetus and neonate than in older children. Nonimmune hydrops fetalis[54,56] can be a presentation of HLH due to either FLH[13] or congenital infections, such as syphilis or rubella. Neonates and young infants with severe herpesvirus (HSV, CMV, or HHV-8) or enteroviral infections,[57] or bacterial or fungal sepsis[58] can develop secondary HLH. This may be a more common complication of severe infection than in older, immunocompetent children, most likely because of developmental limitations in fetal and neonatal host defense mechanisms.[59]

LABORATORY AND PATHOLOGIC FINDINGS

General

Characteristic laboratory abnormalities include pancytopenias, hypertriglyceridemia, hyperferritinemia, hyperbilirubinemia, transaminemia, and hypofibrinogenemia (Table 12-3).[1,43] Platelets are the most consistently depressed blood lineage, and thrombocytopenia may be a useful indicator of disease activity.[60] Approximately 80% to 90% of patients have two depressed blood cell lineages at presentation.[43] Hypofibrinogenemia occurs in the majority of patients, and can occur in the absence of disseminated intravascular coagulation. Serum ferritin level is consistently elevated, and in approximately 90% this concentration exceeds 4000 μg/L. A ferritin level >10,000 μg/L is 90% sensitive and 96% specific for HLH.[61] Hyponatremia and low serum protein and albumin concentrations are common.[43]

TABLE 12-2. Clinical Manifestations of Hemophagocytic Lymphohistiocytosis

Symptoms	Present at Time of Diagnosis (%)
Fever	91–100
Hepatomegaly	89–97
Splenomegaly	61–98
Lymphadenopathy	17–52
Skin rash	6–65
Respiratory distress	33–88
Hypotension	85
Jaundice	72
Gastrointestinal	44
Neurologic	20–47

Adapted from references 43–47.

PART II   Clinical Syndromes and Cardinal Features of Infectious Diseases: Approach to Diagnosis and Initial Management

SECTION A   Septicemia, Toxin- and Inflammation-Mediated Syndromes

TABLE 12-3. Laboratory Findings in Hemophagocytic Lymphohistiocytosis

Laboratory Finding	Present at Time of Diagnosis (%)
Anemia	89–94
Thrombocytopenia (<100,000 platelets/mm³)	82–100
Neutropenia (<1000 cells/mm³)	58–100
Leukopenia	39–87
Hypertriglyceridemia	80–100
Hypofibrinogenemia	65–85
Elevated serum alanine aminotransferase level	33–92
Hyperbilirubinemia	33–74
Hyponatremia	79
Cerebrospinal fluid pleocytosis	52–91

Adapted from Arico M, Janka G, Fischer A, et al. Hemophagocytic lymphohistiocytosis. Report of 122 children from the International Registry. FHL Study Group of the Histiocyte Society. Leukemia 1996;10:197–203; Henter JI, Elinder G, Soder O, et al. Incidence in Sweden and clinical features of familial hemophagocytic lymphohistiocytosis. Acta Paediatr Scand 1991;80:428–435; Janka GE. Familial hemophagocytic lymphohistiocytosis. Eur J Pediatr 1983;140:221–230.

Clinical Immunology

In primary HLH due to FHL, GS type II, and CHS, a function defect in killing by CD8⁺ T lymphocytes and NK cells occurs, and the circulating levels of CD4⁺ and CD8⁺ T lymphocytes and NK cells usually are normal or elevated.[21,62] NK-cell mediated cytotoxicity is decreased only moderately or even is normal in some cases of primary HLH, including FHL,[63] whereas CD8⁺ T-lymphocyte-mediated cytotoxicity is more uniformly impaired. In cases of secondary HLH, such as from severe EBV infection, the circulating number of NK cells often is reduced; transiently, most patients have reduced NK cell activity if blood is used as a source of NK cells for the assay.[9] The reason for this depression of circulating NK-cell numbers is unclear, but may reflect NK-cell sequestration in the tissues away from the circulation. Circulating invariant NK T lymphocytes, which have features of NK cells and T lymphocytes, are absent in XLP disease,[64] but are present in normal numbers in patients with XFHL disease.[65] A decreased number of B lymphocyte is common in HLH, including from secondary causes,[66] which can pose challenges in diagnosing certain primary immunodeficiency disorders.[27] There are no consistent abnormalities of quantitative immunoglobulin levels.

Although cytokine assays are not routinely used diagnostically, HLH patients tend to have marked elevations of IFN-γ and interleukin (IL)-10 and only moderately increased IL-6, whereas patients with bacterial septicemia often have markedly elevated levels of IL-6 and only moderate elevations of IL-10 and IFN-γ.[67]

Pathology

The classic histopathology is diffuse infiltration of the bone marrow, liver, spleen, lymph nodes, lungs, and brain with CD8⁺ T lymphocytes and activated non-Langerhans (lacking expression of CD1a) histiocytes that are actively phagocytosing blood cells. Hepatic portal and sinusoidal infiltration with CD8⁺ T lymphocytes expressing granzyme B, and with CD68⁺ CD1a histiocytes, is characteristically found in children with primary HLH. The degree of infiltration correlates with clinical disease severity.[68] Bile duct damage and endotheliitis with preservation of the hepatic parenchyma is frequent.[68] CNS tissue typically shows lymphohistiocytic infiltration of the parenchyma and perivascular

space, and hemophagocytosis in the leptomeninges, choroid plexus, or perivascular areas.[1] Importantly, the characteristic pathologic findings may not be present on an initial biopsy and the demonstration of hemophagocytosis is not required to make the diagnosis (see "Diagnosis" below).

Evaluation for Infectious Diseases

Initial evaluations should include bacterial and fungal cultures of blood, urine, and in most cases, CSF, throat and rectal swabs for viral culture, and a chest radiograph. Serologic evaluation for viruses and fungi should be pursued, although these may not be sensitive in immunocompromised hosts. PCR-based nucleic acid tests for EBV, CMV, parvovirus B19, HHV-6, and HIV infection should be performed; an elevated viral load supports the diagnosis of a poorly controlled viral infection. Specific epidemiologic factors, such as exposure to tuberculosis, travel, and animal exposure should guide further testing.

DIAGNOSIS

The diagnosis requires either confirmation of primary HLH, e.g., by genomic DNA sequencing *or* presence of ≥5 of the following 8 clinical criteria (Box 12-1): (1) fever; (2) splenomegaly; (3) thrombocytopenia, anemia, and/or neutropenia (two or more); (4) hypertriglyceridemia and/or hypofibrinogenemia; (5) histopathologic evidence of hemophagocytosis in bone marrow, spleen, or lymph nodes; (6) low or absent NK-cell cytotoxicity; (7) serum ferritin level of >500 μg/L; and (8) serum level of CD25 (an IL-2 receptor protein derived from T lymphocytes) of ≥2400 U/mL.

Hemophagocytosis may not be evident in bone marrow biopsies obtained early in the disease, and repeat bone marrow aspirates or analysis of other tissues may be required.[1,21] The diagnosis is supported by CSF mononuclear cell pleocytosis and elevated

BOX 12-1. Diagnostic Criteria for Hemophagocytic Lymphohistiocytosis (HLH)

The diagnosis of HLH can be established if either:
- **A molecular diagnosis consistent with HLH, or**
- **Diagnostic criteria are fulfilled (5 of 8)**

Original diagnostic criteria

Clinical:
1. Fever
2. Splenomegaly

Laboratory:
3. Cytopenia (≥2 cell lineages in the peripheral blood)
   Hemoglobin <9.0 g/dL (less than 4 weeks <10 g/dL)
   Platelets <100,000/mm³
   Neutrophils <1000/mm³
4. Hypertriglyceridemia and/or hypofibrinogenemia
   Fasting triglycerides ≥265 mg/dL
   Fibrinogen ≤1.5 g/L

Histopathologic:
5. Hemophagocytosis in bone marrow, spleen, or lymph nodes without evidence of malignancy

New diagnostic criteria

Laboratory:
6. Low or absent natural killer cell activity
7. Ferritin >500 μg/L
8. Soluble interleukin-2-receptor⁻ᵅ chain (CD25) ≥2400 U/mL

Adapted from Henter JI, Samuelsson-Horne A, Arico M, et al. Treatment of hemophagocytic lymphohistiocytosis with HLH-94 immunochemotherapy and bone marrow transplantation. Blood 2002;100:2367–2373 and HLH-2004 protocol: www.histio.org/society/protocols/trails-protocols.html.

protein or a liver biopsy showing chronic persistent hepatitis. Other findings that are suggestive include: meningitis or cerebritis; lymphadenopathy; elevation of serum hepatic enzymes, jaundice; edema, hypoproteinemia; hyponatremia; increased serum level of very low density lipoproteins (VLDL) and decreased level of high density lipoproteins (HDL).[1]

NK-cell cytotoxicity, in which peripheral blood mononuclear cells containing NK cells are incubated with chromium-labeled K562 erytholeukemia target cells, should be evaluated in inflammatory conditions. NK-cell cytotoxicity is markedly decreased or undetectable in most cases of primary or secondary HLH.[9,62,66] Circulating NK cells (CD56+/CD16+/CD3− lymphocytes) are usually present in normal or elevated numbers but are functionally defective in patients with primary HLH.[69] In secondary HLH, particularly in association with EBV infection, the numbers of NK cells often are markedly depressed, accounting for impaired cytotoxicity;[9] activity may return to normal with the recovery of NK-cell numbers. Normal or borderline low NK-cell activity can occur in certain forms of FHL and some cases of XLP disease. Flow cytometric evaluation for cytotoxic granule release based on surface staining of lymphocytes for the CD107a/b proteins[12] may be particularly useful in classifying FHL cases.[3,12]

Clinical flow cytometry assays are available for the determination of T-lymphocyte and NK-cell intracellular perforin, SAP, and XIAP, which are encoded by genes that are mutated in FHL2, XLP disease, and XLFH disease, respectively.[12,70] Genomic DNA sequencing is important in the initial evaluation for primary HLH, as normal flow cytometric protein assays do not exclude the diagnosis (see http://www.ncbi.nlm.nih.gov/sites/GeneTests).[12] Clinical FHL can occur in the absence of any of the known genetic causes of primary HLH, suggesting that other genetic etiologies remain to be defined. Thus, without a previous family history or genetic confirmation, the diagnosis of primary HLH is provisional, and it is essential to exclude malignancy or autoimmune disease as HLH precipitants.

DIFFERENTIAL DIAGNOSIS

The nonspecific nature of the most prominent features of HLH, i.e., fever, hepatosplenomegaly, and cytopenias, leads to a broad differential diagnosis, which includes leukemia, lymphoma, aplastic anemia, myelodysplasia, and Langerhans cell histiocytosis. In the fetus and neonate other etiologies of liver failure, hepatitis, and hydrops fetalis should be considered. Differential diagnosis of neurologic disease includes autoimmune and acute disseminated encephalomyelitis, other CNS demyelinating disease,[52] and vasculitis.

TREATMENT

General

Aggressive supportive care with transfusions, antibiotics, and nutrition typically is indicated. An integrated physician team approach with expertise in hematology/oncology, immunology, infectious diseases,[43] critical care, neurology, and nephrology is ideal. Close monitoring for secondary bacterial and fungal infections and for adequate hemostasis is important, as infections and bleeding are important causes of HLH mortality.[71]

Immunosuppression and Chemotherapy

Aggressive immunotherapy of primary HLH, prior to definitive genetic diagnosis, which may take months, may be necessary because a delay may have adverse consequences.[5] The natural course of untreated primary HLH due to early-onset FHL is progressive multiorgan failure and CNS disease, with a mean survival of only 2 months.[60] Secondary HLH also can have a high mortality, especially if EBV-induced,[21] although some cases can resolve spontaneously without therapy.[72] The type of treatment for children with HLH is determined by disease severity, age of onset, and

history of familial disease.[1,73] The updated HLH-2004 protocol serves as a treatment guide for cases of primary HLH and severe, persistent, or recurrent secondary HLH, particularly EBV-associated HLH,[1,5,74] with the goal being to induce remission, and, where indicated, to bridge to hematopoietic stem cell transplantation (HSCT). For patients with primary HLH and those with severe secondary disease, especially EBV-HLH, treatment includes etoposide, glucocorticoid, and cyclosporine A (CSA) for 8 weeks. For all cases of primary HLH and for secondary HLH that do not respond to initial therapy, intrathecal methotrexate may be used. If neurologic symptoms persist, recur, or progress, intrathecal glucocorticoid therapy may be useful. These agents help control HLH by inducing apoptosis of lymphocytes and histiocytes (mainly an effect of etoposide) and by inhibiting cytokine/chemokine production (mainly an effect of glucocorticoids and CSA). Relapses are common as treatment is reduced, especially in FHL, and may require re-escalation of therapy.[1] Etoposide usually is not used in cases of secondary HLH complicating HIV infection or iatrogenic immunosuppression. Etoposide therapy often results in prolonged neutropenia and is associated with a risk of later acute myeloid leukemia. FHL has been treated with etoposide-free regimens, such as the combination of antithymocyte globulin, glucocorticoids, CSA, and intrathecal methotrexate.[75]

For EBV-associated HLH, which can have a highly variable course,[72] relatively conservative therapies, such as glucocorticoids and CSA with or without immune globulin intravenous can be considered, reserving etoposide for nonresponsive cases.[76] In EBV-associated HLH and primary HLH in XLP disease, rituximab (CD20 monoclonal antibody) has been used.[77,78]

Hematopoietic Stem Cell Transplantation

Patients with primary HLH ultimately require allogeneic HSCT for cure.[1] Reduced intensity non-myeloablative conditioning regimens having had particularly favorable results.[79] Patients with primary HLH who have early relapse of HLH or persistent CNS involvement may benefit from early HSCT.[80] HSCT also has been used for EBV-associated HLH, particularly for those who have had recurrent disease.[81]

PROGNOSIS

If untreated, primary HLH, particularly FHL, is almost uniformly fatal.[1] Increased survival is associated with prompt response to initial therapy and with older age at presentation.[82] Secondary HLH can be a self-limited process with recovery after only supportive measures. Long-term remission is uncommon with CNS disease or in those >30 years of age;[83] early aggressive therapy for severe or recurrent cases appears to be beneficial.[84] A soluble CD25 serum level ≥10,000 U/mL[85] also has been associated with mortality.[37] HLH patients who have a ≥96% drop in serum ferritin with therapy have a reduced risk of mortality.[86]

MACROPHAGE ACTIVATION SYNDROME

Systemic-onset juvenile idiopathic arthritis (soJIA) is a frequent cause of MAS in childhood,[87] and the presence of defective NK-cell function due to NK-cell lymphopenia is similar to that associated with other causes of secondary HLH.[87,88] Clinical and laboratory findings of MAS include persistent fever, hepatosplenomegaly, neurologic abnormalities, marked cytopenias, and coagulopathy.[9] As some diagnostic criteria for HLH also can occur with exacerbations of soJIA, i.e., lymphadenopathy, splenomegaly, and hyperferritinemia, a marked elevation of serum CD25 and CD163 levels[89] can help in diagnosis of MAS in this context. MAS can be managed in most cases using immunosuppression without chemotherapy. The optimal regimen remains controversial and may depend on the underlying disorder; e.g., IL-1 and IL-6 appear to play a central role in soJIA inflammation and MAS,[90] which may account for some patients responding to inhibitors of IL-1 (e.g., anakinra) or IL-6.[90]

SECTION B: Cardinal Symptom Complexes

13 Mucocutaneous Symptom Complexes

Sarah S. Long

Generally, in differentiating between bacterial and viral causes of febrile illnesses in children, the more mucous membranes involved in the patient's illness (e.g., conjunctiva, throat, respiratory, gastrointestinal tract), the more likely the cause is viral. When multiple mucous membranes are involved and an exanthem (i.e., mucocutaneous complex) is present, a self-limited viral cause is likely, but other important diagnoses must be considered. These commonly include inflammatory or immunologically mediated conditions, such as Kawasaki disease (KD), Stevens–Johnson syndrome (SJS), and drug hypersensitivity, and bacterial toxin-mediated diseases, including staphylococcal and streptococcal toxic shock, streptococcal scarlatiniform disorders, and staphylococcal exfoliative toxin syndromes (toxic epidermal necrolysis and staphylococcal scalded-skin syndrome). A "best," if not the definitive, diagnosis can be deduced through careful assessment of: (1) the dominant features of the illness; (2) prodromal events and exposures; (3) specific characteristics of the exanthem and abnormality at each affected mucous membrane; and (4) the cadence of the developing constellation. Laboratory features are of secondary importance, heightening or diminishing the fitness of the clinical assessment.

Table 13-1 shows useful differentiating features of commonly considered causes of mucocutaneous symptom complexes. Features distinguishing streptococcal toxic shock due to streptococcal pyrogenic exotoxin (SPE) A or B from staphylococcal toxic shock associated with toxic shock syndrome toxin-1 (TSST-1) are shown in Table 13-2, and are described in the discussion where pertinent.

Less common conditions share certain clinical features of the mucocutaneous syndromes shown in Table 13-1 but usually can be distinguished on the basis of circumstances of occurrence, such as recurrences/periodicity of febrile episodes in periodic fever with aphthous stomatitis, pharyngitis, and adenitis (the PFAPA syndrome)[1] and chronicity and additional findings in Behçet syndrome.[2] Although the ulcerative gingivitis and pseudomembrane of mucositis associated with neutropenia and anticancer chemotherapy[3] can be indistinguishable from the confluent denuding ulcers of SJS, the clinical setting of the former as well as the absence of conjunctivitis and rash distinguishes mucositis from SJS. Stevens–Johnson syndrome most commonly is associated with antibiotics or anticonvulsant drugs, and *Mycoplasma* infection.[4–6] Paraneoplastic vasculitis complicating myeloproliferative disorders can cause urticaria, erythema multiforme, or palpable purpura. This diagnosis is suspected because of the associated malignancy and is confirmed by skin biopsy.[7]

Rocky Mountain spotted fever (RMSF), an infective vasculitis caused by *Rickettsia rickettsii*, shares many features of other mucocutaneous syndromes (i.e., high fever, progressive serious illness, conjunctival hyperemia and suffusion, peripheral edema despite hypovolemia, and hyponatremia), but the presence of unremitting headache, peripheral petechial rash (if present), season, and exposure to ticks usually set RMSF apart.[8] Ehrlichiosis and anaplasmosis occur in a similar setting; leukopenia may be a clue.[9] Empiric treatment for RMSF or ehrlichiosis sometimes is required because the diagnosis cannot be reasonably or quickly excluded. Leptospirosis is indistinguishable from RMSF except possibly for a biphasic illness and disproportionate organ involvement of the kidney or liver in leptospirosis.[10] Drug hypersensitivity reactions can cause a variety of mucocutaneous abnormalities.[11] For the previously healthy child or adolescent who comes to medical attention in shock, septic shock from unrecognized ruptured appendix, urosepsis, invasive meningococcal or pneumococcal infection (especially if petechiae, purpura, or purpura fulminans is present), and disseminated staphylococcal and group A streptococcal infection must also be considered. *Streptococcus pneumoniae* and group B streptococcus also can cause toxic shock-like manifestations, which probably are related to cytokine stimulation.[12]

SPECIFIC DISTINGUISHING CHARACTERISTICS

Fever and Prodrome

The sequence of events and duration of fever when the child comes to medical attention provide useful clues to diagnosis. Although children with KD and bacterial toxin-mediated syndromes ultimately share many mucocutaneous features, the cadence of the prodrome is distinct. The child with staphylococcal toxic shock usually has profuse diarrhea and severe prostration within hours of onset of fever, whereas the child with KD begins with fever and crankiness, sometimes with unilateral cervical lymphadenitis, not unlike the beginning of a common viral illness.[13,14] Concern about the clinical state of the child with KD usually does not heighten for several days, when fever and crankiness persist and the symptom complex evolves rather than abates, as might be expected in self-limited viral infection.[15,16] An important exception occurs in <10% of children with KD who have more rapidly progressive disease with hypotension requiring admission to an intensive care unit and are misdiagnosed as having septic or toxic shock.[17] The younger the child with a staphylococcal exfoliative toxin syndrome, the more rapidly progressive and dramatic the skin manifestations, with constitutional illness usually secondary.[18,19]

Initial manifestations of SJS can be urticaria, with subsequent progression to the fixed tissue lesions of erythema multiforme, and evolution of mucous membrane inflammation and systemic illness.[4,20] Enteroviruses and respiratory viruses that cause mucocutaneous findings evolve over 3 to 5 days; nasal symptomatology, rhinorrhea, hoarseness, or cough is present in >75% of cases, distinguishing these viral infections from KD. High fever (39.2°C or more) or persistent fever (5 days or more) does not eliminate viral etiology, because viruses commonly considered in such patients (adenovirus, influenza A and B viruses) typically cause high fever, and at least a third of affected children have fever beyond 5 days.[21–23]

Conjunctiva

To ascribe conjunctival findings accurately, the examiner must pay particular attention to: (1) presence of inflammation and exudate versus erythema alone; (2) relative involvement of bulbar versus palpebral and tarsal sites; (3) presence or absence of photophobia, pain on movement, and itching; and (4) presence of uveitis, destructive keratitis, and panophthalmitis versus superficial inflammation.

Ocular manifestations of many infectious, inflammatory, allergic, and toxin-mediated conditions begin with bilateral conjunctival erythema.[24] The earliest ocular findings of

TABLE 13-1. Differentiating among Causes of Mucocutaneous Symptom Complexes

	Kawasaki Disease	Toxic Shock[a]	Staphylococcal Exfoliative Toxin Syndromes	Streptococcal Scarlatina	Stevens–Johnson Syndrome	Viral Infection
CLINICAL FEATURES						
Fever	+++ ≥5 days	+++ <2 days	+ 2–3 days	+ 2–3 days	++ 5 days	++ 3–5 days
Conjunctiva	+++ Bilateral hyperemia (bulbar > palpebral); anterior uveitis	+++ Bilateral hyperemia (bulbar > palpebral)	++ Unilateral or bilateral purulent conjunctivitis (palpebral > bulbar); or normal	– Normal	++ Bilateral purulent conjunctivitis, chemosis; keratitis, panophthalmitis	+/+++ Unilateral or bilateral purulent conjunctivitis (palpebral > bulbar); cobblestone lymphoid hyperplasia
Lips	+++ Erythema, fissures	++ Erythema	– Normal or desquamation	– Normal, with circumoral pallor	+++ Erythema and edema, fissures, denudation; bleeding, black eschar	– Normal
Oropharynx	+++ Mucosal erythema; strawberry tongue	++ Mucosal erythema; strawberry tongue	– Normal, or mucosal erythema	++ Tonsillar erythema, exudate; palatal petechiae; strawberry tongue	++ Panmucosal erythema, confluent ulceration, denudation; pseudomembrane	+/+++ Erythema; anterior or posterior discrete ulceration; tonsillar exudate or follicular hyperplasia; palatal petechiae; each dependent on specific virus
Exanthem	+++ Polymorphous, vasoactive and changing; morbilliform, symmetric; exaggerated or solely in groin	++ Erythroderma	+++ Indurative or papular erythroderma; tender; Nikolsky sign and desquamation during acute phase	+++ Papular erythroderma (sandpaper); Pastia sign	+++ Erythema multiforme; polymorphous, fixed; bullae	+/++ Maculopapular (discrete or confluent), vesicular, or petechial; each dependent on specific virus
Extremities	++ Symmetric, indurative edema distally; painful erythema, palms and soles; stocking/glove distribution; occasional digital cyanosis	++ Symmetric distally; erythema on palms and soles	– Normal, or edema contiguous with exanthem	– Normal	– Normal, or edema contiguous with exanthem	– Normal, or palmar vesicles (enteroviruses, herpesviruses), socks/gloves erythema (parvovirus); other exanthem
Other	+++ Unremitting crankiness; cervical lymphadenopathy; arthralgia/arthritis; meningismus, cranial nerve palsy; abdominal pain, distension, tenderness; hydropic gallbladder	+++ Profuse prodromal diarrhea; dizziness, headache, confusion; hypotension, shock; hydropic gallbladder	+ Infected tissue site	+ Sore throat, odynophagia; cervical lymphadenitis; malaise, vomiting	++ Malaise, arthralgia; urethral/anal ulceration and symptoms; abdominal pain, diarrhea	++ Headache, malaise, myalgia, cough, rhinorrhea; pneumonitis; lymphadenopathy, splenomegaly; each dependent on specific virus

Continued

PART II Clinical Syndromes and Cardinal Features of Infectious Diseases: Approach to Diagnosis and Initial Management

SECTION B Cardinal Symptom Complexes

TABLE 13-1. Differentiating among Causes of Mucocutaneous Symptom Complexes—cont'd

	Kawasaki Disease	Toxic Shock[a]	Staphylococcal Exfoliative Toxin Syndromes	Streptococcal Scarlatina	Stevens–Johnson Syndrome	Viral Infection
Predominant feature(s)	+++ Persistent fever and unremitting crankiness	+++ Fever and prostration	+++ Desquamating skin lesions	++ Exanthem and sore throat	+++ Edematous bloody lips and oral pseudomembrane	+ Variable; respiratory tract and/or constitutional symptomatology
Convalescent clinical features	+++ Desquamation periungually to palms and soles (full-thickness); minimal desquamation elsewhere; hair loss, nail abnormalities; coronary artery aneurysms/thrombosis	+++ Desquamation hands and feet (full-thickness); mild desquamation elsewhere; hair loss, nail abnormalities	+++ Desquamation extensive during acute and convalescent periods	+++ Desquamation hands and feet (full-thickness); desquamation extensive elsewhere	++ Desquamation at sites of exanthem, lips, perineum; recurrences; serious ophthalmologic sequelae	+ Desquamation at sites of exanthem (mild)
LABORATORY FEATURES	Elevated peripheral neutrophils, platelets, sedimentation rate; pyuria ± electro- or echocardiographic abnormalities	Thrombocytopenia, left shift of neutrophils; coagulopathy; hyponatremia; multiorgan dysfunction related to hypoperfusion; acute respiratory distress syndrome	Left shift of neutrophils; hypovolemia in young infant; bacteremia/septicemia related to infected site	Elevated peripheral neutrophils	Elevated peripheral neutrophils, sedimentation rate	Normal or low peripheral neutrophils, or elevated lymphocytes; normal or low platelets
DIAGNOSIS	Clinical, with exclusion of others and supportive laboratory findings; response to IGIV; ectasia, aneurysm, or thrombosis of coronary arteries	TSST-1 producing *Staphylococcus aureus* recovered (from mucosa/infected site); response to aggressive fluid support, antibiotic	Exfoliatin producing *S. aureus* recovered (usually from skin); response to antibiotic	Erythrogenic toxin-producing *Streptococcus pyogenes* recovered (usually from throat); response to antibiotic	Clinical; slow improvement; recurrences	Clinical; rapid improvement
TREATMENT	IGIV 2 g/kg	Crystalloid, colloid, then pressor agents; penicillinase-resistant antibiotic (or vancomycin) plus clindamycin; IGIV not proven	Pencillinase-resistant antibiotic (consider vancomycin or clindamycin); supportive fluids	Penicillin	Supportive; discontinue inciting drug; corticosteroid, IGIV not proven	Supportive; occasional specific antiviral agent

IgE, immunoglobulin E; IGIV, immune globulin intravenous; TSST, toxic shock syndrome toxin; +++, prominent, expected finding; ++, frequent finding; +, variable finding; –, not present.

[a]*Features of staphylococcal toxic shock (i.e., related to TSST-1); see text and Table 13-2 for differences in streptococcal toxic shock.*

Kawasaki disease, measles, SJS, RMSF, and leptospirosis, for example, cannot be distinguished. However, in KD, toxic shock syndromes, leptospirosis and many cases of RMSF, nonedematous, nonexudative erythema of bulbar conjunctivae is the complete evolution. In sharp contrast, adenoviral conjunctivitis is unilateral in 65% of cases, is predominantly palpebral (frequently with follicular lymphoid hyperplasia), and is associated with keratitis, purulent exudate, and photophobia in approximately half of cases and with concurrent pharyngitis in 55%.[25] Conjunctivitis due to other viruses usually is bilateral, palpebral, and exudative.

Bacterial conjunctivitis (especially that due to nontypable *Haemophilus influenzae, S. pneumoniae,* or *Staphylococcus aureus*) is purulent, and usually bilateral; other mucocutaneous symptoms are not present (except with exfoliative toxin-producing *S. aureus* infection). Concurrent acute otitis media is common when nontypable *H. influenzae* is causative.[26] Orbital and periorbital cellulitis manifest predominantly with eyelid edema, erythema, and chemosis. Ocular itching, tearing, and photophobia accompany the "red eye" of allergic disorders; papillary hypertrophy of the palpebral conjunctivae is characteristic. Normal conjunctivae (as well as normal lips and circumoral skin) are somewhat distinctive in streptococcal scarlet fever.

The findings of light sensitivity, ocular pain, and decreased vision suggest uveitis, which is characteristic of juvenile idiopathic arthritis (JIA) and Behçet syndrome. Such forms of JIA generally are not associated with fever and rash. Anterior uveitis is common in KD, being present in 83% of children examined in the first week and in 66% examined after the first week in one study.[27] Unlike in other causes of uveitis, the inflammation in KD is mild and transient and is associated with minimal photophobia or pain.

TABLE 13-2. Comparative Features of Toxic Shock Syndrome[a]

Feature	Staphylococcal Toxic Shock	Streptococcal Toxic Shock
Primary toxin	TSST-1	SPEA, B
Prodrome	Vomiting, diarrhea	Flu-like illness
Duration prodrome	Hours	Hours–days
Severity prodrome	+++	+
Focal infection	+	++
Extreme pain/ hyperesthesia at focal site	–	+++
Rash	Erythroderma	Scarlatina/none
Shock	Predictable	Unpredictable, related to clotting
	Treatable	Sometimes untreatable
Multiorgan failure	Predictable, related to blood pressure	Unpredictable
	Treatable	Sometimes untreatable
Positive blood culture	–	++
Coagulopathy	+	+++
Complicated hospitalization	+	+++
Gangrene	±	+++
Mortality	+	++

SPE, streptococcal pyrogenic exotoxin; TSST, toxic shock syndrome toxin; ±, not an expected occurrence; +, occurs, but infrequently; ++, occurs with some frequency; +++, occurs commonly; –, does not occur.

[a]*Differences represent general comparisons rather than clinical findings or outcomes in individual patients.*

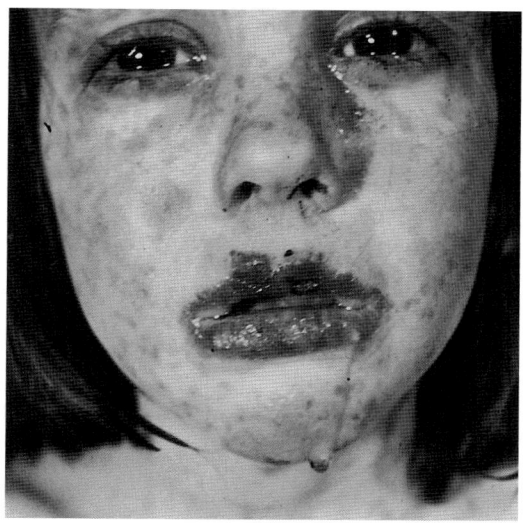

Figure 13-1. Ten-year-old girl with Stevens–Johnson syndrome and characteristic denudation of mucocutaneous junctions of the lips.

SJS frequently is associated with severe anterior-segment involvement, with exudative conjunctival discharge and sloughing of epithelium as well as pseudomembrane formation, and has the potential to cause subsequent severe corneal and eyelid scarring.[28] Anterior uveal inflammation can occur with measles and leptospirosis but is not expected with other mucocutaneous syndromes (e.g., streptococcal or staphylococcal toxin-mediated diseases, enteroviral or adenoviral infection, rickettsial diseases). Ophthalmologic evaluation with slit-lamp examination is valuable in children with evolving conjunctival findings and a mucocutaneous syndrome to uncover intraocular disease and aid in the diagnosis and management of SJS.

Lips

In infants, the lips (and frequently the ears) are brightly colored when fever is high, returning to normal with even transient defervescence. The lips infrequently are involved in mucocutaneous syndromes due to viruses, except during primary herpes simplex stomatitis, when diagnosis is apparent. Measles and influenza may be other exceptions, in which lips can be red, edematous, and cracked after several days of high fever.[29] The lips are noticeably red and are sometimes cracked and fissured in KD and toxic shock, however, providing important clues to diagnosis. The swollen, denuded, bleeding lips with black eschar of SJS are pathognomonic (Figure 13-1), the mucocutaneous junctions of lips, conjunctivae, urethra, and anus being primary target sites of the pathologic process.

Oropharynx

Examination is performed to detect: (1) diffuse erythema, sometimes with uvulitis (KD and toxic shock); (2) hypertrophied or dilated papillae on the tongue to give the appearance of "strawberry tongue" (KD, toxic shock, streptococcal scarlatina); (3) confluent buccal and gingival ulceration with pseudomembrane

formation (SJS and mucositis of neutropenia and antineoplastic drug therapy); (4) palatal petechiae (*Streptococcus pyogenes* and Epstein–Barr virus); (5) discrete ulcers (enteroviruses, herpes simplex virus); (6) Koplik spots (rubeola); and (7) exudative enanthem (*S. pyogenes*, respiratory tract viruses, Epstein–Barr virus). The singular (or few) deep, large ulcerative lesions of aphthous stomatitis and Behçet disease characteristically are found on the buccal or lingual mucosa or the lateral tongue.

Exanthem

The exact characteristics, distribution, pattern of evolution, and timing and manner of resolution of exanthematous lesions are extremely helpful in differentiating among causes of mucocutaneous syndromes. Vesicular skin eruptions are almost unique to herpesviruses and enteroviruses.[30] Bullae are the typical initial lesions of staphylococcal exfoliative toxin syndrome, as is sloughing of sheets of epidermis with gentle pressure or minor trauma – Nikolsky sign. Localized hemorrhagic bullae can form in the skin overlying necrotizing cellulitis, myositis, or fasciitis especially due to toxin-producing *S. pyogenes*.[31] Bullous erythema multiforme, the hallmark of SJS, occurs first in localized areas, evolves at the site over days, and commonly progresses to other sites. Usually, the lesions are symmetric, on extensor surfaces of extremities as well as the trunk, with a predilection for sun-exposed areas. Typical target or iris lesions of erythema multiforme with bullae are expected in SJS, with urticarial lesions as well (see Chapter 72, Vesicles and Bullae).

Vesicular, bullous, or petechial lesions are distinctly rare in KD. The rash of KD is polymorphous (patchy macular, maculopapular, infrequently papular) and is indistinguishable in individual cases from the exanthem of viral infection, drug, or food allergy, SJS, or toxin-mediated disease; however, characteristically, the rash in KD is fiery red, morbilliform (confluent), symmetric (involving both hands, feet, knees, and elbows), and changeable from hour to hour, rather than fixed as in viral infection or SJS. Although urticarial and erythema multiforme-like lesions can occur in KD, they are not fixed. Rashes in KD characteristically spare the head, whereas exanthems in many viral infections, SJS, and staphylococcal toxin diseases commonly begin on, or involve, the face. Exaggeration or confinement of exanthem at the groin is characteristic of KD,[32] although this feature can occur in streptococcal scarlatiniform eruptions, staphylococcal exfoliative toxin syndrome, influenza,[29] and bacterial cellulitis in the neonate (in which primary umbilical colonization is usual). Erythema, induration of the scrotum, and pain in testicles can occur in KD, and RMSF; a hydrocele can appear acutely.[33]

PART II Clinical Syndromes and Cardinal Features of Infectious Diseases: Approach to Diagnosis and Initial Management

SECTION B Cardinal Symptom Complexes

Viral exanthems are not painful or tender. The skin of children with diffuse staphylococcal exfoliative toxin syndrome, however, is erythematous and edematous, sometimes has a sandpaper quality, and usually is painful and tender.[34] In KD, specific sites of exanthem are not painful except on the hands and feet, where edema (and probably vasculitis) causes pain, frequently leading to refusal to bear weight. An important clue to soft-tissue infection due to streptococci (usually β-hemolytic group A organisms, but also group B, C, and G organisms on occasion, and *S. pneumoniae*, the last especially in individuals with connective tissue diseases)[35] and necrotizing *S. aureus* infections is that the patient complains of exquisite pain, sometimes with hyperesthesia or hypoesthesia out of proportion to objective abnormality.[31,36]

Epidemiologic features, such as season, exposure, incubation period, and associated findings, are frequently more helpful in distinguishing viral infections than is the exanthem itself. Enteroviruses are the leading cause of exanthematous diseases, with more than 30 types associated with rash illnesses, some of which also cause mucosal lesions.[30,37,38] Although neonates and young infants can have diffuse macular or blotchy rashes, exanthem at peak ages for enteroviral exanthematous diseases (especially due to echoviruses 4, 9, and 16 as well as coxsackieviruses A9 and B5) usually consists of rubelliform (maculopapular discrete, nonconfluent) lesions beginning on the face and upper trunk and spreading down to the extremities.[38] An important exception is hand–foot–mouth disease (usually due to coxsackievirus A16, followed by A5, A9, A10, B1, and B3, and enterovirus 71), in which peripheral distribution of vesicular or rubelliform lesions is characteristic. Rashes during viral infections due to influenza A and B, parainfluenza, and respiratory syncytial virus (especially in young children) probably occur more than occasionally, are always rubelliform, are frequently present for less than 24 hours, and spread from the head to the trunk and extremities.[30]

Rash occurs in 2% to 8% of adenoviral infections, and adenovirus types 1, 2, 3, 4, 7, and 7a have been isolated most frequently;[38] lesions are distributed as with influenza and usually are rubelliform, occasionally are morbilliform (maculopapular confluent patches), and rarely are erythema multiforme like. Mucocutaneous and systemic manifestations of measles can simulate KD initially, the rash being least differentiating; prominent cough, coryza, and eventual purulent conjunctivitis distinguish measles. Similarly, the prominent respiratory tract symptoms caused by *Mycoplasma pneumoniae* distinguish this infection; maculopapular rashes (5% to 15% of cases), consisting of vesicular or bullous, papular, petechial, urticarial or erythema multiforme-like lesions, have been described.[39]

Classically, staphylococcal toxic shock is associated with diffuse erythroderma, a flushed, sunburned appearance (without discrete lesions, tenderness, or induration) especially on the face, trunk, and proximal extremities. Streptococcal scarlet fever of scarlatina is associated with a diffuse, fine maculopapular rash, which is palpable, sandpaper-like, and prominent on the trunk and proximal extremities; exaggeration of erythema in skinfolds (Pastia sign) is characteristic and in groin is dramatic when present. Children with staphylococcal exfoliative toxin syndrome commonly have crusted, exudative, infective conjunctivitis, or paranasal lesions, in addition to generalized nonexudative exfoliation (Figure 13-2). Frequently, toxin-mediated exanthems overlap, presumably because more than one toxin is encoded.

Extremity Changes

Indurative erythroderma with frank edema of the distal extremities probably is the most helpful differentiating physical finding in some mucocutaneous syndromes, reflecting inflammatory vasculitis (KD), vascular dilatation (toxic shock syndromes), or infective vasculitis (RMSF). It does not occur in viral infections or SJS, except contiguous to sites of erythema multiforme in the latter. The demarcated, socks or gloves distribution of erythema and induration in KD is dramatic on occasion, as are digital cyanosis and gangrene (Figure 13-3). The latter are distinguished easily from the peripheral ischemia of toxic or septic shock by low blood pressure, weak pulse, and pale, cool extremities in shock. Parvovirus B19 and some herpesviruses also cause socks and gloves syndrome (especially in older children) with initial erythema and edema of dorsal and palmar/solar surfaces of hands and feet with progression to papules and purpura, which is well demarcated at ankles and wrists.[40]

Evolution and Resolution

The exanthem of KD evolves, waning, waxing, and migrating over days; that of toxic shock and exfoliative syndromes is rapid in onset and is progressive; viral exanthems characteristically appear days after onset of systemic illness and evolve at one site while progressing to others. Desquamation occurs during the crescendo phase of staphylococcal exfoliative toxin syndrome (as maximal disease manifestations evolve) but during the decrescendo phase of KD (typically days 10 to 20 after onset, beginning in the periungual region), and only during the convalescent phases of staphylococcal and streptococcal toxic shock and scarlet fever. Desquamation of palms and soles is likely to be a full-thickness loss (as if molted) after KD, streptococcal scarlet fever, and toxic shock. In KD, unlike bacterial toxin-mediated diseases, total body desquamation does not occur or is fine and superficial, occurring

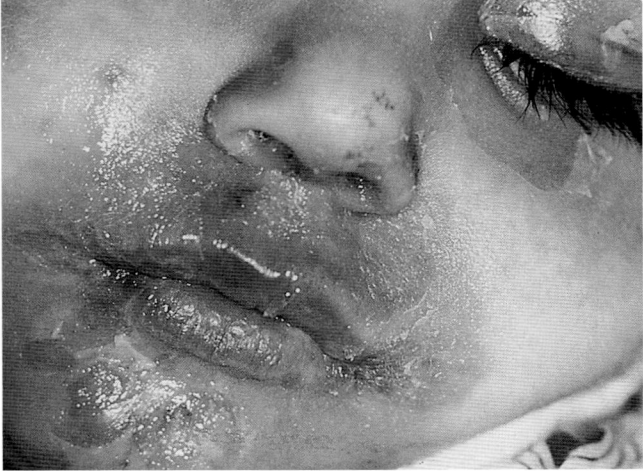

Figure 13-2. Four-year-old boy with staphylococcal exfoliative toxin disease. Note characteristic paper-thin desquamation of skin on eyelid and impetiginous infection around the nose and chin.

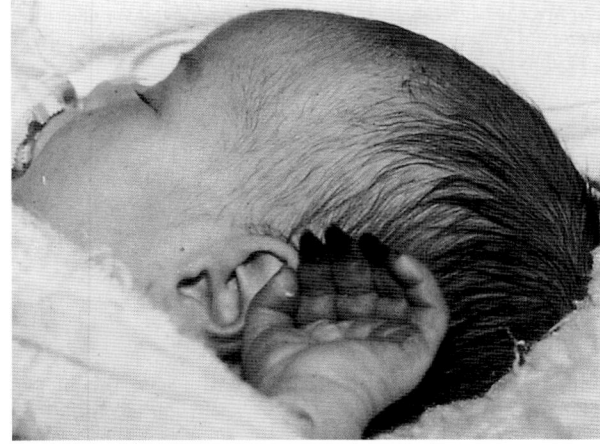

Figure 13-3. Six-week-old boy with the infantile polyarteritis nodosa form of Kawasaki disease. Note the dusky fingers with distal gangrene.

in only about 10% of patients, particularly in the groin and perineal area. Hair loss and nail bed deformities, i.e., grooves (Beau lines), pits, transverse (red) lines, are well described after KD but can occur after other highly febrile illnesses, or with hypotension or ischemia, such as invasive bacterial infection, toxic shock, and RMSF.

Other Clinical Features and Cardinal Feature

Clinical features other than mucocutaneous signs or symptoms, alone or in combination, can provide valuable clues to diagnosis. A partial listing is given in Table 13-1. Inflammation at multiple sites is typical of KD, anterior uveitis being quite specific among diagnoses considered. Transient hydrops of the gallbladder manifesting as right upper quadrant abdominal pain, tenderness and fullness is a common but nonspecific finding in KD that also occurs in staphylococcal toxic shock,[13] streptococcal scarlet fever,[41] and other systemic infectious and inflammatory diseases, such as enteric fever,[42] leptospirosis, Epstein–Barr virus mononucleosis,[43] neonatal group B streptococcal septicemia, asphyxia, and during parenteral alimentation.[44]

Infants younger than 6 months of age with KD are especially prone to a rapidly progressive course and severe vascular complications.[15,45,46] They frequently lack classic diagnostic findings, such as exanthem and erythematous conjunctivae. Extremely high fever, anxious appearance, inconsolable irritability, respiratory distress, and cardiac gallop murmur with hepatomegaly can be clues. Aneurysmal dilation of multiple vessels can occur; pulsatile masses in the axillae or groin can sometimes be appreciated acutely, within days of onset of fever.

Delineating the predominant complaint, or cardinal feature, of the child's illness aids in establishment of a correct diagnosis (see Table 13-1). Unremitting crankiness is almost universal in KD, probably related to the multiple sites of vasculitis and painful edema or ischemia; unilateral, remarkable cervical lymphadenitis is sometimes a dominant feature.[47] Prodromal fever, diarrhea, and then profound prostration and hypotension are predominant in staphylococcal toxic shock but also can occur in streptococcal toxic shock. The prodrome is frequently nonspecific in streptococcal toxic shock; the clinical picture is dominated by extreme painfulness of apparent minor soft-tissue infection (if present), followed by sudden inexorable shock and coagulopathy.

Children with staphylococcal exfoliative toxin syndrome have variable degrees of illness, depending on age and presence of bloodstream or focal infection; the rapidly evolving exanthem with loss of skin in sheets as well as purulence around eyelids and nose dominate the clinical picture. Edematous, bleeding, black eschared lips and oral mucosal denudation are dramatic findings in SJS; in some cases, inflammatory necrosis of respiratory or intestinal tract mucosa causes wheezing, odynophagia, and other symptoms. In viral illnesses, the mucocutaneous features broaden the differential diagnosis, but other symptoms (such as cough, hoarseness, sore throat) commonly dominate the patient's or parent's complaints; general debilitation is usually modest, and the epidemiologic setting heightens the likelihood of a specific diagnosis.

Table 13-2 summarizes the differentiating features of classic staphylococcal toxic shock (associated with TSST-1 and enterotoxin B) and streptococcal toxic shock (associated with SPE A or B and, possibly, proteases). Although these syndromes are superficially similar, the evolution of clinical symptoms, the complications, and the outcomes frequently are distinctive. Staphylococcal toxic shock usually has a dramatic onset and rapid progression. Focal infection is present in most nonmenstrual pediatric cases but can be relatively minor (e.g., sinusitis, surgical wound).[48,49] Streptococcal toxic shock usually has a less abrupt onset of symptoms, with initial malaise, myalgia and then complaints of severe pain, hyperesthesia, or hypoesthesia at an apparently minor soft-tissue site of infection.[35,36,50] Nonexudative pharyngitis is the occasional primary site of streptococcal infection, with a complaint of sore throat out of proportion to the findings.[51] Many

children with streptococcal toxic shock have been brought for medical attention one or more times before the onset of catastrophic multiorgan system failure and shock.[52] A possible potentiating role of nonsteroidal anti-inflammatory drugs in invasive streptococcal disease has been questioned[53] and not excluded by case-control studies.[54,55]

DIAGNOSIS AND EMPIRIC THERAPY

The best working diagnosis, barring the presence of pathognomonic features, is made on clinical grounds. Laboratory findings infrequently confirm a diagnosis at the time therapy must be given. Brisk elevations of acute-phase reactants are supportive laboratory findings in KD (and are variably present in SJS); white blood cell count <15,000/mm^3, erythrocyte sedimentation rate <40 mm/hour, C-reactive protein <3 mg/dL, or platelet count <200,000/mm^3 are negative indicators for KD[15] (with important exception of low platelets in patients with severe shock-like presentation[17]). Leukemoid reaction with neutrophil count exceeding 30,000/mm^3 frequently occurs in very young infants with the infantile polyarteritis presentation of KD; anemia is universal.[45] These can be important clues to the diagnosis when mucocutaneous features are absent.

Leukocytosis is not expected in enteroviral infections. Leukocyte counts are <15,000/mm^3 in 90% of children hospitalized with influenza; leukopenia occurs in approximately 25%.[22,29] Adenoviral infection can be associated with a brisk inflammatory response, probably owing to cytokine stimulation.[56] In a study of 105 children hospitalized with adenoviral infection, the mean peripheral leukocyte count was 13,300/mm^3 (10% had counts >20,000/mm^3), and almost 30% had an erythrocyte sedimentation rate >40 mm/hour.

Thrombocytosis is universal in KD but not until after the first week of illness. Thrombocytopenia is described in rare cases of KD, usually unassociated with consumption coagulopathy.[17,57] Thrombocytopenia is common in invasive bacterial infection and toxic shock syndromes and occurs in the early stages of RMSF and ehrlichiosis;[9] modest thrombocytopenia can occur with uncomplicated enteroviral infections. A normal or low, rather than high, neutrophil count with extreme left shift is a typical effect of bacterial toxins;[58] thrombocytopenia and consumption coagulopathy (with extremely low erythrocyte sedimentation rate) also are common. Pyuria without hematuria is common in KD but infrequent in other conditions except SJS.

Empiric therapies are shown in Table 13-1, and conditions other than Stevens–Johnson syndrome are discussed in depth in specific chapters. Prompt and aggressive antibiotic and supportive therapies are lifesaving in invasive bacterial infections and in staphylococcal exfoliative toxin syndrome in young infants. Antibiotic therapy may be beneficial in staphylococcal toxic shock, especially to treat focal infection and to prevent recurrence, but aggressive reversal of hypovolemia and cardiovascular shock is paramount. The important challenges in streptococcal toxic shock are: (1) halting microbial replication and toxin production; (2) reversing tissue ischemia, acidosis, hypovolemia, and hypotension; and (3) supporting multiorgan failure related to diffuse thromboemboli. Data from animal models of streptococcal necrotizing myositis, as well as clinical observations suggest that clindamycin is superior to β-lactam agents for treatment.[50,59]

Corticosteroid therapy is contraindicated as initial treatment of KD, is not indicated in staphylococcal exfoliative toxin syndrome, or staphylococcal or streptococcal toxic shock, and is controversial in SJS.[60] Aggressive care in burn units for children with SJS or toxic epidermal necrolysis with more than 10% skin loss improves outcome.[61] Many experts would give a 5-day trial of corticosteroids to a subset of children with SJS who are toxic and have mucosal involvement in addition to the mouth, skin eruption for 3 days or less, and less than 20% skin denudation.[19] Excess rate of infections[62] and mortality in drug-induced toxic epidermal necrolysis[61] have been reported with use of corticosteroids in uncontrolled studies.

PART II Clinical Syndromes and Cardinal Features of Infectious Diseases: Approach to Diagnosis and Initial Management

SECTION B Cardinal Symptom Complexes

Therapy with immune globulin intravenous (IGIV) is critical for optimal outcome in patients with KD[15,16] and is lifesaving for very young infants.[45] No randomized prospective study with adequate power has been performed to evaluate IGIV therapy in staphylococcal or streptococcal toxic shock. Case reports and retrospective, matched case-control studies in adults suggest a potential benefit. Dosage used was 500 mg/kg per day × 5 days for staphylococcal disease and 2 g/kg once for streptococcal disease.[63] A European randomized, double-blind, placebo-controlled trial of IGIV (1 g/kg on day 1 followed by 500 mg/kg on days 2 and 3) for streptococcal toxic shock[64] showed trend of benefit[65] but a multicenter retrospective study in U.S. children did not.[66] Anecdotal reports and predominantly retrospective case series of use of IGIV for severe SJS suggest possible beneficial effect but are conflicting.[60,67,68]

14 Fever without Localizing Signs

Eugene D. Shapiro

The vast majority of young children with fever and no apparent focus of infection have self-limited viral infections that resolve without treatment and are not associated with significant sequelae. However, a small proportion of them who do not appear to be seriously ill may be in the early stages of a serious bacterial infection or may have occult bacteremia. A very small proportion of the latter group may subsequently develop a serious focal infection such as meningitis. Despite numerous studies that attempted both to identify the febrile child who appears well but who actually has a serious infection and to assess effectiveness of potential interventions, no clear answers have emerged.[1-4] Studies show that parents generally are more willing than are physicians to assume the small risk of serious adverse outcomes in exchange for avoiding the short-term adverse effects of invasive diagnostic tests and antimicrobial treatment.[5,6] The best approach to the management of the febrile child combines informed estimates of risks, careful clinical evaluation and follow-up of the child, and judicious use of diagnostic tests.[7]

ETIOLOGIC AGENTS

The list of microbes that cause fever in children is extensive. Relative importance of specific agents varies with age, season, and associated symptoms. The focus of this chapter is the febrile child with occult bacterial infection.

Table 14-1 shows the most common causes of serious bacterial infection in children younger than 3 months.[8,9] The division at 1 month is not absolute; considerable overlap exists. Also, certain viruses, notably herpes simplex and enteroviruses, can cause serious infections in neonates, mimicking septicemia.

In children 3–35 months of age, most bacterial infections with no apparent focus are caused by *Streptococcus pneumoniae* (in unimmunized children), *Neisseria meningitidis*, or *Salmonella* spp. (the latter often occurring in association with symptoms of gastroenteritis). *Haemophilus influenzae* type b has become rare and incidence of *Streptococcus pneumoniae* infection has fallen substantially since universal administration of effective vaccines began.[10,11] Other common causes of invasive bacterial infections, such as *Staphylococcus aureus*, are usually associated with identifiable foci of infection.

EPIDEMIOLOGY

Children Younger than 3 Months

Risk of serious bacterial infection varies with age. Although longitudinal studies indicate that during their first 3 months only 1% to 2% of children come to medical attention for fever, a greater proportion of such febrile infants have serious bacterial infections than do older children.[12-15] Risk is greatest during the immediate neonatal period and through the first month (and is heightened in the infant born prematurely).

In a prospective study, researchers in Rochester identified factors associated with a low risk of serious bacterial infection in febrile infants younger than 3 months.[16] Among 233 infants who were born at term with no perinatal complications or underlying diseases, who had not received antibiotics, and who were hospitalized for fever, 144 (62%) were considered unlikely to have a serious bacterial infection and fulfilled all of the following criteria: (1) no clinical evidence of infection of the ear, skin, bones, or joints; (2) white blood cell (WBC) count between 5000 and 15,000/mm³; (3) <1500 band cells/mm³; and (4) normal results

TABLE 14-1. Age-Related Causes of Serious Bacterial Infections in Very Young Infants

BACTEREMIA/MENINGITIS	
<1 month	*Escherichia coli* (and other enteric gram-negative bacilli)
	Group B streptococcus
	Listeria monocytogenes
	Streptococcus pneumoniae
	Haemophilus influenzae
	Staphylococcus aureus
	Neisseria meningitidis
	Salmonella spp.
1–3 months	*Streptococcus pneumoniae*
	Group B streptococcus
	Neisseria meningitidis
	Salmonella spp.
	Haemophilus influenzae
	Listeria monocytogenes
OSTEOARTICULAR INFECTIONS	
<1 month	Group B streptococcus
	Staphylococcus aureus
1–3 months	*Staphylococcus aureus*
	Group B streptococcus
	Streptococcus pneumoniae
URINARY TRACT INFECTION	
0–3 months	*Escherichia coli*
	Other enteric gram-negative bacilli
	Group D streptococcus (including *Enterococcus* species)

of urinalysis. Only 1 of these 144 infants (0.7%) had a "serious" bacterial infection (*Salmonella* gastroenteritis), and none had bacteremia. By contrast, among the 89 infants who did not meet these criteria, 22 (25%) had a serious bacterial infection *(P<0.0001)* and 9 (10%) had bacteremia *(P<0.0005)*.

Subsequent investigations largely have corroborated results of the Rochester study.[17–20] Although investigators have used slightly different criteria to define young febrile infants at low risk of serious bacterial infection, all found that the risk of a serious bacterial illness in the group defined as being at low risk is, indeed, very low. In a meta-analysis of studies of febrile children younger than 3 months, the risks of "serious bacterial illness," bacteremia, and meningitis were 24.3%, 12.8%, and 3.9%, respectively, in "high-risk" infants and 2.6%, 1.3%, and 0.6%, respectively, in "low-risk" infants.[15] The negative predictive value for serious bacterial illnesses of infants fulfilling low-risk criteria ranged from 95% to 99% (and was 99% for bacteremia and 99.5% for meningitis).[15] Thus, clinical and laboratory assessment can be used to identify the slightly more than 50% of febrile infants <3 months of age at very low risk of serious bacterial infections.

An observational study of more than 3000 infants <3 months of age with fever >38°C treated by practitioners and reported as part of the Pediatric Research in Office Settings network found that the majority (64%) were not hospitalized.[3,21] Practitioners individualized management and relied on clinical judgment; "guidelines" were followed in only 42% of episodes.[3,21,22] Outcomes of the children were excellent. If the guidelines had been followed, outcomes would not have improved but there would have been both substantially more laboratory tests performed and more hospitalizations.[3]

Risk of serious bacterial infection has fallen further with the marked reduction in early-onset group B streptococcal infections because of effective peripartum antimicrobial prophylaxis of colonized pregnant women.[23] Risk of serious bacterial infections also is lower in febrile children who have an identified viral infection.[24]

Children 3 Months and Older

During the 1970s, reports of occult pneumococcal bacteremia began to appear.[25] Some children aged 3 months or older with fever who did not appear to be toxic and who had no apparent focus of infection had bacteremia, most often due to *Streptococcus pneumoniae* but occasionally due to *H. influenzae* type b or *N. meningitidis*.[25–32] Moreover, in some instances, serious focal infections such as meningitis developed in children with occult bacteremia.

The overall rates of bacteremia reported in studies of these febrile children range from 3% to 8%.[33] Fever alone is not associated with an excessive risk of bacteremia; the two largest studies of children 3 to 36 months of age with fever ≥39°C and no apparent focus of infection documented bacteremia in 2.8% (27 of 955) and 2.9% (195 of 6733) of children, respectively.[34,35] Frequency of occult bacteremia in disadvantaged urban populations and in suburban populations served by private practitioners is similar.[36,37] Risk of bacteremia is greater when very high fever is associated with high total WBC count.[22,27,33,38,39]

Most children with occult bacteremia have transient infection and recover (even without antimicrobial therapy) without having a serious complication such as meningitis or septic shock.[22,40–46] Risk of meningitis complicating occult bacteremia varies with bacterial species. Compared with the risk of developing meningitis with occult pneumococcal bacteremia (4 of 225; 1.8%), the odds of developing meningitis was 15 times greater for children with occult *H. influenzae* type b bacteremia and 81 times greater for children with occult *N. meningitidis* bacteremia.[32]

Risk of meningitis among children with occult bacteremia decreased substantially when occult bacteremia due to *H. influenzae* type b was virtually eliminated with introduction of the conjugate vaccine;[10,47] among children aged 3 to 35 months who are evaluated for high fever without a focus, it was estimated that bacterial meningitis would develop subsequently

in approximately 1 of 1000 to 1500 untreated children.[6] Consequently, even if "expectant" antimicrobial treatment of febrile children were 100% effective, it would have been necessary to treat 1000 to 1500 children to prevent 1 case of meningitis. In the United States, after introduction in 2000 of the polysaccharide–protein conjugate vaccine against 7 serotypes of pneumococci, substantial reduction in incidence of invasive disease has been documented in vaccinated children.[7,11] However, during this time there was a small increase in pneumococcal infections caused by serotypes not included in the vaccine, many of which, while less likely to be associated with bacteremia and meningitis than were some of the types in the vaccine, were still able to cause serious infections such as pneumonia and empyema.[7] In 2010, replacement of the 7-valent vaccine with a 13-valent conjugate pneumococcal vaccine promises to lead to additional decreases in serious bacterial infections in children caused by pneumococci and to further reduction of occult bacteremia and its consequences.[48]

LABORATORY FINDINGS AND DIAGNOSIS

Various diagnostic tests to quantify the risk of bacteremia and its complications have been assessed including the WBC count and differential, microscopic examination of buffy coat of blood, erythrocyte sedimentation rate, C-reactive protein, procalcitonin serum levels, morphologic changes in peripheral blood neutrophils, and quantitative cultures of blood.[22,38,49–55] In addition, clinical scales have been developed to help identify the febrile child with a serious illness.[56]

Unfortunately, no test has sufficient sensitivity and positive or negative predictive value to be clinically useful for an individual patient. In one prospective study of children with a temperature >40°C, those with a WBC count of ≥15,000/mm^3 had three times greater risk of bacteremia than did those with a WBC count of <15,000/mm^3.[27] However, the positive predictive value of this test for bacteremia was only 14%; thus, more than 85% of highly febrile children with a WBC count of ≥15,000/mm^3 did not have bacteremia. Others have reported similar results.[38,57] Subsequent to these studies, the prevalence of occult bacteremia diminished markedly because of introduction of vaccines effective against common causes of occult bacteremia and serious bacterial infections, so the positive predictive value of such test results is now substantially lower. Consequently, such testing as a routine can no longer be justified.[4,7,58]

The outcome of primary concern is not occult bacteremia but meningitis. An ideal diagnostic test would specifically identify febrile children at risk of a serious complication, because many focal infections after bacteremia (e.g., most cases of either pneumonia or cellulitis) can be treated when they become apparent and are not usually associated with serious sequelae. Unfortunately, there is no such test. Lowering the risk of serious complications by preventing infections through use of conjugate vaccines has proven to be the most effective strategy.

MANAGEMENT

Although there is no single correct approach to the management of febrile infants without localizing signs who appear well, studies have provided data upon which informed decisions can be based.[7] There is general agreement that febrile children who are "very young" (variably considered to be younger than 3, 2, or 1 month of age) should be managed differently from the way in which older children are managed.

Children Younger than 3 Months

Because of the substantially greater risk of serious infections in very young infants with fever and the difficulty in assessing degree of wellness accurately, pediatricians have approached the management of such infants conservatively. Some clinicians adhere to a protocol of treating all young infants with fever and no apparent focus of infection with broad-spectrum antimicrobial agents administered intravenously in the hospital until the results of

PART II Clinical Syndromes and Cardinal Features of Infectious Diseases: Approach to Diagnosis and Initial Management

SECTION B Cardinal Symptom Complexes

cultures of the blood, urine, and cerebrospinal fluid (CSF) are known.[59] Although sometimes perceived as the "safe" approach, such management incurs considerable financial cost and risk of iatrogenic complications and of diagnostic misadventures associated with hospitalization.[60-62] These risks include errors in the type and dosage of drugs, complications of venous cannulation (such as phlebitis and sloughing of the skin), and nosocomial infections. In addition, hospitalization of a young infant is a major disruption for the family and may potentiate the development of the "vulnerable child" syndrome.[63]

Investigators have found that selected young infants with fever can do well without hospitalization.[3,7,17,18,21,64] Consequently, many experts believe that febrile infants from 2 to 3 months of age with no apparent focus of infection who appear well and/or who have a laboratory-documented viral infection can be managed without either additional laboratory tests or hospitalization, provided that careful follow-up is ensured.[7] Others require laboratory criteria predictive of low risk (some include normal CSF analysis in the criteria). Some would simply observe the patient very closely without giving antimicrobial therapy; others would treat all such infants for 2 days with a single daily dose of ceftriaxone while awaiting the results of the cultures. Either approach can be defended.

If an antimicrobial agent is to be administered, cultures of the blood, urine, and CSF should be obtained first. Rapid tests for specific viral pathogens, which now are widely available, may aid decisions about managing patients and may reduce the need for and/or the duration of hospitalization.[7,65] Febrile infants at low risk of serious bacterial infection for whom adequate home observation and follow-up cannot be ensured should be hospitalized and can be observed without antimicrobial treatment. Doing so (if the child appears well) is reasonable and avoids the adverse side effects of antimicrobial agents and intravenous cannulation, shortens the duration of hospitalization, and saves money without placing the child at significant risk of complications.[18,21,64]

Most febrile infants with no apparent focus of infection who are younger than 1 month should be hospitalized and treated with antimicrobial therapy, although, in selected instances, hospitalization without antimicrobial treatment, or management as an outpatient (after laboratory evaluations, including analysis of CSF), may be reasonable. If a decision is made to administer antimicrobial agents intravenously, ampicillin plus gentamicin provides a suitable spectrum of activity until results of cultures permit discontinuation or alteration of treatment. Ampicillin plus a third-generation cephalosporin such as cefotaxime could be chosen, but there is no proven benefit in children without meningitis. Before initiating antimicrobial treatment, cultures of the blood, urine (obtained by either urethral catheterization or suprapubic aspiration of the bladder), and CSF should be obtained.

Children Older than 3 Months

Children older than 3 months of age who appear well and have no apparent focus of infection can be followed clinically without laboratory tests or treatment with antimicrobial agents; risk of occult or of serious bacterial infection is extremely low. For febrile children (i.e., those with a temperature ≥39°C) aged 3 to 35 months, there has been controversy about whether and which diagnostic tests should be performed and whether "expectant" antimicrobial treatment should be initiated.[6,7,22] Although results of a complete WBC count and differential may help to identify children at increased risk of occult bacterial infection, these tests have no direct therapeutic impact, and their positive predictive value is poor. Substantial evidence suggests that obtaining blood cultures routinely in these children has little impact on outcome (although false-positive blood culture results lead to substantial unnecessary costs).[66,67] The authors of a carefully conducted decision analysis concluded that a strategy of obtaining blood cultures in all such febrile children did more harm than good, in part because many children in whom bacteremia spontaneously clears are hospitalized and treated unnecessarily.[1] With the further decrease in the frequency of occult bacteremia and its

complications since introduction of conjugate pneumococcal vaccine, the balance is shifting even further away from benefit for routine testing of these children.[7] Indeed, isolates from cultures of the blood of are now substantially more likely to be contaminants than to be pathogens.[7]

Furthermore, it is not clear that "expectant" therapy of febrile children prevents serious complications such as meningitis. Two large randomized clinical trials were conducted of the efficacy of "expectant" antimicrobial treatment in preventing focal complications in all febrile (temperature of ≥39°C) children 3 to 36 months of age with no apparent focus of infection.

In the first trial, 955 children were randomized to receive either amoxicillin or placebo in a double-blind manner; no statistically significant difference in outcomes was observed.[34] However, because of the rarity of focal complications of bacteremia, 2 of 10 (10%) patients in the amoxicillin group and 1 of 8 (12.5%) patients in the placebo group, there was insufficient statistical power to exclude the possibility that amoxicillin is effective.

In the other clinical trial, 6733 children aged 3 to 36 months with a temperature of ≥39°C and no apparent focus of infection (or with otitis media) were randomized to receive 1 dose of ceftriaxone (50 mg/kg) or amoxicillin (20 mg/kg per dose) three times a day for 2 days.[35] Among children with occult bacteremia, no statistically significant difference was observed in the frequency of definite and probable complications (ceftriaxone, 3 of 101 (3.0%) patients; amoxicillin, 6 of 91 (6.6%) patients). Although the investigators seemed to endorse routine use of ceftriaxone, their methods and conclusions have been criticized.[6,68] Criticisms have included biased definition of the outcomes (a positive culture at follow-up is less likely in patients treated with ceftriaxone if focal infection was incipient or already present at enrollment), incomplete follow-up, and inappropriate statistical analyses. Furthermore, 4 of 5 children in whom meningitis developed were infected with *H. influenzae* type b, a disease that now has been virtually eliminated. Consequently, even if one accepted the investigators' conclusions, these data no longer apply.

Routine antimicrobial treatment of febrile children for possible occult bacteremia is not without risk.[6,7,69] In addition to substantial financial costs, antimicrobial agents have predictable as well as idiopathic adverse side effects. Widespread use of antibiotics selects for resistant organisms. In addition, loss of clinical improvement as a marker of natural history of infection in a partially treated child, difficulty in interpreting mildly abnormal CSF at follow-up, and frequent contaminated blood cultures all lead to increased frequency of unnecessary hospitalization and increased use of laboratory tests and of antimicrobial therapy. Perhaps most important, thoughtful assessment, individualized management, and close follow-up of the febrile child may be forgotten.

In view of current data, including the marked reduction in the incidence of invasive infections with vaccine-preventable pathogens in children, the following approach seems appropriate: The febrile child should be carefully assessed for foci of infection and, if found, should be treated according to likely pathogens. If the child appears toxic, appropriate cultures and diagnostic tests should be performed and antimicrobial treatment, usually with ceftriaxone, should be initiated (some would add vancomycin); most such children should be hospitalized. If no focus is found and the child does not appear toxic, no diagnostic tests are indicated routinely. Parents should be instructed to look for signs that a more serious problem is developing (e.g., persistent irritability or lethargy, inattentiveness to the environment). Serial observations should be planned that will permit subsequent clinical and laboratory evaluation and antimicrobial treatment as indicated.

Other Considerations

This chapter focuses on invasive bacterial infections (particularly bacteremia) as a cause of fever without apparent focus. It should not be forgotten that urinary tract infection is an important cause of fever in young children.[70] Indeed, urinalysis may be a more appropriate diagnostic test in the febrile infant than complete blood count or blood culture.[6,7,71] In addition, viral infections are the major cause of fever in infants and toddlers. Human herpesvirus 6 (and, to a lesser extent, human herpesvirus 7), influenza, respiratory syncytial virus, rhinovirus, and enteroviruses have been implicated as common causes of fever in young children.[7,72–74]

Although other serious illnesses, such as autoimmune diseases and inflammatory bowel disease, can manifest as fever without a focus, they are rare and come to attention because of persistence or recurrence of fever (see Chapter 15, Prolonged, Recurrent, and Periodic Fever Syndromes).

15 Prolonged, Recurrent, and Periodic Fever Syndromes

Sarah S. Long and Kathryn M. Edwards

Diagnosing and managing patients with prolonged, recurring, or periodic fever requires extensive review of symptoms and systems to establish onset and cardinal feature(s) of illness, to define the exact fever pattern, and to understand the context of illness within the patient's family and past medical history. Temperature is interpreted with the use of norms for age and sex (Figure 15-1).[1] At 18 months of age, mean rectal temperature for males is 37.7°C with a standard deviation (SD) of 0.38°C; thus, a rectal temperature of 38.5°C is <2 SD above the mean.

Defining fever patterns (such as shown in Box 15-1) is useful to prioritize differential diagnosis and investigation.[2] A disciplined physical examination is aimed at identifying target organ abnormalities of potential infectious and noninfectious diseases. In children with prolonged fever, laboratory testing should include simple screening and then targeted investigation is performed into specific organ systems as identified by history, physical examination, or prioritized clinical differential diagnosis (Box 15-2).[2] In children with periodic fever, the main goal of performing screening laboratory tests is to confirm normal organ system function, to lead the clinician toward a specific disorder (e.g., recurrent urinary tract infection), or to support the diagnosis of a noninfectious periodic fever syndrome. In evaluating children with any fever pattern, casting a broad net of antibody testing for unusual infectious agents is rarely fruitful in the absence of a specific exposure history or clinical finding.

FEVER OF UNKNOWN ORIGIN (FUO)

Definition and Approach

Criteria for FUO in Petersdorf and Beeson's landmark study in adults in 1961[3] were: (1) illness of more than 3 weeks' duration; (2) fever higher than 38.3°C on several occasions; and (3) uncertain diagnosis after 1 week of study in the hospital. Applying these criteria resulted in a high incidence of serious disease with infections accounting for 36% of cases, neoplastic diseases for 19%, collagen vascular diseases for 13%, and no diagnosis in 7% of cases. In a separate assessment of individuals with "fever" that did not exceed 38.3°C (even if protracted), diagnosis of significant illness was rare. A prospective, population-based study conducted in the 1990s in adults in the Netherlands used fixed epidemiologic entry criteria and a specific diagnostic protocol.[4,5] The classic definition of FUO was adjusted: immunocompromised patients were excluded, and 1 week of hospitalization was replaced with 1 week of intensive evaluation (usually including computed tomography

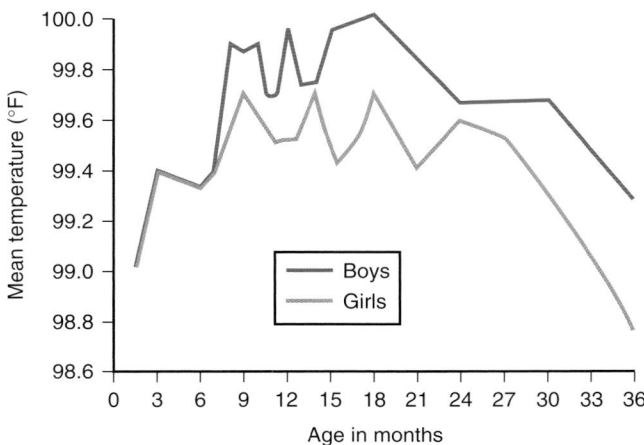

Figure 15-1. Normal mean rectal temperature is shown for boys and girls through 36 months of age. 100°F (37.8°C). Data from Bayley M, Stolz HR. Maturational changes in rectal temperature of 61 infants from 1 to 36 months. Child Dev 1937;8:195.

> **BOX 15-1.** Fever Patterns of Illness (for Purpose of Defining an Approach to Diagnosis)
>
> **Prolonged fever:** A single illness in which duration of fever exceeds that expected for the clinical diagnosis (e.g., >10 days for viral upper respiratory tract infections; >3 weeks for mononucleosis)
> *Or*
> A single illness in which fever was an initial major symptom and subsequently is low-grade or only a perceived problem
> **Fever of unknown origin:** A single illness of at least 3 weeks' duration in which fever >38.3°C is present on most days, and diagnosis remains uncertain after 1 week of intense evaluation
> **Recurrent fever:** A single illness in which fever and other signs and symptoms wax and wane (sometimes in relationship to discontinuation of antimicrobial therapy)
> *Or*
> Repeated unrelated febrile infections of the same organ system (e.g., sinopulmonary, urinary tract)
> *Or*
> Multiple illnesses occurring at irregular intervals, involving different organ systems in which fever is one variable component
> **Periodic fever:** Recurring episodes of illness for which fever is the cardinal feature, other associated symptoms are similar and predictable, duration of episodes is days to weeks, with intervening weeks to months of complete wellbeing. Episodes can have either "clockwork" or irregular periodicity

PART II Clinical Syndromes and Cardinal Features of Infectious Diseases: Approach to Diagnosis and Initial Management

SECTION B Cardinal Symptom Complexes

BOX 15-2. Physical Examination and Screening Laboratory Testing in Children with Prolonged, Recurrent, or Periodic Fever

PHYSICAL EXAMINATION
- Growth chart
- Thorough general examination
- Careful organ-specific examination
- Notation of mouth ulcers, exanthem, joint abnormalities, lymph nodes

TESTS
- Complete blood count with manual differential count of white blood cells[a]
- Erythrocyte sedimentation rate and C-reactive protein[a]
- Screening serum chemistry tests (and uric acid level if prolonged fever)
- Serum quantitative immunoglobulin levels
- Urinalysis
- Urine culture
- Chest plain radiograph (if prolonged or recurrent fever)
- Other imaging only as directed by examination/other screening tests
- Blood culture (if prolonged fever)

[a]Perform during episode and interval if periodic fever.

(CT) of the abdomen) and pursuit of potentially diagnostic clues without diagnosis. Infections accounted for 26% of cases, neoplasms for 13%, and noninfectious inflammatory diseases for 24%. No diagnosis was made in 30% of patients, three-quarters of whom recovered spontaneously. In another prospective multicenter study in adults in the Netherlands, using the structured diagnostic protocol, 51% of patients had no cause of FUO found.[6]

Limiting factors of published case series of FUO in children include small numbers, variability in definition of FUO and investigation of subjects, study methodologies, years and sites of study, and subspecialty referral biases.[7] In multiple studies of FUO in children, decreasing stringency of entry criteria correlates with increased likelihood of self-limited conditions.[8-14] When fever approaches 4 weeks' duration without a definable source, the rate of life-altering diagnoses, such as malignancy, collagen vascular disease, and inflammatory bowel disease, rises to 40% in some series.[9-11] In a Greek study of adults, C-reactive protein (CRP) >6 mg/dL, eosinophils <40/mm^3, ferritin <500 µg/L were independently associated with infection, with positive predictive value of ≥2 of these findings of 86% for infectious diagnoses and negative predictive value of 95% when ≥2 findings were absent.[8]

For purposes of management, FUO in children is only considered after a minimum of 14 days of daily documented temperature of 38.3 °C or greater without apparent cause after performance of repeated physical examinations and screening laboratory tests. This definition assumes exclusion of: (1) protracted but waning symptoms from acute, self-limited respiratory tract infections; (2) well-documented periodic fever; and (3) repeated but unrelated episodes of fever with identifiable causes. Almost one-half of children referred for FUO do not meet fever and exclusion criteria. In those who do, careful reassessment of history and physical examination often reveals potentially diagnostic clues that should be pursued with targeted testing.[15] FUO is more likely an unusual presentation of a common disease than an uncommon disease.[16] A chest radiograph (regardless of symptoms) and CT of the sinuses (with symptoms) are viewed as "early studies" in the workup. Chest CT may be indicated when granulomatous or embolic disease is suspected. In an evaluation of 28 children with prolonged fever by abdominal CT, 86% of children in whom clinical features directed suspicion to the abdomen had positive CT findings; the yield of the procedure in others was low.[17] In another study of 109 children with FUO, multiple modalities, including

radioisotope scans, rarely led to an unsuspected diagnosis.[18] Performing imaging studies in absence of signs or symptoms of involvement of that organ system generally is not helpful. Furthermore, "definite normal" interpretation of imaging studies is unusual, and often, any "abnormality" leads to further studies, all of which can divert focus from a correct diagnosis.

In a rigorous prospective study of FUO in adults in whom no potentially diagnostic clues were gleaned from the history or physical examination, the diagnostic yield of scintigraphy, other imaging modalities, liver or bone marrow biopsy, and screen for endocrine abnormalities was nil.[5] Fluorodeoxyglucose position emission tomography (FDG-PET) was thought to be an "early", useful test in FUO in adults in the Netherlands[6] and in one meta-analysis.[19] FDG-PET is not adequately studied in children with FUO. Biopsy of enlarged lymph nodes confined to cervical and inguinal areas (in a patient with normal findings on chest radiograph and abdominal ultrasonography) also was fruitless.[5] The investigators of this study recommend repeating a thorough exploration of the history, physical examination, and "first-level" laboratory tests and waiting for potential diagnostic clues to appear.[5] This approach is appropriate in children as well, unless there is progression of weight loss, or of an abnormality on examination or simple screening tests.

Etiology

A systematic review in 2011 of 18 studies published since 1968 divided studies into those performed in developed countries (8

TABLE 15-1. Reported Infectious Causes of Fever of Unknown Origin in 832 Children in Developed and Developing Countries[7]

Infection	Developed Countries[a] (N = 275)	Developing Countries[b] (N = 557)	Most Common Agents/ Infections (in descending order of frequency)
Bacteria	56%	61%	Developed: Urinary tract, osteomyelitis, tuberculosis, *Bartonella*, septicemia (not specified), *Salmonella*, *Brucella* Developing: *Brucella*, urinary tract, *Salmonella*, tuberculosis, abscess (not specified), septicemia (not specified)
Viruses	15%	3%	Developed: Epstein–Barr virus, cytomegalovirus, enterovirus Developing: Epstein–Barr virus, cytomegalovirus, human-immune deficiency virus
Fungi	1%	0.2%	Developed: *Blastomyces*, *Histoplasma*
Parasites	2%	14%	Developed: *Leishmania* Developing: *Leishmania*, *Plasmodium*
Infectious syndrome without pathogen	26%	22%	Developed: Viral syndrome (not specified), pneumonia, meningitis Developing: Pneumonia, respiratory tract (not specified), infectious mononucleosis, viral syndrome (not specified)

[a]U.S., Germany, and Spain.

[b]Tunisia, India, Turkey, Poland, Argentina, Serbia, Georgia, and Kuwait.

studies from just three countries, all published more than one decade ago) and in developing countries (10 studies, 8 published since 2000).[7] A total of 1638 children were reported, the majority of whom had fever of 2 to 3 weeks' duration; at least 80% were inpatients during at least part of their investigation. Overall, categories of diagnoses in developed and developing countries were remarkably similar: infection in 51%, malignancy in 6%, collagen

vascular diseases (CVD) in 9%, miscellaneous noninfectious conditions in 11%, and no diagnosis in 23%. Infectious causes were slightly more common in developing countries (56% vs. 42%), while no diagnosis was more common in developed countries (31% vs. 18%). Infections diagnosed in 832 children are shown in Table 15-1.

Box 15-3 summarizes noninfectious causes of FUO. In the systematic review, leukemia and lymphoma were the most common malignancies, and juvenile idiopathic arthritis and systemic lupus erythematosus the most common CVDs. Inflammatory bowel disease and non-specified autoimmune disease were the most common miscellaneous diagnoses in developing countries and Kawasaki disease the most common miscellaneous diagnosis in developed countries.[7]

Table 15-2 displays some discriminating features of infectious and noninfectious causes of FUO.[22-62] Generally, for infections, the agents, sites, and clinical manifestations are typical but are subtle and overlooked, or are associated with an insidious or prolonged course.[2,20,21] In older series, almost half the patients with infections had upper or lower respiratory tract infections exclusive of granulomatous disease. In the latest prospective series of children in the United States, none of the children had respiratory tract infection.[12] Agents that produce granulomatous infections (e.g., *Bartonella*, *Mycobacterium*, *Salmonella*, *Brucella*, and *Francisella* species) cause FUO disproportionately and frequently involve the visceral organs, reticuloendothelial system, and bone marrow.[21]

BOX 15-3. Noninfectious Causes of Fever of Unknown Origin

- Kawasaki disease
- Autoimmune diseases
- Autoinflammatory disorders
- Inflammatory bowel disease
- Malignancy
- Drugs, other medicinal and nutritional products
- Munchausen syndrome by proxy
- Dysautonomia
- Central thermoregulatory disorder
- Diabetes insipidus
- Anhidrotic ectodermal dysplasia
- Hyperthyroidism
- Hematoma in a closed space
- Pulmonary embolus

TABLE 15-2. Discriminating Features of Infectious and Noninfectious Causes of Fever of Unknown Origin

	Exposure/Condition	Features	Diagnostic Method
INFECTIOUS CAUSES			
Salmonella species[22-25]	Exposure to endemic; immigration; turtles, animals, foodstuffs	High spiking fever; overlooked or mild abdominal pain	Culture blood, stool; culture bone marrow (if antibiotic given)
Bartonella henselae[12,26-29]	Kitten; healthy and immunocompromised persons	Mild abdominal complaints, headache; lymphadenopathy usually absent; hepatic/splenic, bone marrow granulomas	Serology; histology
Epstein–Barr virus[12,30]		"Typhoidal" course without classic mononucleosis symptoms/signs; malaise; pneumonia	Serology; plasma PCR
Yersinia enterocolitica[31]	Animals, especially pigs; pork chitterlings	Abdominal pain; hepatic/splenic granulomas/ abscess; exanthems	Culture blood, stool, biopsy specimen; serology
Mycobacterium tuberculosis[32-34]	Exposure to symptomatic adults; endemic; immigration; HIV	Extrapulmonary, miliary, disseminated disease	Chest radiograph; tuberculin skin test; culture gastric aspirate, bone marrow, biopsy specimen
M. non-*tuberculosis*[35]	HIV, malignancy, cystic fibrosis; occasionally healthy toddler	Respiratory/gastrointestinal symptoms; mediastinal lymphadenopathy	Culture gastric aspirate, blood, stool, mediastinal/enteric biopsy specimen; histology
Plasmodium species[7,22]	Exposure to mosquitoes in endemic; rare in U.S. mosquito, blood transfusion	Persistent (early) or remitting spiking fever, splenomegaly; anemia	Wright stain blood smears
Brucella species[36,37]	Unpasteurized dairy products; farm animals	High spiking fever, arthralgia, hepatomegaly; elevated hepatic transaminases; Coombs-positive anemia	Serology
Coxiella burnetii[38]	Unpasteurized dairy products; aerosol parturient cat	Fever persistent 5–10 days or relapsing over months; elevated hepatic transaminases	Serology
Francisella tularemia	Tick/flea/mite/deer fly; airborne or direct contact animal	Ulceroglandular, "typhoidal", pleuropneumoniae	Serology
Leptospira species	Rodents, domestic animals	Persistent or biphasic fever, aseptic meningitis; hepatitis	Serology
Leishmania	Exposure to endemic; immigration	Insidious onset (2–6 months); hepatosplenomegaly; Coombs-positive anemia	Giemsa or Wright stain biopsy/aspirate specimen; culture bone; serology

Continued

PART II Clinical Syndromes and Cardinal Features of Infectious Diseases: Approach to Diagnosis and Initial Management

SECTION B Cardinal Symptom Complexes

TABLE 15-2. Discriminating Features of Infectious and Noninfectious Causes of Fever of Unknown Origin—cont'd

	Exposure/Condition	Features	Diagnostic Method
Rickettsia, Ehrlichia, Anaplasma[12]	Exposure to ticks in endemic	Absent or atypical rash; headache	Serology; PCR; Wright stain of blood/CSF (morulae of *Anaplasma, Ehrlichia*)
Neisseria meningitidis (chronic)		Petechial exanthema	Culture of blood
Toxocara canis, T. catis	Dog and cat feces; pica	Hepatosplenomegaly; eosinophilia; hypergammaglobulinemia	Serology
Human immunodeficiency virus	Sexual/vertical acquisition	Hepatosplenomegaly; mononucleosis syndrome; hypergammaglobulinemia	PCR; serology
Endocarditis	Congenital or acquired heart disease, central venous catheter; occasionally no underlying condition	Splenomegaly, new heart murmur; immune-complex exanthems; anemia; HACEK organism from blood culture; persistent positive blood culture	Blood culture; echocardiogram; consideration of uncultivatable pathogens
Intra-abdominal retroperitoneal abscess[7,39-41]	Appendicitis; surgery; urinary tract infection; *Staphylococcus aureus* bloodstream infection	Localized pain/tenderness; elevated inflammatory markers; positive blood culture	Computed tomography
Pelvic/vertebral osteomyelitis		Localized pain/tenderness; elevated inflammatory markers; positive blood culture	Magnetic resonance imaging
Odontogenic infection[42]	Dental caries	Painful teeth, discomfort with chewing/biting on tongue depressor; lung abscess; submandibular/submental lymphadenopathy; swelling, tenderness face/jaw	Dental radiography
Kikuchi–Fujimoto disease[43,44]		Regional or generalized lymphadenopathy; elevated inflammatory markers	Biopsy/histology
Inflammatory pseudotumor[45-47]	History of prior nonspecific illness (presumed host-controlled infection)	Insidious; malaise, weight loss, vague abdominal pain/tenderness; anemia; elevated inflammatory markers	Abdominal computed tomography; biopsy/histology
NONINFECTIOUS CAUSES Kawasaki disease (incomplete)[48,49]		Asynchronous or incomplete features Kawasaki disease; elevated inflammatory markers; thrombocytosis	Clinical constellation; echocardiogram
Juvenile idiopathic arthritis[13,50]	Familial, sporadic	Hepatosplenomegaly, lymphadenopathy, exanthem; anemia, elevated inflammatory markers	Clinical constellation
Systemic lupus erythematosus	Familial, sporadic	Malaise, weight loss; then multisystem involvement (kidneys, joints, skin)	Serum anti-nuclear antibody, anti-double-stranded DNA, anti-smooth muscle antibody
Hemophagocytic lymphohistiocytosis[51,52]	Virus-associated; familial; rheumatologic disorder	Severe, rapidly progressive illness; hepatomegaly, lymphadenopathy, exanthem; cytopenias; extreme elevations inflammatory markers	Ferritin, triglyceride levels, other diagnostic criteria; macrophage phagocytosis blood cells; natural killer cell, CD8+ T-lymphocyte dysfunction
Vasculitis syndromes	Familial, sporadic	Specific hallmarks (renal, neurologic, stomatitis/perianal ulcers, uveitis, pulmonary)	Clinical constellation; specific autoantibodies; biopsy/histology
Sarcoidosis[53]	Geography; race	Fatigue, weight loss, leg pain; anemia, elevated inflammatory markers; mediastinal lymphadenopathy; uveitis	Clinical constellation; biopsy/histology
Inflammatory bowel disease	Familial; sporadic	Linear growth failure, subtle gastrointestinal symptoms/abdominal tenderness; perirectal skin tag; iron-deficiency anemia; elevated inflammatory markers	Abdominal computed tomography; barium study
Lymphoreticular malignancy[7,54,57]		Weight loss, fatigue; nonarticular bone pain; lymphadenopathy; cytopenias	Bone marrow/tissue biopsy
Drug hypersensitivity[58,59]	Prescription/nonprescription drug exposure	Preserved sense of wellbeing; exanthems; eosinophilia; organ dysfunction (renal, cardiac, pulmonary)	Clinical constellation; withdrawal of drug
Factitious fever/Munchausen syndrome by proxy[60]	Predisposing parent–patient dynamic	Discordant temperature-vital signs; discordant parent-measured temperature and urine temperature; normal inflammatory markers	Clinical constellation; medical validation temperature
Hypothalamic dysfunction/diabetes insipidus/dysautonomia/absent corpus callosum[61,62]	Underlying condition; genetic syndrome; anatomic abnormality	Normal inflammatory markers; hypernatremia; no response to nonsteroidal anti-inflammatory drugs	Clinical constellation; laboratory tests and imaging

PROLONGED INSIGNIFICANT FEVER, PROLONGED ILLNESS WITH RESOLVED FEVER, FATIGUE OF DECONDITIONING

One of the most frequent referrals to pediatric infectious disease subspecialists for "prolonged fever" is an adolescent with low-grade or falsely perceived fever, or whose fever has resolved who generally feels unwell and is unable to attend school and social activities. Such patients require the same disciplined performance of history and examination as those with true FUO. For the sub-specialist to offer a definitive opinion, the family must perceive that a thorough and thoughtful consultation has occurred. All laboratory test results, actual imaging studies, and biopsy slides should be reviewed. The findings listed in Box 15-4, evaluation of complaints, review of systems, and laboratory test results taken together suggest that no cryptogenic infection or serious medical condition is present.[2]

The discordance of lengthy list of complaints with the normal findings of examination and laboratory tests is typical. The family's modus operandi centers around the patient. Prodded recitation of a typical 24-hour period of activity reveals a feeling of tiredness but no prolongation of actual time asleep. There is frequently a parental model of chronic illness, or a recent change in extended-family dynamics (e.g., divorce, serious medical diagnosis, death). Deconditioning (i.e., diminution of physical strength, stamina, and vitality), loss of self-esteem, fear of failure to perform at previous expectation, and secondary gain may all play into the clinical state. The patient should be queried privately about potential abuse and other insights. Depression should be considered. Clues in depressed individuals include a feeling of sadness all the time, lack of self-worth, dislike of or wanting to hurt oneself, anger, marginalization, and feeling of being disliked by others.[63] Fatigued individuals generally do not have these feelings, but instead have increased somatic complaints and a tendency to internalize stress.[64] In the last decade, neurally mediated hypotension and postural tachycardia have been postulated as mechanisms of persistent fatigue. Two studies in adults published in 2005 suggest that orthostatic instability is a common finding in healthy as well as in fatigued individuals,[65] and that among military recruits with orthostatic intolerance, endurance exercise training significantly improved the physiologic findings and symptoms.[66] In a formal study of 14 adolescents with orthostatic hypotension, symptoms and findings were attenuated by static hand grip[67] (see Chapter 200, Chronic Fatigue Syndrome).

Management of patients with fatigue of deconditioning begins with a precise review of findings and conclusions of what the

diagnosis is and is not.[2] Management is outlined in Box 15-5. It is a disservice to diagnose "chronic fatigue syndrome," support home tutoring, or refer the patient to additional subspecialists for minor findings. The primary care pediatrician should set the tempo for reconditioning and monitoring. A personal fitness trainer may introduce a new positive relationship with the patient that separates the patient effectively from an illness-enabling family dynamic.

RECURRENT, PERIODIC, AND HEREDITARY PERIODIC FEVER SYNDROMES

Recurrent Fever

When history is carefully obtained, most children who are referred to subspecialists for recurrent fever have multiple self-limited infections. Relapsing infection is an unusual cause of recurring fevers,[68] unless malaria is a possibility. Fever, in the absence of respiratory tract symptoms, which abates repeatedly during antibiotic therapy can occasionally be due to endocarditis or renal infection in predisposed hosts. *Borrelia recurrentis* is a rare cause of tickborne relapsing fever distinguished by history of travel through forested areas. Periodic fever syndromes are uncommon but must be considered.

Periodic Fever Syndromes

For purposes of clinical approach to diagnosis, periodic fever is defined as recurring episodes of illness in which fever is the cardinal feature; episodes have a predictable onset, symptom complex and duration; and episodes are separated by symptom-free intervals. Some syndromes are characterized by "clockwork" periodicity (i.e., multiple calendar-documented recurrences with the same duration of episodes and the same duration of wellness intervals). Differentiating features of periodic fever syndromes likely to be encountered by an infectious diseases subspecialist are shown in Table 15-3. Most are due to autoinflammation, many of which have a genetic basis. PFAPA and cyclic neutropenia are not included as autoinflammatory periodic fever syndromes because PFAPA

TABLE 15-3. Differentiating Features of Periodic Fever Syndromes

	PFAPA	Cyclic Neutropenia	FMF	HIDS/MVK Deficiency	TRAPS	CAPS
OMIM	–	162800	249100	260920	142680	FCAS, 120100 MWS, 191900 NOMID, 607115
Usual inheritance	Sporadic	Autosomal dominant	Autosomal recessive	Autosomal recessive	Autosomal dominant	Autosomal dominant, or de novo (NOMID)
Genetic locus/gene	–	19p13/*ELA2*	16p13/*MEFV*	12q24/*MVK*	12q13/*TNFRSF1A*	1q44/*CIAS1*
Protein	–	Neutrophil elastase	Pyrin/marenostrin	Mevalonate kinase	p55 TNFR1	Cryopyrin
Onset <5 years	Expected	Usual; often <1 year old	Common; peak onset middle of first decade	Expected; median 6 months	Variable; severe form <1 year old	Expected, almost always <6 months
Length of fever episode	3–6 days	5–7 days	1–3 days	3–7 days	7–21 days	<24 h (FCAS); 1–2 days (MWS); short fevers, almost continuous other manifestations (NOMID)
Periodicity of episodes	q3–6 wk (mean 28 days)	q14–28 days (most 21 days)	Irregular intervals: weeks, months, or occasionally years	q4–8 wk or irregular intervals; immunization trigger	Irregular intervals: weeks to years	Cold trigger (FCAS); irregular intervals (MWS); no interval/continuous (NOMID)
Associated symptoms/signs	Pharyngitis, aphthous stomatitis, cervical adenopathy, chills, headache (each > ⅔); abdominal pain, nausea/vomiting (each ⅓)	Ulcers, gingivitis, periodontitis; otitis media, sinusitis, cellulitis; rare peritonitis; rare gram-negative bacillary or clostridial septicemia	Polyserositis; erysipelas-like rash; scrotal pain and swelling	Headache, chills, abdominal pain, diarrhea in young; arthralgia; small macules, papules, nodules, especially on extremities; splenomegaly	Migratory myalgia and pseudocellulitis; conjunctivitis; periorbital edema; other	Urticaria-like rash (FCAS); erythematous and edematous papules → plaques (MWS, NOMID)
Laboratory findings	Mild neutrophilia, ESR elevated <60 mm/h (during episode only)	Absolute neutrophil count <200 cells/mm³ for 3–5 days in cycle	Elevated acute-phase response	Elevated acute-phase response; variable ↑IgA and IgD	Elevated acute-phase response	Elevated acute-phase response, ±eosinophilia

OMIM, Online Mendelian Inheritance in Man;[101] ESR, erythrocyte sedimentation rate; G-CSF, granulocyte colony-stimulating factor. See text for other abbreviations and treatment.

cases usually are non-familial, innate immune defects have not been established, and the etiology is unknown. Clinical manifestations in cyclic neutropenia are related more to absence of neutrophil protection than to autoinflammation.

Periodic Fever, Aphthous Stomatitis, Pharyngitis, and Cervical Adenitis (PFAPA)

Epidemiology and Cardinal Clinical Features

PFAPA was first described in 1987 in 12 children from Tennessee and Alabama.[69] More than 700 cases from multiple continents and racial backgrounds have been reported; there are undoubtedly exponentially more cases not reported. PFAPA appears to be predominantly a sporadic disorder. However, history of recurrent fevers or PFAPA-like illnesses (in parent or sibling) is as high as 20%[70] and 45%,[71] and cases in monozygotic twins are reported.[72] In one study, blood samples from PFAPA patients during flares (12) compared with those during asymptomatic intervals (21) and from healthy controls (21) showed overexpression of complement genes during PFAPA attacks, suggesting an infectious trigger with a strong IP-10, and IL-1/IL-18-mediated response of the innate immune system.[73] Activation and probable recruitment of T lymphocytes to peripheral tissues suggest involvement of adaptive immunity in the pathogenesis of PFAPA. Shortening of asymptomatic interval in up to 50% of steroid-treated PFAPA patients[70,74] also is compatible with partial infectious pathophysiology.[75]

Multiple studies attempting to identify a pathogen of PFAPA have been negative.

Table 15-4 shows features of PFAPA patients followed through a Nashville registry.[76] Clockwork cycle and abrupt onset after 1 to 2 hours of "glassy eyes" and clinging behavior followed by fever >39°C (which persists at that height for most of the duration of the episode) are cardinal features, overshadowing others. There are no recognizable triggering events. Respiratory symptoms are absent. Typically, mouth ulcers are small, shallow, scattered or solitary, seemingly not painful; and frequently only are noted in episodes subsequent to the query. "Pharyngitis" usually includes tonsils that are normal or moderately enlarged, erythematous but are not exudative (a discrepant characteristic finding between U.S. case series and some others[77–79]). Cervical lymph nodes wax and wane with episodes, are mildly tender bilaterally but are not erythematous or larger than 3 to 4 cm. Description of the syndrome generally is similar across countries and has not changed over 2 decades.[74,75,80–82]

Absent or minimal response to acetaminophen, nonsteroidal anti-inflammatory drugs, or antibiotics is typical of PFAPA. Use of a corticosteroid abruptly aborts an episode, but this should not be used as a diagnostic test since patients with hyperimmunoglobulinemia D syndrome (HIDS), tumor necrosis factor receptor-associated periodic fever syndrome (TRAPS), and many infectious diseases can have similar response.[70] Children with PFAPA are completely well and fully energetic between episodes, seem to have fewer symptomatic infectious diseases than siblings, are viewed as healthy by parents, and grow and gain milestones normally.

TABLE 15-4. Characteristics of Cases at Diagnosis of Periodic Fever, Aphthous Stomatitis, Pharyngitis, and Cervical Adenopathy (PFAPA)

Demographic and Clinical Features		Percent with Signs and Symptoms at Episodes[a]	
Male : Female	1.2	Fever + >1 cardinal feature	97%
Onset of PFAPA	2.8 years (2.4–3.3 years)[b]	Cervical lymphadenopathy (77%)	
Maximum temperatures	40.5°C (40.4–40.6°C)	Aphthous stomatitis (67%)	
Duration of fever	3.8 days (3.5–4.1 days)	Pharyngitis (65%)	
Duration of episode	4.8 days (4.5–5.1 days)	Chills	80%
Episodes/year	11.5 (10.5–12.5)	Headache	65%
Wellness interval	28.2 days (26.0–30.4 days)	Nausea	52%
Mean white blood cell count at episode	13,000/mm^3 (range 2–37 × 10^3)	Abdominal pain	45%
Mean erythrocyte sedimentation rate at episode	41 (range 5–190 mm/hour)	Diarrhea	30%
		Coryza	18%
		Rash	15%

[a]*Although 94 children were included in the original registry, parents did not always answer all queries (frequently citing inability to assess because of age).*

[b]*Mean (95% confidence interval).*

Modified from Thomas KT, Feder HM, Lawton AR, et al. Periodic fever syndrome in children. J Pediatr 1999;135:15–21.[76]

Treatment and Outcome

Data on >200 children with PFAPA followed for >2 years[74,76] and 60 children followed for 12 to 21 years have been published.[82] More than 50% of children with PFAPA have fever episodes for >2 years[74] and >3 years.[76] In the very long follow-up study, 83% had complete resolution of PFAPA (mean duration 6.3 years); 15% continued to have persistent PFAPA for a mean duration of 18.1 years.[82] Symptoms at onset of PFAPA for those without resolution were similar to others with PFAPA, although over time persisters had shorter duration of fever (1.8 days) and longer symptom-free interval (29 to 59 days). Of 60 patients, 1 patient was diagnosed with Behçet disease and another with familial Mediterranean fever. Episodes of PFAPA are expected to retain characteristics as at diagnosis. Families should be queried at follow-up for development of additional features. If such occurs, a differential diagnosis should be reconsidered. Lengthening of the wellness interval frequently precedes resolution of PFAPA.

Cimetidine therapy is associated with resolution or amelioration of fever attacks in approximately one-third of patients.[76] Prednisone (most often given as one or two doses of 1–2 mg/kg/day) characteristically aborts an attack of PFAPA.[74,76,82] In a single medical center experience, a lower dose of prednisone (mean 0.6 mg/kg/day) also was effective.[83] It is not our practice to use prednisone as routine management of episodes of PFAPA, as mean frequency of 11.5 episodes annually could lead to substantial corticosteroid exposure and risk of adverse effects.

Tonsillectomy was first noted to benefit patients with PFAPA in 1989.[84] A systematic review was published in 2011 evaluating the benefit of tonsillectomy with or without adenoidectomy in resolution at PFAPA.[85] Studies totaled only 15 and treated children only 149; 13 studies were observational, non-comparative (of which 11 were retrospective) and 2 were prospective, randomized controlled trials (RCT).[86,87] Other limitations were variability in criteria for diagnosis of PFAPA, type of surgical procedure performed (tonsillectomy with or without adenoidectomy), and duration of follow-up. Using complete resolution as the primary outcome, resolution following surgery was 83% (95% CI, 77–89%) for all studies combined, and odds ratio for complete resolution following surgery for the two RCTs was 13 (95% CI, 4–43).[85]

It is our practice to discuss these data with parents at the time of diagnosis, assess with them the degree to which episodes interfere with the child's and family's quality of life, and recommend commencement of a diary and follow-up to accrue a history of multiple episodes over one year before a surgical decision is made. With this approach, some patients do not have PFAPA-fulfilling courses; many families are comfortable with following the natural history; and a few evolve to symptoms of a genetic autoinflammatory disease. PFAPA resolves spontaneously in childhood in most cases with no known long-term adverse effects.

History of recurrent fever episodes after a hiatus of years after a PFAPA diagnosis should lead to investigation for other diagnoses. Padeh reported 14 adults in Israel with PFAPA-like conditions with onset in adolescence or early adulthood; episodes all responded to a single dose of prednisone. All had exudative tonsillitis and 40% had arthralgia or myalgia; genetic and rheumatologic testing was not reported.[88]

Cyclic Neutropenia

Epidemiology and Etiology

Cyclic neutropenia is an autosomal dominantly inherited hematologic disorder characterized by regular cycling of the peripheral blood neutrophil count to nadir of <500 cells/mm^3 (usually <200 cells/mm^3), and a symptom complex manifesting during the neutrophil nadir. Cyclic neutropenia was first recognized more than a century ago. Favorable response to granulocyte colony-stimulating factor was reported in 1989 and mutations in the *ELA2* gene encoding neutrophil elastase (in cyclic as well as severe congenital neutropenia) were reported in 1999.[89] There are multiple confirming reports, as well as long-term treatment and outcome data of >200 patients from multiple continents entered into the Severe Chronic Neutropenia International Registry.[90] Mutations in *HAX1* and *CSF3R* genes also have been identified in severe congenital neutropenias, suggesting a spectrum of possible genotypes and phenotypes.[91] Currently the favored hypothesis is that mutations encoding the protease neutrophil elastase lead to destabilization of a proteoglycan, which induces unfolding, which in turn increases the transcription of chaperone-encoding, endoplasmic reticulum-associated protein degradation and pro-apoptotic genes that leads ultimately to neutrophil apoptosis, i.e., "mutation arrest", as seen in bone marrow.[91]

Cardinal Clinical Features

Diagnosis of cyclic neutropenia usually is established early in childhood. Cardinal features are recurrent fever with clockwork periodicity, pharyngitis, mouth ulcers, and lymphadenopathy. Some cases are diagnosed because of recurrent bacterial cellulitis at sites of minor trauma. Gingivitis and periodontitis are remarkable and persistent into the second week following a fever episode; mouth ulcers are deep and painful. Periodontal disease can lead to deciduous tooth loss in childhood. Recurrent bacterial infections – cellulitis, otitis media, sinusitis, pharyngitis – distinguish cyclic neutropenia from the periodic autoinflammatory syndromes. Some patients have few or relatively minor associated bacterial infections, while others can have spontaneous bacterial peritonitis, overwhelming gram-negative or *Clostridium* septicemia or septic shock resulting from ileocolonic ulceration during

PART II Clinical Syndromes and Cardinal Features of Infectious Diseases: Approach to Diagnosis and Initial Management

SECTION B Cardinal Symptom Complexes

neutropenic episodes. Although oral manifestations linger, these children usually are well between episodes.

During the neutropenic period, peripheral blood neutrophils characteristically fall to <200 cells/mm³ for 3 to 5 days. The count then usually rises and remains at approximately 2000 cells/mm³. At the time that clinical symptoms of fever, stomatitis, and lymphadenopathy appear, neutropenia may be resolving – typically with immature myelocytic cells present in peripheral blood. Children with clockwork periodicity of fevers plus *any* family or clinical feature (as noted above) compatible with cyclic neutropenia should have twice-weekly complete blood counts performed during the interval of wellness and continuing through the next febrile episode. Alternatively or additionally, genetic testing for *ELA2* mutations can be performed. Although inheritance is autosomal dominant, manifestations can be mild and the parental inheritance unrecognized.

Course, Treatment, and Outcome

Granulocyte colony-stimulating factor (G-CSF) administered subcutaneously daily is effective treatment of cyclic neutropenia. G-CSF is thought to affect intracellular signaling as well as stimulate production. Adverse effects associated with G-CSF include osteopenia and osteoporosis; anecdotal evidence suggests beneficial effect of bisphosphonate therapy. Although there is a substantial risk of myelodysplasia and acute myelogenous leukemia in children with severe congenital neutropenia compared with cyclic neutropenia, many experts in the field believe that with increasing survival of patients receiving G-CSF, such cases will occur in cyclic neutropenia.[90] The causal role of G-CSF therapy in development of myelodysplasia and acute myelogenous leukemia versus the genetic defect is uncertain.

Hereditary Periodic Fever Syndromes

The term *autoinflammatory syndrome* was used in the late 1990s to describe a group of systemic inflammatory diseases apparently different from infectious, autoimmune, allergic, and immunodeficiency-associated diseases.[92,93] Unlike autoimmune disorders that require development of targeted antibodies and activation of T lymphocytes, autoinflammatory diseases result from genetically predisposed dysregulation of innate immune signaling. The characterization of patients with recurring autoinflammatory illnesses into distinct clinical phenotypes provided clues to the mode of inheritance of these conditions and facilitated subsequent identification of causative gene mutations. An excellent review and updated classification scheme based on molecular insights is proposed to replace clinical classification.[94] The proposed categories of autoinflammatory diseases are: IL-1β activation disorders (inflammasomopathies), NF-κB activation syndromes, protein misfolding disorders, complement regulatory diseases, disturbances of cytokine signaling, and macrophage activation syndromes. Surprisingly many identified mutations result in gain of function and manifest with inflammation that seemingly is unprovoked and systemic. Diagnosis and management are changing rapidly.[94-100] Those conditions known to be hereditary result from gene mutations and are registered in the Online Mendelian Inheritance in Man (OMIM) database (http://www.ncbi.nlm.nih.gov/sites/entrez?db=OMIM).[101] Genotyping analyses also are registered for familial periodic fever syndromes (http://fmf.igh.cnrs.fr/infevers).[102,103]

Diagnostic genetic testing for major mutations of hereditary autoinflammatory diseases is now available commercially using a buccal smear specimen (http://www.genedx.com). Since the *Infevers* database was established in 2002, approximately 300 sequence variants in related genes have been identified.[94] In a European study of 228 consecutive patients with a history of periodic fever, clinical features were collected and genetic screening was performed to detect mutations in *MVK*, *TNFRSF1A*, and *MEFV* genes.[104] In patients with clinical manifestations consistent with an autoinflammatory syndrome, the rate of detection of mutations in these 3 genes was <20%.[104] A diagnostic score was developed from clinical features of mutation-positive and mutation-negative

patients and applied to an independent validity set of 77 patients. Clinical features of young age at onset, positive family history of periodic fever, abdominal pain, thoracic pain, and diarrhea were significantly associated with gene defects.

For purposes of initial evaluation by infectious diseases subspecialists, clinical syndromic classification may still be useful (Table 15-3). Certain dermatologic manifestations can be typical.[105] PFAPA is by far the most commonly encountered periodic fever syndrome. The likelihood of seeing a patient with a hereditary periodic fever syndrome among those with PFAPA is small (e.g., <5% in practice), but could be higher depending on the patient population served and referral patterns.[69,76,77,80] In a genetic study in Italy of 210 children with PFAPA syndrome diagnosis, 43 children carried diagnostic mutations (*MVK*, 33; *TNFRSF1A*, 3; *MEFV*, 7).[78] Mutation-positive patients had significantly higher frequency of abdominal pain, vomiting, and cutaneous rash and arthralgia; a diagnostic score for risk of genetic mutations was proposed.[79] In a study of 49 U.S. children with PFAPA who had genetic testing for major mutations in genes noted above as well as *ELA2* genes, 18% had mutations; more than one-half of mutation-positive patients had more unusual characteristics of attacks including loss of appetite, headache, myalgia, and abdominal pain.[70]

It is our practice to perform genetic testing for hereditary autoinflammatory diseases if any of the following is present: onset <12 months of age, positive family history, migratory rash, arthralgia/arthritis, remarkable abdominal pain, substantial vomiting or diarrhea with episodes. We evaluate for cyclic neutropenia by repeated white blood cell counts or genetic testing or both if there is any clinical clue (lingering gingivitis, history of recurring simple infections such as cellulitis or otitis media), any invasive infection, or laboratory clue (e.g., neutrophil count during episode <6000 cells/mm³). Since hereditary autoinflammatory diseases have symptom complexes that evolve with age, follow-up of children with PFAPA diagnosis is important. The goals of diagnosis of a chronic autoinflammatory disorder are to intervene to relieve symptoms and to prevent amyloidosis.

Familial Mediterranean Fever (FMF)

Epidemiology and Etiology

Familial Mediterranean fever (FMF) is the prototypic autoinflammatory disease, and the most common. In 1997, two consortia independently identified mutations in a single gene, denoted *MEFV*, that cause the disease.[106,107] *MEFV* encodes a protein product alternatively termed *pyrin* (Greek *pyrus* for "fever") or *marenostrin* (Latin for "our sea"). Mutations causing FMF are present in very high frequency in several populations: for this reason the disease is more prevalent (but is not exclusively found) in the Mediterranean basin and Middle East. More than 50 disease-associated mutations have been identified in *MEFV* and most are nucleotide substitutions localized in exon 10. Homozygous *M694V* genotype is the most common in that region and is associated with young onset, severe course, and high risk of amyloidosis. The pyrin protein is a member of the death domain superfamily, which provides critical biochemical pathways of apoptosis and innate immunity. There is general consensus that through complex intracellular mechanisms, pyrin plays a role in modulating caspase-1 activity and subsequent IL-1β release; its net effect on levels of IL-1β, however, is debated.[108] Pyrin interacts with tubulin and co-localizes with microtubules, suggesting a rationale for the highly efficacious treatment of FMF using colchicine, a microtubular-destabilizing agent.[94]

Cardinal Clinical Features

Classic manifestations of FMF are recurring episodes of fever, polyserositis (involving synovia, pleura, peritoneum), and erysipelas-like rash, but clinical manifestations are highly variable. Most patients have had episodes of undiagnosed fevers in childhood; disease onset has been reported in various studies to occur before 10 years of age in 25% to 60% of cases, and before 20 years of age in 64% to 90% of cases. Mean delay in diagnosis is 7 years.[98]

More specific manifestations frequently develop over time with approximately 90% having had recurring abdominal pain, and 40% thoracic pain, by 20 years of age.[104] Episodes do not have clockwork periodicity, with weeks to years between episodes, and can be triggered by stress or minor trauma. High fever has short duration, a few to 72 hours. Abdominal pain (sterile peritonitis) ranges from mild and localized, to severe and diffuse with abdominal rigidity. Well-demarcated erysipelas-like lesions are distinctly associated with FMF, typically developing below the knees anteriorly to the dorsum of the feet, bilaterally (symmetrically) or unilaterally.[105] Histology reveals dermal infiltration of neutrophils. Children also may exhibit purpuric lesions of the face, trunk and extremities. Vasculitides such as leukocytoclastic vasculitis, Henoch–Schönlein purpura, and polyarteritis nodosa are described in FMF.[96] Arthritis usually is monoarticular, involving the knee, ankles, or hips; fluid pleocytosis is neutrophilic. Mouth ulceration is distinctly absent. Children are well between episodes, but inflammatory markers persist. Genetic testing is diagnostic.

Course, Treatment, and Outcome

The most serious complication of FMF is the development of amyloidosis. Prior to effective therapy with colchicine, endstage renal disease occurred in many patients by the age of 40 years. Oral colchicine is the treatment of choice for both children and adults, reducing both the frequency and severity of attacks and the risk of amyloidosis. The vast majority of patients benefit from colchicine. In others, adjunctive therapy with the IL-1 receptor antagonist anakinra has proved beneficial.

Hyperimmunoglobulinemia D Syndrome (HIDS) also Known as Mevalonate Kinase (MVK) Deficiency

Epidemiology and Etiology

Hyperimmunoglobulinemia D and periodic fever syndrome (HIDS) was first described in several Dutch patients by van der Meer in 1984;[109] decreased mevalonate kinase (MVK) activity in skin fibroblasts and increased mevalonate in urine was demonstrated in 1999,[110] and in the same year, the causative *MVK* gene was localized on the long arm of chromosome 12.[111] The HIDS registry in the Netherlands (www.hids.net) currently has data on more than 200 patients worldwide. Although the majority of patients are white and from northern European countries, genetic testing has confirmed broader populations affected, including the Mediterranean basin and Asia.[98]

HIDS is due to autosomal recessively inherited mutations of the *MVK* gene; MVK deficiency may be a more accurate name for the condition. More than 35 mutations have been reported (http://fmf.igh.cnrs.fr/infevers), mapped to chromosome 12q24. Most HIDS patients are compound heterozygotes for missense mutations, resulting in residual MVK activity 1% to 8% of normal. Mutations in *MVK* also are responsible for mevalonic aciduria, in which mutations cluster around the active sites of the enzyme, and result in total absence of enzyme activity and a catastrophic disease characterized by dysmorphic features, failure to thrive, mental retardation, ataxia, recurrent fever attacks, and death in early childhood. Five adults with neurologic signs and symptoms and MVK deficiency have been described, suggesting that there may be overlapping syndromes and a spectrum of disease.[112]

MVK is an essential enzyme in the isoprenoid biosynthesis pathway and cholesterol cascade. The pathogenic mechanisms leading to autoinflammatory disease remains poorly understood. Shortage of a metabolic product downstream to MVK, rather than excess of mevalonate, is likely to cause increased IL-1β secretion by peripheral blood mononuclear cells as observed in these patients in response to LPS stimulation.[98]

Cardinal Clinical Features

Clinical features and long-term follow-up of 103 patients from 18 different countries with recurrent attacks of fever and at least one mutation in the *MVK* gene have been reported from the International HIDS database.[113] The median age of first attack is 6 months (range 0–120 months) but the median period from onset of disease to diagnosis is 9.9 years. A typical attack starts with prodromal symptoms such as malaise and headache, followed by a rapid rise in temperature (often >40°C), chills, enlargement and pain in cervical lymph nodes, abdominal pain and vomiting or diarrhea or both, and arthralgia of large peripheral joints (with arthritis in 50%). Skin lesions accompany attacks in more than two-thirds of patients. Although small macules, papules and nodules are the usual exanthem, urticaria, purpura, and erythema nodosum have been reported.[97,105] Histology of lesional skin usually shows mild vasculitis, but can show dense dermal infiltrate of neutrophils.[96] Oral aphthous ulcers without or with accompanying genital ulcers are reported in almost one-half of patients.[113] One-third to one-half of patients have splenomegaly during attacks.[96,113]

In the HIDS registry report, childhood vaccinations induced the first attack in two-thirds of patients.[98] Others have noted this triggering event as well as injury, physical exercise, or emotional stress.[96,114] Similarities between HIDS and PFAPA sometimes are remarkable, with 4- to 8-week cycles, 3- to 6-day episodes, and complete wellbeing between episodes. Differentiating features of HIDS, such as severe headache (sometimes with aggressive personality change), recurring gastrointestinal complaints, rash, genital ulceration, and arthralgia, can evolve over years after onset of febrile episodes.[114] Dramatic response to corticosteroids occurs in HIDS and does not distinguish HIDS from infections or other autoinflammatory syndromes.[96,98]

Elevation of serum IgD level has been considered a hallmark of the disease, the median concentration of the highest IgD measured in HIDS registry patients being 400 IU/mL (range <0.8–5300 IU/mL). IgD level usually is normal until 3 years of age;[115] 10% to 22% of patients never have IgD level above normal (>100 IU/mL).[115,116] Most patients with elevated IgD level and no *MVK* mutation have no definite diagnosis.[116] Elevation of IgA level has been reported in HIDS patients, even at a young age.[117] IgA concentration was above the upper limit of normal of 260 mg/dL in 64% of HIDS registry patients, but median IgA was only 405 mg/dL. Mevalonic acid concentrations in urine are elevated only during febrile episodes. B-lymphocyte cytopenia has been described in two brothers with HIDS.[118] Genetic testing for mutations in *MVK* is the best confirming test for HIDS. In a French and Dutch study the most discriminatory clinical composite was onset <5 years of age, or complaint of joint pains plus length of attacks <14 days (sensitivity 100%, specificity 28% for HIDS).[119]

Course, Treatment, and Outcome

The HIDS registry showed decreasing frequency of attacks with age; 44% in the first decade of life had >12 attacks per year, whereas 30% did in the second decade. HIDS impairs several aspects of quality of life.[114] Amyloidosis occurred in 3 of 103 (2.9%) patients in the HIDS registry; all patients had recurring fevers for >20 years before the manifestation of amyloidosis. Abdominal adhesions and joint contractures also were reported. Specifically targeted anti-inflammatory therapies are under study.[99] The p75 TNF receptor fusion protein, etanercept, has demonstrated clinical benefit, as has the IL-1 receptor antagonist, anakinra. In 20 patients in the HIDS registry given etanercept or anakinra, 80% had at least some response.[114]

Tumor Necrosis Factor Receptor-Associated Periodic Fever Syndrome (TRAPS)

Epidemiology and Etiology

TRAPS was first described in 1982 in a large Irish family with recurrent fever and localized inflammation, and called familial Hibernian fever.[120] A wider range of northern European and virtually every ethnic origin subsequently has been reported. TRAPS

PART II Clinical Syndromes and Cardinal Features of Infectious Diseases: Approach to Diagnosis and Initial Management

SECTION B Cardinal Symptom Complexes

is an autosomal dominant disease with variable penetrance; sporadic cases can occur.

In 1998, linkage studies placed the susceptibility locus of a subset of individuals to a region of chromosome 12p13,[121,122] and within a year, mutations in the *TNFRSF1A* gene were identified as the causative.[92] Although there are some general genotype/phenotype associations, the exact pathophysiology of TRAPS remains unclear. TNF stimulates TNFR1, which recruits several proteins to form a complex that results in activation of nuclear factor-κB, at the same time activating the apoptosis pathway. Some patients with TRAPS have been shown to have defective shedding of cleaved soluble TNFR1 at the cell surface, which acts as a decoy for TNF; others have a ligand-independent abnormality in which mutant TNFR1 is unable to traffic appropriately from the endoplasmic reticulum to the cell surface, indirectly or directly (by macroaggregation) causing a proinflammatory response.[99] Mutant TNFR1 also may result in prolonged survival of inflammatory cells through impaired TNF-mediated apoptosis.

Cardinal Clinical Features

Disease symptoms vary from person to person, and kindred to kindred probably based in part on specific gene defect(s). The classic disease is characterized by recurrent attacks of fever, migratory myalgia and tender erythematous plaques, abdominal pain, and periorbital edema or other ocular complaints (due to conjunctivitis, uveitis, iritis).[94,97] Chest pain (due to pleuritis or pericarditis) or mouth ulcers each occurs in <20% of patients. Disease manifestations also can be milder and nonspecific. Attacks last 7 to 21 days and usually do not have clockwork periodicity. Injury, immunizations, and stress can trigger episodes. Mean age of onset for "severe" TRAPS was 18 months and for "mild" TRAPS was 58 months in one study.[104] In a known TRAPS kindred, the first febrile attack of a subsequently affected infant occurred at 4 days of age, and was associated with irritability, lethargy, and diarrhea.[123]

Almost two-thirds of patients develop distinctive cutaneous lesions of localized erythematous macules (1 cm) or patches (up to 28 cm).[97,105] Lesions appear to undergo a set progression – from solitary or grouped macules and papules, to lesions that expand and coalesce – resulting in annular and serpiginous patches and plaques, which migrate distally and are associated with underlying myalgia.[96,97] A third of cutaneous lesions resolve with an ecchymotic appearance. Purpuric lesions, including Henoch–Schönlein purpura, have been reported.[73]

Microscopy of skin lesions reveals superficial and deep perivascular infiltrate of lymphocytes and monocytes.[8] Small vessel vasculitis and recurrent panniculitis can lead to misdiagnosis of TRAPS as Weber–Christian disease. Systemic inflammatory responses during episodes (raised ESR, CRP, fibrinogen, ferritin), neutrophilia, thrombocytosis, low hemoglobin, and polyclonal gammopathy are expected and are not distinctive among autoinflammatory diseases. Genetic testing for mutations of *TNFRS1A* is diagnostic.

Course, Treatment, and Outcome

The most severe complication of TRAPS is amyloidosis, which is said to occur in 8% to 10% of patients.[96] Etanercept, which binds serum TNF, thus preventing engagement with cell surface TNFR1, has been beneficial in some patients, but limitations have become clear;[99] infliximab was successful in one patient who failed etanercept therapy.[124] The IL-1 receptor antagonist, anakinra, has been safe and associated with sustained effectiveness in small numbers of cases reported, which supports increasing use as a first-line agent.[125,126]

Cryopyrin-Associated Periodic Syndromes (CAPS)

Epidemiology and Etiology

CAPS includes familial cold autoinflammatory syndrome (FCAS, previously called familial cold urticaria, FCU), Muckle–Wells syndrome (MWS), and neonatal-onset multisystemic inflammatory disease syndrome (NOMID) also known as chronic infantile neurologic, cutaneous, and articular (CINCA) syndrome. The three syndromes represent a spectrum of disorders, sharing episodic fever, urticaria-like skin rash, and varying degrees of joint and neurologic involvement. FCAS generally is considered the mildest, NOMID the most severe, and MWS intermediary.[95–97,99] CAPS is an autosomal dominantly inherited disease, with new mutations arising. Although most patients have been reported from the U.S. and Europe (predominantly in persons of northern European origin), patients from other origins (including the Mediterranean basin) have been described.[127]

Independent linkage studies placed the susceptibility locus for both MWS and FCAS on chromosome 1q.[128,129] In 2001, mutations in a 9-exon gene were identified in both FCAS and MWS families[130] and in 2002, mutations in the same gene were identified in patients with NOMID.[131,132] The gene, named *CIAS1* (for cold-induced autoinflammatory syndrome 1), encodes the protein cryopyrin (also known as NALP3). Cryopyrin belongs to a group of interacting proteins that form a macromolecular complex called the *inflammasome*; CAPS is classified as an intrinsic inflammasomopathy.[99] Inflammasone assembly leads to activation of caspase 1, which cleaves pro-IL-1β into its bioactive form. More than 50 missense mutations in *CIAS1* have been identified in patients with CAPS. The overlapping yet wide spectrum of phenotypes (FCAS, MWS, NOMID) suggests presence of combinations of genetic mutations as well as other genetic factors. Additionally, 40% of 18 patients from multiple U.S. sites with the clinical diagnosis of NOMID have not had *CIAS1* mutations found, yet have indistinguishable phenotypes from those with mutations.[132]

Cardinal Clinical Features

CAPS is characterized by episodes of fever, urticaria-like eruption,[82] and limb pain. Onset in CAPS is almost always in the first 6 months of life. FCAS episodes are induced by generalized exposures to cold temperatures (and not necessarily contact with cold objects or drinking cold liquids).[96] Symptoms often are delayed an average of 2.5 hours after exposure and last approximately 12 hours. MWS is not necessarily triggered by changes in temperature and episodes last longer (1–2 days). Microscopic examination of skin lesions reveals perivascular infiltrate of neutrophils, without vasculitis, mast cells or mast cell degranulation.[96] Systemic symptoms of fever, headache, nausea, sweating, drowsiness, extreme thirst, conjunctivitis, blurred vision, ocular pain, and polyarthralgia can be present during episodes. MWS can manifest this constellation plus abdominal pain or progressive sensorineural hearing loss or both. Confusion with other autoinflammatory syndromes, Weber–Christian disease, and autoimmune disorders has occurred.[127]

NOMID manifests within the first 6 weeks of life with an urticaria-like rash, other manifestations of MWS, chronic arthritis, and a characteristic bony overgrowth predominantly involving the knees in most children.[133] Central nervous system manifestations are inexorable and include chronic aseptic meningitis, increased intracranial pressure, cerebral atrophy, ventriculomegaly, chronic papilledema, optic atrophy and loss of vision, mental retardation, seizures, and sensorineural hearing loss. Other manifestations include hepatomegaly; elevated neutrophil count, sedimentation rate and CRP; and short stature.

Course, Treatment, and Outcome

Amyloidosis occurs in a substantial percentage of patients with CAPS (FCAS, MWS, and NOMID). Corticosteroids and nonsteroidal anti-inflammatory drugs can alleviate fever and pain but not disease progression. Drugs targeting TNF also have been somewhat successful,[99] but inflammation persists and 20% of NOMID patients die before adulthood.[133] Use of the IL-1 receptor inhibitor, anakinra, has been highly successful in treatment of all three syndromes. In a study of 18 patients with NOMID, anakinra therapy resulted in complete remission in both peripheral and central nervous system inflammation in most patients. Discontinuation of therapy was associated with rapid relapse, and reintroduction with remission.[133] Fourteen patients newly enrolled in the Italian registry of CAPS were treated with anakinra; follow-up reported at mean of 37.5 months showed significant and persistent improvement in clinical manifestations and overall quality of life.[134]

16 Lymphatic System and Generalized Lymphadenopathy

Mary Anne Jackson and P. Joan Chesney

ANATOMY AND FUNCTION OF LYMPHOID TISSUE

The lymphoid system is composed of an extensive capillary network that collects lymph into elaborate systems of collecting vessels. These collecting vessels merge to empty lymph into the bloodstream by way of the thoracic duct, at its entry into the left subclavian vein, or the right lymphatic duct, which empties into the right subclavian vein. Interspersed along the collecting vessels are specialized lymphatic structures, including the tonsillar tissues of the Waldeyer ring, mucosa-associated lymphoid nodules, spleen, thymus, and lymph nodes (Table 16-1).

The Waldeyer ring of lymphoid tissue that surrounds the oropharyngeal isthmus and the opening of the nasopharynx into the oropharynx is uniquely positioned to interact with foreign material entering the nose or mouth. The ring is formed superiorly by the midline pharyngeal tonsil, which is located in the roof of the nasopharynx (adenoid), and inferiorly by the lingual tonsil in the posterior third of the tongue. On either side of the pharynx, the lateral pharyngeal bands of lymphoid tissue connect the adenoid to the tubal tonsils of Gerlach at the openings of the eustachian tubes and to the faucial (palatine) tonsils. Smaller aggregates of lymphoid tissue in this area include the posterior pharyngeal granulations and the lymphoid tissue within the laryngeal ventricle. Small submucosal lymphoid nodules, located throughout the respiratory, gastrointestinal, and genitourinary tracts, are composed of phagocytic and lymphoid cell collections without a connective tissue capsule. These nodules are ideally situated to respond to mucosal antigens. The thymus, which is located over the superior vena cava in the anterior mediastinum, is relatively protected from antigens. Surrounded by a thin connective tissue capsule, the thymus is uniquely composed of both epithelial and lymphatic elements. The spleen is the largest lymphatic organ in the body and the only lymphatic tissue specialized to filter blood. Similar to the lymph nodes, the spleen is a component of the peripheral lymphoid system and is composed of red pulp (red blood cells) and the interior white pulp, which contains lymphoid nodules with germinal follicles.

Normal lymph nodes are small oval or bean-shaped bodies that are strategically located along the course of lymphatic vessels to filter lymph on its way to the bloodstream. Lymphatic vessels enter around the periphery of the nodes. Lymph filters through the cortex to the medulla of the node and exits through the hilum. Blood vessels enter and leave through the hilum, connected to capillaries that course through the node. During this process, lymphocytes can leave the blood and re-enter the lymphatic circulation. Nodes are densely packed with lymphocytes that are organized loosely into cortical nodules and medullary cords by connective tissue trabeculae and lymphatic sinuses. The juxtaposition of phagocytic cells, antigen-processing cells, and lymphocytes in an area of sluggish blood flow is ideally suited to provide the first line of defense against pathogens. As lymph slowly filters through the rich reticular network, organisms are trapped and can be ingested by phagocytic cells, thus stimulating cytokine release, which in turn recruits lymphocytes into immunologic responses.

The lymph node groups in the body can be divided into the superficial and peripheral nodes, which generally are easily palpable, and the deeper groups adjacent to major vessels and viscera (see Table 16-1).

TABLE 16-1. Anatomic Types and Locations of Lymphoid Tissue

Type of Tissue	Location	Distinguishing Features
Discrete lymph node groups	Occipital, preauricular, postauricular, submandibular, submental, facial, parotid, cervical, supraclavicular, para-aortic, axillary, epitrochlear, inguinal, iliac, popliteal, mediastinal, hilar, pelvic, mesenteric, celiac	Nodes have discrete capsules; afferent lymphatic flow enters from periphery; efferent lymphatic flow exits and blood vessels enter and exit through hilum of node
Waldeyer ring	Pharyngeal (adenoid), palatine (faucial), lingual and tubal (Gerlach) tonsils; lateral pharyngeal bands; posterior pharyngeal granulations	Aggregates of lymphoid nodules are partially encapsulated; there are no afferent lymphatics and no lymphoid sinuses; efferent lymphatic flow is not as structured as for lymph nodes
Lymphoid nodules	Small, submucosal lymphoid collections throughout the intestinal (Peyer patches), respiratory, and genitourinary tracts (mucosal-associated lymphoid tissue, or MALT)	Lymphatic flow is not encapsulated or structured; tissue responds to mucosal antigens with phagocytosis and immunoglobulin A production
Thymus	Anterior mediastinum	Organ is composed of lymphoid and epithelial cells; no afferent lymphatic vessels; protected from antigen; essential for development and maturation of peripheral lymphoid tissues
Spleen	Abdomen	Lymphatic tissue is uniquely specialized to filter blood; largest lymphatic organ in the body; no afferent lymphatic vessels and no lymphatic vessels within spleen; sinusoid structure is similar to lymph node but lymph empties into splenic vein

PART II Clinical Syndromes and Cardinal Features of Infectious Diseases: Approach to Diagnosis and Initial Management

SECTION B Cardinal Symptom Complexes

DEVELOPMENTAL CHANGES

Lymphoid tissue, including the thymus, forms a significantly larger percentage of total body weight in infants and children than in adults. Considerable lymphoid activity is present at birth, and continuing exposure to environmental antigens results in an increase in lymphoid mass that reaches a peak between ages 8 and 12 years. Atrophy of lymphoid tissue begins during adolescence. In children, the thymus can weigh 40 g; in adults, it is replaced by fibrous and fatty tissue and can weigh only 10 g. By adult standards, almost all children have "lymphadenopathy," because palpable nodes, particularly in the cervical, axillary, and inguinal areas, are common in children of all ages, including neonates (Table 16-2). Prominent palatine tonsils are common in preadolescent children, whereas in infants <1 year old and adults, the palatine tonsils usually are not visible.

Aside from, or because of, their normally hyperplastic nodes, the response of children to antigenic, infectious, or neoplastic stimuli is much more rapid, prolific, and exaggerated than that in adults. Lymph nodes can increase in size as much as 15-fold within 5 to 10 days of antigen exposure. Increased size of mediastinal and mesenteric nodes can be particularly pronounced.

TABLE 16-2. Frequency and Location of Palpable Peripheral Lymph Nodes in Healthy Children

Palpable Node	Neonate[a]	Age <2 years[b]	Age >2 years[b]
Cervical	+	++	++
Postauricular	–	+	–
Occipital	–	++	+
Submandibular	–	+	++
Supraclavicular	–	–	–
Axillary	+	+++	+++
Epitrochlear	–	–	–
Inguinal	+	+++	+++
Popliteal	–	–	–
None	++	++	++

+++, Normally present in >50% of children; ++, normally present in 25% to 50%; +, normally present in 5% to 25%; –, normally present in <5%.

[a]Data from Bamji M, Stone RK, Kaul A, et al. Palpable lymph nodes in healthy newborns and infants. Pediatrics 1986;78:573.

[b]Data from Herzog LW. Prevalence of lymphadenopathy of the head and neck in infants and children. Clin Pediatr 1983;22:485.

CHARACTERISTICS OF LYMPHADENOPATHY

Lymphadenopathy (enlarged lymph nodes) can be characterized by size, location, consistency, rate of growth, tissue inflammation, and fixation. In all ages and lymph node groups, a node is considered enlarged if it measures (in the longest diameter) >10 mm. There are two exceptions to this rule. In the epitrochlear region, nodes >5 mm are abnormal, and in the inguinal region, only nodes >15 mm are considered abnormal.

In healthy neonates, lymph nodes ranging from 3 to 12 mm can be found in the cervical, axillary, and inguinal regions.[1] Most children examined when healthy have palpable lymph nodes.[2] In the child <2 years old, palpable nodes can be present at any peripheral location, except in the epitrochlear, supraclavicular, and popliteal areas, where palpable lymph nodes always are abnormal. In the child >2 years, palpable lymph nodes in these areas and in the posterior auricular and suboccipital areas are considered abnormal.

Characteristics of lymph nodes are determined by palpation (Table 16-3). Soft, discrete, nontender, small (<2 cm) nodes that are found bilaterally or generally with no periadenitis, cellulitis, or abscess formation usually result from hyperplasia secondary to viral infection. Unilateral, large (>2 cm), warm, tender, poorly defined nodes with surrounding edema, erythema, or abscess formation usually are infected with pyogenic bacteria.

Moderately large, unilateral nodes, with discrete margins and minimal inflammation, that progress slowly to become erythematous (but not warm), fluctuant, and adherent to overlying skin are characteristic of chronic, usually bacterial, infections.

Enlarged nodes resulting from lymphoma generally are firm, discrete, freely movable, nontender, and rubbery and have no surrounding inflammation. Nodes increase in size over time and adjacent nodes can become matted together and lose individual characteristics. Suppuration and fixation to skin or deeper structures, as seen in inflammatory lymphadenopathy, are not expected in lymphoma. Lymphomatous nodes can wax and wane in size over weeks to months, and lymphomatous changes can develop (or become more apparent) in nodes for which a biopsy specimen initially showed only hyperplasia.[1-3] Enlarged nodes that result from metastatic tumors are described as being hard and bound to each other and to surrounding tissues.

Enlarged nodes can be single or multiple and contiguous when confined to one region, the condition is referred to as regional lymphadenopathy. Enlargement of a single node or regional nodes can be the result of localized disease or the first manifestation of generalized lymphadenopathy. Generalized lymphadenopathy is defined as the simultaneous presence of ≥2 enlarged nodes in noncontiguous groups; enlargement need not be present in every body site of lymph nodes. Thus, the simultaneous presence

TABLE 16-3. General Characteristics of Enlarged Lymph Nodes According to Cause

Characteristic	Causes of Enlargement			
	Acute Bacterial	Chronic Bacterial	Acute Viral	Malignant
Large size	+++	+++	+	++/+++
Erythema	+++	++	–	–
Tenderness	+++	++	+	++
Consistency	Soft/firm	Firm	Soft	Firm/rubbery
Discrete	++	+++	+++	+++
Matted	++	++	–	++
Fixed	+++	+	–	–
Fluctuant	+++	+++	–	–
Associated with cellulitis	+++	+	–	–
Unilateral	+++	+++	–	+

+++, Common finding; ++, less common; +, occasional; –, rare.

of mesenteric and hilar adenopathy is considered generalized lymphadenopathy. Splenomegaly also can be present but is not included in the definition.

PATHOGENESIS OF LYMPHADENOPATHY AND LYMPHADENITIS

Microorganisms reach lymph nodes directly by lymphatic flow from the inoculation site or by lymphatic spread from adjacent nodes. If initial involvement of regional nodes does not contain infection adequately, organisms can reach noncontiguous nodes by hematogenous spread. Lymph node enlargement can result from a variety of mechanisms (Box 16-1).

In acute pyogenic lymphadenitis, the initial inflammatory response in the node, including complement activation and cytokine release, causes recruitment of neutrophils and mononuclear phagocytes. Vascular engorgement and intranodal edema, as well as cellular replication in response to the antigenic stimulus, lead to rapid enlargement of the node. Involvement of adjacent lymph nodes and surrounding soft tissues, including skin, can result in cellulitis, suppuration, necrosis, and fixation to adjacent tissues. Once purulence occurs, lymph node architecture (and antibiotic access) is destroyed. Healing occurs by fibrosis.

For microorganisms that cause subacute or chronic granulomatous changes, the increase in node size and tenderness and adjacent inflammatory response usually are modest. Formation of granulomas and, in some cases, caseating necrosis also destroy nodal architecture; drainage or removal may be required to relieve pain or hasten resolution.

With local or generalized viral infections, the nodal response primarily is one of hyperplasia without necrosis, and this resolves as infection abates without sequelae.

Enlarged lymph nodes, lymphoid nodules, or lymphoid tissue, such as the Waldeyer ring, can result in obstruction, compression, or erosion of important structures, rupture of nodal contents, or inflammation of adjacent structures. Generalized hyperplasia of the Waldeyer ring can result in obstruction of the posterior nares, eustachian tube, or oropharynx. Extensive mediastinal lymphadenopathy can lead to obstruction or erosion of the airways, esophagus, superior vena cava, recurrent laryngeal nerve, or lymphatics (see Chapter 18, Mediastinal and Hilar Lymphadenopathy, Table 18-2). Gastrointestinal inflammation of Peyer patches (e.g., *Salmonella* Typhi infection) can lead to intestinal perforation and hemorrhage or may serve as lead point for intussusception. Infectious mesenteric lymphadenitis can lead to an intraabdominal abscess. Perinodal inflammation of muscles in the neck results in torticollis, and spread of infection in the neck can lead to deep fascial space infections.

HISTOPATHOLOGY OF LYMPHADENITIS

Nonspecific hyperplasia is the most common histopathologic finding in biopsy specimens of enlarged lymph nodes. The etiology is not determined in most children, and the condition usually resolves. For 17% to 25% of cases, however, a pathologic process ultimately develops, most often a lymphoreticular disease.[3–5]

In acute pyogenic infection, lymph nodes are filled with neutrophils, microorganisms, edema, and necrotic debris. Granuloma formation along with caseating necrosis is typical of infections caused by *Mycobacterium tuberculosis, Histoplasma capsulatum, Coccidioides immitis,* and some nontuberculous mycobacteria. Stellate abscesses surrounded by palisading epithelioid cells are typical for lymphogranuloma venereum (caused by *Chlamydia trachomatis*) and infections caused by *Bartonella henselae* and *Francisella tularensis* (with most extensive granuloma formation in the latter). Toxoplasmosis produces characteristic nodal histologic findings of reactive follicular hyperplasia with scattered clusters of epithelioid histiocytes in cortical and paracortical zones, blurring of margins of germinal centers, and focal distention of subcapsular and trabecular sinuses by monocytoid cells. *Yersinia* spp. can cause necrotizing lymphadenitis in cervical, mediastinal, and mesenteric nodes. Brucellosis is characterized by noncaseating granulomas that are indistinguishable from those of sarcoidosis.

LYMPHOCUTANEOUS AND OCULOGLANDULAR SYNDROME

For several infections resulting in regional and, with extension, generalized lymphadenopathy, a characteristic (often granulomatous) inflammatory reaction develops at the site of inoculation. Regional adenopathy often develops from lymphatic spread of organisms before the inoculation site has healed. When the initial inoculation site is in the conjunctiva, the constellation is called Parinaud oculoglandular syndrome (see Chapter 17, Cervical Lymphadenitis and Neck Infections) and, when in the skin, the lymphocutaneous syndrome. Organisms that cause these syndromes are shown in Table 17-4.

INFECTIOUS CAUSES OF GENERALIZED LYMPHADENOPATHY

Distinction of local or generalized lymph node enlargement due to self-limited conditions from potentially life-threatening disorders, such as a neoplasm, histiocytic proliferation, or autoimmune disease, is essential.[6,7] Such distinctions usually can be made on the basis of history, lymph node examination (see Table 16-3), the presence of other systemic manifestations, and a limited number of laboratory tests (Box 16-2).

PART II Clinical Syndromes and Cardinal Features of Infectious Diseases: Approach to Diagnosis and Initial Management

SECTION B Cardinal Symptom Complexes

Systemic infections are the most common causes of generalized lymphadenopathy. Many conditions characterized by generalized adenopathy also cause hepatic or splenic enlargement or, initially, regional adenopathy. Differentiating features of characteristic syndromes are presented in Table 16-4.

Spirochetal Infection

Rash and generalized, painless lymphadenopathy are present in 90% of patients with secondary syphilis. Enlargement of the epitrochlear nodes is a unique and common finding. In 70% of patients, rash and lymphadenopathy are accompanied by constitutional symptoms of fever, malaise, anorexia, and weight loss.

In leptospirosis, generalized lymphadenopathy and hepatosplenomegaly, in addition to constitutional symptoms of muscle tenderness, conjunctival injection, and skin rashes, are present in the first septicemic stage.

The first clinical manifestation of Lyme disease is the typical annular rash, erythema migrans. Untreated, nearly 25% have dissemination that leads to secondary lesions of erythema migrans. Patients also complain of fever, headache, myalgia, malaise, and arthralgia; nontender regional or generalized lymphadenopathy also can be present.

Bartonella Infections

In the mountain valleys of Peru, Ecuador, and southwest Colombia, between the altitudes of 600 and 2760 meters, *Bartonella bacilliformis* infection can be transmitted by the sandfly vector (or by blood transfusion), causing Oroya fever. In the acute stage, cells of the reticuloendothelial system contain many organisms following phagocytosis and destruction of infected, deformed red cells. Fever, headache, and muscle and joint pain are accompanied by anemia and generalized, painless lymphadenopathy. Splenomegaly is present only in patients with intercurrent infection. *B. henselae* infection (cat-scratch disease) on occasion manifests with generalized lymphadenopathy, splenomegaly, and granulomatous hepatitis (especially in the immunocompromised host). In most instances of generalized lymphadenopathy, only two or three sites are involved, suggesting that, in some cases, separate inoculations may have occurred.

Enteric Infections

Enteric fever caused by *Salmonella* spp. primarily affects the lymphoid tissue in Peyer patches in the ileum, the lymphoid follicles of the cecum, and the mesenteric nodes. About 50% of patients have hepatosplenomegaly. Occasionally, generalized lymphadenopathy is present, particularly involving cervical nodes. Lymphoid tissue undergoes consecutive stages of hyperplasia, necrosis, ulceration and healing. Suppurative lymphadenitis has been described.

Yersinia pseudotuberculosis and *Y. enterocolitica* infection has been associated with terminal ileitis and mesenteric adenitis, in which mesenteric lymph nodes are enlarged and can become necrotic and intensely suppurative. Concurrently enlarged inguinal and, rarely, cervical and hilar nodes have been described.

Pulmonary Infections

Although rare, legionellosis in children can manifest with nonspecific symptoms and occasionally with findings of rash, splenomegaly, and lymphadenopathy. Pneumonia caused by *Mycoplasma pneumoniae* infection is accompanied by lymphadenopathy, particularly cervical, in about 25% of cases; mediastinal and hilar lymphadenopathy also can occur.

Tuberculosis usually is characterized by mediastinal and occasionally cervical lymphadenopathy. Protracted hematogenous disease can cause high fever, hepatosplenomegaly, and generalized lymphadenopathy.

Symptomatic, disseminated coccidioidomycosis occurs, rarely, within weeks or months following the initial localized pulmonary infection; most frequently, extrapulmonary spread is to bone, soft tissue, lymph nodes, and meninges. Tissue reaction primarily is granulomatous but can be accompanied by acute inflammation.

In acute disseminated histoplasmosis in infants, the reticuloendothelial system has a high density of yeast forms compared with mycelial forms. Hepatosplenomegaly and intra-abdominal lymphadenopathy are common, and one-third of patients have peripheral lymphadenopathy. In acute pulmonary histoplasmosis, lymphohematogenous spread involves lymph nodes in the neck (where suppuration of supraclavicular or cervical nodes can occur), mediastinum, liver, and spleen.

Paracoccidioidomycosis is endemic in most countries of Latin America, particularly Brazil. The disease almost always is disseminated, with predilection for the reticuloendothelial system. Peripheral lymphadenopathy is present in 75% of children with the acute or subacute forms. Cervical, inguinal, mesenteric, or mediastinal lymphadenopathy is present almost universally. Lymph nodes vary in size, number, and consistency; over time, abscesses and fistulas form. Masses of lymph nodes (frequently with caseation) can be present; hepatosplenomegaly usually is present.

Other Bacterial Infections

Acute onset of symptoms occurs in 50% of patients with brucellosis. As organisms are ingested by mononuclear phagocytes, disease is localized primarily to the lymph nodes, liver, spleen, and bone marrow. Noncaseating granulomas that are indistinguishable from sarcoidosis are the usual finding in liver biopsy specimens.

Lymphadenitis is a common manifestation of tularemia. Although regional involvement (with the site depending on whether acquisition was oropharyngeal or tick related) is the most common presentation, involvement of multiple sites can occur. Hepatosplenomegaly was present in 35% of infected children in one series.[8]

Generalized lymphadenopathy is rarely described as a feature of scarlet fever. It may be more typical of the severe toxic form of the disease.

Exanthematous Syndromes

Studies of rubella virus inoculation in adolescents and young adult volunteers demonstrated that suboccipital and posterior auricular lymphadenopathy is most characteristic, but generalized involvement can occur.[9]

Pharyngitis and cervical lymphadenopathy are common in measles during the exanthematous period. Generalized lymphadenopathy with suboccipital, posterior auricular, and mediastinal involvement and splenomegaly are common.

Generalized lymphadenopathy is an uncommon manifestation of varicella-zoster viral infection and is more often related to secondary bacterial infections.

Clinically, parvovirus B19 infection most often causes erythema infectiosum, but a mononucleosis-like syndrome with generalized lymphadenopathy and hepatosplenomegaly also is described.

Mononucleosis Syndromes

Lymphadenopathy in Epstein–Barr virus (EBV)-associated mononucleosis most prominently involves anterior and posterior cervical nodes, but diffuse lymphadenopathy often is present and involves the occipital, supraclavicular, axillary, epitrochlear, inguinal, and mediastinal lymphatic chains. Enlarged nodes usually are not tender (or minimally tender) and have no overlying erythema, and are most prominent during the second to fourth week of illness. Splenomegaly is present in 50% and hepatomegaly in 30% to 50% of cases.

In children, cytomegalovirus (CMV) is a less common cause of mononucleosis than is EBV, but lymphoid manifestations are similar. In one study of 124 children with the mononucleosis

TABLE 16-4. Diseases and Organisms That Cause Generalized Lymphadenopathy and Accompanying Predominant Regional Involvement

Disease	Organism	Generalized	Hepatosplenomegaly	Mediastinal	Cervical	Other
			Lymphadenopathy — Regional			
SPIROCHETAL SYNDROMES						
Syphilis, secondary	*Treponema pallidum*	++++	–	+	++	++
Leptospirosis	*Leptospira* spp.	++++	++++	–	++	++
Lyme disease	*Borrelia burgdorferi*	+	+(H)	–	–	++
***BARTONELLA* SYNDROMES**						
Bartonellosis (Oroya fever; verruga peruana)	*Bartonella bacilliformis*	++++	–	–	–	–
Cat-scratch disease	*Bartonella henselae*	+	+(S)	++	+++	++++
MESENTERIC LYMPHADENOPATHY SYNDROMES						
Typhoid fever	*Salmonella* Typhi	++++	++++(S)	+	+	+
Yersiniosis	*Yersinia enterocolitica*	+	–	+	+	+++
PULMONARY SYNDROMES						
Mycoplasma infection	*Mycoplasma pneumoniae*	+	–	++	++	–
Legionnaire disease	*Legionella pneumophila*	+	+(S)	–	–	–
Primary tuberculosis	*Mycoplasma tuberculosis*	++	++++	++++	++	+
Histoplasmosis (disseminated)	*Histoplasma capsulatum*	+	++++	+++	++	++
Coccidioidomycosis (disseminated)	*Coccidioides immitis*	+	–	++	–	+
Paracoccidioidomycosis	*Paracoccidiodes brasiliensis*	++++	++	+++	++++	+
MISCELLANEOUS BACTERIAL SYNDROMES						
Scarlet fever	*Streptococcus pyogenes*	+	+	–	++++	+++
Brucellosis	*Brucella melitensis*	+++	+++	–	++	+
Tularemia	*Francisella tularensis*	++	++	–	+++	++
EXANTHEMATOUS SYNDROMES						
Measles	Measles virus	+++	++(S)	+++(A)	+++	+
Rubella	Rubella virus	++	+(S)	–	++++	+
Chickenpox	Varicella-zoster virus	++	–	–	–	–
MONONUCLEOSIS SYNDROMES	Epstein–Barr virus	++++	+++	+	++++	++
	Cytomegalovirus	+++	+++	–	+++	++
	HIV	++++	+++	+	++	++
	HHV-6	++++	+++	–	++	+
	Parvovirus B19[19]	++	++	–	–	+++
	Hepatitis A virus	+	+++(H)	–	+++	+
	Toxoplasma gondii	++	+	–	++++	++
CASTLEMAN DISEASE	HIV, HHV-8	++++	+++	+++	+++	+++
MISCELLANEOUS VIRAL SYNDROMES						
Pharyngoconjunctival fever	Adenovirus	++	+++	–	++++	++
Nonspecific febrile illness	Enterovirus	+	+	–	+	+
RICKETTSIA*/*CHLAMYDIA						
Scrub typhus	*Rickettsia tsutsugamushi*	++++	+++	–	+++	++++
Lymphogranuloma venereum	*Chlamydia trachomatis*	+	–	–	–	++++
Ehrlichiosis	*Ehrlichia sennetsu*	++++	–	–	–	–
	Ehrlichia chaffeensis	+++	–	–	–	–
TROPICAL SYNDROMES						
Chagas disease (American trypanosomiasis)	*Trypanosoma cruzi*	++++	++	–	+	+
African sleeping sickness (African trypanosomiasis)	*Trypanosoma brucei*	++	++	–	++++	+
Kala-azar (leishmaniasis)	*Leishmania* spp.	++	++++	–	+	+
Filariasis	*Wuchereria bancrofti* *Brugia* spp.	+++	–	–	–	+++
Schistosomiasis (Katayama fever)	*Schistosoma* spp.	+++	+++	–	+	+
Dengue fever	Dengue virus	++	+	–	+	+
Chikungunya disease	Chikungunya virus	+++	–	–	++++	–
Lassa/Ebola fever	Lassa and Ebola viruses	+++	++	–	–	–
West Nile fever	West Nile virus	++	–	–	–	–

Continued

TABLE 16-4. Diseases and Organisms That Cause Generalized Lymphadenopathy and Accompanying Predominant Regional Involvement—cont'd

Disease	Organism	Lymphadenopathy Generalized	Regional Hepatosplenomegaly	Mediastinal	Cervical	Other
CONGENITAL SYNDROMES	HIV	++++	+++	–	+++	+
	Rubella virus	+++	++++	–	–	+
	Cytomegalovirus	+	++++	–	–	–
	Toxoplasma gondii	+++	++++	–	+	+
	Treponema pallidum	+++	++++	–	+++	+++
	Trypanosoma cruzi	+++	++++	–	–	–
MISCELLANEOUS SYNDROMES						
IAHS	Varied	++++	++++	–	+++	+++
Sarcoidosis	–		++++	+++	+++	+
Gianotti–Crosti syndrome	–	++++	++++	–	+	+
Chronic granulomatous disease	–	+++	++	++	+++	+++
Chronic atopic eczema	–	++	+	–	+++	+++
Typhoid immunization	*Salmonella* Typhi (inactivated)	++	–	–	++	++

A, atypical; H, predominantly hepatomegaly; HHV, human herpesvirus; HIV, human immunodeficiency virus; IAHS, infection-associated hemophagocytic syndrome; S, predominantly splenomegaly; ++++, characteristic association; +++, frequent association; ++, occasional association; +, rare association.

syndromes, fever, hepatosplenomegaly, rashes, and upper-airway obstruction were found with equal frequency in infection caused by EBV or CMV. Cervical lymphadenopathy was more common with EBV (93% of cases) than CMV (75%).

Clinical disease caused by human immunodeficiency virus (HIV) in infants and young children is characterized by generalized lymphadenopathy, hepatosplenomegaly, failure to thrive, intermittent fever, chronic or recurrent diarrhea, parotitis, chronic dermatitis, and recurrent infections. In older children and adults, a mononucleosis-like syndrome (so-called seroconversion syndrome) can occur weeks after HIV infection and includes generalized lymphadenopathy, fever, malaise, myalgia, headache, sore throat, diarrhea, and rash. Lymphadenopathy can involve several sites and can persist for months. Lymph nodes are discrete, nontender, and nonsuppurative; biopsy reveals follicular hyperplasia. With progression to acquired immunodeficiency syndrome (AIDS), lymphocyte depletion occurs; a biopsy specimen of rapidly enlarging nodes should be examined to exclude malignancy. Multicentric Castleman can occur in HIV-infected patients (see below).

Patients with anicteric hepatitis A or B can manifest a mononucleosis-like syndrome, commonly characterized by posterior cervical lymphadenopathy. Generalized lymphadenopathy is unusual; splenomegaly is present in 15% of cases.

The most common findings in symptomatic acquired toxoplasmosis are fatigue and lymphadenopathy without fever. Nodes are discrete, may or may not be tender, and do not suppurate. The cervical, suboccipital, supraclavicular, axillary, and inguinal nodes are most often involved. Lymphadenopathy can be localized or generalized, including involvement of the retroperitoneal and mesenteric nodes. Lymphadenopathy can simulate lymphoma.

Miscellaneous Viral Infections

The usual onset of adenoviral pharyngoconjunctival fever is abrupt, with sore throat, headache, generalized aches and pains, eye irritation or pain, and fever. Some degree of anterior and posterior cervical lymphadenopathy occurs in most patients. Preauricular lymphadenopathy is surprisingly uncommon, and generalized lymphadenopathy is found in 10% to 20% of patients. Hepatosplenomegaly is common.

Generalized lymphadenopathy occasionally occurs in nonspecific illnesses caused by enteroviruses.

Rickettsia, *Ehrlichia*, and *Anaplasma* Infections

In patients with scrub typhus, after an incubation period of 1 to 2 weeks, the initial mite bite lesion and necrotic eschar are noted. This coincides with the onset of the main characteristic features of the disease, which are fever, headache, rash, and generalized lymphadenopathy. Lymphadenopathy is particularly prominent in the axilla, neck, and inguinal areas. Hepatosplenomegaly and conjunctival injection are common.

Sennetsu fever caused by *Ehrlichia sennetsu* appears to be confined to western Japan. Abrupt onset of fever, chills, headache, malaise, sore throat, and muscle and joint pains is accompanied by generalized, tender lymphadenopathy. Posterior auricular and posterior cervical adenopathy are particularly prominent.

Generalized lymphadenopathy is not found in other rickettsial infections (e.g., *R. ricketsii* infection) and is present inconsistently in *Ehrlichia* and *Anaplasma* infections.

Tropical Syndromes

During the acute phase of symptomatic Chagas disease (*Trypanosoma cruzi*), generalized lymphadenopathy, moderate hepatosplenomegaly, rash, vomiting, diarrhea, and neurologic and cardiac changes are present. At various stages of African trypanosomiasis, the hemoflagellate trypanosomal protozoans (*T.b. rhodesiense* and *T.b. gambiense*) can be found in lymphatics and lymph nodes. Fever and posterior cervical lymphadenopathy can be present, along with the local chancre.

In visceral leishmaniasis, or kala-azar, principal histopathology is the result of macrophage infection and reticuloendothelial hyperplasia. Massive splenomegaly and generalized lymphadenopathy with pancytopenia are present.

In filarial infections, lymphangitis with involvement of regional nodes is more common than is generalized lymphadenopathy. Hematogenous dissemination by way of the thoracic duct, however, can lead to generalized adenopathy.

Katayama fever (acute schistosomiasis) occurs with severe schistosomal infestation. Generalized, nontender lymphadenopathy, splenomegaly, and hepatomegaly with tenderness are common, in addition to fever, headache, myalgia, weakness, and gastrointestinal symptoms.

Generalized lymphadenopathy is an integral part of several tropical viral hemorrhagic fever syndromes (see Table 16-4).

Congenital Syndromes

One-third of infants who have congenital toxoplasmosis show signs and symptoms of acute infection. In these infants, splenomegaly (90%), hepatomegaly (70%), and generalized adenopathy (68%) are present. Hepatosplenomegaly is present in 50% to 75% and generalized lymphadenopathy in 20% to 50% of infants with congenital rubella. These manifestations usually resolve over a few weeks. Generalized lymphadenopathy is uncommon in congenital herpes simplex and CMV infections. Infants with intrauterine HIV infection have generalized painless lymphadenopathy; lymph node biopsy results can demonstrate a variety of patterns, including follicular hyperplasia, angioimmunoblastic changes, or atrophy.

Hepatosplenomegaly is present in almost all infants with early congenital syphilis. Generalized lymphadenopathy is described in 50% of patients. Nodes can be ≥1 cm and usually are nontender. Enlarged epitrochlear nodes are relatively unique to congenital syphilis.

OTHER CAUSES OF GENERALIZED LYMPHADENOPATHY

Hodgkin and Non-Hodgkin Lymphoma

Lymphadenopathy can result from malignant transformation of cells intrinsic to the node or from metastatic spread of cells extrinsic to the node (Box 16-3). Primary neoplasms of lymph nodes include the lymphomas and histiocytosis.[10] Data from the American Cancer Society for 2005 show that lymphomas account for approximately 8% of cancers in children less than 15 years old, and leukemia and central nervous system tumors account for 30% and 21% respectively.

Hodgkin lymphoma (HL) and non-Hodgkin lymphoma (NHL) occur; HL in children under age 16 years accounts for 10% to 15% of the approximate 7880 total HL cases diagnosed annually in the United States. NHL in children makes up about 5% of the 53,370 cases of the total cases of NHL diagnosed each year. Among childhood NHL, lymphoblastic lymphomas (30%), Burkitt lymphoma (30% to 40%), anaplastic large-cell lymphoma (10%), and large B-lymphocyte lymphoma (20%) are most common. The cure rate for lymphoma in children is as high as 90% for certain categories; lymphoma is among the most curable of all cancers – this makes early diagnosis important.

The most common first clinical manifestation of both HL and NHL is painless lymph node enlargement, most often in the cervical (in 60% to 90% of cases) or supraclavicular chains. Onset typically is subacute and prolonged in HL, but can occur rapidly over a few days or weeks in NHL. HL is primarily a disease of adolescents and young adults. Of childhood cases, 60% occur in children 10 to 16 years of age, with fewer than 3% of cases in children <5 years of age. Constitutional symptoms of fever, weight loss, drenching night sweats, generalized pruritus, and pain are present in only 30% of children at the time of presentation. For patients with HL, 90% come to medical attention with an unusual mass or swelling and enlarged painless supraclavicular or cervical nodes. Up to 70% of patients have mediastinal lymphadenopathy at presentation, making a chest radiograph valuable if the diagnosis is suspected. Involvement of the Waldeyer ring should be considered if high cervical nodes are enlarged.

Hepatosplenomegaly occurs in patients with advanced disease. Left-sided or bilateral cervical or supraclavicular involvement is more common in extramediastinal para-aortic and splenic spread. Mediastinal disease more often accompanies right-sided cervical or supraclavicular disease.

Other Lymphoproliferative Disorders

Children with congenital or acquired immunodeficiency syndromes (including HIV infection and immunosuppression following organ transplantation) have risk of developing lymphoproliferative disorders that is 100 to 10,000 times that of age-matched controls. The lymphoproliferative disorders are a heterogeneous group of B-lymphocyte proliferations that range from polyclonal hyperplasia to true monoclonal malignant lymphoma. The child's underlying condition (inherited, iatrogenic, or acquired) permits expansion of lymphoid cell populations that would be more strictly regulated in the healthy child. Defects in immune regulation and surveillance result in unchecked proliferation of subpopulations of cells with new, irreversible cytogenetic aberrations, eventuating in NHL (Box 16-4). A mononucleosis-like syndrome with fever, pharyngitis, and generalized lymphadenopathy resulting from lymphoproliferation develops. In early stages, this syndrome can mimic mononucleosis, and EBV infection plays an etiologic role.

Drug-Induced Hyperplasia Related to Hypersensitivity

Localized or generalized lymphadenopathy can appear 1 to 2 weeks after beginning phenytoin or other anticonvulsant medications such as carbamazepine. A severe, pruritic, maculopapular rash, along with fever, hepatosplenomegaly, jaundice, anemia, leukopenia, and plasmacytosis in blood and bone marrow, occurs concurrently with or after lymphadenopathy. This often is referred to as DRESS syndrome – drug rash accompanied by eosinophilia and systemic symptoms. DRESS syndrome is recognized as a great clinical mimicker as the major clinical features also occur in other systemic disorders.[11] Other drugs that have been associated with generalized lymphadenopathy include pyrimethamine,

---

BOX 16-3. Noninfectious Causes of Generalized Lymphadenopathy

- **Inherited immunodeficiency syndromes**
  Chronic granulomatous disease
  Wiskott–Aldrich syndrome
  Chédiak–Higashi syndrome
- **Papular acrodermatitis (Gianotti–Crosti syndrome)**
- **Sarcoidosis**
- **Hyperthyroidism**
- **Drug-induced hyperplasia/hypersensitivity**
- **Autoinflammatory and autoimmune disorders**
- **Lipid storage diseases**
- **Other lymphoid hyperplasia syndromes**
  Infection-associated hemophagocytic syndrome
  Rosai–Dorfman disease
  Kikuchi–Fujimoto disease
  Multicentric Castleman disease
- **Cancers**
  Primary lymphomas and metastatic neoplasms
  Non-Hodgkin lymphoproliferative disorders
  Childhood histiocytoses

BOX 16-4. Lymphoproliferative Disorders Associated with Immunodeficiency

- **Inherited immunodeficiency syndromes**
  Ataxia–telangiectasia syndrome
  Wiskott–Aldrich syndrome
  Combined immunodeficiency syndromes
  X-linked lymphoproliferative syndrome
- **Immunodeficiency resulting from solid-organ and stem-cell transplant therapy**
- **Viral infections causing immunodeficiency syndromes**
  Epstein–Barr virus infection
  Retrovirus infection

PART II Clinical Syndromes and Cardinal Features of Infectious Diseases: Approach to Diagnosis and Initial Management

SECTION B Cardinal Symptom Complexes

anti-leprosy and anti-thyroid drugs, isoniazid, aspirin, barbiturates, penicillin, tetracycline, iodides, sulfonamides, allopurinol, and phenylbutazone.

Metastatic Neoplasms

Metastatic involvement of lymph nodes occurs in a variety of non-lymphomatous cancers, including neuroblastoma, the leukemias, and malignancies of the head and neck (rhabdomyosarcoma, lymphosarcoma, and sarcoma of the parotid gland, thyroid, and nasopharynx).

Histiocytosis

Childhood histiocytoses are a rare and diverse group of disorders that can cause generalized lymphadenopathy. Diagnosis and treatment are difficult. The histiocytoses are characterized by infiltration and accumulation of macrophages formed from histiocytic stem cells. Cells of the histiocytic system consist of antigen-processing (phagocytic) and antigen-presenting (dendritic) cells. Both are found in normal and reactive lymph nodes. Langerhans dendritic cells primarily are located in the skin but can be found in lymph nodes. Sinus histiocytes are the principal cells involved in phagocytosis of foreign particulate matter and are primarily located in lymph node sinuses.

The pathophysiology of histiocytoses is thought to be uncontrolled immunologic stimulation of normal antigen-processing cells, rather than malignant transformation. Lymphadenopathy is a frequent manifestation.

Infection-Associated Hemophagocytic Syndrome

Infection-associated hemophagocytic syndrome (IAHS) is characterized by reactive histiocytic hyperplasia with leukoerythrophagocytosis in a variety of organs. Children with IAHS usually are critically ill, with fever, pancytopenia, generalized lymphadenopathy, and hepatosplenomegaly.[12,13] Laboratory abnormalities include cytopenia, disseminated intravascular coagulation, elevated levels of tissue enzymes, transferrin and triglycerides, and extremely high levels of cytokines.[13] Bone marrow examination reveals excessive proliferation of benign-appearing histiocytes that are phagocytosing white blood cells, red blood cells, and platelets. IAHS has been associated with viruses, bacteria including *Chlamydia pneumoniae*, fungi, and parasites, although the pathophysiology is unknown.[14] IAHS is more commonly associated with immunodeficiency autoimmune syndromes but can occur in otherwise healthy children. The mortality rate is high (20% to 40%). IAHS should be distinguished from malignant histiocytosis and familial erythrophagocytic lymphohistiocytosis (see Chapter 12, Hemophagocytic Lymphohistiocytosis and Macrophage Activation Syndrome).

Inherited Immunodeficiency Syndromes

Generalized lymphadenopathy often is characteristic of inherited immunodeficiency syndromes (e.g., Wiskott–Aldrich syndrome and common variable immunodeficiency) (see Box 16-4). Detection of dysregulated lymphoproliferation in these patients with underlying chronic generalized lymphadenopathy can be difficult. Over 85% of patients with Chédiak–Higashi syndrome have an accelerated phase of disease with generalized lymphadenopathy and hepatosplenomegaly.

Lymphadenopathy, with or without dermatitis, is a common early feature of chronic granulomatous disease and occurs in almost all patients. Although cervical lymphadenopathy is most common, femoral, inguinal, hilar, mediastinal, and generalized adenopathy also are observed. Typically, early signs of inflammation, such as fever, pain, and local inflammation, are lacking and affected nodes suppurate chronically (cold abscesses). Such nodes demonstrate caseating or noncaseating granulomas with central necrosis, a reaction to inadequate killing of intracellular and extracellular organisms.

Sinus Histiocytosis with Massive Lymphadenopathy (Rosai–Dorfman Disease)

Sinus histiocytosis with massive lymphadenopathy (Rosai–Dorfman disease) is characterized by generalized proliferation of sinusoidal histiocytes.[15] A rare disease that occurs in the first two decades of life, the cause of Rosai–Dorfman disease is unknown but is thought to be the result of dysregulated immune system or response to a presumed infectious agent or both. All patients have a history of bilateral cervical lymphadenopathy, often of several months' duration. Lymphadenopathy can be asymmetric, and in 80% of patients, involves other nodal groups, including the axillary, inguinal, hilar, and mediastinal nodes. In 30% of patients, extranodal disease occurs, involving the nasal and oral cavities, salivary glands, pharynx, tonsils, paranasal sinuses, trachea, orbit, bone, or skin. Systemic manifestations usually include fever, anemia, leukocytosis, elevated sedimentation rate, and hypergammaglobulinemia. The course usually is indolent with spontaneous regression, but immune-modulating therapy may be required for extensive or progressive disease.

Histiocytic Necrotizing Lymphadenitis (Kikuchi–Fujimoto Disease)

Histiocytic necrotizing lymphadenitis (Kikuchi–Fujimoto disease) is a benign cause of lymphadenopathy, which is accompanied in 20% of patients by systemic symptoms such as fever, nausea, weight loss, night sweats, arthralgia or hepatosplenomegaly, and leukopenia.[16] The most common manifestation is regional or generalized lymphadenopathy, with or without fever. The median age of onset is 30 years, but cases in children 2 to 18 years of age occur. Lymph node histologic examination reveals reactive histiocytes and large immunoblastic lymphoid cells. Focal necrotic lesions are present in the paracortical areas of lymph nodes. The cause is thought to be dysregulation of the disordered immune system. The prognosis is excellent, with spontaneous resolution of lymphadenopathy within 4 months.

Multicentric Castleman Disease

Castleman disease is an atypical lymphoproliferative disorder characterized by hyperplasia of lymph nodes in which plasma cell predominance and marked capillary proliferation are noted histologically. It may be identified as a localized, indolent disease that can be cured by local excision or, particularly in HIV-infected individuals, as a rapidly progressive disease with a poor prognosis. The multicentric form has been associated strongly with HIV and human herpesvirus 8 (HHV-8).[17-19] Symptoms include fever, myalgia, and weight loss; patients have diffuse lymphadenopathy, splenomegaly and rhabdomyolysis. An HIV-infected adult with Castleman disease (with HHV-8 identified in lymph nodes, peripheral blood, and mononuclear cells) responded well to foscarnet therapy with concomitant antiretroviral therapy.[20]

Autoinflammatory and Autoimmune Disorders

Forty percent of children with juvenile idiopathic arthritis of systemic onset have generalized lymphadenopathy, often preceding joint involvement. Splenomegaly and, less often, hepatomegaly are present. Seventy percent of children with systemic lupus erythematosus have lymphadenopathy, which is generalized in one-third of these children. Hepatosplenomegaly is common. Serum sickness (a hypersensitivity reaction to foreign proteins, often drugs) is characterized by fever, urticaria, edema, polyarthralgia, and generalized lymphadenopathy. In Sjögren syndrome, a rare disease in children, lymphadenopathy and splenomegaly can be present along with parotid and lacrimal gland involvement. Lymphadenopathy in Kawasaki disease usually is not generalized.

Papular Acrodermatitis (Gianotti–Crosti Syndrome)

Papular acrodermatitis of childhood is a distinctive eruption in children aged 6 months to 12 years, associated with malaise, low-grade fever, generalized lymphadenopathy, and hepatomegaly (when accompanied by hepatitis B viremia). The discrete, 1- to 5-mm, flat-topped, firm papules that appear in groups on the face, buttocks, limbs, palms, and soles resolve spontaneously within 3 weeks, whereas lymphadenopathy and hepatomegaly can persist for months. This eruption has been associated with a number of viral syndromes, including hepatitis B and C infection.

Sarcoidosis

Sarcoidosis is a multisystem granulomatous disease of unknown cause, affecting young adults, and most commonly manifesting as asymptomatic bilateral hilar and paratracheal adenopathy, often with parenchymal lung involvement. Generalized lymphadenopathy with prominent cervical involvement is the most common finding in children. Enlarged nodes are discrete, painless, and freely movable. Characteristic histologic findings are epithelioid cell tubercles with little or no necrosis. Other findings result from local granuloma formation and include changes in the eyes, skin, liver, spleen, and parotid glands. Biopsy results of a supraclavicular node are diagnostic in 85% of cases.

Lipid Storage Diseases

In Niemann–Pick, Gaucher, Wolman, and Farber diseases, lipid-laden histiocytes accumulate in lymph nodes, liver, or spleen, resulting in detectable enlargement. Diagnosis is made on the basis of bone marrow examination or lymph node biopsy.

Miscellaneous Disorders

Hyperthyroidism is associated with generalized lymphoid hyperplasia. Beryllium exposure can result in granulomatous lymphadenopathy, which can be generalized.

17 Cervical Lymphadenitis and Neck Infections

Emily A. Thorell

EPIDEMIOLOGY

Neck masses in children, unlike those in adults, seldom represent ominous disease. Most (95%) masses are enlarged or inflamed lymph nodes and are acute in nature. Other masses are congenital cysts and sinuses (3%), vascular malformations, salivary and thyroid anomalies, benign and malignant neoplasms, traumatic injuries, and non-lymphatic infections. Of those children admitted to the hospital for evaluation of a persistent neck mass, malignancy is present in about 15%.[1,2]

Although cervical lymphadenopathy (enlargement) and lymphadenitis (inflammation) are very common, only a few original studies of etiology are recent and represent a minority of cases. Attempts to delineate the causes and causative agents of acute lymphadenitis have been based on analysis of specimens obtained through needle aspiration and surgical biopsy, or by serologic testing. In 40% to 80% of culture-positive cases, aspiration of acutely inflamed, unilateral nodes reveals *Staphylococcus aureus* or *Streptococcus pyogenes* infection.[3,4] In more recent years, community-acquired methicillin-resistant *S. aureus* (CA-MRSA) has emerged, making empiric therapy more challenging.[5,6] As anaerobic organisms outnumber aerobic and facultative organisms in normal oropharyngeal flora by 10 to 1, anaerobic bacteria are common as well. In a study from 1980, anaerobic bacteria were isolated in 38% of cases, and were the only isolate in one-half.[7] Depending on many factors, especially pretreatment with antimicrobial therapy, no pathogen is isolated in at least 25% of cases of acutely inflamed nodes.[4,7]

For persistent cervical masses, biopsy may be needed for diagnosis. One large study from 1963 examined the biopsy results of persistent cervical masses in 267 children.[2] Congenital cyst or cystic hygroma accounted for 60% of masses; malignant tumors accounted for 15.7%, and benign tumors for 7%. Nonspecific lymphoid hyperplasia was found in 10%, and tuberculous granuloma in 7%. Of the 46 malignant tumors, 20 were lymphosarcoma or Hodgkin disease; 11, neurogenic tumors (neuroblastoma, neurofibroma, neurofibrosarcoma); 11, thyroid; and 4, parotid tumor.

In a review of peripheral lymph node excisional biopsy in 239 children, a specific cause was found in only 41% of cases.[8] Of all excised nodes, 76% were located in the neck. Reactive hyperplasia accounted for 52% of cases, granulomatous diseases for 32%, neoplasia for 13% (cases suggestive of lymphoma prior to biopsy were excluded), and chronic lymphadenitis for 3%. Of the 31 cases of malignancy, Hodgkin lymphoma and non-Hodgkin lymphoma (NHL) accounted for 24, neuroblastoma for 4, and rhabdomyosarcoma for 3 cases. In this series, generalized lymphadenopathy was associated most often with reactive hyperplasia. Close follow-up of patients with a diagnosis of nonspecific reactive hyperplasia is important, as studies indicate that up to 25% of such patients ultimately develop severe lymphoreticular disease.[1,5,9,10]

More recently, the use of polymerase chain reaction (PCR) testing of surgical specimens has improved diagnostics in persistent, culture- or serology-negative cases. In a 2009 study, of 60 children treated surgically for suspected infectious persistent cervical lymphadenitis, an etiology was identified in 82%.[11] Methods combining conventional stain and culture with PCR to amplify the eubacterial 16S ribosomal RNA followed by more specific pathogen amplification were used. Organisms identified were both tuberculous and nontuberculous *Mycobacterium* species

TABLE 17-1. Age-Specific Causes of Cervical Lymphadenitis

	Patient Age			
Organism	Neonate	2 Months–1 Year	1–4 Years	5–18 Years
Group A streptococcus	–	–	+	++
Group B streptococcus	++	+	–	–
Staphylococcus aureus	+	++	++	++
Nontuberculous *Mycobacterium*	–	–	++	+
Bartonella henselae	–	+	++	++
Toxoplasma gondii	–	–	+	+
Anaerobic bacteria	–	–	+	++

++, Frequent cause; +, occasional cause; –, rare cause or never a cause.

PART II Clinical Syndromes and Cardinal Features of Infectious Diseases: Approach to Diagnosis and Initial Management

SECTION B Cardinal Symptom Complexes

TABLE 17-2. Physiology of Lymph Flow in the Head and Neck

Lymph Node Group	Areas Drained
HEAD	
Postauricular (mastoid)	Temporal and parietal scalp; posterior wall of ear canal; upper half of pinna
Occipital	Posterior scalp; skin of upper, posterior side of neck
Preauricular	Anterior and temporal regions of scalp; anterior ear canal and pinna; lateral conjunctivae
Parotid	Root of nose; eyelids; temporal scalp; exterior auditory meatus; parotid glands; middle ear; floor nasal activity; posterior palate
Facial	Eyelids, conjunctivae; skin and mucous membranes of nose and cheek; nasopharynx
NECK	
Submental	Central lower lip; floor of mouth; skin of chin; tongue tip
Submandibular (submaxillary)	Buccal mucosa; side of nose; medial palpebral commissure; upper lip; lateral part of lower lip; gums, anterior part of tongue margin, teeth
Superficial cervical	Anterior: superficial anterior neck tissues including skin, lower larynx, thyroid, cranial trachea
	Posterior: lower ear canal; parotid region
Superior deep cervical	Tonsil, adenoid; posterior scalp and neck; tongue, larynx, palate; thyroid; nose, nasopharynx; esophagus; paranasal sinuses; all nodes of head and neck except inferior deep cervical
Inferior deep cervical (scalene, supraclavicular)	Dorsal scalp and neck; superficial pectoral region of arm; superior deep cervical nodes; larynx, trachea; thyroid
	Right: left lower lobe, lingula, right lung and pleura
	Left: left upper lobe; entire abdomen

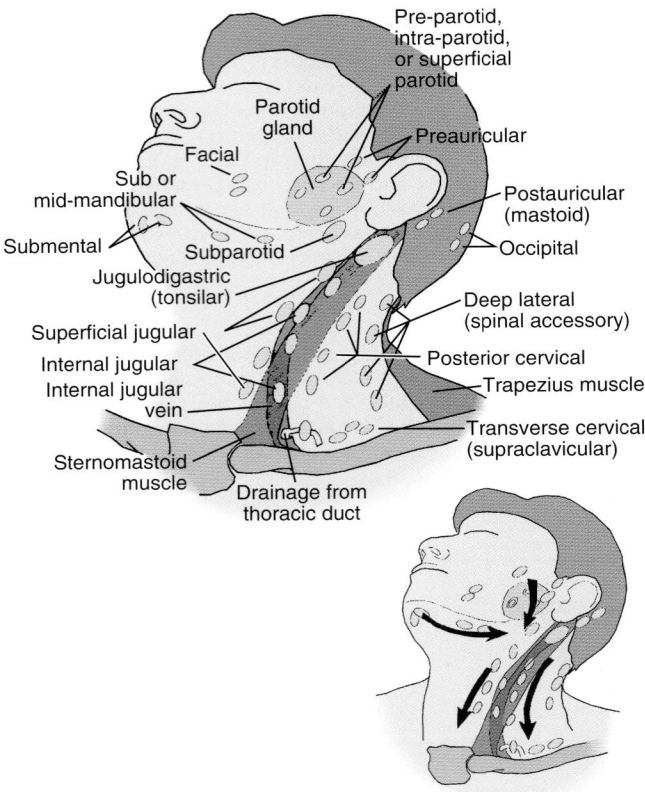

Figure 17-1. Lymphatic flow in the head and neck.

(62%) followed by *Bartonella* species (10%) and *Legionella* species (10%). Interestingly, this is the first case series describing *Legionella* as a cause of persistent cervical lymphadenitis, and diagnosis was made with PCR.

Surgical biopsy results from children in developing countries show a slightly different spectrum of disease. A review of 1332 patients younger than 15 years of age over a 23-year span in South Africa shows 48% reactive nodes, 25% *Mycobacterium tuberculosis*, 11.6% neoplasm, and 11.5% chronic granuloma. Miscellaneous etiologies included syphilis, yaws, toxoplasmosis, sinus histiocytosis, and Kaposi sarcoma.[12]

Age is useful in predicting etiology of infection (Table 17-1). Group B streptococcus commonly cause lymphadenitis in young infants; *S. aureus* infects infants and children; and *S. pyogenes*, *S. aureus*, and nontuberculous *Mycobacterium* species in children 1 to 4 years old. Acute cervical lymphadenitis may be more common in the young child because of an inability to localize the organism to the initial nasal or pharyngeal site of attachment. In children 5 to 15 years old and adults, anaerobic bacteria, toxoplasmosis, cat-scratch disease, and tuberculosis are important considerations.

LYMPHATIC FLOW AND FASCIAL SPACES OF THE HEAD AND NECK

A complex and efficient lymphatic system has evolved to defend against microbial invasion of the head, neck, nasopharynx, and oropharynx, as shown in Table 17-2 and Figure 17-1. There are three interrelated lines of defense. The ring of Waldeyer is composed of a circle of adenoidal, tonsillar, and lingual lymphoid tissue (see Chapter 16, Lymphatic System and Generalized Lymphadenopathy). A collar of superficial satellite lymph nodes runs along the lower margins of the jaw and encircles this ring. This outlying collar of nodes of the head consists of the occipital, postauricular, preauricular, parotid, and facial groups. Finally, the

nodes of the neck are the salivary gland-associated submaxillary and submental nodes and the vertically oriented superficial and deep cervical chains.

Occipital nodes are often enlarged when generalized lymphadenopathy is present; regional enlargement is almost always infectious and is due to tinea capitis, pediculosis capitis, seborrheic dermatitis, or scalp cellulitis or abscess. Enlargement of preauricular nodes reflects local skin or conjunctival infection. Asymptomatically enlarged parotid glands raise the possibility of malignancy.

Specific Lymph Node Groups

Superficial Cervical Nodes

The superficial cervical nodes in the neck are a disparate group composed roughly of three vertical chains. The deep lateral or spinal accessory chain runs behind the posterior border of the sternocleidomastoid (SCM) muscle and along the spinal accessory nerve. The superficial cervical chain follows the external jugular vein, which runs obliquely across the surface of the SCM muscle to empty into the subclavian vein in the supraclavicular triangle. The superficial anterior chain runs in the midline from the chin to the suprasternal notch and comprises, in descending order, the infrahyoid, prelaryngeal, pretracheal, and anterior cervical nodes. "Posterior cervical nodes" is a nonspecific term referring to nodes of the spinal accessory chain and those of the superficial cervical chain that lie over and behind the SCM muscle; lymph nodes in and anterior to the muscle are designated as lying in the anterior triangle and those behind the muscle lie in the posterior triangle.

Deep Cervical Nodes

The deep cervical chain of lymph nodes runs from the base of the skull to the root of the neck in close approximation to the internal jugular vein on the carotid sheath, and under the SCM muscle. This chain contains numerous large nodes and is divided into superior and inferior deep cervical groups. The superior group is above, and the inferior group below, the point low in the neck where the omohyoid muscle crosses the internal jugular vein. The lymphatic channels and nodes in the head and neck are linked, and ultimately all empty into the thoracic duct on the left or the lymphatic duct on the right, each of which in turn immediately empties into the respective subclavian vein.

The superior deep cervical group of nodes consists of the tonsillar or jugulodigastric node located at the angle of the mandible just below the posterior belly of the digastric muscle. The lymphoid tissue of the palatine tonsil drains into this gland. Other nodes of this group, which lie under the SCM muscle along the length of the internal jugular vein, drain the adenoid, larynx, trachea, thyroid, palate, esophagus, paranasal sinuses, nasopharynx, occipital scalp, back of the neck, pinna, and much of the tongue. The large jugulo-omohyoid node that drains the tongue lies just above the omohyoid muscle, at the point where it crosses the internal jugular vein, which separates the superior and inferior deep cervical nodes.

Because the majority of lymphatics of the head and neck drain to the submaxillary and deep cervical nodes, it is not surprising that these nodes are involved in more than 80% of cases of cervical lymphadenitis in young children.

The inferior deep cervical nodes lie low in the neck, below the omohyoid muscle and under and posterior to the anterior clavicular insertion of the SCM muscle. They lie in close approximation to the brachial plexus and to the entrance sites of the thoracic duct and right lymphatic duct into the left and right subclavian veins. All lymph from the head and neck, arms, superficial thorax, lungs, mediastinum, and abdomen passes through these nodes. The left supraclavicular nodes (Virchow–Troisier nodes) drain the left upper lobe of the lung, left mediastinum, stomach, small intestine, kidney, and pancreas. Enlargement of these nodes in the absence of cervical adenopathy suggests intraabdominal tumor or inflammation (Troisier sign) or intrathoracic disease. The right supraclavicular nodes drain the left lingula and lower lobes as well as the entire right lung, pleura, and right mediastinum. Enlargement of these nodes most often indicates thoracic lesions. Both Hodgkin lymphoma and NHL are common causes of enlargement of these nodes, and prompt biopsy is indicated in the absence of easily documented pulmonary or cervical infection.

Deep Neck Infections

The fascial system of the neck is complex, but a general anatomic description is useful to understand the deep neck infections. The neck fascia is divided into two layers: the superficial layer and the deep layer. The deep fascia is further divided into the superficial, middle, and deep layers of the deep fascia (Figure 17-2). There are 11 deep neck spaces that can all communicate with each other. These are the lateral pharyngeal (parapharyngeal),

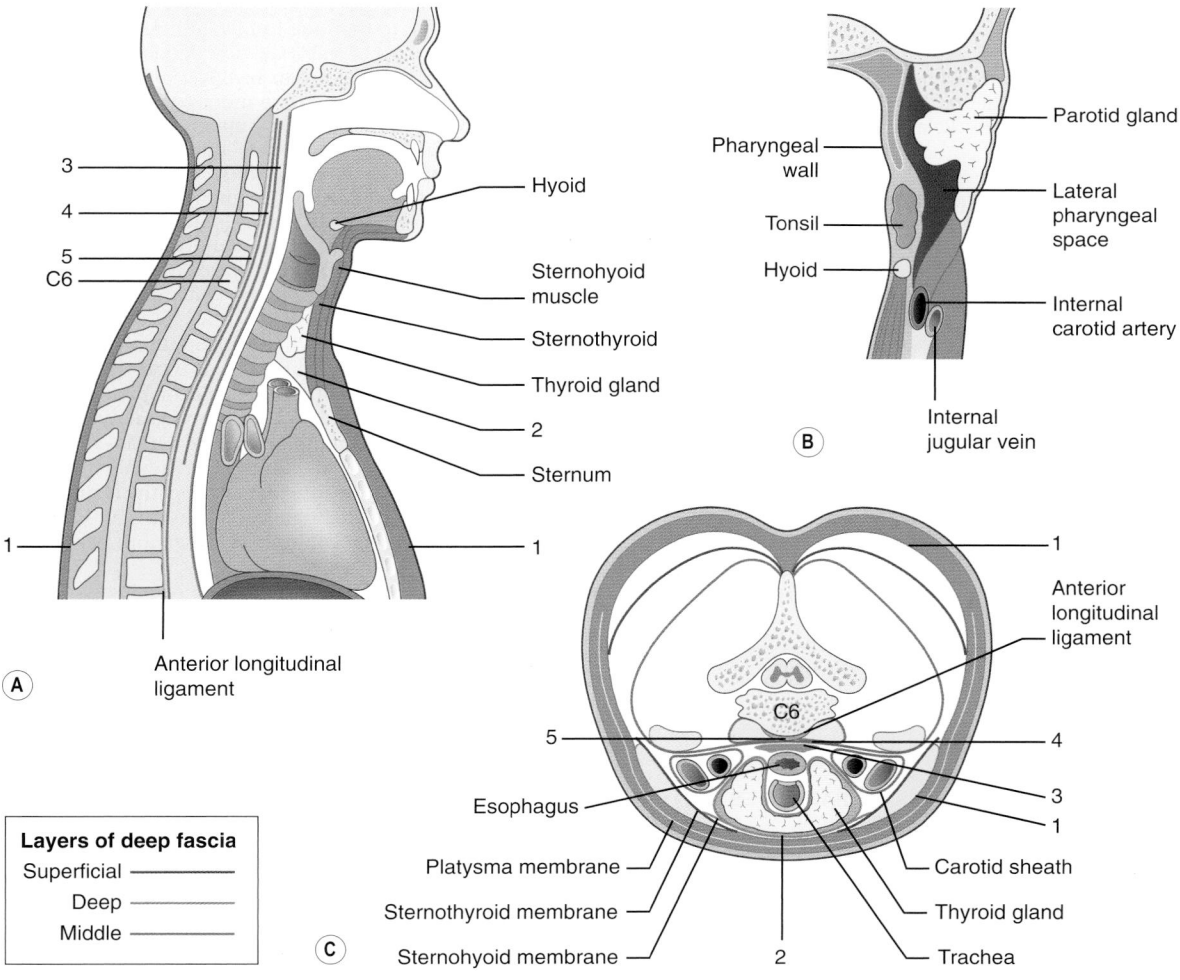

Figure 17-2. Relation of the lateral pharyngeal, retropharyngeal, and prevertebral spaces to the posterior and anterior layers of the deep cervical fascia. **(A)** Midsagittal image of the head and neck. **(B)** Coronal image in the suprahyoid region of the neck. **(C)** Cross-section of the neck at the level of the thyroid isthmus. In all illustrations, 1: superficial space; 2: pretracheal space; 3: retropharyngeal space; 4: danger space; 5: prevertebral space. (From Mandell, Principles and Practice of Infectious Disease, 7th Edition, 2009, Reproduced with permission of Elsevier.)

PART II Clinical Syndromes and Cardinal Features of Infectious Diseases: Approach to Diagnosis and Initial Management

SECTION B Cardinal Symptom Complexes

retropharyngeal, prevertebral, "danger", masticator, submandibular, carotid, pretracheal, peritonsillar, parotid, and temporal spaces.[13]

The most clinically relevant deep neck spaces include the submandibular, peritonsillar, retropharyngeal, and lateral pharyngeal spaces. Infection in the submandibular space is known as Ludwig angina. Ludwig angina is a bilateral, brawny cellulitis that originates in the floor of the mouth. Infection of the retropharyngeal space is most common in children aged 2 to 4 years. The space and thus involvement in infection is age limited as it contains several small lymph nodes that atrophy by adolescence. Infection in this space in older children and adults usually is secondary to direct trauma rather than to lymphatic spread. Cervical adenitis is not a common presentation as these nodes drain into the prevertebral space; however, mediastinitis and empyema can occur. The peritonsillar space surrounds the palatine tonsil. Peritonsillar abscess is the most common deep neck infection, accounting for 50% of cases, and is more common in adolescents and young adults. Abscess usually is unilateral but can be bilateral. Cervical and submandibular adenopathy also can occur from drainage of the superior deep cervical nodes.[14,15]

The lateral pharyngeal space is a central connection for all other neck spaces and thus infections can follow infection at multiple sites. Presentation with unilateral cervical adenitis is common given this circumstance. The lateral pharyngeal space is divided into anterior and posterior compartments. Suppurative jugular thrombophlebitis (Lemierre syndrome) is a well-described complication of *Fusobacterium* infection of the posterior compartment, most commonly spread from primary tonsillitis. Along with sepsis because of proximity to the carotid sheath, swelling around the SCM muscle or "bull neck," neck pain and stiffness, and torticollis are common.[14,15] More detailed descriptions regarding neck space infections are found in Chapter 25, Infections of the Oral Cavity, and Chapter 28, Infections Related to the Upper and Middle Airways.

OCULOGLANDULAR SYNDROME OF PARINAUD

The oculoglandular syndrome of Parinaud consists of unilateral, chronic granulomas or ulcers of the conjunctivae associated with preauricular and submaxillary lymphadenitis.[16] Causes are listed in Box 17-1, with the most common being *Bartonella henselae* infection. Primary conjunctival inoculation causes grey or yellow granulomatous nodules or areas of focal necrosis, often surrounded by significant conjunctival chemosis and palpebral inflammation. Recovery without sequelae (except for occasional mild conjunctival scarring) occurs within 2 to 3 months. Antimicrobial therapy usually is given but has not been proven to alter the course.[17]

BOX 17-1. Organisms Associated with Lymphocutaneous and Oculoglandular (Parinaud) Syndromes

VIRUSES

Herpes simplex

BACTERIA

Treponema pallidum
Mycobacterium tuberculosis
Bartonella henselae
Francisella tularensis
Corynebacterium diphtheriae
Spirillum minor
Chlamydia trachomatis
Bacillus anthracis
Nocardia brasiliensis
Yersinia enterocolitica
Listeria monocytogenes

FUNGI

Histoplasma capsulatum
Coccidioides immitis
Paracoccidioides spp.

PARASITES

Trypanosoma spp.

RICKETTSIA

Rickettsialpox

INFECTIOUS CAUSES OF LYMPHADENITIS

For purposes of predicting etiology, most cases of infectious cervical lymphadenitis can be divided into the following three categories (with some overlap): (1) acute bilateral lymphadenitis; (2) acute unilateral lymphadenitis; and (3) subacute (chronic) lymphadenitis.

Acute Bilateral Lymphadenitis

Acute bilateral lymphadenopathy/lymphadenitis most often is a localized response to acute pharyngitis or part of a generalized lymphoreticular response to systemic infection in older children. Usually, lymph nodes are small and soft, may or may not be tender, and are not associated with erythema or warmth of the overlying skin. Viral upper respiratory tract infection is the most common cause, followed by pharyngitis due to *Streptococcus pyogenes* and *Mycoplasma pneumoniae*.

Epstein–Barr virus. Although generalized lymphadenopathy is common in Epstein–Barr virus (EBV) infection, cervical adenopathy is most prominent and is present in 93% of infected children.[18] Enlargement is usually bilateral and most prominent in the posterior cervical chain, followed by the anterior cervical chain. Lymph nodes are enlarged singly or in groups; vary from 5 to 25 mm in diameter; and are firm, discrete, and minimally tender. Moderate splenomegaly occurs in 75% of patients. Significant enlargement of the lymphoid tissue in Waldeyer ring can result in nasopharyngeal and oropharyngeal airway obstruction.

Cytomegalovirus. Mononucleosis due to cytomegalovirus (CMV) is similar to that due to EBV, although it is more frequent in children <4 years of age.[18] Cervical adenopathy is less common in CMV infection (75%) than in EBV (95%) infection. Tonsillopharyngitis and sore throat are more common in EBV infection, whereas hepatosplenomegaly, upper-airway obstruction, and rashes are more common in CMV infection.

Herpes simplex virus infections. Cervical, submaxillary, and submental nodes frequently are enlarged and tender during the course of primary gingivostomatitis due to herpes simplex virus (HSV). Primary infections of the conjunctivae and lids are accompanied by preauricular adenopathy. Localized or regional necrotizing lymphadenitis from primary HSV infection also has been reported as a rare occurrence.[19]

Adenoviral syndromes. Pharyngoconjunctival fever, caused by adenovirus, is characterized by abrupt onset of fever, pharyngitis, and granular conjunctivitis (unilateral or bilateral). Hyperplasia of the tonsillar, adenoidal, and pharyngeal lymphoid tissue is present. A study from Spain showed that 32% of children with positive pharyngeal cultures for adenovirus had cervical node enlargement.[20] Preauricular adenopathy is surprisingly infrequent. Generalized adenopathy is present in 10% to 20% of patients with pharyngoconjunctival fever, and hepatosplenomegaly is common.

Preauricular adenitis occurs in 90% of patients with epidemic keratoconjunctivitis. Half of patients with the usually unilateral, acute, follicular conjunctivitis also have pharyngitis and rhinitis.[21]

Acute respiratory disease due to adenoviruses generally has significant constitutional as well as localized respiratory symptoms. Bilateral cervical adenopathy is present almost always.

Enteroviruses. Nonspecific febrile illness due to coxsackieviruses and echoviruses generally has an abrupt onset. Manifestations include fever, malaise, sore throat, nausea, vomiting, and abdominal pain. Minimal conjunctival and pharyngeal erythema with bilateral cervical adenopathy is present.

Human herpesvirus 6 and 7 (roseola). In one reported series of human herpesvirus 6 (HHV-6) infections in 688 children, mild bilateral cervical adenopathy was present in 31% of cases. Typically, the occipital, posterior auricular, and posterior cervical nodes are involved, but enlargement is modest.[22] HHV-7 also can cause roseola; however, the complete clinical picture of disease has not been defined.[23]

Human herpesvirus 8. HHV-8 generally is thought of as the etiologic agent of Kaposi sarcoma in severely immunosuppressed patients with human immunodeficiency virus infection. It has also been associated with primary effusion lymphoma and multicentric Castleman disease. Fever, sore throat, morbilliform rash, and cervical lymphadenopathy, however, can occur with primary infection in immunocompetent children.[24,25]

Rubella virus. In patients with experimentally induced rubella, lymph node enlargement begins as early as 7 days before the onset of the rash. Although generalized lymphadenopathy occurs, the nodes most commonly involved are the posterior auricular, suboccipital, and cervical nodes. Tenderness and swelling are most severe on the first day of the rash. Although tenderness of nodes subsides within 1 to 2 days, enlargement persists for weeks.

Parvovirus B19. A mononucleosis-like syndrome due to parvovirus B19 infection can be associated with bilateral cervical and intraparotid lymphadenopathy. Generalized lymphadenopathy and hepatosplenomegaly also can be present. Facial palsy and parotitis can accompany intraparotid lymphadenopathy.[26]

Mycoplasma pneumoniae. Physical examination of children and adults with pneumonia due to *M. pneumoniae* reveals cervical adenopathy in 25%, pharyngitis in 50%, and auscultatory findings in 75%. In patients in whom pharyngitis is the major manifestation, 43% have exudative tonsillitis and 50% have cervical adenopathy.

Corynebacterium diphtheriae. Cervical adenitis is variable in tonsillar and pharyngeal diphtheria. In some cases, adenitis is associated with edema of the soft tissues of the neck ("erasive edema") so severe as to appear as to cause a bull-neck appearance. In other cases, lymphadenitis is minimal.

Acute Unilateral Lymphadenitis

Table 17-3 summarizes clinical clues to and diagnostic tests for selected causes of unilateral cervical lymphadenitis.

Staphylococcus aureus and Streptococcus pyogenes. *S. aureus* or *S. pyogenes* infections account for 40% to 80% of cases of acute unilateral cervical lymphadenitis.[3,4] Typically, the patient is a 1- to 4-year-old child with a history of recent upper respiratory tract symptoms (sore throat, earache, coryza) or impetigo and signs of pharyngitis, tonsillitis, or acute otitis media. Few clinical findings distinguish streptococcal from staphylococcal infection.

The infected nodes, usually in the submaxillary or superior deep cervical chain, are 2.5 to 6 cm in diameter, tender, and often the overlying skin is erythematous and warm. Systemic symptoms, bacteremia, or metastatic foci of infection can occur. Occasionally, suppuration and periadenitis are so severe that torticollis is present and individual nodes cannot be palpated. Systemic symptoms such as high fever, toxicity, tachycardia, and flushed facies may be present. In up to a third of cases that come to medical attention, lymph node suppuration and fluctuation develop. Infection caused by *S. aureus* tends to have a longer duration of disease before diagnosis, a higher likelihood of suppuration, and slower resolution (Figure 17-3).

The role of *S. aureus* as a sole cause of acute unilateral lymphadenitis has been questioned. In a study from 1979, node aspirates from 65% of the patients yielded pure growth of *S. aureus*; 41% of these patients exhibited an immune response to one or more of the extracellular antigens of *S. pyogenes*.[27] Additionally, it has been observed that many children improve clinically with penicillin or ampicillin therapy alone, which would not be effective against β-lactamase-producing *S. aureus*. Recent studies suggest a predominant role of *S. aureus* (including CA-MRSA) compared with *S. pyogenes* when etiology is confirmed; however, recent serologic studies have not been performed.[5,6,28]

Streptococcus agalactiae (group B streptococcus). Typically, the young infant with group B streptococcal cellulitis–adenitis (submandibular/cervical) syndrome has abrupt onset of fever, poor feeding, and irritability associated with unilateral facial or submandibular swelling that is erythematous and tender.[29] Bacteremia usually is present, and the organism is isolated from the aspirate of cellulitis or a lymph node. Ipsilateral otitis media is common. Meningitis is present in as many as 24% of infants with cellulitis–adenitis.[30] Suppurative submandibular lymphadenitis

TABLE 17-3. Clinical Clues and Diagnostic Test(s) for Selected Causes of Unilateral Cervical Lymphadenitis

Organisms	Clinical Clues	Diagnostic Test(s)
Staphylococcus aureus *Streptococcus pyogenes*	Acute unilateral adenitis; ages 1–4 years; 2–6-cm nodes, frequent associated cellulitis; 25–33% become fluctuant For *Staphylococcus aureus*, suppuration is rapid; without therapy, 85% of nodes suppurate	Throat culture for *Streptococcus pyogenes*; needle aspirate of node for Gram stain and culture
Group B streptococcus	Ages 2–6 weeks; cellulitis–adenitis syndrome; facial or submandibular cellulitis; ipsilateral otitis media	Blood culture and aspirate of node or soft tissue for Gram stain and culture CSF evaluation if cellulitis–adenitis syndrome
Anaerobic bacteria	Older children; dental caries; periapical or periodontal disease present, Lemierre Syndrome	Needle aspiration of node for Gram stain and culture; blood culture
Bartonella henselae	Most common cause of chronic unilateral adenopathy; contact with kittens; oculoglandular syndrome; inoculation papule present	Serologic analysis; culture of tissue with granulomas with stellate abscesses on biopsy, PCR
Nontuberculous *Mycobacterium*	Age 1–5 years; no systemic symptoms; no exposure to TB; unilateral submandibular node: normal chest radiograph and ESR; TST usually <15 mm	Characteristic granulomatous reaction; culture of excised node, PCR
Mycobacterium tuberculosis	Age >5 years; systemic symptoms with history of exposure to TB; bilateral lower cervical node involvement; elevated ESR	Positive TST and chest radiograph; culture of gastric aspirate, PCR
Toxoplasma gondii	Fever, fatigue, myalgia, sore throat; discrete <3 cm localized anterior cervical, suboccipital, or supraclavicular nodes; ± mediastinal adenopathy	Serologic analysis (laboratory with special expertise)

CSF, cerebrospinal fluid; ESR, erythrocyte sedimentation rate; PCR, polymerase chain reaction; TST, tuberculin skin test; TB, tuberculosis.

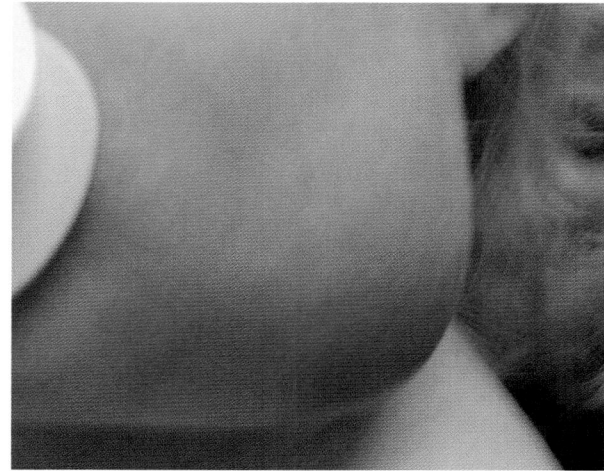

Figure 17-3. *Staphylococcus aureus* neck abscess in a toddler.

PART II Clinical Syndromes and Cardinal Features of Infectious Diseases: Approach to Diagnosis and Initial Management

SECTION B Cardinal Symptom Complexes

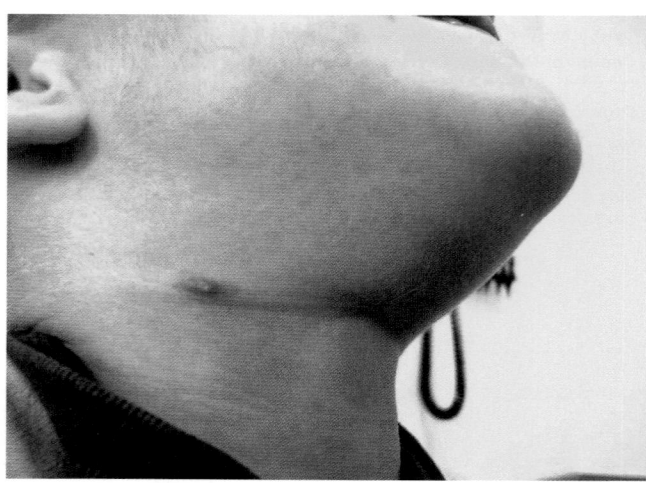

Figure 17-4. Ulceroglandular tularemia. Note adenopathy relative to papular lesion at the site of the tick bite.

caused by *S. aureus* sometimes is distinguishable because of manifestation as a discrete mass and the propensity for suppuration.

Anaerobic bacteria. In older children with the acute onset of unilateral adenitis, an anaerobic infection secondary to periodontal or dental abscesses should be considered. Such infection can lead to septic thrombophlebitis of the jugular vein, septic pulmonary emboli, and central nervous system infection (Lemierre syndrome; see Chapter 25, Infections of the Oral Cavity; Chapter 28, Infections Related to the Upper and Middle Airways). Presentation is with bull neck, severe inflammatory response, systemic toxicity, and several positive blood cultures with isolation of *Fusobacterium* spp. or less commonly viridans streptococci.

Francisella tularensis. Cervical lymphadenopathy alone or concurrent with other regional adenopathy was common in tularemia. In one series, lymphadenopathy (especially cervical nodes) was the most common manifestation, being present in 96% of patients; in 4 of 28 children, cervical nodes were the only enlarged nodes (Figure 17-4).[31] One-third of the children had late suppuration after antibiotic therapy. In untreated cases, the skin over the involved nodes is inflamed, and about 50% of nodes suppurate and drain. In the remainder of cases, the nodes remain firm, enlarged, and tender for several months.

In oculoglandular tularemia, the eyelids become edematous, and the conjunctivae are inflamed and painful, with nodules and ulcers. Preauricular, submaxillary, and cervical nodes are enlarged, tender, and painful.

Pasteurella multocida. After an animal bite or scratch on the head, neck, or upper chest, acute unilateral cellulitis due to *P. multocida* can be associated with tender cervical lymphadenitis.

Yersinia pestis. Fleas from wild mammals, cats, and dogs in the western United States serve as the vectors for *Y. pestis* (bubonic plague). Organisms are carried in lymphatics to the nearest node, usually causing acutely enlarged, edematous, exquisitely tender, unilateral lymphadenitis with overlying erythema (bubo). As animal bites occur more commonly on the extremities than around the head and neck, cervical adenopathy is the third most common site of involvement. Fever and other systemic manifestations accompany the appearance of buboes. Untreated, the nodes suppurate and ulcerate.

Unusual organisms. Rarely, gram-negative bacilli, *Streptococcus pneumoniae*, group C streptococci, *Nocardia brasiliensis*, *Yersinia enterolitica*, *Staphylococcus epidermidis*, α-hemolytic streptococci, *Legionella,* or endemic fungi such as *Histoplasma* or *Coccidioides* are isolated from a node. Immunodeficiencies such as Job syndrome and chronic granulomatous disease should be considered if a catalase-producing gram-positive or gram-negative organism is causative.

Subacute or Chronic Unilateral Lymphadenitis

Mycobacterial infections, cat-scratch disease, and toxoplasmosis are most commonly associated with subacute lymphadenitis. Typical finding is a painless or minimally tender, unilateral, swollen cervical or submaxillary node. If the lymph nodes enlarge and the disease progresses, the overlying skin becomes taut and effaced, with pinkish discoloration (although there is no increase in skin temperature). Skin becomes attached to the underlying mass. If the infection is untreated, fluctuation and spontaneous drainage (with or without formation of sinus tracts) usually follow. Suppuration from toxoplasmosis is rare.

Cat-scratch disease. Cat-scratch disease is regional lymphadenitis that follows inoculation of *B. henselae* into damaged skin or mucosal membrane. The most common sites of lymphadenopathy are the axilla (52%) and neck (28%), presumably from scratches on the extremities and cuddling an animal, respectively. Classically, adenopathy begins 5 days to 2 months after inoculation. Generally, the affected node is solitary, often >4 cm in diameter, and tender. Constitutional symptoms usually are mild and include fever in up to 25% of cases. Overlying skin is not red or warm, but suppuration occurs in 30% to 50% of patients brought to medical attention. The oculoglandular syndrome of Parinaud, initially described in cat-scratch disease, is common.[12] Supraclavicular nodes can be involved from scratches on the neck or upper chest. Nonsuppurative nodes diminish in size after 4 to 6 weeks. Treatment probably aborts suppuration of larger nodes (see Chapter 160, *Bartonella* Species).

Toxoplasmosis. In the 10% of patients with acquired toxoplasmosis who are symptomatic, lymphadenopathy and fatigue without fever are the most common manifestations.[32] The nodes most commonly involved are the cervical, suboccipital, supraclavicular, axillary, and inguinal. The involved nodes are discrete, may or may not be tender, and do not suppurate. Adenopathy is localized or involves multiple areas.

Nontuberculous Mycobacterium (NTM). Infection due to NTM occurs in children 1 to 4 years old and cervical adenitis is the most common manifestation in this age group. Organisms are ubiquitous in soil and probably are ingested; infection is localized to a submandibular or single tonsillar node. Bilateral involvement is rare. A recognizably enlarged node is usually the superficial marker of a large, deeper cluster. Initial appearance can be rapid (over 24 hours), with gradual increase in node size over 2 to 3 weeks. Most enlarged nodes are ≤3 cm in diameter, although enlargement to >5 cm can occur. Pain, tenderness, and constitutional illness are minimal. Approximately 50% of children with recognized lymphadenitis have fluctuant lesions, and in 10%, spontaneous drainage and sinus tract formation occur (Figure 17–5A). The skin changes from pink to a distinctive lilac red, with the overlying skin developing a thin, parchment-like quality. In some cases, fluctuation without skin changes develops. Signs and symptoms of *Mycobacterium tuberculosis* adenitis and NTM adenitis are identical (Figure 17–5B). Other clinical and epidemiologic features are distinctive. Chest radiograph is normal in children with NTM infection, and an intermediate Mantoux tuberculin skin test results in <15 mm induration (usually 5 to 9 mm). Surgical excision generally is recommended unless proximity to nerves is concerning or cosmetic outcome is undesirable. Incisional drainage is not recommended as the development of sinus tracts is possible. Therapy with antimicrobial agents active against NTM as adjunctive therapy may be useful in some situations.[33–35] (see Chapter 135, *Mycobacterium* Species Non-*tuberculosis*).

Mycobacterium tuberculosis. Striking enlargement of the superficial regional lymph nodes is an integral part of the primary lower respiratory tuberculous complex. Involvement of the cervical nodes is most often the result of extension from the paratracheal nodes to the tonsillar and submaxillary nodes or from the apical pleurae and upper lung fields by direct spread to the inferior deep cervical (supraclavicular) nodes. Rarely, superficial lymph nodes are enlarged secondary to generalized adenopathy during the course of lymphohematogenous spread of infection

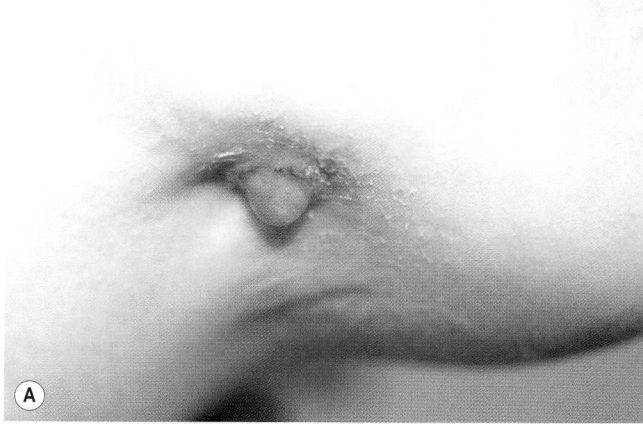
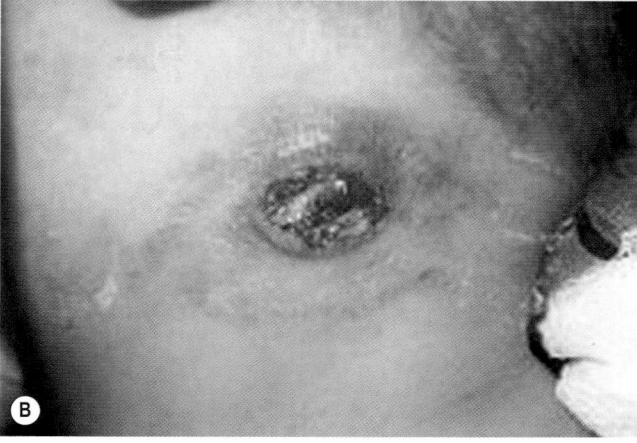

Figure 17-5. (A) Draining lymph node due to nontuberculous *Mycobacterium* infection (courtesy of J. Christenson, Indianapolis, IL). **(B)** Draining lymph node due to *Mycobacterium tuberculosis* infection. These are clinically indistinguishable.

(Figure 17-5B). Reactivation of quiescent tuberculous infection can manifest initially as localized or generalized adenopathy.

When superficial nodes are involved early in the infection, nodes usually are enlarged, painless and rubbery.[36] Bilateral enlargement is the rule, but right-sided involvement can predominate. Acute nontuberculous respiratory tract infections can precipitate or aggravate tuberculous lymphadenitis, resulting in local pain and perilymphadenitis. Rarely, the patient is seen with a fluctuant mass and shiny, erythematous overlying skin. These nodes can rupture and drain chronically. Secondary infection with other pyogenic bacteria can occur. In general, clinical features do not distinguish tuberculous and nontuberculous mycobacterial infections and diagnosis may be difficult if exposure to *M. tuberculosis* is suspected.[36] Surgical excision frequently is avoided with infection due to *M. tuberculosis* as infection usually extends into the mediastinum and responds to antituberculous therapy.

***Actinomyces* and *Nocardia* species.** In cervicofacial actinomycosis, *Actinomyces israelii* causes a chronic, granulomatous suppurative infection of the soft tissues in and around the mandible. Although lymph nodes usually are not involved, chronic tissue induration can mimic chronic lymphadenopathy. Tissue destruction can be considerable without proper therapy.

The lymphocutaneous syndrome due to *Nocardia* spp. in children begins with a facial papular lesion followed by fever and an enlarged, tender, unilateral, submaxillary gland.[37] *N. brasiliensis* is the most common species causing the skin and lymph node cervicofacial syndrome. Lymphadenitis was associated with the skin lesions in 58% of children in Texas with nocardiosis.[38] Lymphocutaneous nocardiosis can occur in healthy children, and an

exhaustive search for an immunodeficiency is not necessary if there is a prompt response to trimethoprim-sulfamethoxazole therapy.

BCG vaccination. When vaccination using Calmette-Guérin bacillus is given, painless enlargement of regional nodes (axillary, rarely cervical) can occur and presumably is due to multiplication of bacilli and formation of granulomas. Calcification or abscess formation with breakdown can occur, particularly in infants.[39] Rarely, regional adenitis can develop years after vaccination, especially if the individual becomes immunocompromised. Treatment is controversial and spontaneous resolution of nonsuppurative lesions generally occurs without antimicrobial therapy in young children.[40]

NONINFECTIOUS CAUSES OF LYMPHADENOPATHY

Kawasaki disease. Lymph node swelling is the least common of the principal diagnostic criteria of Kawasaki disease, occurring in 50% to 75% of patients. Lymphadenitis, one of the earliest manifestations, usually is unilateral and confined to the anterior triangle; the node is moderately tender. The enlarged node or mass of nodes usually is >1.5 cm in diameter and nonfluctuant, sometimes with overlying erythema. The ultrasound appearance of an acutely enlarged node due to Kawasaki disease differs from that of bacterial lymphadenitis, and can be a useful diagnostic tool.[41] Suppuration does not occur, and adenopathy usually resolves early in the course of disease.

Periodic fever, aphthous stomatitis, pharyngitis, and cervical adenitis (PFAPA). First described in 1987,[42] PFAPA usually affects children younger than 5 years. Bilateral modestly enlarged and tender cervical nodes are typical during febrile episodes; other lymph nodes are not affected (see Chapter 15, Prolonged, Recurrent, and Periodic Fever Syndromes).

Sarcoidosis. The most common physical finding in children with sarcoidosis is peripheral lymphadenopathy. Involved cervical nodes are enlarged bilaterally and are discrete, firm, and rubbery. More than 80% of children have involvement of the supraclavicular nodes; bilateral hilar adenopathy is almost always present, along with nonspecific symptoms and other multisystem manifestations.

Sinus histiocytosis with massive lymphadenopathy (Rosai–Dorfman disease). Rosai–Dorfman disease is a rare non-Langerhans cell histiocytosis that manifests in the first decade of life with mobile, discretely and asymmetrically enlarged lymph nodes, initially usually located in the neck.[43] With progression, the nodes become massively enlarged bilaterally and are painless and adherent to surrounding tissues. Other nodal groups (e.g., axillary, inguinal, and hilar nodes) and extranodal sites can be involved. Systemic manifestations of fever, leukocytosis, neutrophilia, anemia, elevated inflammatory markers, and hypergammaglobulinemia frequently are present. Histopathologic analysis demonstrates florid follicular hyperplasia, marked histiocytic proliferation, and prominent plasmacytosis. Resolution occurs spontaneously after 6 to 9 months, but therapy may be required for extensive or progressive disease.

Histiocytic necrotizing lymphadenitis (Kikuchi–Fujimoto disease). Kikuchi–Fujimoto disease is a benign, rare entity of unknown etiology that manifests in older children with bilaterally enlarged, firm, painful cervical nodes, most often in the posterior cervical triangle, which are unresponsive to antibiotic therapy. Perinodal inflammation is common. Associated findings in 50% of patients include skin lesions, fever, leukopenia with atypical lymphocytosis, and an elevated erythrocyte sedimentation rate. Those with prolonged fever are more likely to develop leukopenia.[44] Splenomegaly, nausea, weight loss, and night sweats can be present. Nodal histology showing necrosis and exuberant histiocytic infiltration is characteristic but can be confused with that of malignant lymphoma. No other diagnostic test is available. Symptoms resolve in most patients a few days after excisional biopsy. Viral etiology is suspected based on a few reports of serologic

PART II   Clinical Syndromes and Cardinal Features of Infectious Diseases: Approach to Diagnosis and Initial Management

SECTION B   Cardinal Symptom Complexes

studies suggesting EBV, CMV, human T-lymphotropic virus (HTLV), HHV-6, and parvovirus B19 infection.[45] Kikuchi–Fujimoto disease also has been shown to occur in association with or preceding systemic lupus erythematosus in some cases. In the majority of cases the prognosis for spontaneous resolution of Kikuchi–Fujimoto disease is excellent.[46,47]

Kimura disease. Kimura disease is a chronic, benign, but potentially disfiguring unilateral, localized cervical lymphadenopathy of Asians, most often males of Chinese or Japanese descent. Insidious onset of painless, subcutaneous nodules overlying the affected lymph nodes occurs. Eosinophilia and a marked increase in serum immunoglobulin E are present. Renal involvement may occur, with proteinuria present in 12% to 16% of cases.[48] Resection, irradiation, or corticosteroid therapy can be associated with recurrences.[49,50]

NECK MASSES NOT INVOLVING LYMPH NODES

Tumors of the Head and Neck

The differential diagnosis of neck masses includes congenital cysts and sinuses, vascular malformations, salivary and thyroid anomalies, and benign and malignant neoplasms of nonsquamous origin.

Malignancy should be considered, particularly in older children with a painless, firm, cervical mass >3 cm in diameter that is fixed to the deep cervical tissues, has grown rapidly, or is located in the supraclavicular area or posterior triangle of the neck. Such masses can be multiple and can extend across the anterior and posterior triangles. The incidence of all pediatric cancer has increased in the last few decades; however, the incidence of pediatric neck masses over the same timeframe has increased at a greater rate. Teenagers 15 to 18 years old are the most frequently affected (39%), followed by children aged 4 years and younger (27%).[51]

Fifty percent of masses in the posterior triangle are malignancies, most of lymphoid origin. Fifty percent of all malignant neck masses in children are Hodgkin lymphoma or NHL; neuroblastoma is the next most common, accounting for 15%, followed by thyroid tumors. Soft-tissue sarcomas, including primary rhabdomyosarcoma and carcinoma of salivary glands and the nasopharynx, also occur. Age is predictive of diagnosis; in children younger than 6 years, the most common malignancies, in order of decreasing frequency, are neuroblastoma, NHL, rhabdomyosarcoma, and Hodgkin lymphoma. In patients 7 to 15 years old, Hodgkin lymphoma and lymphosarcoma occur with equal frequency, followed by thyroid carcinoma, rhabdomyosarcoma, and parotid adenocarcinoma.

Soft-tissue sarcomas manifesting in the neck are primary rhabdomyosarcoma and undifferentiated sarcomas. Rhabdomyosarcoma accounts for 18% of all solid carcinomas in children; of these, 36% manifest in the head and neck region, usually as an asymptomatic mass or with symptoms related to location.

Hodgkin lymphoma most commonly manifests as an asymptomatic cervical or supraclavicular mass. Upper cervical nodes are three to four times more likely to be involved than supraclavicular nodes. NHL is more likely to be associated with systemic symptoms, including fever and leukocytosis with pronounced neutrophilia, and cervical lymph node involvement, which can be unilateral and associated with massive swelling. Cervical adenopathy is a primary symptom in only 11% to 35% of patients with Hodgkin lymphoma, and extranodal head and neck masses are unusual.[52]

Congenital Cysts and Sinuses

Multiple congenital cysts and sinuses related to embryologic development can manifest as infection or as the sudden appearance of a mass as if infected.[53] Recurrence of a suppurative mass in exactly the same location should lead to evaluation for an underlying congenital lesion.[54] Table 17-4 delineates noninfectious causes of neck masses in children.

TABLE 17-4. Noninfectious Causes of Neck Masses[a]

Condition	Comments
CONGENITAL ANOMALIES	
Thyroglossal duct cyst	Most common congenital neck mass; discrete 1-cm midline nodule that may elevate with tongue protrusion; elective excision best; may contain only existing thyroid tissue
Second pharyngeal (branchial) cleft anomaly	Second most common congenital neck mass; anterior to upper or middle one-third of sternomastoid muscle; external sinus opens anterior to sternal head of muscle; tract needs to be excised; cyst associated with lymphatic tissue
Cystic hygroma	Third most common congenital neck mass; occurs along jugular lymphatic chain in posterior supraclavicular fossa; failure of mesenchymal clefts to fuse; varies from few centimeters to massive collar-like lesions; may extend into mediastinum
Dermoid or epidermoid cysts	Midline, deep to mylohyoid muscle; soft, fluid-filled midline mass; may elevate with tongue protrusion; contain caseous material or epithelial debris
NONLYMPHOMATOUS MALIGNANCIES	
Neuroblastoma	Second most common malignant neck mass in children (first in younger children)
Thyroid cancer	Third most common neck malignancy (first in 11–18 years); high incidence of malignancy in thyroid nodules; prompt biopsy required
Rhabdomyosarcoma	Most common nasopharyngeal malignancy in children
Nasopharyngeal carcinoma	Cervical adenopathy often initial and only symptom; arises most often in fossa of Rosenmüller
Parotid tumors	Vascular anomalies most common; asymptomatic node may be malignant and should be excised
MISCELLANEOUS	
Sternocleidomastoid tumor	Fibrous mass within muscle; detected at 2–4 weeks of age in 0.4% of infants; head turned away from mass; ipsilateral facial hypoplasia
Sinus histiocytosis with massive lymphadenopathy (Rosai–Dorfman disease)	Bilateral, painless cervical nodes; generalized lymphadenopathy may develop; systemic manifestations include fever and hypergammaglobulinemia; self-limited
Giant lymph node hyperplasia (Castleman disease)	Asymptomatic lymphadenopathy in mediastinum or neck; systemic symptoms include fever and hypergammaglobulinemia; surgical removal curative (see Ch. 18)
Histiocytic necrotizing lymphadenitis (Kikuchi–Fujimoto disease)	Asymptomatic cervical or generalized adenopathy; skin lesions, fever, and leukopenia; spontaneous resolution; recurrences possible
Kimura disease	Benign, chronic, unilateral lymphadenopathy; adjacent subcutaneous nodules, peripheral eosinophilia and increased serum immunoglobulin E, proteinuria and renal involvement possible

[a]For review of lymphomas, see Chapter 16, Lymphatic System and Generalized Lymphadenopathy; Chapter 18, Mediastinal and Hilar Lymphadenopathy.

Branchial Cleft Cysts and Sinuses

During the fifth week of embryologic development, four endodermal pharyngeal pouches fuse with four ectodermally derived clefts and are obliterated. Rarely, they are not completely obliterated, and persistence of the cleft can result in a cystic mass or sinus tract that is prone to infection. Persistence of the first pharyngeal cleft results in a sinus tract opening just behind the ramus of the mandible. Cystic components of the tract, which extends to the external ear canal, often are more extensive than is apparent clinically. Persistence of the second cleft is most common, the opening of which is just anterior to the sternal attachment of the SCM muscle. The unseen tract extends the length of the SCM muscle, beginning at the tonsillar bed. Cysts, with potential for acute enlargement, can occur anywhere along the length of the tract. Anomalies of the second and third cleft are indistinguishable. Because the thymus also is derived from the third cleft, thymic duct remnants can be seen as soft, fluctuant, mobile paratracheal masses low in the neck. Surgery usually is required to remove the sinus tract or cyst to prevent recurrences.

Midline Sinuses and Cysts

Dermoid or epidermoid cysts are embryologic defects in fusion. They occur as painless, soft, fluid-filled midline masses.

Thyroid tissue originates embryologically at the base of the tongue and descends the thyroglossal duct to its usual site anterior to the proximal end of the trachea. Although the tract usually is obliterated, cysts can form along its course, appearing as 1-cm midline nodules. Retaining attachment to the base of tongue, such cysts elevate on tongue protrusion. It is important to determine the presence and position of thyroid tissue, because cysts may contain the only functional gland. Nodules within the thyroid gland have a high incidence of malignancy in children. A thyroid mass in the neonate most often is a congenital goiter or a teratoma.

Lymphangiomas

In the sixth embryologic week, clefts develop in the cervical mesenchyma, which subsequently fuse to form lymph channels and lymph nodes. Sequestration, or failure to communicate with the rest of the lymphatic system, leads to tumor-like masses of lymph channels most commonly found along the external jugular chain of lymphatics in the lateral cervical region. Lymphatic masses vary in size from a few centimeters to massive collarlike lesions with extension into the mediastinum. In the larger lesions, lymphatic channels dilate into cystic spaces and the lesion is called a cystic hygroma. Most cystic hygromas are posterior to the sternomastoid muscle in the supraclavicular fossa. Sixty-five percent are present at birth and gradually increase in size as a result of obstructed flow or bleeding; the remainder almost always appears before age 2 years (Figure 17-6).

Salivary and Thyroid Gland Masses

Parotid Gland Masses

Parotid tumors are rare. The most common parotid masses are vascular anomalies, usually capillary hemangiomas and rarely cavernous hemangiomas. Large cavernous hemangiomas can disfigure and destroy tissue, whereas capillary hemangiomas usually resolve by the age of 4 to 5 years without any permanent findings. Parotid gland enlargement in childhood can result from calculus formation or recurrent sialectasia, in which case the parotid gland becomes rubbery, firm, and tender but has no signs of inflammation. Parotid infections are discussed in Chapter 25, Infections of the Oral Cavity.

Thyroiditis

Infection of the thyroid gland is rare but potentially is life-threatening. Infection can arise via the hematogenous route or

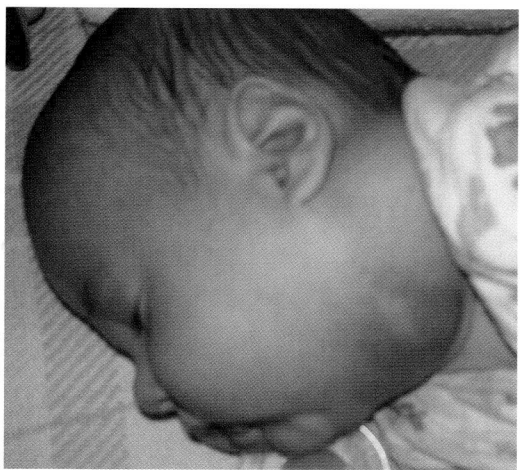

Figure 17-6. Cystic hygroma in a 2-month-old child, infected secondarily with group B streptococcus.

directly from an adjacent fascial space infection, from a patent foramen cecum and infected thyroglossal duct cyst, or from anterior esophageal perforation. Suppuration usually results from infection of pyriform sinus fistula or thyroglossal duct remnant. The most common aerobic pathogens are *S. aureus*, group A streptococci, pneumococci, and viridans streptococci. Anaerobic bacteria also are isolated, with the most common being gram-negative bacilli including *Prevotella* spp. and *Peptostreptococcus* spp. Other pathogens are *Haemophilus influenzae*, *Eikenella corrodens*, *Actinomyces* spp., with rare reports of enteric gram-negative bacilli, mycobacteria, and fungi.[55,56]

History and physical examination identify acute onset of fever, chills, sore throat, dysphagia, hoarseness, and an extremely tender, red, warm, and enlarged gland. Involvement can be unilateral or bilateral; pain can be referred to the ear or chest. Results of thyroid function tests usually are normal. Laboratory investigation of thyroiditis should include ultrasonography, radionuclide scan, or computed tomography to detect paratracheal extension; needle aspiration is performed for diagnostic microbiology. With prompt and aggressive therapy, complete resolution without abscess formation is expected.

Subacute (de Quervain) thyroiditis is a poorly defined, self-limited condition characterized by an insidious onset with tenderness and marked induration of the gland. The sedimentation rate is high, and biopsy reveals acute and chronic inflammation with granulomatous changes. In most cases, the cause is a virus, such as mumps virus, influenza virus, enterovirus, adenovirus, echovirus, EBV, or, rarely, St. Louis encephalitis virus.[56] Mild and transient manifestations of hypermetabolism and elevated thyroid hormone levels can be present. Differentiation from bacterial thyroiditis can be difficult.

DIAGNOSTIC APPROACH TO CERVICAL LYMPHADENOPATHY

The assessment and specific evaluation and management of cervical lymphadenopathy and lymphadenitis are directed by integration of the history and initial examination (Table 17-5). In young infants with acute unilateral involvement and systemic manifestations, causative agents can be expected to be *S. aureus*, group B streptococcus, or gram-negative organisms. Blood as well as aspirate of the node or cellulitis is obtained for culture. Examination of cerebrospinal fluid should be considered in young infants if the etiology is group B streptococcus. Isolated finding of discrete small cervical nodes in a healthy infant is likely to be normal (see Table 14-1). Associated findings may lead to evaluation for congenital infection in other patients.

PART II Clinical Syndromes and Cardinal Features of Infectious Diseases: Approach to Diagnosis and Initial Management

SECTION B Cardinal Symptom Complexes

TABLE 17-5. Mode of Onset and Characteristics of Lymph Nodes Infected by Selected Organisms

Pathogen	Mode of Onset		Characteristics		
	Acute	Subacute/Chronic	Suppuration	Cellulitis	Generalized Adenopathy
BACTERIA					
Staphylococcus aureus	++++	–	++++	++++	–
Streptococcus pyogenes	++++	–	+++	++++	+
Anaerobic bacteria	+++	–	+++	++	–
Bartonella henselae	–	++++	+++	+	+
Francisella tularensis	+++	++	+++	+++	–
Yersinia enterocolitica	++	++	+++	+	+
Pasteurella multocida	+++	–	+	+++	–
Yersinia pestis	++++	–	++++	++	–
Nontuberculous *Mycobacterium*	+	++++	+++	+	–
Mycobacterium tuberculosis	+	++++	+++	+	+++
Group B streptococcus	+++	–	+	+++	–
Calmette-Guérin bacillus	+	++	++	–	–
Mycoplasma pneumoniae	+	+	–	–	–
Nocardia brasiliensis	++	++	++	–	–
Actinomyces israelii	–	++	++	–	–
VIRUSES					
Epstein–Barr	+++	++	–	–	++++
Cytomegalovirus	++	++	–	–	+++
Hepatitis A, B	+	+	–	–	+
Herpes simplex	++++	–	–	++	–
Human immunodeficiency	–	++	–	–	+++
Adenovirus	+++	–	–	–	+
Rubella	+++	–	–	–	+++
Rubeola	+++	–	–	–	+++
Influenza	+++	–	–	–	–
Human herpesvirus 6	++	–	–	–	–
Enterovirus	++	–	–	–	+
Parvovirus B19	+++	–	–	–	+++
PROTOZOA					
Toxoplasma gondii	++	+++	–	–	+

++++, characteristic; +++, frequently associated; ++, occasionally associated; +, rarely associated; –, not known to be associated.

The older child with bilateral, soft, discrete, minimally tender, and minimally enlarged (<2 cm) nodes high in the neck who has had respiratory tract symptoms and fever usually has a viral infection, or may have streptococcal pharyngitis or *M. pneumoniae* infection. In roseola, rubella, adenoviral, or enteroviral infections, cervical adenopathy is frequently in the suboccipital, posterior auricular, or superficial posterior cervical areas (Table 17-6).

If nodes are large and minimally tender, with no overlying cellulitis, mononucleosis due to EBV or CMV is likely. For protracted or unusual cases, sarcoidosis, Kikuchi–Fujimoto and Rosai–Dorfman diseases are considered.

When acute unilateral or bilateral adenopathy is associated with an obvious site of infection, diagnostic studies are focused on the site. Obvious sites of infection include herpes simplex ulcerations, infected abrasions, scalp infections, animal bites or scratches, and conjunctival granulomas.

Acutely inflamed, unilateral, tender large nodes with associated periadenitis and cellulitis, fever, and constitutional symptoms, often with poor node definition and torticollis, are usually due to *S. aureus* or *S. pyogenes* in the young child[57] (see Tables 17-3 and 17-5). In older children and adolescents, a dental focus with resulting anaerobic infection should be considered. Failure to respond to antibiotic therapy after 48 hours leads to evaluation for antimicrobial resistance, an abscess or a more unusual cause, such as Kawasaki disease, and infected or uninfected congenital cysts and sinuses.

The most challenging problem is the patient with a unilateral, asymptomatic, initially noninflamed, nontender, firm node of acute or subacute onset. Some such nodes become fluctuant and develop the characteristic findings of cat-scratch disease or nontuberculous mycobacterial disease, while others do not change over time.

It is important to identify toxoplasmosis, tuberculosis, and lymphoma or another malignancy as soon as possible to initiate appropriate therapy if indicated. Accurate measurements of the size and consistency of such nodes should be performed once or twice a week in order to determine whether malignancy should be considered. The presence of systemic symptoms, hepatosplenomegaly, pneumonia, or mediastinal adenopathy (see Chapter 18, Mediastinal and Hilar Lymphadenopathy) is suggestive of tuberculosis or malignancy.

Guidance for biopsy of lymph nodes to rule out a malignancy is provided in Box 17-2. If an excisional biopsy is performed and nonspecific hyperplasia is reported, the patient must be followed carefully, because 25% of patients with such findings are ultimately found to have a lymphoreticular malignancy.

Needle Aspiration

Needle aspiration of the infected node is a valuable diagnostic tool for acute and subacute lymphadenitis and also can be therapeutic. In 60% to 90% of patients with acute cervical

TABLE 17-6. Associations of Selected Organisms with Involvement of Specific Lymph Node Groups in the Neck

Pathogen	Preauricular	Postauricular	Occipital	Submaxillary	Tonsillar	Anterior Cervical	Posterior Cervical	Superior Deep Cervical	Supraclavicular
BACTERIA									
Staphylococcus aureus	–	–	++	++	++++	+++	–	+++	+
Streptococcus pyogenes	–	–	++	++	++++	+++	–	+++	+
Anaerobic bacteria	–	–	–	++++	++	++	–	–	–
Arcanobacterium haemolyticum	–	–	–	+	+++	+++	–	++	–
Mycoplasma pneumoniae	–	–	–	++	++	++	++	–	–
Francisella tularensis	++	–	–	++	+	++	++	+	–
Mycobacterium tuberculosis	–	–	–	+++	+++	–	–	–	+++
Nontuberculous Mycobacterium	++	–	–	+++	+++	–	–	+	–
Bartonella henselae	++++	–	–	+	+++	+++	++	+	+
Nocardia brasiliensis	–	–	–	++++	+	–	–	–	–
VIRUSES									
Herpes simplex	–	–	–	+++	+++	+	+	+	–
Rubeola	–	++	++	–	–	–	–	–	–
Rubella	–	+++	+++	–	–	–	++	–	–
Human herpesvirus 6	–	++	++	–	–	++	++	–	–
Epstein–Barr	–	–	++	++	++	++	++	+	–
Keratoconjunctival fever	++++	–	–	–	–	–	–	–	–
Pharyngoconjunctival fever	±	–	–	–	–	++	++	–	–
Parvovirus B19	++	–	–	+	+	+	–	+	–
PROTOZOA									
Toxoplasma gondii	–	–	–	–	–	–	+++	–	–
Trypanosoma cruzi	+	–	–	–	–	–	+++	–	–
FUNGI									
Tinea capitis	–	+	++++	–	–	–	+	–	–
Histoplasma capsulatum	–	–	–	–	–	++	–	+	+++
Coccidioides immitis	–	–	–	–	–	–	–	–	+++

++++, characteristic site of adenopathy; +++, additional site, often associated; ++, occasional site; +, rare site; –, not described.

lymphadenitis in whom needle aspiration is performed for bacterial and mycobacterial culture, an etiologic agent is recovered.[3,4,9,58] The procedure is safe and easy to perform and has no serious complications. Controversy exists as to whether a persistently draining fistula is precipitated by aspiration if the lymphadenitis is due to mycobacterial infection. The preponderance of data suggests that aspiration is not contraindicated and is greatly useful to direct definitive therapy. As tuberculous and nontuberculous diseases are difficult to distinguish clinically, needle aspiration is a useful diagnostic tool if M. tuberculosis exposure is possible. Laboratory polymerase chain reaction diagnosis also is being evaluated as a diagnostic tool using needle aspiration samples.[59,60]

The specimen is obtained from the largest and most fluctuant node. If no material is aspirated, saline is injected into the node and repeat aspiration performed. Gram and acid-fast stain should be performed, and the specimen should be inoculated onto media for growth and isolation of anaerobic and aerobic bacteria, fungi, and mycobacteria. If no visible specimen is obtained, the needle and syringe can be flushed into a blood culture flask.

Lymph Node Biopsy

If the diagnosis remains in doubt and the enlarged lymph node fails to regress, enlarges further, is hard, or is fixed to adjacent structures, biopsy should be performed. An accelerated schedule for biopsy is appropriate in the presence of persistent fever or weight loss (in the absence of confirmed diagnosis) or if firm lymph nodes are found in the posterior cervical triangle or supraclavicular area (if M. tuberculosis and B. henselae are excluded). These settings are associated with greater possibility of malignancy.

Excisional biopsy (to establish lymph node architecture and complete histologic character) is preferred to incisional biopsy of lymph nodes, although there are a few retrospective studies that support the use of fine-needle aspiration as an initial diagnostic mechanism; negative or nonspecific findings do not exclude malignancy.[61,62] Yield from biopsy is maximized through careful choice of tissue site and proper handling of resected tissue. Generally, the largest, firmest nodes should be excised. Whenever possible, more than one node should be obtained. When several

PART II Clinical Syndromes and Cardinal Features of Infectious Diseases: Approach to Diagnosis and Initial Management

SECTION B Cardinal Symptom Complexes

BOX 17-2. Settings that Prompt Early Consideration of Biopsy of Enlarged Cervical Lymph Node to Rule Out Malignancy

SITE

Supraclavicular

Posterior cervical (particularly with extension across sternomastoid muscle to involve anterior and posterior triangles)

Deep to fascia

SIZE

>2 cm diameter

Continued enlargement after 2 weeks

No significant decrease in size after 4–6 weeks

Not normal in size after 8–12 weeks

CONSISTENCY

No inflammation

Nontender (unless rapidly enlarging)

Firm, rubbery, or matted (may be fixed to underlying structures)

Ulceration

POTENTIAL LOCAL OR SYSTEMIC SPREAD EVIDENCED BY

Mediastinal or generalized adenopathy

Bone marrow involvement

Fever, weight loss, hepatosplenomegaly

Recurrent epistaxis, progressive nasal obstruction, facial paralysis, or otorrhea

NO EVIDENCE TO SUPPORT AN INFECTIOUS ETIOLOGY

Negative results of evaluation for infectious causes

No response to empirically chosen antibiotics

---

groups of nodes are involved, biopsy specimens taken from the lower neck and supraclavicular area (or a region other than the neck) have higher diagnostic yield than those taken from high cervical nodes. If EBV or toxoplasmosis is expected, biopsy is carefully considered because of the difficulty of discrimination of such diseases from malignancy and the ability to confirm both diagnoses by serologic testing. If lymphoma is suspected, needle biopsy or frozen section is unreliable for excluding the diagnosis. When nontuberculous mycobacterial infection is suspected and surgery is required for diagnosis and therapy, excisional dissection of deep nodes may be necessary. The individual situation dictates specific evaluations of excised tissue, but evaluation commonly consists of flow cytometry, special stains, including Giemsa, periodic acid–Schiff (PAS), methenamine silver, and Warthin–Starry silver stains and, in selected cases, testing by in situ hybridization, PCR, or electron microscopy. Culture for facultative and anaerobic bacteria, mycobacteria, and fungi is appropriate.

Many reactive processes simulate malignant histology and may make definitive diagnosis impossible. Examples are dysregulated inflammatory responses as with rheumatoid arthritis, phenytoin-induced adenopathy, dermatopathic adenitis, and infections such as toxoplasmosis and EBV mononucleosis. A thorough history and a second series of evaluations, including serologic tests, are essential for making a correct diagnosis of these cases.

MANAGEMENT

Initial Therapy

Children with bilaterally enlarged cervical lymph nodes (<3 cm in size) that are not erythematous or exquisitely tender are observed without evaluation or therapy. If the initial findings are typical of acute bacterial lymphadenitis (unilateral node, >2 to 3 cm, erythematous, and tender) without systemic symptoms, empiric therapy is given for *S. aureus* and *S. pyogenes* infection unless the course or findings are typical for *S. pyogenes* (Table 17-7). Therapy usually is given for 10 days or at least 5 days beyond resolution of acute signs and symptoms, whichever is longer. Knowledge of local resistance patterns is important when choosing empiric therapy. Antimicrobial resistance or alternative pathogens should be considered if empiric antimicrobial therapy fails. If a primary focus of infection is identified elsewhere, the mode and duration of therapy are directed in reference to that site as well. Impetigo and other skin infections usually are caused by *S. aureus* and *S. pyogenes*. Dental or periodontal disease leads to lymphadenitis due to anaerobic bacteria. A culture should be obtained from suppurative sites whenever possible. Aspiration of the inflamed site should be performed if moderate to severe adenitis with cellulitis and constitutional symptoms is present or if no improvement occurs after 48 to 72 hours of therapy. In the latter instance, additional diagnoses are considered, including viral infection, Kawasaki disease, nontuberculous mycobacterial infection, and more unusual causes of adenitis. If cat-scratch disease is suspected, *Bartonella* specific antimicrobial therapy is given if a node is >3 cm, in an attempt to avoid abscess formation. See Chapter 160, Bartonella Species (Cat-Scratch Disease).

Routine antituberculous therapy generally is ineffective for nontuberculous mycobacterial infections. In cases in which removal of the node is not advised (e.g., because of size or proximity to the facial nerve), combination NTM therapy generally is given (see Chapter 135, *Mycobacterium* Species Non-*tuberculosis*).

Patients with marked lymph node enlargement, moderate to severe systemic symptoms, and cellulitis frequently require parenteral therapy for the first several days. This route provides a higher concentration of drug in inflamed tissue, halts bacteremia if present, and may promote more rapid localization. Although a decrease in fever, inflammation, and tenderness is expected within 48 to 72 hours after appropriate treatment of bacterial lymphadenitis, lymph node regression may be slow, requiring 4 to 6 weeks, and suppuration despite appropriate therapy is not unusual.

Abscess Drainage

Ultrasonography or computed tomography can be helpful in cases in which abscess is suspected in the absence of fluctuation on physical examination.[58] For abscesses due to *S. aureus* or *S. pyogenes*, incision and drainage are the procedures of choice. Needle aspiration can be therapeutic. For abscesses from suspected mycobacterial or *Bartonella* infection, aspiration (with an 18- or 19-gauge needle) initially is preferred to avoid fistula formation. Installation of saline may facilitate aspiration when pus is very thick. Surgical excision is required infrequently for cat-scratch disease.

Surgical Excision and Long-Term Therapy

Surgical excision is the most effective treatment for nontuberculous mycobacterial cervical adenitis.[63,64] Excision of the largest and necrotic mass or masses is usually adequate, because the remaining adenopathy resolves spontaneously over ensuing months. Excision of all affected nodes (especially as documented by imaging studies) requires extensive and difficult surgery, and is not warranted as a first procedure; adjunctive antimicrobial therapy usually is given. When infection has ruptured into soft tissue, resection of inflamed overlying skin and sinus tracts, followed by primary closure without leaving a drain, is advocated. A decision to begin combination therapy for *M. tuberculosis* infection is based on the clinical setting and tuberculin skin test results. The clinical response of *M. tuberculosis* infection to antituberculous therapy usually is rapid, with resolution of symptoms and marked regression of the lymph nodes within 3 months; prolonged therapy is required. *Actinomyces* infections of the neck require very prolonged antimicrobial therapy; osteomyelitis of the jaw may require aggressive debridement as well.

TABLE 17-7. Treatment of Acute Bacterial Cervical Lymphadenitis

Presumed Pathogen and Setting	Empiric Therapy (consult local antibiogram)	Route/Duration	Diagnostic Test(s)
STAPHYLOCOCCUS AUREUS* OR *STREPTOCOCCUS PYOGENES			
No prominent systemic symptoms, cellulitis, or suppuration	Amoxicillin-clavulanate, cephalexin, or clindamycin (TMP-SMX if MRSA known, not for *S. pyogenes*)	PO/10 days or 5 days past resolution of symptoms, whichever is longer	Routine culture (+ PCR for MRSA)
With cellulitis, marked enlargement, moderate or severe symptoms	Nafcillin, cefazolin, or clindamycin; vancomycin or clindamycin for MRSA	IV/10 days or 5 days past resolution of symptoms, whichever is longer. Consider PO after clinical improvement	Routine culture (+ PCR for MRSA)
	Needle aspiration if no improvement after 48 hours		
With suppuration	Parenteral antibiotics as above and incision and drainage	IV/10 days or 5 days past resolution of symptoms, whichever is longer. Consider PO after clinical improvement	Routine culture (+ PCR for MRSA)
GROUP B *STREPTOCOCCUS* OR *STAPHYLOCOCCUS AUREUS			
Infant <2 months with cellulitis with or without systemic symptoms or adenitis	Nafcillin or oxacillin	IV/10–14 days	Routine culture (+ PCR for MRSA)
	Vancomycin if MRSA rates high (evaluate for meningitis if Group B strep)		
ANAEROBIC BACTERIA			
Associated dental or periodontal disease, bull neck	Clindamycin or penicillin plus metronidazole	PO or IV, depending on severity/duration depends on anatomic locations and severity of disease	Anaerobic culture
	(Alternative piperacillin/tazobactam or carbapenem if severe disease)		
BARTONELLA HENSELAE			
Fluctuant or draining node; systemic manifestations	Needle aspiration of node; consider use of azithromycin, rifampin, ciprofloxacin, TMP-SMX, or gentamicin (see Chapter 160)	PO, IV/optimal duration not known	Serologic analysis, PCR, granulomas on tissue, Warthin–Starry silver stain of tissue
NONTUBERCULOUS *MYCOBACTERIUM			
TB ruled out; node not draining	Excision of node or see Chapter 135		TST, Mycobacterial culture, tissue PCR, granulomatous reaction
MYCOBACTERIUM TUBERCULOSIS	See Chapter 134		TST, Mycobacterial culture, tissue PCR, granulomatous reaction, Interferon-γ release assays
FRANCISELLA TULARENSIS			
Acute onset, fever; diagnosis reasonably certain	Streptomycin (gentamicin/amikacin)	IM, IV/10 days or longer for severe illness	Serologic analysis, PCR, culture of blood or tissue (alert laboratory personnel with clinical suspicion)
	Alternative: ciprofloxacin, doxycycline See Chapter 171		
PASTEURELLA MULTOCIDA			
Onset within 24 h of animal bite	Amoxicillin-clavulanate or nafcillin until diagnosis confirmed; then penicillin	PO, IV depending on severity/7–10 days for local infections and 10–14 days for severe infections	Routine culture

IM, intramuscular; IV, intravenous; MRSA, methicillin-resistant Staphylococcus aureus; PCR, polymerase chain reaction; PO, oral; TB, tuberculosis; TMP-SMX, trimethoprim-sulfamethoxazole; TST, tuberculin skin test.

COMPLICATIONS

Complications of pyogenic neck infections, such as mediastinal abscess, purulent pericarditis, thrombosis of the internal jugular vein, and pulmonary emboli or disseminated septic emboli, have become uncommon since the availability of effective antimicrobial therapy. *Fusobacterium* species infection is an exception. Rapid progression or failure to treat adenitis due to *S. aureus* or *S. pyogenes* can result in cellulitis, bacteremia, septicemia, or toxin-related symptoms. Poststreptococcal acute glomerulonephritis occurs occasionally.

Acknowledgment

The authors acknowledge re-use of Figure 17-1 from a previous edition as provided by P. Joan Chesney, Memphis, TN.

18 Mediastinal and Hilar Lymphadenopathy

Mary Anne Jackson, P. Joan Chesney, and Sarah J. Fitch

ANATOMY OF THE MEDIASTINUM

The mediastinum is the space between the pleural cavities that contains the heart and all chest viscera except the lungs. Consisting of loose areolar tissue and organs, it is more a potential space than an actual body cavity. It is bounded laterally by the parietal pleurae, anteriorly by the sternum, posteriorly by the ribs and paravertebral gutters, superiorly by the thoracic inlet, and inferiorly by the diaphragm. The anterior mediastinum contains everything anterior and superior to the heart, including the thymus, aortic arch and its major branches, innominate veins, and lymphatic tissue (nodes and vessels). Most masses here are of thymic origin, a teratoma, lymphoma, or angiomatous tumor. The middle mediastinum is triangular with the apex at the fourth thoracic vertebra. It contains the heart, pericardium, trachea, pulmonary hilar and mediastinal lymph nodes and vessels, and phrenic and vagus nerves. Masses in this compartment usually are infectious or are malignant lesions of lymph nodes. The posterior mediastinum extends from the first rib to the diaphragm, behind the heart and lung roots. It contains the esophagus, descending aorta, paravertebral lymph nodes, lower portion of the vagus nerve, and sympathetic nerve chains. Neurogenic tumors and duplication cysts are the most common lesions encountered.

Although the delicacy of mediastinal tissue planes offers little resistance to the spread of disease between compartments, tumors and inflammation tend to extend within compartments. Infections within the mediastinum are relatively uncommon, but their proximity to many vital structures makes accurate diagnosis essential.

LYMPHATIC DRAINAGE OF THE LUNGS AND PLEURA

As shown in Figure 18-1, lymph from the thoracic viscera (heart, pericardium, lungs, pleura, thymus, and esophagus) traverses one of three possible sets of nodes before entering the thoracic duct or right lymphatic duct. Anterior mediastinal nodes are located anterior to the aortic arch, innominate veins, and large arterial trunks leading from the aorta. They receive afferents from the thymus and pericardium, the sternal nodes, and the thyroid gland.

Posterior mediastinal nodes lie dorsal to the pericardium and adjacent to the esophagus and descending aorta. They receive afferents from the esophagus, dorsal pericardium, diaphragm, and convex surface of the liver. Middle or mediastinal nodes drain the lungs and pleura. Lymphatic drainage of the lungs is composed of superficial and deep plexuses. The superficial plexus lies beneath the visceral pleura. Lymph flows around the border of the lung to enter the bronchopulmonary (hilar) nodes. The deep plexus accompanies branches of the pulmonary vessels and ramifications of the bronchi throughout the lungs.

Lymphatic drainage of the lung passes through four sets of lymph nodes (Table 18-1). Intrapulmonary lymph nodes are located within the lung, chiefly at the bifurcations of the larger bronchi. Bronchopulmonary or hilar nodes are located at the pulmonary hilus at the site of entry of the main bronchi and vessels. Tracheobronchial nodes are divided into superior and inferior groups. The superior group lies in the obtuse angle between the trachea and bronchi on both sides. The inferior, or subcarinal, group lies under the carina at the tracheal bifurcation. The fourth group, the tracheal or paratracheal nodes, lies beside and somewhat anterior to the trachea. A fifth group of lymph nodes of importance in the drainage of the lungs is the inferior

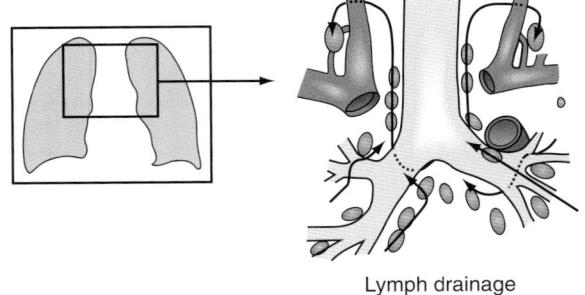

Lymph drainage patterns

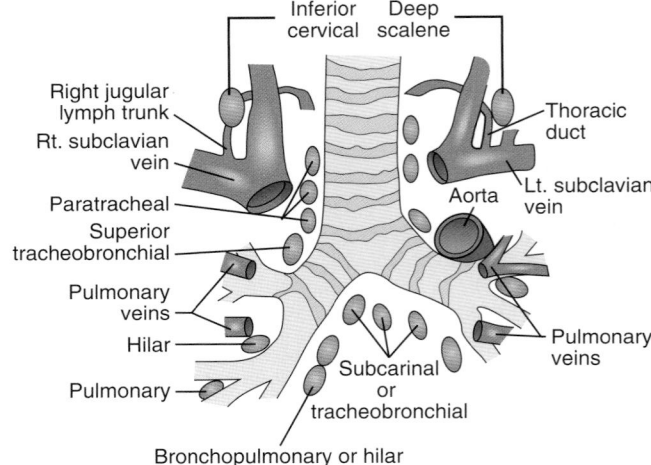

Figure 18-1. Lymphatic drainage of the thorax.

TABLE 18-1. Lymphatic Drainage of the Lung and Pleura

Lymph Node Group	Areas Drained
Intrapulmonary	Pulmonary vessels, bronchi, and parenchyma
Hilar (bronchopulmonary)	Intrapulmonary nodes and superficial plexus of visceral pleural lymphatics
Tracheobronchial: superior and inferior (subcarinal)	
Right side	All hilar nodes of right lung and hilar nodes of left lower lobe and lingula
Left side	Left upper lobe hilar nodes
Paratracheal nodes	
Right side	Right tracheobronchial nodes
Left side	Left tracheobronchial nodes
Supraclavicular nodes	
Right side	Right apical pleura, right paratracheal nodes, head, neck, arms, and upper thorax
Left side (Virchow node)	Left apical pleura, left paratracheal nodes, intra-abdominal nodes, head, neck, arms, and upper thorax

deep cervical (scalene or supraclavicular) chain, which is located over the lower portion of the internal jugular vein, just above the clavicle and usually under the scalenus anterior muscle. The apical pleurae drain directly to these deep cervical nodes, as do the paratracheal chains. A finding of supraclavicular lymphadenopathy should lead to investigation for intrathoracic or intra-abdominal pathology.

Ultimately, all lymph from the lungs and pleurae reaches the tracheobronchial and paratracheal lymph nodes. As a general rule, lymph from the lungs flows from left to right, a probable explanation for the pre-eminence of right upper paratracheal and supraclavicular lymphadenopathy in infectious pulmonary processes, particularly tuberculosis. Lymph from the left lower lobe (and usually also the lingula) flows from the hilar nodes to the lower tracheobronchial nodes, and then to the right paratracheal nodes. Lymph from the right hilar nodes travels to the right paratracheal nodes (see Table 18-1).

Lymph vessels from the paratracheal nodes join with lymph trunks from the anterior mediastinum to form the right and left bronchomediastinal trunks. These trunks then join with the lymphatic trunks from the supraclavicular nodes to form the right lymphatic duct and left thoracic duct.

EPIDEMIOLOGY

At least one-third of all mediastinal masses occur in children younger than 15 years; one-half of such masses are symptomatic. Among children with mediastinal masses, 50% who present with symptoms of airway compression have malignant tumors, whereas 90% of those who have noncompressive symptoms have nonmalignant conditions. The greater proportion of symptomatic masses in children compared with adults may be due to smaller thoracic size, resulting in symptoms of compression, or to a higher frequency of malignant lesions.[1] The overall incidence of tumors (excluding metastatic disease) and cysts in the mediastinum is 1 per 100,000 people.

In series of biopsies of only anterior and middle mediastinal masses in children (thus excluding neurogenic tumors), 1% to 57% are reported to be due to histoplasmosis. This extreme variance in rate is due to prevalences of *Histoplasma capsulatum* in the geographic areas in which studies are done. For example, at St. Jude Children's Research Hospital in Memphis, histoplasmosis was a relatively common complication in children with cancer, and a reason for referral of children without cancer.[2] Fever

with pulmonary infiltrates (frequently nodular) and hilar or mediastinal mass/lymphadenopathy were the usual presentation. Blastomycosis, coccidioidomycosis, and tuberculosis also are associated with infectious mediastinal disease. A variety of other pathogens, including *Pneumocystis jirovecii* and *Mycoplasma*, can lead to mediastinal lymphadenitis associated with pulmonary infiltrates. Cysts and tumors predominate as the cause of posterior mediastinal lymphadenopathy (Table 18-2). Overall, neurogenic tumors are the most common cause of mediastinal masses; lymphomas are second, and germ cell tumors are third in frequency.

CHARACTERISTICS OF LYMPHADENOPATHY

Lymph nodes are readily identifiable on computed tomography (CT) and can be categorized according to size, shape, coalescence, replacement by tumor mass, presence of calcium, abscess cavities, and parenchymal lung involvement. Most authorities use a 10-mm diameter as the upper limit of normal size for lymph node.[3,4] Mediastinal lymph nodes >20 mm virtually are always abnormal; this statement may not be true for hilar nodes. Mediastinal nodes have the potential to become much larger than any other nodes in the body.

Densely calcified bilateral nodes are typical of histoplasmosis and, occasionally, of blastomycosis, coccidioidomycosis, or sarcoidosis. Unilateral densely calcified nodes are typical of prior or late-diagnosed tuberculosis. Benign mediastinal tumors also can be calcified (i.e., teratoma, cystic thymoma, and thyroid adenoma). Childhood lymphomas can cause bilateral hilar adenopathy but usually do not become calcified until after therapy.

In general, mediastinal mass lesions require a tissue diagnosis. Situations in which a biopsy may not be necessary include: (1) certain granulomatous lesions that show dense calcification and are not increasing in size, as shown by consecutive imaging studies; (2) lymphomatous lesions diagnosed by biopsy of tissue outside the thorax; and, most importantly, (3) tuberculosis or histoplasmosis, which should be confirmed with other diagnostic testing.

CLINICAL MANIFESTATIONS

Mediastinal lymphadenopathy frequently is asymptomatic until compression or erosion through a mediastinal structure occurs. Table 18-3 delineates findings associated with mediastinal disease.

TABLE 18-2. Relative Frequencies of Noninfectious Mediastinal Masses in Children[a]

	Study			
	Silverman & Saleiston[30]	Filler et al.[31]	Woods et al.[15]	Gaebler et al.[32]
Number of children	437	429	68	37
FREQUENCY OF MASS (%)				
Neurogenic tumor	40	33	–	–
Lymphoma	18	14	68	43
Leukemia	–	–	17	–
Germ cell tumor	11	9.8	–	–
Mesenchymal tumor	7	6.8	–	–
Bronchogenic cyst	7	7.5	–	–
Lymph node infection	–	4.4	9	57
Other cysts or malignancy	14	25	6	–

[a]Anterior and middle mediastinal masses only.

TABLE 18-3. Symptoms of Compression Resulting from Mediastinal Adenopathy

Structure	Symptom or Sign
Airway	Cough, wheezing; recurrent respiratory infections, bronchitis, atelectasis, unresolved pneumonia; hemoptysis; chest pain, sudden death
Esophagus	Dysphagia (interruption of peristalsis); hematemesis (fistula formation)
Superior vena cava	Dilation of collateral veins of the neck and upper thorax; chemosis of conjunctiva, edema of face, neck, upper chest, and arm; cyanosis; headaches, visual disturbances; epistaxis, tinnitus
Lymphatic channels	Pleural effusion
Recurrent laryngeal nerve	Hoarseness, inspiratory stridor (paralysis of vocal cord)
Phrenic nerve	Paralysis of left diaphragm
Sympathetic ganglia	Horner syndrome
Vertebrae, ribs	Pain secondary to bony erosion; symptoms of spinal cord compression

Respiratory symptoms result from airway obstruction or erosion. If the obstruction is significant enough, distal obstructive emphysema, atelectasis, pneumonia, or chronic, recurrent respiratory tract infections can result. Obstruction of the superior vena cava is a rare complication most commonly associated with rapidly growing malignant mediastinal tumors. The superior vena cava is particularly vulnerable to obstruction because of its thin wall, low intravascular pressure, and confinement by lymph nodes and other rigid structures. Older children with mediastinal masses may describe feeling intrathoracic discomfort or pain, which probably is due to pressure on intercostal nerves or pleura. Vertebral erosion secondary to posterior mediastinal tumors can cause a boring, interscapular pain. Most children with mediastinal disease caused by histoplasmosis present with chest pain or cough.

The finding of mediastinal widening, regardless of symptoms, leads to evaluation by CT. The diagnosis of lymphoma is considered first. If granulomatous lung disease is present, the diagnosis of tuberculosis is considered as is histoplasmosis in endemic regions. History of travel, foreign birth, consumption of unpasteurized milk, or farm or bird exposure is sought.

DIAGNOSIS

Traditionally, the differential diagnosis of mediastinal masses evident on chest radiograph has been considered according to location within one of the four mediastinal compartments. Use of CT has largely supplanted the need for this classification because distinct tissue groups are now defined: fat, lymph nodes, vessels, airways, thymus, esophagus, and paraspinal tissues.

Imaging Studies

CT is the imaging study of choice for children with mediastinal mass. Unenhanced CT augments recognition of calcification. CT with administration of contrast material is useful to define anatomy better and distinguish vessels from lymph nodes.

TABLE 18-4. Causes of Mediastinal Lymphadenopathy

Etiology	Frequency	Associated Pneumonia	Node Abscess	Node Calcification	Method of Diagnosis
INFECTIOUS CAUSES					
Bacteria					
Mycobacterium tuberculosis	++	++	++	++	Tuberculin skin test; chest radiograph; culture of gastric aspirate or bronchial washing
Nontuberculous mycobacteria	±	–	+	–	Culture and histopathologic analysis of tissue
Mycoplasma pneumoniae	+	++	–	–	Serology; cold agglutinin
Bartonella henselae	±	–	+	–	Serology; culture; histopathology
Yersinia enterocolitica	±	–	+	–	Culture; serology
Actinomyces species	±	–	+	–	Culture; histopathology
Melioidosis	+	–	+	–	Culture
Fungus					
Histoplasma	++	+	+	++	Serology; antigen detection; culture
Coccidioides	+	+	±	+	Serology; culture
Blastomyces	+	++	+	+	Culture
Paracoccidioides	±	+	++		Culture
Cryptococcus	±	±	–	–	Culture
Viruses					
Epstein–Barr virus	±	–	–	–	Serology
Protozoa					
Toxoplasma	±	–	–	–	Serology
Chronic infection					
Cystic fibrosis	++	++	±	–	Sweat test; gene identification
Bronchiectasis	+	+	±	–	Radiograph; culture
Lung abscess	±	+	–	–	Radiograph
NONINFECTIOUS CAUSES					
Malignancy					
Hodgkin lymphoma	++	±	–	±[a]	Biopsy
Non-Hodgkin lymphoma	++	–	–	±[a]	Biopsy
Leukemia	+	–	–		Bone marrow
Other					
Chronic granulomatous disease	+	+	++	–	Neutrophil function assay
Sarcoidosis	++	–	–	–	Biopsy
Rosai–Dorfman disease	+	–	–	–	Biopsy; histopathology
Castleman disease	+	–	–	–	Biopsy; histopathology
Lymphoproliferative syndromes	++	–	–	–	Epstein–Barr virus serology; biopsy
Graves disease	±	–	–	–	Thyroid hormone measurement

++, frequent cause; +, occasional cause; ±, rare cause, consider under special circumstances.

[a]After treatment.

Identification of a solid, homogeneously enhancing soft-tissue mass distinguishes lymphoma from cavitating lesions of histoplasmosis and tuberculosis, which are peripherally enhancing with low attenuation centrally. With the widespread use of multidetector helical CT, multiplanar imaging now is routine and allows definition of mediastinal structures in all planes. Magnetic resonance imaging (MRI) is required infrequently to evaluate the mediastinum, since most lesions are visualized well on multidetector helical CT. In addition, MRI usually requires sedation (which can be dangerous in the presence of intrathoracic mass) and cooperation of the child to hold the breath (lest there be motion artifact). MRI is used for specific problem-solving, such as evaluation of soft-tissue masses of the chest wall, and when neurogenic lesions are suspected, to evaluate extension into the spinal canal.

Although CT and MRI are highly sensitive in detecting enlarged lymph nodes, neither reliably distinguishes between benign and malignant causes. Both can show displacement or compression of trachea or esophagus, but neither distinguishes invasion. MRI has the limitation of not being able to demonstrate calcium and is highly sensitive to motion (breathing or heart contraction) artifact.

Tissue Diagnosis and Biopsy

In general, mediastinal mass lesions require a tissue diagnosis because of likely causes and their proximity to vital structures. In some cases, diagnosis can be made without obtaining mediastinal tissue. Supraclavicular nodes (whether enlarged or not) or other enlarged extrathoracic nodes can provide diagnostic tissue. In one-half of children with mediastinal malignancy, at least one lymph node in the cervical, supraclavicular, or infraclavicular or axillary area is larger than 2 cm, and can be biopsied. Tissue biopsy from other sites along with serologic testing can confirm sarcoidosis. Bronchoscopy with bronchoalveolar lavage or gastric aspirates may identify an infectious cause.

INFECTIOUS CAUSES

Table 18-4 shows differentiating features of the causes of mediastinal lymphadenopathy. Mycobacteria and the endemic fungal organisms, *Histoplasma* and *Coccidioides*, commonly cause hilar and mediastinal adenopathy. Although mediastinal infection without significant pulmonary infection is rare, the degree of adenopathy frequently is disproportionate to degree of parenchymal involvement. Pneumonia due to *Mycoplasma pneumoniae*, *Bartonella henselae*, *Yersinia enterocolitica*, or *Francisella tularensis* can be associated with hilar adenopathy, as can bronchiectasis and cystic fibrosis. Adenopathy is rare in other acute bacterial and viral pneumonias.

Bacterial Causes

Mycobacterium tuberculosis. Primary pulmonary infection with *M. tuberculosis* has the following three elements: the primary parenchymal focus, intraparenchymal lymphangitis, and regional lymphadenitis (Figures 18-2 and 18-3). At least 70% of primary pulmonary foci are subpleural, with spread through lymphatics to the regional lymph nodes. After several weeks, hypersensitivity develops, with regional node enlargement and the potential for caseating necrosis. Caseating lesions have a high density of actively multiplying bacilli, which spread rapidly to adjacent lymphatics. The hallmark of early tuberculosis is excessive unilateral mediastinal lymphadenitis compared with the relatively insignificant focus in the lung. Hilar adenopathy is unilateral in ≥80% of cases of tuberculosis.

Infection can spread beyond the hilar and tracheobronchial nodes to the more distant right upper paratracheal nodes (the ones most often affected) and deep cervical (supraclavicular) nodes.[5] Additionally, apical subpleural primary infections can drain directly to the supraclavicular nodes. In one series of patients,

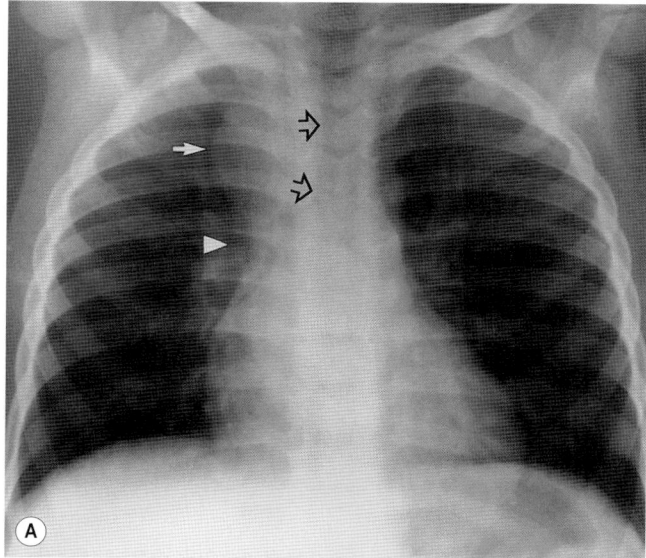

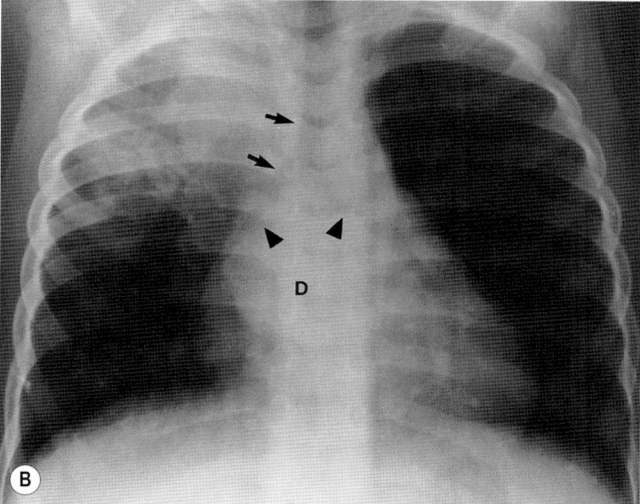

Figure 18-2. (A) Chest radiograph of a child with tuberculosis shows right paratracheal adenopathy (closed arrow) and right tracheobronchial adenopathy (arrowhead), causing effacement of the right lateral aspect of trachea (open arrows). **(B)** Chest radiograph of the same patient 4 months later (without therapy) shows right upper lobe pneumonia with subtle effacement of the right lateral aspect of the trachea and right mainstem bronchus, indicating right hilar and right paratracheal adenopathy (arrows). There is splaying of the carina (arrowheads) and double density (D) of the lower mediastinum centrally, indicating subcarinal adenopathy.

14 of 54 patients with a primary lesion in the right upper lobe had ipsilateral enlargement of deep cervical nodes.[6]

Enlargement of hilar nodes adjacent to bronchi can cause bronchial obstruction with the collapse or consolidation or fan-shaped segmental lesion typical of childhood tuberculosis. Infection and inflammation of the bronchial wall can occur, and obstruction of the lumen rarely can result in sudden death or in obstructive hyperaeration, segmental atelectasis, or secondary pneumonia. Multiple segmental lesions can occur, usually in the same lung.

Calcification follows caseous necrosis and occurs more often in children and in the regional lymph nodes than in the primary pulmonary focus. Extensive calcification is uncommon with early treatment, which prevents caseation.

In one series, CT of 23 young adults presenting with tuberculous mediastinal or hilar lymphadenitis demonstrated pulmonary involvement in 14 patients.[7] There was remarkable preponderance

PART II   Clinical Syndromes and Cardinal Features of Infectious Diseases: Approach to Diagnosis and Initial Management

SECTION B   Cardinal Symptom Complexes

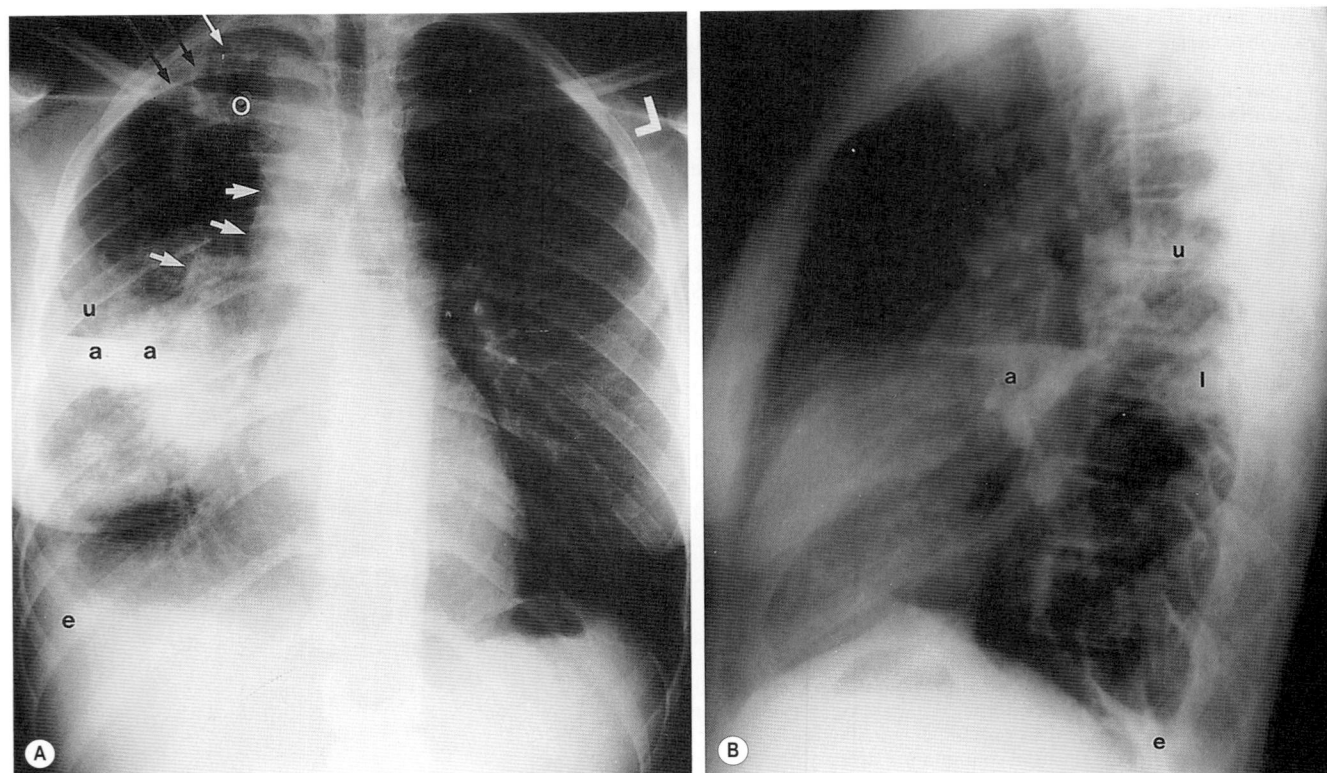

Figure 18-3. (A and B) Chest radiographs of a child with reactivated tuberculosis show cystic changes in the apex of the right upper lobe (open circle), and pleural thickening in the superior hemithorax (long arrows). There is a right pleural effusion (e); right paratracheal, tracheobronchial, and hilar adenopathy (short arrows); and atelectasis or pneumonia in the right middle lobe (a), right upper lobe (u), and right lower lobe (l).

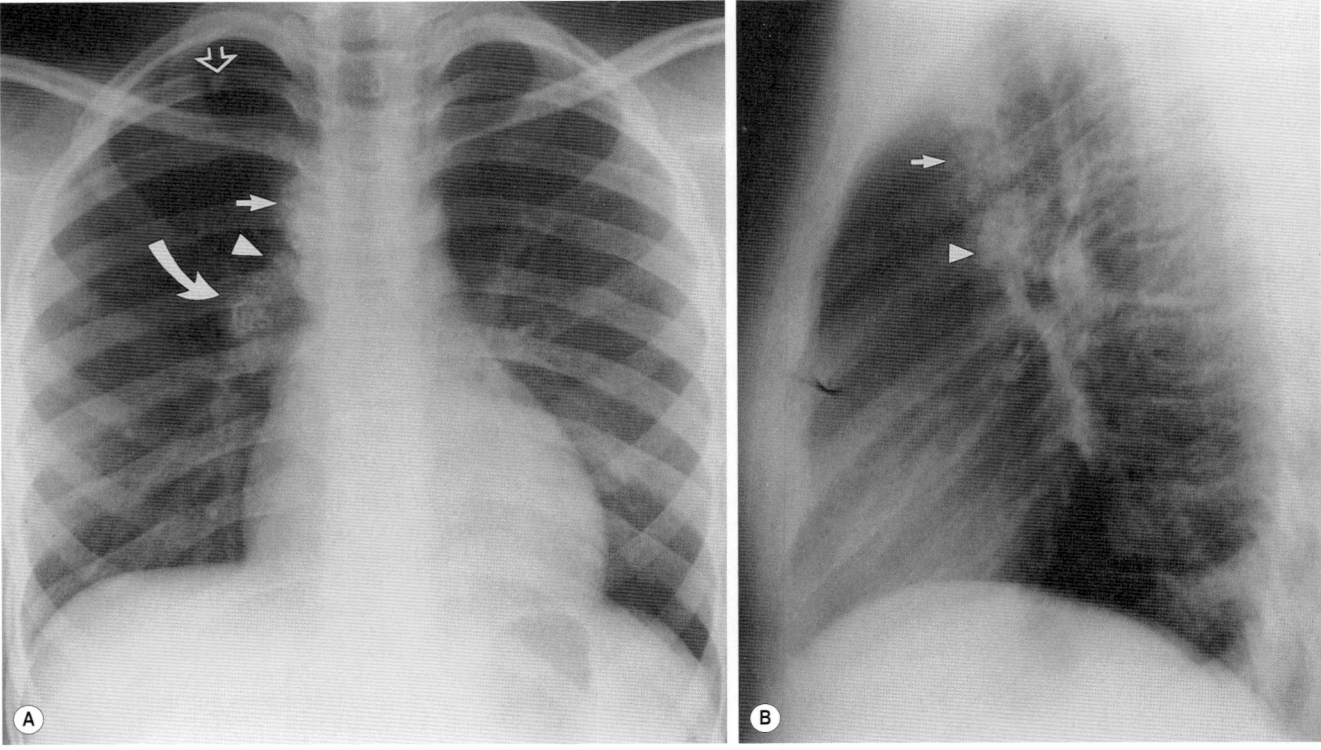

Figure 18-4. (A and B) Chest radiographs of a child with healed histoplasmosis shows granuloma in right upper lobe (open arrow), calcified paratracheal nodes (straight arrow), tracheobronchial nodes (arrowhead), and calcified right hilar nodes (curved arrow).

of involvement of the right paratracheal and tracheobronchial nodes. Nodes >2 cm in diameter invariably showed central areas of relatively low density and peripheral rim enhancement that was irregular in thickness.

Nontuberculous mycobacteria. In immunocompromised children (and occasionally in normal young children), nontuberculous mycobacteria can cause: (1) extensive hilar and paratracheal lymphadenopathy with or without parenchymal disease; and (2) endobronchial disease with atelectasis.[8] In all reported patients in one series, the organism was isolated from lymph node, lung, or bronchoalveolar lavage. Lymphadenopathy can be unilateral or bilateral, and nodes undergo extensive caseating necrosis.

Mycoplasma pneumoniae. Radiographic findings in 56 patients with pneumonia (21 younger than 20 years) due to *M. pneumoniae* revealed that 22% of patients had hilar or paratracheal node enlargement, and 14% had pleural effusions.[9,10]

Bartonella henselae. A few patients with cat-scratch disease have been described with mediastinal and peripheral lymphadenopathy. Mediastinal node biopsy in one patient revealed granuloma with microabscesses.[11]

Yersinia enterocolitica. Significant bilateral self-limited hilar adenopathy without pneumonia due to *Y. enterocolitica* has been described in several adults. All patients recovered without therapy. The diagnosis was based on results of culture or serum agglutination titers.[12]

Lung abscess. Lung abscess frequently is associated with anaerobic infections but can occur in the course of any necrotizing pneumonia. Mediastinal lymphadenopathy is not unusual.

Bronchiectasis. In children and adults, bronchiectasis of any etiology (e.g., associated with congenital anomaly, foreign body), and especially that associated with cystic fibrosis in children, can cause mediastinal lymphadenopathy. In one study of CT in patients with bronchiectasis, mediastinal lymphadenopathy (nodes >1 cm in diameter) was present in 29% of patients.[13]

Fungal Causes

Histoplasma capsulatum. Infection due to *Histoplasma capsulatum* has multiple clinical forms (Figures 18-4 and 18-5). In the immunocompetent host, histoplasmosis most frequently is subclinical, recognized incidentally. In symptomatic infection, cough or chest pain is most common. Mediastinal lymphadenopathy, an uncommon finding in disseminated infection, is the most common manifestation in healthy children with self-limited infection. Of 35 children hospitalized with histoplasmosis between 1968 and 1988, 29 (83%) had pulmonary infection, mediastinal infection, or both. Chest radiograph was abnormal in 31 (91%), revealing adenopathy in 25 (74%) and infiltrates in 19 (56%).[14] Isolated mediastinal adenopathy can be difficult to distinguish from lymphoma.[15,16] Rarely, massive inhalation of fungus causes disseminated, symptomatic primary infection with fever, cough, and massively enlarged mediastinal lymph nodes. The differentiation is important as, in most cases, histoplasmosis is mild and self-limited in most immunocompetent people. Antifungal therapy is reserved for those with acute diffuse pulmonary infection, chronic pulmonary infection, progressive disseminated disease, and mediastinal adenitis associated with obstructive symptoms.

In the otherwise healthy host, marked enlargement of mediastinal lymph nodes can cause obstruction of bronchi, the superior vena cava, or the esophagus. Additionally, a group of large nodes can become necrotic and matted to form a large single mediastinal mass known as an acute mediastinal granuloma. Most such masses resolve spontaneously; the effect of antifungal therapy has not been studied.

In the transplant population, pulmonary histoplasmosis can be a difficult diagnosis, mainly because it is not often considered. It generally occurs sporadically, manifesting as a prolonged febrile illness with subacute pulmonary symptoms.[17] Disseminated histoplasmosis in patients with an underlying disease treated with anti-TNF-α is well described. Pulmonary symptoms are not

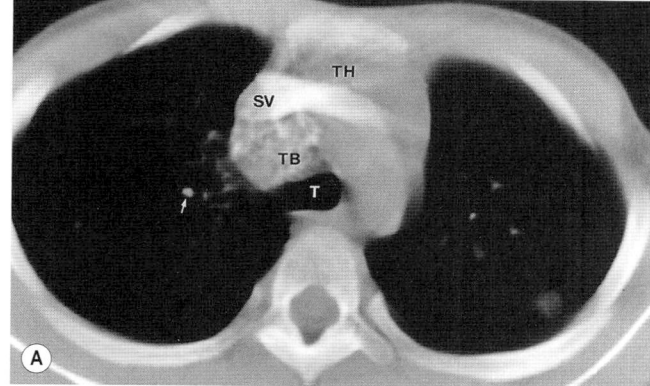
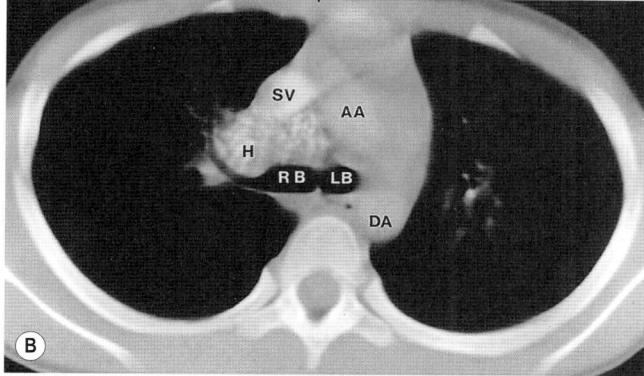
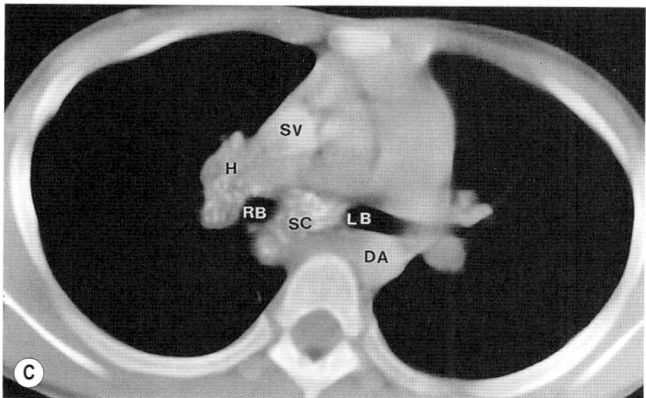

Figure 18-5. (A through C) Enhanced computed tomography scan of the patient in Figure 18-4 shows extensive right tracheobronchial, right hilar, and subcarinal lymphadenopathy. Particulate calcification within the nodes is characteristic of healed histoplasmosis. Arrow indicates calcified granuloma in right upper lobe. AA, ascending aorta; DA, descending aorta; H, calcified right hilar node; LB, left mainstem bronchus; RB, right mainstem bronchus; SC, calcified subcarinal nodes; SV, superior vena cava; T, trachea; TB, calcified tracheobronchial nodes; TH, thymus.

prominent, however, and the patient often is thought to have a flare of the underlying disease. Diagnosis in this setting as well as those in the transplant population requires detection of *Histoplasma* antigen in the serum and urine.[18] Disseminated disease previously noted frequently in people with advanced HIV infection living in endemic areas is rarely seen now due to the early diagnosis and treatment of HIV infection.

Coccidioidomycosis immitis. Coccidioidomycosis occurs primarily in the southwestern United States. It is subclinical in children in 60% of cases. An insignificant flu-like illness or severe respiratory infection with lobar pneumonia and pleural effusions can occur. Radiographic findings are nonspecific; bronchopneumonic

PART II Clinical Syndromes and Cardinal Features of Infectious Diseases: Approach to Diagnosis and Initial Management

SECTION B Cardinal Symptom Complexes

infiltrates often are associated with enlargement of hilar nodes. Cavitation, nodule formation, or calcification occurs in a minority of patients.

Parenchymal infiltrates commonly are associated with hilar lymphadenopathy. More extensive mediastinal adenopathy is not considered part of the primary complex and may represent dissemination. Rarely, bilateral hilar adenopathy occurs without apparent pulmonary disease.

Paracoccidioides brasiliensis. A progressive chronic disease due to *P. brasiliensis,* paracoccidioidomycosis preferentially involves the lungs and reticuloendothelial system. It occurs predominantly in a few Latin American countries. Only about 2% of cases occur in children. Pulmonary lesions can be infiltrative, fibrotic, fibrocaseous, or cavitary. Enlargement of hilar and mediastinal lymph nodes is observed. Enlargement of liver, spleen, and other lymph nodes (e.g., cervical, inguinal, and mesenteric) also occurs. Complications include suppuration and fistula formation and scarring of affected nodes with residual pulmonary fibrosis.

Pneumocystis jirovecii. A patient with acquired immunodeficiency syndrome (AIDS) and *P. jirovecii* pneumonia with calcified hilar and mediastinal nodes has been reported.[18]

Other. An immunocompetent child with fever, pneumonia and a posterior mediastinal mass with hilar and subcarinal lymphadenopathy was originally thought to have lymphoma but at biopsy, a granuloma with broad septated fungal hyphae with right angle branching compatible with zygomycosis was found.[19]

Viral Causes

Epstein–Barr virus. Generalized lymphadenopathy secondary to extensive lymphocytic hyperplasia can include the mediastinum.[19,20] In transplant recipients undergoing immunosuppression, lymphoproliferative disease related to Epstein–Barr virus can manifest as generalized lymphadenopathy, including involvement of the mediastinal nodes.

Rubeola. Pulmonary infiltrates and hilar adenopathy appearing early in the course of measles are well described. In one series of 130 children with measles, 55% had pulmonary infiltrates, and 74% had hilar adenopathy.[21]

NONINFECTIOUS CAUSES

Malignancy

Lymphomas (Figures 18-6 and 18-7) characteristically occur in the anterior and middle mediastinum and are the third most common cause of mediastinal masses in children. The most common manifestation of Hodgkin lymphoma or non-Hodgkin lymphoma is painless lymph node enlargement, most often in the cervical or supraclavicular chains. Fifty percent to 60% of patients with Hodgkin lymphoma have mediastinal lymphadenopathy (usually bilateral) and evidence of tracheobronchial compression at the time of diagnosis. Involved nodes are hilar ($\geq$25%), subcarinal (22%), posterior mediastinal (5%), and cardiophrenic angle (8%). Ipsilateral pulmonary parenchymal involvement is present in 10% of patients.

Childhood non-Hodgkin lymphoma is a rapidly proliferating malignancy, usually affecting adolescent males and often with a duration of symptoms of only 4 to 6 weeks. Lymphoblastic lymphoma and the closely related acute lymphoblastic leukemia often manifest indistinguishably, with mediastinal adenopathy and compression. Dissemination is present in 70% of children at the time of diagnosis. Non-Hodgkin lymphoma can arise in any lymphoid tissue and in numerous extralymphatic sites. Painless, rapidly progressive enlargement of cervical, supraclavicular, and axillary nodes is a common presenting complaint. With involvement of these nodes, an anterior mediastinal tumor is common (50% to 70%), as are pleural effusions.

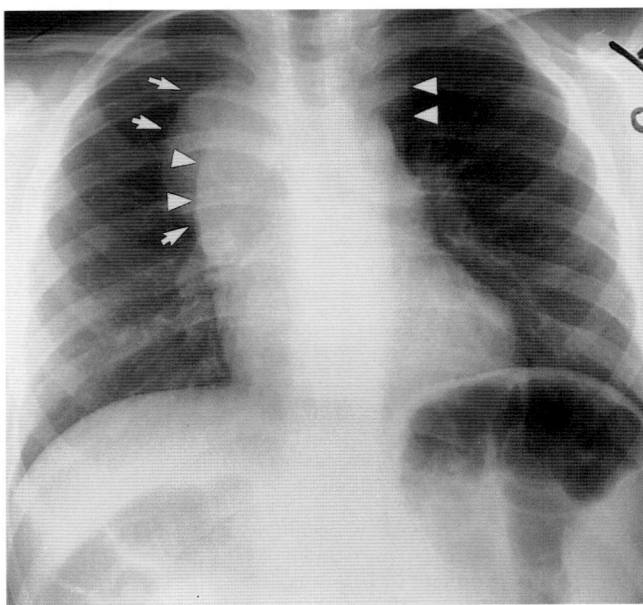

Figure 18-6. Chest radiograph of a child with mixed-cell Hodgkin disease shows right paratracheal (arrows) and tracheobronchial lymphadenopathy (arrows). The superior mediastinum is widened on the left as well, indicating enlargement of anterior mediastinal nodes (arrowheads).

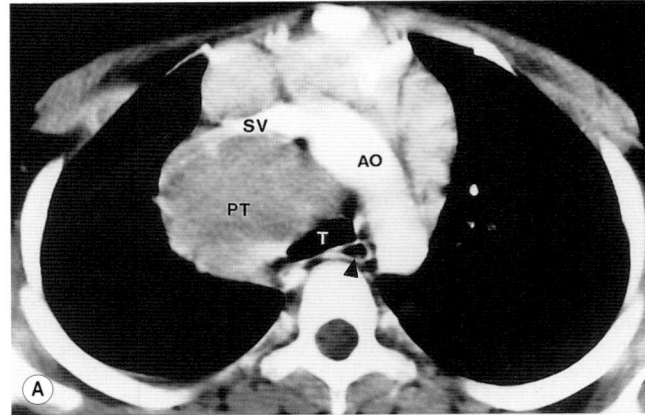

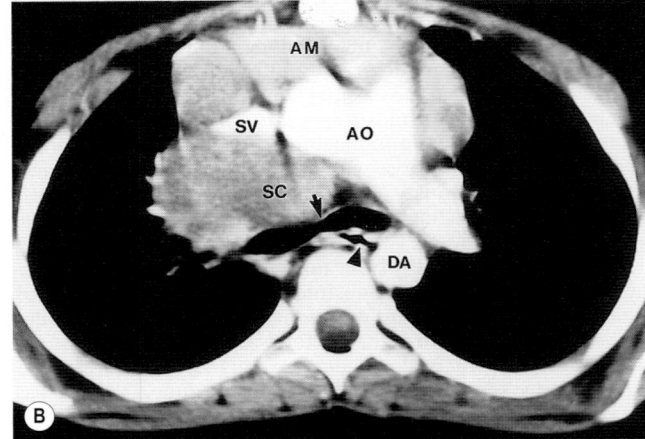

Figure 18-7. (A and B) Enhanced computed tomography scans of a child with mixed-cell Hodgkin disease show extensive mediastinal adenopathy. Arrow indicates carina, and arrowhead indicates esophagus containing air. AM, anterior mediastinal nodes; AO, aortic arch; DA, descending aorta; SC, subcarinal nodes; SV, superior vena cava; T, trachea.

Other Causes

Sarcoidosis. Sarcoidosis is a multisystem granulomatous disease of unknown cause that is relatively uncommon in children; it has two age group incidence peaks, between 9 and 16 years of age and in young adults. Sarcoidosis most commonly involves the lungs, lymph nodes, eyes, skin, liver, and spleen. Nonspecific symptoms consist of fever, weight loss, cough, fatigue, lethargy, lymphadenitis, visual disturbances, and rashes. In large series of children and adults, 90% of patients have bilateral involvement of the lungs and hilar lymph nodes.[22,23] In children, bilateral hilar lymphadenopathy, occasionally involving the paratracheal nodes, was associated with parenchymal involvement in 50% of cases.[23] Patients should be evaluated for ocular involvement as well as other visceral sites of disease.

Giant lymph node hyperplasia (Castleman disease). Castleman disease, a rare disease in children younger than 14 years, can manifest as an asymptomatic mass in the mediastinum or neck, along the aorta or in the abdomen.[24,25] Some patients have prolonged fever, anemia, weight loss, splenomegaly, hypergammaglobulinemia, elevated erythrocyte sedimentation rate (ESR), bone marrow plasmacytosis, and a poor outcome. Microscopically, the large, well-circumscribed ovoid nodes 3 to 8 cm long are characterized by lymphoid follicular hyperplasia with and without germinal center formation and marked capillary proliferation with endothelial hyperplasia. Human herpesvirus 8 (HHV-8) has been found in the nodes of affected patients. Surgical removal of localized nodes for diagnosis and therapy may relieve systemic symptoms. Recurrences have not been reported in children. In a patient infected with human immunodeficiency virus, foscarnet and antiretroviral agents resulted in dramatic improvement.[26]

Wegener granulomatosis. Mediastinal adenopathy with tracheal and bronchial stenosis associated with Wegener granulomatosis has been reported rarely in children. In these cases, disease was limited to the airways and sinuses.

Chronic granulomatous disease. Hilar adenopathy in association with pneumonia raises suspicion of chronic infection or granuloma formation. Patients with chronic granulomatous disease frequently have mediastinal adenopathy in conjunction with pneumonia.

Graves disease. Thymic enlargement simulating an anterior mediastinal mass has been noted in adults and adolescents with Graves disease. In such cases, thyrotropin-receptor autoantibodies stimulate the thyroid and some extrathyroid tissues including the thymus. Clinical findings of hyperthyroidism may be subtle but measurement of thyroid hormone levels are diagnostic.[27]

DIAGNOSTIC APPROACH

The diagnostic approach depends on the age of the patient, exposures, presence and progression of symptoms, associated physical findings, and specific abnormalities of imaging studies (see Table 18-4). Results of serologic tests (e.g., for *Bartonella*, *Mycoplasma*, *Histoplasma* infection) and the tuberculin skin test frequently confirm the diagnosis, averting the need for tissue diagnosis. *H. capsulatum* antigen detection in serum, urine, or bronchoalveolar lavage fluid can confirm the diagnosis. Antigen detection is most sensitive for disseminated disease and can be negative in pulmonary histoplasmosis. Rapidly enlarging masses, in the absence of a confirmed, compatible diagnosis, require prompt biopsy. Optimal therapy depends on rapid and accurate diagnosis.[27,28]

Subacute infections associated with hilar lymphadenopathy can be difficult to distinguish from lymphoreticular malignancy. In one study of 37 children with anterior and middle mediastinal masses, 16 had lymphomas and 21 had histoplasmosis.[29] The two entities could not be distinguished on the basis of patient age or sex, fever, weight loss, duration of illness, anemia, ESR, or lung infiltrates and calcifications. Anterior mediastinal masses were due to lymphoma in 81% of cases and histoplasmosis in 5%. Of the patients with lymphomas, only 7% had *Histoplasma* complement fixation titers of ≥1:8 but 67% of patients with histoplasmosis had titers of ≥1:32. The authors of this study concluded that anterior mediastinal masses should be biopsied. Immunodiffusion testing for *H. capsulatum*, however, is highly specific. The finding of H bands is highly suggestive of acute infection (see Chapter 250, *Histoplasma capsulatum* (Histoplasmosis)).

19 Abdominal and Retroperitoneal Lymphadenopathy

Angela L. Myers and Mary Anne Jackson

Lymphadenopathy, the abnormal enlargement of lymph nodes, can result from a wide variety of infectious and noninfectious causes. Acute enlargement of superficial lymph nodes caused by infection can occur over a period of days, accompanied by pain and tenderness to palpation, resulting in lymphadenitis. Alternatively, the enlargement of nodes can occur over weeks to months, with little tenderness, representing a more chronic inflammatory process. Abdominal and retroperitoneal lymphadenopathy is a diagnosis made by imaging techniques such as ultrasonography (US), computed tomography (CT), or magnetic resonance imaging (MRI). Without sequential imaging studies, it can be uncertain whether enlargement represents a new, rapidly evolving process or a more prolonged, chronic, relatively stable one. Without the ability to examine the lymph nodes directly, the clinician must rely on clues from the history and physical examination to formulate a diagnosis.

Inflammation in lymph nodes may be the direct result of infection in the tissues (or other lymph nodes) that the nodes drain or a consequence of bloodstream dissemination of organisms. Tissues and organs of the abdomen and retroperitoneal space can be infected by a variety of pathogens through various routes (see Chapter 68, Appendicitis; Chapter 69, Intra-Abdominal, Visceral, and Retroperitoneal Abscesses).

EPIDEMIOLOGY AND DIFFERENTIAL DIAGNOSIS

Abdominal and retroperitoneal lymphadenopathy in children can have infectious and noninfectious causes. Malignant processes and serious infection are the primary concerns; malignant tumors may account for up to 25% of cases.[1-6] A systematic approach to evaluation for infection requires consideration of selected factors from the history and clinical examination (Box 19-1).

The regional lymph nodes that drain the organs and tissues from the abdomen, retroperitoneal space, and lower extremities are shown in Figure 19-1.[4,7] Focal, deep lymphadenopathy

PART II Clinical Syndromes and Cardinal Features of Infectious Diseases: Approach to Diagnosis and Initial Management

SECTION B Cardinal Symptom Complexes

BOX 19-1. Evaluation of Patients with Lymphadenopathy of Suspected Infectious Etiology

SYMPTOMS

Duration of symptoms: acute (days) or chronic (weeks to months)

Presence of weight loss, fever

Presence of organ system-specific symptoms: diarrhea, abdominal pain, jaundice, dysuria, flank pain, hip pain

EXPOSURES

Exposure to animal bites or scratches: cats, rodents, farm animals

Travel to areas endemic for enteric bacterial or parasitic pathogens, fungal pathogens: *Histoplasma, Coccidioides, Mycobacterium,* or *Plasmodium*

Ingestion of unpasteurized dairy products

Risk factors for HIV infection

UNDERLYING DISORDERS

Concomitant infection elsewhere in the patient

History of previous or chronic infection of liver or gallbladder, spleen, pancreas, bowel, kidney or ureters, bladder, ovaries or uterus, iliopsoas muscle, or vertebral bodies

Presence of underlying immunocompromising disorders: malignant tumors, chemotherapy, corticosteroid therapy, HIV infection

Congenital immunodeficiencies: chronic granulomatous disease, severe combined immunodeficiency

Transplantation: immunodeficiency and posttransplant lymphoproliferative disorders

Crohn disease

Celiac disease

PHYSICAL EXAMINATION

Lymphadenopathy: focal versus regional or systemic

Evidence of infection in tissues or organs drained by lymph nodes

Evidence of systemic infection: Epstein–Barr virus infection, cat-scratch disease, tuberculosis

HIV, human immunodeficiency virus.

---

suggests infection in the adjacent draining structures or lymph node groups; generalized adenopathy suggests a disseminated process that is likely to involve other lymph nodes, which may be palpably enlarged, as well as the liver and spleen.

Infectious causes of enlarged superior or inferior mesenteric lymph nodes include most of the bacterial, viral, and parasitic pathogens that cause gastroenteritis. Mesenteric lymph node enlargement in association with an acute, symptomatic febrile illness that most often manifests as abdominal pain is referred to as mesenteric lymphadenitis. *Yersinia, Salmonella* and *Shigella* ssp., *Escherichia coli,* adenoviruses, enteroviruses, and *Entamoeba histolytica* are important causes of mesenteric lymphadenitis and each has a characteristic constellation of clinical and laboratory findings (see Chapter 68, Appendicitis).[4,8-13] Associated inflammation of the terminal ileum and ileocecal junction suggests infectious causes, such as *Yersinia,*[10] *Mycobacterium tuberculosis* or *M. bovis,* as well as Crohn disease.[12,14] *M. tuberculosis* is considered especially if the child was born in an endemic region, has traveled to tuberculosis-endemic areas, or may have ingested contaminated food products (e.g., homemade unpasteurized cheese).[14-16]

Epstein–Barr virus (EBV) and *Bartonella henselae* infection are the most commonly reported infectious causes of abdominal lymphadenopathy in otherwise healthy children. In mononucleosis, the accompanying malaise, pharyngitis, systemic lymphadenopathy, and hepatosplenomegaly often lead to the diagnosis.[17] Peripheral findings of a papule at the site of inoculation and of regional peripheral lymphadenopathy frequently are present in patients with cat-scratch disease. However, fever, with or without abdominal pain, in the absence of peripheral findings, can be the presentation of *B. henselae* infection of the liver, spleen, or abdominal lymph nodes.[18,19] Other less common systemic infections include malaria, toxoplasmosis, and pentastomiasis.[20-22]

Tuberculosis in children can manifest with abdominal lymphadenopathy as the sole anatomic manifestation of systemic infection. Lymphadenopathy can occur during primary infection or during reactivation of a previous infection. Both *M. tuberculosis* and *M. bovis* can cause symptomatic infection of the intestines, lymph nodes, peritoneum, omentum, liver, or spleen.[15,16,23,24] Additionally, a newly recognized mycobacterium species, *M. gastri,* has been reported to cause disseminated infection with extensive abdominal lymphadenopathy.[25] Children can have symptoms of weight loss, fatigue, and intermittent abdominal pain in the absence of abdominal physical findings. The clinical presentation can mimic inflammatory bowel disease.[26] Since low numbers of organisms

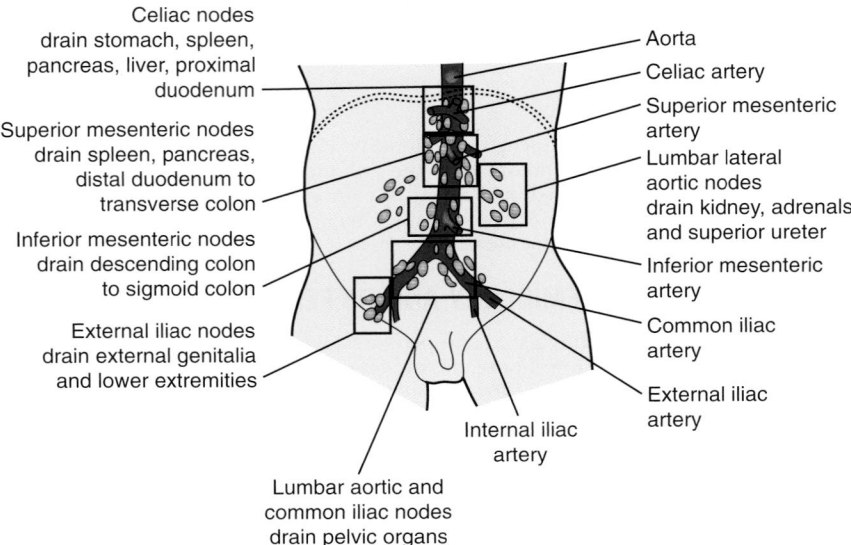

Celiac nodes drain stomach, spleen, pancreas, liver, proximal duodenum

Superior mesenteric nodes drain spleen, pancreas, distal duodenum to transverse colon

Inferior mesenteric nodes drain descending colon to sigmoid colon

External iliac nodes drain external genitalia and lower extremities

Aorta

Celiac artery

Superior mesenteric artery

Lumbar lateral aortic nodes drain kidney, adrenals and superior ureter

Inferior mesenteric artery

Common iliac artery

External iliac artery

Internal iliac artery

Lumbar aortic and common iliac nodes drain pelvic organs

Figure 19-1. Location and drainage patterns of deep abdominal lymph nodes.

typically are present, polymerase chain reaction (PCR) is a more reliable test than mycobacterial stain or culture. If the infection is caused by *M. tuberculosis,* hilar adenopathy also may be detected on chest radiograph but, in most cases, abdominal tuberculosis occurs in the absence of pulmonary disease.

Lymphoproliferative syndromes caused by EBV and characterized by abdominal lymphadenopathy have been well described.[17,27] At one center approximately 8% of pediatric transplant recipients developed lymphoproliferative syndrome.[27] Approximately one-half of children with an EBV-related abdominal lymphoproliferative disorder have abdominal pain; one-quarter have enlarged liver or spleen, or present with an abdominal mass. Evidence of EBV infection of B lymphocytes is usually present.

In children with symptomatic human immunodeficiency virus (HIV) infection, abdominal lymphadenopathy can signify the underlying HIV infection, an HIV-related cancer, or secondary infection.[2,28] In particular, *M. avium* complex (MAC) infection can cause massive systemic lymphadenopathy, including the mesenteric and retroperitoneal lymph nodes.[29] Congenital immunodeficiencies, such as chronic granulomatous disease, also rarely can be characterized by mesenteric lymphadenopathy.[30]

Mesenteric lymphadenopathy can accompany noninfectious inflammation of the bowel, such as that due to Crohn disease[12] or celiac disease.[31] Abdominal lymphadenopathy can be a systemic manifestation of a number of disorders of unknown cause, including sarcoidosis,[32] Castleman disease,[33] Rosai–Dorfmann disease,[3] or familial Mediterranean fever.[34]

DIAGNOSTIC TESTS

Imaging Studies

US has been used to assess the significance and degree of abdominal lymphadenopathy in both infectious and noninfectious conditions,[35,36] including cat-scratch disease[37] and abdominal tuberculosis.[38,39] Subtle differences detectable by US can help differentiate between infectious causes of enlarged nodes. In studies in which US and CT have been compared, CT is more sensitive for detecting abdominal lymphadenopathy,[38] aiding in the diagnosis of both abdominal and retroperitoneal lymphadenopathy.[12,40] MRI has been used to evaluate lymphadenopathy in both the abdominal and retroperitoneal spaces and has advantages over other imaging techniques for the detection of vascular lesions and tumors.[16,41,42]

Clinical Findings and Laboratory Tests

Clues to the cause of lymphadenopathy are based on physical findings that can include systemic lymphadenopathy or hepatosplenomegaly. Other physical findings of infection of the respiratory tract, gastrointestinal tract, skin, skeletal system, cardiovascular system, or genitourinary system also can provide clues to the primary site of infection.

In the immunocompetent child, a tuberculin skin test (TST) remains one of the most sensitive and specific techniques for diagnosis of infections caused by *M. tuberculosis* or *M. bovis.* False-negative test results have been seen in conjunction with disseminated tuberculosis and immunocompromising conditions. Diagnostic assays based on production of interferon-γ by cultured peripheral blood lymphocytes following in vitro exposure to purified proteins from *M. tuberculosis* are useful in adults, but are not reliable in children <5 years of age.[43,44] These tests can differentiate *M. tuberculosis* infection from *M. bovis,* bacille Calmette-Guérin and most nontuberculous mycobacterial infections.

Biopsy

Many infections that lead to abdominal lymphadenopathy can be detected by specific serologic tests, including infections caused by *B. henselae,* EBV, cytomegalovirus, *Toxoplasma* sp., and HIV. The types of cultures obtained from blood, urine, stool, or biopsy specimens should be directed toward the suspected pathogens, noting the particular lymph node group affected, pertinent history and clinical findings, and associated or underlying disease(s).

When tissue samples are required for accurate diagnosis, particularly in the case of tumors, the techniques discussed in Chapter 69 (Intra-Abdominal, Visceral, and Retroperitoneal Abscesses) are useful for the diagnosis not only of organ disease but also of lymph node disease. Options include open surgical biopsy and laparoscopic biopsy or fine-needle biopsy, directed by US or CT. Considerations for choosing the optimal technique in individual cases include the volume of tissue required for diagnosis, the urgency for arriving at a diagnosis, institutional procedural experience, and the ancillary support services available. In general, histologic diagnosis of specific tumors requires larger amounts of tissue than are required for diagnosis of infection.

Special stains and cultures can be used to identify bacteria, fungi, mycobacteria, or viruses. Biopsy samples are examined histologically for evidence of acute or chronic inflammation, abscess or granuloma formation, or primary or metastatic tumors. Pathogens generally produce a characteristic histopathologic findings. For example, caseating granuloma characterizes tuberculosis, but stellate granuloma is more suggestive of infection due to *B. henselae.*

THERAPY

Although many infectious causes of abdominal and retroperitoneal lymphadenopathy are benign and self-limiting, antimicrobial therapy can be beneficial depending on the pathogen implicated. The chapters that discuss each specific pathogen in detail should be consulted.

---

20 Localized Lymphadenitis, Lymphadenopathy, and Lymphangitis

Angela L. Myers and Mary Anne Jackson

LYMPHADENOPATHY AND LYMPHADENITIS

Lymphadenopathy is defined as disease of the lymph nodes, but the term is more commonly used to denote lymph node enlargement. Enlarged lymph nodes can arise in association with a wide variety of infectious, inflammatory, or neoplastic disease processes. *Lymphadenitis* refers to a localized inflammatory process within a given lymph node or group of nodes, usually of bacterial etiology. Lymphadenitis can develop acutely or chronically and can be pyogenic or granulomatous in nature. Other chapters in this textbook are

PART II Clinical Syndromes and Cardinal Features of Infectious Diseases: Approach to Diagnosis and Initial Management

SECTION B Cardinal Symptom Complexes

specifically devoted to the evaluation and management of generalized lymphadenopathy (see Chapter 16, Lymphatic System and Generalized Lymphadenopathy) and lymphadenopathy of the cervical nodes (see Chapter 17, Cervical Lymphadenitis and Neck Infections), hilar nodes (see Chapter 18, Mediastinal and Hilar Lymphadenopathy), inguinal nodes (see Chapter 52, Skin and Mucous Membrane Infections and Inguinal Lymphadenopathy), and abdominal nodes (see Chapter 19, Abdominal and Retroperitoneal Lymphadenopathy) groups. The current discussion focuses on regional lymph node disease encountered in the remaining superficial locations.

Pathogenesis

Lymph nodes can enlarge as a result of: (1) intrinsic proliferation of lymphocytes or reticuloendothelial cells; or (2) infiltration by cells from an extrinsic source. Lymphocytes or lymphoblasts proliferate upon recognition of antigenic stimuli, producing lymph node enlargement, which recedes upon antigen clearance. Infectious organisms able to survive intracellularly can represent persistent stimuli and can be associated with chronic lymphatic cellular hyperplasia. Extrinsic invasion of lymph nodes occurs with neutrophils in response to bacteria and bacterial toxins, with histiocytes in histiocytosis and certain storage diseases, and with malignant cells in leukemia, lymphoma, and metastatic solid tumors.

Etiologic Agents

The pyogenic bacteria *Staphylococcus aureus* and *Streptococcus pyogenes* account for greater than 95% of acute bacterial lymphadenitis.[1] Lymph node infection usually can be attributed to spread from an adjacent skin infection or inoculation site; occasionally, no clear origin is evident. Acute localized lymphadenitis with overlying cellulitis can develop in an infant as a manifestation of late-onset bacteremic group B streptococcal disease.[2] Subacute development of localized lymph node enlargement in healthy children is found with cat-scratch disease (*Bartonella henselae* infection) and with nontuberculous mycobacterial infection. Adenitis with fungal pathogens such as *Aspergillus* or *Candida* can occur in immunosuppressed patients, such as those with leukemia who are undergoing chemotherapy.[3] Unusual pathogens can produce lymphadenitis in otherwise healthy people after specific environmental exposures (e.g., *Francisella tularensis* after tick bite/animal skinning or *Corynebacterium pseudotuberculosis* in sheep handlers).

History and Clinical Findings

Certain clinical features may be useful in guiding the evaluation of localized lymph node infections (Table 20-1). Small inguinal, cervical, or axillary lymph nodes can be palpated in about a third of healthy neonates.[4] Subsequent antigenic stimulation leads to steady enlargement of lymphoid tissue from infancy through puberty. As a result, the vast majority of healthy children have palpable cervical, inguinal, and axillary nodes.[5] In contrast, other peripheral node groups (e.g., posterior auricular, supraclavicular, epitrochlear, iliac, and popliteal) are always considered abnormal if they can be palpated on examination.[6]

A careful history must be obtained regarding the time of onset and rate of lymph node enlargement (Box 20-1). The skin and soft-tissue areas drained by the enlarged nodes should be examined for signs of infection and disruption. History of exposure to animals should be detailed. Occurrence of bites (including tick bites) or traumatic scratches or other papular or ulcerative skin lesions is elicited. Weight loss, protracted fever, rash, generalized lymphadenopathy, or hepatosplenomegaly suggests a systemic disease.[7] Lymph nodes associated with viral infection tend to be small, bilateral, freely mobile, and variably tender.[8] The presence of erythema, warmth, and tenderness overlying a node typically indicates a pyogenic acute inflammatory response related to a bacterial pathogen. Fluctuation of the lymph node is suggestive of acute pyogenic bacterial adenitis but also can be seen with more indolent pathogens, including nontuberculous mycobacteria (NTM); and presence of overlying violaceous hue raises suspicion of the latter. Most acutely infected lymph nodes in children are rubbery or firm in consistency and freely mobile. Fixation of the node to underlying tissue raises concern for a neoplastic process.

Differential Diagnosis

Knowledge of lymphatic drainage patterns is essential to identification of the primary focus of infection and the most likely etiologic agents in the child with localized lymphadenopathy. The regions drained by specific lymph node groups are listed in Table 20-1, along with the associated infections encountered in each case.

TABLE 20-1. Infections Associated with Localized Lymphadenopathy

Lymph Node Group	Area of Drainage	Palpable Nodes	Infectious Etiologies	
			Common	**Less Common**
Occipital	Back of scalp and neck	5% of healthy children	Impetigo Pediculosis (head lice) Tinea capitis Seborrheic dermatitis	Rubella Toxoplasmosis
Preauricular	Lateral portion of eyelids Lateral conjunctivae Skin above cheek, temple	Only with disease	Adenoviral conjunctivitis Parinaud syndrome secondary to cat-scratch disease	*Chlamydia* conjunctivitis Parinaud syndrome secondary to tularemia or herpes simplex virus infection
Axillary	Hand and arm	70–90% of healthy children	Local pyogenic infection	Calmette-Guérin bacillus vaccine, fever, tuberculosis (scrofuloderma), hidradenitis suppurativa
	Chest wall, breast Upper lateral abdominal wall		Cat-scratch disease	
Epitrochlear	Ulnar aspect of hand and forearm	Only with disease	Local pyogenic infection	Tularemia, cat-scratch disease, secondary or congenital syphilis
Iliac	Lower abdominal viscera Urinary and genital tract Lower extremities	Only with disease	Abdominal infection such as appendicitis, following abdominal trauma, urinary tract infection	Pyogenic infection of lower extremity
Popliteal	Skin of lateral foot and lower leg, knee joint	Only with disease	Severe local pyogenic infection	–

Occipital Nodes

The occipital lymph nodes drain the posterior scalp and can become enlarged in association with impetigo, pediculosis capitis, tinea capitis, or inflamed seborrheic dermatitis. Tularemia often involves occipital nodes because a common site for tick bite in children is on the parieto-occipital scalp. Occurrence of the tick bite itself may be unknown or forgotten as often the bite occurred a week or more prior. The history of exposure to a tick-infested area should raise suspicion. The scalp should be inspected carefully for a papule or an ulcer although glandular tularemia is more common than ulceroglandular disease and is most common in those under 2 years of age.[9] Less often, rubella infection or toxoplasmosis can produce isolated occipital lymphadenopathy.

Preauricular Nodes

Preauricular nodes drain the lateral eyelid and conjunctivae, along with skin overlying the cheek and temple. Severe conjunctivitis associated with ipsilateral preauricular lymphadenopathy is known as Parinaud or oculoglandular syndrome. Oculoglandular syndrome is a relatively common complication of *Bartonella henselae* infection (cat-scratch disease), affecting approximately 8% of symptomatic patients (Figure 20-1).[10] The differential diagnosis also includes tuberculosis, tularemia, and nontuberculous lymph node infection. Chlamydial neonatal inclusion conjunctivitis can appear 5 to 10 days after birth, and the presence of lymph node enlargement helps distinguish it from gonococcal ophthalmia neonatorum.[11] Trachoma, which is a chronic form of chlamydial eye infection, causes an oculoglandular syndrome with potential blindness as a result. It is rare in the United States, but endemic in many developing countries. Epidemic keratoconjunctivitis[12] and pharyngoconjunctival fever[13] are adenoviral infections that can be associated with preauricular adenopathy.

Axillary Nodes

The axillary nodes drain the upper extremity, chest wall, and upper lateral abdominal wall. Localized axillary lymphadenopathy most often represents a response to a pyogenic infection of the upper extremity. *B. henselae* infection is commonly associated with localized axillary lymphadenopathy after a cat scratch on the arm, and rat-bite fever due to *Spirillum minor* can cause axillary node enlargement and tenderness.[14] Regional cutaneous tuberculosis (scrofuloderma) can be associated with axillary node enlargement.[15] The most common complication of bacille Calmette–Guérin (BCG) vaccination is granulomatous lymphadenitis of the ipsilateral axillary region, which sometimes heals spontaneously but can have a protracted course. Disease responds poorly to isoniazid therapy and can require surgical excision.[16,17] This diagnosis should be kept in mind when evaluating internationally adopted

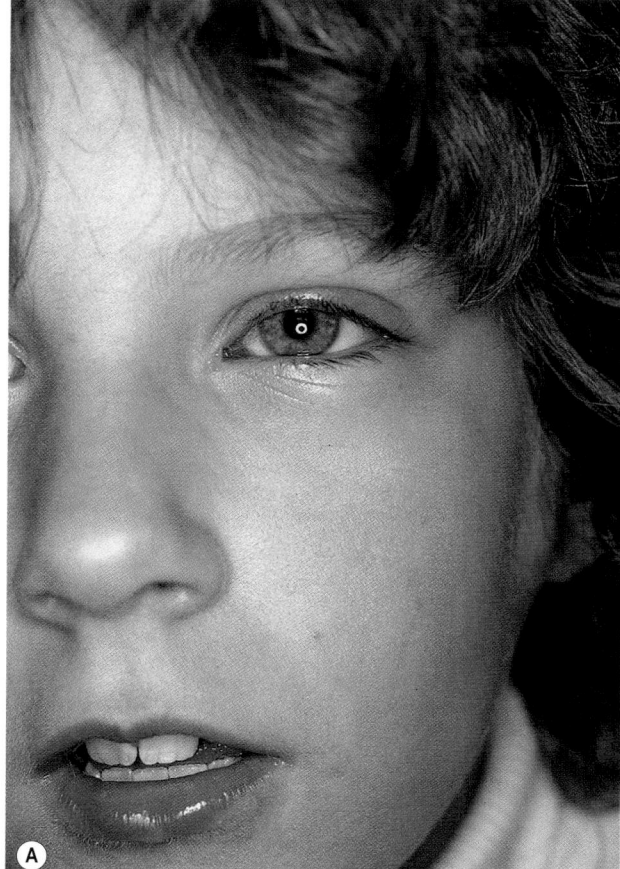

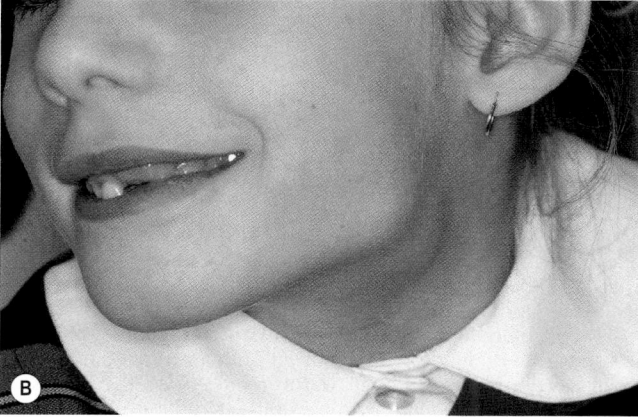

Figure 20-1. Two school-aged girls with granulomatous conjunctivitis and lymphadenopathy due to *Bartonella henselae* infection. One girl has associated preauricular lymphadenopathy **(A)** and the other has facial and anterior cervical lymphadenopathy **(B).** (Courtesy of Sarah Long, MD.)

children. Hidradenitis suppurativa is a defect of terminal follicular epithelium, often affecting obese adolescent girls, which leads to recurrent polymicrobial axillary node abscesses, fistulas, and scarring.[18] Although gram-positive organisms predominate as causes of axillary skin and lymph node abscesses, *Proteus mirabilis* was an unexpected pathogen in 28% of axillary skin abscesses in adolescent girls in a single-center study.[19] Noninfectious causes of axillary lymphadenopathy must be considered, because steadily enlarging nodes in the absence of an obvious focus are worrisome for lymphoma or other neoplasms. Rheumatologic diseases with inflammation of the wrists or finger joints also can produce axil-

PART II Clinical Syndromes and Cardinal Features of Infectious Diseases: Approach to Diagnosis and Initial Management

SECTION B Cardinal Symptom Complexes

lary lymph node swelling, though this is not generally isolated to axillary nodes.

Epitrochlear Nodes

The epitrochlear nodes drain the distal arm and the middle, ring, and fifth fingers. Isolated enlargement typically is a result of a local skin lesion infected with *Staphylococcus* or *Streptococcus*. Epitrochlear lymphadenopathy also can follow cutaneous inoculation of *B. henselae, F. tularensis,* or (rarely) *Sporothrix schenckii*. Chronic enlargement of epitrochlear nodes is known to occur in cases of secondary syphilis and can be a clue to congenital syphilis. Hodgkin disease can present with epitrochlear adenopathy.[20]

Iliac and Femoral Nodes

Enlarged iliac nodes can be detected by deep palpation over the inguinal ligament, and enlarged femoral nodes by deep palpation below the inguinal ligament, on the leg in the fossa between the adductor and rectus muscles. Suppurative iliac lymphadenitis is an important cause of retroperitoneal abscess and can result from abdominal trauma, appendicitis, urinary or genital tract infection, or infections of the lower extremity.[21] Femoral lymphadenitis results from superficial or deep infection of the lower extremity. *S. aureus* and *S. pyogenes* are implicated most commonly, but *B. henselae* also can cause prominent femoral or iliac lymphadenitis. Additionally, *Yersinia enterocolitica, Salmonella,* and tickborne *F. tularensis* can infect the inguinal nodes.

The child with iliac lymphadenitis can manifest fever and limp, abdominal or hip pain, and spasm of the psoas muscle. The patient typically prefers to lie with the hip flexed and the thigh abducted, because hip extension is extremely painful. The distinction of iliac lymphadenitis from appendicitis is facilitated by the lack of nausea and vomiting, and from pyogenic arthritis by demonstration of fuller range of motion of the hip on examination.[22] Computed tomography is the favored imaging modality when more extensive evaluation of iliac lymph node abnormalities is required.

Popliteal Nodes

The popliteal lymph nodes are difficult to palpate unless they are substantially enlarged. Consequently, popliteal lymphadenopathy is appreciated only in association with severe pyogenic infections of the distal lower extremity or knee joint, or noninfectious diseases of the reticuloendothelial system.

Management and Therapy

Definitive therapy of localized lymphadenopathy or lymphangitis requires identification of the most likely pathogen involved. The history of antecedent trauma, presence of a skin lesion or infection in the region drained by the involved node or nodes, along with rapid development of a large, warm, tender mass, is highly suggestive of acute pyogenic lymphadenitis. Needle aspiration of a fluctuant node can provide therapeutic benefit, rapid presumptive diagnosis (with use of Gram stain), and a sample for culture and antibiotic susceptibility testing. Children with nonfluctuant nodes whose symptoms are otherwise consistent with acute bacterial infection can be treated empirically and closely monitored for clinical response. Timely needle aspiration is increasingly important with the rise in community-associated methicillin-resistant *S. aureus* (CA-MRSA) infection. The child with significant fever or systemic symptoms should be further evaluated with a blood culture, complete blood cell count, and measurement of inflammatory markers (e.g., C-reactive protein).

Treatment of acute lymphadenitis should be based on presumed etiologic agent (Box 20-2). Specimen from node should be obtained to guide definitive therapy. Because acute pyogenic lymphadenitis can be staphylococcal or streptococcal in origin, the use of a cephalosporin (e.g., cephalexin 50 mg/kg per day) or clindamycin (30 mg/kg per day) is appropriate initial therapy for an outpatient. It is imperative to consider local prevalence of

> **BOX 20-2.** Treatment of Common Infections Associated with Isolated Lymphadenitis
>
> **EMPIRIC THERAPY**
>
> Cephalexin, cefadroxil, clindamycin (consider local *Staphylococcus aureus* antibiogram)
>
> **PERIODONTAL ABSCESS**
>
> Penicillin V or clindamycin
>
> **CAT-SCRATCH DISEASE**
>
> Macrolides, rifampin, trimethoprim-sulfamethoxazole (TMP-SMX)
>
> **TULAREMIA**
>
> Gentamicin, doxycycline (high relapse rate), ciprofloxacin

CA-MRSA, and of clindamycin resistance among MRSA as well as methicillin-susceptible *S. aureus* (MSSA).[23] Linezolid, a newer oxazolindinone with excellent bioavailability, could be considered but should be reserved for MRSA infections that are clindamycin-resistant. Trimethoprim-sulfamethoxazole is ineffective against *S. pyogenes*. Macrolide antibiotics, such as erythromycin and azithromycin, should not be used in the setting of acute bacterial adenitis given the high rate of resistance of *S. aureus,* occasional resistance of *S. pyogenes,* and lack of data supporting use for deeper infections. Azithromycin is an option if cat-scratch infection is considered likely.[24] In patients who appear systemically ill and in young infants at higher risk for bloodstream infection (BSI), initiation of parenteral therapy with similar agents (e.g., nafcillin, clindamycin or both in areas where both MRSA and clindamycin resistance of MSSA are prevalent) is indicated. Nodes with significant suppurative changes are likely to respond more promptly to therapy after percutaneous aspiration or incision and drainage. A total antibiotic (parenteral plus oral) course of 2 to 3 weeks' duration is often required for complete resolution of bacterial lymphadenitis. In the setting of bacteremia or for life-threatening disease, vancomycin should be given (60 mg/kg per day) in addition to an antistaphylococcal β-lactam and clindamycin, after collection of specimens likely to yield a microbiologic diagnosis.[25]

Localized lymph node enlargement lacking the characteristic features of acute pyogenic lymphadenitis and enlarged nodes that do not respond to antibiotic therapy merit careful further evaluation. Any clue regarding possible exposure to unusual pathogens should be pursued diagnostically. A tuberculin skin test (TST) should be performed, realizing that both *M. tuberculosis* and nontuberculous strains of mycobacteria (NTM) can be associated with a positive test result, the latter typically an intermediate response. The interferon-gamma release assay (IGRA) can be useful to differentiate between infection due to *M. tuberculosis* versus NTM, as the test result is negative in the latter.[26] However, the IGRA is approved for use only in children ≥5 years of age, and may not distinguish between *M. tuberculosis* and certain NTM, such as *M. kansasii*.[26,27] *B. henselae* infection can be evaluated by serologic testing. Cat-scratch lymphadenitis typically is a self-limited infection requiring no antibiotic therapy in some cases, antibiotic therapy is beneficial and aspiration of suppurative nodes may be required. Follow-up is important as unusual systemic complications, such as hepatic involvement and encephalopathy, can occur.[28] Tularemia can be diagnosed by serologic testing and initial testing usually is diagnostic if lymphadenopathy has been present for ≥2 weeks. Hidradenitis suppurativa can be temporized by antibiotic therapy (e.g., with clindamycin and rifampin), although wide surgical excision is considered most effective; healing by granulation follows.[29,30]

In patients in whom history, associated physical findings, and screening laboratory tests fail to lead to a diagnosis, and one suspects but cannot confirm a diagnosis of neoplasm or an unusual infection, lymph node biopsy is indicated. In a series of 75 children who underwent excisional biopsy of a peripheral lymph node, nonspecific reactive hyperplasia was found in 55%, noncaseating granulomas (e.g., cat-scratch disease) in 21%, lymphoreticular malignancy in 17%, and caseating granulomas in 7%.[31] Studies also suggest that fine-needle aspiration, perhaps guided by ultrasound, is a safe and effective alternative to excisional biopsy for discriminating infection from malignancy in lymph nodes of children, with one study revealing diagnostic sensitivity of 86% and specificity of 96%.[32,33] However, excisional biopsy should be utilized in the setting of suspected malignancy and inconclusive aspiration results, and is the preferred method of therapy in the setting of suspected or presumed NTM infection.[34] Any specimen from an excised node or needle aspirate should be submitted for Gram stain, acid-fast stain, and culture for bacteria (except when tularemia is suspected when culture poses risk for laboratory personnel), mycobacteria, and fungi; staining with Warthin–Starry reagents for *Bartonella* is sometimes performed but a positive result is not specific.

LYMPHANGITIS

Lymphangitis refers to inflammation of subcutaneous lymphatic channels, typically in an extremity, and can represent an acute bacterial infection or a more chronic, indolent process due to a fungal, mycobacterial, or parasitic pathogens.

Etiologic Agents

Infections that cause lymphangitis are summarized in Table 20-2. *S. pyogenes* is the leading cause of acute lymphangitis. Less commonly, *S. aureus* or other streptococci can cause lymphangitis, as can *Pasteurella* species after cat or dog bite and *Spirillum minor* after a rat bite. When inoculated cutaneously, a variety of organisms are capable of producing chronic, nodular lymphangitic infection.[35,36] They include the dimorphic fungus *Sporothrix schenckii*, *Nocardia* spp., *Mycobacterium marinum* and certain other mycobacteria, and *Leishmania* spp. In the case of *Nocardia* or NTM, the antecedent history of trauma often is elicited; a foreign body, often wood, can be present. Arthropod-borne filariasis due to *Wuchereria bancrofti* or *Brugia* spp., which is endemic in the tropics and subtropics, manifests as acute lymphangitic inflammation or chronic lymphatic obstruction with lymphedema.

Clinical Manifestations

Acute bacterial lymphangitis can accompany cellulitis or can occur in association with minor or inapparent skin infection. Lymphangitis is recognized from the rapid appearance of tender, red, linear streaks proceeding from the site of cutaneous (frequently minor) infection toward the regional lymph nodes. Tender lymphadenopathy typically is present, as are systemic symptoms such as fever, chills, and malaise. BSI is present in approximately 5%.[37] Nodular lymphangitis, also known as lymphocutaneous syndrome, has distinctive clinical features and expected pathogens.[38] Most often infection manifests on the hands and upper extremities; sporotrichosis is the prototypical lymphocutaneous infection (Figure 20-2). The disease often begins with a shallow ulcer at the site of inoculation. Subcutaneous nodules varying from 2 to 20 mm in size appear indolently as the infection advances along the course of the lymphatic channel. These nodules are either small and freely mobile or adherent to the superficial skin. Larger nodules often exhibit overlying erythema, but rarely are painful. Nodules sometimes ulcerate, releasing serosanguineous fluid. In contrast to acute bacterial lymphangitis, systemic symptoms of infection and regional adenopathy typically are absent in chronic nodular lymphangitis. Most patients do not come to medical attention until several weeks into the clinical illness. Biopsy and culture of lesions establish the diagnosis.

Differential Diagnosis

Acute lymphangitis is a clinical diagnosis made in the febrile patient with tender, linear red streaking that extends proximally from a site of peripheral infection or traumatic inoculation. Thrombophlebitis is the major differential diagnostic consideration, but this condition lacks the characteristic inciting lesion (unless it is associated with an intravascular cannula) and the tender regional lymphadenopathy associated with acute lymphangitis. The precise etiologic agent (usually *S. pyogenes*) can be identified with Gram stain and culture of a specimen from the cutaneous lesion or, not uncommonly, by culture of the blood.[37] Acute lymphangitis develops in about 20% of patients with animal bites infected with *Pasteurella canis* (dogs) or *P. multocida* (cats).[39,40] Finally, *Spirillum minor* infection should be considered in a child living in a crowded urban dwelling that is prone to rat infestation, because the superficial bite wound often completely heals during the 1- to 3-week incubation period before development of acute lymphangitis.

The origin of nodular lymphangitis usually is established through careful history of potential exposure to causative pathogens. The incubation period between inoculation and development of lymphangitic nodules can vary from 1 to 8 weeks, depending on the infecting organism.[36,38] *S. schenckii* is found in soil and botanical debris, and infection follows contact with thorned material such as rose bushes or sphagnum moss.[41] *M. marinum* is a ubiquitous

TABLE 20-2. Causes of Lymphangitis

Etiologic Agent	Exposure	Onset	Clinical Features
ACUTE BACTERIAL LYMPHANGITIS			
Streptococcus pyogenes (less commonly, *Staphylococcus aureus*)	Localized skin infection	Acute (<24–48 hours)	Red streaking, tender regional nodes, fever, chills, malaise
Pasteurella multocida	Dog or cat bite	Acute (<24–48 hours)	Red streaking, tender regional nodes, fever, chills, malaise
Spirillum minor	Rat bite	Acute, after 1–3-week incubation period	Red streaking, tender regional nodes, fever, chills, malaise, headache
NODULAR LYMPHANGITIS (LYMPHOCUTANEOUS SYNDROME)			
Sporothrix schenckii (sporotrichosis)	Soil, peat moss, thorned flowers	Insidious, 1–12-week incubation period	Inoculation site papule, proximal spread of reddish nodules, systemic symptoms rare
Mycobacterium marinum (occasionally *Mycobacterium chelonae*)	Fish, shellfish, aquarium, ponds	Insidious, 2–4-week incubation period	Nontender nodules at inoculation site and spreading proximally, systemic symptoms rare
Nocardia brasiliensis	Soil botanicals	Insidious, 2–4-week incubation period	Localized chronic granuloma with nodular spread, drainage with "sulfur granules," regional adenopathy
Leishmania brasiliensis (also *Leishmania mexicana*)	Travel to endemic area, sandfly bite	Insidious, 2–8-week incubation period	Primary ulcer with surrounding nontender nodules, no adenopathy or systemic symptoms
Wuchereria bancrofti (also *Brugia* spp.)	Travel to endemic area, mosquito bite	Acute or chronic	Acute: red streaking, adenopathy, fever rare Chronic: lymphatic obstruction, elephantiasis

PART II Clinical Syndromes and Cardinal Features of Infectious Diseases: Approach to Diagnosis and Initial Management

SECTION B Cardinal Symptom Complexes

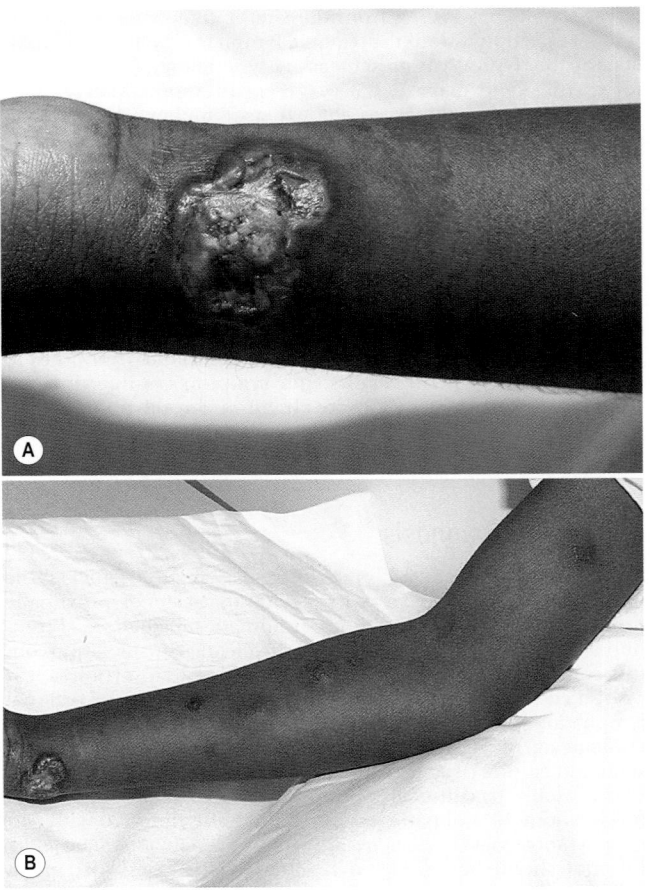

New World cutaneous leishmaniasis is a protozoal disease seen in travelers to rural Central or South America who encounter the sandfly vector. After development of a shallow ulcer at the location of the insect bite, nodular lymphatic spread with superficial scale, discharge, and crusting is not uncommon.[45]

The histopathologic changes associated with chronic nodular lymphangitis typically are granuloma formation with epithelioid and giant cells and varying degrees of neutrophilic infiltration. Diagnosis of sporotrichosis is made through identification of fungal spores surrounded by eosinophilic material ("asteroid bodies") or inoculation of a specimen from tissue drainage on Sabouraud agar. *M. marinum* often is not detected on acid-fast stain of lymphatic biopsy specimens, but culture on appropriate media incubated at 30°C is highly sensitive. *Nocardia* species appear as delicate, beaded, branching, gram-positive bacilli that can be grown on simple media but may take several days to display characteristic colonial morphology.[46] Pathognomonic sulfur granules are sometimes seen in exudate from lesions. Diagnosis of cutaneous leishmaniasis is made by direct visualization of amastigotes within histiocytes from a biopsy specimen or scraping.

Therapy

Since *S. pyogenes* is the predominant cause of acute lymphangitis, penicillin is the preferred initial treatment. Children with mild disease can be treated with oral penicillin V (50 mg/kg per day). Patients with *S. pyogenes* disease and concurrent BSI should be treated with intravenous penicillin G (100,000 to 400,000 U/kg per day), depending upon illness severity; resistance to penicillin has never been documented. Penicillin also is the drug of choice for *Pasteurella* lymphangitis and *S. minor* rat-bite fever. Those with prominent systemic symptoms and unknown or possible bacteremia should receive intravenous therapy with an antibiotic that also provides adequate coverage for *S. aureus*.

Lack of familiarity with the syndrome of nodular lymphangitis often leads to delays in correct diagnosis and inappropriate antibiotic therapy directed at pyogenic bacteria. Conservative measures, such as local application of a heating pad, may contribute significantly to resolution of lesions associated with sporotrichosis, *M. marinum* infection, or cutaneous leishmaniasis. Itraconazole (100 to 200 mg/day) is the drug of choice for lymphocutaneous sporotrichosis, supplanting saturated solution of potassium iodide (SSKI) because of lower toxicity.[41] Treatment should be continued for 4 weeks beyond resolution of lesions (2 to 3 months total). Antimicrobial agents (e.g., trimethoprim-sulfamethoxazole, minocycline, rifampin plus ethambutol) are variably effective against *M. marinum* lymphangitis, and surgical excisional debridement often is required. *Nocardia* infection generally responds readily to a sulfa drug; amoxicillin-clavulanate is an option for patients allergic to sulfa, and linezolid has been used successfully in some cases. Cutaneous leishmaniasis often heals spontaneously with topical care, but therapy with pentavalent antimony should be used if lesions evolve to the mucocutaneous form.

Figure 20-2. An adolescent girl with a 4-month history of an ulcerating skin lesion on her wrist **(A)** and nodular lymphangitis **(B)**. *Sporothrix schenckii* was isolated. Her only exposure to roses was from a florist. (Courtesy of Sarah Long, MD.)

organism in marine and freshwater environments as well as aquariums and swimming pools. A reddish blue primary lesion develops at the site of trauma (e.g., the fingers and hands in "fish-handlers' granuloma", or elbows or knees in "swimming-pool granuloma"). Ulceration with purulent drainage can occur, and the disease can spread centripetally to produce sporotrichoid-like nodular lymphangitis.[42] The rapidly growing soil and water mycobacteria *M. chelonae* can produce a similar constellation.[43]

Nocardia brasiliensis can gain access to lymphatics through minor wounds contaminated with soil and can produce nodular lymphangitis with suppurative ulceration, occasionally accompanied by regional adenopathy and systemic symptoms.[44]

---

21 Respiratory Tract Symptom Complexes

Sarah S. Long

MUCOPURULENT RHINORRHEA

Mucopurulent rhinorrhea, or purulent nasal discharge, denotes nasal discharge that is thick, opaque, and colored. It occurs at any age, usually as a manifestation of self-limited, uncomplicated viral upper respiratory tract infection (URI). Mucopurulent rhinorrhea is most problematic in children younger than 3 years because of: (1) protracted course and frequent recurrence, especially in those in out-of-home child care;[1] (2) parental concern about and misperception of etiology; and (3) overprescription of antibiotics

TABLE 21-1. Causes of Mucopurulent Rhinorrhea

Acute	Chronic or Recurrent	
	Underlying Conditions	**Obstructing Lesions**
Viral nasopharyngitis	Allergy[a]	Polyps
Bacterial sinusitis	Medications[a]	Congenital nasal anomalies (choanal
Acute otitis media	(antihypertensives, oral	atresia or stenosis,
Streptococcal nasopharyngitis	estrogens, aspirin and nonsteroidal	Tornwaldt cyst, deviated septum)
Anaerobic bacterial nasopharyngitis (nasal foreign body)	anti-inflammatory drugs) Pregnancy[a] Hypothyroidism[a]	Neuroembryonal mass (dermoid, encephalocele,
Adenoiditis	Rhinitis medicamentosa[a]	glioma, teratoma)
Syphilis	(α_1-adrenergic	Tumor (hemangioma,
Pertussis	agonists)	angiofibroma,
	Immunoglobulin	neurofibroma,
	deficiency	lipoma,
	Human immunodeficiency	craniopharyngioma)
	virus infection	Neoplasm (lymphoma,
	Cystic fibrosis	rhabdomyosarcoma,
	Ciliary dyskinesia	nasopharyngeal carcinoma)

[a]*Rhinorrhea is characteristically clear, but opaque white discharge is not unusual.*

by healthcare providers.[2-5] Occasionally, this symptom is a clue to diagnosis of a treatable bacterial infection or underlying condition.

Acute, sporadic mucopurulent rhinorrhea has an infectious cause and almost always is the manifestation of the uncomplicated "common cold" due to rhinovirus, coronavirus, or other circulating viruses.[6] When the problem is chronic or recurrent, or persistent and unilateral, broader underlying anatomic, obstructive, immunologic, and allergic disorders are considered (Table 21-1).[7-10] Onset in an infant younger than 3 months heightens suspicion of anatomic anomaly, ciliary dyskinesia, or cystic fibrosis. Accompanying sinusitis, otitis media, or pneumonia raises consideration of an immunologic deficiency (especially immunoglobulin deficiency or dysfunction, as in hypogammaglobulinemia or human immunodeficiency virus (HIV) infection), neutrophil defect, cystic fibrosis, or ciliary dyskinesia. URIs are conspicuously severe in such instances, with recrudescence almost immediately after discontinuation of antibiotic therapy. Unilateral nasal discharge and obstruction should prompt investigation for a foreign body, mass lesion, or unilateral posterior choanal atresia.

Table 21-2 shows differentiating features of important or common causes of acute mucopurulent rhinorrhea; allergic rhinitis is included because it is frequently part of the differential diagnosis in older children and adolescents.

Causes of Acute Mucopurulent Rhinorrhea

Viral Nasopharyngitis

In uncomplicated viral nasopharyngitis or rhinitis, nasal discharge is initially clear but can become white, yellow, or green (related to mucous secretions, dryness, blood, exfoliation of damaged epithelial cells and cilia, and leukocytic inflammatory response). Presence of high fever and persistence of discharge depend on the specific viral cause but are more common in uncomplicated infection than generally perceived.

In a study of hospitalized children, more than 50% of those with uncomplicated adenovirus, influenza, parainfluenza, or respiratory syncytial virus infection had temperatures >39°C, and 12% had temperatures >40°C; height of fever in these children was not different from that in children with serious bacterial infection.[11] Fever persisted for 5 days or longer in 37% of the children

in the study; 20% to 30% of those with adenovirus or influenza A infection had fever for 7 days or longer. In another study, nasal discharge or congestion associated with uncomplicated URI persisted for 6.6 days in 1- to 2-year-old children who were in home care and for 8.9 days in children younger than 1 year in out-of-home childcare centers.[1] In this study, 13% of 2- to 3-year-old children in out-of-home childcare had symptoms for more than 15 days.

The bacteriology of nasopharyngeal flora in children with uncomplicated viral respiratory illnesses, mucopurulent rhinorrhea, acute otitis media, and sinusitis has been evaluated and compared with that in normal children.[6,12-23] Viral infection is associated with acquisition of new serotypes of *Streptococcus pneumoniae* and with temporally increased risk of acute otitis media.[21] Quantitative, and some qualitative, differences in nasopharyngeal flora have been found in children with purulent nasopharyngitis (and uncomplicated viral upper respiratory illnesses), with excessive isolation rates reported for *S. pneumoniae* and *Haemophilus influenzae*,[13,18] *Peptostreptococcus* spp., *Fusobacterium* spp., and *Prevotella melaninogenica*.[18,19] The significance of such findings is unclear; isolation of such organisms may reflect exuberant proliferation in virus-induced inflammatory mucus or acquisition of a more robust specimen than is collected in healthy subjects. Furthermore, "high" rates of isolation of *S. pneumoniae* in 25% to 46% of subjects do not exceed those in healthy young children when fastidious technique is used.[22]

Only two systematically performed studies on the course of mucopurulent rhinorrhea have been published. In one study, prospective evaluation showed that there was no difference in duration of illness or complications in children with clear or purulent nasal discharge.[14] In a placebo-controlled, blinded study of 142 children 3 months to 3 years old with mucopurulent rhinorrhea of any duration, antibiotic therapy (cephalexin), systemic use of an antihistamine-decongestant, or both had no effect on the course or complications of mucopurulent rhinorrhea.[12] In a small pilot study of 13 children younger than 2 years whose purulent nasal discharge had persisted for at least 10 days without improvement, amoxicillin-clavulanate (40 mg/kg per day divided into 3 doses for 10 days) was significantly associated with resolution of symptoms in comparison with placebo.[15]

Response to antimicrobial therapy does not necessarily validate an entity of bacterial nasopharyngitis, however; it seems more likely that some children with such responses have an incomplete symptom complex of ethmoid sinusitis. Acute bacterial adenoiditis is postulated to be another cause of purulent nasal discharge when: (1) tympanic membranes are normal; (2) *S. pyogenes* is not found in culture specimens; and (3) radiographs show an enlarged adenoid shadow but no sinus abnormality.[23,24] Critical study has not been performed to validate this entity.

Bacterial Sinusitis

Mucopurulent rhinorrhea or daytime cough (which frequently is worse at night), or both of 10 or more days' duration without improvement (or recrudescence after improvement or new onset of fever) is highly suggestive of paranasal bacterial sinusitis and responsive to antibiotic therapy.[17,25,26] Sinus radiographs show significant abnormalities in nearly 90% of children 2 to 6 years old with uncomplicated upper respiratory tract illness (see Chapter 32, Sinusitis), and thus are nonspecific in this age group, supporting a clinical approach to diagnosis without imaging.

Streptococcal Nasopharyngitis

In children younger than 3 years, *S. pyogenes* has been associated with high fever, toxicity, and clear rhinorrhea or indolent infection with irregular fever and purulent nasal discharge, sometimes with associated excoriation of nares or tender anterior cervical lymphadenitis.[13,18,25] In a streptococcal outbreak studied in a childcare facility for school-aged and young children, 26% of children younger than 3 years were affected, but pharyngitis was predominant, with no case of nasal streptococcosis.[27]

PART II Clinical Syndromes and Cardinal Features of Infectious Diseases: Approach to Diagnosis and Initial Management

SECTION B Cardinal Symptom Complexes

TABLE 21-2. Differentiating Among Causes of Nasal Discharge[a]

	Viral Nasopharyngitis[1,11–15]	Acute Bacterial Sinusitis[16,17,24]	Streptococcal Nasopharyngitis[25]	Foreign Body-Related Rhinitis (Bacterial)[18]	Allergic Rhinitis[10]
HISTORY					
Peak age	Peak in first 2 years after "new recruitment" into childcare or school	Any	<3 years	<3 years	>2 years; peak in adolescence
Onset	Dryness, burning in nose or nasopharynx	Insidious, with cough day and night; occasionally, acute, febrile, toxic	Insidious; occasional acute, febrile, toxic	Insidious	Seasonal; precipitants
Associated symptoms	Nasal congestion, sneezing, malaise	Malodorous breath; head or facial pain, edema		Malodorous breath ± hyponasal voice	Sneezing; nasal or palatal pruritus; tearing; snoring
Fever	Yes/no	No/yes	Low/high	No	No
Duration of discharge	3–8 days	≥10 days	>5 days	Chronic	Chronic, recurrent
PHYSICAL EXAMINATION					
Associated findings	Red, excoriated nares; sometimes, acute otitis media	Periorbital swelling, facial tenderness; mucopurulent postnasal discharge	Anterior cervical lymphadenitis; impetiginous lesions below nose	Mouth-breathing	Transverse nasal or lower eyelid crease; periorbital hyperpigmentation; cobblestone conjunctivae or posterior pharynx
Character of discharge	Clear or colored, watery or thick	Thick, colored	Thick, colored	Unilateral, purulent, putrid bloodstained	Watery, clear, or white
Rhinoscopy	Hyperemic mucosa; dry or glazed early, edematous later; crusted discharge	Normal mucosa; discharge from middle meatus	Normal, hyperemic, or excoriated mucosa	Identifiable object (button, pit, nut), boggy mass (vegetable), or rhinolith	Pale or blue, edematous turbinates
DIAGNOSTIC TESTS	None; nasal smear shows neutrophils and mononuclear cells ± inclusion bodies, pyknotic epithelial cells	None; sinus radiograph (>6 years of age)	Nasopharyngeal culture for streptococcus only	Rhinoscopy	Nasal smear shows goblet cells and eosinophils; skin test or radioallergosorbent test (RAST)
CAUSE	Multiple agents, depending on age and seaso	*Streptococcus pneumoniae, Haemophilus influenzae, Moraxella catarrhalis*	*Streptococcus pyogenes*	Normal nasopharyngeal facultative and anaerobic bacteria	Allergens in predisposed individual
THERAPY	Saline nasal drops, humidification; amoxicillin if acute otitis media	Amoxicillin; amoxicillin-clavulanate (14:1 formulation)	Penicillin V	Removal of obstruction; amoxicillin-clavulanate if tissue or sinus complication	Avoidance; oral antihistamine/ decongestant; or topical corticosteroid; cromolyn

[a]Superscript numbers indicate references.

Other Infectious Causes

Bacterial nasopharyngitis associated with nasal foreign body is typified by the young age of the patient and putrid, commonly bloodstained, unilateral nasal discharge. Fever is unusual unless infection has spread to contiguous sinuses or distant sites. *Prevotella, Fusobacterium,* and *Peptostreptococcus* spp. as well as facultative flora are responsible. Nasal discharge can be the first manifestation of congenital syphilis and a later finding in nasal diphtheria, in which discharge is putrid and sanguineous and contains pieces of pseudomembrane.

Allergic Rhinitis

Allergic rhinitis typically begins in the second decade of life, is uncommon before age 3 years, and incidence appears to be increasing in children between these ages. Diagnosis can be suspected because of the season, environmental precipitants, personal and family history of allergy, other associated symptoms and physical findings, and the response to specific interventions of avoidance or pharmacotherapy (see Table 21-2). Nasal secretions usually are clear or whitish. Diagnostic usefulness of nasal cytologic analysis is controversial;[10,28] relative eosinophilia (above 20%) is suggestive but not diagnostic of allergic rhinitis.

Management of Acute Mucopurulent Rhinorrhea

In the vast majority of children with purulent nasal discharge (even if thick and green) of up to 1 week in duration, history and setting of illness, associated symptoms, and physical findings suggest uncomplicated viral URI. Antimicrobial therapy is inappropriate unless acute otitis media or sinusitis is diagnosed from additional findings (see Chapter 32, Sinusitis). Symptomatic therapy with saline nose drops or lavage facilitates expulsion of secretions and provides humidification. Its effectiveness reduces parental pressure to prescribe an antibiotic.[29]

If mucopurulent rhinorrhea persists for more than 5 days, and especially if some findings (e.g., anterior cervical lymphadenitis, scarlatiniform rash, excoriation around nostrils) or the epidemiology heightens the likelihood of group A streptococcal disease, nasopharyngeal specimens should be obtained for culture of *S. pyogenes* only. If culture is positive, penicillin V is given for 10 days. Routine culture for, or recovery of, *S. pneumoniae, H. influenzae, Moraxella catarrhalis,* or *Staphylococcus aureus* has no meaning and is an opportunity for misinterpretation.

If mucopurulent rhinorrhea persists for more than 10 days without diminution, and especially if other symptoms are present, paranasal sinusitis is likely. Nasal mucosa is examined after use of single or second (5 minutes after the first) application of a topical vasoconstrictor such as oxymetazoline.[15] If purulent secretions flow from the middle meatus, the diagnosis of acute sinusitis is confirmed. Signs of allergic rhinitis also can be confirmed. Radiographs may be helpful in patients older than 6 years to confirm sinusitis (or possibly to suggest adenoiditis). Many clinicians would treat children who have purulent nasal discharge of greater than 10 days' duration as for acute sinusitis, usually with amoxicillin initially. When antimicrobial therapy is effective, substantial improvement of symptoms is expected within 48 to 72 hours. Therapy is continued for 1 week beyond complete resolution of respiratory symptoms.

STRIDOR

Characteristics

Stridor is a rough, crowing sound caused by passage of air through a narrowed upper airway, which includes the extrathoracic trachea, larynx, and hypopharynx. Because the extrathoracic airway normally narrows during the inspiratory phase of respiration, stridor due to upper-airway disease occurs during inspiration (or is more pronounced during inspiration if severe narrowing causes obstruction during inspiration and expiration). Because the intrathoracic trachea normally narrows during expiration, obstruction of the intrathoracic trachea, such as that due to extrinsic compression of vascular ring or intraluminal obstruction of foreign body, inflammation, or tracheomalacia, causes a loud noise, acoustically like stridor, heard during both phases of respiration but is more pronounced on expiration. Extrathoracic obstruction (inspiratory stridor) is associated with prolonged inspiration and underaeration of the chest, whereas intrathoracic obstruction (expiratory stridor or wheezing) is associated with prolonged expiration and overinflated chest. Stridor can be associated with mild tachypnea, but a respiratory rate >50 breaths/minute should not be ascribed to upper-airway obstruction alone.

The timbre of the stridulous sound provides a clue to etiology: for example, (1) the high-pitched, fixed, dry sound of congenital subglottic stenosis; (2) the wet, rhonchal changing sound of inflammatory laryngotracheitis; and (3) the low-pitched, vibratory, positionally variable sound of laryngomalacia. Associated voice changes are useful in specifying disease as well. Vocal cord paralysis causes a weak, dysphonic cry; supraglottic obstruction, a muffled voice; and laryngotracheitis, hoarseness or aphonia, frequently with a barking cough.

Etiology

Categorization of the setting and duration of stridor as acute, persistent, or recurrent or episodic provides a framework for considering likely causes (Table 21-3).[30-34] Infectious agents cause most acute upper-airway obstruction, from intraluminal, epithelial inflammation or by encroachment on the airway by reactive or infected lymphoid tissue in parapharyngeal or paratracheal spaces. Fungal or viral tracheobronchitis must be considered when stridor occurs in an immunocompromised child; odynophagia and dysphagia also are present commonly.[31] Congenital anatomic abnormalities are considered, especially in infants whose persistent stridor began neonatally. Acquired obstruction can have abrupt onset and an obvious cause (such as foreign-body aspiration or necrotizing tracheobronchitis in ventilated neonates) or more insidious onset and inapparent cause (such as expanding laryngotracheal papillomas or hemangioma or an extrinsic compressing mass). The younger the infant, the more likely that sudden obstruction, apnea, or feeding difficulties overshadow a singular complaint of stridor.

Clinical Features of Acute Infectious Causes

Recognition, care to avoid precipitating sudden airway occlusion, and urgent, expert intervention to establish an airway when indicated are paramount to avert disastrous outcomes of acute upper-airway obstruction. Table 21-4 shows characteristic features of

TABLE 21-3. Causes of Upper-Airway Obstruction and Stridor[a]

Acute	Persistent[30]
INFECTIOUS	**CONGENITAL**
Viral laryngotracheitis (croup)	Laryngotracheal web, cleft, cyst, hemangioma
Bacterial tracheitis	Tracheal stenosis
Epiglottitis, supraglottitis	Vascular ring
Peritonsillar, retropharyngeal, or parapharyngeal abscess	Laryngotracheal malacia
Tracheobronchitis associated with immunodeficiency[31]	Neuromuscular disorder
	Cystic hygroma
NONINFECTIOUS	**ACQUIRED**
Angioedema	Posttraumatic tracheal stenosis
Foreign body	Foreign-body aspiration
Necrotizing tracheobronchitis in neonates[32,33]	Mediastinal mass (tumor, lymphatic, vascular)
Recurrent/episodic	Papilloma (perinatally acquired)
Spasmodic croup	Posttraumatic spinal cord, vagal or glossopharyngeal nerve, or vocal cord damage
Gastroesophageal reflux[34]	Bulbar neuropathy (infectious, postinfectious, malignant)

[a]*Superscript numbers indicate references.*

infectious causes of stridor and acute airway obstruction.[35-42] Viral laryngotracheitis (infectious croup) or laryngotracheobronchitis due to parainfluenza viruses is by far the most common.[35,36] Influenza viruses, respiratory syncytial virus, adenoviruses, and other viruses typically cause symptomatic disease elsewhere in the respiratory tract, but during epidemic seasons, stridor is the predominant feature in a minority of infected children. Bacterial tracheitis is usually a complication of viral laryngotracheitis (with concordant peak age and season) but can occur at any age or as a complication of oropharyngeal surgery.[43] *Staphylococcus aureus* is the most common cause, followed by *Streptococcus pyogenes*; the role of anaerobic bacteria is less clear.[41,43] With the universal use of *H. influenzae* b vaccine, epiglottitis is a rare cause of stridor; current cases of supraglottitis are more likely to affect the aryepiglottic region and to be caused by streptococci. Parapharyngeal and retropharyngeal infections in young children must also be considered; their incidence is increasing[42,44,45] (see Chapter 28, Infections Related to the Upper and Middle Airways).

The history surrounding the onset of stridor and the patient's age and demeanor are the most helpful clues to the likely site and cause of infection. The child with viral laryngotracheitis usually has had 2 to 3 days of typical upper respiratory tract illness when cough worsens and stridor begins. The child with bacterial tracheitis usually has had a similar background illness and then has sudden high fever, toxicity, and rapid progression of airway obstruction. The young child with retropharyngeal abscess or adolescent with peritonsillar abscess has less stridor but refuses to swallow, has a muffled voice, and a guarded posture to maximize the oropharyngeal airway. Trismus is an expected and useful finding in patients with peritonsillar abscess as well as in some with lateral pharyngeal space infections of odontogenic origin.[38] Epiglottitis and supraglottitis cause the patient to guard anxiously in a sitting posture with arms back, jaw forward, and chin raised ("sniffing dog") to maximize "lift" of the epiglottis away from the airway. In contrast, subglottic, tracheal obstruction cannot be lessened by position; patients with laryngotracheitis or bacterial tracheitis thrash about with the anxiety of suffocation.

The expected course[36,46,47] and sequelae of acute infectious airway obstruction are shown in Table 21-5. Children with viral laryngotracheitis are less prone to sudden complete obstruction; hourly course is predictable by degree of stridor and adequacy of aeration; response to racemic epinephrine and corticosteroid therapy usually averts intubation. Establishment of an artificial airway is urgently required for almost all patients with stridor due to acute supraglottic and bacterial tracheal infection, and for many with retropharyngeal infection. The course of disease in children

TABLE 21-4. Differentiating among Infectious Causes of Upper-Airway Obstruction[a]

	Viral Laryngotracheitis[35–37]	Supraglottitis[38,39]	Bacterial Tracheitis[40,41]	Retropharyngeal Abscess[38,40,42]
HISTORY				
Peak age	1–2 years	3–6 years, any	2–4 years, any	<3 years
Peak season	Late fall, late spring	Any	Late fall, late spring; any	Any
Prodrome	Viral illness	Uncommon	Viral illness	Uncommon
Onset of stridor	Gradual	Abrupt	Abrupt	Abrupt
PHYSICAL EXAMINATION				
Peak temperature (°C)	38–39	>39	>39	>39
Predominant findings	Brassy cough, stridor	Toxicity, stridor	Toxicity, stridor	Toxicity, stridor
Associated findings	Bark, rhinorrhea	Sore throat, odynophagia, dysphagia, anxiety, drooling	Brassy cough, anxiety	Lethargy
Voice	Hoarse, raspy	Normal, muffled, mute	Hoarse, raspy	Muffled, mute
Position	Any; thrashing	"Sniffing dog"; still	Any; thrashing	"Sniffing dog"; still
Airway occlusion	Predictable from degree of stridor	Sudden	Sudden	Sudden
Response to racemic epinephrine?	Yes, with rebound	No	No or partial	No
LABORATORY TESTS				
Peripheral neutrophils	Normal or low	High	Immature	Immature
RADIOGRAPH				
Hypopharynx	Distended	Distended	Distended	Anteriorly displaced
Airway	Subglottic narrowing; edema cords	Swollen epiglottitis, aryepiglottic folds	Subglottic narrowing; irregular trachea ± intraluminal mass	Prevertebral soft-tissue mass with anterior displacement of airway (not valid sign if expiratory film, flexed neck)
Chest	Underaerated ± cardiomegaly	Underaerated ± cardiomegaly	Patchy parenchymal peribronchial infiltrate	Underaerated ± cardiomegaly
ENDOSCOPY	Red, edematous subglottis; crusting pseudomembrane	Red, edematous supraglottic structures	Red, edematous, eroded trachea and bronchi; purulence, pseudomembrane	Bulging mass in posterior pharyngeal wall; purulence
CAUSE	Parainfluenza viruses (epidemic); other viruses (sporadic)	Streptococcus pyogenes, Streptococcus pneumoniae, Haemophilus influenzae b	Staphylococcus aureus, Streptococcus pyogenes, Streptococcus pneumoniae	Streptococcus pyogenes; Staphylococcus aureus; rare Streptococcus pneumoniae

[a]Superscript numbers indicate references.

TABLE 21-5. Expected Course and Sequelae of Acute Infectious Upper-Airway Obstruction

	Viral Laryngotracheitis	Supraglottitis, Epiglottitis	Bacterial Tracheitis	Retropharyngeal Abscess
Artificial airway (% of cases)	<20	>90	>75	≥75
Median intubation period	4 days	2 days	6 days	2 days
Airway occlusion after intubation	Rare	No	Yes	No
Death during hospitalization	No	No	Yes	No
Airway sequelae (% of cases)	<3	Rare	<3	No

with bacterial tracheitis can be further complicated, because infection (and obstructive consequences) commonly extends the length of the trachea and below.

COUGH

Characteristics

Cough is a critical protective mechanism to expel particulate matter from the larynx and trachea as well as a cardinal sign of infectious and noninfectious respiratory tract and nonrespiratory tract disorders. Occasional acute life-threatening infectious and noninfectious causes may be overlooked unless the clinician adopts a disciplined approach. Careful assessment of a pathologic cough – its onset, duration, clinical context, and association with other findings as well as its specific timbre, pattern, and productivity

– frequently predicts the site of pathophysiology and narrows the differential diagnosis to a limited number of entities. Cough usually is defined as acute (<3 weeks), subacute (3–8 weeks), or chronic (>8 weeks). A "wet" or "moist" cough in children, frequently referred to as *productive* (although young children rarely expectorate), is associated with detectable secretions by bronchoscopy and can be reported accurately by parents and clinicians.[47]

Etiology

A dry cough is expected in allergic rhinitis/sinusitis or asthma while a wet cough is typical in infectious sinusitis, bronchitis, bronchiectasis, and pneumonia. The vast majority of coughs are related to self-limited viral upper respiratory tract illness (URI) with up to 40% of school-aged children still coughing 10 days after onset of a common cold, and 10% of preschool-aged children coughing 25 days after a URI.[48] Isolated subacute cough (in absence of other symptoms), which usually is dry and follows viral infection, frequently is related to increased cough receptor sensitivity.[49] Chronic cough is pathologic. Differential diagnosis also can be focused by age, history, and clinical findings; algorithm for sequential evaluation and management is specific and sometimes complex[50] – best performed by a pediatric pulmonologist. Most common causes of chronic cough evaluated in older (mean 8–9 years) U.S.[51] and Turkish[52] children were: allergic or nonallergic rhinitis and sinusitis, asthma, protracted bacterial bronchitis, and gastroesophageal reflux disease. An important minority of children have cystic fibrosis, non-CF bronchiectasis, or ciliary dyskinesia syndrome. The focus of management is etiology. No

evidence supports the use of medications aimed at symptomatic relief of acute or chronic cough and some data suggest potential harmful effects.

Cough should not be accepted as a sign of self-limited URI in infants younger than 3 months. The mnemonic CRADLE may be useful to call to mind important considerations for such patients:[53] C, cystic fibrosis; R, respiratory tract infections (especially pneumonia and pertussis); A, aspiration (swallowing dysfunction, gastroesophageal reflux, tracheoesophageal fistula); D, dyskinesia of cilia; L, lung, vascular, or airway malformations; E, edema (heart failure, pulmonary lymphangiectasia).

Table 21-6 provides a framework for consideration of cough illnesses. Comments on certain infections follow. There is

TABLE 21-6. Differentiating among Causes of Cough

	Peak Age	Nature of Cough	Cough Dominant Feature?	Anticipated/Associated Findings
INFECTIONS OF THE RESPIRATORY TRACT				
Viral laryngotracheitis	>5 years	Brassy, painful	Yes	Hoarse, raspy voice; viral URI complex[a]
Viral laryngotracheitis/laryngotracheobronchitis	4 months–3 years	Barking, brassy	Codominant with stridor	Stridor, hoarseness, viral URI complex[a]
Mycoplasmal tracheobronchitis	Adolescent	Hacking, paroxysmal, painful	Yes	Prodromal, fever, headache, myalgia; then gradual worsening cough
Pertussis	Infancy, adolescence	Sudden paroxysm of explosive machine-gun bursts (15–30 per breath)	Yes	Bulging, watering eyes during paroxysm, posttussive emesis; skin and conjunctival hemorrhages; afebrile, without lower respiratory tract symptoms or symptoms between paroxysms
Chlamydia trachomatis pneumonia	1–3 months	Staccato, dry (single cough per breath)	Yes	History can include conjunctivitis; afebrile, tachypnea, rales
Bronchiolitis	4 months–2 years	High-pitched or grunt	No	Wheezing, rhinorrhea, respiratory distress; ± fever
Pneumonia (bacterial or viral)	Any	Wet, productive or nonproductive	Codominant with respiratory distress	Tachypnea, rales, respiratory distress; fever
Pleurodynia	Any	Inspiratory hitch; expiratory grunt	Codominant with chest pain	Chest pain; costochondral tenderness
Sinusitis	Any	Irritative; occurs in day and worsens at night	Sometimes	Mucopurulent rhinorrhea, postnasal discharge; facial pain, swelling, or tenderness; headache; ± fever
Tracheoesophagitis (fungal or viral)	Any	Irritative	No	Odynophagia or dysphagia; immune-compromised host; hoarseness; oropharyngeal lesions
Cystic fibrosis	<2 years; any	Wet, productive; paroxysmal, hacking	Sometimes	Poor growth; persistent and recurrent sinusitis, pneumonia; digital clubbing
Protracted bacterial bronchitis	Any, mean 8–9 years	Wet, productive; >8 weeks	Yes	Bronchoscopy; neutrophils, bacteria, cytokines; response to antibiotic
OTHER CONDITIONS				
Purulent pericarditis	Any	Grunt	Sometimes	Fever, toxicity, respiratory distress/dyspnea; displaced point of maximum impulse; muffled heart sounds
Myocarditis	Any	Grunt	Sometimes	Fatigue, dyspnea, tachypnea; ± fever
Congestive heart failure	Any	Grunt, wet, or brassy	Sometimes	Fatigue, dyspnea, sweating, tachycardia, tachypnea; ± fever; distended neck veins, liver
NONINFECTIOUS AIRWAY ABNORMALITIES				
Gastroesophageal reflux	6 weeks–6 months	High-pitched, dry	Codominant with other symptoms	Stridor, choking, gagging, irritability, arching (Sandifer syndrome) ± regurgitation, pneumonia
Reactive airway, asthma	6 months–adolescence	Irritative dry, repetitive (not paroxysmal); night especially	Sometimes	Atopic, precipitants, seasonal; ± wheezing; response to β-agonist
Congenital vascular rings, pulmonary sling	Infancy	Brassy	No	Stridor; onset of symptoms in first month of life
Compression on airway or glossopharyngeal or phrenic nerve	Any	Irritative, dry	Sometimes initially	Can be positional (tumors, other masses), associated with other neuropathies, stridor, changes in phonation
Habit cough	Adolescence	Vibratory, low-pitched, honking; disappears with sleep	Yes, sole feature	"La belle indifference"; family dynamics and other somatization

[a]Viral upper respiratory tract infection (URI) complex consists of fever, rhinorrhea, sore throat, conjunctivitis, exanthem, enanthem.

PART II Clinical Syndromes and Cardinal Features of Infectious Diseases: Approach to Diagnosis and Initial Management

SECTION B Cardinal Symptom Complexes

considerable overlap in symptomatology of cough caused by certain infectious agents, such as *Bordetella pertussis* or *Mycoplasma pneumoniae* in adolescents,[54] because of a common tracheobronchial site of pathophysiology and frequent dual infection by microbes.[55] *B. pertussis* causes a dramatic, debilitating paroxysmal cough without airway or lower tract abnormalities (unless secondary pneumonia occurs, leading to fever and toxicity), whereas *C. trachomatis* causes pneumonia with prominent tachypnea: the cough is only important because it brings the child to medical attention (see Chapter 162, *Bordetella pertussis* (Pertussis) and

Other *Bordetella* Species; Chapter 167, *Chlamydia trachomatis*). Diagnosis of pneumonia is based on signs of lower respiratory tract involvement, such as tachypnea and retractions, in addition to cough, and the likely causative agent is determined from the constellation of clinical findings (Tables 21-7 and 21-8).

Protracted bacterial bronchitis is inadequately studied but may be an underdiagnosed cause of chronic wet cough, or misdiagnosed as asthma.[56] Diagnosis rests on clinical bronchoscopy findings, i.e., presence of dense bacteria and neutrophilic acute inflammatory response,[57] normal imaging of the chest, and response to antimicrobial therapy. Commonly implicated organisms are *Streptococcus pneumoniae*, *Haemophilus influenzae*, and *Moraxella catarrhalis*. In attempts to avoid bronchoscopy, some pulmonologists prescribe a trial of amoxicillin-clavulanate (14:1 formulation) for 2 weeks in patients with typical isolated episode of chronic cough.

TACHYPNEA AND OTHER SIGNS OF LOWER RESPIRATORY TRACT DISORDERS

Tachypnea can be a voluntary or involuntary response to anxiety, fright, or pain; an abnormal breathing pattern related to central nervous system dysfunction; or the physiologic response to increased temperature or metabolic state. It is most usually the response to respiratory acidosis or hypoxemia of acute infection or the attempt to restore pH balance during metabolic acidosis (e.g., diabetes, salicylate poisoning, dehydration). Metabolic causes should not be forgotten, while the clinician pursues the

TABLE 21-7. Symptoms and Signs of Pneumonia

Symptoms	Signs	Physical Examinations
Fever	Fever	Rales
Cough	Cough	Wheezes
Rapid breathing	Tachypnea	Diminished breath sounds
Difficulty breathing	Dyspnea	Tubular breath sounds
Vomiting	Retractions	Dullness to percussion
Poor feeding	Nasal flaring	Decreased tactile and vocal fremitus
Irritability	Grunting	Meningismus
Lethargy	Splinting	Ileus
Chest pain	Apnea	Pleural friction rub
Abdominal pain		
Shoulder pain		

TABLE 21-8. Clinical Features of Pneumonia in Infants Younger than 3 Months

	Respiratory Syncytial Virus	Other Respiratory Viruses	Chlamydia trachomatis	Cytomegalovirus	Pertussis[a]
HISTORY					
Season	Winter	Unique to each	Any	Any	Any; peak July–October
Onset	Acute, days	Acute, days	Insidious	Insidious	Progressive, days
Illness in others	URI	URI, "flu," croup	No	No	Cough
Fever	Half of cases	Majority of cases	No	Unusual	No
Cough	Yes	Yes	Yes/staccato	Yes	Yes/paroxysmal
Associated features	Apnea, URI	URI, croup, conjunctivitis	Conjunctivitis (prior or current)	Failure to thrive, hepatosplenomegaly	Apnea, cyanosis, posttussive vomiting
PHYSICAL EXAMINATION					
Predominant feature	Respiratory distress	Respiratory distress	Cough	Failure to thrive	Cough
General appearance	Ill, not toxic	Ill, not toxic	Well, tachypneic	Chronically ill	Well between paroxysms
Degree of illness: respiratory findings	Degree of illness = findings	Degree of illness = findings	Findings > degree of illness	Ill general appearance > respiratory illness	Ill only during cough
Auscultation	Wheezes, coarse crackles	Crackles, wheezes	Diffuse crackles	Crackles, ± wheezes	Clear
LABORATORY STUDIES					
Chest radiograph	Hyperaeration, sub-segmental atelectasis	Hyperaeration, ± peribronchial thickening, ± diffuse interstitial infiltrates	Hyperaeration, diffuse alveolar and interstitial infiltrates	Diffuse interstitial infiltrates	Normal or perihilar infiltrate
White blood cell count	Normal or lymphocytosis	Normal, lymphocytosis, neutropenia	Eosinophilia	Normal, eosinophilia, lymphocytosis neutropenia	Lymphocytosis; eosinophilia unusual
Other findings	Hypoxemia		Increases in IgG, IgA, IgM	Increases in IgG, IgA, IgM; thrombocytopenia	
Diagnostic tests	Nasal wash EIA, DFA, PCR, culture	Nasal wash EIA, DFA, PCR, culture	Conjunctival, NP DFA, EIA	Throat, bronchoscopy, lung biopsy, or urine culture	NP DFA, culture, PCR

DFA, direct fluorescent antibody (test); EIA, enzyme immunoassay; Ig, immunoglobulin; NP, nasopharyngeal specimen; PCR, polymerase chain reaction; URI, upper respiratory tract infection.

[a]*Pertussis is included in this table because it should be considered in young infants with cough and respiratory distress, although pneumonia is characteristically absent.*

much more likely primary pulmonary causes. Additionally, tachypnea can result from primary cardiac abnormalities (congestive heart failure, cyanotic congenital heart disease), pulmonary vascular abnormalities (cardiac shunts, capillary dilatation, hemorrhage, obstructed return to the heart, or infarction), impaired lymphatic flow (congenital lymphangiectasia, tumor), or pleural fluid collections (hemorrhagic, purulent, transudative, or lymphatic fluid or a misplaced infusion from a vascular catheter).

Clinical practice guidelines for management of community-associated pneumonia in infants and children have been published from the Pediatric Infectious Diseases Society and the Infectious Diseases Society of America, and include excellent literature review of clinical findings.[58] Table 21-7 shows symptoms and signs of pneumonia in infants and children. Tachypnea is thought to be the best clinical predictor of lower respiratory tract infection in children. The World Health Organization defines pneumonia primarily as cough or difficult breathing and tachypnea, which definition is age-related: respiratory rate (RR) in breaths/minute >60 in infants 0–2 months of age, >50 in infants 2 to 12 months, >40 in children 1 to 5 years, and >20 in children >5 years of age.[59] Tachypnea has sensitivity of 50% to 85% for diagnosis of lower respiratory tract infection with specificity of 70% to 97%.[60,61] The younger the patient under 24 months of age, the less likely that pneumonia is present if tachypnea is absent. In one study, for infants younger than 2 months, respiratory rate of 60 breaths/minute, retractions, or nasal flaring had sensitivity for diagnosis of pneumonia of 91%.[61] Tachypnea also can be a response to fever, dehydration, or metabolic acidosis. In a study from a U.S. emergency department of children younger than 5 years of age who were undergoing chest radiography for possible pneumonia, respiratory rates in those with and without documented pneumonia did not differ significantly. However, 20% of those with WHO-defined tachypnea had pneumonia confirmed compared with 12% in those who did not.[62] Performance of a chest radiograph in febrile infants without an apparent focus of infection to exclude pneumonia "missed" by physical examination has low yield in the absence of tachypnea.[63,64] Cough is a more sensitive but nonspecific symptom of pneumonia. Other symptoms and signs associated with pneumonia, such as nasal flaring, intercostal retractions, and cyanosis, have less sensitivity (25%, 9%, and 9%, respectively) but high specificity (87%, 93%, and 94%, respectively).[60] Although fever, cough, and tachypnea are cardinal features, any or all of them can be overshadowed or overlooked in patients who come to medical attention for pneumonia-associated stiff neck, abdominal pain, or chest pain or for nonspecific symptoms of illness, such as feeding difficulty in infants. While chest radiograph is not necessary routinely in children with any of these complaints, it should be considered if the patient has fever and cough or tachypnea.[65,66] Classic symptoms of pneumonia reported in adolescents and adults are fever, chills, pleuritic chest pain, and cough productive of purulent sputum, with less noticeable tachypnea.[67]

Grunting is an expiratory sound produced in the larynx when vocal cords are adducted to generate positive end-expiratory pressure (self-induced PEEP) and increased resting volume of the lung. Its causes are myriad but never trivial. Grunting can be a sign of surfactant deficiency in the neonate, or of pulmonary edema, foreign-body aspiration, severe pneumonia, mediastinal mass or severe mediastinal shift from any cause, pleuritic or musculoskeletal chest pain, or myopericarditis or other cardiac abnormalities at any age.[68] Retractions (intercostal, subcostal, or suprasternal) and grunting have been associated with severe pneumonia; and nasal flaring and head bobbing with hypoxemia.

Adventitial respiratory sounds usually indicate lower respiratory tract disease, pulmonary edema, or hemorrhage. *Wheezes* are musical continuous sounds present predominantly on expiration and are a sign of airway obstruction. Widespread bronchiolar narrowing, as most commonly occurs with the inflammation of virus-associated lower respiratory tract infection, produces heterophonous high-pitched, sibilant wheezes of variable pitch and presence in different lung fields. Fixed obstruction in a larger airway, as from

foreign body or anomaly, produces homophonous, monotonous wheeze. The rate of radiographically confirmed pneumonia among children with wheezing is low, <5% overall, and 2% in the absence of fever.[65] *Rhonchi*, sometimes also termed low-pitched wheezes, or coarse crackles, are nonrepetitive, nonmusical, low-pitched sounds frequently present on early inspiration and expiration; they are usually a sign of turbulent airflow through secretions in large airways. *Fine crackles* (the term preferred by pulmonologists for rales, which has a variety of meanings across languages) are high-pitched, low-amplitude, end-inspiratory, discontinuous popping sounds indicative of the opening of peripheral air–fluid interfaces. Fine crackle is the auscultatory finding suggestive of the diagnosis of pneumonia. Auscultatory abnormalities of crackles and wheezing have disparate diagnostic usefulness among various studies, depending on the categorization of bronchiolitis. Tachypnea is a more sensitive finding than crackles for bacterial pneumonia; wheezing is more sensitive than tachypnea for bronchiolitis.

Diminished or distant breath sounds, dullness to percussion, and decreased vocal fremitus indicate peripheral pulmonary consolidation, pleural mass, or fluid collection. *Tubular breath sounds* (low-pitched sound of similar intensity throughout inspiration and expiration, as normally heard in the intrascapular area), dullness to percussion, and increased vocal fremitus indicate parenchymal consolidation, atelectasis, or the presence of another continuous tissue or fluid density abutting both a bronchus and the chest wall.

Radiographic infiltrates have been reported in 5% to 19% of children with fever in the absence of symptoms or signs of lower respiratory tract infection.[69,70] Rate of pneumonia deemed as occult fell from 15% to 9% after universal vaccination with 7-valent pneumococcal conjugate vaccine (PCV7) in one study.[70] Clinical features associated with occult pneumonia in another study included presence of cough, fever greater than 5 days' duration, high fever (>39°C) and leukocytosis >20,000 cells/mm³; only 5% of children without cough had radiographically confirmed pneumonia.[69]

DIFFERENTIATING FEATURES OF PNEUMONIA

Pneumonia in Young Infants

In young infants, acute infection with bacterial and nonbacterial respiratory tract pathogens frequently leads to lower respiratory tract infection. Except in the first few days of life, when pneumonia is due predominantly to bacteria acquired from the mother's genital tract or to organisms acquired transplacentally, nonbacterial pathogens are overwhelmingly predominant.[68] As perinatally acquired agents persist, community exposures increase, and maternally derived antibody protection wanes, the infant between 3 weeks and 3 months old is vulnerable to a unique array of lower respiratory tract pathogens.[71] Clinical setting, specific symptom complex, and severity of illness in proportion to findings on physical examination aid distinction of likely causes and guide the diagnostic and therapeutic approach (see Table 21-8). Although the pathogens listed in Table 21-8 frequently are referred to as causing "afebrile pneumonia," this is a misnomer, because *Bordetella pertussis* infrequently causes lower respiratory tract abnormalities, and respiratory syncytial virus and especially other respiratory viruses frequently cause fever.[11,68,72,73] A causal role for *Ureaplasma urealyticum* is not completely defined, because the situation is confounded by the asymptomatic presence of this organism in women and young infants. Pneumonia due to *Pneumocystis jirovecii* probably is confined to infants with severe debilitation or immune defects.

Pneumonia in Older Infants, Children, and Adolescents

Table 21-9 categorizes the features of acute pneumonia in older infants, children, and adolescents by etiology. No single fact

TABLE 21-9. Clinical Features of Acute Pneumonia in Children and Adolescents

	Bacteria	Virus	Mycoplasma	Tuberculosis
HISTORY				
Age	Any; infants especially	Any	School age	Any; <4 years and 15–19 years especially
Temperature (°C)	Most ≥39	Most <39	Most <39	Most <39 (unless empyema)
Onset	Abrupt	Gradual	Worsening cough	Insidious cough
Others in home ill	No	Yes, concurrent; upper respiratory tract infection, rash, conjunctivitis	Yes, weeks apart; pharyngitis, "flu," cough	Yes, persistent cough
Associated signs, symptoms	Toxicity, rigors	Myalgia, rash, mucous membrane involvement	Headache, sore throat, chills, myalgia, rash, pharyngitis, myringitis	Weight loss, night sweats (late)
Cough	Wet, productive	Nonproductive	Hacking, paroxysmal, usually nonproductive	Irritative or productive
PHYSICAL EXAMINATION				
Predominant feature	Toxicity, respiratory distress	Respiratory distress	Cough	Persistent cough
Degree of illness: respiratory finding	Degree of illness > findings	Degree of illness ≥ findings	Degree of illness < findings	Well → no findings (± cough); ill → findings
Pleuritic chest pain	No/yes	No	No	No/occasional
Auscultation	Unilateral, anatomically confined or no crackles; dullness, diminished or tubular sounds	Diffuse, bilateral crackles, wheezes	Unilateral, anatomically confined crackles; ± wheezes	Most normal; or unilateral crackles ± dullness
LABORATORY STUDIES				
Chest radiograph	Hyperaeration, patchy alveolar infiltrate or consolidation in lobe, segment, subsegment	Hyperaeration, interstitial infiltrate in diffuse or perihilar distribution; "wandering" atelectasis	Patchy alveolar and/or interstitial infiltrate in single or contiguous, usually lower lobe(s), unilaterally; perihilar adenopathy	Patchy alveolar infiltrate in single or contiguous lobes with disproportionate hilar adenopathy; or miliary or lobar consolidation
Pleural fluid	No/yes → large	No/yes → small	No/yes → small	No/yes → small, large
Peripheral white blood cell count (cells per mm³)	Majority >15,000; neutrophils ± bands	Majority <15,000; lymphocytes	Majority <15,000; neutrophils	Majority <15,000; neutrophils, monocytes
Sedimentation rate >40 mm/hour	Usual	Infrequent	Infrequent	Frequent
Sputum	Copious, purulent; neutrophils, abundant bacteria	Scant mucoid; epithelial, mononuclear cells	Scant mucoid; mixed mononuclear cells/neutrophils	Scant → copious; neutrophils (if copious)
Diagnostic tests	Sputum Gram stain, culture; blood culture	Nasal wash, throat, bronchoscopy specimen for antigen detection, culture; acute and convalescent serology	Cold agglutinin; acute and convalescent specific serology; throat culture, antigen detection, DNA techniques	Gastric aspirate; sputum stain and culture

in history or finding on examination is unique for any agent, but when they are taken together, a working diagnosis emerges and guides intervention or further diagnostic testing. Chest radiography and laboratory tests usually are reserved for patients who are ill and hospitalized or whose clinical picture is not compelling for a category of etiologic agents. A number of studies using complex diagnostic methodologies have confirmed the specific cause of pneumonia in 45% to 85% of cases.[72–76] Viral etiologies predominate, and, currently, most are amenable to diagnosis.[72] The efficacy trial and postmarketing studies of PCV7 infers *Streptococcus pneumoniae* as a relatively common cause of pneumonia with patchy or consolidative infiltrates.[77,78] Urine antigen detection test in children with lobar pneumonia also supports the important role of *S. pneumoniae*;[79] however, the test is positive in >15% of children with asymptomatic colonization.[80] Testing for *Mycoplasma pneumoniae* using IgM enzyme immunoassay serologic test is problematic because of false-positive tests, and may be best utilized in school-aged children and adolescents with findings consistent with mycoplasma infection in those whose pretest

probability is moderate or higher.[58,81] Currently, ascribing a causal role of pneumonia to *Chlamydophila pneumoniae* is confounded by the findings of prolonged asymptomatic carriage and inconsistent serologic results among studies.[82]

HEMOPTYSIS

Hemoptysis, defined as coughing up of blood that originated below the larynx, is uncommon in children; most commonly, supposed episodes are due to a posteriorly draining nosebleed. Mechanisms of hemoptysis include bleeding from: (1) congenital or acquired abnormal bronchial or pulmonary blood flow, venous obstruction, or vascular abnormalities; (2) immune-mediated endothelial damage; or (3) infectious or traumatic erosion of tracheal, bronchial, or bronchiolar epithelium. Hemorrhage can be mild (tracheitis, tracheobronchitis) or massive (congenital malformations, foreign body, bronchiectasis, pulmonary hemosiderosis). Causes of hemoptysis in children are listed in Table 21-10. Infection is

TABLE 21-10. Causes of Hemoptysis in Children

Epithelial Damage	Vascular Abnormality/Damage
Acute infection (bacterial and fungal)	Congenital heart disease or pulmonary vascular anomalies (venous obstruction, arteriovenous fistulae)
Bronchiectasis (cystic fibrosis, non-CF, immunodeficiency, retained foreign body)	Congenital malformation (pulmonary sequestration)
Trauma (airway or chest)	Autoimmune vasculitis (systemic lupus erythematosus, sarcoidosis, Wegener granulomatosis, inflammatory bowel disease, Goodpasture syndrome)
Foreign body	Sickle-cell disease
Tumor (primary airway or pulmonary, metastatic)	Pulmonary hemosiderosis
	Nonspecific endothelial damage (chemical, drug)

the most common cause of mild hemoptysis. Panton–Valentine leukocidin-producing *Staphylococcus aureus* pneumonia is specifically associated with hemoptysis.[83] Epstein–Barr virus was implicated in a single case.[84] For more severe hemoptysis, bronchiectasis associated with cystic fibrosis accounts for as many cases as all other causes combined.[85]

Rigid bronchoscopy, computed tomography, and magnetic resonance imaging are useful diagnostic modalities in most cases of hemoptysis. Digital subtraction angiography and, occasionally, cardiac catheterization or arteriography are required.

22 Abdominal Symptom Complexes

Matthew B. McDonald, III and Robert S. McGregor

To simplify the clinical approach to abdominal symptom complexes, abdominal pain is usually classified as acute or chronic/recurrent abdominal pain. Acute abdominal pain demands rapid diagnosis and appropriate intervention so that catastrophic outcomes can be avoided.

ACUTE ABDOMINAL PAIN

Signs and symptoms of medical and surgical conditions that cause acute abdominal pain have considerable overlap. Even though Scholer and associates[1] determined that only 1.5% of 1141 non-scheduled healthcare visits for acute abdominal pain resulted in a surgical diagnosis, rapid diagnosis and intervention should always be a primary goal to avoid an adverse outcome. Cope,[2] in a classic monograph, pointed out that the first principle in approaching the patient with acute abdominal pain is the necessity of coming to a "best," albeit not "certain," diagnosis because severe abdominal pain of 6 hours' duration occurring in a previously well child frequently is caused by a condition of surgical importance.

History

The history and character of the patient's acute abdominal pain are elicited with specific consideration of anatomy, embryology, and physiology. Diaphragmatic irritation, for example, causes shoulder pain, because the diaphragm, a high thoracic structure embryologically, shares cervical nerve innervation with the shoulder. History of therapies already provided is elicited, and potential effects integrated. Anti-inflammatory agents, especially corticosteroids, can alter expected clinical findings substantially, and potent analgesics or pretreatment with antimicrobial agents can mask otherwise clarifying symptoms. Regimentation in history-taking is essential. The three features of pain of particular importance are location, migration, and radiation sites.

Location of Pain

Pain over the entire abdomen suggests a diffuse peritoneal process. Pain relative to disease in the small intestine is chiefly felt in the epigastric and umbilical areas, and because innervation of the appendix is similarly derived embryologically, the initial pain of acute appendicitis is located periumbilically. Pain relative to

disease in the large intestine usually is felt in the hypogastrium or over the site of colonic abnormality. Pain of pelvic structures also is appreciated in the hypogastrium.

Migration of Pain and Radiation Sites

Migration of pain and sites of radiation are useful clues.[3] The early epigastric pain of appendiceal obstruction is carried by visceral pain fibers. Once the inflamed appendix irritates or adheres to the abdominal wall, somatic pain fibers in the parietal peritoneum cause migration of pain to the right lower quadrant. Similarly, biliary colic begins with epigastric pain but moves to the right upper quadrant when the inflamed gallbladder contacts parietal peritoneum. Because the eighth thoracic nerve innervates both the bile ducts and the infrascapular area of the posterior thorax, pain of biliary colic is often perceived just inferior to the right scapula. Renal and ureteral colic radiates to the ipsilateral testicle. Vertebral pain, as in osteomyelitis, radiates to the corresponding site of abdominal innervation.

Associated Symptoms

The presence, timing, and nature of associated symptoms, especially vomiting, provide important clues to diagnosis. Pancreatitis can cause severe, repeated vomiting, because the inflamed pancreas directly irritates the celiac nerve plexus. Bowel obstruction causes vomiting; the more proximal the obstruction, the more severe the vomiting. High small-bowel obstruction causes intractable bilious emesis early in the course, whereas distal small-bowel obstruction allows delayed onset of emesis with longer periods between episodes (which can progress to feculent emesis). Large-bowel obstruction is associated with late-onset emesis or no emesis. Nausea and loss of appetite can replace vomiting as a symptom in patients with less sensitive triggering of emesis. In children with acute abdominal pain, sudden loss of appetite heightens concern, whereas preserved hunger lessens concern.

Character and Relative Severity of Symptoms

The younger the patient, the less helpful the character of the pain. A sense of wellbeing between waves of pain is helpful, however. The child with crampy pain from gastroenteritis is playful and

PART II Clinical Syndromes and Cardinal Features of Infectious Diseases: Approach to Diagnosis and Initial Management

SECTION B Cardinal Symptom Complexes

active intermittently, whereas children with appendicitis, obstruction, or intussusception do not experience complete relief. Factors that either exacerbate or alleviate pain can be useful clues. The relative importance of symptoms is also helpful. Nausea, vomiting, and diarrhea are cardinal features of gastroenteritis, and abdominal pain is secondary. Abdominal pain is the initial and unremitting feature of acute appendicitis or peritonitis, with other symptoms being variable and less significant.

Physical Examination

The physical examination must not be supplanted by imaging studies or laboratory tests.

Vital Signs and Habitus

Vital signs often are normal until the pathologic condition causing abdominal pain is advanced; however, an elevated respiratory rate (out of proportion to temperature) is a clue to thoracic causes of pain referred to the abdomen. Abdominal processes that cause splinting of the diaphragm lead to shallow tachypnea and the appearance of a respiratory tract condition. Acidosis related to compromised bowel or infection causes increases in both respiratory rate and tidal volume (Kussmaul breathing). Fever is not a discriminating feature, although high temperatures (39.5°C or higher) at the onset of abdominal pain in the absence of vomiting and diarrhea suggest a renal or pulmonary process or primary peritonitis. When the abdominal pain and high temperature are associated with vomiting, diarrhea, or both, primary infectious gastrointestinal disease (e.g., salmonellosis, shigellosis) is a primary consideration.

The patient's preferred position and degree of movement provide diagnostic information. The child with intussusception lies anxiously, anticipating a paroxysm of pain that causes the child to writhe. The patient with pain due to Henoch–Schönlein purpura (HSP) tosses and turns, trying to find comfort, whereas the child with appendicitis flexes at the waist, and the child with peritonitis lies motionless.

Examination of Abdomen

Careful observation may reveal abdominal distention, swelling, or masses. Limited diaphragmatic movement implicates an upper abdominal process, including pancreatic or hepatobiliary disease. While distracting the child, the physician should palpate the abdomen with warmed hands and a light touch, beginning at the site most distant from the reported location of pain. Palpation can reveal a mass (intussusception, tubal pregnancy, ovarian cyst, malignancy, hydronephrosis) or a site of tenderness, or can confirm abdominal rigidity (sign of parietal peritoneal inflammation). Persistent palpation, as an attempt to overcome localized or generalized abdominal rigidity, elicits greater pain and rigidity unless disease is in the thorax. A rectal examination is necessary and may identify heme-positive stool or mucus, a mass, fullness, or localization of tenderness. It also can raise consideration of gynecologic disease.

Percussion of the abdomen is generally not helpful in differentiating among abdominal processes; however, dullness suggests the presence of peritoneal fluid or helps delineate edges of the liver or spleen. Auscultation distinguishes ileus but rarely adds diagnostic specificity.

Other Findings

Physical findings of importance outside the abdomen include: (1) evidence of respiratory distress (nasal flaring, retractions, and adventitial auscultatory findings); (2) rashes (HSP, gonococcemia); (3) vaginal discharge; (4) pelvic girdle tenderness; and (5) hip pain on testing range of motion. The patient with abdominal pain who holds one hip flexed and externally rotated is likely to have acute appendicitis or primary inflammation of the iliopsoas muscle.

Specific Causes and Approach

Conditions in which acute abdominal pain is the cardinal feature are discussed here, with focus on early clinical approach and intervention. Abdominal pain as part of fever of unknown origin and malignancy is discussed in Chapter 14, Fever without Localizing Signs. Specific diagnostic studies are discussed elsewhere.

Appendicitis

Acute appendicitis in its classic, most common form can be diagnosed readily before appendiceal rupture. Wagner et al.[4] described the characteristic sequence of symptoms (rather than the presence of any particular symptom) in acute appendicitis and recognized that the sequence reflects pathophysiologic events. Interruption of this order should increase suspicion of an alternative diagnosis. The expected sequential events or findings in appendicitis are shown in Box 22-1. Atypical localization of tenderness and pain can occur, depending on the position of the appendix. If the organ lies retrocecally and cephalad, the serosa abuts the iliopsoas muscle, causing pain that results in a preferred position of flexion at the waist with flexion and external rotation of the right hip. If the appendiceal tip is directed inferiorly, then pelvic, left lower quadrant, or urinary symptoms can predominate. Occasionally, pelvic appendicitis can inflame rectal tissue and cause painful defecation, spasms of diarrhea, or rectal obstruction. Presence of a mass or tenderness on palpation of the right or anterior rectal wall during rectal examination can clarify the diagnosis. Left-sided appendicitis, sometimes associated with thoracic situs inversus, can cause all of the presentations seen in right-sided appendicitis, but in mirror image.

Appendicitis generally evolves from first symptoms to rupture in less than 24 hours.[5] The diagnosis remains a clinical one, although ultrasonography may add specificity and computed tomography both sensitivity and specificity.[6] Clinical scoring systems can be helpful in identifying children at low risk for appendicitis and potentially avoid radiation exposure.[7] Except in cases of altered anatomy, diagnosis and appendectomy are expected to be achieved before rupture. Infants and toddlers present a diagnostic challenge; preoperative ruptures occur in >50% of cases in such patients because of their inability to communicate classic signs or symptoms and because of lack of distinction from acute gastroenteritis, which is frequent in this age group.[8]

Mesenteric Adenitis

A diagnosis often made by surgeons during an otherwise normal laparotomy performed for suspected appendicitis, mesenteric adenitis has been illuminated with the use of improved imaging

---

BOX 22-1. Expected Sequence of Events or Findings in Appendicitis

1. **Pain, usually epigastric or umbilical:** Appendiceal obstruction and distention stimulate visceral afferent nerves of T8 to T10, referring pain to the epigastrium and periumbilical area
2. **Anorexia, nausea, and vomiting:** Further obstruction and distention of the appendix lead to colicky pain and reverse peristalsis
3. **Abdominal tenderness:** Serosal inflammation follows, with irritation of the parietal peritoneum. Pain shifts to somatic fibers, resulting in the localization of tenderness to deep palpation and, later, localization of pain, to the right lower quadrant
4. **Fever:** Arterial supply of the appendix is compromised, leading to gangrene and rupture. Fever precedes rupture and frank peritonitis and is usually mild (39°C or less)
5. **Leukocytosis:** Development of localized peritonitis triggers neutrophilia (a relatively late event)

techniques. Often >1 cm, inflamed nodes typically cluster in the mesentery in groups of 5 to 8. The mesentery itself also can be inflamed and thickened. Mesenteric adenitis manifests clinically as symptoms of severe localized abdominal pain that mimics pain of other regional pathologic processes. Mesenteric adenitis has been associated with positive culture of sampled lymph node for *Yersinia* spp. and has preceded classic Epstein–Barr virus mononucleosis. Unfortunately, the diagnoses of mesenteric adenitis and of acute abdominal processes are not mutually exclusive, often making the diagnosis of mesenteric adenitis one of exclusion despite visualization of nodes on ultrasonography or computed tomography.[8,9] Improper order of symptoms for acute appendicitis, milder pain, disproportionately high fever, and preserved appetite may permit judicious avoidance of surgery. Mesenteric adenitis occurs with appendicitis in up to 49% of cases, and can occur in association with inflammatory bowel disease, acute pancreatitis, *Bartonella* infection, and multiple enteric and systemic viral infections.[10]

Pneumonia

When abdominal pain is associated with high fever, cough, nasal flaring, tachypnea, respiratory distress, and abnormal auscultatory findings, the diagnosis of pneumonia is obvious. More subtle manifestations make differentiation more challenging, but careful attention to severity of fever and initial signs (especially respiratory rate, retractions, and nasal flaring), and meticulous auscultation over all lung fields permits differentiation. The theory of referred abdominal pain secondary to diaphragmatic irritation has been refuted by the reports of isolated upper and middle lobe pneumonia causing similar pain syndromes.[11] Typical bacterial causes of community-acquired pneumonia are expected.

Pyelonephritis

Specificity of symptoms of urinary tract infection (UTI) is age-related. In the neonate and infant, the disease can cause decreased appetite alone or intermittent fussiness. Previous UTI, temperature higher than 40°C and suprapubic tenderness are positive predictors of UTI in infants.[12] The toddler often has nonspecific abdominal pain (presence of dysuria being variable). The older child and adolescent are most likely to have dysuria, flank pain, tenderness at the costo-vertebral angle, and hypogastric pain. Pyuria is not uncommon during acute appendicitis. Pelvic appendicitis, or pelvic abscess from any source, can cause dysuria and pyuria, mimicking UTI.

Pancreatitis

The incidence of acute pancreatitis in children is rising.[13] Identifiable causes of pancreatitis remain variable. Systemic illness, biliary disease, trauma, and medications commonly are identified while many cases are idiopathic.[14] Pancreatitis also occurs in association with endocrinopathies, with multiple organ failure, and with metabolic disorders. Alcohol consumption is rarely implicated in pediatric cases.

Anatomic relationships predict the symptomatology of acute pancreatitis. The gland lies close to the celiac plexus and semilunar ganglion; consequently, pancreatic inflammation causes nausea, intractable vomiting (never feculent), and severe epigastric pain. The head of the pancreas is surrounded by duodenum, whereas the body overlies the lumbar vertebrae, and the tail reaches the left flank; inflammation occasionally causes pain only in the left hypochondrium or flank. Because of the organ's proximity to the diaphragm, pain can occasionally be referred simultaneously to the left scapula and the left supraspinous fossa (phrenic pain).

Fever commonly is present, typically 38.5°C to 39.2°C; its presence does not presuppose bacterial superinfection. Epigastric tenderness is expected, but muscular rigidity is variable. Jaundice is common and usually is due to swelling of the head of the pancreas rather than to obstructing gallstones.

Hemorrhagic pancreatitis, a life-threatening form of pancreatitis, can have either of two pathognomonic signs, bluish discoloration in the flank (Grey Turner sign) or around the navel (Cullen sign). Carbohydrate intolerance can occur as pancreatic islet cells are destroyed.

Acute pancreatitis is a clinical diagnosis supported by elevated serum levels of pancreatic amylase and lipase and abnormal findings on ultrasonography or computed tomography. Edema and para-pancreatic fluid collections are typical and should not be over-interpreted as abscess. Serum amylase concentration alone is neither sensitive nor specific. Combining the use of amylase and lipase tests increases sensitivity and specificity.[15]

Gallbladder Disease

Acute cholecystitis and infection of the gallbladder are rarely seen in children, except when predisposing conditions exist (e.g., porto-enterostomy for biliary atresia, obstructing anomalies). Cholelithiasis, the usual antecedent of cholecystitis in adults, typically occurs without cholecystitis in children. In two pediatric series consisting of 85 patients with gallstones, only 2 patients developed cholecystitis.[16,17] Children with cholelithiasis typically have an identifiable precipitating cause, such as hemolysis, total parenteral nutrition, or adolescent pregnancy. The usual sequence of symptoms is: (1) fever; (2) colicky epigastric abdominal pain that shifts to the right upper quadrant; and (3) tenderness over the right upper quadrant. An elevated serum concentration of γ-glutamyltranspeptidase and bilirubin (out of proportion to elevation of aminotransferase) is expected. Enterococci, *Escherichia coli*, and other Enterobacteriaceae and oropharyngeal flora occasionally are isolated from blood, hepatic biopsy, or as ascitic fluid specimen.

Biliary dyskinesia is increasingly described in the pediatric literature. In one series of consecutive pediatric patients with cholecystectomies, biliary dyskinesia was implicated in 16% of the patients.[18] Biliary dyskinesia symptoms mimic those of cholelithiasis, with right upper quadrant pain and fatty food intolerance. The diagnosis is considered when ultrasonography fails to identify gallstones despite a high clinical suspicion of gallbladder disease. Ultrasonography may demonstrate gallbladder wall-thickening or sludge. The diagnosis is confirmed with hepatobiliary nuclear imaging scans using cholecystokinin stimulation.[19] The spectrum of disorders of functional motility can blur the separation of acute and recurrent abdominal pain.

Pelvic Inflammatory Disease

Adolescent women are at higher risk of pelvic inflammatory disease (PID) than adult women. Higher infection rates with *Chlamydia trachomatis* and *Neisseria gonorrhoeae* in general, combined with biologic factors such as immaturity of the menstrual cycle, lack of antibodies to sexually transmitted infectious agents, and extent of cervical ectropion, contribute to the explanation.[20]

Some women with PID are asymptomatic, and others have only mild or nonspecific symptoms or signs (abnormal bleeding, dyspareunia, or vaginal discharge). Because of this wide variability, PID must be considered with even mild lower abdominal pain in a sexually active adolescent. Because of the difficulty of confirming PID and the possible consequence of long-term decreased fertility if the diagnosis is missed, a low threshold for diagnosis and treatment of PID is recommended. Diagnostic criteria are listed in Box 22-2.[21]

Classic physical findings are fever, lower abdominal pain, pelvic tenderness, or both, and vaginal discharge. The constellation of abnormal vaginal discharge, a tender mass on bimanual examination, and elevated erythrocyte sedimentation rate predicts laparoscopically proven PID; however, only 20% of patients with PID have the triad.

Henoch–Schönlein Purpura (HSP)

In its most common presentation, the following four features distinguish HSP: (1) purpura due to leukocytoclastic vasculitis, classically palpable and present below the waist (in young

PART II Clinical Syndromes and Cardinal Features of Infectious Diseases: Approach to Diagnosis and Initial Management

SECTION B Cardinal Symptom Complexes

BOX 22-2. Criteria for Clinical Diagnosis of Pelvic Inflammatory Disease

Minimum Criteria (if no other cause of illness is identified) Include <u>One</u> of the Following

Uterine/adnexal tenderness
or
Tenderness on motion of the cervix

Additional Supportive Criteria (enhancing specificity of minimum criteria)

Oral temperature >38.3°C
Abnormal cervical or vaginal mucopurulent discharge
Abundant number of white blood cells (WBCs) on saline
  microscopy of vaginal secretions
Elevated erythrocyte sedimentation rate or C-reactive protein
Laboratory documentation of chlamydial or gonococcal
  infection

Specific Criteria

Endometrial biopsy showing endometritis
Transvaginal sonography or MRI demonstrating thickened,
  fluid-filled fallopian tubes with or without free pelvic fluid or
  tubo-ovarian complex, or Doppler study suggesting pelvic
  inflammation (e.g. tubal hyperemia)
Laparoscopic abnormalities characteristic of pelvic
  inflammatory disease

From Centers for Disease Control and Prevention. Sexually transmitted diseases treatment guidelines 2010, MMWR 2010;59(RR-12):63–67.

---

children, especially nonambulatory children, the distribution can be atypical – often involving face and scalp); (2) glomerulonephritis, with a spectrum from microscopic hematuria, with or without proteinuria, to renal failure with severe hypertension; (3) arthritis affecting larger joints and with pain out of proportion to synovial fluid accumulation; and (4) abdominal pain, caused by the leukocytoclastic vasculitis. The abdominal pain in HSP usually is midline and is colicky; intestinal mucosal purpura causes gastrointestinal bleeding or can initiate intussusception.

Abdominal pain can precede purpura by days (rarely weeks) in 14% to 36% of patients.[22] Because many patients with HSP have fever and abdominal pain (which can be severe) at onset, intra-abdominal infections and appendicitis often are considered before the typical purpuric rash appears.

Enteric and Other Infections

Enteric infections rarely cause abdominal pain and fever as cardinal features. In the relative absence of gastrointestinal symptoms, *Salmonella, Shigella, Escherichia coli* O157:H7, and *Clostridium difficile* infections can cause severe pain due to intestinal spasm before diarrhea; dysenteric stool with mucus and blood clarifies the pathophysiology. *Campylobacter jejuni* infection can mimic inflammatory bowel disease with myalgia and arthralgia in association with bloody stools. Infections due to *Yersinia enterocolitica* and *Y. pseudotuberculosis* most closely mimic acute appendicitis when they cause mesenteric adenitis. Appendicitis has rarely been associated with shigellosis.[23] Typhoid fever, visceral abscesses,[24] intestinal granuloma in chronic granulomatous disease, yersiniosis, visceral *Bartonella henselae* infection, cryptococcal infection, *Toxocara* infection, and brucellosis each can manifest as fever with a predominant complaint of abdominal pain. Acute hepatitis can cause abdominal pain, but disproportionate nausea, right upper quadrant tenderness, and hepatomegaly provide clues to the correct diagnosis. Epstein–Barr virus infection can cause predominant abdominal symptomatology with severe splenic enlargement. *Enterobius vermicularis* is occasionally found in the appendix of a patient with acute symptomatology.

Streptococcus pyogenes causing acute pharyngitis also can cause abdominal symptoms ranging from pain to nausea and vomiting, thought to be related to extracellular enzymes produced by the organism. One prospective study failed to identify abdominal pain as a positive predictor of *S. pyogenes* infection as a singular symptom or combined with other predictive factors.[25] *S. pyogenes* can cause retroperitoneal abscess, necrotizing fasciitis, and tubo-ovarian abscess, all of which manifest as severe abdominal pain.

Intussusception

Intussusception in childhood is most often idiopathic, with peak incidence in the United States at 5 to 9 months of age. Typically, infants have no demonstrable intestinal lead point. Hypertrophy of Peyer patches or mesenteric lymphadenopathy may initiate intussusception. Adenovirus has been recovered in stool or mesenteric node cultures in idiopathic cases.[26] Historically, the rotavirus vaccine of the late 1990s was implicated rarely as causal.[27] Older children are more likely to have a pathologic lead point, identified in 8% of cases,[28] the most common identifiable cause being a Meckel diverticulum.[29]

Regardless of cause, the clinical manifestations of intussusception are similar. Midline abdominal pain occurs in paroxysms as each peristaltic wave advances the intussusception. An apathetic presentation is seen in approximately 5% of patients; children appear "drugged" and inattentive rather than writhing in pain. Primary intracranial disease or intoxication can be incorrectly pursued before a palpable abdominal mass or "currant jelly stool" focuses attention on the intestinal tract. It has been speculated that this peculiar presentation may be due to high levels of endogenous opiates released in response to the painful process of intussusception.

Volvulus

Volvulus, generally occurring in infants with congenital malrotation, is a life-threatening event. Abdominal pain is unusual without associated emesis, which becomes bilious in the acute presentation. Because vascular compromise is present, infection is a common secondary event. Treatment for septicemia is indicated but should never be considered as sole treatment in the ill infant with bilious emesis.

Occasionally, postprandial pain can be a prominent feature of the subacute or chronic presentation of volvulus. Volvulus occasionally can occur in infants with apparently normal intestinal anatomy and in older children. Volvulus and internal hernia with strangulation also should be considered in children with a history of prior abdominal surgery, because adhesions can predispose to these entities.

CHRONIC OR RECURRENT ABDOMINAL PAIN

Unlike acute abdominal pain, chronic (CAP) or recurrent abdominal pain (RAP) requires an inclusive, thorough consideration of the medical, psychosocial, and family history. Both CAP and RAP are a subset of functional gastrointestinal disorders. The term functional abdominal pain (FAP) is preferred in recent literature. The approach to patients with CAP, RAP, or FAP can involve days to weeks of data collection with only selective use of laboratory tests. Constipation, a common cause of recurrent abdominal pain, is not discussed here.

RAP, as defined by Apley,[30] required the occurrence of 3 episodes of pain severe enough to affect activities, over a period of 3 months and occurring during the year before investigation. Peak incidence of RAP is in 9- and 10-year-old girls. The pain is characterized as paroxysmal, periumbilical, and lasting less than 60 seconds. Its character often is vague but has been described as dull, crampy, or sharp but not temporally related to activity, meals, stress, or bowel habits. Prevalence of RAP in 1000 unselected schoolchildren has been reported to be as high as 25% in girls. Family histories of children with RAP showed a higher incidence of migraine, psychiatric disorders, and peptic ulcer disease than those of controls.[31] In uncontrolled observations from a wide range of practice settings, socioeconomic status correlated directly with the prevalence of RAP.

In 2006, consensus guidelines for the diagnosis of FAP were published from the Rome III group meeting. These guidelines essentially shorten the duration of symptoms establishing chronicity at 2 months. Symptoms may be episodic or continuous, lack evidence of inflammatory, anatomic, metabolic or oncologic process to explain symptoms, and lack criteria for a more specific functional diagnosis.[32]

Differentiating Causes

FAP disorders are considered more broadly in the bio-psychosocial model. While respecting the complex interplay of genetic, psychological variables (stress, role modeling, intrinsic, and extrinsic supports), and physiologic variables (inflammatory mediators, motility, hyperresponsiveness of environmental stimuli), the clinician must still have a pragmatic approach to the individual patient and family. Diagnostic studies of choice are a thorough history, physical examination (both between and during episodes of pain), and simple laboratory tests. Extensive use of laboratory testing usually fails to make a diagnosis and heightens the family's fear and pursuit of missed disease. Distinguishing features of RAP of nonorganic origin are characteristic enough that the clinical diagnosis is not simply a diagnosis of exclusion (Table 22-1). For children who meet Apley criteria for RAP, an organic disease, which if treated, eliminates the symptoms, is identified in fewer than 10%.[33] In the largest follow-up study, tracking 161 patients over 5 years, only 3 of 161 patients were found eventually to have organic disease, which was Crohn disease in all 3.[34]

TABLE 22-1. Features of Nonorganic Versus Organic Causes of Abdominal Pain

Findings	Nonorganic Causes	Organic Causes
Pain		
Location	Periumbilical	Peripheral
Character	Dull, crampy	Colicky, penetrating, burning, boring
Pattern	Not progressive	Progressive
	Follows precipitating event in one-third of cases, normal between events, better on weekends	Associated with meals, or fluid bolus
		Nocturnal symptoms, daily, persistent
Associated signs	Normal abdominal examination, little objective findings	Retching, writhing
		Distended abdomen, abdominal tenderness
		Mouth ulcers, digital clubbing
Associated symptoms	Multiple, vague, often unrelated	Focused, one or two related symptoms, including fever, weight loss, poor growth, arthritis, diarrhea, vomiting, dysuria
	Headache, "dizzy," fatigued	
	Fever absent	
Family history	Can be positive for depression, anxiety, migraine	Can be positive for pancreatitis, peptic ulcer, inflammatory bowel disease
Social history	Frequent school absence; high socioeconomic status	
Screening laboratory tests	Normal ESR, CRP, complete blood count, and urinalysis	Anemia, high ESR and CRP
		Stool positive for occult blood
		Abnormal urinalysis

CRP, C-reactive protein; ESR, erythrocyte sedimentation rate.

Nonorganic Causes

The pain of FAP is located centrally, most often periumbilical, and vague in character. Associated phenomena such as headache, diarrhea, nausea, pallor, and sleepiness after attacks are common. Fever with the first painful episode is not uncommon, and a few children have recurrent low-grade fever with episodes. Persistent fever or fevers >38.3°C raise suspicion of possible infection or inflammatory process. Vomiting is common, but only rarely occurs with each episode. Recurrent vomiting with painful episodes, particularly if postprandial and associated with bloating, prompts concern for intermittent volvulus. An imaging study performed at the time of an attack may be the only means of clarifying the diagnosis.

Compared with controls, children with RAP are described as fussy, excitable, anxious, timid, or apprehensive. Patients and their parents are described as overly conscientious. The child is indrawn and is more likely to express features of emotional disturbance.[31] With open-ended history-taking, precipitating events can be identified at the onset of RAP in one-third of cases. In a study of adults by Campo et al.,[35] 28 former RAP patients were significantly more likely than controls to describe anxiety symptoms and disorders, to demonstrate hypochondriacal beliefs, to have greater perceived vulnerability to physical impairment, to exhibit poor social functioning, to be receiving current treatment with psychoactive drugs, and to have a family history of generalized anxiety. Within these studies,[31,35] there were trends suggesting associations between childhood RAP and lifetime psychiatric disorder, depression, family history of depression, and migraine. Similarly a prospective cohort study confirmed these findings in a cohort of patients meeting the Rome III, FAP definition. In addition to the increased anxiety, depression, and somatic comorbidities, these students had increased school absenteeism, and parental work absences.[36] This study noted no gender difference in frequency in this preadolescent population, but did note seasonality, with increased pain in the winter months.[36]

Bakker et al. demonstrated in a cohort of patients referred for CAP an increased auditory startle reflex versus controls, supporting a theory of generalized hyperresponsiveness to sensory stimuli even outside of the gastrointestinal tract.[37]

Organic Causes

Table 22-2 lists the organic disorders to be considered in the evaluation of patients with RAP. UTI is the most common organic cause. Obstructive uropathy is less frequent. When pain in the flank and an abdominal mass are present, abdominal ultrasonography should be performed; hydronephrosis is most likely. The absence of hematuria and lateralizing pain has been documented in more than one-half of the patients younger than age 8 who ultimately had urolithiasis as the etiology for their RAP; almost 80% had diffuse or central abdominal complaints.[38]

Gastroesophageal reflux (GER) has been demonstrated in a few studies to be more prominent than previously thought. A study of patients with atypical RAP demonstrated that 56% of consecutively evaluated patients had significant GER as detected by pH probe; 71% of cases were responsive to histamine-receptor type 2-blocking agents and prokinetic agents.[39] Similarly, a Norwegian study prospectively used pH probe as part of a diagnostic scheme to evaluate children with RAP and demonstrated GER in 21%. This study did not describe effects of treatment of the GER on RAP symptoms.[40]

Inflammatory bowel disease can manifest as RAP. Weight loss, poor linear growth, pubertal delay, digital clubbing, perirectal abnormalities (fistulae or skin tags), joint symptoms, and nocturnal bowel movement raise suspicion of inflammatory bowel disease. Interruption of linear growth can precede overt gastrointestinal symptoms and signs by years.

Peptic ulcer disease can cause RAP. A history of recurrent emesis and a pattern of nocturnal pain that awakens the child suggest peptic ulcer disease.[41] Helicobacter pylori is the primary cause of peptic ulcer disease in adults[42,43] and in children.[44] RAP and H.

PART II Clinical Syndromes and Cardinal Features of Infectious Diseases: Approach to Diagnosis and Initial Management

SECTION B Cardinal Symptom Complexes

TABLE 22-2. Chronic or Recurrent Abdominal Pain – Expanded Diagnosis

Common Causes	Less Common Causes	Rare Causes	
Psychophysiologic Recurrent abdominal pain Irritable-bowel syndrome Conversion reaction Task-induced phobia	**Genitourinary** Dysmenorrhea Pelvic inflammatory disease Mittelschmerz	**Genitourinary** Urolithiasis Tumors (ovarian, renal) Endometriosis Hematocolpos	**Neurologic** Intracranial mass Radiculopathy Spinal cord tumor/injury
Gastrointestinal Nonulcer dyspepsia Gastroesophageal reflux Constipation	**Gastrointestinal** Inflammatory bowel disease	**Gastrointestinal** Angioedema Malrotation Cystic fibrosis Mesenteric cyst Recurrent pancreatitis Cholelithiasis Gallbladder dysmotility Recurrent intussusception Meckel diverticulum Chronic appendicitis Abdominal wall hernia	**Cardiovascular** Chronic dysrhythmias Familial dysautonomia Superior mesenteric artery syndrome **Miscellaneous** Abdominal epilepsy Abdominal malignancy Abdominal migraine Acute intermittent porphyria Addison disease Collagen vascular disease Familial Mediterranean fever Heavy-metal intoxication Hyperthyroidism Wegener granulomatosis
Genitourinary Urinary tract infection			

Adapted from McGregor RS. Chronic complaints in adolescence. Chest pain, chronic fatigue, headaches, abdominal pain. Adolesc Med 1997;8:15–31.

pylori[45] have been linked in some select populations, in which eradication of *H. pylori* was associated with resolution of RAP.[46] Evaluation for *H. pylori* infection is currently limited to children with symptoms of peptic ulcer disease.

Abdominal migraine, although rare and challenging to diagnose, is worth addressing because of evidence-based efficacy of treatment with an anti-migraine medication; in one small trial, pizotifen therapy was the only intervention demonstrated to reduce days of abdominal pain.[47]

Chronic pancreatitis, although uncommon, can mimic RAP. Measurement of serum amylase and lipase concentrations is justifiable in the evaluation of RAP.

Although celiac disease is included as a cause of RAP, incidence of positive antibodies was no more frequent among children with RAP than age-matched controls in one study.[48]

Approach to Diagnosis and Management

As seen in Table 22-1, the clinical features of RAP of nonorganic origin are sufficiently characteristic that the diagnosis often is established after an open-ended history and thorough physical examination. Screening laboratory tests to eliminate more common organic causes (UTI, inflammatory bowel disease, pancreatitis) can contribute to physician and family confidence in the diagnosis. Screening tests include urinalysis, urine culture, erythrocyte sedimentation rate, C-reactive protein (CRP) level,

complete blood count and differential leukocyte count, stool test for occult blood, and serum albumin, amylase, and lipase measurements. Investigation for gastroesophageal reflux may be moving to first-line evaluation. Endoscopy and radiographic evaluation are performed only to evaluate specific leads from the history, physical examination, or screening laboratory test results, or if pain is atypical (e.g., right upper quadrant pain and fatty food intolerance, or atypical location of pain).

Multiple treatment regimens for FAP including RAP have failed to demonstrate efficacy in systematic reviews. These have included dietary fiber supplements, lactose restriction and probiotic supplementation,[49] and pharmacologic interventions.[50] Data support the use of psychological therapies including cognitive-behavioral therapy and hypnosis.[51]

Management of RAP must involve: (1) confirmation of the legitimacy of the patient's complaints; (2) expression of empathy for the family's concerns; (3) reduction of the child's stresses and family's unrealistic expectations; (4) resetting of the family's focus on wellness; and (5) normalization of the patient's activities and the family's response to the pain syndrome. Confident reassurance of the patient and family is the treatment for most children with RAP. Assisting the family to gain insight into psychosocial influences on the patient's symptoms is very important. Nonselective use of multiple consultants may be detrimental. Poor outcome has been associated with use of more than three consultants.[52]

23 Neurologic Symptom Complexes

Geoffrey A. Weinberg

The child manifesting symptoms referable to the nervous system is worrisome, and requires a thoughtful approach and evaluation. Often the presence of an infectious disease is not readily apparent. This chapter focuses on the most common presenting neurologic symptoms and features of the history and

physical examination that are characteristic of infections, as well as those that distinguish infectious from noninfectious causes. Management, complications, and prognosis are discussed briefly; more details are found in relevant chapters on infectious etiologies.

HEADACHE

Headache occurs in up to 35% to 70% of school-aged children and adolescents.[1-4] It is severe enough to be brought to medical attention in a small fraction of cases, although 1% of pediatric emergency department visits are for headaches.[1] Most children evaluated in primary care settings or in a pediatric emergency department with an acute headache and a normal neurologic examination have an acute viral illness, sinusitis, or migraine. Chronic headaches that gradually but progressively worsen in frequency and severity over time, are associated with seizures or focal abnormalities on examination, occur early in the morning or cause awakening at night, or occur in children <3 years of age are more ominous than acute single or acute recurrent headaches separated by periods of normalcy.[1-4]

History

Important characteristics that aid in differentiating causes of headache are: (1) pattern, duration, severity, location, and frequency of pain; (2) associated symptoms, such as fever, sinus pain, and rhinorrhea; (3) family history, triggering events, and efficacy of medications; and (4) presence of any underlying condition that predisposes to infection (Table 23-1). Children who have headache coincident with other complaints in which headache is not the cardinal feature rarely have intracranial disease. Although fever is perhaps the most helpful clue in ascribing an infectious origin, its absence does not preclude serious infection. Fever is present in 95% of children with meningitis, but in only 30% to 70% of children with brain abscess.[5,6]

Persisting focalization of head pain in children is unusual and is commonly associated with primary intracranial disease. Additional clues to intracranial disease (in approximate order of importance) include: (1) abnormal neurologic examination (especially abnormalities in eye movement or gait); (2) papilledema; (3) headache worsened by cough, Valsalva maneuver, or change in position; (4) forceful vomiting after prolonged period of recumbency; (5) headache that awakens the child from sleep or is most severe on awakening; (6) change in prior headache

pattern, especially headaches of recent onset with progressive severity and frequency; and perhaps (7) lack of family history of migraine. Questions regarding appetite, activity level, hydration, and mental status also may help identify the seriously ill child.

Physical Examination

Physical examination is directed to exclude life-threatening intracranial disease and begins with evaluation of mental status. Nonspecific terms, such as lethargy and fussiness, should be augmented or replaced by notation of interaction with the environment, consolable irritability, verbalization, and sense of wellbeing. Specific responses to verbal stimulation should be observed and recorded. If the examiner can elicit a smile from an infant or engage an older child in conversation, acute meningitis or meningoencephalitis is unlikely, although subacute brain abscesses or tumors are not excluded.

Meticulous attention to abnormalities in vital signs helps assess the diagnosis, pace of illness, and need for immediate intervention. Examples are tachycardia, hypotension, or orthostatic hypotension in the child with moderate to severe dehydration, toxic or septic shock, or the combination of bradycardia, systolic hypertension (wide pulse pressure), and slow, deep, respirations (Cushing triad) indicating increased intracranial pressure. Overt signs of impending herniation, such as hyperventilation, Cheyne–Stokes respiration (pattern of progressive increase in depth and sometimes rate of breaths followed by apnea) or ataxic respiration (chaotic gasping and apnea), bulging fontanel, fixed pupils or anisocoria, must be identified quickly. The presence of papilledema is a specific but insensitive sign of intracranial disease. It is rare in children with bacterial meningitis, given the relative rapidity of disease, but is notable in 40% to 70% of children with brain abscess.[5,7] Abnormalities of cranial nerve function, asymmetry in strength, tone, or reflexes, gait changes, and papilledema help define an existing lesion; the vast majority of children with a brain tumor have some abnormality demonstrable on careful neurologic examination.[1-4]

Nuchal rigidity is present in a quarter of patients with brain abscess[7] and in >95% of children beyond the neonatal period with

TABLE 23-1. Differentiating Features of Causes of Headaches in Children

Feature	Meningoencephalitis and Meningitis	Brain Abscess	Sinusitis	Brain Tumor	Migraine and Tension	Pseudotumor Cerebri
SYMPTOMS						
Fever	+++	++	++	+	−	−
Onset	Acute	Subacute	Subacute	Subacute	Acute	Subacute
Location	Diffuse	Localized to site	Frontal or diffuse	Localized to site	Unilateral, diffuse, or occipital	Diffuse
Frequency	Single	Daily	Daily	Daily	Variably recurrent	Daily
Duration	Hours	Weeks	Days	Weeks	Hours	Days–weeks
PREDISPOSING CONDITIONS AND ASSOCIATED FEATURES	Preceding illness; epidemic disease; seasonality	Mastoiditis, otitis, sinusitis; facial cellulitis; cyanotic heart disease; empyema; immunodeficiency; gram-negative bacterial meningitis	Allergic rhinitis	Morning severity; forceful emesis; awakens from sleep; increased severity with change of position	Family history	Obesity; menses; vitamin A; corticosteroids; Lyme disease
PHYSICAL EXAMINATION						
Altered mental status	++[a]	+	−	+	−[b]	−
Focal deficits	++[a]	++	−	++	−[b]	+[c]
Nuchal rigidity	+++	++	+	−	−	−

+++, expected; ++, frequent; +, occasional; −, rare or not associated.

[a]In meningoencephalitis.

[b]Can occur with basilar artery or complicated migraine.

[c]Especially abducens nerve palsy.

PART II Clinical Syndromes and Cardinal Features of Infectious Diseases: Approach to Diagnosis and Initial Management

SECTION B Cardinal Symptom Complexes

meningitis,[8] but can occur with posterior fossa tumors as well. Fever, headache, and nuchal rigidity can occur with acute bacterial pneumonia, especially that involving the upper lobes; tachypnea is almost invariably present but may have been overlooked.

Sinusitis is a relatively uncommon cause of headache in children (10% to 15%);[1] data from studies of adults reveal that many "sinus headaches" are likely migraine,[9] but in up to 25% of children with sinusitis, headache is the chief complaint. The constellation of fever, purulent nasal discharge, frontal location of dull pain, and sinus tenderness usually identifies these patients.[9]

Evaluation

If examination reveals overt signs of increased intracranial pressure or focal deficits, brain imaging (computed tomography and/or magnetic resonance imaging) is warranted urgently as the first study. Electroencephalogram is not recommended in the routine evaluation of headaches in children.[3]

Much discussion has centered on whether a brain imaging study must be performed prior to lumbar puncture in the child with probable bacterial meningitis, in order to diagnose increased intracranial pressure (ICP) which might induce brain herniation after lumbar puncture.[10] Herniation after lumbar puncture for bacterial meningitis certainly has been reported, but such reports are retrospective in design or anecdotal, and often involve a study population including the most critically ill patients, who sometimes have had herniation even without lumbar puncture.[8,10–18] Thus, the published incidence of herniation in bacterial meningitis of 4% to 6% is likely biased by both study design and publication bias.[10–12,14,16] It is clear that increased ICP does accompany bacterial meningitis, but in general, the diffusely increased ICP of meningitis, with or without performance of lumbar puncture, is much less likely to lead to brain herniation than the differentially increased (focal) ICP associated with intracranial mass lesions. Unfortunately, even a normal result of brain imaging study does not exclude the uncommon-to-rare likelihood of herniation.[16,18] A large prospective study of the utility of brain imaging in adults with suspected meningitis showed that imaging is overutilized, and that clinical features alone may suffice to choose which patients can proceed to lumbar puncture without imaging.[19,20] Similar prospective pediatric data are lacking, but several case series show that clinical signs are more accurate than head imaging in prediction of impending herniation in children. In current practice, few children with suspected bacterial meningitis have intracranial pressure measured at the time of lumbar puncture; recent data suggest that the normal ranges of pressure are wider than once thought.[10,21]

Thus, in general, if meningitis is suspected in a child without papilledema or focal neurologic findings, a lumbar puncture can be performed without obtaining brain imaging.[8,10] Additional important but less common contraindications to lumbar puncture include clinically important cardiorespiratory compromise in a neonate or older child; infection in the skin, soft tissue, or epidural area overlying lumbar puncture site; and severe bleeding diathesis.[8]

In the uncommon child with suspected bacterial meningitis and signs of impending herniation or focal neurologic signs, blood cultures are obtained, antibiotics are administered, and an imaging study of the brain is performed urgently. Lumbar puncture is postponed until signs of herniation (as judged by both imaging studies and physical examination) have resolved.

A written and videographic review of lumbar puncture methods is available.[22]

Therapy

Antibiotic therapy for infectious causes of headaches is that which is appropriate for the relevant infection, e.g., sinusitis, meningitis, or brain abscess. In addition, brain abscesses >2.5 cm in size generally require therapeutic drainage procedures beyond simple diagnostic aspiration.

ALTERED MENTAL STATUS

Diagnostic evaluation of the child with altered mental status focuses on quickly identifying the likely cause or causes and initiating appropriate treatment, which usually is determined empirically. The causes of altered mental status in children are shown in Table 23-2, and differentiating features in Table 23-3. Diagnostic evaluation in the emergency department typically involves rapid testing for hypoglycemia, abnormalities of electrolytes or renal function, and, perhaps, intoxications. The differential diagnosis at the time of infectious diseases consultation usually has been narrowed beyond these noninfectious illnesses.

Encephalitis or meningoencephalitis in the United States most often is caused by viruses, especially enteroviruses, arboviruses (including St. Louis encephalitis virus, California group encephalitis viruses, eastern equine encephalitis virus, and in the older child and adult, West Nile virus), Epstein–Barr virus, varicella-zoster virus, and herpes simplex virus (HSV, being the one agent clearly treatable with antiviral therapy).[23–28] Bacterial causes of encephalitis or meningoencephalitis include *Bartonella henselae* (cat-scratch disease encephalitis), *Mycoplasma pneumoniae* (although somewhat controversial as diagnosis has often relied upon imperfect IgM antibody assays), and rarely, *Listeria monocytogenes*.[29–31] Other notable infectious causes of pediatric acute encephalitis or meningoencephalitis of unknown origin include influenza virus, rotavirus, bacteremia, toxic shock syndrome, and rabies. (See Chapter 44, Encephalitis.)

Acute disseminated encephalomyelitis (ADEM) is a presumed postinfectious inflammatory demyelinating illness with acute or subacute onset, which affects multiple areas of the CNS.[32–35] ADEM appears to be common in children than in adults. Clinical symptoms most often include behavioral changes, alterations in consciousness, and monoparesis or even hemiparesis. The CSF protein and white cell count generally are both elevated without the presence of oligoclonal bands. Cranial MRI usually reveals large, multifocal, hyperintense lesions on FLAIR or T_2-weighted images in the white matter of the brain, but also often in the grey matter of the thalamus and basal ganglia as well. However, published consensus definitions have emphasized diagnosis based more on clinical changes than on abnormal MRI abnormalities.[36,37] (See Chapter 45.)

Recently, it has become clear that one form (if not the majority) of "paraneoplastic limbic encephalitis" occurs more commonly than was once thought, and is likely an autoimmune disease caused by the presence of autoantibodies to the neuronal cell

TABLE 23-2. Causes of Altered Mental Status

Intracranial	Systemic
INFECTION	**METABOLIC ENCEPHALOPATHY**
Meningitis	Endogenous
Meningoencephalitis (enterovirus, HSV, WNV, other arboviruses)	Hypoglycemia
	Hyperammonemia
Postinfectious encephalitis (ADEM)	Hypercarbia
Brain abscess	Hypoxia
Bartonella encephalopathy	Uremia
Mycoplasma pneumoniae encephalopathy	Exogenous
	Acute poison ingestion
	Chronic heavy metal exposure
TRAUMA	
POSTICTAL STATE	**INTUSSUSCEPTION**
COMPLEX PARTIAL STATUS EPILEPTICUS	**HYPOTENSION**
INTRACRANIAL MASS	
AUTOIMMUNE	
NMDAR antibodies	
CNS vasculitis	

ADEM, acute disseminated encephalomyelitis; CNS, central nervous system; HSV, herpes simplex virus; NMDAR, N-methyl-D-aspartate receptor; WNV, West Nile virus.

TABLE 23-3. Differentiating Features of Causes of Altered Mental Status in Children

Feature	Encephalitis	Toxic Ingestion	Space-Occupying Lesion	Reye Syndrome
Predominant age	Variable	Toddlers, adolescents	Variable	1–14 years
Fever	++	+	+	–
Prodrome	Headache, fever, irritability, personality change	–	Headache	Upper respiratory tract infection days before protracted vomiting, stupor, coma
Seizures	++	+	++	–[a]
Focal neurologic signs	++	–	++	–
Other associated findings	Rhinorrhea, rash	Altered pupils or vital signs ↑, ↓ sweating ↑, ↓ saliva		Hepatomegaly

++, frequent; +, occasional; –, rare; ↑, increased; ↓, decreased.

[a]Can occur with markedly increased intracranial pressure.

membrane *N*-methyl-D-aspartate receptor (NMDAR).[38–40] Encephalitis with NMDAR antibodies originally was described to occur primarily in young women with ovarian teratomas, but it is now known that most NMDAR encephalitis is found in patients without associated tumors in men, women, and children. The characteristic illness consists of the acute onset of behavioral and neuropsychiatric changes and seizures, followed by progressive coma, orofacial and upper limb choreoathetoid movement disorder, and dysautonomia. Laboratory findings include CSF lymphocytic pleocytosis (70–90% of patients), CSF oligoclonal bands (40% of patients), and abnormal EEG findings (50–100% of patients), yet rather unremarkable MRI scans of the head (70–80% of scans normal); all in association with elevated serum anti-NMDAR antibodies.[38–40]

History

Important features in the history of altered mental status include age, past medical history, presence of fever, convulsions, or antecedent illness, immunizations, length and progression of illness, medications in the home, length of time the child or adolescent was unobserved prior to the change in mental status, and, for the adolescent, any recent change in disposition at home or school.

Physical Examination

The degree of alteration in consciousness should be measured specifically. Coma scales, particularly the Glasgow Coma Scale, at times fall short in assessing consciousness in children, because the scales require an adult level of neurodevelopment and often have a high degree of interobserver variability.[41] Delineation of the patient's neurologic examination is most useful. Identifying signs of increased intracranial pressure or focal neurologic deficit are of utmost importance. A record of normal blood pressure is important and excludes hypertensive encephalopathy.

The remainder of the physical examination focuses on recognition of a toxic syndrome or identification of a systemic illness. Toxic ingestion is supported by abnormalities in vital signs, skin (flushing or sweating), mucous membranes (sparse or excessive saliva), and pupillary size and reactivity. Physical examination of the child with hepatic encephalopathy usually reveals other obvious signs, most notably icterus and decreased liver span, and, in the case of Reye syndrome, hepatomegaly without icterus. Infants with intussusception may present with remarkable lethargy, fluctuating consciousness, or hypotonia instead of, or in addition to, the more familiar features of severe, paroxysmal, colicky abdominal pain and bloody stools, perhaps secondary to release of neuroactive endotoxins or central endorphins.[42] Neuropsychiatric changes and seizures can mark HSV encephalitis or NMDAR encephalitis.

An infectious etiology of altered mental status also is likely if there is fever with systemic signs, such as involvement of multiple mucous membranes (e.g., conjunctivitis, mucositis, or pharyngitis), diarrhea, abnormal lung findings, or rash (see Table 23-2).

Evaluation

Unless steps taken to this point determine a likely extracranial cause of the altered mental status, a brain imaging study is performed to identify focal lesions or evidence of intracranial hypertension and assess the size of ventricles. MRI is superior to CT in making an earlier diagnosis of HSV encephalitis, and in assessing the white matter for changes indicative of ADEM. Lumbar puncture is performed if no mass lesion is identified, opening pressure is measured, and specimens of CSF are sent for multiple tests (see Chapter 44, Encephalitis). Not infrequently, these study findings also are normal, or show only a mildly elevated CSF protein concentration and mononuclear pleocytosis; the remaining differential diagnosis still may include toxic encephalopathy and encephalitis. Oligoclonal band analysis may help if NMDAR encephalitis (40% of patients positive) or multiple sclerosis (essentially all patients positive) are in the differential diagnosis, as opposed to ADEM (oligoclonal bands not expected). Electroencephalography may be helpful in determining a seizure focus and identifying periodic lateralizing epileptiform discharges (which finding increases the likelihood of but is not pathognomonic for HSV encephalitis), or focal slowing; however, absence of abnormality does not narrow the differential diagnosis significantly. It is noteworthy that complex partial status epilepticus can manifest with only alteration in mental status. Normal values of serum hepatic enzymes and ammonia exclude Reye syndrome (which virtually has disappeared since routine aspirin use in children was halted).[43–45] Close monitoring of neurologic status, so as to recognize the necessity to intervene to manage intracranial hypertension, and monitoring of cardiac function for dysrhythmia associated with intoxications are indicated.

Therapy

Infectious causes of altered mental status in which antimicrobial therapy is critical include HSV encephalitis, listeriosis, bacterial meningitis, and brain abscess (along with surgical intervention if large). Empiric therapy for HSV encephalitis is given if no other diagnosis is likely, after appropriate specimens have been collected for culture and molecular identification. Delay in obtaining CSF for PCR testing for HSV does not reduce its sensitivity. Antimicrobial therapy sometimes is given for possible *Bartonella* and *Mycoplasma* encephalopathy/itis, although the effect of antimicrobial therapy in these conditions is unproven. ADEM, NMDAR encephalitis, and CNS vasculitis are treated with anti-inflammatory

PART II Clinical Syndromes and Cardinal Features of Infectious Diseases: Approach to Diagnosis and Initial Management

SECTION B Cardinal Symptom Complexes

medications, generally glucocorticoids, (along with removal of ovarian tumor if present in NMDAR). Enterovirus and West Nile virus encephalitis are treated with supportive therapy.

ATAXIA

Ataxia is a disorder of impaired balance and poor coordination of intentional movement. Ataxia results from cerebellar dysfunction due to damage to either the afferent sensory nerve pathways to the cerebellum, or to the motor fibers to or from the cerebellum. The differential diagnosis of ataxia in children is broad and includes infectious etiologies primarily when onset is acute or subacute (see Chapter 44, Encephalitis; Chapter 132, *Listeria monocytogenes*). Before universal childhood immunization against varicella, acute cerebellar ataxia was recognized to be a not infrequent complication of chickenpox. Other uncommon viral causes of acute cerebellar ataxia include Epstein–Barr virus and mumps virus.[32,46] *Listeria* CNS infection sometimes causes rhomboencephalitis with prominent feature of ataxia. Whether postinfectious acute cerebellar ataxia is actually a form of ADEM is uncertain.[32] Differentiating features of acute ataxia are shown in Table 23-4.

History

History for a patient with ataxia focuses on: (1) the child's age; (2) presence of fever, recent illness, immunization, trauma, medications in the home and ingestion or intoxication; (3) progression, duration, and frequency of the ataxia if intermittent; (4) presence of constitutional symptoms; and (5) family history of migraine headache. Fever and ataxia have only rarely been reported as sole findings in patients with acute bacterial meningitis.[47]

Physical Examination

In considering the differential diagnosis, the clinician should first distinguish cerebellar dysfunction and ataxia from other disorders of gait (muscular or neuromuscular disorders, primary hip or limb disease) and incoordination (neuromuscular or neurosensory disorders, chorea). The verbal child with middle-ear or inner-ear disease leading to disequilibrium complains of dizziness; this is not usually the case in the child with ataxia due to cerebellar or posterior column disease. The ataxic child generally is not weak, and the Romberg test is positive with eyes both opened and closed. Ataxia due to posterior column disease is associated with a positive Romberg test result only when the eyes are closed.

Once disease is localized to the cerebellum, initial evaluation targets life-threatening causes. Central nervous system tumor, particularly brainstem glioma, usually is associated with chronic, intermittent ataxia but rarely can cause acute ataxia. Signs of increased intracranial pressure can be but are not invariably present. On the other hand, increased intracranial pressure from whatever cause can manifest initially as ataxia.

The general physical examination should be thorough and should be directed at distinguishing etiologies (see Table 23-4). Fever and new or healing rash (e.g., chickenpox) can be clues to acute infectious or postinfectious cerebellitis. Careful examination of skin and scalp for ticks (wood or dog ticks) is warranted, because the initial signs of tick paralysis are ataxia and nystagmus; motor weakness and ascending paralysis follow within 48 hours.[48,49] Middle-ear disease can result in vestibular dysfunction and ataxia (with complaints of dizziness and vertigo). The paraneoplastic syndrome of opsoclonus–myoclonus–ataxia occurs in only 2% to 3% of all children with neuroblastoma, but 50% to 80% of children identified with opsoclonus–myoclonus–ataxia are found to have neuroblastoma.[50] Despite a relative increase in survival with treatment of children with neuroblastoma, chronic ataxia and severe neurodevelopmental delay usually persist.[50]

Unless the ataxia is very short-lived, as with basilar artery migraine syndrome and benign paroxysmal vertigo, further evaluation (including cranial imaging, followed by lumbar puncture and perhaps other studies) is necessary, as summarized in Table 23-4 (see also Chapter 45).

Therapy

Empiric therapy with ampicillin for *Listeria* is considered depending on the clinical setting and CSF findings. Postinfectious acute cerebellar ataxia generally resolves spontaneously. Tick paralysis and its initial ataxia is rapidly reversed by removal of attached ticks.

HYPOTONIA AND WEAKNESS

Tone and strength are distinctly different, but intimately related, properties of skeletal muscle. Muscle tone is the least resistance generated against passive movement of the muscle and is best evaluated in the wakeful, relaxed state. Strength is the greatest force that a muscle can generate actively against an opposing force and requires the patient's maximal effort.

Hypotonia can occur without accompanying weakness when the upper motor neuron is the site of disease. Weakness often is accompanied by a decrease in muscle tone in conditions with acute onset, but not necessarily in chronic conditions (e.g., children with cerebral palsy may have weakness and hypertonia; stroke may cause acute hypotonia followed by weakness and hypertonia). In children, hypotonia is a cardinal feature of disease almost exclusively in infancy, whereas weakness is a complaint

TABLE 23-4. Differentiating Features of Causes of Acute Ataxia in Children

Feature	Infectious or Postinfectious Cerebellitis	Toxic Ingestion	Neuroblastoma	Basilar Artery Migraine	Benign Paroxysmal Vertigo
Predominant age	<10 years	Toddler	<5 years	Any	<4 years
Fever	– to ++	–	+	–	–
Onset	Acute to subacute	Acute	Subacute	Acute	Acute
Frequency	Single	Single	Single	Recurrent	Recurrent
Duration	Days–weeks	Hours	Months	Minutes–hours	Seconds–minutes
Associated symptoms and signs	Resolving antecedent illness (e.g., chickenpox)	Altered mental status	Opsoclonus, myoclonus	Disturbed vision; vomiting; headache; vertigo; ataxia; dysarthria	Suddenly reaches for support; refuses to walk
Results of evaluation	Normal or modest ↑ protein, cells in CSF	Abnormal serum, urine toxin screen	↑ Urine HVA, VMA; abnormal imaging of abdomen and chest		

CSF, cerebrospinal fluid; HVA, homovanillic acid; VMA, vanillylmandelic acid; ++, frequent; +, occasional; –, absent; ↑, increased.

TABLE 23-5. Differentiating Features of Causes of Hypotonia in Infancy

Feature	Infant Botulism	Myasthenia Gravis	Spinal Muscular Atrophy	CNS Injury/ Genetic Syndrome	Peripheral Neuropathy	Myopathy
SITE OF DISEASE	Neuromuscular junction	Neuromuscular junction	Anterior horn cell	Central nervous system	Peripheral nerve	Muscle
HISTORY						
Prenatal, perinatal	Normal	Decreased fetal movement, polyhydramnios; short umbilical cord, abnormal fetal lie, low Apgar scores can occur in all				
Onset	1–12 months	Birth	Birth; more obvious with time	Birth	Birth	Birth; more obvious with time
Course	Deficits peak at 1–5 days. Recovery 3–12 weeks	Deficits peak at birth. Recovery in passive form	Death in infancy	Not progressive	Not progressive	Not progressive
Family history	–	Myasthenic mother in passive form	Autosomal-recessive	Variable	Variable	Variable
Other	Breastfed; constipation; loss of facial expression; poor suck; weak cry	Fatigability; loss of facial expression; poor suck	Preserved facial expression	–	–	–
PHYSICAL EXAMINATION						
General	Normal–flushed skin; ptosis; poor suck; weak cry	–	Paucity of movement; frog-legged position; expressive face	Abnormal head size; dysmorphic features	–	–[a]
Cognition	Normal	Normal	Normal	Abnormal	Normal	Normal
Strength	↓	↓	↓	Normal	↓	↓
Reflexes	Normal–↓	Normal–↓	↓–Absent	↑–Normal	↓–Absent	Normal–↓
Muscle bulk	Normal	Normal	Proximal atrophy	Normal	Distal atrophy	Proximal atrophy
Fasciculations	–	–	++	–	+	
Sensation	Normal	Normal	Normal	Normal	Normal–↓	Normal
Other	Oculomotor ↓; bulbar findings; descending symmetrical paralysis, always including cranial nerves; autonomic signs	Oculomotor ↓; bulbar findings; fatigability	Facial muscles, diaphragm spared	Apnea; seizures; abnormal fundi	–	Facial diplegia
EVALUATION	Stool toxin assay	EMG. Edrophonium chloride	EMG. Muscle biopsy	Brain imaging. Chromosomes	EMG. Nerve conduction study	EMG muscle biopsy

CNS, central nervous system; EMG, electromyography; ++, frequent; +, occasional; –, absent; ↑, increased; ↓, decreased.

[a]Hepatomegaly in Pompe disease (glycogen storage disease IIa).

TABLE 23-6. Differentiating Features of Causes of Weakness in Older Children and Adults

Feature	Guillain–Barré Syndrome	Transverse Myelitis	Paralytic Poliomyelitis[b]	West Nile Virus Acute Flaccid Paralysis	Spinal Cord Tumor	Conversion Disorder	Tick Paralysis
SITE OF DISEASE	Peripheral nerve root	Spinal cord	Anterior horn cell	Anterior horn cell	Spinal cord	Psyche	Peripheral nerve and neuromuscular junction
HISTORY							
Onset	Subacute	Subacute (50 h to maximum deficit)	Acute or subacute	Acute	Insidious	Acute	Subacute
Progression	Ascending	Paresthesias, leg weakness, then sensory deficit	Biphasic paralysis 3–5 days after fever	Acutely progressive with febrile meningoencephalitis	Weeks–months	Variable	Ataxia, then ascending paralysis
Duration	Weeks–months	Weeks–months	Days–weeks	Weeks–months	Variable	Variable	Days

Continued

PART II Clinical Syndromes and Cardinal Features of Infectious Diseases: Approach to Diagnosis and Initial Management

SECTION B Cardinal Symptom Complexes

TABLE 22-6. Differentiating Features of Causes of Weakness in Older Children and Adults—cont'd

Feature	Guillain–Barré Syndrome	Transverse Myelitis	Paralytic Poliomyelitis[b]	West Nile Virus Acute Flaccid Paralysis	Spinal Cord Tumor	Conversion Disorder	Tick Paralysis
Recovery	+++	64% of cases	Dependent on degree/extent of paralysis	+	Dependent on tumor type, location, intervention	++++	Recovery if tick is removed
Predominant age	Adolescence	Adolescence	Any	Predominantly adults	Any	School age–adolescence; rarely <5 years	2–5 years
Paresthesias	++++	+++	++	–	++, if dorsal columns involved	++	+
Back pain	+	+++	20%	–	++ Dull, aching	++	–
PHYSICAL EXAMINATION							
Autonomic dysfunction	60%	++	20%	–	+	–	–
Fever	+	+++	+++	+++	+	–	–
Distribution	Ascending, symmetric[a]	Usually symmetric; motor/sensory level	Patchy	Asymmetric	Below level of tumor	Varies moment to moment	Ascending, symmetric
Bowel, bladder dysfunction	+	95%	20%	+++	+++	–	–
Sensation abnormality	+ (proprioception)	95% (pain and temperature)	+	–	++++	++	++
Reflexes	Absent	30% ↑ initially; 65% ↓ overall	↓ or absent on affected side	↓	↓ if corticospinal tract involved	Normal	Absent
ASSOCIATED FEATURES	Antecedent URI or diarrheal illness (e.g., *Campylobacter*)	Abdominal pain; antecedent trauma 30%; URI 30%	Intense muscle pain; URI symptoms; nuchal rigidity; headache	Headache; dyskinesia (e.g., parkinsonism); meningoencephalitis	Change in posture, Valsalva accentuate pain; abnormal gait	Subconscious stress; model for symptom; secondary gain	*Dermacentor andersoni* and *D. variabilis* ticks
CSF	↑ Protein 0–few cells	↑ Protein ↑ cells	↑ Protein ↑ cells	↑ Protein ↑ cells	Not applicable	Normal	Normal

CSF, cerebrospinal fluid; URI, upper respiratory tract infection; ++++, expected; +++, frequent; ++, occasional; +, rare; –, absent; ↑, increased; ↓, decreased.

[a]*The less common Miller–Fisher variant consists of ophthalmoplegia, ataxia, areflexia, and weakness that is less pronounced than in the classic form.*

[b]*Paralytic poliomyelitis-like syndrome can also occur with other enteroviruses, especially enterovirus 71.*

more often found in the toddler and older child. The spectrum of disease causing diminished tone and strength varies within these age groups, and includes infectious,[26,27,51] postinfectious,[52–55] malignant, and other causes. For these reasons, the features and causes of hypotonia and weakness are considered separately in Tables 23-5 and 23-6.

Therapy

Infant botulism is treated with botulism-specific human immune globulin (see Chapter 189). Guillain–Barré syndrome and transverse myelitis generally are treated with immune globulin intravenous (IGIV) and glucocorticoids (see Chapter 45).[52–55]

24 Musculoskeletal Symptom Complexes

Kathleen Gutierrez

Musculoskeletal pain is a common presenting complaint in young children and adolescents. The usual cause of musculoskeletal pain is trauma or strain to joint, bone, or muscle. Often, the etiology is never determined and symptoms resolve with symptomatic treatment. The challenge for the clinician is to rule out serious disease, including infection, as a cause of symptoms. This chapter focuses on the illnesses responsible for three different categories of musculoskeletal symptoms – extremity pain, back pain, and chest pain – and the distinguishing features of each of these illnesses.

HISTORY

Because the differential diagnosis of musculoskeletal pain is extensive, a comprehensive history must be obtained. Important information includes the acuity of onset of illness and presence or absence of fever. Symptoms that are acute, persistent, and accompanied by fever are more likely to be caused by infection. Chronic or subacute symptoms often are the result of noninfectious illnesses.

Important information obtained in the history of the present illness includes the onset and location, description of the progression and severity of the musculoskeletal pain, and whether pain medication has been used and has been helpful. History is elicited of change in gait, ability to bear weight or move the affected area, joint or soft-tissue swelling, and presence of induration, erythema, and warmth. A history of trauma, previous or recent illnesses, growth and development, family history, travel, animal exposures, and medication use is important. A review of systems, including history of fever, skin or mucous membrane lesions, pharyngitis, eye inflammation, lymphadenopathy, respiratory or cardiac symptoms, abdominal pain, vomiting or diarrhea, recent sexually transmitted diseases, or neurologic symptoms is crucial in determining whether a systemic disease is associated with the musculoskeletal abnormalities.

PHYSICAL EXAMINATION

The primary focus of the physical examination is to pinpoint the location of symptoms in order to generate an accurate differential diagnosis and facilitate diagnostic testing. Examination of infants or young children is difficult as they are unable to verbalize the exact location of discomfort. Since musculoskeletal pain is a result of disease affecting a variety of structures, including joints, bones, muscles, nerves, or blood vessels, careful examination of each of these systems is necessary.

Vital signs document the presence or absence of fever, hypothermia, or cardiovascular instability. Height, weight, head circumference, and general appearance of the child should be noted. Poor growth or weight loss could be consistent with inflammatory bowel disease (IBD) or other chronic inflammatory processes, malignancy, or chronic infections such as tuberculosis. Examination of the eyes may reveal conjunctival hyperemia consistent with Kawasaki disease. Mucous membranes are examined for the presence of ulcers (IBD, Behçet, systemic lupus erythematosus (SLE)), an enanthem (group A streptococcal infection, enterovirus infection), or hyperemia (Kawasaki disease). Lymphadenopathy can be seen in juvenile idiopathic arthritis (JIA) and malignancy and is a feature of Kawasaki disease. The chest is palpated for bone pain (malignancy, multifocal osteomyelitis, pleurodynia); palpated for decreased (pleural effusion), and increased (consolidated lung) tactile fremitus during vocalization; and percussed for dullness (pleural effusion or consolidation). Auscultation can reveal decreased breath sounds, rales or rhonchi or wheezing (pneumonia associated with hematogenous dissemination of bacteria to bones, joints, or muscles), or decreased breath sounds such as in pleural effusion (occasionally seen with JIA and SLE). Cardiac examination may reveal a new murmur (endocarditis or acute rheumatic fever (ARF)) or muffled heart sounds (pericarditis). The abdomen should be assessed for tenderness, masses (psoas abscess, tumor), hepatomegaly, or splenomegaly (JIA, malignancy, endocarditis). Exanthems are noted (viral infections, associated bacterial infections/intoxications, Kawasaki disease).

Careful examination of bones, joints, muscles, and nervous system is particularly important. The examiner should note how the patient holds the affected limb and whether areas of skin or soft tissue appear swollen or red. Gait and stance are observed carefully. The bones and muscles in the affected limb should be palpated carefully, and passive and active range of motion of joints evaluated. Pain in the lower extremities can be referred from the back, pelvis, abdomen, or hip. A careful examination of the back and pelvis is necessary to rule out diskitis, vertebral osteomyelitis,

pelvic osteomyelitis, or abscess. Bones of the spine and pelvis are palpated and the spine is assessed for abnormalities in flexion or extension. Skin overlying the vertebral bodies should be examined for the presence of a hemangioma, hair, pit or mass associated with spinal dysraphism. Infection or structural abnormalities of the hip can cause pain referred to the knee. Careful examination of the hip joint must be performed in all children with a symptom or sign referable to the lower extremity. Neurologic examination includes evaluation for presence and symmetry of deep tendon reflexes, evaluation for clonus, and sensory examination and estimation of muscle strength. Foot deformities may suggest underlying neurologic conditions.

LABORATORY EVALUATION AND IMAGING

The laboratory and radiologic evaluation of musculoskeletal pain is guided by findings on history and physical examination. If infection is suspected, attempts should be made to obtain blood cultures and joint, bone, or tissue culture (depending on location of disease) prior to initiation of antibiotic therapy. Synovial fluid cell count and cultures are recommended, particularly for patients with monoarticular arthritis, fever, and no other sites/signs of systemic disease. Inflammatory markers (erythrocyte sedimentation rate (ESR) and C-reactive protein (CRP)) and white blood cell (WBC) counts can be abnormal with infection, inflammatory disease, and hematologic malignancy. Use of other diagnostic tests depends on the differential diagnosis generated on the basis of the history and physical examination.

If a bone or joint disease is suspected, a plain radiograph of the affected area generally is indicated. Both anteroposterior and lateral views should be obtained since abnormalities sometimes can be missed with a single view. Depending on suspected site of problem, specialized views sometimes are required (Figure 24-1). Plain radiographs can identify fracture, chronic bone infection, joint effusion, soft-tissue swelling, tumor, and structural abnormalities of bone. Ultrasound is useful in identifying joint effusions, particularly in the hip. Magnetic resonance imaging (MRI) or radionuclide scans may be necessary to diagnose bone infections, particularly in the acute phase. These scans also are useful in establishing the diagnosis and extent of bone involvement with

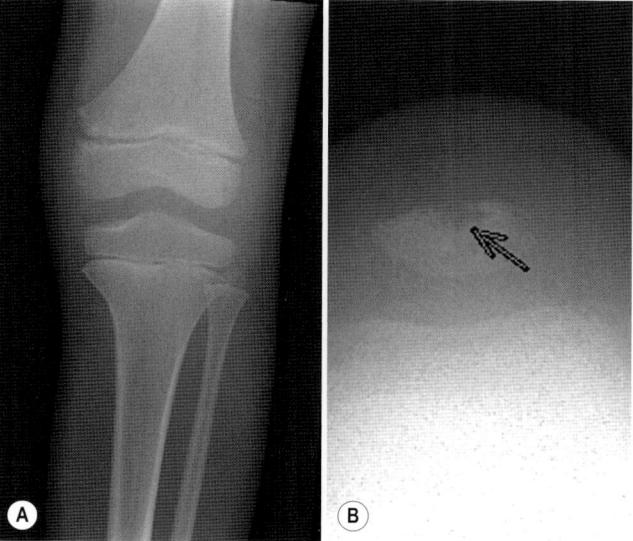

Figure 24-1. Radiographs of an 8-year-old boy with fever, limp, and anterior knee pain. Routine PA view **(A)** is normal, with lytic lesion of patellar osteomyelitis seen on the sunrise view **(B)**. Arrow shows lytic lesion. (Courtesy of Feja KN and Tolan RW, Jr, The Children's Hospital at Saint Peter's University Hospital, New Brunswick, NJ, reprinted with permission of Pediatrics in Review.)

malignancies. Radionuclide bone scans are useful if multifocal disease is suspected.

LIMB PAIN

The causes of limb pain in children are extensive and include the broad categories of infection, inflammatory disease, malignancy, trauma, and "orthopedic" problems (Box 24-1). These conditions may involve the joints, bones, muscles, or soft tissue of the affected limb.

Disease Involving the Joints

Arthritis is a common cause of limb pain in children and can have multiple etiologies (Table 24-1). Infection of the joints can be caused by bacterial, and, less often, viral or fungal infection.

Pyogenic Arthritis

Pyogenic arthritis usually is the result of hematogenous dissemination of bacteria to the joint space, and less likely the result of direct extension from infected bone, soft tissue, or muscle. The usual bacterial causes vary depending on age (see Chapter 79, Infectious and Inflammatory Arthritis); *Staphylococcus aureus* is the most common cause of pyogenic arthritis in all age groups. Pathogens typically causing infection in neonates should be considered in infants less than 2 months old. *Neisseria gonorrhoeae* should be considered in sexually active adolescents. Arthritis caused by

Borrelia burgdorferi is considered in children who live in or who have traveled to areas where Lyme disease is endemic. Bacterial arthritis can affect any joint, but the joints of the lower extremity are involved most commonly. Pyogenic arthritis generally is monoarticular, but *N. gonorrhoeae* and occasionally *S. aureus* can infect multiple joints. Infants are particularly at risk for infection of multiple joints. Pyogenic arthritis in children is characterized by acute onset of fever, joint pain, redness, and swelling. Physical examination shows markedly decreased range of motion of the affected joint, except in Lyme disease when effusion characteristically is large and range of motion is relatively preserved.

Pyogenic arthritis of the hip may be difficult to diagnose, since associated overlying redness and swelling frequently is not apparent. Pain often is referred to the groin, thigh, or knee. To decrease intracapsular hip joint pressure, the child prefers to hold the affected leg in a flexed, abducted, and externally rotated position. Examination for prone internal rotation is helpful in diagnosing intra-articular hip pathology.[1] The child is placed in a prone position with the pelvis flat on the table and with knees and ankles flexed and falling away from the body. The examiner tests for pain and limitation of internal rotation. Prompt diagnosis of pyogenic arthritis of the hip is necessary to prevent vascular compromise to the femoral head due to increased intracapsular pressure. Joint effusion can be detected by ultrasonography. If pyogenic hip arthritis is suspected, surgical drainage of infected fluid is indicated urgently.

Transient Synovitis

Transient synovitis is a common cause of limp and hip pain in children 18 months to 12 years of age (mean age 5 to 6 years) and typically involves a hip joint unilaterally (see Chapter 81, Transient Synovitis). Transient synovitis often is seen in association with a viral respiratory or gastrointestinal illness and may be the result of either direct viral infection of the synovium or a postinfectious response. Although illness is self-limited and resolves with supportive therapy, differentiation from pyogenic arthritis can be challenging. Typically, children with pyogenic arthritis are more likely to have a history of fever, are unable to bear weight, and have modestly elevated ESR, CRP, WBC count or an increased hip joint space (>2 mm) on plain radiographs or fluid identified by ultrasonography.[2,3] There is, unfortunately, overlap in clinical and laboratory findings between transient synovitis and pyogenic arthritis and therefore careful clinical reassessment is necessary when transient synovitis is suspected until the diagnosis is clear.

Other Noninfectious Causes

Reactive arthritis is inflammation of the joint space that occurs in response to an infection elsewhere in the body. Noninfectious inflammatory causes of arthritis generally are more subacute or chronic in presentation. The usual organisms associated with noninfectious reactive arthritis include gastrointestinal pathogens such as *Salmonella* spp., *Campylobacter* spp., *Shigella* spp., *Yersinia* spp., *Clostridium difficile*, sexually transmitted infections such as *Chlamydia trachomatis* and *Neisseria gonorrhoeae*, and occasionally *Streptococcus pyogenes*.

JIA is considered in children less than 16 years of age when symptoms of joint inflammation have been present for 6 weeks or more and other causes have been excluded.[4] Categories of JIA include systemic arthritis, oligoarthritis, and polyarthritis.[5] Systemic JIA typically manifests with high fever, an evanescent rash, hepatosplenomegaly, generalized lymphadenopathy, and occasionally pleuritis and pericarditis. These symptoms can precede joint involvement by several weeks to months. Symmetrical involvement of large or small joints is typical. The WBC, ESR, and CRP usually are briskly elevated. Rheumatoid factor is negative and antinuclear antibodies generally are not seen. Oligoarthritis is characterized by involvement of one to four joints within the first 6 months of disease; iridocyclitis often is associated. Polyarthritis is inflammation of five or more joints during the first 6

BOX 24-1. Causes of Limb Pain and/or Limp in Children

INFECTIOUS DISEASES
Bacterial arthritis
Viral arthritis
Mycoplasma arthritis
Mycobacterial arthritis
Fungal arthritis
Lyme disease
Disseminated *Neisseria gonorrhoeae*
Hepatitis B infection
Subacute bacterial endocarditis
Psoas/obturator internus muscle abscess
Spinal/paraspinal infection
Osteomyelitis
Skin/soft-tissue infection

POSTINFECTIOUS/ REACTIVE DISEASES
Acute rheumatic fever
Enteric/sexually transmitted infection
Neisseria meningitidis
Haemophilus influenzae b
Immunization
Transient (toxic) synovitis

NEOPLASTIC DISEASES
Bone/soft-tissue tumors
Leukemia/lymphoma
Metastatic neuroblastoma

HEMATOLOGIC DISEASES
Sickle-cell anemia
Hemophilia

RHEUMATIC DISEASES
Juvenile idiopathic arthritis (JIA)
Systemic lupus erythematosus (SLE)
Spondyloarthropathy
Dermatomyositis

VASCULITIS
Henoch–Schönlein purpura
Serum sickness
Kawasaki disease

ORTHOPEDIC CONDITIONS
Trauma
Congenital hip dislocation/ dysplasia
Slipped capital femoral epiphysis (SCFE)
Legg–Calvé–Perthes disease
Osgood–Schlatter disease
Chondromalacia patellae
Osteochondritis dissecans
Foreign-body synovitis
Physical overuse syndromes

MISCELLANEOUS CONDITIONS
Inflammatory bowel disease (IBD)
Reflex sympathetic dystrophy
Familial Mediterranean fever
Behçet disease
Sarcoidosis
Neurologic/neuromuscular disease
Fibromyalgia syndrome
Psychogenic disorders

TABLE 24-1. Diseases Associated with Joint Pain

Etiology	Joints Involved	Associated Findings	Laboratory Studies	Ancillary Studies
Pyogenic arthritis	Any joint, more often joints of lower extremities, usually monoarticular	Fever, joint pain, redness, swelling, decreased range of motion	Elevated WBC, CRP, ESR. Synovial fluid WBC >50,000/mm^3, predominantly PMN. Blood or joint fluid cultures may be positive	Joint space widening. US shows fluid in joint space
Transient synovitis	Unilateral hip	Recent viral infection, afebrile or low-grade fever, decreased range of motion of hip joint	CBC <12,000/mm^3. ESR <40 mm/hour. CRP <2 mg/dL	US shows fluid in joint space, cannot differentiate infected versus noninfected fluid
Reactive arthritis	Usually large joints of lower extremities, occasionally small joints, wrists, and elbows. Sacroiliac joint involvement in adults	Enteric infection, sexually transmitted diseases, occasionally *Streptococcus pyogenes*, *Neisseria meningitidis*. Urethritis, mucous membrane ulcers, conjunctivitis may be present	Elevated ESR, CRP. Synovial fluid WBC <50,000 cells/mm^3	HLA-B27-positive
Juvenile idiopathic arthritis (JIA):				
Systemic	Large or small joints, symmetrically	High fever, evanescent rash, hepatosplenomegaly, lymphadenopathy	Elevated WBC, ESR and CRP. RF and ANA are negative	
Oligoarthritis	Involvement of ≤4 joints within the first 6 months of illness	Iridocyclitis can be present		
Polyarthritis	Involvement of >4 joints within the first 6 months of illness		Subdivided into RF-positive and RF-negative forms	
Systemic lupus erythematosus	Painful symmetric arthritis involving 2 or more joints, may be migratory	Fever, malar or discoid rash, photosensitivity, oral ulcers, serositis, neurologic abnormalities	Abnormal urinalysis (casts, proteinuria), leukopenia, anemia, thrombocytopenia. Positive anti-DNA or anti-Sm antibody	Radiograph can show pleural effusion. ECG can show pericardial effusion
Acute rheumatic fever	Painful, migratory polyarthritis	Fever, carditis, erythema marginatum, chorea, subcutaneous nodules	Elevated ESR, CRP. Evidence of *Streptococcus pyogenes* infection (positive culture, ASO titer, or anti-DNase)	Abnormal ECG

ANA, antinuclear antibodies; anti-Sm, antismooth muscle; CRP, C-reactive protein; ECG, electrocardiogram; ESR, erythrocyte sedimentation rate; HLA, human leukocyte antigen; PMN, polymorphonuclear cells; RF, rheumatoid factor; US, ultrasound; WBC, white blood cell count.

months of illness and is further divided into rheumatoid factor-negative or -positive forms. SLE is a multisystem autoimmune disease often associated with arthralgia and arthritis. Although children of any age can develop SLE, it most commonly develops in females around the time of puberty or during pregnancy. Children and adolescents can come to medical attention with constitutional symptoms of fatigue, weight loss, hair loss, lymphadenopathy, and hepatosplenomegaly. Nonerosive painful, symmetric arthritis involving two or more joints is seen commonly. Criteria for diagnosis of SLE include the presence of at least four of the following: (1) malar rash; (2) discoid rash; (3) photosensitivity; (4) oral ulcers; (5) arthritis; (6) serositis (pleural or pericardial effusion); (7) renal dysfunction (proteinuria or cellular casts); (8) neurologic derangement; (9) hematologic disorder (anemia, leukopenia, lymphopenia, or thrombocytopenia); (10) presence of anti-DNA antibody or anti-smooth muscle antibody; and (11) presence of antinuclear antibody.[6,7]

Acute rheumatic fever is a nonsuppurative complication of *S. pyogenes* infection.[8,9] Diagnosis is based on clinical and laboratory findings. Exquisitely painful migratory polyarthritis typically involving the elbows, knees, and ankles is a major criterion for diagnosis of ARF. Arthritis occurs early in the course of illness and does not result in chronic joint disease. Other major criteria of ARF include carditis, erythema marginatum, chorea, and subcutaneous nodules. Minor criteria of ARF include fever, arthralgia, elevated ESR, or CRP, and prolonged P-R interval on

electrocardiogram. Two major criteria of ARF or one major and two minor criteria plus laboratory evidence of a preceding *S. pyogenes* infection are necessary to establish the diagnosis of ARF. Chorea alone can be used to diagnose ARF if other causes have been ruled out.

Hip and knee pain also can be the result of noninfectious and noninflammatory structural abnormalities. Hip pain in boys 2 to 12 years old (mean 7 years) can be secondary to Legg–Calvé–Perthes (LCP) disease. LCP occurs when blood supply to the proximal femoral epiphysis is disrupted, resulting in necrosis and infarction of the femoral epiphysis. Predisposing factors are not completely known but cardiolipin antibodies and thrombophilic coagulation disorders increase the risk of LCP.[10] The most common clinical complaint is limp or vague chronic pain in the groin or anterior thigh. Findings include antalgic gait (shortened stance and prolonged swing phase), muscle spasm, and mild limitation range of motion of the hip. Diagnosis is made by plain radiographs of the hip and pelvis.

Slipped capital femoral epiphysis (SCFE) also must be considered.[11] SCFE occurs when there is displacement of the proximal femur head anterolaterally and superiorly. Sometimes there is a history of associated trauma or chronic pain. Pain often is referred to the anterior thigh or knee. Affected adolescents often are obese but SCFE can occur in children of normal weight. Both hips are involved in a substantial number of cases. Physical signs of an acute slip include severe pain when range of motion is attempted.

PART II Clinical Syndromes and Cardinal Features of Infectious Diseases: Approach to Diagnosis and Initial Management

SECTION B Cardinal Symptom Complexes

A child with a chronic stable SCFE complains of vague intermittent dull aching pain involving the hip and groin over a period of several weeks. Diagnosis is made by plain radiographs of the hips and pelvis.

Knee pain can be caused by a variety of processes, including Osgood–Schlatter disease, patellofemoral pain syndrome, and osteochondritis dissecans. Osgood–Schlatter disease is an inflammatory disorder of the proximal tibial physis where the patellar tendon inserts on the tibia. Pain is most pronounced over the tibial tubercle. Osteochondritis dissecans of the knee occurs when an area of bone adjacent to cartilage separates. The cause is unclear but possibly is related to repetitive trauma.[12] Children complain of nonspecific aching knee pain exacerbated by exercise. Tenderness of the anterior medial aspect of the knee can be noted. Plain radiography shows lesions most often in the medial distal femoral condyle. Patellofemoral knee syndrome is one of the most common causes of knee pain. Pain may be the result of trauma to the patella or peripatellar tissues, overuse, or abnormal patellar tracking. Risk factors include quadriceps weakness and tightness of patellar soft tissue.[13] Symptoms include dull aching pain during activity and with prolonged sitting, joint stiffness, and crepitus. Diagnosis is based upon physical examination.

Other causes of joint pain in children include hematologic malignancies and trauma.

Diseases Involving Bone

Infectious Causes

Osteomyelitis is an important cause of limb pain in children (see Chapter 78, Osteomyelitis). Osteomyelitis in children generally is caused by hematogenous dissemination of bacteria to the bony metaphysis. Infection usually is well localized. Multifocal bone involvement is reported in infants. Most cases of osteomyelitis involve the long bones. However, a substantial number of bone infections involve bones in the pelvis. Pelvic osteomyelitis can be difficult to diagnose, since pain often is poorly localized and may be referred to the hip, groin, or buttock.[14] Onset of fever and bone pain generally is acute, although in some cases fever can be low grade with intermittent bone pain evolving over a few weeks. Children can come to medical attention with limp or extremity pain. Physical examination can reveal tenderness, redness, warmth, and swelling over the affected bone. Children with pelvic osteomyelitis have pain upon compression of the bones of the pelvis. A draining fistula can occur in patients with chronic osteomyelitis. Plain radiographs in acute osteomyelitis show deep soft-tissue swelling within a few days after onset of symptoms. Changes consistent with bone destruction typically are not visible for 2 or 3 weeks after onset of symptoms. Bone scan or MRI is useful for early diagnosis of osteomyelitis. WBC, CRP, and ESR are frequently elevated and blood culture often is positive.

Noninfectious Causes

Noninfectious causes of bone pain include trauma (accidental and nonaccidental), stress fractures, "growing pains," malignancies, and hemoglobinopathies. Trauma generally is diagnosed by history. "Growing pains" are characterized by bilateral leg pain typically occurring at night, with no symptoms during the day. Malignant tumors associated with bone pain include osteosarcoma, Ewing sarcoma, and hematologic malignancies such as lymphoma and leukemia.[15,16] Night pain severe enough to awaken a child from sleep, diffuse or migratory bone pain, and pain out of proportion to findings on physical examination raise concern for a malignant process. Vaso-occlusive crises in patients with sickle-cell disease manifest with fever and bone pain and can be difficult to differentiate from osteomyelitis. Finally, chronic recurrent multifocal osteomyelitis (CRMO) can be a cause of limb pain. CRMO is characterized by periodic episodes of bone pain and fever. CRMO may be associated with febrile neutrophilic dermatosis and pustulosis palmaris and plantaris.[17]

Muscle Diseases

Infectious Causes

Pyomyositis is a bacterial infection of skeletal muscle that can cause limb pain, particularly in the lower extremities.[18,19] Muscle infection probably occurs when bacteria are seeded hematogenously to injured muscle. The most common bacterial causes of pyomyositis are *S. aureus* and *S. pyogenes*, although a number of gram-negative and anaerobic organisms also can infect muscle. Presentation can be subacute and symptoms include fever, pain, swelling of the affected extremity, and limp (if the lower extremity is involved). Initial symptoms of pyomyositis include malaise and cramping muscle pain. The overlying skin can appear normal; the muscle involved feels firm on palpation. As the infection progresses, abscesses form in the muscle and the affected area becomes more tender, red, and swollen. Untreated, pyomyositis can progress to septicemia, shock, and, rarely, death. The WBC, ESR, and CRP generally are elevated. The causative bacteria are usually isolated from abscess culture; blood cultures also can be positive, and persistent bloodstream infection can occur especially with *S. aureus*. Ultrasound, CT, and MRI have been used to diagnose and determine the extent of infection. The differential diagnosis of pyomyositis includes cellulitis, fasciitis, osteomyelitis, pyogenic arthritis, thrombophlebitis or deep-vein thrombosis (all which can coexist with pyomyositis), muscle strain, malignancy, or compartment syndrome.

Viral infection of muscles also can cause inflammation and severe pain. Viruses most commonly reported include influenza, enteroviruses, and human immunodeficiency virus. Myositis associated with influenza infection is manifest as acute pain and tenderness of the gastrocnemius and soleus muscles, making it difficult for the patient to walk.[20,21] Symptoms appear as influenza infection is resolving. On physical examination localized tenderness and swelling of calf muscles are noted. Serum creatinine kinase levels are elevated. Rhabdomyolysis occurs in rare circumstances and is more common in girls and with influenza A infection.

Parasitic causes of myositis include *Trichinella* spp., *Taenia solium* (cysticercosis), and *Toxoplasma gondii*[22] (see Chapter 77, Myositis, Pyomyositis, and Necrotizing Fasciitis).

Noninfectious Causes

Noninfectious illnesses that are associated with muscle inflammation generally present less acutely than infections of muscles. Dermatomyositis is nonsuppurative inflammation of striated muscle and is the most frequently diagnosed inflammatory myopathy in children.[23,24] Onset of illness is insidious and symmetrical weakness of proximal muscle groups, rather than pain, usually is the presenting symptom. The illness is associated with a characteristic malar rash and/or blue purple discoloration of the upper eyelids. The skin over extensor surfaces of joints can be scaly and erythematous. Affected muscles often are stiff and tender to palpation. Associated clinical findings include joint contractures, dysphagia, and cardiac arrhythmias. Serum creatinine kinase levels are elevated. Diagnosis is confirmed by electromyography; muscle biopsy typically reveals perivascular inflammation.

Fibromyalgia syndrome is a chronic pain syndrome characterized by chronic musculoskeletal pain in the absence of any other underlying medical condition or elevation of serum inflammatory markers.[25] Criteria for diagnosing fibromyalgia syndrome are not well defined in children or adolescents. In adults, symptoms include diffuse musculoskeletal pain in at least three areas of the body for at least 3 months, and a physical examination showing pain over at least 11 of 18 previously defined trigger points. Associated symptoms include nonrestorative sleep, fatigue, chronic anxiety, chronic headache, the feeling of soft-tissue swelling, irritable bowel syndrome, extremity numbness, and modulation of pain by stress, weather, or physical activity.

Diseases of Soft Tissue and Fascia

Limb pain can be the result of cellulitis or infections involving the deeper levels of the dermis and superficial muscle fascia. The most serious of these infections is necrotizing fasciitis.[26-29] Necrotizing fasciitis is a bacterial infection that spreads rapidly along fascial planes, causing necrosis, thrombosis, and extensive tissue damage. Bacterial causes of necrotizing fasciitis include methicillin-susceptible and methicillin-resistant *S. aureus*, *S. pyogenes*, gram-negative bacteria, and anaerobic organisms, including *Clostridium* spp. and *Bacteroides* spp. Infection can be polymicrobial. Predisposing factors include trauma, burns, omphalitis, varicella infection, and immunosuppression. Most patients with *S. aureus* or *S. pyogenes* previously were healthy. Symptoms are rapid in onset and the patient often appears to have pain out of proportion to findings on physical examination. The patient can have high fever and tachycardia and appear very uncomfortable. Blisters or bullae can be present over the affected area and skin can appear dusky and the underlying tissue is exquisitely tender. Crepitus is present in some cases. Untreated, infection spreads rapidly, progressing to hypotension, shock, and multisystem organ failure. Diagnosis requires a high index of suspicion. WBC >15,000 cells/mm^3 and serum sodium less than 135 mmol/L may help distinguish necrotizing fasciitis from cellulitis.[30] One group of investigators has developed a laboratory scoring system of risk indicators for necrotizing fasciitis using CRP, WBC, hemoglobin, serum sodium levels, serum creatinine, and glucose to estimate risk of necrotizing fasciitis.[31] This scoring system needs prospective validation. MRI is the preferred imaging modality for ascertaining involvement of the fascia. Computed tomography is somewhat less sensitive but may be available more readily and expeditious for a critically ill patient.[28] Biopsy of the affected area is useful in determining depth of infection. Management of necrotizing fasciitis involves surgical debridement, empiric broad-spectrum antibiotics, and supportive care in an intensive care unit. The differential diagnosis includes pyomyositis and cellulitis.

BACK PAIN

Back pain is a common complaint in children, particularly in adolescents,[32,33] and can have multiple etiologies including uncommon but serious problems such as primary infection or tumor (Box 24-2). Infection can be present in the disk space, vertebral body, epidural space, or a paravertebral or psoas muscle (Table 24-2). Mild trauma may be a predisposing factor but frequently none is determined. Upper-back or neck pain can be associated with meningitis, retropharyngeal abscess, or Ludwig angina.

Infectious Causes

Diskitis

Diskitis is inflammation of the intervertebral disk and the vertebral body endplates (see Chapter 78, Diskitis). Children under the age of 6 years are affected most often.[34] The rich vascular anastomosis between vertebral bodies in the young child may account for the higher incidence of inflammation localized to the disk space and vertebral endplates with relative sparing of vertebral body. Infection and destruction of the vertebral body are more frequent in older patients. Diskitis usually involves the lower thoracic or lumbar spine. *S. aureus* is most frequently isolated when cultures are positive, although *Kingella kingae*, enteric gram-negative bacteria, and *S. pneumoniae* occasionally have been isolated from blood or disk space cultures. Clinical findings in children with diskitis vary depending on age. Symptoms are subacute and increase in severity over several days. The young child is likely to manifest nonspecific signs of irritability or refusal to walk.[35] Older children may be able to localize pain to their back, or complain of abdominal symptoms, leg pain, or hip pain. On physical examination, the child may refuse to walk or walk with a limp. Hip flexion causes pain. Loss of normal lordosis of the spine is typical. Plain radiographs of the back are normal initially,

---

> **BOX 24-2.** Causes of Back Pain in Children
>
> **INFECTIOUS DISEASES**
> Diskitis
> Vertebral osteomyelitis
> Spinal epidural abscess
> Sacroiliac joint infection
> Paraspinal myositis/abscess
>
> **RHEUMATIC DISEASES**
> Juvenile ankylosing spondylitis
>
> **MECHANICAL DISORDERS**
> Muscle strain
> Spondylolysis/spondylolisthesis
> Scheuermann disease
> Herniated nucleus pulposus
>
> **HAMARTOMATOUS AND NEOPLASTIC DISEASES**
> Osteoid osteoma
> Osteoblastoma
> Aneurysmal bone cyst
> Hemangioma
> Eosinophilic granuloma
> Ewing sarcoma
> Lymphoma, leukemia
> Glioma
> Neurofibroma
> Ganglioneuroma
> Neuroblastoma

---

but after approximately 2 to 4 weeks, narrowing of the affected disk and irregularity of the vertebral endplates are observed. ESR and CRP usually are elevated modestly. Blood cultures usually are negative, but should be obtained as a positive culture will help guide antibiotic therapy.

Vertebral Osteomyelitis

Infection of the vertebral bodies is relatively rare in children compared with adults.[36] Infection is the result of hematogenous seeding or spread from contiguous infection of muscle or soft tissue.[37] *S. aureus* is isolated most commonly, although infections with gram-negative enteric bacteria are reported. If the process appears chronic, infection with *Mycobacterium tuberculosis* should be considered. Children with vertebral osteomyelitis generally have fever. Pain can be localized to the affected area of the back or referred to the chest, abdomen, and legs. Spasm of paraspinous muscles often is present as is loss of normal curvature of the spine. The neurologic examination is abnormal in some cases. Blood culture is positive in 30% of cases and WBC, ESR, and CRP often are elevated. Plain radiographs or MRI show involvement of the disk space and also destruction of adjacent vertebral bodies. If the blood culture is negative, biopsy of the affected vertebral body should be considered.

Spinal Epidural Abscess

Spinal epidural abscess is a rare but potentially catastrophic infection in children.[38] Most epidural abscesses are located posteriorly in the thoracic and lumbar spine and result from hematogenous seeding.[39] Anterior epidural spinal abscesses also can result from extension of infection from a vertebral body or disk space, or from the retropharyngeal or retroperitoneal space. Predisposing factors include trauma, previous spinal surgery, and immunodeficiency. Epidural abscesses have been reported in young children with congenital abnormalities such as a neuroenteric fistula[40] or Currarino triad (congenital sacral abnormality, anorectal

PART II Clinical Syndromes and Cardinal Features of Infectious Diseases: Approach to Diagnosis and Initial Management

SECTION B Cardinal Symptom Complexes

TABLE 24-2. Diseases Associated with Back Pain

	Clinical Features	Clinical Findings	Laboratory Studies	Ancillary Studies
Diskitis	Children <6 years. Subacute presentation. Nonspecific signs: refusal to walk, difficulty sitting, abdominal pain	Low-grade fever, limp, pain with hip flexion, loss of normal spine lordosis	Elevated ESR and CRP. Blood cultures or disk space cultures are rarely positive	After 2–4 weeks plain radiographs show narrowing of disk space and irregularity of vertebral endplate
Vertebral osteomyelitis	Older children. Signs can be subacute	Fever, pain in back, chest, abdomen; tenderness over involved vertebral body, paraspinous muscle spasm; loss of normal spine curvature; neurologic deficits in 15–20%	Elevated ESR and CRP. Blood cultures positive in 30%	Plain radiographs show narrowing of affected disk space and lucency of the affected vertebral bodies. MRI delineates extent of disease
Spinal epidural abscess	Anterior abscess results from spread of vertebral body or disk space infection. Posterior abscess results from hematogenous source. History can include surgery to spine, trauma, immune dysfunction, congenital anomaly of spine	Fever, back pain, malaise, limp; as infection progresses: radicular nerve pain, muscle weakness, bowel and bladder dysfunction; soft-tissue swelling over back	Elevated WBC, ESR and CRP. Blood and abscess cultures positive	MRI delineates extent of abscess, bone, or muscle involvement
Psoas muscle abscess	Primary abscess results from hematogenous source. Secondary abscess results from underlying bowel pathology	Fever, abdominal pain, hip pain, limp, and back pain; psoas sign; if abscess is large, a mass may be palpated in the abdomen	Elevated WBC, ESR, and CRP	Abdominal US or CT can confirm the diagnosis

CRP, C-reactive protein; CT, computed tomography; ESR, erythrocyte sedimentation rate; MRI, magnetic resonance imaging; US, ultrasound; WBC, white blood cell count.

malformation, and a presacral mass).[41] *S. aureus* is most often isolated but other gram-positive, gram-negative, and anaerobic organisms have been identified from culture of abscess material.

Initial clinical findings include back pain, malaise, fever, and difficulty walking. As the abscess increases in size, sensory and motor abnormalities typically appear. Untreated, radicular nerve pain, muscle weakness, and bladder or bowel dysfunction can develop. Local tenderness may be noted and, in young children, soft-tissue swelling over the lower back may be observed. Blood cultures are positive in 60% of cases and the WBC count usually is elevated. Diagnosis is made by gadolinium-enhanced MRI. Patients should be managed with a pediatric neurosurgeon since surgical decompression is necessary urgently in most cases to prevent sequelae.

Muscle Abscess

Psoas muscle abscess can cause back pain, limp, hip pain, or abdominal pain.[42,43] Psoas muscle abscess is classified as primary or secondary. Primary abscess is more common in children compared with adults and occurs without an obvious intra-abdominal focus of infection. Most primary psoas muscle abscesses are caused by *S. aureus*, although older reports emphasize the importance of *M. tuberculosis*. Secondary psoas abscesses arise as a complication of gastrointestinal conditions (e.g., appendicitis or IBD) or pelvic, renal, or urologic infection. Inflammation of the psoas muscle can result in pain elicited on extension of the thigh ("psoas sign"), which may not be useful consistently, particularly in the young, frightened, irritable child.[42] If the abscess is large, an abdominal mass may be palpated. Inflammatory markers and WBC count generally are elevated. Diagnosis can by confirmed by ultrasound or CT.

Noninfectious Causes

Spondylosis is a defect in the lamina of the vertebra between the posterior articular facets, usually at L4 or L5.[44,45] This defect may occur as a result of trauma or genetic predisposition. When the defect is bilateral, the vertebral body can slip forward (spondylolisthesis). Patients complain of low-back pain and leg pain. Lumbar flexion and extension are limited and hyperextension of

the lumbar spine exacerbates pain. Muscle spasm of the hamstring and paravertebral muscles can be present. Standing lateral and supine oblique radiographs of the lower back are diagnostic.[45]

Scheuermann kyphosis manifests in late childhood and is hypothesized to result from defects in ossification of the anterior portion of the vertebral body or vertebral body wedging due to abnormal biomechanical stress.[46] Progressive wedging of the vertebral body produces kyphosis. Back pain is more common in adults than in adolescents. On physical examination an angular deformity of the back is noted when the patient bends forward. With postural kyphosis, the back deformity is more rounded and less angular. Diagnosis is made by anteroposterior and lateral radiographs of the back.

Children with malignant spinal cord tumors present with back pain that typically is worse at night,[33,35] abnormal gait, and scoliosis. Tumors are classified by location. Intramedullary tumors generally are located in the cervical region of the spinal cord. Lymphoma, neuroblastoma, and sarcomas can metastasize to extramedullary sites, in either intradural or extradural locations. Neurologic abnormalities, including muscle weakness and sensory deficits, commonly are seen.[35,47] Deep tendon reflexes can be diminished at the level of tumor infiltration and increased below the level of the lesion. Bowel and bladder function can be impaired. Although plain radiographs show vertebral body destruction, MRI generally is used for diagnosis.

CHEST PAIN

Most children who present with chest pain have either a musculoskeletal cause of pain or the etiology is never determined (Box 24-3).[48–50] Musculoskeletal symptoms often are a result of trauma or strain. Infection involving the muscles or bones of the chest wall, lungs, heart, or mediastinum can cause chest pain. Less common causes of chest pain include other types of pulmonary disease, gastrointestinal disease and, in fewer than 10% of cases, cardiac disease (Table 24-3).

Bony and Cartilaginous Causes

Osteomyelitis of the ribs or sternum is uncommon but causes chest pain. Extension of infection from the lung with organisms

MUSCULOSKELETAL DISORDERS

Costochondritis
Muscle strain/trauma
Slipping-rib syndrome
Tietze syndrome
Precordial catch
Gynecomastia

CARDIAC DISEASES

Myocarditis
Pericarditis
Endocarditis
Dysrhythmia
Mitral valve prolapse
Hypertrophic cardiomyopathy
Aortic stenosis
Coronary arteritis
Coronary artery anomaly
Coronary artery atherosclerosis

RESPIRATORY DISORDERS

Pneumonia
Pleuritis
Pleural effusion
Asthma
Pneumomediastinum
Pneumothorax
Cough

GASTROINTESTINAL DISORDERS

Gastroesophageal reflux
Esophagitis
Gastritis
Esophageal spasm
Esophageal foreign body
Caustic ingestion

MISCELLANEOUS CONDITIONS

Shingles (varicella zoster)
Pleurodynia
Sickle-cell crisis
Hyperventilation
Cocaine abuse
Psychogenic
Idiopathic

such as *Aspergillus* spp. *or Actinomyces* spp. occasionally can cause infection of the contiguous bones and soft tissue.

Bacterial pyomyositis and necrotizing fasciitis occasionally involve muscle and fascial tissue of the chest wall.

Enterovirus infection (usually coxsackieviruses or echoviruses) can cause inflammation of the intercostal muscles, upper abdominal muscles, and pleura. The patient often has nonspecific symptoms of a viral illness, fever, and acute onset of sharp chest or abdominal pain. Pain is worse with inspiration and cough. Diagnosis is made by identifying virus in respiratory secretions or stool.[51,52]

Costochondritis is an inflammatory process involving the costochondral or costosternal joints. Rarely, biopsy and culture of cartilage reveal a bacterial pathogen. Patients manifest anterior chest wall pain and tenderness over the costochondral junction of affected ribs. In contrast to Tietze syndrome, swelling, erythema, and warmth generally are not noted. The sedimentation rate can be elevated. Plain radiographs are normal or show soft-tissue swelling, and occasionally cartilage calcification and destruction.

Tietze syndrome is distinguished from costochondritis by the presence of swelling in the area of pain.[53] It is not often reported in children, being more common in the second to fourth decade of life. The etiology is unknown and symptoms resolve over time with supportive care. Usually only one site of swelling and tenderness is noted. Because of the rarity of this diagnosis in children, other causes of anterior chest pain and swelling, such as tumor, soft-tissue infection, or osteomyelitis, must be excluded.

Pulmonary Causes

Pulmonary causes of chest pain include pneumonia[54] and reactive airways disease. Patients with pneumonia usually are febrile, tachypneic, and may have pleural effusion, pneumothorax, or pneumomediastinum. Signs and symptoms of pulmonary disease include decreased breath sounds, dullness to percussion, rales, rhonchi, wheezes, and, rarely, chest wall crepitus.

Pulmonary embolus is rare but should be suspected in patients with any predisposing factor: central venous catheter, methicillin-resistant *S. aureus* infections, obesity, surgery or trauma, cancer, pregnancy, use of oral contraceptives, or inherited hypercoagulable state.[55,56] History of previous venous thrombosis also is a risk factor. Symptoms of pulmonary embolus include sudden onset of dyspnea, pleuritic chest pain, cough, and hemoptysis. Findings on physical examination include tachypnea and tachycardia, rales, and an audible S4 and a loud S2 heart sound. Chest radiographic findings are nonspecific. A number of tests have been utilized to diagnose pulmonary embolus, including serum D-dimer levels, ventilation/perfusion scanning, pulmonary angiography, helical CT, and MR angiography.

Cardiac Causes

Pericarditis with pericardial effusion caused by bacterial, viral, fungal, or inflammatory disease is often associated with chest pain. Pain can be located over the precordium or referred to the neck, shoulder, or left arm. Pain often is relieved if the child bends forward. Physical examination reveals distant heart sounds (if a large effusion is present) and a pericardial friction rub. Pulsus paradoxus is seen with cardiac tamponade. Echocardiogram is used to assess pericardial disease.

Myocardial infarction is rare in childhood.[57] Myocardial ischemia may occur as a result of anatomic or acquired heart lesions or arrhythmias. Anatomic lesions are often associated with a heart murmur. Myocardial ischemia can be seen with acquired heart disease caused by ARF, endocarditis, or viral myocarditis, trauma, or cocaine abuse. Children with Kawasaki disease and coronary artery aneurysms are at risk for coronary artery thrombosis with subsequent myocardial infarction. Symptoms of myocardial infarction in children may be nonspecific, with young children unable to describe the character of pain. Presenting symptoms include shock, vomiting, irritability, dyspnea, or abdominal pain. Older children are more likely to complain specifically of squeezing chest pain that may or may not radiate and shortness of breath. Diagnosis is made by electrocardiogram changes which include ventricular arrhythmias, ST segment changes, and wide Q waves. Elevation of cardiac enzymes is noted in most cases, but is not as reliable an indicator of myocardial ischemia in children as in adults.

Other Causes

Gastrointestinal causes of chest pain include gastrointestinal reflux, presence of an esophageal foreign body, and caustic ulceration from oral medications (especially tetracyclines and nonsteroidal anti-inflammatory drugs) taken without sufficient fluid or just before recumbency.

Marfan disease is an inherited disorder of connective tissue. Associated clinical findings include a history of subluxation of the lens of the eye, increased height and arm span, narrow fingers and toes, hypermobility of the joints, anterior chest wall deformities, and scoliosis. The most common cardiovascular complication is

PART II Clinical Syndromes and Cardinal Features of Infectious Diseases: Approach to Diagnosis and Initial Management

SECTION C Oral Infections and Upper and Middle Respiratory Tract Infections

TABLE 24-3. Diseases Associated with Chest Pain

	Clinical Features	Clinical Findings	Laboratory Studies	Laboratory Studies
Osteomyelitis	Infection of the ribs or sternum uncommon; can result from contiguous infection from lungs (fungal or actinomycoses), or previous surgery or trauma	Fever, tenderness, erythema, and warmth over affected bone, sinus tract or poorly healing surgical site	Elevated WBC, ESR, CRP. Blood or tissue cultures can be positive	Plain radiographs show bone destruction. Bone scan can be useful if multifocal disease suspected
Pleurodynia	Acute onset of sharp chest or upper abdominal pain. Preceding respiratory or enteric illness	Fever, pain worse on inspiration, mild chest wall tenderness	Enterovirus can be identified in respiratory secretions or stool	
Costochondritis	Acute or subacute onset of anterior chest wall pain	Tenderness over the costochondral or costosternal junctions (usually 2nd to 5th costal cartilages); unilateral	Elevated ESR in some patients	Radiograph normal; occasionally soft-tissue swelling at costochondral junction or cartilage calcification
Pneumonia	Acute onset. Preceding URI, cough	Fever, hypoxia, tachypnea, decreased breath sounds, dullness to percussion, rales, rhonchi	Elevated WBC, ESR, CRP. Blood and sputum cultures can be positive	Radiograph abnormal
Pulmonary embolus	Risk factors include the presence of a central venous catheter, immobility (and other, discussed in text). Acute onset of dyspnea, pleuritic chest pain, cough	Tachypnea, tachycardia, rales, loud S2 and S4	Positive D-dimers	Radiograph nonspecifically abnormal
Pericarditis	Precordial pain, can be referred to neck or arm	Fever, distant heart sounds, pericaridial friction rub; relief of pain if patient bends forward		ST segment elevation, PR segment depression, T wave changes, low voltage with effusion. Radiograph can show increased heart size
Myocardial infarction	Rare in children, usually underlying anatomic heart disease or acquired heart disease (Kawasaki disease)	Hypotension, shortness of breath, cyanosis, anxiety	Elevated cardiac enzymes (reliability in children not well evaluated)	ECG changes: arrhythmias, ST segment changes, wide Q waves
Aortic dissection	Patient may have clinical features of Marfan disease. Acute onset of pain that can radiate to the back	Tachycardia, soft murmur over the aorta, hypotension		Echocardiogram confirms diagnosis

CRP, C-reactive protein; ECG, electrocardiogram; ESR, erythrocyte sedimentation rate; URI, upper respiratory infection; WBC, white blood cell count.

progressive enlargement of the aortic root predisposing to aortic aneurysm, dissection, or rupture.[58] Symptoms of a dissecting aortic aneurysm include sudden onset of substernal chest pain that radiates to the back or shoulders. Findings on physical examination can include a soft murmur over the aorta, tachycardia, hypotension, and poor perfusion. Echocardiography establishes the presence of dilatation of the aortic root and ascending aorta and aortic or mitral valve insufficiency. Spontaneous pneumothorax also can be a feature of Marfan disease and an additional cause of chest pain.

SECTION C: Oral Infections and Upper and Middle Respiratory Tract Infections

25 Infections of the Oral Cavity

Jana Shaw

Normally, the oral cavity is sterile just before birth but becomes colonized shortly thereafter.[1] The mouth has a substantial microflora living in symbiosis with a healthy host. Molecular methods of 16S DNA amplification reveal a tremendously diverse bacterial environment, largely uncharacterized.[2]

ODONTOGENIC INFECTIONS

Tooth Infections

In the healthy oral cavity, *Streptococcus, Peptostreptococcus, Veillonella* species, and diphtheroids account for more than 80% of the total recoverable flora. Quantitative studies indicate that anaerobes occur in numbers as great as eight times those of facultative bacteria. Facultative gram-negative bacilli are uncommon in the healthy child but may be more prominent in seriously ill patients.[3] In addition, certain sites tend to favor certain bacteria. For example, *Streptococcus salivarius* and *Veillonella* species have a predilection for the tongue and buccal mucosa and predominate before eruption of teeth.[4] In contrast *Streptococcus sanguis, Streptococcus mutans* as well as *Actinomyces viscosus* preferentially colonize the tooth surface while *Fusobacterium*, pigmented *Bacteroides,* and anaerobic spirochetes appear to be concentrated in the gingival crevices.[4]

Dental Caries

In the United States, caries are the most common chronic disease of childhood and are five times more common than asthma.[5] Caries of primary teeth commonly are referred to as caries of early childhood.[6]

Plaque-related bacteria colonize the tooth surface and produce a weak acid during their carbohydrate metabolism.[7] Acid production lowers local pH and results in demineralization of the tooth with efflux of calcium, phosphorus, and carbonate.[8] Tooth colonization with cariogenic bacteria is a key factor for development of caries. Bacterial 16S sequence analysis has shown association of *S. mutans* with early stages of caries and progression.[9] With progression there also is loss of microbial community diversity. The major reservoir from which infants acquire *S. mutans* is from their primary caregiver, usually the mother.[10] Caries can affect any part of the tooth. In children, coronal caries typically have been found in the pits and fissures of the occlusal surfaces of molars and premolars. Food retention occurs less frequently at interproximal sites and the gingival margins except in infants who fall asleep with a bottle of milk or juice. In early childhood the disease develops over smooth surfaces. Treatment consists of restoration of the affected tooth augmented by preventive methods such as fluoride treatments, flossing, tooth brushing, meticulous removal of the biofilm, and placement of sealants.

Pericoronitis

Pericoronitis is an acute localized infection associated with operculum of the gum overlying partially erupted teeth or impacted wisdom teeth. The third molars (wisdom teeth) often are affected especially when their eruption is hindered by a lack of space. The tissue around the tooth becomes red, edematous, and tender to touch but the underlying bone usually is not involved. The patient will report continuous pain that ranges from dull to throbbing to intense, often radiating to the mouth, ear, throat, or the floor of the mouth. Other symptoms can include swelling of the cheek, trismus, and dysphagia. Systemic manifestations can include fever, chills, and submandibular, submental or cervical lymphadenopathy. Treatment consists of gentle debridement, irrigation under the operculum and a systemic antibiotic effective against mouth flora, along with incision and drainage if infection spreads into soft tissue.[11]

Pulpitis and Periapical Abscess

Pulpal infection most frequently results from caries. Demineralization and destruction of the enamel is followed by invasion of the pulp to produce localized or generalized *pulpitis*. In early stages of infection patients typically complain of tooth sensitivity to percussion, heat, and cold. Pain stops abruptly when the stimulus is withdrawn. In the late stage of pulpitis the tooth is exquisitely tender to hot stimuli, but cold provides relief. If drainage of the pulp is obstructed, infection progresses rapidly to pulpal necrosis, which leads to *periapical abscess* or invasion of the alveolar bone. The most common organisms isolated are *Bacteroides* spp., anaerobic gram-positive cocci, *Fusobacterium* spp., and *Actinomyces* spp. Facultative isolates include *Streptococcus salivarius*, other α-hemolytic streptococci, and non-hemolytic streptococci. β-Lactamase production is noted in 33% of the *Prevotella* spp.[12] Treatment consists of elimination of infected pulp (root canal treatment) or extraction of the tooth. Antibiotic therapy is indicated if drainage cannot be performed or the infection has spread to surrounding soft tissues. Penicillin usually is adequate; amoxicillin-clavulanate or clindamycin are effective against β-lactamase-producing anaerobic bacteria. Serious complications of periapical infections are rare.[13] However, in some cases the infection spreads, causing abscesses in the submaxillary triangle or in the parapharyngeal or submasseteric space.[11] In the maxilla, periapical infection can manifest in the soft tissues of the face. Infection also can extend to the infratemporal space including the

sinuses and from there to the central nervous system, causing subdural empyema, brain abscess, or meningitis.[13]

Periodontal Infections

Periodontitis is inflammation that extends deep into the tissues and causes loss of supporting connective tissue (periodontium) and alveolar bone. Severe periodontitis can result in loosening of teeth, impaired mastication, and even tooth loss. Bacterial species reproducibly associated with disease include *Porphyromonas gingivalis*, *Tannerella forsythensis*, *Aggregatibacter* (formerly *Actinobacillus*) *actinomycetemcomitans*, and *Treponema denticola*.[14] Histologically, nonprogressive inflammatory foci tend to be composed predominantly of T lymphocytes and macrophages, suggesting that the cell-mediated response can control disease. Destructive lesions are dominated by B lymphocytes and plasma cells, suggesting that humoral immunity is not always effective.[2]

Early-Onset Periodontitis

Juvenile (aggressive) periodontitis is a particularly destructive form of periodontitis seen in adolescents. Its localized form is characterized by rapid bone loss affecting the first molar and incisor teeth. The generalized form is rapidly progressive, affecting other teeth. Plaque is minimal, and specific defects in neutrophil chemotaxis and phagocytosis were demonstrated among 75% of patients. Subgingival cultures have revealed *A. actinomycetemcomitans* and gram-negative capnophilic, and anaerobic bacilli. Treatment consists of systemic antibiotics, tetracycline or metronidazole, combined with local periodontal treatment.

MUCOSAL INFECTIONS

Gingivitis

Gingivitis is the most common periodontal disease during childhood with peak incidence around adolescence.[15] Inflammation is initiated by local irritation and bacterial invasion.[16] Bleeding of the gums after eating or brushing and fetor oris can be early signs of gingivitis. There usually is no pain. Treatment consists of plaque removal and good oral hygiene.[11]

Other Oral Infections and Conditions

Differentiating features of oral infections and other conditions encountered frequently are shown in Tables 25-1 and 25-2.

Herpes Simplex Virus (HSV) Gingivostomatitis

HSV gingivostomatitis is the most recognized viral infection of the oral cavity. Primary infection with HSV-1 occurs throughout childhood, most commonly between the ages of 6 months and 5 years, and during adolescence and results in protective antibodies in up to 90% of all adults.[17,18] In children with primary HSV infection, up to 90% are asymptomatic.[19] Recrudescent disease has been estimated to occur in up to 40% of seropositive individuals in the U.S.[20] HSV infection is ubiquitous and transmitted from symptomatic and asymptomatic people with primary or recurrent infection. Infections with HSV-1 usually result from direct contact with infected oral secretions. The incubation period for HSV infection beyond the neonatal period is usually 2 days to 2 weeks.[21] Primary symptomatic infections are accompanied by fever, lymphadenopathy, malaise, pharyngitis, and anorexia. Gingiva are red, swollen, and bleeding. Small vesicles on the gingiva and anterior lingual and buccal mucosa rapidly rupture giving rise to ulcerations. In primary infection, vesicles appear on the first day of illness in 85% of affected children and can persist for 7–18 days.[22] HSV gingivostomatitis is painful and children commonly refuse to swallow, resulting in drooling. Differential diagnosis includes coxsackievirus infection (herpangina), erythema multiforme, pemphigus vulgaris, acute necrotizing ulcerative gingivitis, and most commonly aphthous stomatitis.

PART II Clinical Syndromes and Cardinal Features of Infectious Diseases: Approach to Diagnosis and Initial Management

SECTION C Oral Infections and Upper and Middle Respiratory Tract Infections

TABLE 25-1. Viral Infections of the Oral Cavity in Immunocompetent Individuals[a]

Agent	Acquisition	Usual Intraoral Site	Oral Manifestations
HERPES SIMPLEX VIRUS TYPE 1 AND 2			
Primary gingivostomatitis	Saliva; direct contact with active lesions (oral, perioral, genital)	Anterior gingiva and mucosa, hard palate, tongue, lips	Vesicles, ulcers covered with yellowish exudates; gingival edema/erythema
Herpes labialis	Saliva; direct contact with active lesions (oral, perioral, genital)	Lips	Vesicles, ulcers and crusting
Recurrent intraoral herpes	HSV reactivation	Gingiva, hard palate	Vesicles, ulcers
Erythema multiforme	HSV reactivation	Buccal and labial mucosa, tongue, lips	Erythematous macules, vesicles, ulcers
VARICELLA ZOSTER VIRUS			
Chickenpox	Saliva, direct contact with active lesions	Hard and soft palate, buccal mucosa, tongue, lips	Vesicles, ulcers
Zoster	VZV reactivation	Palate, lips, tongue, buccal mucosa, gingiva	Unilateral vesicles, ulcers, bone necrosis, tooth exfoliation; pain along trigeminal nerve
EPSTEIN–BARR VIRUS			
Infectious mononucleosis	Saliva	Hard and soft palate, gingiva	Lymphadenopathy, palatal petechiae, gingival necrosis, ulcers, edema of uvula
Oral hairy leukoplakia	Established EBV infection	Lateral borders of the tongue	Vertical white, hyperkeratotic lesions
Burkitt lymphoma	Not known	Maxilla, molar-premolar area	Tumors; loosening and displacement of teeth
Nasopharyngeal carcinoma	Not known	Nasopharynx	Keratinizing squamous carcinoma; non-keratinizing squamous carcinoma; undifferentiated carcinoma
CYTOMEGALOVIRUS	Congenital; breastfeeding; saliva	Teeth	Enamel hypoplasia, dental attrition, discoloration
HUMAN HERPESVIRUS 8	Possibly sexual transmission	Hard and soft palate	Kaposi sarcoma
COXSACKIEVIRUSES			
Hand-foot-mouth disease	Saliva	Buccal and labial mucosa, tongue	Vesicles, ulcers
Herpangina	Saliva	Soft palate	Vesicles, ulcers
HUMAN PAPILLOMAVIRUSES			
Condyloma acuminata	Direct contact with lesions	Tongue, gingiva, labial mucosa, palate	Soft, broad-based papules with a pebble-like surface
Focal epithelial hyperplasia (Heck disease)	Direct contact with lesions; self-inoculation	Alveolar mucosa, lips	Soft, flat, non-pedunculated papules, usually with a pebble-like surface
Squamous cell papilloma	Transformation chronic infection	Uvula, hard and soft palate, tongue, frenulum, lips, buccal mucosa, gingival	Soft, pedunculated, exophytic papules with cauliflower-like surface
Verruca vulgaris	Direct contact with lesions, self-inoculation	Lips, tongue, labial mucosa, gingiva	Firm, broad-based elevated papules with cauliflower-like surface
MOLLUSCUM CONTAGIOSUM	Direct contact with lesion	Lips	Waxy, dome-shaped papules
MEASLES	Saliva, respiratory droplets	Buccal and labial mucosa; teeth	Bluish-white macules surrounded by erythema (Koplik spots); pitted enamel
MUMPS	Saliva, respiratory droplets	Salivary glands	Swelling of salivary glands; erythema and edema of Wharton and Stensen duct openings; oral dryness
RUBELLA	Saliva, respiratory droplets	Hard and soft palate	Petechiae; small dark-red papules (Forchheimer sign)
HEPATITIS C VIRUS	Blood, sexual transmission	Buccal mucosa	Lichen planus

[a]Reproduced from Glick M, Siegel MA. Viral and fungal infections of the oral cavity in immunocompetent patients. Infect Dis Clin North Am 1999:13;817–831.

Complications of HSV gingivostomatitis include dehydration, herpetic whitlow or herpetic keratitis from autoinoculation, and secondary bacteremia with oral flora.[23,24] Recurrent HSV orolabial lesions occurs in one-third of individuals with prior HSV infection. Reactivation lesions typically are found around the gingiva, the hard palate, and vermilion border of the lip ("cold sore"). A prodrome of tingling, burning, and itching occurs 12 to 36 hours prior to the eruption of the vesicles at the site. Viral shedding persisted for a mean of 7 days (range 2–12 days) among 36 untreated immunocompetent children in one study.[22]

Treatment of HSV gingivostomatitis usually is palliative, with hydration and pain control. Topical application of diphenhydramine, aluminum hydroxide and magnesium hydroxide (Maalox), and viscous lidocaine is frequently prescribed. However, their usefulness and benefit have been questioned.[25] Treatment with oral acyclovir during early stages reduced the duration of symptoms, improved healing, and reduced infectivity among 61 children[26] (See Chapter 204, Herpes Simplex Virus). Only one trial in a systematic review showed weak evidence that oral acyclovir offered treatment benefit.[27] In general, most experts would treat patients who come to attention early or who have severe disease. Chronic suppressive therapy is recommended rarely to reduce recurrences, such as in patients with facial, periorbital or ocular lesions or very frequent episodes.[21] Topical acyclovir is ineffective even in immunocompetent hosts, and is not recommended.

Oral Candidiasis (Thrush)

The usual causative agent of oral candidiasis is *Candida albicans*. Affected neonates typically are colonized during passage through the birth canal. Other sources of transmission to neonates include colonized skin of breasts (for breastfed infants), hands, and/or improperly cleaned bottle nipples. *Candida* spp. are asymptomatically carried in the gastrointestinal tract of many healthy children

TABLE 25-2. Oral Mucosal Manifestations of Local and Systemic Infection and Other Conditions

Cause	Lesion	Site	Disease Course/Comment
BACTERIA			
Scarlet fever (*Streptococcus pyogenes*)	Strawberry tongue	Tongue	Reddened edematous papillae project through white coating; coating peels off to leave red glistening tongue with prominent papillae
	Punctiform and petechial lesions	Palate	Intraoral erythema; uvula and free margin of soft palate red and edematous; lips uninvolved
Toxic shock syndrome (*Staphylococcus aureus*)	Intraoral erythema, edema, and desquamation	Lips, all intraoral mucous membranes	Can progress to painful desquamation
Treponema pallidum	Painless ulcer with rolled edges	Anywhere on oral mucous membranes	Primary chancre heals over 5–10 days; followed by systemic manifestations if untreated
Gingivitis	Edema, thickening, erythema, and easy bleeding; usually painless	Gingiva and interdental papillae	Subgingival plaque always present; common in children, particularly during puberty
Acute necrotizing ulcerative gingivitis (ANUG)	Pseudomembranes (necrosis of papillae)	Gingiva	Necrosis of interdental papillae results in marginated, punched-out, eroded appearance; grey necrotic pseudomembranes; fusiform bacilli and spirochetes consistently found
Cystic gingival lesions	Red, cystic lesion, 4–10 mm	Gingival ridge	Infants <10 months with pneumococcal bacteremia
Glossitis	Swollen, red, painful	Tongue	*Streptococcus pyogenes, Staphylococcus aureus, Haemophilus influenzae b*
Uvulitis	Red, edematous	Uvula	*Streptococcus pyogenes, Haemophilus influenzae b;* can cause respiratory compromise
FUNGUS			
Candida species	Pseudomembranes of creamy white plaques on erythematous mucosa	Tongue, gingiva, buccal mucosa; rarely, pharynx, larynx, esophagus; cheilitis	Lesions can be painless, can burn, or can feel sore or dry
Histoplasma capsulatum	Ulcers	Oropharynx	Occurs with subacute or chronic disseminated disease
UNKNOWN			
Kawasaki disease	Strawberry tongue; mucosal erythema; erythema, cracking peeling, bleeding lips	Tongue, oropharynx, lips	Mucositis present in all but atypical forms
Recurrent oral ulcerations (aphthous stomatitis)	Shallow, circular painful ulcer <5 mm on erythematous base with pseudomembrane	Nonkeratinized movable labial and buccal mucosa; tongue and floor of mouth	Healing occurs after 4 days; common (incidence 20%); recurrences 12 times/year; etiology unknown; symptomatic therapy
	Deep ulcers of >5 mm diameter; painful	All areas of oral cavity	Lasts 6 weeks–3 months; heals with scarring (Sutton scarring aphthae)
	Small cluster of vesicles; extremely painful; no erythematous border	Tip and lateral margins of tongue	Herpetiform ulcers with no relationship to HSV
PFAPA syndrome	Small ulcers	Oral mucosa	Syndrome of recurrent fever, aphthous stomatitis, pharyngitis, and cervical adenitis; affects children <5 years; recurrence every 2–9 weeks
Gangrenous stomatitis (noma)	Focal, destructive lesions	Gingiva and deeper structures	Rare, acute, fulminating in severely debilitated and malnourished children; spirochetes and other anaerobic bacteria may be involved
Cyclic neutropenia and agranulocytosis	Small ulcers	Oral mucosa	
Drug- or radiation-induced stomatitis	Ulcers and pseudomembrane formation; painful	Nonkeratinized labial and buccal mucosae soft palate; floor of mouth; ventral and lateral tongue surfaces	Microbiologic diagnosis important to rule out viral reactivation or bacterial superinfection
Behçet syndrome	Ulcers	Oral mucosa	Multisystem disease that can involve many mucous membranes
Stevens–Johnson syndrome	Macules, papules, vesicles, bullae	Buccal mucosa and vermilion border of the lips; relative sparing of gingivae	Erythema multiforme exudativum; 25% of cases confined to oral mucosa; lesions appear in crops; complete healing 4–6 weeks; can cause recurrent stomatitis and labiitis
Inflammatory bowel disease	Ulcers (aphthous-like)	Oral mucosa	Manifestation of multisystem disease

PFAPA, periodic fever with aphthous stomatitis, pharyngitis, and adenitis.

and premature infants as well as patients treated with antibiotics or who are receiving chemotherapy, radiation therapy, or inhaled glucocorticoids. Thrush that is more than mild, which occurs beyond 6 months of age in the absence of risk factors, should prompt evaluation for HIV infection, cell-mediated immunodeficiency, neutropenia, or other phagocytic defect.[28] The pseudomembranous form of candidiasis is most common and is characterized by white plaques on the buccal mucosa, palate, tongue, or oropharynx. The plaques can be wiped off to reveal a red, raw, painful surface. Many patients with oral candidiasis are asymptomatic. Symptomatic patients can complain of feeling of "cotton" in the mouth, loss of taste, and sometimes pain during eating and swallowing. The diagnosis of oropharyngeal candidiasis usually is suspected clinically and is readily confirmed by scraping the lesions with a tongue depressor and preparing a slide for Gram stain or KOH preparation. Thrush is the most common oral manifestation of HIV, with reported prevalence ranging between 20% and 72%.[29-31] Thrush (which usually is extensive) can be the initial indication of HIV infection in a patient who appears otherwise healthy.[32] Topical agents (nystatin oral suspension or clotrimazole troches) are recommended for initial therapy of oral candidiasis. Systemic therapy, such as with oral fluconazole or itraconazole should be considered for patients with severe disease or those who fail to improve with topical treatment.[33,34]

Acute Necrotizing Ulcerative Gingivitis (ANUG)

ANUG, also known as Vincent disease or trench mouth, has a sudden onset with gingiva showing punched-out crater-like ulcerations, covered with a whitish pseudomembrane, surrounded by a demarcated zone of erythema. Any area of the mouth can be affected. There is spontaneous bleeding and breath has fetid odor. The patient's chief complaint is pain. Bacterial overgrowth of *Borrelia vincenti* and *Bacillus fusiformis* contribute to the infection. However, other factors are believed to contribute to the disease.[35] Penicillin and metronidazole are commonly used systemic therapy in addition to an oral antiseptic rinse such as chlorhexidine.[36]

Periodontitis, Gingivitis, and Mucositis in Immunocompromised Hosts

HSV infection in immunocompromised hosts has a higher risk of dissemination and longer duration of outbreaks and is less responsive to therapy.[37] Complications include esophagitis, tracheobronchitis, pneumonitis, bacteremia, hepatitis, and pancreatitis.[22,23,38-40] Parenteral therapy with acyclovir is given, augmented by topical acyclovir.[41]

Chemotherapy/radiotherapy-induced mucositis is the result of breakdown of the mucosal epithelium, ulceration, and bacterial overgrowth in the presence of granulocytopenia. Gram-negative bacteria or α-hemolytic streptococci are important causes of complicating septicemia in patients with mucositis.[42] A Cochrane systematic review and meta-analysis of randomized trials of nine interventions (allopurinol, aloe vera, amifostine, cryotherapy, IV glutamine, honey, keratinocyte growth factor, laser, and polymixintobramycin-amphotericin antibiotic pastille/paste) showed some statistically significant evidence of benefit (albeit weak) for preventing and reducing severity of mucositis in cancer patients.[43] Trial of a novel drug, palifermin,[44] as well as a randomized control trial of visible-light therapy in hematopoietic stem cell transplant patients also showed benefit.[45]

HIV-Associated Oral Lesions

The pathogenesis of oral lesions in children with HIV is not well characterized. Combination of lymphopenia, low CD4+ lymphocyte counts, humoral dysregulation, and phagocytic defect most likely contribute to the array of infectious complications. In 1992 a European and U.S. expert panel developed a classification system, and diagnostic criteria for HIV-associated lesions.[46] A simplified summary is provided in Box 25-1.

BOX 25-1. Classification of HIV-Associated Oral Lesions[a]

LESIONS STRONGLY ASSOCIATED WITH HIV INFECTION

Candidiasis
  Erythematous
  Pseudomembranous
Hairy leukoplakia
Kaposi sarcoma
Non-Hodgkin lymphoma
Periodontal disease
  Linear gingival erythema
  Necrotizing ulcerative gingivitis
  Necrotizing ulcerative periodontitis

LESIONS LESS COMMONLY ASSOCIATED WITH HIV INFECTION

Bacterial infections (*Mycobacterium avium* complex)
Mycobacterium tuberculosis
Melanotic hyperpigmentation
Necrotizing (ulcerative) stomatitis
Salivary gland disease (xerostomia, swelling of major salivary glands)
Thrombocytopenic purpura
Ulceration (not otherwise specified)
Viral infections (herpes simplex virus, human papillomavirus, varicella-zoster virus)

[a]Modified from Kline WM. Oral manifestations of pediatrics human immunodeficiency virus infection: a review of literature. Pediatrics 1996;97:380–388.

Besides oral candidiasis, parotid enlargement occurs commonly in HIV infection, with prevalence of 47% reported from a large study of HIV-infected children from the U.S.[47] Periodontal disease, hairy leukoplakia, and aphthous ulcers have been reported rarely.[48] Several forms of periodontal disease such as linear gingival erythema and necrotizing ulcerative gingivitis are strongly associated with HIV infection.[33]

COMPLICATIONS OF ODONTOGENIC AND MUCOSAL INFECTIONS

Ludwig Angina

The classic description of Ludwig angina includes rapidly spreading indurated cellulitis of the submandibular and sublingual spaces bilaterally without abscess formation. Infection starts in the floor of the mouth. Dental infection is found in 50% to 90% of reported cases.[11,49] Trauma to the oral cavity, piercing, or laceration preceded infection in a number of reported cases. Clinically, patients demonstrate brawny, board-like swelling in the submandibular spaces that does not pit on pressure. The mouth is held open and the floor is elevated, pushing the tongue to the roof of the mouth. Eating and swallowing are difficult and respiration can be impaired by obstruction of the tongue. Rapid progression can result in edema of the neck and glottis and can precipitate asphyxiation. Fever and toxicity usually are present. Treatment requires high doses of antibiotics active against oral flora, airway monitoring, early intubation or tracheostomy when required, dental care, soft-tissue decompression, and surgical drainage.

Suppurative Jugular Thromblophebitis (Lemierre Disease)

The incidence of Lemierre disease decreased dramatically since its original description by Andre Lemierre in 1936[50] but has had an apparent resurgence. The syndrome includes septic thrombophlebitis of the internal jugular vein (IJV), usually secondary to an acute oropharyngeal infection, and frequently is complicated by blood-stream and metastatic infection. The usual agent is *Fusobacterium necrophorum*; however, *Staphylococcus aureus* and *Streptococcus pyogenes* are occasional causes. Most cases occur in adolescents and young adults with tonsillopharyngitis as the primary infection. Odontogenic infections, sinusitis, and otitis externa have been reported as primary infections in a few patients with Lemierre disease. Infection from the neck can spread hematogenously by septic embolization into the lungs, joints, liver, spleen, or kidneys, as well as rostrally to cause brain and extra-axial infection and intracranial venous thromboses.[51] Patients come to attention with fever, neck pain, swelling and tenderness of the anterior border of the sternocleidomastoid muscle, headache, increased intracranial pressure, torticollis, and stiff neck. Diagnostic methods to detect IJV thrombosis include magnetic resonance venography or contrast-enhanced computed tomography of the neck. Aerobic and anaerobic blood cultures should be collected promptly and properly. The mainstay of treatment is prolonged intravenous antibiotic therapy (3 to 6 weeks) effective against anaerobic organisms. For *Fusobacterium* spp., >95% are susceptible to ampicillin-sulbactam, third-generation cephalosporins, and carbapenems; ≤85% are susceptible to fluoroquinolones and none are susceptible to vancomycin. The role of anticoagulant therapy remains controversial. Mortality remains high (18%) even with appropriate therapy.[51]

INFECTIONS OF THE SALIVARY GLAND

Bilateral asymptomatic enlargement of the parotid gland usually is due to a noninfectious cause. The differential diagnosis includes metabolic and endocrine disorders such as malnutrition (vitamin B6 and C deficiencies), chronic pancreatitis, obesity, cystic fibrosis, thyroid disease, and diabetes mellitus. Infections of the salivary glands (including the parotid) are discussed below.

Acute Suppurative Sialadenitis (ASS)

In contrast to adults, children commonly incur repeated episodes of acute sialadenitis.[52] The parotid gland is affected more commonly than the submandibular gland, and more than one gland can be affected during a single episode.[53] Primary etiology appears to be salivary stasis. Predisposing factors may include calculi, duct stricture, dehydration, infancy, autoimmune disease, and congenital sialectasia. Clinical manifestations include local pain, tenderness, and edema of the soft tissue overlying the affected gland. A purulent discharge can be seen draining from the duct of the involved gland. Most children remain nontoxic during acute episodes.[52] Residual induration and enlargement of the gland can persist for months after the initial infection. Treatment consists of systemic antibiotics, local heat and massage, fluids, and sialagogues. *Staphylococcus aureus* is the most common infectious cause. In addition, direct needle aspiration has confirmed α-hemolytic streptococci, *Haemophilus influenzae*, *S. pyogenes*, *S. pneumoniae*, *Moraxella catarrhalis*, *Escherichia coli*, and anaerobic bacteria as causative.[53,54] Mycobacterial and fungal parotitis also have been described rarely. Acute sialadenitis infrequently progresses to abscess formation. The patient should be monitored closely for spread of infection into contiguous fascial spaces of the neck.[55]

Recurrent parotitis is associated with poor oral hygiene and underlying disease such as abnormal ductal architecture, allergies and IgA deficiency, and HIV.[56–58] *S. pneumoniae* was isolated from parotid gland pus in a patient with HIV infection.[56] Empiric therapy should include a penicillinase-resistant antistaphylococcal antibiotic, as well as consideration of local prevalence of methicillin-resistant *S. aureus*. Purulent discharge from the gland's duct on the buccal mucosa should be cultured to guide antimicrobial therapy.

Neonatal Sialadenitis

Neonatal suppurative sialadenitis is an uncommon but recognizable disease with a prevalence of 3.8/10,000 hospital admissions in one report.[59] Neonatal sialadenitis much more commonly affects the parotid gland than the submandibular gland. Presence of calculi or anatomic deformities of the oral cavity, dehydration, and prematurity are established risk factors in sialadenitis in this age group. Horovitz and co-authors reviewed 12 reports over the previous 30 years, which included 32 cases of neonatal parotitis.[59] Approximately 40% of neonates with parotitis were born prematurely. The most common causative organism was *S. aureus*. Other organisms identified included viridans streptococci, *E. coli*, *Pseudomonas aeruginosa*, and *M. catarrhalis*, peptostreptococci, and coagulase-negative staphylococci. Taken together, facultative gram-positive cocci and gram-negative bacilli caused 94% of infections.[59] Salivary secretions should be cultured and Gram stain obtained. Disease usually is limited to one gland and signs and symptoms of systemic disease may not be present. Physical examination reveals a warm, tender, erythematous mass; pus can be expressed from the parotid/salivary duct. Laboratory test abnormalities are nonspecific. Leukocytosis with neutrophil predominance was found in 70% of the 32 cases reported but sedimentation rate was elevated in only 2 of 10 cases tested.[59] Serum amylase was measured in 9 of 32 cases and was elevated in only 4 (45%) of cases.[60] Adequate hydration and antibiotic therapy was successful in 78% of the cases. If prompt clinical improvement does not occur, surgical intervention is considered. In resistant cases, ultrasonography of the infected gland may demonstrate the presence of an intraparotid abscess.

Viral Parotitis

The most common cause of viral parotitis is mumps virus. The disease is seen most frequently during spring and winter months. The incubation period is 14 to 21 days, and the contagious period includes 1 to 2 days prior to until 5 days after the onset of parotid swelling.[24] The prodrome includes malaise, fever, and sore throat with chills. The major salivary glands become tender. The patient may have trismus and difficulty chewing. The duct orifice may be swollen; saliva is clear. White blood cell count is normal or slightly elevated with lymphocytosis. The diagnosis is based on clinical manifestations, but culture and serologic tests can be used for the diagnosis. Differential diagnosis includes other viral infections such as influenza, parainfluenza 1 and 3, coxsackievirus A and B, echoviruses, Epstein–Barr virus, cytomegalovirus, lymphocytic choriomeningitis virus, HSV-1, HIV, HHV-6, and bacterial causes (see above). Noninfectious causes of parotitis include Sjögren syndrome and metabolic, endocrine, and neoplastic disorders. People with parotitis lasting for more than 2 days should undergo diagnostic testing to confirm mumps infection.[61] Viral cultures of Stensen duct fluid, saliva, or throat washing should be obtained within 1 to 3 days after the onset of parotitis to maximize recovery of virus. Elevated mumps-specific IgM antibody is diagnostic, but a negative IgM antibody test should lead to repeated testing 2 to 3 weeks after the onset of symptoms. A delayed IgM response has been documented in patients with confirmed mumps, especially among an immunized population.[62] Treatment is symptomatic; swelling usually resolves over 2 to 3 week period. Complications include sialectasia, orchitis, meningoencephalitis, and sensorineural hearing loss.

Mumps is a preventable disease, two doses of MMR vaccine resulting in approximately 88% vaccine effectiveness.[6] In 2006, multiple states reported mumps cases initially among college students. By the end of the outbreak, 2597 cases were reported to the CDC, the largest number in a single year since 1991.[61] Although the initial source of the cases was never identified in the outbreak, highlighting the importance of vaccination, early recognition of the disease, and use of reliable laboratory diagnostic tests. RT-PCR test for mumps virus is available through many state laboratories.

Juvenile Recurrent Parotitis (JRP)

JRP is the second most common salivary gland disease in children. A variety of causative factors have been proposed, including ductal congenital malformations, hereditary-genetic factors, viral or bacterial infection, allergy, and local manifestation of an autoimmune disease. A review of published literature shows all cases before puberty.[63,64] Clinical symptoms of JRP include recurrent, nonobstructive, nonsuppurative parotid inflammation. JRP is usually unilateral, but bilateral exacerbations can occur. Patients with HIV infection can manifest recurrent or chronic sialadenitis; cytomegalovirus and *S. pneumoniae* have been associated. Treatment of an acute episode generally includes early antibiotic therapy to prevent further parenchymal damage, adequate fluid intake, massage and warm compresses, and use of gum and other sialagogues. Performing sialography with dilatation and hydrocortisone lavage along with parenteral amoxicillin-clavulanate therapy was reported to be useful in relieving symptoms in 26 children reported with JRP.[64]

Granulomatous Parotitis

Granulomatous diseases can be associated with chronic inflammatory parotitis. Children are affected infrequently.[55] Patients usually have localized nodules, which should be distinguished from malignancy. The mass usually is painless, slowly progressive, and often has no surrounding erythema. Saliva is normal in color. Sialography demonstrates extrinsic pressure on the ductal system without intrinsic abnormalities. Possible causes include sarcoidosis, cat-scratch disease, actinomycosis, tuberculosis, and nontuberculous mycobacterial infection. Excision of the gland is diagnostic and therapeutic. Tuberculous infection of the gland is part of a systemic disease and requires systemic antimycobacterial therapy.

OSTEOMYELITIS

Mandibular Osteomyelitis

Osteomyelitis of the mandible is rare. Clinical manifestations include fever, facial swelling, jaw pain, and usually are accompanied by the finding of a carious tooth. Surgical drainage of dental abscess along with antibiotic therapy usually results in a clinical cure. Treatment is given for a minimum of 4 weeks.[11]

Actinomycosis is an infrequent cause of mandibular osteomyelitis. Compilation of 19 pediatric cases over three decades showed a median age of the patients to be 7 years, and 58% were females. Nearly 50% of patients had a history of recent tooth extraction,

loss of a tooth with periodontitis, tooth abscess, or trauma with a pencil.[65] All cases presented with firm painful mass over the mandible. All cases required at least 1 surgical debridement in addition to prolonged antibiotic courses (several months).[65] Unfortunately, relapses are common. In such instances, additional debridement and cultures should be performed to direct antibiotic therapy. Penicillin, clindamycin, and amoxicillin-clavulanic acid are safe and effective choices for prolonged therapy.

Infantile Maxillary Osteomyelitis

Infantile maxillary osteomyelitis is rare, usually occurring in infants <12 weeks of age.[66] It is an acute bacterial infection of the maxilla with necrosis and sequestration of the surrounding structures. Clinical findings can simulate orbital cellulitis, including chemosis, fever, proptosis, with purulence at the inner or outer canthus. The palate on the affected side is swollen and the alveolar dental ridge is markedly thickened.[66] *S. aureus* is the usual pathogen. The condition can be mistaken for orbital cellulitis. Correct diagnosis is imperative for proper management and the prevention of complications, such as extension intracranially, optic nerve damage, disfiguring scarring of the face, and damage to the developing teeth. Surgical drainage and antibiotic therapy are mainstays of management.

Garré Osteomyelitis

Garré osteomyelitis, also known as "nonsuppurative ossifying periostitis" and "periostitis ossificans," is a chronic nonsuppurative, sclerosing osteomyelitis. This condition usually is associated with carious tooth, periodontal defect, or other type of low-grade inflammatory process (erupting molars).[67] The disease usually appears as an asymptomatic, unilateral swelling of the mandible in children and adults. Clinical and radiographic findings, frequently showing laminated or onion-skin appearance, are suggestive but not pathognomonic. Differential diagnosis includes cortical hyperostosis (Caffey disease), osteosarcoma, and Ewing sarcoma. Histologic examination is necessary to establish a definite diagnosis. In general, the clinical course usually has sudden onset, with progression, spontaneous regression, and remodeling. Resolution is enhanced by the dental extraction(s) and removal of the inflamed tissue.

---

26 The Common Cold

Diane E. Pappas and J. Owen Hendley

The common cold, also known as upper respiratory tract infection (URI), is an acute, self-limited viral infection of the upper airway that may involve the lower respiratory tract as well. The characteristic symptom complex consisting of rhinorrhea, nasal congestion, and sore or scratchy throat is familiar to all adults. Colds are the most common cause of human illness and are responsible for significant absenteeism from school and work. Children are especially susceptible because: (1) they have not yet acquired immunity to many of the viruses; (2) they have poor personal hygiene practices; and (3) they have frequent close contact with other children who are excreting virus.

ETIOLOGY

Colds are common because some of the causative viruses do not produce lasting immunity after infection and some viruses have

numerous serotypes (Table 26-1). Cold viruses that do not produce lasting immunity include respiratory syncytial virus (RSV), parainfluenza viruses (PIVs), and coronaviruses (HCoVs). Cold viruses that have numerous serotypes but produce lasting serotype-specific immunity after infection include rhinoviruses, adenoviruses, influenza viruses, and enteroviruses.[1]

Rhinoviruses, with at least 100 serotypes, are the most common cause of URIs in children and adults. At least 50% of colds in adults are caused by rhinoviruses. Other viruses that cause URIs are HCoVs, RSV, human metapneumovirus, influenza virus, parainfluenza viruses, adenoviruses, echoviruses, and coxsackieviruses A and B. Human bocavirus (HBoV), discovered in 2005, has been reported in children with symptomatic upper respiratory tract infection (>10%) and may also be present in asymptomatic children, making its role in causing illness unclear.[2-4] Some of these viruses cause characteristic syndromes; for example, RSV

TABLE 26-1. Immunity to Common Cold Viruses

Virus	No. of Serotypes
LONG-LASTING IMMUNITY NOT PRODUCED BY INFECTION (REPEATED INFECTION WITH SAME SEROTYPE USUAL)	
Respiratory syncytial virus (RSV)	1
Parainfluenza virus	4
Human coronavirus	2
IMMUNITY PRODUCED BY INFECTION (REINFECTION WITH SAME SEROTYPE UNCOMMON)	
Rhinovirus	>100
Adenovirus	≥33
Influenza	3[a]
Echovirus	31
Coxsackievirus group A	3
Coxsackievirus group B	6

[a]Type A subtypes change.

Modified from Hendley JO. Immunology of viral colds. In: Veldman JE, McCabe BF, Huizing EH, et al. (eds) Immunobiology, Autoimmunity, Transplantation in Otorhinolaryngology. Amsterdam, Kugler Publications, 1985, pp 257–260.

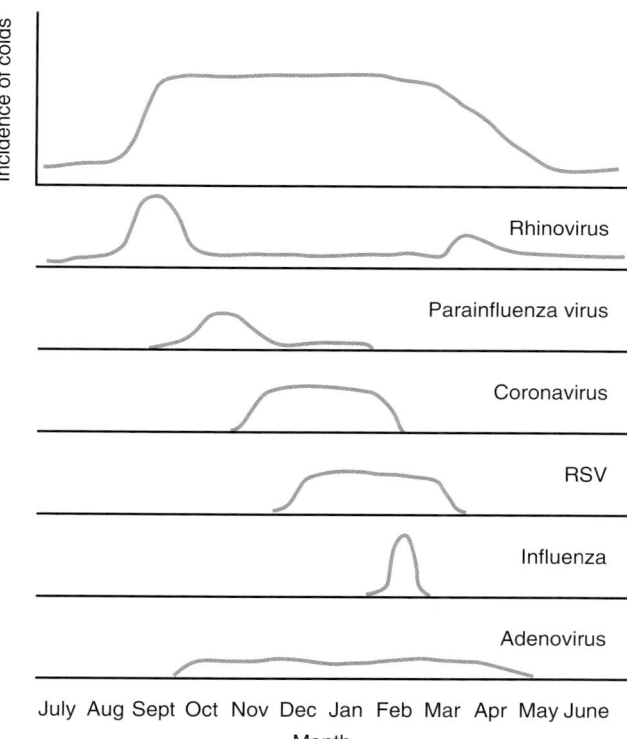

Figure 26-1. Schematic diagram of the incidence of colds and frequency of causative viruses. RSV, respiratory syncytial virus. (Redrawn from Hendley JO. The common cold. In: Goldman L, Bennett JC (eds) Cecil Textbook of Medicine, 21st ed. Philadelphia, WB Saunders, 2000, pp 1790–1793.)

causes bronchiolitis in children 2 years or younger, influenza viruses cause febrile respiratory illness with severe lower respiratory tract involvement, adenoviruses cause pharyngoconjunctival fever, parainfluenza viruses cause croup in young children, HBoV is associated with wheezing, and enteroviruses cause a variety of illnesses, including aseptic meningitis and herpangina.

EPIDEMIOLOGY

In temperate climates in the northern hemisphere, the predictable yearly epidemic of colds begins in September and continues unabated until spring. This sustained epidemic curve is a result of successive waves of different respiratory viruses moving through the community (Figure 26-1). The epidemic begins with a sharp rise in the frequency of rhinovirus infections in September (after children return to school), which is followed by PIVs in October and November. RSV and HCoVs circulate during the winter months, whereas infection due to influenza virus peaks in the late winter. The epidemic finally ends with a small resurgence of rhinovirus infections in the spring. Adenovirus infection occurs at a constant rate throughout the cold season.[5]

The frequency of colds varies with age. A 10-year study of families with children who did not attend a childcare facility showed that the peak incidence of colds occurs in preschool children 1 to 5 years old, with a frequency of 7.4 to 8.3 colds per year. Infants younger than 1 year averaged 6.7 colds per year, and teenagers averaged about 4.5 colds per year. Mothers and fathers experienced about 4 colds per year.[6] With the greater exposure of children to other preschool children in childcare facilities, the frequency of colds in children younger than 6 years has increased. Thus, the typical preschool child experiences at least one URI per month throughout the cold season.

Viral transmission occurs primarily in the home setting, although the exact mechanism of spread has not been clearly established. Colds can be spread by: (1) small-particle (<5 μm in diameter) aerosol, which infects when inhaled; or (2) large-particle (>10 μm in diameter) droplets, which infect by landing on nasal or conjunctival mucosa; or (3) direct transfer via hand-to-hand contact.[7] Small-particle aerosol is an effective method of transfer for influenza virus[8] and coronavirus[9] but not for RSV.[10] Rhinoviruses are most likely spread by large-particle droplets or direct transfer. Rhinoviruses can survive as long as 2 hours on human hands and up to several days on other surfaces. Studies in young adults have shown that infected individuals commonly have rhinovirus on their hands, which can be efficiently

transferred to the hands of uninfected individuals during brief contact; infection then results when the uninfected person transfers the virus from the hands on to his or her nasal or conjunctival mucosa. Sneezing and coughing are ineffective modes of rhinovirus transmission,[11] although there is some evidence that virus could also be transmitted by aerosols generated by coughing, talking, and breathing.[12] Inoculation of the oral mucosa with rhinovirus[13] or RSV[14] does not result in infection.

PATHOGENESIS

Symptoms of the common cold do not appear to result from destruction of nasal mucosa, because nasal biopsy specimens from young adults with both natural and experimentally induced colds show intact nasal epithelium during symptomatic illness.[15,16] Study by in situ hybridization of nasal biopsy specimens obtained during rhinovirus infection indicates that replication occurs in only a small number of epithelial cells.[17,18] Furthermore, in vitro studies have shown that rhinovirus and coronavirus produce no detectable cytopathic effect when replicating in a cultured monolayer of nasal epithelial cells, whereas influenza virus A and adenovirus produce obvious damage.[19]

The symptoms of the common cold appear to result from release of cytokines and other mediators from infected nasal epithelial cells as well as from an influx of polymorphonuclear cells (PMNs). Nasal washings of volunteers experimentally infected with rhinovirus showed a 100-fold increase in PMN concentration 1 to 2 days after inoculation.[20] This influx of PMNs coincides with onset of symptoms and correlates with the presence of a colored nasal discharge.[21] A yellow or white nasal discharge may result from the higher number of PMNs, whereas the enzymatic activity of PMNs (due to myeloperoxidase and other enzymes) may cause a green nasal discharge. A potent chemoattractant for PMNs is produced by cells in culture infected with rhinovirus.[22] This chemoattractant has been identified as interleukin-8 (IL-8).[23] Elevated levels of IL-8 and other cytokines (IL-1β, IL-6) also have been demonstrated in the nasal secretions of infected individuals.[24,25] Furthermore, elevated levels of albumin and kinins (predominantly bradykinin) in nasal secretions have been shown to coincide with the onset of symptoms in experimental rhinovirus infection.[20] The elevated concentration of albumin and kinins likely results from exudation of plasma proteins due to greater vascular permeability in the nasal submucosa. The method by which viral infection initiates this vascular leak has not yet been determined. The release of kinins resulting from plasma exudation may augment the symptoms of the cold; bradykinin alone can cause rhinitis and sore throat when sprayed into the noses of uninfected individuals.[26]

The paranasal sinuses usually are involved during an uncomplicated cold. In one study, computed tomographic (CT) scans obtained during the acute phase of illness revealed abnormalities of one or more sinuses in 27 (87%) of 31 young adults.[27] Without antibiotic therapy, there was complete resolution or marked improvement of the sinus abnormalities in 11 (79%) of the 14 subjects in whom second CT scans were obtained 2 weeks later. In another study, MRI revealed that 60% of children with upper respiratory tract infections had major abnormalities in their paranasal sinuses; these tended to resolve without antibiotic therapy.[28] It is not known whether these sinus abnormalities result from viral infection of the sinus mucosa or from impaired sinus drainage secondary to viral rhinitis. Nose-blowing can generate enough pressure to force fluid from the nasopharynx into the paranasal sinuses, suggesting that nose-blowing may force mucus containing viruses, bacteria, and inflammatory mediators into the paranasal sinuses during a cold.[29]

The middle ear can also be involved during uncomplicated colds. Studies in school-aged children have shown that two-thirds will develop abnormal middle-ear pressures within 2 weeks after onset of a cold.[30] Otitis media was not diagnosed during the study, as ears were not examined and none of the children sought medical care. It is not known whether the abnormal middle-ear pressures result from viral infection of the mucosa of the middle ear and eustachian tube or from viral nasopharyngitis with secondary eustachian tube dysfunction.

CLINICAL MANIFESTATIONS

Symptoms of the common cold do not vary by specific causative virus. In older children and adults, rhinorrhea, nasal obstruction, and sore or scratchy throat are typical. The rhinorrhea is initially clear but may become colored as the illness proceeds. Cough or sneeze may be present. Fever (>38°C) is uncommon in adults. Other symptoms are malaise, sinus fullness, and hoarseness. Objective findings are minimal except for mild erythema of the nasal mucosa or pharynx. Symptoms resolve in 5 to 7 days.

Compared with adults, infants and preschool children with colds are more likely to have fever (>38°C) and moderate enlargement of the anterior cervical lymph nodes (Table 26-2).[1] Rhinorrhea may not be noticed until the nasal discharge becomes colored. Nasal congestion can disrupt sleep and can lead to fatigue and irritability. The illness often persists in infants and preschool children for 10 to 14 days.[31]

TABLE 26-2. Characteristics of Viral Colds in Adults and Young Children

Characteristic	Adults	Children <6 years
Frequency	2–4 per year	One per month, September–April
Fever	Rare	Common during first 3 days
Nasal manifestations	Congestion	Colored nasal discharge
Duration of illness	5–7 days	14 days

Modified from Hendley JO. Epidemiology, pathogenesis, and treatment of the common cold. Semin Pediatr Infect Dis 1998;9:50–55.

DIFFERENTIAL DIAGNOSIS

The differential diagnosis of a cold includes allergic rhinitis, vasomotor rhinitis, intranasal foreign body, and sinusitis. A diagnosis of allergic rhinitis is suggested by a seasonal pattern of clear rhinorrhea, absence of associated fever, and family history of allergy. Possible associated conditions are asthma and eczema. Physical findings consistent with allergic rhinitis include allergic "shiners" and "nasal salute." The detection of numerous eosinophils upon microscopic examination of the nasal mucus using Hansel stain confirms the diagnosis of allergic rhinitis. A diagnosis of vasomotor rhinitis is suggested by a chronic course without fever or sore throat. The diagnosis of bacterial sinusitis is suggested by persistent rhinorrhea or cough or both for greater than 10 days.[32]

CLINICAL APPROACH

The diagnosis of a cold is based on history and physical examination; generally, laboratory tests are not useful. The rapid test for detecting RSV, influenza, parainfluenza, and adenovirus antigens in nasal secretions can be used to confirm the diagnosis. RSV, rhinovirus, influenza viruses, parainfluenza viruses, and adenoviruses also can be isolated in cell culture. HCoV cannot be detected reliably in cell culture, so serologic titer rise can be used for diagnosis, if necessary. Polymerase chain reaction assays for diagnosis of all the respiratory viruses are available in research laboratories and increasingly in clinical laboratories; there is lack of standardization and validation for many tests offered. Other methods of detection can be used but are rarely needed.

MANAGEMENT

At present, no antiviral agents are available that are effective for treatment of the common cold. Although an array of medications may be used to relieve symptoms, there is little scientific evidence to support the use of symptomatic treatments in children. Because the common cold is a self-limited illness with symptomatology that is largely subjective, a substantial placebo effect can suggest that various treatments have some efficacy. Inadequate blinding of placebo recipients in a study can make an ineffective treatment appear effective.

In adults with colds, first-generation antihistamines (i.e., chlorpheniramine) have been shown to provide modest symptomatic relief, with decreases in nasal discharge, sneezing, nose-blowing, and duration of symptoms.[33] This effect is presumably due to the anticholinergic effects of these medications. A randomized, double-blind, placebo-controlled study in preschool children with URIs showed that treatment with an antihistamine–decongestant combination (brompheniramine maleate and phenylpropanolamine hydrochloride) produced no improvement in cough, rhinorrhea, or nasal congestion, although a larger proportion of the treated children (47% versus 26%) were asleep 2 hours after treatment.[34]

Numerous decongestants, antitussives, and expectorants are available over the counter, but there is no evidence to support their use in children. A study of phenylephrine, a topical decongestant, in children 6 to 18 months old showed no decrease in nasal obstruction with its use during a URI.[35] In a study comparing placebo, dextromethorphan, and codeine for cough suppression in children 18 months to 12 years old, cough decreased in all patients within 3 days, but there was no difference in cough reduction among the three treatment groups.[36] Guaifenesin, an expectorant, has not been shown to change the volume or quality of sputum or the frequency of cough in young adults with colds.[37] Echinacea preparations, commonly believed to be effective in the treatment of the common cold, have been shown to have no effect on the prevention or treatment of rhinovirus infection[38] as has intranasal zinc gluconate for treatment of colds[39] or prevention of experimental rhinovirus colds.[40] In January, 2008, the U.S. Food and Drug Administration issued an advisory strongly recommending that over-the-counter cold and cough medications not be given to infants because of the risk of life-threatening side effects.

Antibiotics have no role in the treatment of uncomplicated URIs in children. Antibiotic therapy does not hasten resolution of the viral infection or reduce the likelihood of occurrence of secondary bacterial infection.[41] Antibiotics are only indicated in cases of secondary bacterial infection, such as sinusitis and acute otitis media.

Thus, supportive measures remain the mainstay of treatment of the common cold in children. Bulb suction with saline drops (about 1 teaspoon salt in 2 cups of water) may help relieve nasal congestion and remove secretions. A recent study suggests that honey given at bedtime may help reduce cough in children with upper respiratory tract infections, although honey is not recommended for children under the age of 12 months because of the risk of exposure to *C. botulinum* spores.[42]

COMPLICATIONS

The common cold usually resolves in about 10 to 14 days in infants and children. New-onset fever and earache during this period may herald the development of bacterial otitis media, which occurs in about 5% of colds in preschool children. Persistence of nasal symptoms for longer than 10 days has been thought to signify the development of a secondary bacterial sinusitis. However, a recent study found that 20 children hospitalized for preseptal or orbital cellulitis, indicative of bacterial sinusitis, had symptoms of acute respiratory tract infection for 7 days or less prior to hospitalization, suggesting that the complications of rhinosinusitis can occur during the first few days of a cold.[43] Bacterial pneumonia is an uncommon secondary infection. For children with underlying reactive airways disease, wheezing is common during the course of a viral URI; at least 50% of asthma exacerbations in children are associated with viral infection. Children who experience more than one *lower* respiratory tract infection (such as croup or bronchiolitis) during their first year of life have an increased risk of asthma thereafter.[44] Other complications are epistaxis, eustachian tube dysfunction, conjunctivitis, and pharyngitis.

RECENT ADVANCES

The symptoms of the common cold appear to result from effects of inflammatory mediators released in response to the viral infection of the respiratory tract. As the determinants of this process are further elucidated, treatments may be developed that can interrupt or ameliorate release of inflammatory mediators and thus prevent or reduce the symptoms of the common cold. Vaccines are unlikely to be useful for prevention, given the large number of serotypes of some cold viruses as well as the lack of lasting immunity to others. The use of alcohol-based hand gels has been suggested as a means of reducing secondary transmission of respiratory illnesses in the home,[45] but this was not shown to be effective in one field trial.[46] Also, virucidal tissues have been shown to be effective in preventing viral passage and transmission, and may reduce secondary transmission by about 30%.[47,48] Until new methods are developed, prevention of the common cold is limited to avoiding self-inoculation (transfer of virus from contaminated fingers to nasal or conjunctival mucosa) by removing virus through handwashing or by killing virus with application of a virucide to the hands.

---

27 Pharyngitis

John C. Arnold and Victor Nizet

Acute pharyngitis is one of the most common illnesses for which children in the United States visit primary care providers; pediatricians make the diagnosis of acute pharyngitis, acute tonsillitis, or "strep throat" more than 7 million times annually.[1]

A partial list of the more common microorganisms that can cause acute pharyngitis is presented in Table 27-1. Most cases in children and adolescents are caused by viruses and are benign and self-limited. Group A β-hemolytic streptococcus (GAS, *Streptococcus pyogenes*) is the most important bacterial cause. Strategies for the diagnosis and treatment of pharyngitis in children and adolescents are directed at distinguishing the large group of patients with viral pharyngitis that would not benefit from antimicrobial therapy from the significantly smaller group of patients with GAS pharyngitis for whom antimicrobial therapy would be beneficial. Making this distinction is extremely important in attempting to minimize the unnecessary use of antibiotics in children and adolescents.

ETIOLOGY

Viruses are the most common cause of acute pharyngitis in children and adolescents. Respiratory viruses (e.g., influenza virus, parainfluenza virus, rhinovirus, coronavirus, adenovirus, and respiratory syncytial virus), enteroviruses (including coxsackievirus and echovirus), herpes simplex virus (HSV), and Epstein–Barr virus (EBV) are frequent causes of pharyngitis. EBV pharyngitis often is accompanied by other clinical findings of infectious mononucleosis (e.g., generalized lymphadenopathy, splenomegaly), and can be exudative and indistinguishable from GAS pharyngitis. HSV pharyngitis often is associated with stomatitis in children, and tends to affect the entire oral mucosa including the gingival, buccal mucosa, and tongue. Enteroviral pharyngitis can be an isolated finding (herpangina), or part of the spectrum of hand-foot-and-mouth disease, and has a typical appearance. Systemic infections with other viruses (e.g., cytomegalovirus, rubella virus, and measles virus) also can include pharyngitis.

GAS is the most common bacterial cause of acute pharyngitis, accounting for 15% to 30% of the cases in children. Other causative bacteria include groups C and G β-hemolytic streptococci (GCS, GGS). *Arcanobacterium haemolyticum* is a rare cause in adolescents and *Neisseria gonorrhoeae* can cause acute pharyngitis in sexually active adolescents. Other bacteria such as *Francisella tularensis*, *Yersinia enterocolitica*, and *Corynebacterium diphtheriae* as well as mixed infections with anaerobic bacteria (e.g., Vincent angina) are rare causes. *Chlamydophila pneumoniae* and *Mycoplasma pneumoniae* have been implicated rarely, particularly in adults. Although other bacteria such as *Staphylococcus aureus*, *Haemophilus influenzae*, and *Streptococcus pneumoniae* frequently are isolated from throat cultures of children and adolescents with acute pharyngitis, their etiologic role is not established. *Fusobacterium necrophorum*, the typical etiologic agent of Lemierre syndrome, also may cause uncomplicated pharyngitis.[2] Non-infectious cases of recurrent or prolonged pharyngitis and sore throat include the periodic fever, adenitis, pharyngitis, and aphthous ulcers (PFAPA) syndrome, gastroesophageal reflux and/or laryngopharyngeal reflux, and allergic rhinitis.

TABLE 27-1. Etiology of Acute Pharyngitis

Etiologic Agent	Associated Disorder(s) or Clinical Findings(s)
Bacterial	
Streptococci	
Group A	Scarlet fever
Groups C and G	
Mixed anaerobes	Vincent angina
Neisseria gonorrhoeae	
Corynebacterium diphtheriae	Diphtheria
Arcanobacterium haemolyticum	Scarlatiniform rash
Yersinia enterocolitica	Enterocolitis
Yersinia pestis	Plague
Francisella tularensis	Tularemia
Fusobacterium necrophorum	Lemierre syndrome (jugular vein septic thrombophlebitis)
Viral	
Rhinovirus	Common cold
Coronavirus	Common cold
Adenovirus	Pharyngoconjunctival fever; acute respiratory disease
Herpes simplex virus types 1 and 2	Gingivostomatitis
Parainfluenza virus	Common cold; croup
Coxsackievirus A	Herpangina; hand, foot, and mouth disease
Epstein–Barr virus	Infectious mononucleosis
Cytomegalovirus	Cytomegalovirus mononucleosis
Human immunodeficiency virus (HIV)	Primary HIV infection
Mycoplasmal	
Mycoplasma pneumoniae	Acute respiratory disease; pneumonia
Chlamydial	
Chlamydophila psittaci	Acute respiratory disease; pneumonia
Chlamydophila pneumoniae	Pneumonia
Non-Infectious Etiologies	
Gastroesophogeal reflux disease	Heartburn
Laryngopharyngeal reflux	Cough, hoarseness
PFAPA syndrome	Periodic fever, aphthous ulcers, adenitis
Allergic pharyngitis	Scratchy serration, post-nasal drip, hoarseness

HIV, human immunodeficiency virus.

Modified from Bisno AL, Gerber MA, Gwaltney JM, et al. Practice guideline for the diagnosis and management of group A streptococcal pharyngitis. Clin Infect Dis 2002;35:113–125, with permission.

EPIDEMIOLOGY

Most cases of acute pharyngitis occur during the colder months of the year when respiratory viruses are prevalent. Spread among family members in the home is a prominent feature of the epidemiology of most of these agents, with children being the major reservoir. GAS pharyngitis is primarily a disease of children 5 to 15 years of age, and, in temperate climates, prevalence is highest in winter and early spring. Enteroviral pharyngitis typically occurs in the summer and early fall.

Gonococcal pharyngitis occurs in sexually active adolescents and young adults. The usual route of infection is through orogenital sexual contact. Sexual abuse must be considered strongly when N. gonorrhoeae is isolated from the pharynx of a prepubertal child. Widespread immunization with diphtheria toxoid has made diphtheria a rare disease in the U.S., with <5 cases reported annually in recent years.

GCS and GGS express many of the same toxins as GAS, including streptolysins S and O, and GCS pharyngitis can have clinical features similar to GAS and can cause elevation of serum antistreptolysin-O (ASO) antibody.[3] GCS is a relatively common cause of acute pharyngitis among college students and adults who seek urgent care.[4,5] Outbreaks of GCS pharyngitis related to consumption of contaminated food products (e.g., unpasteurized cow milk) have been reported in families and schools.[6] Although there also are several well-documented foodborne outbreaks of GGS pharyngitis, the etiologic role of GGS in acute, endemic pharyngitis remains unclear. A community-wide outbreak of pharyngitis in children was described in which GGS was isolated from 25% of 222 consecutive children with acute pharyngitis seen in a private pediatric office; results of DNA fingerprinting suggested that 75% of isolates belonged to the same GGS clone.[7]

The role of GCS and GGS in acute pharyngitis may be underestimated. Laboratories may use bacitracin susceptibility to identify GAS; many GCS and GGS are bacitracin-resistant. Additionally, rapid antigen detection tests (RADTs) recognize the GAS cell wall carbohydrate, but are nonreactive with GCS or GGS.[8]

CLINICAL MANIFESTATIONS

Group A Streptococcus

The presence of certain clinical and epidemiologic findings suggests GAS as the cause of an episode of acute pharyngitis (Box 27-1). Patients with GAS pharyngitis commonly present with sore throat (usually of sudden onset), severe pain on swallowing, and fever. Headache, nausea, vomiting, and abdominal pain also can be present. Examination typically reveals tonsillopharyngeal erythema with or without exudates, and tender, enlarged anterior

---

BOX 27-1. Clinical and Epidemiologic Characteristics of Group A β-Hemolytic Streptococci (GAS) and Viral Pharyngitis

FEATURES SUGGESTIVE OF GAS ETIOLOGY

Sudden onset
Sore throat
Fever
Scarlet fever rash
Headache
Nausea, vomiting, and abdominal pain
Inflammation of pharynx and tonsils
Patchy discrete exudates
Tender, enlarged anterior cervical nodes
Patient aged 5–15 years
Presentation in winter or early spring
History of exposure

FEATURES SUGGESTIVE OF VIRAL ETIOLOGY

Conjunctivitis
Coryza
Cough
Hoarseness
Myalgia
Diarrhea
Characteristic exanthems

Modified from Bisno AL, Gerber MA, Gwaltney JM, et al. Practice guideline for the diagnosis and management of group A streptococcal pharyngitis. Clin Infect Dis 2002;35:113–125, with permission.

cervical lymph nodes. Other findings can include a beefy, red, swollen uvula; petechiae on the palate; and a scarlatiniform rash. No finding is specific for GAS. Many patients with GAS pharyngitis exhibit signs and symptoms that are milder than a "classic" case of this illness. Some of these patients have bona fide GAS infection (i.e., have a rise in ASO antibodies), whereas others are merely colonized and have an intercurrent viral infection. GAS pharyngitis in infants is uncommon, and is difficult to differentiate from viral infections because nasopharyngitis, with purulent nasal discharge, and excoriated nares frequently accompany pharyngitis.

Scarlet fever is associated with a characteristic rash that is caused by a pyrogenic exotoxin (erythrogenic toxin)-producing GAS, and occurs in individuals who lack prior antitoxin antibodies. Although less common and less severe than in the past, the incidence of scarlet fever is cyclical, depending on the prevalence of toxin-producing strains of GAS and the immune status of the population. The modes of transmission, age distribution, and other epidemiologic features are otherwise similar to those of GAS pharyngitis.

The rash of scarlet fever appears within 24 to 48 hours of the onset of signs and symptoms and can be the first sign. The rash often begins around the neck and spreads over the trunk and extremities. It is a diffuse, finely papular (sandpaper-like), erythematous eruption producing bright red discoloration of the skin that blanches with pressure. Involvement often is more intense along the creases in the antecubital area, axillae, and groin, and petechiae along the creases can occur (Pastia lines). The face usually is spared, although the cheeks can be erythematous with pallor around the mouth (Figure 27-1). After 3 to 4 days, the rash begins to fade and is followed by fine desquamation, first on the face, progressing downward. Occasionally, sheet-like desquamation occurs around the fingernails periungually, the palms, and the soles. Pharyngeal findings are the same as with GAS pharyngitis. In addition, the tongue usually is coated and the papillae are swollen. With desquamation, the reddened papillae are prominent, giving the tongue a strawberry appearance.

Viruses

The presence of certain clinical findings (e.g., conjunctivitis, cough, hoarseness, coryza, anterior stomatitis, discrete ulcerative lesions, viral exanthema, myalgia, and diarrhea) suggests a virus rather than GAS as the cause of an episode of acute pharyngitis (see Box 27-1).

Adenovirus pharyngitis typically is associated with fever, erythema of the pharynx, enlarged tonsils with exudate, and enlarged cervical lymph nodes. Adenoviral pharyngitis can be associated with conjunctivitis, when illness is referred to as *pharyngoconjunctival fever;* pharyngitis can persist up to 7 days and conjunctivitis

up to 14 days, when both resolve spontaneously. Outbreaks of pharyngoconjunctival fever have been associated with transmission in swimming pools; widespread epidemics and sporadic cases also occur.

Enteroviruses (coxsackievirus, echovirus, and enteroviruses) are associated with erythematous pharyngitis but tonsillar exudate and cervical lymphadenopathy are unusual. Fever can be prominent. Resolution usually occurs within a few days. Herpangina is a specific syndrome caused by coxsackieviruses A or B or echoviruses and is characterized by fever and painful, discrete, grey-white papulovesicular/ulcerative lesions on an erythematous base in the posterior oropharynx (Figure 27-2). Hand-foot-and-mouth disease is characterized by painful vesicles and ulcers throughout the oropharynx associated with vesicles on the palms, soles, and sometimes on the trunk or extremities. Enteroviral lesions usually resolve within 7 days.

Primary oral HSV infections usually occur in young children and typically produce acute gingivostomatitis associated with ulcerating vesicular lesions throughout the anterior mouth including the lips, sparing the posterior pharynx. HSV gingivostomatitis can last up to 2 weeks and often is associated with high fever. Pain can be intense and the poor oral intake can lead to dehydration. In adolescents and adults HSV also can cause mild pharyngitis that may or may not be associated with typical vesicular, ulcerating lesions.

EBV pharyngitis during infectious mononucleosis can be severe, with clinical findings identical to those of GAS pharyngitis (Figure 27-3A). However, generalized lymphadenopathy and hepatosplenomegaly also can be present. Posterior cervical lymphadenopathy and presternal and periorbital edema are distinctive if present. Fever and pharyngitis typically last 1 to 3 weeks, whereas the lymphadenopathy and hepatosplenomegaly resolve over 3 to 6 weeks. Laboratory findings include the presence of atypical lymphocytosis (Figure 27-3B), heterophile antibodies, viremia (by PCR), and specific antibodies to EBV antigens. If amoxicillin has been given, an intense maculopapular rash is expected (Figure 27-3C).

Other Bacteria

A. haemolyticum pharyngitis can resemble GAS pharyngitis, including the presence of a scarlatiniform rash. Rarely, *A. haemolyticum* can produce a membranous pharyngitis that can be confused with diphtheria.

Pharyngeal diphtheria is characterized by a greyish brown pseudomembrane that can be limited to one or both tonsils or can extend widely to involve the nares, uvula, soft palate, pharynx, larynx, and tracheobronchial tree. Involvement of the tracheobronchial tree can lead to life-threatening respiratory obstruction.

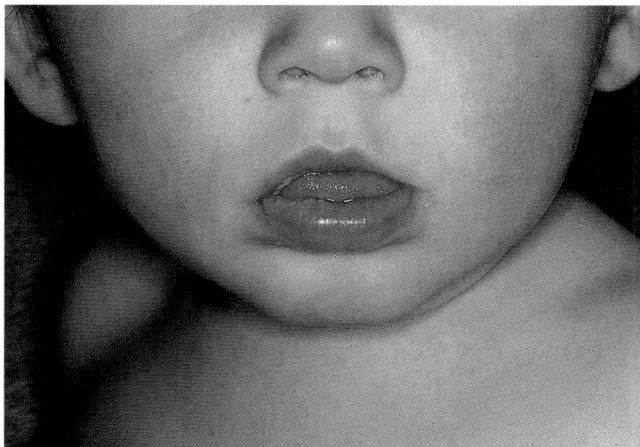

Figure 27-1. Child has group A streptococcal pharyngitis and scarlatiniform rash, with characteristic circumoral pallor. (Courtesy of J.H. Brien©.)

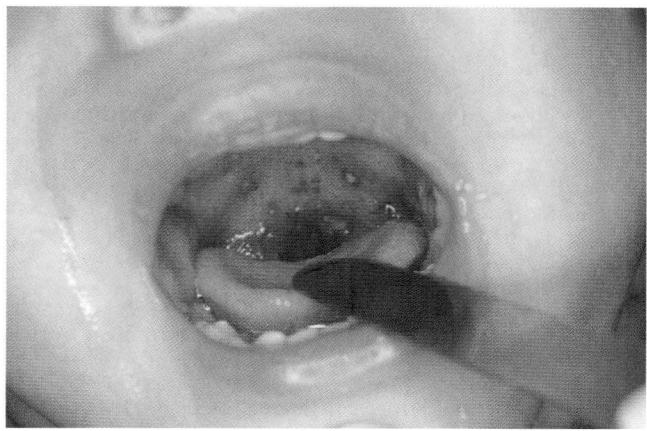

Figure 27-2. Child with posterior pharyngeal grey-white papulovesicular lesions characteristic of enteroviral herpangina. (Courtesy of J.H. Brien©.)

PART II   Clinical Syndromes and Cardinal Features of Infectious Diseases: Approach to Diagnosis and Initial Management

SECTION C   Oral Infections and Upper and Middle Respiratory Tract Infections

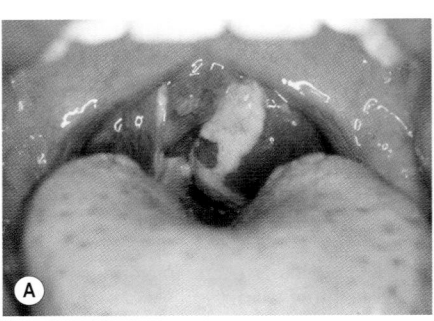
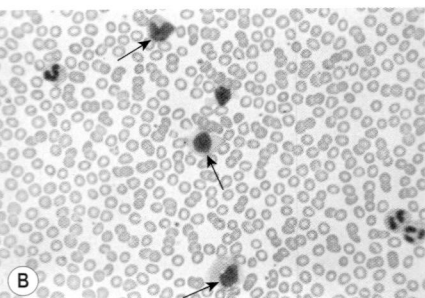
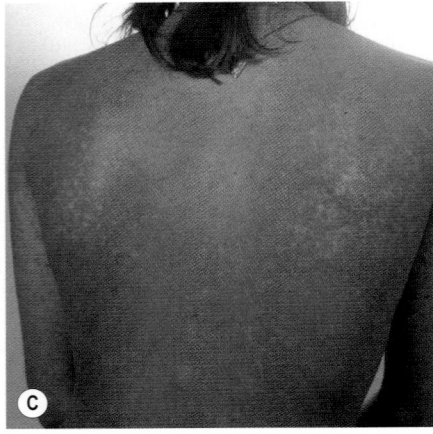

Figure 27-3. (A) Pharyngeal erythema and exudate of Epstein–Barr virus (EBV). **(B)** Peripheral blood smear showing atypical lymphocytes (arrows) in a patient with EBV mononucleosis. Note the abundant cytoplasm with vacuoles, and deformation of cell by surrounding cells. **(C)** Diffuse erythematous raised rash in adolescent with EBV mononucleosis who received amoxicillin; note predominance on trunk and coalescence. (Courtesy of J.H. Brien©.)

Soft-tissue edema and prominent cervical and submental lymphadenopathy can cause a bull-neck appearance.

Fusobacterium necrophorum may be a common cause of non-streptococcal pharyngitis, occurring in as many as 10% of adolescents and young adults with pharyngitis.[9] *F. necrophorum* appears to cause typical signs of bacterial pharyngitis (high fever, odynophagia, lymphadenopathy, and exudative tonsillitis), and can cause concomitant bacteremia.[10] The frequency of progression from tonsillitis to Lemierre syndrome is unknown.

DIAGNOSIS

Distinguishing between GAS and viral pharyngitis is key to management in the U.S. Scoring systems that incorporate clinical and epidemiologic features attempt to predict the probability that the illness is caused by GAS.[11,12] Clinical scoring systems are helpful in identifying patients at such low risk of GAS infection that a throat culture or RADT usually is unnecessary. However, in a 2012 systematic review of 34 articles with individual symptoms and signs of pharyngitis assessed and 15 articles with data on prediction rules, no symptoms or signs individually or combined into prediction rules could be used to diagnose GAS pharyngitis with a probability of ≥85%.[13] Adding to the complexity of diagnosis is the ability to distinguish between GAS pharyngitis and other bacterial pathogens such as GCS, which have very similar clinical manifestations.[3] Therefore, recent guidelines from the Infectious Diseases Society of America (IDSA),[14] as well as guidelines from the American Academy of Pediatrics (AAP)[15] and the American Heart Association (AHA),[16] indicate that microbiologic confirmation (either with a throat culture or RADT) is required for the diagnosis of GAS pharyngitis.

The decision to perform a microbiologic test on a child or adolescent with acute pharyngitis should be based on the clinical and epidemiologic characteristics of the illness (see Box 27-1). A history of close contact with a documented case of GAS pharyngitis or high prevalence of GAS in the community also can be helpful. More selective use of diagnostic studies for GAS will increase not only the proportion of positive test results, but also the percentage of patients with positive tests who are truly infected rather than merely GAS carriers.

Because adults infrequently are infected with GAS, and rarely develop rheumatic fever, 2001 practice guidelines from the Centers for Disease Control and Prevention (CDC), the American Academy of Family Physicians (AAFP), and the American College of Physicians–American Society of Internal Medicine (ACP–ASIM) recommend the use of a clinical algorithm without microbiologic confirmation as an acceptable approach to the diagnosis of GAS pharyngitis in adults only.[17] Although the goal of this algorithm-based strategy was to reduce the inappropriate use of antibiotics in adults with pharyngitis, such an approach could result in the administration of antimicrobial treatment to an unacceptably large number of adults with non-GAS pharyngitis.[18]

According to a study intended to assess the impact of six different guidelines on the identification and treatment of GAS pharyngitis in children and adults,[19] guidelines that recommended selective use of RADTs and/or throat culture and treatment based only on positive test results significantly reduced the inappropriate use of antibiotics in adults. In contrast, the empiric strategy proposed in the CDC/AAFP/ACP–ASIM guidelines resulted in the administration of unnecessary antibiotics to an unacceptably large number of adults. Therefore, diagnosis of adults by symptom-complex only has been discouraged by the latest AHA scientific statement.[16]

Throat Culture

Culture on sheep blood agar of a specimen obtained by throat swab is the standard laboratory procedure for the microbiologic confirmation of GAS pharyngitis.[20] If performed correctly, a throat culture has a sensitivity of 90% to 95%.[21] A negative result can occur if the patient has received an antibiotic prior to sampling.

Several variables impact on the accuracy of throat culture results. One of the most important is the manner in which the swab is obtained.[22,23] Throat swab specimens should be obtained from the surface of both tonsils (or tonsillar fossae) and the posterior pharyngeal wall. Other areas of the pharynx and mouth are not acceptable sampling sites and should not be touched during the procedure.

Anaerobic incubation and the use of selective culture media have been reported to increase the sensitivity of throat cultures.[24,25] However, data regarding the impact of the atmosphere of incubation and the culture media are conflicting, and, in the absence of definite benefit, the increased cost and effort associated with anaerobic incubation and selective culture media are difficult to justify.[25-28]

Duration of incubation can impact the yield of throat cultures. Cultures should be incubated at 35°C to 37°C for at least 18 to 24 hours prior to reading. An additional overnight incubation at room temperature, however, identifies substantially more positive cultures. In a study performed in patients with pharyngitis and negative RADT, 40% of positive GAS cultures were negative after 24 hours of incubation but positive after 48 hours.[29] Therefore, although initial therapeutic decisions can be guided by negative result at 24 hours, it is advisable to wait 48 hours for definitive results.

The clinical significance of the number of colonies of GAS present on inoculated agar is controversial. Although density of bacteria is likely to be greater in patients with bona fide acute GAS pharyngitis than in GAS carriers, there is too much overlap in the colony counts to permit differentiation on the basis of degree of positivity alone.[26]

The bacitracin disk test is the most widely used method in physicians' offices for the differentiation of GAS from other β-hemolytic streptococci on a sheep blood agar plate. This test provides a presumptive identification based on the observation that >95% of GAS demonstrate a zone of inhibition around a disk containing 0.04 units of bacitracin, whereas 83% to 97% of non-GAS are not inhibited by bacitracin.[26] An alternative and highly specific method for the differentiation of β-hemolytic streptococci is the performance of a group-specific cell wall carbohydrate antigen detection test directly on isolated bacterial colonies for which commercial kits are available. Additional expense for the minimal improvement in accuracy may not be justified.[26]

Rapid Antigen Detection Tests

RADTs developed for the identification of GAS directly from throat swabs are more expensive than blood agar cultures, but offer speed in providing results. Rapid identification and treatment of patients with GAS pharyngitis can reduce the risk of the spread of GAS, allow the patient to return to school or work sooner, and speed clinical improvement.[21,30] In addition, in certain environments (e.g., emergency departments) the use of RADTs compared with throat cultures has significantly increased the number of patients appropriately treated for GAS pharyngitis.[31,32]

The majority of currently available RADTs have specificities of ≥95% compared with blood agar cultures.[33] Therapeutic decisions, therefore, can be made with confidence on the basis of a positive RADT result. However, the sensitivity of RADTs is between 70% and 90%.[33] Although some patients with falsely negative RADT results merely are GAS carriers, a large proportion truly are infected with GAS.[34]

The first RADTs utilized latex agglutination methodology, were relatively insensitive, and had unclear endpoints.[33] Subsequent tests based on enzyme immunoassay techniques had a more sharply defined endpoint and increased sensitivity. RADTs using optical immunoassay (OIA) and chemiluminescent DNA probes may be more sensitive than other RADTs and perhaps even as sensitive as blood agar plate cultures,[33] but because of conflicting and limited data about the OIA and other commercially available RADTs, advisory groups still recommend a confirmatory blood agar culture for children and adolescents who are suspected on clinical grounds of having GAS pharyngitis and have a negative RADT result.

The relative sensitivities of different RADTs can only be determined by direct comparisons in the same study. There have been only five reports of direct comparisons of different RADTs.[35-39] Only a handful of studies have investigated the performance of RADTs in actual clinical practice and physician investigators have concluded differently about adequacy of test performance.[29,36-41] In one study,[29] performed over three winter periods and using on-site office testing in a pediatric group practice, RADT had a sensitivity of approximately 85% compared with a single blood agar plate culture. Investigators in a different pediatric group practice reviewed their experience with 11,427 RADTs performed between 1996 and 1999.[42] Only 2.4% of specimens negative by RADT were positive by culture.[42] A retrospective review of over 19,000 clinical RADTs performed in a heterogeneous inpatient and outpatient group demonstrated a negative predictive value (NPV) ranging from 90% to 96% and a maximum sensitivity of 77% to 86%.[39] Physicians electing to use any RADT in children and adolescents without culture backup of negative results should do so only after demonstrating with adequate sample size calculation that the RADT is as sensitive as throat culture in their own practice.[14,15]

Neither blood agar culture nor RADT accurately differentiates individuals with GAS pharyngitis from carriers. However, use facilitates withholding antimicrobial therapy in the great majority of patients with GAS sore throat. There are an estimated 6.7 million visits to primary care providers by adults who complain of sore throat each year in the U.S.; antimicrobial therapy historically was prescribed at 73% of these visits.[43] With encouragement for judicious use of antibiotics, trends show a modest decline in the use in children and adolescents diagnosed with pharyngitis to 69% in one study in 1999 to 2000,[44] and to 54% in another study in 2003.[45]

Follow-up Testing

The majority of asymptomatic persons who have a positive throat culture or RADT after completing a course of appropriate antimicrobial therapy for GAS pharyngitis are GAS carriers,[46] therefore follow-up testing is not indicated routinely. Follow-up throat culture (or RADT) for an asymptomatic individual should be performed only in those with a history of rheumatic fever, and should be considered in patients who develop acute pharyngitis during outbreaks of acute rheumatic fever or poststreptococcal acute glomerulonephritis, and in individuals in closed or semi-closed communities during outbreaks of GAS pharyngitis.[46]

Other Diagnostic Considerations

Antistreptococcal antibody titers have no value in the diagnosis of acute GAS pharyngitis, but are useful in prospective epidemiologic studies to differentiate true GAS infections from GAS carriage. Antistreptococcal antibodies are valuable for confirmation of prior GAS infections in patients suspected of having acute rheumatic fever or other non-suppurative complications.

Polymerase chain reaction (PCR) testing for GAS from tonsillar tissue has been shown to be highly sensitive,[47] but is not currently available clinically, and expense likely will restrict its use in clinical practice.

The need to definitively diagnose non-GAS causes of pharyngitis occurs rarely and generally only in those who are very ill or have prolonged symptoms. A. haemolyticum will not be identified using standard throat culture methods (intended to identify only GAS), and requires use of standard respiratory culture methods. N. gonorrhoeae can be identified either by selective growth media or by using nucleic acid amplification tests. EBV is routinely diagnosed using the heterophile antibody (monospot), but low sensitivity in younger children necessitates the use of specific antibody testing or serum PCR. Other common viruses such as HSV, adenoviruses, and enteroviruses could be identified in general viral cultures and/or by PCR.

TREATMENT

Antimicrobial therapy is indicated for individuals with symptomatic pharyngitis after the presence of GAS has been confirmed by throat culture or RADT. In situations in which the clinical and epidemiologic findings are highly suggestive of GAS, antimicrobial therapy can be initiated while awaiting microbiologic confirmation, provided that such therapy is discontinued if culture or RADT is negative. Antimicrobial therapy for GAS pharyngitis shortens the clinical course of the illness.[30] However, GAS pharyngitis usually is self limited, and most signs and symptoms resolve spontaneously within 3 or 4 days of onset.[48] In addition, initiation of antimicrobial therapy can be delayed for up to 9 days after the onset of GAS pharyngitis and still prevent the occurrence of acute rheumatic fever.[49]

Antimicrobial Agents

Penicillin and its congeners (such as ampicillin and amoxicillin), as well as numerous cephalosporins, macrolides, and clindamycin, are effective treatment for GAS pharyngitis. Several advisory groups have recommended penicillin as the treatment of choice for this infection.[14,15,50] GAS has remained exquisitely susceptible to β-lactam agents over five decades.[51] Amoxicillin often is used because of acceptable taste of suspension; efficacy appears to equal penicillin. Orally administered macrolides (clarithromycin and

PART II   Clinical Syndromes and Cardinal Features of Infectious Diseases: Approach to Diagnosis and Initial Management

SECTION C   Oral Infections and Upper and Middle Respiratory Tract Infections

erythromycin) or azalides (azithromycin) also are effective (see below). Sulfa drugs, including trimethoprim/sulfamethoxazole, and tetracyclines are not effective and should not be used for GAS pharyngitis.

Following a meta-analysis of 35 clinical trials completed between 1970 and 1999 in which a cephalosporin was compared with penicillin for the treatment of GAS tonsillopharyngitis, it was first suggested that cephalosporins should be the treatment of choice for GAS tonsillopharyngitis.[52] However, several methodologic flaws (most notably, the inclusion of GAS carriers) have led to controversy regarding this conclusion.[53] Indirect evidence of the superiority of cephalosporins over penicillins to prevent treatment failures and relapses continues to appear;[54,55] however, there has not been a prospective study to clarify the issue beyond doubt. Although the use of cephalosporins for GAS pharyngitis could reduce the number of persons (especially chronic carriers) who harbor GAS after completing therapy, empiric first-line use would be associated with substantial economic and possibly ecologic cost. There are compelling reasons (e.g., its narrow antimicrobial spectrum, low cost, and impressive safety profile) to continue to use penicillin as the drug of choice for uncomplicated GAS pharyngitis. Selected use of a first-generation cephalosporin as the drug of choice may be appropriate for patients at high risk of complications (such as a history of rheumatic fever), with severe symptoms, or with a suspected treatment failure or relapse.

Dosing Intervals and Duration of Therapy

Oral penicillin must be administered multiple times a day for 10 days in order to achieve maximal rates of GAS eradication. Attempts to treat GAS pharyngitis with a single daily dose of penicillin have been unsuccessful.[56] Reduced frequency of dosing and shorter treatment courses (<10 days) may result in better patient adherence to therapy. Several antimicrobial agents, including clarithromycin, cefuroxime, cefixime, ceftibuten, cefdinir, and cefpodoxime, are effective in GAS eradication when administered for ≤5 days[57-62] and effective eradication with once-daily dosing has been described for amoxicillin, azithromycin, cefadroxil, cefixime, ceftibuten, cefpodoxime, cefprozil, and cefdinir.[14,58,61,63-66] However, the endpoints of these studies generally are eradication of GAS, not symptomatic improvement or prevention of rheumatic fever (the two main clinical reasons for treatment). In addition, many agents have a broader spectrum of activity and, even if administered for short courses, can be more expensive than standard therapy.[58] Therefore, additional studies are needed before these short-course or once daily-dose regimens can be recommended routinely.[14]

Table 27-2 gives recommendations for several regimens with proven efficacy for GAS pharyngitis.[14] Intramuscular benzathine penicillin G is preferred in patients unlikely to complete a full 10-day course of therapy orally.

Macrolide and Lincosamide Resistance

Although GAS resistance to penicillin has not occurred anywhere in the world,[67] there are geographic areas with relatively high levels of resistance to macrolide antibiotics.[68,69] The rate of GAS resistance to macrolides in the U.S. generally has remained <5%. In an investigation of 245 pharyngeal isolates and 56 invasive isolates of GAS obtained between 1994 and 1997 from 24 states and the District of Columbia, only 8 (2.6%) isolates were macrolide-resistant.[51] A prospective, multicenter, U.S. community-based surveillance study of pharyngeal GAS isolates recovered from children 3 to 18 years of age during three successive respiratory seasons between 2000 and 2003 found macrolide resistance of <5% and clindamycin resistance of 1%,[70] and no evidence of increasing erythromycin minimum inhibitory concentrations over the 3-year study period. There was, however, considerable geographic variability in macrolide resistance rates in each study year, as well as year-to-year variability at individual study sites.[70]

Higher resistance rates have been reported occasionally. For example, 9% of pharyngeal and 32% of invasive GAS strains collected in a San Francisco study during 1994 to 1995 were

TABLE 27-2. Antimicrobial Therapy for Group A β-Hemolytic Streptococci (GAS) Pharyngitis

Route of Administration, Antimicrobial Agent	Dosage	Duration
ORAL		
Penicillin	Children: 250 mg bid or tid	10 days
	Adolescents and adults: 250 mg tid or qid	10 days
	Adolescents and adults: 500 mg bid	10 days
INTRAMUSCULAR		
Benzathine penicillin G	6.0×10^5 U (for patients ≤27 kg)	1 dose
	1.2×10^6 U (for patients >27 kg)	1 dose
Mixtures of benzathine and procaine penicillin G	Varies with formulation[a]	
ORAL, FOR PATIENTS ALLERGIC TO PENICILLIN		
Erythromycin	Varies with formulation	10 days
First-generation cephalosporins[b]	Varies with agent	10 days

bid, twice daily; tid, three times daily; qid, four times daily.

[a]*Dose should be determined on basis of benzathine component.*

[b]*These agents should not be used to treat patients with immediate-type hypersensitivity to β-lactam antibiotics.*

Modified from Bisno AL, Gerber MA, Gwaltney JM, et al. Practice guideline for the diagnosis and management of group A streptococcal pharyngitis. Clin Infect Dis 2002;35:113–125, with permission.

macrolide-resistant.[71] During a longitudinal investigation of GAS disease in a single elementary school in Pittsburgh, investigators found that 48% of isolates of GAS collected between 2000 and 2001 were resistant to erythromycin; none was resistant to clindamycin.[72] Molecular typing indicated that this outbreak was due to a single strain of GAS. Clinicians should be aware of local resistance rates.

OTHER TREATMENT CONSIDERATIONS

There is currently no evidence from controlled studies to guide therapy of acute pharyngitis when either β-hemolytic group C or group G streptococcus is isolated. If one elects to treat, the regimen should be similar to that for GAS pharyngitis, with penicillin as the antimicrobial agent of choice.[8]

Acyclovir treatment of HSV gingivostomatitis initiated within 72 hours of the onset of symptoms shortens the duration of illness and decreases the number of lesions.[73] Use of antiviral medications for primary EBV pharyngitis has been shown to interrupt viral replication temporarily, but symptomatic relief is negligible and does not justify the use of acyclovir. Corticosteroids are recommended for EBV pharyngitis only when tonsillar enlargement threatens airway patency.[15] Several reviews of the large group of heterogeneous studies of use of corticosteroids for GAS and non-GAS pharyngitis conclude a small but measurable benefit in pain reduction, especially when initiated early in the course of severe illness.[74-77] While no adverse outcomes related to corticosteroids were reported, the modest and short-lived benefit of treatment versus potential for harm weigh against their use.

Treatment Failures, Chronic Carriage, and Recurrences

Antimicrobial treatment failure for GAS pharyngitis can be classified as either *clinical* or *bacteriologic failure*. The significance of *clinical treatment failure* (usually defined as persistent or recurrent signs or symptoms suggestive of GAS pharyngitis) is difficult to determine without repeated isolation of the infecting strain of GAS (i.e., true bacteriologic treatment failure).

Bacteriologic treatment failures can be classified as either *true* or *apparent*. True bacteriologic failure refers to the inability to eradicate the specific strain of GAS causing an acute episode of pharyngitis with a complete course of appropriate antimicrobial therapy. No penicillin-resistant strains of GAS have ever been identified. The following factors have been suggested but not established definitively: (1) penicillin tolerance (i.e., a discordance between the concentration of penicillin required to inhibit and to kill the organisms);[78,79] (2) enhancement of colonization and growth of GAS by pharyngeal flora or inactivation of penicillin by production of β-lactamases;[67] (3) resistance of intracellular organisms to antimicrobial killing.[80]

Apparent bacteriologic failure can occur when newly acquired GAS isolates are mistaken for the original infecting strain, when the infecting strain of GAS is eradicated but then rapidly reacquired, or when adherence to antimicrobial therapy is poor. However, most bacteriologic treatment failures are manifestations of the GAS carrier state. *Chronic carriers* have GAS in their pharynx but no clinical illness or immunologic response to the organism, can be colonized for 6 to ≥12 months, are unlikely to spread GAS to close contacts, and are at very low (if any) risk for developing suppurative or nonsuppurative complications.[81,82] During the winter and spring in temperate climates, as many as 20% of asymptomatic school-aged children carry GAS.[81] GAS carriers should not be given antimicrobial therapy; the primary approach to the suspected or confirmed carrier is reassurance. A throat culture or RADT should be performed whenever the patient has symptoms and signs suggestive of GAS pharyngitis, but should be avoided when symptoms are more typical of viral illnesses (see Box 29-1). Each clinical episode confirmed with a positive throat culture or RADT should be treated. Identification and eradication of the streptococcal carrier state are desirable in certain specific situations. When antimicrobial therapy is employed, oral clindamycin (20 mg/kg per day up to 450 mg, divided into 3 doses) for 10 days is preferred,[51] but intramuscular benzathine penicillin (alone or in combination with procaine penicillin) plus oral rifampin (20 mg/kg per day divided into 2 doses; maximum dose, 300 mg for 4 days beginning on the day of the penicillin injection)[37] also is effective. Chronic carriage can recur upon re-exposure to GAS.

In a patient with symptoms suggesting GAS following treatment, a throat culture (or RADT) usually is performed and, if positive, many clinicians would elect to administer a second course of penicillin therapy.

The patient with repeated episodes of acute pharyngitis associated with a positive throat culture (or RADT) is a common and difficult problem for the practicing physician. The fundamental question is whether this patient is experiencing repeated episodes of GAS pharyngitis or is a GAS carrier experiencing repeated episodes of viral pharyngitis. The latter situation is by far the more common. Such a patient is likely to be a GAS carrier if: (1) clinical and epidemiologic findings suggest a viral etiology; (2) there is little clinical response to appropriate antimicrobial therapy; (3) throat culture (or RADT) is positive between episodes of pharyngitis; and (4) there is no serologic response to GAS extracellular antigen (e.g., ASO, anti-deoxyribonucleases B). In contrast, the patient with repeated episodes of acute pharyngitis associated with positive throat cultures (or RADTs) for GAS is likely to be experiencing repeated episodes of bona fide GAS pharyngitis if: (1) clinical and epidemiologic findings suggest GAS pharyngitis; (2) there is a demonstrable clinical response to appropriate antimicrobial therapy; (3) throat culture (or RADT) is negative between episodes of pharyngitis; and (4) there is a serologic response to GAS extracellular antigens. If determined that the patient is experiencing repeated episodes of true GAS pharyngitis, some physicians have suggested use of prophylactic oral penicillin V. However, the efficacy of this regimen has not been proven, and antimicrobial prophylaxis is not recommended except to prevent recurrences of rheumatic fever in patients who have experienced a previous episode of rheumatic fever. Tonsillectomy may be considered in the rare patient whose symptomatic episodes do not diminish in frequency over time and in whom no alternative explanation for the recurrent GAS pharyngitis is evident. However, tonsillectomy has been demonstrated to be beneficial for a relatively small group of these patients, and any benefit is relatively short-lived.[83,84]

COMPLICATIONS

GAS pharyngitis can be associated with suppurative and nonsuppurative complications (See Chapter 118, *Streptococcus pyogenes* Group A Streptococcus). Suppurative complications result from the spread of GAS to adjacent structures and include peritonsillar abscess, para- and retropharyngeal abscess, cervical lymphadenitis, sinusitis, otitis media, and mastoiditis. Before antimicrobial agents were available, suppurative complications of GAS pharyngitis were common; however, antimicrobial therapy has greatly reduced the frequency of such complications.

Acknowledgments

The authors are indebted to the scholarship of Michael Gerber who wrote this chapter in prior editions that have served as a comprehensive template upon which we have provided updated information.

---

28 Infections Related to the Upper and Middle Airways

Marc Tebruegge and Nigel Curtis

Supraglottic infections comprise peritonsillar abscess, retropharyngeal abscess, parapharyngeal abscess and epiglottitis. Infections of the middle airways include croup (laryngotracheitis) and bacterial tracheitis. All these conditions share the potential for respiratory compromise and airway obstruction. Table 28-1 summarizes the typically affected age groups, common clinical features at presentation, and the most commonly implicated organisms. Differentiation from other airway infections is discussed in Chapter 21, Respiratory Tract Symptom Complexes (see Table 21-4).

PERITONSILLAR ABSCESS (QUINSY)

Peritonsillar abscess is the most common deep oropharyngeal infection,[1] and albeit rare, usually is a complication of pharyngotonsillitis. The infection primarily affects adolescents and young adults, but can occur at any age.

Etiologic Agents

Streptococcus pyogenes is the most commonly isolated aerobic bacterium in cases with peritonsillar abscess.[2–9] Other streptococci,

TABLE 28-1. Clinical Features of Infections of the Upper and Middle Airways

Disease	Typical Age Group	Potential Initial Infection	Key Clinical Findings	Typical Organism(s)
Peritonsillar abscess	Adolescents	Pharyngotonsillitis	Sore throat, odynophagia, dysphagia, peritonsillar swelling, uvular deviation to contralateral side, muffled voice	*Streptococcus pyogenes*
Retropharyngeal abscess	<5 years of age	Pharyngitis, tonsillitis, adenitis	Sore throat, odynophagia, dysphagia, neck pain and swelling, limited neck mobility, torticollis	*Streptococcus pyogenes*, viridans streptococci, *Staphylococcus aureus*, *Haemophilus* and *Neisseria* species, anaerobic bacteria; often polymicrobial
Parapharyngeal abscess	All age groups	Pharyngitis, tonsillitis, adenitis, otitis media	Sore throat, odynophagia, dysphagia, neck pain and swelling, torticollis, deviation of the lateral wall of the oropharynx to the midline	As for retropharyngeal abscess
Lemierre disease (primary oropharyngeal infection; septicemia; thrombophlebitis of the internal jugular vein; metastatic infection at distant site(s))	Adolescents	Pharyngitis, tonsillitis, adenitis, otitis media, mastoiditis	High-grade fever, neck pain and swelling, dysphagia, nausea and vomiting, hypotension; pulmonary involvement: dyspnea, hemoptysis, pleuritic chest pain	*Fusobacterium necrophorum*
Epiglottitis	In Hib-unimmunized populations: children <4 years of age; in Hib-immunized populations: school age children	–	Unwell-looking, high-grade fever, stridor, drooling, muffled voice, tripod position with neck extension	*Haemophilus influenzae* type b
Croup (laryngotracheitis)	6 months to 2 years of age	–	Inspiratory stridor, barking cough, hoarseness; symptoms typically worsen during nighttime	Parainfluenza virus, influenza virus, respiratory syncytial virus
Bacterial tracheitis	2 to 10 years of age	–	Moderate- to high-grade fever, cough, stridor, dyspnea, retractions; rapid deterioration is common	*Staphylococcus aureus*

Staphylococcus aureus, and *Haemophilus influenzae* are less frequently implicated. Anaerobic bacteria, including *Prevotella, Bacteroides,* and *Peptostreptococcus* species, also are common isolates. Polymicrobial infection is not uncommon.

Epidemiology and Pathogenesis

The peak incidence of peritonsillar abscess is in adolescence and early adult life.[1,3,7,10-13] However, although uncommon, peritonsillar abscess can occur in very young children, including infants.[14-16] There is no clear gender predilection in most reports.

Peritonsillar abscess traditionally has been regarded invariably to be the result of extension of acute exudative pharyngotonsillitis. However, there is some evidence to suggest that this condition also can result from abscess formation within Weber salivary glands located in the supratonsillar fossa.[17]

Clinical Manifestations and Diagnosis

The patient almost invariably presents with severe sore throat and odynophagia.[7,10,12] Difficulty with swallowing often leads to decreased oral intake, potentially resulting in dehydration.[12] Symptoms may worsen and the patient may become unable to swallow saliva, leading to drooling. Fever is reported in the majority of cases but is not universal.[12] Common clinical signs at initial presentation include peritonsillar swelling, muffling of the voice, cervical lymphadenopathy, trismus, and uvular deviation towards the contralateral tonsil.[10,12] Bilateral disease is very rare.[11,18]

Inflammatory markers, including white blood cell (WBC) count and C-reactive protein, frequently are elevated.[10,12] In cases where there is doubt about the diagnosis, transcutaneous or intraoral ultrasound, or computed tomography (CT), can be useful for confirmation.[19-21]

Management

Peritonsillar abscess requires drainage, which can be achieved by needle aspiration, incision and drainage, or (quinsy) tonsillectomy.[12,13] Pus obtained during the procedure should be sent for Gram stain and routine and anaerobic culture. The choice of the intervention partly depends on the extent of patient cooperation and locally available expertise. Local practices vary widely,[22] and currently there are no convincing data to suggest that one approach is superior to another.[23-26]

There is no general consensus regarding the optimal choice of antibiotics for empiric antibiotic treatment. However, empiric therapy should provide sufficient coverage for anaerobic and β-lactamase-producing bacteria. Regimens that have been suggested include penicillin combined with metronidazole, amoxicillin-clavulanate, ampicillin-sulbactam, ticarcillin-clavulanate, cefoxitin, and clindamycin.[7,27-31]

The role of adjuvant corticosteroid treatment remains controversial.[10,23,32] Data from one randomized controlled trial in adults suggest that corticosteroids may expedite symptomatic improvement.[33]

The choice whether to manage a case of peritonsillar abscess as an outpatient or inpatient is made on an individual basis, taking into account the patient's age, coexisting morbidities, and the need for intravenous hydration, pain control, and airway monitoring.[12]

Complications and Prognosis

Only a relatively small proportion of patients require intensive care support, usually for management of airway compromise.[10] The course of the illness can be complicated by contiguous invasive spread of the infection with extension to the retropharyngeal or parapharyngeal space.[10,11] Other potential complications include aspiration pneumonia and mediastinitis.

The prognosis of appropriately managed peritonsillar abscess is good. Fatal outcome is rare. Relapse or recurrence occurs in approximately 5% to 10% of cases.[10–12,18]

RETROPHARYNGEAL ABSCESS

The retropharyngeal space extends from the base of the skull to the upper thoracic spine. The anterior border of this space is formed by the constrictor muscles of the pharynx, the lateral borders by the carotid sheaths and the posterior border by the prevertebral fascia.

Etiologic Agents

Polymicrobial infection is common; mixed aerobic and anaerobic infection occurs frequently.[34–39] Commonly implicated aerobic bacteria include: S. pyogenes, viridans streptococci, S. aureus, as well as Haemophilus and Neisseria species.[7,27,34,36,37,40–43] Although relatively uncommon, cases due to methicillin-resistant S. aureus have been described.[37,38] Common anaerobic isolates include Peptostreptococcus, Prevotella, Bacteroides, and Fusobacterium species.

Epidemiology and Pathogenesis

Retropharyngeal abscess can occur at any age, but most commonly affects children younger than 5 years of age.[7,34,41,44–46] In the majority of reports there is male predominance.[34,37,38,41,44,46–48] In the United States the incidence peaks during the winter and spring months.[41,42,47] Some data suggest that the incidence of retropharyngeal abscess has increased in the U.S. over the last decade.[34,37,39]

Retropharyngeal abscess in children predominately results from infection and suppuration of the retropharyngeal chains of lymph nodes, which drain the nasopharynx, the paranasal sinuses, and the adenoids.[34,36–39,42] Common primary infectious foci include pharyngitis, tonsillitis, adenitis, and less frequently sinusitis, otitis media, mastoiditis, and dental infections. Unlike in adults, local trauma and foreign body ingestion play a relatively minor role.[7,37,39,40,42,44]

Clinical Manifestations and Differential Diagnosis

Common presenting features include fever, sore throat, dysphagia, odynophagia, neck pain, neck swelling, limited neck mobility (particularly on extension), and torticollis.[7,34,37–42,44–46,48] Trismus and drooling are less common. The majority of patients have evidence of pharyngitis or tonsillitis and cervical lymphadenitis on examination.[40,46] In most reports the proportion of cases with symptoms indicative of airway obstruction, such as difficulty in breathing and stridor, is relatively small.[37,39–42,44,46] Airway obstruction in the context of retropharyngeal abscess predominately occurs in infants and very young children.[37–39]

Peripheral blood leukocytosis is common.[7,34,37,42,44,46] C-reactive protein (CRP) and erythrocyte sedimentation rate (ESR) generally are elevated.[46] In the majority of cases an enlargement of the retropharyngeal space/prevertebral tissue can be seen on plain lateral neck radiographs (Figure 28-1).[34,37,40,49] However, CT imaging has been shown to be the most sensitive imaging technique in cases with suspected retropharyngeal abscess, and therefore is considered the investigation of choice.[39,41,44,49–55]

Management

There is no consensus regarding the optimal empiric antibiotic treatment. Penicillin or ampicillin alone provide insufficient coverage, as S. aureus and mixed infections are common, and β-lactamase-producing organisms are isolated in a significant proportion of cases. Empiric antibiotic regimens include: a combination of a second- or third-generation cephalosporin and clindamycin; a combination of a second- or third-generation cephalosporin and

metronidazole, amoxicillin-clavulanate; ampicillin-sulbactam, or piperacillin-tazobactam.[34,41,42,53,56–59] Some authors have suggested that clindamycin alone may be sufficient.[36,48] Local patterns of susceptibility of S. aureus as well as clinical state of the patient should be taken into account. (A combination of antibiotics that includes clindamycin or vancomycin may need to be considered.)

The role of surgical drainage remains controversial.[34,37,39,42,44,46,54,60] Patients with significant respiratory distress require urgent airway management and surgical drainage. However, there is debate whether a trial of conservative management with intravenous antibiotics for a 24- to 48-hour period in conjunction with close monitoring is appropriate for patients who are stable and have no respiratory distress.[34,40–42,44] The reported success rates with conservative management alone vary considerably between different studies, and there are no data from randomized trials.[34,40–42,44,46,48] Surgical drainage usually is performed via the transoral approach, and less commonly via the transcervical route.[37–39,41,42,48,53,54]

Complications and Prognosis

Potential complications include internal jugular vein thrombosis, mycotic aneurysm of the carotid artery, aspiration pneumonia, mediastinitis, and sepsis, although these are rare overall.[37–39,41,44,45] Only a small proportion of patients require repeated surgical intervention.[39,41] The vast majority of patients have an uncomplicated course and can be discharged on oral antibiotics within a few days.[37,38] Fatal outcomes are rare in recent studies.

PARAPHARYNGEAL ABSCESS

The lateral pharyngeal space (or parapharyngeal space) is shaped like an inverted cone extending from the base of the skull to the hyoid bone, bounded medially by the superior pharyngeal constrictor muscle and laterally by the internal pterygoid muscle.[61] The lateral pharyngeal space contains the following anatomical structures: the internal carotid artery, the internal jugular vein, the cranial nerves IX–XII, the sympathetic chain, and lymph nodes. This space is separated from the retropharyngeal space only by the alar fascia, which provides little barrier against the spread of infection.[61] Consequently, simultaneous infection of both compartments is common, and some authors believe that a distinction between parapharyngeal and retropharyngeal abscess is clinically not meaningful.[42,58,61–63]

Etiologic Agents, Epidemiology, and Pathogenesis

The spectrum and frequency of causative organisms are similar to those reported in retropharyngeal abscess.[27,64] Studies on deep neck space infections in children suggest that parapharyngeal abscesses are less common than retropharyngeal abscesses.[7,28,41,46] In contrast to retropharyngeal abscess, parapharyngeal abscess occurs in all age groups without predilection for younger children.[45,65] Parapharyngeal abscess is thought primarily to result from infection and subsequent suppuration of lymph nodes in the lateral pharyngeal space, which are part of the lymphatic drainage of the nasopharynx and the middle ear.[65–68] In a large proportion of cases there is a history of preceding pharyngitis or tonsillitis.

Clinical Manifestations and Differential Diagnosis

The clinical features of parapharyngeal abscess closely resemble those associated with retropharyngeal abscess.[61] Fever and neck swelling are common features; dysphagia, odynophagia, torticollis, or trismus also can be present.[45,58,59,61,63–65,67–70] A key distinguishing feature from retropharyngeal abscess is the frequent finding on oral inspection of deviation of the lateral wall of the oropharynx to the midline.[65,69–71]

Peripheral blood leukocytosis and CRP elevation are common.[59,66] Contrast-enhanced CT is considered to be the imaging modality of choice in cases with suspected parapharyngeal abscess.[41,45,46,58,61,62,69,72] Unlike in retrophayngeal abscess, plain lateral neck radiographs are not useful.[41]

PART II Clinical Syndromes and Cardinal Features of Infectious Diseases: Approach to Diagnosis and Initial Management

SECTION C Oral Infections and Upper and Middle Respiratory Tract Infections

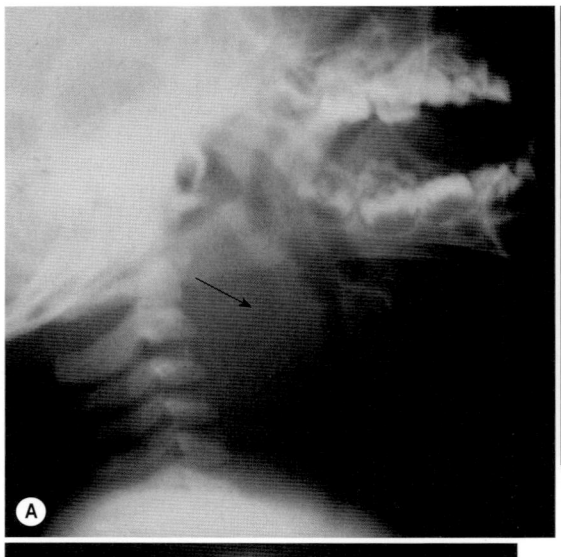

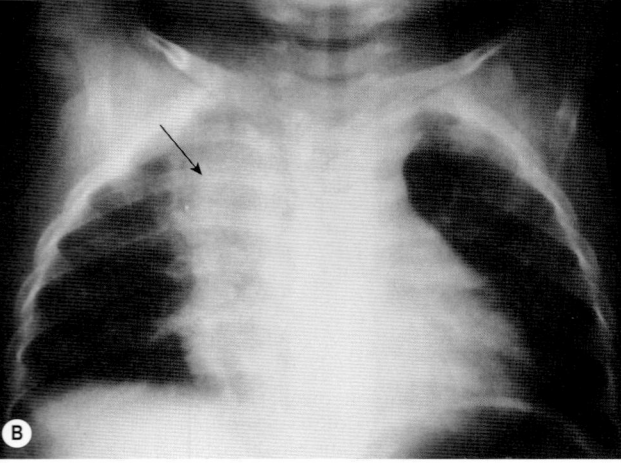

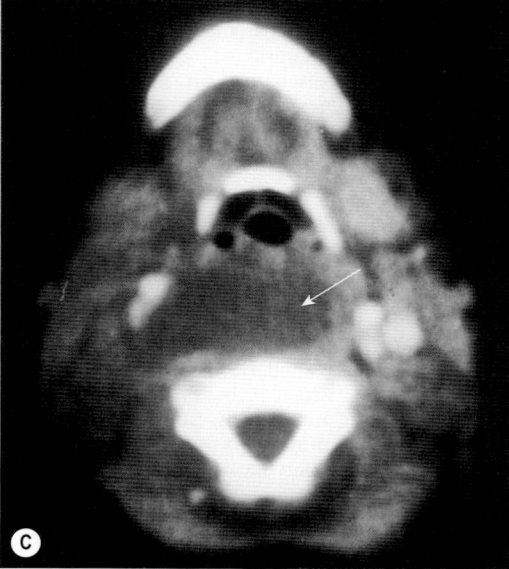

Figure 28-1. (A) Lateral neck radiograph of an 18-month-old toddler with retropharyngeal abscess due to *Staphylococcus aureus* infection. Note marked retropharyngeal soft-tissue density (arrow) with anterior displacement of the hypopharynx and the laryngotracheal airway. Note the normal appearance of the epiglottis, glottis, and subglottic airway. **(B)** Chest radiograph. Note extension of the infection into the mediastinum (arrow). **(C)** Computed tomography scan without contrast of the upper cervical region. Note abscess in the retropharyngeal space (arrow) with anterior displacement and compression of the airway and lateral displacement of the great vessels. Bony structures are the mandible (top), hyoid bone, and the cervical vertebrae.

Management, Complications, and Prognosis

The management of parapharyngeal abscess is similar to that of retropharyngeal abscess. There is ongoing controversy among experts about whether surgery is mandatory in all patients.[42,46,58,59,62,63,65,67,68,70] Traditionally, an external cervical approach has been used for the drainage of parapharyngeal abscesses.[7,53,73] More recently, transoral drainage has been reported to be safe and effective in selected cases with abscess location medial to the great vessels.[61,63,68,69,73] The transoral approach has cosmetic advantages, and the intraoperative time generally is shorter.[73]

Potential complications comprise internal jugular vein thrombosis, erosion of the carotid artery, airway obstruction, aspiration pneumonia, pleural empyema, mediastinitis, pericarditis, and septic shock.[7,45,62,64,65,68,74,75] Fatal outcome and long-term sequelae are rare.[28,62,65]

LEMIERRE DISEASE

The first description of this clinical syndrome was published in 1900 by Courmont and Cade,[76] followed by a report by Schottmuller in 1918.[77] However, the syndrome, also referred to as "necrobacillosis," is named in honor of André Lemierre, who described a series of 20 cases of "postanginal septicemia" in 1920.[78] Classically, Lemierre disease is characterized by the following features: (1) primary infection of the oropharynx; (2) blood-culture confirmed septicemia; (3) evidence of thrombophlebitis of the internal jugular vein; and (4) metastatic infection at one or more distant sites.[79]

Etiologic Agents

Fusobacterium necrophorum is by far the most commonly implicated etiologic agent.[79–82] *F. necrophorum* is an obligate anaerobic gram-negative bacillus that is part of the normal flora of the oral cavity and the gastrointestinal and female genital tract. Most strains are susceptible to second- and third-generation cephalosporins, clindamycin, and metronidazole; a significant proportion of clinical isolates produce β-lactamase.[83–85] Other causative bacteria described in association with Lemierre syndrome include other *Fusobacterium* species, *Bacteroides* and *Prevotella* species, streptococci (mainly non-group A), and infrequently staphylococci.[79,80,82,86,87] Mixed infections are not uncommon.[81,87]

Epidemiology and Pathogenesis

Despite the absence of solid epidemiologic data, most experts agree that the incidence of the disease has declined considerably during the antibiotic era. Lemierre syndrome currently is an uncommon disease, with an estimated incidence of approximately 1 per million persons per year.[88] However, there are some data suggesting that the incidence may have increased in recent years, potentially as a result of more judicious antibiotic prescribing practices for cases of upper respiratory tract infection.[89] The disease typically affects teenagers and young adults,[79,80,86,87,89,90] although a few cases in infancy have also been described.[83,91] There appears to be some male predominance.[79,92] The vast majority of cases have no predisposing illness.

In the majority of cases the disease process begins with a primary focus of infection in the oropharynx (e.g., palatine tonsils or peritonsillar tissue). Other infections in the head and neck area, including sinusitis, otitis, mastoiditis, parotitis, and odontogenic infections, are less common sources.[79,83,86–88,91–93] The infection subsequently spreads to the lateral pharyngeal space (or parapharyngeal space). Further progression results in infectious thrombophlebitis of the internal jugular vein, which in turn results in septic pulmonary emboli and metastatic infection at other distant sites. The lungs are by far the most commonly involved secondary site, followed by joint and soft-tissue infections.[79,80,87,92] Other manifestations, such as skin infection, osteomyelitis, liver abscess, splenic abscess, and meningitis, are relatively rare.[79,83,92,94–97]

Clinical Manifestations and Differential Diagnosis

The presenting features depend partly on the primary site of infection. Most cases come to medical attention within 7 days of onset of the primary infection.[79] In patients with an oropharyngeal source, inspection may reveal exudative tonsillitis, hyperemia, or greyish pseudomembranes. Importantly, an unremarkable oropharyngeal appearance at the time of septicemia does not rule out Lemierre syndrome.[79,98] Patients with otitis media or mastoiditis as the primary focus can present with otorrhea or postauricular fluctuation.[83,99] The majority of patients have high fever (>39.5°C), although fever can be absent. Neck swelling and tenderness is present in the majority of cases. Other symptoms and signs that may be present include trismus, dysphagia, dyspnea, hemoptysis, pleuritic chest pain, nausea and vomiting, jaundice, hepatomegaly, and hypotension. Severe shock and renal failure are relatively uncommon, despite the septicemic state.[79,86] Auscultation and percussion of the chest may reveal crepitus and evidence of pleural effusions in cases with pulmonary involvement.

Inflammatory markers, including WBC count, CRP, and ESR, often are markedly elevated.[80,87,89,91,92,100–103] Thrombocytopenia occurs in approximately a quarter of patients.[100] Serum-hepatic enzymes and bilirubin are not infrequently elevated.[79,87] Blood

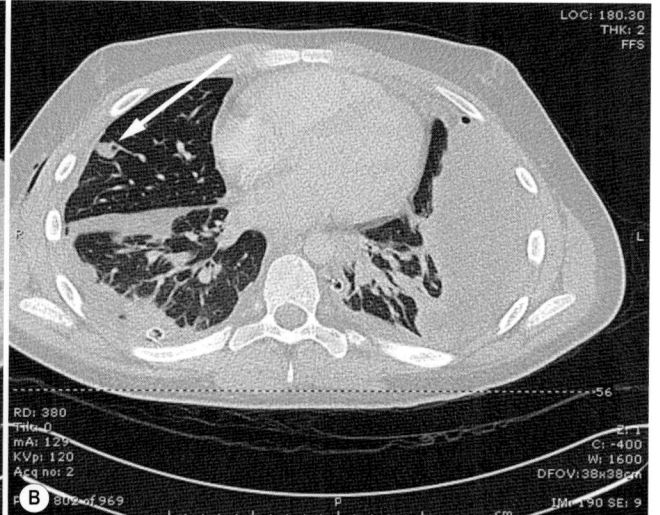

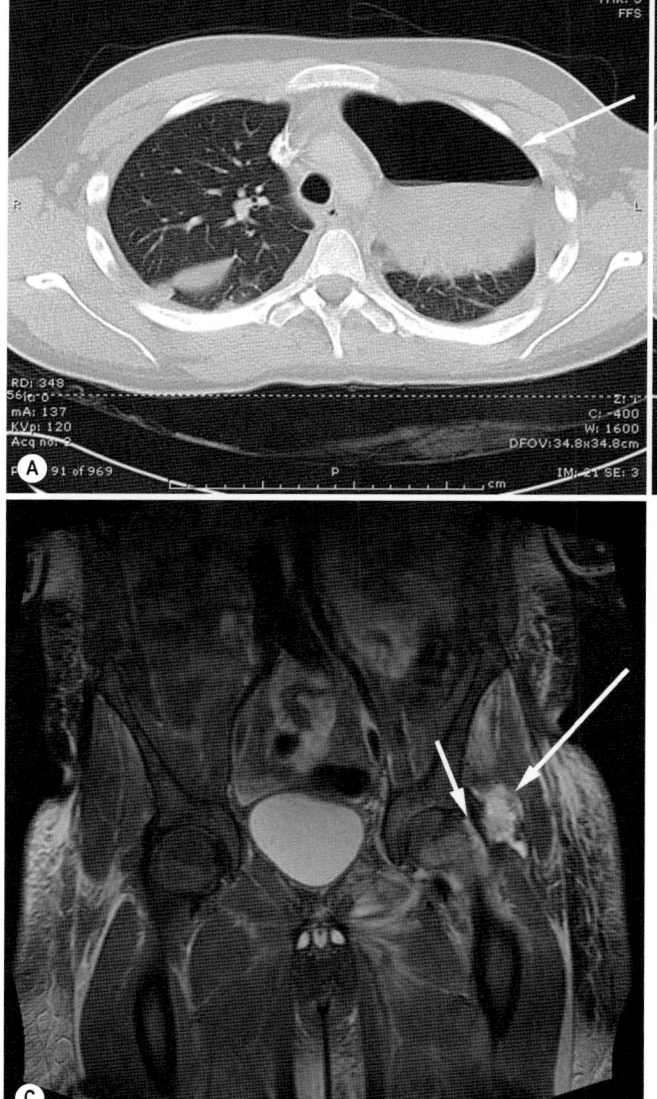

Figure 28-2. (A) Chest computed tomography scan of a 16-year-old patient with Lemierre syndrome with marked pulmonary involvement showing a large left sided pneumothorax (arrow) and adjacent empyema. **(B)** Chest computed tomography scan of the same patient showing widespread bilateral pulmonary consolidation and nodular foci. Note the central cavitation in the lesion marked by the arrow. **(C)** Coronal magnetic resonance image of the hip region in the same patient, who also developed septic arthritis of the left hip joint and abscess formation in the adjacent muscles. Note the synovial enhancement and joint effusion (small arrow) and the adjacent fluid collection (large arrow), which extends anteriorly between the iliopsoas, the rectus femoris medially, and the gluteus muscles laterally.

cultures typically are positive, but can be sterile in patients who have taken antibiotics prior to presentation. Contrast-enhanced CT of the neck is considered to be the most useful investigation. Possible CT findings include distended neck veins, intraluminal filling defects, and soft tissue swelling.[87,91,101,103,104] Doppler ultrasonography or MRI are further useful imaging modalities in this setting. Chest radiographs and chest CT may reveal pulmonary infiltrates, pulmonary cavitation, or pleural effusions (Figure 28-2).

Management

Antibiotic treatment is the mainstay of therapy. Empiric regimens commonly suggested by experts include: high-dose penicillin in combination with metronidazole; clindamycin; ticarcillin-clavulanate, and ampicillin-sulbactam.[82,87,89,98,100–102,105] Due to the endovascular nature of the infection, prolonged intravenous therapy for several weeks is required. Surgical debridement of necrotic tissues, and drainage of abscesses or empyemas often is required in conjunction with medical therapy. Ligation or resection of the internal jugular vein was a common therapeutic intervention in the pre-antibiotic era. However, this is rarely necessary now, and should be restricted to unstable patients who fail to respond to conservative therapy.[89,100,101,106] The role of routine anticoagulation therapy in Lemierre syndrome continues to be controversial.[81,86,87,89,91,100,106]

Complications and Prognosis

Metastatic infections can cause complications depending on their location. Pleural effusions, empyema, lung abscesses, and pulmonary cavitation are not uncommon manifestations. Pneumatocele and pneumothorax also have been described. Pyogenic arthritis typically affects larger joints, such as the shoulder, elbow, and hip joints (Figure 28-2).[79,92] Renal involvement can be associated with proteinuria or hematuria.

In the pre-antibiotic era the prognosis was poor, with fatality rates as high as 90% in some historical reports.[78,93] Recent reviews of the literature suggest that fatal outcome is now uncommon, and likely to be between 5% and 10%.[79,80]

ACUTE EPIGLOTTITIS (SUPRAGLOTTITIS)

Since introduction of effective vaccines against *Haemophilus influenzae* type b (Hib), and their inclusion in routine childhood immunization programs in many countries, the incidence of invasive Hib disease has decreased dramatically, and epiglottitis has become a rare disease.[107–118] Necrotizing epiglottitis is an extremely rare variant, which has predominately been reported in immunocompromised patients.[119]

Etiologic Agents

Haemophilus influenzae type b accounted for approximately 75% to 90% of epiglottitis cases in the pre-Hib vaccination era.[108,115,120] Since the introduction of Hib conjugate vaccines, the proportion of cases caused by Hib has declined considerably, although cases related to vaccination failure have continued to be reported.[108,111,115,120–124] Other organisms implicated in epiglottitis are *S. pyogenes*, *S. pneumoniae*, *S. aureus*, nontypable *Haemophilus influenzae*, *H. parainfluenzae*, *Pseudomonas* species, *Klebsiella* species, and *Moraxella catarrhalis*.[108,115,120,125–128]

Epidemiology and Pathogenesis

In the pre-Hib vaccination era the incidence of epiglottitis peaked in early childhood, typically affecting children younger than 4 years of age.[120,125] Since the introduction of universal Hib vaccination, the peak incidence has shifted towards an older age group, with a simultaneous increase in the proportion of adult cases.[108,114,118,124,125,128–130] Many studies show no gender predominance, while others report some male predominance.[111,120,130–132] In temperate climates, there is little seasonal variation in the incidence.[118,130–133]

Acute epiglottitis is a localized, invasive bacterial infection of the supraglottic area, comprising the epiglottis, the arytenoid cartilages, aryepiglottic folds, and false vocal cords. Inflammation results in airway edema and narrowing, which leads to airway obstruction manifesting as stridor and respiratory distress. The localized infection can evolve into phlegmon and abscess formation. Bacteremia is common in cases caused by Hib, but dissemination to distant sites (e.g., causing arthritis or meningitis) is rare.

Clinical Manifestations and Diagnosis

Children with epiglottitis typically look systemically unwell, and have high fever and stridor.[111,125,132] Aphonia and a muffled ("hot potato") voice are common features.[118,125] Odynophagia is very common, and drooling frequently is observed. The majority of patients assume an upright position (e.g., "tripod position") with extension of the neck.[134] Cervical lymphadenopathy is also a common feature.[125]

Peripheral blood leukocytosis is present in the majority of cases.[118,125,128,133] Lateral neck radiographs, demonstrating epiglottic enlargement or a classic "thumb sign," have relatively high sensitivity, but should only be attempted in stable patients in a safe environment (Figure 28-3).[121,125]

Management

Effective airway management is the most critical component of management of epiglottitis. Causing upset to the child and attempts at oral/pharyngeal inspection can potentially result in complete airway obstruction. Nebulized epinephrine (adrenaline) may provide some transient improvement in patients with respiratory distress, but also can cause agitation and precipitate respiratory obstruction. Unstable patients should be urgently intubated via direct laryngoscopy/bronchoscopy in a controlled setting (i.e., operating room or intensive care unit). Although rarely required, facilities to perform a tracheostomy must be available in case intubation attempts fail.[111,118,125,130] There

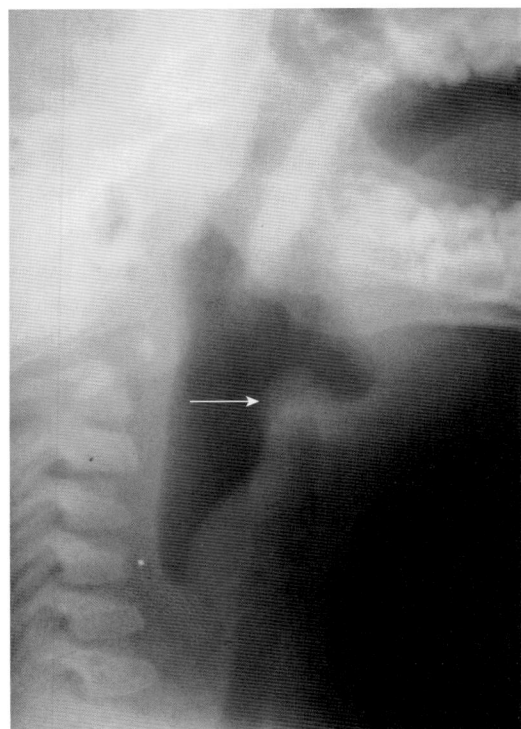

Figure 28-3. Lateral neck radiograph of a 4-year-old child with acute epiglottitis. Note characteristically distended hypopharynx and "thumbprint" edematous epiglottis and aryepiglottic folds (arrow).

continues to be controversy about whether cases at the mild end of the disease spectrum without significant respiratory distress can be managed safely without intubation while being closely monitored.[118,125,135]

Blood cultures and throat/epiglottic swabs (in intubated cases) should be obtained for culture and susceptibility testing. Empiric antibiotic therapy, such as a third-generation cephalosporin or ampicillin-sulbactam, should be commenced promptly.[108,111,120,123,135,136] The routine use of corticosteroids, intended to reduce airway edema, remains controversial; there are no randomized controlled trial data available at present;[118,128,135] however, uncontrolled studies have not shown a clear benefit regarding the need for intubation, duration of ventilation, or duration of hospital stay.[125,128,133] In cases with confirmed Hib epiglottitis, prophylaxis with rifampin should be considered for household contacts according to American Academy of Pediatrics recommendations.[137]

Complications and Prognosis

Potential complications include complete airway obstruction and cardiac arrest, epiglottic abscess, deep neck infection, pneumonia, and seizures.[111,118,120,125]

Most patients require only a short period of intubation and ventilation, and can be extubated within 24 to 72 hours.[111,118,120,132] Fatal outcome is relatively rare (less than 5%) in settings where good intensive care support is available.[118,120,125,130]

CROUP (LARYNGOTRACHEITIS)

Viral croup is the commonest cause of infectious upper-airway obstruction in young children. Some authors prefer to divide croup into spasmodic croup and laryngotracheitis (also commonly referred to as laryngotracheobronchitis).[138] However, in a clinical setting this distinction is not particularly meaningful, and croup is therefore used as a summative term in this chapter.

Etiologic Agents and Epidemiology

Parainfluenza virus types 1, 2, and 3 are the most common causative agents of croup, accounting for 50% to 80% of cases, followed by influenza A, influenza B, and respiratory syncytial virus.[139-144] Other, less common etiologic agents include adenoviruses, rhinoviruses, coxsackieviruses, and echoviruses.[139,140,144,145] More recent studies have documented human metapneumovirus, human bocavirus, and human coronavirus NL63 as further causative agents of croup.[145-152] There are some data suggesting that the clinical course of croup caused by influenza virus is more severe than croup caused by parainfluenza virus.[139]

Epidemiology and Pathogenesis

Croup is a very common disease; one study from Seattle estimated the annual incidence in children under the age of 6 years to be as high as 7 per 1000 children.[144] The incidence of croup is highest in children aged 6 months to 2 years.[140,142-144] Typical croup symptoms are rarely observed in children older than 6 years of age, likely owing to the increase in airway diameter.[143] The incidence is higher in boys.[138-140,142,153] In temperate climates the incidence typically peaks in late autumn and winter.[140,142,144,153]

Inflammatory edema and mucus production result in airway narrowing in the subglottic region, resulting in stridor.[134,138,154,155] Inflammation of the vocal cords results in hoarseness, and sometimes aphonia.

Clinical Manifestations and Differential Diagnosis

The typical features of croup are inspiratory stridor, a barking cough, and hoarseness. The symptoms often start abruptly, and typically worsen during the nighttime.[156] Nonspecific coryzal symptoms frequently precede the illness. The majority of patients have low-grade or moderate fever.[141,142] Less than 3% of cases presenting

in a primary care setting require hospitalization.[141,142] (Infectious and noninfectious causes and clinical features of upper-airway obstruction, including croup, are delineated in Chapter 21, Respiratory Tract Symptom Complexes, and highlighted in Tables 21-3, 21-4, and 21-5.) Noninfectious differential diagnosis includes foreign body aspiration, vocal cord dysfunction, laryngeal web, allergic or hypocalcemic laryngospasm, subglottic stenosis (e.g., after prolonged intubation), tracheomalacia, H-type tracheoesophageal fistula, gastroesophageal reflux, and vascular ring.[138,156-159] Laryngeal diphtheria, now a very rare but potentially life-threatening infection, can present as severe croup.[156,160,161]

The diagnosis of croup primarily is made on clinical grounds. Airway or chest radiographs are not indicated in cases with uncomplicated croup.[156,162,163] However, radiologic investigation can be useful if an alternative diagnosis is suspected. Similarly, laboratory tests, including rapid antigen tests and viral cultures, are not indicated routinely as they rarely help in case management.[156]

Management

Treatment with mist or humidified air has been a key component of croup management for much of the twentieth century.[138] However, there are few published randomized controlled trials (RCTs) investigating the effectiveness of humidified air.[164-167] All of these studies have been conducted in a hospital environment, and there are no published data on the effectiveness of warm humidified air in the home environment – a measure frequently recommended to parents.[168] A recent Cochrane review that included pooled data from three RCTs found that there was some, but statistically nonsignificant, improvement in the croup severity score of patients receiving humidified air compared with patients remaining in room air during the first hour of treatment; there was no difference between treatment groups for other outcome measures.[168]

Treatment with corticosteroids is indicated routinely.[138] A recent Cochrane review, which included 31 RCTs, showed that corticosteroid treatment was associated with significant improvement in croup severity score at 6 and 12 hours compared with placebo.[169] In addition, corticosteroid treatment was associated with a shorter duration of stay in the emergency department or hospital, fewer admissions, and fewer return visits. However, a variety of corticosteroids (dexamethasone, budesonide, methyl-prednisolone, and fluticasone), different routes of administration (orally, intramuscular, inhaled) and doses were used in the trials included. Most experts currently recommend the use of either oral or intramuscular dexamethasone (at a dose of 0.6 mg/kg) or nebulized budesonide (at a dose of 2 mg).[138,162,170-172] It currently remains unclear whether repeated doses over the first 48 hours improve outcome.

Multiple studies have shown that nebulized epinephrine (adrenaline) is effective for achieving symptomatic improvement in children with moderate to severe croup.[173-178] In addition, there are data to suggest that the use of nebulized epinephrine has resulted in a considerable reduction in the need for intubation or tracheostomy.[179] The drug can be administered as racemic epinephrine (2.25%; 0.5 mL in 2.5 mL of saline) or L-epinephrine (1 : 1000 solution; 5 mL). The treatment is safe and side effects, such as pallor and tachycardia, generally are mild and transient.[180]

In children with moderate croup (i.e., with stridor and chest wall indrawing at rest) who fail to improve sufficiently within 4 to 6 hours of administration of a corticosteroid, hospitalization should be considered. Children with severe croup should receive a dose of a corticosteroid and be treated with nebulized epinephrine; repeated administration of nebulized epinephrine may be necessary. Intensive care support should be considered if there is insufficient response. It is important to remember that the effect of nebulized epinephrine only lasts for 1 to 2 hours.[173] Once the drug effect wears off clinical symptoms can return to baseline, or even become more severe (so-called "rebound effect").[170]

Children with oxygen saturation below 92% in room air should be given supplemental oxygen. Several reports have described the use of heliox in croup, with some promising results.[181-183]

PART II Clinical Syndromes and Cardinal Features of Infectious Diseases: Approach to Diagnosis and Initial Management

SECTION C Oral Infections and Upper and Middle Respiratory Tract Infections

However, a recent Cochrane review concluded that there is currently insufficient evidence to support its use in this setting.[184] The use of antitussive and decongestant agents is not recommended.[138,170] Treatment with antibiotics is not indicated, unless clinical features or laboratory results indicate secondary bacterial infection.[138,157,170] In cases of severe croup caused by influenza A or B virus, treatment with a neuraminidase inhibitor should be considered, although currently there are insufficient efficacy data in this setting.[138,185-187]

Complications and Prognosis

Only a small proportion of cases with croup require intubation and ventilation.[139,140] Contiguous spread of the viral infection is not uncommon, which can result in otitis media, bronchiolitis, or pneumonia. Bacterial superinfection can lead to bacterial tracheitis (see below) or bronchopneumonia.

The prognosis of uncomplicated croup is very good. Symptoms largely resolve within 48 to 72 hours in the majority of patients.[156] Fatal outcome is very rare.

ACUTE LARYNGITIS

Isolated, acute laryngitis is primarily a disease described in adolescents and adults.

Etiologic Agents

Acute laryngitis is most commonly caused by viral infections; the spectrum of causative viral agents is very similar to that described in croup.[188-192] Bacterial organisms that have been implicated in acute laryngitis include *S. pneumoniae*, *H. influenzae*, and *M. catarrhalis*.[193-195]

Clinical Manifestations and Management

The key features of acute laryngitis are a change in the normal pitch of the voice and hoarseness, which typically lasts for 3 to 7 days. Coexistence of nonspecific upper respiratory tract infection symptoms, such as coryza, sore throat, and cough, is common.

Acute laryngitis in previously healthy individuals is a self-limiting disease. Given that the majority of cases are due to viral infection, treatment with antibiotics is not routinely indicated. Notably, a recent Cochrane review on this topic, which included two RCTs evaluating penicillin V and erythromycin versus placebo, concluded that routine antibiotic treatment is of no proven benefit.[196]

BACTERIAL TRACHEITIS

The term "bacterial tracheitis" was first used in a publication by Jones et al. in 1979.[197] However, earlier reports describe cases of "laryngotracheobronchitis" that closely resemble descriptions of bacterial tracheitis, suggesting that this entity existed previously.[198,199]

Etiologic Agents

S. aureus is by far the most common causative organism.[114,200-202] Other bacteria commonly implicated in bacterial tracheitis are *S. pyogenes*, *S. pneumoniae*, *H. influenzae*, and *M. catarrhalis*. Cases attributed to a variety of other bacteria, including *Pseudomonas aeruginosa*, *Bacillus cereus*, *Escherichia coli*, *Prevotella*, and *Bacteroides* species, also have been reported in the literature, although these appear to be uncommon.[200-207]

Epidemiology and Pathogenesis

Bacterial tracheitis is a rare disease, with an estimated incidence below 0.1/100,000 children per year in the United Kingdom and in Australia.[201] No incidence data have been published for other countries. Some data suggest that the incidence peaks during autumn and winter.[201] Bacterial tracheitis predominately affects young children, although a few adult cases have been described.[208-210]

The pathogenesis of bacterial tracheitis remains unclear. It has been postulated that viral infection of the upper respiratory tract may facilitate secondary bacterial infection and invasion of the airways, resulting in inflammation and edema, which ultimately leads to narrowing of the trachea.[200] This concept is supported by the fact that the peak incidence of bacterial tracheitis coincides with the peak season for viral respiratory pathogens. In one large case series, coinfection with influenza virus was identified in almost one-third of cases.[202] Coinfection with parainfluenza virus, respiratory syncytial virus, or adenovirus has been described in other reports.[114,201,204,211]

Clinical Manifestations and Differential Diagnosis

The majority of patients with bacterial tracheitis report prodromal symptoms suggestive of a minor upper respiratory tract infection, which typically are present for 2 to 5 days prior to the onset of stridor. Once stridor and dyspnea develop, patients often deteriorate rapidly, frequently requiring intubation to overcome increasing upper-airway obstruction within the first 24 hours.[197,201,212,213] Other common features at presentation include fever (often moderate to high grade), hoarse voice or aphonia, cough, as well as intercostal and subcostal retractions. Drooling is uncommon. Most cases show little or no response to nebulized epinephrine.[214]

The main differential diagnoses are epiglottis and viral croup. Unlike cases of bacterial tracheitis, children with epiglottitis typically refuse to speak, have drooling, and adopt an upright position with extension of the neck. Cases with croup typically have only low-grade fever, do not appear toxic, and generally respond to nebulized epinephrine.

Inflammatory markers, such as CRP and WBC count, are elevated in the majority of cases at presentation.[201,214] Radiographs may demonstrate narrowing of the tracheal air shadow and tracheal membranes, although these are not universal findings (Figure 28-4).[204,211] Coexisting pulmonary changes, including infiltrates and atelectases, are relatively common.[201,214-217] Direct visualization of the airways reveals an unremarkable or only mildly inflamed epiglottis, but marked subglottic inflammation, edema of the tracheal mucosa, and copious purulent endotracheal secretions.[197,214] Endotracheal aspirates should be obtained and sent for bacterial culture and susceptibility testing. Blood cultures are positive infrequently.

Management

Proactive airway management is critical in bacterial tracheitis, in order to prevent complete airway obstruction and consequent respiratory arrest. In most larger published case series, 80% to 100% of the cases required intubation or tracheostomy and mechanical ventilation.[200] Intubation of these cases generally is challenging, and usually requires the use of an endotracheal tube of considerably smaller diameter than would be expected based on the patient's age. It is important that the capability to conduct a tracheostomy is available, in case conventional intubation attempts fail.

There is no consensus among experts regarding the most appropriate empiric antibiotic treatment, although there is agreement that this must include effective anti-staphylococcal coverage. Based on published data on the frequency and range of causative organisms, a combination of a third-generation cephalosporin (e.g., cefotaxime) and a penicillinase-resistant penicillin (e.g., cloxacillin or nafcillin) intravenously is a suitable choice. In areas where community-acquired methicillin-resistant *S. aureus* infections are common, vancomycin should replace the latter. Although good quality evidence is lacking, many centers use systemic corticosteroids in the first few days of the illness with the intention to reduce airway edema.

The majority of patients require ventilatory support for a relatively short period of time, typically for 2 to 5 days, unless complications occur. The optimal duration of antibiotic treatment is unknown, but it generally is recommended for a minimum of 10 days.

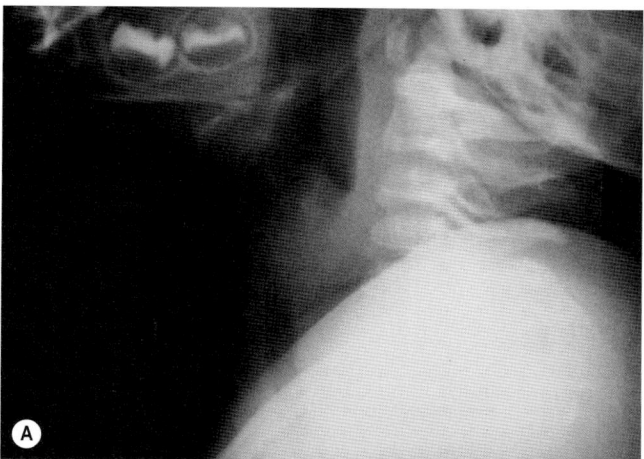

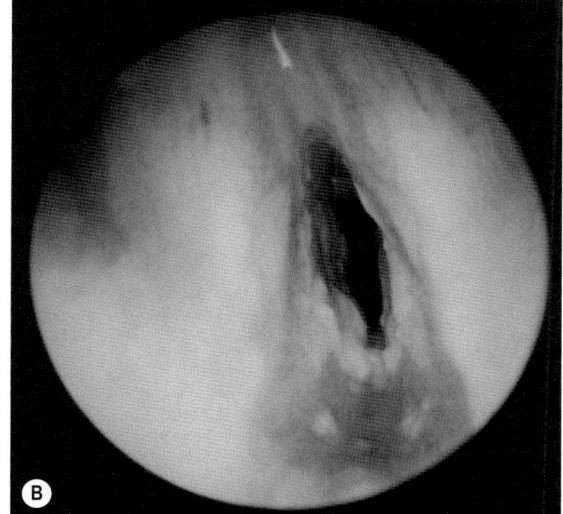

Figure 28-4. (A) Lateral neck radiograph of a 22-month-old boy with bacterial tracheitis caused by *Staphylococcus aureus* showing subglottic haziness (similar to croup). **(B)** Endoscopic view of the trachea shows mucosal denudation, intraluminal debris, and purulent laryngotracheal secretions.

Complications and Prognosis

Complications of bacterial tracheitis include pneumothorax, pulmonary edema, acute respiratory distress syndrome, hypotension, and cardiorespiratory arrest.[204,211,214,218] In addition, a few cases with toxic shock syndrome have been described.[211,213,219] Neurologic sequelae are common in patients who experience cardiores-

piratory arrest. Subglottic stenosis and subglottic polyps are further potential long-term sequelae, albeit rare.[211,220]

Bacterial tracheitis is a potentially life-threatening condition, with some of the earlier publications reporting case fatalities in excess of 20%.[211,218] However, fatal outcomes are uncommon in reports published during the last decade, likely reflecting improvements in recognition and intensive care support.[114,201,202]

ACUTE BRONCHITIS

Acute bronchitis predominately occurs in adolescents and adults. Data from the U.S. National Health Interview Survey suggest that approximately 5% of all adults experience one or more episodes of bronchitis per year.[221] The incidence peaks in autumn and winter.[222]

Etiologic Agents

Most cases of bronchitis are nonbacterial in nature. However, in a large proportion of patients no causative organism can be identified. Viral infections appear to account for the majority of cases.[223,224] Viruses commonly implicated in acute bronchitis include influenza virus, parainfluenza virus, respiratory syncytial virus, rhinovirus, adenovirus, and human metapneumovirus.[223-228] Infection due to bacterial organisms, including *Bordetella pertussis*, *Chlamydophila pneumoniae*, and *Mycoplasma pneumoniae*, is less common.[223-225]

Clinical Manifestations and Management

The illness typically begins with nonspecific upper respiratory tract infection symptoms, which usually last for a few days. This is followed by a second phase characterized by persistent cough, frequently with sputum production or wheezing, which typically lasts for 1 to 3 weeks.[222,223]

Antibiotic therapy is not routinely indicated in previously healthy individuals with acute bronchitis.[222,229] A recent Cochrane review that included nine RCTs showed that antibiotic treatment on average reduces the duration of cough only by less than one day compared with placebo; simultaneously adverse effects were significantly more common in the antibiotic-treated patients.[230] Recent guidelines for management of acute bronchitis by the American College of Physicians and the American College of Chest Physicians have discouraged the routine use of antibiotics, inhaled bronchodilators, and mucolytic agents.[231,232] Nevertheless, patients diagnosed with pertussis should receive antibiotics, primarily to limit transmission.[222]

Acknowledgments

The authors wish to acknowledge the use of figures and legends (Figures 28-1, 28-3, and 28-4) contributed by Richard H. Schwartz from the 3rd edition.

29 Otitis Media

Stephen I. Pelton

Otitis media is a disease of early childhood. Its relevance to child health has evolved from an association with suppurative complications, such as mastoiditis and brain abscess, to the current concern of prolonged conductive hearing loss as well as language or cognitive delays. Furthermore, the current frequency of diagnosis and treatment of acute otitis media (AOM) results in >12 million antibiotic prescriptions annually, as well as

significant family disruption.[1] Recent re-evaluation of criteria for diagnosis and management of AOM have been influenced by selective pressure on colonization with otopathogens from universal administration of pneumococcal conjugate vaccine and concern over the widespread use of antibiotics for treatment of AOM that has contributed to the emergence of antibiotic resistance.[2]

ACUTE OTITIS MEDIA

Pathogenesis

AOM generally is considered to be a bacterial infection because bacterial otopathogens are isolated from middle-ear culture in 70% of cases,[3] but most frequently it is a coinfection, with a viral upper respiratory tract infection (URI) enhancing the ability of bacterial otopathogens to ascend from the nasopharynx to the middle ear. Respiratory tract viruses alone can, on occasion, elicit signs and symptoms of AOM and are recovered without evidence of bacterial coinfection from a small proportion of tympanocenteses (2% to 20%).[4] Eustachian tube dysfunction (as indicated by the presence of negative pressure with tympanometry) has been demonstrated to occur in 75% of children with viral URI and is a major contributing factor to the development of bacterial AOM.[5] Additionally, influenza A infection suppresses neutrophil function[6] and macrophage recruitment, which likely contributes to the high attack rate for AOM observed in children with influenza A infection.[7] Viral URI in animal models and as observed in children enhances the frequency and density of nasopharyngeal colonization with otopathogens in children.[8–10] Figure 29-1 represents a synthesis of these important pathophysiologic mechanisms.

Microbiology and Antimicrobial Susceptibility

A limited number of viral and bacterial pathogens are recovered from culture of the middle ear. Table 29-1 and Figure 29-2 provide data on the relative frequency of recovery of viral[4] and bacterial pathogens. Four bacterial otopathogens – *Streptococcus pneumoniae* (Sp), nontypable *Haemophilus influenzae* (NTHi), *Moraxella catarrhalis*, and *Streptococcus pyogenes* (group A streptococcus: GAS) – consistently are recovered from middle-ear cultures. Although the proportion of disease due to each pathogen varies with geography and age, remarkable consistency has been observed in microbiologic studies of symptomatic middle-ear disease. Jacobs and

associates[3] reported on otopathogens recovered from 917 episodes of AOM in Eastern European, Israeli, and United States children. In the U.S., since 7-valent pneumococcal conjugate vaccine (PCV7) was begun in 2000, the microbiology of AOM has shifted, with increasing importance of nonvaccine serotypes of *S. pneumoniae*

TABLE 29-1. Virus Detected Alone or in Combination with Bacterial Pathogens from Middle-Ear Fluid in 128 Children with Acute Otitis Media

Virus	No. of Children	%
Respiratory syncytial	72	49.0
Parainfluenza (types 1, 2, and 3)	20	13.6
Influenza (A and B)	19	12.9
Enterovirus	10	6.8
Rhinovirus	10	6.8
Cytomegalovirus	8	5.0
Adenovirus	7	4.8
Herpes simplex	1	0.7
Total	147	100

Adapted from Chonmaitree T. Viral and bacterial interaction in acute otitis media. Pediatr Infect Dis J 2000;19:S24–S30.

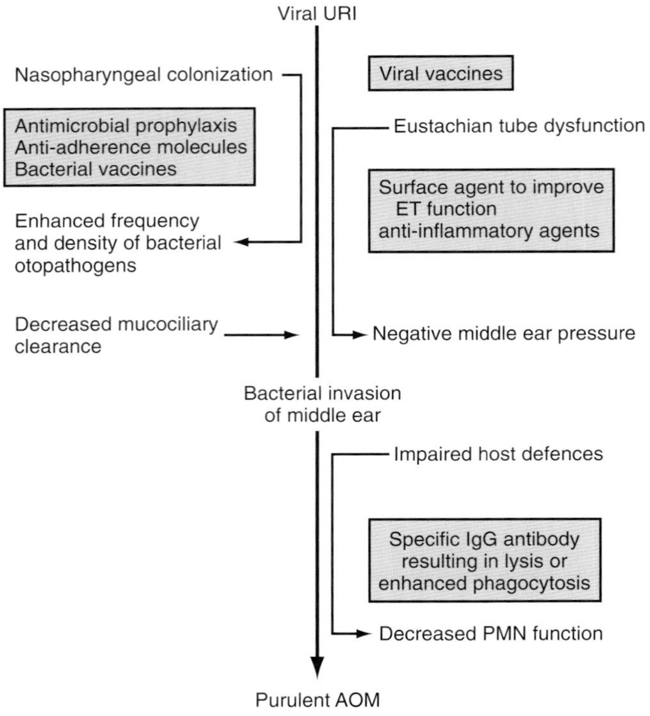

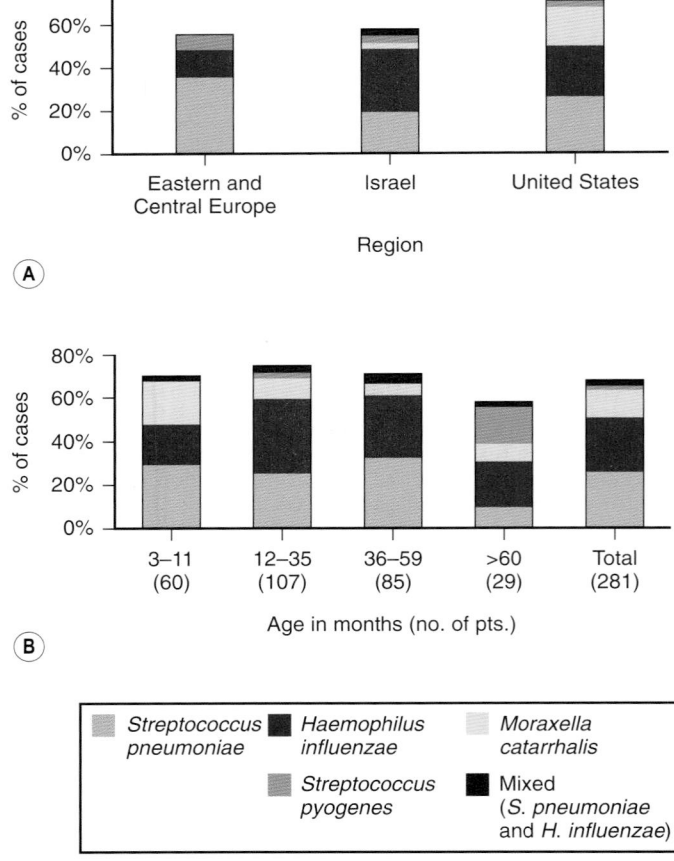

Figure 29-2. (A) Microbiology of acute otitis media in the United States, eastern and central Europe, and Israel, 1998. **(B)** Age distribution of middle-ear pathogens in U.S. children. (Redrawn from Jacobs MR, Dagan R, Appelbaum PC, et al. Prevalence of antimicrobial-resistant pathogens in middle ear fluid. Multinational study of 917 children with acute otitis media. Antimicrob Agents Chemother 1998;42:589–595.)

Figure 29-1. Schema of events in viral-bacterial pathogenesis of acute otitis media (AOM), with potential intervention strategies (shown in boxes). ET, endotracheal tube; Ig, immunoglobulin; PMNL, polymorphonuclear leukocyte; URI, upper respiratory tract infection.

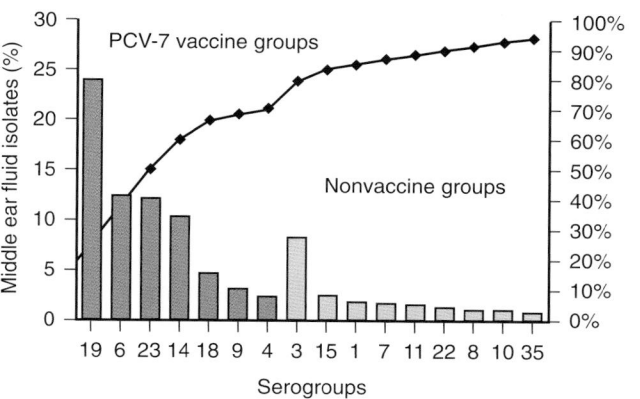

Figure 29-3. Serogroups of *Streptococcus pneumoniae* causing acute otitis media in North American children, 2000. (Redrawn from Hausdorff WP, Bryant J, Kloek C, et al. The contribution of specific pneumococcal serogroups to different disease manifestations: implications for conjugate vaccine formulation and use. Part II. Clin Infect Dis 2000;30:122–140.)

(NV-Sp), and emergence of NTHi as the most common otopathogen in children failing initial therapy.[11–13]

Streptococcus pneumoniae

The pneumococcus is recovered from 30% to 50% of children with AOM.[14–18] In the U.S. prior to the introduction of PCV7, 70% of episodes of pneumococcal otitis media were due to seven serotypes (Figure 29-3).[19] Following universal PCV7 immunization of infants in 2000, a shift in serotypes recovered from middle-ear cultures of children with AOM was observed. This is consistent with the understanding that differences in capacity of Sp serotypes to produce AOM are small.[20] NV-Sp are nearly as likely as V-Sp to cause AOM. From 1985 through 1999 increasing penicillin and multidrug resistance emerged among isolates of Sp. Resistance was most common among 5 to 7 serotypes,[21] which were included in PCV7. Vaccination was associated with decline in carriage of V-Sp and replacement with NV-Sp; an initial decrease in disease due to penicillin-resistant and multidrug-resistant Sp (as well as initial decline in treatment failures) was followed by increasing resistance among NV-Sp.[2,22]

Haemophilus influenzae

NTHi causes a substantial proportion of cases of AOM in children.[23] A well-recognized clinical syndrome, otitis–conjunctivitis, is associated with recovery of NTHi from both the middle ear and the conjunctiva.[24] Several investigators have reported an increased proportion of disease due to NTHi, specifically among immunized children who have persistent or recurrent disease after initial treatment.[12,13] The majority of these isolates of NTHi are β-lactamase-producing and amoxicillin-resistant. In Japan, isolates of NTHi with high-level resistance to amoxicillin due to alterations in the penicillin-binding proteins have been recovered from children with AOM.[25] Such isolates are also observed in France and although uncommon in US, are increasing.[26]

Moraxella catarrhalis

M. catarrhalis has been recognized only recently as a bona fide pathogen in AOM, with isolation from middle-ear cultures of children with AOM and development of a humoral immune response.[27] The organism appears to be more prevalent in certain geographic areas as well as in the first year of life.

Groups A and Group B Streptococcus

Otitis media due to GAS was common in the preantibiotic era. Currently, these organisms are most often AOM pathogens in school-aged children (>5 years of age). Jacobs and associates[3] reported a greater proportion of cases in eastern European children than in U.S. children.

Staphylococcus aureus and Staphylococcus epidermidis

The role of *Staphylococcus aureus* as a pathogen in AOM remains controversial. In Japan and South Africa, *S. aureus* is reported as a primary pathogen of AOM in children, recoverable from tympanocentesis.[28] In the U.S., *S. aureus* is recovered from <3% of middle-ear cultures from children with AOM and intact tympanic membrane. *S. aureus* and recently community-associated methicillin-resistant *S. aureus* (CA-MRSA) are identified pathogens in children with acute otorrhea associated with a tympanostomy tube.[29,30]

Epidemiology

Otitis media is virtually universal in childhood. By 2 years of age, 90% of children have had at least one symptomatic or asymptomatic episode.[31] The age-specific incidence peaks between 6 and 18 months in the U.S. and somewhat later in Europe. Risk factors for AOM are: young age,[32] exposure to young children (group childcare attendance or siblings in household),[33] and positive family history. Studies evaluating features such as race,[34] breast-feeding,[35] use of pacifier,[36] and exposure to cigarette smoke[37] have identified associations with AOM less consistently.

Recognition of the otitis-prone child has been important in the development of strategies for reducing the burden of AOM and otitis media with effusion (OME). Onset of disease in the first few months of life is a sentinel event, either as a summation of risk features or possibly as an event that itself creates enhanced susceptibility. Unfortunately, trends in the U.S., as reported by Block et al. in 2001,[38] suggest that early onset of AOM and the proportion of children with >3 or >6 episodes before their first birthday are increasing compared with observations by Teele and colleagues in 1989.[39]

In the last decade, several studies of insurance claims document a decline in the number of OM-related visits in the U.S., Canada, and United Kingdom, although no prospective birth cohort studies have been published.[40–42] The relationship between the decline in visits and the introduction of PCV7 is entangled in the secular changes in diagnostic criteria, expanded use of influenza vaccine, and adoption of initial observation for some children. Both Grijalva et al.[40] and de Wals et al.[42] provide evidence that the decline in AOM preceded the introduction of PCV7 and was potentially accelerated with its introduction.[40,42] Although clinical trials demonstrated only a modest reduction in AOM episodes or visits, some investigators speculate that prevention of early pneumococcal otitis media may have compounding benefits that results in a more substantial decline than observed in short-term clinical trials.

Treatment

Multiple issues require evaluation in order to determine the appropriate strategy for treatment of AOM: (1) What is the natural history of AOM, and does antibiotic therapy alter the natural history? (2) Should the outcome be measured by clinical or microbiologic endpoints? (3) Does the emergence of multiple-drug-resistant *S. pneumoniae* affect the outcome and choice of therapy for AOM? (4) What guidelines have been established for the treatment of AOM? (5) Does initial observation increase the risk of development of suppurative complications such as mastoiditis?

Natural History

In the preantibiotic era, mastoiditis was a common complication of AOM; the use of antimicrobial therapy for the treatment of AOM has resulted in a dramatic decline in incidence. Similarly, in special populations such as Alaska Eskimos, chronic otorrhea occurred in ~30% of children prior to the routine use of

PART II Clinical Syndromes and Cardinal Features of Infectious Diseases: Approach to Diagnosis and Initial Management

SECTION C Oral Infections and Upper and Middle Respiratory Tract Infections

antimicrobial agents.[43] In 1999, Baxter[44] reported a substantial decline in chronic otorrhea over a 30-year period that was associated with the introduction of routine antimicrobial therapy for the treatment of AOM. During this same period, socioeconomic conditions also improved, blurring the specific contribution of medical management in reducing chronic otorrhea.

In general, an episode of AOM resolves in the majority of children with or without antimicrobial therapy. Antibiotic treatment does not benefit the 20% to 30% of episodes of middle-ear disease with negative culture results. Additionally, some children with bacterial AOM clear the pathogen spontaneously.[45]

Therapeutic trials that include placebo groups consistently report excess failure rates in children who receive only symptomatic treatment; however, the significance of these differences is fiercely debated. Little and coworkers[46] compared the outcome of AOM in children initially treated with amoxicillin with those given a prescription to be filled only if symptoms persisted for 72 hours. Children treated with antibiotics improved more quickly. McCormick and colleagues[47] evaluated the strategy of "watchful waiting" for children with perceived mild disease as defined by a structured assessment. Children assigned to the delayed treatment group had increased treatment failures and persistent symptoms (Table 29-2). More frequent mild adverse events as well as the emergence of multidrug-resistant isolates of *S. pneumoniae* in the nasopharynx occurred in the early-treatment group. Evaluating outcomes within the first 3 to 5 days provides the best evidence for more rapid resolution in antibiotic-treated compared with placebo-treated cohorts as well as differences between antibiotic regimens.[48,49] Effective antimicrobial therapy sterilizes the middle ear, resulting in a more rapid resolution of clinical signs (bulging and erythema) and symptoms (fever, earache, irritability). Two recent clinical trials described the magnitude of the benefit of antibiotic treatment in children residing in industrialized countries.[50,51] One study reports a substantial benefit for amoxicillin-clavulanate compared with placebo for resolution of fever, irritability, decreased activity, and poor appetite.[51] In the other, treatment with amoxicillin-clavulanate was associated with a lower symptom score over the first 7 days.[50] If recurrence within 30 days is the outcome measured, small but statistically significant differences are reported between children given effective antimicrobial therapy and those given placebo or ineffective therapy.[52]

A substantial proportion of children (30% to 50%), especially younger children, have persistent middle-ear effusion (OME) 30 days after an acute episode of AOM, long after resolution of acute signs and symptoms.[53] In a study by Teele and associates[54] of resolution of OME, 40% of children had OME at 1 month, 20% at 2 months, and 10% at 3 months. OME is part of the morbidity of OM because of its association with conductive hearing loss of up to 50 decibels (dB).[55]

TABLE 29-3. Correlation Between Microbiologic Outcome at Day 4/5 and Clinical Outcome in Acute Otitis Media

Clinical Outcome	Culture Negative at Day 4/5		Culture Positive at Day 4/5	
	No.	%	No.	%
Success	236	93	25	60
Failure	17	7	15	40

Adapted from Carlin SA, Marchant CD, Shurin PA, et al. Host factors and early therapeutic response in acute otitis media. J Pediatr 1991;118: 178–183.

Pharmacodynamic Principles of Antimicrobial Selection

In 1992, the Infectious Disease Society of America established guidelines for evaluation of new agents for AOM.[56] Guidelines require both clinical and microbiologic studies as well as outcome measures 3 to 5 days after initiation of antimicrobial therapy. Guidelines are consistent with the principles established by Carlin and colleagues,[57] and confirmed by Dagan and associates,[58] that middle-ear concentration of antibiotic has a high correlation with clinical success (Table 29-3).

The selection of antimicrobial therapy should be based on pharmacodynamic principles and results of clinical trials using microbiologic endpoints. β-Lactam agents and trimethoprimsulfamethoxazole (TMP-SMX) depend on time that drug concentration is above the minimum inhibitory concentration (MIC) for efficacy.[59] In Craig's studies,[60] efficacy (sterilization of middle-ear fluid) for β-lactam agents is predictable when the drug concentration exceeds the MIC for ~40% of the dosing interval; for azalides (azithromycin) and fluoroquinolones, ratios of AUC_{24} (area under the antibiotic concentration curve per 24 hours):MIC or peak concentration to MIC are relevant; and for azithromycin, AUC_{24}:MIC ratio of 25 predicts efficacy. Although these principles are well established, controversy persists regarding whether extracellular or intracellular concentrations of antibiotics are necessary. For β-lactam agents, there is no enhanced intracellular accumulation; however, for azalides and ketolides, intracellular concentrations of drug exceed extracellular (serum) concentrations up to

TABLE 29-2. Clinical Outcome by Treatment Assignment and Age

Age Cohort	Failure (Day 0–12)		Recurrence (Day 13–33)		Cure	
	No.	%	No.	%	No.	%
<2 YEARS						
Antibiotic immediately	4	6	11	17	50	77
Watchful waiting	12	24	10	20	28	56
Total	16	14	21	18	78	68
>2 YEARS						
Antibiotic immediately	1	2	9	21	34	77
Watchful waiting	9	18	3	6	38	76
Total	10	14	12	16	72	76

From McCormick DP, Chonmaitree T, Pittman C, et al. Nonsevere acute otitis media: a clinical trial comparing outcomes of watchful waiting versus immediate antibiotic treatment. Pediatrics 2005;115:1455–1465.

TABLE 29-4. 2000 Clinical and Laboratory Standards Institute (CLSI) Breakpoints and Pharmacodynamically Derived Breakpoints for Selected Antimicrobial Agents and Otopathogens

Antibiotic	CLSI Breakpoints (μg/mL)		Pharmacodynamic Breakpoints (μg/mL)
	Streptococcus pneumoniae	*Haemophilus influenzae*	
Amoxicillin	2	4	2
Amoxicillin-clavulanate	2	4	2
Cefuroxime	1	4	1
Cefprozil	2	8	1
Cefixime	0.5	1	1
Cefaclor	1	8	0.5
Loracarbef	2	8	0.5
Azithromycin	0.5	4	0.12
Clarithromycin	0.25	8	0.25

Data from National Committee for Clinical Laboratory Standards (now the Clinical and Laboratory Standards Institute (CLSI)). Performance Standards for Antimicrobial Susceptibility Testing. Tenth Informational Supplement. Wayne, PA, NCCLS, 2000.

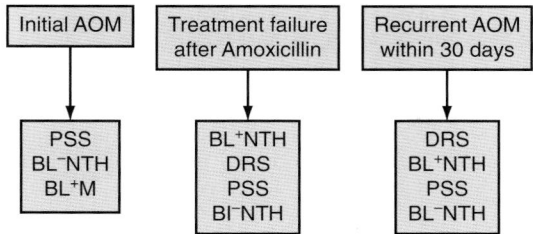

Figure 29-4. Presumptive pathogens in acute otitis media (AOM). BL⁺ or BL⁻, NTHi, β-lactamase-positive or -negative nontypable *Haemophilus influenzae*; DRSP, drug-resistant *Streptococcus pneumoniae*; Mc, *Moraxella catarrhalis*; PSSp, penicillin-susceptible *Streptococcus pneumoniae*.

TABLE 29-5. Proportion of Antibiotic Resistance Among 2008–2009 Pneumococcal Isolates from Children <7 Years of Age in Massachusetts

Antibiotic	Total Isolates (%) (N = 290)
PNSP[a]	98 (34)
PCN-I[b]	64 (22)
PCN-R[c]	34 (12)
Erythromycin-NS[a]	83 (29)
Clindamycin-NS[a]	29 (10)
Trimethoprim-sulfamethoxazole-NS[a]	58 (20)
Ceftriaxone-NS[a]	30 (10)
MDR1[d]	81 (28)
MDR2[e]	55 (19)

[a]Antibiotic abbreviations are as follows: PNSP (penicillin nonsusceptible Streptococcus pneumoniae), PCN (penicillin), I (intermediate-susceptibility), R (resistant), NS (nonsusceptible). The following breakpoints were used: PNSP (>0.06), erythromycin-NS (>0.25), clindamycin-NS (>0.5), trimethoprim-sulfamethoxazole-NS, (>0.5), and ceftriaxone-NS (>1.0).

[b]Based upon pre-2008 breakpoint for penicillin intermediate susceptibility (MIC >0.06–1.0 mg/L).

[c]Based upon pre-2008 breakpoint for penicillin resistance (MIC ≥2.0 mg/L).

[d]MDR1 refers to multidrug resistance defined as nonsusceptibility to penicillin, plus one other antibiotic class.

[e]MDR2 refers to multidrug resistance defined as nonsusceptibility to 3 or more classes of antibiotics.

Adapted from Wroe FC, Lee GM, Finkelstein JA, et al. Pneumococcal carriage and antibiotic resistance in young children before 13-valent conjugate vaccine. Pediatr Infect Dis 2012;31:249–254.

100-fold. Results from animal models and clinical trials suggest that extracellular concentrations are the critical factor.[61]

The acceptance of these principles led the Clinical and Laboratory Standards Institute (CLSI) to identify specific breakpoints for susceptibility versus resistance relative to sites of infection. Table 29-4 summarizes both CLSI-specific breakpoints and those derived from pharmacodynamic analysis for *S. pneumoniae* and NTHi.[62]

In the majority of cases of AOM, the specific pathogen is unknown, and presumptive therapy is based on the likely pathogens and their in vitro susceptibility (Figure 29-4). The proportion of isolates of NTHi-producing β-lactamase has risen to 40% over a 25-year period.[63] A limited number of β-lactamase-producing, amoxicillin-clavulanate-resistant isolates also have emerged. The spread of pneumococci with altered penicillin-binding proteins and reduced susceptibility to β-lactam agents occurred rapidly in the U.S.[64–66] Recently the CLSI has re-evaluated breakpoints for *S. pneumoniae* and has redefined resistant as isolates with penicillin MIC ≥8 μg/mL. These new breakpoints are more consistent with pharmacokinetic/pharmacodynamic (PK/PD) principles and translate to few isolates interpreted as resistant to penicillin and other β-lactams. Resistance to macrolides and azalides also has become common and is mediated by an efflux pump mechanism that decreases intracellular accumulation of antibiotic, or by a mutation in ribosomal methylase that affects binding between drug and target site, or both.[67,68] Susceptibility of nasopharyngeal isolates of *S. pneumoniae* in Massachusetts children from 2008/2009, based on 2000 guidelines, are shown in Table 29-5.

Risk factors for the presence of isolates of *S. pneumoniae* with reduced susceptibility are age <2 years, recent treatment with antibiotics, season (late winter to early spring), and attendance in group childcare.[69,70] For most isolates with penicillin MIC >2 to <8 μg/mL, a 10-day course of high-dose (90 mg/kg per day) amoxicillin or a three-dose regimen of ceftriaxone (50 mg/kg per day) has proven efficacy.[49,71] There is anecdotal evidence and PK/PD support for efficacy of clindamycin for susceptible isolates. Animal studies suggest that linezolid also may be effective against drug-resistant *S. pneumoniae* (DRSP);[72] however, linezolid has no efficacy against *Haemophilus influenzae*.

Clinical Failure, Relapse, and Recurrence

Rosenfeld and coworkers[48] reviewed seven clinical trials comparing antibiotic and placebo treatments and identified persistence of symptoms in 15.4% of cases at 2 to 3 days, in 10.5% at 6 to 7 days, and in 8.6% at 7 to 14 days. The failure of AOM to respond to initial antimicrobial therapy is related to both the severity of the initial symptoms and the age of the patient.[57,73] Kaleida and associates[73] observed that 12.1% of "severely" symptomatic patients younger than 2 years were unchanged, but only 4.1% of children older than 2 years with similar severity of symptoms showed no improvement; in children with "nonsevere" otitis, only 6.5% of those younger than 2 years and 0.5% of those older than 2 years showed no change after 24 hours of therapy.

Leibovitz and colleagues[74] reported on 16 children whose disease did not respond to high-dose amoxicillin. In studies performed prior to the PCV7 era or in countries where PCV7

immunization is not universal, β-lactamase-positive NTHi was isolated from tympanocentesis specimens in 50%, and DRSP in 25% of cases of AOM. In the U.S., post PCV7, studies initially reported that disease in children with severe or refractory AOM was more often caused by β-lactamase-positive NTHi than Sp;[12,13] however, in the most recent years both SP and NTHi have been found with equal frequency.[13] Antimicrobial treatment for such children must include agent(s) active against both organisms. Ceftriaxone, high-dose amoxicillin-clavulanate, high-dose amoxicillin in combination with cefixime or ceftibuten, or standard-dose amoxicillin in combination with amoxicillin-clavulanate are appropriate. Studies of gatifloxacin and levofloxacin demonstrate in vitro activity against all NTHi and >95% of Sp; clinical trials demonstrate rapid sterilization and clinical resolution of middle-ear infection due to both pathogens.[75,76] However, fluoroquinolones are not licensed for use in children for treatment of AOM.

Recently, MDR pneumococci, resistant to all oral antimicrobial agents licensed for the treatment of AOM, have been isolated from children failing outpatient therapy. These isolates predominantly have been serotypes 19A and 35B.[77,78] Pichichero and Casey reported successful treatment with vancomycin or levofloxacin and tympanostomy tube insertion;[77] linezolid also has been successful treatment for infections due to MDR 19A pneumococci.[79]

Relapse and *recurrence* have been defined as occurrence of episodes of disease after an initial symptomatic response to antibiotic treatment, either during treatment or within some defined period after completion of therapy. Discriminating relapse from recurrence requires defining the microbiology of both episodes. Leibovitz and colleagues demonstrated that the majority of such events are due to new pathogens or different serotypes of the same pathogen.[74] Two other studies found that after treatment of AOM with ceftriaxone or other β-lactam antibiotics, susceptible isolates of *S. pneumoniae* are eliminated from the nasopharynx but there is little effect on resistant strains.[80,81] Newly acquired *S. pneumoniae* in children who are receiving antimicrobial therapy frequently demonstrate resistance.[82] These events appear to begin as early as 3 to 4 days into the course of treatment.[81] Thus, the likelihood

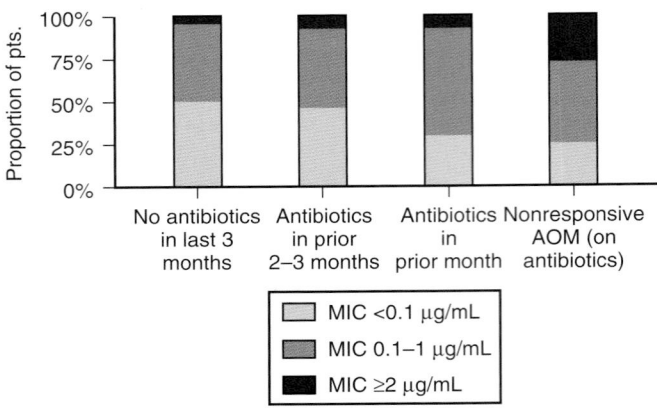

Figure 29-5. Correlation between recent antibiotic therapy and likelihood of drug-resistant *Streptococcus pneumoniae* in acute otitis media (AOM). MIC, minimum inhibitory concentration. (Redrawn from Jacobs MR. Increasing antibiotic resistance among otitis media pathogens and their susceptibility to oral agents based pharmacodynamic parameters. Paediatr Infect Dis J 2000;19:S47–S55.)[83]

of nasopharyngeal colonization with a resistant otopathogen increases during and after antibiotic therapy if resistant isolates are present in the community;[47] recurrent episodes of AOM are more likely due to resistant pathogens. Figure 29-5 demonstrates that the chance of recovering penicillin-nonsusceptible pneumococcus correlates with time since last receipt of antibiotics.[83] Data support the recommendation from the American Academy of Pediatrics (AAP) that treatment of recurrent episodes within 30 days of a prior event may necessitate use of antibiotic agents (such as ceftriaxone or high-dose amoxicillin-clavulanate) that target resistant otopathogens.[84]

American Academy of Pediatrics (AAP) Guidelines for the Diagnosis and Treatment of AOM

The AAP guidelines, published in 2004, define the presence of middle-ear effusion as detected by physical examination or tympanometry as the critical criterion for diagnosis.[84] Classification as AOM also requires recent onset of signs and symptoms of acute inflammation such as earache, ear-tugging, or a bulging tympanic membrane. The AAP guidelines recommend amoxicillin at 90 mg/kg per day administered twice daily for initial therapy in most children with AOM (Tables 29-6 and 29-7).[84] Among β-lactam antibiotics, only oral "high-dose" amoxicillin or intramuscular ceftriaxone achieves middle-ear concentrations that fulfill PK/PD requirements for penicillin-nonsusceptible Sp and β-lactamase-nonproducing NTHi. Cefuroxime axetil, cefprozil, and cefpodoxime represent alternatives to high-dose amoxicillin; however, each only achieves sufficient middle-ear concentration

to be effective against <50% of penicillin-nonsusceptible Sp. Also, cefprozil has limited activity against NTHi.[85] Macrolide efficacy at currently recommended dosage is limited to disease due to susceptible Sp. Extracellular middle-ear fluid concentrations of macrolides are below the MIC for almost all NTHi and Sp isolates with efflux or ribosomal mechanisms of resistance. Amoxicillin is ineffective against β-lactamase-producing isolates of NTHi. Because amoxicillin-clavulanate resists destruction by the β-lactamase, it effectively eradicates middle-ear infection caused by virtually all NTHi. However, isolates of NTHi with altered penicillin-binding proteins (referred to as β-lactamase negative, ampicillin resistant (BLPNAR)) are common in Japan and have been reported in the U.S.[86] Isolates with both altered penicillin binding proteins and β-lactamase production also have been identified (referred to as β-lactamase producing, amoxicillin-clavulanate resistant (BLPACR)). Such isolates can have MICs for amoxicillin that are at the breakpoint for effective eradication even with the recommended high-dose strategy. Although the AAP guidelines recommend the consideration of amoxicillin-clavulanate as initial therapy only for children with severe disease (temperature >39 °C) and substantial otalgia, the increasing prevalence of AOM due to NTHi associated with universal PCV7 immunization may warrant broader use of amoxicillin-clavulanate as first-line therapy. Guidelines are in the process of revision and are expected to be available in 2011/2012.

Initial therapy for the child with type I allergy to penicillin (urticaria, laryngeal spasm, wheezing, or anaphylaxis) remains challenging. The choice of alternatives to β-lactams is limited by the substantial prevalence of resistance (Table 29-7). Macrolides, including azithromycin and clarithromycin, are ineffective for 25% to 40% of Sp. Resistance to TMP-SMX among Sp and NTHi also is substantial.[87] AAP guidelines acknowledge the potential limitations of these agents but recommend their use as best alternative. For the child with "severe" disease, a combination of agents such as clindamycin (for SP) and sulfisoxazole (for NTHi) may be effective. Unlike other macrolides, clindamycin may be effective against isolates of Sp with the efflux mechanism of resistance and therefore maintains activity against approximately 80% to 90% of Sp isolates in the U.S. However, the proportion of isolates of Sp with ribosomal mechanisms of resistance is increasing and local-community antimicrobial susceptibility patterns provide the best information about the predicted efficacy of clindamycin.[88] AAP guidelines emphasize that "watchful waiting" includes providing analgesia for children suffering from AOM. A limited number of studies suggest that ibuprofen or acetaminophen is effective.[89] Topical agents such as auralgan also may offer temporary symptomatic relief.[90] For children with severe pain, myringotomy is an effective method to attain relief.

Evaluation of the Child with Recurrent Otitis Media

In clinical practice, most children with recurrent otitis media (ROM) do not have a quantifiable immunologic abnormality.[91,92]

TABLE 29-6. Recommendations for Treatment of Acute Otitis Media in the Child without Penicillin Allergy

Temperature >39°C and/or Severe Otalgia	Diagnosis, Day 0 (when initial management includes antibiotic)	Clinical Failure, Day 3 (when initial management was observation)	Clinical Failure, Day 3 (when initial management was antibiotic)
No	High-dose amoxicillin, (80–90 mg/kg per day)	High-dose amoxicillin (80–90 mg/kg per day)	High-dose amoxicillin-clavulanate (90 mg/kg per day amoxicillin; 6.4 mg/kg per day clavulanate)
Yes	High-dose amoxicillin-clavulanate (90 mg/kg per day amoxicillin; 6.4 mg/kg per day clavulanate)	High-dose amoxicillin-clavulanate; or ceftriaxone IM, 1 or 3 days	Ceftriaxone IM, 3 days

IM, intramuscularly.

From Lieberthal AS, Ganiates TG, Cox EO, et al. Clinical practice guidelines: diagnosis and treatment of acute otitis media. Pediatrics 2004;13:1451–1465.

TABLE 29-7. Recommendations for Treatment of Acute Otitis Media in Children with Penicillin Allergy

Temperature >39°C and/or Severe Otalgia	Diagnosis, Day 0 (when initial management includes antibiotic)	Clinical Failure, Day 3 (when management was observation)	Clinical Failure, Day 3 (when management was antibiotic)
No	Nontype I: cefdinir, cefuroxime, or cefpodoxime Type I: azithromcyin, clarithromycin	Nontype I: cefdinir, cefuroxime, cefpodoxime Type I: azithromycin, clarithromycin	Nontype I: ceftriaxone IM, 3 days Type I: clindamycin
Yes	Nontype I: ceftriaxone IM, 1 or 3 days Type I: clindamycin	Nontype I: ceftriaxone IM, 1–3 days Type I: clindamycin	Tympanocentesis: clindamycin

IM, intramuscularly.

When an immune defect is detected, the abnormality usually is limited to IgG subclasses or IgA deficiency.[91,93] These disorders often are maturational and therefore when laboratory values support such a diagnosis in infants, repeated testing after 4 years of age is indicated. In children with recurrent serious infections in addition to ROM, more serious immunologic defects must be considered.

Recurrent AOM is very common in children with HIV infection.[94-97] In general, additional signs of immunodeficiency such as recurrent thrush, lymphadenopathy, hepatomegaly or splenomegaly, failure to thrive, or chronic diarrhea are present, although ROM can be the presenting or dominant feature early in the course of disease. Marchisio et al.[98] defined the bacterial etiology of AOM in 60 episodes in 21 HIV-infected children. *S. pneumoniae*, NTHi, and GAS were recovered from the middle ear in 56% of cases, a proportion similar to that seen in immunocompetent children. *S. aureus* was identified in HIV-infected children with severe immunosuppression.

In general, an immunologic evaluation for the child whose infections are limited to ROM, in the absence of additional concerns for enhanced susceptibility to infection, signs or symptoms such as failure to thrive, chronic diarrhea, lymphadenopathy, or organomegaly, is unlikely to reveal a serious immune deficiency. Even when the diagnosis of an IgA or IgG subclass deficiency is suggested from the measurement of immunoglobulins and immunoglobulin subclasses, the disorder often is maturational.

Prevention of Recurrent Acute Otitis Media

Decreasing the morbidity of otitis media has potential implications for decreasing antimicrobial use and the associated emergence of resistance, reducing healthcare costs and surgical procedures, and preventing the language and cognitive delays that occur in some children with recurrent AOM and prolonged conductive hearing loss. In Paradise and colleagues' study,[31] >45% of urban children in the first year of life, and 30% in the second year, spent more than 3 months of each year with middle-ear effusion; 10% of children spent >50% of each year with middle-ear effusions.

Prevention of recurrent bacterial AOM can be achieved by preventing nasopharyngeal colonization with otopathogens, preventing viral respiratory tract infection, and providing specific antibacterial immunity. Several interventions such as breastfeeding, avoidance of supine bottle feeding and bottle propping, limiting pacifier use in the first 6 months of life, and improved hand hygiene with use of alcohol-based disinfectants are low-technology interventions that have variable benefit for prevention of respiratory tract infection and/or AOM. Specific interventions such as insertion of tympanostomy tubes do not reduce the frequency of acute episodes substantially; however, their presence shortens the duration of middle-ear effusion.[99] Antimicrobial prophylaxis lowers the frequency of colonization with respiratory otopathogens and decreases the number of acute episodes.[100] The greatest benefit occurs in children at highest risk for recurrent AOM (age 6 to 24 months) and in otitis-prone children who have multiple episodes per year and in whom the problem does not abate with increasing age.

Chemoprophylaxis

Chemoprophylaxis offers short-term benefits only. Most otitis-prone children continue to have recurrent episodes once prophylaxis is discontinued, until their immune systems and eustachian tube function have matured.[100] A five-carbon sugar alcohol, xylitol, has been demonstrated to reduce episodes of AOM in group childcare attendees (3.03 versus 2.01 episodes per child year).[101,102]

Viral respiratory tract illness is a cofactor in the pathogenesis of AOM. Influenza vaccine has been associated with a reduction in AOM episodes, in febrile AOM, and in myringotomy and insertion of tympanostomy tubes over a winter season.[103]

Vaccination

Three pneumococcal conjugate vaccines (PCV$_{CRM}$, PCV$_{OMP}$, and PHiD-CV), administered at 2, 4, and 6 months with a booster at 12 to 15 months of age with either conjugate vaccine or the 23-valent pneumococcal polysaccharide vaccine, have been shown to reduce AOM due to vaccine serotypes of *S. pneumoniae* by approximately 60% (Table 29-8).[104-106] However, the overall reduction in episodes of AOM (6% to 10%) was modest in two clinical trials of PCV7. Initial results with an 11-valent pneumococcal polysaccharide vaccine conjugated to protein D from *Haemophilus influenzae* (PHiD-CV) demonstrated that protection against AOM could be extended to include NTHi and vaccine serotypes of Sp.[106] PHiD-CV has been reformulated as a 10-valent pneumococcal vaccine with 8 of the polysaccharides conjugated to protein D. PHiD-CV is licensed in multiple countries (not in the U.S.) and further clinical trials are ongoing to determine if comparable efficacy is observed with the new formulation.

Follow-up studies of cohorts of the original clinical trials of infant immunization with PCV7 in California and Finland have identified significant reductions in tympanostomy tube insertions in immunized children.[107,108] Studies of PCV7 immunization in children with frequent ROM have failed to demonstrate a significant reduction in episodes.[109] Post-marketing studies have confirmed an increase in the proportion of AOM disease due to NV-Sp. and NTHi.[13] Studies evaluating the change in OM episodes or visits using claims data comparing the pre- and post-PCV7 era

TABLE 29-8. Efficacy of 7-Valent Pneumococcal Conjugate Vaccine (PCV7) for the Prevention of Pneumococcal Otitis Media

Etiology of Otitis Media	No. of Episodes		Difference (%)
	PCV7	Control	
All pneumococcal episodes	269	420	↓36
Vaccine serotypes	107	254	↓57
Vaccine serogroups	143	325	↓56
Nonvaccine serogroups	126	95	↑34

Data from Eskola J, Kilpi T, Palmu A, et al. For the Finnish Otitis Media Study. Efficacy of a pneumococcal conjugate vaccine against otitis media. N Engl J Med 2001;344:403–409.

have reported larger declines than observed in the Finnish and U.S. Kaiser Permanente clinical trials.[40,41] These studies are unable to disentangle the reduction due to the direct and indirect effect of PCV7 from the secular changes in diagnostic criteria and management of AOM that have occurred over the decade.

Complications of Acute Otitis Media

Perforation of the tympanic membrane is the most common complication of AOM and is observed most frequently in younger children. Certain ethnic groups, such as Alaska Eskimos and Native Americans, have a higher proportion of spontaneous perforation with AOM. Differentiation between AOM with perforation and acute otitis externa can be difficult. The microbiology of AOM in children with acute perforation demonstrates a higher proportion of episodes due to GAS and *S. aureus*.[29] The natural history of AOM with perforation usually is complete resolution with healing of the tympanic membrane. A small proportion of patients have persistent dry perforation or chronic suppurative otitis media (persisting for more than 6 to 12 weeks). *S. pneumoniae* and NTHi are the most common pathogens in infants and toddlers, whereas *S. aureus* and *Pseudomonas aeruginosa* are frequent pathogens in older children and during the summer months.[110] Amoxicillin generally is effective for the therapy of acute otorrhea through a tympanostomy tube and, compared with placebo, results in rapid clearing of bacterial pathogens and a shortened duration of otorrhea.[111] An alternative to oral antimicrobial therapy is topical otic suspensions, either ofloxacin or ciprofloxacin.[112,113] When CA-MRSA is the pathogen, oral trimethoprim-sulfamethoxazole or topical fluoroquinolone preparations have transient benefits, but drainage often recurs.[114,115]

Facial palsy as a complication of AOM is uncommon.[116] Facial weakness and earache are the predominant symptoms. Antibiotic therapy and myringotomy (with or without tube insertion) are usually sufficient to achieve complete resolution.

Mastoiditis, once commonplace, has decreased dramatically since the routine use of antimicrobial therapy. However, mastoiditis still remains the most common suppurative complication of AOM.[117] *Streptococcus pneumoniae*, GAS, and NTHi are most common pathogens of acute mastoiditis but *P. aeruginosa* was found in 29% and *S. epidermidis* in 31% of cases in one large series.[117] These pathogens should be suspected when a history of otorrhea precedes development of acute mastoiditis (see Chapter 31, Mastoiditis).

Labyrinthitis develops when AOM spreads (through the round window) into the cochlear space. The process can be suppurative or serous (due to bacterial toxins). The onset of labyrinthitis often is sudden, with vertigo and hearing loss being characteristic. Acute surgical intervention (myringotomy with tube insertion) with antimicrobial therapy is the treatment of choice.

Additional rare complications of AOM are brain abscess, epidural abscess, and otic hydrocephalus, which can result from transverse, lateral, or sigmoid sinus thrombosis.

BOX 29-1. Comorbid Conditions Associated with Increased Risk for Developmental Difficulties in Children with Otitis Media with Effusion (OME)

- Permanent hearing loss separate from OME
- Suspicion of speech language delay or disorder
- Autism spectrum disorders
- Uncorrectable visual disorders or blindness
- Cleft palate
- Congenital syndromes associated with cognitive, speech, or language delays
- Documented developmental delay of unknown etiology

From Rosenfeld RM, Culpepper L, Doyle KJ, et al. Clinical practice guideline: otitis media with effusion. Otolaryngol-Head Neck Surg 2004;130:s95–s118.

OTITIS MEDIA WITH EFFUSION

OME is the relatively asymptomatic presence of middle-ear effusion, which often is associated with conductive hearing loss and can persist for months. The pathogenesis most often reflects a postinfectious event that results from the presence of cytokines and other inflammatory mediators. Several investigators have suggested that biofilm formation and persistence by bacterial otopathogens, individually or in combination, may be responsible for the ongoing inflammatory response that provokes persistence of middle-ear effusion.[118,119]

In most children, OME resolves without specific intervention within a few months.[120] When OME persists beyond this period and there is a substantial conductive hearing loss (>20 dB), intervention with tympanostomy tubes and adenoidectomy may be considered. Consequences of tube placement can include recurrent otorrhea, persistent perforation, development of granulation tissue, chronic otitis media, and cholesteatoma.[121] Repeated insertions of tympanostomy tubes also have been associated with mild hearing loss, including a sensorineural component.[122] Guidelines from the AAP and American Academy of Otolaryngology[120] stress the need to identify children at risk for speech, language, and cognitive impairment early in the course of disease. The guidelines focus on children with sensory, physical, cognitive, or behavioral features that are likely to increase the risk of developmental difficulties (Box 29-1) and therefore warrant earlier hearing and language assessment and tympanostomy tube insertion. For otherwise healthy children, watchful waiting for up to 6 months, with hearing evaluation at 3 months, is suggested. The primary intervention for OME is surgical; antihistamines and decongestants are ineffective and therapy with antibiotics or corticosteroids does not result in lasting benefit.[123,124]

---

30   Otitis Externa and Necrotizing Otitis Externa

Thomas G. Boyce

OTITIS EXTERNA

Epidemiology and Clinical Manifestations

Otitis externa is infection of the skin of the hairy and glabrous parts of the ear canal. Acute otitis externa ("swimmer's ear") is usually unilateral and is associated with head immersion in water. In temperate climates, the disease peaks in the summer. When the skin of the ear canal is wet for prolonged periods, local defense mechanisms are impaired. Cerumen, which has antimicrobial properties,[1] is washed away, the thickness of the keratin layer is reduced, the pH of the canal increases, and microscopic fissures develop. This can cause itching of the ear canal that may predispose to further trauma from cotton-tipped buds.[2] Gram-negative bacteria, most commonly *Pseudomonas* spp., flourish in the moist environment and invade superficial layers of skin.[3–5]

The ensuing inflammatory dermatitis progresses through three stages.[6,7] Each is associated with pain and tenderness exaggerated by movement of the tragus. In *mild otitis externa*, pain is ameliorated by simple analgesics. Skin of the hairy part of the ear canal is erythematous but not edematous. In *moderate otitis externa*, there is increasing pain. The patient actively resists insertion of anything into the ear canal. The skin of the hairy part of the ear canal is intensely red under the macerated pieces of desquamated skin. The canal lumen is narrowed to less than 50% of its normal diameter, obscuring the tympanic membrane. *Severe otitis externa* is characterized by: (1) intense pain, often requiring narcotics; (2) inflammatory edema, which narrows the external auditory meatus to barely admit a nasopharyngeal swab; and (3) desquamated debris that precludes visualization of the tympanic membrane. The auricle can be swollen and painful.[7]

In advanced cases, tender preauricular or postauricular lymphadenopathy, protrusion of the auricle, and contiguous cellulitis of the skin overlying the mastoid area can be present. Unlike acute mastoiditis, the entire auricle is not only protruding but is edematous and the posterior auricular sulcus is preserved. Suctioning of the ear canal is difficult to perform without adequate analgesia. Such cases are difficult to differentiate from necrotizing otitis externa, which is a perichondritis of the cartilaginous outer third of the ear canal.[8–10] Severe otitis externa also can be difficult to distinguish from noninfectious disorders involving the ear canal, such as rhabdomyosarcoma, Langerhans cell histiocytosis, and Wegener granulomatosis.

Etiologic Agents

In healthy individuals, the microbial flora of the ear canal includes coagulase-negative staphylococci, corynebacteria, and micrococci. With prolonged exposure to water, gram-negative bacteria predominate.[3] *Pseudomonas aeruginosa* is responsible for the majority of cases of otitis externa associated with swimming or due to persistent otorrhea from a patent tympanostomy tube. Other gram-negative bacteria occur less commonly. *Staphylococcus aureus* may be increasing in incidence.[11] *S. aureus* and *Streptococcus pyogenes* are the usual causes of acute otitis externa that occurs as an extension of a focal infection.[12]

Fungi are uncommon causes of otitis externa, in most series comprising fewer than 5% of cases.[13] However, in some studies fungi comprise a higher proportion of isolates.[14] *Aspergillus* spp. account for about two-thirds and *Candida* spp. account for the remainder.[15] Prolonged use of topical antibacterial agents appears to be a risk factor for otomycosis.[15,16]

Viruses rarely cause otitis externa. Reactivation of latent varicellazoster virus in the seventh cranial nerve results in Ramsay Hunt syndrome, which is characterized by unilateral otalgia, auricular vesicles, and peripheral facial paralysis.[17]

Management

Mild cases can be treated with instillation of topical otic antibiotic drops. Culture of otorrhea is usually unnecessary. The patient can enter the swimming pool as long as prolonged submersion is avoided. Excess water should be drained from the ear canal and the ear canal dried thoroughly with a hairdryer.

In addition to adequate analgesia, moderate or severe otitis externa usually requires aural lavage of the ear canal to permit contact of the antibiotic drops with infected skin. This is best accomplished by referring the patient to an otorhinolaryngologist. Lavage may have to be performed daily in some cases. Sometimes a wick is inserted into the canal to allow topical antibiotic drops to remain in contact with the wall. Individuals with moderate or severe otitis externa should avoid swimming until inflammation subsides.

Available topical otic antibiotic drops include: ofloxacin, ciprofloxacin with either hydrocortisone or dexamethasone, and polymyxin B-neosporin-hydrocortisone. The use of corticosteroids is empiric. Topical steroid alone is inferior to antibiotic-steroid combinations.[18] A Cochrane database review found that the topical antibiotic preparations available were equally effective, and that all were superior to placebo.[19] Systemic antibiotics are unnecessary for uncomplicated cases.[20] Neomycin is an aminoglycoside and is ototoxic; it should not be administered unless the tympanic membrane is known to be intact. Neomycin also can cause a contact dermatitis in some patients. However, in a trial comparing ciprofloxacin-dexamethasone to polymyxin B-neomycin-hydrocortisone, adverse events were uncommon and were not different in the two groups.[21] Polymyxin B-neosporin-hydrocortisone is administered three to four times daily, ciprofloxacin-containing drops are administered twice daily, and ofloxacin drops can be administered once daily with equivalent cure rates.[22] Most patients can be treated with a 7-day course. Symptoms improve within 3 to 6 days of starting therapy. In patients who do not respond, consideration should be given to the possibility of necrotizing otitis externa, particularly in immunocompromised hosts.

Another consideration in the patient who fails to respond to empiric therapy is fungal infection. A Gram stain of exudate may reveal the hyphae of *Aspergillus* spp. or the budding yeast of *Candida* spp. Clotrimazole 1% solution is the most commonly used agent for otomycosis.[23] It has excellent activity against both *Aspergillus* and *Candida*.[24] Nontuberculous mycobacteria rarely can be the cause of persistent tympanostomy tube otorrhea.[25] Furunculosis and local cellulitis respond best to the application of warm compresses and an orally administered antibiotic directed against *S. aureus*.

Prevention

Swimmers prone to recurrent otitis externa may benefit from thorough drying of the ear canals with a hairdryer after immersion. The prophylactic instillation of 2% acetic acid can be used to reduce *Pseudomonas* colonization.[26]

NECROTIZING OTITIS EXTERNA

Epidemiology and Clinical Manifestations

Necrotizing ("malignant") *otitis externa* results from invasive infection of the cartilage and bone of the external ear canal. A more accurate term is skull base osteomyelitis secondary to otitis externa.[27] Infection begins in the external auditory canal and spreads to the skull base through the fissures of Santorini – small perforations in the cartilaginous portion of the canal.[28] Infection then spreads along venous channels and fascial planes. The compact bone of the skull base becomes replaced with granulation tissue, leading to bone destruction. Mastoid involvement is common.

Necrotizing otitis externa occurs most frequently in adults with diabetes mellitus. In a review of 46 adult cases, two-thirds of patients were diabetic.[29] In contrast, a series of 14 pediatric cases reported only 21% with diabetes.[30] Other predisposing factors include immune deficiency, especially due to AIDS, chemotherapy-induced neutropenia, or functional neutrophil disorders.[31,32] It can be the presenting manifestation of malignancy.[33] Rarely, patients without risk factors are affected.[34]

The presenting symptoms are severe otalgia and otorrhea, both occurring in more than 90% of patients.[29] About 25% of patients will have facial nerve palsy at presentation.[28] On physical examination, there is purulent otorrhea with a swollen, tender external auditory canal. Granulation tissue or exposed bone is seen on the floor of the canal at the bone–cartilage junction.[28] Patients often are afebrile and have a normal leukocyte count, although the erythrocyte sedimentation rate usually is elevated. The presentation in children is more acute, and they are more often febrile.

The initial presentation can mimic otitis externa; thus, clinicians must maintain a high index of suspicion in the high-risk host. The

PART II Clinical Syndromes and Cardinal Features of Infectious Diseases: Approach to Diagnosis and Initial Management

SECTION C Oral Infections and Upper and Middle Respiratory Tract Infections

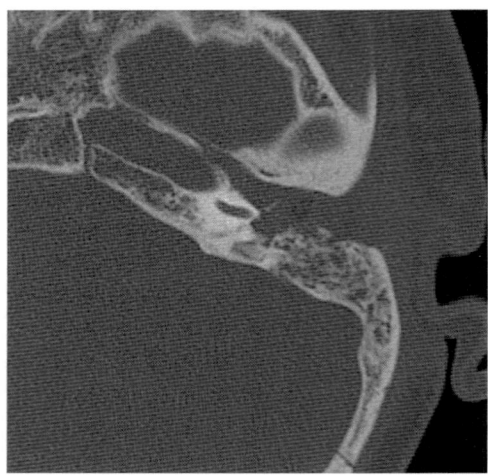

Figure 30-1. A 21-year-old man with medulloblastoma and chemotherapy-induced neutropenia presented with a 10-day history of severe left ear pain, otorrhea, and facial palsy. Axial noncontrast CT depicts soft tissue opacification of the left external auditory canal and opacification of the left middle ear and mastoid air cells. Irregularity and erosion of the posterior margin of the osseous portion left external auditory canal suggests osseous invasion and mastoid osteomyelitis consistent with necrotizing otitis externa. Intraoperative cultures obtained during debridement of the left mastoid grew *P. aeruginosa*.

diagnosis in a patient not known to have risk factors should engender testing for diabetes and immune deficiency.

Imaging studies used include computed tomography (CT), magnetic resonance imaging (MRI), bone scan, and gallium scan. CT is sensitive in detecting bone erosion and decreased skull base density.[28] CT also is sensitive in diagnosing abscess formation and involvement of the mastoid (Figure 30-1). However, it is inadequate for demonstrating intracranial extension and marrow involvement. MRI is superior in showing soft-tissue changes, dural enhancement, and involvement of the medullary bone spaces.[35] Technetium bone scan is highly sensitive, including early in the course of infection, but it is nonspecific. Gallium scan has similar sensitivity and is more useful for following the response to therapy.[36]

Complications occur from contiguous spread to nearby structures. Spread to the stylomastoid foramen results in facial nerve palsy. Less commonly, involvement of the jugular foramen results in palsies of the glossopharyngeal, vagus, and accessory nerves. Septic thrombophlebitis of the internal jugular vein and of the sigmoid sinus can occur. Intracranial extension can result in meningitis, cerebral abscess, or dural sinus thrombosis, all of which portend a poor prognosis.[27]

Etiologic Agents

P. aeruginosa is by far the most common cause, especially in patients with diabetes.[29] *S. aureus* is the second most common cause. *Aspergillus* spp., most commonly *A. fumigatus*, are sometimes isolated, particularly in patients with advanced AIDS.[29]

Management

In the past, necrotizing otitis externa was managed surgically. Currently, most cases are effectively treated with prolonged courses of antibiotics. However, surgery still plays a critical role in two aspects: obtaining tissue samples for culture and histology; and local debridement of necrotic tissue. Initial empiric therapy should be directed toward coverage of *P. aeruginosa* and *S. aureus*. Using two agents with antipseudomonal activity, such as cefepime and gentamicin, is prudent initially. Fluoroquinolones should be avoided if the patient recently received topical fluoroquinolone therapy, as the incidence of resistance is high.[29,37] Vancomycin can be used for initial staphylococcal coverage. If the patient fails to improve on initial therapy, and adequate debridement has occurred, imaging to assess for extension of infection should be considered. In addition, the possibility of infection by a filamentous fungus should be suspected and empiric antifungal therapy started with liposomal amphotericin or voriconazole. The duration of therapy generally is at least 6 weeks, although some patients are transitioned to oral therapy toward the end of the course.[28]

Prognosis

Once a condition with a case-fatality rate of 50%,[38] patients with necrotizing otitis externa are now cured in approximately 95% of cases.[29] Poor prognostic factors include intracranial extension, advanced underlying disease, and infection with *Aspergillus* spp.[27] In contrast to adults with necrotizing otitis externa, facial nerve paralysis in children usually is not reversible; children also are more likely to experience permanent hearing loss from ossicular destruction.[10,30]

31 Mastoiditis

Ellen R. Wald and James H. Conway

ACUTE MASTOIDITIS

Acute mastoiditis is exclusively a complication of acute otitis media (AOM). Previously, only a third of cases occurred in the context of a first episode of otitis media;[1] more recently, acute mastoiditis has been the first evidence of otitis media in at least 50% of children.[2,3] The incidence of mastoiditis declined remarkably after the introduction of antibiotics. Where antibiotic use for AOM has been explicitly restricted, there is a higher incidence of acute mastoiditis, though it remains a relatively unusual occurrence.[4-6] However, frequent intracranial and extracranial complications are observed in the cases of acute mastoiditis that do occur.[3,7,8]

Pathogenesis

Knowledge of the anatomy of the middle ear and mastoid is essential to understand the clinical presentation of mastoiditis and its complications. Figure 31-1 demonstrates the relationship between the eustachian tube, middle ear, and mastoid. At birth, the mastoid consists of a single cell, the antrum, connected to the middle ear by a narrow channel, the aditus ad antrum.[9] As the child grows, the mastoid bone becomes pneumatized, resulting in a series of interconnected air cells, lined by modified respiratory epithelium.

When AOM develops as a result of eustachian tube dysfunction, there is an acute inflammatory response of the mucosa lining the

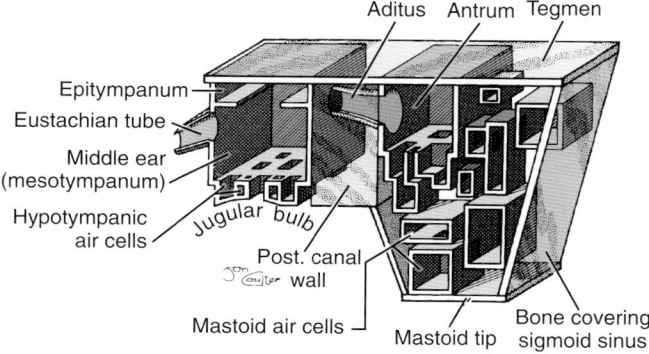

Aditus Antrum Tegmen

Epitympanum
Eustachian tube
Middle ear
(mesotympanum)
Hypotympanic
air cells
Jugular bulb
Post. canal
wall
Mastoid air cells
Mastoid tip
Bone covering
sigmoid sinus

Figure 31-1. Schematic representation of the anatomy of the middle ear and mastoid air cell system. The aditus ad antrum is the narrow connection between the two; it may be a site of obstruction inhibiting drainage into the middle ear. (From Bluestone CD, Klein JO. Intratemporal complications and sequelae of otitis media. In: Bluestone CD, Stool SE, Kenna M (eds) Pediatric Otolaryngology, 3rd ed. Philadelphia, WB Saunders, 1996, pp 583–647.)

BOX 31-1. Complications of Mastoiditis

EXTRACRANIAL	INTRACRANIAL
Subperiosteal abscess	Meningitis
Bezold abscess	Temporal lobe or cerebellar abscess
Facial nerve paralysis	
Osteomyelitis	Epidural empyema
Deafness	Subdural empyema
Labyrinthitis	Venous sinus thrombosis

middle ear and, in many cases, the mastoid as well.[10] Almost all episodes of AOM respond to antibiotic therapy; eustachian tube dysfunction resolves, and the mucosa of the middle ear and mastoid recovers. In rare cases of newly diagnosed AOM, or in cases of inadequate or inappropriate treatment, inflammation of the middle ear and mastoid persists. Histopathologic specimens from children who undergo mastoidectomy for acute or chronic mastoiditis demonstrate similar subacute/chronic infectious changes.[11] Serous and then purulent material accumulate within the mastoid cavities. As the pressure increases, the thin bony septa between air cells may be destroyed – so-called acute coalescent mastoiditis.[9] This may be followed by formation of abscess cavities and ultimately the dissection of pus into adjacent areas.

The direction in which purulent material dissects determines the clinical presentation and complications associated with acute mastoiditis (Box 31-1). Pus traversing the aditus ad antrum reaches to the middle ear and empties either through the eustachian tube (with resolution of the process) or via perforation of the tympanic membrane. If the pus erodes the lateral cortex of the mastoid, a subperiosteal abscess is produced. The abscess results in swelling or fluctuation either above the auricle in infants (when erosion comes from the zygomatic mast cells) or behind the lower earlobe

over the mastoid process in older children.[7] Rarely, erosion occurs through the medial aspect of the mastoid tip, resulting in a neck abscess beneath the attachment of the sternocleidomastoid and digastric muscles (Bezold abscess).[12] Pus can dissect medially to the petrous air cells (in the 20% of the population in which there is pneumatization), resulting in petrositis, or posteriorly to the occipital bone, resulting in osteomyelitis of the calvarium (Citilli abscess).[9] Purulent material can spread to the labyrinth and facial nerve. Finally, pus within the mastoid can dissect toward the inner cortical bone, causing suppurative complications in the central nervous system, such as meningitis, epidural, subdural, temporal lobe or cerebellar abscesses, and venous sinus thrombosis.

Clinical Presentation

The clinical presentation of the patient with mastoiditis depends on age of the patient and the stage of the osteitis (i.e., whether uncomplicated or already evolved to a subperiosteal abscess). Uncomplicated infection in a child younger than 2 years manifests as fever, otalgia or irritability, retroauricular pain, swelling, erythema, and a downward and outward deviation of the auricle (Figure 31-2A and B).[7] In most cases, otorrhea or a bulging, immobile, opaque tympanic membrane is observed. There may be sagging of the posterosuperior wall of the external auditory canal. In rare instances, with obstruction at the aditus ad antrum, middle-ear infection clears via the eustachian tube but the mastoid, unable to drain, continues to suppurate.

In children older than 2 years, the pinna usually is deviated upward and outward, because the inflammatory process frequently concentrates over the mastoid process. When subperiosteal pus has accumulated, a fluctuant, erythematous, and tender mass can be found overlying the mastoid bone in all age groups.

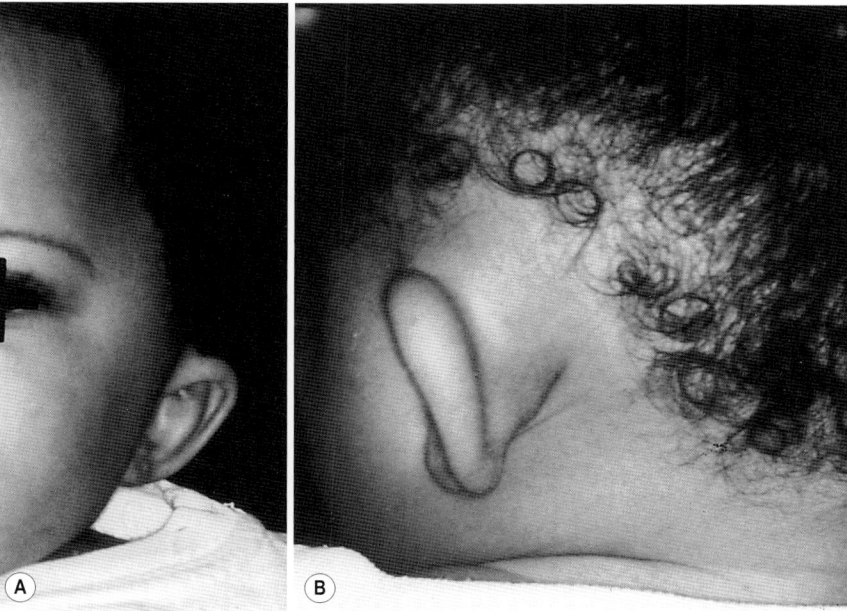

Figure 31-2. A 13-month-old toddler with a 10-day history of acute otitis media unresponsive to amoxicillin therapy. **(A and B)** There is erythema and edema above the left ear with downward, outward, and anterior displacement of the pinna.

PART II Clinical Syndromes and Cardinal Features of Infectious Diseases: Approach to Diagnosis and Initial Management

SECTION C Oral Infections and Upper and Middle Respiratory Tract Infections

Considerable attention has been given in the past two decades to the entity "masked mastoiditis" or "subacute mastoiditis."[13] In this presentation, the patient typically has had persistent middle-ear effusion or recurrent episodes of acute otitis media without sufficient antimicrobial therapy. In either case, there is low-grade but persistent infection in the middle ear and mastoid with osteitis. Masked mastoiditis can manifest as fever, otalgia, and an abnormal tympanic membrane or, occasionally, with an extracranial or intracranial complication.

Microbiology

The most recent prospective study of the microbiology of acute mastoiditis in children was published in 1987.[14] Precise delineation of the microbiology has been hampered by routine antibiotic therapy before clinical presentation. Most existing series published in the antibiotic era are retrospective reviews.[1–3,7,13,15–24]

Clinical specimens should be obtained from the middle ear either by tympanocentesis or by aspiration through a tympanostomy tube or perforation after careful sterilization of the surrounding structures. Cultures obtained from the external canal without careful sterilization can be contaminated with *Pseudomonas aeruginosa, Staphylococcus aureus,* and other colonizing organisms. Culture of the cerebrospinal fluid is valuable when bacterial meningitis is present. Blood cultures rarely are positive. Percutaneous aspiration of a subperiosteal abscess should be undertaken, particularly if definitive surgery will be delayed. Any material from abscesses (brain, epidural, or subdural) that are drained or aspirated should be submitted for Gram stain and aerobic and anaerobic cultures.

In contrast to the usual pathogens that cause AOM (i.e., *Streptococcus pneumoniae, Haemophilus influenzae,* and *Moraxella catarrhalis*),[25] the bacterial species most often implicated in acute mastoiditis are *S. pneumoniae, S. pyogenes, P. aeruginosa,* and *S. aureus* (Table 31-1). *P. aeruginosa* rarely is a true pathogen in acute mastoiditis. Exaggerated rates of recovery may reflect the sampling method for culture from the external canal.[21] Except for a single prospective study in which anaerobic bacteria predominated,[14] *H. influenzae,* Enterobacteriaceae, mycobacteria, and anaerobic organisms are only recovered occasionally. Although all patients in that study were described as having acute mastoiditis, 37% had a history of otorrhea, implying a chronic etiology.[14]

Interestingly, the introduction of heptavalent pneumococcal conjugate vaccine (PCV7) has not affected the proportion of acute mastoiditis cases caused by *S. pneumoniae,*[23] related almost entirely to increase in serotype 19A as the predominant serotype isolated from mastoid cultures.[26] The effect of PCV13 on the incidence and microbiology of mastoiditis will require ongoing study.

Diagnosis

The diagnosis of mastoiditis usually is made clinically, without need for imaging studies (Box 31-2). Recent studies have shown that outcomes are similar in patients with acute mastoiditis regardless of whether computed tomography (CT) scans are performed.[27] A recent systematic review of >1000 articles in the published literature identified the clinical signs most frequently used to diagnose acute mastoiditis as post-auricular swelling, erythema, tenderness, and protrusion of the auricle.[28] High-grade fevers and elevated inflammatory markers such as absolute neutrophil counts and C-reactive protein levels may suggest more complicated infections.[24]

If plain radiographs are obtained, they often show clouding of the mastoid or coalescence of air cells (i.e., dissolution of thin bony septa from increased pressure and ischemia). Clouding of the mastoid is not diagnostic of acute mastoiditis and is observed in at least 50% of patients with uncomplicated AOM. Coalescent mastoiditis is a diagnostic radiographic finding, but is seen in a minority of patients. Plain radiographs in acute and even complicated mastoiditis can be reported to be normal.[1,29]

CT imaging generally is more helpful when there are intracranial complications or in patients suspected of having masked mastoiditis.[12,21] Evidence of mastoiditis by CT consists of: (1) haziness or destruction of the mastoid outline; and (2) loss of or decrease in sharpness of bony septa that define the mastoid air cells (Figure 31-3).[9] Cloudiness in areas normally pneumatized,

---

BOX 31-2. Diagnosis of Acute Mastoiditis

- Fever, otalgia, postauricular swelling + redness
  Older child: ear up and out
  Infant: ear down and out
- Tympanic membrane: acute otitis media
- Radiograph: mastoid air cells coalescent or clouded
- Computed tomography, magnetic resonance imaging, or bone scan as needed

---

TABLE 31-1. Bacteriology of Cases of Acute Mastoiditis in Children (1955–2009)[a]

Bacterial Species	Number	Percent
Streptococcus pneumoniae	230	32
Streptococcus pyogenes	121	17
Staphylococcus aureus	62	9
Other gram-positive cocci[b]	26	4
Haemophilus influenzae	34	5
Pseudomonas aeruginosa	119	16
Other gram-negative bacilli[c]	29	4
Anaerobic bacteria[d]	72	10
Mycobacterium tuberculosis	31	4
Total isolates	724	100

[a]Data from references 1–3, 7, 11, 15–24; many patients received antimicrobial therapy before specimens were obtained for culture. Isolates were obtained from blood, myringotomy aspirate, external auricular drainage, subperiosteal aspirate, cerebrospinal fluid, or surgical specimens.

[b]Viridans streptococci, Enterococcus, coagulase-negative staphylococci sp.

[c]Citrobacter freundii, Escherichia coli, Enterobacter sp., Acinetobacter sp., Klebsiella sp.

[d]Bacteroides spp., Fusobacterium nucleatum, microaerophilic streptococci.

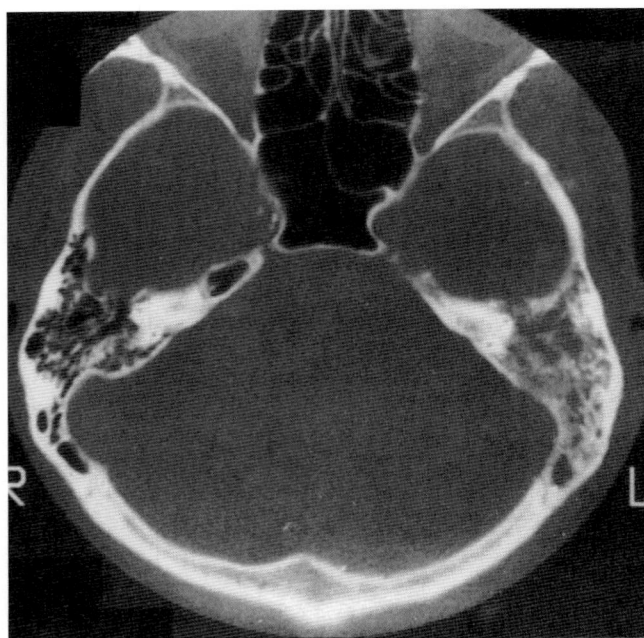

Figure 31-3. Computed tomography of a child with acute mastoiditis showing coalescence/destruction of septa between the mastoid air cells.

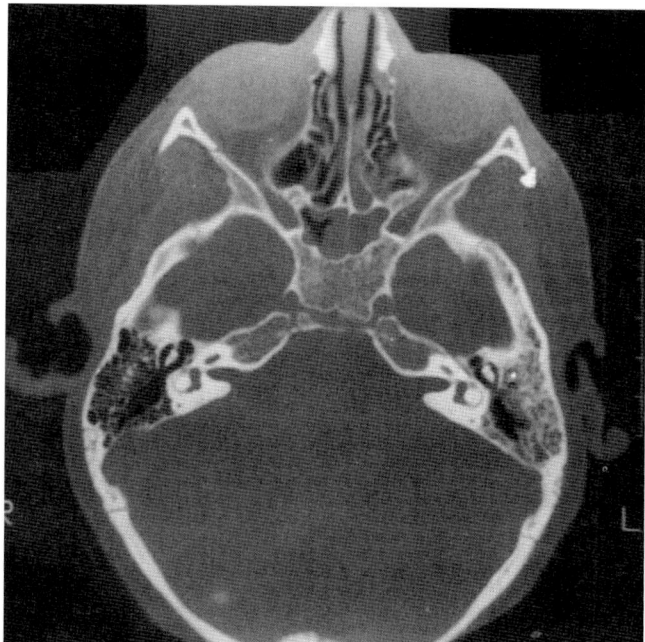

Figure 31-4. Computed tomography of a child with acute otitis media showing clouding of the mastoid without bony destruction.

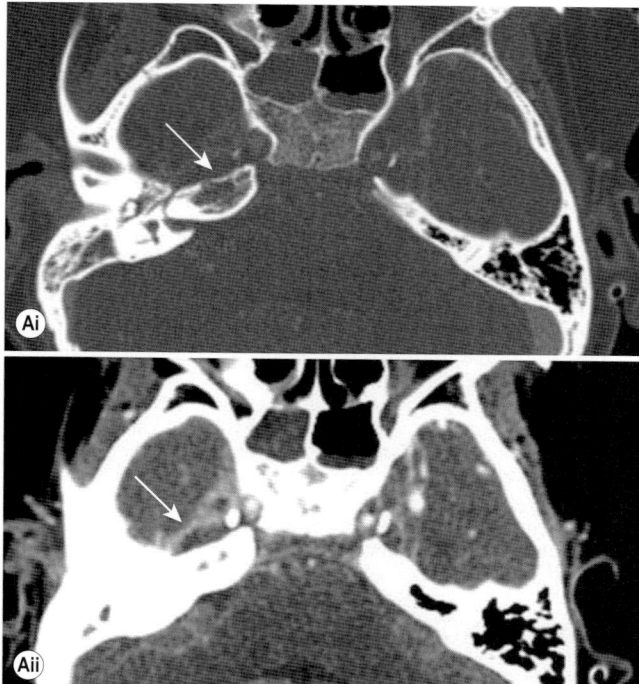

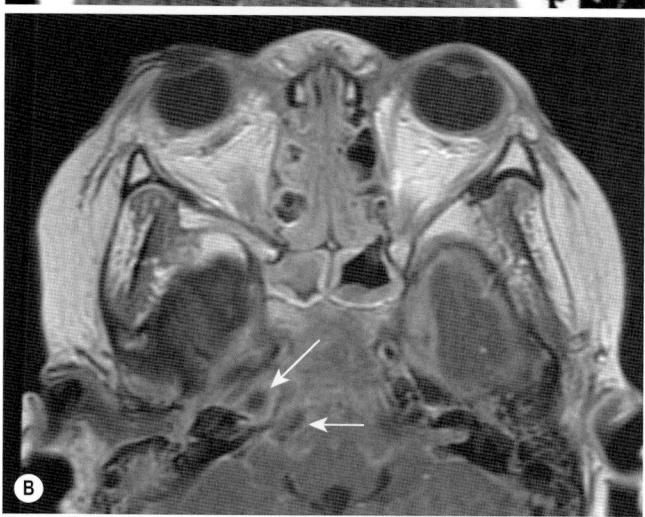

Figure 31-5. Case of a 6-year-old boy with Gradenigo syndrome. Non-contrast computed tomography **(Ai)** shows expansion and erosion of apex of the petrous portion of the right temporal bone *(arrow)* and mastoid coalescence. Contrast-enhanced CT **(Aii)** shows rim-enhancing abscess along the superior border of the petrous apex with anterior extension *(arrow).* Contrast-enhanced, T₁-weighted axial magnetic resonance imaging **(B)** shows hypointense lesions with rim enhancement (abscesses) around the petrous bone *(long arrow)* as well as in the right anterior pons *(short arrow).* (Courtesy of Faerber EN, St. Christopher's Hospital for Children, Philadelphia, PA.)

which can be seen in uncomplicated AOM, is not diagnostic of mastoiditis (Figure 31-4). Lytic lesions of the temporal bone and soft-tissue abscess sometimes can be seen (Figure 31-5). In order for bony destruction to be appreciated, 30% to 50% of bone must be demineralized. In cases in which the CT shows cloudiness, a technetium-99 bone scan, which is more sensitive to osteolytic changes, may be useful.[30]

CT with enhancement or magnetic resonance imaging (MRI) is recommended in patients with suspected vascular thrombosis as a complication of mastoiditis. MRI with gadolinium enhancement confirms the diagnosis and delineates the extent of suspected disease[31] because of higher sensitivity for detection of extra-axial fluid collections and associated vascular complications.[32]

Complications

Complications of mastoiditis are related to the spread of infection or inflammation from the middle ear or mastoid to contiguous structures and occur in 7% to 16% of cases.[17,21] Suppurative labyrinthitis (resulting in deafness), Bezold abscess, and cranial osteomyelitis are infectious complications. Facial paralysis can result from infection or inflammation of the facial nerve as it traverses the petrous bone. If infection spreads to the petrous bone, Gradenigo syndrome can follow, characterized by sixth-nerve palsy, pain in the distribution of the trigeminal nerve (eye pain), and otorrhea. Intracranial complications include epidural or subdural empyema, cerebellar or temporal lobe abscess, meningitis, and venous thrombosis.

Management

Treatment of uncomplicated mastoiditis includes intravenous antimicrobial therapy and usually myringotomy, with or without placement of a tympanostomy tube. Whenever possible, tympanocentesis should be performed if there is an intact tympanic membrane in order to ascertain microbiology and antimicrobial susceptibility.[9] The same treatment is appropriate when facial paralysis occurs as an isolated complication.[9] If the child does not improve in 48 hours (evidenced by diminution in systemic and local findings), a simple mastoidectomy may be required. Simple mastoidectomy in combination with antimicrobial therapy and

tympanostomy tube placement usually is indicated as initial management when a subperiosteal abscess is noted. Radical mastoidectomy only is performed when there is no response to simple mastoidectomy, as evidenced by continued otorrhea.[9]

Several different agents are appropriate for intravenous treatment of acute mastoiditis. Empiric antibiotic therapy should provide coverage for frequent bacterial pathogens (Table 31-1). Cefepime 150 mg/kg per day in divided doses every 12 hours, ceftazidime 150 mg/kg per day in divided doses every 8 hours, or piperacillin-tazobactam 240 to 300 mg/kg per day (piperacillin component) in divided doses every 6 to 8 hours (not approved for use for such in patients younger than 12 years), is suitable. In a penicillin-allergic patient, clindamycin, at 40 mg/kg per day in divided doses every 6 hours plus aztreonam (120 mg/kg per day in divided doses every 8 hours), will provide coverage for both gram-positive and gram-negative pathogens. The addition of vancomycin 60 mg/kg per day in divided doses every 6 hours should be considered for children who are severely ill with concerns about secondary bacterial meningitis, as well as those at high risk for resistant pneumococcal infection caused by penicillin resistant pneumococci or methicillin-resistant *S. aureus*. Immunization history and consideration of local resistance data are important in determining optimal antibiotic choices.

If Gram stain of aspirated material demonstrates an unexpected finding, additional antimicrobial agents are considered (such as for brain abscess). When results of culture and susceptibility tests are available, therapy is adjusted. Intravenous treatment should be maintained for at least 7 to 10 days. If the clinical response to treatment has been satisfactory, oral antimicrobial therapy can be substituted to complete a 4-week course. Prolonged courses of intravenous therapy generally are unnecessary in the absence of CNS extension of infection. Placement and maintenance of indwelling vascular catheters increase the cost of therapy significantly, and come with associated risks.[33]

CHRONIC MASTOIDITIS

Pathogenesis

Chronic mastoiditis almost always is a result of chronic suppurative otitis media (CSOM)[9] and, less frequently, the result of inadequate management of acute mastoiditis. CSOM is characterized by long-standing (>3 weeks), painless otorrhea through a nonintact tympanic membrane (either a spontaneous perforation or a patent tympanostomy tube) that is not responsive to the antibiotics customarily prescribed for patients with AOM (Box 31-3).[9,34] (See Chapter 30, Otitis Externa and Necrotizing Otitis Externa.)

A nonintact tympanic membrane is essential for pathogenesis, providing microbial species that colonize the external auditory canal access to the middle ear and, ultimately, the mastoid. These organisms cause a low-grade, persistent inflammatory response that is typically unaltered by conventional therapeutic agents for AOM. Although the inflammatory process is painless and patients rarely are febrile, CSOM can lead to chronic osteitis of the mastoid and complications such as hearing loss, cholesteatoma, facial nerve paralysis, meningitis, and brain abscess.

The microbiology of CSOM and chronic mastoiditis has been documented during the 1980s–1990s (Table 31-2).[9,35–39] *P. aeruginosa* is most common, followed by gram-negative enteric bacilli and *S. aureus*. *P. aeruginosa* and *S. aureus* occur together frequently.[9,35,40] With the exception of a single study, anaerobic flora are isolated only occasionally.[41] Rarely, *S. pneumoniae* or *H. influenzae* is causative.

TABLE 31-2. Bacteriology of Chronic Suppurative Otitis Media in 200 Children (1983–1992)

Bacterial Species	Number	Percent
Pseudomonas spp.	176	58
Pseudomonas aeruginosa	171	
Other species	5	
Enteric gram-negative rods	50	16
Escherichia coli	8	
Enterobacter spp.	9	
Proteus spp.	17	
Others	16	
Staphylococcus spp.	41	13
Staphylococcus aureus	38	
Staphylococcus epidermidis	3	
Streptococcus pneumoniae	10	3
Haemophilus influenzae	10	3
Others	19	6

Data from references 35 to 39.

Mycobacterium tuberculosis was a common cause of mastoiditis, manifesting as a chronically draining ear, in the early 1900s. This organism now is recovered rarely from patients with long-standing otorrhea.[42] Nontuberculous mycobacteria and *M. bovis* can produce an identical clinical syndrome. Most nontuberculous mycobacterial infections are suspected to occur through introduction of organisms through perforated tympanic membranes, emphasizing the need for good hygiene after tympanostomy tube placement.[43] *M. bovis*, not easily distinguished from *M. tuberculosis*, should be considered in patients who consume unpasteurized dairy products.[44]

Diagnosis

The diagnosis of CSOM usually is based on typical clinical presentation of painless otorrhea unresponsive to conventional antibiotic therapy. The patient with CSOM is readily distinguished from the patient with a spontaneous perforation due to AOM, in whom systemic and local symptoms are prominent and response to antimicrobial management is brisk. Distinction also must be made from the child with otorrhea due to otitis externa, in whom pressure on or movement of the tragus causes discomfort and the tympanic membrane is normal.

An otomicroscopic examination of the tympanic membrane should be undertaken by the otolaryngologist in the initial evaluation of chronic otorrhea.[40] This procedure, which may require general anesthesia, provides an opportunity to detect cholesteatoma, retraction pocket, granulation tissue, polyp, or foreign body. A specimen should be obtained from the middle-ear cavity without contamination from the external auditory canal and sent for Gram and acid-fast stains and culture for aerobic, anaerobic, and mycobacterial pathogens. A biopsy should be performed of any suspicious tissue protruding through the perforation or tympanostomy tube, because rhabdomyosarcoma and neuroblastoma can manifest as CSOM or chronic mastoiditis, usually with associated cranial nerve palsies. The tuberculin skin test (TST) should be performed when CSOM does not respond to standard antimicrobial therapy.

Management

Failure of response to oral antibiotics is important in defining CSOM and suggests *P. aeruginosa* as the probable cause. Treatment of patients with CSOM often is initiated with topical antimicrobial agents and vigorous aural toilet, which consists of daily suctioning of the external auditory canal to permit delivery of topical therapy. When otorrhea is copious, ototopical therapy cannot be

---

BOX 31-3. Diagnosis of Chronic Mastoiditis

- Otorrhea ≥3 weeks
- Nonintact tympanic membrane (perforation or patent tympanostomy tube)
- Nonresponsive to usual antibiotics
- Etiology
  - Pseudomonads
  - Staphylococci
  - Other gram-negative bacilli
- Complications
  - Cholesteatoma
  - Progressive mastoiditis
  - Deafness (eighth nerve or ossicular)

effective unless the external canal is cleared. Topical therapy is chosen because the bacteria isolated from patients with CSOM often are resistant to commonly prescribed oral antibiotics.

Ofloxacin otic solution (0.3%), a topical fluoroquinolone approved for use in children in 1999, has excellent activity against virtually all microbial species likely to be found in patients with CSOM.[34,45] Importantly, it has shown no ototoxic effects when administered to adults or children.[46] A Cochrane database of systematic reviews performed to assess effect of topical antibiotics without corticosteroids for patients with chronically draining ears and underlying eardrum perforations found topical quinolones significantly better for CSOM than antiseptics and no drug. Studies were inconclusive regarding differences between quinolone and nonquinolone antibiotics.[47] The aural discharge frequently clears within several days to 1 week after appropriate topical therapy is started.

If the CSOM does not respond to topical therapy, a course of antimicrobial therapy intravenously is appropriate. Comparison of regimens for the treatment of CSOM is confounded by differences in patient selection, causative agents, use of topical agents in conjunction with systemic therapy, frequency of aural toilet, and use of prophylactic antibiotics after completion of initial therapy. An appropriate choice for intravenous therapy is an antipseudomonal penicillin (e.g., piperacillin and tazobactam at 240–300 mg/kg per day in divided doses every 6 hours; not approved for use in children younger than 12 years) or a third- or fourth-generation cephalosporin with antipseudomonal activity (e.g., ceftazidime at 150 mg/kg per day in divided doses every 8 hours or cefepime at 100 mg/kg per day in divided doses every 12 hours, respectively).[34] Daily aural toilet is instituted for debridement and to assess cessation of drainage. In general, intravenous therapy should be continued at least 1 week after drainage has ceased, because the middle-ear mucosa is still likely to be inflamed, and immediate relapse is possible.[48,49] At the end of intravenous therapy, antimicrobial prophylaxis with amoxicillin for several months should be considered.[34] If otorrhea persists despite parenteral therapy or recurs shortly after the cessation of intravenous therapy, a simple tympanomastoidectomy is required.

Several investigators have reported effectively treating CSOM in children with intravenous or intramuscular antibiotics (such as ceftazidime) on an outpatient basis, with daily return to the otolaryngologist for aural toilet.[39]

32 Sinusitis

Ellen R. Wald

Upper respiratory tract infections (URIs) are the most common medical condition evaluated by the primary practitioner who cares for children. It has been estimated that approximately 5% to 10% of URIs in early childhood are complicated by acute bacterial sinusitis (ABS).[1] Children average 6 to 8 colds per year; accordingly, sinusitis is a common problem in clinical practice.

PATHOGENESIS

The respiratory mucosa that lines the nose is continuous with the mucosa that lines the paranasal sinuses. Secretions produced within the sinus cavities are delivered via the sinus ostia to the nose by normal mucociliary function. The maxillary, anterior ethmoid, and frontal sinuses drain to the middle meatus; the sphenoid and posterior ethmoid sinuses drain to the superior meatus.

The three key elements important to the normal physiology of the paranasal sinuses are: (1) patency of the ostia; (2) function of the ciliary apparatus; and, integral to the latter (3) quality of the secretions.[2] Retention of secretions in the paranasal sinuses usually is due to one or more of the following conditions: obstruction of the ostia, reduction in number of or impairment in the function of the cilia, and overproduction of or change in the viscosity of secretions.

Most cases of ABS are thought to be bacterial complications of viral URIs. The viral infection affects the mucosa of the nose, causing rhinitis, and often the mucosa of the sinuses as well. In most instances, the inflammatory response subsides spontaneously. In some cases, however, mucositis results in obstruction of the sinus ostia, impairment of the mucociliary apparatus, and alteration in the volume and quality of secretions.

The narrow caliber of the individual ostia that drain the maxillary and ethmoid sinuses sets the stage for obstruction to occur easily and often during the course of a viral URI. When obstruction occurs, there is a transient increase in intrasinal pressure. This is followed quickly by the development of negative pressure within the sinus cavities as the oxygen component of the intrasinus air is rapidly absorbed by a metabolically active mucosa.

When the pressure in the sinuses is negative relative to normal atmospheric pressure in the nose, conditions favor aspiration of mucus heavily laden with bacteria from the nose or nasopharynx into the presumably sterile paranasal sinuses.

Under ordinary circumstances, these contaminating bacteria would be swept out again by normal ciliary function. However, when ciliary function is impaired and sinus ostia are obstructed, bacteria multiply to high density and initiate an intense inflammatory response. Alternatively, sneezing, sniffling, and nose-blowing alter intrasinus pressure and facilitate bacterial contamination of the paranasal sinuses. Intranasal pressures are extremely high during nose-blowing, and nasal fluid has been shown to enter the maxillary sinus at that time.[3]

The factors predisposing to ostial obstruction can be divided into those that cause mucosal swelling, consequent to either systemic illness or local insults, and those due to mechanical obstruction (Table 32-1). Although many conditions can lead to ostial closure, viral URI and allergic inflammation are by far the most common and most important.

TABLE 32-1. Factors Predisposing to Sinus Ostial Obstruction

Mucosal Swelling	Mechanical Obstruction
SYSTEMIC DISORDER	Choanal atresia
Viral upper respiratory tract infection	Deviated septum
Allergic inflammation	Nasal polyps
Cystic fibrosis	Foreign body
Immune disorders	Tumor
Immotile cilia	Ethmoid bulla
LOCAL INSULT	
Facial trauma	
Swimming, diving	
Drug-induced rhinitis	
Gastroesophageal reflux	

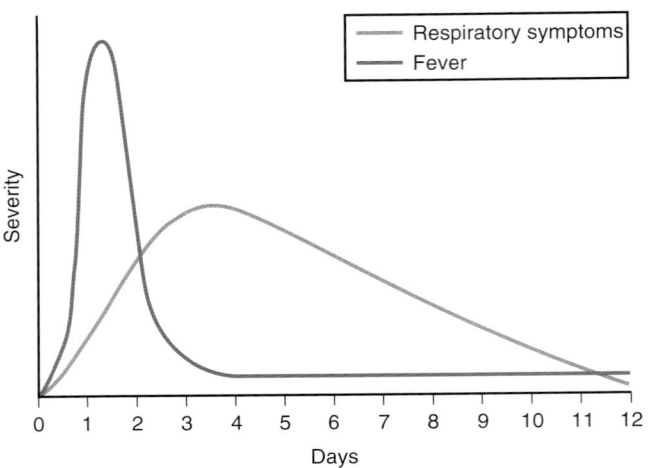

Figure 32-1. Timeline of course of fever and respiratory tract symptoms in uncomplicated viral upper respiratory tract illness.

BOX 32-1. Clinical Manifestations of Acute Sinusitis

PERSISTENT SYMPTOMS

Nasal discharge, cough, or both present >10 days and not improving

SEVERE SYMPTOMS

High fever (temperature ≥39°C) and purulent nasal discharge together for >3 days

WORSENING SYMPTOMS

Resolving upper respiratory symptoms
Worsening on day 6 or 7 with new or recurrent fever or exacerbation of nasal symptoms and/or cough

---

CLINICAL MANIFESTATIONS

Viral Upper Respiratory Tract Infections

To develop criteria to be used in distinguishing episodes of ABS from other common respiratory infections, it is helpful to describe an uncomplicated viral URI (depicted schematically in Figure 32-1). The course of most uncomplicated viral URIs is 5 to 10 days.[4] Although the patient may not be free of symptoms on the 10th day, almost always the respiratory symptoms have peaked in severity on days 3 to 6 and begun to improve. Most patients with uncomplicated viral URIs do not have fever. However, if fever is present, it tends to be present early in the illness, often in concert with other constitutional symptoms such as headache and myalgia. Typically, the fever and constitutional symptoms disappear in the first 24 to 48 hours and the respiratory symptoms become more prominent.

Viral URIs usually are characterized by nasal symptoms (discharge and congestion/obstruction) or cough, or both. Patients also may complain of a scratchy throat. Usually the nasal discharge begins as clear and watery. Often, however, the quality of nasal discharge changes during the course of the illness. Most typically, the nasal discharge becomes thicker and more mucoid and can become purulent (thick, colored, and opaque) for several days. Then the situation reverses, with the purulent discharge becoming mucoid and then clear again, or simply drying. The transition from clear to purulent to clear again occurs in uncomplicated viral URIs without the intervention of antimicrobial therapy.

Clinical Presentations of Acute Bacterial Sinusitis

With the clinical picture of an uncomplicated viral URI in mind, three clinical presentations of ABS can be described (Box 32-1).[5] The most common clinical presentation is onset with persistent symptoms.[6,7] The cardinal clinical features are nasal symptoms (anterior or posterior nasal discharge/nasal obstruction/congestion) or cough or both for more than 10 but fewer than 30 days that is not improving. This last qualifier is extremely important. Some individuals with uncomplicated viral URIs still have residual respiratory symptoms at the 10-day mark. To be considered a sign of ABS, these respiratory symptoms must be persistent without improvement. The nasal discharge in patients with persistent symptoms can be of any quality, thick or thin, serous, mucoid, or purulent, and the cough, which may be wet or dry, must be present during the daytime, although it is often described as worse at night. Malodorous breath often is reported by parents of preschool children. Complaints of facial pain and headache are

rare, although painless morning swelling of eyelids occurs occasionally. The child may not appear very ill, and usually, if fever is present, it is of low grade. It is not the severity of the clinical symptoms but their persistence that calls for attention. In clinical practice, strict observance of this presentation results in a diagnosis of acute sinusitis in 6% to 7% of children with upper respiratory tract symptoms who are evaluated by primary care providers.[8,9]

The second presentation is characterized as onset with severe symptoms. Severity is described as a combination of high fever, a temperature of at least 38.5°C and a particular quality of nasal discharge, a purulent nasal discharge, concurrently for at least 3 to 4 consecutive days.[7] The presence of persistent fever for at last 3 to 4 days distinguishes this presentation from an uncomplicated viral URI (in which fever usually is present for less than 48 hours).

The third presentation is described as worsening symptoms or presentation with a biphasic illness (in the Scandinavian literature, this is referred to as "double sickening").[5,10] This illness begins similarly to an uncomplicated viral URI from which the patient seems to be recovering. On the 6th or 7th day of illness, the patient becomes substantially worse again. The worsening symptoms can be manifest as an increase in respiratory symptoms (exacerbation of nasal discharge or nasal congestion or daytime cough) or the new onset of fever or a recurrence of fever if it had been present at the outset.

Patients with subacute or chronic sinusitis have a history of protracted (>30 days and not improving) respiratory symptoms. Nasal congestion (obstruction) and cough (day and night) are most common. Sore throat is a frequent complaint resulting from mouth breathing secondary to nasal obstruction. Nasal discharge (of any quality) and headache are less common; fever is rare.

On physical examination, the patient with ABS can have mucopurulent discharge in the nose or posterior pharynx. The nasal mucosa usually is erythematous but can occasionally be pale and boggy; the throat can show moderate injection. Examination of the tympanic membranes can show evidence of acute otitis media or otitis media with effusion; this occurs more often in chronic than acute sinusitis. The cervical lymph nodes usually are not enlarged significantly or tender. Occasionally, there is either tenderness, as the examiner palpates over or percusses the paranasal sinuses, or appreciable periorbital edema, with soft, nontender swelling of the upper and lower eyelid and discoloration of the overlying skin. Unfortunately, facial tenderness is neither a sensitive nor a specific sign of sinusitis. Malodorous breath (in the absence of pharyngitis, poor dental hygiene, or a nasal foreign body) can suggest bacterial sinusitis. None of these characteristics, however, differentiates rhinitis from sinusitis.

DIAGNOSTIC METHODS

Imaging

In cases of uncomplicated sinusitis, no confirmatory imaging is recommended. Imaging studies were recommended in the past. However, many studies have documented that when images of any kind (plain x-rays, computed tomographic (CT) studies or magnetic resonance imaging (MRI)) are performed in children or adults with uncomplicated viral upper respiratory tract infections, most will exhibit the same findings that we have in the past associated with acute sinusitis (i.e., diffuse opacification, mucosal swelling, or an air–fluid level).[11-15] Accordingly, while normal images can assure the practitioner that the patient's respiratory symptoms are not attributable to sinusitis, abnormal images cannot confirm a diagnosis of sinusitis and are not indicated in uncomplicated infections. By contrast, when patients present with complications of acute sinusitis, either subperiosteal abscess or intracranial disease or have protracted or non-responsive symptoms, imaging (usually CT and occasionally MRI) is extremely helpful in clarifying the precise diagnosis and informing the necessity for surgical interventions.[7]

Sinus Aspiration

Maxillary sinus aspiration can be performed safely by a skilled otolaryngologist in the ambulatory setting using a transnasal approach. Sedation or general anesthesia may be required for adequate immobilization in the young child. Current indications for maxillary sinus aspiration are: (1) lack of response of sinusitis to multiple courses of antibiotics; (2) severe facial pain; (3) orbital or intracranial complications; and (4) evaluation of an immunocompromised host.

There must be careful decontamination and anesthesia of the area beneath the inferior turbinate through which the trocar is passed. Material aspirated from the maxillary sinus should be sent for Gram stain and quantitative aerobic and anaerobic cultures. The recovery of bacteria in a density of at least 10^4 colony-forming units (CFU) per milliliter is considered to represent true infection.[16] The finding of at least one organism per high-power field on Gram stain of sinus secretions correlates with the recovery of bacteria in a density of 10^5 CFU/mL.

MICROBIOLOGY

Data on the microbiology of sinusitis in pediatric patients are best organized according to the duration of clinical symptoms (Table 32-2). However, literature review is complicated by varying definitions of acute, subacute, and chronic sinusitis. Several studies of ambulatory patients with acute (duration, 10 to 30 days) and subacute (30 to 120 days)[17,18] illnesses have shown the important bacterial pathogens to be *Streptococcus pneumoniae*, *Haemophilus influenzae*, and *Moraxella catarrhalis*. *S. pneumoniae* has been most common in all age groups, accounting for 30% to 40% of isolates. *H. influenzae* and *M. catarrhalis* are similar in prevalence and each accounts for approximately 20% of cases. In the last decade there has been a variable prevalence of penicillin-resistant *S. pneumoniae* (depending on the use of conjugate pneumococcal vaccine and

emergence of non-vaccine serotypes) and many of the *H. influenzae* (35% to 50%) and *M. catarrhalis* (55% to 100%) are β-lactamase-producing and also resistant to penicillin.[19,20] Other less frequently recovered bacterial species are group A streptococcus, group C streptococcus, viridans streptococci, *Peptostreptococcus* spp., other *Moraxella* spp., and *Eikenella corrodens*.[16] Neither staphylococci nor anaerobic respiratory flora are recovered commonly from patients with acute or subacute sinusitis. Respiratory viruses, including adenovirus, parainfluenza virus, influenza virus, and rhinovirus, are identified in approximately 10% of patients (both with and without bacterial species). This percentage would be higher if nasal samples were obtained earlier in the course of respiratory symptoms.

Unfortunately, there are no data that have been generated regarding the microbiology of ABS in children since 1984.[21] However, because of the similarity of the pathogenesis and microbiology of acute otitis media and ABS, it is acceptable to regard recent data from cultures of middle-ear fluid, obtained by tympanocentesis, from children with acute otitis media as a surrogate for cultures of the paranasal sinuses.[22] Attributable in large part to the near-universal use of pneumococcal conjugate vaccine (PCV7) in the United States, licensed in 2000, several reports in 2004 initially highlighted a decrease in isolates of *S. pneumoniae* and an increase in isolates of *H. influenzae* recovered from middle-ear aspirates.[23,24] This change in microbiology relates to the decrease in recovery of vaccine strains of *S. pneumoniae* from the nasopharynx of immunized children.[19] However, after several years, the emergence of non-vaccine strains of *S. pneumoniae* restored temporarily the relative proportion of *S. pneumoniae* and *H. influenzae* to those observed before 2000.[20,25] Presumably, these changes are occurring in the paranasal sinuses as well. Fortunately, the licensure of PCV13 in 2010 has once again resulted in a decrease in the recovery of *S. pneumoniae* from children with ABS.

In patients with very protracted (years) or severe sinus symptoms (requiring surgical intervention), *S. aureus* and anaerobic organisms are recovered more frequently. Commonly recovered anaerobic bacteria are anaerobic gram-positive cocci (such as *Peptococcus* and *Peptostreptococcus* spp.) and *Bacteroides* or *Prevotella* spp.[26] In addition, viridans streptococci and *H. influenzae* are recovered frequently.

MEDICAL MANAGEMENT

Antimicrobial agents are mainstays in the medical management of sinusitis.[7,9] Table 32-3 shows a list of agents potentially useful in patients with ABS. Amoxicillin has been the treatment of choice for many cases of uncomplicated sinusitis in children. It is effective most of the time, narrow spectrum, inexpensive, and safe. Concern about penicillin-resistant *S. pneumoniae* (in children <2 years of age, those attending group childcare, and those who have recently been treated with an antimicrobial agent) should prompt the use of high-dose amoxicillin (90 mg/kg per day).[7] However, amoxicillin at any dose does not cover β-lactamase-producing *H.*

TABLE 32-2. Bacteriology of Sinusitis

Bacterial Species	Acute (10–29 days)	Subacute (30–120 days)	Chronic (>120 days)
Streptococcus pneumoniae	+++	++	+
Haemophilus influenzae	+++	++	+
Moraxella catarrhalis	++	++	+
Staphylococcus aureus			+
Anaerobic bacteria[a]			+

[a]*Respiratory anaerobic cocci*, Bacteroides *spp.*, Prevotella spp., Veillonella spp. +++, most common; ++, common; +, less common.

TABLE 32-3. Antimicrobial Agents and Dosage Schedules for the Treatment of Sinusitis in Children

Antimicrobial Agent	Dosage
Amoxicillin	45–90 mg/kg per day in 2 divided doses
Amoxicillin/potassium clavulanate	45/10 mg/kg per day in 2 divided doses
Amoxicillin/potassium clavulanate (high dose)	90/6.4 mg/kg per day in 2 divided doses
Cefpodoxime proxetil	10 mg/kg once daily
Cefuroxime axetil	30 mg/kg per day in 2 divided doses
Cefdinir	14 mg/kg per day in 1 or 2 daily doses
Cefprozil	30 mg/kg per day in 2 divided doses

PART II Clinical Syndromes and Cardinal Features of Infectious Diseases: Approach to Diagnosis and Initial Management

SECTION C Oral Infections and Upper and Middle Respiratory Tract Infections

influenzae and *M. catarrhalis*. Accordingly, amoxicillin should be reserved for children with mild illness, early in the respiratory season, who have no risk factors for infection with resistant bacterial species.

A broader-spectrum regimen is appropriate in the following clinical situations: (1) lack of symptom improvement with amoxicillin therapy in 48 to 72 hours; (2) the presence of any risk factors for resistant bacterial species (young age, attendance at day care, or recent treatment (either the index case or a close contact) with an antibiotic); (3) the occurrence of frontal or sphenoidal sinusitis; (4) the occurrence of complicated ethmoidal sinusitis (the presence of even minimal eye swelling); and (5) the presence of protracted (>30 days') symptoms. Antimicrobial agents with the most comprehensive coverage for patients with sinusitis are "high-dose" amoxicillin-potassium clavulanate (amoxicillin 90 mg/kg per day and clavulanate 6.4 mg/kg per day in 2 divided doses; maximum dose 8 g amoxicillin per day), cefuroxime axetil (30 mg/kg in 2 divided doses), and cefpodoxime proxetil (10 mg/kg once daily). For patients with chronic sinusitis, amoxicillin-potassium clavulanate is an attractive choice, especially because the mode of amoxicillin resistance in the pathogens causing chronic sinusitis is β-lactamase production.

Other antimicrobial agents that are available for the management of respiratory infections but are considerably less potent or adequate in spectrum are: cefdinir, cefprozil, clarithromycin, and azithromycin. In general, clarithromycin and azithromycin should be reserved for children who have lower respiratory tract disease suggestive of *Mycoplasma* infection or have a type 1 hypersensitivity reaction to β-lactam agents.

Infections due to penicillin-resistant pneumococci are a persistent problem. Organisms are classified as *susceptible* when the minimum inhibitory concentration (MIC) of the drug is <0.1 μg/mL; *moderately resistant* when the MIC is between 0.1 and 1.0 μg/mL; and *resistant* when the MIC is ≥1 μg/mL for oral beta-lactams. The frequency of penicillin-resistant pneumococci varies geographically, and many isolates of pneumococci are resistant to other commonly used antimicrobial agents, such as trimethoprim-sulfamethoxazole, erythromycin-sulfisoxazole, and the macrolides (azithromycin and clarithromycin). Therapeutic options include high-dose amoxicillin, an advanced-generation cephalosporin (for some pneumococci with moderate resistance), clindamycin, linezolid, and rifampin. Selection of an antimicrobial agent should be guided by susceptibility test results when available.

Patients with ABS may require hospitalization because of systemic toxicity or inability to take antibiotics orally. These patients can be treated with intravenous cefotaxime at 200 mg/kg per day in 4 divided doses, intravenous ceftriaxone at 100 mg/kg per day given once daily, or intravenous ampicillin-sulbactam, at 200 mg/kg per day of ampicillin component in 4 divided doses (not approved for such indications in children younger than 12 years).

Clinical improvement is prompt in nearly all children treated with an appropriate antimicrobial agent. Patients febrile at the initial encounter become afebrile, and there is a remarkable reduction of nasal discharge and cough within 48 to 72 hours. If the symptoms either do not improve or worsen in 48 to 72 hours, clinical re-evaluation is appropriate. If amoxicillin was prescribed initially, an antimicrobial agent effective against β-lactamase-producing bacterial species and penicillin-resistant pneumococci should be prescribed. If amoxicillin-clavulanate was prescribed originally and the patient has not improved, clindamycin or linezolid and cefixime is a reasonable second line drug combination. If the patient is still not improved, parenteral therapy should be considered as well as sinus aspiration for precise bacteriologic identification.

The appropriate duration of antimicrobial therapy for patients with ABS has not been investigated systematically. For patients whose respiratory symptoms improve dramatically within 3 to 4 days of commencement of therapy, 10 days of treatment is adequate. For cases that respond more slowly, it is reasonable to treat until the patient is symptom-free plus an additional 7 days.

Adjuvant therapies, such as antihistamines, decongestants, and anti-inflammatory agents, have received little systematic

---

BOX 32-2. Major Complications of Sinusitis

ORBITAL

Inflammatory edema[a]
Subperiosteal abscess
Orbital abscess
Orbital cellulitis
Optic neuritis

INTRACRANIAL

Epidural empyema
Subdural empyema
Cavernous or sagittal sinus thrombosis
Meningitis
Brain abscess

OSTEITIS

Frontal (Pott puffy tumor)

[a]Inflammatory edema is not a true orbital complication of sinusitis. Infection is confined to the paranasal sinuses; periorbital swelling is due to impedance of venous blood flow.

---

evaluation. The overall impact of intranasal budesonide as an adjunct to oral antibiotic therapy for children with acute sinusitis is extremely modest and it is not recommended.[27]

Some children experience recurrent or chronic episodes of sinusitis. The most common cause of recurrent sinusitis is recurrent viral URI, often a consequence of attendance at out-of-home childcare or the presence of a school-aged child in the household. Other predisposing conditions are allergic and nonallergic rhinitis, cystic fibrosis, an immunodeficiency disorder (insufficient or dysfunctional immunoglobulins), ciliary dyskinesia, gastroesophageal reflux, and an anatomic abnormality (see Table 32-1). Evaluation of children with recurrent or chronic sinusitis should include consideration of consultation with an allergist, performance of a sweat test, quantitative measurements of serum immunoglobulin levels, and a mucosal biopsy to assess ciliary structure and function.

If specific allergens are identified or an allergic diathesis is documented, therapy might include desensitization, antihistamine, or topical intranasal steroid therapy. If a treatable immunodeficiency is identified, specific immunoglobulin therapy is initiated. Antimicrobial prophylaxis has not been studied in patients with recurrent acute sinusitis, although it has proved to be a useful strategy in reducing symptomatic episodes of acute otitis media in patients with frequent recurrences. Concerns regarding antibiotic resistance have discouraged recent use of antibiotic prophylaxis. If sinusitis does not respond to maximal medical therapy, surgical intervention may be appropriate.

The major complications of acute sinusitis are shown in Box 32-2. Subperiosteal abscess of the orbit and intracranial abscess (subdural and epidural empyema) are the most common.[28,29] Signs of orbital infection are eyelid swelling, proptosis, and impaired extraocular eye movements. With intracranial spread of infection there may be signs of increased intracranial pressure, meningeal irritation, and focal neurologic signs. CT or MRI is essential for diagnosis. Antibiotic therapy and surgical drainage usually are required for successful treatment.

SURGICAL MANAGEMENT

Patients with acute sinusitis rarely require surgical intervention in the absence of orbital or central nervous system complications. An appreciation for the fact that a large group of pediatric patients with chronic sinusitis have underlying allergic rhinitis or other medical problems such as gastroesophageal reflux has led to more aggressive medical management and less enthusiasm for surgical solutions.[30] Occasionally, sinus aspiration is required to ventilate a sinus in a patient with no response to aggressive antimicrobial therapy.

In the rare child who has failed conventional treatment with oral antibiotics and an array of local and systemic adjuvants to therapy, antibiotic therapy delivered via a percutaneous intravenous catheter may be a worthwhile trial.[31] This can be combined with adenoidectomy, or adenoidectomy may be undertaken either as a solo intervention or performed in conjunction with functional endoscopic surgery.[32,33]

When functional endoscopic sinus surgery is performed, the focus is on the ostiomeatal complex, highlighted in Figure 32-2. This is the area between the middle and inferior turbinates that represents the confluence of drainage areas of the frontal, ethmoid, and maxillary sinuses. In the ostiomeatal complex, there are several areas in which two mucosal layers come into contact, predisposing to local impairment of mucociliary clearance. Using an endoscope, the natural meatus of the maxillary outflow tract is enlarged by excising the uncinate process and the ethmoid bullae and performing an anterior ethmoidectomy. Ramodan reported a group of 66 children undergoing either adenoidectomy or endoscopic surgery for chronic rhinosinusitis.[32] The group undergoing endoscopic sinus surgery had the greatest improvement in overall symptom scores. As our understanding of the pathogenetic factors predisposing to sinusitis expands and our therapy of these mucosal diseases becomes more effective, the pediatric candidates for surgical management of their sinus disease will continue to decrease. Judicious use of surgery in young children with chronic rhinosinusitis is strongly recommended.[34]

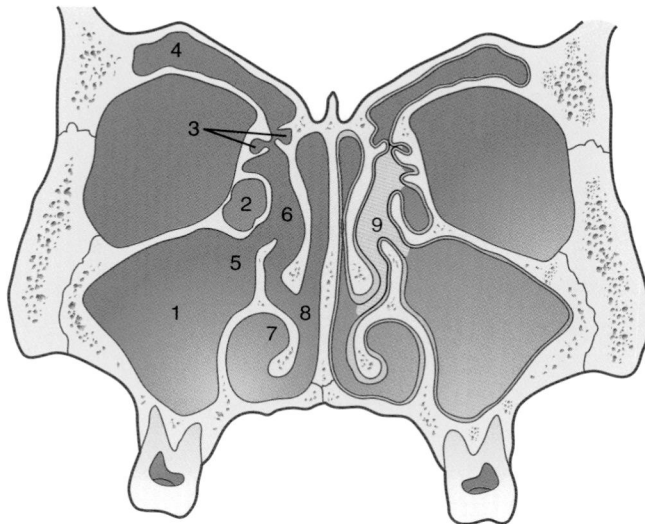

Figure 32-2. Coronal section of the nose and paranasal sinuses. 1, Maxillary sinus; 2, ethmoidal bursa; 3, ethmoidal cells; 4, frontal sinus; 5, uncinate process; 6, middle turbinate; 7, inferior turbinate; 8, nasal septum; 9 (blue area), ostiomeatal complex. (From Wald ER. Sinusitis in children. N Engl J Med 1992;326:319–323.)

SECTION D: Lower Respiratory Tract Infections

33 Bronchiolitis

H. Cody Meissner

Bronchiolitis, a disease primarily of the first 2 years of life characterized by signs and symptoms of obstructive airway disease, is caused most commonly by viruses.[1] Approximately 2% to 3% of infants in the first 12 months of life are hospitalized with bronchiolitis, accounting for approximately 125,000 hospitalizations and 200 to 500 deaths annually in the United States.[2] Data from the Centers for Disease Control and Prevention (CDC) indicate that the number of yearly hospital admissions attributable to bronchiolitis increased more than twofold between 1980 and 1996.[3] Increasing survival rates for premature infants as well as infants with compromised cardiac, pulmonary, and immune status increase the number of children at risk for severe bronchiolitis.

ETIOLOGIC AGENTS

Many viruses can cause bronchiolitis, although respiratory syncytial virus (RSV), human metapneumovirus, and parainfluenza virus type 3 are the most common etiologic agents.[1-7] Other viruses are implicated less frequently (Table 33-1).[8-10] During the winter months, RSV is identified as the etiologic agent by cell culture or antigen detection assays in up to 80% of children hospitalized with bronchiolitis or pneumonia. Epidemics of bronchiolitis in early spring and fall often are caused by parainfluenza virus type 3.[11-14] The yearly cycles of these respiratory viruses are depicted in Figure 33-1. Other viral causes of bronchiolitis include rhinoviruses and coronaviruses.

Bordetella pertussis, Mycoplasma pneumoniae, measles, influenza, and adenovirus have been associated with a severe form of bronchiolitis, bronchiolitis obliterans.[15-18] This uncommon obstructive pulmonary disease is characterized histologically by the progression of acute airway inflammation to necrosis of the cells lining the lumen with severe obliterative fibrosis in the final stages. The pathogenesis of bronchiolitis obliterans probably differs from that of simple viral bronchiolitis.

EPIDEMIOLOGY

Bronchiolitis may be defined as an episode of obstructive lower airway disease precipitated by a viral infection in infants younger than 24 months of age. The peak incidence of severe disease occurs between 2 and 6 months of age.[1,19,20] Rates of hospitalization are higher in boys and among infants living in industrialized urban settings rather than in rural settings.[21] Hospitalization rates are about 5 times higher among infants and children in high-risk groups than among non-high-risk infants. High-risk groups include premature infants (<35 weeks' gestation), infants born with hemodynamically significant congenital heart disease, as well as infants with chronic lung disease of prematurity (previously called bronchopulmonary dysplasia).[22-27] Although mortality has been reduced in recent years, morbidity among high-risk patients can be high, with average hospital length of stay and intensity of care several times that of previously healthy infants.[2,28]

Occurrence of the respiratory virus season is predictable, even though the severity of the season, the date of onset, the peak of activity, and the end of the season cannot be predicted with precision. There can be variation in timing of community outbreaks of disease due to RSV from year to year in the same community and among neighboring communities, even in the same season. In the U.S., communities in the south tend to experience the earliest

PART II Clinical Syndromes and Cardinal Features of Infectious Diseases: Approach to Diagnosis and Initial Management

SECTION D Lower Respiratory Tract Infections

onset of RSV activity and the midwest tends to experience the latest onset.[29] The duration of the season for the west and the northeast is typically between that in the south and the midwest. Nevertheless, these variations occur within the overall pattern of RSV outbreaks, usually beginning in November or December, peaking in January or February, and ending by the end of March or April.

Limited numbers of cases of bronchiolitis occur during summer and early fall, and they are likely to be caused by viruses other than RSV, such as rhinovirus and parainfluenza viruses. These cases are generally milder than RSV-related cases. In tropical countries, the annual epidemic of RSV coincides with the rainy season or "winter," although sporadic cases can occur throughout the year.[10]

RSV can be divided into A and B strains, each with numerous subtypes or genotypes. Type A strains may be associated more commonly with epidemics, severe disease, and a higher hospitalization rate than type B strains, although not all studies are consistent with regard to differences in severity.[30-33] Both strains may circulate during the same season, and infants may be reinfected within the same year.

A progressive increase in hospitalization rates for bronchiolitis in the U.S. has occurred since the late 1980s.[3,22] This increase may be related to a greater ability to identify hypoxic infants through the use of pulse oximetry. Alternatively, the increase in hospitalization may reflect increased use of daycare centers or changes in criteria for admission.[3] Household crowding is an important risk factor for severe viral lower respiratory tract illness due to RSV as well as other respiratory viruses.[34,35] Generally it is recognized that as the number of household members increases, the risk of exposure to infectious respiratory secretions also increases. Childcare attendance has been correlated with an increased risk of bronchiolitis in some studies. Unlike other respiratory virus infections, exposure to passive household tobacco smoke has not been associated with an increased risk of RSV hospitalization on a consistent basis. In contrast to the well-documented beneficial effect of breastfeeding against some viral illnesses, existing data are conflicting regarding the specific protective effect of breastfeeding against RSV infection.[35-39] Parental history of bronchiolitis or

TABLE 33-1. Infectious Causes of Bronchiolitis

Infectious Agent	Occurrences
Respiratory syncytial virus	++++
Human metapneumovirus	++
Parainfluenza virus 3	++
Parainfluenza virus 1	+
Parainfluenza virus 2	+
Coronaviruses	+
Adenovirus	+
Influenza virus (A or B)	+
Mycoplasma pneumoniae	+
Enterovirus	+
Rhinovirus	+

++++, *most common cause;* ++, *causes substantial percentage of cases in some studies;* +, *occasional cause. Relative importance varies with season and epidemic disease (see text).*

Data from references 7, 8, 11, 13, 15.

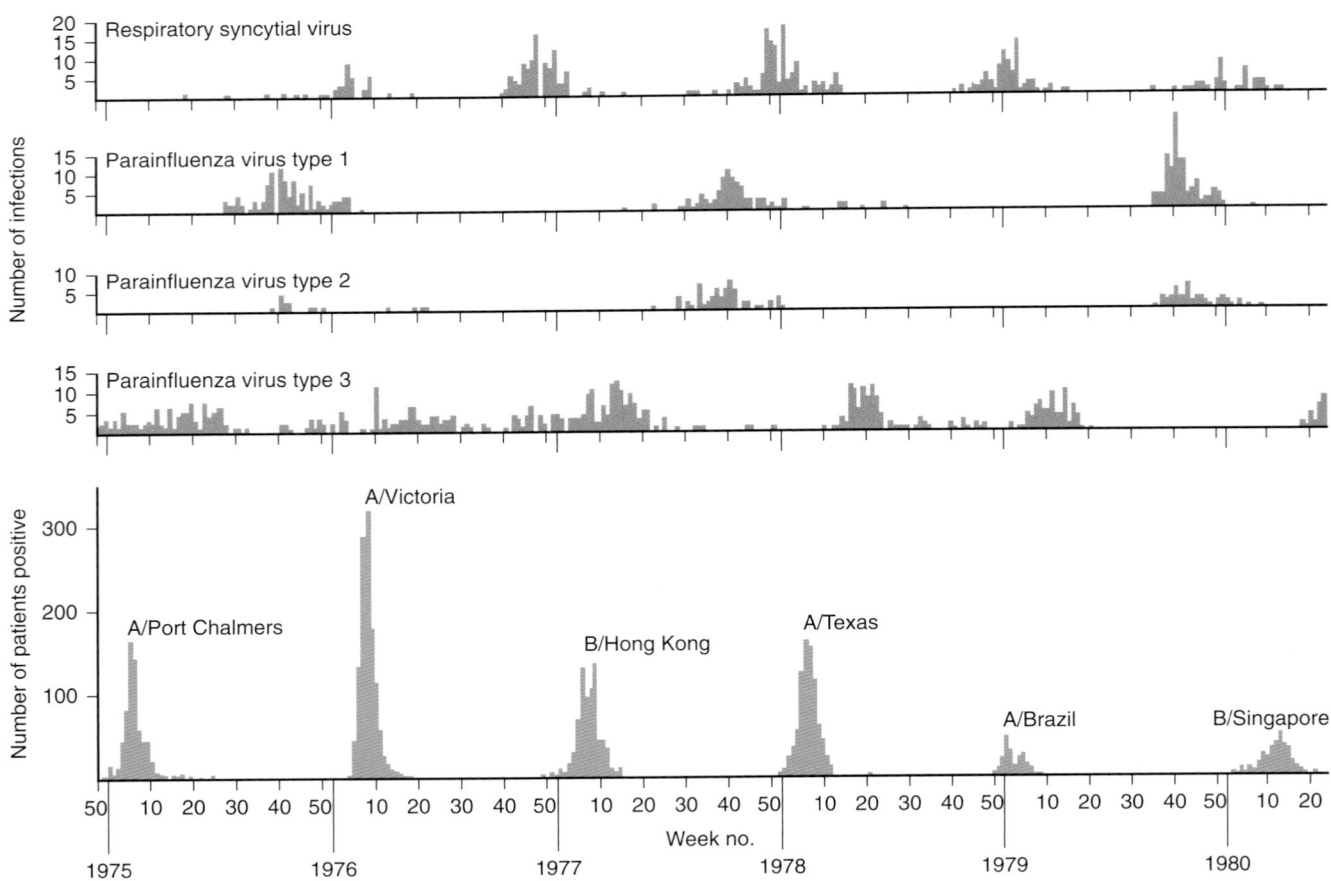

Figure 33-1. Patterns of occurrence of respiratory syncytial virus and parainfluenza virus in Houston, Texas. (From Couch RB. Viral respiratory diseases. In: Stringfellow DA (ed) Virology. Kalamazoo, MI, Scope, 1983, p 65.)

asthma is associated with a higher risk for the development of lower respiratory illness in offspring.[40,41]

Young chronologic age at the beginning of the RSV season is a consistent risk factor for RSV hospitalization. Several reasons may account for this increase in risk. Most severe RSV disease occurs in the first 6 months of life so that birth shortly before or early after the onset of the RSV season will result in a longer period of exposure to RSV earlier in life. Second, maternal antibody concentrations to RSV show seasonal variation and infants born early in the RSV season are more likely to be born to mothers with low serum antibody concentrations to the F (fusion) protein of RSV.[42,43] Low concentrations of RSV antibody correlate with susceptibility to severe RSV disease in infants.

PATHOGENESIS AND PATHOLOGIC FINDINGS

Acute bronchiolitis generally implies disease of infectious etiology, usually due to viruses with specific tropism for bronchiolar epithelium. Because most healthy infants recover from bronchiolitis without incident, information regarding the pathologic changes caused by infection is inferred from animal studies and from biopsy or autopsy materials in severe cases. Viral infection causes profound alterations in the epithelial cell and mucosal surfaces of the human respiratory tract. The characteristic histopathology in bronchiolitis is a lymphocytic infiltration of the bronchiolar walls and edema of the surrounding tissue. Disease progression is associated with proliferation and necrosis of the bronchiolar epithelium. The sloughed necrotic epithelium and the increased mucus production lead to obstruction of the lumen of the infant's small airways. Air movement is restricted during inspiration and expiration but is more restricted during expiration when the lumen is further compromised by positive expiratory pressure, resulting in expiratory wheezing. The obstruction results in air trapping and the characteristic appearance of hyperinflation on chest radiographs. As this air is absorbed, the radiographic pattern evolves to show atelectasis.[44–49]

The presence of high serum concentrations of immunoglobulin IgG antibodies to RSV (whether transplacentally acquired or administered intramuscularly) ameliorates RSV illness.[50–54] Severe obstructive illness may be related to stimulation of virus-specific IgE-mediated hypersensitivity responses or altered cell-mediated immune responses.[55–60]

CLINICAL MANIFESTATIONS

Bronchiolitis represents the late stage of a respiratory disease that progresses over several days. Upper respiratory tract symptoms consisting of nasal discharge and mild cough begin about 3 to 5 days after onset of infection. Approximately 30% to 40% of RSV-infected infants have progression of disease to involve the lower respiratory tract. Spread to the lower airway occurs either by aspiration of RSV-infected epithelial cells or by cell-to-cell spread of the virus. Lower-airway involvement is marked by a sudden increase in the work of breathing, cough, tachypnea, wheezing, crackles, use of accessory muscles, and nasal flaring.[61,62] The respiratory rate often exceeds 60 to 70 breaths/minute in young infants, and expiration is prolonged. Intercostal and subcostal retractions with wheezing are evident. Initially, wheezing occurs during the expiratory phase only and is only audible through a stethoscope. As wheezing progresses, it can be heard without a stethoscope. The chest becomes hyperexpanded and hyperresonant, respirations more labored, and retractions more severe. Hypoxemia out of proportion to clinical distress is typical of RSV infection. Mild hypoxemia occurs even in otherwise well-appearing infants, the so-called happy wheezers. Respiratory failure can be due to hypoxemia (an early and sometimes sudden occurrence) or progressive hypercapnia due to fatigue. The small airways of young infants can become so narrowed that wheezing is inaudible. In this setting disease severity is recognized by the absence of audible air exchange, flaring of the alae nasae, expiratory grunting, severe subcostal, supraclavicular, and intercostal retractions, and hypoxemia. Progressive illness often is accompanied by a rapid fall in oxygen saturation after minimal manipulation. A child with these findings usually requires intubation and ventilatory support. Apnea can be an early manifestation of RSV infection, at times resulting in respiratory failure.[63] RSV-related apnea is mediated by the central nervous system, occurring in young, often prematurely born infants.[64] Because the severity of bronchiolitis often waxes and wanes prior to consistent improvement, assessment of respiratory status can vary markedly over a short period. The ability of the young infant to breast- or bottle-feed without distress over time often provides a practical guide to disease severity and management. An infant who has substantial difficulty feeding as a result of respiratory distress has moderate or severe illness and usually requires hospitalization.

Otherwise healthy infants younger than 2 months of age, infants born prematurely (less than 35 weeks' gestation), and infants with chronic lung disease of prematurity (previously called bronchopulmonary dysplasia) or infants born with congenital heart disease have the highest morbidity and mortality rates due to bronchiolitis.[65,66] Infants born with congenital heart disease at greatest risk of hospitalization due to bronchiolitis include those with moderate to severe pulmonary hypertension and infants with cyanotic heart disease. RSV-infected infants and children with the following hemodynamically insignificant heart disease are generally not considered to be at increased risk of hospitalization: secundum atrial septal defect, small ventricular septal defect, pulmonic stenosis, uncomplicated aortic stenosis, mild coarctation of the aorta, and patent ductus arteriosus, as well as infants with lesions adequately corrected by surgery (unless they continue to require medication for management of congestive heart failure).[67,68] Severe respiratory distress with bronchiolitis can be the presenting manifestation of previously unrecognized congenital heart disease.

Once hospitalized, the RSV-infected infant may have a highly variable course of illness.[69–73] Among otherwise healthy infants, intensive care unit admission because of respiratory deterioration is uncommon.[74] A decision to admit to the intensive care unit is based on the possible need for intubation because of progressive hypercapnia, increasing hypoxemia despite supplemental oxygen, or apnea. The typical course for a previously healthy infant older than 6 months is one of improvement over 2 to 5 days, as evidenced by decreases in respiratory rate, retractions, duration of expiration, and oxygen requirement. The median duration of symptoms in 95 infants with first-time bronchiolitis who came to medical attention at an emergency department in Wisconsin was 15 days and one-quarter of the infants remained symptomatic after 3 weeks.[75] Pulmonary function abnormalities and evidence of mild desaturation (oxygen saturations in the range of 93% to 95%) can persist for several weeks.[76] The differential diagnosis of bronchiolitis includes airway hypersensitivity to environmental irritants, anatomic abnormality of the airway, cardiac disease with pulmonary edema, cystic fibrosis, foreign-body aspiration, and gastroesophageal reflux.

DIAGNOSIS

The diagnosis of bronchiolitis is based on clinical criteria with supporting radiographic findings. Typical chest radiographic findings are hyperinflation, with flattening of the diaphragms and hyperlucency of the lungs, and patchy atelectasis, especially involving the right upper lobe (Figures 33-2 and 33-3).[74,76] Atelectasis is due to airway narrowing or mucous plugging and is associated with volume loss; it may be confused with lobar consolidation or aspiration pneumonia, both of which are generally volume-expanding lesions. Bacterial pneumonia infrequently occurs as a complication of bronchiolitis but should be suspected in the infant with fever persisting for more than 2 to 3 days and lack of response to supportive management.

Establishing a specific etiologic diagnosis is helpful in predicting the clinical course, in cohorting in the hospital, and may become increasingly useful as more antiviral agents effective against respiratory viruses become available. Although viral culture of respiratory secretions has been the "gold standard" for

PART II Clinical Syndromes and Cardinal Features of Infectious Diseases: Approach to Diagnosis and Initial Management

SECTION D Lower Respiratory Tract Infections

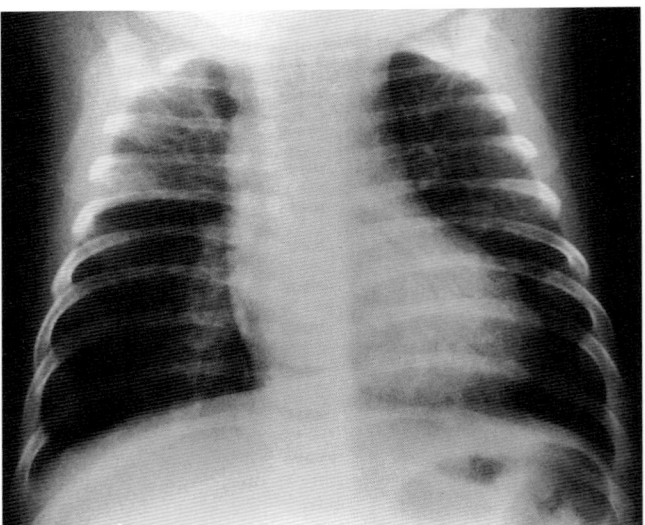

Figure 33-2. Typical radiographic appearance of bronchiolitis. Hyperinflation, hyperlucency, and flattened diaphragms are most characteristic. Peribronchiolar infiltrates are common, and parenchymal infiltrates are less common. (Courtesy of Richard Heller, MD, Vanderbilt University Children's Hospital, Nashville, TN.)

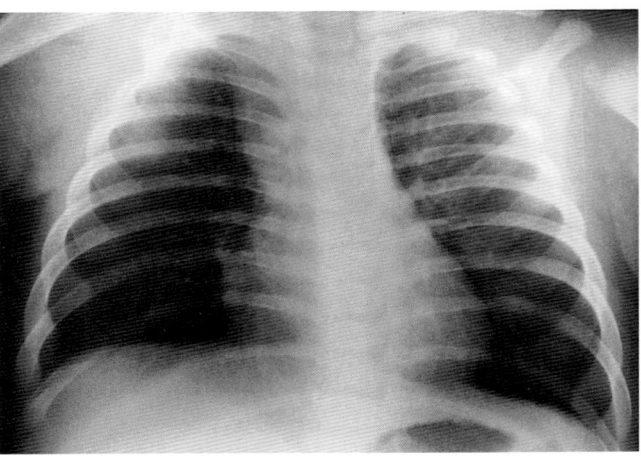

Figure 33-3. Atelectasis, particularly of the right upper lobe, is a not uncommon feature of bronchiolitis. This should not be confused with pneumonia, which manifests as volume expansion, not volume loss. (Courtesy of Richard Heller, MD, Vanderbilt University Children's Hospital, Nashville, TN.)

diagnosis of RSV infection, it often is too slow a method to be clinically useful. Enzyme immunoassays and direct fluorescent antibody (DFA) techniques for the identification of RSV, influenza virus, parainfluenza viruses, and adenoviruses permit rapid and accurate diagnoses.[77-81] Nasal wash is the preferred method of specimen collection. The DFA test permits evaluation of adequacy of the specimen's number of epithelial cells for antigen detection. A respiratory screening of nasal secretions using pooled monoclonal antibodies to the common agents of bronchiolitis, followed by specific identification for a positive reaction, is a cost- and time-saving procedure compared with standard tissue culture isolation. Amplification of virus using the shell vial method, followed by use of specific monoclonal agents, and amplification of viral genome by the polymerase chain reaction offer the promise of improved sensitivity for rapid detection but are not as widely available nor as rapid as enzyme immunoassay and fluorescent antibody techniques.[82,83] A multitest system for quantitative

reverse transcription–polymerase chain reaction–enzyme hybridization assay (Hexaplex) is available to test a single nasopharyngeal sample for RSV, influenza A and B viruses, parainfluenza virus, and adenoviruses.[84]

Antigen detection tests are useful in diagnosing certain viral infections, but, as with all tests, the positive predictive value decreases as disease incidence goes down. Specificity of antigen detection assays are lowest during the off season and at the onset and end of the respiratory virus season.

MANAGEMENT

General Measures

Most infants with bronchiolitis can be managed at home with supportive care, but hypoxia or inability to feed adequately necessitate hospitalization. Once hospitalized, most infants respond to administration of supplemental oxygen and replacement of fluid deficits.[1] The value of mist inhalation by vaporizer or tent is not proven; its use can provoke reflex bronchoconstriction. The specific treatment strategies used differ widely across children's medical centers.[71] Fewer than 10% of previously healthy infants hospitalized for bronchiolitis require intubation and mechanical ventilation because of respiratory failure or apnea; the percentage is higher for prematurely born infants and infants with chronic lung disease or congenital heart malformations.

Bronchodilator Therapy

The therapeutic role of bronchodilator agents in bronchiolitis is controversial.[1,85] Bronchodilator therapy is not recommended for routine management of first time wheezing associated with RSV bronchiolitis. Occasionally, a single administration of an aerosolized bronchodilator elicits a response, but this improvement is not seen in most infants with bronchiolitis and is not generally reproducible with subsequent doses.[86-92] Modest improvement in clinical scores and in tests of pulmonary function have been reported with use of inhaled racemic epinephrine [91-93] and β-adrenergic agents, principally salbutamol and albuterol.[92-94] However, clinical improvement following repeated doses of epinephrine is not sustained and favorable response to β-adrenergic agents, as measured by clinical score and oxygenation, is inconsistent.[95-100] Flores and Horwitz[101] performed a meta-analysis of eight studies with similar designs. Overall, their analysis supported a beneficial effect in certain infants, but identifying those infants could not be consistently accomplished at the time of initial presentation. On balance, an initial trial of bronchodilator therapy for the hospitalized infant with bronchiolitis is reasonable, although brief episodes of hypoxia can be precipitated by adrenergic agents. Bronchodilator therapy should only be continued if consistent improvement in respiratory distress or oxygen saturation is observed. Racemic epinephrine should not be continued beyond one or two doses.

Corticosteroid Therapy

Although corticosteroids reduce the inflammatory changes observed with bronchiolitis, they may increase viral replication and prolong shedding. Most studies examining the role of corticosteroids alone in the treatment of bronchiolitis have not demonstrated a consistent clinical benefit.[102-110] Although one meta-analysis of previously published reports of corticosteroid use in bronchiolitis concluded that there may be slight improvements in duration of symptoms, length of hospital stay, and clinical scores, these benefits appear to be limited.[111] The routine use of corticosteroids in bronchiolitis is not recommended. However, a national collaborative, blinded, placebo-controlled trial conducted in Canada demonstrated that the combination of nebulized epinephrine and oral dexamethasone treatment for children with bronchiolitis evaluated in emergency departments reduced the subsequent rate of hospitalization by 9% compared with placebo or either treatment alone (P=0.07) and was less costly.[112,113]

Antiviral Therapy

Ribavirin is a nucleoside analogue with in vitro activity against RSV, adenovirus, influenza A and B viruses, and parainfluenza viruses. Early trials indicated that ribavirin therapy was associated with modest improvement in clinical scores, oxygenation, and duration of mechanical ventilation for infants with severe bronchiolitis due to RSV infection. These studies were challenged on the basis that control groups received water aerosols, which may produce bronchospasm in individuals with hyperreactive airways. Clinical trials with ribavirin have not demonstrated a consistent decrease in need for mechanical ventilation, decrease in length of stay in the intensive care unit, or reduction in days of hospitalization. Conflicting results from efficacy trials, concern about potential toxic effects among exposed healthcare professionals, aerosol route of administration, and high cost have all resulted in limited use of ribavirin.[114-116] Guidelines for the use of ribavirin in RSV disease are presented in Chapter 225, Respiratory Syncytial Virus.

Potential options for the treatment of bronchiolitis, if caused by influenza A or B viruses, are discussed in Chapter 229, Influenza Viruses.[117-121]

Immune Globulins and Other Therapies

Antibody preparations containing high titers of neutralizing antibody against RSV as well as a preparation of monoclonal antibodies directed against one of the two major RSV surface glycoproteins (fusion glycoprotein) reduce the risk of hospitalization due to RSV infection.[50,51] Used therapeutically, they result in more rapid clearing of virus from the respiratory tract but do not alter the course of illness and should not be used for the treatment of RSV infection.[122-126] Although vitamin A levels have been demonstrated to be low in infants with RSV bronchiolitis, a therapeutic benefit of vitamin A therapy has not been demonstrated.[127-129]

PROGNOSIS, COMPLICATIONS, AND SEQUELAE

Most otherwise healthy infants recover completely from acute bronchiolitis, although subtle pulmonary abnormalities can persist for weeks.[38] An important question is whether bronchiolitis

in infancy increases the likelihood of childhood asthma. Numerous studies have defined a higher risk of recurrent wheezing throughout childhood after bronchiolitis in infancy, and abnormalities of small-airway function have been identified in school-aged children with a history of bronchiolitis in infancy. However, each of these findings may simply be a reflection of hereditary tendencies that are expressed both at the time of bronchiolitis and upon allergen exposure in later childhood.[130-134] Moreover, by adolescence, the rate of recurrent wheezing in subjects who had bronchiolitis in infancy appears to fall to the rate observed in subjects without a history of bronchiolitis.[134] Thus, it is uncertain whether bronchiolitis is causally associated with long-term respiratory morbidity.

PREVENTION

Strategies that reduce contact of vulnerable infants with individuals with respiratory tract infections, minimizing passive exposure to cigarette smoke, and limiting nosocomial transmission of causative agents offer immediate opportunities to reduce bronchiolitis morbidity. Monthly administration of monoclonal anti-F antibody (palivizumab) throughout the RSV season reduces the incidence of hospitalization due to RSV infection in infants with bronchopulmonary dysplasia, congenital heart disease, and prematurity by about 50% (see Chapter 225, Respiratory Syncytial Virus). The high cost and modest effect of palivizumab limit its use for passive immunoprophylaxis to the most medically fragile infants.

No vaccine to prevent infection with RSV or parainfluenza viruses, the most common causes of bronchiolitis, is licensed or near licensure. Trivalent influenza vaccine is recommended for all infants older than 6 months of age during the influenza season. Because this is not approved for use in infants younger than 6 months, routine influenza vaccination is important for family members and caregivers of these young patients. Potential RSV vaccine candidates currently being evaluated include inactivated preparations of the purified fusion protein of RSV, DNA vaccines coding for the major immunogenic proteins of the virus, and replicating mutants of the virus that replicate in the upper respiratory tract but are inactivated at the higher temperatures of the lung.[135]

---

34 Acute Pneumonia and Its Complications

Chitra S. Mani and Dennis L. Murray

Pneumonia (Greek word meaning "inflammation of the lungs") is one of the most common illness affecting infants and children globally, causing substantial morbidity and mortality.[1] Community-acquired pneumonia (CAP) designates acquisition in the community whereas hospital-associated or nosocomial pneumonia (HAP) is acquired during or after hospitalization.

ACUTE PNEUMONIA

Acute pneumonia is defined as inflammation of the alveoli and interstitial tissues of the lungs by an infectious agent resulting in acute respiratory symptoms and signs.[2] Over 155 million cases of pneumonia and 1.8 million deaths occur annually worldwide, especially affecting children <5 years of age in resource-poor countries.[3] Children in the United States have considerably less morbidity and mortality due to CAP. In the U.S., rates of outpatient visits for CAP are reported to be 74 to 92 per 1000 cases for children <2 years of age and 35 to 52 per 1000 cases in children 3 to

6 years of age;[4] the rate of hospitalization is about 200 per 100,000 cases, with the highest rate seen in infants (>900 cases per 100,000).[5] There were 525 reported deaths due to pneumonia in children <15 years of age in the U.S. in 2006.[6]

Etiologic Agents and Epidemiology (see Table 34-1)

Multiple microbes, predominantly viruses and bacteria, cause lower respiratory tract infection (LRTI) in infants and children. Establishing microbial diagnosis of pneumonia has been problematic in infants and children due to difficulty in distinguishing infection from colonization of the upper airways and lack of availability of dependable diagnostic laboratory tests.[7] In two studies of pneumonia in immunocompetent children, specific etiologic agents were confirmed in only 43% to 66%.[8,9] Identification of more than one pathogen makes it difficult to assign primary pathogenicity.[2] While bloodstream infection (BSI) confirms etiology, BSI occurs in only 1% to 10% of hospitalized children

PART II Clinical Syndromes and Cardinal Features of Infectious Diseases: Approach to Diagnosis and Initial Management

SECTION D Lower Respiratory Tract Infections

TABLE 34-1. Microbial Causes of Community-Acquired Pneumonia in Childhood

Age	Etiologic Agents[a]	Clinical Features
Birth–3 weeks	Group B streptococcus	Part of early-onset septicemia; usually severe
	Gram-negative enteric bacilli	Frequently nosocomial; occurs infrequently within 1 week of birth
	Cytomegalovirus	Part of systemic cytomegalovirus infection
	Listeria monocytogenes	Part of early-onset septicemia
	Herpes simplex virus	Part of disseminated infection
	Treponema pallidum	Part of congenital syndrome
	Genital Mycoplasma or Ureaplasma	From maternal genital infection; afebrile pneumonia
3 weeks–3 months	Chlamydia trachomatis	From maternal genital infection; afebrile, subacute, interstitial pneumonia
	Respiratory syncytial virus (RSV)	Peak incidence at 2–7 months of age; usually wheezing illness (bronchiolitis/pneumonia)
	Parainfluenza viruses (PIV), especially type 3	Similar to RSV, but in slightly older infants and not epidemic in the winter
	Streptococcus pneumoniae	The most common cause of bacterial pneumonia
	Bordetella pertussis	Primarily causes bronchitis; secondary bacterial pneumonia and pulmonary hypertension can complicate severe cases
3 months–5 years	RSV, PIV, influenza, HMPV, adenovirus, rhinovirus	Most common causes of pneumonia
	Streptococcus pneumoniae	Most likely cause of lobar pneumonia; incidence may be decreasing after vaccine use
	Haemophilus influenzae	Type b uncommon with vaccine use; nontypable stains cause pneumonia in immunocompromised hosts and in developing countries
	Staphylococcus aureus	Uncommon, although CA-MRSA is becoming more prevalent
	Mycoplasma pneumoniae	Causes pneumonia primarily in children over 4 years of age
	Mycobacterium tuberculosis	Major concern in areas of high prevalence and in children with HIV
5–15 years	Mycoplasma pneumoniae	Major cause of pneumonia; radiographic appearance variable
	Chlamydophila pneumoniae	Controversial, but probably an important cause in older children in this age group

CA-MRSA, community-acquired methicillin-resistant Staphylococcus aureus; *HIV, human immunodeficiency virus; HMPV, human metapneumovirus.*

[a]*Ranked roughly in order of frequency. Uncommon causes with no age preference: enteroviruses (echovirus, coxsackievirus), mumps virus, Epstein–Barr virus, Hantavirus, Neisseria meningitidis (often group Y), anaerobic bacteria,* Klebsiella pneumoniae, Francisella tularensis, Coxiella burnetii, Chlamydophila psittaci. Streptococcus pyogenes *occurs sporadically or especially associated with varicella-zoster virus infection.*

with bacterial pneumonia.[10-12] Pathogens vary according to age, underlying illnesses, and maturation and function of the immune system.[13] Certain pathogens, particularly respiratory syncytial virus (RSV), rhinoviruses, influenza viruses, and *Mycoplasma*, are seasonal. In other instances, the pattern of family illness provides a clue to the causative agent. Extensive or invasive testing usually is not necessary.

Neonates and Young Infants

Pneumonia in neonates can manifest as early-onset disease (within the first week of life) or late-onset disease (≥7 days of life). Aspiration of either infected amniotic fluid or genital secretions at delivery is the cause of most early-onset infections. Group B streptococcus is the most frequent cause of early-onset pneumonia,[14] but *Listeria monocytogenes, Escherichia coli,* and other gram-negative bacilli can cause severe respiratory distress resembling hyaline membrane disease, usually as a part of a widespread systemic infection. Prenatal and perinatal risk factors, including preterm delivery, maternal chorioamnionitis and prolonged rupture of membranes, increase the risk for development of neonatal pneumonia. Hematogenous dissemination also can occur from an infected mother.

Chlamydia trachomatis pneumonia can occur 2 to 3 weeks after birth in 10% of neonates born to mothers colonized with the organism in their genital tract. *Bordetella pertussis* infection can cause secondary bacterial pneumonia or pulmonary hypertension (simulating pneumonia). Viruses are a less common cause compared with older infants. Congenital or perinatal infection with

cytomegalovirus (CMV), herpes simplex virus (HSV), or *Treponema pallidum* can cause severe pneumonia. Genital *Mycoplasma* species and *Ureaplasma urealyticum* can cause LRTI in very-low-birthweight infants.

Infants, Children, and Adolescents

Viruses have been considered to be the most common cause of acute LRTI in children 1 to 36 months of age. In a study published in 2004 of acute pneumonia in hospitalized, immunocompetent children 2 months to 17 years of age, bacteria were identified in 60%, viruses in 45%, *Mycoplasma* species in 14%, *Chlamydophila pneumoniae* in 9%, and mixed bacterial-viral infections in 23%.[11]

Viruses

Viruses account for approximately 14% to 35% of childhood CAP[11] but for 80% of CAP in children <2 years.[12] RSV is the predominant respiratory tract viral pathogen. Other viruses include human metapneumovirus (HMPV), parainfluenza viruses (PIV) types 1, 2, and 3, influenza viruses (A and B), adenoviruses, rhinoviruses, and enteroviruses.[15] Rhinoviruses have been recovered in 2% to 24% cases of childhood pneumonia.[10,16,17] Varicella-zoster virus (VZV), CMV, and HSV can cause LRTI in immunocompromised children. Human parechovirus 1 (HPeV-1) was identified in the early 2000s, to cause LRTI in young children.[18] In 2003, coronavirus was recognized as the causative agent of severe acute respiratory syndrome (SARS) in adults; however, it caused milder disease with no documented deaths in children.[19-21]

RSV, HMPV, and influenza viruses cause infection during the winter season whereas PIV and rhinoviruses are more common in spring and autumn; adenovirus infections can occur throughout the year. A novel strain of influenza virus (H1N1) in 2009 resulted in a less severe infection in healthy infants and children compared with seasonal influenza virus.[22]

Mycoplasma pneumoniae and Chlamydophila pneumoniae

In one study, *Mycoplasma pneumoniae* was detected in 30% of children with CAP.[23] Harris et al.[24] found that children >5 years of age had a higher rate of *Mycoplasma* infection (42%) compared with children <5 years of age (15%). Coinfections with either *Streptococcus pneumoniae* (30%) or *Chlamydophila pneumoniae* (15%) are common.[25] Infections due to *M. pneumoniae* occur in 2- to 4-year epidemic cycles. Transmission between family members is slow (median interval 3 weeks).[26,27] *C. pneumoniae* was the causative organism of 9% to 20% of CAP in children of all ages (median age 35 months).[11,28] Asymptomatic carriage of *C. pneumoniae* is well documented and confounds assessment of pathogenicity.

Bacterial Pathogens

Bacterial pneumonia is more common in children living in developing countries, presumably due to chronic malnutrition, crowding, and chronic injury to the respiratory tract epithelium from exposure to cooking and heating with biomass fuels without adequate ventilation.[29] Evidence from multiple sources indicates that *S. pneumoniae* is the single most common cause of bacterial pneumonia beyond the first few weeks of life, occurring in all age groups and accounting for 4% to 44% of all cases.[8,10,28,30,31] The serotypes that cause uncomplicated pneumonia in the U.S. generally are similar to those that cause BSI and acute otitis media (AOM). The availability of protein conjugated vaccines against *Hemophilus influenzae* type b (Hib) and *S. pneumoniae* (PCV) has significantly reduced the morbidity and mortality associated with bacterial pneumonia in the U.S.[32,33] Pneumonia due to nontypable *H. influenzae* is uncommon in the U.S. except in children with underlying chronic lung disease, immunodeficiencies, or aspiration. Recently, a virulent strain of community-associated, methicillin-resistant *Staphylococcus aureus* (CA-MRSA) has emerged as an important agent of pneumonia, including life-threatening necrotizing pneumonia.[34-36] *Streptococcus pyogenes* (group A streptococcus or GAS) is not a frequent cause of acute pneumonia. However, both staphylococcal and streptococcal pneumonia are rapidly progressive and severe, frequently leading to hypoxemia and pleural effusion within hours. Other bacteria, especially gram-negative bacilli, are rare causes of pneumonia in previously healthy children. In one study, viral and bacterial coinfection was detected in 23% of the children with pneumonia.[11]

Occasional Pathogens

A variety of epidemiologic and host factors prompt consideration of specific organisms (Table 34-2). The most important of these is *Mycobacterium tuberculosis* (MTB), which should always be suspected if there is a history of exposure, presence of hilar adenopathy, or when pneumonia does not respond to regular therapy. In North America and Europe, risk factors for primary MTB in children are: birth to recent immigrants from countries with a high prevalence of infection, contact with infected adults, or HIV infection.[37]

Residence, and exposures lead to consideration of certain pathogens. *Coccidioides immitis* is endemic in the southwestern U.S., northern Mexico, and parts of Central and South America. *Histoplasma capsulatum* is endemic in the eastern and central U.S. and Canada. *Chlamydophila psittaci* and *Coxiella burnetii* are transmitted from infected birds and animals. *Pneumocystis jirovecii* causes pneumonia in untreated HIV-infected infants at 3 to 6 months of age, in severely malnourished children, and in other immunocompromised hosts. *Legionella pneumophila*, a rare cause of pneumonia in children, is considered with certain environmental exposures and in immunocompromised individuals.

TABLE 34-2. Occasional Causes of Pneumonia in Special Circumstances

Organism	Risk Factors	Diagnostic Methods
Histoplasma capsulatum	Exposure in certain geographic areas (Ohio and Mississippi River valleys, Caribbean)	Culture of respiratory tract secretions; urine antigen; serum immunodiffusion antibody test; and serum histoplasma complement fixation antibody test
Coccidioides immitis	Exposure in certain geographic areas (southwestern United States, Mexico, and Central America)	Culture of respiratory tract secretions; serum immunodiffusion antibody test
Blastomyces dermatitidis	Exposure in certain geographic areas (Ohio, Mississippi, St. Lawrence River valleys)	Culture of respiratory tract secretions; serum immunodiffusion antibody test
Legionella pneumophila	Exposure to contaminated water supply	Culture or direct fluorescent assay of respiratory tract secretions; antigen test on urine (type 1 only)
Francisella tularensis	Exposure to infected animals, usually	Acute and convalescent serology
Pseudomonas pseudomallei (melioidosis)	Travel to rural areas of Southeast Asia	Culture of respiratory tract secretions; acute and convalescent serology
Brucella abortus	Exposure to infected goats, cattle, or their products of conception; consumption of unpasteurized milk	Acute and convalescent serology
Leptospira spp.	Exposure to urine of infected dogs, rats, or swine, or to water contaminated by their urine	Culture of urine; acute and convalescent serology
Chlamydophila psittaci	Exposure to infected birds (often parakeets)	Acute and convalescent serology
Coxiella burnetii	Exposure to infected sheep	Acute and convalescent serology
Hantavirus	Exposure to dried mouse dung in a closed structure (opening cabins after winter closure)	Acute and convalescent serology; PCR test on the respiratory tract secretions

PCR, polymerase chain reaction.

PART II Clinical Syndromes and Cardinal Features of Infectious Diseases: Approach to Diagnosis and Initial Management

SECTION D Lower Respiratory Tract Infections

Pathogenesis and Pathology

Pneumonia occurs in a child who lacks systemic or secretory immunity to a pathogenic organism. Invasion of the lower respiratory tract or lung usually occurs at a time when normal defense mechanisms are impaired, such as after a viral infection, during chronic malnutrition, or with exposure to environmental pollutants. Aerosol exposure or BSI occasionally can cause bacterial pneumonia.

The pulmonary defense mechanisms against LRTI consist of: physical and physiologic barriers, humoral and cell-mediated immunity, and phagocytic activity. Physical barriers of the respiratory tract include the presence of hairs in the anterior nares that can trap particles >10 µm in size, configuration of the nasal turbinates, and acute branching of the respiratory tract. Physiologic protection includes filtration and humidification in the upper airways, mucus production, and protection of the airway by the epiglottis and cough reflex. Mucociliary transport moves normally aspirated oropharyngeal flora and particulate matter up the tracheobronchial tree, minimizing the presence of bacteria below the carina. However, particles less than 1 µm can escape into the lower airways. Immunoglobulin A (IgA), is the major protective antibody secreted by the upper airways; IgG and IgM primarily protect the lower airways. Substances found in alveolar fluid – including surfactant, fibronectin, complement, lysozyme, and iron-binding proteins – have antimicrobial activity. The LRT has distinct populations of macrophages. Alveolar macrophages are the pre-eminent phagocytic cells that ingest and kill bacteria. Viral infection (especially due to influenza virus), high oxygen concentration, uremia, and use of alcohol and/or drugs can impair the function of the alveolar macrophages, predisposing to pneumonia. Cell-mediated immunity plays an important role in certain pulmonary infections such as those caused by *M. tuberculosis* and *Legionella* species.

Viruses

Viral respiratory infections can lead to bronchiolitis, interstitial pneumonia, or parenchymal infection, with overlapping patterns.[38,39] Viral pneumonia is characterized by lymphocytic infiltration of the interstitium and parenchyma of the lungs.[40] Giant cell formation can be seen in infections due to measles or CMV, or in children with immune deficiency. Viral inclusions within the nucleus of respiratory cells and necrosis of bronchial or bronchiolar epithelium can be seen in some fatal viral infections especially, adenoviral pneumonia.[41,42] Air trapping with resultant disturbances in ventilation–perfusion ratio can occur from obstructed or obliterated small airways and thickened alveolar septa.

Bacteria

Five pathologic patterns are seen with bacterial pneumonia: (1) parenchymal inflammation of a lobe or a segment of a lobe (lobar pneumonia, the classic pattern of pneumococcal pneumonia); (2) primary infection of the airways and surrounding interstitium (bronchopneumonia) often seen with *Streptococcus pyogenes* and *Staphylococcus aureus*; (3) necrotizing parenchymal pneumonia that occurs after aspiration; (4) caseating granulomatous disease as seen with tuberculous pneumonia; and (5) peribronchial and interstitial disease with secondary parenchymal infiltration, as seen when viral pneumonia (classically due to influenza or measles) is complicated by bacterial infection.[42] Bacterial pneumonia is associated with diffuse neutrophilic infiltration, resulting in airspaces filled with transudates or exudates, impairing oxygen diffusion. The proximity of alveoli and a rich pulmonary vascular bed increase the risk for complications, such as bacteremia, septicemia, or shock.

Clinical Manifestations

The symptoms of pneumonia are varied and nonspecific. Acute onset of fever, rapid breathing, and cough have been described to be the classic symptom complex of pneumonia.[43] Fever can be absent in very young infants and typically is absent in infections due to *Chlamydia trachomatis*, *B. pertussis*, and *Ureaplasma*. Some children have a prodrome of low-grade fever and rhinorrhea prior to developing LRT symptoms. No single sign is pathognomonic for pneumonia; tachypnea, nasal flaring, decreased breath sounds, and auscultatory crackles (crepitations or rales) are suggestive signs. Guidelines developed by the World Health Organization (WHO) for the clinical diagnosis of pneumonia in resource-poor regions highlight tachypnea (or shortness of breath) and retractions as the two best indicators of LRTI.[44] Palafox et al. observed that, in children <5 years of age, tachypnea (as defined by WHO) had the highest sensitivity (74%) and specificity (67%) for radiologically confirmed pneumonia, but it was less sensitive and specific in early disease.[45] Tachypnea can occur in other conditions such as asthma, cardiac disease, and metabolic acidosis. Crackles and bronchial breathing were reported to have sensitivity of 75% but specificity of only 57% for pneumonia.[46] Crackles can be absent early or in a dehydrated patient. Isolated wheezing or prolonged expiration is uncommon in bacterial pneumonia.[47] The value of clinical findings for predicting the presence of radiographically evident pneumonia has been evaluated in a number of studies.[48–51] In one study, the combination of a respiratory rate >50 breaths/min, oxygen saturation <90%, and presence of nasal flaring in children <12 months of age was highly associated with radiographically confirmed pneumonia.[52] About three-fourths of children with radiographically confirmed pneumonia appear ill. Severity of illness correlates with the likelihood of a bacterial cause. Approximately 6% to 25% of children <5 years of age with fever >39 °C without a source, and a white blood cell (WBC) count >20,000/mm^3 with no symptoms or signs of LRTI have radiographically confirmed pneumonia.[51,53] A systematic review of studies that considered observer agreement of clinical examination suggested that observed clinical signs were better than auscultatory signs;[54] interobserver agreement was low in recognizing crackles, retractions, and wheezing, but high in determining respiratory rate and cyanosis. However, neither respiratory rate nor cyanosis is a specific or sensitive indicator of hypoxia. Oxygen saturation should be measured in any child with respiratory distress, especially if the child has retractions or decreased level of activity.[55]

Neonates and Young Infants

The neonate with bacterial pneumonia usually develops tachypnea and respiratory distress in the first few hours of life with or without septicemia or meningitis or both. In very young, especially premature infants, apneic spells without fever and tachypnea can be the initial finding of LRTI.[54] Infants with *C. trachomatis* pneumonia present insidiously between 3 weeks and 3 months of age with staccato cough, tachypnea and crackles on auscultation.

Infants, Children, and Adolescents

Viruses. The onset of viral pneumonia is usually gradual and occurs in the context of an upper respiratory tract illness (URI) in the patient or family members. Irritability, respiratory congestion, cough, post-tussive emesis and fever follow. Although hypoxia can be marked, the patient may not appear toxic. Auscultation can reveal diffuse, bilateral wheezing and crackles. Adenovirus occasionally can cause severe pneumonia with findings similar to a bacterial infection, especially in immunocompromised hosts.

Bacteria. The onset of bacterial pneumonia usually is abrupt but can follow several days of mild URI. The patient usually is ill and toxic appearing with high fever, rigors, and tachypnea. Cough can occur later in the course of illness when the debris from the involved lung is swept into the upper airway. Unilateral pleuritic chest pain, or abdominal pain in the presence of radiographically demonstrated infiltrate, is a specific sign of bacterial pneumonia. Physical findings usually are focal, limited to an anatomic segment and include decreased tactile and vocal fremitus, diminished air entry, rales and dullness to percussion over the involved area of the lung. Wheezing is an unusual finding in bacterial pneumonia.

Other pathogens. The major symptoms of LRTI due to *M. pneumoniae*, *C. pneumoniae*, and *C. burnetii* (Q fever) are fever and cough that persist for more than 7 to 10 days. The onset of pneumonia caused by *M. pneumoniae* usually is not well demarcated, but malaise, headache, sore throat, fever, and photophobia occur early, and sometimes subside when gradually worsening, nonproductive cough ensues. Although coryza is unusual, AOM with or without bullous myringitis can occur. Findings on physical examination and auscultation can be minimal, most commonly dry or musical crackles. In persons with sickle-cell disease, acute chest syndrome is common. *C. pneumoniae* infection usually causes bronchospasm and can cause an acute exacerbation of asthma. *C. burnetii* has an acute onset with intractable headache, fever, and cough with round parenchymal opacities on chest radiograph.

Differential Diagnosis

Pneumonia is highly probable in children with fever, cough, tachypnea, and shortness of breath in whom chest radiograph demonstrates pulmonary infiltrates. Alternative diagnoses are considered particularly in the absence of fever or with relapsing symptoms and signs, including foreign-body aspiration, asthma, gastroesophageal reflux, cystic fibrosis, congestive cardiac failure, systemic vasculitis, and bronchiolitis obliterans. Children who develop chemical pneumonia after ingestion of volatile hydrocarbons can have severe necrotizing pneumonia with high fever and leukocytosis as seen in bacterial pneumonia.

Laboratory Findings and Diagnosis

Radiograph

In a study evaluating ambulatory children >2 months of age with acute LRTI, routine use of chest radiography did not change clinical outcome in most cases.[56] Antibiotic was prescribed more frequently in those who underwent radiography (61% versus 53%).[57] However, chest radiograph is necessary in the following situations: children <12 months of age with acute LRTI; patients who are severely ill or hospitalized; those who have recurrent disease, fail initial antibiotic therapy, or have chronic medical conditions; those who develop complications; and those in whom the diagnosis is uncertain. Radiograph can appear falsely normal early in the course of pneumonia or in dehydrated patients.[48] Radiograph is insensitive in differentiating bacterial from nonbacterial pneumonia; however, combined with clinical findings, a normal radiograph accurately excludes bacterial pneumonia in most cases.[58,59]

Bilateral diffuse infiltrates are seen with pneumonia caused by viruses, *P. jirovecii*, *L. pneumophila*, and occasionally *M. pneumoniae*. *C. pneumoniae*, *C. psittaci*, *Coxiella burnetii*, and *M. pneumoniae* can cause patchy alveolar infiltrates, which are out of proportion to clinical findings (Figure 34-1). Distinctly confined lobar or segmental abnormality or a large pleural effusion suggests bacterial infection (Figure 34-2) and, rarely, *M. pneumoniae* or adenovirus infections.[60-62] Round appearance of infiltrate, common in children <8 years of age, most often is due to *S. pneumoniae*.

Hilar adenopathy suggests tuberculosis, histoplasmosis, or *Mycoplasma* pneumonia. Tuberculosis is highly likely in an adolescent with epidemiologic risk factors and apical disease or cavitation. Pneumatoceles (thin-walled air–fluid-filled cavities) resulting from alveolar rupture usually are associated with *S. aureus* and rarely, *S. pneumoniae*, *S. pyogenes*, Hib, other gram-negative bacteria, or anaerobic infections. Involvement of the lower lobes, particularly with recurrent infections, suggests aspiration pneumonia, or if confined to the same site, pulmonary sequestration. Recurrent bacterial pneumonia involving the same anatomic area suggests congenital anomaly or foreign body whereas recurrences in different areas suggest an abnormality of host defense, cystic fibrosis, or other causes.

Chest radiography rarely is useful in following the clinical course of a child with acute pneumonia who is recovering as

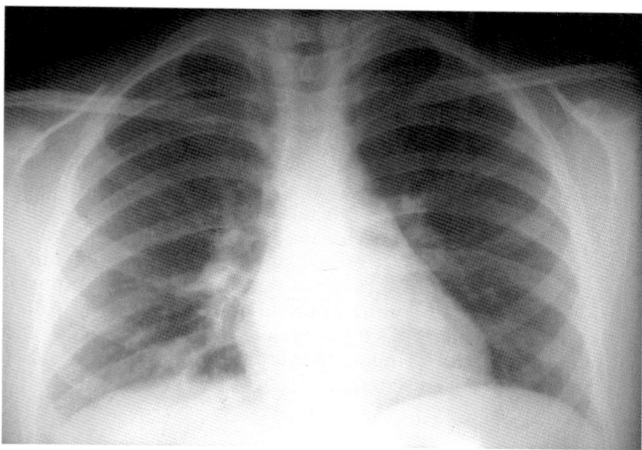

Figure 34-1. Chest radiograph of a 9-year-old girl with a 2-week history of fever, headache and hacking cough. *C. psittaci* infection was confirmed. (Courtesy of S.S. Long, St. Christopher's Hospital for Children, Philadelphia, PA.)

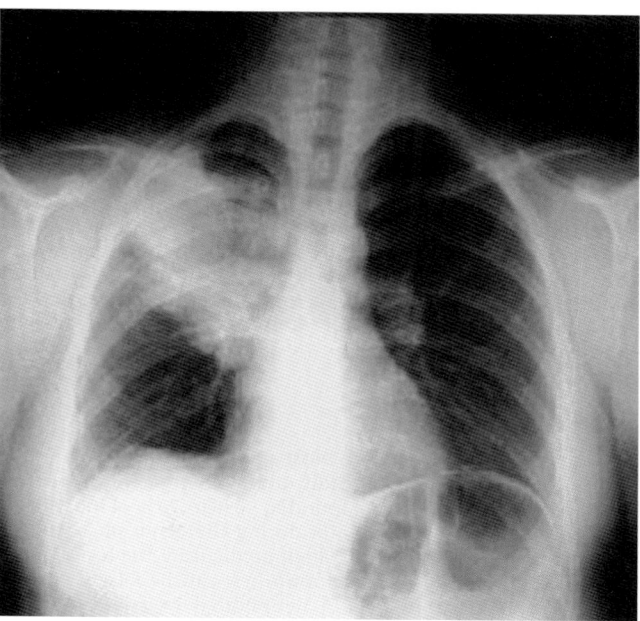

Figure 34-2. Plain radiograph showing consolidative pneumonia in the right upper lobe, typical of acute bacterial pneumonia.

expected. Radiographic improvement significantly lags clinical changes; complete resolution is expected in 4 to 6 weeks after onset. Follow-up radiography is indicated for children with lobar collapse, complicated pneumonia, recurrent pneumonia, foreign body aspiration, and round pneumonia (to exclude tumor as the cause).[61,62]

Laboratory Tests

Peripheral WBC, white blood cell differential, erythrocyte sedimentation rate (ESR), and C-reactive protein (CRP) best detect invasive infections, particularly those caused by bacteria. Viral pneumonia comparatively is associated with a less brisk rise of acute-phase reactants, except with infections due to adenovirus, influenza, and measles virus. Conclusions of prospective study suggest that these tests do not stand alone as indicators of bacterial versus viral pneumonia.[63,64]

Diagnosis of Specific Agents

Viruses

Viral pathogens are best identified by isolation in tissue culture or detection of viral products (antigens or nucleic acid) in respiratory tract secretions. Combined real-time polymerase chain reaction (PCR) can rapidly detect common viral and atypical bacterial agents of CAP.[65] However, both false-positive and false-negative results can occur when specimens are obtained or transported improperly or tests are performed suboptimally. The best specimen is a nasopharyngeal aspirate or wash that contains epithelial cells. The presence of a virus in the upper respiratory tract does not exclude secondary bacterial pneumonia. Testing acute and convalescent sera for rising antibodies to various viruses usually is confined to research settings.

Bacterial Pathogens

In children >10 years of age, sputum is considered appropriate for microbiologic evaluation when Gram stain reveals <10 squamous epithelial cells and >25 neutrophils per low-power field, and a predominant microorganism. Culture of nasopharyngeal specimens does not confirm etiology because many bacterial pathogens also are common commensals. Further, noncommensal organisms residing in the upper airway may not be the cause of LRTI. Tracheal aspiration is useful for culture if performed with direct laryngoscopy. However, culture samples obtained via a catheter directly passed through a tracheostomy, endotracheal tube, or deep nasotracheal tube have limitations due to frequent contamination with upper respiratory tract organisms. (Specimen could be evaluated as for a sputum sample.) Quantitative culture performed on a bronchoalveolar lavage specimen is considered significant when the isolate colony count is >10^4/mL. Blood culture is specific but insensitive. A 2002 study demonstrated that transthoracic needle aspiration (lung tap) in hospitalized children with clinical pneumonia had a high microbiologic yield and was relatively safe; this procedure is not performed widely in the U.S.[32]

Other Pathogens

M. pneumoniae can be detected most effectively by PCR methodology but the test may not be readily available; culture may require 3 weeks. Cold agglutinins are found in 30% to 75% of individuals with *M. pneumoniae* pneumonia during the acute phase of the disease;[66] a titer of ≥1:64 has a high predictive value for *M. pneumoniae* infection. The cold agglutinin test can be falsely positive (certain viral infections and in lymphoma) or falsely negative (mild disease or in young children). Testing for serum IgM and IgA antibodies to *M. pneumoniae* is positive in 80% of cases during the early convalescent period but false-positive and false-negative results occur;[66,67] examining paired sera is the most definitive test.

C. trachomatis infection is associated with eosinophilia and elevated total serum IgM concentration.[68-70] *C. pneumoniae* infection is identified by isolation in tissue culture or PCR.[67] Serology also can confirm infections due to *C. pneumoniae*, *C. psittaci*, and *C. burnetii*.

When tuberculosis is considered, a tuberculin skin test (TST) is performed on the patient, immediate family members, and other significant contacts. In acutely ill patients, the TST can be nonreactive because of general or specific anergy to MTB antigen. When tuberculosis is suspected, multiple respiratory tract specimens, including sputum (spontaneous or induced), gastric aspirate, and/or bronchoalveolar lavage should be obtained for culture. Gastric aspirates are superior to bronchoscopic specimens in infants with primary or military tuberculosis.[71] The interferon-γ release assay (IGRA) on whole blood can be useful in diagnosis of latent infection (LTBI) and disease (TB). Data are limited on the use of IGRA in children <5 years of age, those recently infected, and in immunocompromised hosts.

Management

Indications for Hospitalization

Hypoxemia with SaO_2 <92% is the single most important indication for hospitalization because of increased risk of death.[72] Other indications include cyanosis, rapid respiratory rate (RR >70 breaths/min in an infant or >50 breaths/min in a child), apnea, dyspnea, expiratory grunting, toxic appearance, poor oral intake, dehydration, recurrent pneumonia, underlying medical condition, or uncertain observation at home.

Cyanosis may not be noted in hypoxic infants and children until they are terminally ill. Irritability can be an indication. Sole reliance on pulse oximetry values is hazardous in ill patients because hypercarbia, an important sign of impending respiratory failure, is missed; blood gas should be evaluated in such patients. Rapid breathing, fever, and fatigue increase the fluid requirements in a child with acute LRTI. Frequent oral hydration with small volumes of fluids or intravenous hydration may be necessary. Hydration should be performed cautiously because the syndrome of inappropriate secretion of antidiuretic hormone (SIADH) occurs in approximately one-third of patients hospitalized with probable bacterial pneumonia.[73] Malnutrition has been associated with a worse prognosis of pneumonia. Infants and small children fare better when frequently fed small quantities to prevent pulmonary aspiration.[74] Intubated or very ill children may require enteral feeding tube or parenteral nutrition.

Antimicrobial Therapy

In previously healthy, preschool children with clinical symptoms most consistent with a viral infection, antibiotics are not helpful and may increase drug toxicity or promote the development of antimicrobial resistance.

Optimal antibiotic treatment of pneumonia in infants and children has not been determined by randomized, controlled, clinical trials. Recommendations are based on the most likely etiologic agents at different ages and in various settings. Therapy with ampicillin and gentamicin are appropriate in neonatal pneumonia because the pathogens are similar to those of sepsis. A macrolide antibiotic (preferably azithromycin in infants <1 month of age) is recommended for *C. trachomatis*, *Ureaplasma*, and pertussis.[75] The dose of azithromycin for pertussis is 10 mg/kg per day on each of 5 days.[76] Amoxicillin at 80 to 90 mg/kg per day is effective empiric therapy for pneumonia in febrile children >3 months of age; alternatives include amoxicillin-clavulanate (given 3 times daily), cefuroxime axetil, or cefdinir.[77-79] In older children (>5 years) suspected of having an infection with *Mycoplasma*, *Chlamydophila*, or *Legionella*, treatment with azithromycin, erythromycin, or doxycycline (at age ≥8 years) is recommended.[80] For a hospitalized child beyond the neonatal period with uncomplicated pneumonia, initial parenteral (intravenous) therapy with ampicillin is appropriate, even in areas with penicillin-nonsusceptible *Streptococcus pneumonia*; some experts recommend use of higher doses of cefuroxime, ceftriaxone, cefotaxime, or ampicillin-sulbactam.[77-79] While the use of vancomycin, clindamycin, or linezolid is not recommended for initial treatment of uncomplicated CAP, these agents may be considered for treating suspected CA-MRSA infection, if pneumonia is unresponsive to initial antibiotics, or in those patients allergic to beta-lactam agents.[81] Other antimicrobial agents may be chosen if a likely pathogen is identified, the case has clinical or epidemiologic features strongly suggestive of a particular infection, or the evolution of the disease suggests a more specific cause.

Opinions differ about the frequency with which viral pneumonia is complicated by bacterial superinfection.[11,82] There is a good deal of evidence, however, that withholding antibiotics from hospitalized children with pneumonia clinically compatible with or proven to be of viral origin is safe and is preferable to empiric antibiotic treatment.[83] Use of specific antiviral therapy depends on the pathogen, the severity of the clinical course, and availability of effective nontoxic therapy. Use of aerosolized ribavirin for the

TABLE 34-3. Antiviral Agents for Treating Influenza

Medication	Treatment	Chemoprophylaxis
OSELTAMIVIR		
Infants birth to <3 months	3 mg/kg/dose bid × 5 days[a]	Not usually recommended
Infants 3 to 12 months	3 mg/kg/dose bid × 5 days	3 mg/kg/dose once daily × 10 days
Body weight ≤15 kg	30 mg/dose bid × 5 days	30 mg/ dose once daily × 10 days
≥15 kg to 23 kg	45 mg/dose bid × 5 days	45 mg/ dose once daily × 10 days
≥23 kg to 40 kg	60 mg/dose bid × 5 days	60 mg/dose once daily × 10 days
≥40 kg	75 mg/dose bid × 5 days	75 mg/dose once daily × 10 days
Max dose	75 mg/dose bid × 5 days	75 mg/dose once daily × 10 days
ZANAMAVIR[b]	Only in children ≥7 years 10 mg (two 5 mg puffs) twice daily	Only in children ≥5 years 10 mg (two 5 mg puffs) once daily

[a]*Oseltamivir is not FDA approved in this age group; recommend discussing with an infectious diseases physician before use.*

[b]*Zanamavir cannot be used in individuals with asthma or chronic lung disease.*

From Centers for Disease Control and Prevention. Antiviral agents for the treatment and chemoprophylaxis of influenza. Recommendations of the Advisory Committee on Immunization Practices (ACIP). MMWR 2011;60(RR-1):1–25.

treatment of RSV is guided by recommendations from the American Academy of Pediatrics, although the value of such treatment has been questioned.[84–87]

Although therapy for influenza is most effective when antivirals are started early in the course of infection,[88] recent data, indicate benefit when therapy is begun >48 hours of onset of illness in seriously ill and rapidly deteriorating patients[89,90] (Table 34-3).

Prognosis and Sequelae

Mortality due to CAP is uncommon beyond infancy in Europe and North America because of improved and enhanced immunization rates, early access to medical care, and availability of antimicrobial and supportive therapy. Most healthy children with acute LRTIs recover without sequelae, but some patients, especially premature infants, immunocompromised hosts, or children with chronic lung, neuromuscular, or cardiovascular diseases can develop complications. Complications include necrotizing pneumonia, parapneumonic effusion, empyema, pneumatocele formation, and lung abscess. In the late 1990s, there was a significant increase in complications from bacterial pneumonia in infants and children in the U.S.[91,92] Since universal immunization with pneumococcal conjugate vaccine in children <2 years of age, frequency of complicated pneumococcal pneumonia due to vaccine strains and complications due to presumed bacterial pneumonia have decreased.[93,94]

Bacterial pneumonia usually is not associated with long-term sequelae. Epidemiologic studies have linked viral bronchiolitis, *C. trachomatis*, and *C. pneumoniae* with asthma and other respiratory problems in childhood.[95–100] A study of 35-year-old adults, with history of having pneumonia before age 7 years, demonstrated a significant reduction of forced expiratory volume and forced vital capacity.[97–106] However, several longitudinal studies of lung function in children with bronchiolitis have suggested that lung function abnormalities may have preceded the acute infectious illness.[102–106] It remains unclear whether childhood pneumonia causes subsequent pulmonary abnormalities.

Prevention

Most viral respiratory tract infections are transmitted by direct inoculation from hands contaminated with respiratory secretions onto conjunctival and nasal mucosa. Airborne spread by large droplets also can occur. Hand hygiene is the single most important method of preventing hospital-associated infections. Wearing facemasks and goggles can prevent large droplet transmission. Spread of infection by small droplets can be reduced by placing the patient in a negative-pressure room.

Universal immunization with Hib conjugate vaccine and PCV has eliminated invasive Hib disease and has significantly reduced the incidence of pneumococcal pneumonia, respectively, in children and in contacts of other ages through herd immunity.[93,94,107,108]

RSV bronchiolitis and pneumonia can be reduced in high-risk infants by passive immunoprophylaxis using a monoclonal antibody (palivizumab).[109,110] Annual vaccination against influenza is recommended for all individuals ≥6 months of age.[111] It is anticipated that varicella and influenza vaccination programs will reduce incidence of bacterial pneumonia, especially that caused by *S. aureus* and *S. pyogenes*.

PLEURAL EFFUSION, PARAPNEUMONIC EFFUSION, AND EMPYEMA

Pleural effusion is the presence of demonstrable fluid between the visceral and parietal pleurae. It may be useful to characterize pleural effusions as a *transudate* or an *exudate* based on the relative concentration of pleural fluid protein to serum protein (>0.5 in an exudate versus <0.5 in a transudate), pH, glucose, and lactate dehydrogenase (LDH) concentrations (Table 34-4). Exudates more frequently have an infectious etiology and transudates a noninfectious etiology (Table 34-5).

Parapneumonic effusion (PPE) is a collection of inflammatory fluid adjacent to a pneumonic process. In prospective studies in children with CAP from Europe and the Americas, the incidence of PPE in children was 2% to 12%.[112–115] Hospitalizations for PPE have increased in the U.S. in recent years.[116–118]

Empyema is a purulent or seropurulent parapneumonic fluid. PPE can be complicated (CPPE) or uncomplicated. CPPE and empyema represent a continuum.[119] Estimated incidence of empyema in children is approximately 3.3 per 100,000.[120] Both CPPE and empyema are serious illnesses associated with significant morbidity but with infrequent mortality in the U.S.[121] Seventy percent of complicated pneumonia occurs in children <4 years of age; pneumatoceles occur predominantly in children <3 years of age.[121]

Etiologic Agents

Bacteria account for 40% to 50% of cases of PPE;[120] *S. pneumoniae*, *S. pyogenes*, and *S. aureus* are most common in countries where

TABLE 34-4. Biochemical Characteristics of Parapneumonic Pleural Effusions

Laboratory Value	Uncomplicated Effusion Transudate	Complicated Effusion Exudate
pH	>7.2	<7.1
Glucose level	>40 mg/dL	<40 mg/dL
Lactate dehydrogenase concentration	<1000 IU/mL	>1000 IU/mL
Pleural protein : serum protein	<0.5	>0.5

TABLE 34-5. Noninfectious Causes of Pleural Effusion in Children

Transudate		Exudate
Hypoalbuminemia	Spontaneous chylothorax	Malignancy
Congestive heart failure	Posttrauma or postsurgical	Collagen vascular disease
Cirrhosis with ascites	Postoperative chylothorax	Pancreatitis
Myxedema	Pulmonary lymphangiectasia	Subphrenic or other intra-abdominal abscess
Peritoneal dialysis	Uremic pleuritis	Drug reaction
Central venous catheter leak	Sarcoidosis	Meig syndrome (pelvic tumor)
Fluid mismanagement	Dressler syndrome (postmyocardial infarction)	
Adult respiratory distress syndrome		

Hib vaccination rates are high.[11] During the latter 1990s, *S. pneumoniae*, especially serotype 1, emerged as the most common isolate from children with CPPE.[122] With the introduction of universal PCV in the U.S., the incidence of CPPE due to vaccine-serotype *S. pneumoniae* decreased, although serotypes 1, 19A and other nonvaccine serotypes have emerged.[117,118] CA-MRSA has become an important cause of pneumonia and CPPE in children.[123] In South Asia, *S. aureus* is the most common cause of CPPE or empyema.[124] Less frequently, *S. pyogenes, Pseudomonas aeruginosa,* mixed anaerobic pathogens, *Mycobacterium* species and, rarely, fungi can be etiologic agents.[120] About 20% of cases of PPE are due to *M. pneumoniae* and approximately 10% are due to viruses but such PPEs rarely are large enough to require intervention. In 22% to 58% of cases, PPEs are sterile and etiology is not defined.[116,124] Use of real-time PCR assay on culture-negative PPE significantly increases detection of *S. pneumoniae*, especially for serotypes other than 19A, and raises pathogen detection overall to >80%.[125]

Pathogenesis and Pathologic Findings

Usually the pleural space contains 0.3 mL/kg of fluid, maintained by a delicate balance between secretion and absorption by lymphatic vessels. Various infectious agents induce pleural effusion by different mechanisms including a sympathetic response to a bacterial infection by elaboration of cytokines, extension of infection, an immune-complex phenomenon or as a hypersensitivity reaction (e.g., rupture of tuberculous granuloma). Replication of microorganisms in the subpleural alveoli precipitates an inflammatory response resulting in endothelial injury, increased capillary permeability, and extravasation of pulmonary interstitial fluid into the pleural space. Pleural fluid is infected readily because it lacks opsonins and complement. Bacteria interfere with the host defense mechanism by production of endotoxins and other toxic substances. Anaerobic glycolysis results from further accumulation of neutrophils and bacterial debris. This in turn causes pleural fluid to become purulent and acidic (i.e., empyema). The acidic environment of the pleural fluid suppresses bacterial growth and interferes with antibiotic activity. With disease progression, inflammatory cytokines activate coagulation pathways, leading to deposition of fibrin.

Three corresponding clinical stages are: (1) exudative, in which the pleural fluid has low cellular content; (2) fibrinopurulent, in which pus containing neutrophils and fibrin coats the inner surfaces of the pleura, interfering with lung expansion and leading to loculations within the pleural space; and (3) organizational (late stage), in which fibroblasts migrate into the exudate from visceral and parietal pleurae, producing a nonelastic membrane called the pleural peel. Before the availability of antibiotics, spontaneous drainage sometimes occurred by rupture through the chest wall (empyema necessitans) or into the bronchus (bronchopleural fistula). At present, such events are rare.

Clinical and Radiographic Manifestations

PPE should be suspected by clinical examination, when the response of pneumonia to antibiotic therapy is slow, or if there is

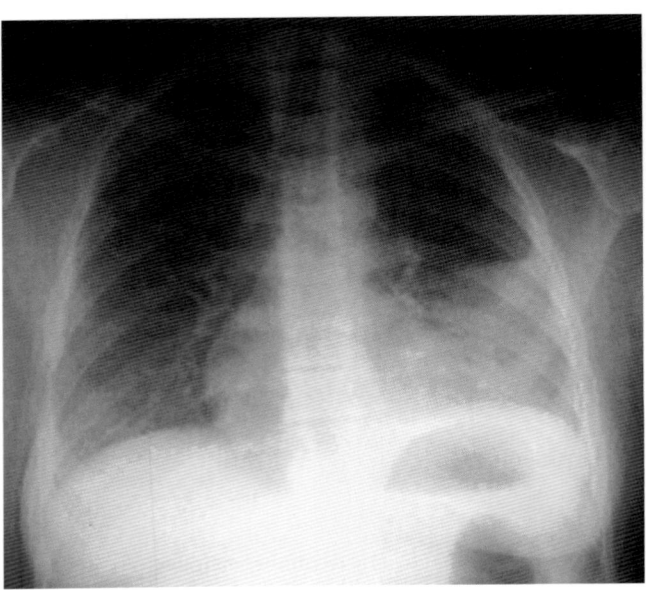

Figure 34-3. Plain radiograph showing left lower lobe pneumonia and a parapneumonic effusion, typical of acute bacterial pneumonia.

clinical deterioration during treatment. Initial symptoms can be nonspecific and include malaise, lethargy, fever, cough, and rapid breathing. Chest or abdominal pain can occur on the involved side, associated with high fever, chills, and rigors.[116,126] Difficulty in breathing (dyspnea) progresses as effusion increases. The patient usually is ill and toxic appearing, with fever and rapid, shallow respirations (to minimize pain). Breath sounds usually are diminished. The percussion note on the involved side is dull when the effusion is free-flowing; by contrast, dullness can disappear as the effusion organizes.

Chest radiography is more sensitive than physical examination, especially in detecting small pleural effusions. Blunting of the costophrenic angle, thickening of the normally paper-thin pleural shadow, or a subpulmonic density suggest pleural effusion (Figure 34-3). Movement and layering of fluid on lateral decubitus films differentiate free effusions from loculated collections, pulmonary consolidation, and pleural thickening. Effusions of >1000 mL compress the lung and shift the trachea. Ultrasonography or computed tomography (CT) aid differentiation of PPE from parenchymal lesion.[127–129]

Laboratory Findings and Diagnosis

Although the majority of PPEs in children are due to bacterial infection, only 25% to 49% of Gram stains or cultures are positive.[116,128] Several studies using nucleic acid or antigen detection methods demonstrate that most culture-negative empyemas, especially in patients pretreated with antibiotics, are due to penicillin-susceptible, non-vaccine serotypes of *S. pneumoniae*.[128,130-134]

Biochemical testing of pleural fluid in children with PPE associated with pneumonia rarely is necessary.[135]

Acid-fast and fungal stains and cultures for *M. tuberculosis* and fungi are performed on pleural fluid (and on sputum or gastric aspirate for TB) in suggestive or confounding clinical settings. TST and IGRA should be considered; anergy is unusual in the presence of pleural effusion.[136]

Management

The optimal management of PPEs in children depends on the size of the PPE. Small to moderate sized effusions, without significant mediastinal shift, rarely require drainage because most of these patients recover on antibiotics alone.[137] Most large effusions (defined as opacification of $>\frac{1}{2}$ of the thorax) fail simple aspiration and drainage, and require continuous pleural drainage.[137,138] While PPE without loculations can be treated with simple placement of a chest tube, loculated PPE is more effectively treated (shortening hospital stay) with chest tube placement, intrapleural fibrinolysis (using urokinase or tissue plasminogen activator), or video-assisted thoracoscopic surgery (VATS).[139–142] Patients with persistent large effusions (worsening respiratory compromise despite 2 to 3 days of chest tube placement and completion of fibrinolytic therapy) may require VATS or rarely, open thoracotomy with decortication; the latter procedure is associated with higher morbidity. Routinely obtained chest radiographs after chest tube placement or VATS are not useful, but re-imaging is indicated for worsening clinical status or if fever persists for >4 days after appropriate pleural drainage. The chest tube typically is removed when there is no intrathoracic air leak and drainage is <1 mL/kg per 24 hours.[139,140]

Antimicrobial Therapy

Probable pathogens, clinical circumstances, Gram stain of the pleural fluid, and radiographic appearance are considered when choosing antibiotic therapy for CPPE or empyema. Is infection community- or hospital-associated, is the patient immunocompetent or immunocompromised, is there an underlying medical condition? The empiric therapy should cover *S. pneumoniae*, CA-MRSA, and *S. pyogenes*. Therapy for anaerobic bacteria is considered if aspiration is likely. A macrolide (<8 years) or doxycycline (≥8 years) is added if atypical pathogens are suspected. Antibiotic therapy is narrowed when a pathogen is identified. Duration of parenteral therapy and total treatment is based on clinical response and adequacy of drainage; optimal duration of therapy is approximately 2 to 4 weeks, or 10 days after resolution of fever. When effusion persists and the microbial etiology is unknown, it is important to remember that fever, anorexia, and toxicity can be prolonged, even with optimal management and choice of antibiotics – due to inflammatory response within the pleural space. Therefore, additions or changes in appropriately selected antibiotic therapy should be avoided.

Prognosis

Most patients with uncomplicated PPE recover without major sequelae; although morbidity can be prolonged, the mortality rate for CPPE in previously healthy children is between 0% and 3%.[143] Mortality is highest in young infants and with *S. aureus* infection. Decortication rarely is indicated. Patients are usually asymptomatic at follow-up but radiograph can show pleural thickening which regresses only over months. Mild abnormalities occur with equal frequency in children treated with and without chest tube drainage.[144]

NECROTIZING PNEUMONIA AND LUNG ABSCESS

Necrotizing pneumonia usually occurs as a consequence of a localized lung infection by particularly virulent, pyogenic bacteria. Necrotizing pneumonia in an otherwise healthy child can resolve without further complications after antimicrobial treatment, or

TABLE 34-6. Microbiology of Lung Abscesses in Children[a]

	Organisms	Percent Cases
Aerobic and facultative bacteria	*Staphylococcus aureus*	19
	Streptococcus pneumoniae	10
	Other streptococci	32
	Haemophilus influenzae	6
	Pseudomonas aeruginosa	13
	Escherichia coli	9
	Other gram-positive organisms	7
	Other gram-negative organisms	6
Anaerobic bacteria	*Bacteroides* species[b]	25
	Prevotella melaninogenica	9
	Peptostreptococcus species	21
	Fusobacterium species	5
	Veillonella species	8
	Other gram-positive organisms	8
	Other gram-negative organisms	3
Fungi		10
Mycobacteria		1

[a]Note: more than one organism can be isolated from a lung abscess.
[b]Includes some Prevotella melaninogenica (formerly Bacteroides melaninogenica).
Data compiled from references 145–147, 149, 150.

can lead to formation of a pneumatocele, lung abscess, or bronchopleural fistula. Lung abscess also can be the consequence of aspiration of heavily infected mouth secretions or a foreign body, secondary to BSI or septic emboli, chronic infection (e.g., cystic fibrosis, chronic granulomatous disease after prolonged intubation, or hospital-associated infection), or an underlying anomaly (e.g., congenital cystic adenomatoid malformation or pulmonary sequestration).

Etiologic Agents (see Table 34-6)

Necrotizing pneumonia can complicate CAP;[145] the pathogen can be *S. pneumoniae*, *S. aureus* (especially CA-MRSA), or *S. pyogenes*, or no pathogen is identified. *S. pneumoniae* or *S. aureus* can cause pneumatoceles; *S. aureus* especially can progress to abscess.[146,147] Severe *M. pneumoniae* pneumonia rarely can result in lung abscess.[148] Lung abscess frequently is accompanied by PPE.

Pneumonia associated with aspiration of bacteria from the oropharynx, or from regurgitated stomach contents, is particularly likely to cause necrosis and abscess formation. Anaerobic bacteria can be isolated from 30% to 70% of lung abscesses, especially *Peptostreptococcus* spp., *Bacteroides* spp., *Prevotella* spp., *Veillonella* spp., and facultative aerobic pathogens including β-hemolytic streptococci (Lancefield groups C and G).[146]

Single or multiple lung abscesses due to *S. aureus*, *Streptococcus anginosus*, or *Fusobacterium necrophorum* can result from right-sided endocarditis, severe septicemia, or endovascular infarction or infection of the large veins in the neck (Lemierre disease).[149] Abscesses in intubated infants and children usually are due to hospital-associated pathogens.[147] Abscesses developing in the later stages of cystic fibrosis secondary to chronic bronchiectasis are caused by *Staphylococcus aureus*, *Pseudomonas aeruginosa*, or mycobacteria.[150] Necrotizing pneumonia in neutropenic and immunocompromised patients can have bacterial or fungal etiology.

Pathogenesis

Necrosis of lung parenchyma as a consequence of inadequate or delayed treatment of severe lobar or alveolar pneumonia often results in abscess formation. Aspiration and obstruction of the airways also predispose to lung abscess, typically developing 1 to

2 weeks after the aspiration episode. Risk factors for aspiration include decreased level of consciousness, neuromuscular disorders depressing the gag reflex, esophageal abnormalities, gastroesophageal reflux, prolonged endotracheal intubation, periodontal disease predisposing to bacterial hypercontamination of aspirated material.[150] Obstruction of the airway can occur from extrinsic or intrinsic masses, lobar emphysema, pneumatoceles, aspirated foreign body, or abnormal drainage as seen in congenital pulmonary sequestration. Impaired immune responses, chronic airway disease, cystic fibrosis, congenital ciliary dysfunction, bronchiectasis, high-grade bacteremia, and pulmonary infarction secondary to septic embolization increase the likelihood of abscess formation.

Clinical Manifestations

Clinical manifestations of necrotizing pneumonia are similar to, but usually are more severe than those of uncomplicated; pneumonia evolution to abscess frequently is insidious.[151,152] Prolonged fever, toxic appearance, and persistent hypoxia despite appropriate antimicrobial therapy frequently are noted. Fever, cough, dyspnea, and sputum production are present in approximately half of patients while chest pain and hemoptysis occur occasionally.[145,152]

The differential diagnosis of typical bacterial lung abscess includes necrotizing infections such as tuberculosis, nocardiosis, fungal infections, melioidosis, paragonimiasis and amebic abscess. Lesions caused by certain noninfectious diseases (malignancy, sarcoidosis, or pulmonary infarction) can mimic abscess on chest imaging.

Diagnosis

Necrotizing pneumonia is suspected in a child when the symptoms do not respond to appropriate antibiotic treatment for pneumonia. Plain film can reveal a radiolucent lesion but CT is more discerning. Decreased parenchymal contrast enhancement on CT correlates with impending necrosis and cavitation.[152] Lung abscess appears as a cavity at least 2 cm in diameter with an air–fluid level and a well-defined wall. Lung abscesses usually are found in either lower lobes or right upper lobe (Figure 34-4).[152]

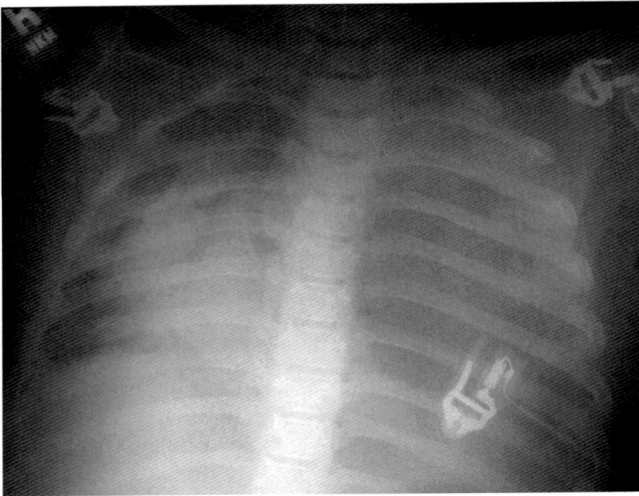

Figure 34-4. Anaerobic pleural empyema in a 5-year-old girl who came to medical attention because of a 1-month history of abdominal pain, tiredness, and constipation, but no history of an aspiration event, fever or respiratory symptoms. This radiograph was obtained after an acute respiratory event during evaluation for constipation. Note complete opacification of the left hemithorax with severe shift of the heart and trachea to the right. Three liters of putrid pus was drained, revealing a left lower lobe abscess. Gram stain and culture revealed polymicrobial anaerobic and facultative oropharyngeal flora. (Courtesy of E.N. Faerber and S.S. Long, St. Christopher's Hospital for Children, Philadelphia, PA.)

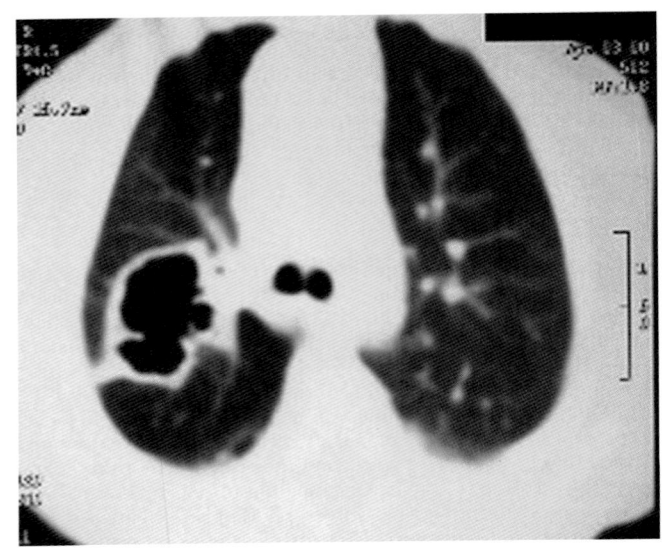

Figure 34-5. Lung windows of computed tomography study showing right sided lung abscess.

CT is useful to define the extent of disease, underlying anomalies, and the presence or absence of a foreign body (Figure 34-5). Bronchoscopy is diagnostic and therapeutic on many occasions to facilitate the removal of a foreign body or to promote the drainage of purulent fluid if this has not occurred spontaneously.[152] Specimens for culture, other than those obtained by bronchoscopy or direct aspiration of the lung, are of limited value. Quantitative culture of bronchoalveolar lavage fluid improves the accuracy of identification of aerobic and anaerobic bacteria as causes of lung abscess.[153] Ultrasound or CT-guided transthoracic aspiration of lung abscess performed on complex cases, successfully identifies the etiologic agent in >90% of cases.[154]

Management

Most cases of necrotizing pneumonia or lung abscess without substantial PPE can be effectively treated with antibiotics without surgical intervention. Parenteral therapy usually is initiated. Clindamycin was determined to be superior to penicillin for the treatment of anaerobic lung abscess in adult studies; however no difference between these two drugs was noted in a clinical trial involving children.[155-157] Parenteral clindamycin is an appropriate empiric therapy for children with suspected *S. aureus* (including MRSA) or anaerobic lung infection. Combination therapy with ticarcillin or piperacillin and a β-lactamase inhibitor, with or without an aminoglycoside, is considered when necrotizing pneumonia occurs in a hospitalized child or in a child for whom an Enterobacteriaceae (e.g., *Escherichia coli*, *Klebsiella*, etc.) or *Pseudomonas aeruginosa* infection is suspected. Duration of total antibiotic therapy is based on clinical response and usually is 4 weeks, or at least 2 weeks after the patient is afebrile and has improved clinically.

Necrotizing pneumonia or abscess is frequently complicated by PPE, which benefits from percutaneous drainage or other invasive procedures. However, percutaneous abscess drainage carries the hazard of bronchopleural fistula with prolonged morbidity or the necessity for surgical repair.[158] Percutaneous drainage is considered in patients with continued systemic illness 5 to 7 days after initiation of antibiotic therapy, in hosts with underlying conditions, and especially if lesions are peripheral or if bronchoscopy fails to drain a more central lesion. Drainage also may be necessary if an abscess is >4 cm in diameter, causes mediastinal shift, or results in ventilator dependency.[159] Surgical wedge resection or lobectomy rarely is required, and is reserved for cases in which medical management and drainage fail or bronchiectasis has occurred.

Prognosis and Complications

Necrotizing pneumonia in otherwise healthy children resolves in 80% to 90% of the cases with antibiotic treatment alone provided airway obstruction is removed.[145] Fever usually persists for 4 to 8 days. The most common complication of lung abscess is intracavitary hemorrhage with hemoptysis or spillage of abscess contents with spread of infection to other parts of the lung.[158] Other complications include empyema, bronchopleural fistula, septicemia, cerebral abscess, and SIADH.[158]

35 Persistent and Recurrent Pneumonia

Dennis L. Murray and Chitra S. Mani

In young adults with community-acquired pneumonia, clinical resolution occurs in more than 85% of cases, and radiographic resolution in approximately 75% of cases by 4 weeks after onset.[1] *Persistent pneumonia* has been defined as continuation of symptoms and radiographic findings beyond this period.[2] In both adults and children with community-acquired pneumonia (CAP), radiologic abnormalities lag behind clinical resolution. Persistent or residual abnormalities occur in 10% to 30% of children with radiographically confirmed CAP 3 to 6 weeks after initial imaging.[3,4] Few studies to date, however, have followed radiographic abnormalities systematically in children over extended periods of time. Up to one-third of adults with uncomplicated pneumococcal pneumonia have radiographic abnormalities for 6 to 8 weeks.[1,5] While pneumonia due to respiratory syncytial virus (RSV) or parainfluenza virus clears within 2 to 3 weeks,[6] pneumonia due to adenovirus can cause persistent abnormalities for up to 12 months.[7] Thus, in children making an uneventful clinical recovery from an episode of uncomplicated CAP a repeat chest radiograph is not recommended routinely.

Recurrent pneumonia has been defined as occurrence of two or more episodes of pneumonia in a 1-year period or more than three episodes in any period, with radiographic resolution between episodes.[2] Using this definition, approximately 8% of children requiring hospitalization for pneumonia would be identified as having recurrent pneumonia.[8] In children with underlying conditions such as cystic fibrosis (CF) or pulmonary sequestration, complete resolution does not occur between exacerbations. Radiographic documentation of episodes is essential for categorization, because precise clinical distinctions are made infrequently and "pneumonia" is the diagnosis sometimes conveyed to the parent (or the parent perceives) for conditions such as bronchiolitis, bronchitis, asthma, or persistent cough.

Although a chest radiograph is not necessarily indicated to confirm the diagnosis of acute pneumonia in previously healthy outpatients, nor indicated routinely at the end of treatment of the first episode of acute pneumonia requiring hospitalization, a history of prior episodes, especially in the same lobe, and persistence or recurrence of symptoms are indications for initial and follow-up radiographic evaluations.[9,10] In a child with a history of "recurrent pneumonia," documenting a normal radiographic appearance 2 months after an acute episode (the time at which radiographic findings are expected to be normal in more than 90% of cases) is the most useful step in shaping a differential diagnosis. Before investigations are initiated for persistent or recurrent pulmonary infection, radiographs should be obtained and reviewed with a radiologist experienced in disorders of children to define the abnormalities precisely and to consider both infectious and noninfectious processes as well as underlying conditions.[2]

The differential diagnosis for and clinical approach to recurrent pneumonia in children are distinct from those for persistent pneumonia and also depend on: (1) whether the site of parenchymal disease is the same or different with each episode; and (2) whether the infiltrate is, on the one hand, dense, focal, and consolidated, or, on the other, atelectatic, patchy, diffuse, nodular, or interstitial. The specific approach to children whose pneumonia is associated with hospitalization, human immunodeficiency virus (HIV) infection, or some other form of immunologic deficiency is addressed in other chapters in this book.

PERSISTENT OR PROGRESSIVE PNEUMONIA AT A SINGLE SITE

Pathogen-Related Causes

Unresolved or untreated acute infection usually is responsible for persistent pneumonia (Table 35-1). In a patient receiving empiric antibiotic therapy, the cause is: (1) infection by an organism not eliminated by the chosen antibiotic, either because of antimicrobial resistance of a common bacterial pathogen (β-lactamase-producing *Haemophilus influenzae*, *Prevotella melaninogenica*, penicillin-resistant *Streptococcus pneumoniae*, methicillin-resistant

TABLE 35-1. Diagnostic Considerations for Pneumonia at a Single Site

Persistent or Progressive	Persistent or Recurrent
Untreated common acute infection	Atelectasis
Unresolved common acute infection	Segmental bronchiectasis
	Intraluminal obstructing lesions
Complication of acute infection	Foreign body
Tuberculosis	Granuloma (infective or foreign body)
Uncommon infection	Right middle lobe syndrome
	Bronchial tumor (adenoma, papilloma, lipoma)
	Extrinsic obstructing lesions
	Lymph nodes (infective or malignant)
	Tumor
	Enlarged heart, pulmonary arteries
	Vascular ring, sling
	Congenital abnormalities
	Bronchial anomalies (bronchomalacia, bronchial stenosis or web, tracheal bronchus)
	Tracheobronchial cysts (cyst adenomatoid malformation, lobar emphysema, bronchogenic cyst)
	Pulmonary sequestration

PART II Clinical Syndromes and Cardinal Features of Infectious Diseases: Approach to Diagnosis and Initial Management

SECTION D Lower Respiratory Tract Infections

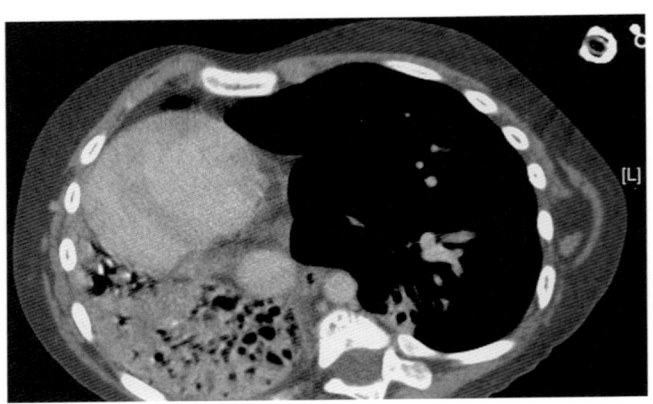

Figure 35-1. Computed tomography of a 9-year-old boy with severe cerebral palsy, seizures, aspiration, and recurrent right lower lobe pneumonia showing severe bronchiectasis. Surgical resection was necessary. (Courtesy of J.H. Brien©.)

Staphylococcus aureus (MRSA), resistant gram-negative bacilli); or (2) more commonly, infection with organisms for which the chosen antimicrobial therapy was ineffective (most often *Mycobacterium tuberculosis*, but also *Mycoplasma* or *Chlamydophila* spp., *Francisella tularensis*, viruses, fungi, protozoa, or parasites).[11] Complications of appropriately treated bacterial pneumonia, such as necrotizing pneumonia, pleural effusion, and progression to lung abscess or empyema, or bronchiectasis also must be considered. The clinical, radiographic, and other imaging findings as well as the context of the patient's illness help prioritize possible causes (Figure 35-1).

Tuberculosis always should be considered in children with persistent pneumonia or subacute presentation even if exposure is not obvious. Immigration from a region of the world with a high prevalence of tuberculosis (Asia, Africa, Latin America, or eastern Europe) or contact with individuals at high risk for tuberculosis (immigrants from regions in which tuberculosis is endemic; Native Americans; homeless persons; individuals with history of drug abuse or imprisonment; or persons with HIV infection) heightens the likelihood of tuberculosis.[12] A history of weight loss, cough, and/or fever is not always present. The radiographic abnormality generally is more impressive than the limited clinical findings, although occasional patients can manifest hectic fever, respiratory distress, and toxicity simulating acute pyogenic pneumonia. The presence of enlarged thoracic lymph nodes is a suggestive, but inconsistent, finding.

Coxiella burnetii (Q fever) and *Chlamydophila psittaci* infections are considered in patients with persistent fever, malaise, and myalgia, hacking cough, persistent parenchymal infiltrate, and exposure to farm animals or psittacine birds. Systemic illness usually overshadows pulmonary symptoms in young children with Q fever; psittacosis is rare in young children.

The likelihood of fungal pneumonia in a previously healthy child depends on place of residence or unusual environmental exposure. Nodular or miliary densities are more common than lobar consolidation, but not consistently. *Histoplasma capsulatum* is endemic to the Ohio and Tennessee River valleys, as well as eastern and central Canada. Subacute presentation with fatigue and a persistent cough is usual, and hilar lymphadenopathy is a clue. *Blastomyces dermatitidis* is a rare cause of persistent pneumonia in children. Endemic areas partially overlap those of histoplasmosis, including parts of the Mississippi, Ohio, Missouri, and St. Lawrence waterways. Older children with *Blastomyces* pneumonia may produce purulent sputum and often have failed at least one course of treatment with an antibacterial agent prior to the etiology being identified correctly. *Coccidioides immitis* is endemic to the southwestern United States, including west Texas, Arizona, New Mexico, California, Utah, and Nevada, as well as northern Mexico and parts of Central and South America. Erythematous rashes and erythema multiforme are frequent early in the course

and erythema nodosum (also seen in *Blastomyces* or *Histoplasma* infection) can accompany pneumonia. Since environmental exposure often is a cause of fungal pneumonia, clusters of cases within the same family or in other persons exposed simultaneously can occur with *Histoplasma*, *Blastomyces*, and *Coccidioides* infections. Rarely, a previously healthy child with or without undue exposure to dust, pigeon excreta, model terrarium, construction, or home renovation develops pneumonia due to *Cryptococcus* or *Aspergillus* spp. that leads to a protracted infection.

In adolescents at risk for HIV infection, *Pneumocystis jirovecii* should be considered, especially when persistent pneumonia is bilateral, interstitial, and associated with hypoxemia disproportionate to the severity of clinical illness or physical findings. Risk factors for HIV infection (injection drug use, multiple sexual partners, bisexual partner) need to be evaluated. In the infant with HIV infection, *P. jirovecii* pneumonia, especially when not properly treated, is rapidly progressive and has a very high mortality.

Diffuse lower respiratory tract inflammation caused by some respiratory viruses can predispose to bacterial superinfection. In fact, viral-bacterial coinfection as a cause of pneumonia in children has been recognized in 23% of children evaluated at a tertiary children's hospital.[13] Thus, for those children with laboratory-confirmed viral respiratory infection for whom symptoms persist or progress, a viral-bacterial coinfection deserves consideration. Several viruses, including influenza, can cause a rapidly progressive pneumonia nonresponsive to antibacterial therapy. Hantavirus can act similarly and also can involve other organs. Adenovirus can cause a necrotizing lobar pneumonia unresponsive to antibiotics.

Host-Related Causes

Multiple congenital or acquired anatomic abnormalities also are considered in children whose pneumonia: (1) fails to resolve; (2) responds symptomatically to antimicrobial therapy but does not resolve radiographically; or (3) resolves and then recurs at the same site (see Table 35-1). Atelectasis (parenchymal volume loss) should be differentiated from persistent infiltrate or consolidation (without volume loss). Atelectasis occurs commonly with RSV bronchiolitis, airway hyperreactivity in infants and toddlers, asthma, and complete bronchial obstruction from intrinsic or extrinsic causes. Except with fixed obstructing lesions, atelectasis is expected to be transient or migratory; if atelectasis persists, the affected lung segment can become infected secondarily.

Bronchiectasis, with dilatation of the bronchi, arises most commonly from damage to bronchial walls by infection and/or chronic inflammation. The bronchial wall then is susceptible to further dilatation and distortion during breathing. Severe acute viral, bacterial, or fungal infection or recurrent infection related to CF, immunodeficiency, or local obstruction are known causes of bronchiectasis.[14] Adenovirus and measles virus infections, retained foreign body, and tuberculosis are associated most commonly with segmental bronchiectasis in the healthy host. In children with untreated or poorly controlled HIV infection or congenital immunodeficiency, lymphocytic interstitial pneumonia or recurrent bronchitis or pneumonia can progress to bronchiectasis.[15] Lower respiratory tract *Mycoplasma pneumoniae* infections also can be a cause occasionally.[16] Once bronchiectasis has developed, impaired ciliary function and bronchial mechanics predispose to recurrent pneumonia. Children with extensive bronchiectasis often are fatigued easily, may have slower growth, and commonly have digital clubbing.

Intraluminal Obstructing Lesions

In otherwise healthy children, aspirated foreign body (or granulation tissue resulting from presence of a foreign body) is the most common cause of incompletely resolved or recurrent pneumonia at the same site.[2] In one-third of cases, an aspirated foreign body is not detected in the week after the event.[17] The diagnosis is apparent if history of an event is elicited or a foreign body is visualized radiographically. Neither finding is present in most cases, but frequently the event is remembered by older children once the object (e.g., timothy grass or other barbed twig) is retrieved at bronchoscopy. Spontaneous hemorrhage from the lower respiratory tract suggests foreign body (or pulmonary sequestration) and can be life-threatening.

Pneumonia at a single anatomic site can be related to particular positional vulnerability in children who are relatively immobile and who aspirate oropharyngeal material because of impaired neuromuscular function or coordination. A dependent segment or segments of lung is/are involved usually.

Other intraluminal bronchial obstructions can cause associated single-site pneumonia, including bronchial adenoma, lipoma, papilloma, foreign-body granuloma (e.g., peanut, other vegetable matter), granuloma of *M. tuberculosis* or atypical *Mycobacterium* spp., or segmental bronchomalacia or bronchial stenosis.

The right middle lobe is predisposed to persistent atelectasis and subsequent infection or delayed resolution of pneumonia because of the acute angle and length of its bronchus, the proximity of its bronchus to hilar nodes, and poor to no collateral ventilation compared with other regions of the lung. The right middle lobe also is a site of aspiration in the upright position. Recurrent right middle lobe pneumonia and atelectasis make up the so-called right middle lobe syndrome. Right middle lobe syndrome in children can have an intraluminal cause secondary to a primary ventilation disorder and chronic inflammation; asthma and foreign body aspiration are two such causes. Extraluminal compression from anatomic abnormalities and compression via lymph nodes from infectious causes, such as fungi and *M. tuberculosis*, also can be responsible. Evaluation of children with recurrent abnormalities of the right middle lobe should include bronchoscopy with direct visualization of the airway and sampling for cultures and cytology.[18]

Extrinsic Obstructing Lesions

Extrinsic airway compression most commonly is due to lymph node enlargement. Tuberculosis is most common, causing hilar, carinal, and other superior mediastinal airway compression, leading to secondary bacterial pneumonia. Pulmonary histoplasmosis, blastomycosis, and coccidioidomycosis also are important causes of hilar adenopathy.[2] Tumors can cause compression of the airway directly or through lymph node involvement. Congenital or acquired heart disease associated with an enlarged heart can cause compression of left lower lobe bronchus especially, leading to pneumonia. Shunting procedures that cause excessive pulmonary blood flow can lead to airway compression or segmental congestion and impaired drainage, predisposing to localized infection.

Congenital Abnormalities of the Respiratory Tract

Congenital abnormalities of airways or pulmonary parenchyma or the diaphragm can cause localized persistent or recurrent pneumonia (Figure 35-2). Tracheal bronchus, an abnormal bronchus arising from the trachea, leads to impaired drainage of the right upper lobe and persistent collapse. Congenital cystic anomalies of the tracheo-bronchial tree include cystic adenomatoid malformation (CCAM), congenital lobar emphysema, and bronchogenic cysts[19] (Figure 35-3). CCAM and congenital lobar overinflation usually cause respiratory distress in infancy (and cystic abnormality on radiographs), whereas bronchogenic cysts and pulmonary sequestrations can manifest as chronic or recurrent pneumonia later in childhood. More than three-fourths of bronchogenic cysts become infected.[20] Radiographically, bronchogenic cysts usually appear as round or oval lesions with air–fluid levels in the perihilar area.[21,22]

Pulmonary sequestrations are masses of ectopic pulmonary tissue with a vascular connection but aberrant or no communication with the airways. Usually sequestrations occur in the lower lobes, more commonly on the left side, with blood supply arising from the aorta.[19,23] Although frequently asymptomatic, pulmonary sequestrations can manifest as recurrent infection because of

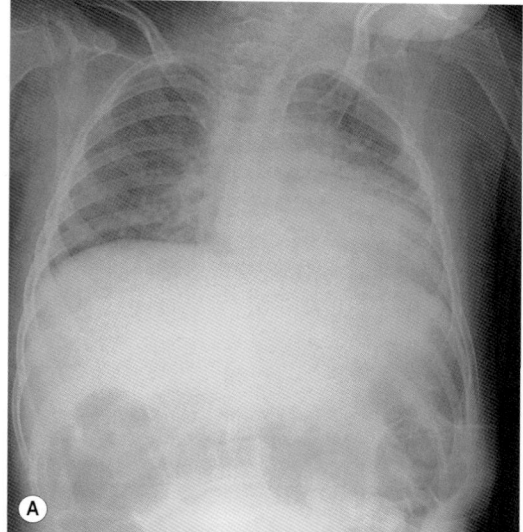

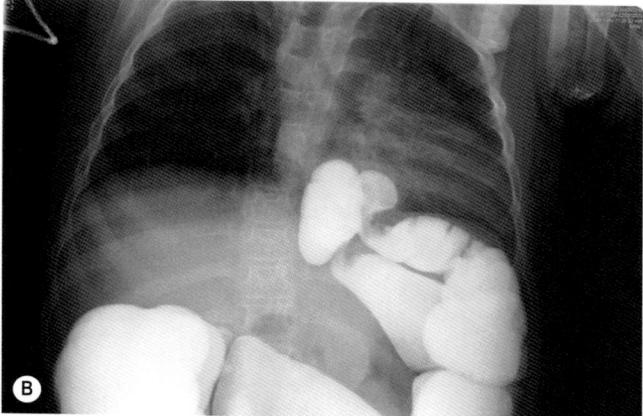

Figure 35-2. A 9-year-old girl with microcephaly had multiple episodes over multiple years of left lower lobe pneumonia **(A)** when barium study revealed congenital diaphragmatic hernia as the cause of persistent "consolidation" **(B)**. (Courtesy of J.H. Brien©.)

poor drainage of secretions.[20] Patients with a secondary abscess due to an underlying pulmonary anomaly such as CCAM or sequestration require surgical consultation for considerations of long-term management.[24]

Congenital pulmonary cysts are located in the periphery of the lung. They arise during alveolar development and, unlike bronchogenic cysts, usually communicate with airways.[20,21] Pulmonary cysts can cause respiratory distress in the neonatal period or manifest later in life as recurrent infections.

Approach to Diagnosis

The history of illness, associated symptoms, and environmental or contact exposures, judgment about adherence to prescribed therapy, the possibility of partial improvement, and re-evaluation of the appropriateness of prescribed therapy usually identify children with incompletely or inadequately treated uncomplicated acute pneumonia. Continued therapy or change in therapy with follow-up to document resolution is appropriate in many situations.

A tuberculin skin test (TST) should be performed in all patients (with anergy assessment in selected individuals). In infants and young children, serial first-morning gastric aspirates are obtained for testing; they may be superior to specimens obtained by bronchoscopy. Sputum is obtained from older children and adolescents. The use of an interferon-γ release assay (IGRA), especially

PART II Clinical Syndromes and Cardinal Features of Infectious Diseases: Approach to Diagnosis and Initial Management

SECTION D Lower Respiratory Tract Infections

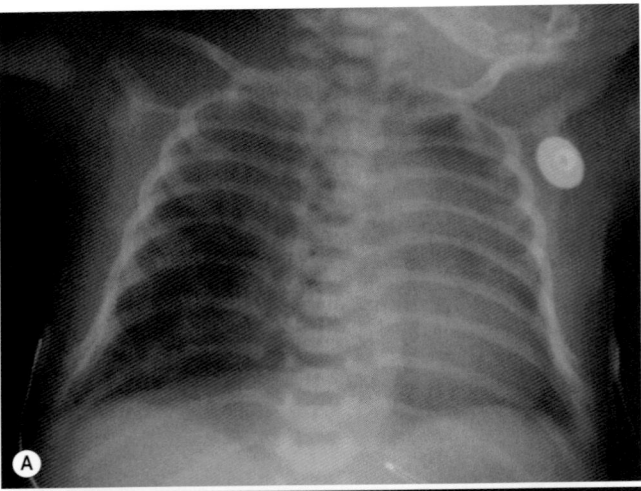

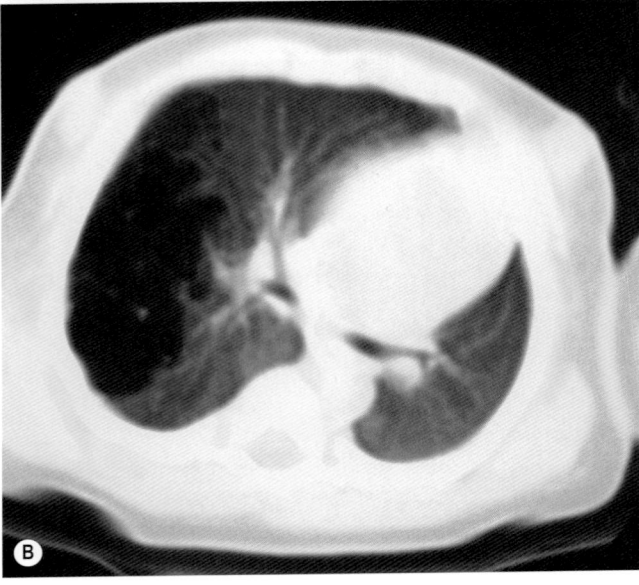

Figure 35-3. Congenital cystadenomatoid malformation (CCAM) in a term neonate who was evaluated because of respiratory distress. Plain radiograph **(A)** and lung window of axial computed tomography **(B)** show typical cluster of cysts, varying in size. Note superiority of computed tomography in demonstrating sites and extent of pathology. (Courtesy of E.N. Faerber.)

for children ≥5 years of age, should be considered for assessing *M. tuberculosis*. HIV testing is indicated for all individuals in whom tuberculosis is diagnosed.

Serologic tests for Q fever, psittacosis, mycoplasmal infection, histoplasmosis, coccidioidomycosis, or blastomycosis are useful when the setting and clinical findings are compatible. Cross-reactivity can cause false-positive test results, tests do not include all pathogens, are insensitive, and may not be available easily. Molecular-based methods, such as polymerase chain reaction (PCR) assays, are available for some organisms. Fungal pneumonia due to *Candida, Cryptococcus,* or *Aspergillus* can be difficult to diagnose. Serologic testing for cryptococcal and galactomannan antigen sometimes can be helpful. Bronchoalveolar lavage (BAL) usually is the next diagnostic modality for persistent pneumonia, and has been reported to confirm the etiology of persistent pneumonia (including *Blastomyces, Histoplasma,* viruses, bacteria, and obstructing lesions) in 30% of immunocompetent children,[25] in 27% of children with cancer,[26] and in 70% of children with acquired immunodeficiency syndrome (AIDS).[27]

If *Pneumocystis* pneumonia (PCP) is suspected in an adolescent, diagnosis can be attempted through identification of the organism

with methenamine silver staining of an induced sputum specimen. If the result is negative or a specimen cannot be obtained, BAL is performed. If PCP pneumonia is confirmed an underlying immunodeficiency must be sought.

Patients with documented recurrent pneumonia, segmental bronchiectasis, suspected anatomic or obstructing lesions, or pneumonia that persists beyond 8 weeks of appropriate therapy require further evaluation. Poor weight gain, weight loss, digital clubbing, polycythemia, or anemia validates a history of chronicity and the need to proceed aggressively. Bronchoscopy is performed to: (1) exclude, or detect and remove, a foreign body; (2) detect extrinsic compression or intraluminal anomaly; (3) obtain a biopsy specimen of a mass; or (4) obtain a specimen for microscopy and culture.

Computed tomography (CT) is useful to evaluate more distal airways (including for bronchiectasis), mass lesions, tracheal bronchus, and congenital cystic anomalies, and to define precise relationships of cysts with surrounding structures before surgical excision.[20,28,29] Additionally, CT is better than chest radiography to detect parenchymal lung complications (cavitary necrosis, abscess, bronchopleural fistula) and loculation of pleural fluid, and can better define pleural versus parenchymal disease.[30] CT, magnetic resonance imaging, or Doppler ultrasonography can confirm the specific blood supply to sequestered pulmonary tissue, obviating invasive studies such as angiography before lobectomy.[16,19] Bronchiectasis can be diagnosed with CT as well; compared with bronchography, CT has a sensitivity of 98% and a specificity of 99%.[31]

PERSISTENT OR RECURRENT PNEUMONIA NOT CONFINED TO A SINGLE SITE

Causes of Dense Focal or Multifocal Infiltrates

Primary pulmonary as well as a variety of nonpulmonary disorders can lead to recurrent and chronic pneumonia affecting multiple areas of the lungs (Table 35-2). Primary pulmonary disorders include inflammatory diseases (such as asthma), congenital and acquired causes of epithelial dysfunction (ciliary dyskinesia, CF, viral infection), and congenital and acquired structural abnormalities (laryngeal and tracheal anomalies, chronic lung disease in infancy). Nonpulmonary disorders that cause pneumonia are myriad, comprising: (1) conditions that impair or overcome normal pulmonary clearance mechanisms, such as impaired cough or gag reflex, neuromuscular disorders, and gastroesophageal reflux; and (2) conditions that increase the risk of infections in the lung, such as congenital and acquired immunodeficiency states and sickle-cell hemoglobinopathies.

Respiratory Tract Disorders and Aspiration

Asthma. Asthma causes most cases of recurrent pulmonary atelectasis or infiltrates in children by inducing diffuse inflammation or mucus plugging of airways (Figure 35-4);[32] common manifestations include recurrent wheezing and cough.[32,33] Environmental stimuli (e.g., allergens, passive smoke) or infectious agents (e.g., viruses, *Mycoplasma* or Chlamydiaceae spp.) enhance inflammation and bronchial hyperreactivity. The majority of asthma exacerbations are associated with occurrence of viral infections.[34] Nocturnal cough, protracted coughing after upper respiratory illnesses, and, even if not acutely ill, exercise-induced cough are important historical clues to asthma, especially in older children. Wandering atelectasis, segmental overaeration, and nonconsolidated, perihilar, peribronchial, and interstitial infiltrates are helpful radiographic clues that asthma is the underlying cause.

Cystic fibrosis. CF is the most frequently inherited disorder, affecting approximately 1 in 2000 to 2600 white children.[35] More than 1500 mutations of the CF gene on chromosome 7 have been identified. Genetic screening of newborns for CF is now available routinely throughout the United States. CF is characterized by mucoviscid respiratory tract secretions that impair ciliary clear-

TABLE 35-2. Diagnostic Considerations for Recurrent or Chronic Pneumonia not Confined to a Single Site

Dense Focal or Multifocal Infiltrates[a]	Diffuse Interstitial Infiltrates[b]
RESPIRATORY TRACT DISORDERS AND ASPIRATION	**MISCELLANEOUS CONDITIONS**
Asthma	Bronchopulmonary dysplasia
Cystic fibrosis	Pulmonary lymphangiectasia
Ciliary dyskinesia	Hypersensitivity pneumonitis
Bronchiolitis obliterans	Allergic bronchopulmonary aspergillosis
Recurrent aspiration (drugs, seizures, cricopharyngeal incoordination, neuromuscular disorders)	Vasculitis syndromes
	Desquamative interstitial pneumonitis
Gastroesophageal reflux	Lymphocytic interstitial pneumonitis
Laryngotracheal anomalies (laryngeal or submucosal cleft)	Histiocytosis
Esophageal obstruction or dysmotility (webs, stricture, achalasia)	Metastatic malignancies (neuroblastoma, Kaposi sarcoma)
Tracheoesophageal fistula	Alveolar proteinosis
Congenital abnormalities of heart and vessels	Idiopathic pulmonary fibrosis
	Drug, chemotherapy, radiation, or physical agent (smoke inhalation, kerosene, etc.) injury
IMMUNOLOGIC ABNORMALITIES[c]	
Agammaglobulinemia	
Common variable immunodeficiency	
Immunoglobulin G subclass deficiency	
Cellular immunodeficiency	
Complement deficiency	
Phagocytic defects	
Immunodeficiency secondary to disease or drug	
OTHER DISEASES	
Sickle-cell disease	
Pulmonary hemosiderosis[b]	

[a]Most pneumonitis is infectious.
[b]Most pneumonitis is noninfectious.
[c]Infiltrates can also be diffuse interstitial or nodular, depending on pathogen.

ance, malabsorption due to failure of the exocrine pancreas, and increased salt loss in sweat. Chronic cough, poor weight gain, digital clubbing, sinusitis, and nasal polyposis at a preadolescent age are distinctive characteristics. Early colonization with *Staphylococcus aureus, Haemophilus influenzae,* and *Streptococcus pneumoniae* is followed by chronic infection of the lower respiratory tract due to *Pseudomonas aeruginosa.* Chronic infection with *Burkholderia cepacia, Stenotrophomonas maltophilia,* and MRSA also can occur. Chest radiograph can be abnormal in infancy and is never normal again, with multiple persistent and new areas of parenchymal consolidation, overinflation, and eventual bronchiectasis. Measurement of chloride concentration in sweat obtained by iontophoresis after pilocarpine stimulation is the diagnostic method of choice; most affected patients have a value >60 mEq/L.[36] Ability to detect CF mutations by direct DNA analysis for the CF transmembrane conductance regulator (*CFTR*) gene on chromosome 7 has advanced the diagnosis and detection of heterozygotes. Although 67% of cases are due to F508del deletions, hundreds of mutations account for the remainder, none of which is responsible for >2% of cases.

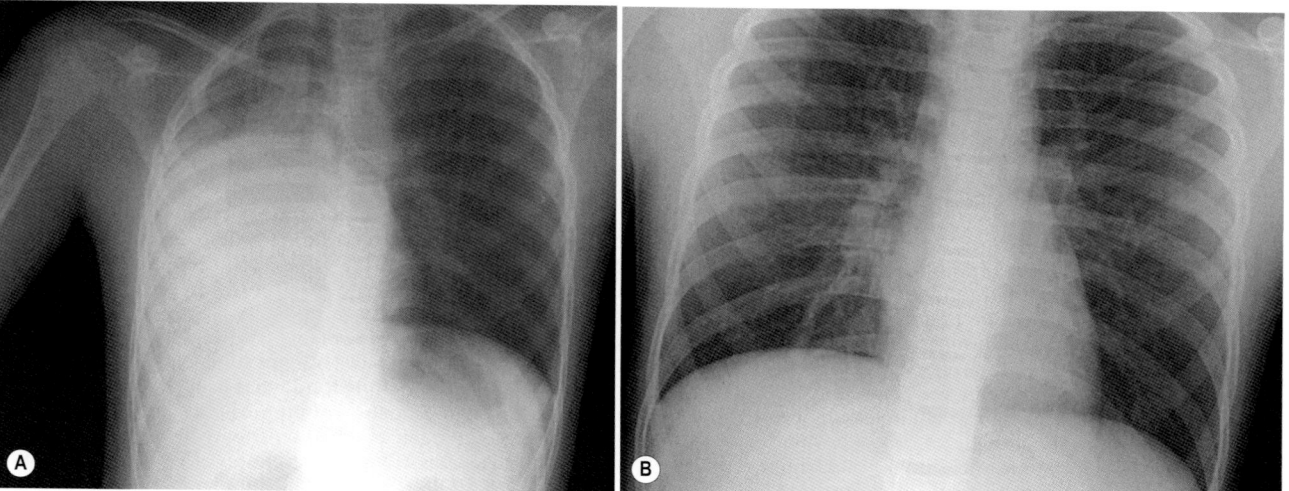

Figure 35-4. A 9-year-old girl with asthma was hospitalized for treatment of "pneumonia." Chest radiograph on admission shows dense right lung consolidation **(A).** Note decreased volume of right side of chest with deviation of trachea and heart to the right, suggesting atelectasis. Chest radiograph 2 days later, following chest physical therapy and treatment of asthma **(B).** Course is most compatible with mucus plug. (Courtesy of J.H. Brien©.)

PART II Clinical Syndromes and Cardinal Features of Infectious Diseases: Approach to Diagnosis and Initial Management

SECTION D Lower Respiratory Tract Infections

Primary ciliary dyskinesia. Normal ciliary motility is necessary for adequate clearance of fluid and foreign materials from both the upper and lower respiratory tracts. Originally described as the Kartagener triad, consisting of dextrocardia, sinusitis, and bronchiectasis, primary ciliary dyskinesia always leads to recurrent sinopulmonary infections. Affected patients have a chronic productive cough, and repeated sinusitis and otitis media; only half have situs inversus. Affected males have reduced fertility. Ultrastructural abnormalities of tubules forming the cilia prevent normal ciliary beating. The most common structural abnormality is absence of one or both dynein arms. Diagnosis is confirmed by histologic examination of specimens of respiratory tract columnar cells obtained by nasal brush biopsy or mucosal scraping.[37] Samples should be obtained when the patient is not infected acutely. Chronic infection can cause replacement of areas of columnar epithelium on mucosal surfaces by squamous cells, which are not useful in making the diagnosis. Morphologic abnormalities are accompanied by reduced frequency of ciliary beat. This can be tested with use of the saccharin transit time as a direct measure of ciliary function; delayed tasting of saccharin placed in the inferior nasal turbinate confirms dyskinesia.[38]

Epithelial damage. Damage of epithelium due to infection by viruses, *Bordetella pertussis*, and *Mycoplasma pneumoniae* can lead to impairment of defense mechanisms and recurrent pneumonia.[39] Additionally, exposure to cigarette smoke and other environmental pollutants impairs ciliary function.

Bronchiolitis obliterans. Bronchiolitis obliterans is a chronic lung disease, which in the majority of cases in children follows lower respiratory tract infection, usually caused by adenovirus. The incidence is highest when children are infected between 6 months and 2 years of age. Certain populations of Native Americans and Maoris (New Zealand) have a higher incidence of chronic lung disease following pulmonary adenovirus infection in childhood. Bronchiolitis obliterans also occurs after inhalation of various acids, as a late complication following lung transplantation, and in bone marrow transplant patients associated with graft-versus-host disease. Bronchiolitis obliterans organizing pneumonia (BOOP) arises from masses of granulation tissue in alveolar ducts that obliterate airspaces. Dyspnea and cough, combined obstructive and restrictive functional abnormalities, radiographic hyperaeration, and airspace consolidation are typical. In occasional cases, the obliterative process is confined to one lung, which then can result in unilateral hyperlucent lung or Swyer–James syndrome. Patients with bilateral, diffuse obliterative disease often have pulmonary edema. While the clinical course, chest radiograph, and CT are suggestive, the diagnosis is confirmed by lung biopsy.[40] Corticosteroid therapy appears to be beneficial in some forms and stages of bronchiolitis obliterans.[41]

Neurologic dysfunction. Neurologic dysfunction is the most common nonpulmonary cause of recurrent pneumonia. Dysfunction predisposes to pneumonia as a result of pharyngeal incoordination or muscle weakness, which leads to failure of the gag, cough, or swallow reflex to protect the airway. Lesions of upper motor neurons, seizures, and decreased level of consciousness are common predisposing conditions. Children who aspirate frequently lose their cough reflex.[18] Pneumonia tends to occur in dependent lobes, e.g., the middle lobe or lung bases when aspiration occurs in the upright position, and the upper lobes when in the supine position.[42] Fluoroscopic examination during a barium meal can be performed to examine upper pharyngopalatal coordination. Although gastric fundoplication and placement of a gastrostomy tube frequently are performed in such patients for convenience of feeding, aspiration of oropharyngeal secretions continues. Chronic pulmonary aspiration results in progressive pulmonary disease, bronchiectasis, and respiratory failure eventually. Chronic pulmonary aspiration is the leading cause of death in children with severe neurologic disorders.[43] The diagnosis of chronic pulmonary aspiration in children is challenging, and no gold-standard diagnostic test exists. Radionuclide salivagram using technetium-sulfur colloid[44] has been used primarily in adults, and has poor correlation with other studies to assess swallowing, functional anatomy, gastroesophageal reflux, etc.[45]

Gastroesophageal reflux. Gastroesophageal reflux (GER) can cause pneumonia in infants by spillover of gastric acid, particulate matter, or both into the trachea. A history of postprandial emesis, irritability accompanied by arching of the back (Sandifer syndrome), and stridor are recognized manifestations, but recurrent wheezing or pneumonia can dominate the clinical picture.[42,46–48] In children, recurrent pneumonia from aspiration in association with GER most commonly occurs in those younger than 2 years of age.[8,18] The most frequent method for diagnosis is 24-hour intraesophageal pH monitoring[42] but false-positive test results occur. Esophageal impedance monitoring may become the future gold standard for diagnosis of GER.[45] Barium swallow, esophageal manometry, and esophagoscopy are alternative diagnostic modalities, but are less sensitive than pH probe and do not measure pathological reflux. A barium swallow study has a sensitivity of approximately 50% for diagnosis.[49] Correlation of findings with causation of clinical pulmonary disease and the relative merits of medical or surgical therapies are controversial.[50–52]

Congenital anomalies. H-type tracheoesophageal fistula is a rare developmental abnormality that can escape recognition in the neonatal period and manifest later as recurrent pneumonia. Respiratory distress with feeding is typical. Radiographic demonstration of caudad-to-cephalad fistula to the trachea during retrograde filling of the esophagus with barium is diagnostic. Recurrent aspiration can persist after surgical repair because of esophageal dysmotility and pooling of secretions above the surgical anastomotic site.[53] Clues to other congenital anomalies of the trachea, great vessels, or esophagus that cause recurrent pneumonia are usually present in associated symptoms or signs (positional respiratory distress, cough, stridor, feeding disorders).

Ventilator-associated pneumonia. Ventilator-associated pneumonia (VAP) is defined as healthcare-associated pneumonia in ventilated patients that develops >48 hours after initiation of mechanical ventilation.[54] In adults, VAP is responsible for both significant morbidity and mortality, and prolonged hospital stay.[55] Mortality associated with and the overall cost of VAP are not as well known in children. In one pediatric series, only 1% of patients admitted to a pediatric intensive care unit (PICU) acquired a nosocomial bacterial pneumonia, but the mortality rate for those patients was 8%. VAP is considered to be the second most common nosocomial infection in the PICU.[56] Underlying comorbidities in children differ substantially from those of adults. Risk of VAP in the neonatal intensive care unit (NICU) generally increases as the postconceptual age decreases. In one study, birth at <28 weeks and NICU stay >30 days were significant risk ractors.[57] In a limited number of prospective studies involving neonates, infants, and children, important risk factors for VAP were immunodeficiency, neuromuscular blockade, transportation out of PICU (for imaging or surgery), prior antibiotic use, enteral feeding, and narcotic use.[58] Rates of VAP also vary by institution and investigator.[58] Bacteria that colonize the oropharynx can evade host defenses more easily in the presence of endotracheal intubation and neuromuscular blockade. *Pseudomonas aeruginosa*, *Staphylococcus aureus* (including MRSA), and enteric gram-negative bacilli (especially *Klebsiella* and *Enterobacter* species) are the most frequently recovered organisms from endotracheal aspirates in both premature infants and older children with VAP.[57,59]

The diagnosis of VAP is made using criteria developed by the National Nosocomial Infection Surveillance System, now the National Healthcare Safety Network (NHSN).[56] Clinical criteria differ by age; separate criteria exist for children <1 year, 1 through 12 years, and ≥13 years. No in-depth diagnostic test data exist for VAP in neonates, older infants, and children.[60] Endotracheal aspirate cultures are sensitive, but not sufficiently specific for diagnostic purposes.[61] One study found that using both BAL and blind protected brush specimens, culture positivity plus the identification of intracellular bacteria had sensitivity of 90% and sensitivity of 88% for diagnosis of VAP.[60] Prevention of VAP has been studied extensively in adults, whereas few comparable pediatric studies exist.[56] The role of selective digestive decontamination or sucralfate for prevention in adults remains controversial.[62] Intermittent enteral feeding compared with continuous feeding, while intubated, is associated with lower gastric pH and a lower risk of VAP in some studies.[56] Aspiration is important in the pathogenesis of VAP in children. Elevation of the head of the bed 30° to 45°, in-line subglottic suctioning, and use of noninvasive positive pressure ventilation may be effective in preventing VAP in children, as they have been in adults.[56]

Immunologic Abnormalities

Immunologic abnormalities constitute an uncommon cause of recurrent pneumonia. The characteristic pattern of pulmonary involvement is recurrent, dense focal infiltrates at different sites, but diffuse interstitial or alveolar and interstitial infiltrates can occur, depending on the pathogen and defect. Qualitative or quantitative defects in phagocytic function, immunoglobulin synthesis, cellular immune function, or complement activity can lead to recurrent pneumonia.[42] The etiologic agents of pneumonia and involvement of the sinopulmonary system exclusively, or in concert with other organ involvement, predict the presence and type of immune defect.

Immunoglobulin and complement deficiency. Recurrent pulmonary infections caused by encapsulated organisms such as *S. pneumoniae* and *H. influenzae* suggest a quantitative or qualitative abnormality in immunoglobulins. Nontypable *H. influenzae*, *S. aureus*, and *P. aeruginosa* also are pulmonary pathogens associated with X-linked agammaglobulinemia and other antibody deficiency syndromes. Dysfunctional hypergammaglobulinemia of HIV infection is associated with sinopulmonary and invasive infection due to *S. pneumoniae* and other encapsulated organisms. Complement deficiency, although rare, can predispose to recurrent pulmonary pyogenic infection.

Phagocytic cellular defects. Abnormalities in the number or function of phagocytic cells predispose to recurrent pyogenic infection, including pneumonia. Recurrent skin and soft-tissue infections, and other invasive infections, also occur commonly. The most common neutrophil disorder resulting in recurrent infections is chronic granulomatous disease (CGD), a microbicidal neutrophil defect preventing production of peroxidase. In the national registry of CGD patients, 80% had at least one episode of pneumonia.[63] Infections are caused exclusively by catalase-producing organisms and can be a clue to the defect. In the national registry, *Aspergillus*, *S. aureus*, and *Burkholderia cepacia* were the most common causes of pneumonia in CGD patients. Other organisms, such as *Serratia marcescens*, *Nocardia* spp., and nontuberculous mycobacteria, occasionally can be involved.

Cellular immune defects. Abnormalities of T lymphocytes, such as those due to congenital combined immunodeficiency, DiGeorge anomalad, HIV infection, or immunodeficiency secondary to disease or therapeutic agents, predispose to recurrent and progressive persistent infections, frequently pneumonia. Progressive disseminated viral, fungal, or mycobacterial infection and *P. jirovecii* pneumonia are suggestive of cellular immune defects.

Other Conditions

Acute thoracic, bony infarction or pulmonary infarction in a patient with sickle-cell hemoglobinopathy can lead to the "acute chest syndrome," which can be difficult to distinguish from pneumonia and commonly is precipitated or complicated by pneumonia (see Chapter 108, Infectious Complications in Special Hosts). Pulmonary hemorrhage with hemosiderosis can masquerade as recurrent pneumonia with alveolar, anatomically confined, "lobar" densities. Occurring predominantly in infants younger than 1 year and postulated to be related to cow's milk protein allergy in some cases and exposure to molds in others, pulmonary hemorrhage with hemosiderosis is signaled by a characteristic abrupt onset of respiratory distress and panting with concurrent pallor and drop in hematocrit.[64–66] Additional clues are rapid resolution of pulmonary infiltrate over 3 to 5 days (uncharacteristic of pneumonia related to infection) and the presence of hemosiderin-laden alveolar macrophages in BAL specimens. In older children,

hemosiderosis and diffuse pulmonary disease are associated with collagen vascular diseases.

Causes of Diffuse Interstitial Infiltrates

A variety of noninfectious entities cause chronic or recurrent lower respiratory tract symptoms and diffuse interstitial or alveolar infiltrates on chest radiographs that can be difficult to distinguish from pneumonia (see Table 35-2).[67] Many of the chronic interstitial or diffuse lung diseases of children (ChILD, children with interstitial lung disease) are rare, idiopathic disorders characterized by adventitious breath sounds, diffuse infiltrates, restrictive functional defect, and disordered gas exchange.[68] Cardiac abnormalities include congestive heart failure, anomalous pulmonary venous return, and congenital or acquired inequality of pulmonary artery blood flow. Congenital lymphangiectasia or pulmonary veno-occlusive disease can be misdiagnosed as recurrent pneumonia or pulmonary edema.[69] Idiopathic or autoimmune disorders that cause infiltrates include hypersensitivity pneumonitis, allergic aspergillosis, fibrosing alveolitis, Hamman–Rich syndrome, desquamative and lymphocytic interstitial pneumonitis, sarcoidosis, vasculitis syndromes, Wegener granulomatosis, and Goodpasture syndrome.

Reticulonodular infiltrate suggests a differential diagnosis that includes Kaposi sarcoma, histiocytosis, metastatic neuroblastoma, and lymphoma.[70] Children with HIV infections and chronic lung disease most commonly have lymphoid interstitial pneumonitis (see Chapter 111, Diagnosis and Clinical Manifestations of HIV Infection), but infiltrates also can be nonspecific, perhaps related to HIV itself.[71]

Many children with ChILD have symptoms that go unrecognized for years. Typical symptoms include cough, dyspnea, chronic tachypnea, exercise intolerance, and recurring respiratory infections. Although not forms of ChILD, cystic fibrosis and ciliary dyskinesia can manifest with similar symptoms.[72] Diagnostic evaluation includes pulmonary function tests, high-resolution CT, and BAL. Testing for mutations in surfactant proteins, such as SP-B, SP-C and others, may be necessary.[72] Lung biopsy often is required to determine the primary cause.

Approach to Diagnosis

Clues from history, physical examination, growth and development, radiographic pattern, and confirmed causes of pneumonia or other infections should guide investigation and permit a staged evaluation. For example, stridor suggests tracheal anomalies; chronic cough productive of purulent sputum suggests bronchiectasis possibly due to disorders of antibody or phagocytic function, CF, or ciliary dyskinesia; severe and complicated sinusitis or otitis media suggests antibody deficiencies or ciliary dyskinesia; wheezing commonly indicates asthma but can be present in a variety of respiratory tract disorders (e.g., foreign body, CF, bronchiolitis obliterans). A history of recurrent problems confined exclusively to the respiratory tract makes cellular immune defects and phagocytic defects unlikely. Infections involving other organ systems, such as recurrent boils or soft-tissue abscesses, raises the possibility of phagocytic defects. Involvement of the central nervous system, gastrointestinal tract and, in some conditions, development of arthritis, in addition to recurrent pneumonia, suggests the possibility of various forms of antibody deficiency.

Confirmation of specific infectious agents heightens suspicion of certain disorders. Examples of sentinel organisms are: catalase-producing agents for CGD; *P. aeruginosa* for CF; *B. cepacia*, for CF or CGD; and *P. jirovecii*, for cellular defects or HIV infection.

A complete blood count is used to assess anemia or polycythemia; abnormal numbers, appearance, or differential makeup of leukocytes; and thrombocytopenia (associated with immunologic disorders such as Wiskott–Aldrich syndrome, primary hematologic cytopenias, or suppression by disseminated virus infection) or thrombocytosis (associated with an acute inflammatory response). Tuberculin skin test, with anergy assessment, should be performed routinely.

An underlying medical condition is identified in more than 90% of cases of recurrent pneumonia requiring hospital admission.[8] In the otherwise healthy child, asthma is the most common diagnosis identified.[8] The following pattern makes the diagnosis of asthma more likely: recurrent wheezing, coughing exaggerated at night or early morning, positive family history, prolonged expiratory phase of respiration, radiograph showing air-trapping, and scattered peribronchial infiltrates or atelectasis. Findings such as poor linear growth and digital clubbing should not be ascribed to asthma. Spirometric measurement of reduced air flow, beneficial response to β_2-agonist drugs, or $\geq 20\%$ reduction in forced expiratory volume in 1 second (FEV_1) with methacholine or histamine challenge documents small-airway hyperreactivity typical of asthma. Assessment of clinical response to therapeutic interventions and follow-up examination including spirometry are appropriate first steps.

In a 10-year retrospective review involving 238 children with recurrent pneumonia,[8] the most common causes for recurrence of pneumonia were: (1) oropharyngeal muscular incoordination and the resulting difficulty in handling respiratory tract secretions; (2) seizure disorders; and (3) neurologic abnormalities (Table 35-3). A pattern of pneumonia in dependent pulmonary segments suggests aspiration. For other patients, certainly those with impaired growth or digital clubbing, and those with radiographs showing lobar or segmental infiltrates, thoracic adenopathy, or bronchiectasis, a specific diagnosis must be pursued. Testing for CF should be performed routinely. If infections are confined to the respiratory tract in infants, a barium swallow study is a useful initial test for vascular rings, duplication, cysts, gastroesophageal reflux, and tracheoesophageal fistula. Further diagnostic tests, including fluoroscopy, bronchoscopy, CT, and magnetic resonance imaging (to define vascular structures), are selected according to the likely etiology. Evaluation of columnar cells from scraping nasal turbinates and/or a bronchial mucosa biopsy to assess ciliary structure and function, should be considered if the child has a documented history of recurrent sinusitis, otitis media, and pneumonia, especially when bronchiectasis is present.

Host defense defects are rare. When appropriate, screening tests should include testing for HIV, quantitative measurement of immunoglobulins (Igs) including IgG subclasses, total hemolytic complement, and functional white blood cell tests, such as a dihydrorhodamine reduction (DHR) for CGD. Measurement of specific antibody responses to proteins (tetanus IgG antibody), and polysaccharide antigens (IgM isohemagglutinins; and pre- and postpneumococcal polysaccharide vaccination IgG antibodies in children ≥ 2 years of age) are more reliable measurements for B-lymphocyte function than is quantity of immunoglobulins,

TABLE 35-3. Underlying Causes of Recurrent Pneumonia

Cause	Percent of Cases
Aspiration syndrome	48
Immune disorder	10
Malignant neoplasm	5
Dysgammaglobulinemia	2
Human immunodeficiency virus infection	2
Autoimmune pancytopenia	<1
Congenital heart disease	9
Asthma	8
Airway or lung anomaly	8
Tracheoesophageal fistula	3
Cyst adenomatoid anomaly	1
Vocal cord paralysis	1
Subglottic stenosis	1
Tracheomalacia	1
Other	1
Gastroesophageal reflux	5
Sickle-cell anemia	4
No identified predisposing cause	7

Data from Owayed AF, Campbell DM, Wang EE. Underlying causes of recurrent pneumonia in children. Arch Pediatr Adolesc Med 2000;154: 190–194.

especially for suspected IgG subclass deficiency states. Using a battery of skin tests to detect delayed hypersensitivity can be used when/where available to screen for cellular immune function.

Bronchoscopy with BAL (or in older, larger children obtaining a protected brush specimen) can confirm underlying conditions and/or specific infectious causes of pneumonia. Lung biopsy is the definitive test required to establish the etiology or pathophysiology of many causes of chronic, recurrent pneumonia when specific pathogens are not otherwise confirmed, especially when the pattern of involvement is interstitial and a noninfectious cause is suspected.

Acknowledgment

The authors acknowledge the past contributions of Kenneth McIntosh and Marvin Harper to the development of this chapter.

---

36   Pneumonia in the Immunocompromised Host

Kenneth McIntosh and Marvin B. Harper

Pneumonia is a common disease in naturally occurring states of immunologic incompetency, such as congenital immunodeficiencies, malnutrition, and human immunodeficiency virus (HIV) infection as well as in iatrogenically induced immunodeficiency, as occurs during chemotherapy for cancer, treatment of rheumatologic diseases, or after tissue transplantation. The clinical findings are diverse, the potential for extended morbidity and mortality is great, and there is a broad range of causative microorganisms.

ETIOLOGIC AGENTS AND EPIDEMIOLOGY

The etiologic agents of pneumonia in the immunocompromised host consist not only of the same agents that cause pneumonia in the immunocompetent host but also of a large number of opportunistic agents. The importance of agents in various forms of immunologic incompetence depends on the particular part of the immune system that is deficient as well as the part of the immune system that normally defends against that microorganism (Table 36-1).

TABLE 36-1. Microorganisms Associated with Severe Pneumonia in Immunodeficiency States

Deficiency	Viruses	Pyogenic Bacteria	Mycobacteria	Fungi
B-lymphocyte deficiency	Enteroviruses Adenoviruses	Streptococcus pneumoniae Haemophilus influenzae Meningococcus	None	None
T-lymphocyte deficiency (including tumor necrosis factor-alpha deficiency)	Varicella-zoster virus Rubeola virus Herpes simplex virus Cytomegalovirus Adenovirus Respiratory syncytial virus Parainfluenza virus Human metapneumovirus	Neisseria meningitidis Listeria monocytogenes Pseudomonas aeruginosa Stenotrophomonas spp. Burkholderia spp. Legionella spp. Other opportunistic bacteria	Mycobacterium tuberculosis Mycobacterium avium complex Mycobacterium fortuitum Calmette-Guérin bacillus Other opportunistic mycobacteria	Pneumocystis jirovecii Candida albicans Cryptococcus neoformans Nocardia spp.
Neutrophil dysfunction	None	Staphylococcus aureus Burkholderia cepacia Serratia marcescens	Mycobacterium tuberculosis Calmette-Guérin bacillus Nontuberculous mycobacteria	Aspergillus spp. Nocardia spp. Candida spp.
Neutropenia	None	Pseudomonas aeruginosa Stenotrophomonas spp. Burkholderia spp. Other opportunistic bacteria	None	Aspergillus spp. Pseudallescheria boydii Agents of mucormycosis

In conditions in which the normal quantities of functional antibody are deficient, such as hypogammaglobulinemia,[1] or in the functional B-lymphocyte deficiency that accompanies HIV infection in infants and children,[2] bacterial pneumonias are common. They are largely caused by *Streptococcus pneumoniae*, various species of *Haemophilus*, and other encapsulated bacteria. Pneumonia due to respiratory viruses is not more frequent or more severe in antibody deficiency states.

In conditions of relatively pure deficiency in cell-mediated (lymphocyte) immunity, such as severe malnutrition, the late stages of AIDS, and some congenital immunodeficiencies (DiGeorge syndrome being a prototype of this form of immunodeficiency), certain viral infections are more severe, produce life-threatening pneumonia, and require careful prophylaxis and potent treatments. These viruses include the herpesviruses, especially cytomegalovirus, varicella-zoster virus (VZV), herpes simplex virus (HSV), and, occasionally, human herpesvirus 6 (HHV-6),[3] all of which are unusual causes of clinically significant pneumonia in healthy children. In areas of the world where measles remains endemic, pneumonia is a common complication of infection in the malnourished child and can be severe and life-threatening. Common respiratory viruses, particularly respiratory syncytial virus (RSV), parainfluenza viruses, and adenovirus, can cause prolonged and, on occasion, severe infection.[4,5] Lymphocyte deficiencies also predispose to pneumonia due to many bacteria (see Table 36-1) as well as several fungi, including *Pneumocystis jirovecii* (formerly *P. carinii*).

Epstein–Barr virus (EBV) is a special case. A form of subacute pneumonia characterized by micronodules of proliferating lymphoid tissue, known as lymphocytic interstitial pneumonitis (LIP), is frequently (although not exclusively) associated with infection by EBV in several states of immunologic dysregulation, particularly in children with HIV infection.[6–8] LIP usually manifests as a slowly developing, afebrile pulmonary disease associated with progressive hypoxia, and generalized lymphadenopathy, with characteristic diffuse micronodular infiltrates apparent on chest radiography (see Figure 112-2). In HIV-infected children, LIP usually develops between 18 months and 6 years of age and often is accompanied by striking hyperglobulinemia.[6] This disease has become uncommon in children treated with antiretroviral drugs. In its early forms it is responsive to treatment with corticosteroids.

In states of neutrophil dysfunction or profound neutropenia, an entirely different spectrum of organisms is commonly implicated in pneumonia. In chronic granulomatous disease as well as pure neutropenia, pneumonia is frequently caused by *Staphylococcus aureus* (including methicillin-resistant strains) and

opportunistic bacteria and fungi such as *Pseudomonas aeruginosa*, *Burkholderia cepacia*, *Nocardia* spp., *Mycobacterium tuberculosis*, particularly in areas where it is widespread,[9] nontuberculous mycobacteria, and *Aspergillus* spp.[10] Neutropenia alone does not appear to predispose to either viral or *P. jirovecii* pneumonia.

Defects in innate immunity, either genetic or drug-induced, add an additional layer of complexity to this picture. IRAK-4 and Myd88 deficiencies present very much like B-lymphocyte defects, with frequent pyogenic pneumonias in childhood.[11] Common genetic polymorphisms in the mannose-binding lectin gene may contribute to susceptibility to opportunistic pneumonias in the posttransplant period.[12] Innate immunity can also be inhibited pharmacologically, and drugs that block tumor necrosis factor-α predispose to mycobacterial and fungal infections as well as other infections for which cellular immunity is important.[13]

Immunodeficiencies that are drug-induced, particularly those that occur during cancer chemotherapy or after organ or stem cell transplantation, are complex. Often, at different times and with different drug regimens, there is a combination of neutropenia or neutrophil dysfunction, which can be profound, with associated innate or drug-induced defective lymphocyte function. In addition, during both cancer chemotherapy and bone marrow transplantation, drug-induced compromise of the oral and intestinal mucosal barriers allows resident bacteria to invade the bloodstream with ease. In this setting, pneumonia is commonly due to opportunistic bacteria and fungi, acquired nosocomially or from resident mucosal flora, such as *Pseudomonas aeruginosa* and *Stenotrophomonas maltophilia*, α-hemolytic streptococci and other oral bacteria, *Nocardia*, *Candida*, *Aspergillus* spp., and other yeast and filamentous fungi.[14–16] Although antibody levels are not extremely low in children undergoing cancer chemotherapy, and may be supplemented by periodic infusions of immune globulin intravenous, mixtures of lymphocyte and neutrophil deficiencies are common. In addition, even though total immunoglobulin (Ig) levels are normal, children and adolescents may be susceptible to encapsulated bacteria (*Streptococcus pneumoniae*, *Haemophilus influenzae*) after solid-organ transplantation, demonstrating that the defense against many microorganisms is multifaceted.[17,18]

The most common viral infections in these drug-induced immunodeficiency states are those due to the same viruses that cause pneumonia in children with pure lymphocyte deficiencies: cytomegalovirus (CMV), VZV, HSV, and, in endemic areas, rubeola.[19,20] As in children with congenital deficiencies of lymphocyte function, pneumonia associated with HHV-6 has also been described.[21] Viruses that commonly cause pneumonia in healthy hosts, such as RSV, influenza, parainfluenza viruses, human metapneumovirus, and adenovirus, display greater

PART II Clinical Syndromes and Cardinal Features of Infectious Diseases: Approach to Diagnosis and Initial Management

SECTION D Lower Respiratory Tract Infections

virulence in both children and adults after solid-organ or human stem cell transplantation, particularly when cellular immunity is profoundly suppressed.[22–28] This probably was demonstrated in the recent pandemic of H1N1 2009 influenza.[29] In the posttransplant setting, EBV can cause progressive pulmonary disease, but this is usually in the form of posttransplantation lymphoproliferative disease, with enlarging masses of lymphoid tissue in the mediastinum and parenchyma of the lung rather than diffuse LIP, as was described earlier.[30]

Because patients with iatrogenically imposed states of immunodeficiency tend to spend long periods in hospital, organisms that cause significant pneumonia in such patients are often nosocomially acquired. In addition, they reflect the epidemiology and antimicrobial resistance patterns of hospital-associated organisms, whether through carriage on the hands of caregivers (as, for example, methicillin-resistant *S. aureus* or multidrug-resistant gram-negative enteric organisms), through the hospital's water supply (as, for example, *Legionella* species), or through the spread of small-particle aerosols (as, for example, *Aspergillus* spp.).

The frequency of pneumonia after solid-organ transplantation, as well as the causes identified, vary greatly by transplant center and the organ transplanted. Some of this variation is likely due to differences in the definition of pneumonia and the intensity of microbial investigation. Nonetheless, certain etiologic patterns emerge. CMV pneumonia occurs in 12% to 45% of renal,[17] liver,[31,32] lung,[33] and allogeneic bone marrow transplant recipients.[34,35] Anticipatory strategies,[36] or prophylaxis with ganciclovir or valganciclovir have reduced, but not eliminated this problem.[37,38] Nosocomially acquired viruses and bacteria remain major causes of pneumonia among transplant recipients, with incidences varying widely among centers.[31–35,39,40] *Aspergillus* has been identified as the cause of up to 35% of pneumonia following bone marrow or solid-organ transplantation.[17,31–35,39,40] Tuberculosis is a high risk following renal transplantation in endemic areas. The causes of pneumonia, as well as other infections, often follow a temporal pattern specific to the chemotherapy used or tissue transplanted. For example, after solid-organ transplantation, nosocomially acquired bacteria predominate as a cause of pneumonia in the first month; later, viruses, especially CMV and adenovirus, and to a lesser extent *Listeria*, *Nocardia*, and *Aspergillus*, may be the etiology. More than 6 months after solid-organ transplantation the agents of community-associated bacterial pneumonia become more common.[41]

PATHOGENESIS AND PATHOLOGIC FINDINGS

The pathogenesis of pneumonia in the immunocompromised host is similar to that of pneumonia in the healthy host, except that defects in host defense play a critical part in the spread of microorganisms from the upper respiratory tract, where they reside as commensals or have recently been acquired from the environment, to the lower respiratory tract and then within the lung itself. Many states of systemic immunodeficiency are accompanied by mucosal immunodeficiency. In the upper respiratory tract, mucosal immunity is primarily mediated by IgA, but in the lower respiratory tract, IgG is more important (see Chapter 34, Acute Pneumonia and Its Complications). There is probably also a role in the healthy host for mucosal cellular immunity along the respiratory tract (the bronchus-associated lymphoid tissue or BALT), as there is in the lining of the gastrointestinal tract.[42] Finally, because the function of macrophages, including alveolar macrophages, depends on interleukins secreted by T lymphocytes, the normal phagocytic and microbicidal activities of these important defenders are impaired when cell-mediated immunity is deficient or when critical interleukins are blocked.[13] Clearly, neutrophils also play an important part in the defense of the airway and lung.

In addition, patients with congenital or acquired immunodeficiencies often develop structural abnormalities that compromise the airways, such as ciliary damage and bronchiectasis due to recurrent bronchitis,[37] or intubation in the hospital setting. These defects lead to more rapid and extensive spread of microbes from the upper to the lower respiratory tract. Often, such patients have

been exposed to multiple antimicrobial agents and nosocomial organisms, with resultant colonization and subsequent infection by resistant bacteria, yeast, or fungi.

CLINICAL DIAGNOSIS AND RADIOGRAPHIC MANIFESTATIONS

The diagnosis and management of pneumonia in the compromised host overlap in time. A flow diagram is shown in Figure 36-1 to serve as a rough guide for decisions.

Clinical manifestations of pneumonia in the immunocompromised host are variable. Fever, with or without cough, may be the only sign of a potentially life-threatening disease.[18] Conversely, a chronic cough without fever also can signal significant lower respiratory tract disease. Certain infections, such as *Pneumocystis* pneumonia (PCP), and interstitial viral pneumonia, caused by RSV, parainfluenza viruses, CMV, or other herpesviruses, impair oxygenation and commonly manifest as hypoxia. Pleural chest pain indicates localized pneumonia at the periphery of the lung and, in this setting, may be due to either bacterial or fungal infection.

Radiographic imaging is critical to both the diagnosis and management of pneumonia in immunocompromised children. Conventional radiographs, computed tomography (CT), or both should be performed. While not generally required, magnetic resonance imaging may be more sensitive than CT for the early recognition of necrotizing pneumonia.[43] High-resolution CT has been shown to have high sensitivity and specificity for the characterization of pneumonia following pediatric bone marrow transplantation.[44] Among iatrogenically immunocompromised patients, the differential diagnosis often includes noninfectious disorders, such as an underlying malignancy or drug-induced pulmonary disease.[18]

The pattern of abnormality on chest radiograph or CT often is helpful in narrowing the differential diagnosis and guiding further investigations and treatment (Table 36-2). If an interstitial pattern is present, viruses and atypical bacteria such as *Mycoplasma pneumoniae* should be sought by sampling of the nasopharynx and the use of rapid identification methods. A positive test result for respiratory viruses or *M. pneumoniae* in nasopharyngeal specimens may be useful evidence of their causative role in pneumonia; such simple tests can spare the patient an invasive procedure such as bronchoscopy or lung biopsy. Definitive diagnosis of *P. jirovecii* pneumonia depends on finding "cysts" in pulmonary secretions. In older children, these "cysts" can sometimes be identified in an induced sputum sample, but the most useful procedure is bronchoscopy with bronchoalveolar lavage (BAL) or brush biopsy. In the proper clinical setting, however, a positive β-D-glucan test or *P. jirovecii* PCR can provide sufficient evidence for the presumptive diagnosis of *P. jirovecii* pneumonia. Diagnosis of CMV pneumonia often is difficult, because CMV can colonize the upper respiratory tract asymptomatically, and its isolation from BAL fluid may not be meaningful. The definitive diagnosis can be made by the presence of characteristic inclusion bodies in biopsy tissue. In the proper clinical setting, identification of CMV in circulating white blood cells by fluorescence testing or at high levels in plasma or serum by polymerase chain reaction suggests CMV as the cause of pneumonia.[45]

Determining the cause of consolidative or nodular pneumonia can be difficult. Blood should be obtained for culture and, in the appropriate setting, quantitative tests for EBV and CMV. A positive test for galactomannan in the blood is important information in support of a diagnosis of invasive *Aspergillus* infection.[46] β-D-glucan is also a useful marker for *Pneumocystis jirovecii* infection, as previously noted, but also can be elevated in other pulmonary fungal infections, including *Aspergillus*.[47] Pleural fluid, if present, should be sampled; often it is sterile, however, when patients have been receiving antimicrobial treatment. Bronchoscopy can be helpful, but organisms causing consolidative infiltrates can colonize the upper respiratory tract, and results of culture may be misleading. Gram stain of deep tracheal secretions or BAL fluid

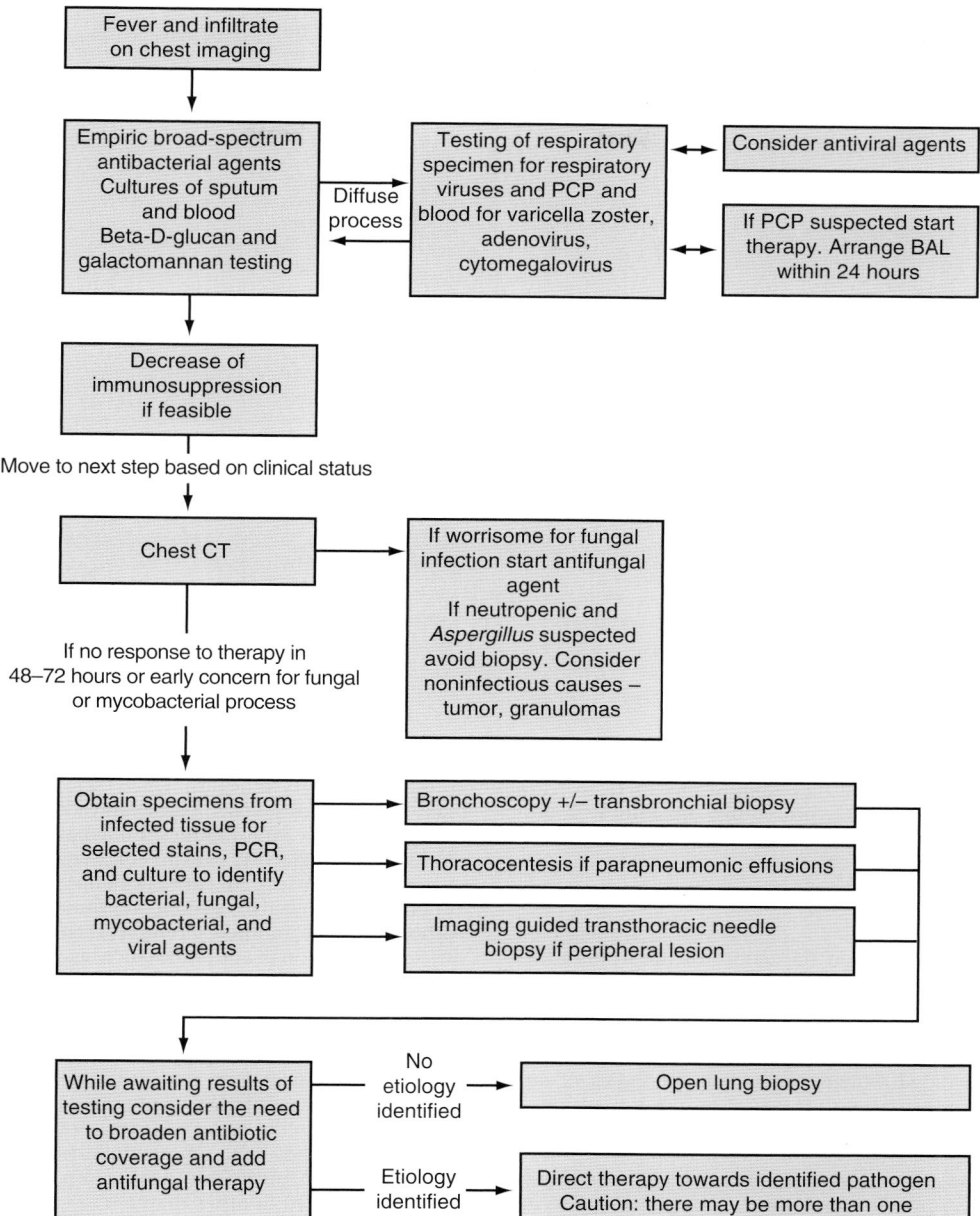

Figure 36-1. Approach to evaluation of the immunocompromised patient with pulmonary infiltrates. The pace of working through the algorithm will depend on the overall clinical status of the patient, prior therapy, and likelihood of finding a pathogen at each step. Invasive procedures are likely to carry higher risk in the neutropenic patient, and therefore a longer trial of empiric therapy and a delay before biopsy may be appropriate for these patients. At any step, if the clinical picture, early tests, or imaging point to a specific etiology the treatment may be tailored and there may be no need to continue the algorithm. PCP, *Pneumocystis* pneumonia; BAL, bronchoalveolar lavage.

often is helpful in indicating density of bacteria in the lower respiratory tract and in guiding therapy. Definitive diagnosis may require lung biopsy. There is a role for empiric antimicrobial treatment of pneumonia in the immunocompromised patient, particularly if the immunocompromised state is likely to be temporary. However, an aggressive approach to definitive microbiologic diagnosis of pneumonia in highly immunocompromised patients often is indicated, because appropriate therapy may be complex, prolonged, and toxic, as well as life-saving.[48]

MANAGEMENT AND THERAPY

Empiric treatment should be guided by the radiologic, clinical, and epidemiologic circumstances. The presence of diffuse pulmonary infiltrates, particularly with hypoxia, generally should prompt

early investigation for respiratory viruses and consideration for bronchoscopy to identify *Pneumocystis jirovecii*. Empiric therapy should include trimethoprim-sulfamethoxazole for *P. jirovecii*, as infection is potentially life-threatening. In addition, macrolide therapy for *Mycoplasma* or *Legionella* should be considered. Although it is clearly preferable to perform diagnostic tests *before* therapy has been started, *P. jirovecii* usually can be identified for several days after treatment has been started.[49] Decision concerning adjunctive corticosteroid therapy for treatment *of P. jirovecii* pneumonia, however, should await definitive diagnosis.

Localized infiltrates more likely are due to bacterial infection, and empiric antibiotic therapy should include agents that effectively treat resident flora and nosocomial organisms, including methicillin-resistant *Staphylococcus aureus*. Nodular infiltrates can suggest fungal infection,[35] or, especially if associated with

TABLE 36-2. Radiographic Patterns and Pathogens of Pneumonias in Immunocompromised Hosts

Radiographic Pattern	Likely Pathogens	Diagnostic Approach
Diffuse, interstitial	Viruses (CMV, RSV, parainfluenza, HSV) *Mycoplasma pneumoniae*,[a] *Chlamydia*[a] *Pneumocystis jirovecii*	Rapid viral, mycoplasmal, or chlamydial diagnostic tests on upper-airway secretions; beta-D-glucan for *Pneumocystis*; bronchoscopy with PCR or immunofluorescence for viruses, and methenamine silver stain for *Pneumocystis*
Focal, consolidative	Pyogenic bacteria (*Streptococcus pneumoniae*, *Haemophilus influenzae*, others) Nosocomial bacteria *Legionella* spp. (Also consider fungi and mycobacteria)	Blood cultures Gram stain and culture of deep respiratory tract secretions *Legionella* antigen in urine *Cryptococcus* antigen (blood) *Histoplasma* antigen (urine) Galactomannan (blood) Acid-fast smears Bronchoscopy Biopsy
Micronodular	Viruses (adenovirus, VZV, EBV (LIP)) Mycobacteria *Histoplasma*, *Candida* spp., *Cryptococcus*	Rapid viral diagnostic tests on upper respiratory tract secretions Acid-fast smears, cultures of lower respiratory tract secretions *Histoplasma* antigen (urine); *Cryptococcus* antigen (blood)
Nodular	*Aspergillus* spp., other fungi, agents of mucormycosis *Nocardia* spp. EBV lymphoproliferative disease	Galactomannan (blood); *Histoplasma* antigen (urine); *Cryptococcus* antigen (blood); EBV PCR (blood); bronchoscopy; biopsy(transbronchial, fine-needle, VATS, or open)

CMV, cytomegalovirus; EBV, Epstein–Barr virus; HSV, herpes simplex virus; LIP, lymphocytic interstitial pneumonitis; PCR, polymerase chain reaction. RSV, respiratory syncytial virus; VATS, video-assisted thoracoscopic surgery; VZV, varicella-zoster virus.

[a]Can also cause patchy infiltrate in less compromised individuals.

lymphadenopathy, lymphoproliferative disease. None of these "rules," however, is completely reliable, and further clinical and epidemiologic information always should be used to guide decisions. Aggressive diagnostic procedures are indicated more urgently if the illness is severe and the immunosuppressed state is likely to be of longer duration.

PREVENTION

Preventive strategies depend on the nature of the immunodeficiency, the consequent anticipated threats, and the circumstances under which these threats occur (after organ transplantation, during chemotherapy, or in an evolving immunodeficiency, such as with HIV infection). All preventive modes are important. Pathogens should be avoided whenever possible. Examples of such simple preventive measures are the use of barrier precautions in the hospital environment, influenza immunization of family contacts, avoidance of *Salmonella*-contaminated foods or reptiles at home, and, most importantly, maintenance of good hand hygiene by family caregivers, medical personnel, and patients. Vaccines

should be administered in such a way as to optimize response (for example, *before* solid-organ transplantation, or early in the life of an infant with HIV infection, when CD4+ lymphocyte counts are likely to be highest). When particular vaccines are contraindicated (for example, live viral vaccines immediately after stem cell transplantation), ineffective (as in children with many congenital immunodeficiencies), or not available, and it is known that antibody is protective, generic immune globulin intravenous, pathogen-specific immune globulin (such as CMV immune globulin), or monoclonal antibody (such as palivizumab to prevent severe disease due to RSV in infants and, possibly, in young children) should be administered. In selected circumstances, chemoprophylaxis is extremely effective in preventing important and potentially life-threatening pneumonias, such as those due to *P. jirovecii*, HSV, and CMV. In certain diseases, such as chronic granulomatous disease, interferon-gamma, given by injection three times per week, reduces the occurrence of serious infections by as much as two-thirds.[50] Recommendations for prevention of infection by specific organisms depend on clinical circumstances, which are detailed in other chapters.

SECTION E: Cardiac and Vascular Infections

37 Endocarditis and Other Intravascular Infections

Stéphanie Levasseur and Lisa Saiman

The American Heart Association (AHA) Committee on Rheumatic Fever, Endocarditis, and Kawasaki Disease and the European Society of Cardiology provide updated scientific statements on many of the topics discussed in this chapter.[1–5] Readers are encouraged to review these consensus statements and seek new documents by these authoritative groups as updates are written.

INFECTIVE ENDOCARDITIS

Infective endocarditis is a well-described, but relatively rare, infection of the cardiac endothelium. In this disease process, pathogens become enmeshed in fibrin and platelets to form *vegetations* that are attached to heart valves, mural endocardial surfaces, or papillary muscles. The historical risk factors of rheumatic heart disease and unrepaired congenital heart disease remain relevant, particularly in the developing world, but in developed countries, endocarditis more often occurs following surgery for congenital heart disease, as a result of complications of intravenous drug abuse, use of indwelling central venous catheters, or as healthcare-associated infections (see Chapter 102, Clinical Syndromes of Device-Associated Infections).[6-11]

Endocarditis was uniformly fatal in the preantibiotic era, but the rate of cure in referral centers is as high as 88% to 90% with appropriate treatment.[12-14] Similarly, a mortality rate of 5% was reported from an administrative dataset of patients hospitalized with endocarditis from 2784 institutions.[15] However, the crude mortality rate when including endocarditis diagnosed postmortem may be as high as 21% to 24%.[12,16]

Etiologic Agents and Associated Risk Factors

The pathogens causing endocarditis in children from representative case series are shown in Table 37-1. Streptococci, especially viridans streptococci, e.g., *Streptococcus sanguis, S. mitis, S. salivarius, S. mutans,* and *S. oralis,* are frequent causes of endocarditis. These pathogens generally are associated with infection following rheumatic fever and unrepaired congenital heart disease, and with late postoperative endocarditis.[17-19] Staphylococci are more common than streptococci in some series.[12,15,20] Coagulase-negative staphylococci (CoNS) can cause endocarditis after cardiac surgery, and *S. aureus,* including community-acquired methicillin-resistant *S. aureus* (CA-MRSA), cause endocarditis in normal hearts as well.[21] *Candida* and *Aspergillus* species[19,22] increasingly are common causes of healthcare-associated endocarditis, particularly among patients in the neonatal intensive care unit (NICU),[23] those with central venous catheters, or following prosthetic valve surgery. Gram-negative enteric bacilli and gram-negative oropharyngeal flora, the so-called AACEK (formerly HACEK) organisms, an acronym for *Aggregatibacter* (formerly *Haemophilus*) *parainfluenzae, Aggregatibacter* (formerly *Actinobacillus*) *actinomycetemcomitans, Cardiobacterium hominis, Eikenella corrodens,* and *Kingella kingae,* are uncommon causes of endocarditis in children. Among the AACEK group, *K. kingae* and *A. parainfluenzae* are the most common causes of endocarditis in children.[24] In the preantibiotic era, *Streptococcus pneumoniae* caused 15% of cases of endocarditis. Today, pneumococcal endocarditis is rare, but is associated with a high rate of mortality.[25]

Culture-negative endocarditis seems to be less common in children than in adults. Approximately 5% to 10% of children with endocarditis have sterile blood cultures. Previous treatment with antibiotics is a common cause of negative blood cultures[26,27] but fastidious pathogens that require special culture conditions or non-culture techniques also can cause culture-negative endocarditis. Other causes of culture-negative endocarditis include fastidious AACEK organisms and other rare fastidious pathogens such as *Bartonella, Brucella, Mycoplasma,* and *Legionella* spp., as well as *Coxiella burnetii.* Non-AACEK pathogens are more easily detected by serologic or polymerase chain reaction testing as described below.[28-30] Endocarditis in children is rarely caused by mycobacteria, *Chlamydia psittaci,*[31] and *Tropheryma whipplei.*[32]

Epidemiology

The true incidence of endocarditis in children is difficult to ascertain as the literature primarily derives data from referral centers. Between 1930 and 1972, 1:2000 to 1:5000 pediatric hospital admissions were due to endocarditis and during the 1960s to 1980s, 1:500 to 1:1000 hospitalizations were due to endocarditis.[33-36] In 2003, 1:3500 randomly selected hospital admissions from a national database were attributed to endocarditis.[15]

The risk factors for endocarditis in children have changed over the past several decades. As shown in Table 37-2, congenital heart disease is the most common predisposing condition in the United States. While surgical correction of ventricular septal defects or patent ductus arteriosus substantially reduces the risk of endocarditis, other interventions such as palliative shunts, valve replacement, and placement of pacemakers, or defibrillators or both, can increase the risk of endocarditis due to the introduction of foreign material in the bloodstream.[37] Advances in surgical techniques and supportive care now permit earlier repairs of certain lesions (e.g., tetralogy of Fallot)[38] as well as neonatal palliation of previously inoperable lesions.[39] This has been associated with endocarditis, including early postoperative endocarditis,[16] occurring in younger patients; in some series the median age at presentation is ≤2 years.[16,20] Of note, 18% to 31% of patients with endocarditis in the developed world have no previously known cardiac defect.[12,14,16,20]

Neonatal endocarditis is well described and appears to be increasing.[17,19,33,40,41] In this population, endocarditis usually is a complication of extreme prematurity, major surgery, or prolonged use of indwelling central venous catheters (CVCs). Fewer than 30% of neonates with endocarditis have congenital heart disease and most endocarditis is right sided.[19,42] Older children without cardiac defects also can develop right-sided endocarditis,[15,16] including adolescents with intravenous drug abuse, those with pacemakers,[43,44] or critically ill patients with long-term presence of CVCs.[33,45-51]

TABLE 37-1. Trends in Agents of Infective Endocarditis

Period of Data Collection	1950–1992[14,16,37,156,157]	1990–2008[136,142,158-160]
Number of cases	421	202
Streptococci		
Viridans streptococci	158 (38%)	58 (29%)
Streptococcus pneumoniae	11 (3%)	3 (1%)
Group B streptococci	3 (<1%)	1 (<1%)
Other	2 (<1%)	1 (<1%)
Enterococci	16 (4%)	20 (10%)
Staphylococci		
Staphylococcus aureus	113 (27%)	46 (23%)
Coagulase-negative staphylococci	22 (5%)	25 (12%)
Gram-negative bacilli	26 (6%)	19 (9%)
Fungi	9 (2%)	17 (8%)
Other organisms	5 (1%)	–
Polymicrobial	4 (1%)	12 (6%)
Culture negative	58 (14%)	21 (10%)

TABLE 37-2. Trends in Underlying Cardiac Diseases in Children with Infective Endocarditis

Reference	Series 1[34]	Series 2[12]	Series 3[14]	Series 4[16]
YEARS OF STUDY	1930–1972	1977–1992	1990–2002	1992–2004
NUMBER REPORTED	266	62	57	85
CARDIAC DEFECT *n* (%)				
CONGENITAL CARDIAC DEFECT (*n, %*)	208 (78%)	40 (64%)	46 (81%)	68 (80%)
Acyanotic (*n*)	NA	18	15	48
Cyanotic (*n*)	NA	22	31	20
RHEUMATIC HEART DISEASE	37 (14%)	3 (5%)	0 (0%)	1 (1%)
NO CARDIAC DEFECT	21 (8%)	19 (31%)	11 (19%)	13 (18%)

NA, not available.

PART II Clinical Syndromes and Cardinal Features of Infectious Diseases: Approach to Diagnosis and Initial Management

SECTION E Cardiac and Vascular Infections

Pathogenesis/Pathologic Findings

Native Valve Endocarditis

The most important factor in the pathogenesis of endocarditis is disruption of the endothelium, typically caused by turbulent blood flow or foreign body in contact with the endocardium or both. Turbulence generally is from an area of high pressure to an area of low pressure, i.e., across a ventricular septal defect or regurgitation through an incompetent valve.[11,17,35,36,40,52] Turbulent flow causes erosion of endothelium, facilitating deposition of platelet-fibrin thrombi on the mural surface or on an abnormal valve on the down-pressure side of turbulent flow.

Important bacterial factors in the pathogenesis of endocarditis include bacteremia/bloodstream infection (BSI) or fungemia and bacterial adhesins. The peptidoglycan surface of oral streptococci facilitates adherence to endothelial cells (see Chapter 121, Viridans Streptococci, *Abiotrophia* and *Granulicatella* Species, and *Streptococcus bovis*). Similarly *S. aureus* binds to collagen, fibronectin, laminin, vitronectin, and fibrinogen.[1,53] Microbial surface components that recognize adhesive matrix molecules (MSCRAMMS) are thought to be virulence factors of *S. aureus*.[8] Patients with *S. aureus* endocarditis have higher serum levels of adhesin molecules than patients with *S. aureus* BSI without endocarditis.[54] The bacterial adhesins of CoNS are less well understood, but may be capsular polysaccharides.[55]

The rate of bacteremia associated with common events and medical procedures is shown in Table 37-3.[56] Dental procedures, such as drainage of an abscess, gingival surgery, and tooth extraction, are particularly likely to cause bacteremia. Transient bacteremia also is common during usual daily activities.[2] Thus, an antecedent event clearly responsible for endocarditis is rarely identified.[2]

Right-sided endocarditis due to a CVC extending into the structurally normal heart is well described. An experimental model of endocarditis in rabbits confirms this pathophysiology; endocarditis only develops when bacteremia is preceded by placement of an intravenous polyethylene catheter across the tricuspid valve into the right ventricle.[46] The catheter acts as a foreign body, abrading endocardial and valvular surfaces and resulting in sterile vegetations that serve as a nidus for infection.

Postoperative Endocarditis

The pathogenesis of endocarditis occurring ≤6 months after surgery (early postoperative endocarditis) and endocarditis occurring more than 6 months after surgery (late postoperative endocarditis) differ. In the early postoperative period, denuded endothelium and exposed sutures are adjacent to prosthetic material; thrombi can form at these sites with fibrin deposition. Endocarditis can result if bacteremia or fungemia occurs due to contamination of intravenous solutions or the cardiac bypass pump (less common), a surgical wound infection, a central line-associated bloodstream infection (CLABSI), or infection of exposed pacemaker wires or intracardiac catheters (also less common). In addition, bacterial or fungal contamination of the operative site can occur due to infected homografts[57,58] or the colonized hands of healthcare personnel.[59] Late postoperative endocarditis occurs after re-endothelialization of cardiac and vascular surfaces. Thus, the natural history and etiology of late postoperative endocarditis more closely resembles that of native valve endocarditis.

Pacemaker and Ventricular Assist Device Infections

While placement of pacemakers and cardioverter-defibrillators in children and adolescents is rare, the use of these devices is increasing in both children and adults.[60,61] Infections of these devices usually occur from contamination during placement and involvement of the pulse-generator pocket. Endocarditis is relatively rare and accounts for approximately 10% of implantable device-associated infections,[3,62] although younger patients may have more frequent lead-wire infections than older patients.[61,63] Complete removal of the device is recommended when a deep pocket infection occurs due to the high risk of relapse and the potential for contaminating the intravascular portion of the device.[44,62,64]

Ventricular assist devices (VADs) are increasingly being used to support patients awaiting heart transplantation, although there are limited data for VAD-related infections in pediatrics.[65] The rate of infectious complications of VADs is high, occurring in 18% to 59% of patients.[66] Infectious complications include surgical site infections, BSIs, and endocarditis presenting as relapsing BSI.[67,68]

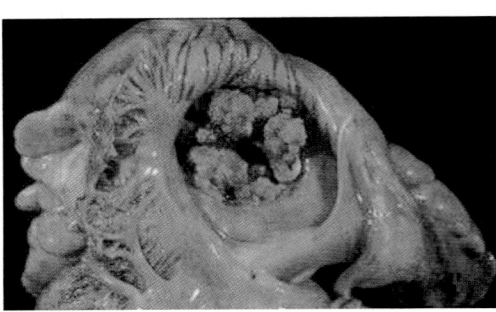

Figure 37-1. Infective endocarditis of the surface of the mitral valve. Note the healing masses at 10:00 and 2:00; this is "subacute" endocarditis with healing granulation tissue and fibrosis microscopically. No exophytic acute vegetation is present. (Courtesy of Charles Marboe, MD, Department of Pathology, Columbia University.)

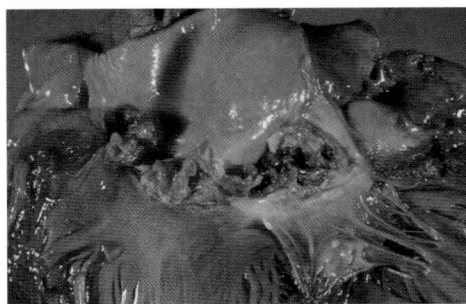

Figure 37-2. Infective endocarditis of the aortic valve. The LV outflow tract is below the severely damaged valve and the aorta is above. The anterior leaflet of the mitral valve is to the right and below the aortic valve. The aortic valve leaflets are almost entirely destroyed by the multiple vegetations of acute endocarditis. (Courtesy of Charles Marboe, MD, Department of Pathology, Columbia University.)

TABLE 37-3. Rate of Bacteremia following Various Procedures

Procedure	Episodes of Bacteremia Per Episode[a]	
	Mean Percent	**Range Percents**
Tooth extraction	60%	18–85
Periodontal surgery	88%	60–90
Tonsillectomy	35%	33–38
Rigid bronchoscopy	15%	
Tracheal intubation	<10%	0–16
Urinary tract catheter insertion or removal	13%	0–26
Upper endoscopy	4%	0–8
Barium enema	10%	5–11
Colonoscopy	5%	0–5
Cardiac catheterization	2%	0–5

[a]*Data from reference 56.*

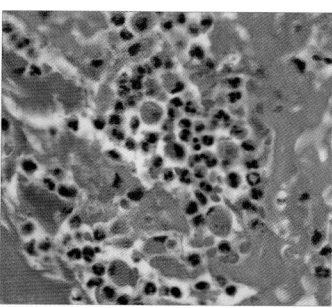

Figure 37-3. The histopathology of infective endocarditis. Vegetations are composed of neutrophils, macrophages and fibrin (red). Organisms are present in acute, untreated endocarditis. (Courtesy of Charles Marboe, MD, Department of Pathology, Columbia University.)

TABLE 37-4. Frequency of Symptoms Associated with Pediatric Infective Endocarditis

Symptom	% Frequency[a]
Fever	75–100
Malaise	50–75
Anorexia/weight loss	25–50
Heart failure	25–50
Arthralgia	17–50
Chest pain	0–25
Neurologic symptoms (focal neurologic deficit, aseptic meningitis)	0–25
Gastrointestinal symptoms	0–50

[a]Data from references 12, 18, 35, 36, 40, 69, 136

Management of VAD-related infections is highly complex due to the critical need for the device, the presence of intravascular and intracardiac foreign material, and high risk of relapse.

Pathologic Lesions

Gross findings. Vegetations can be single or multiple and vary in size from 1 to 2 mm to several centimeters (Figures 37-1 and 37-2).[1] Endocarditis can destroy the underlying valve or perforate valve leaflets; rupture the chordae tendineae, papillary muscle, interventricular septum; or lead to abscess of the valve ring. Healing can result in fibrosis and calcification. Myocardial abscesses and pericarditis also can be a gross pathologic finding.
Microscopic findings. Vegetations consist of fibrin, platelets, and bacteria. Neutrophils and red blood cells also can be seen (Figure 37-3).
Embolic findings. Pathologic processes following emboli to distal organs consist of abscesses or infarction or both. In the kidney, the lesions of glomerulonephritis are characterized by subepithelial deposits containing IgG, IgM, IgA, or complement. Mycotic aneurysms are detected most commonly in the central nervous system and arise from direct bacterial invasion, embolic occlusion or immune complex deposition within the arterial wall. Intracerebral or subarachnoid hemorrhage can result from emboli. Emboli to the lung can result in pneumonia, empyema, or effusion.

Clinical Manifestations

Symptoms

The clinical presentations of endocarditis have been categorized as either subacute or acute. Subacute endocarditis generally manifests as a prodrome of moderate illness with nonspecific symptoms for several weeks. Acute endocarditis generally has a short prodrome and a sepsis-like presentation. However, individual cases can have mixed features and the presentation is not always predictive of the infecting microorganism.

Common symptoms of endocarditis in children are shown in Table 37-4. The subtle and nonspecific nature of symptoms can delay diagnosis for weeks.[17,40,69,70] Endocarditis should be suspected in patients with: (1) congenital heart disease or other risk factors for endocarditis with unexplained fever and fatigue (or anemia) that can remit temporarily when oral antibiotics are prescribed; (2) congenital heart disease with new onset of congestive heart failure or conduction abnormalities especially if accompanied by fever; (3) abrupt onset of septicemia or appearance of vascular lesions in soft tissues or mucous membranes; and (4) structurally normal hearts in whom CVC has been removed but blood cultures are persistently positive.

As vegetations, especially those on valve leaflets, increase in size, they can break off into the circulation. Significant morbidity can result from infectious emboli to the lungs (right-sided endocarditis), or to the central nervous system, spleen and extremities (left-sided endocarditis). Embolic events can be the predominant clinical feature in some patients.[71,72] Thus, patients with fever and neurologic symptoms or with pneumonia or pulmonary emboli should be promptly evaluated for endocarditis.

Physical Examination

Table 37-5 provides the physical findings that can be present in endocarditis.[4] Subtle changes in an existing murmur or detection of a new murmur in a febrile and tachycardiac child may be difficult to appreciate. In patients with rapidly progressive infection, physical examination may not reveal the usual signs of endocarditis, and thus, endocarditis is suspected due to underlying heart disease or persistently positive blood cultures. Signs due to deposition of immune complexes composed of bacterial antigens, antibodies, and complement are rare in children.[1] These include Osler nodes, i.e., small (2 to 15 mm), painful, purplish lesions in the pulp of the fingers or toes that persist for hours or days; Janeway lesions, i.e., painless hemorrhagic macular plaques on the palms or soles due to emboli that persist for days; or Roth spots, i.e., small hemorrhagic retinal lesions with a pale center, usually near the optic disk. In addition, splinter hemorrhages, i.e., dark linear streaks in the nail beds, can result from microemboli.

Differential Diagnosis

When the onset of endocarditis is abrupt, the differential diagnosis includes septicemia, septic shock, and other acute cardiac inflammatory diseases, such as myocarditis, pericarditis, or rheumatic fever. Persistent BSI can arise from suppurative thrombophlebitis as described below. If the onset of endocarditis is insidious, with prolonged or intermittent fever, the differential

TABLE 37-5. Frequency of Signs Associated with Infective Endocarditis in Children

Sign	% Frequency[a]
Fever	75–100
Splenomegaly	50–75
Petechiae	21–50
Embolic phenomenon	25–50
New or changed murmur	21–50
Clubbing	0–10
Osler nodes	0–10
Roth spots	0–10
Janeway lesions	0–10
Splinter hemorrhages	0–10
Conjunctival hemorrhages	0–10

[a]Data collated from references 12, 18, 35, 36, 40, 69, 136.

PART II Clinical Syndromes and Cardinal Features of Infectious Diseases: Approach to Diagnosis and Initial Management

SECTION E Cardiac and Vascular Infections

TABLE 37-6. Relative Frequency of Common Laboratory Findings Associated with Pediatric Infective Endocarditis

Abnormal Laboratory Finding	% Frequency[a]
Positive blood culture	75–100
Elevated erythrocyte sedimentation rate	75–100
Anemia	75–90
Presence of rheumatoid factor	25–50
Hematuria	25–50
Low serum complement	5–40

[a]Data collated from references 12, 18, 35, 36, 40, 69, 136.

diagnosis includes fever of unknown origin, prolonged viral illness, and collagen vascular disorders, such as juvenile idiopathic arthritis or systemic lupus erythematosus (SLE). In patients with SLE or the antiphospholipid syndrome, sterile, verrucous vegetations called Libman–Sacks vegetations can be misdiagnosed as infective endocarditis.[73] Other echocardiographic findings that can mimic endocarditis include ruptured chordae and flail leaflet, severe myxomatous valvular changes, and some cardiac tumors.

If the complications of endocarditis are the main clinical presentation, the differential diagnosis includes strokes, vasculitis, or cerebral vascular malformations. Glomerulonephritis also can be the predominant presenting pathology and endocarditis must be distinguished from other causes of nephritis such as vasculitis.[74,75]

Laboratory Findings and Diagnosis

Ancillary Laboratory Tests

The laboratory tests that support the diagnosis of endocarditis are presented in Table 37-6. However, with the exception of positive blood cultures, these tests are nonspecific and are not diagnostic criteria for endocarditis. In contrast, immunologic phenomena, including presence of rheumatoid factor, hematuria, nephritis, and low serum complement associated with glomerulonephritis,

are considered minor diagnostic criteria.[76] Laboratory evidence of cardiac injury, i.e., elevated serum levels of troponin I and B-type natriuretic peptide, is associated with worse outcomes in adults and may play a role in identifying patients who would benefit from surgical intervention.[77,78]

Microbiologic Evaluation

Persistent bacteremia or fungemia is the most helpful laboratory test in endocarditis. In streptococcal endocarditis, 96% and 98% of the first versus second blood cultures were found to be positive.[79] In endocarditis caused by other species, 82% to 94% and 100% of the first versus second blood cultures yielded the diagnosis.[80] Nevertheless, it is recommended that 3 to 5 blood culture specimens be collected from separate venipuncture sites to optimize recovery of a pathogen, particularly if the pathogen is a fastidious microorganism. If recent antibiotics have been received and the patient is clinically stable, antimicrobial therapy should be suspended for 24 hours to improve the yield of blood cultures.

The clinical significance of a single positive blood culture, particularly with a possible contaminant (e.g., CoNS or occasionally viridans streptococci) can be difficult to assess. However, if multiple blood cultures are obtained and only one is positive, endocarditis is unlikely. Ideally both anaerobic and aerobic bottles are inoculated with 3 to 5 mL per bottle from smaller children and 10 mL per bottle from larger children to optimize detection of pathogens, particularly in the setting of low level bacteremia.[81] If limited blood is available for culture, the aerobic bottle should be inoculated.

The clinical microbiology laboratory should be alerted that endocarditis is being considered. Modern blood culture technologies can detect nutritionally variant streptococci and the AACEK organisms. Prolonged incubation or specialized media are rarely required. As shown in Table 37-7, serologic tests (e.g., for *Coxiella*, *Chlamydia*, *Bartonella*, *Legionella* antibody), urine antigen tests (e.g., *Legionella*), and molecular technologies, i.e., polymerase chain reaction testing for 16S rDNA performed on excised valves and serum specimens (e.g., *Bartonella*) are important adjunctive tests available in reference laboratories in difficult, "culture-negative" cases.[1,29,82] However, with the exception of *C. burnetii*

TABLE 37-7. Adjuvant Diagnostic Testing for Culture-Negative Endocarditis[29,30]

Pathogen	Test	Comment
Aspergillus species	Serology	Indirect hemagglutination assay
Bartonella henselae, *Bartonella quintana*	Blood culture	Direct inoculation of blood agar, 5% CO_2 and shell vial
	Valve culture	Indirect immunofluorescent antibody test; titer ≥1:800
	Serology	Western immunoblot
Brucella melitensis	Serology	IgG ≥1:200[a]
Chlamydia species	Serology?	Serologic cross-reactivity with *Bartonella* spp.
		Role as pathogen in endocarditis remains uncertain
Coxiella burnetti	Blood/valve culture	Routine or heparinized blood inoculated in shell vials to detect bacteria by immunofluorescence[a]
	Serology	Anti-phase I immunoglobulin G antibody titer >1:800 is major criterion
	Polymerase chain reaction	IgG, IgA, IgM to phase I and phase II[a]
		htpAB-associated repetitive element[a]
Legionella pneumophila	Serology	Indirect immunofluorescent antibodies ≥1:256
	Urine antigen	Available for serogroup 1
Mycoplasma pnemoniae	Serology	IgG ≥1:200[a]
Tropheryma whipplei	See below	Etiologic agent of Whipple disease
Unknown	16S rDNA blood	Universal primer to identify bacteria by amplification and sequencing[a]
	16S rRNA valve	Universal primer for yeast
	18S rDNA blood	
	18S rRNA valve	
	Pathology of valve	Immunoenzymatic assay with polyclonal specific antibodies for *Coxiella*, *Bartonella*, *Chlamydia*, *Tropheryma*[a]

[a]Available in reference laboratories.

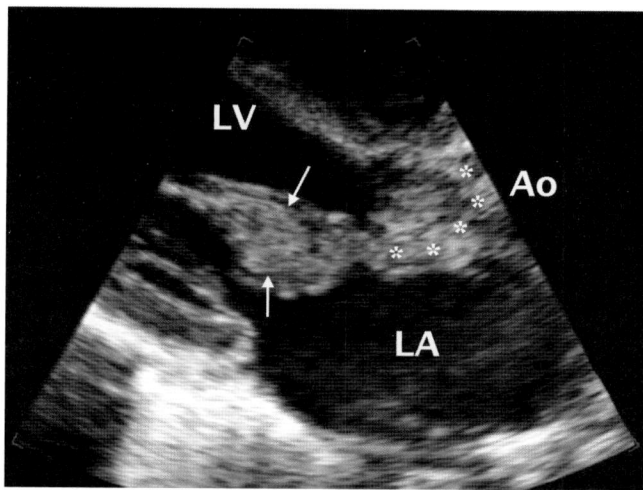

Figure 37-4. A large vegetation (arrows) involving the mitral valve. The primary lesion originated from a bicuspid aortic valve with direct extension to the intervalvular fibrosa. The associated large aortic root abscess is marked by the asterisks (*). The aortic valve is not seen on this particular image. Ao, aorta; LA, left atrium, LV, left ventricle.

antibodies, these diagnostic assays are not standardized or available widely and hence are not yet diagnostic criteria in the modified Duke classification.[1,83]

Diagnostic Imaging

Echocardiography is the main diagnostic imaging modality to identify the pathology and cardiac complications of endocarditis and must be performed early to insure rapid diagnosis and appropriate treatment. Two-dimensional imaging can visualize vegetations as small as 2 mm, intracardiac abscesses and other perivalvular abnormalities, valvular dehiscence and insufficiency as shown in Figure 37-4. However, echocardiography can be

falsely negative early in the disease process due to small vegetations or embolization[1] and should be repeated within 7 to 10 days if there is continuing suspicion for endocarditis.[5] Color and spectral doppler imaging can demonstrate flow through cardiac structures and the hemodynamic consequences of pathological lesions.

In adult populations, transthoracic echocardiography (TTE) has significantly lower sensitivity (40% to 63%) compared with transesophageal echocardiography (TEE) (≥90%).[84–88] However, in pediatrics, TEE is used less frequently because of the relative invasiveness of TEE, technical limitations in very small children, and the higher sensitivity of TTE (≥80%).[1,89–93] Nevertheless, TEE does have a role in pediatrics to evaluate prosthetic valves, to assess certain complications, particularly abscesses,[4] and to evaluate patients with complex anatomy with previous cardiac surgery. Intraoperatively, TEE is invaluable to improve visualization of lesions and to assess surgical results.

Echocardiography also plays a central role in the treatment of patients with endocarditis.[94,95] Serial echocardiograms are used to monitor heart function and enlarging vegetations as well as to detect complications that may require surgery such as perivalvular extension and abscesses. Echocardiography can be used to assess the risk of embolization as vegetation size (>10 mm), location

---

BOX 37-1. Modified Duke Clinical Criteria for Diagnosis of Infective Endocarditis[a]

DEFINITE INFECTIVE ENDOCARDITIS
Pathologic Criteria
1. Microorganisms demonstrated by culture or histology in a vegetation, embolized vegetation, or intracardiac abscess
2. Pathologic lesions (vegetation or intracardiac abscess) with active endocarditis confirmed by histology

Clinical Criteria
1. 2 major criteria
2. 1 major and 3 minor criteria
3. 5 minor criteria

POSSIBLE INFECTIVE ENDOCARDITIS
1. 1 major criterion and 1 minor criterion
2. 3 minor criteria

REJECTED
1. Firm alternative diagnosis for manifestations of endocarditis
2. Resolution of endocarditis manifestations with antibiotic therapy ≤4 days
3. No pathologic evidence of infective endocarditis at surgery or autopsy with antibiotic therapy for ≤4 days
4. Does not fulfill criteria above

[a]Modified from reference 83. Any one of the numbered findings listed above are taken as evidence.

BOX 37-2. Definitions of Major and Minor Criteria Used in the Duke Schema for the Diagnosis of Infective Endocarditis (IE)[a]

MAJOR CRITERIA
1. Positive blood culture for IE
   a. Typical microorganism consistent with IE from two separate blood cultures:
      (i) Viridans streptococci[b]
      (ii) *Streptococcus bovis*
      (iii) AACEK group (see group)
      (iv) *Staphylococcus aureus*
      (v) Community-acquired enterococci (without a primary focus)
   b. Microorganism consistent with IE from persistently positive blood cultures if:
      (i) At least 2 positive blood cultures sampled more than 12 hours apart
      (ii) All 3 or a majority of more than 4 blood cultures
   c. Single positive blood culture for *Coxiella burnetii* or IgG antibody titer >1:800
2. Evidence of endocardial involvement by positive echocardiogram for IE, defined as:
   (i) Oscillating intracardiac mass on valve or supporting structures, in the path of regurgitant jets, or on implanted material
   (ii) Abscess
   (iii) New partial dehiscence of prosthetic valve
   (iv) New valvular regurgitation (worsening or changing of pre-existing murmur not sufficient)

MINOR CRITERIA
1. Predisposing heart condition or intravenous drug abuse
2. Fever: temperature ≥38.0°C
3. Vascular phenomena: major arterial emboli, septic pulmonary infarcts, mycotic aneurysm, intracranial hemorrhage, conjunctival hemorrhages, Janeway lesions
4. Immunologic phenomena: glomerulonephritis, Osler nodes, Roth spots, rheumatoid factor
5. Microbiologic evidence: positive blood culture but does not meet major criteria or serologic evidence of active infection with organism consistent with IE

[a]Modified from reference 83.
[b]Includes nutritionally variant strains (*Abiotrophia* species).

PART II Clinical Syndromes and Cardinal Features of Infectious Diseases: Approach to Diagnosis and Initial Management

SECTION E Cardiac and Vascular Infections

TABLE 37-8. Antimicrobial Agents for Treatment of Pediatric Infective Endocarditis Caused by Gram-positive Cocci

Definitive Therapy	Agent	Prosthetic Material or Artificial Valves	
		Duration, if Absent	Duration, if Present
STREPTOCOCCI			
Highly susceptible to penicillin (MIC ≤0.12 μg/mL) includes most viridans, and nonenterococcal group D (*Streptococcus bovis*)	Penicillin G (or ampicillin) *or*	4 weeks	6 weeks
	Cetriaxone *or*	4 weeks	6 weeks (±2 weeks gentamicin)
	Penicillin G *plus* gentamicin *or*	2 weeks	Not applicable
	Ceftrixone *plus* gentamicin *or*	2 weeks	Not applicable
	Vancomycin[a]	4 weeks	6 weeks
Relatively resistant to penicillin (MIC >0.12 to ≤0.5 μg/mL)	Penicillin G *or*	4 weeks	6 weeks (±6 weeks gentamicin)
	Cetriaxone *plus* gentamicin *or*	4 weeks (gentamicin 2 weeks)	6 weeks (± 6 weeks gentamicin)
	Vancomycin[a]	4 weeks	6 weeks
Resistant to penicillin (MIC >0.5 μg/mL) (*Abiotrophia, Granulicatella, Gemella* spp.)	Penicillin G (or ampicillin) or Ceftriaxone *plus* gentamicin *or*	4–6 weeks	6 weeks (+ 6 weeks gentamicin)
	Vancomycin[a]	6 weeks	6 weeks
ENTEROCOCCI			
Susceptible to penicillin, vancomycin, gentamicn[c]	Ampicillin (or penicillin) *plus* streptomycin	4–6 weeks	4–6 weeks (+4–6 weeks gentamicin[c])
	Vancomycin[a] *plus* gentamicin[c]	6 weeks	6 weeks (+6 weeks gentamicin[c])
Resistant to penicillin, susceptible to vancomycin			
B-lactamase-producer	Ampicillin-sulbactam *plus* gentamicin[b]	6 weeks	6 weeks
Intrinsic resistance	Vancomycin *plus* gentamicin[b]	6 weeks	6 weeks
Resistant to penicillin, vancomycin, aminoglycoside *E. faecium*	Linezolid or Quinupristin-dalfopristin	≥8 weeks	≥8 weeks
STAPHYLOCOCCI			
Staphylococcus aureus or coagulase-negative staphylococci			
Susceptible to oxacillin	Oxacillin (or nafcillin) *plus* (optional gentamcin)	6 weeks (3–5 days)	≥6 weeks *plus*
	Cefazolin *plus* (optional gentamcin)	6 weeks (3–5 days)	≥6 weeks rifampin *plus* 2 weeks gentamcin
Resistant to oxacillin	Vancomycin	6 weeks	≥6 weeks *plus* ≥6 weeks *plus* rifampin *plus* 2 weeks gentamcin

MIC, minimal inhibitory concentration.

[a]If unable to tolerate β-lactam agent.

[b]If susceptible to gentamicin.

[c]If resistant to gentamicin, use streptomycin.

Table modified from reference 1.

(mitral valve anterior leaflet), and increased mobility may predict clinically important embolization.[71,96,97]

In adult populations, three-dimensional echocardiography can improve characterization of the pathology associated with endocarditis.[98–100] Cardiac magnetic resonance imaging (MRI) and computerized tomography (CT) also have been introduced as adjunctive imaging strategies.[101–103]

Diagnostic Criteria

The diagnosis of endocarditis is obvious in the setting of new murmur or new valvular vegetations and blood cultures that yield an organism that commonly causes endocarditis. However, the diagnosis of endocarditis can be more difficult in high-risk patients with negative blood cultures, intermittently positive blood cultures, or with blood cultures positive for unusual or fastidious pathogens. Thus diagnostic criteria have been developed and revised; the Von Reyn (or Beth Israel) criteria[104] were replaced by the Duke criteria,[105,106] which were followed by the modified Duke

criteria (Boxes 37-1 and 37-2).[83] The last is widely accepted for diagnosing endocarditis[1,94] and can be used in children[4,107,108]

Management

When endocarditis is suspected, urgent evaluation of hemodynamic status is critical. If signs and symptoms of heart failure are present, an echocardiogram and several closely spaced blood cultures are obtained quickly. Empiric antibiotic therapy and hemodynamic support must be provided without delay. Patients with heart failure often require urgent cardiac surgery, which can be life-saving.

Empiric Antibiotic Therapy

Presumptive antibiotic therapy is based on patient age, clinical presentation, pre-existing cardiac status, recent surgery, prior episodes of BSI or endocarditis, community versus healthcare acquisition, and local antimicrobial susceptibility patterns. Antimicrobial

TABLE 37-9. Doses of Commonly Used Antibiomicrobial Agents Recommended to Treat Infective Endocarditis

Antimicrobial Agent	Total Daily Dose[a]		
	Children	Adults[b]	Dose Interval
Ampicillin	300 mg/kg	12 g	4–6 hours
Cefazolin	100 mg/kg	6 g	8 hours
Ceftriaxone	100 mg/kg[b]	2 g[c]	24 hours
Penicillin G			
If native valve and PCN-susceptible (MIC ≤0.12 μg/mL)	200,000 U/kg	12–18 million U	4–6 hours
If native valve and PCN-resistant (MIC >0.12 μg/mL)	300,000 U/kg	24 million U	
If prosthetic material	300,000 U/kg	24 million U	
If enterococci PCN-susceptible	300,000 U/kg	18–30 million U	
Gentamicin[c]	3 mg/kg	3 mg/kg	8 hours *or* as single dose q 24 hours
Oxacillin, nafcillin	200 mg/kg	12 g	4–6 hours
Streptomycin	20–30 mg/kg	15 mg/kg	Div 12 hours
Vancomycin[c]	40 mg/kg	30 mg/kg Max: 2 g/day	Children 8 hours Adults 12 hours

MIC, minimal inhibitory concentration; PCN, penicillin.

[a]Doses are recommended for normal renal function.

[b]Calculate maximum dose for large children and adolescents.

[c]Dosage adjustment is necessary when renal insufficiency exists.

treatment for endocarditis in children is derived from recommendations developed for adults (Tables 37-8 and 37-9). High doses of bactericidal antibiotics are strongly preferred; penetration of bioactive cells and substances into the infected vegetation can be difficult and bacteriostatic agents are less effective. When combinations of agents – generally a β-lactam agent plus an aminoglycoside – are used to provide synergistic effects, these should be delivered close together temporally to maximize potential activity.[1] If blood cultures are sterile, but symptoms respond to therapy, the initial regimen can be continued while pursuing other diagnostic strategies (described above).

Definitive Antibiotic Therapy: Drug, Dose, Duration

Recommendations for treatment of endocarditis depend on the pathogen, in vitro susceptibility test results, presence of a foreign body (e.g., prosthetic valve), the need for surgery either to remove the vegetation or to replace a dysfunctional valve, or because of embolic complications or combinations thereof (Tables 37-8 and 37-9).[1,109,110] When clinical experience is limited, such as with endocarditis caused by multidrug-resistant organisms, recommendations are based on case reports, expert opinion, or data from animal models. Endocarditis caused by *S. pneumoniae* or group A, B, C, or G streptococci requires 4 weeks of treatment with penicillin if susceptible (*S. pneumoniae* minimal inhibitory concentration (MIC) ≤0.1 μg/mL). Relatively resistant (MIC >0.1–1.0 μg/mL) or resistant (≥2.0 μg/mL) strains can be treated with high-dose penicillin or a third-generation cephalosporin agent.[1]

Endocarditis due to enterococci generally is treated with a combination of ampicillin plus an aminoglycoside.[1,111,112] Gentamicin is prescribed as a single dose every 24 hours to achieve a trough concentration <1 μg/mL. Some enterococcal spp., as well as rarer causes of endocarditis such as *Abiotrophia defectiva*, *Gemella* spp., and *Granulicatella* spp. (formerly known as nutritionally variant streptococci), are inherently less susceptible to penicillin (MIC >0.5 μg/mL) and are treated using the regimens described for enterococci.[1,111,113] If the enterococcal isolate is resistant to ampicillin or the patient is allergic to penicillin, vancomycin plus an aminoglycoside is used and trough levels of vancomycin should be 10–15 μg/mL. Vancomycin-resistant enterococcal endocarditis is treated with multiple-drug regimens,[114,115] linezolid,[116,117] or quinupristin/dalfopristin.[65]

Patients with *S. aureus* or *S. epidermidis* resistant to oxacillin should be treated with vancomycin (Table 37-8). The addition of a second agent for treatment of staphylococcal endocarditis (generally gentamicin for 3 to 5 days for left-sided endocarditis) is optional, except in patients with endocarditis of prosthetic valves or failing to respond to antimicrobial therapy.[1] Compared with streptococcal endocarditis, the treatment response of children with staphylococcal endocarditis is more protracted, with a mean of 2 days to sterile blood cultures, and mean of 7 days to defervescence including more than 14 days of fever in 17% of cases.[18] To date, glycopeptide-intermediate *S. aureus* (GISA), heterogeneous GISA, and glycopeptide-resistant *S. aureus* are rarely associated with endocarditis; such strains also are resistant to daptomycin.[110] Treatment of endocarditis caused by such strains is challenging.

For endocarditis caused by enteric gram-negative bacilli, two bactericidal agents are chosen on the basis of in vitro susceptibility and generally include an expanded-spectrum β-lactam agent and an aminoglycoside.[1] The AACEK organisms frequently express β-lactamases and are slow growing, which makes susceptibility testing more difficult to perform. Thus, treatment with a third-generation cephalosporin or ampicillin-sulbactam is recommended.[1]

Management of endocarditis caused by *Candida* and *Aspergillus* spp. generally includes both medical and surgical approaches (discussed below) to optimize cure. Rare cases of fungal endocarditis have been managed successfully with fungicidal therapy alone.[118,119] Traditionally, amphotericin or lipid amphotericin products have been used,[120] but caspofungin[121,122] and voriconazole[123] may be less toxic therapeutic alternatives. Unfortunately, pharmacokinetic studies with these newer agents have not been performed in neonates. "Lifelong" (long-term) fluconazole prophylaxis has been advocated in patients with fungal endocarditis to prevent relapses or as suppressive therapy in patients not deemed to be surgical candidates.[1]

Duration of treatment is based on the pathogen and antimicrobial susceptibility, the presence of prosthetic cardiac material, and the clinical course. In children with native valve endocarditis due to viridans streptococci, 4 weeks of penicillin G alone is effective and may be preferred because of limited experience with the 2-week regimen in children. Treatment for 6 weeks generally is recommended in "high-risk" situations, including infection due to relatively resistant streptococci or to enterococci, staphylococci,

PART II Clinical Syndromes and Cardinal Features of Infectious Diseases: Approach to Diagnosis and Initial Management

SECTION E Cardiac and Vascular Infections

gram-negative bacilli, and in patients with intravascular prosthetic material. For the AACEK organisms, 4 weeks (if native valve) or 6 weeks (if prosthetic valve) of treatment is recommended. At least 6 weeks of therapy is recommended for patients with enterococcal endocarditis who have had a longer duration of symptoms, i.e., >3 months.[1] Even more prolonged courses are recommended for complicated endocarditis (e.g., intracardiac abscess) and in patients who have a slow response to therapy. Regardless of surgical intervention, fungal endocarditis should be treated with prolonged courses (≥6 weeks) of parenteral antifungal agents followed by oral fluconazole as describe above.

There is a role for outpatient management for endocarditis. Although there are not controlled trials documenting safety of such an approach, careful selection of clinically stable patients at low risk for complications (specifically heart failure and/or embolic phenomena) is possible, providing that meticulous catheter care and close follow-up is ensured.[124]

Antibiotics are almost always administered intravenously. Although there are reports of successful oral treatment of endocarditis, including with linezolid[116,125] and voriconazole,[123] this strategy has not been studied systematically and is generally not recommended. In addition, there are reports of successful management with antibiotics given orally for *S. aureus* endocarditis in intravenous drug abusers who are not candidates for parenteral therapy.[1]

Surgery

Timely surgical intervention can be critical to optimal management of endocarditis.[126] Guidelines for surgical intervention have been advised by the AHA expert advisory panel[1] and the European Society of Cardiology.[5] While these guidelines emphasize the need to individualize management of endocarditis, they provide guidance for adjunctive surgery that can reduce the risk of mortality. Surgery should be strongly considered early in patients with congestive heart failure, at high risk for embolization, and with prosthetic valve endocarditis. Generally, removal of prosthetic material

TABLE 37-10. Potential Indications for Surgical Intervention for Endocarditis and Recommendations for Timing of Surgery[a]

Indication	Timing[b]
Heart failure	
(1) Heart failure (valvular regurgitation, obstruction, fistula) with refractory pulmonary edema or shock	Emergent
(2) Persistent heart failure or echocardiographic signs of poor tolerance such as early mitral closure or pulmonary hypertension	Urgent
(3) Severe aortic or mitral regurgitation without heart failure	Elective
Uncontrolled infection	
(1) Evidence of perivalvular extension (abscess,[c] false aneurysm, fistula, complete heart block) or enlarging vegetation with treatment	Urgent
(2) Persistent fever and positive blood culture for more than 7–10 days	Urgent
(3) Fungi/mold/multidrug-resistant organisms	Urgent
Prevention of left-sided embolism from aortic or mitral valve endocarditis with:	
(1) Large vegetation (>10 mm) following 1 or more embolic events	Urgent
(2) Large vegetation (>10 mm) with other predictors of complicated course including heart failure, persistent infection, or abscess	Urgent
Very large vegetation (>15 mm)	Urgent

[a]*Adapted from references 1 and 5.*

[b]*Emergency, <24 hours; Urgent, within a few days; Elective, >1 week of treatment.*

[c]*In some instances, small abscesses or pseudoaneurysms can be treated medically.*

(e.g., a patch or conduit) in children is not necessary, with the exception of pacemaker wires. A summary of these recommendations is included in Table 37-10.[93,127–129] The European guidelines also recommend preservation of the native valve, particularly the mitral valve if possible,[130] and resection of vegetations >10 mm after one or more embolic events.

Following embolic complications, surgical resection of an enlarging mycotic aneurysm in the cerebral vasculature is necessary if neurologic symptoms or bleeding ensue. Delayed splenic rupture due to emboli is a potentially fatal complication of endocarditis. Large emboli to major blood vessels can lead to cold, painful, and pulseless extremities and require immediate surgical intervention. Major embolic events are associated especially with fungal endocarditis.

Anticoagulation

There is no evidence that anticoagulation therapy with either aspirin or other agents is beneficial in endocarditis. However, controversy exists regarding management of patients receiving anticoagulation therapy who subsequently develop endocarditis, particularly with *S. aureus* or in the setting of prosthetic valve endocarditis; such patients have a very high risk of hemorrhagic stroke.[1,5,131,132] There is increasing evidence that, during cardiopulmonary bypass for urgent surgery following an embolic stroke, anticoagulation is not absolutely contraindicated.[133–135]

Complications

Complications of endocarditis include direct valvular damage, perivalvar extension of infection, or heart failure. Infection can disrupt valvular structure and cause leaflet fenestrations and chordae rupture, which can result in secondary valvular incompetence and heart failure. Heart failure also can be caused by obstructive vegetations or new shunt lesions leading to extensive damage to cardiac structures. Perivalvar extension can lead to endocardial abscesses, secondary fistulas, or pseudoaneurysms. Most abscesses in children are associated with native aortic valve and *S. aureus* endocarditis.[95] Clues to possible abscess formation include persistent fever and BSI; conduction abnormalities occur less frequently than is reported in adults with abscesses.

Emboli from right-sided endocarditis can cause necrotizing pneumonia and prolonged fever, although outcomes following complications of right-sided endocarditis generally are good with prolonged therapy. Emboli from left-sided endocarditis cause systemic emboli to the brain, visceral organs, limbs, and coronary arteries. The greatest risk of emboli is associated with *S. aureus*, *Candida*, the AACEK organisms, and *Abiotrophia*.[1] Large (>10 mm) left-sided vegetations, particularly of the mitral valve, are associated with a higher risk of significant embolic events.[13,71,89,136–140] Septic emboli can result in hemorrhage, infarct, or abscess of the involved viscera. Emboli to the central nervous system can result in stroke and/or mycotic aneurysms. The risk of neurologic events has not been well defined in children, but 6% of pediatric patients with endocarditis were reported to have a stroke.[141] Most embolic events occur before or within the first 2 weeks of appropriate therapy.[140] Acute renal failure can occur from immune complex deposition, renal infarction, hemodynamic instability, adverse effects of antibiotic therapy, or combinations of these factors.

Prognosis

Cure rates for endocarditis depend on the infecting organism, the site of endocarditis, embolic phenomena, and the underlying clinical state of the host. More than 90% of children with native valve endocarditis due to viridans streptococci are cured.[12,69,70,136,142] Enterococcal endocarditis, if synergistic antibiotics are available, has a cure rate of 75% to 90%. The cure rate for methicillin-susceptible *S. aureus* (MSSA) endocarditis may be as low as 60% to 75%, but the cure rate does not appear to be lower for MRSA. For gram-negative bacilli, the cure rate is even lower, particularly for left-sided disease. Fungal endocarditis due to yeasts and filamentous fungi have the poorest prognosis, with cure rates <50% and <20%, respectively.

Features associated with a poorer prognosis include heart failure; presence of prosthetic cardiac material, especially artificial heart valves; extremes of age (infants and the elderly); and the formation of large vegetations >10 mm. Persistence of fever for ≥2 weeks has been shown to be associated with increased morbidity (myocardial abscesses, urgent cardiac surgery, healthcare-associated complications) and mortality.[143]

In some series, the prognosis of endocarditis, including crude mortality, has not improved in the modern era.[16,144] In contrast, a significant reduction in mortality was achieved when a therapeutic protocol was implemented by an interdisciplinary team of infectious disease and microbiology specialists, cardiologists, and cardiac surgeons for adults with endocarditis; one year mortality decreased from 18.5% to 8.2%.[145]

Prevention

In 2007, the AHA modified antibiotic prophylaxis guidelines as existing evidence does not support widespread prophylaxis (see Chapter 7, Chemoprophylaxis).[146] The procedures for which prophylaxis is recommended have been reduced and the antibiotic regimens have been simplified.[5] In fact, the National Institute for Health and Clinical Excellence of England and Wales (NICE) is no longer recommending prophylaxis for dental procedures.[147]

OTHER "ENDOCARDITIS-LIKE" INTRAVASCULAR INFECTIONS

Other types of infection can present as persistent BSI (bacterial or fungal). These include septic (or suppurative) thrombophlebitis or, more commonly, CLABSI.[148] Septic thrombophlebitis is rare in children; 0.12% of hospital admissions were associated with this entity and the rate is likely to be lower today due to improvements in catheter insertion and maintenance strategies.[149]

Risk factors for septic thrombophlebitis include prolonged use (>96 hours) of intravascular catheters, surgical manipulation of a vessel, extension of infection from adjacent nonvascular structures, or severe burns.

The pathogenesis of septic thrombophlebitis is as follows: sterile thrombi or fibrin clots form on catheters, generally at the distal tip, or at the site of a surgical anastomosis or vascular prosthesis. Phlebitis results from trauma or irritation of the vessel wall, e.g., from infused particles during intravenous drug abuse. The clot or inflamed vessel is infected during bacteremia, from contaminated infusates, or from infected adjacent structures.[150] Suppurative thrombophlebitis develops if the vessel wall becomes infected. Progression of infection and inflammation can occlude the vessel, leading to a painful, enlarged, thickened, and tortuous vessel.

Nonvascular infections at adjacent sites can cause well-described septic thrombophlebitis syndromes. Pharyngitis or peritonsillar abscess can cause Lemierre syndrome, i.e., internal jugular vein septic thrombophlebitis.[151] Appendicitis, intra-abdominal infection, or abdominal surgery can cause pylephlebitis, i.e., portal vein septic thrombophlebitis.[148] Septic abortions, pelvic surgery, or pelvic abscesses can cause pelvic vein thrombosis and infection.

Symptoms of superficial thrombophlebitis include fever, chills, induration, warmth, erythema, and tenderness of the infected vessel. In contrast, only about half of patients with central thrombophlebitis have signs of inflammation and symptoms may not occur until several days after catheter removal.[152] Symptoms of portal vein thrombophlebitis include fever, right upper quadrant pain, anorexia, weight loss, and malaise.

The diagnosis of septic thrombophlebitis can be delayed, particularly if the symptoms and signs are not at the site of infection. CT, MRI, and/or ultrasound may demonstrate thrombophlebitis while radionuclide scans are not generally useful.

Blood cultures usually are positive persistently, but pathogens also can be cultured from pus at the exit site, aspiration of the thrombosed vein, or the surgically resected vessel. S. aureus is the most common etiology of suppurative thrombophlebitis, but Enterobacteriaceae or fungi also can cause this entity. Vaginal flora, including Bacteroides spp., streptococcal spp., and gram-negative bacilli cause pelvic thrombophlebitis; and intestinal flora, including gram-negative bacilli and enterococci, cause intra-abdominal thrombophlebitis. Lemierre syndrome usually is caused by Fusobacterium necrophorum in singular or polymicrobial pathogenesis.

Septic thrombophlebitis can be life-threatening, particularly if diagnosis and treatment are delayed. Like cardiac vegetations, these lesions are not vascularized, and penetration of antibiotics into such lesions can be poor. Thus, principles of therapy are similar to those for endocarditis (described above). A fluctuant mass along the course of a previously catheterized vein can be aspirated, and frequently halts persistent BSI. Otherwise, treatment of suppurative thrombophlebitis requires antimicrobial therapy and catheter removal, ligation of the infected vessel, and excision of the infected segment.[148–150,153] If this management fails, further surgical resection or removal of an infected vascular prosthesis may be necessary.

Complications of septic thrombophlebitis can mimic those of endocarditis and include sepsis, hypotension, and septic emboli. The latter can provide the clue to the diagnosis. Lemierre syndrome can present with embolic cavitating pulmonary lesions. Superficial thrombophlebitis can be complicated by subperiosteal abscesses of the long bones that present as bony tenderness and inflammation.[154] Deep-vein thrombophlebitis can be complicated by pulmonary emboli or osteomyelitis.[155] Septic thrombophlebitis of the thoracic central veins following catheterization can lead to the superior vena cava syndrome.

---

38 Myocarditis

Craig A. Shapiro and Joseph A. Hilinski

Myocarditis can manifest in a variety of ways, ranging from nonspecific systemic symptoms such as fever and myalgia, to fulminant heart failure or sudden death. The condition is defined as "inflammation of the heart muscle," and generally refers to diseases not associated solely with valvular abnormalities. There is continued debate regarding appropriate diagnosis, classification, and management of myocarditis.[1,2]

ETIOLOGY

Myocarditis can be a manifestation of almost every infectious agent. For most cases in routine clinical practice, a specific etiology is not found. Viruses remain the most common cause in North America and Europe, and often are presumed to be causative in cases without a proven etiology. Initial studies using serologic

PART II Clinical Syndromes and Cardinal Features of Infectious Diseases: Approach to Diagnosis and Initial Management

SECTION E Cardiac and Vascular Infections

assays implicated enteroviruses as common causes of myocarditis, particularly coxsackievirus B serotypes 1 through 5.[3,4] Studies using molecular techniques such as polymerase chain reaction (PCR) assays of endomyocardial biopsy specimens confirm the importance of enteroviruses as causative agents of acute myocarditis (25% to 35%), as well as of idiopathic dilated cardiomyopathy (10% to 30%).[5-7] In addition, using PCR techniques, other viruses such as adenovirus[7] and parvovirus B19[5,8] have been identified in myocardium. However, assigning a true causal role to these viruses may be difficult.[9,10] Influenza, cytomegalovirus, and Epstein–Barr virus also have been implicated, and myocarditis is recognized as a complication during outbreaks of mumps, measles, influenza, and poliovirus.[7,11,12] Case reports from the 2009/2010 influenza pandemic cite the H1N1 strain of influenza as a possible cause of myocarditis.[13,14] Human immunodeficiency virus and hepatitis C virus have been implicated as causes of myocarditis; however, the exact role each virus plays in causing disease is unclear.[2]

Bacteria less frequently cause myocarditis than viruses. Invasion of the bloodstream by any bacterial pathogen can result in myocardial seeding and microabscesses, such as in complications of *Staphylococcus aureus*, *Neisseria meningitidis*, *Salmonella*, and other bloodstream infections.[15-17] Myocarditis can be a toxin-mediated complication of tetanus or diphtheria, or can be caused by other bacteria such as *Borrelia burgdorferi* (occurring in up to 10% of adults with Lyme disease), *Rickettsia* spp. (especially scrub typhus), and *Mycoplasma pneumoniae*.[18-20]

Parasites are a major cause of myocarditis worldwide, with *Trypanosoma cruzi* (the causative agent of Chagas disease) being the principal cause in South America, with as many as 20% of infected patients developing chronic heart failure.[21] Many additional agents have been reported to cause myocarditis in immunocompromised hosts, most importantly cytomegalovirus, *Toxoplasma gondii*, *T. cruzi*, *Cryptococcus*, *Candida*, and *Aspergillus* species.

EPIDEMIOLOGY

The incidence of myocarditis can coincide with the occurrence of epidemic enterovirus infections. Enteroviruses cause approximately 5 to 10 million symptomatic infections annually in the United States, and occur in all human populations. The rates of infection vary by geographic location, season of the year, and age. In the U.S. enterovirus activity peaks from June through November, although in other parts of the world transmission is year round.[22] Young children are most susceptible, probably because they lack cross-reacting immunity from prior infections.[23] Serologic studies show higher rates of enteroviral illness among people with myocarditis and controls with similar exposures than among people without common exposures.[4] Chagas disease is endemic in South and Central America, and is a leading cause of myocarditis in those regions.[1]

Autopsy series are helpful in demonstrating the incidence of myocarditis as a cause of mortality. Myocarditis has been implicated in 6% to 20% of sudden cardiac deaths in autopsy series of young previously healthy adults.[24,25] Other studies using PCR techniques highlight the possible role of myocarditis in sudden infant death syndrome (SIDS).[26,27] Enteroviruses, parvovirus B19, and adenoviruses were among the most commonly detected viruses in cases associated with SIDS, although Epstein–Barr virus, cytomegalovirus and *Toxoplasma gondii* have also been detected.[28]

PATHOPHYSIOLOGY

Pathogenesis

The pathogenesis of myocarditis has been gleaned in large part from animal models. Both direct myocardial invasion by viruses and host immune responses are important in the pathogenesis of disease. Direct myocyte invasion by infectious agents can initiate the process, which in later stages results in development of both CD4[+] helper and CD8[+] cytotoxic T-lymphocyte responses.[29] Additionally, circulating antiheart antibodies directed against

contractile, structural, and mitochondrial proteins have been described.[2,30] Mouse models show that exercise,[31] cold exposure, malnutrition, pregnancy, and immune suppression can worsen clinical disease in disseminated enteroviral infections, which also can occur in humans.[32] A common coxsackievirus-adenovirus receptor (CAR) on cardiac myocytes has been described, which may offer a partial explanation for the prominence of these viruses as causes of myocarditis.[33] The significance of CAR may be explained by data showing that a decrease in CAR leads to a concomitant decrease in myocardial viral titers in a mouse model.[34]

Pathologic Findings

Several standardized criteria have been developed to classify myocarditis using histopathology. The Dallas pathologic criteria divide conventionally stained heart-tissue biopsy findings into those of active myocarditis (inflammatory cellular infiltrate with evidence of myocyte necrosis), borderline myocarditis (inflammatory cellular infiltrate without evidence of myocyte injury), and no myocarditis. Inflammatory infiltrates are then described as lymphocytic, eosinophilic, or granulomatous; with mild, moderate, or severe inflammation; and focal, confluent, or diffuse distribution.[35] Other pathologic classifications exist using more specific markers and features.[36-38] Regardless of which classification system is used, pathologic guidelines likely underestimate cases of myocarditis for several reasons, most notably biopsy sampling site error, and interobserver variability.

Myocarditis from bacterial, parasitic, and fungal causes can show specific findings. Bacterial and fungal infection result in polymorphonuclear cell infiltrates, which can be focal or organized into microabscesses. Trypanosomes often can be visualized in the biopsy specimens from patients with chronic Chagas disease. Giant-cell myocarditis is a rare disorder in which multinucleated giant cells in the absence of granulomas are found on biopsy; an autoimmune process is suspected.[2]

CLINICAL MANIFESTATIONS

Manifestations of myocarditis can be highly variable, but usually arise in the setting of a systemic infection. Cardiac manifestations range from an asymptomatic state with electrocardiogram (ECG) abnormalities to cardiogenic shock. A viral prodrome is often reported by patients. The prodrome consists of influenza-like complaints including fevers, myalgia, gastroenteritis, chest pain, dyspnea, and tachypnea.[39] This can be followed abruptly by hemodynamic collapse. Sudden death can be a presenting sign of myocarditis at any age, but particularly in infants and children.[40]

Infants and children frequently have nonspecific findings such as feeding difficulties, irritability, respiratory distress, and newonset murmur or cardiac findings. Typical findings of heart failure also can be present. In a retrospective review of 31 children with biopsy confirmed or probable myocarditis, emergency department findings included: preceding "viral illness" (77%), tachypnea or other respiratory difficulty (68%), chest pain (29%), symptoms related to hypoperfusion (23%), Kawasaki-associated symptoms (10%), and gastrointestinal tract complaints (7%). Chest pain in acute myocarditis usually results from associated pericarditis or, occasionally, from coronary artery spasm. Decreased ventricular function seen on echocardiography was present in 73% of cases and ST-T-wave changes were noted on ECG in 67% of cases. Chest radiography abnormalities were observed in 55% of cases.[41]

DIFFERENTIAL DIAGNOSIS

Many conditions mimic infectious myocarditis. Most involve systemic inflammatory conditions, including autoimmune diseases, toxic or hypersensitivity drug reactions, envenomation, endocrinopathies, radiation, and transplant rejection (Box 38-1). Several cardiac diseases can present similarly to or in conjunction with infectious myocarditis. Endocarditis should be distinguishable by primary valvular abnormalities in the presence of positive blood cultures and echocardiographic evidence of vegetations.

INFLAMMATORY DISEASES

Inflammatory bowel disease
Systemic lupus erythematosus
Polymyositis/dermatomyositis
Mixed connective tissue disease
Kawasaki disease
Rheumatic fever
Rheumatoid arthritis
Sarcoidosis
Thyrotoxicosis
Transplant rejection
Giant-cell myocarditis

DRUG REACTIONS

Adriamycin
Alcohol
Amitriptyline
Amphetamines and methamphetamines
Arsenic
Catecholamines
Cefaclor
Cocaine
Cyclophosphamide
Daunorubicin
Furosemide
Isoniazid
Lead
Lithium
Methyldopa
Penicillins
Sulfonamides
Tetracyclines

BITES AND STINGS

Bee
Scorpion
Snake
Spider
Wasp

IDIOPATHIC CAUSES (LYMPHOCYTIC)

PERIPARTUM PERIOD

PHEOCHROMOCYTOMA

RADIATION THERAPY

higher sensitivity compared with other enzymes tested. Given this sensitivity for myocardial damage, a low-level elevation in the cardiac enzymes indicates ongoing, low-grade myocardial necrosis that often accompanies active viral infection.[42-44]

ECG findings are highly variable in myocarditis; however, suggestive changes include ST-segment elevations in two contiguous leads (54%), T-wave inversions (27%), widespread ST-segment depressions (18%), and pathologic Q waves (18% to 27%).[2] Low-voltage complexes can be observed commonly in standard and precordial leads. Other related findings can include tachycardia out of proportion to fever, arrhythmias, and conduction disturbances. Occasionally ST-segment and T-wave abnormalities can be associated with events other than myocarditis, including fever, hypoxia, electrolyte disturbances, and minor childhood viral infections.[45] Many ECG abnormalities resolve in 1 to 2 months.

Echocardiography is useful to confirm and quantify impaired systolic cardiac function. The loss of right ventricular function is the most powerful predictor of death or need for a cardiac transplant. In addition, exclusion of other causes of cardiac dysfunction such as valvular vegetations or pericardial effusion is important diagnostically and therapeutically. Common echocardiographic findings are segmental or global abnormalities of motion of the heart wall due to inflammation and edema of the myocardium.[46] Repeated echocardiograms are useful to follow evolution of disease, with persistent abnormalities suggesting development of dilated cardiomyopathy.

Other imaging techniques useful for diagnosis of myocarditis include nuclear imaging with gallium[67]-labeled or indium[111]-labeled antimyosin antibodies, and magnetic resonance imaging (MRI). Nuclear imaging techniques with gallium[67] or indium[111] detect the extent of myocardial inflammation and myocyte necrosis, respectively, and may be highly sensitive for detecting myocarditis and for predicting outcomes.[2,47] MRI is now a widely used modality for both diagnostic and prognostic purposes. Consensus criteria have been published for use of MRI in myocarditis.[48]

Endomyocardial biopsy remains the gold standard for establishing the diagnosis of myocarditis, despite its limited sensitivity and specificity. In large series of patients with cardiomyopathies using the Dallas criteria, positive biopsy results are reported in approximately 10% of patients.[49,50] In general, biopsies performed within weeks of symptom onset have a higher yield than biopsies performed later. Studies have demonstrated the usefulness of biopsy to identify possible causative agents.[5,7,8,51] In many cases the risk of biopsy outweighs the potential clinical and diagnostic gains from the procedure. Consensus guidelines have been published on the diagnostic role of endomyocardial biopsy and usefulness to determine whether myocarditis is active, healing, or healed.[52]

Specific diagnosis of infectious agents causing myocarditis can be made in several ways. Agents can be isolated directly from myocardial tissue, visualized using specific stains, or amplified with molecular techniques such as PCR. Indirect associations can be made by demonstration of likely infectious agents from other tissue or body fluids, such as positive nasopharyngeal, throat, or stool assays for viral pathogens or blood cultures for agents such as *Neisseria meningitidis*. In the acute setting, blood can be obtained for PCR analysis for common viruses such as enteroviruses, adenovirus, cytomegalovirus, Epstein–Barr virus, and others. Serologic assays showing a fourfold rise of titer in paired sera, or a single positive immunoglobulin M assay can implicate infectious causes, but have limited usefulness in the immediate workup and management of myocarditis. Epidemiologic clues such as time of year and geographic location may be helpful in evaluating for etiologies, such as in the midst of an influenza or enteroviral epidemic, or to suspect Chagas disease in a patient from South America.

Pericarditis can be distinguished by the findings of precordial chest pain, signs of pericardial fluid, and absence of arrhythmia. Myocardial infarction can have findings similar to myocarditis, whether infarction is due to coronary artery atherosclerosis, or is secondary to drug ingestions such as cocaine and methamphetamine. The term *idiopathic* (or *lymphocytic* if characteristic lymphocytic infiltrates are seen) myocarditis is used to describe cases in which no causative agent is found.

LABORATORY FINDINGS AND DIAGNOSIS

A high index of suspicion is required to establish the diagnosis of myocarditis accurately in children. If the diagnosis is considered, useful initial tests include chest radiography, ECG, and echocardiography. Nonspecific laboratory findings are leukocytosis, elevated sedimentation rate, eosinophilia, or an elevation in the cardiac fraction of creatine kinase (CK-MB). Measurements of troponin I and T may be useful in the diagnosis because of the

MANAGEMENT

Supportive therapy is the most important initial management of patients with myocarditis. Many patients have mild myocarditis as a complication of systemic infection and can be managed with minimal intervention. Patients with symptoms of congestive heart failure or fulminant disease require careful management in an intensive-care setting. Diuretic and vasodilator agents may be necessary to lower ventricular filling pressures. If congestive heart failure is present, an angiotensin-converting enzyme inhibitor agent should be used to decrease vascular resistance, and a beta-blocking agent or diuretics also may be indicated.[1] Digoxin should be used with caution and only at low doses, because a mouse model of myocarditis indicated increased mortality with its use.[53] Arrhythmias may require pharmacologic therapy, or placement of a defibrillator. Bedrest should be recommended for most patients because exercise can exacerbate disease. Retrospective studies and case reports have shown a benefit from use of ventricular assist devices or extracorporeal membrane oxygenation (ECMO) when necessary.[54–56]

Specific infectious agents such as bacteria, fungi, or parasites should be treated with appropriate antimicrobial agents. Diphtheric myocarditis should be treated with a combination of antitoxin and antimicrobial therapy. Clinical trials have not been done to evaluate efficacy of specific antiviral agents for viral myocarditis. However, if a treatable viral cause of myocarditis is established, antiviral therapy seems prudent.

Many studies have been performed to evaluate immune-modulating agents including systemic corticosteroids, immune globulin intravenous (IGIV), interferons, and other immunosuppressive drugs for treatment of myocarditis; results are controversial. The high incidence of spontaneous recovery after myocarditis necessitates studies that include a control group for accurate analysis of efficacy. In one of the largest trials of use of immunosuppressant agents, the Myocarditis Treatment Trial, 111 adults with biopsy-proven myocarditis were randomized to receive placebo or an immunosuppressive regimen consisting of prednisone plus either cyclosporine or azathioprine. No difference in mortality was found between the two groups, and improvement in left ventricular function was identical at the 28-week follow up.[49] Another controlled trial using prednisone (60 mg daily) for unexplained dilated cardiomyopathy in adults showed initial improvement in left ventricular ejection fraction at 3 months of follow-up in the treated group, which was not sustained at 6 or 9 months.[57] A meta-analysis, performed to review the use of immunosuppressive regimens for acute myocarditis in children, concluded that immunosuppressive therapy does not significantly improve outcomes in children.[58] For these reasons, and findings in other similar studies, immunosuppression should not be used routinely in treatment of myocarditis.

Use of IGIV as therapy for myocarditis also has been controversial. One pediatric trial suggested benefit of high-dose IGIV (2 g/kg) in 21 children compared with historic controls, but other larger, randomized controlled studies in adults do not support a consistent clinical benefit.[59,60] Therefore, the long-term benefit of this treatment remains unknown. Single-center trials of interferon-α and interferon-β have been performed showing benefit in patients with dilated cardiomyopathy and myocarditis. Data need to be confirmed in a large-scale, multicenter trial.[61,62]

COMPLICATIONS AND PROGNOSIS

Complications of myocarditis include congestive heart failure, arrhythmias, cardiac rupture, sudden death, and progression to dilated cardiomyopathy, which is the major long-term sequela of myocarditis.[63] One study using echocardiograms to evaluate risk factors for developing unremitting severe cardiac failure showed higher likelihood of poor outcomes in patients with ejection fractions less than 30%, shortening fractions less than 15%, left ventricular dilatation, and moderate to severe mitral regurgitation.[64] Elevated serum C-reactive protein level, elevated serum creatine kinase concentration, decreased left ventricular ejection fraction, and intraventricular conduction disturbance(s) at the time of admission, also have been associated with poor outcomes.[65] Follow-up data are available from a series of 41 children with suspected myocarditis, of whom 66% made a complete recovery, 10% had incomplete recovery, 12% died, and 12% underwent cardiac transplantation. Medical management of this cohort varied significantly, with some patients receiving corticosteroid therapy, some receiving IGIV, and some receiving neither therapy.[66]

PREVENTION

Prevention of acute infectious myocarditis relies on prevention of underlying microbial causes. Since most cases are caused by viruses including enteroviruses and adenoviruses, targeting prevention of infection with these agents is problematic. Frequent hand hygiene after contact with infectious body fluids, covering the mouth while coughing, and food and water sanitation are important. Some causes of myocarditis are preventable with adherence to the standard immunization schedule including annual seasonal influenza immunization.

39   Pericarditis

Craig A. Shapiro and Joseph A. Hilinski

Pericarditis is inflammation of the pericardium and the proximal great vessels. Pericarditis can be acute, subacute, or chronic in presentation. Pericarditis can have an infectious or noninfectious cause; in either case, pericarditis can be the sole manifestation of a disease or part of a multisystem disorder. Pericarditis can manifest as cardiac tamponade with a fulminant, life-threatening process, constrictive pericarditis from chronic disease, or an incidental finding of pericardial fluid in an asymptomatic person. Extensive guidelines have been published by the European Society of Cardiology on the diagnosis and management of pericardial diseases.[1]

ETIOLOGY

Pericarditis caused by infection can be classified as purulent, "benign," or granulomatous. Purulent pericarditis is caused by bacterial infection; benign pericarditis is caused by viral infection or hypersensitivity, postinfectious, or postpericardiotomy syndromes; and granulomatous pericarditis usually is caused by *Mycobacterium tuberculosis* and, occasionally, by fungal infection. Up to 90% of acute cases are "idiopathic" or presumed to be of viral origin. Noninfectious causes include cardiac injury, uremia, radiation, neoplasia, collagen vascular disease, sarcoidosis, inflammatory bowel disease, and drug hypersensitivity.

Viral pericarditis is more common in adults than children. This condition can be clinically subtle, detected because of an enlarged heart on a routine chest radiograph, or fulminant, with severe hemodynamic manifestations. A viral cause is assumed if pericardial fluid is not purulent and spontaneous resolution occurs. Enteroviruses, especially the coxsackieviruses, are the most common causes of viral pericarditis, and can be associated with seasonal epidemics, or can occur in clusters.[2] Other viral causes (often associated with myocarditis) also have been implicated,

TABLE 39-1. Causes of 163 Cases of Purulent Pericarditis, 1950–1977

Causative Organism	Number of Isolates (%)
Staphylococcus aureus	72 (44)
Haemophilus influenzae type b	35 (22)
Neisseria meningitidis	14 (9)
Streptococcus pneumoniae	9 (6)
Salmonella spp.	4 (3)
Escherichia coli	3 (2)
Other[a]	7 (5)
Unknown	17 (10)

[a]*Includes isolates of* Klebsiella *spp.,* Streptococcus pyogenes, *"Paracolon spp.,"* Pseudomonas aeruginosa, Staphylococcus epidermidis, Bacteroides *spp., anaerobic streptococci, singly or in combination.*

Data from Feldman WE. Bacterial etiology and mortality of purulent pericarditis in pediatric patients: a review of 162 cases. Am J Dis Child 1979;133:641.

and include adenovirus, influenza A and B, herpes simplex, cytomegalovirus, Epstein–Barr virus, mumps, lymphocytic choriomeningitis, varicella-zoster, and human immunodeficiency virus (HIV). Cytomegalovirus is an important cause of pericarditis in immunocompromised and HIV-infected people.[3]

Bacteria invade the pericardium as a result of bacteremia or contiguous spread from the lungs or pleural space. *Staphylococcus aureus* and *Haemophilus influenzae* type b (Hib) historically were the most frequent causes of purulent pericarditis in children (Table 39-1).[4,5] Both pathogens usually cause pericarditis in children under 5 years of age, although occasionally older children and adults are infected.[6] The frequency of pericarditis caused by Hib has decreased due to routine vaccination of infants. Other bacteria including group A streptococcus (GAS), *Streptococcus pneumoniae* and *Neisseria meningitidis* also have been identified as causes.[7–9] Purulent pericarditis rarely can be caused by anaerobic bacteria, either by contiguous spread (especially pulmonary actinomycosis)[10] or bacteremic spread (especially *Bacteroides fragilis*).[11] HIV infection is an important predisposing factor worldwide for pericarditis, especially for bacterial and mycobacterial causes.[12]

Pericarditis caused by *M. tuberculosis* is uncommon, occurring in about 1% of cases of tuberculosis, either by direct extension from a pulmonary focus or spread from lymphatic or bacteremic origin. Although an uncommon cause of pericarditis in developed countries, *M. tuberculosis* can cause up to 70% of cases of pericarditis in areas where tuberculosis remains a major public health problem, especially in patients with AIDS.[13]

Pericarditis occasionally is caused by fungal infection after surgery, instrumentation, immunosuppression, or neutropenia.[14] Fungi associated with pericarditis include *Candida* species, *Aspergillus, Blastomyces, Histoplasma, Cryptococcus,* and *Coccidioides* species. Less common causes of pericarditis include *Rickettsia* spp., *Mycoplasma pneumoniae,*[15] *M. hominis, Ureaplasma urealyticum, Entamoeba histolytica, Toxoplasma gondii,* and *Toxocara canis.* Pericarditis also can result from inoculation at surgery, invasion associated with instrumentation of the genitourinary tract, and immunosuppression.

EPIDEMIOLOGY

Pericarditis is not a reportable disease, and population-based studies are not available. Pericarditis commonly occurs in the late summer and fall concurrent with epidemics of enteroviruses. Pericarditis occurs in people of all ages, although viral pericarditis is more common in adults than in children. In contrast, purulent pericarditis is common in children; one-half of all cases reportedly occur in children under 13 years of age, with equal incidence in males and females. Tuberculous pericarditis is more common in poor urban populations and among immigrants from countries where tuberculosis is endemic, and is the most common cause of pericarditis in high-risk regions.[13]

PATHOGENESIS

The pericardium consists of two layers, the inner layer, or visceral pericardium, which is continuous with the outer tissue of the myocardium, and the parietal pericardium, which lines the surrounding mediastinal structures and has attachments to the sternum, the diaphragm and adventitia of the great vessels. The two layers are 1 to 2 mm thick, with a space between them that contains 10 to 15 mL of clear fluid in healthy children and 15 to 35 mL in adults. The pericardium is semitransparent. There is independent blood supply from the internal mammary arteries, and innervation from the phrenic nerve, explaining the severe pain and vagally mediated reflexes that sometimes occur with inflammation. With inflammation, there is influx of fibrin, polymorphonuclear and mononuclear cells, and exudation of fluid into the pericardial space. Pericardial inflammation results in proliferation of fibrous tissue, neovascularization, and scarring, with consequent loss of elasticity and restriction of cardiac filling.

Purulent pericarditis frequently results from contiguous extension of pneumonia, empyema, suppurative mediastinal lymphadenitis, liver abscess, or cardiac conditions, such as myocarditis, myocardial abscess, and infectious endocarditis. Bacterial pericarditis can result from inoculation during bacteremia, which commonly is the pathogenesis in pericarditis due to *S. aureus.* Pericarditis can complicate placement of pacemaker devices or during sternal osteomyelitis/mediastinitis postoperatively. *S. aureus, S. epidermidis, Candida,* and nonenteric and enteric gram-negative bacilli usually are responsible.[16,17]

Enteroviruses are transmitted primarily by the fecal-oral route. After initial proliferation in the lymphoid tissues of the intestine, viremia can lead to disseminated or focal infection in skin, brain, meninges, heart, and pericardium. Pericarditis can be the sole manifestation of enteroviral infection or part of multiorgan infection.

Regardless of cause, acute pericarditis results in collection of fluid in the space between the visceral and parietal pericardium. Small increases in fluid production are clinically insignificant because they are reabsorbed. Large increases in fluid secretion that exceed resorptive capacity can result in significant cardiac dysfunction. As a result of the ability of the heart to dilate in response to long-standing stress, slowly accumulating collections of 1 liter or more of fluid in adults may not interfere with cardiac function. However, 200 to 300 mL of rapid fluid accumulation can exceed maximal distensibility of the pericardial sac. When this occurs, small incremental fluid accumulation causes a sharp increase in intracardiac pressure, which interferes with cardiac filling, leading to decreased stroke volume (cardiac tamponade). Death from low cardiac output occurs if fluid is not removed urgently.

Tuberculous pericarditis results from lymphatic spread from a focus in the lung or lymph nodes, or by hematogenous spread from a distant site. Granulomas of the pericardium containing *M. tuberculosis* develop initially and are followed by a serous or serosanguineous effusion containing lymphocytes and monocytes. Healing of tuberculous pericarditis results in deposition of fibrin and collagen, often leading to constrictive pericarditis.

CLINICAL MANIFESTATIONS

The presentation of acute pericarditis varies depending on the cause. Precordial chest pain is the most common symptom of pericarditis. Pain is often unrecognized in young children, in whom manifestations are irritability and a grunting expiratory sound as they splint the thoracic cage. Exercise intolerance and fever are common but are nonspecific manifestations of pericardial infection. Enteroviral infection often is characterized by fever, malaise, and rash. Pericarditis frequently follows an upper respiratory tract infection, thus fever, weakness, and chest pain after nonspecific febrile or upper respiratory tract illnesses should suggest consideration of the diagnosis of pericarditis.

Pain is felt over the entire precordium, to the left side over the trapezius ridge, and over the scapula; pain sometimes radiates down the arm and can be aggravated by movement. Pain generally

PART II Clinical Syndromes and Cardinal Features of Infectious Diseases: Approach to Diagnosis and Initial Management

SECTION E Cardiac and Vascular Infections

is worse when supine, and can be relieved by sitting. Pain also can be referred, because pericardial pain fibers are located in the diaphragmatic reflection of the pericardium. Pain is more common in acute infectious pericarditis than in more indolent forms.

Examination of the heart can reveal muffled heart sounds caused by the surrounding effusion and increasing tachycardia as the effusion impinges on the volume of chambers. A pericardial friction rub can be audible, especially when the effusion is small. The rub is best heard during deep inspiration and with the patient kneeling or in the knee-chest position, leaning forward. The rub is typically a to-and-fro, high-pitched loud rasping or creaking sound, heard throughout the cardiac cycle, although it can be limited to systole. Pleural rubs can be differentiated because they occur in timing with the respiratory cycle.

Clinical manifestations of tamponade include tachycardia, peripheral vasoconstriction, reduced arterial pulse pressure, and pulsus paradoxus. Pulsus paradoxus represents a drop of greater than 10 mmHg in systolic blood pressure during inspiration from decreased venous return to the heart. Pulsus paradoxus is not pathognomonic for pericardial tamponade, and can occur in the presence of chronic lung disease and in pericarditis without tamponade. Other findings described in pericarditis include the Kussmaul sign (a rise or failure to fall of jugular venous pressure with inspiration), and Beck triad (hypotension, muffled heart sounds, and raised jugular venous pressure).

DIFFERENTIAL DIAGNOSIS

Chest pain and fever occur with pneumonia, empyema, myocarditis, or pleurodynia. Myocardial infarction is rare in children. Dressler syndrome is a form of pericarditis that can occur weeks to months after infarction. Myocardial ischemia can follow use of crack cocaine and crystal methamphetamine ("ice") in adolescents and adults.[18] Noninfectious causes of pericardial effusion include blunt trauma, malignant tumors, irradiation, uremia, sarcoidosis, collagen vascular disease, and inflammatory bowel disease. Any direct injury can cause pericarditis. Postpericardiotomy syndrome is considered in the 6 weeks after cardiac surgery. Systemic inflammatory disorders associated with pericarditis, include collagen vascular diseases, Kawasaki disease, rheumatoid arthritis, rheumatic fever, scleroderma, and polyserositis (such as can follow meningococcemia). Metabolic diseases, including uremia and myxedema, and exposure to certain drugs, including hydralazine, procainamide, and phenytoin, also can cause pericarditis.

LABORATORY FINDINGS AND DIAGNOSIS

The diagnosis of pericarditis is made on the basis of history, physical examination, and imaging studies. All patients with suspected pericarditis should undergo electrocardiogram (ECG), chest radiography, and echocardiography.[1] The specific cause of pericarditis is best determined by examination of pericardial fluid. Some authors have advocated risk-based assessment in adult patients to decide the need for invasive testing to determine a specific etiology;[19] children more frequently require therapeutic and diagnostic aspiration. Complete cell count and morphology, glucose level, lactate dehydrogenase, and protein concentrations are useful to support likely causes. Serosanguineous or hemorrhagic fluid is suggestive of tumor, trauma, tuberculosis, toxoplasmosis, or GAS infection. Systemic leukocytosis and elevated acute-phase reactants are common. Troponin I can be elevated in some patients, although studies of its use in children are lacking.[20]

An increase in the size of the cardiac shadow on chest radiograph, especially in the absence of pulmonary congestion, suggests presence of pericardial fluid. The epicardial fat pad can be visualized within the left borders of the cardiopericardial silhouette in about 15% of patients with pericardial effusion. Concomitant findings of pneumonia or findings suspicious for tuberculosis can be helpful etiologic clues.

Typical ECG features of pericarditis are generalized ST elevation without reciprocal ST depression, except in leads V1 and aVR. A few days into illness, elevated ST segment returns to baseline. At this time there is flattening or inversion of the T wave. Low-voltage QRS complexes may be evident without the pathologic Q wave of myocardial infarction; these findings result from damping of electrical activity by effusion. With resolution of disease ECG results normalize, although T-wave abnormalities can persist.

Echocardiographic examination of the heart and its surroundings is the most valuable tool for diagnosis and assessment of the severity of pericarditis, and can differentiate between pericarditis, myocarditis, and endocarditis. When pericardial fluid is present, both M-mode and two-dimensional echocardiography demonstrate a sonolucent space between the two layers of pericardium. M-mode is the more sensitive procedure and can estimate reliably the volume of effusion. Two-dimensional echocardiography can be used to direct catheter placement for drainage. Transesophageal echocardiogram may be necessary in certain cases, including when transthoracic views are suboptimal, or there is evidence of complex diastolic dysfunction or suspected constrictive pericarditis. Imaging with computed tomography (CT) or magnetic resonance imaging (MRI) has an important role in the assessment of complications of pericarditis. CT is useful to delineate extracardiac masses and other causes of an enlarged cardiac silhouette. Combined studies with flow imaging by MRI are useful to delineate intracardiac masses.[21]

Microbiologic evaluation of pericardial fluid obtained by pericardiocentesis is the best method for determining the specific cause of pericarditis. In one report on patients with large pericardial effusions undergoing subxiphoid pericardial biopsy, a diagnosis was established in 93% of cases, whether or not the cause was infectious.[22] In another study of patients undergoing pericardiocentesis without suspicion of purulent pericarditis, the diagnostic yield was under 10%.[23] Evaluation of fluid should include Gram, acid-fast, and fungal stains and culture for bacteria, viruses, mycobacteria, and fungi. Special attention to rapid transport under anaerobic conditions is necessary to optimize recovery of anaerobic bacteria. Blood cultures should be obtained and are positive in up to 70% of patients with purulent pericarditis.[24] If pericarditis results from extension from a contiguous focus, cultures of sputum, pleural fluid, and mediastinal fluid or tissue may identify the causative organism.

Viral causes of pericarditis may be determined by culture, rapid antigen tests, serologic tests, and molecular genetic techniques. Tissue culture should be inoculated for recovery of viruses; suckling mouse inoculation enhances recovery of certain enteroviruses. Consideration should be given to polymerase chain reaction (PCR) assays for common viral agents, such as enteroviruses, directly from pericardial fluid, or indirectly from blood. A study performed on 106 pericardial fluid and biopsy specimens using PCR identified an etiologic agent more often than culture alone.[25] However, even with these procedures, identification of virus in pericardial fluid is unusual. Paired sera can be tested for antibody to prevalent enterovirus serotypes. A fourfold rise between acute and convalescent serum titers for enteroviruses or the presence of specific immunoglobulin M antibody is considered diagnostic. Virus detected from a site other than the pericardial fluid, such as stool, respiratory tract, or throat, often can be considered the likely cause of concomitant pericarditis. A rise in serum antibody to an isolate confirms active infection. Serology also offers the best opportunity for diagnosis of *Rickettsia* and *Mycoplasma* species infection.

Recovery of mycobacteria and fungi is uncommon, but appropriate cultures for these agents should be performed in cases of granulomatous pericarditis. When these agents are suspected, biopsy of the pericardium for histologic examination and culture has a higher yield than direct stain or culture of pericardial fluid alone. If tuberculous pericarditis is suspected, a tuberculin skin test or use of an interferon-γ release assay should be performed. PCR for *M. tuberculosis* directly from pericardial fluid can offer the advantage of rapid diagnosis; however, larger studies may be needed to determine sensitivity and specificity of PCR.[26,27] Adenosine deaminase and interferon-γ levels also have been used to make a diagnosis of tuberculous pericarditis using pericardial fluid.[28,29]

Postcardiotomy syndrome occurs in up to one-third of children and one-fifth of adults following open-heart surgery.[30] This syndrome is characterized by fever, chest pain, and pericardial friction rub. An autoimmune process, triggered by virus replication (especially cytomegalovirus) or surgical trauma, is the postulated mechanism of disease.

MANAGEMENT

Patients who have a small pericardial effusion of apparent viral cause can be managed with close monitoring, bedrest, and symptomatic relief of pain. The presence of a large effusion with tamponade or impending tamponade requires immediate removal of fluid by pericardiocentesis or open drainage, possibly with resection of the anterior pericardium (pericardiectomy). Patients with suspected bacterial or fungal pericarditis should undergo pericardiocentesis promptly. Echocardiographically guided pericardiocentesis provides immediate improvement of acute clinical deterioration. Pericardiectomy, the definitive procedure, is indicated if the fluid is too thick to withdraw through a small-bore tube, if fluid persists after pericardiocentesis, or if the process is chronic and constrictive.[1] A comprehensive review of the literature concluded that pericardiectomy should be limited to patients with persistent restrictive pericarditis and patients with hemodynamically unstable restrictive pericarditis. Pericardiectomy in recurrent pericarditis is not indicated unless there is cardiac tamponade or concern for corticosteroid toxicity.[31] Performance of pericardiectomy limited to producing a small subxiphoid "window" versus resection of the whole anterior pericardium is controversial. In selected pediatric patients, complete pericardiectomy has been performed with good outcomes.[32] For cases of purulent pericarditis, irrigating the pericardial cavity is mandatory. A small case series and case reports indicate that irrigation with streptokinase may help liquefy the exudate.[11,33]

Therapy with broad-spectrum antimicrobial agents is initiated empirically if purulent pericarditis is suspected (Table 39-2).

Bacterial pericarditis usually is treated for 3 to 4 weeks with parenteral antimicrobial agents. Given high rates of methicillin-resistant *S. aureus* in most communities (CA-MRSA), empiric therapy for presumed purulent pericarditis should include vancomycin.[34] Candidal pericarditis almost always requires combined medical and surgical treatment.[14] Fungal pericarditis caused by disseminated *Aspergillus* spp. or dimorphic fungi (*Histoplasma, Coccidioides, Blastomyces*) usually is treated for several months with antifungal agents (see chapters on specific pathogens). Empiric antituberculous therapy using three or four drugs should be initiated if tuberculous pericarditis is suspected; corticosteroids also may be indicated.

Drainage of purulent pericardial fluid is mandatory to decrease the immediate risk of death. Use of antimicrobial agents and drainage has improved outcomes for patients with pericarditis. Of 162 children with purulent pericarditis reported in 1979,[4] mortality was 82% in children who were given only antimicrobial therapy treatment and 22% in children who had both antimicrobial therapy and drainage. Young age was an independent risk factor for poor outcome. Children <1 year of age who were infected with either *S. aureus* or *Haemophilus influenzae* had a mortality rate of 63%, which is substantially higher than the mortality rate (26%) for children >1 year of age.[4] In a 1994 report,[24] 42 of 43 patients with purulent pericarditis treated with both antimicrobial agents and drainage recovered completely.

The major long-term complication of pericarditis is thickening and stiffening of the pericardial membrane leading to constrictive pericarditis, which usually necessitates surgical stripping of the pericardium. In one series, surgical pericardiectomy was required in 8 of 24 (33%) patients with tuberculous, purulent, or neoplastic pericarditis, versus only 1 of 203 (<1%) patients with idiopathic, viral, or *Toxoplasma* pericarditis.[35] Pericarditis can recur in 15% to 30% of people in whom the disease is idiopathic. Fever and pericardial fluid collections in patients with the postpericardiotomy syndrome usually resolve with aspirin, nonsteroidal anti-inflammatory agents, or corticosteroid therapy.[36]

TABLE 39-2. Antimicrobial Therapy of Major Causes of Pericarditis

Causative Agent	Antimicrobial Agent	Dosage (mg/kg per day)
Enterovirus and other viruses	None[a]	–
Empiric therapy for purulent pericarditis	Vancomycin *or*	60
	Nafcillin[b] *or*	200
	Oxacillin[b] *plus*	200
	Cefotaxime *or*	200
	Ceftriaxone	80 (qd) or 100 (divided bid)
Therapy when agent is confirmed		
Staphylococcus aureus or *S. epidermidis* (susceptible to methicillin)	Oxacillin *or*	200
	Nafcillin	200
S. aureus or *S. epidermidis* (resistant to methicillin)	Vancomycin[c]	60
Haemophilus influenzae	Ampicillin (if susceptible) *or*	200–300
	Cefotaxime *or*	200
	Ceftriaxone	80–100 (divided bid)
Streptococcus pneumoniae (susceptible to penicillin) or *S. pyogenes*	Penicillin G	200,000–300,000 units
S. pneumoniae (intermediate to penicillin)	Cefotaxime	300
S. pneumoniae (highly resistant to penicillin)	Vancomycin	60
Mycobacterium tuberculosis[d]	Isoniazid	10–15 mg for 6 months
	+	
	Rifampin	10–20 mg for 6 months
	+	
	Pyrazinamide	30–40 mg for 2 months
	±	
	Ethambutol	20–25 mg until susceptibility studies are available

[a]Cytomegalovirus may respond to ganciclovir or valganciclovir.

[b]Nafcillin or oxacillin should only be used if community rates of methicillin-resistant Staphylococcus aureus (MRSA) are low.

[c]Linezolid would be an alternative; some community-associated MRSA are susceptible to clindamycin.

[d]Addition of corticosteroids to antibiotic regimen is recommended (e.g., prednisone 1 mg/kg per day for 6–8 weeks); in communities where isoniazid-resistant Mycobacterium tuberculosis has been encountered, a four-drug initial treatment is recommended.

SECTION F: Central Nervous System Infections

40   Acute Bacterial Meningitis beyond the Neonatal Period

Carla G. Garcia and George H. McCracken, Jr

ETIOLOGIC AGENTS AND EPIDEMIOLOGY

In otherwise healthy children, the three most common organisms causing hematogenously acquired acute bacterial meningitis worldwide are *Streptococcus pneumoniae, Neisseria meningitidis,* and *Haemophilus influenzae* type b (Hib). Although Hib was the most common bacterial cause before availability of the Hib conjugate vaccine, the current likelihood of Hib meningitis in a child who has received at least two doses of vaccine is extraordinarily low. In surveillance studies conducted by the Centers for Disease Control and Prevention (CDC), the incidence of Hib disease declined by 95% from 1987 to 1993 in children younger than 5 years (41 cases per 100,000 in 1987 to 2 per 100,000 in 1993) (Figure 40-1).[1] Similar data from 1997 indicated a further decline to 1.3 cases per 100,000 (97% reduction),[2] and there was a further decline, to approximately 0.11 cases per 100,000, by 2008.[3] The incidence also has decreased markedly in other areas of the world where Hib conjugate vaccines have been implemented for universal use in

infants.[4,5] Currently, Hib meningitis occurs primarily in children who have not completed the primary immunization series.[3,6]

Meningitis caused by Hib has a peak incidence in the fall and winter and occurs more commonly in African Americans. Pneumococcal meningitis and meningococcal meningitis also occur more commonly during the winter; meningococcal disease can be endemic or epidemic. The annual incidence of bacterial meningitis in children younger than 5 years, as assessed by the CDC, has been relatively stable for *N. meningitidis* (about 4 to 5 cases per 100,000 since 1980). For *S. pneumoniae* the incidence was about 2.5 per 100,000 before 2000. Seven of the >90 pneumococcal serotypes (4, 6B, 9, 14, 18F, 19F, and 23F) accounted for >80% of invasive disease in children from developed countries; serotypes 5 and 1 also are prevalent in developing countries.[7] The incidence of invasive disease, including meningitis, caused by vaccine strains of *S. pneumoniae* fell by greater than 90% after the implementation of universal heptavalent conjugate vaccination (PCV7) in U.S. infants in 2000.[8] Recent studies, however, have shown an increase in invasive pneumococcal disease caused by nonvaccine serotypes. In the U.S., the incidence of disease caused by serotype 19A has increased, and these isolates have been reported to be resistant to β-lactam antibiotics, including penicillin and third-generation cephalosporins.[9,10] The recently implemented 13-valent pneumococcal vaccine (PCV13) includes the 19A serotype as well as types 1 and 5 that are more common in the developing world.

Serogroups B and C are the most common serogroups of *N. meningitidis* causing invasive infections in North America, although group Y strains can account for up to 20% to 25% of cases. A conjugated vaccine against meningococcal serogroup C was introduced in 1999 in the United Kingdom's routine immunization schedule, showing an approximate 80% reduction of serogroup C disease within 2 years of implementation.[11] In 2005, the quadrivalent meningococcal (A/C/Y/W-135) polysaccharide-protein conjugate vaccine (MCV4) was licensed and is recommended currently for all U.S. adolescents beginning at 11 to 12 years of age and for persons 2 through 54 years of age who have elevated risk for invasive meningococcal disease.[12,13] Insufficient time since implementation precludes estimation of the impact of this immunization in the U.S.[14]

Underlying conditions can be associated with increased risk of meningitis or particular bacterial species or both (Table 40-1). Children with a basilar skull or cribriform fracture and a cerebrospinal fluid (CSF) leak have greater risk for pneumococcal meningitis, as do children with asplenia (anatomic or functional) or human immunodeficiency virus (HIV) infection. Deficiencies in terminal components of complement lead to greater risk for meningococcal infection. Common causes of meningitis after penetrating head trauma or neurosurgery are *Staphylococcus aureus* and coagulase-negative staphylococci, streptococci, and gram-negative enteric bacilli, especially *Escherichia coli, Klebsiella* spp., and *Pseudomonas aeruginosa*. These organisms also are associated with meningitis related to a dermal sinus or embryopathy of the neurenteric canal. Nontypable *H. influenzae* meningitis is associated with immunoglobulin deficiencies and *Listeria* meningitis with cellular immune defects; *Listeria* meningitis occurs occasionally in immunocompetent infants and children as well. *Salmonella* spp. rarely cause meningitis in immunocompetent children beyond early infancy, and some cases have been linked to reptile pets. The presence of a ventriculoperitoneal shunt is a risk factor

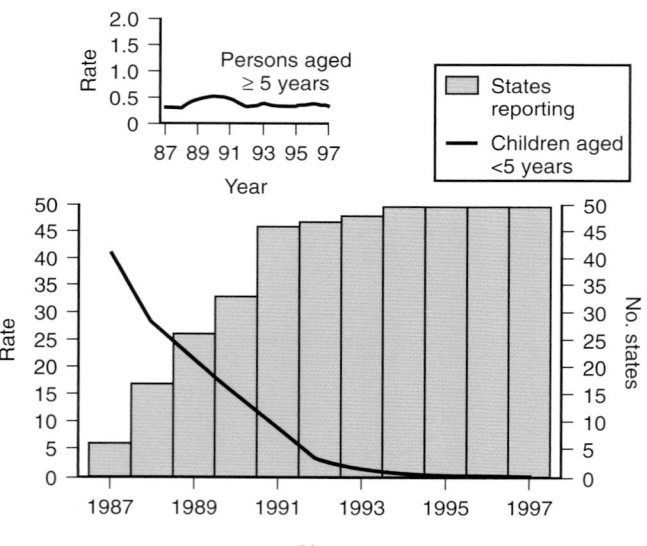

* Per 100 000 children aged <5 years
† Per 100 000 persons aged ≥5 years
§ Because of the low number of states reporting surveillance data during 1987–1990, rates for those years were race-adjusted using the 1990 U.S. population

Figure 40-1. Incidence of invasive *Haemophilus influenzae* disease among children younger than 5 years and the number of states reporting *H. influenzae* surveillance data to the National Notifiable Diseases Surveillance System, 1987–1997, United States. Insert represents the incidence of invasive *H. influenzae* disease among persons 5 years or older. Rate is expressed as cases per 100,000 population. (From Centers for Disease Control and Prevention. Progress toward eliminating *Haemophilus influenzae* type b disease among infants and children – United States, 1987–1997. MMWR 1998;47:993.)

TABLE 40-1. Underlying Conditions and Organisms Commonly Associated with Bacterial Meningitis

Condition	Organism
Cerebrospinal fluid leak (otorrhea, rhinorrhea)	*Streptococcus pneumoniae*, *Haemophilus influenzae*
Dermal sinus tracts meningomyelocele	Staphylococci, gram-negative enteric bacilli, intestinal bacteria (related to site of defect)
Persistent complement deficiency	*Neisseria meningitidis*
Asplenia (anatomic or functional)	*S. pneumoniae*, *N. meningitidis*, *Salmonella* spp.
Renal transplantation, T-lymphocyte deficiency	*Listeria monocytogenes*
Otic fistula (stapes footplate, oval window; cochlear implant)	*S. pneumoniae*
Ventriculoperitoneal shunt	Staphylococci (coagulase-negative and *Staphylococcus aureus*), *S. pneumoniae*, *H. influenzae*, *N. meningitidis* (hematogenous), diphtheroids (e.g., contaminated shunt)
Antibody deficiency state (including HIV infection)	*S. pneumoniae*, *N. meningitidis*, *H. influenzae* type b
Penetrating trauma	Varies with nature and site of trauma (e.g., *Pasteurella multocida* after dog or cat bite, skin organisms after skull trauma, nasopharyngeal organisms after orbital or sinus trauma)
Surgery	Skin organisms, nosocomial pathogens

HIV, human immunodeficiency virus.

for meningitis; ventriculitis often is related to shunt contamination with skin organisms at the time of surgery. Isolation of an organism other than pneumococcus, meningococcus, or Hib from the CSF of a child older than 2 months requires an explanation with possible evaluation for unusual host susceptibility such as an anatomic abnormality or immunologic disorder. Children with recurrent pneumococcal or meningococcal infections also should undergo thorough investigation, including neuroimaging studies. Patients with cochlear implants, especially using a positioner device, have >30-fold increased incidence of pneumococcal meningitis[15] and increased risk of Hib meningitis.

PATHOGENESIS AND PATHOLOGY

Development of bacterial meningitis progresses through the following five related steps: (1) bacterial colonization of the nasopharynx (or skin), (2) mucosal invasion (or breach in skin barrier) and penetration into the bloodstream, (3) intravascular multiplication and entrance through the blood–brain barrier (BBB) usually via the choroid plexus, (4) generation of inflammation within the subarachnoid space, and (5) induction of neuronal and auditory cell damage.[16]

The three common meningeal pathogens colonize the nasopharyngeal mucosa in 5% to 40% of young children at any given time; for Hib and *N. meningitidis*, fimbriae mediate adherence to epithelial cells; for *S. pneumoniae*, specialized surface components, such as surface adhesion proteins, may be important. These encapsulated organisms are able to evade local host defenses and either invade between epithelial cells (Hib) or pass through epithelial cells (*N. meningitidis*) to reach the subepithelial tissues, where the organisms can invade small blood vessels to enter the bloodstream.[16] A viral upper respiratory tract infection can facilitate this process. Increased hospitalization for invasive pneumococcal disease has been correlated with the viral respiratory season.[17,18] Intravascular replication leads to bacteremia and, with sufficient

density of organisms, egress through the endothelium of the choroid plexus and cerebral capillaries into the ventricular fluid. A complex interplay between endothelial cells and microbial gene products appears to orchestrate the traversal of bacteria across the blood–brain barrier – transcellularly, paracellularly, or through infected phagocytes. For organisms that invade transcellularly, including *E. coli*, group B streptococcus, and *S. pneumoniae*, the process is mediated by interactions with host receptors in the human brain microvascular endothelial cells.[19] For *N. meningitidis*, invasion is mediated by the outer membrane protein Opc invasin binding to human fibronectin to attach and invade human brain endothelial cells.[20] Organisms multiply quickly and spread throughout the subarachnoid space because of the lack of host defenses within the CSF. The host inflammatory response to organisms leads to many of the alterations in CNS function and in the CSF that are characteristic of meningitis.

Communications between mucosal surfaces or skin and CSF that result from trauma or congenital malformations can lead to direct invasion of the CNS by bacteria. A fracture through the cribriform plate (CSF rhinorrhea), paranasal sinuses, or temporal bone (CSF otorrhea) provides entrance for respiratory tract organisms into the CNS. Penetrating injuries of the skull by sharp objects (toys, teeth) in younger infants or children can precede bacterial meningitis. Bacteria also can reach the CNS through congenital defects, such as a dermoid sinus tract, meningomyelocele, or fistula through the stapes footplate, oval window, or cochlear aqueduct. These defects should be sought in patients with recurrent bacterial meningitis or meningitis due to unexpected bacteria.[21] Bacterial meningitis also can be a complication of neurosurgery, spinal anesthesia, or placement of a ventricular shunt or external ventriculostomy device (Table 40-1).[22]

The pathology of Hib meningitis has been described in detail.[23,24] Increased brain weight and flattened convolutions are evidence of cerebral edema. Temporal lobe or cerebellar herniation can occur. The brain and spinal cord are covered with a purulent subarachnoid exudate that consists primarily of neutrophils, which also infiltrate the perivascular spaces of blood vessels in the outer layers of the cortex of the brain and connective tissue sheaths of cranial and spinal nerves. Endothelial cells of small subarachnoid arteries and veins are swollen, leading to narrowing of the lumen and microscopic changes within brain parenchyma consistent with ischemia. The interstitial tissue of the plexus is infiltrated with neutrophils (choroid plexitis). Phlebitis, venous thrombosis, arteritis, and brain necrosis are pathologic changes noted at necropsy in children who had untreated bacterial meningitis for less than 3 weeks. The foramina of Magendie and Luschka can be obstructed by exudate, resulting in obstructive hydrocephalus; however, communicating hydrocephalus is more common. This exudate, rich in bacterial products and proinflammatory substances, also can traverse the cochlear duct to involve the auditory tissue. Ongoing research is focusing on delineation of the complex molecular events taking place at the cellular level that can potentially explain the precise mechanisms of the brain damage resulting from bacterial meningitis.[16] It is currently believed that neuronal death is caused mainly by apoptosis through caspase-dependent and independent pathways.[25]

CLINICAL MANIFESTATIONS

Symptoms and signs of bacterial meningitis depend, in part, on the age of the patient and duration of the illness. Often, clinical manifestations are nonspecific and are not readily distinguished from those of self-limited viral infection. Inconsolable crying is a nonspecific symptom of serious infection in infants. In many patients, the initial symptoms consist of fever, irritability, nausea, vomiting, and diarrhea. An infant may become progressively more irritable and lethargic, may refuse feedings, and may manifest increasingly less interaction with caregivers. Grunting respirations indicate a critically ill infant.

Older children may complain of headache, vomiting, back pain, myalgia, and photophobia; may be confused or disoriented; and may verbalize specifically that the neck is stiff or sore. Seizures are

PART II Clinical Syndromes and Cardinal Features of Infectious Diseases: Approach to Diagnosis and Initial Management

SECTION F Central Nervous System Infections

noted in up to 20% to 30% of patients before or soon after hospital admission and tend to occur more frequently in pneumococcal or Hib meningitis than in meningococcal disease. The level of consciousness at the time of treatment is an important prognostic sign; outcome for children who are irritable or lethargic is superior to that for children who are comatose.[26]

On physical examination, the fontanel of an infant may be bulging, presumably indicating increased intracranial pressure; this sign is neither highly sensitive nor specific for meningitis but requires evaluation. The infant demonstrates diminished activity and may show little interest in the environment during the examination. More specific physical findings of meningeal inflammation are Kernig and Brudzinski signs and neck stiffness. These occur more commonly in children older than 12 to 18 months. A sixth cranial nerve palsy suggests increased intracranial pressure; seventh and third cranial nerve dysfunctions also have been observed. Papilledema is uncommon in a child with uncomplicated meningitis and, if present, suggests another diagnosis (brain abscess, epidural or subdural empyema, another cause of increased intracranial pressure) or a complication of meningitis (venous sinus thrombosis). Unilateral weakness (hemiparesis) often is a result of ischemia or infarction, usually associated with vasculitis or spasm of a cerebral artery. Occasionally in an older child, ataxia is the major complaint.

A petechial or purpuric rash and shock classically are associated with meningococcal meningitis but also can occur occasionally in infection due to Hib or *S. pneumoniae*. A maculopapular rash, which is difficult to distinguish from a more common enteroviral exanthem, can occur in up to 15% of children with meningococcemia. Focal infections such as pneumonia, pyogenic arthritis, buccal cellulitis, pericarditis, and endophthalmitis can be present concurrently with bacterial meningitis; their presence should not discourage evaluation of CSF unless the severity of the condition warrants deferral of the test.

Children with bacterial meningitis present with one of three basic patterns of illness:[27] (1) the most common, an insidious form with nonspecific symptoms that progress over 2 to 5 days before meningitis is diagnosed; (2) a more rapid form, in which symptoms and signs of meningitis progress over the course of 1 or 2 days; and (3) a fulminant form, with rapid deterioration and shock early in the course of illness. Host and bacterial factors influence the type of presentation.

Recognizing the infant or child with meningitis or other invasive bacterial infection among the large numbers of children with febrile illnesses due to viral or uncomplicated bacterial infections of the upper respiratory tract requires expertise as well as careful observation and examination. The differential diagnosis in children with fever and alteration in CNS function includes other infections, such as viral meningitis, encephalitis, brain abscess, and subdural or epidural abscess; Lyme disease; rickettsial or *Mycoplasma* infections, and leptospirosis. Noninfectious conditions affecting the central nervous system, such as Kawasaki disease, collagen vascular disease and other disorders characterized by vasculitis, hypersensitivity to drugs (trimethoprim-sulfamethoxazole, immune globulin intravenous, antithymocyte globulin), and Reye syndrome, also can be confused initially with bacterial meningitis.

LABORATORY FINDINGS AND DIAGNOSIS

A lumbar puncture to obtain CSF is necessary when the diagnosis of bacterial meningitis is considered. Although the typical CSF white blood cell (WBC) count in bacterial meningitis is >1000 cells/mm^3, few or no WBCs can be present in CSF in the early phase (usually of rapidly progressive infection). WBCs are predominantly neutrophils; presence of immature neutrophils is suggestive of bacterial infection. Normally, CSF in children older than 6 months contains <6 WBCs/mm^3 (no polymorphonuclear leukocytes), glucose >45 mg/dL, and protein <45 mg/dL.[28] Values for 677 infants <90 days of age with febrile illness but without meningitis were studied recently.[28] In months 1, 2, and 3 of life, respectively, mean CSF WBCs were 6, 3, and 3 cells/mm^3 and

protein 75, 59 and 40 mg/dL.[29] Effects of traumatic lumbar puncture of CSF values also have been studied, showing presence of approximately 2 WBCs/mm^3 and 1.1 mg/dL protein for every 1000 RBCs.[30] Only 2 of 122 children with proven bacterial meningitis in one study had CSF with <6 WBCs/mm^{7,31} The protein concentration is elevated (mean, 100 to 200 mg/dL), and the glucose concentration usually is depressed (CSF-to-serum ratio less than 0.6), but the relative severity of abnormalities depends on the offending organism as well as the cadence and duration of infection. Depending on the observer, the CSF Gram stain smear is positive in up to 80% of patients with untreated bacterial meningitis. Table 40-2 offers a differential etiologic diagnosis based on usual CSF findings of various meningeal pathogens.

Detection of polysaccharide antigen in CSF by latex agglutination is most sensitive for Hib (85% to 95%), followed by *S. pneumoniae* (50% to 75%) and *N. meningitidis* (33% to 50%); false-positive tests also can occur.[26] Antigen is detected readily only in urine of children with Hib meningitis but also can be detected after immunization with Hib conjugate vaccines, and pneumococcal antigen after PCV. There is no reliable method to detect the polysaccharide of *N. meningitidis* serotype B. Thus, in the Hib vaccine era, rapid antigen tests have limited value in untreated patients, are infrequently more discriminating than Gram stain, and cannot be used to direct specific therapy.

Many children with bacterial meningitis receive oral or parenteral antibiotics before diagnosis. In general, prior oral therapy in standard doses does not alter CSF findings to a point that prevents a final diagnosis of bacterial meningitis. The most comprehensive information about the impact of oral antibiotics on CSF abnormalities, however, relates to Hib meningitis.[32] Similar data for large numbers of patients with pneumococcal or meningococcal meningitis are not available; the impact could be greater for exquisitely susceptible pathogens, such as meningococci, and when a parenteral dose of a cephalosporin is administered. Positive results of antigen detection tests are most helpful in pretreated patients in whom CSF is abnormal, but results of Gram stain and culture are negative.

Although measurement of serum C-reactive protein concentration can be useful to distinguish bacterial from viral meningitis in many patients, the main value of this inflammatory marker appears to be related to the detection of complications or treatment failures after serial measurements. A CSF leukocyte aggregation test has been suggested to help distinguish between bacterial and aseptic causes. One study has indicated that this test might be of value as a sensitive adjunctive screening tool for the timely diagnosis of bacterial meningitis,[33] but the test has the limitation of low specificity.

Polymerase chain reaction (PCR) assay performed on CSF has been employed to detect microbial DNA in patients with bacterial meningitis. Primers are available for the simultaneous detection of *N. meningitidis*, *S. pneumoniae*, and Hib. One study detected species-specific amplicons in 87 of 98 CSF samples (sensitivity of 89%) from patients with meningitis caused by any of these pathogens, with no false-positive results.[34] Another group used a PCR-based assay developed to amplify a conserved region of the pneumococcal autolysin gene.[35] The amplified product was tagged and detected with a biotin-labeled probe in an enzyme immunoassay (EIA). This test was performed on CSF samples from 11 patients with culture-negative meningitis, five of which yielded positive results. The researchers suggested that the PCR-EIA test might be useful when results of CSF culture, Gram stain, and latex agglutination are negative because of prior antibiotic treatment. Real-time PCR is a promising sensitive and specific technique that likely will have future usefulness in the clinical setting.[36] It has shown improved detection of bacterial pathogens,[37,38] and is particularly helpful in diagnosing enteroviral meningitis, which is common in many areas during the summer months.

Lumbar puncture for collection of CSF is contraindicated in certain situations. For children with hypotension, respiratory distress, or cardiac disorder, the positioning for lumbar puncture can further compromise ventilation and blood flow, so is deferred until the child's condition is stable. Likewise for children with

TABLE 40-2. Usual Cerebrospinal Fluid (CSF) Findings in Children with Meningitis Caused by Various Microbial Etiologies

CSF Finding	Viral	Bacterial	Partially Treated Bacterial	Lyme	Fungal	TB
Leukocytes/mm³	<1000	>1000[a]	>1000	<500	<500	<300
Neutrophils	20–40%[b]	>85–90%	>80%	<10%	<10–20%	<10–20%[b]
Protein (mg/dL)	N or <100	>100–150	60 to >100	<100	>100–200	>200–300
Glucose (mg/dL)	N[c]	UD to <40	<40	N	<40	<40
Blood-to-glucose ratio	N	<0.4	<0.4	N	<0.4	<0.4
Positive smear[d]	–	>85%[e]	≥80%	–	<40%	<30%
Positive culture	Rare	>95%	<90%	–	>30%[f]	<30%
PCR or other methods	Enterovirus, herpesvirus	16S RNA, bacterial DNA	16S RNA, bacterial DNA	Borrelia burgdorferi antibodies	Histoplasma and Cryptococcus antigen, India ink for Cryptococcus	Mycobacterium tuberculosis

CSF, cerebrospinal fluid; PCR, polymerase chain reaction; TB, tuberculosis; UD, undetectable.

[a]*Fewer than 500 leukocytes can be seen in severe/rapid onset pneumococcal meningitis.*

[b]*Neutrophil predominance can be observed in early stages of meningitis.*

[c]*Low glucose concentration can occur in meningitis caused by mumps and herpesviruses.*

[d]*Gram or acid-fast bacilli staining for bacteria or Mycobacterium, respectively.*

[e]*Fewer positive smears in Listeria meningitis due to lower bacterial inoculum.*

[f]*Better culture isolation rates for Candida than for Histoplasma or Cryptococcus organisms.*

profound thrombocytopenia or a clotting disorder, the lumbar puncture is deferred until the condition is corrected. An older child or any child with an underlying predisposing condition (cyanotic heart disease or chronic sinusitis) who manifests fever and evidence of increased intracranial pressure or focal neurologic deficit should have an imaging study performed before lumbar puncture to exclude a brain abscess, other mass lesion, or other cause of increased intracranial pressure. Occasionally, the skin overlying the lumbar vertebrae is infected or inflamed by cellulitis or an abscess associated with an infected dermal sinus, precluding a lumbar puncture. Empiric antibiotic therapy is begun without delay in all of these situations.

Blood culture results are positive in most children with bacterial meningitis, especially in cases due to Hib or *S. pneumoniae*. The diagnostic yield of blood culture can be increased in meningococcemia by inoculation of broth without sodium polyanethol sulfonate (see Chapter 287, Laboratory Diagnosis of Infection Due to Bacteria, Fungi, Parasites, and Rickettsiae). Aspiration of an inflamed joint, cellulitis (particularly of the cheek), purpuric lesion, or purulent middle-ear fluid maximizes identification of the infecting organism and provides a pathogen for susceptibility testing. In children with meningitis after surgery or trauma, culture of a specimen protected from infected wounds is useful. Culture specimens obtained from puncture of sinus, middle-ear cavity, or mastoid bone can be useful when meningitis complicates these infections.

MANAGEMENT

Empiric treatment of children with possible or proven bacterial meningitis is guided by knowledge of likely pathogens and their most current antimicrobial susceptibility. In addition, antibiotics and dosages should be selected to produce CSF drug concentrations likely to be at least 8- to 10-fold greater than those required to inhibit and kill the pathogen in vitro (minimal inhibitory concentration, or MIC), a level in animal models that predicts successful treatment.[39] For β-lactam antibiotics and vancomycin, the time during which the drug concentration exceeds the MIC appears to determine drug effectiveness. Concentrations in CSF should surpass the MIC for at least 50% to 60% of the dosing interval (concentration-independent activity). For

aminoglycosides and fluoroquinolones, effectiveness is determined by the ratio between the peak concentration or area under the curve of the antibiotic and the MIC of the pathogen (concentration-dependent activity).[40]

Antimicrobial Resistance

National surveillance conducted by the CDC in 1986 showed that 32% of Hib isolates recovered from children with invasive infections were resistant to ampicillin because of β-lactamase production;[41] by the mid 1990s, the rate of resistant organisms had increased to 40%.[42] Occasional additional isolates are ampicillin resistant as a result of alterations in penicillin-binding proteins, or are chloramphenicol resistant because of production of chloramphenicol acetyltransferase enzyme.[41] Cefotaxime and ceftriaxone have excellent activity against all Hib strains and are comparable in efficacy but superior in rapidity of CSF sterilization compared with chloramphenicol for treatment of ampicillin-resistant Hib meningitis.[43–45]

The penicillin resistance of *S. pneumoniae* is a growing problem worldwide.[46] Before the mid 1980s, there were only scattered reports of bacterial meningitis due to resistant *S. pneumoniae* throughout the world, including the U.S. In some areas of the U.S., however, as many as 40% of pneumococcal isolates are penicillin nonsusceptible,[47] whereas in other countries, rates of resistance as high as 60% have been noted. In January 2008, the Clinical and Laboratory Standards Institute (CLSI) established the latest breakpoints for *S. pneumoniae* depending on clinical site of infection (Table 40-3). For meningitis, strains are defined as susceptible if MIC is ≤0.06, and nonsusceptible if MIC is ≥0.12 μg/mL.[48] *S. pneumoniae* with relative or high-level resistance to penicillin have alterations in penicillin-binding proteins and also can have reduced susceptibility to other β-lactam antibiotics. Pneumococcal serotypes 6B, 23F, 14, and 19 are the most common serotypes associated with penicillin resistance and also are the serotypes most frequently isolated from children with systemic infection, although this varies worldwide and is influenced by PCV immunization. Furthermore, pneumococcal isolates can be resistant to multiple classes of antibiotics (penicillins and cephalosporins, trimethoprim-sulfamethoxazole, chloramphenicol, and macrolides). In children's hospitals in the U.S. >20% of

PART II Clinical Syndromes and Cardinal Features of Infectious Diseases: Approach to Diagnosis and Initial Management

SECTION F Central Nervous System Infections

TABLE 40-3. Clinical and Laboratory Standards Institute Guidelines for Interpretation of Susceptibility Testing of *Streptococcus pneumoniae* for Meningitis

Interpretation	Minimal Inhibitory Concentration (µg/mL)					
	Penicillin	Cefotaxime/Ceftriaxone	Meropenem	Vancomycin[a]	Rifampin	Chloramphenicol
Susceptible	≤0.06	≤0.5	≤0.25	≤1	≤1	≤4
Intermediate	–	1.0	0.5	–	2	–
Resistant	≥0.12	≥2.0	≥1	–	≥4	≥8

[a]*Absence or rare occurrence of resistant strains precludes defining results catergories.*

pneumococci recovered from children with invasive infections can be expected to show penicillin resistance. Penicillin or ampicillin is inappropriate therapy for meningitis caused by pneumococci that are relatively or highly resistant to penicillin; treatment failures have been documented in such cases.

Pneumococcal isolates that are tolerant to β-lactam antibiotics and vancomycin also have been documented.[49] Because of defective autolysis, tolerant bacteria produce fewer cell wall–derived substances that cause meningeal inflammation, so CSF abnormalities can be mild.[50] As a result of tolerance, organisms can persist in CSF, and cause relapse after treatment is stopped.

Cefotaxime and ceftriaxone remain active against many penicillin-resistant pneumococci; however, treatment failures have occurred in some cases of meningitis.[51] The MIC for cefotaxime or ceftriaxone in treatment failures usually is ≥0.5 µg/mL. Guidelines for interpreting MIC values of antibiotics for *S. pneumoniae* meningitis are shown in Table 40-3.[52] Vancomycin and rifampin are active against cefotaxime- or ceftriaxone-resistant *S. pneumoniae*. Microbiology laboratories routinely should test all pneumococcal isolates from normally sterile sites for penicillin susceptibility. Screening can be accomplished with several methods, including oxacillin disc, E-test, and commercial microtiter methods.[53]

Aqueous penicillin G remains the agent of choice for meningococcal meningitis, although ampicillin and third-generation cephalosporins also are effective and can be easier to administer. Clinical isolates of *N. meningitidis* with relative resistance to penicillin (MIC ≥0.125 µg/mL) have been reported.[54] Resistance is associated not with β-lactamase production but with alterations in penicillin-binding proteins. The clinical significance of this type of resistance in the treatment of meningococcal meningitis is unclear. Ceftriaxone resistance is rare.

Antimicrobial Therapy

Initial empiric therapy using cefotaxime or ceftriaxone plus vancomycin (60 mg/kg/day divided q6h) is prudent for infants ≥1 month and children with suspected bacterial meningitis.[55,56] Limited pediatric clinical data preclude recommendations regarding use of rifampin combined with a cephalosporin as initial therapy. In the Hib vaccine era, ampicillin plus chloramphenicol is not an optimal combination for initial therapy because of its likely inadequacy or potential antagonism against pneumococci.

Once an organism has been identified and the antimicrobial susceptibility pattern is known, antibiotic therapy can be simplified or modified (Table 40-4). Penicillin G or ampicillin can be used to complete therapy for pneumococcal or meningococcal meningitis due to susceptible organisms. Cefotaxime or ceftriaxone is continued for penicillin-nonsusceptible pneumococci that are susceptible to these agents (MIC ≤0.5 µg/mL).[57] Although many patients with isolates having third-generation cephalosporin MIC of 0.5 to 1.0 µg/mL have been treated successfully, treatment with cephalosporin alone is usually not recommended. It is prudent to repeat the CSF examination after 24 to 48 hours of therapy in patients with infection caused by β-lactam-resistant pneumococci to document a sterile culture and negative Gram stain. This is relevant particularly for patients who have not shown clinical improvement. If results of the second CSF Gram stain or culture are positive, or a pneumococcal isolate has an MIC of ≥1.0 µg/mL for extended-spectrum cephalosporins, vancomycin (if not begun previously) with or without rifampin should be added.[58] Rifampin should be added if the patient is already receiving vancomycin. Vancomycin penetration into CSF during meningitis can be unpredictable, and thus, peak serum and trough values

TABLE 40-4. Recommendations for Pathogen-Specific Antimicrobial Therapy of Children with Bacterial Meningitis

Bacteria	Antibiotic of Choice	Other Useful Antibiotics
Neisseria meningitides	Penicillin G or ampicillin	Cefotaxime or ceftriaxone
Haemophilus influenzae	Cefotaxime or ceftriaxone	Ampicillin or chloramphenicol[a]
Streptococcus pneumoniae[b]		
1. Penicillin-susceptible	Penicillin G or ampicillin	Cefotaxime or ceftriaxone
2. Penicillin-resistant	Cefotaxime or ceftriaxone[b] *plus* vancomycin	Cefepime[c] or meropenem
3. Cephalosporin-nonsusceptible	Cefotaxime or ceftriaxone[b] *plus* vancomycin	Add rifampin to antibiotics of choice Meropenem + vancomycin New fluoroquinolones[d]
Listeria monocytogenes	Ampicillin ± gentamicin	Trimethoprim-sulfamethoxazole
Streptococcus agalactiae	Penicillin G ± gentamicin	Ampicillin ± gentamicin
Enterobacteriaceae	Cefotaxime or ceftriaxone *with/without* aminoglycoside	Cefepime or meropenem
Pseudomonas aeruginosa	Ceftazidime + amikacin	Cefepime or meropenem

MIC, minimal inhibitory concentration.

[a]*In areas with economic constraints: ampicillin for susceptible strains and chloramphenicol for ampicillin-resistant* Haemophilus influenzae *type b isolates.*

[b]*Higher dosages might be helpful.*

[c]*CLSI MIC breakpoints for cefepime for meningitis are S ≤ 0.5, I 1, R ≥ 2.*

[d]*These drugs currently are under investigation.*

should be in the upper therapeutic range (35 to 40 and 10 to 15 μg/mL, respectively).

Although rarely used today in developed countries, chloramphenicol is an option for treatment of bacterial meningitis caused by ampicillin-resistant Hib or in the child with a history of anaphylaxis or respiratory distress associated with penicillin or other β-lactam antibiotics. Because the pharmacokinetics of chloramphenicol are variable, serum concentrations should be monitored to ensure that safe and effective concentrations are achieved.[59] Ideal peak values are 15 to 30 μg/mL at 60 to 120 minutes after the completion of infusion. Values exceeding 30 μg/mL are associated with bone marrow suppression; concentrations greater than 50 to 80 μg/mL have been associated with "grey baby" syndrome (which is not confined to infants) and impaired myocardial contractility. Chloramphenicol is best avoided in children with septic shock. Additionally, several drugs affect the metabolism of chloramphenicol; concurrent administration of phenobarbital and rifampin lowers the chloramphenicol metabolism, whereas administration of phenytoin raises it.

Other potentially useful antimicrobial agents for the treatment of bacterial meningitis are cefepime and meropenem, both of which have been shown to be equivalent to third-generation cephalosporins in treatment of children infected with common meningeal pathogens.[60-63] The efficacy of these antibiotics against β-lactam-resistant pneumococci has not been defined, although they appear not to be superior to cefotaxime or ceftriaxone. The use of imipenem-cilastatin is not recommended in children with CNS infection because of potential epileptogenic activity of imipenem in the pediatric population. Because of the increasing rate of isolation of multiple-drug-resistant pneumococci worldwide, there is an urgent need to develop antibiotics with different mechanisms of action against these strains. Accordingly, fluoroquinolones (including newer agents like gemifloxacin and moxifloxacin) and other novel antibiotics (including glycopeptides like oritavancin and teicoplanin, as well as daptomycin, linezolid, and telavancin) need to be evaluated in clinical trials of children with bacterial meningitis. Linezolid appears to enter the central nervous system adequately, based on limited data in both children and adults.[64,65]

Monitoring During Therapy

Performance of complete blood counts during therapy is helpful for early detection of neutropenia, which is associated with β-lactam antibiotics and chloramphenicol; the neutropenia is readily reversible when antibiotics are discontinued. Anemia is common in children with bacterial meningitis and also can be exacerbated by chloramphenicol. Ceftriaxone has been associated with immune-mediated, rapidly fatal hemolysis in patients with sickle-cell disease, human immunodeficiency virus infection, and leukemia.[66,67] Thrombocytosis (platelet count >750,000/mm^3) occurs frequently in patients with meningitis, has no apparent adverse clinical effect, and platelet counts need not be monitored. Diarrhea is the most common adverse effect of ampicillin and the extended-spectrum cephalosporins. Rashes, eosinophilia, and mild elevation in serum hepatic transaminase values can occur with any of these agents as well. Ceftriaxone occasionally has been associated with abdominal discomfort and pseudolithiasis ("sludge") in the gallbladder, as seen on ultrasonography;[68] this process can be reversed with discontinuation of the drug. Routine performance of computed tomography or magnetic resonance imaging of the head during antimicrobial therapy has no therapeutic benefit; monitoring with these modalities is most useful if the course is complicated or the pathogen is unusual.[69]

Duration of Therapy

The duration of antibiotic therapy for meningitis varies with the organism and the clinical response.[70] For otherwise uncomplicated cases, meningitis due to *S. pneumoniae* is treated for 10 to 14 days; that due to *N. meningitidis*, for 4 to 7 days; and that due to Hib, for 7 to 10 days. When possible, therapy should be completed in the hospital to permit careful assessment of the response to treatment and to prevent complications of disease or therapy. Parenteral therapy can be completed at home for carefully selected patients if meningitis is due to a fully susceptible organism and the patient has resumed normal activity. Ceftriaxone is approved for a once-daily dosing schedule, making it more convenient and perhaps less expensive than other agents for treatment of fully susceptible organisms. It is essential, however, to calculate and administer each dose correctly so that the patient is not treated inadequately for 24 hours because of a dosage or administration error.

MENINGITIS DUE TO UNUSUAL ORGANISMS

E. coli and *Klebsiella* spp. are the most common gram-negative enteric organisms that cause bacterial meningitis in children other than neonates.[71] A combination of an extended-spectrum cephalosporin or ampicillin plus an aminoglycoside administered intravenously is reasonable empiric therapy for suspected gram-negative meningitis, with consideration of susceptibility patterns of nosocomial organisms in hospital-associated cases.[72] Modifications are made once antimicrobial susceptibility information is available. Ceftazidime (cefepime, meropenem, ticarcillin or piperacillin) generally is given with an aminoglycoside for *Pseudomonas* meningitis. Aminoglycoside peak serum concentrations should be close to the upper safe limit in treatment of meningitis. Meningitis due to multidrug-resistant gram-negative bacilli other than *Pseudomonas* may require the treatment with other agents, such as meropenem or cefepime.

For patients with meningitis caused by gram-negative organisms a repeat CSF specimen is obtained for culture at 24 to 48 hours after commencement of therapy and approximately every 48 hours thereafter until sterilization of CSF is documented. Occasionally, CSF does not become sterile unless an aminoglycoside is instilled directly into the ventricles (almost exclusively in postoperative or posttraumatic cases). This is best done through an Ommaya reservoir. Systemic treatment is continued for a minimum of 21 days or at least 2 weeks beyond the first documented sterile CSF culture, whichever is longer.

Surgical drainage of wound infections after trauma or neurosurgery also is required, as is removal of contaminated devices. Imaging studies are performed in patients with gram-negative bacillary meningitis before the decision to terminate therapy, to assess the nature of cerebral involvement and the need for surgical intervention.

Meningitis caused by *S. aureus* is treated with nafcillin when the organism is susceptible (oxacillin does not adequately penetrate into CSF). Vancomycin is an alternative for patients who are allergic to penicillin or have a methicillin-resistant isolate. Adding rifampin to the antistaphylococcal regimen may be necessary if CSF Gram stain or culture results remain positive despite the use of agents active in vitro. Ampicillin plus an aminoglycoside is recommended for patients with meningitis due to susceptible strains of *Enterococcus* species. Vancomycin (with aminoglycoside) is used for ampicillin-resistant *Enterococcus* spp. Scattered case reports of successful therapy with linezolid and daptomycin in adults with meningitis caused by resistant staphylococci and enterococci have been published.[73-75] Ampicillin is also the drug of choice for *Listeria monocytogenes* infection; data support the possible beneficial role of concurrent aminoglycosides, at least for the first few days of therapy. When infection occurs in a patient with a ventriculoperitoneal shunt, bacterial eradication is best accomplished by removal of the device coupled with antimicrobial therapy.

SUPPORTIVE CARE

Unless the patient is only mildly affected, initial supportive care of the child with bacterial meningitis is best provided in an intensive care setting, where the patient can be observed and monitored continuously.[76] Typically, most life-threatening complications of bacterial meningitis (septic shock, herniation, infarctions,

---

BOX 40-1. Causes of Prolonged or Recurrent Fever in Children with Bacterial Meningitis

- Inadequate treatment
- Nosocomial infection
- Transient elevation after discontinuing dexamethasone
- Phlebitis
- Suppurative complication
- Pericarditis
- Pneumonia
- Pyogenic arthritis
- Subdural empyema
- Immune-mediated arthritis
- Drug fever (rare)
- Unknown

---

seizures, and inadequate ventilation) occur early in the course of treatment and require urgent interventions for optimal outcome.

Maintenance of blood pressure within the normal range for age may require infusion of a vasoactive agent, such as dopamine or dobutamine. Initially, the patient is not fed orally. Fluid restriction is advised only in patients without clinical evidence of dehydration who have hyponatremia (i.e., suspicion of inappropriate antidiuretic hormone secretion). If the patient is hypovolemic or in shock, additional intravenous fluids must be given accordingly. There is no evidence that fluid restriction reduces cerebral edema in children with bacterial meningitis. A recent Cochrane meta-analysis found that fluid restriction in bacterial meningitis can be associated with poorer neurologic outcome compared with maintenance of adequate intravenous fluids.[77]

Increased intracranial pressure is a major component of the pathophysiologic alterations of meningitis. In addition to elevation of the patient's head, some clinicians administer mannitol (0.5 to 2 g/kg) if clinical signs (apnea, bradycardia, sluggish pupils, or pupillary dilation) of extremely high intracranial pressure are detected. Immediate intubation and hyperventilation can be life-saving if cerebral herniation develops. Seizures are controlled with standard anticonvulsants, such as phenobarbital and phenytoin. Most seizures occur early in the illness, and are generalized, and usually can be controlled easily. Seizures that occur early in the course of meningitis and are controlled easily usually have no prognostic significance. However, seizures that are focal, occur 48 or more hours after admission, or are difficult to control imply an underlying vascular disturbance, such as venous thrombosis or infarction, and are associated with development of epilepsy and other neurologic sequelae.[78]

Once adequate therapy begins, the duration of fever typically is 4 to 6 days. Children with meningitis due to Hib tend to have a relatively longer febrile period. Recurrence of fever or persistence of fever beyond 8 days can be caused by several conditions (Box 40-1). Fever patterns should be evaluated carefully, although a specific explanation often is not found. It is unlikely that uninfected subdural effusions cause prolonged fever.

ADJUNCTIVE MEASURES

Modulating the host response to infection may be beneficial in decreasing some sequelae of meningitis. Prospective studies have shown that dexamethasone therapy initiated just before or concurrently with the first dose of intravenous antibiotics significantly diminishes the incidence of neurologic and audiologic deficits due to Hib meningitis.[42,79–82] Although the benefit of dexamethasone in meningitis due to other pathogens has not been evaluated as extensively as for Hib disease, three meta-analyses of published data indicated that early administration of dexamethasone can improve outcome in pneumococcal disease, in both children and adults.[83–85] For pneumococcal meningitis, it is crucial to administer dexamethasone before or concomitantly with parenteral antibiotics, particularly in emergency departments of both developed and developing countries.[86,87] Because of the intrinsically better prognosis of meningococcal meningitis, it is likely that thousands of patients would need to be studied to assess reliably the role of corticosteroid therapy. Dexamethasone can decrease the penetration of antibiotics into the CSF and, theoretically, jeopardize

bacterial eradication of β-lactam-resistant pneumococcal strains. Although some clinical reports have indicated that dexamethasone does not affect the bactericidal activity of a third-generation cephalosporin combined with vancomycin against highly resistant pneumococci,[88] a careful clinical assessment and second CSF evaluation are warranted in this situation.

Dexamethasone administration is associated with a rapid resolution of fever (i.e., 1–2 days) in treated patients, but a secondary transient rise in body temperature is observed in up to 40% of cases once the drug is discontinued. Its administration has been associated rarely with severe gastrointestinal bleeding. To minimize potential, albeit infrequent, adverse events while maintaining therapeutic anti-inflammatory effect, the currently recommended dosing regimen is 0.6 to 0.8 mg/kg daily in 2 or 3 divided doses for 2 days.

The response to adjunctive anti-inflammatory therapy may be suboptimal in children with underlying conditions including malnutrition and infection with human immunodeficiency virus (HIV). Similarly, response may be altered if there is a delay in time of starting antibiotics or in those treated with suboptimal antibiotics. In developing countries, novel adjuvant therapies are needed. A meta-analysis that included trials performed in developing countries showed that patients who received dexamethasone had lower occurrence of hearing loss. In this meta-analysis, however, dexamethasone was not associated with significant reduction of death or other neurologic sequelae.[89] A recent multicenter study performed in different countries of Latin America showed that administration of oral glycerol to children with meningitis reduced the occurrence of some neurologic sequelae and performed comparably or better than dexamethasone.[90]

PROGNOSIS AND SEQUELAE

With modern management, the mortality rate for bacterial meningitis in children caused by the three common pathogens is less than 5% to 10% in most studies. Case-fatality rates and incidence of neurologic sequelae are greatest with pneumococcal meningitis. The neurologic sequelae of meningitis are listed in Box 40-2. Sensorineural hearing loss is the most common readily identifiable sequela. Hearing loss occurs in approximately 20% to 30% of previously healthy children after meningitis due to S. pneumoniae and in 5% to 10% of patients after meningitis caused by Hib or N. meningitidis. Balance disturbances are common in these children because the vestibular portion of the inner ear also is affected. Hearing loss is more likely if the admission CSF glucose concentration is <20 mg/dL. Hearing should be tested before discharge or within 1 month after discharge in all children with bacterial meningitis, so that if hearing loss is detected, appropriate management can be instituted as soon as possible. Reversible deafness has been documented in some children tested at discharge and 4 to 6 months later.

Acute hydrocephalus as well as many sequelae related to vascular compromise can improve with time. Hemiparesis can resolve several months to years after the event. Imaging studies demonstrate evidence of infarction in such patients, although these findings usually do not affect or change management.

Behavioral and academic problems are more subtle consequences of bacterial meningitis that may not be apparent for several years after infection. Although formal testing generally

---

BOX 40-2. Neurologic Sequelae of Bacterial Meningitis

- Sensorineural hearing loss
- Ataxia
- Vascular compromise
- Hemiparesis
- Quadriparesis
- Epilepsy
- Spinal cord infarction
- Cortical blindness
- Diabetes insipidus
- Hydrocephalus
- Behavioral disorder
- Intellectual deficits

---

is not necessary, careful assessment over time is essential; any concerns regarding school performance warrant further investigation.

PREVENTION

Close contacts of patients with meningococcal disease should receive chemoprophylaxis with rifampin (5 mg/kg if <1 month of age, 10 mg/kg if ≥1 month of age; maximum dose 600 mg) twice daily for 2 days, started ideally within 24 hours of the exposure. A single large oral dose of ciprofloxacin (20 mg/kg, maximum 500 mg) or azithromycin (10 mg/kg, maximum 500 mg) or a parenteral dose of ceftriaxone (125 mg IM if <15 years, 250 mg IM if ≥15 years) are suitable alternatives; the last is preferred for pregnant women. Rifampin prophylaxis also is recommended for all household contacts of an index case with Hib disease when at least one household contact is younger than 4 years and is unimmunized or incompletely immunized.

Undoubtedly, the greatest advance regarding this disease is the introduction of conjugated vaccines to prevent meningitis due to the most common microorganisms. The formidable impact of the conjugate Hib vaccines has been documented extensively. PCV7 tested in a large-scale trial conducted in the U.S. showed a 97% per-protocol efficacy against invasive infections caused by the pneumococcal serotypes contained in the vaccine.[91] A marked reduction of pneumococcal meningitis in vaccinated U.S. children has been documented postmarketing.[92,93] A trial of PCV9 conducted in African children with or without HIV infection was associated with reduced incidence of a first episode of invasive pneumococcal disease caused by vaccine serotypes by 65% and 83%, respectively.[94] In 2010, PCV13 was licensed in the U.S. In addition to PCV7 serotypes, PCV13 includes serotypes 1, 3, 5, 6B, 7F, 19A.

Epidemiologic studies identifying cases of invasive pneumococcal disease through Active Bacterial Core surveillance (ABCs) of the CDC before and after the implementation of PCV7 have shown significant decrease in pediatric cases of pneumococcal meningitis.[95] Since routine infant immunization in 2000, cases of invasive pneumococcal disease due to any serotype decreased by 76% in the U.S.[96] A decline in cases of meningitis in children <2 years of age also was evident in Europe following implementation of PCV. However, an increase in meningitis cases in children >2 years of age was noted.[97] Children >2 years of age who are at high risk of developing invasive pneumococcal disease, such as patients with sickle-cell disease and nephrotic syndrome, or meningitis, such as children with cochlear implants, also should receive the 23-valent polysaccharide vaccine (PPSV23).

Children at high risk for meningococcal infection, such as those with asplenia or persistent complement deficiencies, should receive MCV4 at 2 years of age and every 5 years thereafter. All adolescents should receive MCV4 at 11 to 12 years of age, with a booster at 16 years of age.[98] An MCV against serogroup C was used in the U.K. in 1999. A study performed 4 years after implementation in the U.K. showed that, at 1 year post vaccination, vaccine effectiveness was 93% (95% CI, 67% to 99%); however, a decline was seen >1 year post vaccination.[99] In 2006, a booster dose was recommended at 1 year of age (see Chapter 125, *Neisseria meningitidis*). Currently, work is ongoing to develop an effective vaccine against group B meningococcus, particularly targeting the outer-membrane vesicle.

---

41 Chronic Meningitis

Douglas Swanson and Christopher J. Harrison

Chronic meningitis is defined arbitrarily as persistent or progressive signs and symptoms of meningeal irritation and cerebrospinal fluid (CSF) pleocytosis lasting for at least 4 weeks without improvement. The symptoms of chronic meningitis vary, but most patients have a gradual onset of fever, headache, and vomiting. The 4-week timeframe is intended to avoid extensive evaluation for individuals with self-limiting processes (e.g., acute or subacute meningoencephalitis, resolving acute meningitis). In most cases of prolonged meningitis, diagnosis and treatment occur before clinical symptoms have continued for 4 weeks; thus, chronic meningitis is relatively rare.

ETIOLOGY AND EPIDEMIOLOGY

There are many infectious (Table 41-1[1-29]) and noninfectious (Box 41-1[30-40]) causes of chronic meningitis. Several parameningeal infections also can manifest as chronic meningitis. The most common entities are shown in Box 41-2. The etiology and epidemiology of chronic meningitis can vary considerably, depending on a patient's geographic locality or underlying medical condition. Individuals with an impaired immune system are at increased risk for developing chronic meningitis, and they have more potential etiologies. The overall incidence of chronic meningitis is unknown due to limitations of the medical literature; and it is different for each etiologic agent. The literature consists primarily of case reports and case series, which contain demographic and diagnostic bias.[41-43] Furthermore, most case reports are of adults. Except for tuberculosis, there is a paucity of information regarding children with chronic meningitis. The history, physical examination findings, and laboratory test results may help identify the cause of chronic meningitis; however, an etiology is not found in about one-third of cases.[41,42]

MAIN FEATURES OF AGENTS CAUSING CHRONIC MENINGITIS

Mycobacterium tuberculosis

Epidemiology. Most tuberculous meningitis occurs in children between 6 months and 4 years of age.[44-49] Risk factors include close contact with contagious cases, travel to or residence in tuberculosis (TB) endemic areas, HIV infection, other viral infections (i.e., measles), malnutrition, and immunosuppression. Close contact with an adult with pulmonary TB disease can be established in 45% to 75% of children; however, the exposure history may not be elucidated initially.[44-50] African Americans and immigrants from countries where tuberculosis is endemic account for a disproportionate number of cases of tuberculous meningitis in the United States. Large epidemiological studies including children and adults find that about 1% of tuberculosis disease involves the central nervous system (CNS).[51,52] However, children are at a higher risk for developing CNS tuberculosis. A review of pediatric tuberculosis cases in the U.S. from 1993 to 2006 shows that meningeal infection accounted for 3.1% of all cases,[53] and depended on age: 7.5% in those <1 year old, 3.5% for 1 to 4 years old,[5] 1.4% for 5 to 9 years old, and 1.8% for 10 to 14 years old.[53]

Pathogenesis. Tubercle bacilli are inhaled, enter the lung alveoli, are filtered into draining lymph nodes, and then are

TABLE 41-1. Infectious Causes of Chronic Meningitis

Agent	Reference No.
BACTERIA	
Mycobacterium tuberculosis	1
Treponema pallidum	2
Brucella spp.	3
Borrelia burgdorferi	4
Nocardia spp.	5
Actinomyces (or Arachnia) spp.	6
Leptospira spp.	7
Tropheryma whipplei	8
Mycoplasma or Ureaplasma spp.	9
VIRUSES	
Human immunodeficiency virus	10
Lymphocytic choriomeningitis virus	11
Enterovirus[a]	12
Cytomegalovirus[b]	13
FUNGI	
Blastomyces dermatitidis	14
Histoplasma capsulatum	15
Coccidioides immitis	16
Cryptococcus neoformans or gattii	17
Candida spp.	18
Aspergillus spp.	19
Pseudallescheria boydii (asexual form, Scedosporium apiospermum)	20
Zygomycetes	21
Cladosporium spp.	22
Sporothrix schenkii	23
OTHERS	
Toxoplasma gondii	24
Taenia spp. (cysticercosis)	25
Acanthamoeba spp.	26
Balamuthia	27
Angiostrongylus spp.	28
Baylisascaris spp.	29

[a]In patients with agammaglobulinemia.

[b]In patients infected with the human immunodeficiency virus.

BOX 41-1. Noninfectious Causes of Chronic Meningitis

Sarcoidosis[30]
Neoplasm (e.g., non-Hodgkin lymphoma)
Systemic lupus erythematosus
Polyarteritis nodosa
Rheumatoid arthritis
Granulomatous angiitis[31]
Other forms of vasculitis[32]
Behçet syndrome[33]
Sjögren syndrome[34]
Neonatal-onset multisystem inflammatory disease (NOMID)[35]
Uveomeningoencephalitis syndrome[36]
Chronic benign lymphocytic meningitis[37]
Subarachnoid hemorrhage
Subdural hematoma
Drug-induced (e.g., ibuprofen, cyclooxygenase-2 inhibitor, trimethoprim)[38,39]
Wegener granulomatosis[40]

BOX 41-2. Parameningeal Infections That Can Manifest as Chronic Meningitis

- Encephalitis
  - Viral
- Brain abscess
- Subdural empyema
- Cranial osteomyelitis
- Mastoiditis
- Sinusitis

---

spread lymphohematogenously throughout the body. Meningitis develops when caseous lesions in the brain cortex or leptomeninges rupture into the subarachnoid space.[54,55]

Clinical manifestations. The clinical onset of CNS tuberculosis can be acute, but more often is a gradual progression of symptoms. CNS tuberculosis usually manifests as meningitis, and less frequently as intracranial tuberculoma or a brain abscess.[44–50] Association with disseminated (miliary) tuberculosis is not uncommon. A compilation of 913 children from 6 retrospective case series of CNS tuberculosis identifies common presenting symptoms to be fever (72%), altered mental status (62%), vomiting (61%), seizure (47%), and headache (37%).[44–46,48–50] About 29% of children develop cranial nerve paresis.[44,46–50] In outcome studies totaling 847 children with CNS tuberculosis, 18% died and 46% had neurologic sequelae.[44–50]

Laboratory findings and diagnosis. A careful history for tuberculosis risk factors in concert with clinical findings suggests the diagnosis. Abnormalities on chest radiograph consistent with TB are present in ~75% of cases, and tuberculin skin test (TST) is positive in ~50% of children.[44–50] Cranial computed tomography (CT) frequently reveals hydrocephalus and basilar enhancement.[46–50] CSF abnormalities can be modest initially but become progressively more abnormal with increasing duration of symptoms. The CSF leukocyte count typically ranges from 10 to 500 cells/mm^3, and can briefly show polymorphonuclear cell predominance, but usually there is lymphocytic predominance. The CSF glucose level typically is low (frequently <20 mg/dL), and the protein level often is very elevated (>400 mg/dL). Reported positivity of acid-fast bacilli (AFB) stains of CSF have ranged from 5% to 51%. The likelihood of detecting organisms on AFB stain depends on the volume of CSF sampled and the diligence of microscopic evaluations;[56] large volumes (5 to 10 mL) of centrifuged CSF and ≥30 minutes of microscopic inspection yield better results. Growth of M. tuberculosis from CSF occurred in 155 of 374 (41%) children with TB meningitis reported, and yields as high as 70% have been reported when up to 10 mL of CSF is sampled.[44–48,50] Gastric aspirate or sputum AFB smear and culture can increase the probability of diagnosis in children. Nucleic acid amplification (NAA) tests, such as polymerase chain reaction (PCR), are commercially available to detect mycobacterial DNA from CSF. A meta-analysis of the accuracy of NAA for diagnosing tuberculous meningitis revealed a sensitivity of 56% (negative predictive value, 44%) and a specificity of 98% (positive predictive value 35.1%) among commercially available assays.[57] The PCR test can remain positive for several weeks after treatment is initiated.

Treponema pallidum

Epidemiology. Chronic syphilitic meningitis is rare and occurs in <1% of patients with syphilis; the incidence of meningitis is greatest in the first 2 years after T. pallidum infection.[2] In recent years, the incidence of syphilis has declined in the U.S., but continued attention to populations with increased risk (e.g., HIV-infected individuals) and early treatment mitigates severe consequences. Although neurosyphilis rarely manifests as chronic meningitis, partially treated neurosyphilis can imitate chronic meningitis.

Pathogenesis. Congenital syphilis usually occurs by transplacental transmission of T. pallidum from the mother directly into the fetal circulation.[58] Postnatally acquired syphilis develops when the mucous membranes or abraded skin are penetrated by *T. pallidum* by direct contact with ulcerative lesions of infected people. The organism disseminates lymphohematogenously and can invade the CNS.

Clinical manifestations. In children, syphilis usually is congenitally acquired. Most infants are asymptomatic at birth although those with syphilitic meningitis are more likely to be symptomatic than those without meningitis. Common clinical features of congenital infection include one or more of the following: hepatosplenomegaly, mucocutaneous lesions, lymphadenopathy, and osteochondritis.[59] About 50% of infants with symptoms of congenital syphilis and 10% of asymptomatic but infected infants have CSF abnormalities: a reactive Venereal Disease Research Laboratory (VDRL) test, elevated white blood cell (WBC) count, and/or elevated protein level. Even with abnormal CSF, usually there are no detectable clinical neurologic signs or symptoms.[60] Without treatment, congenitally infected infants can develop acute leptomeningitis between 3 and 6 months of age with one or more signs: stiff neck, vomiting, bulging fontanel, and hydrocephalus.[59] If untreated, chronic meningovascular syphilis with progressive hydrocephalus, cranial nerve palsies, and intellectual deterioration develops toward the end of the first year. About one-third of patients with the early stage of postnatally acquired syphilis have CNS involvement that may or may not lead to acute meningovascular neurosyphilis. If untreated, one-half develop symptomatic or asymptomatic late neurosyphilis. Features of symptomatic late neurosyphilis include dementia, tabes dorsalis, meningovascular disease, seizures, and optic atrophy.

Laboratory findings and diagnosis. The diagnosis of syphilitic meningitis can be difficult. A serum fluorescent treponemal antibody absorption (FTA-ABS) test is positive in more than 95% of patients. If the serum FTA-ABS test result is negative, the probability of syphilitic meningitis is very low (except in patients with poorly controlled HIV infection, who may fail to produce antibodies).

Useful tests for CSF samples include specific treponemal immunoglobulin (Ig) M antibodies, VDRL, and FTA-ABS.[61] The specificity of the VDRL test on CSF is high, but sensitivity is low (30% to 70%). A nonreactive result does not exclude the diagnosis. False-positive reaction can be due to blood contamination or high CSF protein. In contrast, a negative result of FTA-ABS test on CSF rules out neurosyphilis, but a positive test does not confirm the diagnosis because false-positive results can occur as a result of CSF contamination with blood or small amounts of antibodies from the serum.

The best indicator of CNS infection in neonates is an abnormal physical examination, anemia, thrombocytopenia, CSF abnormalities, and abnormal bone radiographs. A positive PCR test for *T. pallidum* DNA in the blood or CSF is highly predictive of neurosyphilis.[60] The PCR technique has been shown to be sensitive for diagnosis of acute neurosyphilis but to be less useful in chronic cases.[62]

Brucella Species

Epidemiology. Brucellosis is a zoonotic disease, associated particularly with sheep, goats, swine, and cattle. Humans become infected by direct contact with infected animals or by ingestion of unpasteurized milk products. There does not appear to be an increased risk for patients with underlying diseases.[63] Brucellosis is an uncommon disease in the U.S., with about 100 cases occurring annually, and less than 10% occurring in children.[64] Brucellosis is a common disease worldwide. Thus, a history of travel and consumption of unpasteurized dairy products is important, especially travel in the Mediterranean region, India, or Latin America. Meningitis occurs in fewer than 5% of patients with brucellosis and is the first manifestation of the disease in about 1%. The incubation period varies from <1 week to several months, with an average of 3 to 4 weeks.

Pathogenesis. *Brucella* are facultative intracellular pathogens that can survive and multiply within phagocytes and other cells. It is postulated that infected leukocytes carry the organism into the CNS.[65] Another hypothesis is that bacteria enter the CNS through direct endothelial cell invasion.

Clinical manifestations. Meningitis is the most common presentation of neurobrucellosis. Symptoms are nonspecific and include fever, headache, vomiting, and meningeal irritation.[3,66,67] CSF findings include lymphocytic pleocytosis with a low to normal glucose concentration and high protein concentration. Systemic manifestations of brucellosis may be present. If treated, the prognosis usually is good; however, cases with serious neurologic sequelae have been reported.[66]

Laboratory findings and diagnosis. Because neurobrucellosis has nonspecific symptoms, it is important to obtain a careful history regarding travel, diet, and animal exposures. CSF lymphocytic pleocytosis with low to normal glucose and elevated protein concentrations is typical. The CSF Gram stain usually is negative. CSF culture is positive in fewer than 25% of patients; cultures of blood and, especially, bone marrow increase the diagnostic yield. The laboratory should be instructed to maintain the cultures for at least 4 weeks. The diagnosis can be confirmed by detection of specific *Brucella* antibodies in the CSF or serum by agglutination or enzyme immunoassay (EIA) with Western blot.[68] PCR detection of *Brucella* DNA in the CSF or serum is a promising tool.[69,70]

Borrelia burgdorferi

Epidemiology. *Borrelia burgdorferi* should be considered in endemic areas, which includes the northeast, upper midwest, and northern Pacific coast of the U.S. Approximately 2% of children with Lyme disease develop clinical evidence of meningitis.[71] Chronic meningitis with serious neurologic sequelae is rare.[4]

Pathogenesis. The spirochete enters the host from a bite of an infected tick: *Ixodes scapularis* in the northeast and upper midwest of the U.S. or the *Ixodes pacificus* in the west. *Borrelia* multiplies locally in the skin at the site of the tick bite. Local inflammation typically results in erythema migrans. In days to weeks, the spirochete can spread lymphohematogenously to other sites, including the CNS.

Clinical manifestations. Meningitis usually presents during the early disseminated phase of disease with acute onset of symptoms similar to viral meningitis: fever, headache, stiff neck, and malaise. However, clinical symptoms with Lyme meningitis usually are prolonged compared with viral meningitis.[72-74] In addition, about half of patients develop cranial neuropathies, with facial palsy being the most common. The prognosis usually is very good with therapy. If untreated, symptoms can last for many months.

Laboratory findings and diagnosis. Residence in or travel to an endemic area and a history of erythema migrans are important clues to the diagnosis. The CSF typically shows a modest monocytic and lymphocytic pleocytosis with modestly elevated protein concentration. In the absence of a history of erythema migrans, the features of prolonged headache, cranial neuropathy, and predominance of CSF mononuclear cells can help distinguish Lyme meningitis from other forms of aseptic meningitis.[72-74] Spirochetes can only rarely be isolated from CSF using a specific culture medium.[75-77] Intrathecal antibodies specific to *B. burgdorferi* can be measured by EIA, although the sensitivity and specificity of the test in uncertain.[76,77] Paired serum antibodies should be obtained so that the CSF:serum antibody ratio can be determined.[75,77] An elevated CSF:serum antibody ratio might reflect past CNS infection, but in conjunction with a CSF pleocytosis and elevated protein can be used to support the diagnosis of active infection. DNA PCR detection of *B. burgdorferi* from the CSF has good specificity, but poor sensitivity – ranging from 20% to 50% in acute cases to 0 to 25% in chronic cases.[77,78] Because of limited studies, the advantage of immunoassays over PCR for diagnosing Lyme meningitis has not been demonstrated conclusively. If the result for the immunoassay is negative and there is a high suspicion of Lyme neuroborreliosis, PCR testing may be considered.

Other Bacteria

Leptospirosis is a rare cause of chronic meningitis because the clinical signs and symptoms of meningitis generally disappear within 7 to 21 days.[7] Other rare bacterial causes include *Nocardia*,[5]

Actinomyces,[6] and *Tropheryma whipplei*.[8] Both *Mycoplasma hominis* and *Ureoplasma urealyticum* can cause chronic meningitis in preterm infants associated with development of hydrocephalus.[9]

Cryptococcus Species

Epidemiology. *Cryptococcus neoformans* is a yeast-like fungus with worldwide distribution and is probably the most common cause of fungal meningitis in immunocompromised adult patients. Although *Cryptococcus* can infect normal hosts, it more commonly develops in patients with risk factors of primary impaired cellular immunity, high-dose corticosteroid treatment, leukemia, lymphoma, or HIV infection. Cryptococcal meningitis develops in up to 10% of adults with AIDS; it is the most common life-threatening fungal infection in patients with poorly controlled HIV infection and, in 40% of those affected, is the first AIDS-defining opportunistic infection.[79] However, cryptococcal meningitis is relatively rare in children. Abadi et al. retrospectively compiled 30 cases of *Cryptococcus neoformans* infections in HIV-infected children from 1985 to 1996, and estimated a 1% 10-year point prevalence of cryptococcosis among children with AIDS.[80] *Cryptococcus gattii* was historically found more often in tropical and subtropical geographic regions, although it is now being reported in temperate areas, mostly on the west coast of California and British Columbia.[81] *C. gattii* meningitis is associated with progressive CNS disease in immunocompetent patients, suggesting that genotypic or phenotypic differences of the fungus, or both, may explain its virulence in immunocompetent hosts.[81]

Pathogenesis. *C. neoformans* is found in bird droppings and soil and *C. gattii* is found in certain trees and soils. Humans become infected by inhaling airborne fungi into the lungs, where organisms can spread lymphohematogenously to the meninges.

Clinical manifestations. The most common presenting signs and symptoms are insidious onset of headache, fever, vomiting, nuchal rigidity, changes in mental status, and seizures.[79,80] Focal neurologic signs are not uncommon. The clinical presentation can be very similar to tuberculous meningitis. However, some patients can be completely asymptomatic.[82]

Laboratory findings and diagnosis. CSF typically shows lymphocytic pleocytosis and low glucose concentration; however, patients with AIDS can have normal CSF findings.[79] Nevertheless, most patients have confirmatory findings from CSF India ink or calcofluor white fluorescent stains, CSF or serum cryptococcal antigen, and CSF fungal culture. Fungal cultures of the blood, urine, and sputum (if available) should be obtained, even in patients without clinical manifestations of specific organ involvement. Repeated large volumes (5 to 10 mL) of CSF sampling may be needed to confirm the diagnosis. The possibility of capsule-deficient cryptococcal meningitis should be considered in the rare event that the diagnosis is suspected strongly but the staining and antigen detection tests are negative. In such cases, the diagnosis can be established by indirect immunofluorescence staining or reformation of the capsule by inoculation into mice although the latter is not available readily.[83]

Histoplasma Species

Epidemiology. *Histoplasma capsulatum* is a dimorphic fungus found in soil, and is endemic in the Mississippi, Ohio, and Missouri River valley regions of the U.S. CNS infection is rare and usually occurs in immunocompromised or malnourished individuals or infants. Neurologic involvement is reported in 8% to 18% of cases of disseminated disease,[15] but an incidence of 55% has been found in AIDS patients with disseminated histoplasmosis.

Pathogenesis. Humans become infected by inhaling spores into the lungs, which then spread lymphohematogenously to the meninges or brain.

Clinical manifestations. In a report of 18 cases and review of 86 cases from the literature, chronic meningitis was the most common form of CNS *Histoplasma* infection, with about 40% of patients coming to medical attention with accompanying disseminated histoplasmosis, and 25% with isolated chronic meningitis.[15]

Clinical symptoms are nonspecific among chronic meningitis cases, and included headache (24%), depressed level of consciousness (29%), confusion (22%), and cranial neuropathy (19%). Personality changes and seizures occur in 10% to 15% of patients. Fever typically is present. The onset of symptoms is at least 2 months before diagnosis in more than 70% of cases.

Laboratory findings and diagnosis. CSF reveals an elevated protein concentration, modestly low glucose concentration, and 50 to 500 WBC/mm^3 (predominantly mononuclear cells).[15] CSF culture for *Histoplasma* is positive in 30% to 50% of cases. Culturing a large volume (>10 mL) of CSF is recommended for optimal yield.[84] Blood culture is positive in about 50% of cases. *Histoplasma* antigen can be assayed in blood, urine, and CSF. In earlier reports, the sensitivity of antigen detection in chronic meningitis was 38% in blood, 71% in urine, and 38% in CSF. However, a new assay with improved sensitivity is available commercially, but performance in CSF samples has not been evaluated sufficiently. The antigen test can cross-react in cases of blastomycosis. CSF and serum antibody tests are approximately 90% sensitive, but can reflect past infection. In addition, the antibody response can be impaired in immunosuppressed individuals and the test may have false-positive results due to cross-reactions caused by infection with other fungi, including *Cryptococcus neoformans*. Current recommendations to evaluate for CNS histoplasmosis are to perform multiple tests, including: (1) fungal culture, antigen and antibody tests on CSF; (2) fungal culture, antigen and antibody tests on blood; and (3) antigen test on urine.[84] CSF specimens should be obtained repeatedly if there is no diagnosis and suspicion for histoplasmosis remains. Chest radiographs may provide a clue to the diagnosis; one-half of cases have abnormalities consistent with histoplasmosis.[84]

Coccidioides Species

Epidemiology. *Coccidioides* species are dimorphic fungi found in the soil of southwestern U.S., northern Mexico, Central America, Venezuela, Argentina, and Paraguay. Primary infection develops from the inhalation of airborne spores, and occurs most frequently in the summer and fall. The incidence of coccidioidomycosis appears to increase when rainy summers are followed by dry winters and windstorms.[85] Although respiratory infection with *Coccidioides* is common, disseminated disease develops in only 1% of persons. Approximately one-third of patients with disseminated disease develop meningitis. Those at increased risk for disseminated disease and meningitis include immunosuppressed hosts, African American and Filipino people, pregnant women, neonates, and elderly people.[86]

Pathogenesis. Airborne spores are inhaled into the lungs, where organisms then can spread lymphohematogenously to the meninges or brain.

Clinical manifestations. Symptoms with the primary respiratory infection often are absent, but may include fever, malaise, cough, myalgia, headache, and chest pain. Case series of adults with coccidioidal meningitis indicate that the most common presenting symptoms include headache (75%), nausea and vomiting (52%), and fever (50%). Meningismus and focal neurologic symptoms occur in one-third and one-fourth of patients, respectively.[16]

Laboratory findings and diagnosis. A history of travel or residence in endemic areas provides an important clue to the diagnosis. Cranial CT or MRI are abnormal in more that one-half of cases, with basilar enhancement, hydrocephalus, or infarctions being the most common findings.[16] Visualization of *Coccidioides immitis* in CSF samples is rare, and although the organism is not fastidious in growth requirements, only about one-third of patients with meningitis have a positive CSF culture. Sampling of large volumes of CSF followed by sterile filtration and culture of the filter increases the yield. Detection of antibodies to *Coccidioides* by EIA has a sensitivity of 93% on serum and 75% on CSF specimens.[16]

Other Fungi

The usual course of *Candida albicans* meningitis is acute. Chronic meningitis is an uncommon manifestation of disseminated

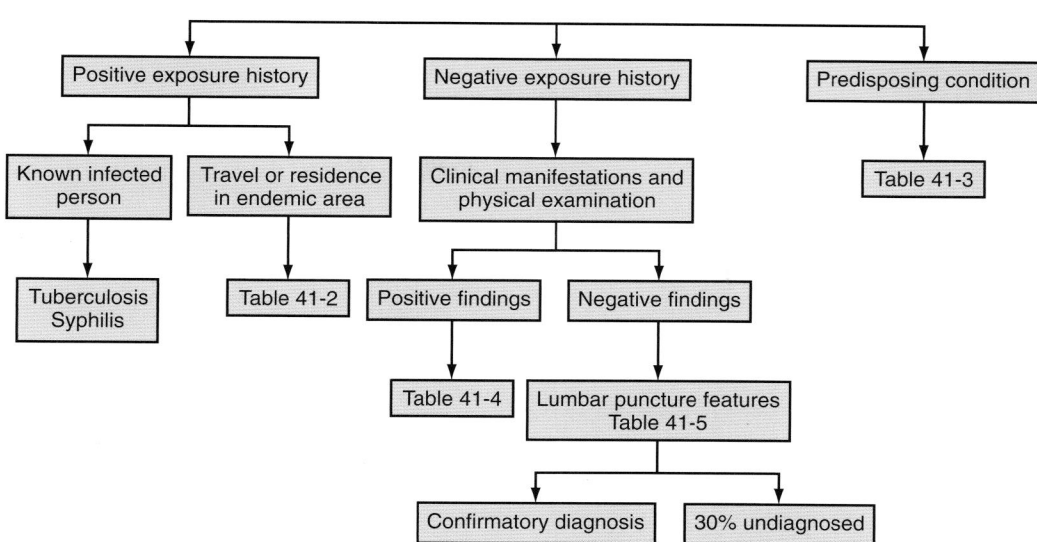

Figure 41-1. Algorithm for evaluation of patients with signs and symptoms of chronic meningitis.

candidiasis that can be seen in premature infants and children with congenital immunodeficiencies. CNS *Candida* infection also can occur in children with a ventriculoperitoneal shunt. Chronic meningitis due to *Blastomyces dermatitidis* is uncommon, but should be considered in the immunocompetent host from an endemic area (i.e., the Mississippi and Ohio River valley regions and regions along the Great Lakes and the St. Lawrence River of the U.S.). Other fungi, such as *Aspergillus, Sporothrix, Cladosporium,* and *Allescheria* spp., and agents of mucormycosis and phaeohyphomycosis are rare causes of chronic meningitis. Disseminated aspergillosis often involves the CNS, but usually as a focal brain lesion, and not as isolated chronic meningitis.

Parasites

Protozoa and parasites can cause chronic meningitis, including *Toxoplasma,*[24] *Taenia,*[25] and rarely *Acanthamoeba,*[26] *Balamuthia,*[27] *Baylisascaris,* and *Angiostrongylus* species.[28] Reactivation of *Toxoplasma gondii* is a rare cause of CNS infection in children with immunosuppression, and usually causes focal brain lesions rather than meningitis. *Taenia* are tapeworms endemic to Latin America, Asia, and East Africa that can form cysts in the brain (neurocysticercosis) that most commonly result in acute onset of afebrile seizures; neurocysticercosis rarely presents as chronic meningitis.

Viruses

HIV itself is probably the most common viral cause of chronic meningitis,[10] but patients with poorly controlled HIV infection also can develop chronic cytomegalovirus (CMV) meningitis. In patients with agammaglobulinemia, enteroviruses can cause persistent meningitis.[12] Another rare viral cause of chronic meningitis is lymphocytic choriomeningitis virus.[11] Diagnosis based on viral isolation from the CSF or demonstration of specific antibody responses (in blood or CSF) can require 4 to 6 weeks and is insensitive. PCR assays offer rapid detection (within hours if necessary) for many viruses (e.g., enteroviruses, CMV) with excellent sensitivity and specificity. In chronic meningitis viral replication can be low; PCR especially is valuable.

EVALUATION

Before testing for the myriad infectious causes of chronic meningitis (see Table 41-1), noninfectious and parameningeal conditions should be considered (see Boxes 41-1 and 41-2). In addition, cases of recurrent meningitis (i.e., repeated episodes of acute meningitis separated by symptom-free periods) should be distinguished from chronic meningitis (see Chapter 42, Recurrent

Meningitis). Figure 41-1 is an algorithm to guide differential diagnosis.

History

Although the exact cause of chronic meningitis may not be found in up to one-third of cases,[41,42] close attention to details can provide important clues to the diagnosis, or at least help narrow the differential diagnosis. A history of environmental exposure (travel, drugs, unusual foods, animals, insects, etc.) or exposure to persons infected with pathogens spread by person-to-person contact (e.g., tuberculosis, syphilis, HIV) should be sought (Table 41-2). Concomitant symptoms, such as rash or chronic cough, can

TABLE 41-2. Agent Causing Chronic Meningitis and Likely Exposure History in Patient

Agent	Exposure History
Brucella spp.	Ingestion of unpasteurized dairy products, especially in the Mediterranean, India, or Latin America
Leptospira spp.	Occupational (farmer) or recreational (camper, swimmer) exposure to urine of wild and domestic mammals during summer and fall
Borrelia burgdorferi	T/R[a] in northeast United States, Wisconsin, Minnesota, California, and Oregon, especially during late summer and early fall, or in Europe, China, Japan, and Australia, with consequent tick exposure
Blastomyces spp.	T/R in Ohio and Mississippi River valleys or North Carolina
Histoplasma sp.	T/R as for *Blastomyces*, plus Appalachian mountains and Virginia
Coccidioides sp.	T/R in southeastern United States, Mexico, Central America, Venezuela, Argentina, or Paraguay
Sporothrix sp.	T/R in tropical and subtropical Americas, or a prick from a rose thorn
Cysticercosis	T/R in Latin America, Southeast Asia, Africa, eastern Europe, and southwestern United States
Angiostrongylus sp.	T/R in Hawaii, Australia, Southeast Asia, or Philippines
Baylisascaris sp.	Exposure to raccoon feces

[a]*T/R, travel or residence.*

PART II Clinical Syndromes and Cardinal Features of Infectious Diseases: Approach to Diagnosis and Initial Management

SECTION F Central Nervous System Infections

TABLE 41-3. Causes of Chronic Meningitis with Predisposing Conditions

Causative Organism	Indwelling Catheter	Trauma or Surgery	Illicit IV Drug Use	Long-term Corticosteroid	Cancer	Transplant	HIV Infection
Candida	•	•	•	•	•	•	•
Aspergillus	•	•	•	•	•	•	•
Cryptococcus				•	•	•	•
Cladosporium		•					
Zygomycetes		•	•				
Histoplasma					•	•	•
Coccidioides				•	•	•	•
Blastomyces					•	•	
Toxoplasma					•	•	•
Nocardia				•	•	•	
Mycobacterium tuberculosis[a]				•	•	•	•

HIV, human immunodeficiency virus; IV, intravenous.

[a]Also occurs in immunocompetent host.

assist in determining the etiology. Although in most cases, signs and symptoms of illness develop within a short time after the exposure (such as in brucellosis, Lyme disease, and blastomycosis), a long incubation period (such as for cysticercosis) or reactivation of a dormant focus several years after exposure (such as in tuberculosis, histoplasmosis, and toxoplasmosis) can occur.

A careful history also can reveal predisposing conditions that increase the risk of opportunistic infections (Table 41-3). For example, prematurity, prolonged usage of corticosteroid therapy, cancer, HIV infection, intravenous drug abuse, or use of indwelling catheters facilitates invasion and dissemination of *Candida* spp. Direct extension of *Aspergillus* spp. infection from an adjacent

sinus, ear, or orbit or after head trauma or surgery can lead to infection of the CNS.

Physical Examination

A thorough and careful physical examination is important because, occasionally, the physical findings suggest the diagnosis (Table 41-4).

Skin. The skin examination can reveal a typical lesion, such as the erythema migrans of Lyme disease, or provide a source for culture or biopsy to identify an etiology. Erythema nodosum is seen in some diseases, and nonerythematous nodules can be

TABLE 41-4. Etiology of Chronic Meningitis Relative to Clinical Manifestations

Skin Lesions	Erythema Nodosum	Lung Involvement	Chorioretinitis	Endophthalmitis	Cranial Neuropathy	Hepatomegaly
Blastomyces	Mycobacterium tuberculosis	Blastomyces	Candida	Candida	Cranial	Brucella
Candida	Histoplasma	Coccidioides	Histoplasma	Cryptococcus	Mycobacterium tuberculosis[a]	Leptospira
Coccidioides	Coccidioides	Cryptococcus	Mycobacterium tuberculosis	Coccidioides	Treponema pallidum[b]	Histoplasma
Cryptococcus	Behçet disease	Histoplasma	Treponema pallidum	Sporothrix	Borrelia	Sarcoidosis
Zygomycetes (e.g., mucormycosis)	Sarcoidosis	Paracoccidioides	Toxoplasma	Pseudallescheria	Histoplasma	
Sporothrix	Systemic lupus erythematosus	Mycobacterium tuberculosis	CMV	Treponema pallidum	HIV	
Treponema pallidum		Sarcoidosis	Sarcoidosis	Actinomyces	Cancer	
Borrelia burgdorferi				Mycobacterium tuberculosis	Sarcoidosis	
Nocardia					Peripheral	
Taenia					Borrelia	
					Brucella	
					Sarcoidosis	
					Systemic lupus erythematosus	
					CMV[c]	

AIDS, acquired immunodeficiency syndrome; CMV, cytomegalovirus; HIV, human immunodeficiency virus

[a]Especially cranial nerve VI.

[b]Especially cranial nerves VII and VIII.

[c]In AIDS patients.

found in patients with systemic candidiasis, blastomycosis, and nocardiosis. Although uncommon, the umbilicated nodules of cryptococcal infection in HIV-infected patients and the characteristic palmar lesions of secondary syphilis can guide investigations.

Lungs. The lungs are the portal of entry for many of the pathogens that cause chronic meningitis, including *Blastomyces, Cryptococcus, Coccidioides, Histoplasma,* and *M. tuberculosis.* Careful physical examination and selective laboratory evaluations (chest radiography, microscopy, sputum culture, and, occasionally, lung biopsy) can be useful.

Eye. An examination by an ophthalmologist can sometimes identify important ocular lesions suggestive of an etiology. Findings of endophthalmitis can support the diagnosis of infection with *Candida, Cryptococcus,* and rarer infections. Chorioretinitis can be indicative of CMV, histoplasmosis, or toxoplasmosis. Uveitis might suggest a possible noninfectious etiology, such as systemic lupus erythematosus (SLE). If mental status changes or papilledema are present, cranial CT should precede performance of the lumbar puncture.

Neurologic examination. The neurologic examination is of limited use in identifying a specific etiology, because a variety of neurologic abnormalities can be seen with most causes of chronic meningitis. Cranial neuropathy is more commonly seen with syphilis, tuberculosis, and Lyme disease. Peripheral neuropathy and chronic meningitis may indicate Lyme disease, CMV infection, or SLE.

Liver. Hepatomegaly, not a common finding in patients with chronic meningitis, should direct the diagnosis toward a relatively few pathogens that cause this complication (see Table 41-4).

Imaging Studies

CT or MRI with contrast material should be performed before lumbar puncture to exclude space-occupying lesions, hydrocephalus, or increased intracranial pressure. Imaging also can help to identify a parameningeal infectious site, meningeal inflammation, focal brain lesions, or cerebral infarction. Because the lungs often are the primary site of infection for many organisms that cause chronic meningitis, chest radiograph is obtained routinely.

Cerebrospinal Fluid Analysis

Most infectious causes of chronic meningitis elicit similar CSF abnormalities (i.e., pleocytosis <500 WBC/mm^3 with lymphocyte predominance, low or normal glucose concentration and elevated protein concentration), but CNS can help to direct the differential diagnosis (Table 41-5). An infectious cause other than early *M. tuberculosis* is rare when CSF has <50 WBC/mm^3; in such cases, noninfectious causes should be considered.

CSF pleocytosis with predominance of neutrophils is uncommon in chronic meningitis, but can be seen in infection due to *Actinomyces, Nocardia., Aspergillus,* or *Candida* species and early in tuberculous meningitis. A suppurative parameningeal focus, such as brain abscess, subdural or epidural empyema, cranial osteomyelitis, mastoiditis, or sinusitis, can cause sympathetic inflammation in the CSF, causing mild pleocytosis, mild elevation of protein, typically without hypoglycorrhachia. Noninfectious causes of neutrophilic pleocytosis in CSF include SLE, exogenous chemicals (e.g., radiographic contrast material, chemotherapeutic agents, povidone iodine), and drugs (i.e., isoniazid, ibuprofen, or sulfa drugs).

Eosinophilic pleocytosis in chronic meningitis occurs rarely, and possible etiology includes parasites, such as *Angiostrongylus cantonensis, Taenia solium,* and *Baylisascaris procyonis* (ascarid of raccoons). Neurosyphilis, tuberculous meningitis, and coccidioidal meningitis rarely can cause mild CSF eosinophilia (<10% of WBCs). Noninfectious processes, such as Hodgkin disease, chemical meningitis, drug hypersensitivity, and complications of ventriculoperitoneal shunts also should be considered in the differential diagnosis of CSF eosinophilia.

Stains for bacteria, fungi, and acid-fast organisms should be performed. Special staining (using monoclonal antibodies) of lymphocytes in CSF should be considered if leukemia or lymphoma is suspected. Culture of a CSF sample is important and should include appropriate techniques for isolation of aerobic,

---

TABLE 41-5. Predominant Leukocyte Found in CSF for Various Causes of Chronic Meningitis

Causative Agent	Predominant Leukocytes in CSF		
	Lymphocytes	**Neutrophils**	**Eosinophils**
Bacteria	Mycobacterium tuberculosis	Nocardia	Mycobacterium tuberculosis
	Treponema pallidum	Actinomyces	Treponema pallidum
	Borrelia	Brucella	
	Brucella	Leptospira	
Fungi	All	All	Coccidioides
Parasite	Taenia	Entamoeba histolytica	Angiostrongylus
	Toxoplasma		Taenia solium
			Baylisascaris
Viruses	LCMV	Mumps	
	CMV	CMV^c	
Other	Parameningeal focus^a	Suppurative parameningeal focus^a	Hodgkin disease
	Sarcoidosis^b	Systemic lupus erythematosus	Chemical meningitis
	Chronic idiopathic meningitis	Chemical meningitis	Drug hypersensitivity
	Malignant process	Drug hypersensitivity	
	Behçet disease	NOMID/CINCA	

AIDS, acquired immunodeficiency syndrome; LCMV, lymphocytic choriomeningitis virus; CMV, cytomegalovirus; NOMID/CINCA, neonatal-onset multisystem inflammatory disease/chronic infantile neurologic cutaneous articular syndrome.

^{a}*See Box 41-2.*

^{b}*See Box 41-1.*

^{c}*In AIDS patients.*

TABLE 41-6. Commercially Available Diagnostic Tests for Causative Agents of Chronic Meningitis[a]

Agent	CSF					Blood	
	Stain	Culture	Antigen	Antibody	PCR	Ab	Ag
Mycobacterium tuberculosis	+	++			++		
Treponema pallidum	+/−			+++	++	+++	
Brucella	+/−	+		++		++	
Borrelia burgdorferi	+/−	+/−		++	+	+++	
Nocardia	+/−	++					
Actinomyces	+/−	++					
Leptospira		+/−				++	
Mycoplasma		++			+++		
Ureaplasma		++			+++		
Blastomyces	+/−	+/−		+		+	
Histoplasma	+/−	+/−	++	+		+	++
Coccidioides	+/−	+	++	+		+	++
Cryptococcus	++	+	+++			++	++
Candida	++	+++					
Aspergillus	+/−	+			++		++
Sporothrix	+/−	+		+	++	+	
Toxoplasma	+/−	+/−		++	+++	++	
Angiostrongylus	+		++				
Taenia				++		+++	
Viruses		+		+	+++	+	

Ab, antibody; Ag, antigen; CSF, cerebrospinal fluid; PCR, polymerase chain reaction.

[a]*+++ Test of choice; ++ modestly useful; + occasionally useful; +/− rarely useful.*

facultative anaerobic, and fastidious bacteria (e.g., increased CO_2 to enhance growth *of Actinomyces, Nocardia,* and *Brucella* spp.); fungi; and mycobacteria. Cultures should be incubated for an extended time because growth of some bacteria and fungi is slow.

CSF and serum for cryptococcal antigen should be performed in most instances. When indicated, testing for CSF antibodies to agents, such as *Treponema pallidum, Borrelia burgdorferi, Histoplasma capsulatum, Coccidioides immitis, Sporothrix schenckii, Toxoplasma gondii,* and *Taenia* spp., is performed with concurrent serum specimen testing. Measurement of antigen in CSF or blood and PCR testing are available for some pathogens (Table 41-6). Lumbar puncture may need to be repeated for cultures, additional studies, and to follow the course of meningeal inflammation.

Additional Evaluations

Many patients with chronic meningitis also have disseminated disease, therefore fungal and mycobacterial blood and urine cultures should be considered. With an appropriate exposure history, serologic tests for some pathogens (see Table 41-6) can be diagnostic. Because immunodeficiency greatly modifies the differential diagnosis, HIV testing should be performed for all patients with chronic meningitis. If immune suppression is considered likely, PCR assays may be more reliable than antibody testing. A Mantoux tuberculin skin test or, in children 5 years of age or older, an interferon-γ release assay (IGRA) is indicated to evaluate for tuberculosis. Repeat testing may be helpful if tuberculosis remains a concern. Brain biopsy should be considered when the diagnosis remains elusive and radiographic imaging identifies a focal lesion or meningeal enhancement.[87]

EMPIRIC THERAPY

When the initial evaluation of the patient identifies the cause of chronic meningitis, specific therapy should be instituted. When choosing the antimicrobial agent or agents, the drug's ability to penetrate the blood–brain or CSF barrier in order to achieve consistent and adequate drug levels is of paramount importance. Chapters on specific pathogens contain specific recommendations.

After the initial evaluation, the cause of chronic meningitis remains unknown in many patients. In these situations, decisions regarding use of empiric treatment and preferred antimicrobial agents are controversial. Because tuberculous meningitis is probably the most common cause of chronic meningitis, an empiric trial with antituberculous drugs is favored by many clinicians. Such an approach was not found to be beneficial in one study from the Mayo Clinic.[88] If empiric antituberculous therapy is initiated, further studies should be done in patients who are seriously ill or who deteriorate rapidly. Corticosteroid therapy should only be added if the patient continues to deteriorate on antituberculous therapy or if fungal meningitis is reasonably excluded. Several adult patients with idiopathic chronic meningitis in the Mayo Clinic study were treated with empiric corticosteroid, and had a favorable response.[88] The mean length of symptoms before starting corticosteroids was 17 months. Corticosteroid therapy should be considered cautiously because of the potential catastrophic outcome when given to patients with unrecognized tuberculous or fungal meningitis. If fungal meningitis is a possibility, empiric antifungal treatment should be considered, recognizing the potential adverse drug effects, and that response to therapy may be difficult to determine because patients with fungal meningitis often respond slowly to treatment. Choice of antifungal agent should be made on the basis of the suspected fungus and the degree of CSF penetration of the agent.

In previously healthy patients who have had symptoms of meningitis for several weeks and who are not seriously ill, it is reasonable to investigate the cause of meningitis without initiating treatment. If the cause cannot be found and the patient is not improving, empiric therapy should be considered. If antituberculous medications are initiated and the patient does not improve within a few weeks, antifungal therapy should be considered.

Acknowledgment

The authors acknowledge substantial use of some tables from previous editions contributed by Ram Yogev.

42 Recurrent Meningitis

Robyn A. Livingston and Christopher J. Harrison

Recurrent meningitis typically is defined as two or more separate episodes of meningitis weeks to months apart with full recovery between events. This is in contrast to recrudescence or relapse of meningitis, which represents persistence of the original infection resulting from treatment failure.[1] Recurrent meningitis is a relatively uncommon diagnosis, and its etiology often is difficult to ascertain. When the cause is detected, most cases are bacterial in origin although recurrent episodes can be characterized by negative cerebrospinal fluid (CSF) cultures.

ETIOLOGIC AGENTS

Streptococcus pneumoniae is the infectious agent identified in more than 50% of patients with recurrent bacterial meningitis and most often is associated with an underlying anatomical abnormality or immunodeficiency. *Neisseria meningitidis* is the second most common bacterial pathogen, accounting for approximately 25% of cases of recurrent bacterial meningitis,[1] and occurs predominantly in patients with complement deficiency. Recurrent *Haemophilus influenzae* meningitis has been reported rarely in countries where the conjugate vaccine has been introduced. *Staphylococcus aureus* and gram-negative bacilli such as *Escherichia coli* can be associated rarely with recurrent meningitis; the recurrent isolation of any of these organisms suggests a communication between the subarachnoid space and the paranasal sinuses, skin (such as a dermal sinus), or intestine if gram-negative organisms are isolated (such as posterior neurenteric fistula or anterior meningomyelocele). Other bacteria, such as oral streptococci, *Proteus* spp., enterococci, *Klebsiella* spp., and group B streptococcus have been sporadically reported to cause recurrent meningitis. In cases in which bacteria cannot be detected, the differential diagnosis of recurrent aseptic meningitis should be considered (Box 42-1).[2–14]

EPIDEMIOLOGY

Recurrent episodes of meningitis are rare, and the prevalence for each of the predisposing causes varies. A 1999 review of 463 cases of bacterial meningitis in children identified 6 patients with confirmed recurrent episodes, representing 1.3% of bacterial meningitis cases.[15] The most common predisposing condition is a communication between the subarachnoid space and the base of the skull (CSF leak or fistula) resulting from head trauma, surgery,

or a congenital defect; immunologic defects are less common. CSF rhinorrhea or otorrhea occurs after approximately 1% to 2% of all head injuries, but either condition is more frequent in selected presentations, i.e., 11% of basilar skull fractures,[16] and 25% of fractures involving the paranasal sinuses.[17] Most CSF leaks resolve spontaneously within a few days. Persistent CSF leaks are associated with an increased risk of meningitis.[18]

The risk of development of meningitis at a particular time after injury is variable. About one fifth of cases of posttraumatic meningitis occur within a week or two after head trauma,[19] one third within the first month, and half within 6 months. However, almost 50% of patients have the first episode of meningitis 7 months or longer after the traumatic event causing the CSF leak, and delay of as long as 34 years has been reported.[20] Procedures such as intracranial surgery, nasal and paranasal sinus surgery, and otologic surgery also can predispose to recurrent meningitis.[17] On average, post-neurosurgical meningitis develops within 10 days of the procedure with an incidence of 0.3% to 8.9%;[21] gram-negative bacteria frequently are isolated.

A variety of congenital defects in the bony structure of the skull contributes to the development of CSF fistulas and thus predispose to recurrent meningitis (Box 42-2). The incidence of recurrent meningitis in patients with a congenital defect is unknown but probably is low, although the defects themselves are not uncommon. For example, in children with idiopathic sensorineural hearing loss, computed tomography (CT) of the temporal bone revealed that 21% had an inner-ear malformation.[22] Mondini dysplasia (a developmental arrest at the seventh week of gestation characterized by hypoplasia of the cochlear labyrinth resulting in 1 to 1.5 turns instead of the normal 2.5 turns) is commonly cited as contributing to recurrent meningitis (Figure 42-1).[23] Although deafness frequently is associated with Mondini dysplasia, it is unilateral and therefore often unrecognized. Additionally, trauma can precipitate a fistulous connection in milder defects and lead to meningitis. Epidermoid and dermoid cysts

---

BOX 42-1. Conditions Associated with Recurrent Aseptic Meningitis

Mollaret syndrome[2]
Familial Mediterranean fever (FMF)[3]
Intracranial or intraspinal cyst[4]
Dermoid or epidermoid tumor[5]
Behçet syndrome[6]
Sarcoidosis[7]
Systemic lupus erythematosus[8]
Intracranial tumors[9]
Drug-induced (e.g., penicillins, cephalosporins, trimethoprim-sulfamethoxazole, NSAIDs, IGIV, OKT3)[10,11]
Herpes simplex type 1 or 2 infection[12]
Enterovirus[13]
Migraine syndrome[14]

BOX 42-2. Congenital Anomalies Associated with Recurrent Bacterial Meningitis

ANOMALIES OF THE ANTERIOR FOSSA

Encephalocele
Meningocele
Defects of the cribriform plate
Enlarged subarachnoid space
Intracranial cyst

ANOMALIES OF THE TEMPORAL BONE

Mondini dysplasia
Stapedial anomalies
Klippel–Feil syndrome
Pendred syndrome
Petromastoid fistula
Widened cochlear aqueduct
Hyrtl fissure

SPINAL DEFECTS

Dermoid or epidermoid cyst
Neuroenteric fistula

PART II Clinical Syndromes and Cardinal Features of Infectious Diseases: Approach to Diagnosis and Initial Management

SECTION F Central Nervous System Infections

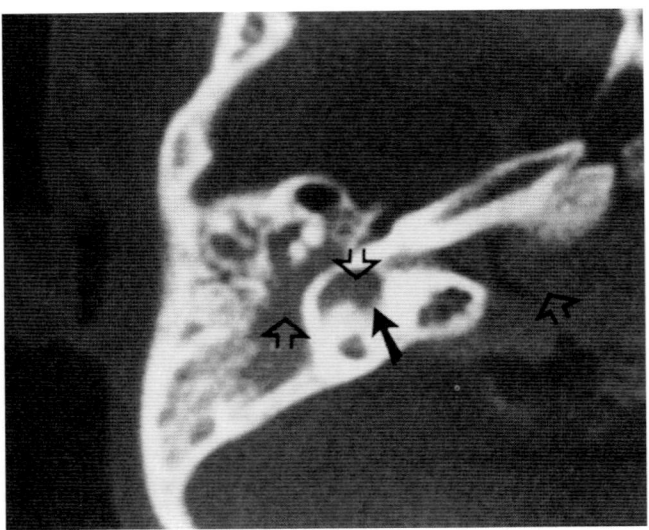

Figure 42-1. Computed tomography with intravenous contrast enhancement of the right middle ear showing a dysplastic cochlea (black arrow) consistent with Mondini dysplasia. (Courtesy of N.M. Young, MD, Children's Memorial Hospital, Chicago.)

BOX 42-3. Parameningeal Foci of Infection Associated with Recurrent Meningitis

---

Sinusitis
Mastoiditis
Brain abscess
Subdural empyema
Central nervous system shunt infection
Infected dermoid sinus
Infected porencephalic cyst
Cranial or vertebral osteomyelitis
Neurenteric fistula
Anterior meningomyelocele

---

with dermal sinus tract are well-known causes of recurrent meningitis with many cases coming to attention due to a new-onset neurologic deficit or infection or both.[24] Lymphangiomatosis of the skull is a rare cause for CSF leak and recurrent meningitis.[25] The incidence of recurrent bacterial or culture-negative meningitis after a parameningeal focus of infection (Box 42-3) or related to more distant foci (e.g., endocarditis) is unknown, but these entities should be considered in the differential diagnosis of recurrent meningitis.

Immunologic Defects

Several disorders of the immune system can predispose to recurrent meningitis, particularly meningitis caused by encapsulated bacteria. These include antibody immunodeficiencies (X-linked agammaglobulinemia, common variable immunodeficiency, IgG subclass deficiencies), HIV infection, splenic dysfunction (i.e., surgical splenectomy, congenital asplenia, sickle-cell disease, or hemoglobinopathies), properdin deficiency, and complement deficiencies (see Chapter 105, Infectious Complications of Complement Deficiencies, and Chapter 108, Infectious Complications in Special Hosts).

The frequency of a persistent complement deficiency in the general population is most likely <0.03%.[26] Deficiency of properdin (the molecule that stabilizes the C3bBb complex) and terminal components of complement are associated with recurrent

meningococcal infection. Meningitis occurs in approximately 39% of patients with terminal complement deficiencies and 6% of those with properdin deficiency.[27] Recurrent bacterial meningitis (especially due to *N. meningitidis*) occurs in patients with deficiency of one of the terminal complement components (i.e., C5 to C9) and can be mild.

In contrast recurrent meningococcal meningitis is rare in individuals with properdin deficiency because the initial infection usually is fatal.[28]

Bacterial infections are less frequent in C4 deficiency, presumably because affected individuals can compensate via the alternative pathway. In general, C5 deficiency is associated with a higher incidence of bacterial meningitis than deficiencies in more terminal components, probably because C5 promotes chemotaxis that localizes infection. Almost 50% of individuals with C6 deficiency and 40% with C7 deficiency experience bacterial meningitis. Specific defects in the trimeric C8 molecule are associated with race. Deficiency of the C8-α and C8-γ subunits (the portion responsible for membranolytic function) is seen in African American and Hispanic populations whereas deficiency of the C8-β subunit (the portion responsible for attachment of C8 to C5b67) is seen in white populations. Most patients with C9 deficiency are healthy and rarely have meningococcal meningitis. Reported complement deficiencies in African Americans involve terminal components almost exclusively.[26]

Persons with a complement deficiency have a 42% lifetime risk of any meningococcal infection compared with 0.0072% in the general population.[26] An estimated 10% to 15% of all patients with single or recurrent systemic infections due to *Neisseria* spp. have a complement deficiency.[26,29] The median age for the first episode of meningococcal infection in the general population is 3 years (peak age, 3 to 8 months), compared with 17 years in individuals with complement deficiency. In addition, recurrent meningococcal infection is rare in the general population, and relapsing infection is uncommon, with a rate of about 0.6%. In contrast, the recurrence rate in patients with complement deficiencies is high, approximately 45%, and the relapse rate is 10 times higher than in the general population, about 6%. The mortality rate for meningococcal infection with meningococcemia is estimated to be 25% in the general population, but only 6.9% for all complement-deficient patients, and 4.5% for those with terminal complement deficiencies.

Deficiency in some immunoglobulin (Ig) subclasses (such as IgG2 and IgG3 subclasses) is associated rarely with recurrent meningitis, as are mutations in mannose-binding lectin (MBL).[30–32]

PATHOGENESIS

Trauma and Congenital Defects

Recurrent meningitis after head trauma only occurs if, in addition to fracture, there is a tear of the dura. Because the dura is bound more tightly to the base of the skull in children than in adults, a higher incidence of CSF leak occurs after head trauma in children. CSF leak is a portal of entry for bacteria comprising the normal flora of the nasopharynx into the central nervous system (CNS). Fracture through the paranasal sinuses can manifest as an apparent CSF leak only transiently or not at all, with recurrent bacterial meningitis perhaps as the only indication of the abnormal communication. Fracture of the temporal bone is the most common cause of CSF leak into the middle ear.[33] After fracture of the petrous bone, CSF can leak into the nasopharynx, but the expected rhinorrhea may not be detected externally. Meningitis or recurrence can occur years or even decades after the initial skull fracture occurred. Obtaining a detailed history for previous head trauma is crucial.[34]

Encephalocele is a rare cause of CSF leak that predisposes to recurrent meningitis. The probable etiology is a small congenital defect in the skull bone that allows cerebral tissue to protrude, but trauma, intracranial infections, tumor, or a surgical procedure can be the cause. In patients with congenital abnormalities of the inner ear, several mechanisms contribute to the communication between the CSF and the middle-ear space.[35] First, the cochlear aqueduct (i.e., the perilymphatic duct), which normally connects the subarachnoid space with the inner ear, can be abnormally wide, allowing CSF to flow freely to the inner ear. (Cochlear implant using a spacer can provide the same connection.) Second, a Hyrtl fissure (an embryonic cleft connecting the posterior fossa and the middle ear), which usually is obliterated during normal ossification of the petrous bone, can remain patent. Third, there may be an abnormal communication between the internal acoustic canal (traversed by the eighth nerve) and the perilymph of the vestibule. CSF leakage from the vestibule to the middle ear occurs most commonly through the oval window. A hole in the stapes footplate with CSF leakage through the oval window due to increased vestibular perilymph pressure that displaces the stapes footplate has been described.[36,37]

In Pendred syndrome (congenital perceptive hearing loss with thyroid enlargement and abnormal perchlorate test result), a cochlear defect that resembles Mondini dysplasia predisposes to recurrent meningitis.[38] In Mondini dysplasia, the CSF leaks into the middle ear through a defective foramen ovale.[39] In Klippel–Feil syndrome (low hairline with short neck and limitation of neck movement), several anomalies can predispose to recurrent meningitis.[40] The most common are inner-ear abnormalities, including fistulas through the oval window, the stapes footplate, the round window, or along the facial nerve. Anomalies of vertebral bodies with neuroenteric cyst or fistulas or a dermoid cyst, with or without dermal sinus tract, also have been described in children with Klippel–Feil syndrome and can serve as portals for entry of bacteria.

Occult CNS abnormalities should be suspected in any patient who has recurrent meningitis who does not have predisposing CNS abnormalities or underlying immunologic defects. A dermal sinus tract ending intracranially (Figure 42-2) or intraspinally (Figure 42-3) in a dermoid cyst can permit entry of skin flora into the subarachnoid space.[41] Thus, meningitis caused by skin organisms (i.e., *Staphylococcus* spp., gram-negative bacilli) should prompt a careful search for such a lesion. Other abnormalities, such as an enteric cyst contained within a meningocele,[42] continuous sequestration of bacteria on a CNS shunt or in paraventricular sites (i.e., brain abscess[43]), or a neuroenteric fistula, can serve as the entry points. Rare cases of recurrent meningitis also have been reported secondary to migration of a ventriculoperitoneal shunt through the bowel wall into the gastrointestinal tract, or associated with procedures to dilate the rectum or esophagus or after spinal arthrodesis for scoliosis.[44,45]

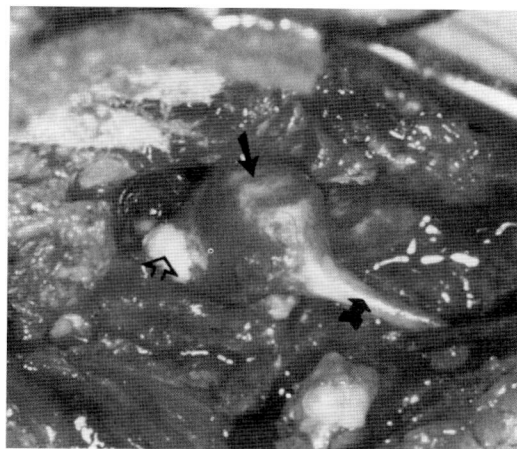

Figure 42-3. A lumbosacral dermal sinus tract (broad black arrow) leading into a dermal cyst (thin black arrow). Note the white material extruding from the cyst, which may cause chemical meningitis (open arrow). (Courtesy of J. Grant, MD, Children's Memorial Hospital, Chicago.)

Immunologic Defects

The pathogenesis of bacterial infections in patients with complement deficiencies is not understood fully. In individuals with complement deficiency, as in the general population, specific antibodies against pathogenic bacteria develop after exposure early in life. Complement defect, however, precludes full bactericidal activity of antibodies, and affected individuals experience a lifelong susceptibility to these pathogens. Although this process explains recurrent infections, it fails to explain adequately the unique susceptibility to *N. meningitidis* but not to other gram-negative bacteria, such as *H. influenzae* or *E. coli*, or other encapsulated bacteria such as *S. pneumoniae* in such people. Additional factors that influence the activation of the complement system (e.g., the presence of sialic acid on the bacterial surface) also may be important in the unique susceptibility of these patients, and could explain the excessive occurrence of *N. meningitidis* group Y infection in patients with complement deficiency compared with the general population (44% versus 11%, respectively).[26] The lower rate of mortality may be the result of lower virulence of infecting organisms or more effective recruitment of other host defense mechanisms, such as the C3b complement pathway, or less disturbance of clotting systems or less activation of systemic cytokine release.

Drug-Induced

Drug-induced recurrent meningitis has been reported in connection with several antibiotics (e.g., trimethoprim-sulfamethoxazole, penicillin, and cephalosporins), nonsteroidal anti-inflammatory drugs (e.g., ibuprofen, naproxen), cytotoxic drugs (e.g., azathioprine, cytosine arabinoside), OKT3 monoclonal antibody, and immune globulin intravenous (IGIV).[10,11,46] The likely pathogenesis of meningitis in these situations is either a direct chemical irritation by the drug or a hypersensitivity reaction. In the case of ibuprofen-induced meningitis, immune complexes have been found in the CSF.[47] The onset of drug-induced meningitis varies from a few minutes to several months after drug intake. The onset of IGIV-induced meningitis generally is <24 hours after administration. The CSF findings typically resemble those of bacterial or aseptic meningitis (a polymorphonuclear predominant pleocytosis, normal-to-low glucose concentration, and modestly increased protein level).[10]

Mollaret Meningitis

Mollaret meningitis is characterized by recurrent episodes of aseptic meningitis lasting 3 to 5 days followed by spontaneous

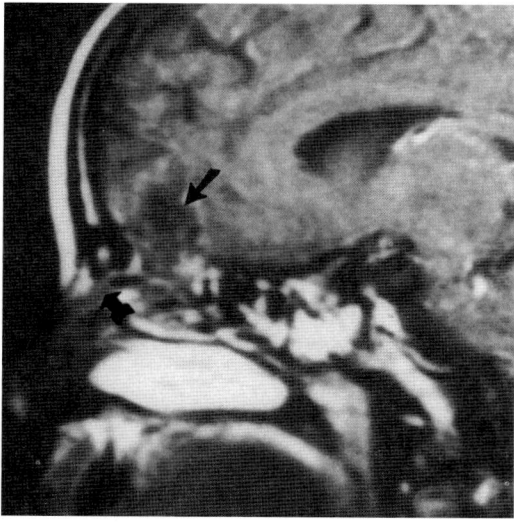

Figure 42-2. Sagittal T1 weighted MRI image showing dermal cyst (long arrow) with sinus tract (short arrow) extending to the skin surface of the nose. (Courtesy of T.T. Tomita, MD, Children's Memorial Hospital, Chicago.)

PART II Clinical Syndromes and Cardinal Features of Infectious Diseases: Approach to Diagnosis and Initial Management

SECTION F Central Nervous System Infections

recovery.[2] Symptom-free periods vary from weeks to months, and the period of recurrences usually is 3 to 5 years, although longer durations have been reported. Symptoms include fever, headache, and meningismus with occasional transient neurologic findings. CSF analysis reveals a polymorphonuclear pleocytosis up to several thousand cells per mL early in the course of illness followed by a lymphocytic predominance later. Early in the course of illness, large "endothelial" cells (Mollaret cells) with distinct nuclear shapes often with deep nuclear clefts are seen commonly in the CSF, but can be absent. Further ultrastructural and immunohistochemical studies suggest that these cells are of monocyte/macrophage lineage.[48] The protein level is moderately increased, and glucose concentration is normal or slightly decreased.

Several etiologies have been postulated for Mollaret meningitis. Eosinophilia in a few patients has suggested a possible allergic or hypersensitivity mechanism. Elevated CSF cytokines levels may cause the symptoms. The occurrence of uveitis or transient facial paralysis suggests that Behçet syndrome or sarcoidosis may be related etiologically. The resemblance of Mollaret meningitis to familial Mediterranean fever (FMF), specifically the pattern of recurrent attacks and the response to colchicine, suggested the possibility that FMF was a cause.[3] Intracranial and intraspinal epidermoid cysts can produce chemical meningitis upon release of contents into the subarachnoid space.[4,49] However, since the development of polymerase chain reaction (PCR) technologies, recent studies have shown that the CSF of many patients with benign recurrent lymphocytic meningitis, including Mollaret meningitis, contain herpes simplex virus (HSV) DNA.[12] In most cases, HSV-2 DNA was detected, in the absence of cutaneous lesions, suggesting that recurrent lymphocytic meningitis may be a unique presentation of HSV-2 infection of the CNS.[50]

CLINICAL MANIFESTATIONS

In most patients the signs and symptoms of recurrent meningitis are suggestive of classic acute bacterial meningitis although the intensity may be milder, resembling aseptic meningitis. Physical examination otherwise is normal. History of trauma, congenital abnormalities, or recent surgery should prompt a detailed physical examination for a CSF leak including a detailed examination for skull fracture or congenital bony malformations. Anosmia, hearing loss, otitis media with effusion, or hemotympanum are important clues to the potential presence of congenital or acquired CSF fistula or head trauma. CSF rhinorrhea or otorrhea can be intermittent and can cease when increasing pressure during an acute episode of meningitis occludes fistulas. Certain maneuvers, such as coughing, sneezing, Valsalva maneuver, or bending the head forward, may initiate or exacerbate CSF rhinorrhea. The cranispinal axis (especially the occipital, lumbosacral, and midline face) is examined carefully for a dimple or bulge, tract, tuft of hair, nevus, or hemangioma. Some patients note recurring fluid discharges from sites of a mucosal or cutaneous lesion (Figures 42-4 to 42-6). Examination of the nasal cavity may reveal granulation tissue or a meningocele at the site of the leak.

DIAGNOSIS

If history of recurrent episodes of meningitis is obtained, special attention is given to any history of head injuries or cranial surgery, multiple serious non-CNS bacterial infections, family history of recurrent infections, splenectomy, fluid leakage from ears or nostrils, and medication use. In addition, any child who experiences meningitis and has known deafness or a family history of anomalies of the ear should be evaluated for anatomic abnormalities. So also should individuals whose deafness is discovered during meningitis after trauma. Evaluation of children with recurrent meningitis requires coordinated efforts, frequently between neuroradiologist and neurosurgeon. An algorithm has been proposed for diagnostic tests for children with recurrent meningitis of unknown origin.[15]

The results of tests performed on CSF from episodes of meningitis help differentiate bacterial causes from aseptic causes (see

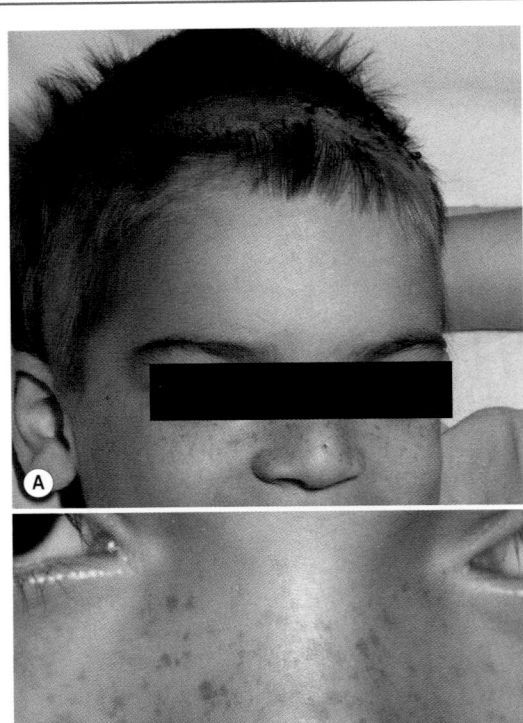

Figure 42-4. Dermoid cyst. A 6-year-old boy had a 3-week history of severe headache and then seizure, hemiparesis, and obtundation. *Enterobacter agglomerans* was isolated from a frontal lobe brain abscess and subarachnoid space. Postoperatively a midline "comedone" was noted **(A),** which on closer inspection was a pit with a tuft of hair **(B)** overlying a dermoid cyst and tract to the subarachnoid space. The family recalled that the nose lesion had periodically discharged fluid over the child's lifetime. (Courtesy of E.N. Faerber and S.S. Long, St. Christopher's Hospital for Children, Philadelphia, PA.)

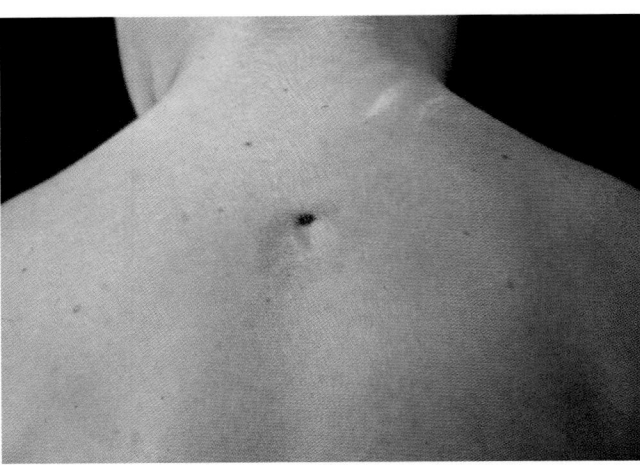

Figure 42-5. Dermoid cyst. "Pit and pucker" on the midline of the back of a boy with a dermoid cyst connecting to the subarachnoid space. (Courtesy of J. Bass, through J.H. Brien.)

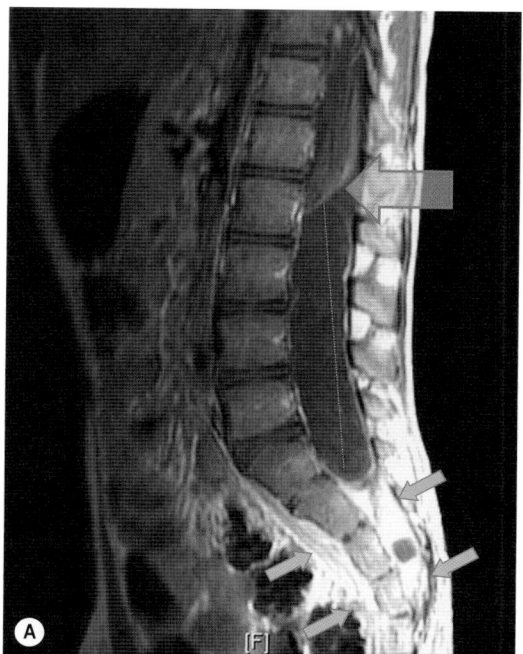

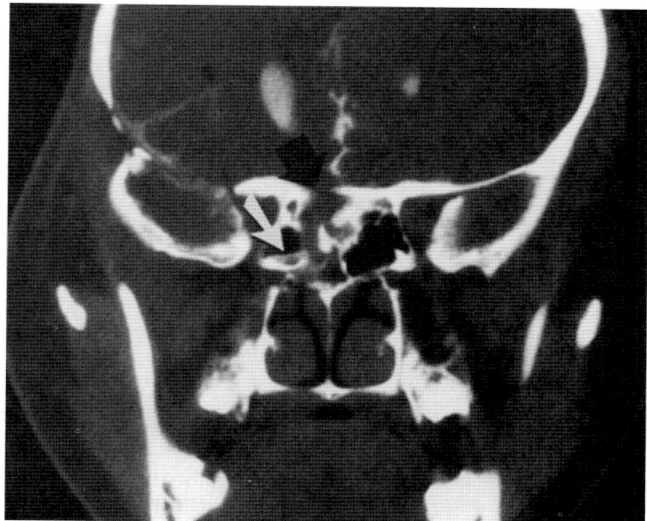

Figure 42-7. Coronal computed tomography with intravenous contrast enhancement showing defect in the bone (black arrow) and collection of contrast material with fluid level (white arrow) in the sphenoid sinus. (Courtesy of S.E. Byrd, MD, Children's Memorial Hospital, Chicago.)

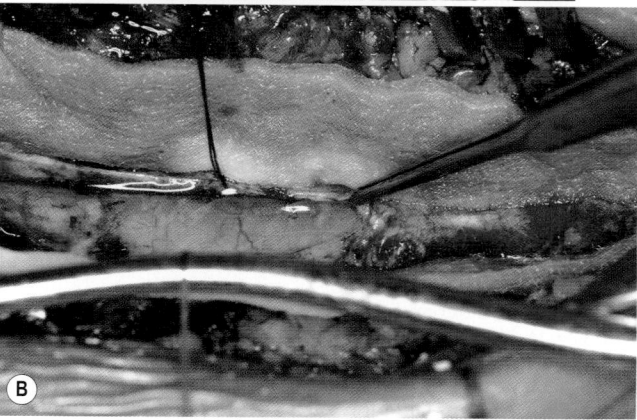

Figure 42-6. Arachnoid cyst with sinus tract. A 5-year-old boy came to medical attention for draining sacral osteomyelitis. His parents had throughout his life repeatedly "popped" a pustule over his sacrum. Sagittal magnetic resonance image **(A)** and operative field **(B)** show a large sausage-shaped arachnoid cyst (dotted line within) occupying the entire bony central canal from L2 to S1. Note the tip of the spinal cord conus at L1–L2 level (large arrow) and enhancing soft tissue, bone, and bony canal in the sacral region (small arrow). (Courtesy of J.H. Brien©.)

Boxes 42-1 and 42-2). The type of bacteria isolated can lead to suspicion of the site of the predisposing condition. For example, *S. pneumoniae* or *H. influenzae* (or oral streptococci or anaerobic bacteria of oropharyngeal flora) is more common in patients with head trauma or congenital CSF communication to the middle ear, nose, or sinuses, whereas *N. meningitidis* suggests a complement deficiency. Recurrent pneumococcal infection, including meningitis, can occur in individuals with agammaglobulinemia, IgG subclass deficiency, early complement deficiency (C2–C4), HIV infection, and asplenia.[1] If *Staphylococcus aureus,* coagulase-negative staphylococci or *Corynebacterium* species; enteric or environmental gram-negative bacteria; anaerobic bacteria; or a combination of such organisms is isolated, a dermal sinus should be suspected. For polymicrobial gram-negative or anaerobic infections, a neurenteric defect or sequestration of bacteria in the CNS should be suspected.

Fluid suspicious for CSF rhinorrhea or otorrhea can be tested for glucose and protein using multireagent strips. However,

glucose testing often is unreliable with both false-negative and false-positive results reported. Recently, testing for β₂-transferrin has become more common in the clinical setting. This assay reportedly has high specificity as the protein is found only in the CSF, vitreous humor, and inner ear perilymph.[51]

Several imaging methods are available for the evaluation of suspected CSF fistulas and other anomalies. Plain radiography can detect large defects or abnormalities. CT and magnetic resonance imaging (MRI) are more precise for localizing smaller lesions; multiple thin-cut coronal views must be obtained, because small defects can be missed in axial views. Use of dyes or contrast material (Figure 42-7) is helpful in visualizing smaller bony defects.[52] Radionuclide cisternography (RC) alone or in combination with pledgets placed in the nostrils or ears is considered by some to be the method of choice for localizing occult CSF fistulas in the skull.[16] RC using diethylenetriamine penta-acetic acid (DTPA), labeled with either ⁹⁹ᵐTc or ¹¹¹In, allows for up to 72 hours of observation, increasing the detection of slow or intermittent CSF leaks.[53]

The initial screening test for complement deficiencies is the total hemolytic complement (CH50) assay. A low CH50 assay value suggests that one or more of the classic or terminal components is missing. CH50 may be within normal range if only C3 or C4 are abnormal. If there is high suspicion for complement deficiency, individual components may need to be tested despite a normal CH50. If the complement cascade is intact, analysis of quantitative serum immunoglobulins and subclasses is warranted. Imaging of the abdomen (e.g., ultrasound or splenic scan) can be performed to rule out hyposplenism or asplenia. If Mollaret meningitis is suspected, CSF PCR for HSV is useful. In addition, serum-to-CSF ratio of antibodies for HSV can be done if PCR is negative.[54]

TREATMENT

For recurrent bacterial meningitis due to head trauma, congenital malformations, or complement deficiency, the choice of empiric antibiotic therapy should be similar to that for single-episode meningitis. For patients with a known dermal sinus or history of meningitis due to staphylococcal or gram-negative bacteria, an antibiotic with a broader spectrum of activity targeting the identified pathogen(s) is required. In rare cases when multidrug-resistant infections have not responded to treatment intravenously,

PART II Clinical Syndromes and Cardinal Features of Infectious Diseases: Approach to Diagnosis and Initial Management

SECTION F Central Nervous System Infections

antibiotic has been administered intraventricularly,[55] although adverse effects can be related to such installations.

The length of therapy is similar to that for sporadic cases; there is no advantage to longer courses of therapy. Time to sterilization may be prolonged and should be documented in cases of gram-negative bacillary infections associated with dermoid or epidermoid cysts because squamous collections can act like foreign bodies. Meticulous examination and diagnostic evaluation (occasionally including exploratory surgery) to identify and perform primary repair of the site of CSF fistula are most important. In the case of otorrhea, packing of the middle ear with fat is inadequate because it fails to close the fistula permanently. Even packing with muscle or fascia alone seems to be insufficient; additional grafting of the vestibule is needed. For CSF rhinorrhea, extracranial surgery may be the preferred technique, because of lower morbidity; the few disadvantages of this procedure are cranial nerve paralysis and postoperative sinusitis. In patients with Mollaret meningitis, initial anti-HSV therapy followed by long-term suppression (e.g., acyclovir) may be helpful.

Fresh frozen plasma has been given as replacement therapy to patients with complement deficiency. Although this may be reasonable in the few patients who suffer from life-threatening disease, routine administration of plasma can stimulate the production of antibodies against the missing component. Additionally, the short half-life of complement proteins makes this approach impractical. Monthly immunoglobulin infusions for patients with immunoglobulin subclass deficiency should be individualized according to the severity of the disease (i.e., recurrent bacterial versus aseptic meningitis).

PREVENTION AND PROPHYLAXIS

Imaging of the temporal bone should be considered in children with idiopathic sensorineural hearing loss to identify those who have an inner-ear anomaly. Parents of children with proven inner-ear anomaly should be educated about the risk of recurrent meningitis from middle-ear infection, contact sports, and activities that may increase the inner- or middle-ear pressure (e.g., diving, prolonged Valsalva maneuver). Suspected middle-ear infections should be treated promptly and aggressively and in patients with common cavity abnormalities, exploratory tympanotomy should be considered. If cochlear implantation is considered in patients with inner-ear malformation, the type of implant, the risk for meningitis, and pre-procedure immunization should be discussed.[56] All efforts should be made to identify and seal CSF leaks because continued leakage increases the risk for postoperative meningitis.[57]

Although prophylactic antibiotics often are given to patients with recurrent meningitis, their efficacy in preventing further episodes is questionable. Antibiotic prophylaxis has been prescribed to prevent meningitis associated with basilar skull fracture. However, a 2006 Cochrane review concluded that prophylactic antibiotics had no effect on the prevention of meningitis in these patients.[58] In addition, one review suggested that antibiotic prophylaxis after basilar skull fracture could be harmful because of increased risk of infection due to antibiotic-resistant organisms.[59] Prophylactic antibiotics have been used in patients with complement or significant immunoglobulin subclass deficiency. In some cases, such treatment markedly reduced the incidence of infection, yet the clinical failure of penicillin prophylaxis against meningococcal disease suggests that long-term prophylaxis may have limited value.[28] The advisability of antibiotic prophylaxis in patients with recurrent meningitis should be made on a case-by-case basis; firm guidelines are not available.

Limited data suggest that chronic oral acyclovir (for one year or more) may prevent recurrences of Mollaret meningitis.[60]

The quadrivalent A, C, Y, W-135 meningococcal conjugate vaccine (MCV4) is recommended for children ≥2 years of age who have terminal complement component deficiencies and for those who have anatomic or functional asplenia (i.e., groups at high risk for recurrent meningococcal meningitis).[61] A 2003 study found that quadrivalent polysaccharide vaccine (MPSV4) substantially decreased the incidence of meningococcal disease in patients with terminal complement deficiency when compared to similar patients who were unvaccinated.[62] MCV4 is preferred to MPSV4 because of enhanced immunogenicity and absence of vaccine-induced tolerance to serogroup C. A 2-dose series of MCV4 given 2 months apart and then a booster every 5 years is recommended for people at increased risk of *N. meningitidis* infection.[61] MCV4 may even be advantageous in individuals 2 years or older with previous meningococcal infections who do not have deficiency of the terminal complement pathway and in those with properdin deficiency.

Pneumococcal conjugate vaccine (PCV13) currently is recommended for prevention of invasive pneumococcal disease in all children beginning at 2 months of age.[63] In addition, children 2 years of age or older and adults in high-risk groups (e.g., patients with CSF leaks) also should receive pneumococcal polysaccharide vaccine (PPSV23). Ideally, children should complete age-appropriate pneumococcal vaccines (PCV13 plus PPSV23) at least 2 weeks before implantation of a cochlear device.[64] Failure of pneumococcal vaccines to prevent recurrent episodes of meningitis in predisposed individuals can occur.[65] Education of families to seek immediate medical attention for illness is critical.

---

43 Aseptic and Viral Meningitis

José R. Romero

The term "acute aseptic meningitis" was introduced in 1925 to describe a self-limited central nervous system (CNS) syndrome characterized by acute onset of fever and meningeal irritation in which the cerebrospinal fluid (CSF) exhibited a mononuclear pleocytosis and was bacteriologically sterile.[1] With advances in diagnostic methodologies it is now recognized that multiple infectious agents, drugs, heavy metals, as well as localized and systemic inflammatory conditions can cause aseptic meningitis (AM) syndrome (Box 43-1).[2,3]

Viral meningitis can be described as a CNS infection that is associated with signs of meningeal irritation (i.e., neck stiffness, Kernig and/or Brudzinski signs) but not neurologic dysfunction as a result of brain parenchymal involvement. In contrast, viral encephalitis is a CNS disorder with evidence of brain parenchymal dysfunction as manifest by an altered state of consciousness or other objective signs of neurologic dysfunction (e.g., seizures, cranial nerve palsies, abnormal reflexes, paralysis or both). While commonly discussed as separate syndromes, overlap

COMMON

Human enteroviruses A–D (echoviruses, coxsackieviruses, other enteroviruses) and parechoviruses
Arboviruses (western equine encephalitis virus, St. Louis encephalitis virus, Colorado tick fever, La Crosse encephalitis virus, West Nile virus, tickborne encephalitis virus)
Borrelia burgdorferi
Partially treated bacterial meningitis

UNCOMMON

Herpes simplex 2
Mumps virus
Human immunodeficiency virus
Mycobacterium tuberculosis
Parameningeal bacterial infection
Fungi (*Cryptococcus, Coccidioides, Histoplasma, Blastomyces*)

RARE

Respiratory viruses (adenovirus, influenza, parainfluenza)
Lymphocytic choriomeningitis virus
Other herpesviruses (herpes simplex 1, human herpesvirus 6, Epstein–Barr, varicella-zoster, cytomegalovirus)
Measles virus
Miscellaneous viruses (parvovirus B19, rotavirus)
Bartonella sp. (cat-scratch disease)
Spirochetes
Leptospira sp.
Brucella sp.
Parasites (e.g., *Taenia solium* (cysticercosis), *Toxoplasma gondii*, *Trichinella spiralis* (trichinosis))
Mycoplasma pneumoniae
Rickettsia

NONINFECTIOUS CAUSES

Drugs (e.g., nonsteroidal anti-inflammatory agents, agents instilled into cerebrospinal fluid)
Biologic products (e.g., immune globulin, OKT3)
Systemic immunologically mediated diseases (e.g., rheumatologic diseases, Behçet disease)
Neoplastic diseases

enteroviruses (EV). Using cell culture in addition to animal inoculation and serology, the etiology of AM could be established in ~55% to 70% of cases.[9–11] Cell culture clearly established EV as the dominant etiology of AM, accounting for ~55% to 90% of all identifiable causes.[4,9–12] Use of vaccines for prevention of mumps and polio led to nonpolio-enteroviruses becoming the overwhelming dominant cause of AM.[4,9–12] Nucleic acid amplification tests (NAATs) continue to support their significant etiologic role.[13–15]

Enteroviruses and Parechoviruses

Enteroviruses are members of the Picornaviridae family of viruses.[16] Four species (human enteroviruses A to D), encompassing ~100 confirmed or putative serotypes, are recognized within the genus.[16,17]

Enteroviruses have a worldwide distribution. Although ~100 serotypes comprise the genus, only a few cause disease each year. Furthermore, the dominant serotypes vary geographically and temporally.[17–21] In regions with temperate climates, EV infections exhibit a strong seasonal epidemiology, occurring primarily in the summer and fall.[17–19] In topical and subtropical regions, infections occur year-round with increased incidence during the rainy season.

The use of NAAT has demonstrated that >70% of AM cases in children for which an etiology is identified are attributable to EV.[13–15,22] Given their significant contribution as causes of AM it is not surprising that the seasonal occurrence of AM parallels activity of these viruses (Figure 43-1).

Parechoviruses, also in the family Picornaviridae, are recognized causes of AM.[23–25] Initially classified as enteroviruses, biologic, antigenic, and genomic differences led to their reclassification into a novel genus.[16,26–29] The majority of human parechovirus (HPeV) infections occur during the summer and fall. HPeV type 3 is most frequently associated with AM and has been identified in an average of 5% to 7% of enterovirus-negative archival CSF specimens.[23,24]

Arboviruses

The arboviruses comprise a group of >500 viruses from multiple viral families transmitted by an arthropod vector.[30] Human-to-human transmission is rare and is the result of blood, organ, or maternal-fetal/infant transmission. Mosquitoes are the vectors for the majority of clinically significant arboviruses endemic to North America. Notable exceptions include Colorado tick fever (CTF)

(meningoencephalitis) occurs frequently. This chapter focuses on viral agents more commonly associated with acute AM.

ETIOLOGIC AGENTS AND EPIDEMIOLOGY

Because AM is not a reportable disease in the United States, the total annual cases and incidence are unknown. The estimated annual number of AM cases is believed to be at least 75,000. In Olmsted County, Minnesota the incidence of AM over 32 years was found to be 10.9 per 100,000 person years.[4] The highest rates occurred in infants, toddlers, and children. The Centers for Disease Control and Prevention (CDC) reported that over a 10-year period the incidence of AM ranged from 1.5 to 4 per 100,000.[5] The differences in incidences may be the result of underreporting due to a passive reporting system used by the CDC. In Finland, a 14-year birth cohort study found the annual incidence of viral meningitis to be 27.8 per 100,000.[6] The highest rates were observed in infants and children <4 years of age.

Prior to the advent of cell culture, a specific etiology of AM was identifiable in only 25% of cases.[7,8] The principal agents identified were lymphocytic choriomeningitis virus (LCMV), mumps virus, herpes simplex virus (HSV), and polioviruses.

Cell culture led to a substantial improvement in the identification of viral causes of AM, primarily due to identification of

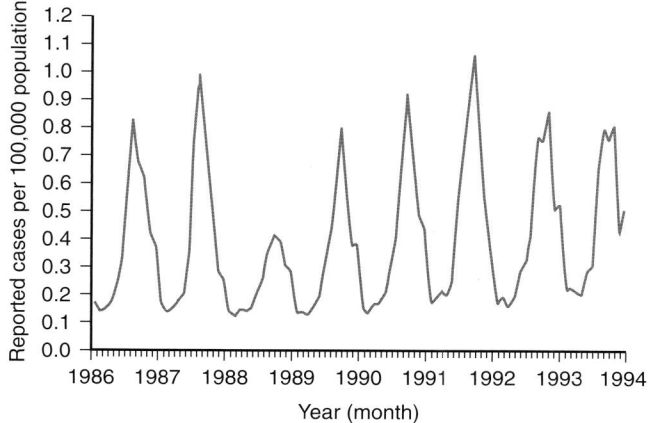

Figure 43-1. Seasonal incidence of aseptic meningitis in the United States from 1986 to 1993, as reported to the Centers for Disease Control and Prevention. The summer predominance reflects the role of enteroviruses as the leading cause of the aseptic meningitis syndrome. (Redrawn from Centers for Disease Control and Prevention. Summary of notifiable diseases, United States, 1993, MMWR 1994;42:69.)

and Powassan (POW) viruses, as well as, in Eurasia, tickborne encephalitis virus (TBEV), which are transmitted by ticks.[31,32] TBEV infection also can occur via consumption of infected unpasteurized milk.[32] The peak incidence of arboviral infections coincides with the periods of maximal activity of their respective vectors. In North America this is summer and fall.

The majority of arboviruses associated with AM in North America are members of the Flaviviridae family. Neurotropic Flaviviridae fall into either the Japanese encephalitis (Japanese encephalitis (JE), West Nile (WN), St. Louis encephalitis (SLE), and Murray Valley encephalitis viruses) or tickborne encephalitis (POW, CTF, TBE viruses) complexes.

West Nile virus (WNV) is the most common cause of arboviral infection in North America. However, <1% of infections in adults and children result in CNS disease. In the U.S., children account for 3% of WNV neuroinvasive disease (WNND). Meningitis is the most common manifestation in children, accounting for ~50% of cases.[33] Pediatric cases of WNND have been reported from most states in the U.S. and multiple countries worldwide.[33,34] The median annual incidence is 0.07 cases per 100,000 children.[33] South Dakota, Wyoming, New Mexico, and Nebraska, in decreasing order, have the highest median annual incidence (0.45 to 1.02/100,000 children).

SLE virus was first recognized in 1933 and is widely distributed throughout the American continent.[35,36] Epidemics or sporadic cases have been reported in virtually every state in the U.S. A mean of 4.25 cases of SLE neuroinvasive disease (SLEND) were reported annually from 2006 to 2008.[37] The reported rate of SLE in 2008 for children aged 1 to 14 years was 0.02 per 100,000.

Three neurologic syndromes have been reported with SLEND: encephalitis, AM, and febrile headache.[38] AM accounts for ~40% of SLEND cases in children. In Japan and Asia, a related flavivirus, JE virus, can cause AM in children.[39]

In Europe, TBEV is an important cause of AM.[32] Three subtypes exist: European, Siberian, and Far Eastern. The European and Siberian subtypes can cause meningitis, encephalitis, or myelitis. AM constitutes ~60% to 70% of pediatric TBEV CNS disease.[40,41] TBE occurs primarily from March to November. The reported incidence in Swiss children is 1.0 per 100,000.[40] In Slovenia, the annual incidence varies from 3.7 to 24.6 per 100,000; 12% to 27% of cases occur in children <15 years of age.[42] Although not endemic to North America, cases have occurred in persons returning from Europe and China.[43]

In North America, POW virus, a related virus, causes occasional cases of AM.[31] The tickborne CTF virus in the Reoviridae family also can cause AM.[44]

La Crosse (LACV) virus is in the family Bunyaviridae. AM accounts for 15% of LACV CNS disease.[45,46] In the U.S., 80% of LACV infections occur from July to September and >80% of cases occur in children <15 years of age.[45] Based on probable and confirmed cases from the eastern U.S., the calculated mean incidence risk for children <15 years is 30.2 per 100,000 persons.

Paramyxoviruses

Multiple Paramyxoviridae (measles, mumps, parainfluenza viruses, etc.) can cause CNS infection.[47] In mumps, AM occurs as complication in 0.5% to 15% of cases and CSF pleocytosis is seen in >50% of patients with mumps parotitis.[48,49] In North America, prior to mumps vaccine, mumps caused 2.5% to 15% of all AM cases and 17.5% to 22% of known causes of meningitis.[4,9–12,50] In countries where mumps remains endemic, meningitis continues to occur.[51,52] During each of 2 recent U.S. outbreaks, cases of meningitis were reported.[53,54] There are >10 mumps vaccine strains used around the world.[55] Although the Jeryl Lynn and its related vaccine strains (used exclusively in the U.S.) rarely, if ever, cause AM, other vaccine strains have been associated with varying incidences of AM.[55]

Parainfluenza viruses can cause AM.[47] The dominant serotype identified has been PIV type 3. Measles infection can be associated with pleocytosis usually without signs or symptoms of meningitis.[56]

Arenaviruses

The arenavirus LCMV was identified as a cause of AM in 1935.[57,58] Although previously a major cause of AM,[8,9] due to undefined epidemiologic factors or, perhaps, lack of testing, LCMV meningitis is now uncommon. Rodents, particularly the common house mouse, are its natural reservoirs; hamsters and guinea pigs also are capable hosts.[58] LCMV is shed in rodent excreta and secretions throughout the animal's life. Human infection occurs via contact with LCMV-contaminated fomites or inhalation/ingestion of aerosolized virus. The highest incidence of infections occurs during the late fall and winter.

Herpesviruses

Virtually every member of the human herpesviruses has been associated with AM in children.[59] Notable among these are varicella-zoster virus (VZV) and HSV type 2 (HSV-2). VZV-related meningitis has been reported in immunocompetent children during primary infection.[60] The use of NAAT has allowed the identification of VZV-associated meningitis in zoster cases lacking cutaneous lesions.[61,62]

Use of NAATs has documented HSV-2 and, less commonly, HSV-1 as causes of meningitis in children and adolescents.[63–66] HSV-2 infection can cause primary or recurrent AM. The latter occurs more frequently in women.

Other Viruses

Various other viruses occasionally have been identified as causes of AM: parvovirus B19,[67] adenovirus AM,[10] rotavirus,[68,69] influenza A and B viruses,[70] and human immunodeficiency virus.[71]

Other Etiologies

Less commonly, certain bacteria not readily visualized in stains of CSF or grown in standard culture systems, such as Borrelia, Treponema, and Rickettsia, mycoplasma, and fungi can cause AM syndrome) (see Box 43-1). Additionally, various parameningeal processes, neoplasms, systemic illnesses, drugs, and noninfectious etiologies can result in an AM syndrome.[3,72]

PATHOGENESIS AND PATHOLOGY

The majority of what is known regarding the pathogenesis of enterovirus infections has been derived from the study of the polioviruses.[73,74] Enteroviruses are transmitted primarily via the fecal–oral route and, less commonly, by respiratory droplets and transplacentally. Following ingestion, infection and replication occurs in the nasopharynx and lower gastrointestinal (GI) tract. Replication at these sites results in a minor or primary viremia that seeds multiple organs including the CNS, liver, lungs, and heart. Replication at these sites produces a major or secondary viremia. If the CNS was not seeded during the initial viremic phase, spread there can occur during the major viremia. Viremia continues until the host develops type-specific antibodies.

The exact means by which polioviruses and other enteroviruses enter the CNS is unclear and multiple routes have been proposed.[73,74] Infection of endothelial cells expressing specific receptors may facilitate CNS entry. Infection of mononuclear cells may allow CNS access via a "Trojan horse" mechanism. Lastly, access to the CNS may occur via axonal retrograde transport from the peripheral nervous system.

The pathogenesis of arbovirus infections begins with vector-mediated intradermal inoculation of the virus.[32,75] Viral replication occurs at the site of inoculation. For some flaviviruses replication occurs in Langerhans dendritic cells, which migrate to the regional lymph nodes. Virus reaching the regional lymph nodes leads to further replication resulting in a viremia that seeds the entire reticuloendothelial system, allowing for further amplification of viremia. Viremia results in infection of multiple organs including the brain. The mechanism by which all arboviruses enter the CNS is yet unknown. For some, infection of cerebral microvascular endothelial cells or transneural spread following infection of the olfactory bulb are modes of entry. Viremia persists until the host develops type-specific antibodies.

Due to the generally favorable outcome of aseptic and viral meningitis, histopathologic data are scarce. A report of a child who died of coxsackievirus B5 myocarditis with concomitant meningitis describes choroid plexus inflammation of the lateral and fourth ventricles, fibrosis of the vascular walls with focal destruction of the ependymal lining, and fibrosis of basal leptomeninges.[76] Parenchymal findings were limited to moderate symmetric ventricular dilatation and an increase in number and size of subependymal astrocytes. The choroid plexus inflammatory reaction supports the concept of viremic spread to the CNS. In an adolescent who died of systemic coxsackievirus B3 infection, the dura was grossly distended, with swelling of the leptomeninges and brain parenchyma.[77] Microscopically, round cell infiltrates were noted in the meninges overlying the cerebellum; the brain parenchyma was congested, with increased numbers of oligodendrocytes. Lymphocytic infiltration was most prominent around blood vessels in the cerebral white matter and in the basal ganglia. Focal areas of necrosis and hemorrhage also were seen. The occasional fatalities from mumps meningitis demonstrate pathologic findings of demyelination near blood vessels (suggesting an autoimmune process) and evidence of acute parenchymal involvement.[78]

CLINICAL MANIFESTATIONS

The clinical presentation and manifestations of enteroviral meningitis vary with age of the patient. Additionally, regardless of age, clinical findings of meningitis can coexist with clinical findings of other syndromes (e.g., myocarditis, pericarditis, pleurodynia, hand-foot-and-mouth syndrome).

Neonates can present with abrupt onset of fever and irritability. Poor feeding and lethargy may occur. Physical examination can reveal a bulging or full fontanel. Exanthems occasionally can be present. Nuchal rigidity is uncommon.[79–81] In severe cases, evidence of involvement of other organ systems can be dominant (i.e., hepatitis, myocarditis, pneumonitis, disseminated intravascular coagulopathy).[81]

In infants and children, fever of abrupt onset is the most common presenting sign.[82–85] In some, the fever pattern and clinical course is biphasic.[82,86] In infants, nonspecific symptoms such as irritability, lethargy, poor feeding, emesis, or diarrhea can be present.[84,87,88] In older children, additional nonspecific findings include generalized malaise, sore throat, abdominal pain, nausea, myalgia, and exanthems. Physical findings include nuchal rigidity and Brudzinski and Kernig signs. Less than 10% of infants <3 months of age exhibit these findings, which increase in frequency with advancing age.[83,87] In children able to report it, headache is almost always present and may be temporarily relieved by the performance of a lumbar puncture.[88,89] Photophobia is common and some patients complain of phonophobia. Seizures occur in <5%.[87,90] When the presentation exhibits a biphasic course, nonspecific signs and symptoms are followed by a brief period of improvement and then with evidence of neurologic involvement.[82,91]

In adolescents and adults, headache usually is present.[92–95] Fever, photophobia, signs of meningeal irritation, nausea, emesis, and neck stiffness occur in the majority of patients. Myalgia is common. Abdominal pain and exanthems also are reported occasionally.

Although limited information is available, the clinical presentation of HPeV AM in infants and children appears to parallel that of the enteroviruses.[24]

Typically, in children with mumps parotitis, the onset of meningitis occurs during the first week of illness. However, AM can precede parotitis by a week or follow it by as many as 3 weeks.[47] Fever, headache, emesis, and meningeal signs are common.[8,96,97] Approximately 50% of patients have no evidence of parotitis. Additional symptoms include abdominal pain, diarrhea, and sore throat.

The clinical findings of arbovirus meningitis are not unique enough to distinguish them from other viral meningitides. The signs and symptoms of WNV meningitis in children are similar to those reported in adults.[33] The onset is abrupt with fever, headache, and neck stiffness and Kernig and Brudzinski signs. Photophobia, phonophobia, and weakness can be present. Additional symptoms can include nausea, vomiting, diarrhea, sore throat, cough, rash, and lymphadenopathy.

TBEV meningitis has a biphasic course in approximately two-thirds of children.[41,42] Onset is abrupt with fever, headache, malaise, abdominal pain, emesis, and arthralgia lasting 3 to 5 days. The second, symptomatic phase follows a 6- to 10-day period of recovery and is characterized by fever, headache, fatigue, emesis, and signs of meningeal irritation.

A biphasic illness also can be seen with CTF.[44] The initial phase consists of sudden onset of high fever, headache, emesis, and flu-like constitutional symptoms lasting 2 to 3 days. After 1 to 2 days of improvement, fever returns in association with nuchal stiffness and signs of meningeal irritation.

In HSV meningitis and HSV-2 recurrent benign lymphocytic meningitis (RBLM), the onset of illness is acute with severe headache, neck stiffness, fever, photophobia, and emesis.[63,64,66] The majority of patients can provide no history of genital HSV infection.[64] Each episode lasts 1 to 3 days.[66] Multiple recurrences can occur.

The onset of LCMV meningitis is preceded by nonspecific symptoms suggestive of a viral upper respiratory tract illness and, occasionally, a rash. A brief period of improvement precedes the sudden onset of severe headache, nausea, emesis, photophobia, and myalgia. Physical examination reveals nuchal stiffness and signs of meningeal irritation.[2,8,57]

DIFFERENTIAL DIAGNOSIS

Borrelia burgdorferi (Lyme) meningitis is not clinically distinguishable from viral meningitis. Endemicity, time of year, and history of erythema migrans or tick exposure are helpful in considering Lyme disease. Children with Lyme meningitis are more likely to be afebrile and have a subacute presentation. Cranial neuropathy can be present.[98] CSF findings are similar to viral meningitis.

A small proportion (1% to 2%) of children with untreated *Mycobacterium tuberculosis* infection will develop meningitis.[99] Because symptoms early in the illness are vague and nonspecific, a high index of suspicion is required in order to make the diagnosis.

Treponema pallidum can cause AM during the secondary or tertiary phases of syphilis. Headache and signs of meningeal irritation can be present or the patient can be asymptomatic.[100]

Meningitis associated with leptospirosis occurs during the immunologic phase of illness. In addition to typical signs of meningeal irritation, patients can exhibit rash, uveitis, conjunctival suffusion, and hepatosplenomegaly.[2] AM can complicate brucellosis in 5% of cases.[101] *Mycoplasma pneumoniae, Chlamydophila pneumoniae, M. hominis,* and *Ureaplasma urealyticum* infections have been associated with AM.[102–105]

Parameningeal infectious foci (sinusitis, mastoiditis, vertebral osteomyelitis, epi- or subdural empyema, etc.) can manifest as AM. Endocarditis may result in CSF abnormalities suggestive of AM.[106]

AM occurs in up to 26% of children with Kawasaki disease.[107] Urinary tract infections in children have been associated with CSF pleocytosis in the absence of bacteria in the CSF.[108] Pleocytosis also can occur following complex migraines and prolonged seizures.[109,110] AM has been associated with systemic illnesses such as sarcoidosis, systemic lupus erythematosus, Behçet disease, other connective tissue/vasculitis syndromes, and malignancies.[72]

Multiple medications and biological agents can cause AM.[3] The major groups of drugs associated with drug-induced AM are non-steroidal anti-inflammatory drugs (NSAIDs), immune globulin intravenous (IGIV), and immunomodulating agents. AM related to NSAIDs is more commonly seen in women. Trimethoprim alone or in combination with sulfamethoxazole is the most

PART II Clinical Syndromes and Cardinal Features of Infectious Diseases: Approach to Diagnosis and Initial Management

SECTION F Central Nervous System Infections

common cause of antibiotic-induced AM. Multiple reports describing AM in children receiving IGIV exist, making this, perhaps, the most common cause of drug-induced AM in children.[3] Immunomodulating agents, most notably OKT3, chemotherapeutic agents, and intrathecal agents also are associated with AM.

LABORATORY FINDINGS AND DIAGNOSIS

Key to the diagnosis of AM is the cytochemical analysis of the CSF. Pleocytosis is a prerequisite and typically is lymphocytic in character, ranging from 100 to 1000 cells/mm[3].[8,41,42,47,63,64,79,84,87,90,96] Count can exceed 2000 cells/mm[3] in some cases of LCMV, EV, and mumps meningitis.[59,82,111] If the CSF is examined early in the illness, particularly with enteroviral meningitis, polymorphonuclear pleocytosis can predominate.[86,87,90,111] Re-examination several hours to days later reveals a shift towards lymphocytic predominance.[86,91,112] Eosinophilic pleocytosis has been reported with EV meningitis.[113]

The CSF protein concentration generally is mildly to moderately increased while the glucose concentration is normal. Hypoglycorrhachia occurs in up to a quarter of LCMV and mumps meningitis cases as well as sporadic cases of EV and HSV-2 meningitis.[47,59,85,90,96,111,113]

Traditionally, the diagnosis of EV meningitis has relied on cell culture detection of virus from CSF.[114] NAATs are significantly more sensitive and rapid; they have become the standard for detection of EV in CSF, and timely results can reduce length of hospital stay and antibiotic use.[114–116]

In neonates with suspected EV meningitis, blood, CSF, and rectal swab/stool samples can be submitted for cell culture. Viral shedding from mucosal sites infers recent infection. The same is not true in older patients, who can shed EV from mucosal sites for weeks to months after infection.

Serologic confirmation of enteroviral infection generally is impractical and not useful in acute management.[114]

NAATs are the methodology of choice for the diagnosis of parechovirus meningitis.[24]

Because the sensitivity of CSF culture for HSV is too low to be of clinical utility, NAAT detection should be used.[63,64,66] Detection of HSV antibodies in CSF should not be used to confirm the diagnosis of HSV meningitis.[65] Inflammation of the blood–brain barrier can permit serum HSV antibodies to cross into the CSF resulting in a false-positive assay. CSF NAAT also should be used to detect other herpesviruses (VZV, EBV, CMV, HHV-6).

The diagnosis of arbovirus meningitis relies on the detection of virus-specific antibodies.[30–31] IgM or IgG capture immunoassays or immunofluorescence typically are used; antibody capture format is more sensitive than other methods for IgM detection. Hemagglutination inhibition and complement fixation tests mainly are used for research.

The approach to the diagnosis of any arbovirus meningitis generally follows that used for WNV.[30–31] Because the presence of arbovirus-specific IgM antibodies in CSF infers intrathecal production, this test should be performed to diagnose WNV meningitis. WNV-specific IgM antibodies usually are present in the CSF by days 3 to 5 of illness.[30] Serum IgM appears 3 days later. While the finding of specific IgM in CSF is considered diagnostic, detection in serum is not because IgM anti-WNV can be present for >2 years following infection.[117] Prolonged false-positive result of serum IgM anti-WNV also can occur with SLE. Because of cross-reactions with related viruses, a positive IgM anti-WNV assay result should be followed by a virus-specific neutralization test.

If only serum is available for testing, an arbovirus-specific cause can be established by documenting rising titers. While serum NAAT can detect WNV early in infection, by the time CNS symptoms appear NAATs are less sensitive than antibody tests because of rapid clearance of the virus.[30]

The appearance of antibodies to CTF virus occurs late in the illness (10 to 14 days after onset of symptoms), rendering serology less useful for diagnosis.[31,118] NAAT permits early (within 5 days of onset) detection of CTF virus. Detection of intra-erythrocyte CTF virus using immunofluorescence staining is possible but

interpretation is subjective. Virus isolation using cell culture or animal inoculation is possible. However, the latter is rarely used.

The diagnosis of mumps meningitis can be made by virus isolation, documentation of significant convalescent antibody titers, presence of mumps-specific IgM antibodies, or NAAT detection of mumps genome.[119] Mumps virus can be isolated from saliva, blood, urine, and CSF. The virus may be present in saliva 9 days prior to and 8 days after the onset of parotitis and in urine for up to 2 weeks after the onset of symptoms. Serum IgM anti-mumps virus is present within 3 to 4 days of the onset of symptoms and can persist for up to 3 months.[119] A single serum sample obtained within 10 days of the onset of illness documenting the presence of IgM anti-mumps virus is sufficient to establish the diagnosis. IgG antibodies are detectable 7 to 10 days after symptom onset and persist for life. Antibodies to other paramyxoviruses can cross-react with mumps serologic assays, leading to false-positive results.

MANAGEMENT, EMPIRIC AND DEFINITIVE THERAPY

When it is not possible to exclude a bacterial etiology or if the patient is an infant or child it may be decided to hospitalize and initiate empiric antibiotic therapy while awaiting results of bacterial cultures of blood and CSF and/or NAAT. Adolescents and adults who appear well and whose CSF findings are not suggestive of a bacterial infection may not require hospitalization.

Treatment of viral meningitis is supportive. Antipyretics, intravenous fluids, and narcotic analgesic may be indicated. Anticonvulsants may be required to manage seizures should they occur, but a need for prolonged use is uncommon.

No antiviral therapies approved by the Food and Drug Administration (FDA) are available for the majority of viral causes of meningitis. Reports of the use of immune serum globulin (ISG), maternal serum or plasma, or commercial IGIV in severe neonatal enteroviral disease have been published.[81] No definitive conclusions can be derived from these reports.[81]

Pleconaril, an antiviral compound that inhibits enterovirus uncoating and blocks viral attachment to host cell receptors,[120] failed to meet criteria for FDA licensure for uncomplicated AM.[74] However, post hoc analysis found pleconaril to be beneficial in accelerating the resolution of headache.[95]

The role of acyclovir in the therapy of HSV-related meningitis (unlike HSV encephalitis) remains unproven.[66] Use has been associated with rapid resolution of symptoms. Valacyclovir and famciclovir have been used in the treatment of RBML.[66]

COMPLICATIONS, PROGNOSIS, AND SEQUELAE

Reported complications of enterovirus meningitis occur in ~10% of infected patients and include coma, increased intracranial pressure, and inappropriate secretion of antidiuretic hormone (ADH).[87,121] Enteroviruses require antibody-mediated mechanisms for their elimination. EV in individuals with agammaglobulinemia or hypogammaglobulinemia can lead to chronic meningitis or meningoencephalitis that persists and progresses over many years, often with a fatal outcome.[122]

Beyond the neonatal period, EV meningitis rarely has a poor outcome, but short-term morbidity can be substantial and prolonged.[80,92,95,123] The incidence of morbidity and mortality due to perinatal EV infections may be as high as 73% and 10%, respectively.[81] Death usually is the result of hepatic failure or myocarditis. The long-term prognosis for young children with EV meningitis is good; no differences in neurodevelopmental testing between patients and controls were reported in a large study.[87] In children and infants the duration of illness is generally ≤1 week. In adolescents and adults the time to complete recovery is 2 to 3 weeks.[92,95]

Mumps meningitis is benign with minimal risk of mortality or long-term sequelae. A review of ~200 cases of mumps AM revealed that all recovered without sequelae with none developing deafness.[47] Hydrocephalus complicating mumps meningitis has been reported but occurs rarely.[47] Occasional deaths have occurred in children with mumps meningoencephalitis.[78]

Arboviral meningitis in children generally is associated with an excellent prognosis. The mortality rate for reported cases of WNND in the U.S. over a 10-year period was <1%.[34] Recovery from WNV meningitis appears to be complete.[33] Long-term sequelae in Western forms of TBEV are infrequent and virtually all pediatric patients with meningitis recover fully.[32,41,42]

Individuals with HSV-2 primary meningitis or RBLM can exhibit transient neurologic findings that include seizures, hallucinations, diplopia, and cranial nerve palsies.[64,66] Less commonly, patients may be drowsy or have altered mental status. Failure of any of these symptoms to resolve should call into question the diagnosis. Recurrent episodes can occur but recovery occurs without sequelae.[63,65]

Meningitis due to LCMV has a benign course lasting 10 to 14 days with complete recovery in immunocompetent individuals.[57]

PREVENTION

The use of vaccines for the prevention of poliomyelitis and mumps has dramatically reduced these agents as causes of AM. Several effective vaccines for prevention of TBE are available in Europe and Russia.[32]

Handwashing prevents the spread of EVs. In patients with inherited antibody deficiency, maintenance supplementation with IGIV limits the risk of development of chronic EV meningitis.

Use of insect repellents and appropriate clothing as well as avoidance of areas known to be mosquito- or tick-infested help decrease the risk of arbovirus infection. Routine maintenance of screens and house integrity will decrease the risk of exposure to mosquito-borne arboviruses and murine LCMV.

Suppressive therapy with acyclovir, valacyclovir, and famciclovir have been used to control HSV-associated RBLM. Regardless of a history of genital lesions, individuals with HSV-2 meningitis should receive counseling regarding genital herpes and the possibility of transmission of infection; prepubertal children should be evaluated for sexual abuse.[66]

44 Encephalitis

Carol Glaser and Sarah S. Long

Encephalitis generally refers to inflammation of the brain parenchyma and clinically presents as fever, headache, and alteration in consciousness. Alteration in consciousness distinguishes encephalitis from the more common entity of uncomplicated meningitis, whose features typically include fever, headache, and nuchal rigidity but lack global or focal neurologic dysfunction. Encephalitis is one of the most challenging conditions for clinicians to diagnose, treat, and manage because of the severity of illness, the vast number of potential etiologies, ineffective treatment options for many causes, and the lack of an identifiable etiology in most cases. Without the identification of a neurotropic agent or analysis of brain tissue, the diagnosis of encephalitis is presumptive and is based on clinical features. Patients with encephalitis can manifest parenchymal brain findings alone, but most have associated meningeal inflammation, thus representing the overlap with the syndrome termed meningoencephalitis. For the purposes of this chapter, the terms encephalitis and meningoencephalitis are used interchangeably. This chapter focuses predominantly on viral causes of encephalitis in the immunocompetent host, but other pertinent agents and special hosts also are considered.

ETIOLOGIC AGENTS AND EPIDEMIOLOGY

Although the term encephalitis often is used in conjunction with a viral etiology, other agents and entities can cause encephalitis or encephalitis symptomatology. Infectious causes of encephalitis, include viruses, bacteria, fungi, and parasites (Table 44-1). Additionally, a number of noninfectious conditions can mimic encephalitis (Box 44-1). Despite the multitude of infectious and noninfectious etiologies of encephalitis, no etiology is identified in more than 50% of cases.

The reported incidence of acute encephalitis varies throughout the world and ranges between 1.5 and 7.4/100,000 population.[1,2] Most studies find that the incidence of encephalitis is higher in the pediatric age group than in adults.[1] Data from hospitalizations in England over a 10-year period show an overall incidence of 1.5/100,000 population, and a rate of 2.8/100,000 in children and 8.7/100,000 in infants.[2] Similar rates in children were found in

Finland where the incidence was 8.8/100,000 from 1973 to 1987[3] and in Slovenia where the incidence was 6.7/100,000 from 1979 to 1991.[4]

In countries where vaccines are used widely to prevent measles, mumps, rubella, and varicella infections, the spectrum of causative agents of encephalitis has changed over time.[3-6] For example, because vaccine preventable diseases such as measles, mumps, and rubella have decreased dramatically in the past few decades in the United States, the incidence of encephalitis due these viruses also has decreased. However, there has been an increase in the identification of new pathogens, including West Nile virus, Nipah virus, enterovirus 71, *Balamuthia mandrillaris*, *Baylisascaris procyonis*, and Chandipura virus.

Viruses

Most cases of viral encephalitis are uncommon complications of common infections or expected presentations of newly emerging or rare pathogens.

Enteroviruses

Enteroviruses (EVs), nonenveloped RNA picornaviruses, cause approximately 10-15 million symptomatic infections per year in the U.S.[7] Encephalitis is a rare complication of EV infection, but because EV infections are ubiquitous, they are a leading cause of encephalitis in children and are responsible for 10-15% of encephalitis cases for which an etiology is identified.[8] Outside the U.S., outbreaks involving substantial numbers of EV 71 encephalitis cases have been observed among young children in some countries.[9,10]

Human Parechoviruses

The reclassification of former enteroviruses, echovirus 21 and echovirus 22, was the genesis of the new human parechovirus (HPeV) genus. Echoviruses 21 and 22 are now classified as HPeV-1

Text continued on page 302.

PART II Clinical Syndromes and Cardinal Features of Infectious Diseases: Approach to Diagnosis and Initial Management

SECTION F Central Nervous System Infections

TABLE 44-1. Exposures Associated with Agents Causing Encephalitis and Encephalitis-Like Syndrome

Risk Factor/Exposure	Agent	Epidemiology
ARTHROPODS		
Mosquito	**Alphaviruses**	
	Chikungunya virus	Tropical Africa and Southeast Asia, Indian Ocean and parts of Europe
	Western equine encephalitis virus	Summer and early fall onset; western U.S. and Canada, Central and South America; rare cause of encephalitis, with 640 cases reported in the U.S. from 1964 to 1999. There have been only 4 cases of neuroinvasive disease due to WEE since 1989, with no cases reported in the last 10 years (through 2009)
	Eastern equine encephalitis virus	Eastern and southern coastal states; children and elderly disproportionately affected; rare cause of encephalitis, with 260 cases reported in the U.S. from 1964 to 1999
	Venezuelan equine encephalitis virus	Mexico, Central and South America; rarely in border states of U.S. (Texas, Arizona)
	Semliki Forest virus	Africa
	Flaviviruses	
	West Nile virus	Emerging cause of epidemic encephalitis throughout U.S., Europe; endemic in Middle East; cases also found in Africa, Caribbean, India, Australia, Russia, and Southeast Asia; peak incidence adults >50 years
	Japanese encephalitis virus	Most common worldwide cause of encephalitis, endemic throughout Asia; vaccine preventable
	St. Louis encephalitis virus	Endemic to western U.S.; with periodic outbreaks in central/eastern U.S., peak incidence in adults >50 years
	Murray Valley encephalitis virus	Australia and New Guinea
	Bunyaviruses	
	California/La Crosse virus	Endemic in midwestern and appalachia in North America, with an average of 79 cases reported annually since 1964; peak incidence in school-aged children
	Phleboviruses	
	Rift Valley Fever virus	Africa and Arabia
Tick	Powassan virus	In the U.S., endemic in the Upper Midwest, Great Lakes, New England, New York, and in eastern Canada
	Anaplasma phagocytophila	Endemic to New England, north central and western U.S.
	Ehrlichia ewingii	Endemic to southeastern and central U.S.
	Ehrlichia chaffeenesis	Endemic to northeastern U.S. and Midwest
	Rickettsia rickettsii	Rocky Mountain spotted fever has been reported throughout the U.S. with the exception of Hawaii and Vermont; states with highest incidence are Oklahoma and North Carolina
	Tickborne encephalitis virus	Endemic to Eastern and Central Europe, East and Southeast Asia
	Borrelia burgdorferi	Encephalitis in early disseminated Lyme disease; encephalopathy in late disease
	Kyasanur Forest disease virus	India
Sandflies	*Bartonella bacilliformis*	Southwestern Colombia, Ecuador, and Peru
	Toscana virus	Italy, Mediterranean
	Chandipura virus	India
Tsetse flies	*Trypanosoma brucei gambiense*	West Africa and India; CNS illness can occur years after infection
	Trypanosoma brucei rhodesiense	East Africa; CNS illess can occur years after infection
WILD OR DOMESTIC ANIMALS		
Bats	Rabies virus	Vaccine preventable. Between 1995 and 2009, 43 rabies cases were recognized in the U.S.; 10 of these cases were imported (usually from a canine strain), and the remaining cases were acquired in the U.S. mostly related to bat exposures and often with an unknown bite event
	Nipah virus	Epidemics in Southeast Asia; also found in Bangladesh and India. Reservoir host is fruit bat but humans generally acquire disease through direct contact with infected swine
	Histoplasma capsulatum	Eastern and central U.S.; occupational or recreational activities where there is exposure to disturbed soil, such as gardening, playing in barns, hollow trees, bird roosts or caves, and examination, demolition, or renovation of contaminated buildings
Deer	*Borrelia burgdorferi*	Deer is reservoir host but infection usually is transmitted to humans via tick vector
	Anaplasma phagocyophila	Deer is reservoir host but infection usually is transmitted to humans via tick vector
Dogs	Rabies virus	Vaccine preventable; dogs important in developing countries; worldwide distribution
	Toxocara canis	Dogs, especially puppies, shed eggs in feces and organism survives in soil for prolonged period

Continued

TABLE 44-1. Exposures Associated with Agents Causing Encephalitis and Encephalitis-Like Syndrome—cont'd

Risk Factor/Exposure	Agent	Epidemiology
Cats	*Bartonella henselae*	Typically follows scratch or bite from cat or kitten; highest incidence in children
	Toxoplasma gondii	Cats and other felines are reservoir hosts; they shed oocytes in feces, and the soil becomes contaminated. Sheep, goats, swine, cattle serve as intermediate hosts
	Rabies virus	Vaccine preventable; most common vector in the U.S. is bat, and bites often unrecognized, cats are second to dogs in importance in developing countries; worldwide distribution
	Toxocara cati	Cats, especially kittens, shed eggs in feces and organism survives in soil for prolonged period
Rodents	Lymphocytic choriomeningitis virus	Peak incidence in fall and winter; chronic infection in laboratory or house mice, hamsters, and guinea pigs; humans infected by inhalation or ingestion of dust or food contaminated by urine, feces, blood, nasopharyngeal secretions of infected rodents
	Leptospira spp.	Rodents (and other animals) excrete organism in urine, and the organism remains viable in soil or water for weeks to months
Raccoon	*Baylisascaris procyonis*	Pica, particularly near raccoon latrine
	Rabies virus	"Raccoon strain" extends along eastern seaboard of the U.S. and has reached as far north as Ontario and New Brunswick in Canada
Sheep/goats	*Brucella melitensis*	Direct contact with infected animals or their secretions
	Coxiella burnetii	Inhalation; either direct exposure to animal or exposure to contaminated materials (e.g., wool, straw)
Birds	*Cryptococcus neoformans*	Inhalation of soil contaminated with bird feces
	Chlamydophila psittaci	Healthy and sick birds can harbor and transmit organism to humans; usually acquired via inhalation of fecal dust/sections of birds
	West Nile virus	Birds are reservoir host but infection usually is transmitted to humans via mosquito vector
Old World Monkeys	Herpes B virus	Bite of Old World monkey (e.g., macaque)
Horses	Hendra virus	Endemic in Australia; associated with excretions/tissues from horses
Swine	Nipah virus	Epidemics in Southeast Asia; close contact with pigs
Skunks	Rabies virus	Skunk populations are widely distributed in the U.S.; cases found in California, Arizona, north central U.S., eastern coast of U.S.
Parturient animals (especially farm animals)	*Coxiella burnetii*	Humans generally acquire via inhalation; either direct exposure to animal or exposure to contaminated materials (e.g., wool, straw)
INGESTION OR INHALATION		
Fresh water	*Naegleria fowleri*	Swimming or diving in warm, natural bodies of water (rarely poorly chlorinated pools reported)
	Leptospira spp.	Organisms excreted in animal urine or placental tissue and can remain viable for weeks to months in soil or water; recreational exposure associated with wading or swimming in contaminated water (particularly after floods)
Soil	*Balamuthia mandrillaris*	Contact with soil seems to be important risk factor, presumably through inhalation or inoculation
	Acanthamoeba spp.	Contact with soil seems to be important risk factor, presumably through inhalation or inoculation
	Baylisascaris procyonis	Pica, particularly near raccoon latrine; raccoons infected with *B. procyonis* appear to be common in many parts of the U.S.; human cases reported in California, Oregon, New York, Pennsylvania, Illinois, Michigan, Georgia, Minnesota, and Missouri
	Coccidioides spp.	Also known as "Valley fever." Infection is seasonal and is acquired by inhalation of soil or dust or laboratory acquired; endemic in certain areas of Arizona, California, Nevada, New Mexico, Texas, Utah, and northwestern Mexico. Also found in northern Argentina, northwest Brazil, Colombia, Paraguay, Venezuela, and Central America
	Histoplasma capsulatum	Inhalation of airborne spores from soil. Outbreaks have occurred in endemic areas with exposure to bird, chicken, or bat droppings or recently contaminated soil. Globally distributed, with the Ohio and Mississippi River basin, Mexico, and Central and South America being endemic areas in which as many as 80% of children have been infected. Also found in Africa, East Asia, Australia, and rarely in Europe
	Blastomyces dermatitidis	Endemic areas include the midwest, southwestern, and south central U.S. and the Canadian provinces near the Great Lakes or St. Lawrence Seaway
	Toxocara canis/T. cati	Eggs in sandboxes and playgrounds; organisms survive long periods in soil
Undercooked pork or beef (rarely chicken)	*Toxoplasma gondii*	Consuming raw or undercooked infected meat; worldwide

Continued

PART II Clinical Syndromes and Cardinal Features of Infectious Diseases: Approach to Diagnosis and Initial Management

SECTION F Central Nervous System Infections

TABLE 44-1. Exposures Associated with Agents Causing Encephalitis and Encephalitis-Like Syndrome—cont'd

Risk Factor/Exposure	Agent	Epidemiology
Undercooked freshwater fish, chicken, or pork	Gnathostoma spp.	Southeast Asia and Mexico
Freshwater crayfish or crabs	Paragonimus westermani	Mostly in Asia but some reports from Africa and South America
Raw or undercooked meat	Trichinella spp.	Mostly associated with pigs but has been found in other mammals (e.g., horses, bear, foxes)
Frogs, snakes	Gnathostoma spinigerum	Southeast Asia and some areas in South and Central America
Raw or undercooked freshwater prawns, crabs, or frogs, or unwashed produce (with snails or slugs)	Angiostrongylus cantonensis	Reported in Louisiana, Hawaii, the South Pacific, Pacific Islands, Southeast Asia, Asia, Australia, and the Caribbean
Raw vegetables	Toxoplasma gondii	Consumption of raw, unwashed, vegetables
Unpasteurized milk	Coxiella burnetii	Animal exposures (particularly placenta and amniotic fluid)
	Tickborne encephalitis virus	Tick bite or ingestion of unpasteurized milk; endemic to Eastern and Central Europe, East and Southeast Asia
	Listeria monocytogenes	Can be found in about 5% of unpasteurized milk samples and products
	Toxoplasma gondii	Consumption of raw goat milk
SEASON		
Fall	Enteroviruses	Peak incidence in late summer and early fall; enterovirus 71 a cause of large outbreaks in Asia, with children primarily affected
	Arthropod-borne pathogens	Geographically specific agents/risks
Winter	Influenza virus, other respiratory viruses	Sporadic cases in children, with most reports from Japan and Southeast Asia
Spring	Enteroviruses	Peak incidence in late summer and early fall; enterovirus 71 a cause of large outbreaks in Asia, with children primarily affected
	Arthropod-borne pathogens	
Summer	Enteroviruses	Peak incidence in late summer and early fall; enterovirus 71 a cause of large outbreaks in Asia, with children primarily affected
	Naegleria fowleri	Swimming or diving in brackish, fresh water lakes or ponds
	Arthropod-borne pathogens	Geographically specific agents/risks
RECREATION		
Camping or hunting	Arthropod-borne pathogens	Geographically specific agents/risks
Spelunking	Rabies virus	Airborne transmission has been reported rarely in caves inhabited by millions of bats
	Histoplasma capsulatum	Inhalation of spores from soil contaminated with bat guano
Sexual activity	Human immunodeficiency virus	Global risk
	Treponema pallidum	Global risk
	Herpes simplex virus 2	Herpes simplex virus 1 also can be transmitted by sexual activity
Water sports	Naegleria fowleri	Swimming or diving in brackish, freshwater lakes or ponds
	Leptospira spp.	Exposure to water contaminated with urine of infected animals via swallowing water or skin contact
BLOOD TRANSFUSION OR ORGAN TRANSPLANT		
	Toxoplasma gondii	Infection can occur through blood transfusion or organ transplantation
	Rabies virus	Rare case reports of transmission via organ transplantation
	Balamuthia mandrillaris	Rare case reports of transmission via organ transplantation
	Lymphocytic choriomeningitis virus	Rare case reports of transmission via organ transplantation
FOREIGN TRAVEL		
Global	West Nile virus	Geographically specific risks
	Rabies virus	Dog bites are the most common mode of acquisition in developing countries
	Herpes simplex virus 1 and 2	Sporadic
	Influenza	Seasonal by region
	Measles	Measles SSPE can occur despite history of immunization (child generally had unrecognized infection before measles vaccine)
	Enteroviruses	Seasonal by region
	Human immunodeficiency virus	Sexual activity and bloodborne
	Plasmodium spp.	Tropical and subtropical areas
Africa	Chikungunya virus	Particularly Tanzania
	Poliovirus	Wild poliovirus transmission still occurs in Afghanistan, India, Pakistan, Nigeria
	Histoplasma capsulatum	Microfoci throughout Africa
	Taenia spp.	East Africa, particularly in underdeveloped communities with poor sanitation and where people eat raw or undercooked pork

Continued

TABLE 44-1. Exposures Associated with Agents Causing Encephalitis and Encephalitis-Like Syndrome—cont'd

Risk Factor/Exposure	Agent	Epidemiology
Asia	Chikungunya virus	Particularly India, Indonesia, Thailand, and Indian Ocean islands
	Japanese encephalitis virus	Including Southeast Asia
	Tickborne encephalitis virus	Central Europe to Japan
	Borrelia burgdorferi	Temperate forested regions throughout northern Asia
	Histoplasma capsulatum	Microfoci throughout eastern Asia
	Gnathostoma spinigerum	Southeast Asia, particularly Thailand, and Japan
	Nipah virus	Southeast Asia, particularly Malaysia
	Taenia spp.	Southeast Asia, particularly in underdeveloped communities with poor sanitation and where people eat raw or undercooked pork
Australia	Murray Valley encephalitis virus	Also in New Guinea
	Japanese encephalitis virus	Northern Australia
	Histoplasma capsulatum	Microfoci throughout Australia
	Hendra virus	Exposure to body fluids and excretions of infected horses is important
Caribbean	Venezuelan equine encephalitis virus	Trinidad
Europe	Tickborne encephalitis virus	Central Europe to Japan
	Chikungunya virus	Italy (northeastern)
	Anaplasma phagocytophila	Temperate zones, particularly Germany, Portugal, and Denmark
	Toscana virus	Italy, Mediterranean
	Borrelia burgdorferi	Temperate forested regions throughout Europe, particularly eastern and central Europe
	Taenia spp.	Eastern Europe, particularly in underdeveloped communities with poor sanitation and where people eat raw or undercooked pork
Mediterranean	Toscana virus	Central Italy, France, Spain, Portugal, Greece, Cyprus
North America	Powassan virus	Northeastern and central U.S., Canada
	California/La Crosse virus	Midwestern and eastern U.S.
	St. Louis encephalitis virus	Geographic range extends from Canada to Argentina, but most human cases in the western U.S., with periodic outbreaks in central and eastern U.S.
	Ehrlichia chaffeensis	Southern and central U.S., and mid-Atlantic and coastal states
	Anaplasma phagocytophila	Wooded areas of the north and northeastern U.S., mid-Atlantic, Midwest, west coast
	Rickettsia rickettsii	Throughout southern Canada and North America, with peak incidence in southeast and south central U.S., northern and southwestern Mexico, Costa Rica and Panama
	Eastern equine encephalitis	Highest incidence in Atlantic and Gulf states
	Venezuelan equine encephalitis virus	Florida and southwestern U.S., rarely in border states (Texas, Arizona); tropical latitudes of Mexico and Central America
	Western equine encephalitis virus	Most cases occur in western U.S. and prairie provinces in Canada, but also occurs in Mexico and Central America; infection associated with residence in rural areas and with agricultural occupations and other outdoor activities that lead to contact with the vector mosquito
	Borrelia burgdorferi	Eastern U.S., upper midwest states, and Pacific northwest; epidemics in summer months when ticks actively seek hosts and human outdoor activity is greatest
	Coccidioides spp.	Semiarid regions of southwestern U.S. and Mexico
	Blastomyces dermatitidis	Southeastern and central states, midwestern states bordering the Great Lakes; thrives in decaying vegetation or wet soil
	Histoplasma capsulatum	Endemic in Mississippi, Ohio and Missouri River valleys in U.S. and other microfoci throughout U.S., Mexico, and Central America
	Balamuthia mandrillaris	Highest number of cases reported from Arizona, California and Texas in U.S.; also occurs in Mexico and Central America
	Taenia spp.	Mexico and Central America, especially in underdeveloped communities with poor sanitation and where people eat raw or undercooked pork
	Gnathostoma spinigerum	Mexico and Central America; humans become infected by eating undercooked fish or poultry containing third-stage larvae, or reportedly by drinking water containing infective second-stage larvae
Russia	*Taenia* spp.	More prevalent in underdeveloped communities with poor sanitation and where people eat raw or undercooked pork
	Tickborne encephalitis virus	Eastern Russia

Continued

PART II   Clinical Syndromes and Cardinal Features of Infectious Diseases: Approach to Diagnosis and Initial Management

SECTION F   Central Nervous System Infections

TABLE 44-1. Exposures Associated with Agents Causing Encephalitis and Encephalitis-Like Syndrome—cont'd

Risk Factor/Exposure	Agent	Epidemiology
South America	Venezuelan equine encephalitis virus	Tropical latitudes, particularly Colombia, Venezuela, Peru, and Ecuador
	St. Louis encephalitis virus	From Canada to Argentina, but most human cases occur in the U.S.
	Western equine encephalitis virus	Associated with residence in rural areas and with agricultural occupations and other outdoor activities that lead to contact with the vector mosquito
	Rickettsia rickettsii	Brazil and Argentina
	Coccidioides spp.	Semiarid regions
	Histoplasma capsulatum	Microfoci throughout South America
	Gnathostoma spinigerum	Consuming undercooked fish or poultry containing third-stage larvae, or reportedly by drinking water containing infective second-stage larvae
	Bartonella bacilliformis	Middle altitudes of Andes Mountains
	Taenia spp.	More prevalent in underdeveloped communities with poor sanitation and where people eat raw or undercooked pork

and HPeV-2 respectively. At least 10 HPeV serotypes have been described to date; nearly all have been associated with encephalitis, most often in children younger than 2 years of age.[11] The relative frequency of HPeV encephalitis is unknown; encephalitis due to HPeV would have been missed in the past because polymerase chain reaction (PCR) testing for EVs does not detect HPeVs.

Herpesviruses

Herpesviruses are a large group of enveloped DNA viruses, and at least eight herpesvirus types are known to infect humans. Similar to EVs, herpesviruses are a frequent cause of human disease. Herpes simplex virus (HSV-1) is the most commonly identified cause of encephalitis in adults and follows EV as the most commonly identified cause of encephalitis in children.[12,13] Most but not all herpes simplex encephalitis (HSE, referring to disease

outside of the neonatal period) in children is a consequence of primary HSV-1 infection, while most HSE in adults is the result of reactivation. In a large cohort of 322 pediatric encephalitis cases over a 12-year period, 5% were due to HSE.[14] Other herpesviruses, including varicella-zoster virus (VZV), Epstein–Barr virus (EBV), and human herpesvirus 6 (HHV-6) also cause encephalitis.

Arboviruses

Arboviruses are viruses transmitted by an arthropod vector and are well-recognized causes of encephalitis. Three arbovirus families are known to cause encephalitis in humans: Togaviridae, Flaviviridae, and Bunyaviridae. Of these families, the viruses responsible for most clinically significant disease in the U.S. include eastern equine encephalitis virus (EEE) and western equine encephalitis virus (WEE) (Togaviridae family); West Nile virus (WNV), St.

BOX 44-1. Conditions Mimicking Encephalitis

IMMUNE MEDIATED

Anti-*N*-methyl-D-aspartate receptor-associated (NMDAR) encephalitis
Other neuronal antibody-associated encephalitis[a]
Rheumatologic (systemic lupus erythematosus, Sjögren, Behçet, sarcoidosis)
Small-vessel vasculitis
Corticosteroid-responsive encephalopathy associated with Hashimoto thyroiditis
Acute disseminated encephalomyelitis (ADEM)
Acute necrotizing encephalopathy (ANE)
Periarteritis nodosa

TOXIC ENCEPHALOPATHY

Bacterial toxins (*Shigella* spp., *Campylobacter jejuni*, *Salmonella* spp.)
Reye syndrome
Acute toxic ingestion
Lead intoxication
Hyperpyrexic encephalopathy and shock syndrome

INBORN ERROR OF METABOLISM

Ornithine transcarbamylase deficiency, heterozygote
Glutaric acidemia type 1
Medium-chain acyl coenzyme A dehydrogenase deficiency
Mitochondrial encephalopathy with lactic acidosis and stroke syndrome
Acute intermittent porphyria

ACQUIRED METABOLIC

Electrolyte disturbances
Renal disorder
Liver disorder
Endocrine disorder
Vitamin deficiency

TUMOR

Brainstem glioma
Other neoplasms (primary or metastatic; paraneoplastic disease)

OTHER CENTRAL NERVOUS SYSTEM CONDITIONS

Stroke
Pseudotumor cerebri
Acute confusional migraine
Brain malformations
Psychosis
Epilepsy
Bacterial meningitis
Brain or parameningeal abscess
Endocarditis complicated by brain embolism
Chronic encephalitis
Neuroborreliosis with peripheral facial palsy
Venous sinus thrombosis
Subdural/epidural hematoma
Head injury
Connective tissue disorder

[a]Two broad categories of antigens: (1) intracellular paraneoplastic antigens, including Hu, Ma2, CV2 CRMP5, and (2) cell surface antigens, such as voltage-gated potassium channels and others.

Louis encephalitis virus (SLE), and to a lesser extent Powassan virus (Flaviridae family); and La Crosse virus (LACV) from the California (CAL) serogroup (Bunyaviridae family).

Historically, arboviruses have been cited as one of the most common causes of encephalitis in children; however, recent studies in the U.S. found arboviruses to be relatively uncommon in the pediatric age group.[15,16] WNV was detected for the first time in the Western hemisphere in 1999 and currently is the leading cause of arboviral encephalitis in the U.S.[17] From 1999 to 2007, over 27,000 cases of WNV were reported in the U.S., but only 4% of all reported West Nile neuroinvasive disease (WNND, which includes encephalitis, aseptic meningitis, and acute flaccid paralysis) cases were in children. The Centers for Disease Control and Prevention (CDC) reports a WNND incidence of 0.05/100,000 in persons less than 10 years of age compared with 1.35/100,000 in persons 70 years of age and older.[18]

La Crosse virus is the second most common cause of arboviral infections in the U.S. Unlike WNV, 90% of LACV neuroinvasive disease occurs in children rather than adults.[19] In fact, the incidence of pediatric WNND is similar to the incidence of all neuroinvasive disease due to LACV. Powassan virus, a tickborne arbovirus in the northeastern U.S. and Canada, is rarely identified in children.[20]

Other Viruses

Other less frequent but important viral causes of encephalitis include lymphocytic choriomeningitis (LCM) virus and rabies virus. LCM is an arenavirus acquired from infected house mice, hamsters, and guinea pigs. Infections occur when feces, saliva, or urine from LCM-infected rodents are inhaled or ingested. Infections are reported more frequently in the winter months when rodents typically migrate indoors.[21] The incidence of LCM is unknown but it is likely that infection is underdiagnosed.

Rabies is rare in the U.S., but 55,000 deaths occur annually worldwide, primarily from contact with rabid dogs.[22] These cases occur mostly in Asia, Africa, and Latin America where animal rabies control and postexposure prophylaxis (PEP) are limited. Rabies is unique among encephalitis viruses in that the incubation period can be several years. The incubation period generally is between 20 and 60 days but can range from a few days to 6.5 years.[23] In the U.S., 43 rabies cases were recognized between 1995 and 2009; 10 of these cases were imported (usually a canine strain), and the remaining cases were acquired in the U.S. Most U.S. cases were related to bat exposures and often the bite event was unrecognized. Bats have very small teeth and, therefore, bites may not be noticed and marks may not be visible (Figure 44-1).

Other viruses important outside the U.S. include Japanese encephalitis virus (JEV), Nipah virus, and measles virus. In hyperendemic areas, JEV causes several thousand cases annually, primarily in children in Asia, Southern Asia east of Pakistan, and Southeast Asia.[24] Nipah virus has been associated with outbreaks of encephalitis in Malaysia,[25] Singapore,[26] Australia,[27] Bangladesh,[28,29] and India.[29] There are an estimated 30 million cases of measles worldwide annually and acute encephalitis occurs in 1 of 1000 cases. Subacute sclerosing panencephalitis (SSPE) is an indolent, progressive, and fatal form of measles encephalitis that becomes manifest usually several years after infection. Because measles vaccination is universal in the U.S. and some other countries, a history of vaccination is common in patients with SSPE. Infection likely occurred at an early age in such cases prior to immunization and was not recognized.[30] Genetic analysis of virus from brain specimens in cases of SSPE identifies wild measles virus endemic at the time and geographic site of the patient's earlier acquisition and not vaccine virus.[31]

Influenza-associated encephalitis (IAE) and encephalopathy have been described sporadically and follow the seasonal influenza pattern with illnesses typically occurring during winter months in temperate climates. Most cases of IAE, especially acute necrotizing encephalopathy, have been reported from Japan,[32] but cases of encephalitis and encephalopathy have been reported throughout the world, including the U.S.[33]

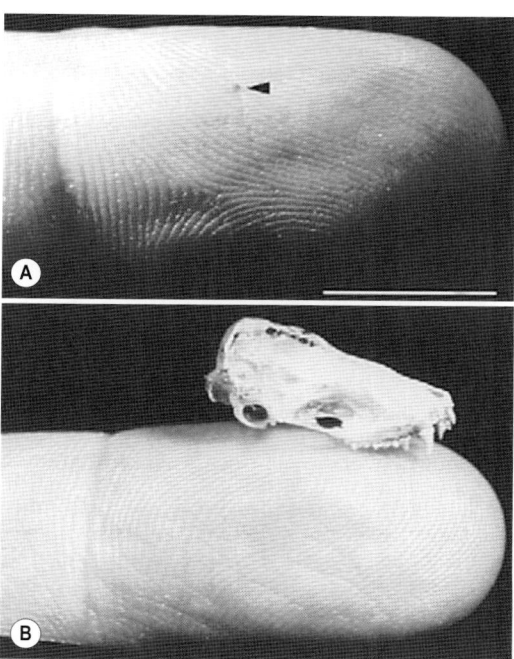

Figure 44-1. (A) Puncture wound of a bite from a silver-haired bat and **(B)** skull of silver-haired bat. (Reprinted from The Lancet, Jackson AC and Fenton MB. Human rabies and bat bites 2001;357:1714, with permission from Elsevier.)

Bacteria

Important bacterial causes of encephalitis include Rocky Mountain spotted fever (RMSF), *Borrelia hermsii* and *Borrelia recurrentis*, *Bartonella henselae* (and other *Bartonella* species), *Anaplasma phagocytophila* and *Ehrlichia* spp., and *Mycobacterium tuberculosis* (MTB). Importantly, *Neisseria meningitidis* and *Streptococcus pneumoniae* infections sometimes can cause clinical manifestations that are indistinguishable from encephalitis.

Bacterial tickborne diseases follow a seasonal pattern. RMSF, for example, occurs during the warm months when ticks are most active and when there typically is an increase in human outdoor recreational activity. Both RMSF and Lyme disease occur primarily in the eastern U.S., although reservoirs of *Borrelia burgdorferi* occur in the upper midwest states and the Pacific northwest, and the geographic area is expanding. Neuroborreliosis follows erythema migrans by 3 to 10 weeks and thus can manifest in cooler months.

Fungi

Fungal central nervous system disease generally manifests as meningitis and brain abscesses but some patients have encephalitis-like symptoms. Important fungal causes in the U.S. include *Coccidioides* spp., *Histoplasma capsulatum*, and *Blastomyces dermatitidis* (see Table 44-1 for endemic areas).

Free-Living Amebas and Parasites

The free-living amebas causing encephalitis classically are divided into two clinical entities: (1) primary amebic meningoencephalitis (PAM), a fulminant infection occurring in children and young adults due to *Naegleria fowleri* (also known as "the brain-eating ameba"); and (2) granulomatous amebic encephalitis, typically associated with *Acanthamoeba* spp. or *Balamuthia mandrillaris*. These three pathogens are dispersed in soil and water. *N. fowleri* infects immunocompetent hosts, *Acanthamoeba* spp. chiefly causes infections in immunocompromised hosts, and *B. mandrillaris* infections are described in both host groups. The importance of *Balamuthia* as a causative agent of encephalitis has been recognized increasingly.[34]

Significant protozoan parasites associated with encephalitis include *Toxoplasma gondii* and *Plasmodium falciparum*. *T. gondii* typically is acquired through foodborne contact or through direct contact with cat feces containing oocysts.[35] Most cases of *P. falciparum*-causing malaria in the U.S. are imported in people returning from endemic areas in Africa, Asia, and the Americas.[36]

Baylisascaris procyonis, the common raccoon roundworm, is an important cause of encephalitis, especially in the U.S. Other important neurotropic helminths include *Gnathostoma spinigerum* and *Angiostrongylus* spp. *G. spinigerum* is endemic in Southeast Asia and is being recognized increasingly in Central and South America.[37,38] *Angiostrongylus* spp. have been reported in Louisiana and Hawaii as well as the South Pacific, Asia, Australia, and the Caribbean.[39,40]

Other Causes

Hundreds of additional infectious agents have been associated with encephalitis, but the relevance and frequency of many of them is unknown. In particular, when a non-neurotropic agent is identified in a patient with encephalitis, particularly when identified only outside the central nervous system (CNS), the significance is unknown. For example, several case reports and large case series have identified *Mycoplasma pneumoniae* as one of the most commonly diagnosed infections among children with encephalitis.[41] However, even when IgM antibody to *M. pneumoniae* is identified in a patient, the significance of the finding is unclear given the high background incidence of acute infection and the limitations of serologic testing.[42] *M. pneumoniae* is a ubiquitous pathogen and up to 80% of the human population has evidence of past exposure. Other examples include parvovirus B19, rotavirus, and human metapneumovirus.[43-46] Common noninfectious illnesses can mimic infectious encephalitis, including neoplasms, vasculitis, stroke, drug reactions, paraneoplastic syndromes, and autoimmune disease (see Box 44-1). A newly recognized form of immune-mediated encephalitis, anti-*N*-methyl-D-aspartate receptor (NMDAR) encephalitis, has been described and is a relatively frequent cause of encephalitis syndrome.[47] The initial syndrome was first described in young women with ovarian teratomas who presented with acute psychosis and personality changes that progressed to include decreased level of consciousness, dyskinesia, autonomic instability, and hypoventilation.[47] As awareness of this disorder has increased, there have been a striking number of cases of anti-NMDAR encephalitis identified in children and young adults.[48] Unlike adult patients, pediatric patients are less likely to have a tumor identified.[49]

PATHOGENESIS

The pathogenesis of acute viral encephalitis is not well understood and is highly variable depending on the causative agent. EVs, HPeVs, HSV-1, arboviruses, and rabies are examples of neurotropic viruses in which the virus directly infects the grey matter of the brain. Measles, EBV, and rubella are examples of viruses that can trigger an autoimmune reaction with a resultant postinfectious encephalitis, acute disseminated encephalomyelitis (ADEM), in which the white matter of the brain is involved predominantly (discussed in Chapter 45). Encephalitis symptoms in bacterial meningitis and rickettsial infections, on the other hand, are caused by the vasculitis and toxins of the surrounding infection. Inflammatory response to bacteria, fungi, and parasites especially can lead to hydrocephalus.

Infectious agents enter the CNS by different pathways. The most common route of invasion is via the bloodstream, as is the case for EVs, HPeVs, and arboviruses as well as several bacteria, rickettsia, and fungi agents. Once the agent reaches the CNS, it penetrates the blood–brain barrier via the choroid plexus or through vascular endothelium.[50] An intraneuronal route is used by some other viruses such as rabies and HSV-1. HSV-1 can cause encephalitis after primary infection or reactivation of the latent virus.

Once inside the CNS, the offending pathogen may target only certain cells and, depending on the region involved, variable clinical manifestations develop. Cortical infection or reactive parenchymal swelling can lead to an altered level of consciousness. Agents with specific predilection to areas such as the brainstem can lead rapidly to coma or respiratory failure. Arboviruses primarily affect the cortical grey matter, brainstem, and thalamic nuclei. HSE is characterized by hemorrhagic and necrotizing lesions which are characteristically located in the temporal lobes, orbital frontal lobes cortex, and limbic structures.[51]

The histology typically seen in viral encephalitis includes perivascular mononuclear cell inflammation, phagocytosis of neurons, and microglial nodules. Distinctive histopathologic features can be seen in certain viral infections; the herpesviruses often are associated with intranuclear inclusion bodies while Negri bodies are pathognomonic for rabies.

Viruses such as influenza are known to be associated with CNS manifestations, but the mechanisms by which they cause neurologic signs and symptoms are not always well understood. In most studies of IAE, the virus is not found in the brain or cerebrospinal fluid (CSF), and there is bilateral symmetrical edema and apoptosis of neurons with absence of pleocytosis, suggesting a different pathogenesis, such as that mediated by cytokines.

Rickettsial agents generally cause CNS manifestations affecting the integrity of the small vessels in the brain. Subsequent meningeal irritation with perivascular mononuclear infiltrates develops. Characteristic pathologic lesions within the CNS include multifocal glial nodules and arteriolar microinfarctions.[52] In tuberculous, fungal, or partially-treated bacterial meningitis, a chronic basilar meningeal inflammation can cause a subarachnoid exudate leading to obstruction of CSF reabsorption with resultant communicating hydrocephalus and cranial nerve palsies. Vasculitis of the vessels within the brain leads to infarcts and focal neurologic deficits.

N. fowleri causes hemorrhagic destruction of grey matter and devastation of the olfactory bulbs.[53] The hallmark of *B. mandrillaris* and *Acanthamoeba* infections is granulomatous amebic encephalitis (GAE) characterized by multinucleated giant cells, focal necrosis, and hemorrhage. The pathology of *Baylisascaris procyonis* is characterized by CNS larval migration with histology demonstrating inflammation and necrosis with "track"-like spaces.[54]

CLINICAL MANIFESTATIONS AND DIFFERENTIAL DIAGNOSIS

The clinical manifestations of encephalitis are extremely variable and reflect the degree and specific area of brain involvement and the inherent pathogenicity of the offending agent (Table 44-2). Most patients with encephalitis have fever and headache, followed by an altered level of consciousness. Other findings can include seizures, impaired cognition, behavioral changes, speech disturbances, hemiparesis, and other focal neurologic signs. Arboviruses are associated with global involvement resulting in global neurologic dysfunction with vomiting, obtundation, and coma. Most EVs also often cause global impairment, but some, such as EV 71, can lead to focal manifestations. Focal symptoms generally are seen in HSE as HSV-1 typically involves the temporal and frontal lobes. Physical findings outside the CNS also can provide important clues to etiology.

The characteristic presentation of EV encephalitis includes mental status changes ranging from lethargy and mild disorientation to coma. A unique form of encephalitis can be seen with some enteroviruses, including EV 71 and coxsackievirus A16. In a Taiwan epidemic of EV 71, nearly 90% of cases had a biphasic illness where either hand-foot-and-mouth disease or herpangina preceded the onset of myoclonus, tremor, or ataxia.[55] Of the hospitalized patients, brainstem encephalitis was a common feature and the case fatality rate was 14%.

The classic presentation of HSE includes fever, altered level of consciousness, visual field defects, dysphasia, focal motor seizures, and hemiparesis. Over 90% of adults have classic signs and symptoms. Children, however, are more likely to come to medical attention with atypical manifestations. In one study, 25% of children with HSE had atypical features of ataxia, decreased visual acuity, or generalized tonic-clonic seizures.[14] Aphasia and altered

TABLE 44-2. Associated Manifestations for Specific Agents in Encephalitis

Clinical Features	Agents	Neurologic Features	Agents
Chronic meningitis	*Coccidioides* spp. *Cryptococcus neoformans* *Histoplasma capsulatum*	Cranial nerve palsies	*Balamuthia mandrillaris* *Borrelia burgdorferi* *Coccidioides* spp. Epstein–Barr virus *Histoplasma capsulatum* *Mycobacterium tuberculosis* *Naegleria fowleri* *Toxoplasma gondii*[a]
Hepatitis	*Coxiella burnetii* West Nile virus		
Hepatosplenomegaly	*Histoplasma capsulatum*	Paralysis[b]	Enteroviruses 71 Japanese encephalitis virus La Crosse virus Tickborne encephalitis virus West Nile virus
Hydrophobia	Rabies virus		
Insidious onset	*Acanthamoeba* spp. *Balamuthia mandrillaris* *Coccidioides immitis* *Histoplasma capsulatum* Measles virus (SSPE) *Mycobacterium tuberculosis*		
		Cognitive or psychiatric abnormalities	Herpes simplex virus 1
		Myoclonus/jerks	Measles virus (SSPE) Nipah virus
Lymphadenopathy	*Bartonella henselae* Cytomegalovirus[a] Epstein–Barr virus Human immunodeficiency virus *Mycobacterium tuberculosis* *Toxoplasma gondii*[a] West Nile virus	Sensorineural hearing loss	Mumps virus
		Visual loss	JC virus (PML)[a] *Baylisascaris procyonis*
		Laboratory Features	
Parotitis	Human immunodeficiency virus Mumps virus Parainfluenza virus	CSF atypical lymphocytes	Cytomegalovirus[a] Epstein–Barr virus West Nile virus
Pneumonia	Adenovirus Influenza virus *Mycoplasma pneumoniae*	CSF eosinophils can be mistaken for neutrophils in CSF; Wright or Giemsa stain is needed to identify eosinophils)	*Angiostrongylus* spp. *Baylisascaris procyonis* *Coccidioides* spp. *Gnathostoma* spp.
Respiratory symptoms	Adenovirus *Histoplasma capsulatum* Influenza virus *Mycoplasma pneumoniae* *Mycobacterium tuberculosis* Parainfluenza virus	Morulae in WBC	*Anaplasma phagocytophila* *Ehrlichia* spp.
		CSF lymphocytic pleocytosis with hypoglycorrhachia	*Mycobacterium tuberculosis*
Retinitis	*Bartonella henselae* Cytomegalovirus[a] *Toxoplasma gondii*[a] *Treponema pallidum* West Nile virus	**Neuroimaging Abnormality**	
		Acute necrotizing encephalopathy (ANE)	Influenza virus (and other respiratory viruses)
Exanthems		Arteritis	*Rickettsia* spp. *Treponema pallidum* Varicella-zoster virus
Hand-foot-mouth	Enterovirus		
Macules/papules on trunk	West Nile virus	Basal ganglia	Influenza virus (ANE) Enteroviruses Epstein–Barr virus
Petechiae	*Rickettsia rickettsii* (and other rickettsia)		
Recent macular exanthem	Human herpesvirus 6	Brainstem	Enteroviruses Epstein–Barr virus Herpes simplex virus 1 Influenza virus (ANE) *Listeria monocytogenes* *Mycobacterium tuberculosis* West Nile virus
Salmon-colored macules/papules	Rubella virus		
Vesicles	Herpes B virus Varicella-zoster virus		
Neurologic Features			
Ataxia	Epstein–Barr virus *Listeria monocytogenes* *Mycoplasma pneumoniae* Varicella-zoster virus	Calcifications (neonate)	Cytomegalovirus Lymphocytic choriomeningitis virus *Toxoplasma gondii*
Change in taste or smell	*Naegleria fowleri*	Cerebellar	Epstein–Barr virus *Mycoplasma pneumoniae* Varicella-zoster virus West Nile virus

Continued

PART II Clinical Syndromes and Cardinal Features of Infectious Diseases: Approach to Diagnosis and Initial Management

SECTION F Central Nervous System Infections

TABLE 44-2. Associated Manifestations for Specific Agents in Encephalitis—cont'd

Neuroimaging Abnormality	Agents	Neuroimaging Abnormality	Agents
Corpus callosum	West Nile virus	Temporal lobe	Enteroviruses
			Herpes simplex virus 1
Frontal lobe	Enteroviruses		La Crosse virus
	Herpes simplex virus 1		*Treponema pallidum*
	Herpes simplex virus 2	Thalamus	Enteroviruses
	Treponema pallidum		Epstein–Barr virus
Hydrocephalus	*Balamuthia mandrillaris*		Influenza virus (ANE)
	Coccidioides immitis	White matter (different than	*Balamuthia mandrillaris*
	Histoplasma capsulatum	ADEM)	*Baylisascaris procyonis*
	Mycobacterium tuberculosis		HPeV-3 (especially neonate)
	Toxoplasma gondii (neonate)[a]		Human immunodeficiency virus
Infarctions	*Rickettsia* spp.		JC virus[a]
	Treponema pallidum		Measles virus (SSPE)
	Varicella-zoster virus		West Nile virus
Microcephaly	Cytomegalovirus[a]	**EEG Abnormality**	
	Lymphocytic choriomeningitis virus	Perio dic lateralizing epileptiform discharges (PLEDS)	Herpes simplex virus 1
	Toxoplasma gondii (neonate)[a]		Epstein–Barr virus
Myeloencephalitis	*Gnathostoma* spp.		La Crosse virus
Parietal lobe	West Nile virus		Measles virus (SSPE)
Space-occupying lesions	*Balamuthia mandrillaris*		
	Toxoplasma gondii[a]		

SSPE, subacute sclerosing panencephalitis.

[a]*Causes encephalitis primarily in immunocompromised patients or the neonate or both.*

[b]*Testing should be performed on serum at acute phase of disease and then later when sera in acute and convalescent phase of disease are available.*

olfactory perception along with behavioral disturbances may be suggestive particularly of HSE. Symptoms of EBV encephalitis can include distinguishing features such as "Alice in Wonderland" syndrome (micropsia, macropsia, and/or size distortion of other sensory modalities), movement disorders, or cerebellar ataxia. Individuals with HHV-6 encephalitis can have focal features similar to HSV-1 or multifocal areas of demyelination,[56,57] which are found more commonly in immunocompromised hosts.

The majority of children infected with WNV are asymptomatic initially or have a mild febrile illness. Clinical manifestations of WNV encephalitis (WNE) include fever, headache, seizures, confusion, paralysis, tremors, facial palsy, photophobia, ataxia, and dysphasia. In addition to neurologic complications, other complications include hepatitis, myocarditis, pancreatitis, cardiac dysrhythmia, rhabdomyolysis, orchitis, uveitis, vitritis, and optic neuritis. Brainstem encephalitis, seizures, movement disorders, cranial neuropathies, cerebellitis, and optic neuritis also have been described as accompanying clinical features of WNV.[58] Clinical manifestations of LACV can be similar to WNE, but also can mimic HSV encephalitis with seizures, increased intracranial pressure, focal neurologic signs, and possibly cerebral herniation.

Rabies always should be considered in patients with rapidly progressive encephalitis. Paresthesia at or near the site of bite (inoculation site) is a unique feature of rabies. A small percentage of patients with rabies come to attention with the "paralytic" form with ascending paralysis, followed by confusion and then coma. The "furious" form of rabies is more common and is characterized by agitation, hydrophobia, delirium, and seizures.

Initial symptoms of IAE include fever, cough, and headache followed within a few days with altered level of consciousness and seizures.[59] One of the best recognized and most serious type of encephalitis associated with influenza and similar viruses is acute necrotizing encephalopathy (ANE).[60-62] Diagnostic criteria for ANE include the acute-onset encephalopathy with seizures, absence of CSF pleocytosis, normal blood ammonia levels and characteristic neuroimaging and exclusion of an alternative etiology (Box 44-2). Neuroimaging is characterized by symmetric

BOX 44-2. Clinical Characteristics of Acute Necrotizing Encephalopathy

CLINICAL AT ONSET

Typical age <5 years, rarely >10 years

Onset *during* the peak of febrile illness

Rapid development of encephalopathy often with seizures

Variable elevation of serum amintotransferases, normal blood ammonia

Normal CSF (± increased pressure, or mildly elevated protein level)

Exclusion of other causes (e.g. hypoxia, intoxication, hemolytic uremic syndrome, metabolic disorder)

CRANIAL MRI

Diffuse, bilateral, symmetric high-intensity signal on T_2-weighted images

Unremarkable T_1-weighted images

Involvement of periventricular and deep white matter (thalamus, brainstem tegmentum, cerebellum, medulla)

No enhancement with gadolinium

SECONDARY CLINICAL

Disseminated intravascular coagulopathy/SIRS that *follows* CNS signs

Multiorgan failure that *follows* CNS signs

AUTOPSY

Edema, apoptosis/necrosis of neurons

No vasculitis

No inflammation

CSF, cerebrospinal fluid; HUS, hemolytic uremic syndrome, MRI, magnetic resonance imaging; PCR, polymerase chain reaction; SIRS, systemic inflammatory response syndrome.

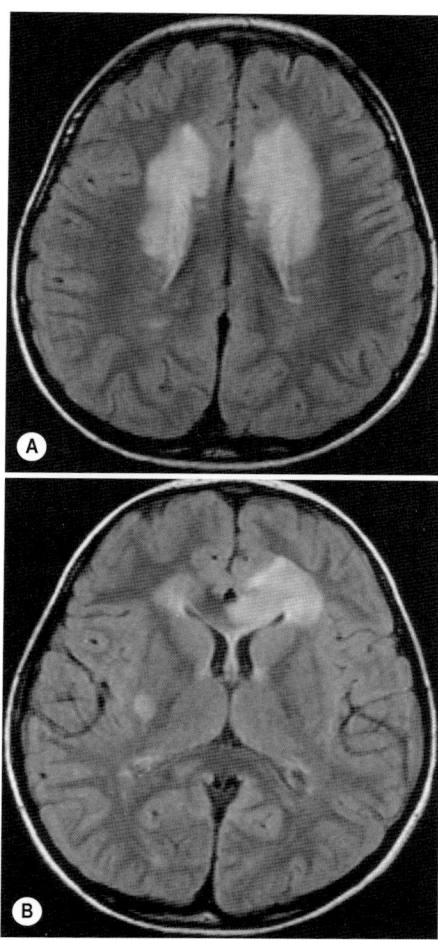

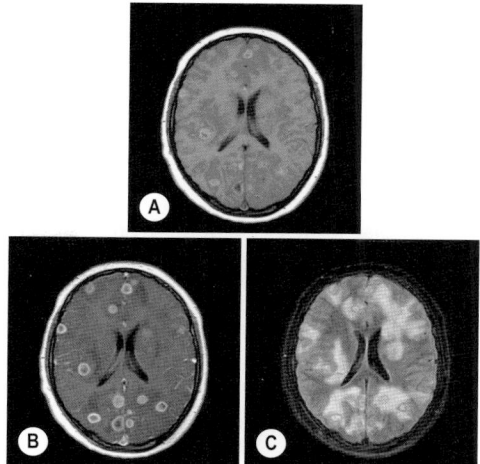

Figure 44-3. Magnetic resonance imaging of a patient with widely disseminated amebic encephalitis from *Balamuthia mandrillaris* (1.5 Tesla scanner) using axial T₁ (pre- and post-contrast) **(A and B)** and FLAIR sequences **(C).** Images demonstrate numerous ring-enhancing lesions seen within the cerebral cortex, subcortical white matter, and deep grey matter including the thalami and basal ganglia. The T₂ hyperintensity seen on the FLAIR images is consistent with perilesional edema and contributes to the lesions having mild local mass effect. (Courtesy of D. Michelson, Loma Linda University School of Medicine, Loma Linda, CA.)

Figure 44-2. Acute necrotizing encephalopathy in a 3-year-old with influenza B Sichuan group/Shanghai-like. On the third day of fever and influenzal symptoms he had acute onset of diminished arousal and recognition, mutism, ataxia, and left-sided increase in tone and reflexes. Axial fluid-attenuated inversion recovery (FLAIR) magnetic resonance imaging shows bilateral symmetrical, extensive hyperintense lesions in the centrum semiovale with periventricular involvement **(A)** and in the white matter anterior to the frontal horns, in the corpus callosum, and right globus pallidus **(B).** (Courtesy of E.N. Faerber and S.S. Long, St. Christopher's Hospital for Children, Philadelphia, PA.)

seizures, cranial nerve palsies (particularly third and sixth cranial nerves), and diplopia.[34,64,65] Neuroimaging in patients with *B. mandrillaris* almost always is abnormal, with variable findings, including meningeal enhancement, edema, hydrocephalus, or ring-enhancing lesions[34,66] (Figure 44-3). Patients with CNS complications of *B. procyonis* have clinical manifestations similar to other encephalitides but also can have ocular disease and eosinophils in the CSF. Neuroimaging in patients with *B. procyonis* often shows diffuse periventricular white matter changes[67] (Figure 44-4).

Noninfectious entities that can mimic encephalitis may have suggestive clinical features. Early symptoms of anti-NMDAR encephalitis, for example, include behavioral changes, seizures, and abnormal movements. Recognition of this syndrome is important because, despite the severity, improvement can occur

multifocal brain lesions, particularly in the thalamus, internal capsule, cerebellum and sometimes brainstem (Figure 44-2).[62] Most cases of ANE occur in previously healthy children younger than 5 years of age, many of whom are of Asian descent.[62] ANE mortality approaches 30% with mortality highest in patients with abnormal serum hepatic enzyme levels and low platelet counts.

The clinical descriptions of *M. pneumoniae*-associated encephalitis include a wide variety of neurologic (e.g., lethargy, seizures, hallucinations, and focal neurologic findings) and non-neurologic (e.g., respiratory and gastrointestinal) symptoms. Severity of illness also is extremely variable.[41,42] Fungal and *M. tuberculosis* infections of the CNS generally manifest with subacute meningitis. However, acute fulminant presentations with encephalitis-like features have been described.[63]

The clinical manifestations of parasitic infections are highly variable depending on the agent involved. For *N. fowleri*, patients typically have headache, nausea, vomiting, and nuchal rigidity, which rapidly progresses to irreversible coma. Individuals may also experience a change in taste or smell. *B. mandrillaris* and *Acanthamoeba* spp. typically have a less fulminant course characterized by fever, headache, vomiting, ataxia, hemiparesis, tonic-clonic

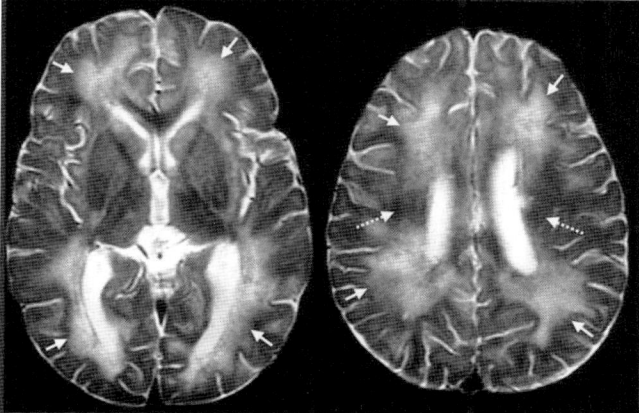

Figure 44-4. Magnetic resonance images of a 13-month-old boy with *Baylisascaris procyonis* encephalitis, showing abnormally high signal throughout the central white matter compared with darker signal expected for age. (Courtesy of Sorvillo F, Ash LR, Berlin OGW, et al. *Baylisascaris procyonis:* an emerging helminthic zoonosis. Emerg Infect Dis 2002;8:355–359.)

PART II Clinical Syndromes and Cardinal Features of Infectious Diseases: Approach to Diagnosis and Initial Management

SECTION F Central Nervous System Infections

with immunosuppressive therapy and the removal of tumor, if present.[47] Several disease processes must be considered in the differential diagnosis of acute encephalopathy, including immune-mediated, toxic ingestions, inborn errors of metabolism, acquired metabolic disorders, mass lesions (tumor or abscess), and other CNS conditions (see Box 44-1).

CLINICAL APPROACH

With a thorough diagnostic evaluation a treatable cause may be identified. More frequently a cause is not found or, if an agent is found, there may be no specific treatment. However, the following clinical approaches are important and can be helpful for prognosis, potential postexposure prophylaxis of contacts, counseling of patients and families, and public health interventions. Additionally, the identification of a specific agent may lead to withdrawal of unnecessary antimicrobial and antiviral agents. There are many important caveats to laboratory testing in patients with encephalitis (Table 44-3).

A thorough history is very important and should include an assessment of exposures as outlined in Table 44-1, with an emphasis on ill contacts, vector and animal exposures, outdoor activities, ingestion, and travel history. Any current or recent antecedent respiratory, gastrointestinal illness, or rash should be explored.

The initial evaluation for a patient with suspected encephalitis should include a complete blood count, tests of renal function and hepatic enzyme levels, and coagulation studies (Box 44-3). A baseline chest radiograph also should be obtained as focal infiltrates would be suggestive of certain pathogens (e.g., fungal or mycobacterial infections), and might prompt other diagnostic studies (e.g., bronchoscopy). An eye examination by an ophthalmologist also is suggested as chorioretinitis may be identified in the newborn infant, or a migratory nematode in older individuals.

Neuroimaging is an important part of the evaluation for encephalitis. Cranial computed tomography (CT) is helpful to identify abnormalities, such as ventriculomegaly, an abscess or tumor, and can help determine whether it is safe to perform a lumbar puncture (LP). However, magnetic resonance imaging (MRI) is more sensitive than CT for detecting the more subtle changes often seen in encephalitis.[68,69] Electroencephalography (EEG) is an informative test early in the course of encephalitis to assess seizure activity, which is not always obvious, and can help identify the region of the brain affected.

An LP with measurement of the opening pressure and CSF analysis (cell count with differential analysis, glucose and protein concentrations) should be performed unless there is a specific contraindication.[70] Results from the LP offer some of the best clues as to whether the patient has an infectious or noninfectious etiology and, within the infectious realm, whether the cause is viral, bacterial, fungal, or parasitic. CSF cultures for bacteria should be performed in all cases. Fungal and mycobacterial testing should be performed in cases suggestive of those etiologies. CSF viral culture is no longer recommended as its sensitivity is extremely low and may unnecessarily deplete the CSF sample. PCR testing is more rapid and generally is more sensitive than culture for viral CNS infections,[71] including herpesviruses and EV.[72] There are important limitations, however, both in terms of sensitivity and specificity for CSF PCR testing as outlined in Table 44-3. The diagnostic test for HSE is CSF HSV DNA PCR testing. If initial testing is negative and HSE is strongly suspected, the test should be repeated on a second CSF specimen within a few days after the first LP. For HSV and VZV, intrathecal antibodies can be performed to supplement nucleic acid testing.[73] For many of the arboviruses, antibody testing of serum is preferred to PCR testing as peak viremia generally occurs prior to symptom onset.

In patients with respiratory symptoms, a viral culture from respiratory specimens should be performed early in the hospitalization to optimize the recovery of virus. If a particular agent, such as influenza, is suspected but the viral culture is negative, then agent-specific PCR testing should be performed. Similarly, if diarrhea is present, a stool culture for viral and bacterial pathogens should be obtained. In a young child, a stool viral culture and/or enterovirus PCR should be performed to optimize enterovirus detection, regardless of presence of diarrhea.

For serologic testing an extra red-top serum tube should be drawn in the acute phase of illness and held for later studies. A convalescent serum should be collected 10–21 days later. Although results from acute and convalescent studies may not be helpful in the immediate management of the patient, testing ultimately may be helpful in determining the diagnosis (see Box 44-3).

Brain biopsy is rarely performed today but still has value because of limitations in both molecular and serologic methods. The utility of targeted biopsy was illustrated in a series of 16 patients with unknown CNS illness in that brain biopsy detected bacterial abscess (6), toxoplasmosis (3), HSV (1), *Aspergillus* infection (2), and *M. tuberculosis* infection (2) that were not detected

Text continued on page 312.

TABLE 44-3. Laboratory Testing with Focus on Pathogens Found in the U.S.

Agent	Recommended Diagnostic Studies	Caveats
VIRUS		
Adenovirus	• CSF, respiratory, brain tissue for PCR or culture	• Pathogen of unknown neurologic potential
Arboviruses	• Serology is the most useful assay for most arboviruses: CSF IgM, serum IgM and IgG (paired sera if possible) for specific viruses as suggested by geography: – West Nile virus (WNV) – St. Louis encephalitis virus (SLE) – California serogroup viruses (e.g., La Crosse virus (LACV)) – Eastern equine encephalitis virus (EEE) – Powassan virus (POW) – Western equine encephalitis virus (WEE)	• Acute viremia stage often over by the time of clinical presentation; however, polymerase chain reaction (PCR) is sometimes positive in very acute specimens • PCR can be helpful in immunocompromised host because of prolonged viremia and delayed antibody response • Knowledge of geographic and seasonal variation of arboviruses important and can limit unnecessary testing • CSF IgG for specific arbovirus usually not helpful because of blood–brain barrier integrity; CSF blood contamination can cause false-positive results for both IgM and IgG • High rate of serologic cross-reactivity among arbovirus (WNV, SLE, and POW; individual with prior dengue infection will test positive for WNV IgG) • Antibody typically positive early in presentation but if negative, repeat on later specimen • WNV: Predominance of polymorphonuclear cells in CSF can persist beyond the first 24 hours in contrast to other viral encephalitides

Continued

TABLE 44-3. Laboratory Testing with Focus on Pathogens Found in the U.S.—cont'd

Agent	Recommended Diagnostic Studies	Caveats
		• WNV: Abnormal appearing reactive lymphocytes including plasma cell-like and Mollaret-like cells • EEE: CSF WBC counts can be very high, with counts up to 4000/mm^3 • POW: Testing only available at CDC and a few state laboratories
Cytomegalovirus (CMV)	• CSF for PCR • Shell vial on urine, saliva (neonate)	• Serology can be problematic especially due to false-positive results • Rare causes of encephalitis in immunocompetent host • Atypical lymphocytes in CSF
Enteroviruses (EV)	• CSF for PCR • Respiratory swab for PCR • Stool for PCR or culture	• PCR on CSF alone can be negative as EV present only transiently in CSF; test non-CNS site (respiratory sample PCR, viral stool culture) to increase yield
Epstein–Barr virus (EBV)	• CSF for PCR • Serum for anti-VCA IgM/IgG, anti-EBNA • Serum heterophile antibody	• Both serology (serum) and PCR (CSF) is recommended • False negatives and false positives can occur with EBV PCR. False positives occur because EBV DNA is found in peripheral blood mononuclear cells • Atypical lymphocytes in CSF or peripheral blood is consistent but not always present
Hepatitis C virus	• CSF for PCR	• Pathogen of unknown neurotropic potential
Herpes simplex virus 1 (HSV1)	• CSF for PCR • CSF for antibody if >1 week of symptoms • Neonate: – CSF for culture and/or PCR – Nasopharyngeal (NP) swab for culture and/or PCR – Conjunctival swab culture and/or PCR – Rectal swab for culture and PCR – Skin lesion swab for culture and/or PCR	• Outside neonatal period, HSV-1 causes the majority of HSE. In neonatal period, most infections due to HSV-2 • Approximately 5–10% of HSE patients have a normal CSF in first LP, particularly in children. HSV PCR can be negative in first LP. For cases where HSE is highly suspected (e.g., temporal lobe involvement), a second LP should be performed for CSF PCR and intrathecal HSV antibody testing • Presence of either HSV IgG or IgM antibody can indicate CNS infection; however, diminished blood–brain barrier and possible CSF contamination with blood should be considered when interpreting results
Herpes simplex virus 2 (HSV2)	• CSF for PCR • CSF for antibody if >1 week of symptoms • Neonate: – CSF culture and/or PCR – NP swabs, conjunctival, rectal swab – culture and/or PCR – Skin lesion PCR and culture	• Neonatal period, HSV-2 important cause of HSE. Beyond neonatal period, HSV-2 causes primarily meningitis syndrome but has been associated with encephalitis • Presence of either HSV IgG or IgM antibody can indicate CNS infection; however, blood–brain barrier issues and possible CSF contamination of blood need to be considered when interpreting results
Human herpesvirus 6 (HHV6)	• CSF for PCR	• Pathogen of unknown neurologic potential • Not all HHV-6 CSF PCR positive results correlate with disease; when positive, important to consider chromosomal integration or latent infection
Human immunodeficiency virus (HIV)	• Serum EIA and Western blot • Plasma and CSF for PCR	
Human metapneumovirus	• Respiratory tract (NP or throat swab) for PCR	• Pathogen of unknown neurologic potential • CSF PCR rarely positive
Influenza A/B virus	• Respiratory secretions for viral culture • Respiratory secretions for viral antigen test • Respiratory secretions for PCR	• Most cases are encephalopathy (vs. encephalitis) • CSF PCR rarely is positive
JC polyomavirus	• CSF for PCR	• A positive result correlates with diagnosis; negative result does not rule it out
Lymphocytic choriomeningitis virus (LCM)	• CSF for LCM IgM/IgG antibody • Serum for LCM IgM/IgG antibody • Neonate: – Serology on both infant and mother (neonate)	• One of the few viruses that can cause low glucose in CSF
Measles virus – acute	• CSF for measles virus antibodies • CSF for measles virus PCR • Serum IgG/IgM (paired serum samples if possible) • Brain tissue (if available) for measles virus PCR	• Measles PCR and antibody testing (both serum and CSF)

Continued

PART II Clinical Syndromes and Cardinal Features of Infectious Diseases: Approach to Diagnosis and Initial Management

SECTION F Central Nervous System Infections

TABLE 44-3. Laboratory Testing with Focus on Pathogens Found in the U.S.—cont'd

Agent	Recommended Diagnostic Studies	Caveats
Measles virus – SSPE	• CSF IgG antibodies • Serum IgG antibodies • Brain tissue (if available) PCR	• Since SSPE is result of long-standing infection, measles IgM is negative; IgG levels in CSF and serum very high
Mumps virus	• CSF for culture or PCR • CSF for IgM/IgM antibodies • Serum for IgM/IgG antibodies (paired serum samples if possible) • Throat swab for PCR	• One of few viruses that can cause low glucose in CSF
Parvovirus B19	• Serum for IgM antibody • CSF for PCR	• Pathogen of unknown neurologic potential

Rabies virus	• Antemortem: serum for antibodies
	  – Saliva for PCR
	  – Nuchal biopsy for PCR and DFA
	  – Brain tissue (if available) for DFA
	• Postmortem:
	  – Brain tissue for culture; or antigen detection
		• Antemortem testing is challenging but possible
		• Multiple samples and different assays should be performed. Negative tests antemortem do not rule out rabies
		• Coordinate testing with local and state health department

Respiratory syncytial virus (RSV)	• Respiratory secretions or PCR antigen	• Pathogen of unknown neurologic potential • CSF PCR rarely positive
Rotavirus	• Stool for antigen detection • CSF PCR (CDC)	• Pathogen of unknown neurologic potential • Typically young child with history of diarrhea; mechanism of CNS illness unclear
Rubella virus	• Serum for antibody • CSF for antibodies	• One of few viruses that can cause low glucose in CSF
Varicella-zoster virus (VZV)	• CSF for PCR • CSF for antibody if >1 week of symptoms • Serum for IgM/IgG • Skin lesions for DFA or PCR	• Since some CNS VZV infections are reactivation, IgM not always positive • Positive test on VZV skin lesions does not prove CNS etiology, but may be suggestive
West Nile virus	• See Arboviruses (above)	
FUNGUS *Coccidioides* spp.	• CSF culture (large volume) • CSF for antigen • CSF for antibody • Serum for antigen • Serum for antibody	• Warn laboratory that coccidiomycosis is being considered if culture ordered • Eosinophils sometimes present in CSF • "EDTA-heat" treated antigen test reported to increase sensitivity for CSF and serum samples
Histoplasma capsulatum	• CSF for culture (large volume) • CSF for serum and urine for antigen detection • CSF for antibody • Serum for antibody	• May need to do multiple tests • Isolated CNS disease can be difficult to diagnose because of insensitive assays • "EDTA-heat" treated antigen test reported to increase sensitivity for CSF and serum samples
Blastomyces dermatitidis	• CSF for culture (large volume) • CSF, serum, urine for antigen detection • CSF for antibody • Serum for antibody	• May need to do multiple tests • "EDTA-heat" treated antigen test reported to increase sensitivity for CSF and serum samples
FREE-LIVING AMOEBAS AND PARASITES *Naegleria fowleri*	• Wet mount of warm CSF • Brain (if available) histopathology	• Demonstration of motile ameba on wet mount • CSF often demonstrates very high WBC (often with neutrophil predominance), high protein (>100 mg/dL), and low glucose (<<50 mg/dL)
Balamuthia mandrillaris	• Serum for antibody • CSF and/or brain for PCR • Brain (if available) histopathology (special stains)	• Serology and PCR available at specialized laboratories • Brain tissue can show necrotic and hemorrhagic meningoencephalitis • CSF often shows high WBC (lymphocyte or neutrophil predominance), high protein (>100 mg/dL), resembling tuberculous meningitis
Acanthaemeba spp.	• Serum for antibody • CSF and/or brain for PCR • Brain (if available) histopathology (special stains)	• Serology and PCR available at specialized laboratories

Continued

TABLE 44-3. Laboratory Testing with Focus on Pathogens Found in the U.S.—cont'd

Agent	Recommended Diagnostic Studies	Caveats
Baylisascaris procyonis	• CSF for antibody • Serum for antibody	• Serology available in specialized laboratories (Parasitic Disease Branch, CDC) • Eosinophils almost always present in CSF and peripheral blood
Toxoplasma gondii	• Neonatal: serum for IgG, IgM, IgA, IgE antibodies. Older child: serum for IgG, IgM; CSF for PCR	• Serology can be falsely negative; important to test mother and infant • Often reactivation of disease, so IgM may not be positive, IgG titers persistently high
BACTERIA		
Bartonella henselae	• Serum for indirect fluorescent antibody • Lymph node for PCR	• Utility in performing both serology and CSF PCR (if available) • CSF often negative
Borrelia burgdorferi	• Serum for antibodies sequential (EIA and Western blot) • CSF for serum:CSF antibody index	• CSF for *Borrelia;* may be delay in CNS intrathecal synthesis • CSF PCR rarely positive (in contrast to synovial fluid) but may be useful in some cases
Brucella spp.	• CSF for IgG and IgM • CSF for culture • Serum for IgG and IgM	• Perform serology on both CSF and serum; culture increases sensitivity • PCR available in some research settings; unknown sensitivity
Leptospira spp.	• Serum IgM and IgG • Urine culture	• If serology negative on acute serum, important to repeat on convalescent serum
Listeria monocytogenes	• Routine bacterial culture	• May also be helpful to test CSF for *Listeria* antibody since detection of CSF antibody can indicate CNS infection
Mycobacterium tuberculosis	• CSF for AFB smear, culture, PCR, direct examination • Respiratory for culture highly suggestive	• CSF PCR is insensitive; important to test multiple samples • Should be considered in patients with lymphocytic pleocytosis (but neutrophilic predominance can occur), with CSF protein >100 mg/dL or CSF glucose <50 mg/dL
Mycoplasma pneumoniae	• Nasopharyngeal swab or respiratory secretion for culture or PCR • Serum for IgM • Serum for IgG paired	• Pathogen of unknown neurologic potential • Perform PCR on respiratory samples, serology on acute/convalescent serum • CSF PCR rarely positive • Single IgG titer is not helpful • Single IgM test can have false-positive results
Treponema pallidum	• CSF for VDRL • CSF for fluorescent treponemal antibody (FTA) • CSF for PCR • Serum for VDRL and FTA	• Multiple tests as well as clinical findings are important for definitive diagnosis • CSF VDRL is specific but CSF FTA is more sensitive • FTA does not distinguish between syphilis and other treponematoses such as pinta and yaws • Non-treponemal tests can have a prozone phenomenon resulting in false-negative FTA • Infection with *Borrelia burgdorferi* can cause false-positive FTA
RICKETTSIA		
Anaplasma phagocytophila	• Peripheral blood for morulae in neutrophils • Whole blood for PCR • Serum IgG/IgM (paired sera if possible)	• If serology negative on acute serum, important to repeat on convalescent serum
Coxiella burnetii	• Serum for acute and convalescent antibody	• Utility of PCR for *Coxiella burnetii* PCR for Q fever encephalitis unknown
Ehrlichia chaffeensis	• Morulae in peripheral blood monocytes • Whole blood for PCR • Serum for IgG/IgM (paired sera if possible)	• If serology negative on acute serum, important to repeat on convalescent serum
Ehrlichia ewingii	• Morulae in peripheral blood granulocytes • Whole blood for PCR • Serum for IgG/IgM antibodies	• If serology negative on acute serum, important to repeat on convalescent serum
Rickettsia spp.	• Serum for indirect fluorescent antibody • Skin biopsy of rash for PCR or immunohistochemical staining	• If serology negative on acute serum, important to repeat on convalescent serum

PART II Clinical Syndromes and Cardinal Features of Infectious Diseases: Approach to Diagnosis and Initial Management

SECTION F Central Nervous System Infections

BOX 44-3. Initial Diagnostic Evaluation for Patients with Encephalitis

GENERAL STUDIES

CBC with differential analysis
Renal function tests
Serum hepatic enzyme
Chest radiograph
Ophthalmologic examination

LUMBAR PUNCTURE

Opening pressure
CSF WBC count and differential, protein, and glucose
Culture for bacteria
PCR for herpes simplex virus
PCR for enterovirus
± PCR for human parechovirus
± Culture for fungus
± Culture for *Mycobacterium* (PCR is insensitive)

SERUM FOR ANTIBODY

Arboviruses (seasonal)
Epstein–Barr virus
Human immunodeficiency virus

RESPIRATORY SECRETIONS/STOOL SPECIMEN

PCR on respiratory tract specimen for enterovirus
PCR or culture on stool specimen for enterovirus
If respiratory symptoms:
    Rapid test, PCR, culture for influenza if season
Other respiratory viruses according to seasonality (rapid test or PCR)

NEUROIMAGING

Computed tomography
Magnetic resonance imaging
Electroencephalogram

CSF, cerebrospinal fluid; PCR, polymerase chain reaction; CBC, complete blood count; WBC, white blood cell.

TABLE 44-4. Differential Diagnosis of Encephalitis in the Neonate

Infection/Disorder	Frequency
PERINATAL INFECTION	
Herpes simplex virus	++
Enterovirus[a]	+++
Adenovirus	+++
Group B streptococcus[b]	+
Listeria monocytogenes[b]	+
Citrobacter spp.[b]	+
CONGENITAL INFECTIONS	
Cytomegalovirus	+++
Lymphocytic choriomeningitis virus	+
Toxoplasmosis	+
Rubella virus	+
Syphilis	+
GENETIC/INBORN ERRORS OF METABOLISM	+[c]
Aicardi–Goutiere syndrome	
Leigh disease (subacute necrotizing encephalomyelitis)	
Maple syrup urine disease	
Organic acidopathies (methylmalonic acidemia, propionic acidemia)	
Urea cycle defects	
PRIMARY CENTRAL NERVOUS SYSTEM DISORDER	
Nonconvulsive status epilepticus	+
Hemorrhage	+
Hypoxic ischemic encephalopathy	++

+++, *most frequent;* ++, *frequent;* +, *occasional.*

[a]*Includes aseptic meningitis.*

[b]*Cerebritis.*

[c]*Combined incidence.*

by other methods.[74] Biopsies also are helpful for the diagnosis of noninfectious entities such as small-vessel vasculitis and intravascular lymphoma.[75] In the unfortunate event of the death of a patient with an unknown illness, an autopsy should be encouraged to determine the cause of death.

LABORATORY FINDINGS

General laboratory studies (see Box 44-3) infrequently help to identify specific etiologies but can indicate the overall health of the patient.

Most patients with viral encephalitis have CSF mononuclear cell pleocytosis, with cell counts ranging from 10 to 200 mg/dL.[1] However, early in the disease course, pleocytosis can be absent or there can be an elevation in neutrophils. A repeat LP in 1–2 days may be useful.[76] The CSF protein generally is elevated but usually less than 100 mg/dL, while the glucose level is almost always normal with a few important exceptions (LCM and mumps), and when depressed, nonviral agents should be considered.

Neutrophilic pleocytosis (particularly in cases where CSF WBC count is >1000 cells/mm^3, protein >200 mg/dL, or CSF glucose level <⅔ of blood levels) is suggestive of a nonviral entity. In fungal infections moderate lymphocytic pleocytosis usually is found. *Naegleria* infections generally elicit a very high CSF cell count with predominance of neutrophils. Eosinophils in the CSF are suggestive of a helminth-parasitic infection (e.g., *Baylisascaris procyonis*, *Angiostrongylus* spp., and *Gnathostoma spinigerum*) and coccidiomycosis. As noted in Table 44-4, there are important caveats about detection of eosinophils in spinal fluid.

MANAGEMENT

Clinicians first should focus on treatable and common causes of encephalitis. Empiric treatment for bacterial meningitis (vancomycin plus a third-generation cephalosporin) should be started since the clinical presentation may overlap with encephalitis. Therapy with ampicillin is considered additionally when rhombencephalitis is expected or CSF is suggestive of *Listeria* infection. HSE is one of the few treatable causes of viral encephalitis; therapy with acyclovir should be started and continued until HSV-1 has been reasonably excluded as a diagnosis, which may require serial CSF samples (see prior discussion). Antiviral therapy generally is restricted to treatment of herpesviruses (especially HSV-1 and VZV), and the unusual instance of HIV infection.[77] Therapy for tuberculous or fungal meningitis should be initiated when clinical and laboratory testing is compatible. If rickettsial or *Ehrlichia* infections are suspected, doxycycline should be initiated empirically. For influenza-associated encephalitis, oseltamivir, while not proven to be efficacious, usually is given and may be beneficial.[78] There is no evidence that treatment of presumed CNS *Mycoplasma* infection alters outcome. Corticosteroids and immune globulin intravenous also may be helpful in some influenza-associated encephalitis cases since a mechanism of hyperintense cytokine response is suggested.[78]

In addition to directed therapy, aggressive supportive care is critical, and minimizing secondary brain injury should be made a high priority. Cerebral edema is an important complication of encephalitis and encephalopathy and should be monitored closely in patients who are not improving. Physicians frequently neglect to measure CSF opening pressure, although this test can give clues as to etiologies and cue prevention of impending complications. Repeat neuroimaging to monitor for cerebral edema is particularly important in comatose patients. Typical indicators of elevated intracranial pressure, such as poorly reactive dilated pupils, decorticate or decerebrate posture, or Cushing triad (systolic hypertension, bradycardia, and shallow respirations) are late findings. Patients also should be monitored for the syndrome of inappropriate secretion of antidiuretic hormone. If hyponatremia is present, it is important to correct sodium levels slowly in order to avoid the complication of extra-pontine osmotic myelinolysis (EPM). SIADH and EPM illustrate how acquired metabolic derangements can both complicate, and mimic, encephalitis.[79]

Conditions that mimic infectious encephalitis should be considered, particularly if no etiology is identified in the first week of hospitalization. Metabolic and toxic disorders causing encephalopathy and seizures should be excluded. Anti-NMDAR encephalitis is of particular importance given its apparently high incidence, and when identified, immunotherapy and removal of the tumor, if present, have been associated with improvement.[47] As outlined in Chapter 45, in patients suspected to have postinfectious encephalitis/ADEM, often with characteristic MRI showing prominent white mater of deep grey nuclei inflammation, corticosteroid, or other immunotherapy often is recommended.

COMPLICATIONS AND PROGNOSIS

In general, the prognosis of encephalitis is highly dependent on the underlying cause, when known. Rabies and *Naegleria fowleri,* for instance, have an almost 100% fatality rate. Two of the best-studied viral causes of encephalitis include HSV-1 and enterovirus. HSV-1 encephalitis has been reported to have a worse prognosis than EV with greater than 35% of patients with HSE suffering severe sequelae or death.[80,81] Other viral etiologies are less well studied with information limited to case reports and small series. Persistent neurologic deficits after EBV encephalitis are reported to be rare.[81,] Influenza has been associated with a severe type of encephalitis with high mortality particularly in Japan and Taiwan, including several case reports of acute necrotizing encephalopathy (ANE).[82,83] In the U.S., cases appear to be less severe with better outcomes although further studies are needed.[84]

Deaths and complications caused by arboviruses are better documented as a result of reporting to the CDC. Although a common and feared cause of arboviral encephalitis, WNV has a much better prognosis in children than in adults. Children accounted for only 4% of WNV neuroinvasive disease (WNND) reported to the CDC from 1999 to 2007, with 63% of cases older than 10 years and only 15% under 4 years. There were only 3 pediatric fatalities over this time period (1% of all cases of WNND), a case fatality rate substantially lower than for older adults (14% for adults ≥50 years).[85] La Crosse virus and EEE are more severe in children than WNV.[86] In a study of 127 children with LACV, 12% had neurologic deficits at discharge.[86] EEE also is known to have a higher mortality (almost 30%) and potentially severe neurologic complications.

Bacterial infections also have variable outcomes. Both *Listeria monocytogenes* and tuberculous meningitis may have high morbidity and mortality. *L. monocytogenes* has been linked with rhombencephalitis in case reports.[87,88] In a French study, these two etiologies accounted for the majority of fatalities due to encephalitis (together 12 of 26 fatalities);[89] *L. monocytogenes* infections seem to be less common in the U.S.[15] Both infections are reported to cause severe and potentially fatal sequelae. In a recent study, tuberculous meningitis had the worst outcome with 30% mortality and 40% sequelae with moderate or severe disabilities.[90] On the other hand, bacterial agents such as *Bartonella* spp., which typically causes encephalopathy rather than encephalitis, have an excellent outcome; over 90% of patients recover completely without sequelae.[91]

There are limited studies reporting outcomes specifically on encephalitis of unknown etiology. One study, however, reported significant sequelae in up to 53% of survivors hospitalized with unknown causes of encephalitis.[92] The dearth of information on this subset of patients likely is due to the heterogeneous nature of diseases. In children, some cases of unknown etiology may be due to postinfectious demyelinating disease, multiple sclerosis, or idiopathic epilepsy syndromes.

FUTURE DIRECTIONS IN TREATMENT

Although few specific treatments are routinely available for encephalitis, progress is being made toward treatment of some infections once considered to be universally fatal. In 2004, for example, an unvaccinated adolescent survived rabies encephalitis after a novel therapy was used.[93] Similarly, good outcomes were achieved with various combination drug regimens for *B. mandrillaris* and *B. procyonis*.[94–96] Other treatment considerations include ribavirin intravenously for La Crosse virus and Nipah virus, and interferon-α or monoclonal antibody for WNV.[58,97–99]

PREVENTION

Since the majority of cases do not have a known etiology, recommendations on prevention are difficult. Routine immunizations decrease encephalitis related to diseases such as measles, mumps, rubella, varicella, and influenza. For the immunocompromised host, passive postexposure prophylaxis for varicella and measles also is available. Avoidance of exposure to arthropod vectors is an effective means of preventing arbovirus encephalitis.

SPECIAL HOSTS
Neonates

The epidemiology and clinical presentation of agents causing congenital or neonatal encephalitis differ from those of older children (Table 44-4). Identifying infants with CNS infections can be particularly problematic because the clinical features are extremely vague during the early phase of illness. Congenital infection with cytomegalovirus (CMV), VZV, rubella virus, LCM virus, and *Toxoplasma gondii* can cause CNS infection with structural brain damage and neurologic symptoms present at birth. If infection occurs during the first trimester there is an increased risk of spontaneous abortion.[100] Later in gestation, congenital infection can lead to chorioretinitis, intracranial calcifications, hydrocephalus, microcephaly or macrocephaly, mental retardation, and seizures.[101,102] West Nile virus also has been associated, albeit rarely, with neurologic manifestations secondary to congenital infections.[103]

HSV-1 and HSV-2, EV, HPeV, and HIV are viruses acquired primarily in the perinatal period. Meningoencephalitis may be the sole manifestation of HSV infection or it can be associated with skin, eye and mucous membrane (SEM) disease, and/or disseminated disease. Recognition of HSV is particularly important because of beneficial treatment with acyclovir. Prior to the availability of antiviral therapy, the mortality associated with disseminated HSV disease was 85% and 50% for infants with CNS disease. Presentation of neonatal HSV CNS disease is a spectrum including nonspecific signs and symptoms, apnea, lethargy, focal or generalized seizures, and paralysis.

In neonates, a variety of EVs and HPeVs have been associated with serious complications including encephalitis and death.[104,105] HPeV-3 is noteworthy in the neonatal period because it appears to be a major cause of neonatal encephalitis, possibly three times more common than EV.[106] The typical presentation is fever, rash, irritability, seizures, and occasionally hepatitis. Notably, the CSF is normal in most cases (90%), which suggests that the diagnosis of encephalitis could be overlooked easily.[11,106] Further, neuroimaging of HPeV-3 often demonstrates distinctive white matter involvement that may be thought erroneously to be periventricular leukomalacia (PVL). Unlike PVL, however, the white matter abnormalities in neonatal HPeV-3 involve the subcortical white matter and entire fiber tracts including the corpus callosum, optic radiation, as well as grey matter regions such as the posterior thalamus.[106]

As outlined in Table 44-3, workup of neonates is somewhat different from that of older patients for the same agents. Acyclovir should be administered empirically to ill infants with signs compatible with CNS HSV infection and no other likely diagnosis.

PART II Clinical Syndromes and Cardinal Features of Infectious Diseases: Approach to Diagnosis and Initial Management

SECTION F Central Nervous System Infections

Immunocompromised Hosts

In addition to all the agents that can cause encephalitis in the immunocompetent host, many other agents must be considered in the immunocompromised host, particularly because some require specific treatment.

Several herpesviruses (CMV, EBV, HHV-6, VZV), can reactivate to cause encephalitis. *Toxoplasma gondii* and JC viruses also can reactivate to cause encephalitis. CMV is particularly problematic

in organ transplant recipients and HIV-infected individuals. CMV encephalitis can manifest as a diffuse encephalopathy with confusion, disorientation, psychomotor slowing, and cranial nerve palsies. JC virus typically causes multifocal demyelinating disease, progressing to multifocal leukoencephalopathy. Fungal infections of the CNS are relatively rare but are being recognized increasingly as the immunocompromised population grows. Similarly, the free-living ameba, *Acanthamoeba* spp. and *B. mandrillaris*, also can cause encephalitis in the immunocompromised host.

45 Para- and Postinfectious Neurologic Syndromes

Carol Glaser and Jonathan B. Strober

Inflammation of the central and/or peripheral nervous system can produce a myriad of symptoms depending on site. The inflammation often arises during, or in response to, an infection. However, the same syndrome can be seen when there have been no signs of a preceding illness and occasionally the syndrome can develop

after vaccination. The presentation can be localized to one structure, such as in optic neuritis, or affect multiple structures, such as in acute disseminated (or demyelinating) encephalomyelitis (ADEM). Inflammation typically causes temporary demyelination, although it can cause injury to the underlying parenchyma

TABLE 45-1. Etiologies of Para- and Postinfectious Syndromes of the Central Nervous System

ACUTE DISSEMINATED ENCEPHALOMYELITIS	Viruses	Bacteria	Noninfectious
	Enteroviruses	*Bartonella henselae*	Adrenoleukodystrophy
	Epstein–Barr virus	*Borrelia burgdorferi*	Behçet syndrome
	Herpes simplex virus 1 and 2	*Streptococcus pyogenes*	CNS lymphoma
	Influenza A and B	*Leptospira* sp.	Langerhans cell histiocytosis
	Measles virus	*Mycoplasma pneumoniae*	Metachromatic leukodystrophy
	Mumps virus	**Parasites**	Mitochondrial disorders
	Parainfluenza viruses	*Plasmodium falciparum*	Multiple sclerosis
	Rubella virus		Primary CNS vasculitis
	Varicella zoster virus		Systemic lupus erythematosus
	Variola virus		Sjögren syndrome
			Sarcoidosis
			Vaccines
TRANSVERSE MYELITIS	Viruses	Bacteria	Noninfectious
	Enterovirus	*Bartonella henselae*	Anti-phospholipid antibody syndrome
	Epstein–Barr virus	*Borrelia burgdorferi*	Ischemic myopathy
	Herpes simplex virus 1 and 2	*Streptococcus pyogenes*	Neuromyelitis optica (Devic)
	Influenza A and B	*Leptospira* sp.	Spinal cord tumor
	Measles virus	*Mycoplasma pneumoniae*	Sjögren syndrome
	Mumps virus	**Parasites**	Systemic lupus erythematosus
	Parainfluenza viruses	*Plasmodium falciparum*	
	Rubella virus	*Schistosoma* spp.	
	Varicella zoster virus	*Toxocara canis*	
	Variola virus		
CEREBELLITIS	Viruses	Bacteria	Noninfectious
	Adenovirus	*Borrelia* spp.	Antineuronal antibodies (e.g., anti-Hu)
	Cytomegalovirus	*Coxiella burnetii*	Methadone ingestion
	Enterovirus	*Rickettsia* spp.	Systemic lupus erythematosus
	Herpes simplex virus 1 and 2	*Salmonella* Typhi	Tick paralysis
	Human herpes virus 6		Vaccines
	Human immunodeficiency virus		
	Influenza virus		
	Mumps virus		
	Rotavirus		
	Varicella zoster virus		
	West Nile virus		

TABLE 45-2. Etiologies of Para- and Postinfectious Syndromes of the Peripheral Nervous System

Guillain–Barré syndrome	Viruses	Bacteria	Noninfectious
	Cytomegalovirus	*Campylobacter* spp.	Chronic progressive external ophthalmoplegia
	Epstein-Barr virus	**Mimicking**	Heavy metal poisoning
	Herpes simplex virus 1 and 2	Infant botulism	Myasthenia gravis
	Varicella zoster virus	Poliovirus	Tick paralysis
		West Nile virus	Vaccines
Facial nerve palsy (Bell)	Viruses	Bacteria	Noninfectious
	Herpes simplex virus 1	*Borrelia* spp.	Aneurysm of vertebral, basilar or carotid arteries
	Epstein–Barr virus	*Mycobacterium tuberculosis*	Cholesteatoma of the middle ear
	Human herpesvirus 6	*Mycobacterium leprae*	Drugs (e.g., linezolid)
	Human immunodeficiency virus	**Mimicking**	Leukemic meningitis
	Parvovirus B19	Acute otitis media	Parotid tumors
	Varicella zoster virus	Intraparotid lymphadenitis	Sarcoidosis
		Necrotizing otitis externa	Fracture of base of the skull
		Osteomyelitis of the skull base	Fracture of the temporal bone
		Parotid gland abscess	Trauma
Optic neuritis	Viruses	Bacteria	Noninfectious
	Chikungunya virus	*Bartonella henselae*	ADEM
	Varicella zoster virus	**Parasites**	Autoimmune (IBD, SLE)
	West Nile virus	*Angiostrongylus cantonensis*	Copper deficiency
		Baylisascaris procyonis	Diabetes mellitus
		Toxocara canis/catii	Drugs (e.g., ethambutol)
		Treponema pallidum	Neuromyelitis optica (Devic disease)
			Multiple sclerosis
			Vasculitis
Oculomotor neuropathy	Viruses	Infectious	Noninfectious
	Varicella zoster virus	Brain abscess	Aneurysm
		Meningitis	Congenital palsy
			Diabetes mellitus
			Myasthenia gravis
			Sarcoidosis
			CNS tumor
			Trauma

ADEM, acute disseminated encephalomyelitis; CNS, central nervous system; IBD, Inflammatory bowel disease; SLE, systemic lupus erythematosus.

or axons, leading to more permanent injury. The focus of this chapter is the more common syndromes seen in the pediatric population, their various etiologies, diagnostic evaluation, and management (Tables 45-1 and 45-2).

CRANIAL NERVE PALSIES

Facial Nerve Palsy (Bell Palsy)

The most common parainfectious neurologic syndrome is inflammation of the peripheral facial nerve (cranial nerve (CN) VII). When no etiology is identified, the condition often is referred to as Bell palsy. One study reported an incidence of 4.2 per 100,000 children under the age of 10 years, increasing to 15.3 per 100,000 in children aged 10 to 20 years.[1] There are no seasonal or sex differences. It typically is unilateral and acute in onset and often develops after a preceding illness. Facial nerve palsy also can occur in conjunction with peripheral nervous system involvement.

There are two proposed pathologic mechanisms, both leading to edema and entrapment of the nerve in the facial canal. The most likely explanation is direct inflammation of the nerve. MRI can show gadolinium enhancement of the nerve,[2] and pathologic studies describe lymphocytic infiltration and associated demyelination or axonal degeneration.[3] Another, less plausible, possibility is that increased capillary permeability, as occurs in diabetes, leads to edema and compression of the nerve's microcirculation. This mechanism is supported by the finding that diabetics are 2.5 times more likely to develop Bell palsy than nondiabetics.[4]

Herpes simplex virus (HSV) has been the most frequent virus associated with Bell palsy[5] although other viruses, including Epstein–Barr virus (EBV) and hepatitis B virus, have been implicated. Ramsay Hunt syndrome, a rare complication of latent varicella-zoster virus (VZV) infection, is defined as an acute peripheral facial neuropathy associated with an erythematous vesicular rash of the skin of the ear canal, auricle (also termed herpes zoster oticus), and/or mucous membrane of the oropharynx. *Borrelia burgdorferi* infection also can cause facial palsy, which can develop without a history of antecedent tick bite or erythema migrans.[6] In one study of facial palsy in a Lyme disease endemic area, 34% of people ≤20 years of age who were evaluated in the emergency department of a large urban pediatric tertiary care center with a facial palsy were found to have Lyme disease.[7] Predictors of facial palsy due to Lyme disease included headache, fever, bilateral involvement, lack of herpetic lesions, and presentation from June through October.

Treatment is aimed at the underlying etiology, but good eye care is important to protect the cornea. Bacterial causes should be treated with appropriate antibiotics. Cases due to Lyme disease should be treated with 21 to 28 days of doxycycline or amoxicillin for children <8 years of age, to help shorten the duration and stop progression.[8] Most Bell palsies resolve without treatment. A meta-analysis of adults and children with Bell palsy demonstrated a 17% improvement with corticosteroid treatment compared with no treatment.[9] There is controversy whether acyclovir or valacyclovir should be used in the treatment of acute Bell palsy, since a high percentage of cases are due to HSV

PART II Clinical Syndromes and Cardinal Features of Infectious Diseases: Approach to Diagnosis and Initial Management

SECTION F Central Nervous System Infections

infection. The addition of an antiviral agent to corticosteroid therapy, even when used in the first 72 hours of onset of illness, does not appear to improve outcome.[10] The extent of facial nerve recovery does not necessarily relate to the severity of the initial nerve involvement.[11]

Optic Neuritis

The second most common cranial nerve to be affected by para-infectious demyelination is the optic nerve. Optic neuritis (ON) has been reported to have an incidence of 0.2/100,000 in Canadian children,[12] similar to that of ADEM and transverse myelitis (TM). ON typically manifests with reduced vision (e.g., blurred or "foggy" vision) and pain with eye movement. ON can be accompanied by other neurologic signs or symptoms, as is seen in ADEM, or can be the heralding manifestation of multiple sclerosis (MS) or neuromyelitis optica (NMO; Devic disease). Therefore, brain MRI is recommended for patients with isolated ON. Up to 85% of cases are preceded by an infection or vaccination and the vast majority regain at least 20/40 vision.[13]

Females are more commonly affected than males;[12,14,15] however, female sex does not necessarily increase the risk of subsequently developing MS. ON often is unilateral, but can be bilateral.[15] On fundoscopic examination, the head of the optic nerve may be swollen but can appear normal even to an experienced ophthalmologist. The presence of white matter lesions on MRI disseminated in space and time is the strongest predictor for developing MS;[14,15] a normal MRI at first-episode ON does not preclude the development of MS.[16] The presence of NMO antibodies are highly specific for the diagnosis of Devic disease; their sensitivity is approximately 80%.[17] Brain MRI often is normal in this condition.

Bartonellosis is one of the most common infectious cause of isolated ON as well as when accompanied by lymphadenopathy and fever. Arboviruses, including West Nile virus (WNV)[18] and chikungunya,[19,20] also have been associated with ON. Animal roundworms, e.g., *Toxocara canis* and *Baylisascaris procyonis*, are rare causes of ON. When these nematodes invade the eye, a neuro-retinitis also can occur and the worm itself is sometimes visualized in the retina. *Angiostrongylus cantonensis* (a cause of eosinophilic meningitis) is found in Southeast Asia, the South Pacific, Australia, the Caribbean and sometimes in the United States (Hawaii and Louisiana), and also can cause ON.

The typical treatment for ON is a 3-day course of high-dose corticosteroid administered intravenously followed by a short oral taper, regardless of underlying cause. Additional treatment with specific antimicrobial therapy may be needed depending on the cause. In 1992, the Optic Neuritis Treatment Group found that treatment with corticosteroid intravenously hastened recovery over placebo, but did not change long-term outcome.[21] Treatment with oral corticosteroid did not seem to affect outcome although patients receiving oral therapy relapsed more frequently than those receiving IV therapy. Prognosis is good, with visual acuity at or near baseline in at least 70% of patients.

Ocular Motor Nerve Palsies

Isolated neuropathies affecting one of the three nerves that move the eye, the oculomotor nerve (CN III), trochlear nerve (CN IV), and abducens nerve (CN VI), have been reported to occur as a postinfectious entity.[22] These are rare conditions that often do not require treatment. However, more common causes of these neuropathies, such as trauma, increased intracranial pressure, tumor, and vascular causes should be excluded. Ocular motor palsies also are associated with the Miller–Fisher variant of Guillain–Barré syndrome (GBS).

CEREBELLITIS

Apart from affecting individual nerves in the central nervous system (CNS), the cerebellum can become inflamed due to an

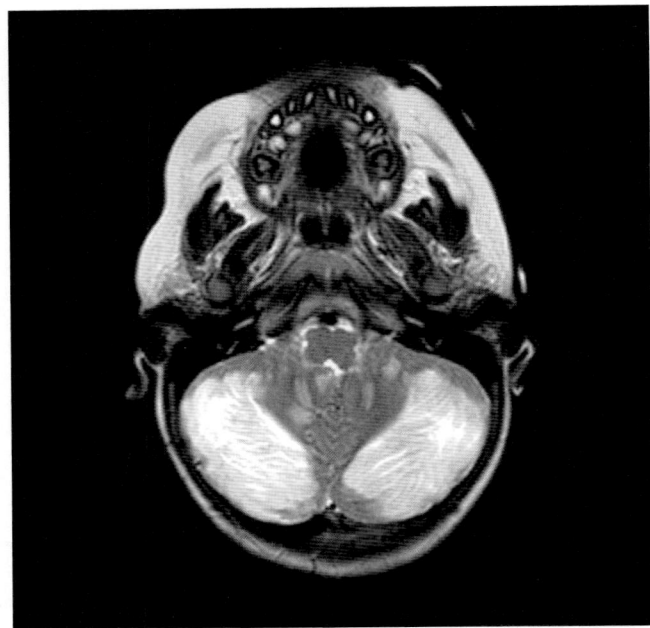

Figure 45-1. Brain MRI from patient with cerebellitis and diffusely increased FLAIR T_2 signal. (Courtesy of Brian Lee, MD, Children's Hospital & Research Center Oakland.)

infectious or postinfectious process, commonly known as cerebellitis or acute cerebellar ataxia. It typically presents with acute-onset ataxia and often is self-limiting with complete recovery. It is estimated to occur in approximately 1 per 100,000 to 500,000 children,[23] although it is difficult to determine an accurate incidence since many children with mild disease may not come to medical attention or may be evaluated only by their primary care physician.

Cerebellitis often presents concurrently with a viral illness, with VZV having the best recognized association. Cerebellitis also has been reported in association with EBV, *Mycoplasma pneumoniae*, mumps and enterovirus, as well as vaccinations.[23,24] Pathologic studies have shown inflammation, primarily composed of T lymphocytes, of the leptomeninges and molecular layer of the cerebellum. Imaging typically shows enhancement of the cerebellum, localized mostly to the leptomeninges (Figure 45-1).[24] Cerebrospinal fluid analysis can be normal or show mild mononuclear pleocytosis and elevated protein concentration.

Management is supportive; however, due to its location, cerebellar swelling can lead to acute and severe hydrocephalus eventually causing herniation and brainstem compression. In severe cases, corticosteroid therapy is indicated[25] to help minimize swelling and prevent complications.

ACUTE DISSEMINATED ENCEPHALOMYELITIS (ADEM)

ADEM usually is a monophasic polysymptomatic disorder that can affect any part of the brain and spinal cord. ADEM has an estimated incidence of 0.4 to 0.8 per 100,000, accounting for about 10% to 15% of cases of encephalitis in the U.S.[12,26,27] Neurologic symptoms often develop 2 to 4 weeks after an infection or vaccination and typically progress quickly, often over hours to days.[27] Up to 75% of cases of ADEM have an identifiable trigger. Historically, vaccine-preventable diseases such as measles and mumps were common precedents of ADEM. Measles virus can cause direct viral encephalitis and also is considered one of the most important triggers of ADEM. In countries where vaccines are widely used to prevent

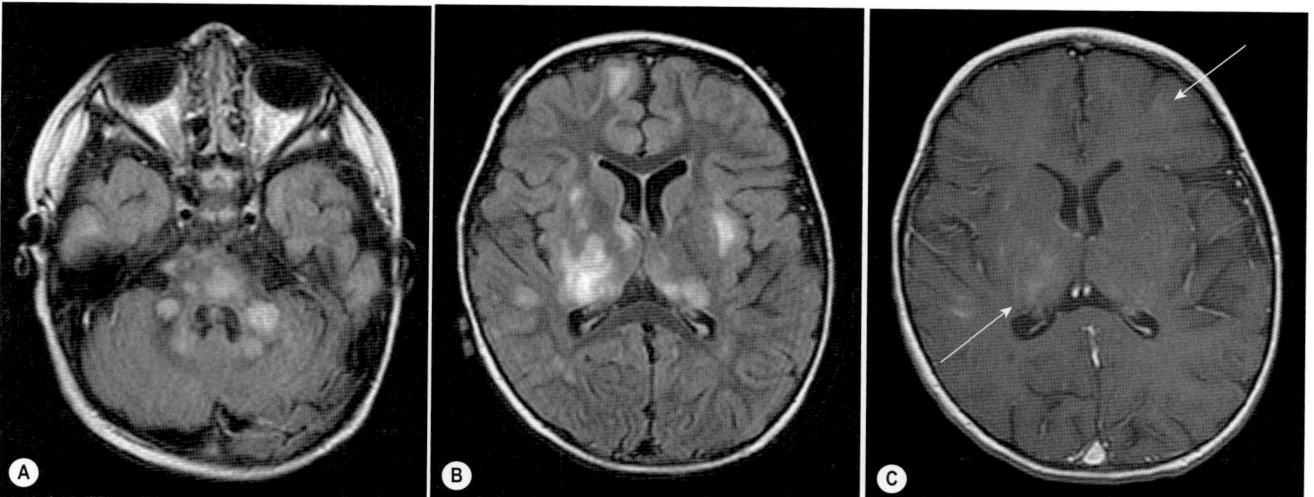

Figure 45-2. Brain MRI from patient with acute disseminated encephalomyelitis showing multiple hyperintense lesions in the cerebellum and brainstem **(A)** as well as deep and superficial white matter and deep grey matter **(B)** with subtle patchy enhancement (arrows in **C**).

measles, mumps, rubella, and varicella infections, upper respiratory infections are the most common illnesses preceding ADEM. Vaccines also can trigger ADEM. The incidence of measles vaccination associated ADEM is reported to be 0.1 per 100,000, compared with 0.2 to 0.3 per 100,000 following wild-type measles infection.[28] ADEM also has been reported to occur after exposure to the human papillomavirus (HPV) vaccine.[29]

Clinical manifestations of ADEM include altered mental status in 50% to 75% of cases and seizures in 10% to 35% of cases.[27] The presenting symptoms vary according to the regions of the CNS that are affected, which differ substantially from patient to patient. Motor weakness (e.g., acute hemiparesis), ataxia, decreased verbal output or mutism, cranial neuropathies, and urinary disorders are common.[30] Recovery often is full, although residual deficits can occur in up to 30% of patients.

Less than one-third of patients with ADEM have a recurrent or multiphasic course, which can be difficult to distinguish from MS in some instances.[27] Recurrent ADEM is defined as a new event with recurrence of initial symptoms ≥3 months after the first event and ≥1 month after discontinuing corticosteroid therapy.[31] MRI does not show new lesions in ADEM although original lesions may have enlarged. Involvement of the deep grey structures such as basal ganglia and thalamus can occur in ADEM whereas these structures rarely are involved in MS.

Many disorders can appear radiologically similar to ADEM on MRI. These include systemic immunologic and inflammatory disorders such as systemic lupus erythematosus (SLE), sarcoidosis, Behçet syndrome, and Langerhans cell histiocytosis, which often have multisystem involvement. Meningitis, meningoencephalitis, brain abscesses, or tumors usually are easy to differentiate from ADEM. However, some infectious agents, such as *Balamuthia mandrillaris* and *Baylisascaris procyonis*, can have MRI changes that can be confused with ADEM due to T_2 signal changes in the white matter. Metabolic disorders, such as adrenoleukodystrophy and metachromatic leukodystrophy, tend to present more insidiously while mitochondrial disorders can present with acute T_2 signal lesions on neuroimaging, but tend to have more of a relapsing and remitting course.

The diagnosis of ADEM is based primarily on the clinical course and MRI findings (Figure 45-2). Lumbar puncture (LP) should be performed to exclude infectious etiologies. The most common cerebrospinal fluid (CSF) abnormalities are a mild pleocytosis (usually with lymphocyte predominant) and elevation in protein concentration. Evaluation for the presence of oligoclonal bands

should be performed when MS is considered. However, the presence of oligoclonal bands does not confirm a diagnosis of MS as they can be found in up to almost 30% of patients with ADEM.[32]

High-dose corticosteroids are considered first-line therapy for ADEM.[33] Intravenously administered immunoglobulin (IGIV) or plasmapheresis often are utilized, if there is no response to corticosteroid. Immunomodulating agents, such as cyclophosphamide, sometimes are used in refractory cases.

TRANSVERSE MYELITIS

Transverse myelitis (TM) can occur in association with ON, neuromyelitis optica, cerebral lesions (ADEM) or in isolation. Approximately 1400 new cases of isolated TM occur each year in the U.S., 20% of which occur in children <18 years of age.[34] In a Canadian cohort, the incidence was reported as 0.2 per 100,000, which is similar to incidence of ADEM and ON.[12] Incidence is approximately equal in males and females. TM has been reported in infants as young as 6 months of age. Approximately 50% to 75% of cases have a history of a preceding illness, often a presumed respiratory tract infection, or vaccination.[34,35]

Diagnosis of TM is based on evidence of spinal cord inflammation, such as CSF pleocytosis, increased CSF IgG index or gadolinium enhancement on MRI (Figure 45-3), and lack of an alternative etiology. Presenting symptoms depend on the affected area, but often begin with back pain with progression to loss of bowel and bladder function as a result of autonomic dysfunction and lower extremity weakness and sensory loss. MRI is abnormal in 80% to 95% of patients, typically showing involvement of >3 vertebral bodies in length[35]. CSF is abnormal in up to 70% of patients, often showing elevated protein and less often an increased white blood cell count.

A number of different infections, similar to those associated with ADEM, have been implicated as causes of TM (see Table 45-1). Enteroviruses are one of the most frequently implicated causes.[36]

The mainstay of treatment of TM is corticosteroids. IGIV and plasma exchange also sometimes are used. Recovery often is not complete and treatment has not been associated with improved outcome. The most common neurologic deficit is impaired bladder control,[34] but >25% of children with TM require ongoing assistance with self-care activities. Younger age, longer time to diagnosis, and larger lesions were associated with poorer prognosis.

PART II Clinical Syndromes and Cardinal Features of Infectious Diseases: Approach to Diagnosis and Initial Management

SECTION F Central Nervous System Infections

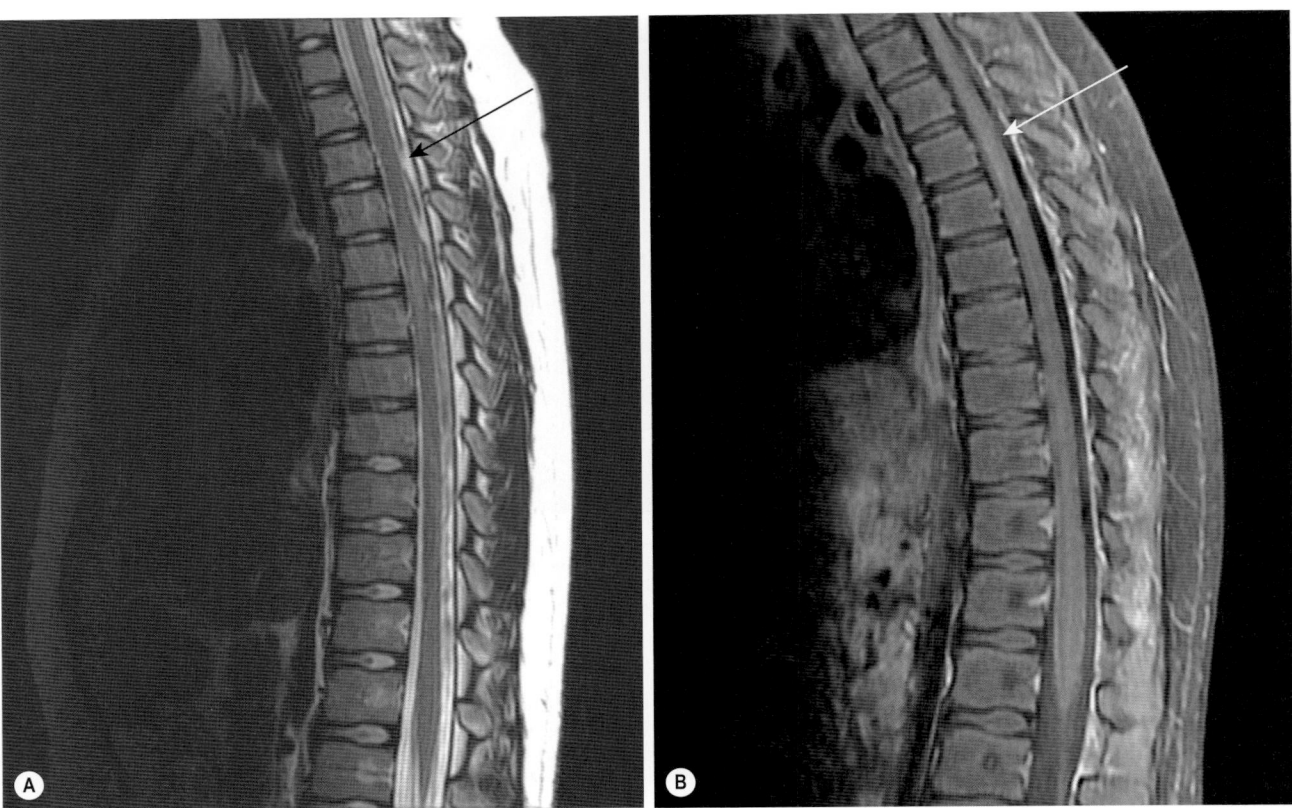

Figure 45-3. Thoracic spine MRI from patient with transverse myelitis showing increased T_2 signal (arrow in **A**) and patchy gadolinium enhancement (arrow in **B**).

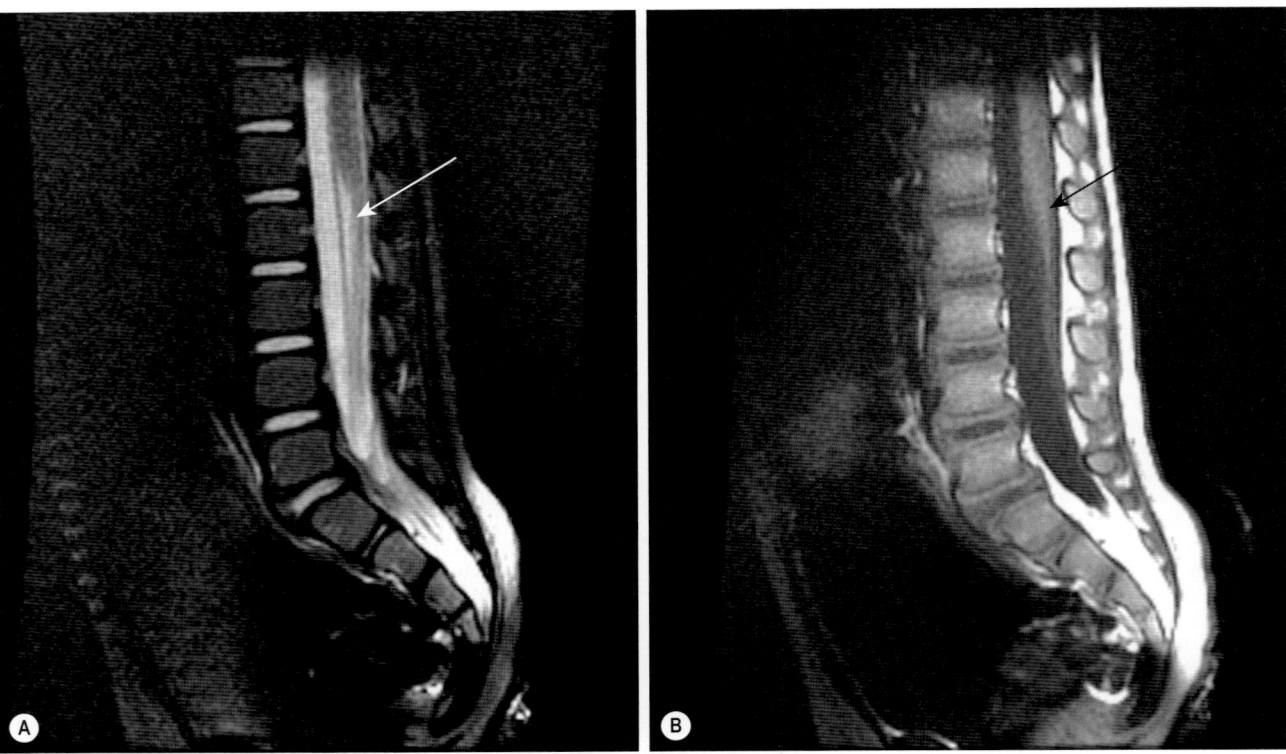

Figure 45-4. MRI of lumbar spine from patient with Guillain–Barré syndrome showing increased T_2 signal in the cauda equina (arrow in **A**) with smooth enhancement (arrow in **B**).

ACUTE INFLAMMATORY DEMYELINATING POLYRADICULONEUROPATHY (GUILLAIN–BARRÉ SYNDROME)

Acute inflammatory demyelinating polyradiculoneuropathy (AIDP), better known as Guillain–Barré syndrome (GBS), typically is an acute to subacute disorder leading to ascending paralysis. There are several variants. In the post-polio era, GBS is the most common cause of acute motor paralysis in children, with an estimated incidence of 0.5 to 1.5 per 100,000 people <18 years of age,[37] with a slight male predominance.

In the classic form of GBS, extremity weakness is accompanied by areflexia and occurs in an ascending pattern. Sensory and autonomic symptoms, including urinary retention, cardiac arrhythmias, and autonomic instability, are common. Radicular back pain is a frequent initial complaint. These symptoms often are preceded by symptoms consistent with a gastrointestinal or upper respiratory tract illness. *Campylobacter jejuni* infection[38] and influenza vaccine are the most commonly identified specific precipitants of GBS.[39] Ninety-five percent of GBS cases in the U.S. are the classic demyelinating sensorimotor neuropathy form.[40] Other forms include axonal forms (both acute motor and sensorimotor), which account for up to 30% of cases in China and Latin America, and the Miller–Fisher variant, characterized by ataxia and ophthalmoplegia. Cranial nerve involvement also can occur in the classic form.

Electromyography/nerve conduction studies (EMG/NCS) can be helpful in diagnosing GBS, being consistent with the diagnosis in almost 70% of cases in one pediatric series.[40] However, electrophysiology can be normal for up to a week into the illness, with the initial abnormality often being prolongation of the F wave, a measure of proximal nerve conduction. EMG/NCS can be helpful in excluding other conditions, such as infant botulism and myasthenia gravis, if ophthalmoparesis is present, and other neuropathies, such as heavy metal poisoning. The most typical CSF finding is albuminocytologic dissociation, i.e., elevated protein without white blood cells (WBCs). However, CSF pleocytosis, with WBCs >50/mm^3 has been observed.[40] MRI can be helpful diagnostically, occasionally showing hyperintensity of the anterior nerve roots (Figure 45-4).

Clinically, GBS symptoms plateau eventually and then recovery begins. Respiratory support may be necessary during the nadir of the illness. Expert guidance, published in 2003, recommends plasma exchange (PE) for nonambulatory patients within 4 weeks of onset or for ambulatory patients within 2 weeks of onset.[41] IGIV was considered to be equivalent to PE and was recommended for patients who required aid to walk, within 2 to 4 weeks of onset. Unlike a number of the other parainfectious conditions, corticosteroids are not recommended for treatment of GBS.

Overall, children with GBS have a good prognosis. Up to 95% of children are asymptomatic or have symptoms that do not affect daily functioning 2 years after disease.[42,43] Mortality in GBS is low, occurring in <10% of patients,[42] mostly from respiratory failure, often in association with cardiac arrhythmia or autonomic dysfunction.

---

46 Focal Suppurative Infections of the Nervous System

Christopher J. Harrison

Diverse microorganisms cause focal suppurative nervous system infections; however, a majority are due to a few species, mostly gram-positive bacteria.

Risk factors for suppurative nervous system infections include cyanotic congenital heart disease (CCHD), penetrating trauma, hematogenous dissemination from distant persistently infected sites, from instrumentation, or from contiguous sinus, middle ear or mastoid infection.

Risk factors for fungal infections are altered immune capabilities, receipt of broad-spectrum antibacterial agents and long-term indwelling foreign material. As more children have conditions requiring iatrogenic prolonged neutropenia or cell-mediated suppression, more invasive fungal nervous system infections are likely.

ETIOLOGY

Overall, gram-positive cocci are the most common pathogens of brain abscess. The *Streptococcus milleri* group *(S. constellatus, S. intermedius,* and *S. anginosus)* are isolated in 50% to 70% and staphylococci in 10% to 30% of cases. Although *Streptococcus pneumoniae* commonly causes meningitis, it rarely causes brain abscess.[1] Up to 30% of brain abscesses are polymicrobial, often including nutritionally variant streptococci (e.g., *Abiotrophia* species[2]) or anaerobes (e.g., *Bacteroides, Prevotella,* and/or *Peptostreptococcus* spp.); their detection requires specific culture techniques.[3]

Gram-negative bacteria are isolated from 10% to 25% of brain abscesses or subdural empyemas (Table 46-1), mostly in young infants[4,5]. *Citrobacter,*[6,7] *Salmonella,*[8] *Serratia,*[9] *Proteus* spp.,[10] *Cronobacter* species (previously *Enterobacter sakazakii*),[11] or *Bacteroides fragilis*[12] are most frequent. *Citrobacter koseri* and *Cronobacter sakazakii* are associated with multifocal brain abscesses, and *Cronobacter* with powdered formula ingestion. Rarely, *Mycoplasma* or *Ureoplasma* species cause neonatal brain abscess.[13]

Chronic middle-ear infections, uncontrolled diabetes mellitus, and chemotherapy-induced neutropenia are risks for *Pseudomonas aeruginosa.*[14] Impaired cell-mediated immune function, e.g., macrophage- or T-lymphocyte-related defects, or neutrophil phagocytic defects predispose to *Listeria monocytogenes*[15] or *Nocardia* spp.[16]

Fungal brain abscesses occur with congenital or acquired neutrophil abnormalities, stem cell[17] or solid organ transplantation,[18] or poorly controlled acquired immunodeficiency syndrome (AIDS), particularly after broad-spectrum antibacterial treatment. Over 90% of brain abscesses after bone marrow or stem cell transplantation are due to fungi, usually *Candida* or *Aspergillus* spp.[19]

Although *Cryptococcus* usually manifests as meningitis, it can cause brain abscess. Other pathogens rarely causing brain abscess include *Blastomyces,*[20] *Histoplasma,*[21] *Pseudallescheria,*[22] Zygomycetes,[23] *Coccidioides,*[24] *Dactylaria, Fonsecaea, Ramichloridium, Bipolaris, Exophiala, Curvularia,* and *Xylohypha (Cladosporium)* spp.

Toxoplasma gondii commonly causes brain abscess in adults with AIDS, but is rare in children.[25] *Entamoeba histolytica* brain abscess is rare even with amebiasis. Other protozoa causing brain abscess include *Acanthamoeba, Schistosoma,* or *Paragonimus* spp. Helminthic migration (*Strongyloides stercoralis, Trichinella,* or *Taenia*) can cause brain abscesses or masses.[26] Neurocysticercosis is a relatively frequent cause of single or multiple central nervous system (CNS) masses that can be ring enhancing and can be misconstrued as bacterial brain abscesses among patients from endemic areas, e.g., Mexico.

PART II Clinical Syndromes and Cardinal Features of Infectious Diseases: Approach to Diagnosis and Initial Management

SECTION F Central Nervous System Infections

TABLE 46-1. Likelihood (% of cases) of Bacterial Pathogen in Focal Suppurative Nervous System Infections

Bacteria	Brain Abscess	Subdural Empyema	Epidural Abscess Cranial	Epidural Abscess Spinal
Mixed	20–40	5–10	5–10	5–10
Alpha streptococci, not pneumococcus[a]	50–70	20–30	40–60	5–10
Anaerobic bacteria[b]	20–30[b]	5–10[b]	10–20	5–10
Staphylococci	10–30	10–20	10–20	60–80
Enterobacteriaceae	10–25	5–10	5–15	5–20
Pathogens of meningitis[c]	5–10	30–50	5–10	<1
Sterile[d]	10–25	20–30	20–30	5–10

[a]*Aerobic, anaerobic, or microaerophilic (e.g.,* Streptococcus anginosus *group).*

[b]*Mostly anaerobic streptococci.*

[c]Streptococcus pneumoniae, Haemophilus influenzae *type b, or* Neisseria meningitidis. *Much less common in countries with routine use of pediatric conjugate vaccines.*

[d]*More common with antibiotic pre-treatment or in children <5 years of age.*

Table 46-2 includes additional uncommon pathogens.[27–30] *Mycobacterium tuberculosis* brain abscess[31] differs from tuberculoma, which is a granulomatous mass containing epithelioid and giant cells. Tuberculous abscesses are purulent collections containing acid-fast bacilli. Magnetic resonance imaging (MRI) differentiates these two conditions.

Lesion location or distribution can suggest the pathogen. Frontal lobe abscess (usually a complication of sinusitis) suggests oral flora, i.e., *Streptococcus* spp. (aerobic, microaerophilic, anaerobic), staphylococci, and/or anaerobic bacteria[32] (Table 46-3). Penetrating trauma increases the risk for *Staphylococcus aureus* (increasingly methicillin-resistant *S. aureus,* MRSA) but *Streptococcus* spp. remain common. Temporal lobe or cerebellar abscesses suggest middle-ear pathogens in addition to oral flora (mostly anaerobic and microaerophilic streptococci plus anaerobes, and less often Enterobacteriaceae).

Hematogenous spread due to endocarditis, septic thrombophlebitis, lung abscess, pleural empyema, bronchiectasis (in cystic fibrosis), osteomyelitis, or skin infections classically produces multiple lesions in the distribution of the middle cerebral artery. However, hematogenous abscesses can occur in any pattern.

Common hematogenous pathogens are *Staphylococcus aureus,* aerobic or anaerobic streptococci, and, rarely, *Nocardia* or *Actinomyces* spp. With CCHD, *Aggregatibacter* (formerly *Haemophilus*) *aphrophilus* is relatively common, whereas *S. aureus* is more frequent with prosthetic valve endocarditis or prolonged bloodstream infection (BSI) (de novo or associated with intravascular catheter).

Clues to causative pathogens in subdural empyemas relate to the pathogenesis. In young children, subdural empyema usually accompanies bacterial meningitis; pathogens are *Haemophilus influenzae* type b (Hib), pneumococcus, or rarely meningococcus[33,34] (see Table 46-2).

Subdural empyemas not accompanying meningitis have the same pathogens as brain abscesses. Aerobic and anaerobic streptococci (e.g., *S. intermedius* and *S. anginosus* group) predominate when associated with sinusitis. *S. aureus* is traditionally more common postoperatively or post trauma, but now occurs after sinus or middle ear disease. Cultures are sterile in 20% to 30%, likely due to one or more of the following: antibacterial pretreatment; nonviability of fastidious or anaerobic bacteria, or nonoptimal collection, transportation, and isolation procedures.[35]

Rare subdural pathogens include nontyphoid *Salmonella,*[36] *S. pyogenes,*[37] *Burkholderia,*[38] *Brucella melitensis,*[39] *Propionibacterium,*[40] *Prevotella,*[41] or fungi (e.g., *Candida albicans,*[42] *Pseudallescheria boydii*).[43] *Mycobacterium tuberculosis* rarely causes subdural empyema.[44] Gram-negative organisms are increasingly detected in both subdural empyema and epidural abscess.[45]

S. aureus is the most common pathogen causing both cranial and spinal epidural abscess.[46,47] However, *S. pneumoniae*[48] or *S. agalactiae*[49] also cause cranial epidural abscesses. *Pseudallescheria,*[43] *Aspergillus,*[50,51] or *Candida* spp.,[52] Zygomycetes or *M. tuberculosis* cranial epidural abscesses occur in immunocompromised hosts.[53] Spinal epidural abscess rarely is due to *Brucella melitensis* (Middle Eastern and Mediterranean area),[54] *Nocardia asteroides* group,[55] *Actinomyces israelii,*[56] *Cryptococcus neoformans,*[57] or *Aspergillus.*[58]

TABLE 46-2. Uncommon Pathogens in Brain Abscesses or Focal Ring Enhancing Lesions

Bacteria Aerobic	Anaerobic	Fungi	Parasites
Aggregatibacter aphrophilus	Propionibacterium	Mucormycosis	Taenia solium
S. pneumoniae	Fusobacterium	Pseudallescheria boydii	Toxoplasma
Eikenella	Peptostreptococcus	Scedosporium	Entamoeba
Enterococcus	Bacteroides	Curvularia	Schistosoma
Moraxella	Clostridium	Histoplasma	Trichinella
Pasteurella	Actinomyces	Blastomyces	Strongyloides
Bacillus cereus		Coccidioides	Paragonimus
Nocardia		Cladosporium	Acanthamoeba
S. pyogenes[a]			
Listeria			
Brucella[b]			

[a]Streptococcus pyogenes *usually concurrent with acute mastoiditis.*

[b]Brucella melitensis *occurs mostly in the Middle East and Mediterranean areas.*

TABLE 46-3. Relative Importance of Organisms by Site of Focal Lesion

Site	Most Common Pathogens
SOLITARY LESION	
Frontal lobe with sinusitis or oral/dental infection	Oral and/or nasopharyngeal aerobic and/or anaerobic flora, e.g. streptococci, *Staphylococcus aureus*
Temporal lobe area, posterior fossa or cerebellum contiguous with middle ear/mastoid infection	Streptococci (aerobic and anaerobic), anaerobic oral flora, Enterobacteriaceae
Post trauma	*Staphylococcus aureus*, non-pneumococcal alpha streptococci, *propionibacterium*, Enterobacteriaceae
MULTIPLE LESIONS	
Underlying congenital heart disease	Non-pneumococcal alpha streptococci (aerobic and/or anaerobic), *Haemophilus* spp.
With endocarditis	Non-pneummococcal alpha streptococci, *Staphylococcus aureus*
With lung infection	Oral flora including anaerobes, *Nocardia* spp.
No known risk	*Staphylococcus aureus*
Immunocompromised host	*Toxoplasma*, fungi, *Nocardia*, Enterobacteriaceae

Epidural and other paravertebral abscess can complicate *Bartonella henselae* vertebral osteomyelitis.[59,60]

Septic intracranial thrombophlebitis mostly is due to *S. pneumoniae*,[61] *S. pyogenes*, or *S. aureus* associated with sinusitis, mastoiditis, or facial infections. Other middle-ear pathogens or non-group A streptococci also are reported.[59] Anaerobes (e.g., *Fusobacterium* species[62]) are rare (most often associated with Lemierre disease) but have severe complications. Polymicrobial infections can occur.[63]

EPIDEMIOLOGY

Brain abscess is uncommon in developed countries, but remains relatively common among socioeconomically disadvantaged people in developing countries. Risks also vary geographically; e.g., chronic otitis media is the primary risk in 60% of brain abscesses in China,[64] but only 30% in Europe.[65] Overall nearly 25% of brain abscesses occur before 15 years of age, peaking between 4 and 7 years of age. Neonatal brain abscess is associated predominantly with gram-negative bacterial meningitis. In immunocompetent hosts, most brain abscesses are solitary. Multiple brain abscesses are more frequent from hematogenous spread and in immune compromised patients.[66] Brain abscesses of immunocompetent hosts are multiloculated in 10% to 20%.

Intracranial subdural empyema occurs in both sexes equally in young children, but males predominate (3:1) among older children. Frequency is similar in young children to bacterial meningitis,[67] being least frequent where Hib and pneumococcal conjugate vaccines are used routinely. In older children, the source is paranasal sinuses or the middle ear/mastoid in ~85% and hematogenous in 5% to 10%. Intracranial subdural empyema after neurosurgical procedures (e.g., craniotomy) is infrequent (0.04%).[45]

Spinal subdural abscess is rare in children.[68] Because obesity is a risk factor in adults and obesity is increasingly prevalent in children, an increase in cases of spinal subdural abscess is likely.

Intracranial epidural abscess is the most common CNS suppurative complication of middle ear, mastoid, or temporal bone infection. Posterior fossa epidural abscesses are extensions from the middle ear/mastoid infection after osseous erosion of the petrous pyramid or over the sigmoid sinus plate.[69] Intracranial epidural abscesses also result from orbital abscesses or frontal sinusitis via valveless emissary veins, or are concurrent with subdural empyema or cavernous sinus thrombosis.[70] Intracranial epidural abscess is 10 to 40 times more frequent than intracranial subdural empyema after neurosurgical procedures, but remains uncommon (0.43% to 1.8% of procedures).[45]

Spinal epidural abscess accounts for 6 per 100,000 hospital admissions,[71] with fewer than 100 reported pediatric cases,[72] the largest series being 58 cases.[48]

Suppurative intracranial thrombophlebitis usually accompanies another intracranial infection, usually extradural, as a complication of mastoiditis or paranasal sinusitis. However, 10% to 20% of cases originate from facial (typically the middle third) or dental infections.

PATHOGENESIS

Brain Abscess

Hematogenous brain abscesses are most common, the most common risk factor being CCHD (Box 46-1). Approximately 6% of patients with unrepaired CCHD develop brain abscess. Brain infarction or emboli lead to infection, the risk increasing with time until repair. Any lesion with right-to-left shunting, e.g., ventricular septal defect or patent foramen ovale,[73] allows transient venous BSI to bypass the reticuloendothelial filter in the lung. Classically, uncorrected tetralogy of Fallot or transposition of the great vessels was the most common predisposing anomaly, but routine early surgical repair has reduced such brain abscesses.

Endocarditis predisposes to brain abscess, especially acute left-sided endocarditis because septic embolization is more common. Increased magnitude and duration of BSI increase the risk of CNS infection. Septic embolization from deep neck phlebitis associated with para-pharyngeal infection (Lemierre disease) produces brain abscess, and usually is polymicrobial, especially oral flora, including anaerobes such as *Fusobacterium* spp.[74] Brain abscesses also occur metastatically from distant pyogenic infections, e.g., bone, teeth, skin, abdomen, chronic lung abscess, empyema, bronchiectasis.[75]

BOX 46-1. Risk Factors for Brain Abscess[a]

HEMATOGENOUS

Uncorrected cyanotic congenital heart disease
Septic thrombophlebitis
Lung infections, bronchiectasis
Cystic fibrosis[75]
Esophageal/rectal dilatation or endoscopy[b,77]
Hereditary hemorrhagic telangiectasia
Pulmonary arteriovenous malformation[77]
Hepatopulmonary syndrome[78]
Septic abortion[80]

CONTIGUOUS SPREAD

Middle ear and/or mastoid infection
Sinusitis
Meningitis
Other focal infections (e.g., teeth, orbit, bone)
Penetrating head trauma
Ventriculoperitoneal shunt infection[89]
Postoperative intracranial surgery
Halo device to immobilize cervical spine[8]

[a]Within Hematogenous and Contiguous Spread, conditions are listed in order by relative frequency.
[b]It is unclear whether some infections result from direct spread from mucosal site via local drainage through the Batson plexis.

PART II Clinical Syndromes and Cardinal Features of Infectious Diseases: Approach to Diagnosis and Initial Management

SECTION F Central Nervous System Infections

Chronic pyogenic lung disease due to IgA or IgG deficiency or bronchiectasis in longstanding cystic fibrosis also are risks for brain abscess.[76] Rarely brain abscess occurs with pulmonary arteriovenous malformations,[77] aspirated foreign body or hepatopulmonary syndrome.[78] Endoscopy-associated brain abscess results from translocation of intestinal bacteria to paravertebral veins and from there into the cavernous sinus.[79] Septic abortion and in situ intrauterine devices are associated with brain abscess.[80]

Extension from nearby infection (middle ear, mastoid, sinus, orbit, face, or scalp) is the second most common cause of brain abscess; extension from middle ear is most frequent in young children and from paranasal sinuses in adolescents.[81-83] In the second decade of life, frontal, ethmoid, and sphenoid sinuses have thin bony/cartilaginous walls abutting the dura, allowing erosion (osteomyelitis) and ingress into the CNS. Other portals include pre-existing or posttraumatic anatomic cranial openings or diploic/emissary veins.

Bacterial meningitis rarely causes brain abscess except in neonates. Thrombophlebitis, venous stasis, and/or ischemia likely contribute to the pathogenesis. Focal deep cerebritis, deep infarcts, and pathogen virulence, e.g., *S. aureus* or *Cronobacter*, appear important for brain abscess formation. Rarely pyogenic infection between the lateral ventricles occurs due to anatomical communication with the ventricular system.[84]

Brain abscess following neurosurgery or head trauma is relatively rare, but penetrating skull injuries, such as dog bite,[85] pencil puncture,[86] lawn darts,[87] or open skull fracture, increase the risk. Oral flora can be injected via intraoral punctures (such as chopsticks).[88] Gut-associated ascending infection along a ventriculoperitoneal shunt or an untreated shunt infection can cause brain abscess.[89] Other rare causes are orthopedic halo devices[90] or intracranial migration of foreign bodies (e.g., sublaminar or interspinous wires in the cervical spine).[91] Pre-existing intracerebral hematoma, necrosis, or neoplasm rarely can serve as the nidus of infection.

Subdural Empyema

In young children, subdural empyema is a sequela of meningitis. In older children subdural empyema usually results from extracranial infection (e.g., middle ear, sinus, or calvarium).[33] Risk increases with post-mastoidectomy bone defects, prior craniotomy,[35] skull trauma,[35] septic phlebitis of emissary veins,[82] ventriculoperitoneal shunt,[89,92] pre-existing hematoma,[93] halo-pin traction,[94] BSI from lung abscess, or endoscopic procedures.[95]

Epidural Abscess

Intracranial epidural abscesses usually are extensions from infected sinuses,[96] middle ear, or orbit. Rarely, penetrating head injuries, fetal monitoring,[97] or wrestling injury[98] can be the source. The tightly adhering dura usually impedes expansion of epidural abscesses causing insidious clinical presentations. Epidural abscesses can extend (e.g., to the subdural space, brain) causing coexistent intracranial infections. MRSA is observed in epidural abscesses associated with deep lower extremity or pelvic septic venous thrombosis.[99]

Source of spinal epidural abscess usually is hematogenous (e.g., infected skin, soft tissue, bone, respiratory or urinary tract). Other sources are: nearby infections (bacterial meningitis, osteomyelitis, retropharyngeal, retroperitoneal, or abdominal abscess); iatrogenic introductions (post spinal fracture,[100] penetrating injury, spinal surgery, spinal fusion, spinal rod placement, lumbar puncture, steroid injection,[101] or epidural analgesia[102]); fistulas (Crohn disease),[103] midline neuroectodermal defects, dermal sinuses; or intradural tumors (e.g., lipoma). Almost one-third of cases of epidural abscess have no source identified.

Intracranial Septic Venous Thrombosis

Intracranial septic thrombosis can follow bacterial meningitis (especially thrombosis of the superior sagittal sinus), or arise from contiguous infections (sinuses, ear, face, or oropharynx) via emissary veins.[104] Lateral venous sinus involvement usually is otogenic, but cavernous sinus thromboses originate from teeth, paranasal/sphenoid sinuses, or face.[105] Septic venous sinus thrombosis can occur near an epidural abscess or by hematogenous spread. Certain conditions increase the risk for nonseptic thrombosis, e.g., sickle-cell disease, dehydration, or certain malignancies.

CLINICAL MANIFESTATIONS

Brain Abscess

The abscess location affects presenting signs and symptoms (Box 46-2). Frontal lobe abscesses may have prolonged asymptomatic

---

BOX 46-2. Signs and Symptoms in Relation to Site of Brain Abscess

ANY SITE
- Signs of increased intracranial pressure (often late signs)
  Headache, nausea, emesis, papilledema
  Depressed consciousness
- Behavioral changes
  Confusion, decreased attentiveness

FRONTAL LOBE
- Behavioral changes
  Personality changes, emotional lability, impulsive behavior
- Motor abnormalities
  Motor speech disorder (apraxia), forced grasping and sucking
  Focal weakness, hemiparesis

TEMPORAL LOBE
- General
  Ipsilateral headache
- Cranial nerve dysfunction
  Upper homonymous hemianopia, ipsilateral third cranial nerve palsy
- Motor abnormalities
  Speech dyspraxia, aphasia[a]
  Motor dysfunction of face and arm

PARIETAL LOBE
- Visual abnormalities
  Homonymous hemianopia, visual field defects in inferior quadrant
- Motor abnormalities
  Dysphasia,[a] speech dyspraxia[b]
- Perceptive abnormalities
  Contralateral spatial neglect[b]

INTRASELLAR
- Visual field defects
- Endocrine imbalance via altered pituitary function

CEREBELLAR
- Balance/perception abnormalities
  Lateral nystagmus (fast component toward lesion)
  Dizziness or central vertigo, ipsilateral ataxia, tremor
  Vomiting aggravated by motion
- Cranial nerve dysfunction
  Sixth cranial nerve palsy

BRAINSTEM
- Dysphasia
- Facial and multiple cranial nerve palsies
- Hemiparesis

[a]If abscess is in dominant hemisphere.
[b]If abscess is in nondominant hemisphere.

TABLE 46-4. Clinical Manifestations of Focal Suppurative Infections of the Central Nervous System by Percentage of Cases

Signs or Symptoms	Brain Abscess (%)	Subdural Empyema (%)	Cranial Epidural Abscess (%)	Septic Venous Thrombosis		
				Superior (%)	Lateral (%)	Cavernous (%)
Headache	60–70	60–80	100	70–90	80–90	75–90
Emesis	50–60	60–70	20–30	50–80	60–80	30–50
Fever	40–60	80–90	80–90	60–70	75–90	70–85
Focal neurologic deficit	35–50	30–40	10–20	40–60	60–75	75–90
Mental status change	30–40	60–80	50–60	55–75	20–45	15–30
Papilledema (usually late)	30–40	35–50	<5	40–60	25–40	65–80
Seizures	25–40	50–60	20–30	50–60	15–25	15–25
Meningeal signs	25–35	50–60	10–20	60–70	30–40	25–40
Hemiparesis	20–30	60–70	15–30	45–55	<5	<5
Coma	15–20	20–30	<5	60–80	25–45	10–15

periods, producing symptoms and signs only when mass effect increases intracranial pressure (ICP). Parietal lobe abscesses often remain silent until extending to the sensorimotor cerebral cortex. Pathogen virulence and host immune status also affect the clinical acuity. While the mean duration of bacterial brain abscess symptoms before diagnosis is 2 weeks, range is up to 4 months.[4]

The initial presentation of brain abscess in ~50% of cases includes headache, fever, and vomiting (Table 46-4). Lateralized headache in children should raise suspicion for organic intracranial pathology. Mental status changes or generalized seizures occur in fewer than 50% of cases of brain abscess. Focal neurologic abnormalities occur in 35% to 40%. Papilledema and meningismus occur in 30% of affected children. Coma, a late sign, occurs in 15% to 20%.

While fever, headache, and focal neurologic deficit suggest brain abscess, this triad occurs in fewer than 30%. Thus, pediatric brain abscesses often have nonspecific clinical presentations, and must be distinguished from other CNS processes (Table 46-5). Sudden clinical deterioration with meningismus suggests rupture of abscess into the ventricles or subarachnoid space.[106]

Intracranial Subdural Empyema

In infants, subdural empyema can evolve during appropriate antimicrobial therapy of bacterial meningitis, presenting with

bulging fontanel, persistent fever beyond 5 days of treatment, or new onset of neurologic findings (e.g., depressed responsiveness, seizures). Persistent meningismus plus fever also suggest subdural empyema.[35,107] Signs of increased ICP (vomiting, depressed responsiveness, enlarging head circumference, or papilledema) should trigger investigation for subdural empyema.[108]

In older children, subdural empyema mimics brain abscess, with fever or vomiting, or both but headache often is absent. Diagnosis sometimes is not made until the onset of hemiparesis or hemiplegia. After surgery or trauma, an overlying wound infection plus focal neurologic signs suggests subdural empyema.

Intracranial Epidural Abscess

Onset is insidious, with nonspecific symptoms (fever, headache sometimes with localized pain with tenderness, and mental status changes). Additional signs that are common in other intracranial suppurative processes (vomiting, seizures, focal neurologic deficits, papilledema, or meningeal signs) are relatively rare, developing only if mass effect or increased ICP occurs.

Unilateral facial pain with weakness of the ipsilateral ocular rectus muscle (Gradenigo syndrome) indicates an epidural abscess near the petrous bone. Confusion progressing rapidly to coma with focal or generalized seizures (symptoms of obstructed superior sagittal sinus) suggests an occipital epidural abscess.

Since 2000, MRSA has been the most common pathogen in epidural abscesses accompanying orbital cellulitis and acute sinusitis.[109]

Spinal Epidural or Subdural Abscess

Initially, spinal epidural abscess presents as localized or generalized back/flank pain exaggerated by movement, particularly spinal rotation. Local edema or tenderness to percussion also can occur, followed by nerve root pain, which can assist in abscess localization. Focal neurologic deficits (usually sensory and motor) develop early, progressing to weakness and impaired sensation. Signs then progress to paraparesis, bladder and/or bowel dysfunction, or altered consciousness. Early intervention prevents paralysis/paraplegia, which can occur in as few as 4 days from onset of nerve root pain or one week from initial back pain.

Spinal subdural abscess manifests similarly to epidural abscess, but can be differentiated by meningismus without focal spine tenderness to percussion.

Septic Venous Thrombosis

Clinical presentations vary based on the involved venous sinus. With complete thrombosis plus obstruction of blood flow in the superior sagittal sinus, severe generalized headache is common, but can be frontal. Soon, nausea, vomiting, and

TABLE 46-5. Differential Diagnosis of Brain Abscess

Infectious Etiologies	Noninfectious Etiologies	
	Vascular	Other
Meningitis	Hemorrhage	Primary tumor
Encephalitis[a]	Parenchymal	Metastatic tumor
Meningoencephalitis	Intracerebral	Multiple sclerosis
Subdural empyema	Subarachnoid	Acute disseminated
Mycotic aneurysm[b]	Subdural (chronic)	encephalomyelitis
Epidural abscess	Venous sinus	(ADEM)
Cranial osteomyelitis	thrombosis[d]	
Suppurative thrombosis	Cerebral infarction	
Cysticercosis	Migraine	
Tuberculoma[c]	Central nervous system	
Cryptococcosis	vasculitis	

[a]Especially when the etiologic agent is herpes simplex virus.

[b]As a result of septic embolus (e.g., endocarditis).

[c]Or tuberculous abscess.

[d]Nonseptic.

PART II   Clinical Syndromes and Cardinal Features of Infectious Diseases: Approach to Diagnosis and Initial Management

SECTION F   Central Nervous System Infections

meningismus develop, sometimes progressing rapidly to coma. Focal or generalized seizures or hemiparesis can occur. If venous obstruction is incomplete, symptoms are less severe and progress more slowly.

Cavernous sinus thrombosis can manifest with cranial nerve deficits (usually III and VI), plus prominent headache often localizing to the orbit or second branch of the trigeminal nerve. When present, unilateral periorbital edema quickly becomes bilateral.[105] Papilledema or dilated retinal veins occurs in 50% and meningismus in up to 33% of cases. Ptosis with ophthalmoplegia can cause impaired vision or blindness.

Septic thrombosis of the lateral sinus manifests subacutely, usually with temporal or occipital headache, followed by nausea, vomiting, and/or vertigo. The otogenic source often is detected via middle-ear examination (e.g., ruptured tympanic membrane or even cholesteatoma). Meningismus is less frequent than with cavernous sinus thrombosis, but altered mental status is more common. Soft-tissue swelling behind the auricle (Griesinger sign) or Gradenigo syndrome raise suspicion for lateral sinus thrombosis.

DIFFERENTIAL DIAGNOSIS

Extracranial foci often are sources for CNS suppurative infection, e.g., orbital suppurative complications of sinusitis. Simultaneous orbital and intracranial infection also can occur.[32,110] Multifocal intracranial or parameningeal CNS infection is not uncommon. For example, subdural empyema or brain abscess can accompany meningitis. With an orbital complication of sinusitis, rapidly progressing symptoms (e.g., changes in neurologic status) or poor response to antimicrobial therapy or to surgical drainage suggest a concurrent intracranial focus. Pott puffy tumor (with frontal sinusitis) (Figure 46-1) requires imaging studies to assess for an intracranial suppurative focus.[111]

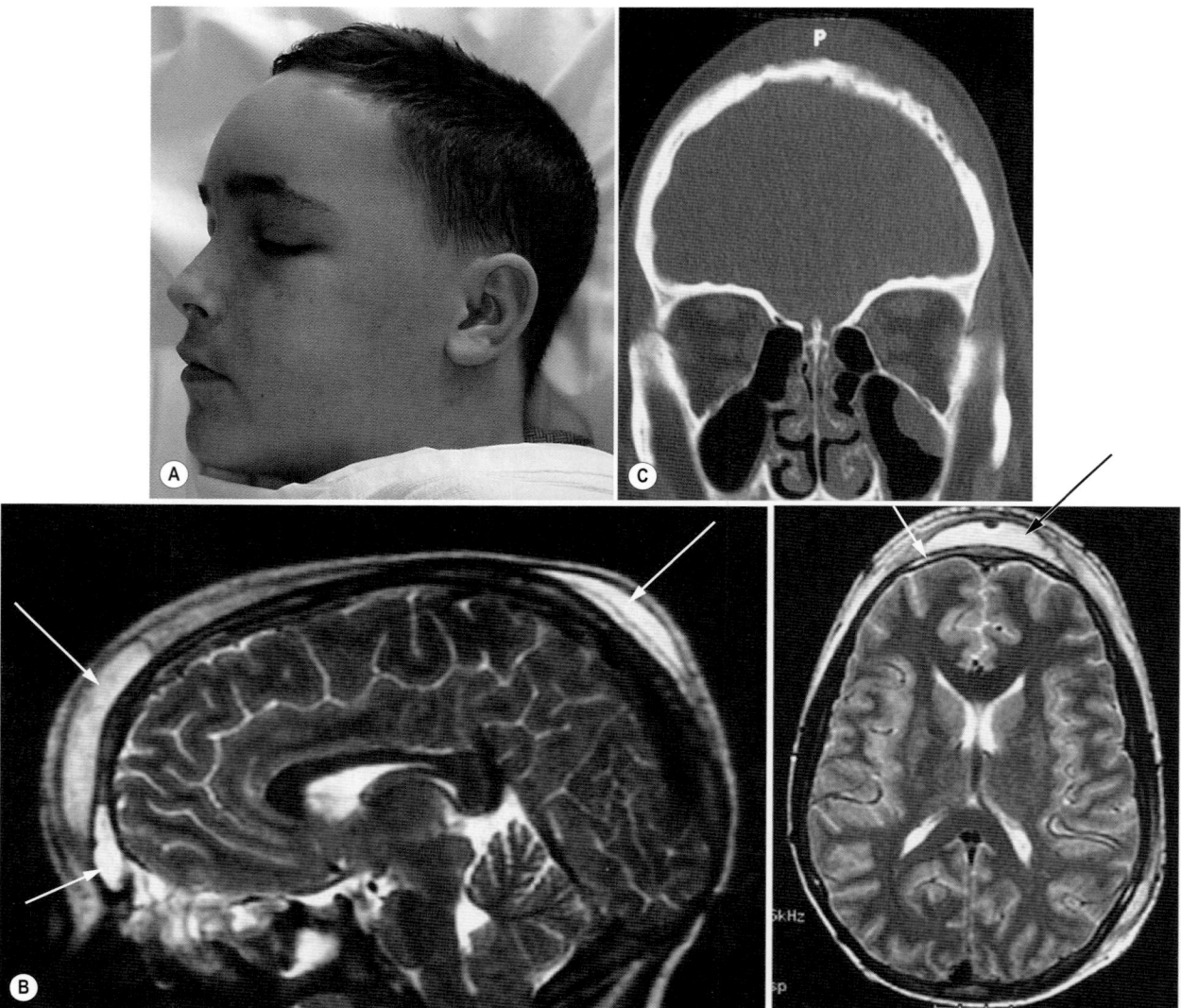

Figure 46-1. A 14-year-old presents with 1 week of high fever and chills, followed by facial and forehead pain and swelling. There is an edematous, tender, fluctuant mass over forehead and occiput **(A).** Computed tomography (CT) showed pansinusitis. Sagittal and axial, T$_2$-weighted MRI **(B)** revealed increased signal in extracranial frontal and occipital masses (long arrows), the frontal sinus (medium arrow), and frontal bone (short arrow). Blood culture yielded *Fusobacterium necrophorum.* Coronal CT after drainage confirmed osteomyelitis of the frontal bone **(C).** Prolonged antibiotics yielded complete recovery. (Courtesy of E.D. Thompson and S.S. Long, St. Christopher's Hospital for Children, Philadelphia, PA.)

Brain Abscess

The broad differential diagnosis of brain abscess includes infectious and noninfectious conditions (see Table 46-5), vascular and oncologic diagnoses being the most common noninfectious causes. Postinfectious acute disseminated encephalomyelitis should be considered if there is altered consciousness, seizures, headache, nausea, and emesis.

Focal suppurative CNS infection should be considered when any three of the following are present: fever, headache, nausea/emesis, increased ICP, altered consciousness, seizures (focal or generalized), or cranial nerve abnormality. However, these CNS symptoms/signs also can reflect nonpurulent conditions, infectious or otherwise, that mimic purulent brain abscess.

Extracerebral Intracranial Infections

Signs and symptoms usually are nonspecific, failing to differentiate among extracerebral and intracranial suppurations. However, the differential diagnosis of suppurative infection outside the brain resembles brain abscess, with some specific signs possibly narrowing the possibilities. With confirmed bacterial meningitis, focal neurologic signs warrant brain imaging for a focal complication. Meningismus is expected with meningitis, but if meningismus persists for >3 days into antibiotic therapy or the initial CSF was not fully compatible with purulent bacterial meningitis, a parameningeal suppurative focus should be considered. Persisting meningismus rarely indicates parenchymal brain abscess unless rapid clinical deterioration occurs due to abscess rupture into ventricles or parameningeal spaces. The exception is neonatal meningitis due to certain pathogens, e.g., *Cronobacter* or *Citrobacter* spp.

Cranial epidural abscess can be the result or the origin of other suppurative extra-CNS infections, e.g., orbital abscess or phlegmon, or of other CNS infections, such as meningitis, brain abscess, venous thrombophlebitis, or subdural empyema. Thus, clinical differentiation usually is not possible without neuroimaging.

The broad differential diagnosis of septic thrombosis of dural venous sinuses includes any cause of spontaneous, inflammatory, or posttraumatic thrombosis. These include disseminated intravascular coagulopathy, hypercoagulopathy (e.g., protein S and antithrombin III deficiency), polycythemia, sickle-cell anemia, dehydration, congenital heart disease, malformation of the vein of Galen, nephrotic syndrome, use of oral contraceptives, pregnancy, trauma, neoplasm, asphyxia, brain infarction, and pseudotumor syndrome. Other intracranial infections, such as brain abscess, subdural empyema, and meningitis, also are in the differential diagnosis. Cavernous sinus septic thrombosis can mimic orbital cellulitis or ophthalmoplegic migraine.

Spinal Infections

Symptoms and signs of spinal epidural abscess (or subdural empyema) can mimic diskitis, syphilis (tabes dorsalis), vertebral or spinal tuberculosis, bacterial or vertebral osteomyelitis, particularly *Bartonella henselae* vertebral infection. Acute transverse myelitis, spinal cord tumor, lymphoma, hematoma in the epidural space, subdural space or spine, as well as vascular malformation must be considered. A larger differential diagnosis is listed in two reviews of the literature.[112,113]

LABORATORY FINDINGS AND DIAGNOSIS

Routine Tests

Blood tests reveal nonspecific inflammation. Peripheral white blood cell (WBC) counts are >10,000 cells/mm³ in nearly 50% of children with brain abscess, but only 30% exceed 20,000/mm³ and only 25% exhibit a left shift (band forms >10%). The erythrocyte sedimentation rate (ESR) is insensitive, being normal in up to 40% of brain abscesses, particularly when associated with CCHD.[114] C-reactive protein (CRP) is more sensitive but is not specific.[115] Both ESR and CRP appear to be elevated more often when intracranial suppurative foci complicate sinusitis.[116] In spinal infection neither the ESR nor CRP is abnormal reliably.[117]

Blood cultures yield a pathogen in approximately 10% of brain abscesses.[3] Low-frequency delta waves on electroencephalogram are compatible with brain abscess.[4,118]

Cerebrospinal Fluid

With suspected focal intracranial suppuration, lumbar puncture is contraindicated until increased ICP is excluded by CT or MR to prevent significant morbidity, brainstem herniation, or even death.[3]

Completely normal CSF is found in up to 20% of cases of brain abscess. Elevated CSF protein (>40 mg/dL) occurs in 70% to 85%; mild to moderate pleocytosis (<500/mm³) occurs in 60% to 80%, with neutrophil predominance in 40% to 60%. Hypoglycorrhachia (<40 mg/dL) occurs in fewer than 33%. Pathogen growth from CSF cultures is low (<10%) except with coexisting meningitis or rupture of brain abscess into subarachnoid spaces. PCR testing of brain abscess material can provide rapid pathogen identification,[119] but is not widely available and sensitivity/specificity is not defined fully.

CSF findings with spinal epidural abscess or subdural empyema are nonspecific, with normal to moderately elevated neutrophil and protein values. Lumbar puncture through infection around the lumbar area, e.g., spinal epidural abscess, inadvertently can inoculate the CSF. Partial or complete obstruction of flow around the spinal cord by infection or tumor can elevate CSF protein concentration (>100 mg/dL), but usually fluid shows 100 to 300 WBC/mm³ (mostly lymphocytes) and normal glucose concentrations.

Imaging Studies

Imaging of brain, sinuses, middle ears, and orbits is critical to identify intracranial infections and potential sources and to formulate management.

Specific Considerations

Brain abscess. For suspected brain abscess, use of contrast-enhanced CT or MRI reduces mortality rates from brain abscess by 90% because lesions are diagnosed earlier, localized more accurately, and surgically drained more safely and completely.

Contrasted CT shows enhanced vascularity related to inflammation.[120] Typically, a hypodense signal from brain tissue edema surrounds a bright ring of signal enhancement, which in turn surrounds a central hypodense signal of the abscess core (Figure 46-2). Cerebritis appears similarly but components are not as well demarcated. CT findings can lag clinical manifestations by several days; an initially normal CT (particularly non-contrast-enhanced) does not exclude brain abscess. Further, neutropenia and corticosteroid therapy can diminish the intensity of ring enhancement.[121] Tumors, granulomas, resolving hematomas, or infarcts can produce ring enhancement.

Subdural empyema. Open fontanels can permit use of high-resolution ultrasonography to detect and differentiate subdural empyema from subdural effusion.[122] Intralesional particulate or shifting material suggest an empyema. CT is more specific and does not require an open fontanel. Non-contrast-enhanced CTs can demonstrate hypodense pus collections, but contrast-enhanced CT is superior at delineating the inflamed meninges or cerebral cortex (Figure 46-3). Higher resolution of MRI makes it superior to CT in detecting smaller lesions, extra-axial fluid near bones, and rim enhancement.[123] Neither CT nor routine MRI always definitely distinguished subdural empyema from reactive subdural effusion (the more common complication of

PART II Clinical Syndromes and Cardinal Features of Infectious Diseases: Approach to Diagnosis and Initial Management

SECTION F Central Nervous System Infections

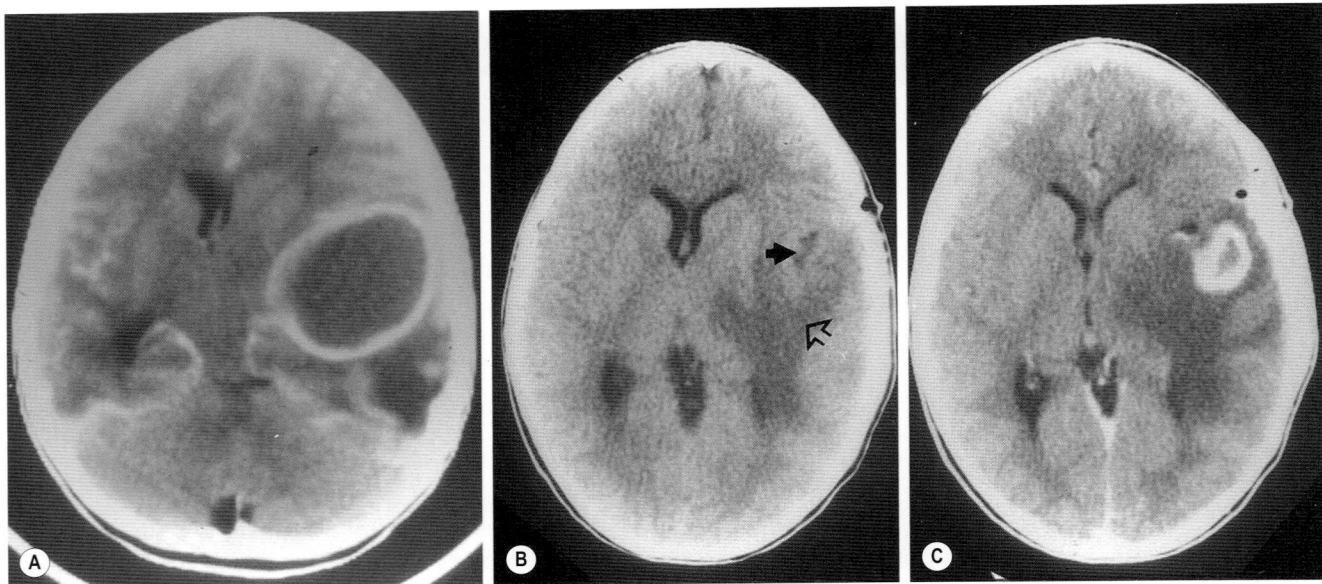

Figure 46-2. Computed tomography (CT) in a child with headache for 6 weeks and temporal lobe brain abscess. **(A)** CT with contrast at diagnosis shows intense ring enhancement and edema. **(B)** CT without contrast following surgical drainage shows a much smaller abscess cavity (solid arrow). Marked edema persists (open arrow). **(C)** Postsurgical contrasted CT reveals an abscess cavity with air, enhanced abscess wall, and marked edema. (Courtesy of M.A. Radkowski, MD, Children's Memorial Hospital, Chicago.)

meningitis). Diffusion-weighted imaging can improve characterization of subdural fluid.[124]

Epidural abscess. Cranial epidural abscesses show focal hypodense pus collections between the dura and calvarium on CT. Contrast-enhanced CT shows an enhanced rim around abscesses, displacing the dura (Figure 46-4). MRI reveals subdural abscesses in more detail, and otherwise undetected concomitant epidural abscesses.

Venous sinus thrombosis. Sagittal venous sinus thromboses in infants can be detected by ultrasonography.[125] Filling defects in thrombosed sinuses are visible in contrast-enhanced CT, e.g., in superior sagittal sinus thrombosis, as hypodense triangular areas surrounded by a hyperintense ring (the delta sign).[59] MRI seems even better for detecting diminished venous flow (Figure 46-5).

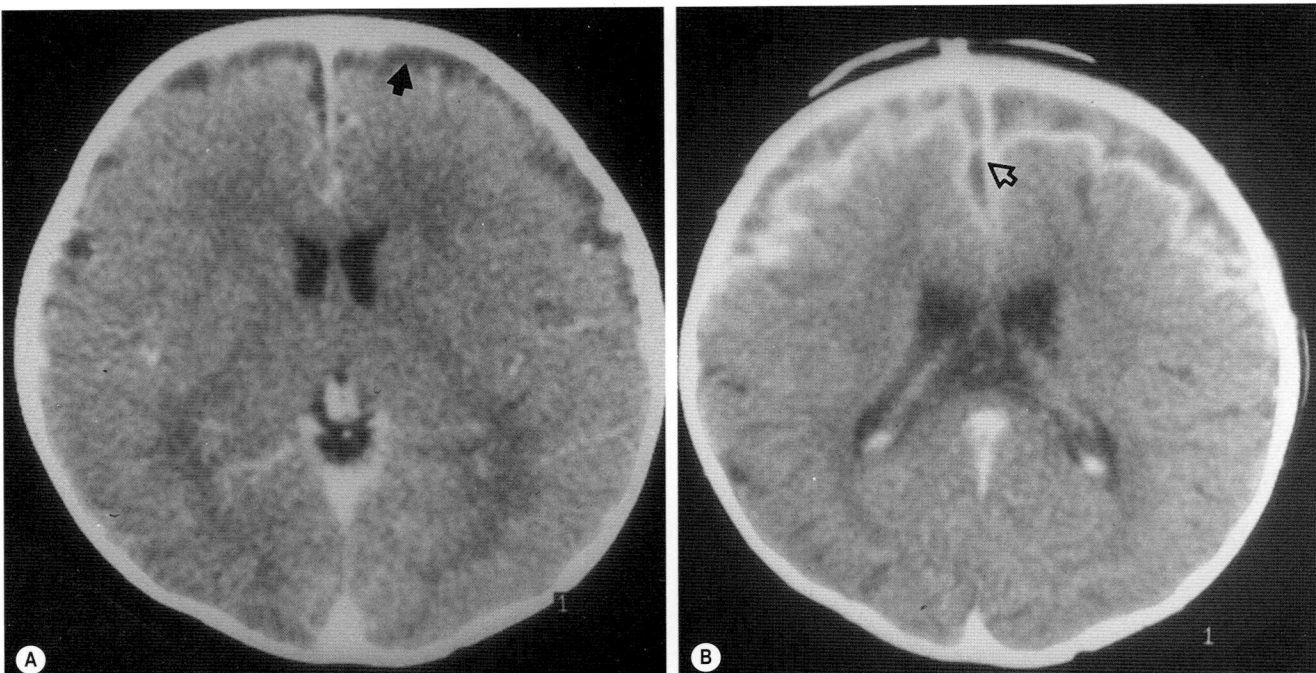

Figure 46-3. CT in an 8-month-old with meningitis and seizures during therapy **(A)** shows bilateral extra-axial fluid collections in the frontal region (solid arrow), suggesting early subdural empyema. **(B)** One week later, there is increased extra-axial fluid extending to the anterior interhemispheric fissure (open arrow) and enhanced membrane consistent with subdural empyema. (Courtesy of M.A. Radkowski, MD, Children's Memorial Hospital, Chicago.)

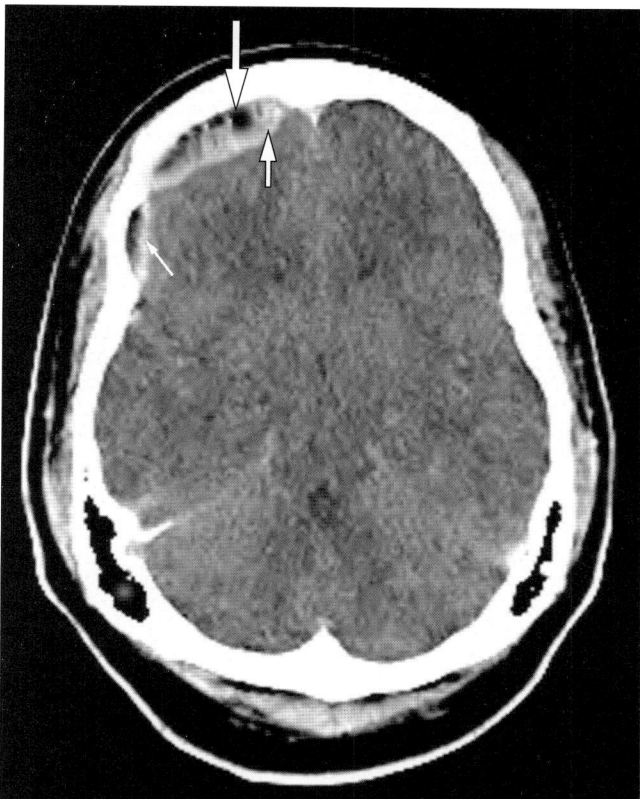

Figure 46-4. Contrast-enhanced CT of a 16-year-old with sinusitis and persistent fever despite therapy shows collections in the frontal region (large arrow), which is relatively large and has epidural abscess, and subdural extension (medium arrow). There is an additional small extra-axial collection consistent with epidural abscess (small arrow) in the parietal area. (Courtesy of Lisa Lowe, MD, Children's Mercy Hospitals and Clinics, Kansas City, MO.)

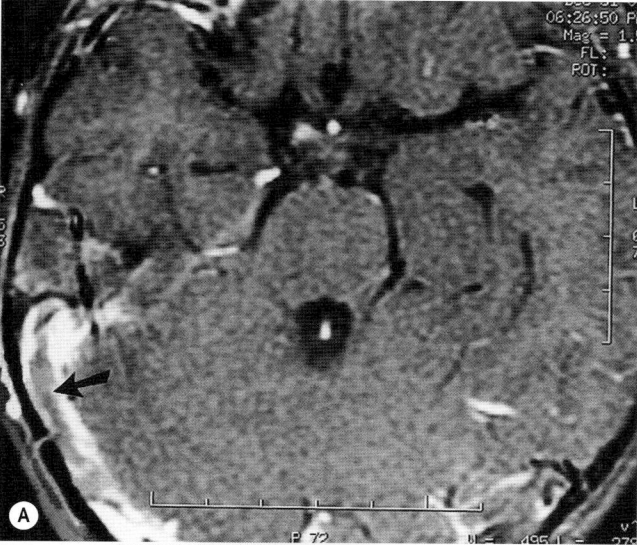

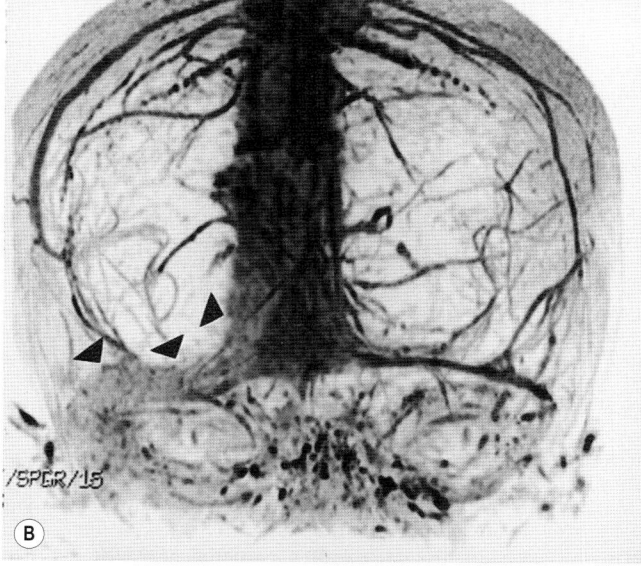

Figure 46-5. (A) T_1-weighted MRI with contrast shows thrombosis of the transverse (lateral) sinus. The greyish area (arrow) represents the thrombus itself. **(B)** Three-dimensional, time-of-flight MR angiography in the same patient shows complete blockage of the sinus, with extension of thrombus into the superior sagittal sinus (arrows). (A, courtesy of C. Darling, MD, Children's Memorial Hospital, Chicago.)

General Considerations

MRI is considered the most sensitive diagnostic test for intracranial suppurative infections because of superior soft-tissue detail compared with CT.[126] Lesions are detected earlier, and smaller lesions undetectable by CT can be apparent. Contrast-enhanced CT performed in both axial and coronal planes and extending through frontal bone and sella can avoid missing suppurative processes (e.g., epidural or interhemispheric abscess) not seen with standard maxillofacial or orbital CT.

Contrast-enhanced MRI differentiates abscess fluid from CSF and is more accurate for detecting possible abscess rupture.[127] If conventional and diffusion MRI does not differentiate abscess from cystic tumor, perfusion-weighted images may be useful. Because abscess capsules are hypovascular compared with tumor capsules, relative blood signal is different.[128] Although MRI is superior to CT for venous thrombosis and surrounding inflammation, magnetic resonance with angiography (MRA) can demonstrate diminished flow in occluded veins. MR spectroscopy also may distinguish bacterial brain abscess from necrotic brain tumor.[129]

MRI is superior to CT for epidural or subdural spinal abscesses, which are isointense on T_1-weighted but hyperintense on T_2-weighted images. Concomitant diskitis, osteomyelitis, or paraspinal abscess is identified easily. Further, MRI differentiates active inflammation from chronic granulation. MRI also is superior in differentiating the more common reactive subdural effusions from empyema, and subdural from epidural abscess. Because of intense radiation exposure from CT, MRI is the preferred follow-up test, particularly if MRI was the initial examination.

MANAGEMENT

Medical-Surgical Management Versus Medical Therapy Alone

CT- or MRI-guided stereotactic techniques revolutionized management of intracranial suppurative infections,[130] being minimally invasive and performed using local anesthesia with minimal risk of hemorrhage or complications. Pathogen detection in aspirates using Gram, acid-fast, India-ink, or specialized immunohistochemical stains as well as by aerobic/anaerobic, fungal, and mycobacterial culture allows specific antimicrobial therapy.

Brain Abscess

Antibiotic therapy plus open surgical drainage has been standard management. However, antimicrobial therapy without aspiration/

surgery is preferred (1) when concomitant bacterial meningitis is due to a confirmed pathogen; (2) when abscess is deep-seated or is in critical or high-risk anatomic sites; and (3) in poor surgical candidates. Nonsurgical therapy, even in ideal candidates, can fail. Follow-up is necessary, with repeated imaging studies if signs/symptoms do not resolve as expected, or if deterioration occurs. Improved findings (reduced ring enhancement, less edema, and less mass effect) generally occur within 1 to 2 weeks of initiating therapy in patients responding favorably to nonsurgical management. Reduced abscess size usually occurs within 2 to 4 weeks.

Antibiotics plus aspiration of the lesion are successful with small (<3 cm) well-encapsulated brain abscesses in alert, clinically stable patients without signs of increased ICP.[131] It may not be possible to sample each of multiple abscesses, but aspiration of at least one abscess by CT-guided technique should be helpful.

Identification of the antibiotic susceptibilities of pathogen/s from blood (10% or less of patients), CSF culture (<10% of patients), or CT-guided aspiration of abscess material (65%) improve likelihood of treatment success in the absence of open surgery.

Patients failing nonsurgical management or with large abscesses require intervention, either closed stereotactic aspiration, or craniotomy hopefully with excision. Disadvantages of stereotactic aspiration can be the need (in some cases) for repeated aspirations (possibly more tissue damage or bleeding) and the relative inaccessibility of posterior fossa lesions. Excision is preferred for: (1) fungal or helminthic abscesses not responding to medical therapy; (2) posterior fossa abscesses, especially with coma or brainstem compression;[132] (3) failure despite aspiration of multiloculated abscesses; and (4) re-accumulation following repeated aspirations.[133]

Reports suggest cure rates of >90% from combining: (1) surgical aspiration or removal of all abscesses >2.5 cm in diameter; (2) ≥6weeks of effective antibiotics; and (3) repeat neuroimaging to ensure abscess cavity resolution prior to cessation of antibiotics.[132]

Decision on duration of therapy, as well as intravenous versus oral formulations, is individualized. With expected improvement in clinical and imaging findings, antibiotics are continued for 3 to 6 weeks. The shorter 3- to 4-week course is reasonable if complete surgical excision of the brain abscess is possible.[134] Follow-up imaging studies near the end of the proposed treatment duration should provide evidence of lesion improvement before stopping therapy, and provide a baseline in the case of later symptoms/signs suggesting relapse. The endpoint should be resolution of the abscess cavity, not absence of enhanced signal. Repeat imaging in asymptomatic patients beyond this is not necessary and can be misleading, because enhanced signal persists beyond resolution of infection.

Corticosteroid treatment for brain abscess is controversial and is used infrequently because of potential disadvantages including reduced antibiotic penetration through the steroid-stabilized blood–brain barrier. However, small series have not shown increased mortality, or significant outcome differences, related to corticosteroid use.[135] Corticosteroids directly decrease ring enhancement out of proportion to improvement in infection, and "rebound" of enhancement can occur upon discontinuation, compromising interpretation of repeated imaging. Corticosteroids should be used only with severe or progressively increased ICP or neurologic deterioration, when reduction of edema may be life-saving. A short course (3 to 6 days) of high-dose dexamethasone (1 to 2 mg/kg per day divided q6 hours) generally is considered safe.

Extracerebral Abscesses

Antibiotics alone are sufficient for relatively small subdural empyemas (<3 cm in diameter) or neurologically stable patients rapidly responding to empiric therapy.[35,136] Appropriate antibiotic therapy plus aspiration of subdural empyemas accompanying bacterial meningitis are sufficient because of known antimicrobial susceptibilities for the pathogens. Subdural empyema from other

causes (e.g., contiguous site infection or after penetrating trauma) may not be aspirated easily, necessitating burr holes or craniotomy. The empyema's location and extent dictate the type of drainage procedure. Although craniotomy provides better evacuation of pus from larger empyemas, burr holes plus irrigation can be effective.[137] Irrigating empyema cavities with antibiotics is not recommended or supported by current data. As little as 2 weeks of intravenous antibiotics can be sufficient in patients with subdural empyema completely drained by craniotomy.[138]

Unless cranial epidural abscess is <1 cm in diameter or close to critical structures making intervention dangerous, drainage and debridement plus appropriate antibiotic systemically usually is recommended. Exceptions are isolated epidural abscesses with minimal mass effect complicating sinusitis, in which case adequate sinus drainage plus appropriate antibiotics can be sufficient.[139,140] Repeat MRI should show reduced abscess size and absence of subdural extension. Decreased abscess size may occur only after 2 weeks of therapy. Total antibiotic therapy for 3 to 4 weeks is adequate except with concomitant osteomyelitis (when total therapy usually is 4 to 6 weeks).

In most cases of infection with suppurative complete venous thrombosis, appropriate antibiotics plus surgical drainage of the suppurative source is performed.[105] Anticoagulant therapy is controversial because of the fear of hemorrhage[141] but is becoming standard care, particularly with incompletely thrombosed obstruction of a lateral sinus. The risk of hemorrhage appears to be low, and early anticoagulant treatment appears beneficial, in patients when no existing hemorrhagic complications are seen by CT or MRI.[142] Internal jugular vein ligation is not necessary, but repeated MRI/CT monitoring for progression of thrombosis is important.

For spinal epidural or subdural abscess, urgent drainage and appropriate antibiotics are critical to halting progressive permanent neurologic deficits. Endoscopy is the procedure of choice instead of open laminectomy.[143] Antibiotics alone can be successful in patients with localized pain but without progression of root pain or spinal cord compression, or in patients stable for more than 3 days without radiculopathy or signs of partial cord compression.[144] Frequent MRI studies are important to document regression.

Antibiotic regimen for spinal epidural/subdural abscess should be designed to adequately penetrate to the site and generally is given for 3 to 4 weeks, unless osteomyelitis is present when therapy may be as long as 8 weeks. The duration of intravenous antibiotics depends on the extent of the epidural or subdural abscess, accompanying foci of infection (e.g., myositis or osteomyelitis), and drug susceptibility of identified pathogens and bioavailability of oral forms of drug. Adequate CSF penetration is important with subdural abscesses, but is not as critical with epidural abscesses without a concomitant intradural or brain focus. Intravenous therapy for as few as 5 to 7 days can be effective, if therapy can be completed using oral agent(s) having sufficient bioavailability (fluoroquinolones, linezolid, clindamycin, rifampin).

Specific Antimicrobial Regimens

Recommended empiric antibiotics (Table 46-6) are based on likely pathogens, predisposing conditions, expected susceptibility patterns, and concentration of antibiotic(s) at infected sites.[145] Recommendations are based on clinical experience or case series (mostly in adults) because there are no well-controlled pediatric trials.

Ceftriaxone (or cefotaxime) plus metronidazole had been appropriate empiric therapy for brain abscess and subdural empyema accompanying otitis media, mastoiditis, sinusitis, or CCHD until newly emerged serotype 19A pneumococci became resistant to third-generation cephalosporins. Vancomycin is added to empiric regimens for coverage of resistant pneumococci and MRSA. Small numbers of patients with brain abscesses have been treated successfully with alternative antibiotics, such as imipenem,[146] meropenem,[147] and ciprofloxacin[148] but these have no MRSA activity. Approximately 25% of S. pneumoniae 19A strains are carbapenem-resistant, so carbapenem use requires confirmed

TABLE 46-6. Empiric Therapy for Brain Abscess Based on Predisposing Factors

Predisposing Factor	Antibiotic (Dose)
Congenital heart disease	Vancomycin (60 mg/kg per day) *plus* ceftriaxone (100 mg/kg per day)[a] *plus* metronidazole (30 mg/kg per day)[b]
Dental pathology	Penicillin (300,000 U/kg per day) *plus* metronidazole[b] (as above); *or* Ampicillin-sulbactam (300–400 mg/kg per day)[c]
Sinusitis, mastoiditis, and/or otitis media[d,e]	Vancomycin (as above) *plus* ceftriaxone (as above) *plus* metronidazole[a] (as above)[b]
Penetrating trauma or post surgery	Vancomycin (60 mg/kg per day) *plus* ceftriaxone (100 mg/kg per day)[a] or cefepime (150 mg/kg per day)
Meningitis	
Neonates	Cefotaxime (50 mg/kg/dose) *plus* ampicillin (100 mg/kg/dose) with dosing interval for each drug being q12h in first week of life, q8h from 8 to 28 days of life and q6h >28 days of life)
Infants and children	Ceftriaxone[a] (as above) *plus* vancomycin[b] (60 mg/kg per day)
Endocarditis	
Natural valve	Ampicillin[f] (as above) *plus* aminoglycoside (maximum doses); *or* Ceftriaxone (as above) *plus* vancomycin (as above)
Prosthetic valve	Vancomycin (as above) *plus* gentamicin
Unknown or immunocompromised[g]	Vancomycin (as above) *plus* ceftazidime (see below) *plus* metronidazole

[a]*Cefotaxime (300 mg/kg per day), can be substituted.*

[b]*If anaerobic bacteria are resistant to metronidazole, change to meropenem (120 mg/kg per day), or in countries where still available, use chloramphenicol (80–100 mg/kg per day).*

[c]*Ampicillin-sulbactam (≥300–400 mg/kg per day of ampicillin) acceptable only if MRSA or penicillin-resistant pneumococcus is not a risk.*

[d]*When staphylococci or penicillin-resistant* Streptococcus pneumoniae *is suspected, add vancomycin.*

[e]*With chronic otitis media or sinusitis, change to ceftazidime (150–200 mg/ kg per day) or cefepime 100 mg/kg per day.*

[f]*Penicillin (300,000–400,000 U/kg per day) can be substituted.*

[g]*If no response within 1 week and organism is unknown, consider amphotericin B.*

TABLE 46-7. Antifungal Therapy for Central Nervous System Focal Infections

Pathogen	Therapy	Alternative Therapy
Candida spp.	Amphotericin B + flucytosine	Liposomal amphotericin or fluconazole
Aspergillus spp.	Voriconazole	Amphotericin B + flucytosine or liposomal amphotericin or caspofungin[a]
Agents of mucormycosis	Amphotericin B[b]	Liposomal amphotericin + itraconazole or amphotericin + rifampin[a]
Coccidioides immitis	Amphotericin B	Fluconazole or liposomal amphotericin or caspofungin[a]
Cryptococcus neoformans	Amphotericin B + flucytosine	Liposomal amphotericin or fluconazole
Blastomyces dermatitidis	Amphotericin B	Liposomal amphotericin or fluconazole
Histoplasma capsulatum	Amphotericin B	Liposomal amphotericin or fluconazole
Pseudallescheria spp.	Voriconazole[a]	Itraconazole[a] or caspofungin[a]

[a]*Limited experience.*

[b]*While hyperbaric oxygen has been used as adjunct therapy, results have been controversial.*

Doses: Amphotericin B, 1.0–2.0 mg/kg per day; liposomal amphotericin, 5 mg/kg per day starting dose; fluconazole, 10–12 mg/kg per day; itraconazole, 10–12 mg/kg per day; flucytosine, 100–150 mg/kg per day; rifampin, 20 mg/kg per day; voriconazole, 8–10 mg/kg per day; caspofungin, 70 mg/m^2 per day (maximum 70 mg/day).

susceptibility. Pneumococcal 19A strains are rarely (<3% in the United States) resistant to fluoroquinolones, but only anecdotal data exist for use in intracranial abscesses. Likewise vancomycin will likely be needed empirically due to increasing MRSA in complicated sinusitis and orbital infections or coagulase-negative staphylococci in focal CNS infections (penetrating head trauma, ventriculoperitoneal shunts, or prosthetic valve endocarditis).

Vancomycin, a third-generation cephalosporin plus anaerobic coverage is the recommended empirical regimen for CNS infections because of their polymicrobial nature. Some experts use cefepime as the third-generation cephalosporin when *Pseudomonas* spp. is considered, i.e., with chronic otitis media or sinusitis, following neurosurgery or in immunocompromised patients.

In neonates, cefotaxime plus ampicillin is preferred because *S. pneumoniae* is rare, whereas *Listeria monocytogenes* or enterococci remain potential pathogens.

For brain abscess associated with α-streptococcal endocarditis on a natural valve, high-dose combination therapy recommended for endocarditis (e.g., penicillin plus aminoglycoside) is useful although aminoglycosides in purulent collections can be relatively ineffective (low pH and low oxygen content reduces binding to ribosome). Therapy with a third-generation cephalosporin appears to be a reasonable alternative.

Nocardia brain abscesses are rare and are treated with trimethoprim-sulfamethoxazole (15 to 20 mg of trimethoprim/kg per day divided every 6 or 8 hours). If local TMP-SMX resistance is present, or response is inadequate, carbapenems or a third-generation cephalosporin plus amikacin or minocycline may be effective. Linezolid was reported effective against multiple *Nocardia* brain abscesses.[149] CSF/CNS penetration of linezolid is 44% to 69% in adults.[150,151]

Prevalence of fungal species in brain abscesses parallels other invasive fungal disease. In one review[152] including all ages, *Candida* spp. were most common (42%), followed by *Aspergillus* (29%), other molds (14%), and *Cryptococcus* (4% and mostly in adults). Endemic fungi (*Histoplasma, Blastomyces, Coccidioides*, 3%) occur mostly in defined endemic geographic areas. *Scedosporium* spp. is seen increasingly, particularly in stem cell transplant recipients.

Antifungal therapy for focal CNS infection is challenging, and is based on fungicidal activity against confirmed pathogen and pharmacodynamics (Table 46-7). Data from double-blind well-controlled treatment trials in CNS fungal infections are scant for single agents, let alone myriad possible combinations given four classes of drugs (polyenes, pyrimidine analogues, imidazoles, and echinocandins) and multiple class members (see pathogen-specific chapters and Chapter 293, Antifungal Agents).

COMPLICATIONS AND PROGNOSIS

About two-thirds of brain abscess patients recover without sequelae. Pediatric mortality fell from over 30% in the preimaging era to 3% to 15% after standard use of CT.[153] A higher mortality occurs with rapid onset (<4 days), severe mental status changes at diagnosis, or rapidly progressing neurologic impairment.[135] Higher mortality is associated with multiple abscesses,[4] and with rupture of abscess into ventricles (40% mortality despite aggressive management).[154] Seizures develop in 10% to 30% of

PART II Clinical Syndromes and Cardinal Features of Infectious Diseases: Approach to Diagnosis and Initial Management

SECTION F Central Nervous System Infections

patients following treatment of brain abscess, with onset sometimes several years after treatment.[155] Frontal or temporal lobe abscess, or any large abscess, is associated with a higher incidence of seizures. Other sequelae include hemiparesis (10% to 15%), cranial nerve palsy (5% to 10%), hydrocephalus (5% to 10%), and behavioral and intellectual disorders (more serious in children <5 years of age[156]). Less common sequelae include spasticity, ataxia, optic atrophy, and visual deficits.

Outcomes for patients with subdural empyema also improved with CT/MRI use and improved surgical techniques;[35] mortality is <2%.[157] Mortality is lowest (<10%) if the patient is alert at presentation and highest (>50%) if the patient is comatose at presentation. The 5% to 10% of patients with venous sinus thrombosis accompanying subdural empyema have increased morbidity and mortality. Patients with subdural empyema have more persistent neurologic problems (15% to 40%), e.g., seizures or hemiparesis.[35]

Uncomplicated intracranial epidural abscesses, e.g., no accompanying subdural empyema or brain abscess, have excellent prognoses. However, delay in diagnosis can produce long-term neurologic sequelae similar to those after subdural empyema or brain abscess.

Suppurative septic sinus thrombosis is associated with 25% to 35% mortality despite improved diagnostic tools and antibiotic therapy.[61] With superior sagittal sinus involvement, complete occlusion has the highest mortality while anterior segment thrombosis commonly is associated with complete recovery.[61] Lateral sinus thrombosis is associated with sequelae in up to 20%, e.g., hearing loss, decreased visual activity, brain abscess, or rarely meningitis.[105] Cavernous sinus thrombosis is associated with sequelae in up to 33%, e.g., blindness, oculomotor paralysis, hemiparesis, or pituitary insufficiency.[158]

The prognosis with spinal epidural or subdural abscess is excellent if therapy begins before radicular symptoms appear. The overall mortality is <10%.[159] Long-term sequelae correlate with the duration of paralysis before surgery, the degree of thecal sac compression, and younger age.[72,160] Common neurologic sequelae include sphincter disturbance, spasticity, and paraparesis.

47 Eosinophilic Meningitis

Marian G. Michaels and Klara M. Posfay-Barbe

The finding of even a few eosinophils in human cerebrospinal fluid (CSF) raises suspicion of certain pathologic states. Helminthic infestation of the central nervous system (CNS), particularly with the rat lungworm *Angiostrongylus cantonensis*, is the most common cause of eosinophilic meningitis worldwide.[1-6] The differential diagnosis of CSF eosinophilia, however, is broad and includes infestation by other parasites, such as the raccoon ascarid *Baylisascaris procyonis*;[7-16] reaction to placement, malfunction or infection of a ventriculoperitoneal shunt;[17-19] medications;[20-22] malignancies;[23,24] hypereosinophilic syndrome;[25] and an unusual manifestation of a more common fungal, bacterial, or viral infection of the CNS.[26-30] Table 47-1 lists the causes of eosinophilic meningitis to be considered.

Eosinophilic meningitis is defined as: (1) at least 10 eosinophils/mm³ in CSF; or (2) eosinophils making up at least 10% of the white blood cells in CSF, but the presence of eosinophils in the CSF should always be considered as an abnormal finding.[5] Diagnostic examination of CSF should always include Giemsa, Wright, or other stain of a cytocentrifuged specimen to delineate the exact composition of pleocytosis, as well as routine CSF examination, including Gram stain, quantitative cell count, and biochemical tests.[5]

INFECTIOUS CAUSES

Helminths

Angiostrongylus cantonensis

The rat lungworm, *A. cantonensis*, is the most common cause of eosinophilic meningitis worldwide. Although no cause is predominant in the United States, it is important that clinicians consider parasitic infections in cases of eosinophilic meningitis on one hand, and warn travelers to endemic areas about the risks of dietary indiscretions on the other hand. *Angiostrongylus* infestation has been the subject of several reviews.[1-4,31,32] CNS migration is characteristic of the lungworm's normal life cycle in the rat as well as in the accidental human host. Adult worms live in the rat pulmonary arteries and lay eggs in the lung. After

hatching, larvae make their way through the alveolar spaces and up the trachea, from which they are swallowed and then excreted in rat feces.

Many species of slugs and snails serve as intermediate hosts, in which the larvae develop into infectious third-stage larvae. When third-stage larvae are ingested by rats, the definitive host, larvae migrate across the intestinal wall and are carried by the circulatory system to the brain. Juvenile worms have been found in the eyes, brain, and spinal cord in human infections.[33] In the CNS, larvae undergo two more moltings and mature into adult worms; the worms return to the pulmonary arteries to renew the cycle. Human infection occurs after consumption of raw snails, shrimp, or fish that have fed on infected snails. Likewise, infectious larvae can be ingested accidentally on raw vegetables, raw vegetable juice, or fomites contaminated with snail slime.[3,4,31,34,35] CNS tropism is retained in human infection; however, the life cycle is disrupted, and generally, the disease is self-limited, with larvae dying in the CNS.

Human infection by *A. cantonensis* probably is more widespread than believed and has been found in Asia, notably in Thailand, Malaysia, and China; the South Pacific, including Taiwan, Hawaii, American Samoa, New Guinea, Indonesia, and Australia; India, Egypt, Brazil, and the Caribbean.[1-4,32,36] Worms can migrate on ships within their natural hosts (the rat) to distant countries, including mainland U.S.[35] The first reported, nonimported case in the U.S. was a child from New Orleans who reported eating a raw snail "on a dare."[37] The child had meningitis that abated with supportive care.

In adults, symptoms classically begin 2 to 35 days after infection, with acute onset of headaches.[1-4] Other common complaints are nausea, and vomiting, weakness, paresthesias or hyperesthesias, pruritus, somnolence, and cranial nerve palsies, especially optic nerve and nerves VII and VIII.[1-4,35,38] About 20% of patients also have a stiff neck.[33] Fever is usually of low grade if present. Hearing loss has been reported, as has retinal detachment or hemorrhage.[15,39] Most patients recover completely, with symptoms beginning to abate within several weeks of the initial neurologic manifestations. Headaches and paresthesias can be more persistent.[3,38] Neurologic symptoms may not be due only to mechanical

TABLE 47-1. Causes of Eosinophilic Meningitis (EM)

Cause	Association with EM	Possible Transmission	Country	Comments
NEMATODES (ROUNDWORMS)	Most common causes			
Angiostrongylus cantonensis		Contact with rat lungworm; consumption of snail, slug, crustacean, mollusk, crab; frogs, fish, lizards; lettuce and vegetable	South Pacific, Africa, Australia, Caribbean, Hawaii, U.S. port cities	Neurotropic Usually self-limited
Baylisascaris procyonis		Contact with raccoon or feces; rarely dogs, rodents, small mammals, birds	U.S.	Neurotropic Prolonged, profound encephalitis Young children with pica are typical patients
Gnathostoma spinigerum		Contact with dog, cat; consumption of raw fish, poultry, crustaceans, amphibians	Southeast Asia, Japan, China, Mexico, Central and South America, Africa, and the Middle East	Peripheral eosinophilia common
Ascaris lumbricoides		Exposure to embryonated eggs in human feces	Worldwide	Rarely associated with EM
Trichinella spiralis		Consumption of raw or undercooked meat	Worldwide; endemic in Japan and China	Larvae usually found in skeletal muscle Rarely associated with EM
CESTODES (TAPEWORMS)	Occasional causes			
Taenia solium		Exposure to eggs in human feces	Worldwide	Neurocysticercosis is a rare cause of EM
Echinococcus granulosus		Exposure to eggs in feces sheep; wolves, dogs, moose, reindeer	Europe; northern North America and Eurasia	Rarely infects CNS and associated with EM
OTHER PARASITES	Rare			
Toxoplasma gondii		Consumption of undercooked meat; exposure to oocyst in cat feces	Worldwide	Anecdotal report
Schistosoma japonicum		Contaminated water	Worldwide, tropical and subtropical; most cases Africa	
Paragonimus westermani		Contaminated water	Far East	Lung fluke but can invade CNS and other sites
Fasciola hepatica		Contaminated water	Worldwide; southeast Asia	
FUNGI	Occasional			
Coccidioides immitis		Exposure to aerosolized arthroconidia	Southwestern U.S., Mexico, South America	Low level of CSF eosinophils common; true EM also reported
Cryptococcus neoformans		Environmental exposure		Diabetes is a risk factor
BACTERIA AND VIRUSES	Case reports			
Treponema pallidum		Exposure to infected person	Worldwide	EM rarely associated with neurosyphilis
Mycobacterium tuberculosis		Exposure to infected person	Worldwide	Questionable association with direct CNS infection versus treatment
Rickettsia rickettsii		Tick bite	North, Central and South America	Rare
Lymphocytic choriomeningitis virus		Exposure to rodents	Worldwide	Association made through serologic studies
Ventricular shunt bacterial infections				Same pathogens as in shunt infections without eosinophils
NONINFECTIOUS ETIOLOGIES	Occasional or case reports	Not applicable	All or not applicable	
Ventricular shunt complications/reaction to shunt material				No infection and improvement with removal of shunt
Systemic drugs				Reported with fluoroquinolones, nonsteroidal anti-inflammatory drugs and illicit drugs intravenously
CNS neoplasms				Reported with Hodgkin lymphoma, acute lymphoblastic leukemia, and primary CNS tumors
Hypereosinophilic syndrome				Reported in patients without other cause
Immunologic/hypersensitivity reaction				Reported with sarcoidosis or rabies vaccine

CNS, central nervous system; CSF, cerebrospinal fluid; EM, eosinophilic meningitis.

damage caused by worm migration in the brain, but also to the neurotoxicity of eosinophil-derived basic proteins.

Infected children may not complain of headache. Clinical manifestations in younger patients can be more insidious, with upper respiratory symptoms, cough, and fever preceding mental status changes, seizures, or focal neurologic abnormalities.[2,6,34] Psychiatric changes also have been reported.[40] One series of 16 young adults consuming raw infected great African *Achatina fulica* snails in American Samoa was notable for the absence of headache as a major complaint.[41] All of the patients experienced severe radiculomyeloencephalitis; one died. Unlike other intermediate hosts or contaminated vegetables, *A. fulica* snails can contain thousands of parasites, possibly accounting for the more fulminant course in patients who acquire parasites from consuming these snails. Other reported fatalities or sequelae are observed primarily in young children, who are at risk for acquiring a relatively higher infectious load.[2,34,42]

CSF examination reveals pleocytosis typically between 150 and 2000 WBCs per mm^3.[1,2,41] Peak eosinophilia occurs between 2 and 4 weeks of illness, with CSF eosinophils representing a median of 49% of the total WBCs (range, 15% to 97%).[1-4,6,34,42] The CSF protein value often is elevated, and the glucose value is normal or mildly decreased.[1,2] Peripheral eosinophilia is common but does not correlate with the extent of CNS eosinophilia.[1,2,4] Coincident infections with other parasites may contribute to peripheral eosinophilia.

A diagnosis of eosinophilic meningitis is usually made on the basis of clinical presentation in patients who are from or are traveling from an area enzootic for *A. cantonensis* and have a consistent dietary history. Consumption of Caesar salad was strongly associated in a Jamaican outbreak.[35] The history of eating raw seafood can be absent in young children who have a propensity for pica.[6,34,42] On occasion, worms are found in the CSF, especially if a large-bore cannula is used for removal of CSF or if CSF is aspirated rather than allowed to flow by gravity.[2] Enzyme immunosorbent assays to detect antibody in serum or CSF have been developed and are available in enzootic areas and can be facilitated by contact with the Centers for Disease Control and Prevention Disease Surveillance Division of Parasitic Infections (770-488-7775).[3,4]

Baylisascaris procyonis

The ascarid parasite of the raccoon, *Baylisascaris procyonis*, is found in 20% to 90% of both rural and urban raccoons in the U.S.[8,43-45] Evidence of raccoon latrines near human habitation[44] increases the concern for this emerging infection, which has been highlighted in several reviews.[12,46] Like *A. cantonensis*, this ascarid migrates through the CNS during its normal life cycle and is neurotropic in humans.[7,8,12,46] The ascarid causes little disease in the raccoon, but ingestion of eggs by aberrant hosts, such as foxes, rabbits, birds, and humans, can result in migration of larvae, which cause severe CNS damage. Experimental disease in nonhuman primates consists of eosinophilic meningitis, neurologic deterioration, coma, and death (discussed in references 8, 12, 46). Despite the high prevalence of this parasite in raccoons, *B. procyonis* is rarely documented in humans. In the U.S., just over a dozen clinical cases have been reported, most commonly in young children, resulting in eosinophilic meningoencephalitis with dramatic eosinophilic CSF pleocytosis, severe neurologic devastation, and, in 6 patients, death.[7,8,12,46-49] Ocular larva migrans and visceral larva migrans also can occur.[12,50] Exposure to raccoon droppings near nesting sites is the expected mode of acquisition. Recently, however, behavior related to substance abuse has been identified as a possible risk factor.[51] Because clinician awareness of this parasite is limited, and diagnosis is not straightforward, it is possible that the disease is more widespread and that less severe symptoms remain undiagnosed.[52] Asymptomatic infection has been suspected by finding a low level of seropositivity in otherwise healthy children (reviewed in references 12 and 46). As improved serodiagnostic assays become more readily available, the true incidence and clinical array will become more apparent. Currently

serologic testing of serum and CSF is only available from the Department for Veterinary Pathobiology at Purdue University, West Lafayette, IN (765-494-7558).

Gnathostoma spinigerum

The nematode of dogs and cats, *Gnathostoma spinigerum*, is commonly found in Thailand and other parts of Southeast Asia, but its prevalence is increasing in Mexico and Central and South America.[38] *Gnathostoma* can cause visceral larva migrans when it infects humans who consume raw or undercooked fish, frogs, pigs, snakes, fowl, eels, or poultry containing third-stage larva or, rarely, have direct larval penetration of the skin.[19,31,38] Gnathostomiasis typically presents as cutaneous, visceral, or CNS forms. Gnathostomiasis most often is characterized by migratory subcutaneous nodules, but larvae can wander to organs and cause local symptoms[53] or enter the CNS via the nerve root, causing a myeloencephalitis.[15,53,54] Patients can manifest disease over a period of a year with intermittent intense nerve root pain followed by paralysis or sudden deterioration in mental status.[15,53] The CSF shows a striking eosinophilia but can often also have many red blood cells or xanthochromia. Frequently, *G. spinigerum* infection is associated with concurrent peripheral eosinophilia, which is pronounced.[31,53,54] Infection can be severe and results in death more often than infection with *A. cantonensis*.[1,5] Diagnosis is challenging; blood eosinophilia may be lacking, or head CT can show nodular lesions, area of hemorrhage, or hydrocephalus.[38]

Other Infectious Causes

Other parasites can invade the CNS, including *Taenia solium*, *Toxocara canis*, *Toxoplasma gondii*, *Paragonimus westermani*, *Fasciola hepatica*, *Trichinella spiralis*, *Ascaris lumbricoides*, *Echinococcus granulosus*, *Schistosoma japonicum*, and *Onchocerca volvulus*. Associated CSF eosinophilic pleocytosis characteristically is mild.[3,5,10,31,55]

Bacteria occasionally have been associated with mild degrees of CSF eosinophilic pleocytosis. The first descriptions of eosinophilic meningitis were in patients with neurosyphilis.[5] Other implicated agents are *Mycobacterium tuberculosis*, group B streptococcus, and *Rickettsia rickettsii*.[28,29,56,57]

A retrospective review of 27 adults in the southwestern U.S. with *Coccidioides immitis* meningitis noted eosinophils in the CSF of 70% of patients; 30% of instances met the definition of eosinophilic meningitis.[30] Other fungal infections of the CNS, such as those due to *Histoplasma capsulatum* or *Cryptococcus neoformans*, and *Aspergillus* species are occasionally associated with CSF eosinophilia.[58,59] Rarely, viral infections of the CNS (lymphocytic choriomeningitis virus, coxsackieviruses B3 and B4, measles virus, echovirus 6, and varicella-zoster virus) have been associated with eosinophilic pleocytosis of CSF.[26,27,57] In some of these cases, diagnosis was suggested by results of serologic testing or by isolation of the virus from sites other than the CNS.[26,27]

Noninfectious Causes

Review of series of children with complications of ventriculoperitoneal shunts have shown varying rates of eosinophilic pleocytosis associated with bacterial infection,[19,57] intraventricular administration of antibiotics,[21] antibiotic-impregnated ventriculostomy catheters,[22] or without any risk factor other than the shunt itself.[17] In one series evaluating 558 shunt insertions; 36 (6.5%) were found to have more than 8% eosinophils in the CSF.[17] Affected children characteristically had experienced excessive numbers of shunt revisions and shunt infections. A recent study demonstrated activation of eosinophils in CSF related to shunt obstruction.[18]

A study from Bulgaria likewise found that 6.4% of 404 children with ventriculoperitoneal shunts had transient CSF eosinophilia.[18] However, in most of these children, the eosinophilia value was no more than 3% or eosinophils were present prior to placement of the shunt. Vinchon and associates[19] reported finding eosinophilic meningitis associated with 27 of 81 presumed bacterial shunt infections; CSF culture results were positive in 63% of cases, and the microbes found did not differ from the types of organisms found in patients with noneosinophilic shunt infections. Persistent eosinophilic pleocytosis, failure to isolate infectious agents in many cases, and an association with eventual extrusion of subcutaneous tubing in some populations suggest that hypersensitivity to shunt material occasionally occurs. Replacement of the shunt with one of a different material sometimes is undertaken and sometimes is curative. A recently reported case noted an association between the use of a minocycline- and rifampin-impregnated ventricular drain in a child with a shunt malfunction and the development of eosinophilic pleocytosis; eosinophilia resolved coincident with corticosteroid administration and removal of the tubing.[22]

Several other noninfectious possibilities are included in the differential diagnosis of eosinophilic meningitis. Systemic drug administration has been associated on occasion with aseptic meningitis, and, more rarely, fluoroquinolone and nonsteroidal anti-inflammatory agents have been associated with eosinophilic meningitis.[20,31] In addition, CNS involvement with Hodgkin primary lymphoma[23] or acute lymphoblastic leukemia[24] has caused eosinophilic meningitis. Other primary CNS tumors (as well as aseptic meningitis after resection of tumors) can be associated with mild eosinophilic pleocytosis.[57] Patients with sarcoidosis and hypereosinophilia syndrome have been reported to have accompanying eosinophilic meningitis.[25,57] Eosinophilic meningitis has also been described in two intravenous drug users who were negative for human immunodeficiency virus or other identifiable infections.[60] The authors postulate that this might represent an eosinophilic response to systemically injected drug adulterants that were used as cut substances for street drugs.

DIAGNOSIS AND TREATMENT

Careful attention to the clinical setting (i.e., occurrence, history of exposure or travel) and findings on physical examination almost invariably narrow possible causes of eosinophilic meningitis to one or two categories. Careful examination of large amounts of CSF for parasites and malignant cells and culture of CSF for fungus can yield a diagnosis.

Examination of stool for ova and parasites is often unrewarding, because most human neurotropic parasites do not complete the life cycle in humans. However: (1) parasitic infestations often occur concurrently; and (2) on occasion, *Ascaris lumbricoides*, *Schistosoma japonicum*, *Taenia solium*, and *Fasciola hepatica* have been associated with eosinophilic meningitis. Therefore, stool evaluation is justified. Serologic tests of the CSF and serum for *Cryptococcus neoformans* (CSF antigen test), *Angiostrongylus cantonensis*, or *Baylisascaris procyonis*, when epidemiologically indicated, are appropriate. However, for angiostrongyliasis, the sensitivity and specificity of serologic assays vary greatly, rarely exceed 80%, and may present cross-reactivity with other microorganisms, such as

Gnasthostoma spp.[33,38] Reliable antigen-specific immunoassays are still needed. CSF often is cloudy, with increased opening pressure and protein concentration, but normal glucose concentration. Neuroimaging can be of benefit and can guide biopsy of the meninges or brain if other tests do not confirm a diagnosis. Approximately half of the patients have an abnormal MRI with leptomeningeal enhancement, and lesions in the brain parenchyma or hydrocephalus.[38,61]

The treatment and prognosis of parasitic and infectious causes of eosinophilic meningitis or meningoencephalitis depend on the cause, underlying conditions, and extent of involvement at time of diagnosis. Recommendations for specific therapies can be found in chapters addressing individual pathogens.

No systematic study of treatment with antiparasitic agents has been undertaken for *A. cantonensis*, and treatment is primarily supportive. A multicenter study prospectively evaluated patients between 2 and 65 years of age with eosinophilic meningitis; 19% of patients were younger than 20 years. Treatment was not dictated by the study; however, no difference was noted in course or outcome among patients who received 5 days of corticosteroid therapy, antibiotics, or analgesics alone.[1] Uncontrolled studies have reported the use of corticosteroids to be beneficial.[62,63] A randomized controlled trial in adults in Thailand showed no benefit of prednisolone plus albendazole compared with prednisolone alone.[22,62] Another group reported in a placebo-controlled trial that albendazole decreased the duration of headache in adult patients. In mice, anti-CCR3 monoclonal antibodies decreased significantly the eosinophil infiltration of the brain, and may offer new possibilities for future treatment in human. Observations that clinical improvement occurs after (repeated) lumbar puncture or is temporally related to use of corticosteroid and mannitol suggest that some symptoms may be a consequence of the inflammatory response, raised intracranial pressure, or both.[1,2,25]

Children with severe eosinophilic meningitis due to *Baylisascaris* have not been shown to benefit from treatment; however, experimentally infected mice were protected from neurologic disease if treated with albendazole or diethylcarbazine prior to larvae entering the brain (reviewed in reference 12). In some cases, antipsychotic drugs have been used as well in specific cases.[40] Because of the potential for severe, even fatal, outcome, particularly in young children, some experts recommend treatment of children exposed to raccoon excrement with albendazole to prevent disease.[12,44,46]

Educating the public about potential dangers from exposures to raccoons and their feces is the most important component of prevention. Raccoons have adapted readily to human habitats and are attracted to areas with sources of water and food. Therefore their presence should be discouraged by cleaning up areas and ensuring that food is not left out unwittingly. Parents, of toddlers in particular, should be mindful of potentially contaminated play areas, encourage good handwashing after playing outside, and discourage pica.

---

48 Prion Diseases

Leonel T. Takada and Michael D. Geschwind

Transmissible spongiform encephalopathies (TSEs), or prion diseases, are a group of neurodegenerative diseases caused by prions. The term "prion" is derived from "*pro*teinaceous *in*fectious particle" and was coined by Stanley Prusiner,[1] who won the 1997 Nobel Prize in Physiology or Medicine for his work on it. Prion diseases are unique as they occur via three mechanisms: spontaneous, genetic, and acquired (infectious/transmitted). For many

years, prion diseases were thought to be caused by slow viruses,[2] but Prusiner and others showed that these diseases were due to a normal cellular protein, the prion-related protein (PrP), that misfolds into a disease-causing form, called the prion.

The majority of human prion diseases (85% to 90%) consist of sporadic forms, called sporadic Creutzfeldt–Jakob disease (sCJD). The second most common group are genetic (10% to 15%) and the least frequent are acquired forms (<1%). CJD was first described by Alfons Jakob in 1921 (the case described by Hans Creutzfeldt in 1920 was not prion disease).[3] The disease should thus probably be referred to as Jakob or Jakob–Creutzfeldt disease, but the acronym JCD can be confused with the JC virus. Nonetheless, the eponym including Creutzfeldt's name remains and is currently used to designate most forms of human prion diseases. As some forms of prion disease are not always transmissible and/or do not have significant spongiform changes, the authors of this chapter prefer the term prion disease to TSE. Thus, the terms Jakob–Creutzfeldt (CJD) and prion disease will be used in this chapter.

The normal function of the prion protein, PrP^C ("C" denoting the normal cellular form) is not entirely known, but it probably plays a role in neuronal development and function.[4] The abnormal disease-causing form, the prion, is referred to as PrP^{Sc} ("Sc" deriving from scrapie). PrP^C and PrP^{Sc} essentially have identical amino acid sequences (except in genetic prion diseases), but have different conformations. Prions are characterized by their infectious properties and PrP^{Sc} has an intrinsic ability to act as a template for conversion of PrP^C to PrP^{Sc}. So when PrP^{Sc}, which has mostly β-pleated sheet structure, comes in contact with PrP^C, which has mostly α-helical structure, PrP^C is misfolded into PrP^{Sc}. This new PrP^{Sc} then becomes a template for conversion of existing PrP^C, initiating an exponential, cascade reaction that leads to neuronal injury and death.[2,5]

In sporadic CJD (sCJD), the misfolding of PrP^C to PrP^{Sc} is thought to occur spontaneously. In genetic prion diseases, mutations in the human prion gene, PRNP, probably make the PrP^C more susceptible to misfolding into PrP^{Sc}.[6] In acquired forms, PrP^{Sc} is transmitted accidentally, iatrogenically, or orally. In the orally acquired prion diseases, it is believed that prions taken up through intestinal epithelium accumulate in lymphoid tissue before being transported via sympathetic and parasympathetic nerves to the central nervous system.[7]

The PRNP gene is located in chromosome 20p13 and encodes a 253 amino acid protein. Several polymorphisms also have been found in PRNP, a few of which can affect the risk for manifesting nongenetic forms of prion disease and also affect the way genetic and nongenetic prion diseases present.[8,9] The most acknowledged polymorphism is at codon 129, which can carry either methionine (M) or valine (V) alleles. In a normal white population, 50% are heterozygous (MV), 40% have MM, and less than 10% have VV.[10] The codon 129 polymorphism frequencies in each prion disease form will be addressed in the corresponding sections. PRNP mutations will be discussed in the genetic prion diseases section.

Although prion diseases occur in species other than humans (namely scrapie in sheep and goat, bovine spongiform encephalopathy (BSE) in cattle, chronic wasting disease in cervids, and others[2]), this chapter focuses on human prion diseases. BSE is the only nonhuman form currently believed to be transmissible to humans.[11,12]

EPIDEMIOLOGY

The incidence of human prion diseases is about 1 to 1.5 per million per year in most developed countries. Annually, there are ~6000 human prion cases worldwide and about 250 to 400 in the United States. The peak age of onset of sporadic CJD occurs around a unimodal relatively narrow peak of about 68 years,[13] with an age of onset range of 14 to 98 years.[14,15]

CLINICAL MANIFESTATIONS OF HUMAN PRION DISEASES

Acquired Prion Diseases

Kuru

Kuru is a disease of the Fore ethnic group of Papua New Guinea and was transmitted through a practice in which deceased relatives were honored by ritualized endocannibalism.[16] The clinical picture was of a pure cerebellar ataxia and an illness duration of 6 to 36 months primarily in women and children, who consumed tissues with highest prion concentration.[17] The practice of cannibalism stopped in the late 1950s, and since then the incidence of Kuru has decreased dramatically.[18] The mean incubation period was estimated to be ~12 (range 5 to 56) years.[18]

Iatrogenic CJD (iCJD)

More than 400 cases of iatrogenic CJD (iCJD) have been reported since the 1950s.[19] As with other forms of prion disease, homozygosity at the polymorphism at codon 129 in PRNP (the prion protein gene) is a risk factor for iCJD (the distribution is roughly 20% MV, 25% VV, and 55% MM).[19,20] The number of reported cases has been decreasing in the past few years,[19] but new iCJD cases are still occurring from past exposures, so continuous surveillance and preventive measures still are needed.[21]

Human Pituitary Hormones

Two forms of cadaveric-derived human pituitary hormones (hPHs), human growth hormone (hGH) and human pituitary gonadotropic hormone (hPG), have been implicated in iCJD. From the late 1950s until mid-1985, cadaveric hGH was used as a treatment for short stature in children. Unfortunately, a few batches contained hPH from cadavers that unknowingly had CJD, and approximately 30,000 patients were potentially exposed.[17] In 1985, a report first mentioned the occurrence of CJD in a 20-year-old man and its association with hGH,[22] which soon led to the suspension of its use. As of May 2011, more than 200 cases of iCJD due to hGH have been reported (115 in France, 65 in the United Kingdom, and 28 in the U.S.).[19,23-25] The mean incubation period is ~15 (range 4 to 36) years, and the youngest case was 10 years of age at onset.[19,26] As the last known contaminated batches were given in the mid-1980s, new hGH iCJD cases would be manifest in adulthood. The clinical presentation for the majority of cases is progressive ataxia, with dementia occurring later.[17]

Similarly contaminated cadaveric hPG was used as an infertility treatment in Australia in the 1970s, resulting in four women developing iCJD in the early 1990s. It is estimated that ~2100 persons treated with hPH still could be at risk in Australia;[19,23,27] no new iCJD cases have been reported there in the past 20 years, however.[23] As of July 2011, the last deaths reported in hormone recipients in the U.S., France and the U.K. were in 2007, 2009, and 2010, respectively.[23-25]

Dura Mater Grafts

iCJD caused by the use of cadaveric dura mater grafts was first recognized in 1987,[17,28] and by 2006, 196 cases had been reported worldwide. The majority of cases occurred in Japan, but a few were in France, Spain, Germany, the U.K., and the U.S.[19] Most cases (>90%) were linked to Lyodura® brand grafts processed before May, 1987.[17,29,30] Due to changes in the disinfection protocol,[19] no cases have been reported from patients who received grafts after 1993.[29]

As of 2008, 132 cases were reported in Japan,[29] with the mean age at symptom onset of 55 (range 15 to 80) years and a median incubation period 12.4 years (range 1.2 to 24.8 years). In most cases, except for the earlier age of onset, the clinical manifestations, neuroimaging, cerebrospinal fluid (CSF), and neuropathology findings reportedly were similar to sCJD.[31] The estimated risk of developing CJD from Lyodura® grafts is calculated as 1 case per 1250 recipients. Homozygosity at codon 129, particularly VV, is a strong risk factor for this form of iCJD.[19,31]

Other Sources of iCJD

Two young-onset (ages 17 and 23) cases of CJD were reported in 1977 after the patients had been implanted, 20 and 16 months previously, respectively, with stereotactic electroencephalographic

(EEG) depth electrodes that had been used in a patient with CJD.[32] Prion-contaminated neurosurgical instruments also have been implicated in a few cases of transmission of CJD.[17,19,33] Despite cornea being considered a low prion infectivity tissue,[34] in at least two (and possibly three) cases corneal transplantation is considered the source for iCJD.[17,19,35,36] A few isolated reports have claimed association between bone graft, liver transplant, or pericardial graft and subsequent development of CJD. It is thought, however, that those cases probably are sporadic and not iatrogenic.[37] To date, blood products have been linked to prion transmission only in variant CJD cases (discussed below) and no other form of human prion disease.[38]

Variant CJD

Variant CJD (vCJD) was first identified in 1995 in the U.K.[11] and received worldwide attention because it affected adolescents and younger adults and was linked with BSE (i.e., mad cow disease). As of March 2011,[39] 224 cases had been reported officially. The vast majority occurred in the U.K. (78%), followed by France (11%). A few cases were documented in other European countries (Ireland, Italy, Netherlands, Portugal, and Spain), Asia (Japan, Taiwan, and Saudi Arabia) and North America (U.S. and Canada). The five North American cases are all believed to have been acquired in the U.K. or Saudi Arabia. (M.D. Geschwind personal communication, manuscript in preparation.) The incidence of vCJD peaked in 2000 and has since been consistently on a downward curve.

It is believed that BSE occurred from the practice of feeding scrapie-infected sheep products to cattle. More than 280,000 cattle suffered from BSE, the majority in the U.K. (and 22 cases in North America[40]). Although the incidence of BSE has declined dramatically since 1992, a few isolated cases still have been reported over the past few years.[41]

Clinically, vCJD differs from sCJD in several ways. Patients with vCJD generally are much younger, with a median age of onset ~27 years (range 12 to 74 years).[42,43] The mean disease duration is longer, about 14.5 months. Although psychiatric symptoms can occur early in sCJD,[44] in vCJD, profound psychiatric symptoms often are the initial symptoms for several (typically >6) months

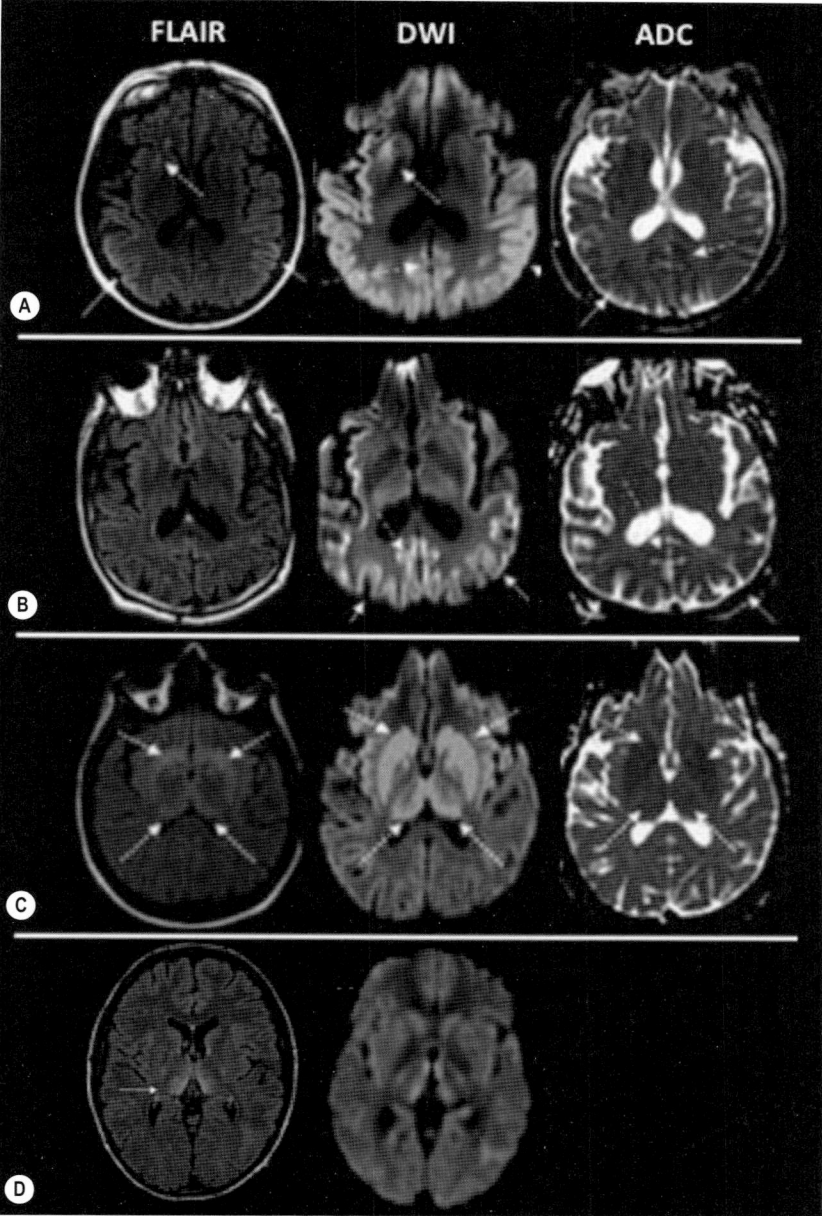

Figure 48-1. Magnetic resonance findings in CJD. Three common variations of sporadic CJD presentation on MRI **(A, B, C)** and MRI findings in variant CJD **(D)**. **(A)** Neocortical (solid arrow), limbic and subcortical grey matter (dotted arrow). **(B)** Neocortical and limbic. **(C)** Subcortical and limbic. Note that the DWI abnormalities are more easily seen than in FLAIR sequences. ADC hypointensities are most easily identified in the basal ganglia. **(D)** Variant CJD – bilateral thalamic hyperintensities in the mesial and posterior parts of the thalamus (double hockey stick sign). Pulvinar sign (arrow); posterior thalamus (pulvinar) hyperintensity. CJD, Creutzfeldt–Jakob disease; MRI, magnetic resonance imaging; DWI, diffusion-weighted imaging; FLAIR, fluid-attenuated inversion recovery; ADC, apparent diffusion coefficient. (Modified from Vitali et al., Neurology 2011;76(20):1711–1719 and Vitali et al., Semin Neurol 2008;28:467–483.)

PART II Clinical Syndromes and Cardinal Features of Infectious Diseases: Approach to Diagnosis and Initial Management

SECTION F Central Nervous System Infections

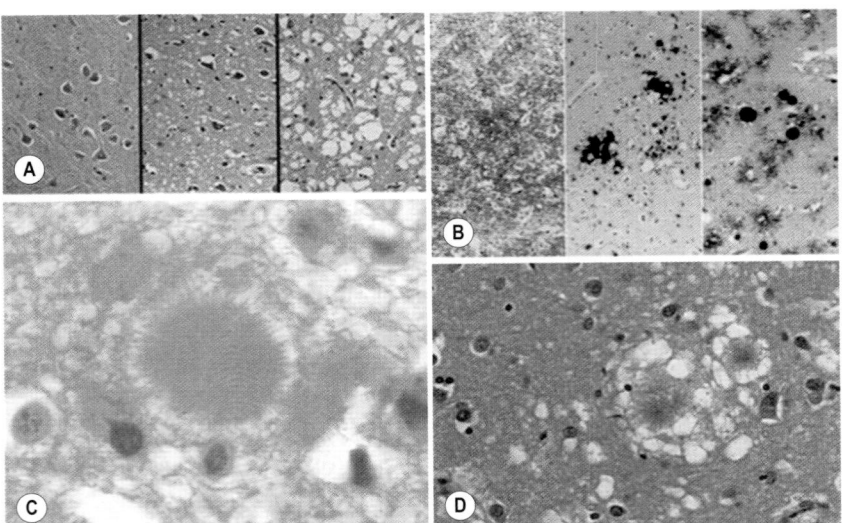

Figure 48-2. Neuropathologic findings in prion diseases. Neuropathology of prion disease **(A)** in sporadic CJD, in which some brain areas may have no (hippocampal end plate, left), mild (subiculum, middle), or severe (temporal cortex, right) spongiform change. Hematoxylin and eosin (H & E) stain. **(B)** Cortical sections immunostained for PrP^{Sc} in sporadic CJD showing synaptic (left), patchy/perivacuolar (middle), or plaque type (right) patterns of PrP^{Sc} deposition. **(C)** Large Kuru-type plaque, H & E stain. **(D)** Typical "florid" plaques in vCJD, H & E stain. (Modified from Budka H, Br Med Bull 2003;66:121–130 Copyright © 2003 Oxford University Press.)

before obvious neurologic symptoms begin. EEG only very rarely shows periodic sharp wave complexes (PSWCs).[45] Brain MRI usually shows the "pulvinar sign," in which the posterior thalamus is brighter than the anterior putamen on T_2-weighted or diffusion-weighted imaging (DWI) MRI (and was found in more than 85% of cases in the first examination) (Figure 48-1);[46] this finding is extremely rare in other human prion diseases.[47] Diagnostic criteria for probable vCJD require a progressive neuropsychiatric syndrome and duration of illness >6 months, as well as manifestations such as painful paresthesias, ataxia, myoclonus, chorea, dystonia, and/or dementia, which are reported to have sensitivity of 83% and specificity as high as 100%.[42]

Definitive diagnosis of vCJD requires pathologic evidence of the variant form of PrP^{Sc} in brain. Unlike other human prion diseases, in PrP^{Sc} vCJD also is found outside the central nervous system, in the lymphoreticular system, including tonsillar tissue.[48] Brain pathology of vCJD shows abundant PrP^{Sc} deposition, particularly multiple fibrillary PrP plaques surrounded by a halo of spongiform vacuoles ("florid" plaques) and amorphous pericellular and perivascular PrP deposits, especially prominent in the cerebellar molecular layer (Figure 48-2).[49] Virtually all vCJD cases to date have been 129MM. Two definite vCJD cases (see blood product transfusion cases below) and one dietary-acquired possible vCJD case have been 129MV.[50]

TABLE 48-1. Sporadic CJD in Individuals 20 Years of Age or Younger at Onset[63,65]

Reference	Sex	Age of Onset (years)	Duration (months)	First Symptom(s)	EEG	Brain MRI	Neuropathology	*PRNP* Codon 129 Polymorphism
Murray et al., 2008[65]	F	15	15	Forgetfulness and nervousness	Slow waves, no PSWC	N/A (CT – progressive ventricular enlargement)	c/w sCJD. PrP staining +	N/A
Monreal et al., 1981[66]	M	16	28	Forgetfulness and slowness of thought	PSWC +	N/A	c/w sCJD + white matter changes	N/A
Brown et al., 1985[67]	F	19	4	Lethargy, aggressive behavior	PSCW +	N/A	c/w sCJD + white matter gliosis (temporal cortex fragment)	N/A
Berman et al., 1988[15]	F	14.5	≈24	Incoordination, forgetfulness, labile temperament	Paroxysmal slow wave activity	Severe cerebral atrophy	c/w sCJD + white matter changes	N/A
Kulczycki et al., 1991[68]	F	19	10	Loss of memory, confusion	Generalized slowing	N/A (CT brain atrophy)	c/w sCJD	N/A
Murray et al., 2008[65]	F	15	54	Choreiform movements, lethargy, emotional lability, altered personality, poor concentration	Slow waves	High signal in caudate and putamen	c/w sCJD + white matter abnormalities	MV
Petzold et al., 2004[47]	F	19	24	Dysesthesias, insomnia, depressive mood, apathy, forgetfulness	Slowing	Pulvinar hyperintensities (5 months after onset)	sCJD	VV1
Meissner et al., 2005[69]	F	19	21	N/A	N/A; no PSWC	Cortical signal increase, not in basal ganglia	N/D	VV1

PRNP, prion protein gene; N/A, not available; PSWC, periodic sharp wave complexes; M, methionine; V, valine; VV, valine homozygosis at PRNP codon 129; CT, computed tomography scan; EEG, electroencephalogram; MRI, magnetic resonance imaging; N/D, not done; c/w, consistent with.

Through June 2011, 5 cases of vCJD have been reported to be acquired through blood or blood product transfusion (two of these died from non-neurological causes, but were found to have vCJD in lymphoreticular tissue).[51-55] Four patients acquired vCJD through blood transfusions received before 1999; three (all codon 129MM) died from definite vCJD with incubation periods of about 6 to 9 years, whereas a fourth (heterozygous at codon 129) died from non-neurologic causes 5 years after receiving a contaminated blood transfusion. Since then, additional measures were taken to prevent transmission of vCJD through blood products; these measures include universal leukoreduction of donated blood, donor selection, and efforts towards developing methods to detect PrP in blood.[41] The fifth case of vCJD associated with blood products was a British patient with hemophilia (129MV) who received pooled factor VIII (in addition to plasma) in the 1990s (from a batch that contained material from a donor who later developed vCJD) and was found to have positive prion testing in the spleen.[41,55] It is not known if platelets transmit vCJD.[56]

Latent or asymptomatic vCJD (i.e., individuals harboring vCJD) is of great concern, as individuals might pose a higher risk for spread through blood transfusions and surgical procedures. Cases acquired from blood transfusion show that transmission from asymptomatic blood donors occurs years before the onset of symptoms;[57,58] exposed individuals with 129MV or 129VV genotype also might have longer incubation times than those with 129MM. Two studies in the U.K. have found an unexpectedly high frequency of latent vCJD. In one study, prions were found by immunostaining in 3 of 11,246 appendix samples collected from 1995 to 2000.[59] In another similar study from the National Anonymous Tonsil Archive, 1 sample was positive among a subset of 10,000 tested.[60] Repeat analysis of this positive tonsil specimen by other methods for detecting PrP^{Sc} was negative, however. Estimates of population prevalence of latent vCJD in the U.K. population (particularly those in the highest risk cohort born between 1961 and 1985), are about 109 to 237 per million, with a wide 95% confidence interval of 0 to ~600 per million depending on whether or not these cases are falsely positive.[60-62]

Sporadic Prion Disease (Sporadic CJD)

Sporadic CJD is characterized by rapidly progressive dementia, with a median survival of 7 to 8 months (>90% of patients die within the first year of manifestations). The mean age of onset is 68 (range 14 to 98) years. Occurrence of sCJD before age 40 or later than mid-70s is uncommon.[48,63] Clinical presentation is highly variable, and most commonly the first symptoms are cognitive or cerebellar.[13,44] Onset typically is subacute, but rarely is acute or stroke-like.[64] Often under-recognized first symptoms are subtle

behavioral or psychiatric symptoms and constitutional symptoms (i.e., vertigo, fatigue, headache, etc.).[44]

Cases of sCJD with onset <20 years of age are rare,[65] with 8 cases reported to date (Table 48-1). In a review of cases <50 years at disease onset, and comparing clinical features with older-onset sCJD,[70] patients with younger onset had longer duration of illness, more frequent neuropsychiatric symptoms, less frequent typical EEG and MRI findings, but had earlier onset of severe dementia.

Among all patients with sCJD, about 70% to 80% are homozygotes (mainly 129MM),[9,10] and one study showed that a disproportionately high percentage of subjects <50 years had codon 129VV in *PRNP*, suggesting this polymorphism might predispose to younger onset.[71]

Typical neuropathologic features of sCJD (see Figure 48-2) include neuronal loss, gliosis, vacuolation, and deposition of PrP^{Sc}.[49] Inflammatory changes characteristically are absent.[72] Ancillary tests and their typical findings in sCJD are discussed below.

Genetic Prion Disease

The discovery that the purified scrapie-causing protein was encoded by a human gene,[73] and subsequent finding that mutations in the *PRNP* cause prion diseases provided strong evidence that prion diseases were caused by a protein.[74,75] Currently, there are more than 40 mutations identified in the *PRNP* gene (Figure 48-3), inherited in an autosomal-dominant pattern and with penetrance close to 100%, depending on the mutation. Most mutations are point mutations and insertions (particularly of octapeptide repeat insertions, OPRI). The most frequent mutations worldwide are E200K, V210I, P102L, and D178N.[76,77] It is important to point out that although genetic prion diseases (gPrD) sometimes are referred to as "familial," this term can be a misnomer as up to 60% of patients with gPrD do not have a positive family history of CJD, although upon further inspection often there may a family history of other neurologic illness that probably had been misdiagnosed.[77] As with other dementing or neuropsychiatric genetic diseases, sometimes families keep the disease a secret, even from other branches of the family. Genetic prion diseases often are divided according to their genetic, clinical, and pathologic characteristics into three forms: familial CJD (fCJD), Gerstmann–Sträussler–Scheinker (GSS) syndrome, and fatal familial insomnia (FFI).

Familial CJD (fCJD)

More than 15 *PRNP* mutations manifest as fCJD. Depending on the mutation, most patients are indistinguishable clinically from sCJD in age of onset, clinical symptoms, disease duration, and

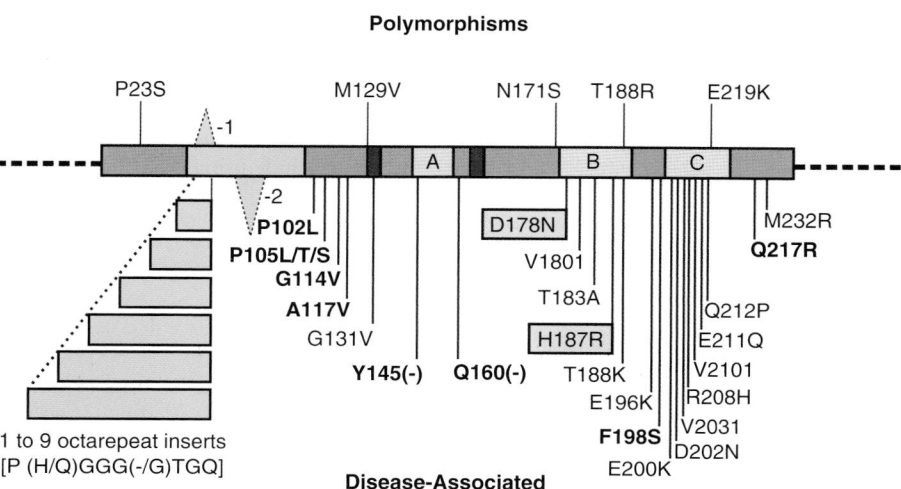

Figure 48-3. *PRNP* gene polymorphisms and mutations. Schematic representation of the *PRNP* gene, with the major polymorphisms and prion disease-associated mutations. All mutations are associated with a Creutzfeldt–Jakob disease (CJD) phenotype except those in bold (Gerstmann–Sträussler–Scheinker syndrome), D178N (fatal familial insomnia or CJD, depending on codon 129 genotype), and H187R (CJD phenotype but variable pathology). (From Mastrianni JA. The genetics of prion diseases. Genet Med 2010;12:187–195.)

neuropathology. This is particularly true for the most common gPrD worldwide, E200K.[72,77] Younger age of onset (in the 30s or 40s) might be seen in mutations such as D178-129V, 7- or 9-OPRI, or T183A.[72] A P105T mutation carrier with positive family history has been described with onset at 13 years of age with anxiety as the initial symptom, followed by ataxia and pyramidal signs.[78] Other gCJD cases with onset earlier than 20 years of age have been reported.[79] Ancillary tests, such as EEG and MRI, might not be as helpful in the diagnosis as they are in sporadic cases.[9]

Gerstmann–Sträussler–Scheinker (GSS) Syndrome

GSS syndrome usually presents as subacute progressive ataxia and/or parkinsonian disorder with later onset of cognitive impairment. Onset usually is in the fourth to sixth decades, but can occur as early as the third decade.[72,77] There is considerable phenotypic variability within and between mutations and families,[9] and at least 15 *PRNP* mutations have been shown to cause GSS syndrome.[80] GSS neuropathology is distinct from most other prion diseases, with large plaques of PrP^{Sc} amyloid plaques, called Kuru plaques (these plaques also can be seen in ~10% of sCJD cases[81]) (see Figure 48-2).[49]

Familial Fatal Insomnia (FFI)

Fatal familial insomnia (FFI) is a rare disorder that usually manifests with progressive, severe insomnia and dysautonomia, with motor and cognitive problems appearing later. Onset usually occurs in the fifth and sixth decade (but has been reported in individuals as young as 19 years[77]) and duration is around 1 to 1.5 years.[9] Although brain MRI usually is normal, FDG-PET imaging reveals thalamic and cingulate hypometabolism. Both sporadic (a subtype of sCJD) and familial forms of fatal insomnia are recognized. FFI is caused by a single *PRNP* point mutation, D178N, with codon 129M on the same chromosome (cis) (patients with D178N-129V usually present as fCJD).[82] Neuropathology of FFI is primarily characterized by thalamic gliosis and neuronal loss.[9,49]

LABORATORY FINDINGS AND DIAGNOSIS

Some diagnostic laboratory test findings have been discussed above for specific forms of human prion disease. CSF typically is normal in human prion disease, perhaps with a mildly elevated protein (typically <75 mg/dL). CSF pleocytosis (>10 WBC cells/mm^3), an elevated IgG index, or the presence of oligoclonal bands is unusual in sCJD and should lead to consideration of other conditions, particularly infectious or autoimmune disorders. Several currently used CSF biomarkers are 14-3-3 protein, total tau (t-tau), neuronal specific enolase (NSE), and S100β.[83] The reported sensitivities and specificities of each marker vary greatly. A large European study has found the sensitivity and specificity of the 14-3-3 to be 85% and 84%, t-tau (cut-off >1300 pg/mL) 86% and 88%, NSE 73% and 95%, and S100β 82% and 76%, respectively.[84] Thus far, t-tau might be the best CSF diagnostic protein for sCJD but it still does not approach the utility of brain MRI.[85]

A typical EEG in sCJD has periodic sharp, or triphasic, wave complexes (PSWCs) occurring about once every second; however, this EEG finding is found in only about two-thirds of sCJD patients, usually only after serial EEGs and often not until later stages of the illness.[86] Often the only finding is focal or generalized slowing. These EEG findings are relatively specific but PSWCs sometimes are seen in other conditions, including toxic-metabolic and anoxic encephalopathies, progressive multifocal leukoencephalopathy, and Hashimoto encephalopathy.[87,88]

MRI has been shown to be highly sensitive and specific (92% to 95%) for sCJD. Typical findings are T$_2$-weighted and DWI basal ganglia (e.g., caudate/putamen) and cortical gyral hyperintensities (often called "cortical ribboning")[85,89,90] (see Figure 48-1). Hyperintensities in sCJD typically are more evident on DWI sequences than on fluid-attenuated inversion recovery (FLAIR) images,

and show diffusion restriction with concomitant apparent diffusion coefficient (ADC) map hypointensities (see Figure 48-1). Basal ganglia hyperintensities, when present, typically have an anterior to posterior gradient, with greater hyperintensity anteriorly.[85] Basal ganglia or thalamic hyperintensities on DWI and/or FLAIR MRI also have been described, however, in non-prion conditions, including Wilson disease, Wernicke encephalopathy, vasculitis, strokes, seizures, lymphoma, and metabolic perturbations.[91–93] Cortical ribboning on DWI sequences might occur with seizures (particularly prolonged), vasculitis or autoantibody syndromes, but the neuroanatomical pattern of hyperintensity and temporal progression usually is different from that of sCJD.[91,93]

Several diagnostic criteria exist for sCJD. Criteria were created mostly for surveillance purposes, and so are not particularly useful for the early stages of diseases (as most patients fulfill criteria only at later stages of disease). The most commonly used criteria for probable sCJD are the revised WHO criteria,[94] which require progressive dementia, and two other signs among myoclonus, visual or cerebellar disturbance, pyramidal or extrapyramidal signs and/or akinetic mutism, as well as positive CSF 14-3-3 and/or PSWCs in EEG. More recently, diagnostic criteria that utilize MRI have been proposed.[95,96]

In the pediatric population prion disease only seldom is considered among differential diagnostics, unless epidemiologic data suggest plausibility (e.g., family history of CJD or history of possible exposure to prions). Among the possible alternative diagnoses, subacute sclerosing panencephalitis (SSPE) shares several overlapping features with sCJD including the presence of periodic activity in EEG, relatively rapid onset, and myoclonus. Periodic EEG activity in sCJD, however, typically is short-interval, whereas in SSPE there are long-interval periodic activities.[97] Although SSPE occurs predominantly in children, there is overlap in age of onset among older adolescents and young adults for vCJD.[98] Clinically, myoclonus is perhaps more frequent in SSPE and early psychiatric features more common in vCJD. The pulvinar sign on MRI, however, is absent in SSPE, and elevated CSF immunoglobulins and oligoclonal bands are characteristic of SSPE.

TREATMENT AND PREVENTION

In spite of active efforts, there are no currently available treatments to slow or stop the progression of human prion diseases. Two large studies have found oral quinacrine to not improve survival in human prion disease[99,100] (M. Geschwind, personal communication). Trials with doxycycline are underway currently in 2011 in Europe (M. Geschwind, personal communication). Intraventricular administration of pentosan polysulfate (PPS) has been used in several patients, with somewhat prolonged survival in a few cases, but no clinical improvement,[101,102] so many consider PPS of little if any benefit. Although there are no approved treatments, medications to treat specific symptoms often are used. For example, SSRIs often are used for depression and agitation, atypical antipsychotics to treat agitation and psychoses, and clonazepam, levetiracetam, or valproic acid to treat severe myoclonus.

Decontamination of prions requires methods that will denature proteins, as prions resist normal inactivation methods used to kill viruses and bacteria. Methods include using higher than normal temperatures, pressure and time, with or without denaturing agents (many of which are caustic and might damage medical equipment and instruments).[21,103,104] When feasible, many hospitals dispose of surgical or invasive equipment potentially exposed to prions by incineration.

Acknowledgments

The authors would like to thank Suzanne Solvyns (President, CJD Support Group Network, Australia), J.B. Matthieu (President MCJ-HCC, France), and Jennifer Cooke for their input on human pituitary hormones and iCJD. MDG was supported by NIH R01 AG031189 and the Michael J. Homer Family Fund.

49 Urinary Tract Infections

Jen-Jane Liu and Linda Marie Dairiki Shortliffe

Bacterial urinary tract infection (UTI) is the most common cause of childhood urinary tract inflammation. Recognition that bacteriuria can cause renal parenchymal and functional loss has prompted recommendations for rapid diagnosis and evaluation of UTI with genitourinary imaging techniques. In infants, UTI is a common cause of fever and is the most common cause of renal parenchymal damage.

ETIOLOGIC AGENTS

The most common bacteria infecting the urinary tract are gram-negative Enterobacteriaceae, primarily *Escherichia coli,* and then *Klebsiella, Proteus, Enterococcus, Pseudomonas,* and *Enterobacter* spp. UPEC (uropathogenic *E. coli*) or ExPEC (extraintestinal *E. coli*) are serotypes that contain specific cell wall O antigens and commonly cause UTI in children.[1-3] *Staphylococcus saprophyticus* accounts for ≥15% of UTIs in female adolescents. *S. aureus,* including methicillin-resistant *S. aureus* (MRSA), rarely causes pyelonephritis or cystitis; thus, recovery of *S. aureus* from the urine suggests a bloodstream infection (BSI). Although occasionally isolated from neonates and adolescents, group B streptococcus is an unusual urinary tract pathogen. Occasionally, gastrointestinal pathogens such as *Salmonella, Shigella,* and *Campylobacter* infect the urinary tract.[3] *Lactobacillus* spp., *Corynebacterium* spp., and α-hemolytic streptococci are periurethral flora and usually are contaminants when recovered from urine. Protozoa, significant in some areas of the world, are rare uropathogens in the United States. Enterobiasis can be associated with entry of pinworms into the urethra, causing dysuria, frequency, and pyuria.

Mycobacterium tuberculosis infection of the urinary tract should be considered when sterile pyuria is present. Organisms such as *Haemophilus* spp., which can be associated with UTI in patients with abnormal urinary tracts,[4] and *Trichomonas, Chlamydia,* micro-aerophilic microorganisms, and viruses will not be isolated from standard media, but should be considered when evaluating sterile pyuria. Viral cystitis is associated with bone marrow transplantation and other immunosuppressed conditions. Adenovirus is the most common cause of viral acute hemorrhagic cystitis in children. BK virus has been found in the urine of bone marrow transplant recipients and other immunosuppressed patients with hemorrhagic cystitis.[5,6]

EPIDEMIOLOGY AND PATHOGENESIS

Only during the first year of life are males more affected by UTI than females,[2,7] and during that year the risk of UTI in uncircumcised boys is about ten times that of circumcised boys.[8,9] The incidence of UTI drops below 1% in school-age boys and rises to 1% to 3% in school-age girls,[10-12] with sexually active females having more UTIs than sexually inactive ones.[13] UTI accounts for 2.4% to 2.8% of physician visits for children with commercial insurance or Medicaid, and cost for hospitalization of children with UTI is $180 million a year.[14]

UTI begins with bacterial adherence to host epithelial cells following a fecal–perineal–urethral route and retrograde ascent of bacteria.[15] While risk factors and bacterial virulence influence this course, they do not predict pyelonephritis, renal scarring, or parenchymal and functional loss. Of the 3% of girls and 1%

of boys who contract a UTI prepubertally, ≥17% will have infection-related renal scarring. Of those with scarring, 10% to 20% may become hypertensive, but only rarely does damage progress to renal dysfunction culminating in end-stage renal disease.[2] Bacteria overcome urethral defenses of urethral washout, epithelial shedding, and paraurethral glandular secretion.[16] Host defenses include bacterial lipopolysaccharide triggering of toll-like receptors (TLRs) and the urinary Tamm–Horsfall protein adhering to UPEC to help wash out urethral bacteria.[17] Two important markers for *E. coli* virulence are mannose-resistant hemagglutination characteristics and P blood-group-specific adhesins (P-fimbriae or P-pili).[18-20] Attachment between the uroepithelial cell and bacteria via type 1 pili and fimbriae initiates a molecular interaction that triggers bacteria uptake into bladder surface umbrella cells.[21] The intracellular bacteria transform into biofilms that allow microbial adaptation and systemic infection, anti-microbial resistance via plasmid exchange, endotoxin production, and increased resistance to host immune systems.[22] Once bacteria are in the bladder, host immune mechanisms, impaired ureteral peristalsis, vesicoureteral reflux, and organism-specific uropathogenicity determine retrograde ascent.

RISK FACTORS FOR BACTERIURIA AND RENAL DAMAGE

Age. UTI prevalence for both males and females is higher below the age of 1 year than at other times during childhood due to host factors such as periurethral colonization and immature immune status.

Genetic predisposition. Risk factors for recurrent UTI in young women are age at first UTI and UTI in the mother.[23] Blood group phenotypes such as P1 blood group, ABO and Lewis secretor phenotypes, and host genetic polymorphisms of adhesion molecules (ICAM-1), transforming growth factor-β, TLR, and vascular endothelial growth factor influence susceptibility to UTI.[24-26]

Race and ethnicity. Epidemiologic studies show racial variance in prevalence and complications of UTI. One study of children <2 years of age showed that UTI in girls was more prevalent in white and Hispanic compared with black races, but in boys was most common in Hispanic, white, and then black races. These studies show that African Americans have fewer UTIs, and perhaps less reflux nephropathy than Hispanic or white children.[27-29] In Chinese children, UTI and vesicoureteral reflux (VUR) with renal scarring are more common in boys than girls.[30] However, recent studies show that Asian females and African American and Hispanic males are more likely to be hospitalized for pyelonephritis.[31] Circumcision status confounds racial predisposition data.

Colonization. In the first few months of life, the incidence of UTI in otherwise healthy infants may be high due to dense colonization of the periurethral area with *E. coli,* enterococci, and staphylococci.[32] Colonization density decreases over the first year and is not a factor in children >5 years of age without recurrent infections.

For the first 6 months of life periurethral uropathogenic organisms are more frequent in uncircumcised than circumcised boys,[33] and the majority (70% to 86%) of male neonatal UTIs occur in uncircumcised boys.[34-36] Controversy exists regarding the

PART II Clinical Syndromes and Cardinal Features of Infectious Diseases: Approach to Diagnosis and Initial Management

SECTION G Genitourinary Tract Infections

advantages and disadvantages of circumcision.[37] Current data do not support routine neonatal circumcision solely for UTI prevention in children. Calculations from meta-analysis suggest that only boys having recurrent UTI or who are at high risk for renal damage from UTI may benefit from circumcision.[38] Since most bacterial UTIs result from fecal–perineal–urethral ascent, neonatal fecal colonization is important, with subsequent bacteriuria or pyelonephritis occurring up to several months later.[39]

Immune status and infancy. Serum IgG and IgA levels are lowest between age 1 and 3 months,[40] when periurethral colonization is highest.[41,42] Case-control studies suggest that breastfeeding is protective against UTI during the first 6 months of life.[43] Immunoglobulins and oligosaccharides in human milk may inhibit *E. coli* adherence to the uroepithelium.[44]

Sexual activity. Sexual activity is a risk factor for UTI and, as such, may serve as a marker for sexual activity in adolescents.[45] Adolescent females with dysuria and frequency should be evaluated for both UTI and sexually transmitted infection (STI). It is estimated that 50% of high school students have had at least one sexual encounter. The prevalence of *Chlamydia* is 13% to 26% and *Neisseria gonorrhoeae* about 2% to 10% in this population.

Genitourinary anatomic abnormalities. Most studies on rate of urinary tract abnormalities discovered secondary to investigation after a UTI were performed before routine use of prenatal ultrasonography (US). A recent study of children with first febrile UTI showed that 56% have urinary tract abnormalities (vesicoureteral reflux 30%; renal hypodysplasia 2%; hydronephrosis 34%; hydroureter 3%).[46]

Discovering UTI-associated urinary tract abnormalities may permit (1) surgical correction of a potential renal-damaging anomaly, (2) discovery of an abnormality that requires further management, and (3) location of a site of recurrent UTI due to bacterial persistence because of poor antimicrobial penetration. Management of these UTIs and patients depends on the specific abnormality uncovered.

Vesicoureteral reflux. VUR is found commonly in children with UTI, but no correlation between reflux and susceptibility to UTI is evident.[2] VUR usually is congenital and is caused by ureteropelvic muscular inadequacy/dysfunction that permits retrograde flow of urine from the bladder into the ureter and pelvicaliceal system. While VUR raises risk of pyelonephritis with bacteriuria, it correlates poorly with UTI-induced renal scarring.[47]

CLINICAL MANIFESTATIONS

UTI should be suspected in any seriously ill infant or young child, even if other clinical signs and symptoms are absent or point elsewhere. Children with pyelonephritis can have classic symptoms of fever, chills, and unilateral or bilateral flank pain with or without accompanying lower tract symptoms of dysuria, frequency, incontinence, and urgency. In febrile infants from birth to 8–10 weeks of age, neither clinical symptoms nor laboratory tests predict UTI well. Risks for infant UTI include lack of circumcision, and fever >24 hours.[48] The prevalence of UTI in febrile infants (<8 weeks of age) is ~14%, with the majority occurring in males.[49] In adolescent males, UTI can be associated with structural abnormalities and lower urinary tract symptoms with voiding dysfunction. Adolescents with dysuria and frequency should be evaluated for both UTI and STI. In the older child, fever, and abdominal or upper quadrant pain may be present; suprapubic and flank palpation may induce pain. Palpation of a renal mass may indicate a gross abnormality, such as severely infected hydronephrosis and pyonephrosis or xanthogranulomatous pyelonephritis.

DIAGNOSTIC TESTS

Urinary specimens. Reliable urinary specimens from which to make the diagnosis of UTI may be hard to obtain. Ranked from most to least reliable, urine collection methods are: (1) suprapubic bladder aspiration, (2) urethral catheterization, (3) midstream

voided collection, and (4) "bagged" (plastic bag attached to the perineum) specimen collection. Even after extensive skin cleansing, a bagged specimen usually reflects perineal and rectal flora. A midstream-voided specimen in a circumcised boy, older girl, or older uncircumcised boy who can retract his foreskin can be reliable. A catheterized specimen is most reliable when the first portion of urine that may contain urethral organisms is discarded. Disadvantages to catheterization are trauma and the potential of introducing urethral organisms into a sterile bladder. Suprapubic bladder aspiration is the most reliable method as urethral or periurethral organisms are absent and skin contamination can be avoided with careful skin preparation. Organisms present in a suprapubic aspirate are indicative of bacteriuria. Plastic bag specimens are unreliable for diagnosis of UTI in high-risk populations and infants <2 months old, and when antimicrobial therapy must be instituted. A negative culture of a bagged specimen eliminates the possibility of a bacterial UTI.[50,51]

Urinalysis. Urinalysis determinants that support presence of a UTI are: (1) pyuria – usually defined as >5 white blood cells/high power field (WBC/hpf) in a centrifuged specimen, (2) any bacteria per hpf in the unstained uncentrifuged urinary sediment, (3) positive urinary leukocyte esterase test, and (4) positive urinary nitrite test. Finding red and white cell casts in the urinary sediment is unreliable. Sensitivity of routine urinalysis for UTI is calculated to be 82% in children <2 years of age.[52,53] Urinary leukocyte esterase is produced by the breakdown of white cells in the urine. Dietary nitrates present in the urine, which are reduced by many gram-negative bacteria, are measured by the urinary nitrite test. Gram-positive bacteria and many non-Enterobacteriaceae and non-enteric gram-negative bacteria do not reduce nitrate. Children who lack renal concentrating ability or who receive large amounts of fluids intravenously and infants (who void frequently) may not have bladder dwell-time to break down WBCs or reduce nitrate. Among urinalysis tests, nitrite is the least sensitive (53%) and leukocyte esterase is the least specific (72%).[54]

In a general pediatric population, when urinary specimens are properly collected and promptly processed, the combined use of testing for leukocyte esterase, nitrite, and microscopic bacteria has almost 100% sensitivity for detection of UTI by positivity of one or more tests (with mean specificity of one or more positive tests of 70%, range 60% to 92%).[54] When all (or leukocyte esterase and nitrite tests) are negative, the negative predictive value approaches 100%, and may be sufficient to avoid culture in many situations.[51,55]

Serum tests indicating UTI severity. C-reactive protein (CRP) >7 mg/dL has been associated with serious bacterial infection in febrile children 1 to 36 months of age.[56] Serum procalcitonin, a hormonally inactive precursor of calcitonin, is elevated in the systemic circulation during early, severe inflammation. Serum procalcitonin may correlate better with pyelonephritis than erythrocyte sedimentation rate (ESR) or CRP and predict renal scarring.[57,58] Overall, none of these tests is reliable enough to detect early UTI or to differentiate upper from lower tract infection.

Urinary culture. The gold standard for the diagnosis of UTI is quantitative urinary culture. Although ≥100,000 colony-forming units (CFU)/mL of voided urine is the traditional definition for a clinically significant UTI,[59] studies have shown that ≤10,000 CFU/mL occasionally can indicate a significant UTI.[60,61] In febrile children <2 years of age, ≥50,000 CFU/mL from a catheterized specimen is evidence of a UTI.[62] Even lower numbers of bacteria may justify UTI diagnosis, especially if obtained by suprapubic needle aspiration, or in patients with obstructive uropathy. In one emergency department study of 185 febrile children <36 months of age, 14% of specimens obtained by urethral catheterization were contaminated (i.e., had negative urinalysis plus multiple pathogens, nonpathogens or CFU/mL growth of <10,000; odds ratio for contamination were increased for age <6 months, uncircumcised boys and difficult catheterization procedure.[63] Since routine viral cultures are performed infrequently, children with symptoms of acute hemorrhagic cystitis most often have no growth on routine urinary culture.

MANAGEMENT OF PEDIATRIC URINARY TRACT INFECTIONS

Antimicrobial Treatment

Children <90 days of age can have a rapidly changing course of disease. Those <1 month of age are usually hospitalized for diagnosis and treatment. One study showed that ampicillin-resistant gram-negative bacteria are the most common cause of serious bacterial infection in infants <3 months.[64] In children ≤30 days of age with presumptive serious bacterial infection, antimicrobial coverage should include activity against *Listeria monocytogenes* (perinatally acquired) and *Enterococcus* (usually postnatally acquired). Thus, ampicillin and gentamicin frequently are recommended in this age group.[65] Cetriaxone, administered intramuscularly, can be used for infants >30 days of age with a presumptive febrile UTI if they are able to take fluids and have caregivers who will assure adequate follow-up.[66] However, as enterococcal UTI still occurs under 2 months of age, ceftriaxone therapy alone may not be adequate.[67] A multicenter randomized clinical trial showed that oral cefixime appeared as effective as initial cefotaxime intravenously in hospitalized children aged 1 to 24 months with febrile UTI.[68] Initial treatment orally or intravenously is equally efficacious; choice of administration is based on practical considerations.[54] Young children (2 to 5 years of age) with presumptive UTI who are systemically ill with a fever and flank or abdominal pain and are unable to take fluids, or immune compromised children should be treated with broad-spectrum antimicrobial agents, administered parenterally, (e.g., aminoglycoside and ampicillin, third-generation cephalosporin, aminoglycoside and cephalosporin, or aminopenicillin/clavulanic acid) because of widespread ampicillin resistance.[69] For those who are not taking adequate fluids, parenteral treatment continues for 2 to 4 days until defervescence and bacterial susceptibility test results are available to allow treatment with an oral drug with narrower spectrum, usually for 7 to 14 days.[54]

School-age children who are not systemically ill and have symptoms of lower tract infection can be treated with one of many well-tolerated oral broad-spectrum antimicrobial agents for 3 to 5 days.[70-72] In these children single dose treatment, particularly with intramuscular aminoglycoside, could be curative and cause less fecal antimicrobial resistance,[73] but in unselected children single doses may not be as effective as 3 to 5 days of treatment.[73,74]

In a large series of children from 3 months to 5 years of age with febrile UTI, intravenous gentamicin 5 mg/kg/day once daily until afebrile (2 to 4 days) in a day treatment center, followed by oral antibiotic for a total of 10 days, was successful.[75,76]

Selection of Parenteral Antimicrobial Therapy

Most third-generation cephalosporins have broad-spectrum activity against Enterobacteriaceae, and conveniently require only once-or twice-daily dosing. *Enterococcus* is resistant to most cephalosporins.[77,78] Aminoglycosides can provide excellent coverage for UTI, and meta-analysis of available randomized evidence recommends adoption of a once daily dosing in children for potential outpatient treatment.[79] There is little evidence that gentamicin treatment permanently damages those with reduced residual renal function.[80]

Selection of Oral Antimicrobial Therapy

Common community-associated uropathogens are increasingly resistant to trimethoprim-sulfamethoxazole and ampicillin, making these agents less attractive choices for empiric therapy even for first UTIs; second- or third-generation cephalosporins have activity against >90% of bacteria causing first UTI in children. Predictors of pathogen resistance to commonly used agents are recent hospitalization, recent use of antibiotics especially trimethoprim-sulfamethoxazole,[81] and presence of urinary

malformations or urethral catheters.[82] Nitrofurantoin attains high urinary concentrations and low serum concentrations, and thus is a poor choice to treat systemic or renal infection; however, nitrofurantoin is ideal for treating a bladder UTI in patients with a normal urinary tract. Resistance rates to nitrofurantoin have changed little over the past decade.[83] In adults, fluoroquinolones are useful because of their activity against *Pseudomonas aeruginosa,* but in children, use of this drug is limited because of studies showing adverse musculoskeletal events in animals. With careful monitoring, studies of fluoroquinolone usage in children have shown little or no indication of musculoskeletal events. Fluoroquinolones are not approved by the Food and Drug Administration for routine treatment of pediatric UTI. In situations such as an abnormal urinary tract or resistant organisms such as *Pseudomonas aeruginosa,* usage may be indicated.[84]

Prophylaxis

Daily use of antimicrobial agents to prevent recurrent UTI in children who have a 30% to 40% annual chance of recurrence is rational if this prevents significant morbidity and renal damage. Multiple systematic reviews suggest, however, that there is not definitive evidence that prophylaxis prevents recurrent symptomatic UTI;[85-87] infections that occur are more likely due to resistant pathogens. Furthermore, long-term patient compliance with daily prophylaxis may be difficult, and once prophylaxis is initiated, the duration is unclear.[88] After completing the therapeutic regimen for acute UTI, a daily prophylactic antimicrobial agent usually should be given until imaging evaluation of the urinary tract can be performed. Until further data are available, prophylaxis is limited to those with high-grade reflux and underlying obstructive/complex uropathies. The ideal prophylactic agent should have low serum and high urinary concentrations, minimal effect on the normal fecal flora, be easily administered and tolerated, and be cost-effective. In children with normal urinary function, useful agents for urinary prophylaxis are nitrofurantoin, cephalexin, or trimethoprim-sulfamethoxazole.

IMAGING EVALUATION

Radiologic imaging can: (1) evaluate and localize an acute urinary infection, (2) detect renal damage from the acute UTI, (3) identify genitourinary anatomy that increases the risk of future renal damage from UTI, and (4) evaluate change in the urinary tract over time.

Imaging During Acute Infection

Early urinary tract imaging is important in a seriously ill and/or febrile child in whom the site of infection is unclear. US is recommended in guidelines of the United Kingdom National Institute for Health and Clinical Excellence when a child does not respond to antimicrobial treatment within 48 hours or if the UTI is "atypical," defined as a child being seriously ill, having poor urinary flow, abdominal mass, elevated creatinine, or infection with a non-*E. coli* organism.[89] Obstructive lesions are found in 5% to 10% of children and reflux is found in 21% to 57%.[7,90,91] Detection of obstructive abnormalities would merit imaging.

Urinary tract imaging evaluation consists of renal and upper collecting system evaluation (usually renal and bladder US, RBUS) and at times voiding cystourethrogram (VCUG). Current AAP recommendations for imaging for first febrile UTI in children between 2 months and 2 years reflect more selective imaging using RBUS alone as standard management, with VCUG performed in children: (1) whose RBUS reveals hydronephrosis, scarring or other findings that would suggest either high-grade VUR or obstructive uropathy; (2) whose clinical course or findings are atypical or complex; (3) who have recurrent febrile UTI.[54]

In presumed hemorrhagic viral cystitis with a negative bacterial culture, RBUS should be considered to evaluate for other causes of hematuria.

Imaging Findings

Focal or general renal enlargement or swelling can be seen in acute pyelonephritis by RBUS, nuclear scans (e.g., dimercaptosuccinic acid, DMSA), computed tomography (CT), and magnetic resonance imaging (MRI); focal hypo- or hyperechoic areas can indicate focal pyelonephritis (lobar nephronia). The latter represents a localized, severe nonliquefactive infection of one or more renal lobules.[92,93] Other findings on US include thickening of the renal pelvis, hypoechogenicity, and focal or diffuse hyperechogenicity and ureteral dilation.[94]

Follow-up imaging. When urinary tract imaging is normal during acute UTI, but kidneys show massive generalized or focal edema with areas of hypoperfusion, a study 3 to 6 months later may reveal renal scarring or shrinkage. If a child with no VUR on previous VCUG has a subsequent febrile UTI, a nuclear VCUG may be more sensitive at revealing reflux although less likely to characterize it.[95,96]

Generally when a child has no abnormality found after initial imaging of the urinary tract, no subsequent studies are necessary.

COMPLICATIONS

Recurrent pyelonephritis, especially that associated with reflux nephropathy, can result in delayed hypertension and progressive renal dysfunction without further observed UTI. While end-stage renal disease caused by UTI alone is rare, end-stage renal disease related to reflux nephropathy is commonly associated with UTI and is estimated to account for 7% to 17% of end-stage renal disease worldwide, but only about 2% in the U.S.[97]

OTHER GENITOURINARY TRACT INFECTIONS AND COMMON ASSOCIATED PROBLEMS

Funguria

Fungal UTI is an increasing healthcare-associated infection (HAI), especially in patients who have received antimicrobial agents or have a urethral catheter.[98] Other predisposing factors include prematurity, and intravenous or umbilical artery catheterization, parenteral nutrition, and immunocompromised status.[99] Prophylactic use of oral nystatin or fluconazole in very low birthweight infants (<1500 g) has been reported to decrease colonization and invasive fungal infection.[100] C. albicans is the most common species and is responsible for one-half of fungal infections. The second most common is C. glabrata, which is important to recognize because of common resistance to fluconazole.[98,101] Renal US can be helpful in evaluating the extent of fungal infection. Fungal bezoars can form in the renal pelvis, causing obstruction, and anuria in infants with bilateral involvement.[99,102-104] Urinary alkalinization or antifungal therapy (intravenously or orally) can result in resolution of fungus balls. In infants, however, fungus balls can obstruct the small urinary tract, requiring percutaneous or open removal of the bezoars and drainage so that both local irrigation and systemic therapy can be given. The decision regarding treatment of asymptomatic funguria in the setting of an indwelling urethral catheter is controversial, but progression to disseminated candidemia is uncommon.[98,105] Treatment is considered when cultures repeatedly yield growth of >10,000 to 15,000 CFU/mL.[106] Management of candiduria includes: (1) stopping unnecessary antimicrobial agents; (2) removing or changing the indwelling catheter; (3) urinary alkalinization; and when persistent, (4) irrigating the bladder with intravesical amphotericin B or administering oral fluconazole (if susceptibility confirmed) or both. Recurrences are common.[107,108]

Catheter-Associated UTI (Cauti)

The urinary tract is the most common site of nosocomial infection. Nosocomial UTIs complicate pediatric hospitalization especially when urethral catheterization is performed.[28,109] Infectious complications associated with catheterization are acute epididymitis-orchitis, pyelonephritis, periurethral abscess, and struvite and renal calculi. Cultures taken from urethral catheter tips correlate poorly with urine cultures.[110,111]

When urethral catheters remain indwelling for >4 days, bacteriuria is almost inevitable; biofilms form and cause resistance of organisms to routine antimicrobial treatment.[112] During urethral catheter placement, the patient risks urethral injury and potential BSI from catheter manipulation, especially in the presence of bacteriuria. Adult studies show that in 95% of open drainage systems, bacteriuria occurs by 4 days,[59] and daily risk of bacteriuria in closed drainage systems is 5% to 10%.[113] Prophylactic antimicrobial drug therapy to prevent infection during insertion or while indwelling is inappropriate. Full implementation of the "bundle" of infection prevention practices for CAUTI is expected as a safety initiative in healthcare. Guidelines from the Centers for Disease Control and Prevention were updated in 2009 and are available (www.cdc.gov/hicpac/pubs.html). In 2007, the American Heart Association removed recommendation for antibiotic prophylaxis for the purpose of preventing endocarditis during genitourinary (GU) tract procedures.[114] Urethral catheter drainage for bladder emptying must be differentiated from catheter or stent drainage following urethral, bladder, or renal surgical procedures. In these situations bacteriuria often is expected and the reason for drainage may be surgical or reconstructive.

Covert or Asymptomatic UTI

Whether asymptomatic UTIs truly are symptom free is debated. Children may have nocturnal and/or diurnal enuresis, squatting, and urgency, and at least 20% have history of UTI,[11,115] even when symptoms are not the reason for urinalysis or culture. About 50% of children have normal urinary tracts on imaging.

Most infants who have covert bacteriuria clear bacteriuria without treatment;[116] about 30% of asymptomatic school-age girls clear bacteriuria without treatment.[117,118] If the urinary tract is evaluated and found to be normal, treatment or screening for subsequent asymptomatic UTI is unnecessary – obtaining urinary screening cultures is not supported.[119,120] Studies of older children with asymptomatic bacteriuria suggest that more than one-half will have recurrent bacteriuria whether or not treated; the risk of renal damage in these children is low.[11,116,117]

Recurrent UTI With a Normal GU System

Recurrent UTI from reinfection differs from recurrent from persistence. Reinfection often occurs with a different organism or new retrograde infection, whereas recurrence indicates ongoing presence of the original infection (e.g., with an infected stone).[121] Recurrent UTIs occur in ~20% of patients, the majority of whom are girls, regardless of whether the urinary tract is normal.[122] For a girl who has a UTI, the risk of another UTI within a year is proportional to the number of previous infections, regardless of the severity of the original UTI.[2] If the child has frequently recurring infections (≥2 episodes over a 6-month period) prophylactic antimicrobial treatment over a limited period can be considered. When prophylaxis is halted, however, the child often returns to a pattern of increased susceptibility to UTI.[2,123] Nocturnal and diurnal incontinence are common in children with recurrent UTI. In addition to voiding dysfunction, children with recurrent UTI frequently have constipation. Treatment of constipation and/or abnormal voiding behaviors can result in decreased UTIs.[124]

BACTERIOLOGIC ECOLOGY AND ANTIMICROBIAL RESISTANCE

The development of potent antimicrobial agents permits improved and less morbid treatment of UTI. Simultaneously, however, resident flora and infecting bacteria frequently become resistant to standard antimicrobial agents.[125] Widespread injudicious use of antibiotics leads to reservoirs and "epidemic outbreaks" of transmission of multidrug-resistant organisms. To mitigate this global problem, prescribing antimicrobial agents for treatment of UTI must be done in a socially conscious manner. Recommendations by the CDC and the Infectious Disease Society of America (IDSA) include: (1) optimal use of antimicrobial agents, (2) restriction of classes or specific agents, (3) rotational or cyclic usage, and (4) use of combination antimicrobial therapy to decrease resistance.[126]

50 Renal Abscess and Other Complex Renal Infections

Jen-Jane Liu and Linda Marie Dairiki Shortliffe

Pyelonephritis can progress to more complex renal infections (Figure 50-1), such as pyonephrosis, renal abscess, perinephric and paranephric abscess, and xanthogranulomatous pyelonephritis (XGP) that may require surgical intervention. In addition to ultrasonography (US), which is commonly used in the evaluation of simple urinary tract infections (UTIs), axial imaging with computed tomography (CT) or magnetic resonance imaging (MRI) often is helpful to characterize the extent of these infections. In the pre and early antibiotic era, gram-positive organisms commonly caused renal and perinephric abscesses, originating from organisms found in skin and soft-tissue infections (SSTIs). With current rapid antibiotic treatment of SSTIs, organisms causing more severe renal and perinephric infections usually are the pathogens of uncomplicated UTIs and pyelonephritis. These complex genitourinary infections are more likely to be associated with underlying conditions (Box 50-1), especially congenital genitourinary (GU) abnormalities, thus warranting additional evaluation. Furthermore, these infections frequently result in bloodstream infection (BSI) and require complex medical and sometimes surgical management for control.

PYONEPHROSIS

Pyonephrosis is characterized by accumulation of purulent debris and sediment in the renal pelvis and urinary collecting system. Children with pyonephrosis have symptoms similar to those of acute pyelonephritis, but frequently symptoms are more severe or persistent, or there are additional signs of hydronephrosis. Pyonephrosis usually implies bacterial infection and obstruction (infection under elevated pressure), so rapid diagnosis and treatment

are essential to avoid BSI or parenchymal loss or both. The majority of obstructed pyonephrotic kidneys are either nonfunctioning or poorly functioning. The renal US may show shifting fluid–debris levels with changes in the patient's position, persistent echoes from the lower collecting system, air in the collecting system, or decreased echogenicity secondary to pus in a dilated poorly transonic renal collecting system.[1] When pyonephrosis and obstruction are present together, penetration and efficacy of antimicrobial agents can be impaired. The treatment for pyonephrosis is administration of appropriate antimicrobial drugs and prompt drainage of the infected pelvis by either retrograde catheterization or nephrostomy tube placement.

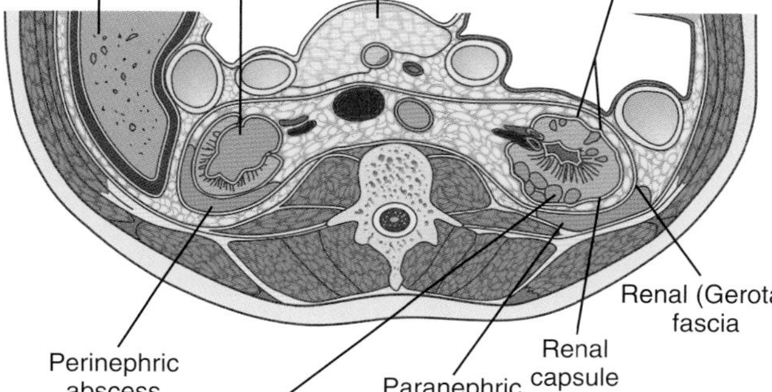

ACUTE FOCAL BACTERIAL NEPHRITIS (ACUTE LOBAR NEPHRONIA)

Severe pyelonephritis can evolve into an inflammatory mass that does not contain drainable pus, known as acute focal bacterial

Figure 50-1. Anatomy and sites of focal infections related to the kidneys.

BOX 50-1. Conditions That Increase Risk for Renal Abscesses

URINARY TRACT CONDITIONS

Infection
Anomalies (reflux, obstruction, duplications)
Neurogenic bladder
Urinary tract stones
Tumor
Polycystic disease
Peritoneal dialysis

PRIMARY INFECTION ELSEWHERE WITH BACTEREMIA

Skin and soft tissue
Dental
Respiratory tract
Gastrointestinal tract
Intra-abdominal
Cardiac
Genital
Intravascular catheter-related
Intravenous illicit drug-related

SURGERY

Urinary tract, including transplantation
Intra-abdominal

OTHER

Immunodeficiency states
Trauma in area of kidney
Diabetes mellitus

PART II Clinical Syndromes and Cardinal Features of Infectious Diseases: Approach to Diagnosis and Initial Management

SECTION G Genitourinary Tract Infections

nephritis (AFBN) or acute lobar nephronia, which is an intermediate stage between pyelonephritis and intrarenal abscess. Similar to renal abscess, AFBN results from ascending or hematogenous infection, and more commonly is observed in patients with genitourinary malformations such as vesicoureteral reflex (VUR), or intrarenal abnormalities such as in sickle-cell disease or polycystic kidney disease. AFBN can be distinguished from renal abscess by CT, which commonly shows a focal, i.e., lobar or wedge-shaped, distribution of hypointensity lesions.[2] Lesions can appear hyper- or hypoechoic on US.[3] No clear abscess wall is seen. Differentiating between AFBN and abscess is important because AFBN can be treated with parenteral antibiotics alone, while renal abscess requires drainage. Complications of AFBN include renal cyst or scarring.[4] Treatment duration is 14 to 21 days, with therapy tailored to culture and susceptibility test results.

PERINEPHRIC OR RENAL ABSCESS

Improvements in imaging of the genitourinary tract and widespread use of potent antimicrobial agents have decreased the incidence and changed the natural history and evaluations of perinephric and renal abscesses.[5,6] In the past, the high mortality rate from perinephric abscesses related in part to diagnostic delay. Abscesses arise either from hematogenous seeding from extragenital sites of infection or renal extension of ascending UTIs. Children with renal and perinephric abscesses usually have severe pyelonephritis – fever, flank pain, leukocytosis, and sometimes BSI. Occasionally the preceding UTI was subclinical, unrecognized, or partially treated as an incorrect diagnosis for a febrile illness (e.g., otitis media), and the patient comes to attention for fever of unknown origin with or without vague abdominal complaints. Perinephric and renal abscess also can be the consequence of seeding from BSI, especially *Staphylococcus aureus* BSI; sepsis can dominate the clinical features.

Since most abscesses have a fluid component, perinephric collections usually appear lucent on US; diagnostic aspiration of this area usually carries minimal morbidity. CT can delineate extent of abscess, presence of perirenal fluid or gas, renal distortion, and involvement of the retroperitoneum[7] (Figure 50-2). Although hematogenous seeding by *S. aureus* was the most common cause of renal abscesses in children and adults more than 2 decades ago,[8] and still occurs, gram-negative bacilli (GNB) (especially *Escherichia coli* and other enteric GNB) are now the most common cause. GNB renal abscesses can occur as retrograde extension of lower UTI, usually in association with severe pyelonephritis and genitourinary anomalies.[8–11] Anaerobic bacteria, usually as part of

a polymicrobial infection, can cause perinephric or renal abscesses in association with previous abdominal surgery, renal transplantation, malignancy, and oral or dental infection.[12]

Some renal and perinephric abscesses can be managed using antimicrobial therapy alone, usually parenterally for a minimum of 2 to 3 weeks, if collections are relatively small or multiple, and microbiology is established by urine or blood culture. In many cases, however, percutaneous or surgical drainage combined with appropriate antibiotic therapy is required.[8,9,11]

XANTHOGRANULOMATOUS PYELONEPHRITIS (XGP)

Under certain circumstances, chronic bacterial pyelonephritis and obstruction are associated with a distinct severe inflammatory process known as xanthogranulomatous pyelonephritis (XGP). While this occurs in only about 1% of cases of pyelonephritis, XGP is diagnosed more frequently recently due to increased use of imaging.[13,14] XGP is important because of confusion with childhood renal tumors (Wilms tumor, multilocular cystic nephroma, congenital mesoblastic nephroma, malignant rhabdoid tumor, and clear cell sarcoma) and need for surgical management. Although the cause is unknown, the process usually is associated with both infection and obstruction.

XGP occurs mainly in adults, but children also can be affected. Symptoms in children and adults are similar and include flank pain, fever, chills, and chronic bacteriuria; vague symptoms such as malaise, malnutrition, weight loss, and failure to thrive can be predominant. Lower tract irritative symptoms (frequency, urgency, dysuria) are uncommon. Most patients with XGP have symptoms for longer than a month before coming to medical attention, or diagnosis.[13,15]

Proteus species (which are overrepresented as cause of XGP considering their infrequent causal role in UTI) and *E. coli* are the most common infecting organisms. Urinalysis usually shows white blood cells and protein, and peripheral blood counts often show anemia reflecting the chronic nature of the disease. XGP usually is unilateral and can involve pericalyceal tissue alone (focal) or the kidney diffusely (diffuse), with extension into the perinephric fat, and even the retroperitoneum with encasement of the great vessels.[14,16]

XGP is most common in adults >40 years of age, but the age range is 21 days to 90 years. XGP in children most frequently affects children ≤8 years of age and boys; the left kidney is the predominantly affected site in most but not all series. While the diffuse form is more common, children are more likely than adults to have the focal form (17% to 25% of cases in children).[15] Contralateral renal hypertrophy can occur.[17] While multiple obstructive calculi containing calcium usually are present in both children and adults, obstruction sometimes is associated with congenital genitourinary abnormalities in children. Obstruction is present in 70% to 80% of children with diffuse XGP and seldom in those with focal XGP.[15]

Radiologic findings include renal calculi in 38% to 70% of patients, nonfunctioning renal segments in 27% to 80%, and a visualized mass in as many as 62% of patients.[14,18] US can show an enlarged kidney with hypoechoic areas that represent areas of necrosis and pus-filled calyces. CT with contrast shows areas of low attenuation that do not enhance and may show extension of the mass into the perinephric fat. Grossly the kidney shows yellow-white nodules and evidence of pyonephrosis. The diagnostic histologic feature is the xanthoma cell – a foamy lipid-laden histiocyte that can simulate the renal carcinoma cell. Xanthoma cells also can appear in other conditions of chronic inflammation and obstruction such as obstructive pneumonia.[19] Consequences of recurrent pyelonephritis include hypertension, progressive renal dysfunction, and even end-stage renal disease.

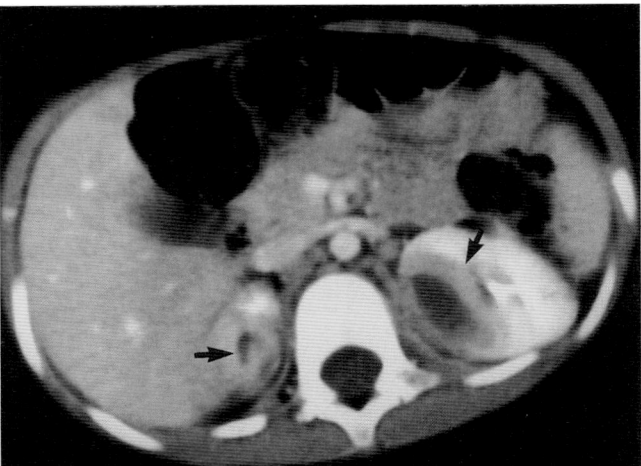

Figure 50-2. Renal abscess in a 5-year-old, ill-appearing girl with a 5-week history of fever and abdominal pain following treatment of *E. coli* urinary tract infection. Contrast-enhanced CT shows a large renal abscess on the left as a large hypodense oval (arrow) representing nonenhancing liquefied center of the abscess. There is a smaller abscess (arrow) on the right.

APPROACH TO DIAGNOSTIC IMAGING

While seldom used to evaluate acute renal inflammatory processes, more extensive imaging by CT or MRI is required for the more complex UTI spectrum of potential pyonephrosis, abscesses,

TABLE 50-1. Relative Radiation Exposures

Examination	Average Effective Dose (mSv)	Equivalent Chest Radiograph	Equivalent Background Radiation
Background radiation in a year	3	150	1 year
U.S. coast–coast airline flight	0.03	1.5	3.6 days
Chest radiograph	0.1	1	10 days
Abdomen radiograph	1	50	125 days
VCUG (infant)	0.8	40	90 days
VCUG (5–10 years)	1.6	80	180 days
Intravenous urogram (IVU)	1.6	80	180 days
Abdomen/pelvis CT (pediatric parameters)	3–5	250	1 year 260 days
Abdomen/pelvis CT with and without contrast (pediatric parameters)	6–10	500	3 years 155 days
Abdomen/pelvis CT (adult parameters)	15–20	750–1000	5–6 years
Renal scan DMSA (99 m-Tc)	1	50	125 days

VCUG, voiding cystourethrogram; CT, computed tomography; DMSA, dimercaptosuccinic acid.

Data from Gaca,[26] American College of Radiology and Radiological Society of North America,[25] Wein AJ, Kavoussi LR, Novick AC, et al. Campbell-Walsh Urology, 10th Edition, 2011, with permission from Elsevier.

calculi and infection. These modalities are indicated when US suggests unusual or complicating anatomic configurations in patients with pyelonephritis, and are useful in distinguishing between inflammatory, neoplastic, and other renal masses.

Acute inflammatory changes of the kidney can be: (a) unilateral or bilateral, (b) focal or diffuse, (c) with or without focal swelling, and (d) with or without renal enlargement. Other distinguishing features are cortical hypoattenuation, wedge defects, and poor corticomedullary differentiation during the cortical and parenchymal nephrographic phases, and linear bands of alternating hyper- and hypoattenuation parallel to the tubules and collecting ducts creating a striated effect during the excretory phase of the study. Scans delayed ≥3 hours can help to differentiate renal abscess from hypofunctioning parenchyma in severe pyelonephritis.[20] Acute focal pyelonephritis (lobar nephronia) has been misinterpreted as a renal abscess by CT, because of the appearance of decreased perfusion in the early phase of the study, and at times MRI- or CT-guided needle aspiration may be needed to clarify the clinical situation.

Risks of Ionizing Radiation and Responsible Imaging

Recommendations for imaging evaluation after UTI have changed in part from greater knowledge of the epidemiology of UTI and in part from evolving imaging technologies. While technology has wrought newer imaging modalities with improved tissue and organ resolution, patient radiation exposure must be considered. Use of CT is the main cause in one country for increased exposure to medical ionizing radiation by almost 25% (1.59 to 1.98 mSv per capita) from 1994 to 2002.[21] There is now evidence for a linear increase in risk of excess lifetime solid cancer and leukemia for radiation exposure from 1 to 150 mSv, with highest risks for those exposed as children.[22,23] Radiation exposure is of particular concern in children because (1) childhood radiation has a longer timespan during which effects can become manifest, (2) developing cells have greater potential of developing direct damage from radiation exposure, and (3) the amount of radiation for medical and diagnostic procedures appropriate for adults often is not adjusted for children, leading to disproportionately high radiation exposure.

The measure of effective radiation dose is the millisievert (mSv), which denotes radiation dosage averaged over the entire body compared with tissue exposure by natural background radiation.[24] Most common background radiation is from cosmic rays at ground level, primordial radionuclides, or ingested potassium. Average background radiation is estimated to be 3 mSv per year,[25] and estimated radiation exposure of common pediatric urologic procedures is shown Table 50-1. CT with and without contrast in a child using appropriate pediatric exposures yields an effective radiation dose of 6 to 10 mSv, equivalent to almost 3.5 years of background radiation,[26] and the estimated lifetime cancer mortality from a pediatric abdominal CT in a 1-year-old is 0.18%.[27]

Radiation risk to children can be limited in 2 ways: (1) decreased exposure through technologic imaging advances and (2) practitioner decision analysis in which imaging studies with risk of ionizing radiation exposure are selected only when information gained is likely to alter management. Such considerations in children should lead to usage where possible of modalities that do not confer ionizing radiation, such as US and MRI.

51 Sexually Transmitted Infection Syndromes

Laura M. Kester, Gale R. Burstein, and Margaret J. Blythe

Many people become sexually active during middle and late adolescence. Reported sexually acquired infections rates remain highest in the 15- through 19- and 20- through 24-year-old populations.[1] Surveys indicate that confidentiality is extremely important for adolescents seeking sexual healthcare. Healthcare personnel (HCP) must feel comfortable discussing behaviors that place teens at risk for sexually transmitted infections (STIs) as well as provide confidential testing, appropriate treatment,

PART II Clinical Syndromes and Cardinal Features of Infectious Diseases: Approach to Diagnosis and Initial Management

SECTION G Genitourinary Tract Infections

immunizations, and counseling on partner notification.[2] Adolescents are concerned about STIs and benefit from interactive, non-judgmental, and developmentally and culturally appropriate counseling about potential risks and consequences.[3,4] This chapter reviews possible presentations of clinical symptoms and syndromes of STIs. STIs diagnosed in prepubertal patients require assessment for sexual abuse; infections acquired during infancy can be the result of sexual abuse or perinatal acquisition (see Chapter 56, Infectious Diseases in Child Abuse).

ASYMPTOMATIC INFECTION

Most *common* STIs usually are asymptomatic. Thus, regular screening for infections in sexually active people is required to improve early detection and treatment of infections, as well as minimize risk of adverse medical consequences. In particular, the United States Preventive Services Task Force (USPSTF) and Centers for Disease Control and Prevention (CDC) recommend annual screening in sexually active adolescent/young adult females for *Chlamydia trachomatis* and *Neisseria gonorrhoeae*.[5,6] People who test positive should be retested approximately 3 months after treatment or whenever they next present for medical care, regardless of partner treatment. Providers may consider more frequent screening for asymptomatic patients who report a partner change, participate in high-risk sexual behaviors, or live in communities with high *Chlamydia* prevalence.[7] Results of a 2004 study from a nationally representative sample of adolescent/young adult men and women indicate an overall prevalence for *Chlamydia* of 4% and for gonorrhea of 0.4%. More than 95% of infected people in this survey denied symptoms in the 24 hours prior to testing.[8] Less than two-thirds of infected people thought they were at risk for infection and less than one-third had been tested for STIs in the prior 12 months.[9]

SYMPTOMATIC INFECTION

Adolescents and young adults manifesting STI symptoms can be divided into six clinical syndromes due to a variety of infectious agents: (1) discharge/dysuria syndrome; (2) anal discharge/proctitis syndrome; (3) genital ulcer/lymphadenopathy syndrome; (4) pelvic or scrotal pain syndrome; (5) pharyngeal infection; and (6) dermatologic syndromes (Table 51-1). Office and laboratory tests used to determine the etiology of STI syndromes are shown in Table 51-2.

Discharge/Dysuria Syndrome

The genital discharge/dysuria syndrome generally is caused by one or more of the following genital infections: *C. trachomatis*, *N. gonorrhoeae*, and *Trichomonas vaginalis*.[8,10] Studies indicate that 30% to 70% of young adults diagnosed with gonorrhea are coinfected with *Chlamydia*.[8,11,12] In addition to these major causes, there also is an increased incidence of urethritis caused by *Mycoplasma genitalium* in certain populations; the high infection rates found among sexual partners of people infected with *M. genitalium* suggest sexual transmission.[7,13,14] Nucleic acid amplification testing (NAAT) demonstrates that the *Ureaplasma urealyticum* and *M. genitalium* prevalences are higher among males with urethritis symptoms compared with males without urethritis symptoms.[7,13–16] Other less commonly identified organisms associated with discharge/dysuria syndrome include viruses such as herpes simplex virus (HSV), *Mycoplasma hominis* or enteric organisms from insertive anal sex.[7] Other non-STI conditions associated with vaginal discharge include bacterial vaginosis and vaginal candidiasis (Table 51-1).

Clinical features, including color, smell, presence of pruritus, and discharge quantity, are not reliable predictors of the microbiologic etiology of genital discharge/dysuria. Young women can

TABLE 51-1. Sexually Transmitted Infection (STI) Syndromes in Adolescents and Young Adults

STI Syndrome	Primary Organisms	Other Causal Organisms
GENITO-URINARY SYNDROMES		
Discharge/dysuria	Chlamydia trachomatis	Ureaplasma urealyticum
	Neisseria gonorrhoeae	Mycoplasma hominis, Mycoplasma genitalium
	Trichomonas vaginalis	Herpes simplex 1, 2
	Females: Candida albicans, anaerobes	
Discharge/proctitis/proctocolitis/enteritis	Chlamydia trachomatis	Shigella species
	Neisseria gonorrhoeae	Campylobacter species
	Treponema pallidum	Salmonella species
	Herpes simplex 1, 2	Giardia lamblia
		Entamoeba histolytica
Genital ulcer/lymphadenopathy	Herpes simplex 1, 2	Haemophilus ducreyi
	Treponema pallidum	Lymphogranuloma venereum
		Calymmatobacterium granulomatis
Pelvic pain (pelvic inflammatory disease)	Chlamydia trachomatis	Mycoplasma hominis, Mycoplasma genitalium
	Neisseria gonorrhoeae	Mixed aerobic/anaerobic bacteri
Scrotal pain (epididymitis)	Chlamydia trachomatis	Ureaplasma urealyticum
	Neisseria gonorrhoeae	Mycoplasma genitalium
PHARYNGITIS	Neisseria gonorrhoeae	Treponema pallidum
	Herpes simplex 1, 2	Human papillomaviruses
DERMATOLOGIC SYNDROMES		
Genital warts	Human papillomaviruses	
Molluscum contagiosum	Molluscum contagiosum virus	
Rash, alopecia	Treponema pallidum	
Arthritis/dermatitis syndrome	Neisseria gonorrhoeae	
	Chlamydia trachomatis	
Jaundice/hepatitis	Hepatitis A, B, C	
Scabies	Sarcoptes scabiei	
Pubic lice	Phthirus pubis	

TABLE 51-2. Office and Laboratory Tests to Determine Etiology of Sexually Transmitted Infection (STI) Syndromes in Adolescents and Young Adults

STI Syndrome	Office Tests	Laboratory Tests
GENITO-URINARY SYNDROMES		
Discharge/dysuria	Females: wet prep of vaginal secretions; LET, pH paper, rapid tests for TV, test cards for BV Males: Gram stain urethral discharge, LET	NAATs for GC, CT, TV and Culture for yeast (recurrent yeast infections)
Discharge/proctitis/proctocolitis/enteritis	Gram stain of anorectal secretions	NAAT for GC, CT Cultures for gram-negative pathogens, ameba
Genital ulcer/lymphadenopathy	Females, males: Darkfield examination for syphilis	Cultures for HSV-1, -2 or PCR or HSV; serology for type-specific glycoprotein G (gG) for HSV-2; RPR or VDRL and confirmatory tests for syphilis if positive or treponemal EIA or CIA chemiluminescence immunoassays and confirmatory nontreponemal test (RPR or VDRL) if positive; nucleic acid detection for *C. trachomatis;* PCR genotyping or serology for LGV (complement fixation or microimmunofluorescence); Gram stain and culture for chancroid; staining for Donovan bodies on tissue biopsy
Pelvic pain (pelvic inflammatory disease)	Wet prep and Gram stain of vaginal secretions; pH paper, rapid tests for TV; Gram stain endocervical fluid, LET; urine pregnancy test	NAATs for GC, CT, TV
Scrotal pain (epididymitis)	Gram stain of urethral discharge; leukocyte esterase on first-void urine	NAATs for GC, CT
PHARYNGITIS	Rapid strep test	NAAT for GC; culture or PCR for HSV-1, -2; PCR assay for HSV DNA; RPR or VDRL and confirmatory tests if positive
DERMATOLOGIC SYNDROMES		
Genital warts	Characteristic lesions	
Molluscum contagiosum	Characteristic lesions	Wright or Giemsa staining for intracytoplasmic inclusions
Rash/alopecia		RPR or VDRL and confirmatory tests if positive
Arthritis/dermatitis syndrome	Males: Gram stain urethral discharge, LET Females: wet prep of vaginal secretions; pH paper; LET	NAAT or culture for GC from rectum, pharynx, genital; or NAATs of genital secretions or urine
Jaundice/hepatitis		Appropriate laboratory tests for hepatitis
Scabies	Microscopic examination of skin and hair	
Pubic lice	Identification of eggs, nymphs and lice with naked eye or microscopy	

BV, bacterial vaginosis; CT, Chlamydia trachomatis; GC, Neisseria gonorrhoeae; HSV-1, -2, herpes simplex-1,-2; LET, leukocyte esterase test of urine; LGV, lymphogranuloma venereum; NAATs, nucleic acid amplification tests; RPR, rapid plama reagin; TV, Trichomonas vaginalis; VDRL, Venereal Disease Research Laboratory. EIA, enzyme immunoassay; CIA, chemiluminescence immunoassay.

have dysuria and white blood cells (WBCs) in their urine but have a negative urine culture ("sterile pyuria"). Sterile pyuria can accompany cervicovaginal infection due to meatal irritation or urethral infection. Other symptoms can accompany vaginal discharge/dysuria in females, including abnormal vaginal bleeding, dyspareunia, vulvovaginal pruritus, and mild pelvic pain.

Among males, characteristics of the urethral discharge are useful but are not reliable to distinguish chlamydial from gonococcal infections. In general, urethral discharge caused by *N. gonorrhoeae* is more purulent and profuse compared with discharge caused by *C. trachomatis*. A majority of symptomatic males with gonococcal infections complain of both discharge and dysuria; only about 2% complain of dysuria alone. Urethritis due to *C. trachomatis* or *M. genitalium* can be associated with dysuria alone, that may only occur with the initial phase of urination. Other findings can include hematuria, meatal pruritus, and edema of the glans and head of the penis.

Anal Discharge/Proctitis/Proctocolitis/ Enteritis Syndrome

Anorectal discharge and pain associated with tenesmus with or without anorectal bleeding is an STI syndrome occurring in both young men and women. Infections without a history of anal sex can occur in females but not males.[7] Proctitis primarily is

a result of receptive anal intercourse and is most commonly associated with *N. gonorrhoeae*, *C. trachomatis* (including lymphogranuloma venereum (LGV) serovars), *Treponema pallidum*, and HSV.[7,17] Asymptomatic infections are common, although the exact prevalence is not known since population-based screening studies have not been done.

Proctocolitis manifests similarly to proctitis with additional symptoms of abdominal pain, diarrhea, and bloating. These infections are acquired from receptive anal intercourse and caused by *Shigella* species, *Campylobacter* species, *Salmonella* species, *Entamoeba histolytica*, and *C. trachomatis* (including serovars associated with LGV). In HIV-infected immunocompromised people, these organisms along with CMV must be considered as possible opportunistic infections.[7] Unlike proctitis, sexually acquired proctocolitis and enteritis also can result from anal–oral contact and is most commonly associated with *Giardia lamblia*.[7] In addition, sexually transmitted enteritis can be caused by HIV infection or can arise as an HIV-opportunistic infection.[7]

Genital Ulcer/Lymphadenopathy Syndrome

Genital HSV

In the U.S., the most common cause of genital ulcers is HSV-2 or HSV-1. In the past, genital herpes typically was associated with

HSV-2, with a small proportion of incident cases associated with HSV-1. Recently, the proportion of genital herpes in the U.S. due to HSV-1 has risen and is estimated to be 30% to 50% of new cases.[18] Data from national studies indicate that the prevalence of HSV-2 positive serology among people 14 through 19 years of age is 1% and increases to 11% for people 20 through 29 years of age.[19] Overall, 25% of females and 20% of males ≥12 years of age are seropositive for HSV-2. Up to 81% of people with positive HSV-2 serology indicate that they had no previous diagnosis of genital herpes.[19] Over two-thirds of the U.S. population has antibody to HSV-1, specifically, 44% of people 12 to 19 years of age and 56% of people 20 though 39 years of age.[20] The most common transmission of genital herpes occurs from asymptomatic viral shedding among people who are unaware that they are infected.[7]

HSV infections are classified by HSV serologic status at time of infection and by history of symptomatic episodes. A *primary infection* occurs in a patient who is seronegative for both HSV-1 and HSV-2 antibody. A *first episode* is the first clinical manifestations of genital herpes due to HSV-1 or HSV-2 infection. A first genital herpes episode can be a primary infection (seronegative for HSV-1 and HSV-2 antibody) or a nonprimary infection (HSV-2 infection in a person with pre-existing HSV-1 antibody or HSV-1 infection in a person with pre-existing HSV-2 antibodies). A *recurrent episode* is a clinical HSV genital outbreak in a patient with a previous genital herpes episode from the same HSV type.

A first clinical episode is more likely to be associated with systemic symptoms such as headache, myalgia, photophobia, fever, and malaise, particularly if a primary infection. Approximately 10% of first clinical episodes occur among people with antibody to the same HSV type.[21] Initial symptoms can be limited to pain, burning, or pruritus in the area where lesions eventually appear. Development of single or small groups of vesicles typically follows within a few hours. Vesicles often are quite painful, and progress to ulcers over a period of a few days. Tender, usually bilateral, inguinal lymphadenopathy can appear at this time. New lesions can appear, leading to finding of lesions in various stages of development. The length of viral shedding and time required to heal depend on whether the infection is primary, nonprimary, or recurrent; for primary infections, viral shedding continues for 10 to 12 days and healing requires up to 3 weeks; for recurrent infections, shedding occurs for up to 4 days, with healing in 5 to 7 days. Dysuria and urethral or vaginal discharge also are common. In people with HSV-2, intermittent, frequent asymptomatic shedding usually occurs.

Syphilis

Primary syphilis is an important cause of genital ulcer/lymphadenopathy syndrome, although relatively uncommon among adolescents in the U.S. The classic primary syphilis lesion is a single, deep, indurated, painless ulcer associated with unilateral, nonfluctuant, ipsilateral inguinal lymphadenopathy. Multiple chancres occur in approximately 25% of cases. These lesions occur about 3 weeks (10 to 90 days) after sexual contact with an infected person; untreated infections heal spontaneously without treatment in 1 to 6 weeks. Lesions can occur almost anywhere in the genital/rectal area, with perianal and rectal chancres usually the result of rectal intercourse.

Clinical presentation of genital lesions due to HSV can appear similar to a primary *Treponema pallidum* infection. Classic findings for genital herpes (multiple, shallow, tender ulcers) and for primary syphilis (deep, indurated, painless ulcers) are clinical indicators, but only with an estimated 35% sensitivity for a confirmed diagnosis.[22]

Other Causes

Other causes of genital ulcer disease are rare in the U.S., with sporadic outbreaks of LGV occurring primarily among HIV-infected men who have sex with men (MSM) in both Europe and the U.S.[17] LGV is caused by *C. trachomatis* serovars L1, L2, L3, with an incubation of 3 to 12 days or longer. Most infections begin as an asymptomatic ulcer, papule, or erosion at the site of infection and can be associated with nonspecific urethritis. Lesions typically progress to tender femoral or inguinal unilateral lymphadenopathy. Another rare cause of lymphadenopathy/genital syndrome in the U.S. is *Haemophilus ducreyi* (chancroid), a gram-negative anaerobic bacillus.[23] Incubation usually is 4 to 7 days with no prodromal symptoms; lesions are tender papules surrounded by erythema that become pustular, erode, and then form painful ulcerations over 14 to 48 hours, ultimately progressing to painful suppurative lymphadenopathy. Granuloma inguinale (donovanosis), caused by *Klebsiella (Calymmatobacterium) granulomatis*, can be considered as a possible etiology of genital ulcerative disease if the infection was acquired in a developing country or by sexual contact with someone traveling from a developing country. Lesions typically are painless, highly vascular, and "beefy red", and gradually progress to ulcerations without regional lymphadenopathy; subcutaneous nodules also can be associated.[7]

Pelvic or Scrotal Pain Syndrome

Pelvic or scrotal pain often is associated with an STI. Pelvic pain is common in females presenting with pelvic inflammatory disease (PID). Although *N. gonorrhoeae* and *C. trachomatis* are the most common infections associated with PID, these pathogens are identified in less than one-third of PID cases. Other organisms, including anaerobes representing endogenous vaginal flora, such as *G. vaginalis*, *Haemophilus influenzae*, enteric gram-negative rods, and *Streptococcus agalactiae*, also have been isolated from the endometrium and fallopian tubes and thereby linked to PID.[7,24,25] Some studies have identified *M. genitalium*, *M. hominis*, and *U. urealyticum* with PID.[7,26-29]

PID symptoms can be mild or severe. Mild or subclinical PID episodes can go unrecognized. The clinical diagnosis of PID is imprecise and relies on history and clinical indicators. Currently, there are no single pieces of data (history, physical examination, or laboratory finding) that are both sensitive and specific for diagnosis.[7] Due to the significance of disease sequelae, empiric therapy for PID should be initiated in sexually active young females experiencing pelvic or lower abdominal pain, without an identifiable cause, and who meet minimum criteria of cervical motion tenderness *or* uterine tenderness *or* adnexal tenderness present on examination. Specificity can be further increased with evidence of associated lower-genital tract infection/inflammation, specifically, mucopurulent cervical discharge on examination and/or WBCs on microscopic evaluation of a vaginal fluid saline preparation.[7] Additional supportive criteria include oral temperature >38.3°C, elevated erythrocyte sedimentation rate (ESR) or C-reactive protein, or laboratory documentation of *N. gonorrhoeae* or *C. trachomatis* infection. Minimum criteria should be present, but supportive criteria need not be present to initiate treatment. A urine pregnancy test, urinalysis, and culture always should be performed since ectopic pregnancy and urinary tract infection/pyelonephritis can cause pelvic pain.

Scrotal pain in young men at risk for STIs most often represents epididymitis. Presentation usually is insidious with onset of unilateral scrotal pain, tenderness, and swelling in the affected area. Presentations can be chronic or acute. Torsion of the testicle first must be excluded with imaging evaluation. History of dysuria and urethral discharge is often, but not invariably, present. Fever or bilateral involvement is infrequent. Alleviation of pain with gentle manual elevation of the affected side (Prehn sign) is supportive of the diagnosis. Presence of WBCs and gram-negative intracellular diplococci (*N. gonorrhoeae*) on a Gram stain are helpful, as is the presence of positive leukocyte esterase on a urine dipstick or WBCs on urinalysis. Among young men, *C. trachomatis* and *N. gonorrhoeae* are the most commonly identified microbiologic etiologies and can occur concurrently. *U. urealyticum* and *M. genitalium* likely cause some cases but their exact role as agents of epididymitis is poorly defined.[30] Cases of epididymitis also have been associated with *Escherichia coli* and other gram-negative enteric organisms, although this presentation is most common with insertive anal sex and among men older than 35 years of age. Chronic epididymitis can be secondary to *Mycobacterium tuberculosis,* with suspicion based on appropriate history and possible acquisition of infection.[7]

Pharyngeal Infection

Gonococcal infections occur on mucosal surfaces lined with columnar epithelium, and can include the cervix, urethra, rectum, pharynx, and conjunctiva. Gonococcal infection of the pharynx can manifest as an asymptomatic infection or as mild symptoms with pharyngeal erythema. Gonococcal infection of the pharynx can lead to disseminated gonococcal infection (DGI).

HSV-1 and HSV-2 can infect the pharynx, with clinical manifestations of sore throat, fever, malaise, myalgia, headache, and tender anterior cervical lymphadenopathy. Mild ulceration and diffuse erythema can be the initial manifestation. Oral syphilis can cause painless chancres on the lips, buccal mucosa, tonsils, and pharynx; lesions on the tonsils and pharynx may be painful. Oral and laryngeal papillomas due to human papillomavirus (HPV) can appear after oral–genital contact.[7]

Dermatologic Syndromes

Dermatologic syndromes that occur in adolescents and young adults include genital warts, molluscum contagiosum, dermatologic manifestations of secondary syphilis, the arthritis/dermatitis syndrome associated with DGI, jaundice/hepatitis associated with several sexually transmitted viruses, and the parasites scabies and pubic lice acquired during sexual contacts.

Of the 100 types of HPV identified, approximately 40 infect the anogenital region.[7] HPV subtypes 6 and 11 are responsible for 90% of exophytic genital warts (condyloma acuminata)[16] along with other low-risk types, including 42 and 43. Additionally oncogenic subtypes 16, 18, 31, 33, and 35 can be associated with genital warts, but are thought usually to be coinfections with types 6 and 11.[7] Genital warts can occur at almost any squamous epithelial site within the genital tract. In young men, common sites of warts are the glans, prepuce, urethral meatus, and shaft of the penis, as well as the perianal area. In young women, warts are found in almost any area of the vulva, perianal area, vagina, and cervix. HPV types 6 and 11 also have been associated with warts in nasal, conjunctival, oral, and laryngeal regions. A quadrivalent HPV vaccine protects against the HPV types that cause 90% of genital warts (types 6 and 11).[31]

Molluscum contagiosum can be acquired during sexual contact and can be confused with genital warts. Lesions typically are 1 to 2 mm, smooth, skin-colored papules. Infections can be transmitted by any skin-to-skin contact; lesions on nongenital skin are common. Lesions usually are asymptomatic.

Lesions of secondary syphilis occur 2 to 6 weeks after initial infection. Often, the primary lesion has not been noticed, or has been ignored. Secondary syphilis has a number of potential dermatologic presentations. Diffuse maculopapular and papulosquamous rashes of the trunk, arms, and legs are most common. A papulosquamous rash involving the palms and soles also occurs. Wart-like growths, typically in the perianal or posterior vulvar area, are manifestations of secondary syphilis, referred to as condyloma lata, and initially can be confused with genital warts.

The arthritis/dermatitis syndrome of DGI classically includes dermatitis, tenosynovitis, and migratory polyarthritis. Knee, ankle, wrist, and metacarpophalangeal joints are involved most commonly. Dermatitis usually is a painless, maculopapular rash typically occurring on the trunk and limbs. Tenosynovitis usually involves the hands and fingers, and can be asymmetric. Dissemination of infection can occur from any primary *N. gonorrhoeae* infection of the genitalia, anus, or pharynx. DGI is more common among young women than young men.

For many adolescents, jaundice associated with acute viral hepatitis could be the result of sexually acquired hepatitis A or B virus, cytomegalovirus, or Epstein–Barr virus.

Scabies is caused by the mite *Sarcoptes scabiei.* Acquisition during sexual contact is common, although close personal contact such as sharing a bed can lead to transmission in the absence of sexual contact. Genital infestations are common, although concentration of mites is more common on the hands and fingers. The rash associated with scabies, however, is caused in part by sensitization and can occur at body sites other than those directly infested. Pruritus typically is worse at night.

Pubic lice *(Phthirus pubis)* are associated with close interpersonal contact, not necessarily sexual contact. Symptoms are related to itching and irritation: lice and/or nits are often visible.

52 Skin and Mucous Membrane Infections and Inguinal Lymphadenopathy

Kimberly A. Workowski

GENITAL ULCER WITH LYMPHADENOPATHY

Infections that cause lymphadenopathy with and without genital ulcer disease (GUD) are frequently transmitted sexually and can manifest as unilateral or bilateral inguinal lymphadenopathy. Genital ulcerations due to sexually transmitted infections (STI) pose complex clinical problems because of the multiple possible etiologies, diverse clinical presentations, and challenges to making a definitive diagnosis.[1-3]

Etiologic Agents and Epidemiology

The most common infectious causes of genital ulceration are herpes simplex viruses (HSV-2 and HSV-1), *Treponema pallidum* (syphilis), *Chlamydia trachomatis* serovars L1, L2, and L3 (lymphogranuloma venereum), *Haemophilus ducreyi* (chancroid), and *Klebsiella granulomatis* (donovanosis or granuloma inguinale).[1-3] Associated with genital ulceration, regional lymph nodes may become involved and lead to femoral or inguinal adenopathy or ulceration.

Infrequently, scabies and pubic lice can result in GUD, as can pyoderma, *Entamoeba histolytica,* and *Capnocytophaga* spp. infections. Genital, anal, or perianal lesions also can be associated with conditions that are not transmitted sexually (fixed drug eruption, psoriasis, aphthae).

In general, GUD is a common presentation of a sexually transmitted infection, particularly in developing countries. In the United States, most young sexually active people with genital, anal, or perianal ulcers have either genital herpes or syphilis.[1] The frequency of each condition differs by geographic area and

PART II Clinical Syndromes and Cardinal Features of Infectious Diseases: Approach to Diagnosis and Initial Management

SECTION G Genitourinary Tract Infections

population. Genital herpes also has become a leading cause of genital ulceration in some developing countries.[4]

There is marked variation in prevalence of syphilis and chancroid by city, region, and risk group in North America.[5,6] In the late 1980s and early 1990s, syphilis and chancroid were found to be the cause of 40% to 90% of GUD in crack cocaine users.[7,8] Following a decline in reported syphilis incidence in the 1990s, several large syphilis outbreaks have been identified in North America and Europe.[5,9,10]

Granuloma inguinale occurs rarely in the U.S., although the disease is endemic in several geographic locations including India, the Caribbean, northern Australia, and South Africa. Lymphogranuloma venereum (LGV) can manifest as either inguinal or femoral adenopathy or proctocolitis. LGV proctitis has been reported in men who have sex with men in the U.S. and Europe. Most men with LGV proctitis have been HIV-coinfected and have participated in high-risk sexual behaviors.[11,12]

Prior to the HIV epidemic in Africa, Southeast Asia, and India, GUD was more commonly due to chancroid than HSV.[13] However, an increasing proportion of GUD in developing countries is now due to genital HSV.[4] For example, in Botswana the proportion of GUD due to HSV increased from 35% in 1998 to 61% in 2002, whereas there was substantial decline in the proportion due to *T. pallidum* (52% to 5%) and *H. ducreyi* (33% to <1%).[14] This pattern is believed to be similar in other sub-Saharan countries.[15]

GUD due to HSV and the interaction with HIV has been the topic of considerable research.[16,17] HSV infections are chronic; many people are not aware they are infected and may have unrecognized or only mild symptoms. The majority of genital HSV infections are transmitted by people unaware that they have the infection. People with HSV-2 infections shed virus intermittently in the genital tract, at which time they can transmit HSV-2 to sexual partners.[1] While the majority of recurrent GUD is due to HSV-2, infection caused by HSV-1 in the United States may be increasing.[18] The course of symptoms can be modified by therapy with acyclovir (or its analogues) if treatment is started during the prodrome or within 24 hours of symptom onset.[1] Genital, especially vulvar, ulcers are uncommon but well-described manifestations of primary varicella-zoster virus infection and zoster, Epstein–Barr virus infection, cytomegalovirus infection in immunocompromised hosts, and as a manifestation of Crohn and Behçet disease.[19-21]

GUD increases the risk of transmission of HIV.[22] Further, even in the absence of ulceration, HSV-2 infection increases the risk of HIV transmission to a sex partner and can increase HSV shedding among HIV-infected persons.[17] Suppressive or episodic therapy with antiviral agents is effective in decreasing the clinical manifestations of HSV among HIV infected persons.[1]

Clinical Manifestations and Differential Diagnosis

Identification of the etiology of GUD presents several challenges. Experienced clinicians are unable to distinguish between GUD etiologies based upon clinical presentation only.[1,3] Obtaining a specific etiologic diagnosis frequently requires specialized testing. The specimen collection materials, testing equipment, and trained personnel required to conduct and interpret some of tests are typically not available in many laboratories, especially in the developing world.

The classic clinical features of the major causes of GUD are described in Table 52-1. In clinical practice, distinctions are not necessarily apparent, because lesions of different etiologies may

TABLE 52-1. Classic Clinical Features[a] of Sexually Transmitted Genital Ulcer Disease Syndromes

Feature	Herpes simplex (Herpes)	Treponema pallidum (Syphilis)	Haemophilus ducreyi (Chancroid)	Chlamydia trachomatis (Lymphogranuloma Venereum)	Klebsiella granulomatis (Granuloma Inguinale)
Incubation period estimates	2–7 days	14–28 days	1–14 days	3–42 days	8–80 days
Site					
Male	Glans/prepuce, penis, anus/rectum	At site of inoculation	At site of inoculation	At site of inoculation (urethal/rectal)	90% involve genitalia
Female	Cervix, vulva, perineum, buttocks/legs, anus/rectum	At site of inoculation	At site of inoculation	At site of inoculation (urethal/rectal)	90% involve genitalia
Typical primary lesion presentation	Vesicle (variable, depending upon lesion duration, host immune status, etc.)	Papule (ulcerates)	Papule or pustule	Papule, vesicle, vesiculopustular lesion	Subcutaneous nodule that erodes; occasionally verrucous
Number of lesions	Usually multiple; can coalesce, especially in immunocompromised host	Usually single, can be multiple	Often multiple; can coalesce	Usually single	Single or multiple
Ulcer appearance	Small, superficial, smooth; with erythematous edge, circular	Superficial, medium size, well demarcated; with elevated edge, circular/oval	Deep, small to large; undermined, with ragged edge, irregular shape	Variable depth, small to medium size; elevated edge, round/oval	Small to large lesions; with elevated edge and beefy base, irregular shape
Induration	None	Firm	Soft	Occasionally firm	Firm
Pain	Exquisitely	Typical painless	Variable	Variable	Not typical
Lymphadenopathy characteristic	Firm, tender, often bilateral	Firm, nontender, bilateral	Tender, can suppurate; unilateral; superinfection	Large, tender, unilateral; can suppurate	Pseudobuboes; regional lymphadenopathy with superinfection
Treatment	Acyclovir, famciclovir or other acyclovir analogues	Penicillin (dose and duration depend upon clinical stage)	Azithromycin, ceftriaxone, doxycycline, or erythromycin	Doxycycline (alternative: erythromycin)	Doxycycline (alternative: erythromycin)

[a]*Typical but not universal clinical presentation.*

coexist, GUD clinical presentations are less distinctive for each etiology than previously believed, and immunocompromising conditions, such as HIV infection, can further modify clinical manifestations. Careful examination of the entire genital region, including the perineum and anus, facilitated by a good light source and a handheld magnifying lens, may improve the clinical assessment and guide selection of appropriate diagnostic tests. Additionally, due to the asymptomatic nature of several of these infections, anorectal manifestations may be overlooked by the patient as well as the clinician. Performing an anoscopic examination can assist in the identification of lesions and improve GUD diagnosis and treatment.

Laboratory Diagnosis and Management

Confirmation of etiology is usually possible with appropriate specimen collection and testing (Table 52-2). A discussion with local laboratory personnel before collection and submission of a specimen can facilitate optimal testing.

A clinical diagnosis of genital HSV should be confirmed by laboratory testing.[1] The prognosis and type of counseling messages depends on the type of genital herpes (HSV-1 or HSV-2) causing the infection. Recurrences and subclinical shedding are less frequent for genital HSV-1 than genital HSV-2. Both virologic tests and HSV type-specific serologic tests should be available in clinical settings that provide care for persons with sexually transmitted infections or those at risk for these infections. Viral detection of HSV in cell culture or by the polymerase chain reaction (PCR) are the preferred tests for people who seek medical treatment for genital ulcers or other mucocutaneous lesions. However, the sensitivity of culture is low, especially for recurrent lesions, and declines rapidly as lesions begin to heal. Failure to detect HSV by culture or PCR does not indicate an absence of HSV infection, because viral shedding is intermittent. The use of cytologic detection of cellular changes due to HSV infection is insensitive and nonspecific for genital lesions and for cervical Papanicolaou smears and should not be used. Accurate, type-specific HSV serologic assays are based on the HSV-specific glycoproteins G2 (HSV-2) and G1 (HSV-1). These assays first became commercially available in 1999, but older assays that do not accurately distinguish HSV-1 from HSV-2 antibody remain on the market. Therefore, the serologic type-specific glycoprotein G (gG)-based assays should be requested when serology is performed.[1] Repeat testing might be indicated in some settings, especially if recent

acquisition of genital HSV is suspected. IgM testing for HSV is not useful, because these tests are not type specific and can be positive during recurrent episodes.[1]

Optimal management of GUD should include empiric treatment for the most likely diagnosis based on the clinical presentation and epidemiologic circumstances (see Table 52-1). If no clinical improvement is evident following treatment, the clinician must consider if the diagnosis is correct, coinfection with a concurrent STI or HIV, reinfection, adequacy of partner treatment, antimicrobial resistance, or noninfectious etiology.[1]

Because concurrent infections may be present in people diagnosed with GUD, testing for other sexually transmitted infections is recommended. A thorough risk assessment, counseling, and testing for HIV infection are important in all persons diagnosed with a sexually transmitted infection and for those at ongoing risk of infection. Partner counseling and treatment (if indicated) is also recommended as part of comprehensive care.

Diagnosis of sexually transmitted infection in a child should trigger a thorough evaluation for sexual abuse.[1]

INGUINAL ADENOPATHY WITHOUT GENITAL ULCERS

While infections associated with GUD often cause inguinal adenopathy (see Table 52-1), some pathogens cause inguinal adenopathy without ulcers (Table 52-3). In these infections, inguinal lymphadenopathy typically is bilateral, although a chancroid bubo usually is unilateral. Inguinal lymphadenitis associated with pyogenic infections of the lower extremities, lower abdominal wall, or perineum is usually unilateral and frequently is of acute onset; progression to local abscess formation can occur (see Table 52-3), typically due to *Staphylococcus aureus* or group A streptococcus.

Retrocecal appendicitis can cause an unexplained limp with right-sided inguinal lymphadenopathy which is then followed by fever. Back and hip pain become increasingly prominent with abscess formation, and extension of the upper leg produces pain. Cat-scratch disease (see Chapter 160, *Bartonella* Species) and mycobacterial infections occasionally can manifest with inguinal adenopathy (see Chapter 134, *Mycobacterium tuberculosis*, and Chapter 135, *Mycobacterium* Species Non-*tuberculosis*). In bubonic plague, if the fleabite initiating the infection occurs on the leg, inguinal or femoral buboes can occur (see Chapter 148, *Yersinia* Species). *Yersinia enterocolitica* intestinal infection can manifest as lymphadenopathy of mesenteric or inguinal nodes, and sometimes is suppurative.[23] Tularemia can mimic plague but is more likely to cause ulceroglandular syndrome than glandular symptoms alone (see Chapter 171, *Francisella tularensis*).

Management of isolated inguinal lymphadenopathy depends on the suspected etiology (see Table 52-2). Aspiration of lymph nodes with smear examination and culture is useful in pyogenic infections. Further diagnostic investigations, such as ultrasonography or computed tomography, are helpful if osteomyelitis or retrocecal appendicitis is suspected. Specific antimicrobial therapy is directed against the inciting pathogen.

GENITAL DERMATOSIS

Yeast Infections

Many skin infections affect the genitals and genitocrural folds, especially infections of the diaper region and perineum caused by *Candida albicans* or *C. glabrata* (see Chapter 243, *Candida* Species). In diapered infants, eruption often starts in the perianal area and spreads to involve the perineum and upper thighs. Onset can be acute, with scaly macules or papules that coalesce to form well-demarcated, erythematous lesions with irregular borders and frequently with satellite lesions. Treatment consists of keeping the area as dry as possible and applying a topical antifungal cream.

In older children and adolescents, genital candidal infection can involve the vagina or the penis. Symptoms of vulvovaginitis

TABLE 52-2. Specimen Selection and Laboratory Tests for Diagnosis of Genital Ulcer with Lymphadenopathy Syndrome

Condition	Specimen Type	Test
Herpes	Scraping from ulcer base	Tissue cell culture, PCR
	Serology	HSV-1 and HSV-2 antibody
Syphilis	Exudate from ulcer	Darkfield microscopy
	Serology	Nontreponemal (with titer quantification); if positive, confirm with treponemal test
Chancroid	Swab from ulcer base or aspirate from bubo	Semiselective media, PCR
Lymphogranuloma venereum	Aspirate from bubo	Tissue culture
	Lesion or swab from ulcer base	Direct immunofluorescence, nucleic acid detection for *C. trachomatis* approved
Donovanosis (Granuloma inguinale)	Crush preparation from lesion	Giemsa or Wright stain for Donovan bodies

HSV, herpes simplex virus; PCR, polymerase chain reaction.

PART II Clinical Syndromes and Cardinal Features of Infectious Diseases: Approach to Diagnosis and Initial Management

SECTION G Genitourinary Tract Infections

TABLE 52-3. Differential Diagnosis of Inguinal Lymphadenopathy

Condition	Organism	Pattern of Lymphadenopathy	Associations
WITHOUT ULCER(S)			
Pyogenic bacteria	Group A streptococcus, *Staphylococcus aureus*	Suppurative, unilateral, and tender; can progress to abscess	Retrocecal appendicitis; osteomyelitis, pyogenic arthritis; infection of skin or abdominal wall
Tuberculosis	*Mycobacterium tuberculosis*	Caseating, can be unilateral, nontender	Miliary tuberculosis, osteomyelitis
Cat-scratch disease	*Bartonella henselae*	Unilateral, tender, slowly progressive	Scratch lesion on lower limb
Plague	*Yersinia pestis*	Large cluster, very tender nodes	Exposure to fleas, rodents, or rabbits
WITH ULCERS			
Herpes	Herpes simplex virus		
Syphilis	*Treponema pallidum*		
Chancroid	*Haemophilus ducreyi*	Bilateral nodes (see text for details)	Sexually transmitted
Lymphogranuloma venereum	*Chlamydia trachomatis* (L1, L2, L3)		
Granuloma inguinale (donovanosis)	*Klebsiella granulomatis*		
Tularemia	*Francisella tularensis*	Large, very tender lymph nodes with ulcerated skin lesions	Exposure to rabbit, squirrel, coyote
Mononucleosis	Epstein–Barr virus	Vulvar ulcers with regional adenopathy	
Yersiniosis	*Yersinia enterocolitica*	Inguinal (unilateral or bilateral)	Fecal–oral; or consumption of pork chitterlings

pruritus, include pain, and a whitish milky discharge (see Chapter 53, Urethritis, Vulvovaginitis, and Cervicitis). Balanoposthitis can be associated with pruritus, and erythematous lesions with whitish patches can be seen on the glans, prepuce, and shaft of the penis. Topical antifungal therapy is effective, but relapses can occur.

Dermatophyte Infections

Excessive perspiration and friction in intertriginous areas such as the groin predispose to superficial infections with dermatophytes including *Trichophyton rubrum*, *T. mentagrophytes*, or *Epidermophyton floccosum* (see Chapter 254, Dermatophytes and Other Superficial Fungi). These infections are more common in hot weather and occur more in males than in females. The infection, although often symmetric, can be asymmetric with extension from the crural areas to the upper thigh. Lesions can be erythematous scaly patches with papular or vesicular margins. The lesions typically

are pruritic; scratching can lead to lichenification. Treatment consists of use of a topical antifungal agent. Systemic therapy (e.g., fluconazole) occasionally is used if lesions are widespread or recalcitrant, a common manifestation of candidiasis in immunocompromised patients, until the infection is resolved.

Genital Warts (Condyloma Acuminatum)

Genital warts are caused by infection of the epidermis with a human papillomavirus (HPV), especially types 6 and 11 (see Chapter 211, Human Papillomaviruses) (Figure 52-1).[1] Among adolescents and adults, anogenital warts most often are transmitted sexually. In children, the mode of acquisition is more difficult to assess (see Chapter 56, Infectious Diseases in Child Abuse).[1] Pre-exposure vaccination is the most effective method for preventing HPV. Details regarding human papillomavirus vaccines are available at http://www.cdc.gov/std/hpv.

Molluscum Contagiosum Infection

Molluscum contagiosum is caused by parapoxvirus, and can be transmitted sexually and nonsexually (see Chapter 202, Poxviridae). Diagnosis usually is based on clinical appearance. The mean incubation period is 2 to 3 months. Unlike genital warts, which occur predominantly on external genitalia and the perianal area, lesions of molluscum contagiosum most often occur on thighs, inguinal region, buttocks, and lower abdominal wall. Children more typically have lesions on the face, trunk, and extremities, but some children can have genital lesions. Lesions begin as small papules and can grow to 10 to 15 mm. They become smooth, firm, and dome-shaped with central umbilication, from which caseous material can be expressed. Lesions can be removed mechanically with curettage or through induction of local inflammation, as with application of podophyllin. In adolescents with multiple facial molluscum lesions, and in children with multiple lesions, concurrent HIV infection should be considered. Lesions associated with HIV infection can be atypical and extensive. Treatment of extensive infections is challenging, and patients with this condition should be referred to a dermatologic specialist for treatment.

OTHER CONDITIONS

Scabies and pubic lice also can be transmitted sexually and can cause skin lesions in the genital area.

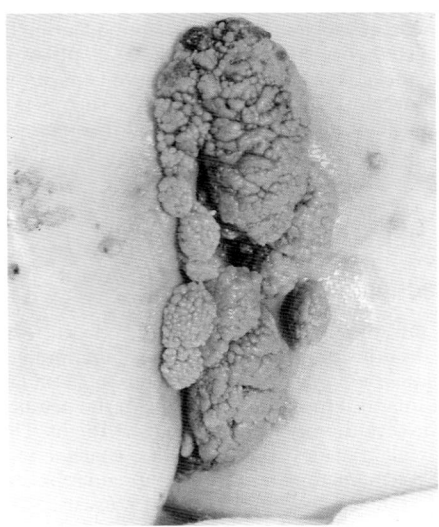

Figure 52-1. A 3-year-old girl with large cauliflower-like genital warts with satellite lesions due to human papillomavirus.

53 Urethritis, Vulvovaginitis, and Cervicitis

Paula K. Braverman

URETHRITIS

Urethritis is inflammation of the urethra. Clinical presentation includes dysuria, urinary frequency, and urethral discharge or itching. Neutrophils usually are found in urethral secretions.[1] According to the Centers for Disease Control and Prevention (CDC), urethritis is documented by presence of one of the following: visibly abnormal urethral discharge; positive leukocyte esterase (LE) test in a male <60 years of age without other urinary tract disease that could cause pyuria; Gram stain of urethral smear showing ≥5 white blood cells per high-powered field (WBCs/hpf); positive leukocyte esterase test on first-void urine or ≥10 WBCs/hpf in first-void urine sediment.[2,3] However, studies have demonstrated that symptoms of urethritis can occur without microscopic evidence of pyuria on Gram stain of urethral swab specimens or in first-void urine samples.[4,5]

It is somewhat easier to establish the diagnosis in men than in women because some pathogens simultaneously infect multiple genital areas, making it difficult for women to localize symptoms.[6] In the absence of a documented urinary tract infection, dysuria in a female can represent vulvar inflammation from vaginitis or vulvar dermatoses or urethral infection with a sexually transmitted infection (STI). *Urethral syndrome* is a term used for females who have dysuria in the presence of sterile urine cultures for bacterial cystitis.[6,7]

Etiologic Agents

Infectious Causes

Organisms associated with STIs are the most significant etiologic agents in urethritis. With the advent of newer, more sensitive molecular diagnostic testing modalities for STIs, there have been advances in the understanding of specific pathogens that cause urethritis.

Males. *Chlamydia trachomatis* and *Neisseria gonorrhoeae* are common causes of urethritis in men.[1] *N. gonorrhoeae* has been estimated to cause approximately one-third of the cases of acute urethritis and is differentiated from other causes, which are referred to as nongonococcal urethritis (NGU).[8] NGU is the most common clinical STI syndrome in men. Rates of specific etiologic agents vary by geography, socioeconomic factors, age, race, and sexual orientation or sexual practices.[1,5,8-14] Coinfection with multiple pathogens can occur and, in 25% to 40% of cases, no pathogen is identified.[15] Approximately 15% to 40% of NGU in men is caused by *C. trachomatis*, 15% to 25% by *Mycoplasma genitalium*, 10% to 20% by *Trichomonas vaginalis*, and 10% to 20% by *Ureaplasma urealyticum*.[15]

There has been confusion in the literature regarding the role of *U. urealyticum* as a cause of nongonococcal, nonchlamydial infection in men, with conflicting reports.[5,11,15-21] Upon further analysis, it appears that the genus *Ureaplasma* has two types: biovar 1 (*U. parvum*) and biovar 2 (*U. urealyticum*). Biovar 2 is the biotype most likely associated with urethritis.[15-21] In addition, further analysis has revealed that within biovar 2, only specific subtypes may be independently associated with NGU.[17]

T. vaginalis traditionally was considered a less frequent cause of urethritis in men. However, nucleic acid amplification testing (NAAT), such as polymerase chain reaction (PCR), demonstrate that *T. vaginalis* is associated with 10% to 20% of cases of urethritis.[10,15,22,23] *T. vaginalis* can be demonstrated in males without

clinical signs of urethritis and commonly is associated with other STIs.[15,24-26]

Herpes simplex virus (HSV) is a less frequent cause of urethritis in men.[5,11,27] Urethritis develops in 30% of men with primary HSV infection, and is found in 2% to 3% of cases of NGU.[15] Studies reported in 2006 found that HSV-1 was responsible for more cases of NGU than HSV-2, and HSV-1 was more likely to be associated with men engaging in oral–genital sex as well as men having male partners.[5,11] Infrequent causes of urethritis in men include adenoviruses, *Haemophilus* species, and *Neisseria meningitidis*; coliforms can be an etiologic agent in men who have sex with men (MSM).[1,5,11,15] The presence of some of the pathogens associated with urethritis suggests that infection with oropharyngeal flora, which are normal nonpathogenic organisms in monogamous partners, is possible.[11] Nonsexually transmitted NGU is associated with urinary tract infection (UTI), bacterial prostatitis, urethral stricture, phimosis, and urethral catheterization.[1] In 25% to 40% of cases, the etiology of NGU in males remains unknown.[15]

Females. Urethritis in females can be caused by *N. gonorrhoeae*, *C. trachomatis*, HSV, and *M. genitalium*. *T. vaginalis* typically causes vaginitis in women but is known to infect the urethra and is associated with pyuria.[6,7,10,25,28,29]

Noninfectious Causes

In both males and females, urethritis can accompany noninfectious systemic diseases, such as Stevens–Johnson syndrome, or can result from chemical irritation.[1,6]

Epidemiology

Although people 15 to 24 years of age comprise one-quarter of the sexually experienced population, they acquire approximately one-half of new STIs.[3] Population-based data derived from urine-based NAAT among 18- to 26-year-old subjects who participated in the Add Health study in 2001 showed a rate of *C. trachomatis* of 3.7% in males and 4.7% in females, a rate of *N. gonorrhoeae* of 0.4% in both males and females, and a rate of *T. vaginalis* of 1.7% in males and 2.8% in females.[30] Prevalence rates of *T. vaginalis* infection increased with age, were highest among black women, who had a prevalence of 10.5%, lower among black men (3.3%), and lowest among whites (1.1% for women and 1.3% for men).[30,31] Similar ethnic/racial differences have been found for *C. trachomatis* and *N. gonorrhoeae*.[3] Data from several studies including the CDC's 2008 Sexually Transmitted Disease Surveillance Report illustrate that the STI rates vary by specific populations.[3,22,30,32] Youth in correctional facilities have among the highest STI rates.[3,32] These data should be considered when evaluating patients.

Sexual practices and behavior can influence the epidemiology of urethritis. Urethritis due to *C. trachomatis*, *N. gonorrhoeae*, or HSV among adolescent women is correlated with having new sex partners.[6] Adenovirus and HSV-1 have been associated with oral–genital contact and having a male partner, whereas *M. genitalium* and *C. trachomatis* have been associated with vaginal sex.[5] In one study, *N. gonorrhoeae* and *U. urealyticum* urethritis were found in heterosexual men while *C. trachomatis* urethritis was associated with MSM, and *T. vaginalis* was more common in men >30 years of age.[33]

Urethritis due to STI pathogens also can occur in prepubertal boys and, less frequently, in prepubertal girls. In this age group, transmission commonly results from sexual abuse with

PART II Clinical Syndromes and Cardinal Features of Infectious Diseases: Approach to Diagnosis and Initial Management

SECTION G Genitourinary Tract Infections

TABLE 53-1. Clinical Manifestations of Nongonococcal and Gonococcal Urethritis

	Nongonococcal Urethritis	Gonococcal Urethritis
Incubation period	2–3 weeks	2–6 days
Onset	Insidious	Abrupt
Dysuria	+; may wax and wane	++; continuous
Discharge	Scant to moderate; may be absent	Profuse; absent in <10%

+, Modest discomfort; ++, more severe discomfort.

genital-to-genital contact (see Chapter 56, Infectious Diseases in Child Abuse).

Clinical Manifestations and Differential Diagnosis

Symptomatic urethritis in adolescent males is characterized by dysuria, urethral discharge, and/or urethral pruritus. Discharge can be mucoid, mucopurulent, or purulent. Gonococcal urethritis compared with NGU usually has a shorter incubation period, more acute onset, and more profuse discharge (Table 53-1).[1,34] Discharge in patients with NGU can be so scant that it is only noted in the morning or is apparent as crusting on the meatus or as stains in underwear.[1] Urethral infection with *N. gonorrhoeae* and the various organisms causing NGU also can be asymptomatic.[35]

Urethritis must be differentiated from UTI, particularly in adolescent boys with dysuria but no discharge. In contrast to UTI, frequency, hematuria, and urgency are uncommon in urethritis. However, if the adolescent male is sexually active, pyuria is more likely to be due to urethritis than to UTI, since UTI is uncommon in this age group. A focused STI history (see Chapter 51, Sexually Transmitted Infection Syndromes) and past medical history can help establish relative risk of urethritis versus UTI.

In adolescent girls, dysuria is the cardinal feature of urethritis. The urethral syndrome must be differentiated from acute bacterial cystitis and vulvovaginitis (Table 53-2). The literature describes differentiation between "internal" and "external" dysuria. Internal dysuria is pain that is felt internally during voiding. External dysuria is discomfort that is felt as urine passes over the labia.[7] Internal dysuria, urinary frequency, and isolation of >10^2 uropathogens per milliliter of voided urine suggest acute bacterial cystitis; isolation of ≤10^2 uropathogens per milliliter suggests acute urethritis due to STI pathogens.[6,36] Pain that is felt internally only at the end of urination is consistent with bacterial cystitis.[7] External dysuria can occur with vulvovaginitis. Adolescent females can have

vaginitis alone or a concurrent UTI, and may not be able to adequately distinguish between internal and external dysuria.[7,37] Any female suspected of having urethritis requires an STI-directed history and physical examination to determine whether other STI or STI syndromes (e.g., pelvic inflammatory disease (PID)) are present.

In prepubertal boys and girls, urethritis due to STI pathogens can manifest with dysuria and urethral or vaginal discharge. There may be vague lower abdominal pain, unwillingness to void, and, in boys, irritation in the distal urethra or meatus. Dysuria in a prepubertal child is much more likely to be due to UTI than urethritis associated with STI. Urethritis is more probable in the presence of a discharge or a history of sexual abuse, especially if genital-to-genital contact has occurred.

Laboratory Findings and Diagnosis

Males

In males, specimens are obtained both to document urethritis and to detect common causes, *N. gonorrhoeae* and *C. trachomatis*. Definitive diagnosis is enhanced if the patient has not voided recently; examination in the morning before voiding is ideal.[1] When discharge is present, a meatal swab specimen can be taken for Gram stain; presence of gram-negative intracellular diplococci of the typical kidney-bean morphology pattern (Figure 53-1A), or ≥5 neutrophils per oil immersion field (×1000) is diagnostic of urethritis.[1] Gram-stain smear is sensitive and specific in diagnosing gonococcal urethritis if intracellular diplococci are detected. If Gram stain is equivocal or negative, culture of the specimen or NAAT for *N. gonorrhoeae* is indicated.

In all patients, regardless of whether *N. gonorrhoeae* is suspected by Gram stain, an intraurethral specimen should be obtained for detection of *C. trachomatis* by culture, antigen detection, or NAAT; or a first-voided urine specimen should be tested by NAAT (see Chapter 167, *Chlamydia trachomatis*). Although culture previously was the "gold standard" for diagnosing *C. trachomatis* infection, NAATs (e.g., polymerase chain reaction (PCR), strand displacement amplification, or transcription-mediated amplification (TMA)) are more sensitive and are the preferred diagnostic method.[38] The urinary LE dipstick technique for detecting pyuria has been used as a screening tool for identifying asymptomatic urethritis in adolescent males, but is not sensitive enough to be considered reliable.[39–41] The availability of NAATs for *N. gonorrhoeae* and *C. trachomatis* now provide noninvasive tests on urine with excellent sensitivity and specificity. LE testing may be useful in situations in which the new tests are cost prohibitive.[41]

The diagnosis of *T. vaginalis* in men is more challenging than in women. Studies have shown that the use of NAATs (TMA and PCR) to diagnose *T. vaginalis* in males is superior to culture or wet

TABLE 53-2. Distinguishing Features of Urethritis, Acute Bacterial Cystitis, and Vulvovaginitis in Adolescent Females

	Urethritis	Acute Bacterial Cystitis	Vulvovaginitis
Symptoms	Internal dysuria	Internal dysuria, frequency, urgency, hematuria	External dysuria, vaginal discharge, vulvar burning, itching
Duration of symptoms	Often ≥7 days	Usually ≤4 days	Varies with cause
Signs	Mucopurulent cervicitis Vulvar lesions	Suprapubic tenderness	Vulvar lesions and inflammation; vaginal discharge
Epidemiologic associations	New sex partner Previous STI Sexual partner with STI	Previous cystitis Onset of symptoms within 24 hours of intercourse Use of diaphragm Use of a spermicide	History of genital herpes Sex partner with genital herpes Antibiotic use Previous vulvovaginitis Candidiasis

STI, sexually transmitted infection.

Adapted from Holmes KK, Stamm WE, Sobel JD. Lower genital tract infection syndromes in women. In: Holmes KK, Sparling PF, Mardh P-A, et al (eds) Sexually Transmitted Diseases, 4th ed. New York, McGraw-Hill, 2008, pp 987–1016.

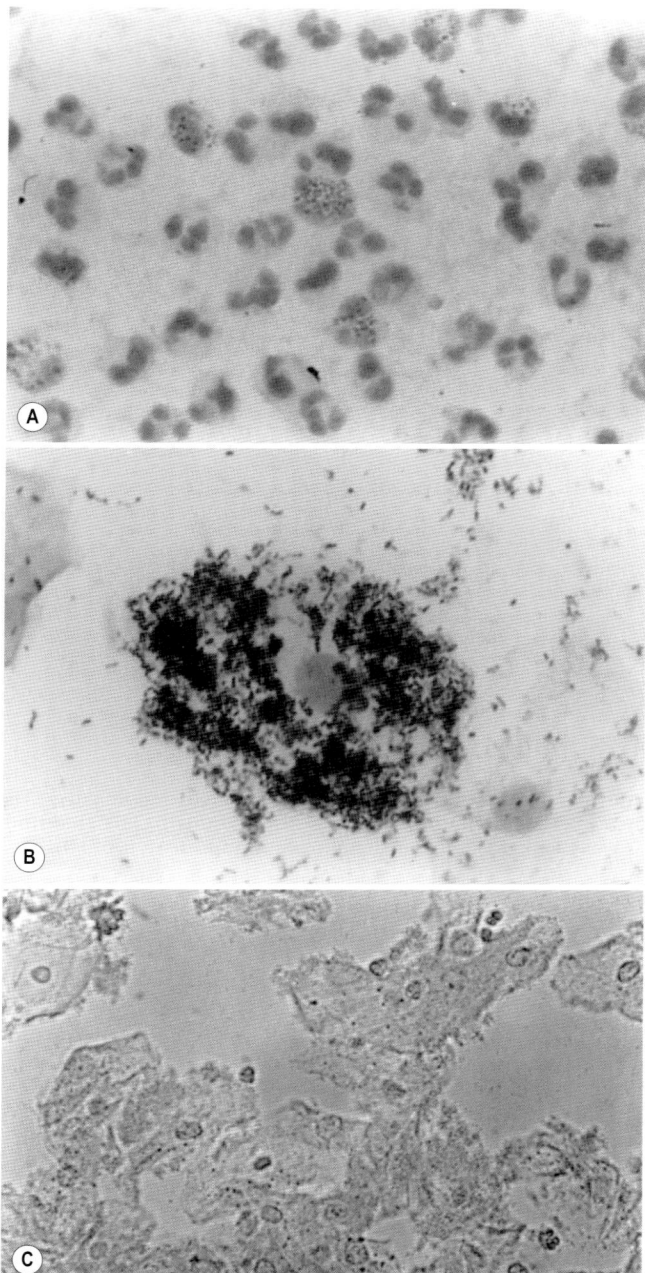

Figure 53-1. (A) Gram stain of urethral discharge from an adolescent male with urethritis showing multiple neutrophils and intracellular diplococci with kidney-bean morphology typical of *Neisseria gonorrhoeae* (magnification ×1000). **(B)** Gram stain of vaginal fluid from an adolescent with bacterial vaginosis showing clue cells and squamous vaginal epithelial cells covered with coccobacilli, which gives them a stippled or granular appearance. Note the absence of rods with blunt ends (lactobacilli) (magnification ×2000). **(C)** Wet mount of vaginal secretions in an adolescent female with bacterial vaginosis showing clue cells. Note stippled epithelial cells with ragged (bacteria-covered), ill-defined borders (magnification ×200).

mount preparation.[10,23–25,42,43] An advantage of PCR and TMA is that they can be performed on a urine specimen: however, at this time, PCR remains a research tool and is not commercially available and the TMA test is available only as an analytic specific reagent for laboratory research validation. In males, the diagnosis of *T. vaginalis* must rely on wet mount examination of a urethral smear or culture. Wet mount detects only 30% of *T. vaginalis*

infections in men.[24] Culture can be performed on either urine or urethral specimens and appears to yield better results if both are tested.[25] The InPouch culture system (BioMed Diagnostics, San Jose, CA) is equivalent to the gold-standard Diamond media and urethral or urine sediment specimens can be inoculated.[22] However, several studies have demonstrated that InPouch remains less likely than PCR testing to detect *T. vaginalis* in males.[23,42]

Cultures for *U. urealyticum* are not available readily and *M. genitalium* is difficult to isolate.[1,28,44] In research studies, both are diagnosed and evaluated utilizing NAATs. At this time, NAATs are not available commercially for either organism and management relies on the clinical presentation and exclusion of other etiologies. Because of the strong correlation between *M. genitalium* and symptomatic urethritis, use of the LE test has recently been debated in the literature as a means of identifying cases of NGU due to *M. genitalium*.[45,46]

Females

Endocervical and urethral specimens should be obtained for culture or NAAT for both *N. gonorrhoeae* and *C. trachomatis* in adolescent girls with urethritis, because concurrent infection is common.[6] Urinalysis and urine culture also are indicated, because simultaneous UTI and STI can occur in sexually active females.[7] Urine testing using NAAT for *C. trachomatis* and *N. gonorrhoeae* may not be as sensitive as endocervical specimen testing in females.[38,47] Although studies using NAAT testing of vaginal specimens have shown good correlation with cervical specimens, not all NAATs are approved by the U.S. Food and Drug Administration for use on vaginal specimens.[38,47] NAAT is not recommended for testing of specimens obtained by rectal or pharyngeal swabs. *T. vaginalis* can be diagnosed by a variety of methods, including wet mount, culture, nucleic acid probe, or immunochromatographic capillary flow dipstick technology.[2,22,48,49] As in males, wet mount microscopy has poor sensitivity compared with other methods. NAATs for *T. vaginalis* including PCR and TMA are not readily available at this time to most clinicians outside of the research environment.[43,48,50,51]

In prepubertal children, some experts recommend meatal, rather than intraurethral, specimens because the former are less painful to obtain.[52]

Management/ Empiric and Definitive Therapy

Initial treatment in males can be based on Gram stain results (Table 53-3).[2] Patients with Gram-stain evidence of *N. gonorrhoeae* should be treated with single-dose therapy with a cephalosporin, orally or intramuscularly. All patients should be tested for *C. trachomatis* and treated if positive. If *C. trachomatis* testing is not possible, empiric treatment is indicated because coinfection is common. Routine co-treatment of people diagnosed with *N. gonorrhoeae* for *C. trachomatis* is recommended since this may reduce development of antimicrobial resistant *N. gonorrhoeae* and optimize treatment for pharyngeal infection when using oral cephalosporins. For NGU, single-dose azithromycin therapy may be preferred over one-week therapy with doxycycline in adolescents because of adherence.[2] Alternative treatments include erythromycin or a fluoroquinolone. In addition, confirmed cases of *N. gonorrhoeae* or *C. trachomatis* must be reported to the local health authorities, and sexual partners should be contacted for assessment and treatment.

Immediate follow-up and repeat testing for *N. gonorrhoeae* or *C. trachomatis* urethritis in adolescents are not recommended routinely if appropriate treatment is completed, symptoms and signs disappear, and no re-exposure to an untreated partner occurs. However, because of the high rate of reinfection within 6 months of initial treatment, repeat testing for *N. gonorrhoeae* and *C. trachomatis* is recommended in 3 to 6 months.[2] If symptoms persist despite good adherence and no re-exposure, culture of an intraurethral specimen or first-void urine for *T. vaginalis* should be performed because of the high prevalence of *T. vaginalis* infection in men with nongonococcal, nonchlamydial urethritis as well as

PART II Clinical Syndromes and Cardinal Features of Infectious Diseases: Approach to Diagnosis and Initial Management

SECTION G Genitourinary Tract Infections

TABLE 53-3. Treatment of Urethritis

	Gram Stain	Suggested Treatment
RESULTS AVAILABLE		
Increased neutrophils	**Gram-negative intracellular diplococci**	
Present	Present	Treat for gonococcal and chlamydial urethritis.
		For *Neisseria gonorrhoeae*: for children >45 kg and adolescents, ceftriaxone, 250 mg IM once, *or* cefixime, 400 mg PO once; for children ≤45 kg, ceftriaxone 125 mg IM once[a]
		For *Chlamydia trachomatis*: for children ≥8 years and adolescents, azithromycin, 1 g PO once, *or* doxycycline, 100 mg bid PO for 7 days. For children <8 years of age, erythromycin base or ethylsuccinate, 50 mg/kg per day in four divided doses for 14 days; for children <8 years but ≥45 kg, azithromycin, 1 g PO once
Present	Absent	Treat for nongonococcal urethritis. Azithromycin once, *or* doxycycline for 7 days, *or* ofloxacin 300 mg PO twice a day for 7 days *or* levofloxacin 500 mg PO once a day for 7 days *or* erythromycin base 500 mg PO four times a day for 7 days *or* erythromycin ethylsuccinate 800 mg PO four times a day for 7 days; for children <8 years of age, erythromycin for 14 days
Absent	Absent	Defer treatment until microbiologic results are available; or if patient is high-risk by history and follow-up cannot be ensured, treat for gonococcal and chlamydial urethritis
RESULTS NOT AVAILABLE		
Urethral discharge		Treat for gonococcal and chlamydial urethritis
No urethral discharge		Defer treatment until microbiologic results are available; or, if patient is high-risk and follow-up cannot be ensured, treat for gonococcal and chlamydial urethritis
RECURRENT/PERSISTENT URETHRITIS		Metronidazole 2 g PO once *or* tinidazole 2 g PO once and azithromycin 1 g PO once if not used for initial episode

IM, intramuscularly; PO, orally.

[a]*Because of escalating resistance, fluoroquinolones are no longer recommended as first-line therapy.*[2]

coinfection with *N. gonorrhoeae* and *C. trachomatis.* Treatment for *T. vaginalis* as part of the initial treatment for male urethritis has been suggested,[26] but that recommendation is not part of the CDC's 2010 STI treatment guidelines. If *T. vaginalis* is diagnosed, metronidazole or tinidazole therapy is prescribed (see Chapter 274, *Trichomonas vaginalis*). However, *T. vaginalis* culture is insensitive; current CDC guidelines recommend treatment with metronidazole or tinidazole plus azithromycin (if azithromycin was not used for the initial episode) in all cases of persistent urethritis.[1,2,12]

U. urealyticum can be difficult to eradicate and resistance to tetracyclines has been demonstrated.[1,44] Studies also have shown persistence of *M. genitalium* urethritis in men treated with doxycycline, tetracycline, erythromycin, and fluoroquinolones. Studies also have demonstrated resistance to azithromycin.[44,53] A single dose of 1 g of azithromycin has been shown to be more effective than multidose doxycycline in the treatment of *M. genitalium.*[54] However, other studies have shown that rate of clinical cure was superior using a 5-day course of azithromycin (loading dose of 500 mg on the first day and 250 mg on subsequent days) compared with a single 1 g dose.[12,28,55–57] In cases in which azithromycin is ineffective, moxifloxacin (400 mg daily for 7–10 days) has been shown to eradicate *M. genitalium.*[2,57] Patients who do not respond to therapy should be referred to a urologist.

Females with findings suggestive of bacterial cystitis can be treated presumptively for UTI. However, if urethritis is suspected, a single dose of azithromycin (1 g) or a 7-day course of doxycycline (100 mg twice a day) would be indicated pending results of urine culture and STI testing. If symptoms of dysuria are found to be secondary to vulvovaginitis, treatment should be directed at the etiology (see below).

Complications

Complications of urethritis in males include epididymitis (1% to 2%), and in both males and females disseminated gonococcal infection (0.5% to 3%), and reactive arthritis syndrome (Reiter syndrome). The frequency of reactive arthritis syndrome as a complication of NGU is not well known. Urethral strictures and prostatitis are rare.[1] Females with *N. gonorrhoeae* and *C. trachomatis*

infection also are at risk for PID.[7] In both males and females, STIs associated with urethritis increase susceptibility to HIV infection as well as increasing viral shedding and transmission of HIV.[58]

Prevention

Correct and consistent use of condoms is the most effective means of preventing and reducing transmission of the STIs associated with urethritis.

VULVOVAGINITIS

Vulvovaginitis (inflammation of the vagina or vulva, or both) is a common gynecologic problem in both prepubertal and adolescent females. The etiology, pathogenesis, and management differ substantially between these two age groups.[7] Vaginitis and vulvitis are a continuum in young children, whereas they are distinct clinical entities in adolescents.

Vulvovaginitis in Prepubertal Females

Etiologic Agents and Epidemiology

Prepubertal girls can have specific or nonspecific vaginal infections; 25% to 75% of cases in prepubertal girls who come to attention at referral centers for suspected vulvovaginal infections have nonspecific vulvovaginitis.[7] Several factors predispose young girls to vulvovaginal irritation, including close proximity of the vagina to the rectum, poor hygienic practices, lack of protective labial fat pads and pubic hair, and lack of estrogen effect on vaginal mucosa.[7,59,60] Prepubertal girls are more likely than postpubertal girls to experience vulvar irritation and trauma from soaps, bubble baths, and clothing.[7] The lack of estrogen effect in prepubertal girls promotes an environment with a neutral pH, predisposing to overgrowth with a variety of potential pathogens.[6,59,60] Vaginal microbial infections that are not STIs usually are due to respiratory tract and enteric pathogens.

T. vaginalis is rare in prepubertal children because lack of estrogen makes the vagina resistant to this infection.[7] The role of *Gardnerella vaginalis* in prepubertal vaginitis is controversial.[7]

Candida vulvovaginitis is not common in prepubertal girls unless there are other risk factors, such as antibiotic use, diabetes mellitus, immunosuppression, or use of diapers; 3% to 4% of prepubertal girls have *Candida* spp. as part of normal vaginal flora.[7,59] Although prepubertal vulvovaginitis often is not sexually transmitted, sexual abuse must be considered if pathogens such as *C. trachomatis, N. gonorrhoeae, T. vaginalis,* human papillomavirus (HPV), or HSV are identified.[7,59] Attributing HPV to sexual abuse versus vertical transmission or inoculation from caregivers and autoinoculation is challenging because of the lack of studies in this age group regarding incubation, latency to clinical presentation, and cutoff ages for vertical transmission.[59] Similar to the cervical epithelium of postpubertal girls, the cuboidal vaginal epithelium of prepubertal girls is susceptible to *N. gonorrhoeae* and *C. trachomatis.*[6] Other causes of vulvovaginitis include foreign body, vulvar skin disorders, or allergic reactions (Box 53-1).

Clinical Manifestations, Differential Diagnosis, and Clinical Approach

The clinical features of vulvovaginitis in children include vaginal discharge, vulvar irritation, pruritus, dysuria, bleeding, genital inflammation, and foul smell.[7,59,60] When associated with a foreign body, discharge can be profuse, foul-smelling, and blood-tinged.[7] Parents often are unaware that the child has inserted something into the vagina. In *Enterobius vermicularis*-associated vulvovaginitis, recurrent symptoms and vulvar and/or anal pruritus are common. Discharge is bloody in more than one-half of cases of vulvovaginitis caused by *Shigella* spp. and also can occur with *Streptococcus pyogenes* infection.[6,7,59,61] Bleeding also should raise concern about trauma. Diffusely hyperemic vulvar mucosa is suggestive of streptococcal vulvovaginitis. Discharge associated with gonococcal infection is commonly green and purulent, whereas discharge is less frequent with chlamydial infection.

All prepubertal children with vulvovaginitis require a careful interview and history, and physical examination. History may reveal recurrent infections or onset of symptoms after a day at the beach. Vaginitis due to *S. pyogenes* can occur after a pharyngeal or skin infection in the patient or family members. Finding a sibling with an STI raises concern about sexual abuse by someone associated with the family.[7,59] Gynecologic examination includes abdominal inspection and palpation. In a gentle supportive manner, inspection of the perineal skin, vulva, and perirectal and genital areas is performed to detect excoriation, erythema, ulcers, or structural abnormalities. Visualization of the vagina and cervix without instrumentation usually is possible with the patient in the knee–chest position.[7] This facilitates detection of a foreign body, especially if a magnifying lens or otoscope head is used. Examination with the patient under anesthesia may be necessary in some cases.

Laboratory Findings and Diagnosis

When vaginal discharge is present, samples are obtained (Box 53-2) using a sterile saline-moistened swab for potassium hydroxide (KOH) preparation, Gram stain, and culture.[59] A vaginal wash using nonbacteriostatic saline or vaginal aspiration using an eyedropper are alternative methods of specimen collection.[59,62] However, these latter specimens may not be as sensitive for identification of *C. trachomatis* if few epithelial cells are collected (which are necessary because the organism is an obligate intracellular pathogen). Culture confirmation of *N. gonorrhoeae* and *C. trachomatis* are the most admissible legal evidence for cases of suspected sexual abuse. NAAT may be an alternative if confirmatory test is available and culture systems for *C. trachomatis* are unavailable. Confirmation test should consist of a second U.S. FDA-cleared NAAT that targets a different sequence from the first test.[63] *T. vaginalis* can be detected in vaginal wash specimens or by culture.[7,49] If *Enterobius* infestation is suspected, the parent is instructed to examine the perianal region at night for the small white pinworms, and a Scotch tape swab or paddle specimen is collected from the perianal area immediately on the child's awakening. Samples for culture for yeast should be considered if itching persists or the history suggests risk factors for candidal infection.[7,59]

PART II Clinical Syndromes and Cardinal Features of Infectious Diseases: Approach to Diagnosis and Initial Management

SECTION G Genitourinary Tract Infections

Management/ Empiric and Definitive Treatment

The mainstay of treatment for nonspecific vulvovaginitis is education, attention to personal hygiene, and avoidance of agents such as bubble baths and tight nylon undergarments that provoke the problem.[59] Sitz baths in warm water without soap may be helpful. Vitamin A and D ointment or petroleum jelly (Vaseline) can protect the vulva, and a short course of 1% hydrocortisone cream can alleviate acute exacerbations of irritant vulvitis.[7,59] Occasionally, in severe cases, an estrogen cream is applied for several weeks to ameliorate symptoms.[59,60] If a foreign body is detected, prompt removal usually resolves the problem.

Treatment of vulvovaginitis due to specific pathogens is initiated on the basis of the Gram stain or wet mount findings and/or culture results. Treatments are ceftriaxone for *N. gonorrhoeae*; erythromycin for *C. trachomatis* for patients <8 years of age and <45 kg; azithromycin for those <8 years of age and >45 kg; and azithromycin or doxycycline for older females; an antifungal agent such as clotrimazole for *Candida* or oral fluconazole if topical therapy is not effective; and penicillin for group A streptococcus. Other antimicrobial agents are chosen on the basis of vaginal bacterial culture results.[2,7,59]

Prognosis and Sequelae

The follow-up of children with vulvovaginitis depends on the etiology. Fortunately, gonococcal and chlamydial vulvovaginitis rarely are associated with upper tract disease, especially if treated early.[7] Thus, impairment of fertility is unlikely if adequate treatment is given. When recurrences are due to *S. pyogenes*, pharyngeal colonization in the patient or carriage in family members is considered.[59]

Vaginitis in Pubertal Females

Etiologic Agents and Epidemiology

Under the influence of estrogen at puberty, the vaginal epithelium shifts from cuboidal to a glycogen-containing stratified squamous epithelium.[6,7] There is an associated increased growth of lactobacilli, which produce lactic acid from glycogen. This results in a decrease in vaginal fluid pH from a prepubertal level of about 7.0 to 4.0 to 4.5. The lower pH, associated with hydrogen peroxide production by lactobacilli, is important in the regulation of vaginal flora.[6,7] Changes in the type of epithelium and colonizing flora render the vaginal environment relatively resistant to infection caused by *C. trachomatis* and *N. gonorrhoeae*. Thus, in adolescents, these two organisms cause cervicitis, rather than vulvovaginitis. Leukorrhea, the normal white mucous vaginal discharge that represents the effect of estrogen on the vaginal mucosa in adolescents, must be distinguished from pathologic discharge. Saline wet-mount examination of vaginal secretions would reveal sheets of epithelial cells without inflammatory cells, yeast, clue cells, or trichomonads. Leukorrhea sometimes is considered excessive by patients, and they need reassurance.[7]

The major causes of vaginitis in adolescents are bacterial vaginosis (BV), candidiasis, and *T. vaginalis* infection. *Bacterial vaginosis* has replaced the term *nonspecific vaginitis*, because this condition generally is not inflammatory but arises from a change in the vaginal flora.[7,64] Less common causes of vaginitis in adolescents include ulceration and infection associated with tampons, cervical caps, vaginal contraceptive ring, and other foreign bodies; chemical agents such as those found in douches and spermicides; and toxin-producing *Staphylococcus aureus*.[6,7,65]

Bacterial vaginosis. BV is the most common cause of vaginitis in postpubertal women, affecting approximately one-third of women.[66] BV represents a disruption in the normal vaginal flora, with a decrease in lactobacilli and overgrowth of a variety of organisms that can include *G. vaginalis*, genital mycoplasmas (*M. hominis*), and anaerobic bacteria, particularly *Bacteroides* (*Prevotella* and *Porphyromonas*), *Peptostreptococcus*, *Fusobacterium*, and *Mobiluncus* species.[64,66] Although many patients with BV have moderate-to-heavy concentrations of vaginal *Gardnerella* species, detection of this organism is not diagnostic because vaginal colonization with small numbers is common in both sexually active (30% to 60%) and nonactive (20% to 30%) adolescents without BV.[64,67,68] New technologies using amplification of ribosomal DNA are being utilized to characterize bacterial species that are not identified by culture.[64,66,69,70] An anaerobic bacterium, *Atopobium vaginae*, has demonstrated resistance to metronidazole and also has been found in the upper genital tract in women.[22,64]

Risk factors for BV include a higher number of lifetime sex partners, a female sex partner, douching, poverty, smoking, low educational achievement, high body mass index, being non-Hispanic black, and previous pregnancy.[64,71-74] Although BV is more common in adolescents and young adults who are sexually active and have multiple sexual partners, designating BV as an STI has been controversial because BV can be found in sexually inexperienced females.[64,66-68,71-77] The prevalence of BV among women attending STI clinics is higher (24% to 37%) than among college women attending student health clinics for routine annual examination (4% to 15%).[7,67] One study of women entering the military found that 19% of subjects denying a history of vaginal intercourse met criteria for BV compared with 28% who had been active sexually.[72] Further, studies have shown a concordance between the presence of *G. vaginalis* in the urethra of male sex partners of women diagnosed with BV but did not find this organism in male controls.[64] Sexual transmission remains controversial because although sexual activity, multiple sexual partners, receptive oral sex, vaginal insertion of sex toys that were not cleaned are associated with BV,[73-76,78,79] while use of condoms appears to be protective,[64,76] treatment of sex partners does not appear to prevent recurrence.[64]

Up to one-third of women experience recurrent episodes of BV within 3 months of treatment.[66] In one study, factors associated with recurrence over a 12-month period included a past history of BV and a having female sex partner or a regular sex partner.[80] Studies also have identified a biofilm that adheres to the epithelial cells in women with BV. The two organisms most associated with the biofilm are *G. vaginalis* and *A. vaginae*. Some investigators have postulated that the recurrence of BV is related to persistence of the biofilm that provides protection from systemic and topical antibiotics.[70] In one study, *G. vaginalis* was detected in 100% and *A. vaginae* in 75% of women with recurrent BV. Those individuals with both organisms were more likely to have a recurrence.[81] Recurrence also may be related to reinfection from an infected partner, or to failure to reestablish lactobacilli dominance with persistence of pathogenic bacteria.[66,70]

Candidiasis. Vulvovaginal candidiasis has an estimated lifetime incidence of up to 75%.[82] Candidal colonization of the vagina usually originates from the gastrointestinal tract, and sexual transmission is not an important mode of acquisition.[68,82] As many as 30% of healthy asymptomatic women are colonized with yeast and *Candida albicans* is the organism found in most uncomplicated cases.[66] Risk factors include pregnancy, poorly controlled diabetes, receptive oral sex, use of estrogen and various contraceptives including intrauterine devices, diaphragm, vaginal ring, and possibly spermicides.[65,66,82] Antibiotic use is mentioned frequently, but it is not a major cause of infection in most women. Rather, colonization by a more virulent species of *Candida* may place a subpopulation of women at higher risk for symptomatic infection.[66,82,83] In approximately one-half of females, no risk factors are identified.[66]

Most women experience uncomplicated vulvovaginal candidiasis (VVC), with infrequent episodes that are mild or moderate clinically and are caused by *C. albicans*.[82] However, 10% to 20% have VVC that is "complicated," i.e., more severe, recurrent (RVVC), or secondary to *C. non-albicans* species. These women are more likely to have underlying medical risk factors.[82] Approximately 5% of women have RVVC, defined as ≥4 episodes in a 12-month period.[84] RVVC is more likely to be associated with *C. non-albicans* species compared with uncomplicated infections.[66,82] The most common *C. non-albicans* species reported is *C. glabrata*.[82] Although most women with RVVC do not have diabetes mellitus or immunosuppression, these conditions increase the risk. It is postulated that some patients may have a genetic predisposition to RVVC or an aberrant Th2-dominant profile of the vaginal T lymphocytes.[66,82]

Trichomonas vaginalis. *T. vaginalis* has worldwide distribution with prevalence in community-based studies ranging from 2% to 46% in women.[10] The prevalence and incidence of *T. vaginalis* is difficult to assess since it is not a reportable disease and in the absence of screening guidelines, clinical evaluation commonly is focused on symptomatic people. In addition, there is wide variation depending on whether the least sensitive (wet mount) or more sensitive (culture or NAAT) methods are used for diagnosis.[48] Studies utilizing PCR testing of urine or vaginal swabs in 14- to 26-year-old women have shown *T. vaginalis* prevalence rates of approximately 2% to 3%, which was higher than the rate for gonorrhea in these same people.[48] Certain populations may have higher prevalence as demonstrated in studies from adolescent clinics (up to 18%) and college health programs (10%)[10,48] and in incarcerated women (up to 47%).[10,48] Other risk factors include being African American, smoking, using alcohol and drugs, having multiple partners, and among adolescents, having an older sexual partner.[10] *T. vaginalis* facilitates transmission and acquisition of HIV and commonly is associated with other STIs.

Clinical Manifestations and Differential Diagnosis

Clinical presentations that help distinguish BV from candidal vulvovaginitis and trichomonal vaginitis are shown in Table 53-4.

In the sexually active adolescent, cervicitis also must be excluded because cervicitis can occur as a coinfection or as the sole cause of the vaginal discharge.[85] Symptomatic BV presents with a thin white-grey homogeneous vaginal discharge that adheres to the vaginal walls and has a fishy odor.[64,66] Women with symptomatic candidal infection commonly complain of vaginal pruritus and burning, dysuria, and dyspareunia. Discharge can be thick and white with a "cottage cheese" appearance but also can be watery and homogeneous. Discharge usually is not malodorous and in many cases, women do not notice a change in vaginal discharge.[66,82] Patients with symptomatic trichomoniasis often have pruritus and a malodorous, frothy yellow or greenish discharge and can present with dysuria, abdominal pain, vulvar erythema and edema, and bloody vaginal discharge; cervicitis can occur, with "strawberry cervix" (punctuate hemorrhages) and friability. Asymptomatic *T. vaginalis* infection occurs commonly.[10]

Laboratory Findings and Diagnosis

Laboratory features that help distinguish BV from candidal vulvovaginitis and trichomonal vaginitis are shown in Table 53-4.

Bacterial vaginosis. The diagnosis of BV is commonly established in the clinical setting by the presence of ≥3 of the following (Amsel criteria): (1) thin, homogeneous vaginal discharge; (2) vaginal pH >4.5; (3) characteristic fishy "amine" odor released

TABLE 53-4. Characteristics and Recommendations for Treatment of Vaginitis in Adolescents

	Bacterial Vaginosis	Candidal Vaginitis	Trichomonal Vaginitis
SYMPTOMS	Malodorous discharge	Vaginal discharge Usually not malodorous Vulvar itch or discomfort Dysuria Dyspareunia Often exacerbated symptoms just prior to menses	Vaginal discharge May be malodorous Vulvar itch Dysuria Dyspareunia
SIGNS			
Discharge	Thin, homogeneous, white, clings to vaginal wall; ± frothy	Thick, curdlike	Heavy, grey or yellow-green; frothy
Other signs	None	Vulvar and vaginal erythema, vulvar edema	Vulvar and vaginal erythema
LABORATORY FINDINGS			
pH	>4.5	<4.5	>4.5
KOH preparation	"Fishy," amine odor when mixed with 10% KOH (positive-whiff test)	Hyphae or pseudohyphae	Occasionally positive-whiff test
Saline preparation	"Clue cells," few neutrophils	Neutrophils and epithelial cells in equal numbers	Motile trichomonads, neutrophils
Gram stain	Few gram-positive bacilli; abundant mixed flora	Hyphae or pseudohyphae or blastospores	Trichomonads visualized rarely
Culture	Not useful	Can be useful if KOH-negative	Culture more sensitive than wet mount

TREATMENT	**Oral**
	Metronidazole, 500 mg bid for 7 days, *or*
	  Clindamycin, 300 mg bid for 7 days, *or*
	  Tinidazole 2 g once daily for 3 days, *or*
	  Tinidazole 1 g once daily for 5 days
	Topical intravaginal
	Clindamycin cream 2%, one full applicator amount per vagina at bedtime for 7 days *or* clindamycin ovules 100 mg per vagina at bedtime for 3 days
	Metronidazole, 0.75% gel, one full applicator amount per vagina once a day for 5 days
		Topical intravaginal[a]
		Butoconazole cream
		Clotrimazole cream
		Nystatin vaginal tablet
		Miconazole cream or vaginal suppository
		Terconazole cream or vagina suppository
		Tioconazole ointment
		Oral
		Fluconazole, 150 mg once
			Oral
			Metronidazole, 2 g for 1 dose, *or*
			  500 mg bid for 7 days *or*
			Tinidazole 2 g orally in a single dose

KOH, potassium hydroxide.

[a]Intravaginal therapies are available in 1- to 14-day regimens.

PART II Clinical Syndromes and Cardinal Features of Infectious Diseases: Approach to Diagnosis and Initial Management

SECTION G Genitourinary Tract Infections

when alkali (10% KOH weight/volume) is added to the vaginal fluid specimen (positive whiff test); and (4) ≥20% of epithelial cells having the appearance of "clue cells." Clue cells are stippled epithelial cells whose borders are obscured by adherent bacteria, e.g. *G. vaginalis* and others (Figure 53-1B and C).[64] Accuracy of diagnosis increases with use of Amsel criteria.[22] Alternative tests include use of Gram stain to group bacteria into morphologic types (Nugent scoring). Amsel criteria and Nugent scores show good correlation.[86]

Alternative testing includes nonmicroscopic point-of-care testing. Some tests detect the metabolic products of BV-related organisms such as sialidase and prolineaminopeptidase.[64] A DNA probe for *G. vaginalis* ribosomal RNA (Affirm VP III DNA probe, Becton Dickinson, Franklin Lakes, NJ) is available but not useful if rapid results are needed. This test is most helpful as a supplemental marker to detect the presence of high concentrations of *G. vaginalis*.[22,86] Routine aerobic and anaerobic vaginal cultures are not helpful.

Usually, BV does not produce an inflammatory response; presence of WBCs on vaginal smear indicates concurrent vaginitis or cervicitis due to another etiology.[86,87]

***Candida* species.** *Candida* vaginitis is diagnosed by demonstrating hyphae, pseudohyphae, and/or blastospores on microscopic examination of a saline or 10% KOH preparation.[88] This technique has a sensitivity of about 50%. *C. glabrata* only produce blastospores and are missed more easily.[88] If the KOH preparation is negative, culture can confirm the diagnosis. Culture of vaginal, rather than cervical, specimens is more sensitive and may be particularly helpful in patients with ongoing nonspecific symptoms in whom BV and trichomoniasis have been excluded.[82,89] In cases of complicated vulvovaginal candidiasis, culture is important in identifying the species of the organism because therapy may be different or longer.[88,90] Culture can also demonstrate eradication of the organism and in cases where there are persistent symptoms, another etiology should be investigated.[90] It is useful to measure vaginal pH since, unlike BV or trichomoniasis, the vaginal pH remains low in vaginal candidiasis.[82]

***Trichomonas vaginalis*.** Diagnosis of trichomoniasis can be made by visualizing the motile protozoa on a wet mount preparation; however, the test is negative in 30% to 50% of cases. Culture using Diamond media or the InPouch *T. vaginalis* culture system is more sensitive; the latter is more available and is easier to store and transport.[22,91] Culture can be performed on vaginal specimens, including patient self-collected specimens. Conventional Papanicolaou (Pap) smear identification has a high false-positive rate.[92,93] However, liquid-based Pap smear appears to be more accurate, and compared with culture in one study had a positive predictive value of 96% and a negative predictive value of 91%.[94] A DNA probe test (Affirm VP, Becton Dickinson, Franklin Lakes, NJ) is sensitive (80% to 90%) and specific (95%) compared to wet mount and culture, but generally is best performed in the laboratory rather than the office setting because the test is moderately complex and requires about 45 minutes to complete.[10,22,51,95] One point-of-care test takes 10 minute to complete and utilizes an immunochromatographic capillary flow assay with monoclonal antibodies (OSOM *Trichomonas* Rapid Test, Genzyme Diagnostics, Cambridge, MA). This Clinical Laboratory Improvement Amendments (CLIA) waived test has been shown to be 83% to 90% sensitive and 99% to 100% specific in studies that included NAAT and culture comparison.[51] PCR has excellent sensitivity and specificity (85% to 100%) but is not available commercially.[10] TMA has sensitivity of >96% and specificity of >97% using vaginal swab specimens.[43,96] Although available commercially, TMA currently is not FDA-approved and must be validated in individual laboratories.

Vaginal specimens collected without use of a speculum, compared with specimens obtained during speculum examination, have comparable sensitivity to detect trichomoniasis, BV, and vulvovaginal candidiasis. Because NAAT for *N. gonorrhoeae* and *C. trachomatis* can be performed on urine and vaginal swabs, it may be possible to avoid the more invasive speculum examination to determine etiology for vaginitis in adolescents.[97]

Management/ Empiric and Definitive Treatment

Bacterial vaginosis. Metronidazole administered orally for 7 days is the recommended therapy for BV,[2] and preferred over single-dose therapy because of superior efficacy.[2,22,64] Alternative regimens are outlined in Table 53-4. Topical treatments have fewer gastrointestinal tract side effects but increase the risk for vaginal candidiasis.[22] Oral therapy is preferred in pregnant women because of the possibility of existing subclinical upper-genital tract infection.[2] Furthermore, use of 2% clindamycin cream intravaginally has been associated with onset of premature labor. Clindamycin cream should not be used when condoms are used because the oil base weakens the latex.[2,22] Although metronidazole and clindamycin regimens yield equivalent clinical responses the antibiotics may differ in ability to eradicate specific organisms associated with BV.[64,66,98,99]

Alternate therapeutic regimens have included use of tinidazole, which has fewer side effects than metronidazole.[2,66,100,101] A Cochrane Review found insufficient evidence to recommend for or against probiotics but use in combination with metronidazole may be promising.[101] Short-term prophylaxis with a vaginal probiotic capsule over a 3-week period reduced the risk of recurrent BV through 11 months of follow-up.[102]

Antimicrobial therapy for BV is further complicated by newly identified noncultivatable organisms, whose susceptibility is unknown.[81,99] There are no current recommendations for treatment of recurrent BV infection. However, a large multicenter study demonstrated 70% efficacy of twice-weekly maintenance therapy using metronidazole vaginal gel. For many subjects, suppression of BV only occurred while on this regimen, and vaginal candidiasis was a complication.[103] Oral nitroimidazole followed by intravaginal boric acid and metronidazole gel as well as a regimen involving a combination of monthly oral metronidazole and fluconazole have been evaluated.[2] It is not clear that treatment of asymptomatic BV in nonpregnant women is useful. One randomized, placebo-controlled, double-blind study comparing metronidazole gel and placebo found no statistically significant differences in retrospective assessments of vaginal discharge or odor.[104]

***Candida* species.** Topical therapy with azoles, such as clotrimazole, terconazole, miconazole, butoconazole, and tioconazole, is effective for vulvovaginal candidiasis. Single-dose fluconazole (150 mg) therapy has efficacy to comparable topical therapy.[2,66,105] Sexual partners usually do not require therapy unless candidal balanitis is present. Recurrent or chronic candidal vulvovaginitis merits investigation for predisposing conditions and may require a longer duration of topical (7 to 14 days) or oral therapy including a non-fluconazole imidazole drug.[2,66,82] Topical boric acid in the form of suppositories (600 mg in a gelatin capsule) and topical flucytosine have been useful in patients with *Candida* non-*albicans* species and imidazole-resistant *C. albicans*. Resistance to imidazole agents is uncommon among *C. albicans* and more likely in *C.* non-*albicans* species. Alternative therapies are useful, especially in cases of *C. glabrata* and *C. tropicalis*.[66,82,106,107] When using fluconazole, patients with RVVC can be treated initially with a dose of 150 mg every three days for a total of three doses followed by 100 mg, 150 mg, or 200 mg once a week. In women who cannot take fluconazole, repeated topical imidazole therapy has been effective.[2,66] Suppressive therapy usually is continued for 6 months, but recurrence is common after therapy is discontinued because organisms are suppressed rather than eradicated; prophylaxis can be reinstituted.[82] Fluconazole resistance and clinical failure is uncommon but in patients with breakthrough *Candida* infection, susceptibility testing may be helpful.[107,108]

***Trichomonas vaginalis*.** Systemic therapy with oral metronidazole or tinidazole is indicated for treatment of trichomoniasis.[2] Metronidazole has a 90% to 95% cure rate with either a 7-day course (500 mg twice daily) or a large single dose (2 g orally). Although uncommon, metronidazole resistance has been reported in approximately 1% to 9% of cases.[2,22,48,92] Treatment using higher doses, longer courses of metronidazole as well as using tinidazole (tinidazole, 2 g orally in a single dose) is reported.[2,10,22,48,109] Single-dose tinidazole has an 86% to 100%

cure rate and studies comparing single 2 g dosing regimens of metronidazole and tinidazole show tinidazole to be equivalent or superior for cure and symptom resolution.[2] One study found a 92% cure rate utilizing a combination of oral and vaginal tinidazole in patients unresponsive to metronidazole.[109] Tinidazole appears to be better tolerated than metronidazole and has fewer gastrointestinal tract and central nervous system side effects. Topical therapy with metronidazole gel is not effective because the gel does not penetrate the urethral and perivaginal glands adequately.[2,10] Sexual partners should be evaluated for STIs and treated for trichomoniasis.

Complications

BV has been associated with chorioamnionitis, postpartum endometritis, posthysterectomy vaginal cuff cellulitis, postabortion PID, premature rupture of membranes, preterm labor and delivery, low birthweight, spontaneous abortion, and intraamniotic infection.[22,64,77,110] The risk of preterm delivery is restricted to a small subset of women; risk may be related to genetic host response to inflammation and cytokine production.[22,64,77] Additionally, vaginal microorganisms can ascend to the upper tract causing infection and inflammation in the decidua, chorioamnion or amniotic fluid.[64] Data are conflicting whether treatment of pregnant women for BV prevents these complications.[22,64,77,111–113] A Cochrane Review[113] and another analysis[112] found little evidence that screening and treating all pregnant women (i.e., including women at low or average risk for preterm delivery with asymptomatic BV) prevents preterm birth and the sequelae. The results for women with high risk for preterm delivery were conflicting, with some studies showing a benefit and one demonstrating harm.[112]

Some of the conflicting data may be a result of inadequate understanding of the vaginal ecosystem. Women with preterm birth are more likely to have absent or decreased lactobacilli compared with the predominance of lactobacilli expected during pregnancy. Further, some authors have described an entity named aerobic vaginitis in which *Escherichia coli*, group B streptococci and enterococci predominate. Aerobic vaginitis is associated with vaginal proinflammatory cytokines; women with preterm labor may have a flora composition more consistent with aerobic vaginitis than BV.[114] Although screening of all pregnant women is not recommended, the 2010 CDC guidelines recommend testing and treatment of all symptomatic pregnant women.[2,64,77,112]

Studies have shown an association between BV and cervicitis and PID but a causal relationship remains unproven.[64,66] Organisms associated with BV have been found in the upper genital tracts of women with PID. In addition, studies utilizing endometrial biopsies have found an association between BV and endometritis, which either may be silent clinically or manifest as intermenstrual or increased bleeding.[64] Women with BV are more likely to have PID, and women with PID are more likely to have BV.[22,64,77] Treatment of BV has been associated with decreased PID in women undergoing abortion, and decreased postoperative cuff cellulitis.[64,77] Further, intravaginal treatment of BV has been associated with improved rates of resolution of cervicitis.[64] However, the relationship between BV and PID for women not undergoing abortion or uterine instrumentation is not clear.[22,77,115] There is no current recommendation for treatment of nonpregnant asymptomatic women as a standard clinical practice.[2,64]

Trichomoniasis has been associated with premature rupture of membranes and preterm delivery.[22] *T. vaginalis* also may play a role in the development of PID and has been postulated to act as a vehicle transporting other pathogens to the upper genital tract.[7,22,48] Controversy exists about treatment of *T. vaginalis* during pregnancy, since treatment does not appear to reduce complications. Furthermore, although treatment eliminates the organism, a few studies have shown an increased risk of preterm birth in treated women, which raises concern for treatment of all pregnant women, including women who are symptomatic.[2,10,24,25,111,116,117] All symptomatic pregnant women should be considered for treatment, but current CDC guidelines recommend discussing the option of deferring treatment until after 37 weeks' gestation for asymptomatic pregnant women. Although a single dose (2 g) of metronidazole has been demonstrated to be safe at all stages of pregnancy, more studies are needed regarding use of tinidazole.[2]

Both BV and *T. vaginalis* enhance acquisition of HIV and transmission to a partner.[22,25,48,64,77] Vulvovaginal candidiasis has been associated with increased HIV seroconversion in HIV-negative women and higher levels of cervicovaginal HIV shedding in HIV-positive women. Treatment of *T. vaginalis* reduces HIV viral shedding in vaginal secretions. However, there are no studies that have demonstrated similar effects on viral shedding in subjects with BV or vulvovaginal candidiasis.[2,22]

Vulvitis in Adolescents

Inflammation of the vulva in adolescents most commonly is due to HSV and yeasts (see Table 53-4). HSV often causes painful genital ulcers, along with vulvar inflammation and inguinal lymphadenopathy (see Chapter 52, Skin and Mucous Membrane Infections and Inguinal Lymphadenopathy).[118] Occasionally, inflammation can be associated with *T. vaginalis* infection.

CERVICITIS

Cervicitis is inflammation of the endocervix or ectocervix, or both. Both are common problems among adolescents, but neither is common in prepubertal girls. Under the influence of estrogens following puberty, the vaginal epithelium and ectocervix become cornified and thus relatively resistant to infection with a number of pathogens, including *N. gonorrhoeae* and *C. trachomatis*.[7] By contrast, the endocervix continues to be lined with columnar epithelium and remains susceptible to infection with these organisms. Therefore, in adolescent and adult women, these organisms usually cause endocervicitis in the absence of vaginitis.

A normal developmental finding in adolescents is the presence of the ectropion, which appears as an erythematous area surrounding the os. This represents the area of the squamo-columnar junction, with the erythematous area corresponding to the columnar epithelium and the surrounding pink area corresponding to the stratified squamous epithelium. During adolescence, the ectropion recedes as the result of squamous metaplasia. Although some adolescents with a large ectropion may have significant vaginal discharge, this is not a pathologic or infectious process. The ectropion usually is not friable; the presence of edema or friability suggests infection.[6]

Ectocervicitis

Ectocervicitis represents infection of the stratified squamous epithelium of the ectocervix. Ectocervicitis can occur in conjunction with candidal vulvovaginitis, trichomonal vaginitis, and HSV infection. HSV causes both ectocervicitis and endocervicitis.[6,118–122]

Endocervicitis

Etiologic Agents and Epidemiology

Endocervicitis represents infection of the endocervical columnar epithelium and can produce mucopurulent cervicitis. Common pathogens that cause endocervicitis are *N. gonorrhoeae* and *C. trachomatis*.[120,121] Other agents include HSV, which often causes concurrent exocervicitis.[6,119–122] Studies utilizing NAAT demonstrate an association between *M. genitalium* and mucopurulent cervicitis.[29,120,121,123–126] There also is a possible association with BV since cervicitis was more likely to resolve when patients also were treated for BV.[22,120,121,123] Possible theories for this relationship include the presence of proinflammatory vaginal cytokines in patients with BV and the presence of glucosidases and proteinases produced by BV-associated organisms that may degrade cervicovaginal mucus.[120]

PART II Clinical Syndromes and Cardinal Features of Infectious Diseases: Approach to Diagnosis and Initial Management

SECTION G Genitourinary Tract Infections

STI agents are not solely responsible for clinically apparent cervicitis. Other entities include tuberculosis and noninfectious causes such as sarcoidosis and Behçet disease, as well as local insults due to chemical douches, spermicides, and foreign bodies.[120–122]

Clinical Manifestations/Differential Diagnosis

Endocervicitis often is overlooked and underdiagnosed because symptoms and signs can be mild or absent. PID is one consequence of untreated mucopurulent cervicitis.[6] Sexually active adolescents with vaginal discharge; lower abdominal pain of recent onset; inter-menstrual, postcoital, or prolonged abnormal vaginal bleeding; or deep dyspareunia should be evaluated promptly for endocervicitis.[127,128] Evaluation also is indicated if a sexual partner has an STI.

Cervical abnormalities associated with endocervicitis range from subtle changes to the presence of intensively hyperemic, erythematous, raised, irregular, friable lesions.[127] There is no consensus definition for mucopurulent cervicitis, which makes evaluation of the research literature difficult.[120] Current definitions include inflammation of the endocervix with possible edema; yellow-green endocervical discharge; increased numbers of neutrophils on microscopic examination of cervical secretions; and inducible endocervical bleeding. Mucopurulence is characterized by a yellow or green color on a cotton-tipped applicator obtained from the endocervix. The number of neutrophils considered significant varies in different studies from ≥30 cells per 400× magnified microscopic field to >10 cells per 1000× microscopic field. The use of 30-cell cutpoint provides greater specificity.[2,6,119–122]

Laboratory Findings and Diagnosis

Specific microbiologic diagnosis informs appropriate treatment. Patients should be tested for *N. gonorrhoeae*, *C. trachomatis*, and *T. vaginalis*. Gram-negative intracellular diplococci are seen on Gram stain in about one-half of cases of gonococcal endocervicitis.[6] Given the poor sensitivity of the Gram stain and the possibility of infection in the absence of any abnormality, evaluation for gonococcal endocervicitis must include an appropriate culture or NAAT. Inflammatory changes can be even less remarkable with endocervicitis caused by *C. trachomatis*. Therefore, NAAT, chlamydial culture, or other chlamydial detection tests are recommended

in all cases of suspected infection.[2,6,7,120] NAAT is the most sensitive test available for *C. trachomatis*. Saline wet mount can be used to diagnose *T. vaginalis* and to help establish the diagnosis of BV.[2,6,7,119,120] Because of the poor sensitivity of wet mount, further testing for *T. vaginalis* by culture or antigen-based tests should be conducted if the wet mount is negative. If HSV is suspected, a culture should be obtained. Typing HSV strains differentiates between HSV-1 and HSV-2 isolates. NAAT testing for *M. genitalium* is not available commercially.

Management/Empiric and Definitive Therapy

The initial management of endocervicitis varies depending on the clinical findings and the risk of the adolescent for certain STIs (Table 53-5). A positive laboratory test for *N. gonorrhoeae*, *C. trachomatis*, *T. vaginalis*, or HSV defines treatment. However, empiric treatment can be considered if there is a high suspicion of *N. gonorrhoeae* or *C. trachomatis*, based on high prevalence of either microbe in the community or a concern that the patient may be at risk for loss to follow-up.[2,123] Treatment of BV also can be considered since higher rates of resolution of endocervicitis occurred with treatment of BV in some studies.[120]

More data are needed regarding treatment of *M. genitalium* cervicitis. The antibiotics directed at treating *N. gonorrhoeae* and *C. trachomatis* are not adequate to treat cervicitis caused by other organisms and the standard treatment regimen for PID with cefoxitin and doxycycline has been shown to be ineffective for women with *M. genitalium* associated with PID.[123,129,130] Although *M. genitalium* theoretically is susceptible to macrolides, fluoroquinolones, and tetracyclines, a 5-day course of azithromycin may be more effective in eradicating it and, to date, moxifloxacin is the only antibiotic without treatment failure.[130,131] The need to consider *M. genitalium* in the adolescent population was demonstrated in several studies. One study showed a cumulative rate over a 27-month period among 14- to 17-year-old females to be 14%, which was concordant with their male partners.[132] Another study in women 14 to 21 years old found a rate of 22%.[133]

Follow-up after completion of therapy is recommended for adolescents with persistent symptoms.[2] The management of mucopurulent cervicitis also requires evaluation and treatment of all sexual partners for STIs, and provides an opportunity to reinforce STI prevention measures.

TABLE 53-5. Treatment of Cervicitis in Adolescents

Results	Suggested Treatment
Mucopurulent endocervical discharge and smear with many neutrophils on Gram stain or saline wet mount	Treat for *Chlamydia trachomatis* Azithromycin, 1 g in a single dose, *or* doxycycline, 100 mg PO bid for 7 days. Concurrently treat for *Neisseria gonorrhoeae* if prevalence is high (>5%) in patient population
Gram-negative intracellular diplococci on smear regardless of presence or absence of endocervical discharge or neutrophils on smear	Treat for *Neisseria gonorrhoeae* and *Chlamydia trachomatis*
Mucopurulent endocervical discharge and smear without neutrophils	Defer therapy until further microbial results are available *or* If patient is high-risk by history (e.g., known contact, new and/or multiple sex partners, age ≤25, unprotected sex), consider treatment for *Neisseria gonorrhoeae* and *Chlamydia trachomatis* unless follow-up can be ensured
Trichomonas seen on wet mount or identified on rapid test	Treat with oral metronidazole or tinidazole
Bacterial vaginosis diagnosed	Treat with oral metronidazole or tinidazole or intravaginal metronidazole or clindamycin
RESULTS NOT AVAILABLE	
Clinical presentation suggestive of herpes simplex virus infection	Consider oral acyclovir or famciclovir or valacyclovir
No endocervical discharge	Defer therapy until further microbial results are available If patient is high-risk by history; consider treatment for *Neisseria gonorrhoeae* and *Chlamydia trachomatis* unless follow-up can be ensured and also treat for *Neisseria gonorrhoeae* if prevalence is >5%

Complications

Sequelae from untreated mucopurulent cervicitis include PID as well as possible long-term sequelae of ectopic pregnancy and infertility. The relationship between *N. gonorrhoeae* and *C. trachomatis* and PID is well established and there is increasing evidence that *M. genitalium* also is associated with PID.[6,121,131,134–138] Cervicitis also increases the risk of transmission and acquisition of HIV infection. Viral shedding of HIV-1 decreases with effective treatment for cervicitis.[2,6,121]

Prevention

Consistent use of condoms will reduce transmission of STI pathogens associated with cervicitis.

---

54 Pelvic Inflammatory Disease

Eloisa Llata, Harold C. Wiesenfeld, and David E. Soper

Pelvic inflammatory disease (PID) is a clinical infection of the upper genital tract, often due to sexually transmitted infection (STI) pathogens such as *Chlamydia trachomatis* or *Neisseria gonorrhoeae*. PID is a spectrum of infections that can include endometritis, salpingitis, tubo-ovarian abscess, and pelvic peritonitis. Morbidity from PID includes chronic pelvic pain, ectopic pregnancy, and infertility. Published data suggest overall declining rates of women diagnosed with PID in the United States in both hospital and ambulatory settings.[1,2] While no single factor explains this trend, some have suggested increases in *Chlamydia* screening, use of more sensitive diagnostic technologies, and availability of single-dose therapies for uncomplicated lower genital tract infections could be impacting PID rates.[1–3] Despite declining trends, sexually active adolescents have among the highest age-specific rates of PID[1,4] of all sexually active females, potentially impacting fertility for decades of reproductive potential among this young population. Risk factors such as anatomic and behavioral predispositions, barriers to healthcare, poor compliance, and issues surrounding confidentiality make this age group especially vulnerable.[5]

EPIDEMIOLOGY

Approximately 750,000 cases of PID occur annually in the U.S., with 20% occurring among sexually active females <19 years of age.[4] Both acute PID and long-term sequelae have a significant economic impact, with annual U.S. expenditures estimated at 1.88 billion dollars.[6] Risk factors among adolescents for PID are multiple and are often interrelated.[7,8] Because many cases of PID result from complications of a first STI, risk factors for PID include risk factors for the acquisition of an initial infection such as engaging in unprotected sex, having multiple sex partners, age discrepancy of partners, early sexual debut, drug/alcohol abuse, or having serially monogamous relationships of short duration and high frequency.[9–11]

Contraceptives play an important role in predisposing women to the acquisition of PID. Non-use of contraception is a risk factor for PID, whereas barrier methods decrease the risk of STI acquisition and subsequent development of PID.[12,13] The use of oral contraceptives (OCs) may result in greater exposure of the endocervical tissue onto the ectocervix, clinically referred to as ectopy (Figure 54-1). Cervical ectopy is believed to increase susceptibility to *Chlamydia* and may improve detection of *C. trachomatis* antigen.[14,15] In contrast, OCs have been shown to reduce the risk of symptomatic PID, which may be due to changes in cervical mucus, shorter duration of menses, and decreased "receptivity" of the endometrium to infection.[16–19] The role of OCs on the acquisition of *N. gonorrhoeae* is less defined, although one study investigated the influence of OC on gonococcal infection in women exposed to males with gonococcal urethritis and found that combined OCs were associated with lower gonorrhea rates.[20] Intra-uterine devices (IUDs) have had limited use among the adolescent population due to concerns of increased risk of PID and STIs. However, more recent studies indicate that the risk of PID among women with IUD ranges from 0% to 2% when no infection is present at the time of insertion and 0% to 5% when insertion occurred during a documented infection.[21–23] Recent guidance encourages providers to consider the IUD, among other top tier methods of contraception, as first-line choices for adolescents.[23a]

A prior history of PID or other STI increases a woman's risk for future PID. The increased risk observed may be due to reinfection from untreated partners, relapse from inadequate therapy for the first infection, increased vulnerability to subsequent gram-negative or anaerobic bacterial infection, and/or continued presence of risk factors. In a prospective longitudinal study over the course of a 4-year period of 110 adolescent females diagnosed with PID, nearly one-third of females who returned for follow-up were diagnosed with a subsequent STI or PID or both within 6 months of initial PID diagnosis.[24]

ETIOLOGIC AGENTS

C. trachomatis and *N. gonorrhoeae* have been isolated from both the lower and upper genital tract in women with PID and are accepted universally as etiologic agents of PID. Estimates from the

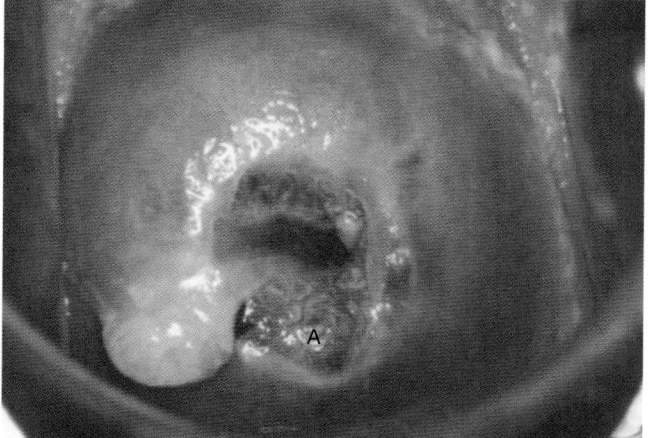

Figure 54-1. Examination of an adolescent girl shows an area of cervical ectopy (A), where the columnar cells that line the inner area of the cervix extend to the outer area.

PART II Clinical Syndromes and Cardinal Features of Infectious Diseases: Approach to Diagnosis and Initial Management

SECTION G Genitourinary Tract Infections

PID Evaluation and Clinical Health (PEACH) Study found that approximately 40% of women diagnosed with PID had cervical *C. trachomatis* or *N. gonorrhoeae* infection.[25] *Chlamydia* is the most commonly reported STI in the U.S., with >900,000 reported female cases in 2009.[26] Females aged 15 to 19 years had the highest incidence of reported *Chlamydia* infection (3329 per 100,000 females) and women aged 20 to 24 had the second highest incidence (3274 per 100,000).[26] *Chlamydia* infection has been associated with tubal scarring, obstruction, and peritubal adhesions.[27–29] Recent evidence demonstrates that *C. trachomatis* infection is particularly important in subclinical (or "silent") PID, a term used to describe women with lower genital tract infections and concurrent endometritis and/or salpingitis but with mild to no symptoms. Subclinical PID is estimated to account for at least one-half of all PID cases.[19] *N. gonorrhoeae* is the second most commonly reported bacterial STI in the U.S., with incidence reaching 569 per 100,000 among girls aged 15 to 19 years.[26] Women <25 years of age are at the highest risk for acquiring gonorrhea and between 10% to 20% of women with inadequately treated gonococcal cervicitis will develop PID.[30] Between 75% to 90% of gonococcal infections in women are asymptomatic.

In addition to isolation of both STI pathogens, endogenous microorganisms associated with bacterial vaginosis (BV), a disruption of the normal vaginal microflora leading to an overgrowth of anaerobic and facultative bacteria, have been recovered from the upper genital tract in women with acute PID. Multiple investigations have demonstrated an association between BV and acute PID,[25,31–37] and many conclude that BV not only facilitates ascending spread of vaginal microorganisms by interfering with the host's defenses but also provides an inoculum of potentially pathogenic microorganisms.[38] *Mycoplasma genitalium* also has emerged as a possible causative agent for PID[39,40] but further research is needed to further investigate the importance of this organism.

PATHOGENESIS AND PATHOLOGIC FINDINGS

The ascent of *C. trachomatis* and *N. gonorrhoeae* from the cervix through the endometrium to the fallopian tubes is the most common antecedent to PID. Once infection-induced inflammation reaches the fallopian tube, a complex interaction of epithelial degeneration, edema, and other inflammatory responses occurs leading to scarring of the involved fallopian tube.[41] The presence of other bacteria may be explained by priming of tissue by the STI organisms (mono-microbial phase) for opportunistic invasion by facultative and anaerobic bacteria from the lower genital tract (polymicrobial phase).[42] This "priming" could result from either alteration of local mucosal defenses, or anatomic interference with mechanical host defenses that drain secretions from the upper genital tract mucosa.

DIAGNOSIS

Despite diagnostic guidelines (Box 54-1), the clinical diagnosis of PID presents diagnostic challenges because of the variations in clinical presentation that often lead to under- or misdiagnosis. Diagnosing PID in female adolescents can pose unique challenges as they may be unable to recognize their symptoms as indications of a possible medical illness, may be reluctant to reveal their sexually active status for fear of disclosure to their parents, and may limit or forgo the use of medical care because of the stigma of having an STI. In a recent study, nearly 25% of young women 12 to 21 years of age diagnosed with PID were diagnosed inaccurately.[43] Clinicians need to recognize the implication of mild or nonspecific findings, particularly in a young female giving a challenging history and undergoing her first pelvic examination.[44]

Although laparoscopy is considered the gold standard for the diagnosis of PID, the diagnosis of PID usually is based on clinical findings. Pelvic pain is the most common symptom of PID, although it may be mild in some women. Other symptoms associated with acute PID are listed in Box 54-2. A directed approach to the history, including assessment of symptomatology, risk factors, sexual and menstrual history, and prior STI, is critical in making

---

BOX 54-1. CDC Guidelines for the Clinical Diagnosis of Pelvic Inflammatory Disease (PID)

MINIMAL CRITERIA

Empiric treatment of PID should be initiated in sexually active young women and others at risk for STIs if ≥1 of the following minimum criteria are present and no other cause(s) for the illness can be identified: Cervical motion tenderness *or* uterine tenderness *or* adnexal tenderness

ADDITIONAL CRITERIA

Oral temperature >38.3°C (>101°F)
Abnormal cervical or vaginal mucopurulent discharge
Presence of abundant numbers of WBCs on saline microscopy of vaginal secretions
Elevated erythrocyte sedimentation rate
Elevated C-reactive protein
Laboratory documentation of cervical infection with *C. trachomatis* or *N. gonorrhoeae*

DEFINITIVE CRITERIA FOR DIAGNOSING PID

Endometrial biopsy with histopathologic evidence of endometritis
Transvaginal sonography or magnetic resonance imaging techniques showing thickened, fluid-filled tubes with or without free pelvic fluid or tubo-ovarian complex, or doppler studies suggesting pelvic infection (e.g., tubal hyperemia); and
Laparoscopic abnormalities consistent with PID

From the Centers for Disease Control and Prevention, 2010 guidelines for treatment of sexually transmitted infections. MMWR 59:RR-12, 2010.

BOX 54-2. Symptoms Associated with Clinically Suspected Pelvic Inflammatory Disease

Abdominal pain
Abnormal purulent discharge
Metrorrhagia (uterine bleeding at irregular intervals)
Postcoital bleeding
Fever
Dysuria
Nausea/vomiting

---

an accurate diagnosis. A pelvic examination should be performed to assess for signs of cervical inflammation (cervicitis) including mucopurulent discharge, cervical erythema or friability (easy bleeding to touch). After the speculum examination, with collection of the appropriate microbiologic samples (see below), a bimanual examination should be performed to assess for cervical, uterine, or adnexal tenderness or masses. Microscopy of the vaginal secretions should be performed looking for leukorrhea (more than 1 leukocyte per epithelial cell).

When the diagnosis of PID is in doubt, there is concern for a tubo-ovarian abscess, or the patient is not responding to conventional therapy for PID, further diagnostic evaluation using ultrasonography can be helpful. Although other causes of pelvic or abdominal pain should be explored (Box 54-3 and Table 54-1), the rarity of some of these conditions in adolescence helps to narrow the diagnosis. Providers should maintain a low threshold for treating PID in at-risk populations (such as the sexually active adolescent) and empiric therapy should be initiated in all adolescents unless another etiology is discovered.

LABORATORY FINDINGS AND DIAGNOSIS

A cervical test for *C. trachomatis* and *N. gonorrhoeae* should be obtained in all patients with suspected PID.[45,46] Nucleic acid amplification tests (NAATs) are preferred because of their increased

BOX 54-3. Differential Diagnosis of Pelvic Inflammatory Disease

GYNECOLOGIC CAUSES

Pregnancy (ectopic, or septic or threatened abortion)
Ovarian cyst (intact, ruptured, or torsed)
Endometriosis
Mittelschmerz (pain associated with ovulation)
Dysmenorrhea

GASTROINTESTINAL CAUSES

Appendicitis
Constipation
Diarrhea
Gastroenteritis
Inflammatory bowel disease
Irritable bowel syndrome

URINARY TRACT CAUSES

Cystitis
Urethritis
Urinary calculus
Pyelonephritis

Adapted from Shrier LA. Bacterial sexually transmitted infections: gonorrhea, chlamydia, pelvic inflammatory disease, and syphilis. In: Emans SJH, Laufer MR, Goldstein DP (eds) Pediatric and Adolescent Gynecology, 4th ed. Philadelphia, Lippincott-Raven, 1998, p 480; updated 5th ed, 2005, p 591.

sensitivity to detect infection compared with culture. Laboratory confirmation of an STI is helpful because it provides diagnostic corroboration and guidance in therapy, and serves as a baseline for subsequent testing of the patient for microbiologic cure, but is not necessary to justify initiation of therapy for PID.

Patients can be assessed for the presence of other vaginal infections such as BV (vaginal pH, clue cells, and whiff test) and *Trichomonas* vaginitis. All women diagnosed with acute PID should have a pregnancy test and be offered HIV testing.[46,47] Male partners of women with PID should be referred for diagnosis and treatment of both *N. gonorrhoeae* and *C. trachomatis*, regardless of the test results in the female partner diagnosed with PID. Serum testing for elevated white blood cell count, erythrocyte sedimentation rate and/or C-reactive protein generally is reserved for women with clinically severe PID.[38] While an endometrial biopsy offers an acceptable approach to documenting inflammation of the upper genital tract, biopsy generally is not performed among adolescents and delay between biopsy and final histopathologic report makes this test most appropriate in cases in which there is diagnostic uncertainty.

MANAGEMENT

The principles of management and criteria for hospitalizations are outlined in Box 54-4. The severity of disease generally dictates whether a patient is managed as an inpatient or an outpatient. The vast majority of women with clinically suspected PID are treated with antimicrobial therapy as outpatients. Among women with mild to moderate PID, there is no difference in clinical course, recurrent PID, chronic pelvic pain, or infertility between women hospitalized for PID and those treated as outpatients.[25]

TABLE 54-1. Comparative Clinical Characteristics of Pelvic Inflammatory Disease, Ectopic Pregnancy, and Acute Appendicitis

	Pelvic Inflammatory Disease	Ectopic Pregnancy	Acute Appendicitis
HISTORY			
Age	Any after puberty	Risk increases with age	Any
Onset of symptoms	75% within 7 days of menses	At 4 weeks' gestation or later; rupture at 6–10 weeks' gestation	Any
Abdominal pain	Dull, crampy, localized to lower abdomen; right upper quadrant pain (perihepatitis) can be present	Before rupture: localized or diffuse dull abdominal pain. After rupture: severe, poorly localized pain, rectal pressure	Poorly localized periumbilical or epigastric pain with shift to right lower quadrant after 4–6 hours; increasing severity
Vaginal discharge	55%	Not associated	Not associated
Menstrual pattern	Metrorrhagia; missed menstruation not associated	Intermittent bleeding or spotting; often missed or late menstruation	No change in usual pattern
Fever	>38°C in up to 35%	>38°C in up to 20%	Usually <38°C; >38°C after perforation
Nausea and vomiting	Uncommon	Uncommon	50–60%
SIGNS			
Cervicitis	Purulent exudate in 80%	Not associated	Not associated
Cervical motion tenderness	>95%	Can be present; not as pronounced as in salpingitis	Usually none; can be present with perforation if appendix adjacent to adnexa
Adnexal mass	5–50%	35–50%	Not associated
LABORATORY EVALUATION			
Anemia	Not associated	Significant (hematocrit <25%) after rupture	Not associated
Leukocyte count	Normal or elevated	Usually elevated	Mildly elevated
Pregnancy test	Usually negative	Positive 1–2 weeks after conception	Usually negative, but pregnant patients can have appendicitis as well
Ultrasonography	Common findings: cul-de-sac fluid, adnexal enlargement, complex adnexal mass	Intrauterine gestational sac absent	Can detect inflamed appendix
Laparoscopy	Inflammation of fallopian tubes	Fallopian tube pregnancy with or without rupture	Normal fallopian tubes; inflamed appendix

Adapted from Paradise JE, Grant L. Pelvic inflammatory disease in adolescents. Pediatr Rev 1992;13:216–223.

PART II Clinical Syndromes and Cardinal Features of Infectious Diseases: Approach to Diagnosis and Initial Management

SECTION G Genitourinary Tract Infections

BOX 54-4. Principles of Management of Pelvic Inflammatory Disease

- Exclude pregnancy and appendicitis
- Use minimal criteria to guide diagnosis[a]
- Err on the side of over diagnosis
- Perform testing for *C. trachomatis* and *N. gonorrhoeae*
- Consider screening and treating for lower genital tract infections, including bacterial vaginosis and *Trichomonas vaginalis*
- Offer HIV testing to all women diagnosed with acute PID
- Treat early and with broad-spectrum antibiotics
- Reassess patient 48–72 hours after initiating therapy
- Criteria for hospitalization:
  - Surgical emergency (e.g., appendicitis cannot be excluded)
  - Patient is pregnant
  - Patient does not respond clinically to oral antimicrobial therapy
  - Patient is unable to follow or tolerate an outpatient oral regimen
  - Patient has severe illness, nausea and vomiting, or high fever
  - Patient has a tuboovarian abscess
- Identify, evaluate, and treat sex partners. In settings where only women are treated, male sex partners should be referred for appropriate treatment
- Educate patient about STI prevention (see Chapter 51, Sexually Transmitted Disease Syndromes), including abstinence, encouraging the use of barrier methods of protection, and regular assessment for STIs

HIV, human immunodeficiency virus; PID, pelvic inflammatory disease; STI, sexually transmitted infection.
[a]See Box 54-1.

TABLE 54-2. Centers for Disease Control and Prevention Treatment Guidelines for Acute Pelvic Inflammatory Disease

Parenteral Regimens	Oral Regimens
Regimen A	**Recommended regimen**
Cefotetan 2g IV every 12 hours	Ceftriaxone 250 mg IM in a single dose
Or	
Cefoxitin 2 g IV every 6 hours;	Plus
Plus	Doxycycline 100 mg orally twice a day for 14 days
Doxycycline 100mg orally or IV every 12 hours	With or without
	Metronidazole 500 mg orally twice a day for 14 days
	Or
Regimen B	Cefoxitin 2 g IM in a single dose and probenecid, 1 g orally administered concurrently in a single dose
Clindamycin 900 mg IV every 8 hours	
Plus	Plus
Gentamicin loading dose IV or IM (2 mg/kg of body weight) followed by a maintenance dose (1.5 mg/kg) every 8 hours. Single daily dosing (3–5 mg/kg) can be substituted	Doxycycline 100 mg orally twice a day for 14 days
	With or without
	Metronidazole 500 mg orally twice a day for 14 days
	Or
Alternative parenteral regimens	Other parenteral third-generation cephalosporin (e.g., ceftizoxime or cefotaxime)
Ampicillin-sulbactam 3 g IV every 6 hours	
Plus	Plus
Doxycycline 100 mg orally or IV every 12 hours	Doxycycline 100 mg orally twice a day for 14 days
	With or without
	Metronidazole 500 mg orally twice a day for 14 days

Adapted from Centers for Disease Control and Prevention, 2010 guidelines for treatment of sexually transmitted infections. MMWR 2010;59:RR-12.

A critical component to the outpatient management is short-term follow-up, especially in the adolescent population. Adolescents may be reluctant to disclose their diagnosis of PID and because of their dependence on adults for financial and logistical support, they may not be able to obtain prescriptions and/or keep follow-up appointments.

PID treatment regimens provide broad-spectrum coverage of likely pathogens. Current guidelines recommend that empiric treatment for PID be initiated in sexually active young women and other women at risk for STIs if they are experiencing pelvic or lower abdominal pain, if no cause for the illness other than PID can be identified, and if ≥1 of the following criteria are present on pelvic examination: cervical motion tenderness, uterine tenderness, or adnexal tenderness (see Table 54-1).[46] Additional supportive criteria are intended to help clinicians recognize when PID should be suspected and when additional information is needed to increase diagnostic certainty.[46]

Recommended treatment regimens for PID are outlined in (Table 54-2). Limitations in coverage of anaerobic bacteria by recommended cephalosporins may require the addition of metronidazole. Due to increased fluoroquinolone resistance of *N. gonorrhoeae*, fluoroquinolones should not be used in the treatment of acute PID. Concerns over compliance and tolerability issues, especially among adolescents, have prompted interest in searching for alternative regimens that demonstrate efficacy equal to currently recommended regimens. Multiple clinical trials have examined the efficacy of azithromycin alone or azithromycin plus metronidazole in the treatment of PID. While each of the studies found similarly high rates of clinical success, further research is needed to determine optimal dosing. Comparison studies with currently recommended regimens also are needed.

COMPLICATIONS AND SEQUELAE

Several factors influence a woman's risk for developing adverse reproductive outcomes after an episode of PID. These include the number of episodes of PID, the severity of infection as measured by inflammatory reaction, and the duration of the interval between the development of PID and the administration of appropriate antimicrobial therapy. At least one-fourth of women with PID experience ≥1 serious long-term sequela, including increased risk of ectopic pregnancy (6- to 10-fold increased rate), infertility (approximately 10% after first episode, approximately 20% after second episode), chronic abdominal pain (3-fold increased rate), and recurrent infection (2- to 3-fold increased rate).[48–50] Women treated within 3 days of onset of illness have improved fertility compared with women whose treatment is delayed, reinforcing the importance of early, often empiric, treatment. Mortality from PID is <1% and usually is secondary to rupture of a tubo-ovarian abscess or to ectopic pregnancy.[42]

PREVENTION

Adolescents should be queried about their sexual activity and risk factors for STIs/PID, and should be educated about the symptoms and signs of STIs/PID. Sexually active adolescents should be screened routinely for STIs and offered treatment according to accepted guidelines. The U.S. Preventive Services Task Force recommends chlamydial screening for all sexually active females ≤24 years of age at routine healthcare visits, as well as older asymptomatic women at risk for *C. trachomatis*.[51] There is evidence that screening and treating for *C. trachomatis* reduces the incidence of PID and its sequelae.[51,52] The rate of PID among an asymptomatic study population undergoing risk-based enhanced screening for *C. trachomatis* was reduced by 66% compared with controls.[52] Since STIs play a major role in PID, empiric treatment of male sexual partners is critical to prevent reinfection and to improve the long-term health of young women.[19,46]

55 Epididymitis, Orchitis, and Prostatitis

Noni E. MacDonald and William R. Bowie

EPIDIDYMITIS

Epididymitis is an inflammatory reaction or infection of the epididymis, the coiled convoluted tubular structure attached to the upper posterior part of each testicle that collects, stores, and matures sperm.

Etiology, Epidemiology, and Pathogenesis

For young adult males, epididymitis is common, causing suffering and days lost from work.[1] In prepubertal boys, the incidence in a prospective population-based study in 2000 was noted to be 1.2 per 1000 boys, with peaks for hospital admissions in summer and winter.[2,3] The age distribution in boys is bimodal with a peak <5 years of age and then again in early puberty.[4] Acute epididymitis in boys is more common than testicular torsion.[5,6]

Epididymitis can occur as an inflammatory postinfectious reaction to a number of bacterial and viral pathogens,[1,3] or as a complication of urethral infections caused by sexually transmitted pathogens,[1,7] by genitourinary tract pathogens (especially if predisposing obstructive anatomic,[6,8–10] neurologic genitourinary abnormalities,[10,11] or anorectal malformations[12] exist), or, more rarely, through hematogenous spread to the epididymis from a primary focus of infection (e.g., *Haemophilus influenzae* b, *Salmonella* spp., *Streptococcus pneumoniae*, or *Mycobacterium tuberculosis*). The microbial etiology and predisposing factors (Table 55-1) in acute bacterial epididymitis in children and adolescents vary with age. Occasionally, epididymitis is not caused by inflammation or infection but is related to trauma, systemic diseases such as Henoch–Schönlein purpura or Kawasaki disease, or to medication such as amiodarone.[2,3,12–15]

TABLE 55-1. Microbial Etiology and Predisposing Factors in Acute Epididymitis in Children and Adolescents

Predisposing Factors	Etiology	Incidence
PREPUBERTAL CHILDREN		
Underlying structural or neurologic abnormalities of the genitourinary tract	Enterobacteriaceae *Pseudomonas aeruginosa*	Uncommon
Hematogenous spread from primary focus	*Haemophilus influenzae* b *Streptococcus pneumoniae* *Neisseria meningitidis* *Salmonella* spp. Other	Uncommon
ADOLESCENTS		
Urethritis	*Chlamydia trachomatis* *Neisseria gonorrhoeae*	Related to frequency of sexual activity
Underlying genitourinary tract pathology	Enterobacteriaceae *Pseudomonas aeruginosa*	Uncommon
Hematogenous spread from primary focus	*Streptococcus pneumoniae* *Neisseria meningitidis* *Mycobacterium tuberculosis* Other	Rare

Clinical Manifestations and Differential Diagnosis

Epididymitis, whether inflammatory or infectious in etiology, typically has an acute onset, with unilateral scrotal pain and swelling that increases over 1 or 2 days. Commonly associated symptoms include dysuria and other lower urinary tract symptoms. Sexually transmitted epididymitis usually is accompanied by urethritis, which frequently is asymptomatic. Differentiation of epididymitis from testicular torsion, which requires immediate surgical intervention, is critical.[16,17] Bacterial orchitis, an extension of epididymitis, is another important consideration in the differential diagnosis, especially in prepubertal children. Table 55-2 compares the clinical and laboratory differences among these disorders. The presence of Prehn sign, i.e., relief of pain with testicular elevation, supports the diagnosis of epididymitis but is not definitive.[18] The cremasteric reflex usually is present in epididymitis but absent in testicular torsion. Presence of urethral discharge is suggestive but not diagnostic of epididymitis. In prepubertal boys with acute scrotal pain, urinalysis and urine culture frequently are performed; positive yield in epididymitis is low.[19] Ultrasonography, radionuclide scan, and occasionally, magnetic resonance imaging[13,17–24] are helpful in differentiating among entities (see Table 55-2). For the diagnosis of acute epididymitis, radionuclide scan is the most accurate radiologic method but is not available routinely. Color duplex doppler ultrasonography has a sensitivity of 70% and a specificity of 88% in acute epididymitis.[25]

Laboratory Findings and Diagnosis

Organisms responsible for infectious epididymitis usually can be isolated from urine and urethral specimens. When a sexually transmitted infection (STI) is suspected, a Gram stain of urethral exudate or intraurethral swab specimen and a culture of intraurethral exudate or a nucleic acid amplification test (NAAT) (either on intraurethral swab or first-void urine) for *Chlamydia trachomatis* and *Neisseria gonorrhoeae* is indicated.[1,25] As with any STI syndrome, testing for other STIs, including HIV, should be considered based upon the patient's sexual history and risk factors. (Chapter 51, Sexually Transmitted Infection Syndromes).

Management and Complications

Empiric therapy is indicated before laboratory test results are available. Early treatment of STI epididymitis cures the infection, improves the symptoms and signs, and prevents transmission of these STI microbes to others, and decreases potential complications.[1,25] For epididymitis most likely caused by gonococcal or chlamydial infection, the recommended treatment regimen is ceftriaxone (single 250 mg intramuscular dose) plus doxycycline (100 mg orally twice a day for 10 days) while awaiting laboratory test results.[25] For acute epididymitis most likely caused by enteric organisms such as *Escherichia coli* or *Pseudomonas*, levofloxacin or ofloxacin is recommended.[25] In young children with presumed hematogenous infection, broad-spectrum therapy is used initially. In addition to antimicrobial therapy, bedrest, scrotal elevation, and administration of analgesics are recommended until fever and local inflammation resolve.[1] Failure of symptoms to improve within 3 days requires re-evaluation of the diagnosis and therapy, and may require hospitalization. If an STI is identified, the sexual partner(s) is contacted for assessment and treatment.

PART II Clinical Syndromes and Cardinal Features of Infectious Diseases: Approach to Diagnosis and Initial Management

SECTION G Genitourinary Tract Infections

TABLE 55-2. Comparison of Clinical Manifestations and Laboratory Findings in Acute Epididymitis, Acute Orchitis, and Testicular Torsion in Children and Adolescents

		Acute Orchitis		
	Acute Epididymitis	**Bacterial**	**Viral**	**Torsion Testes**
CLINICAL FEATURES				
Most common age	Adolescence	Rare in childhood	Adolescence	Peripubertal
Predisposing factors	Postpuberty: urethritis (sexually transmitted infection)	Epididymitis	Failure to be immunized against mumps	None
	Prepuberty: structural abnormality			
PAIN				
Onset	Gradual	Gradual	Acute/occasionally gradual	Acute
Severity	Mild–severe	Moderate–severe	Mild–severe	Severe
Fever	Moderate	Moderate–high	Low–high	Uncommon
SYSTEMIC SYMPTOMS				
Anorexia, vomiting, malaise	May occur with severe infection, uncommon	Common	Can occur	Uncommon
Dysuria	Common	Common	Can occur	Uncommon
SCROTAL FINDINGS				
Testicular lie	Vertical (normal)	Vertical	Vertical	Possibly horizontal
Swelling	++; usually unilateral	++	++ to +++	+
Prehn sign	Pain ↓	Pain ↓	No change in pain	Pain unchanged or ↓
Cremasteric reflex	Usually present	Usually present	Usually present	Usually absent
Tenderness				
Testes	± epididymis tender	++	+ to ++ (can be unilateral)	++
Spermatic cord	++	++	++	–
Presence of hydrocele	Common	Common	–	± (~30%)
Skin inflammation	++	+	–	–
Urethral discharge	Possible	Possible	–	–
LABORATORY FINDINGS				
Peripheral blood leukocytosis	++	++	±	±
C-reactive protein	++	+	++	normal
Pyuria (>10 WBC/hpf)	++	±	Usually negative	Usually negative
IMAGING FINDINGS				
Epididymis				
Doppler blood flow	↑ or normal vascularity	↑ vascularity	↑ vascularity	↓ vascularity or avascular
Sonogram	Enlarged and thickened	↑ perfusion	Increased perfusion	Enlarged with increased echotexture vs. opposite side
Testis				
Doppler blood flow	↑ or normal vascularity	↑ vascularity	↑ vascularity	↓ vascularity or avascular
Sonogram	Enlarged, hypervascular ↑ perfusion	Testicluar masses or swollen testicles with hypoechoic and hypervascular areas	Testicluar masses or swollen testicles with hypoechoic and hypervascular areas	No change in echotexture unless late

+, mild to moderate; ++, moderate to severe; ±, variably present; –, absent; ↑, increased; ↓, decreased.

Patients in whom gram-negative organisms are isolated also may need investigation for underlying anatomic or neurologic abnormalities that may be causing urinary tract obstruction. Direct aspiration of the epididymis for specimen collection may be done if other testing does not provide the answer and/or there is evidence of an abscess.

In patients with inflammatory postinfectious reactive epididymitis, treatment includes analgesics and supportive care; antimicrobial therapy is not indicated.[3,19] In these patients there is even a question whether urinalysis and urine culture are of value.[19]

Complications of epididymitis include testicular abscess, chronic epididymitis, testicular infarction, and infertility. Drainage of scrotal abscesses or orchiectomy is seldom needed if the condition is diagnosed and treated promptly and close follow-up is performed.

ORCHITIS

Orchitis, inflammation of the testis, rarely occurs in prepubertal patients. While bacterial epididymo-orchitis does occur, usually infection has spread from the epididymis to include the testicle.[26] Primary orchitis is uncommon except with certain viral diseases, with mumps being the most common pathogen.[27,28] Less frequently, enterovirus[29] or, rarely, adenoviruses,[30] varicella-zoster virus,[31] or West Nile virus[32] are responsible.

When associated with mumps, orchitis usually follows parotitis by 4 to 8 days, but can develop up to 6 weeks after parotid gland involvement or in the absence of parotitis.[27,28] The onset of viral orchitis can be gradual but usually is abrupt with mumps[28] and is heralded by fever, chills, nausea, and lower abdominal pain (see Table 55-2). When the right testis is involved, appendicitis can be suspected erroneously if the scrotum has not been examined carefully. The affected testis is warm, swollen and tender, and the adjacent skin is edematous and red. Patients with mumps orchitis appear to have higher serum levels of C-reactive protein than do patients with mumps meningitis.[28,33] The mumps virus can be detected in the semen for 14 days and mumps RNA can be detected for up to 40 days.[34] Mumps orchitis is associated with a transient but significant reduction in sperm count and abnormal sperm morphology, which may account for the long-term adverse effect on fertility in some patients.[28] While anti-sperm antibodies can be detected, they do not seem to play a role in mumps orchitis nor in the subsequent infertility.[28]

Bacterial epididymo-orchitis usually occurs as a consequence of contiguous spread from bacterial epididmitis and is due to organisms such as *E. coli, Pseudomonas aeruginosa,* and *Klebsiella* or from hematogenous seeding from another source. Signs and symptoms are similar to those accompanying epididymitis (see Table 55-2). *Toxoplasma gondii* is a rare cause of orchitis, usually in the presence of widely disseminated disease or in a patient with immunodeficiency.[35]

Management of viral orchitis is supportive and symptomatic, consisting of bedrest and analgesia. Corticosteroid therapy is not recommended as there is no evidence that therapy speeds resolution and it might contribute to testicular atrophy.[28] A small randomized controlled trial suggests that early treatment of mumps orchitis with interferon-α_{2B} may lead to earlier symptom resolution and return to normal sperm count and motility but there may be prolongation of abnormal sperm morphology.[36] Bacterial epididymo-orchitis is treated with antimicrobial therapy (see Epididymitis, above). Surgery may be necessary if testicular abscess or pyocele of the scrotum occurs. Infertility can result from viral or bacterial orchitis, but is uncommon even after bilateral disease due to mumps.[27,28]

PROSTATITIS

Prostatitis, inflammation of the prostate, encompasses a group of poorly defined clinical entities associated with pelvic and genital pain or discomfort and variable voiding and sexual complaints[37,38]

Etiology, Pathogenesis, and Epidemiology

Prostatitis is classified into four syndrome categories according to the National Institutes of Health consensus classification: (1) acute bacterial; (2) chronic bacterial; (3) chronic prostatitis/chronic pelvic pain syndrome; and (4) asymptomatic inflammatory prostatitis.[39] Prostatitis does not occur in prepubertal boys and is unusual in adolescents and young adults.[38] Suggested risk factors for bacterial prostatitis include urinary tract instrumentation, urethral strictures, and urethritis.[37] Pathogens reach the prostate by reflux of infected urine, hematogenous spread, or lymphatic spread. The most commonly associated pathogen is *E. coli,* which is found in 65% to 80%, with *P. aeruginosa, Klebsiella* spp., *Serratia* spp., and *Enterobacter aerogenes* accounting for 10% to 15%.[37,38] In adolescents, sexually transmitted pathogens are not a cause of bacterial prostatitis except when prostatitis accompanies Reiter syndrome precipitated by *Chlamydia trachomatis.* Reflux of sterile urine, which incites an inflammatory reaction, can contribute to noninfectious prostatitis.

Clinical Manifestations and Differential Diagnosis

Acute bacterial prostatitis typically manifests abruptly, although occasionally insidiously, with voiding symptoms and poorly localized pain, and often with fever and malaise. In adolescents, the sudden onset of chills, fever, and malaise with voiding difficulties is much more likely to be caused by urinary tract infection, epididymitis, or urethritis than by acute bacterial prostatitis. With acute bacterial prostatitis, rectal examination usually is painful, with a warm, tense, and swollen prostate. Prostatic massage is not recommended because this can precipitate bacteremia.

In adolescents, scrotal or pelvic pain variant also is a possibility. In these cases, there is a history of vague scrotal pain with or without voiding symptoms but no fever and on examination no objective physical findings. Adults with chronic bacterial prostatitis have symptoms of recurring episodes of pain or discomfort in the perineum, groin, lower back, or scrotum, and voiding dysfunction and usually have a history of recurrent urinary tract infection. Prostatic examination often is not helpful because findings are variable.

Nonbacterial (inflammatory) prostatitis and chronic pelvic pain syndrome also are seen in adults. The presentation is similar to chronic bacterial prostatitis but without the history of preceding urinary tract infection. On examination, the prostate is either boggy with nodular areas caused by inflammation or is fibrous and difficult to massage. Whether chronic prostatitis occurs in adolescents is unclear but a study of 16- to 19-year-olds using the National Institutes of Health Chronic Prostatitis Symptom Index[38] reported chronic prostatitis-like symptoms in 6% to 8%.[40]

Laboratory Findings and Diagnosis

When acute bacterial prostatitis is suspected based upon clinical findings, a urinalysis, urine culture, and STI screening are indicated as well as blood cultures and a complete blood count.[37] In patients in whom chronic prostatitis or nonbacterial prostatitis is suspected, prostate fluid is cultured and examined for leukocytes. Examination of expressed prostate secretions has been the definitive test for differentiating the prostatitis syndromes since introduction of the prostate localization 4-cup urine collection test.[38] This method, however, is cumbersome, time-consuming, expensive and has not been well validated.[37] A study of a simpler 2-cup screening test using urine collected before and after prostatic massage reported accuracy similar to the traditional 4-cup test.[41] The specimens are sent for quantitative bacterial culture, and Gram stain of the urinary sediment for examination for leukocytes.

Management

Treatment of bacterial prostatitis can be difficult because of limited penetration and activity of antibiotics in acidic prostatic fluid.[37] Parenteral antibiotics, usually a broad-spectrum β-lactam agent with or without an aminoglycoside, are recommended for acute bacterial prostatitis if the patient is systemically ill with the duration of therapy for 2 to 4 weeks.[37] Therapy for less acute cases includes trimethoprim-sulfamethoxazole, a macrolide, doxycycline, or a fluoroquinolone for 2 weeks. If mechanical obstruction is contributing to the problem, correction is required.

There are no formal guidelines for treatment of nonbacterial chronic prostatitis/chronic pelvic pain syndrome and no proven therapies.[38] Antibiotic therapy is not indicated.

Complications

Abscess of the prostate and stone formation are rare complications of acute bacterial prostatitis.[42]

PART II Clinical Syndromes and Cardinal Features of Infectious Diseases: Approach to Diagnosis and Initial Management

SECTION G Genitourinary Tract Infections

56 Infectious Diseases in Child Abuse

Kirsten Bechtel

Sexual abuse is the persuasion or coercion of a child to engage in sexually explicit conduct.[1] In 2007, of the 794,000 children in the United States found to be abused or neglected, sexual abuse accounted for 7.6%.[2] More than half of these victims were girls between 4 and 15 years old.[2] Federally mandated reporting laws require that all healthcare workers report cases of suspected sexual abuse to child protective service agencies.[3]

MEDICAL EVALUATION

In most cases of sexual abuse, the diagnosis is based on the child's statements; rarely are there physical residua from the abuse.[4-6] The following also can be used to confirm the diagnosis:

- sexually reactive behaviors
- penetrating genital trauma without history of unintentional genital trauma
- presence of seminal products in a child
- pregnancy
- presence of a sexually transmitted infection (STI) beyond the incubation period of vertical transmission (*N. gonorrhoeae, C. trachomatis, T. pallidum*).

The decision to perform screening tests for STIs in pediatric victims of sexual abuse depends on the type of abusive exposure, the regional prevalence of STIs in the adult population, prior consensual sexual activity (in adolescents), and most importantly for prepubertal children, the presence of genital symptoms or an abnormal genital examination. The presence of one STI in a child or adolescent should prompt an evaluation to exclude other STIs.

INFECTIOUS AGENTS

Neisseria gonorrhoeae and *Chlamydia trachomatis*

Prevalence rates for *N. gonorrhoeae* and *C. trachomatis* are from 0.7 to 3.7% in prepubertal children who have been sexually abused.[7-11] The majority of children with such infections are girls with genital complaints (vaginal discharge) or with abnormal genital examinations.[8-12] Routine screening for *N. gonorrhoeae* and *C. trachomatis* in otherwise asymptomatic prepubertal girls after sexual abuse has low diagnostic utility[10,13] and is not recommended. Adolescent females with sexual abuse have higher rates of infection, up to 14% in some studies.[7,8] While most with STI have a history of consensual peer sexual activity, this prevalence is higher than in a non-abused adolescent population.[14]

The use of nucleic acid amplification tests (NAATs) in children and adolescents who have been sexually abused has not been studied extensively. Using NAATs may be beneficial in young children because less biological sample is required, the specimen is less susceptible to environmental changes, and can be obtained in a less invasive manner by using a urine specimen.[15] There are potential negative implications of using NAATs.[16-19] Even with its relatively high sensitivity (97%) and specificity (99%), NAATs may have low positive predictive values in prepubertal children because of the low prevalence rates of *N. gonorrhoeae* and *C. trachomatis* in this population.[18] Falsely positive NAATs in prepubertal children could erroneously lead to the diagnosis of sexual abuse.[17,19] Thus, the Centers for Disease Control and Prevention (CDC) advocates evaluating children and adolescents who have been sexually abused for *N. gonorrhoeae* and *C. trachomatis* by culture methods only and if NAATs are used, positive tests should be confirmed by a second NAAT that targets a different genomic sequence[14] (Figure 56-1).

Several studies have evaluated NAATs in children who have been sexually abused. Matthews-Greer et al.[20] found that PCR and culture were equivalent to detect *C. trachomatis*. Kellogg et al.[21] found that while agreement between ligase-chain reaction (LCR), PCR, and culture for *N. gonorrhoeae* was poor, there was 84% agreement for urine and vaginal PCR for *C. trachomatis*. These authors concluded that urine PCR can be substituted for vaginal PCR for the detection of *C. trachomatis* in children and adolescents evaluated for sexual abuse. In neither of these studies was a

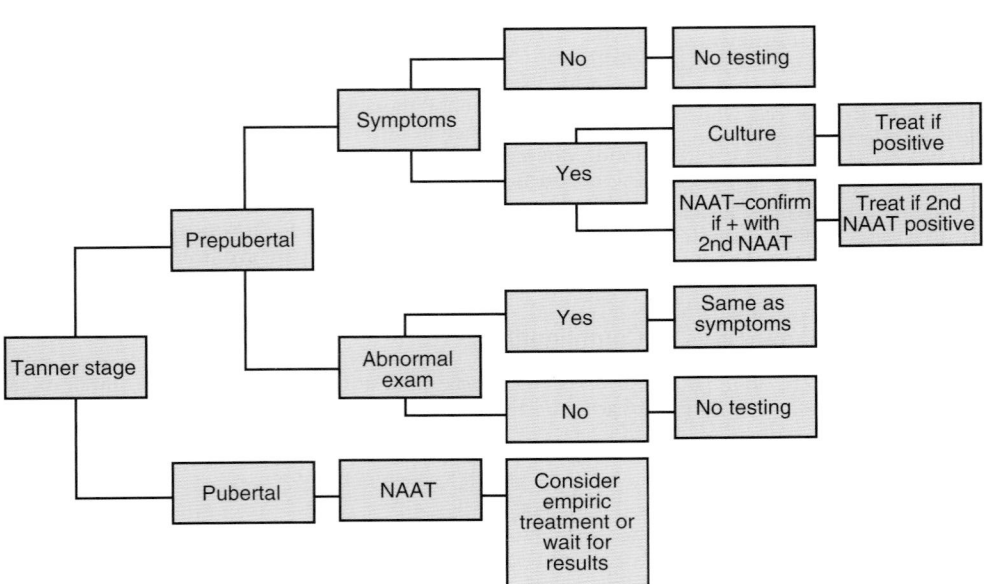

Figure 56-1. Algorithm for evaluation of sexually abused girls for *N. gonorrhoeae* and *C. trachomatis*. NAAT, nucleic acid amplification test.

positive test confirmed by a second NAAT targeting a different genomic sequence.

Black et al. compared urine and genital swabs for *N. gonorrhoeae* and *C. trachomatis* by using PCR confirmed by a second PCR with an alternative target. The sensitivity of urine NAATs relative to vaginal culture was 100% and resulted in a 33% increase in detection of infection.[22] These results suggest that NAATs performed on urine, with confirmation, may replace culture diagnosis of *N. gonorrhoeae* and *C. trachomatis* in children who have been sexually abused.

As there are many other non-abusive causes of vulvovaginitis in prepubertal girls, empiric antibiotic treatment is not indicated after sexual abuse.[23–28] If NAATs are used, any positive test should be confirmed by a second NAAT that targets a different genomic sequence before empiric antibiotics are administered. One could consider empriric treatment of adolescents after cultures/NAATs are obtained, as the prevalence is higher than in the non-abused population and false-positive tests are less of a problem. Alternatively, since many of these adolescent patients are under supervision of child protective service agencies, follow-up can be arranged more easily for treatment and test of cure.

Treponema pallidum

Syphilis is an uncommon infectious complication of child abuse and should not be treated empirically.[29,30] Sexual transmission should be assumed in children who develop syphilis unless another mode of acquisition is identified.[31] Determining the mode of acquisition of syphilis in preverbal children can be challenging. Both Horowitz and Chadwick[29] and Christian et al.[32] described 5 such children who presented with signs of secondary syphilis, including condyloma lata (3 children), syphilitic nephropathy (1 child), and corymbiform rash (1 child). In the child with syphilitic nephropathy, there had been a history of genital rashes consistent with a primary chancre and condyloma lata that were missed by medical providers.[24] In none of these cases was there a history from the child or caregivers of sexual abuse. In cases in which the mode of transmission of an STI is likely to be sexual abuse, but there is no confirmatory history, a comprehensive investigation is needed to insure that the child has no other STI and that no other children in the home have a history of sexual abuse or an STI.[29,32]

Human Papillomavirus (HPV)

The most common HPV subtypes that cause genital warts are 6, 11, 16, and 18. The methods by which children acquire genital warts are unclear. Sexual abuse is the most worrisome form of transmission. Vertical acquisition at delivery may not become clinically apparent for years and may not be the sole source of HPV infection in infants. Horizontal mother-to-child transmission may occur during childhood. Marais et al.[33] evaluated the likelihood of vertical maternal-to-child transmission by measuring serum antibodies to HPV-16 and HPV-18. The prevalence of antibodies was higher in children of seropositive mothers compared with seronegative mothers, but these differences were not statistically significant. Castellsague et al.[34] found that 19.7% of infants born to mothers with cervical HPV and 16.9% of those born to HPV-negative mothers tested HPV-positive at some point during infants' follow-up. Dunne et al.[35] evaluated the prevalence of antibodies to HPV-16 in a sample of children 6 to 11 years of age. Overall, 2.4% of 1316 children were seropositive. Seroprevalence was higher in boys than in girls (3.5% vs. 1.2%), and in children >7 years of age than in younger children (3.3% vs. 0.4%). Further study is needed to fully explain HPV-16 seropositivity in this population.

Several authors have evaluated the mode of acquisition of genital warts in children. Marcoux et al.[36] concluded that the modes of acquisition in children cannot be identified either by the clinical appearance of the lesions or by human papillomavirus typing. Thus the best way to identify possible sexual abuse as the mode of transmission is by the history, physical examination, and family assessment. Sinclair et al.[37] evaluated the likelihood of sexual abuse in 55 children with HPV anogenital infection; 31%

provided a history of sexual abuse. The risk of sexual abuse increased with the child's age at presentation with genital warts (odds ratio of 12.1 in children 8 years of age). The positive predictive value of HPV for possible sexual abuse was 36% for children 4 to 8 years of age at diagnosis and 70% for children >8 years of age. There were no differences in history of parental genital or hand warts in HPV-infected children with and without a history of sexual abuse.

Herpes Simplex Virus (HSV)

Infection with herpes simplex virus in children can indicate sexual abuse. It can also result from non-abusive hand-to-genital contact (autoinoculation in a child with primary oral HSV, or from caregivers during bathing and toileting).[14] The potential value of typing HSV to determine if sexual abuse was the mode of transmission is limited by the fact that up to 20% of adult cases of genital HSV infection are due to HSV-1.[14] There is also a low prevalence of antibodies to HSV-2 in children and adolescents with a history of sexual abuse and thus routine screening for HSV-2 antibodies is not useful.[38]

It is more helpful to conduct a careful clinical history in children with genital HSV to determine if sexual abuse has occurred. A review of several case series in children found that over half of reported cases of genital HSV had a sexual mode of transmission; this was reported more commonly in children ≥5 years of age, those with genital lesions only, and those with HSV-2.[39] A careful assessment for sexual abuse should be performed in any child with genital HSV.

Human Immunodeficiency Virus (HIV)

HIV seroconversion after sexual abuse is rare. Gellert et al.[40] found that only 28 (0.4%) of 5622 children who had been sexually abused were HIV seropositive. The mean age of children at the time of diagnosis was 9 years and 75% provided a clear history of sexual abuse, with 50% describing genital–genital contact. Of the perpetrators, 67% were HIV seropositive, 42% were a parent, 25% were a relative, and 33% had another STI at the time of the child's evaluation.[40] Giardet et al. found that of 1750 children screened for HIV at the time of evaluation for sexual abuse, only one patient (0.06%) contracted HIV after the abusive contact.[41] In children who have been sexually abused, HIV testing and postexposure prophylaxis (PEP) should be considered in those with a concurrent STI or with mucosal injury resulting in bleeding, those in whom the perpetrator either is HIV positive or high risk for HIV seropositivity (e.g., concurrent infection with hepatitis B or C, high-risk behaviors (intravenous drug abuse, incarceration)), those living in an area with high regional disease prevalence in adults, those whose sexual abuse involved multiple perpetrators, and adolescents with a history of sexual assault by an unknown perpetrator.[42,43]

The rationale for HIV PEP is that there may be a window during which the viral load can be controlled by the immune system. The addition of antiretrovirals during this window would then end replication. HIV PEP ideally should be initiated within 72 hours of exposure, with 1 hour being optimal.[44] Within this time frame, PEP would be beneficial for children who have been sexually abused.[45] PEP should also only be given to patients without a suspicion of current HIV infection, when they and their guardians clearly understand the risks and benefits of PEP, and agree to comply with a follow-up program including serologic testing.[44] However, since many cases of child and adolescent sexual abuse present long after this 72-hour period, PEP usually is not indicated.

Even if a child or adolescent presents at a time when PEP may be beneficial, there is no consensus as to the number or type of antiretrovirals that should be used. Some authors recommend 3 drugs only with exposures most likely to transmit HIV infection and to use zidovudine-lamivudine as the base;[46] other authors suggest that it is important to consider local resistance patterns, and to consider a regimen containing zidovudine or stavudine.[47]

PART II Clinical Syndromes and Cardinal Features of Infectious Diseases: Approach to Diagnosis and Initial Management

SECTION H Gastrointestinal Tract Infections and Intoxications

PEP efficacy after sexual exposure has not been formally evaluated. Recent literature documenting seroconversion after PEP in adults suggests it may not be completely effective, perhaps due to ongoing exposure.[48]

Even when pediatric patients are provided PEP, it is often not administered in a timely fashion nor are the appropriate drugs provided.[49] Another difficulty is compliance and follow-up.[50-53] Even with outpatient support teams and provision of the full course, very few adolescents finish the entire course of PEP.[42,43] Uncertainty about exposure, low follow-up rates, intolerance of side effects, and psychiatric comorbidity also may limit adherence.[52,53]

SECTION H: Gastrointestinal Tract Infections and Intoxications

57 Approach to the Diagnosis and Management of Gastrointestinal Tract Infections

Larry K. Pickering and Andi L. Shane

Most infections of the gastrointestinal tract manifest as *diarrhea*, a clinical syndrome of diverse etiology associated with frequent loose or watery stools often accompanied by emesis, fever, and abdominal bloating or pain and occasionally by extraintestinal manifestations. Infectious diarrhea can have a bacterial, viral, or parasitic etiology (Table 57-1); most enteropathogens are associated with specific epidemiologic factors or clinical manifestations.[1] Establishing an etiologic diagnosis for a specific episode sometimes is difficult because of the wide array and complexity of potential agents. Therapy is directed at fluid and electrolyte replacement and maintenance, and dietary considerations in all cases, and at specific antimicrobial therapy in some cases.[2-4] Pathogen-specific chapters also should be consulted. Licensed vaccines for prevention of diarrhea are available in the United States only for *Salmonella* Typhi and rotavirus.[5-8]

EPIDEMIOLOGY

Enteropathogens are acquired through the fecal–oral route from person-to-person contact or via contaminated food or water. Enteric pathogens acquired via person-to-person transmission generally require a low-dose inoculum. People with certain host defects may be more susceptible to infection with various enteric pathogens and may suffer greater mortality or severe morbidity. Table 57-2 shows the inocula of various enteric pathogens necessary to cause diarrhea in adult volunteers. This table also lists outbreaks of diarrhea due to person-to-person transmission reported in childcare centers (see Chapter 3, Infections Associated with Group Childcare). Because volunteer studies are not performed in children, outbreaks of diarrhea in childcare centers can be used as a surrogate for organisms associated with low-inoculum disease in this population.[9]

There are 20 to 35 million episodes of diarrhea in the U.S. annually, resulting in 2.1 to 3.7 million healthcare visits, 220,000 hospitalizations (accounting for almost 1 million hospital days), and 300 to 400 deaths.[5,10,11] The majority of episodes of severe diarrhea worldwide in children <5 years of age are due to rotavirus,[12,13] but the number of children hospitalized in the U.S. with diarrhea due to rotavirus has decreased since licensure of two rotavirus vaccines.[14,15] In 2009, the World Health Organization recommended inclusion of rotavirus immunization in all national immunization programs.[16] This is expected to lower the global disease burden of rotavirus.[13,16,17] Children at higher risk of death due to diarrhea include young infants who were born prematurely, infants residing in crowded settings where dehydration may not be recognized, infants born to mothers who have had little or no prenatal care, and children with underlying immune deficiencies. In the U.S., the incidence of diarrhea in children <3 years of age is estimated to be 1 to 3 episodes per child per year, with higher rates in children attending group childcare.[9,18] Worldwide, diarrheal diseases are a leading cause of pediatric morbidity and

TABLE 57-1. Causative Agents of Gastroenteritis

Bacteria	Parasites	Viruses
Aeromonas species	Cryptosporidium parvum	Astroviruses
Bacillus cereus		Enteric adenoviruses
Campylobacter jejuni	Cyclospora cayetanensis	Noroviruses
Clostridium difficile		Rotaviruses
Clostridium perfringens	Entamoeba histolytica	
Escherichia coli	Giardia intestinalis	
Listeria monocytogenes	Cystoisospora belli	
Plesiomonas shigelloides	Microsporidia (including Enterocytozoon bieneusi and Encephalitozoon intestinalis)	
Salmonella species		
Shigella species		
Staphylococcus aureus		
Vibrio cholerae		
Vibrio parahaemolyticus		
Vibrio vulnificus		
Yersinia enterocolitica		

TABLE 57-2. Inoculum Required to Cause Diarrhea in Adult Volunteers and Association of Agents with Outbreaks of Diarrhea Due to Person-to-Person Transmission in Childcare Centers

Organism	Inoculum	Outbreaks Reported in Childcare Centers
Shigella	10^{1-2}	Yes
Escherichia coli O157:H7	Unknown	Yes
Cryptosporidium	132 oocysts	Yes
Rotavirus	Unknown	Yes
Enteric adenovirus	Unknown	Yes
Astrovirus	Unknown	Yes
Giardia intestinalis	10^{1-2} cysts	Yes
Entamoeba histolytica	10^{1-2} cysts	No
Campylobacter jejuni/coli	10^{2-6}	Rare
Salmonella	10^6	No
Vibrio cholerae	10^8	No
Escherichia coli	10^8	Yes[a]

[a]Limited to enteropathogenic and enterohemorrhagic strains.

mortality, with 1.5 billion episodes and 1.5 to 2.5 million deaths estimated annually among children <5 years of age.[13,16,17,19,20] Repeated early-childhood enteric infections result in long-term disability, including stunted growth.[21]

GENERAL CONSIDERATIONS AND ETIOLOGY BY EXPOSURE

Evidence-based recommendations, reviews, and meta-analyses that provide guidance for management of people with diarrhea are available and include information about the following: (1) administration of fluid and electrolyte solutions; (2) clinical and epidemiologic evaluation in immunocompetent and immuno-compromised hosts; (3) ordering of selective studies on stool specimens; (4) use and avoidance of antimotility agents; (5) insti-tution of selective antimicrobial therapy; (6) prevention of disease by immunization; and (7) prevention of travelers' diarrhea.[1–8,22–27] Considering diarrhea by exposure category assists in evaluation (Figure 57-1). Etiologies overlap among the various categories, but specific agents are responsible for most episodes in each category. (See pathogen-specific chapters.)

Foodborne and Waterborne Disease

Foodborne and waterborne diseases, including infections and intoxications, are acquired by consumption of contaminated food.[22–30] including unpasteurized milk[30,31] at a variety of locations including at home and in restaurants.[32] Major causes of foodborne disease are: a diverse group of chemical contaminants (heavy metals and organic compounds), bacterial toxins (enterotoxins of *Bacillus cereus*, *Staphylococcus aureus*, *Clostridium perfringens*, *Clostridium botulinum*, *Escherichia coli*), products accumulated in

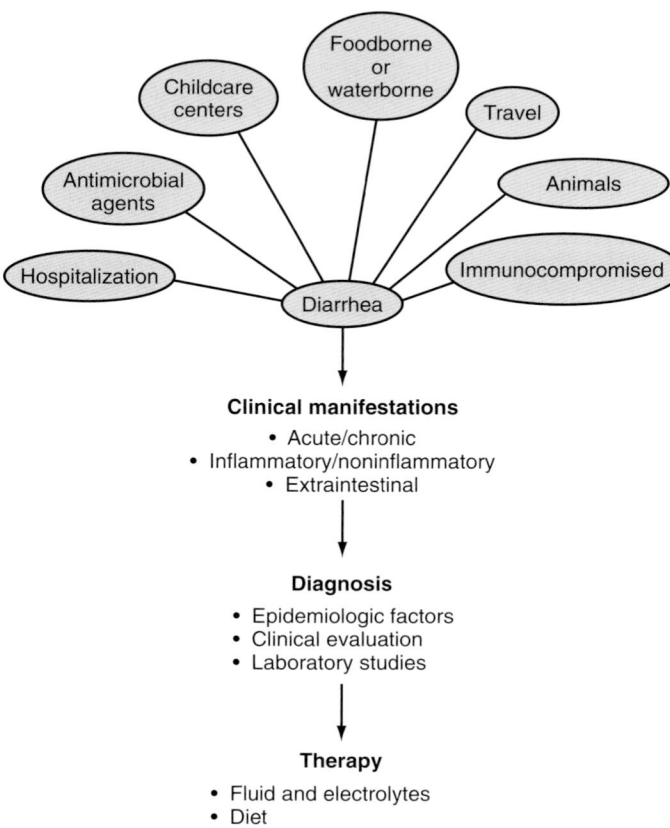

Figure 57-1. Steps in assessment of likely causative agents and management of diarrhea in children.

the food chain of fish and shellfish (scombroid, ciguatera, myco-toxins, neurotoxic and paralytic shellfish poisoning, pufferfish tetrodotoxin, and domoic acid), and disease due to other bacteria (*Salmonella*, *Shigella*, *E. coli*, *Brucella*, *Yersinia*, *Campylobacter*, *Vibrio*, and *Listeria*), viruses (norovirus, rotavirus, and hepatitis A virus), and parasites (*Giardia*, *Cyclospora*, *Cryptosporidium*, *Taenia*, *Toxo-plasma*, and *Trichinella*) (see Chapter 61, Foodborne and Water-borne Disease).[22,23] Viruses are the most common cause of foodborne illness.[22,23] Cryptosporidiosis and giardiasis are the most common gastrointestinal tract illness reported to the U.S. Waterborne Disease and Outbreak Surveillance System and are associated with water intended for drinking, water not intended for drinking, and water of unknown intent.[24]

An *outbreak of foodborne disease* is defined as the occurrence in ≥2 people of a similar illness, usually involving the gastro-intestinal tract, following consumption of a common food.[22,23] The incubation period, duration of the resultant illness, clinical manifestations, and population involved in the outbreak are helpful in establishing a diagnosis, but prompt and thorough laboratory evaluation of involved people and implicated food or water is critical for definitive diagnosis. Individual cases are diffi-cult to identify unless a distinct clinical syndrome exists, such as occurs with botulism.

Most people with "food poisoning" respond to supportive care, because most illnesses are self-limited. Exceptions include botu-lism (which causes constipation rather than diarrhea), paralytic shellfish poisoning, long-acting mushroom poisoning, Shiga toxin-producing *E. coli* infections, and typhoid fever, all of which can result in significant morbidity and mortality in previously healthy people. Prevention and control of these diseases, regardless of the specific cause, are based on avoidance of food contamina-tion, or destruction/denaturation and prevention of further spread or multiplication of contaminants. A suspected case of foodborne illness should be reported to public health officials as it could represent the sentinel case of a widespread outbreak. Detailed information on food safety issues and practices, including steps consumers can take to protect themselves can be obtained online at the following sites: (1) www.foodsafetyworkinggroup.gov, (2) www.foodsafety.gov, (3) www.fightbac.org, and (4) www.cdc.gov/foodborneoutbreaks/. Nationally notifiable enteric diseases can be found at www.cdc.gov/ncphi/disss/nndss/phs/infdis2011htm/.

Revised recommendations for responding to fecal accidents in swimming venues can be found at http://www.cdc.gov/healthyswimming/pdf/fecal_accident_response_recommendations_for_pool_staff.pdf.

Travelers' Diarrhea

Diarrhea is the most common illness encountered among inter-national travelers to resource-poor countries, affecting approxi-mately 40% of people in the first 2 weeks of travel.[25,26,33,34] Most studies of diarrhea in travelers have been performed in adults.[35] Diverse enteric pathogens are associated with travelers' diarrhea. Bacteria are implicated most frequently, especially enterotoxigenic *E. coli*, *Campylobacter jejuni*, *Salmonella* species, and *Shigella* species; parasites account for a smaller percentage of cases. In 10% to 50% of episodes in older studies, no pathogen was identified. With the widespread availability of specific diagnostic assays, noroviruses now are recognized as an important cause of travelers' diarrhea.[36,37]

Risk factors for travelers' diarrhea are young age, season, eating in restaurants, and short duration of stay (travel) in a developing country.[38–40] Etiologic diagnosis is complex in developing coun-tries because of the diversity of potential pathogens, requirements for specialized testing for some agents, and lack of local laboratory facilities. Clinical illness is variable, reflecting the diversity of causative agents.[26,27,33,34,41] Because most diarrheal episodes are bacterial in origin, travelers to developing countries should be given area-specific advice on how to diagnose and treat a diarrheal illness empirically with an antimicrobial agent if they cannot obtain medical care. Most experts recommend that all people traveling from a low-risk to such high-risk settings should carry one of three antibiotics for self-treatment: ciprofloxacin (or

PART II Clinical Syndromes and Cardinal Features of Infectious Diseases: Approach to Diagnosis and Initial Management

SECTION H Gastrointestinal Tract Infections and Intoxications

levofloxicin), rifaximin, or azithromycin (which is preferred for children).[26] Use of antimicrobial agents as a preventive measure is not recommended routinely,[42] although it may be beneficial in high-risk people.

Travelers should be informed about: (1) the ubiquitous exposure to pathogens during travel; (2) safe foods and beverages and the often unsafe items, which may depend on travel destination; (3) the need to follow appropriate rules of hygiene, including proper preparation of food, and use of hand hygiene; and (4) the importance of fluid replacement if diarrhea occurs. Children who travel may have a higher risk of disease and a greater severity of diarrhea if disease occurs (see Chapter 9, Protection of Travelers).

Antimicrobial-Associated Diarrhea

Diarrhea occurs commonly in people receiving antimicrobial agents. Antimicrobial-associated diarrhea can result from changes in small-bowel peristalsis or from alterations in the intestinal microflora, including overgrowth by *Clostridium difficile*. In one prospective study, 29% of 76 children who received amoxicillin-clavulanate for therapy of otitis media experienced diarrhea, which led to discontinuation of therapy in 5 children (23%).[43] In 10 (13%) of the 76 children, *C. difficile* toxins were identified in post- but not pre-therapy stools. A *C. difficile* strain with variations in toxin genes, which has become more resistant to fluoroquinolones, has emerged as a cause of outbreaks of *C. difficile*-associated diarrhea (CDAD).[44-47]

Many reports have shown increases in incidence of CDAD, changes in clinical presentation and epidemiology, and risk factors.[47] Interpretation of studies can be difficult because 25% to 65% of infants <1 year of age without diarrhea can be colonized with toxin-producing *C. difficile*[48,49] with no correlation with acute community- or healthcare-associated diarrhea.[50] Colonization rates of toxigenic *C. difficile* are 0 to 10% in older children; diagnosis of antimicrobial-associated *C. difficile* diarrhea and colitis can be established more easily in this population. There is an increasing trend of *C. difficile*-related hospitalizations in children,[51-53] but rates of colectomy and in-hospital death have not increased in affected children as they have among adults.[53] Increased risk of *C. difficile* disease occurs in children with medical conditions including inflammatory bowel disease and immunosuppression, or conditions requiring antibiotic administration or administration of gastric-protective agents that alter intestinal flora. The Society for Healthcare Epidemiology of America and the Infectious Diseases Society of America (IDSA) has published clinical practice guidelines for *C. difficile* infection in adults.[54]

Diarrhea in Immunosuppressed Children

Diarrhea in children, adolescents, and adults with primary or secondary immune deficiencies is caused by enteropathogens of healthy hosts as well as enteropathogens unique to this population.[55-61] In 1995, the U.S. Public Health Service and the IDSA developed guidelines for preventing opportunistic infections among children, adolescents, and adults infected with human immunodeficiency virus (HIV). Guidelines were revised in 1997, 1999, and 2002.[56] The Centers for Disease Control and Prevention (CDC), National Institutes of Health, and IDSA published new guidelines including treatment recommendations for adults and children in 2004,[61] which were updated in 2009.[57,59] Gastrointestinal tract disease in children with acquired immunodeficiency syndrome (AIDS) can be due to enteric infection, malignancy, chronic disease, and to invasion by HIV.[57] Clinical manifestations and ease of eradication depend on location of involvement in the gastrointestinal tract, immune status of the host, severity of intestinal tract injury, and availability and effectiveness of therapy. Organisms and diseases of the gastrointestinal tract that fulfill the surveillance case definition of the CDC for AIDS have been published.[58] Prior to use of highly active antiretroviral therapy, both acute and persistent episodes of diarrhea and death from these episodes were frequent among HIV-infected infants.[62] The overall incidence of opportunistic infections (including

cryptosporidiosis) declined from 14.4 cases per 100 patient years before the introduction of highly active antiretroviral therapy (HAART) to 1.1 cases per 100 patient years post HAART.[63] Guidelines have been published for prevention of opportunistic infections, including gastrointestinal tract infections, in HIV-infected people and among recipients of hematopoietic stem cell transplantation.[60]

Diarrhea in Out-of-Home Childcare Settings

The greater use of out-of-home childcare has had a significant impact on the epidemiology of diarrheal disease in the U.S. (see Chapter 3, Infections Associated with Group Childcare).[9,18] After respiratory tract illness, diarrhea is the most common disease among children in childcare facilities, occurring at a rate of approximately 3 cases per year among children <3 years of age.[9] Acute infectious diarrhea in childcare settings can be due to bacterial, viral, and parasitic enteropathogens. Rotavirus, norovirus, enteric adenoviruses, astroviruses, *Shigella*, *Cryptosporidium*, *E. coli* O157:H7, and *Giardia intestinalis* are the most frequently identified organisms associated with outbreaks of diarrhea in childcare centers. The major route of transmission is person-to-person. Risk factors include gathering of children (specifically children <3 years of age), new enrollment in a center, centers that house large numbers of children, centers without an exclusion policy for diarrheal disease, and inadequate hand hygiene.[9,18] The single most important procedure for minimizing fecal or oral transmission of enteric pathogens is frequent hand hygiene combined with education, training, and monitoring of staff regarding infection control procedures.[64]

Healthcare-Associated Diarrhea

Diarrhea can develop in children as a result of infections acquired before or during healthcare/hospitalization encounters. Healthcare-associated infections (HAIs) are caused by a wide variety of common and unusual bacteria, fungi, and viruses. As defined by the CDC, healthcare-associated gastroenteritis must meet ≥1 of 2 criteria: (1) acute onset of diarrhea (liquid stools for >12 hours) with or without vomiting or fever (>38°C) and no likely noninfectious cause (e.g., diagnostic procedure, therapeutic regimen other than antimicrobial agents, acute exacerbation of a chronic condition, or psychologic stress); (2) ≥2 signs or symptoms (nausea, vomiting, abdominal pain, fever (>38°C), or headache) with no other recognized cause *plus* ≥1 of the following confirmations of enteric pathogen by: culture of stool or rectal swab; detection by routine or electron microscopy; antigen or antibody assay or molecular testing on blood or feces; cytopathic changes in tissue culture (toxin assay); or diagnostic single pathogen-specific antibody titer (IgM) or 4-fold increase in paired sera (IgG).[65,66]

Reports by the CDC as part of the National Nosocomial Infections Surveillance (NNIS) system from 1985 to 1991 demonstrated that nosocomial diarrhea occurred in general pediatric care units at a rate of 11 cases per 10,000 discharges and in newborn nurseries at a rate of 3 cases per 10,000 discharges. Rate of diarrhea is higher in neonatal intensive care units (NICUs), averaging 20 per 10,000 discharges, and accounting for 8% of all NICU-associated infections.[67] Viral agents are the most common pediatric nosocomial enteropathogens, with rotavirus and norovirus identified most frequently.[36,68] Hospitalization following rotavirus infection has decreased since licensure and use of rotavirus vaccine,[5,6,15] but HAIs due to *C. difficile* appear to be increasing.[51-53] Guidelines for prevention of HAIs can be found at www.cdc.gov/hai/.

Several important factors affect transmission of enteric organisms in hospitals: (1) patient-to-patient transmission via hands of hospital personnel, generally after contact with a child who has diarrhea; (2) asymptomatic carriers; (3) hospital personnel with gastroenteritis; (4) contaminated food, medications, or medical instruments; (5) hospital crowding; and 6) improper cleaning procedures. Host risk factors are immunocompromised states, prolonged hospitalization, young age, and antibiotic use. Prevention of nosocomial gastrointestinal tract infection is best accomplished by surveillance of methods to improve hospital infection prevention and control procedures. Contact isolation is recommended for children with diarrhea to prevent transmission between children and among staff and children.[66,69] Guidelines for isolation precautions in healthcare settings are available (www.cdc.gov/hicpac/pdf/isolation/Isolation2007.pdf).

PATHOGENESIS

The gastrointestinal tract is barraged constantly by foreign material, including bacteria, viruses, parasites, and toxins. Numerous protective host factors include gastric acidity, intestinal motility, enteric microflora, glycoconjugates, and specific immune components (cells and humoral compounds). Host age, personal hygiene, intestinal receptors, past exposures, and food intake (including human milk) influence these protective factors and are major determinants of colonization and disease.

The effect of microbial factors is influenced by the size of the inoculum and specific virulence traits of the enteropathogen. *E. coli*, for example, can cause gastrointestinal tract disease depending on the presence of transmissible plasmids or phages that encode for virulence traits, producing secretory heat-stable or heat-labile enterotoxins and cytotoxins, promoting invasiveness, or aggregability.[70–77] In addition, some bacteria (such as *C. botulinum*, *S. aureus*, and *B. cereus*) produce neurotoxins while others have variations in toxin genes that enhance virulence.[44,45] Generally, all bacteria that cause gastrointestinal tract disease possess one or more of these virulence traits.[4,70]

Enteric viruses can cause diarrhea through selective destruction of absorptive cells (villus tip cells) in the mucosa, leaving secretory cells (crypt cells) intact. Infections with rotavirus, noroviruses, astroviruses, and enteric adenoviruses alter absorptive fluid balance and also reduce brush-border digestive enzymes;[5,36,77] *E. coli* pathotypes and many parasitic infections induce similar changes.[36,70,71,76–80]

CLINICAL MANIFESTATIONS

Clinical manifestations consist of primary gastrointestinal tract and systemic manifestations as well as intestinal or extraintestinal complications. Clinical manifestations localized to the gastrointestinal tract can be categorized for diagnostic and therapeutic considerations into several groups:

- Watery diarrhea (enteric viruses, enterotoxin-producing bacteria, and protozoa that infect the small intestine)
- Purging, watery diarrhea (*Vibrio cholerae* and enterotoxigenic *E. coli*)
- Dysentery with scant stools that contain blood and mucus (pathogens that invade the large intestine)
- Persistent diarrhea that lasts for 14 days or longer
- Vomiting with minimal or no diarrhea (chemical contaminants and toxins associated with foodborne and waterborne outbreaks and viral enteropathogens)

Extraintestinal manifestations result from infection and immune-mediated mechanisms. Extraintestinal infections related to bacterial enteric pathogens can include local spread, e.g., vulvovaginitis and urinary tract infection. Remote spread can result in endocarditis, arteritis, osteomyelitis, arthritis, meningitis, pneumonia, hepatitis, peritonitis, chorioamnionitis, soft-tissue infection, keratoconjunctivitis, and septic thrombophlebitis.[81–84] Immune-mediated extraintestinal manifestations of enteric pathogens are shown in Table 57-3. Signs and symptoms usually occur after diarrhea has resolved. In a population-based cohort study, an increased risk of inflammatory bowel disease was demonstrated in people with an episode of *Salmonella* or *Campylobacter* gastroenteritis.[84]

DIAGNOSIS

Laboratory studies can be performed to identify the cause of diarrhea, to guide therapy, and for surveillance, but often are not

TABLE 57-3. Immune-Mediated Extraintestinal Manifestations of Enteric Pathogens

Manifestation	Related Enteric Pathogen(s)
Erythema nodosum	*Yersinia*, *Campylobacter*, *Salmonella*
Glomerulonephritis	*Shigella*, *Campylobacter*, *Yersinia*
Guillain–Barré syndrome	*Campylobacter*
Hemolytic anemia	*Campylobacter*, *Yersinia*
Hemolytic uremic syndrome	Shiga-toxin producing *Escherichia coli*
Immunoglobulin A nephropathy	*Campylobacter*
Reactive arthritis	*Salmonella*, *Shigella*, *Yersinia*, *Campylobacter*, *Cryptosporidium*
Reiter syndrome	*Shigella*, *Salmonella*, *Campylobacter*, *Yersinia*

required because most episodes of diarrhea are self-limited. The approach to a child with acute diarrhea aims to: (1) assess the degree of dehydration and provide fluid and electrolyte replacement; (2) determine if the episode is part of an outbreak; (3) prevent spread; and (4) maintain nutrition in select episodes, determine the etiologic agent and provide specific therapy if indicated. In some children, additional laboratory tests on stool specimens may be indicated. Additional evaluation includes observation of stool, microscopy, rapid diagnostic tests, culture, and use of specialized laboratory tests.

History

The following recent history should be obtained to narrow etiologic possibilities: childcare center attendance; travel to a diarrhea-endemic area; hospitalization; visitation to a farm or petting zoo, or contact with reptiles or other animals;[85,86] use of antimicrobial agents; exposure to contacts with similar symptoms; intake of seafood, unwashed vegetables, unpasteurized milk, contaminated water, or uncooked meats; and status of the immune system (see Figure 57-1). Information also should be sought regarding how and when the illness began; duration and severity of diarrhea; stool frequency and consistency; presence of mucus and blood; and associated signs and symptoms, such as fever, vomiting, abdominal pain, headache, and seizures.

The occurrence of fever suggests an inflammatory process, usually involving the large intestine (see Chapter 59, Inflammatory Enteritis, and Chapter 60, Necrotizing Enterocolitis), but fever also can result from dehydration and systemic spread of an organism. Nausea and emesis are nonspecific symptoms, although vomiting suggests upper intestinal tract infection, as occurs with infection due to enteric viruses, enterotoxin-producing bacteria, *Giardia*, *Strongyloides*, and other protozoa. As a general rule, in people with inflammatory diarrhea, fever is common, abdominal pain is more severe, and tenesmus can occur in the lower abdomen and rectum. In noninflammatory diarrhea, emesis is common; fever usually is absent or low-grade; pain is crampy, periumbilical, and not severe; and diarrhea is watery, indicating upper intestinal tract involvement (see Chapter 58, Viral Gastroenteritis). History of underlying primary or secondary immunodeficiency or chronic disease leads to consideration of special pathogens. *Persistent diarrhea*, defined as diarrhea lasting more than 14 days, occurs as a result of multiple consecutive infections, the post-gastroenteritis syndrome, or persistent infection.

Examination of Stool

Stool should be examined for mucus, blood, and leukocytes, the presence of which indicates colitis. Fecal leukocytes are produced in response to bacteria that invade the colonic mucosa diffusely. A positive fecal leukocyte examination or stool lactoferrin assay indicates presence of an invasive or cytotoxin-producing organism such as *Shigella*, *Salmonella*, *Campylobacter jejuni/coli*, invasive *E.*

coli, Shiga toxin-producing E. coli (STEC), C. difficile, Yersinia enterocolitica, Vibrio parahaemolyticus, Balantidium coli, Trichuris trichiura and, possibly, Aeromonas hydrophila or Plesiomonas shigelloides.[87] Not all patients with colitis have leukocytes in stool or a positive lactoferrin assay result; ingestion of human milk can interfere with the lactoferrin assay.

Not all children with acute diarrhea require performance of a stool culture;[1,88,89] however, when indicated specimen should be obtained as early in the course of disease as possible. Culture should be performed when the diagnosis of hemolytic uremic syndrome is suspected, stools contain blood or fecal leukocytes, during outbreaks, in people who are immunosuppressed,[1,4,57,73] and for public health surveillance. All stools submitted for routine testing from patients with acute community-acquired diarrhea should be cultured for E. coli O157:H7 and assayed for Shiga toxin to identify non-O157 STEC.[73] Fecal specimens that cannot be inoculated immediately can be transported to the laboratory in a non-nutrient-holding medium such as Cary–Blair transport medium to prevent drying or overgrowth of specific organisms.

Identification of Y. enterocolitica, diarrhea-causing E. coli organisms, Vibrio cholerae, V. parahaemolyticus, Aeromonas spp., C. difficile, and Campylobacter spp. require modified laboratory procedures and often are overlooked in routine stool cultures. Laboratory personnel should be notified when one of these organisms is suspected. For further characterization of E. coli, serotype and toxin assays are available in reference and research laboratories.

Proctosigmoidoscopy may be helpful in establishing a diagnosis in patients in whom symptoms of colitis are severe or the etiology of an inflammatory enteritis syndrome remains obscure after initial laboratory evaluation. Non-culture diagnostics, such as enzyme immunoassay and DNA probes, are becoming increasingly available and are highly sensitive for bacterial, viral, and parasitic enteropathogens.[36,73,79,80]

TREATMENT

All patients with diarrhea require some level of fluid and electrolyte therapy and attention to diet, a few need other nonspecific support, and some may benefit from specific antimicrobial therapy.

Fluid and Electrolyte Therapy

Oral rehydration therapy (ORT) is the preferred treatment for fluid and electrolyte losses due to diarrhea in children with mild to moderate dehydration.[2,90] Surveys show that healthcare providers do not always follow such recommended procedures.[91] Stool losses of water, sodium, potassium, chloride, and base must be restored in children with dehydration to ensure effective rehydration.[92,93] In the mid-1960s, discovery of coupled transport of sodium and glucose (or other small organic molecules) provided scientific justification for oral rehydration as an alternative to intravenous therapy.[94] In initial studies, conducted in patients with cholera in Bangladesh and India in the late 1960s, oral glucose-electrolyte solutions compared favorably with standard intravenous therapy.[95,96] Solutions used were similar to the oral rehydration salt solution recommended by the World Health Organization (WHO) and United Nations Children's (Emergency) Fund (UNICEF), which has been used successfully throughout the world for more than 30 years.

Since the early 1980s, a series of studies from developed countries have proved the effectiveness of ORT compared with intravenous therapy in children with diarrhea from causes other than cholera,[97–101] showing a reduction in subsequent unscheduled follow-up visits.[97] These studies evaluated glucose-electrolyte ORT solutions with sodium concentrations ranging from 50 to 90 mmol/L compared with rapidly administered intravenous therapy. ORT solutions were successful in rehydration for >90% of dehydrated children and had complication rates lower than rates for intravenous therapy.[102] Additional benefits of ORT are lower expense, avoiding hospitalization, and ease of

TABLE 57-4. Composition of Representative Glucose-Electrolyte Solutions

Solutions	CHO[a] (g/L)	Na	CHO:Na	K	Base	Osmolality (mosm/L)
CeraLyte-50	40	50	3.1	20	30	220
Pedialyte	25	45	3.1	20	30	250
Enfalyte	30	50	1.4	25	30	200
Rehydralyte	25	75	1.9	20	30	310
WHO (1975)	20	90	1.2	20	30	310
WHO (2002)	13.5	75	1.2	20	30	245

CHO, carbohydrate; WHO, World Health Organization.

[a]All commercial oral rehydration salts solutions except Ceralyte contain glucose. Ceralyte contains a complex mixture of rice CHOs and proteins.

administration in many settings.[99] The frequency and volume of stools, duration of diarrhea, and rate of weight gain are similar with the two therapies.[97–101] In 2002 the WHO and the UNICEF recommended a reduced-osmolarity formulation of ORT for treatment of diarrhea[2,103] to avoid risk of hyponatremia.

Most oral solutions available in the U.S. (Table 57-4) have sodium concentrations ranging from 45 to 50 mmol/L, which is at or just below the lower concentration of the solutions studied. Although these products are best suited for use as maintenance solutions, they can be used to rehydrate otherwise healthy children who are mildly or moderately dehydrated.[98,104,105] Glucose-electrolyte solutions such as these, which are formulated on physiologic principles, must be distinguished from other popular but nonphysiologic liquids that have been used inappropriately to treat children with diarrhea, including cola, apple juice, sports beverages, and chicken broth. These beverages have inappropriately low electrolyte concentrations and are hypertonic because of their carbohydrate content.[106]

Dietary Intake

Early feeding of age-appropriate foods to children with diarrhea after rehydration should be an integral component of management. When used with glucose-electrolyte ORT, early feeding can reduce stool output as much as can cereal-based ORT.[104,107] Studies of early-feeding regimens including human milk,[108–111] dilute or full-strength animal milk or animal milk formulas,[109,110] dilute or full-strength lactose-free formulas,[97,108,112] and staple-food diets with milk[111,113–115] have shown that unrestricted diets do not worsen the course of symptoms of mild diarrhea[110,111] and can decrease stool output[114,115] compared with rehydration therapy alone. Studies on early refeeding from developed countries[109,115–117] indicate reduction in duration of diarrhea by 0.43 days (95% confidence interval, −0.74 to −0.12).[2] Although these beneficial effects are modest, the added benefit of improved nutrition with early feeding has major importance.[93,113]

One meta-analysis showed that >80% of children with acute diarrhea can safely tolerate full-strength nonhuman milk.[113] Although reduction in intestinal brush-border lactase levels often is associated with diarrhea,[118] most infants with decreased lactase levels do not have clinical signs or symptoms of malabsorption.[118] Infants fed human milk can be nursed safely during an episode of diarrhea.[108] If children are monitored to identify the few who demonstrate signs of malabsorption, a regular age-appropriate diet, including full-strength milk, can be used safely.

During the re-feeding period, certain foods, including complex carbohydrates (rice, wheat, potatoes, bread, and cereals), lean meats, yogurt, fruits, and vegetables, are better tolerated than other foods.[102,107,113,114] Fatty foods and foods high in simple sugars (including juices and soft drinks) should be avoided.[2]

TABLE 57-5. Medications Used to Relieve Symptoms in Patients with Acute Diarrhea

Mechanism	Generic Name	Trade Name
Alteration of intestinal motility	Loperamide	Imodium
		Imodium A-D
		Maalox Antidiarrheal
		Pepto Diarrhea Control
	Difenoxin and atropine	Motofen[a]
	Diphenoxylate and atropine	Lomotil[a]
	Tincture of opium	Paregoric[a]
Alteration of secretion	Bismuth subsalicylate	Pepto-Bismol
		Kaopectate
Adsorption of toxins and water	Attapulgite	Diasorb
		Donnagel Rheaban
Alteration of intestinal microflora	*Lactobacillus*	Pro-Bionate
		Superdophilus

[a]Requires prescription.

Nonspecific Therapy

A variety of pharmacologic agents have been used as nonspecific therapy for people with acute infectious diarrhea (Table 57-5). These compounds can be classified according to the following mechanisms of action: (1) alteration of intestinal motility; (2) alteration of secretion; (3) adsorption of toxins or fluid; and (4) alteration of intestinal microflora. Many of these compounds, especially agents that alter motility, have systemic toxic effects that are augmented in infants and children or in people with diarrheal disease. Most are not approved for children <2 or 3 years of age. Few published data are available to support use of most antidiarrheal agents to treat acute diarrhea, especially in children.[2,119,120] Use of probiotics has been shown to be modestly effective in randomized clinical trials for (1) treating acute viral gastroenteritis in healthy children and (2) preventing antibiotic-associated diarrhea in healthy children.[121] Human milk is a source of prebiotic compounds and probiotic organisms. Breastfeeding during episodes of diarrhea may result in delivery of human-milk-containing prebiotics and probiotics, resulting in anti-inflammatory effects on intestinal epithelia. Continued evaluation of specific probiotic products, in well-designed clinical trials involving infants and children, will be needed to develop definitive recommendations for applications of prebiotics and probiotics.[122-124]

Antimicrobial Therapy

Antimicrobial agents are of no benefit and may have deleterious effects in children infected with enteric viruses, including rotavirus, enteric adenovirus, astrovirus, and norovirus. Patients with diarrhea associated with certain bacterial and protozoal agents may benefit from therapy. Limited benefit can be achieved with therapy of people infected with *Aeromonas* species (trimethoprim-sulfamethoxazole), *Blastocystis hominis* (metronidazole or iodoquinol), *Campylobacter jejuni* (erythromycin or azithromycin, if given early in the course of therapy), *Cryptosporidium* (nitazoxanide), and intestinal microsporidia (albendazole).[3] Antimicrobial therapy of immunocompetent children with intestinal salmonellosis and *Y. enterocolitica* is given for extraintestinal infection but is of no known gastrointestinal benefit, except possibly for infants <3 months of age. A meta-analysis of antibiotic therapy of children with *E. coli* O157:H7 did not show a higher risk of hemolytic uremic syndrome associated with antibiotic administration,[125] but therapy of children with STEC infection is not recommended.

PREVENTION

The most important aspect in prevention and control of diarrheal disease is hygiene, both public and personal. Public issues are clean water, clean food, and appropriate sanitation facilities. Despite the high-quality water and food supplies available in the U.S., outbreaks of foodborne and waterborne disease continue to occur,[22-24] as illustrated by the large outbreak of cryptosporidiosis in 1993 involving >400,000 people in Milwaukee due to contamination of the public water supply.[126] Personal measures include careful personal hygiene, especially hand hygiene,[64] and limited use of antacids, antimotility drugs, and antimicrobial agents. Appropriate diaper-changing facilities and techniques should be available and implemented in childcare centers.[18] Written infection control policies must be in place and adhered to in all healthcare facilities, and childcare facilities. Guidelines for preventing opportunistic infections in children with HIV and among hematopoietic stem cell transplant recipients are published,[57,60] as are guidelines to prevent disease associated with pets in the home and exposure to animals in public settings.[85,86]

Currently, vaccines against *Salmonella* Typhi[8] and rotavirus[5,6] are the only vaccines against enteric disease commercially available in the U.S. Hepatitis A vaccines are part of the recommended childhood and adolescent immunization schedule.[127] There are no effective vaccines against enteric parasitic infections. New and improved vaccines against enteric pathogens are under study and are directed against the organisms themselves, adherence factors, cytotoxins, or enterotoxins.[128]

Other nonspecific agents that may interfere with microbial adherence or with the virulence mechanisms of toxins are being developed and evaluated, as are compounds that serve as competitors for binding of organisms or toxins to receptors in the intestine. Applications of glycoconjugates and probiotics in disease prevention are under investigation.[121,129,130]

Breastfeeding provides young infants with significant protection against morbidity and mortality due to diarrheal disease.[130] Breastfeeding protects against diarrhea in part through decreased exposure of breastfed infants to organisms present on or in contaminated bottles, food, or water. In addition, immunologic components in human milk protect infants against disease after exposure to an infectious agent.

58 Viral Gastroenteritis

Ben A. Lopman and Joseph S. Bresee

Viruses are the most common cause of gastroenteritis – a syndrome of acute vomiting and diarrhea associated with inflammation of the stomach and large and small intestines. Viral gastroenteritis remains a leading cause of pediatric morbidity and mortality worldwide. With the discovery of both norovirus[1] and rotavirus[2] in the early 1970s, and subsequent improved diagnostic testing,[3] the importance of viruses as causes of diarrheal disease has been increasingly appreciated. The most important agents

TABLE 58-1. Relative Distribution of Viral Pathogens as Causes of Acute Gastroenteritis among Children under the Age of 5 Years

Agent	Hospitalizations[a] (%)	Community Disease[a] (%)
Rotaviruses	25–50	5–40
Noroviruses	5–30	10–25
Sapoviruses	<5	5–10
Astroviruses	5–10	5–10
Adenoviruses 40/41	5–12	5–10

[a](% of all viruses detected). Other viruses often found in stool samples account for the remainder, including coronaviruses, toroviruses, picornaviruses, enteroviruses, and others.

in children include rotaviruses, human caliciviruses (noroviruses and sapoviruses), adenovirus 40/41, and astroviruses (Table 58-1). Many other viruses (parvovirus B19, enteroviruses, coronaviruses, toroviruses, picobirnaviruses, and bocaviruses) occasionally have been associated with acute vomiting and diarrhea, but none is likely to be a common cause. Viral gastroenteritides share similar clinical presentations, modes of transmission, and treatment; many causes remain clinically undiagnosed.

ETIOLOGIC AGENTS

A small group of viruses account for most cases of acute gastroenteritis among children. These include rotaviruses, caliciviruses, astroviruses, and adenoviruses.

Rotaviruses. Rotaviruses (family Reoviridae) are 100-nm, triple-layered particles comprised of an outer capsid, inner capsid, and core.[4] The double-stranded RNA genome is composed of 11 segments which code for 6 structural proteins (VP1 to VP4, VP6, and VP7) and 6 nonstructural proteins (NSP1 to NSP6). The outer capsid is composed of 2 proteins, VP7 (G protein, for glycoprotein) and VP4 (P protein, for protease-cleaved protein). These proteins are the principal antigens to which neutralizing antibodies are directed and are the proteins that account for the classification scheme for rotavirus strains. The middle layer is made up of the VP6 protein, which is the most abundant protein in the virus and is the protein to which common immune diagnostics are directed. Rotaviruses commonly are classified according to group and serotype. Six groups of rotavirus have been described (A to F), and are based on differences in the VP6 protein. Only viruses in groups A, B, and C are known to cause disease in humans, with group A viruses being the principal cause of human disease. Groups B and C rotaviruses also cause gastroenteritis but are uncommon, and may disproportionately affect adults[5–8] (see Chapter 216, Rotaviruses). Group A rotaviruses are further classified by serotype based on their VP7 (G) and VP4 (P) proteins. While more than 10 P types and G types have each been described,[9] 5 G types (G1 to G4 and G9) and 3 P types (P[4], P[6], and P[8]) predominate globally.[9] Over 40 P–G combinations have been detected, but only 5 combinations of these common types generally account for more than 90% of circulating viruses: P[8]G1, P[4]G2, P[8]G3, P[8]G4, and P[8]G9. P[8]G1 strains are the dominant strain worldwide, accounting for 50% to 90% of seasonal strains characterized in most large reviews.[10–12] Less common strains, such as G8, G12, and G5 strains, may be of public health importance and may even predominate in any given season.[13,14]

Caliciviruses. Caliciviruses are nonenveloped, 27- to 40-nm single-stranded RNA viruses in the family Caliciviridae.[15] Human caliciviruses are divided into two genera, norovirus and sapovirus. Noroviruses include a number of genetically related viruses, of which Norwalk virus is the prototype. Noroviruses – discovered in 1972[16] – previously have been referred to by a variety of names, including "small round-structured viruses" and "Norwalk-like viruses." Likewise, sapoviruses have been referred to as "classic caliciviruses" and "Sapporo-like viruses" in reference to location of detection of the prototype strain in Japan. When viewed by

electron microscopy, sapoviruses have characteristic cup-shaped depressions over the surface of the virion (Greek, calyx = cup), but the noroviruses, have rough, nondistinct borders and lack the calyx appearance (Figure 58-1). Noroviruses are further divided into five genogroups (I to V), three of which (I, II, and, rarely, IV) cause human disease. At least 8 and 19 genotypes, respectively, have been identified for genogroups I and II.[17,18] Genogroup II genotype 4 (GGII.4) viruses have been the most common cause of outbreaks in recent years; the emergence of new GGII.4 strains has been associated with a global increase in gastroenteritis outbreaks.[19,20]

Astroviruses. Astroviruses, first discovered in 1975,[21,22] are non-enveloped, single-stranded RNA viruses in the family Astroviridae. Astroviruses are 28 nm in diameter with a smooth edge, and may have a characteristic 5- or 6-pointed star-like appearance in the center (Greek, astron = star). Eight distinct serotypes of human astroviruses (HastV 1 to 8) have been described. Serotype 1 is detected most commonly, but more than one serotype usually circulates in communities during each season. Non-serotype 1 viruses can predominate in a season, and greater serotype diversity may be found in developing countries.[23,24]

Adenoviruses. Adenoviruses are 70- to 80-nm, nonenveloped, double-stranded DNA viruses in the family Adenoviridae.[25] While six subgenus of adenoviruses, containing at least 51 different serotypes, can cause human infection, subgenus F (serotypes 40 and 41) adenoviruses cause gastroenteritis.[26] Certain serotypes of the subgenus A and C also have been detected in acute diarrhea, but there role is likely to be minor.[27–29]

Other viruses. Other viruses are associated with gastroenteritis, including human coronaviruses and toroviruses within the virus family Coronaviridae, and picobirnavirus. Human coronaviruses and toroviruses have been detected in studies in several countries, but their association with gastroenteritis remains unclear.[30] Reports of the clinical characteristics of patients infected with the severe acute respiratory syndrome-coronavirus have described diarrhea in approximately one-fourth of cases.[31] Human bocavirus – classified in the Parvoviridae family – has been detected in diarrheal stools in children, more frequently than in control samples,[32,33] although their role in gastroenteritis has not been evaluated fully. Pestiviruses, some picornaviruses, and parvo-like viruses, reoviruses, enteroviruses, and other unclassified small round viruses have been identified in fecal specimens and implicated in sporadic cases and single outbreaks of gastroenteritis. Data are inconclusive regarding their pathogenicity.

EPIDEMIOLOGY

Two distinct epidemiologic patterns are associated with viral gastroenteritis – endemic and epidemic disease. Rotavirus, astrovirus, enteric adenovirus, and sapovirus infections occur primarily as endemic disease, while norovirus infections commonly occur both as endemic illnesses and outbreaks (Table 58-1). All common viral gastroenteritis viruses have no geographic limits. Rotavirus, astrovirus, and sapovirus infections occur in wintertime seasonal peaks in temperate countries,[24,34–37] while they often circulate year-round in tropical settings, with peaks during dry seasons.[38,39] Seasonality of adenoviruses is less distinct.[40] Noroviruses circulate year-round in most areas, but there is a clear wintertime seasonality to outbreaks in temperate locations, particularly in healthcare settings.[41,42] Rotaviruses historically had a distinct seasonal "traveling wave" of occurrence in the United States, first in the southwest, with later peaks in the northeast.[43] However, this pattern has become less evident in recent years, possibly due to demographic changes,[44] as well as the impact of vaccination. Since introduction of routine vaccination in the U.S., the rotavirus season has diminished substantially in magnitude, and also has been delayed by 2 to 4 months in some years.[45,46] In the U.S., summertime rotavirus infections are rare (with most positive test results falsely positive), but can occur among immunocompromised children.[47]

The highest rates of rotavirus infection occur in the first 2 years of life, with most hospitalizations and severe dehydrating disease

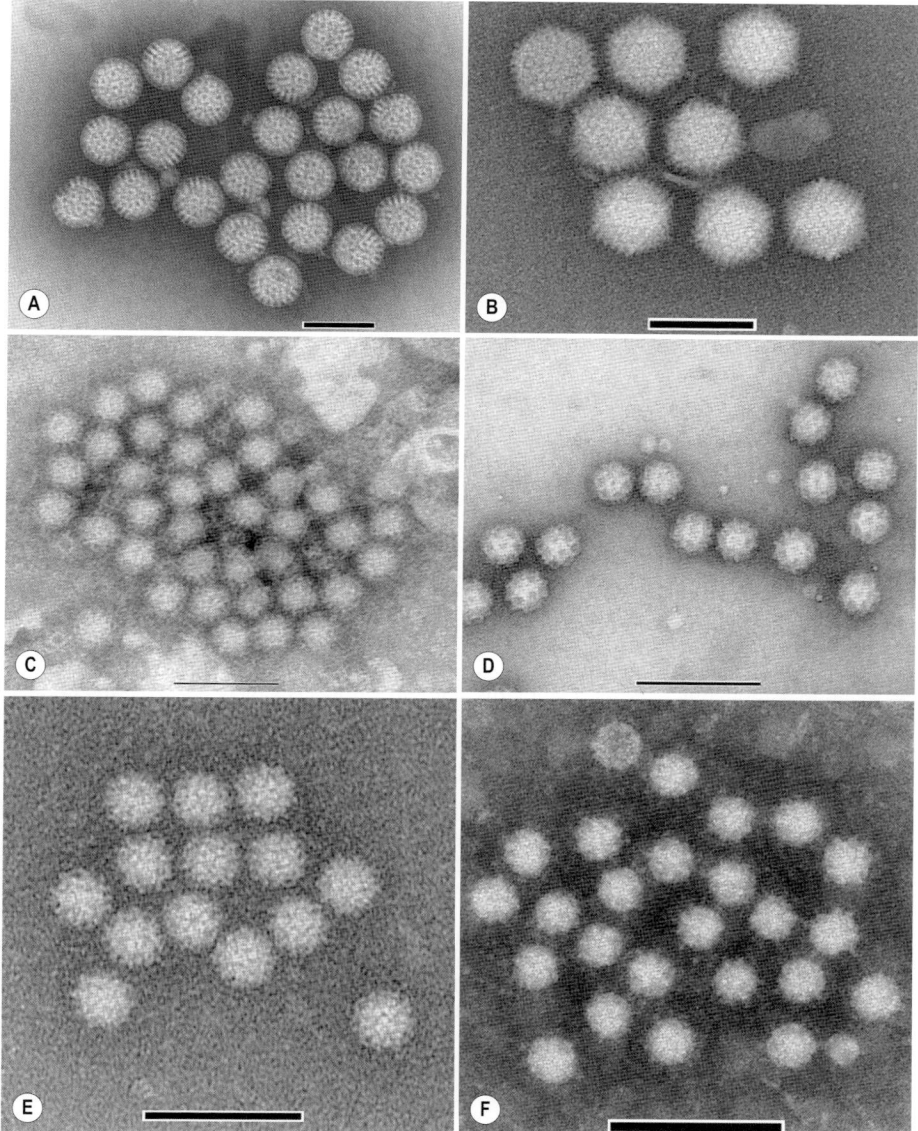

Figure 58-1. Electron micrographs of four viruses that are known to cause gastroenteritis. **(A)** Rotaviruses are 70- to 80-nm multi-shelled particles; the inner shell has a visible "wheel and spoke" character. **(B)** Adenoviruses are 70- to 90-nm icosahedral structured viruses with fiber extensions on their vertices. The fibers are fragile and not always seen on cell culture prepared adenovirus or on virus seen in fecal suspensions. **(C–E)** Noroviruses and sapoviruses are 33- to 40-nm viruses. Fecal suspension particles often are coated with gastrointestinal derived antibodies as shown in panel **C.** Human noroviruses and sapoviruses are fastidious but virus-like particles (VLPs) formed of capsid proteins can be produced in recombinant-based cultures, as shown in panels **D** and **E.** The calicivirus VLPs may be slightly larger (37 to 41 nm) than their respective viruses but have typical calicivirus structure. Panel **D** VLPs were derived from sapovirus and panel **E** from norovirus. The "star of David" image associated with caliciviruses is readily apparent on sapovirus VLPs **D** but is not visible on norovirus VLPs **E.** **(F)** Astroviruses are 25–30 nm, have a smooth edge, and a distinctive 5- or 6-pointed star on some particles in fecal-suspension derived virus. The smooth surface is not always present on astroviruses grown in culture and can resemble miniature versions of noroviruses. Scale bars = 100 nm. (Courtesy of Charles D. Humphrey, PhD, CDC, Atlanta, GA.)

occurring between 4 and 23 months of age.[48,49] Infections in the first 3 months are less common and often asymptomatic because of protection from maternally acquired antibodies.[48,50] Rotavirus infections can occur more than once, with each subsequent infection becoming less severe as a result of developing immunity.[48] Illness among older children and adults is less common, but can occur in people exposed to younger children in group childcare and schools. Without immunization, rotaviruses account for 25% to 50% of gastroenteritis hospitalizations among children <5 years of age and 5% to 20% of milder cases in people who seek care in clinics.[49,51] Globally, rotavirus causes approximately 450,000 deaths per year in children less than 5 years of age, with deaths among children in the poorest countries accounting for >85% of the total.[49,51b] In the U.S., rotavirus caused 55,000 to 70,000 hospitalizations annually prior to vaccine introduction,[52,53] but mortality is rare in developed countries.[54,55]

Noroviruses are now recognized as the most common cause of both endemic disease among all ages and outbreaks of gastroenteritis,[3] with an estimated 21 million illnesses a year in the U.S.[56] Norovirus may be the most common cause of pediatric gastroenteritis in the community,[57] but because disease is less severe, it is second to rotavirus as a cause of hospitalizations. Globally, norovirus is estimated to cause 12% of severe diarrheal disease in children <5 years of age.[58] In the U.S., norovirus also is the most commonly reported cause of foodborne disease while in international settings, estimates vary widely.[56,59,60] Common foods associated with outbreaks include uncooked products contaminated by ill foodhandlers who are shedding virus, and shellfish harvested from contaminated water. Healthcare facilities, including nursing homes and hospitals, are the most common settings of norovirus outbreaks, with other closed environments such as childcare facilities and cruise ships frequently affected. The emergence of new variants of norovirus (genogroup II type 4) may be associated with unusual seasonal activity and a surge in outbreaks.[19,20,61] All age groups can be infected with noroviruses, but serosurveys document that first infection is acquired at an early age.[3]

Sapoviruses most commonly are associated with sporadic gastroenteritis, usually among young children.[62,63] Sapoviruses were detected in approximately 10% of all gastroenteritis episodes in England and Finland and 4% of hospitalized cases in Finland among children <2 years of age.[64,65] Sapovirus infections tend to be less severe than norovirus;[65] outbreaks are less common and tend to occur in the elderly.[66]

Although astroviruses have been detected in all age groups, most infections are in children <2 years of age and tend to be less severe than rotavirus.[67] Serosurveys in the U.S. have shown that

PART II Clinical Syndromes and Cardinal Features of Infectious Diseases: Approach to Diagnosis and Initial Management

SECTION H Gastrointestinal Tract Infections and Intoxications

>90% of children have antibody to human astroviruses by 6 to 9 years of age.[68] Disease in adults is uncommon, but can occur in outbreak settings.[69] Generally, astroviruses are detected in <10% of young children treated for gastroenteritis in outpatient clinics or in hospitals, but occasionally are found at higher frequencies.[40,70] While astroviruses primarily cause sporadic disease, outbreaks have been reported in a range of settings including nosocomial gastroenteritis in children's hospitals.[71]

Most enteric adenovirus infections occur in children <2 years of age year-round, and less often are causes of gastroenteritis among adults.[72,73] Enteric adenoviruses account for 5% to 10% of hospitalizations for acute gastroenteritis in children and may be a common cause of healthcare-associated diarrhea.[74] Enteric adenoviruses generally are detected in 1% to 4% of children with community-associated diarrhea.[75,76] Enteric adenoviruses compared with other viral agents appear to account for a smaller proportion of diarrheal disease in economically developing than in developed countries.

PATHOGENESIS

All the major enteric viruses are transmitted primarily through close person-to-person contact via the fecal–oral route.[77] Noroviruses, in addition, are spread easily through contaminated food and water, and therefore are a major cause of foodborne disease.[41,56,78] Noroviruses are present in vomitus of ill people, and droplet spread through exposure to vomitus is an efficient mechanism of spread both in healthcare and public settings, including airplanes.[79–81] The modes of transmission of adenovirus are less well understood, but transmission is presumed to be primarily through close contact by fecal–oral spread. Spread through fomites is possible for each of the agents, and may play an important role in disease acquired in institutional settings and group childcare.[82]

After oral inoculation, viruses infect mature villous enterocytes (which have both digestive and absorptive functions) of the small intestine,[83] leading to cell death, sloughing, and villus blunting. Rotavirus infection likely results in osmotic diarrhea due to loss of absorptive enterocytes. Rotavirus infections also can cause secretory diarrhea due to the opening of calcium channels, which results in an influx of calcium and efflux of sodium and water (associated with a nonstructural viral protein, NSP4).[84,85] The intraenterocyte calcium concentration also leads to cell death. In a normal host, infection resolves as the number of susceptible mature enterocytes decreases due to cell death and as the host

generates an immune response. While viral gastrointestinal tract infections generally are confined to the intestine, rotavirus and norovirus infections can result in antigenemia and presence of nucleic acid in blood of ill patients,[86,87] but extraintestinal disease is rare.

Following infection, viruses are shed in large amounts in stool during the acute illness. However, rotaviruses, noroviruses, and astroviruses can be shed for 1 to 2 days prior to illness and for several days following resolution of symptoms, facilitating transmission.[77,82] Asymptomatic infection is common, especially for norovirus,[64] although the role of asymptomatic infection in transmission is unknown.

Immunity to rotavirus is acquired and multiple infections typically are required until a child is protected against disease.[48,88,89] After a primary infection, homotypic immunity is stronger, but immunity seems to broaden to other serotypes with subsequent infections.[48] Immunity to norovirus is short-lived (months to a year) and heterotypic immunity is limited, so disease occurs in older children and adults.[90] There also is a correlation between expression of histo-blood group antigens (HBGAs) and susceptibility to norovirus infection.[91–94] The expression of histo-blood group antigens (HBGAs), as determined by the *FUT2* gene, has been associated with strain-specific susceptibility to norovirus infection, and mutations in the *FUT2* gene leading to the absence of HBGA expression have been associated with resistance to infection.[91–98] However, HBGA status does not explain completely the differences among infected and uninfected people for all strains of norovirus. Because diarrheal disease caused by astrovirus, adenovirus, and sapoviruses is largely restricted to children, immunity is believed to be long-lasting.

CLINICAL MANIFESTATIONS

After a short incubation period, infections with any of the viruses lead to an acute onset of gastroenteritis (Table 58-2). Clinical characteristics of illnesses caused by the different viruses generally are indistinguishable. Vomiting often is an early sign, common in rotavirus, and particularly pronounced in norovirus infections.[99] Stools are frequent, watery, and without blood or visible mucus. Fever occurs in approximately half of children and often is an early sign. Vomiting and fever often cease within 1 to 3 days, whereas diarrhea can persist, especially in rotavirus infections. Other symptoms include abdominal cramps and malaise. Stools generally do not contain hemoglobin or fecal leukocytes.

TABLE 58-2. Epidemiologic Features of Viral Agents of Gastroenteritis

Feature	Rotavirus	Noroviruses	Sapoviruses	Astroviruses	Adenoviruses
Age of illness	<5 years	All ages	<5 years	<2 years	<2 years
Mode of transmission	Person-to-person via fecal–oral route, fomites	Person-to-person via fecal–oral route, fomites, food/water	Person-to-person via fecal–oral route	Person-to-person via fecal–oral route	Person-to-person via fecal–oral route
Incubation period	1–3 days	12–48 hours	12–48 hours	1–4 days	3–10 days
SYMPTOMS					
Diarrhea	Explosive, watery (5–10 episodes/day)	Watery with acute onset	Watery; milder than rotavirus	Watery; milder than rotavirus	Watery; milder than rotavirus; can be prolonged
Vomiting	80–90%	>50%; often dominant symptom	Less common than rotavirus	Less common than rotavirus	Less common than rotavirus
Fever	Frequent	Less common, usually mild	Less common, usually mild	Less common, usually mild	Less common, usually mild
Illness duration	2–8 days	1–5 days	1–4 days	1–5 days	3–10 days
PRINCIPAL METHODS OF CLINICAL DIAGNOSIS	Stool EIA or LPA	RT-PCR	RT-PCR	Stool EIA (not available in the United States)	Stool EIA

EIA, enzyme immunoassay; EM, electron microscopy; IEM, immune electron microscopy; LPA, latex particle agglutination; RT-PCR, reverse transcriptase-polymerase chain reaction.
Modified from Peck AJ, Bresee JS. Viral gastroenteritis. In: McMillan JA, Feigin RD, De Angelis CD, Jones MD (eds) Oski's Pediatrics, 4th ed. Philadelphia, PA, Lippincott, Williams and Wilkins, 2006, pp 1288–1294.

The most important and common complication of viral gastroenteritis is dehydration, often with electrolyte abnormalities. Malabsorption can occur during the illness and persist for weeks. Respiratory tract symptoms if present are likely due to concurrent wintertime respiratory tract viral infections. Extraintestinal complications are rare, but encephalitis, acute myositis, hemophagocytic lymphohistiocytosis, acute flaccid paralysis, and sudden infant death syndrome have been described rarely in children with rotavirus infections;[4] relationship to rotavirus infection remains unclear. Prolonged diarrhea associated with each agent has been reported among children with malnutrition and among immunocompromised people.[100] The severity and duration of norovirus gastroenteritis has been shown to be greater in vulnerable populations.[101]

Unlike in individual cases, clinical characteristics of cases in outbreak settings can predict etiology. Outbreaks that meet simple epidemiologic and clinical criteria are likely to be due to noroviruses: (1) failure to detect a bacterial or parasitic pathogen in stool specimens; (2) the occurrence of vomiting in >50% of patients; (3) mean duration of illness of 12 to 60 hours; and (4) mean incubation period of 24 to 48 hours.[99] These "Kaplan" criteria have been validated[102] widely and are used by local health departments for diagnosis of outbreaks in the absence of laboratory testing for norovirus.

DIAGNOSIS

Laboratory diagnosis of viral gastroenteritis is best made by detection of viral antigen or nucleic acid in fresh, whole stool samples obtained during the acute illness. Commercially available assays to detect rotavirus antigen in stools offer an easy and inexpensive method for diagnosis, and include enzyme immunoassay (EIA) or latex particle agglutination test for group A rotaviruses, designed to detect the VP6 protein.[4] Antigen detection tests generally have a <90% sensitivity and <95% specificity.[93] Other methods for rotavirus detection include electron microscopy, viral isolation, and polyacrylamide gel electrophoresis (PAGE) of RNA extracted directly from stool. Reverse transcriptase-polymerase chain reaction (RT-PCR) has high analytical sensitivity and can detect virus when it is not disease-causing; RT-PCR rarely is used clinically. Serologic testing for rotavirus infection is possible but impractical in clinical applications.

Commercial antigen detection kits are available for caliciviruses, but are not recommended for use in clinical settings in the U.S. because of poor sensitivity; however, testing may be useful in outbreak investigations.[103–105] RT-PCR has become the standard diagnostic assay used for caliciviruses, but seldom is used clinically. Real-time (quantitative) RT-PCR has become widely available in public health laboratories for outbreak investigations, and sequencing of the PCR product from clinical samples can permit linking cases to each other and to a common source.[106] Given the exquisite sensitivity of RT-PCR for norovirus and the high frequency of finding norovirus in healthy people,[64,107] test results must be interpreted carefully. Caliciviruses have not been propagated in cell cultures, which has hampered development of simple diagnostic tests and evaluation of disinfectants/hand sanitizers.

Commercial EIAs for detection of astrovirus antigen in stool are available in Europe, but not in the U.S.[108] RT-PCR (highly sensitive and specific), serologic assays, and electron microscopy primarily are used in research settings. Similarly, EIA and latex particle agglutination kits are available commercially and provide highly sensitive and specific antigen detection of enteric adenoviruses. All viral gastroenteritis agents are detectable by electron microscopy and immune electron microscopy, but these tests are seldom used because of relatively low sensitivity and specificity, expense, and required expertise.

TREATMENT

No specific therapies are available for viral gastroenteritis. Case management depends on accurate and rapid assessment, correction of fluid loss and electrolyte disturbances, and maintenance of adequate hydration and nutrition.[109] Oral rehydration therapy with appropriate glucose-electrolyte solutions is sufficient in most cases. Intravenous rehydration may be required for children with severe dehydration with shock or intractable vomiting. Breastfed infants should continue to nurse on demand. Infants receiving formula should continue their usual formula upon rehydration. Children taking solid foods should continue to receive their usual diet during episodes of diarrhea, although substantial amounts of foods high in simple sugars should be avoided because the osmotic content might worsen diarrhea. Use of antimicrobial agents in patients with acute gastroenteritis should be severely restricted.

Some evidence exists to support use of oral probiotics, such as *Lactobacillus* species, that reduce the duration of diarrhea caused by rotavirus.[110,111] Zinc, used both as supplement and treatment, may reduce severity, duration, and incidence of diarrhea in some populations.[112,113] Human or bovine colostrums and human serum immunoglobulin that contain antibodies to rotavirus may be beneficial in decreasing or preventing rotavirus diarrhea, but are not used routinely.

PREVENTION

Except for rotavirus, prevention of viral gastroenteritis is limited to nonspecific strategies. Breastfeeding confers some protection against rotavirus infection, and probably other viral etiologies of infections, in young infants; protection likely is mediated through antibodies and other nonimmunologic factors in human milk. Good hygiene, including hand hygiene practices, is an effective prevention strategy and should be encouraged, particularly in institutional settings, such as childcare facilities and hospitals.[114] Hand hygiene adherence in school-age children has been shown to reduce environmental contamination with norovirus.[115] Noroviruses are relatively resistant to environmental disinfection, but cleaning contaminated surfaces and food preparation areas with cleaners approved by the U.S. Environmental Protection Agency can decrease spread of viruses and likely is effective in settings where rotavirus and astrovirus outbreaks occur.[114]

Adequate reduction of transmission of viral agents of gastroenteritis is difficult because the infectious dose is low, viruses are excreted in high quantity in stool (and often vomitus) of infected people, and the agents are quite stable in the environment. Indeed, improvements in sanitation and hygiene have not reduced rates of disease from enteric viral agents to the same extent that they have reduced disease from bacterial and parasitic agents.

The best option for preventing rotavirus morbidity and mortality is use of live, oral rotavirus vaccines in routine immunization programs. Rotavirus vaccines are attenuated strains given in multiple doses designed to replace a child's initial exposures to wild-type rotavirus with strains that will not cause disease but will generate an adequate immune response to confer protection.[116] Two rotavirus vaccines are licensed. Additional vaccines are in development and may be available within the next several years. While most vaccines in clinical development are live, orally administered vaccines, parenterally administered vaccines also are being investigated.

Rotavirus vaccines are incorporated into routine immunization programs in the U.S., Australia, and several Latin American and European countries.[117,118] With introduction of vaccination, pediatric hospitalizations have declined substantially in these populations[45,119–121] and – in Mexico – a reduction in diarrhea-associated mortality has been observed.[122] Vaccine effectiveness in the field is high. Although vaccine trials show reduced efficacy (40% to 75%) in low/middle-income populations,[123–125] impact still is substantial due to the higher burden and adverse outcomes of disease. The World Health Organization has issued global recommendations for the use of rotavirus vaccines, including universal introduction in countries where diarrheal deaths account for ≥10% of mortality among children aged <5 years.[126]

Vaccines against noroviruses are in development.[127] No vaccines against other caliciviruses, astroviruses, or enteric adenoviruses are in human trials.

59   Inflammatory Enteritis

Ina Stephens and James P. Nataro

Inflammatory enteritis is a pathologic diagnosis characterized by ileal and/or colonic inflammation, which can range from small, superficial patches of leukocyte infiltration amid relatively normal mucosa to deep, exudative ulcerations with involvement of the entire intestinal wall.[1] The large number of infectious and noninfectious causes of inflammation results in a wide range of manifestations. Inflammatory enteritis should be considered in the differential diagnosis of patients with abdominal pain, dysentery, or watery diarrhea, particularly when patients present with fever and blood or mucus in stool.

CLASSIFICATION

Inflammatory enteritides can be classified into several distinct clinical entities, the recognition of which facilitates suspicion for etiologic agents (Table 59-1) diagnosis and management. However, many patients with inflammatory enteritis do not easily fit into any of these categories, thereby broadening their differential diagnosis.

Acute dysentery is defined by the presence of fecal blood and mucus, associated with frequent, small loose bowel movements. Fever often is present. Dysentery is the result of microbial invasion of the colonic mucosa, with mucosal and submucosal inflammation and destruction. Shigellosis is a prototype of acute dysentery.

Chronic inflammatory enteritis typically is an indolent and slowly progressive illness. The patient can manifest fever, abdominal pain, and weight loss over several weeks. Recurring, relapsing symptoms commonly occur. *Mycobacterium tuberculosis* is a classic cause of chronic inflammatory enteritis; children in the United States with chronic inflammatory enteritis are more likely to have inflammatory bowel disease.

Ulcerative proctitis is characterized by severe anorectal pain, purulent discharge, tenesmus, hematochezia, constipation, and fever. Erythematous, friable mucosa is visualized in the rectal vault.[2–4] Severe disease can lead to rectal abscesses or fistulas. This condition, which occurs primarily in men who have sex with men (MSM) and in immunocompromised patients, can be caused by a variety of sexually transmitted and other infectious agents[4] (Table 59-1).

Necrotizing enterocolitis (NEC) of the newborn is characterized by varying degrees of mucosal necrosis.[5–8] NEC occurs almost exclusively in premature infants, who typically demonstrate a sepsis-like illness with abdominal distention and, commonly, grossly bloody stools. Although many factors contribute to development of intestinal necrosis, a common pathway features ischemia, followed by disruption of the mucosal barrier, bacterial invasion, proliferation, and gas formation within the bowel wall.[5,6] Gram-negative bacteria of the normal flora may be important factors in triggering the injury process in a setting of a paucity of bacterial species and possible lack of protective gram-positive organisms.[7] Although outbreaks of NEC ascribed to single pathogens are described, prospective studies have failed to implicate a specific infectious cause in most cases (see Chapter 60, Necrotizing Enterocolitis).[8]

Antimicrobial-associated colitis (AAC) is characterized by the presence of multiple yellow plaque-like ulcerative lesions (1 to 5 mm in size) overlying an erythematous, friable, colonic mucosa. In severe cases, lesions become confluent, resulting in sloughing of necrotic tissue and formation of the characteristic pseudomembrane.[9–11] Clinical presentation of AAC varies from mild watery diarrhea (with or without crampy abdominal pain) to fulminant colitis that can progress to toxic megacolon, colonic perforation, shock, and death. Overgrowth of toxigenic *Clostridium difficile* with release of potent cytotoxins is responsible for almost all cases.[9,10] *C. difficile* colitis in the absence of antibiotic therapy is unusual; however, use of both proton pump inhibitor (PPI) and H_2-receptor agonist drugs is associated with increased risk of community-associated *C. difficile*-associated disease.[11] Data suggest that the incidence and severity of *C. difficile*-associated disease (CDAD) are increasing in the United States,[11,12] and that increase may be associated with the emergence of newer strains with increased virulence, antimicrobial resistance, or both. These "hypervirulent" strains, which carry variations in toxin genes and also are more resistant to the fluoroquinolones, erythromycin, and tetracycline, have emerged as a cause of CDAD outbreaks.[12–14] *C. difficile* colitis is common in patients with HIV, in whom *C. difficile* can account for up to 54% of cases of bacterial diarrhea.[15] Even in the age of highly active antiretroviral therapy (HAART), large-bowel infections frequently are due to opportunistic pathogens such as cytomegalovirus (CMV), cryptosporidiosis, *Mycobacterium avium* complex (MAC), and spirochetosis.[16]

Noninfectious causes of inflammatory enteritis include ulcerative colitis, Crohn disease, Henoch–Schönlein purpura, eosinophilic gastroenteritis, enterocolitis complicating Hirschsprung disease, Behçet disease, and allergic colitis.[17,18] Intussusception can cause acute onset of bloody, diarrheal stools, but inflammatory exudate is not expected.

TABLE 59-1. Differential Diagnoses of Inflammatory Enteritis

Acute Inflammatory Enteritis	Chronic Inflammatory Enteritis (≥2 Weeks)	Proctitis
BACTERIAL	**BACTERIAL**	*Chlamydia trachomatis*
Aeromonas hydrophila	*Campylobacter jejuni/coli*	*Entamoeba histolytica*
Campylobacter jejuni/coli	Enteroaggregative *Escherichia coli*	Herpes simplex virus
Enteroaggregative *Escherichia coli*	*Mycobacterium tuberculosis*	*Neisseria gonorrhoeae*
Enterohemorrhagic *Escherichia coli*	*Salmonella* spp.	*Shigella* spp.
Enteroinvasive *Escherichia coli*	*Shigella* spp.	*Treponema pallidum*
Plesiomonas shigelloides	**FUNGAL**	Other enteric pathogens[a]
Salmonella spp.	*Candida* spp.	
Shigella spp.	*Histoplasma capsulatum*	
Vibrio parahaemolyticus	*Paracoccidioides brasiliensis*	
Yersinia enterocolitica	Phycomycosis agents[a]	
PARASITIC		
Balantidium coli		
Cryptosporidium parvum[a]		
Entamoeba histolytica		
Schistosoma species		
Strongyloides stercoralis		
Trichinella spiralis		
VIRAL		
Cytomegalovirus[a]		
Enteroviruses[a]		

[a]*Primarily in immunocompromised patients.*

PRINCIPAL ETIOLOGIC AGENTS

A variety of infectious agents classically are considered as causes of acute inflammatory enteritis (Table 59-1). Patients come to medical attention with fever, abdominal pain, blood or mucus in stool, or a combination of these findings. However, many of these pathogens can cause clinical illnesses without overt characteristics of inflammation. Absence of clinical signs of inflammation does not therefore rule out these agents. In the U.S., most cases of inflammatory enteritis in children are caused by bacterial pathogens, whereas parasitic agents are common among travelers to or indigenous populations in developing areas. Generally, differentiation among bacterial enteropathogens on clinical grounds alone is not possible; pathogenesis and potential complications associated with these agents are shown in Table 59-2. Detailed description can be found in pathogen-specific chapters.

***Shigella* species.** All four *Shigella* species can elicit prototypic acute bacillary dysentery, but *S. sonnei* most often elicits an uncomplicated watery diarrhea and is most prevalent in developed countries.[19,20] *Shigella* spp. have no known animal reservoir. Organisms are highly contagious and have a low infectious dose (as low as 10^2 colony-forming units), a feature hypothesized to be related to the organism's acid resistance.[21,22] Person-to-person and foodborne transmissions are most common in childhood infections;[20] environmental contamination also can be a source of transmission.

***Salmonella* species.** Nontyphoidal *Salmonella* serotypes cause a spectrum of illness that includes mild diarrhea, dysentery-like inflammatory enteritis, and disseminated disease, including septicemia, enteric fever, and focal seeding (especially in immunocompromised hosts).[23] Most infections due to *Salmonella* in the U.S. are foodborne,[24] and most commonly via contaminated animal products such as unpasteurized milk, eggs, and improperly cooked meat.

***Escherichia coli*.** Diarrheagenic *E. coli* are divided into five major pathogenic categories on the basis of mechanism of pathogenesis.[25] Categories are: (1) enterotoxigenic (watery diarrhea in infants and travelers); (2) enteroinvasive (dysentery identical to that of *S. sonnei*); (3) enteropathogenic (acute and chronic watery diarrhea in infants and children); (4) enterohemorrhagic (hemorrhagic colitis associated with the hemolytic–uremic syndrome); and (5) enteroaggregative (acute or persistent watery diarrhea, prevalent in developing countries, and in the immunocompromised host). Each type of *E. coli* except enterotoxigenic strains can cause inflammatory enteritis. Both enterohemorrhagic and enteroaggregative *E. coli* pathotypes occur commonly in the U.S.

***Yersinia enterocolitica*.** *Yersinia enterocolitica* typically causes acute diarrhea, fever, and abdominal pain.[26] Other manifestations include septicemia in infants and immunocompromised hosts, mesenteric lymphadenitis (mimicking appendicitis) in older children and young adults, dysentery, and postinfectious syndromes, including reactive arthritis, Reiter syndrome, glomerulonephritis, and erythema nodosum.[27,28] In the U.S., most *Y. enterocolitica* transmissions are foodborne, with outbreaks often due to unpasteurized milk and contaminated pork or chitterlings.[29]

***Campylobacter jejuni*.** *Campylobacter jejuni* is one of the most commonly documented bacterial causes of diarrhea among people of all ages in the U.S. and Canada.[30] Inflammatory enteritis and acute dysentery with severe abdominal pain and fever are common manifestations.[30] Bacteremia or dissemination is rare. The reservoir for *C. jejuni* is the gastrointestinal tract of wild and domestic birds and, to a lesser extent, animals, allowing for foodborne outbreaks via ingestion of contaminated water, raw milk, or undercooked meat and poultry. Person-to-person spread has been documented, although such transmission is less likely than with shigellosis as the infectious dose of *C. jejuni* is considerably higher (10^{4-6} organisms).[30]

***Aeromonas hydrophila*.** *Aeromonas* species are found in soil and in fresh and brackish waters worldwide. *A. hydrophila* has been associated with acute gastroenteritis, soft-tissue infection, and bacteremia, especially in immunocompromised hosts. *A. hydrophila* is a significant cause of infections in the wake of natural disasters (hurricanes, tsunamis, and earthquakes) and has been linked to emerging illnesses, including prostatitis and hemolytic uremic syndrome.[31] Diarrhea due to *A. hydrophila* also is associated with the consumption of seafood.[32] Mechanism of intestinal disease is unknown.

***Vibrio parahaemolyticus*.** *Vibrio* spp. other than *V. cholerae* can elicit acute inflammatory enteritis with explosive, watery diarrhea.

TABLE 59-2. Pathogenesis and Complications of Principal Infectious Causes of Inflammatory Enteritis

Agent	Pathogenesis	Intestinal Complications	Extraintestinal Complications
Shigella spp. and enteroinvasive *Escherichia coli*	Invasion of colonic enterocytes with lateral spread through mucosa and submucosa;[96] enterotoxins possibly involved[49]	Colonic perforation, protein-losing enteropathy	Seizures Septicemia HUS Immune-mediated disease (reactive arthritis, Reiter syndrome)
Salmonella spp.	Invasion of distal ileal mucosa; can spread to reticuloendothelial system[97]	Colonic perforation (enteric fever), chronic carriage	Septicemia Meningitis, disseminated foci
Campylobacter jejuni/coli	Invasion of colonic enterocytes[98]	Chronic disease	Dissemination Immune-mediated disease (Guillain–Barré syndrome, reactive arthritis)
Yersinia enterocolitica	Invasion of ileal mucosa with inflammatory response; enterotoxins possibly involved[26,50]	Mesenteric adenitis	Dissemination with septicemia, suppurative foci
Enterohemorrhagic *Escherichia coli*	Attaching and effacing lesions of colonic mucosa; production of Shiga-like toxins linked to HUS[39]	Toxic megacolon, colonic perforation	HUS Seizures
Clostridium difficile	Cytotoxin production	Toxic megacolon, colonic perforation	Septicemia
Entamoeba histolytica	Contact-dependent and contact-independent cytotoxicity; proteases; secretory factors possibly involved[36]	Chronic disease, toxic megacolon, colonic perforation	Ameboma, liver abscess, disseminated foci

HUS, hemolytic uremic syndrome.

PART II   Clinical Syndromes and Cardinal Features of Infectious Diseases: Approach to Diagnosis and Initial Management

SECTION H   Gastrointestinal Tract Infections and Intoxications

Illness usually is caused by *V. parahaemolyticus* acquired through consumption of undercooked seafood.[33] Some non-O1 *V. cholerae* also have been implicated in inflammatory enteritis.[34,35]

Entamoeba histolytica.   The classic clinical manifestation of *Entamoeba histolytica* enteritis is amebic dysentery, which can be acute and fulminant (especially in children), or mild and insidious with only abdominal pain, tenesmus, and small, frequent bowel movements.[36,37] Illness often follows an intermittent or waxing and waning course over weeks to months. Long incubation periods (1 week to 1 month) allow onset of symptoms long after return from travel to a developing country where infection was acquired. Dissemination, most frequently to the liver, can occur after resolution of untreated amebic dysentery. Examination of the colonic mucosa of people with dysentery often reveals shallow, flask-like ulcers.[36] Trophozoites characteristically are found in stools of patients with dysentery or diarrhea; cysts more commonly are found in asymptomatic people.

EPIDEMIOLOGY

The epidemiology of infectious inflammatory enteritis is determined by the specific causative agent and susceptibility of the host. Predictive epidemiologic associations should be explored in the patient's history, including foreign travel, childcare or institutional exposure, swimming and other exposure to water sources, receipt of antibiotics, diet, animal exposure, and underlying conditions. Risk factors and associated agents are shown in Table 59-3.

Infectious inflammatory enteritis often occurs in outbreaks related to person-to-person, foodborne, or waterborne transmission. Etiology of outbreaks of enteric disease can often be predicted from the incubation period.[38] Cases with onset between 1 and 16 hours of source event usually are not inflammatory in nature and are toxin-mediated; those with onset between 16 and 72 hours can be caused by infection, such as due to *Salmonella* or *Shigella* spp., *C. jejuni*, enteroinvasive *E. coli*, *V. parahaemolyticus*, and *Y. enterocolitica*; an incubation period >72 hours suggests enterohemorrhagic *E. coli* O157:H7.[38,39] The implicated vehicle of transmission also can be helpful in predicting the cause. Cysts of parasites, including *Cryptosporidium parvum*, *Balantidium coli*, and *E. histolytica*, resist chlorination and thus contaminate municipal water supplies. Some pathogens are associated with specific foods,

e.g., *Salmonella* spp. (undercooked poultry, produce and eggs), *C. jejuni* (undercooked poultry), *V. parahaemolyticus* (raw and undercooked seafood), and *Y. enterocolitica* (pork, chitterlings, milk). *N. gonorrhoeae*, herpes simplex virus, *C. trachomatis*, and *T. pallidum* are sexually transmitted agents of ulcerative proctitis in MSM; MSM also have increased risk for colitis caused by typical enteric pathogens.

PATHOGENESIS

All inflammatory enteritides share common features of mucosal damage and accompanying release of inflammatory mediators. The mechanism of such damage elicited by infectious agents follows one of two general paradigms, cytotoxin elaboration or mucosal invasion, although some organisms are able to execute both mechanisms. The cytotoxic mechanism is exemplified by *Clostridium difficile* colitis. Two *C difficile* exotoxins (toxin A, a 308-kd enterotoxin, and toxin B, a 250- to 270-kd cytotoxin) damage enterocytes, leading to mucosal necrosis, and also may be responsible for secretion of fluid into the intestinal lumen.[40-42] Both toxins act by catalyzing glycosylation of Rho proteins (guanosine triphosphate-binding proteins) in target eukaryotic cells, thereby inducing derangement of the cytoskeleton and altering multiple cellular processes.

In addition, *C difficile* toxins induce release of cytokines from epithelial cells, monocytes, macrophages, and neuronal cells of the lamina propria; these cytokines contribute to the toxin-mediated inflammation, apoptosis of colonocytes, and damage of colonic mucosa with formation of colonic ulcers and pseudomembranes.[10,43,44]

The invasive mechanism of bacterial enteritis is exemplified by shigellosis, yersiniosis, and salmonellosis, which penetrate mucosa of the ileum and colon. The role of inflammation in these infections is not entirely clear, but apparently is complex and may benefit both host and pathogen.[45] For example, experimental evidence suggests that migration of neutrophils into the intestinal lumen can exacerbate both *Shigella* and *Salmonella* diarrhea.[46,47] Moreover, mice who are deficient in the apoptotic (and proinflammatory) enzyme caspase 1 are resistant to *Salmonella* infection. However, mice deficient in certain cytokine responses also are unable to limit *Salmonella* infection to the intestine and are more likely to succumb to systemic disease. A great deal is known about the molecular events underlying *Salmonella* pathogenesis (reviewed in reference[48]). The clinical manifestations of inflammatory enteritis may be the result of a finely tuned co-evolution between host and parasite, the result of which favors the survival of both species. In addition, invasive pathogens can secrete enterotoxins.[49-51] A summary of pathogenic mechanisms for principal pathogens is shown in Table 59-2.

DIAGNOSTIC EVALUATION

Before embarking on diagnostic evaluation of a patient with enteric disease, one should consider whether determining the causative agent will affect management. Most gastrointestinal tract infections in the U.S. are caused by viruses, for which there is no specific therapy. Most viral infections do not elicit an inflammatory syndrome, and therefore, the presence of acute inflammatory enteritis suggests a bacterial or parasitic etiology. Some bacterial agents of inflammatory enteritis can be treated to benefit the patient, potential contacts, or both, whereas other agents, like nontyphoid *Salmonella* confined to the gut, are not responsive to antimicrobial therapy. A practical, selective diagnostic approach to the patient with enteritis should be cost-effective and likely to yield information helpful for management.

By far the most common infectious causes of acute inflammatory enteritis in U.S. children are the bacterial enteropathogens. Relevant epidemiologic factors (see Table 59-3), disease patterns in the community, and patient characteristics are useful in assessing the likelihood of a bacterial etiology.[52-54] Suggestive signs and symptoms include fever, abrupt onset of diarrhea, >4 stools per

TABLE 59-3. Epidemiologic Risk Factors Associated with Infectious Agents of Inflammatory Enteritis

Risk Factor	Infectious Agents
Travel	Enterotoxigenic and enteroaggregative *Escherichia coli*, *Shigella*, *Salmonella*, *Campylobacter* spp., *Entamoeba histolytica*
Beef consumption	Enterohemorrhagic *E. coli*, *Salmonella*
Poultry consumption	*Salmonella*, *Campylobacter*
Pork consumption	*Yersinia enterocolitica*, *Salmonella* spp.
Seafood consumption	*Vibrio parahaemolyticus*, *Aeromonas hydrophilia*
Water contamination	*Shigella*, *Salmonella*, *Campylobacter*, *Cryptosporidium* spp.
Institutional exposure/ childcare	*Shigella*, *Cryptosporidium*, *Giardia lamblia*, enterohemorrhagic *E. coli*
Sexual transmission	*Treponema pallidum*, herpes simplex virus, *Neisseria gonorrhoeae*, *Chlamydia trachomatis*, *Shigella*, *E. histolytica*
Unpasteurized milk consumption	*Salmonella*, *Campylobacter*, *Y. enterocolitica*, *Mycobacterium* spp.
Antimicrobial therapy	*Clostridium difficile*

TABLE 59-4. Association of Fecal Leukocytes with Intestinal Pathogens

Present	Variable	Absent
Campylobacter	Clostridium difficile	Bacillus cereus
Enteroinvasive	Salmonella	Clostridium perfringens
Escherichia coli	Schistosoma	Entamoeba histolytica
Shigella	Vibrio parahaemolyticus	Enteric viruses
	Yersinia enterocolitica	Enteropathogenic
		Escherichia coli
		Enterotoxigenic
		Escherichia coli
		Giardia intestinalis
		Vibrio cholerae

TABLE 59-5. Diagnostic Studies for Enteropathogens

Organism	Diagnostic Studies
ACUTE DISEASE	
Balantidium coli	Stool examination, microscopic examination of mucosal scrapings
Campylobacter	Stool culture
Cryptosporidium	Modified acid-fast/auramine or fluorescein-labeled monoclonal antibody stain of stool, duodenal aspirate, or small-bowel biopsy specimen
Entamoeba histolytica	Stool examination; serology for invasive disease; proctosigmoidoscopy with scrapings or biopsy
Escherichia coli	Stool culture followed by gene probes, adherence assays, or serotyping
Salmonella	Stool, blood, bone marrow cultures
Schistosoma	Stool examination
Shigella	Stool culture
Yersinia enterocolitica	Stool culture, blood culture
Cytomegalovirus	Endoscopic mucosal biopsy for microscopy (viral inclusions), immunochemical staining, shell-viral culture, pp65 antigen
CHRONIC DISEASE	
Candida	Potassium hydroxide stain, culture
Enteroaggregative Escherichia coli	Stool culture, DNA probe, adherence to human laryngeal cell line (HEp-2)
Mycobacterium	Acid-fast examination and stool culture, blood culture; microscopic examination of biopsy specimens
PROCTITIS	
Chlamydia trachomatis	Culture, gene probe
Herpes simplex	Culture, enzyme immunoassay or direct fluorescent antibody test
Neisseria gonorrhoeae	Culture
Treponema pallidum	Darkfield microscopy examination of mucosal scrapings, serology
Entamoeba histolytica	Microscopic examination of stool or intestinal biopsy tissue; serology
OTHER	
Antimicrobial-associated colitis	Toxin assays, sigmoidoscopy with rectal biopsy
Necrotizing enterocolitis	Abdominal radiograph

day, absence of vomiting before onset of diarrhea, and presence of blood or mucus in stool. The patient with none of these features is unlikely to have a bacterial pathogen. A scoring system for predicting bacterial enteritis has been proposed, in which risk is weighted for each feature.[53] However, such a quantitative approach is unlikely to determine the precise risk of inflammatory enteritis in all locales.

The leukocyte assay of stool mucus is a practical, inexpensive screening test that could be used to predict probable inflammatory enteritis, helping to limit performance of stool culture.[52,55,56] Sensitivity and specificity of this test in predicting bacterial enteritis have been reported to be >80% (for ≥5 white blood cells/high-power field);[52] however, the reported values vary widely among studies, in part owing to differences in the definition of a positive result. Moreover, the predictive value of the assay depends on the likelihood of bacterial inflammatory enteritis as indicated by historical factors and clinical signs. Most leukocytes detected in stool are neutrophils (mononuclear cells also can be associated with *Salmonella* infection).[56] Presence of leukocytes is not always indicative of bacterial inflammatory enteritis (Table 59-4), as leukocytes can be present in inflammatory bowel diseases such as ulcerative colitis and Crohn disease, and fecal neutrophils occasionally can be present in cases of viral enteritis.[57]

Fecal lactoferrin, detected with a commercially available rapid agglutination test, correlates closely with the presence of fecal leukocytes.[58] In one study, 94% (16 of 17) of patients for whom smears of fecal mucus had >1 neutrophil/high-power field also had a positive lactoferrin test result, whereas 16% (3 of 19) of patients with diarrhea without neutrophils in smears and none of 7 healthy controls had positive test results. In another study, the fecal lactoferrin test had a better positive predictive value than fecal leukocyte smear or occult fecal blood detection for the detection of bacterial pathogens.[59] Lactoferrin is stable in fecal specimens and can be detected even when leukocytes disintegrate during transport or storage. Fecal lactoferrin tests can have false-positive results in infants who are breastfed. Fecal calprotectin, an early predictor of acute bacterial versus viral gastroenteritis, is another valuable noninvasive marker in young children, with a diagnostic accuracy of 92%. In one study, combined fecal calprotectin and serum C-reactive protein tests improved diagnostic accuracy to 94% for acute bacterial gastroenteritis.[60]

Selection of Tests to Confirm Etiology

When performance of stool culture is indicated on the basis of history, physical examination, or fecal leukocyte assay, specimens should be inoculated into culture medium adequate for recovery of *Shigella, Salmonella, Y. enterocolitica,* and *C. jejuni.* In the U.S., all bloody stool specimens should be inoculated onto sorbitol–MacConkey agar for detection of enterohemorrhagic *Escherichia coli* O157:H7 and tested with an assay that detects Shiga toxins to

detect non O157 STEC.[60a] In addition, all stool specimens from patients with diarrhea who have a known human contact or who have exposure to a contaminated vehicle should be cultured for *E. coli* O157:H7. If certain epidemiologic risk factors are present, such as a history of seafood ingestion or exposure to brackish water, specialized media should be requested for isolation of *Vibrio, Aeromonas,* and *Plesiomonas* spp. Other specialized tests are sometimes indicated in evaluation of patients with diarrhea; preferred diagnostic methods for etiologic agents of inflammatory enteritis are shown in Table 59-5. (See Chapter 287, Laboratory Diagnosis.)

Direct microscopic examination of stool specimens can reveal protozoal trophozoites, cysts, or oocysts; fungal spores; or helminthic larvae. Although parasitic diseases are not as common in the U.S. as elsewhere and rarely cause inflammatory enteritis, their presence should be suspected, and direct examination for them performed, in the following high-risk situations: (1) recent travel to a developing country; (2) persistent diarrhea (>14 days); (3) immunocompromised status; (4) contact with a person with intestinal parasitic disease; and (5) occurrence of diarrhea in the presence of an outbreak of undetermined cause. Eosinophilia in a patient with inflammatory enteritis may indicate strongyloidiasis.[61] If amebic dysentery is suspected on the basis of risk factors, at least three fresh stool specimens should be examined using the iodine-trichrome method. Yield can be increased by examining stool concentrates stained with iron-hematoxylin.[36] Diagnosis is made visually by detection of hematophagous trophozoites or characteristic cysts in stools. Serum antibody to *Entamoeba histolytica* is present in 85% to 95% of patients with invasive disease but is likely to be absent in asymptomatic cyst excreters and persons with mild diarrhea.[36]

Intestinal biopsy (for histology, special staining for microscopic identification of pathogen, and culture) should be considered in cases of persistent inflammatory enteritis or in an immunocompromised host when diagnosis cannot be made by noninvasive methods. Specimens obtained at biopsy generally have better yield for parasites such as *E. histolytica*. Certain entities, such as enteropathogenic *Escherichia coli*, exhibit characteristic histopathology on electron microscopy.

Diagnosis of *Clostridium difficile* colitis is established by detection of *C. difficile* in stool by tissue culture assay for cytotoxin A and B, or detection of antigens in stool by rapid enzyme immunoassays.[9,62,63] However, problems with these tests include relatively slow turnaround times for stool culture and cell cytotoxin assay, and lack of sensitivity for the enzyme immunoassay.[62,64] Stool culture results can be misleading (especially in infants), because they do not distinguish toxigenic from nontoxigenic strains of *C. difficile*.[62–64] At least four FDA-approved nucleic acid amplification assays are available to clinical laboratories; because these assays detect a gene that encodes toxin and not the toxin itself, only symptomatic patients should be tested to avoid overtreatment of those carrying the organism or its DNA.[64] The best approach may be a combination of diagnostic tests used only in patients in whom there is clinical suspicion of *C. difficile* enteritis. Sigmoidoscopic findings of pseudomembranous colitis are beneficial in confirming diagnosis of antibiotic-associated colitis due to *C. difficile*.

INFLAMMATORY ENTERITIS IN THE IMMUNOCOMPROMISED HOST

Clinical Approach

Diarrhea is a symptom in up to 50% to 60% of patients with the acquired immunodeficiency syndrome (AIDS) in the U.S.[15,65] Although hospital admissions attributable to diarrhea have declined, diarrhea still is a debilitating symptom in patients infected with human immunodeficiency virus (HIV), even in the era of HAART.[15,16,66] Digestive tract disease in children with AIDS and other immunodeficiencies can be produced by a variety of infectious agents, including HIV.[15,16,65,67–70] Depending on the specific cause and the immunologic status of the patient, clinical manifestations can be acute or chronic. Patients with CD4+ T-lymphocyte counts <50 cells/mm^3 and low serum albumin levels are more likely to have an infectious etiology.[71] Signs and symptoms include diarrhea, vomiting, anorexia, failure to thrive, weight loss, and malabsorption. The histopathologic changes in immunocompromised patients usually are similar to changes in healthy patients, although often are more severe. In addition to typical enteric pathogens, opportunistic agents cause acute and chronic inflammatory enteritis in immunocompromised patients; disease due to the following agents fulfill AIDS-defining criteria of the Centers for Disease Control and Prevention (CDC): *Candida, Cryptosporidium, Histoplasma, Cystisospora* (formerly *Isospora*) spp., MAC, *Salmonella* infection with septicemia, CMV, and herpes simplex virus.[15,65,68]

BOX 59-1. Diagnostic Evaluation of Immunocompromised Patients with Inflammatory Enteritis

1. Routine stool culture for *Shigella, Salmonella,* and *Campylobacter jejuni/coli*
2. Specialized stool culture for *Mycobacterium avium* complex, other *Campylobacter* species, *Yersinia enterocolitica, Escherichia coli*
3. Assay for *Clostridium difficile* toxin if patient is receiving antibiotics
4. Microscopic stool examination:
   a. Fecal leukocytes/fecal lactoferrin test for assessment of invasive bacterial etiology
   b. Ova, cysts, and parasites such as *Giardia intestinalis, Strongyloides, Entamoeba histolytica* (see Table 59-1)
   c. Acid-fast stain for *Mycobacterium, Cryptosporidium, Cyclospora, Isospora*
5. Blood culture for bacteria; mycobacteria; detection of cytomegalovirus
6. If symptoms persist, if results of preceding workup are negative, and/or if patient is severely ill:
   a. Obtain abdominal radiographs to detect pneumatosis intestinalis (present in severe cytomegalovirus colitis)
   b. Consider esophagogastroduodenoscopy or colonoscopy with intestinal biopsy for histology, culture, special stains, molecular diagnosis

---

In early studies, no infectious etiology of enteric disease was found in a large proportion of patients with AIDS. Subsequent studies demonstrate that aggressive workup, including endoscopy with biopsy, substantially improves diagnostic yield.[69,70] These data, coupled with the broad range of pathogens seen in this compromised population (even in the era of HAART), support an intensive diagnostic approach when reasonable empiric therapy fails.[72]

NEC of the cecum and surrounding tissues (typhlitis) is a life-threatening condition that occurs in profoundly neutropenic patients, usually people undergoing aggressive chemotherapy (with or without irradiation) for malignancy.[73] Typhlitis also has been described in patients with AIDS.[68] Typhlitis manifests as fever, abdominal pain, tenderness (especially right-sided, lower-quadrant tenderness mimicking that of acute appendicitis), and diarrhea. Evidence of right-sided colonic inflammation can be obtained using computed tomography, ultrasonography, and plain radiography.[73]

An approach to evaluation of the immunocompromised host with inflammatory enteritis is summarized in Box 59-1.

Specific Agents

Cytomegalovirus. Gastrointestinal tract disease due to CMV occurs almost exclusively in the setting of immunodeficiency, including AIDS, organ transplantation, cancer chemotherapy, and corticosteroid therapy.[74–76] Colitis, the most common manifestation of enteric CMV disease, is characterized by fever, diarrhea, abdominal pain, and hematochezia. Abdominal radiographs can reveal pneumatosis intestinalis or free peritoneal air.[67] Endoscopic findings in patients with CMV-associated inflammatory colitis range from localized hyperemia to deep ulceration with overlying exudate and necrosis; the most common finding is mild patchy colitis. If CMV is suspected, biopsy should be performed even if the mucosa appears normal grossly. Pp65 antigen detection and/or CMV DNA detection with polymerase chain reaction technology can aid diagnosis.[76,77] Complications of CMV colitis include intestinal perforation, severe hemorrhage, peritonitis, small-bowel obstruction, and toxic megacolon. Ganciclovir therapy has been shown to be beneficial for CMV colitis when initiated early in the disease.[74,76] Ganciclovir induction therapy should be administered for 3 to 6 weeks, depending on the degree of involvement and immunologic state of the patient; maintenance therapy may be required thereafter.[78]

Cryptosporidium. Cryptosporidial infection is one of the most common causes of enteric disease in patients with AIDS, occurring in 10% to 20% of adults with AIDS in the U.S.[79,80] It may be less common in children and has been decreasing in frequency in the age of ART.[81] Typical AIDS-related diarrheal syndromes consist of profuse, watery, and often bloody diarrhea associated with anorexia and weight loss; death is common.

***Mycobacterium avium* complex.** MAC infections are common in patients with AIDS and low CD4+ T-lymphocyte counts.[82] Signs and symptoms usually are nonspecific and include fever, night sweats, malaise, and diarrhea. The small intestine appears to be involved more commonly than the colon. Mucosal changes include erythema, edema, friability, and, occasionally, small erosions and fine white nodules.

Fungi. Local or systemic fungal infections can cause chronic inflammatory enteritis.[83,84] Fungal pathogens include *Candida* spp., which can cause chronic, bloody, or nonbloody diarrhea; *Paracoccidioides brasiliensis* (South American blastomycosis), which causes a granulomatous or ulcerative lesion in the gastrointestinal tract; *Histoplasma capsulatum*, which can manifest with ulceration, bleeding, or obstruction; and the phycomycoses, which can cause abdominal pain, diarrhea, gastrointestinal tract bleeding, and peritonitis.

MANAGEMENT

Fluid loss is the most important consequence of acute gastroenteritis. The primary aims of management are aggressive rehydration and replacement of electrolytes by oral or intravenous routes, maintenance of blood volume and acid–base balance, and replacement of ongoing diarrheal losses. Nutritional support also is important, especially in immunocompromised and malnourished patients, who are prone to persistent illness. Early feeding minimizes caloric deficit and stimulates repair of the intestinal brush border.[85] Breastfeeding of infants should be continued, especially in developing countries, adding the benefit of passively acquired protective factors. In severe persistent inflammatory enteritis in which absorption is compromised, parenteral nutrition is considered.

Antimicrobial therapy is reserved for the small numbers of patients with suspected or proven bacterial causes of diarrhea in whom benefit is likely.[38] Empiric antibiotic therapy is appropriate in the following patients with inflammatory enteritis: (1) the severely ill patient in whom there is a strong suspicion of bacterial dysentery; (2) immunocompromised people, including patients with AIDS and recipients of immunosuppressive drugs; (3) infants <3 months of age with *Salmonella* infection (who are at high risk of bloodstream infection (BSI)); (4) patients with hemoglobinopathy or asplenia; and (5) people with a high likelihood of a treatable cause according to history, physical findings, or epidemiologic factors. Antibiotics not recommended in patients in whom Shiga toxin-producing *E. coli* infection is suspected (typically presenting afebrile with bloody diarrhea), because such therapy may increase the risk of hemolytic–uremic syndrome,[86] although this is controversial.[87]

Antibiotics hasten clinical improvement in people with shigellosis and severe, *Campylobacter* enteritis if given early in the disease.[87] Therapy also shortens duration of fecal shedding of these organisms and of *Y. enterocolitica*. In developed countries, trimethoprim-sulfamethoxazole has long been effective empiric treatment for suspected shigellosis in children. However, increasing antibiotic resistance renders this agent ineffective in many cases. Antibiotic susceptibility testing should be performed on patient isolates, and clinicians should be aware of susceptibility patterns in their area. Cefixime has in vitro activity against most

TABLE 59-6. Use of Antimicrobial Therapy in Inflammatory Enteritis

Antimicrobial Therapy	Enteropathogen
Effective clinically	*Shigella*, enteroinvasive *Escherichia coli*
Decreased excretion	*Shigella*, enteroinvasive *E. coli*, *Yersinia enterocolitica*, *Campylobacter jejuni*
Indicated in certain hosts[a]	*Salmonella*, *Campylobacter*, enteropathogenic *E. coli*, enterotoxigenic *E. coli*, *Clostridium difficile*, *Yersinia enterocolitica*
Unclear effect	Enteroaggregative *E. coli*, *Aeromonas*, noncholera *Vibrio* spp.
Controversial[b]	Enterohemorrhagic *E. coli*

[a]Antimicrobial agents warranted for patients with severe colitis or with increased risk of disseminated disease: infants <3 months of age, persons with immunodeficiency disorders (including acquired immunodeficiency syndrome, hemoglobinopathy, and asplenia) as well as recipients of immunosuppressive drugs.
[b]See text.

strains of *Shigella* that are resistant to ampicillin or trimethoprim-sulfamethoxazole and is safe for use in children.[88] One dose of ciprofloxacin usually is adequate for treatment of all *Shigella* species except *Shigella dysenteriae* 1; however, fluoroquinolones are approved by the U.S. FDA for use only in people ≥18 years of age. A Scientific Working Group of the World Health Organization has raised the possibility that the efficacy of fluoroquinolones for shigellosis may outweigh the small risk of adverse effects in selected children.[89] The role of antibiotics in treating people with specific causes of bacterial gastroenteritis is summarized in Table 59-6.

Nonspecific therapies other than antimicrobial agents are available for symptomatic treatment of patients with diarrhea. Bismuth subsalicylate has some effect in decreasing stool volume and illness in travelers' diarrhea.[90] One study showed a decrease in frequency and volume of diarrhea in children.[91] Antiperistaltic agents (loperamide and diphenoxylate hydrochloride) and antiemetic agents can be effective in the management of diarrhea in adults; however, their use is not recommended in infants and young children as safety and efficacy data are lacking.[92] Antiperistaltic agents have been demonstrated to worsen the clinical course of disease due to *Shigella* spp., *C. difficile*, and *E. coli* O157:H7.

Infants with Inflammatory Enteritis

An infant <3 months of age with inflammatory enteritis should be managed cautiously, because of the propensity of *Salmonella* strains to cause BSI with disseminated suppurative foci in this age group.[93,94] Although the precise frequency of BSI is not known, a prospective study of children with gastroenteritis due to *Salmonella* spp. reported BSI in 6 of 91 (2 of the 6 infants were ≤3 months of age).[93] Infants who appear toxic with diarrhea as the prominent feature of illness should be hospitalized, cultures of blood and cerebrospinal fluid should be obtained, and intravenous antibiotics with a spectrum of activity against enteric pathogens, as well as common invasive pathogens, should be given. In the infant ≤3 months of age who does not appear toxic, one panel of experts recommended obtaining blood or stool cultures if the stool contains blood or leukocytes.[94] Cefotaxime, ceftriaxone, and sometimes ampicillin are effective for treatment of invasive focal *Salmonella* infections.[95] If stools contain blood or leukocytes, antimicrobial therapy may be initiated pending culture results. The value of antimicrobial therapy for *Salmonella* gastroenteritis without BSI has not been established. There is no evidence of clinical benefit of antimicrobial therapy in otherwise healthy children and adults with nonsevere *Salmonella* diarrhea.

60   Necrotizing Enterocolitis

C. Michael Cotten and Daniel K. Benjamin, Jr

Necrotizing enterocolitis (NEC) is the most common neonatal gastrointestinal emergency. NEC results in substantial morbidity and mortality, particularly in premature infants. Less commonly, NEC is observed in older children. Incomplete gastrointestinal development and underlying gastrointestinal pathology likely allow bacterial translocation and concurrent infection with enteric organisms.

EPIDEMIOLOGY

NEC affects predominantly premature infants in neonatal intensive care units (NICUs). Incidence of NEC is 1 to 3 cases per 1000 live births. Prevalence among very-low-birthweight (VLBW, <1500 grams at birth) infants is approximately 10%, and has not changed significantly in recent years. Incidence among VLBW infants varies by geographic location, ranging from 0.3% to 22%. Incidence of NEC increases with lower gestational age and birthweight, and is lower among infants fed human milk.[1] NEC does not have seasonal, geographic, or sex predilection.[2,3] In the most recent report on hospital morbidity and mortality among very preterm infants from the National Institutes of Child Health and Human Development (NICHD) Neonatal Research Network, 11% of infants born at tertiary centers, at or earlier than 28 weeks of gestation, had NEC, approximately one-half requiring surgery.[4]

NEC is associated with prolonged hospital stay[1,5] and increased risk of neurodevelopmental impairment, particularly in survivors of severe NEC that required surgical treatment.[6,7] The overall mortality of VLBW premature infants has remained steady, and is approximately 50% for infants with NEC requiring surgery.[1,8,9]

NEC in full-term infants often occurs in the first postnatal week, and associated factors suggest that mucosal injury and ischemia are important (Table 60-1).[10–12] Cyanotic congenital heart disease has been a known risk factor for NEC for over 30 years, with the highest risk among infants with hypoplastic left heart syndrome.[13] In a multicenter review of 30 term and near term infants with NEC, affected infants were highly likely to have congenital heart disease, polycythemia, or documented early-onset sepsis (and longer antimicrobial courses); only one infant was fed human milk.[14]

Focal isolated gastrointestinal perforation (FIP) without NEC occurs in the first few postnatal days of extremely-low-birthweight (ELBW, <1000 grams at birth) infants. The usual site is the distal ileum. Perforation has been associated with the combination of treatment with corticosteroids and indomethacin.[15,16] Microbiology of peritonitis is distinctive, with predominant organisms being *Candida* species or *Staphylococcus epidermidis*. Hypotheses regarding pathophysiology of isolated perforation focus on risk factors related to vascular and developmental signaling pathways. FIP should be considered a separate entity from NEC.[17]

PATHOLOGIC FINDINGS AND PATHOGENESIS

The pathophysiology of NEC is not completely understood, but multiple factors likely contribute without any one being both necessary and sufficient alone. The combination of immature and highly immunoreactive intestine with poor motility, an imbalance in perfusion, and variations in extent and diversity of microbial colonization all likely contribute[18,19] (Box 60-1).

The most common sites of NEC in preterm infants are the watershed areas of the intestine, the distal ileum and proximal colon, although lesions occur throughout the intestine.[20] The earliest pathologic lesions are superficial mucosal ulceration, submucosal hemorrhage and edema. The initially trivial infiltration of acute inflammatory cells speaks against primary infection as causative. More likely, suboptimal barrier function of the immature intestinal mucosa allows passage of bacteria and undigested food antigens.[21] In addition, histologic evaluation of resected bowel in patients with NEC indicates that loss of intestinal epithelia through apoptosis or necrosis precedes inflammation and may be a key to pathogenesis in some individuals. Immature intestinal epithelia may be more susceptible to apoptotic injury, further compromising an already immature structural barrier.[18,22] Hepatobiliary gas or intramural gas (pneumatosis intestinalis) appearing as bubbles or linear lucencies, likely produced by bacteria invading the submucosa, are pathognomonic for NEC (Figure 60-1). In severe cases, coagulative transmural necrosis and perforation are noted. If the disease does not progress to transmural necrosis and perforation, healing can occur by epithelialization and proliferation of fibroblasts and granulation tissue. Strictures can follow.[23,24]

TABLE 60-1. Factors and Conditions Associated with Necrotizing Enterocolitis

Premature	Full-Term
Lower gestational age	Cyanotic congenital heart disease
Feeding	Polycythemia
H2 blocking agents	Exchange transfusions
Empiric antibiotics	Perinatal asphyxia
	Small for gestational age/intrauterine growth restriction (IUGR)
	Umbilical catheters
	Maternal pre-eclampsia
	Antenatal cocaine
	Premature rupture of membranes
	Milk allergy
	Gestational diabetes

BOX 60-1. Limitations of the Preterm Infant's Intestine That May Contribute to Risk of Necrotizing Enterocolitis

IMMUNOLOGIC FACTORS

Decreased secretory immunoglobulin A
Decreased intestinal lymphocytes
Poor antibody response
Immaturity of innate immune system

LUMINAL FACTORS

Lower H^+ output in stomach
Lower proteolytic enzyme activity

IMMATURE INTESTINAL BARRIER

Less protective mucin barrier
Less protective microvillous membrane
Higher permeability

LOWER/LESS ORGANIZED MOTILITY

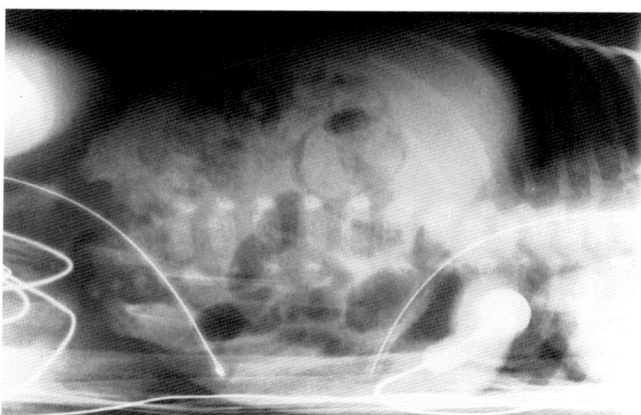

Figure 60-1. Abdominal radiograph of an infant with necrotizing enterocolitis and pneumatosis intestinalis. (From Willoughby RE Jr, Pickering LK. Necrotizing enterocolitis and infection. Clin Perinatol 1994;21:307–315.)

Clinical NEC is likely the "final common pathway" of multiple combinations and interactions of immaturity, injury, bacteria, and substrate.[20,21,25] The pathogenesis of NEC in preterm infants likely involves contributions of the presence of some substrate (more likely formula than human milk) in an immature intestine. Intestinal immaturity is characterized functionally by poor motility, digestion, and absorption, an imbalance in microvascular tone, accompanied by a strong likelihood of abnormal microbial colonization in the context of weak barrier function and suboptimal immune defenses and a highly immunoreactive intestinal mucosa.[18,19,26]

Most investigators think that major perinatal hypoxic–ischemic events are not likely to contribute substantially to NEC pathogenesis in preterm infants, but hypoxia and ischemia influence microvascular tone related to the relative production of vascular regulators such as nitric oxide and endothelin, which probably play a downstream role in the pathogenic cascade resulting in NEC.[19,27] More weight is given to processes allowing microbial invasion of intestinal epithelia and submucosa.

The human intestine adapts to gradual colonization and increased microbial stimulation by modifying the epithelial innate immune response. Innate immunity factors must exhibit balanced response to colonization, with proinflammatory aspects preventing bacterial overgrowth and invasion, and anti-inflammatory factors preventing overwhelming inflammation responding to inevitable colonization that weakens barrier function and may move intestinal cells towards apoptosis.[18,28]

Toll-like receptor 4 (TLR4) appears to be a key pattern recognition receptor of the innate immune system in developing intestine. It is located on intestinal cell surfaces in larger numbers in newborns than adults. It responds to stimulation by lipopolysaccharide (LPS), a bacterial cell wall component. Signal via TLR4 initiates synthesis of proinflammatory mediators. TLR4 is increased in fetal cells compared with adult cells,[29] and IκB, which regulates the proinflammatory transcription factor nuclear factor κB (NF-κB), is developmentally underexpressed.[30] Such differences between the fetal and the mature intestine in immune balance may be a basis for the excessive and potentially damaging inflammatory response that leads to NEC. These observations suggest that enterocytes in the preterm infant, which have resided in a germ-free intrauterine environment, are not prepared for the excessive stimulation of initial postnatal colonization and antigen exposure.[19]

Epidemiologic observations support an important but not singular role for microbes. Clustered cases have been observed in NICUs.[31,32] Associations have been noted between clinical practices likely to modify colonization, including prolonged antibiotic exposure and antacid exposure.[33,34] "Inappropriate" colonization is one hypothesis for NEC,[35] but molecular methodologies to

characterize intestinal flora in preterm babies with and without NEC have failed to find consistent pathogens. NEC, however, is associated with less microbial diversity, as evidenced by culture or molecular methodologies such as 16S-ribosomal DNA with PCR-denaturing gradient gel electrophoresis (PCR-DGGE).[36–38] No single pathogen has been associated consistently with NEC, although gram-negative enteric species predominate.[39] Bacterial toxins (e.g., hemolysins of staphylococci, enterotoxins of *Escherichia coli*, and exotoxins of clostridia) have been associated with NEC. In one center, clostridia species were more likely to be found in stool of infants with NEC compared with others;[40] however, bacteria identified from stool, blood, or peritoneal fluid of infants with NEC also colonize the gastrointestinal tract of asymptomatic infants in NICUs.[41]

Viruses (e.g., rotavirus, norovirus, and cytomegalovirus) have been identified in ill infants during NEC clusters, but case-control studies sometimes have demonstrated similar rates in well infants. NEC outbreaks have been associated with illness in caregivers, reinforcing the need for infection control practices.[42,43] Evidence for cytomegalovirus as one cause of NEC-like illness is strong, with identification by immunoperoxidase staining of cytomegalovirus-positive intracytoplasmic viral inclusions in resected intestinal tissues.[44,45]

CLINICAL MANIFESTATIONS, DIFFERENTIAL DIAGNOSIS, CLINICAL APPROACH

Although there has been progress in understanding mechanisms involved in NEC pathogenesis, diagnostic and therapeutic approaches have not progressed to alter prevalence or severity of outcomes. NEC's clinical course can vary from a slow indolent process to a fulminant course with lethal progression over hours. Classic signs usually follow initiation of feedings and include abdominal distention, sometimes with abdominal wall discoloration or erythema, and bloody stools. However, bloody stools are not always present in infants with NEC, especially in the most premature infants.[43] Many patients have less specific signs indicative of generalized sepsis (Box 60-2). Thrombocytopenia and low or high white blood cell counts are common. Systemic hypotension and falling leukocyte and platelet counts combined with worsening metabolic acidosis suggest worsening disease.[19]

Differential diagnoses include medical conditions associated with decreased intestinal motility, such as bacterial or viral infection, metabolic disorders including hypothyroidism, and congenital heart disease. NEC is suspected when gastrointestinal signs predominate. Infectious enterocolitis, small-bowel volvulus, isolated gastrointestinal perforation, colonic aganglionosis with enterocolitis, and other surgical diseases of the intestinal tract should be considered.[19,43]

Confirmation of NEC depends on radiographic findings (see Figure 60-1). Pneumatosis intestinalis can be subtle, but is pathognomonic. Intestinal distention with thickened and dilated loops of small bowel is common, but is nonspecific. Pneumoperitoneum (best assessed on a cross-table or left lateral decubitus

---

BOX 60-2. Initial Signs of Necrotizing Enterocolitis

Feeding intolerance (decreased oral intake, vomiting, increased gastric residual fluid)
Lethargy
Temperature instability
Apnea
Metabolic acidosis
Shock
Disseminated intravascular coagulation
Ileus
Clinitest-positive stools
Heme-positive stools or heme-positive vomitus

PART II Clinical Syndromes and Cardinal Features of Infectious Diseases: Approach to Diagnosis and Initial Management

SECTION H Gastrointestinal Tract Infections and Intoxications

TABLE 60-2. Modified Bell Staging for Necrotizing Enterocolitis

Stage	Classification	Systemic Signs	Intestinal Signs	Radiograph
IA	Suspected NEC	Temperature instability, apnea, bradycardia, lethargy	Increased pregavage residuals, midabdominal distention, emesis, heme-positive stool	Normal or intestinal dilatation, ileus
IB	Suspected NEC	Same as above	Bright-red blood from rectum	Same as above
IIA	Proven NEC – mildly ill	Same as above	Same as above, plus absent bowel sounds, with or without abdominal wall tenderness	Intestinal dilation, ileus, pneumatosis intestinalis
IIB	Proven NEC – moderately ill	Same as above, plus mild metabolic acidosis and mild thrombocytopenia	Same as above, plus absent bowel sounds, definite tenderness, with or without abdominal cellulitis or right lower-quadrant mass	Same as stage IIA, plus definite ascites
IIIA	Advanced NEC – severely ill, bowel intact	Same as stage IIB, plus hypotension, bradycardia, severe apnea, combined respiratory and metabolic acidosis, disseminated intravascular coagulation, and neutropenia	Same as above, plus signs of generalized peritonitis, marked tenderness, and distention of the abdomen	Same as stage IIA, plus definite ascites
IIIB	Advanced NEC – severely ill, bowel perforated	Same as stage IIIA	Same as stage IIIA	Same as stage IIB, plus pneumoperitoneum

radiograph) or presence of intra-abdominal fluid is a serious sign indicating need for immediate surgical intervention. Although increased exhaled breath hydrogen, elevated serum levels of interleukin 6, neutrophil CD64, C-reactive protein (CRP), endotoxin, α-antitrypsin, stool-reducing substances and specific short-chain fatty acid profiles, and ultrasound have been suggested as early findings associated with NEC, none has been introduced into clinical practice.[46–48] Diagnostic criteria for NEC were originally developed by Bell and Conorkers. Modified criteria provide uniformity for therapeutic decision-making[49] (Table 60-2).

Blood and peritoneal fluid cultures are positive in approximately 30% of preterm infants with advanced NEC. Isolates usually reflect intestinal bacterial flora, e.g., *Enterococcus*, *Enterobacter*, and *Klebsiella* species. Coagulase-negative staphylococci (CoNS) or *Candida* species are isolated from peritoneal cultures in <20% of NEC cases.[8,50] In 96 cases of neonatal culture-positive peritonitis, Enterobacteriaceae were recovered from 75% of cases with NEC, whereas *Candida* species and coagulase-negative staphylococci were found in 44% and 50% of cases with focal intestinal perforation, respectively.[50]

MANAGEMENT

Management largely is supportive and is directed at preventing progression, restoring homeostasis, and minimizing complications. Oral feedings should be withheld, and a large-bore nasogastric tube placed with intermittent suction applied. Intravenous access is required to provide fluid, electrolytes, nutrition, and antimicrobial therapy. The duration of restriction of enteral feeding should be based upon radiographic findings and clinical status. Many patients whose signs resolve and whose NEC does not progress beyond stage I (see Table 60-2) are fed after 48 to 72 hours. If the period of enteral restriction is longer (e.g., >7 days, common if ≥stage II), total parenteral nutrition should be considered. Usually low volumes of elemental formula or mother's milk are used initially to allow optimal nutrient absorption and avoid osmolar challenge and further potential injury to the intestinal mucosa; however, few randomized clinical trials have been performed to guide feeding strategies after NEC.[51] In a prospective observational study, serial CRP levels in the days following NEC diagnosis had apparent value.[52] When less severe disease was observed and radiographs normalized, CRP was persistently low. These infants were safely fed earlier and antibiotics stopped sooner (at 48 hours if cultures were negative) than those whose CRP remained elevated. Abnormal CRP values in infants with stage II NEC returned to normal at a mean of 9 days from onset, except in 7 infants, 4 of whom required exploratory surgery for stricture formation and 3 for intra-abdominal abscesses and peritonitis.[52]

Because microorganisms have been implicated in NEC pathogenesis, and can invade intestinal epithelium and enter the bloodstream, and because NEC clinically can resemble septicemia, blood, stool, urine, and cerebrospinal fluid cultures usually are obtained, and antibiotics are administered intravenously. Recommendations for empiric therapy vary among experts.[19,53] Initial therapy with ampicillin and gentamicin is common. Some experts also recommend the addition of an antibiotic active against *Bacteroides* species (e.g., metronidazole or clindamycin), especially if perforation is likely. Vancomycin may be used if infection with a *Staphylococcus* species is suspected.[54] Clindamycin has been associated with increased strictures following stage II NEC in one small randomized study.[55] The empiric use of vancomycin for possible coagulase-negative staphylococci must be balanced against the risk of selecting vancomycin-resistant enterococci. Reinforcement of strict handwashing is essential. Infection control measures such as barrier isolation and cohorting of affected infants and personnel may abort epidemics.

Abdominal radiography is used to assess NEC progression and to identify perforation or other indications for surgery. Radiographic studies usually are repeated every 6 hours during escalation of signs. Progressive neutropenia or thrombocytopenia may be useful to identify worsening conditions and provide indications for exploratory surgery. Fluid and electrolyte status is monitored strictly because third-space losses can occur with intestinal inflammation and edema. Severe metabolic acidosis can result from poor perfusion and often is difficult to control. Indications for surgery include pneumoperitoneum or cellulitis of the anterior abdominal wall, which are signs of perforation or a gangrenous bowel. The classic operative strategy is conservative, with resection of grossly gangrenous bowel and creation of a proximal enterostomy. Drain placement rather than extensive laparoscopic surgery also is used. A prospective observational trial that compared use of drains with laparotomy, and a randomized trial comparing the two strategies have been completed.[7,56] Neither strategy appears to provide clear benefit. In a multicenter observational trial of infants with surgical NEC, mortality was not different for management by laparotomy vs. placement of a drain, but neurodevelopmental outcome was better among those managed with laparotomy.[9] A clinical trial that includes long-term follow-up is ongoing.

OUTCOME

NEC exerts major impact on developing infants, most likely due to the significant immunologic stimulation in the inflamed intestine. Preterm infants with NEC, particularly surgical NEC, have markedly higher risk for developmental delay than those without NEC.[57] Approximately 50% of neonates with NEC requiring surgery die.[1,8,58] Morbidity related to long-term effects on the gastrointestinal tract occurs in 10% to 30% of affected children, especially among those with NEC requiring surgery. Acute and chronic complications are listed in Box 60-3. One of the most serious complications is short-bowel syndrome, which in the mildest form requires extensive parenteral nutrition (with attendant infectious risks from prolonged venous access) and in the extreme form requires bowel transplant.[59] Serious nutritional consequences result if >70% of the intestine is removed. Preservation of the terminal ileum and the ileocecal valve improves long-term enteral nutrition and function, but predilection of NEC to injure this area makes preservation difficult.

Bacterial overgrowth is a common consequence of short-gut syndrome. Gastric hypersecretion is characteristic in short-gut syndrome. Treatment with antacids and histamine antagonists leads to increased colonization by oral flora in the stomach and upper intestine. Bacterial overgrowth can be exacerbated when resection of the ileocecal valve eliminates the distal barrier to colonic bacteria, which then reflux into the small intestine. Bacterial overgrowth can result in decreased mucosal hydrolases, causing carbohydrate malabsorption and osmotic diarrhea. Deconjugation of bile salts in the small intestine by bacteria leads to malabsorption of fat and fat-soluble vitamins. Bacterial overgrowth also can result in decreased intestinal transit time.

The diagnosis of bacterial overgrowth requires the isolation of >10^5 colony-forming units/mL of bacteria from small intestinal fluid specimen; isolation of strictly anaerobic bacteria, such as the *Bacteroides fragilis* group, also establishes the diagnosis. The hydrogen breath test after a lactulose challenge is the most reliable noninvasive marker of bacterial overgrowth. If available, a fasting breath hydrogen screening test can be helpful; values of hydrogen >40 ppm are indicative of bacterial overgrowth. An empiric trial of antibiotics sometimes is given when adverse intestinal signs are present. No single regimen has proved effective for overgrowth. Although some clinicians may perceive a potential benefit of use of probiotics after a lengthy course of antibiotics in infants with short gut after NEC, bacteremia with probiotic agents used in this situation has been reported.[60]

RECENT ADVANCES

Three recent reviews present advances in understanding of developing intestinal immunology, the importance of the innate immune system, and the importance of local nitric oxide production.[18,19,43] Advances in clinically available diagnostic tests and clear-cut better prevention strategies and therapies derived from enhanced understanding of underlying pathophysiology, beyond supporting use of human milk, antimicrobial stewardship, and infection control, are still in development.

PREVENTION

Over years, the large-scale practice of encouraging use of human milk as the primary nutritional source has resulted in reduced rates of NEC in large cohorts when mother's milk is used versus formula.[61,62] In a single multicenter randomized clinical trial in which a human milk-derived human milk fortifier was compared with bovine milk-derived fortifier, NEC was significantly reduced among those receiving an exclusively human milk-derived diet.[63] The biologic basis for protective effect of human milk includes presence of substances that modify bacterial colonization; immune and growth factors, including lactoferrin, platelet-activating factor (PAF) acetyl-hydrolase; and coincident intestinal colonization with commensal bacteria.[21] Omega-3 fatty acids, found in human milk, appear to have anti-inflammatory effects, with a reduction in the levels of PAF and leukotrienes in the intestinal mucosa.

A meta-analysis of controlled studies has suggested a reduction in the incidence of NEC when antenatal corticosteroids were used, and animal models suggest that corticosteroid administration is associated with maturation of the intestinal barrier, limitation of bacterial colonization, and reduced inflammation.[20]

Although timing of NEC in preterm infants, i.e., after initiation of feedings, implies that feeding, even with human milk, plays a substantial role, slow advancement of feeding may be better tolerated than a long delay before feedings are initiated; however, it is unknown whether slower vs. faster advancement of feeding reduces the risk of NEC.[64] Long periods of not feeding can cause intestinal cell atrophy and worsened inflammatory responses that predispose to NEC.[18]

The authors of one single-center study suggest that L-arginine supplementation may reduce NEC risk by increasing intestinal nitric oxide synthesis.[29] However, additional appropriately powered studies are needed. Recombinant PAF acetyl-hydrolase, the enzyme found in human milk that degrades PAF, has been proposed as a preventive agent.[30] In a double-blind placebo-controlled study in septic neonates, the immunomodulating agent pentoxifylline was shown to have reduced NEC incidence,[31] but this study needs replication. In a multicenter trial of glutamine (micronutrient thought to mitigate intestinal stress), there was no reduction observed in the incidence of infection or death (the primary outcome variables) or NEC.[65]

Multiple strategies of alteration of intestinal flora have been studied. Prophylactic use of antibiotics has been evaluated in small studies, with conflicting results.[66] Supplementing formula with an immunoglobulin A (IgA)-IgG preparation was shown to reduce NEC in one study,[2] but this has not been replicated.[67,68] Lowering intestinal pH may reduce NEC risk,[33,69] and in support of this hypothesis, use of antacids was associated with increased odds of NEC in a large multicenter cohort.[33]

Direct manipulation of the intestinal flora with probiotics has been considered, with some experts believing that the published clinical trials warrant change in practice.[70] Others recommend caution until a multicenter trial is performed in a population of extremely preterm infants using a probiotic product with preclinical testing that validates product consistency. The U.S. Food and Drug Administration has not approved the administration of a microorganism in preterm infants, and probiotic products have not been subjected to rigorous quality control during manufacturing. The contents of probiotic products, although appearing safe in individual studies, may not be reproducible according to drug or pharmaceutical standards.[19] The debate intensifies because of growing understanding of the importance of microbial colonization and host response, and the persistence of NEC among extremely preterm infants despite other advances in care.

Investigators also are assessing the potential value of prebiotics (compounds that enhance growth of potentially beneficial microbes) in NEC. Human milk contains >200 human milk oligosaccharides, comprising the third largest component of milk after lactose and lipid. Oligosaccharides contribute to innate immunity by preventing attachment of potential pathogens to intestinal lining and by promoting colonization by a healthy gut microbiota.[71] It may be possible to add individual human milk oligosaccharides to milk to reduce the risk of NEC.[72]

PART II Clinical Syndromes and Cardinal Features of Infectious Diseases: Approach to Diagnosis and Initial Management

SECTION H Gastrointestinal Tract Infections

61

Enteric Diseases Transmitted Through Food, Water, and Zoonotic Exposures

Laura B. Gieraltowski, Sharon L. Roy, Aron J. Hall, and Anna Bowen

More than 200 known pathogens can be transmitted through ingestion of food or water contaminated with viruses, bacteria, parasites, microbial or chemical toxins, metals, and prions, or through contact with animals or their environments.[1] One of the most common illness types resulting from foodborne, waterborne, or zoonotic transmission is enteric disease. Symptoms of enteric illness range from mild gastroenteritis to life-threatening sepsis, neurologic, hepatic, ocular and renal syndromes. Despite improvements in water, sanitation and hygiene, foodborne, waterborne, and zoonotic enteric diseases remain major public health problems in developed as well as developing countries.

EPIDEMIOLOGY

Foodborne Disease

The epidemiology of enteric disease is changing rapidly. Large-scale industrialized production of food products and rapid national and international distribution of food have been introduced without failsafe hygienic precautions. These processes have led to the emergence of new food vehicles for recognized pathogens.[2] Antimicrobial resistance has become increasingly prevalent among strains of *Salmonella, Campylobacter,* and *Shigella* due in part to widespread use of antimicrobial agents administered to humans and feed animals.

From 1998 to 2008, 5059 single confirmed outbreaks of enteric disease affecting 156,469 people in the United States were reported to the Centers for Disease Control and Prevention (CDC).[3] The annual number of foodborne illnesses in the U.S. was estimated to be approximately 48 million illnesses, with 128,000 hospitalizations and 3000 deaths in 2007.[4,5] The highest reported rates for several important foodborne enteric pathogens, including *Salmonella* spp., *Campylobacter* spp., *E. coli* O157:H7, and *Shigella* spp., occur in children <5 years of age, suggesting that children are at higher risk for foodborne diseases than adults.[3] However, the highest rate of hospitalizations associated with norovirus, the leading cause of foodborne disease in the U.S.,[4] occurs in the elderly aged ≥65 years.[6] Overall, norovirus causes approximately 50% of recognized foodborne illnesses associated with outbreaks in the U.S. (Table 61-1).

Waterborne Disease

Enteric waterborne disease resembles disease resulting from contamination of food and can be caused by many of the pathogens generally associated with foodborne transmission. Large waterborne outbreaks resulting in enteric illness have been caused by *Campylobacter jejuni, E. coli* O157:H7, *Salmonella* Typhi, nontyphoid *Salmonella* spp., *Shigella* spp., chemical agents, hepatitis A, norovirus, *Giardia intestinalis,* and other agents.[7-19] Although *Cryptosporidium* spp. were implicated in only 15 (2.1%) enteric drinking-water outbreaks between 1971 and 2006, a single outbreak in Milwaukee accounted for an estimated 403,000 cases.[8,17] Agents most commonly reported to the CDC from 1971 to 2006 as the etiologies of drinking water-associated outbreaks are listed in Table 61-2. Between 1971 and 2006, 714 drinking water-associated outbreaks resulting in enteric illness, including gastroenteritis and hepatitis, were identified, comprising more than 576,000 illnesses and 76 deaths (CDC unpublished data).

While the annual number of reported drinking water-related outbreaks in the U.S. declined from 1980 through 2006, the annual number of reported recreational water-associated outbreaks increased during the same period. In 2006, the number of reported recreational water-associated outbreaks was >2.5-fold the number of reported drinking water-related outbreaks.[18,19] Recreational water illnesses (RWIs) are caused by pathogens transmitted by ingesting, inhaling aerosols of, or having contact with contaminated water in pools, hot tubs, interactive fountains, lakes, rivers,

TABLE 61-1. Foodborne Disease Outbreaks, Cases, and Deaths of Confirmed Etiology Reported to the Centers for Disease Control and Prevention 1998 to 2008

Disease Type	No. of Outbreaks (Total = 4779)	No. of Cases (Total = 153,392)	No. of Deaths
BACTERIAL			
Bacillus cereus	56	881	0
Brucella	4	14	0
Campylobacter	167	5012	0
Clostridium botulinum	29	106	5
Clostridium perfringens	253	13,182	5
Escherichia coli O157:H7	265	5644	21
Listeria monocytogenes	38	348	48
Salmonella	1291	37,394	58
Shigella	118	6103	1
Staphylococcus aureus	167	4818	3
Streptococcus group A	1	4	0
Vibrio cholerae O1	1	6	0
Vibrio parahaemolyticus	37	1056	0
Yersinia enterocolitica	11	100	0
Other bacteria	2	69	0
CHEMICAL			
Ciguatoxin	152	615	1
Histamine (scombroid)	28	166	0
Mushrooms	11	72	2
Paralytic shellfish	9	28	0
Other chemicals	17	485	1
PARASITIC			
Cryptosporidium spp.	13	354	
Cyclospora cayetanensis	28	1571	0
Giardia intestinalis	15	354	0
Trichinella spiralis	9	40	0
Other parasites	1	18	0
VIRAL			
Hepatitis A	75	2138	8
Norovirus	1974	72,337	22
Other viruses	7	489	0

Modified from Centers for Disease Control and Prevention. CDC Foodborne Disease Outbreak Surveillance System, Unpublished data, downloaded: April 26, 2011.

Etiologic Agent	Outbreaks	
	Number	%
Giardia	129	32.9
Chemicals	57	14.5
Shigella species	4	11.5
Norovirus	37	9.4
Campylobacter species	30	7.7
Hepatitis A	29	7.4
Cryptosporidium species	16	4.1
Nontyphoid *Salmonella*	16	4.1
Escherichia coli O157:H7	12	3.1
Salmonella Typhi	5	1.3
Entamoeba histolytica	3	0.8
Enterotoxigenic *Escherichia coli*	3	0.8
Plesiomonas shigelloides	2	0.5
Vibrio cholerae	2	0.5
Yersinia enterocolitica	2	0.5
Cyclospora cayetanensis	1	0.3
Entamoeba species	1	0.3
Helicobacter canadensis	1	0.3
Rotavirus	1	0.3
Total	392	100%

[a]*A total of 714 drinking water outbreaks associated with enteric illness, including acute gastroenteritis and hepatitis A, were reported to CDC during 1971–2006. Of these, 346 had an unidentified etiology. The remaining 368 outbreaks had at least one etiologic agent identified; of these, 19 had multiple etiologic agents per outbreak.*[CDC unpublished data]

oceans, etc. RWIs also can be caused by chemicals in the water or those that volatilize from the water and cause indoor air quality problems. Enteric illness is the most commonly reported RWI, and more than 4000 cases were reported in the U.S. during 2005. *Cryptosporidium* has become the leading cause of enteric illness outbreaks associated with treated recreational water (e.g., pools and interactive fountains). *Cryptosporidium*, which is chlorine tolerant, accounted for approximately 68% of the outbreaks associated with treated recreational water reported to CDC during 1997–2006. In contrast, *Cryptosporidium* was implicated in only 13% of enteric illness outbreaks associated with untreated recreational water during this time period; other implicated pathogens in untreated recreational water outbreaks included norovirus (21%), all *E. coli* (19%), *Shigella* spp. (13%), and *Giardia* (5%).[19]

Zoonotic Disease

Enteric infections can also be acquired by direct and indirect contact with wild or farm animals, chicks, reptiles, amphibians, and occasionally, pets such as dogs and cats. Exposure to animals can occur in many venues, including in the wild and in farms, zoos, fairs, animal swap meets, petting zoos, camps, shopping malls, schools, and homes. Most households in the U.S. have one or more pets.[20] Additionally, the number of households with nontraditional pets, such as imported non-native species, indigenous wildlife, and wildlife hybrids, has increased over time. Among nontraditional pets, reptiles pose a particular risk for zoonotic disease because of their high *Salmonella* carriage rates.[21] Outbreaks due to a number of pathogens, including *Salmonella*

spp., *E. coli* O157:H7 and other Shiga-toxin-producing *E. coli* (STEC); *Campylobacter* spp., *Giardia intestinalis*, and *Cryptosporidium* spp.,[22–41] have resulted from various routes of zoonotic exposure. Direct contact with animals, particularly young animals; contamination of food, water, or the environment; and inadequate hand hygiene have all been cited as reasons for zoonotic infection. Children often are disproportionately affected and children <5 years of age are at higher risk for serious infections, as are pregnant women, the elderly, and people of all ages with immunodeficiencies.[21] Public health officials, physicians, and families should be aware of the potential for animals to serve as a source of enteric illness in humans.

PATHOGENESIS AND CLINICAL SYNDROMES

Enteric diseases are often classified according to the mechanism of pathogenesis: ingestion of various classes of chemicals or preformed toxins, in vivo production of bacterial toxins, direct pathogen attachment and local invasion, or disseminated infection. Considering the clinical syndrome is more useful for diagnosis of enteric illness. The cause of an enteric illness is suggested by the clinical symptoms, the incubation period, and epidemiologic clues. Laboratory testing is required to confirm the identity of specific pathogens. An outbreak should be suspected when ≥2 people who have shared a common exposure (e.g., food, water, or animal) develop the same acute illness, most often characterized by nausea, vomiting, diarrhea, systemic, or neurologic symptoms. For additional information, refer to Table 61-3 and pathogen-specific chapters.

DIAGNOSIS

Epidemiologic Clues

The incubation period, clinical syndrome, and exposure history – including foods consumed and how they were prepared, as well as water and animal exposures – provide clues to the pathogenic etiology of enteric disease, but a definitive diagnosis requires laboratory confirmation. The incubation period often is underestimated or unknown. Patients and clinicians may focus incorrectly on the most recent meals and fail to consider water or animals as potential sources of disease transmission. Young children can become infected through person-to-person transmission or transmission via fomites without eating the implicated food, ingesting the implicated water, or directly handling animals. A careful exposure history should include animal contact, drinking water source, recreational water use, and food and beverages consumed during at least the previous 4 days.

It is rare that a food, water, or animal source can be implicated definitively using data from a single ill patient. Interviews with several ill people might identify a shared exposure and permit calculation of the median incubation period. However, incrimination of the responsible vehicle might require performing a case-control or a cohort study and also may be supported by laboratory testing of the implicated vehicle. Interviewing both ill and non-ill people can yield information to support an epidemiologic association between specific exposures and developing illness.

Foods

Foods commonly associated with foodborne microbial pathogens are shown in Table 61-4. Foodborne *Salmonella* outbreaks most often are caused by foods of animal origin, including beef, poultry, pork, dairy products, and eggs. Inadequate cooking or cross-contamination from raw food is often implicated. Internal contamination of intact eggs with *Salmonella* Enteritidis has led to marked increases in these infections in many countries.[42,43] Foodborne infections due to *Y. enterocolitica* have been caused by consumption of raw pork, contaminated milk, and by cross-contamination of infant formula during the preparation of pork chitterlings in the household.[44] *Clostridium perfringens* spores are frequently found in raw meat, poultry, fish, and gravies, but

TABLE 61-3. Characteristics of Enteric Illnesses Caused by Microbes and their Toxins

Organism	Median Hours Incubation (Range)	Symptoms				Duration
		Emesis	Diarrhea	Fever	Other	
Bacillus cereus toxin						
Emetic syndrome	2 (1–6)	+++	+/++	0		2–12 hours
Diarrheal syndrome	9 (6–16)	+	+++	0	C	12–24 hours
Campylobacter jejuni	48 (24–168)	+	+++	+++	C, BD, MA	2–14 days
Clostridium perfringens toxin	12 (6–24)	+	+++	0	C	12–24 hours
Cryptosporidium parvum	168 (48–240)	+++	+++	++	C, weight loss	1–2 weeks +/– remitting-relapsing course up to 30 days
Cyclospora cayetanensis	168 (48 to ≥336)	+	+++	+	Anorexia, weight loss, fatigue, cramps, flatus	1–4+ weeks +/– remitting-relapsing course
Enteroaggregative *Escherichia coli* (EAEC)	(20–48)	+	+++	+	C	Unknown
Enteroinvasive *Escherichia coli* (EIEC)	(20–48)	+	+++	++	C, BD	Unknown
Enteropathogenic *Escherichia coli* (EPEC)	(9–12)	+	+++	+	C	Prolonged
Enterotoxigenic *Escherichia coli* (ETEC)	(10–72)	+	+++	+	C	1–5 days
Giardia intestinalis	168 (168–504)	0	+++	0	C, weight loss, anorexia, flatus	Prolonged +/– remitting-relapsing course
Listeria monocytogenes	31 (11–70)	+	+	+++	Meningitis, bacteremia	Unknown
Vibrio parahaemolyticus	15 (4–96)	++	+++	++	C, HA, BD (rare)	1–7 days
Norovirus	24 (12–48)	+++	+++	++	HA, My	1–2 days
Salmonella spp.	36 (12–72)	+	+++	++	C, HA, My	3–10 days
Shiga-toxin producing *Escherichia coli* (STEC)	96 (48–120)	++	+++	+	C, BD, HA, HUS	2–12 days
Shigella spp.	(7–168)	+	+++	+++	C, BD	2–10
Staphylococcus aureus toxin	3 (1–6)	+++	++	0		12–24 hours
Vibrio cholerae O1 or O139	48 (6–120)	++	+++	+	Dehydration	1–7 days
Vibrio cholerae non-O1, non-O139	11 (5–96)	+	+++	+++	C, BD (25%)	1–12 days
Vibrio parahaemolyticus	15 (4–96)	++	+++	++	C, HA, BD (rare)	1–7 days
Yersinia enterocolitica	96 (48–240)	+	+++	+++	C, HA, pharyngitis, MA	3–20 days

BD, bloody diarrhea; C, abdominal cramps; HA, headache; HUS, hemolytic–uremic syndrome; MA, mesenteric adenitis; My, myalgias.

0, rare (<10%); +, infrequent (11%–33%); ++, frequent (33%–66%); +++, classic.

disease is most likely to occur when food is cooked and then held for many hours at room temperature allowing germination of spores and elaboration of toxin.[45] The epidemiology of long-incubation diarrheal illness due to *B. cereus* is similar, but a wider variety of foods have been implicated, including vegetable dishes, milk products, dried foods such as seasoning mixes, spices, dried potatoes, dried beans, and cereals.[46,47] Likewise, norovirus outbreaks have resulted from nearly all food commodities,[48] although norovirus contamination of meat and poultry generally occurs during handling by an ill food handler after cooking.

Fresh produce increasingly has been implicated in foodborne outbreaks due to *Salmonella, E. coli* O157:H7 and other STEC, *Shigella* spp., *Cryptosporidium,* and *Cyclospora cayetanensis.* Lettuce, sprouts, and tomatoes are among the most commonly implicated foods.[48] In some outbreaks, the produce may have become contaminated through the use of contaminated irrigation water.[49,50] Norovirus is the leading cause of outbreaks attributed to fresh produce, with leafy greens and fruits most often implicated.[51] During 2006–2007, there were 51 produce-associated norovirus outbreaks reported in the U.S., resulting in at least 1529 illnesses.[51] Many outbreaks of salmonellosis have been associated with fresh fruits, including melons, unpasteurized orange juice, and vegetables, including tomatoes and alfalfa sprout.[52–57] Outbreaks of *Cyclospora* infection have been linked to imported fresh raspberries, mesclun lettuce, basil, and snow peas.[58,59] Additionally, between 1995 and 2004 there were 26 juice- or cider-associated

outbreaks causing 1384 illnesses, 149 hospitalizations, and 1 death.[3] These outbreaks were caused by bacteria and parasites such as *Salmonella, E. coli* O157:H7, and *Cryptosporidium.*

Dairy products are an effective vehicle for a number of pathogens.[60] Despite its risk, raw milk continues to be sold legally in many states and sometimes is given to school groups who visit farms. Eighty-five outbreaks associated with unpasteurized milk or cheese were reported in the U.S. between 1998 and 2008;[51] etiologic agents commonly include *Salmonella, Campylobacter, Listeria, Mycobacterium bovis,* and STEC. Raw milk and undercooked poultry are most often implicated in outbreaks of *Campylobacter jejuni* infections.[61] Formula-fed infants have a heightened risk of salmonellosis and infections due to *Cronobacter* spp. compared with breastfed infants, perhaps because they are not receiving immunologic protection from human milk, or because of contamination of formula in the bottle.[62]

Recently, several commercial products such as prepackaged cookie dough,[63] salami made with contaminated pepper,[64] and frozen microwaveable meals[65] were implicated in outbreaks of *Salmonella* infection. Commercial carrot juice[66] and canned hot dog chili sauce[67] were implicated in recent outbreaks of botulism. Typically, however, botulism outbreaks are associated with consumption of low-acid home-canned vegetables, fruits, and fish. Honey has been implicated as the source of *Clostridium botulinum* spores in some cases of infant botulism.[68] Norovirus also can cause outbreaks associated with commercial products, as demon-

TABLE 61-4. Epidemiologic Clues to Bacterial, Parasitic, and Viral Foodborne and Waterborne Illnesses

Organism	Implicated Vehicles	Season	Comments
Bacillus cereus			
Emetic syndrome	Fried rice	Year-round	Inadequate reheating of cooked rice
Diarrheal syndrome	Beef, pork, chicken	Year-round	Advance preparation and inadequate holding temperature
Campylobacter jejuni	Poultry, raw milk	Late spring through early fall	
Clostridium perfringens	Beef, poultry, gravy	Fall through spring	Advance preparation and inadequate holding temperature
Cryptosporidium spp.	Contaminated swimming pools, hot tubs, water parks, lakes, rivers or oceans, contaminated drinking water from untreated shallow unprotected wells	Year-round but peak in warm season	Children who attend out-of-home childcare centers, childcare workers, international travelers, backpackers or campers, swimmers, people who handle infected cattle
Cyclospora cayetanensis	Fresh raspberries, mesclun lettuce, basil, snow peas	Year-round but peak in spring and summer	
Giardia intestinalis	Untreated water, contaminated drinking water, childcare settings	Year-round but peak in summer	International travelers, people in childcare settings, backpackers or campers
Listeria monocytogenes	Soft cheeses, hot dogs, cold cuts, milk, coleslaw, chicken	Year-round but peak in summer	Risk increased in people with cancer, diabetes mellitus, pregnancy, renal failure, HIV, neonatal period
Norovirus	Shellfish, salads, ice	Year-round	
Salmonella species	Beef, poultry, pork, eggs, dairy products, vegetables, fruit	Summer	*Salmonella* Enteritidis (egg-associated)
Shiga toxin-producing *Escherichia coli*	Beef (especially hamburger), raw milk, cider, lettuce, sprouts	Summer, fall	Secondary transmission relatively common
Shigella species	Egg salad, lettuce	Summer	Secondary transmission common
Staphylococcus aureus	Ham, poultry, cream-filled pastries, potato and egg salads	Summer	Inadequate refrigeration
Vibrio cholerae non-O1	Oysters	Summer, fall	Contaminated oyster beds
V. cholerae O1	Shellfish	Summer, fall	Most common in Gulf Coast states, international travelers
Vibrio parahaemolyticus	Fish, shellfish	Spring through fall	Most common in Gulf Coast states
Yersinia enterocolitica	Pork, chitterlings, tofu, raw milk	Winter	Risk increased with iron overload (i.e., thalassemia)

HIV, human immunodeficiency virus.

strated by an outbreak involving packaged delicatessen meat contaminated during processing.[69]

Foods that undergo handling are at risk of contamination with a variety of pathogens.[70] Given widespread norovirus infections in the community,[60] outbreaks often result through contamination of foods by an ill food handler.[71] Ready-to-eat foods, such as salads and sandwiches, as well as self-service food items often are implicated in norovirus outbreaks.[72] Staphylococcal food poisoning usually is associated with such foods that also have a high protein content, including cooked meats, fish, and poultry; custard or cream-filled baked goods; dairy products; and potato and egg salads.[73] Foodborne shigellosis outbreaks are most often associated with potato and egg salads as well as fresh produce from salad bars.[74-77] Norovirus or raw shellfish outbreaks appear to occur most frequently after food has been contaminated by an ill food handler.[70]

Histamine fish poisoning outbreaks are associated with scombroid fish, the most common of which are tuna, mackerel, bonito, and skipjack. Ciguatera fish poisoning has been associated with more than 400 species of fish, including barracuda, red snapper, amberjack, and grouper.[78] Shellfish, especially bivalve mollusks, are important vehicles of foodborne illness, particularly because they are often consumed raw.[79] Shellfish can be colonized naturally with pathogenic *Vibrio* organisms, including *V. vulnificus, V. cholerae* non-O1, *V. parahaemolyticus,* and *V. mimicus.* As filter feeders, shellfish concentrate pathogens from contaminated water, including hepatitis A, norovirus, toxigenic *V. cholerae* O1, *Shigella,* and *Plesiomonas.*[80,81]

Most outbreaks of the short-incubation "emetic syndrome" of *B. cereus* food poisoning are associated with rice, particularly fried rice, that has been cooked and then held at warm temperatures.

Foodborne outbreaks of heavy-metal poisoning are most often associated with acidic beverages such as lemonade, fruit punch, and carbonated drinks that have been stored in corroded metallic containers.[82]

Water

A recent review of all 780 drinking water-associated outbreaks in the U.S. reported to CDC during 1971–2006,[83] including but not limited to those resulting in enteric illness, identified a shift in the types of drinking water systems involved in waterborne outbreaks during this period, with a decreasing proportion of outbreaks due to public water systems (680, 87%) and an increasing proportion due to individual, privately owned water systems (82, 10.5%). Privately owned systems tend to serve fewer people and do not fall under the drinking water regulations established by the U.S. Environmental Protection Agency (EPA) to protect water quality in public drinking water systems. Water system contamination resulting in drinking water outbreaks occurred at a variety of points, including the water source, treatment processing, storage, distribution system, premise plumbing, and point of use, the latter of which included 12 outbreaks associated with water contaminated in containers, pitchers, bottles, hoses, and hose bibs.

PART II Clinical Syndromes and Cardinal Features of Infectious Diseases: Approach to Diagnosis and Initial Management

SECTION H Gastrointestinal Tract Infections

This 36-year review of drinking water-associated outbreaks also revealed a changing epidemiologic trend in the water sources associated with these outbreaks.[83] From 1989 to 2006, a decreasing proportion of reported drinking water outbreaks due to public water systems was associated with contaminated, untreated, or improperly treated surface water sources such as lakes or rivers.

However, the annual proportion of outbreaks in public water systems associated with contaminated, untreated, or improperly treated ground water remained unchanged over time.[9] In recent studies of public systems using ground water, human enteric viruses, such as enteroviruses and norovirus, have been isolated from aquifers that might have been contaminated from surface water intrusion or sewage discharges.[84] The broader public health impact of such contaminated ground water could be substantial since approximately 45% of the U.S. population is supplied by ground water, either through public or individual water systems.[85]

Cryptosporidium is most commonly implicated in outbreaks associated with treated recreational water. Because *Cryptosporidium* is extremely tolerant to chlorine levels used in treated water, these outbreaks can occur even in well-maintained facilities and have the potential to expand community-wide, starting in recreational water transmission and moving by person-to-person transmission into childcare programs and other settings.[86,87] Outbreaks of gastrointestinal illness associated with untreated water primarily are caused by bacteria and viruses and usually are linked to swimming in lakes or ponds. This suggests that swimmers themselves might be important sources of water contamination.[88]

Zoonotic Exposures

Zoonotic transmission of enteric pathogens can occur from exposures to pets and other animals. Enteric pathogens can contaminate the environment (e.g., water sources, soil) and persist in animal housing areas for long periods. Contact with animals in public settings (e.g., fairs, farm tours, and petting zoos) provides opportunities for pathogen transmission to visitors, especially children, in these settings. Reports of illness and outbreaks among visitors to fairs, farms, and petting zoos are documented. A 2004 review identified >25 human infectious disease outbreaks during 1990–2000 associated with visiting animal exhibits.[89] The primary mode of transmission in these outbreaks is the fecal–oral route. Because animal fur, hair, skin, and saliva can become contaminated with fecal organisms, transmission might occur when persons pet, touch, or are licked by animals.[90] Outbreaks have also resulted from contaminated animal products used for educational activities in schools.[25-28]

Outbreaks of salmonellosis have been associated with dissection of owl pellets and with frozen mice.[25] Turtles and other reptiles, rodents, and baby poultry (e.g., chicks, ducklings, or goslings) have long been recognized as sources of human *Salmonella* infections.[30-39,91] Since 2006, at least three large multistate outbreaks have been linked to contact with small turtles.[33-35] Since 2009, at least four multistate outbreaks linked to baby poultry birds have been identified; ill persons included those who reported

contact with baby poultry birds at feed stores, school classrooms, fairs, and petting zoos.[26-32] During 2006–2008, a total of 79 human *Salmonella* infections were linked to multiple brands of contaminated dry dog and cat food.[40,41] Human *Salmonella* infections have been linked to contaminated pig ear treats and pet treats containing beef and seafood,[89,92-94] and to contact with home aquariums containing tropical fish and aquatic frogs.[95,96]

Cryptosporidium and *Giardia* are the most common enteric protozoa in the U.S. that are associated with zoonotic transmission. Zoonotic transmission of *Cryptosporidium* has been associated with domestic animals, more commonly young animals. Pre-weaned calves[97] are the most commonly linked animals linked to human cryptosporidiosis through zoonotic transmission. Other animals, including sheep,[98] horses,[99] pigs,[100] dogs,[101] cats, goats, and birds, have also been implicated as well through the use of molecular diagnostic tools and epidemiologic investigations.[102] The molecular and epidemiologic understanding of the potential for zoonotic transmission of *Giardia* is evolving, and it is not known presently how frequently zoonotic transmission occurs. However, molecular testing has indicated that wild and domestic animals, including dogs, cats, sheep, cattle, pigs, beavers, muskrats, rats, pet rodents, rabbits, and nonhuman primates, among other animals, might be hosts of *Giardia* that can infect humans.[102]

Geographic Location and Seasonality

Foods

Geographic location can provide useful clues for diagnosis, although modern distribution of foods is making this information less valuable. *E. coli* O157:H7 infections appear to be most common in the northern and western U.S. and Canada.[103] Seafood-related illnesses tend to occur near specific reservoirs of pathogens (Table 61-5). *Vibrio* infections are most common in the Gulf Coast states. Ciguatera outbreaks occur in tropical and subtropical regions and are more common in Puerto Rico, Virgin Islands, Hawaii, and Florida.[104,105]

The seasonal distribution of common causes of foodborne illness is useful in differential diagnosis (Tables 61-4 and 61-5). Norovirus infections occur year-round, although there is increased activity during the winter.[106] *Y. enterocolitica* outbreaks have a distinct winter peak, which probably is related to preparation of traditional holiday foods, in contrast to many other bacterial infections. Mushroom poisoning occurs most often in the spring, late summer, and fall and is associated with species-specific syndromes (Table 61-6).[107,108]

Water

Drinking water-associated outbreaks occur across the country without a noticeable geographic distribution associated with water system type, water source, or agent causing enteric illness. Most detected cases associated with drinking water outbreaks are confined geographically to the service area, and

TABLE 61-5. Characteristics of Poisoning Syndromes Caused by Fish and Shellfish

Syndrome	Vehicles (Toxin-Producing Dinoflagellate)	Incubation Period	Duration	Region	Season
Ciguatera	Snapper, grouper, barracuda, amberjack (*Gambierdiscus toxicus*)	1–6 hours	Days to months	35°N–35°S latitude	Feb–Sept
Domoic acid	Mussels (*Nitzschia pungens*)	15 minutes–38 hours	Indefinite	Prince Edward Island, Pacific Northwest	Nov
Histamine (scombroid)	Tuna, mackerel, bonito, mahi-mahi, bluefish	5 minutes–1 hours	Hours	Temperate tropical coasts (especially Hawaii, California)	Year-round
Neurotoxic shellfish poisoning	Shellfish (*Gymnodinium breve*)	5 minutes–4 hours	Hours to days	Gulf coast, Atlantic coast of Florida	Spring, fall
Paralytic shellfish poisoning	Shellfish (*Gonyaulax catenella, Gonyaulax tamarensis*)	5 minutes–4 hours	Hours to days	New England, US west coast, Alaska, Guatemala	May–Nov

TABLE 61-6. Mushroom Poisoning Syndromes

Syndrome	Mushroom Species	Toxins
SHORT INCUBATION		
Delirium	Amanita muscaria, Amanita pantherina	Ibotenic acid, muscimol
Disulfiram reaction	Coprinus atramentarius	Disulfiram-like substance
Hallucination	Psilocybe spp. Paneaolus spp.	Psilocybin, psilocin Psilocybin
Parasympathetic hyperactivity	Inocybe spp. Clitocybe spp.	Muscarine Muscarine
Gastroenteritis	Many	?
LONG INCUBATION		
Gastroenteritis, hepatorenal failure	Amanita phalloides Amanitavirosa Amanita verna Galerina autumnalis Galerina marginata Galerina venenata	Amatoxins, phallotins Amatoxins Amatoxins Amatoxins Amatoxins Disulfiram-like substance
Gastroenteritis, hepatic failure, hemolysis, seizures, coma	Gyromitra spp.	Gyromitrin

multistate outbreaks are rare.[83] In contrast, while recreational water outbreaks also occur across the country, their geographic dispersion varies. Illnesses associated with recreational water that does not attract patrons from a large geographic area (e.g., a local community pool) tend to be confined to one community; conversely, illnesses associated with recreational water that attracts patrons from more geographically dispersed area (e.g., waterparks and oceans) can involve residents of a wide area. Dispersion of affected people might decrease the likelihood that the outbreak will be detected.[18]

Drinking water outbreaks occur throughout the year but are reported most frequently during the summer months.[83] Similarly, although enteric illness associated with recreational water outbreaks can occur throughout the year, the 48 outbreaks reported during 2005–2006 were clustered in the summer months, with 40 (83%) occurring during June–August.[18]

Zoonotic Exposures

Zoonotic enteric diseases do not have a noticeable geographic trend. However, cases appear to be more common in the spring and summer. Outbreaks of human salmonellosis associated with baby chicks and ducklings have occurred repeatedly in the spring months.[36–39] Also, people have more contact with wildlife and animals at petting zoos and fairs during the summer months, particularly in August and September.[48]

Laboratory Diagnosis

Appropriate collection and processing of clinical specimens and environmental samples are essential for confirming the cause of foodborne, waterborne, and zoonotic diseases. Because of the large number of different specimens, techniques, and culture media needed to evaluate all potential causes, it is most efficient to plan the laboratory investigation based on clinical or epidemiologic suspicion. Stool specimens (placed in agent-appropriate transport media) and sera can be obtained early in the investigation and stored for later studies. Table 61-7 summarizes the principal laboratory tests recommended for diagnosis.[109–112]

Confirmation of food poisoning due to *Staphylococcus aureus*, *Bacillus cereus*, and *Clostridium perfringens* usually is limited to outbreak investigations. Confirmation of a staphylococcal food-poisoning outbreak requires isolation of *S. aureus* from vomitus or feces of patients, the implicated food, or hands or nares of a food handler. Because a large proportion of healthy people are colonized with *S. aureus*, strains should be demonstrated by phage typing or pulsed-field gel electrophoresis (PFGE) methods to be identical to strains from vomitus or feces.[113] Staphylococcal enterotoxin can be demonstrated in food by enzyme immunoassay (EIA) or radioimmunoassay (RIA).[114] A *B. cereus* outbreak can be confirmed by isolation of the organism from ≥2 ill people who shared the same meal or by isolation of ≥10⁵/gram *B. cereus* organisms from implicated food. Serotyping and plasmid analysis can be useful for confirmation because 14% of healthy adults have transient colonization with *B. cereus*.[115] To confirm food poisoning due to *C. perfringens*, colony counts of ≥10⁶/gram of stool or identification of enterotoxin in stool must be demonstrated, because at lower levels the organism can be part of normal flora in healthy people. Demonstration of ≥10⁵/gram *C. perfringens* in implicated food also confirms etiology.

Salmonella spp., *Shigella* spp., *Campylobacter* spp., *Vibrio* spp., and *Y. enterocolitica* are confirmed by isolation of organisms from stools of ill people. Serotyping is available through state public health laboratories and often provides additional information. Molecular subtyping at state public health laboratories has become a critical component of disease surveillance and identifies outbreaks that would otherwise not be detected. *Campylobacter* spp., *Y. enterocolitica*, *Vibrio* spp., and *E. coli* O157:H7 require use of selective media for optimal recovery (see Table 61-7). *E. coli* O157:H7 can be identified presumptively by screening sorbitol-negative colonies on sorbitol MacConkey (SMAC) media, an inexpensive screening procedure that should be implemented in all laboratories. Detection of other STEC requires identification of Shiga toxins or detection of toxin genes; a commercial EIA is available widely, and polymerase chain reaction (PCR) test is available in some reference and state or federal public health laboratories. Enterotoxigenic *E. coli* infections are confirmed using a commercial latex agglutination assay or by PCR to identify the production of heat-stable (ST) or heat-labile (LT) toxin by *E. coli* isolated from stool. All *Salmonella* spp., *Shigella* spp., STEC, *Vibrio* spp., and *Listeria monocytogenes* isolates should be forwarded to the state public health laboratory for full characterization for surveillance and outbreak detection purposes.[116]

Botulism outbreaks can be confirmed by demonstration of botulinum toxin in serum or stool of ill people or in implicated food by use of the mouse neutralization test.[117] Outbreaks caused by heavy metals, chemicals, histamine fish poisoning, ciguatera and shellfish poisoning may be documented by demonstration of the offending toxin in the implicated food. If chemical food poisoning is suspected, a urine specimen can yield evidence of the chemical.

Identification of norovirus has been enhanced by availability of PCR-based assays available in many public health laboratories. Ideally, stool samples to be tested for virus should be collected within 5 days of illness onset and kept refrigerated but not frozen. Identification of norovirus outbreaks in the U.S. has improved with the advent of Calicinet, a national network of public health laboratories that contribute to a database of norovirus genetic sequences obtained during investigations of disease clusters.

If *Cryptosporidium* infection is suspected, specific testing of serial stool specimens should be requested. Diagnostic techniques for *Cryptosporidium* include acid-fast staining, direct fluorescent antibody (DFA), and EIA for detection of *Cryptosporidium* antigens. Tests for *Cryptosporidium* are not performed routinely in most laboratories during standard ova and parasite testing; therefore, healthcare providers should request specific testing for this parasite.[97] EIA and immune chromatography (point-of-care rapid tests) for detecting antigen in stool are available commercially. Genotyping and subtyping tools are used increasingly to differentiate *Cryptosporidium* species for outbreak investigations and infection/contamination source tracking, although *Cryptosporidium* isolates cannot be reliably genotyped/subtyped if stool is preserved in formalin. *Giardia* infections are best diagnosed with immunodiagnostic techniques such as DFA testing or EIAs of stool

TABLE 61-7. Laboratory Tests for Diagnosis of Foodborne, Waterborne, and Zoonotic Enteric Diseases

Organism	Laboratory Tests	
	People	Food
Bacillus cereus	Isolation from stool (patients + controls)	Isolation of >10 CFU/g in food
Campylobacter jejuni	Stool culture by selective media (e.g., Campy-BAP, Skirrow, Butzler)	Culture (selective media)
Ciguatera		Demonstration of ciguatoxin by bioassay or EIA
Clostridium perfringens	Isolation of >10^6 CFU/g stool	Isolation of >10^5 CFU/g in food
Cryptosporidium spp.	Stool examination (acid-fast stain; enzyme immunoassays, direct fluorescent antibody (DFA))	Not established
Cyclospora cayetanensis	Stool examination (e.g., bright-field microscopy with differential interference contrast (DIC); UV fluorescence microscopy; modified acid-fast or safranin staining)	Not established
Giardia intestinalis	Stool examination (direct fluorescent antibody (DFA); enzyme immunoassays)	Not established
Histamine fish poisoning		Demonstration of 100 mg histamine per 100 g of fish
Listeria monocytogenes	Blood culture; stool culture (cold enrichment)	Culture (cold enrichment)
Norovirus and other enteric viruses	Reverse transcriptase PCR of stool	Reverse-transcriptase PCR
PSP and NSP		Demonstration of toxin by bioassay
Salmonella species	Stool culture, serotyping	Culture
Shiga toxin-producing Escherichia coli	Stool culture (SMAC agar), serotyping; toxin-testing by EIA; serology	Culture (selective media), toxin testing
Shigella species	Stool culture, serotyping; stool culture of food handlers	Culture
Staphylococcus aureus	Isolation from vomitus, feces; culture of nares, hands of food handlers	Isolation of >10 CFU/g in food; demonstration of enterotoxin
Vibrio parahaemolyticus, Vibrio cholerae O1	Stool culture (TCBS agar); serology	Culture (TCBS agar)
Yersinia enterocolitica	Stool culture (CIN agar); serotyping	Culture (cold enrichment)

BAP, Brucella agar-amphotericin B-polymyxin; CFU, colony-forming unit; CIN, cefsulidin-Irgasin-novobiocin; EIA, enzyme immunoassay; NSP, neurotoxic shellfish poisoning; PCR, polymerase chain reaction; PSP, paralytic shellfish poisoning; SMAC, sorbitol MacConkey; TCBS, thiosulfate-citrate-bile salt-sucrose.

specimens.[118] Molecular methods (e.g., PCR) for both Cryptosporidium and Giardia are used increasingly in reference diagnostic laboratories to determine species and genotypes of these parasites and thus enhance outbreak investigations. Molecular testing can be performed on nonpreserved, refrigerated, or frozen stool specimens.[119] Cyclospora testing must be specifically requested of the laboratory and is best diagnosed with examination of at least three stool specimens. Following stool concentration, bright-field microscopy with differential interference contrast (DIC), UV fluorescence microscopy, modified acid-fast staining, or safranin staining can be used.

Water testing, both in the context of drinking water and recreational water outbreaks, also is useful during outbreak investigations. Ultrafiltration methods have been developed by which large volumes of water can be filtered in a relatively short time, and the filtrate and filter can then be shipped to reference diagnostic laboratories for analysis.[119] Other water-related media, such as filter cartridges and filter backwash from swimming pools, can also be tested.

Additional information on collection of specimens for diagnosis and investigation of enteric disease outbreaks is available at http://www.cdc.gov.foodborneoutbreaks/guide_sc.htm and http://www.cdc.gov/healthywater/emergency/toolkit/.

MANAGEMENT

Supportive care is central to the management of acute foodborne, waterborne, or zoonotic diarrheal disease. Careful replacement of fluid and electrolyte losses is crucial, particularly in infants. For mild to moderate dehydration, even with some vomiting, oral replacement with appropriate electrolyte solutions is the preferred treatment.[120] Antiemetics may be useful for patients with severe or prolonged vomiting. Antiperistaltic agents are not recommended for young children or for patients with signs of enteroinvasive disease, such as fever or bloody diarrhea.[120] Bismuth subsalicylate provides symptomatic relief;[121,122] however, some pediatricians have raised concerns about the possibility of precipitating Reye syndrome by using bismuth subsalicylate. Certain strains of probiotics have been found useful in hastening the recovery of children from acute diarrheal episodes.[123,124]

Specific antimicrobial therapy is indicated for severe infections due to certain confirmed infections, notably listeriosis, shigellosis, enterotoxigenic and enteroinvasive E. coli, typhoid fever, cholera, cyclosporiasis, giardiasis, and cryptosporidiosis. The efficacy of the single drug currently approved by the U.S. Food and Drug Administration to treat cryptosporidiosis (nitazoxanide) is somewhat limited.[125-127] Antimicrobial agents usually are not indicated for salmonellosis, except in very young children, persons with an immunodeficiency, or in cases of invasive salmonellosis. Recent outbreaks of salmonellosis and shigellosis have been caused by bacterial strains resistant to multiple antimicrobial agents; thus, antimicrobial therapy for these patients should be tailored to the specific susceptibility profile of the pathogen. The role of antimicrobial therapy is less clear for treatment of diarrheal illness due to Y. enterocolitica, Campylobacter, V. parahaemolyticus, Aeromonas, and Plesiomonas, but therapy may have a role in severe or prolonged gastrointestinal tract illness caused by these pathogens. The association between antimicrobial agents and increased risk of hemolytic uremic syndrome (HUS) is not clear.[125-130] Therefore, antimicrobial agents are not recommended for children with E.

coli O157:H7 and other STEC infections. Additional information about antimicrobial therapy is available in the pathogen-specific chapters.

Medical care providers who suspect botulism should immediately contact their state health department's 24-hour emergency telephone line. The state health department will contact the CDC to arrange for clinical consultation by telephone and, if indicated, release of botulinum antitoxin. The California Infant Botulism Treatment & Prevention Program provides consultation and BabyBig for suspected cases of infant botulism (510-231-7600). For cases of suspected botulism among older children, CDC's 24-hour telephone number for state health departments to report possible botulism cases, obtain emergency consultation, and request botulinum antitoxin is 770-488-7100. Most pediatric botulism cases are infant botulism. Patients with ciguatera, paralytic shellfish poisoning (PSP), or botulism must be observed closely for evidence of respiratory compromise. Preliminary data suggest that intravenously administered mannitol may ameliorate the acute neurologic symptoms of severe ciguatera, and tocainide may improve the dysesthesias.[104,105] Symptoms of histamine fish poisoning may respond to antihistamines and H_2-receptor antagonists. In cases with bronchospasm, epinephrine may be required.

For most patients with mushroom poisoning, supportive care is adequate.[107,108] Removal of unabsorbed mushroom should be attempted by induced emesis or use of cathartics or enemas. Uneaten mushrooms should be saved, and mycologists or experts in poison control should be consulted for species identification and possible use of specific antidotes. Pyridine hydrochloride and methylene blue may be useful in cases of *Gyromitra* ingestion. Thioctic acid is an experimental antidote for *Amanita* poisoning; a regional or nationwide (1-800-222-1222) poison control center should be contacted for information on availability. Liver transplantation has been used successfully in severe *Amanita* poisoning.

Therapy for acute heavy-metal poisoning is supportive. Antiemetics are contraindicated, and emesis should be induced if it does not occur spontaneously. Very severe cases of toxicity may require use of specific antidotes, but this is rarely necessary.

COMPLICATIONS

The most common complications of foodborne, waterborne, and zoonotic diarrheal illnesses are dehydration, electrolyte abnormalities, and hypoglycemia. Children and elderly people are more susceptible to these complications. Severe vomiting can result in subconjunctival hemorrhage, syncope, or Mallory–Weiss esophageal tears. Enteric infection with *Salmonella* spp., *Y. enterocolitica*, *Vibrio* species other than *V. cholerae*, and *Campylobacter* spp. can be complicated by bloodstream infection (BSI) or focal extraintestinal infections, such as osteomyelitis, meningitis, endocarditis, or endarteritis. Infants also are at increased risk for BSI and metastatic infections due to common bacterial pathogens, particularly *Salmonella* spp. People with defects of cellular immunity (e.g., HIV infection, leukemia, lymphoma), reticuloendothelial function (e.g., sickle-cell disease, malaria), and iron overload syndromes also have increased risk of *Salmonella* and *Campylobacter* BSI. People with immunosuppressing conditions are also at risk for disseminated disease, malabsorption, or death due to *Cryptosporidium*. Postinfectious syndromes have been recognized as important consequences of enteric infections, including HUS after infections with *E. coli* O157:H7;[131] reactive arthritis after salmonellosis, shigellosis, and giardiasis;[132] and Guillain–Barré syndrome after campylobacteriosis.[61] Norovirus infections have been associated with necrotizing enterocolitis in neonates, chronic diarrhea in immunosuppressed patients, and postinfectious irritable bowel syndrome.

PREVENTION

Food and Water

The risk of foodborne disease can be minimized by careful attention to selection of foods, cleaning of cooking surfaces used for preparation of raw foods, personal hygiene of food handlers and others while preparing food, thorough cooking immediately before serving, and proper storage at temperatures too low (<4 °C) or too hot (>60 °C) to support bacterial growth. Raw foods of animal origin require particular attention, including poultry, beef, pork, unpasteurized (raw) milk, uncooked eggs, and uncooked shellfish. People at greatest risk of severe disease (i.e., young infants and people with chronic liver disease, decreased gastric acidity, and acquired or congenital immunodeficiency) as well as people who seek to minimize their risk of illness should avoid foods such as uncooked shellfish, raw sprouts, raw milk, or incompletely cooked eggs or meat. Cross-contamination of cooked foods from raw foods via contaminated surfaces and food preparation equipment is a common but avoidable error. Attention to the source of fish and shellfish may help avoid acquiring an infection or developing food poisoning. Widespread use of hepatitis A vaccine will reduce foodborne transmission of hepatitis A virus. Several websites provide up-to-date educational information about foodborne diseases (cdc.gov/foodnet/, cdc.gov/foodsafety/, nal.usda.gov/foodborne/, and fightbac.org).

The risk of waterborne disease can be minimized by appropriate drinking water treatment and proper hygiene, particularly at childcare facilities and recreational water venues such as pools and beaches. Enteric illnesses due to recreational water exposures can be prevented by adequately training pool operators and enforcing pool codes through pool inspections;[133] through provision of appropriate hygiene infrastructure, such as conveniently placed, well-stocked and maintained showers, toilets, diapering stations, and handwashing facilities at recreational water venues; and through public education. Persons with diarrhea, including aquatics staff, should not swim or participate in water play; all others should shower with soap immediately before entering the water and should wash hands thoroughly after using the toilet or changing diapers. The U.S. CDC also recommends checking diapers every 30–60 minutes while children are swimming to help prevent fecal contamination of the water. Diapered children should be changed at a diapering station (not poolside). Children should be taught not to swallow water while swimming or playing at splash parks. Limiting water play in childcare facilities may also prevent enteric disease.[134] Additional information is available at http:// www.cdc.gov/healthywater/swimming/.

Much of foodborne and waterborne illness prevention lies in reducing contamination of food and water before it reaches the consumer. Major revision of meat inspection procedures and revised requirements for drinking water treatment began in the 1990s in the U.S. For food and water that still may be contaminated with dangerous pathogens, a systematic disinfection or pathogen reduction, such as pasteurization of milk and chlorination of water, is required. Meats, seeds for sprouting, spices, shell eggs, and some produce items may also be irradiated before sale in commercial markets in the U.S. Such regulatory and industry efforts have been successful in decreasing the incidence of infection with several foodborne pathogens. For example, in comparison with 1996–1998, rates of infection in 2009 were lower for *Listeria* (decreased by 26%), *Campylobacter* (decreased by 30%), and *E. coli* O157:H7 (decreased by 26%).[135] Likewise, EPA regulations that protect public water supplies, such as the Surface Water Treatment Rule, coincide with a decrease in the proportion of drinking water outbreaks associated with public water systems and surface water supplies.[83] However, foodborne and waterborne illnesses remain important public health concerns. Clinicians have the important role of providing education and appropriate counseling to high-risk patients, including parents of infants and young children and persons with immunocompromising conditions, about the health hazards of food and waterborne pathogens, vehicles of transmission, and prevention measures.

Zoonotic Exposures

Zoonotic enteric infections can be prevented through careful hygiene and by limiting interaction of some populations with animals and their environments. Children <5 years old and those with immunocompromising conditions should avoid contact with reptiles, amphibians, baby poultry, puppies and kittens <6 months old, pets with diarrhea, and petting zoos or farm animals.[22–41,136,137] Children should not be allowed to kiss animals or to put their hands or other objects into their mouths while interacting with animals. Careful handwashing with soap and water as soon as possible after contact with animals, their feces, their cages/pens, and their food can help prevent infection. Additional information is available at http://www.cdc.gov/healthypets/.

Prompt diagnosis and reporting of enteric infections can aid recognition and mitigation of outbreaks. Currently, many enteric illnesses go undetected because they often are misinterpreted as illnesses caused by person-to-person spread (such as "stomach flu"). Stool examinations may not be performed because they are not considered to be cost-effective for an individual patient or might not lead to specific therapy, despite providing a public health benefit. Reporting may be incomplete or delayed, or public health departments may not have adequate resources to conduct an investigation. However, laboratory diagnosis of enteric illness, along with timely reporting, public health investigation, and use of rapid subtyping methods, can identify outbreaks, detect emerging pathogens, identify new vehicles and modes of transmission, and prevent additional illness. Recognition of an outbreak can lead to removal of contaminated food items from the marketplace or correction of contaminated drinking water systems or recreational water venues and enhance industry and regulatory control measures to prevent contamination in the future. A list of nationally notifiable infectious conditions in the U.S. can be found at: http://www.cdc.gov/ncphi/disss/nndss/PHS/infdis.htm. State health departments can provide additional information about reporting infectious diseases within their jurisdictions.

SECTION I: Intra-Abdominal Infections

62 Acute Hepatitis

Laurie S. Conklin and John D. Snyder

Acute hepatic inflammation in children can be caused by many infectious and noninfectious causes (Table 62-1). Because the liver has limited mechanisms by which to manifest acute injury, diverse disease states can present initially with similar patterns of hepatic injury. This chapter presents a systematic approach to the evaluation and diagnosis of acute liver injury in immunocompetent children. The pathogenesis of many infectious causes is covered more fully in pathogen-specific chapters in this book.

APPROACH TO EVALUATION

Signs and symptoms associated with acute hepatic injury usually include jaundice, vomiting, poor feeding, lethargy, hepatomegaly, and right upper quadrant pain. Assessment of the multiple possible etiologies begins with the patient's age and a detailed history and physical examination with special emphasis on potential exposures, evolution of symptoms, concomitant health problems, and family history. The physical examination must include a careful evaluation for extrahepatic manifestations of disease as well as a thorough assessment of the abdomen.

Elevated serum hepatic enzyme levels, and often bilirubin levels, are present in people with acute hepatitis, but the pattern of elevations rarely is diagnostic.[1–3] The initial diagnostic tests required to evaluate acute liver injury by age are shown in Box 62-1 and in Table 62-2. In most cases, a core group of tests, common for all age groups, is ordered initially (Table 62-2). Evaluation for infectious causes is always a central component but requires tailoring for age. The core set of tests given in Box 62-1 usually are ordered simultaneously to provide a complete initial assessment of the disease process. Depending on the age of the child, several additional tests are considered (Table 62-2). The severity of the child's illness can influence the pace and extent of testing. For example, in a mildly affected child, results of tests for infectious diseases often are evaluated before metabolic disorders are pursued.

INFECTIOUS CAUSES

A variety of infectious agents have been implicated in hepatic inflammation in neonates, including bacterial, parasitic, and especially viral pathogens.[3–6] Hepatitis in neonates caused by specific agents usually is distinguished from the category of neonatal hepatitis, which has been used to designate hepatic inflammation of no known cause.

Disseminated Infections

Disseminated systemic and extrahepatic bacterial and viral infections must always be considered when jaundice is present, especially in the newborn infant.[5] Gram-negative bacterial infections, disseminated herpes simplex virus (HSV) infection, and enterovirus infection are important causes in neonates that require immediate, appropriate therapy.[7,8] The pathogenesis of hepatic dysfunction in sepsis is not understood completely but the cholestatic effects of endotoxins and endotoxin-induced mediators appear to be important.[7,8] Jaundice also can occur in the absence of severe illness, as in gram-negative bacillary urinary tract infection.[6] Disseminated infection caused by gram-positive organisms and viruses also can be associated with cholestasis.[8] The diagnosis usually is made because infected children appear severely ill. A clue to diagnosis is an elevation of serum levels of conjugated bilirubin greatly out of proportion to elevation of aminotransferases or alkaline phosphatase.[4] In the absence of hemolysis associated with mild liver disease, this pattern suggests septicemia.

Many viruses in addition to the primary hepatotropic viruses (hepatitis A, B, C, D, E, and G) must be considered when hepatitis occurs in children. Viruses which can cause hepatic injury as part of a disseminated, multisystem illness include Ebstein–Barr virus (EBV), cytomegalovirus (CMV), enteroviruses, adenoviruses, rubella, HSV, and human immunodeficiency virus (HIV)[3,5] In neonates, HSV and enterovirus can cause massive necrosis of liver, profound coagulopathy, and fulminant sepsis-like syndrome; a clue is the disproportionate hepatic insult. A few cases of survival have been associated with use of extracorporeal life support or liver transplantation or both.[9–11] Congenital viral infections cause milder hepatitis and often are associated with prematurity and growth retardation, and rubella is associated with congenital malformations.[3] Other causes of disseminated infection and associated hepatitis (which usually is mild) in neonates include congenital syphilis, disseminated candidiasis, and toxoplasmosis.[3,5] Infection caused by these agents can involve skin, central nervous, cardiorespiratory, and musculoskeletal systems.[3,5]

A wide spectrum of hepatic dysfunction, ranging from mild to fulminant disease, can occur with any of the infectious agents listed above.[3–5] Fulminant hepatitis is characterized by rapid progression to very high hepatic enzyme levels, decreased production of coagulation proteins, elevated ammonia, hypoglycemia from loss of glycogen reserves, shock, coma, or death.

TABLE 62-1. Age of Onset of Infectious and Noninfectious Causes of Acute Hepatitis

Etiology	Neonates and Infants	Children	Adolescents
INFECTION			
Primarily hepatotropic			
Hepatitis A	–	+	+
Hepatitis B	+	+	+
Hepatitis C	+	+	+
Hepatitis D	+	+	+
Hepatitis E	–	+	+
Hepatitis G	+	+	+
Generalized infection			
Adenovirus	+	–	–
Arbovirus	+	–	–
Coxsackievirus	+	–	–
Cytomegalovirus	+	+	+
Enterovirus	+	–	–
Epstein–Barr virus	+	+	+
Herpes simplex virus	+	–	–
Human immunodeficiency virus	+	+	+
Rubella	+	–	–
Varicella	+	+	+
ANATOMIC			
Biliary atresia	+	–	–
Choledochal cyst	+	+	+
Congenital hepatic fibrosis	+	+	+
AUTOIMMUNE	–	+	+
Autoimmune hepatitis	–	+	+
Sclerosing cholangitis	+	+	+
METABOLIC DISORDERS			
α_1-Antitrypsin deficiency	+	+	+
Cystic fibrosis	+	+	+
Disorders of carbohydrate metabolism			
Galactosemia	+	–	–
Glycogen storage diseases	+	+	–
Hereditary fructose intolerance	+	–	–
Disorders of protein metabolism			
Urea cycle deficiencies	+	–	–
Organic acidemias	+	–	–
Tyrosinemia	+	–	–
Disorders of metal metabolism			
Neonatal hemochromatosis	+	–	–
Indian childhood cirrhosis	–	+	–
Wilson disease	–	+	+
Lipid storage diseases			
Gaucher disease	+	+	+
Nieman–Pick disease	+	+	+
Wolman disease	+	–	–
Errors of bile acid metabolism	+	–	–
TOXINS/DRUGS			
Acetaminophen, alpha-methyldopa, alcohol, amiodarone, chlorpromazine, dilantin, oral contraceptives, halothane, isoniazid, total parenteral nutrition, and amanita toxin	+	+	+
TUMORS	+	+	+
IDIOPATHIC			
Byler syndrome	+	–	–
Neonatal hepatitis	+	–	–
Reye syndrome	+	+	+

+, Recognized or usual age of occurrence; –, unexpected or not an age of occurrence.

BOX 62-1. Initial Diagnostic Evaluation for Suspected Hepatitis in All Age Groups

BLOOD
Tests of hepatic cell injury and function
Bilirubin, total and direct
Alanine aminotransferase
Aspartate aminotransferase
Gamma-glutamyltranspeptidase
Albumin
Prothrombin time
Ammonia
Fasting glucose

Tests for infectious causes
Serology for hepatotropic viruses (see Table 62-2)
CMV antigen
Human immunodeficiency virus
Serology for Epstein–Barr virus
Serology, antigen or molecular tests for cytomegalovirus
Serology or molecular tests for human immunodeficiency virus

Metabolic screening lists
Alpha-1-antitrypsin level and protease inhibitor type

URINE
Shell vial culture for cytomegalovirus

RADIOLOGY
Ultrasound

Hepatitis Viruses

The six hepatotropic viruses, hepatitis A, B, C, D, E, and G, which cause hepatitis as the primary disease manifestation, play a limited role in symptomatic hepatitis in neonates.[6]

Hepatitis A virus (HAV). HAV infection continues to be the most common cause of acute hepatitis reported in the United States.[12,13] Infection primarily is spread through direct human fecal–oral contamination or by contaminated food and water.[13,14] HAV is common in early childhood especially in developing countries with poor conditions of sanitation and hygiene. Almost all children in these countries become seropositive before 5 years of age.[12,14] In the U.S., transmission often occurs in childcare facilities, but with inclusion of hepatitis A vaccine in the childhood immunization schedule in the U.S., a significant decrease in rates of disease has occurred.[6,14] Illness usually is mild or unrecognized in young children and often manifests with symptoms of an influenza-like illness.[6,12,14] Outbreaks in childcare facilities are recognized usually by illnesses with jaundice in staff or parents of attendees (see Chapter 3, Infections Associated with Group Childcare).

Hepatitis B virus (HBV). HBV is the only hepatotropic virus that is not directly cytopathic; it causes disease through the host's immune response against virus-infected hepatocytes. The severity of infection is related inversely to the effectiveness of the immune system to diminish viral replication.[15] Two main patterns of transmission occur. In endemic areas like China, Southeast Asia, and sub-Saharan Africa, transmission usually occurs at birth or through horizontal transmission among children <5 years of age.[15,16] In the U.S., the most common routes of transmission are injection drug use, sexual contact, and nosocomial infection; no risk factor is found in about 30% of cases.[13,15–17] Incidence of HBV infections in neonates is declining in countries with neonatal immunization programs.[15–18] Most neonatal infections are not associated with clinically evident disease but chronic infection develops in infants not treated immediately after birth with hepatitis B immune globulin and vaccine.[16,17] Children and adolescents are more likely to

PART II Clinical Syndromes and Cardinal Features of Infectious Diseases: Approach to Diagnosis and Initial Management

SECTION I Intra-Abdominal Infections

TABLE 62-2. Additional Age-Specific Evaluation for Patients with Suspected Hepatitis

	Age Group		
	Neonates	**Children**	**Adolescents**
BLOOD TESTS			
Infectious	HBsAg	HBsAg	HBsAg
	Anti-HBc IgM	Anti-HBc IgM	Anti-HBc IgM
		Anti-HAV IgM	Anti-HAV IgM
	Anti-HCV, HCV PCR	Anti-HCV, HCV PCR	Anti-HCV, HCV PCR
	Toxoplasmosis titer: mother and child	Anti-HCV	Anti-HCV
	Plasma HSV PCR, virus culture mucosal strips	Anti-HDV	Anti-HDV
	Plasma enterovirus PCR, virus culture mucosal samples	Anti-HEV (if travel history)	Anti-HEV (if travel history)
Metabolic	Cystic fibrosis screen or sweat test, serum amino acids	Same as for neonates	Same as for neonates
		Ceruloplasmin	Ceruloplasmin
		24-hour urine copper	24-hour urine copper
Autoimmune		ESR, quantification of serum immunoglobulins; antinuclear antibody; LKM and smooth-muscle antibodies	Same as for children
URINE TESTS			
Metabolic	Reducing substances Organic acid screen	Same as for infants	

HBcAg, hepatitis B core antigen; HA (_C, _D, _E) V, hepatitis A (_B, _C, _D, _E) virus; HBsAg, hepatitis B surface antigen; ESR, erythrocyte sedimentation rate; LKM, liver–kidney–microsomal.

develop clinical illness if infected with HBV, usually acquired by close contact with an infected adult, sexual contact, or use of intravenous drugs.[15–17] Viral genotypes are important predictors of clinical outcome, drug responses, and mutations.[15] Implementation of the national vaccination strategy to eliminate HBV transmission has greatly reduced the disease burden in the U.S.[13,17,18] HBV is potentially a vaccine-preventable disease but only if all countries establish effective vaccination programs for several generations and at-risk adults also are vaccinated.[19] There are now 7 medications approved for treatment of HBV in the U.S. but only 3 are approved for use in children.[20]

Hepatitis C virus (HCV). HCV infection in young children is acquired primarily by perinatal transmission in the U.S., but the use of unsafe injections and medical procedures is an important cause in resource-poor countries.[21] In older people, the great majority of cases are caused by injection drug use (68%) or sexual contact with an infected partner (18%).[21] Because of major improvements in serologic diagnosis, HCV infection now is rarely caused by blood transfusion or organ transplantation. In contrast to HAV and HBV, no effective HCV vaccine is available.[21] The efficiency of perinatal transmission appears to be low in the general population but greatly increases if the mother is coinfected with (HIV) or has a high titer of HCV RNA.[21,22] HCV infections usually are mild or asymptomatic in children, but a high proportion of those infected progress to develop fibrosis, cirrhosis, and hepatocellular cancer.[20–22] Until recently, the standard in HCV treatment in adults has been a combination regimen of pegylated interferon-α with ribavirin.[23] This combination has been shown to be effective in randomized trials in children, and is approved by the FDA for use in children.[24] Two new direct-acting antiviral agents, telapravir and boceprevir, have been approved for use in adults; studies of safety, dosing, and treatment response in children will be forthcoming.[24a]

Hepatitis D virus (HDV, delta virus). HDV infections, which can occur only in conjunction with HBV infection, have been described rarely in neonates and are infrequent in all age groups in the U.S.[24,25] The importance of perinatal transmission appears to be minimal.[23] In older infants and children, the disease is uncommon and usually occurs in people with chronic HBV infection.[23,24]

Hepatitis E virus (HEV). HEV is common in endemic areas of developing countries outside of the U.S. and in travelers to those areas, especially the Middle East and Asia. However,

autochthonous (locally acquired) HEV infection also is emerging in industrialized countries where HEV is thought to be a zoonosis transmitted by pigs.[26] HEV has not been reported as a cause of neonatal hepatitis.[27] However, pregnant women with jaundice and acute viral hepatitis caused by HEV infection have a higher mortality rate and worse obstetric and fetal outcomes than pregnant women with other types of viral hepatitis.[28] HEV disease is similar to HAV except that HEV primarily affects older children and adults and has been associated with neurologic disorders.[26,29] An HEV vaccine has been shown to be safe and effective in phase 3 trials.[30]

Hepatitis G virus (HGV). HGV, the most recently identified hepatitis virus, appears to produce the mildest illness of the hepatotropic viruses.[31] Although most infected people have evidence of persistent viremia, histologic evidence of HGV infection is rare and serum aminotransferase values usually are normal. Currently, there is no conclusive evidence that HGV causes fulminant or chronic disease and it appears that HGV may not be a pathogen.[31]

Diagnostic Approach

Hepatitis virus infection should be suspected in patients with predominant or severe hepatocellular dysfunction and in fulminant hepatitis. The evaluation for infectious causes of hepatitis in children relies on serologic tests to identify antibodies (usually IgM) or antigens or the use of molecular diagnostic techniques, especially polymerase chain reaction (PCR), to diagnose infection.[1–3,7] The series of tests ordered, beyond the core group, should be individualized and based on the child's age and exposures (Table 62-2). For example, neonates are not evaluated for hepatitis A, D, E, or G except in unusual circumstances. Rubella testing rarely is required since maternal testing is included in routine prenatal care. The "TORCH" serologic screen is inappropriate as certain agents are unlikely to cause hepatitis as a cardinal feature (toxoplasmosis and rubella) and CMV may be diagnosed more efficiently by other techniques.[3] Liver biopsy rarely is required to make the diagnosis of infectious hepatitis.

ANATOMIC CAUSES

Biliary Atresia

Biliary atresia is the most common cause of neonatal cholestasis and usually is manifest by one month of life.[32] Biliary atresia is a process affecting both intrahepatic and extrahepatic ducts which leads to ongoing fibrosis and eventual obliteration of the biliary tract. Even in children who are treated surgically, this process eventually progresses to cirrhosis.[32] Although no clinical or laboratory findings are diagnostic of biliary atresia, the majority of infants are healthy and well grown at birth and are asymptomatic for the first several weeks of life.[2,3,32] By contrast, infants with neonatal infections are more likely to be born prematurely, small for gestational age, and ill appearing at birth.[2,3] The finding of situs inversus, splenic abnormalities, and congenital cardiac defects associated with cholestasis should suggest the possibility of biliary atresia.[32]

Paucity of Bile Ducts

Paucity of bile ducts is a histologic diagnosis made when the ratio of ducts to portal tracts is less than one.[33] Paucity of bile ducts can be grouped into the syndromic or nonsyndromic varieties; both usually are manifest in infancy with jaundice and hepatomegaly. Children with the syndromic type (Alagille syndrome) have a variety of associated anomalies including peculiar facies (broad forehead, hypertelorism, small chin) and cardiac (most commonly peripheral pulmonic stenosis), ocular (posterior embryotoxon), and vertebral arch (butterfly vertebrae) abnormalities.[33] The nonsyndromic form of paucity of bile ducts does not include such anomalies.[33]

Choledochal Cysts

Choledochal cysts often become manifest in infancy but can become symptomatic in any age group.[34] The spectrum of disease is wide, ranging from solitary lesions involving the extrahepatic biliary tree to diffuse intrahepatic involvement (Caroli disease).[33,34]

Congenital Hepatic Fibrosis

Congenital hepatic fibrosis, a syndrome that includes hepatomegaly, cholestasis, cystic disease of the kidneys, and portal hypertension, varies in clinical manifestation depending on the age of the child.[33,34] The renal form of disease (autosomal recessive polycystic disease) usually predominates in infancy, whereas the hepatic-related form is more common in older children and adults.[33,34]

Genetic Intrahepatic Cholestasis

Several forms of genetic intrahepatic cholestasis have been identified, in which molecular defects can lead to abnormalities in bile synthesis, transport, and excretion.[35] The most common presentation is as jaundice in neonates. Some diseases, such as bile salt export pump (BSEP) abnormalities and MDR3 deficiency, are liver-specific disorders. Others, such as FIC1 deficiency, are systemic disorders with multisystem involvement.[35]

Diagnostic Approach

The diagnosis of most anatomic lesions is made by ultrasound (e.g., choledochal cyst) or liver biopsy (e.g., intrahepatic cholestasis, congenital hepatic fibrosis, and sclerosing cholangitis).[1–3] Endoscopic retrograde cholangiopancreatography (ERCP) and magnetic resonance cholangiopancreatography (MRCP) may be helpful in diagnosing biliary tract lesions, especially in older children.[1–3]

AUTOIMMUNE CAUSES

Autoimmune Hepatitis

Autoimmune hepatitis usually presents with the insidious onset of malaise, anorexia, and fatigue in adolescents, with a striking female predominance (see Chapter 63, Chronic Hepatitis). However, the disease can occur in younger children, in both sexes,

and with acute manifestations precipitated by another event, such as an intercurrent viral illness.[36] The diagnosis of autoimmune hepatitis is made using the clinical and serologic criteria included in a scoring system developed by a group of experts.[37] The constellation of findings in autoimmune hepatitis include hypergammaglobulinemia, autoantibodies, and evidence for other disorders known to be associated with disturbances in immunoregulation.

Primary Sclerosing Cholangitis

Primary sclerosing cholangitis (PSC) is rare in young children, usually manifesting in adolescence or adult life.[38] Jaundice and right upper quadrant pain are the most common signs.[35] The disease often is associated with inflammatory bowel disease, especially ulcerative colitis or Crohn colitis.[38] Patients with PSC are at risk for developing associated cholangiocarcinoma.[39]

METABOLIC CAUSES

Metabolic conditions include a large group of disorders that must be considered in every infant with hepatitis, especially children in whom usual infectious causes have been excluded.[2,3,40] Initial manifestations including jaundice, lethargy, vomiting, hepatomegaly, and failure to thrive, mimicking many other causes of hepatic dysfunction. Developmental delay can be an important clue to metabolic disease. Diagnostic tests indicated for the initial evaluation for metabolic disease are included in Box 62-1 and in Table 62-2. Many of the metabolic diseases occur in early childhood so that extensive testing for these disorders usually is not required when previously healthy children and adolescents present with hepatic dysfunction.

α_1-Antitrypsin Deficiency

α_1-Antitrypsin deficiency can cause a hepatitis-like illness in children of any age group, including neonates.[41] Approximately 10% to 20% of people with α_1-antitrypsin deficiency develop signs and symptoms of liver dysfunction at some time.[41] Neonatal liver disease is almost always limited to infants with homozygous protease inhibitor phenotype zz.[41,42] The clinical presentation is not distinctive; disease should be considered in any infant, child, or adolescent with jaundice or abnormal liver function tests.[41,42] The condition frequently is unmasked by an intercurrent infection or hepatic insult.

Cystic Fibrosis

Cystic fibrosis is associated with a wide range of hepatobiliary tract disease, including steatosis, focal biliary cirrhosis, cholelithiasis, and intrahepatic duct stones or sludge. Clinically significant hepatobiliary tract disease occurs in about one-third of children with cystic fibrosis, but accounts for only about 2–3% of mortality.[43,44] In the neonatal period, severe cholestatic disease can occur in the absence of pulmonary involvement. The "gold standard" test for diagnosis remains the sweat test.[43] However, serologic genetic screening can be helpful in suspected patients of European descent because they often have the most common mutations, including δ-F508.[40] If the genetic screening is negative, a sweat test still is required to rule out the diagnosis. Genetic screening can be especially valuable in neonates, in whom a sweat test often is unreliable due to difficulties in obtaining an adequate sample. Since there is no phenotypic association between the incidence of liver disease and specific mutations, genetic testing cannot be used to predict the development of liver disease.[43]

Carbohydrate Metabolism

Several disorders of carbohydrate metabolism can cause hepatic dysfunction in infants and children.[45] A family history of liver disease always should be sought since disorders of carbohydrate metabolism are inherited disorders and the pattern of symptom onset can help to guide the diagnosis. For example, the onset of

PART II Clinical Syndromes and Cardinal Features of Infectious Diseases: Approach to Diagnosis and Initial Management

SECTION I Intra-Abdominal Infections

diarrhea and liver dysfunction occurring after ingestion of fructose (e.g., in fruit juices) raises the likelihood of fructosemia. Galactosemia must be ruled out by testing the urine for reducing substances in any neonate with liver dysfunction who receives lactose. In addition, fasting hypoglycemia, in the absence of liver failure or endstage hepatic disease, is an important clue to the possibility of disorders of carbohydrate metabolism, including six of the eight forms of glycogen storage disease.[44] Splenomegaly is not common in these disorders and usually occurs only in amylopectinosis disease (type IV glycogen storage disease.)[45]

Protein Metabolism

Disorders of protein metabolism often manifest in infancy, but some diseases, such as the chronic form of tyrosinemia, can occur later in life.[40] Developmental delay and seizures often are associated with these disorders, but may not be manifest initially; laboratory evaluation or biopsy may be required to establish the diagnosis.[2,3] Hyperammonemia can be an important clue to disorders involving protein metabolism including disorders of the urea cycle and organic acidemias.[2,3] Many of these disorders are apparent at birth or shortly thereafter.

Metal Metabolism

Consideration of disorders of metal metabolism is influenced by the age of the child. For example, Wilson disease, which can present as acute, chronic, or fulminant liver dysfunction, rarely presents in children <4 years of age.[46,47] By contrast, Indian childhood cirrhosis typically occurs in children <3 years of age and hepatic insufficiency develops in the first week of life in neonatal hemochromatosis.[2,3]

Lipid Storage Diseases

The lipid storage diseases usually are associated with hepatosplenomegaly and progressive central nervous system deterioration. Signs and symptoms can be apparent early in the first year and can progress quickly to death (Wolman disease); or onset can occur throughout childhood and even into adulthood (Niemann–Pick and Gaucher diseases).[40]

Disorders of Mitochondrial Fatty Acid Oxidation

A growing number of disorders of fatty acid oxidation are being discovered. Children with these disorders can present in infancy but often do not develop symptoms until later in life when prolonged fasting, often in conjunction with an acute infection,

causes a Reye-like syndrome.[48] Cardinal features include hypoglycemia, acidosis, and hepatic injury, often with little elevation in bilirubin levels.

Disorders of Bile Acid Metabolism

An increasing number of disorders that cause errors in metabolism of bile acids are being discovered; these disorders routinely cause cholestasis and hepatitis in neonates.[49] These rare disorders previously were placed in the category of neonatal, or idiopathic, hepatitis. Clinical manifestations usually are not diagnostic, but infants often have low serum bile acids, low γ-glutamyl-transpeptidase (GGT) levels, and have no pruritus, which findings are otherwise rare in conditions of hepatic dysfunction and chronic cholestasis.[49]

TOXINS AND MEDICATIONS

A variety of hepatotoxins, including medications and chemicals, can be associated with a hepatitis-like picture.[50] The clinician should obtain a history about exposure to medications including acetaminophen, valproic acid, tegretol, isoniazid, sulfonamides, phenytoin, carbamazine, and phenobarbital. Drug-related hepatitis in neonates is rare but exposure to these compounds must be considered in older infants and children, since the diagnosis usually is made on clinical grounds.[50] Children receiving total parenteral nutrition, especially prematurely born infants, are at risk of developing hepatic injury.[51] Since there is no diagnostic test for this disorder, it must be considered as a diagnosis of exclusion following rigorous evaluation. A rare but important toxic cause of severe hepatic injury in children is ingestion of *Amanita* mushrooms.

TUMORS

Hepatic tumors can present with hepatomegaly and abnormal serum hepatic tests but usually are identified by initial imaging studies. The liver often has a hard, rock-like feel on palpation.

IDIOPATHIC CAUSES

Age helps in differentiating disorders in the idiopathic category. *Neonatal hepatitis* (also called *giant cell hepatitis*) is defined as a group of disorders of unknown etiology associated with cholestasis in the neonate and young infant. The presentation can be similar to that of biliary atresia but usually is distinct from neonatal infectious hepatitis, which is characteristically part of an illness affecting multiple organ systems.[2,3]

63 Chronic Hepatitis

Parvathi Mohan and John D. Snyder

Chronic hepatitis is a clinical and pathologic syndrome associated with a wide variety of diseases and conditions[1,2] (Table 63-1). Continuous activity for 6 months is used as a definition for chronic hepatitis in adults and this provides definite proof of the persistent nature of hepatitis. However, the impact of inflammation can vary greatly so that a combination of clinical, laboratory, and histologic findings now are sought routinely that can establish the diagnosis sooner and enable earlier treatment.[1,3,4] The goal of this chapter is to provide a practical approach to evaluation of a child with chronic hepatitis.

APPROACH TO EVALUATION

A careful history and physical examination is important and can be challenging since onset often is insidious and many patients are asymptomatic.[2] Signs and symptoms, when present, are variable and can include hepatitis, fatigue, abdominal pain, anorexia, weight loss, dark-colored urine, clay-colored stools, and fever.[2] Some patients may be diagnosed after months or years of puzzling symptoms such as relapsing jaundice. Alternatively, variceal bleeding or organomegaly can be the presenting sign. A history of

TABLE 63-1. Causes of Chronic Hepatitis by Age of Onset

Causative Factor	Age of Onset		
	Neonates, Infants	Children	Adolescents
HEPATOTROPIC INFECTION			
Hepatitis B	+	+	+
Hepatitis C	+	+	+
Hepatitis D	+	+	+
GENERALIZED INFECTION			
Cytomegalovirus	+	+	+
Epstein–Barr virus	+	+	+
Human immunodeficiency virus	+	+	+
Rubella virus	+	–	–
Varicella virus	+	+	+
ANATOMIC ABNORMALITIES			
Biliary atresia	+	–	–
Congenital hepatic fibrosis	+	+	–
Sclerosing cholangitis	–	+	+
Primary biliary cirrhosis	–	–	+
AUTOIMMUNE DISORDERS	–	+	+
METABOLIC DISEASES			
α_1-Antitrypsin deficiency	+	+	+
Cystic fibrosis	+	+	+
Carbohydrate, protein, and lipid disorders	+	+	+
Obesity	–	+	+
Wilson disease	–	+	+
Errors of bile acid metabolism	+	–	–
TOXINS AND DRUGS	+	+	+
IDIOPATHIC			
Cryptogenic	+	+	+
Neonatal hepatitis	+	–	–

+, Recognized or usual age of occurrence; –, unexpected age or never an age of occurence.

BOX 63-1. Laboratory Evaluation of Children with Chronic Hepatitis

INITIAL TESTS

Blood

Tests of hepatic injury and function
Bilirubin, total and direct
Alanine aminotransferase
Aspartate aminotransferase
Alkaline phosphatase or gamma-glutamyltranspeptidase
Total protein and albumin
Prothrombin time
Ammonia
Fasting glucose
Platelet count

Tests for infectious agents
Hepatitis B surface antigen
Hepatitis B core antibody
Hepatitis C virus antibody
Hepatitis D virus antibody
Epstein–Barr antibody
Cytomegalovirus antibody
Human immunodeficiency virus antibody

Urine
Shell vial culture for cytomegalovirus for neonates

Imaging
Ultrasonography of the liver

FURTHER EVALUATIONS IF TEST RESULTS FOR INFECTIOUS CAUSES ARE NEGATIVE

Blood
Erythrocyte sedimentation rate
Quantitative serum immunoglobulin levels
Antitissue transglutaminase and serum immunoglobulin A level
Autoantibody tests
• Antinuclear antibody
• Liver–kidney–microsomal antibody
• Anti-smooth-muscle antibody
• P-antinuclear cytoplasmic antibody
Metabolic tests
• α_1-antitrypsin level with protease inhibitor type
• Ceruloplasmin level
Sweat test

Urine
Quantification of copper in 24-hour specimen

Radiology
Magnetic resonance imaging (MRI, MRCP, MRS)

Liver biopsy

exposure to blood products, use of intravenous drugs, or maternal infection are important clues to viral hepatitides.[4] The presence of thyroiditis, Sjögren syndrome, or idiopathic colitis, especially in a female, raises the possibility of autoimmune hepatitis (AIH).[3] History of exposure to drugs and toxins also must be sought.

The pattern of biochemical abnormalities usually is not diagnostic for a specific etiology. Serum levels of serum aminotransferases often are elevated but can be intermittently normal in hepatitis C infection.[4] Often, levels of serum aminotransferases do not reliably reflect the severity of disease by liver biopsy.[4] Patients with chronic hepatitis can progress to cirrhosis with normal serum levels of aminotransferases.[1,4,5] Bilirubin elevations and levels of other serum enzymes such as alkaline phosphatase and γ-glutamyltranspeptidase can be variable.

In contrast to acute hepatitis, liver biopsy often is an essential tool in the diagnosis and management of patients with chronic hepatitis. Liver biopsy also is used to assess prognosis by grading the severity of disease and its progression. The terms *chronic active, chronic persistent,* and *chronic lobular* hepatitis have been replaced by new terminology that grades the severity of liver inflammation and fibrosis from minimal to severe.[1,3]

The list of diagnostic possibilities for a patient with chronic hepatitis is shown in Table 63-1 and the approach to the initial evaluation in Box 63-1. Infectious causes are most common and should be included in the initial evaluation. If the testing, which can be completed in a few days, is negative, the second stage of testing is undertaken.[4,5]

ETIOLOGIES

Infectious Causes

Hepatitis B virus (HBV) infection is one of the most common causes of chronic hepatitis in children worldwide but the incidence has decreased in the United States due to universal vaccination and blood donor screening.[2,4,5] Chronic HBV infection still is encountered in the U.S. in children infected perinatally or in adoptees from endemic areas such as the Far East.[2] The risk of developing chronic HBV infection is related directly to the age of acquisition. Perinatal infection is associated with a 90% to 95% risk of chronic hepatitis in infants born to mothers who are hepatitis B e-antigen-positive, whereas infection in adults results in a less than 10% incidence of chronic hepatitis.[2,5,6] Exposure to

PART II Clinical Syndromes and Cardinal Features of Infectious Diseases: Approach to Diagnosis and Initial Management

SECTION I Intra-Abdominal Infections

infected blood products (now rare), intravenous drug use, and institutionalized settings increase the risk of HBV infection and subsequent chronic hepatitis.[6,7] Hepatitis D virus (HDV) is an incomplete virus that only occurs in conjunction with HBV infections. Perinatal transmission is rare, and most cases of HDV infection occur as superinfections in patients who are long-term carriers of HBV, leading to a more severe form of hepatitis.[8] The signs and symptoms of chronic HBV infections are variable; many children have a mild or asymptomatic course.[6,7] The diagnosis usually is made on serologic criteria; a liver biopsy is performed primarily for prognosis or for evaluation of efficacy of therapy.[9] Treatment involves use of interferon, or oral antiviral agents such as nucleoside analogues.[2,10] In the U.S., interferon and lamivudine are approved for use in younger children and adolescents with chronic HBV; adefovir dipivoxil is effective for children over 12 years of age.[10,11] Interferon given for 24 weeks offers a beneficial initial response in about 20% to 50% of patients but clearance of surface antigen occurs only in about 10% of cases; therapy is associated with significant adverse effects. Use of oral agents is safe and initially can clear HBeAg in 15% to 35% of cases, but disadvantages include the indefinite length of treatment, minimal clearance of HBsAg and viral resistance and relapse in a substantial number of patients.[10,11]

Hepatitis C virus (HCV) has emerged as a leading cause of chronic hepatitis in the U.S., but only a small proportion of cases occur in the pediatric population.[12] The estimated seroprevalence of HCV antibody in children is about 0.6 % based on data from the Centers for Disease Control and Prevention.[10] Prior to the advent of effective screening techniques in the early 1990s, children who had received blood products were at greatest risk for infection.[10,12,13] Now most new pediatric cases are caused by vertical transmission, with an approximate 5% risk of infection in infants born to seropositive mothers.[10] Diagnosis usually is made by detection of antibodies to core and nonstructural antigens but detection of active infection is best established by molecular diagnostic techniques, using polymerase chain reaction (PCR). Diagnosis of hepatitis C by PCR in infants should be confirmed after the first year of life, because transient viremia has been observed in neonates.[10,11] Laboratory findings of chronic HCV infection are most notable for a fluctuating pattern of serum aminotransferase values.[10,11] A liver biopsy often is performed to assess the severity of liver disease or to evaluate the efficacy of antiviral therapies.[10-12] Over one-half of children and adults infected with HCV develop chronic hepatitis.[7,10,12] Progression of the disease appears to be slower in children than in adults although advanced fibrosis, cirrhosis, and hepatocellular carcinoma can be encountered in chronically infected children.[11,13] Treatment of chronic HCV infection in children above 3 years of age with pegylated interferon and ribavirin has been approved by the FDA, and a sustained viral response of 50% to 80% has been reported depending on the genotype.[14]

Cytomegalovirus and Epstein–Barr virus infections can cause chronic hepatitis, although progression of these infections to cirrhosis and liver failure is rare.[15]

Nonalcoholic Fatty Liver Disease

Nonalcoholic fatty liver disease (NAFLD) refers to a spectrum of conditions associated with fatty infiltration of the liver.[16] Findings range from simple fatty infiltration to nonalcoholic steatohepatitis (NASH), a condition in which inflammation or fibrosis can progress to advanced liver disease and cirrhosis.[16] The potential for NAFLD and NASH to become even more common causes of chronic liver disease in children is linked directly to the current obesity epidemic; more than 20 million children worldwide are estimated to fulfill criteria for obesity.[16,17] Since the prevalence of NAFLD is estimated to be 2% to 3% among adolescents, NAFLD may be the most common cause of chronic liver disease in pediatrics.[16-18] Patients often are asymptomatic except for obesity and come to attention when elevated aminotransferase levels are noted incidentally. The physical examination usually is remarkable only for excess weight (body mass index >85% for age) and

hepatomegaly.[16] Acanthosis nigricans also can be present as a sign of associated insulin resistance. Several factors are implicated in development of NAFLD, including hyperinsulinemia, insulin resistance, associated free fatty acid hepatotoxicity, and oxidant stress.[17] Sonography demonstrates a homogeneous pattern of increased echogenicity in the liver in these patients. Since these findings are subjective and observer-dependent, magnetic resonance imaging (MRI) or MR spectrography is accepted as a more specific diagnostic modality.[16] A liver biopsy almost always is required to exclude other causes of liver diseases and to confirm the diagnosis of NAFLD.[16,17] Hepatic dysfunction usually normalizes if the body mass index can be improved with a low glycemic diet and exercise.[17] Pharmacologic agents such as vitamin E and metformin are under investigation but are not yet validated in children.[16]

Autoimmune and Autoinflammatory Disorders

Autoimmune liver disease is a heterogeneous group of diseases consisting of AIH, primary sclerosing cholangitis (PSC), and primary biliary cirrhosis (PBC).[19-22] AIH causes a diffuse pattern of hepatocellular injury whereas PSC and PBC primarily involve injury to the biliary tract, with secondary cholestasis and hepatocyte injury leading to acute liver failure or cirrhosis if untreated.

AIH primarily occurs in children under 18 years of age with a mean age of onset from 6 to 10 years of age, but has been diagnosed as early as 6 months of age.[19,20] AIH should always be considered in patients who have the distinctive clinical and serologic findings including female sex, coexistent autoimmune disease, low ratio of albumin to total protein, elevated immunoglobulins, and a relative elevation of serum transaminases compared with alkaline phosphatase.[19] In addition, elevated titers of nonorgan-specific autoantibodies are characteristic of AIH, and are used to identify subgroups of disease. In type 1 AIH, antinuclear (ANA) or antismooth-muscle (SMA) antibodies usually are present, whereas in type 2 AIH, antiliver-kidney-microsomal (LKM) antibodies or anticytosol antibodies (LAC) are seen.[3,19,20] Although clinical, laboratory, and histologic findings are helpful in suggesting the diagnosis, there is no single diagnostic test for AIH, and careful exclusion of infectious, toxic, and metabolic causes is critical. Autoantibody-negative AIH also has been reported.[20] A widely applied scoring system has been developed to improve diagnostic consistency among clinicians and researchers.[3,20] Treatment usually involves use of corticosteroids initially, followed by long-term immunosuppressive agents including azathioprine and mycophenolate. In some cases cyclosporine or tacrolimus have been used.[19,20] Liver transplantation can be required and can be complicated by recurrence of AIH in the transplanted liver.[3]

PSC is a rare cause of chronic liver disease in children and adolescents, and most commonly occurs in children with colitis caused by inflammatory bowel disease.[18,20,21] PSC is characterized by progressive fibrosis obliterating intra- and extrahepatic bile ducts.[20,21] The presence of jaundice, fatigue, and right upper quadrant pain is the most common presentation.[20,21] Diagnosis often requires endoscopic retrograde cholangiopancreatography (ERCP) and a liver biopsy. The continuing improvements in MR cholangiopancreatography (MRCP) may allow this technique to supplant use of the more invasive ERCP.[21] Treatment with ursodeoxycholic acid and immunosuppressive agents is unsatisfactory and many patients ultimately require liver transplantation.[20,21]

PBC is primarily a disease of middle-aged females but it has been identified in adolescents. This disease is characterized by the presence of antimitochondrial antibodies.[22]

Metabolic Disorders

Metabolic disorders are uncommon causes of chronic hepatitis but should be considered, especially when initial testing for infectious causes does not yield a diagnosis.[2] The clinical presentation of these disorders usually is not distinctive enough to permit diagnosis without laboratory testing, including a liver biopsy.

Although α_1-antitrypsin deficiency most commonly affects lungs, it can cause chronic liver disease in all age groups, including neonates who usually manifest with cholestatic jaundice.[23] Liver involvement in some infants progresses to cirrhosis and early death, but many people lead active lives through childhood before developing signs of chronic liver failure in late adolescence.[23] Liver disease developing later in childhood or adolescence can be associated with a wide spectrum of histologic findings, ranging from mild portal fibrosis to cirrhosis or hepatoma.[23] Diagnosis is established by measuring the serum α_1-antitrypsin level and the protease inhibitor (PI) type of the affected person.[23] Usually the most severe disease develops in people who are homozygous (PI type ZZ), but disease also occurs in heterozygotes having MZ, SZ, and Z null phenotypes.[23] There is no specific treatment for the liver disease except a liver transplant. Protein replacement therapy has been advocated for the lung disease.[23]

Chronic hepatic dysfunction occurs in as many as one-half of children with cystic fibrosis and can include steatosis, cholelithiasis, focal biliary cirrhosis, and portal hypertension.[24,25] Except in the first year of life, liver disease rarely is the initial manifestation of cystic fibrosis, so diagnostic difficulties usually are not encountered. The diagnosis of cystic fibrosis can be made by newborn screening, sweat test or genetic screening for the most common mutations.[24,25]

Disorders of carbohydrate (e.g., glycogen storage disease), protein (e.g., chronic form of tyrosinemia), and lipid (e.g., Niemann–Pick and Gaucher disease) metabolism rarely manifest after the neonatal period as chronic hepatitis.[15] These diseases often require liver biopsy as well as laboratory evaluation for diagnosis. They usually are not included in the initial evaluation unless the patient has signs and symptoms such as hypoglycemia, seizures, or developmental delay.

Wilson disease (WD) can manifest as acute, chronic, or fulminant hepatitis, and since it is potentially treatable, it must be part of the differential diagnosis of chronic hepatitis in children and adolescents.[26,27] WD rarely is reported in children <3 years of age, but in older children WD should be considered when liver disease is associated with hemolytic anemia, renal disease, or neuropsychological deterioration.[26] The finding of a Kayser–Fleischer ring on ophthalmologic examination is the most distinctive finding on physical examination but may not be present in younger children or children with liver involvement alone.[26] The diagnosis is suggested by low serum ceruloplasmin level and elevated urinary copper level (especially after penicillamine treatment) and is confirmed by elevated levels of copper in the liver biopsy specimen.[26] The abnormal gene has been identified and mutation analysis by gene sequencing can be a valuable tool in the diagnosis of indeterminate or difficult-to-diagnose cases.[27] Treatment requires the lifelong use of chelating agents such as D-penicillamine, trientine, or zinc. Liver transplantation often is required for decompensated disease or acute liver failure.

Liver disease, though seldom severe, has been observed in association with celiac disease (gluten-sensitive enteropathy). The diagnosis should be considered in all cases of hepatitis when no other cause can be found.[28]

Toxins and Drugs

Patients should always be questioned for a history of exposures to toxins and intake of drugs, since a number of agents can cause chronic hepatic injury.[29] These agents include α-methyldopa, nitrofurantoin, isoniazid, dantrolene, propylthiouracil, valproic acid, and sulfonamide.[30] Affected people often have markers of autoimmune diseases, including positive lupus erythematosus slide preparation test and elevated ANA level.[29] Discontinuation of the drug usually results in improvement or resolution of the clinical and biochemical abnormalities. The timing of toxic drug reactions is unpredictable; reactions can occur after years of regular use of a medication. The toxic effect of long-term use of total parenteral nutrition also can be an important cause of chronic hepatitis in children, particularly in children with short bowel syndrome.[31]

Idiopathic and Anatomic Causes

Cryptogenic hepatitis (hepatitis of unknown cause) is a diagnosis of exclusion when all of the above etiologies have been excluded. Depending on location and age of the population studied, cryptogenic hepatitis accounts for about 25% of the cases of chronic hepatitis.[15,32] Analysis of risk factors in adults suggests that silently progressive fatty liver may be an underrecognized cause of cryptogenic cirrhosis.[32]

Neonatal hepatitis, defined as a group of disorders of unknown etiology that cause cholestasis in neonates, also is a diagnosis of exclusion. This diagnosis usually is made early in the neonatal period; patients rarely go unrecognized and unevaluated until later infancy. The number of cases of neonatal hepatitis is decreasing as more sophisticated methods of diagnosis identify new diseases, especially errors in bile salt metabolism.[33]

The anatomic causes of hepatitis listed in Chapter 62 (Acute Hepatitis) can be associated with chronic hepatitis, but diagnosis is almost always made before hepatitis becomes chronic.

64 Granulomatous Hepatitis

Nada Yazigi and Beverly L. Connelly

The presence of histologically evident granulomas in the liver is referred to as granulomatous hepatitis. Patients may or may not be symptomatic and serum hepatic enzymes usually are normal or only minimally abnormal.[1] Granulomas have been reported as an incidental finding in liver tissue specimens obtained from adults at the time of screening for living-related liver donation[2] and in 2% to 10% of liver biopsy specimens overall in adults.[3-6] In one review of 521 liver biopsy specimens from pediatric patients, 4% showed granulomas.[7] It is estimated that granulomatous hepatitis in children accounts for 5% to 7% of hepatitis cases overall.[8] Increased utilization of computed tomography (CT) and magnetic resonance imaging (MRI) in patient evaluations has led to an increasing recognition of granulomatous hepatitis and increased search for the cause(s).

PATHOGENESIS AND PATHOLOGIC FINDINGS

The epithelioid cell is the hallmark of hepatic granulomas. Granuloma formation is initiated when monocyte-macrophages migrate into an area of inflammation. Various stimuli can cause the macrophage to transform into an epithelioid cell. It is well established in some disorders that immunomodulatory molecules, such as proinflammatory cytokines, chemokines, and other cytokines, regulate T-lymphocyte function and lead to the formation and maintenance of granuloma.[9,10] In most situations more than one mechanism is involved. The triggers are varied, and include intracellular microbial antigens, foreign-body reactions, and host immunologic hypersensitivity responses.

Hepatic granulomas vary in size (50 to 300 mm in diameter) and morphology (from clusters of epithelioid cells to well-developed granulomas rimmed by lymphocytes).[1] Epithelioid cells can merge to form multinucleated giant cells. Central caseation or abscess formation can occur. Distribution of epithelioid cells often is patchy, and the small granulomas can only be identified with serial tissue section analysis. The quantity and distribution of granulomas are best established with the periodic acid–Schiff stain.[11]

Some histologic features are associated with specific diagnoses.[11] In tuberculosis, the granulomas display central caseation and the epithelioid cells are in a radial array at the periphery; Langhan giant cells can be seen. In sarcoidosis, the granulomas are large and loose, the epithelioid cells show no pattern and there is no central caseation, but there can be central eosinophilic necrosis and multinucleated giant cells.[12] In chronic granulomatous disease of childhood, pigmented macrophages are found in architecturally normal liver, and necrotizing granulomas are found in areas of active inflammation.[13] *Bartonella henselae* causes granulomas typically with stellate microabscess. *Toxocara canis* and *T. catis* cause palisading granulomas with numerous eosinophils;[8] caseation is rare.[14] Eosinophilic infiltrates distinguish hepatic granulomas caused by visceral larva migrans. A portion of the larva can be seen within the granulomatous inflammation.[8] Eosinophilic granules also are seen often with histoplasmosis.

Special histologic stains and techniques should be used when an infectious cause is suspected. Acid-fast bacilli (AFB) are demonstrated in fewer than 10% of cases of granulomatous hepatitis caused by *Mycobacterium tuberculosis*, whereas large numbers of AFB usually are present in patients with the acquired immunodeficiency syndrome (AIDS) who are infected with *M. avium* complex.[15] Immunohistochemistry techniques can aid in identifying viruses, especially cytomegalovirus (CMV) and Epstein–Barr virus (EBV). Nucleic acid amplification techniques can be useful to identify bacteria, viruses, fungi, and rickettsiae in tissues.

CLINICAL MANIFESTATIONS AND DIFFERENTIAL DIAGNOSIS

Hepatic granulomas generally reflect a systemic disease.[1] In a comprehensive review of 6000 liver biopsies, only 4% reflected a disease limited to the liver.[16] When granulomas are limited to the liver, primary biliary cirrhosis is an important diagnosis.[5]

Clinical manifestations vary with the underlying disease. Fever and chills often are primary symptoms. In 44% of patients with granulomatous hepatitis in one series, diagnosis was pursued because of fever of unknown origin.[17] Mild right upper quadrant abdominal pain and tenderness are common. Serum hepatic enzyme levels generally are normal or mildly abnormal.[1]

Granulomatous inflammation of the liver is induced by numerous infectious agents. Drugs and toxins (including chemotherapy and radiation), inert materials and chemicals, as well as noninfectious conditions of the host can also lead to granulomatous hepatitis. The differential diagnosis is broad and, despite aggressive evaluation, no etiology can be established in many cases.[18,19]

Infectious Causes

The leading causes of granulomatous hepatitis in children are infections,[7] which are listed in Table 64-1. Geographic variability and host immunocompetence influence the prevalence of the various causes. Mycobacteria are the most frequent bacterial cause of granulomatous hepatitis.[19,20] In one review of 63 patients with granulomatous hepatitis, 9 of 11 patients younger than 20 years had tuberculosis.[17] In a large biopsy series in India, 55% of cases of granulomatous hepatitis were due to tuberculosis.[6] The liver is probably seeded during the initial lymphohematogenous dissemination of *M. tuberculosis*; involvement can occur at any stage of the infection.[21] In patients with AIDS, *M. avium* complex and other nontuberculous mycobacteria can be associated with granulomatous hepatitis. Disseminated bacillus Calmette-Guérin (BCG)

TABLE 64-1. Agents and Conditions Associated with Granulomatous Hepatitis

Infectious Agents	Noninfectious Agents/Conditions
Bacteria	**Immune dysregulation**
Bartonella henselae	Autoimmune hepatitis
Brucella spp.	Biliary cirrhosis, primary
Coxiella burnetii	Chronic granulomatous disease
Francisella tularensis	Common variable immunodeficiency
Listeria monocytogenes	Inflammatory bowel disease
Mycobacterium tuberculosis	Juvenile idiopathic arthritis
Nontuberculous mycobacteria	Sarcoidosis
Nocardia spp.	Systemic lupus erythematosus
Pasteurella multocida	Wegener granulomatosis
Treponema pallidum	
Yersinia enterocolitica	**Drugs/Chemicals**
	Allopurinol
Viruses	Barium
Cytomegalovirus	Carbamazepine
Epstein–Barr virus	Mebendazole
Hepatitis C virus	Methyldopa
Human immunodeficiency	Antimicrobial agents: norfloxacin,
virus	penicillin
	Chemotherapeutic agents
Fungi	Phenytoin
Candida spp.	Pyrazinamides
Coccidioides immiti	Sulfasalazine
Histoplasma capsulatum	Talc
	Quinine
Parasites and protozoa	
Amebas	**Neoplasms**
Schistosoma spp.	Hodgkin disease
Strongyloides spp.	Lymphoma
Toxocara spp.	
Toxoplasma gondii	**Idiopathic**

infection can cause granulomatous hepatitis in adults who receive BCG instillation into the bladder for therapy of bladder carcinoma.[22,23]

Among other bacteria, *B. henselae* infection is undoubtedly a major and underdiagnosed cause of granulomatous hepatitis in healthy and immunosuppressed children, often manifesting with abdominal pain and fever.[24] Infection with *B. henselae* leads to granulomatous hepatitis in 11% of infected patients presenting with atypical disease.[25] Histologically, necrotizing granulomas, with or without periportal and retroperitoneal lymphadenopathy and splenomegaly, are evident.[26,27]

Progress in diagnostic testing in the 1990s led to the recognition that chronic hepatitis C may be a leading cause of viral-induced granulomatous hepatitis.[4,28] In a review in the United Kingdom, hepatitis C accounted for 10% of all cases, surpassing tuberculosis more than twofold.[28] Characteristically, in chronic hepatitis C, granulomas are noted in the portal tracts.[4] Chronic infection with hepatitis A, hepatitis B, CMV, or EBV has been implicated in granulomatous hepatitis as well.

Several tickborne infections, including ehrlichiosis, tularemia, Q fever, and Lyme disease, rarely have been associated with granulomatous hepatitis.[29]

Among parasites and protozoa, schistosomiasis is a leading cause of hepatobiliary disease worldwide, particularly where the pathogens are prevalent in tropical and subtropical regions of Asia, the Caribbean, South America, and Africa.[30] Histopathologic examination of biopsy tissue reveals granulomatous inflammation in the portal vessels in response to schistosomal ova. The inflammatory reaction ultimately leads to fibrosis, portal hypertension, and massive splenomegaly.[31] Migrating larvae of *T. canis* and *T. cati* lead to hepatic or splenic granulomatous disease associated with visceral larva migrans.[32] Peripheral eosinophilia is often significant and organ enlargement can be severe.

Histoplasmosis is the most common fungal infection reported in association with granulomatous hepatitis in immunocompetent as well as immunocompromised patients.[6,7,33] Hepatic and

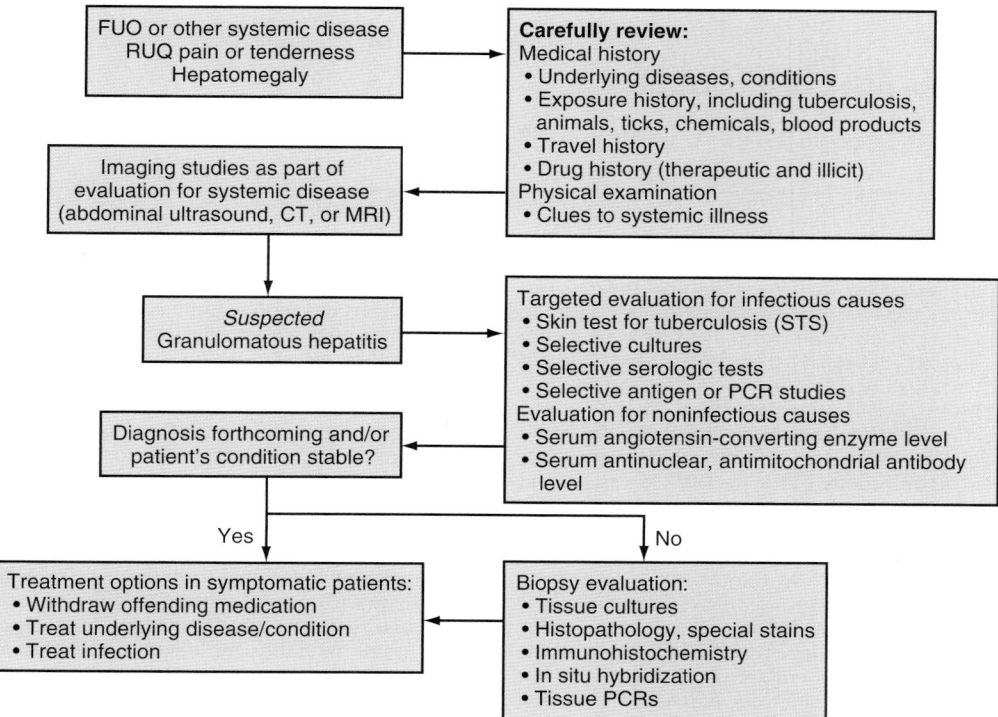

Figure 64-1. An approach to the diagnosis of granulomatous hepatitis. CT, computed tomography; FUO, fever of unknown origin; MRI, magnetic resonance imaging; PCR, polymerase chain reaction; PPD, purified protein derivative; RUQ, right upper quadrant.

splenic granulomas and abscesses due to *Candida* species are well-recognized complications in the neutropenic and otherwise immunocompromised population, and occasionally in children with bloodstream infection related to a central venous catheter.

Noninfectious Causes

Noninfectious causes of hepatic granulomas are noted in Table 64-1. Systemic conditions with abnormal immune regulation are most associated.[34] Sarcoidosis is by far the most frequently encountered entity that causes granulomatous hepatitis with multisystem manifestations.[6,17,18,35,36] In chronic granulomatous disease of childhood, the liver is one of a number of organs that are infected chronically, containing abscesses or noncaseating granulomas.[37] Hepatic granulomas can occur in a variety of lymphoreticular disorders, such as Hodgkin disease.[3,28,38]

Primary biliary cirrhosis, affecting mostly adult women, is the most common cause of granulomas isolated to the liver.[5,28] When present in primary sclerosing cholangitis, hepatic granulomas have been associated with more severe systemic immune dysregulation and linked to worse outcome.[39]

Numerous drugs and toxins have been associated with noncaseating granulomatous hepatitis.[39,40] Chemotherapeutic agents, antibiotics, anticonvulsants, and anti-inflammatory agents are associated most frequently. It has been speculated that many of the "idiopathic" cases of granulomatous hepatitis may be drug-related.[40]

Hepatic granulomas can occur as an extraintestinal manifestation of inflammatory bowel disease (Crohn), in chronic inflammatory systemic disorders such as juvenile idiopathic arthritis,[1,8] and in individuals with abnormal immune function such as common variable immunodeficiency.[34] In all of these individuals with immune dysfunction, any of the infectious causes can occur as well.

DIAGNOSIS

Granulomatous hepatitis should be suspected in any patient with fever of unknown origin or with a systemic disorder in which right upper quadrant abdominal pain or tenderness, hepatomegaly, or a mild elevation of serum concentration of hepatic enzymes is seen. Granulomas also are seen sometimes on imaging studies as part of the evaluation of such symptoms. Ultrasonography, but mostly CT and MRI, are sensitive screening diagnostic modalities; MRI may allow differentiation between caseating and noncaseating granulomas.[41] The role of FD6 PET/CT in detection of granulomas in the liver is growing but remains to be defined.[42] As depicted in Figure 64-1, testing, guided by a careful history to capture epidemiologic clues, and the physical examination, paying attention to clues for underlying systemic disease, often can lead to the diagnosis, and guide the treatment without having to perform a liver biopsy. Because of the prevalence of viral infections such as EBV, CMV, and hepatitis C, testing for these in the absence of tissue examination may not be specific. In immunocompromised individuals and those with progressive symptoms without a compelling diagnosis, a tissue diagnosis should be sought. Tissue from a lymph node or skin lesion in a patient with systemic disease may provide the diagnosis, avoiding the more invasive liver biopsy. Tissue cultures may yield an offending pathogen. Histopathologic clues from routine and special stains can guide immunohistochemistry (in situ hybridization) and nucleic acid amplification testing (PCR) of tissue specimens and substantially increase detection of most infectious agents.[43] Further serologic studies and serum PCR studies then may be indicated. Thorough investigation for all possible causative diseases should be performed before the condition is labeled idiopathic.

MANAGEMENT AND OUTCOME

Granulomatous hepatitis of infectious origin regresses with appropriate targeted therapy. Treatment of any underlying disease, however, is the cornerstone of management. Empiric therapy with corticosteroids has been advocated in idiopathic cases in adults, although illness may resolve without therapy in these patients.[44] There are no collective data regarding the outcome of children with idiopathic granulomatous hepatitis. Thus, empiric therapy with corticosteroids is rarely indicated in children in view of the predominance of infectious causes of pediatric cases.

65 Acute Pancreatitis

Nada Yazigi and Beverly L. Connelly

Acute pancreatitis is a rare disorder in children. In its mild form, pancreatitis is likely underdiagnosed in pediatrics, and resolves spontaneously with no sequelae. The etiologic factors leading to pancreatitis cover a wide variety of disorders that vary in incidence by age. In adults, alcohol and biliary tract disease are the major causes of acute pancreatitis.[1] In children, pancreatitis is most often due to trauma (22% to 25% of cases); structural anomalies, systemic disease (e.g., cystic fibrosis, metabolic disorders), drugs and toxins each account for 10% to 15% of cases; the remainder of cases are attributed to infections (10% to 15% of cases), and increasingly recognized hereditary forms.[2–7]

PATHOGENESIS

Inflammation of the pancreas in response to a variety of insults is due to autodigestion of the organ by pancreatic enzymes. The precise circumstances and chronology of events leading to enzyme activation vary by etiology.[8] The end result, however, is that enzymes are activated within the pancreatic parenchyma, leading to local inflammation and damage. The inflammatory cascade that follows pancreatic injury results in the systemic inflammatory response syndrome.[9] Interleukin 1 (IL-1) and tumor necrosis factor (TNF) mediate this response. These agents, in turn, increase production of platelet-activating factor (PAF), nitric oxide, IL-6, and IL-8. Inflammatory mediators are responsible for the clinical findings of severe acute pancreatitis: adult respiratory distress syndrome, vascular leakage, renal dysfunction, hypovolemia, and shock. Other factors, such as activated complement (C) 5 and IL-10, may act to dampen the inflammatory response.[10]

CLINICAL MANIFESTATIONS

Abdominal pain is the predominant symptom in most patients, and can be isolated. The pain is typically in the epigastric area and is continuous and dull in nature. It begins abruptly, increases in severity, and peaks in a few hours. Sometimes the pain is mild, is localized elsewhere in the abdomen, or radiates to the middle of the back. Nausea and vomiting occur in 70% of patients. The child's position of comfort is usually one with the knees flexed on the abdomen. Compared with older children with pancreatitis, infants and toddlers in one study had significantly fewer signs and symptoms of abdominal pain, epigastric tenderness, or nausea.[11] Epigastric or midabdominal tenderness with guarding often is found on physical examination. Bowel sounds disappear as ileus develops. An abdominal mass can develop as a manifestation of a pancreatic pseudocyst. Rigid abdomen or cutaneous signs of hemorrhagic pancreatitis, such as bluish flank (Grey Turner sign) and periumbilical discoloration (Cullen sign), are rare and represent signs of severity.[12] Care should be taken to identify complications such as shock. In pediatrics, the vast majority of pancreatitis remains mild, and has spontaneous resolution.

DIAGNOSIS

The diagnosis of acute pancreatitis relies on clinical symptoms and should be considered in any child manifesting upper or diffuse abdominal pain or shock.[13] No single definitive diagnostic test is available. A comprehensive history highlighting potential causes should be elicited. The diagnosis is usually confirmed by the finding of elevated serum pancreatic enzymes. Elevated total serum amylase has a sensitivity of 95% to 100% if tested within the first 24 hours after onset of symptoms; serum amylase level tends to fall within 48 hours of onset. Specificity (70%) and positive predictive value (15% to 72%) of elevated serum amylase level are low.[14] Serum lipase is more specific for pancreatic inflammation and is more sensitive in later stages of the disease.[15] When used together, elevated serum amylase and serum lipase values yield a specificity of 90% to 95%.[16] Persistence of elevated amylase beyond 48 hours after the onset of symptoms raises the possibility of the development of pancreatic pseudocyst.

Abdominal ultrasonography is the best initial imaging study when pancreatitis is suspected. Ultrasonography can show swelling of the pancreas, but most importantly helps exclude surgically treatable causes of pancreatitis such as gallstones, and extrapancreatic masses. A plain film of the abdomen is useful to exclude other causes of abdominal pain; pancreatic calcification can occur in patients with acute recurrent or chronic pancreatitis. Intravenous contrast-enhanced abdominal computed tomography is the most useful modality for diagnosis of significant abdominal trauma, necrotizing pancreatitis, and pseudocyst.[17] It should be done in all cases of severe pancreatitis to guide therapy. Endoscopic retrograde cholangiopancreatography or magnetic resonance cholangiopancreatography can be useful in selected cases, particularly when therapeutic intervention is needed.

DIFFERENTIAL DIAGNOSIS

The differential diagnosis of acute pancreatitis varies with the severity of the pancreatitis attack. In its mild forms (the most frequent presentation in children), pancreatitis can mimic acute gastroenteritis. Mild acute pancreatitis also can occur during acute viral gastroenteritis. Biliary tract disease (cholelithiasis, choledocholithiasis, choledochal cyst), peptic ulcer disease (penetrating or perforated peptic ulcer), intestinal obstruction, and factitious pancreatitis should be excluded. Renal failure and diabetic ketoacidosis can be responsible for falsely elevated serum amylase levels and should be excluded as well.

Infectious Causes

Although many infectious agents have been implicated in acute pancreatitis (Box 65-1), evidence supporting their causality is usually indirect, based on results of serologic assays or epidemiologic association. Undiagnosed but self-limited viral illnesses likely account for many "idiopathic" cases of acute pancreatitis.

BOX 65-1. Common Infectious Causes of Acute Pancreatitis in Children

VIRUSES	PARASITES
Mumps virus	*Ascaris lumbricoides*
Group B coxsackieviruses	*Clonorchis sinensis*
Other enteroviruses	*Cryptosporidium parvum*
Hepatitis A	*Echinococcus granulosus*
Hepatitis B	
Epstein–Barr virus	**OTHER**
Cytomegalovirus	*Mycoplasma pneumoniae*
Human immunodeficiency virus	
Influenza A virus	
Rotavirus	

Viral agents, particularly mumps, are the most common infectious pathogens.[2] Mild pancreatitis occurs in up to 15% of patients with mumps. Parotitis usually precedes abdominal pain and vomiting by 4 to 5 days; pancreatitis rarely occurs alone. Enteroviruses, especially group B coxsackieviruses, also are implicated frequently.[18,19] Epstein–Barr virus (EBV) infection has been associated with pancreatitis in multiple case reports.[20,21] Hepatitis B surface and core antigens (HBsAg and HBcAg) have been detected in pancreatic acinar cells, a finding that may explain the pancreatitis associated with hepatitis B infection.[22] A report from Brazil documented 4 cases of pancreatitis associated with measles infection; 3 of the 4 patients were immunosuppressed.[23] Pancreatitis in patients with human immunodeficiency virus (HIV) infection is attributed to direct HIV infection, superinfection with cytomegalovirus or another opportunistic agent (e.g., *Toxoplasma gondii*), tumor, or drug therapy (e.g., pentamidine or dideoxyinosine).[24-27] Pancreatitis unrelated to antiretroviral therapy is a poor prognostic indicator in HIV-infected children.

Ascaris lumbricoides, Clonorchis sinensis, and *Cryptosporidium parvum* cause pancreatitis via physical obstruction of the pancreatic duct as they migrate from the intestinal lumen into the biliary or pancreatic ducts or both.[28-30] Bacteria are unusual causes of acute pancreatitis, but enteric organisms complicate necrotizing pancreatitis and worsen the prognosis. Fungal pathogens have not been reported as causative agents in pancreatitis, but can infect a necrotic pancreas.

Noninfectious Causes

The many noninfectious causes of pancreatitis are shown in Box 65-2. Traumatic pancreatitis occurs in association with blunt abdominal trauma, child abuse, or penetrating wounds or after surgery. Systemic inflammatory disorders such as Kawasaki disease,[31] juvenile idiopathic arthritis, systemic lupus erythematosus, Crohn disease, and toxic epidermal necrolysis[32] have been associated with acute pancreatitis. Prescription medications as well as the accidental ingestion of the drugs listed in Box 65-2 can

---

BOX 65-2. Common Noninfectious Causes of Acute Pancreatitis in Children

TRAUMA

ANATOMIC

Congenital duct anomalies
Annular pancreas
Biliary duct stones
Tumor (blocking pancreatic duct)

DRUGS

Corticosteroids
L-Asparaginase
Thiazides
Furosemide
Dideoxyinosine
Azathioprine
Valproic acid
Others

INFLAMMATORY DISEASE

Kawasaki syndrome
Other vasculitic disorders
Juvenile idiopathic arthritis
Crohn disease
Systemic lupus erythematosus
Henoch–Schönlein purpura
Toxic epidermal necrolysis
Stevens–Johnson syndrome
Major burns

METABOLIC DISORDERS

Hyperlipidemia (type I, IV, V)
Type 1 diabetes
Glycogen storage disease
Cystic fibrosis
Mitochondrial disorder

HEREDITARY

IDIOPATHIC

---

be causal.[33] Corticosteroids are the most commonly implicated drugs causing pancreatitis in children. Pancreatitis in infants and toddlers is associated more often with multisystem infection or disease, especially hemolytic uremic syndrome.[34] Pancreatitis following bone marrow transplantation can occur during graft-versus-host disease,[35] possibly as a consequence of corticosteroid treatment. Acute pancreatitis following liver transplantation is thought to be multifactorial.[36]

Hereditary pancreatitis, which manifests first in infancy or adolescence, is an autosomal-dominant disorder described in more than 40 kindreds, and linked to chromosome 7q35 in a kindred from the United States.[37] Juvenile tropical pancreatitis, which occurs in Africa and Asia, manifests as recurrent abdominal pain in childhood. Both entities characteristically progress to chronic pancreatitis. Specific CFTR genotypes are significantly associated with pancreatitis in patients with cystic fibrosis[38] and in some patients with idiopathic pancreatitis.[39]

TREATMENT

Therapy for acute pancreatitis is primarily supportive. Gut rest is only indicated if pain continues or a complication arises. Withdrawing an offending agent is important whenever possible and is particularly relevant for drugs causing cholelithiasis. Pancreatitis may signal the need for treatment of an underlying systemic inflammatory disorder.

Supportive care is dictated by the severity of the multiorgan dysfunction that can complicate pancreatitis. Meperidine hydrochloride is usually selected for pain control because it has less of a constrictive effect on the sphincter of Oddi than does morphine. Nasogastric suction is only used in patients with ileus or severe vomiting, for symptomatic relief.[40] If fasting is required for more than 3 days and no improvement is seen, parenteral nutrition or jejunal feeding is indicated. Clinical trials suggest a possible role for early enteral antimicrobial therapy (given by oral and rectal routes) to prevent systemic infection in severe pancreatitis.[41-43] The administration of broad-spectrum antibiotics to patients with severe, necrotizing pancreatitis results in improved mortality and morbidity.[44] The use of agents to inhibit pancreatic secretion, such as cimetidine, somatostatin, calcitonin, glucagon, and fluorouracil, has proven to be ineffective in improving outcomes. Testing of protease inhibitors, PAF antagonist, and cholecystokinin A receptor antagonist have yielded mixed results.[45-47]

CLINICAL COURSE

Most children recover completely from acute pancreatitis; mortality rates in children are not defined clearly. In one series in children, 21% died, but all had serious underlying multisystem disorders.[6] Other series report 2% to 20% mortality.[3,13] Death or complications are more likely in those with pancreatic or peripancreatic hemorrhage or necrosis, which presages a complicated acute course that can include hemodynamic instability, serious biochemical abnormalities, and multiorgan failure. Local complications include formation of abscess or pseudocyst. Development of a secondary fever indicates a possible complication; abdominal ultrasonography or computed tomography is indicated, and drainage of abscess or guided-needle aspiration of necrotic tissue is required. In a Dutch randomized multicenter study of patients with necrotizing pancreatitis, step-up approach of percutaneous drainage followed, if necessary, by minimally invasive retroperitoneal necrosectomy had superior outcomes to open necrosectomy.[48] There is now consensus that the best outcomes for intervention are achieved when debridement is delayed until approximately 4 weeks after onset of pancreatitis.[49]

66   Cholecystitis and Cholangitis

Nada Yazigi and Beverly L. Connelly

Cholecystitis and *cholangitis* refer to inflammation of the gallbladder and extrahepatic bile ducts, respectively. They are much more common in adults than in children but occur often enough to be important to clinicians caring for children with acute abdominal illnesses.

PATHOGENESIS

Most cases of cholecystitis and cholangitis are initiated by obstruction of normal bile flow through the cystic duct and common bile duct, respectively, by biliary stones, anatomic abnormalities, or devices such as stents. Biliary stones can be composed of pure pigment produced by hemolysis as a complication of hemoglobinopathies (e.g., spherocytosis, thalassemia, and sickle-cell anemia), or in infants after extracorporeal membrane oxygenation support.[1] Biliary stones more often are cholesterol based; these stones occur in association with sudden weight loss, overweight problems, prolonged total parenteral nutrition and with no enteral feeding, chronic liver disorders (affecting the integrity of bile acids secretion), and prolonged use of medications that can result in biliary sludge (i.e., some diuretics and antibiotics). Some patients have a familial predisposition to stone formation, particularly as young adults; in these instances the prevalence is higher in women.

Portoenterostomy (Kasai procedure), the classic surgical procedure performed for biliary atresia, predisposes children to recurrent cholangitis. In one study, 46 of 101 infants who underwent a portoenterostomy had one to eight episodes of postoperative cholangitis, despite restoration of bile flow.[2] Most of the 105 episodes of cholangitis occurred during the first 3 postoperative months; only a few children had cholangitis after 1 year of age.[2] Late cases, occurring more than 5 years after successful surgical repair, also are reported.[3] Use of the intestinal conduit to restore bile flow from the liver to the small intestine is thought to lead to the ascent of intestinal flora and cholangitis.[4,5] Because of this well-recognized risk, patients are usually given antibiotic prophylaxis for 6 to 12 months. Similarly, cholangitis occurs, although less frequently, in children who have undergone orthotopic liver transplantation using a Roux-en-Y procedure for a biliary conduit.

Other rare causes of impaired biliary drainage predisposing to cholangitis include choledochal cyst, Caroli disease, primary sclerosing cholangitis, biliary stricture after abdominal trauma, prior duct surgery, cystic fibrosis, and tumors of the extrahepatic ducts (e.g., rhabdomyosarcoma, neuroblastoma). Infection of the biliary tree also can occur during instrumentation for percutaneous cholangiography or endoscopic retrograde cholangiopancreatography (ERCP).

In Asia, biliary obstruction can result from migration into the bile ducts by the Chinese liver fluke *Clonorchis sinensis* or the roundworm *Ascaris lumbricoides*. Rarely, bile ducts are partially obstructed by daughter cysts from hepatic hydatid disease. *Echinococcus granulosus*, the dog tapeworm, is prevalent in sheep-raising communities in southern Europe, Australia, and New Zealand.

Ductal obstruction from any cause results in increased intraductal pressure and/or distention of the gallbladder. Superinfection of the stagnant bile with gut flora organisms follows, along with edema and congestion, further compromising blood supply and lymphatic drainage. Tissue necrosis follows, favoring further bacterial proliferation. In cholangitis, the risk of bacteremia and septicemia is very high,[6] accounting for the high morbidity and mortality of this condition, and making cholangitis a medical and surgical emergency.

Although obstruction to biliary drainage remains the most frequent cause for cholecystis, occasionally this entity can be seen without obstruction. This condition, known as acalculous cholecystitis, occurs in critically ill patients after trauma, burns, and major surgery – notably following spinal instrumentation and fusion for scoliosis.[7] Cholecystitis also has been reported in children with infections caused by *Mycoplasma pneumoniae*, *Salmonella* Typhi and non-Typhi spp., *Shigella* spp., and *Giardia lamblia*.[8] Infectious causes of acute cholecystitis have been reviewed recently.[9] Acute acalculous distention (hydrops) of the gallbladder can occur acutely in infants and children, and is associated with a variety of infections and inflammatory conditions (notably Kawasaki disease, streptococcal pharyngitis, septicemia, toxic shock syndrome, and Henoch–Schönlein purpura), and during prolonged fasting and total parenteral nutrition. The affected patient can have pain or a palpable mass or both; ultrasonography shows markedly distended echofree gallbladder without dilatation of the biliary tract. The course usually is self-resolving.

ETIOLOGY

Bile normally is sterile. However, in patients with obstructed biliary drainage, bacteria commonly are found in the bile and in the gallbladder wall. The likelihood of bactibilia is greater when obstruction results from gallstones or benign stricture than when it results from malignancy.[10] The explanation of this phenomenon is not clear, although the likelihood of a complete obstruction with malignancy is higher, which may prevent the passage of bacteria from the intestinal tract into the biliary system. A few clinical settings and symptoms predict bactibilia: acute cholecystitis, fever, rigors, history of biliary tract intervention, jaundice, and diabetes mellitus.[10]

Organisms isolated from bile usually are part of the intestinal flora, namely enteric gram-negative bacilli, enterococci, and anaerobes. Common gram-negative bacilli include *Escherichia coli*, *Klebsiella pneumoniae*, *Enterobacter* spp., and *Proteus* spp. Common anaerobes include *Bacteroides* spp., *Clostridium* spp., and *Fusobacterium* spp. When present, anaerobes usually are part of polymicrobic infections. In one study predominantly of adults with cholecystitis, bacterial growth was observed in 85% of 145 biliary tract specimens processed for both aerobic and anaerobic bacteria.[11] Aerobic and facultative bacteria were present in 48% of the culture-positive specimens, aerobic bacteria alone in 3%, and mixed growths of anaerobic and aerobic or facultative bacteria in 49%. The six most common bacterial isolates were *E. coli* (71), *Enterococcus* spp. (42), *Klebsiella* spp. (29), *Bacteroides* spp. (28), *Clostridium* spp. (27), and *Enterobacter* spp. (16).[11] Anaerobic infections are more common in patients who have had biliary tract surgery, biliary-intestinal anastomosis, or chronic biliary tract infections. *Candida* species occur predominantly in association with intestinal disease (e.g., necrotizing enterocolitis) or surgery, prolonged antibiotic therapy, total parenteral nutrition, proton-pump inhibitor therapy, and immune suppression.[12]

Bacteria isolated from the blood of patients with cholangitis are the same as those isolated from bile, except that bloodstream infection (BSI) caused by enterococci or anaerobic organisms is uncommon. BSI is reported in 21% to 70% of patients with acute cholangitis. Bacteria also have been isolated from the liver in patients with acute cholangitis; isolates correlate with those found in the bile.[13]

CLINICAL AND LABORATORY MANIFESTATIONS

Patients with cholecystitis or cholangitis usually have an antecedent history compatible with biliary tract disease, surgery with or without endoprosthesis, or predisposing factors such as a hemoglobinopathy, prolonged total parenteral nutrition, chronic liver disease, cystic fibrosis, or a family history of gallstone formation. Clinical manifestations of cholecystitis typically are milder than those of cholangitis, but there can be substantial overlap. The clinical triad of fever, right upper quadrant pain, and jaundice classically alerts for the presence of biliary tract disease. Cholecystitis usually is heralded by mild epigastric pain with nausea and vomiting, followed by a shifting of the pain to the right upper quadrant, sometimes with radiation to the right shoulder or scapula. Pain usually is aggravated by movement or deep breathing. The gallbladder is palpable in less than 50% of cases. Moderate temperature elevation and mild icterus can be evident, but high spiking fevers, chills, prominent jaundice, circulatory collapse, and other findings of gram-negative BSI are more suggestive of cholangitis. There also can be signs of localized peritonitis, including guarding, rigidity, and rebound tenderness.

The white blood cell count is normal or slightly elevated in the presence of cholecystitis and, typically, is substantially increased with a "shift" to immature forms with cholangitis. In patients with cholecystitis, serum levels of bilirubin and aspartate aminotransferase (AST) are elevated in about 50%, and alkaline phosphatase in about 25%. By contrast, most patients with cholangitis have elevated bilirubin, AST, and alkaline phosphatase levels; the degree of abnormality is greater in those with cholangitis than in those with cholecystitis. Serum amylase concentrations can be elevated in both disorders. Disseminated intravascular coagulopathy can occur with cholangitis.

Blood cultures rarely are positive in children with cholecystitis, whereas about 50% of children with cholangitis have bacteremia. Culture of liver biopsy specimens also can be positive.[13]

DIAGNOSIS

The differential diagnosis of cholecystitis and cholangitis includes appendicitis, pancreatitis, perforating ulcer, acute pyelonephritis, biliary colic without cholecystitis, hepatitis, perihepatitis (Fitz-Hugh–Curtis syndrome), and right lower lobe pneumonia.

Ultrasonography (US) is the most useful diagnostic test and should be obtained in suspected cases. US is expected to demonstrate thickening and edema of the gallbladder wall and surrounding tissue in cholecystitis and dilatation of bile ducts in cholangitis. US also can uncover the underlying cause of biliary tract disease by demonstrating stones, a choledochal cyst, or other obstruction to bile flow.

Radionuclide hepatobiliary scanning can demonstrate obstruction of the common bile duct or cystic duct (excluding the gallbladder). Percutaneous transhepatic cholangiography and ERCP also are valuable in evaluating and treating obstructions of the biliary tract. Magnetic resonance cholangiopancreatography (MRCP) is emerging as a noninvasive diagnostic modality but does not have the advantage of being therapeutic.

Since the advent of the above testing modalities, use of cholecystography has declined in the diagnostic evaluation of suspected cholecystitis or cholangitis. Oral cholecystography is time-consuming and cannot be used in patients with jaundice or vomiting. Intravenous cholecystography is more rapid and is not affected by vomiting, but is not sensitive if the serum bilirubin concentration is >4 mg/dL, a level often present in patients with cholangitis. Furthermore, cholecystography is less sensitive than US or radionuclide scans.

Culture of a liver biopsy specimen is the most definitive diagnostic procedure for cholangitis. Nonetheless, even in the presence of cholangitis, biopsy specimen culture results can be negative. Blood cultures can be diagnostic and appear to be especially sensitive when performed immediately after liver biopsy (such as in cases in children after liver transplantation). Bile culture sometimes can be useful to guide therapy and is diagnostic when the specimen is obtained at the time of a percutaneous or endoscopic biliary drainage procedure.

TREATMENT

The initial treatment of cholecystitis and cholangitis in children consists of supportive therapy and use of broad-spectrum antibiotic therapy effective against enteric gram-negative bacilli and anaerobic bacteria. Drainage of the obstructed biliary tract is the mainstay of treatment for patients with cholangitis who are severely ill. Percutaneous or endoscopic drainage has replaced surgical intervention as the method of choice for emergent re-establishment of bile flow.

Antibiotics are complementary to biliary drainage when there is a high index of suspicion for acute gallbladder infection and may circumvent surgery in patients who are not critically ill; guidelines have been published.[14] Appropriate initial antimicrobial therapy employs an aminoglycoside such as gentamicin or a cephalosporin in combination with an agent active against anaerobic bacteria, such as clindamycin or metronidazole, or an agent combined with a β-lactamase inhibitor. Cefazolin, cefoperazone, ceftriaxone, trimethoprim-sulfamethoxazole (TMP-SMX), mezlocillin, or piperacillin-tazobactam sometimes is selected because of each agent's high biliary concentration.[10,12,15,16] Ampicillin often is included because of the possibility of enterococcal infection. Patients who receive TMP-SMX prophylactically are likely to have resistant enteric bacilli. Antibiotic prophylaxis with piperacillin, cefazolin, cefuroxime, cefotaxime, or ciprofloxacin before therapeutic ERCP has been shown to reduce the risk of bacteremia and cholangitis.[16,17] If organisms are isolated from cultures, the antibiotics are adjusted according to susceptibility test results and then continued for 7 to 10 days.

In most cases of treated cholecystitis and cholangitis, symptoms and signs resolve promptly with medical treatment. If the symptoms do not respond to initial medical management, and if gallstones or obstructing lesions are demonstrated by US, biliary drainage is indicated. Generally, current practice is immediate establishment of biliary drainage via endoscopic cholangiography, followed by nonemergent laparoscopic cholecystectomy once the active inflammatory process has subsided.[18,19] Cholecystectomy with exploration and drainage of the common bile duct or percutaneous transhepatic drainage now are performed only infrequently.

COMPLICATIONS

Perforation occurs in up to 15% of cases of cholecystitis;[20] sometimes peritonitis results, but more often, the perforation is spontaneously localized by surrounding omentum and serosa of contiguous viscera. When localized, perforation results in persistent fever, a palpable mass, and, occasionally, a friction rub over the liver. Pancreatitis and cholangitis also can complicate cholecystitis.

Cholangitis is a high level medical-surgical emergency. Complications include perforation, macroscopic hepatic abscesses, pancreatitis, and septicemia.

CHOLECYSTITIS AND CHOLANGITIS IN SPECIAL CLINICAL CONDITIONS

Biliary Atresia

Recurrent episodes of bacterial cholangitis occur in about 50% of patients with biliary atresia after a successful Kasai procedure.[2,4,5] Repeated bouts of cholangitis result in progression of the liver disease to cirrhosis. The causative organisms are usually susceptible to TMP-SMX or third-generation cephalosporin agents during the initial episode but are likely to be resistant after repeated episodes of cholangitis and courses of antibiotic therapy.[2]

Chronic antibiotic prophylaxis can reduce the frequency of recurrent attacks of cholangitis; however, no definitive, placebo-controlled evaluation has been conducted. Although the Roux-en-Y loop (which retains adherence properties of intestinal mucosa) is likely to become colonized with enteric flora despite long-term antibiotic therapy, there may be sufficient suppression of bacterial growth to reduce the concentration of bacteria below the threshold that results in symptoms of recurrent cholangitis.[10]

TMP-SMX is used commonly for the prevention of recurrent episodes of cholangitis.[12,20] TMP-SMX is active against most common biliary pathogens, has low toxicity even after prolonged use, is relatively inexpensive, has excellent bioavailability after oral administration, and is excreted in substantial concentrations into bile.[21] Breakthrough infections and superinfections due to resistant Enterobacteriaceae, *Pseudomonas*, or *Candida* organisms can occur.[17] When cholangitis recurs multiple times despite prophylaxis, percutaneous drainage and/or liver transplantation are considered.

Sickle-Cell Disease

The incidence of gallstones in individuals with sickle-cell disease (SCD) is reported to be between 17% and 33% in those younger than 18 years and >50% in the adult population. A report of gallstone disease in sickle-cell patients in Jamaica who were studied prospectively from birth to age 17 to 24 years revealed that approximately 30% of homozygously affected individuals developed gallstones, whereas only 11% of patients with mixed sickle-cell hemoglobinopathy developed gallstones.[22] Of the 99 patients with SCD and gallstones, only 7 became symptomatic, requiring cholecystectomy; no patient with mixed sickle-cell hemoglobinopathy had symptoms. The risk of gallstones in patients with SCD correlated with higher reticulocyte counts and higher mean corpuscular volume; the risk correlated minimally with elevated unconjugated bilirubin levels and low fetal hemoglobin levels. When gallbladder sludge was noted, gallstones developed within 1 to 2 years in most patients, none of whom had symptoms. One case report of a patient with SCD in whom hepatic duct strictures developed raises the possibility that hypoxic injury to the biliary system results in gallstone formation in patients with chronic anemia.[23] Patients with sickle-cell disease who have gallstones and experience repeated bouts of abdominal pain have generally been treated with elective cholecystectomy, and reports have indicated a resultant decrease in frequency of hospitalization for abdominal pain.[24]

Management of acute cholecystitis or cholangitis in the patient with SCD is the same as that for other patients.

Orthotopic Liver Transplantation

In children, the biliary anastomosis for liver transplantation is often done via an intestinal Roux-en-Y, which predisposes patients to ascending cholangitis.

A chronic subclinical form of cholangitis can occur and manifest as chronic graft dysfunction. This entity, felt to be due to poor drainage of the Roux-en-Y limb, is difficult to diagnose. With improved surgical technique, this chronic situation currently is rare. It would be unlikely to occur in patients with pre-existing Roux-en-Y (for biliary atresia) who did not have recurrent cholangitis prior to transplantation. Chronic cholangitis should only be considered as the cause of hepatic graft dysfunction when all other causes have been ruled out, and the liver biopsy still suggests acute biliary tract inflammation. A hepatobiliary nuclear scan could be helpful to support the diagnosis. No prospective studies exploring this entity, its diagnosis, or treatment are available.

Acute cholangitis is more commonly seen with, and is a hallmark of, liver graft bile duct stenosis. BSI due to biliary sepsis can be the initial presentation of bile duct stenosis or the condition can be unmasked by a liver biopsy for graft dysfunction; in the latter situation, the diagnostic liver biopsy typically is followed within 12 hours by symptomatic BSI. Right upper quadrant pain is notably absent in these patients due to lack of innervation of the liver graft. The absence of dilated intrahepatic bile ducts by US does not exclude the diagnosis; CT often is more sensitive to demonstrate dilated biliary ducts in liver grafts. As the viability of liver graft bile ducts depends on the integrity of hepatic arterial flow, documentation of blood flow is critical. Another common cause of biliary stenosis after liver transplantation is chronic rejection.

After transplantation, patients have higher risk of BSI due to their immunosuppression. Clinical presentation initially can be subtle, followed by a quick and severe deterioration if not treated promptly. Primary biliary BSI or BSI secondary to hepatic artery thrombosis occurs most frequently in the early posttransplantation time, but also can occur many years posttransplantation, raising the additional possible cause of chronic rejection. Therefore special attention and high index of suspicion for biliary sepsis should always be exercised in this special population, and addressed as a medical emergency.

67 Peritonitis

Samuel E. Rice-Townsend, R. Lawrence Moss, and Shawn J. Rangel

Peritonitis is an inflammatory process involving the peritoneum, a specialized lining of the abdominal cavity which functions to lubricate the abdominal organs and clear the cavity of infectious particles and other debris. Infectious peritonitis classically has been described as primary or secondary in etiology, depending upon on the continuity of the gastrointestinal (GI) tract. Primary, or spontaneous, bacterial peritonitis (SBP) is a relatively rare infection that develops in the presence of a continuous GI tract without an apparent source of inoculation. Secondary bacterial peritonitis is much more frequent and arises from the inoculation with bacteria and other inflammatory debris following intestinal perforation or postoperative anastomotic leak. Catheter-related infections (e.g., peritoneal dialysis catheters and ventriculoperitoneal shunts)

comprise a third category, in which infections arise following direct or indirect contamination of the indwelling foreign body.

EPIDEMIOLOGY

The overall incidence of infectious peritonitis in children is difficult to estimate due to the heterogeneity in diagnostic criteria and the multiple underlying disease processes associated with the infection. Spontaneous bacterial peritonitis plus catheter-related peritonitis together account for approximately 10% of cases of peritonitis in children.[1-4] A decreasing incidence of catheter-related cases of peritonitis has resulted from improvements in catheter and connecting hardware technology used for continuous ambulatory peritoneal dialysis (CAPD) and a decrease in the frequency of touch contamination.[5–8]

The incidence of SBP in children peaks between the ages of 5 and 9 years, and affects males and females equally. Although SBP is reported in previously healthy children, this is rare.[9] In a 22-year review of peritonitis in children without pre-existing illness, only seven cases of SBP occurred compared with 1840 cases of secondary peritonitis from acute appendicitis alone.[10] Immunocompromised children are at greater risk for developing primary and catheter-related peritonitis than healthy children. Children with ascites due to portal hypertension are at relatively high risk for developing SBP, with incidence rates exceeding 20% in some series.[11,12] The most common predisposing condition for SBP is nephrotic syndrome (NS). The first episode of SBP typically occurs during the first 2 years following diagnosis of NS, and the overall incidence of SBP in these children may be as high as 5%.[13–19]

Catheter-related peritonitis remains a major complication in children receiving CAPD.[20,21] Data from the United States Renal Data System indicate that infectious complications are the most frequent cause for hospitalization among children receiving CAPD.[22] Up to two-thirds of all children receiving CAPD will experience at least one episode of peritonitis. CAPD-associated peritonitis in the U.S. has decreased over the past several decades from one episode per 3 to 6 patient months of dialysis to one episode per 14 to 24 months.[23–30] Similar decreases in CAPD-associated peritonitis have been reported in Europe, and a remarkably low incidence of peritonitis has been observed in Japanese children (one episode in every 29 months of dialysis).[29–31] These results have been attributed to an intensive CAPD training program and the rigorous attention to hygiene practiced in the Japanese culture.

Despite the overall decrease in CAPD-associated peritonitis worldwide, incidence in the pediatric population has remained persistently higher than that observed in adults.[32] CAPD-associated peritonitis is especially common in children under 6 years of age with the highest incidence in children less than 1 year of age.[23,25,33] This relatively high rate of infection may be due to the proximity of the catheter exit site to gastrostomy tubes and diapers, the frequent use of single-cuffed catheters in children, and their shorter tunnel lengths.

PATHOPHYSIOLOGY

Peritonitis can be caused by a variety of infectious and noninfectious insults that produce an inflammatory response involving the visceral and parietal peritoneum. The initial inflammatory response of the peritoneum to bacterial infection is characterized by vasodilation, tissue edema, transudation of fluid, and the influx of inflammatory macrophages and leukocytes. Lymphatic channels located in the undersurface of the diaphragm facilitate the clearance of bacteria, endotoxin, and other infectious particles from the peritoneal cavity. This drainage provides an important adjunctive defense mechanism to the local cellular immune response. Impairment of this process by fibrin and inflammatory debris can result in accumulation of peritoneal fluid and dilution of immunoglobulins and opsonins. This may be particularly relevant to the pathophysiology of peritonitis in children with pre-existing ascites, in which serum and peritoneal concentrations of these immunoreactive compounds are lower than that seen in healthy children.[34,35] Selective IgG subgroup deficiencies have been described in infants undergoing CAPD, which may further predispose this cohort to a more severe course of peritonitis.[36,37]

Infectious peritonitis can be exacerbated by inflammation due to concomitant intra-abdominal hemorrhage, urine extravasation, or leakage of gastrointestinal contents due to perforation. Adynamic ileus can lead to bacterial stasis and secondary infection through translocation of intestinal flora.

ETIOLOGY

Primary Bacterial Peritonitis

Seeding from a hematogenous source is the proposed pathophysiology in most cases of primary bacterial peritonitis. Other mechanisms include lymphatic seeding, retrograde inoculation from a genitourinary source, and translocation of intestinal flora (Table 67-1). The bacteriologic profile of peritoneal infections largely depends upon the source of infection and underlying comorbidities (Table 67-2).

Primary peritoneal infections in healthy children often are mono-microbial and in the majority of cases are caused by *Streptococcus pneumoniae*. There is a close association between peritonitis caused by *Streptococcus* species and kidney disease, with over two-thirds of culture-positive cases being reported in children with nephrotic syndrome.[13,16] In the past few decades, an increasing incidence of peritoneal infections caused by gram-negative organisms (especially *Escherichia coli*) has been observed.[38,39] Immunocompromised patients with advanced blood cell cancers (e.g., leukemia) and those receiving high-dose corticosteroid therapy are at an increased risk for gram-negative peritonitis. Gram-positive organisms (particularly group B streptococcus) predominate as the cause of primary peritoneal infections in the neonate. These infections, also known as "neonatal idiopathic primary peritonitis," are likely caused by hematogenous seeding in the majority of cases, although the infection also has been associated with oomphalitis.[40–43]

Mycobacterium tuberculosis (TB) is a rare cause of peritonitis but should be considered if the history suggests exposure to a known infected individual. Abdominal TB accounts for nearly 12% of extrapulmonary disease and approximately 1% to 3% of all TB-associated infections.[44–46] The widespread practice of dairy

TABLE 67-1. Proposed Mechanisms and Associated Conditions Leading to the Development of Peritonitis in Children

Primary Bacterial Peritonitis	Catheter-Associated Peritonitis	Secondary Bacterial Peritonitis
Hematogenous seeding (sepsis)	Poor sterile technique during dialysis	Neonatal period
Direct extension of localized process	Migration of skin flora along catheter	Necrotizing enterocolitis
Ascending urinary tract infection	Direct extension of local infection	Spontaneous gastric perforation
Genital/pelvic infection	Exit-site infection (with CAPD)	Feeding tube perforation (iatrogenic)
Mesenteric adenitis (TB)	CNS infection (with VPS)	Intestinal volvulus
Omphalitis	Hematogenous seeding of dialysate/CSF	Hirschsprung disease
Lymphogenous seeding		Postneonatal period and childhood
Translocation of intestinal flora		Acute appendicitis
		Intestinal volvulus
		Intussusception
		Incarcerated hernia

CAPD, continuous abdominal peritoneal dialysis; CNS, central nervous system; CSF, cerebrospinal fluid; TB, tuberculosis; VPS, ventriculoperitoneal shunt.

PART II Clinical Syndromes and Cardinal Features of Infectious Diseases: Approach to Diagnosis and Initial Management

SECTION I Intra-Abdominal Infections

TABLE 67-2. Organisms Commonly Associated with Peritonitis in Children[a]

Primary Bacterial Peritonitis	Catheter-Associated Peritonitis	Secondary Bacterial Peritonitis
Previously healthy children	**CAPD-associated**	**Proximal GI perforations**
Streptococcus pneumoniae	Staphylococcus epidermidis	Facultative organisms
Group A streptococcus	Staphylococcus aureus	Escherichia coli
Staphylococcus aureus	Pseudomonas spp.	Klebsiella sp.
Gram-negative bacilli	Other enteric gram-negative bacilli	Enterobacter sp.
	Fungi	Pseudomonas sp.
Neonatal idiopathic primary peritonitis		Gram-positive cocci
Group B streptococcus	**VPS-associated**	
Streptococcus pneumoniae	Coagulase-negative staphylococci	**Anaerobic organisms**
Staphylococcus aureus	Staphylococcus aureus	Bacteroides sp.
Enteric gram-negative bacilli	Escherichia coli (late)	Clostridium sp.
	Other gram-negative bacilli (late)	Peptostreptococcus sp.
Nephrotic syndrome		
Coagulase-negative staphylococci		**Colonic perforations**
Streptococcus species		Bacteroides fragilis
Staphylococcus aureus		Gram-negative rods (E. coli)
Enteric gram-negative bacilli		Other anaerobic organisms
		Enterobacter sp. (NEC)
Cirrhosis		
Escherichia coli		
Klebsiella sp.		
Streptococcus pneumoniae		

CAPD, continuous abdominal peritoneal dialysis; GI, gastrointestinal; NEC, necrotizing enterocolitis; VPS, ventriculoperitoneal shunt.

[a]Organisms are listed in the order of relative incidence by category, although there may be substantial variation in microbiological data over time and between different published series.

pasteurization in the U.S. and other developed countries has effectively eliminated infection caused by *Mycobacterium bovis*.[47]

Peritoneal infection with *Haemophilus influenzae*, *Neisseria gonorrhoeae*, and other encapsulated organisms is uncommon, but should be considered in previously healthy children who have had a splenectomy. Gonococcal peritonitis can occur in otherwise healthy adolescent girls from ascending genital/pelvic infection. Infection can lead to inflammation of the liver capsule, resulting in gonococcal perihepatitis (Fitz-Hugh–Curtis syndrome).

Catheter-Associated Peritonitis

Cultures of peritoneal fluid are positive in approximately 80% to 85% of children with clinically apparent peritonitis occurring during peritoneal dialysis.[48] Between one-half and two-thirds of all episodes are caused by gram-positive organisms, and the majority of the remainder are caused by gram-negative bacteria.[25,33,49–52] In the U.S., coagulase-negative staphylococci (CoNS) and *Staphylococcus aureus* each account for about 15% of cases. Relative importance of gram-negative bacteria is increasing due to improved connection technology, exit-site care, and antibiotic prophylaxis that reduces gram-positive bacterial contamination.[25,26,53] Gram-negative infections usually are associated with touch contamination and can be caused by a variety of organisms including *Pseudomonas*, *Enterobacter*, *E. coli*, and *Klebsiella*, among others.[25,30,51,54] In the U.S., the most commonly isolated gram-negative organism is *Pseudomonas*.[52] *Pseudomonas* species are isolated from approximately 10% to 20% of catheter exit-site infections, suggesting a mechanism for bacterial migration along the catheter tunnel. Although gram-negative peritonitis in patients receiving CAPD can be caused by a secondary source (e.g., ruptured appendicitis), isolation of a single organism strongly suggests a catheter-associated etiology.

Fungal peritonitis is a rare but serious complication of CAPD and is associated with substantial morbidity and mortality.[55–60] Although fungal pathogens account for only 3% to 6% of all CAPD-associated cases of peritonitis in children, the incidence of fungal peritonitis appears to be increasing.[56–59] Many patients with fungal peritonitis have had catheter-related infection(s) treated with antibiotics, suggesting that these infections may be opportunistic. Compared with bacterial peritonitis, fungal peritonitis can be particularly difficult to treat, resulting in a greater likelihood of catheter loss and conversion to hemodialysis.[55,57–60] *Candida* species are the most commonly isolated fungi in culture-positive cases.

Infectious peritonitis is a rare complication in children with indwelling ventriculoperitoneal (VP) shunts, affecting less than 1% of all patients.[61] Peritonitis can arise from contamination of intra-abdominal cerebrospinal fluid (CSF) by either hematogenous seeding or bacterial translocation, or from contamination of the peritoneal cavity by an infection originating in the central nervous system. In a patient with a VP shunt and abdominal pain, bacterial peritonitis must be distinguished from the more common, simple, CSF-containing pseudocyst. VP-shunt-associated peritoneal infections in the first several months after placement usually are caused by gram-positive cocci (CoNS and *S. aureus*), while late infections are more likely to be due to gram-negative organisms.[61] Secondary peritonitis following erosion of the VP catheter into the colon also can occur in children.

Secondary Bacterial Peritonitis

Secondary peritonitis can arise from any condition that results in the loss of GI tract continuity (Table 67-1). In the neonatal period, secondary peritonitis most often results from conditions that lead to intestinal ischemia and perforation, such as necrotizing enterocolitis (most common), gastric perforation, meconium ileus, intestinal atresia, and Hirschsprung disease.[40] Acute appendicitis is the most common condition resulting in secondary peritonitis in older children.[62] Other conditions that can lead to perforation and secondary peritonitis include volvulus, intussusception, and incarcerated hernia.[40]

In contrast to primary and catheter-related peritonitis, secondary infections tend to be polymicrobial and the bacteriology is more dependent on the location of perforation than associated comorbidities. Aerobic and facultative gram-negative enteric organisms including *E. coli*, *Klebsiella*, *Pseudomonas*, and others are frequently isolated from perforations of the proximal GI tract.

The colon contains predominately anaerobic organisms, with *Bacteroides* species being the most commonly isolated organism following colonic perforations. In neonates with distal intestinal perforations facultative enteric gram-negative rods are more commonly isolated than anaerobes, although *Bacteroides* and clostridia often are isolated.[63] In a large review of neonates with necrotizing enterocolitis, *Enterobacter* species was the most common organism isolated, with anaerobes isolated in only 6% of cases.[63]

CLINICAL PRESENTATION

The clinical presentation of peritonitis depends on many factors, including age, underlying cause of infection, associated comorbidities, and immune status. The clinical presentation of the neonate frequently is nonspecific due to a paucity of localizing signs. The neonate generally appears ill, with marked abdominal distention, hypothermia, emesis, and respiratory distress.[40,41,43] The abdominal wall can appear erythematous or edematous when there is severe peritoneal inflammation. Fever is not a common sign of peritonitis in the neonate, present in <20% of documented cases.[40,41,43]

The presentation of older children with peritonitis can include abdominal pain and tenderness, distention, vomiting, hypoactive bowel sounds, and varying degrees of systemic toxicity. Neutropenic children and those receiving high doses of corticosteroids (e.g., as for chronic nephrotic syndrome) can have benign presentations. These children often are afebrile and have minimal abdominal tenderness, leading to a misdiagnosis of gastroenteritis or another less serious ailment.

The presence of fever or abdominal pain in any child undergoing CAPD should alert the clinician to the possibility of catheter-associated peritonitis, especially in the context of cloudy dialysis effluent. The clinical presentation of VP-shunt-associated peritonitis can be subtle, with the only symptoms being mild abdominal pain and low-grade fever. Peritonitis associated with tuberculosis often is insidious in onset, characterized by weight loss, chronic weakness, fever, night sweats, and anorexia.[46] Approximately 40% of patients with tuberculous peritonitis have symptoms/signs of active pulmonary infection.

The specific organism causing infection can affect clinical presentation and course. Presentation of peritonitis caused by *S. aureus* generally is more severe than that caused by CoNS and infection tends to resolve more slowly.[64] Gram-negative peritonitis often causes intense abdominal pain and is associated with dramatic alterations in the peritoneal membrane transport capacity.[23,65]

DIAGNOSIS

Laboratory Evaluation

Laboratory findings in a child with peritonitis usually are nonspecific, often suggesting the presence of a systemic inflammatory process rather than a specific diagnosis. Analysis of peritoneal fluid aspirates should be performed and can aid in differentiating primary from secondary peritonitis. The presence of stool, amylase, and bile is indicative of intestinal perforation, while the presence of blood can be seen with both primary and secondary peritonitis. In children undergoing CAPD, the presence of cloudy effluent with WBC >100 cells/mm^3 and a neutrophil predominance is adequate for the diagnosis of peritonitis and an indication to begin antibiotics empirically.[66,67]

Imaging

The primary utility of imaging in patients with suspected peritonitis is to help determine the etiology (i.e., primary vs. secondary causes) and the necessity of urgent laparotomy. While plain films of the abdomen and ultrasound may provide useful information (e.g., free air), computed tomography (CT) is the most useful imaging modality in the evaluation of the child with an acute abdomen. The finding of complex ascites, with or without visualization of the appendix, is strongly suggestive of perforated appendicitis in older children. In the case of primary or catheter-related peritonitis, typical imaging findings include simple ascites, high-attenuation characteristics of peritoneal fluid, and nodular irregularity of the peritoneal lining.[68–70] CT findings in patients with abdominal tuberculosis can include lymphadenopathy, splenomegaly, and focal mesenteric calcifications.[71]

MANAGEMENT

Primary Peritonitis

In a child with an anatomically normal peritoneal cavity who develops primary bacterial peritonitis, antibiotic treatment should be directed at the most likely organisms, which include gram-positive cocci and gram-negative rods (Table 67-2). Both gram-positive and gram-negative organisms have been implicated as causative organisms in children with nephrotic syndrome, while enteric gram-negative infections are much more common in children with cirrhosis.[12,38,39] With the emergence of resistant strains of gram-positive organisms and the increasing incidence of gram-negative rods (particularly in children with ascites), empiric coverage with cefotaxime or another third-generation cephalosporin is indicated. Antibiotic coverage can be narrowed subsequently based on culture results from the peritoneal aspirates. Aggressive removal of infected peritoneal fluid has not been shown to improve outcomes and therefore is not recommended.

Catheter-Associated Infections

Empiric antibiotics should be initiated when the diagnosis of bacterial peritonitis is suspected (Figure 67-1). The wide variability of organisms associated with peritonitis in children treated with CAPD warrants the use of broad-spectrum agents until culture results dictate otherwise. The combined intraperitoneal administration of a third-generation cephalosporin such as ceftazidime and a first-generation cephalosporin is recommended as initial therapy (Table 67-3).[29,66,72–74] In a systematic review of therapies, intermittent or continuous administration regimens were equivalent,[75] but failures of intermittently administered ceftazidime for gram-negative bacillary peritonitis are excessive, questioning such practice.[74] Substitution of a glycopeptide for the first-generation cephalosporin in children should be restricted to those at high risk for resistant organism (such as young age, history of *S. aureus* infection, recent catheter-related infection).[74] Ceftazidime generally is preferred over aminoglycosides if *P. aeruginosa* is suspected due to the potential for ototoxicity and nephrotoxicity with aminoglycosides in the setting of high cumulative exposure.

Antibiotics should be adjusted once culture results are available (see Figure 67-1). If initial culture results reveal only gram-positive organisms, the third-generation cephalosporin (e.g., ceftazidime) should be discontinued. A first-generation cephalosporin should be used for methicillin-susceptible *S. aureus*, and vancomycin for resistant strains. Clindamycin can be used as an alternative to vancomycin, in the absence of inducible resistance. Ampicillin is sufficient to treat most strains of *Enterococcus* and *Streptococcus* spp. Antibiotic treatment for gram-positive organisms should continue for 2 to 3 weeks.[66]

If culture and susceptibility test results identify only gram-negative organisms susceptible to ceftazidime, gram-positive coverage should be discontinued. *Pseudomonas/Stenotrophomonas* species are effectively covered by ceftazidime, but the addition of a second agent is recommended for double coverage by some experts. If cultures identify anaerobic organisms or multiple gram-negative bacilli, metronidazole should be added and an intra-abdominal source for secondary peritonitis should be sought. Antibiotic treatment should be continued for a total of 2 to 3 weeks. If the patient improves on empiric therapy and the initial cultures remain negative, the initial combination of antibiotics should be continued for a total of 2 weeks.

Fungal peritonitis has historically been treated with either intravenous amphotericin B or a combination of an imidazole/

PART II Clinical Syndromes and Cardinal Features of Infectious Diseases: Approach to Diagnosis and Initial Management

SECTION I Intra-Abdominal Infections

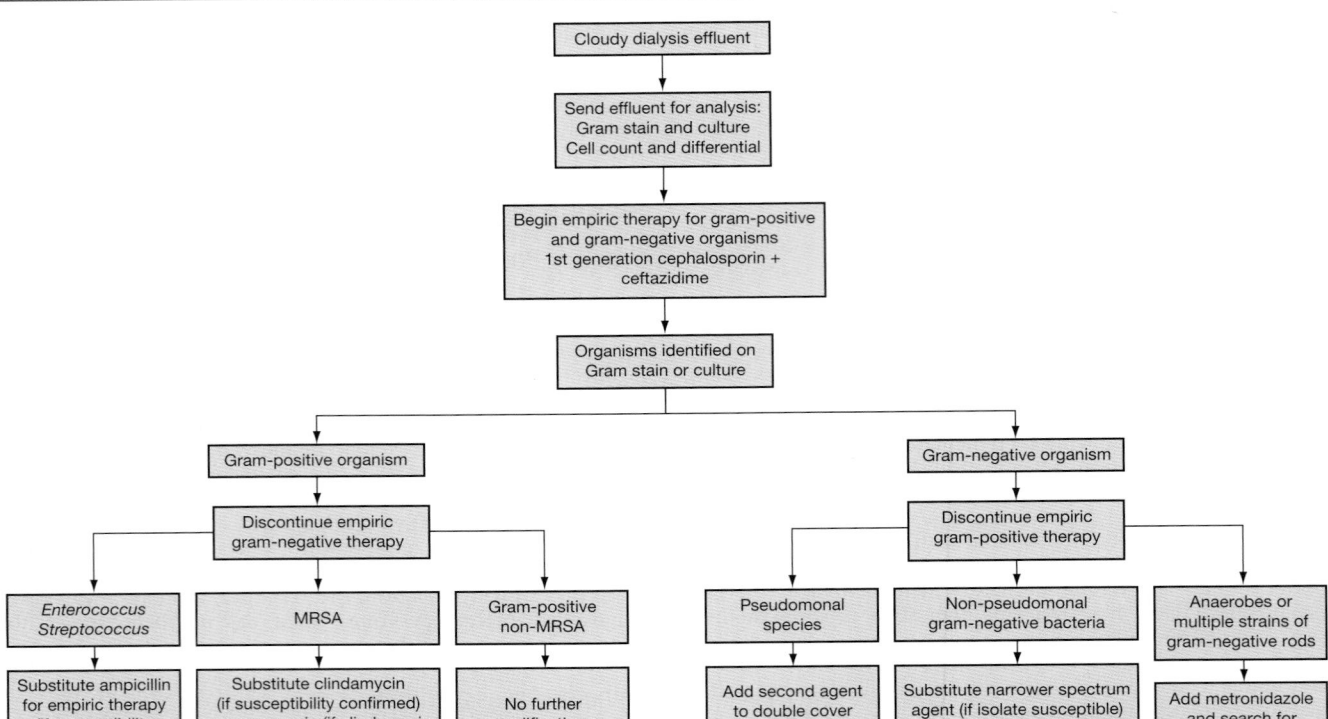

Figure 67-1. Algorithm for the management of CAPD-associated peritonitis. MRSA, methicillin-resistant *Staphylococcus aureus*.

TABLE 67-3. Recommended Antibiotic Dosing of Common Therapy for Catheter-Associated Peritonitis; Route is Via Intraperitoneal Unless Otherwise Specified[23,66]

| Antibiotic | Continuous Therapy[a] | | Intermittent Therapy[b] |
	Loading Dose[c]	Maintenance Dose	
Cefazolin	500 mg/L	125 mg/L	15 mg/kg every 24 h
Ceftazidime	250 mg/L	125 mg/L	15 mg/kg every 24 h
Vancomycin	1000 mg/L	25 mg/L	30 mg/kg every 3–7 days[d]
Gentamicin	8 mg/L	4 mg/L	–
Ampicillin	–	125 mg/L	–
Clindamycin	300 mg/L	150 mg/L	–
Metronidazole	–	–	35–50 mg/kg/day by mouth in 3 doses

[a]Concentration-dosing assumes approximately 1100 mL/m^2 or usual patient specific fill volume.

[b]Intermittent administration should occur over ≥6 h in one bag per day for continuous ambulatory peritoneal dialysis patients or over a full fill volume daytime dwell for automated peritoneal dialysis.

[c]Loading dose should be administered during a 3 to 6 h dwell period.

[d]Redosing should occur when blood level is <12 mg/L.

triazole (fluconazole) and flucytosine.[55] Fluconazole is considered the preferred agent (when isolated *Candida* species is proved to be susceptible) over amphotericin due to superior peritoneal penetration and bioavailability.[23,76] The dialysis catheter should be removed if no improvement is evident after the first 72 hours of therapy.[77] If clinical improvement is observed and the dialysis catheter is not removed, antifungal treatment should be continued for at least 4 to 6 weeks following complete resolution of clinical symptoms. With removal of the catheter, treatment should be continued for at least 2 weeks following resolution of clinical symptoms. Temporary hemodialysis should be used while therapy is completed and until a new peritoneal dialysis catheter can be placed.[55,66,78]

With appropriate antibiotic coverage, improvement (i.e., reduction in fever, abdominal pain, and the cloudiness of the peritoneal effluent) should be observed within 72 hours of initiating therapy. Subsequent aspirates of dialysate in a patient responding to antibiotics should reveal a decrease in WBCs by at least 50%. Other potential sources of infection should be sought if no clinical improvement is seen with empiric treatment. Further treatment may include additional modifications of antibiotic coverage and removal of the dialysis catheter.[66,78] With the exception of cases involving pseudomonal species, removal and replacement of the catheter usually can be performed simultaneously once the patient has responded clinically and effluent leukocyte counts are less than 100/mm^3.

Relapsing peritonitis is defined as the recurrence of peritonitis with the same organism within 4 weeks of treatment. Empiric treatment is the same as for the initial infection, with further modifications guided by culture results. Relapsing peritonitis can occur in up to 20% of gram-positive infections initially responsive to antibiotic therapy.[79] Coagulase-negative staphylococci can survive antibacterial treatment within a biofilm secreted on the catheter surface, and *P. aeruginosa* can prove difficult to treat due to the formation of biofilm and microabscesses within the catheter tunnel. Catheter removal is not recommended universally after the first recurrence but removal should be considered strongly with the second recurrence and in all cases associated with *Pseudomonas* species. Catheter removal also is suggested when the source of reinfection is thought to originate from within the catheter tunnel. Relapsing peritonitis should be treated with intraperitoneal antibiotics for a total of 3 weeks.

It is important to note that the recommendations for the treatment of catheter-associated peritonitis are based largely on expert opinion and convention rather than randomized controlled trials. Wiggins et al. examined 36 randomized controlled trials (2089 adults and children) to assess the evidence for current recommendations and could only conclude from the available data that intraperitoneal administration of antibiotics is superior to intravenous dosing and that use of routine peritoneal lavage or urokinase was not supported.[75] Moreover, there has been considerable variability in antibiotic susceptibility of pathogens secondary to regional uses of different antibiotic regimens. A plan of therapy should take into account institutional patterns of antibiotic resistance.[64,80]

Secondary Peritonitis

Patients with secondary peritonitis require urgent laparotomy to identify and control the source of peritoneal contamination. All infectious debris should be removed and necrotic tissue debrided. Indwelling foreign bodies should be removed. Intraoperative peritoneal irrigation has been shown to decrease the bacterial burden and reduce postoperative infectious complication. Irrigation with antibiotic solutions does not confer any benefit and should be avoided.[81] Inadequate control of the source of infection at initial laparotomy can lead to recurrent peritonitis and is associated with increased mortality and morbidity. Early recognition of tertiary peritonitis and having a low threshold for prompt re-exploration are critical when the possibility of continued contamination is high. This includes situations in which there is massive contamination (fecal peritonitis) or when intestinal viability is questionable at the time of abdominal closure (necrotizing enterocolitis). Mandatory re-exploration 24 to 48 hours after the initial laparotomy (so-called "second-look" operation) is practiced by many and has been shown to decrease morbidity and mortality compared with selective re-exploration.[81]

Empiric antibiotic treatment for secondary peritonitis should cover enteric pathogens including anaerobes and gram-negative bacilli. Treatment of secondary peritonitis with ampicillin, gentamicin, and flagyl has long been the gold standard, but does not confer any benefit over broad-spectrum monotherapy options (e.g. piperacillin-tazobactam). Clindamycin and second-generation cephalosporins were used in the past as first-line therapy, but should no longer be used due to increasing resistance of *Bacteroides fragilis* to these agents. There are no consensus guidelines for the length of antibiotic treatment once the source of infection has been controlled with operative management, although most would favor continuing therapy for 7 to 10 days following complete resolution of clinical and laboratory indicators of infection.

COMPLICATIONS AND PROGNOSIS

Infectious peritonitis has been associated with many life-threatening complications, including mesenteric vein thrombosis, adult respiratory distress syndrome, progressive multi-organ failure, and death. Severe complications are associated more often with secondary peritonitis, although immunocompromised children have increased risk regardless of source of peritonitis. Other complications include prolonged ileus, surgical wound infection, intra-abdominal abscess, enteric fistula, and the development of inflammatory adhesions. Inflammatory thickening of peritoneal surfaces and compartmentalization of the peritoneal cavity can limit the subsequent effectiveness of peritoneal dialysis. Short-term hemodialysis may be required in these patients.

The prognosis of peritonitis largely depends on the etiology of the infection, associated comorbidities, and the host response to the inflammatory process. Mortality rates for healthy children who develop perforated appendicitis should be very low, while mortality associated with necrotizing enterocolitis in low-birthweight neonates remains in excess of 30% to 50%.[82–84] Contemporary estimates of case-fatality rates for patients receiving chronic peritoneal dialysis are approximately 6%, with peritoneal infections comprising over 15% of all-cause mortality and 69% of infection-related mortality in this cohort. Fungal peritonitis carries a particularly poor prognosis in children, with some series reporting case-mortality rates exceeding 25%.[85]

Mortality rates for primary peritonitis in children can approach 10%, varying by etiology and associated comorbidities. Estimates of case-fatality rates for spontaneous bacterial peritonitis in children with nephrotic syndrome are around 9%.[13] Spontaneous peritonitis in a child with cirrhosis and portal hypertension carries a much worse prognosis, with mortality rates exceeding 30% to 40% at one month following diagnosis.[86] The observation that overall survival at 6 months following the first episode of SBP is less than 30% suggests that the diagnosis may be a marker of rapidly progressing hepatic dysfunction. This has led some to consider the first episode of SBP in these children as a relative indication for liver transplantation.

PREVENTION

Strategies to prevent bacterial peritonitis in children largely have focused on patients undergoing CAPD. The use of strict sterile technique during the dialysis process is crucial to prevent contamination-associated peritonitis.[87] Double-bag disconnect systems, which take away the need for "spiking" dialysis bags, have been associated with a significant reduction in peritonitis caused by touch contamination.[23] The competency of CAPD training appears to be critical in this regard, and studies suggest a strong correlation between the duration and quality of training and low incidence of peritonitis.[88,89] In this regard, the typical 6- to 7-week intensive training period employed in Japan is noteworthy.[90]

Observational studies conducted from registry data and a few controlled trials have associated decreased rates of peritonitis and exit-site infections with specific techniques during catheter placement.[91] These include the use of a double-cuffed Dacron catheter (versus a single-cuffed model) and directing the peritoneal opening inferiorly (versus cephalad).[92–94] However, a systematic review of data by the Cochrane Collaboration failed to demonstrate a significant benefit with any specific catheter design or insertion technique with respect to the incidence of peritonitis, tunnel-site infections, or need for catheter removal.[95]

Nasal carriers of *S. aureus* have been identified in up to 45% of families of children treated with CAPD.[96] The use of mupirocin applied to the nares or catheter exit site in patients (and family members) who are known carriers has been shown to decrease the incidence of exit site infections and peritonitis in several studies.[96–98] Not all community-associated MRSA are susceptible to mupirocin or carried solely in the nose. Topical aminoglycoside has been used with promising results to decrease *Pseudomonas*-related infections, although related resistance is a problem.[99]

Prophylactic antibiotic therapy with a first-generation cephalosporin at the time of catheter insertion significantly decreases the incidence of postoperative peritonitis.[100] Children with a history of MRSA colonization should receive vancomycin. A short course (24 to 48 hours) of a first-generation cephalosporin also is recommended when there is suspected contamination of the dialysate or connecting hardware, and prior to procedures involving the gastrointestinal or genitourinary tract.[101] Prophylactic systemic long-term antibiotics are not indicated in patients receiving CAPD.

Following placement of a catheter, initiation of peritoneal dialysis should be delayed for a minimum of 2 weeks to allow wound healing and dressing changes should be conducted by trained dialysis staff ideally no more than once per week.[102]

68   Appendicitis

Marion C.W. Henry and R. Lawrence Moss

Appendicitis is the most common reason for emergent abdominal surgery in children and accounts for 80,000 hospitalizations and more than one-third of hospital days for abdominal pain annually in people <18 years of age in the United States.[1] Although rarely fatal, morbidity associated with appendicitis remains substantial. Efforts to decrease morbidity focus on improving methods of diagnosis, optimizing surgical management, and improving post-operative care.

EPIDEMIOLOGY

Appendicitis can affect children of all ages, including infants <1 year of age; however, the peak incidence is at 12 to 18 years. The incidence increases from 1 to 2 cases per 10,000 in children <4 years of age to 25 cases per 10,000 in older children.[2] There is a slight male predominance with an 8.7% lifetime risk for boys compared with 6.7% risk for girls.[2] Epidemiologic factors that may increase the risk for appendicitis include summer months,[3] a low fiber intake,[4] and possibly a positive family history.[4,5]

The rate of perforation at the time of operation ranges from 20% to 76%.[6] The incidence of perforation is highest in infancy, occurring in 70% to 95% of cases,[7] and decreases with age to 10% to 20% in adolescents.[4,7,8] Perforation rates are increased among minorities and economically disadvantaged children.[3,9–11]

Appendicitis resulting in perforation is associated with a more severe clinical illness, high morbidity, and a longer hospital course than non-perforated appendicitis. An elapsed time of >36 hours from first reported symptoms to the time of surgery correlates with an increased rate of perforation.[4,12,13] Contributing factors may include difficulty in access to care or diagnostic uncertainty.[14,15]

PATHOGENESIS

The pathogenesis of appendicitis is clear.[16,17] An initial event leads to occlusion of the lumen of the appendix between the cecal base and the tip. This may be caused by a foreign body, such as an appendicolith, or by inflamed mucosa due to an infectious process or hyperplasia of intramural lymphoid tissue. Luminal occlusion is followed by increased intraluminal pressure leading to swelling, congestion, and distention of the mucosa and appendiceal wall. Overgrowth and translocation of bowel flora leads to an acute inflammatory infiltrate in the wall of the appendix; full-thickness inflammation, and localized peritonitis. If untreated, necrosis and frank gangrene of the appendiceal wall results. Rupture of the appendix leads to spread of peritonitis and the development of an inflammatory phlegmon, an intra-abdominal abscess, or gen-eralized peritonitis.

ETIOLOGY

The most common pathogens associated with appendicitis and subsequent intra-abdominal infections are shown in Box 68-1.

BOX 68-1. Most Common Organisms in Perforated Appendicitis

E. coli
Alpha streptococci
Bacteroides group
Bacteroides fragilis
Bilophila wadsworthia
Peptostreptococcus species

Although the cost-effectiveness of obtaining cultures of the peri-toneal fluid at the time of operation has been questioned,[18,19] increasing rates of antibiotic resistance underscore their potential utility.[20] The most commonly isolated organisms are anaerobes: *Bacteroides fragilis*, clostridia, *Peptostreptococcus*, and gram-negative rods including *Escherichia coli*, *Pseudomonas*, *Enterobacter*, and *Klebsiella*.

CLINICAL MANIFESTATIONS AND DIAGNOSIS

Although the classically described symptoms of appendicitis are periumbilical pain that migrates to the right lower quadrant, fol-lowed by nausea, occasional vomiting and low grade fever, the clinical presentation depends upon the location of the appendix, the host response to infection, and most prominently the age of the patient (Table 68-1).

In children <2 years of age, the most common symptoms are vomiting, abdominal pain, fever, abdominal distention, diarrhea, irritability, right hip pain, and limp.[15] In children 2 to 5 years of age, abdominal pain precedes vomiting and usually is associated with fever and anorexia. Tenesmus, which can be perceived as diarrhea, is common in infants and toddlers and may lead to misdiagnosis.[7] School-aged children describe abdominal pain that is constant and worse with movement or coughing.[15] Nausea, vomiting, anorexia, tenesmus, and dysuria also occur in this age group.[15] Older children sometimes report that they are hungry.[1] A few studies have attempted to determine the sensitivity and spe-cificity of these symptoms. Two retrospective studies of children[21,22] and one prospective study of children and adults[23] found that vomiting has a low sensitivity (0.43) and specificity (0.64).[24] Fever has better sensitivity and specificity: 0.75 and 0.78, respectively. Anorexia and pain migration have low sensitivities (0.64 for ano-rexia, 0.41 for pain migration) and specificities (0.43 for anorexia, 0.54 for pain migration).[24] In older children the most sensitive symptom is increased pain with coughing and movement (0.8), but the specificity is low (0.52).[24]

Physical findings also vary by patient age. In those <2 years of age, nonspecific signs such as fever and diffuse tenderness are the most common findings. Preschool children aged 2 to 5 years demonstrate right lower quadrant tenderness, fever, and involun-tary guarding. School-aged children are more likely to have local-ized right lower quadrant tenderness, or diffuse guarding and

---

TABLE 68-1. Clinical Signs or Symptoms in Appendicitis by Age of Patient[14,21]

Clinical Sign or Symptom	Age of Children with Finding (%)		
	≤2 years	2–5 years	6–12 years
Abdominal pain	35–77	89–100	100
Right lower quadrant pain	<50	58–85	>90
Diffuse tenderness	55–97	19–28	15[a], 83[b]
Vomiting	85–90	66–100	68–95
Fever	40–60	80–87	64
Anorexia	NR	53–60	47–75

NR, not reported.

[a]Without perforation.

[b]With perforation.

Infectious gastroenteritis
Pneumonia
Urinary tract infection
Mesenteric adenitis
Intussusception
Inflammatory bowel disease
Meckel diverticulum
Hernia
Primary peritonitis
Orchitis
Testicular torsion
Blunt abdominal trauma
Ovarian cyst

rebound tenderness, if the appendix has perforated.[24] Two studies[25,26] have examined rebound tenderness in children and found low sensitivity (50%) and specificity (60%). The sensitivity and specificity of signs equated with appendicitis in adults, including Rovsing sign (pressure palpation in left lower quadrant induces pain at McBurney point), obturator sign, and psoas sign, have not been critically evaluated in children.[24]

Differential Diagnosis

Appendicitis can mimic many disorders (Box 68-2). Other inflammatory diseases, most commonly gastroenteritis, can produce signs and symptoms similar to appendicitis.[1,27] In girls, ovarian pathology such as ruptured ovarian cyst and ovarian torsion can cause right lower quadrant pain and peritoneal irritation. In neutropenic patients, differentiating appendicitis from typhlitis or neutropenic enterocolitis can be difficult and imaging studies often are necessary.[1,28]

Laboratory Studies

The white blood cell count (WBC) typically is mildly elevated to 11,000 to 16,000/mm^3. Great variability in sensitivity (19% to 88%) and specificity (53% to 100%) for appendicitis have been reported.[24]

The sensitivity of C-reactive protein (CRP) in appendicitis ranges from 48% to 75% and specificity from 57% to 82%.[24,29] While in adults, the combination of a normal WBC and normal CRP makes the diagnosis of appendicitis very unlikely, this is not true in children.[30] CRP levels must be interpreted with caution in obese children, as the mean levels in these patients are substantially higher than in non-obese children and specificity and positive predictive values substantially lower.[31] In a study of 212 children the sensitivity of a procalcitonin level >0.5 ng/mL for gangrene or perforation was 73%, and specificity 95%.[32] However, in the majority of children with simple acute appendicitis, the procalcitonin level was <0.5 ng/mL.[32]

Urinalysis can show pyuria and hematuria in as many as 30% of children with appendicitis.[33-35] Pyuria especially occurs when the inflamed appendix is adjacent to the ureter or bladder.

Diagnostic Imaging

In the past, plain abdominal radiographs were the most common imaging study performed in patients with suspected appendicitis. However, plain abdominal radiographs have been found to be normal or misleading in up to 82% of children with appendicitis.[15] Although the presence of a fecalith is suggestive of appendicitis,[36] fecaliths occur with low frequency.[24] Fecal loading in the cecum appears to be a sensitive and specific radiographic finding for appendicitis in adult and pediatric patients.[37]

Ultrasound (US) findings are well documented in appendicitis. Diagnostic criteria include: appendiceal diameter >6 mm, a target sign with 5 concentric layers, distention or obstruction of the appendiceal lumen, high echogenicity surrounding the appendix, an appendicolith, fluid surrounding the appendix, enlarged and thickened bowel wall and lack of peristalsis.[24] Sensitivity of US ranges from 71% to 92% and specificity from 96% to 98%.[38-41] Patient characteristics that limit US utility include obesity and gaseous distention of bowel loops.[42] Value of US also is dependent on the experience of the ultrasonographer. Many authors recommend US as the first study for children with suspected appendicitis due to its low cost, freedom from ionizing radiation, and its superiority to clinical judgment in equivocal cases.[43-46]

In adults with appendicitis, computed tomography (CT) has higher specificity and sensitivity than US.[47] Studies in children also have shown high sensitivity (94% to 99%) and specificity (87% to 99%) of CT for the diagnosis of appendicitis.[40,47,48] Several of these studies have been prospective, although not blinded. Limitations of CT include: cost, the need for oral contrast and possible sedation, and exposure to ionizing radiation.[49]

The false-negative rate of an imaging study is increased if the study is performed in a child with a high clinical suspicion of disease; the false-positive rate is increased if the study is performed in a child with a low clinical suspicion of disease.[50] Imaging studies are most useful when used only in children with clinically equivocal presentations. Further indications for CT scan may be in the evaluation of children with suspected complicated appendicitis, as this diagnosis can influence the management strategy, directing the surgeon toward initial nonoperative therapy.[51] In one study, an approach based on selective imaging for equivocal cases, using US, followed by CT for inconclusive studies, has been shown to be accurate and cost-effective,[50,52] with sensitivity 99%, specificity 92%, and accuracy 97%.[53]

Some studies have shown that CT offers no increased accuracy over history, physical examination, and laboratory analysis.[54,55] Observation with serial examinations can be a cost-effective method of determining appendicitis with <2% of patients perforating during observation.[56]

Scoring Systems

The Alvarado (MANTRELS) scoring system for the diagnosis of appendicitis was developed from a large cohort of mostly adults (Table 68-2). Its use has been tested in children and renamed the Pediatric Appendicitis Score (PAS). Although some authors have found the scores to be accurate,[57] most studies in young children show only moderate sensitivity (76% to 90%) and specificity (50% to 81%) when the score is ≥7. In older children (over 16 years), a score of ≥7 has a sensitivity of 100% and a specificity of 93%.[24,58] Another study found the PAS most useful when ≤4, to exclude appendicitis (without need for imaging), and ≥8, to confirm appendicitis (without imaging).[59]

TABLE 68-2. MANTRELS Score[108]

Symptoms	Migration of abdominal pain from the epigastrium to the right lower quadrant	1
	Anorexia	1
	Nausea/vomiting	1
Signs	Right lower quadrant tenderness	2
	Rebound tenderness	1
	Elevated temperature	1
Investigation	Leukocytosis	2
	Left shift	1
Total possible score	Appendicitis unlikely	<5
	Appendicitis possible	5–6
	Appendicitis likely	>6

PART II Clinical Syndromes and Cardinal Features of Infectious Diseases: Approach to Diagnosis and Initial Management

SECTION I Intra-Abdominal Infections

MANAGEMENT

While some aspects of management of appendicitis have become standardized over the past 25 years, great variability remains,[6,60] and there may be major regional variations.[61]

Uncomplicated Appendicitis

In cases of acute, uncomplicated appendicitis, prompt appendectomy is the mainstay of treatment. Appendectomy following 12 hours of antibiotic treatment does not result in increased perforation rates or clinical morbidity compared with immediate appendectomy.[62,63]

Laparoscopic and open techniques for appendectomy are both utilized widely. Some studies suggest that laparoscopic procedures lead to a shorter hospital course, less pain, and better cosmetic result. A randomized trial in Europe of laparoscopic and open appendectomy found only marginal differences in cost but a quicker return to activities in children who had laparoscopic appendectomy.[64] Another randomized comparative trial found that children undergoing laparoscopy had less pain, and shorter duration of hospitalization. While operating times and costs were slightly increased with laparoscopy, there was an overall reduction in costs because of the decreased length of hospital stay.[65,66]

In perforated appendicitis, some studies have suggested an increased rate of developing an intra-abdominal abscess following laparoscopy.[67-71] A large study of four centers treating children with perforated appendicitis, however, found no difference in the rate of abscess between those treated by laparoscopic or open appendectomy.[72]

Preoperative antibiotics, administered with the goal of preventing postoperative infections, are commonly prescribed. Although several studies have challenged the use of routine preoperative antibiotics, these studies are limited by small sample size.[73-76] One prospective, randomized study found no effect of antibiotics in complication rates in patients with simple appendicitis. However, among the one-third of patients in this study who had gangrenous appendicitis at operation, those who did not receive preoperative antibiotics had a significantly higher rate of postoperative infection.[77] Unfortunately, there is no reliable way to differentiate between simple and complicated appendicitis preoperatively. A Cochrane review suggests that routine antibiotic prophylaxis for any type of appendicitis helps prevent infectious complications.[78] The Surgical Infection Society guidelines suggest that children with appendicitis routinely should receive preoperative antibiotics, consisting of either a single agent, or combination of agents, that provide adequate coverage for gram-negative bacilli and anaerobic bacteria.[79]

The value of the routine use of postoperative antibiotics for either simple or complicated appendicitis has not been established.

Many institutions have adopted clinical algorithms for the management of appendicitis. The majority of the data to support these algorithms is derived from retrospective reviews. Studies examining the benefit of these guidelines generally have shown a reduction in cost and length of stay for patients treated under guidelines.[80] Some studies also have reported lower readmission rates, despite increased disease severity, following implementation of a care pathway.[81,82]

Complicated Appendicitis

Most of the controversies and the majority of the variability in care of children with appendicitis surround cases of complicated appendicitis. Controversy exists on definition of complicated appendicitis, as some surgeons opine that gangrenous and perforated appendicitis cannot be differentiated. There is inconsistency among surgeons in describing the severity of appendicitis.[83] The distinction is important, however, as gangrenous appendicitis is associated with outcomes and morbidity rates more consistent with simple appendicitis than perforated appendicitis. Inconsistency in the definition of perforation limits the validity of

observations based on retrospective studies. Future studies will benefit from a strict, evidence-based definition of perforation.[84]

The use of nonoperative management for children with perforated appendicitis is controversial and under investigation. If peritonitis is present, many surgeons advocate immediate appendectomy. However, some surgeons treat these patients with intravenous antibiotics followed by interval appendectomy.[85-87] Surgeons in favor of this approach cite the high rate of complications when operating during a period of intense inflammation and peritonitis. However, high failure rates of the nonoperative approach are reported. If a child does not respond clinically within 24 to 72 hours of beginning intravenous antibiotic therapy, an appendectomy is recommended.

Persistence of fevers beyond 24 hours and band counts >10% to 15% have been associated with failure of nonoperative management.[87,88] Patients who do not respond to nonoperative treatment and undergo delayed appendectomy often have high complication rates and prolonged hospitalizations.[86,89]

Reduced morbidity rates have been reported for a nonoperative approach for patients presenting with a long duration of symptoms (so called "missed appendicitis").[89] A prospective randomized trial of initial nonoperative management versus early appendectomy for children presenting with a well-defined abscess found no difference in total length of hospitalization, recurrent abscesses, dose of narcotics, or total hospital charges.[90]

As nonoperative management of perforated appendicitis becomes more prevalent, distinguishing between perforated and acute appendicitis preoperatively is more critical. Such a scoring system has been developed (Table 68-3). A cutoff score of ≥9 improved the likelihood ratio and the post-test probability of having perforated appendicitis compared with the surgeon's clinical impression alone.[91] However, one of the elements in this scoring system is findings of CT, which has attendant risk of exposing children to radiation.

Some proponents of nonoperative management question the necessity of performing an interval appendectomy. These surgeons note an insignificant rate of recurrence[92] and argue that after perforation, the lumen of the appendix is obliterated. A randomized controlled trial of 60 patients showed a 10% recurrence rate of appendicitis in patients managed nonoperatively.[93] Other cohort studies have reported a similar recurrence rate.[92,94-96] In one study with an average of 7.5 years of follow-up, 80% of cases recurred within 6 months, and there were no recurrences after 3 years.[96] A major limitation of these studies, is the length of follow-up. A survey of members of the American Pediatric Surgical Association found that 86% of surgeons perform an interval appendectomy.[60]

In a survey of pediatric surgeons, postoperative antibiotics were routinely used for complicated appendicitis;[60] however, there was variation in what type of antibiotics and duration of treatment. Common antibiotic regimens have included multidrug therapy, most frequently ampicillin plus gentamicin plus clindamycin or metronidazole. Monotherapy with a broad-spectrum antibiotic such as piperacillin-tazobactam appears to be equally effective.[97] The length of antibiotic treatment is variable and controversial. In one randomized trial, there was no difference in infectious complications between those patients who were treated for a minimum of 5 days of antibiotics compared with those treated for variable durations, based on clinical factors.[98] Other studies have shown that children can be discharged safely on outpatient parenteral

TABLE 68-3. Ruptured Appendicitis Scoring System[91]

Finding	Points
Generalized tenderness	4
Abscess by computed tomography	3
Duration symptoms >48 hours	3
Peripheral leukocyte count >19,400 cells/mm³	2
Fecalith by computed tomography	1

antibiotics[99] or on oral antibiotics after a course of intravenous antibiotics.[100,101] One literature review did not observe a difference in infectious complication rates between those treated with 3 days of antibiotics compared with those treated for longer periods.[102] Prescribing antibiotics until the patient has been afebrile for 24 hours and the WBC has returned to normal has been shown to be an effective strategy.[103] A randomized trial found that completing the antibiotic course with oral antibiotics once a child was afebrile for 12 hours and tolerating a regular diet decreased the length of hospitalization without increasing the risk of postoperative abscess.[104]

Traditionally it has been thought that the natural history of appendiceal rupture was within the control of the physician and that a high rupture rate reflected a failure of care. In order to decrease the rupture rate, early surgical intervention has been the gold standard and high rates of negative exploration have been acceptable in order to decrease the likelihood of rupture. Despite many efforts to decrease the rates of complicated appendicitis, though, rates of preoperative rupture in children range from 30% to 74%.[10] These high rupture rates may not be related to the medical care provided but to delay in presentation to a health care provider. Several studies have linked race with an increased risk of perforation.[10,105] In a review of a national pediatric discharge database, the likelihood of perforation differed by race, after controlling for age and health insurance status.[105] A review of a large pediatric health systems database revealed that the rate of rupture

in school-aged children was associated with race and insurance status and not with negative appendectomy rate.[10,106,107] Examination of a statewide database also revealed that children with Medicaid or no insurance were more likely to develop appendiceal perforation than children with private insurance.[106] Efforts focusing on improved access to healthcare would be more beneficial to reducing rates of complicated appendicitis than altering hospital management. Additionally, in a large retrospective cohort study, a lower hospital volume was associated with increased risk of misdiagnosis, but not increased risk of appendiceal perforation.[105]

FUTURE DIRECTIONS

Several studies have shown considerable variability in the care of children with appendicitis. A survey of pediatric surgeons showed that most surgeons base their management strategy on "individual surgeon's preference" with 24% using informal guidelines and only 17% with formal clinical practice guidelines.[60]

Discrepancies in practice patterns and treatment styles suggest that efforts to develop standardized evidence-based guideline may be a worthwhile effort. Quality improvement processes such as pathway development, refinement of guidelines and feedback to providers could improve the care of children with appendicitis. The evaluation of comparative data among centers would allow for the identification and adoption of best practices that could lead to improved outcomes and more economic use of resources.

---

69 Intra-Abdominal, Visceral, and Retroperitoneal Abscesses

Karen A. Diefenbach and R. Lawrence Moss

Intra-abdominal abscesses in children are not infrequent occurrences. When they occur, they are sometimes difficult to diagnose and even more difficult to treat. Even when managed appropriately, morbidity can be high. If not managed appropriately, the results can be devastating. Abdominal abscesses are categorized into three types, with the first being the most common: intra-abdominal (intraperitoneal), visceral, and retroperitoneal abscesses.

Bacteria from the original site of colonization or infection can travel hematogenously, by regional lymphatics, or directly to form an abscess. In intra-abdominal abscesses, mixed flora of facultative and anaerobic bacteria frequently is present, but in visceral and retroperitoneal abscesses, single organisms are more common. The types of bacteria isolated can indicate the origin of the infection. The most common facultative bacteria isolated in intra-abdominal abscesses are *Escherichia coli*, *Staphylococcus aureus*, and *Enterococcus* spp.[1,2] Anaerobic bacteria include *Bacteroides fragilis* group, *Peptostreptococcus* spp., *Clostridium* spp., and *Fusobacterium* spp.[1,2] These enteric organisms might also cause visceral abscesses, but this type of abscess also can be caused by the gram-positive bacteria of a systemic infection, or by fungi in immune-compromised hosts. Retroperitoneal abscesses contain organisms specific to the site of the primary infection.[3] For example, a perinephric abscess usually is caused by organisms that cause pyelonephritis, whereas an iliopsoas abscess (IPA) usually is caused by bacteremic *S. aureus*.[3-5]

The tenets of management of an abscess include drainage, appropriate antibiotic therapy, and correction, if possible, of any underlying pathology that can cause recurrence. Drainage can be accomplished in a variety of ways, including open surgical exploration, laparoscopic surgical exploration, and percutaneous, image-guided drainage. Empiric antibiotic therapy should be initiated immediately upon diagnosis considering likely abscesses by site (Table 69-1), and changed, if necessary, to definitive therapy when

culture and susceptibility test results become available. Coordinated management by the surgical, interventional radiology, and infectious diseases specialists, as well as the child's primary care physician will facilitate optimal care.

INTRA-ABDOMINAL ABSCESSES

Etiology and Clinical Manifestations

Complicated appendicitis is the most common cause of intra-abdominal abscesses in children. Patients can come to medical attention with an abscess after perforation of the appendix or can develop an abscess postoperatively.

TABLE 69-1. Summary of Common Organisms in Abscesses by Site[1-3,7,25-30,34,37]

Site	Organisms
Intra-abdominal	*Escherichia coli*, *Enterococcus* spp., *Bacteroides* spp., *Peptostreptococcus* spp., *Clostridium* spp., *Fusobacterium* spp., *Staphylococcus aureus*, *Klebsiella* spp., and *Pseudomonas* spp.
Visceral (liver, spleen, and pancreas)	*Staphylococcus aureus*, *Escherichia coli*, *Enterococcus faecalis*, *Klebsiella* spp., *Enterobacter* spp., *Pseudomonas* spp., *Streptococcus* spp., *Salmonella*, *Bartonella*, and *Candida* spp.
Retroperitoneal (iliopsoas, other)	*Staphylococcus aureus*, *Streptococcus* spp., *Escherichia coli*, *Klebsiella* spp., and *Candida* spp.

PART II Clinical Syndromes and Cardinal Features of Infectious Diseases: Approach to Diagnosis and Initial Management

SECTION I Intra-Abdominal Infections

Several other potential causes of intra-abdominal abscesses originate from the gastrointestinal tract, but rates are much lower. Any operation on the GI tract, whether elective or emergent, has the potential for causing a postoperative abscess. Elective operation on the bowel carries the risk of contamination of the peritoneum at the time of surgery or later from a complication such as an anastomotic leak. Emergent surgery for perforation is performed in the setting of contamination and has an even higher risk of abscess formation. Other emergent causes of a perforated viscus and resultant abscess include necrotizing enterocolitis, inflammatory bowel disease, peptic ulcer, Meckel diverticulum, and trauma.[1] Location of an abscess within the abdominal cavity, such as subphrenic and pelvic sites, can predict an underlying disease as can the isolation of certain pathogens. The bacteria most frequently isolated in abscesses after bowel disease or surgery include *Escherichia coli*, *Bacteroides* species, and *Enterococcus* species, but any enteric organism can be present.[2] Brook studied the microbiology of intra-abdominal abscesses in children and found that 8% of cultures yielded only facultative bacteria, 17% only anaerobic bacteria, and 75% mixed flora.[1,6]

A postoperative patient with persistent fever and abdominal pain must be evaluated for the possibility of an abscess. Symptoms from compression of the abscess on adjacent structures, such as early satiety for abscesses near the stomach, urinary frequency or urgency for those near the bladder, or diarrhea or tenesmus for abscesses near the colon or rectum associated with anorexia and weight loss are common findings in patients with abscesses.

Although not common, the incidence of biliary tract disease in children is increasing. Children with hemolytic disorders such as sickle-cell anemia and hereditary spherocytosis are at increased risk of cholelithiasis and biliary tract disease. Although most cases of cholelithiasis in children are managed electively, some patients present with complicated disease and associated cholecystitis. These patients are at risk for postoperative abscess, and this complication should be suspected in a patient who has undergone a recent cholecystectomy and has persistent fever and right upper-quadrant pain. Additional symptoms can include nausea, vomiting, and back or shoulder pain. Elevated white blood cell count and abnormal hepatic enzymes often are present. Bilirubin levels usually are normal, but if elevated should prompt an evaluation for ascending cholangitis. Hyperbilirubinemia in children can result from obstruction of the common bile duct by a retained stone or as a result of obstruction following a Kasai procedure or liver transplantation, or due to congenital anomaly or malignancy. If identified, urgent decompression of the biliary tree is required. Bilirubin levels also can be elevated in the presence of a postoperative bile leak. This usually occurs at the raw surface of transplanted partial liver in the gallbladder fossa. The resulting collection of bile can become infected and require drainage. A retained gallstone in the peritoneal cavity following cholecystectomy is another source of intra-abdominal abscess.[7] The most common pathogens associated with cholecystitis are *E. coli*, *Klebsiella*, *Pseudomonas*, and *Bacteroides* species.[7] Empiric antibiotic therapy in a patient with a history of cholecystitis presenting with a postoperative abscess should be directed against these organisms.

When an intra-abdominal abscess from any cause is suspected, imaging is indicated. Plain radiographs of the abdomen can show indirect evidence of abscess such as a pleural effusion or ileus. The diagnosis is confirmed by cross-sectional imaging using ultrasound or computed tomography (Figure 69-1). These imaging studies can facilitate treatment by providing guidance for aspiration of material for culture and placement of drainage catheters.

In general, one must maintain a high index of suspicion for abscess in patients with known risk factors, including recent surgery or trauma, immunocompromising condition, and a chronic illness, such as Crohn disease.

Management

Broad-spectrum antibiotics directed against facultative and anaerobic bacteria should be initiated empirically.[1,6] Therapy should be based on location and presumed etiology. Continued therapy

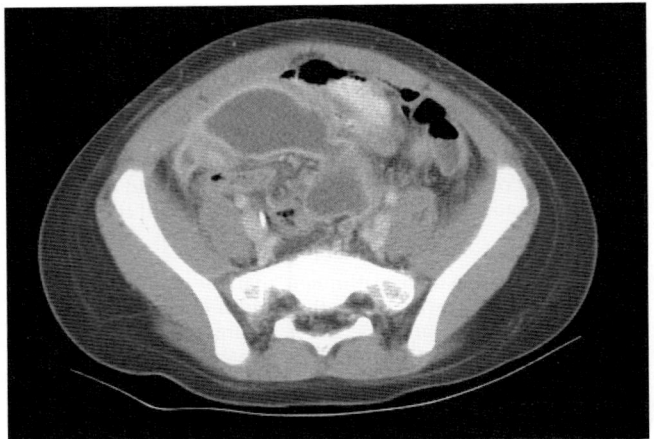

Figure 69-1. A postoperative abscess visualized by computed tomography. This rim-enhancing fluid collection has the typical appearance of an abscess.

should be guided by culture and susceptibility tests. Guidelines from the Surgical Infection Society recommend limiting the duration of intravenous antibiotics to 7 days if there is adequate control of source/drainage of abscess; otherwise antibiotic therapy parenterally may be required for an extended period of time.[8]

The manner in which an intra-abdominal abscess is managed should be individualized. Antibiotics alone can be effective with fluid collections <2 cm in diameter. Patients with a large inflammatory mass of fibrinous material with small fluid pockets are considered to have a phlegmon and are usually best treated with antibiotics alone. When imaging reveals a collection of fluid >2 cm or when a smaller collection has failed to respond to antibiotics, drainage combined with antibiotics is indicated.

Percutaneous drainage with image guidance has become a mainstay of therapy for children with abscesses (Figure 69-2). Different modalities have been used to facilitate drainage, such as ultrasound and CT guidance for placement of the drain with fluoroscopy and CT to re-evaluate and confirm adequate drainage of the abscess cavity.[2,9] Percutaneous drainage is desirable because it is well tolerated, less invasive than laparotomy, and provides accurate confirmation of response to therapy[2,9–11] (Figure 69-3). Although percutaneous drainage frequently requires general anesthesia, the risks of bowel manipulation, visceral injury, and the probability of adhesive small-bowel obstruction are reduced. Clinical setting, location, size, organization, and number of abscesses all play a role in determining the patient's eligibility for percutaneous drainage.[9,10] Factors associated with reduced success of percutaneous drainage include presence of complex abscesses, loculated or poorly organized abscesses, or those with multiple or extensive collections.[1,9] One study assessed indicators of the outcome of attempted percutaneous procedures.[10] Although the sample size was small, abscesses with less viscous contents, as indicated by the presence of air–fluid levels or peripheral air bubbles, were drained successfully by percutaneous methods in 95% of cases. Thicker fluid collections, as evidenced by deep air bubbles, had only a 66% success rate of percutaneous drainage.[10]

Some intra-abdominal abscesses are best managed by operative or reoperative laparotomy. Indications for surgical intervention include uncontrolled septicemia, a cause of the abscess that requires surgical correction (i.e., an anastomotic leak), abscess(es) not amenable to percutaneous drainage, and unsuccessful percutaneous drainage. Surgical drainage can be performed by open or laparoscopic technique. There is no clear evidence that one method is better than the other.[12] Proponents for laparoscopic drainage cite better visualization of the entire abdominal contents and ability to irrigate the area adequately. In other cases, the need for a concomitant surgical procedure, such as to form a stoma or revise an anastomosis, is an indication for an open procedure. Several case series have suggested laparoscopy is an adequate method to drain abscesses.[12–15]

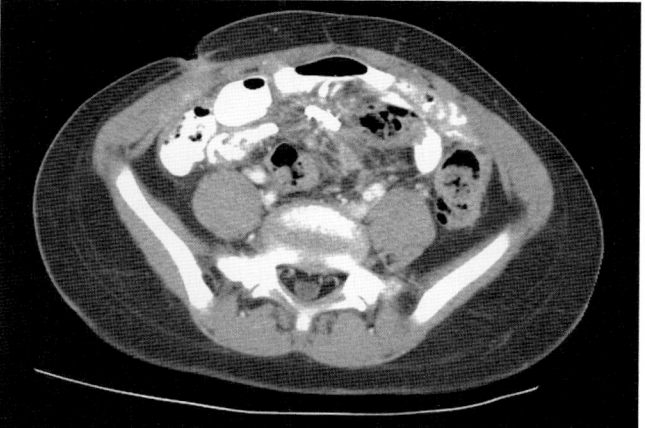

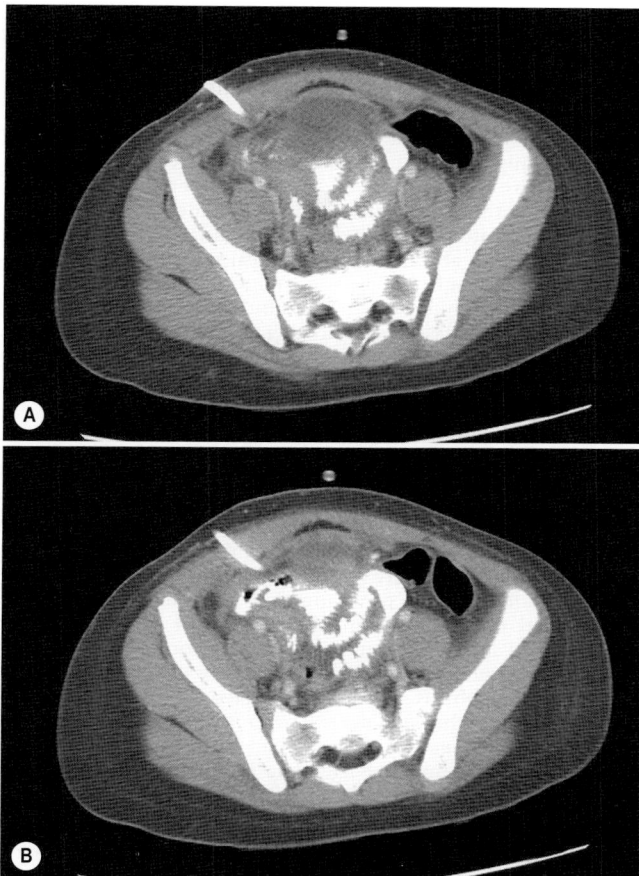

Figure 69-3. Resolution of the fluid collection, catheter still visualized next to small bowel.

Figure 69-2. (**A** and **B**) Computed tomography-guided placement of a drainage catheter into the abscess.

VISCERAL ABSCESSES

Etiology and Clinical Manifestations

Prior to the availability of antibiotics, abscesses in the liver were not uncommon in otherwise healthy children. However, with the development of appropriate antimicrobial therapies, most liver abscesses that occur currently are seen in underdeveloped countries where antibiotics are less available or in immunocompromised patients such as those receiving chemotherapy, or children with chronic granulomatous disease or acquired immunodeficiency syndrome (AIDS).[1,16] Immunologically normal children who develop pyogenic liver abscesses usually have had a recent episode of appendicitis or cholecystitis.[17]

Pyogenic liver abscesses in children are caused by aerobic, facultative or anaerobic bacteria, or a mixture of bacteria.[1,3,18,19] The bacteria associated with these infections include *S. aureus, E. coli, Enterococcus faecalis,* or *Klebsiella, Enterobacter, Pseudomonas,* or *Salmonella* species. Cat-scratch disease also has been associated with multiple microabscesses of the liver and spleen in otherwise healthy children and in immunocompromised children with cancer or HIV.[1,20] Abscesses in the liver can be single or multiple, simple or complex. They can occur as a result of direct extension from local infection, such as cholecystitis or cholangitis. They also can result from hematogenous spread through the hepatic artery or through the portal vein from sources within the abdominal cavity. Pyelophlebitis, for example, occurs when enteric organisms access the liver through the portal system.

Amebiasis is frequently discussed as a cause of liver abscess, although some argue that it is not a true abscess.[1] This parasite reaches the liver through the portal venous system, and usually causes a single large abscess. Other types of parasitic infections, including ascariasis, have been associated with hepatic abscesses. The granulomas induced by these infections are recognized as a predisposing factor for pyogenic liver abscesses in children in endemic areas.[17]

Traumatic injury to the liver has been associated with liver abscess in about 1% of cases.[21] Abscess associated with trauma is most common in patients managed operatively and in those with concurrent injury to a hollow viscus.

Symptoms of hepatic abscesses include fever; abdominal pain, which can be localized in the right upper quadrant or diffuse; nausea; vomiting; and anorexia.[22] Jaundice is less common, but can be present if the abscess is compressing the biliary tree and when parasitic infections, such as ascariasis, cause obstruction of the lumen of the bile ducts. The white blood cell count and serum hepatic enzymes can be elevated. A detailed history is important, including kitten exposure, travel in endemic areas of parasitic infestation, recent trauma, infection, or surgery. Ultrasonography or CT can be used to confirm the presence of the abscess(es). Specific antibody tests can be helpful if a parasitic infection is suspected, such as the hemagglutination test which usually is positive with amebic abscesses, or serum antibodies for *Bartonella henselae,* if cat-scratch disease is suspected.

The incidence of splenic abscesses appears to be increasing, although it is unclear whether this is a true increase in number of cases or a higher index of suspicion coupled with better diagnostic tools.[23–25] Some reports indicate that the increasing number of immunocompromised patients is contributing to the changing pattern of splenic abscesses.[25] Aggressive cancer chemotherapy, numbers of patients with HIV/AIDS, and immunosuppression for organ transplantation may be responsible.[25] Other populations at risk are patients with hemolytic disorders such as sickle-cell anemia and those with a history of splenic trauma.

Splenic abscesses can be large or small, solitary or multiple. Infections can be due to single organisms or can be polymicrobial. Organisms frequently identified include *S. aureus, E. coli,* and *Salmonella, Streptococcus, Candida,* and *Klebsiella* species.[25–28]

The triad of fever, leukocytosis, and left upper-quadrant pain is common. Nausea and vomiting also can be present as well as splenomegaly and tenderness on physical examination. The diagnosis can be suspected on chest radiograph, when the left hemidiaphragm is elevated or a left pleural effusion is present. Ultrasonography or CT confirms the diagnosis.

Renal and perinephric abscesses are visceral abscesses found in the retroperitoneal space that result from urogenital pathology such as pyelonephritis, urinary obstruction from ureteral stone, or seeding from systemic infections causing bacteremia or fungemia. Renal and perinephric abscesses are discussed elsewhere (see Chapter 50, Renal (Intrarenal and Perinephric) Abscesses).

PART II   Clinical Syndromes and Cardinal Features of Infectious Diseases: Approach to Diagnosis and Initial Management

SECTION I   Intra-Abdominal Infections

Pancreatic abscesses in children are rare, and can be the result of acute pancreatitis or trauma. Injuries of the pancreas due to blunt or penetrating trauma can precipitate an abscess in the presence of either devitalized, necrotic tissue or a leak of the pancreatic duct. If not diagnosed preoperatively or identified at the time of exploration, the resulting fluid collection can be infected secondarily. Mortality associated with pancreatic abscesses is 15% to 50%, with morbidity rates as high as 75% to 80%.[29,30] The most common organisms include *E. coli* and *Klebsiella*, *Enterococcus*, *Staphylococcus*, *Streptococcus*, and *Pseudomonas* species, as well as fungi.[29,30]

Symptoms include fever, epigastric or left upper-quadrant pain, and hemodynamic instability. Laboratory tests show an elevated white blood cell count with variable elevation of serum amylase and lipase levels. CT with rapid contrast injection is the most sensitive test for pancreatic abnormalities and can show a nonenhancing portion of the pancreas or a fluid collection in or near the pancreas.[29]

Management

Antibiotic therapy should be broad-spectrum, with activity against the most common organisms associated with the type of abscess identified. In immunocompromised patients, the addition of antifungal therapy should be considered. Decisions regarding drainage are made based on the clinical presentation, condition of the patient, and need for microbiologic confirmation.

Multiple microabscesses of the liver have been treated successfully with antibiotics alone, especially in cases of cat-scratch disease.[20,22] Abscesses <4 cm in diameter can be successfully treated by aspiration, with antibiotic therapy continued until the patient's clinical status improves and CT shows resolution of the abscess. However, in patients with abscesses >4 cm or recurrence after aspiration, continuous drainage using a CT- or ultrasound-guided percutaneous catheter is indicated in addition to antibiotic therapy.[22] Surgical drainage is recommended in patients with liver abscesses that do not resolve with percutaneous drainage, those who present with rupture of the abscess into the peritoneal cavity, and in patients with chronic granulomatous disease who have persistent or recurrent liver abscesses.[16,22]

The management of splenic abscesses is similar to that of liver abscesses. Although salvage of the spleen is preferable and usually is possible, the primary goal is eradication of infection. Splenectomy should be considered in patients who do not respond to drainage and antibiotics. Splenectomy also should be considered in patients who are immunocompromised and have ongoing septicemia, in patients with sickle-cell disease or other hemoglobinopathies, in those who present with rupture of the abscess into the peritoneal cavity, and in those who have an abscess following a traumatic splenic injury.[25–27,31]

Pancreatic abscesses should be managed with drainage. In cases of pancreatic fluid collections that may not be infected or in cases of pancreatic phlegmon, CT-guided aspiration of pancreatic or peri-pancreatic fluid can provide specimens for culture to guide antibiotic therapy. Percutaneous drainage catheters can be left in place if the fluid appears purulent or Gram stain is positive for organisms. Percutaneous drainage has reported success rates ranging from 69% to 86%.[29,30] In patients who have ongoing septicemia or whose fluid collections are not amenable to percutaneous drainage, open operative exploration is required.[29,30,32] In those patients who ultimately require surgery, percutaneous drainage often is a good temporizing measure in patients who are too unstable to undergo surgery due to severe sepsis.

RETROPERITONEAL ABSCESSES

Etiology and Clinical Manifestations

In addition to abscesses of the kidney and pancreas, other causes of abscesses in the retroperitoneum include traumatic duodenal injury and intra-psoas abscess. Traumatic duodenal injury may be a result of penetrating trauma or blunt trauma associated with "handlebar" injuries of bicycles or motorcycles. Several cases of penetrating trauma to the duodenum have been reported in which retroperitoneal abscess followed the ingestion of a sharp foreign body such as a needle, toothpick, or fish bone.[33] Abscesses associated with duodenal injuries or perforations are difficult to manage and have a high rate of morbidity and mortality.[34–36] Evacuation of the abscess cavity is difficult, and the underlying problem, a disruption of the duodenal wall, must be addressed to prevent further complication, such as duodenal fistula.

Retroperitoneal abscess should be suspected in a patient with right upper-quadrant or epigastric pain, fever, nausea and vomiting, an elevated white blood cell count, and, in many cases, an elevated serum amylase level following trauma. Findings on physical examination suspicious for duodenal injury include a contusion of the upper abdomen with signs of peritonitis. Plain radiographs of the abdomen may not be diagnostic unless free air is present. An upper intestinal contrast study or CT usually is diagnostic.[34,35] Organisms reported in these abscesses include *Staphylococcus* and *Streptococcus* species, *Escherichia coli*, *Klebsiella*, and *Candida* species.[3,34,37]

Intra-psoas abscess (IPA) is either primary or secondary.[38] Primary IPA has no detectable source, and is the most common type in children. Secondary IPA is associated with a known source of infection. Because the psoas muscle is intimately related to the ureter, renal pelvis, spine, appendix, terminal ileum, pancreas, jejunum, and sigmoid colon, an infectious process deriving from any of these structures can cause a secondary IPA.[15,39,40] Examples include pyelonephritis, appendicitis, osteomyelitis, pancreatitis, and inflammatory bowel disease. The most common organism in primary IPA is *S. aureus*, indicating that an unidentified, mucocutaneous source leading to bacteremia is most likely.[15,39,41] Other etiologies include *Streptococcus pneumoniae* (the most common causative organism in patients with a history of recent respiratory tract infection) and gram-negative organisms, such as *E. coli* (in patients with a history of appendicitis or other gastrointestinal infection or surgery). Underlying illness such as diabetes mellitus, HIV infection, or connective tissue disease increase risk in adults; case reports of IPA in neonates suggest a predisposing event of femoral venous catheterization or omphalitis.[5,39,40] The most common organism is *S. aureus*, especially methicillin-resistant *S. aureus*.

Presenting symptoms of IPA include fever, leg pain or swelling, and decreased range of motion in the ipsilateral hip.[38] The degree of dysfunction of the hip joint varies widely, from no apparent dysfunction to complete pseudoparalysis. A positive psoas sign, inguinal swelling, or lymphadenopathy can be present on physical examination.

Septic arthritis of the hip must be distinguished from IPA. Laboratory testing often demonstrates an elevated white blood cell count and an elevated erythrocyte sedimentation rate in both conditions. Plain radiographs may reveal obscuring of the sacroiliac joint or an effusion of the hip in IPA, which is sympathetic effusion due to the surrounding inflammatory process. Because a delay in treatment of pyogenic arthritis must be avoided, an aspiration of the joint is the safest approach to exclude this diagnosis.[38] Ultrasonography or CT is the best diagnostic tool to characterize an IPA and can assist in obtaining samples for culture, placement of drains, and follow up for resolution.

Management

Several factors should be considered when deciding the best approach for the management of retroperitoneal abscesses resulting from duodenal pathology. These include time since injury, clinical presentation and hemodynamic stability of the patient, as well as concurrent injuries or illnesses. Any approach should accomplish drainage of the retroperitoneal abscess cavity and address the primary pathology of the duodenum.[34–36] Possible surgical approaches include primary repair and drainage with or without pyloric exclusion versus a more aggressive approach of a pancreaticoduodenectomy. Successful percutaneous drainage also has been reported.[35] Nutritional support is important as enteral feeding will be precluded in the postoperative period.[34,36]

IPAs are managed by drainage and antibiotic therapy. Except in the case of a known prior infection, empiric antibiotic therapy should cover *S. aureus*, since this is the most common organism.

Recently, drainage has been accomplished by ultrasound-guided aspiration or drainage using a percutaneous catheter.[42,43] A retroperitoneoscopic approach as well as an open operative approach have been used when percutaneous drainage is not successful.[28]

SECTION J: Skin and Soft-Tissue Infections

70 Superficial Bacterial Skin Infections and Cellulitis

Hillary S. Lawrence and Amy Jo Nopper

Providing a permeability barrier, which prevents both the loss of water and electrolytes and the invasion of pathogens, the skin has a primary protective function. Intact skin is resistant to colonization and invasion of bacteria via a number of mechanisms.[1-3] The outermost layer of the epidermis, the stratum corneum, constitutes the principal barrier against infection. The stratum corneum consists of corneocytes (anucleated keratinocytes or skin cells), and an outer lipid matrix. Corneocytes fit together in an overlapping fashion, making penetration by organisms difficult; they are shed from the skin after approximately 14 days, thus pathogenic organisms have limited time to invade further into the epidermis. The lipid matrix surrounding corneocytes is acidic, providing antimicrobial activity against pathogenic organisms, including *Staphylococcus aureus* and *Streptococcus* species.[1,2] Keratinocytes also participate in innate immunity via secretion of antimicrobial peptides (AMPS) such as human β-defensins, canthelicidin, psoriasin, and dermicidin. AMPs are small peptides with broad-spectrum antimicrobial activity against bacteria, viruses and yeast.[2,4-6] Production of AMPs by keratinocytes is stimulated by inflammatory cytokines produced in the skin as a result of injury or inflammation and by invasive organisms via pathogen-associated molecular patterns (PAMPs).[6] Resident bacteria on the skin provide additional protection against infection by preventing colonization with pathogenic organisms via competitive binding to cell surface receptors, and by the production of toxic substances called bacteriocins that inhibit the growth of similar bacteria.[1,3,7]

Skin microflora generally can be categorized into two groups: resident flora and transient flora. Resident florae establish secure attachments to the skin, are present in stable numbers, and are able to tolerate an acidic environment. Transient florae are introduced from the environment and only attach if the skin is disrupted.[1,8] Group A streptococcus (GAS, *Streptococcus pyogenes*) and *S. aureus* are the most common transient bacteria on the skin that cause infection.[1,3]

Many different bacteria are considered to be normal, resident flora, and each organism has a predilection for specific anatomic locations and for hosts of a particular age.[1,3,7] The skin becomes colonized with microorganisms during the birth process and through contact with the environment. Infants born vaginally acquire *Staphylococcus epidermidis* during passage through the vaginal canal; and within hours, coryneform bacteria also are found on neonatal skin.[1] The dry surface of the stratum corneum is colonized by micrococci and coagulase-negative staphylococci (CoNS),[1,7] while coryneform organisms and gram-negative bacilli prefer moist, intertriginous areas.[1,3,7,9] *Propionibacterium* spp. grow in hair follicles and sebaceous glands, and are mainly found after puberty, when sebaceous activity increases.[1-3,7,9] Hair follicles are colonized by micrococci and CoNS superficially;[8] *Corynebacterium* and *Propionibacterium* spp. are found deep in follicular canals.[10]

Transient colonization of the skin by pathogens is facilitated by factors that harm the resident flora, including elevated temperature, humidity, and antibiotic therapy.[1-3,8] When a pathogen achieves successful colonization of the skin, the other cutaneous defense mechanisms must also be overcome before infection commences. Therefore, the main determinant of cutaneous infection is the balance between the virulence of the organism and the defense mechanisms of the host.[11] Compromised cutaneous barrier function occurs in patients with chronic dermatitis and premature infants, making their skin more susceptible to pathogenic colonization and cutaneous infection.[1]

Primary bacterial infection of the skin can involve the epidermis, dermis, or subcutaneous tissue, whereas soft-tissue infections extend deeper, to the fascia or muscle. Superficial skin infections are mainly limited to the epidermis and dermis; although secondary inflammation can involve the subcutis.[11] Several types of lesions can form in the skin as the result of a primary infectious process (Table 70-1); however, a pathogen usually produces a characteristic primary lesion with a characteristic pattern of spread. When cutaneous bacterial infection occurs, recognition of the type and depth of lesion produced are helpful in determining the likely causative agent. Primary, superficial bacterial infections of the skin and cellulitis are the focus of this chapter (Table 70-2). Other infectious agents (viruses, fungi) that sometimes resemble these bacterial infections are discussed briefly.

SUPERFICIAL INFECTIONS

Impetigo

Impetigo is a common skin infection caused by *S. aureus* and GAS. Impetigo occurs in two forms: bullous and nonbullous, and is highly contagious. Children aged 2 to 5 years are affected most often,[12,13] and infection rates peak in the summer and late fall.[14] Impetigo can be a primary infection or a secondary infection involving skin compromised by dermatitis or trauma.[15] Factors that predispose to infection include poor hygiene, crowded living conditions, humidity, pre-existing dermatitis, and minor skin trauma.[10,14,16]

TABLE 70-1. Primary Skin Lesions

Lesion	Description
Macule	Flat lesion, <1 cm
Patch	Flat lesion, >1 cm
Papule	Elevated lesion, <1 cm
Plaque	Elevated broad flat lesion, >1 cm
Nodule	Dome-shaped or rounded lesions, >1 cm. Arising from the dermis or subcutis
Pustule	Pus-filled lesion
Vesicle	Elevated lesion, <1 cm. Filled with serous fluid
Bulla	Elevated lesion, >1 cm. Filled with serous fluid

TABLE 70-2. Primary Superficial Cutaneous Bacterial Infections

Disease Entity	Skin Lesions	Infectious Agent(s)
Anthrax	Papule, vesicle, bulla	*Bacillus anthracis*
Blistering distal dactylitis	Vesicle	*Streptococcus pyogenes*, group B streptococcus, *Staphylococcus aureus*
Cellulitis	Plaque	*Streptococcus pyogenes*, *Staphylococcus aureus*
Diphtheria	Papule, pustule, ulcer	*Corynebacterium diphtheriae*
Ecthyma	Pustule, ulcer	*Streptococcus pyogenes*
Ecthyma gangrenosum	Papule, vesicle, ulcer	*Pseudomonas aeruginosa*
Erysipelas	Plaque, sometimes vesicles/bullae	*Streptococcus pyogenes*, groups B, C, G streptococci
Erysipeloid	Patch, plaque	*Erysipelothrix rhusiopathiae*
Folliculitis	Pustule, papule	*Staphylococcus aureus*, *Malassezia* spp.
Sycosis barbae	Pustule, papule	*Staphylococcus aureus*
Gram-negative folliculitis	Pustule, papule	*Klebsiella* spp., *Enterobacter* spp., *Escherichia coli*, *Pseudomonas aeruginosa*
	Pustule, nodule	*Proteus* spp.
Hot-tub folliculitis	Pustule, papule	*Pseudomonas aeruginosa*
Erythrasma	Patch	*Corynebacterium minutissimum*
Furuncles, carbuncles	Nodule	*Staphylococcus aureus*
Impetigo	Vesicle, bulla, pustule, plaque, erosion	*Staphylococcus aureus*
Intertrigo	Patch, plaque, erosion	*Streptococcus* spp., *Staphylococcus aureus*, *Candida albicans* *Streptococcus pyogenes*
Paronychia	Patch	Mixed flora (see text)
Perianal dermatitis	Patch	*Staphylococcus aureus*, *Streptococcus pyogenes*
Pitted keratolysis	Erosion	*Kytococcus sedentarius*, *Dermophilus congolensis*, *Corynebacterium* spp.

Nonbullous impetigo is the most common form of the infection, accounting for more than 70% of cases of impetigo.[10,15] Lesions of nonbullous impetigo typically form on traumatized skin and are most often located on the exposed skin of the face and extremities.[10,12] Lesions initially begin as small vesicles or pustules that rupture, forming an adherent, honey-colored crust.[10,12,14,16,17] Impetigo is associated with minimal pain or erythema, and constitutional symptoms generally are absent. Pruritus, regional adenopathy, and leukocytosis are commonly associated with nonbullous impetigo. The differential diagnosis of nonbullous impetigo includes contact dermatitis, as well as viral, fungal, and parasitic (scabies, pediculosis) infections, all of which can be complicated by secondary infection with impetigo. If left untreated, most cases of nonbullous impetigo resolves in approximately 2 weeks without scarring.[15]

The bacterial etiology of lesions of nonbullous impetigo cannot be predicted clinically.[15] The predominant cause of nonbullous impetigo in the United States is *S. aureus*, though infection can also be attributed to GAS[10,12-14,16,18] or mixed pathogens.[14,16,18] Anaerobic bacteria also have been isolated from lesions of nonbullous impetigo, although a pathogenic role is unclear.[18] *S. aureus* causes impetigo in children of all ages, and the bacteria usually are present in the nose, perineum, axillae, or underneath the fingernails prior to causing cutaneous infection. In contrast, infections due to GAS are unusual before 2 years of age, except in highly endemic areas;[10] and GAS colonizes the skin an average of 10 days before development of impetigo via inoculation of organisms into a break in the skin.[10,12] Several types of GAS can cause nonbullous impetigo and they are different from the strains implicated in streptococcal pharyngitis.[10]

Bullous impetigo occurs mainly in infants and young children. It is caused by strains of *S. aureus*, usually from phage group 2,[10,16] capable of producing an exfoliative toxin that disrupts cell-to-cell adhesion in the superficial epidermis, leading to superficial blister formation.[12,13,17] Since the lesions of bullous impetigo are a manifestation of localized toxin production, they develop on intact

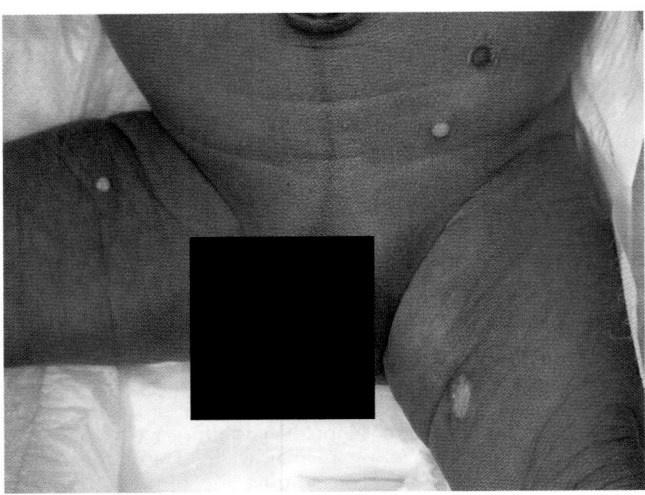

Figure 70-1. Scattered pustules on the abdomen and thighs of an infant with bullous impetigo caused by *S. aureus*. One lesion has ruptured, leaving an erosion with a collarette of scale.

skin.[10] The flaccid bullae and pustules of this form of impetigo occur beneath the stratum corneum and are easily ruptured, leaving shallow erosions with a collarette of scale (Figure 70-1).[10,15-17] Bullae can be single or clustered; regional adenopathy and systemic symptoms are unusual. The differential diagnosis of bullous impetigo in the neonate includes transient neonatal pustular melanosis, epidermolysis bullosa, bullous mastocytosis, and herpetic infection. Insect bites, contact dermatitis, burns, erythema multiforme, and autoimmune bullous dermatoses must be considered in older children, particularly if the lesions are unresponsive to therapy.

Complications of impetigo are rare, and include invasive infections such as pneumonia, osteomyelitis, pyogenic arthritis, and septicemia. Cellulitis can complicate nonbullous impetigo but rarely is associated with the bullous form. Streptococcal impetigo can be followed by lymphangitis, suppurative lymphadenitis, scarlet fever, and acute glomerulonephritis. Acute poststreptococcal glomerulonephritis occurs after skin and pharyngeal infections with nephritogenic strains of *S. pyogenes* (M groups 2, 49, 53, 55, 56, 57, and 60 for epidemics associated with impetigo). Symptoms develop an average of 18 to 21 days following skin infection, and children aged 3 to 7 years old are most commonly affected.[10] The anti-DNAase B titer is the best serologic test for detecting preceding streptococcal impetigo as the etiology of acute glomerulonephritis.[10,12] Strains of *S. pyogenes* associated with endemic impetigo in the U.S. have little or no nephritogenic potential and acute rheumatic fever does not occur as a result of impetigo.[10]

Localized impetigo can be treated with topical antimicrobial agents. Topical mupirocin has been demonstrated to be as effective as oral erythromycin for the treatment of impetigo, and may be associated with fewer side effects.[19,20] Retapamulin is a newer topical antibiotic, which like mupirocin, is approved by the U.S. Food and Drug Administration for treatment of impetigo caused by methicillin-susceptible *S. aureus* (MSSA) and *S. pyogenes*.[13,21] Systemic therapy is recommended for patients with widespread lesions and for lesions associated with fever or evidence of deeper involvement (cellulitis, furunculosis, abscess formation, suppurative lymphadenitis).[10] An agent effective against both staphylococcus and streptococcus, such as a first-generation cephalosporin, penicillinase-resistant penicillin, macrolide, or clindamycin, usually is utilized when systemic antimicrobial therapy is indicated.[10,12,14,17] Antibiotic selection should be based on local resistance patterns to ensure coverage for methicillin-resistant *S. aureus* (MRSA) when appropriate. Antibiotic therapy does not prevent acute glomerulonephritis resulting from streptococcal impetigo, but will help prevent the spread of nephritogenic strains of the bacteria.[10,12] Patients with recurrent impetigo sometimes are evaluated for carriage of *S. aureus*; decolonization can be attempted.[10] Frequent handwashing and attention to personal hygiene should be emphasized to patients to prevent spread of infection.[14]

Perianal Bacterial Dermatitis

Perianal bacterial dermatitis usually occurs in children between the ages of 6 months and 10 years,[22] and peaks between the ages of 3 and 5 years.[23] The infection is most commonly due to GAS, but *S. aureus* also can cause infection.[24] Physical examination characteristically reveals superficial, well-demarcated, circumferential erythema extending around the anus and surrounding skin (Figure 70-2).[22,25,26] Vulvovaginitis, vaginal discharge, and vulvar redness can be seen in girls and penile involvement in boys.[22,25] *S. aureus* is the likely pathogen when small papules and pustules on the buttocks and inguinal area are seen in addition to the characteristic findings, or when there is extension of erythema onto the buttocks.[24] Additional manifestations include irritability,[26] pruritus, painful defecation (at times associated with refusal to defecate), blood-streaked stools, fissures, mucoid discharge, and yellow crust.[22,23,27] Familial spread of perianal dermatitis is common.[22,25] Perianal streptococcal dermatitis is reported to be an infectious trigger for guttate psoriasis, and patients presenting with guttate psoriasis should be examined for asymptomatic GAS infection.[27]

The differential diagnosis of perianal bacterial dermatitis includes psoriasis, irritant contact dermatitis, candidiasis, and pinworm infestation. Diagnosis of perianal bacterial dermatitis often is delayed due to misdiagnosis and lack of awareness of the condition,[23] with patients frequently undergoing treatment with topical antifungal agents or topical corticosteroids before the correct diagnosis is made.[22,23] Isolation of *S. pyogenes* or *S. aureus* from culture of perianal swab specimens confirms the diagnosis.[22] A 10–14-day course of systemic antibiotics, often penicillin or

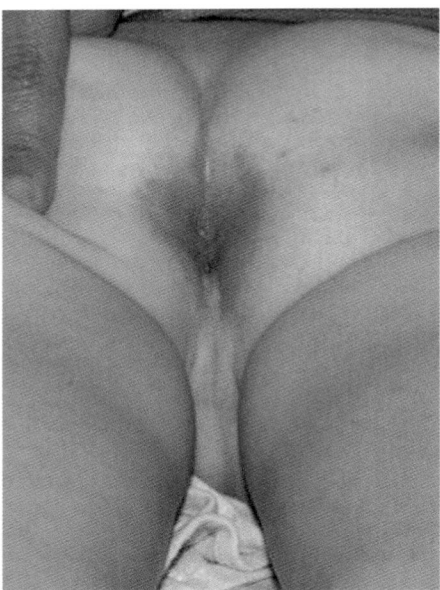

Figure 70-2. Brilliant erythematous perianal dermatitis due to group A streptococcus.

erythromycin, is recommended.[25] Clindamycin, a β-lactamase resistant penicillin, or a cephalosporin may be useful in cases due to *S. aureus*;[24] therapy is guided by culture results and susceptibility test results. Topical erythromycin[28] and mupirocin[24] are reportedly as effective as solitary treatment; however, topical antibiotics generally are used as an adjunct to systemic therapy.[27]

Intertrigo

Intertrigo is a disorder of the skin folds resulting from the friction created by opposing skin surfaces, combined with a moist environment. Because infants tend to have deep skin folds as a result of their short necks, generally flexed posture, and chubbiness, and due to their tendency to drool, infants are particularly susceptible to intertrigo.[29] Secondary infections with *Candida albicans*, GAS, *S. aureus*, and mixed organisms can occur. Bright red, well-demarcated weeping patches and plaques are seen in the folds of the neck, axillae, antecubital fossa, inguinal area, or popliteal fossae (Figure 70-3). The presence of satellite lesions is suggestive of *Candida*

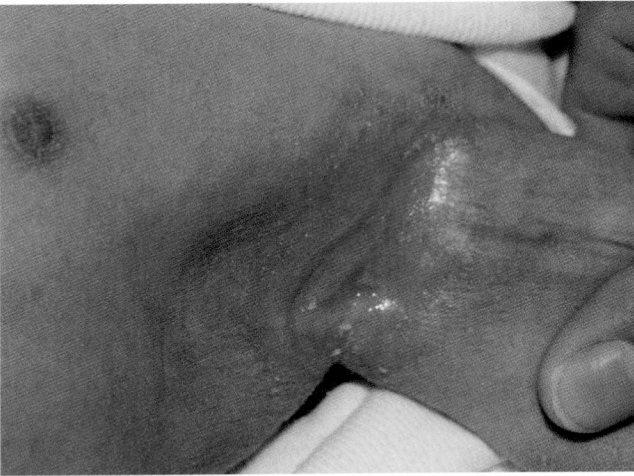

Figure 70-3. Erythematous weeping patch of intertrigo in the axillae of a 2-month-old girl, who had similar lesions on the fold of her neck and inguinal creases. Bacterial culture of the lesion grew both group A streptococcus and *Staphylococcus aureus*.

PART II Clinical Syndromes and Cardinal Features of Infectious Diseases: Approach to Diagnosis and Initial Management

SECTION J Skin and Soft-Tissue Infections

infection, while streptococcal intertrigo commonly is associated with a foul odor. Affected infants usually appear well, but can have associated fever, fussiness, or malaise.[29,30]

In addition to intertrigo, the differential diagnosis of intertriginous dermatitis includes seborrheic dermatitis, atopic dermatitis, irritant or allergic contact dermatitis, erythrasma, "inverse" psoriasis, scabies and Langerhans cell histiocytosis. Diagnosis is confirmed by culture of a lesion. Treatment of candidal intertrigo consists of topical antifungal agents such as nystatin, econazole, or ketoconazole, while streptococcal intertrigo can be treated with a 10-day course of penicillin or cephalexin, in combination with topical mupirocin. Anti-inflammatory agents, like topical hydrocortisone 1%, can be used for associated erythema. Use of barrier ointments and ensuring that skin folds are completely dry will reduce the friction and moisture of intertriginous areas, helping to prevent intertrigo.[29]

Erythrasma

Corynebacterium minutissimum is the causative agent of erythrasma. This cutaneous infection is manifest as well-demarcated reddish-brown patches and plaques located in moist intertriginous zones. The condition may be asymptomatic or associated with pruritus and involved skin may be thin with a "cigarette paper" quality.[31] Commonly affected sites include the groin, axillae, intergluteal folds, submammary region, and interdigital spaces of the toes. Heat, humidity, obesity, diabetes mellitus, hyperhidrosis, and poor hygiene are predisposing factors.[31,32]

Erythrasma can be confirmed with Wood lamp examination. *C. minutissimum* produces porphyrins that fluoresce a brilliant coral-red color under ultraviolet light; however, bathing within 20 hours before the Wood lamp examination can remove the water-soluble porphyrins. When Wood lamp examination is negative, a potassium hydroxide examination is useful to exclude dermatophyte infection and skin scrapings can be stained with periodic acid–Schiff, methenamine silver, or Gram stain to evaluate for coccobacilli.[31]

The treatment of choice is erythromycin 250 mg four times daily for 2 weeks. Topical clindamycin twice daily also can be used. For severe cases, a combination of oral erythromycin and topical antibiotics may be needed. Recurrence can be minimized by the use of an antibacterial soap.[32]

Pitted Keratolysis

Pitted keratolysis is a skin infection affecting the thick stratum corneum of the plantar surface of the feet and less commonly the palms. Characteristic findings include white, hyperkeratotic areas studded with multiple 1 to 7 mm pitted or erosive lesions on the soles, particularly over pressure-bearing sites (Figure 70-4).[31,33]

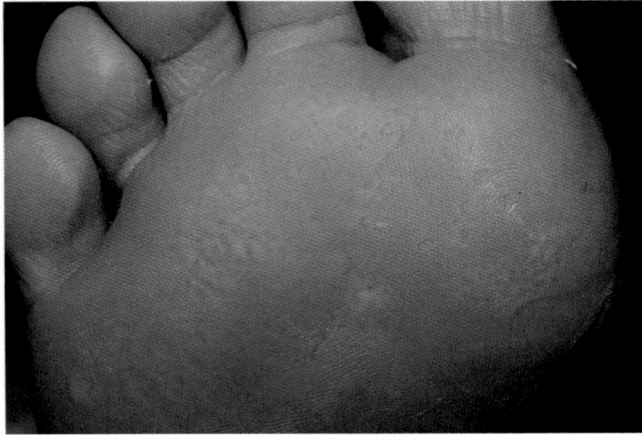

Figure 70-4. White plaques with numerous shallow pits on the plantar surface of the foot of a patient with pitted keratolysis.

Ringed erythematous lesions that coalesce can be seen on non-hyperkeratotic areas.[31] The condition can be asymptomatic or associated with hyperhidrosis, malodor, pain, and sliminess of the skin. People whose feet are moist for prolonged periods due to hyperhidrosis, immersion in water, or use of occlusive shoes are most frequently affected. Males are affected more often than females.[31,33]

Kytococcus sedentarius (formerly *Micrococcus* spp.), the suspected causative agent of pitted keratolysis, produces serum proteases capable of degrading keratin in calloused skin.[34] *Dermophilus congolensis* and *Corynebacterium* spp. also have been implicated as pathogens.[31,33] Diagnosis is based on characteristic clinical findings. Effective therapeutic regimens include topical or systemic erythromycin, miconazole, fusidic acid, and control of hyperhidrosis with topical aluminum chloride or botulinum toxin. Improved hygiene and use of adequately fitting shoes also may help.[31]

Trichobacteriosis

Trichobacteriosis (formerly trichomycosis) is an asymptomatic infection of the axillary and less commonly the pubic hair shafts caused by *Corynebacterium tenuis* and other coryneform species.[31,35] A bacterial biofilm encases the hair, creating yellow or white concretions distributed along the length of the hair shaft. Hyperhidrosis and a foul odor can be associated with the condition. The diagnosis is clinical, though a pale yellow fluorescence may be seen with Wood light examination. Treatment consists of shaving the affected area, applying topical antibiotics like clindamycin or erythromycin, and use of antiperspirants to control hyperhidrosis.[31]

ADNEXAL AND FOLLICULAR INFECTIONS

Folliculitis

Bacterial folliculitis is a superficial infection of the hair follicle manifest by discrete 2 to 5 mm papules and pustules on an erythematous base. The papules and pustules can be single or grouped, and often a hair shaft is seen in the center of the lesion (Figure 70-5).[17] Lesions usually are located on the scalp, buttocks, or extremities,[15,17] but can occur on any hair-bearing area.[15] Folliculitis can be asymptomatic or accompanied by pruritus; systemic symptoms usually are absent.[17] Gram stain and culture of purulent material from the follicular orifice can identify the causative organism of folliculitis. *S. aureus* is the predominant pathogen[15,17,36] and affected patients often are chronic carriers of *S. aureus* in the nares, perineum, or axillae;[36] however, gram-negative bacteria also can cause folliculitis (see below). The differential diagnosis of bacterial folliculitis includes inflammation of the hair follicle due to physical injury or chemical irritation, eosinophilic folliculitis, insect bites, scabies, pseudofolliculitis barbae, and infection due to *Malassezia* species. Simple bacterial folliculitis often resolves spontaneously without scarring.[17] When treatment is desired, topical antibiotic cleansers, such as chlorhexidine, topical antibacterial agents (mupirocin, erythromycin, clindamycin), or benzoyl peroxide usually are effective for mild infections.[17,36] Systemic antibiotic therapy with a first-generation cephalosporin, penicillinase-resistant penicillin, clindamycin, macrolide, or fluoroquinolone (depending on local resistance patterns) is used in severe or refractory cases.[17]

Less common forms of bacterial folliculitis include sycosis barbae, gram-negative folliculitis, and hot tub folliculitis. Sycosis barbae is a severe, recurrent form of facial folliculitis due to *S. aureus*. Painful erythematous, follicular papules and pustules involving the entire depth of the follicle develop on the chin, upper lip, and angle of the jaw, primarily in young black males. Papules can coalesce into plaques, and healing may occur with scarring. Treatment includes warm saline compresses and a topical antibiotic such as mupirocin. Extensive or recalcitrant cases may require therapy with a systemic antistaphylococcal antibiotic with attempted eradication of *S. aureus* carriage.[36]

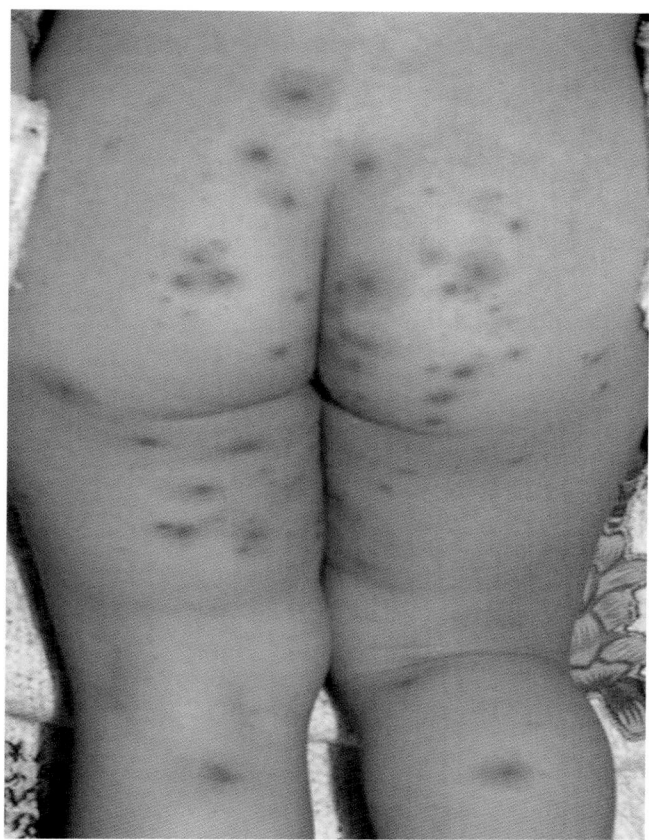

Figure 70-5. Erythematous follicular papules and pustules on the buttocks and posterior legs of a young child with folliculitis due to *Staphylococcus aureus*.

Gram-negative folliculitis primarily occurs in patients with treatment-resistant acne vulgaris who have received long-term therapy with broad-spectrum systemic antibiotics.[37,38] It is felt that prolonged use of antibiotics alters the balance of normal nasal flora, allowing colonization with gram-negative organisms;[37] however, gram-negative folliculitis may also be observed in patients without a history of prolonged antibiotic use.[38] In most patients, lesions consist of perioral and perinasal papules and pustules most often due to *Klebsiella* spp., *Enterobacter* spp., or *Escherichia coli*. A deeper form consisting of inflamed, painful nodules on the face and trunk caused by *Proteus* spp. occurs less commonly. Culture of infected follicles is necessary to establish the diagnosis. Treatment consists of an oral antibiotic, whose selection is based on susceptibility test results.[37] Isotretinoin is an effective treatment option for severe, recalcitrant cases; however, because of the potential for severe side effects, use should be limited to experienced providers.[17]

Hot-tub folliculitis is caused by *Pseudomonas aeruginosa*. This infection is seen in patients who bathe in contaminated water or use objects contaminated with *P. aeruginosa,* and occurs when the bacterium gains entry into the skin via hair follicles or breaks in the skin.[39] Outbreaks of *Pseudomonas* folliculitis have been associated with exposure to under-chlorinated swimming pools, whirlpools, hot tubs, and saunas.[39,40] Follicular erythematous macules, papules, and pustules develop in areas of skin exposed to water and abrasive garments (bathing suits, diving suits); onset generally is 6 to 48 hours after exposure. Fever, malaise, and lymphadenopathy develop occasionally. The eruption usually resolves spontaneously within 1 to 2 weeks,[39,41] often leaving postinflammatory hyperpigmentation.[41] Diagnosis is based on history and isolating the organism from culture of purulent lesions. Sometimes, topical agents with antipseudomonal activity, such as gentamicin cream, can be used

to treat the infection. Consideration should be given to the use of a systemic antibiotic, such as ciprofloxacin, in patients with constitutional symptoms. *Pseudomonas* hand–foot syndrome, which manifests as painful, red nodules on the palms and/or soles, may be seen in conjunction with hot-tub folliculitis or as an isolated infection; the disease course and treatment are similar to *Pseudomonas* folliculitis.[39] *Aeromonas hydrophila* folliculitis is an eruption that mimics *Pseudomonas* folliculitis and has been reported in children exposed to contaminated water while swimming.[42]

Malassezia (*Pityrosporum*) folliculitis is a follicular infection caused by the fungus *Malassezia furfur* and is included in the differential diagnosis of infectious folliculitis and truncal acne vulgaris. *Malassezia* folliculitis manifests as pruritic, 2 to 3 mm, monomorphic, erythematous, perifollicular papules and papulopustules on the back, chest, and upper arms.[43–45] Predisposing factors include diabetes mellitus, malignancy, HIV/AIDS, organ transplantation, or other causes of immunosuppression and prolonged oral antibiotic therapy.[43,44,46] *Malassezia* also has been implicated in the form of eosinophilic folliculitis associated with advanced HIV infection.[43,46] Diagnosis is made by microscopic examination of a potassium hydroxide-treated scraping from a lesion, which reveals budding yeast and spores.[43–45] Skin biopsies of *Malassezia* folliculitis show dilated follicular ostia with budding yeast and spores and a mixed inflammatory infiltrate; however, a biopsy rarely is necessary for diagnosis.[43,44,46] Isolation of the organism in culture requires use of a special lipid-containing medium.[44,45] Mild cases can be treated with topical imidazoles or selenium sulfide. Systemic antifungal agents (ketoconazole, fluconazole, or itraconazole) are indicated for immunosuppressed patients or those with extensive lesions.[43,46] Since recurrence of *Malassezia* folliculitis is common, maintenance regimens of either oral or topical antifungal agents often are prescribed following effective treatment.[44,45]

Furuncles and Carbuncles

A furuncle (or "boil") is an infection of the hair follicle; however, unlike folliculitis in which the infection remains in the epidermis, the inflammation in furuncles extends deep into the dermis.[12,36] Furuncles can originate from a preceding folliculitis and manifest as tender, deep-seated, erythematous, perifollicular nodules with an overlying pustule (Figure 70-6). With time, the inflammatory mass becomes fluctuant and often opens to the skin surface, draining purulent material.[17] Lesions are found on hair-bearing areas, with the face, neck, axillae, buttocks, and groin being common sites of involvement. A carbuncle is a painful infection involving an aggregate of contiguous follicles, with multiple drainage points, and inflammatory changes in the surrounding connective tissue. Carbuncles commonly are found on the posterior neck and in persons with diabetes mellitus.[12] While individuals with furuncles usually have no constitutional symptoms, fever, leukocytosis, and bacteremia can accompany carbuncles. Both lesions tend to heal with scarring.

The causative agent of furuncles and carbuncles is almost always *S. aureus*. The staphylococcal isolates (both MSSA and MRSA) associated with furunculosis often possess the virulence factor Panton–Valentine leukocidin, a pore-forming toxin that targets neutrophils.[13,36,47] Conditions that predispose to furuncle formation include obesity, immunosuppression, diabetes mellitus, hyperhidrosis, maceration, friction, and pre-existing dermatitis.[36] Outbreaks of furunculosis have been reported in sports teams, families, and other populations with close contact.[12,48] Recurrent furunculosis frequently is associated with carriage of *S. aureus* at multiple sites (nares, axillae, perineum) or with sustained close contact with someone who is a carrier. Rarely, children with recurrent furunculosis may have an underlying immunodeficiency.[12] Other bacteria or fungi occasionally cause furuncles or carbuncles; therefore Gram stain and culture of the purulent exudate are indicated. The differential diagnosis of furuncles includes epidermal cysts, cystic acne, and hidradenitis suppurativa.

Treatment consists of frequent application of a hot, moist compress to lesions to promote drainage. Large furuncles and most

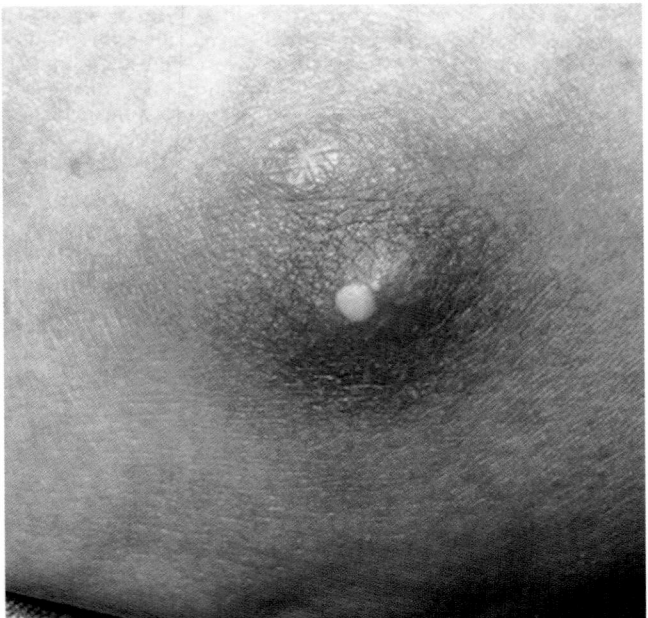

Figure 70-6. Furuncle due to *Staphylococcus aureus*. (Courtesy of J.H. Brien©.)

carbuncles require surgical drainage, with disruption of any existing loculations and wound packing as appropriate.[12,13,36] When lesions are large, multiple, there is extensive surrounding cellulitis, or fever is present, treatment with an oral antistaphylococcal agent is indicated. For recurrent furunculosis, attempts to eradicate staphylococcal carriage can be undertaken. Attention to personal hygiene, bleach baths, or use of chlorhexidine soap may be beneficial.

HAND AND NAIL INFECTIONS

Paronychia

Acute paronychia is an infection of the soft-tissue folds surrounding a fingernail or toenail. The infection occurs when minor trauma allows bacteria to enter the cuticle or nail fold. Paronychia is seen most commonly in children who suck their fingers, bite their nails or cuticles, or have poor hygiene; and also is associated with dishwashing, manicures, and use of artificial nails. The lateral nail fold becomes warm, erythematous, edematous, and painful; purulent fluid can accumulate underneath the nail plate. Usually only one nail is affected. In most cases, the infection is caused by *S. aureus* or mixed aerobic and anaerobic flora.[49,50] The most common aerobic organisms are *S. aureus*, *S. pyogenes*, and *Eikenella corrodens*; anaerobic pathogens include *Bacteroides* spp., *Fusobacterium* spp., and gram-positive cocci.[51] Diagnosis of acute paronychia is based on clinical examination. Both aerobic and anaerobic cultures of purulent material are recommended to identify the causative pathogen(s) and perform susceptibility testing of *S. aureus*. Warm compresses generally are curative for superficial lesions. Antibiotic therapy with an oral antistaphylococcal agent, in addition to incision and drainage, is needed for treatment of deeper lesions with abscesses. When exposure to oral flora is suspected (nail biting), a broad-spectrum oral antibiotic effective against anaerobes (clindamycin or amoxicillin-clavulanate) is indicated.[49]

The differential diagnosis of acute paronychia includes chronic paronychia, psoriasis, and herpetic whitlow. Chronic paronychia can be distinguished from acute infection by the duration of symptoms. Chronic paronychia often is associated with *C.*

albicans, and usually is seen in people whose hands are frequently exposed to water (finger sucking, dishwashers, house cleaners, bartenders, food handlers, nurses).[49,50] Like bacterial paronychia, herpes simplex virus infection of the fingers can occur after sucking or parental nail-trimming by biting. Herpetic whitlow can resemble staphylococcal infection. Multiple coalescing vesicles of the digit associated with edema and a dusky appearance are typical of whitlow. Direct fluorescent antibody testing and viral culture can confirm the diagnosis. Herpetic lesions should not be incised or debrided; instead, oral antiviral therapy should be given.[49,52]

Blistering Distal Dactylitis

Blistering distal dactylitis is an acral infection caused by *S. pyogenes*, and less commonly *S. aureus* or CoNS.[53,54] It usually is seen in children aged 2 to 16 years, but has been reported in infants and adults. This infection manifests as a tense nontender bulla with an erythematous base involving the distal volar fat pad of the phalanges.[53–56] Dark discoloration of the surrounding skin may be associated.[53] One or more digits can be affected, as can the nail fold, the volar surfaces of the proximal phalanges, the toes, and the palm.[54–56] Systemic symptoms generally are absent.[53–56] The blisters are filled with a thin purulent fluid containing neutrophils and the infecting organisms.[53,54] Infections caused by *S. aureus* may be more likely to be associated with pain and involvement of more than one digit.[55] The diagnosis is based on examination and culture. Treatment consists of incision and drainage or a 10-day course of systemic therapy or both using an agent with staphylococcal and streptococcal coverage.[53,55,56]

ULCERATIVE INFECTIONS

Anthrax

Bacillus anthracis causes inhalational, gastrointestinal, meningeal, and cutaneous infections. Cutaneous anthrax in the U.S. is limited mainly to individuals who work with contaminated animals or animal products, including carcasses, hair, and wool; however, cases due to acts of bioterrorism have been reported. Cutaneous infection occurs 1 to 7 days after exposure/inoculation of an endospore into the skin, usually at the site of a cut or abrasion.[57] The primary lesion is a small, painless, pruritic papule that transforms over a few days into a 1- to 2-cm bulla, which can be associated with satellite vesicles. Characteristic brawny, nonpitting edema surrounds the lesion. The bulla ruptures, forming an ulcer with a central black eschar.[57,58] (Figure 70-7) Malaise, low-grade fever, and regional lymphadenopathy frequently are noted.[57] Differential diagnosis includes ecthyma, ecthyma gangrenosum, a furuncle, and necrotic arachnidism. Diagnosis is based on Gram-stained smear and culture of vesicular fluid, eschar, or tissue.[57,59] Incision and drainage of the lesion can precipitate bacteremia; however, skin biopsy of a lesion while administering antibiotic therapy likely confers minimal risk.[57,60] Treatment of mild naturally occurring cutaneous anthrax consists of penicillin for 7 to 10 days. Cutaneous anthrax associated with bioterrorism in children is treated with ciprofloxacin or doxycycline for 60 days due to the risk of inhalational exposure to the spores; therapy can be modified based on results of antimicrobial susceptibility test results.[57,59]

Diphtheria

Cutaneous infection with *Corynebacterium diphtheriae* is rare in developed countries, and is seen mainly in travelers to endemic tropical areas,[35,61–63] the immunosuppressed, and those living in crowded, unsanitary conditions.[35,61] Infection can occur despite adequate immunization for the organism.[35,62] Cutaneous diphtheria occurs in three forms: primary infection, which consists of a tender pustule that evolves into a punched-out ulcer with an adherent membrane and erythematous, edematous rim;

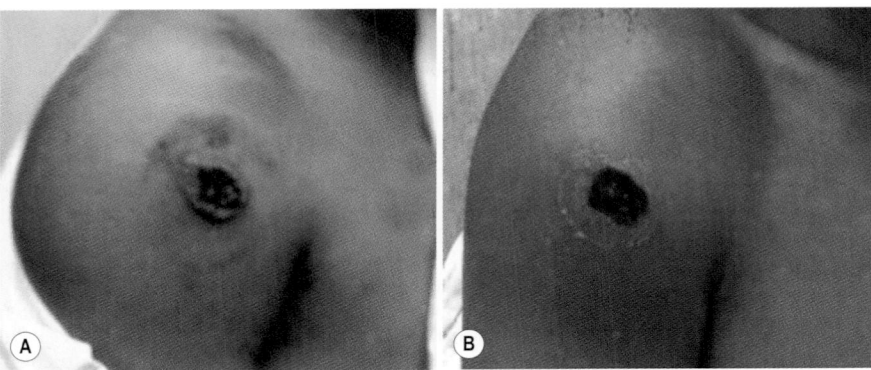

Figure 70-7. Cutaneous anthrax. Note ulcer with vesicular ring, induration and erythema **(A)**. As eschar forms, induration lessens; surrounding desquamation occurs, but erythema persists **(B)**. (Source: http://www.bt.cdc.gov/agent/anthrax/anthrax-images.)

secondary infection of a pre-existing ulcer or wound; and super-infection of eczematous skin lesions.[61,63] Lesional skin sheds bacteria for 2 to 6 weeks without treatment, and thus is an important reservoir for person-to-person transmission and environmental contamination of pathogenic organisms, which can cause both cutaneous and respiratory disease.[35,62,63] Systemic complications, including neurologic symptoms and myocarditis, are rare in immunized patients[62,63] and more often are associated with the respiratory tract than cutaneous diphtheria.[35]

Culture of a lesion or its overlying membrane confirms the diagnosis, and laboratory personnel must be notified when *C. diphtheriae* is suspected. Treatment consists of cleansing the affected skin and systemic antibiotic therapy with penicillin or erythromycin for 10 days.[35,63] The use of antitoxin in addition to systemic antibiotics is controversial,[35,61] since cutaneous lesions are either nontoxigenic or produce small amounts of toxin.[63] To document eradication of the organism, two negative cultures should be obtained after treatment concludes.[35]

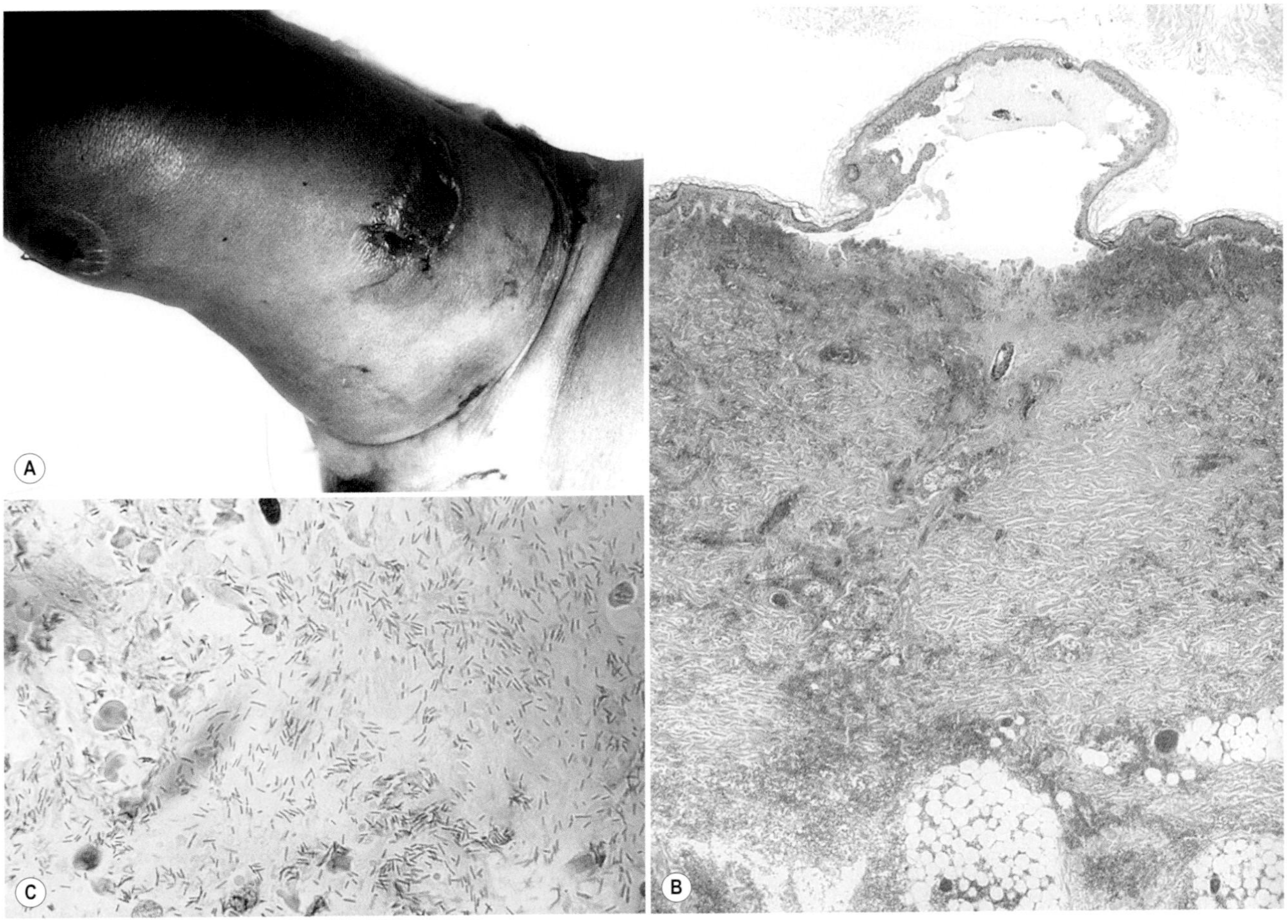

Figure 70-8. *Pseudomonas aeruginosa* septicemia and ecthyma gangrenosum in a young male with severe neutropenia **(A)**. Microscopic appearance of ecthyma gangrenosum in fatal *P. aeruginosa* septicemia in an infant with leukemia **(B)**. Haematoxylin–eosin stain shows superficial necrosis and elevation as well as bland ischemic necrosis beneath. Gram stain of fluid from bullous lesion **(B)** shows dense gram-negative bacilli with rare inflammatory cells **(C)**. (Courtesy of J.H. Brien©.)

PART II Clinical Syndromes and Cardinal Features of Infectious Diseases: Approach to Diagnosis and Initial Management

SECTION J Skin and Soft-Tissue Infections

Ecthyma

Ecthyma is a deep ulcerative infection of the skin that penetrates down to the dermis and is most commonly caused by *S. pyogenes*. Initially a vesicle or vesicopustule with surrounding erythema is noted; over time the lesion evolves into a crusted ulcer with an elevated rim. Lesions usually are located on the legs, and frequently are seen in association with pruritic conditions such as insect bites or scabies. Lymphangitis, cellulitis, and poststreptococcal glomerulonephritis are potential complications of ecthyma. Systemic antibiotic therapy with an agent effective against streptococci is recommended.[11]

Ecthyma Gangrenosum

Ecthyma gangrenosum is the characteristic skin lesion found in association with *Pseudomonas aeruginosa*. *Pseudomonas* septicemia usually is seen in the setting of neutropenia or congenital neutrophil dysfunction, but also has been described in healthy patients; often less than one year of age.[64,65] Cutaneous findings are the result of a necrotizing bacterial vasculitis affecting small veins in the skin. Lesions begin as erythematous, indurated papules, vesicles, and nodules that progress, over hours to days, into a necrotic ulcer with a black eschar and an erythematous rim (Figure 70-9). Lesions are commonly observed on the gluteal and perineal areas, but may be found all over the body.[64,66] Ecthyma gangrenosum also can manifest in a localized form, usually on the buttocks and legs, after inoculation of the organism into the skin. This localized form of ecthyma gangrenosum usually is not associated with bacteremia[11,66,67] and can occur in healthy children or those with occult immunodeficiency.[67] Culture of the lesions, and blood cultures, confirm the diagnosis. Effective treatment requires prompt initiation of an antibiotic effective against *P. aeruginosa*. Ecthyma gangrenosum-like lesions can develop as a result of infection with other agents, usually in the setting of immunosuppression. Etiologic agents include gram-negative bacteria other than *P. aeruginosa*,[12,66] MSSA, MRSA[66] *Streptococcus* species,[67] *Candida* species, fungi (*Aspergillus, Mucor*, and *Fusarium* species),[12] and herpes viruses.[66]

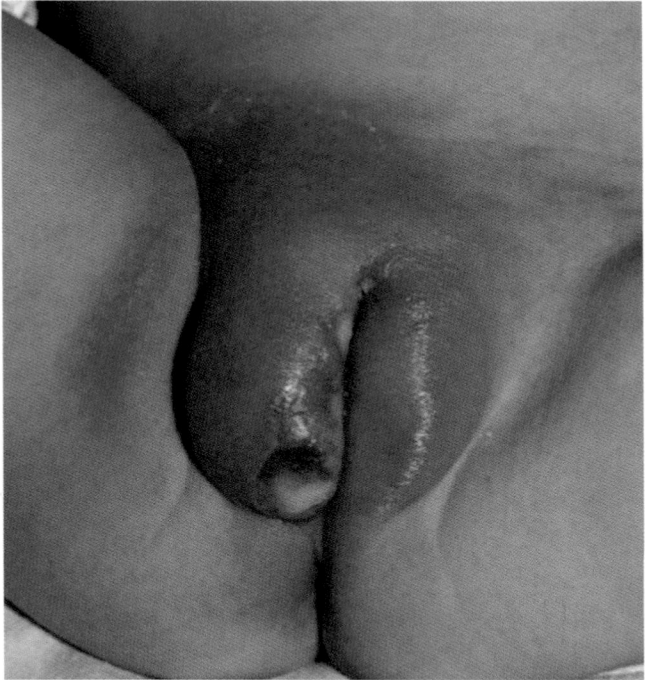

Figure 70-9. Ecthyma gangrenosum due to *Pseudomonas aeruginosa*: necrotic ulcers with surrounding erythema and edema forming on the labium majus of a young girl with neutropenia and leukemia.

SOFT-TISSUE INFECTIONS

Erysipelas

Erysipelas is a superficial skin infection affecting the upper dermis and the lymphatic system. In most cases, GAS is the cause of erysipelas;[12,13,17,68] however, group B, C, and G streptococcus occasionally can cause the infection,[12,68] and rarely, *S. aureus, Streptococcus pneumoniae, Klebsiella pneumoniae, Yersinia enterocolitica,* and *Haemophilus influenzae* are implicated as pathogens.[68] Erysipelas has a bimodal distribution, being seen most often in young children and older adults.[12,68] Infection occurs when disruption of the skin barrier allows entry of organisms into the skin, and often is associated with abrasions, leg ulcers, intertriginous or pedal fungal infections, insect bites, venous or lymphatic obstruction, and chronic edema.[12,13,68,69] In neonates, infection can originate at the umbilical stump and spread to the abdominal wall.[68]

The onset of erysipelas is abrupt and is characterized by a painful, bright red, shiny, edematous plaque with well-demarcated and slightly raised borders. In severe cases, bullae and necrosis can occur. Infection usually occurs on a lower extremity (most often), or the face, and can be associated with regional lymphadenitis.[12,13,17,68] Fever, chills, and malaise can precede the onset of cutaneous findings. Potential systemic complications of erysipelas include septicemia, streptococcal toxic shock syndrome, endocarditis, and meningitis; however, complications are rare with prompt diagnosis and appropriate treatment. The differential diagnosis includes contact dermatitis, burns, cellulitis, ecthyma gangrenosum, and urticaria.[68] Diagnosis of erysipelas is made primarily on clinical grounds.[13,68] Blood cultures, skin biopsies, and needle aspirations are of low yield.[12]

Treatment for erysipelas in immunocompetent patients consists of oral penicillin for 10 to 14 days, with follow-up after 48 to 72 hours to ensure the infection is improving. Patients with severe infections, young infants, and the immunosuppressed initially may require hospitalization for parenteral therapy.[68] For penicillin allergic patients, macrolide therapy usually is effective;[12,68] and if the presence of staphylococci is a concern, an antistaphylococcal antibiotic should be used.[12] Local wound care and attention to predisposing factors (treating tinea pedis, elevating edematous legs) also are important aspects of treatment. Prophylactic therapy is considered infrequently for patients with recurrent disease.[12,68]

Cellulitis

Cellulitis is an acute infection of the skin involving the dermis and subcutaneous tissues. Cellulitis is manifested by edema, warmth, erythema, and tenderness of the skin. The lateral margins of cellulitis tend to be indistinct, unlike the well-demarcated borders of erysipelas (Figure 70-10). Vesicles, bullae, and petechiae can occur on involved skin. The lower legs are affected most commonly, but infection can occur at any site. Associated findings include lymphangitis, regional lymphadenopathy, fever, chills, and malaise. When cellulitis occurs in a periorbital distribution, and especially in the absence of a break in the skin, orbital cellulitis should be considered. Predisposing factors for cellulitis include pre-existing skin infections (ecthyma, impetigo), breaks in the skin due to trauma or insect bites, lymphatic obstruction or other causes of edema, leg ulcers, and obesity.[12,13]

The most common etiologic agents of cellulitis are *S. pyogenes* and *S. aureus*.[12,36] When facial cellulitis in children is associated with a portal of entry such as a tooth abscess or cutaneous trauma, the etiology may also be due to oral anaerobic bacteria.[70] *H. influenzae* capsular type b (Hib) was an important cause of periorbital[13] and facial cellulitis in children aged 3 months to 3 years of age prior to the introduction of the Hib conjugate vaccine. This form of cellulitis has a characteristic bluish discoloration resembling a bruise and often is associated with bacteremia.[71] Bacteremic *S. pneumoniae* also can cause facial cellulitis in children resembling that due to *H. influenzae*.[72] In patients who are immunocompromised or have been exposed to animals or special conditions, a

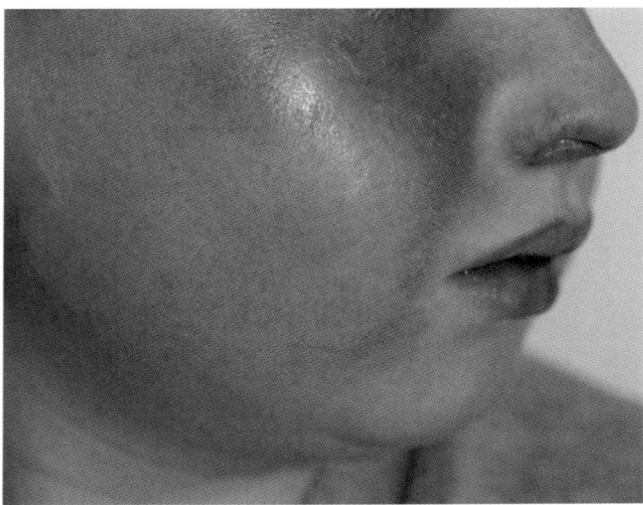

Figure 70-10. Ill-defined erythema and edema on the cheek of a boy with cellulitis. (Courtesy of Brandon Newell, MD.)

TABLE 70-3. Special Causes of Cellulitis

Exposure	Etiology
Cat/Dog bites	*Pasteurella* species, *Capnocytophaga canimorsus*
Penetrating trauma	*Staphylococcus aureus*
Freshwater immersion	*Aeromonas hydrophila*
Saltwater immersion	*Vibrio* species
Freshwater, saltwater fish	*Streptococcus iniae*
Swine, poultry, fish	*Erysipelothrix rhusiopathiae*
Periorbital/Facial cellulitis	*Haemophilus influenzae, Streptococcus pneumoniae*
Neutropenia	*Pseudomonas aeruginosa,* other gram-negative bacilli
HIV infection	*Helicobacter cinaedi*
Acute varicella	*Streptococcus pyogenes*
Immunosuppression	*Cryptococcus neoformans*

number of other bacterial or fungal agents have been implicated in causing cellulitis (Table 70-3).

Diagnosis of cellulitis is based on physical examination and a detailed history to determine if there are any factors predisposing to cellulitis caused by one of the less common pathogens. Attempts to determine the specific etiology of the infection may be of low yield. Blood culture should be performed in the setting of young age or systemic illness; otherwise yield is low.[73] Culture of an aspirate from the site of inflammation yields a pathogen in 10% of patients,[74] with an aspirate taken from the point of maximum inflammation yielding the causal organism more often than does a leading-edge aspirate.[75] Tissue culture is positive in 18% to 20% of patients and the density of organisms present is low,[74,76] although a higher density of organisms has been noted in specimens taken from a site near an ulcer.[76] Culture of a primary lesion (ulcer, abrasion) corresponds to that of a tissue culture;[74] therefore culture of a primary lesion can avoid a more invasive procedure. Due to their low yield, aspirates and tissue cultures usually are reserved for cases of severe or atypical cellulitis or when patients are immunocompromised or are not responding to empiric therapy.

Uncomplicated cellulitis in immunocompetent patients should resolve with antimicrobial therapy targeting streptococci and staphylococci. If fever and lymphadenopathy are absent, outpatient treatment using a penicillinase-resistant penicillin, first-generation cephalosporin, or macrolide is appropriate.[12,13] The need for an agent providing coverage for CA-MRSA should be guided by local prevalence and antibiotic susceptibilities. Parenteral therapy is instituted if fever, rapid progression, lymphangitis, or lymphadenitis is present. When erythema, warmth, edema, and fever have decreased substantially in uncomplicated cases, a 10-day course

of treatment can be completed with oral therapy. Adjunctive therapies include elevation of the affected extremity, analgesics for pain, and tetanus immunization when appropriate.[17]

Erysipeloid

Erysipeloid is a rare acute cutaneous infection resulting from traumatic inoculation of *Erysipelothrix rhusiopathiae* into the skin. Infection usually occurs in patients with occupational exposure to raw fish, poultry, and meat products [77,78] or to contaminated animals, especially swine.[77] Localized cutaneous infection manifests as a well-demarcated erythematous-to-purple inflammatory plaque with raised borders on the dorsal aspect of one hand and/ or fingers; and typically occurs 2 to 7 days after inoculation. The lesion spreads peripherally and can display central clearing.[77,78] Vesicles, bullae, and edema of the fingers sometimes are seen; and lesions can be asymptomatic or associated with pain, pruritus, or fever.[77] Untreated limited cutaneous infection can resolve spontaneously after 2 to 3 weeks, but can recur weeks to months later.[78] Rarely a diffuse cutaneous form of infection occurs, manifesting as lesions over several areas of the body,[77,78] and may be associated with fever, lymphadenopathy, myalgia, and arthralgia. Rare systemic complications of erysipeloid include encephalitis, meningitis, endocarditis, pyogenic arthritis, and sepsis.[77] *E. rhusiopathiae* is difficult to isolate, although tissue culture of the advancing edge of the lesion might identify the organism.[78] Diagnosis is based mainly on the patient's occupation or exposure history, clinical findings, and rapid improvement with antibiotic therapy. The recommended treatment for localized cutaneous infection is penicillin or a cephalosporin for 7 days, with improvement generally seen after 2 to 3 days.[77]

---

71 # Erythematous Macules and Papules

Sara Jane Heilig and Andrea L. Zaenglein

Many of the classic exanthems, such as measles, rubella, and erythema infectiosum, are associated with macules or papules on the skin. Differentiating common and uncommon causes of infectious rashes often is difficult as the patterns are not always unique

to a specific infectious agent. Detailed and accurate history taking is vital to making a correct diagnosis. The patient's age and preexisting conditions are important as many infectious rashes occur predominantly within a specific age range or in the context of

PART II   Clinical Syndromes and Cardinal Features of Infectious Diseases: Approach to Diagnosis and Initial Management

SECTION J   Skin and Soft-Tissue Infections

BOX 71-1. Questions That Can Elucidate Possible Etiologies of Exanthems

- What time of year did the rash start?
- Where on the body did the rash start and how has it evolved?
- Is the eruption localized or generalized?
- Does the rash come and go? Over what timeframe? Is the rash worse at a specific time of day? Is the rash made worse by the sun?
- Is there an associated enanthem?
- Is the rash pruritic? Painful? Or asymptomatic?
- What other symptoms are present? Joint swelling? Fever? Adenopathy? Vomiting? Cough? Headache? Photophobia?
- Is there a recent history of use of any medications, including over-the-counter medications?
- Has there been recent illness?
- Has there been recent exposure to another person with a similar illness? Is the child in group childcare or school?
- Are immunizations up-to-date?
- Is there an immunocompromising condition/drug?
- Where was the child born? Has there been recent travel?
- Has there been recent exposure to pets, wildlife, or biting insects?
- What evaluation has been done already? Laboratory studies? Cultures?
- Has treatment been given? Was the treatment effective?

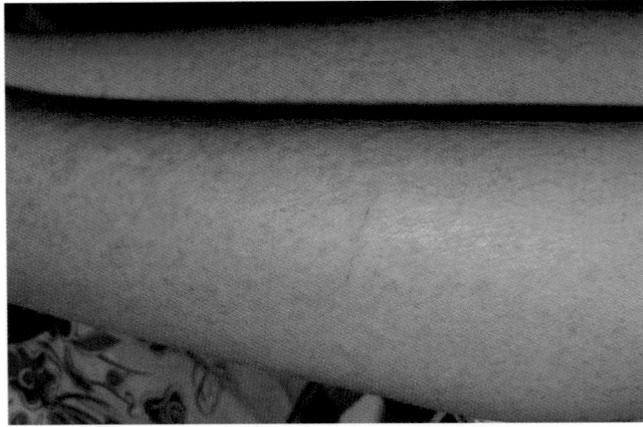

Figure 71-2. Discrete and confluent erythematous pink, blanchable papules associated with enterovirus infection.

another illness. When investigating the cause of a rash, and whether an infectious agent is responsible, it is important to question the patient and the parents thoroughly (Box 71-1).

Oftentimes, a careful and complete physical examination can establish a diagnosis. The child's sense of wellbeing or degree of illness is assessed. Mucous membranes are examined to note an associated enanthem, eye or genital involvement. Distribution of the rash, and areas of accentuation or sparing, are noted. Recognizing primary skin lesions and using the correct terminology for their description is essential in differentiating cutaneous presentations of infectious disease. *Macules* are lesions in the same plane as the skin; there is a change in color but the lesion is not palpable (Figure 71-1). *Papules* are discrete, raised lesions that are less than 1 cm in size (Figure 71-2). If a raised lesion is larger than 1 cm and flat-topped, the term *plaque* is used. At times, papules can coalesce into plaques. *Purpura* (see Chapter 73), caused by

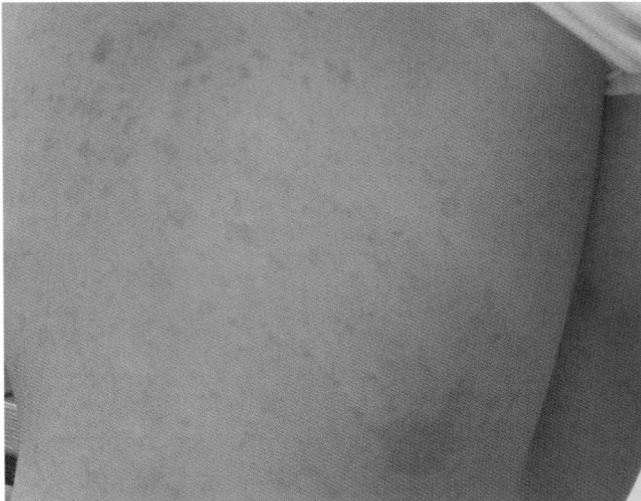

Figure 71-1. Nonspecific viral exanthem; generalized, pink erythematous macules on the trunk of a 7-year-old with a mild upper respiratory infection.

extravasated red blood cells, often is macular but does not blanch with pressure. Early purpuric, vesicular, or ulcerative eruptions can begin as macular erythema then progress to their characteristic morphology.

The commonly used, and often overused, term *maculopapular* describes a rash that has both macular and papular components at some time during the course of the disease. *Morbilliform* (measles-like) is used to describe uniform lesions that have coalesced. *Scarlatiniform* is used when the exanthem resembles scarlet fever, i.e., has a sandpaper feel and is confluent in the flexural areas. If lesions are generalized but remain discrete, the term *rubelliform* may be used. Secondary characteristics should be added to help to further describe the exanthem; *annular, lacy, reticulated, evanescent, urticarial, petechial,* and *purpuric* are useful descriptors. Color is described in shades and erythema can range from faint pink to violaceous red.

Macular and papular exanthems can result from numerous infectious causes. An extensive list of viral and nonviral causes is shown in Table 71-1. In children, enteroviruses are by far the most common cause of morbilliform rash with febrile illness, especially under the age of one.[1] Enteroviruses have a marked seasonality, with an increase in prevalence in the summer and a large peak in August and fall. Parvovirus B19, the etiologic agent of erythema infectiosum, is the macular and papular rash most commonly identified in children aged 4 through 10 years of age.[2] The exanthem is typified by bright red macules on the cheeks that spare the nasolabial folds (Figure 71-3), followed by the development of reticulated lacy pink macules and thin papules on the extremities that can persist for up to 3 weeks. Fever and joint pain can occur concomitantly, especially in adults. This is an important eruption to recognize, as pregnant women exposed to parvovirus B19 during the 20 to 28th week of gestation risk transplacental infection and possible hydrops fetalis.

Macular and papular rashes in children also can be indirectly related to an infectious agent. It is estimated that between 1.2% and 12% of children develop cutaneous adverse reactions to medications, especially antibiotics.[3] Many drug eruptions can be confused with viral exanthems as they have similar morphology and course. In the case of Epstein–Barr mononucleosis virus, the administration of an antibiotic (classically ampicillin) can lead to a florid maculopapular rash. Common noninfectious causes of macular and papular exanthems are listed in Table 71-2. These disorders should be considered in the differential diagnosis.

The vast majority of exanthems related to infections in childhood are mild and self-limited; however, there are a few exceptions. For example, Rocky Mountain spotted fever can be associated with encephalitis and many enteroviral infections can be associated with myopericarditis. It is important that the clinician uses cutaneous clues as well as the patient history to differentiate the many infectious causes of macular and papular rashes.

TABLE 71-1. Infectious and Common Noninfectious Conditions That Can Cause Macular and Papular Exanthems

Viruses					Likely Viral Cause
Human herpesvirus	**Poxvirus**	**Picornavirus**	**Paramyxovirus**	**Arbovirus**	Gianotti–Crosti syndrome
Erythema multiforme	Smallpox	(coxsackievirus and echovirus)	Measles	West Nile fever	Unilateral laterothoracic exanthem
Varicella	Vaccina	Nonspecific exanthems	Rubella	Dengue	Viral-associated trichodysplasia
Shingles	Orf	Hand foot and mouth disease	**Parvovirus**	Alphavirus	
Mononucleosis	Milker's nodules	Boston exanthem	Erythema infectiosum	**Papovavirus**	
Pityriasis rosea	Cowpox	Eruptive pseudoangiomatosis	Papular purpuric gloves and socks syndrome	Warts	
Roseola infantum	Molluscum contagiosum			**Retroviruses**	
				Human T-lymphotropic virus 1	

Bacteria	Rickettsia	Protozoa	Helminths	Fungi
Impetigo	Epidemic typhus	Amebiasis cutis	**Trematodes**	**Dermatophytes**
Folliculitis	Endemic typhus	Leishmaniasis	Freshwater swimmers' itch	Tinea capitis
Paronychia	Rocky	Trypanosomiasis	Saltwater marine dermatitis	Tinea corporis
Staphylococcal scalded skin syndrome	Mountain spotted fever	Toxoplasmosis		Tinea faciei
Toxic shock syndromes	Mediterranean spotted fever		**Nematodes**	Tinea cruris
Scarlet fever	African tick bite fever		Pinworms (can cause generalized papules)	Majocci granuloma
Erysipelas	Yucatan spotted fever		Hookworms	**Early cutaneous, or deep fungal infections**
Cellulitis	Japanese spotted fever		Larva migrans	Blastomycosis
Perineal dermatitis	North Asian tick-bite fever		Onchocerciasis	Histoplasmosis
Rheumatic fever	Queensland tick typhus			Coccidioidomycosis
Erythrasma	Scrub typhus			Phaeohyphomycosis
Actinomycosis	Rickettsialpox			Chromomycosis
Echthyma	Q fever			Sporotrichosis
Hot tub folliculitis				Fusariosis
Meningococcemia				Aspergiillosis
Gonococcemia				*Alternaria* infection
Salmonellosis				
Glanders				**Yeast**
Cat-scratch disease				Candidiasis
Bacillary angiomatosis				Tinea versicolor
Rat-bite fever				
Tularemia				
Brucellosis				
Ehrlichiosis				
Anaplasmosis				
Leptospirosis				
Lyme disease				
Secondary syphilis				
Yaws				
Pinta				

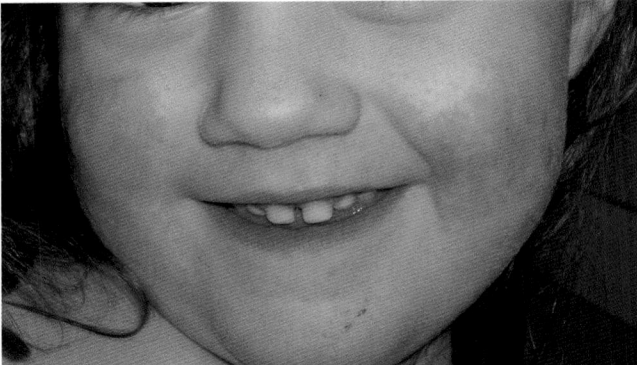

Figure 71-3. Bilateral, bright red macular erythema of the cheeks typical of parvovirus infection.

TABLE 71-2. Common Noninfectious Causes of Macular and Papular Exanthems

Predominantly Papules	Predominantly Macules	Both Macules and Papules
Insect bites	Sunburn	Adverse drug eruption
Acne	Dermatomyositis	Atopic dermatitis
Keratosis pilaris	Systemic lupus erythematosus	Contact dermatitis
Miliaria		Polymorphous light eruption
Granuloma annulare		
Cnidarian stings		

PART II Clinical Syndromes and Cardinal Features of Infectious Diseases: Approach to Diagnosis and Initial Management

SECTION J Skin and Soft-Tissue Infections

72 Vesicles and Bullae

James Treat

Vesicles and *bullae* (blisters) result from a disturbance of epidermal or basement membrane connections creating spaces which allow fluid collection. Blisters can be caused directly by bacterial, viral, and fungal infections or be a reactive phenomenon to an infection. Diagnosis of vesiculobullous eruptions must be made promptly because, although some conditions are benign, others are rapidly progressive and life-threatening.

The skin consists of epidermis, composed primarily of keratinocytes, and an underlying dermis of connective tissue (Figure 72-1). The stratum corneum is held together tightly relative to the keratinocytes of the spinous layer. The basement membrane zone anchors the epidermis to the dermis. Cohesion between layers of the skin is weakest at the stratum corneum–spinous cell transition zone and particularly within the least electron-dense region of the basement membrane zone, called the lamina lucida. A plane of cleavage, or blister, therefore is most apt to develop at these levels (Figure 72-1). Application of a lateral, sliding force to nonblistered skin (usually at a site adjacent to a bullous lesion) that produces a plane of cleavage is the *Nikolsky sign*. This maneuver can be useful in the clinical recognition of a blistering disorder but cannot be used to judge the depth of the blister within the skin.

Vesicles and bullae are circumscribed, elevated lesions filled with clear fluid. Depending on the mechanisms responsible for their formation, blisters can contain a combination of edematous or lymphatic fluid, serum proteins, antigen–antibody complexes, and soluble inflammatory mediators. Cellular elements also often are present, including inflammatory cells, erythrocytes, detached epidermal cells, and infectious agents. Vesicles measure <1 cm in diameter and bullae measure ≥1 cm. Vesicles and bullae associated with infection can be any of the following: (1) solitary, such as the lesion of streptococcal blistering dactylitis; (2) localized, as in staphylococcal bullous impetigo; (3) grouped or clustered, as in herpes simplex virus (HSV) infection; (4) arranged in a dermatome, as in zoster; or (5) generalized, as in chickenpox.

A vesicle or bulla that is located in the epidermis tends to be *flaccid* and to rupture easily. When located subepidermally, more often they are *tense*, have greater structural integrity, and rupture less easily. As a vesicle or bulla matures, an influx of leukocytes and accumulation of cellular debris can occur, leading to

development of a *pustule*. Depending on the cause of the inflammatory response, a pustule can be infected or sterile. Rupture and detachment of the roof of a subcorneal or intraepidermal blister can form a moist, slightly depressed erosion. Erosions do not extend below the epidermal–dermal junction and heals without scarring. Postinflammatory pigmentary changes, however, can be present for weeks to months. When an unroofed blister extends into the dermis or subcutaneous tissue, it forms an *ulcer*. Scarring or postinflammatory pigmentary changes can follow healing of a wound that involves the dermis. Erosion or ulceration is accelerated in areas of friction or maceration, such as in the axillae or perineum, and on the mucous membranes of the oropharynx and vagina. *Crusts*, or *scabs*, are the dried remnants of serum, blood, and cellular debris; they form quickly over denuded areas.

It is not unusual for several types of lesions to be present at the same time in an individual. For example, the eruptions caused by varicella can comprise a variety of lesions in various stages of evolution, including macules, papules, vesicles, and pustules, mixed with erosions, ulcers, crusts, and self-induced linear excoriations. Bullae can form if staphylococcal superinfection occurs (Figure 72-2).

ETIOLOGY AND CLINICAL MANIFESTATIONS

Although the list of infectious agents capable of causing vesiculobullous rashes is lengthy, the most common agents are enteroviruses, varicella-zoster virus (VZV), HSV, *Staphylococcus aureus*,

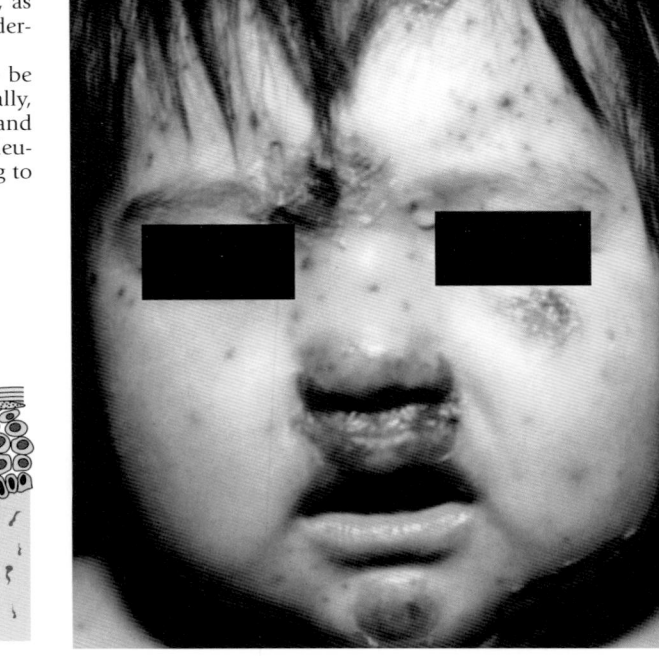

Figure 72-2. Chickenpox lesions, infected secondarily with *Staphylococcus aureus*, forming crusted plaques and bullae on the face of an infant.

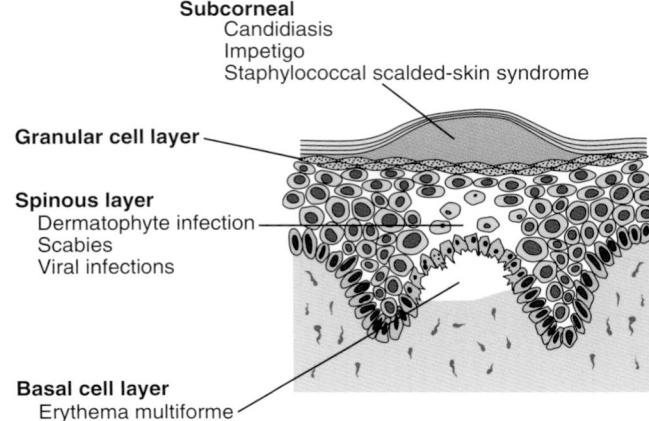

Subcorneal
Candidiasis
Impetigo
Staphylococcal scalded-skin syndrome

Granular cell layer

Spinous layer
Dermatophyte infection
Scabies
Viral infections

Basal cell layer
Erythema multiforme

Figure 72-1. Sites of vesiculobullous diseases in the skin.

TABLE 72-1. Clinical Features of Blistering Skin Disorders by Etiologic Agent

Infection or Reaction Pattern	Type of Blister	Size	Usual Locations	Other Clinical Signs/Symptoms
Herpes simplex virus	Tense	Vesicles	Most often mucosal or perimucosal	Clustered and painful
Zoster (varicella-zoster virus reactivation)	Tense	Vesicles	Any dermatome	Clustered in a dermatome or disseminated in immunocompromised
Hand-foot-and-mouth disease (enterovirus infection)	Tense	Vesicles	Palms, soles, oral mucosa, and buttocks	Vesicles tend to be oval and on the hands and feet following dermatoglyphics
Bullous impetigo	Flaccid	Vesicles or bullae	Perioral or perineal	Honey-colored crusting
Staphylococcal scalded skin syndrome	Flaccid, very superficial epidermis only	Large bullae	First manifests in intertriginous areas, then can be widespread	Age <5 years
Dactylitis	Tense	Bullae	Digits	Painful and red
Vibrio vulnificus infection	Tense	Bullae	Feet	Purple edematous (typically on extremity) with tense bullae
Necrotizing fasciitis	Tense	Bullae	Any site	Hyperesthetic or anesthetic purpuric skin
Bullous tinea	Tense	Vesicles or bullae	Feet	Annular or interdigital scaling
Stevens–Johnson syndrome	Flaccid, full thickness of epidermis	Vesicles or bullae	Face and orofacial, any site	Exuberant mucosal involvement (lips, oral mucosa, eyes, perineum)

and *Streptococcus pyogenes*. The list of noninfectious conditions that closely mimic the eruption caused by these organisms also is lengthy, often leading to difficult or delayed diagnosis.[1-3] The cause of a vesiculobullous infection frequently can be established by consideration of the epidemiologic context. Season, patient age, history of recent exposure to infectious agents or medications, previous disease, and concurrent symptoms, as well as the morphology, distribution, and evolution of the eruption aid in diagnosis. Categorization based on depth (tense or flaccid) and the predominant size (vesicles or bullae) can also aid in diagnosis (Table 72-1).

Infections Associated with Vesicles

Cutaneous HSV typically manifests as 1- to 4-mm vesicles that appear in clusters corresponding to the distribution of the infected nerve or primary inoculation site. Mucosa and perioroficial areas tend to have microabrasions and thus be more susceptible to infection. Primary HSV infections can be exuberant and lead to extensive vesiculation especially in the mouth "primary herpetic gingivostomatitis". Recurrences of HSV more often are localized and may lead only to edematous crusted papules (Figure 72-3). HSV infecting digits (whitlow) usually causes one tense larger bulla made of many individual vesicles that are held together by

the very thick acral skin. Recurrent, clustered vesicles, crusts, or pustules in a fixed spot even if not mucosal should alert the clinician to the possibility of HSV infection. Long-standing crusted ulcerations are a common presentation in immunocompromised patients when the HSV infection cannot be adequately cleared.

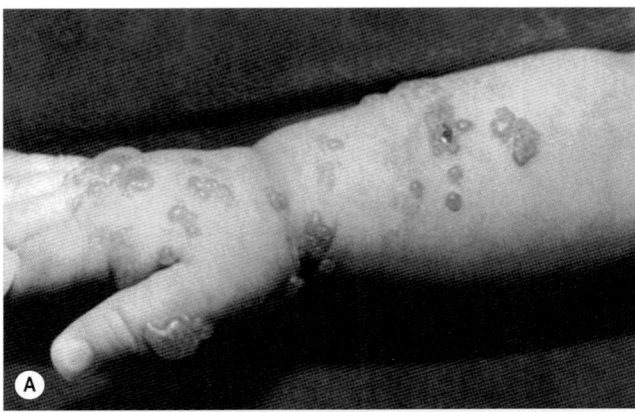

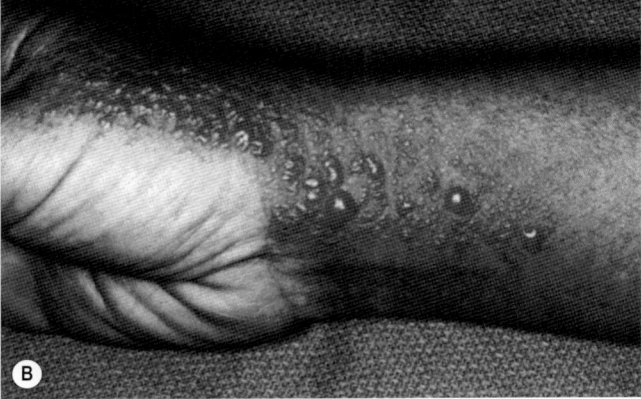

Figure 72-4. (A) Bullae on the dorsal hand and forearm of an infant resulting from reactivation of varicella-zoster virus, without superinfection. **(B)** Vesicles and bullae on the hand and wrist of a girl with contact dermatitis caused by poison oak.

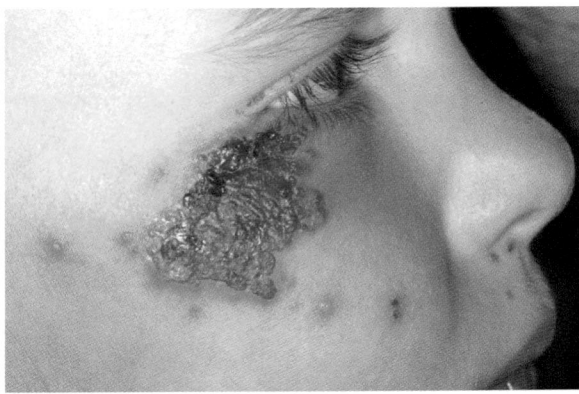

Figure 72-3. A young girl hospitalized for febrile pneumonia had reactivation herpes simplex virus 1 in a dermatomal distribution on her face. (Courtesy of J.H. Brien©.)

PART II Clinical Syndromes and Cardinal Features of Infectious Diseases: Approach to Diagnosis and Initial Management

SECTION J Skin and Soft-Tissue Infections

Zoster is cutaneous reactivation of the VZV virus that corresponds to the sensory nerve in which VZV had been dormant. The initial presentation may be with painful red papules clustered in a plaque that then vesiculate over a few days and finally crust and leave erosions. The key to diagnosis is the dermatomal distribution (Figure 72-4).

Primary varicella (chickenpox) and disseminated VZV in immunocompromised patients both manifest as widely disseminated crusted papules and vesicles on a red base "dew drops on a rose petal." Dissemination from an initial dermatomal cluster should alert the clinician to the possibility of underlying immunosuppression.

Hand-foot-and-mouth disease is caused by enteroviruses (including coxsackievirus A16 and enterovirus 71) and presents with vesicles anywhere in the mouth (including the tongue) as well as on the palms, soles, and also commonly the buttocks. The oral mucosa has very thin epithelium without stratum corneum so vesicles rupture easily, thus it is more common to see only erosions. Conversely, the palms and soles have very thick epidermis and therefore the vesicles may appear as red macules and it can be difficult to detect the fluid inside. Vesicles on the palms and soles tend to be oval and follow the dermatoglyphics (fingerprint markings).

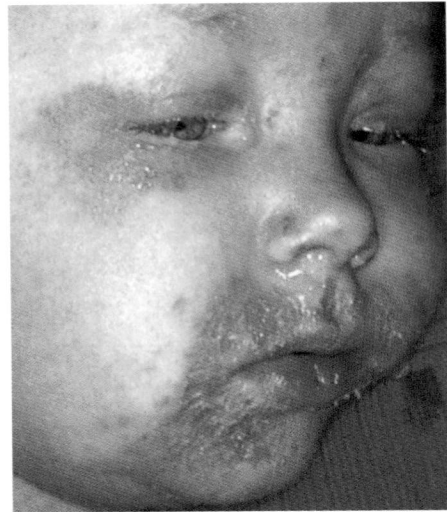

Figure 72-5. Staphylococcal scolded skin syndrome in a toddler. (Courtesy of J.H. Brien©.)

Infections Associated with Flaccid Bullae

Bullous impetigo is an acute blistering infection caused by *S. aureus* group II, typically phage 71 infection. This strain of *S. aureus* carries exfoliative toxin A, which specifically targets and disrupts the intraepidermal keratinocyte connection desmoglein 1 (DSG1).[4] DSG1 is most important for intracellular keratinocyte adhesion in the top layers of the epidermis so lesions in bullous impetigo tend to be flaccid and rupture easily. When the ruptured blister and serous fluid dries, it results in honey-colored crusting. The function of DSG1 is duplicated in the mucosa by coexpression of DSG3. DSG3 is not targeted by exfoliative toxin and thus there is no mucosal blistering in bullous impetigo or in *staphylococcal scalded skin syndrome* (SSSS) (see below).

If the exfoliative toxin A becomes disseminated it can cause cleavage of DSG1 which is distant from the initial infection SSSS. Clinically the cleavage presents as bright red patches of painful skin which, with friction, easily shear off because bullae are very superficial. The most common sites for bullae include the neck, axillae, inguinal folds, and periorofacial areas (Figure 72-5). SSSS is more common in children <5 years of age.

Infections Associated with Tense Bullae

Blistering distal dactylitis classically is due to *S. pyogenes* infection and manifests as tense firm single or multiple vesicles and bullae typically on the volar surface of the fingers.

Gram-negative septicemia can lead to *purpura fulminans*, which is a clinical phenotype characterized by large purpuric patches with hemorrhagic, sometimes tense bullae due to vascular damage and epidermal necrosis.

Necrotizing fasciitis also comes to medical attention with large tense bullae (often hemorrhagic) due to underlying dermal necrosis.

Dermatophyte infections most typically are round, scaling plaques but if there is enough burden of fungus and inflammation a split can occur typically deep in the epidermis or at the dermoepidermal junction, leading to tense bullae. This is most common on the feet but can occur on the trunk or extremities as well.

Vesiculobullous Disease Induced by Infection

Stevens–Johnson syndrome (SJS) is a severe, life-threatening, necrotic mucocutaneous reaction. The hallmark is severe mucosal involvement typically involving the lips and oral mucosa, conjunctivae, and sometimes the urethra, anus and vagina (Figure 72-6A–C). The classic cutaneous lesion is a "target" appearance characterized by a red-purple macule or patch with central duskiness, which can vesiculate or form large bullae. Traumatized areas can shear off and leave only deep erosions. Medications are the most common cause of SJS. *Mycoplasma pneumoniae* also can induce typical SJS or SJS with a predominant mucosal involvement with very few if any cutaneous lesions.[5] SJS is differentiated from SSSS by the predominance of mucosal involvement and the full-thickness epidermal necrosis leading typically to tense bullae and deeper wounds in SJS.

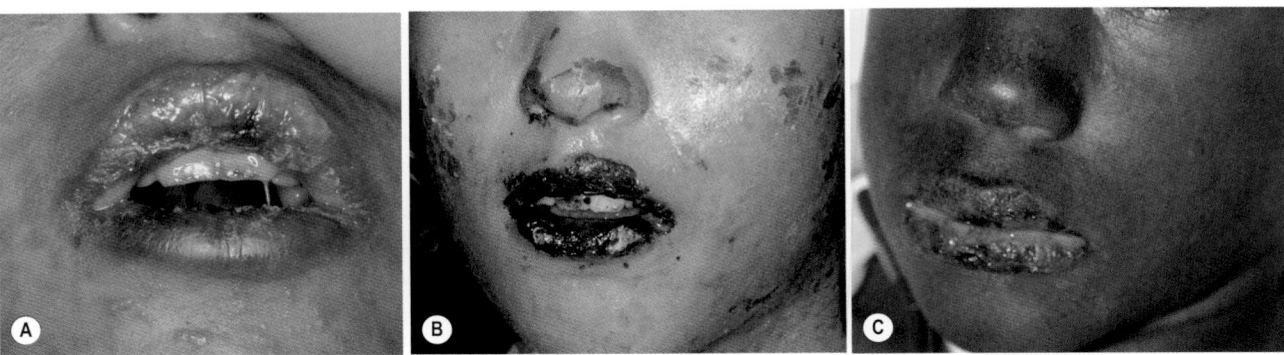

Figure 72-6. Adolescents with Stevens–Johnson syndrome in stages of development **(A)** and resolution **(B and C)**. (Courtesy of J.H. Brien©.)

DIAGNOSIS

In order to diagnose an infectious cause of a blister, an intact blister can be cleansed with alcohol, the edge incised and the fluid collected for Gram stain and culture. If there are no intact blisters, the base of an erosion can be swabbed and cultured; growth of normal skin flora must be interpreted in context. A potassium hydroxide preparation or fungal culture from the unroofed blister can be done if dermatophyte infection is suspected. The viral causes of blisters can be diagnosed by culture, polymerase chain reaction (PCR), or direct fluorescent antibody testing. A Tzanck smear showing multinucleated giant cells with nuclear molding can rapidly diagnose HSV and VZV infection but is less sensitive than other tests. The flaccid bullae in SSSS typically is sterile because the blister is caused by the toxin distant from the primary infection. A primary site of infection or colonization can be investigated.

The diagnosis of SJS can be made rapidly by a frozen section on a skin biopsy to evaluate histologically for full-thickness epidermal necrosis. If there is no inciting medication, *Mycoplasma*

serology or PCR can be used to investigate a causative relationship. The differential diagnosis of noninfectious vesiculobullous eruptions in children includes (1) autoimmune blistering disorders such as linear IgA (chronic bullous disease of childhood), (2) epidermolysis bullosa (EB), (3) thermal or friction injury, (4) contact dermatitis, (5) bullous mastocytoma, and (6) incontinentia pigmenti. After discontinuing an offending drug, the management of SJS, especially with reference to corticosteroid use and immune globulin intravenous, is controversial and has been reviewed recently.[6]

When the cause of vesicular lesions remains in doubt, culture, biopsy for histopathologic evaluation, and immunofluorescence staining are helpful, particularly to exclude noninfectious bullous disorders.[1]

Acknowledgment

The author acknowledges use of parts of chapter of previous editions by J. Browning and M. Levy.

73 Purpura

Melissa A. Reyes and Lawrence F. Eichenfield

Purpura can be a significant finding, especially as it is associated with multiple infectious etiologies, some of which are life-threatening. Purpura results from trauma to blood vessels in the skin leading to hemorrhage into the surrounding tissue. Vessel damage can be the result of direct trauma (physical, chemical, infectious/toxic), vessel occlusion, immune complex deposition, platelet depletion or dysfunction, or other conditions that cause vascular leakage of erythrocytes into the skin, mucous membranes, conjunctivae, or retina. The clinical appearance of purpuric lesions depends on the size of the affected vessels, location of the vessels, extent of hemorrhage, and the coagulation status of the patient. There are a substantial number of noninfectious causes of purpura. Morphology and clinical presentation can be useful in discriminating among likely etiologies. Purpuric lesions can be divided into six subtypes based on size and morphology of the lesions[1]: *petechiae, macular purpura, ecchymoses, palpable purpura, noninflammatory retiform purpura*, and *inflammatory retiform purpura*.

TYPES OF PURPURIC LESIONS AND PATHOGENESIS

Petechiae, macular purpura, and *ecchymoses* are all superficial flat cutaneous lesions of varying sizes, ≤4 mm, 5 to 9 mm, and ≥1 cm, respectively. *Palpable purpura* is raised, partially blanching, erythematous to purple, typically round lesions. *Retiform purpura* appears lace-like in pattern as the affected vessels are larger and exist in the dermis and subcutis. *Inflammatory retiform purpura* initially is erythematous before evolving into purpura. All purpuric lesions share similar changes in color based on the age of the lesion. Lesions initially are bright red or deep red and become purple as the heme pigments break down and progress to green and yellow-brown before fading. The amount of time to fading depends on the amount of extravasated blood.

Petechiae, macular purpura, and ecchymoses are considered *macular* or *flat purpura* and result from simple extravasation of blood into the skin. Histologically, there is minimal inflammation, in contrast to the inflammatory hemorrhage seen in microvascular occlusion or cutaneous small-vessel vasculitis, which

results in *palpable purpura*.[1] *Inflammatory purpura* occurs secondary to occlusion by a clot with resulting ischemia and necrosis of the vessel, in the case of microvascular occlusion syndromes. *Vasculitis* is caused by immune complexes deposited on the vessel lumen, which attracts neutrophils that destroy the complexes as well as injure the vessel wall. *Retiform purpura* and *inflammatory retiform purpura* result from both occlusion and vasculitis, respectively, of larger, slow-flow vessels.

In patients with septicemia, purpura can arise from five main etiologies: (1) disseminated intravascular coagulation (DIC) and coagulopathy, (2) direct vascular invasion and occlusion by organisms, (3) infective vasculitis, (4) emboli, such as seen with endocarditis, and (5) vascular changes due to toxins.[2] Many infections are associated with thrombocytopenia with development of petechiae or ecchymoses, with or without DIC. Invasion of microorganisms into capillaries can occur especially with bloodstream infection (BSI) due to *Neisseria meningitidis, Neisseria gonorrhoeae*, and *Pseudomonas aeruginosa* (Figure 73-1). Diffuse vasculitis with pathologic evidence of *Rickettsiae* in vascular endothelial cells is seen with Rocky Mountain spotted fever (RMSF) and epidemic typhus. Immune mediated vasculitis is associated with a broad set of petechial rashes associated with atypical measles, hepatitis B, and chronic meningococcemia. Intravascular catheter-associated infections and acute and subacute endocarditis can manifest with infectious embolization, complicated by infarction, tissue hemorrhage, and necrosis. Endocarditis also can be associated with immune-mediated vasculitis and petechiae. The scarlatiniform petechial eruptions of *Streptococcus pyogenes* (group A streptococcus, GAS) are an example of toxin-mediated rashes, also known as toxic erythemas.

CAUSES OF PURPURA

Petechiae and Macular Purpura

Petechiae are small, ≤4 mm in diameter, non-blanching purpuric macules that can appear on the skin, conjunctiva, retina, and mucous membranes. Lesions of *macular purpura* are larger than

PART II Clinical Syndromes and Cardinal Features of Infectious Diseases: Approach to Diagnosis and Initial Management

SECTION J Skin and Soft-Tissue Infections

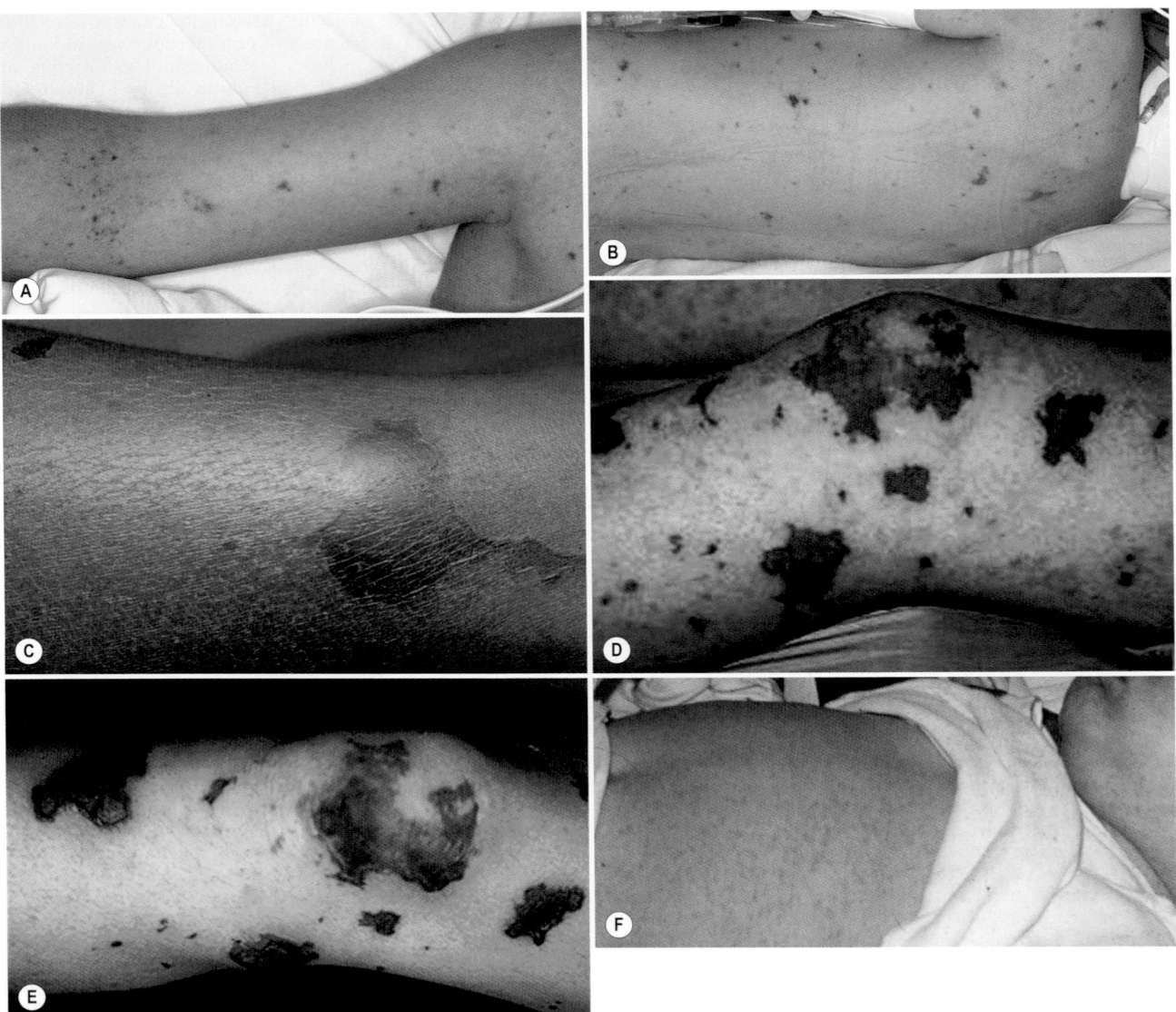

Figure 73-1. Skin manifestations of meningococcemia. Rapidly progressive disease with first examination showing one patient with petechiae on the arm with exaggeration distal to the site of a tourniquet **(A)** and petechiae and purpura on the back **(B)**; and another patient with a purpuric plaque on the distal leg **(C)**. Purpuric lesions around the knee in a patient at the time of admission **(D)** and 4 days later **(E)**. Early manifestations of rapidly progressive, fatal meningococcemia with predominantly non-petechial, macular lesions **(F)**. (A, B, D, and E, courtesy of J.H. Brien©; C and F, courtesy of S.S. Long.)

petechiae but smaller than ecchymoses. Both are the result of extravasation of blood from capillaries. For the remainder of the chapter, "petechiae" will be used to include all macular purpuric lesions <1 cm in size.

Petechiae resolve in 2 to 3 days also but can evolve into macular purpura, ecchymoses, palpable purpura, vesicles, pustules, or necrotic ulcers, depending on the underlying etiology and clinical course. In certain cases, petechiae can be difficult to differentiate from telangiectases and angiomas. Because these latter lesions are not the result of extravasated blood, applying pressure with a glass slide to blanch the vessels (diascopy) can help differentiate petechiae from other vascular lesions.

The appearance of petechiae or purpura in a febrile patient raises the concern for an infectious etiology (Box 73-1). Petechiae can occur in "crops", are seen commonly in BSIs, and usually occur with fever and as an early clinical sign in BSI.[3] When petechiae occur on the nail bed, they appear as red-brown, longitudinal discolorations under the nail plate and are called "splinter hemorrhages".

Historically, the presence of fever and petechiae in a child required evaluation for meningococcal infection. Early studies focused on hospitalized children reported an incidence of meningococcal disease in 7% to 11% of children with fever and petechiae and a case-fatality rate of 10%.[4] More recently, it has been recognized that bacterial causes of fever and petechiae are relatively uncommon.[5,6] In a retrospective review of 129 hospitalized children with fever and petechiae, 20% had culture-proven bacterial infection, one-half of which was due to *N. meningitidis* (11%) and a smaller percentage due to *Haemophilus influenzae* type b (6%).[7] The majority of cases, almost 60%, were attributed to viral causes, while the remainder was attributed to other infectious and non-infectious causes. A prospective study including 190 children hospitalized with fever and petechiae documented 7% with meningococcal disease and 10% with GAS disease.[8] Three patients had clinical sepsis and purpura fulminans with negative blood cultures. In the study, children with invasive bacterial infections were more likely to appear ill, to have meningeal irritation, and to have petechiae below the nipple line. Non-bacteremic patients

BOX 73-1. Major Infectious Causes of Purpura in Children and Neonates

CHILDREN

Bacteria

Arcanobacterium haemolyticum, Bacteroides fragilis, Bartonella hensleae, Borrelia spp., *Brucella* spp., *Campylobacter jejuni, Capnocytophaga canimorsus,*[a] *Enterococcus* spp., *Escherichia coli, Francisella tularensis, Haemophilus influenzae* type b, *Klebsiella* spp., *Leptospira* spp., *Listeria monocytogenes, Moraxella catarrhalis, Mycobacterium leprae, Mycobacterium tuberculosis, Neisseria meningitidis,*[a] *Neisseria gonorrhoeae,*[a] *Pseudomonas aeruginosa,*[a] *Salmonella typhimurium, Staphylococcus aureus, Streptobacillus moniliformis, Streptococcus pneumoniae, Streptococcus pyogenes,*[a] viridans streptococci, *Yersinia pestis, Yersinia enterocolitica*

Fungus

Candida, Aspergillus, Rhizopus, Fusarium species and agents of mucormycosis

Helminths

Ascaris spp., *Strongyloides stercoralis* (hyperinfection syndrome), *Trichinella spiralis*

Mycoplasma

Mycoplasma pneumoniae

Protozoa

Plasmodium falciparum

Rickettsiae

Ehrlichia canis, Ehrlichia chafeensis, Ehrlichia equi, Anaplasma phagocytophilum, Rickettsia akari, Rickettsia prowazekii (epidemic typhus),[a] *Rickettsia rickettsii* (Rocky Mountain spotted fever),[a] *Rickettsia typhi*

Viruses

Adenoviruses; Colorado tick fever virus; coxsackievirus A4, A9, B2–B5; cytomegalovirus,[a] echovirus 3, 4, 7, 9, 18; dengue fever virus; Epstein–Barr virus; hantavirus; hepatitis virus A, B,[a] C;[a] human immunodeficiency virus; parvovirus B19; respiratory syncytial virus; rotavirus; rubella virus; rubeola virus (typical and atypical measles); varicella-zoster virus; yellow fever and other hemorrhagic fever viruses (e.g., Ebola, Marburg and Lassa viruses)

NEONATES

Bacteria

Gram-positive and gram-negative bacteria associated with septicemia[a]

Treponema pallidum

Protozoa

Toxoplasma gondii

Viruses

Enteroviruses; cytomegalovirus; herpes simplex virus types 1, 2; rubella virus

[a]Most common.

(15% with a confirmed viral etiology) had higher white blood cell counts (WBCs) and absolute band counts. Another prospective study attempted to capture a broader cohort of patients by evaluating 411 consecutive pediatric patients presenting to a hospital emergency department with both fever and petechiae.[3] Of the 53 ill-appearing patients ("toxic appearance", inconsolable crying or screaming, or lethargy), 6 had invasive bacteremial infection while none of the 357 well-appearing children had positive blood cultures or cerebrospinal fluid bacterial cultures. In this study of 411 patients with fever and petechiae, only 2 patients had *N. meningitidis* (0.5%), 2 had *Streptococcus pneumoniae*, and 1 had GAS invasive infection. The study also found that WBCs ≥15,000 was predictive of severe BSI. Thus, a febrile patient with petechiae who is well-appearing, has normal laboratory workup, petechiae above the nipple line, and documented streptococcal pharyngitis has low risk of invasive bacterial disease. Petechiae in febrile patients is more commonly associated with viral infections, given their high prevalence, but also because viruses tend to damage small cutaneous vessels.[9]

Petechiae on the palate are characteristic of streptococcal pharyngitis,[10] but also can be seen in Epstein–Barr virus infection, *Arcanobacterium haemolyticum* pharyngitis, rubella, roseola, viral hemorrhagic fevers, thrombocytopenia, and palatal trauma.[10] Palmar and plantar petechiae can be seen in the "gloves and socks" syndrome caused by parvovirus B19. In this condition, there is confluent erythema of the distal extremities with pinpoint macules evolving into petechiae on the palms and soles with concurrent fever and leukopenia.[11] Parvovirus B19 also has been reported to cause a generalized petechial eruption,[12] and petechiae in a "bathing suit" distribution.[13] Clusters of patients with generalized petechial eruptions are reported during community outbreaks of erythema infectiosum, apparently associated with the viremic phase of parvovirus B19 infection.[14] Other reported infectious causes of generalized petechiae include scarlet fever, RMSF, parainfluenza, influenza, respiratory syncytial virus, enterovirus,

rotavirus, atypical measles, rubella, dengue, and adenovirus infections.[6]

Petechiae or purpura also can be due to noninfectious causes, such as secondary to drug eruptions, acute leukemia,[6] low platelet count, and mechanical causes (Box 73-2). Severe coughing or vomiting can increase intrathoracic pressure, causing petechiae in areas perfused by the superior vena cava, approximately corresponding to skin above the nipple line. This distribution of petechiae is not always benign – a reported 25% of patients with fever and petechiae confined to the upper torso had bacterial infection in one study.[7] Petechiae also can form distal to tourniquet placement and are of no clinical significance without other findings. In contrast, the tourniquet test can cause distal petechiae in patients with dengue fever and is positive in most patients with dengue hemorrhagic fever.[15] In newborns, petechiae can occur at sites of pressure as they progress through the birth canal, but petechiae also can result from acquired infection or maternal antiplatelet antibodies; thus appropriate evaluation should be performed. Older children with petechiae and no fever should be evaluated for blood dyscrasias.

Ecchymoses

Ecchymoses are purpuric flat patches on the skin, commonly known as bruises. Ecchymoses typically are ≥1 cm in size and are caused by a greater volume of extravasated blood than in petechiae. Thus, ecchymoses tend to take longer to resolve (1 to 3 weeks). Petechiae in a patient with an underlying coagulopathy can quickly evolve into ecchymoses, sometimes within minutes.

Ecchymoses resulting from infection are uncommon in children. When ecchymoses occur, they are most frequently due to *N. meningitidis* BSI with coagulopathy.[16] Other reported causes include other gram-negative bacteria, gram-positive bacteria (*Staphylococcus aureus, S. pyogenes,* and *S. pneumoniae*), viruses

PART II Clinical Syndromes and Cardinal Features of Infectious Diseases: Approach to Diagnosis and Initial Management

SECTION J Skin and Soft-Tissue Infections

BOX 73-2. Major Noninfectious Causes of Purpura

PLATELET DISORDERS[a]

Thrombocytopenia

Decreased production of platelets: drugs, marrow infiltration or aplasia, toxins

Decreased survival of platelets: disseminated intravascular coagulation, drugs, hemolytic–uremic syndrome, idiopathic and autoimmune thrombocytopenic purpura, prosthetic heart valve, hypersplenism, sequestration

Platelet dysfunction (inherited or acquired)

Thrombocytosis

VASCULAR DISORDERS

Noninflammatory purpura

Amyloidosis, angiokeratoma corporis diffusum, antiphospholipid syndrome, atrophie blanche, corticosteroid therapy, Cushing disease, Ehlers–Danlos syndrome, fat embolism, hereditary hemorrhagic telangiectasia, increased capillary pressure (choking, coughing, forced restraint, tourniquet, vomiting), Langerhans cell histiocytosis, progressive pigmentary dermatosis (pigmented purpura), scurvy, trauma

Vasculitis and inflammatory purpura

Behçet disease, Churg–Strauss syndrome, cystic fibrosis, dermatomyositis, drug- or toxin-induced hypersensitivity vasculitis (nonsteroidal anti-inflammatory drugs, penicillin, quinidine, propylthiouracil, sulfonamides, allopurinol, diphenylhydantoin, phenothiazines, thiazides), dysproteinemias (Waldenström Adom hyperglobulinemic purpura, Waldenström Adom macroglobulinemia, essential mixed cryoglobulinemia, paraproteinemia), Henoch–Schönlein purpura, inflammatory bowel disease, Kawasaki syndrome, leukemia, lymphoma, pityriasis lichenoides, polyarteritis nodosa, pyoderma gangrenosum, rheumatoid arthritis, sarcoidosis, scleroderma, primary and acquired immunodeficiencies (graft-versus-host disease, human immunodeficiency virus infection), second component of complement deficiency, serum sickness, Sjögren syndrome, Sweet syndrome (acute febrile neutrophilic dermatosis), systemic lupus erythematosus, urticarial vasculitis, Wegener granulomatosis

COAGULATION DISORDERS[b]

Clotting factor deficiencies

Depletion of clotting factors through increased use or proteolysis, inadequate production, presence of inhibitor of coagulation, synthesis of abnormal form of clotting factor

Thrombotic disorders

Antiphospholipid syndrome, antithrombin III deficiency, plasminogen deficiency, protein C deficiency, protein S deficiency

[a]Primarily petechiae.
[b]Primarily ecchymoses.

(dengue and other hemorrhagic fevers), and *Rickettsia rickettsii* (RMSF).[16–19]

Ecchymosis occurring acutely and in an ill-appearing patient is called *purpura fulminans*. In this setting, ecchymoses rapidly evolve, are usually symmetric in distribution, and develop necrotic patches and eschars.[3] Purpura fulminans is caused by abnormalities in coagulation secondary to infection. Purpura can occur 7 to 10 days after an otherwise benign infection (idiopathic purpura fulminans) and in the setting of acute infection such as gram-negative infection caused by *N. meningitidis*.[16] Idiopathic purpura fulminans has been associated with varicella, scarlet fever, streptococcal tonsillopharyngitis, viral exanthem, rubella, measles, upper respiratory tract infection, and gastroenteritis.[16] A variant called symmetric peripheral gangrene results in ischemic necrosis of the distal parts of two or more extremities without large-vessel obstruction. This variant is associated with higher mortality and morbidity, such as amputation, in patients with purpura fulminans.[20] Both purpura fulminans and symmetric peripheral gangrene occur more frequently in infants and children than in older individuals.[2] In neonates, purpura fulminans can be a manifestation of inherited homozygous protein C, or rarely protein S, deficiency. In older children, BSIs in patients with these underlying deficiencies (as well as properdin deficiency, splenic dysfunction, or neutropenia) can lead to purpura fulminans.

Palpable Purpura

Unlike, petechiae and ecchymoses, *palpable purpura* are raised purpuric papules and plaques that can range in size from a few millimeters to a few centimeters. Palpable purpura favors dependent areas such as the lower extremities, but in the supine patient can occur on the back, buttocks, and distal arms. Palpable purpura can evolve into nodular, vesicular, pustular, necrotic, or ulcerative lesions.

Palpable purpura is classically associated with leukocytoclastic vasculitis, an inflammatory process injuring the vessel.[21] Histopathologically, fibrin deposition in vessel walls, neutrophilic debris, and perivascular lymphocytes are present. Palpable purpura also can occur with *S. aureus* BSI or bacterial endocarditis as the result of infectious microemboli occluding the vascular lumen. Osler nodes and Janeway lesions found in bacterial endocarditis are types of microembolic-induced palpable purpura. Osler nodes are tender nodules on the palms, soles, and pads of the fingers/toes. Janeway lesions are nontender, purpuric macules, papules or nodules usually on the palms and soles. Lesions similar to Osler nodes have been reported in typhoid fever, polyarteritis nodosa, systemic lupus erythematosus, Churg–Strauss syndrome, mixed cryoglobulinemia, and Wegener granulomatosis.[1,2]

Palpable purpura can have a variety of causes, including infection (10% to 15%), drug exposure, immunization, and autoimmune disease. The most common infectious causes of palpable purpura include *N. meningitidis*, *S. aureus*, and *N. gonorrhoeae* but cases have been reported due to *Mycobacterium*, *Rickettsia*, *Mycoplasma*, and rarely *Bartonella*, *Treponema pallidum*, *Salmonella*, *Campylobacter*, *Yersinia*, and *Brucella* species. Viral causes include hepatitis viruses (hepatitis C more common than hepatitis B, and hepatitis B more common than hepatitis A), hepatitis virus vaccines, HIV, parvovirus, and rarely cytomegalovirus, varicella, and influenza.[1]

Retiform Purpura

Retiform purpura is due to occlusion of dermal and subcutaneous vessels, which causes a lace-like pattern of purpura, also known as *livedo reticularis*. A complete reticulate pattern is not usually seen, but rather a "puzzle piece"-like or "branching" pattern occurs because of the angulated or sometimes serpentine pattern of the purpura. Vascular invasion by fungi (*Mucor*, *Aspergillus* in immunocompromised patients), gram-negative organisms (*Pseudomonas*) that multiply in arterioles, and *Strongyloides* can cause noninflammatory retiform purpura while vasculitis during BSI can cause inflammatory retiform purpura.[1]

74 Urticaria and Erythema Multiforme
Kara N. Shah

Urticaria and erythema multiforme are common cutaneous hypersensitivity reactions seen in children that may be triggered by infection, although noninfectious causes are prevalent as well. Although distinctly different entities, acute urticaria often is misdiagnosed as erythema multiforme. Although urticaria is usually an isolated finding, urticaria and urticarial dermatoses can be seen in a number of syndromes and disorders such as papular urticaria, urticarial vasculitis, and the cryopyrin-associated periodic syndromes (CAPS). Of note, the use of the historical and confusing terms erythema multiforme minor to refer to classic erythema multiforme and erythema multiforme major to refer to Stevens–Johnson syndrome (SJS) has been abandoned.

URTICARIA

Etiologic Agents

Both acute and chronic urticaria have been attributed to numerous bacterial, viral, fungal, and other infectious agents (Box 74-1). However, the data in support of causality are circumstantial at best, in particular as the use of antibiotics and other medications is common in the context of infection and urticaria. Noninfectious etiologies and associations include foods, physical stimuli, and systemic diseases (Box 74-2). In infants younger than 6 months, urticaria largely is due to cow milk allergy; in older infants, food allergy, infection (particularly viral), and medications predominate.[1-3]

In acute urticaria in children, an infectious etiology can be demonstrated in up to 60% of cases.[2,4] Viral upper respiratory tract and gastrointestinal tract infections are the primary infectious triggers of acute urticaria in children, with rhinovirus, adenovirus, rotavirus, and *Streptococcus pyogenes* the most commonly associated infectious agents.[5]

In contrast, chronic urticaria in children is idiopathic or autoimmune in etiology in the majority of cases.[6,7] When an etiology is found, physical urticaria is the most common cause, although chronic urticaria also has been reported to occur in association with a variety of infections.[2,7–10] In one study of 226 children ages 1 to 14 years with chronic urticaria, an etiology was identified in 20%; infection accounted for 4.4% of these cases.[11] The relevance of occult dental, sinus, or ear infections remains controversial.[12] Based on the lack of resolution of most cases of chronic urticaria after treatment of the purported infectious trigger, some experts argue that there is no relationship between chronic infection and chronic urticaria.[13] Some evidence suggests that patients with chronic autoimmune urticaria may, however, manifest an infection-associated autoreactive response.[14] There is no demonstrated association between chronic urticaria and malignancy.[15]

Epidemiology

Urticaria is a common problem, developing in 20% to 25% of the population over a lifetime.[16,17] In children and adolescents, the prevalence estimates range from 2% to 20%.[2,18,19] The majority of cases of urticaria in children are acute and self-limiting. In children, chronic urticaria is uncommon, with a prevalence of only 0.1% to 0.3%.[20] There is no known sex, ethnic, or racial predisposition. Controversy exists as to whether there is an increased prevalence of urticaria in people with a personal or family history of atopic disease.

Pathogenesis/Pathologic Findings

Urticaria results from degranulation of mast cells and basophils with release of histamine and other vasoactive mediators.[21] Histamine acts via both H_1 and H_2 receptors to produce vasodilation and altered vascular permeability, which result in fluid extravasation and dermal edema. Together with the axonal reflex, which produces the associated cutaneous flare, these features comprise the triple response of Lewis. Other mediators of urticaria include kinins, prostaglandins, leukotrienes, cytokines, chemokines, and neuropeptides.

The pathophysiology of urticaria can be defined as immunologic or nonimmunologic. Immune-mediated urticaria results from an IgE-mediated type I hypersensitivity reaction; from the development of autoantibodies against IgE or the high-affinity IgE FceR1 receptor (type II hypersensitivity reaction); through the

---

BOX 74-1. Infectious Agents Associated with Urticaria

BACTERIA

Borrelia burgdorferi (erythema chronicum migrans), *Chlamydophila pneumoniae, Escherichia coli, Helicobacter pylori, Neisseria gonorrhoeae, Neisseria meningitidis, Pseudomonas aeruginosa, Shigella sonnei, Streptococcus pyogenes,*[a] *Yersinia enterocolitica*

FUNGI

Candida albicans, Cladosporium spp., *Coccidioides immitis, Histoplasma capsulatum, Candida glabrata, Trichophyton* spp.

HELMINTHS

Ancylostoma duodenale, Anisakis simplex, Ascaris lumbricoides, Echinococcus spp., *Enterobius vermicularis, Fasciola hepatica, Necator americanus, Onchocerca volvulus, Schistosoma* spp., *Strongyloides stercoralis, Toxocara canis, Trichinella spiralis, Trichobilharzia* spp. (avian blood flukes), *Wuchereria bancrofti*

MYCOPLASMA

Mycoplasma pneumoniae

PROTOZOA

Blastocystis hominis, Entamoeba histolytica, Giardia lamblia, Plasmodium spp., *Trichomonas vaginalis*

RICKETTSIA

Coxiella burnetii

TREPONEME

Treponema pallidum

VIRUSES

Adenovirus;[a] coxsackieviruses A9, A16, B4, B5;[a] cytomegalovirus, echovirus 11;[a] Epstein–Barr virus;[a] hepatitis viruses A, B, C; influenza B virus;[a] human immunodeficiency virus; measles virus, attenuated; mumps virus; parvovirus B19, respiratory syncytial virus[a]

[a]Most common.

PART II Clinical Syndromes and Cardinal Features of Infectious Diseases: Approach to Diagnosis and Initial Management

SECTION J Skin and Soft-Tissue Infections

BOX 74-2. Differential Diagnosis of Urticaria and Urticarial Eruptions in Infants and Children

ARTHROPOD BITES (PAPULAR URTICARIA)

Ants (Solenopsis saevissima), bedbugs (Cimex lectularius), bees,[a] body lice (Pediculus humanus),[a] caterpillars, fleas (Pulex irritans),[a] chiggers (Trombicula irritans), flies, gypsy moths, kissing bugs (Triatoma sanguisuga), mosquitoes, scabies mites (Sarcoptes scabiei),[a] scorpions, spiders, wasps

ANNULAR ERYTHEMAS

Erythema multiforme, annular erythema of infancy, acute hemorrhagic edema of infancy, erythema annulare centrifugum/gyrate erythema

AUTOIMMUNE/CONTACT

Animal dander, caterpillars and moths (Lepidoptera), chemicals, cosmetics, epoxy resins, fish, coral, jellyfish, hedgehog, foods, medications, nickel, parabens, saliva, wood dust

DERMAL HYPERSENSITIVITY REACTIONS

Eosinophilic cellulitis
Exanthematous drug eruptions

DRUGS

Acetylsalicylic acid,[a,b] allopurinol, amoxicillin,[a] barbiturates, cephalosporin antibiotics, tetracycline, codeine, curare, meperidine, morphine,[a] nonsteroidal anti-inflammatory agents (e.g., indomethacin),[a,b] penicillin,[a] phenytoin, polymyxin B, procainamide, quinidine, iodinated radiocontrast media,[b] sulfa-derived antibiotics,[a] sulfonylureas, thiamine, thiazides, vancomycin, zidovudine

FOOD ADDITIVES, PRESERVATIVES, AND DYES (PSEUDOALLERGIC REACTION)

Azo dyes (e.g., sunset yellow, tartrazine[a]), butylhydroxyanisole, butylhydroxytoluene, 4-hydroxybenzoic acid,[a] sodium benzoate,[a] sodium metabisulfite

FOOD ALLERGY

Chocolate, egg,[a] fish,[a] fresh berries, milk,[a] nuts,[a] peanuts,[a] shellfish,[a] tomatoes

AUTOINFLAMMATORY SYNDROMES

Schnitzler syndrome; cryopyrin-associated periodic syndromes (CAPS) (neonatal-onset multisystem inflammatory disease (NOMID), familial cold autoinflammatory syndrome, Muckle–Wells syndrome)

INHALANT ALLERGENS

Animal danders, mold spores, pollens

PHYSICAL AND EMOTIONAL CAUSES

Aquagenic; cholinergic stimuli, including emotional stress (psychogenic), exercise, heat; cold;[a] dermatographism;[a] pressure; sunlight; sweating; vibration

SYSTEMIC DISEASE

Autoimmune thyroid disease, celiac disease, bullous pemphigoid, juvenile idiopathic arthritis, Kawasaki disease, acute rheumatic fever (erythema marginatum), hypocomplementemic urticarial vasculitis (associated with systemic lupus erythematosus and other connective tissue diseases), serum sickness, serum-sickness-like reactions, common variable immunodeficiency

OTHER

Cutaneous mastocytosis (urticaria pigmentosa, solitary mastocytoma)

[a]Most common.
[b]Can cause pseudoallergic reaction.

---

binding of circulating immune complexes to mast cells expressing Fc receptors for IgG and IgM (type III hypersensitivity reaction); and rarely through T-lymphocyte-mediated activation of mast cells (type IV hypersensitivity reaction).[21] In nonimmunologic (pseudoallergic) urticaria, direct degranulation of mast cells and basophils occurs because of exogenous factors such as pressure and cold; via activation of membrane receptors involved in innate immunity such as by opioids; via direct mast cell toxicity as occurs with iodinated radiographic contrast agents, drugs such as aspirin and NSAIDs, and foods; or through inhibition of kinin breakdown by inhibitors of angiotensin-converting enzymes. The mechanism of urticaria due to infectious agents is postulated to involve either the formation of immune complexes with activation of complement and release of anaphylotoxins or the development of IgE antibodies to microbial antigens.[22,23]

Clinical Manifestations/Differential Diagnosis/Clinical Approach

Commonly referred to as "hives" or "welts," urticaria is characterized by the appearance of wheals with or without angioedema. Nearly all cases of urticaria in infants and most cases in children are acute; by definition, resolution occurs within 6 weeks. Chronic urticaria is diagnosed when urticaria persists daily or almost daily, with or without angioedema, for more than 6 weeks.

The hallmark clinical features of urticaria include the acute onset of edematous papules and plaques, which often manifest central clearing and are surrounded by erythema; pruritus or a burning sensation; and an evanescent duration of 1 to 24 hours.[10] Individual wheals can vary in size from a few millimeters to several centimeters in diameter. Although classically annular or circular, individual wheals can assume a bizarre, serpiginous morphology (Figure 74-1). Occasionally, wheals can have a

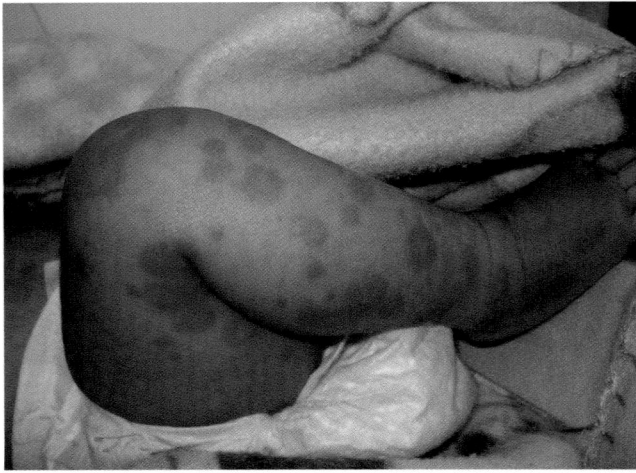

Figure 74-1. Acute urticaria. Migratory, edematous, erythematous plaques with central clearing associated with edema of the hands and feet.

transient, dusky, violaceous center, which can be confused with erythema multiforme; this variant of acute urticaria has been referred to as "urticaria multiforme" or acute annular urticaria.[24,25] Associated dermatographism, a form of pressure-induced urticaria, often is seen.

Angioedema, defined by the presence of edema of the deep dermis and subcutis that classically involves the mucous membranes and acral areas (hands, feet, and face), occurs in about 5% to 10% of children with urticaria. Angioedema usually resolves more slowly that urticaria and can last for up to 72 hours. A burning or stinging sensation can be present, but pruritus usually is not prominent.

When urticaria is associated with anaphylaxis, systemic symptoms develop as a result of the release of vasoactive mediators, and swelling of viscera can occur. Systemic symptoms and signs include hoarseness, respiratory distress, emesis, diarrhea, abdominal pain, arthralgia, flushing, syncope, hypotension, and cardiovascular collapse.

The clinical approach to urticaria in children involves establishing a definitive diagnosis of spontaneous urticaria and identifying a plausible trigger. In most cases, the diagnosis and likely etiology can be established through a thorough and pertinent history and physical examination. The history should include information on the frequency and duration of wheals; associated symptoms such as pruritus or burning; presence of systemic symptoms such as fever, arthralgia, or respiratory or gastrointestinal symptoms; and recent medication exposures. On physical examination, attention should be paid to the morphology, distribution, and progression of wheals; their transient nature can be documented through serial examination with marking of individual wheals if necessary. Presence or absence of angioedema and mucous membrane abnormalities and specific findings such as lymphadenopathy, hepatospenomegaly, and arthritis should be noted. The differential diagnosis of urticaria includes other annular erythemas, such as erythema multiforme; autoinflammatory syndromes, in particular the cryopyrin-associated periodic syndromes (CAPS); exanthematous drug eruptions; and urticarial eruptions associated with systemic disease such as systemic lupus erythematosus (Box 74-2).

Laboratory Findings and Diagnosis

The diagnosis of urticaria usually is established from the history and clinical examination. Skin biopsy can be helpful in equivocal cases or when a diagnosis other than urticaria such as urticarial vasculitis is suspected. Histologically, urticaria demonstrates dermal edema, dilatation of postcapillary venules and lymphatic vessels, and a sparse, mixed perivascular infiltrate with variable numbers of eosinophils and neutrophils; an increase in mast cells also can be found.[26] In some cases, the histology of urticaria can be nonspecific or appear as "normal skin."

Specific diagnostic tests in a child with acute urticaria generally are recommended only when the history and physical examination suggest a specific, treatable etiology (e.g., streptococcal pharyngitis, bacterial enteritis, food allergy) or when the diagnosis is uncertain or unlikely to be urticaria. For mild chronic urticaria under pharmacologic control and in the absence of corroborating physical examination findings or suggestive history, extensive laboratory evaluations generally are not indicated.[27]

Skin prick testing combined with RAST testing as clinically indicated can be performed if food and environmental allergy is suspected to be the cause. Oral food challenges and elimination diets, if clinically indicated, should be performed under the guidance of an experienced allergist. Provocation testing may be performed to validate a diagnosis of physical urticaria. If a specific infectious etiology is suspected, directed testing should be performed; examples include oropharyngeal culture for *S. pyogenes* and/or serum for antistreptolysin O titer; nasopharyngeal swab for antigen detection/PCR for common respiratory viruses, including adenovirus and rhinovirus; Epstein–Barr virus serology and/or blood PCR; serology for hepatitis viruses; vaginal smear for *Candida* and *Trichomonas*; urinalysis and urine culture; stool examination for

ova and parasites; stool for culture, antigen detection for rotavirus and antigen detection/PCR for adenovirus. Additional laboratory evaluations considered in selected cases of urticaria in which the history and physical examination are suggestive of systemic disease include a complete blood cell count with differential count, sedimentation rate and C-reactive protein; serum hepatic enzyme levels, thyroid function tests, ANA, tryptase, quantitative immunoglobulins, and complement (C3, C4, CH50). Imaging studies such as chest or sinus radiography are considered in selected patients. The autologous serum skin test and basophil histamine release assay are specialized diagnostic tests used to confirm a diagnosis of chronic autoimmune urticaria.

Management

In cases in which an etiology can be identified, the primary management is focused on providing symptomatic relief and eliminating or avoiding the known cause(s) or trigger(s). Factors that may aggravate urticaria include heat, exercise, emotional stress, and certain medications such as aspirin and NSAIDs.[28] Infection, if present, should be treated, although treatment of the associated infection results in an improvement in urticaria in only a minority of patients.

The most successful approach to treating the symptoms of urticaria is with medications that block the effect of histamine at the level of its receptor on cutaneous blood vessels. Antihistamines that block H_1 receptors have been considered as first-line therapy for urticaria. Hydroxyzine hydrochloride is the most effective of the classic H_1 antihistamines for suppression of the wheal-and-flare response, pruritus, and dermatographism.[29-31] Because of significant sedative and anticholinergic effects of the first-generation antihistamines, however, newer nonsedating H_1 antihistamines such as fexofenadine, loratadine, and cetirizine are recommended as first-line therapeutic agents. These agents are as efficacious as first-generation antihistamines and have a longer duration of action.[32] Levocetirizine has been demonstrated to be safe and effective in reducing the duration of acute urticaria in infants as young as 12 months of age.[33] Antihistamine therapy should be initiated at the upper end of the recommended dosage range and then gradually increased as needed until symptoms are relieved or until side effects, particularly sedation, become prohibitive. Use of antihistamines at 2–4 times that recommended by the manufacturer may be required.[34] Administering most of the daily dose just before bedtime can minimize sedation. The therapeutic response to the H_1 antihistamines can be improved with the addition of an H_2 receptor antagonist such as cimetidine or ranitidine.[35] H_2 receptor antagonists should not be used as monotherapy because of their insufficient H_1 blockade.

Topical corticosteroid agents generally are of limited utility in the treatment of urticaria. Use of systemic corticosteroids rarely is indicated in children and discouraged for use in chronic urticaria due to concerns for significant adverse effects. A short course of oral corticosteroids generally is reserved for children with severe unremitting symptoms, especially asthma, laryngeal edema, or anaphylaxis, or when angioedema is particularly severe on the face.

Rarely, chronic urticaria is severe enough that despite the use of oral antihistamines, additional systemic therapy is warranted. Alternative or adjunctive therapies include mast cell stabilizers, leukotriene antagonists, tricyclic antidepressants (in particular doxepin), dapsone, cyclosporine, mycophenolate mofetil, and omalizumab.[34,36]

Complications, Prognosis, Sequelae, and Prevention

Complications are rare but can result from associated angioedema or anaphylaxis. By definition, acute urticaria resolves within 6 weeks, and most cases resolve within 1 to 2 weeks, either with or without therapy. Over 50% of all cases of chronic urticaria resolve within 6 months, although patients with associated angioedema

PART II   Clinical Syndromes and Cardinal Features of Infectious Diseases: Approach to Diagnosis and Initial Management

SECTION J   Skin and Soft-Tissue Infections

are more likely to have persistent disease.[37] Approximately one-half of children with chronic urticaria have remission within 1 to 3 years.[2,7,38]

The development of urticaria is an unpredictable hypersensitivity reaction and, as such, it is not preventable. If an etiology has been found, avoidance is recommended, if possible, to prevent recurrence.

ERYTHEMA MULTIFORME

Etiologic Agents and Epidemiology

Although numerous infections have been reported in association with erythema multiforme (EM), herpes simplex virus (HSV) is by far the most common and best documented (Box 74-3).[39,40] Recurrent EM also is significantly associated with infection with HSV.[41,42] Demonstration of prior exposure to HSV by serology and documentation of a cutaneous recurrence of HSV infection was noted in a series of patients with recurrent EM and was less common in patients with a single episode.[42]

Epidemiologic data on the prevalence of EM in children are lacking, and although typically a disease of young adults 20 to 40 years of age, an estimated 20% of cases are seen in children and adolescents.[43–45] There is no clear sex, ethnic, or racial predisposition. Recurrent EM occurs more commonly in the spring.[45] The presence of the human leukocyte antigens B62, B35, and DR53 have been associated with a higher risk of HSV-induced disease, particularly the recurrent form.[46]

BOX 74-3.   Infectious Agents Associated with Erythema Multiforme

BACTERIA

Bartonella henselae, Corynebacterium diphtheriae, Francisella tularensis,[a] *Legionella pneumophila, Mycobacterium leprae, Mycobacterium tuberculosis,*[a] *Neisseria gonorrhoeae, Proteus mirabilis,*[a] *Pseudomonas aeruginosa, Salmonella* spp.,[a] *Staphylococcus aureus,*[a] *Streptococcus pneumoniae, Streptococcus pyogenes,*[a] *Vibrio parahaemolyticus,*[a] *Yersinia* spp.[a]

CHLAMYDIA

Chlamydophila psittaci, Chlamydia trachomatis (lymphogranuloma venereum)

FUNGI

Coccidioides immitis, Histoplasma capsulatum[a]

IMMUNIZATIONS

Calmette-Guérin bacillus, diphtheria and tetanus toxoid, hepatitis B, measles, mumps, rubella, poliomyelitis

MYCOPLASMA

Mycoplasma pneumoniae

PARASITES

Trichomonas vaginalis

TREPONEME

Treponema pallidum

VIRUSES

Adenovirus[a] 7; coxsackieviruses A10, A16, B5; echovirus 6; Epstein–Barr virus;[a] hepatitis viruses A, B; herpes simplex viruses 1, 2;[a] human immunodeficiency virus; influenza A virus; measles virus; mumps virus; orf virus; paravaccinia virus[a] parvovirus B19; varicella-zoster virus

[a]Most clearly established.

Pathogenesis and Pathologic Findings

The pathogenesis of EM is incompletely understood, but evidence increasingly implicates a host-specific, cell-mediated immune response to an antigenic stimulus that targets keratinocytes at the dermal-epidermal junction.[44,45] Cytokines released by activated mononuclear cells and keratinocytes contribute to necrosis of keratinocytes. Although circulating and tissue-bound immune complexes can be demonstrated, they do not appear to play a central role in the pathogenesis of erythema multiforme. HSV antigens and DNA have been documented in skin lesions from patients with EM but are absent in unaffected skin of such patients.[40,47–49]

Histologically, EM demonstrates mild spongiosis, lymphocytic exocytosis, variable papillary dermal edema, a perivascular and interstitial mononuclear infiltrate, and basal vacuolization with liquefactive degeneration of the basal layer of the epidermis; the feature of satellite cell necrosis is a hallmark of EM.[26] An increased number of eosinophils and/or nuclear dust may be seen. Subepidermal blisters and necrosis of the entire epidermis can be seen in more severe cases.

Clinical Manifestations, Differential Diagnosis, and Clinical Approach

As the name suggests, EM has variable cutaneous manifestations. EM is characterized by the acute onset of a symmetric, fixed cutaneous eruption of erythematous macules, papules, vesicles, and/or bullae most commonly distributed on the palms, dorsal surfaces of the hands and feet, and extensor surfaces of the arms and legs with relative sparing of the face, trunk and mucous membranes.[44] Lesions can expand and evolve over several days to assume the classic annular "target" appearance with a dusky, necrotic center surrounded by a ring of edema and pallor and an erythematous border (Figure 74-2). The development of new lesions 72 hours after onset is unusual. The isomorphic phenomenon, which refers to the development of lesions at sites of prior skin trauma, is common. Lesions usually are asymptomatic, although a burning sensation or pruritus can be present. Photoaccentuation is common. Prodromal symptoms generally are absent, although low-grade fever, malaise, and upper respiratory tract symptoms can occur. Cervical lymphadenopathy can occur in association with oral involvement, which occurs in about 25% of cases and usually includes localized erosions involving the gingival, tongue, or buccal mucosa (Figure 74-3). Rarely, more extensive involvement can be seen but extensive hemorrhagic crusting such as is seen with Stevens–Johnson syndrome does not

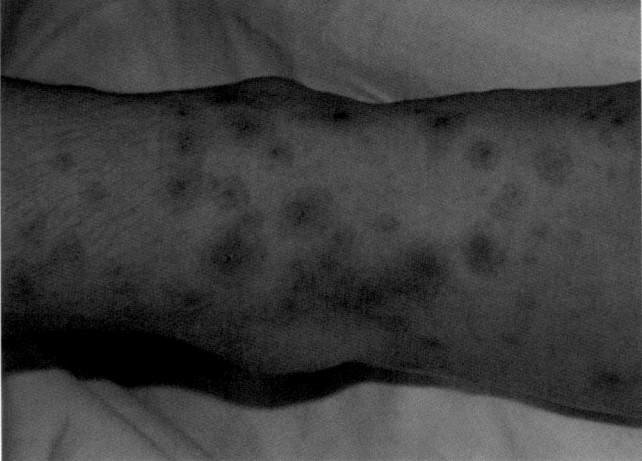

Figure 74-2. Erythema multiforme. "Target" lesions manifest as edematous papules with dusky, necrotic centers and erythematous annular borders.

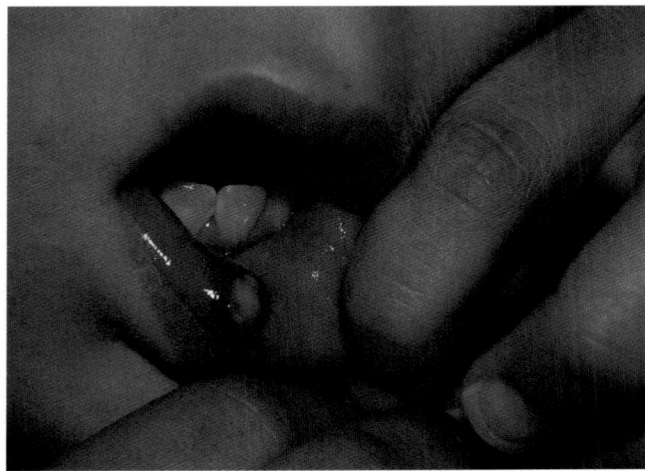

Figure 74-3. Oral aphthae in a child with HSV-associated recurrent erythema multiforme.

occur.[44,45] Ocular or other mucous membrane involvement is not seen and, if present, should raise the possibility of Stevens–Johnson syndrome (see Chapter 72, Vesicles and Bullae).

Lesions of HSV-induced recurrent EM typically develop 10 to 14 days after the onset of recurrent mucocutaneous lesions or occur after asymptomatic reactivation of HSV. EM has a similar morphology and distribution from episode to episode, but can vary considerably in frequency and duration in a given patient. Oral mucous membrane involvement is common in recurrent EM.[50]

The differential diagnosis of EM includes acute urticaria, vasculitis, viral exanthem, exanthematous drug eruption, Stevens–Johnson syndrome, acute hemorrhagic edema of infancy, systemic lupus erythematosus, and polymorphous light eruption.

Laboratory Findings and Diagnosis

Although typically a clinical diagnosis, skin biopsy can be helpful to confirm the diagnosis. There are no typical laboratory abnormalities, although elevated ESR, moderate leukocytosis, and mildly elevated serum hepatic transaminases can be seen in some patients. In cases where HSV infection is suspected, PCR or direct fluorescent antigen (DFA) testing on primary or recurrent cutaneous lesions can be performed.

Management

In most cases of EM, supportive treatment is all that is necessary. Use of oral antihistamines and analgesics, both oral and topical in the case of oral mucosal involvement, may be helpful in addressing associated pruritus and pain, respectively. Debridement of necrotic skin is not recommended, and blisters should be left intact when possible. Areas that have eroded, blistered, or crusted should be monitored for infection; re-epithelialization of denuded areas is facilitated by application of bland emollients or antibiotic ointments and use of petrolatum-impregnated gauze or hydrocolloid or foam dressings. No controlled, prospective studies support the use of corticosteroids.[45,51] Acyclovir given orally early with episodes of primary or recurrent EM may lessen the severity of the clinical course.[50,52]

Complications, Prognosis, Sequelae, and Prevention

Complications are unusual, but secondary bacterial skin infections can occur. EM typically resolves within 2 to 4 weeks. Significant postinflammatory hyperpigmentation can result, but scarring is unusual unless secondary bacterial infection of the skin has developed. Recurrent EM usually remits after several years.

Primary episodes of EM are unpredictable and therefore not preventable. Preventive measures for recurrent EM include sun protective measures such as routine use of sunscreen, use of protective clothing, and avoidance of excess exposure. Use of acyclovir or valacyclovir (in adolescents over 12 years of age) for 6 to 12 months can be considered at suppressive doses for children and adolescents with more than 3–4 recurrences per year (see Chapter 204, Herpes Simplex Virus)

Acknowledgments

The author acknowledges use of the work of previous authors G.L. Darmstadt, John Browning, and Moise Levy.

---

75 Papules, Nodules, and Ulcers

Christine T. Lauren and Maria C. Garzon

Papules, nodules, and ulcers are primary lesions of the skin that can be caused by a variety of infectious and noninfectious agents (Tables 75-1 and 75-2). A *papule* is a raised superficial lesion that is <1 cm in size whose surface may be smooth, scaly, or hyperkeratotic. A larger, >1 cm raised often flatter-topped lesion is called a *plaque*. A *nodule* is a solid palpable lesion that is >1 cm in size; an *ulcer* is a loss of skin to the level of the dermis or deeper. A particular type of cutaneous lesion can be associated with a specific organism (e.g., umbilicated papule of molluscum contagiosum or hyperkeratotic papule of human papillomavirus), or multiple morphologic lesions can occur within the natural history of infection due to a single organism. For example, in tuberculosis or sporotrichosis, an initial papule can enlarge to form a nodule and then break down to an ulcer. These papular or nodular lesions can consist of a proportionately large volume of the infectious agent (e.g., poxvirus of molluscum contagiosum), or almost exclusively of inflammatory cells (e.g., histiocytes within well-controlled primary cutaneous tuberculosis), or frequently a combination of the inciting agent and inflammatory reaction. *Nodular lymphangitis* is a distinctive, underrecognized pattern resulting from cutaneous inoculation of a limited number of agents characterized by a linear pattern of lymphadenopathy often proximal to the site of the primary inoculation (e.g., *Sporothrix schenckii*, *Nocardia brasiliensis*, *Mycobacterium marinum*, other *Mycobacterium* species, *Leishmania*, and *Francisella*).[1–4] Chronic nodular lymphangitis due to any etiology can become ulcerative.[3,4]

A variety of nonspecific reactive lesions can manifest in the skin as a result of an infectious process elsewhere (e.g., erythema nodosum as a sign of streptococcal pharyngitis). These eruptions result from a disordered immune response after infection; at the time of development of these lesions, infectious organisms

PART II Clinical Syndromes and Cardinal Features of Infectious Diseases: Approach to Diagnosis and Initial Management

SECTION J Skin and Soft-Tissue Infections

TABLE 75-1. Primary Infectious Causes of Papules, Nodules, and Ulcers

Disease Entity	Skin Lesions[a]	Infectious Agent	Disease Entity	Skin Lesions[a]	Infectious Agent
ARTHROPODS			Mycetoma	P, N, U	Multiple organisms
Cutaneous myiasis	P, N	*Dermatobia hominis*	Phaeohyphomycosis	N	Multiple organisms
Scabies	P	*Sarcoptes scabiei*	Sporotrichosis	P, N, U	*Sporothrix schenckii*
Tungiasis	P	*Tunga penetrans*	Tinea barbae, tinea	P, N	*Trichophyton* spp.
BACTERIA			capitis	P, N	*Microsporum* spp.
Actinomycosis	P, N, U	*Actinomyces israelii*	Tinea corporis	P	*Trichophyton* spp.
Anthrax	P, U	*Bacillus anthracis*		P	*Microsporum canis*
Bartonellosis	P, N	*Bartonella bacilliformis*	Zygomycosis	U	*Absidia, Rhizopus, Mucor*
Brucellosis	P, N	*Brucella* spp.	**HELMINTHS**		
Cat scratch disease	P, N	*Bartonella henselae*	Dracunculosis (guinea	U	*Dracunculus medinensis*
Chancroid	P, U	*Haemophilus ducreyi*	worm)		
Diphtheria	P, U	*Corynebacterium diphtheriae*	Larva currens	P	*Strongyloides stercoralis*
Ecthyma	U	*Streptococcus pyogenes*	Cutaneous larva migrans	P	*Ancylostoma braziliense*
Ecthyma gangrenosum	P, U	*Pseudomonas aeruginosa*		P	*Ancylostoma caninum*
Folliculitis	P	*Enterobacter* spp.	Cysticercosis	N	*Taenia solium*
	P	*Escherichia coli*	Ground itch	P	*Necatur americanus*
	P	*Klebsiella* spp.	Loiasis	N	*Loa loa*
	P, N	*Proteus* spp.			*Ancylostoma duodenale*
	P	*Pseudomonas aeruginosa*	Onchocerciasis	P, N	*Onchocerca volvulus*
	P	*Staphylococcus aureus*	Cercarial dermatitis	P	*Trichobilharzia* spp.
Furunculosis, carbunculosis	N	*Staphylococcus aureus*	Schistosomiasis	P	*Schistosoma* spp.
Granuloma inguinale	P, N, U	*Calymmatobacterium granulomatis*	**MYCOBACTERIA**		
			Nontuberculous	P, N, U	*Mycobacterium marinum*
Hidradenitis suppurativa	N	Mixed skin flora	mycobacteriosis	N, U	*Mycobacterium kansasii*
Impetigo	P, U	*Staphylococcus aureus*		N, U	*Mycobacterium scrofulaceum*
	P, U	*Streptococcus pyogenes*		N, U	*Mycobacterium ulcerans*
Lyme disease	P, U	*Borrelia burgdorferi*		P, N, U	*Mycobacterium avium* complex
Lymphogranuloma venereum	P, U	*Chlamydia trachomatis*		P, N, U	*Mycobacterium fortuitum, Mycobacterium chelonae*
Malacoplakia	P, N, U	Multiple organisms		P, N, U	*Mycobacterium leprae*
Melioidosis	N, U	*Pseudomonas pseudomallei*	Cutaneous tuberculosis	P, N, U	*Mycobacterium tuberculosis*
Meningococcemia, chronic	P	*Neisseria meningitidis*		P, N, U	*Mycobacterium bovis*
				P, N, U	Calmette-Guérin bacillus
Nocardiosis	P, N	*Nocardia brasiliensis*	**PROTOZOA**		
	P, N	*Nocardia asteroides*	Amebiasis	N, U	*Entamoeba histolytica*
Pyomyositis	N	Multiple organisms	Leishmaniasis	P, N, U	*Leishmania* spp.
Rhinoscleroma	N, U	*Klebsiella rhinoscleromatis*	**TREPONEMES**		
Sycosis barbae	P	*Staphylococcus aureus*	Pinta	P	*Treponema carateum*
Septic emboli	P, U	Multiple organisms	Syphilis	P, N, U	*Treponema pallidum*
Tularemia	U	*Francisella tularensis*	Yaws	P, N, U	*Treponema pertenue*
FUNGI			**VIRUSES**		
Blastomycosis	P, N, U	*Blastomyces dermatitidis*	Epidermodysplasia verruciformis	P	Human papillomaviruses
Candidiasis	P, N, U	*Candida albicans*	Herpes simplex	N, U	Human herpes virus 1, 2
	P, N, U	*Candida tropicalis*	Herpes zoster	N, U	Varicella zoster virus (HHV-3)
Coccidiomycosis	P, N, U	*Coccidioides immitis*	Milker's nodule	P, N	Paravaccinia virus
Cryptococcosis	P, N, U	*Cryptococcus neoformans*	Molluscum contagiosum	P, N	Molluscum contagiosum virus
Folliculitis	P	*Candida albicans*	Orf	P, N	Orf virus
	P	*Malassezia furfur*	Parvovirus	P	Parvovirus B19
Histoplasmosis	P, N, U	*Histoplasmosis capsulatum*	Warts	P, N	Human papillomaviruses
Hyalohyphomycosis	N	Multiple organisms			

[a]N, nodule; P, papule; U, ulcer.

generally are not recoverable (Table 75-3 and Box 75-1). Drug reactions in children also can manifest as papules or rarely nodules, often in the setting of a concurrent viral infection, and this may be confused with a response to the infection.

This chapter contains a brief discussion of selected disease entities that can cause papules, nodules, or ulcers. Infections in which skin lesions do not develop primarily but are manifestations of systemic disease (e.g., bartonellosis, tularemia, and trypanosomiasis) are discussed elsewhere.

MOLLUSCUM CONTAGIOSUM

Molluscum contagiosum (MC) is one of the most common cutaneous infections arising in childhood and produces a papule in the skin in which viral particles can be identified easily.[5,6] MC differs from common warts caused by human papillomavirus (HPV) in that molluscipoxvirus is as a rule found in abundance within the lesions. In contrast, HPV is present in variable quantities within the cutaneous lesions of common warts depending upon

TABLE 75-2. Major Noninfectious Causes of Papules, Nodules, and Ulcers

Disease Entity	Skin Lesions[a]	Disease Entity	Skin Lesions[a]
Acne vulgaris	P, N	Mastocytoma	P, N
Amyloidosis	P, N	Melanoma	P, N, U
Arthropod bite hypersensitivity reaction	P, N	Metastasis, cutaneous	P, N, U
Autoimmune disease (SLE, dermatomyositis, Behçet)	P, N, U	Miliaria rubra	P
Calcinosis cutis	P, N, U	Milium	P
Dermatofibroma	P, N	Necrobiosis lipodica diabeticorum	N, U
Dermoid cyst	P, N	Neuroblastoma	N
Drug hypersensitivity reaction	P	Neurofibroma	P
Eczema, follicular	P	Neutrophilic dermatosis (Sweet syndrome)	P, N, U
Elastosis perforans serpiginosa	P	Nevus	P
Epidermal cyst	P, N	Panniculitis	N, U
Eruptive vellus hair cyst	P	Pilar cyst (trichilemmal cyst)	P, N
Erythema induratum	N, U	Pilomatricoma	P, N
Erythema multiforme	P, U	Pityriasis rubra pilaris	P
Erythema nodosum leprosum	N	Polyarteritis nodosa	N, U
Factitial panniculitis	N	Polymorphous light eruption	P
Foreign-body reaction	P, N	Prurigo nodularis	P, N
Fox–Fordyce disease	P	Pseudoxanthoma elasticum	P
Gout	P, N, U	Psoriasis	P
Granuloma annulare	P, N	Pyoderma gangrenosum	N, U
Juvenile xanthogranuloma	P, N	Pyogenic granuloma	P
Kawasaki disease	P	Rheumatoid nodule	N
Keloid/hypertrophic scar	P, N	Sarcoidosis	P, U
Keratosis follicularis (Darier disease)	P	Spitz nevus	P, N
Keratosis pilaris	P	Steatocystoma multiplex	P, N
Langerhans cell histiocytosis	P, N, U	Subcutaneous fat necrosis	N
Leukemia	P, N	Superficial thrombophlebitis	N
Lichen nitidus	P	Trichoepithelioma	P, N
Lichen planus	P, U	Tuberous sclerosis	P
Lipoma	N	Urticaria	P
Lupus erythematosus	P, U	Urticaria pigmentosa	P, N
Lupus panniculitis	N	Vascular malformation	P, N
Lymphoma	P, N	Vasculitis	P, U
Lymphomatoid granulomatosis	N, U	Xanthoma	P, N

[a]N, nodule; P, papule; U, ulcer.

the HPV type. Papular lesions in MC develop largely from hyperproliferation of basal cells and retention of upper epidermal keratinocytes.

The poxvirus that causes MC is a double-stranded DNA virus that replicates in the cytoplasm of host epithelial cells (see Chapter 202, Poxviridae). The disease is acquired through direct contact with an infected person or from fomites and is spread by autoinoculation. School-aged children who are otherwise well and people with impaired cellular immune function are affected most commonly.[7] Children with a history of atopic dermatitis and impaired skin barrier function appear to be at greater risk for the development and spread of lesions. Moreover the pruritic nature of the underlying dermatitis makes children more likely to scratch the affected areas and autoinoculate through breaks in the skin. The incubation period is estimated to be 2 to 8 weeks but can be longer. One mechanism the MC virus uses to evade host mechanisms for killing virus-infected cells is its viral flice-like inhibitory protein (FLIP). Viral FLIPs inhibit apoptotic mediated cell death.[8,9]

The lesions of MC are discrete, pearly-pink, or skin-colored, dome-shaped papules varying in size from 1 to 5 mm (Figure 75-1), which upon close inspection have central umbilication. Lesions can coalesce into larger papules or become erythematous and inflamed. In some cases, a plug of cheesy whitish material can extrude from the center and may be mistaken for purulence. Papules can occur anywhere on the body, but there is predilection for the face, trunk, and sites where skin is in contact with other skin surfaces such as the thighs and axillae. When the lesions are found in clusters on the genitalia or in the groin of a sexually active adolescent, other sexually transmitted infections should be sought. Lesions commonly involve the genital area in children and frequently are not acquired by sexual transmission; however, an interview and examination for other signs that would suggest sexual abuse should be performed. Mild surrounding erythema or an eczematous dermatitis can accompany the papules. Lesions in children with the acquired immunodeficiency syndrome (AIDS) tend to be large and numerous, particularly on the face, and can have an atypical appearance which includes coalescent crusted lesions and large separate lesions on an erythematous base; exuberant lesions also occur in children with leukemia or other immunodeficiency.[10]

The diagnosis of MC often is made by the clinical finding of typical umbilicated papules; however, if lesions are clinically atypical, histologic confirmation may be warranted. On microscopic examination, the papule of MC consists of a lobulated mass of virus-infected epidermal cells. These eosinophilic viral inclusion bodies (Henderson–Patterson or molluscum bodies) become more prominent as infected keratinocytes move upward from the basal layer to the stratum corneum. This central plug of material, which is composed of virus-laden cells, can be shelled out from a lesion and examined under the microscope with 10% potassium hydroxide or with Wright or Giemsa stain. The rounded, cup-shaped mass of homogeneous cells, often with identifiable lobules, is diagnostic.

PART II Clinical Syndromes and Cardinal Features of Infectious Diseases: Approach to Diagnosis and Initial Management

SECTION J Skin and Soft-Tissue Infections

TABLE 75-3. Conditions with Sterile Papular, Nodular, or Ulcerative Skin Lesions After Infection

Disease Entity	Skin Lesions[a]	Infectious Agent
Autosensitization	P, N	See Box 75-3
Erythema elevatum diutinum	P, N	*Streptococcus pyogenes*
Erythema multiforme	P	See Chapter 74 (Urticaria and Erythema Multiforme)
Erythema nodosum	N	See Box 75-1
Gianotti–Crosti syndrome	P	See Box 75-2
Guttate psoriasis	P	*Streptococcus pyogenes*
Henoch–Schönlein purpura	P, N	*Streptococcus pyogenes*, cocksackievirus
Polyarteritis nodosa	P, N, U	*Streptococcus pyogenes*
Postscabitic nodule	P, N	*Sarcoptes scabiei*
Reiter disease		
Circinate balanitis	U	—[b]
Keratoderma blenorrhagicum	P, N	—[b]
Rheumatic fever	N	*Streptococcus pyogenes*
Unilateral laterothoracic exanthema	P	Multiple viral etiologies[c]
Urticaria	P	See Chapter 74 (Urticaria and Erythema Multiforme)
Common exanthem	P	Multiple viral etiologies[d]

[a]N, nodule; P, papule; U, ulcer.

[b]Sexually transmitted form follows infection with Chlamydia trachomatis. Postdysenteric form follows infection due to Salmonella and Shigella species, Yersinia enterocolitica, Yersinia pseudotuberculosis, Campylobacter fetus, and Clostridium difficile.

[c]Implicated agents Epstein–Barr virus, parainfluenza virus (PIV), adenovirus.

[d]Associated viruses include enteroviruses, EBV, human herpesviruses 6 and 7, and respiratory viruses such as RSV, PIV and adenovirus.

BOX 75-1. Infectious Agents Associated with Erythema Nodosum

BACTERIA

Bartonella henselae,[a] *Brucella* spp., *Campylobacter jejuni, Corynebacterium diphtheriae, Francisella tularensis, Haemophilus ducreyi, Leptospira interrogans, Neisseria meningitidis, Salmonella* spp., *Streptococcus pyogenes,*[a] *Yersinia enterocolitica,*[a] *Yersinia pseudotuberculosis*

CHLAMYDIA

Chlamydophila psittaci, Chlamydia trachomatis (lymphogranuloma venereum)

FUNGI

Blastomyces dermatitidis, Coccidioides immitis,[a] dermatophytoses (tinea capitis), *Histoplasma capsulatum, Sporothrix schenckii*

HELMINTHS

Ancylostoma duodenale, Necator americanus

MYCOBACTERIA

Mycobacterium leprae, M. marinum, M. tuberculosis[a]

MYCOPLASMA

Mycoplasma pneumoniae

PROTOZOA

Toxoplasma gondii

TREPONEME

Treponema pallidum

VIRUSES

Epstein–Barr virus; hepatitis viruses B, C; herpes simplex virus; mumps virus; paravaccinia virus

[a]Most common.

The differential diagnosis of molluscum contagiosum in an immunocompetent child includes noninfectious papules such as pilomatricoma, trichoepithelioma, ectopic sebaceous glands, syringoma, hidrocystoma, or an atypical melanocytic proliferation. In immunosuppressed individuals such as those with HIV infection, disseminated deep fungal infections such as cryptococcosis and histoplasmosis can be indistinguishable clinically from MC.

MC is a self-limited, epidermal disease. The average duration is 6 to 12 months, although lesions can persist for years,[11] can spread to distant sites, can become secondarily infected with bacteria, and can be transmitted to others. Affected persons should be advised to avoid sharing baths and towels until the infection has cleared. Infection can spread rapidly and produce hundreds of lesions in children with atopic dermatitis or immunodeficiency.[7] Treatment should be considered to eliminate symptoms of pruritus or discomfort in cases of molluscum dermatitis, to eliminate visible lesions, to prevent scarring, superinfection, acquisition of additional lesions, and spread to contacts. There are few randomized controlled studies to assess the effectiveness of various treatment modalities for molluscum contagiosum in children and the majority of reports are anecdotal. Common therapies include destructive, immunomodulatory, or antiviral measures. Spontaneous resolution or active management can result in postinflammatory pigment changes or a residual shallow atrophic scar. Cantharidin therapy is considered by many physicians to be a very effective therapy for lesions in certain locations due to its usually painless in-office application by a trained physician/provider as well as significant efficacy.[12,13] After application, treated lesions develop a superficial blister or significant enough inflammation to result in the loss of the infectious molluscum body. Additional in-office

destructive therapies include cryotherapy and curettage prior to which application of topical anesthetic is indicated to reduce discomfort. A brief, 6- to 9-second topical application of liquid nitrogen also is effective. The molluscum body also can be expressed with a needle, a sharp curette, or a comedo extractor. Once-daily topical application of retinoic acid product can incite an inflammatory response, which may lead to resolution of lesions. Cidofovir (both intravenous and topical) has been reported for the

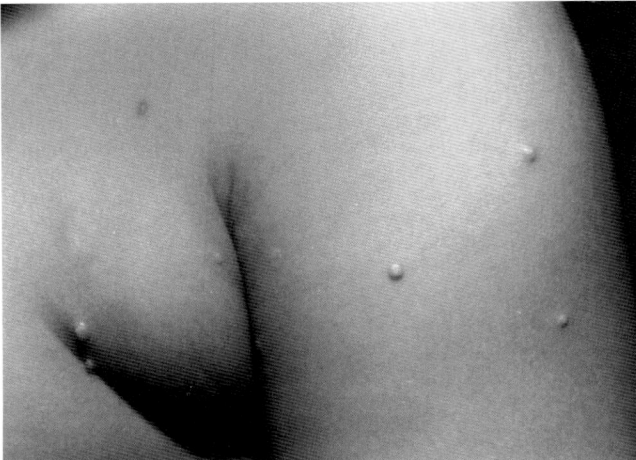

Figure 75-1. Umbilicated papules on the upper arm and chest of a child with molluscum contagiosum.

treatment of immunocompromised adults with severe recalcitrant MC. Due to significant side effects/toxicity, cidofovir is not indicated in healthy children with self-limited infections.[14] The role of topical application of imiquimod in children currently is under investigation.[15]

ERYTHEMA NODOSUM

Erythema nodosum is a form of panniculitis that typically manifests as the sudden appearance of tender, erythematous, 1- to 10-cm nodules usually located symmetrically on the extensor surfaces of the legs[16] (see Figure 160-1K). Less commonly, lesions can arise at other sites, including the trunk, upper extremities, and head and neck. Erythema nodosum is rare in children younger than 2 years and arises most frequently in the pediatric population during adolescence. Nodules typically enlarge over a few days, remain stable for 1 to 2 weeks, and then resolve gradually over 3 to 6 weeks with color changes that mimic a bruise. Ulceration, suppuration, and scarring do not occur, but residual hyperpigmentation can persist for weeks to months. Fever, chills, malaise, leukocytosis, and elevated erythrocyte sedimentation rate often are present.

Erythema nodosum is a hypersensitivity reaction caused by a variety of etiologies; however, in children in the United States it is most commonly associated with group A streptococcal pharyngitis (see Box 75-1). Infection precedes onset of erythema nodosum by approximately 3 weeks. A variety of other infectious agents have been associated with the erythema nodosum, most notably tuberculosis (worldwide),[17] coccidioidomycosis (in the southwestern U.S.), *Yersinia enterocolitica* (in Europe), cat-scratch disease *(Bartonella henselae)*, and tularemia. Erythema nodosum also can be associated with: (1) use of drugs, such as sulfonamides and oral contraceptive agents; (2) sarcoidosis and, occasionally, malignancies such as leukemia and lymphoma; and (3) systemic diseases, including Behçet disease, reactive arthritis, systemic lupus erythematosus, and inflammatory bowel disease. Differential diagnosis includes insect bite hypersensitivity reaction, lupus panniculitis, factitial panniculitis, superficial thrombophlebitis, polyarteritis nodosa, necrobiosis lipoidica diabeticorum, erythema induratum, erythema nodosum leprosum, and sarcoidosis. Sweet syndrome (painful, indurated cutaneous plaques accompanied by fever and leukocytosis) also should be considered. Sweet syndrome can be associated with hematologic malignancies or chronic recurrent multifocal osteomyelitis.[18,19]

The pathogenesis of erythema nodosum is poorly elucidated. Erythema nodosum is classified as a septal panniculitis without vasculitis and is regarded as an immunologic reaction to etiologic antigenic stimuli, most commonly group A streptococcal antigens in children.

Diagnosis usually is made clinically; however, skin biopsy can be useful to confirm the diagnosis and exclude other conditions. Histopathology reveals septal panniculitis without vasculitis, with inflammation and thickening of the fibrous septa of the subcutaneous fat. In early lesions the inflammatory infiltrate is predominantly composed of neutrophils. Lesions in a later stage show an infiltrate composed of lymphocytes, giant cells, and granulation tissue;[20] however, the changes of leukocytoclastic and lymphocytic angiitis are not present. Foreign body-type giant cells are typical.

Erythema nodosum is self-limited and usually resolves within 3 to 6 weeks. Recurrent erythema nodosum exists in children and can be due to repeated streptococcal infections. Attention should be directed to identifying and treating potential causes of the reaction. Nonsteroidal anti-inflammatory agents may provide symptomatic relief. Leg elevation and bedrest may minimize lower-extremity edema and, thus, decrease discomfort. Potassium iodide treatment may hasten resolution of the nodules.[21]

GIANOTTI–CROSTI SYNDROME

Gianotti–Crosti syndrome, also known as *papular acrodermatitis of childhood* (PAC), is characterized by erythematous papules which are distributed symmetrically on the extremities, buttocks, and

---

BOX 75-2. Infectious Agents Associated with Gianotti–Crosti Syndrome

IMMUNIZATIONS

Calmette-Guérin bacillus, diphtheria, tetanus, pertussis, MMR, Haemophilus b, hepatitis B, hepatitis A, oral poliomyelitis, Japanese B encephalitis, influenza

VIRUSES

Adenoviruses[a]; coxsackievirus A16, B4, B5[a]; cytomegalovirus; echovirus 7, 9[a]; Epstein–Barr virus[a]; hepatitis virus A, B[a]; HHV6; human immunodeficiency virus; parainfluenza viruses[a]; parvovirus B19; poliovirus; respiratory syncytial virus[a]; rotavirus

[a]Most common.

---

face of children. The syndrome initially was reported in association with hepatitis B (HBV) infection. However, since then a variety of viral infections, frequently infections of the upper respiratory tract. as well as immunizations have been associated (Box 75-2). In the U.S., the eruption is not commonly associated with HBV and the association has become rare since universal HBV immunization during infancy. In the U.S., Epstein–Barr virus infection typically is reported as the most common cause of Gianotti–Crosti syndrome.[22]

The disorder classically presents with the sudden eruption of symmetric, flat-topped, discrete, erythematous, 2- to 10-mm papules on the face, upper and lower extremities, and buttocks. The trunk and antecubital and popliteal fossae usually are spared. Pruritus and the Koebner phenomenon (accentuation of lesions at sites of trauma) can be present. Peak incidence is between 1 and 4 years of age. Differential diagnosis includes lichen planus, lichen nitidus, lichenoid dermatitis or drug eruption, and Langerhans cell histiocytosis.

The pathogenesis of the syndrome has been suggested to involve an immune-reactive process, perhaps mediated by immune complexes or due to a delayed hypersensitivity response.[23] In the form associated with HBV infection, however, lesions have not yielded evidence of immune complex vasculitis, and the surface antigen has not been demonstrated in skin lesions.

The syndrome generally is self-limited, resolving within 3 to 6 weeks. Lesions occasionally can persist for a few months, and relapses, although rare, have been reported. Treatment is supportive and will not shorten the course of the skin lesions. Orally administered antihistamines may provide symptomatic relief.

OTHER EXANTHEMATOUS INFECTIONS

Although beyond the scope of this chapter, it deserves mention that numerous infectious etiologies can manifest in the skin with a papular, or less commonly, ulcerative eruption. The classic bilaterally symmetric exanthem or "morbilliform" eruption classically progresses cephalocaudad and often is due to one of a variety of viral etiologies[24] (see Chapter 71, Erythematous Macules and Papules). Often careful history and review of systems can elicit the necessary signs and symptoms to determine the underlying infectious agent. Morphologically unique eruptions such as unilateral laterothoracic exanthem (asymmetric periflexural exanthem) deserve recognition with thought to possible underlying infectious causes. In addition, exanthems may present atypically in an ulcerative fashion, as in the setting of bacterial superinfection of primary vesicular lesions of HSV or VZV infections. In addition to viral etiologies, bacterial infections, such as group A streptococcus, can be associated with exanthems, such as the papular eruption of scarlet fever.

AUTOSENSITIZATION/ID REACTION

A symmetric papular or papulovesicular cutaneous eruption can arise at a site distant to the site of primary dermatitis and is known

---

BOX 75-3. Infectious Agents Associated with a Papular or Nodular Autosensitization ("Id") Reaction

FUNGI

Blastomyces dermatitidis, Candida albicans, Coccidioides immitis, Epidermophyton floccosum, Histoplasma capsulatum, Sporothrix schenckii, Trichophyton mentagrophytes,[a] *T. rubrum,*[a] *T. tonsurans*[a]

MYCOBACTERIA

Mycobacterium bovis, M. leprae, M. tuberculosis

PROTOZOA

Leishmania spp.

TREPONEMES

Treponema carateum

[a]Most common.

---

as autosensitization or "*id*" reaction. This reaction is felt to be due to hematogenously circulating products and/or the resultant host immune response. Most commonly triggered by noninfectious etiologies such as a contact dermatitis, id reaction can occur in response to infectious processes such as dermatophyte or bacterial infections.

Id reactions are inflammatory autosensitivity reactions of the skin thought to occur in association with dermatophytosis but at sites distant from infection (Box 75-3).[24,25] Epidermal cytokines released from sites of skin infection have been implicated as causing the heightened sensitivity of skin, at sites distant from the site of infection, to a variety of stimuli that would usually be innocuous. Culture and potassium hydroxide examination of id lesions do not reveal the organism, but *Trichophyton* skin reactivity is positive. The most common dermatophyte infection triggering a dermatophytid reaction is tinea pedis, although id lesions also can occur in the setting of tinea capitis and tinea corporis.

Tuberculid reactions are another example of autosensitization;[17] these reactions, however, appear to differ in genesis from dermatophytid reactions. Skin lesions are rare, usually appearing in a host who: (1) has moderate to strong tuberculin reactivity; (2) has a history of previous tuberculous infection of other organs; and (3) usually, but not always, has shown a therapeutic response to antituberculous therapy. Lesions exhibit tuberculoid features histologically but do not contain detectable mycobacteria, although organisms may be detected with methods such as polymerase chain reaction. Tuberculid reactions are postulated to result from hematogenous dissemination of bacilli during a transient waning of immunity; they represent the paucibacillary pole of disease.[17] Rapid local destruction may account for the absence of bacilli within lesions.

The most commonly observed tuberculid is *erythema induratum*, a panniculitis associated with tuberculosis infection. Unlike erythema nodosum, erythema induratum has a predilection for the posterior aspect of the lower extremities, and is more common in female patients. Both erythema induratum and the papulonecrotic tuberculid (vesicular eczema) form often are associated with pulmonary tuberculosis. In papulonecrotic tuberculid, recurrent crops of symmetrically distributed, asymptomatic, firm, sterile, dusky red papules appear on the extensor aspects of the limbs, the dorsum of the hands and feet, and the buttocks. They may represent the paucibacillary form of intravascular dissemination. Papules can undergo central ulceration and eventually heal, leaving sharply delineated, circular, depressed scars. Lesions are characterized histopathologically by a wedge-shaped area of upper dermal necrosis, with the broad base toward the epidermis, surrounded by a tuberculoid inflammatory infiltrate. Obliterative vasculitis is noted in the deep dermis. The duration of the eruption is variable, but lesions usually disappear promptly after treatment of the primary infection.

Lichen scrofulosorum, another form of tuberculid, is characterized by asymptomatic, grouped, pinhead-sized, often follicular, pink or red papules that form plaques, mainly on the trunk. Healing occurs without scarring. On histopathologic examination, granulomas are seen in the superficial dermis, often surrounding follicles and ducts of sweat glands. The inflammatory infiltrate contains epithelioid cells, giant cells, and a rim of lymphocytes. Caseation generally is absent. These lesions can be difficult to distinguish both clinically and histopathologically from lichenoid sarcoidosis.

In addition to dermatophytids and tuberculids, autosensitization has been reported with bacterial (e.g., pharyngitis), spirochetal (e.g., syphilis), and viral infections (e.g., molluscum contagiosum).[26] These reactions also can occur in response to noninfectious stimuli. One common pediatric example is an id reaction occurring with severe contact dermatitis to nickel. In this particular example, an eczematous dermatitis can occur at sites distant from the affected area of contact dermatitis.

Acknowledgment

The authors acknowledge significant use of the work of G.L. Darmstadt, J. Browning, and M. Levy from previous editions.

---

76 Subcutaneous Tissue Infections and Abscesses

Catalina Matiz and Sheila Fallon Friedlander

Infection of soft tissues can involve the skin, subcutaneous tissues and fascia, skeletal muscle, or a combination of these structures. The *subcutaneous compartment* is continuous over the entire body and consists of fat and loose connective tissue containing blood and lymphatic vessels, underlying the dermis.[1] The *fascia* is subdivided into superficial and deep components. The *superficial fascia*, between the dermis and the deep fascia, is further subdivided into two layers. The outer layer, of variable thickness, contains loose collagenous tissue and fat. The inner layer of the superficial fascia is a thin membrane that has relatively little fat but is rich in elastic tissue. Superficial arteries, veins, nerves, and lymphatics lie within the superficial fascia. The *deep fascia* is a membranous sheet surrounding muscles and separating them into functioning units and forming the deepest boundary of the subcutaneous tissue compartment.

Infections of the skin and subcutaneous tissues can be classified by site of involvement (Box 76-1) and as primary, secondary, or tertiary depending on the mechanism of infection. *Primary*

BOX 76-1. Subcutaneous Tissue Infections and Abscesses

CUTANEOUS/SUBCUTANEOUS ABSCESSES
Breast abscess
Carbuncle[a]
Furuncle[a]
Paronychia[a]
Periporitis (sweat gland abscess)
Perirectal abscess

SCALP ABSCESS
NON-NECROTIZING SUBCUTANEOUS TISSUE INFECTIONS
Cellulitis
Erysipelas
Secondarily infected ulcers: decubitus, diabetic
Folliculitis

NECROTIZING SUPRAFASCIAL INFECTIONS
Anaerobic cellulitis
- Clostridial
- Nonclostridial
Bacterial synergistic gangrene
- Meleney ulcer
Gangrenous cellulitis
Necrotizing fasciitis
- Type I: mixed flora (85% polymicrobial)
- Type II: *Streptococcus pyogenes* and *Staphylococcus aureus*
- Other monomicrobial infections (see text)
Fournier gangrene
- Nomab
- Tropical ulcer

NECROTIZING DEEP FASCIAL AND MUSCLE INFECTIONS
Synergistic necrotizing cellulitis
Myositis[b]
Pyomyositis[b]

BOX 76-2. Predisposing Factors for Subcutaneous Tissue Infections and Abscesses

Alteration of normal skin flora
Burn wound
Chronic dermatoses
Corticosteroid therapy
Foreign body
Immunodeficiency diseases
Chédiak–Higashi syndrome[a]
Chronic granulomatous disease[a]
Congenital neutropenia[a]
Cyclic neutropenia[a]
Griscelli syndrome
Hyperimmunoglobulin E syndrome[a]
Leukocyte adhesion deficiency[a]
Leukocyte alkaline phosphatase deficiency[a]
Neutrophil-specific granule deficiency[a]
Transient hypogammaglobulinemia of infancy[a]
Wiskott–Aldrich syndrome[a]
X-linked hypogammaglobulinemia[a]
Multiple innate immune defects
Intravenous drug abuse
Malnutrition
Peripheral vascular disease
Obstruction of drainage
Ischemia
Skin trauma
Surgical wound
Circumcision
Umbilical cord stump
Systemic disease
Cachexia
Cirrhosis
Diabetes mellitus
Neoplasia
Leukemia, lymphoma
Solid tumor
Organ transplantation
Renal tubular acidosis
Renal failure

ᵃAssociated with abscess formation.

infections originate directly in skin that appears to be clinically normal, although minor breaks in the integrity of the barrier function may be required (see Chapter 70, Superficial Skin Infections and Cellulitis). Some infections, such as folliculitis, furunculosis, carbunculosis, and paronychia, evolve into abscesses and occasionally extend from the epidermis or dermis to involve deeper subcutaneous tissues. *Secondary* infections, which occur in previously diseased or wounded skin, include infection of cysts (e.g., epidermal inclusion or pilar cyst), ulcers (e.g., decubitus ulcer), wounds (e.g., surgical or traumatic wound, burn, scalp electrode site, arthropod, animal, or human bite, or burrow due to scabies, flies, or fleas), and dermatitis (e.g., atopic dermatitis, psoriasis). These infections also can spread contiguously to deeper subcutaneous tissue. *Tertiary* infection develops when pathogens are spread hematogenously or via lymphatics to soft tissues from a distant focus (e.g., *Clostridium septicum* necrotizing fasciitis or myonecrosis, *Staphylococcus aureus* abscess). These infections can involve any of the deeper soft tissues, but generally they spare direct involvement of the epidermis. Compromise of blood flow of nutrient vessels or extension of an infectious and inflammatory nidus to the epidermis and dermis, however, can result in cutaneous disease. Multiple conditions predispose to subcutaneous tissue infections and abscesses (Box 76-2).

ETIOLOGY

The exact etiology of abscesses and subcutaneous infections in children is not always clear. A study of 242 hospitalized infants and children 1 to 180 months of age with soft-tissue infections found that 10% had subcutaneous abscesses, most commonly occurring in the cervical, scalp, and perirectal area. The most commonly identified abscess pathogens in this study were *S. aureus* and *Streptococcus pyogenes*.[2] Identification of the pathogen(s) causing a particular subcutaneous soft-tissue infection or, in some cases, exclusion of a variety of noninfectious conditions in the differential diagnosis of subcutaneous tissue infections (Box 76-3), requires proper use of diagnostic tests and interpretation of results. If the surface of a wound or site of infection is sampled with a swab, a number of organisms can be isolated that are colonizing the area but are not contributing to the disease process. If an organism is identified on both Gram stain (or special stains in the case of fungi) and culture, the likelihood of its pathogenicity is increased. Chances of identifying the true pathogen are improved further if culture specimens are obtained by

PART II Clinical Syndromes and Cardinal Features of Infectious Diseases: Approach to Diagnosis and Initial Management

SECTION J Skin and Soft-Tissue Infections

BOX 76-3. Noninfectious Diseases in the Differential Diagnosis of Subcutaneous Tissue Infections in Infants and Children

Acne conglobata
Acne fulminans
Hidradenitis suppurativa
Majocchi granuloma
Jellyfish, scorpion, snake, spider (brown recluse) bites
Factitial disease
Panniculitis
Polyarteritis nodosa
Purpura fulminans
Pyoderma gangrenosum
Sweet syndrome (acute febrile neutrophilic dermatosis)

BOX 76-4. Agents of Subcutaneous Abscesses and Decubitus Ulcers in Infants and Children

BACTERIA

Common

Staphylococcus aureus (CA-MRSA and CA-MSSA)
Streptococcus pyogenes, streptococci (α-hemolytic, nonhemolytic), group B streptococcus

Infrequent and rare

Aeromonas hydrophilia
Actinomyces
Bacteroides fragilis
Brucella
Clostridium
Eikenella corrodens
Enterococcus
Fusobacterium
Haemophilus parainfluenzae
Mycobacterium
Neisseria gonorrhoeae
Nocardia
Peptococcus
Peptostreptococcus
Porphyromonas
Prevotella
Propionibacterium acnes
Pseudomonas aeruginosa
P. mallei
P. pseudomallei

FUNGI

Aspergillus
Candida
Histoplasma capsulatum
Hyalohyphomycoses
Penicillium marnefei
Phaeohyphomycoses
Pseudallescheria boydii
Rhizopus

MYCOPLASMA

Mycoplasma hominis

PROTOZOA

Entamoeba histolytica

decontaminating the skin and then swabbing the exudate from a site of suppuration, by fine-needle aspiration, or by excisional biopsy.[3] Cultures should be obtained for both routine and fastidious, aerobic and anaerobic organisms when appropriate. Susceptibility testing should be performed to guide antibiotic therapy except for anaerobes and *S. pyogenes* (unless therapy other than with a β-lactam agent is contemplated).

This chapter describes infections that lead to abscess formation and tissue necrosis involving subcutaneous tissues as deep as the inner layer of the superficial fascia. Infections that commonly extend into the deep fascia and muscle are covered elsewhere (e.g., see Chapter 77, Myositis, Pyomyositis, and Necrotizing Fasciitis).

ABSCESSES

An *abscess* is a localized, usually inflamed, "walled-off" collection of pus formed by disintegration or necrosis of tissue. An abscess is recognized clinically by the presence of a firm, tender, erythematous nodule that is fluctuant. The initial skin lesion commonly can be mistaken for a "spider bite." A subcutaneous abscess most commonly evolves by local extension of a primary infectious process in the epidermis or dermis, such as a cutaneous abscess originating from a skin appendage (e.g., furuncle, carbuncle, infundibular cyst, periporitis) or secondarily from a site of skin disease or injury. A subcutaneous abscess also can arise by direct traumatic implantation or invasion of pathogens into subcutaneous tissue or, occasionally, by hematogenous spread.

In the patient with an abscess, constitutional symptoms generally are absent, unless the process has extended into deeper tissues or the bloodstream. Often, no predisposing factor can be identified, although a number of processes that disrupt the integrity of the barrier function of the skin or the integrity of local immunologic processes, particularly neutrophil function, are associated with abscess formation. Despite the extensive list of immunodeficiency diseases associated with abscess formation, the vast majority of individuals with recurrent abscesses lack evidence of immunodeficiency.

Pathogenesis

The principal pathogens of subcutaneous abscesses in children are shown in Box 76-4 and vary with body site. The single most common pathogen is *S. aureus*.[4] Community-associated methicillin resistant *S. aureus* (CA-MRSA) is responsible for >60% of the cases of abscesses in children in certain centers in the United States.[5,6] CA-MRSA possesses the staphylococcal cassette chromosome mec (SCCmec) (type IV–V), which contains the *mecA* gene complex responsible for antibiotic resistance. The USA300 clone is the most common clone in the U.S. that causes skin and soft-tissue infections.[7] CA-MRSA abscess formation is thought to be associated with the presence of Panton-Valentine leukocidin (PVL), which causes leukocyte destruction and tissue necrosis, as well as α type phenol-soluble modulins (PSM). The

presence of the type I argine catabolic mobile element (ACME) promotes growth and survival of clone US300 within the skin and enables this bacteria to colonize human skin.[8,9] Table 76-1 shows groups at risk for CA-MRSA skin and soft-tissue infections. As the epidemic of CA-MRSA spread, many affected children have no risk factors.

Occasionally, anaerobic bacteria appear to act alone to cause abscesses. Encapsulated anaerobic bacteria generally appear to be most important.[10] This finding contrasts markedly with observations in superficial skin infections in children, in which anaerobic bacteria play little pathogenic role.[11] Likewise, anaerobic bacteria do not appear to be capable of acting alone to cause necrotizing soft-tissue infections in immunocompetent people.[12] In general, cultures from perineal or perioral abscesses and ulcers in both children and adults contain organisms that reside normally on adjacent mucous membranes rather than skin, whereas lesions remote from the rectum or mouth primarily contain organisms that reside normally on skin at that site.[4,13–19]

TABLE 76-1. Antibiotic Therapy for Cutaneous Abscesses in Era of Community-Associated Methicillin-Resistant *Staphylococcus aureus* Infections[a] [99-103]

	Antibiotic	Clinical Remarks
Empiric therapy	Clindamycin	Depending on geographic rates of resistance
	Trimethoprim-sulfmethoxazole	TMP-SMX alone has no coverage against group A streptococcus. Could be used in combination with a β-lactam agent
	Doxycycline	For children ≥8 years of age
	Minocycline	For children ≥8 years of age
	Linezolid	
Hospitalized patients	Vancomycin	Gold standard for hospitalized patients
	Linezolid, PO and IV	
	Daptomycin	For patients intolerant to vancomycin or for vancomycin-resistant *Staphylococcus aureus*
	Clindamycin	Depending on low rate of resistance (<10%)

[a]*Modified from reference 22.*

Overall, the most common aerobic and facultative bacteria isolated from cutaneous and subcutaneous abscesses and decubitus ulcers in children are CA-MRSA and CA-MSSA and *S. pyogenes*. Streptococci (α-hemolytic and nonhemolytic), *Enterococcus* spp., enteric gram-negative bacilli, *Pseudomonas aeruginosa*, and anaerobes are associated especially with decubitus ulcers.[4,18] Immunocompromised hosts are at risk of abscess formation due to a broader spectrum of pathogenic microbes, including fungi (Box 76-4).[20]

Management

Incision and drainage (I&D) of abscesses less than 5 cm in a healthy host may be the only therapeutic approach necessary.[21] Systemic antibiotic therapy also is recommended if the abscess is larger than 5 cm or the patient has signs and symptoms of illness, rapid progression, associated comorbidities or immunosuppression, abscess in an area difficult to drain (e.g., face, hand, genitalia), or associated phlebitis.[22] Because of the prevalence of CA-MRSA, clindamycin is the initial treatment of choice in geographic areas where CA-MRSA generally is susceptible to clindamycin. Trimethropim-sulfamethoxazole often is used, but may be inferior; antistaphylococcal therapy is not an option if streptococcal infection is suspected. Guidelines for treatment of CA-MRSA skin and soft-tissue infections from the Infectious Diseases Society of America and endorsed by the American Academy of Pediatrics are shown in Table 76-1.[22] More aggressive therapy for skin abscesses is recommended in immunocompromised patients, patients with recurrent furunculosis, very young patients, or patients who appear ill. Intravenous therapy should be reserved for those with moderate to severe disease, or those unable to tolerate oral medications.

Considerations by Clinical Site

Breast Abscess

Breast abscess is an uncommon infection of neonates usually due to *S. aureus* and occasionally caused by group A or B streptococcus, *Escherichia coli*, *Salmonella* spp., *Proteus mirabilis*, or *P. aeruginosa*.

Although anaerobic organisms can be isolated from up to 40% of infections, their pathogenic role in neonates is questionable, and therapy directed specifically against anaerobes usually is unnecessary.[23,24]

Breast abscess develops in full-term neonates during the first 6 weeks of life, most commonly during the second to third week.[23-27] Incidence of breast abscess is twofold higher in girls overall, but is approximately equal in boys and girls during the first 2 weeks of life.[25] Physiologic breast enlargement, which is more common in infant girls than in boys after, but not before, 2 weeks of age,[28] is probably a factor in the pathogenesis, as also is evidenced by the absence of both breast enlargement and breast abscess in premature infants.[25] Other factors are involved, however, because a relatively large retrospective review of neonates with breast abscess found that only about one-half had breast enlargement before development of abscess.[25] It is likely that organisms from the nasopharynx or umbilicus colonize the skin of the nipple and move retrograde via glandular ducts of physiologically enlarged breasts.[29]

Breast enlargement, accompanied by varying degrees of erythema, induration, and tenderness, is present initially and can progress to fluctuation, depending in part on how promptly antibiotic therapy is initiated. Bilateral infection is extremely rare. Fever or constitutional symptoms, such as irritability and toxicity, are present in approximately one-third of cases, although leukocytosis (WBC >15,000 cells/mm^3) is found in approximately one-half to two-thirds.[23] Breast abscess due to *S. aureus* is accompanied by cutaneous pustules or bullae on the trunk, particularly in the periumbilical or perineal region, in 25% to 50% of patients.[25] The symptoms, age at presentation, and clinical findings for infections due to gram-negative bacilli or anaerobes are similar to those for staphylococcal abscesses, except that infants infected with *Salmonella* spp. also can have gastrointestinal symptoms.[27]

The most common complication of breast abscess is cellulitis, which develops in approximately 5% to 10% of affected infants.[25] Cellulitis generally is localized but rarely can extend rapidly over the shoulder or abdomen.[26] Other complications, such as bloodstream infection (BSI), pneumonia and osteomyelitis, are unusual. Scar formation leading to decreased breast size after puberty can be a late sequela.[25]

Results of Gram stain and culture of material expressed from the nipple or obtained by needle aspiration or incision and drainage help guide antibiotic therapy. If the lesion is fluctuant, the abscess must be drained; antibiotic therapy is adjunctive. If fluctuation is absent, antibiotic therapy alone may be curative. Warm compresses also may be beneficial. In areas with a high incidence of MRSA infections, systemic vancomycin or clindamycin is given; otherwise, nafcillin (or cefazolin if there is no concern for BSI or meningitis) is an option for MSSA. If gram-negative bacilli or no organisms are seen on Gram stain or if the infant appears ill, initial therapy also should include an aminoglycoside agent or other antibiotic with gram-negative bacillary coverage. In most instances, a 5- to 7-day course of therapy is sufficient, although total course of therapy sometimes is 10 to 14 days; duration of parenteral therapy depends on the isolate, the presence of BSI and the clinical course.

Sweat Gland Abscess (Periporitis)

Sweat gland abscesses develop rarely in neonates, most often in association with malnutrition or debilitation.[30] The infection also has been termed *periporitis staphylogenes* because of the almost uniform presence of *S. aureus* in the lesions. It appears that lesions of miliaria become infected secondarily, followed by extension of the infection into the sweat gland apparatus and, occasionally, into the adjacent subcutaneous tissue. Miliaria-like lesions, however, are not a constant feature. The 1- to 2-cm, round to oval nodular abscesses occur most commonly on the neck, occiput, back, and buttocks, and unlike furuncles and carbuncles of follicular origin, they are nontender, nonpointing, and cold. Constitutional symptoms can accompany numerous large abscesses, and

PART II Clinical Syndromes and Cardinal Features of Infectious Diseases: Approach to Diagnosis and Initial Management

SECTION J Skin and Soft-Tissue Infections

lymphangitis or cellulitis occurs rarely. Therapy consists of control of factors such as skin occlusion or fever that predispose to miliaria, correction of malnutrition, local care of abscesses, and use of antistaphylococcal antibiotics. Healing occurs over several weeks, generally without scarring.

Axillary abscesses occur predominantly in adolescents, accounting for 6.7% of 564 culture-positive abscesses in patients evaluated in one urban emergency department. In this report 76% were female; although 46% of axillary abscesses were due to CA-MRSA and 24% to MSSA, a surprising 22% were caused by *Proteus mirabilis*.[31]

Perineal Abscess

Most abscesses of the perineal (inguinal, buttock, perirectal, vulvovaginal) region contain multiple species of facultative and anaerobic fecal organisms, particularly *Bacteroides* spp. In recent years, CA-MRSA has become a prevalent cause of superficial genitourinary abscesses in children. Perineal abscesses generally require surgical debridement, cure rates are high and morbidity is low.[32] Antibiotic therapy is adjunctive.

Perirectal Abscess

Perirectal abscesses most commonly affect children <2 years of age, with an incidence that can reach 4%, and a notable predilection to affect males. This is thought to occur because of a congenital anomaly of the anal crypts, an imbalance of the androgen:estrogen ratio or an excess of the former. Others have postulated that perirectal abscesses occur secondary to local infection of a crypt following trauma to the area.[33]

There may be no apparent predisposing factor, or the abscess can develop after minor abrasions or fissures, particularly in association with diarrhea or constipation. Older children who experience perirectal abscess more frequently have a predisposing condition: Crohn disease, neutropenia (in association with cancer, autoimmunity, or chemotherapy), neutrophil dysfunction due to immunodeficiency, acquired immunodeficiency syndrome, diabetes mellitus, corticosteroid therapy, ulcerative colitis, hidradenitis suppurativa, or prior rectal surgery. In those with neutropenia, the risk of perirectal abscess or cellulitis increases with the presence of perirectal mucositis, hemorrhoids, rectal fissure, or manipulation. A break in the mucosal barrier or occlusion of anal crypts usually initiates infection.

The predominant organisms in perirectal abscesses are mixed anaerobic and aerobic flora of the intestine and skin of the anal verge. The most common agent identified is *E. coli* alone or in combination with streptococci, enterococci or anaerobes, followed by *S. aureus*. Other implicated organisms include *S. pyogenes*, *P. aeruginosa*, *Klebsiella* spp., *Proteus* spp. Anaerobic bacteria include *Bacteroides*, *Peptococcus*, *Peptostreptococcus*, *Porphyromonas*, *Fusobacterium*, and *Clostridium* species.[34-38] Perirectal abscess rarely can be due to *Entamoeba histolytica*, *Mycobacterium* spp., *Nocardia* spp., and *Actinomyces* spp. Buttock abscesses are most commonly due to *S. aureus*, even in the neonate.[34]

Superficial buttock abscess in the infant usually manifests as pain on defecation, sitting, or walking and the presence of redness, swelling, and tenderness in the perianal region. A superficial abscess in the epithelium potentially can extend in any of the following directions: inferiorly along the anal sphincter to exit next to the anus on the buttock (fistula in ano), laterally through the external sphincter to the ischiorectal fossa to form a deep abscess, or superiorly to the deep space between the internal sphincter and the levator ani muscles.[39-41] An abscess in deeper tissues can be accompanied by poorly localized, deep pain and constitutional symptoms. An anorectal abscess may not be apparent externally, but pain generally is elicited upon rectal examination.

In immunocompetent infants, a superficial perianal abscess can drain spontaneously (and can be self-limited) or may need to be drained surgically. Exploration of the abscess for fistula depends on clinical circumstances and isolation of organisms other than *S. aureus*. Empiric therapy with antibiotics to cover anaerobic and aerobic gram-negative bacilli and *S. aureus* may prevent regional spread of the infection and decrease the incidence of complications.[35] A 7- to 10-day course of therapy is recommended. Children with granulocytopenia may have delayed development of erythema, induration, and fluctuation. In the absence of fluctuation, extensive soft-tissue disease, or BSI, a trial of parenteral antimicrobial therapy alone may be initiated. Perirectal abscess in young children is less likely associated with underlying anatomic anomalies, and more amenable to complete resolution with conservative nonoperative therapies. However, if progression of disease or fluctuation becomes apparent, surgery should be undertaken. Complications, which occur more commonly in children with underlying disease, include anorectal fistula, recurrence of abscess, BSI, and necrotizing fasciitis. There is some evidence that conservative treatment with systemic antibiotics rather than drainage may be associated with a decreased risk of fistula formation in infants <12 months of age.[42] A chronic fistula may require a fistulotomy.[40]

Scalp Abscess

Scalp abscess appears as a localized, erythematous area of induration 0.5 to 2 cm in diameter usually at the insertion site of a fetal scalp monitoring electrode. The site can become fluctuant, pustular, or suppurative. Presentation occurs most commonly on the third or fourth day of life (range, 1 day to 3 weeks).[43] Regional lymphadenopathy can be present, but other, more serious complications, such as cranial osteomyelitis, subgaleal abscess, and necrotizing fasciitis of the scalp, are uncommon. Death associated with a complication of fetal scalp electrode placement has been described in a premature infant who had *E. coli* scalp abscess and BSI.[44]

The incidence of scalp abscess after placement of a spiral fetal scalp electrode (the type used since the early 1970s) ranged from 0.1% to 1.0% in retrospective studies of approximately 18,000 neonates;[43] prospective studies have reported the incidence to be 0.6%[45] and 4.5%.[46] Reported presence of predisposing factors is conflicting. Okada and associates[46] found significant association with longer duration of placental membrane rupture and of monitoring; monitoring for high-risk indications, particularly prematurity; and nulliparous birth, possibly because of a higher risk of infection of an edematous, hypoxic caput succedaneum. Scalp trauma and compression per se, however, are questionable factors in the pathogenesis of scalp abscess, because most reports have not noted abscess formation at sites of scalp trauma and abrasion due to forceps or vacuum extraction, at sites of fetal blood sampling, or in association with hematomas.[43,47] There are exceptions, because cephalohematomas can become infected,[48] and similar rates of scalp abscess have been reported among infants who were monitored with scalp electrodes and those who were not monitored but were delivered by forceps or vacuum extraction.[49] A threefold greater but not statistically significant rate of scalp abscess has been noted among infants delivered by vacuum extraction compared with those born by spontaneous vaginal delivery.[46] In one study,[50] but not another,[45] an association with prolonged rupture of membranes and development of scalp abscess was found. Risk factors in the latter study included number of vaginal examinations, concurrent monitoring with an intrauterine pressure catheter, use of more than one spiral electrode, fetal scalp blood sampling, maternal diabetes, and endomyometritis.[45]

Scalp abscess typically is a polymicrobial infection. Cultures from abscesses reveal aerobic or facultative organisms alone in approximately one-third, anaerobic isolates alone in 10% to 25% and mixed aerobic or facultative and anaerobic bacteria in 40% to 60%.[43,46,51] The most common aerobic isolates are *S. aureus*, groups A, B, or D streptococci, *S. epidermidis*, and, occasionally, *Haemophilus influenzae*, *E. coli*, *K. pneumoniae*, *Enterobacter* spp., *P. aeruginosa*, and *Neisseria gonorrhoeae*. The role of *S. epidermidis* as a pathogen is questionable. Common anaerobic isolates are *Peptococcus*, *Peptostreptococcus*, and *Bacteroides* species, *Propionibacterium acnes*, and *Clostridium* spp. The anaerobic flora in the abscesses reflects that found in cervical flora during labor. Neonatal necrotizing fasciitis of the scalp has been reported in association with intrapartum fetal scalp electrode monitoring.[52]

The primary differential diagnostic concern in fetal scalp abscess is herpes simplex virus (HSV) infection.[43] The time of appearance of herpetic lesions (peak incidence, 4 to 10 days) overlaps with that for scalp abscess, and the lesions occasionally can be indistinguishable clinically. Mucocutaneous HSV can be associated with central nervous system or disseminated disease or both.[53] If suspicion of HSV exists, complete evaluation and therapy with acyclovir should be initiated while awaiting results of diagnostic tests.

Infants who are subjected to scalp electrode monitoring during birth should be followed closely during the first weeks of life for evidence of infection. Parents should be instructed in surveillance. If weeping, vesiculopustular lesions or abscess is noted, specimens should be obtained by needle aspiration or swabbing of the exudates from the puncture site for direct testing and culture obtained for both aerobic and anaerobic organisms and HSV. Many bacterial infections of the fetal scalp resolve spontaneously, but if fluctuance develops without spontaneous suppuration, incision and drainage may be necessary; extensive debridement, however, should not be performed. If surrounding cellulitis is present, a 5- to 7-day course of parenteral antibiotic therapy usually is sufficient, with culture results guiding antibiotic choice. HSV scalp lesions can also heal spontaneously, but reactivation or dissemination or both can occur, with serious consequences; therefore parenteral acyclovir therapy always should be administered.

NECROTIZING CELLULITIS AND SUBCUTANEOUS TISSUE INFECTION

Clinical Distinction and Etiology

Necrotizing soft-tissue infections are potentially life-threatening conditions characterized by rapidly advancing, local tissue destruction and systemic toxicity. Tissue necrosis distinguishes them from cellulitis (see Chapter 70, Superficial Skin Infections and Cellulitis), in which an inflammatory infectious process involves but does not destroy subcutaneous tissues. Unlike an abscess, necrotizing soft-tissue infections involve diffuse tissue necrosis and lack localized purulence, although a subcutaneous abscess occasionally can form. Such infections can occur anywhere on the body, the most common locations being the extremities, abdomen, and perineal region. Risk is highest in immunocompromised hosts, either systemic or of localized compromise, particularly in those who have diabetes mellitus, neoplasia, peripheral vascular disease, have undergone recent surgery, or are receiving immunosuppressive treatment (especially with corticosteroids). Necrotizing soft-tissue infections also can occur in healthy individuals at enterostomy sites or after: minor puncture wounds, abrasions, or lacerations; vesicular viral infections; blunt trauma; surgical procedures, particularly of the abdomen, gastrointestinal, or genitourinary tracts, or perineum; or needle injections. Since the mid-1980s, there has been a resurgence of fulminant necrotizing soft-tissue infections due to S. pyogenes and most recently due to Panton–Valentine leukocidin-positive S. aureus, often in healthy individuals with little (e.g., varicella-zoster virus infection) or no apparent immunologic deficiency or compromise of skin integrity. Bacterial virulence factors as well as absence of specific host resistance factors appear to be important in the pathogenesis.[54]

Necrotizing soft-tissue infections form a continuum, some developing primarily in the more superficial layers of the subcutaneous tissues and others typically extending to the deep fascia and muscle. Although the rapidity and extent of tissue destruction as well as the causative agent vary, patients characteristically manifest a paucity of early cutaneous signs relative to the rapidity and extent of destruction of the subcutaneous tissues. Early clinical findings include ill-defined cutaneous erythema and edema that extends beyond the area of erythema. In some circumstances the contiguous surface may be anesthetic or develop bullae. In

distinction to clinical findings of cellulitis, which may have a more distinct border, the patient with necrotizing soft-tissue infection has pain, tenderness, and constitutional signs that often are out of proportion to the cutaneous findings. This is particularly true with involvement of the deeper tissues, such as deep fascia and muscle.

In general, patients with involvement of the superficial or deep fascia or muscle tend to be more acutely and systemically ill and have more rapidly advancing disease compared with those with infection confined to subcutaneous tissues above the fascia. Other cutaneous signs, such as vesiculation, bullae formation, ecchymoses, crepitus, anesthesia, and necrosis, are ominous and indicative of advanced disease.[55]

Classification of necrotizing soft-tissue infections has undergone multiple revisions over the years, often with more than one name for the same condition, and resulting in a confusing body of literature. Failure to recognize differences among these infections can lead to suboptimal therapy, because of the need for aggressive surgical intervention and optimal antibiotic therapy varies. The most important question is whether the soft-tissue infection is necrotizing or non-necrotizing; the former requires prompt surgical removal of all devitalized tissue in addition to antimicrobial therapy, whereas the latter responds to antibiotic therapy alone. If the distinction is in doubt, magnetic resonance imaging or incisional biopsy can be helpful.[56,57] These procedures, however, should not delay surgical exploration and intervention in the course of destructive or potentially fulminant infection. Ultimately, precise determination of the planes of tissue involved in the infection cannot be made on clinical examination, but rather must be made definitively in the operating room.

Current classification schemes for necrotizing soft-tissue infections focus on the depth of soft-tissue destruction and the etiologic agent.[58] Disease entities that involve primarily the subcutaneous tissues (sparing fascia and muscle) include clostridial and nonclostridial anaerobic cellulitis, bacterial synergistic gangrene, and Meleney ulcer. Other conditions that can evolve secondarily into subcutaneous tissue infection are infected decubitus or diabetic ulcers or tropical ulcers.

When infection involves the deep layer of the superficial fascia but largely spares the adjacent skin, deep fascia, and muscle, it is termed necrotizing fasciitis. Necrotizing fasciitis encompasses a variety of clinical presentations, ranging from subacute to fulminant, and can be due to a number of pathogens, sometimes apparently acting alone and sometimes synergistically. Synergistic necrotizing cellulitis is indistinguishable clinically from necrotizing fasciitis in most cases, but it frequently extends to involve the deep fascia and muscle.[59] (e.g., see Chapter 77, Myositis, Pyomyositis, and Necrotizing Fasciitis).

Relatively few organisms possess sufficient virulence to cause necrotizing soft-tissue infections when acting alone (Box 76-5). Fulminating infections are caused by S. pyogenes, although a clinically indistinguishable infection of necrotizing fasciitis can be caused by S. aureus (including MRSA), Clostridium perfringens, C. septicum, P. aeruginosa, Vibrio spp. (particularly Vibrio vulnificus), and fungi of the order Mucorales, particularly Rhizopus, Mucor and Absidia spp.[54,60-63]

Necrotizing soft-tissue infections often are polymicrobial. In most cases, a mixture of anaerobic, aerobic, and facultative anaerobic bacteria appears to act together to cause tissue necrosis.[12] Anaerobic isolates are similar to those found in subcutaneous abscesses, consisting of Bacteroides, Peptostreptococcus, Peptococcus, Prevotella, Porphyromonas, Clostridium, and Fusobacterium species.[12,64] The most common aerobic or facultative bacteria are E. coli, Enterobacter spp., and a variety of other Enterobacteriaceae, Pseudomonas spp., several species of hemolytic or nonhemolytic non-group A streptococci, and S. aureus. Bacterial synergistic gangrene is due to microaerophilic streptococci and either S. aureus or a gram-negative bacillus, particularly Proteus spp., acting together to cause tissue damage.[65,66] Entamoeba histolytica and nontuberculous mycobacteria (particularly Mycobacterium kansasii and M. chelonae), in corticosteroid-treated patients can cause an identical clinical syndrome.[65,67] No particular combination of organisms,

PART II Clinical Syndromes and Cardinal Features of Infectious Diseases: Approach to Diagnosis and Initial Management

SECTION J Skin and Soft-Tissue Infections

BOX 76-5. Agents of Necrotizing Soft-Tissue Infections in Infants and Children

MONOMICROBIAL

Bacteria

Streptococcus pyogenes, Staphylococcus aureus, Clostridium perfringens, Clostridium septicum, Haemophilus influenzae type b, *Mycobacterium chelonae, Mycobacterium kansasii, Pseudomonas aeruginosa, Streptococcus agalactiae,* streptococci (groups C, G, and F), *Streptococcus pneumoniae, Vibrio alginolyticus, Vibrio cholerae* (nonserogroup 01), *V. parahaemolyticus, V. vulnificus*

Fungi

Absidia spp., *Aspergillus* spp., *Fusarium* spp., *Mucor* spp., *Rhizopus* spp., *Saksenaea* spp.

Protozoa

Entamoeba histolytica

POLYMICROBIAL

Anaerobic bacteria

Bacteroides, Clostridium, Fusobacterium, Peptococcus, Peptostreptococcus, Porphyromonas, Prevotella

Aerobic or facultative bacteria

Aeromonas, Enterobacter, Escherichia coli, Klebsiella, Proteus, Pseudomonas, S. aureus, streptococci (hemolytic, nonhemolytic nongroup A).

---

however, is diagnostic for any given clinical entity that involves necrotizing soft-tissue infection.

Gas in tissue in association with infection is a hallmark of clostridial infection, but most soft-tissue infections with gas production are due to facultative gram-negative bacilli, such as *E. coli, Klebsiella* spp., *Proteus* spp., and *Aeromonas* spp.[68] Crepitant anaerobic cellulitis due to *Clostridium* spp. also is more common than life-threatening clostridial myonecrosis (i.e., gas gangrene) (see Chapter 77, Myositis, Pyomyositis, and Necrotizing Fasciitis).

Tertiary or hematogenous infections of the subcutaneous tissues occur most commonly in immunocompromised hosts and can lead to abscess or necrotizing soft-tissue infection. Although a wide range of organisms, including bacteria and fungi, can be involved, the most common are *S. aureus* and *P. aeruginosa*.

Pathogenesis

Some of the same organisms that cause necrotizing soft-tissue infections sometimes cause cellulitis, with involvement of fascia or tissue necrosis. Responsible factors are poorly understood, involving a complex interaction among predisposing tissue factors such as local trauma, anaerobic wound environment, systemic and local host defense, and bacterial virulence factors and synergy.

Compromise of immune defense is a primary predisposing factor for development of subcutaneous infections. This process can occur locally, through trauma or surgery that compromises the barrier function of the skin, or can involve systemic immunodeficiency, especially in individuals with defective neutrophil function. Systemic immunodeficiency is especially important for the development of necrotizing infections due to *P. aeruginosa* or fungi. Innate cutaneous defenses, including the physical barrier afforded by the lipids and the cross-linked cornified envelope in the stratum corneum, appear to be sufficient most often to prevent infection. Through trauma to skin or mucosal surfaces, however, a pathogen may be able to adhere to a previously unexposed receptor or a receptor that is newly synthesized in the injured skin.

In some infections, such as those due to *Clostridium* spp., the depth of the initial injury is the most important determinant of depth of infection.[31,68] Other infections, such as necrotizing fasciitis due to *S. pyogenes*, can spread rapidly from superficial layers of the skin to deeper subcutaneous tissues, aided by as yet poorly understood virulence factors. In infections that follow varicella, access to tissue beneath the stratum corneum at sites of chickenpox lesions may allow initiation of local infection.[69-73]

In diabetes, both compromised blood flow to the skin due to small-vessel vasculopathy and impaired function of neutrophils may predispose to necrotizing infection. The relatively high incidence of subcutaneous infections in those with peripheral vascular disease due to other causes supports this concept of pathogenesis, as does the fact that thrombosis of vessels is a major histologic feature of many necrotizing infections.[74,75] Furthermore, a higher degree of vascular thrombosis has been correlated with more acute presentation of necrotizing fasciitis.[74] The cause of vascular thrombosis is not understood completely, but probably involves direct cytolytic or thrombogenic factors released from bacterial pathogens, immune-mediated vascular damage due to the inflammatory infiltrate surrounding the blood vessels, or noninflammatory intravascular coagulation.[75] Disease in the dermis and epidermis occurs secondarily, following thrombosis of deeper vessels.

Synergy of microorganisms does not appear to be necessary for abscess formation, but it does appear to be operative in many necrotizing soft-tissue infections, because anaerobic or facultative organisms rarely are found alone in these infections.[12] The concept of bacterial synergy in the pathogenesis of soft-tissue infection, as advanced in the 1920s by Brewer and Meleney,[76] involved microaerophilic (probably anaerobic) streptococci and *S. aureus,* causing a progressive, chronic subcutaneous tissue infection called "bacterial synergistic gangrene." Since then, numerous combinations of organisms have been found to act synergistically in subcutaneous infections.[77] Even streptococcal necrotizing fasciitis or clostridial anaerobic cellulitis, in some cases, involves more than one agent acting synergistically, *S. aureus* being isolated from the infected tissue of some patients who have streptococcal necrotizing fasciitis.[12,64,74]

Synergistic pathogenesis of anaerobic, aerobic, and facultative bacteria is supported by clinical data and animal models, including studies in tropical ulcer showing synergistic associations of *Fusobacterium* spp., other anaerobic bacteria, and spirochetes.[78,79] In an animal model of necrotizing fasciitis, *S. aureus* or crude staphylococcal α-lysin potentiated the pathogenesis of *S. pyogenes*.[80] The mechanism of synergy appears to vary according to the organisms present, but it may result from mutual protection from phagocytosis and intracellular killing, promotion of bacterial capsule formation, production of essential growth factors or energy sources, and utilization of oxygen by facultative bacteria, thus lowering tissue oxidation reduction potential to facilitate growth of anaerobic organisms.[77,81,82]

Extracellular bacterial toxins and enzymes are important factors in the destruction of subcutaneous tissue.[83] In necrotizing soft-tissue infections due to *Clostridium* spp. and *S. pyogenes* in children, few acute inflammatory cells can be identified in necrotic fascia and subcutaneous tissue. Necrotizing tissue infections appear to be related to production of a variety of potent toxins and enzymes.[84]

Initiation of necrotizing streptococcal infection appears to require a break in the skin or mucous membrane, although the injury is often blunt, trivial, or inapparent.[55] Adherence of *S. pyogenes* to respiratory tract epithelium has been postulated to involve a two-step mechanism: a relatively weak, nonspecific hydrophobic binding followed by high-affinity, specific attachment.[85] The mechanism of adherence of the bacterium to the skin is not well understood.[86-88] Keratinocyte differentiation promotes adherence of *S. pyogenes*,[86] whereas the primary epidermal cytokines tumor necrosis factor-α (TNF-α) and interleukin-1α (IL-1α) decrease adherence.[87] The hyaluronic acid capsule of *S. pyogenes* impedes adherence, and modulation of capsule expression may be important in the pathogenesis of skin infections.[88] The molecular interactions (i.e., bacterial adhesin and keratinocyte receptor) involved in initial attachment to the skin, however, remain unknown. After attachment, invasion of *S. pyogenes* is related to numerous extracellular enzymes and toxins, and membrane-bound proteins that function as virulence factors.[89,90]

Patients with streptococcal necrotizing infections also can experience toxic shock-like syndrome, associated with the presence of the streptococcal pyrogenic exotoxins A, B and/ or C.[91] These toxins, as well as certain M-protein fragments, appear to have the ability to interact simultaneously with the major histocompatibility complex (MHC) class II antigen on antigen-presenting cells as well as specific Vβ regions of T-lymphocyte receptors, inducing massive synthesis and release of monokines, including TNF-α, IL-1β, IL-6, and the lymphokines TNF-β, IL-2, and interferon-γ.[73] These cytokines, particularly TNF, may mediate, at least in part, the rapid, massive tissue destruction seen in necrotizing fasciitis.[55] Protease activity and production of PVL are postulated to correlate better with the ability of *S. aureus* to cause invasive disease and may be a mechanism for invasion of pyogenic bacteria from a cutaneous site.[62,63,92,93] A central feature of necrotizing soft-tissue infections is vascular injury and thrombosis of the arteries and veins passing through the fascia.[56,74] A possible mechanism for the vascular injury leading to tissue ischemia and necrosis is greater adherence of neutrophils to vascular endothelium as a result of streptolysin O-induced upregulation of receptors.[94]

ANAEROBIC NECROTIZING SUBCUTANEOUS SUPRAFASCIAL INFECTIONS

Anaerobic Cellulitis

Anaerobic cellulitis can be caused by *Clostridium* spp. or by nonclostridial pathogens.[95] *Clostridium* spp. are associated with a spectrum of clinical infections, ranging from wound contamination to anaerobic cellulitis to myonecrosis (gas gangrene). Contamination occurs when clostridia grow in devitalized tissue but do not invade surrounding healthy tissue. Contamination can progress to cellulitis, which spares the fascia and muscle. Cellulitis is usually due to *C. perfringens* or sometimes other *Clostridium* spp. The incidence of anaerobic cellulitis due to *Clostridium* is several-fold greater than that of clostridial myonecrosis.[96] Nonclostridial anaerobic cellulitis also spares the fascia and underlying muscle. Nonclostridial anaerobic cellulitis is generally due to *Bacteroides*, *Peptostreptococcus*, or *Peptococcus* species acting synergistically with facultative streptococci and staphylococci, or with facultative or aerobic gram-negative bacilli such as *E. coli*, *K. pneumoniae*, and *Aeromonas* spp.

Anaerobic cellulitis develops in devitalized subcutaneous tissues after spread of a local primary infection or introduction of the pathogen into subcutaneous tissues by trauma or during surgery. It is most prevalent on areas of the body subject to fecal soiling, such as the perineum, abdominal wall, buttocks, and lower extremities. In one series, 5 cases of penetrating wound trauma that did not involve any aquatic environment were complicated by rapidly progressive infections.[95] Rarely, anaerobic cellulitis occurs as a tertiary infection after BSI with *C. septicum* in an immunocompromised patient who has a solid tumor or hematologic malignancy and neutropenia.[96] In this setting, progression to myonecrosis usually is rapid.

Onset of nonclostridial anaerobic cellulitis is relatively gradual, after an incubation period of several days, with development of localized, ill-defined erythema, edema, and tenderness. Once infection is established, destruction of subcutaneous tissue can occur rapidly, but the usual course is indolent compared with that of clostridial myonecrosis, with little tissue edema, necrosis, or pain, and few constitutional symptoms. Generally, there is minimal cutaneous discoloration, even late in the infection.

By contrast, as clostridial myonecrosis advances, the skin becomes bronze-colored, with dark bullae and patches of necrosis.

Gas formation with tissue crepitus usually is remarkable in anaerobic cellulitis, out of proportion to the clinical appearance of the skin, and beyond that seen with myonecrosis. Gas in tissue usually is visible on plain radiograph. A thin, dark, foul-smelling exudate may drain from the wound. Gram-stained smears of tissue or exudate may help distinguish clostridial from nonclostridial infection. In addition, the inflammatory infiltrate often is more substantial with nonclostridial anaerobic cellulitis, particularly early in the course of the disease, because tissue damage with *Clostridium* infection appears to be due in large part to histotoxic exotoxins.

Culture of aspirates or tissue specimens obtained during surgery is definitive. Identification of *Clostridium* species in a patient without acute, severe illness is reassurance that myonecrosis has not occurred. Surgical exploration is necessary, however, to distinguish this entity definitively from clostridial myonecrosis. At the time of surgery (usually required repeatedly), all areas of necrotic tissue must be exposed and debrided. Recommended initial antibiotic therapy consists of intravenous penicillin or ampicillin along with clindamycin or metronidazole. An aminoglycoside or an extended spectrum cephalosporin should also be given if Gram-stained specimens suggest the presence of gram-negative bacilli. Final antibiotic selection can be tailored according to results of cultures and antibiotic susceptibility testing.[97]

Bacterial Synergistic Gangrene

Bacterial synergistic gangrene is a rare, chronic gangrenous infection of the skin and subcutaneous tissue that occurs almost uniformly on the trunk after abdominal surgery. The most common sites are at the exit of a fistulous tract, particularly after appendectomy or drainage of empyema, and in association with an ileostomy or colostomy.[65] Occasionally, bacterial synergistic gangrene develops in close proximity to chronic ulceration on an extremity. A related lesion, chronic undermining ulcer of Meleney, occurs most commonly after lymph node surgery in the neck, axilla, or groin or occasionally after colonic or gynecologic surgery.

Bacterial synergistic gangrene is due to microaerophilic or anaerobic streptococci in combination with *S. aureus* or, occasionally, *Proteus* spp. or other gram-negative bacilli.[66,98–103] Identical lesions, from both clinical and histopathologic points of view, can be caused by cutaneous amebiasis due to *Entamoeba histolytica*.[65]

Bacterial synergistic gangrene is characterized by severe pain and slow but inexorable progression of gangrenous ulceration. It begins with localized tenderness, erythema, and edema, which progresses to ulceration. The ulcer characteristically has a central floor of red granulation tissue with grey to yellow exudate, and a sharply demarcated gangrenous serpiginous border. A raised, dusky red to purple margin surrounds the ulcer, with a peripheral ring of erythema and edema. Meleney ulcer is characterized by burrowing necrotic sinus tracts that emerge at distant sites to form additional ulcers. Systemic signs are minimal in both conditions.

Without treatment, these lesions have minimal tendency to heal, ultimately destroying large areas of skin and subcutaneous tissue. Although antimicrobial therapy alone has been curative in some cases, nutritional support, local surgical debridement, and antibiotic therapy (e.g., with clindamycin plus gentamicin, or another agent for facultative and aerobic bacteria, plus metronidazole) are recommended.[66] Broad-spectrum antibiotic therapy should be initiated and then adjusted according to results of culture and susceptibility testing of facultative and aerobic organisms recovered from surgical material.

Acknowledgment

The authors acknowledge use of some work of recent authors (Moise Levy, MD and John Browning, MD) and G.L. Darmstadt, who wrote this chapter in the first edition, and Alice Pong, MD for her collaboration with this chapter.

PART II Clinical Syndromes and Cardinal Features of Infectious Diseases: Approach to Diagnosis and Initial Management

SECTION J Skin and Soft-Tissue Infections

Key Points. Subcutaneous Abscesses in Children

EPIDEMIOLOGY

Groups at risk
- Defects of skin barrier (e.g., trauma, intravenous drug abuse, secondarily infected eczema, surgical wound, burns)
- Defects in innate and acquired defense (immunodeficiencies and immunosuppressed hosts)
- For CA-MRSA:
  - Athletes in contact sports (wrestling, soccer)
  - Patients with a family or personal history of MRSA infection or colonization
  - Children with cancer
  - Neonates in intensive care units
  - Military personnel
  - Native Americans
  - Canadian aboriginals
  - Pacific Islanders
  - Contact with healthcare facilities and personnel

ETIOLOGY
- CA-MRSA 66%
- MSSA 18%
- Other organisms 9.5% (*Streptococcus pyogenes* most common; other groups predictable by host, site, underlying conditions)

CLINICAL FEATURES
- Can occur at any age
- Commonly mistaken for a "spider bite"
- Firm, tender, erythematous nodule that becomes fluctuant
- Generally without constitutional symptoms

DIAGNOSIS
- Culture of exudate for confirmation of pathogen and susceptibilities

TREATMENT
- Uncomplicated abscesses sometimes can be treated with incision and drainage alone
- Complicated abscesses (see text) are treated with systemic antibiotics chosen on the basis of local rates and resistance patterns of CA-MRSA (Table 76-1)

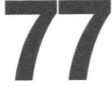

77 Myositis, Pyomyositis, and Necrotizing Fasciitis

Donald E. Low and Anna Norrby-Teglund

Skin and soft-tissue infections (SSTIs) are common in children and usually are recognized easily and treated, with few residual long-term problems. However, although rare, myositis, pyomyositis, and necrotizing fasciitis soft-tissue infections can be difficult to diagnose in their early stages and despite appropriate antibiotic therapy are associated with substantial morbidity and mortality. The epidemiology of SSTIs is evolving, and incidence in children is increasing. Community-associated methicillin-resistant *S. aureus* (CA-MRSA) first emerged among children in the 1990s. Since then CA-MRSA has become the predominant cause of purulent SSTIs in the United States. Coincident with this epidemic, the incidence of pediatric ambulatory visits for SSTIs has nearly tripled.[1] Also in immunocompromised children SSTIs can be atypical and/or more severe.[2]

MYOSITIS

Myositis is defined as inflammation of a muscle, especially a voluntary muscle, characterized by pain, tenderness, swelling, and/or weakness. Etiologies of myositis include infection, autoimmune conditions, genetic disorders, medications, electrolyte disturbances, and diseases of the endocrine system.[3] Infectious myositis can be due to bacteria, fungi, parasites, and viruses (Table 77-1).[3] The clinical course can be acute, subacute, or chronic. Although identification of the causative microbe requires specific diagnostic testing (e.g., cultures), some clinical findings suggest the general category of the agent. For example, bacterial myositis usually causes focal muscle infection, whereas viruses and parasites often cause generalized myalgias or multifocal myositis. Also, bacterial myositis often occurs in the setting of muscular injury, surgery, ischemia, or the presence of a foreign body.

Bacterial Myositis

Acute bacterial myositis, defined as a diffuse muscle infection without an intramuscular abscess, occurs less commonly than pyomyositis and psoas abscess formation. Myositis compared with pyomyositis is seen more typically in adults rather than children.

Staphylococcus aureus. Although *S. aureus* myositis is uncommon, incidence has increased in adults and children in recent years, largely due to the emergence of CA-MRSA.[4,5] In the U.S., the USA300 clone of CA-MRSA accounts for most infections. It appears that virulence has evolved in this strain through the increased expression of core-genome-encoded virulence determinants, such as α-toxin and phenol-soluble modulins, and acquisition of the phage-encoded Panton–Valentine leukocidin (PVL) genes. All these toxins impact disease progression in animal models of USA300 infection. In contrast, the basis of virulence in other CA-MRSA epidemics, which include PVL-negative strains, is less well understood.[5–7]

Streptococcus pyogenes. *S. pyogenes* (group A streptococci; GAS) also can cause myositis. The most severe form is necrotizing myositis, also called streptococcal myonecrosis or spontaneous streptococcal gangrenous myositis. Cases typically occur among men (2 : 1) and young adults; the disease usually occurs spontaneously without a history of penetrating trauma or underlying immunosuppression. The portal of entry often is unknown. Some cases begin with a sore throat, suggesting that pharyngitis may have led to bacteremia and seeding of the muscle; however, most cases occur without an antecedent illness. The clinical presentation includes an initial prodromal stage with flu-like symptoms, which may include rash and myalgias. This evolves to intense local

TABLE 77-1. Common Infectious Causes of Myositis[a]

Organism Group	Organism(s)
Gram-positive bacteria	Staphylococcus aureus
	Streptococcus pyogenes (group A streptococcus)
	Streptococcus (groups B, C, and G; S. pneumoniae; S. anginosus)
Gram-negative bacteria	Aeromonas hydrophila
	Citrobacter freundii
	Enterobacter spp.
	Escherichia coli
	Proteus spp.
	Pseudomonas spp.
	Salmonella spp.
	Vibrio vulnificus
Anaerobic bacteria	Bacteroides spp.
	Clostridium spp.
	Streptococcus spp. (anaerobic, e.g., Peptostreptococcus)
Mycobacterium spp.	Mycobacterium tuberculosis
Fungi	Candida spp.
Parasites	Trachipleistophora
	Plasmodium spp.
	Sarcocystis spp.
	Taenia solium
	Trichinella spp.
Viruses	Enteroviruses (coxsackie B virus and ECHO virus)
	HIV
	HTLV-1
	Influenza A and B viruses

[a]Modified from reference 3.

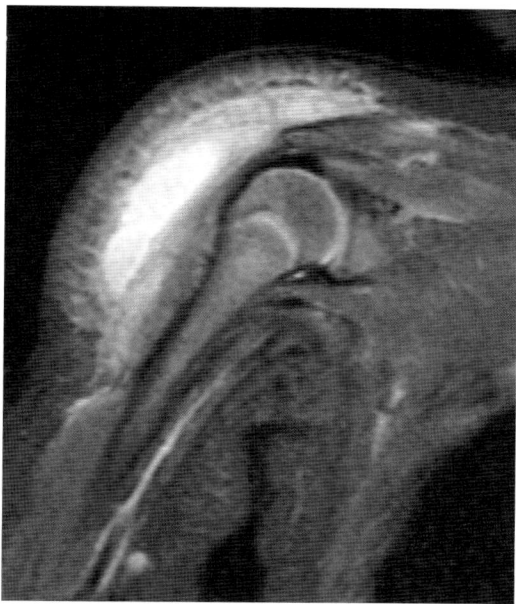

Figure 77-1. Necrotizing pyomyositis due to *Streptococcus pyogenes* in a 6-month-old infant with acute onset of fever, erythema, swelling, and pain of her right shoulder, and decreased use of her arm. There was no break in the skin. Coronal fluid-attenuated inversion recovery (FLAIR) magnetic resonance imaging shows diffuse hyperintensity of the deltoid muscle with associated subcutaneous inflammatory stranding and edema. Osseous and fascial structures are normal. (Courtesy of E.N. Faerber and S.S. Long, St. Christopher's Hospital for Children, Philadelphia, PA.)

muscle pain that is disproportionate to clinical findings as well as local tense swelling and fever.[8] The course can evolve rapidly over several hours (Figure 77-1).

***Clostridium* species.** Clostridial gas gangrene (i.e., myonecrosis) most commonly is caused by *C. perfringens*, *C. novyi*, *C. histolyticum*, and *C. septicum*. *C. perfringens* is the most frequent cause of trauma-associated gas gangrene.[9] This infection occurs in a variety of settings: traumatic wounds with soil contamination, surgery involving the bowel or biliary system, septic abortions, vascular disease with arterial insufficiency, and in association with injection of medications (e.g., epinephrine) or illicit drugs (e.g., heroin). Common characteristics of inciting events include contamination of the site with *Clostridium* spp. (which exist in the soil and as part of the gastrointestinal flora of humans) and the presence of devitalized tissue. The presence of a foreign body is a risk factor. In contrast to traumatic gas gangrene, spontaneous gangrene principally is associated with the more aerotolerant *C. septicum* and occurs predominantly in patients with underlying gastrointestinal conditions, including occult colon cancer, bowel infarction, or neutropenic enterocolitis.

C. septicum infections occur in children in three major predispositions: neutrophil dysfunction (including malignancies, congenital or cyclic neutropenia, aplastic anemia), bowel ischemia (hemolytic-uremic syndrome, intussusception), and trauma.[9] Malignancy underlies >50% of cases, with acute myelocytic and lymphocytic leukemias the most common. Cyclic and congenital neutropenia is present in 20% of the published pediatric cases. Clinical features associated with *C septicum* infections in children include fever, vomiting, diarrhea, blood per rectum, anorexia, and acute abdomen and/or distention. Despite treatment with surgery and parenteral antibiotics, mortality rates of children with *C. septicum* infections remain >50%.[9]

Presenting symptoms for clostridial myonecrosis include intense pain, edema, and a sweet-odorous discharge which occur several hours to a few days after injury. The wound initially is pale but can evolve to a bronze color with hemorrhagic bullae. Classic findings include the presence of gas in the tissues detected by either gas bubbles emitted from the wound or noted on radiographic films. Although gas often is considered to be a sine qua non for gas gangrene, the absence of crepitus or gas on examination should not deter consideration of this diagnosis. The failure of the muscle to contract on stimulation and the lack of bleeding of the wound during operation are characteristic findings. Typical laboratory findings include leukocytosis and a hemolytic anemia due to clostridial α-toxin. Bacteremia is noted in 15% of cases. Gram stain evaluation of the wound exudate usually shows a lack of neutrophils and an abundance of gram-positive bacilli with blunt ends.

Nonclostridial myositis. Anaerobic streptococcal myositis has similar clinical characteristics of clostridial myonecrosis, including a foul copious exudate, gas in infected tissues, and extensive necrosis of the involved muscle(s). Specific etiologies include anaerobic streptococci (e.g., *Peptostreptococcus* spp.), GAS, and *S. aureus*. Synergistic nonclostridial myonecrosis is an infection of the subcutaneous tissues and fascia that can extend into the muscle. The infection often is polymicrobial, consisting of aerobic and anaerobic organisms, such as streptococci (including *Peptostreptococcus* spp.), *Bacteroides* spp., *E. coli*, *Enterobacter* spp., and *Klebsiella* spp. *Aeromonas hydrophila* myonecrosis usually occurs after penetrating trauma in a freshwater environment or tissue injury in association with contact with aquatic animals. Progression can be rapid and gas may form within the tissues.

Vibrio vulnificus is an opportunistic human pathogen that is highly lethal.[10] The bacterium is a part of the natural flora of coastal marine environments worldwide and has been isolated from water, sediments, and a variety of seafood. Of all *Vibrio* infections reported in the U.S. annually, 25% to 30% are non-foodborne *Vibrio* infections (NFVIs).[11] *V. vulnificus* infections are the most common (accounting for 35% of NFVIs), with 72% of *V. vulnificus*

PART II Clinical Syndromes and Cardinal Features of Infectious Diseases: Approach to Diagnosis and Initial Management

SECTION J Skin and Soft-Tissue Infections

infections reported from residents of Gulf Coast states. SSTIs due to *V. vulnificus* result in amputation and death in 10% and 17% of cases, respectively.[11] Clinicians should consider *Vibrio* species as an etiologic agent in infections occurring in persons with recent seawater exposure, even if the individual was only exposed during recreational activities.

Other forms of bacterial myositis. Lyme disease can cause localized myositis of the orbits and other sites, often near areas of erythema migrans or joint involvement.[12] *Mycobacterium* spp. causes myositis either by direct extension from a contiguous source (e.g., an infected joint, bone, or abscess) or less commonly via bacteremia. The most common site is a tuberculous psoas muscle abscess that forms by extension from vertebral osteomyelitis (i.e., Pott disease). Other examples include involvement of the intercostal muscles through extension from the lung or striated muscles of the leg through extension from the knee.

Fungal Myositis

Fungal myositis is uncommon with most cases occurring in immunocompromised patients. Fungal myositis can be due to *Candida* spp. (most commonly), *Cryptococcus neoformans*, *Histoplasma capsulatum*, *Coccidioides* spp., *Aspergillus* spp., *Pneumocystis jirovecii*, and *Fusarium* spp. Biopsy with culture usually is required to confirm the diagnosis. Often the diagnosis is not considered initially and is discovered by histopathology or culture of muscle tissue.

Parasitic Myositis

A variety of parasites can encyst in muscle. The most common are *Trichinella* spp. (trichinosis), *Taenia solium* (cysticercosis), and *Toxoplasma gondii* (toxoplasmosis). The presence of eosinophilia and a travel history to an endemic area suggest a possible parasitic etiology of myositis.

Infection with *Trichinella spiralis* occurs after ingestion of larval cysts in undercooked pork or the meat of certain wild carnivores. The adult worm develops in the gastrointestinal tract and releases larvae that circulate via lymphatics and the bloodstream to striated muscle, where they become encysted and survive for several years. The vast majority of infections are subclinical; autopsies reveal *Trichinella* cysts in >4% of randomly selected diaphragms.[13] Typical manifestations of symptomatic disease include fever, extreme malaise, muscle pain, weakness, and periorbital edema.[14] Serum muscle enzymes are elevated, and eosinophilia is present. Serodiagnostic testing is available and can preclude the need for biopsy. Most mild cases respond to analgesic therapy. In severe cases, anthelmintic therapy with thiabendazole or mebendazole is effective.[15]

After ingestion of eggs of the pork tapeworm *Taenia solium* larvae migrate to excyst within skeletal muscle leading to granulomatous nodules and calcific densities. Although fever, myalgia, and eosinophilia can occur, most cases of muscular cysticercosis, except those involving extraocular muscles, are asymptomatic. For infections that involve extraocular muscles, treatment with albendazole plus a corticosteroid or surgical removal of the encysted parasites may be necessary to preserve vision.[16–18] During acute *Toxoplasma gondii* infection, widespread dissemination of tachyzoites can occur, and skeletal muscle frequently is infected. The vast majority of cases of acquired toxoplasmosis are asymptomatic, although some patients experience a mononucleosis-like syndrome with nonspecific myalgia. Chronic inflammatory myositis associated with *T. gondii* has been reported in human immunodeficiency virus (HIV-1)-infected and other immunocompromised people.[19] Weakness, muscle wasting, and high serum levels of creatine kinase are characteristic features. Infection in the acute phase may be responsive to pyrimethamine plus sulfadiazine, whereas in the chronic phase, corticosteroid therapy may be beneficial.[20]

Viral Myositis

Many viruses can cause myalgias, polymyositis, or virus-associated rhabdomyolysis. Often the symptoms of myositis are diffuse in nature, and patients have other symptoms and signs attributable to the causative viral pathogen. Influenza A and B viruses are the most commonly reported causes of viral myositis. Enteroviruses, HIV, human T-cell leukemia-lymphoma virus (HTLV-1), and hepatitis viruses (B and C) also can cause myositis.

Influenza-associated myositis (IAM) has been reported only sporadically since its first description in 1957. IAM appears to be more common in children than in adults, but its age-specific incidence during influenza epidemics is unknown.[21] IAM is characterized in children by severe lower-extremity myalgia and reluctance to walk. As IAM is associated with the influenza B virus, incidence may depend on circulating strains during an epidemic. IAM typically occurs with a 2:1 male predominance among children aged <14 years and is characterized by abrupt onset of severe myalgia in calf muscles, inability to walk, and elevated serum creatine kinase levels, usually within 1 week of influenza onset, when respiratory symptoms are improving. Whereas the link between influenza and IAM is clearly established, its pathogenesis is not well understood. Two proposed mechanisms are viral invasion of muscle tissue and immune-mediated muscle damage triggered by the respiratory tract infection. Treatment is symptomatic, as myositis is self-limited, usually resolving within a mean of 3 days (range, 1 to 30 days). Influenza virus-associated rhabdomyolysis has been described in children and adults. Rhabdomyolysis is associated more frequently with influenza type A than type B, and occurs more frequently in girls. The 2009 pandemic triple-reassortant influenza A (H1N1) virus was associated with neurologic and muscular syndromes that affected primarily children and included myositis.[22] Rhabdomyolysis can be complicated by renal failure and the development of a compartment syndrome.

Enteroviruses, including coxsackieviruses (group A and B) and enteric cytopathogenic human orphan (ECHO) viruses, also cause myositis. Coxsackievirus B infection manifesting as pleurodynia is most common. Typically children come to attention in the summer or fall with paroxysms of severe, sharp chest pain. The costochondral muscles may be tender on palpation. In addition to pleurodynia, cases of rhabdomyolysis due to coxsackieviruses and ECHO viruses have been reported. The pathogenesis of myositis is uncertain, but muscle biopsies have shown degenerative necrosis of the muscle fibers and picornavirus-like structures. Therapy is symptomatic; the disease usually resolves in several days, but recurrences of pleurodynia have been described in up to one-fourth of cases.

HIV infection can cause a wide range of skeletal disorders including myopathy, polymyositis, and rhabdomyolysis. Generalized myalgia, proximal muscle weakness, and elevated serum creatine kinase are frequent features.[23] Muscle biopsy shows lymphocytic infiltration and necrosis of muscle fibers. These histologic findings are distinct from the mitochondrial myopathy associated with extended zidovudine therapy.[24] Although one study has shown that proviral DNA can be detected in myocytes and muscle macrophages by polymerase chain reaction,[25] other researchers have concluded that the disease probably represents a dysfunctional T-lymphocyte-mediated process.[26] Corticosteroid therapy may be beneficial.[27]

Chronic Inflammatory Myositis

A number of parasitic and other pathogens can cause a chronic inflammatory reaction in skeletal muscle. In these disorders, persistence of the infectious agent appears necessary to cause chronic myopathy, either by direct tissue damage or as a consequence of the normal immunologic response directed toward the infected tissue. In other disorders, such as juvenile dermatomyositis (JDM) and polymyositis, an immunologic dysregulation is the hypothesized mechanism of disease.[28]

JDM is the most common form of pediatric idiopathic inflammatory myopathy, with incidence ranging from 1.9 to 3.2 per million children.[29,30] The two major clinical features of JDM are a characteristic rash and symmetric proximal muscle weakness.[31] The gastrointestinal tract and lung also often are involved.[31]

Compared with the adult form of the disease, JDM more frequently has vasculitis features, skin ulceration, and calcinosis.[32] Patients with JDM often experience a flu-like illness approximately 3 months prior to the onset of the disease. Coxsackievirus B and other enteroviruses are the most frequent infectious agents temporally associated with the onset of JDM.[33–36] Coxsackievirus B1 can induce chronic myositis of the proximal hindlimbs in a murine model.[37] Serologic responses consistent with acute coxsackievirus B infection were found in patients in some studies[33] but not in others.[38] Although picornavirus-like particles have been observed on electron-microscopic examination of muscle biopsy samples from some children with JDM, immunofluorescence, polymerase chain reaction,[39] in situ nucleotide hybridization,[40] and tissue culture[35] have failed to identify a virus. If an infectious agent precipitates JDM, it is hypothesized that immunologically mediated injury (possibly through molecular mimicry), rather than direct infection, is the mechanism of injury. This pathogenic mechanism is supported by gene expression profile analyses of untreated JDM muscle biopsies, demonstrating an intense interferon α/β-induced response typical of that seen during an immune response to a viral antigen.[41]

Several reports have demonstrated an association between the human leukocyte antigen (HLA)-DQA1*0501 and JDM.[41–43] This association has been linked to an enhanced cytokine response partly contributed to by the tumor necrosis factor-alpha (TNF-α)-308A allele,[41,44] which is known to promote TNF-α synthesis. Enhanced TNF-α production was demonstrable in both circulation[44] and in muscle biopsies[45] from untreated JDM patients positive for the TNF-α-308A allele. This allele has been shown to be associated with pathologic calcifications and disease chronicity.[44,46] The pathogenesis of JDM following group A streptococcal infection has been suggested to involve cytotoxic and cytokine responses elicited by specific epitopes of the streptococcal M-protein homologues of human skeletal myosin.[47]

PYOMYOSITIS

Pyomyositis is as an acute intramuscular infection secondary to hematogenous spread of the microorganism into the body of a skeletal muscle. By definition, it is not secondary to a contiguous infection of the soft tissue or bone, nor due to penetrating trauma. Pyomyositis has a predilection for large-muscle groups and often results in localized abscess formation. Pyomyositis often is called tropical myositis because of its prevalence in tropical areas, where pyomyositis accounts for 3% to 5% of hospital admissions.[48–50] The first case of tropical pyomyositis reported from a temperate region was in 1971.[51] Since then many cases have been reported from various parts of the world.[52–54] Within North America, the highest incidence of pyomyositis is in southern regions.[55] Pyomyositis occurs most often in children and young adults,[56,57] exhibits a 2 : 1 male preponderance, and has been reported in the neonatal period.[58] Methicillin-susceptible *S. aureus* (MSSA) was isolated from the purulent material in approximately 90% of cases in tropical areas and 75% of cases from temperate countries prior to the 1990s.[52] CA-MRSA (especially the USA300 clone) has since emerged as an important/dominant cause in temperate climates.[59] Group A streptococcus accounts for 1% to 5% of cases. Other causes include streptococci (group B, C, and G), *E. coli, Citrobacter freundii, Serratia marcescens, Yersinia enterocolitica, Klebsiella* spp., and *Salmonella* spp. Individuals infected with HIV-1 are at increased risk for development of bacterial pyomyositis, sometimes with multifocal involvement.[60]

Staphylococcal pyomyositis most frequently affects the quadriceps, hamstring, or gluteal muscles but also can affect the paraspinus, shoulder girdle, psoas, and other muscles.[57] Symptoms generally begin insidiously, with low-grade fever, muscle aches, and cramping evolving over several days. Abscesses are multiple in about 25% of patients. In the early stages, examination may reveal only a hard, rubbery firmness to the muscle belly, with no other superficial signs of inflammation. Within days to 3 weeks, boggy swelling, erythema, tenderness, and warmth appear, and the lesion becomes fluctuant. Although substantial muscle

destruction can develop with delayed treatment, serum levels of muscle enzymes generally are normal. Pyomyositis occasionally is complicated by metastatic infection such as empyema, pericarditis, or lung abscess. In rare cases, fulminant septicemia or toxic shock syndrome occurs.[61]

Pyogenic abscess in the psoas muscle produces a distinct clinical syndrome with lower abdominal or back pain radiating to the hip.[62] The febrile child may limp or hold the hip in fixed flexion because of muscle spasm. Confusion with pyogenic arthritis is common. Pain on hyperextension or abduction of the hip is elicited on examination. *S. aureus* is the most common cause, but psoas abscess occasionally can develop as an extension of an abdominal process such as a ruptured appendix.[62] In such cases, a mixed infection with anaerobic and facultative bowel flora is likely.

Group A streptococci are an increasingly important cause of pyomyositis.[63,64] GAS infection of skeletal muscle can present as a localized phlegmon, an abscess, or more fulminant necrotizing myositis.[65,66] Intense pain is the most common presenting symptom, often out of proportion to clinical signs of inflammation. The child may refuse to bear weight or to move an extremity. Ultimately, high fever, localized swelling, and overlying erythema are observed. Tachycardia, hypotension, oliguria, confusion, lethargy, and scarlatiniform eruptions are early signs of associated streptococcal toxic shock syndrome. Mild to moderate leukocytosis with immature neutrophils (often more than 50%) and elevation of blood urea nitrogen, creatinine, and creatine kinase are common.[8]

Although a portal of entry is not always evident, the exanthem of primary varicella and various forms of minor skin trauma are important predisposing factors to the development of GAS deep-tissue infection in children. A prospective population-based active surveillance for pediatric invasive GAS disease in Ontario revealed that varicella-zoster virus infection is associated with a 58-fold increased risk of invasive GAS disease in children.[63] Although the attack rate of invasive GAS was relatively low (5.2/100,000), 15% of all pediatric invasive GAS infections, including 50% of cases of necrotizing fasciitis, followed varicella infection.

NECROTIZING FASCIITIS

Necrotizing fasciitis (also known as hospital gangrene or hemolytic streptococcal gangrene) was described as early as the fifth century BC by Hippocrates.[67] Necrotizing fasciitis is a rapidly progressive, deep-seated bacterial infection of the subcutaneous soft tissue that can involve any area of the body. The course often is fulminant and has a high mortality rate, ranging from 25% to 75%.[68,69] Many terms have been used to describe necrotizing soft-tissue infections. A simplified classification is provided in Table 77-2.

Although more than 500 cases of necrotizing fasciitis have been reported in North America, it is an uncommon disease and the true incidence is not known.[70,71] Males are affected slightly more commonly than females.[68,69,72] An increased frequency is associated with diabetes mellitus, intravenous drug use, chronic alcohol consumption, immunosuppression, and peripheral vascular disease.[69,70,72] Necrotizing fasciitis also occurs in young, previously healthy children and adults, in whom mortality rates are lower than among the elderly and those with underlying disease.[70] Patients may report a history of recent surgery, trauma, eczema, or varicella infection.[68,73,74] Other precipitating factors include insect bites, perirectal abscess, incarcerated hernia, and subcutaneous insulin injection. Necrotizing fasciitis is reported as a complication of varicella infection.[70,73,75] Necrotizing fasciitis can also occur with a preceding GAS pharyngitis or without any previous evidence of trauma or infection. The association between the use of nonsteroidal anti-inflammatory drugs and necrotizing fasciitis was not supported definitively by a prospective, multicenter case-control study carried out among children hospitalized with primary varicella complicated by invasive GAS infection or necrotizing soft-tissue infection.[73,76–78] In neonates, necrotizing fasciitis can complicate omphalitis or circumcision.

PART II Clinical Syndromes and Cardinal Features of Infectious Diseases: Approach to Diagnosis and Initial Management

SECTION J Skin and Soft-Tissue Infections

TABLE 77-2. Necrotizing Infections of the Soft Tissues

Type	Usual Etiologic Agent	Predisposing Causes	Clinical Manifestations
Meleney synergistic gangrene	*Staphylococcus aureus*, microaerophilic streptococci	Surgery	Slowly expanding ulceration confined to superficial fascia
Clostridial cellulitis	*Clostridium perfringens*	Local trauma or surgery	Gas in skin, fascial sparing, little systemic toxicity
Nonclostridial anaerobic cellulitis	Mixed aerobes and anaerobes	Diabetes mellitus	Gas in tissues
Gas gangrene	Clostridial species (*Clostridium perfringens*, *Clostridium histolyticum,* or *Clostridium septicum*)	Trauma, crush injuries, epinephrine injections; spontaneous cases related to cancer, neutropenia, cancer chemotherapy	Myonecrosis, gas in tissues, systemic toxicity, shock
Necrotizing fasciitis type 1	Mixed anaerobes, gram-negative aerobic bacilli, enterococci	Surgery, diabetes mellitus, peripheral vascular disease	Destruction of fat and fascia; skin may be spared; involvement of perineal area in Fournier gangrene
Necrotizing fasciitis type 2	Group A streptococcus	Penetrating injuries, surgical procedures, varicella, burns, minor cuts, trauma	Systemic toxicity, severe local pain, rapidly extending necrosis of subcutaneous tissues and skin; gangrene, shock, multiorgan failure

Adapted from Bisno AL, Stevens DL. Streptococcal infections of skin and soft tissues. N Engl J Med 1996;334:240–245. with permission from Massachusetts Medical Society.

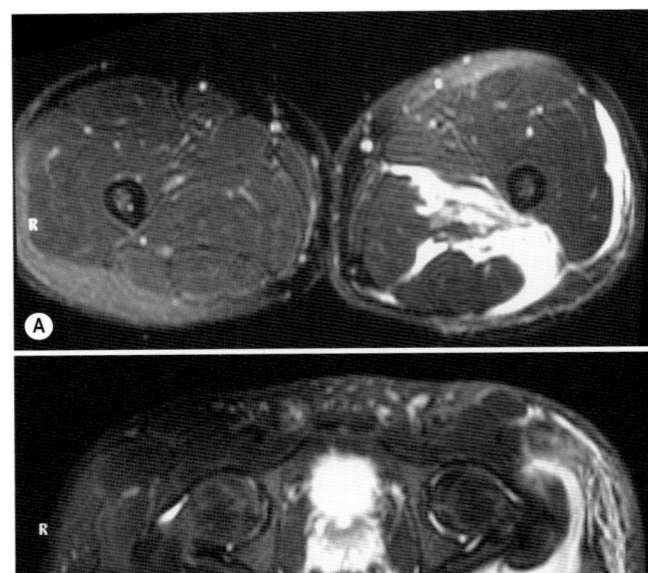

Figure 77-2. Pyomyositis and necrotizing fasciitis due to methicillin-resistant *Staphylococcus aureus* in a 17-year-old male with a 1-day history of fever, poor appetite, and left hip pain, precluding ambulation. Physical examination showed fullness and exquisite tenderness of the buttock and posterior thigh, without a break in the skin or erythema. Axial T_2-weighted magnetic resonance imaging **(A, B)** shows hyperintensity of the fascia surrounding the tensor fascia lata and biceps femoris muscles from midthigh to the pelvic girdle. Surgery revealed necrotizing fasciitis. (Courtesy of E.N. Faerber and S.S. Long, St. Christopher's Hospital for Children, Philadelphia, PA.)

Necrotizing fasciitis often is classified into three types. The polymicrobial form of the disease is described as necrotizing fasciitis type 1 and often occurs postoperatively or in patients with diabetes mellitus or peripheral vascular disease.[68,69,79] Pathogens include gram-negative bacilli, enterococci, streptococci, S. aureus and anaerobes includes *Bacteroides* spp., *Peptostreptococcus* spp., and *Clostridium* spp. (see Table 77-2). Necrotizing fasciitis type 2 is due to GAS infection that can occur postoperatively or as a result of penetrating trauma, varicella infection, burns, or minor cuts; and is characterized by rapidly extending necrosis and severe systemic toxicity. Type 2 disease is the most common form of necrotizing fasciitis in children.[70,72,80] Necrotizing fasciitis type 3 is rare and is caused by marine *Vibrio* spp., which enter through skin lesions that have been exposed to seawater or marine animals.

In children, necrotizing fasciitis often occurs 1 to 4 days after trauma, with soft-tissue swelling and pain over the affected area. Patients may appear well at initial presentation. When associated with varicella, the findings typically begin 3 to 4 days after onset of the exanthem.[74] Infants and toddlers may be fussy or irritable. Toddlers and young children may limp or refuse to bear weight. Initially, pain with manipulation of the affected extremity often is out of proportion to the cutaneous signs of infection.

Induration and edema generally are apparent within the first 24 hours and are followed rapidly by blistering and bleb formation.[64,75,81] Infection spreads in the plane between the subcutaneous tissue and the superficial muscle fascia, which results in progressive destruction of fascia and fat (Figure 77-2). Pain and tenderness in the subcutaneous space are exquisite, but destruction of the nerves that innervate the skin eventually can lead to anesthesia of the overlying skin. The rapidly progressing infection can lead to toxic shock syndrome and severe systemic toxicity, including renal and hepatic failure, acute respiratory distress syndrome, and decreased myocardial contractility.

Extension of the infection along fascial planes leads to necrosis of the superficial fascia and the deeper layers of the dermis. Destruction and thrombosis of the small blood vessels in the area lead to necrosis of the surrounding tissues. The extensive tissue damage often leads to systemic symptoms, including multiorgan failure and shock.

Although white blood cell counts can be normal or elevated, there often is a pronounced shift to immature neutrophils. Thrombocytopenia and coagulopathy can occur. Attempts to identify causative organisms should be made through collection of anaerobic and aerobic blood cultures.[69,75] Cultures of the wound and surgically debrided tissue should be obtained. Frozen section biopsies can be helpful in making a timely diagnosis.

PATHOGENESIS

Skeletal muscle tissue is intrinsically resistant to bacterial infections, likely due to sequestration by myoglobin of iron that is required for proliferating bacteria. Staphylococcal muscle infections appear to be a complication of transient bacteremia and typically develop without penetrating injury or other clear portal of entry. Blood cultures frequently are negative.[82] Muscular trauma, strain, or vigorous exercise may be predisposing factors.[55,83] The

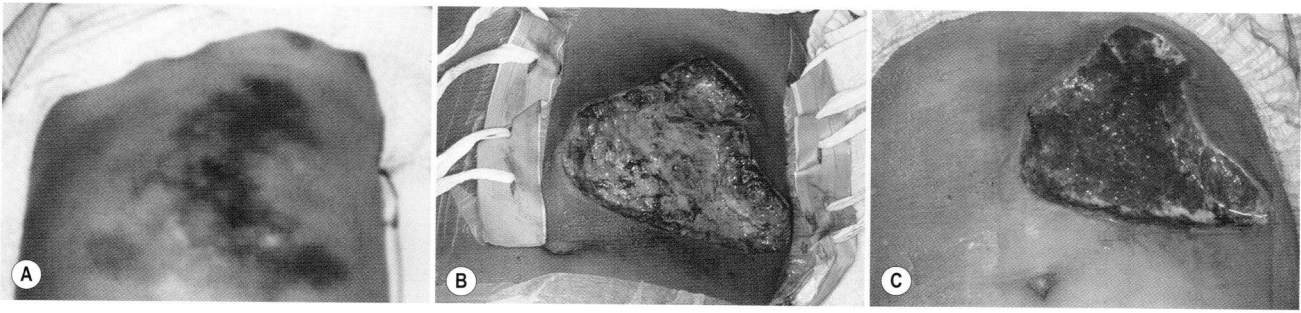

Figure 77-3. Necrotizing fasciitis of the abdominal wall due to *Streptococcus pyogenes* as a complication of chickenpox in a 7-year-old girl. Note duskiness, ecchymosis, purpura, and edema of the abdominal wall **(A).** There was full-thickness necrosis of skin, subcutaneous tissue, and fascia **(B).** After multiple surgical debridements, the patient is ready for grafting **(C).** (Courtesy of J.H. Brien©.)

high prevalence of the disease in the tropics has led to speculation that in patients with migrating parasitic infections, such as toxocariasis, microscopic foci of necrotic muscle develop that predispose to bacterial seeding.[84] Alternatively, a viral infection can be the precipitant; ultrastructural studies of nonsuppurating lesions in some patients with tropical pyomyositis reveal intracellular particles and a lymphocytic infiltrate.[85]

Group A streptococcal infection of skeletal muscle can take the form of a localized phlegmon, an abscess, or more fulminant necrotizing myositis or fasciitis,[65,66] associated with septicemia and toxic shock syndrome. The association of invasive GAS with primary varicella infection may simply result from the full-thickness skin lesion of chickenpox, serving as a portal of entry for the organism (Figure 77-3).[75,86,87] Varicella also produces a transient immunologic derangement, predisposing to secondary bacterial infection. A potential mechanism underlying the association of blunt trauma and streptococcal myonecrosis was provided by Bryant et al.,[88] who reported that muscle injury resulted in increased cellular vimentin expression, which enhanced colonization of GAS to the site of injury.

Both *S. aureus* and GAS express virulence factors, including adhesins, cytotoxins, superantigens, and immunomodulatory proteins, which contribute to the pathogenesis of infection. Although specific virulence factors are implicated in certain disease manifestations, such as superantigens as mediators of systemic toxicity and tissue injury,[89–91] no single virulence factor is sufficient to provoke a severe staphylococcal or streptococcal infection. Rather a coordinated action of virulence factors is required in order for the bacteria to colonize successfully and spread within the host.[92–94] Tissue injury and systemic toxicity are largely due to excessive inflammatory responses. A direct relation between the magnitude of the inflammatory response and severity of invasive GAS infections has been demonstrated. Although GAS usually is considered an extracellular organism, macrophages can be a reservoir for GAS during acute deep tissue infections.[95] This may explain partially the persistent massive bacterial load despite adequate intravenous antibiotic therapy for a prolonged time in many patients.

Clostridium perfringens elaborates at least two exotoxins (α-toxin and perfringolysin O) that are cytolytic to host tissues and are lethal when purified and injected into animals.[96] *C. septicum* also expresses a pore-forming cytolysin, α-toxin, which triggers fulminant myonecrosis as well as inhibition of leukocyte influx into the lesion.[97] Exotoxin-induced microvascular dysfunction is an important factor producing the anaerobic environment that favors *C. perfringens* replication and ischemic necrosis.[38] By contrast, *C. septicum* is relatively aerotolerant, a feature that may partially explain its ability to spread through the bloodstream and establish infection in otherwise healthy muscle.[98]

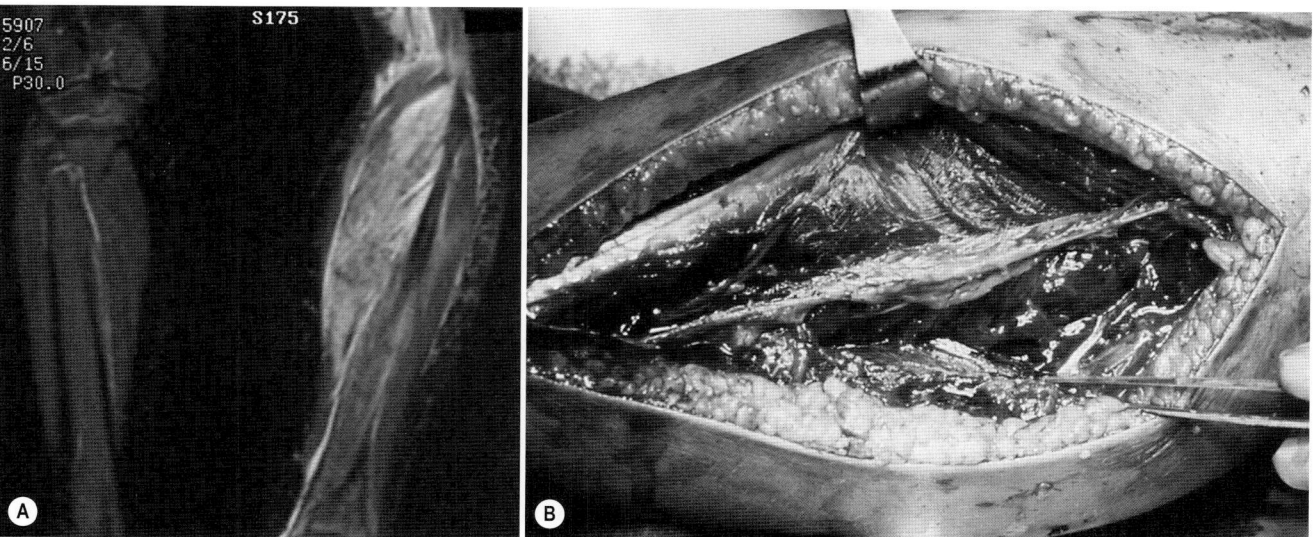

Figure 77-4. A 5-year-old girl experienced severe left posterior calf pain, tenderness, and swelling 1 week after onset of primary varicella. **(A)** With magnetic resonance imaging technique in which fat signal intensity is suppressed, marked signal enhancement is seen diffusely in the calf musculature, indicative of a widespread inflammatory process. **(B)** Operative exploration of the calf revealed liquefaction necrosis of the soleus muscle and the lateral head of the gastrocnemius muscle, which were radically debrided. Group A streptococcus was isolated from culture of tissue and blood. (Courtesy of J.H.T. Waldhausen, MD.)

PART II Clinical Syndromes and Cardinal Features of Infectious Diseases: Approach to Diagnosis and Initial Management

SECTION J Skin and Soft-Tissue Infections

DIAGNOSIS

Early in the course, myositis, pyomyositis, or necrotizing fasciitis can be difficult to distinguish from a number of noninfectious disorders. Plain radiographs usually are normal, but other imaging techniques can be useful in defining the extent of muscle involvement. Although computed tomography (CT) may be useful in defining the extent of soft-tissue involvement, magnetic resonance imaging (MRI) is the preferred modality. MRI can reveal extension of inflammation along the fascial plains and distinguish compartments and structures (bone, muscle, fascia, fat) involved (see Figure 77-2).[99–101] Ultrasonography (US) is helpful in the suppurative phase.[99,102,103]

CT or US may delineate a low-density (or hypoechoic) fluid collection, thereby facilitating diagnostic aspiration or percutaneous drainage.[104,105] Diagnostic MRI findings include hyperintense signal within the muscle with edema in pyomyositis, and a hyperintense rim on unenhanced T1-weighted images and peripheral enhancement after intravenous infusion of gadolinium if abscess has formed[100] (see Figure 77-1). CT or MRI also can detect marked skeletal muscle abnormalities in GAS necrotizing myositis (Figure 77-4).[105,106] Infrared thermography may help reveal the extent of tissue viability in clostridial myonecrosis.[107]

TREATMENT

Therapeutic interventions for SSTIs include incision, drainage, debridement, compartment release, and antibiotic therapy. Recommendations from both the Centers for Disease Control and Prevention[108] and the American Academy of Pediatrics[109] emphasize performing incision and drainage as the primary treatment of abscesses, sending purulent material for culture, and targeting CA-MRSA when empiric antibiotics are prescribed (Table 77-3). Effective surgical drainage of fluid collections or abscesses often can be accomplished percutaneously with ultrasound or CT guidance,[110] but an open surgical procedure may be required.

Surgical debridement usually is necessary for GAS necrotizing pyomyositis once the patient has been stabilized medically.[111] Fasciotomies are performed if there is evidence of increased compartment pressures. GAS uniformly is susceptible to penicillin and other β-lactam antibiotics, and penicillin remains an appropriate antibiotic treatment of GAS infections. However, in patients with aggressive GAS infections, such as myositis and necrotizing fasciitis, a β-lactam antibiotic should be combined with clindamycin (40 mg/kg per day) because of pharmacokinetic properties, activity at the ribosomal level, and inhibition of toxin production.

Therapy of clostridial gas gangrene consists of prompt and radical debridement of involved muscles; amputation may be required. Because 5% of strains of *C. perfringens* are clindamycin resistant, the recommended antibiotic treatment is penicillin plus clindamycin.[112] Although the role of hyperbaric oxygen is

controversial, therapy may serve an adjunctive role by retarding growth of *C. perfringens*, inhibiting α-toxin production, and increasing oxidative killing by host neutrophils.[113] Patients who survive may require amputation, skin grafting, or reconstructive surgery.

In severe GAS infections, the use of high-dose immune globulin intravenous (IGIV) has been proposed as adjunctive therapy. The mechanism of action of IGIV in this setting is believed to include inhibition of the superantigen activity through neutralizing antibodies, opsonization through M-specific antibodies, and a general anti-inflammatory effect.[114] Large controlled studies of IGIV therapy in patients with severe invasive GAS infections have not been conducted, but case reports and small controlled studies have reported use of IGIV in GAS toxic shock syndrome, necrotizing fasciitis, and necrotizing myositis (Table 77-4). A favorable outcome was reported for invasive GAS infections in an observational cohort study of Canadian patients identified through active surveillance[115] and in one European multicenter placebo-controlled trial.[116] Data on the efficacy of IGIV for necrotizing fasciitis are limited (see Table 77-4).[111,117,118] In one study, mortality was 10% among IGIV-treated patients, compared with 37% in non-treated control subjects.[117] In an observational case study, the use of an aggressive medical regimen including high-dose IGIV appeared to mitigate the need for aggressive surgical intervention.[81] Seven patients with severe GAS soft-tissue infection (6 patients with toxic shock syndrome) were treated with antibiotics parenterally and high-dose IGIV; surgery was either not performed or limited to exploration; all patients survived. This limited study suggests that an initial conservative surgical approach combined with the use of immune modulators, such as IGIV, may reduce the morbidity associated with extensive surgical exploration in hemodynamically unstable patients.

Excellent guidelines available online from the Infectious Diseases Society of America provide empiric therapeutic options for specific clinical scenarios, i.e., dog bite, and specific pathogens of SSTIs.[112]

TABLE 77-4. Intravenous Polyspecific Immunoglobulin (IGIV) as Adjunctive Therapy in Severe Invasive Group A Streptococcal Infections

Study Design	No. of Patients[a]	Case-Fatality Rate (%)
NF and myonecrosis, case series identified through active surveillance[118]	IGIV: 10 No IGIV: 4	19 25
NF, case series identified through active surveillance[117]	IGIV: 10 No IGIV: 67	10 37
Severe soft-tissue infections, observational cohort study[111]	7	0
STSS + NM, case report[119]	1	0
STSS + NF, case report[120]	1	0
STSS + NF, case report[121]	1	0
STSS + NF, case report[122]	1	0
STSS, case report[123]	1	0
STSS, case report[124]	1	0
STSS, case report[125]	1	0
STSS, case report[126]	1	0
STSS, case series[127]	5	20
STSS, multicenter placebo RCT[b,116]	IGIV: 10 Placebo: 11	10 36
STSS, case-control study[115]	IGIV: 21 No IGIV: 32	33 66

NF, necrotizing fasciitis; NM, necrotizing myositis; STSS, streptococcal toxic shock syndrome; RCT, randomized control trial.

[a]*All received IGIV unless otherwise specified.*

[b]*Trial prematurely terminated due to slow patient recruitment.*[116]

TABLE 77-3. Antimicrobial Agents for Treatment of Community-Acquired Methicillin-Resistant *Staphylococcus aureus* Infections in Children

Antimicrobial	Daily Dosage
Daptomycin[1]	4–6 mg/kg per day q24 hours
Linezolid	30 mg/kg per day divided q8 hours
Vancomycin	40 mg/kg per day divided q6 hours
Clindamycin	10–30 mg/kg per day divided q6–8 hours
Trimethoprim/sulfamethoxazole	20 mg/kg per day divided q6 hours
Linezolid	30 mg/kg per day divided q8 hours

Daptomycin should not be used to treat pneumonia; not approved by the Food and Drug Administration for the treatment of children.

78 Osteomyelitis

Kathleen Gutierrez

Osteomyelitis is inflammation of bone. Bacteria are the usual etiologic agents, but fungal osteomyelitis occurs occasionally. Osteomyelitis in children primarily has hematogenous origin, occurring less commonly as a result of trauma, surgery, or infected contiguous soft tissue. Osteomyelitis due to vascular insufficiency is rare in children.

ACUTE HEMATOGENOUS OSTEOMYELITIS

Pathogenesis

Acute hematogenous osteomyelitis (AHO) is primarily a disease of young children, presumably because of the rich vascular supply of their rapidly growing bones.[1-3] Infecting organisms enter the bone through the nutrient artery and then travel to the metaphyseal capillary loops, where they are deposited, replicate, and initiate an inflammatory response (Figure 78-1). Metaphyseal localization results from sluggish blood flow, the presence of endothelial gaps in the tips of growing metaphyseal vessels, and lack of phagocytic cells lining the capillaries.[3-6] Bacteria proliferate, spread through vascular tunnels, and are anchored to areas of exposed cartilaginous matrix. Large colonies of bacteria surrounded by glycocalyx obstruct capillary lumens, impairing phagocytosis and antibiotic penetration.[7]

Age-related differences in the anatomy of the bone and its blood supply influence the clinical manifestations of osteomyelitis.[2,3] Transphyseal vessels are present in most children younger than 18 months, providing a vascular connection between the metaphysis and the epiphysis.[8] As a result, in infants, infection originating in the metaphysis can spread to the epiphysis and joint space. The risk of ischemic damage to the growth plate is greater in the young infant with osteomyelitis.[9] Before puberty, the periosteum is not firmly anchored to underlying bone. Infection in the metaphysis of a bone can spread to perforate the bony cortex, causing subperiosteal elevation and extension into surrounding soft tissue. Bony destruction can spread to the diaphysis. By age of 2 years, the cartilaginous growth plate usually prevents extension of infection to the epiphysis and into the joint space. When the metaphysis of the proximal femur or humerus is involved, however, infection can extend into the hip or shoulder joint at any age, because at these sites, the metaphysis is intracapsular.

Histologic features of acute osteomyelitis include localized suppuration and abscess formation, with subsequent infarction and necrosis of bone. Segments of bone that lose blood supply and become separated from viable bone are called *sequestra*. An *involucrum* is a layer of living bone surrounding dead bone.[10] A *Brodie abscess* is a subacute, well-demarcated focal infection, usually in the metaphysis but sometimes in the diaphysis of bone.

Epidemiology

Approximately half of all cases of AHO occur in the first 5 years of life.[11] Boys are affected twice as frequently as girls, except in the first year of life.[11,12] One-third of patients have minor trauma to the affected extremity before infection, but the specific importance of this history is unclear, because virtually all young children experience frequent mild trauma.[13]

The relative risk of developing osteomyelitis appears to be higher in some populations. In one study, Polynesian and Maori children were more likely to develop complicated osteomyelitis with *Staphylococcus aureus* than other children in the same New Zealand community.[14] It is unclear whether genetic or socioeconomic or environmental factors accounted for this difference.

Microbiology

S. aureus is the most common cause of AHO.[1,13,15-21] *Kingella kingae*, *Streptococcus pneumoniae*,[22] and *S. pyogenes*[23] are the organisms isolated in most other cases of AHO in children. *K. kingae* and *S. pneumoniae* infections are most common in children less than 3 years of age. *S. pneumoniae* accounts for a relatively small proportion of infections, especially in the context of widespread immunization with the pneumococcal conjugate vaccine.[24,25] *K. kingae* can be associated with small outbreaks of bone and joint infections in childcare centers.[20,26] Coagulase-negative staphylococci (CoNS) (almost exclusively as a complication of medical intervention), enteric gram-negative bacilli, and anaerobic bacteria are uncommon causes of AHO. *Bartonella henselae* can cause granulomatous infection of bone.[27-29] *Actinomyces* spp. cause facial and cervical osteomyelitis.[30] Infection with *Serratia* spp. and *Aspergillus* spp. should be considered in children with chronic granulomatous disease.[31] Before widespread use of *Haemophilus influenzae* type b (Hib) conjugate vaccines, 10% to 15% of cases of osteomyelitis in children younger than 3 years were caused by this organism.[15,18] Invasive disease is rare in immunized children.[32]

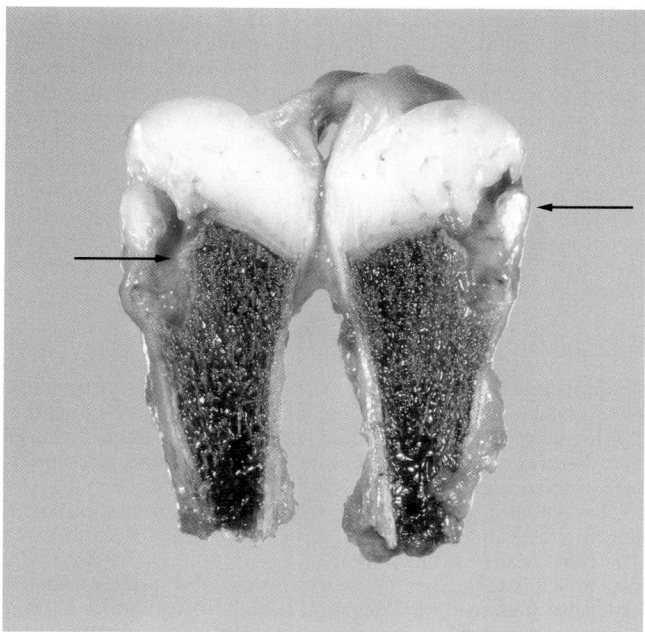

Figure 78-1. Gross specimen showing osteomyelitis of the proximal humerus in a 6-week-old infant. Note metaphyseal location and bony destruction (arrows). (Courtesy of S.S. Long.)

PART II Clinical Syndromes and Cardinal Features of Infectious Diseases: Approach to Diagnosis and Initial Management

SECTION K Bone and Joint Infections

Community-acquired methicillin-resistant *Staphylococcus aureus* (CA-MRSA) AHO has been increasing dramatically.[33-36] Some CA-MRSA isolates causing osteoarticular infection carry the genes for Panton–Valentine leukocidin (PVL), a virulence factor or marker for complicated infections.[33,37,38]

Clinical Characteristics and Differential Diagnosis

Most patients with AHO have symptoms for <2 weeks before they are brought to medical attention, although a small proportion have low-grade fever and intermittent bone pain for several weeks.[13,17] The most common manifestations are fever, pain at the site of infection, and reluctance to use an affected extremity.[18,39] Less common complaints are anorexia, malaise, and vomiting. Physical findings consist of focal swelling, tenderness, warmth, and erythema (usually over the metaphysis of a long bone). Rarely, a draining fistulous tract develops over the affected bone.[13] Tenderness out of proportion to soft-tissue findings suggests osteomyelitis rather than soft-tissue infection or cellulitis. Exaggerated immobility of the joint and lack of point tenderness over the metaphysis suggest pyogenic arthritis. Other causes of bone pain are fracture, bone infarction secondary to hemoglobinopathy, leukemia, vitamin deficiency, and bony neoplasms such as metastatic neuroblastoma and Ewing sarcoma.

Osteomyelitis most frequently occurs in the long bones (Figure 78-2), although in some series, 10% to 25% of cases involve short or nontubular bones, including the pelvis, clavicle, calcaneus, skull, ribs, and scapula.[17,18,40] Multiple bones are involved in about 5% of cases.

Compared with methicillin-sensitive *S. aureus* (CA-MSSA), patients with CA-MRSA infections have more protracted courses of fever, as well as hospitalization, multiple foci of infection, pyomyositis, and subperiosteal and intraosseous abscesses.[36,38,41,42] A recent retrospective study demonstrated that four independent predictive factors (temperature 38°C, hematocrit <34%, WBC count >12,000 cells/mm³ and C-reactive protein level >1.3 mg/dL) were useful in differentiating MRSA from MSSA osteomyelitis. Prospective validation of this scoring system is pending.[42a] Patients with PVL-positive CA-MRSA are at increased risk for deep-vein thrombosis or septic emboli to the lungs.[33,35-37] Compared with infection due to PVL-negative organisms, infection with PVL-positive *S. aureus* also appears more likely to result in chronic osteomyelitis.[33]

Laboratory Diagnosis

Bacteriologic diagnosis can be confirmed in 50% to 80% of cases of AHO; the yield is highest when multiple specimens, including blood, bone, and joint fluid, are sampled.[3,12,13,17,18,39] Cultures obtained by imaging-guided bone biopsy are more likely to be positive if larger volumes (>2 mL) of purulent material are aspirated.[43] Diagnosis of *K. kingae* infection is enhanced with intraoperative inoculation of culture material directly into liquid media or onto agar plates or when polymerase chain reaction (PCR) analysis is performed;[20,21,44] cultures should be held for at least 7 to 10 days.

The erythrocyte sedimentation rate (ESR) is elevated in up to 90% of cases of osteomyelitis, and the C-reactive protein (CRP) level in 98%.[17,18,38,45] The mean ESR is 40 to 60 mm/h, but levels >100 mm/h can occur. ESR generally peaks 3 to 5 days after initiation of therapy and returns to normal in approximately 3 weeks. CRP levels peak by the second day (mean, 8.3 mg/dL) and return to normal (<2.0 mg/dL) after approximately 1 week of therapy.[45] Patients infected with PVL-positive versus PVL-negative *S. aureus* are more likely to have positive blood cultures and higher ESR and CRP levels at presentation.[38] Higher levels of CRP at diagnosis may predict greater risk of sequelae.[46,47] The peripheral white blood cell count can be elevated or normal; thrombocytosis can be noted, especially if symptoms have been present for more than 1 week.

Radiologic Diagnosis

Plain Radiographs

Radiographic abnormalities in osteomyelitis reflect inflammation, destruction, and new formation of bone.[3,48] The earliest abnormalities, seen within the first 3 days of onset of symptoms, are deep soft-tissue swelling and loss of the normally visible tissue planes around the affected bone. Osteopenia or osteolytic lesions from destruction of bone usually are not visible until approximately 50% of bone has been demineralized. Lytic lesions, periosteal elevation due to subcortical purulence, and periosteal new bone formation appear approximately 10 to 20 days after onset of symptoms. Sclerosis of bone is seen when infection has been present for longer than a month. If deep soft-tissue swelling is noted on plain radiograph in a patient with a short history of symptoms and with point tenderness over the affected metaphysis, no further imaging studies are necessary to support the diagnosis of osteomyelitis.

Radionuclide Scanning

Radionuclide scans are useful in the early diagnosis of osteomyelitis, even when plain radiographs are normal. Technetium-labeled methylene diphosphonate isotope is most frequently used because its uptake by infected bone is enhanced when osteoblastic activity is increased.

The reported sensitivity of technetium-99 bone scanning is between 80% and 100% (Table 78-1),[49-53] (Figures 78-3 and 78-4). The bone scan can be normal in 5% to 20% of children with osteomyelitis in the first few days of illness.[52,54-56] Bone scan is less expensive than MRI, and sedation usually is not required. Bone scan is particularly useful when multifocal bone involvement is suspected.[57]

A variety of disorders, including malignancy, deep soft-tissue infection, cellulitis, pyogenic arthritis, trauma, fracture, and bone

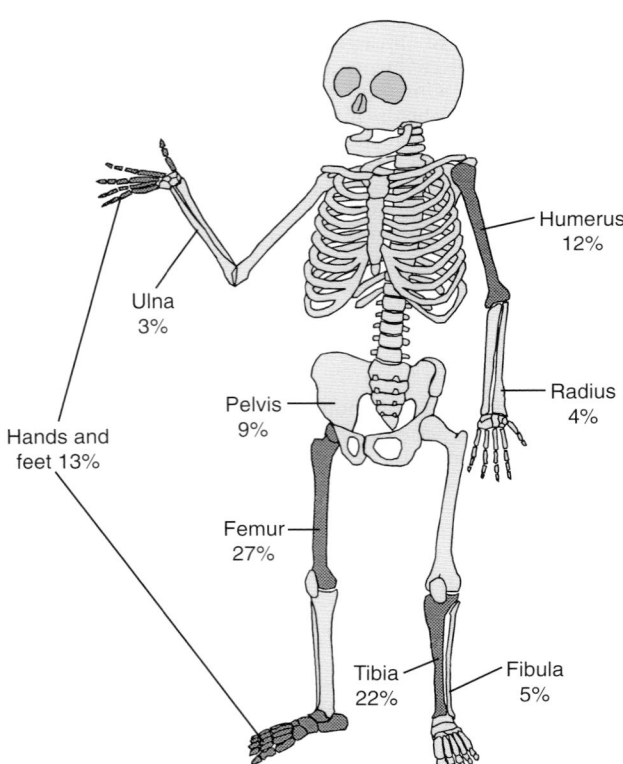

Figure 78-2. Sites of acute osteomyelitis in 657 children in whom a single bone was involved. Shaded areas constitute sites of approximately 75% of cases. Miscellaneous sites accounting for 5% are not shown. (Data collated from references 12, 17, 18, and 39.)

Humerus 12%

Ulna 3%

Radius 4%

Pelvis 9%

Hands and feet 13%

Femur 27%

Tibia 22%

Fibula 5%

TABLE 78-1. Technetium Bone Scans for Osteomyelitis in Children

Study[a]	Year	Patient Age	Sensitivity (%)
Tuson et al.[49]	1994	6 months–13 years	92
Hamdan et al.[50]	1987	6 months–14 years	89
Howie et al.[51]	1983	6 weeks–13 years	89
Sullivan et al.[52]	1980	3 weeks–15 years	81[b]
Bressler et al.[53]	1984	<6 weeks	100

[a]Superscript numbers indicate references.

[b]The 2 patients younger than 6 weeks of age had normal scans.

infarction, can result in positive scan results. Metaphyseal site of maximal uptake and lack of uptake in bone on both sides of a joint support the diagnosis of AHO, rather than pyogenic arthritis. Diaphyseal uptake suggests tumor, trauma, or infarction.

In some cases of osteomyelitis, bone scans show areas of decreased technetium uptake ("cold scans"), probably reflecting compromised vascular supply to the bone from ischemia or thrombosis;[49,58] such findings make differentiation of osteomyelitis from infarction associated with sickle-cell disease difficult. Patients with osteomyelitis and decreased uptake on bone scan may have more complicated infection, frequently with thrombosis and ischemic necrosis.[58]

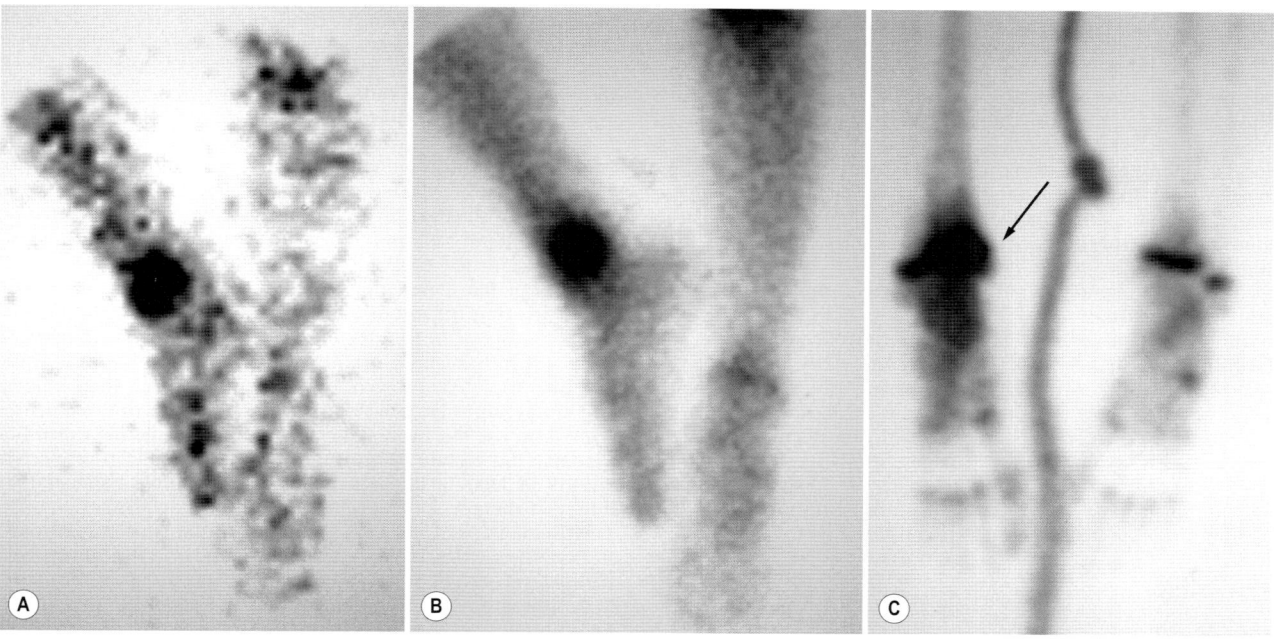

Figure 78-3. Typical technetium-99 bone scan findings of acute osteomyelitis in a 4-year-old girl who had a 2-day history of fever, ankle pain, and swelling, and refusal to bear weight. Plain radiograph was unremarkable. Triple-phase anterior images of bone scan show increased tracer activity in the region of the right ankle in the angiographic (immediate) phase **(A)**, increased tracer activity in the soft tissues in the region of the ankle in the blood pool (15-minute) phase **(B)**, and localization of tracer in the distal tibial metaphysis (arrow) without periarticular distribution in the delayed (2.5-hour) phase **(C)**. Diagnosis was confirmed at surgery with finding of subperiosteal pus; *Streptococcus pyogenes* was isolated. (Courtesy of E. Geller and S.S. Long, St. Christopher's Hospital for Children, Philadelphia, PA.)

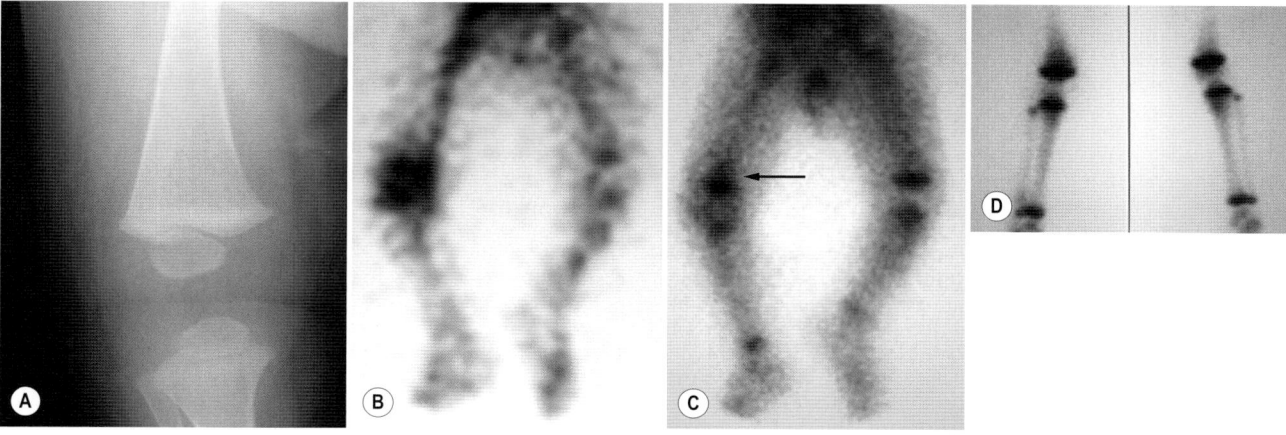

Figure 78-4. Plain film and technetium-99 bone scan of acute osteomyelitis and pyogenic arthritis in a 7-month-old boy who had a 3-day history of high fever, fussiness and redness, and swelling of the lateral right leg from the thigh to the lower leg, with limitation of motion of the knee. Aspiration of the knee revealed 169,000 white blood cells/mm² and gram-positive cocci. Plain film shows obscuration of right lateral subcutaneous fat–muscle plane, from the thigh to the lower leg **(A)**. Triple-phase bone scan shows increased tracer activity in the region of the right knee in the angiographic phase **(B)** and in the periarticular soft tissues in the blood pool phase **(C)**, as well as localization of tracer in the distal femur (arrow) but not in the proximal tibia in the delayed phase **(D)**. Diagnosis of osteomyelitis of the femur was confirmed at surgery. Methicillin-susceptible *Staphylococcus aureus* was isolated from blood, joint and bone specimens. (Courtesy of E. Geller and S.S. Long, St. Christopher's Hospital for Children, Philadelphia, PA.)

PART II Clinical Syndromes and Cardinal Features of Infectious Diseases: Approach to Diagnosis and Initial Management

SECTION K Bone and Joint Infections

Nuclear scanning using gallium-67 citrate or indium-111-labeled leukocytes is positive in diseases characterized by increased bone turnover and, thus, have limited specificity for osteomyelitis.[59] Indium scanning, which reflects migration of white blood cells into areas of inflammation, can be useful in the diagnosis of osteomyelitis associated with trauma, surgery, chronic ulcers, or prosthetic devices,[60] but is limited by poor localization of infection (i.e., bone versus soft tissue), decreased sensitivity in diagnosing infection in the central skeleton, and relatively high radiation exposure. Simultaneous performance of a technetium bone scan sometimes increases specificity.[61]

Magnetic Resonance Imaging

Magnetic resonance imaging (MRI) is a sensitive bone–imaging test.[62,63] Its reported sensitivity for detection of osteomyelitis ranges from 92% to 100%. Normal red and fatty portions of the bone marrow have a characteristic appearance on MRI. Fatty marrow produces a bright signal on T_1-weighted images.[64] Changes in marrow caused by infection and inflammation produce an area of low signal intensity within the bright fatty marrow. Areas of low signal intensity in infected marrow seen on a T_1-weighted image change to bright signal intensity on a T_2-weighted image. These changes are not specific for osteomyelitis and can be seen with malignancy, fracture, and bone infarction.

MRI can detect signal alterations in soft tissue and is particularly useful in differentiating cellulitis from osteomyelitis. MRI also may differentiate acute from chronic osteomyelitis.[65]

Gadolinium-enhanced MRI can be particularly useful in the diagnosis of soft-tissue, muscle, or bone abscesses associated with infection.[41] The use of contrast agents can increase confidence in the diagnosis of osteomyelitis in cases which bone and soft-tissue edema are seen on unenhanced images.[66] MRI has been used to identify bone marrow infection in cases of *Bartonella henselae* infection, particularly when plain films and computed tomography (CT) of the affected bones appear normal.[28]

TREATMENT

Antibiotic Choice

Considerations in choosing a specific antimicrobial regimen include the age of the child, underlying medical conditions, suspected pathogens and their susceptibility pattern, antibiotic pharmacodynamics, and the safety and efficacy of the antibiotic.

Most β-lactam antibiotics achieve therapeutic concentrations in bone.[67,68] Clindamycin has particularly good bone penetration, attaining a high bone-to-serum ratio.[67,69–71] Vancomycin has excellent penetration into the bones of experimental animals.[67] Aminoglycoside agents theoretically have poor bactericidal activity in bone because of local tissue hypoxia and acidosis. Although ciprofloxacin penetrates well into bone, fluoroquinolones are not recommended routinely for use in young children.[72]

Most cases of AHO in any age group are caused by *S. aureus.* Empiric therapy should include coverage for this organism. Parenterally administered nafcillin, clindamycin, or a first-generation cephalosporin historically have been the usual choices for empiric therapy; however, the increase in CA-MRSA infections has made the choice of initial antibiotic therapy challenging. Direct sampling of bone for culture is increasingly important. Clindamycin remains a good choice for empiric therapy in communities where resistance (both constitutive and inducible) occurs in fewer than 10% of *S. aureus* isolates.[41] In communities where CA-MRSA resistance to clindamycin and methicillin is greater than 10% to 15%, vancomycin is the drug of choice for empiric therapy.[72a] Clindamycin and vancomycin are active against most isolates of *S. pyogenes* and *S. pneumoniae*. Neither offers coverage for *K. kingae* infection, which is susceptible to most β-lactam antibiotics. Ampicillin-sulbactam should be considered in addition to clindamycin or vancomycin, especially in young children.

Empiric therapy for young children who have not been immunized against *Haemophilus influenzae* type b should include a third-generation cephalosporin in addition to antistaphylococcal coverage. A second-generation cephalosporin such as cefuroxime alone is a reasonable alternative if suspicion for MRSA is low.[73] However, with the dramatic reduction of cases of Hib disease in the United States, it is reasonable to use only an antistaphylococcal–antistreptococcal antibiotic in the fully immunized and immunocompetent child.

Neonates with osteomyelitis should be treated with antibiotics active against *S. aureus*, group B streptococcus (GBS), and gram-negative enteric organisms. Suggested initial empiric parenteral antibiotic therapy for neonates and children with AHO is outlined in Table 78-2.

Antibiotic therapy should be modified according to results of culture and susceptibility testing. Nafcillin, oxacillin, a first-generation cephalosporin, or clindamycin (if susceptible) are the drugs of choice for infections caused by MSSA. Clindamycin is a good definitive choice for susceptible MRSA and MSSA[73a] but should not be used if inducible resistance is detected because of reports of treatment failure under this circumstance.[74,75]

There are few antibiotic choices for clindamycin-resistant CA-MRSA infection in children. Recently published guidelines by the Infectious Disease Society of America (IDSA) recommend vancomycin plus/minus rifampin for the treatment of MRSA osteomyelitis in children. Linezolid is suggested as an alternative choice.[72a] Limited data support efficacy of linezolid.[76,77] In one group of pediatric patients, linezolid was as effective as vancomycin in treating infections caused by MRSA, although efficacy in treating bone or joint infections was not specifically evaluated.[77] Linezolid has excellent oral bioavailability and offers an alternative to prolonged intravenous therapy. However, it is expensive and many children object to the taste of the oral suspension. Long-term use has been associated with neutropenia, thrombocytopenia, and elevated serum transaminase levels.[78] There are rare reports of lactic acidosis and optic neuropathy associated with linezolid therapy.[79,80]

Most CA-MRSA isolates are susceptible to trimethoprim-sulfamethoxazole, tetracyclines, and rifampin. Clinical experience with these drugs for osteoarticular infections is limited.[81,82] Rifampin should not be used as a single agent because of rapid development of resistance. Although daptomycin and tigecycline have activity against MRSA, neither is approved for use in children. The IDSA guidelines suggest that daptomycin may be used in children in selected circumstances.[72a] If no organism is isolated, and the symptoms are resolving, initial empiric therapy should be continued. Most cases of culture-negative osteomyelitis respond to therapy with antistaphylococcal antibiotics.[83]

Management of children with osteomyelitis should include concurrent care by an orthopedic surgeon. Indications for surgery include desirability of specific pathogen diagnosis; prolonged fever, erythema, pain, and swelling; persistent bacteremia despite adequate antibiotic therapy; soft-tissue or periosteal abscess; formation of a sinus tract; and presence of necrotic, nonviable bone.[16,84–86]

Duration of Therapy

Duration of antibiotic therapy depends on the cause and extent of infection as well as the clinical course. The usual duration ranges from 3 to 6 weeks and should be individualized on the basis of severity of illness and clinical response. Historical evidence suggests that <3 weeks of treatment is associated with higher rates of relapse or recurrence than longer duration of therapy.[13] Plain radiographs obtained at the end of therapy may be useful as a marker of maximal anticipated destruction, a baseline for further studies, and a guide to possible complications.

Peripherally inserted or tunneled central venous catheter (PICC/CVC) often is placed to continue intravenous antibiotics at home. Use of PICC or CVC for >2 weeks in children with osteomyelitis can be associated with an increase in catheter-related complications,[87] including catheter malfunction, thrombosis and catheter-associated bloodstream infections.[88]

TABLE 78-2. Antibiotic Selection for Initial Treatment of Osteomyelitis

Patient Age	Likely Pathogen	Antibiotic Selection	Dosage	
			mg/kg per day	Doses/Day
>3 years	Staphylococcus aureus	Nafcillin	150	4
		or		
		Clindamycin[c]	30–40	3–4
		or		
		Vancomycin	45–60	3–4
<3 years	S. aureus	Nafcillin	150	4
	Haemophilus influenzae type b[a]	or		
	Kingella kingae[b]	Clindamycin[c]	30–40	3–4
		or		
		Vancomycin	45–60	3–4
		plus		
		Cefotaxime	100–150	4
		or		
		Ceftriaxone	100	2
		or		
		Cefuroxime	75–150	3
		or		
		Ampicillin-sulbactam	300	4
Neonate	S. aureus	Nafcillin	100	4
	Group B streptococcus	or		
	Enteric gram-negative bacteria	Vancomycin	30	2
		plus		
		Gentamicin	5–7.5	3
		OR		
		Nafcillin	100	4
		or		
		Vancomycin	30	2
		plus		
		Cefotaxime	150	3

[a]If patient is fully immunized against Haemophilus influenzae type b, consider using only antistaphylococcal coverage.

[b]If patient is treated with either clindamycin or vancomycin, consider adding an ampicillin or cephalosporin agent for Kingella kingae.

[c]Clindamycin 40 mg/kg/day recommended for treatment of susceptible MRSA osteomyelitis.

Sequential parenteral–oral antibiotic regimens can be successful.[89-94] Early transition to oral therapy was not associated with a higher risk of treatment failure in a recent study.[87] The change to oral antibiotics is generally made when fever, pain, and signs of local inflammation have resolved and laboratory values, especially CRP, are normalizing. The willingness of the child to take oral medication and the likelihood of adherence to the regimen also must be assessed. The oral antibiotic should have the same spectrum of coverage as the parenteral drug. If a β-lactam agent is used, dosage required is generally two to three times the usual oral dose (Table 78-3).

TABLE 78-3. Dosage of Antibiotics Commonly Used in the Oral Phase of Treatment of Osteomyelitis[a]

Antibiotic	Dosage	
	mg/kg per day	Doses/Day
Dicloxacillin	75–100	4
Cephalexin	100–150	4
Clindamycin	30–40[b]	3–4

[a]In general, the dose of β-lactam antibiotics used for osteomyelitis is 2–3 times the usual dose.

[b]Clindamycin 40 mg/kg/day is recommended for treatment of susceptible MRSA osteomyelitis.[72a]

Once the change to oral therapy is made, the child should be monitored to ensure continued clinical improvement. The CRP level is expected to return to normal 7 to 10 days after initiation of appropriate therapy, and the ESR normalizes within 3 to 4 weeks.[45,93]

SPECIAL CLINICAL SITUATIONS

Neonatal Osteomyelitis

Osteomyelitis is uncommon in the neonatal period. The incidence is estimated to be approximately 1 to 3 cases for every 1000 intensive-care nursery admissions.[95]

Associated risk factors include prematurity, low birthweight, preceding infection, bacteremia, exchange transfusion, and the presence of an intravenous or umbilical catheter.[96-99] Osteomyelitis of the skull secondary to contiguous spread of infection has occurred as a complication of fetal scalp electrode monitoring[100-102] and in association with infected cephalohematoma.[103,104] Osteomyelitis of the calcaneus has complicated heel lancet puncture.[97,105]

The diagnosis of osteomyelitis in neonates often is delayed because of nonspecific symptoms.[106] Signs and symptoms include fever, irritability, swelling or decreased movement of a limb (pseudoparalysis), erythema, and tenderness over the affected bone.[95-97,107] Preterm infants are more likely than term infants to manifest symptoms of septicemia.[108]

PART II Clinical Syndromes and Cardinal Features of Infectious Diseases: Approach to Diagnosis and Initial Management

SECTION K Bone and Joint Infections

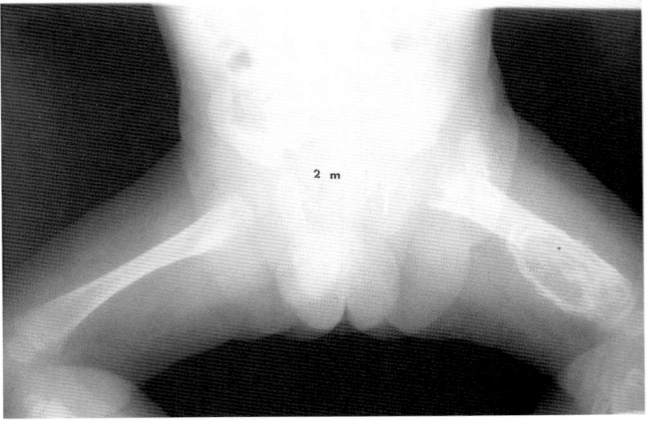

Figure 78-5. Plain radiograph of an infant at 2 months of age who had *Staphylococcus aureus* bloodstream infection during a stay in the neonatal intensive care unit in the first month of life. He had multiple sites of infection, including the proximal and distal femur and hip joint. Note widespread destruction of femur, acetabulum, and joint. (Courtesy of S.S. Long, St. Christopher's Hospital for Children, Philadelphia, PA.)

Approximately 20% to 50% of neonates with osteomyelitis have infection of multiple bones,[95,96,109] and about 75% have suppurative arthritis of contiguous joints[96] (Figure 78-5).

S. aureus (including CA-MRSA[110]), GBS, and enteric gram-negative bacilli are the most common causes (Table 78-4); fungi,[111] *Ureaplasma urealyticum*,[112] CoNS,[113] *Neisseria gonorrhoeae*,[107] and anaerobic[100] bacteria are unusual causes.

Infants with GBS bone infection usually have had an uncomplicated neonatal course and have infection of a single bone. There is a predilection for involvement of long bones on the right, particularly the right proximal humerus,[113,114] which may be related to trauma during vaginal delivery.[113] Misdiagnosis of bone infection as trauma in these mildly ill infants is common. Since the release of the 1996 consensus guidelines for prevention of GBS disease, the incidence of early-onset perinatal GBS disease but not late-onset disease has declined in the U.S.[115]

The white blood cell count commonly is normal; ESR and CRP often are elevated.[116] In most infants, an osteolytic lesion is visible on plain radiograph 10 to 12 days after onset of symptoms (frequently the time of diagnosis).[86,96,97,107,117,118] Radionuclide bone scans can be positive[53,95,106] but sometimes are less sensitive than plain radiographs.[97]

Neonatal osteomyelitis can lead to permanent joint abnormalities or disturbance in skeletal growth secondary to damage to the cartilaginous growth plate, including arthritis, decreased range of motion, limb length discrepancy, and gait abnormalities.[119] The reported incidence of permanent sequelae varies from 6% to 50%.[96,97,108,113]

Vertebral Osteomyelitis

Vertebral osteomyelitis accounts for approximately 1% to 3% of cases of osteomyelitis in children.[13,18,120,121] Boys are affected twice as frequently as girls.[122] Infection usually occurs as a result of hematogenous seeding of the vertebral bodies by arterial or venous vessels. Osteomyelitis also can result from extension of soft-tissue infection or as a complication of a surgical procedure.[16,123]

Clinical manifestations can be indolent and nonspecific, leading to delayed diagnosis. Young infants can have nonspecific signs of septicemia.[124] Symptoms in older children include back, chest, abdominal, or leg pain as well as loss of normal curvatures.[120,125] Rarely, children manifest dysphagia secondary to a paravertebral or retropharyngeal abscess or acute spinal cord paresis/paralysis due to paraspinal compression.[120,126] Fever is common, and tenderness over the involved vertebrae is expected. Neurologic deficits are found in 15% to 20% of cases.[120,122]

S. aureus is isolated in most cases.[16,120,122,127] In one review, *Salmonella* spp. caused 12% of cases of childhood vertebral osteomyelitis.[120] Gram-negative bacilli such as *Escherichia coli* cause vertebral osteomyelitis in adults, particularly those with a history of recent urinary tract infection or instrumentation. Vertebral osteomyelitis in intravenous drug users is commonly caused by *Pseudomonas aeruginosa* and less commonly by *S. aureus, Serratia* spp., *Klebsiella* spp., *Enterobacter* spp., or *Candida* spp.[128,129] Tuberculosis and brucellosis should be considered if symptoms and radiographs suggest chronic infection.[130,131]

Characteristic findings on plain radiograph consist of narrowing of the involved disk space, lucency of the adjacent vertebral bodies, and, eventually, reactive sclerosis of the bone with fusion of vertebral bodies.[16,120,127] Vertebral osteomyelitis is differentiated from diskitis radiographically by the minimal vertebral endplate involvement associated with diskitis (see Chapter 80, Diskitis). MRI is reported to be highly sensitive (96%) and specific (92%) for diagnosis of vertebral osteomyelitis.[132,133]

Blood culture results are positive in only about 30% of acute cases. When blood culture results are negative, strong consideration should be given to obtaining a biopsy specimen from the vertebral body for culture and histologic examination.[133]

Children with uncomplicated vertebral osteomyelitis and no evidence of abscess formation should be treated with at least 4 weeks of antibiotic administered parenterally.[120] Surgical decompression or debridement or both are indicated in the presence of spinal epidural abscess, signs of spinal cord compression, or extensive bony destruction.

Complications of vertebral osteomyelitis include neurologic deficits secondary to epidural abscess,[134] paravertebral abscess,[135] and infected aneurysms of the aorta.[136]

Pelvic Osteomyelitis

Approximately 6% to 9% of all cases of hematogenous osteomyelitis involve the bones of the pelvis.[40,137,138] The ilium and ischium are most commonly involved;[137] infection of the sacrum, acetabulum, or pubic symphysis is rare.[137–140] Risk factors (not always present) include a history of pelvic trauma, intravenous drug use, and genitourinary procedures.[137,140]

Most patients with pelvic osteomyelitis have fever, gait abnormalities, and pain that is often localized to the hip, groin, or buttock.[137,140–143] Pain with hip movement and point tenderness over the affected bone often is observed. Clinical features can mimic those of pyogenic arthritis of the hip;[137] however, in pelvic osteomyelitis there is more likely to be near-normal range of motion of the hip, absence of referred pain to the knee, specific point tenderness over the affected bone (or pain on rocking of the pelvic girdle), and abnormal rectal findings.[143] Responsible pathogens are similar to those that cause osteomyelitis of long bones.

TABLE 78-4. Frequency of Organisms Causing Neonatal Osteomyelitis (*n* = 128)

Single Organism	%
Staphylococcus aureus	60.6
β-Hemolytic streptococcus	
Group B	16.5
Group A	3.1
Enteric gram-negative bacilli	8.7
Staphylococcus epidermidis	2.4
Nonhemolytic streptococcus	2.4
Streptococcus pneumoniae	0.8
Neisseria gonorrhoeae	0.8
Multiple organisms	4.7

Plain radiographs of the pelvis often are normal. Technetium scanning,[137,138,141–143] MRI, or CT can suggest the correct diagnosis and may be useful for differentiating osteomyelitis from bacterial infection of the muscles of the pelvic girdle. MRI has the advantage of identifying abscesses associated with pelvic osteomyelitis and is the imaging technique of choice.[144]

Patients should be treated for at least 4 weeks with antibiotics parenterally.[137–140,143] Surgical drainage or debridement should be considered in cases of extraosseous abscess formation or in patients whose symptoms do not respond to intravenous antibiotic therapy.

Children with Sickle Hemoglobinopathies

Children with sickle-cell disease have increased susceptibility to bacterial infections, including osteomyelitis.[145] The suspected pathogenesis is primary microscopic infarction in the intestinal mucosa and bone, resulting in bacteremia and focal bone infection. Splenic hypofunction, impaired opsonization, impaired macrophage function, and microembolism as well as tissue infarction are likely contributing factors in osteomyelitis.[146,147]

Salmonella spp. plus other gram-negative enteric bacilli were the cause of >70% of cases of osteomyelitis in children with hemoglobinopathies in past decades.[148–151] *S. aureus* currently is an important/dominant cause of osteomyelitis in this population. Other organisms causing osteomyelitis in children with sickle hemoglobinopathies are listed in Box 78-1.

Distinctive features of osteomyelitis in children with sickle-cell disease are frequent involvement of the diaphyses of long bones, flat bones, and small bones of the hands and feet as well as multifocal, symmetrical bone involvement.[146,152] Manifestations of osteomyelitis are difficult to differentiate from those of acute vaso-occlusive crisis. Fever, bone pain, and leukocytosis are common to both conditions. Temperature >39° C, toxic appearance, and an absolute band count >500 cells/mm^3 are more consistent with infection; however, there is considerable clinical and laboratory overlap.[148]

Plain radiograph, technetium scanning, and MRI cannot differentiate infarction from infection.[152,153] Therefore, if fever and bone pain have not improved after supportive care has been given for vaso-occlusive crisis, needle aspiration of the affected area of bone for Gram stain and culture should be performed.

A prolonged course of parenteral antibiotic therapy (6 to 8 weeks) may be necessary for treatment of osteomyelitis in patients with sickle hemoglobinopathy. Oral therapy can be substituted for parenteral treatment once a pathogen has been confirmed and there is clinical improvement; therapy may need to be very protracted. Relapses especially when due to *Salmonella* are not infrequent.[146,148]

OSTEOMYELITIS DUE TO UNUSUAL ORGANISMS

Fungal Osteomyelitis

Fungal osteomyelitis is unusual in healthy children, occurring occasionally in neonates, immunocompromised patients, and intravenous drug users.[111,154–157] Osteomyelitis caused by *Candida* spp. is reported in intravenous drug users and in prematurely born neonates.[111,154–158] *Aspergillus* spp. cause osteomyelitis in children with chronic granulomatous disease, often resulting from contiguous spread of pulmonary infection.[159] *Blastomyces dermatitidis, Coccidioides immitis, Histoplasma capsulatum,* and *Cryptococcus neoformans* cause osteomyelitis in indigenous geographic regions and in immunosuppressed hosts.[160–163]

Tuberculous Osteomyelitis

Skeletal lesions occur in approximately 1% of children with tuberculosis.[130,164] Bones and joints are infected through hematogenous or lymphatic dissemination of *Mycobacterium tuberculosis.* Infection can smolder for years before clinical signs are apparent. The most commonly involved bones are the vertebrae (tuberculous spondylitis), femur, long bones around knees and ankles, and small bones of the hands and feet.[165] Other sites less frequently infected are the ribs, mandible, sternum, clavicle, and other long bones. Multifocal osteomyelitis is reported in 10% to 15% of cases.[166,167]

Clinical signs and symptoms of skeletal tuberculosis include low-grade fever, weight loss, pain, and soft-tissue swelling at the site of infection. Vertebral involvement begins in the anterior vertebral body, eventually causing disk space collapse and anterior wedging of vertebral bodies, and sometimes gibbus deformity. The lower thoracic spine is the usual site of involvement (Pott disease), followed by the lumbar spine.

The Mantoux tuberculin skin reaction is usually positive. The role of interferon-γ release assays in the diagnosis of Pott disease is currently being evaluated. Plain radiographic findings include periarticular osteopenia, lytic lesions in the body of the vertebra, joint space narrowing, and soft-tissue swelling.[168] The chest radiograph often is normal. CT is useful for the evaluation of bone destruction, adjacent soft-tissue abscess formation, and calcification, and in guiding percutaneous biopsy.[169,170] MRI is helpful in determining extent of bone and soft-tissue disease.[171] Biopsy specimens should be obtained in an attempt to demonstrate the organism with stains and culture.

Antituberculous therapy includes 2 months of therapy with four drugs, followed by 7 to 10 months of isoniazid and rifampin (for susceptible organisms) daily or twice weekly (see Chapter 134, *Mycobacterium tuberculosis*).[172] Surgical intervention is indicated in cases of spinal instability and neurologic impairment secondary to paravertebral abscess formation and for drainage of soft-tissue abscesses. Nontuberculous *Mycobacterium* spp. infrequently cause osteomyelitis in immunocompromised individuals.

Anaerobic Bacterial Osteomyelitis

Anaerobic bacteria are associated with chronic and nonhematogenously acquired osteomyelitis.[173–175] Risk factors include surgery, trauma, diabetes mellitus, human bites, chronic otitis media or sinusitis, dental infection, fibrous dysplasia of bone, presence of a prosthesis, and decubitus ulcers (Figure 78-6). Children are more likely than adults to experience anaerobic osteomyelitis of the skull and facial bones.[173] Osteomyelitis of ribs follows contiguous spread from aspiration lung infection; *Actinomyces* spp. are the primary pathogens. Soft-tissue swelling or abscess can be the presenting abnormality. Similarly, *Actinomyces* spp. can cause osteomyelitis of the maxilla or mandible, frequently without dental pathology.

Infection usually is polymicrobial; gram-positive cocci, *Bacteroides* spp., *Prevotella* spp., and *Fusobacterium* spp. are the most common anaerobes, and *S. aureus* is the most commonly associated aerobic isolate.[174] Therapy consists of treatment of underlying conditions, surgical debridement of necrotic bone, and appropriate antibiotic therapy. Examples of effective antibiotics are clindamycin, metronidazole, imipenem, and amoxicillin-clavulanate.

PART II Clinical Syndromes and Cardinal Features of Infectious Diseases: Approach to Diagnosis and Initial Management

SECTION K Bone and Joint Infections

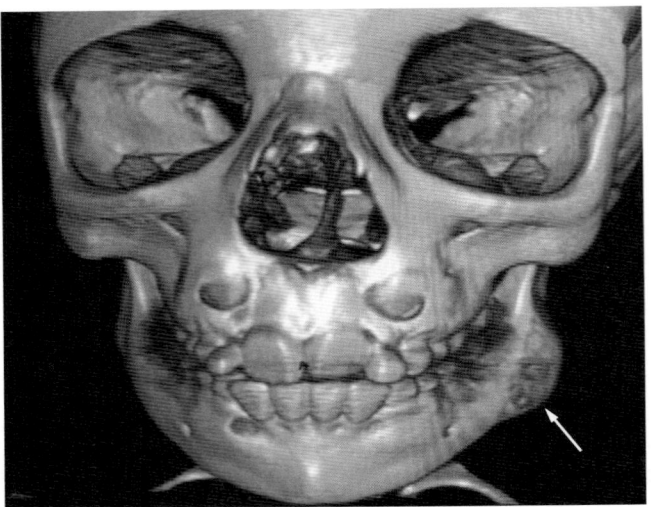

Figure 78-6. Actinomycosis of the mandible in a 9-year-old girl with history of painless expansion of the jaw over several months. Reconstructed spiral computed tomography shows expansion of bone with complex lytic and sclerotic mass (arrow). Surgical biopsy confirmed *Actinomyces* osteomyelitis and fibrous dysplasia of bone. (Courtesy of L. Kaban and M. Pasternack, Massachusetts General Hospital; and S.S. Long, St. Christopher's Hospital for Children, Philadelphia, PA.)

Many anaerobic isolates are susceptible to penicillin. The choice of antibiotic depends on the specific organisms isolated and their potential for β-lactamase production. Therapy is protracted, frequently exceeding 1 year of oral penicillin or amoxicillin plus probenecid for actinomycosis.

NONHEMATOGENOUS OSTEOMYELITIS

Contiguous Infection

Factors associated with the development of nonhematogenous osteomyelitis include open fractures requiring surgical reduction,[176,177] implanted orthopedic devices, decubitus ulcers,[173] and neuropathic ulcers.[178,179] Facial osteomyelitis usually is secondary to untreated mastoiditis, sinusitis, or periodontal abscess.[173,177] Osteomyelitis can occur after local soft-tissue infection or direct inoculation of bone from human and animal bites.[180,181] Puncture wounds can lead to osteomyelitis of the foot (e.g., stepping on a nail or toothpick[182]) or the patella (e.g., kneeling on a needle).

Indolent presentation is common among children with nonhematogenous osteomyelitis. Fever is present in less than half of patients.[183] Persistent drainage or ulceration of the soft tissue over the affected bone is typical. Plain radiograph shows bony destruction. Peripheral white blood cell count often is normal, and ESR and CRP can be normal.

Nonhematogenous osteomyelitis often is caused by *S. aureus*, although coinfection with gram-negative and anaerobic organisms occurs.[174] Examination of specimens from an associated sinus tract is unreliable in defining the etiology of osteomyelitis.[184] Biopsy with culture of the affected bone is the best method of determining appropriate antibiotic therapy. Therapy should be prolonged if infection is chronic, sometimes with parenteral therapy followed by oral therapy for a total of 4 to 6 months.

The rate of recurrence in nonhematogenous osteomyelitis is as high as 40%, even with prolonged courses of antibiotic therapy.[183] Aggressive surgical debridement or other interventions are required in addition to antibiotic therapy. Implanted devices commonly must be removed for cure. Debridement followed by muscle flap procedure to re-establish the blood supply in decubitus ulcer-associated osteomyelitis frequently is beneficial.[185]

PUNCTURE WOUND OSTEOCHONDRITIS OF THE FOOT

Bacterial osteochondritis is a complication of puncture wounds of the foot, occurring in approximately 1.5% of such injuries.[182,186–188] Symptoms of osteochondritis, which appear several days to weeks after the initial injury, include increasing tenderness, erythema, and swelling at the site of the puncture.

Infection usually is caused by *Pseudomonas aeruginosa*,[189] often as a result of inoculation from the colonized moist soles of tennis shoes.[190] *S. aureus* is the usual pathogen if symptoms began within 3 to 5 days of injury. Obtaining specimens from bone for microbiologic diagnosis is desirable.

Empiric antibiotic therapy should include coverage for *P. aeruginosa* and *S. aureus*. Ticarcillin-clavulanate, piperacillin-tazobactam, ceftazidime or cefepime, with or without an aminoglycoside, would be appropriate empiric therapy if MRSA is not likely. With appropriate surgical debridement, short-duration (7 to 10 days) parenteral antibiotic therapy has been effective for *P. aeruginosa*,[189,191] as has 3 to 4 weeks of antibiotic therapy without debridement.[190] Treatment with oral ciprofloxacin in conjunction with surgical debridement also is successful[192] (see Chapter 292, Antimicrobial Agents).

CHRONIC RECURRENT MULTIFOCAL OSTEOMYELITIS

Chronic recurrent multifocal osteomyelitis (CRMO) is an inflammatory disease of children and young adults characterized by recurring episodes of low-grade fever, swelling, and pain over affected bones and by radiologic abnormalities suggestive of osteomyelitis.[193,194] Females are more frequently affected than males.[195] The median age of onset of illness is 10 years. CRMO sometimes is associated with palmoplantar pustulosis,[196] psoriasis, arthritis, sacroiliitis, inflammatory bowel disease,[197] and Sweet syndrome.

Radiographic abnormalities occur most commonly in the metaphysis of long bones and are characterized by radiolucent bone lesions with reactive sclerosis and soft-tissue swelling.[195,198,199] The sternal end of the clavicle, the vertebral bodies, and the smaller bones of the hands and feet often are involved. Radiographic changes are similar to those seen in acute osteomyelitis, but multiple, often symmetrical lesions are present in CRMO. Bone scanning and MRI are useful in determining the extent and evolution of disease.[199–201] An infectious cause of CRMO has not been determined.

The course of CRMO consists of prolonged bone pain with remissions and relapses over several years; the mean duration of disease is 6 years.[202] In a long-term follow-up study of 23 patients with CRMO, 26% had active disease at a median of 13 years after diagnosis.[197] Although the clinical outcome in most patients is good, approximately 20% of patients have a prolonged and severe course. Young age at onset and multiple sites of involvement predict less favorable outcome.[203] Treatment with a variety of antibiotics has no apparent effect on the course or outcome. Some experts have advocated the use of corticosteroids or nonsteroidal anti-inflammatory agents for relief of symptoms.[195,198] Other therapies utilized in small numbers of patients have included colchicine, INF-γ, IFN-α, and infliximab.[197,203,204]

Because multifocal bone lesions in childhood can occur with neuroblastoma, histiocytosis X, leukemia, and staphylococcal osteomyelitis, histologic examination and culture of bone specimens should be performed. Histologic findings in CRMO are nonspecific acute and chronic inflammatory changes; in the chronic phase of the disease, granulomatous changes can be seen.[205]

CHRONIC OSTEOMYELITIS

Chronic osteomyelitis develops in fewer than 5% of cases of AHO;[12,206] it more often follows nonhematogenous osteomyelitis.[183]

Chronic osteomyelitis is characterized by alternating periods of quiescence and recurrent pain, swelling, and sinus tract drainage, persisting for years despite prolonged antibiotic therapy. Infections are often polymicrobial, and the original metaphyseal infection, with skeletal growth, moves to become a lytic lesion in the diaphysis.[175,185]

Surgical debridement of necrotic bone is primary management. Alternative therapeutic approaches include the use of antibiotic-impregnated polymethyl methacrylate beads,[207,208] local antibiotic delivery via implantable pumps,[209] and suction vacuum devices or bone grafts, skin grafts, and muscle flaps to eliminate dead space and improve vascularity.[210–212]

79 Infectious and Inflammatory Arthritis

Kathleen Gutierrez

Infectious arthritis in children can be caused by bacteria, viruses, fungi, or mycoplasma. Pyogenic arthritis is characterized by a purulent inflammatory response, usually caused by bacterial infection. Reactive (inflammatory) arthritis is inflammation of one or more joints that can result from a response to infection elsewhere in the body or from a systemic inflammatory or autoimmune disorder.

INFECTIOUS ARTHRITIS

Pyogenic (Bacterial) Arthritis

Epidemiology

The incidence of pyogenic arthritis is less than that of transient synovitis and varies substantially (from 1/100,000 to 37/100,000 children) depending on the population studied.[1,2] Although pyogenic arthritis occurs in all age groups, the peak incidence of disease is in children under 3 years of age.[3–5] A history of trauma temporally related to the onset of arthritis caused by *Staphylococcus aureus* is common.[6,7] Upper respiratory tract infection frequently precedes pyogenic arthritis caused by *Haemophilus influenzae* type b (Hib) and *Kingella kingae*.[7–9] Gastroenteritis and aphthous stomatitis also can precede arthritis with *K. kingae*.[10]

Although most children have no underlying disorder, risk factors for pyogenic arthritis include immunodeficiency, hemoglobinopathy, diabetes, intravenous drug abuse, and rheumatoid arthritis.[11–13]

Pathophysiology

Most cases of pyogenic arthritis in childhood follow hematogenous spread of organisms to the vascular synovium of the joint space.[14] Animal models of Hib bacterial arthritis illustrate possible mechanisms of articular damage.[15] Bacterial endotoxin within the joint space stimulates release of tumor necrosis factor and interleukin-1.[16,17] These cytokines stimulate production of proteinases by synovial cells and chondrocytes, enhancing leukocyte migration. Neutrophil elastases augment destruction of cartilage matrix within the joint.[18,19]

Bacteria also can spread to joints from contiguous osteomyelitis.[20] The presence of transphyseal blood vessels in the child younger than 18 months facilitates spread of infection from the metaphysis across the growth plate to the epiphysis and adjacent joint space.[21] In addition, the joint capsule of the hip and shoulder overlies the bony metaphysis of the femur and humerus, allowing direct extension of bone infection into these joint spaces. Primary pyogenic arthritis rarely extends into the bone to cause a secondary osteomyelitis.

Joints also can be infected from penetrating wounds, intra-articular injections of medications, arthroscopy, and prosthetic joint surgery.[22]

Etiology

Age is the most important predictor of etiology of pyogenic arthritis.[3,7,23–26] *S. aureus*, enteric gram-negative organisms, and group B streptococcus (GBS) are the most frequent causes of pyogenic arthritis among neonates. *S. aureus* (methicillin-susceptible (MSSA) and community-associated methicillin-resistant (CA-MRSA)), *Kingella kingae*, *Streptococcus pyogenes*, and *Streptococcus pneumoniae* cause pyogenic arthritis in children younger than 5 years of age. In one series, *K. kingae* was the most common cause of pyogenic arthritis in children younger than 36 months.[25] *K. kingae* is being reported with increasing frequency as a cause of pyogenic arthritis in the United States.[27–30] Hib infection now is rare in immunized immunocompetent children.[31–33] Approximately one third of bone and joint infections caused by *S. pneumoniae* are caused by strains with decreased susceptibility to penicillin.[34] Although *S. pneumoniae* caused approximately 6% of cases of pyogenic arthritis prior to universal conjugate vaccination,[35] cases of invasive disease due to vaccine serotype now have been reduced dramatically.[36,37] *S. aureus* and *S. pyogenes* are the most common causes of pyogenic arthritis in children older than 5 years.

CA-MRSA osteoarticular infections are now common,[38] and are more aggressive than MSSA infections involving multiple bones and joints[39] and sometimes are associated with venous thrombosis and pulmonary disease.[38,40] *S. aureus* isolates (either MRSA or MSSA) possessing Panton-Valentine leukocidin appear to cause particularly severe infections.[41]

Other organisms reported to cause pyogenic arthritis in children include *K. kingae*,[9,10] *Neisseria meningitidis*,[42] *Salmonella* spp.,[43,44] β-hemolytic streptococci other than serogroups A or B,[45] and rarely, anaerobic bacteria.[46,47]

Joint infections caused by *Pseudomonas aeruginosa* and *Candida* spp. are reported in intravenous drug abusers.[12] *Brucella* spp. infection should be considered if a history of travel to endemic areas, contact with livestock, or consumption of unpasteurized dairy products is elicted.[48,49] Arthritis related to *Bartonella henselae* infection has been reported.[50]

Clinical Manifestations

Fever, malaise, poor appetite, and irritability are heralding systemic symptoms. Pain in the affected joint usually occurs early in the course of the illness. As infection progresses, the joint becomes swollen and the overlying skin red. Limp or refusal to walk occurs with infection of a lower extremity. If the affected joint is in the upper extremity, "pseudoparalysis" or refusal to use the affected joint is seen; manipulation causes pain. The infected joint is swollen, red, warm, and tender on palpation. Range of joint motion is decreased.

The joints of the lower extremities, especially the knees, are the most common sites of pyogenic arthritis[3,8] (Table 79-1). More than

PART II Clinical Syndromes and Cardinal Features of Infectious Diseases: Approach to Diagnosis and Initial Management

SECTION K Bone and Joint Infections

TABLE 79-1. Frequency of Joint Involvement in 1050 Children with Pyogenic Arthritis

Site	No.	%
Knee	467	41
Hip	287	25
Ankle	143	13
Elbow	116	10
Shoulder	53	5
Other[a]	70	6
Total[b]	1136	100

[a]*Includes sacroiliac joint, joints of hands and feet, sternoclavicular joint.*

[b]*Some children had more than one joint affected.*

Data from references 3, 4, 6, 8, 96, 98.

90% of cases of pyogenic arthritis are monoarticular.[3,23] However, multiple joints can be involved, particularly with infections caused by *Neisseria gonorrhoeae*, *N. meningitidis*, and *Salmonella* spp.

The diagnosis of pyogenic arthritis of the hip can be difficult because often there is no obvious joint swelling, and signs and symptoms are nonspecific, especially in infants and young children. Infants with pyogenic arthritis of the hip are irritable when the hip is moved (e.g., during diaper changes); soft-tissue swelling around the hip joint occasionally is noted and can extend to involve the entire leg.[51] The affected hip often is held in a flexed, externally rotated and abducted position.[52] Older children with pyogenic arthritis of the hip limp or refuse to walk and complain of pain, which sometimes is referred to the knee.[53] Range of motion of the hip joint is decreased markedly.

Diagnosis

The erythrocyte sedimentation rate (ESR) is more than 20 mm/hour (mean, 44 to 65 mm/hour) in most patients with pyogenic arthritis.[3,54,55] Similarly, the level of C-reactive protein (CRP) often is increased (mean, 8.5 mg/dL).[47,55,56] A normal CRP is a good negative predictor for pyogenic arthritis. In one study, the probability that the patient did not have pyogenic arthritis was 87% if the CRP was <1.0 mg/dL.[57] Excellent sensitivity for diagnosis of osteoarticular infections is obtained by utilizing both ESR and CRP.[56]

Analysis of joint fluid is helpful in differentiating bacterial and other causes of arthritis (Table 79-2). Joint fluid in bacterial arthritis typically has a cloudy appearance. A leukocyte count >50,000 cells/mm³, with a predominance of neutrophils, is strongly suggestive of bacterial infection, even if culture of the

joint fluid is negative.[58,59] However, synovial fluid white blood cell (WBC) counts of less than 50,000/mm³ can occur in bacterial arthritis, particularly in cases of infection caused by *K. kingae*.[10,23,52,60] WBC counts >50,000/mm³ with neutrophil predominance can occur in children with juvenile rheumatoid arthritis or Lyme disease.[61,62] Synovial fluid glucose and protein levels do not differentiate reliably among most infectious and inflammatory processes and, therefore, have limited value.[63]

Blood culture should be obtained and synovial fluid sent for Gram stain, culture, and WBC count. Isolation of *K. kingae* is enhanced when synovial fluid is inoculated directly into fluid blood culture medium.[30] Use of 16S ribosomal DNA polymerase chain reaction (PCR) increased the identification of *K. kingae* in one series of children with osteoarticular infections.[64]

In the adolescent, specimens also should be obtained from the cervix or urethra, throat, skin lesions, and rectum for isolation of *N. gonorrhoeae*.

When appropriate cultures are obtained, the bacterial cause is confirmed in 60% to 70% of cases of pyogenic arthritis.[3,23] Blood cultures are positive in 40%[4,22] of cases and joint fluid culture is positive in 50% to 60%.[3,4,8,23]

Imaging Studies

Children with suspected pyogenic arthritis should have plain radiographic studies to exclude osteomyelitis or other osseous abnormalities. Soft-tissue swelling and widening of the joint can be observed in children with pyogenic arthritis. Erosion of subchondral bone may be evident 2 to 4 weeks after onset of infection.[65]

Swelling of the hip capsule and lateral displacement or obliteration of the gluteal fat planes are early radiographic findings in pyogenic arthritis of the hip.[65] With continued swelling of the hip capsule, the femoral head is displaced upward and outward, and lateral subluxation can occur. Concomitant osteomyelitis of the femur may be present.[52] These findings are particularly common in infants, although in this age group, radiographic findings are difficult to interpret because of minimal ossification of the proximal femur. Plain radiograph sometimes is normal in children with proven pyogenic arthritis of the hip.[66]

Ultrasonography (US) should be performed in suspected pyogenic arthritis of the hip. If fluid is present in the joint, a diagnostic aspiration should be performed under US guidance.[67,68] False-negative US results are reported in children later diagnosed with pyogenic arthritis; these are the result of either inadequate imaging or imaging performed very early (<24 hours) after onset of symptoms.[69]

Although technetium phosphate radionuclide scan generally is not used in the diagnosis of pyogenic arthritis, a scan can be valuable in evaluating involvement of deep joints, such as the hip or sacroiliac joint. A characteristic finding is increased activity in the early (blood pool) phase and increased bony uptake on both sides of the joint (which would be uncharacteristic in osteomyelitis). Similarly, computed tomography (CT) may be helpful in the diagnosis of arthritis in areas of complex anatomy, such as the shoulder, hip, and sacroiliac joint.

Magnetic resonance imaging (MRI) is highly sensitive for the early detection of inflamed/infected joints.[70] Abnormal MRI findings in pyogenic arthritis include periarticular high-intensity signal and periarticular abscesses in some cases. MRI can delineate abnormalities of adjacent bone, soft tissue, and the extent of cartilage destruction. Compared with patients with transient synovitis, those with pyogenic arthritis are more likely to have MRI findings of high intensity in the bone marrow[71] and decreased signal in the femoral epiphysis on fat-suppressed gadolinium-enhanced T_1-weighted images.[72]

Treatment

Children with pyogenic arthritis should be managed in conjunction with an orthopedic surgeon experienced in treating children. Goals of therapy include decompression, sterilization of the joint space, and removal of inflammatory debris.

TABLE 79-2. Characteristic Synovial Fluid Findings

Diagnosis	WBC/mm³ (Typical)	WBC/mm³ (Range)	% PMNs (Typical)
Normal	<150	–	<25
Bacterial arthritis	>50,000	2000–300,000	>90
Tuberculous arthritis	10,000–20,000	40–136,000	>50 (10–99)
Lyme arthritis	40,000–80,000	180–140,000	>75
Candidal arthritis	–	7500–150,000	>90
Viral arthritis	15,000	3000–50,000	<50 (variable)
Reiter syndrome	15,000	10,000–22,000	>70 (37–98)
Rheumatoid arthritis	–	2000–50,000	>70
Rheumatic fever	25,000	2000–50,000	>70

PMNs, polymorphonuclear cells; WBC, white blood cells.

Data from references 59, 61, 62, l48, 152, 180.

All children with pyogenic arthritis of the hip require prompt surgical drainage and irrigation of the joint space.[24,73,74] Delay in drainage increases the likelihood of permanent damage because increased intra-articular pressure can compromise blood supply, resulting in avascular necrosis of the femoral head; muscle spasms also can occur, predisposing the patient to dislocation. Open surgical drainage of joints other than the hip usually is not required. However, aspiration must be performed promptly to decompress the joint and obtain synovial fluid for analysis. Repeated aspirations often are necessary when fluid reaccumulates. Concurrent osteomyelitis can be associated with the need for repeated debridements of the joint.[75] Debridement by arthroscopy has been undertaken in some cases of pyogenic arthritis of the knee and hip.[76,77]

The initial choice of antibiotics is based on age, clinical history, and physical examination. Adequate penetration into the joint is essential. Penicillin, ampicillin, nafcillin, methicillin, dicloxacillin, some first- and third-generation cephalosporins, clindamycin, vancomycin, and aminoglycosides attain acceptable concentrations in joints after intravenous or intramuscular administration. Agents that are well absorbed from the gastrointestinal tract attain adequate joint space concentrations after oral administration.[78-85] Because antibiotics achieve high synovial fluid-to-serum ratios,

there is no role for intra-articular instillation of antibiotics, which can produce chemical irritation and inflammation.

Parenterally administered therapy is used initially (Table 79-3). Antistaphylococcal therapy should be given for a child of any age. Infants younger than 3 months of age should be treated with antibiotics active against *S. aureus*, gram-negative enteric organisms, and GBS. Children 3 months to 5 years of age should receive empiric therapy for *S. aureus*, *K. kingae*, *S. pneumoniae*, and *S. pyogenes*. Although Hib infection is uncommon in immunized children, other serotypes of *Haemophilus* occasionally cause pyogenic arthritis.[84] Children older than 5 years are treated for the most likely pathogens, *S. aureus* or streptococci. Empiric therapy for *N. gonorrhoeae* is indicated for the sexually active adolescent.[85]

Empiric therapy with vancomycin or clindamycin is indicated where CA-MRSA isolates exceed 10%.[86] Resistance to clindamycin may preclude its use as empiric therapy in many communities. Most *S. pyogenes* and *S. pneumoniae* isolates are susceptible to vancomycin and clindamycin, though susceptibility testing should be performed for both organisms. Neither of these drugs is effective in treating infection caused by *K. kingae*. Most β-lactam antibiotics, including ampicillin, ampicillin-sulbactam and second- and third-generation cephalosporins, have activity against *K. kingae*.[26]

TABLE 79-3. Empiric Antibiotic Therapy for Pyogenic Arthritis in Children

Age	Likely Pathogen	Antibiotic	Dosage mg/kg per day	Doses/day
Neonate (doses are for infants >2000 g and >7 days old with normal serum creatinine)	*Staphylococcus aureus*[a] Group B streptococcus Gram-negative bacilli	Nafcillin *or* Vancomycin *or* Clindamycin *plus* Cefotaxime *or* Gentamicin	100 30 20–30 100–150 5–7.5	4 2 3 3 3
Child, ≤5 years	*S. aureus*[a] *Haemophilus influenzae*[b] *Kingella kingae*[c] *Streptococcus pyogenes* *Streptococcus pneumoniae*	Nafcillin *or* Vancomycin *or* Clindamycin[d] *plus* Cefotaxime *or* Cefuroxime *or* Ampicillin-sulbactam[e]	150 45–60 30–40 100–150 150 300 Unasyn	4 3 3 3–4 3 6
Child, >5 years	*S. aureus*[a] *Streptococcus pyogenes*	Nafcillin *or* Vancomycin *or* Clindamycin[d]	150 45–60 30–40	4 3 3
Adolescent (sexually active)	*Neisseria gonorrhoeae* (consider)	Ceftriaxone[f]	50	1

[a]If more than 10% of community-acquired isolates are methicillin-resistant Staphylococcus aureus, consider empiric therapy with either vancomycin or clindamycin until culture and susceptibility results are available. If infection is confirmed to be caused by MRSA, see Clinical Practice Guidelines by the Infectious Diseases Society of America for treatment of MRSA infections in adults and children for specific dosing recommendations.[86a]

[b]Children who have been completely immunized are less likely to have Haemophilus influenzae type b infection.

[c]If empiric therapy with vancomycin or clindamycin is used, consider adding a second- or third-generation cephalosporin for Kingella kingae coverage in patients <36 months of age.

[d]Maximum oral dose of clindamycin is 1.8 g/day; adult dose is 600 mg/dose PO/IV given every 8 hours.

[e]The dose is for the drug Unasyn (300 mg Unasyn = 200 mg ampicillin plus 100 mg sulbactam). Sulbactam dose in an adult should not exceed 4 g. Unasyn is not approved for infant <1 year of age, or for this indication.

[f]The dose of ceftriaxone for children ≥45 kg is 1 g/day, given in a single dose.

PART II Clinical Syndromes and Cardinal Features of Infectious Diseases: Approach to Diagnosis and Initial Management

SECTION K Bone and Joint Infections

Nafcillin, oxacillin, or a first-generation cephalosporin remain the drugs of choice if MSSA is isolated. Choices of antibiotics for MRSA infections in children are limited. Vancomycin is effective, but no absorbable oral formulation exists. If MRSA is susceptible to clindamycin (including no inducible resistance), clindamycin is an excellent choice as an oral agent. Linezolid and daptomycin have been used in some patients with serious MRSA infection, although data regarding daptomycin use in children is limited. Linezolid has excellent oral bioavailability, however thrombocytopenia, anemia, and leukopenia can occur after 2 or 3 weeks; and lactic acidosis has been reported. Longer-term use is associated with peripheral and optic neuropathy. Linezolid is a weak reversible monoamine oxidase inhibitor and serotonin syndrome has occurred in children who also are receiving a serotonin-receptor inhibitor. The Infectious Diseases Society of America has published guidelines for the management of MRSA infections.[86a]

Specific therapy based on culture results and susceptibility testing is continued parenterally until the child is afebrile; joint pain, swelling, and erythema have decreased; and joint mobility has increased. In addition, markers of acute phase response should decrease. Because CRP normalizes more quickly than ESR (which typically is elevated for up to 2 weeks), CRP is used to monitor early response to therapy.[56] Open drainage of any joint (with lysis and irrigation of loculated collections) should be undertaken when aspirations yield samples that are persistently positive on culture.

Orally administered antibiotic therapy can be substituted for parenteral treatment after adequate control of infection and inflammation has been achieved, if an oral antibiotic with appropriate coverage is available and if adherence and careful monitoring can be ensured[87-91] (Table 79-4). Use of clinical practice guidelines have been successful in decreasing the number of days parenteral antibiotics are given and duration of hospitalization, without increasing complications or sequelae.[92]

For children in whom oral therapy is not feasible, outpatient parenteral antibiotic therapy administered through a tunneled central venous catheter or a peripherally inserted central catheter has been successful. Catheter-related mechanical and infectious complications may occur with prolonged intravenous administration of antibiotics and the risk versus benefit of prolonged central venous access should be considered carefully.[93]

Duration of antimicrobial therapy remains a subject of considerable debate. Duration generally is determined by the specific pathogen, clinical and laboratory response, and whether adjacent osteomyelitis is present. Joint infections caused by *S. aureus* and gram-negative enteric organisms generally are treated for at least 3 to 4 weeks; a longer course of therapy may be necessary for pyogenic arthritis of the hip.[52] Arthritis caused by *H. influenzae*, *S. pneumoniae*, *S. pyogenes*, and *K. kingae* is treated for 2 to 3 weeks, depending on clinical response. Therapy for less than 2 weeks in children in Finland with culture-positive arthritis was successful in most cases.[91] Notably, none of the children in this study had MRSA infection and several children with hip infections required longer courses of treatment. A larger, controlled, prospective study is necessary to more adequately evaluate the adequacy of short-course antibiotic therapy.[94]

TABLE 79-4. Dosage of Antibiotics Commonly Used in Oral Treatment of Pyogenic Arthritis[a]

| Agent | Dosage | |
	mg/kg per day	Doses/day
Dicloxacillin	75–100	4
Cephalexin	100–150	4
Clindamycin	30–40	3–4

[a]Doses can be modified depending on results of serum bactericidal levels. In general, the oral dose of β-lactam antibiotics used for osteoarticular infections is two to three times the usual dose.

Prognosis

Sequelae of pyogenic arthritis in children include abnormalities of bone growth, limitation of joint mobility, unstable articulation, and chronic dislocation of the joint. Joint dysfunction may not become apparent for months to years after infection.[95] An estimated 10% to 25% of children with pyogenic arthritis have residual dysfunction.[3,95]

A number of risk factors for development of sequelae have been identified and include: (1) age younger than 6 months;[3-8] (2) infection of the adjacent bone, which is evident in 10% to 16% of children with pyogenic arthritis and increases the likelihood of sequelae to approximately 50%;[3,24,40,96,97] (3) infection of the hip or shoulder;[3,95,98] (4) a delay of ≥4 days before decompression and antibiotic therapy;[13,52,99-101] and (5) prolonged time to sterilization of synovial fluid.[102] Staphylococcal and gram-negative bacillary infections carry a high risk of sequelae, whereas meningococcal and gonococcal infections carry a low risk.

SPECIAL SITUATIONS AND PATHOGENS

Neonatal Arthritis

Risk factors for pyogenic arthritis in the neonate include umbilical vessel catheterization, presence of a central venous catheter,[103] femoral vessel blood sampling,[51,104,105] and possibly fetal breech presentation.[106] Pyogenic arthritis often is a complication of osteomyelitis, and the onset may be insidious (see Chapter 94, Bacterial Infections in the Neonate). The hip and knee are the most frequently involved joints.[105] *S. aureus*, *N. gonorrhoeae*, and *Candida* spp. frequently cause polyarticular infection.

If infection is contracted in the hospital, MRSA and MSSA, enteric gram-negative organisms, and *Candida* spp. are common. GBS, *S. aureus*, and *N. gonorrhoeae* are the pathogens most commonly isolated from neonates who develop joint infections after hospital discharge.[107]

Gonococcal Arthritis

Arthritis caused by *N. gonorrhoeae* must be considered in sexually active adolescents.[85] The incidence of disseminated gonococcal infection in individuals with urethritis or cervicitis is approximately 1%.[108] Disseminated gonococcal infection is characterized by mild fever, polyarthralgia, rash, tenosynovitis, and suppurative arthritis, and is more common in girls, often during menstruation. Suppurative arthritis most often involves the knee. The hand, wrist, ankle, elbow, and foot are involved less often, and infection of the shoulder or hip is uncommon.[109] Skin lesions occur in approximately 40% of patients. Lesions typically are few in number, and represent vasculitis. Lesions occur most frequently on extremities or over affected joints, are papular with a hemorrhagic component, and evolve into vesiculopustular lesions on an erythematous base.[42] Other skin lesions, including bullae and purpura, have been described.[13]

Culture of joint fluid is positive in only 25% to 35% of cases. Cultures of blood, cervix, urethra, rectum, vagina, skin lesions, or throat specimens may be positive when joint fluid is negative. Cultures obtained from normally sterile sites should be inoculated onto chocolate agar. Cultures from nonsterile sites should be inoculated immediately onto Thayer–Martin agar and incubated in carbon dioxide. *N. gonorrhoeae* also can be detected by PCR or other DNA amplification tests on first-voided urine specimens and urethral and cervicovaginal swab samples.

Because of the increasing prevalence of penicillin-resistant *N. gonorrhoeae*, 7 days of treatment with a parenterally administered third-generation cephalosporin, such as ceftriaxone or cefotaxime, is recommended.[109-111] Marked improvement in fever and joint pain usually occurs 1 to 2 days after beginning therapy. Sequelae are rare.

Polyarthritis, Fever, and Rash

Bacterial causes of the clinical syndrome of fever, polyarthritis, and rash include infection with *N. meningitidis* and *N. gonorrhoeae*, rat bite fever *(Streptobacillus moniliformis* or *Spirillum minus)*, bacterial endocarditis, and rheumatic fever;[112] multiple viruses also are considered (see below). Noninfectious causes include Kawasaki disease, serum sickness, erythema multiforme, and other autoinflammatory and autoimmune diseases.

Lyme Arthritis

Lyme disease is caused by the tickborne spirochete *Borrelia burgdorferi.*[113] Arthralgia occurs early in the course of infection and is recurrent in 18% of individuals. Approximately one half of patients with Lyme disease have arthritis,[114] with typical onset 1 to 2 months after erythema migrans with sudden onset of monoarticular or oligoarticular joint pain. Joints involved, in descending order of frequency, include the knee, shoulder, elbow, temporomandibular joint, ankle, and wrist. Involvement of the hip or small joints is unusual.[62] Patients characteristically are not ill, although about one half have fever. Affected joints are warm and swollen, have large effusions but motion typically is not severely limited. The peripheral white blood cell count often is normal, but the ESR and CRP usually are modestly elevated.[115] Synovial fluid leukocyte counts range from 180 to 140,000/mm^3; polymorphonuclear cells predominate.[62] *B. burgdorferi* DNA has been detected by PCR of synovial fluid of patients with Lyme arthritis.[116] Patients with Lyme arthritis are more likely to have MRI findings of myositis, lymphadenopathy, and lack of subcutaneous edema compared with children with pyogenic arthritis (P < 0.01).[117]

Lyme arthritis is treated with amoxicillin or doxycycline, depending on age (see Chapter 185, *Borrelia burgdorferi* (Lyme Disease)). Duration of therapy usually is 4 weeks. Children with multiple recurrences or persistent arthritis sometimes require intravenous or intramuscular ceftriaxone or intravenous penicillin for 14 to 28 days. Prognosis in children is excellent.[118] Rupture of fluid from knee joint into the popliteal space (popliteal cyst, Baker cyst) is described.[119]

If untreated, recurrences of arthritis are common. Recurrences usually are separated by months to years. Frequency and duration of attacks decrease over time. Chronic synovitis develops in approximately 11% of untreated individuals.

Viral Arthritis

Arthritis as a result of viral infection can occur by direct viral invasion of the synovium or through immune complex deposition (Box 79-1). The viruses most commonly associated with the development of arthritis include rubella, parvovirus B19, certain arboviruses, and hepatitis B.

BOX 79-1. Viruses that Cause Arthritis

TOGAVIRIDAE	**RETROVIRIDAE**
Rubella virus	Human immunodeficiency virus
Ross River virus	type 1
Chikungunya virus	Human T-lymphotropic virus
O'nyong-nyong virus	type 1
Mayaro virus	
Sindbis virus	**HERPESVIRIDAE**
Barmah Forest virus	Herpes simplex virus 1
	Varicella-zoster virus
PARVOVIRIDAE	Cytomegalovirus
Parvovirus B19	Epstein–Barr virus
PARAMYXOVIRIDAE	**FLAVIVIRIDAE**
Mumps virus	Hepatitis C virus
PICORNAVIRIDAE	**HEPADNAVIRIDAE**
Echovirus	Hepatitis B virus
Coxsackie B virus	

Rubella virus. Arthritis following rubella infection is uncommon in childhood but is reported in 30% of women and 15% of men. Arthritis usually develops 1 to 2 days after onset of rash, although it has preceded the rash in a few cases. Symmetrical involvement of small joints of the hands is most common. Wrists and knees are sometimes affected. Analysis of joint fluid shows a predominance of mononuclear cells. Rubella virus has been isolated from synovial fluid. Symptoms resolve after several days, and long-term sequelae do not occur. Arthralgia and arthritis occur in approximately 25% of postpubertal females who receive live attenuated rubella vaccine. Joint symptoms begin 7 to 21 days after vaccination and usually are mild and self-limited.[120,121]

Parvovirus. Symptoms of arthritis or arthralgia were reported in 80% of adults and 8% of children during an outbreak of erythema infectiosum,[122] and arthritis can occur in the absence of rash. Infection often is symmetric and polyarticular, and the joints of the hands, wrists, and knees are involved most commonly. Children are more likely to have asymmetric involvement of a few joints. Levels of total hemolytic complement are low in some individuals with parvovirus B19 arthritis, suggesting an immune complex-mediated pathogenesis. Arthritis associated with parvovirus B19 infection usually is self-limited; resolution of symptoms occurs within 1 to 2 months.

Hepatitis viruses. Arthralgia can occur as a prodromal symptom of infection with hepatitis A or B viruses, but arthritis occurs only with hepatitis B infection.[123,124] Joint symptoms precede the onset of icterus by 1 or 2 weeks. Multiple small joints of the hands usually are involved. In addition, sometimes symmetric involvement of knees, elbows, ankles, and shoulders is seen. An urticarial or maculopapular rash, usually involving the lower extremities, appears simultaneously with the joint findings in 30% to 40% of patients with arthritis. Hepatitis C viral infection has been associated with development of polyarthralgia and polyarthritis in a few patients.[125]

Arboviruses. Several arboviruses in the family Togaviridae, genus alphavirus, found in Australia, Africa, Asia, and South America cause systemic illness in which arthritis is a predominant manifestation. All are transmitted by bites of mosquitoes or ticks.

Epidemic polyarthritis caused by Ross River virus occurs most frequently in Australia.[126] Clinical manifestations include fever, papular, petechial or morbilliform skin rash, adenopathy, and polyarthritis. Small joints of the hands and feet are affected most commonly. Most patients recover spontaneously within 2 weeks. Barmah Forest virus, also endemic to Australia, causes fever, polyarthritis, and rash.[127]

Chikungunya virus infection is endemic in Africa, India, and Southeast Asia and imported cases occur worldwide.[128] Illness is biphasic, heralded by abrupt onset of fever, nausea, vomiting, and intense pain in one or more joints. The first phase of illness lasts 1 to 6 days, the patient becomes afebrile for 3 days, and then fever recurs. The second phase of illness is characterized by pharyngitis, rash, lymphadenopathy, and persistent arthritis. Children sometimes have febrile seizures and severe hemorrhagic manifestations.

O'nyong-nyong virus (East Africa), Sindbis virus (Africa, Australia, Asia, Europe, and the Middle East), and Mayaro virus (Central and South America) infections cause febrile illnesses that are characterized by rash, adenopathy, arthralgia, and arthritis.

Other viruses. Other viruses less commonly associated with arthralgia or arthritis include Epstein–Barr virus,[129] enteroviruses (echovirus and coxsackie B),[130] mumps virus,[131] varicella-zoster virus,[132-135] cytomegalovirus, and herpes simplex virus.[136]

Persistent or intermittent arthralgia involving the knee or shoulder has been reported in 35% to 45% of adults with human immunodeficiency virus infection[137,138] but in only 15% of children with this infection.[139]

Mycoplasma Species

Mycoplasma pneumoniae, M. hominis, M. salivarium, and *Ureaplasma urealyticum* have been identified in joint fluid of patients with arthritis.[140-145] Most patients are immunocompromised or have suffered trauma to the joint. Characteristically, onset is insidious, with minimal systemic signs and a mildly affected, boggy joint with relative preservation of movement.

Mycobacterium Species

Skeletal tuberculosis occurs in 1% to 6% of all cases of tuberculosis. Isolated tuberculosis of the joint is uncommon.[146] Articular infection can represent reactivated or primary infection. The knees and hips are affected most commonly, but infection of other joints can occur. Chronic swelling or pain of the affected joint without systemic symptoms is common. The skin test for tuberculosis (STS) is expected to be positive.[147] Synovial fluid WBC count typically ranges between 10,000 and 20,000 cells/mm^3, and neutrophils predominate. Synovial fluid cultures are positive in 79% of cases; synovial biopsy is diagnostic in more than 90%.[148] MRI shows joint effusion with high-intensity signal on T$_2$-weighted images, and post contrast enhancement on T$_1$-weighted images. Hypointense internal debris, synovial thickening, and cartilage destruction also may be noted.[149]

Nontuberculous mycobacteria can cause osteoarticular infections in immunocompromised hosts.[150,151]

Fungi

Fungal arthritis is unusual in healthy children, except in areas endemic for specific fungi. Chronic monoarticular arthritis is typical of most fungal joint infections. The diagnosis of arthritis usually requires microscopic evaluation of synovial biopsy specimens and culture of synovial tissue and fluid.

Candida species. Arthritis caused by *Candida* spp. occurs by hematogenous spread or, rarely, by direct inoculation of the organism into the joint space.[152] Risk factors in neonates include prematurity, use of broad-spectrum antibiotics, intravenous alimentation, and presence of an intravascular catheter.[103,107] Risk factors in older children include immunosuppression and intravenous drug use. Clinical manifestations vary. Children with disseminated disease have an acute onset of fever, systemic illness, and joint symptoms. In other cases, systemic symptoms are mild or absent. Joint symptoms may persist for months to years before a diagnosis is established. Neonates often have polyarticular involvement, but monoarticular infection is typical in older children. The knee is most frequently affected. Arthritis caused by *Candida* spp. in intravenous drug users often occurs in fibrocartilaginous joints, such as the sacroiliac joint, costochondral joints, and intervertebral disks.[153]

Synovial fluid WBC counts range from 7500 to 150,000 WBCs/mm^3, with neutrophil predominance. Diagnosis of fungal arthritis is confirmed by culture of synovial fluid or tissue. Culture of blood, urine, or cerebrospinal fluid may be positive in cases of systemic disease and especially in neonates.[152]

Amphotericin B or liposomal amphotericin B followed by prolonged (at least 6 weeks) treatment with fluconazole has been successful.[154,155] An echinocandin antifungal may be used as an alternative therapy.[155] *Candida* spp. should be tested for susceptibility to fluconazole if this drug is considered. Adequate debridement of the joint is necessary for successful therapy.

Sporothrix schenckii is a dimorphic fungus found worldwide in soil and decayed plant material. Individuals at risk for infection include those whose occupations place them in frequent contact with plant debris and moist soil. Infection in children is rare. *S. schenkii* causes both cutaneous and extracutaneous infection. Osteoarticular sporotrichosis is the most common manifestation of extracutaneous infection.[156] Joints most frequently involved include the knee, ankle, wrist, and elbows. Itraconazole is the treatment of choice, with amphotericin B recommended as alternative therapy.[157]

Aspergillus species. *Aspergillus* infection of the joint is uncommon and usually occurs secondary to extension of infection from adjacent bone. Children at risk include those with chronic granulomatous disease, chronic neutropenia, underlying cancer, and prolonged immunosuppression.[158]

Coccidioides immitis is found in soil in the southwestern U.S. and northern Mexico. Infection usually is asymptomatic or associated with localized pulmonary disease. Extrapulmonary manifestations include cutaneous lesions, lymphadenopathy, central nervous system infection, and osteoarticular infection. Joint involvement usually is unifocal and often adjacent to sites of osteomyelitis.[159]

Cryptococcus neoformans is found in soil contaminated by bird droppings. Infection typically involves the lungs, skin, or the central nervous system. Although bone lesions are found in 5% to 10% of cases, joint involvement is rare and usually secondary to infection in adjacent bone.[160]

Histoplasma capsulatum is endemic to the central and southeastern U.S., where large quantities of fungus are found in soil contaminated by bat or bird droppings. Infection usually is asymptomatic. Symptomatic infection is characterized by fever, chills, headache, cough, and chest pain. Approximately 10% of symptomatic patients have arthritis or severe arthralgia accompanied by erythema nodosum. Arthritis and arthralgia can be prolonged. Antifungal therapy is not always indicated in the immunocompetent host (see Chapter 250, *Histoplasma capsulatum* (Histoplasmosis)).[161,162] Nonsteroidal anti-inflammatory drugs are recommended for relief of joint pain.[162]

Blastomyces dermatitidis is found commonly in warm moist soil containing decayed vegetation east of the Mississippi River. Blastomycosis typically involves the lungs, skin, and genitourinary system. Skeletal disease occurs in 10% to 15% of cases.[163] Arthritis usually results from extension of osteomyelitis from adjacent bone and usually is monoarticular but can be oligoarticular.[164] Fungi are identifiable on a wet preparation of synovial fluid.[165] Itraconazole or other imidazoles have been used to treat blastomycoses.[166]

Other fungal organisms, such as *Scedosporium* spp., are rare causes of arthritis.[167]

REACTIVE ARTHRITIS

Reactive arthritis is defined as inflammation in one or more joints related to an infection at a site distant from the joint.[168] Infections of the gastrointestinal, genitourinary, and respiratory tract are associated with reactive arthritis and an increasing number of pathogens are implicated.[169-174] Children are less likely than adults to develop reactive arthritis after enteric infection. Organisms most commonly associated with reactive arthritis are listed in Box 79-2.[168-170,172,173,175,176] Immune-complex associated arthritis occurs in 2% to 16% of cases of meningococcal disease.[177]

A genetic susceptibility exists for development of reactive arthritis due to distant infection; individuals who are HLA-B27 antigen-positive have an increased incidence of disease.[178]

Reiter syndrome consists of arthritis, urethritis, and bilateral conjunctivitis. In children, symptoms usually follow a diarrheal illness.[179] In adults, Reiter syndrome also can follow an episode of

---

BOX 79-2. Bacteria Associated with Reactive Arthritis

GASTROINTESTINAL PATHOGENS

Shigella spp.
Salmonella spp.
Yersinia enterocolitica
Campylobacter spp.
Clostridium difficile

SEXUALLY TRANSMITTED PATHOGEN

Chlamydia trachomatis

PYOGENIC AND REACTIVE ARTHRITIS-CAUSING ORGANISMS

Streptococcus pyogenes
Neisseria gonorrhoeae
Neisseria meningitidis

nongonococcal urethritis. Although Reiter syndrome and reactive arthritis are sometimes used interchangeably, reactive arthritis is diagnosed in many children who do not have the triad of symptoms.

Reactive arthritis usually is polyarticular and involves the large joints of the lower extremities. Small joints, wrists, and elbows are involved less frequently. Sacroiliitis is more common among adults than children. Urethritis, if present, manifests with dysuria and pyuria. Mucous membrane ulcers (in the mouth, rectum, or vagina or on the glans penis) sometimes are present. Abnormalities of the eye include keratitis, uveitis, and corneal ulcerations.

WBC count and ESR usually are elevated. Synovial fluid WBC count is less than 50,000 cells/mm³, with a predominance of neutrophils.[180] ESR ranges from 20 to >100 mm/hour. Responsible pathogens are sometimes identified in stool or urethral specimens.

Nonsteroidal anti-inflammatory agents are useful in controlling symptoms. Antibiotic treatment of the predisposing bacterial organism may be appropriate when cultures are positive at the

time of onset of joint symptoms.[177,181] In children, joint symptoms persist for 1 to 12 months and recurrences are rare. The long-term prognosis of the disease is unknown.

Some bacteria cause both direct infection of the joint and reactive arthritis. For example, *S. pyogenes* causes infective pyogenic arthritis and also is associated with postinfectious reactive arthritis and rheumatic fever.[182] Poststreptococcal reactive arthritis typically occurs 3 to 14 days after streptococcal infection, and is differentiated from the arthritis of acute rheumatic fever in that arthritis generally is symmetric, can involve both large and small joints, and is nonmigratory.[183] Similarly, *N. meningitidis*, *N. gonorrhoeae*, and *Salmonella* spp. sometimes are isolated from synovial fluid but, in other cases, infection at another site is associated with reactive arthritis. In addition to being a response to a pathogen, reactive arthritis can occur in association with a more generalized autoinflammatory or immunologic disorder, such as Crohn disease, ulcerative colitis, rheumatoid and rheumatic disorders, Kawasaki disease, hereditary autoinflammatory disorders, serum sickness, or Henoch–Schönlein purpura.

80 Diskitis

Kathleen Gutierrez

Diskitis is an inflammatory process involving the intervertebral disks and the endplates of the vertebral bodies, and is associated with characteristic clinical and radiologic findings. Our understanding of diskitis is primarily derived from retrospective studies and case reports of small numbers of patients. Diskitis has been reported under a variety of other names, including spondylodiskitis, pyogenic infectious spondylitis, spondylarthritis, acute osteitis of the spine, intervertebral disk space infection, and benign osteomyelitis of the spine.[1-6] The definition of diskitis varies among studies, and often it is difficult to distinguish disk space inflammation alone from vertebral osteomyelitis. In fact, disk space inflammation likely is part of a spectrum of disease that includes vertebral osteomyelitis; however, diskitis appears to have a more benign clinical course.[7,8]

There has been no consistent approach to the diagnosis, treatment, and long-term follow-up of patients with diskitis. Thus, knowledge of incidence, causes, and optimal treatment of this infection remains limited.

EPIDEMIOLOGY AND ETIOLOGY

Although the incidence of diskitis is unknown, it appears to be uncommon. In one center, diskitis was reported to occur at a rate of approximately 1 to 2 per 30,000 clinic visits per year.[1] Most cases occur in children aged 6 years and younger,[1,9-13] although cases have been reported in older children and adolescents. Disk space infection in adults most commonly occurs in the postoperative setting. Spontaneous diskitis is uncommon in adults,[14,15] but when reported it has been associated with older age, diabetes mellitus, and systemic infection.[16]

Diskitis is probably the result of low-grade bacterial infection of the disk space.[2-4,17,18] Some investigators believe that intervertebral disk inflammation is noninfectious and the result of antecedent trauma to the spine.[19]

Most blood cultures obtained from patients with diskitis are negative. If positive, *Staphylococcus aureus* is the most common isolate (Table 80-1). Other organisms isolated from either blood culture or disk aspirate from affected children have included *S. epidermidis*,[20] *Kingella kingae*,[6,14,21-24] anaerobes,[25] gram-negative

enteric organisms,[20,26,27] *Streptococcus pneumoniae*,[2] and *Brucella* species.[28] In most cases, cultures of intervertebral disk specimens are sterile (Table 80-2).

Viruses have not been isolated from disk space cultures. *Mycobacterium* species and *Candida* species have been isolated by disk space aspiration from older patients.[29]

PATHOGENESIS AND PATHOLOGIC FINDINGS

The lumbar or lower thoracic spine is involved in most cases.[30] There are rare reports of diskitis involving the cervical spine.[3,26] Usually only one disk space is involved, although patients with involvement of two intervertebral disk spaces have been reported.[13]

The difference in blood supply to the vertebral bodies and disk spaces in children compared with adults may explain the age-related incidence of diskitis.[31-34] In the young child, there are widespread anastomoses between intraosseous arteries supplying the vertebrae. These vessels begin to involute at about 8 months of age and are few in number by the age of 7 years. By the third decade of life, the anastomoses have atrophied fully and peripheral periosteal arteries develop. As a result of this rich blood

TABLE 80-1. Results of Blood Cultures in Children with Diskitis

Author	No. of Patients	Blood Cultures No.	Blood Cultures No. of Positive Results
Smith & Taylor (1967)[13]	20	24	0
Wenger et al. (1978)[3]	41	22	10ª
Scoles & Quinn (1982)[26]	29	9	0
Crawford et al. (1991)[44]	36	28	2ᵇ
Ryoppy et al. (1993)[12]	18	0	0
Brown et al. (2001)[45]	11	11	0

ªStaphylococcus aureus (9); diphtheroids (1).
ᵇStaphylococcus aureus (2).

PART II Clinical Syndromes and Cardinal Features of Infectious Diseases: Approach to Diagnosis and Initial Management

SECTION K Bone and Joint Infections

TABLE 80-2. Results of Disk Space Aspirates in Children with Diskitis

Author	No. of Patients	No. of Biopsies/ Aspirates	No. of Positive Culture Results
Smith & Taylor (1967)[13]	20	3	1/3[a]
Spiegel et al. (1972)[2]	48	15	5/15[b]
Wenger et al. (1978)[3]	41	9	6/9[c]
Scoles & Quinn (1982)[26]	29	6	2/6[d]
duLac et al. (1990)[9]	12	8	6/8[e]
Crawford et al. (1991)[44]	36	3	0/3
Ryoppy et al. (1993)[12]	18	17	0/17
Brown et al. (2001)[45]	11	3	0/3
Garron et al. (2002)[6]	42	35	22/35[f]

[a]*Staphylococcus aureus (1).*

[b]*Moraxella spp., Staphylococcus aureus, Streptococcus pneumoniae, diphtheroids, and micrococcus (1 each).*

[c]*Staphylococcus aureus (6; 1 also a-hemolytic streptococcus).*

[d]*Klebsiella spp., Staphylococcus aureus (1 each).*

[e]*Moraxella spp. (1), Staphylococcus aureus (5).*

[f]*Staphylococcus aureus (12), Kingella kingae (6), Staphylococcus epidermidis (1), Clostridium clostridiiforme (1), Streptococcus sp. (1), Coxiella burnetii (1).*

TABLE 80-3. Frequency of Presenting Symptoms in Patients with Diskitis (n = 165)

Symptoms	%
Limp, leg pain, or refusal to walk[a]	41
Back pain	41
Abdominal pain	15

[a]*Children whose presenting symptom was refusal to bear weight or walk were younger (≥5 years) at time of presentation.*

Data from references 2, 3, 20, 26, 38, 44.

supply to the vertebral endplates, a septic embolus in a child leads only to small areas of vertebral endplate infarction or infection, with disproportionate involvement of the intervertebral disk. A septic embolus in an adult results in a much larger area of vertebral body infarction and subsequent infection, which leads to vertebral osteomyelitis.[1,32]

The intervertebral disk is composed of the cartilaginous plate, the annulus fibrosus, and the nucleus pulposus.[31] Examinations of cadavers have demonstrated that blood vessels are present in the cartilaginous endplates until 7 years of age and in the annulus fibrosus until 20 years of age.[33] This may explain the finding of disk space inflammation or infection with relative sparing of the vertebral body that is seen in children. An ovine animal model of diskitis demonstrates that infection of the disk impedes disk development but does not seem to affect vertebral body growth.[35]

Magnetic resonance imaging (MRI) findings in children with diskitis suggest a pathophysiologic sequence in which infection or inflammation begins in the metaphyseal bone near the vertebral endplates, with anterior spread to the disk region and the adjacent vertebral endplate.[5,36] Histologic examination of disk biopsy specimens from children with diskitis reveals subacute or chronic nonspecific inflammation. In some children with the characteristic clinical and radiologic findings of diskitis, histologic results are normal.[2,12]

CLINICAL MANIFESTATIONS

The clinical manifestations of diskitis vary, depending on the age of the child.[2,3,9,11,13,26] Onset is gradual, with symptoms often present for several days to weeks before coming to medical attention. Younger children are more likely to have a history of irritability and reluctance to walk or bear weight. Older children complain of back pain, hip pain, abdominal pain, or pain with walking. Some patients have abdominal complaints, such as anorexia, vomiting, abdominal pain, and constipation (Table 80-3).

On physical examination, the child frequently has a low-grade fever and appears well. Comfortable when lying still, the child refuses to bear weight or walks with a limp. Irritability with sitting or with flexion of hips and pain with palpation over the lower back are common. Spasm of paraspinous muscles can occur. Alterations in the normal curvature of the spine sometimes are noted, with loss of the normal lumbar lordosis.[10,20,37,38] Gower sign (use of hand "push-off" rather than pelvic girdle to rise from sitting)

can be present in children with diskitis and disappears following treatment.[39,40] Abnormal neurologic findings are uncommon; however, one retrospective case series described decreased muscle tone, muscle weakness, and decreased tendon reflexes in 7 of 17 children diagnosed with diskitis.[41] Therefore, neurologic abnormalities do not exclude a diagnosis of diskitis; however, when present, imaging studies are needed to exclude intraspinal involvement or an alternative diagnosis.

Failure to consider a diagnosis of diskitis, to examine the lower back carefully, and to order the appropriate radiologic studies often results in delay in diagnosis and inappropriate use of tests.[42]

DIFFERENTIAL DIAGNOSIS

The differential diagnosis of diskitis includes vertebral osteomyelitis or osteomyelitis of the pelvis, pyogenic arthritis of the hip or sacroiliac joint, abscess of psoas muscle or pelvic structures, spinal epidural abscess, meningitis, appendicitis, malignant processes, pyelonephritis, and tuberculosis of the spine. If a child appears to be ill and has a high fever, marked leukocytosis, neurologic abnormalities, or extensive involvement of the vertebral body, diskitis is not the likely diagnosis.[43] Immediate workup to rule out a more serious cause of symptoms should be initiated.

DIAGNOSIS

The erythrocyte sedimentation rate (ESR) is almost always elevated (rarely more than 60 mm/h) in children with diskitis.[10,11,26] Peripheral white blood cell (WBC) count is normal or slightly elevated.[11,44] C-reactive protein (CRP) can be elevated.[45] Blood culture is obtained, but the result usually is negative. Skin test for tuberculosis and chest radiograph are useful in circumstances where tuberculosis is possible. When culture results are positive, therapy can be specifically targeted to the causative pathogen.

Early in the course of diskitis, findings of plain film of the spine may be normal. Two to 4 weeks after onset of symptoms, the involved disk space is narrow and the margins of the vertebral endplates exhibit demineralization and irregularity (Figure 80-1). Two to 3 months after onset of symptoms, the disk space remains narrow and remineralization of vertebral endplates has occurred. Long-term follow-up in most patients shows persistence of a narrow disk space and sclerotic changes at the vertebral endplates (Figure 80-2). In some cases, fusion of involved vertebral bodies or changes in their shape is noted.[10,11,26,46,47]

Other imaging modalities are useful if plain film results are normal. Technetium bone scan has been used in the past and frequently shows increased uptake at the disk space.[37,44] Computed tomography (CT) can demonstrate narrowing of disk space and vertebral body involvement early in the course of disease.[20] MRI is the most sensitive technique for confirming the diagnosis of diskitis.[5,9,35,38,48] MRI is particularly useful to detect paravertebral abscess, epidural abscess, severe protrusion of the disk, or significant vertebral body involvement.[45,49]

Aspiration of the disk space for culture in cases with compatible clinical findings and supportive imaging is controversial. Some investigators have reported a good yield from culture of material obtained from aspiration.[9,17,18] Identification of an organism, especially an unusual one, such as *K. kingae,* may affect choice of

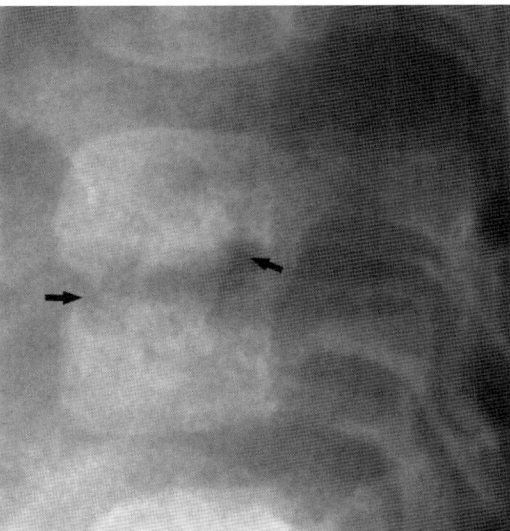

Figure 80-1. Diskitis involving the L4 to L5 space in an 18-month-old girl. Note the narrowed disk space and irregularities of the adjacent vertebral endplates. (Courtesy of Bruce Parker, MD.)

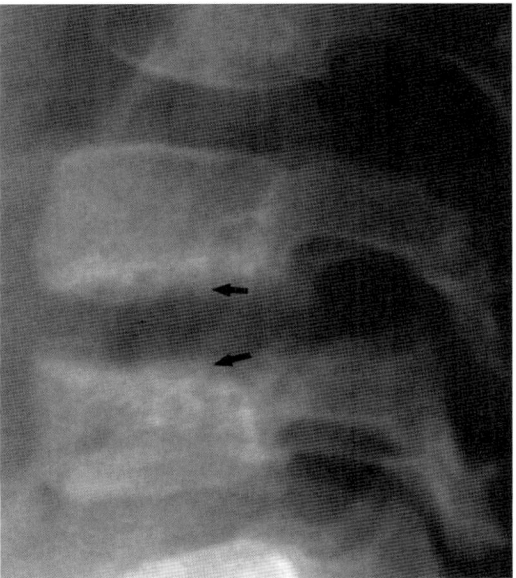

Figure 80-2. Follow-up films of the same patient as in Figure 80-1, 6 months after onset of symptoms. Some narrowing of disk space persists. Note sclerotic changes of the adjacent vertebral endplates. (Courtesy of Bruce Parker, MD.)

therapy. In many studies, most aspirates from a disk space are sterile (even when antibiotics have not been administered).[2,13,26,44] Therefore, aspiration of disk space may be limited to cases in which there is no response to immobilization or empiric antibiotic therapy, cases with extensive involvement of the vertebral body, or cases that have other atypical features.[4,13,27,29,44] Aspirate or biopsy of the disk space should be cultured for bacteria, mycobacteria, and fungus.

MANAGEMENT

Most children with diskitis respond promptly to bedrest, with decreased pain within 48 hours. Immobilization of the spine sometimes is required. Failure to respond to immobilization suggests that the diagnosis is incorrect. Optimal duration of immobilization is unknown. There has been no study correlating long-term outcome and duration of immobilization.

Some investigators suggest the use of antibiotic therapy only if culture results are positive or the child appears to be systemically ill or has not responded promptly to immobilization.[2,12,23,26,37,44] Although antibiotic therapy for diskitis does not appear to alter the long-term prognosis, one retrospective analysis of 47 patients showed that use of a short course of parenterally administered antibiotic agents, followed by oral therapy, hastened resolution of symptoms.[5] Because a number of cases have been associated with positive culture results, particularly for *S. aureus*, antibiotic treatment for an arbitrary length of time seems prudent.[1,3-5] In the absence of a positive culture result, empiric therapy for

staphylococci and *K. kingae* is appropriate. Antibiotic agents can be administered intravenously for several days, until fever and pain have resolved and the ESR is decreasing, and then given orally. Optimal duration of therapy is unknown, but it should be continued until the patient is asymptomatic and the ESR or CRP is normalizing.

OUTCOME

Most children with diskitis have persistently abnormal radiographic findings long after clinical symptoms have resolved.[12,35,46] The involved disk space may never regain its original height, and sclerotic changes in the vertebral endplates persist. There are reported cases of recurrence of symptoms.[2] Although reports of follow-up of patients with diskitis have included small numbers of patients and relatively short periods of time, most patients are asymptomatic with no limitation of activity.[2,3,12,50] Younger children appear to have a lower rate of bony ankylosis compared with older children, presumably as a result of the presence of vascular channels that may promote more rapid healing.[50] Some patients have mild, chronic back pain.[12,37] A study of 35 patients who were followed for an average of 17 years found that 42% complained of persistent backache. Extension of the spine was restricted in 30 patients. Most patients had been treated with bedrest or with a lengthy course of antibiotic agents and immobilization.[47]

81 Transient Synovitis

Kathleen Gutierrez

Transient synovitis (TS) is a self-limited, unilateral inflammation of the synovium, usually of the hip joint. TS is a common cause of limp in childhood. Synonyms for this condition include toxic synovitis, "observation" hip, irritable hip, and "benign aseptic" arthritis.[1-3]

ETIOLOGY AND EPIDEMIOLOGY

The cause of transient synovitis is unknown. In the few cases for which biopsy specimens of synovial membrane have been obtained, histologic examination shows a nonspecific

PART II Clinical Syndromes and Cardinal Features of Infectious Diseases: Approach to Diagnosis and Initial Management

SECTION K Bone and Joint Infections

inflammation.[4,5] Considering that many children with transient synovitis have had a recent or concurrent upper respiratory or gastrointestinal viral infection and that elevated serum interferon levels have been demonstrated in some patients, transient synovitis is likely to represent either a self-limited infection involving the synovial membrane or a postinfectious inflammatory response.[6–8] Some investigators have noted positive results on throat culture for group A streptococcus or elevated anti-streptolysin O (ASO) titer, or both, in a small number of children with toxic synovitis.[7,9] However, no single organism has been implicated consistently as the cause of TS. In one series, an increase in antibody concentrations against rubella, enterovirus, Epstein–Barr virus, or *Mycoplasma* was demonstrated in 67 of 80 children with TS, but there was no unaffected control group; results of viral culture for synovial fluid were negative; and culture samples were not obtained from other sites.[10] In other reports, including one prospective study in which a control group was included and one study in which serologic evidence of acute parvovirus B19 or human herpesvirus 6 infection was sought, no evidence of viral or streptococcal causes was found.[4,11–14] Parvovirus B19 DNA has been detected by PCR in serum of a small number of children with TS.[15]

TS occurs predominantly in children from 18 months to 12 years of age, with the mean age of occurrence being 5.6 to 5.9 years.[3,11,13,16] Boys are affected approximately twice as often as girls.[3,7,11,13,14,16–18] Although the annual incidence in the United States is unknown, TS frequently is referred to as the most common cause of hip pain in children.[19] The average annual incidence in one study of Swedish children was 0.2%.[18]

CLINICAL MANIFESTATIONS

The usual manifestation is acute onset of leg pain or limp in an otherwise healthy child. Symptoms are unilateral, with right and left hips affected equally. There have been rare reports of children with involvement of both hips.[3,11]

Leg pain can be localized to the hip, thigh, or knee. The intensity of pain ranges from mild to severe enough to awaken the child.[2,18] Most children are afebrile or have minimal temperature elevation.[20,21] The child usually appears minimally ill, with pain on movement of the knee, thigh, or hip on the affected side and limited internal rotation and adduction of the affected hip.[3,7]

Duration of symptoms ranges from 1 day to 3 weeks. Most children become asymptomatic approximately 1 week after onset of symptoms.[12,13,22] Prolonged hip pain suggests another diagnosis.

DIAGNOSIS

Laboratory and imaging studies are helpful only to distinguish TS from more serious causes of hip pain. The white blood cell (WBC) count usually is normal, and the erythrocyte sedimentation rate (ESR) is normal or mildly elevated (no greater than 30 mm/h). The mean C-reactive protein (CRP) level in one study of 64 patients with transient synovitis was 1.0 mg/dL.[23] There can be overlap in inflammatory markers between pyogenic (bacterial) arthritis and transient synovitis.[21,23] Blood and joint fluid cultures are helpful because a positive culture rules out transient synovitis.

Plain radiographs of the pelvis and hip often are normal,[17,18,24] and are obtained to rule out osteomyelitis, cancer, or Legg–Calvé–Perthes (LCP) disease.[9,24,25] Ultrasound (US) is a useful noninvasive method for delineating the presence of joint effusion,[22,26–29] which is found in approximately 70% of children with TS.[11] US is helpful in guiding joint aspiration, particularly in children <8 years, because cartilaginous structures are visualized well; in older children fluoroscopic guidance is preferred.[25] Bone scan is normal or shows increased uptake, especially in the blood pool phase.[30–32] Magnetic resonance imaging (MRI) results are normal or reveal abnormal thickening of the articular surfaces and joint effusion.[33,34] Signal intensity alterations detected by MRI in bone marrow may help differentiate pyogenic arthritis and transient synovitis. Low-signal-intensity alterations on fat-suppressed T_1-weighted images and high-signal-intensity alterations on fat-suppressed T_2-weighted images are seen in bone marrow of the affected joint in many of patients with bacterial arthritis and not seen in patients with TS.[35,36]

DIFFERENTIAL DIAGNOSIS

TS is a diagnosis of exclusion.[8,18] The differential diagnosis includes bacterial arthritis of the hip; osteomyelitis of the proximal femur, acetabulum, or sacroiliac joint; pyomyositis, psoas muscle or intra-abdominal abscess; trauma; pauciarticular arthritis; rheumatic fever; malignant tumor; slipped capital femoral epiphysis; LCP disease; fracture, or reactive arthritis.

Early differentiation between transient synovitis and bacterial arthritis of the hip is crucial, because delay in surgical decompression for pyogenic arthritis can result in increased morbidity.[20,21] An evidence-based clinical prediction algorithm using four independent multivariate predictors, including fever ≥38.5°C, non-weight-bearing, an ESR of >40 mm/h, and a peripheral WBC count of >12,000 cells/mm³, was proposed by Kocher et al. to estimate the probability of pyogenic arthritis.[37] Presence of 3 or 4 predictors had positive predictive value (PPV) for pyogenic arthritis of 93% and 99.6% respectively.[37] Studied prospectively by the same investigators on a new cohort of children, the performance was comparatively diminished; in the new cohort, the area under the receiver operating characteristic curve was 0.86 compared with 0.96 in the original study.[38] In a subsequent study of five independent clinical and laboratory markers (temperature >37°C, ESR >20 mm/h, CRP ≥2 mg/dL, WBC >11,000 cells/mm³, and a difference of joint space distance >2 mm) presence of 4 predictors had a PPV for pyogenic arthritis of 99%, presence of 0 or 1 predictor had PPV of 0.1 to 1.7%.[39] A prospective study utilizing the variables in a Kocher algorithm in addition to CRP found that fever was the best predictor of pyogenic arthritis, followed by an elevated CRP, ESR, refusal to bear weight and an elevated WBC.[40] Finally in a retrospective application of 5 factors (with temperature ≥38.5°C, ESR ≥40 mm/h and CRP ≥2 mg/dL) in a general hospital, presence of all 5 factors had a PPV of only 60%, and fever was the best predictor.[41] It is important to consider that the validity of clinical prediction algorithms can vary substantially between institutions and that to date no clinical prediction rule has been validated by large prospective studies in different populations.[42,43]

Aspiration of fluid from the joint space frequently is attempted in patients with suspected TS, because this is the most reliable method of excluding the diagnosis of pyogenic arthritis. The procedure also relieves pain. With TS, fluid is expected to be clear or slightly turbid, usually is <5 mL in volume, and contains <1000 WBC/mm³.

LCP disease frequently manifests as a limp in an otherwise healthy 5- to 9-year-old afebrile child who has a normal peripheral WBC count and ESR. Boys are affected four times more frequently than girls. Initially, the clinical features, laboratory test results, and US findings may be indistinguishable from findings in TS. Plain films, bone scan, and MRI are all useful differentiating tests; LCP disease shows ischemic necrosis of the head of the femur.[18,25,31,33,44] In addition, in children with LCP disease, bone age often is delayed from 6 months to 3 years.[2]

TREATMENT AND PROGNOSIS

The treatment of TS of the hip is bedrest. The usual duration of symptoms ranges from 5 to 7 days. One small double-blind placebo-controlled trial of ibuprofen versus placebo demonstrated that ibuprofen shortened the duration of symptoms from 4.5 to 2 days in children with clinical TS.[45] Close follow-up is necessary to detect development of signs and symptoms of pyogenic arthritis or osteomyelitis, which is especially challenging if patients have received anti-inflammatory drugs. Children who are older than 6 years or who have protracted symptoms require careful evaluation and follow-up to distinguish LCP disease and other disorders.

TS is self-limited and resolves with supportive therapy. Symptoms recur in a small number of children.[4,7,8] In some series, up to 30% of children who were followed for 1 to 30 years after an initial episode developed asymptomatic overgrowth (coxa magna)

of the femoral head.[1,16] The long-term significance of this finding is unknown.

Some investigators suggest that children with TS are at a higher risk for developing LCP disease,[6,8,17] whereas others have found no relationship between the two entities other than the similarity in initial clinical presentation.[13]

SECTION L: Eye Infections

82 Conjunctivitis in the Neonatal Period (Ophthalmia Neonatorum)

Douglas R. Fredrick

Ophthalmia neonatorum is defined as conjunctivitis occurring within the first month of life. It is the most common eye disease of neonates, with an incidence ranging from 1.6% to 12.0%.[1-3] Incidence is directly related to the prevalence of sexually transmitted diseases in adults. One hundred years ago, *Neisseria gonorrhoeae* was the most common pathogen and a major cause of blindness among children. With the advent of Credé prophylaxis (instillation of silver nitrate at time of birth) and changing trends in sexually transmitted diseases, *Chlamydia trachomatis* has become the most common pathogen (Table 82-1).[4-14] In general, offspring of women who receive prenatal care have a lower incidence of infectious conjunctivitis.[12-14] In the absence of maternal sexually transmitted disease, neonatal conjunctivitis is acquired postnatally and is caused by *Staphylococcus aureus, Streptococcus pneumoniae, Haemophilus* spp., and viridans streptococci. Viruses, with the exception of herpes simplex virus (HSV), are less common pathogens in this age group.

Hospital-associated infection can occur in neonatal intensive care units due to *Staphylococcus aureus*, gram-negative bacilli (especially *Pseudomonas aeruginosa*), and adenovirus. Significant predictors of conjunctivitis include low birthweight, use of ventilator or nasal cannula, and continuous positive airway pressue.[15] Ophthalmologic examination has been associated with nosocomial

bacterial conjunctivitis, and most notably adenovirus conjunctivitis (sometimes with dissemination and fatal outcome).[15,16]

PATHOGENESIS

Microbial pathogens can be transmitted to the eye by a variety of routes. Premature rupture of placental membranes allows for the retrograde spread of organisms to the fetal conjunctiva and cornea. Hematogenous spread can occur transplacentally as well. During vaginal delivery, the neonate's eyes can become infected by contact with infected maternal genital secretions. After birth, caregivers can transmit pathogens to the neonate's eyes through direct contact or aerosolization.

In addition to the immaturity of the immune system, the neonate has local risk factors for ocular infections. The secretory rate of tears under basal conditions in premature infants is about 20% of that in full-term infants,[17] and the blink frequency is decreased. The concentration of lysozyme, the enzyme in tears that catalyzes the breakdown of the bacterial cell wall, is also diminished in premature infants compared with full-term infants and adults.[18] A final reason for increased susceptibility of the neonatal eye is a lack of immunoglobulin secretory (Ig) A in the tears of neonates.[19]

TABLE 82-1. Prevalence of *Chlamydia trachomatis*, *Neisseria gonorrhoeae*, and Other Bacterial Pathogens as Causes of Neonatal Conjunctivitis

Country of Study	Year	No. of Infants	Chlamydia trachomatis (%)	Neisseria gonorrhoeae (%)	Other Bacterial Pathogens[a,b] (%)	Reference
United States	1977	302	28	15	22	4
U.S.	1979	100	13	0	39	5
United Kingdom	1982	42	1	0	33	2
U.S.	1984	61	8.2	0	31	6
U.S.	1985	90	44	0	NS	7
U.S.	1986	100	46	0	50	8
Kenya	1986	149	13	43	9	9
U.K.	1986	73	51	1	10	10
Sweden	1987	107	12.2	0	66	11
Belgium	1987	42	10	0	80	12
Kenya	1988	169	11	5	NS	13
U.S.	1993	109	2	0	44	14

NS, not stated.

[a]*Percentages represent approximations, because most studies show total number of isolates, and multiple isolates were recovered from individual patients.*

[b]*Excludes* coagulase-negative staphylococci, *Corynebacterium* spp., Propionibacterium acnes, *and diphtheroids.*

PART II Clinical Syndromes and Cardinal Features of Infectious Diseases: Approach to Diagnosis and Initial Management

SECTION L Eye Infections

ETIOLOGIC AGENTS

Chlamydia trachomatis

Epidemiology

C. trachomatis is the most common cause of infective neonatal conjunctivitis (see Table 82-1). Frequency of conjunctivitis reflects a high prevalence of maternal genital infections, ranging from 18% to 23%.[20,21] The likelihood of transmission from untreated infected mothers to infants ranges from 18% to 61% (Table 82-2).[22-28]

Clinical Manifestations

Chlamydial conjunctivitis is usually clinically evident within 5 to 14 days of birth, although it may appear as early as 3 days, especially after premature rupture of membranes, or as late as 60 days.[22,29] Typical findings are eyelid swelling, erythema, and unilateral or bilateral mucopurulent conjunctivitis; the cornea usually is not involved. On occasion, pseudomembranes and (rarely) true membranes develop. Because neonates lack lymphoid tissue, the expected follicular response of the conjunctiva does not appear unless the infection persists beyond 6 weeks of age. In treated cases, healing usually occurs without sequelae. Infection in untreated or inadequately treated cases can persist for 2 to 12 months, and some cases remain clinically apparent for years. Persistent infection can lead to conjunctival scar formation and corneal micropannus.[30,31]

The major nonocular complication of chlamydial conjunctivitis is pneumonia. Pneumonia develops in 11% to 20% of infected infants and typically manifests at 1 to 3 months of age.[29,32,33] Infants usually are afebrile but have nasal congestion, prolonged cough, tachypnea, and rales. Hyperinflation with interstitial or alveolar infiltrates is evident radiographically. Total serum IgG and IgM antibody values are elevated, and eosinophilia sometimes occurs. Antibodies to *C. trachomatis* are detectable in tears and serum. Although infection usually is self-limited, systemic treatment is recommended because it shortens the duration of ocular and respiratory tract illness and because treatment of ocular infection prevents pneumonia.[33-35]

Diagnosis

In the past, *C. trachomatis* conjunctivitis was diagnosed by Giemsa staining of conjunctival scrapings showing blue-stained intracytoplasmic inclusions within epithelial cells. The sensitivity of Giemsa staining ranges widely, from 22% to 95%, reflecting varied technical and examiner skill.[5,6,36] Staining has been replaced by use of nucleic acid amplification tests performed on conjunctival swabs. These tests are available widely and provide rapid results with high sensitivity.[37] Organism detection by direct fluorescence has lower sensitivity and is difficult to standardize but is less costly.[8,38-42] Cultivation of organisms in yolk sac or tissue culture is a sensitive means of confirming the diagnosis, but these techniques are laborious, slow and are used only in special circumstances.

Treatment

Systemic therapy for conjunctivitis due to *C. trachomatis* is recommended in all cases to prevent pneumonia. Erythromycin estolate or ethylsuccinate, 50 mg/kg per day in four divided doses for 14 days, is curative in about 80% of cases.[34] A second course may be required for those who fail to respond. Preliminary studies suggest that a short course of azithromycin (20 mg/kg), given as a single dose or daily for 3 days, also is effective, and may be less associated with idiopathic hypertrophic pyloric stenosis.[25] Although topical erythromycin may be effective clinically for chlamydial conjunctivitis, therapy does not eradicate nasopharyngeal colonization or prevent pneumonia.[26] Topical corticosteroid therapy is contraindicated because it can prolong the infection and possibly lead to conjunctival scarring.

Neisseria gonorrhoeae

Epidemiology

In the past, *N. gonorrhoeae* was the most serious cause of ophthalmia neonatorum because of this organism's capacity to damage the eye; this infection accounted for 24% of children enrolled in schools for the blind between 1906 and 1911.[43] After the widespread use of perinatal ocular prophylaxis, the incidence of gonococcal ophthalmia neonatorum decreased, and the proportion of admissions to schools for the blind as a result of this infection dropped to 0.6% by 1959. In the United States, the emergence of penicillin-resistant gonococci and the increase in frequency of asymptomatic genital gonococcal infection resulted in a higher prevalence of infections.[44,45] In developing countries, the estimated incidence of gonococcal ophthalmia neonatorum is much higher than in the U.S., ranging from 15% to 34%. In Kenya, where ocular prophylaxis was discontinued in the mid-1970s and the prevalence of penicillinase-producing *N. gonorrhoeae* has risen to 60%, gonococcal ophthalmia has reached epidemic proportions.[9]

Clinical Manifestations

The clinical manifestations of gonococcal ophthalmia neonatorum typically appear 2 to 7 days after birth, although initial manifestations in the second week are not uncommon (Table 82-3). Later onset suggests postnatal exposure to the organism. Most neonates have edema of the eyelid and purulent conjunctivitis; however, some have a mild or catarrhal response.[46] The inflammatory response of the external ocular surface in infants tends to be less severe than that in the older child or adult. Even with treatment, exudative conjunctivitis can continue for 7 to 14 days before subsiding, contributing to the common complication of conjunctival scarring.

Corneal involvement is the most serious complication, because ulceration with resultant scarring is the major cause of visual impairment.[47] Initially, superficial keratitis gives the corneal surface a dull appearance. Subsequently, marginal and central infiltrates can appear, which then ulcerate, sometimes forming a

TABLE 82-2. Prevalence of Chlamydial Conjunctivitis among Infants Born to Mothers with Chlamydial Cervicitis

Country of Study	No. of Infants	Neonates Infected (%)	Reference
United States	18	44	22
U.S.	18	61	23
Sweden	23	22	24
U.S.	60	20	25
U.S.	95	28	20
U.S.	131	18	27
U.S.	120	25	28
Kenya	201	31	13

TABLE 82-3. Differential Diagnosis of Neonatal Conjunctivitis

Cause of Conjunctivitis	Time of Onset	Discharge	Corneal Involvement
Chemical	24 hours	Serous	No
Neisseria gonorrhoeae	2–7 days	Mucopurulent	Infiltrate
Chlamydia trachomatis	5–14 days	Mucopurulent	No
Herpes simplex virus	6–14 days	Serous	Dendrite, epithelial ulcer

ring abscess. Corneal perforation leads to abnormal apposition of the iris against the posterior cornea, which can persist as an adherent leukoma. The ulcerated or perforated cornea also can be the portal for invasion by other organisms, resulting in endophthalmitis. Prompt use of antibiotic therapy to treat gonococcal ophthalmia neonatorum can prevent such ocular complications.

Extraocular gonococcal infection may coexist with ocular infection and is more common than previously thought. Fransen and colleagues[9] reported that N. gonorrhoeae was isolated from pharyngeal specimens in 15% of infants with gonococcal ophthalmia. Although gonococcal pneumonia is not well documented, pharyngeal colonization can lead to bacteremic spread to distant sites, especially joints.[48,49]

Diagnosis

Gram stain of ocular exudate shows predominance of neutrophils with intracellular gram-negative diplococci. Moraxella catarrhalis and Neisseria meningitidis can be confused with N. gonorrhoeae on Gram stain.[50–53] Diagnosis of gonococcal ophthalmia is confirmed by culture on chocolate agar or Thayer–Martin media incubated at 37°C in humidified carbon dioxide. Appropriate culture specimens also should be obtained from the mother and testing for Chamydia, syphilis, and HIV should be performed. Blood and cerebrospinal fluid cultures (in an infant who is febrile or otherwise not behaving normally) also are obtained, as are tests for concurrent C. trachomatis infection.

Treatment

Although ocular prophylaxis is effective in preventing gonococcal conjunctivitis, topical therapy is ineffective in the treatment of established infection and does not prevent disseminated disease. Neonates with gonococcal ophthalmia should be hospitalized and treated with parenteral therapy. Because of the increased prevalence of penicillin resistance in N. gonorrhoeae, penicillin cannot be used as the initial therapy. The treatment of choice is ceftriaxone (25 to 50 mg/kg, not to exceed 125 mg, given once intravenously or intramuscularly).[54] Ceftriaxone should not be given to neonates with hyperbilirubinemia; a single 100 mg dose of cefotaxime given intravenously or intramuscularly is an alternative.[54] In addition, the eye should be irrigated with saline solution at first hourly and then every 2 to 3 hours until discharge is eliminated. Instillation of topical antibiotic is not necessary once diagnosis is confirmed and appropriate systemic antibiotic therapy has been initiated. It is imperative that the mother of the child and all sexual partners be referred for testing for Chlamydia and other sexually transmitted infections. Gonococcal infections are designated as a notifiable disease.

Herpes Simplex Virus

Epidemiology

HSV can infect and seriously damage a neonate's eye. Prior to the availability of antiviral therapy, many infants with isolated herpetic conjunctivitis or skin or other mucous membrane infection progressed to more serious infection.[55,56] Infants usually contract the infection when their abraded skin or mucosal surfaces come in contact with infected maternal genital secretions at delivery. Most neonatal infections are caused by HSV type 2, for which there is an estimated prevalence of nearly 25% among adults in the U.S.[57]

Clinical Manifestations

Ophthalmia neonatorum due to HSV typically becomes evident 6 to 14 days after birth, although infants born after prolonged rupture of placental membranes can have manifestations at birth.[58] Conjunctivitis, which can be unilateral or bilateral, is associated with ipsilateral eyelid edema and serous discharge. In the absence of herpetic lesions of the cornea or skin, herpetic conjunctivitis is indistinguishable from ophthalmia from other causes. Depending on the duration and severity of infection, examination of the cornea can reveal superficial keratitis, epithelial dendrite, geographic ulcer, or disciform stromal keratitis.[59] Although keratoconjunctivitis can be the sole manifestation of HSV infection in the neonate, it more commonly appears in association with other manifestations of systemic infections.[55,56] Most corneal infections in the neonate are detected with the use of a speculum to hold the eyelids apart and a cobalt blue light to illuminate the corneal surface, stained with a fluorescent dye.

Diagnosis

The diagnosis of HSV infection is confirmed by culture of specimens obtained from skin vesicles or conjunctival or corneal lesions. All neonates suspected as being infected with HSV should have a lumbar puncture performed and the CSF tested for HSV DNA using PCR. Direct immunofluorescence assay or enzyme immunoassays also can be performed on swabs from the conjunctiva, but sensitivity and specificity is lower than PCR.

Treatment

All infections caused by HSV in the neonatal period are treated with systemically administered acyclovir (60 mg/kg per day in three divided doses intravenously for 14 days; duration may be longer if other sites are involved. The presence of keratoconjunctivitis requires the addition of topical therapy. Trifluridine (Viroptic) 1% drops are given every 2 to 3 hours for 1 week, and then the dosage is tapered. Alternative medications are 3% vidarabine ointment and idoxuridine, 0.5% ointment or 0.1% solution, each given five times per day. Topical ganciclovir has been produced, but it has not been tested on children. If treatment failure occurs with one medication, another topical regimen can be tried. Topical cycloplegics are indicated for relief of ciliary spasm if keratitis is present. Topical corticosteroid agents should be avoided, because they may augment corneal damage.

Other Infectious Causes

The predominant bacterial pathogens recovered from young infants with nonchlamydial, nongonococcal conjunctivitis include Haemophilus influenzae, Streptococcus pneumoniae, and coagulase-negative staphylococci (see Table 82-1).[2–6,8–12,14,60] Although less common, various gram-negative organisms, such as Escherichia coli, Klebsiella pneumoniae, and Pseudomonas aeruginosa (especially in nosocomial settings), and Neisseria cinerea, collectively account for a sizable proportion of cases of conjunctivitis. Isolation of these bacteria from conjunctival specimens is not a priori evidence of causation. Demonstration of neutrophils and a single bacteria organism (especially with some present intracellularly) supports a pathogenic role.

Staphylococci have been implicated in ophthalmia neonatorum, but in most cases it is unclear whether the organisms resided on the conjunctiva or the eyelid (where they may be part of normal flora).[61,62] S. aureus can be acquired postnatally from the skin or nares of hospital personnel or from family members. Infection usually manifests as mild catarrhal conjunctivitis with mucoid or mucopurulent discharge. Potential ocular complication of such as corneal infiltrates and ulcers is perforation and resulting endophthalmitis. Systemic complications include infection at contiguous or distant sites (sinusitis, pneumonia, osteomyelitis, septicemia) or toxin-mediated disease (scalded-skin syndrome).[63] Localized staphylococcal conjunctivitis can be treated with topical erythromycin, bacitracin ointment, or polymyxin/trimethoprim eye drops. Susceptibility tests should be performed as community-associated and hospital-associated S. aureus can be multiply resistant.

P. aeruginosa is a rare but important cause of neonatal conjunctivitis in hospitalized infants. Prematurity, ventilatory support, and receipt of systemic antibiotic therapy are risk factors. Conjunctivitis can be self-limited and associated with moderate discharge or can progress rapidly, resulting in corneal abscess and endophthalmitis followed by septicemia and death.[64-66] The diagnosis should be suspected when Gram stain of exudate reveals slender gram-negative bacilli. Treatment is topical tobramycin or amikacin drops, initially instilled every 3 hours. Some experts advocate the addition of subconjunctival tobramycin because of its high intraocular penetration.[67] Lack of response to therapy or progression to endophthalmitis or periocular infection requires systemic or intraocular antibiotic therapy or both (see Chapter 86, Endophthalmitis).

PROPHYLAXIS

In 1881, Credé introduced ocular prophylaxis, consisting of cleansing of the eyelids immediately after birth followed by instillation of 2% silver nitrate drops into the conjunctival sac. This simple treatment successfully prevented most cases of ophthalmia neonatorum due to *N. gonorrhoeae*. The combined results of 24 studies conducted in North America and Europe between 1930 and 1979 indicated that only 0.06% of infants receiving topical silver nitrate experienced gonococcal ophthalmia.[68] Reported incidence was similar in the U.S. among 12,431 infants born between 1986 and 1988.[69] However, use of silver nitrate is limited by its ocular toxicity and failure to prevent all cases of gonococcal ophthalmia.[70-72] Chemical conjunctivitis lasting up to 72 hours can occur after instillation of silver nitrate and corneal scarring after inadvertent use of a high concentration of silver nitrate has been reported. The introduction of single-use wax ampules of silver nitrate, designed to prevent evaporative loss and to maintain the concentration of silver nitrate at 1%, has reduced the incidence

and severity of these complications. Changes in the epidemiology of ophthalmia to a predominance of *C. trachomatis* in the early 1970s, however, prompted consideration of alternate prophylactic strategies.[73] Topical erythromycin and tetracycline were proposed because of their activity against *C. trachomatis*.[24] Two U.S. studies have shown that, although silver nitrate, erythromycin, and tetracycline preparations are each effective prophylaxis against gonococcal ophthalmia, none prevents chlamydial ophthalmia.[13,69]

The American Academy of Pediatrics and the Centers for Disease Control and Prevention recommend the use of 1% silver nitrate solution, 1% tetracycline ointment, or 0.5% erythromycin ointment for prophylaxis against *N. gonorrhoeae*.[54] Although this treatment is highly effective when administered properly and within 1 hour of birth, infants born to mothers who have gonococcal infection at parturition also should be treated with a single dose of ceftriaxone given intravenously or intramuscularly (25 to 50 mg/kg; maximum dose 125 mg).[54] In developing countries, a single application of a 2.5% solution of povidone-iodine can be considered for ocular prophylaxis because it is inexpensive and has been shown to be more effective and less toxic than erythromycin and silver nitrate.[74] A second application of 2.5% povidone-iodine was found to be no more efficacious than a single application.[75] Reducing sexually transmitted infections and treating infected mothers before parturition are the best means of preventing infection in neonates.[76]

Acknowledgment

The author acknowledges substantial use of material from previous editions by Avery Weiss.

83   Conjunctivitis beyond the Neonatal Period

Douglas R. Fredrick

Conjunctivitis is the most common infectious disease of the eye in childhood. It is useful to separate conjunctivitis into acute infection (abrupt onset, lasting less than 10 to 14 days) and chronic infection (insidious onset, often persisting for several weeks, months, or even years). The vast majority of acute conjunctivitis is self-limited and can be managed by primary care physicians and providers. Evaluation and successful management of chronic conjunctivitis, however, usually require consultation with an ophthalmologist for specialized diagnostic techniques and to prevent eventual vision-threatening damage.

Organisms can be transmitted to the ocular surface in a number of ways, but direct contact with contaminated fingers is the most common. Bacterial pathogens usually are found in nasopharyngeal secretions as well. Viral pathogens have specific tissue tropism, some rarely affecting conjunctival mucosa (e.g., influenza, respiratory syncytial virus), with others having a proclivity for conjunctival mucosa (e.g., adenovirus, herpes simplex). Organisms can be inoculated into the conjunctiva by airborne droplets produced by coughing and sneezing and, because many viruses can remain viable on dry surfaces for several hours, infection can result from exposure to infected fomites. Vector-borne ocular infections occur in some developing countries. For example, the filarial parasite *Onchocerca volvulus* is transmitted to the eye by the bite of an infested blackfly.

Conjunctivitis is a clinical diagnosis based on the presence of conjunctival hyperemia and ocular discharge. Typically, the palpebral conjunctiva is more inflamed than the bulbar conjunctiva, and the area surrounding the cornea (limbus) is spared. Thus, pulling down the lower lid and noting the predominant area of

inflammation enables one to distinguish conjunctivitis from keratitis, uveitis, and other causes of red eye.[1] Conjunctival hyperemia associated with Kawasaki disease or bacterial toxin-mediated syndrome is distinguished by predominant involvement of bulbar conjunctivae and lack of exudate. The concurrent presence of a serous or purulent discharge confirms the diagnosis of conjunctivitis. Scant amounts of conjunctival discharge are best confirmed by asking the patient about the presence of eyelid crusting upon awakening, because dried exudate accumulates along the lid margins during sleep.

ACUTE CONJUNCTIVITIS

Etiologies

Bacteria and viruses cause acute conjunctivitis. An epidemiologic study of 99 children with conjunctivitis published in 1981 observed that 65% of cases of acute conjunctivitis were caused by bacteria and 20% of cases were caused by a virus.[2] A similar study of 95 children published in 1993 confirmed that the majority (78%) of infections were caused by bacteria.[3] Differentiating features of bacterial conjunctivitis and viral conjunctivitis are shown in Table 83-1.

Bacterial Causes

***Haemophilus influenzae* and *Streptococcus pneumoniae*.** Nontypable *Haemophilus influenzae* is the predominant organism isolated from infected conjunctivae. *Streptococcus pneumoniae*, other

TABLE 83-1. Clinical Findings in Acute Bacterial and Viral Conjunctivitis

Clinical Finding	Bacterial Disease	Viral Disease
Bilateral disease at onset	50–74%	35%
Conjunctival response[a]	Papillary[b] or nonspecific	Follicular[c]
Conjunctival discharge	Mucopurulent	Watery
Conjunctival membrane	Late onset	Early onset
Preauricular adenopathy	No[d]	Yes
Concurrent otitis media	20–73%	10%

[a]Conjunctival response *refers to conjunctival appearance on slit-lamp examination.*

[b]Papillary response *denotes focal area of inflamed conjunctiva centered on a blood vessel.*

[c]Follicular response *represents: focal accumulation of lymphocytes encircled by blood vessels.*

[d]Except granulomatous bacterial infection.

Data from Gigliotti F, Williams WT, Hayden FG, et al. Etiology of acute conjunctivitis in children. J Pediatr 1981;98:531–536; Weiss A, Brinser JH, Nazar-Stewart V. Acute conjunctivitis in childhood. J Pediatr 1993;122: 10–14.

streptococcal species (particularly *S. mitis*), and *Moraxella catarrhalis* are other commonly isolated bacteria.[2,3] Collectively, these organisms are responsible for 55% to 72% of acute bacterial infections of the conjunctivae.[4,5] An outbreak of 698 cases of acute conjunctivitis on a college campus in 2002 was caused by an atypical, unencapsulated strain of *S. pneumoniae* that was identical to strains that had caused outbreaks two decades previously.[6]

Staphylococci. *Staphylococcus aureus* and *S. epidermidis* often are recovered from "eye" cultures but are infrequently a cause of acute conjunctivitis.[3] Studies in which the lids and conjunctivae are sampled separately show that staphylococci can be recovered in relatively large numbers from lids, whereas few organisms are recovered from conjunctivae. Although staphylococci commonly colonize the lids without causing disease, they can cause blepharoconjunctivitis, a chronic infection of the lid margins.

Gram-negative bacilli. Gram-negative bacilli other than *H. influenzae* occasionally cause conjunctivitis. Special clinical circumstances usually are pertinent, such as: (1) exposure to broad-spectrum antibiotics that promote the emergence of gram-negative nasopharyngeal flora; (2) circumstances of poor hygiene in which children rub their eyes with fingers contaminated by feces or urine; and (3) prolonged hospitalization, especially in intensive care settings, where immobilization, exposure keratitis, and dragging of a tracheal suction catheter across the face raise the risk of direct inoculation.[7]

Neisseria gonorrhoeae. *Neisseria gonorrhoeae* rarely causes conjunctivitis but is important to consider because infection can lead to corneal ulceration and blindness.[8,9] The organism binds avidly to surface receptors on the conjunctivae and cornea, triggering the release of bacterial toxins and inflammatory cell-degradative enzymes that damage the corneal epithelium and underlying collagenous stroma. Clinical hallmarks of infection are the onset of purulent conjunctivitis after an incubation period of less than 7 days and the presence of corneal opacification. Unusual cases of infection after incubation periods of up to 19 days and infection associated with minimal symptoms have been reported.[10,11] Beyond the neonatal period, gonococcal conjunctivitis is a result of sexual activity or abuse.[12] *N. gonorrhoeae* can be isolated from the pharynx, rectum, or genital mucosa as well as conjunctivae.

Neisseria meningitidis. *Neisseria meningitidis*, a rare cause of conjunctivitis, is important because it can be complicated by meningococcemia and meningitis.[13–16] In a report of 21 cases and a review of 63 previously reported cases, Barquet and colleagues[15] noted that 18% of patients with conjunctivitis due to *N. meningitidis* experienced meningococcemia. Systemic infection was more common among those treated with topical antibiotics alone.

Bilateral hyperacute conjunctivitis is typical. Conjunctival scrapings show the presence of gram-negative intracellular diplococci.

Haemophilus aegyptius. *Haemophilus aegyptius* deserves special mention because it can cause a meningococcal-like illness (see Chapter 173, Other *Haemophilus* Species). In South America, this organism is the cause of Brazilian purpuric fever.[17,18] Especially prominent in children younger than 10 years, this catastrophic illness typically begins as hyperacute conjunctivitis, which is followed by fever within 3 to 5 days. Disseminated purpura, hypotensive shock, and death ensue within 48 hours. Molecular studies show that all isolates causing Brazilian purpura fever are related genetically.[19] Initially, all reported cases came from São Paulo, Brazil, and the neighboring state of Parana, but new strains emerged in other regions, raising concern about the disease's potential to spread worldwide.[20] The genome of pathogenic *H. aegyptius* is larger than that of nonpathogenic strains. Frequent gene exchange between bacterial species has been shown to underlie this genetic addition.[21,22] In the United States *H. influenzae* biotype *aegyptius* (a nontypable *H. influenzae*) is associated with simple acute seasonal conjunctivitis.

Viral Causes

Viral conjunctivitis has an acute onset, spreading from one eye to the other within a week, and the inflammation lasts 4 days to 2 weeks, depending on severity. Involvement of the second eye usually is less severe than the first affected eye and this pattern helps distinguish viral from bacterial causes. Conjunctival discharge is watery, and slit-lamp examination shows follicular hyperplasia of conjunctivae. Inflammatory membranes over the conjunctival surface can develop. Lid swelling can be minimal or marked. Invasion of the corneal epithelium (punctate keratitis) is associated with pain and photophobia. Superficial keratitis usually is transient but can evolve into an immune-mediated stromal keratitis that reduces vision. Ipsilateral preauricular adenopathy is common. Acute follicular conjunctivitis can be caused by a number of viruses, with associated ocular and nonocular clinical manifestations (Table 83-2).

Adenovirus. Pharyngoconjunctival fever is characterized by the concurrent presence of fever, pharyngitis, and conjunctivitis.[23,24] It is caused by adenovirus (serotypes 3 and 7) and usually affects children younger than 10 years. Although direct contact with airborne droplets is the usual mode of transmission, prolonged fecal excretion of the virus may be responsible for epidemics associated with swimming pools.[24]

Epidemic keratoconjunctivitis is the most common ocular infection due to adenovirus (usually serotypes 8, 19, and 37) in older children.[25,26] Unassociated with fever or pharyngitis, conjunctivitis often is associated with corneal inflammation. The epithelium of the cornea and conjunctiva share a membrane cofactor protein (CD46) that attaches to and promotes entry of adenovirus type 37.[25] Diffuse punctate lesions of epithelial keratitis evolve over 7 to 10 days into circumscribed subepithelial opacities that can impair vision and result in local discomfort for weeks to months. Resolution occurs without scarring. In young children, adenovirus conjunctivitis often causes ocular adnexal inflammation, eyelid edema, and erythema simulating periorbital cellulitis; an inflammatory pseudomembranous or palpebral conjunctivitis is distinctive.[27] Direct contact with infected individuals is the usual mode of transmission,[28,29] but indirect spread by common-use instruments, particularly those used by ophthalmologists, also can occur.[30,31] Adenoviral conjunctivitis can be associated with an acute respiratory infection that can be mild or severe. Faden et al. reported an outbreak of adenovirus 30 disease in a neonatal nursery in which 6 infants with pre-existing respiratory disease expired and ophthalmologic procedures were the infectious source.[32,33]

Herpes simplex virus. Both primary and recurrent herpes simplex virus (HSV) infections can result in unilateral follicular conjunctivitis or blepharoconjunctivitis.[26] Single or multiple clusters of vesicles characteristically appear on the eyelid and progress through pustular and crusted stages before healing

PART II Clinical Syndromes and Cardinal Features of Infectious Diseases: Approach to Diagnosis and Initial Management

SECTION L Eye Infections

TABLE 83-2. Diagnostic Features of Acute Follicular Conjunctivitis

Clinical Syndrome	Etiologic Agent	Eyelid Lesions	Corneal Lesions	Nonocular Findings
Pharyngoconjunctival fever	Adenoviruses 3 and 7	None	Punctate epithelial keratitis	Fever, pharyngitis
Epidemic keratoconjunctivitis	Adenoviruses 8, 19, and 37	Lid swelling	Early: epithelial keratitis Late: subepithelial opacities	None
Herpetic keratoconjunctivitis	Herpes simplex virus	Vesicles	Punctate epithelial keratitis Dendritic keratitis	None
Acute hemorrhagic conjunctivitis	Enterovirus 70, coxsackievirus A24	None	Punctate epithelial keratitis	Neurologic sequelae Facial palsy Radiculomyelitis
Newcastle disease	Newcastle disease virus	None	Punctate epithelial keratitis	Usually occurs in poultry workers or veterinarians
Rubella, rubeola	Rubella and rubeola viruses	Skin exanthem	Punctate epithelial keratitis	Fever, diffuse exanthem, cough, rhinorrhea; occipital, postauricular adenopathy (rubella); Koplik spots (rubeola)

Modified from Dawson CR, Sheppard JD. Follicular conjunctivitis. In: Tasman W, Jaeger EA (eds) Duane's Clinical Ophthalmology, vol 4. Philadelphia, Lippincott-Raven, 1991, pp 1–26.

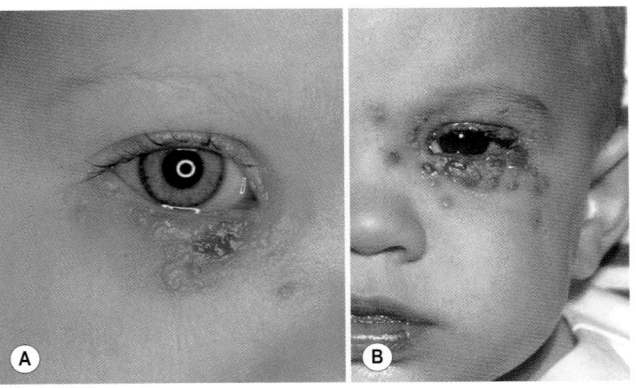

Figure 83-1. (A, B) Typical herpetic skin lesions of the eyelids associated with conjunctivitis in various stages of development and healing. (Courtesy of J.H. Brien©.)

(Figure 83-1A, B). When present, accompanying corneal ulcers manifest as marginal infiltrates, punctate epithelial defects, or classic dendrites. Whenever a child or adult has had an episode of herpetic blepharoconjunctivitis it is imperative that subsequent episodes of conjunctivitis be promptly evaluated by an ophthalmologist, as recurrent episodes usually involve the cornea. Prompt antiviral treatment of herpetic keratoconjunctivitis can prevent blinding consequences of corneal scarring.

Picornaviruses. Acute hemorrhagic conjunctivitis is a highly contagious illness usually caused by the picornaviruses, especially enterovirus 70 and coxsackievirus A24. Infection is characterized by the sudden onset of bilateral conjunctivitis associated with profuse watery discharge, lid edema, and fine, punctate epithelial keratitis.[34-36] A prominent distinguishing feature is the presence of subconjunctival hemorrhage, which can be pinpoint or confluent. The disease lasts for 3 to 5 days and resolves without adverse ocular sequelae. However, this pandemic infection can be accompanied by neurologic involvement, in particular radiculomyelitis with extremity weakness, unilateral facial nerve palsy, or other cranial neuropathies.[37,38]

CONJUNCTIVITIS–OTITIS SYNDROME

The frequent association of conjunctivitis with otitis media has received increased attention. Because 20% to 73% of children with conjunctivitis have otitis media, children presenting with conjunctivitis should have otoscopic examinations. Nontypable *H. influenzae* is the major pathogen implicated.[39-42] In one study from France, 16% of children with acute otitis media had concurrent

conjunctivitis; conjunctival exudates yielded growth of nontypable *H. influenzae* in 89% of 419 cases.[42]

Diagnosis

Most cases of acute conjunctivitis occurring in pediatric patients do not require confirmation of bacterial cause because empiric therapy is cost effective and efficacious. Conjunctival swabs should be obtained for microbiologic evaluation from affected neonates, immunocompromised children, hospitalized children, and those in whom herpetic disease is suspected. Etiologic agent usually cannot be predicted clinically. Bacterial cultures are more useful than viral cultures, because their diagnostic yield is higher and their costs are lower. The combination of sterile culture of conjunctiva and low density of organisms from lid cultures is strong indirect evidence of a viral infection.[3] Molecular detection of adenovirus with real-time, polymerase chain reaction assay is rapid and is an acceptable alternative to viral cultures.[43,44] When HSV is a diagnostic consideration, viral cultures should be performed.

Although rarely necessary, conjunctival scraping can be helpful.[3,45] Specimens should include conjunctival epithelial cells to allow detection of intracellular pathogens. The conjunctival surface is scraped gently with a spatula after the instillation of topical anesthetic drops; swabbing of surface exudate with a cotton-tipped applicator is more likely to yield an amorphous mixture of fibrin and cellular debris than intact cells. Gram stain of the scraping provides preliminary information about the presence and relative quantity of bacteria. Giemsa stain can help to differentiate bacterial infections from viral infections; predominance of neutrophils typically is present in bacterial infections and a predominance of lymphocytes suggests viral infection.

Treatment

Bacterial Disease

Acute conjunctivitis usually is self-limited. Topical antibiotic treatment is recommended because it speeds eradication of the offending pathogen and shortens the duration of symptoms.[46] Clinical factors for low risk of bacterial conjunctivitis, such as lack of discharge causing eyelid closure, age greater than 6 years, and occurrence from April through November are commonly associated with negative bacterial culture, making treatment with antibiotics less indicated.[47,48] In general, treatment is empiric because cultures and cytologic examinations are not performed routinely. When the decision to treat with antibiotics is made, topical antibiotic therapy should be broad spectrum, nontoxic, and of low cost.

For infants, erythromycin ointment or polymyxin-bacitracin ophthalmic ointment instilled 3 times a day for 5 to 7 days is well tolerated and covers most pathogens.[4,46] Ointments and solutions containing neomycin should be avoided, as there is a high incidence of allergic sensitization with these agents, which can lead to chronic conjunctivitis. For older children, ophthalmic solutions should be used, with polymyxin-trimethoprim solution or sodium sulfacetamide 5% solution being good choices for broad-spectrum coverage.[49–51] Tobramycin 3% solution is used commonly, but resistance of *Streptococcus* species limits effectiveness. Topical fluoroquinolones such as ciprofloxacin, ofloxacin, and norfloxacin are effective but expensive. The widespread use of topical fluoroquinolones has led to the emergence of resistant organisms, therefore their use should be restricted to infections involving the cornea or to those caused by gram-negative organisms in hospitalized patients.[52–61] Azithromycin 1.5% ophthalmic solution is well tolerated and has good coverage, especially against *Haemophilus* and many *Streptococcus* species.[62]

Systemic antibiotics are effective in the treatment of bacterial conjunctivitis. Their use is recommended when there is concurrent acute otitis media (AOM), pharyngitis, or bronchitis that requires systemic therapy. Oral therapy also may prevent the development of AOM. In one study, 11 of 42 (26%) patients treated with topical antibiotics alone, but only 2 of 41 (5%) patients treated with topical and systemic antibiotics, had evidence of AOM at a 2-week follow-up visit.[40] In another study, however, oral cefixime was no more effective than topical polymyxin-bacitracin for either the eradication of conjunctival colonization or prevention of AOM.[4]

Intravenous antibiotics attain levels in the conjunctiva that are sufficient to eradicate potential pathogens. Efficacy of oral therapy is less clear, because the conjunctival concentrations of drugs are considerably lower. In one study, 46 of 48 (96%) children with acute conjunctivitis treated with oral antibiotics alone had negative bacterial cultures after 3 to 5 days of therapy.[63] A controlled study by Isenberg et al.[64] indicates that topical solution of 1.25% povidone-iodine is as effective as neomycin-polymyxin-gramicidin in the treatment of acute conjunctivitis. Low cost and lack of microbial resistance make this an attractive option, especially in developing countries.

Herpes Simplex Virus

Treatment of HSV eye infections usually should be undertaken in collaboration with an ophthalmologist. Treatment with orally administered acyclovir or topical trifluridine are both effective, but intravenous therapy should be used when treating a patient with a history of atopy, a child with disseminated disease, an immuno-compromised child, or a neonate.[65] Topical ganciclovir is available for the treatment of herpetic eye disease, but clinical trials are still ongoing to determine efficacy. Topical corticosteroid agents are contraindicated in suspected conjunctivitis and superficial keratitis due to HSV but are used by ophthalmologists on occasion, in conjunction with antiviral agents, for immune-mediated disease of the corneal stroma.

Adenovirus and Other Viruses

Treatment is supportive and may include cool compresses, use of artificial tears, and topical vasoconstrictors. Topical ketorolac 0.5%, a nonsteroidal anti-inflammatory agent, used 4 times daily is no better than artificial tears.[66] Topical cidofovir, a broad-spectrum antiviral agent, is not effective at 0.2% concentration, and the 1% concentration is limited by local toxicity.[67,68] Corticosteroid drops are contraindicated because they predispose to corneal involvement and can prolong viral shedding, as observed in an animal model.[69]

CHRONIC CONJUNCTIVITIS

Nasolacrimal Duct Obstruction

Nasolacrimal duct obstruction is the most common cause of chronic or recurrent eye infection of infants.[70] Although usually a developmental anomaly, sometimes obstruction can be acquired

(as following local adenovirus or bacterial infection). Persistence of an imperforate membrane along the nasolacrimal duct blocks tear drainage and predisposes to secondary infection of retained tears. Consequently, tears pool in the conjunctival cul-de-sac and then spill over the lid margins, flowing onto the cheek (epiphora). At night or during sleep, spillage of infected material leads to accumulation of crusted exudate along the lid margins.

Digital compression of the lacrimal sac region usually elicits reflux of mucopurulent discharge. When reflux cannot be elicited, delayed clearance of 5% fluorescein dye instilled onto the eye confirms the diagnosis of a blocked tear duct. The conjunctiva appears normal or only minimally inflamed. The lower eyelid skin frequently becomes red and inflamed due to chronic wetness and rubbing, but the tissue is not edematous, painful or tender, differentiating this condition from cellulitis. Topical antibiotics and digital massage of the lacrimal sac are the initial treatments of choice. Because 95% of obstructions resolve by 12 months of age, lacrimal duct probing is reserved for patients in whom obstruction persists beyond this age.

Staphylococcal Blepharitis

Blepharitis is a primary infection of the eyelid with secondary inflammation of the conjunctiva. Blepharitis is the most common cause of chronic conjunctivitis in older children.[70,71] *S. aureus* or coagulase-negative staphylococci (CoNS) are the usual pathogens. Affected children come to medical attention because of red eyes, ocular irritation, chronic eye rubbing, and pulling of the eyelashes. Photophobia is a sign of corneal involvement.

Clinically, it is useful to separate blepharitis into anterior and posterior types. Anterior blepharitis is accompanied by crusting along the lid margin because of the build-up of epithelial debris and fibrin centered on the eyelashes (cilial collarettes). Close inspection reveals superficial excoriations of the lid margin and telangiectatic vessels. Chronic rubbing of the eyelid and eyelash pulling lead to breakage and partial loss of eyelashes. In posterior blepharitis, the meibomian gland orifices, located along the posterior lid margin, are blocked, causing retention of sebum and predisposing to meibomian cysts, chalazion, and secondary infections. The incidence of meibomitis peaks in young children[72] and during adolescence, when the sebaceous glands undergo hormonal stimulation. Examination reveals inspissation of meibomian glands, from which exudative material can be expressed by gentle compression of the lids with cotton applicators. Although blepharitis is a clinical diagnosis, the recovery of relatively more staphylococcal species from lid cultures than conjunctival cultures, as well as cytologic evidence of neutrophils on Giemsa stains of conjunctival scrapings, helps to confirm the diagnosis.

The most common complication of blepharitis is chalazion formation. This results from obstruction of the meibomian gland orifices by debris and secondary infection. Blepharitis should be suspected in any child who demonstrates recurrent or multiple chalazia. Toxic epithelial changes of the cornea (punctate keratitis), immune-mediated subepithelial infiltrates, and marginal ulcerations can result from corneal contamination with exotoxins of staphylococci. Chronic staphylococcal keratitis can lead to corneal neovascularization and visual loss.

Blepharitis cannot be cured, but symptoms can be controlled through the use of eyelid hygiene and topical antibiotics. Lid hygiene entails applying a washcloth presoaked in warm water at least 2 to 4 times a day and scrubbing the lid margin with a cotton-tipped applicator presoaked in a 50:50 mixture of a nonirritating shampoo (or soap) and water. Attention to personal hygiene and avoidance of chronic eyelid rubbing are helpful in preventing contamination of the lids. Topical antibiotics should be used to treat secondary infection. Bacitracin or erythromycin ointments are appropriate choices. They should be applied 1 to 4 times daily for 1 to 2 weeks and then once daily for 4 to 8 weeks. Treatment is continued for 1 month after all signs of inflammation abate. Topical corticosteroids sometimes are required to suppress the inflammatory component, but should be used only with the supervision of an ophthalmologist. Indiscriminate use of

PART II Clinical Syndromes and Cardinal Features of Infectious Diseases: Approach to Diagnosis and Initial Management

SECTION L Eye Infections

corticosteroids could lead to glaucoma and exacerbation of unrecognized herpetic eye disease. Systemic erythromycin in children under the age of 8 years and systemic tetracycline in older children are effective treatment options in severe cases of blepharoconjunctivitis.[72,73] Erythromycin and tetracycline appear to accumulate in the meibomian glands where they inhibit bacterial protein synthesis and lipase breakdown of sebum.

Ulcerative and Angular Blepharitis

Herpes simplex infections can cause ulcerative blepharitis. The presence of grouped vesicles is suggestive of herpetic infections. Diagnosis is confirmed by viral culture. Angular blepharitis refers to an infection localized to the lateral canthal region and, less frequently, to the medial canthal area. The involved area is erythematous, with eczematous changes, maceration, and fissuring of affected skin. It is most common among adolescents living in warm climates. *S. aureus* and *S. pneumoniae* are the most commonly implicated bacteria. Treatment is administration of topical antibiotics.

Chlamydial Infections

Trachoma

Trachoma is the most important ocular infection worldwide because it is a major, preventable cause of blindness.[74] *Chlamydia trachomatis*, usually serotype A, B, or C, is the usual cause of infection. Trachoma has an insidious onset in infants and young children, in whom the organism attaches to and invades the conjunctival and corneal epithelium, eliciting the formation of lymphoid follicles. Chronic inflammation causes a loss of conjunctival goblet cells with resulting mucin deficiency and subconjunctival fibrosis (particularly of the upper lid). As lymphoid follicles of the limbus regress, semilunar areas of thinned cornea, known as Herbert pits, appear and are pathognomonic of the disease. Progressive cicatrization of the conjunctiva can pull the lid margin inward, causing the eyelashes to rub on the cornea (trichiasis). The combined effects of chronic inflammation, mucin deficiency, and trichiasis can lead to corneal scarring, neovascularization, and blindness.

Trachoma is treated with topical erythromycin or tetracycline, or sulfacetamide ointment applied either twice daily for 2 months or twice daily for the first 5 days of the month for 6 months. Oral erythromycin or tetracycline therapy for 40 days is given if infection is severe. Single-dose azithromycin (20 mg/kg) also is effective and can be beneficial, especially in hyperendemic areas.[75-79] In one large study, the prevalence of infection fell from 9.5% before introduction of single-dose azithromycin therapy to 0.8%

24 months after introduction.[79] On the basis of a chlamydial recurrence rate of 11% at 6 months, one study proposed that repeat single-dose treatment biannually potentially could eliminate ocular *Chlamydia trachomatis*.[80]

Inclusion Conjunctivitis of the Adolescent

Chlamydia trachomatis (serotypes D through K) is the most common sexually transmitted infection with disproportionate occurrence in sexually active adolescents.[81,82] The clinical hallmark of eye involvement is a unilateral follicular conjunctivitis with mucopurulent discharge, eyelid swelling, and ipsilateral preauricular adenopathy. Photophobia and severe irritation are symptoms consistent with corneal involvement. The organism invades the corneal epithelium, resulting in a superficial keratitis that can progress to subepithelial infiltrates and micropannus formation. If untreated, the disease can persist for months to years. Diagnosis is based on positive cultures, detection of chlamydial antigens, or molecular techniques. Treatment consists of systemic tetracycline, doxycycline, or erythromycin for 7 days or longer.

Parinaud Oculoglandular Syndrome

Parinaud oculoglandular conjunctivitis is a syndrome characterized by the presence of granulomatous conjunctivitis and ipsilateral preauricular or submandibular adenopathy. Usually unilateral, there may be one or more granulomas of the upper or lower palpebral conjunctiva. Fever, malaise, and other systemic signs can be present. *Bartonella henselae* is the most common cause,[83] but oculoglandular syndrome also can be associated with tularemia, sporotrichosis, tuberculosis, syphilis, and infectious mononucleosis.

Viruses

Viruses rarely cause chronic conjunctivitis, with the exception of molluscum contagiosum, a poxvirus infection. One or more umbilicated papules of varying size on the eyelid are the cardinal features. Rupture of lesions on the eyelid margin releases molluscum bodies onto the conjunctiva, inciting a follicular response.[84] Molluscum contagiosum of the eyelids can be a manifestation of human immunodeficiency virus infection.[85] Diagnosis is based on the presence of typical lesions on the lid and elsewhere on the skin. Treatment consists of excision, curettage, or cryopexy of individual lesions.[86]

Acknowledgments

The author acknowledges substantial use of material from previous editions by Avery Weiss.

84 Infective Keratitis

Douglas R. Fredrick

Infective keratitis is an uncommon but important infection because it has the potential to cause blindness. It can be caused by a wide variety of microorganisms. Most children with corneal infections come to medical attention because of a painful red eye. Distinguishing infectious keratitis from other causes of red eye accurately and promptly is extremely important.

PATHOGENESIS

The cornea is susceptible to microbial invasion because of its exposed position, avascularity, and limited inflammatory repertoire. Apart from epithelial Langerhans cells, the normal cornea lacks white cells, which must be recruited from the tear film,

Risk Factors for Bacterial Keratitis in Children

TRAUMA

Corneal foreign body
Corneal abrasion/laceration
Contact lens wear
Trichiasis/dystichiasis
Prior ocular or eyelid surgery

CORNEAL EXPOSURE

Congenital and acquired disorders of the eyelids
Globe proptosis
Facial palsy
Moribund or sedated state

ABNORMALITIES OF THE OCULAR SURFACE

Dry-eye syndrome
Mucin deficiency from loss of goblet cells
Malnutrition
Corneal anesthesia
Ocular rosacea

IMMUNODEFICIENCY STATES

Topical corticosteroid therapy
Immunosuppressive therapy
Immune deficiency syndrome
Atopy

limbal lymphoid aggregates, and perilimbal circulation.[1,2] The epithelium and its basement membrane serve as a relative barrier to most infectious agents, but, once breached, the hypocellular stroma is vulnerable to infection, often with organisms of low virulence. Release of proteases, collagenases, and oxygen-derived free radicals from invasive organisms and infiltrating neutrophils degrades collagen and proteoglycans, the major constituents of the corneal stroma.

Trauma caused by the use of contact lenses is the most common factor predisposing to bacterial and fungal keratitis in children (Box 84-1).[3-7] Trauma from contact lenses can cause epithelial damage and corneal hypoxia. The risk of bacterial keratitis is 10- to 15-fold greater in subjects who wear contact lenses overnight compared with users of daily-wear lenses.[8] Orthokeratology, a procedure for reshaping the cornea by wearing nocturnal contact lenses, is popular among teenagers and predisposes to corneal infections.[9] Dry eyes, related to a deficient tear film or abnormality of the ocular surface, corneal anesthesia, and prior treatment with topical corticosteroid agents are other factors increasing the risk of bacterial keratitis. In developing countries, malnutrition, vitamin A deficiency, poor hygiene, and trachoma also predispose to corneal infections.[10]

Inadequate eyelid closure is another important risk factor for infective keratitis. Corneal exposure in the severely ill or sedated child predisposes to breakdown of the epithelium, and secondary infection.[3] Children with eyelid defects, facial nerve weakness, and proptotic globes as well as those in intensive care under pharmacologic paralysis are prone to exposure keratopathy and secondary infection. Protocols must be in place to assure eyelid closure and lubrication in these patients. Premature infants and older children receiving mechanical ventilators are particularly susceptible to conjunctival colonization with *Pseudomonas aeruginosa* and keratitis.[11-13]

CLINICAL PRESENTATION

Severe pain is the hallmark of infective keratitis. Reflex tearing, redness of the eye, photophobia, and decreased vision are prominent symptoms. Keratitis usually is distinguished by the presence of greyish corneal opacification. Loss of the epithelium over the

corneal infiltrate dulls the corneal light reflex and permits topically applied fluorescein dye to stain the area. Progressive destruction can lead to corneal thinning and eventual perforation. The anterior chamber can contain dispersed inflammatory cells or visible aggregates of neutrophils layering inferiorly (hypopyon). In an uncooperative child examination of the eye is facilitated by the use of a topical anesthetic and a lid speculum.

ETIOLOGIC AGENTS

Herpes Simplex Virus

Keratoconjunctivitis caused by herpes simplex virus (HSV) usually is mild and is indistinguishable from other causes of viral conjunctivitis, except by the presence of skin or corneal lesions. The most common manifestations are unilateral follicular conjunctivitis, watery ocular discharge, and preauricular adenopathy.[14] Inspection of the swollen lids often reveals the presence of vesicles or lid margin ulcerations. Initially, the cornea is spared, but within a few days to 2 weeks mild punctate keratitis or dendritic keratitis develops in about one-half of infected children (Figure 84-1). Primary herpetic keratitis is self-limited in most children beyond the neonatal period.

Most episodes of herpetic keratitis represent recurrent disease following primary infection that has resulted in latent infection of the cornea or trigeminal ganglion. Most recurrent episodes are not accompanied by vesicular skin lesions, but manifest as red eye, photophobia, watery discharge, and blurred vision. Only 20% of recurrences appear during childhood; their number, frequency, and type are highly variable.[14,15] The spectrum of recurrent HSV keratitis includes epithelial dendrites (Figure 84-2), large geographic defects, immune-mediated diskiform edema (Figure 84-3), necrotizing keratitis complicated by corneal thinning or perforation, and chronic neurotrophic ulcerations. There are few serious sequelae if infection remains confined to the corneal epithelium, but if stromal disease ensues, progressive corneal scarring can result in permanent visual loss.

Varicella-Zoster Virus

Infection caused by varicella-zoster virus (VZV) may be associated with small vesicular or papular eruptions at the limbus. These lesions usually resolve without sequelae, but the affected conjunctiva often is red and painful. Less frequent corneal manifestations of VZV infection include superficial punctate epithelial defects, linear dendrites, and diskiform or necrotizing keratitis with ulceration. Recurrent epithelial or stromal keratitis also occurs.[14,16]

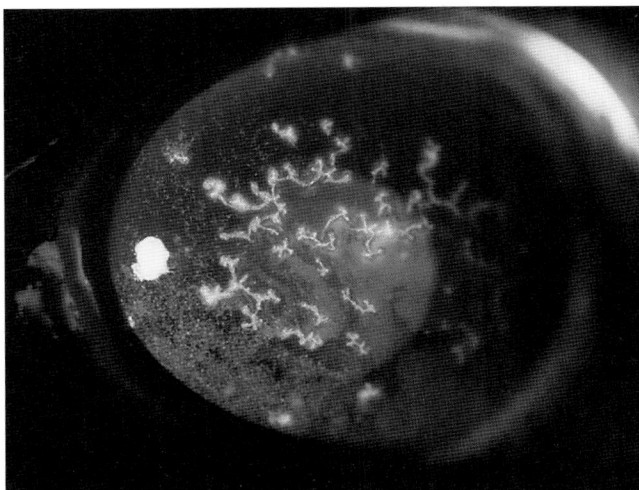

Figure 84-1. Classic appearance of primary herpes simplex virus keratitis stained with 1% fluorescein, showing multiple epithelial dendrites.

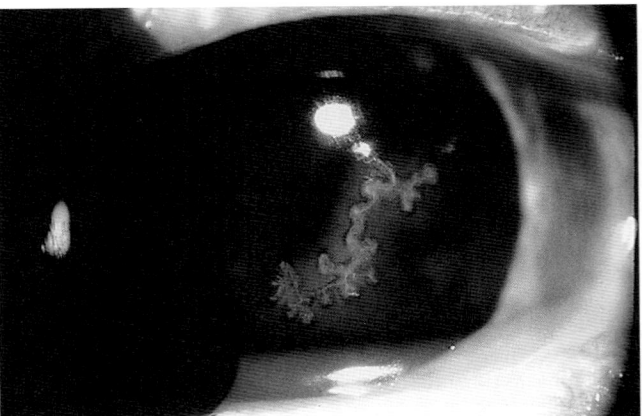

Figure 84-2. Slit-lamp appearance of recurrent dendritic keratitis due to herpes simplex virus stained with 1% fluorescein.

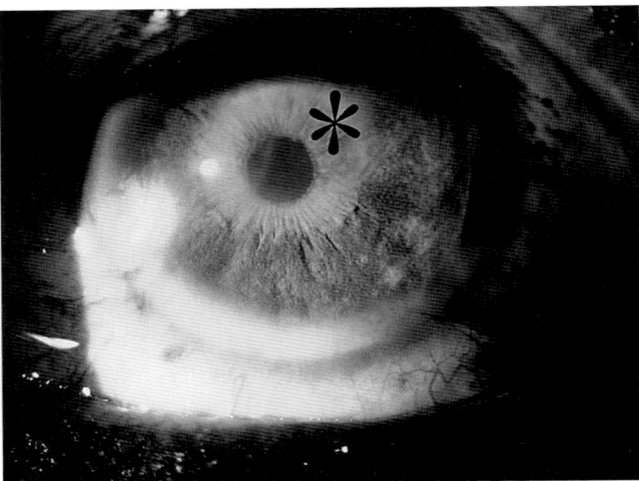

Figure 84-3. Herpes simplex virus diskiform keratitis, consisting of a disk-like area of stromal edema (asterisk) believed to be a cell-mediated immune response to residual herpes simplex virus antigen.

Herpes zoster ophthalmicus refers to reactivation of VZV along the sensory distribution of the ophthalmic division of the trigeminal nerve. Although uncommon in childhood, it can occur because of immunosuppression or following infection contracted during the first year of life.[17] A vesicular eruption is confined to the branches of the ophthalmic nerve. Uveitis and keratitis are the most common ocular manifestations. In the acute infectious stage, examination of the cornea can reveal punctate, dendritic, or geographic epithelial inflammation, which can progress to necrotizing stromal keratitis.[14,18] An immune-mediated response to zoster-related antigens appears as a delayed-onset diskiform or nummular (coin-shaped) keratitis. A chronic and recurrent epithelial or stromal keratitis can occur.[19] All children with zoster ophthalmicus must receive a funduscopic examination, as chorioretinitis can lead to permanent vision impairment. Although herpes zoster infections in previously vaccinated children tend to be mild, some children can have severe sclerokeratitis and anterior uveitis, which can lead to increased intraocular pressure and glaucoma.[20]

Other Viruses

Measles, mumps, rubella, adenovirus, coxsackievirus A24, and enterovirus 70 are associated commonly with a self-limited punctate epithelial keratitis; however, there are important exceptions. Epithelial lesions associated with adenovirus infections sometimes progress over 10 to 14 days to subepithelial opacities that can persist for months.[21] Measles keratitis usually is mild but can cause severe corneal disease when contracted by malnourished, immunocompromised, or vitamin A-deficient children.[22,23] Localized edema of the corneal stroma can, on occasion, be a delayed complication of mumps.[24]

Epstein–Barr virus can invade all layers of the cornea. Superficially there can be multiple epithelial dendrites. Stromal disease is more common and is characterized by multiple coin-shaped lesions in the anterior and mid-stroma or recurrent infiltrate of the deeper layers associated with vascularization.[25–27] The condition resolves spontaneously without ocular sequelae; symptomatic treatment with artificial tears is sufficient.

Bacteria

Bacterial infection of the cornea is considered a medical emergency because it can progress rapidly and lead to severe visual loss. The presence of a dense greyish infiltrate and surface ulceration in an actively inflamed eye should be considered bacterial infection until proven otherwise (Figure 84-4). Infection can be caused by a wide range of gram-positive and gram-negative organisms.[3–6] *Staphylococcus aureus* and streptococcal species are among the most common gram-positive isolates, especially in cooler climates. *S. epidermidis* frequently is isolated from corneal cultures, but this often represents contamination from the eyelids. *Pseudomonas aeruginosa* is the most common gram-negative isolate, especially among contact lens wearers. Ulcerative keratitis also can complicate bacterial conjunctivitis due to *Haemophilus influenzae* and *Moraxella catarrhalis*. *Shigella* and other enteric pathogens can cause keratitis following transfer to the eyes by fingers contaminated from extraocular sites of infection.

Fungi

Fungal keratitis is rare in childhood and usually is the consequence of ocular trauma, especially with vegetable matter. The prior use of topical corticosteroid agents, systemic immunosuppression, pre-existing corneal disease, and tropical environment increase the risk of fungal infection. *Fusarium* species were isolated in an outbreak of corneal ulcers associated with the use of a specific contact lens solution.[28] Typically, the ulcer has a subacute onset and progresses insidiously. Slit-lamp examination typically reveals a yellow-white infiltrate with feathery edges, a dry, raised surface, and satellite lesions.[29,30] A wide range of fungi can be corneal pathogens. *Aspergillus* and *Fusarium* species are the most common pathogens worldwide.[3–6,30,31] In the United States, *F. solani* is the most common pathogen in southern states, whereas

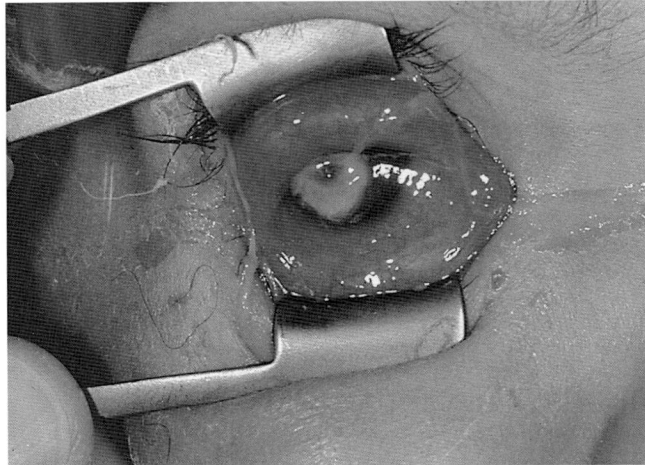

Figure 84-4. Perforated keratitis due to *Streptococcus pneumoniae* in a 3-year-old child after an eye injury.

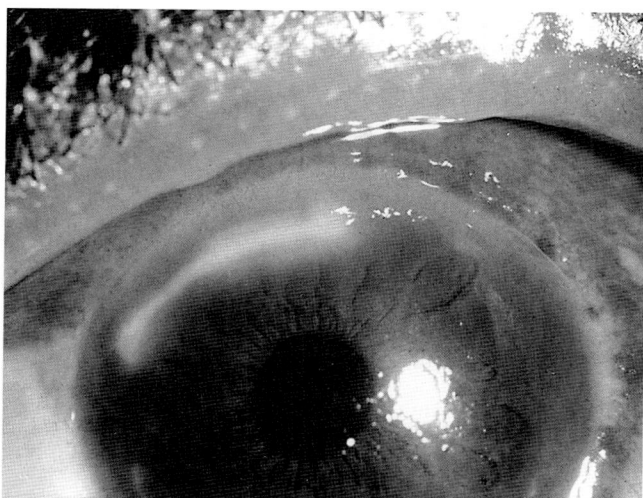

Figure 84-5. Extensive marginal keratitis in a child secondary to staphylococcal lid disease. Note the characteristic lucid interval between arcuate infiltrate and corneal limbus.

Aspergillus species and *Candida albicans* are most common elsewhere.[32,33] Dematiaceous (pigmented) fungi, particularly *Curvularia* species, are emerging as important corneal pathogens.[30]

Acanthamoeba

Acanthamoeba causes a recalcitrant keratitis that frequently leads to visual loss. It usually occurs in contact lens wearers or in persons exposed to contaminated water.[34,35] Severe pain, out of proportion to the severity of the keratitis, is common. This seems to be related to a propensity of the organism to infiltrate corneal nerve endings.[36] Initially, corneal epithelium is involved, and later a stromal infiltrate develops. As the infection progresses the infiltrate becomes most dense at the periphery, giving rise to a very characteristic ring-shaped lesion.[37–39]

Interstitial and Marginal Keratitis

Interstitial keratitis usually is a delayed manifestation of a systemic infection from a variety of bacterial, viral, and parasitic pathogens. Congenital syphilis formerly was the predominant cause of interstitial keratitis.[40,41] More recently, *Mycobacterium tuberculosis*, nontuberculous mycobacteria, *Borrelia burgdorferi*, herpesviruses, and onchocerciasis have become more common causes. Interstitial keratitis represents an immune-mediated reaction to retained microbial antigens rather than active infection. Pain, photophobia, and reflex tearing are the major symptoms. Examination reveals an intact corneal epithelium with underlying cellular infiltration of the superficial or deep stroma. Limbal blood vessels often proliferate and extend into the opacities. Once the inflammation subsides, the opacities and blood vessels regress, leaving stromal scars and ghost vessels. Depending on the severity of scarring, final visual acuity ranges from 20/20 to 20/200.[42]

Staphylococcal lid disease is associated with a marginal keratitis in which infiltrates form in the peripheral cornea, often where the lid margins cross the limbus (at 2, 4, 8, and 10 o'clock). Cultures of the infiltrates are sterile, suggesting that they result from hypersensitivity reactions to staphylococcal antigens or exotoxins deposited on the ocular surface (Figure 84-5). Ocular rosacea can lead to corneal ulceration and should be considered in patients with eyelid disease and recurrent keratitis.[43]

DIAGNOSTIC PROCEDURES

Evaluation of infectious keratitis should include corneal scrapings for smears and cultures. Children often require sedation or examination under anesthesia to allow thorough evaluation and collection of appropriate specimens. Corneal specimens are obtained by scraping the leading edge and base of the ulcer with a sterilized Kimura spatula or Calgi swab.[44,45] Specimens from the lids and conjunctiva should be collected and cultured separately. Ideally, specimens should be inoculated directly onto the culture media since corneal scrapings contain small numbers of fastidious organisms. Amies transport media without charcoal is a useful alternative in the clinical setting.[46] Culture media should include blood and chocolate agar, anaerobic blood agar, Sabouraud dextrose agar (without cycloheximide), and enriched thioglycolate broth. Tissue culture is inoculated for isolation of viruses. *Acanthamoeba* species can be isolated using nonnutrient agar plates overlaid with a dried broth culture of *Escherichia coli*.

Staining of corneal scrapings is important for the early identification of bacteria, fungi, and *Acanthamoeba* and may provide the sole etiologic evidence in culture-negative cases.[44,45] Multiple specimens should be taken for Gram, Giemsa, and other specialized stains. Methenamine silver, acridine orange, and Calcofluor white stains are useful for the detection of fungi and *Acanthamoeba*.[47,48]

Microbial antigens can be detected using immunodiagnostic methods. Enzyme immunoassays and fluorescein-labeled monoclonal antibodies are especially useful in the diagnosis of chlamydial, herpetic, and other viral infections. Recombinant DNA methods have been applied to the detection of corneal fungi, herpes and other viruses, and *Acanthamoeba*.[49–51] Fungi and *Acanthamoeba* can be visualized directly in the cornea with confocal slit-lamp microscopy.[52]

Lumbar puncture should be performed in neonates with suspected herpetic eye disease. Testing CSF for HSV by PCR is the diagnostic test of choice.

TREATMENT

The mainstay of treatment for corneal infections is the intensive use of topical anti-infective agents.[53] Corneal ulcers are medical emergencies. Although some children with keratitis can be managed successfully in an outpatient setting,[54] most require inpatient care. Mydriatic drops should be used to avoid pupillary synechiae and provide comfort; ciliary spasm contributes to photophobia.

Viruses

With the exception of herpetic eye disease, the treatment of viral infections, is symptomatic because infections are self-limited and no effective therapy is currently available. Epithelial HSV infections can be debrided or treated with topical antiviral drugs, either vidarabine ointment (Vira-A) or trifluorothymidine (Viroptic) drops or systemic acyclovir. Drops are administered while the patient is awake every 2 hours during the first week and every 6 hours during the second week, and then rapidly tapered since these drugs are toxic to the corneal epithelium.[14] Acyclovir systemically is equally effective in the treatment of herpetic keratitis and represents an alternative to topical therapy.[55,56] Topical ganciclovir also is available, but multicentered controlled trials comparing clinical equivalency have not yet been conducted. Children with recurrent episodes of herpetic keratitis may benefit from long-term prophylactic use of acyclovir to prevent recurrence, but resistance to acyclovir can develop over time.[57] Stromal HSV disease may require the addition of topical corticosteroid agents, but concomitant use with topical antiviral agents is necessary to prevent the reactivation of epithelial infection. Herpes zoster keratouveitis is unresponsive to available topical antiviral agents and is best managed with frequent application of corticosteroid topically and acyclovir (80 mg/kg per day) orally.

Bacteria

The mainstay of treatment for bacterial keratitis has been a combination of a cephalosporin (50 mg/mL) drops and a fortified aminoglycoside, either tobramycin (15 mg/mL) or gentamicin

PART II Clinical Syndromes and Cardinal Features of Infectious Diseases: Approach to Diagnosis and Initial Management

SECTION L Eye Infections

(14 mg/mL).[45] Cefazolin is selected for gram-positive coverage and ceftazidime when there is concern about *P. aeruginosa*. Toxicity, drug instability, and variability of concentration and pH of fortified antibiotics led to the use of topical fluoroquinolone antibiotics, including ciprofloxacin, ofloxacin, and norfloxacin. Several studies have shown ciprofloxacin to be an effective single agent in the treatment of bacterial keratitis.[58,59] Increasing resistance of gram-positive cocci, *Actinomyces*, and *Pseudomonas* species to ciprofloxacin prompted the concurrent use of a cephalosporin and treatment of bacterial keratitis with a newer generation of fluoroquinolones.[60-64] Levofloxacin penetrates ocular tissues effectively and has superior gram-positive coverage; however, increasing resistance to this agent is reported.[64,65] Moxifloxacin has lower minimum inhibitory concentrations for gram-positive organisms and gatifloxacin for gram-negative organisms. Both are active against methicillin-susceptible *Staphylococcus aureus* isolates.[66] The newer fluoroquinolones are reported to have better in vitro activities, increased ocular penetration, and potentially lower rates of development of resistance than other fluoroquinolones.[67] Severe cases of bacterial keratitis should be treated with a cephalosporin combined with a fluoroquinolone or aminoglycoside. Choices for methicillin-resistant *S. aureus* are limited to gentamicin and vancomycin.

Because of their rapid clearance, topical antibiotics should be administered frequently, beginning with 1 drop every minute for 5 minutes, followed by doses every 15 to 30 minutes until culture results are available.[68] Subsequent therapy is modified according to culture results and clinical course, but treatment usually is continued for 7 to 14 days. A favorable therapeutic response is indicated by diminished pain, healing of the epithelium, decrease in size and density of the corneal infiltrate, and decrease in corneal edema and inflammation in the anterior chamber.

Fungi

Fungal keratitis is treated with topical natamycin, flucytosine, amphotericin B, miconazole, or flucytosine.[29,30] Frequent (hourly) initial instillation is slowly reduced over several weeks. Adequate treatment requires 6 to 12 weeks owing to poor corneal penetration and the slow growth of fungi. Lack of a therapeutic response should prompt the addition of parenteral therapy or consideration of excisional keratoplasty.[69] Deep fungal keratitis requires parenteral therapy from the outset because of the risk of fungal endophthalmitis. Subconjunctival fluconazole can be helpful in severe fungal keratitis unresponsive to topical and systemic therapy.[70]

Acanthamoeba

Treatment of *Acanthamoeba* keratitis often is complicated by delayed diagnosis. Early and aggressive therapy with cationic disinfectants (polyhexamethylene biguanide or chlorhexidine) combined with propamidine isethiocyanate (Brolene) and neomycin can be curative.[71-76] Both cationic compounds result in rapid killing of the trophozoites and cysts at concentrations that are not toxic to corneal cells.[77] Clearance of *Acanthamoeba* trophozoites and cysts requires months of treatment.[78] Corneal transplantation is only recommended when the infection continues, and anti-infectives will be required long term to prevent recurrence in the graft.

COMPLICATIONS

Long-term complications usually are related to loss of corneal transparency and refractive changes. Central corneal scars (leukomas) that obstruct the visual axis can cause serious visual loss. Although the severity of scarring tends to diminish over time, even short periods of visual deprivation in children younger than 8 years of age can result in development of amblyopia. Although corneal transplants can restore vision,[78] corneal grafting in children may fail due to graft rejection. Performing an optical iridectomy can lead to improved visual function without the risk of corneal rejection. This is an excellent option in emerging nations, where rates of blindness from corneal infection are high and availability of transplantation is low.

Acknowledgments

The author acknowledges substantial use of material from previous editions by Avery Weiss.

85 Uveitis, Retinitis, and Chorioretinitis

Douglas R. Fredrick

Uveitis refers to any intraocular inflammation. Anterior uveitis is characterized by inflammation of the iris and ciliary body (iridocyclitis). Intermediate uveitis includes inflammation of the pars plana and vitreous (pars planitis, vitritis). Posterior uveitis features inflammation of the retina and choroid (retinitis, choroiditis). Uveitis is an uncommon disorder in childhood; among affected children, the anterior form is more common than the posterior form.

ANTERIOR UVEITIS

Table 85-1 summarizes the important pathogens and disorders responsible for anterior uveitis, with distinguishing features of each. At least one-half of children with an identifiable cause of anterior uveitis have juvenile idiopathic arthritis or human leukocyte antigen (HLA)-B27-related spondyloarthropathy.[1,2]

Clinical Manifestations

Patients with anterior uveitis come to attention because of ocular pain, photophobia, and blurred vision. The whole eye looks red, but closer inspection reveals that the predominant area of hyperemia is at the corneal limbus owing to the vascular engorgement of the underlying ciliary body. Slit-lamp examination allows visualization of: (1) cells floating in the anterior chamber or adherent to the corneal endothelium (keratic precipitates); and (2) turbidity of the normally optically clear aqueous humor resulting from the spillover of protein (flare). Distortion of the pupil is related to formation of inflammatory scars between the iris and lens surface (synechiae). Dystrophic calcification of the epithelial basement membrane (band keratopathy), iris nodules, lens opacities, and phthisis bulbi can occur.

TABLE 85-1. Common Causes of Anterior Uveitis

Organism or Condition	Duration	Associated Ocular Findings	Associated Systemic Findings
Varicella	Acute	Iris atrophy (rare)	Vesicular skin rash
Herpes simplex	Acute	Keratitis	None
Mumps	Acute	NS	Fever, headache, parotitis
Influenza	Acute	NS	Febrile respiratory illness
Infectious mononucleosis	Acute	NS	Fever, pharyngitis, lymphadenopathy
Measles	Acute	NS	Fever, coryza, Koplik spots
Kawasaki disease	Acute	NS	Fever, mucocutaneous findings, peripheral edema, unilateral lymphadenopathy
Herpes zoster	Chronic	Iris atrophy (common), KP	Fever, vesicular skin rash
Syphilis	Chronic	Iris nodules, chorioretinitis, optic neuritis	Maculopapular skin rash (palms and soles)
Tuberculosis	Chronic	Iris nodules, granulomatous KP, choroidal granulomas	Pulmonary lesions
Lyme disease	Chronic	Keratitis, optic neuritis	Erythema migrans, arthritis
Leprosy	Chronic	"Iris pearls" of iris atropy	Peripheral neuropathy, skin lesions

KP, keratitic precipitates that represent aggregates of inflammatory cells on the corneal endothelium; NS, nonspecific.

Etiologies

Viruses

Many viruses are associated with an acute nongranulomatous uveitis that is mild and self-limited.[3,4] Varicella-zoster virus (VZV) demonstrates the spectrum of disease involvement. Anterior uveitis resulting in mild inflammation occurs in up to 25% of patients with chickenpox.[5,6] It tends to be self-limited, resolving within 10 to 14 days. By contrast, uveitis associated with herpes zoster ophthalmicus is more severe and usually requires aggressive treatment with a topical corticosteroid, cycloplegic agents, and systemic acyclovir. Devastating visual complications can occur when there is concurrent involvement of structures of the posterior segment. Uveitis associated with herpes simplex virus (HSV) infection usually is a complication of a deep keratitis but can occur without antecedent keratitis.[7]

Mycobacterium tuberculosis. Chronic granulomatous uveitis, sometimes in association with iris nodules, once was caused commonly by *Mycobacterium tuberculosis*.[8] It is now uncommon, except in developing countries and in patients with acquired immunodeficiency syndrome (AIDS).

Treponema pallidum. The incidence of congenital syphilis parallels the incidence of syphilis among heterosexual persons in the United States. Congenital syphilis also remains a problem in developing countries. Chorioretinitis is a classic sign of early congenital syphilis, "salt-and-pepper" pigmentary changes of the peripheral retina being the most common finding.[9,10] Although

anterior uveitis is a common presentation, some patients predominantly have an intense posterior uveitis with necrotizing retinitis, retinal vasculitis, or optic neuritis.[11,12]

Borrelia burgdorferi. *Borrelia burgdorferi*, the organism responsible for Lyme borreliosis, can invade the cornea (keratitis) and uveal tract (iridocyclitis), and infection of the vitreous retina and choroid is documented with growing frequency.[13,14] Lyme uveitis can be a late manifestation of Lyme disease.[15,16]

Kawasaki disease. Anterior uveitis is common in Kawasaki disease. In one prospective study, anterior uveitis was found in 83% of 41 patients with Kawasaki disease in the first week of the disease.[17] Iridocyclitis and periorbital vasculitis also have been described. Conjunctival hyperemia is present in >90% of cases.

POSTERIOR UVEITIS (RETINITIS)

Table 85-2 summarizes the predominant ocular manifestations and associated findings for the infectious agents most commonly implicated in retinitis.

Etiologies

Bacteria and Fungi

Prior to the advent of effective antibacterial and antifungal therapies the prevalence of septic emboli and secondary retinitis from bloodstream infection (BSI) was high. The presence of Roth spots (white centered intraretinal hemorrhages, once believed to be pathognomonic for septic emboli) was a sign of endocarditis. In fact, white centered hemorrhages are nonspecific and can be seen with septic emboli, clotting abnormalities, trauma, vascular occlusive disease, and vasculitis.[18] The white center can be composed of a fibrin aggregate, or can be a mixture of inflammatory cells, bacteria, or fungal organisms. In patients with BSI from infective endocarditis or catheter-related infection, the presence of septic emboli can be used to monitor antibacterial therapy.

The incidence of positive retinal findings in patients with fungal BSI ranges from 7% to 20%, with a higher incidence in neutropenic patients receiving chemotherapy or following organ or bone marrow transplantation.[19-22] The incidence in children is lower than in adults.[23] In premature infants, fungal emboli to the crystalline tunica vasculosa lentis can cause inflammatory ocular disease that mimics retinopathy of prematurity, congenital cataracts, or conjunctivitis. Systemic treatment of *Candida* and other fungi with amphotericin, caspofungin, or voriconazole usually results in resolution of chorioretinal infection; the need for intravitreal injections and surgical vitrectomy has decreased in recent years.[24] For patients with BSI whose initial examination is negative but whose BSI persists, serial examinations must be performed to make certain that there are not new lesions.[25]

Toxoplasma gondii. Toxoplasmosis is the most common cause of posterior uveitis in immunocompetent individuals. Infection can be contracted prenatally or postnatally;[26-29] the proportion of

TABLE 85-2. Common Infectious Causes of Retinitis

Organism	Predominant Manifestation	Associated Findings
Toxoplasma gondii	Necrotizing retinitis	Vitritis, optic neuritis
Rubella virus	Pigmentary retinopathy	Cataract, microphthalmia
Cytomegalovirus	Hemorrhagic retinitis	Cottonwool spots
Herpes simplex virus	Necrotizing retinitis	Vitritis, vasculitis, optic neuritis
Varicella-zoster virus	Necrotizing retinitis	Occlusive vasculitis, vitritis
Toxocara canis	Retinal granuloma	Vitritis, endophthalmitis

PART II Clinical Syndromes and Cardinal Features of Infectious Diseases: Approach to Diagnosis and Initial Management

SECTION L Eye Infections

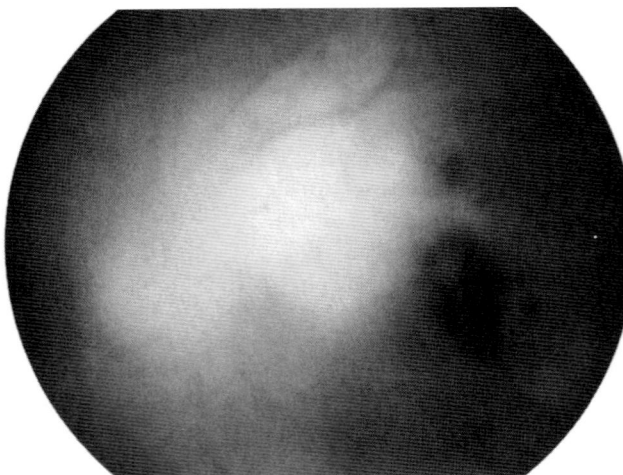

Figure 85-1. Fundus photograph shows active toxoplasmic lesion situated at the edge of a pigmented chorioretinal scar; the view is hazy because there are inflammatory cells in the overlying vitreous.

prenatal versus postnatally acquired infections varies geographically. Evidence of congenital infection may be identified at birth as active retinal lesions or inactive chorioretinal scars, or may not become clinically evident until months or years later.[30,31] Acquired infections can have an acute or delayed onset of ocular disease. Peak occurrence of acquired infection is between the second and fourth decades of life. Active lesions appear as fluffy, white areas of focal necrotizing retinitis attributable to proliferation of live parasites and reactive inflammatory cells in the overlying vitreous.[31] In some cases, the vitreal reaction is so severe that it obscures the underlying retina, giving the so-called "headlight-in-a-fog" appearance (Figure 85-1). Healing of these lesions leaves atrophic chorioretinal scars, which can be located in the macula or the peripheral retina (Figure 85-2). In addition to focal retinitis there are atypical presentations. Punctate outer retinal toxoplasmosis is characterized by the presence of grey-white lesions of the outer retina with little or no overlying vitritis.[32] Healed lesions appear as granular white opacities. Neuroretinitis features optic disk swelling with macular exudates and visual loss, and multifocal retinal infiltrates.[33] Optic neuritis can occur with infections of the nerve or surrounding retina.

Trapping of organisms within the terminal branches of the perifoveal capillaries probably explains the high incidence of macular involvement and visual loss. Additional causes of visual loss in toxoplasmosis are tractional distortion of the macula, optic atrophy, cataract, and retinal detachment. Recurrences usually appear at the edge of a quiescent scar, where dormant encysted organisms reactivate.[30,31]

Toxoplasmosis acquired postnatally often manifests with isolated ocular involvement.[29,34,35] Solid organ transplant recipients can have evidence of toxoplasmosis infection that is delayed in onset due to the protective effect of trimethoprim-sulfamethoxazole prophylaxis.[36] Although necrotizing retinochoroiditis is the major sequela, early manifestations can be limited to vitritis, anterior uveitis, or retinal vasculitis.[36] Patients with AIDS commonly have multiple active lesions or extensive retinitis.[37]

The clinical diagnosis of ocular toxoplasmosis is confirmed in 50% to 80% of cases by demonstration of *Toxoplasma*-specific immunoglobulin (Ig) G, IgM, and IgA in the serum.[38,39] Detection of specific IgG and IgA in serum or aqueous humor by immunoblotting is the most sensitive method, providing confirmatory evidence in 70% of cases.[39] Identification of *Toxoplasma*-specific gene sequences by polymerase chain reaction (PCR) testing of aqueous humor has reported specificities of 83% to 100% and sensitivities ranging from 28% to 53%.[40,41] Invasive procedures to obtain aqueous humor or ocular tissue may be indicated in severe cases.

Although active infections usually are treated with antiparasitic drugs, toxoplasmosis is a self-limited disease in immunocompetent individuals. Therefore the long-term benefits of treatment for acute and recurrent toxoplasmic chorioretinitis are uncertain. Current regimens include the following: (1) pyrimethamine plus sulfadiazine and folinic acid; (2) trimethoprim-sulfamethoxazole; and (3) adjunctive clindamycin for coverage against the encysted form.[42-47] In murine models the combination of atovaquone and sulfadiazine is effective.[48] Systemic corticosteroid therapy is indicated when there is visual loss due to inflammation involving the optic nerve or macula.[31] Local destruction of solitary lesions with photocoagulation, cryotherapy, or surgical vitrectomy to remove preretinal membranes or relieve retinal traction may be beneficial in selected cases.[31,49]

Rubella

The most common ocular manifestations of congenital rubella are retinitis, cataract, microphthalmos, and glaucoma.[50-52] Retinitis is characterized by pigmentary mottling of the retinal pigment epithelium (RPE) due to viral invasion, which gives the fundus a "salt-and-pepper" appearance (Figure 85-3). At birth, the fundi can be normal or can show pigmentary changes. Persistent infection of the RPE causes the pigmentary disturbances to develop or

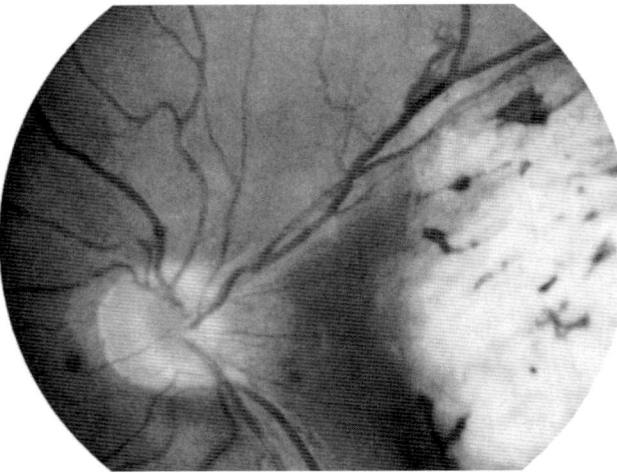

Figure 85-2. Fundus photograph shows portion of toxoplasmic chorioretinal scar centered on the macula with scattered clumping of retinal pigmentation.

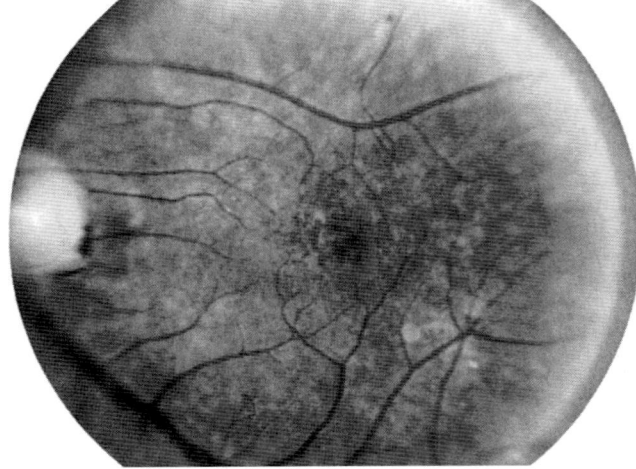

Figure 85-3. Fundus photograph shows "salt-and-pepper" retinopathy typical of congenital rubella.

to progress during the first few years of life, after which they tend to remain stable.[51,53] Visual function is normal in patients with involvement of RPE alone. Choroidal neovascularization, macular detachment, and visual loss rarely can be late complications of rubella retinopathy.[54,55] Despite newer technology, cataract surgery is frequently associated with poor visual outcomes owing to postoperative inflammatory complications, glaucoma, and cortical visual impairment.[51,52] Virus can be isolated from lens material for several years after intrauterine infection.[56]

Rubella can contribute to the development of Fuch heterochromic cyclitis, a chronic, unilateral uveitis with mild inflammation that leads to iris atrophy. Assay of aqueous humor revealed IgG rubella antibodies in all 52 patients in one study, and the presence of rubella-specific gene sequence in 18% of patients.[57]

Cytomegalovirus

Chorioretinitis is the major ocular sequela in infants congenitally infected with cytomegalovirus (CMV).[58–60] Postinfectious scars appear as geographic areas of chorioretinal atrophy with surrounding hyperpigmentation (Figure 85-4). Lesions vary in size from 0.5 to 5.0 mm (½ to 5 disk diameters) and are located in the macula or peripheral retina. Chorioretinal scars are present in 10% to 21% of symptomatic infants but are uncommon in asymptomatic infants. Typically, chorioretinitis in congenital CMV is inactive, but individual cases with late onset and reactivation of chorioretinitis are reported.[61] Visual loss is associated with macular scarring but can be due to optic atrophy or cortical visual impairment.

CMV retinitis also can be an acquired infection in immunosuppressed children, such as transplant recipients, those receiving chemotherapy for malignancy, and those with congenital or acquired immunodeficiencies, such as HIV/AIDS.[62–66] In the era of highly active antiretroviral therapy (HAART) for HIV, the incidence of CMV retinitis has decreased and the rates of visual loss, retinal detachment, and mortality have decreased.[67–70] The clinical characteristics of CMV retinitis are similar for patients with and without HIV infection.[71] Early retinitis appears as small white lesions that can be mistaken for cottonwool spots. The white lesions correspond histologically to areas of intracellular and extracellular edema and necrosis of the retina. These inflammatory changes frequently are associated with intraretinal hemorrhage and vasculitis of nearby retinal vessels, but the overlying vitreous is clear. As infection spreads, the size of the lesions increases along the course of the vessels, and new lesions develop (Figure 85-5). When lesions heal, the necrotic retina is replaced by glial scar tissue with associated pigmentary clumping.[72–74] Visual loss is

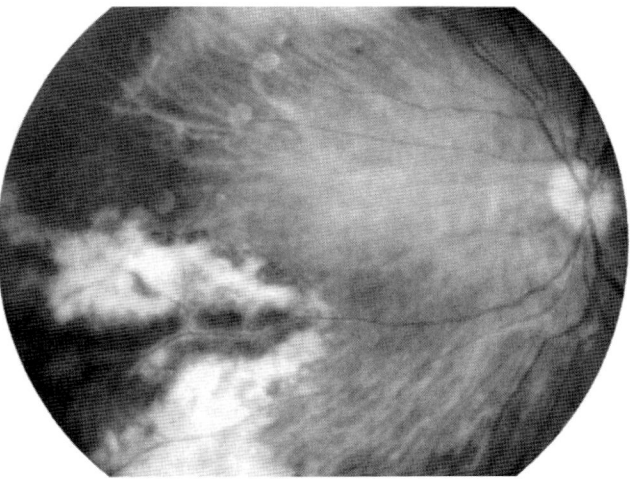

Figure 85-5. Fundus photograph shows localized area of cytomegalovirus retinitis in the peripheral retina; necrotizing lesion has spread along the course of a retinal vessel and is surrounded by hemorrhage.

correlated with the location of retinitis. Involvement in the region of the optic nerve and macula is associated with decreased visual acuity and a central visual field defect. Peripheral retinitis causes loss of peripheral visual field but acuity can be normal.

Both neonates and immunosuppressed children with CMV-induced chorioretinitis should be treated, because active CMV infection can progress relentlessly to blindness.[74–76] Ganciclovir, foscarnet, and cidofovir are parenteral therapies approved for initial induction and maintenance therapy of CMV retinitis.[77–87] Oral ganciclovir may be an alternative to intravenous medications for maintenance, with fewer side effects.[88] For patients with progressive retinitis or drug-related toxicity (neutropenia, renal disease), local therapy given as an intravitreal injection or surgically implanted "pellet" should be considered.[89] Local treatment is combined with a systemic antiviral agent to prevent systemic disease and to protect the second eye. Current drugs are virostatic and must be given long term to prevent progression or recurrence of disease. Maintenance anti-CMV therapy can be discontinued in patients with immune reconstitution.[90] Human monoclonal antibody directed against CMV appears to enhance the benefit of standard antiviral therapy.[91,92]

A subset of patients who become immunologically reconstituted with CD4+ T-lymphocyte counts >100 cells/mm^3 after initiation of HAART develop floaters due to vitritis, the incidence of which varies between centers. Complications include papillitis, macular abnormalities, and visual loss.[93,94]

Herpes Simplex Virus

Keratoconjunctivitis can be a manifestation of localized neonatal HSV infection, acquired during passage through the birth canal. HSV retinitis in neonates generally indicates disseminated or CNS disease.[95,96] The presence of skin lesions, chorioretinitis, and brain abnormalities at birth is suggestive of intrauterine infection.[97] The lesions consist of yellowish areas of necrotizing retinitis, which can be localized or diffuse. Marked vitritis, retinal vasculitis, and persistent fetal vasculature can occur; full-thickness necrosis can lead to optic atrophy and blindness.[98–100] Opsoclonus can be an early sign of encephalitis.[101] Acyclovir is the treatment of choice.

Congenital Varicella

During the first 20 weeks of pregnancy, approximately 2% of fetuses whose mothers have chickenpox develop an embryopathy.[102,103] Damage is mediated by direct neuropathic effects of the virus or by secondary vasculitis. Clinical features include skin

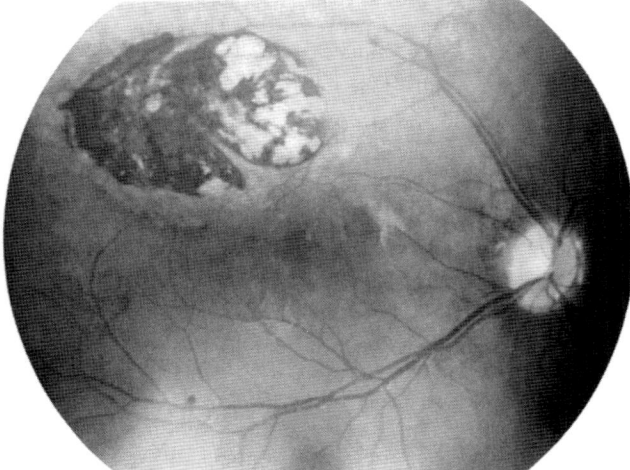

Figure 85-4. Fundus photograph shows geographic chorioretinal scar related to congenital cytomegalovirus infection.

PART II Clinical Syndromes and Cardinal Features of Infectious Diseases: Approach to Diagnosis and Initial Management

SECTION L Eye Infections

scarring (76%), eye defects in 51% (chorioretinitis, cataracts, and microphthalmia), skeletal anomalies (49%), and microcephaly and other neurologic deficits (60%).[104,105] Chorioretinitis associated with VZV is indistinguishable ophthalmoscopically from that due to other intrauterine infections. Reduced visual acuity is common because lesions frequently involve the macula.

Herpesvirus Retinochoroiditis and the Acute Retinal Necrosis Syndrome

Primary varicella or herpes zoster ophthalmicus can be associated with optic disk swelling, macular exudates, multifocal retinitis, and retinal vascular occlusion.[106-108] Acute retinal necrosis (ARN) is an uncommon disease that can occur in immunocompetent or immunocompromised individuals due to VZV, HSV type 1 (HSV-1) or type 2 (HSV-2), CMV or, rarely, Epstein–Barr virus.[109-114] HSV-2 is the most frequently identified cause of ARN in childhood,[115] and often is attributed to reactivation of congenital or neonatal HSV infection.[112,115,116] Characteristic features include multifocal necrotizing retinitis, occlusive arteritis, panuveitis, and rapidly deteriorating vision. Thinning and atrophy of the retina in necrotic areas combined with vitreous organization and traction predispose to retinal detachment. Inflammatory optic neuropathy and panuveitis with visual loss can precede the retinopathy.[117] Diagnosis is based on detection of virus-specific gene sequence in aqueous or vitreous samples using the PCR assay. Disease progression is so rapid that visual loss often is irreversible despite aggressive antiviral treatment. However, early treatment with antiviral therapy can prevent further visual loss and the development of ARN in the second eye.[118]

In patients with AIDS, and, less frequently, in immunocompetent individuals, the retinopathy can be atypical, featuring a rapidly progressive necrotizing retinitis and severe bilateral visual loss.[119-122] Although progressive outer retinal necrosis has been emphasized, there is histopathologic evidence of panretinal necrosis.

West Nile Virus

West Nile virus (WNV) is an important cause of arboviral infections of the central nervous system (CNS) in the U.S.[123] The combined presence of acute encephalitis with multifocal chorioretinitis and vitritis should prompt consideration of WNV or other arbovirus infections. Detection of IgM antibody to WNV in serum confirms the diagnosis.[124,125]

Toxocara canis

Systemic migration of the nematode *Toxocara canis* usually occurs in 1- to 4-year-old children and results in the clinical syndrome of visceral larval migrans.[126,127] Ocular involvement is not concurrent with the visceral larva migrans stage and usually is detected between 4 and 8 years of age. Ocular toxocariasis takes one of the three forms: (1) inflammatory granuloma of the posterior pole; (2) diffuse endophthalmitis; and (3) solitary granuloma of the peripheral retina.[128,129] Common clinical findings include decreased vision, white pupil (leukocoria), and strabismus. The diagnosis is confirmed by the enzyme immunosorbent assay test. The specificity of this assay is high but sensitivity is low, unless a specimen from the aqueous humor is tested.[130] Treatment with periocular or systemic corticosteroids is directed at the inflammatory response incited by the death of the worm.[131] Surgical removal of vitreal membranes and reattachment of the retina can improve vision in individual cases.[132]

Diffuse Unilateral Subacute Neuroretinitis

Diffuse unilateral subacute neuroretinitis is an infection of the eye caused by nematodes endemic to the southeastern and midwestern regions of the U.S. Although the organisms have not been isolated, migratory worms have been visualized directly in the subretinal space. One possible worm is *Ancylostoma caninum*, a dog hookworm, which is a common cause of cutaneous larval migrans. Initially, acute visual loss in one eye is noted. Examination of the fundus reveals grey-white lesions in the outer retina that fade over a few days and then reappear elsewhere. Invariably, cells are present in the vitreous, and the optic disk is swollen. Progressive involvement leads to further visual loss, diffuse pigmentary changes, and optic atrophy. Diminution of electroretinographic responses confirms retinal damage and probable visual loss.[133,134] *Baylisascaris procyonis*, a common intestinal raccoon roundworm, is another cause of neural larva migrans and ocular larva migrans. Although neurologic deterioration predominates the clinical syndrome, ophthalmologic findings include a diffuse unilateral neuroretinitis and choroidal infiltrates.[135,136] Treatment of active vitritis consists of either oral thiabendazole or ivermectin or direct photocoagulation of the worm.[137-139]

Histoplasma capsulatum

Histoplasmosis of the choroid is believed to be due to invasion by *Histoplasma capsulatum*. Supporting evidence is largely epidemiologic, because the organism has never been isolated from choroidal lesions.[140,141] Recent evidence for persistence of *H. capsulatum* DNA sequences in the lesions suggests that these products serve as immunogens and incite chronic inflammation.[142] Viable organisms have been isolated only from immunocompromised patients with endophthalmitis accompanying disseminated infection.[143,144]

This syndrome is characterized by the presence of multiple areas of atrophy in the peripheral retina, referred to as "histo spots." Curvilinear areas of clumped pigment and hypopigmentation surround the disk.[145] Focal scars do not contain viable organisms, but recurrent lymphocytic infiltration predisposes to the development of neovascular membranes and hemorrhagic macular detachment. Treatment options include laser photocoagulation, photodynamic therapy with verteporfin, and intravitreal instillation of corticosteroid, particularly when the macula is threatened.[146-148] Antifungal therapy has no role in treatment of this disease because there are no actively replicating organisms.

Focal and Multifocal Choroiditis

Infectious organisms that spread hematogenously are more likely to become trapped in the choroid than in other parts of the eye because of high choroidal blood flow and the large number of fenestrated capillaries. Choroidal infiltrates can be single or multiple (Figure 85-6). Tuberculosis can be associated with a focal

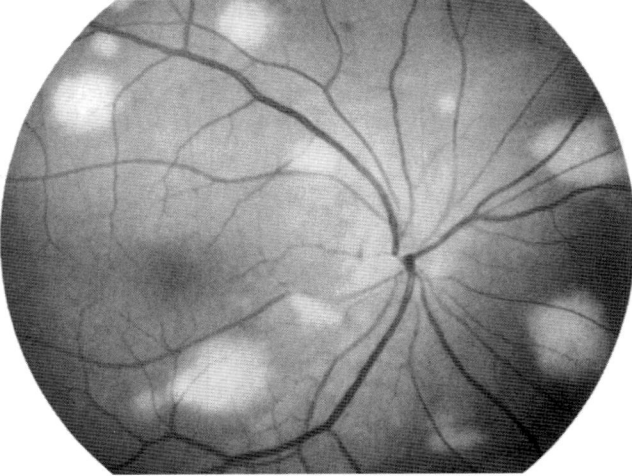

Figure 85-6. Fundus photograph shows multifocal choroidal infiltrates deep to the retina; there are no inflammatory cells in the overlying vitreous.

choroidal mass, multiple choroidal masses, diffuse or multifocal choroiditis, or retinal vasculitis.[149] Additional infections associated with choroiditis include coccidioidomycosis, cryptococcosis, and nocardiosis.

Multifocal choroiditis occurring in the context of AIDS deserves special mention because of its association with life-threatening systemic infections. Etiologic agents include *Pneumocystis jirovecii*,

Cryptococcus neoformans, *M. tuberculosis*, *Candida*, *Mycobacterium avium* complex, and *H. capsulatum*.[149–151]

Acknowledgments

The author acknowledges substantial use of material from previous editions by Avery Weiss.

86 Endophthalmitis

Douglas R. Fredrick

The term *endophthalmitis* is applied to bacterial or fungal infection involving intraocular tissues (retina, uveal tract, or lens) or fluids (vitreous or aqueous). Two broad categories of infectious endophthalmitis are distinguished. *Exogenous* infection results from introduction of organisms into the eye through a surgical or traumatic penetrating wound; *endogenous* (or metastatic) infection is caused by organisms that enter the eye via the bloodstream. Both categories of infection are extremely serious, threatening sight and even loss of the globe.[1–3] Whereas most cases of endophthalmitis in adults occur post surgically or by endogenous routes, most cases of endopthalmitis in children occur following penetrating ocular trauma.[4]

ETIOLOGIC AGENTS

A wide variety of microorganisms can cause endophthalmitis. Gram-positive cocci (both staphylococci and streptococci) are leading pathogens for both exogenous and endogenous endophthalmitis. In recent years gram-positive isolates have become increasingly resistant to antibiotics, including early-generation fluoroquinolones, but fortunately resistance to vancomycin and fourth-generation fluoroquinolones remains uncommon.[5,6] *Staphylococcus epidermidis* is the organism most often identified in the postoperative setting and is a frequent agent of posttraumatic endophthalmitis as well.[1,2] Often, *S. epidermidis* infection has a subacute onset 1 week to 1 month after surgery. Neonatal group B streptococcal septicemia can be associated with endogenous endophthalmitis.[3]

The gram-positive anaerobic bacillus *Propionibacterium acnes* is one of the most common causes of endophthalmitis after cataract surgery. Characteristically (although not invariably), *P. acnes* endophthalmitis develops one to several months postoperatively and follows a chronic smoldering course.[7] In contrast, *Bacillus cereus* is the most virulent organism inside the eye, capable of destroying the entire retina within hours of introduction by trauma or hematogenous seeding.[8]

Neisseria meningitidis was the most common cause of endogenous endophthalmitis before the advent of antibiotics and still must be recognized as having a predilection for intraocular localization.[3] Nontypable *Haemophilus influenzae* can cause endophthalmitis after accidental trauma and surgery.[9] Over the past decade, *Klebsiella pneumoniae* has emerged as the predominant cause of endogenous endophthalmitis in east Asia.[8,10,11] Numerous other gram-negative bacilli (notably *Pseudomonas aeruginosa* and *Escherichia coli*) have been associated with both exogenous and endogenous endophthalmitis, especially following trauma or surgery, and in people with underlying conditions.[1,3,12]

Candida albicans bloodstream infection (BSI) remains the most common fungal precursor of endogenous endophthalmitis, although this complication appears to be decreasing in frequency with earlier initiation of systemic treatment for candidemia and

invasive candidiasis.[1,13–15] Meta-analysis of neonatal *Candida* BSI showed 3% prevalence of endophthalmitis.[14] Non-*albicans Candida* spp. and a variety of other fungi (notably *Aspergillus* and *Fusarium*, *Alternaría*, and *Scedosporium* spp.) have been implicated in both endogenous and exogenous endophthalmitis, especially in posttraumatic cases or immunocompromised hosts.[16,17] Fungal endophthalmitis tends to follow a more indolent course than that of most bacterial infections.

EPIDEMIOLOGY AND HOST FACTORS

Postoperative endophthalmitis most often follows cataract extraction but can be associated with any form of intraocular procedure or extraocular operations, such as strabismus repair (in which organisms presumably are introduced into the globe by inadvertent needle perforation of the sclera).[18,19] The rate of endophthalmitis after pediatric intraocular surgery is similar to that found in adults – approximately 1 in 1000 cases.[20–22] Extracapsular cataract surgery with intraocular lens implantation (increasingly being performed in childhood) predisposes particularly to chronic endophthalmitis caused by *P. acnes*.[7] A recent trend in cataract surgery toward use of unsutured "self-sealing" incisions through temporal clear cornea (as opposed to the superior limbus) has been associated with a small but significant increase in the frequency of postoperative endophthalmitis.[23]

Filtering operations for glaucoma (which produce a fistulous connection for aqueous flow through the corneoscleral limbus between the anterior chamber and a conjunctival bleb) lower the physical resistance of the globe to invasion by microorganisms, creating a higher risk of intraocular infection that can persist for decades if the drainage tract remains patent. The frequency of late bleb-related endophthalmitis appears to have grown considerably in children as well as in adults because of increasing use of intraoperatively or postoperatively administered periocular antifibrotic agents (mitomycin C or 5-fluorouracil). These drugs improve the rate of successful lowering of intraocular pressure after filtering surgery but tend to result in blebs that are large and thin-walled and, thus, are particularly vulnerable to bacterial invasion.[9,24]

A recently recognized inflammatory condition that occurs following intraocular surgery, toxic anterior segment syndrome, can be confused with postoperative infectious endophthalmitis.[25] In this condition, toxins on surgical instruments that have been improperly sterilized lead to an inflammatory reaction within days after the anterior segment surgery. The diagnosis is made only after appropriate diagnostic aqueous and vitreous samples have been obtained for culture and sensitivity and intraocular empiric antibiotics have been administered, as the consequence of not treating an infectious process could be devastating.

Endophthalmitis is a major concern after any penetrating trauma to the globe, especially in childhood, when contamination

PART II Clinical Syndromes and Cardinal Features of Infectious Diseases: Approach to Diagnosis and Initial Management

SECTION L Eye Infections

of the causative instrument with soil, saliva, or fecal material is relatively common.[16,26,27] Occult penetration of the globe by a needle, thorn, or similarly shaped object can be unsuspected in a nonverbal child until days later when infection leads to obvious inflammatory signs. In a child with posttraumatic endophthalmitis, the possibility of an intraocular foreign body (which must be removed surgically) must be considered, and should be excluded, if necessary, with ultrasonographic or radiographic imaging.

Endogenous endophthalmitis usually occurs in a host already known to have BSI or who is immunocompromised, but occasionally, ocular involvement is the first indication of the underlying problem.[3] Endocarditis and meningitis are the most important localized infections associated with endophthalmitis. Diabetic patients have the propensity for retinal spread (often bilaterally) of *K. pneumoniae* from hepatic abscesses and of *E. coli* from an infected urinary tract.[11,12] Intravenous drug abusers have increased risk for intraocular fungal infection and also for devastating *B. cereus* endophthalmitis.[3,8]

Although otherwise healthy persons are occasionally affected, most cases of endogenous candidal endophthalmitis are nosocomial, occurring in association with indwelling intravascular catheters, use of broad-spectrum antibiotics, or immunosuppressive or major surgical treatment. Infants with intraocular candidiasis usually have a history of premature birth and pulmonary disease.[13]

PATHOPHYSIOLOGY

Microbial proliferation begins and remains concentrated in the aqueous or vitreous fluid in most cases of exogenous endophthalmitis. Damage to the retina and other intraocular structures occurs secondarily from exposure to toxins elaborated by the organisms and inflammatory cells.

By contrast, endogenous endophthalmitis typically originates in tissue within which a septic embolus has lodged.[3] When this process occurs in a small terminal branch of a vessel, ocular infection begins as either a microabscess in the iris or a focal lesion of retinitis or choroiditis. Diffuse involvement of the anterior ocular segment can develop rapidly after invasion of the iris, but posterior extension usually remains limited in such cases. Spillover of organisms and inflammatory cells from infected tissues of the posterior ocular segment leads to involvement of the vitreous, which subsequently can remain localized or become diffuse, extending ultimately to the anterior segment, sclera, and orbit (panophthalmitis). With initial occlusion of the central retinal artery by a relatively large embolus, initial ischemia followed by massive dissemination of organisms directly into the retina can lead to irreversible blindness within a short time.

CLINICAL MANIFESTATIONS

The first external sign of endophthalmitis usually is injection of conjunctival vessels, which can be striking and is associated with marked conjunctival and eyelid edema or can be so mild that it scarcely attracts attention, particularly in postoperative or posttraumatic settings in which some degree of inflammation is expected. Endophthalmitis must therefore be included in the differential diagnosis of every "red eye." Careful inspection of the anterior segment with a hand light usually permits identification of a whitish *hypopyon*, which results from layering of abundant leukocytes from aqueous fluid on to the surface of the iris or in the most dependent portion of the anterior chamber (Figure 86-1). Sometimes, however, the only readily identifiable sign in the anterior segment is blue-grey haziness or loss of clarity in visualization of the iris and the pupil (which typically shows absence of or diminished reactivity to light as well). Vision usually is reduced.

Low-grade endophthalmitis localized to the posterior segment (including most cases of intraocular candidiasis) may produce no external signs. Typically there is decreased clarity of ophthalmoscopic visualization and dimming of the fundus red reflex (resulting from vitritis), and visual acuity is reduced significantly. In some cases, however, the problem only becomes evident when

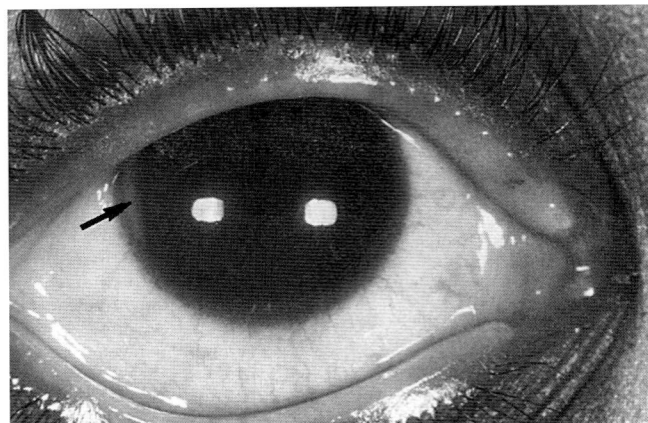

Figure 86-1. Right eye of a 15-year-old girl with acute meningococcal meningitis and bilateral endophthalmitis. Note the small hypopyon (arrow), layered temporally in the anterior chamber because she had been lying on her right side.

detailed examination of the fundus through a dilated pupil reveals the presence of one or more small whitish chorioretinal or vitreal infiltrates with indistinct borders.

DIAGNOSTIC EVALUATION

Suspicion of endophthalmitis mandates consultation with an ophthalmologist, who can confirm the diagnosis, quantify the vision loss, and determine the extent of posterior-segment involvement (employing B-scan ultrasonography if the fundus cannot be visualized).

In the context of well-defined systemic infection with an identifiable organism, generally it is not necessary to perform additional microbiologic studies when making the diagnosis of endophthalmitis.[2] Otherwise, aspiration of ocular fluid for culture is required. If the patient is cooperative or immobilized easily, aqueous fluid (about 0.1 mL) can be obtained at the bedside with the use of a 27- or 30-gauge needle on a 1 mL syringe. Aspiration of the vitreous is a surgical procedure best performed in the operating room for pediatric patients (Figure 86-2), despite increasing performance in the outpatient setting in adults. Vitreous culture has a substantially higher yield than aqueous culture in exogenous and posteriorly localized endogenous infection.[3,28,29] When fungal infection is suspected, polymerase chain reaction

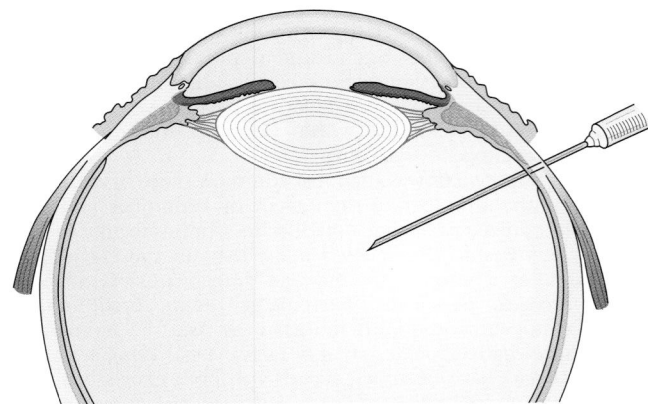

Figure 86-2. Diagrammatic illustration of needle passing through the pars plana of the ciliary body for diagnostic aspiration of vitreous or intravitreal injection of antibiotic. (Adapted from Bohigian GM. Endophthalmitis. In: Krupin T, Kolker AE, Rosenberg LF (eds) Complications in Ophthalmic Surgery, 2nd ed. St. Louis, Mosby, 1999, pp 19–36.)

testing of vitreous aspirate can provide rapid confirmation of the diagnosis.[30,31]

In one-quarter to one-half of cases of presumed infectious endophthalmitis, eye fluid cultures are sterile. For maximum yield, aspirates should be inoculated promptly into appropriate media, including media used for isolation of anaerobic and fungal organisms. Inoculation of fluid specimens into blood culture bottles also has been used successfully.[1]

With endophthalmitis of unknown origin, multiple blood cultures should be performed, followed by an exhaustive search for remote infections (particularly meningitis, endocarditis, hepatic abscess, and urinary tract infection) and predisposing conditions (occult ocular trauma, diabetes, acquired immunodeficiency syndrome, and other immunodeficiency syndromes).

MANAGEMENT

Antimicrobial agents for endophthalmitis can be delivered by a variety of routes. Intravenous antibiotic administration is the mainstay of treatment for endogenous bacterial infection.[3,10] The choice of drugs should be based on known or presumed sensitivities of the documented or suspected pathogens, with dosage and duration at levels appropriate for meningitis (or greater if required for associated infection at another site). Endogenous fungal endophthalmitis usually responds well to treatment with intravenous amphotericin B; however, newer agents such as voriconazole (which can yield therapeutic intraocular concentration after oral as well as intravenous administration) are increasingly viewed as appropriate and possibly preferable alternative therapies.[32,33] If fungal chorioretinitis extends into the vitreous cavity, intravitreal injection with either amphotericin B (5–10 µg) or voriconazole (100 µg) is necessary, and vitrectomy may be required to remove fungal burden and inflammatory cells to minimize risk of retinal damage.

In the past, many cases of exogenous endophthalmitis were cured with combined intravenous, subconjunctival, and topical antibiotics, but intravitreal administration is now regarded as the most important route of drug delivery for this condition (see Figure 86-2).[1,18,19] Initially, only a single injection is given (immediately after aspiration of vitreous for culture), followed by one or more additional injections if response to the first is incomplete. Gentamicin and cefazolin were formerly the intraocular antibiotics most often used, but growing concerns about aminoglycoside retinal toxicity and drug-resistant organisms (mainly among *Staphylococcus epidermidis* and streptococci) have led to a shift toward other agents, particularly ceftazidime and vancomycin (Table 86-1).[34]

Controversy persists regarding the need for concurrent use of multiple routes of therapy.[35] Outcomes reported after combined intravitreal and systemic administration of antibiotics are similar to those seen with intravenous treatment alone in endogenous infections and with intravitreal treatment alone in most exogenous infections.[3,10,36,37] Many experienced clinicians continue to employ both modalities routinely. Fourth-generation fluoroquinolones such as moxifloxacin can achieve therapeutic intraocular levels after oral administration (initial loading dose in an adult of 400 mg twice daily, followed by 400 mg once daily for 1 to 2 weeks) and have a favorable spectrum of coverage, making them an attractive and increasingly used adjunct to intravitreal injection.[38] Moxifloxacin has become the antibiotic of choice for oral administration due to its high intraocular penetration, but caution should be exercised when used in children because of its association with potential tendon rupture. Minimum inhibitory concentrations for methicillin-resistant *S. aureus* are at least 10-fold those for methicillin-susceptible *S. aureus* (MIC_{90} 2 to 16 µg/mL). Subconjunctival antibiotics (given as once- or twice-daily injections) also sometimes are used, although data to indicate incremental benefit are lacking. Cephalosporins often are used for treatment following discharge from the hospital, but intraocular and intravenous therapy will always be required at the time of initial diagnosis. Many clinicians also include corticosteroid agents (intraocular, subconjunctival, topical, systemic, or a combination)

TABLE 86-1. Intravitreal Injection for Endophthalmitis

Drug	Dose[a] (mg)	Comment
Vancomycin	1	Unless gram-positive bacteria can be excluded
Amikacin	0.4	Now seldom used because of potential retinal toxicity
Ceftazidime	2.25	Preferred agent for gram-negative coverage
Amphotericin B	0.005	If fungus suspected
Voriconazole	0.05	Increasingly used alternative to amphotericin
Dexamethasone	0.4	Recommended for anti-inflammatory effect by some authorities

[a]Each drug should be diluted to provide the indicated dose in a volume of 0.1 mL and should be injected using a separate 1 mL syringe.

Recommendations from references 1 and 18, and Hariprasad SM, Mieler WF, Flynn HW, et al. Advances in Endophthalmitis Management. Instruction course syllabus, American Academy of Ophthalmology Annual Meeting, Las Vegas, Nevada 2006.

in the regimen in an attempt to reduce ocular damage from the inflammatory process; no adverse effect on control of infection from this practice has been documented when appropriate antimicrobial therapy is given.[1,2,18]

The role of vitrectomy in the management of exogenous endophthalmitis was clarified by the results of a major multicenter, randomized clinical trial. The investigators compared outcomes from treatment of postoperative endophthalmitis after cataract surgery using intravitreal antibiotics (amikacin and vancomycin) with and without immediate surgical removal of most of the infected vitreous. Vitrectomy provided significant benefit only when initial visual acuity was severely reduced to the level of light perception only. With better initial vision, outcomes were the same with and without vitrectomy.[37] Vitrectomy with removal of infected lens material appears to be required for cure of most cases of chronic endophthalmitis caused by *P. acnes*.[7] Most authorities continue to view vitrectomy as warranted for endophthalmitis associated with penetrating trauma and glaucoma filtering blebs.[2,18]

Occasionally, even after intensive treatment, an eye is left blind and intractably inflamed by endophthalmitis. In such cases, it may be necessary to remove the entire ocular contents surgically (evisceration) or to remove the complete globe (enucleation).

OUTCOME

With current optimal therapy, the prognosis for infectious endophthalmitis is good. Recovery is the rule in: (1) postoperative endophthalmitis due to *S. epidermidis* and *P. acnes*; (2) endogenous *Candida* endophthalmitis; and (3) endogenous bacterial endophthalmitis that shows either primarily anterior-segment or only focal posterior-segment involvement at the time of diagnosis, regardless of organism.[1,3,39] Mild to moderate permanent visual loss is common even in these favorable cases, however.

In situations other than those mentioned, endophthalmitis remains a grave disorder. Cases of bacterial infection due to trauma or to a hematogenous spread from other sites of infection that show diffuse posterior-segment involvement have a particularly poor prognosis, typically leaving the patient with a nonseeing eye or no eye at all.[3,8,16]

Overall, with current therapeutic methods, useful vision (finger-counting or better) is retained in about 60% of eyes treated for acute or subacute exogenous bacterial endophthalmitis and in 40% of eyes treated for endogenous bacterial endophthalmitis. These figures have changed little over several decades.[3,25,40]

PART II Clinical Syndromes and Cardinal Features of Infectious Diseases: Approach to Diagnosis and Initial Management

SECTION L Eye Infections

PREVENTION

Preoperative application of a drop of 5% povidone-iodine (half-strength dilution of the common commercially available solution) to the ocular surface has been shown to reduce the conjunctival bacterial population significantly and appears to lower the incidence of postoperative endophthalmitis.[21,41] It also remains common practice among ophthalmologists to administer a single subconjunctival injection of antibiotic (usually an aminoglycoside or a cephalosporin) at the conclusion of intraocular surgery and to prescribe application of a topical solution several times a day for a week or longer. Use of moxifloxacin topically before as well as after surgery has been increasing. A minority of surgeons add antibiotic to the infusion fluid that circulates through the eye during cataract or vitrectomy surgery. Recent studies support the injection of antibiotic into the anterior chamber at the conclusion of surgery, but this approach has not been widely adopted in North America.[42]

More intensive prophylaxis against endophthalmitis is employed by most ophthalmologists after penetrating trauma. Intravenously administered vancomycin plus ceftazidime has largely replaced the traditional use of a first-generation cephalosporin, with or without an aminoglycoside.[2] Oral administration of a fluoroquinolone (moxifloxacin, currently the preferred agent) can achieve therapeutic drug levels in the vitreous and reasonably good coverage for common infecting organisms.[43]

Some authorities recommend intravitreal injection as a preventive measure in cases of traumatic endophthalmitis that are likely to involve heavy contamination.[2,22,26] Culture of foreign material removed from the eye, aqueous or vitreous, exposed uveal tissue, or the conjunctiva (in roughly descending order of usefulness) at the time of surgical wound repair can provide information of value in optimizing treatment if endophthalmitis develops later.

Because of the risk of endophthalmitis, conjunctivitis that develops in an eye with a glaucoma filtering bleb should be treated promptly and aggressively with topical and, possibly, systemic antibiotics.[9]

Ophthalmologic evaluation to rule out ocular involvement in patients with *Candida albicans* fungemia or deep tissue infection appears to be justified, given the paucity of external signs when it develops in such cases, but the yield is likely to be low if systemic treatment has been started.[15] Ophthalmologic screening has a very low yield in patients who have fever of unknown origin or in whom *Candida* is isolated only from a superficial site or a catheter, and so is no longer generally recommended.

Acknowledgment

The author acknowledges substantial use in this chapter of work of M.J. Greenwald from previous editions.

87 Periorbital and Orbital Infections

Ellen R. Wald

The practitioner frequently has the opportunity to manage the child for whom the chief complaint is a "swollen eye" (Figure 87-1). Some children have trivial or self-limited disorders, but others can have sight- or life-threatening problems.

DIFFERENTIAL DIAGNOSIS

The noninfectious causes of swelling of or around the eye include: (1) blunt trauma (leading to the proverbial "black" eye); (2) tumor; (3) local edema; and (4) allergy. In cases of blunt trauma, history provides the key to the diagnosis. Eyelid swelling continues to increase for 48 hours and then resolves over several days. Tumors that characteristically involve the eye include hemangioma of the lid, ocular tumors such as retinoblastoma and choroidal melanoma, and orbital neoplasms such as neuroblastoma and rhabdomyosarcoma.[1] Other tumors reported to cause orbital involvement are Langerhans cell histiocytosis and granulocytic sarcoma.[2,3] Tumors usually cause gradual onset of proptosis in the absence of inflammation. Orbital pseudotumor, an autoimmune inflammation of the orbital tissues, manifests as eyelid swelling, red eye, pain, and decreased ocular motility.[4] Hypoproteinemia and congestive heart failure cause eyelid swelling due to local edema; characteristic findings are bilateral, boggy, nontender, nondiscolored soft-tissue swelling. Allergic inflammation includes angioneurotic edema or contact hypersensitivity.[5] Superficially, allergic inflammation can resemble acute infection; however, the presence of pruritus and the absence of tenderness are helpful distinguishing characteristics.

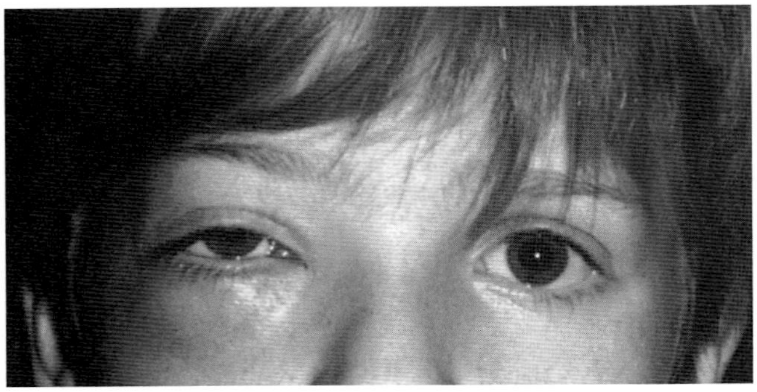

PATHOGENESIS

The anatomy of the eye is important for an understanding of its susceptibility to spread of infection from contiguous structures. Veins that drain the orbit, the ethmoid and maxillary sinuses, and the skin of the eye and periorbital tissues (Figure 87-2) constitute an anastomosing and valveless network.[1] This venous system provides opportunities for spread of infection from one anatomic site to another and predisposes to involvement of the cavernous sinus.

Figure 87-3 demonstrates the relationship between the eye and the paranasal sinuses. The roof of the orbit is the floor of the frontal sinus, and the floor of the orbit is the roof of the maxillary sinus. The medial wall of the orbit is formed by the frontal maxillary process, the lacrimal bone, the lamina papyracea of the ethmoid bone, and a small part of the sphenoid bone.[6] Infection originating in the mucosa of the paranasal sinuses can spread to involve the bone (osteitis with or without subperiosteal abscess) and the intraorbital contents. Orbital infection can occur through

Figure 87-1. A 10-year-old boy with the complaint of swollen eye.

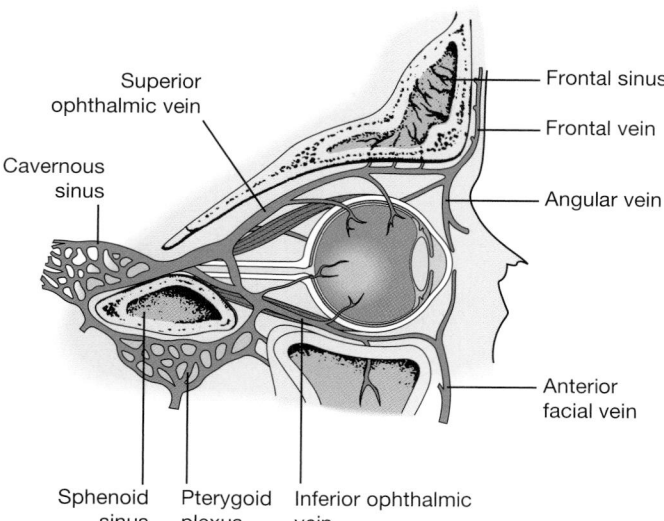

Figure 87-2. The valveless venous system of the orbit and its many anastomoses.

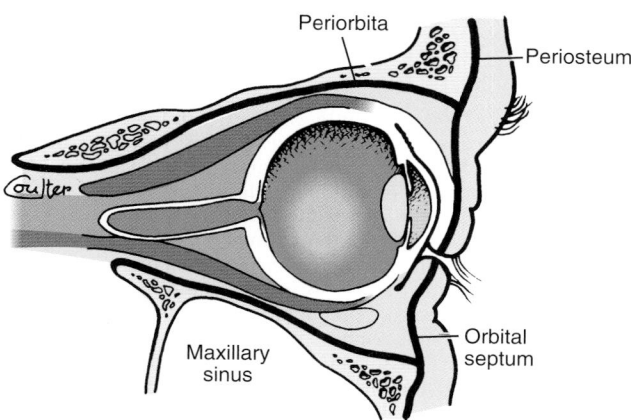

Figure 87-4. The orbital septum is a connective tissue extension of the periosteum that is reflected into the upper and lower lid. (Redrawn from Shapiro ED, Wald ER, Brozanski BA. Periorbital cellulitis and paranasal sinusitis: a reappraisal. Pediatr Infect Dis J 1982;1:91–94.)

natural bony dehiscences in the lamina papyracea of the ethmoid or frontal bones or via foramina through which the ethmoidal arteries pass.[5]

Figure 87-4 shows the position of the orbital septum, a connective tissue extension of the periosteum (or periorbita) that is reflected into the upper and lower eyelids. Infection of tissues anterior to the orbital septum are described as *periorbital* or *preseptal*.[7] The septum provides a nearly impervious barrier to spread of infection to the orbit. Although preseptal cellulitis or periorbital cellulitis (the terms may be used interchangeably), often is considered a "diagnosis," either term is an inadequate diagnostic label unless accompanied by a modifier that indicates likely pathogenesis.

Infectious causes of preseptal cellulitis occur in the following three settings: (1) secondary to a localized infection or inflammation of the conjunctiva, eyelids, or adjacent structures (e.g.,

conjunctivitis, hordeolum, acute chalazion, dacryocystitis, dacryoadenitis, impetigo, traumatic bacterial cellulitis); (2) secondary to hematogenous dissemination of nasopharyngeal pathogens to the periorbital tissue; and (3) as a manifestation of inflammatory edema in patients with acute sinusitis (Box 87-1).[7]

Infections behind the septum that cause eye swelling include subperiosteal abscess, orbital abscess, orbital cellulitis, cavernous sinus thrombosis, panophthalmitis, and endophthalmitis. Although all of these entities can be labeled "orbital cellulitis," a systematic approach allows a more specific diagnosis, thereby directing management. Infections intrinsic to the eye (i.e., conjunctivitis, keratitis, endophthalmitis, and panophthalmitis) are discussed in Chapters 82 through 86.

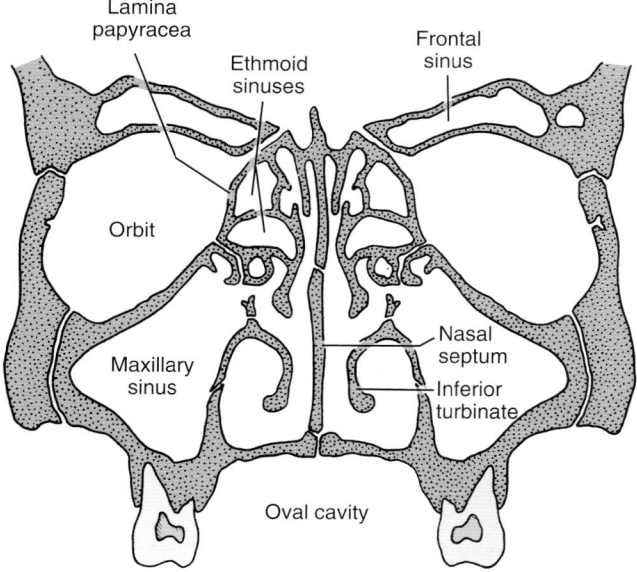

Figure 87-3. The relationship between the eye and the paranasal sinuses is shown schematically. The roof of the orbit, the medial wall, and the floor are shared by the frontal, ethmoid, and maxillary sinuses, respectively. (Redrawn from Shapiro ED, Wald ER, Brozanski BA. Periorbital cellulitis and paranasal sinusitis: a reappraisal. Pediatr Infect Dis J 1982;1:91–94.)

BOX 87-1. Infectious Causes of Preseptal and Orbital Cellulitis

PRESEPTAL CELLULITIS

Localized infection of the eyelid or adjacent structure

Conjunctivitis
Hordeolum
Dacryoadenitis
Dacryocystitis
Bacterial cellulitis (trauma)

Hematogenous dissemination

Bacteremic periorbital cellulitis

Acute sinusitis

Inflammatory edema

ORBITAL CELLULITIS

Acute sinusitis

Subperiosteal abscess
Orbital abscess
Orbital cellulitis
Cavernous sinus thrombosis

Hematogenous dissemination

Endophthalmitis

Traumatic inoculation

Endophthalmitis

PART II Clinical Syndromes and Cardinal Features of Infectious Diseases: Approach to Diagnosis and Initial Management

SECTION L Eye Infections

PRESEPTAL INFECTIONS

Conjunctivitis

Conjunctivitis is the most common disorder of the eye for which children are brought for medical care. In most cases, the lids are crusted and thickened with hyperemic conjunctiva. The usual causes of conjunctivitis in children older than neonates but less than 6 years old are *Haemophilus influenzae* (nontypable) and *Streptococcus pneumoniae*.[8,9] In approximately 20% to 25% of children with conjunctivitis due to *H. influenzae*, acute otitis media is a complicating feature. In this case, systemic antibiotics are preferable to topical ophthalmic preparations. Adenovirus is the most common cause of viral conjunctivitis in children older than 6 years and frequently is associated with pharyngitis.[10] Occasionally young children with adenovirus infection have diffuse swelling of the lids that can be mistaken for a more serious problem.[11] Other viral causes of hemorrhagic conjunctivitis are enterovirus 70 and Coxsackie A24 (see Chapter 82, Conjunctivitis in the Neonatal Period (Ophthalmia Neonatorum)).

Hordeolum and Chalazion

An *external hordeolum*, or stye, is a bacterial infection of the glands of Zeis or Moll (sebaceous gland or sweat gland, respectively) associated with a hair follicle on the eyelid. In most cases, infection is localized and points to the lid margin as a pustule or inflammatory papule. The lid can be slightly swollen and erythematous around the area of involvement. An external hordeolum usually lasts a few days to a week and resolves spontaneously.

An *internal hordeolum* is a bacterial infection of a meibomian gland, a long sebaceous gland whose orifice is at the lid margin.[12] The infection usually causes inflammation and edema of the neck of the gland, which can result in obstruction. If there is no obstruction, infection points to the lid margin. If obstruction is present, infection points to the conjunctival surface of the eye.[12] Sometimes the swelling caused by an acute internal hordeolum is diffuse rather than localized, and a pustule is not obvious on the lid margin. To clarify the cause, it is necessary to evert the eyelid and examine the tarsal conjunctiva. A tiny, delicate pustule is diagnostic of an internal hordeolum.

The usual cause of acute internal or external hordeola is *Staphylococcus aureus*. An antibiotic ophthalmic ointment containing bacitracin can be applied to the site of infection. The main purpose of the topical therapy is to prevent spread of infection to adjacent hair follicles. Warm compresses may facilitate spontaneous drainage.

In contrast to the internal hordeolum, a *chalazion* manifests as a persistent (more than 2 weeks in duration), nontender, localized bulge or nodule (3 to 10 mm) in the lid; the overlying skin is completely normal. It is a sterile lipogranulomatous reaction. When a chalazion is large and causes local irritation, incision may be required.

Dacryoadenitis

Dacryoadenitis is an infection of the lacrimal gland. Sudden onset of soft-tissue swelling that is maximal over the outer portion of the upper lid margin is typical. Occasionally, the eyeball is erythematous and the eyelid swollen, and the patient can have remarkable constitutional symptoms. The location of the swelling is a distinguishing characteristic (Figure 87-5). When dacryoadenitis is caused by viral infection (mumps virus, Epstein–Barr virus,[13] cytomegalovirus, coxsackievirus, echoviruses, and varicella-zoster virus), the area is only modestly tender.[14] By contrast, when the infection is caused by bacterial agents, discomfort is prominent. In addition to *S. aureus*, which is the most common cause of bacterial dacryoadenitis, etiologic agents include streptococci, *Chlamydia trachomatis*, *Brucella melitensis*, and, occasionally, *Neisseria gonorrhoeae*.[15,16] Fungal and rare parasitic infections of the lacrimal gland have been reported, including those with *Cysticercus*

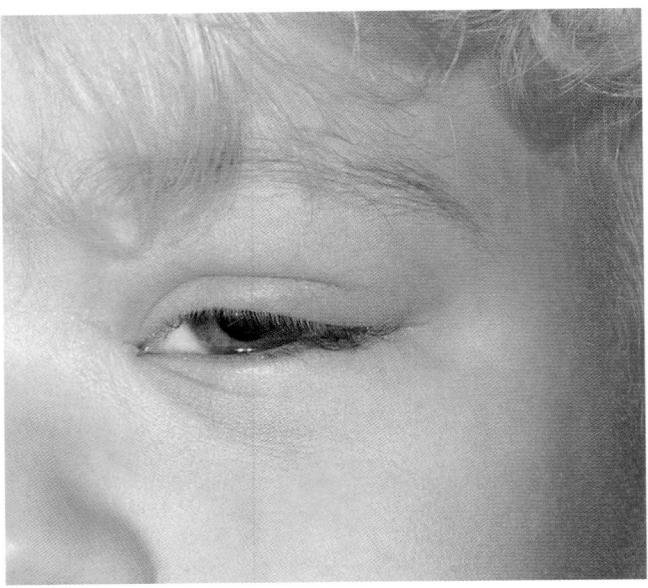

Figure 87-5. A patient with dacryoadenitis during a viral illness. The nontender swelling over the lateral portion of the left upper lid resolved without antibiotic treatment. (Courtesy of J.H. Brien©.)

cellulosae and *Schistosoma haematobium*.[14] If parenteral therapy is required for suspected bacterial dacryoadenitis due to *S. aureus*, nafcillin, at 150 mg/kg per day divided into doses every 6 hours, is appropriate. If methicillin-resistant *S. aureus* (MRSA) is suspected, vancomycin (60 mg/kg divided into doses every 6 hours) should be initiated. Oral treatment of acute dacryoadenitis is undertaken with a semisynthetic penicillin such as dicloxacillin (100 mg/kg per day divided into doses every 6 hours), cephalexin or cefadroxil (100 or 50 mg/kg per day, respectively, divided into doses every 6 or 12 hours, respectively), sulfamethoxazole-trimethoprim (based on 40 mg/kg per day of trimethoprim divided into doses every 12 hours), or clindamycin (40 mg/kg per day divided into doses every 6 hours). Treatment is continued until all signs and symptoms have disappeared.

The differential diagnosis of swelling of the upper outer aspect of the eyelid includes inflammatory noninfectious problems such as Sjögren syndrome and sarcoidosis as well as benign and malignant tumors.[14]

Dacryocystitis

Dacryocystitis is a bacterial infection of the lacrimal sac. Although uncommon, dacryocystitis can occur at any age as a bacterial complication of a viral upper respiratory tract infection (URI). Because of the course traversed by the lacrimal duct, which drains to the inferior meatus within the nose, it is surprising that the duct and sac are not infected more often. Delayed opening of the duct, inspissated secretions, and anatomic abnormalities lead to disproportionate representation of infants younger than 3 months among children with dacryocystitis.

Patients with dacryocystitis usually have had a viral URI for several days. They then experience fever and impressive erythema and swelling in addition to exquisite tenderness, which is most prominent in the triangular area just below the medial canthus[17] (Figure 87-6). Pressure over the lacrimal sac causes considerable discomfort but can result in expression of purulent material from the lacrimal puncta. Common causative organisms are gram-positive cocci. *Streptococcus pneumoniae* is most common in neonates, although *S. aureus*, *H. influenzae*, and *Streptococcus agalactiae* also have been reported.[15,18] *S. aureus* and *S. epidermidis* are most commonly implicated in acquired dacryocystitis in the older patient.[19] It is important to obtain material from the punctum because other organisms (including enteric gram-negative bacilli,

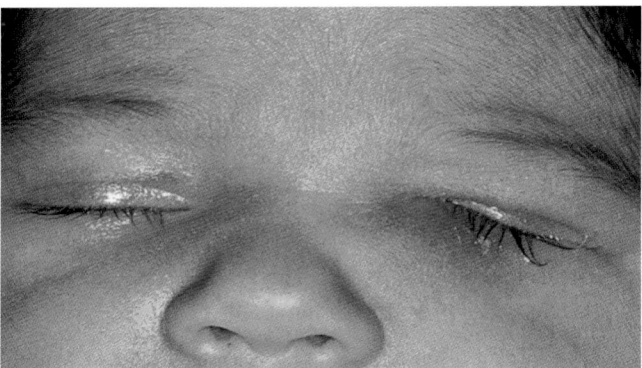

Figure 87-6. Dacrocystitis in an infant. The area at or beneath the medial canthus is erythematous, indurated, and exquisitely tender. (Courtesy of J.H. Brien©.)

anaerobic bacteria, and yeast) occasionally have been observed. Unusual pathogens, such as *Pasteurella multocida* and *Aeromonas hydrophilia,* have been reported rarely.[20]

Most patients with dacryocystitis require admission to hospital. Often they appear ill or toxic. Because of the potential for any case of bacterial facial cellulitis to result in cavernous sinus thrombosis, therapy with parenteral antibiotics is indicated until the infection begins to subside. Nafcillin (at a dose of 150 mg/kg per day divided into doses every 6 hours) or cefazolin (at a dose of 100 mg/kg per day divided into doses every 8 hours) is appropriate. In penicillin-allergic patients, or when MRSA is suspected, vancomycin or clindamycin (40 mg/kg per day divided into doses every 6 hours) suffices. After substantial improvement is observed in local findings, an oral agent can be substituted to complete a 10- to 14-day course of therapy.

The role of nonmedical management of dacryocystitis is controversial. Although surgical manipulation of the lacrimal duct is not necessary for most patients, both probing of the duct and incision and drainage have been reported to be successful in neonates.[18] Incision and drainage and direct application of antibiotics inside the sac have been promoted by some practitioners who care for older children and adults.[21]

Preseptal Cellulitis After Trauma

Occasionally, preseptal cellulitis results from secondary bacterial infection of sites of local skin trauma (including insect bites) or with spread of infection from a focus of impetigo. The traumatic injury can be extremely modest or completely inapparent. Loosely bound periorbital soft tissues permit impressive swelling to accompany minor infection. The overlying skin can be bright red with subtle textural changes, or intense swelling can lead to a shiny appearance (Figure 87-7). Some patients have fever, but many are afebrile despite dramatic local findings. The peripheral white blood cell count is variable. In these cases, cellulitis, similar to that on any other cutaneous area, is caused by *S. aureus* (including MRSA) or group A streptococcus.[22,23]

Several less common causes of lid cellulitis have been reported. Periocular cellulitis and abscess formation have resulted from infection with *Pasteurella multocida* in a healthy child who sustained a cat bite and cat scratch to the eyelid.[24] Ringworm (caused by *Trichophyton* species) also has been recognized as a cause of lid infection (leading to preseptal cellulitis) characterized by redness, swelling, ulceration, and vesicle formation.[25,26] A case of palpebral myiasis was reported in which larvae were extracted from a small draining fistula at the site of an erythematous and edematous lid.[27] Several cases of cellulitis of the eyelid due to *Bacillus anthracis* have been reported from Turkey.[28] The diagnosis was suspected when the erythematous and swollen lid developed an eschar. Scrapings showed the presence of gram-positive bacilli which were confirmed by culture. A primary case of lymphocutaneous *Nocardia*

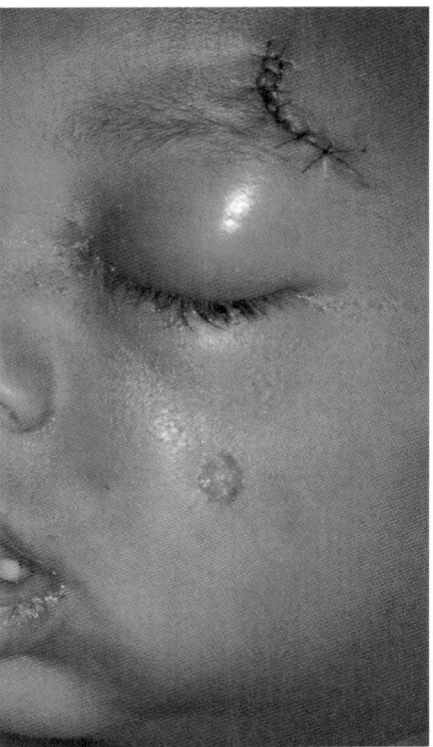

Figure 87-7. An infant with rapid onset of left eyelid swelling and erythema after a small laceration above the eye was sutured. Group A streptococcus was recovered from the wound. (Courtesy of J.H. Brien©.)

brasiliensis of the eyelid has been reported in an adult hunting in England 2 weeks before presentation following a small abrasion on his lower eyelid.[29] In endemic countries, *Mycobacterium tuberculosis* should also be considered in patients who present with a swollen lid; in pediatric cases of tuberculous lesions of the eyelids, presentation usually is relatively indolent (2 days to 2 months) and intermittently draining cutaneous sinuses occur during the course of conventional antibiotic treatment for more typical bacterial disease.[30] Diagnosis is confirmed by a positive tuberculin skin test, the identification of a primary focus of tuberculosis in lung or bone, and response to antituberculous therapy. Intraorbital complications of mycobacterial infection also can occur.[31]

Patients with bacterial cellulitis of traumatized areas rarely have bacteremia. Precise bacteriologic diagnosis is made through culture of exudate from the wound. If there is no drainage, a careful attempt at tissue aspiration is undertaken if this can be done safely (i.e., at a distance far enough from the orbit that there can be no potential damage to the eye). A tuberculin syringe with a 25-gauge needle can be used for aspiration of "tissue juice." Usually, only a minuscule amount of infected material can be aspirated. A small volume of nonbacteriostatic saline (0.2 mL) is drawn into the syringe before the procedure. The saline is not injected into the skin; instead, it is used to expel the small volume of tissue fluid within the needle onto chocolate agar for culture.[32] Parenteral treatment similar to that for dacryocystitis is recommended in patients with bacterial cellulitis (unless an unexpected microbial etiology emerges), to hasten resolution and avoid spread of infection to the cavernous sinus.

Bacteremic Periorbital Cellulitis

The child with bacteremic periorbital cellulitis, which most often is seen in infants younger than 18 months, has had a viral URI for several days. There is a sudden increase in temperature (to >39°C) accompanied by the acute onset and rapid progression of eyelid swelling. Swelling usually begins in the inner canthus of the

PART II Clinical Syndromes and Cardinal Features of Infectious Diseases: Approach to Diagnosis and Initial Management

SECTION L Eye Infections

upper and lower eyelid and can obscure the eyeball within 12 hours. Periorbital tissues are markedly discolored and usually erythematous, although if the swelling has been rapidly progressive, the area may have a violaceous discoloration.[33,34] The child's resistance to examination commonly leads to the erroneous impression of tenderness. Retraction or separation of the lids reveals that the globe is normally placed and extraocular eye movements are intact. If retraction of the lids is not possible, computed tomography of the orbit may be necessary.[35] The young age, high fever, and rapid progression of findings differentiate bacteremic preseptal cellulitis from other causes of swelling around the eye.

In the era before universal *H. influenzae* type b (Hib) immunization, Hib was the most common cause of bacteremic periorbital cellulitis (approximately 80% of cases), *S. pneumoniae* accounted for the remaining 20%. The substantial decline that has been observed in the total number of cases of bacteremic periorbital cellulitis is attributable to the widespread use of the Hib vaccine since 1991 and pneumococcal conjugate vaccine (PCV) since 2000.[36] A precise bacteriologic diagnosis is made by recovery of the organism from blood culture. If a careful tissue aspiration is performed, culture of the specimen can be positive.

The pathogenesis of most of these infections, which usually occur during the course of a viral URI, is hematogenous dissemination from a portal of entry in the nasopharynx. This process is akin to the mechanism of most infections caused by Hib and some infections caused by *S. pneumoniae.*

In patients with bacteremic periorbital cellulitis, radiographs of the paranasal sinuses often are abnormal. However, the abnormalities almost certainly reflect the viral respiratory syndrome that precedes and probably predisposes to the bacteremic event, rather than a clinically significant sinusitis.[7] Bacteremic cellulitis rarely arises from the paranasal sinus cavities, as evidenced by the finding that typable *H. influenzae* organisms are almost never recovered from maxillary sinus aspirates and likewise are rarely recovered from abscess material in patients who have serious local complications of paranasal sinus disease, such as subperiosteal abscess. Although *S. pneumoniae* can cause subperiosteal abscess in patients with acute sinusitis, such patients usually are not bacteremic.

Treatment for suspected bacteremic periorbital cellulitis requires parenteral therapy. *S. pneumoniae* is the most likely cause in a child who has received both the Hib and PCV series. Because this infection usually is bacteremic in the age group in whom the meninges are susceptible to inoculation, it may be prudent to use an advanced-generation cephalosporin such as cefotaxime or ceftriaxone (150 or 100 mg/kg per day, respectively, divided into doses every 8 or 12 hours, respectively). Lumbar puncture should be performed unless the clinical picture precludes meningitis. Addition of vancomycin (60 mg/kg per day divided into doses every 6 hours) or rifampin (20 mg/kg once daily, not to exceed 600 mg/day) is appropriate if cerebrospinal fluid pleocytosis is present. When evidence of local infection has resolved and there is no meningitis, oral antimicrobial therapy is prescribed to complete a 10-day course.

Preseptal (Periorbital) Cellulitis Caused by Inflammatory Edema of Sinusitis

Several complications of paranasal sinusitis can result in the development of swelling around the eye. The most common and least serious complication often is referred to as *inflammatory edema* or a *sympathetic effusion.*[6] This is a form of preseptal cellulitis, although infection is confined to the sinuses.

Typically, a child at least 2 years old has had a viral URI for several days when swelling is noted. Often, there is a history of intermittent early-morning periorbital swelling that resolves after a few hours. On the day of presentation, the eyelid swelling does not resolve typically but progresses gradually (see Figure 87-1). Surprisingly, striking degrees of erythema also can be present. Eye pain and tenderness are variable. Eyelids can be very swollen and difficult to evert, requiring the assistance of an ophthalmologist. However, there is no displacement of the globe or impairment of

extraocular eye movements. Fever, if present, is usually of low grade.

The peripheral white blood cell count is unremarkable, blood culture is sterile, and if a tissue aspiration is performed, culture is sterile. Sinus radiographs or other images show ipsilateral ethmoiditis or pansinusitis. The age of the child, gradual evolution of lid swelling, and modest fever differentiate inflammatory edema from bacteremic periorbital cellulitis.

The pathogenesis of sympathetic effusion or inflammatory edema is attributable to the venous drainage of the eyelid and surrounding structures. The inferior and superior ophthalmic veins, which drain the lower lid and upper lid, respectively, pass through or just next to the ethmoid sinus. When the ethmoid sinuses are completely congested, physical impedance of venous drainage occurs, resulting in soft-tissue swelling of the eyelids, maximal at the medial aspect of the lids. In this instance, infection is confined within the paranasal sinuses. The globe is not displaced, and there is no impairment of the extraocular muscle movements. However, inflammatory edema is part of a continuum with more serious complications resulting from the spread of infection outside the paranasal sinuses into the orbit.[37] Rarely, infection progresses despite initial optimal management of sympathetic effusions.

The infecting organisms in cases of inflammatory edema are the same as those that cause uncomplicated acute sinusitis (i.e., *S. pneumoniae*, nontypable *H. influenzae*, and *Moraxella catarrhalis*). Antibiotic therapy can be given orally if, at the time of the first examination, the eyelid swelling is modest (lid closure <50%), the child does not appear toxic, and the parents will adhere to management. Otherwise, admission to the hospital and parenteral treatment should be undertaken.

The only source of bacteriologic information is that obtainable by maxillary sinus aspiration, which is not usually performed. Appropriate agents for outpatient therapy should have activity against β-lactamase-producing organisms (e.g., amoxicillin-potassium clavulanate, cefuroxime axetil, and cefpodoxime proxetil). Parenteral agents include ceftriaxone (75 to 100 mg/kg per day, given as a single dose, or ampicillin-sulbactam (200 mg/kg per day divided into doses every 6 hours). The latter combination, although not approved for children younger than 12 years, is an attractive choice. Although the use of topically applied intranasal decongestants such as oxymetazoline has not been evaluated systematically, such agents may be helpful during the first 48 hours. After several days, once the affected eye has returned to near normal, an oral antimicrobial agent is substituted to complete a 14-day course of therapy.

A handful of children who present with a swollen eye experience one or more recurrences. In these cases anatomic abnormalities must be considered (natural or acquired bony dehiscences in the lamina papyracea,[38] or uncinate process[39]) in addition to reactivation of herpes simplex infection, sinusitis, allergic inflammation,[40] and orbital cysts derived from lacrimal tissue.[41]

ORBITAL INFECTION

The child or adolescent with true orbital disease secondary to sinusitis usually has sudden onset of erythema and swelling about the eye after several days of a viral URI (Figure 87-8). Eye pain can precede swelling and often is dramatic. The presence of fever, systemic signs, and toxicity is variable. Orbital infection is suggested by proptosis (with the globe usually displaced anteriorly and downward), impairment of extraocular eye movements (most often upward gaze), or loss of visual acuity or chemosis (edema of the bulbar conjunctiva). While most cases of orbital cellulitis secondary to sinusitis originate as a complication of viral URI, a few cases are of odontogenic origin.[42,43] Rarely, orbital abscess can occur without apparent underlying sinus or dental disease and absent acute signs of infection.[44] Occasionally, unusual infections such as cysticercosis, echinococcal disease, or *M. tuberculosis* can involve the orbit.[31,45] In most of these cases the spread of infection to the orbit is via the bloodstream. Fortunately, orbital infection is the least common cause of the "swollen eye."

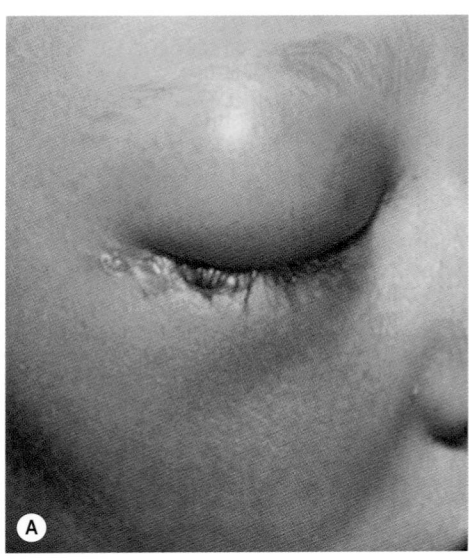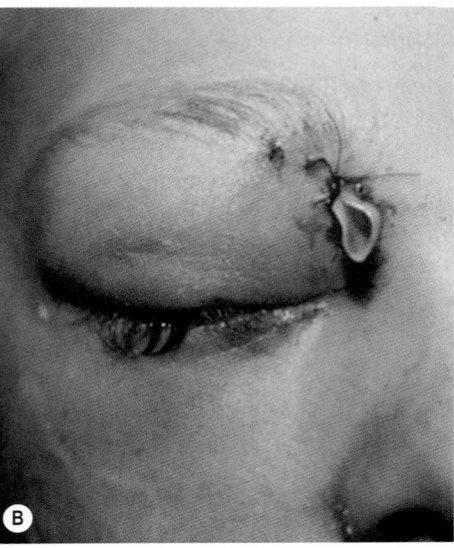

Figure 87-8. A boy with orbital cellulitis complicating sinusitis, pre **(A)** and post drainage **(B)**. He had a 3-day history of eye pain with progressive swelling and erythema of the eyelids. He had proptosis, chemosis, and upward gaze palsy. (Courtesy of J.H. Brien©.)

Most orbital infections involve the formation of a subperiosteal abscess. In young children, such an abscess results from ethmoiditis and ethmoid osteitis. In the adolescent, subperiosteal abscess can be a complication of frontal sinusitis and osteitis. Rarely, orbital cellulitis evolves, without formation of subperiosteal abscess, by direct spread from the ethmoid sinus to the orbit via natural bony dehiscences in the bones that form the medial wall of the orbit.

In addition to proptosis, impaired extraocular movements and loss of visual acuity, other factors including age, extent of periorbital edema, absolute neutrophil count (>10,000/mm³) and previous antibiotic treatment may be used to estimate risk of orbital infection.[46] Imaging studies usually are performed if orbital disease is suspected to help determine whether subperiosteal abscess, orbital abscess, or orbital cellulitis is the cause of the clinical findings (Figure 87-9). In the presence of a large, well-defined abscess, complete ophthalmoplegia, or impairment of vision, prompt operative drainage of the paranasal sinuses and the abscess is performed.[47-49] Subperiosteal abscess frequently can be drained successfully via endoscopy performed through an intranasal approach, thus avoiding an external incision.[50-52] In many cases, inflammatory tissue rather than a well-defined abscess is observed interposed between the lateral border of the ethmoid sinus and the swollen medial rectus muscle. Antimicrobial therapy alone usually is successful in such patients, as well as in patients with small abscesses that responded rapidly.[48,53-55] If the patient and ocular findings do not improve after 24–48 hours, surgical intervention is appropriate. Occasionally, CT can suggest an abscess when only inflammatory edema is present;[37,56] accordingly, the clinical course is the ultimate guide to management.

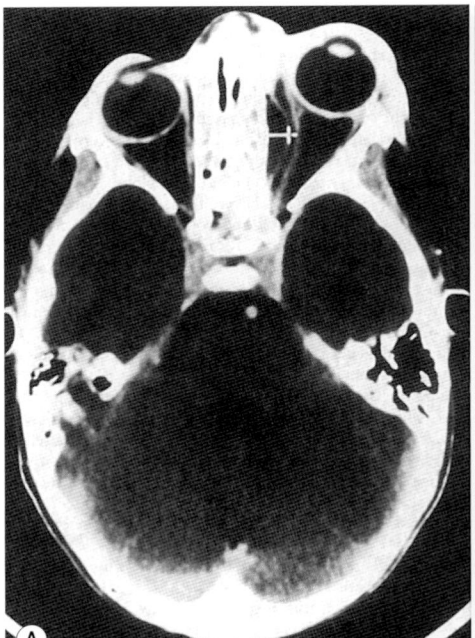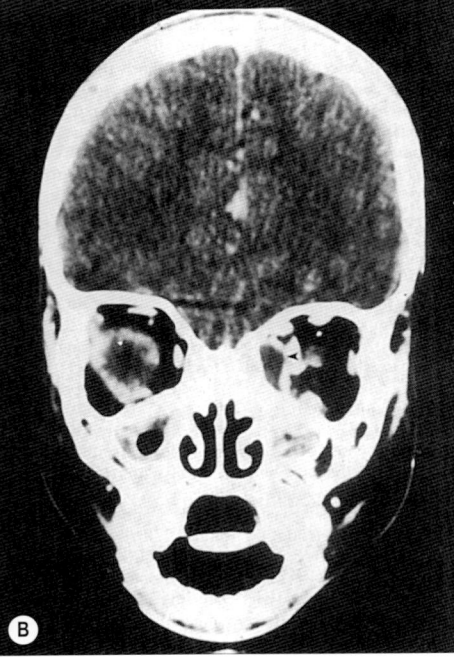

Figure 87-9. Axial **(A)** and coronal **(B)** computed tomography scans show a subperiosteal abscess extending from the left ethmoid sinus.

PART II Clinical Syndromes and Cardinal Features of Infectious Diseases: Approach to Diagnosis and Initial Management

SECTION M Infections Related to Trauma

Empiric antimicrobial therapy should be chosen to provide activity against *S. aureus, S. pyogenes,* and anaerobic bacteria of the upper respiratory tract (anaerobic cocci, *Bacteroides* spp., *Prevotella* spp., *Fusobacterium* spp., and *Veillonella* spp.) in addition to the usual pathogens associated with acute sinusitis (i.e., *S. pneumoniae, H. influenzae,* and *M. catarrhalis*).[52,57,58] An appropriate regimen is ampicillin-sulbactam (200 mg/kg per day divided into doses every 6 hours) plus vancomycin (60 mg/kg per day in 4 divided doses). Vancomycin will provide coverage in the event the causative organism is MRSA or if *S. pneumoniae* is highly resistant to penicillin. If surgery is performed, Gram stain of material drained from the sinuses or the abscess guides consideration of additional drugs or an altered regimen. When final results of culture and susceptibility tests are available, antibiotic therapy may be adjusted if necessary. Intravenous therapy is maintained until the eye appears nearly normal. At that time, oral antibiotic therapy can be substituted to complete a 3-week course of treatment.

SECTION M: Infections Related to Trauma

88 Infection following Trauma

Sarah L. Wingerter

Trauma is a major cause of morbidity in children and the leading cause of death in children older than 1 year. About 90% of childhood injuries are secondary to blunt trauma, often caused by motor vehicle accidents, falls, or abuse.[1,2] Infection that follows trauma can be due to the injury itself or, more commonly, can be a consequence of healthcare procedures and prolonged hospitalization. In one study, 10% of children admitted to a pediatric intensive care unit after trauma experienced infection.[3] The incidence of infection following trauma in adults may be as high as 25%; wound infections or other hospital-associated infections appear to be equally likely.[3] Hospital-associated infections are addressed in detail in Chapter 101 (Healthcare-Associated Infections). Trauma-associated infections, which can cause considerable morbidity, are the focus of this chapter.

PATHOGENESIS

Severe injuries increase a child's susceptibility to infection for several reasons. Breaks in the skin and mucosal barriers allow pathogens to gain entry, and accumulation of blood provides a favorable environment for bacterial growth. Devitalized or necrotic tissue at the injury site can harbor pathogens that can evade the host's defense mechanisms. Foreign bodies introduced by the injury itself or as a consequence of hospitalization (e.g., catheters) allow entry and persistence of pathogens. Risk factors for infection in patients hospitalized for trauma include the severity of the injury, the presence of shock, the number of organs injured, and the amount of blood lost.[4,5] Other potential risk factors are underlying host factors and the number and virulence of organisms introduced as a result of injury.

Trauma can adversely affect host defense mechanisms. Monocyte activation occurs rapidly after severe injury and hemorrhagic shock. After monocyte activation, inflammatory mediators can be released in a dysregulated pattern, leading to the systemic inflammatory response syndrome[6] (see Chapter 11, The Systemic Inflammatory Response Syndrome (SIRS), Sepsis, and Septic Shock). Complement is activated by injured tissue, thus decreasing complement levels, and antibody production also diminishes after blunt trauma.[7] Suboptimal nutrition can further impair immune responsiveness.

GENERAL PRINCIPLES OF MANAGEMENT

Patients who sustain trauma can exhibit signs and symptoms consistent with infection in the absence of infection. Retroperitoneal blood can cause fever, as can atelectasis. Pulmonary contusions can mimic pneumonia radiographically, and the signs and symptoms of hemorrhagic shock can be indistinguishable from those of septic shock. Thorough evaluation may be hampered by a patient's immobility or diminished neurologic status and by dressings that can obscure foci of infection. The decision to begin antibiotic therapy should be made carefully, after acquisition of appropriate microbiologic specimens. Appropriate use of antibiotics can benefit the patient, but inappropriate use has no benefit and can lead to adverse effects and promote the development of resistant organisms.

Measures that prevent infection include rapid surgical intervention when necessary, removal of unnecessary catheters, and strict attention to infection-control procedures and hand hygiene. Prophylactic or presumptive antibiotic therapy may be beneficial in some circumstances.

Immunity to tetanus should be assessed in any patient with an open wound. Tetanus toxoid-containing vaccine should be given to any child in whom the primary vaccination series has been delayed

Table 88-1. Common Pathogens and Recommended Prophylaxis following Trauma

Type of Trauma	Common or Important Pathogens	Recommended Prophylaxis
All trauma	*Clostridium tetani*	Ensure tetanus immunity or give vaccine ± tetanus immune globulin
Penetrating abdominal injuries	Enteric gram-negative bacilli and anaerobic bacteria	Ceftriaxone plus metronidazole, or cefoxitin, or gentamicin plus metronidazole
Splenectomy	Encapsulated organisms, e.g., *Streptococcus pneumoniae, Haemophilus influenzae,* and *Neisseria*	Ensure vaccination against all three organisms. Give penicillin prophylaxis
Basilar skull fracture	Meningitis due to respiratory tract organisms	No prophylaxis recommended
Open fractures (including skull)	*Staphylococcus aureus,* gram-negative bacilli	Nafcillin, or cefazolin, or clindamycin;[a] add gram-negative coverage for grade III fractures
Thoracic trauma requiring chest tube	*S. aureus* and *Streptococcus* species	Nafcillin, or cefazolin, or clindamycin[a]

[a]*Vancomycin may be appropriate if MRSA is prevalent in the community or if the patient is known to be colonized with MRSA.*

or who has not received tetanus vaccine in more than 5 years. Tetanus immune globulin should be used in conjunction with the vaccine in high-risk wounds (e.g., puncture wounds, wounds contaminated with soil, feces, or saliva) if the child has not received adequate prior immunization. Children 11 to 18 years who were vaccinated against tetanus 5 years earlier and require a tetanus toxoid-containing vaccine as part of wound management should receive a tetanus toxoid, reduced diphtheria toxoid, acellular pertussis vaccine (Tdap) if they have not received Tdap previously.[8]

The use of prophylactic or presumptive antibiotic therapy in select situations can reduce the incidence of infection (Table 88-1); however, duration of antibiotic therapy longer than 24 hours has not demonstrated additional benefit, as discussed in detail below.

Nutritional status also can affect infection risk. Patients with trauma who are given enteral nutrition have a lower risk of infectious complications than those given intravenous nutrition.[9,10] There is conflicting evidence whether injured patients fed an enteral diet rich in glutamine, arginine, and omega-3 fatty acids have a lower risk of infection than those fed a standard enteral diet or those who receive no early enteral nutrition.[11-13]

SKIN AND SOFT-TISSUE TRAUMA

Factors associated with a greater risk of infection after injury to the skin and soft tissues are the severity of the wound, shock, and blood loss (Table 88-2)[4,7] Because wounds sustained in trauma are inherently contaminated, thorough cleansing and debridement of

Table 88-2. Infection Risk and Management following Trauma

Type of Trauma	Infection Risk	Intervention
Skin and soft tissue	*Streptococcus pyogenes* (GAS) <2 days Methicillin-susceptible/methicillin-resistant *Staphylococcus aureus* (MSSA/MRSA) ≥2 days	First-generation cephalosporin; wound culture; consider other antibiotics based on local resistance patterns (clindamycin, TMP-SMX, tetracycline, rifampin); vancomycin or linezolid if life-threatening
Animal/human bites	As above, plus *Pasteurella multocida, Eikenella corrodens,* anaerobic bacteria	Blood culture, needle aspirate; extended-spectrum β-lactam, clindamycin plus TMP-SMX if penicillin-allergic
Body piercings, tattoos	Skin flora, *P. aeruginosa*	Ceftazidime or piperacillin-tazobactam
Water-associated Fresh water	*Aeromonas hydrophila*	Third- or fourth-generation cephalosporin or extended-spectrum β-lactam
Salt water or contact	*Vibrio vulnificus*	Third-generation cephalosporin with raw seafood exposure
Fish spines, fishtanks	*Mycobacterium marinum*	Surgical excision; combination antibacterial therapy
Blunt/penetrating trauma Pyomyositis	*S. aureus,* GAS	Surgical drainage, debridement; antibiotics
Necrotizing fasciitis/gas gangrene	*S. aureus,* GAS, *Clostridium* species	Fasciotomy; debridement; penicillin or nafcillin plus clindamycin
Abdominal trauma Penetrating – higher risk of intestinal injury + spillage of bowel contents	Acute: peritonitis (± septicemia) Later: abscess, surgical	Surgical exploration, metronidazole plus aminoglycoside
Blunt – risk of duodenal/pancreatic hematoma (increased risk of infection if large-volume transfusion required)		Aminoglycoside or third-generation cephalosporin; surgical/CT-guided abscess drainage site of infection
Splenic rupture: Nonoperative	Blood transfusions pathogens	
Splenectomy	Post-splenectomy septicemia (encapsulated organisms)	Immunizations: Hib, pneumococcal, meningococcal vaccines; penicillin prophylaxis until at least 5 years of age and 1 year post splenectomy
Head trauma	Meningitis (especially with basilar skull fracture, penetrating trauma, or open wounds); ventriculitis; brain abscess, *S. pneumoniae, H. influenzae, N. meningitidis,* GAS, *S. aureus,* gram-negative bacilli	CSF analysis and culture; antibiotics with good CSF penetration; gram-positive coverage, e.g., vancomycin plus third-generation cephalosporin; gram-negative coverage if contaminated wound or extensive soft-tissue damage; surgical intervention if persistent CSF leak
Fractures Open	Highest risk: grade IIIB or IIIC, internal/external fixation device, involvement of lower leg; *S. aureus, Enterobacter* spp., *Pseudomonas* spp., *Enterobacter* spp., *Pseudomonas* spp.	Surgical debridement; antibiotic therapy. Antibiotic prophylaxis for open fractures: gram-positive coverage for open fractures; gram-negative coverage for grade III; add high-dose penicillin if fecal contamination, or clostridial infection suspected clinically
Puncture wounds of the foot	Cellulitis, abscess, osteochondritis; *Pseudomonas, S. aureus,* GAS, *E. corrodens* (toothpick)	Surgical debridement; antibiotics
Thoracic trauma Pulmonary contusion, hemothorax, pneumothorax	Risk factors for hospital-associated pneumonia: prolonged intubation, poor pulmonary toilet, aspiration	Antibiotics active to cover oro/nasopharyngeal organisms (including anaerobes) and defined gram-negative bacilli by local intensive care unit pathogens and respiratory culture. Empiric choices: clindamycin plus third-generation cephalosporin or aminoglycoside; or β-lactam + β-lactamase inhibitor

PART II Clinical Syndromes and Cardinal Features of Infectious Diseases: Approach to Diagnosis and Initial Management

SECTION M Infections Related to Trauma

devitalized tissue have pre-eminent importance in preventing infection.

Cellulitis can follow minor or major trauma to the skin. Rapidly spreading cellulitis that occurs within 2 days of injury is more likely due to *Streptococcus pyogenes* (group A streptococcus (GAS)), whereas staphylococcal cellulitis may not manifest for several days. Although GAS and *Staphylococcus aureus* are the most common causes of cellulitis, other pathogens should be considered in certain settings. Animal or human bites can lead to infection with *Pasteurella multocida* or *Eikenella corrodens*, respectively, as well as with anaerobes, *S. aureus* and GAS. Body piercings and tattoos, which are increasingly common in adolescents, also can lead to bacterial infection. Although skin flora is usually the cause, *Pseudomonas aeruginosa* is a common cause of infection following piercing of the auricular cartilage[14] and there have been outbreaks of methicillin-resistant *S. aureus* (MRSA) infections in tattoo recipients.[15] Hepatitis B, hepatitis C, and human immunodeficiency virus (HIV) infection also can be transmitted through piercing and tattooing. *Aeromonas hydrophila* infection is associated with lacerations obtained while swimming in fresh water, and *Vibrio vulnificus* can cause skin or soft-tissue wound infections after contact with salt water or drippings from raw seafood. *Mycobacterium marinum* can cause cutaneous infection after freshwater or salt-water injuries from fish spines or marine shellfish, or from contamination during exposure to fishtanks.[16]

Blood culture and needle aspirate have low yield in typical cases of cellulitis, but can be revealing in cases of cellulitis associated with animal bites or other unusual injuries.

For mild to moderate cases of typical wound cellulitis, empiric therapy with a first-generation cephalosporin provides coverage for the most common pathogens, including *S. aureus* and GAS. The emergence of community-associated MRSA (CA-MRSA) in posttraumatic skin and soft-tissue infections makes empiric treatment problematic.[17,18] MRSA-colonized children have a greater risk for developing a wound infection following trauma. For more severe cases of cellulitis, for wound infections requiring hospitalization, or for an infection not responding to initial β-lactam antibiotic therapy, a diagnostic specimen should be obtained and treatment should include coverage of MRSA.[19] While many CA-MRSA are susceptible to clindamycin,[20,21] some have inducible or constitutive clindamycin resistance.[22,23] Most strains also are susceptible to tetracycline (which should be avoided in children <9 years), trimethoprim-sulfamethoxazole, and rifampin. For life-threatening infections possibly due to MRSA, appropriate therapy would include vancomycin or linezolid.[24] Knowledge of local antibiotic resistance patterns should guide empiric therapy.[25]

Pyomyositis can occur after blunt or penetrating trauma and usually is caused by *S. aureus* or GAS. Treatment involves surgical drainage, debridement, and antibiotic therapy. Necrotizing fasciitis, due to GAS or *S. aureus*, and gas gangrene, usually due to *Clostridium* spp., can complicate traumatic wounds and are surgical emergencies. A characteristic symptom is intense pain, often out of proportion to findings on examination, which can include discoloration of the overlying skin, swelling, and crepitus. Patients with necrotizing fasciitis also can have concomitant toxic shock syndrome. Computed tomography (CT) or magnetic resonance imaging may show muscle swelling, fluid collections, or, in the case of gangrene, gas in the muscle. Leukocytosis, thrombocytopenia, a rising creatine kinase level, and hypocalcemia can be seen in these patients.

Therapy for necrotizing fasciitis involves immediate surgical fasciotomy and debridement. Penicillin or nafcillin plus clindamycin should be given for streptococcal and clostridial infections.[26,27] Although penicillin G is the drug of choice for invasive GAS infections, clindamycin also should be used for deep infections such as necrotizing fasciitis. In a mouse model of streptococcal myositis, clindamycin was found to be superior to penicillin.[28,29] The likely explanation is that the high density of GAS leads to reduced replication and decreased expression of penicillin-binding proteins.[29] Clindamycin, which inhibits protein synthesis, maintains its activity against these slowly replicating bacteria and also inhibits the production of bacterial toxins. Clindamycin should

not be used alone until results of susceptibility testing are available because some GAS are resistant.

ABDOMINAL TRAUMA

Trauma to the abdomen can be blunt or penetrating. Penetrating trauma is less common but carries a higher risk for intestinal injury. Either penetrating or blunt trauma can cause intestinal tears that lead to spillage of bowel contents into the peritoneum. Injuries to the colon are associated with a higher risk of infection because of the higher density of organisms in the more distal bowel.[30] Blunt trauma related to physical abuse can cause hematoma of the duodenum and pancreatitis. Requirement for a large volume of transfusion is also a risk factor for infection after abdominal trauma.[5]

Infection can manifest acutely as peritonitis, with or without septicemia, or later, as an abscess or surgical site infection. Diagnosis is aided by CT or, in a patient who cannot be moved, ultrasonography. Needle aspiration of peritoneal fluid is performed in patients with peritonitis to confirm the diagnosis and establish the etiology. Treatment of an established infection requires empiric therapy with antibiotics effective against gram-negative and anaerobic bacteria, and surgical or CT-guided drainage if an abscess is present. Metronidazole plus an aminoglycoside or third-generation cephalosporin, or piperacillin-tazobactam would be appropriate choices. It is not clear that empiric therapy with anti-enterococcal agents improves outcome in these patients; however, anti-enterococcal therapy should be considered for children who have persistent symptoms, or when *Enterococcus* is isolated from peritoneal fluid cultures.

Surgical exploration is part of the routine management of penetrating abdominal injuries and antibiotic therapy should be started as soon as possible. Fullen and associates[31] showed that patients with penetrating abdominal injuries who received antibiotics before surgery had a lower incidence of infection than patients who received the first dose of antibiotics intraoperatively or postoperatively. Because patients with penetrating abdominal injuries are presumed to have bacterial contamination of the peritoneum at the time of injury, antibiotic therapy should be considered presumptive therapy.

The empiric antibiotic regimen should include agents effective against gram-negative enteric and anaerobic bacteria, which play a critical role in intra-abdominal infections after injury.[32] Single-drug therapy with a second-generation cephalosporin, such as cefoxitin, or piperacillin-tazobactam, appears to be as effective as traditional three-drug antibiotic regimens in preventing infection in adults with penetrating abdominal injuries; resistance of anaerobic bacteria to cefoxitin and stimulation of production of extended-spectrum β-lactamases limit current use.[33,34] Other appropriate therapies include a third-generation cephalosporin plus metronidazole or an aminoglycoside plus metronidazole. Patients with trauma have a higher volume of drug distribution, so higher doses of aminoglycosides may be needed.[35,36]

Several studies have evaluated the appropriate length of presumptive therapy for patients with penetrating abdominal injuries. No significant difference in infection rate was found between patients treated for 24 hours and those treated for 5 days.[30,34,37–39] Therefore, current evidence does not support the use of antibiotics beyond 24 hours in patients with penetrating abdominal injuries, even if they have colonic injuries. Longer duration of antibiotic therapy promotes bacterial resistance and fungal overgrowth and may lead to additional side effects without further reducing the likelihood of infection.[40]

Splenic rupture after trauma deserves special consideration (see Chapter 108, Infectious Complications in Special Hosts). If the rupture is managed nonoperatively, multiple blood transfusions may be required, placing the patient at risk for bloodborne pathogens. If splenectomy is performed, the child is at risk for overwhelming post-splenectomy septicemia, especially due to encapsulated organisms. The risk of septicemia in a child who has undergone traumatic splenectomy is as much as 350 times higher than that in a healthy child. Younger children are at higher risk of septicemia than older children. While the period of greatest risk appears to be the first 2 years after splenectomy, septicemia has been reported up to 25 years after splenectomy. Therefore, observation or splenic repair is preferred if the child is clinically stable.[41,42]

If splenectomy is performed, immunizations should be reviewed to ensure that the child has been appropriately immunized with the *Haemophilus influenzae* type b and pneumococcal conjugate vaccines. Meningococcal conjugate vaccine should be administered for children ≥2 years of age. Children 2 years and older who have been adequately immunized with the pneumococcal conjugate vaccine (PCV) also should be given a dose of the 23-valent polysaccharide vaccine (PPSV23). They should receive a second PPSV23 dose 5 years after the first. Partially immunized children older than 2 years should receive one dose of the PCV as well as a dose of the PPSV23 8 weeks and 5 years later. For children 5 years of age and older, most experts recommend the same sequential PCV/PPSV23 vaccine schedule, although either vaccine alone is also acceptable. In addition, penicillin prophylaxis should be considered for all children younger than 5 years, and for at least 1 year after splenectomy in older children.[41]

HEAD TRAUMA

Head trauma is common in children, and central nervous system injury increases mortality among injured children.[1] As many as one-half of patients with head trauma develop an infectious complication, most often a hospital-associated infection.[43] Trauma-related infectious complications include meningitis, ventriculitis, and brain abscess; common pathogens are *Streptococcus pneumoniae* and other upper respiratory tract organisms such as *H. influenzae*, *Neisseria meningitidis*, and GAS. Staphylococcal and gram-negative bacillary meningitis can occur after penetrating trauma, with open wounds, or postoperatively, or associated with devices or after prolonged hospitalization.[44] It is essential to obtain cerebrospinal fluid (CSF) for culture if the diagnosis of meningitis is being considered after head trauma; CSF cell count as well as glucose and protein level can be difficult to interpret in the presence of subarachnoid hemorrhage. Treatment includes antibiotic therapy as well as possible surgical intervention in patients with device in place or following persistent CSF leakage.

Basilar skull fracture accounts for up to 20% of skull fractures and is associated with substantial risk of bacterial meningitis. Meningitis is a consequence of the communication created between the subarachnoid space and the colonized paranasal sinuses, nasopharynx, and middle ear. After basilar skull fracture, the incidence of meningitis can be as high as 17% and approaches 50% in patients who also have a CSF leak. However, a 1998 meta-analysis of 12 studies involving 1241 patients with basilar skull fractures suggested that antibiotic prophylaxis did not prevent meningitis.[45] Even when children and patients with CSF leakage were analyzed separately, there was no evidence that antibiotic prophylaxis decreased the risk of meningitis. In addition, the rate of meningitis in children after basilar skull fracture was only 3%, much lower than rates reported in adults. A 2006 Cochrane Database review found that antibiotic prophylaxis had no significant effect on reducing the frequency of meningitis, all-cause mortality, or meningitis-related mortality in patients with basilar skull fractures.[46] Available data therefore do not support the use of prophylactic antibiotics in children with basilar skull fractures.

Prophylactic antibiotics usually are given following an open skull fracture, although there are few data to guide recommendations. Antibiotics chosen should have good CSF penetration and cover gram-positive organisms. Coverage for gram-negative organisms may be needed if the wound is heavily contaminated or there is extensive soft-tissue damage.

FRACTURES

Fractures are common childhood injuries and can be either closed or open. Open fractures can be graded on a scale of I to III on the basis of wound size and amount of soft-tissue damage. Grade III fractures are further subdivided (IIIA, IIIB, and IIIC) according to vascular injuries and soft-tissue defects. Dellinger and colleagues,[47] evaluating factors associated with infection after open-extremity fractures, found the following independent risk factors: severity of fracture (grade IIIB or IIIC), the placement of an internal or external fixation device, and involvement of the lower leg. Organisms most commonly implicated in fracture-associated infections were *Staphylococcus* spp., *Enterobacter* spp., and *Pseudomonas* spp.[47-49] Therapy consists of surgical removal of infected tissue and antibiotics.

Infection rates associated with open fractures range from as high as 9% for grade I fractures to 50% for grade III fractures. Infection after open fracture can lead to delayed bone healing, prolonged hospitalization, and permanent disability. Open fractures have a higher risk of infection than closed fractures, because bone and soft-tissue contamination likely occurred at the time of injury.

Several studies have demonstrated a reduced risk of infection after open fractures in patients given prophylactic therapy with antibiotics effective against *S. aureus*.[50-52] In addition to *S. aureus*, gram-negative bacilli such as *Pseudomonas* and *Enterobacter* can cause open fracture-associated infections, especially with grade III fractures. The Eastern Association for the Surgery of Trauma (EAST) guidelines revised in 2009 recommend the following: prophylactic antibiotics with gram-positive coverage as soon as possible after injury for all trauma with open fractures; additional coverage for gram-negative organisms for grade III fractures. For grade I and II fractures, antibiotics should be discontinued 24 hours after wound closure. Additionally, for grade III fractures, antibiotics should be continued for only 72 hours after the time of injury or not more than 24 hours after soft-tissue coverage of the wound, whichever comes first. A Cochrane database review from 2010 also found evidence for benefit of antibiotic prophylaxis at the time of surgery for closed long-bone fractures.[53]

The use of antibiotic-impregnated beads, cement, and polymers has shown some promise in reducing open-fracture-associated infections.[49,51,54] Prospective randomized trials are needed to determine effectiveness.

PUNCTURE WOUNDS

The management of infection after a puncture wound to the foot deserves special consideration. Up to 18% of such wounds are complicated by cellulitis or a soft tissue abscess, and up to 2% by osteochondritis. *P. aeruginosa* is responsible for as many as 90% of cases of osteochondritis after a puncture wound to the foot.[34] The liner of used sneakers has been found to contain *Pseudomonas*, making this a likely source; however, *Pseudomonas* can cause infection after a puncture wound through other shoes and even bare feet, and at other sites.[55] Other gram-negative bacilli as well as *S. aureus* and GAS also can cause osteochondritis following a puncture wound. *Eikenella corrodens* and oral anaerobic bacteria have been reported following toothpick puncture injury to the foot.[56,57] Rarely, nontuberculous mycobacteria can be the primary pathogen.[58,59] Surgical debridement is the mainstay of management, both to obtain specimens to determine infectious etiology and to remove necrotic cartilage and any retained foreign body. After debridement, antipseudomonal therapy, if necessary, need only be continued for a week. Osteochondritis due to other organisms should be treated with a conventional course of therapy.

THORACIC TRAUMA

Thoracic injuries are a major cause of death in childhood trauma. Such injuries usually are blunt and often are due to a motor vehicle accident.[1] Significant chest trauma can lead to pulmonary contusion, hemothorax, and pneumothorax. Although any major trauma increases the risk of hospital-associated pneumonia due to prolonged intubation, poor pulmonary toilet, and the risk of aspiration, pulmonary contusions also lead to decreased pulmonary function, thereby further increasing the risk of pneumonia. The diagnosis of pneumonia can be challenging because fever and a pulmonary density can be due to the contusion itself. New fever, leukocytosis, purulent secretions, and the need for increased ventilator settings are clues to the diagnosis. The antibiotic regimen for suspected pneumonia in this setting should take into account knowledge of the pathogens commonly identified in the local intensive care unit as well as results of culture of deep respiratory tract specimens, such as those collected by bronchoalveolar lavage when possible. Therapy consists of agents effective against defined oro/nasopharyngeal or tracheal organisms, including anaerobic and gram-negative bacteria. Clindamycin plus either a third-generation cephalosporin or an aminoglycoside is appropriate, as is a β-lactam plus β-lactamase-inhibiting agent.

Hemothorax due to blunt or penetrating thoracic trauma increases the risk of empyema, as does a thoracostomy tube placed to evacuate a hemothorax or pneumothorax. The risk increases with incomplete drainage of the pleural space or prolonged chest tube placement.[60] S. aureus and gram-negative bacilli predominate in these infections.[61] Prophylactic antibiotic therapy has been studied in the setting of tube thoracostomy after chest trauma. A meta-analysis of 9 prospective trials and 2 earlier meta-analyses found that prophylactic antibiotic therapy reduced the risk of subsequent pneumonia after thoracostomy tube placement.[62] A brief (24-hour) course of an antibiotic with good antistaphylococcal and antistreptococcal activity is appropriate after chest tube placement. Antibiotic prophylaxis for <24 hours also is recommended when open thoracotomy is performed for penetrating chest injury.[63]

89 Infection following Burns

Jane M. Gould and Gail L. Rodgers

In 2007, unintentional injury was the leading cause of death in children 1 to 18 years of age in the United States. Of these deaths, fire/burns were the sixth leading cause in children less than 1 year of age, the third leading cause in children 1 to 4 years of age, and the second leading cause in the 5–9 year age group.[1] Overall the fire/burn nonfatal injury rate per 100,000 population in the age group in 1 to 18 years of age was 158.7 in 2008.[1] Children under 4 years of age and children with disabilities are at the greatest risk of burn-related death and injury.[2] The vast majority of these injuries are preventable. Most young children suffer scald injuries from hot liquids or flame burns from house fires. Older children are more likely to sustain flame burns from accidents with flammable liquids or fireworks and from house fires. On occasion, burn injuries can result from medical therapies, such as therapeutic application of heat, ignition of flammable medications (rubbing alcohol and hot oils), or burns from hot-air vaporizers.[3] In 2006, the U.S. total annual cost of scald burn-related deaths and injuries among children ≤14 years of age was approximately $44 million, with children <4 years of age accounting for 90% of these costs. Total charges for pediatric admissions to burn centers average $22,700 per case.[2]

The survival of children with burns depends on the following factors: (1) age; (2) the percentage of total body surface area (TBSA) burned; (3) the depth of the burn injury; (4) the type of burn; and (5) management. Young children, particularly those <2 years, have a lower survival for the same TBSA burned than older children and adults. Advances in burn care (improvements in resuscitation, intensive care, and care of the burn wound) have narrowed the gap in survival for small children.[4] Currently, the extent of burn associated with a 50% survival in patients older than 1 year is approximately TBSA of 80%.[5] Data suggest that the most common causes of death in burned children are smoke inhalation and hypoxic-ischemic brain injury. The enormous progress in burn survival and therapy is attributable to the following factors: care of patients in centers specializing in the treatment of burns; knowledge of the pathophysiology of shock and aggressive treatment of patients with fluid resuscitation and other adjunctive therapies; recognition of the importance of the caloric needs of the burned patient and its role in wound healing; and advances in the care of the burn wound itself, especially early debridement and excision of the wound, use of topical antimicrobial agents, judicious use of antibiotics systemically, and improved grafting materials and techniques.[6]

TBSA can be estimated either from the Lund and Browder chart or with use of the size of the patient's palm, which roughly is 1% of the TBSA at any age, as a measure.[7] Depth of burn injury is determined by the extent of damage to tissue and is classified by degrees: a first-degree burn involves the epidermis only, is painful, red, and dry, resembling a sunburn; second-degree burn involves the dermis, is severely painful, usually is erythematous, moist, weeps, and may have blisters and bullae; third-degree burn involves the subcutaneous tissue and is usually white or waxy-appearing, dry, avascular, and painless. Depth is alternatively classified as either partial-thickness, involving the epidermis or superficial dermis, or full-thickness, involving the deep dermis and subcutaneous tissue. The larger the percentage of TBSA involved and the deeper the burn, the higher the mortality, both immediately after injury (primarily from shock or occasionally from other associated injuries) and after successful resuscitation (from infectious complications). The type of burn also is important; scald burn is less commonly fatal than flame burn, especially if the latter is associated with pulmonary injury.

Children with burns >30% of TBSA, flame and inhalation injuries, and full-thickness burns are at highest risk of infectious complications.[8] Burn victims are susceptible to a wide variety of infections associated with relative immunosuppression and complications of intensive care. Virtually any organ can become the target of an infection in such patients. The most common infections in burned children are those related to the burn wound and catheter-associated septicemia.[8] Infections related to intravascular and urinary catheters and endotracheal tubes are discussed in Chapter 102 (Clinical Syndromes of Device-Associated Infections). Infection of the burn wound occurs with greatest frequency in children.[9] Burn wound septicemia is associated with at least an 80% mortality in children.

Diagnosis of infectious complications in a burn victim is challenging. Although fever and elevated peripheral white blood cell count with a left shift are usual indicators of infection, their positive predictive value for diagnosis of infectious complications in burn victims is very low because they are commonly seen in uninfected burned children whose wounds are uncovered.[10] Neither severity of fever (frequently >39°C) nor response to antipyretic therapy is a reliable indicator of infection.[10] Peak fever in burned children without infection usually occurs on the second day after the burn, with a second peak around the sixth and seventh days.[11] Fever is probably the result of an increase in metabolic rate and an alteration of hypothalamic temperature regulation. Fever usually subsides without specific therapy, coincident with re-epithelialization of the burn wound or successful grafting of all open areas. Thus, fever alone in the burned child is not a reliable indicator of infection or of the need to investigate for infection or prescribe antibiotic therapy.

Hypothermia usually is a more reliable indicator of infection, although children with burns affecting a high percentage of TBSA who are left uncovered for prolonged periods during dressing changes can have hypothermia that requires external warming. Hypotension due to fluid shifts is common early in the postburn period and usually can be differentiated from infectious causes because of rapid improvement with fluid resuscitation.

Several inflammatory mediators have been evaluated in attempts to distinguish infection from the normal response to thermal injury. They include tumor necrosis factor (TNF)-α,[12–14] interleukin (IL)-1β,[12,14] IL-6,[12,14] and IL-8,[13,15] procalcitonin,[16,17] and C-reactive protein.[18] Levels of mediators in burned patients are higher than those in healthy children, probably secondary to nonspecific inflammation associated with thermal injury. Although several studies have shown significant differences in levels of these inflammatory mediators between burned patients with septicemia and those with uncomplicated thermal injury,[12,13,15–17] none is highly discriminatory. However, changes in serial C-reactive protein levels can occur in septicemia an average of 2.3 days earlier than a decrease in platelet count or clinical manifestations.[18]

Thus, diagnosis of infectious complications is made through evaluation of all clinical signs, examination of the burn wound and all catheter sites, and consideration of supporting laboratory evidence, and results of culture of blood, urine, or quantitative burn wound biopsy specimens.

BURN WOUND INFECTION

Burn wound infection is defined as the invasion of microorganisms into viable tissue under the wound. Local infection can result in prolonged wound healing or sloughing of graft, toxin production leading to distant organ damage, and septicemia and infection at distant sites.[19]

The diagnosis of burn wound infection is made from local signs of wound infection, with or without systemic signs indicating septicemia or toxemia (Box 89-1), in conjunction with histologic and microbiologic evidence of infection in biopsy specimens of burn wounds (Box 89-2). The technique for quantitative biopsy requires a 1-gram specimen of eschar, which is homogenized and cultured.[20] The procedure consists of cleaning the open wound with alcohol and obtaining the specimen with a scalpel or a dermal punch. Processing of the biopsy consists of aseptic weighing, alcohol dip and flaming to remove surface contamination, dilution in fixed-volume thioglycolate broth or saline, homogenization, and inoculation onto nutrient agar.[21,22] Although selection of the biopsy site, retained activity of topical antimicrobial agents, and multistep processing can be sources of error, quantitative

---

BOX 89-1. Clinical Characteristics of Burn Wound Infection

LOCAL SIGNS

Focal areas of discoloration or necrosis
Edema, erythema, discoloration of wound margin
Conversion of partial- to full-thickness burn
Unexpectedly rapid eschar separation
Hemorrhagic discoloration of subeschar tissue
Purulent exudate on burn wound

SYSTEMIC SIGNS

Hyperthermia
Hypothermia
Hypotension
Altered mentation
Glucose instability
Organ dysfunction

Adapted from Pruitt BA Jr, Yurt RW. Treating burn and soft tissue infections. Infect Surg 1983;2:623–650.

BOX 89-2. Biopsy Findings of Burn Wound Infection

HISTOLOGY

Characteristics of tissue underlying burn

Presence of microorganisms
Thrombosis or hemorrhage
Necrosis
Intense inflammatory response

Presence of intracellular viral inclusions

MICROBIOLOGY

Positive quantitative Gram stain reaction
Isolation of single or multiple organisms, each >10^5 colony-forming units per gram of tissue

Adapted from Pruitt BA Jr, McManus AT. Opportunistic infections in severely burned patients. Am J Med 1984;76:146–154.

---

biopsy culture yielding growth of a single or multiple organisms, each with a density of >10^5 colony-forming units per gram of tissue, correlates with infection. Histologic diagnosis of infection is supported by the presence of bacteria invading viable tissue and can be obtained with frozen or permanent sections, the latter of which is thought to be more accurate.[20] Blood culture results are positive in only 40% to 50% of patients with burn wound sepsis.

Factors that influence burn wound infection pertain to the wound, the host, and the causative organisms.

Wound Factors

Skin is a primary, critical local defense mechanism against infection, providing a mechanical barrier to penetration of organisms that normally reside on the surface. Skin saprophytes are thought to inhibit colonization by more pathogenic bacteria. Skin also produces antibacterial substances, such as unsaturated free fatty acids, that inhibit a number of microorganisms, particularly group A streptococcus (GAS).[23] Thermal injury rapidly disrupts normal functions and produces an ideal culture medium.

After burn injury, the wound site rapidly becomes colonized with normal skin flora and gram-positive pathogens, and then by endogenous or environmental gram-negative bacilli and fungi if the course is protracted. Isolation of microbes from a burn wound is not a priori evidence of infection, because invasion into underlying viable tissue must occur for infection to develop.

Adequacy of blood supply to the wound is critical. Avascularity of the burned tissue results from coagulation of vessels and tissue that make a protein-rich eschar and renders the site inaccessible to systemic antibiotics as well as humoral and cellular defenses. Infection in the burn wound can extend into the blood vessels, causing thrombosis that can compromise the blood supply further, converting a partial-thickness burn into a full-thickness burn. Wound factors such as the acidic, anaerobic, moist environment of the avascular burn tissue favor growth of certain pathogens such as fungi and impair activity of aminoglycoside antibiotics. The cooler temperature of the burn wound may influence infection, because lower temperatures restrict blood flow, possibly causing further tissue necrosis and impairing phagocytic cell metabolism.[24] In addition, the location of the wound can contribute to the overall risk of infection, as is seen with exposure of the globe, bones, cartilage, and joints.[20] Likewise, the presence of foreign bodies in the wound also can promote infection.

Host Factors

Several host factors have been identified that influence the likelihood of burn wound infection. Children with underlying medical conditions, such as diabetes mellitus, neurologic disorder, and immunodeficiency, are more likely to experience burn wound septicemia, resulting in very high mortality.

TABLE 89-1. Immunologic Dysfunction in Burned Children

Type of Dysfunction	References
HUMORAL IMMUNE FUNCTION	
Decreased numbers of B lymphocytes	25–27
Decreased total immunoglobulins	27–35
Decreased fibronectin	26, 27, 36–38
Aberrant production of immunomodulators	24, 26, 28, 39, 40
CELLULAR IMMUNE FUNCTION	
Anergy	26, 27, 41
Decreased mitogen and antigen responses	26, 29, 42
Increased suppressor T lymphocytes	27, 28, 42–44
Decreased helper T lymphocytes	28, 42, 43
NEUTROPHIL FUNCTION	
Decreased adherence	36
Decreased phagocytosis	29, 45–47
Decreased killing	27, 29, 45, 46, 48, 49
Decreased chemotaxis	26, 27, 29, 45, 46, 50, 51
OTHER	
Decreased macrophage and monocyte function	52
Complement-induced increase in release of immunosuppressive mediators	27

Immunologic dysfunction is well described in patients who sustain burn injuries of >30% TBSA, with degree correlating directly with TBSA burned (Table 89-1). The mechanism is unknown. It has been suggested that immunosuppression after injury evolves to protect against autoimmunity that might otherwise result from antigenic bombardment after intense tissue injury.[42,53,54] Immunosuppression of burned patients greatly increases their susceptibility to infection. Polymorphisms in the genes that encode toll-like receptor 4 and TNF-α are significantly associated with increased risk for severe septicemia following burn trauma.[55]

Causative Organisms

Organisms causing burn wound infection have changed over the past century. In the 1930s and 1940s, GAS was the predominant pathogen, followed by *Staphylococcus aureus*. In the 1950s and early 1960s, the predominant pathogen in such infections was *S. aureus*. Gram-negative bacilli, especially *Pseudomonas aeruginosa*, became the predominant pathogen in the 1960s and early 1970s. Since then, *S. aureus* has regained prominence (becoming the most common pathogen in many centers[8,56]), including methicillin-resistant *S. aureus* (MRSA), the spectrum of gram-negative bacilli has broadened, and fungal and viral pathogens have become increasingly important. These changes are direct reflections of complications of aggressive therapy and survival of more severely affected patients.

The number of organisms present on the burn wound is an important factor in infectivity. It is theorized that high temperature initially sterilizes the burn wound. However, rapid colonization by normal skin flora and existent pathogens follows. At the time of hospitalization in our pediatric burn unit, routine cultures reveal that 9% and 54% of patients are colonized with GAS and *S. aureus*, respectively. Colonization of the wound surface is not equivalent to infection. Usually, a bacterial density of 10^5 organisms per gram of tissue is required before invasion of underlying viable tissue (burn wound infection) occurs. Infection can occur with lower bacterial densities, but rarely. The most common organisms to cause wound infections are *S. aureus* and *P. aeruginosa*.[20]

An organism's unique virulence, invasiveness, and motility also affect pathogenicity. It has been demonstrated that nonmotile strains of *Pseudomonas* spp. rarely cause infection.[57]

Early Infections

Colonization pattern of burn wounds is somewhat predictable over time. Initially, gram-positive organisms are present; infection that occurs in the first 48 hours after the burn usually is secondary to GAS. Because streptococcal infection can be rapidly invasive and fatal, it was once common practice to administer penicillin prophylactically to all burned patients at the time of admission. The incidence of GAS infections in burned patients has decreased, probably secondary to immediate use of topical antimicrobial therapy. Routine administration of penicillin prophylaxis is not recommended because it can hasten colonization and potential infection with more resistant organisms. *S. aureus* also causes early septicemia. If there is concomitant inhalation injury, organisms that colonize the respiratory tract can cause bacteremia and invade the burn wound.

In the latter part of the first week after injury, environmental and endogenous gram-negative bacilli colonize the wound. *P. aeruginosa* and Enterobacteriaceae are usual. Colonization of the gut is probably the primary event, followed by bacterial translocation and wound colonization. Bacterial translocation is frequent in burned patients because of the disruption of the mucosal barrier from nutritional factors, immunosuppression, disturbance of the normal barrier of bowel flora (from selective pressure of antibiotic administration), and overgrowth of hospital-associated pathogens. Early institution of enteral nutrition satisfies caloric requirements, improves immune function and tissue healing, and preserves the mucosal barrier, thereby decreasing the incidence of septicemia in burn victims.[58] Another proposed mechanism for acquisition of environmental organisms and subsequent infection is immersion of the patient in water or rolling of the patient in soil in an attempt to control the burning at the time of injury.[59]

Complication of burn injuries by tetanus is uncommon in the U.S. In the nonimmune patient who has a wound contaminated with *Clostridium tetani*, neurologic manifestations of tetanus toxin and minor local infection can occur in the first week after injury.[60] Tetanus immunization is administered routinely to burned patients who have not had boosters within 60 months. Tetanus immunoglobulin is given in addition to patients with heavily contaminated wounds whose immunization status is unknown or who have received fewer than three doses of adsorbed tetanus toxoid.[61]

Later Infections

During the second week after injury, gram-negative bacilli continue to be important pathogens, but the burn wound also becomes colonized with fungi. Risk factors associated with fungal wound infection are preceding antibiotic therapy, presence of indwelling central venous catheters, and infusion of parenteral nutrition, especially of solutions containing lipids. Colonization with *Candida* spp. is common in burned patients, but burn wound septicemia is infrequent. When invasive infection occurs, mortality exceeds 90% despite aggressive medical and surgical therapy.[62]

Fungi such as *Aspergillus* spp. and *Fusarium* spp. and members of the Mucoraceae family are rare causes of infection; infection with such organisms is invasive, however, and usually fatal. These infections frequently follow successful treatment of gram-negative bacillary infection with broad-spectrum antibiotics, and they occur in patients with acidosis. Fungi invade tissue rapidly and cause thrombosis, leading to tissue infarction and systemic dissemination. Extremely aggressive surgical measures are indicated urgently, but mortality remains high. Other fungi isolated from burn wounds are *Geotrichum, Rhodotorula, Cephalosporium, Penicillium, Trichosporon, Trichophyton,* and *Fonsecaea* species; these usually do not invade tissue.[63]

Special Sites of Infection

Anaerobic infections are rare in burned pediatric patients. Anaerobic bacteria have been found to colonize burn wounds around the mouth and anus and can have a synergistic role in burn wound infection, however.[64]

Infections of burns involving the ear cartilage can result in suppurative auricular chondritis, which causes pain, fever, and rapidly progressive edema of the auricle followed by liquefaction of cartilage. Avascularity of this tissue makes treatment difficult. Iontophoresis, a technique that uses direct current to drive charged compounds (antibiotics) into local tissues, has been used in conjunction with topical antimicrobial therapy and grafting, with encouraging results.[65,66]

Corneal infections secondary to direct thermal injury, chemical burn, or ectropion and desiccation can cause permanent scarring requiring corneal transplantation. In addition, infected corneal ulcers can perforate and cause herniation of the lens and loss of the eye. Globe exposure secondary to progressive contracture of burned eyelids and facial skin can require acute eyelid release.[67]

Pyomyositis can occur secondary to vascular compromise in deep burns that leads to muscle necrosis or from the unsuspected deep muscle injury in electrical burns. Intracompartmental infection in which there may be associated pyomyositis can result from delayed escharotomy or extravasation of infused fluids or can occur as a complication of splinting and positioning.[68] Treatment is surgical. Osteomyelitis and pyogenic arthritis can occur when bone and joints are exposed.

OTHER INFECTIONS

Respiratory Tract Infections

Pneumonia is the second most common bacterial cause of death in the burned patient.[69] In patients with inhalation injuries, pneumonia occurs most frequently in the first week after injury. Thermal damage produced by inhalation injury predisposes the airway to infection by: (1) producing structural damage to the respiratory tract epithelium; (2) impairing surfactant production, mucociliary transport, and macrophage function; and (3) producing atelectasis. Pneumonia or tracheobronchitis occurs in up to 35% of those with inhalation injury.[20] Less commonly, pneumonia can result from hematogenous spread of infection from other areas, most notably the infected burn wound; this typically occurs late in the postburn period. A chest tube that must be placed through a wound can result in empyema, and should be removed as soon as is practical.[20]

Sinusitis and otitis media are infectious complications of the child requiring nasotracheal intubation for inhalation injury.

Bacteremia

Bacteremia is not uncommon in the burned patient. Risk factors include wound manipulation and the presence of an intravascular catheter. Suppurative thrombophlebitis or infected intravascular thrombus can cause persistent bacteremia. Endocarditis must be considered in any patient with prolonged bacteremia. Bloodstream infections are the most common cause of bacterial related death in patients with severe burns.[69]

Daily dressing changes and surgical wound debridement have been associated with bacteremia in 7.7% to 65% of episodes.[70-73] The greater the percentage of TBSA burned (and thus manipulated), the higher the risk of bacteremia. Use of prophylactic systemic antibiotics before burn wound manipulation, particularly debridement, has been shown to reduce the incidence of bacteremia but has not had a beneficial effect on subsequent clinical course or incidence of burn wound infection.[70,72,73] Bacteremia can occur in the absence of wound manipulation or other identifiable risk factors, presumably from translocation of gut organisms. Bacteremia secondary to burn wound manipulation or gut translocation usually is transient and does not result in infection at distant sites or interfere with graft adherence. It is possible, however, that the higher incidence of endocarditis demonstrated in burned patients is attributable to the increased number of episodes of transient bacteremia. Pyogenic arthritis and brain abscesses secondary to *S. aureus* bacteremia have been described.[74,75]

Catheter-Related Infections

Burned patients have a high risk of acquiring intravascular catheter-related infections. In one study, the rate of catheter-associated infection correlated inversely with the distance of the catheter insertion site from the burn wound; infection occurred more commonly when the insertion site was <30 cm from the burn wound.[76] Suppurative thrombophlebitis, both peripheral and central, also can occur in burned patients and is difficult to diagnose if the affected vein underlies the burn; prolonged antibiotic therapy, systemic anticoagulation, and need for surgery are considered.[20]

Urinary tract infections are common in burned patients, especially associated with urinary catheters commonly used to care for perineal burns or to monitor fluid status. Catheters placed for fluid status monitoring should be removed as soon as the patient's clinical status is stable, and their use should never be prolonged for the convenience of caregivers.

Intra-Abdominal Infections

Acute cholecystitis can occur in older children and adolescents with burns if enteral nutrition is not instituted. Findings include fever without localizing signs and serum hepatic enzyme abnormalities consistent with cholestasis (mimicking findings in septicemia). Acute pancreatitis as well as pancreatic abscess can occur in severely burned patients. Peritonitis, as a result of splanchnic ischemia, increased gastrointestinal permeability, and bacterial translocation can occur.[20] Early enteral feeding decreases the likelihood of these complications.

Central Nervous System Infections

Infectious complications in the central nervous system are infrequent and usually are associated with bacteremia or endocarditis in patients with a burn >30% of TBSA, possibly related to inability to localize infection. In a postmortem review of burned victims, 53% had central nervous system complications, 16% of which were infectious. Microabscess, septic infarction, and meningitis occurred, and most were caused by *S. aureus*, *Candida* spp., or *P. aeruginosa*.[77]

Viral Infections

Viral infections must be considered in any burn victim with unexplained fever whose burn wound is healing adequately.[78-81] Viral infections can occur at any time but are most common in the second week after injury, and can be due to reactivation or acquisition. Herpes simplex virus (HSV) and cytomegalovirus (CMV) have been isolated from up to 30% of pediatric burned patients;[78] infection correlates directly with the TBSA involved.

CMV infection in burn patients is a purported cause of unexplained fever as well as hepatitis, neutropenia, and thrombocytopenia. Other serious manifestations of CMV infections, such as pneumonia, are infrequent. CMV infection can result from reactivation of latent infection or from primary infection. The cell-mediated immune dysfunction experienced by burned patients enhances reactivation of CMV and exacerbates symptomatic infection. Primary infection can be acquired from blood transfusions or cadaveric skin allografts from seropositive donors. CMV infection is associated with greater risk of bacterial infection in patients with burns.

Orolabial reactivation of HSV is common, and the virus can disseminate locally or cause infection of the burn wound, impeding wound healing; disseminated infection also has been described in burned patients.[82,83]

Other viral infections associated with excessive morbidity, delayed wound healing, or unexplained fevers are varicella-zoster virus, Epstein–Barr virus, and adenovirus. One study, performed before testing of the blood supply for hepatitis C virus (HCV), demonstrated that 18% of burned patients acquired HCV. Chronic hepatitis was observed in 83% of burned patients, which is a high rate in comparison with that in other populations.[84] Nosocomially

PART II Clinical Syndromes and Cardinal Features of Infectious Diseases: Approach to Diagnosis and Initial Management

SECTION M Infections Related to Trauma

acquired respiratory syncytial virus, adenovirus, and rotavirus add considerable morbidity during the protracted hospitalization.

TREATMENT

Specialized care in burn centers, the surgical trend toward aggressive early and repeated debridement and wound closure, and the routine use of topical antimicrobial agents contribute immensely to the prevention and control of infections after burns.

Topical antimicrobial therapy is a mainstay of burn care; such therapy has had an enormous impact on the rates of wound infection and septicemia. The general objectives of topical therapy are to decrease water vapor loss, prevent desiccation of exposed viable tissues, contribute to pain control, and inhibit bacterial and fungal growth.[20] Although topical agents do not sterilize the wound, numbers of colonizing organisms decrease, thus reducing the risk of bacterial invasion of underlying tissue. Topical agents commonly used in burned patients differ in their antimicrobial spectrum and side effects (Table 89-2). Other topical agents used in burn care are discussed in Chapter 294 (Topical Antimicrobial Agents). There is no ideal topical antimicrobial agent. An agent is selected on the basis of defined and expected colonizing organisms, time post injury, knowledge of organisms indigenous to the burn unit, and possible adverse reactions. Initially, silver sulfadiazine usually is used, and subsequent choices are based on results of isolation of organisms from the wound. Silver sulfadiazine has fair to poor eschar penetration, unlike mafenide acetate, a carbonic anhydrase inhibitor, which is capable of eschar penetration.[20]

Debridement of the wound is essential. Both enzymatic and chemical means of debridement have been used in the care of burns as alternatives to surgical excision. Proteolytic and mucolytic enzymes rapidly debride nonviable tissue, but have been associated with a higher risk of septicemia.[85] The recently developed Versajet tool, which uses the Venturi effect to create a stream of water for cutting and a vacuum, has been shown to provide more precise excision compared with blade excision and may decrease the time required for excision.[86] Temporary membranes also are available to use on superficial wounds or donor sites to decrease infection and facilitate comfort.[87] Fresh or reconstituted porcine xenograft, synthetic bilaminates, hydrofibers, semipermeable membranes, hydrocolloid dressings, and human allograft are examples, some of which are impregnated with silver to reduce bacterial and fungal growth. Patients with heavily contaminated wounds or septicemia or both are best managed with allografts initially and later with autografts.[20]

Systemic antimicrobial therapy is only used when systemic infection is strongly suspected, but its role is adjunctive and it never replaces aggressive surgical debridement and the use of topical agents. Parenteral agents should be of the narrowest antimicrobial spectrum possible, being directed specifically at known pathogens, to avoid colonization with resistant bacteria or fungi. In burned patients, the pharmacokinetics of antibiotics are altered as a result of the multiple pathophysiologic changes that occur after the burn injury.[88,89] These changes must be considered in selection of agents and optimal dosage.

Aminoglycosides have a short elimination half-life in burned patients, thus requiring increases in both dose and frequency of administration.[90,91] Once-daily aminoglycoside dosing (8 mg/kg) in burned patients (TBSA burned, 18% to 81%) has been evaluated and was associated with elevation of creatinine >0.5 mg/dL in 35% of patients and ototoxicity in 1 of 13 patients.[92] Thus, without further study, once-daily aminoglycoside dosing cannot be recommended in burned patients. Vancomycin clearance is increased in burned patients, possibly because of increased renal tubular secretion; higher dosages may be necessary.[93] Because burned patients may have renal dysfunction, serum levels of aminoglycosides or vancomycin are monitored to allow individual adjustment of dosages.

The pharmacokinetics of ceftazidime, ticarcillin-clavulanate, imipenem-cilastatin, and aztreonam have been evaluated in burned patients.[89,94-97] Alterations were found for ticarcillin-clavulante and ceftazidime (increased total clearance and volume of distribution) and aztreonam (increased volume of distribution). Creatinine clearance does not adequately predict dosage requirements for these drugs; thus, specific dosage recommendations were not made in any study. It seems prudent to use the highest recommended dose in a burned patient who does not have evidence of renal or hepatic impairment.

MANAGEMENT OF OUTPATIENTS

Partial-thickness burns covering a small TBSA (<10% to 15%) can be treated on an outpatient basis in the following circumstances: (1) the burns are not circumferential or do not involve the face, hands, feet, or perineum; (2) no other injuries are present; (3) child abuse is not suspected; and (4) the caregivers are capable of adhering to management and follow-up. Appropriate treatment of smaller burns is imperative, because inadequate care can lead to wound infection, septicemia, poor wound healing, and a poor functional or cosmetic result.

Outpatient management of burns consists of cleaning the wound thoroughly and removing devitalized tissue. Small blisters can be left intact. Because large blisters can interfere with wound healing, most burn surgeons advocate debridement, whereas others believe that this increases the risk of infection.

TABLE 89-2. Topical Antimicrobial Agents Commonly Used in the Treatment of Burns

Agent	Antimicrobial Activity Against				Adverse/Other Effects
	Gram-Positive Organisms	Gram-Negative Organisms	Anaerobes	Fungi	
Silver sulfadiazine (Silvadene, Thermazene)	++	+++	++	++	Allergic reaction in 5% Leukopenia in 5–15%
Mafenide acetate (Sulfamylon)	+	+++	++	+	Allergic reaction in 10% Pain Metabolic acidosis Pulmonary edema
Nanocrystalline silver dressings (Acticoat A.B., Silverlon)	++	+++	++	++	Limited toxicity, less painful than silver nitrate
Nitrofurazone (Furacin)	+++	+++	++	–	Dermatitis Fungal overgrowth

+++, excellent activity; ++, good activity; +, limited activity; –, no activity.

Data from references 110 and 111.

After cleaning and debridement, gauze dressing containing a broad-spectrum topical antibiotic such as silver sulfadiazine is applied. The dressing is changed with new application of antibiotic twice daily, and the parent or caregiver is educated about the expected changes in appearance of the wound. The wound is inspected 24 to 48 hours later to observe the expected healing, to detect signs of local infection, and to assess adequacy of parents' understanding of wound care.

PREVENTION

Prevention of infection in a burn is paramount to prevent mortality and morbidity. Urgent and adequate care of all burns and use of dressings impregnated with topical antimicrobial agents, followed by meticulous care and assessment, usually are successful. Early closure of the burn wound is the most protective treatment against infection. Pulmonary toilet in the patient with inhalation injury and rapid removal of intravenous and urinary catheters are essential in prevention of nosocomial infections. Strict attention to infection control practices is essential.

Routine use of prophylactic systemic antibiotics is not beneficial in prevention of infections and can predispose to colonization with resistant organisms.[98] Replacement therapy with immune globulin intravenous (IGIV) has been studied, because most burned patients show a decrease in serum immunoglobulin (Ig) G concentration immediately after injury (mean values, 300 mg/dL), with a gradual return to normal after 14 to 60 days.[34,35] In one study, patients younger than 4 years had the most severe and prolonged decreases of IgG levels.[30] Patients with persistent serum IgG concentrations of <500 mg/dL may have a higher risk of septic complications.[31] Although IgG levels normalized with administration of IGIV in the patients studied (from mean of 400 mg/dL pre-infusion to >1200 mg/dL post-infusion), no beneficial effect on development of septicemia was evident.[99] Administration of hyperimmune globulin G against *P. aeruginosa* and *S. aureus* decades ago as adjunctive treatment for septicemia caused by these organisms in burned patients showed some beneficial effect.[100–102]

Interferon-γ, because of its ability to enhance macrophage activity and stimulate host immune responses, has been evaluated as prophylaxis for infectious complications in burned patients. In a European multicenter trial of 216 patients with severe burn injuries, administration of interferon-γ did not give protection from infectious complications or affect the mortality from infections.[103]

A vaccine directed against *P. aeruginosa* was developed decades ago and shown to be efficacious.[104–108] In one study of 322 burned patients, administration of maximal-dose vaccine reduced the rate of invasive disease. A lower mortality was only seen, however, in patients who received parenteral antibiotic therapy and adjunctive hyperimmune globulin. Vaccination did not prevent colonization and 90% of the patients had an adverse reaction to vaccination.[105] In 2000 a double-blind, randomized, placebo-controlled clinical trial of a *P. aeruginosa* vaccine involving 95 adult patients with burn injuries of ≥10% TBSA demonstrated high immunogenicity and a significantly lower incidence of *P. aeruginosa* bacteremia in vaccine recipients.[109] Additional controlled studies are required to assess the benefit of immunotherapy, in view of changes in predominant pathogens, improved supportive measures, and the trend toward early excision and wound closure.

90 Infection following Bites

Marvin B. Harper

In the United States, it is estimated that 4.7 million dog bites, 400,000 cat bites, and 250,000 human bites occur every year.[1] Dog bites alone result in approximately 330,000 emergency department visits (42% among children <14 years of age), 13,000 hospitalizations, and 20 deaths annually (mostly children).[2] Dogs, cats, and humans account for >90% of non-insect-related bite injuries, with rabbits and rodents responsible for most of the remainder.[1,3] The trauma caused by these bites can be quite serious, and infection is the most common late complication.

ETIOLOGIC AGENTS

The organisms causing bite wound infections generally derive from the microbial flora of the biting animal's mouth rather than the victim's skin. Therefore, the infecting organisms vary by species. Bite wound infections should be considered polymicrobial infections; in a large, prospective study of infected dog and cat bites, cultures done at a central reference laboratory yielded a median of five bacterial isolates per culture.[4] Mixed aerobic and anaerobic infection occurred in more than 50% of cases. Specimens sent concomitantly to local microbiology laboratories identified significantly fewer organisms, emphasizing the need for careful microbiologic analysis.

Table 90-1 shows the aerobic and anaerobic bacteria isolated from 50 patients with dog, 57 with cat, and 50 with human bite wounds.[4,5] *Pasteurella* species were the most common isolates from both types of bites, with *P. canis* the predominant organism isolated from dog bites and *P. multocida* the most common from cat bites. Other species isolated from these patients included streptococci, staphylococci, and *Moraxella* and *Neisseria* species. Common anaerobic isolates included *Fusobacterium, Bacteroides, Porphyromonas, Prevotella, Propionibacterium,* and *Peptostreptococcus* species. A number of other bacterial isolates previously had not been recognized as bite wound pathogens.

Other studies confirm polymicrobial nature of bite wounds.[6,7] *Pasteurella multocida* is only seen in animal bites, more commonly from cats,[8] whereas *Eikenella corrodens* and *Streptococcus pyogenes* are more closely associated with human bites, although they are sometimes seen with animal bites as well. *Capnocytophaga canimorsus,*[9,10] *C. cynodegmi,*[9] *Neisseria weaveri* (formerly M-5),[11,12] *Bergeyella zoohelcum,*[13] *Neisseria canis,*[14] *Staphylococcus intermedius,*[15] NO-1,[16] and EO-2[17] are all uncommon organisms to recover from general clinical specimens but are isolated from bite wound infections, particularly from dog bites.

The cause of infections resulting from bites of species other than humans, dogs, and cats is less well described. Simian bites appear to be similar to human bites in microbiology.[18] Polymicrobial infections with *Staphylococcus aureus, Streptococcus pyogenes, Pseudomonas aeruginosa,* and *Bacillus* species have been reported with camel bites.[19] Bites of larger cat species such as leopards and tigers are associated with organisms typical of domestic cat bites, with isolation of *P. multocida* and *N. weaveri.*[20] Snake bites do not routinely require antibiotic management unless there is necrosis, in which case aerobic gram-positive cocci and gram-negative bacilli are thought to predominate.[21] A *Pasteurella caballi* infection was seen after a horse bite,[22] *Pasteurella aerogenes* and a *Chryseobacterium*-like organism have been isolated from infected pig bites,[23,24] *Actinobacillus* species have been reported from horse and sheep bite

TABLE 90-1. Frequency of Isolation of Aerobic and Anaerobic Bacteria Following 50 Dog, 57 Cat, and 50 Human Bite Wounds at Presentation for Management of Infection

	Dog	Cat	Human		Dog	Cat	Human
AEROBIC AND FACULTATIVE				Pediococcus	+		
Acinetobacter		+	+	Proteus	+		+
Aggregatibacter (formerly Actinobacillus)		+	+	Pseudomonas aeruginosa	+		
Aerococcus viridans			+	Pseudomonas non-aeruginosa	+	+	
Aeromonas		+	+	Reimerella anatipestifer		+	
Agrobacterium radiobacter			+	Rhodococcus		+	
Alcaligenes		+	+	Rothia		+	+
Bacillus	+	++		Staphylococcus aureus	+++	+	++++
Brevibacterium	+	+		Staphylococcus coagulase-negative	+++++	+++++	++++
Candida			+	Stenotrophomonas maltophilia	+		
Capnocytophaga	+	+	+	Stomatococcus mucilaginosus	+		+
CDC group EF-4a	+			Streptococcus species	+++++	+++++	+++++
CDC group EF-4b	++	++		Streptococcus pyogenes (group A)	++		++
CDC group NO-2			+	Streptococcus agalactiae (group B)	+	+	
Citrobacter			+	Streptococcus group C/G	+		+
Corynebacterium species	++	+++	++	Streptococcus group F		+	
Corynebacterium jeikeium	+	+		Streptococcus viridans group	+++++	+++++	+++++
Corynebacterium pseudodiphtheriticum	+		+	Streptococcus milleri group (Streptococcus intermedius, Streptococcus anginosus, Streptococcus constellatus)	++	+	+++++
Dermabacter hominis	+			Streptomyces		+	
Eikenella corrodens	+	+	++++	Weeksella	+	+	
Enterobacter cloacae		+	+	**ANAEROBIC**			
Enterococcus	++	++	+	Actinomyces			+
Erysipelothrix		+		Arcanobacterium bernardiae			+
Flavimonas	+	+		Bacteroides	++++	+++	+
Flavobacterium	+			Campylobacter			++
Gemella	+	+	++	Clostridium		+	
Haemophilus			+++	Collinsella (Eubacterium) aerofaciens			+
Kingella			+	Dialister pneumosintes			+
Klebsiella	+	+	+	Eubacterium	+	+	++
Kocuria			+	Filifactor villosus		+	
Lactobacillus	+	+	+	Fusobacterium species	++++	++++	++++
Leclercia			+	Fusobacterium necrophorum			+
Micrococcus	+		+	Fusobacterium nucleatum	++	+++	++++
Moraxella	++	++++	+	Lactobacillus	+		
Neisseria	++	++	+	Peptostreptococcus	++	+	+++
Oerskovia	+			Porphyromonas	+++	++++	+
Pantoea endophytica		+	+	Prevotella	+++	++	++++
Pasteurella	+++++	+++++		Propionibacterium	+++	++	+
Pasteurella canis	+++	+		Veillonella		+	+++
Pasteurella multocida ssp. multocida	++	+++++					
Pasteurella multocida ssp. septica	++	+++					

wounds,[25] and *Halomonas venusta* has been isolated from a fish bite.[26] In bites occurring in marine settings, organisms associated with water, such as *Vibrio* species, *Aeromonas hydrophila*, *Plesiomonas shigelloides*, and *Pseudomonas* species, have caused infections from bites of catfish, eel, crocodile, and swan.[27-31] Additionally, systemic diseases have been transmitted by bites, including, tularemia from cats,[32] rat-bite (Haverhill) fever, and sodoku from rats, herpesvirus B infection from monkeys, hepatitis B from humans, and leptospirosis from dogs and rodents. A rare infectious entity acquired from contact with seals, known as seal finger, is likely caused by a marine mycoplasma.[33] Human immunodeficiency virus (HIV) appears to be difficult to transmit by human bite.[34-36]

EPIDEMIOLOGY

Dog bites account for >80% of bite wounds that come to medical attention. The annual incidence of dog bites of children has been estimated at 1 to 3 per 1000 children per year[37-40] in developed countries, to rates as high as 26 per 1000 per year in developing countries.[41] Dog bite injuries alone account for 0.3% to 0.4% of all emergency department visits.[2,37] The incidence and body part involved with dog bites vary by age. Children are more likely than adults to sustain a dog bite, with the highest risk in the second year of life and steadily decreasing each year thereafter (based on data from Austria) or with peak incidence in the 5- to 9-year age group (based on U.S. data).[37,38] Injuries to the face, head, and neck are most common, accounting for two-thirds of dog bite injuries in preschool children (extremities accounting for 27%). Injuries to the extremities (upper more than lower) become more common with increasing age, accounting for 55% beyond 14 years of age (at which age only 9% involve the head or neck).[38] Between 7% and 25% of children sustaining dog bites require hospital admission, depending on use of general anesthesia for primary wound management and the rate of infectious complications.[37,42]

Fatalities from bites occur primarily from massive blood loss after mauling by large dogs, particularly Rottweiler and pitbull-type dogs or as the result of intracranial injury, particularly in smaller children.[43] Children less than 5 years of age are particularly vulnerable to attack and are more likely to sustain injury from smaller dogs. Overall the relative risk of attack is significantly higher from German shepherd, Doberman, pitbull, and Rottweiler breeds than from Labrador/retriever or cross-bred dogs, but because cross-bred dogs are so much more common, they represent the majority of bite injuries. The majority of dog bites are from dogs owned by the family or friends of the family. Approximately 20 deaths occur each year in the U.S. as a result of dog bite attacks. Infectious deaths due to dog bites are uncommon but can occur as the result of septicemia or intracranial infection. In developing countries, rabies remains a significant late cause of death from dog bites. The estimated risk of infection in the otherwise healthy child depends on the location and extent of the dog bite injury, and the initial management, but is estimated to be from 5% to 15%.

Cat bites are spread more evenly across age groups and cause much less overall initial injury because cats have smaller mouths and less biting force, which results in less tearing of the tissues. However, their thin, sharp teeth produce small deep wounds that are difficult to cleanse and are more likely to result in clinical infection, estimated to be from 10% to 50%.

Human bites may be sustained somewhat differently than bites of other animals and are generally defined as any disruption in the skin as a result of contact with the mouth. These can be self-inflicted (e.g., thumb-sucking resulting in skin breakdown, or self-injury as with autism), the result of a punch to the mouth of another person that results in a laceration to the hand, or may be the result of a typical bite but resulting from sexual activity or abuse that might be concealed from the medical provider. One study of human bite wounds in children seen at a single institution over a 6-year period identified 322 patients, representing 0.2% of all emergency department visits. Infection was seen in 9%, and 2%, overall, were hospitalized for treatment of infection.[44]

Table 90-2 displays the site of bite injuries from any source summarized from two studies.[44,45] Each study enrolled subjects at the time of initial presentation to the outpatient setting, allowing a more accurate estimation of the subsequent rate of infection such as cellulitis or abscess. Bites to the hand are significantly more likely to become infected compared with bites at other sites. Wounds to the face are the least likely to become infected, probably because of its extensive vascularity. In one of these studies,[45] 12% of the wounds became infected, and the risk of infection differed on the basis of the biting species. Only 3 (4%) of 80 dog bites became infected, but 6 (16%) of 37 human bites and 11 (50%) of 22 cat bites became infected. The most common organisms causing infection from dog and cat bites are *P. multocida, S. aureus*, streptococci, *C. canimorsus*, and oral anaerobes. Cat bites also have been associated with transmission of cat-scratch disease (*Bartonella henselae*) and sporotrichosis.[46,47] Human bite wound infections additionally can be caused by *Eikenella corrodens* and are not associated with *P. multocida* infections. *Fusobacterium,*

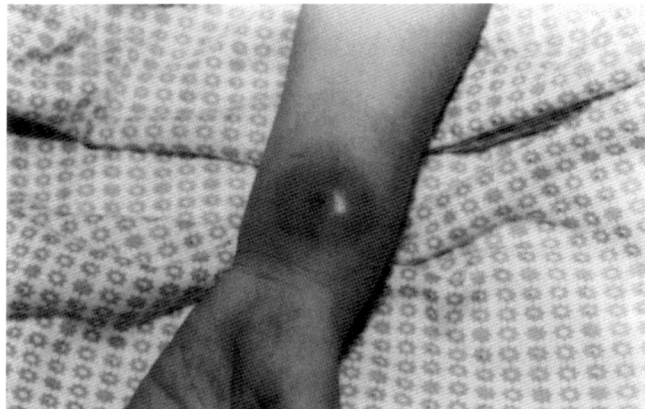

Figure 90-1. Cat-bite abscess of the wrist with presentation for care delayed 1 month after injury. *Pasteurella multocida* was isolated in pure culture.

Prevotella, Peptostreptococcus, and *Candida* also are seen.[5] The paucity of reports regarding infection after rodent or rabbit bites makes the rate difficult to estimate but appears to be small, perhaps related to smaller and less penetrating wounds. Rat bites are associated with *Streptobacillus moniliformis* infections, hamster bites have caused tularemia, and *P. aerogenes* infections[48,49] and guinea pigs have caused *Haemophilus influenzae* infections.[50] Bat bite is important because it can transmit rabies virus. Infections transmitted by biting insects are addressed in other chapters.

PATHOGENESIS

Bite wounds become infected by inoculation of microorganisms into subcutaneous or deeper tissues. Modifying factors include the type and depth of inoculation, the amount of crush injury and devitalized tissue, the involvement of infection-prone structures, the ability to cleanse and debride the wound, and the pathogenicity of the infecting microorganism. Most series show a higher infection rate in bite wounds to the hand. Cat bites have the highest infection rates, probably because they are usually puncture wounds that inoculate bacteria deeply, making wound care more difficult, and because of the high prevalence of *P. multocida* (Figure 90-1). Dog bites are more likely to cause lacerations or avulsion injuries that are easier to clean and debride.

Most infections manifest as local cellulitis or simple abscess. Infection can extend to adjacent areas, particularly if the teeth penetrate structures such as bones or joints in bites to an extremity or the cranium in injuries to the head and face. Regional lymphadenopathy, lymphangitis, fasciitis, toxic shock syndrome, septicemia, and shock also can develop. Septicemia occurs primarily in immunocompromised hosts, particularly asplenic individuals, who are prone to fulminant septicemia and shock with infection caused by *C. canimorsus*,[51-55] or *Eubacterium plautii*[56] after dog bites.

CLINICAL MANIFESTATIONS, DIFFERENTIAL DIAGNOSIS, AND CLINICAL APPROACH

The history and physical examination readily lead to the likely organisms of most bite wound infections (Box 90-1). Signs and symptoms, such as erythema, pain, tenderness, and swelling, almost always become apparent within 24 to 48 hours after the bite. Infections caused by *P. multocida* tend to have a more rapid onset, often within 12 to 18 hours. There may be purulent or serosanguineous discharge. Most patients are afebrile,[4] although fever can occur in patients with severe cellulitis or in the rare instance of bacteremia. The presence of eschariform lesions at bite sites in individuals who appear ill may indicate *C. canimorsus* infection.[54]

The extent of the infection must be determined carefully. Even apparently trivial bites require careful evaluation for penetration

TABLE 90-2. Rates of Infection of Bite Wounds by Body Site

Location of Bite	Rate (%)	# Infected/# Bites
Face/head/neck	6	3/49
Arm/leg	10	7/68
Trunk	10	1/10
Hand	28	21/76
Total	16	32/203

Data from Baker MD, Moore SE. Human bites in children. Pediatrics 1991;88:55; and Aghabian RV, Conte JE Jr. Mammalian bite wounds. Ann Emerg Med 1980;9:79.

PART II Clinical Syndromes and Cardinal Features of Infectious Diseases: Approach to Diagnosis and Initial Management

SECTION M Infections Related to Trauma

HISTORY

The animal

Record type of animal, health of animal, whether attack was provoked or unprovoked, and consider the availability for testing or quarantine for signs of rabies, if applicable. Were local authorities notified (e.g., animal control or police officers)?

The patient

Consider special risks such as immunosuppression, asplenia, diabetes mellitus, antibiotic allergies, and history of tetanus and hepatitis B immunizations

PHYSICAL EXAMINATION

Systemic

Note fever, tachycardia, tachypnea, hypotension, or widened pulse pressure

Local

Note type of wound (e.g., puncture, laceration, avulsion), depth of penetration, involvement of underlying structures (e.g., joint, tendon, bone, cranial contents), extent of edema, erythema, tenderness (with measurements), range of motion, type of drainage (e.g., purulent, serosanguineous, malodorous), neurovascular function, lymphangitic streaking, and regional lymphadenopathy. Consider possibility of retained foreign body (e.g., tooth)

of the skull or other body cavities or possible damage to underlying structures, such as joint spaces, bone, tendons, nerves, and blood vessels. In bite wounds, the physician should consider the size of the mouth of the animal involved and if there are puncture wounds, examine carefully for punctures due to the apposing teeth. For instance, with cosmetically important bite wounds to the face in young children there may be more life-threatening puncture wounds found in the scalp or neck that could be missed easily unless the child is carefully evaluated.[57] The need to assess involvement of deep structures is particularly important for scalp injuries that can penetrate the skull, and for clenched-fist injuries in which joint or tendon injury may be missed.[58] Lacerations sustained when punching and striking teeth most commonly occur on the dorsal aspect of the third metacarpophalangeal joint. Because the injury occurs with a closed fist the injury may not be recognized when examined in the relaxed position; in addition, the initially linear path of injury becomes obstructed, hindering drainage of deep structures.

Paronychial infections, in young children, can result from thumb- or finger-sucking, and oral flora should be considered as a possible cause, especially when a history of injury is lacking. Herpetic whitlow, which can be confused with bacterial infection, should be suspected when erythematous or dusky-appearing vesicular or vesiculobullous lesions are present, particularly in cluster arrangement. Seal finger, which occurs in association with either seal bites or scratches or other contact with seals, has a slightly different clinical presentation. The incubation period is longer (4 to 8 days), edema and severe pain are prominent, and lymphangitis, lymphadenitis, and arthritis occur more frequently than in other bite wound infections.[59] Water organisms, such as *P. aeruginosa* and *Aeromonas* species, should be considered when bites from water animals occur.

LABORATORY FINDINGS AND DIAGNOSIS

Microbiologic confirmation of infection can be highly beneficial in managing bite wound infections regardless of the species causing the bite. Laboratory personnel should be notified that the specimen is from a bite wound, thus allowing consideration of multiple isolates as well as organisms that can be difficult to identify, such as *P. multocida* or *E. corrodens*. Specimens should be sent for both aerobic and anaerobic bacterial culture, taking special care that proper anaerobic transport medium is used. For wounds contaminated by soil or vegetative debris, culture for mycobacteria and fungi should be considered. However, Gram stain and culture of fresh, uninfected bite wounds are not recommended, because they do not predict the risk of subsequent infection or the pathogens that cause them.

Blood specimens for aerobic and anaerobic culture should be obtained from febrile children, particularly if they are immunocompromised or asplenic. Radiographs should be obtained after penetrating injuries overlying bones or joints, when a fracture is suspected, or when a foreign body is suspected.

MANAGEMENT AND PRESUMPTIVE THERAPY

Immediate Postexposure Management

1. Evaluate the Extent of the Injury and Contamination

New, uninfected bites should be carefully examined for foreign bodies, and visible dirt and debris should be sponged or irrigated away.

2. Debride and Cleanse the Wound

The wound should be copiously irrigated with sterile normal saline by high-pressure syringe irrigation, taking care not to inject into the tissue or inflict additional trauma.

a. Consider use of a surgical-type scrub sponge for highly contaminated wounds, especially if particulate matter is present. (Hibiclens or Betadine should not be used, unless diluted to 1%, as these can cause tissue toxicity. Agents such as Pluronic-68 or Shur-Clens are suggested.)

b. Irrigate with ≥250 mL of saline. There is no demonstrated benefit to irrigation with other solutions such as 1% Betadine solution or Pluronic F-68.[60] Antibiotic irrigation has not been shown to have additional benefit; rarely it may be used in special, high-risk circumstances. Animal models suggest high-pressure irrigation reduces bacterial wound counts better and reduces wound infection rates. Irrigation pressures of 5 to 8 pounds per square inch (psi) are recommended clinically and correspond to gentle use of commercially available splash guard shields (e.g., Zerowet) or an 18G catheter/needle attached to a 30 or 60 mL syringe.

c. Perform imaging to establish the presence or absence of foreign material such as embedded teeth or fragments as well as to identify bone damage.

d. Debride devitalized tissue and remove foreign material. Operative exploration and debridement should be considered if there is extensive tissue damage, involvement of a joint space, or cranial injury. There is no role for culture of the wound unless there is clinical evidence of infection.

3. Consider Wound Closure

The role of suturing, in general, is controversial for bite wounds. One study evaluated the practice of primary closure for mammalian bites in a series of 145 consecutive bites (88 dog, 45 cat, 12 human) treated with primary closure. Patients presented a mean of 2 hours after injury. Six percent (95% confidence interval 2% to 9%) experienced wound infections, suggesting that when cosmesis is a primary concern, this rate of infection may be acceptable.[61] Increasing time to closure has been associated with increasing risk for infection but more likely the time to closure is simply a proxy for the time to adequate wound cleansing (often done together with the repair). This has led to specific recommendations against closure for high-risk wounds if more than 8 to 12 hours have passed from the time of injury. This has not been specifically studied in children and there are no prospective data validating this approach with bite wounds. Nonetheless, in the absence of further data, it may be prudent to avoid primary closure if time since trauma is >8 hours or it is difficult to irrigate a deep puncture wound (unless the wound(s) must be repaired for important cosmetic or functional reasons).[1,62] When closure is appropriate, the placement of a drain, microdrains, or only loose approximation of the skin is the optimal approach when feasible. The use of subcutaneous sutures has been associated with increased risk of infection in retrospective studies and their use should be avoided. An underutilized practice is delayed closure (after 48 to 72 hours) of this type of wound. Delayed closure has been recommended for human bites to the head and neck, especially those with exposed cartilage.[63] Elevation and immobilization of the wound are common practice.

4. Consider Postexposure Prophylaxis

a. Antibiotic prophylaxis. The role of antimicrobial prophylaxis is discussed in Chapter 7 (Chemoprophylaxis). Limited data are available from clinical trials. A Cochrane analysis concluded that there is evidence that antibiotic administration significantly reduces infection rates with bites to the hand or human bites.[64] One meta-analysis suggested that antibiotic treatment also lowered

---

BOX 90-2. Indications for Infection Prophylaxis

ANTIBIOTIC RECOMMENDED
Characteristics of the wound

Bite wounds of the face, hands, feet, or genital area
Wounds that cannot be reliably cleansed or completely debrided, e.g., deep punctures
Bite wounds involving tendon, bone, or joint
Wounds with moderate or severe edema, crush injury, or devitalized tissue

Characteristics of the host

Immunocompromised or asplenic host

OTHER POSTEXPOSURE PROPHYLAXIS RECOMMENDED
Hepatitis B

Begin vaccine if a human bite and the patient is not previously immunized. The use of hepatitis B immune globulin is limited to cases in which the biter is known to be hepatitis B surface antigen-positive

Human immunodeficiency virus (HIV)

Prophylaxis is limited to high-risk human bite exposures from known HIV-positive biter (the need for HIV postexposure prophylaxis of bite wounds is uncommon)

Rabies

Administer rabies immune globulin and begin vaccine series for mammalian bites, indicating possible exposure
Administer rabies immune globulin and begin vaccine series

Tetanus

Give DTaP (or DT if not available) DT to those <7 years if primary vaccine series is not up to schedule; give Tdap Td to those 7 years through to 10 years of age whose DTaP series was incomplete; give Tdap to those or Tdap (if not previously received) to these 10 or 11 years of age or older (depending on product licensure) if series is not up to schedule for adolescent dose or if 5 years since last tetanus-containing booster if they have not received Tdap previously. Give tetanus immune globulin to those not known to have received at least three previous doses of tetanus toxoid vaccine or those unlikely to have immune response to the vaccine

---

BOX 90-3. Recommended Antibiotic Therapy

WOUND PROPHYLAXIS IF INDICATED

Amoxicillin-clavulanate; if penicillin-allergic, trimethoprim-sulfamethoxazole plus clindamycin

TREATMENT OF WOUND INFECTION

Oral therapy as above unless febrile, rapidly spreading, or high-risk: then use parenteral therapy
Parenteral therapy if indicated:
- Ampicillin-sulbactam (consider aminoglycoside if reptile or water-related species)
- If penicillin-allergic without anaphylaxis, consider using extended-spectrum cephalosporin or carbapenem (e.g., ceftriaxone, cefipime, or meropenem) *or* if severe allergy, use trimethoprim-sulfamethoxazole plus clindamycin and consider addition of aminoglycoside if reptile or water-associated
- Vancomycin should be considered in severe infections if MRSA, methicillin-resistant *Staphylococcus aureus* is a possibility
- Clindamycin, doxycycline, or trimethoprim-sulfamethoxazole considered for less serious, possible MRSA
- Bite wound infection in the immunocompromised host can include many other pathogens; treatment individualized

---

the risk of infection after dog bites.[65] One small study randomized patients with human bite wounds to placebo or cephalexin/penicillin combination and identified a low rate of infection in both groups (1 of 62 receiving placebo and 0 of 63 individuals receiving antibiotic).[66] Despite limited data regarding efficacy, antibiotic prophylaxis commonly is recommended for infection-prone bite wounds: in moderate to severe wounds (especially if edema or crush injury is present), wounds that are difficult to clean or debride adequately, penetrating cat bite(s), and human bite wounds. On the other hand, less severe wounds or more easily cleansed and dog bite wounds to areas other than the face, hands, feet, or genital area do not require antibiotic prophylaxis routinely. The ability of the host (e.g., immunocompromised patients) to deal with infection, should it occur, should also be taken into consideration (Box 90-2).[1,58] The drug of choice is amoxicillin-clavulanic acid, which is given for 2 to 3 days. All patients with bite wounds should be re-evaluated within 24 to 48 hours for signs of infection (Box 90-3).

b. Tetanus prophylaxis. Bites generally are not tetanus-prone injuries unless there is additional contamination with soil. They are, however, an opportunity to assess the patient's vaccination status. For persons with tetanus-prone injuries who have not completed their primary series, tetanus immune globulin and the vaccine should be administered (see Chapter 188, *Clostridium tetani* (Tetanus)).

c. Rabies prophylaxis. The possibility of rabies must be considered after animal bites (see Chapter 228, Rabies Virus). Bites from bats are considered high risk for rabies in the U.S. and postexposure prophylaxis for these bites is routine. Local public health authorities can assist in determining the need for postexposure rabies prophylaxis.

d. Consideration of systemic infectious agents related to human bites. Hepatitis B, hepatitis C, and HIV could be transmitted potentially by a human bite. Hepatitis B prophylaxis should be considered for human bites. Human bites do not efficiently transmit HIV; postexposure prophylaxis for HIV is not routinely indicated, although it may need to be considered in some special circumstances.[34,35]

e. Consideration of cercopithecine herpesvirus 1 (herpes simiae or B virus) after bites from an Old World macaque monkey. Little is known regarding the risk of infection after a monkey bite but the majority of macaque monkeys are seropositive for herpes simiae by 2 years of age and more than 20 cases of transmission to humans have been reported with development of encephalitis (75% fatal). As a result, copious wound irrigation is recommended; irrigation with diluted sodium hypochlorite (household bleach diluted 1 : 10 with 0.9% saline) is considered as is postexposure antiviral chemoprophylaxis with acyclovir or valacyclovir for 14 days.[67–69]

Most jurisdictions require bite injuries to be reported to the local health department. In cases with multiple or severe bites there is a high risk of posttraumatic stress disorder and referral for counseling should be considered.[70]

EMPIRIC MANAGEMENT WHEN INFECTION OCCURS

When a patient comes to medical attention with an infected bite wound, basic principles of management should be followed. Sutured wounds should be opened, purulent collections should be drained, and necrotic tissue, foreign bodies, and debris removed. Specimens should be obtained for aerobic and anaerobic culture. Infected wounds should not be sutured. If bone or joint penetration has occurred, exploration and debridement of these areas may be necessary.

Empiric antimicrobial therapy for infected wounds should be based on pathogens that are most likely to be associated with the biting species and the clinical setting. Oral antibiotic therapy is appropriate for mild to moderate infections when adherence to the treatment plan is assured. Amoxicillin-clavulanic acid is an excellent choice because it provides activity against all common bite wound pathogens, including anaerobic bacteria, methicillin-susceptible *Staphylococcus aureus*, *S. pyogenes*, *E. corrodens*, and *P. multocida*. Comparable parenteral agents, such as ampicillin-sulbactam or ticarcillin-clavulanic acid, can be used for patients who require hospitalization because of rapidly spreading cellulitis or lymphangitis, large abscesses, bone or joint infection, or suspected sepsis. Appropriate alternative regimens include an extended-spectrum cephalosporin (cefotaxime or ceftriaxone) plus clindamycin. Trimethoprim-sulfamethoxazole has activity against *Pasteurella* and *Eikenella* species, and a combination of trimethoprim-sulfamethoxazole and clindamycin is acceptable for individuals with a history of anaphylactic reactions to penicillins or cephalosporins. Antibiotics commonly used for other skin and soft-tissue infections, such as the antistaphylococcal penicillins, first-generation cephalosporins, vancomycin, clindamycin, and erythromycin, are less active against *Pasteurella* and *Eikenella* species and should not be used as single agents in bite wound infections.[4,71] Azithromycin and fluoroquinolone agents have in vitro activity against the organisms that commonly cause bite wound infections,[72,73] but data on their clinical effectiveness are limited. Tetracycline is the treatment of choice for seal finger and is also active against most aerobic bacteria that cause bite wound infections, including *Pasteurella*;[72] however, tetracyclines generally are not recommended for children under age 8, because they may stain the teeth.

A 7- to 14-day course of antibiotic treatment usually is sufficient for infections limited to the soft tissues. For bone or joint infections, >3 weeks of treatment generally is required. In all cases, the duration and route of antibiotic therapy should be individualized, based on the infected site, culture results, antimicrobial susceptibility testing, and response to treatment.

COMPLICATIONS

The most common complications of bite wound infections are related to tissue destruction. Soft-tissue necrosis can result from infection or from crush injury during the bite. Pyogenic arthritis or osteomyelitis, particularly in cases in which diagnosis is delayed, can result in permanent injury to the joint or bone. Depending on the site of the bite, other complications, such as brain abscess, can develop.[74] Septicemia and meningitis can occur, especially in immunocompromised individuals.

PROGNOSIS AND SEQUELAE

Long-term follow-up studies of children sustaining bite wound infections are not available. In general, soft-tissue infections that are treated promptly and appropriately are expected to heal completely, unless the injury itself has resulted in extensive tissue devitalization. Infections involving underlying bone, tendon, or joint structures have a more guarded prognosis for return to normal function. Goldstein[58] reported residual sequelae in 25% to 50% of patients after clenched-fist injury. In other series, permanent disabilities of the involved extremity were less common and often were related to delayed or inappropriate therapy.[75,76] A delay in therapy, particularly that caused by a failure to recognize deep (bone, joint, or tendon) involvement, may be the most important factor leading to a poor outcome.

PREVENTION

Prevention of bites is the most important measure to decrease bite wounds. This can be accomplished, to some degree, through education of the public to limit exposure of preschool-age children to dogs, selection of specific dog breeds or spaying or neutering dogs, which makes them less likely to bite, and through education of children on proper behavior around animals and the proper respect for dogs. Proper cleansing and debridement of wounds remain the cornerstone for the prevention of wound infections, although antimicrobial prophylaxis also can play an important role in preventing infection for certain bite wounds.

91   Infections Related to Pets and Exotic Animals

Joseph A. Bocchini, Jr and Larry K. Pickering

Contact with animals can provide benefits for children and adults. However, exposure to nontraditional pets in the home and animals in public settings each pose potential risks to children. These risks can be associated with injuries to people that result from changes in physical and behavioral characteristics as young animals reach maturity or from transmission of pathogenic organisms. Potential risks can be minimized or prevented by knowledge and use of educational materials, regulations, and guidelines that have been developed for this purpose.[1,2] Healthcare personnel

(HCP) including pediatricians and veterinarians can provide advice on selection of appropriate pets as well as prevention of disease transmission from nontraditional pets and when children contact animals in public settings.

PET EXPOSURES

The majority of households in the United States include one or more pets. In national surveys conducted by the American Pet

Products Manufacturers Association (APPMA), U.S. households with one or more pets increased from 56% in 1998 to 62% (72.9 million homes) in 2011.[3] Numbers of households in the U.S. owning pets are for dogs, 46.3 million; cats, 38.9 million; freshwater fish, 11.9 million; birds, 5.7 million; small animals (including sloths, porcupines, kinkojous, wallabies, sugar gliders), 5.0 million; reptiles, 4.6 million; horses, 2.4 million; saltwater fish, 0.7 million; and hedgehogs, 0.04 million. Total U.S. expenditures in the pet industry in 2010 was estimated at $48.3 billion.[3] In recent years, the number of families choosing nontraditional pets has increased.

CATEGORIES OF PETS

Animals that become pets can be classified as *traditional* pets and *nontraditional* pets. Traditional pets generally include dogs and cats. Nontraditional pets include exotic animals, defined either as imported, non-native species or species that originally were non-native but now are bred in the U.S.; indigenous wildlife; and wildlife hybrids (wildlife crossbred with domestic animals, producing offspring known as hybrids). The definition of nontraditional pets includes reptiles and certain species of mammals. In addition to exposure to animals in their homes, children may come in contact with animals in a variety of public settings.[2] Although there are many benefits to experiences with animals outside the home, contact with animals in public settings can be associated with substantial risks to children, including infections and injuries. These potential risks are exaggerated when there is inadequate understanding – of disease transmission, methods of transmission prevention, or animal behavior, or lack of appropriate facilities for the care of animals.

Traditional pets. Pets have become part of many families and are often considered to be extended family – living, eating, and even sleeping with human family members.[4] Among dog owners in the U.S., 53% consider their dog to be a member of the family and 56% of dog owners sleep with their dogs next to them. In developed countries, 21% to 23% of dogs and 60% of cats sleep on/in their owners' beds.[4] Transmission of zoonotic agents by close contact between healthy traditional pets and family members through kissing, licking, or biting by pets has been documented,[1,4-6] but is uncommon.

In children, bite injuries are caused by a wide variety of traditional and nontraditional pets, but most wounds result in minor injuries and are not reported. Most systematic studies are limited to dog or cat bites. Bacteria from animal bites are reflective of the oral flora of the biting animal or less commonly of victim's own skin. The oral flora of the biting animal also may contain flora of ingested prey and other foods.[5]

Nontraditional pets. Nontraditional pets are increasing in popularity among families, as lifestyle choices of owners may favor smaller or more unusual pets. Table 91-1 provides examples of animals that are considered nontraditional pets as well as animals to which children may be exposed in public settings.

Since 1998, the number of exotic animals available in the U.S. has increased 75%.[3] In 2005, 87,991 mammals (including 29 species of rodents), 1.3 million reptiles, and 203 million fish were imported legally into the U.S. The U.S. Fish and Wildlife Service estimated that in 2002, 365,000 birds were imported legally. In 2011 reptiles lived in 4.6 million homes.[3] In addition, there is a worldwide illegal trade in exotic animals, estimated at up to $10 billion annually,[7-9] only exceeded by the trafficking of arms and drugs. This illegal trade subverts rules established by regulatory agencies to reduce introduction of disease and potentially dangerous animals through importation restriction, inspection, and/or quarantine.[8]

Human contact with nontraditional pets and, specifically, with exotic animals raises several public health concerns. Most imported non-native species are caught in the wild rather than bred in captivity. Health screening generally is not performed before shipment of these animals to the U.S., and often there is mixing of animal species in holding locations where exposure occurs of healthy animals to animals that might be ill, incubating or carrying potential pathogens. In addition, the significant wildlife black

TABLE 91-1. Animals That Are Considered Nontraditional Pets and/or Animals That Can Be Encountered in Public Settings

Categories	Examples
AMPHIBIANS	Frogs, toads, newts, salamanders
FISH	Many types
MAMMALS	
Wildlife	Raccoons, skunks, foxes, coyotes, civet cats, tigers, lions, bears, kinkajous, coatis, olingos, ringtails, nonhuman primates
Domesticated livestock	Cattle, pigs, goats, sheep
Equines	Horses, mules, donkeys, zebras
Weasels	Ferrets, minks, sables, skunks
Lagomorphs	Rabbits, hares, pikas
Rodents	Mice, rats, hamsters, gerbils, guinea pigs, chinchillas, gophers, lemmings, squirrels, chipmunks, prairie dogs, hedgehogs
Feral animals	Cats, dogs, horses, swine
REPTILES	Turtles, lizards, iguanas, snakes, alligators

Modified from Pickering LK, Marano N, Bocchini JA, et al. Exposure to nontraditional pets at home and to animals in public settings: risk to children. Pediatrics 2008:122;876–886.

market, through which a large number of exotic animals enter the U.S., compounds the risks of introduction of zoonoses.[9] After making the initial decision to acquire a nontraditional pet, owners may discover they are unable to provide the animal with the environment or nutrition required for a healthy life and often subsequently abandon or release the animal into the wild, posing risks for introduction of zoonotic disease and injury to people and other animals.

DISEASES (ZOONOSES) ASSOCIATED WITH NONTRADITIONAL PETS

Zoonotic diseases or zoonoses are infections transmitted between other vertebrate animals and humans. Most emerging infectious diseases in humans are zoonotic in origin.[9-12] Of 1415 human pathogens, 61% are known to be zoonotic, and pathogens with multiple host species are twice as likely to be associated with an emerging infectious disease.[11] From 1980 to 2003, more than 35 new infectious diseases emerged in humans, many of which are zoonoses.[12] The leading causes of their emergence are human behavior and modifications of natural habitats, including expansion of human populations and encroachment on wildlife habitats, changes in food production processes, changes in agricultural practices, and global trade in wildlife.[8,9,12,13] Wild animals also can serve as reservoirs for transmission of zoonotic agents to domesticated animals and to humans.[10] Domestic animals and humans also can acquire zoonotic pathogens from exposure to nontraditional pets. An outbreak of tularemia in wild prairie dogs caught in the U.S. and held in a commercial facility in Texas led to human transmission.[14] Some of the infected animals were distributed to a pet shop in Texas and were exported as far away as the Czech Republic.

Contact between animals from different areas of the world, including exotic animals imported into the U.S. can lead to disease in a new species and establishment of a pathogen in a new geographic area. In 2003, human monkeypox was introduced into the U.S. The source of monkeypox was imported African Gambian rats that were held in close proximity to prairie dogs being sold as pets. The prairie dogs became infected, which ultimately led to infection of humans with whom they had close contact.[15] Prompt recognition and public health efforts controlled this outbreak and may have prevented the establishment of monkeypox in North America.

PART II   Clinical Syndromes and Cardinal Features of Infectious Diseases: Approach to Diagnosis and Initial Management

SECTION M   Infections Related to Trauma

Zoonotic transmission of bacteria, viruses, fungi, and parasites from household pets or animals to children through contact in their homes or public settings is common. Transmission can be direct or indirect – through contact, aerosols, bites or scratches, contamination of the environment, food or water, or disease-carrying vectors. Animals can become ill but more commonly are asymptomatic carriers of specific organisms and can contaminate the environment to which children are exposed. Infants and children younger than 5 years are at greatest risk, in part because they have suboptimal hygiene practices, have attraction to or curiosity about animals, and have developing immune systems, but also because these infections tend to be more severe in infants and young children.[16] People of all ages with primary or secondary immunodeficiencies are at risk of more severe zoonotic disease, as are pregnant women and the elderly.[17]

Reptiles

Reptiles pose a significant risk because of high carriage rates and intermittent shedding of *Salmonella* in their feces, and because of persistence of *Salmonella* organisms in the environment.[16,18–22] A federal prohibition against commercial distribution of turtles with shells <4 inches in diameter was enacted in 1975 after investigations demonstrated that small turtles were a major source of human salmonellosis, particularly in children. This resulted in an important and sustained reduction of human salmonellosis. Despite this ban, however, illegal distribution of small turtles with subsequent human disease continues to occur.[22–24] In addition, young children without direct turtle exposure are at risk for turtle-associated salmonellosis through person-to-person transmission in childcare settings.[22] Amphibians also serve as a source of salmonellosis in households.[16,25] In the U.S. 6% of all sporadic *Salmonella* infections (11% among people <21 years of age) – approximately 74,000 cases annually – are the result of direct or indirect contact with reptiles or amphibians.[16]

Rodents

Contact with hamsters[26] and other rodents[27] purchased from retail pet stores has resulted in multistate outbreaks of salmonellosis. Hamsters also have been associated with outbreaks of disease attributable to lymphocytic choriomeningitis virus (LCMV).[28] Guidelines for minimizing risk for human LCMV infection associated with pet rodents have been published.[29] Hedgehogs, originally from Europe, Asia, and Africa, now are estimated to live in approximately 40,000 U.S. households,[3] and have proven to be an important source of *Salmonella* serotype Tilene in the U.S.[30] *Yersinia pseudotuberculosis, Mycobacterium marinum*, rabies virus as well as other *Salmonella* serotypes also are zoonotic pathogens carried by hedgehogs.

Plague, caused by *Yersinia pestis*, is enzootic among rodents in the western U.S. Humans become infected through bites of infected rodent fleas, inhalation of respiratory secretion from infected animals or humans, and through handling of infected animals, especially rodents, lagomorphs, and domestic cats and dogs.[4,31–33] In parts of the U.S. where plague is endemic, people with rodent-seeking animals can be exposed to *Y. pestis* through direct contact with plague-infected pets or their fleas.[4,32,33] People who live in areas where plague is endemic should follow a flea-control program designed by their veterinarians to keep their cats and dogs free from fleas.

Association with nontraditional pets also can result in skin infections including ringworm, monkeypox, orf, cutaneous anthrax, tularemia, erysipeloid, and ecto- and endoparasites.[34–40] Hedgehogs pose a significant risk, because their spines readily penetrate skin and can be the source of *M. marinum* and *Y. pseudotuberculosis* infections.[30]

Nonhuman Primates

Herpes B virus (Cercopithecine herpesvirus 1) is a naturally occurring infectious agent that is endemic among macaque monkeys (including rhesus macaques, pig-tailed macaques, cynomolgus monkeys, and other macaques). Infected monkeys usually are asymptomatic or have mild oral lesions. Exposure occurs when monkeys are kept as pets or displayed in public settings. Herpes B virus infections in humans have been reported following animal bites, scratches, or percutaneous inoculation with infected material or splashes on mucous membranes. Human infections most often result in fatal meningoencephalitis.[41]

Fish

The major zoonoses transmitted by aquarium fish are mycobacterial infections,[42] but other organisms have been reported following exposure to aquarium water, or tanks, filtration equipment, or other tank contents. Infection usually is sporadic and immunocompromised people have increased risk.[43–45] Typical organisms include *Aeromonas* species, *Vibrio* species, *Edwardsiella* species, *Salmonella* species, *Streptococcus iniae*, and *Erysipelothrix rhusiopathiae*.[46]

Other Sources of Infection

Contact with chicks and other baby poultry purchased at agricultural feed stores have resulted in outbreaks of *Salmonella* infections.[47] Parents who purchase these birds for their children generally are not aware that *Salmonella* can be transmitted from poultry to humans. In addition to direct exposure to animals, exposure to animal-derived pet food treats, such as pig ear chews, and to dry dog and cat food has resulted in human infections attributable to *Salmonella*.[48–50] Animals can become colonized after ingesting contaminated pet food treats, dry pet food, or raw meats. Animals can be asymptomatic and become unrecognized sources of contamination in the household. Handling contaminated pet food treats and pet food by humans also can result in infection.[49] In the U.S., pet treats are regulated by the Food and Drug Administration. *Salmonella*-contaminated pet treats are considered adulterated under the Federal Food, Drug, and Cosmetic Act (21 USC §301-399). The APPMA published guidelines to educate its members about risks of contamination of pet treats.[51] In 2004, the FDA initiated annual nationwide testing of pet treats for *Salmonella* species.

DISEASES ASSOCIATED WITH ANIMALS IN PUBLIC SETTINGS

Certain venues encourage or permit infants and children to come in contact with many different animal species (see Table 91-1) in a variety of public settings (Box 91-1), potentially resulting in millions of human–animal interactions annually. Infectious diseases, rabies exposure, injuries, and other health problems associated with these venues are well documented.[1,2,36,52] Of particular concern are instances in which zoonoses result in many people becoming ill. Infections due to animals' enteric bacteria and parasites pose the highest risk in public settings. Although ruminant livestock (cattle, sheep, and goats) are the major source of infection, live poultry, reptiles, rodents, amphibians, and other domestic and wild animals also are potential sources.[2] These outbreaks have medical, public health, economic, and legal implications.

During 1996 through 2010, approximately 150 outbreaks of human infectious diseases involving animals in public settings were reported to the Centers for Disease Control and Protection (CDC).[2] Most commonly these involved enteric bacteria and parasites.[52] Serious infections with *Escherichia coli* O157:H7 and other Shiga toxin-producing *E. coli* (STEC) have been associated with multiple animals in public settings.[53–69] The primary reservoir of *E coli* O157:H7 and other STEC is ruminant livestock, which are colonized asymptomatically. In many studies, the primary route of transmission has been foodborne,[60] including unpasteurized milk,[61,62] but person-to-person spread, direct animal contact, and contact with environmental items contaminated by animals are common.[55] Some pathogens are shed by animals intermittently

BOX 91-1. Locations Where Contact with Animals in Public Settings Can Occur

Agricultural feed stores
Animal swap meets
Animal displays
Carnivals
Childcare facilities or schools
Circuses
County or state agricultural fairs
Educational farms or farm tours
Feed stores
Fish tanks
Livestock-birthing exhibits
Metropolitan zoos
Nature parks
Pet stores
Petting zoos
Rodeo events
Wildlife photography exhibits
Zoologic institutions

and remain viable in the environment for months or longer.[70] In 2004 and 2005, there were 3 outbreaks in 3 states of *E. coli* O157:H7, accounting for 173 cases associated with direct and indirect animal contact at petting zoos.[56] Outbreaks[18] and sporadic cases of salmonellosis and outbreaks of cryptosporidiosis[71-73] have been described after visits to farms where visitors had either direct or indirect contact with animals. Additional illnesses following exposures in public settings include campylobacteriosis, tuberculosis, rabies, orf virus infection, giardiasis, tularemia, ringworm, and infected bites or wounds.[2,14,19,34,64,66,74,75] Poxvirus has been transmitted from pet rats to humans.[76]

The risk of human infection is increased by certain factors and behaviors, especially in children, including direct contact with animals (especially young animals), contamination of the environment or food or water sources, inadequate handwashing facilities or lack of education about hand hygiene, hand-to-mouth activities, lack of close supervision, and inappropriate layout and maintenance of facilities at animal exhibits.[2] For example, in a study of observations of practices at petting zoos in Canada, hand hygiene facilities were provided but often not used, items that would come into contact with mouths of infants and children (pacifiers, baby bottles, sippy cups) were carried into the petting zoos, and education about hygiene was lacking.[77] The recommendation to wash hands immediately after leaving an animal exhibit is the single most important prevention step for reducing the risk of disease transmission, even if an animal was not touched.

RABIES

People who have contact with rabid animals can be exposed to rabies virus via a bite, or mucous membrane or wound contamination with infected saliva or nerve tissue.[78] New recommendations have been made for postexposure prophylaxis.[78,79] Although human rabies deaths caused by animal contact in public exhibits have not been reported, exposure to rabid mammals at pet stores,[80] county fairs,[81] petting zoos,[82,83] and rodeo events[83] have required extensive public health investigations and medical follow-up. Raccoon-variant rabies in pet rabbits and a guinea pig has led to postexposure prophylaxis of adults and children.[84] Prevention of rabies in domestic cats, dogs, and ferrets can be achieved by regular rabies immunization and reimmunization.[78] Control of rabies among wildlife reservoirs is difficult, and use of licensed oral vaccines for mass immunization of free-ranging wildlife depends on the circumstances surrounding each animal rabies outbreak and is restricted to use through state and federal rabies-control programs.[78] No parenteral rabies vaccine is licensed for use in wild animals or hybrids. Because of the risk of rabies in wild animals (especially raccoons, skunks, coyotes, foxes, and bats), the American Veterinary Medical Association (AVMA), National Association of State and Public Health Veterinarians (NASPHV), and Council of State and Territorial Epidemiologists (CSTE) recommend enactment and enforcement of state laws prohibiting importation, distribution, and/or relocation of these animals. The AVMA has recommended that wild animals or hybrids not be kept as pets (www.avma.org/careforanimals/animatedjourneys/petselection/consider.asp).

INJURIES AND ALLERGIES

Bites, scratches, kicks, falls, and crush injuries of hands or feet or from being pinned between an animal and a fixed object can occur at home or during exposure to animals in a public setting. Serious and fatal injuries can result from a large animal or any animal with aggressive behavior. Some nontraditional pets are chosen when they are young and small without consideration that they may grow into dangerous, aggressive adults. For example, iguanas sold shortly after birth measure <8 inches but by 2 to 3 years grow to several feet, and baby chicks become full-grown chickens and have a lifespan of up to 20 years.

An estimated 4 to 5 million animal bites occur in the U.S. annually.[5] Although approximately 90% of bites are from dogs or cats, severe and fatal bites can occur from large or aggressive nontraditional pets. Animal bites or scratches often become infected. Infectious organisms, depending on the biting animal, include *Pasteurella multocida*, *Francisella tularensis*, *Capnocytophaga canimorsus*, *Staphylococcus* species, *Streptobacillus moniliformis* (rat bite fever), *Bartonella henselae* (cat-scratch disease), *Leptospira*, and herpes B virus. Tularemia occurred in a 3-year-old child bitten by an infected hamster purchased at a pet store.[40] Reptiles can produce injuries by bites, with claws, or with tails. Severe hand injury[39] and cellulitis[36] have been reported following green iguana bites. Unprovoked attacks of children by ferrets, particularly of infants sleeping or lying down, can be severe, with mutilation of the ears or nose.[85,86] Attacks on sleeping infants are similar to those inflicted by rats.[87]

Although the frequency is not known precisely, the potential for having an allergy to nontraditional pets is likely to be substantial. The American Academy of Allergy, Asthma and Immunology estimates that approximately 15% of the population experiences allergies to dogs and cats,[88] usually due to sensitization to their dander, scales, fur, feathers, body waste, or saliva. Flea bites also can lead to allergic manifestations. Hives have been described in people who have contact with hedgehogs.[89] Although scaly animals are not as likely to be as allergenic as furry animals, there are case reports of allergic rhinitis, asthma, and contact hypersensitivity reactions to iguanas.[38] In addition, an iguana bite-induced hypersensitivity reaction has been reported.[39]

REPORTABLE DISEASES ACQUIRED FROM NONTRADITIONAL PETS AND ANIMALS IN PUBLIC SETTINGS

Many national and state notifiable diseases can be transmitted from animals. Public health officials at state health departments and personnel from the CDC collaborate in determining which infectious diseases should be notifiable nationally; states determine which diseases are reportable within states. A disease may be added to the national or state list as a new pathogen emerges, or removed if disease incidence decreases. Because disease reporting varies by state, specific requirements should be obtained from relevant state health departments. Provisional data are published weekly in the *Morbidity and Mortality Weekly Report,* and final data are published each year by the CDC in the annual "Summary of Notifiable Diseases," which can be found online (www.cdc.gov/ncphi/disss/nndss/phs/infdis.htm). These data are necessary for study of epidemiologic trends and development of disease prevention policies. HCP should report suspected cases of human illness to local and state health departments as soon as possible,

PART II Clinical Syndromes and Cardinal Features of Infectious Diseases: Approach to Diagnosis and Initial Management

SECTION M Infections Related to Trauma

including when the patient has a history of visiting an animal exhibit during his or her incubation period.

PREVENTION MEASURES

HCP and veterinarians play an important role in guiding parents and their children about prevention of risks associated with ownership of traditional and nontraditional pets as well as contact with animals in public settings. Parents and pet owners typically lack knowledge about the multiple modes of transmission of zoonotic infectious diseases from pets. Although pediatricians recognize the importance of anticipatory guidance about pet-related hazards, only 5% reported that they regularly educated patients or families about pet-associated salmonellosis or toxoplasmosis.[90]

Pediatricians and veterinarians together can remind parents, children, and pet owners about the importance of measures to avoid illness. Simple and effective advice includes frequent hand-washing and avoiding direct contact with animals and their environments. This is particularly important with animals from which transmission of enteric pathogens is a risk, including young ruminants, young poultry, reptiles, rodents, amphibians, and animals who are ill. Young children always should be supervised closely when in contact with animals in public settings. The NASPHV has developed an excellent compendium with standardized recommendations for use by public health officials, veterinarians, animal venue operators, animal exhibitors, and others concerned with disease control and with minimizing risks associated with animals in public settings.[2]

To reduce the possibility of injury, HCP should remind pet owners about matching the size and temperament of a pet to the age and behavior of an infant or child, providing direct supervision of younger children, and educating all children about appropriate human–animal interactions.

The decision to obtain a nontraditional pet by parents with children in the household is often not discussed with HCP or veterinarians. However, as trusted sources of healthcare information, HCP and veterinarians are in a unique position to offer information and advice to families who already have or are considering the purchase of a nontraditional pet. Informational brochures and posters available for display, or referral to websites can educate parents without significantly increasing time of healthcare visits. Proper pet health maintenance, immunization, flea and tick control, deworming, and diet and activity can minimize the risk

---

BOX 91-2. Guidelines for Prevention of Human Diseases Acquired from Nontraditional Pets at Home and Exposure to Animals in Public Settings

GENERAL

- Wash hands immediately after contact with animals, animal products, or their environment
- Supervise handwashing for children <5 years of age
- Wash hands after handling animal-derived pet treats
- Never bring wild animals home, and never adopt wild animals as pets
- Teach children never to handle unfamiliar, wild, or domestic animals even if the animals appear friendly
- Avoid rough play with animals to prevent scratches or bites
- Do not permit children to kiss pets or put their hands or other objects into their mouths after handling animals
- Do not permit nontraditional pets to roam or fly freely in the house or allow nontraditional or domestic pets to have contact with wild animals
- Do not permit animals in areas where food or drink are prepared or consumed
- Administer rabies vaccine to mammals as appropriate
- Keep animals clean and free of intestinal parasites, fleas, ticks, mites, and lice
- People at increased risk of infection or serious complications of salmonellosis (e.g., children <5 years of age, elderly, and immunocompromised hosts) should avoid contact with animal-derived pet treats

ANIMALS VISITING SCHOOLS AND CHILDCARE FACILITIES

- Designate specific areas for animal contact
- Display animals in enclosed cages or under appropriate restraint
- Do not allow food in animal-contact areas
- Always supervise children, especially those <5 years of age, during interaction with animals
- Obtain a certificate of veterinary inspection for visiting animals and/or proof of rabies immunization according to local or state requirements
- Properly clean and disinfect all areas where animals have been present
- Consult with parents or guardians to determine special considerations needed for children who are immunocompromised or who have allergies or asthma

- Certain animals are not recommended in schools, childcare settings, and hospitals. These include nonhuman primates, inherently dangerous animals (lions, tigers, cougars, bears, wolfdog hybrids), mammals at high risk of transmitting rabies (bats, raccoons, skunks, foxes, and coyotes), aggressive animals or animals with unpredictable behavior, stray animals with unknown health history, reptiles, and amphibians
- Ensure that people who provide animals for educational purposes are knowledgeable regarding animal handling and zoonotic disease issues

PUBLIC SETTINGS

- Venue operators must know about risks of disease and injury
- Venue operators and staff must maintain a safe environment
- Venue operators and staff must educate visitors about the risk of disease and injury and provide appropriate preventive measures

ANIMAL-SPECIFIC GUIDELINES

- Children <5 years of age and immunocompromised people should avoid contact in public settings with reptiles, amphibians, rodents, ferrets, baby poultry (chicks, ducklings), and any items that have been in contact with these animals or their environments
- Reptiles, amphibians, rodents, ferrets, and baby poultry (chicks, ducklings) should be kept out of households that contain children <5 years of age, immunocompromised people, or people with sickle-cell disease and should not be allowed in childcare facilities
- Reptiles, amphibians, rodents, and baby poultry should not be permitted to roam freely throughout a home or living area and should not be permitted in kitchens or other food-preparation areas
- Disposable gloves should be worn when cleaning fish aquariums, and aquarium water should not be disposed in sinks used for food preparation or for obtaining drinking water
- Mammals at high risk of transmitting rabies (bats, raccoons, skunks, foxes, and coyotes) should not be touched by children

Modified from Pickering LK, Marano N, Bocchini JA, et al. Exposure to nontraditional pets at home and to animals in public settings: risk to children. Pediatrics 2008:122;876–886.

of infection or injury and ensure health of the pet. Referral to a veterinarian also can be helpful when parents are contemplating purchase of a nontraditional animal. Veterinarians can provide information about appropriate pet selection, the size of an animal when it attains adulthood, the temperament as well as husbandry needs of an animal, and suitability as a pet.

A history of contact with pets in the home or animals in public settings should be part of every well-child evaluation and especially should be part of an evaluation of a suspected infectious disease. A history of nontraditional pets in the home or contact with animals in public settings can lead to specific testing and additional/optimized management, and occasionally will result in early identification of an unusual infection from another part of the world.

RECOMMENDATIONS AND GUIDELINES

Recommendations dealing with nontraditional pets and exposures to animals in public settings have been developed by several organizations including the American Academy of Pediatrics, whose recommendations are summarized in Box 91-2. The NASPHV and CDC have established recommendations to prevent disease outbreaks associated with animals in public settings.[2] The CDC has issued recommendations for preventing transmission of *Salmonella* from reptiles to humans[22] and information regarding health risks from *Salmonella* posed by contact with baby poultry.[47] Guidelines for prevention of zoonoses in immunosuppressed people also are available.[17,91]

The AVMA supports the view that exotic animals, wildlife, and wildlife–domestic hybrids do not make good pets. These animals are dangerous and are a hazard to human health, other animals, and the environment. The AVMA also recommends that ferret owners have knowledge about the species and stress that no one who is incapable of removing himself or herself from the bite of a ferret should be left unattended with a ferret. Measures to control and prevent psittacosis in humans and birds were published by a committee formed by the NASPHV and were endorsed by the AVMA,[92] the CSTE, and the Association of Avian Veterinarians.

Guidelines for animals that might have contact with children in childcare settings have been published by the National Resource Center for Health and Safety in Child Care and Early Education.[93]

These guidelines state that any pet or animal present at the facility (indoors or outdoors) should be in good health, show no evidence of carrying any disease, be fully immunized, and be maintained on a flea-, tick-, and worm-control program. A current (time-specified) certificate from a veterinarian should be on file in the facility, stating that the specific pet meets these conditions. All contact between animals and children should be supervised by a caregiver who is close enough to remove the child immediately if the animal shows signs of distress or the child shows signs of treating the animal inappropriately. The caregiver should instruct children on safe procedures to follow when in close proximity to animals – for example, not to provoke or startle animals or touch them when they are near their food. Potentially aggressive animals should not be in the same physical space with children. The facility should not keep or bring in turtles, iguanas, lizards, or other reptiles; ferrets; psittacine birds; or any wild or dangerous animals. Recommendations for handwashing by staff, volunteers, and children as well as maintenance of animals housed on the premises are provided in the guidelines.[93] In addition to exposures to animals within a center, childcare and school field trips can result in disease. A field trip to a petting zoo where hand hygiene facilities were not adequate resulted in 44 cases of *E coli* O157:H7 infection in British Columbia.[94] Guidelines for infection control in healthcare facilities are available (www.cdc.gov/ncidod/dhqp/pdf/guidelines/Enviro_guide_03.pdf). (See also Chapter 2, Pediatric Infection Prevention and Control.)

HCP and veterinarians are encouraged to work together to educate one other and to communicate a common message to pet owners regarding the benefits and risks of pet ownership and of contact with animals outside the home. Joint training seminars and joint sponsorship of health communication campaigns in pediatrician and veterinarian offices would greatly increase awareness of pet owners. The "One Medicine" initiative supported by the AVMA to increase veterinary collaboration with counterparts in human medicine is an excellent step forward to benefit clinical medicine and public health and will build and reinforce partnerships between the professions to reduce human illness and injury related to animal contact.[95] A conceptual framework to support "one-health research" for policy on emerging zoonoses has been published.[96]

---

92 Tickborne Infections

Kristina Bryant

The writings of Homer and Pliny suggest that the ancient Greeks recognized ticks as a source of human suffering, although the role of these ectoparasites in transmission of infectious diseases in humans was not established until the early 20th century.[1] These obligate bloodsucking arthropods can transmit a variety of pathogenic organisms including bacteria, viruses, and protozoa, and currently are the most important vectors of human infectious diseases in North America.[2–4]

Along with mites, ticks are arachnids of the subclass Acari. More than 800 species comprise 2 major families within the suborder Ixodida.[1] Hard ticks (Ixodidae) are distinguished from soft ticks (Argasidae) by the presence of a dorsal sclerotized plate or scutum. A third family, the Nuttalliellidae, contains a single species of tick found only in southern Africa. The long lifespan of these bloodsucking arthropods makes them ideal vectors. Hard ticks can survive for several months to 3 years, while soft ticks can live for ≥10 years and are highly resistant to starvation.[1] The longevity of ticks serves to perpetuate the pathogens that they carry.

EPIDEMIOLOGY

While ticks are found throughout the world, individual species have evolved with requirements for specific hosts, habitats, and climates. Thus, most tickborne diseases also have a specific geographic distribution (Table 92-1).[2,3] Common tickborne illnesses are discussed in detail in Chapters 170 (*Ehrlichia* and *Anaplasma* Species), 171 (*Francisella tularensis* (Tularemia)), 178 (*Rickettsia rickettsii* (Rocky Mountain Spotted Fever)), 179 (Other *Rickettsia* Species), 185 (*Borrelia burgdorferi* (Lyme Disease)), 186 (Other *Borrelia* species and *Spirillium minus*), 215 (Coltivirus (Colorado Tick Fever)), 218 (Flaviviruses), and 258 (*Babesia* species (Babesiosis)).

A number of factors influence the incidence of tickborne infections. Human factors include the degree and duration of exposure to tick-infested habitats as well as host immunity. Tick-related factors include the prevalence of ticks and their usual reservoirs and hosts, infection rates, seasonal activity, and the relative

TABLE 92-1. Tickborne Diseases, Their Vectors and Geographic Distribution

Disease	Agent	Principal Vector(s)	Approximate Distribution
Lyme disease	*Borrelia burgdorferi*	*Ixodes scapularis* *Ixodes pacificus* *Ixodes ricinus*	Northeastern and Midwestern U.S. Western U.S. Europe
Babesiosis	*Babesia microti* *Babesia duncani* *Babesia divergans*	*Ixodes scapularis* *Ixodes ricinus*	Northeast and upper midwest U.S. Washington, California Europe
Rocky Mountain spotted fever (RMSF)	*Rickettsia rickettsii*	*Dermacentor variabilis* (American dog tick) *Dermacentor andersoni* (Rocky Mountain wood tick) *Rhipicephalus sanguineus* (brown dog tick)	Widespread in U.S. especially south Atlantic and south central states Mexico, Arizona
Mediterranean spotted fever (MSF)	*Rickettsia conori*	*Rhipicephalus sanguineus*	Mediterranean region, Africa, western Asia
Human monocytic ehrlichiosis	*Ehrlichia chaffeensis*	*Amblyomma americanum* (lone star tick)	South and mid-Atlantic, north/south central U.S.; isolated areas of New England
Human granulocytic anaplasmosis	*Anaplasma phagocytophilum*	*Ixodes scapularis* *Ixodes pacificus*	New England, north central and Pacific states
Ehrlichia ewingii infection	*Ehrlichia ewingii*	*Amblyomma americanum* (lone star tick)	South Atlantic and south central U.S.; isolated areas of New England
Southeastern tick-associated rash illness (STARI)	Not identified	*Amblyomma americanum* (lone star tick)	Southcentral U.S.
Tularemia	*Francisella tularensis*	*Amblyomma americanum* *Dermacentor variabilis* *Dermacentor andersonis*	U.S. (all states except Hawaii), Europe, Asia
Powassan encephalitis	Powassan virus	*Ixodes cookie* *Ixodes marxi* *Ixodes spinipalpus* *Dermacentor andersoni*	Maine, New York, Michigan, Minnesota, Wisconsin, Virginia
Colorado tick fever	Colorado tick virus	*Dermacentor andersoni*	Western U.S. Southwestern Canada (elevations 4000 to 10,000 feet)
Tickborne encephalitis:			
European subtype	Tickborne encephalitis virus	*Ixodes ricinus*	Central and western Europe, Scandinavia, Korea
Siberian subtype	Tickborne encephalitis virus	*Ioxdes persulcatus*	Russia, Finland
Far-eastern subtype	Tickborne encephalitis virus	*Ioxdes persulcatus*	Russia, Far East (China, Japan)
Tickborne relapsing fever	*Borrelia* species[a]	*Onisthodoros* species	Worldwide
Crimean-Congo hemorrhagic fever	Crimean-Congo hemorrhagic fever virus (bunyavirus)	*Hyalomma marginatum* complex	Europe, Asia, Africa

[a]*Borrelia species take their species names from the ticks that transmit them.*

likelihood of individual species to feed on humans. Not all diseases caused by ticks are infectious. Tick paralysis can result after exposure to neurotoxic substances produced by salivary glands of engorged female ticks, generally after attachment of at least 5 to 7 days.[5,6] This rare disease manifests as ataxia or acute flaccid paralysis without sensory loss or pain; symptoms can be confused with botulism or Guillain–Barré syndrome. The ascending paralysis associated with ticks is acute and rapid within 24 to 48 hours whereas in Guillain–Barré syndrome it is slower, occurring over days to weeks. Paralysis in botulism is descending. Most cases occur in children, with girls affected more often than boys.[7] There are no diagnostic tests for tick paralysis. The diagnosis is made by finding and removing an embedded tick and observing resolution of symptoms, generally within 24 hours.[5,6]

Cases of tick paralysis have been reported worldwide and 43 different tick species have been implicated.[8] In North America, most episodes occur in the western United States and Canada and are associated with either *Dermacentor andersoni* and *D. variabilis*.

Cases cluster in April through June when *Dermacentor* ticks emerge from hibernation.[5]

PATHOGENESIS

Three stages – larva, nymph, and adult – comprise the life cycle of a tick. Both larva and nymph must take a blood meal to progress from one stage to the next. Hard ticks feed slowly over several days and only once per stage. In contrast, soft ticks may take up to 10 short blood meals (minutes to hours) that involve multiple hosts. Ticks become infected with microorganisms when blood meal is taken from an infected host. Some pathogens, including recurrent fever *Borrelia* species, spotted fever *Rickettsia* species, and *Francisella tularensis*, also are transmitted transovarially and transtadially (from larva to nymph to adult), allowing ticks to serve as reservoirs as well as vectors. Horizontal transmission when ticks are co-feeding in close proximity on a host has been described but is rare.

Transmission of pathogens to humans generally occurs when ticks attach and feed and the feeding site is contaminated with infected salivary secretions (spotted fever *Rickettsia* species, *B. burgdorferi*, relapsing fever *Borrelia* species, *F. tularensis*), regurgitated midgut contents (*B. burgdorferi*), feces (*R. rickettsii, F. tularensis*) or, in the case of soft ticks, coxal fluid (relapsing fever *Borrelia* species).[2] The duration of tick attachment necessary for transmission is variable. Transmission of bacterial agents generally requires >24 to 48 hours, although *Anaplasma phagocytophilum* can be transmitted more rapidly.[9] Tickborne encephalitis virus, which is the most common arbovirus transmitted by ticks in Europe, is transmitted within minutes of a tick bite and early removal does not decrease transmission.[10,11] Transmission occasionally occurs in the absence of attachment, as can occur when non-intact skin or conjunctiva are touched after crushing an infected tick with one's fingers.

CLINICAL MANIFESTATIONS AND DIFFERENTIAL DIAGNOSIS

A careful travel history can help determine which pathogens should be considered in a patient who manifests signs and symptoms consistent with a tickborne illness. A history of a recent tick bite as well as occupational or recreational exposures that could result in tick exposure should be sought but absence of such a history does not exclude infection with a tickborne illness. Because tick bites usually are painless, people with confirmed tickborne illnesses may be unaware of their exposure to ticks. Recent tick bites were reported only by 60% of people with confirmed Rocky Mountain spotted fever (RMSF)[12,13] and 68% of people with ehrlichiosis.[14] Tick bites can be confused with spider bites, and with chigger bites or other insect bites. Because clustering of some tickborne illnesses is well documented, similar illnesses in family members, other people who share environmental exposures, or pet dogs should prompt consideration of tickborne infection.[15]

Fever, headache, malaise, arthralgia, and myalgia are features common to many tickborne diseases as well as to a variety of infectious and noninfectious conditions. It is therefore not surprising that many tickborne diseases represent a diagnostic challenge. As many as 75% of patients who are proven ultimately to have tickborne rickettsial disease are given another diagnosis when first evaluated by medical personnel.[16,17] Tickborne rickettsioses, for example, must be differentiated from a variety of other illnesses that cause fever and a maculopapular or petechial rash, including infection due to human herpesvirus 6, enterovirus, group A streptococcus, human parvovirus B19, and *Neisseria meningitidis*.[18] Gastrointestinal tract manifestations, including anorexia, nausea, vomiting, and diarrhea, are reported variably with tickborne diseases.[19] Severe abdominal pain mimicking acute appendicitis has been described with RMSF.[20] The erythema migrans skin lesions of *B. burgdorferi* infection and southern tick-associated rash illness (STARI) can be confused with bacterial cellulitis, eczema, tinea corporis, and granuloma annulare, as well as insect or arachnid envenomation.[21] Lyme arthritis must be distinguished from other causes of bacterial arthritis, postinfectious arthritis, and rheumatologic conditions. Ulceroglandular tularemia can mimic cat-scratch disease or bacterial lymphadenitis due to *S. aureus* or group A streptococcus. Concomitant pharyngitis or malaise may suggest Epstein–Barr virus infection. The symptoms of babesiosis overlap with those of malaria. Clinical clues, characteristic skin findings, and common laboratory abnormalities suggestive of tickborne diseases are depicted in Table 92-2.[22,23]

Because some species of ticks serve as vectors for several different pathogens, a single tick bite can result in two or more

TABLE 92-2. Clinical and Laboratory Manifestations of Tickborne Illness

Disease	Clinical Clues	Skin Findings	Common Hematologic Abnormalities	Other Laboratory Abnormalities	Common Diagnostic Strategies	Fatality Rate without Treatment
Lyme disease[24–27]	Monoarticular arthritis Aseptic meningitis Facial nerve palsy	Erythema migrans (single or multiple)	Leukopenia Thrombocytopenia	Serum hepatic transaminase elevation	Serology with confirmatory Western blot	<1%
Babesiosis[28]	Malaria-like illness with fever, hepatosplenomegaly and jaundice	Rash not usually present	Anemia (severe) WBC normal to mildly decreased Elevated reticulocyte count Thrombocytopenia Decreased haptoglobin Positive direct Coombs test	Serum hepatic transaminase elevation (mild) Hemoglobinuria Elevated serum lactate dehydrogenase, BUN, creatinine	Identification of intraerythrocytic parasites in peripheral blood smear PCR assay	Rare in healthy children[a]
Rocky Mountain spotted fever[17,29]	Febrile illness with rash, headache, myalgia	Maculopapular rash in >90% of children, often involving the palms and soles; may become petechial	Thrombocytopenia CSF pleocytosis (<100 cells) with moderate protein elevation	Hyponatremia Serum hepatic transaminase elevation	Acute and convalescent antibody titers Immunohistochemistry of biopsied skin lesion PCR assay	5% to 10%
Mediterranean spotted fever[30–32]	Febrile illness with rash, headache, myalgia and lymphadenopathy	Eschar at site of tick bite (tâche noire) Maculopapular rash on trunk, extremities, palms and soles (96% of children)	Lymphopenia Thrombocytopenia	Serum hepatic transaminase elevation Elevated lactate dehydrogenase	Acute and convalescent serology	1%

Continued

PART II Clinical Syndromes and Cardinal Features of Infectious Diseases: Approach to Diagnosis and Initial Management

SECTION M Infections Related to Trauma

TABLE 92-2. Clinical and Laboratory Manifestations of Tickborne Illness—cont'd

Disease	Clinical Clues	Skin Findings	Common Hematologic Abnormalities	Other Laboratory Abnormalities	Common Diagnostic Strategies	Fatality Rate without Treatment
Human monocytic ehrlichiosis[33-35]	Febrile illness with rash, headache, myalgia	Petechial, maculopapular or diffuse erythema (66% of children)	Leukopenia Thrombocytopenia CSF pleocytosis (<100 cells) with moderate protein elevation	Serum hepatic transaminase elevation	Identification of morulae in peripheral blood smear Acute and convalescent antibody titers	2% to 3%
Human granulocytic anaplasmosis[36]	Febrile illness with headache, myalgia	Rash rare	Leukopenia Thrombocytopenia	Serum hepatic transaminase elevation	Identification of morulae in peripheral blood smear Acute and convalescent antibody titers PCR assay	<1%
Ehrlichia ewingii infection[18]	Febrile illness with headache, myalgia	Rash rare	Leukopenia Thrombocytopenia	Serum hepatic transaminase elevation	Acute and convalescent antibody titers Identification of morulae in peripheral blood smear PCR assay	No documented fatalities
Southern tick-associated rash illness[37-39]	Mild Lyme-like illness presenting outside a Lyme-endemic area	Erythema migrans-like rash	Usually normal	Not reported	Compatible clinical symptoms	No documented fatalities
Tularemia[40-43]	Regional lymphadenopathy Pulse-temperature dissociation	Papule or necrotic ulcer at site of tick bite			Blood, fluid, or tissue culture Acute and convalescent serology[b]	1% to 7%
Powassan encephalitis[44]	Meningitis or meningoencephalitis Profound muscle weakness Hemiplegia			Lymphocytic pleocytosis in CSF		15% (with neuroinvasive disease)
Colorado tick fever[45]	Biphasic febrile illness with fever, myalgia	Maculopapular or petechial rash in 5-12%	Leukopenia Atypical lymphocytosis Thrombocytopenia	Lymphocytic pleocytosis in CSF with elevated protein	Viral isolation from whole blood or red blood cells Immunofluorescent staining of peripheral blood smear PCR assay Acute and convalescent serology	Rare
Tickborne encephalitis[46-48]	Biphasic illness with meningoencephalitis occurring 7 days after self-limited flu-like illness		Initial: Leukopenia Thrombocytopenia Later: Leukocytosis	Serum hepatic transaminase elevation Moderate polymorphonuclear pleocytosis in CSF	Serology Detection of anti-TBEV antibodies in CSF PCR assay (serum and CSF)	<1%
Tickborne relapsing fever[49,50]	Recurring febrile episodes lasting 2-7 days Jarisch-Herxheimer reaction with antibiotic therapy	Petechiae concentrated in the trunk, extremities and mucous membranes	Thrombocytopenia	Hematuria Proteinuria	Blood culture Visualization of spirochetes on peripheral blood smear Acute and convalescent serology	2% to 5%
Crimean-Congo hemorrhagic fever[51,52]	Febrile illness with rash, myalgia and mucosal bleeding Tonsillopharyngitis common	Maculopapular rash Petechiae	Leukopenia Lymphopenia Thrombocytopenia	Elevated serum AST[c] Hematuria Proteinuria	Serology PCR assay Viral cultures[b]	~30%

[a]Mortality rates higher in immunocompromised patients and people with asplenia.

[b]Requires biosafety level 4 facilities.

[c]Aspartate transaminase.

simultaneous infections.[53-55] Concurrent bacterial and viral infections (*A. phagocytophilum* and Powassan encephalitis virus) have been described.[56] Such coinfections can result in atypical clinical manifestations or increased severity of disease.[57,58]

DIAGNOSIS

Because different tick species are known to transmit specific pathogens, the ability to identify ticks can assist with diagnosis. Pictorial guides are available.[59] Estimating the degree of engorgement can suggest the duration of attachment and thus the potential risk of infection. Testing ticks for the presence of pathogens is not recommended routinely for clinical diagnosis. Diagnostic strategies are outlined in Table 92-2.

The clinician should be aware of the limitations of current diagnostic tests, especially serology. Antibody tests can be negative at the onset of symptoms, necessitating testing of acute and convalescent specimens. Asymptomatic or clinically inapparent infection can result in high seroprevalence rates for some tickborne diseases in endemic regions.[60,61] IgG antibodies can persist for years in the absence of any clinical symptoms. Related antigens can exhibit significant cross-reactivity. For example, *A. phagocytophilum* and *E. chaffeensis* have >50% cross-reactivity.[62] Serologic cross-reactivity also has been noted between *B. burgdorferi* and a number of other organisms, including other relapsing fever *Borrelia* species, *Ehrlichia* species, and *Leptospira* species.[63] Knowledge of clinical and ecological factors associated with these diseases is essential for diagnosis.

TREATMENT

Detailed treatment recommendations can be found in pathogen-specific chapters. Because severe or fatal disease can result when treatment is delayed, prompt, empiric antimicrobial therapy with doxycycline is essential for all ages when spotted fever rickettsioses, ehrlichiosis, or anaplasmosis are suspected. Doxycycline is also the preferred treatment for tickborne relapsing fever, and for Lyme disease in children ≥8 years of age. Macrolides, including azithromycin and clarithromycin, are alternatives for the treatment of Mediterranean spotted fever.[64,65] Trimethoprim-sulfamethoxazole therapy has been associated with increased severity of ehrlichiosis and possibly RMSF, and should be avoided when these diagnoses are considered.[66] Intravenous gentamicin is recommended for treatment of tularemia, although fluoroquinolones also are active against *F. tularensis*. Most cases of babesiosis resolve without treatment, but quinine plus clindamycin or atovoquone plus azithromycin are indicated for severe disease and infection in infants. Supportive care is indicated for most viral tick-transmitted diseases. While ribavirin has been used to treat Crimean-Congo hemorrhagic fever, there is limited evidence to support its efficacy.[67]

PROGNOSIS AND SEQUELAE

Tickborne infections may be asymptomatic in children, as has been noted with babesiosis.[68] The outcomes associated with symptomatic tickborne diseases range from mild, self-limited illness (Colorado tick fever) to severe illness and death (untreated tickborne rickettsioses and deer tick virus encephalitis).[69] Case-fatality rates in the absence of treatment are shown in Table 92-2.

PREVENTION

Avoidance of tick-infected areas remains a key strategy for prevention of tickborne illnesses. When tick habitats cannot be avoided, wearing a hat, long-sleeved shirt, pants, socks and closed-toe shoes, can prevent ticks from reaching the skin. Light-colored clothing permits visualization of crawling ticks. Outer clothing can be treated with permethrin. This synthetic pyrethroid should be sprayed onto each side of the fabric in well-ventilated areas only and treated items should be allowed to dry completely before they are worn (at least 2 to 4 hours).[70] This insecticide retains its potency for at least 2 weeks, even if clothing is laundered.

N,N-diethyl-*m*-toluamide (DEET) is an over-the-counter tick repellent used on skin. The product is safe when used as directed in children,[71] although seizures have been reported after excessive application.[72] Preparations containing no more than 30% DEET are recommended for use in children.[73] DEET-containing products are not recommended for children <2 months of age. Picaridin and oil of eucalyptus are potential alternatives to DEET-containing products; both have been approved by the Food and Drug Administration for use as insect repellents.[74]

People living in tick endemic areas should be educated about tickborne diseases and the need to perform routine checks for ticks after possible exposures.[75] Common sites of tick attachment include the scalp, waist, armpits, groin, under socks, and the beltline. After leaving grassy and wooded areas, skin should be inspected for ticks. Prompt removal of ticks may prevent transmission of pathogens. Ideally, attached ticks are grasped with tweezers or fine-tipped forceps and are removed with gentle, steady pulling perpendicular to the skin. Use of folk remedies, including application of gasoline, kerosene, fingernail polish, petroleum jelly, or a lighted match, are not recommended for tick removal.[76]

Controlling tick populations is difficult and may have adverse environmental consequences.[77] In selected areas, populations of black-legged nymphal ticks and lone star ticks have been reduced through use of deer feeding stations that result in transfer of a topical acaricide to the animal.[78] Control of host reservoirs is another potentially important prevention strategy for some tickborne diseases. For example, rodent-proofing homes is recommended in areas where tickborne relapsing fever is endemic.[79] Keeping pet animals free of ticks also has been recommended.

Most tickborne diseases are not vaccine preventable. Distribution of a vaccine developed for prevention of Lyme disease was discontinued in 2002, with the manufacturer citing insufficient consumer demand.[80] Two inactivated vaccines for prevention of tickborne encephalitis virus (TBEV) have been licensed in Europe.[81] The pediatric formulation of FSME-IMMUN (Baxter, Austria) is available for children 1 to 15 years of age, while the pediatric formulation of Encepur (Novartis, Germany) is recommended for children 1 to 11 years of age. Both vaccines are well tolerated and associated with seroconversion rates of at least 87%, although the relationship between seroconversion and clinical protection has not been studied well.[82] A national immunization program in Austria against TBEV has resulted in near-elimination of disease.[83]

The primary series of either vaccine for prevention of TBE consists of three doses. The recommended intervals between doses vary by country and by vaccine. Subsequent boosters are recommended every 5 years for people <50 years of age and every 3 years for those ≥50 years of age. Travelers to TBEV-endemic areas can be vaccinated according to an accelerated schedule that varies by vaccine. FSME-IMMUN can be administered at 0 and 14 days and 5 to 12 months, while the primary series of Encepur can be administered at 0, 7, and 21 days.[84,85] Neither vaccine is licensed or available in the U.S., although FSME-IMMUN is licensed in Canada.

Prophylactic antibiotics after a tick bite to prevent bacterial diseases are not recommended routinely. Even in areas where tickborne diseases are endemic, limited numbers of ticks are infected with pathogenic organisms.[86] The efficacy of preventive antibiotics is variable. For example, antibiotic therapy delays but does not prevent symptoms associated with RMSF.[87]

According to guidelines published by the Infectious Disease Society of America, prophylaxis to prevent Lyme disease may be considered when all of the following criteria are met: (1) the attached tick is reliably identified as an adult or nymphal *I. scapularis* tick that is estimated to have been attached for ≥36 hours based on either the degree of engorgement or certainty about time of exposure; (2) antibiotics can be started within 72 hours of the time the tick was removed; (3) ecological information indicates that the local rate of infection of I. *scapularis* ticks is at least 20%; and (4) doxycycline is not contraindicated.[88] A single dose of doxycycline (200 mg for adults, or 4 mg/kg up to 200 mg) is the only recommended prophylactic regimen. The efficacy of prophylaxis for the prevention of human granulocytic anaplasmosis or babesiosis is unknown. People who develop fever within 4 weeks of a known tick bite should undergo medical evaluation.

Standard precautions are indicated for the care of hospitalized patients with most tickborne infections. A notable exception is Crimean-Congo hemorrhagic fever (CCHF). Blood and body fluids of CCHF patients are highly infectious and healthcare-associated outbreaks have been reported.[89] Strict observation of droplet and contact precautions, along with thorough environmental disinfection, are necessary.

SECTION N: Infections of the Fetus and Newborn

93 Clinical Approach to the Infected Neonate

P. Brian Smith and Daniel K. Benjamin, Jr

Neonates are uniquely susceptible to infection. The immaturity of the neonatal immune system and the environment of the neonatal intensive care unit contribute to the variety of organisms affecting this population. This chapter outlines the clinical approach to the neonate with signs or symptoms consistent with infection. The approach should focus first on supportive measures: respiratory support, correction of metabolic and hematologic derangements, fluid management, and use of inotropic drugs when indicated. The clinician then should obtain diagnostic studies and institute antimicrobial therapy considering the timing of infection and the neonate's previous exposure to maternal and environmental factors.

ETIOLOGIC AGENTS

Timing is one of the most important factors in determining the cause of neonatal infections. Infections can be acquired prenatally,

perinatally, or postnatally (Table 93-1). Detailed discussions of each of these individual infections may be found in Chapter 94, Bacterial Infections in the Neonate; Chapter 95, Viral Infections in the Fetus and Neonate; and Chapter 96, Hospital-Associated Infections in the Neonate.

EPIDEMIOLOGY

Infections acquired in utero result from organisms such as *Toxoplasma gondii*, rubella virus, cytomegalovirus (CMV), herpes simplex virus (HSV), parvovirus B19, and *Treponema pallidum*. These infections typically result from transplacental transmission. Risk of transmission varies depending on trimester of pregnancy during which the maternal infection occurs. For example, *Toxoplasma* transmission rates range from nearly 0% during the first weeks of pregnancy to 60% in the third trimester.[1] Severity of the infection also depends on the stage of pregnancy at which the maternal infection occurred. Congenital toxoplasmosis and rubella acquired during the first trimester often result in stillbirth or severe anomalies. With organisms such as CMV, transmission of infection is dependent on whether the maternal infection is a primary infection or a recurrence. Nearly 40% of neonates born to mothers experiencing a primary CMV infection during the pregnancy are infected whereas only 1% of neonates are infected in pregnancies of seropositive mothers.[2]

Perinatal infections are acquired just prior to birth (often but not always after rupture of membranes) or as the neonate passes through the birth canal. The neonate initially is colonized after exposure to maternal microflora, including with nonpathogenic organisms such as *Lactobacillus*, *Peptostreptococcus*, and *Saccharomyces*. However, the neonate also can be exposed to potential pathogens such as group B streptococcus (GBS), *Escherichia coli*, HSV, human immunodeficiency virus (HIV), and *Candida* species. Perinatally acquired infections can manifest any time from immediately after birth to weeks or months later (e.g., HIV). Early-onset sepsis (sepsis presenting before 7 days of life) almost always is caused by perinatally acquired infections. Risk factors for early-onset sepsis include preterm delivery, prolonged rupture of membranes (>18 hours), maternal fever, and chorioamnionitis.[3] Although GBS is still the most common cause of early-onset sepsis, the institution of intrapartum chemoprophylaxis has decreased the incidence of GBS early-onset sepsis by 70%.[4] Gram-negative bacilli are the most common cause of early-onset sepsis among very low birthweight (VLBW) infants (<1500 g birthweight).[5,6]

Late-onset sepsis (sepsis presenting 7 to 30 days of life) can be caused by perinatally or postnatally acquired infections. The incidence of late-onset sepsis and meningitis caused by GBS has not been reduced with the use of intrapartum chemoprophylaxis.[4] Late-onset and late-late onset (>30 days of life) infections are increasingly found in VLBW neonates.[7] In this population, the organisms are likely to be commensal organisms such as coagulase-negative staphylococci, *Staphylococcus aureus*, *Candida* species, or gram-negative bacilli.[7,8]

TABLE 93-1. Periods of Transmission of Neonatal Pathogens[7,29-32]

Pathogen	Prenatal	Perinatal	Postnatal
VIRUSES			
Cytomegalovirus	×	×	×
Enterovirus	Rare	×	×
Hepatitis B virus	Rare	×	
Herpes simplex virus	Rare		
Human immunodeficiency virus	×	×	×
Parvovirus B19	×		
Rubella virus	×		
Varicella-zoster virus	×	×	×
BACTERIA			
Chlamydia trachomatis		×	
Group B streptococcus	×	×	×
Enterococcus species		×	×
Enterobacteriaceae		×	×
Listeria monocytogenes	×	×	×
Neisseria gonorrhoeae		×	
Staphylococcus species			×
Treponema pallidum	×		
Ureaplasma urealyticum		×	
FUNGI			
Candida species		×	×
PROTOZOA			
Toxoplasma gondii	×		

TABLE 93-2. Characteristic Manifestations of Congenital Infections[33,34]

	Toxoplasma	Rubella	CMV	Treponema	Parvovirus B19	VZV	Herpes	Enterovirus
Anemia				×	×			
Bony abnormalities	×	×		×		×	×	
Cardiac anomalies		×						×
Cataracts	×	×					×	
Chorioretinitis	×	×	×			×	×	
Hearing impairment	×	×	×				×	
Hepatosplenomegaly	×	×	×	×		×	×	×
Hydrocephalus	×	×					×	
Hydrops fetalis				×	×			
Intracranial calcifications	×		×			×	×	
IUGR	×	×	×			×		
Microcephaly	×		×			×	×	
Rash	×	×	×	×		×	×	×
Thrombocytopenia	×	×	×	×		×		

CMV, cytomegalovirus; IUGR, intrauterine growth retardation; VZV, varicella-zoster virus.

CLINICAL MANIFESTATIONS

Although a variety of organisms can cause congenital infections, some aspects of the clinical presentation are common irrespective of the specific etiology (Table 93-2). Findings such as intrauterine growth retardation (IUGR), jaundice, hepatosplenomegaly, rash, intracranial calcifications, microcephaly, chorioretinitis, and thrombocytopenia can occur with several types of infections. Although many sequelae of congenitally acquired infections are present at birth, others (e.g., hearing loss and developmental delay) may not manifest for months or years.

Early-onset bacterial septicemia often is nonfocal and fulminant in onset, in contrast to late-onset sepsis which can progress more slowly and often manifests as a focal infection: meningitis, urinary tract infections, pyogenic arthritis, osteomyelitis, or pneumonia. Over 90% of neonates with early-onset sepsis have clinical manifestations in the first 24 hours, with most of the remainder within 48 hours of birth.[9]

Signs of perinatally and nosocomially acquired septicemia often are nonspecific and subtle, but bacteremia is uncommon in asymptomatic neonates.[9,10] Signs of neonatal systemic infection can include: temperature instability, lethargy, irritability, apnea, respiratory distress, hypotension, bradycardia, tachycardia, cyanosis, abdominal distention, hyperglycemia, hypoglycemia, jaundice, and feeding intolerance.[11] These signs overlap with other diseases in the neonatal period including: anemia, congenital heart disease, respiratory distress syndrome, and metabolic disorders.

LABORATORY FINDINGS AND DIAGNOSIS

If bacterial or fungal infection is suspected, prompt investigation should be accompanied by administration of empiric antimicrobial therapy. Screening tests such as white blood cell counts and acute phase reactants such as C-reactive protein (CRP) have poor positive predictive values in septic neonates (1–2% in asymptomatic neonates at risk for GBS sepsis).[9,12] For bacterial and fungal infections, culture of normally sterile body fluids remains the gold standard for diagnostic purposes. Blood culture sensitivity for candidemia in neonates is poor given the low blood volumes collected. Even in adults, sensitivity of blood cultures is <30% in patients with single organ involvement.[13] There is no consensus as to the recommended number or volume of blood

cultures. Obtaining multiple-site blood cultures increases the ability to distinguish between cultures contaminated with skin flora and those representing true infection.[14] However, the sensitivity increases by only a few percentage points with the addition of a second blood culture. Although a blood culture inoculum of 0.5 mL has demonstrated good sensitivity in neonates, several other studies have shown that 0.5 mL of blood may not detect low-level bacteremia.[15,16] Sensitivity of blood cultures may be further compromised by maternal intrapartum antibiotic administration or recent antibiotic administration to the neonate.

The incidence of bacterial meningitis is higher in the first month of life than at any other time and complicates up to one-third of the cases of septicemia in this population.[17] Diagnosis of meningitis and identification of the offending organisms requires examination of cerebrospinal fluid (CSF). Unless neurologic signs are present at the time of the sepsis evaluation, some clinicians often defer the lumbar puncture until the blood cultures are positive for a pathogenic organism.[18] However, blood cultures can be negative in neonates with meningitis. In one series, blood cultures were negative in 28% (12/43) of neonates with meningitis diagnosed in the first 72 hours of life.[19] In another study, blood cultures were negative in 34% (45/134) of VLBW neonates with culture-proven meningitis.[20] These data suggest that clinicians should continue to include the lumbar puncture as part of the evaluation of neonatal sepsis in symptomatic neonates provided that the infant is stable enough to tolerate the procedure.

Urine culture should be obtained as part of the sepsis evaluation in neonates after day of life 3, but has limited utility before this age.[21] Urine cultures should be obtained by suprapubic aspiration or in-and-out bladder catheterization. Bag specimens are difficult to evaluate due to frequent contamination and can lead to unnecessary antibiotic administration and radiologic studies.

Disseminated HSV can manifest as sepsis without vesicular skin lesions; clues are severe hepatic dysfunction and consumption coagulopathy. Evaluation of neonates suspected of having HSV infection should include surface cultures obtained from swabs of the conjunctivae, mouth, skin, and anus. CSF should be obtained for routine studies and DNA polymerase chain reaction testing.

Characteristics of the clinical presentation and a review of the maternal history may provide additional clues as to which laboratory tests should be obtained. Table 93-3 provides an outline for current diagnostic methods for congenital infections.

PART II Clinical Syndromes and Cardinal Features of Infectious Diseases: Approach to Diagnosis and Initial Management

SECTION N Infections of the Fetus and Newborn

TABLE 93-3. Diagnostic Tests for Congenital Infection[29,32,35]

Pathogen	Method
Cytomegalovirus	Shell vial assay, culture of virus from urine; DNA PCR, detection of IgM antibody
Human immunodeficiency virus	DNA PCR
Parvovirus B19	DNA PCR; IgM antibody
Rubella virus	IgM antibody; culture from nasal specimens
Varicella-zoster virus	IgM antibody; DNA PCR
Herpes simplex virus	DNA PCR of CSF; cell culture of skin lesions, mouth, nasopharynx, eyes
Treponema	Quantitative treponemal test of serum; CSF VDRL; dark-field examination for spirochetes, direct fluorescent antibody test of lesions
Toxoplasma	Detection of IgM or IgA antibody; DNA PCR

CSF, cerebrospinal fluid; IgM, immunoglobulin M; PCR, polymerase chain reaction; VDRL, Venereal Diseases Research Laboratory.

MANAGEMENT/EMPIRIC AND DEFINITIVE THERAPY

A high index of suspicion and timely antimicrobial therapy are important in the management of septicemia in neonates. For newborns with suspected bacterial infections, ampicillin and an aminoglycoside are considered standard empiric therapy.[22] Ampicillin provides coverage for gram-positive infections (GBS and *Listeria monocytogenes*). Gentamicin is active against most gram-negative pathogens of early-onset disease (*E. coli* and other Enterobactericeae) and also provides synergy with ampicillin against GBS and *Listeria*. Cefotaxime, a third-generation cephalosporin with superior CSF penetration compared with gentamicin, may be considered in cases of suspected or proven gram-negative bacillary meningitis. However, the use of empiric cefotaxime versus gentamicin among infants at birth has been associated with increased risk of death among term and preterm infants[23] and development of invasive candidiasis in premature infants.[24] Vancomycin or nafcillin often is substituted for ampicillin for suspected nosocomial infections, especially in the presence of an indwelling central venous catheter. Gram-negative coverage is tailored to the clinical syndrome and to the known susceptibility test results of the infant's prior cultures and other specimens, as well as of bacteria indigenous to the unit. Duration of antibiotic therapy typically is 10 days for confirmed uncomplicated bloodstream infection. Duration for meningitis is longer and is pathogen specific. For meningitis caused by GBS, therapy is given for 14 to 21 days, and, for enteric bacilli, therapy is 14 days after sterilization of CSF or 21 days (whichever is longer).

Although uncommon in term infants, the cumulative incidence of candidemia in extremely low birthweight neonates (ELBW, <1000 g birthweight) is 7%.[8] Empiric therapy for *Candida* should be considered in hospital-associated infection in symptomatic neonates with risk factors for fungal infections, including extreme prematurity, thrombocytopenia, and recent exposure to broad-spectrum antibiotics.[25,26]

Antifungal options for neonates include amphotericin B deoxycholate, lipid products of amphotericin B, fluconazole, and the echinocandins.

Empiric acyclovir therapy should be considered for neonates with elevated hepatic transaminases, skin lesions consistent with herpes infection, maternal peripartum HSV infection, and for those who do not improve with antibiotics and have negative blood cultures at 48 hours.[27,28]

94 Bacterial Infections in the Neonate

Morven S. Edwards and Carol J. Baker

Neonatal sepsis accounts globally for more than 500,000 deaths annually or 6% of all causes of mortality in children younger than 5 years of age.[1] The mortality rate in developed countries is 5% to 10%. Neonatal sepsis is characterized by systemic signs and bloodstream infection (BSI) occurring in the first month of life. The survival of very low birthweight (VLBW) (<1500 grams) and extremely low birthweight (ELBW) (<1000 grams) infants has expanded use of this terminology to infants requiring prolonged hospitalization for complications of prematurity.

ETIOLOGIC AGENTS

Over past decades, the incidence of early-onset sepsis has declined in developed countries and that of later-onset sepsis incidence has increased.[2] The incidence of early-onset group B streptococcal (GBS) infection has declined by 80% to ~0.25 cases per 1000 live births resulting from implementation of maternal intrapartum antibiotic prophylaxis.[3] The predominant pathogens causing early-onset bacterial infections are GBS and *Escherichia coli*, which together account for approximately 70% of infections (Table 94-1).[2,4,5] The remaining early-onset infections are caused by other streptococci, including viridans streptococci and *Enterococcus*; enteric gram-negative bacilli; *Listeria monocytogenes* or other maternal genital flora. Early-onset *Staphylococcus aureus* sepsis is uncommon but in the presence of maternal vaginal colonization during pregnancy with methicillin-susceptible *S. aureus* (MSSA) or community-associated methicillin-resistant *S. aureus* (CA-MRSA), vertical transmission and resultant neonatal infection is possible.[5,6]

In late preterm infants (estimated gestational age 34 to 36 weeks), gram-positive organisms cause most cases of early-onset sepsis.[7] Among VLBW infants, GBS has declined and *E. coli* has increased as a cause of early-onset sepsis.[8,9] More than one-half of early-onset infections in a cohort of VLBW infants at centers of the National Institute for Child Health and Human Development (NICHD) Neonatal Research Network were caused by gram-negative enteric organisms, especially *E. coli*.[10]

Each of the bacteria causing early-onset sepsis can cause late-onset disease. Septicemia due to *E. coli* or GBS remains common (see Table 94-1). The predominant organisms are coagulase-negative staphylococci (CoNS), which often but not always occur in association with a medical device such as an intravascular catheter.[2,11] CoNS accounted for 39% of all late-onset infections and 25% of late, late-onset infections in a contemporary series.[2] Among VLBW infants, a majority of late-onset infections are caused by gram-positive organisms (70%) and CoNS accounted for nearly one-half of infections in the NICHD Neonatal Research Network.[12] Gram-negative enteric bacilli, such as *Enterobacter* and

TABLE 94-1. Bacteria Causing Neonatal Septicemia

Bacteria	Importance of Pathogen	
	Early-Onset	Later-Onset[a]
GRAM-POSITIVE BACTERIA		
Group B streptococcus	+++	+
Viridans streptococci	+	+
Enterococcus spp.	+	++
Coagulase-negative staphylococci	−	+++
Staphylococcus aureus	+	+++
Streptococcus pneumoniae	+	+
Listeria monocytogenes	+	+
GRAM-NEGATIVE BACTERIA		
Escherichia coli	+++	++
Klebsiella spp.	+	++
Enterobacter spp.	+	++
Citrobacter spp.	−	+
Serratia marcescens	−	+
Pseudomonas spp.	−	+
Salmonella spp.	−	+
Haemophilus influenzae	+	−
Neisseria meningitidis	−	+
Other nonenteric gram-negative bacilli	−	+
Other enteric gram-negative bacilli	+	+
ANAEROBIC BACTERIA		
Bacteroides spp.	+	+
Clostridium spp.	−	+
Others	−	+

[a]Includes late- and late, late-onset.

+++, commonly associated; ++, frequently associated; +, occasionally associated; −, rarely associated.

TABLE 94-2. Features Distinguishing Early-Onset from Later-Onset Bacterial Infection in Neonates

Feature	Early-Onset	Late-Onset	Late, Late-Onset
Time of onset (days of age)	<7	≥7–89	≥90
Maternal complications of labor or delivery	Common	Less common	Common
Incidence of prematurity	25%	Less common	Median birthweight <1000 g
Source of organism	Maternal genital tract	Maternal genital tract; nosocomial; community	Nosocomial; community
Usual clinical presentation	Nonspecific or respiratory distress	Focal	Focal
Mortality rate (%)	5–15	2–10	5–60

A number of unusual bacteria have caused infections in neonates.[18] Any bacterial isolate from blood or a normally sterile body site in a clinically ill newborn infant should be considered a true pathogen unless there is sufficient evidence to conclude that it is a contaminant.

EPIDEMIOLOGY

Systemic bacterial infections affect 1 to 5 of 1000 liveborn neonates. These infections are characterized by age at onset. Onset is termed *early* or *late*, reflecting the age at which signs of infection begin (Table 94-2). Neonates with early-onset infection have illness before 7 days of age, but most are ill within 24 to 48 hours of birth. Maternal obstetrical complications are common, and the source of pathogens is the maternal genital tract. Typical clinical presentation is respiratory distress or nonspecific signs, often indistinguishable from those of noninfectious disorders, without evidence of focal infection. For infants with late-onset infection, maternal obstetrical complications other than preterm delivery are uncommon. The source of the causative agent can be the maternal genital tract, the hospital environment if duration of hospitalization exceeds a few days, or the community. The usual clinical presentation is of focal infection, with manifestations such as skin or soft-tissue infection, pneumonia, or meningitis.

The survival of VLBW or ELBW neonates has prompted the use of a third category – *late, late* or *very late* onset. Although such infants are, strictly speaking, no longer neonates, their median gestational age of <28 weeks and their continuing hospitalization for postnatal complications accord them an extended interval as "newborns" on the basis of conceptional age. These infants almost always have intravascular access catheters, and infection often is caused by commensal species. The mortality rate ranges from 5% to 60% depending upon the infecting agent.

PATHOGENESIS

Infants who experience early-onset sepsis, especially preterm infants, usually have one or more risk factors associated with their mother's labor and delivery (Table 94-3). Although most term infants with early-onset sepsis have associated maternal pregnancy and delivery complications, 50% to 70% of those with early-onset GBS sepsis have no identifiable maternal factors. Maternal factors enhancing risk for early-onset septicemia include preterm delivery, premature rupture of membranes (rupture of membranes before onset of labor at any point in gestation), prolonged rupture of membranes >18 hours, chorioamnionitis, GBS bacteriuria during

Citrobacter spp., as well as nosocomial gram-negative pathogens, such as *Pseudomonas aeruginosa* and *Serratia marcescens*, also are encountered. *Streptococcus pneumoniae* and *Haemophilus influenzae* are uncommon causal organisms. Infants with late-onset pneumococcal sepsis usually are full-term and present in the third week of life.[13]

S. aureus is a common cause of healthcare-associated infection, accounting for 8% of late-onset infections in the NICHD Neonatal Research Network.[12] The incidence of late-onset MRSA infections increased >300% among all birth categories between 1995 and 2004 according to data reported by the National Nosocomial Infections Surveillance system.[14] CA-MRSA has emerged as a cause of late-onset sepsis in neonates hospitalized in the neonatal intensive care unit (NICU) since birth.[15] MRSA strains from 75% of infants with late-onset BSI due to *S. aureus* in one large NICU were CA-MRSA USA 300, the dominant CA-MRSA clone in the United States. Outbreaks of CA-MRSA neonatal pustulosis in term babies have been reported from multiple states.[16] Enterococci and *Candida* must be considered in infections that arise from the intestine or with use of intravascular devices. A national point-prevalence survey cited enterococci and fungi as the next most common bloodstream isolates after staphylococci in the NICU setting.[17]

Anaerobic sepsis can result from acquisition of organisms from maternal genital flora especially during chorioamnionitis. Clinical manifestations are similar to those of aerobic infections, except in the setting of late-onset polymicrobial septicemia, in which the intestine is the source of infection (e.g., necrotizing enterocolitis).

PART II Clinical Syndromes and Cardinal Features of Infectious Diseases: Approach to Diagnosis and Initial Management

SECTION N Infections of the Fetus and Newborn

TABLE 94-3. Maternal Peripartum Risk Factors for Early-Onset Bacterial Infection

Risk Factor	Comment
Preterm delivery	Attack rate inversely related to gestation <37 weeks
Premature rupture of membranes	Rupture of membranes >1 hour before onset of labor at any gestation
Chorioamnionitis	Risk of neonatal septicemia is 5–15%
Urinary tract infection	Higher neonatal risk even when mother asymptomatic
Multiple pregnancy	Only noted for group B streptococcal septicemia
Prolonged rupture of membranes	Attack rate directly proportional to duration of rupture of membranes >18 hours
Early postpartum febrile morbidity	Maternal fever (>38°C) during the first 24 hours postpartum
No prenatal care	Higher neonatal risk
Fetal hypoxia	Apgar score <6 associated with higher risk

TABLE 94-4. Clinical Signs of Bacterial Infections in the Newborn

Clinical Sign	Frequency of Sign	
	Septicemia	Meningitis
Hyperthermia	+++	+++
Hypothermia	++	++
Respiratory distress	++	++
Apnea	+	+
Jaundice	++	++
Lethargy	++	+++
Anorexia or vomiting	++	++
Irritability	+	++
Convulsions	−	++
Bulging or full fontanel	−	++
Diarrhea or abdominal distention	+	+
Hypotension	++	+

+++, encountered in ≥50%; ++, frequently associated (25–49%); +, occasionally observed (15–24%); −, rarely associated (<15%).

Adapted from Nizet V, Klein JO. Bacterial sepsis and meningitis. In: Remington JS, Klein JO, Wilson CB, et al. (eds) Infectious Diseases of the Fetus and Newborn Infant, 7th ed. Philadelphia, Elsiever Saunders, 2011, pp 222–275.

pregnancy, multiple pregnancy, early postpartum febrile conditions (including maternal bacteremia, endometritis, and wound infection), and complications of delivery causing or associated with fetal hypoxia. An inverse relationship between the duration of rupture of membranes and the attack rate of GBS septicemia[19] is likely applicable to other pathogens causing early-onset sepsis because this increases the infant's exposure time to potential pathogens.

The pathogenesis of neonatal septicemia is multifactorial and encompasses microbial, host, metabolic and environmental components. Infants with exposure to a high maternal inoculum >10^5 colony-forming units (CFU) per mL) of GBS, for example, are at a greater risk of septicemia than those exposed to a maternal carrier who has low-density colonization. A decreased expression of lectin family proteins is an additional form of neonatal immunodeficiency.[20] Premature neonates are at increased risk of septicemia because of (1) acquisition of lower levels of maternally derived total immunoglobulin (Ig) G and specific antibodies to bacterial pathogens than term neonates; (2) immature function of neutrophils and decreased neutrophil storage pools; and (3) immature immune responses to pulmonary invasion and bacteremia. Metabolic factors such as hypoxia, acidosis, and hyperbilirubinemia further compromise host response. Interruption of mucosal or skin barriers by endotracheal or nasogastric tubes, intravascular access devices, blood sampling, and monitoring equipment promote bacterial invasion, particularly for late, late-onset infection. Prior therapy with broad-spectrum antimicrobial agents increases the likelihood that bacteria resistant to routinely employed antimicrobial regimens will cause late-onset infection.

CLINICAL MANIFESTATIONS

Septicemia and Meningitis

The risk of bacterial infection in healthy-appearing neonates is low.[21] Clinical signs of bacterial infection, however, can be subtle, and even minimal deviation from usual activity can be a possible indication of invasive infection (Table 94-4). In one series of 647 infants, hypoglycemia and hypothermia were the most common findings in both early-onset and late-onset sepsis.[2] In another report, hyperthermia was the most common sign among 455 neonates, but only half of the infants had fever as a sign of septicemia.[18] Temperature elevation without infection in full-term infants is uncommon (except for fever associated with prostaglandin therapy). Only 1% of healthy infants have fever, defined as an axillary temperature in excess of 37.5°C to 37.8°C. Environmentally induced abnormality (e.g., "isolette fever") is rarely persistent.

Infants with a temperature abnormality should be examined closely for other accompanying signs. One-third to one-half of infants with septicemia have signs of respiratory distress, including tachypnea and grunting. Among full-term infants returning for evaluation after the first week of life, jaundice can be a presenting feature. Findings such as lethargy, irritability, abdominal distention, and diarrhea are less common clues, occurring in less than one-fourth of infants.

Neonates with meningitis generally manifest the same signs as those with septicemia (see Table 94-4). In addition, seizures occur in 40%, a bulging or full fontanel in 28%, and nuchal rigidity in 15%.[22] These signs, if present, suggest meningitis, but their absence does not exclude central nervous system involvement.

Infants should be examined for signs suggesting foci of bacterial infection, including otitis media, conjunctivitis, pneumonia, cellulitis, and abdominal findings of distention and diminished bowel sounds (see Chapter 60, Necrotizing Enterocolitis). Extremities should be examined for limitation of motion, swelling, warmth, erythema, and pain with palpation. The signs of osteomyelitis and pyogenic arthritis are subtle. Skin lesions, including pustular lesions consistent with staphylococcal infection, should be sought.

Acute Otitis Media (AOM)

Healthy term infants have otoscopic findings in the immediate neonatal period (e.g., diminution or absence of mobility or a pink appearance) that would suggest middle-ear inflammation in an older infant.[23] These features progressively are less common by age 1 month. In most neonates diagnosis of AOM is established presumptively with pneumatic otoscopy and confirmed by tympanocentesis.[24] Common presenting signs are respiratory signs and fever.[25] The usual pathogens are *Streptococcus pneumoniae* and *Haemophilus influenzae*; gram-negative bacilli and *Staphylococcus aureus* each comprise <10% of isolates. Approximately 40% of middle-ear aspirates are sterile or contain species considered nonpathogenic.

Young infants with isolated pneumococcal AOM usually are full term and often have bilateral disease.[13]

Premature infants in the NICU since birth can have systemic signs associated with bacterial AOM. Fever, abdominal distention, emesis, diarrhea, irritability, and poor feeding are frequent findings, whereas nasal congestion is encountered less often.[26] Nasotracheal intubation for >7 days correlates significantly with the impaired tympanic membrane mobility and risk of AOM. The pathogens commonly encountered are similar to those expected for late-onset sepsis and include *S. aureus*, CoNS, and enteric bacilli.

Conjunctivitis

Infectious conjunctivitis in neonates is caused by *Chlamydia trachomatis*, and various gram-positive and gram-negative bacteria, including *S. aureus*, *S. pneumoniae*, *Enterococcus*, and *Haemophilus* spp.[27] *Neisseria gonorrhoeae*, herpes simplex virus, and adenovirus are infrequent but important pathogens. Regardless of pathogen, eyelid edema, hyperemia of the palpebral conjunctivae, and purulent discharge are common findings. Findings frequently are bilateral. Hospitalized ELBW infants are more likely to have gram-negative enteric bacteria causing conjunctivitis than higher birthweight NICU infants.[28] *Pseudomonas aeruginosa* conjunctivitis can be associated with systemic complications such as BSI and meningitis.[29]

Osteomyelitis and Pyogenic Arthritis

Two clinical syndromes are associated with bone or joint infection in neonates (Table 94-5). The mild or benign form is a consequence of low-grade and transient bacteremia. Edema and swelling of the extremity or joint, usually without warmth or erythema, can be present for several weeks before diagnosis. Pain elicited by lifting the infant or, with femoral involvement, during diaper change, typically is noted. Spontaneous movement is decreased in the involved extremity, as a consequence of pain ("pseudoparalysis") or weakness due to neuropathy, caused by stretching or edema of the nerve plexus. Erb palsy sometimes is diagnosed erroneously when the proximal humerus is involved. Infants with GBS osteomyelitis usually have a benign presentation.

The severe presentation is a consequence of prolonged or intense BSI. Staphylococci, including MRSA or MSSA, are the usual pathogens. Severe systemic signs overshadow early localizing signs of hematogenous seeding of bones. Bone or joint foci can be noted concurrently with BSI or days or weeks after initiation of therapy. Inflammatory changes, such as swelling, tenderness, erythema, and warmth, are prominent. Because of spread across transphyseal vessels, infection in the metaphysis spreads to the contiguous epiphysis and into joint; inflammatory changes characteristically are poorly localized. Multiple bone involvement is common.[30]

The presenting signs of osteomyelitis in 121 neonates consisted of swelling in 64%, pseudoparalysis in 55%, tenderness in 32%, erythema in 30%, fever in 45%, and irritability or lethargy in 36%.[31] Common sites of infection are the femur, humerus, and tibia. Cuboidal bones, primarily bones of the hands or feet, and the flat bones of the ribs, skull, sternum, and scapula, account for one-fourth of sites. Infants with osteomyelitis due to *Candida* spp. have a similar presentation, with subtle signs sometimes involving multiple sites; *Candida* osteomyelitis has become rare with early institution of therapy for *Candida* BSI.

Skin and Soft-Tissue Infections

Bacteremia can occur in association with skin or soft-tissue foci of infection. Pustular lesions can be a presenting feature of staphylococcal BSI, more often with *S. aureus* than with CoNS. Other skin manifestations of infection in the neonate include cellulitis, abscess, impetigo, omphalitis, and necrotizing fasciitis.[13,15,32] These usually are a consequence of gram-positive infection, especially *S. aureus*, but gram-negative bacteria should be considered until excluded by culture. On occasion, infection due to *Candida* spp. can present as soft-tissue abscesses.

LABORATORY FINDINGS AND DIAGNOSIS

Septicemia Screening Tests

The difficulties in early diagnosis of bacterial infection in neonates have prompted development of a number of screening tests. These are useful adjuncts, but no single biomarker or panel is sufficiently sensitive to obviate evaluation of infants with clinical signs of illness.[33,34] Taken in the context of limitations, the total white blood cell (WBC) count with differential count and other screening tests in Table 94-6 can be moderately useful.

A retrospective cross-sectional study of >67,000 term and late preterm newborns who had a complete blood count (CBC) and

TABLE 94-5. Clinical Presentation of Bone and Joint Infections in Newborn Infants

Manifestation	Mild Form	Severe Form
Preceding bacteremia	Low-grade or transient	Prolonged or intense
Duration of signs	Can be several weeks	Simultaneously with bacteremia or in days after initiation of therapy
Physical findings	Subtle	Prominent
Multiple bone involvement	Uncommon	Common

TABLE 94-6. Screening Tests for Septicemia: Uses and Limitations

Test Finding	Finding Supporting Possible Infection	Comment(s)
Total white blood cell count (cells/mm³)	<5000	High likelihood ratio when test performed at ≥4 hours of life
Absolute neutrophil (polymorphonuclear: PMN) count (cells/mm³)	<1000	High likelihood ratio when test performed at ≥4 hours of life
Total immature PMN count (cells/mm³)	>1100 (cord blood) >1500 (12 hours) >600 (>60 hours)	Relatively insensitive; finding unusual in uninfected infants
Ratio of immature PMNs to total PMNs	>0.2	Sensitivity 30–90%; good negative predictive value
Platelet count (cells/mm³)	<100,000	Insensitive, nonspecific, and late finding
C-reactive protein (mg/dL)	>1.0	Sensitivity 50–90% at onset
Interleukin-6 (pg/mL)	>15	Sensitivity >80%; cutoff points vary; serial determinations may be required
Interleukin-8 (pg/mL)	>18	High sensitivity and negative predictive value
Procalcitonin (ng/mL)	>0.5	Promising for early- and late-onset infection
Erythrocyte sedimentation rate (mm/h)	>5 (first 24 hours) > Infant's age in days + 3 (through age 14 days) >20 (>2 weeks of age)	Individual laboratories must establish normal values; normal value varies inversely with hematocrit
Fibronectin (µg/mL)	<120–145	Sensitivity 30–70%
Serum amyloid A (mg/dL)	>0.8–1.0	High sensitivity and negative predictive value; commercial kit available

PART II Clinical Syndromes and Cardinal Features of Infectious Diseases: Approach to Diagnosis and Initial Management

SECTION N Infections of the Fetus and Newborn

blood culture obtained within 1 hour of each other at <72 hours of age determined that optimal interpretation of the CBC requires using interval likelihood ratios for the newborn's age in hours.[35] The WBC and absolute neutrophil counts were most informative when they were low and when testing was performed at ≥4 hours of age. A normal WBC should not preclude evaluation for BSI in an infant with maternal risk factors. Interpretation of WBC and absolute neutrophil counts in VLBW neonates is difficult, especially during the first 72 hours of life, despite published reference ranges.[36]

C-reactive protein (CRP) commonly is used to monitor response to therapy in neonates with bacterial infections. CRP has high sensitivity for infection but can be elevated in many noninfectious conditions (e.g., respiratory distress syndrome, hypoxia, intraventricular hemorrhage, or surgery) associated with tissue injury or inflammation.[37,38] Interleukin-6 has been used for diagnosis of early- or late-onset infection; serial determinations may be needed to avoid overdiagnosis.[39] Procalcitonin is an acute-phase reactant produced by monocytes and hepatocytes; expression increases several hours after exposure to bacterial endotoxin and levels remain elevated for at least 24 hours. The utility of elevated procalcitonin is limited by its rapid postnatal endogenous increase.[34,37,38] Mass spectrometry-based proteomic profiling, a new technology, offers promise in identifying signature host-response biomarkers relevant in neonatal infection.[40]

Microbiologic Techniques

Blood culture is the "gold standard" for diagnosis of BSI. The desired volume of 0.75 to 1 mL has a sensitivity of approximately 90%. Multiple blood cultures do not reliably increase yield and can delay initiation of therapy.[41] Documentation of BSI is absent in approximately 10% of infants with clinical signs; infection is presumed by the clinical course.

It is appropriate to initiate antimicrobial therapy after an evaluation for sepsis. Meningeal dosing should be employed for neonates with suspected BSI until cerebrospinal fluid (CSF) is examined and meningitis is excluded. With computer-assisted automated blood culture systems, virtually all cultures containing clinically relevant bacteria are positive by 24 to 36 hours of incubation, and cultures containing CoNS or yeast are positive within 48 hours.[42] Antibiotic therapy can be discontinued in an infant with a benign clinical course if culture results remain negative at 36 to 48 hours.

A lumbar puncture should be considered in all neonates evaluated for sepsis. If deferred because of clinical instability, CSF should be examined when the infant's condition permits. In one group of 39 infants with confirmed bacterial meningitis, 16% had sterile blood cultures.[43] In the era of intrapartum antibiotic prophylaxis, 20% of infants with GBS meningitis have sterile blood cultures.[44] The yield of lumbar puncture is low among healthy-appearing term neonates evaluated for maternal risk factors and premature infants evaluated for respiratory distress, thus some experts omit lumbar puncture in evaluating these neonates.[45,46] Wiswell[47] observed that meningitis would have been missed or the diagnosis delayed if CSF had not been assessed in up to one-third of neonates <7 days of age. Weighing the benefits of early diagnosis against the minimal procedural risk, we believe CSF should be examined in all neonates evaluated for sepsis.

Urine culture is not required routinely in the evaluation of infants with early-onset infection. Bladder tap or catheter-obtained urine should be obtained for culture for infants >6 days of age. Cultures from foci of apparent infection are obtained for Gram stain and culture. Examples are middle-ear fluid obtained by tympanocentesis, purulent drainage from the eye, joint fluid obtained by arthrocentesis, metaphyseal aspirate for suspicion of osteomyelitis, peritoneal fluid after rupture of an abdominal viscus, and purulent material from pustules or soft-tissue abscesses.

Cultures from surface sites or mucous membranes are not helpful. Isolates from sites such as the ear canal, nasopharynx, axilla, umbilicus, groin, rectum, stomach, and endotracheal tube are uncommonly the same as those from blood, CSF, or other sterile sites and have a positive predictive value of <10%.[48] Screening cultures can be useful in predicting pathogens and susceptibility to antibiotics in certain nosocomial infections (see Chapter 96, Hospital-Associated Infections in the Neonate). Cultures from the placenta or gastric aspirate indicate exposure to a potential pathogen. Positive results of surface sites or placental cultures do not dictate further evaluation if an infant has no risk factors predisposing to, or signs of, septicemia.

MANAGEMENT: EMPIRIC AND DEFINITIVE THERAPY

The choice of empiric antimicrobial therapy is influenced by: (1) likely etiologic agents; (2) susceptibility patterns of isolates from infants in a specific NICU; (3) the antimicrobial agent's CSF penetration; (4) potential toxicity; and (5) the infant's hepatic and renal function. Information concerning dosage schedules by age and birthweight should be available for agents selected.

Empiric Therapy

Early-Onset Sepsis

Empiric therapy for early-onset sepsis, unchanged after three decades of use, consists of ampicillin in combination with gentamicin. Once meningitis is excluded, ampicillin and gentamicin at the doses shown in Table 94-7 are employed. Gentamicin serum levels are not required unless therapy is given for >72 hours, renal function is abnormal or unstable, or birthweight is <1500 g. Combination therapy provides bactericidal activity against GBS and other streptococci, *Enterococcus* spp., *L. monocytogenes*, many *E. coli*, and some other enteric bacilli. A 10-year retrospective review found >90% of isolates from cases of culture-proven early-onset sepsis in term or late preterm infants were susceptible to either ampicillin or gentamicin, or both.[49] Most nonsusceptible isolates were *S. aureus* and infants had an uncomplicated course when therapy was modified appropriately.

Use of maternal intrapartum antibiotic prophylaxis (IAP) for prevention of early-onset GBS infection has raised concern for increasing ampicillin resistance among *E. coli* isolates. Active surveillance from the Centers for Disease Control and Prevention's Active Bacterial Core indicates that the proportion of *E. coli* infections that are resistant to ampicillin has increased significantly among preterm but not full-term infants.[50] Peripartum ampicillin exposure was not associated with a change in the incidence of ampicillin-resistant early-onset sepsis over 18 years.[51] The finding that ampicillin-resistant *E. coli* was the most common cause of serious bacterial infection in febrile infants less than 90 days in Utah led Byington and colleagues[52] to suggest adding a third-generation cephalosporin to the initial treatment of presumed meningitis in young infants. Ongoing surveillance by geographic area will be required to monitor trends in resistance.

Some experts advocate substitution of cefotaxime for gentamicin for empiric treatment of presumed nonmeningeal early-onset infection in neonates. This is inadvisable for the following reasons: (1) superior efficacy to ampicillin and gentamicin has not been demonstrated; (2) third-generation cephalosporins are not active against *Listeria* or *Enterococcus* spp.; (3) routine use of these agents exerts selective pressure for colonization with and BSI caused by multiple drug-resistant gram-negative organisms[53] and (4) for NICU patients, the concurrent use of ampicillin and cefotaxime (or something for which cefotaxime is a surrogate measure) within the first 3 days of life is associated with an increased risk for death, compared with use of ampicillin and gentamicin.[54]

Late-Onset Sepsis

For the term infant up to 8 weeks of age readmitted to the hospital for possible septicemia without an apparent focus of infection, ampicillin and gentamicin are appropriate for empiric therapy unless *S. aureus* infection is suspected. For skin, soft-tissue, bone,

TABLE 94-7. Empiric Antimicrobial Therapy for Neonatal Bacterial Infections

Clinical Presentation	Antibiotic(s) (dose/kg, IV)	Frequency (h)	Expected Duration (days)
SEPTICEMIA			
Early-onset (term infant)	Ampicillin (150 mg) plus gentamicin (4 mg)	q 12 + q 24[a]	10
Late-onset term infant readmitted	Ampicillin (75 mg) plus gentamicin (4 mg) until meningitis excluded; then ampicillin (75 mg)	q 6 + q 24[a]	7–10
Late-onset inpatient	Vancomycin (15 mg) plus gentamicin (4 mg) or amikacin (10 mg)	q 8 + q 24[a] or q 8	10–14
MENINGITIS			
Early-onset	Ampicillin (100 mg) plus gentamicin (4 mg) plus cefotaxime (50 mg)	q 8 + q 8[a] q 12	14–21
Late-onset	Ampicillin (75 mg) plus gentamicin (2.5 mg) or amikacin (15 mg) plus cefotaxime (50 mg)	q 6 + q 8 q 8[a,c]	14–21
BONE OR JOINT INFECTION	Vancomycin[b] plus gentamicin (2.5 mg)	q 8[a]	3–6 weeks
SUSPECTED GASTROINTESTINAL INFECTION	Include clindamycin (10 mg) or piperacillin (50 mg) with aminoglycoside	q 6–8 q 8[a,c]	10–14

[a]For postconception age (PC) <35 weeks, gentamicin dose is 3 mg/kg every 24 hours; for PC age ≥35–44 weeks, gentamicin dose is 4 mg/kg every 24 hours. Serum levels should be monitored if administered for >2 doses to achieve a peak of 5–10 µg/mL and a trough of <1.5 µg/mL.

[b]For postmenstrual age (PM) <30 weeks, vancomycin dose is 20 mg/kg every 24 hours (age ≤7 days) or every 18 hours (age >7 days). For PC age 30–37 weeks, vancomycin dose is 20 mg/kg every 18 hours (age ≤7 days) and 15 mg/kg every 12 hours (>7 days). For PC age >37 weeks, vancomycin dose is 15 mg/kg every 12 hours (age ≤7 days) or every 8 hours (age >7days). At >44 weeks PC age, the dose for meningitis is 15 mg/kg every 6 hours. Serum levels should be monitored to achieve a peak of 20–40 µg/mL and a trough of 15–20 µg/mL.

[c]Serum levels should be monitored to achieve an amikacin peak of 20–35 µg/mL and a trough of <10 µg/mL

or joint infection, vancomycin is substituted for ampicillin. For meningitis, cefotaxime is given either in addition to ampicillin and gentamicin or instead of gentamicin. For infection of suspected gastrointestinal origin, clindamycin or another agent active against anaerobes should be included. For infants previously treated with gentamicin, amikacin could be substituted, but gentamicin-resistant organisms are uncommon outside NICU outbreak settings.

Definitive Therapy

Definitive therapy is based on the susceptibility pattern of an isolated pathogen. Suggested duration is summarized on Table 94-7. The drug of choice for invasive GBS infection is penicillin (see Chapter 119, *Streptococcus agalactiae* (Group B Streptococcus)). Infants with ampicillin-susceptible *E. coli* BSI can receive ampicillin monotherapy when meningitis has been excluded. For ampicillin-resistant isolates, an aminoglycoside or cefotaxime is appropriate for treatment. Combination therapy with a β-lactam and an aminoglycoside should be considered for BSI caused by *Enterobacter, Serratia,* or *Pseudomonas*. Infants with BSI caused by extended spectrum β-lactamase producing and multidrug-resistant gram-negative organisms should receive meropenem.

Topical mupirocin can be considered for mild cases of neonatal staphylococcal pustulosis. For localized pustulosis in a preterm or VLBW infant or more extensive disease in term infants, vancomycin parenterally is recommended, at least until BSI is excluded.[55] Therapy for MSSA infections can be completed with nafcillin. Vancomycin is recommended for completion of therapy for MRSA sepsis and for bone and joint infections with associated BSI. Limited experience indicates that linezolid is well tolerated and is as effective as vancomycin in treatment of resistant gram-positive infections in neonates.[56] Clindamycin sometimes can be used to complete therapy for bone and joint infection if MRSA is susceptible.

Infants with meningitis typically have progression of clinical illness after antimicrobial therapy is initiated. Observation under intensive care is recommended during the first 24 hours of therapy. Bactericidal agents should be chosen, and for gram-negative meningitis, concurrent use of two active agents is ideal (e.g., cefotaxime and gentamicin). Doses used should be high enough to achieve

bactericidal concentrations in the CSF but to avoid associated toxicity (see Table 94-7).

The dose of cefotaxime for suspected meningitis is 50 mg/kg per dose at a frequency of every 12 hours in the first week of life and every 8 hours in weeks 1 through 4 of life. Once the pathogen has been identified, antimicrobial susceptibility determined, and the CSF proven to be sterile, therapy is modified to the most active and least toxic agent(s). For GBS, penicillin G alone at a dose of 450,000 to 500,000 units/kg per day, and for *L. monocytogenes,* ampicillin at 300 mg/kg per day are drugs of choice. For enteric pathogens, combination therapy is suggested for the first 7 to 14 days of treatment, consisting of a β-lactam agent with an aminoglycoside. Some exceptions occur, such as ampicillin-susceptible *E. coli* or *Proteus mirabilis* meningitis, in which ampicillin alone has been efficacious. Meningitis due to multidrug-resistant gram-negative bacilli can necessitate use of meropenem.

Failure of antibiotic therapy to sterilize the CSF within 24 to 36 hours suggests focal involvement, such as cerebritis, ventriculitis (often with obstruction), subdural empyema, or early abscess formation. For meningitis caused by GBS, therapy is administered for a total of 14 to 21 days; for *L. monocytogenes,* 14 days is recommended; and for enteric bacilli, 14 days after sterilization of CSF or 21 total days (whichever is longer) is indicated. For optimal management, sterility of CSF should be tested at 24 to 48 hours after initiation of therapy. The diagnosis of meningitis in the neonate mandates supportive care not routinely given to infants with septicemia, such as careful observation for and control of respiratory failure and seizures, fluid restriction to prevent or treat inappropriate antidiuretic hormone secretion, and care that minimizes elevation of intracranial pressure.

PROGNOSIS/SEQUELAE

The outcome from neonatal bacterial meningitis is guarded. Among infants surviving an episode of GBS meningitis, 22% have neurologic sequelae at hospital discharge, most often persistent seizures, hypertonicity, and dysphagia.[57] Among 88 full-term or near term survivors of meningitis in one report, 17 had moderate or severe disability at one year of age.[58] In a report comparing 5-year outcomes, more children surviving neonatal meningitis

PART II Clinical Syndromes and Cardinal Features of Infectious Diseases: Approach to Diagnosis and Initial Management

SECTION N Infections of the Fetus and Newborn

had serious disability (23%) than did children from a general practice (2%).[59]

RECENT ADVANCES

Ongoing morbidity and mortality from neonatal sepsis despite the use of potent antimicrobial agents and advances in critical care medicine have prompted interest in early pathogen identification through such tools as multiplex polymerase chain reaction (PCR) and multiplex pyrosequencing PCR assays that can identify pathogens directly from whole blood. Real-time PCR and pyrosequencing of the universal 23S rRNA gene has been used successfully in neonatal blood culture samples and holds promise for the future.[60]

Trials assessing the efficacy of immune globulin intravenous (IGIV) in reducing the mortality of neonatal septicemia have documented a reduction in mortality in IGIV-treated patients.[61,62] A meta-analysis showed a significant decrease in mortality for neonates who received IGIV.[63] IGIV is apparently safe when doses of 1 g/kg or less are employed, but there is still insufficient evidence to support routine administration in suspected or documented neonatal bacterial infection.[64] A large, randomized, multicenter placebo-controlled trial found that therapy with intravenous immune globulin had no significant effect on the outcomes of suspected or proven sepsis.[65]

Other potential adjunctive therapies are the use of recombinant granulocyte, monocyte, and granulocyte-macrophage colony-stimulating factors. Recombinant human granulocyte colony-stimulating factor increased the neutrophil count significantly and reduced the incidence of neonatal sepsis in critically ill ventilated neonates with prolonged pre-eclampsia-associated neutropenia compared with conventional therapy.[66] By contrast, a multicenter trial (the PROGRAMS trial) found that early postnatal prophylactic granulocyte-macrophage colony-stimulating factor corrected neutropenia in ELBW infants but did not reduce incidence of sepsis or improve outcomes.[67] The future is bright for the development of adjunctive agents, but their application in practice requires additional investigation.

PREVENTION

Three general approaches for the prevention of neonatal septicemia have been suggested, and the first two have been efficacious: (1) improvement in prenatal care resulting in delivery of infants at term gestation and without maternal risk factors for septicemia; (2) maternal IAP for prevention of early-onset GBS septicemia; and (3) maternal immunization to provide IgG-mediated passive immunity for the infant.

Although the first approach, provision of prenatal care, especially for women younger than 20 years, is self-evident, its achievement continues to elude even urban centers. A decline in the rate of preterm deliveries can reduce the incidence of neonatal septicemia and would eliminate most very late-onset BSI and nosocomial infections in NICUs. The second approach, IAP, targets women who are antenatally identified as carriers of GBS to prevent early-onset neonatal septicemia caused by this organism. Sepsis caused by other organisms is more often associated with preterm birth.[68] Implementation of IAP has been associated with an 80% decrease in the incidence of early-onset GBS infections.[3] For a discussion of this approach, see Chapter 119, *Streptococcus agalactiae* (Group B Streptococcus).

Whereas IAP is a desirable interim approach, prevention of all GBS infections, irrespective of age of onset or presence of maternal risk factors, awaits the development of suitable vaccines. Such capsular polysaccharide-protein conjugate vaccines are immunogenic in experimental animals, and phase I and II clinical trials have been completed. If such vaccines are effective in phase III trials, women of childbearing age could be immunized to protect their neonates against GBS. This approach has been successful in the prevention of tetanus and holds promise to prevent infection caused by other neonatal pathogens.

95 Viral Infections in the Fetus and Neonate

Robert F. Pass

Neonates, like older children and adults, are subject to viral infections acquired by horizontal routes, such as those due to influenza, rotavirus, and enteroviruses. They also are at risk for acquisition of viruses through routes that are unique to the perinatal setting where mother-to-child transmission (MTCT) occurs transplacentally, during birth, or from breast milk. The ability of certain viruses to establish chronic infection in the mother with persistence of infectious virus in blood, mucosa, or milk (herpesviruses, human immunodeficiency virus (HIV), human T-lymphotropic virus 1 (HTLV-1), hepatitis B and C) accounts for the key role vertical transmission plays in their epidemiology and clinical significance. Whether viruses that produce acute, self-limited infections in the mother, such as rubella, varicella-zoster virus (VZV), enteroviruses, and parvovirus B19, are transmitted to the fetus or newborn and produce disease depends on the timing of maternal infection in relation to gestation and parturition. Thus the clinical settings in which fetal and neonatal viral infections must be considered include pregnancy, the newborn nursery, and the evaluation of an ill newborn. This chapter provides an overview of the viral infections that occur in these settings. Detailed discussions of epidemiology, diagnosis, treatment, and prevention are presented in the chapters focused on specific viruses.

PATHOGENESIS

Many viral infections produce disease that is more severe in the fetus or neonate than in adults, children, or infants. Viral infection of the fetus probably follows maternal viremia or viral replication in the placenta. Developmental immaturity of fetal and neonatal cellular and humoral immune function is important in pathogenesis (see review by Lewis and Wilson[1]). Interferon-γ production by T lymphocytes is decreased; CD4+ T lymphocyte antigen-specific responses are delayed compared with adults; and T-cell help for B-cell differentiation is decreased. In addition, neonatal natural killer (NK) cells have an immature phenotype and decreased cytotoxicity against virus-infected cells. Viruses that infect the fetus early in gestation usually result in more damage than those that infect the fetus late in gestation.[2-4] Fetal infection before the third trimester occurs in the absence of substantial concentrations of maternally derived antibodies. Infections early in gestation encounter an immature immune system and developing fetal organs. Tissue damage, organ dysfunction, teratogenicity, and fetal demise are possible consequences of these infections.

Maternal antibody acquired transplacentally and antibody and immunocompetent cells present in colostrum and mother's milk are important components of the neonate's defense against viral infection. A neonate infected by a virus to which the mother lacks immunity is prone to severe infection; neonatal infections caused by herpesviruses are illustrative. Transfusion-acquired CMV infections are rarely evident clinically in term infants of seropositive mothers, but can cause severe illness in small, antibody-negative premature infants. Herpes simplex virus (HSV) and VZV are more likely to cause severe disease in the neonate with absent or low concentrations of maternal antibodies.

EPIDEMIOLOGY

Virus Transmission from Mother to Child

Viruses for which MTCT has well-characterized clinical consequences are listed in Table 95-1 along with the main routes of transmission that result in clinical disease. The likelihood that maternal viral infection spreads to the fetus or neonate is determined by the occurrence of viremia, genital tract viral shedding, or virolactia. Exposure to maternal virus often is a result of chronic infection caused by cytomegalovirus (CMV), HIV, HSV, HTLV-1, hepatitis B, or hepatitis C. For these viruses the prevalence of infection in women of childbearing age and the incidence of new infections during pregnancy contribute to the overall prevalence of fetal or neonatal infection. In contrast, fetal or neonatal infection with VZV, rubella, parvovirus B19, hepatitis E virus, and a number of agents not listed in Table 95-1 is based on the incidence and timing of maternal infection in relation to pregnancy and delivery. MTCT of a number of viruses not listed in Table 95-1 is known to occur. Studies of GB virus C also known as hepatitis G virus, a hepatotropic flavivirus that produces chronic infection, show that 60% to 80% of infants born to mothers with viral RNA

in their blood are infected. Transiently elevated serum alanine aminotransferase concentrations have been noted, but there has been no associated illness in infants with perinatal infection.[5,6] Sporadic reports of congenital disease due to enteroviruses or adenovirus and frequent detection of viral nucleic acid by PCR testing of amniotic fluid suggest that transplacental transmission of these viruses may be more common than is appreciated.[7-10] The proportion of maternal infections that lead to fetal demise, stillbirth, neonatal disease, or asymptomatic infection is not well defined.

Infection of the newborn during birth occurs through exposure to maternal blood or secretions; it is the major route of MTCT for HSV, HIV, hepatitis B, and hepatitis C. Labor and delivery prolong the contact between the neonate's mucosal surfaces and maternal secretions and blood, facilitating transfer of viruses. The newborn who acquires virus during birth typically becomes viremic or sheds virus in other body fluids between 1 and 4 months of age. Intrapartum infection has well-known clinical consequences for the newborn in the case of HSV and HIV. Hepatitis B and hepatic C produce chronic infection that can progress to chronic hepatitis, cirrhosis, and hepatocellular carcinoma. Cytomegalovirus also is commonly spread from mother to infant during birth, but these infections do not appear to be clinically significant except perhaps in very low birthweight premature infants.

Vertical transmission of viruses through ingestion of human milk is important in the epidemiology of CMV, HTLV-1, and HIV. Although the quantity of virus present in human milk usually is low, the nursing infant is exposed to this potential source of infection multiple times per day for months. Breastfeeding is the major route for vertical transmission of CMV. In populations in which mothers nurse their infants routinely and rates of maternal seropositivity are high, most infants acquire CMV during the first year of life.[11] Transmission of CMV through mother's milk rarely causes acute illness or the types of sequelae that follow congenital infection; breast milk-acquired CMV infection in very low birthweight premature newborns is a possible exception (see Chapter 206, Cytomegalovirus). Both HIV and HTLV-1 can be transmitted through human milk, although the onset of infection usually is after the neonatal period.[12-14] Breast milk can also be a significant route of MTCT of GB virus C and TT virus, but neither of these has been proven to cause disease.[5,6,15] Transmission of rubella virus, HSV, and echovirus 18 has been reported when acute maternal infection was present while breastfeeding. It is believed that virolactia occurs during acute infections with these agents.[16-18] Viruses that are transmitted through blood could be transmitted during breastfeeding in the presence of bleeding or cracked nipples even in the absence of virolactia. Because of the consistent association of higher infant mortality with formula feeding, the potential transmission of maternal viral infection rarely should be a reason to interdict breastfeeding in developing countries, with the possible exception of HIV infection. In 2010, the World Health Organization updated recommendations on infant feeding in the context of maternal HIV infection, recommending that national authorities in each country decide which infant feeding practice will be supported.[19] Although the previous recommendation that "… replacement feeding should not be used unless it is acceptable, feasible, affordable, sustainable and safe" remains, the impact of antiretroviral treatment of mother and infant on reducing transmission of HIV through breast milk is acknowledged. The American Academy of Pediatrics Committee on Infectious Diseases has made specific recommendations regarding breastfeeding by mothers known to have certain viral infections (Table 95-2).[20]

Sources of Maternal Infection

The likelihood of maternal viral infections with the attendant risk of MTCT is affected by specific types of exposures. For example, because CMV infection is common in young children who shed CMV chronically, exposure to young children is one of the most important risk factors for maternal CMV infection. Sexual activity is a risk factor for the acquisition of HSV, CMV, HIV, and hepatitis

TABLE 95-1. Routes of Transmission for Selected Viruses for Which Mother-to-Child Transmission Has Well-Characterized Clinical Consequences

Virus	Clinical	Route[a]
Chikungunya virus	Fever, "sepsis," encephalopathy	Transplacental/intrapartum
CMV	Congenital infection syndrome	Transplacental
Dengue virus	Fever, rash, hepatosplenomegaly, thrombocytopenia, pleural effusion	Transplacental/intrapartum
Hepatitis B virus	Chronic liver disease	Intrapartum
Hepatitis C virus	Chronic liver disease	Intrapartum
Hepatitis E virus	Jaundice, hepatitis, liver failure	Transplacental/intrapartum?
HSV	Neonatal herpes	Intrapartum
HIV	Perinatal HIV/AIDS	Intrapartum, breast milk
Human papillomavirus	Laryngeal papillomatosis	Intrapartum
HTLV-1	Adult T cell leukemia	Breast milk
LCMV	Encephalopathy, chorioretinitis	Transplacental
Parvovirus B19	Anemia, hydrops	Transplacental
Rubella virus	Congenital rubella syndrome	Transplacental

CMV, cytomegalovirus; HSV, herpes simplex virus; HIV, human immunodeficiency virus; HTLV-1, human T-lymphotropic virus; LCMV, lymphocytic choriomeningitis virus.

[a]*Principal route responsible for clinical consequences.*

PART II Clinical Syndromes and Cardinal Features of Infectious Diseases: Approach to Diagnosis and Initial Management

SECTION N Infections of the Fetus and Newborn

TABLE 95-2. Summary of American Academy of Pediatrics Committee on Infectious Diseases Recommendations for the U.S. on Breastfeeding (or Provision of Mother's Milk) in the Presence of Maternal Viral Infection

Virus	Recommendation
Cytomegalovirus	Risk for very low birthweight preterm; no clear recommendation
Hepatitis B virus	No restriction
Hepatitis C virus	Discuss theoretical risk with mother
Human immunodeficiency virus	Do not breastfeed
Human T-lymphotropic virus 1	Do not breastfeed
Human T-lymphotropic virus 2	Do not breastfeed
Rubella	No restriction
Varicella	Follow recommendations for VariZig; no recommendations on breastfeeding
West Nile virus	Breastfeeding is recommended in endemic area; no recommendation for breastfeeding during infection

Modified from reference 20.

B virus infections and injecting drug use is a risk factor for HIV, hepatitis B, and hepatitis C. For viruses that cause acute, self-limited infections with seasonal or periodic epidemics such as parvovirus B19, rubella, and VZV, risk of maternal and congenital infection is related to epidemic activity in the community. Success in preventing congenital rubella infection is directly related to wide use of rubella vaccine to prevent outbreaks and thus prevent maternal exposure. In 2005, the Centers for Disease Control and Prevention announced the elimination of domestic rubella and congenital rubella syndrome in the United States.[21] In 2008, there were 11 known cases of rubella in the U.S., all of which were imported or related to imported cases; there was no congenital rubella.[22] Similar success is being achieved in other countries due to incorporation of rubella vaccine into routine childhood vaccine programs, along with national programs that include active surveillance and special efforts to achieve high immunization rates.[22]

Insect vectors and animals can be the source of maternal infections that are spread to the fetus or newborn. Mice excrete lymphocytic choriomeningitis virus (LCMV) and are the source of human infection. Congenital infection due to LCMV is likely underdiagnosed in the U.S. Maternal infection, especially in the first trimester, can lead to fetal infection with subsequent chorioretinitis, micro- or macrocephaly, and intracranial calcifications. Maternal exposure to rodents may be the key epidemiologic clue.[23,24] West Nile virus is a zoonotic pathogen with transplacental and breast-milk transmission reported in the U.S;[25,26] however, MTCT appears to be rare. Chikungunya virus, an emerging cause of febrile illness with arthralgia, myalgia, and rash in Africa, India, and Southeast Asia is transmitted to humans by *Aedes* mosquitoes. Maternal infection has been associated with transmission to the fetus and neonate; a transmission rate of approximately 50% was reported with maternal viremia at term.[27] Although it is unclear whether maternal infection affects the outcome of pregnancy, newborn infection is manifest by a sepsis-like illness, encephalopathy, and high fever and may be associated with central nervous system (CNS) sequelae.[27,28] Dengue virus also is transmitted by *Aedes* mosquitoes and infection is common in tropical areas. Rates of MTCT range from 12% to 60% when maternal infection occurs during pregnancy, and similar to Chikungunya virus, maternal viremia at term is strongly associated with neonatal infection.[29] Infected newborns can have a sepsis-like illness with fever, thrombocytopenia, hepatosplenomegaly, rash, and pleural effusion.

Postnatal Infection: Community Acquired and Nosocomial

Horizontal transmission of viruses to neonates from caregivers or family members occurs primarily through infected droplets or contaminated hands. Neonates are more vulnerable than older hosts because they are immunologically naive and their care requires repeated handling and close contact. In addition, hospitalized neonates are exposed to a continual influx of hospital personnel and new patients, creating multiple opportunities for the introduction and spread of viruses prevalent in the community.

Outbreaks of many different viruses in newborn nurseries have been described; enteroviruses, adenovirus, rotavirus, and respiratory syncytial virus are notable because they are common, difficult to control, and have significant clinical consequences.[9,30] Neonates are infected by the mother, other family members, or hospital personnel. Enterovirus and respiratory virus outbreaks in hospital nurseries usually are associated with community outbreaks. Blood products are a potential source of nosocomial CMV infection that could be clinically significant for premature newborns or babies born to CMV-seronegative mothers. These infections are prevented either by only administering CMV-negative blood to neonates or by using filters to remove leukocytes from blood.

Viruses are the leading cause of illness in patients who present to the hospital with fever prior to 3 months of age.[31] Enteroviruses are particularly common in this age group. Data from the National Enterovirus Surveillance System in the U.S. for the period 1983–2003 showed that 11.4% of all reported enterovirus infections occurred in neonates.[32] During summer and fall, enteroviruses account for the majority of hospitalizations in young infants with suspected sepsis.[9,31] A study of hospitalized, febrile infants reported PCR detection of enterovirus in 28.5% of cerebrospinal fluid samples collected during the enterovirus season (June through October) compared with 11.1% during other months.[33] Parechoviruses (previously echovirus 22 and 23) can cause a sepsis-like illness with rash in newborns.[34] Other viral infections are sporadic or seasonal causes of fever, systemic illness, gastrointestinal disease, and respiratory disease in infants including adenovirus, rotavirus, norovirus, astrovirus, influenza, HSV, respiratory syncytial virus (RSV), and others.[35–38]

CLINICAL MANIFESTATIONS

Prematurity and Low Birthweight

Maternal viral infection can involve the placenta and affect outcome for the infant even if fetal infection does not occur. The proportion of morbidities such as preterm birth or poor fetal growth that can be attributed to viral infection of the mother of fetus is not well defined. A virologic and serologic study of small-for-gestational-age neonates in Sweden did not find evidence that viral infection was causally associated with low birthweight.[39] Maternal herpangina has been associated with premature birth, low birthweight, and poor intrauterine growth.[40] Placental adenovirus infection has been associated with chorioamnionitis and preterm birth.[41] A study of newborn dried blood spots, using PCR to detect enterovirus RNA and herpesvirus DNA, reported an association between detection of CMV DNA and pregnancy-induced hypertension and preterm birth.[42] Adeno-associated virus-2, a member of the parvovirus family, has been reported in association with pre-eclampsia, stillbirth, and preterm birth.[43] Increased risk of prematurity, low birthweight, and other unfavorable pregnancy outcomes have been ascribed to maternal dengue infection; however, a review of 30 published studies concluded that evidence linking maternal infection to adverse pregnancy outcomes was inconclusive.[29]

Spontaneous Abortion and Stillbirth

It is possible that many unexplained spontaneous abortions, intrauterine fetal deaths, and stillbirths are due to unrecognized viral infection, considering that most studies focus on one or a small number of viruses and few studies have employed modern molecular techniques for virus detection. A number of viruses, including poliovirus, measles, rubella, mumps, influenza, parvovirus B19, HSV, CMV, and nonpolio enteroviral infection, have been associated with spontaneous abortion or stillbirth.[44] Studies that have included controls and molecular techniques for virus detection suggest that viral infections probably account for many cases of unexplained fetal death and stillbirth. A histopathologic and molecular study of spontaneous abortions and fetal deaths found evidence of viral infection in 16 of 21 cases and in none of 26 controls; enterovirus/coxsackievirus accounted for 10 of the cases.[45] A study of placental tissue from 62 fetal deaths and 35 control pregnancies found evidence of CMV, parvovirus B19, and HSV in 16%, 13%, and 5% of cases, respectively; only 6% of placentas from control pregnancies were positive for any of these viruses.[46] A Swedish study reported PCR evidence of parvovirus B19 infection in placental or fetal tissue in 7 of 47 (15%) intrauterine fetal deaths, 2 of 37 (5%) miscarriages, and in none of 29 induced abortions and term, normal pregnancies.[47] A German study of 1018 pregnancies complicated by maternal parvovirus B19 infection reported a fetal death rate of 11% when maternal infection occurred prior to 20 weeks' gestation and no fetal demise following infections later in gestation.[48] The extent to which maternal HIV-1 infection in the absence of immune deficiency increases the risk of fetal death or stillbirth is not clear.[44] Declining CD4+ lymphocyte count and comorbidities are associated with increased risk of stillbirth, and in countries with high maternal seroprevalence, HIV-1 could be an important cause of stillbirth.

Syndrome of Congenital Infection

The presence of hepatomegaly, splenomegaly, microcephaly, petechiae, jaundice, dermal manifestations of erythropoiesis, poor intrauterine growth, chorioretinitis, intracranial calcifications, deafness, thrombocytopenia, direct hyperbilirubinemia, or hepatitis in the neonate suggests prenatal infection. Other findings occasionally associated with congenital infection are cardiac defects, hydrocephalus, prematurity, and anemia. Clinical findings suggestive of infection by a specific viral agent are listed in Table 95-3. However, clinical findings alone are not diagnostic; laboratory evaluation is essential in patients with suspected congenital viral infection.

Central Nervous System Infection

Viral encephalitis or meningitis in the neonate can result from prenatal or postnatal infection. Abnormalities suggestive of viral central nervous system disease often are subtle or nonspecific; they include lethargy, hypotonia, irritability, poor feeding, apnea, fever, and seizures. Prenatal viral infections can affect brain growth, leading to microcephaly. Although encephalopathy or encephalitis in the neonate has been noted with a number of viral infections, CMV, enteroviruses, and HSV are the agents most commonly implicated.

TABLE 95-3. Clinical Findings in the Newborn Suggesting a Specific Congenital Viral Infection

Agent	Features
Cytomegalovirus	Microcephaly, hearing loss, petechiae, cholestatic jaundice
Rubella	Cataracts, heart disease, deafness
Varicella-zoster virus	Scarring of skin, limb hypoplasia, ocular abnormalities
Herpes simplex virus	Hydranencephaly, ocular disease, skin scars
Lymphocytic choriomeningitis virus	Micro- or macro-cephaly, chorioretinitis

Sepsis Syndrome

Clinical manifestations suggestive of septicemia sometimes are associated with neonatal enterovirus, coxsackievirus, parechovirus, adenovirus, HSV, RSV, or influenza infections. Neonates with echovirus, parechovirus or coxsackievirus infection can manifest pallor, lethargy, hypotension, apnea, acidosis, and respiratory impairment.[9] Rapid progression of disseminated HSV infection can produce shock, coagulopathy, fulminant hepatitis, and diffuse lung disease.[49] Neonatal RSV and adenovirus infections also can cause nonspecific signs that mimic septicemia, such as apnea, lethargy, irritability, and poor feeding.[50] It is likely that other respiratory viruses have similar effects in the newborn.

Cardiac Insufficiency

Viral infections produce congestive heart failure in the fetus or neonate by causing anemia or by damaging the myocardium directly. Fetal infection with human parvovirus B19 characteristically leads to profound anemia. Although many fetuses appear to recover in utero, hydrops fetalis and fetal death can result.[51] Rare cases of nonimmune hydrops fetalis have been attributed to intrauterine CMV or adenovirus infection.[52,53] Viral myocarditis usually is due to coxsackie B viruses or echoviruses in the neonate and patients often present with cardiac failure or shock.[9]

Pulmonary Disease

Lower respiratory tract disease is an unusual manifestation of congenital or perinatal viral infection; respiratory tract symptoms occur usually as part of multisystem disease in disseminated neonatal HSV or VZV infection. Postnatal lower respiratory infection or pneumonia in the neonate can be due to any of the viruses that cause respiratory tract disease in older children, including RSV, parainfluenza virus, influenza viruses, adenovirus, enteroviruses, rotavirus, rhinovirus, metapneumovirus, and bocavirus. Respiratory virus infection in newborns is likely to produce more severe lung disease than occurs in older children and can manifest more nonspecifically as fever, lethargy, and poor feeding. Outbreaks of respiratory virus disease can cause substantial morbidity in neonatal nurseries.

Ocular Abnormalities

Table 95-4 lists ocular abnormalities that can be found in infants with congenital and neonatal viral infections.[54-57] Careful examination of a neonate's eyes, with the use of indirect

TABLE 95-4. Newborn Ocular Abnormalities Associated with Congenital and Neonatal Viral Infection

Abnormality	Agents
Cataracts	Rubella, CMV, HSV, LCMV, VZV
Chorioretinitis	CMV, HSV, LCMV, VZV, rubella
Optic atrophy	HSV, VZV, rubella, CMV, LCMV
Microphthalmia	CMV, rubella, LCMV
Coloboma	CMV, rubella
Keratoconjunctivitis	HSV
Pigment retinopathy	Rubella
Glaucoma	Rubella
Iritis	HSV, rubella
Anophthalmia	CMV
Peter anomaly[a]	CMV
Horner syndrome[b]	VZV

CMV, cytomegalovirus; HSV, herpes simplex virus; LCMV, lymphocytic choriomeningitis virus, VZV, varicella-zoster virus.

[a]Central corneal/anterior-chamber synechiae, cataract.

[b]Ptosis, meiosis, and ipsilateral absence of facial sweating.

ophthalmoscopy and slit lamp, is an important part of the evaluation of those with suspected congenital or neonatal infection. Abnormalities of the cornea and iris, chorioretinitis, vitritis, optic atrophy, and pigment retinopathy are the abnormalities most often detected in neonates with congenital infection. Chorioretinitis can be evident as scarring or as active lesions, sometimes accompanied by vitritis. Ocular abnormalities usually are associated with evidence of infection of other organs. In addition to association with visual impairment, ocular signs are important in congenital or neonatal viral infection because they may be predictive of central nervous system involvement.

Deafness

Deafness is commonly associated with congenital infection caused by rubella virus and CMV. Newborns with diminished hearing of unknown etiology should be evaluated for congenital infection. Congenital CMV infection accounts for approximately 15–20% of all cases of bilateral moderate to profound sensorineural hearing loss in children in the U.S.[58] Because congenital CMV infection can cause progressive hearing loss, serial hearing evaluations throughout infancy and early childhood are recommended.

APPROACH TO THE NEONATE WITH SUSPECTED VIRAL INFECTION

Differential Diagnosis

The presence, singly but especially in combination, of hepatomegaly, splenomegaly, petechiae, purpura, jaundice, microcephaly, encephalopathy, ocular abnormalities, anemia, thrombocytopenia, conjugated hyperbilirubinemia, or elevated serum hepatic transaminases should prompt the consideration of congenital viral infection. Nonspecific signs, such as fever, lethargy, anorexia, respiratory symptoms, and a sepsis-like syndrome, also suggest the possibility of perinatal viral infection as well as bacterial or fungal infection. Prenatal viral and nonviral infections, especially syphilis and toxoplasmosis, can be indistinguishable clinically from congenital viral infection. Miliary tuberculosis is rare and should be differentiated easily from viral infection, although central nervous system manifestations, hepatomegaly, and splenomegaly might initially suggest congenital infection.

Inborn errors of metabolism can cause encephalopathy, elevation of serum hepatic enzymes, thrombocytopenia, anemia, enlarged liver and spleen, jaundice, retinal pigment defects, and cataracts. Hypoglycemia, acidosis or alkalosis, hyperammonemia, crystalluria, urinary reducing substances, and a positive urine ferric chloride test result are clues to the presence of metabolic disease. Genetic abnormalities can produce CNS and other abnormalities so similar to those seen with congenital infection that the term "pseudo-TORCH" syndrome has been applied.[59–61] Liver disease associated with neonatal giant-cell hepatitis, biliary atresia, choledochal cyst, or intestinal obstruction can lead to hepatomegaly, splenomegaly, elevation of serum transaminases, and cholestatic jaundice. Anemia, hyperbilirubinemia, or hepatosplenomegaly due to rhesus or ABO isoimmunization, red blood cell biochemical defects, red blood cell structural defects, or immunologically mediated thrombocytopenia can be confused with congenital infection.

Fetal exposure to alcohol, anticonvulsants, or cocaine can impair brain growth, leading to microcephaly and neonatal encephalopathy similar to that observed in congenital infection. The prolonged use of intravenous vitamin E in premature infants has been associated with thrombocytopenia, encephalopathy, and cholestatic jaundice that could be confused with signs of congenital or neonatal viral infection. Congenital leukemia and neuroblastoma can present with anemia, thrombocytopenia, and organomegaly.

Laboratory Diagnosis

Laboratory testing should focus on identification of virus by culture or detection of viral nucleic acid or proteins in the appropriate specimens. The most likely etiologies should be selected on the basis of signs, laboratory abnormalities, and clinical context. The specimens required and the approach used for laboratory diagnosis depend on the specific viral infection being considered (see pathogen-specific chapters).

Measurement of maternal or neonatal antibody responses is of limited value but can contribute useful information in certain circumstances. Negative immunoglobulin (Ig) G antibody results for specific agents indicate that maternal infection is not present or is very recent, substantially reducing the likelihood of prenatal MTCT. The accuracy of IgM antibody testing of neonatal serum for viral diagnosis is highly variable, depending on the agent, assay used, and laboratory. Virus culture or PCR testing should be used to confirm specific positive or negative IgM antibody test results. Results of test panels for IgG or IgM antibody to multiple possible causes of infection ("TORCH titers") usually fail to establish an etiologic diagnosis or are not relevant; they should not be used as the sole laboratory diagnostic assay.[62,63]

Prevention and Treatment

Antiviral agents for treatment of congenital and neonatal infections are limited to acyclovir and ganciclovir (or valganciclovir) and antiretroviral agents. Acyclovir treatment of neonates with HSV infection can be life-saving and improves the quality of life for survivors.[49] Acyclovir also is indicated for perinatal VZV infection.[64] Antiviral treatment for severe symptomatic, congenital CMV infection also improves outcome.[65,66] Methods to protect neonates from perinatally transmitted HIV and hepatitis B are critically important. Management of infants with congenital or neonatal viral infection involves provision of supportive care and anticipation of complications, such as hearing loss, mental retardation, cerebral palsy, and chronic liver disease.

96   Hospital-Associated Infections in the Neonate

M. Gary Karlowicz and Laura Sass

As progressively smaller premature infants survive beyond the first few days of life, hospital- (or healthcare-) associated infections (HAI) have emerged as a major cause of morbidity and late mortality in the neonatal intensive care unit (NICU). Effective prevention and treatment of HAI in the NICU require understanding of the distribution of pathogens and various patient-related risk factors for these infections, and the roles of medications and invasive procedures in predisposing to their occurrence.

EPIDEMIOLOGY AND ANATOMIC SITES OF INFECTION

Bloodstream infections (BSIs) are the most common HAI in the NICU, and they can occur in isolation or in association with urinary tract infections[1] and meningitis.[2] Endocarditis, osteomyelitis, septic arthritis, ventilator associated pneumonia, peritonitis, conjunctivitis, and skin abscesses are important, less common HAIs (Table 96-1).

Late-Onset Sepsis

Late-onset sepsis is defined by the National Institute for Child Health and Human Development Neonatal Research Network (NICHD NRN) as BSIs occurring on or after 72 hours of age in neonates. Late-onset sepsis is most common in very-low-birth-weight (VLBW, birthweight <1500 g) infants, in whom HAIs increase hospital length of stay by 19 days and cause 45% of deaths beyond 2 weeks of age.[3] Late-onset sepsis occurred in 21% of VLBW infants who survived beyond 3 days of age in the NICHD NRN study,[3] and similar rates have been reported for the Neonatal Networks in Canada (24%)[4] and Israel (30%).[5]

At the institutional level, the prevalence of late-onset sepsis in VLBW infants is more variable: 11% to 32% in the NICUs of the NICHD NRN[3] and 7% to 74% in the NICUs participating in the Canadian Neonatal Network.[4] Recent data from NICHD NRN confirm risk of late-onset sepsis despite advances in medical care for the extremely premature infant, with 36% of infants born between 22 and 28 weeks' gestation having late-onset sepsis. The rate of late-onset sepsis was strongly and inversely associated with birthweight and gestational age, decreasing from ~60% in neonates with gestational age <25 weeks to 20% in infants born at 28 weeks' gestation.[6] Consequently, institutions caring for more extremely-low-birthweight (ELBW) infants have higher rates. Management practices, particularly those concerning utilization and maintenance care of central venous catheters (CVCs) or peripherally inserted central catheters (PICCs), can further impact these rates of infection.[7]

Most cases of late-onset sepsis in neonates are associated with central catheters (CVCs or PICCs),[3] and are referred to as central line associated bloodstream infections (CLABSIs). The Centers for Disease Control and Prevention (CDC) and National Healthcare Safety Network (NHSN) definition[8] for a CLABSI includes: (1) isolation of a pathogen from one blood culture or of a skin commensal from two blood cultures; (2) one or more clinical signs of infection (e.g., apnea, bradycardia, or temperature instability) that are not related to an infection at another site; and (3) presence of a CVC at the time the blood culture is obtained or within 48 hours

before the development of the infection. A rate of HAI that is linked to device utilization, such as a CLABSI, helps control for variability in management practices from institution to institution, and the preferred unit of measure is infections per 1000 catheter-days. The NHSN continues to recommend that CLABSI be a major focus of surveillance and prevention efforts in NICUs, and to that end, provide summary data on CLABSI rates for different birthweight groups. The NHSN data help individual NICUs assess their CLABSI rate relative to other NICUs. Values at the extremes of the NHSN data indicate problems with effective infection control or underreporting of CLABSI events, respectively. Individual NICUs are encouraged to monitor and compare their CLABSI rates with NHSN data, which are updated annually and usually published in December.[9]

In 2009, data on CLABSI rates from NHSN participating Level III NICUs for the years 2006 to 2008 showed a median number BSI per 1000 catheter-days of 3.2 for infants weighing <750 g, 2.5 for those weighing 751 to 1000 g, and 1.4 for those weighing 1001 to 1500 g at birth.[9] These values represent continuing decline in both CLABSI and device utilization. In addition, data were obtained regarding umbilical catheter-associated BSI for the same time period, which revealed low rates of infection in all weight categories.[9]

Coexistence of endocarditis, osteomyelitis, or pyogenic arthritis should be considered whenever BSIs persist in neonates. *Staphylococcus aureus* is the most common cause of both endocarditis[10,11] and osteomyelitis[12,13] in neonates. These complications are uncommon, but the diagnosis should be considered when multiple blood cultures are positive in a neonate with a CVC.

Late-Onset Meningitis

Until recently, there were few surveillance data on the incidence of late-onset meningitis in the NICU. Consequently, considerable variability has existed in clinical practice concerning performance of a lumbar puncture in neonates with suspected late-onset sepsis. In a prospective study of 9641 VLBW infants who survived >3 days, late-onset meningitis occurred in 134 infants. This represented 1.4% of all infants and 5% of those who had a lumbar puncture performed. Compared with infants without septicemia, VLBW infants with meningitis were more likely to have seizures (25% versus 2%), and were more likely to die (23% versus 2%).[2] Importantly, one-third (45 of 134) of the infants with meningitis had simultaneously drawn blood cultures that were negative. Because meningitis can alter duration of antibiotic therapy and long-term prognosis, all VLBW infants with suspected late-onset sepsis should have a lumbar puncture as part of the initial diagnostic evaluation, unless they are too critically ill to tolerate the

TABLE 96-1. Common Sites and Causes of Healthcare-Associated Infections in the Neonatal Intensive Care Unit

Site of Infection	Anticipated Causal Organisms					
	CoNS	*S. aureus*	Enterococci	GNR	*Candida*	Viruses
BSI	+++	++	++	++	+	−
CLABSI	+++	++	+	++	++	−
Osteomyelitis/septic arthritis	−	+++	−	+	+	−
Endocarditis	+	+++	+	+	+	−
Meningitis	+++	+	+	++	++	+
VAP	−	+	−	+++	+	+[a]
Peritonitis	+	−	+	+++	+	−
UTI	−	−	+	+++	++	−
Conjunctivitis	+	+	−	+	−	−
Skin or subcutaneous tissue	+	+++	−	+	+	+

BSI, bloodstream infection; CoNS, coagulase-negative staphylococci; S. aureus, Staphylococcus aureus; CLABSI, central line-associated bloodstream infection; GNR, gram-negative rods; UTI, urinary tract infection; VAP, ventilator-associated pneumonia.

+++, most common isolate; ++, frequently; +, occasionally; −, rarely or not.

[a]Includes respiratory syncytial virus, influenza virus, parainfluenza viruses, and enterovirus.

PART II Clinical Syndromes and Cardinal Features of Infectious Diseases: Approach to Diagnosis and Initial Management

SECTION N Infections of the Fetus and Newborn

procedure. In the latter case, lumbar puncture should be performed when clinical stabilization is achieved.

Urinary Tract Infection

Urinary tract infection (UTI) is the one of the most common HAIs in adults.[9] The high rate of UTI in hospitalized adults is associated with frequent use of indwelling urinary catheters, which are seldom used in VLBW infants. There is considerable practice variability in performing urine culture and analysis by either suprapubic bladder aspiration or urethral catheterization when late-onset sepsis is suspected.[14] Urine specimens obtained by bag collection from infants have notoriously high rates of contamination – up to 63%[15] – and are not recommended. Clinicians have tended to avoid suprapubic bladder aspiration in neonates because of the risk of serious, albeit rare, complications such as bowel perforation[16] and increased pain.[17] Fortunately, sterile urethral catheterization can be performed easily by experienced nurses, even in ELBW infants, and has a potentially higher rate of success in obtaining urine compared with suprapubic bladder aspiration.[18,19]

Although there have not been prospective studies of UTI, it may be the second most common HAI in the NICU. The reported prevalence in premature infants ranges from 4% to 25%, but these reports are from the 1960s, and do not represent the typical population in NICUs currently. A retrospective study reported an 8% rate of late-onset UTI in 762 VLBW infants in one NICU over an 11-year period.[20] UTI was more common in ELBW infants (12%) than in infants with birthweight 1001 to 1500 g (6%). In a prospective study in one NICU over a one-year period, rate of HAIs was 17.5%, with only 0.7% UTIs.[21] When intervention-associated infections were examined, urinary catheter-associated UTIs (CAUTIs) were up to 17.3%. Again, the highest risk of HAIs was in patients with a birthweight <1000 g (relative risk, 11.8).[21]

Examining paired blood and urine cultures in 189 VLBW infants suspected of having late-onset sepsis, Tamim et al. detected UTIs in 25%.[14] Among the VLBW infants with UTIs, 62% (30 of 48) had negative blood cultures. Phillips and Karlowicz[1] reported a case series of 60 UTIs in NICU patients, primarily documented through specimens obtained by urethral catheterization when late-onset sepsis was suspected. Simultaneous BSIs with the same pathogen were present in 52% of cases of Candida UTI and 8% of cases of bacterial UTI. As most VLBW infants with UTI do not have BSIs, it is our practice to obtain urine for culture (by sterile urethral catheterization or by suprapubic aspiration), whenever late-onset sepsis is suspected.

Ventilator-Associated Pneumonia

It is difficult to diagnosis healthcare-associated pneumonia in any patient population and even more difficult in the NICU population. New definitions from the CDC/NHSN in 2008 attempt to provide reproducible criteria for surveillance, classifying pneumonia into 3 specific types: clinically defined (PNU1), pneumonia with laboratory finding (PNU2), and pneumonia in immunocompromised patients (PNU3).[8] In general, infants and children fall into category 1. Diagnosis of ventilator-associated pneumonia (VAP) is especially difficult in neonates because noninfectious conditions such as respiratory distress syndrome and bronchopulmonary dysplasia are common and frequently cause radiologic abnormalities. The NHSN has published specific guidelines adapted to infants <1 year, but these are not specific to the premature infant. New benchmark data are becoming available through the NHSN. The highest incidence of VAP occurs in infants with a median birthweight of 1.3 per 1000 ventilator days ≤750 grams.[9]

A few investigators have attempted to establish reproducible criteria for VAP specific to the neonatal population. Cordero et al.[22] showed that finding purulent tracheal aspirate with positive tracheal culture in mechanically ventilated neonates in the absence of worsening clinical or radiologic findings is more consistent with clinically insignificant tracheal colonization than with

VAP. Apisarnthanarak et al.[23] performed a prospective cohort study addressing the risk factors, microbiology, and outcomes of VAP in neonates. Their definition of VAP required new and persistent radiologic evidence of focal infiltrates >48 hours after initiating mechanical ventilation and treatment with antibiotics for >7 days for presumed VAP. By this definition, 19 of 67 (28%) of mechanically ventilated VLBW infants developed VAP, with a rate of 6.5 per 1000 ventilator-days.[23] Gram-negative bacteria were isolated from tracheal aspirates in 94% of VAP episodes and most cases were polymicrobial. VAP developed in neonates on a median of day 30 and the risk of VAP increased by 11% for every additional week an infant was mechanically ventilated. VAP was strongly associated with mortality in neonates who required NICU care >30 days.[23]

Intestinal Perforation and Peritonitis

Peritonitis associated with intestinal perforation is another serious HAI infection in the NICU. Coates et al.[24] reported striking differences in the distribution of pathogens associated with peritonitis in 36 infants with focal intestinal perforation (FIP) compared with 80 infants with necrotizing enterocolitis (NEC). Enterobacteriaceae were present in 75% of NEC cases compared with 25% of FIP cases. In contrast, Candida species were found in 44% of FIP cases compared with 15% of NEC cases, and coagulase-negative staphylococci (CoNS) were present in 50% of FIP cases versus 14% of NEC cases. Peritoneal fluid cultures were positive and helped direct antimicrobial therapy in 40% (46 of 116) of cases.[24] Peritoneal fluid culture should be obtained in all neonates with intestinal perforation, regardless of cause.

Other Infections

Conjunctivitis is common in healthy full-term newborns. Few studies address its occurrence in the NICU. Diagnosis can be complicated because conjunctival colonization, especially with CoNS, is common in the NICU.[25] Occurrence rates of conjunctivitis in NICUs vary, with Haas et al.[26] reporting 5% in a prospective study and Couto et al.[27] reporting 12% (although all birthweights were included). The most common pathogens are enteric gram-negative bacilli, but non-enteric flora such as Pseudomonas aeruginosa also can occur.[28]

Most neonatal skin infections are caused by Staphylococcus aureus. Clinical manifestations include impetigo, cellulitis, soft-tissue abscesses, and toxin-mediated diseases such as staphylococcal scaled-skin syndrome and toxic shock syndrome.[29] Methicillin-resistant and methicillin-susceptible S. aureus (MRSA and MSSA) cause similar infections. Carey et al. reported incidence of 4.8% for MSSA and 1.8% of MRSA in ELBW infants' skin infections, with 53% of all NICU skin infections occurring in the ELBW cohort.[30] P. aeruginosa can cause ecthyma gangrenosum lesions even in a VLBW or ELBW infant.[31] Zygomycetes can cause progressive necrotizing skin lesions in neonates, with or without gastrointestinal manifestations.[32]

PATHOGENS OF LATE-ONSET INFECTIONS

Gram-positive organisms are the predominant cause of late-onset sepsis in the NICU (57% to 70% of cases), but gram-negative organisms (19% to 25% of cases) and fungi (12% to 18% of cases) also are important.[3,33] Across many reports the same pathogens cause most episodes: CoNS, Candida species, S. aureus, and Enterobacteriaceae (Table 96-2).

Usual Pathogens

Frequency of pathogens causing late-onset sepsis but also the likelihood that certain pathogens cause rapid progression to severe complications and death (fulminant sepsis) must be considered in choosing empiric therapy. Karlowicz et al.[33] reported that although gram-negative organisms caused only 25% of BSIs in their series, they caused 69% of fulminant late-onset BSIs. Of

TABLE 96-2. Pathogens Commonly Causing Late-Onset Sepsis in the Neonatal Intensive Care Unit (NICU)

Pathogen	Relative Frequency of Isolation	Comment
CoNS	+++	Most common cause of CLABSI
Staphylococcus aureus	++	Highest rate of focal complications; MRSA is a problem in some NICUs
Candida species	++	*Candida albicans* and *Candida parapsilosis* are the most common species
Enteric GNR	++	Most common cause of fulminant sepsis; *Klebsiella* species is the most common GNR
Pseudomonas aeruginosa	+	GNR with highest case-fatality rate
Enterococcus species	+	Increased in importance as a nosocomial pathogen since the 1990s
Group B streptococci	+	Rate of late-onset cases unchanged, in contrast to dramatic decrease in early-onset cases with intrapartum antibiotics

CoNS, coagulase-negative staphylococci; CLABSI, central line-associated bloodstream infection; GNR, gram-negative rods; MRSA, methicillin-resistant Staphylococcus aureus.

+++, most frequent; ++, common; +, occasional.

gram-negative bacilli, *P. aeruginosa* was the most prominent pathogen (42% of fulminant cases) and overall had a case-fatality rate of 56% – in contrast to a case-fatality rate of <1% for CoNS.[33] Similar findings have been reported by others.[3,34]

CoNS are the most common pathogens causing late-onset sepsis, accounting for 35%[29] and 48%[3] of cases. Distinguishing between true BSI and pseudobacteremia can be difficult. The CDC/NHSN defines a laboratory-confirmed bloodstream infection (LCBI) with common skin contaminant flora as ≥2 positive blood cultures drawn on separate occasions.[8] In the report of Stoll et al.[3] of late-onset sepsis, a rate of 48% CoNS would fall to 29% if only LCBSIs were included, a rate similar to the 35% reported by Karlowicz et al.[33]

Emerging Pathogens

Prevalence of pathogens in the community and the healthcare and NICU environment, as well as the selective pressure of antibiotic use, contribute to antibiotic-resistant infections in NICUs.[35] Gram-positive bacteria, including both hospital- and community-associated MRSA[30,36-39] and vancomycin-resistant *Enterococcus faecium*,[40] are serious problems in NICUs. Both gram-negative enteric organisms (extended-spectrum β-lactamase-carrying *E. coli* and *Klebsiella* spp.,[41-43] AmpC β-lactamase-carrying *Enterobacter* spp.,[44] metallo-β-lactamase-carrying enterics,[45] multidrug-resistant *Serratia marcescens*[46,47]) and nonenteric organisms (*P. aeruginosa*,[48,49] *Burkholderia cepacia*,[50] *Chryseobacterium meningosepticum*[51]) and most recently, highly resistant *Acinetobacter* spp. have emerged in NICU environments.[52,53]

In many instances, reservoirs containing the organism are present within the healthcare environment; patients are exposed either through the use of contaminated medical equipment or via the hands of caretakers. The former often results from breakdowns in the cleaning procedures used in the NICU or hospital environment[38,45,47,54] and the latter from ineffective use of hand hygiene by healthcare personnel (HCP).[48,55] Molecular fingerprinting of organisms has been useful for characterizing and controlling some outbreaks.[36,41,45,47,51] Control of NICU outbreaks of antibiotic-resistant organisms frequently requires vigorous application of infection control procedures (surveillance cultures, patient and staff cohorting, hand hygiene education interventions[56,57]) and active education about the factors that predispose to infection. The CDC began a 12-Step Campaign in 2002 to prevent antimicrobial resistance in various healthcare settings; these valuable methodologies can be applied successfully to the NICU.[58]

Viral Infections

HAIs caused by viruses are infrequent in the NICU, with an incidence <1%,[59] but because of patient vulnerability and propensity of viruses to spread patient to patient, impact can be substantial. Respiratory syncytial virus (RSV),[60,61] influenza virus,[62] enteroviruses,[63,64] rotavirus,[65,66] adenovirus,[67] coronavirus,[68] parainfluenza,[69] and norovirus[70,71] have been described in NICU outbreaks, sometimes concurrently.[72] Attack rates can be as high as 33%.[62,64,67] Patients can be asymptomatic or have disease that is lethal,[66] and the attributable costs can be high.[60] Viruses can be introduced into the NICU both by family members and by ill HCPs.

RSV infections can manifest as cough, congestion, apnea, increasing oxygen requirement, or respiratory failure.[59,60] Parainfluenza can present similarly, as can adenovirus, in addition to causing epidemic conjunctivitis.[67] Of note, ophthalmologic procedures can contribute to spread of adenovirus.[67] Coronavirus infection can be associated with respiratory decompensation or abdominal distention and fever.[68] Enteroviruses can be associated with clinical manifestations suggestive of NEC, overwhelming septicemia, rash, or aseptic meningitis.[63] Rotavirus infection is associated with diarrhea that is frequent and watery in term infants, whereas in preterm infants it is more frequently bloody and associated with abdominal distention and intestinal dilatation.[65]

CLINICAL MANIFESTATIONS

The clinical features of sepsis in neonates are nonspecific, with most common clinical features being increased apnea/bradycardia (55%), increased gastrointestinal problems (46%) (feeding intolerance, abdominal distention, or bloody stools), increased respiratory support (29%), and lethargy/hypotonia (23%).[73] Predominant laboratory indicators are abnormal white blood cell count (46%) (e.g., leukocytosis, increased immature white blood cells, or neutropenia), unexplained metabolic acidosis (11%), and hyperglycemia (10%). Unfortunately, the predictive value of features is low, with the best positive predictive value being 31%, for hypotension.[73]

Abnormal heart rate characteristics (reduced variability and transient decelerations) occur early in the course of neonatal sepsis.[74] Although technology has been developed to calculate a heart rate characteristic index (HRCi),[75] Griffin et al. found that HRCi performed similarly to a clinical scoring system in predicting sepsis.[76]

The most common signs of CLABSI in neonates are fever (49%) and respiratory distress (30%),[77] with only 20% of cases showing erythema or purulent discharge at the catheter insertion site.

LABORATORY DIAGNOSIS

The pretreatment diagnostic evaluation of suspected HAI should include at least two blood cultures (such as from any indwelling catheter along with peripheral sites), cerebrospinal fluid (CSF) culture, and urine culture. The isolation of CoNS from a single blood culture generally should be interpreted as a contaminant.

PART II Clinical Syndromes and Cardinal Features of Infectious Diseases: Approach to Diagnosis and Initial Management

SECTION N Infections of the Fetus and Newborn

A definitive diagnosis of a HAI due to bacterial or fungal species requires isolation of the organism from blood or another normally sterile body site or fluid. Exceptions are fungi such as *Aspergillus* and Zygomycetes, which can cause potentially fatal disseminated multiorgan infection but rarely are isolated from blood.[32,78]

When viral infection is suspected, a presumptive diagnosis can be made by rapid diagnostic testing (e.g., a positive direct fluorescent antibody (DFA) test for adenovirus, herpes simplex virus or enzyme immunoassay (EIA) for influenza, respiratory syncytial virus, or rotavirus) and a definitive diagnosis by isolation or polymerase chain reaction testing of nasal wash, tracheal secretions, bronchoalveolar lavage fluid, or stool, as appropriate.

Attempts to identify dependable serum markers for diagnosis, severity, or prognosis have been variably successful, including the use of C-reactive protein (CRP), various proinflammatory cytokines, and/or procalcitonin (PCT) levels. Two recent meta-analysis of PCT showed potential for its use in diagnosis of late-onset sepsis.[79,80] One study found PCT more accurate than CRP,[80] but studies have not had consistent results[81] and it is unlikely that a single test taken out of context and cadence of clinical findings and likely pathogen(s) will have pivotal importance.

TREATMENT

Empiric Therapy

Empiric antimicrobial therapy for suspected HAIs without a clinical focus in neonates should be guided by knowledge of the distribution, case-fatality rates of pathogens, and the local susceptibility patterns of likely pathogens. An empiric antibiotic regimen should effectively treat gram-negative pathogens, particularly *P. aeruginosa*. An aminoglycoside should be used for empiric treatment of possible gram-negative sepsis, the choice of which is determined by the antimicrobial susceptibility patterns of isolates from the NICU. During an outbreak of gentamicin-resistant gram-negative septicemia, amikacin may be the preferred aminoglycoside. Third-generation cephalosporins are not recommended for routine empiric therapy in neonates (unless knowledge of the patient's flora or the NICU pattern of infections specifically dictates) because: (1) they do not have activity against most *P. aeruginosa* and some Enterobacteriaceae; (2) routine use in NICUs has been associated with emergence of cephalosporin-resistant gram-negative bacilli;[82,83] and (3) use has been associated with increased risk of candidemia in VLBW neonates.[84]

Ampicillin may be considered for empiric treatment of possible gram-positive septicemia, especially if *Enterococcus* and *Streptococcus agalactiae* are common pathogens causing late-onset sepsis in the NICU. If MRSA is prevalent in the community or NICU, vancomycin should be used as first-line therapy.[85] If no MRSA is identified, vancomycin should be discontinued. If MSSA is identified, nafcillin is therapeutically superior to vancomycin.

Because CoNS sepsis is common, some advocate broad empiric usage of vancomycin.[86] This creates additional problems. Stoll et al.[3] found it alarming that 44% of all VLBW infants in the Neonatal Research Network were treated with vancomycin whether or not they had CoNS BSI. The Hospital Infection Control and Practices Advisory Committee of the CDC recommend avoiding empiric vancomycin therapy in patients with suspected sepsis to prevent the emergence and spread of vancomycin-resistant enterococci.[87] Karlowicz et al.[33] showed that avoidance of empiric use of vancomycin had no impact on the very low rate of fulminant CoNS sepsis in neonates and that the practice of beginning vancomycin only after CoNS was identified in blood culture did not prolong the duration of BSI. Despite ongoing education, vancomycin continues to be the most commonly used drug in NICUs surveyed and was inappropriately used 32% of the time.[58] It is possible to reduce the empiric use of vancomycin in units that have low levels of MRSA infection without compromising patient care or safety. Chiu et al. demonstrated that the application of guidelines for vancomycin use decreased neonatal vancomycin exposure from 5.2 to 3.1 per 1000 patient-days (40% reduction)

TABLE 96-3. Suggested Duration of Therapy for Selected Healthcare Infections

Site or Manifestation of Infection	Duration of Therapy (days)
BSI	10–14
Meningitis	14–21
CLABSI without removal of CVC	14[a]
Osteomyelitis/septic arthritis	4–6 weeks
VAP	10–14
UTI	10–14
Endocarditis	4–6 weeks
Candidemia, catheter removed, rapidly resolving	10–14
Fungemia, disseminated	~4 weeks
Skin or subcutaneous lesion	7–10

BSI, bloodstream infection; CLABSI, central line-associated bloodstream infection; CVC, central venous catheter; UTI, urinary tract infection; VAP, ventilator-associated pneumonia.

[a]*After first negative blood culture.*

and 10.8 to 5.5 per 1000 patient-days (49% reduction) in two separate NICUs with no change in causes of infection, duration of BSI, or incidence of complications or attributable deaths.[88] Antibiotic stewardship, specific to each NICU, remains critical to prevention of spread of resistant bacteria and avoidance of use of unnecessary medications.

The use of empiric antifungal therapy for VLBW infants at high risk of candidemia is not as standardized as it is in other patient populations. Some studies suggest that empiric therapy may reduce mortality and improve outcomes in this VLBW infants.[89] In a retrospective study, empiric antifungal treatment was given to critically ill neonates <1500 g with additional risk factors for invasive *Candida* infection who had received vancomycin and/or third-generation cephalosporin for 7 days and had ≥1 of the following risks: receipt of total parenteral nutrition, mechanical ventilation, postnatal corticosteroid therapy, or H_2-blocking agent, or mucocutaneous *Candida* infection.[90] No *Candida*-related mortality occurred in patients who received empiric amphotericin B (0 of 6) compared with historical controls (11 of 18).[90] Decision to use an empiric antifungal agent for late-onset sepsis should be made on an individual basis.[91,92]

The suggested duration of therapy for HAIs by anatomic site is summarized in Table 96-3. The duration of treatment for individual patients should be determined by virulence of the pathogen, time it takes for follow-up cultures to become negative, rapidity of clinical response, time to negative blood culture, removal or retention of CVC, and adequate drainage of purulent foci if present.

Adjunctive Therapy

Several adjunctive therapies have been investigated in late-onset sepsis, including immune globulin intravenous (IGIV), hematopoietic growth factors (granulocyte colony-stimulating factor (G-CSF) and granulocyte-macrophage colony-stimulating factor (GM-CSF)), granulocyte transfusions, and pentoxifylline. IGIV,[93] G-CSF and GM-CSF,[94] and granulocyte transfusions[95] have been evaluated by the Cochrane Database of Systematic Reviews, with the conclusion that there is insufficient evidence currently to support routine use in the treatment of neonates with sepsis. Pentoxifylline also has been reviewed by the Cochrane Database as an adjunct to antibiotics for treatment of suspected or confirmed sepsis or NEC, with results, suggesting a decrease in all-cause mortality, but the studies evaluated were small.[96] More research is needed to determine the usefulness of this adjunctive agent. A larger, multicenter trial used GM-CSF for prophylaxis of late-onset sepsis in neonates <31 weeks' gestation and small for gestational age but did not show significant difference in sepsis-free survival.[97] A review of the data from studies of granulocyte transfusions in septic neonates demonstrated improved outcome in the situation of neutropenic depletion of the marrow storage pool, but associated morbidities, including fluid overload, worsening hypoxia and respiratory distress from leukocyte sequestration in the lung, graft-versus-host disease, and risk of transmission of viral infections.[95] Careful assessment of the risks versus the benefits of leukocyte administration is required, as is the use of any of the other adjunctive therapies.[98]

MANAGEMENT OF CENTRAL LINE ASSOCIATED BLOODSTREAM INFECTIONS

Catheters are intravascular foreign bodies; removal is the optimal management when a BSI occurs. Nevertheless, the vital importance of CVCs in critically ill neonates must be acknowledged, especially since successful in situ treatment of CLABSI has become more common.[99] BSIs can occur without being a CLABSI; differentiation of these two conditions can be difficult. There have been no randomized trials to guide management of CLABSI in the NICU; however, several large observational cohort studies have compared outcomes of late-onset sepsis in neonates with CVCs treated with and without CVC removal. Data suggest that management strategies can be different, depending on the pathogen and clinical condition of the infant. If treatment with the CVC in situ is attempted, antimicrobial agents should be administered through the contaminated catheter. The algorithm shown in Figure 96-1 provides a framework for management of CLABSI in neonates until evidence becomes available from randomized trials.

Candida Species

A single-center retrospective study of 104 cases reported that failure to remove CVCs as soon as *Candida* sepsis was detected in neonates was associated with significantly increased mortality in *C. albicans* sepsis (case-fatality risk increase of 39%, number needed to harm of 2.6) and significantly prolonged duration of *Candida* sepsis regardless of *Candida* species (median of 6 days versus 3 days).[100] These findings were confirmed in a retrospective multicenter study of ELBW infants with systemic candidiasis.[89] The Infectious Diseases Society of America (IDSA) guidelines for treatment of catheter-related infections[99] strongly recommend that CVCs be removed as soon as *Candida* sepsis if feasible. Unfortunately, in some neonates, the CVCs are vital lifelines and cannot be removed because of severe generalized skin breakdown or unstable critical condition.

Coagulase-Negative Staphylococci

It has been difficult to interpret clinical studies of CoNS CLABSI in neonates because many studies required only a single positive blood culture for inclusion, thus allowing many cases of pseudobacteremia. In a series of 119 cases[101] of CoNS CLABSI, investigators concluded that in situ treatment often could be successful, but observed it was unclear how long clinicians should wait before abandoning sterilizing attempts and removing the CVC. Karlowicz et al. reported that in situ treatment with vancomycin was successful in 46% of cases with CoNS CLABSI;[100] none of 19 patients with CoNS BSI for >4 days after institution of antibiotic therapy had resolution until the CVC was removed. In contrast, 79% of cases with CoNS BSI for ≤2 days were successfully treated without CVC removal; successful treatment decreased to 44% when BSI persisted for 3 to 4 days.[100] Therefore, when CoNS CLABSI persists in neonates whose catheter is vital to clinical care, it is our practice to administer antibiotic treatment through the CVC for 2 days, perhaps as long as 3 to 4 days in special circumstances, but never beyond 4 days of persistent bacteremia, before removing a CVC.

The use of antibiotic lock therapy for treatment of CoNS CLABSI is part of the IDSA treatment guidelines for both short- and long-term CVC, using 10- to 14-day lock therapy in combination with systemic antibiotic treatment.[99] The role of vancomycin lock therapy in the NICU for treatment is unclear, with more research involving its preventive use.[102]

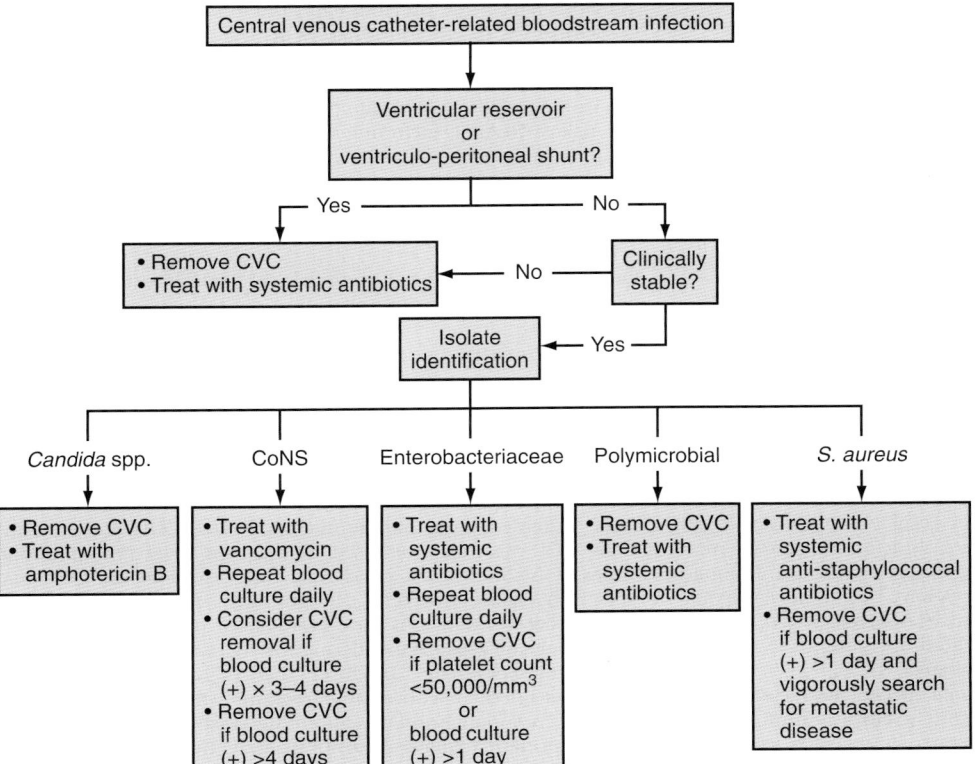

Figure 96-1. Suggested management of central line associated bloodstream infection (CLABSI) in neonates. CoNS, coagulase-negative staphylococci. [a]After commencement of appropriate antibiotic therapy.

PART II Clinical Syndromes and Cardinal Features of Infectious Diseases: Approach to Diagnosis and Initial Management

SECTION N Infections of the Fetus and Newborn

Enterobacteriaceae

Although Enterobacteriaceae are a common cause of late-onset sepsis, data are limited concerning CLABSI. In a report of 53 cases of Enterobacteriaceae CLABSI in neonates, Karlowicz et al. reported resolution of infection in 45% of cases with use of gentamicin or tobramycin without removal of CVCs.[103] In contrast to successful in situ treatment despite several days of CoNS BSI, successful treatment of Enterobacteriaceae with BSIs of >1 day duration was uncommon without removal of CVC. Attempting to treat Enterobacteriaceae BSI with CVC in situ was not associated with observable increase in mortality, morbidity, or recurrence. Severe thrombocytopenia (platelet count <50,000/mm^3) on the first day of Enterobacteriaceae BSI did not resolve until CVCs were removed in 82% of cases.[103] It is our practice to remove CVC in cases associated with severe thrombocytopenia or if Enterobacteriaceae BSI persists >1 day after commencing appropriate antibiotic treatment.

Staphylococcus aureus

In adults, removal of CVC is advised in cases of *S. aureus* BSI, unless there is a *compelling* reason to conserve the catheter.[99] There are few published reports concerning *S. aureus* CLABSI in neonates or children. In a review of 154 cases of *S. aureus* CLABSI in 112 patients in one institution (12 premature neonates),[14] patients had complications related to infection (excluding prolonged bacteremia) with recurrence being most common. The rate of complications was lower in the patients whose catheter was removed <4 days after onset of infection compared with those whose catheter was not removed or was removed >4 days after onset of infection.[104] Data on treating *S. aureus* CLABSI in situ are conflicting, with some showing poor success.[105] Most cases that were treated successfully despite CVC in situ showed resolution of MSSA BSI within 24 hours of starting a penicillinase-resistant penicillin. Focal complications, like soft-tissue abscesses, endocarditis, and osteomyelitis, may be more important risk factors for persistent *S. aureus* BSI than retention of CVC. It is our practice to use a cautious approach, removing CVC immediately if infection persists >1 day after initiation of appropriate antibiotic treatment.

Polymicrobial Infections

Polymicrobial BSI in neonates accounts for about 10% of cases of late-onset sepsis.[106] It occurs generally later than monomicrobial sepsis, in neonates with a severe underlying condition, and among those with longer indwelling CVCs. CoNS is the most common organism recovered from culture and is seen in combination with other gram-positive and gram-negative organisms.[106] It would seem prudent to remove CVCs, as soon as possible, in cases of polymicrobial sepsis.

MANAGEMENT OF PERSISTENT BLOODSTREAM INFECTIONS

The likelihood of adverse outcomes, such as focal complications, increases when BSI persists in neonates. Although it is uncertain whether focal complications are the cause or the consequence of persistent BSI, it is imperative that clinicians obtain serial blood cultures to document resolution of BSI and perform thorough diagnostic evaluations searching for focal complications if BSI persists. In addition, when BSI persists, clinicians must make management decisions concerning timing of CVC removal and changes in antimicrobial therapy. Several cases have been reported of successful treatment of persistent CoNS CLABSIs with CVC in situ, without adverse consequences, by adding rifampin to standard antistaphylococcal antimicrobial therapy.[107,108]

Some pathogens, especially *Candida* species, may continue to be isolated from blood cultures despite prompt removal of CVC and administration of antifungal therapy. In one such series of 96 neonatal cases, candidiasis lasted >7 days in 30% of cases.[109] The risk of focal complications of invasive candidiasis was significantly increased in cases with persistent compared with nonpersistent BSI (48% versus 13%). The most common focal complications were "fungus ball" uropathy (29%), renal infiltration (20%), abscess (19%), and endocarditis (9%).[109] Since more than half of neonates with persistent candidiasis do not have focal complications, Chapman and Faix[109] suggested that aggressive imaging for focal complications be reserved for cases in which blood cultures remain positive despite several days of antifungal therapy, or if there are clinical signs suggesting focal complication. On the other hand, Noyola et al.[110] documented focal complications in 23% of 86 neonates with candidemia, including some with only one positive blood culture, and the authors recommended renal, cardiac, and ophthalmologic diagnostic evaluations in all neonates with candidemia because the presence of focal complications may affect the duration of therapy and outcome.

The prevalence of persistent BSI was reported to be 22% in a series of 335 cases of bacteremia in one NICU.[111] In this case series, the frequent decision to treat bacterial BSI with CVC in situ contributed to the high prevalence of persistent cases. The prevalence of focal suppurative complications (osteomyelitis, septic arthritis, abscess, infected thrombus, or endocarditis) was significantly increased in infants with duration of BSI and with persistent non-CoNS BSI compared with persistent CoNS BSI (28% versus 3%).[111] *S. aureus* caused 50% of persistent non-CoNS BSIs and 67% of the cases with focal complications. The authors recommended that all neonates with persistent BSI undergo extensive evaluation for focal complications, especially for endocarditis, osteomyelitis, and soft-tissue abscesses. This evaluation is especially important in cases of persistent BSI caused by *S. aureus* or Enterobacteriaceae, because the bacteremia will not resolve until the soft-tissue abscesses (sometimes suppurative phlebitis) or bone or joint infections are drained, or the intravascular clot dissolves.

PREVENTION OF HEALTHCARE-ASSOCIATED INFECTIONS

Risk factors for CLABSI have been extensively examined and include use of total parenteral nutrition,[3] mechanical ventilation,[3] previous BSIs,[90] and previous exposure to third-generation cephalosporins.[83] A recent cohort study of monozygotic and dizygotic premature infants concluded that 49% of variance in occurrence of late-onset sepsis may be due to genetic factors and 51% to environmental factors.[112] Manipulation of the central line increases the risk of CLABSI, including the placement of the lines, maintenance of the dressing, and repeated entry into the CVC system. Thus, approaches that minimize these interventions will decrease the rate of CLABSI, with successful programs addressing both technical and contextual factors, often with the use of "bundles" and guidelines.[113] Bizzarro et al. performed a quality improvement initiative designed to reduce their NICU infection rate by implementing several interventions using a multidisciplinary approach, and using guidelines for CVC care.[7] Interventions were associated with a decrease in the rates of CLABSI from 8.40 to 1.28 cases per 1000 central line-days and late-onset sepsis from 5.84 to 1.42 cases per 1000 patient-days.[7]

Hand decontamination by HCP is the most effective means of preventing HAIs,[114] but often is overlooked or performed poorly in the NICU environment.[57,115] Activities such as skin contact, respiratory care, and diaper changes are independently associated with increased hand contamination.[114] The CDC recommends that HCP use alcohol-based hand rubs over antimicrobial soaps.[114] Alcohol-based hand rubs have excellent antimicrobial spectrum against bacteria, fungi, and viruses. In addition, alcohol-based hand rubs have rapid speed of action and are the least likely to cause hand dermatitis in HCP.[114] The institution of a "hand hygiene" taskforce that includes problem-based and task-oriented education programs can help with hand hygiene compliance and concurrent decrease in the infection rate. It is important to have continuous staff involvement to ensure success.[57,116]

The use of chlorhexidine gluconate (CHG) in the NICU for CVC care is increasing, with a recent survey showing 62% of respondents using CHG as off-label use, since it is not approved by the FDA for use in children <2 months of age.[117] At this time, there are no data to support the use of CHG for patient bathing in the neonatal or pediatric population.

Premature infants require respiratory and enteral support. Systemic corticosteroid and H_2-blocking agents have been used to prevent chronic lung disease and enhance gastrointestinal function, respectively. Dexamethasone therapy in VLBW infants is associated with increased risk of late-onset sepsis.[89] Use of H_2-blocking agents in VLBW infants is associated with higher rates of NEC,[118] BSIs,[89] and candidemia.[89,119] Avoiding the use of dexamethasone and H_2-blocking agents should reduce rates of late-onset sepsis.[120]

Human milk contains a number of substances that provide a beneficial effect to the premature infant, including enhancement of innate immunity and enhancement of mucosal barriers. Establishing full enteral feedings with human milk is associated with lower risks of late-onset sepsis in ELBW infants.[121] Human milk also has been found to reduce the development of NEC by 6-fold in a study of 202 VLBW infants who either received >50% compared with <50% human milk in the first 14 days of life.[122] The use of bovine lactoferrin (bLF) also is being studied for prevention of sepsis. The Italian Study Group for Neonatal Infections studied the effect of lactoferrin with and without probiotics (*Lactobacillus* GG) and found a decrease in rate of infection in the infants who were given bLF (5% to 6%) compared with the placebo group (18%).[123] The use of oral lactoferrin was reviewed in a Cochrane Database but only the previously mentioned study was eligible for review. It was shown to be beneficial in infants <1000 g, but more trials are needed.[124]

The American Academy of Pediatrics Red Book 2009 Committee on Infectious Diseases state that the use of fluconazole prophylaxis to prevent invasive candidiasis (IC) in ELBW infants should be considered in nurseries with moderate to high risk of IC after infection control practices are optimized.[125] Kaufman et al. demonstrated a significant reduction in invasive fungal disease in 100 ELBW infants given either fluconazole prophylaxis or placebo, 0% versus 20% respectively, but the level of IC was higher in their NICU than in centers in the Neonatal Research Network at that time.[126] The strongest effect appears to be when prophylaxis is targeted to high-risk patients with birthweight of <1000 g and with use of CVCs. It may be reasonable to use fluconazole with dosing of 3 mg/kg twice per week until intravenous (central or peripheral) access is no longer needed in the high-risk populations, starting in the first 2 days of life.[120] Nystatin prophylaxis also has been studied (but not as extensively) and it also shows potential effectiveness in the same high-risk population but may have increased gastrointestinal side effects compared with fluconazole.[120]

The use of probiotics in the NICU is controversial since probiotics used in studies have varied and not all probiotics can be considered the same. A recent review acknowledges that different strains may have common characteristics and action but also may have unique properties and actions towards specific targets; generalization is difficult.[127] A meta-analysis of 15 randomized controlled trials of enteral probiotic supplementation recommended the use of probiotics in preterm infants if a suitable product is available since the benefits of the reduction of death and NEC disease were clear to the authors.[128] A recent clinical trial using *Bifidobacterium breve* and *Lactobacillus casei* supplementation in human milk fed infants showed reduction of NEC stage >2 in those infants 750 to 1499 g who received the probiotic versus placebo (0 versus 4 cases, respectively).[129] Despite some studies showing benefit, evidence of infection prevention requires further elucidation prior to the universal recommendation of probiotic supplementation, especially with regard to strains used.

SECTION O: Infections and Transplantation

97 Infections in Solid Organ Transplant Recipients

Michael Green and Marian G. Michaels

Solid-organ transplantation (SOT) is now accepted therapy for end-stage disease related to most organs. Accordingly, an expanding number of immunosuppressed children are at risk for developing infection after transplantation.

PREDISPOSING FACTORS

Factors predisposing to infection after SOT can be divided into those that exist before transplant and those secondary to intraoperative and posttransplant events (Box 97-1).

Pretransplantation Factors

The specific organ that is transplanted is the most important determinant of the location of infection, especially during the first 3 postoperative months.[1] The chest, abdomen, and urinary tract are the most common sites of infection after thoracic, liver, and kidney transplantation, respectively. Explanations for these site-specific infections include local ischemic injury and bleeding, as well as potential intraoperative contamination.[2]

The underlying condition causing organ failure also can lead to an increased risk for developing infection after SOT. For example, cystic fibrosis (CF) predisposes to pseudomonal and fungal infections after lung transplantation. Palliative surgery, such as for cardiac, biliary and urologic conditions, before transplantation increases the technical difficulty of the transplant procedure, enhancing the risk of subsequent infection.[3] The severity of disease at the time of transplantation correlates with the risk of postoperative morbidity and mortality.[4] Long-standing malnutrition predisposes children to infections; attempts to correct nutritional deficits with parenteral alimentation carry attendant risks of catheter-associated infection. Finally, mechanical ventilation while awaiting transplantation increases the risk of colonization and infection with nosocomial pathogens, many of which have multidrug resistance.

Age is an important determinant of both susceptibility to and severity of infection after transplantation. Young children undergoing transplantation can experience greater disease severity with certain viruses, such as respiratory syncytial virus (RSV) or parainfluenza virus (PIV) compared with older recipients. Likewise, primary infection with cytomegalovirus (CMV) or Epstein–Barr virus (EBV) is associated with worse outcome compared with reactivation infections.[5,6] By contrast, other pathogens, such as *Cryptococcus* species, rarely are found before young adulthood. Younger age at the time of transplantation also is associated with an increased rate of infection during the first few years after transplantation.[7] Finally, young children who are not fully immunized remain susceptible to vaccine-preventable infections or receive vaccination after transplantation, when their ability to mount an immune response may be hampered by immunosuppression.[8]

PART II Clinical Syndromes and Cardinal Features of Infectious Diseases: Approach to Diagnosis and Initial Management

SECTION O Infections and Transplantation

> **BOX 97-1.** Predisposing Factors for Infections After Organ Transplantation in Children
>
> **PRETRANSPLANTATION FACTORS**
>
> Underlying disease(s), malnutrition
> Specific organ to be transplanted
> Age of patient
> Previous exposures to infectious agents
> Previous immunizations
>
> **INTRAOPERATIVE FACTORS**
>
> Duration of transplant surgery
> Exposure to blood products
> Technical problems
> Organisms transmitted in donor tissue
>
> **POSTTRANSPLANTATION FACTORS**
>
> Immunosuppression
> - Immediate posttransplant immunosuppression
> - Maintenance immunosuppression
> - Augmented therapy for rejection episodes
>
> Indwelling cannulas
> Nosocomial exposures
> Community exposures

Transplant recipients can acquire pathogens from their donors who have active or latent infections at the time of organ harvesting. Examples include CMV,[9-11] EBV, *Toxoplasma gondii, Histoplasma* spp., West Nile virus (WNV), hepatitis B (HBV) and C viruses (HCV), and human immunodeficiency virus (HIV).[12] Screening to preclude donors with HBV or HIV infection is standard practice whereas HCV-positive donors are sometimes used for HCV-positive recipients. Bacteria or fungi colonizing the donor's respiratory tract can cause disease after lung transplantation.[13] Similarly, unrecognized bacteremia or viremia in the donor creates a risk to any recipient.

Intraoperative Factors

Operative factors unique to each SOT procedure can predispose to infection. For example, the type of biliary reconstruction used in liver transplantation influences the likelihood of developing an infectious complication.[14] Surgical events during the operation also alter the risk of infection. Injury to the phrenic, vagal, or recurrent laryngeal nerves affect pulmonary toilet, predisposing a lung transplant recipient to pneumonia.[15] Additional factors, including prolonged operative time, contamination of the operative field, and bleeding at or near surgical sites, also increase the risk of postoperative infections.

Posttransplantation Factors

Immunosuppression is the major risk for infection following transplantation. While immunosuppressive regimens evolve to achieve more specific control of rejection with less impairment of immune function, currently, all regimens interfere with host defenses. Treatment of rejection exacerbates this risk as does use of anti-lymphocyte preparations or other biologic agents.[11,14,16] As newer immunosuppressive agents are introduced, clinicians must be alert for known and unknown infections, risks, and manifestations.[17]

Technical problems after transplantation are major risk factors for infectious complications. Thrombosis of the hepatic artery predisposes to hepatic abscesses and bloodstream infection (BSI) after liver transplantation;[18] vesicoureteral reflux predisposes to graft pyelonephritis in renal transplant recipients;[15,19] and mediastinal bleeding requiring re-exploration predisposes to mediastinitis and BSI in thoracic transplant recipients.[9]

Indwelling cannulas pose a significant risk for infection after transplantation. Central venous catheters are a risk for BSI; urethral catheters predispose to urinary tract infection (UTI); and prolonged endotracheal intubation is associated with pneumonia.

Nosocomial exposures constitute the final group of posttransplant risk factors. All transplant recipients are at risk for transfusion-associated pathogens. Children undergoing transplantation during the winter often are exposed nosocomially to common viruses (e.g., RSV, influenza virus, rotavirus). Areas of the hospital with heavy contamination with pathogenic fungi, such as *Aspergillus* species, increase the risk of invasive fungal disease after SOT. Finally, nosocomial transmission of multiple drug-resistant bacteria predisposes to infection with these pathogens.

TIMING OF INFECTIONS

The timing of specific infections generally is predictable regardless of the type of organ transplanted. Most clinically important infections occur within the first 180 days and tend to present at stereotypical times after transplantation. However, the timing of certain pathogens (e.g., CMV) can be affected by the use of prophylactic strategies, augmentation in immune suppression, or need for additional surgery. In evaluating for the presence of infection, it is useful to divide risk periods posttransplantation into three major intervals: (1) early (0 to 30 days after transplantation); (2) intermediate (30 to 180 days); and (3) late (more than 180 days). In addition, some infections can occur throughout the posttransplant course. While exceptions occur, these divisions provide a useful framework for the approach to and differential diagnosis of a patient with fever after transplantation (Table 97-1).

Early Infections

Early infections (0 to 30 days after transplant) usually are associated with the presence of pre-existing conditions or surgical complications. Bacteria or yeast are the most frequent pathogens recovered.[9,20] Fifty percent or more of all bacterial infections after transplantation occur during the early posttransplant period.[9,20] Superficial or deep surgical wound infections predominate during this period. Technical difficulties, particularly those resulting in anastomotic leaks or stenoses, are important risk factors after most types of SOT.

Intermediate Period Infections

The intermediate period (31 to 180 days after transplant) is the typical time for manifestation of infection due to latent organisms transmitted with donor organs or blood products or reactivation of those already within the recipient. This also is the time of presentation of classic "opportunistic" infections. In the absence of antiviral prophylaxis, CMV infection peaks during this time period.[9-11] Similarly, EBV-associated posttransplant lymphoproliferative disorders (PTLD),[6,21,22] *Pneumocystis jirovecii* pneumonia (PCP),[23-25] and toxoplasmosis[24,26] typically manifest in this period.

Late Infections

Published data on late infectious complications (more than 180 days after transplant) are limited. In general, rates and severity of infection in children ≥6 months after transplantation are similar to those observed in otherwise healthy children.[7] This is likely explained by the fact that the majority of pediatric transplant recipients are maintained on low levels of immunosuppression after this time period. However, chronic or recurrent infections do occur in a subset of transplant recipients who have uncorrected anatomic or functional abnormalities (e.g., vesicoureteral reflux, biliary stricture). Another exception occurs in children experiencing chronic lung rejection manifested as bronchiolitis obliterans syndrome (BOS). These children frequently become infected with *Pseudomonas, Stenotrophomonas,* and *Aspergillus* species.[13,27] Infections due to varicella-zoster virus (VZV) also

TABLE 97-1. Timing of Infectious Complications Following Transplantation[a]

Early Period (0 to 1 month)	Middle Period (1 to 6 months)	Late Period (6 months and later)
BACTERIAL INFECTIONS	**VIRAL INFECTIONS**	**VIRAL INFECTIONS**
Gram-negative enteric bacilli	Cytomegalovirus	Epstein–Barr virus
Small bowel, liver, neonatal heart	All transplant types	All transplant types, but less than middle period
Pseudomonas/Burkholderia spp.	Seronegative recipient of seropositive donor	Varicella-zoster virus
Cystic fibrosis: lung	Epstein–Barr virus	All transplant types
Gram-positive organisms	All transplant types	Community-acquired viral infections
All transplant types	Seronegative recipient	All transplant types
FUNGAL INFECTIONS	Small bowel highest risk group	**BACTERIAL INFECTIONS**
All transplant types	Varicella-zoster virus	*Pseudomonas/Burkholderia* spp.
VIRAL INFECTIONS	All transplant types	Cystic fibrosis: lung
Herpes simplex virus	**OPPORTUNISTIC INFECTIONS**	Lung recipients with chronic rejection
All transplant types	*Pneumocystis jirovecii*	Gram-negative enteric bacilli
Nosocomial respiratory viruses	All transplant types	Small bowel highest risk group
All transplant types	*Toxoplasma gondii*	**FUNGAL INFECTIONS**
	Seronegative recipient of a heart from a seropositive donor	*Aspergillus* spp.
	BACTERIAL INFECTIONS	Lung transplants with chronic rejection
	Pseudomonas/Burkholderia spp. pneumonia	
	Cystic fibrosis: lung	
	Gram-negative enteric bacilli	
	Small bowel highest risk group	

[a]Listed in decreasing order of relative importance.

occur during this later time period.[28] Finally, CMV can manifest late, particularly in children who receive prolonged prophylaxis,[29] and EBV-associated PTLD continues to manifest in the late period.[30]

Infections Occurring Throughout the Postoperative and Posttransplantation Course

Iatrogenic risk factors can occur whenever children require hospitalization. Central venous catheters, percutaneous indwelling catheters, and nasotracheal or endotracheal tubes are maintained for variable periods; increased risk of infection persists for the entire time of cannulation. Likewise the risk of community viruses, such as RSV or influenza, is seasonal. Diagnostic studies should be modified according to these considerations.

BACTERIAL AND FUNGAL INFECTION

With the exception of infections related to the use of indwelling catheters, sites of bacterial infection tend to be at or near the transplanted organ; recovery of bacteria with multidrug resistance is common. Knowledge of prior culture results and local antimicrobial resistance patterns help guide empiric antibiotic use.

Renal Transplantation

Septicemia originating from the urinary tract, the lower respiratory tract, or the transplant wound accounts for most life-threatening infections early after renal transplantation.[15,31] Urinary tract infection (UTI), especially pyelonephritis, is the most common infectious complication, accounting for up to 50% of episodes.[32,33] Gram-negative organisms predominate.[31–33] Reportedly, one-third of pediatric renal transplant recipients experience recurrent UTI.[34] The incidence may be decreased with the use of ureteroneocystostomy and prophylactic use of daily trimethoprim-sulfamethoxazole (TMP-SMX).[19,35] Infection of the lower respiratory tract occurs in 10% to 25% of adult renal transplant recipients and can occur more than a year after transplantation.[31,34] Episodes of pneumonia caused by both gram-negative and gram-positive bacteria can be severe.[36]

Fungal infections are uncommon after renal transplantation. When present, *Candida* spp. predominate, and the urinary tract is the most common site.[15] However, patients also are at risk of infection with opportunistic fungi, such as *Aspergillus* spp.[34,37] Those with fungal infections appear to be at higher risk for graft loss.[38]

Liver Transplantation

Bacterial and fungal infections are common early after liver transplantation.[39–42] Intra-abdominal infection or presence of a central venous catheter predispose to BSI, but it can occur without an obvious source. Enteric gram-negative organisms account for more than 50% of episodes. Bacterial infections involving the abdomen or surgical wound are common. Infectious complications of the transplanted liver also occur. Historically, the most important complication was hepatic abscess, associated with hepatic artery or portal vein thrombosis. However, the introduction of frequent Doppler surveillance studies to assess for thrombosis, coupled with the use of operative thrombectomy and thrombolysis, has essentially eliminated the development of hepatic abscesses in this population.

Ascending cholangitis is common after liver transplantation, and usually is associated with biliary tract abnormalities. Diagnosis is made on clinical grounds in a patient with fever and biochemical evidence of biliary tract inflammation (see Chapter 66, Cholecystitis and Cholangitis). Enteric gram-negative bacilli and enterococcal species predominate. However, cholangitis and acute graft rejection can mimic one another; liver biopsy should be performed to differentiate these processes. Cholangiography is performed to assess the status of the biliary tract for patients with proven cholangitis.

As many as 40% of children develop a fungal infection during the first year following liver transplantation.[41] *Candida* spp. predominate, and infection usually is associated with an intra-abdominal focus or indwelling catheter. Episodes of invasive aspergillosis are uncommon but can be fatal.[43] Children undergoing liver transplantation for CF are at increased risk for infection due to *Aspergillus* spp.[41]

Intestinal Transplantation

An increasing number of children have received intestinal transplants. Many have undergone combined transplantation of liver and intestine or multivisceral transplantation. Bacterial infection

PART II Clinical Syndromes and Cardinal Features of Infectious Diseases: Approach to Diagnosis and Initial Management

SECTION O Infections and Transplantation

occurs frequently in these patients.[20,44,45] Disruption of the mucosal barrier associated with harvest injury or rejection commonly leads to BSI.[44,45] Coagulase-negative staphylococci, enterococci, gram-negative bacilli, and *Candida* account for most episodes. While the majority of BSI episodes occur in the first 3 to 6 months following transplantation, later episodes also occur. Intra-abdominal and wound infections also occur in more than one-third of these patients, and typically are detected early after transplantation.

Heart Transplantation

Infections account for approximately 15% of very early deaths, 19% of deaths within a year, and 7.5% of late deaths after cardiac transplantation.[46] Infection of the lower respiratory tract (including both pneumonia and lung abscess) is most common in these children.[9,47–50] Mediastinitis is an important infection after thoracic transplantation, particularly if re-exploration of the chest is required. Pathogens associated with mediastinitis include *Staphylococcus aureus* and gram-negative bacilli. Young children undergoing heart transplantation are at increased risk for subsequent invasive infection due to *Streptococcus pneumoniae*.[50,51] Infants undergoing heart transplantation represent a unique population and have increased risk of serious bacterial and fungal disease.[50,52,53]

Fungal infections, although uncommon, can be severe after heart transplantation. *Candida* spp. predominate, but serious *Aspergillus* infection can occur.[47]

Lung and Heart–Lung Transplantation

Infection accounts for approximately 46% of all deaths in the first year after pediatric lung transplantation.[54] Infection was the primary or contributing cause of death in the majority of lung and heart–lung recipients who died after the perioperative period in one series[27] and second only to graft failure in the 2007 International Registry data.[54] Recipients of lung transplantation are at high risk for bacterial and fungal infection of the respiratory tract. Pneumonia, the most important infectious complication, is difficult to diagnose definitively because differentiation between chronic colonization and lower respiratory tract infection can be problematic. Gram-negative pathogens and *S. aureus* can be recovered in the presence or absence of disease. Radiographic abnormalities are present almost universally in patients with pneumonia or graft rejection.[55–57] Therefore, bronchoalveolar lavage with transbronchial biopsy often is required to distinguish between causes.

Children undergoing lung transplantation because of CF have a high rate of infectious complications with bacteria and fungi.[58] Patients usually are colonized with *Pseudomonas* or *Aspergillus* spp. Colonization with *B. cenocepacia* (formerly *B. cepacia* genomovar III) has been associated with excessive mortality.[59–61] BSI due to organisms present before transplantation is common after lung transplantation in these patients.[62,63] Because of the importance and difficulty in treating these bacterial complications, protocols at most transplant centers include thorough evaluation of the microbial flora of candidates prior to transplantation, including antibiotic synergy testing and evaluation of isolates of *B. cepacia* complex species at reference laboratories.

Fungal infection frequently complicates pediatric lung transplantation. Infections occur both early and late after transplantation, particularly if patients develop BOS.[64,65] This has prompted many lung centers to institute guidelines for fungal prophylaxis.

VIRAL INFECTIONS

Viral pathogens, especially herpesviruses, are a major source of morbidity and mortality after SOT. Patterns of disease associated with individual viruses generally are similar among all transplant recipients. However, frequency, mode of presentation, and relative severity can differ according to the type of organ transplanted and the pretransplant serologic status of the recipient.

Cytomegalovirus

CMV remains one of the most common and important causes of viral infection after SOT. Infection can be asymptomatic or symptomatic and can be due to primary infection, reactivation of latent CMV, or acquisition of a new CMV strain. Before the use of prophylaxis against CMV, the reported incidence of disease in children after transplantation was 22% for kidney,[59] 40% for liver,[11] and 26% for thoracic[9] organs. Preventive strategies and the use of ganciclovir treatment have resulted in decreased rates and severity of CMV disease.

Primary CMV infection, typically acquired from the donated organ, is associated with the highest rates of morbidity and mortality. Reactivation of latent infection or superinfection with a new CMV strain tends to result in milder illness.[5] Patients treated with high doses of immunosuppressive agents, especially anti-lymphocyte products, have increased rates of CMV disease, regardless of previous immunity.[9,14,59]

CMV disease is characterized by a constellation of fever (which can be high-grade, prolonged, and hectic) and hematologic abnormalities (including leukopenia, atypical lymphocytosis, and thrombocytopenia). Disseminated CMV disease can cause signs and symptoms related to specific organ involvement; common sites include the gastrointestinal tract, liver, and lungs. The site of involvement can vary according to the type of transplant. Of note, CMV chorioretinitis is uncommon in SOT recipients. Before the availability of ganciclovir, fatal, disseminated CMV disease occurred in 4%, 14%, and 19% of infected children after kidney,[59] heart or heart-lung,[9] and liver transplantation,[11] respectively. Although mortality due to CMV has become rare in the ganciclovir era, CMV viremia still is associated with an increased rate of death and retransplantation in pediatric lung transplant recipients.[66,67]

Diagnosis of CMV disease is confirmed in a patient with a compatible clinical syndrome by means of quantitative nucleic acid based or CMV pp65 antigenemia, viral load assays, histopathology, or culture.[68] However, results of viral cultures of urine and respiratory secretions (including bronchoalveolar lavage specimens) can be difficult to interpret because patients frequently shed CMV asymptomatically in these secretions. Quantitative tests have been valuable in predicting which patients are at risk for disease, thus allowing pre-emptive initiation of therapy. Because of multiple methodologies and inter-laboratory variability of results, repeated tests performed in the same laboratory and institutional experience are more useful than single "quantitative cut-point" values for viral load. Histologic examination of involved organs remains the gold standard to confirm the presence of invasive CMV disease.

Antiviral agents with activity against CMV (e.g., ganciclovir, valganciclovir, foscarnet, and cidofovir) have improved the outcome of SOT recipients dramatically. For clinical CMV disease (fever with cytopenia or visceral disease), ganciclovir or valganciclovir therapy is given in conjunction with reduction of immunosuppression, unless there is evidence of concurrent rejection. Clinical response usually occurs 5 to 7 days after treatment is begun. Duration of therapy is guided by serial measurements of CMV viral load using quantitative assays.[29] The role of CMV hyperimmune globulin in combination with ganciclovir in the treatment of CMV disease is controversial, although some evidence for improved outcome with combination therapy has been reported in the treatment of CMV pneumonia in adult transplant recipients.[69] Studies of use of oral valganciclovir in adults have shown it to be comparable with intravenous ganciclovir for clearance of viremia and its use has been recommended for adults with mild to moderate CMV disease.[29,70] However, at the present time data on valganciclovir for treatment of CMV disease in pediatric transplant recipients are limited.[29] The U.S. Food and Drug Administration (FDA) has issued new dosing recommendations to prevent valganciclovir overdose in pediatric transplant patients that has occurred in those with low body weight, low body surface area, and below normal creatinine clearance (www.fda.gov/Drugs/Drug Safety/ucm 225727.htm). Foscarnet and cidofovir use is restricted to patients with apparent or proven resistance to ganciclovir.

Epstein–Barr Virus

EBV is an important cause of morbidity and mortality in pediatric SOT recipients.[10,21,22,71] A wide spectrum of EBV disease is recognized, including nonspecific viral illness, mononucleosis, and PTLD, including lymphoma. Histologic evaluation is important in differentiating among these categories; manifestations can evolve in individual patients. Asymptomatic seroconversion also occurs. Variation in severity and extent of disease is related to the degree of immunosuppression and adequacy of the host immune response. Symptomatic EBV infection in general, and PTLD in particular, is more common after primary EBV infection, thus affecting children disproportionately.[6] In one study, 4% of children undergoing SOT and 10% of children with primary EBV infection developed PTLD between 1 month and 5 years after transplantation.[6] In the absence of preventive interventions, cumulative occurrence can be as high as 12% to 20% by 7 to 12 years after liver transplantation.[30,72] Onset of viral syndrome, mononucleosis, and PTLD occurs primarily within the first year posttransplantation, whereas lymphoma tends to occur later. The introduction of new immunosuppressive agents and regimens invariably impact the incidence and timing of EBV disease.[73,74] Accordingly, careful monitoring is warranted in patients receiving these newer regimens.

The diagnosis of EBV-associated PTLD is made on the basis of clinical, laboratory, and histopathology findings and should be suspected in patients with protracted fever, exudative tonsillitis, lymphadenopathy, organomegaly, leukopenia, and/or atypical lymphocytosis (see Chapter 208, Epstein–Barr Virus (Mononucleosis and Lymphoproliferative Disorders)).[21,22] Gastrointestinal involvement should be suspected in patients with persistent fever and diarrhea. Serologic diagnosis often is confounded by the presence of passive antibody. Quantitative EBV PCR assays to predict risk for, or presence of, EBV viremia or PTLD are used widely.[22,75–77] Although extremely sensitive, these assays lack specificity; viral load often is elevated in asymptomatic patients.[78] Accordingly, every effort should be made to confirm the diagnosis of EBV disease or PTLD histologically. Occult sites of PTLD are assessed by performance of computed tomography of chest and abdomen. Palpable nodes or lesions identified by imaging should be biopsied. Endoscopy should be considered in patients with an elevated viral load and diarrheal illnesses. Histologic evaluation can be augmented through the use of the Epstein-Barr encoded RNA (EBER) probe.[79]

Current guidelines for the management of patients with EBV disease and PTLD recommend a stepwise approach to therapy, starting with reduced immunosuppression; further escalation of treatment is based primarily on the patient's clinical response and the histopathologic characteristics of the PTLD lesion.[80] Although antiviral agents and immune globulin intravenous (IGIV) are used frequently as part of this initial strategy,[75,81] their efficacy in the treatment of EBV/PTLD has not been established. Reduction of immunosuppression, alone or in combination with antiviral therapy, results in an approximate 67% cure rate of EBV-associated PTLD. For patients who fail to respond to this initial approach, two alternative treatment strategies have been proposed. Rituximab, an anti-CD20 antibody, has been used increasingly for the treatment of EBV disease.[80] Experience to date suggests that as many as two-thirds of patients who fail initial withdrawal of immunosuppression respond to a 4-week course of rituximab.[82,83] However, relapse of EBV disease has been observed in 20% to 25% of treated patients 6 to 8 months following completion of therapy at the time the rituximab is no longer present in the body. The second alternative for patients failing initial reduction or withdrawal of immunosuppressive therapy is use of modified doses of cyclophosphamide and prednisone; therapy is successful in approximately two-thirds of patients.[84] Unfortunately, relapse of PTLD has been seen in 22% of treated patients and outright treatment failures have occurred in patients presenting with fulminant disease. Studies comparing these second-line therapies are needed to define the best option for children who fail initial modification of immunosuppression. Finally, cytotoxic chemotherapy should be considered for those patients failing to respond to this stepwise

approach and could be considered as first-line therapy in the setting of T-lymphocyte-associated PTLD, PTLD of the central nervous system, and monomorphic PTLD occurring late in the posttransplant course.[80]

Adenovirus

Adenovirus is the third most important viral infection after pediatric liver transplantation, occurring in 10% of recipients in one large early series.[85] Symptomatic disease (ranging from self-limited fever, gastroenteritis, or cystitis, to devastating illness with necrotizing hepatitis or pneumonia) occurred in over 60% of infected patients. Infections occurred within the first 3 months after transplantation. The frequency of invasive adenovirus infections after pediatric liver transplantation appears to have decreased with the use of tacrolimus-based immunosuppression. This may be due to the ability to decrease the overall amount of immunosuppressive agents.[86,87]

Adenovirus infection in other pediatric organ recipients is less well characterized but can be severe, particularly after lung transplantation, and can be fatal when disease manifests soon after transplantation.[27,88–91] The presence of adenovirus DNA in cardiac biopsies after pediatric heart transplantation was significantly associated with poor graft survival in one series.[92] Adenovirus also has been associated with hemorrhagic cystitis and graft dysfunction in adult renal transplant recipients.[93] High rates of adenovirus infection have been found after pediatric intestinal transplantation, although clinical disease is not always found.[87,94,95] As adenovirus, like CMV, can be latent and can reactivate asymptomatically, ascribing a causative role in the pathologic process can sometimes be difficult.

Varicella-Zoster Virus

Many children have undergone SOT before development of immunity against VZV. Early experience noted severe and potentially fatal disease in children developing varicella after organ transplantation.[96,97] Some fatal cases occurred despite use of intravenous acyclovir and disease developed in approximately 50% of patients who received postexposure varicella-zoster immune globulin (VZIG). Recent reports have shown few or no patients developing significant complications of VZV after SOT.[28,98] In general, these results were achieved in children treated for VZV with intravenous acyclovir, although a small subset thought to be at low risk for severe disease were treated with oral acyclovir or valacyclovir. At present, current recommendations favor an aggressive response to varicella exposure and disease.[99] A VZV immunoglobulin product is recommended within 96 hours of exposure in nonimmune patients. Since production of VZIG has been halted, various recommendations have been made, including the use of an intravenous immunoglobulin emergency investigational new drug (EIND), VariZIG, obtained from FFP Enterprises (800-843-7477). If prompt acquisition is not feasible, oral acyclovir can be given as off-label use starting at day 7 postexposure. If varicella lesions develop, it is prudent to hospitalize patients and administer acyclovir intravenously until fever abates, no new lesions erupt, and existent lesions begin to crust.[99] The use of VZV vaccine after SOT is an area of active research. Limited experience in pediatric renal[100] and liver transplant recipients[101] is encouraging; immunogenicity and safety appear to be acceptable in children who are >1 year out from transplantation and who have stable and relatively low levels of immunosuppression. However, these patients have received vaccine under study protocols with close follow-up and 25% had vaccine-associated rash leading to intervention with antiviral therapy.[101] Additional experience is needed before recommending a standard protocol for VZV vaccination following transplantation.

Common Community-Acquired Viruses

Limited published data suggest that most children who receive SOT experience the usual childhood respiratory and gastrointestinal tract illnesses without significant problems.[7,48] This is especially true when they occur long after transplantation and are not associated with an episode of rejection.[7] However, infections caused by RSV, influenza virus, or PIV have led to more severe disease in young children, especially if they occur soon after transplantation and during periods of maximal immunosuppression.[102,103] A retrospective review of 576 pediatric lung transplant recipients from 14 centers found that 79 (14%) patients who have confirmed respiratory virus infections during the first year had decreased one-year survival.[91] Shirali and colleagues found that the presence of DNA from community-associated viruses such as enterovirus, adenovirus, and parvovirus in heart biopsies of children after cardiac transplantation was associated with increased adverse events but the timing of the biopsies relative to the time of transplantation was not evaluated.[92]

OPPORTUNISTIC INFECTIONS

Pneumocystis jirovecii Pneumonia

Pneumocystis pneumonia (PCP) is a well-documented complication of SOT. Before introduction of prophylaxis, the incidence of PCP was 4% to 35%.[23–25] However, use of TMP-SMX prophylaxis essentially has eliminated this problem. PCP typically occurs after the first month following transplantation, reflecting indolent presence prior to transplantation. Most cases occur within the first year posttransplantation, but PCP can occur later and should remain in the differential diagnosis for patients with fever and lower respiratory tract symptoms, particularly if they are not receiving PCP prophylaxis.

Toxoplasmosis

Toxoplasma gondii can cause significant infection in immunocompromised hosts.[104] A rare cause of disease in renal and liver transplant recipients,[15,105] toxoplasmosis more often is an infectious complication after cardiac transplantation.[26,106] The risk in cardiac recipients may be explained by tropism of the organism for cardiac muscle and subsequent donor transmission. Reactivation of cysts within the graft occurs in the immunosuppressed recipient without previous immunity. This is in contrast to adult patients with AIDS who develop reactivation disease despite the presence of antibody. Clinical manifestations usually occur 2 to 24 weeks after transplantation and include fever, pulmonary disease, chorioretinitis, myocarditis, and neurologic disorders. Use of pyrimethamine or trimethoprim-sulfamethoxazole prophylaxis has been effective in adult patients.[107,108]

Tuberculosis

Tuberculosis is a special concern in immunosuppressed hosts, including SOT recipients. Although the development of tuberculosis is rare in our experience, an incidence of 2.4% was reported from a pediatric liver transplant center in the United Kingdom.[109] While most cases in this series were suspected to represent primary infection acquired after transplantation, transplant recipients with a reactive purified protein derivative (PPD) or who come from areas where tuberculosis is endemic are also at increased risk for symptomatic reactivation after transplantation.[110–112] The risk of reactivation TB appears greatest in patients who received no prior treatment or who had inadequate or incomplete therapy. Accordingly, a careful history of exposure, a PPD, and a chest radiograph are evaluated prior to transplantation. The role of quantiferon assays to diagnose tuberculosis in children remains to be elucidated, but recent studies demonstrate its potential role in differentiating reaction to nontuberculous mycobacteria or reaction to prior BCG vaccination.[113] Patients with latent tuberculosis who received inadequate or no prior treatment should receive isoniazid for at least 9 months after transplant.[109,114] Where possible, treatment should begin prior to transplantation. Attempts at a more definitive diagnosis are indicated in a patient from an endemic area who has a negative PPD test result but a suspicious radiograph. Combination-drug antituberculosis therapy is indicated for

those felt to have disease due to *Mycobacterium tuberculosis*. Evidence of side effects, particularly hepatotoxicity, should be monitored carefully in all pediatric transplant recipients receiving chemotherapy for tuberculosis.

Other Opportunistic Infections

Endemic fungal infections such as coccidioidomycosis and histoplasmosis are of concern in patients with exposure to specific geographic areas. Likewise parasitic infections such as those due to *Trypanosoma cruzi* have occurred in adult recipients. Because patients often travel to transplant centers distant from their homes, physicians caring for SOT candidates or recipients must be cognizant of the environmental risk for each patient. Experience with coccidioidomycosis in transplant recipients suggests that a minimum of 4 months of antifungal therapy, such as fluconazole, should be given to transplant recipients with this history.[115] Similarities between coccidioidomycosis and other fungal infections suggest that such strategies may be necessary for patients with a history of fungal infection with pathogens prone to recurrence after resolution of primary infection.[12]

MANAGEMENT AND PREVENTIVE MEASURES

Pretransplant Evaluation

Pretransplant evaluation permits preventive intervention and anticipation of posttransplantation complications. History and physical examination should be performed, with particular attention to previous infections, exposures, immunizations, and drug allergies. Children with CF or those with a prolonged stay under intensive care just before transplantation may be colonized with antimicrobial-resistant organisms. Pretransplant surveillance cultures are useful in guiding subsequent empiric selection of antimicrobial agents in these patients. Screening for tuberculosis is performed along with serologic studies for CMV, EBV, HSV, VZV, HBV, HCV, HIV, and syphilis. In addition, other serology, such as for *T. gondii*, particularly for heart transplant candidates and hepatitis A serology for liver transplant candidates, should be performed. Donor serology is performed for common microbes that have been proven to be transmitted from blood or organs (Tables 97-2 and 97-3). WNV has been transmitted by organ donation from undiagnosed cases, resulting in severe disease in the recipient. Currently, blood donor screening but not organ donor screening by WNV nucleic acid amplification test is performed routinely.[116] However, screening could be considered in specific geographic areas during periods of WNV activity.

Strategies should be implemented to optimize immunizations during the pretransplant period. This is particularly relevant for young organ transplant candidates who may not have completed their primary vaccination series. These infants should start vaccinations at 6 weeks of age and follow an accelerated schedule.[117] Immunizations sometimes are delayed and often overlooked while these children are waiting for transplantation because of their medical conditions. Despite their underlying illnesses, vaccine responses are likely to be better in the transplant candidate compared with the transplant recipient.[118] Inactivated and purified antigen vaccines are given to maximize protection before immunosuppression. Influenza vaccine should be given to children ≥6 months of age and to all family members. Children expected to have at least 4 weeks before transplantation should be given live virus vaccines at earliest ages recommended. In many centers, immunologic response is assessed by obtaining serology for at least measles, mumps, and varicella. If seroconversion is not documented, revaccination can be attempted if time permits.

Preventive Strategies

Antimicrobial and Immunoglobulin Prophylaxis

Prophylactic regimens for SOT vary by center and type of transplant. Perioperative antibiotics are used for the first 48 to 72 hours

TABLE 97-2. Screening Tests for Transplant Candidates[a]

Test and Pathogen	Comment
SEROLOGIC TEST[b]	
HIV-1 and -2	
HTLV-1 and -2	
Hepatitis A virus	IgG and IgM screening test
Hepatitis B virus	Hepatitis B surface antigen and anti-core antibody indicate active disease; anti-hepatitis B surface antigen indicates serologic conversion after immunization
Hepatitis C virus	
Hepatitis D virus	If Hepatitis B-positive
CMV	IgG test; urine culture if positive
EBV	Antiviral capsid antigen IgG and EBNA
Herpes simplex virus	
Varicella-zoster virus	
Toxoplasma gondii	Obtain for heart and heart–lung transplant candidates in particular; some centers screen all candidates
Measles virus	If serology is negative, consider immunization if ≥3 months anticipated before transplantation
Mumps virus	If serology is negative, consider immunization if ≥3 months anticipated before transplantation
Rubella virus	If serology is negative, consider immunization if ≥3 months anticipated before transplantation
OTHER TESTS	
Mycobacterium tuberculosis	Skin test for tuberculosis (TST) and or interferon release assay
Respiratory tract pathogens	Sputum culture for patients with cystic fibrosis and other lung transplant candidates

CMV, cytomegalovirus; EBNA, Epstein–Barr virus nuclear antigen; EBV, Epstein–Barr virus; HIV, human immunodeficiency virus; HTLV, human T-lymphotropic virus; Ig, immunoglobulin.

[a]All tests performed on all candidates except where noted.

[b]IgG antibody measured except where noted.

TABLE 97-3. Serologic Screening of Organ Donor[a]

Pathogen	Comment
HIV-1 and -2	Positive result contraindicates organ use
Hepatitis A virus	Positive result IgM test contraindicates organ use
Hepatitis B virus	Obtain HBV core antibody and HBV surface antigen; result suggesting current infection contraindicates organ use
Hepatitis C virus	Some centers use positive donor only for positive candidate
CMV	Obtain IgG test; obtain urine culture if positive neonatal donor
EBV	Obtain antiviral capsid IgG and IgM
Toxoplasma gondii	Obtain on heart and heart–lung donors in particular
Treponema pallidum	Obtain reagin test (specific test if positive); positive result contraindicates organ use

CMV, cytomegalovirus; EBV, Epstein–Barr virus; HIV, human immunodeficiency virus; Ig, immunoglobulin.

[a]IgG antibody measured except where noted.

to provide prophylaxis against intraoperative soilage, septicemia, and wound infection. The choice of antimicrobial agents is dictated by the organ being transplanted, patient characteristics, expected flora, and knowledge of the antimicrobial susceptibilities of local pathogens and patient's flora if known. Surveillance cultures of the donor bronchi or trachea also are useful in heart–lung or lung transplantation. CF patients usually require a more prolonged period of prophylaxis.

The frequency and severity of CMV infections in transplant recipients prompt consideration of prophylactic strategies.[119] Although recently published guidelines provide evidenced-based recommendations for adult organ transplant recipients,[29,120–122] definitive data to inform recommendations for pediatric SOT recipients are not available. Accordingly, varying strategies are used.[123,124] The CMV prevention strategies used at the Children's Hospital of Pittsburgh (CHP) vary by organ type and the donor/recipient status. All pediatric recipients deemed to be at risk for developing CMV disease are begun at transplantation on ganciclovir intravenously; oral valganciclovir is considered for those requiring prophylactic therapy beyond 2 weeks. High-risk (donor CMV-positive/recipient CMV-negative) intestinal transplant recipients also receive CMV-IGIV at CHP. At the completion of prophylaxis, many recipients subsequently undergo serial monitoring of CMV load in what some experts have called a "hybrid" prevention approach. Serial monitoring of the blood CMV load with quantitative CMV PCR assays (or less commonly pp65 antigenemia assays) from the time of transplantation to inform the use of pre-emptive antiviral therapy also has been used as an alternative prevention strategy.[125] In this approach, only patients demonstrating an increased viral load are treated. Although this strategy has gained acceptance at some centers, experience in pediatric transplant recipients remains limited.

A number of strategies currently are being explored (e.g., immunoprophylaxis, monitoring, and pre-emptive therapy) to prevent EBV-associated PTLD.[126–128] Relative efficacy of these approaches has not been established. At present, the use of viral load monitoring to inform pre-emptive reductions in immunosuppression appears to be the most promising strategy.[128]

Nystatin suspension can be used in pediatric transplant recipients for the first 3 months after transplantation to prevent oropharyngeal candidiasis. TMP-SMX is used to prevent PCP. When given on a daily basis, the use of TMP-SMX also has been shown to decrease the incidence of posttransplantation UTI in renal transplant recipients.[32] The duration of prophylaxis for PCP is controversial. Most cases occur during the first year after transplantation. However, because late cases occur, TMP-SMX is given indefinitely at some centers. Fungal prophylaxis against *Aspergillus* is used for children undergoing lung transplantation, for variable durations.

Immunizations Following Transplantation

Centers use varying protocols for immunization after transplantation.[129,130] The decision on when to initiate immunizations following organ transplantation should be individualized. For some patients, induction immunosuppression or recurrent treatment of rejection may require a prolonged delay in starting immunizations due to significant ongoing immunosuppression. For others who have a benign posttransplant course, immunizations with inactivated agents may be resumed as early as 3 to 6 months after transplantation depending on baseline immunosuppression. However, earlier use of influenza vaccine should be considered for children who were not immunized before transplantation and who undergo transplantation just before or during the influenza season. Special consideration must be given to live vaccines. In general, live vaccines are not administered after transplantation although several small clinical trials evaluating MMR and varicella vaccines demonstrated promising safety profiles.[101,131,132] In addition, two live rotavirus vaccines are licensed in the U.S. At present, there are insufficient data regarding the efficacy and safety of these vaccines to routinely recommend their use after transplantation, and limitations of age at commencement make most SOT recipients excluded from consideration.[133]

PART II Clinical Syndromes and Cardinal Features of Infectious Diseases: Approach to Diagnosis and Initial Management

SECTION O Infections and Transplantation

98 Infections in Hematopoietic Stem Cell Transplant Recipients

Jorge Luján-Zilbermann

Hematopoietic stem cell transplantation (HSCT) has broad indications in pediatrics, including patients with cancer, primary immunodeficiency syndromes, bone marrow failure syndromes, hemoglobinopathies, and an assortment of genetic conditions, including inborn errors of metabolism, and nonmalignant conditions such as osteopetrosis.[1-3] Patients undergoing HSCT have an increased risk for infectious complications that are somewhat predictable based on the acquired immune deficiencies that occur after HSCT.[4-7]

ETIOLOGIC AGENTS

Patients who have had HSCT have immune deficiencies in the phagocytic, humoral, and cellular arms of the immune system.[4] These immune defects cause disease to occur from infectious agents in three predictable time periods (Figure 98-1).[4] After the conditioning regimen, a period of neutropenia occurs for 3 to 4 weeks. During this period, bacteria and fungi cause most infections; in addition, herpes simplex virus (HSV) and seasonal respiratory viral infections can occur.[4,7,8] The second phase occurs after granulocyte recovery and continues until approximately 100 days after HSCT. Infectious complications during this period are associated with profound impairment of humoral and cellular immunity. Although bacterial and fungal infections still can occur, they are much less frequent than during the neutropenic period. Cytomegalovirus (CMV) is a major infecting agent, but *Pneumocystis jirovecii* disease also can occur. With the advent of effective prophylaxis against both of these agents, the incidence of associated disease has decreased. However, the incidence of infections due to adenovirus and Epstein–Barr virus (EBV) is increasing with the use of mismatched HSCT and T-lymphocyte-depleted

HSCT.[9-11] A third period associated with deficits in humoral immune responses, cellular immune responses, and reticuloendothelial function begins at 100 days after HSCT. Varicella-zoster virus (VZV) and encapsulated bacteria, particularly *Streptococcus pneumoniae* and *Haemophilus influenzae* type b (Hib), are major pathogens during this period.

EPIDEMIOLOGY

Most infecting agents in HSCT patients are derived from the patient's microbial flora or by reactivation of a latent infection. Multiple factors account for the high risk of HSCT recipients for an infectious complication (Box 98-1). Immune deficiency associated with the underlying disease is a determinant of the degree of immune suppression. Allogeneic HSCT recipients (e.g., matched unrelated donor or unrelated cord blood transplantation) are at high risk for graft-versus-host disease (GvHD), which enhances the infection rate by delaying return of normal immune function and by ulceration of the gastrointestinal tract. Moreover, the risk of infection is directly related to the degree of donor–recipient mismatch. To abrogate GvHD, cyclosporine and methotrexate are administered as prophylaxis. Both of these agents increase the risk of infection by depressing the cell-mediated immune response and, in the case of methotrexate, by disrupting mucosal barriers.

The conditioning regimen with or without concomitant irradiation compromises the immune system and also can disrupt mucosal barriers. In addition, purging of the bone marrow in autologous transplants to reduce the load of malignant cells, and T-lymphocyte depletion used in allogeneic transplants to reduce the incidence of GvHD, predispose the host to infection.

The serologic status of the donor and the recipient is important because many infections in patients with transplants are due to reactivation (Table 98-1). This is most notable with the herpesvirus group. CMV is a major cause of pneumonitis in allogeneic transplant recipients. Additionally, other herpesviruses, especially HSV, VZV, and EBV, as well as *Toxoplasma gondii* and adenovirus, are prone to reactivate after the transplant.

All HSCT recipients have a central venous catheter (CVC) placed before transplant, providing a potential nidus for infection. In addition, patients who have other indwelling medical devices (e.g., cerebrospinal fluid shunts) have attendant risk for infection. Patients with a history of invasive aspergillosis who are undergoing HSCT require adequate antifungal prophylaxis and treatment to prevent relapse of aspergillosis.[12]

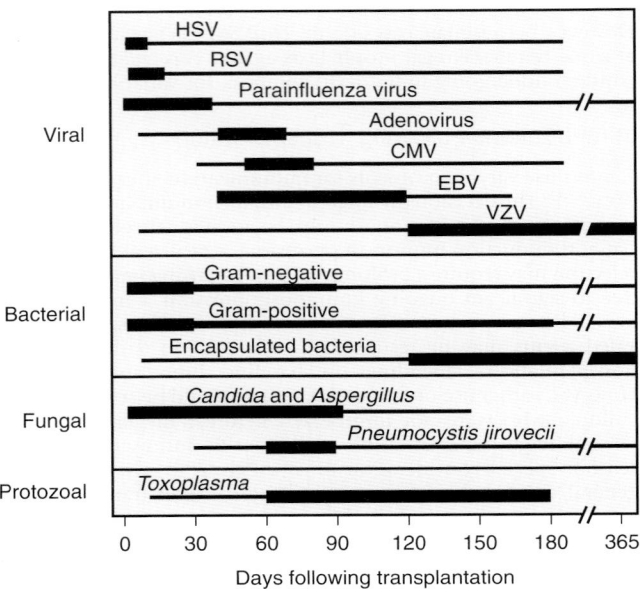

Figure 98-1. Temporal association of infectious agents and hematopoietic stem cell transplantation. Day 0 is the time of stem cell infusion. Boldness of line denotes increasing frequency of infection with offending agent.

BOX 98-1. Predisposing Factors for an Infectious Complication in Hematopoietic Stem Cell Transplant Recipients

- Underlying illness
- Type of transplant
- Conditioning regimen
- Infectious disease history
- Presence of an indwelling medical device
- Occurrence and severity of graft-versus-host disease
- Immunosuppressive regimen administered to prevent graft-versus-host disease
- Epidemiology of infection in hospital or transplant care unit

TABLE 98-1. Pretransplant Evaluation for Patients Undergoing Hematopoietic Stem Cell Transplantation

Study Type	Organism or Test
Serum antibody	CMV
	EBV
	Hepatitis B (HBsAg, HBsAb, HBcAb)
	Hepatitis C
	RPR
	Human immunodeficiency virus
Other laboratory	Serum hepatic enzymes (ALT, AST, bilirubin)
	Renal function tests (BUN, creatinine)
	Complete blood cell count with differential
	Stool for ova and parasites
Skin	Tuberculin skin test (TST)
Radiographic	Chest, posteroanterior and lateral
	Sinus series, if clinically indicated

ALT, alanine aminotransferase; AST, aspartate aminotransferase; BUN, blood urea nitrogen; CMV, cytomegalovirus; EBV, Epstein–Barr virus; RPR, rapid plasma reagin.

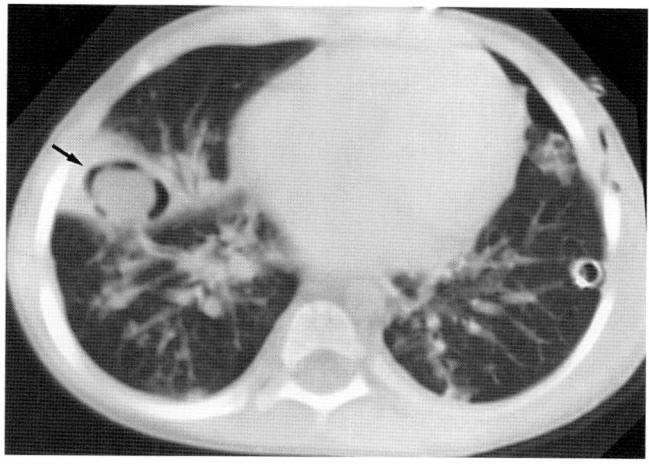

Figure 98-2. Invasive aspergillosis in a patient after hematopoietic stem cell transplantation. Computed tomography of the chest shows bilateral pulmonary involvement, including aspergilloma in the right middle lobe (arrow).

Knowledge of the epidemiology of pathogens associated with the local hospital and the transplant unit allows an assessment of risk for environmental organisms, such as *Aspergillus* and *Legionella* species. Rates of infection can be reduced substantially by preventive mechanisms that inhibit aerosolization of organisms, such as the use of laminar flow rooms or high-efficiency particulate air (HEPA)-filtered rooms.[6]

CLINICAL SYNDROMES, DIFFERENTIAL DIAGNOSIS, AND CLINICAL APPROACH

The approach to a patient who has had HSCT is based on understanding the infections that can occur during each of the risk periods (see Figure 98-1). This provides the framework for matching possible causative agents with the clinical syndrome. Because some of these clinical syndromes are highlighted in Chapters 99 (Fever and Granulocytopenia) and 100 (Infections in Children with Cancer), the following discussion focuses on a clinical approach to the HSCT recipient.

Early Period (Before Engraftment)

Herpes Simplex Virus Gingivostomatitis

HSV infection occurs primarily as a result of reactivation in seropositive patients undergoing HSCT. The diagnosis is difficult because lip lesions are rare and mucosal ulcerations are similar to those that occur as a result of the conditioning regimen.

Central Venous Catheter-Related Bloodstream Infections

During the neutropenic period, HSCT recipients have high risk for bacterial infection, comparable with the risk for patients with cancer who develop chemotherapy-induced neutropenia. Catheter-related bloodstream infections (BSIs) are common because of the uniform use of indwelling CVCs in HSCT patients for administration of medications, hyperalimentation, blood products, and for blood sampling. Measures to prevent CVC-BSIs should be followed.[6,13] *Staphylococcus epidermidis* and other coagulase-negative staphylococci (CoNS) are the most frequent BSIs during the three phases posttransplant.[14–16] Other gram-positive organisms associated with BSI in HSCT recipients include viridans streptococci and *S. aureus.*[14–16] Viridans streptococci infections have been associated with chemotherapy-induced mucositis and poor dental hygiene.[17,18] Most gram-positive catheter-related infections can be treated successfully without removal of the catheter.

Gram-negative bacillary infections occur after mucosal damage with bacterial translocation from the intestinal mucosa into the bloodstream and are the second most frequent cause of BSI. The predominant organisms in this class include *Escherichia coli*, *Klebsiella* spp., and *Pseudomonas aeruginosa*, although other gram-negative organisms (frequently indigenous to the facility) are common.[14,16] Antibiotic resistance among these organisms is common. Catheter-related infections with some gram-negative bacilli, *Candida* spp., and *Bacillus cereus* can be problematic and require catheter removal.

Fungal Infections

The major causes of fungal infection include *Aspergillus* spp., *Candida* spp., and agents of mucormycosis (e.g., *Mucor*, *Absidia*, and *Rhizopus* spp.).[19–21] Additionally, other fungi recognized as pathogens include *Trichosporon* spp., *Fusarium* spp., *Curvularia* spp., and *Alternaría* spp.[21–23] Infection with these organisms usually occurs after a period of antibiotic therapy and is correlated with the degree and duration of neutropenia. Although *Candida albicans* is the most frequent *Candida* spp. causing BSI, *C. tropicalis* may cause more severe disease. Other *Candida* spp., including *C. glabrata*, *C. parapsilosis*, and *C. krusei*, also have emerged owing to resistance to fluconazole, which is used as prophylaxis.[20–22]

The portal of entry for *Aspergillus* and agents of mucormycosis is the respiratory tract, as opposed to that of *Candida* spp., which is the gastrointestinal tract. *Aspergillus* is associated with sinopulmonary disease and dissemination (Figure 98-2), but is rarely recovered from blood cultures. Diagnosis usually depends on tissue histology and culture of material obtained from bronchoscopy, lung aspiration, or open-lung biopsy. The galactomannan assay can be useful in early diagnosis of invasive aspergillosis in high-risk patients.[12,24]

Hemorrhagic Cystitis

Hemorrhagic cystitis is associated with a variety of infectious and noninfectious causes (Box 98-2).[25] The onset can occur at any time during the transplantation period; chemotherapy-induced cystitis occurs soon after commencing the conditioning regimen. The most common infectious causes are polyomaviruses (BK virus and JC virus) and adenovirus.[25–27] Bacterial and fungal pathogens also must be considered.

Enteric Infections

Diarrhea after transplantation is caused most commonly by mucositis and GvHD. Enteric infections can occur throughout the

PART II Clinical Syndromes and Cardinal Features of Infectious Diseases: Approach to Diagnosis and Initial Management

SECTION O Infections and Transplantation

BOX 98-2. Differential Diagnosis of Hemorrhagic Cystitis in Hematopoietic Stem Cell Transplant Recipients

INFECTIOUS CAUSES

Virus

Adenovirus
Cytomegalovirus
Polyomaviruses, especially BK virus and JC virus
Herpes simplex virus

Bacteria

Urinary tract infection, predominantly gram-negative bacilli

Fungus

Urinary tract infection
Fungus ball

NONINFECTIOUS CAUSES

Chemotherapy (e.g., cyclophosphamide)
Graft-versus-host disease
Mechanical trauma from Foley catheter

BOX 98-3. Causes of Pneumonitis in Hematopoietic Stem Cell Transplant Recipients

INFECTIOUS

Bacteria

Enterobacteriaceae
Staphylococcus aureus
Legionella pneumophila

Fungi

Aspergillus species
Mucormycosis
Pneumocystis jirovecii
Candida species

Virus

Parainfluenza types 1–4
Adenovirus
Respiratory syncytial virus
Human metapneumovirus
Cytomegalovirus
Influenza
Human herpesvirus 6
Coxsackievirus and echoviruses
Rhinovirus

NONINFECTIOUS

Pulmonary damage by radiation
Pulmonary damage by chemotherapeutic agents (e.g., bleomycin)
Underlying cancer
Pulmonary edema
Alveolar hemorrhage
Idiopathic interstitial pneumonia
Pulmonary vascular disease
Pneumomediastinum

---

transplantation period. Antibiotic-associated diarrhea, including that due to *Clostridium difficile,* usually occurs during the neutropenic period, when antimicrobial agents are frequently administered. Other infecting agents, including enteric adenovirus, rotavirus, and coxsackievirus, should also be considered.[11,28] The enteric viruses generally are seasonal in occurrence.

Middle Posttransplant Period (Early Engraftment)

The middle period (from days 30 through 100 after transplantation) once was dominated by CMV infection, but the incidence of CMV infection has diminished with the use of ganciclovir as preemptive therapy. Bacterial infections are less problematic during this period, except for those associated with indwelling catheters. Fungal infections still occur in patients with GvHD.

Pneumonitis

Pulmonary infiltrates can have an infectious or noninfectious cause (Box 98-3). Although signs and symptoms can occur throughout the transplantation period, viral infections are more common during the early engraftment period.

CMV manifests at a median time of 40 to 50 days after the transplantation period (see Figure 98-1). CMV most commonly occurs because of reactivation of latent virus in seropositive individuals but also can occur in seronegative patients who receive a transplant from a seropositive donor. Risk factors for CMV pneumonia include seropositivity of donor, type of transplant (allogeneic more than autologous), human leukocyte antigen mismatch transplant, older age of the patient (>10 years of age), and development of acute GvHD.[29] CMV infection occurs in 30% to 50% of patients undergoing HSCT; pneumonia occurs in 10% to 15% of these patients and has a mortality rate of 85%. CMV infection and disease also occur in autologous HSCT recipients, but at a much lower incidence. The clinical manifestations of CMV disease vary from asymptomatic infection to the constellation of fever, hepatitis, and leukopenia, to life-threatening diseases, such as interstitial pneumonitis, esophagitis, and encephalitis.[30]

Other viral causes of respiratory tract infections include adenovirus, respiratory syncytial virus (RSV), the human metapneumovirus, parainfluenza virus, influenza virus, human herpesvirus 6, coxsackie virus, rhinovirus, and echoviruses.[31–37] RSV, influenza virus, and parainfluenza virus can cause sinusitis and life-threatening pneumonia.[31,32]

Pneumocystis jirovecii also causes pneumonia after engraftment.[38] Clinical manifestations are similar to those in other immunocompromised hosts. The incidence of *Pneumocystis* pneumonia (PCP) has been curtailed markedly by routine prophylaxis with trimethoprim-sulfamethoxazole (TMP-SMX).

Adenovirus Infection

Adenovirus infection occurs in approximately 30% of pediatric HSCT recipients and can become latent in lymphoid tissue and kidneys.[39] The most common clinical manifestations of infection include diarrhea, febrile illness, hemorrhagic cystitis, and pneumonia, but also can include hepatitis and encephalitis.[39]

Toxoplasmosis

Toxoplasmosis is a rare but almost always fatal infection after HSCT. Toxoplasmosis usually occurs 2 to 6 months after HSCT, and the central nervous system is affected most often. Symptoms include focal neurologic signs, fever, seizures, and altered mental status. Imaging of the brain typically shows multiple lesions in both hemispheres and the basal ganglia.[40,42]

Encephalopathy

Encephalopathy is a poorly characterized complication of HSCT that has a very poor prognosis in pediatric patients, with a mortality rate of 65% in one study.[41] Several infectious and noninfectious etiologies have been described (Box 98-4).[33,41,42] HHV-6 has been associated with encephalitis and delayed platelet engraftment.[35,36,43]

BOX 98-4. Differential Diagnosis of Meningitis, Encephalitis, and Encephalopathy in Hematopoietic Stem Cell Transplantation Recipients

INFECTIOUS CAUSES

Virus

Adenovirus
Human herpesvirus 6 and 7
Polyomaviruses, especially BK virus and JC virus (progressive multifocal leukoencephalopathy)
Herpes simplex virus
Postviral (acute disseminated encephalomyelitis)

Bacteria

Streptococcus pneumoniae

Fungus

Aspergillus species

Protozoa

Toxoplasma gondii

NONINFECTIOUS CAUSES

Medications (e.g., cyclosporine, amphotericin B)
Nonconvulsive seizures
Thrombotic thrombocytopenic purpura
Multiorgan system failure
Stroke

BOX 98-5. Differential Diagnosis of Hepatitis After Hematopoietic Stem Cell Transplantation

INFECTIOUS CAUSES

Hepatitis viruses A, B, C, D and E
Herpes simplex virus
Cytomegalovirus
Adenovirus
Echovirus
Epstein–Barr virus
Varicella-zoster virus
Human herpesvirus 6

NONINFECTIOUS CAUSES

Veno-occlusive disease
Graft-versus-host disease
Chemotherapy-induced hepatitis
Hepatopathy of total parenteral nutrition
Cholestatic liver injury secondary to septicemia
Nonchemotherapeutic drugs, including acetaminophen and antibiotics

Late Posttransplant Period

At 100 days after transplantation, the late period begins.

Bloodstream Infection

Bacterial infections occur less commonly during this period, but patients continue to be immunosuppressed and susceptible to bacterial infection and BSI. The presence of chronic GvHD augments this immunosuppression. Encapsulated bacteria, especially *S. pneumoniae* and Hib, are the most common agents responsible for bacterial infections that are not related to presence of an indwelling catheter.[4]

Varicella-Zoster Virus Infection

VZV infections occur in 25% to 40% of patients following HSCT.[44] Reactivation occurs more frequently in association with chronic GvHD but also has been described in patients following autologous HSCT. A prodrome of burning or pain over the involved dermatome can occur. Groups of vesicles appear in the distribution of one to three sensory dermatomes. If appropriate therapy with acyclovir is not instituted, dissemination can occur in 36% of infected patients, with a mortality rate of 10%.

Hepatitis

Acute or chronic hepatitis can follow HSCT and has infectious and noninfectious causes (Box 98-5). Hepatitis C virus can infect recipients of HSCT, with activation at the time of discontinuation of immunosuppressive therapy.[45]

LABORATORY FINDINGS AND DIAGNOSIS

Except for microbiologic evaluation, laboratory tests are of limited value. Microbiologic tests include blood cultures for bacteria, fungi, and detection of viruses; specific serologic tests; and special stains. A buffy coat culture for viruses, such as CMV, may improve rate of isolation. Additionally, shell vial techniques (based on a low-speed centrifugation to enhance attachment and monoclonal antibody to detect virus replication) can identify viruses rapidly, including CMV, herpesviruses, and adenovirus, particularly those involving the respiratory tract.

Polymerase chain reaction (PCR) testing is extremely helpful for both screening and diagnosis of viral infections. PCR is available for all the herpesviruses, adenovirus, and polyomaviruses.[11,26,35,46] Real-time PCR of respiratory samples allows the diagnosis of influenza virus, RSV, parainfluenza virus, metapneumovirus, and adenovirus.[47]

Other laboratory tests are of limited value. Complete blood cell counts can be used to assess engraftment status; absolute neutrophil plus count <500/mm^3 is associated with higher incidence of bacterial infections. Serum hepatic enzyme and renal function tests can provide evidence of pathology from an infectious agent or insults from chemotherapy or GvHD (see Boxes 98-2 and 98-5).

MANAGEMENT AND PRESUMPTIVE THERAPY

Initial management of patients with fever and neutropenia is similar to management of patients with chemotherapy-induced fever and neutropenia (see Chapter 99, Fever and Granulocytopenia). One empiric antibiotic therapy regimen may be vancomycin plus ceftazidime.[48] This combination provides effective therapy for penicillin-nonsusceptible viridans streptococci infections, which are common in patients who are given high-dose cytosine arabinoside in the conditioning regimen. In addition, ceftazidime provides adequate therapy for *Pseudomonas aeruginosa* and many other gram-negative bacteria. This combination avoids the use of aminoglycosides in patients who have received nephrotoxic drugs. Consideration of antibiotic regimens should take into account isolates indicating the patient's colonization status, the hospital environment, and the antimicrobial resistance pattern within the community and the hospital. Discontinuation of vancomycin should be considered at 48 hours if blood culture is negative or does not show a gram-positive coccus.

Empiric amphotericin B is begun in the patient who is persistently febrile after 5 to 7 days of antibiotic therapy and who does not have an identified bacterial cause.[48] Lipid or liposomal formulations of amphotericin B can be used as substitutes if nephrotoxicity occurs during use of amphotericin B.[48] Azole agents, such as posaconazole and voriconazole, are effective for the treatment of invasive aspergillosis in immunocompromised hosts.[12,49] The echinocandins, caspofungin and micafungin, alone or in combination therapy with an azole or amphotericin B, are effective therapies for *Candida* spp. infections and invasive aspergillosis.[50-52]

PART II Clinical Syndromes and Cardinal Features of Infectious Diseases: Approach to Diagnosis and Initial Management

SECTION O Infections and Transplantation

Viral infections are treated after a diagnosis is made, if therapy is available. Acyclovir is the treatment of choice for both HSV and VZV infections. Orally administered valacyclovir and famciclovir also can be used to treat HSV infections. CMV pneumonitis is treated with both ganciclovir and immune globulin intravenous (IGIV), to inhibit proliferation of CMV and possibly to abrogate the immune response contributing to the pneumonitis. Foscarnet can be used in cases of ganciclovir-resistant CMV or acyclovir-resistant HSV infections. Cidofovir is a safe and effective therapy for adenoviral infections in pediatric patients, with no dose-limiting nephrotoxicity.[39]

Adoptive immunotherapy, by transferring virus-specific cytotoxic T lymphocytes to patients after allogeneic HSCT, has been used to treat infections caused by EBV and CMV and selectively to reconstitute immune function against these viruses.[53,54] Aerosolized ribavirin can be used for the treatment of parainfluenza virus and RSV infections. Immune globulin or monoclonal antibody for treatment of RSV is not indicated.[55,56]

PREVENTION

Prevention of infectious complications is a high priority for recipients of HSCT. Prophylaxis against PCP using TMP-SMX is started after engraftment and is given orally three times a week until 6 months after the transplant. The dose is 5 to 10 mg/kg per day divided into 2 doses, or 150 mg/m^2 per day divided into 2 doses, for 3 consecutive days per week.

For HSCT recipients with neutropenia, fluconazole, posaconazole, or micafungin are recommended during the period of risk of neutropenia for prophylaxis against candidiasis.[52,57] However, the use of fluconazole has been complicated by the emergence of resistant pathogens, such as *Candida krusei* and some other *Candida* species.[20] Antifungal prophylaxis using posaconazole can be recommended in HSCT recipients with GvHD who are at high risk for invasive aspergillosis.[12]

Primary CMV infection can be decreased in the CMV-seronegative HSCT recipient by using leukocyte-filtered blood products for transfusion.[58] Since the introduction of prophylaxis with ganciclovir for CMV infection, the incidence of CMV disease has been reduced substantially.[30] Pre-emptive therapy with ganciclovir or foscarnet is used in seropositive recipients of HSCT or in patients receiving a transplant from a seropositive donor. The use of ganciclovir as prophylaxis can cause neutropenia with an increased risk of a bacterial infection; however, the risk of CMV pneumonia justifies its use. Pre-emptive ganciclovir prophylaxis administered early in the course of HSCT delays the median time of onset of CMV infection from 1 to 2 months to 4 to 6 months when immune reconstitution is more advanced.[59]

Active Immunizations

Reimmunization is important because most allogeneic and a large proportion of autologous recipients of HSCT lose their immunity to vaccine-preventable diseases. When reimmunizing transplant recipients, recent administration of immunoglobulin preparations (except monoclonal antibody to RSV) must be considered because of interference with the response to live virus vaccine (e.g., measles, mumps, rubella, and varicella). Immunization can be started 12 months after HSCT. One schema is shown in Table 98-2. Transplant recipients and their household contacts should only be given inactivated poliovirus vaccine (IPV). Inactivated influenza vaccine should be administered annually in early autumn to recipients of HSCT beginning 6 months after transplantation. For individuals who are <6 months post-HSCT during the influenza season, chemoprophylaxis should be considered. The live attenuated influenza vaccine should not be administered to HSCT recipients. Insufficient data are available to make recommendations regarding varicella vaccine. Rotavirus vaccine is a live-virus vaccine

TABLE 98-2. Immunization Schedule for Hematopoietic Stem Cell Transplant Recipients

Months after Transplant	Vaccines
12	Td,[a] IPV, Hib, pneumococcal,[b] meningococcal[c] and hepatitis A[d] and B
14	Td,[a] IPV, Hib, and hepatitis B
24	MMR,[e] varicella,[f] Td,[a] IPV, Hib, pneumococcal, and hepatitis A[d] and B

DTaP, diphtheria and tetanus toxoids and acellular pertussis; GvHD, graft-versushost disease; Hib, Haemophilus influenzae type B; IPV, poliovirus vaccine inactivated; MMR, measles, mumps, rubella; Td, diphtheria and tetanus toxoids.

[a]*DTaP or DT if patient <7 years of age; Tdap, if ≥11 years of age and indicated.*

[b]*23-valent pneumococcal vaccine; use of 13-valent conjugate vaccine is considered depending on age and indication (see Chapters 6, Active Immunization, and 123, Streptococcus pneumoniae).*

[c]*Meningococcal conjugate vaccine if indicated by age.*

[d]*Consider for patients who have chronic liver disease or chronic GvHD, or who live in areas with endemic infection.*

[e]*Do not use live virus vaccines in patients with chronic GvHD or in patients receiving corticosteroid therapy. A second dose of MMR should be given 4 weeks or more after the first dose if there is no serologic response to measles after the first dose.*

[f]*Restricted for research protocol.*

indicated in healthy children with dose 1 given by 14 weeks of age and the last dose by 8 months of age. Rotavirus vaccine thus could not be given post-HSCT.[6,60-64] Vaccination of donors prior to transplant and to recipients in the peritransplant period is being investigated in clinical trials.[65] Inactivated vaccines pose no risk to HSCT recipients. There is one study on which to base current recommendations for the use of meningococcal C conjugate vaccine, and no studies regarding acellular pertussis vaccine or post-HSCT transplantation for adults and adolescents or the human papillomavirus vaccine. These vaccines would be expected to be safe and effective as other protein or protein conjugate vaccines in these patients (see Table 98-2). Immunogenicity of a roughly similar vaccine schedule has been shown in a U.K. study; in that study immunizations generally are begun at 12 months after identical sibling, syngeneic and autologous HCST and 18 months after allogeneic HSCT, with MMR given 6 months after the first series.[62]

Passive Immunization and Immunoglobulin Utilization

IGIV, because of its antimicrobial and immunomodulatory effect, has been administered to HSCT recipients with mixed results in infection prevention.[66-68] Differences in dosage, schedule, duration, and preparation used in various studies may contribute to ambiguity of results. IGIV has been reported to decrease the rate of infection and incidence of GvHD in allogeneic transplant recipients.[68] The optimal dose is not known. However, prolonged administration of IGIV can lead to delayed immune reconstitution and an increased incidence of infections after discontinuation. The indications for passive immunization with specific immune globulin preparations (hepatitis B, tetanus, and rabies) in patients post-HSCT are similar to those in otherwise healthy individuals. Passive immunization is recommended for susceptible people with known exposure to varicella[60] (see Chapter 205, Varicella-Zoster Virus).

99 Fever and Granulocytopenia

Andrew Y. Koh and Philip A. Pizzo

Infection remains a major cause of morbidity in children with cancer. The use of empirical antimicrobial regimens in this patient population began with the observation that febrile neutropenic patients with cancer who had potentially fatal infections could not be distinguished from those who had less serious or noninfectious illnesses.

ETIOLOGIC AGENTS

Bacteria

Infections in immunocompromised children can result from bacteria, fungi, viruses, or protozoa, and most organisms arise from the host's endogenous bacterial flora. Studies have documented that with hospitalization and antibiotic therapy (including antineoplastic chemotherapy), there is a shift in normal flora to include potentially pathogenic gram-negative bacteria.[1] The explanations for these microbiologic shifts are unclear, but intuitively, underlying disease and exposure to broad-spectrum antibiotics contribute to changes in microbial populations. Approximately one-half of pathogens responsible for documented infections are acquired by oncology patients after admission to the hospital,[2] including antibiotic-resistant gram-positive and gram-negative organisms.

The relative incidence of gram-negative infections has decreased since the early 1980s while the incidence of gram-positive infections in this population has risen.[3,4] Currently, the gram-positive organisms (particularly coagulase-negative staphylococci, *Staphylococcus aureus* (especially methicillin-resistance *S. aureus*, MRSA), α-hemolytic streptococci, enterococci, and *Corynebacterium* spp.) account for more than half of documented infections in patients with cancer, and *Escherichia coli*, *Pseudomonas* species, and the *Enterobacter–Klebsiella–Serratia* group are identified in a smaller but substantial proportion of patients.[3-6]

Although bloodstream infection (BSI) with gram-positive organisms generally is associated with lower mortality than that associated with gram-negative organisms, the syndrome of α-hemolytic streptococcal septicemia deserves special attention. The α-hemolytic streptococci are normal inhabitants of the oral cavity and have been noted to cause infection in patients receiving cytosine arabinoside.[7] *Streptococcus mitis* and *Streptococcus sanguis* are the most common α-hemolytic streptococci associated with this syndrome, which manifests as septic shock, adult respiratory distress syndrome, and rapid progression to death.[8] Rare cases of secondary myositis also have been reported with α-hemolytic streptococcal bacteremia.[9] Penicillin resistance among these previously susceptible organisms is common.[6,10] Increasing resistance of enterococci, particularly *Enterococcus faecium*, to ampicillin and vancomycin raises the concern of even greater morbidity and mortality due to gram-positive bacteria.[11] Community-acquired MRSA (CA-MRSA) has emerged in adult and pediatric patients with cancer.[12-18] CA-MRSA tends to cause localized skin and soft-tissue infections, although more invasive disease occurs (i.e., sepsis,[16] necrotizing fasciitis,[19] and pneumonia[20]). CA-MRSA isolates often are susceptible to clindamycin, trimethoprim-sulfamethaxazole, and rifampin, but inducible macrolide-lincosamide-streptogramin resistance in a subset of CA-MRSA isolates is well described.[14] An increase in clindamycin resistance among CA-MRSA has been reported recently.[17]

Gram-negative organisms have increasing resistance to a wide range of antibiotics, including all the β-lactam agents (e.g., extended-spectrum penicillins and cephalosporins) as well as the carbapenems, aminoglycosides, and fluoroquinolones. *Enterobacter* and *Serratia* species, especially, are prone to rapid development of resistance due to inducible β-lactamases.

Anaerobic organisms are uncommon causes of bacteremia (<5%) in febrile, neutropenic patients, despite their predominance in normal flora. The most commonly isolated anaerobic organisms are *Bacteroides* spp. and *Clostridium* spp. These organisms have been associated with specific syndromes, such as peritonitis, abdominal or pelvic abscesses, and perirectal cellulitis. Anaerobic bacteria frequently can contribute to infections of the oral cavity, especially necrotizing gingivitis. *Clostridium septicum* can cause a devastating infection characterized by septic shock and rapidly progressive necrotizing fasciitis with myonecrosis. Infection usually arises from a traumatic or surgical wound or spontaneously from necrotic bowel. Pseudomembranous colitis, caused by toxins of *Clostridium difficile*, can result in a spectrum of clinical manifestations, ranging from mild diarrhea and cramping to toxic megacolon and intestinal perforation.

Fungi

With improved treatment of bacterial infections in febrile neutropenic patients, prevention and treatment of fungal infections have assumed greater importance, especially in patients with prolonged neutropenia (i.e., neutropenia lasting >10 days).

Most fungal infections in children with cancer are caused by *Candida* species. Historically, *Candida albicans* was the most common species isolated. However, an increasing proportion of fungal infections are caused by non-albicans *Candida* species (e.g., *Candida tropicalis, Candida parapsilosis, Candida krusei,* and *Candida glabrata*).[21-23] This changing pattern of infections may be due, in part, to the use of oral antifungal agents such as fluconazole.[24]

Aspergillus spp. remain the second most common cause of invasive fungal infections in neutropenic patients. *Aspergillus fumigatus* and *Aspergillus flavus* are the most common species isolated. Other fungi that cause serious infection in neutropenic children are *Mucor* spp., *Fusarium, Trichosporon,* dematiaceous molds, and the phaeohyphomycoses (including *Curvularia, Bipolaris, Alternaria,* and *Exserohilum* species). None of these organisms is part of the normal flora of the respiratory or gastrointestinal tract, but after colonization, organisms can invade barriers when chemotherapy renders the host susceptible. Yeasts such as *Histoplasma, Cryptococcus,* and *Coccidioides* species are more commonly associated with defects of cell-mediated immunity, but they also can cause primary infection or reactivation disease in neutropenic patients.

Pneumocystis jirovecii is a major fungal pathogen in children with cancer.[25] *P. jirovecii* infection generally is due to reactivation of latent organisms in patients with cancer and is associated with a more rapidly progressive pneumonia than that seen in adults and older children infected with human immunodeficiency virus (HIV).[26] The use of corticosteroids is a high risk factor for developing *Pneumocystis* pneumonia (PCP). Because corticosteroids usually are used in the therapy of leukemia, lymphomas, and brain tumors, PCP is especially common in children with these malignancies, and frequently becomes clinically apparent during the tapering and discontinuation of corticosteroids.[27,28]

PART II Clinical Syndromes and Cardinal Features of Infectious Diseases: Approach to Diagnosis and Initial Management

SECTION P   Infections and Cancer

VIRUSES

Herpes simplex and varicella-zoster viruses have been identified consistently as the most common viral pathogens in children with leukemia. Other viruses, such as influenza, parainfluenza, rhinoviruses, cytomegalovirus, human herpesviruses 6 and 8, adenovirus, measles, respiratory syncytial virus, and enteroviruses, also can be associated with substantial morbidity. The incidence of infections is higher in children undergoing induction or during relapse than during remission.[29]

Although some viral illnesses (e.g., dermatomal zoster or herpetic stomatitis) cause clinically recognizable lesions that are accessible to culture, others manifest as nonspecific symptoms or localize to areas that are less accessible (e.g., cytomegalovirus hepatitis or viral encephalitis).

Parasites

Parasites such as *Toxoplasma gondii* and *Cryptosporidium* rarely occur in children with cancer, but infection, if it occurs, can be associated with substantial morbidity. *Toxoplasma gondii* can cause fulminant disseminated disease but most often is localized to the central nervous system (CNS); stem cell transplant patients are at the highest risk of developing CNS toxoplasmosis.[30] *Cryptosporidium* always should be considered in a child with cancer and severe or prolonged diarrhea.[31]

EPIDEMIOLOGY

Studies completed in the late 1970s suggested that more than half of children with fever and neutropenia had a clinically or microbiologically proven infection and that a causative agent could be documented in almost two-thirds of infectious episodes.[32] In more recent studies, the incidence of documented infection is lower. Fever without apparent cause now accounts for two-thirds of febrile episodes, perhaps because earlier, more consistently effective empiric antibiotic therapy masks documentation of infection. Concurrently, the mortality among febrile neutropenic patients has diminished dramatically, with some large series identifying fatal outcomes in only 1% to 5% of cases.[3,33-36]

Pediatric cancer patients differ from their adult counterparts in numerous ways. Children less often have a clinically apparent site of infection and consequently have a higher rate of fever without a source. Also, although the overall incidence of BSI is similar for children and adults, the rate of death during fever and neutropenia is about 1% in children compared with approximately 4% in adults.[3]

PATHOGENESIS AND ETIOLOGY

The interactions of multiple factors are the basis for the higher risk for serious infection in patients undergoing cancer treatment (see Tables 99-1 to 99-4).

Anatomic Disruptions and Devices

Alterations of skin or mucosal integrity or obstruction of an organ or body cavity predisposes to infection (Table 99-1). Cytotoxic chemotherapy often damages gastrointestinal tract mucosa and mucositis has been implicated as a risk factor for development of infections.

Devices that violate skin integrity, such as central venous catheters (CVCs) and peripherally inserted central catheters (PICCs), also lead to a substantial increase (40-fold) in risk of infection.[37] Depending on patient population, techniques of catheter insertion and care, treatment regimens, and the definition of CVC-related infections, such complications are identified in 9% to 80% of patients.[38]

Although some studies have suggested that the incidence of infection is lower for patients with totally implanted devices (e.g., Port-A-Cath) compared with external, tunneled CVCs (Hickman-Broviac type catheters),[39-41] the only prospective, randomized study failed to document a difference in rates of infection.[42] The use of central catheters for delivery of parenteral nutrition increases the risk of infection about 2.4-fold, independent of the type of catheter used.[43]

Devices other than CVCs also have been implicated in the risk of either focal or disseminated infection in immunocompromised patients. Among the most common of these devices are Ommaya (intraventricular) reservoirs, used to deliver chemotherapeutic agents directly into the ventricular space in patients with malignancies of the central nervous system. A review of infections associated with these devices in 61 patients at the National Cancer Institute (NCI) revealed that 75% never experienced a device-related infectious complication. Unlike previously published series of ventricular shunt infections in children with hydrocephalus, this study reported no mortality associated with Ommaya reservoir infections, and many of the infections were cleared without removal of the device.[44]

With any device, the importance of microbial biofilm formation and the mechanisms by which these organisms may perpetuate seeding of the bloodstream and, more importantly, promote emergence of antibiotic resistance warrants emphasis.[45,46]

Limb-sparing procedures for patients with osteosarcoma utilize prosthetic bone–joint hardware that also can be associated with infections. In some institutions, children with such prosthetic devices are not considered candidates for permanent CVCs because of the potential higher risk of bacteremia and seeding of the prosthesis. The relative risk of infection in children with limb prostheses is not known, and optimal management has not been defined.

Neutropenia

The single most important risk factor in the development of infections in children with cancer is neutropenia resulting from cytotoxic chemotherapy. The relationship between neutrophil numbers

TABLE 99-1. Predominant Pathogens Infecting Children with Anatomic Disruptions

Site	Bacteria	Fungi	Other
Oral cavity	α-Hemolytic streptococci Oral anaerobes: *Peptococcus, Peptostreptococcus*	*Candida* spp.	Herpes simplex virus
Esophagus	Staphylococci Other colonizing organisms	*Candida* spp.	Herpes simplex virus Cytomegalovirus
Lower gastrointestinal tract	Gram-positive: group D streptococci Gram-negative: enteric organisms Anaerobes: *Bacteroides fragilis, Clostridium perfringens*	*Candida* spp.	*Strongyloides stercoralis*
Skin (intravenous catheter)	Gram-positive: staphylococci, streptococci, corynebacteria, *Bacillus* spp. Gram-negative: *Pseudomonas aeruginosa*, enteric organisms	*Candida* spp., *Aspergillus* spp., *Malassezia furfur*	
Urinary tract	Gram-positive: group D streptococci Gram-negative: enteric organisms, *P. aeruginosa*	*Candida* spp.	

TABLE 99-2. Predominant Pathogens Infecting Children with Neutropenia

Category	Organisms
Bacteria	Gram-negative enteric organisms
	Escherichia coli, Klebsiella pneumoniae, Enterobacter spp., *Citrobacter* spp., *Pseudomonas aeruginosa, Bacteroides* spp.
	Gram-positive
	Staphylococci: coagulase-negative, coagulase-positive
	Streptococci: group D, α-hemolytic, anaerobic
	Clostridia
Fungi	*Candida* spp. (*C. albicans, C. tropicalis*, other species)
	Aspergillus spp. (*A. fumigatus, A. flavus*)

and the risk of infectious complications in patients with leukemia was first detailed in 1966 by Bodey and colleagues[47] at the NCI. The investigators concluded that (1) the risk of infection clearly was related to the absolute neutrophil count (ANC), severe infections being more prevalent when the absolute neutrophil count fell below 100 cells/mm[3]; (2) relapse of leukemia was associated with higher rates of infection than remission at all levels of neutrophil count; and (3) duration of neutropenia was the single most important factor in predicting risk of infection. Severe neutropenia that lasted longer than 3 weeks was associated with 100% risk of infection and the highest mortality rates.[47] These observations have been confirmed over the ensuing years and have led to the current approach to management of patients with fever and neutropenia. Organisms causing infections in children with neutropenia are listed in Table 99-2.

Normal Microflora

Commensal microbes stimulate the gastrointestinal epithelium to produce antimicrobial proteins (AMPs) that act as a first line of defense against invading pathogenic bacteria.[48] When indigenous commensals are depleted after antibiotic administration, select pathogenic bacteria (e.g., VRE) can overgrow and cause invasive disease.[49] Interestingly, by stimulating intestinal toll-like receptor (TLR) 4 by oral administration of lipopolysaccharide (LPS)[49] or by stimulating TLR5 with purified flagellin,[50] the AMP RegIIIγ can be reinduced and subsequently VRE levels in the gastrointestinal tract are decreased significantly. Thus, methods for maintaining microbial homeostasis during chemotherapy and antibiotic therapy may provide a novel means for preventing colonization and invasion of pathogenic microbes.

Other Defects

Repeated cycles of cytotoxic therapy not only decrease circulating neutrophils but also deplete lymphocytes and natural killer cells.[51] Reduced lymphocyte subset populations have been linked to the occurrence of opportunistic infections in patients receiving dose-intensive chemotherapeutic regimens.[51] Also, TLRs are key components of innate host response that are responsible for recognition of pathogens and cytokine response to surface molecules.[52,53] A study published in 2008 suggested an association between a donor TLR4 haplotype and risk of invasive aspergillosis among recipients of unrelated donor hematopoietic stem cell transplants.[54] Similarly, other TLR4 single-nucleotide polymorphisms have been associated with susceptibility to infections caused by gram-negative bacteria,[55] *C. albicans*,[56] and RSV.[57] Organisms causing infections in children that are related to defects in cell-mediated immunity are listed in Table 99-3. Those related to immunoglobulin and complement abnormalities as well as splenic dysfunction (or absence) are listed in Table 99-4.

TABLE 99-4. Predominant Pathogens Infecting Children with Defects in Immunoglobulins, Complement, and Splenic Function[a]

Defect	Organisms
Immunoglobulin abnormalities	**Gram-positive**
	Streptococcus pneumoniae
	Staphylococcus aureus
	Gram-negative
	Haemophilus influenzae
	Neisseria spp.
	Enteric organisms
	Viruses
	Enteroviruses (including polioviruses)
	Protozoa
	Giardia lamblia
Complement abnormalities C3–C5	**Gram-positive**
	Streptococcus pneumoniae
	Staphylococcus spp.
	Gram-negative
	Haemophilus influenzae
	Neisseria spp.
	Enteric organisms
C5–C9	***Neisseria* spp.**
	Neisseria gonorrhoeae
	Neisseria meningitidis
Splenectomy	**Gram-positive**
	Streptococcus pneumoniae
	Capnocytophaga canimorsus (formerly DF2 bacillus)
	Gram-negative
	Haemophilus influenzae
	Salmonella spp.
	Babesia

[a]See also Chapter 104, *Infectious Complications of Antibody Deficiency*; Chapter 105, *Infectious Complications of Complement Deficiencies*; Chapter 108, *Infectious Complications in Special Hosts.*

TABLE 99-3. Predominant Pathogens Infecting Children with Defects in Cell-Mediated Immunity

Bacteria	Fungi	Viruses	Other
Legionella	*Cryptococcus neoformans*	Varicella-zoster virus	*Toxoplasma gondii*
Nocardia asteroides	*Histoplasma capsulatum*	Herpes simplex virus	*Cryptosporidium*
Salmonella spp.	*Coccidioides immitis*	Cytomegalovirus	*Strongyloides stercoralis*
Mycobacteria	*Candida* spp.	Epstein–Barr virus	Disseminated infection from live virus vaccines (vaccinia, measles, rubella, mumps, yellow fever, or oral poliovirus)
Mycobacterium tuberculosis and nontuberculous mycobacteria	*Pneumocystis jirovecii*	Hepatitis B	
Disseminated bacille Calmette-Guérin			

PART II Clinical Syndromes and Cardinal Features of Infectious Diseases: Approach to Diagnosis and Initial Management

SECTION P Infections and Cancer

CLINICAL APPROACH TO DIAGNOSIS

Many oncology centers have adopted a standardized approach to the evaluation of febrile, neutropenic patients to ensure that all potentially dangerous causes of fever are considered (Box 99-1). For example, for infectious risks, *neutropenia* often is defined as an absolute neutrophil count of fewer than 500 neutrophils/mm³. *Fever* is defined as a single oral-equivalent temperature of 38.3°C (101.0°F) or higher, or a series of three temperatures recorded above 38.0°C (100.4°F) within a 24-hour period. Documentation of fever by the patient or a family member always should be accepted, even if the child is afebrile at the time of medical evaluation. It also is important to remember that some life-threatening infections can occur in the absence of fever in profoundly neutropenic patients.

A careful physical examination should be performed at the time of presentation and repeated frequently throughout the period of observation. Unfortunately, such examinations identify a potential site of serious infection in a minority of patients because the traditional markers of inflammation can be muted or absent in children who lack neutrophils. Thus the usual manifestations of serious infection, such as chills, rigors, and "toxic appearance," may not distinguish patients with BSI or other serious infection from those with an unexplained fever. Physical examination must include examination of the oral cavity and palpation of the perirectal area.

Urine and at least two blood samples for culture should be obtained from all patients before institution of antibiotic therapy. Peripheral blood cultures are not necessary in patients with a vascular access device when two or more sets of blood cultures have been obtained through the catheter. A meta-analysis showed little benefit in two-site culturing in patients with cancer with vascular access devices.[58] During seasonal outbreaks of viral respiratory tract infections, a throat or nasopharyngeal specimen should be obtained (at least in children with respiratory tract symptoms) for antigen or PCR detection or culture.

A chest radiograph frequently is obtained at the time of initial evaluation, but the diagnostic yield in asymptomatic neutropenic patients is small.[59] Chest radiograph at time of initial evaluation, however, can establish a baseline for future comparison in patients anticipated to have prolonged neutropenia (e.g., >7 to 10 days). Pulmonary infiltrates not present initially can become apparent with bone marrow recovery, because neutrophils are recruited to a site of previously "silent" infection.

A number of studies have investigated the potential value of surveillance cultures in patients undergoing chemotherapy. In a survey of 652 episodes of fever and neutropenia at the NCI in which surveillance cultures of nose, throat, urine, and stool were performed, 62% of patients who became bacteremic were found to be colonized with the infecting organism. However, management of these patients generally was not influenced by this information because multiple potential pathogens frequently were isolated from the same site. No single site was predictive of BSI, and the blood isolate frequently was identified before results of the surveillance cultures were available.[60] The cost of routine surveillance is not justifiable for this purpose. Nonetheless, surveillance cultures can be potentially useful in subsets of patients, such as those who have had procedures that increase risk of infection (e.g., nephrostomy, placement of urinary conduit) and patients at centers experiencing a high rate of infections with a resistant or highly virulent organism (such as resistant *Enterococcus, Pseudomonas,* or *Aspergillus*).

MANAGEMENT AND PRESUMPTIVE THERAPY

An empiric antibiotic regimen for febrile neutropenic episodes should (1) provide a broad spectrum of activity against a variety of pathogenic organisms, including but not limited to *Pseudomonas*; (2) be bactericidal in the absence of neutrophils; and (3) have low potential for adverse effects or emergence of resistant organisms.

Empiric Therapeutic Regimens

A number of empiric regimens have been evaluated over the last several decades. Most large comparative clinical efficacy trials have included both adults and children. There is little evidence that children respond differently to this type of infectious process or to the regimens that have been investigated. Many of the regimens studied are equivalent in their efficacy, although study designs and definitions of success have not been uniform. The Infectious Diseases Society of America has published general guidelines for use of antimicrobial agents in neutropenic patients with unexplained fever.[4]

For many institutions, the "standard" antibiotic regimen for a child admitted with fever and neutropenia includes an aminoglycoside and an antipseudomonal β-lactam antimicrobial agent (either an extended-spectrum penicillin or a third-generation cephalosporin). These regimens were developed in the 1970s, when *Pseudomonas* and other gram-negative organisms were the predominant isolates from febrile patients with cancer. They have proved to be effective and generally well tolerated, but the potential for nephrotoxicity and ototoxicity has led many investigators to search for regimens with better safety profiles, because several antineoplastic agents (such as *cis*-platinum) cause renal toxicity. A meta-analysis of randomized controlled trials that compared the ciprofloxacin/β-lactam combination with an aminoglycoside/β-lactam combination for the empiric treatment of febrile neutropenia showed comparable or better outcomes with the ciprofloxacin/β-lactam combination. The authors of this analysis, however, did clarify that this combination of quinolone/β-lactam should only be considered for patients who have not received a fluoroquinolone for prevention of infection and in settings in which resistance is uncommon.[61]

Double β-lactam regimens (usually consisting of an extended-spectrum penicillin and a third-generation cephalosporin) have the advantage of lower toxicity. Coverage for *S. aureus* is less reliable, but the extended-spectrum penicillins have good activity against many enterococci and anaerobic bacteria, organisms generally outside the spectrum of activity of cephalosporins. The major drawback of these regimens is the potential for emergence of β-lactam-resistant gram-negative bacteria.

Monotherapy (using ceftazidime) was pioneered by the NCI in the interest of simplifying antibiotic regimens and reducing toxicity in children who often are receiving complex chemotherapeutic protocols. Monotherapy had equivalent efficacy (i.e., survival of patients with fever and neutropenia) compared with combination regimens regardless of whether a site of infection could be documented. However, many patients required modifications of the initial regimen if they had a documented site of infection or

---

> **BOX 99-1.** Initial Diagnostic Evaluation of Children with Fever and Neutropenia
>
> - Careful medical history
> - Physical examination with attention to the skin, perirectal area, and other mucosal sites (which should be repeated at least daily in febrile neutropenic patients)
> - Specimens for culture
> - Blood: peripheral venipuncture and specimens from every lumen or access port of intravascular catheters
> - Urine
> - Respiratory secretions: for bacteria and viruses if symptoms are present
> - Any site with clinical signs of infection, including *Clostridium difficile* toxin assay if diarrhea present
> - Chest radiograph
> - Other imaging studies or diagnostic procedures as clinically indicated
> - Sinus radiograph or computed tomography
> - Abdominal ultrasonography or computed tomography

more than 7 days of neutropenia. Additional studies evaluating other cephalosporins (e.g., cefepime,[62-64]), the carbapenem imipenem-cilastatin,[33,65] and the carbapenem meropenem[66-68] as single agents for fever and neutropenia typically demonstrate comparable efficacy and provide options for management.

In November 2007, after a meta-analysis investigating the efficacy and safety of cefepime reported that all-cause mortality was higher with cefepime than with other β-lactams,[69] the U.S. Food and Drug Administration (FDA) posted an alert regarding the use of cefepime and the announcement of an investigation to review the safety of administering cefipime. In June 2009, the FDA released a meta-analysis that concluded that there was no statistically significant increase in mortality in cefipime-treated patients compared with comparator-treated patients.[70]

Neither the third-generation cephalosporins nor the carbapenems are effective against methicillin-resistant *S. aureus* and other selected gram-positive bacteria. The increasing frequency of antibiotic-resistant α-hemolytic streptococci,[6,71,72] *S. aureus*, coagulase-negative staphylococci, *Corynebacterium jeikeium*, and enterococci as causes of BSI in neutropenic patients with cancer has led to the inclusion of vancomycin in empiric regimens at some centers. At the NCI, and in randomized trials conducted by the European Organization for Research and Treatment of Cancer (EORTC), delaying administration of vancomycin (i.e., at the time of isolation of the pathogen) had no adverse effect on outcome.[73,74] Vancomycin is recommended for empiric therapy in healthcare environments with high incidence of MRSA. Daptomycin can be used as an alternative, but linezolid is not recommended because of its adverse effects (e.g., bone marrow suppression, specifically thrombocytopenia) and bacteriostatic nature. Antibiotics should be continued for at least 48 to 72 hours. If the pre-antibiotic blood and catheter culture results are negative and no site of infection is determined, the MRSA-specific antibiotic usually should be discontinued. If the cultures are positive, a full therapeutic course is indicated.[75]

Duration and Modification of Therapy

Even when a bacterial pathogen is isolated from a febrile, neutropenic child, broad-spectrum antibiotic therapy should be continued.[76] Specific clinical events that may require modification of the initial treatment regimen are described in Chapter 100, Infection in Children with Cancer; recommendations are summarized in Table 99-5.

The duration of antibiotic therapy depends on a number of factors, including isolation of a pathogen, clinical identification of a presumed infectious process, duration of both fever and neutropenia, and the patient's schedule for chemotherapy. Traditionally, broad-spectrum antibiotic therapy is continued until the absolute neutrophil count has returned to >500 cells/mm³. For patients in whom infection has been documented (either microbiologically or clinically) and resolution of fever and neutropenia has been prompt, the course of antibiotic treatment should be appropriate for the infection identified, which usually should include time to beginning recovery from neutropenia. For patients without a defined site of infection who show signs of bone marrow recovery, antibiotics generally can be discontinued. For patients who remain neutropenic, it is appropriate to continue antibiotics until the patient has been afebrile for at least 7 days.[4]

Empiric Antifungal Therapy

Fungi have emerged as an important cause of superinfection in patients with prolonged neutropenia, occurring in 9% to 31% of this population.[77,78] Traditionally, amphotericin B was the only available systemic antifungal agent. Its use in empiric regimens for prolonged or recurrent fever in neutropenic patients reduced the incidence of documented fungal infections and attributable mortality.[77] It became standard practice to administer amphotericin B empirically in patients who remained neutropenic with persistent or recurrent fever after 4 to 7 days of antibiotic therapy.

The search for alternative antifungal agents has been prompted by the toxicity of amphotericin B and emergence of rare amphotericin-resistant fungi. The azoles represent a less toxic class of antifungal agents. Ketoconazole, fluconazole, itraconazole, and voriconazole are effective in treatment of mucosal candidiasis. Although fluconazole has been reported to be as effective as amphotericin in the treatment of candidemia in patients without neutropenia or other major immunodeficiency,[79] the data are less clear in febrile and neutropenic patients with cancer. Two prospective studies suggest that fluconazole is an equally effective but less toxic alternative to amphotericin B when given as empiric antifungal therapy in patients with cancer who have prolonged fever and neutropenia.[80,81] The azoles, however, may be less active than amphotericin B against some species. Fluconazole has no useful activity against *Aspergillus* and has less activity than amphotericin B against *C. tropicalis*, *C. krusei*, *Candida lusitaniae*, and *C. glabrata*. Itraconazole and voriconazole have activity against all *Candida* spp., *Aspergillus* spp., some of the less common fungi, but no activity against Zygomycetes (the agents of mucormycosis). Voriconazole compared favorably with liposomal amphotericin B in adult cancer patients with fever and neutropenia.[82] In 2006, the FDA approved the use of posaconazole for prophylaxis against the development of invasive *Aspergillus* and *Candida* infections in immunocompromised patients 13 years of age and older. Posaconazole has been successfully used in salvage treatment of infections caused by Zygomycetes but its efficacy as an empiric antifungal agent in febrile and neutropenic cancer patients has not been evaluated.

There is considerable interest in preparations of liposomal or lipid-associated amphotericin because of lower toxicity compared with amphotericin B. In the only randomized, double-blind trial comparing liposomal amphotericin with conventional amphotericin B as empiric antifungal therapy, outcomes were similar with respect to survival, resolution of fever, and discontinuation of study drug because of toxic effects or lack of efficacy.[83] Liposomal amphotericin B was associated with fewer breakthrough fungal infections, less infusion-related toxicity, less nephrotoxicity,[83] and lower hospital costs.[84]

The newest class of antifungal agents are the echinocandins (i.e., capsofungin, micafungin, anidulafungin),which are large lipopeptide molecules that inhibit β (1,3)-glucan synthesis which is essential for fungal cell wall synthesis. The echinocandins are rapidly

TABLE 99-5. Modifications of Antimicrobial Therapy During Fever and Neutropenia

Clinical Event	Possible Modifications in Therapy
Breakthrough bacteremia	If gram-positive isolate, add vancomycin
	If gram-negative isolate (presumably resistant), change regimen
Catheter-associated soft-tissue infection	Add vancomycin (and gram-negative coverage if not already being given)
Severe oral mucositis or necrotizing gingivitis	Add agent active against β-lactamase-producing anaerobic bacteria (clindamycin, piperacillin-tazobactam, metronidazole); consider acyclovir
Esophagitis	Clotrimazole, ketoconazole, fluconazole, voriconazole, caspofungin, or amphotericin B; consider acyclovir
Diffuse or interstitial pneumonitis	Trimethoprim-sulfamethoxazole and erythromycin
New infiltrate in neutropenic patient on antibiotics	If neutrophil count rising, can observe
	If neutrophil count not recovering, pursue biopsy; if biopsy not possible, add amphotericin B
Perianal cellulitis	Add agent active against β-lactamase-producing anaerobic bacteria to broad-spectrum therapy
Prolonged fever and neutropenia	After 1 week of antibiotics, add amphotericin B

fungicidal against most *Candida* spp. and fungistatic against *Aspergillus* spp., but echinocandins are not active against Zygomycetes, *Cryptococcus neoformans*, or *Fusarium* spp.[85] Since the drug target is not present in mammalian cells, adverse events generally are mild, and include (for caspofungin) phlebitis, fever, abnormal serum hepatic enzymes, and mild hemolysis. Oral bioavailability is poor, thereby limiting use to the intravenous route. In a prospective randomized, double-blind trial comparing the efficacy and safety of caspofungin with that of liposomal amphotericin B, as empiric antifungal therapy in patients with persistent fever and neutropenia, caspofungin was as effective and generally better tolerated than liposomal amphotericin B.[86] Caution, however, is warranted in using echinocandins for the treatment of *C. parapsilosis*. Patients who developed *C. parapsilosis* had persistently positive blood cultures when treated with caspofungin but achieved clearance when treated with amphotericin.[87] The optimal caspofungin dosing for pediatric patients is not known. One small prospective study investigated the pharmacokinetics and safety of caspofungin in children and demonstrated that a caspofungin dose of 50 mg/m^2/day provided comparable exposure to that of adult patients treated with 50 mg/day without developing any serious drug-related adverse events or toxicity.[88] The newer echinocandins, micafungin and anidulafungin, also appear to be well tolerated in children with cancer.[89,90] Because of the absence of potential mechanistic antagonism with other antifungal drugs and a mild adverse event profile, echinocandin combination therapy could become a consideration for particular infections such as invasive aspergillosis.

PROGNOSIS AND SEQUELAE

The mortality associated with BSI and other infections during neutropenia has decreased substantially during the past several decades. Several large trials indicate that deaths associated with infectious complications occur in about 5% of cases.[33,34,36]

RISK STRATIFICATION

The prospect of further simplifying the approach to management of low-risk febrile, neutropenic patients continues to be under active investigation. Although there is no consensus about the criteria used prospectively to distinguish high risk from low risk, key factors that affect risk of infectious complications can be surmised from studies that have been conducted: (1) anticipated duration of neutropenia,[91] (2) significant medical comorbidity,[91,92] (3) cancer status and cancer type, (4) documented infection on presentation, (5) evidence of bone marrow recovery,[93,94] and (6) magnitude of fever.[3,93] One small study found that in well-appearing children who had rapid defervescence and negative blood cultures abbreviated hospitalization was safe and cost effective.[95] Another study, however, of early discharge with continued home intravenous therapy found that 4 of 30 patients had medical complications and another 5 required readmission for recurrent or prolonged fever.[96]

Investigations of oral antibiotic therapy have used many antibiotic regimens (pefloxacin,[97] ofloxacin,[98–102] ciprofloxacin,[103–105] cefixime,[106] moxifloxacin[107]) for empiric coverage in low-risk febrile and neutropenic patients with cancer. Although the results of these studies are encouraging, many of the clinical trials were statistically underpowered and were limited by methodologic issues. Two large, prospective randomized studies of low-risk patients have evaluated the efficacy of oral ciprofloxacin plus oral amoxicillin-clavulanate compared with more conventional parenteral antibiotic therapies in an inpatient setting.[108,109] Although the relative efficacies of oral and intravenous regimens were comparable in both of these clinical trials, limited experience precludes this practice as an established standard for treating low-risk patients. When analyzing the spectrum of infections in a very large cohort of low-risk febrile neutropenic patients (757 episodes of fever and neutropenia) at M.D. Anderson Cancer Center, investigators found that episodes of unexplained fever were predominant (58% of episodes), but both clinically documented and microbiologically documented infections were seen with equal frequency (21% each).[110] Among microbiologically documented infections, gram-positive (49%), gram-negative (36%), and polymicrobial (15%) infections were documented. Thus, although these patients were considered at low risk for developing infectious complications, many developed serious infections necessitating broad-spectrum antibiotic therapy.

RECOMBINANT HUMAN COLONY-STIMULATING FACTORS

The use of hematopoietic growth factors, such as granulocyte-macrophage colony-stimulating factor (GM-CSF) and granulocyte colony-stimulating factor (G-CSF), has been implemented widely in the management of neutropenia in patients with cancer and bone marrow transplant recipients. Both G-CSF and GM-CSF have been evaluated as adjuncts to chemotherapy to assist bone marrow reconstitution and to prevent neutropenia and reduce infectious complications. Primary use of G-CSF has been shown to lower the incidence of febrile neutropenic episodes by about 50% in three randomized studies in which the incidence of fever and neutropenia in the control group was >40%. Primary administration of CSFs should be reserved for patients who are expected to experience rates of fever and neutropenia (≥40%) that are comparable to or greater than those seen in the control patients in these randomized trials.

Use of GM-CSF has been less consistently helpful and has been associated with more side effects than G-CSF. No study to date has demonstrated an advantage for use of CSFs in rates of tumor response, fatal infections, or overall survival. Secondary use of G-CSF or GM-CSF in subsequent cycles of chemotherapy has not demonstrated disease-free or overall survival benefits when the dose of chemotherapy was maintained. Therefore, reduction in chemotherapy dose should be considered the primary therapeutic option in a patient who experiences neutropenic fever or severe or prolonged neutropenia after the previous cycle of treatment. Finally, if G-CSF is administered within the first few days of chemotherapy for the initial induction or first post-remission course for acute lymphoblastic leukemia (ALL), the duration of neutropenia of <1000/mm^3 can be shortened by approximately 1 week. These studies and guidelines for the use of hematopoietic growth factors are summarized in a consensus paper by the American Society of Clinical Oncology.[111]

Clinical trials have reported conflicting results when attempting to evaluate whether the addition of CSFs to antibiotics in the treatment of fever and neutropenia improves long-term outcome. A meta-analysis of 13 studies concluded that the use of CSFs in patients with established fever and neutropenia reduces the amount of time spent in the hospital and the neutrophil recovery period. Overall mortality was not influenced by use of CSFs, but a marginally significant decrease in infection-related mortality was noted.[112]

PREVENTION

Preventive strategies have been evaluated, including use of hematopoietic growth factors, isolation measures, active and passive immunization, and prophylactic antimicrobial regimens.

Active Immunization

For children who were not fully immunized before the diagnosis of a malignancy, the American Academy of Pediatrics and Centers for Disease Control and Prevention (CDC) provide guidelines for use of immunizations in healthy and immunocompromised children.[113] In general, live-virus vaccines are not recommended for use in immunosuppressed children. Live-attenuated varicella vaccine previously was used under protocol for children with acute lymphocytic leukemia in remission.[114] Killed virus or subunit vaccines are considered safe for even the most compromised patients, but the efficacy in these individuals may be substantially reduced. Children recovering from allogeneic bone marrow transplantation may acquire the immunity of their donor but generally should be regarded as unimmunized; they are candidates for revaccination with inactivated vaccines. Live-virus vaccines can be administered 2 years after successful transplantation if there is no evidence of graft-versus-host disease.[115]

Passive Immunization

Passive immunization has been evaluated extensively. In certain circumstances, infection-specific or hyperimmune globulins have proved to be particularly helpful, as in the case of postexposure use of varicella-zoster immune globulin (VZIG) in susceptible individuals. VZIG reduced the incidence of primary varicella and its complications in nonimmune individuals if given within 72 hours after exposure. Because protection may be short-lived, repeated doses may be necessary in the setting of community outbreaks of varicella and multiple episodes of exposure. VZIG is no longer produced. VariZIG is available under an investigational new drug protocol (FFF Enterprises, 800-843-7477). If VariZIG is unavailable, IGIV can be used at a dose of 400 mg/kg once. Acyclovir prophylactically also is an option post exposure.[114]

Prophylactic Antimicrobial Therapy

Many clinical trials have focused on use of prophylactic antibiotics to prevent infections in neutropenic patients. The oral fluoroquinolone antibiotics have been investigated because of their good bioavailability and broad antibacterial activity. A meta-analysis of published randomized controlled trials of fluoroquinolone prophylaxis (18 trials with 1408 patients) found that prophylaxis significantly reduced the incidence of gram-negative bacterial infections, microbiologically documented infections, total infections, and fevers but did not alter the incidence of gram-positive infections or infection-related deaths.[116] A large randomized prospective trial evaluating the use of oral levofloxacin (500 mg daily) in adults with cancer (prior to an anticipated chemotherapy-induced neutropenia) showed that the levofloxacin group had a lower rate of microbiologically documented infections,

bacteremia, and single-agent gram-negative BSI compared with placebo recipients. Mortality was similar in the two groups, and the effects of prophylaxis were similar between patients with acute leukemia and those with solid tumors or lymphomas.[117] Two studies have evaluated the use of prophylactic oral levofloxacin (500 mg daily) in patients receiving chemotherapy for either solid tumors or lymphoma[118] or hematologic malignancies;[119] both showed a reduction in documented infections. A recent meta-analysis of antibiotic prophylaxis in neutropenic patients with cancer (95 trials performed between 1973 and 2004) concluded that antibiotic prophylaxis (various antibiotic regimens) significantly decreased the risk for death compared with placebo or no treatment.[120] When trials that utilized fluoroquinolone prophylaxis (52 trials) were analyzed separately, there was a significant reduction in the risk for all cause-mortality, as well as infection-related mortality, fever, clinically documented infections, and microbiologically documented infections. Although these results are encouraging, many of these studies reported increasing rates of antimicrobial resistance.[117,119–121] Thus, if prophylaxis is implemented, vigilant monitoring of the incidence of BSI (specifically gram-negative bacteremia) is critical.

Two large trials using fluconazole as antifungal prophylaxis have been conducted in adult patients with leukemia and bone marrow transplant recipients.[121,122] Although both studies confirmed a decrease in fungal colonization and superficial infections, a reduction in systemic fungal infections and associated mortality was identified only in the patients undergoing bone marrow transplantation. However, in several of the studies investigating fluconazole, infections with fungi known to be resistant to fluconazole (i.e., *Aspergillus* or other molds and non-*albicans Candida* spp.) have been a major cause of morbidity and mortality.[80,123,124]

The incidence of PCP in children with cancer has decreased significantly with the use of trimethoprim-sulfamethoxazole prophylaxis.[125,126] The incidence of recurrent HSV in patients receiving intensive chemotherapy or bone marrow transplantation has been reduced with the use of acyclovir prophylaxis.[127] The use of ganciclovir in preventing cytomegalovirus disease and use of acyclovir or valacyclovir in preventing VZV reactivation after bone marrow transplantation has been shown to be effective.[128,129]

100 Infections in Children with Cancer

Andrew Y. Koh and Philip A. Pizzo

Only approximately one-third of children with cancer, fever, and neutropenia have a clinically or microbiologically proven site of infection. Table 100-1 summarizes documented infections identified in three large clinical trials of empiric antibiotic therapy administered to patients admitted to the National Cancer Institute for fever during episodes of neutropenia.[1–3]

DIAGNOSIS AND MANAGEMENT OF SPECIFIC CLINICAL SYNDROMES OF INFECTION

Catheter-Associated Bloodstream and Soft-Tissue Infections

Several series evaluating the use of central venous catheters in patients with cancer have confirmed that these devices increase the incidence of central line-associated bloodstream infections (CLABSI), regardless of the level of bone marrow suppression.[4] Although gram-positive organisms, particularly coagulase-negative staphylococci, have emerged as the predominant pathogens,

almost any bacteria can be responsible for CLABSI. Fungi, most often *Candida* spp., also can cause catheter-related septicemia and are difficult to eradicate without removal of the device.[5,6] Mixed flora CLABSI should prompt an investigation to identify a causative event (e.g., swimming with the catheter unprotected, dropping of catheter tubing into bathwater, chewing on catheter tubing by young children, disconnection of catheter caps or tubing) so that appropriate education can be provided.

Because of the increased risk of CLABSI, antibiotics may be warranted in non-neutropenic patients with central venous catheters who have fever with no localizing findings. In evaluating children for presumed CLABSI, cultures should be obtained from all lumens of a multilumen device and administration of antibiotics should be rotated through all lumens because the pathogen is sometimes present in only one portion of the catheter. Most episodes of bacterial CLABSI can be treated successfully with the catheter in place, even when multiple organisms are identified.[4,7] The choice of empiric antibiotic therapy in children with cancer should take into consideration organisms that are most likely to cause catheter-related infections and should provide

PART II Clinical Syndromes and Cardinal Features of Infectious Diseases: Approach to Diagnosis and Initial Management

SECTION P Infections and Cancer

TABLE 100-1. Documented Sites of Infection in Patients with Cancer, Fever, and Neutropenia

Site or Type of Infection	Pizzo et al.[1] No. (%)	Pizzo et al.[2] No. (%)	Freifeld et al.[3] No. (%)	Total No. (%)
Bloodstream	81 (43)	109 (27)	20 (17)	210 (29)
Pulmonary	28 (15)	88 (21)	16 (13)	132 (18)
Cutaneous	42 (22)	43 (10)	19 (16)	104 (14)
Head, eyes, ears, nose, throat	11 (6)	69 (17)	28[a] (23)	108 (15)
Gastrointestinal	4 (2)	35 (9)	30 (25)	69 (10)
Urinary tract	22 (11)	29 (7)	NR	51 (7)
Other	2 (1)	38 (9)	7 (6)	47 (7)

NR, not reported separately.

[a]*Includes cases of severe mucositis.*

broad-spectrum activity until an organism is identified. Vancomycin may not be necessary empirically unless there is evidence of catheter-related soft-tissue infection or of a resistant organism.[8] Infections caused by specific organisms that usually require removal of the catheter, include *Bacillus* spp.,[9] the rapidly growing mycobacteria (*Mycobacterium chelonae* and *M. fortuitum*),[10] *Candida* spp.,[5,6] *Pseudomonas aeruginosa*, and vancomycin-resistant enterococci. Polymicrobial infections also usually require removal of the catheter. Other indications for removal of catheters in patients with catheter-associated infections include severe sepsis syndrome, suppurative thrombophlebitis, endocarditis, and failure to clear the infection after several days of appropriate antimicrobial therapy.[11]

Bacteremia can occur in conjunction with a catheter-related soft-tissue infection or without localizing findings. These infections may be confined to the skin immediately surrounding the exit site of a catheter or can involve deeper soft tissue around the subcutaneously tunneled portion of the catheter or access port. Exit site infections, without evidence of purulent discharge or deep subcutaneous involvement, sometimes can be managed with oral antibiotics in children who do not have neutropenia. Erythema, tenderness, or purulent drainage from the site necessitates intravenous antibiotic therapy. Any localizing finding in a neutropenic child should be considered evidence of infection, necessitating the administration of broad-spectrum antibiotics. Infection (induration, erythema, tenderness, or fluctuance) along the subcutaneous tunnel tract of the catheter generally requires removal of the catheter (in addition to antibiotic therapy) and debridement of infected tissue. In the setting of catheter-related soft-tissue infection, inclusion of an empiric antistaphylococcal agent is appropriate.

Skin Infections

Cutaneous infections are common in immunocompromised patients, accounting for 22% to 33% of infections in one series[12] and 16% of infections present at the time of hospitalization for fever and neutropenia in another study.[3] Infections of the skin can be caused by viruses, fungi, or bacteria.

Bacterial skin infections usually are caused by staphylococci or streptococci. In immunocompromised patients, both gram-positive and gram-negative bacteria, including enteric organisms and *Pseudomonas*, can be isolated either from the blood or from material obtained from fine-needle aspiration of the area of cellulitis.[13] *Pseudomonas aeruginosa* infection is associated with the severe necrotic skin lesions of pyoderma gangrenosum (Figure 100-1). Treatment for presumed bacterial cellulitis, therefore, should provide broad-spectrum coverage. Every effort should be made to establish a microbiologic diagnosis; new skin lesions should be biopsied and cultured.

Fungal pathogens including *Candida* spp., *Aspergillus*, *Fusarium*, and Zygomycetes can cause cutaneous lesions either as isolated findings or as manifestations of disseminated infection. Black, rapidly progressing, necrotic eschars should prompt immediate evaluation for fungal infection. Tender, erythematous skin nodules or pustules can develop during candidemia. Superficial cultures of suspicious skin lesions may not provide adequate material for diagnosis of fungal infections; biopsy generally is more useful. Cutaneous fungal infections resulting from *Aspergillus* or other molds require surgical debridement in addition to prolonged courses of antifungal therapy, since often they are a manifestation of hematogenous spread or local angioinvasive infection.

Cutaneous infections secondary to viruses are common in immunocompromised patients. Both herpes simplex virus (HSV) and varicella-zoster virus (VZV) can cause painful or pruritic vesicular lesions that can become secondarily infected. Diagnosis typically is made on the basis of clinical findings of typical skin lesions and can be confirmed by unroofing a fresh vesicle, scraping the base of the lesion, and sending the samples for direct fluorescent antibody staining, specific for each virus or for PCR testing. Diagnostic samples also should be sent for viral culture. Differentiation of the two viruses is important because, although both respond to acyclovir therapy, the therapeutic dose of acyclovir is different.

Patients with cancer who develop primary varicella, especially those actively receiving chemotherapy, are at increased risk of serious disseminated disease, including giant cell pneumonia, encephalitis, hepatitis, and purpura fulminans. Dissemination and subsequent mortality (estimated as 7% to 20% in untreated patients[14]) are reduced by therapy with acyclovir administered intravenously.[15] Although recurrent VZV in the form of zoster is

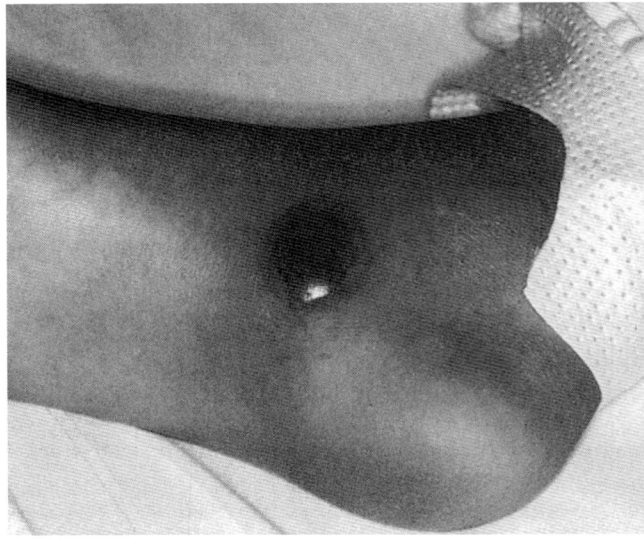

Figure 100-1. Pyoderma gangrenosum in an 8-year-old boy with newly diagnosed acute lymphocytic leukemia, fever, and bacteremia due to *Pseudomonas aeruginosa*.

rarely associated with severe complications when it remains localized to the skin, dissemination occurs in up to 25% of patients with immunocompromising conditions.[16] Severe abdominal pain, back pain, or evidence of inappropriate secretion of antidiuretic hormone may herald multisystem involvement, indicating the need for prompt initiation of acyclovir.[17]

A severe variant of scabies *(Sarcoptes scabiei)*, called Norwegian or crusted scabies, occurs in immunodeficient patients and is characterized by the presence of 10^3 to 10^6 viable mites, resulting in widespread, hyperkeratotic, crusted lesions. Crusted scabies is highly contagious and also can be recalcitrant to standard topical scabicidal therapy (lindane, permethrin, crotamiton, malathion, and benzyl benzoate). Ivermectin orally has been shown to be highly effective in curing both simple and crusted scabies after a single administration, although additional treatment often is employed.[18,19]

Pulmonary Infections

The lungs are the most common site of localized infection in patients with neutropenia. Pulmonary infection in this population produces a wide variety of symptoms, signs, and radiographic appearances. Table 100-2 summarizes causative agents based on specific radiographic findings.

Localized Infiltrates

Acute localized infiltrates at the onset of fever in a patient with cancer, with or without neutropenia, are most often due to bacterial pathogens. Because both community-acquired and nosocomial pathogens can be responsible for pneumonia in neutropenic patients, initial antibiotic therapy should provide coverage for organisms such as *Streptococcus pneumoniae* and *Haemophilus influenzae*, as well as *Pseudomonas* spp. and other gram-negative bacteria. *Legionella* also is considered in immunocompromised patients with patchy infiltrates; antigen test on urine septicemia is sensitive and specific for *L. pneumophila*. *Legionella* organisms have been identified in air conditioning equipment and showerheads and can be spread by aerosolization of contaminated water. Patients with pulmonary metastases also may be at increased risk for postobstructive pneumonia with a variety of pathogens, including anaerobic bacteria. The antibiotic regimens used for empiric therapy of fever without localizing findings in a patient with neutropenia (e.g., a third-generation cephalosporin, an extended-spectrum penicillin in combination with an aminoglycoside, or carbapenem) are appropriate for initial management of pneumonia. In some cases the addition of a macrolide (i.e., erythromycin, clarithromycin, or azithromycin) for possible *Mycoplasma* or *Legionella* infections is warranted. Table 100-3 lists recommendations for empiric antibiotic therapy for most common pathogens in patients with pulmonary infiltrates.

Viruses, such as influenza and parainfluenza viruses, respiratory syncytial virus, and adenovirus, also can cause localized infiltrates in immunocompromised children, although a diffuse process is more common. In one series, respiratory tract viruses were documented in about 25% of episodes of fever in neutropenic patients, but the role of these organisms could not be predicted on the basis of symptoms, radiographic findings, or degree or duration of neutropenia.[9] Consequently, consideration of a viral process does not obviate the need for broad-spectrum antibiotic therapy in a patient with neutropenia, fever, and a pulmonary infiltrate.

Localized infiltrates in patients who fail to respond to broad-spectrum antibiotics also can represent infection resulting from fungi, *Nocardia*, mycobacteria, or antibiotic-resistant bacteria. Tuberculosis also should be considered. Endemic fungi, *Histoplasma*, *Cryptococcus*, and *Coccidioides* can cause localized pneumonia in selected geographic regions and, in compromised hosts, can be associated with extrapulmonary infection as well. The presence of *Candida* in respiratory tract secretions, even in patients with pulmonary infiltrates, correlates poorly with causation because of the high frequency of colonization. Blood cultures positive for *Candida* or presence of ocular lesions (endophthalmitis) are associated with disseminated infection, which can include pneumonia. In the absence of these findings, definitive diagnosis usually requires histopathologic confirmation.

The fungal pathogens of most concern in the patient with neutropenia include *Aspergillus*, *Fusarium*, *Zygomycetes*, *Pseudallescheria boydii*, and *Trichosporon*, since these organisms cause rapidly progressive, extensively destructive infection. Unlikely to be identified at the onset of neutropenia and fever, the finding of a progressive or new infiltrate, accompanied by fever, nonproductive cough or hemoptysis, and pleuritic chest pain, in a persistently neutropenic patient during broad-spectrum antibiotic therapy suggests the possibility of invasive fungal pneumonia. Computed tomography may reveal multiple pulmonary nodules, sometimes with cavitation, that are not readily apparent on routine chest radiograph.[20] The classic histopathologic finding in these infections is invasion of the blood vessels with thrombosis and resulting infarction and hemorrhage. Whereas recovery of *Aspergillus* from the respiratory tract of patients without neutropenia can

TABLE 100-2. Causes of Pulmonary Processes in Patients with Cancer Based on Radiographic Abnormality

Radiographic Manifestation	Infectious Cause	Noninfectious Process
Focal consolidation (lobar or segmental)	Bacteria (routine and nosocomial pathogens) *Legionella* Oral flora (aspiration and postobstructive) *Mycobacterium tuberculosis* *Cryptococcus, Histoplasma, Coccidioides*	Pulmonary hemorrhage Pulmonary infarction Atelectasis Radiation pneumonitis Drug-related pneumonitis Tumor
Diffuse interstitial infiltrate	Viruses *Pneumocystis jirovecii* Miliary tuberculosis Disseminated fungi (*Cryptococcus, Histoplasma, Coccidioides*) *Mycoplasma* *Chlamydia*	Pulmonary edema Adult respiratory distress syndrome Drug-related pneumonitis Radiation pneumonitis Lymphangitic metastasis Lymphocytic interstitial pneumonitis (HIV)
Nodular infiltrate (with or without cavitation)	*Aspergillus*, Mucorales, *Fusarium* *Nocardia* Bacteria (especially *Staphylococcus aureus*, *Pseudomonas*, *Klebsiella*, anaerobic bacteria) *Mycobacterium tuberculosis*	Tumor

HIV, human immunodeficiency virus.

PART II Clinical Syndromes and Cardinal Features of Infectious Diseases: Approach to Diagnosis and Initial Management

SECTION P Infections and Cancer

TABLE 100-3. Approach to Empiric Antibiotic Therapy in Immunocompromised Patients with Extensive Pulmonary Infiltrates

Patient Characteristic	Empiric Regimen	Pathogens Likely to Be Treated
PATIENT WITH DEFICIENT CELL-MEDIATED IMMUNITY (NOT HIV)	Trimethoprim-sulfamethoxazole	*Pneumocystis, Nocardia*
	plus	
	Macrolide	*Legionella, Mycoplasma, Chlamydophila*
	with or without	
	Nafcillin or vancomycin	Aerobic gram-positive cocci
	plus	
	Aminoglycoside or third-generation cephalosporin	Facultative gram-negative bacilli
PATIENT WITH NEUTROPENIA	Trimethoprim-sulfamethoxazole	*Pneumocystis, Nocardia*
	plus	
	Macrolide	*Legionella, Mycoplasma, Chlamydophila*
	plus	
	Nafcillin or vancomycin	Aerobic gram-positive cocci
	plus	
	Aminoglycoside	Facultative gram-negative bacilli, *Pseudomonas aeruginosa*
	plus	
	Ceftazadime or extended-spectrum penicillin	Facultative gram-negative bacilli, *Pseudomonas*
PATIENT WITH HIV	Trimethoprim-sulfamethoxazole	*Pneumocystis*
	plus	
	Macrolide	*Legionella, Mycoplasma*

HIV, human immunodeficiency virus.

represent colonization, isolation of the organism in the setting of a patient with prolonged neutropenia and pulmonary infiltrate is predictive of invasive disease[21] and is sufficient evidence for initiation of antifungal therapy. Because neither bronchoalveolar lavage (BAL), which has a recovery rate of about 50% in biopsy-proven *Aspergillus* pneumonia, nor transbronchial biopsy, which has a yield of about 20%, is sensitive for the diagnosis, open lung biopsy may be required. An enzyme-immunosorbent assay (EIA) for detection of galactomannan antigenemia provides a non-culture diagnostic test for invasive aspergillosis. Sensitivity of galactomannan assays ranges from 50% to 95%, and specificity from 87% to 99% for the diagnosis of invasive aspergillosis;[22-24] piperacillin-tazobactam can cause a false-positive test. Thus, a positive galactomannan assay coupled with computed tomography that is consistent with invasive pulmonary aspergillosis in an immunocompromised host suggest a diagnosis of probable invasive aspergillosis,[25] but a positive culture remains the gold standard. In a meta-analysis of use of (1,3) β-D-glucan (BDG) assay for the diagnosis of invasive fungal infection (not solely pulmonary), pooled sensitivity and specificity for probable proven invasive *Aspergillus* or *Candida* infection was 76.8% and 85.3%.[26] Limitations of BDG are the need for discriminating use and interpretations, and several factors (e.g., cellulose membranes of hemodialysis, blood products, antibiotics, bacterial infections, etc.) that can elevate levels.

Historically, the treatment of choice for *Aspergillus* pneumonia has been amphotericin B at 1.0 to 1.5 mg/kg per day. Based on the findings of an international, randomized, open-label trial demonstrating that voriconazole conferred a significant benefit of survival and overall therapeutic response compared to patients treated with amphotericin, voriconazole is now considered the drug of choice for primary treatment of invasive aspergillosis.[27,28] Caspofungin, an echinocandin, was initially approved for use in cases of refractory aspergillosis. In a prospective study, 90 patients with invasive aspergillosis who were refractory to (86%) or intolerant of amphotericin B, liposomal amphotericin B, or triazoles (14%) were treated with caspofungin. A favorable response to caspofungin therapy was observed in 45% of patients (50% with pulmonary aspergillosis and 23% with disseminated aspergillosis). Only 2 patients discontinued caspofungin therapy because of adverse effects.[29] While successful use of caspofungin as first-line monotherapy for invasive aspergillosis has been reported,[30,31] no randomized controlled trials comparing efficacy to other antifungal agents have been published. Successful therapy with the combination of voriconazole and caspofungin for invasive aspergillosis has been reported.[32-34] Randomized trials are needed in order to determine whether this combination is advantageous (both from a efficacy and safety perspective) over monotherapy or other combination therapy regimens. A randomized trial comparing voriconazole with voriconazole plus anidulafungin is being conducted.[32]

Other fungal pathogens, such as *H. capsulatum, C. immitis,* and *C. neoformans,* also can cause focal infiltrates in patients with neutropenia who are receiving corticosteroid therapy.[35]

Diffuse or Interstitial Infiltrates

Diffuse or interstitial infiltrates most often represent a nonbacterial process although both gram-positive and gram-negative bacteria also can be causative. In children not receiving prophylaxis, *Pneumocystis jirovecii* is the most common organism identified in the setting of diffuse, interstitial infiltrates. *P. jirovecii* should be considered in children receiving corticosteroid therapy or in children with significant deficiency of cell-mediated immunity who have fever, nonproductive cough, tachypnea, and hypoxia. In one review of oncology patients with confirmed *Pneumocystis* pneumonia (PCP), 70% of cases became symptomatic while corticosteroid dosages were being tapered.[36] The chest radiograph typically reveals bilateral perihilar interstitial (or alveolar) infiltrates that spread to involve all lobes (Figure 100-2), but virtually any radiographic pattern can be associated with PCP. The diagnosis of PCP can be established by finding either cysts or trophozoites on smears of respiratory tract secretions obtained by sputum induction, BAL, or open lung biopsy. In non-neutropenic patients with diffuse infiltrates who are unable to undergo BAL or biopsy, an empiric course of trimethoprim-sulfamethoxazole (TMP-SMX) plus a macrolide has been recommended.[37] The treatment of choice for patients with proven or suspected PCP is TMP-SMX at a total daily dose of 15 to 20 mg/kg, divided into 4 doses given every 6 hours, for 14 days. Prednisone usually is given to patients with moderate or severe PCP. Other therapies found to be effective for PCP in patients with human immunodeficiency virus (HIV) infection include pentamidine, trimetrexate, atovaquone, and clindamycin plus primaquine. The incidence of PCP in patients with cancer has been reduced substantially with the use of TMP-SMX in prophylactic regimens. Recurrences of PCP or

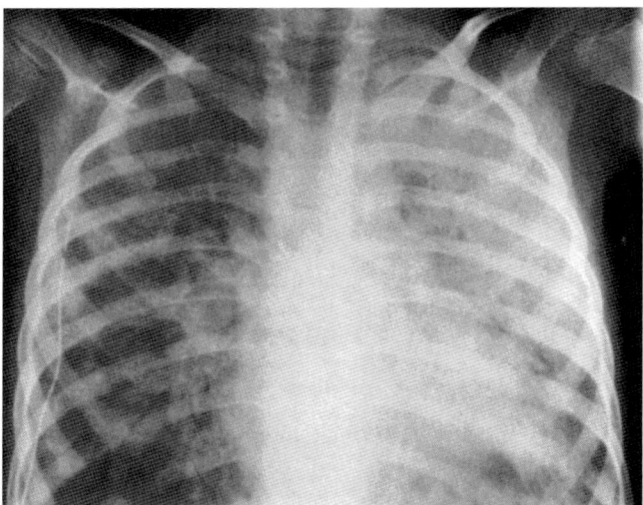

Figure 100-2. Chest radiograph showing bilateral interstitial and alveolar infiltrates in a child with acute lymphocytic leukemia and *Pneumocystis* pneumonia.

breakthrough infections are unusual in children with cancer, although they have been reported in children with HIV infection.[38]

Viral infections also can cause pneumonia with diffuse or interstitial infiltrates. Whereas the common respiratory tract viruses cause more severe disease in immunocompromised patients, the most serious cases are caused by cytomegalovirus (CMV). CMV pneumonia has occurred often in patients receiving allogeneic bone marrow transplants. Onset usually is within the first 3 months of organ or bone marrow transplantation. Clinical presentation includes fever and rapidly progressive diffuse pulmonary infiltrates, often causing pulmonary dysfunction requiring ventilatory assistance. Risk factors identified for development of CMV pneumonia include presence of pretransplant seropositivity for CMV in donor or receipt of total body irradiation as part of the pretransplant regimen, and development of graft-versus-host disease.[39] Historically, CMV pneumonia had a mortality rate of over 80%. Treatment with ganciclovir and high-dose intravenously administered immune globulin has improved survival significantly, but even with this regimen, 50% of patients die.[40,41] Definitive diagnosis requires identification of virus on lung tissue obtained by biopsy. Because of the severity of pulmonary infection caused by CMV, regimens in many transplant centers include preemptive therapy with intravenous ganciclovir for patients who have CMV isolated from any site during the early posttransplant period.[42]

Other herpesviruses, particularly VZV and HSV, can cause diffuse pneumonia in patients with cancer. RSV also can cause severe lower respiratory tract disease with a high mortality rate, notably in patients undergoing therapy for acute myelogenous leukemia or hematopoietic stem cell transplantation.[43,44] Parainfluenza, influenza (including H1N1), adenovirus, and human herpesvirus 6 have been described as causes of interstitial pneumonia in children with cancer.[45,46]

Infections of the Ears and Sinuses

In the neutropenic child, ear infections can be accompanied by pain, with minimal erythema of the tympanic membrane. Patients who have been hospitalized or who are receiving chemotherapy may have altered microbial flora. In addition to the usual bacterial pathogens responsible for otitis media (*S. pneumoniae, H. influenzae, Moraxella catarrhalis*), nosocomial pathogens (such as gram-negative organisms) must be considered. Necrotizing (malignant) otitis externa resulting from invasive infection of the auditory canal with *P. aeruginosa* (and occasionally invasive fungi) occurs more commonly in patients with diabetes mellitus or in those receiving corticosteroids, but necrotizing otitis externa can occur in patients receiving chemotherapy and requires aggressive intravenous antimicrobial therapy and debridement.

Although mastoiditis is an uncommon infection in children with cancer, patients at increased risk include those with anatomic abnormalities of the middle ear and/or prolonged neutropenia. Those with prolonged neutropenia are at risk for developing mastoiditis, not only with the typical bacterial pathogens but also with fungi (particularly *Aspergillus*), which usually requires surgical debridement for cure.[47]

The paranasal sinuses can become infected with typical pathogens or with bacterial flora prevalent in hospitalized patients. Sinusitis was found more commonly in children with hematologic malignancies than in those with solid tumors in one series, and 41% of 91 children with acute lymphoblastic leukemia had abnormal sinus radiographs at the time of induction chemotherapy.[48] Children with tumors involving the sinuses (e.g., nasopharyngeal carcinoma, Burkitt lymphoma, rhabdomyosarcoma) are at particular risk of recurrent or chronic sinusitis; distinguishing between progressive or necrotizing tumor and infection is challenging. Sinus radiograph and computed tomography (CT) are helpful tools in diagnosis. Broad-spectrum antibiotics, including an agent with activity against anaerobic organisms, are indicated in neutropenic patients who demonstrate signs and symptoms of sinusitis. Symptoms not responding to empiric antibiotic therapy within 48 to 72 hours should be further evaluated with aspiration or biopsy of inflammatory material.

Patients remaining neutropenic for more than 7 days are at increased risk of fungal infection, including fungal sinusitis. In one series of fungal sinusitis in children, facial pain or headache, fever, facial swelling, and abnormal findings on sinus radiographs were the most common clinical findings.[48] A 10-year retrospective analysis of invasive fungal sinusitis revealed that the majority of cases were caused by *Aspergillus flavus*, and the most common presenting symptom was periorbital swelling (41% of patients).[49] Other fungi known to cause sinusitis in this setting include Mucorales, *Fusarium, Pseudallescheria boydii, Rhizopus*, and a variety of others. Infection can begin as a small area of blackened eschar within the nose or sinus but can become rapidly progressive with substantial tissue invasion and necrosis secondary to vascular thrombosis, and ultimate extension into the orbits or brain. The utility of surveillance nasal cultures to diagnose invasive *Aspergillus* infection has been shown in some but not all series;[21,48] biopsy material for histopathologic examination and culture is necessary to establish the diagnosis definitively. Therapy for the rhinocerebral syndrome of fungal infection requires aggressive surgical debridement and long-term therapy with voriconazole for sinusitis caused by *Aspergillus* and amphotericin B for infection caused by Zygomycetes.

Gastrointestinal Tract Infections

Infectious complications of the gastrointestinal tract are common in children with cancer. Both the underlying diseases and the cytotoxic and radiation regimens used in therapy predispose to alterations of the mucosal surface, leading to local infections and serving as a portal of entry for the microorganisms residing in the gastrointestinal tract.

Mucositis and Esophagitis

Mucositis as a side effect of cytotoxic chemotherapy can range in severity from isolated small oral ulcers to extensive mucosal sloughing of the oral cavity and more distal gastrointestinal tract. A recognizable complication of this process is necrotizing gingivitis, characterized by a periapical erythema and tenderness. As this complication is presumed to result from anaerobic infection, antibiotic therapy should include an agent effective against anaerobes (e.g., clindamycin, metronidazole, piperacillin-tazobactam, or meropenem). In addition, children who have been hospitalized for a prolonged period or who have received broad-spectrum antibiotics can have oral colonization with resistant gram-negative

PART II Clinical Syndromes and Cardinal Features of Infectious Diseases: Approach to Diagnosis and Initial Management

SECTION P Infections and Cancer

organisms or fungi. Chemotherapy-induced mucositis also can become superinfected with *Candida*, *Aspergillus*,[50] or HSV. A Gram stain of lesions may identify yeast or hyphae; *Candida* infection usually responds to topical treatment with clotrimazole troches; or in more severe cases, fluconazole, voriconazole,[51] caspofungin,[52-54] or amphotericin B may be indicated. Locally invasive or disseminated fungal infection can follow stomatitis. HSV infection can be documented by immunofluorescent staining of scrapings (using a swab or tongue depressor) or culture from swab of the involved area; infection usually responds to acyclovir. Because patients with a past history of HSV infection have a 70% to 80% incidence of reactivation during induction therapy for leukemia or after transplantation, it is recommended that such patients receive prophylactic acyclovir during the high-risk period of leukopenia.[55] Septicemia due to α-hemolytic streptococci with high rates of shock and central nervous system infection also can complicate mucositis. Up to 75% of these organisms can be penicillin nonsusceptible.[56]

Although the differential diagnosis of substernal burning chest pain and odynophagia includes both infectious and noninfectious causes of esophagitis, establishing a specific cause can be difficult. Neither a barium study nor endoscopic visualization reliably distinguishes among *Candida*, HSV, and noninfectious causes (e.g., mucositis secondary to chemotherapy and/or radiation). One study showed that 21 of 22 patients with cancer and a clinical and microbiologic diagnosis of oral candidiasis also had endoscopic findings diagnostic of candidal esophagitis, suggesting that oropharyngeal candidiasis may represent a sensitive marker for esophageal candidiasis in patients with cancer.[57] Definitive diagnosis, however, requires endoscopically performed biopsy and culture. When biopsy is considered too risky (e.g., a patient with a platelet count of <50,000/mm^3), an alternative approach is to begin empiric therapy for *Candida* esophagitis with an azole antifungal agent, and if symptoms fail to respond within 48 hours, institute a trial of amphotericin B or caspofungin. Failure to improve within 48 hours after initiation of amphotericin B or caspofungin suggests that *Candida* is an unlikely cause of esophagitis; endoscopic biopsy should be reconsidered or an empiric trial of acyclovir for presumptive HSV infection should be initiated. In the patient without neutropenia, infectious causes of esophagitis are uncommon; symptomatic treatment with antacids or histamine-blocking agents may be appropriate.

Intra-Abdominal Infections

The immunosuppressed patient with cancer is at increased risk of intra-abdominal infections because of invasion or obstruction of the bowel by tumor, extension of mucosal ulcerations, sloughing caused by chemotherapy, and lack of neutrophil protection. Typhlitis, or neutropenic cecitis, is a necrotizing process involving the cecum and terminal ileum that is seen almost exclusively in patients with profound neutropenia (most often associated with treatment of acute leukemia). Typhlitis manifests with acute right lower quadrant abdominal pain (mimicking appendicitis), which can become generalized and usually is accompanied by fever and systemic symptoms. Because of neutropenia, many patients lack the classic signs of peritonitis. Histopathologic examination of the bowel reveals infiltration of the bowel wall with bacteria, usually gram-negative bacilli (especially *Pseudomonas*), with little or no surrounding inflammation, and progression to necrosis in some areas. In a review of 24 cases of typhlitis over 30 years, bacteremia was documented in 8 of 24 children, and thickening of the bowel wall was seen by CT in 17 of 20 patients studied.[57] Surgical resection of necrotic bowel may be necessary when perforation, abscess formation, uncontrolled bleeding, or septic shock occurs. However, most cases of typhlitis respond to medical management, including use of broad-spectrum antibiotic therapy, and recovery from effects of cancer therapies.[58]

Although uncommon, a specific and devastating variation of typhlitis is caused by *Clostridium septicum*. Peritonitis involving this species classically manifests fulminantly, with rapidly progressive abdominal wall myonecrosis, crepitance, hemolysis, and

shock. Importantly, this devastating syndrome also can occur in the absence of fever. *C. septicum*, which is more aerotolerant than *Clostridium perfringens* and can grow in viable, non-necrotic tissue, can be part of the natural flora of the gastrointestinal tract. Over 80% of patients with this syndrome have an underlying malignant process.[59,60] Steps in pathogenesis are thought to be breaks in mucosal integrity secondary to malignancy or chemotherapy, microbial invasion of the bowel wall, and rapid proliferation in the setting of immunosuppression or granulocytopenia.[61] Additionally, *C. septicum* produces an α-toxin that may play a role in the severity of infection.

Pseudomembranous or antibiotic-associated colitis due to toxins of *Clostridium difficile* has been reported after the use of many of the antibiotics that are part of empiric therapy in febrile neutropenic patients. Many patients become colonized with *C. difficile* during hospitalization. Children with *C. difficile*-associated diarrhea can have symptoms ranging from mild abdominal pain to severe bloody diarrhea. Stool samples should be tested for *C. difficile* toxin whenever diarrhea or abdominal pain develops in a patient with neutropenia. Metronidazole is the drug of choice for the initial episode of mild-to-moderate infections; oral vancomycin (and occasionally colorectal instillation if toxic megacolon is present) is used for more severe infections.[62] Parenteral vancomycin does not provide adequate therapy for *C. difficile* colitis. Treatment of first recurrence is usually with the same regimen as for the initial episode, but additional recurrences should be treated with oral vancomycin therapy using a tapered regimen.[62] The addition of rifampin to metronidazole is an additional therapeutic option.[63] Nitazoxanide[64,65] and teicoplanin[66] may be considered as alternatives to traditional therapy.

Hepatosplenic candidiasis (also referred to as chronic disseminated candidiasis) can occur in patients with cancer, especially patients with prolonged neutropenia. Typical clinical manifestations include persistent fever and neutropenia, unresponsiveness to broad-spectrum antibiotics, right upper quadrant abdominal pain or tenderness, and an elevated serum alkaline phosphatase level. Cultures from blood, urine, and other sites frequently are negative. BDG assay can be useful in certain patients. Besides limitations noted above (in Localized Infiltrates section), inability to distinguish between fungal and non-detection of Mucorales, *Rhizopus*, or *Cryptococcus* infection are a problem.[26,67,68] Confirmation of the diagnosis may require liver biopsy (especially in children with risk factors for hepatic metastasis).

Typical hepatic "bull's eye" lesions visualized by ultrasonography or hypodense lesions by CT can occur as the neutrophil count begins to recover. Magnetic resonance imaging may be the most sensitive study. Before recovery of the inflammatory response, hepatic lesions can be missed by all imaging techniques.

Treatment of hepatic candidiasis is difficult, usually requiring a prolonged course of antifungal therapy. Amphotericin B and amphotericin B lipid complex have been shown to be effective treatment,[69] as has fluconazole in patients in whom amphotericin B failed or who had amphotericin-related toxicities.[20,35,70,71] Treatment failures with fluconazole in this setting have been reported. Antifungal susceptibility tests should be performed when choosing therapy. Fungicidal properties of caspofungin are attractive but data on use in hepatosplenic disease are limited. The appropriate length of therapy is unknown; the endpoint often depends on resolution or calcification of the lesions that were visualized.

Perianal Cellulitis

Although, in general, children have fewer chemotherapy-related perirectal lesions than adults, children are prone to develop mucositis involving the rectal mucosa. These lesions provide a focus for local cellulitis or abscess, usually involving enteric bacteria, particularly gram-negative facultative and anaerobic organisms. Multiple organisms are identified in most cases in which surgical drainage or needle aspiration is performed; anaerobic organisms are isolated most commonly.[72] Most cases can be treated effectively with antibiotics alone. Meropenem, an extended-spectrum penicillin, or third-generation cephalosporin in combination with metronidazole or clindamycin, or piperacillin-tazobactam is appropriate; in some cases, an aminoglycoside also is prescribed.

Central Nervous System Infections

Infections of the central nervous system (CNS) occur infrequently in children undergoing cancer chemotherapy. CNS infection must be considered especially in children who have undergone a neurosurgical procedure. Placement of an intraventricular shunt poses an additional risk of infection; 25% of children experience a related CNS infection, but death is rare.[73] Indolent infections with organisms of low pathogenicity are most common, including coagulase-negative staphylococci and *Propionibacterium acnes*. Because of the vague nature of associated symptoms, any child with a CNS device who has fever and no localizing findings should have fluid sampled for cell count, chemical evaluation, and culture.

One study estimated that <0.9% of infections of febrile neutropenic children with cancer were caused by CNS infections.[74] Patients with fever and a change in mental status should be evaluated promptly. Some studies have reported meningeal signs in a minority of neutropenic patients or in those who develop meningitis following neurosurgical manipulation;[75–77] thus the absence of meningeal signs does not exclude the diagnosis of meningitis. In a retrospective review of 40 cases of bacterial or fungal meningitis in children with cancer, most patients (65%) had recent neurosurgery, placement of a CNS device, or a cerebrospinal fluid leak.[78] Fever and altered mental status were the most consistent signs at presentation, with meningismus notably less frequent in neutropenic patients. *S. aureus* and *Streptococcus pneumoniae* were the most common pathogens. Of the 5 patients with fatal outcomes, all were neutropenic at presentation. Although the incidence of CNS aspergillosis is low, mortality approaches 100%. A retrospective review of 81 patients with definite or probable CNS aspergillosis who were treated with voriconazole found complete or partial response in approximately one-third of patients, and improved survival was seen in those who underwent neurosurgical therapeutic procedures.[79]

Cystitis

Hemorrhagic cystitis, manifesting as bladder pain and significant gross hematuria, has been reported in bone marrow transplant recipients, and both adenovirus (particularly type 11) and polyomavirus (BK virus) have been implicated. PCR detection of adenovirus and BK virus is possible.[80] Successful treatment of adenoviral and polyomaviral hemorrhagic cystitis with intravenous ribavirin, vidarabine, cedofovir, and ganciclovir has been reported, but controlled studies have not been performed.[81–84]

Osteoarticular Infections

Bone and joint infections occurring in patients with cancer are relatively rare. Children with soft-tissue or bone tumors are at risk of infectious complications in areas of destruction by the tumor or following surgery. It may be difficult to distinguish osteomyelitis from tumor or the effects of local radiation. Any organism that can lead to bloodstream infection, including gram-negative and gram-positive bacteria and fungi (e.g. *Aspergillus*[85]), can cause osteomyelitis or arthritis. Diagnosis and treatment can be particularly complex in children who have had limb-sparing procedures involving bone and joint prostheses and in whom long-term stability of the prosthesis is of concern. Serial imaging studies can suggest infection, but biopsy of the involved bone is necessary for definitive diagnosis. Long-term antimicrobial therapy is indicated when infection occurs, and revision of the prosthesis often is required for cure.[86]

---

101 Healthcare-Associated Infections

Susan E. Coffin and Theoklis E. Zaoutis

A *healthcare-associated infection (HAI)* is typically defined as any infection not present or incubating at the time of the patient's initial contact with a healthcare setting. Originally called *nosocomial, hospital-acquired,* or *hospital-onset infections,* the scope of HAI has expanded as patients now receive medical care in a wide variety of healthcare settings. Many HAIs are preventable and thus should be a target for aggressive infection control programs (see Chapter 2, Pediatric Infection Prevention and Control). In 1985, the Study on the Efficacy of Nosocomial Infection Control (SENIC) project found that 5.7% of 169,526 patients hospitalized in 338 randomly selected United States hospitals experienced an infection.[1] The authors of this study estimated that 32% of these hospital-onset infections could have been prevented by the application of known principles and practices of infection control. Recent initiatives by individual institutions, regional and nationwide collaboratives have demonstrated that the majority of HAIs that previously occurred in many institutions are preventable; marked reductions in the rates of central line-associated bloodstream infections (CLABSIs), ventilator-associated pneumonia (VAP), and surgical site infections (SSIs) have been achieved through the scrupulous adherence to evidence-based practices.[2–5]

As in adults, HAIs are common in pediatric patients (Tables 101-1 and 101-2). However, both the rates and microbiology of pediatric HAI differ from those experienced by hospitalized adults.

Children are less likely than adults to have comorbid conditions that increase the risk of specific device-associated HAI. In contrast, children are at far greater risk of developing a nosocomial viral infection than their adult counterparts due to the large reservoir of easily transmissible viruses (such as respiratory syncytial virus (RSV) or norovirus), which is greater in sites where children seek medical care.

The most recognized source of national data on hospital infections in the U.S. is the National Healthcare Safety Network (NHSN), originally named the National Nosocomial Infections Surveillance (NNIS) system. This program was organized in 1970 and is coordinated by the Centers for Disease Control and Prevention (CDC). Neonatal criteria are included in the NHSN definitions of select HAIs, in recognition of differences in the clinical manifestations of certain diseases in infants and adults. For example, two age-based criteria are provided for the definitions of pneumonia and bloodstream infection (BSI); one for infants <12 months and one for patients >12 months. Because the NHSN provides standard surveillance protocols and HAI definitions, these data are among those most commonly used for benchmarking purposes.[5–7] It is important to note that investigators have demonstrated repeatedly that there can be significant differences in the application of these standardized HAI definitions, which may undermine their use for valid inter-institutional comparisons.[8,9]

PART II Clinical Syndromes and Cardinal Features of Infectious Diseases: Approach to Diagnosis and Initial Management

SECTION Q Infections Associated with Hospitalization and Medical Devices

TABLE 101-1. Rates of Pediatric Healthcare-Associated Infections by Site in Hospital, from the National Healthcare Safety Network (NHSN), 2006–2008

Infection Type and Hospital Site	Pooled Mean[a]	Median (25%, 75%)	Device Utilization[b]
CLABSI			
PICU (medical/surgical)	3.0	2.5 (1.1, 4.3)	0.48
Pediatric CICU	3.3	NA	0.62
Pediatric inpatient unit	3.1	0.0 (0.0, 2.7)	0.17
Pediatric hematology/ oncology unit	2.9	NA	0.45
Level III NICU (by birthweight):			
≤750 g	3.9	3.2 (0.0, 5.3)	0.35
751–1000 g	3.4	2.5 (0.0, 4.8)	0.32
1001–1500 g	2.4	1.4 (0.0, 3.5)	0.24
1501–2500 g	2.4	0.7 (0.0, 3.5)	0.16
≥2500 g	1.9	0.0 (0.0, 2.6)	0.20
CA-UTI			
PICU (medical/surgical)	4.2	3.4 (0.8, 5.6)	0.29
Pediatric CICU	4.4	NA	0.23
Pediatric inpatient unit	7.2	2.8 (0.0, 8.6)	0.09
VAP			
PICU (medical/surgical)	1.8	0.7 (0.0, 2.7)	0.42
Pediatric CICU	0.6	NA	0.35
Level III NICU (by birthweight):			
≤750 g	2.2	1.3 (0.0, 3.1)	0.47
751–1000 g	1.8	0.0 (0.0, 3.5)	0.30
1001–1500 g	1.4	0.0 (0.0, 1.4)	0.14
1501–2500 g	0.9	0.0 (0.0, 0.6)	0.09
≥2500 g	0.7	0.0 (0.0, 0.0)	0.14

PICU, pediatric intensive care unit; Pediatric CICU, pediatric cardiac intensive care unit; pediatric inpatient; pediatric medical/surgical inpatient unit; NICU; neonatal intensive care unit.

[a]*Pooled mean rate of device-related infection per 1000 device days.*

[b]*Device utilization = number of device-patient days/number of total patient days × 100.*

TABLE 101-2. Distribution of Pathogens by Infection Type Reported to the National Healthcare Safety Network, 2006–2007[a]

Pathogen	Number	%
CLABSI		
Coagulase-negative staphylococci	3900	34
Enterococcus spp.	1834	16
Staphylococcus aureus	1127	10
Candida albicans	673	6
Klebsiella pneumoniae	563	5
Enterobacter cloacae	443	4
Pseudomonas aeruginosa	357	3
Escherichia coli	310	3
VAP		
Staphylococcus aureus	1456	24
Pseudomonas aeruginosa	972	16
Enterobacter spp.	498	8
Klebsiella pneumoniae	446	8
Acinetobacter baumannii	498	8
Escherichia coli	271	5
CA-UTI		
Escherichia coli	2009	21
Candida albicans	1361	15
Enterococcus spp.	1393	15
Pseudomonas aeruginosa	938	10
Klebsiella pneumoniae	722	8

CLABSI, central line-associated bloodstream infection; VAP, ventilator-associated pneumonia; CA-UTI, catheter-associated urinary tract infection.

[a]*Data include pathogens reported from adult and pediatric patients.*

Rates of HAI among pediatric patients vary according to birthweight, age, underlying diseases, and intensity of medical care. Rates of infection are highest in children <1 year of age and in children who require intensive care, particularly infants in neonatal intensive care units (NICUs).[10-13] These vulnerable patients often have many of the risk factors that predispose patients of all ages to infections, such as severe underlying illness, loss of skin integrity, or the presence of multiple medical devices that breach normal defense mechanisms (e.g., an endotracheal tube bypassing the mucociliary elevator). In addition, pediatric HAIs differ from those seen in adults by site and pathogen. For example, in children BSIs are the most common HAI whereas in adults, catheter-related urinary tract infections (UTIs) predominate.[12,14-16]

BLOODSTREAM INFECTIONS

Device-Associated Infections

BSIs are the most common HAI experienced by pediatric patients (see Table 101-1). Among hospitalized and chronically ill patients, the majority of both CLABSIs and non-CLABSIs are related to the use of intravascular catheters and are discussed in depth in Chapter 102 (Clinical Syndromes of Device-Associated Infections). In addition, pediatric patients are at risk for BSIs as a result of contaminated intravenous fluids or medications, blood or blood products, or dissemination from a distant site of infection.

Infections Associated with the Transfusion of Blood and Blood Products

Epidemiology and Pathogenesis

Transfusion of blood and blood products is a relatively common practice in children. The overall rate of infectious complications of blood transfusions is unknown. The rate of bacterial contamination is thought to be about 1 in every 500,000 units of red blood cells (RBCs) and 1 in every 10,200 units of random-donor platelets.[17] Estimated rates of microbial contamination by bacteria, viruses, and protozoa vary substantially. The contamination rate of unscreened blood has been estimated to be 0% to 0.2% for RBCs, 0% to 5% for single-donor platelets, and 0% to 10% for pooled platelets; the rate of contamination of whole blood is unknown.[18-21] In addition, blood transfusions have been found to be an independent risk factor for a variety of HAIs.[22] Although all fatalities associated with the transfusion of blood and blood products must be reported by law to the U.S. Food and Drug Administration (FDA), some fatalities associated with transfusions may go unrecognized.

Although infectious complications associated with blood transfusion are relatively rare, a wide variety of pathogens can be transmitted (Table 101-3). At present, the American Red Cross Blood Services screen donated blood for the following: rapid plasma reagin antibody for syphilis; hepatitis B virus (HBV) surface antigen and core antibody; nucleic acid amplification test for West Nile virus; antibody to hepatitis C virus (HCV); antibody to human immunodeficiency virus (HIV) types 1 and 2, and HIV p24 antigen; antibody to human T-lymphotropic virus (HTLV), types 1 and 2; enzyme immunoassay (EIA) for *Trypanosoma cruzi* (Chagas disease).[23,24] Since the introduction of screening for bloodborne pathogens and active education programs to pre-screen potential donors, the risk of infection with these agents is extremely low: 1 in 66,000 units for HBV, 1 in 676,000 units for HIV, 1 in 100,000 units for HCV infection.[20,23,25,26] At present, the combined risk of

TABLE 101-3. Predominant Infectious Agents Associated with Specific Blood Products

Blood Component	Storage Conditions	Predominant Organisms
Red blood cells	1–6°C for 35–42 days	Yersinia enterocolitica Pseudomonas spp. Other gram-negative organisms Hepatitis C virus
Platelets	20–24°C for 5 days	Staphylococci Diphtheroids Bacillus spp. Salmonella spp. Escherichia coli Enterococci Flavobacterium spp. Streptococci
Whole blood	1–6°C for 35–42 days	Skin organisms, gram-negative organisms
Plasma	−18°C; thawed, 1–6°C for ≥24 hours	Staphylococcus aureus Pseudomonas aeruginosa

transfusion-related infection with HIV-1 and HIV-2, HTLV-1 and 2, HBV, or HCV is less than the risk of a transfusion-related bacterial infection.[18]

Almost all reported acute infectious complications and most fatalities associated with the transfusion of blood products are caused by bacterial pathogens. The manner in which a blood product is obtained, processed, and stored determines the infectious agents most likely to survive and cause infection upon transfusion.[27] For example, Yersinia enterocolitica and Pseudomonas species are associated specifically with cold storage of red blood cells, while skin flora and gram-negative bacilli are more associated with whole blood and platelet transfusions (Table 101-3). Recommendations by the FDA and the American Association of Blood Banks dictate the safe storage and handling of various blood products.[17] In addition, a wide variety of potential sources for contamination of blood and blood products have been identified, including the donor, the equipment used to obtain and process the blood product, and the procedures used for blood product administration.

Clinical Manifestations and Management

Signs and symptoms associated with the transfusion of contaminated blood or blood products vary according to the characteristics and concentration of the microorganism, the underlying severity of illness, and the immune status of the recipient. Signs and symptoms of transfusion-related BSI range from mild fever to overwhelming septicemia with endotoxic shock.

In a patient who is receiving or has recently received a transfusion, the sudden onset of high fever should raise the suspicion of transfusion-associated BSI. In these situations, the transfusion must be discontinued immediately; the blood product should be visually examined for abnormalities such as hemolysis, clumping, and discoloration, and any residual blood product and the administration set should be saved and refrigerated. Culture-confirmed episodes of transfusion-associated septicemia should be reported to the FDA, Center for Biologic and Evaluation Research (telephone, 301-827-6220; e-mail, fatalities2@cber.fda.gov).

Prevention

Self deferral and appropriate donor screening is essential to identify and exclude donors with potential transmissible diseases.[27] Screening consists of taking an adequate history of recent illnesses and travel, and serologic screening of donor blood. Despite

laboratory-based screening, donors with asymptomatic or incubating infections may be missed. To enhance the safety of transfused blood, potential blood donors are now asked to defer donation if they are known or suspected to have infection with West Nile virus or have recently returned from an area where malaria is endemic. Blood donation also is prohibited by individuals with a history of babesiosis or Chagas disease, or individuals at risk of Creutzfeldt–Jakob disease.[28]

Because episodes of transfusion-related BSI can be caused by normal skin flora, meticulous aseptic technique must be used for the venipuncture. Contamination can occur from introduction of skin surface bacteria during blood collection or through the withdrawal of a skin plug during venipuncture, which introduces skin microflora into the blood bag.[29,30] Even with appropriate skin antisepsis, skin plugs may still harbor normal skin flora that could proliferate (especially in platelet concentrates stored at room temperature) and cause infection upon transfusion. Use of contaminated equipment during the collection or processing of blood also can lead to transfusion infections.[31–34]

RESPIRATORY TRACT INFECTIONS

Epidemiology and Pathogenesis

A variety of hospital-onset respiratory tract infections threaten hospitalized children; these include pneumonia due to aspiration or ventilator-associated pneumonia (VAP). Factors such as the absence of pre-existing immunity, an increased reservoir of viral pathogens in pediatric facilities and units, as well as children's behaviors contribute to an increased risk of viral respiratory tract infection among children, compared with adults. A nasopharyngeal or nasogastric tube can interfere with the normal drainage of the sinuses and the eustachian tubes,[31,35] and has been associated with hospital-onset sinusitis and otitis media.[36,37]

Pneumonia

Pneumonia is the leading cause of death from HAI in the United States[38,39] and is the second most common pediatric infection reported to the NHSN (see Table 101-1). Estimates of the attributable mortality associated with HA pneumonia approach 30% in critically ill adult patients and are related to the severity of illness and the infecting organism.[40–43] Data from pediatric populations are more limited, but mortality appears to be lower in children (<10%).[44–46]

Aspiration pneumonia. Although bacterial pneumonia can occur via hematogenous spread or aerosolization, the majority of cases result from aspiration of bacteria that colonize the upper airway or gastric mucosa of a hospitalized or chronically ill patient.[47–50] Although the most common source of organisms is controversial, studies of ventilated patients have shown that enteric and gram-positive organisms begin to colonize these areas within hours of intubation.[47,50] Microaspiration of bacteria into the trachea is hypothesized to be a primary mode of pathogenesis.[42] Aspiration of gastric or oropharyngeal secretions can lead to serious disease of the lower respiratory tract. Risk factors for aspiration include pre-existing neurologic or neuromuscular conditions, decreased gastric motility, placement of an endotracheal tube, and sedation, which can lead to pooling of oral secretions.[51,52] When oropharyngeal secretions carrying pathogenic bacteria are aspirated into the lower airway, a polymicrobial pneumonia can ensue. In contrast, a noninfectious chemical pneumonitis can follow aspiration of gastric secretions; it typically has a more rapid onset (often developing within 6 hours of aspiration) and often is not accompanied by fever.[53] Nonetheless, it is often difficult to differentiate bacterial from chemical causes of lower respiratory tract disease.

Ventilator-associated pneumonia. Pediatric patients appear to have a lower risk of VAP than adults, likely because they have fewer comorbidities such as chronic heart or lung disease or immunosuppressing conditions. Although the epidemiology of VAP is well described in adults, few data exist for pediatric patients. However, we presume that the pathogenesis of VAP in adults and children is similar. Alterations in the glycoprotein fibronectin, which coats the respiratory epithelium, can occur within hours of hospitalization and enhance the adherence of gram-negative bacilli to the respiratory tract mucosa.[54-56] An endotracheal tube provides a portal for the numerous organisms that colonize the oropharynx to migrate to the lower respiratory tract. An artificial airway inhibits host defenses such as the gag reflex and ciliary function, and provides a substrate for the formation of biofilm.[47,50] Biofilm can be another reservoir of pathogenic bacteria and can be dislodged and delivered directly to the lower respiratory tract through mechanical suctioning or high-pressure airflow.

Pathogenic bacteria that cause VAP can arise from aspirated material from the digestive tract. At normal pH (1.0 to 2.0), the gastric mucosa does not support the growth of bacteria that typically cause HA pneumonia. However, use of proton-pump inhibitors and histamine type 2 (H_2) receptor antagonists for prophylaxis against stress ulcer promotes changes in the colonization of the upper gastrointestinal tract. Studies of critically ill adults repeatedly have shown that patients receiving traditional prophylaxis against stress ulcer have a higher rate of VAP than those who receive the cytoprotective agent sucralfate.[57,58] Thus, the risk of pneumonia must be balanced against the risk of clinically significant gastrointestinal bleeding.

Pediatric risk factors for VAP also include the presence of a genetic syndrome, reintubation, neuromuscular blockade, and immunosuppression.[45] Among neonates, identified risk factors for VAP include antecedent BSI and prolonged intubation.[13,59]

Gram-negative aerobic bacilli, such as *Pseudomonas aeruginosa*, are the most common organisms recovered from critically ill children with VAP.[45,60] NICU patients also have a risk of VAP due to *Enterococcus* spp. and group B streptococcus.[61] In pediatric patients with VAP, viruses such as RSV have been recovered from the lower respiratory tract in the absence of other pathogens.

Viral Respiratory Tract Infections

Viruses are the most common cause of hospital-onset upper and lower respiratory tract infections in children. Unlike aspiration and VAP, which most often are caused by a patient's own microflora, most nosocomial viral infections have exogenous sources (such as from family or other visitors), occur during community outbreaks, and have the potential for widespread transmission within healthcare settings.[62-65] Factors such as visitation (especially of siblings), playroom use, reluctance by healthcare personnel (HCP) to use sick leave, and low influenza vaccination rates among HCP can contribute to an increased risk of nosocomial viral infections in hospitalized children. Both children with underlying diseases and acutely ill patients are at risk for viral pneumonia.[65] Many viruses, including adenovirus, influenza virus, measles virus, parainfluenza virus, RSV, rhinoviruses, and varicella-zoster virus, can cause hospital-onset pneumonia. Among viral respiratory tract pathogens, the modes of transmission of RSV have been studied most carefully.[62,66-68] Both droplet transmission from close contact with infectious individuals and indirect contact transmission via hands or fomites contaminated by secretions occur.[69,70] In hospital-based outbreaks, RSV-contaminated hands are probably the most important means of cross-infection.[69,70] Other respiratory viral pathogens, such as influenza, most often are transmitted by respiratory droplets. However, the possible role of airborne transmission of influenza has led to new recommendations for the use of enhanced respiratory protection and environmental controls when performing aerosol-generating procedures on patients with known or suspected influenza infection.[71]

Clinical Manifestations and Laboratory Diagnosis

Ventilator-Associated Pneumonia

The diagnosis of VAP is difficult to confirm. The classic findings associated with lower respiratory tract infection – fever, cough, production of purulent sputum, and a new or progressive pulmonary infiltrate on chest radiograph – are not present consistently or may represent another process, such as atelectasis or acute respiratory distress syndrome (ARDS).[35,72,73] NHSN has developed guidelines for the diagnosis of VAP in pediatric patients based on clinical and radiographic criteria; sensitivity and specificity of these criteria are poor.[74-77] Accurate diagnosis is more likely when specimens are obtained via bronchoscopy, lung biopsy, lung aspiration, protected specimen brushing (PSB, whether bronchoscopic or nonbronchoscopic), or transtracheal aspiration rather than by aspiration of tracheal contents through an endotracheal tube.[75-78] The isolation of potentially pathogenic bacteria from such specimens is not conclusive, because they can represent lung infection or colonization, or infection at another site (e.g., sinusitis or tracheobronchitis). The use of clinical criteria plus positive sputum or tracheal culture has low specificity for the diagnosis of VAP.[79,80] Recent advances in the diagnosis of VAP in adults have included the use of bronchoscopic bronchoalveolar lavage (BAL) or PSB to obtain secretions of the lower respiratory tract for quantitative bacterial culture. However, these invasive procedures are not used routinely in children because of technical difficulties and the potential for complications. This problem is even more challenging in NICU patients because of the difficulty of obtaining any specimens through the endotracheal tube other than suctioned secretions. In one of the few pediatric studies comparing different diagnostic methods in children, a quantitative culture of lower respiratory tract secretions obtained by blind, protected BAL was the most reliable diagnostic test; a bacterial index (the sum of the log of all species obtained by BAL) of >5 was predictive of VAP.[72]

In 1991, Pugin and colleagues proposed the Clinical Pulmonary Infection Score (CPIS) as a tool to identify adult ICU patients with pulmonary infection and demonstrated good correlation between a threshold score of 6 and quantitative bacteriology of BAL samples.[81] Subsequently, several attempts have been made to validate the CPIS in adult patients, with variable results. This score subsequently was modified and evaluated as a tool to limit unnecessary antibiotic use in an adult ICU. Patients found to be at low risk for infection by the modified CPIS were managed successfully with a short course of empiric antibiotic therapy.[82] Additionally, use of the modified CPIS resulted in significantly lower antimicrobial therapy costs and antibiotic resistance, without adversely affecting patient mortality and length of stay in the ICU. Thus far, clinical scoring systems to establish a diagnosis of bacterial pulmonary infection have not been tested in the pediatric age group. A recent evaluation demonstrated that only 6 of 21 ventilated children with presumed bacterial lower respiratory tract infection had significant concentrations (>10^4 CFU/mL) of bacteria when fluids from a non-bronchoscopic bronchoalveolar lavage were cultured.[73] Many children with presumed VAP may not have significant bacterial infections.

Viral Respiratory Tract Infections

The accurate diagnosis of HA viral respiratory tract infections relies upon the availability of a sophisticated viral diagnostic laboratory. Although some clinicians debate the utility of viral diagnosis when few antiviral therapies exist, accurate diagnosis can uncover a problem and permit the prompt application of appropriate infection control measures and reduce the risk of widespread transmission of common pediatric pathogens, such as RSV and influenza. In addition, identification of viral pathogens also can reduce the inappropriate use of antibiotics.[83,84] Detection of virus (by culture), viral antigen (by immunoassays), or viral genome (by polymerase chain reaction (PCR)) assay in a specimen obtained from the respiratory tract, combined with clinical and radiographic findings consistent with lower respiratory tract infection, generally is accepted as confirmation of viral pneumonia.[64] For viruses that can be shed for prolonged periods (e.g., bocavirus and some adenoviruses) or are latent and can reactivate (e.g., herpes simplex virus or cytomegalovirus), confirmation of a causal role is more difficult and may require histologic examination of tissue.

Management and Outcome

Ventilator-Associated Pneumonia

Empiric management of suspected bacterial pneumonia depends on both patient-specific and hospital-related considerations. All of the following should be considered: the patient's underlying disease, previous antimicrobial therapy, mental status (and other conditions that increase the risk of aspiration), length of hospitalization, and results of Gram stain examination of respiratory tract specimens, and detailed knowledge of the local antimicrobial susceptibility patterns of common bacterial pathogens derived from microbiology surveillance data.

Empiric treatment for VAP generally is given when there is visualization of a new infiltrate on chest radiograph associated with fever, an increase in quantity or purulence of respiratory tract secretions, rising neutrophil count, or an unexplained decrease in oxygen saturation. Gram stain and culture of respiratory tract secretions commonly are used to support the diagnosis. Guidelines for the treatment of adults with HA pneumonia and VAP are available from the Infectious Diseases Society of America (IDSA),[85] but many of the principles apply equally well to children.

The outcome of hospital-onset lower respiratory tract infections varies greatly and is determined by characteristics of both the host and the pathogen. VAP is associated with significant morbidity and mortality, particularly in neonates; the case-fatality rate for neonates with VAP is reported to be 10%, with extremely premature infants having a fatality rate of 27%. Among pediatric ICU patients, the fatality reported rate is approximately 6%. VAP is associated with prolonged ICU stay and prolonged hospital stay in both NICU and pediatric ICU (PICU) patients.[45] Because delays in the initiation of appropriate therapy have been associated with increased morbidity and mortality,[86,87] initial therapy should be broad. Negative lower respiratory tract cultures from specimen(s) taken before a recent change in antibiotic therapy can be used to stop empiric therapy. Short courses (5 to 7 days) of therapy may be adequate in patients with uncomplicated VAP who have a good initial clinical response to treatment.[88]

Viral Respiratory Tract Infections

Children with hospital-onset influenza infection should receive age-appropriate antiviral therapy, ideally within 48 hours of symptom onset. There is limited data among hospitalized patients that antiviral therapy is associated with improved patient outcomes.

The treatment of patients with hospital-onset RSV is more controversial. Although ribavirin has in vitro activity against RSV, it generally is not given.[89,90] Studies have demonstrated that the clinical improvements achieved during aerosolized ribavirin administration are limited or sometimes insignificant. Although several studies have reported that clinical improvement has been seen with subsequent reductions in length of mechanical ventilator support, these findings have been inconsistent, and treatment may not be cost effective in children hospitalized with RSV.[90,91] Treatment may be appropriate in selected patients, such as those who have hemodynamically significant congenital heart disease or are profoundly immunosuppressed.

Immunotherapy with RSV monoclonal antibody has been evaluated for use in therapy; although therapy is associated with reduced viral loads, there is no significant impact on the clinical course or duration of hospitalization.[92-94] RSV monoclonal antibody is not recommended or approval by the FDA for treatment of RSV in any patient group.

Prevention

The Healthcare Infection Control Practices Advisory Committee (HICPAC) of the CDC has published a comprehensive collection of recommendations for the prevention of healthcare-associated pneumonia.[95] The "Guideline for Preventing Healthcare-associated Pneumonia" provides specific recommendations for

---

BOX 101-1. Prevention of Ventilator-Associated Pneumonia (VAP)

GENERAL STRATEGIES
- Conduct active surveillance for VAP
- Pay careful attention to hand hygiene
- Use noninvasive ventilation when possible
- Educate staff on VAP prevention strategies

STRATEGIES TO PREVENT ASPIRATION
- Maintain patients in semi-recumbent position (30–45° elevation)
- Avoid gastric overdistention and unplanned extubation
- Use a cuffed endotracheal tube with in-line or subglottic suction

STRATEGIES TO REDUCE COLONIZATION OF RESPIRATORY MUCOSA
- Perform regular oral care with an antiseptic solution
- Avoid nasotracheal intubation when possible
- Consider using alternative acid-suppressing therapy (e.g. sucralfate) in patients at low risk of gastrointestinal bleeding

STRATEGIES TO MINIMIZE CONTAMINATION OF EQUIPMENT
- Use sterile water to rinse reusable respiratory equipment
- Drain condensate regularly but keep circuit closed when removing condensate
- Change circuit only when visibly soiled
- Store and disinfect respiratory therapy equipment properly

Adapted from Strategies to prevent ventilator-associate pneumonia in acute care hospitals. Infect Control Hosp Epidemiol, 2008.

---

the prevention of bacterial pneumonia, Legionnaire disease, pulmonary aspergillosis, influenza, and RSV. More recently, the Society for Healthcare Epidemiology and the IDSA produced an evidence-based practice recommendation entitled "Strategies to Prevent Ventilator-associated Pneumonia in Acute Care Hospitals."[96] A summary of the recommendations to prevent VAP is given in Box 101-1. Major areas for preventive interventions include avoiding aspiration, minimizing contamination of respiratory mucosa and equipment, and reducing the exposure to mechanical ventilation. Taken together, these interventions, sometimes called "bundles," can reduce the incidence of VAP substantially.[97-99]

Additional study is needed to define the optimal methods to prevent HA viral respiratory tract infection in children. Macartney and colleagues demonstrated that a targeted, multicomponent program designed to reduce nosocomial transmission of RSV was effective and cost efficient.[70] Components include: (1) prompt laboratory confirmation of infection; (2) cohorting of patients and nursing staff; and (3) use of contact precautions (gloves and gowns). However, little is known about the efficacy and cost efficiency of similar programs targeted at other pathogens. Other institutional factors, such as appropriate use of sick leave, consistent visitor screening (or restriction in certain units and seasons), and influenza vaccination of HCP, also are important strategies to prevent transmission of respiratory viruses in the hospital setting.

GASTROINTESTINAL TRACT INFECTIONS

Epidemiology and Pathogenesis

Hospital-onset gastroenteritis has been estimated to occur in a minimum of 10.5 patients per 10,000 discharges.[100] Infants and elderly people are at greatest risk; estimated rates for neonatal, pediatric, and high-risk nursery patients are 3.0, 11.3, and 20.3 per 10,000 discharges, respectively. In the past, an etiologic agent was identified for 97% of episodes of hospital-onset gastroenteritis reported to the NHSN; *Clostridium difficile* and rotavirus were the

PART II Clinical Syndromes and Cardinal Features of Infectious Diseases: Approach to Diagnosis and Initial Management

SECTION Q Infections Associated with Hospitalization and Medical Devices

most common agents, accounting for 91% and 5% of reported infections, respectively. However, several factors suggest that the epidemiology of nosocomial gastroenteritis may be changing. First, the introduction of rotavirus vaccine has led to substantial reductions in community-onset infections and is likely to be associated with similar reduction in nosocomial rotavirus infections. In contrast, recent data suggest that the incidence of *C. difficile* colitis among hospitalized children has risen.[101] Norovirus is emerging as a more commonly recognized cause of both community-onset and healthcare-associated gastroenteritis.[102] Norovirus is highly infective and can survive for long periods on fomites and surfaces; these factors contribute to its ease of spread in the healthcare setting.

Both intrinsic and extrinsic factors raise the risk of gastrointestinal infections in hospitalized patients. Intrinsic factors include impairment of immunity, alterations in gastric acidity, and changes in gastric motility and flora. Several studies have shown that bone marrow transplant recipients and patients with severe immunodeficiencies are at risk of repeated and prolonged episodes of hospital-onset viral gastroenteritis.[103-105] Furthermore, immunocompromised patients excrete large numbers of virus particles for prolonged periods and thus are an important reservoir of infection within the healthcare setting.[100]

Extrinsic factors influencing the risk of hospital-onset gastroenteritis include the adherence to hand hygiene and use of nasogastric tubes or antacids.[106] The most common mode of transmission of gastrointestinal tract pathogens is the fecal–oral route, with pathogens frequently carried from patient to patient on the hands of HCP. Indirect contact via fomites or environmental contamination also can play a role in the transmission of *C. difficile*. Contaminated food or other common vehicles have been associated with the transmission of *Salmonella* spp., *Shigella* spp., *Yersinia enterocolitica*, *Escherichia coli*, noroviruses, and *Cryptosporidium* species.[11,13,107-112]

Viruses

The majority of episodes of hospital-onset gastroenteritis among children are caused by viruses. In the past, rotavirus typically has been the most common and serious cause of viral gastroenteritis among hospitalized children[113] and has been reported to occur in virtually all settings that provide medical care for children.[114-119] The incidence of hospital-onset rotavirus infections parallels that of community-acquired infections; both sporadic and epidemic infections (outbreaks) occur.[105,120] Risk factors associated with transmission include the use of shared toys and poor attention to hand hygiene.[121] Rotavirus vaccine is anticipated to have a major impact on the incidence of hospital-onset gastroenteritis.

Noroviruses have been associated with healthcare-associated outbreaks of gastroenteritis as well as endemic in-hospital transmission.[122-124] Noroviruses can be transmitted through direct and indirect contact, including through food or water sources.[112,122,125,126] Environmental contamination frequently has been implicated as a cause of protracted outbreaks.[127] Immediate cohorting of ill patients, furloughing of ill HCP, and implementation of stringent environmental control measures are necessary to halt transmission.

Adenoviruses and astroviruses also have been reported as causes of hospital-onset gastroenteritis in children. Adenovirus can cause severe gastroenteritis in immunocompromised patients.[128,129] Several clusters of HA adenovirus gastroenteritis have been described. One study specifically surveyed enteric adenoviruses in hospitalized infants with gastroenteritis.[104,130,131]

Clostridium difficile

In both children and adults, *Clostridium difficile* is the most important bacterial pathogen associated with hospital-onset gastrointestinal disease. *C. difficile* was first identified in the stool of neonates in 1935,[132] but initially was not thought to be an important human pathogen. In 1977, however, a *C. difficile* toxin was discovered in the stools of patients with pseudomembranous colitis.[133,134]

The epidemiology of *C. difficile* is complex and somewhat confusing in the pediatric population (see also Chapter 190, *Clostridium difficile*). Up to 50% of healthy neonates may be colonized with toxigenic forms of *C. difficile*.[133,135] After the age of 2 years, colonization rates decrease to adult levels of <5%, although colonization is much more prevalent in hospitalized patients with or without exposure to antimicrobial agents.[136,137] Some studies have questioned the frequency of in-hospital transmission of *C. difficile* in situations other than outbreaks.[138,139] Molecular analysis of isolates has shown that *C. difficile* isolates from asymptomatic or mildly symptomatic hospitalized patients often are polyclonal and likely represent endogenous strains.[140,141]

Clinically apparent disease occurs when the microbial ecology of the gut is upset, such as when a patient is undergoing antimicrobial therapy. With the disruption of normal intestinal flora, *C. difficile* can proliferate and elaborate potent toxins A and B, which stimulate secretory diarrhea and inflammatory colitis.[138,139,142] Although a minority of cases of antibiotic-associated diarrhea (AAD) and not all cases of pseudomembranous colitis are caused by *C. difficile*,[143] *C. difficile* is the most commonly identified pathogen. The major risk factor for pseudomembranous colitis is exposure to a wide variety of antimicrobial agents; risk was associated especially with clindamycin in the past and cephalosporins and fluoroquinolones more recently.[144,145] Other risk factors are underlying gastrointestinal disease, bowel stasis, and anatomic obstruction.[138,146]

Clinical Manifestations and Laboratory Diagnosis

Rotavirus

Rotavirus typically causes a secretory diarrhea, often associated with fever and vomiting, and is more likely than other causes of viral gastroenteritis to lead to dehydration.[147,148] Children between the ages of 6 months and 3 years are most susceptible. However, repeated infections can occur at any age. Case-series of children with hospital-onset rotavirus have demonstrated that hospitalized children of all ages are vulnerable.[105,114,115]

Rotavirus infection typically is diagnosed by detection of rotavirus antigen in the stool of a symptomatic or exposed patient. Alternative methods of diagnosis have included documented seroconversion, detection of viral particles by electron microscopy, or PCR.

Clostridium difficile

Symptoms of uncomplicated AAD usually are mild and resolve with discontinuation of the antibiotics. Symptom onset usually is 1 to 21 days (mean, 4 days) after initiation of antimicrobial therapy. However, occasionally symptoms begin after the agent is discontinued.[138] Associated signs and symptoms include fever, cramping abdominal pain, distention, nausea, and vomiting. Typically, hematochezia does not occur. However, symptoms can progress to pseudomembranous colitis, which usually manifests as the acute onset of profuse watery diarrhea, typically within 1 week of initiation of antimicrobial therapy. The spectrum of disease in pseudomembranous colitis is broad; complications include dehydration, protein-losing enteropathy, ascites, peripheral edema, toxic megacolon, peritonitis, septicemia, and intestinal perforation.[138,139,142,143,146]

Diagnostic tests for *C. difficile* include identification of the organism in stool by culture or glutamate dehydrogenase enzyme, and testing of stool or stool filtrates for toxin using either tissue culture or enzyme immunoassay tests, genetic fingerprinting with serotyping, and PCR.[149] Because the presence of the bacteria or toxin does not necessarily confirm causality of symptoms, endoscopy sometimes is required for definitive diagnosis.[138] On direct examination, lesions in the colon or small bowel are red, edematous, and friable, with multiple raised, yellowish plaques (pseudomembranes) that consist of mucus, fibrin, necrotic cells, and polymorphonuclear cells.

Management, Outcome, and Control

Viral Gastroenteritis

Viral gastroenteritis typically is self-limited. Supportive care with careful attention to hydration status remains the cornerstone of management of infected children.[150] Rotavirus and norovirus have been shown to contaminate the fomites and persist on inanimate objects for long periods of time.[151] Thus, appropriate cohorting of patients and staff, as well as environmental cleaning, are critical to prevent the transmission of viral enteric pathogens in hospitals.[152,153]

Clostridium difficile

AAD is treated by discontinuation of the antibiotic and provision of supportive care; invasive studies are not necessary. Patients with pseudomembranous colitis that persists after discontinuation of antibiotics require specific therapy. Oral metronidazole, bacitracin, or vancomycin all have been documented to ameliorate symptoms and eradicate *C. difficile*.[142,144,146,154,155] In an era of vancomycin-resistant enterococci and growing antimicrobial resistance among other nosocomial pathogens, oral metronidazole is the preferred treatment for patients with mild-to-moderate disease.[156,157] Recent studies in adults demonstrated improved patient outcomes when oral vancomycin was used as initial therapy for severe *C. difficile* colitis;[158] similar studies have not been performed in children. Response to treatment generally occurs within 24 to 48 hours; diarrhea and other symptoms usually resolve within 5 days.

Relapse after therapy occurs in up to 35% of patients and reflects: (1) reinfection; (2) relapse secondary to failure to eradicate the initial organism; or (3) germination of persistent spores.[159,160] Host factors such as pre-existing gastrointestinal disease, immunologic impairment, repeated exposure to antimicrobial agents, as well as the severity of the initial episode may affect the frequency.[161] Adjunctive therapy with probiotic agents, such as *Lactobacillus* and *Saccharomyces boulardii*, has been associated with improved response and reduced recurrence rates,[162,163] although this strategy remains controversial.[164] Antiperistaltic agents are contraindicated because they decrease toxin clearance.

Strict adherence to infection control practices is critical to prevent nosocomial transmission or recurrences of *C. difficile* gastroenteritis. Contact isolation precautions should be instituted for any patient with symptomatic infection. Because *C. difficile* commonly contaminates the inanimate environment, care should be taken to wash hands after all patient contact or after any contact with objects in the patient's room.[159,160] Transmission of *C. difficile* most commonly results from person-to-person transmission after inadequate handwashing by HCP. Soap and water must be used to perform hand hygiene when caring for a patient with *C. difficile*, because alcohol-based hand rubs are not sporicidal.[165] One study demonstrated an increased risk of *C. difficile* among patients placed in a room that had previously housed an infected patient.[166] Careful terminal environmental cleaning of patients' rooms is essential.

SURGICAL SITE INFECTIONS

Epidemiology and Pathogenesis

Data from the NHSN suggest that surgical site infections (SSIs) are among the most commonly reported HAIs, representing 14% to 16% of all infections.[167] Recent data collected by the Pediatric National Surgery Quality Improvement Project have demonstrated that infections are the most common complications experienced by children undergoing a surgical procedure. Using a systematic sample of 3315 patients and detailed investigations to document all 30-day outcomes, investigators found that SSIs occurred after 1.6% of pediatric surgeries.[168] SSI rates for commonly performed procedures in children, calculated with data from January 1992

TABLE 101-4. Selected Surgical Site Infection Rates by Operative Procedure and Risk Index Category, National Healthcare Safety Network, 2006–2008

Procedure	Risk Index[a]	Procedures (*n*)	Pooled Mean Infection Rate (%)
Cardiac surgery[b]	0, 1	21,555	1.1
	2, 3	7130	1.8
Appendectomy	0, 1	5211	1.2
	2, 3	663	3.5
Colon surgery	0	278	4.0
	1	292	5.6
	2	277	7.1
	3	207	9.5
Herniorrhaphy	0	2852	0.7
	1	3348	2.4
	2, 3	1277	5.3
Laparotomy	0, 1	3538	1.7
	2, 3	1561	2.8
Open fracture reduction	0	3600	1.1
	1	5629	1.8
	2, 3	1249	3.4
Spinal fusion	0	20,059	0.7
	1	16,640	1.8
	2, 3	4511	4.1
Ventricular shunt	0	867	4.0
	1, 2, 3	4270	5.9

[a]*Risk index: 1 point is given for each of the following risk factors: an American Society of Anesthesiologists preoperative assessment score of ≥3; an operation classified as contaminated or dirty; and duration of surgery >75th percentile for the particular procedure.*

[b]*Does not include coronary artery bypass graft procedures.*

through April 2000, are presented in Table 101-4.[169] The most significant pediatric SSIs include mediastinitis, ventricular shunt infection, and infection after placement of orthopedic prostheses.

For an SSI to develop, there must be a reservoir of microorganisms, a mode of transmission, and a suitable wound. Surgical infection usually results from intraoperative seeding of the surgical site by endogenous bacteria or by transmission of exogenous bacteria. Almost all microorganisms causing SSIs (Table 101-5) are thought to be acquired during the operation; rarely, small clusters of SSIs may be caused by pre- or postoperative exposures.[170,171] Adults colonized with *S. aureus* have an increased risk of SSI after cardiothoracic surgery.[151,172,173]

The risk of an SSI is influenced strongly by both patient- and procedure-related risk factors. Commonly accepted patient-related risk factors associated with postoperative infections include nutritional status, comorbid conditions, immune status, obesity,[174–176] and extremes of age.[174,177] Procedure-related factors include the type and duration of the procedure,[6,178] appropriate use of perioperative antibiotics,[179] method of hair removal,[180] surgical technique,[174,181,182] and the presence of a remote infection.[174,183]

Clinical Manifestations and Laboratory Diagnosis

A surgical wound is not infected if it heals primarily without discharge. In contrast, a wound can be considered infected if purulent discharge develops, even if microorganisms are not recovered from the discharge.

For surveillance purposes, the NHSN classifies SSIs into incision and organ or space (i.e., involving organs or spaces other than the incision) infections. Incisional infections are subdivided into superficial (involving only the skin and subcutaneous tissue) and

PART II Clinical Syndromes and Cardinal Features of Infectious Diseases: Approach to Diagnosis and Initial Management

SECTION Q Infections Associated with Hospitalization and Medical Devices

TABLE 101-5. Microbiology of Postoperative Infections in Surgical Patients

Nature of Operation	Likely Pathogens
"CLEAN" SURGERY[a]	
Cardiac[b]	
Prosthetic valve, coronary artery bypass, other open-heart surgery, pacemaker implant	Staphylococcus epidermidis, Staphylococcus aureus, Corynebacterium spp., enteric gram-negative bacilli
Vascular	
Arterial surgery involving the abdominal aorta, a prosthesis, or a groin incision	Staphylococcus aureus, Staphylococcus epidermidis, enteric gram-negative bacilli
Lower-extremity amputation for ischemia	Staphylococcus aureus, Staphylococcus epidermidis, enteric gram-negative bacilli, clostridia
Orthopedic	
Total joint replacement, internal fixation of fractures	Staphylococcus aureus, Staphylococcus epidermidis
Ophthalmic	Staphylococcus epidermidis, Staphylococcus aureus, streptococci, enteric gram-negative bacilli, Pseudomonas
Head and neck	
Incisions through oral cavity or pharynx	Anaerobic bacteria, enteric gram-negative bacilli, Staphylococcus aureus
Craniotomy	Staphylococcus aureus, Staphylococcus epidermidis
Abdominal	
Gastroduodenal[c]	Enteric gram-negative bacilli, gram-positive cocci
Biliary tract[d]	Enteric gram-negative bacilli, enterococci, clostridia
Colorectal	Enteric gram-negative bacilli, anaerobic bacteria, enterococci
Appendectomy, nonperforated	Enteric gram-negative bacilli, anaerobes, enterococci
"DIRTY" SURGERY[e]	
Ruptured viscus	Enteric gram-negative bacilli, anaerobes, enterococci
Traumatic wound[f]	Staphylococcus aureus, group A streptococci, clostridia

[a]Parenteral prophylactic antimicrobial agents can be given as a single intravenous dose just before the operation. For prolonged operations, additional intraoperative doses should be given every 4 hours for the duration of the procedure.

[b]An additional dose can be given after patients are removed from bypass during open-heart surgery.

[c]Morbid obesity, decreased gastric acidity, or decreased gastrointestinal motility.

[d]Acute cholecystitis, nonfunctioning gallbladder, obstructive jaundice, or common duct stones.

[e]For "dirty" surgery, therapy usually should be continued for 5 to 10 days.

[f]For bite wounds, likely pathogens can also include oral anaerobic bacteria, Eikenella corrodens (human), and Pasteurella multocida (dog and cat).

Adapted from Antimicrobial prophylaxis in surgery. Med Lett 1999;41:75–80.

deep (involving fascial and muscle layers) categories.[173,184] By definition, a *superficial incisional SSI* must occur within 30 days of the operative procedure and meet at least one of the following criteria: (1) purulent fluid is draining from the incision; (2) an organism is isolated from culture of a specimen that was obtained aseptically from the incision; (3) there is pain, tenderness, localized swelling, redness, or heat, and the incision is opened by the surgeon; or (4) diagnosis of infection is made by the surgeon.

By definition, a *deep incisional SSI* must occur within 30 days after the procedure in the absence of an implanted prosthesis, or within 1 year if prosthetic material was placed. In addition, it must meet at least one of the following criteria: (1) purulent fluid is draining from the deep incision but not from the organ–space component of the site; (2) the deep incision becomes dehiscent or is opened by the surgeon when the patient has fever (>38°C), localized pain, or tenderness, unless the incision is culture-negative; (3) an abscess is found on direct examination, during operation, or by histopathologic or radiographic examination; or (4) diagnosis of infection is made by the surgeon.

An *organ or space infection* involves deeper spaces entered or manipulated during the operative procedure; examples are subdiaphragmatic abscess after an appendectomy, or osteomyelitis after laminectomy. By definition, an organ or space SSI must occur within 30 days after the procedure in the absence of an implanted prosthesis, or within 1 year if prosthetic material was placed. In addition, it must meet at least one of the following criteria: (1) purulent fluid is draining from a drain placed through a stab wound; (2) an organism is isolated from culture of a specimen that was obtained aseptically from the organ or space; (3) an abscess is found on direct examination, during operation, or by histopathologic or radiographic examination; or (4) diagnosis of infection is made by the surgeon.

Management and Outcome

Antimicrobial agents are only one aspect of management of SSIs; considerations of surgical intervention and nutritional support are at least as important. In pyogenic abscesses, clostridial myonecrosis, streptococcal gangrene, or other infections with extensive tissue necrosis, surgical drainage and/or debridement should be considered the primary treatment, with antimicrobial therapy assuming a secondary role. However, in most postoperative infections in which the infected tissues are well vascularized, antimicrobial therapy is paramount. Empiric antimicrobial therapy for SSIs should be based on the location of the initial surgical procedure as well as the known patterns of antimicrobial resistance among pathogens such as *S. aureus*.

Prevention

Key measures to prevent postoperative SSIs were introduced into surgical practice in the last century, and have been the subject of comprehensive reviews.[185,186] These include preoperative measures such as removal of hair and application of antiseptic agents to the patient's skin, performance of surgery in a properly designed and ventilated operating room, and appropriate hand antisepsis by the surgical staff. Finally, the appropriate selection and timing of administration of perioperative antimicrobial prophylaxis has been shown repeatedly to reduce the risk of SSIs.[174,179] Many reviews of antimicrobial prophylaxis have been published, and most have similar recommendations for the procedures in which prophylaxis is desirable.[187–190] The selection of specific antimicrobial agents should take into consideration the most likely pathogens and the antimicrobial susceptibility data of individual facilities.

The efficacy of perioperative antimicrobial prophylaxis in decreasing the incidence of SSIs is well established for a variety of surgical procedures.[188,189,191] Most recommendations for children are extrapolated from studies of adult surgical patients. Such extrapolation may be appropriate for older children, but among neonates and young infants, for whom SSI rates appear to be higher, specific data regarding the optimal agent for, frequency of, and duration of prophylaxis are needed.[192]

Although difficulties exist in establishing evidence-based recommendations for antimicrobial prophylaxis in pediatrics, there remains a core group of well-accepted recommendations for adult patients that can reasonably be applied to children.[187] The American College of Surgeons recommends antimicrobial prophylaxis when (1) prosthetic material is implanted, (2) the rate of infection is relatively high (e.g., clean-contaminated or contaminated), and (3) the consequences of a postoperative infection are severe.[187–189,193,194]

A wide variety of agents have been recommended for perioperative prophylaxis. Selection of a particular agent should be determined by the nature of the procedure and potential pathogens, knowledge of the local antimicrobial susceptibility patterns, and the patient's age, hepatic, and renal function. For most procedures involving the gastrointestinal tract, the agent should have activity against Enterobacteriaceae and the *Bacteroides fragilis* group; cefoxitin (not approved for use in patients younger than 3 months) is the most widely recommended agent in adults. For almost all other operations, the most commonly recommended agent is cefazolin.[188,189,191] Cefazolin has good activity against the common gram-positive pathogens recovered from postoperative infections at these sites (especially methicillin-susceptible *S. aureus*) and has a low incidence of side effects as well as a long serum half-life. Regional changes in the prevalence of methicillin-resistant *S. aureus* colonization among healthy children might require alteration of prophylactic strategies.

Without age-specific guidelines and because of continuing controversy, many centers have developed their own practices based on local consensus and available literature. A review of 43 academic centers performing pediatric cardiothoracic surgery showed that physicians continued prophylactic antimicrobial agents at variable rates after surgery while certain interventions remained in place, as follows: thoracostomy tube (67%), mediastinal tube (72%), transthoracic vascular catheter (51%), central venous catheter (30%), or pacing wire (14%).[195] The general consensus was that first- or second-generation cephalosporins were used as single prophylactic agents and were continued until the removal of transthoracic devices. However, a prospective comparative study demonstrated that discontinuation of antimicrobial agents before removal of all indwelling devices was not associated with higher infection rates.[196]

POSTOPERATIVE MEDIASTINITIS AND STERNAL OSTEOMYELITIS

Mediastinitis is inflammation or infection of the mediastinal area (defined as the extrapulmonary area of the thoracic cavity between the lungs). This area contains the thymus, trachea and bronchi, esophagus, aorta and aortic arch, heart, pericardium, lymph nodes, and nerve tissue. Historically, infections of the mediastinum have been divided into acute (abrupt onset, with or without toxic appearance) and chronic (indolent) processes.[197–199] Although acute mediastinitis is uncommon, it can be serious and life-threatening.

Epidemiology and Pathogenesis

Mediastinitis after cardiac surgery is an infrequent yet serious complication of median sternal incision, with an estimated incidence ranging from 0.15% to >5% of all cardiothoracic operations.[200] In the few studies restricted to children, mediastinitis rates after cardiac surgery varied between 0.1% and 5%, with the highest rates found in neonates.[201–203] Because most pediatric cardiac operations involve correction of congenital anomalies, infection rates and risk factors for infection may differ from those identified from adult studies. Using a large multicenter database, factors that were independently associated with the risk of mediastinitis included: young age, prolonged preoperative hospitalization, preoperative ventilator support, and genetic abnormality.[204] No data are available on whether rates of mediastinitis in children vary according to type of reconstructive surgery or congenital anomaly.

The pathogenesis of infection is multifactorial but generally requires intraoperative introduction of pathogenic bacteria into the operative site; thus, perioperative aseptic technique and surgical technique are critical to prevent mediastinitis.[205,206] Risk factors

for mediastinitis in adults include diabetes mellitus, chronic obstructive pulmonary disease, prolonged duration of perfusion (cardiopulmonary bypass) or time of aortic cross clamping, higher body mass index or obesity, preceding infections (e.g., pneumonia, tracheal infections), and receipt of corticosteroids.[197,199,200,205–209] Outbreaks of mediastinitis have been associated with preoperative colonization, operating room personnel (e.g., anesthesiologist, intraoperative nurses, or surgeons), other intraoperative factors (e.g., contaminated cardioplegia solution or inadequate sterile surgical technique), and postoperative exposures.[170,171,210,211]

Staphylococci are the predominant pathogens causing postoperative mediastinitis.[208,212,213] In children, *S. aureus* accounts for 38% to 96%, and coagulase-negative staphylococci for 10% to 52%, of episodes of mediastinitis in some series.[201,214] Gram-negative organisms and *Candida* spp. are less common pathogens in children.[215,216] A wide variety of pathogens have been reported to cause mediastinitis after cardiac surgery in adults, including staphylococci, *Enterobacter cloacae*, *Escherichia coli*, *Klebsiella* spp., *Pseudomonas* spp., *Proteus* spp., enterococci, *Bacteroides fragilis*, *Corynebacterium xerosis*, *Mycoplasma* spp., nontuberculous mycobacteria, *Aspergillus* spp., *Haemophilus* spp., *Nocardia* spp., and *Rhodococcus bronchialis*.[217,218]

Clinical Manifestations and Laboratory Diagnosis

Common signs and symptoms of postoperative mediastinitis include local tenderness, wound dehiscence, increased erythema of the wound with or without purulence, and an unstable sternum (movable appositional edges). Infants merely can be fussy and display expiratory grunting. Fever occurs on average 5 days after surgery, and local signs occur a mean of 9 days after surgery.[201,216] In older children, signs and symptoms can appear later; in one study, infections were diagnosed at a mean of 15 days postoperatively.[201] Infections due to *Nocardia*, *Rhodococcus*, or *Candida* species, or nontuberculous mycobacteria, can have an indolent onset, sometimes with incubation periods >30 days. Infections associated with these organisms can have minimal local signs (only serosanguineous drainage), and little or no fever.

Laboratory tests usually reveal a moderate leukocytosis with an increased frequency of neutrophils or an elevation in the erythrocyte sedimentation rate or C-reactive protein value. The diagnosis of acute suppurative mediastinitis is suggested by radiographic evidence of widened mediastinum, mediastinal emphysema, and pleural effusions. The presence of gas in the soft tissues is highly suggestive of esophageal perforation. Computed tomography (CT) has been used to differentiate mediastinitis from mediastinal abscess;[219,220] however, in the absence of mediastinal gas, CT may not differentiate mediastinitis from benign postoperative changes. Among heart transplant recipients, gallium scintigraphy has been used to confirm mediastinitis when CT scan is not diagnostic.[221] Gadolinium-enhanced magnetic resonance imaging (MRI) also can help delineate the extent of infection and differentiate among mediastinal tissues, masses, and inflammatory tissue.[222,223] A definitive diagnosis can be made by Gram and acid-fast stains and culture for bacteria, mycobacteria, and fungi performed on specimens obtained via CT-guided aspiration. If esophageal perforation is suspected, fluoroscopy with water-soluble contrast media may aid in the diagnosis of mediastinitis and allow localization of the level of perforation.

Management and Outcome

Aggressive surgical drainage and debridement generally are required to cure mediastinitis after cardiac surgery. For superficial mediastinal infections, incision, drainage, packing of the wound, and antimicrobial therapy may be effective. For deep infections, debridement with removal of infected and devitalized tissue, mediastinal irrigation, and antimicrobial therapy may be necessary. Surgical debridement (with closed-tube irrigation) and systemic antimicrobial therapy usually are sufficient. In severe infections, it may be necessary to leave the wound open, with subsequent secondary closure.[194,224]

PART II Clinical Syndromes and Cardinal Features of Infectious Diseases: Approach to Diagnosis and Initial Management

SECTION Q Infections Associated with Hospitalization and Medical Devices

For postoperative mediastinitis, selection of empiric agents should be based on the prevalent pathogens associated with cardiac SSIs in the institution and the patient's endogenous flora if known; therapy effective for *S. aureus* and coagulase-negative staphylococci must be provided. The combination of vancomycin and a third- or fourth-generation cephalosporin is a common empiric regimen. No studies have been conducted to evaluate the optimal regimen or duration of antimicrobial therapy for mediastinitis; however, 3 to 8 weeks is generally recommended, depending on the severity of the infection and the extent of bone involvement.[225] There is no role for directly instilled (topical) antibiotic therapy.

Sternal osteomyelitis can accompany severe, deep mediastinal infections. These infections most commonly follow surgery involving a median sternotomy. The pathogens responsible for sternal osteomyelitis are similar to those causing mediastinitis, and *S. aureus* and coagulase-negative staphylococci are the predominant organisms. Treatment of sternal osteomyelitis requires debridement of infected bone and a minimum of 4 to 6 weeks of antimicrobial therapy.[202,226,227]

Prevention

Antimicrobial prophylaxis has not been shown in placebo-controlled trials to decrease the risk of mediastinitis; however, because this infection can be catastrophic, perioperative prophylaxis frequently is used. Centers with lower rates of mediastinitis employ: (1) strict perioperative adherence to careful aseptic technique; (2) attention to surgical measures, including hemostasis and precise sternal closure; and (3) interventions targeted to identified risk factors.[196,205,228] Some authorities have proposed the use of intraoperative ultraviolet irradiation, preoperative decolonization, or preoperative chlorhexidine washes of patients who are carriers of *S. aureus* to help prevent infections.[151,172,228]

102 Clinical Syndromes of Device-Associated Infections

Jeffrey S. Gerber and Theoklis E. Zaoutis

The use of medical devices has increased dramatically over the past several years.[1] In children, the most common device-associated infections involve intravascular catheters; cardiac devices, such as prosthetic valves, patches, vascular grafts, pacemakers, and ventricular assist devices; cerebrospinal fluid shunts; peritoneal dialysis catheters; orthopedic implants; and urinary catheters. Such infections contribute to the substantial burden of emergency department visits, hospitalizations, and nosocomial illnesses in children.[2,3] This chapter addresses device-associated infections in children beyond the neonatal period. For device-associated infections in the neonate, see Chapter 96, Hospital-Associated Infections in the Neonate.

Some general principles apply to infections involving medical devices. Factors that influence the risk of developing a device-associated infection include the properties of the device, of potential pathogens, and of the host (Box 102-1).[4] In addition, colonization and subsequent infection associated with medical devices are facilitated by biofilm formation; a complex matrix of colonizing organisms and extracellular proteins.[5,6] Immediately after implantation, biofilms begin to form with the deposition of host proteins on the device surface. Microorganisms adhere, multiply, and contribute additional extracellular proteins to this coating. Properties inherent to biofilms can inhibit host defenses[7,8] and help organisms avoid exposure to antimicrobial agents.[9-11]

The microbiology of device-associated infections varies by device (Box 102-2). Organisms found as part of the normal skin flora are the most common etiologic agents in foreign-body infections in infants and children.[8,12] Certain species are particularly well suited to colonizing devices. *Staphylococcus aureus* adheres specifically to fibrinogen, a component of biofilms.[13,14] Coagulase-negative staphylococci (CoNS), *Pseudomonas aeruginosa*, and *Corynebacterium* spp. produce proteinaceous slime, capsular polysaccharides, and adhesins that enhance adherence and protect the organism from host defenses and the effects of antimicrobial agents.[12,15-17]

Common clinical findings in foreign-body infection include malfunction of the device (e.g., occlusion of catheters and shunts or loosening of prosthetic joints),[18,19] pain at the site of the device, and failure of wound healing after implantation. Fever, leukocytosis, and other systemic signs may be absent; thus, a high index of suspicion is required for timely diagnosis. Cultures are essential

---

BOX 102-1. Determinants of Medical Device-Associated Infections

PROPERTIES OF THE DEVICE

Material: inert, plastic, rubber
Design: hollow, solid
Location: implanted, percutaneous, vascular/nonvascular site

PROPERTIES OF POTENTIAL PATHOGENS

Source: endogenous, environment, contaminated disinfectant/device/solution
Susceptibility: in vitro and in biofilm

PROPERTIES OF THE HOST

Host defenses: skin, mucous membranes, immune system
Medication: anti-inflammatory agents, immunosuppressive agents
Altered flora due to diet, medications (antacids, antimicrobial agents)

BOX 102-2. Pathogens Recovered from Medical Device-Associated Infections

MOST COMMON

Coagulase-negative staphylococci
Staphylococcus aureus
Other skin flora

COMMON

Gram-negative enteric bacilli
Environmental organisms
Candida spp., especially *Candida albicans* and *Candida glabrata*

OCCASIONAL

Other fungi
Nontuberculous mycobacteria

to both establish the diagnosis and guide definitive therapy. Antimicrobial therapy alone sometimes is curative, but frequently the foreign body must be removed. The risk of device-associated infections can be reduced by consistent application of several principles and practices; these practices together are sometimes referred to as "bundles."[20] Devices should only be used in circumstances in which they are essential and, when feasible, removed as soon as possible; strict aseptic technique must be observed during insertion or manipulation of a device; and the frequency of device access or manipulation should be limited to reduce the likelihood of contamination. Although the use of antimicrobial prophylaxis at the time of insertion is commonplace, the efficacy of such measures for many devices has not been established.[21-23] Recent advances in materials used for catheters and prosthetic devices have decreased rates of infection. The use of central venous catheters (CVCs) impregnated with either minocycline and rifampin or chlorhexidine and silver sulfadiazine have been shown to be effective in reducing the incidence of both catheter colonization and catheter-related bloodstream infection (CRBSI) in adult patients;[24-26] however, few efficacy studies of these devices have been performed in children.[27-31]

INTRAVASCULAR CATHETER-RELATED INFECTIONS

Epidemiology and Pathogenesis

Roughly 80,000 CRBSIs occur in intensive care units (ICUs) each year in the United States,[32] and CRBSIs represent the most important healthcare-associated infection experienced by children. Critically ill children who develop CRBSI have longer duration of ICU and hospital stay, and the crude mortality has been estimated to be 19%.[33] In 2005, the attributable cost of a primary nosocomial BSI for a critically ill child was estimated to be $40,000.[34]

The terminology describing catheter-related infections can be confusing. CRBSI identifies the catheter as the source of infection. Central line-associated bloodstream infection (CLABSI), however, is a term used by the National Healthcare Safety Network (NHSN) to facilitate surveillance (and, therefore, has been widely adopted as a surrogate for CRBSI in the literature describing its epidemiology), and may overestimate the true incidence of CRBSI. Also, several different types of CVCs are used in children. A CVC generally is classified by its intended duration of use (short term vs. long term); its site and mode of insertion (peripheral, femoral, subclavian, tunneled vs. non-tunneled); or other specific characteristics (antibiotic-coated, multilumen). Lastly, multiple types of catheter-related infections can be identified. Infection can occur at the exit site, in the subcutaneous tunnel or pocket, or in the bloodstream.[35] Pathogens can be introduced during insertion, manipulation, calibration, and flushing of monitoring devices (all modes of direct contamination influenced by hand hygiene practices), or via contaminated parenteral fluids, flush solutions, or skin antiseptics (Box 102-3).[36-39]

Gram-positive organisms, including CoNS, S. aureus, and enterococci, are most commonly isolated in intravascular

---

BOX 102-3. Routes Medical Device-Associated Infection

INOCULATION AT THE TIME OF INSERTION OF THE DEVICE
Endogenous flora of the host
Environmental flora

INOCULATION DURING MANIPULATION OF THE DEVICE
Breaks in aseptic technique

HEMATOGENOUS SEEDING
Transient bacteremia
Nonintact mucous membranes or gastrointestinal tract

EXTENSION OF LOCAL INFECTION

BOX 102-4. Pathogens Recovered in Vascular Catheter-Related Infections

MOST COMMON
Coagulase-negative staphylococci

COMMON
Enterobacter spp.
Escherichia coli
Klebsiella spp.
Pseudomonas aeruginosa
Staphylococcus aureus
Enterococcus spp.
Candida spp.

OCCASIONAL
Other gram-negative bacilli, including *Acinetobacter* spp. and *Citrobacter* spp.
Nontuberculous mycobacteria
Corynebacterium spp.
Bacillus spp.

---

catheter-associated infections.[32,33,40] Gram-negative bacilli, including *Enterobacter* spp., *P. aeruginosa*, *Klebsiella pneumoniae*, and *Escherichia coli*, have been identified in roughly 20% of infections[41] (Box 102-4). Over the last two decades, *Candida* spp. have become increasingly prevalent and are now the fourth most common cause of nosocomial BSI in the U.S.[41-43] Other relatively common organisms include *Corynebacterium*, *Propionibacterium*, and *Bacillus* spp., *Serratia marcescens*, *Acinetobacter* spp., *Citrobacter* spp., and nontuberculous mycobacteria.[35] The frequency and distribution of these organisms may be influenced by the child's exposure to (or level of illness associated with) the ICU[44] or particular medications, such as IV prostanoid agents.[45] A recent pediatric study in a single center over 7 years of 2592 peripherally inserted central catheter (PICC) placements in 1819 children, which were associated with 116 BSIs, revealed gram-negative organisms in 50 (38%), gram-positive organisms in 49 (37%), and *Candida* spp. in 33 (25%) cases.[44] Children with CVCs managed predominantly in home healthcare settings are at higher risk for nonendogenous (e.g., from water and other environmental sources) gram-negative pathogens, such as *Pseudomonas*, *Acinetobacter*, and *Agrobacterium* spp., particularly during summer months.[46,47]

Catheter-Related Factors

Risk of infection varies by catheter type. Rates are higher for CVCs than for peripheral venous or arterial catheters.[35] Although some studies showed similar infection risks for tunneled and nontunneled catheters,[48,49] later randomized studies showed that tunneling of femoral catheters[50] and internal jugular catheters[51] is associated with lower infection risk (Box 102-5). PICCs now are used more commonly due to their perceived low risk of infection; however, two recent outpatient studies demonstrated a 10% PICC infection rate[52,53] and an analysis of critically ill patients revealed that the risk of catheter infection was similar among patients with a PICC and those with a centrally inserted percutaneous catheter.[54] A correlation between increasing number of lumens and incidence of infection has been noted in some studies, but not others.[55,56] In addition, the presence of multiple venous catheters was found to be an independent risk factor associated with nosocomial BSIs.[33] The site of placement determines the types and burden of organisms in proximity to the catheter entry site, as organisms present at the site of catheter insertion can move from the entry site along the dermal tunnel to the catheter tip within hours.[57] Quantitative cultures of potential catheter sites in adults and neonates show that the upper extremity and chest wall have the lowest burden of bacteria, whereas the groin and jugular areas are more heavily colonized.[58] In adults, catheters placed in the groin

PART II Clinical Syndromes and Cardinal Features of Infectious Diseases: Approach to Diagnosis and Initial Management

SECTION Q Infections Associated with Hospitalization and Medical Devices

---

BOX 102-5. Risk Factors for Vascular Catheter-Related Infections

CATHETER

Site of insertion
Manipulations: entry into the system
Duration of catheterization
Thrombosis
Lumens, stopcocks, monitoring devices
Antiseptic/antibiotic-coated or not
Tunneled or not; implanted or not

INFUSANT

Parenteral nutrition
Lipids
Blood

HOST

Skin integrity
Skin flora
Immune competence

---

are associated with a greater risk of infection than those placed in the neck;[59] however, this does not appear to be consistently supported in pediatric studies,[44,60–62] and recent guidelines do not support preferential placement in children.[32]

The duration of catheter placement is directly related to the risk of infection, a concept that has been substantiated in multiple pediatric studies.[44,63–66] Biofilm formation, which increases with dwell time, clearly increases the opportunity for catheter colonization. In addition, each manipulation of a catheter, stopcock, or needleless device provides an opportunity for the introduction of organisms.[35,67,68] Outbreaks of bacteremia have resulted from contamination of pressure transducers.[59,69–72] Replacing the catheter over a guidewire does not decrease the incidence of infection, and may even increase it.[73] Finally, studies show similar rates of infection when a transparent or a gauze dressing is used.[74,75]

Certain infusates are more likely than others to be associated with BSI. Use of parenteral nutrition fluids increases the risk of CRBSI in multiple pediatric studies.[44,64,76,77] Intrinsically or extrinsically contaminated infusates can cause CLABSI. Although intrinsic contamination of intravenous fluids is rarely reported in the U.S., episodes of extrinsic contamination of intravenous fluids and medications continue to occur.

Host Factors

Host factors can influence the risk of CLABSI. Skin flora varies according to a person's hygiene and medications. Topical antimicrobial agents may alter the nature and density of local flora, and chlorhexidine gluconate is now the preferred agent for preinsertion decontamination and daily maintenance (see Prevention section). Systemic antimicrobial agents alter stool and skin flora and increase the risk of infection by *Candida* spp.[65,78] Factors that lead to a break in the integrity of skin or mucous membranes can increase the risk of catheter infections. Thus, patients with immature skin (premature infants), impaired integrity of the gut epithelium (patients with short-gut syndrome),[79,80] or burn patients may be at risk of bacteremia and subsequent colonization of an indwelling catheter, although the true contribution of these putative mechanisms (as opposed to confounding risks such as illness severity and increased need for line access) remains unclear. Similarly, patients with a distant site of infection (such as an abscess) or who develop a spontaneous bacteremia are also at risk of developing a secondary CRBSI.

Children undergoing cancer chemotherapy are at risk of infection because of neutropenia; infection rates in these patients are increased 2- to 4-fold by the use of indwelling CVCs.[81] In addition, mucositis may raise the risk of bacterial gastrointestinal wall translocation and bacteremia, and may account for differences in the

microbiology of BSIs that occur in neutropenic, compared with non-neutropenic, patients. In a prospective study of over 24,000 episodes of nosocomial BSIs, researchers noted that neutropenic patients were at greater risk of infection due to *Candida* spp., enterococci, and viridans group streptococci.[82] It remains unclear, however, whether the increased infection rate and variable microbiology are attributable to mucositis, or to the associated illness severity, immune suppression, and care environment of such patients. Those with human immunodeficiency virus (HIV) infection are at greater risk for a variety of infections; use of CVCs for nutritional support and for medications increases the risk of bacteremia in HIV-infected and other patients.[83,84] Patients with uremia are at higher risk of CRBSI, particularly those with hemodialysis catheters.[85–87] In patients undergoing hemodialysis, the type of bloodstream access used influences the risk of infection; the risk is lowest with native arteriovenous fistulae, intermediate with artificial arteriovenous grafts, and highest with CVCs.[88,89]

Clinical factors related to the severity of illness also have been found to influence the risk of infection. In a cohort of critically ill pediatric patients, the need for transport out of the unit and for a procedure performed within an ICU were both independently associated with a 3- to 4-fold increase in the risk of developing a nosocomial BSI.[33] Need for ICU exposure, mechanical ventilation, medical cardiac disease, malignancy, metabolic disease, and history of prior CVC also have been associated with CRBSI in children.[44,63,64,76]

Clinical Manifestations and Laboratory Diagnosis

Fever usually is present in patients with catheter-related infections. Patients with localized infection of the exit site, pocket, or tunnel frequently have infection in the absence of fever. When CRBSI is suspected, the exit site should be examined for the presence of local suppuration or cellulitis; however, normal appearance of the exit site does not exclude a local or systemic infection involving the catheter. Any catheter malfunction (including decrease in flow or unidirectional flow) should prompt an evaluation for infection. Findings suggestive of disseminated infection include the presence of emboli in the retina, skin, bone, and viscera (lungs, kidneys, liver, and spleen) and organ dysfunction due to immune complex deposition (e.g., nephritis).

Infections attributable to a CVC include exit, tunnel, and pocket infections as well as CLABSI (Table 102-1).[90] A CLABSI is defined as bacteremia or fungemia in a patient with a centrally placed intravascular catheter in which the catheter is the presumed source of infection. Establishing that the catheter is the source of infection is not always straightforward. For example, a BSI in a patient with an indwelling catheter can originate from an undocumented source of infection (e.g., a postoperative wound infection or a urinary tract infection) rather than from the catheter. In adult patients, only 15% to 20% of CVCs removed in the context of a BSI are implicated ultimately as the primary source of infection.

Several methods have been used to diagnose CLABSI, including simultaneous quantitative cultures of blood obtained through the catheter and a peripheral vein; quantitative and semiquantitative cultures of a catheter segment; and differential time to blood culture positivity[91] (see Table 102-1). Until recently, the most commonly accepted methods of diagnosing a CLABSI have involved either quantitative or semiquantitative cultures of the catheter tip. This strategy relies upon the prompt removal of the catheter and is thus not appropriate in many clinical settings. A positive catheter culture result is defined as growth of at least 15 colonies (CFU) on an agar surface over which the catheter tip was rolled.[92] An alternative method involves sonicating the catheter tip in fluid to dislodge the intraluminal biofilm; this method is associated with a higher rate of positive cultures than the roll technique.[93] A catheter tip culture that yields ≥15 CFU is a valid indication of catheter colonization, which in turn is associated with a higher risk of BSI. However, a relatively small number of patients with colonized catheters have CLABSI.[94] In fact, electron microscopy of

TABLE 102-1. Types of Catheter-Related Infections

Infection	Clinical Diagnosis
Exit site infection	Erythema or induration within 2 cm of catheter exit site
Tunnel infection	Tenderness, erythema, or induration along the subcutaneous tract of a tunneled catheter and more than 2 cm from catheter exit site
Pocket infection	Purulent fluid in the subcutaneous pocket of a totally implanted venous access device. May be accompanied by overlying tenderness, erythema, induration, visible drainage, and skin necrosis
Catheter-associated bloodstream infection	Positive simultaneous blood cultures from the central venous catheter and peripheral vein yielding the same organism in the presence of at least one of the following: • Simultaneous quantitative blood cultures in which the number of CFU/mL isolated from blood drawn through the central catheter is ≥5-fold the number isolated from blood drawn peripherally • Positive semiquantitative (≥15 CFU/catheter segment) or quantitative (≥100 CFU/catheter segment) catheter tip cultures • Simultaneous blood cultures of equal volume in which the central blood culture has growth in an automated system ≥2 hours earlier than the peripheral blood culture

CFU, colony-forming unit.

catheter tips reveals universal colonization with bacteria.[93,95] Thus, the positive predictive value (PPV) of a positive catheter tip culture result is low, ranging in most studies from 5% to 30%, and this method has not been evaluated for antimicrobial agent- or antiseptic-impregnated catheters.

Differential time to positivity of paired blood cultures is an alternative method to evaluate CLABSI. This technique is the simplest of the three methods and does not require specialized laboratory culture methods (other than a continuous-monitoring blood culture system) or catheter removal, but requires that peripheral and central cultures are drawn simultaneously and are of equal volume. If the same organism is isolated from both blood cultures and the time to positivity of the catheter-obtained specimen is >2 hours shorter than the peripherally obtained culture, catheter colonization and CLABSI are likely.[91,96] Compared with quantitative and semiquantitative methods, differential time to positivity of >2 hours had a sensitivity of 93% and a specificity of 75% for catheters in place for >30 days and a sensitivity of 81% and a specificity of 92% for catheters in place for <30 days.[97] Several smaller studies have demonstrated similar results.[98–100] In an analysis of semiquantitative cultures obtained from different lumens of multilumen catheters in pediatric oncology patients with double-lumen catheters in place and no peripheral blood cultures available, the PPV of greater than 5-fold difference in CFU/mL of isolates from samples from the two lumens was 92% predictive of a CLABSI.[101]

Few studies have evaluated the optimal timing of blood cultures. Obtaining multiple samples over a 24-hour period appears to increase the ability to detect intermittent bacteremia compared with obtaining multiple specimens at the same time.[100,102] In patients already receiving antibiotics, samples obtained close to the time that antibiotic concentrations have reached trough levels (i.e., just before next dose) theoretically could improve recovery of organisms in blood cultures;[103] however, this issue has not been studied and may not be practical clinically.

The volume of blood collected also can affect blood culture yield. Studies have demonstrated that the likelihood of growth is lower and the time to detection is delayed when small volumes (<0.5 mL) of blood are used to inoculate blood culture bottles;[104] however, advancements in blood culture detection system technology continue to improve the efficiency of this process. Although multiple cultures enhance the recovery of pathogens, the volume of blood cultured may be more important than the total number of blood cultures obtained. One study found that the pathogen recovery rate at 24 hours was 72% for a large-volume (6 mL) single culture compared with a 47% combined yield of two smaller (2 mL) samples inoculated into separate culture bottles.[105] Similar results were found in studies of adult patients in which standard "adult-volume" cultures (mean, 8.7 mL) had a higher

detection rate (92%) than "low"-volume cultures (mean, 2.7 mL) where the detection rate was only 69%.[106] Investigators estimated that the yield of adult blood cultures increased approximately 3% per mL of blood cultured.

Other technical issues can affect the sensitivity of blood cultures. Diluting the blood into the blood culture broth enhances recovery of pathogens, perhaps by diluting antimicrobial agents (if applicable) and blood components such as phagocytes, antibodies, and complement factors that are known to have bactericidal activity.[107] The ideal blood-to-broth ratio depends on the blood culture system used, but a ratio between 1:5 and 1:10 generally is considered ideal;[108] it is essential to identify the optimal blood volume suitable for the culture system in one's clinical microbiology laboratory. Certain bacteria as well as fungi and mycobacteria require special handling of blood cultures. For example, filamentous fungi require solid media for growth, *Malassezia furfur* requires lipid supplementation, and certain gram-negative species and some mycobacteria need prolonged incubation (see Chapter 286, Laboratory Diagnosis of Infection Due to Bacteria, Fungi, Parasites, and Rickettsiae). Failure of culture to identify a pathogen in the patient with continued clinical evidence of infection should prompt consideration of less common, more fastidious organisms and discussion with microbiology laboratory personnel about additional collection and culture techniques.

Distinguishing between cultures that represent "contamination" from those that represent "true" BSI can be challenging, especially when a skin organism (e.g., CoNS, *Bacillus* species, micrococci) is isolated. Obtaining multiple cultures can clarify most situations. A study using a mathematical model of blood cultures positive for CoNS in patients with a CVC found that the PPV of a single positive culture (if only one culture was obtained) was 55%; however, if only 1 of 2 cultures obtained was positive, the PPV was 20%, and if only 1 of 3 cultures was positive, the PPV was only 5%. Investigators developed a similar model for blood culture positivity depending on sampling site. If 2 of 2 cultures were positive, the PPV was 98% if both samples were obtained from a peripheral vein, 96% if 1 sample was obtained through a catheter and the other was obtained through the vein, and only 50% if both samples were obtained through a catheter.[109] Furthermore, the distinction between pathogen and contaminant is influenced by age and underlying condition(s). Although CoNS often is considered a true pathogen in neonates, this issue remains controversial.[110] Because the isolation of CoNS from a blood culture often results in a clinical intervention and administration of vancomycin, it is particularly important to obtain multiple blood cultures. Overuse of vancomycin has implications for the continued increase of vancomycin resistance among gram-positive organisms.[111–113]

PART II   Clinical Syndromes and Cardinal Features of Infectious Diseases: Approach to Diagnosis and Initial Management

SECTION Q   Infections Associated with Hospitalization and Medical Devices

Repeatedly positive blood culture results despite appropriate antimicrobial therapy suggests the presence of an intravascular focus of infection such as the catheter itself, complicating suppurative thrombophlebitis, or endocarditis (especially if the catheter has been removed).[114,115] Among patients with intravascular catheters, the risk of endocarditis is highest with Swan-Ganz catheters and lowest with peripheral catheters. In an autopsy series, 53% of patients who had undergone pulmonary artery catheterization had right-sided endocardial lesions; 7% had infective endocarditis.[116] Centrally placed catheters often traverse and damage the tricuspid valve, increasing the risk of right-sided endocarditis. Thrombi within the heart can become infected or can obstruct outflow.

Ultrasonography is useful in detecting thrombosis of vessels or formation of vegetations. The value of a negative transcutaneous ultrasonography result is debated; in adults, the use of transesophageal echocardiography increases the likelihood of detecting intracardiac vegetations.[117] Gadolinium-enhanced magnetic resonance venography can be useful in detecting central venous thromboses.[118]

Management and Outcome

Exit site infections can be treated by removal of the catheter and local care. If the catheter remains in place, local topical therapy can be successful in controlling this type of infection; however, systemic antimicrobial therapy and catheter removal usually is required if an exit site infection extends to involve the soft tissues that surround the catheter (i.e., the subcutaneous tunnel or pocket) or is associated with a CLABSI. Limited data guide the management of CLABSI in children. Even in adults, there are insufficient randomized or controlled studies to address optimal management of CLABSI.[91] To help address this uncertainly, the Infectious Diseases Society of America (IDSA) has published guidelines for the diagnosis and management of CLABSI. Although focused on adult patients, this guideline contains recommendations for the management of children with CLABSI, and has been endorsed by the Pediatric Infectious Diseases Society (PIDS).[91]

Empiric therapy in children with suspected CLABSI should include an antimicrobial agent with activity against gram-positive bacteria, such as nafcillin, oxacillin, or vancomycin, and an agent effective against gram-negative bacteria, including *Pseudomonas* species, such ceftazidime or cefipime. The empiric use of both an antipseudomonal β-lactam and an aminoglycoside may be appropriate in severely ill patients or when infection with a resistant gram-negative organism is suspected. In institutions in which methicillin-resistant isolates of *Staphylococcus aureus* (MRSA) are prevalent, the use of vancomycin is appropriate. Aztreonam or fluoroquinolones can be used when β-lactam allergy is present and broad-spectrum gram-negative coverage is required.

Limited data guide clinical decisions regarding the need for catheter removal (Table 102-2). In adults with CLABSI, it is recommended that most nontunneled CVCs should be removed.[91] In children, removal of a catheter may not always be feasible because of the potential for complications associated with reinsertion and limited vascular access sites. Children treated without catheter removal should be monitored closely and additional blood cultures drawn; the catheter should be removed with clinical deterioration or persistent or recurrent CLABSI. In patients with CLABSI associated with a tunneled catheter or implantable device such as a port catheter, the decision to remove the catheter is more complicated; however, good evidence favors the removal of the CVC in patients with evidence of a tunnel infection or pocket infection (the subcutaneous pocket of an implanted device).[91] When culture data are available, treatment decisions can be tailored to the specific organism isolated. Several studies have reported successful treatment of CLABSI without catheter removal, depending on the pathogen identified.[119-122]

Few data exist regarding the duration of antibiotic therapy for CLABSI. The duration of therapy depends in part on the pathogen; whether the catheter is removed; and whether infection is complicated by septic thrombosis, endocarditis, osteomyelitis, or other

TABLE 102-2. Management of the Catheter in Patients with a Central Venous Catheter (CVC)-Related Infection

Type of Infection	Catheter Management
Exit site infection	Remove CVC if: • No longer required • Alternate site exists • Patient critically ill (e.g., hypotension) • Infection due to *Pseudomonas aeruginosa* or fungi
Tunnel infection	Remove CVC
Pocket infection	Remove CVC
Catheter-related bloodstream infection	Remove CVC if: • No longer required • Infection caused by *Staphylococcus aureus*, *Candida* species, or mycobacteria • Patient critically ill • Failure to clear bacteremia in 48–72 hours • Persistent symptoms of bloodstream infection beyond 48–72 hours • Noninfectious valvular heart disease (increased risk of endocarditis) • Endocarditis • Metastatic infection • Septic thrombophlebitis

metastatic foci of bacteria. For complicated infections, the duration of therapy is based on the length of therapy needed to treat the suppurative complication. There are no data to determine the optimal duration of intravenous versus oral antibiotics for the treatment of CLABSI when the catheter is removed. Certain antibiotics with excellent oral bioavailability may be considered an alternative to parenteral therapy once the catheter has been removed (or lock therapy begun), the BSI has cleared, and the patient has shown clinical improvement. Some pathogen-specific recommendations are provided below.

Coagulase-Negative Staphylococci (Other than *S. lugdunensis*)

A relatively low-virulence organism, CoNS infection usually presents with fever alone or with inflammation of the catheter exit site. CoNS CLABSI can resolve with catheter removal alone, although guidelines recommend a short course of antibiotic therapy (3 to 5 days) even after removal of the catheter.[91] If the catheter is retained, the recommended duration of treatment is 10 to 14 days after a negative culture from blood drawn through the CVC has been obtained. In neonates with CoNS BSI, treatment without removal of the catheter can be attempted; however, if a neonate has 3 positive blood cultures despite appropriate antimicrobial therapy, the catheter should be removed because of the increased risk for end-organ damage.[123] (See Chapter 96. Hospital-Associated Infections in the Neonate) The relapse rate in adults with CoNS CLABSI is 20% if the catheter is not removed, compared with 3% if the catheter is removed.[124]

Staphylococcus aureus

Serious complications, including endocarditis and other deep-tissue infections, have been reported in association with *S. aureus* CLABSI.[39,115] Adults with *S. aureus* BSI who have a medical device are at substantial risk for endocarditis; echocardiography is performed routinely as part of management.[125,126] In contrast, the frequency of infective endocarditis is low in children with structurally normal hearts who have *S. aureus* BSI; therefore, echocardiography is not recommended routinely.[127] In a prospective study of 51 children with *S. aureus* BSI, definite or possible endocarditis was diagnosed in 52% of patients with congenital heart disease but in only 3% of children with structurally normal hearts.[127] Echocardiography should be considered in children with (1) prolonged BSI prior to treatment, (2) persistent BSI while receiving appropriate antimicrobial therapy, (3) a new murmur identified on physical examination, or (4) congenital heart disease. Neonates may be more vulnerable than older infants to complications of *S. aureus* BSI.[123] Some experts recommend catheter removal for neonates with a single positive blood culture when *S. aureus* or a gram-negative bacillus is the isolate, as this significantly improves outcome. Two weeks of appropriate antimicrobial therapy, chosen based on susceptibility test results, is recommended for uncomplicated *S. aureus* CLABSI.[90] Longer duration of therapy (4 to 6 weeks) may be necessary for patients with prolonged BSI (>3 days), persistent fever, or complicated infection.[128]

Gram-Negative Bacilli

Few data address the appropriate duration of therapy and the need for catheter removal in patients with CLABSI caused by gram-negative bacilli. In general, for uncomplicated infections, antimicrobial therapy should be administered for 10 to 14 days after documented blood culture negativitiy.[91] Although children with CLABSI caused by gram-negative bacilli have been successfully treated without catheter removal, catheter removal has been shown to be beneficial in the treatment of infections with specific gram-negative bacilli such as *Pseudomonas* spp., *Burkholderia cepacia*, *Acinetobacter baumannii*, and *Stenotrophomonas* spp.[39,90] In a study of adults with CLABSI caused by gram-negative bacilli, catheter removal was associated with a reduced rate of relapse.[129]

Candida Species

Treatment of candidemia without removal of the catheter has been associated with poor outcomes in children and adults;[130–132] however, these studies have not accounted for confounding effects of the severity of illness.[133] Failure to remove the catheter promptly is associated with prolonged candidemia, which in turn has been associated with higher rates of disseminated infection. In a study of 153 children with candidemia, the overall rate of disseminated candidiasis (lung, liver, spleen, eye, brain, heart) was 17%; the crude mortality was 26%.[134] Guidelines recommend that catheters should be removed in patients with candidemia whenever clinically feasible.[135] Patients with candidemia should be treated with amphotericin B, an echinocandin, or fluconazole for at least 2 weeks. Many experts would recommend performance of an ophthalmologic examination to evaluate for candidal endophthalmitis, preferably after the infection is controlled and further disseminated disease is unlikely.[135] Risk of dissemination is multifactorial, depending on the pathogen, host, and duration of candidemia.

Nontuberculous Mycobacteria

Infections due to nontuberculous mycobacteria should be managed by removal of the catheter and antimicrobial therapy. The choice of agent is individualized. The empiric combination of clarithromycin and tobramycin (*M. chelonae*), amikacin and meropenem (*M. fortuitum*)[136,137] or other drugs in combination should be considered depending on the species of pathogen and expected and then proven antimicrobial susceptibility.

Complications

Complications of CRBSI include thrombosis with or without thrombophlebitis, sepsis, septic endocarditis, and metastatic infection with seeding of bone and organs (lung, kidneys, liver, spleen, brain, skin). The prognosis for patients with CRBSI is influenced by factors related to the pathogen, host, and therapy. If the infection is recognized and appropriate antimicrobial therapy is instituted promptly, there can be a high rate of cure, and even salvage of the catheter; delayed treatment is associated with increased morbidity and mortality.[91]

CVC-related thrombosis is common. In one study of children who had CVCs for home parenteral nutrition, venography revealed blockage of central vessels in 66%.[138] In a study of femoral venous catheters, evidence of thrombosis was found in 69% of children. Positive blood culture results were obtained in 38% of patients who had thrombosis versus 3% of patients who did not. The incidence of thrombosis was lower in patients who had heparin-bonded catheters.[139] If a patient with a thrombosed vessel develops BSI, the clot can become infected and lead to thrombophlebitis and persistent BSI.[140] The optimal treatment for septic thrombophlebitis of a CVC is unclear. Phlebitis of peripheral veins is commonly delayed in onset, often becoming apparent ≥24 hours after removal of the catheter.[141,142] Suppurative thrombophlebitis sometimes resolves after catheter removal. Fluctuance at a subcutaneous venous site; persistent erythema, swelling, and tenderness; or persistent BSI despite antimicrobial therapy are clues that aspiration, surgical drainage or resection of the vein may be necessary for cure.[143] Removal of the catheter and prompt therapy with appropriate antimicrobial agents are essential. Although urokinase has been demonstrated to be effective in restoring catheter patency in up to 75% of patients with occluded catheters,[144] the role of anticoagulation or thrombolytic agents in the face of a catheter infection is uncertain.

Overall, fatality rates for CLABSI are 10% to 25%, with rates as high as 50% in critically ill patients and neonates.[145,146] One study demonstrated that only the presence of underlying malignancy or immunodeficiency was independently associated with an increased risk of mortality due to a CLABSI.[147] Relapse of a catheter-associated infection can occur, and reinfection with a new organism is more common in catheters that have been infected previously.[128,136] Frequent recurrences should raise concerns regarding the care of the catheter, particularly in children who are outpatients. Munchausen syndrome by proxy has been implicated as a cause of recurrent central catheter septicemia.[148]

Prevention

The elimination of CRBSI in all patient care areas is the stated goal of many national organizations.[32] Although this target has not been reached in many pediatric settings, considerable progress has been made, particularly within the context of organized initiatives and "care bundles."[20,149] (See Chapter 2, Pediatric Infection Prevention and Control). The simplest way to reduce the risk of CRBSI is to avoid catheterization (Box 102-6). If a catheter is essential, however, a variety of practical measures can be taken to lower the risk of CRBSI.[150,151] Catheters that are no longer needed should be removed promptly. The presence of an idle catheter is very common, accounting for 20% of catheter days in one study, and poses an unacceptable risk to the patient.[152] Strict asepsis and the use of maximal barrier precautions (the wearing of sterile gloves, long-sleeved sterile gown, mask, and cap, and the use of a large sterile sheet drape) during insertion of central catheters help reduce infection risk substantially.[153] These measures have been shown to be cost-effective over a wide variety of clinical conditions.[154]

Careful skin antisepsis before insertion is an important preventive measure. Three randomized trials have demonstrated that 2% chlorhexidine is superior to povidone-iodine for preventing CLABSI,[155–157] and chlorhexidine is now recommended for skin preparation before CVC insertion. Further, 2% chlorhexidine daily skin wash is now recommended for patients with CVCs to decrease the risk of CLABSI.[32] Routine changing of percutaneously inserted lines over guidewires should not be performed to prevent infection[73,150] or to replace a catheter with suspected infection.[32] Systemic antimicrobial prophylaxis prior to insertion of CVC or for catheter maintenance has not been demonstrated to reduce the risk of CRBSI and is not recommended.[32,151,158] Continuous infusion of vancomycin through the CVC was effective in reducing CoNS BSI in neonates in one study, but did not reduce either length of stay in the ICU or mortality.[159] Moreover, routine use of systemic vancomycin for prophylaxis carries the risk of inducing vancomycin resistance and is not recommended.[160]

BOX 102-6. Prevention of Vascular Catheter-Related Infections

GENERAL
- Avoid unnecessary catheter insertion
- Remove unneeded catheters as soon as possible

CATHETER INSERTION
- Apply skin site antisepsis; chlorhexidine for central venous catheter placement
- Use strict aseptic technique
- Use sterile technique and maximal barrier precautions when inserting central venous or arterial catheters

CATHETER CARE
- Minimize manipulation of catheters
- Wash hands before and after palpating, inserting, replacing, or dressing any catheter
- Inspect hub design; avoid preslit cover
- Prepare hub before injection or aspiration through the hub
- Replace end caps frequently

CATHETER SELECTION
- Select a catheter with the fewest lumens needed for management of the patient
- Consider use of antiseptic- or antimicrobial-coated central catheters and silver-impregnated, collagen-cuffed catheters when infection rates remain high despite other measures (e.g., maximal barrier precautions)
- For long-term (>30 days) access in children older than 4 years, consider peripherally inserted central catheters or tunneled or totally implantable devices; for children younger than 4 years, consider totally implantable devices

STOPCOCKS
- Cover all openings
- Minimize use

MONITORING DEVICES (TRANSDUCERS, ETC.)
- Sterilize if being reused; avoid contamination during use

Attention to catheter care is essential to preventing infection. Education and training of staff, as well as insuring appropriate staffing levels, are paramount.[32] Infection rates may be lower when catheter care is provided by a specially trained team.[161] Catheter site dressings should not be changed at fixed intervals but rather when they are loose, soiled, or damaged; the type of dressing (transparent or gauze) is not crucial in determining infection risk.[74,75] Catheter hubs repeatedly have been demonstrated to be common sites of catheter colonization.[162] Thus, the hub of the catheter should be cleansed each time it is accessed. Both 70% ethanol and 1% to 2% tincture of iodine are equally effective;[163] 70% ethanol was found to be superior to 1% chlorhexidine in one study.[164] Intravenous delivery systems need to be changed no more frequently than at 72-hour intervals,[165-167] unless blood- or lipid-containing solutions are administered, in which case tubing should be changed within 24 hours after the infusion is initiated.[150,168]

Several studies suggest that needleless connection systems reduce the risk of needlestick injuries to healthcare personnel, but absent strict infection control practices, such systems may be associated with a higher risk of BSI.[169-173] Practices to reduce such infections include replacing the end cap every 48 to 72 hours; using continuous rather than intermittent infusions;[169] and educating caregivers about aseptic technique and avoiding exposing the catheter to tap water.[171] Hubs should be carefully disinfected before each access.[174] If stopcocks are essential, ports must be covered at all times, and sterile technique used when the bloodstream is accessed via the port. In some studies, infection rates for totally implanted ports have not been lower than those for Hickman or Broviac catheters, whereas in other studies,

patients with implanted CVCs had significantly lower rates of infection.[175-177] Expected frequency and duration of periods of intravenous access are considered when choosing the type of a long-term catheter. No recommendation can be given for the preferred site of a tunneled catheter.[32]

Antimicrobial-based preventive strategies for select populations or individuals at higher risk of CRBSI include antimicrobial catheter lock, antimicrobial-impregnated catheter use, and antimicrobial-impregnated dressings. For an antimicrobial lock, an antimicrobial agent (e.g., antibiotic or 70% ethanol) is confined to the catheter lumen while the CVC is idle. Studies of tunneled catheters[178,179] and nontunneled catheters[180] demonstrated that a vancomycin lock solution was associated with longer time to first episode of BSI by vancomycin-susceptible microorganisms. A large, double-blind randomized trial in 1513 children with tunneled cuffed CVCs or ports showed an 80% reduction in BSIs with routine use of a lock solution containing vancomycin, ciprofloxacin, and heparin.[181] Vancomycin was undetectable in the serum of these patients, and there was no infection or colonization with vancomycin-resistant organisms. Antimicrobial lock therapy should be considered for patients with repeated CLABSI despite optimal adherence to basic preventive measures.[32]

Catheters that are coated or impregnated with antimicrobial or antiseptic agents, such as chlorhexidine-silver sulfadiazine[30] or minocycline-rifampin,[182] can decrease the risk for infection and have been shown to decrease hospital costs, despite the additional expense of these devices.[24] The anti-infective effect of these catheters, however, is not permanent and may be limited to a relatively short period after insertion; data are lacking on the efficacy of these catheters for longer insertion times (e.g., ≥2 weeks).[66] Although the efficacy of these catheters has not been widely demonstrated in children, a single-center study demonstrated that minocycline-rifampin coated CVCs delayed the occurrence of infection in critically ill children,[32] and such catheters are approved by the U.S. Food and Drug Administration for use in patients weighing >3 kg. These catheters are recommended for clinical situations in which the incidence of CLABSI is high despite implementation of other preventive measures.[32,150]

A chlorhexidine-impregnated disk affixed directly to the skin surrounding the catheter was shown in a randomized trial performed in adults to be protective against CLABSI.[183] In a randomized study performed in children with cardiac disease, use of a chlorhexidine-impregnated dressing reduced the rate of catheter colonization but not of catheter-related BSI.[184] Luminal contamination may be reduced through use of closed catheter connection systems[185] or a self-disinfecting CVC hub (containing iodinated alcohol).[186] Use of a chlorhexidine-impregnated dressing is recommended for patients older than 2 months of age when CLABSI rates are not decreasing despite adherence to basic preventive measures.[32]

There are few guidelines for outpatient management of vascular catheters. Issues that require further study include the safety of bathing or swimming; the optimal frequency of dressing, cap, and tubing changes; and optimal care of the insertion site. One study has suggested that children with subcutaneously implanted catheters who swim (while the catheter is not being accessed) are not at higher risk of infection.[187] Nevertheless, when patients are discharged with indwelling venous catheters, they and their caregivers should understand the need to protect the catheter and catheter site and avoid contamination with tap water.

INFECTIONS OF PROSTHETIC VALVES, PATCHES, AND VASCULAR GRAFTS

Epidemiology and Pathogenesis

Prosthetic valve and patch infections are classified as *early* (occurring ≤60 days after implantation) or *late* (occurring >60 days after implantation). Agents causing early infection are presumed to have been introduced at the time of the surgery or soon thereafter (Box 102-7). Early infections are most commonly caused by CoNS or *S. aureus*.[12,188-190] Other pathogens are *Enterococcus* spp., *Corynebacterium* spp., fungi, and gram-negative enteric bacilli;[191,192] and rarely *Mycoplasma hominis*,[193] *Brucella* melitensis,[194] *Legionella* spp.,[195] *Pasteurella multocida*,[196] and *Kingella kingae*.[197]

Late infection typically is the result of bacteremic seeding of the prosthetic material, often caused by oral streptococci. Bacteremia in patients with prosthetic valves often is related to medical devices, particularly vascular catheters. In a prospective study of patients with prosthetic valves and healthcare-associated BSI, 43% had endocarditis.[198] The rate of infection of prosthetic valves is 1% to 4% for early infection and about 1% annually for late infections (after the prosthesis has become endothelialized).[189,190,199] Reported rates of infection of vascular grafts range from 1% to 6%. Grafts in the lower extremities, especially the groin, are more likely to become infected. Hemodialysis grafts and fistulae most often are infected with *S. aureus*. Infection with gram-negative bacilli or nontuberculous mycobacteria often is associated with improper sterilization of hemodialyzers.[200-204]

Clinical Manifestations and Laboratory Diagnosis

Patients with infected prosthetic valves or patches typically come to medical attention with fever. Hemodynamic changes can be present in patients infected with more virulent organisms (Box 102-8).[189,190] Valve ring abscesses can lead to perivalvular leakage. The leakage may be appreciated as a new murmur and can be complicated by congestive heart failure and rhythm disturbances, such as heart block. Late infections generally give rise to the usual signs and symptoms of subacute bacterial endocarditis, but can be more acute and fulminant depending on the pathogen (e.g., *S. aureus*, *Streptococcus pyogenes*).

Blood cultures are essential to optimal management. Bacteremia generally is continuous; however, culture results can be negative because of prior exposure to antimicrobial therapy or the presence of a fastidious organism. Echocardiography is another key component of the evaluation of patients with suspected endocarditis.[205] In children, adequate imaging often can be achieved by transthoracic echocardiography. The sensitivity of transesophageal

echocardiography, however, generally is greater than transthoracic studies.[206] A negative echocardiogram does not exclude endocarditis; negative studies can occur if vegetations are small or have already embolized, or if prosthetic material obscures or distorts the images.

Graft infection can manifest as local wound purulence, pseudoaneurysms at the graft–vessel anastomosis, hemorrhage, or thrombosis. Physical examination often identifies infection in superficially located grafts. Ultrasonography is useful to detect pseudoaneurysms and thromboses. Other studies, such as angiography, computed tomography, and magnetic resonance imaging, are occasionally needed to determine the extent of infection and the presence of complications.[200]

Management and Outcome

Antimicrobial therapy and surgery are the main therapeutic modalities for infections of prosthetic valves and patches. For both early and late infections, combination therapy using synergistic antimicrobial agents is recommended.[189] Because CoNS almost always is resistant to β-lactam agents,[188] vancomycin and an aminoglycoside plus rifampin often are used empirically until culture results are known. Consensus guidelines for the treatment and prevention of endocarditis for patients with prosthetic valves have been published.[207,208]

Surgical consultation is advisable, particularly for patients early in the course and with acute infection. Indications for surgery early in the course of infection include hemodynamic instability, repeated major embolizations, inability to control infection, and relapse of infection. Indications for surgery later in the course of acute infection include new regurgitant murmur, moderate to severe heart failure, or a myocardial abscess unresponsive to medical therapy.[188-190,207] When surgery has been undertaken during acute infection, studies have demonstrated that infection of new valves implanted at this time is relatively uncommon.[188-190,209] A retrospective analysis of *S. aureus* prosthetic valve endocarditis revealed significantly lower mortality when valves were replaced during antimicrobial therapy.[210] Therapy for infected grafts often requires surgical resection or revision for cure.[200] Antimicrobial agents have limited penetration in areas with poor blood flow (i.e., a thrombosed graft).

The role of anticoagulation in infection of prosthetic valves or grafts is still debated. Most patients with prosthetic valves are treated with anticoagulants; discontinuation of this therapy is associated with a higher incidence of thrombosis and embolic phenomena.[189,190] The risk of death, however, from neurologic events is higher if anticoagulation is continued.[211]

Complications of intravascular infections include thrombosis, hemorrhage, embolic infarction and infection, graft dysfunction, heart failure, overwhelming infection, and death. Prognosis of prosthetic valve endocarditis depends on the organism, the condition of the patient at the time of diagnosis, the rapidity and appropriateness of antimicrobial therapy, and the timely use of surgical intervention if appropriate.[207,199,209,210]

Prevention

Important measures to prevent infection of prosthetic valves and grafts include proper timing of surgical procedures (e.g., avoiding elective surgery in a patient with an intravascular device and an active distant infection), appropriate administration of periprocedural prophylactic antibiotics, meticulous attention to surgical asepsis, and prompt removal of catheters and other potential infectious foci (Box 102-9). The common practice of continuing perioperative antimicrobial prophylaxis until catheters or drains are removed is inappropriate and may prevent the timely identification of pathogens in early prosthetic valve endocarditis.

Prevention of graft infection starts with meticulous attention to sterile technique at the time of implantation. Hemodialysis grafts are at risk of contamination and subsequent infection with each dialysis procedure, so good hygiene and care of the graft site with each access are essential.[199] Because *S. aureus* is by far the most

PART II Clinical Syndromes and Cardinal Features of Infectious Diseases: Approach to Diagnosis and Initial Management

SECTION Q Infections Associated with Hospitalization and Medical Devices

> **BOX 102-9.** Prevention of Prosthetic Valve Infection
>
> - Use prophylactic perioperative antimicrobial agents at time of placement and subsequent dental/surgical procedures
> - Minimize intraoperative contamination
> - Remove catheters as soon as possible
> - Use meticulous wound care: handwashing, removal of necrotic tissue, avoidance of contamination
> - Minimize antimicrobial agents to maintain normal flora
> - Avoid antacids to diminish colonization of stomach and subsequent spread to lungs

common pathogen associated with dialysis grafts, attempts have been made to decrease patient colonization through the use of intranasal mupirocin or systemic rifampin and cloxacillin; these attempts have met with some success.[212–215]

If dialyzers are reused, strict adherence to sterilization and reuse protocols is crucial. The Association for the Advancement of Medical Instrumentation and the U.S. Centers for Disease Control and Prevention recommend that hemodialysis fluids be monitored at least monthly with quantitative culture and endotoxin assay. Water used to prepare dialysate must have ≤200 CFU/mL in culture, and water used to reprocess hemodialyzers should have ≤200 CFU/mL in culture and <1 ng/mL of endotoxin on assay. Dialysate colony counts should be ≤2000 CFU/mL.[216]

INFECTIONS ASSOCIATED WITH PACEMAKERS AND LEFT VENTRICULAR ASSIST DEVICES

Epidemiology and Pathogenesis

Temporary pacemaker wires, which generally are inserted percutaneously into the bloodstream, are associated with infection risks similar to those for vascular catheters. In addition, pacemaker wires typically are embedded into the myocardium, posing risk of myocardial abscess. Permanent pacemakers consist of a battery, which is inserted into a soft-tissue pocket, and wires that pass across tissue planes to reach the myocardium. During initial placement either the battery or wires can become contaminated.[217] Soft-tissue infection of the battery pocket and, less commonly, of the wire track occurs in 1% to 7% of patients.[1,218,219] Although most infections are limited to the pocket site, roughly 10% of adult pacemaker infections result in endocarditis.[208]

Left ventricular assist devices (LVADs) consist of a pump with an inflow conduit from the left ventricular apex and an outflow conduit to the ascending aorta. Although original models used bioprosthetic valves to maintain unidirectional flow, newer continuous flow pumps do not require valves.[220] The pump is placed into a pocket formed in the lateral rectus sheath. A driveline, tunneled from the pump, connects to an external power source via an exit site on the lower abdominal wall. LVAD-related infection is a common complication, occurring in 25% to 70% of patients,[221–224] and can include local infection of the driveline or pocket, as well as LVAD-related BSI with or without endocarditis.[223,225]

Clinical Manifestations and Laboratory Diagnosis

Signs of pacemaker infection include tenderness and erythema around the battery pocket, fever, and, occasionally, BSI.[218,226] Most studies of pacemaker and LVAD infections report on relatively few patients and focus on adults. The most common organisms are CoNS (42%) and *S. aureus* (29%), although gram-negative enteric bacilli and yeast can be isolated.[208] Signs of LVAD driveline infection include localized purulent drainage from the abdominal exit site. Device pocket infection is characterized by tenderness and erythema around the pump pocket and purulence within the subcutaneous space. BSI can cause fever, chills, and other constitutional symptoms. The distribution of pathogens identified in LVAD infection is similar to that encountered in pacemaker

infections,[221,222] although recent reports suggest that fungal infections may be becoming more common.[223] Diagnosis is made by culturing relevant purulent drainage and obtaining blood cultures. *Candida* species can be isolated from routine blood culture systems; specialized agar/system is required for isolation of filamentous fungi.

Management and Outcome

Treatment of pacemaker infections depends on the extent of the infection.[217] Localized cellulitis without device involvement often can be managed with systemic antimicrobial therapy without removal of the pacemaker battery. Indications for removal and replacement of the wire include: (1) valvular and/or lead endocarditis or sepsis; (2) pocket infection with abscess formation, device erosion, skin adherence, or chronic draining or recurrent sinus; or (3) occult BSI.[208] The outcome depends on the site of infection, the pathogen, and the condition of the patient. Local infections usually resolve without sequelae; deeper infections are associated with greater morbidity and mortality.

LVAD infections are difficult to eradicate and are associated with significant mortality.[223] Evidence for optimal treatment for LVAD-associated infection is derived largely from single-center case series with relatively few patients, almost entirely adults. Although the optimal duration of therapy for LVAD-associated infection is unknown, continuous antimicrobial therapy before, during, and beyond transplantation may be required. The results of a large single-center study suggested that continuous antimicrobial therapy is associated with fewer relapses than a limited course of therapy.[222] The potential benefits of prolonged antimicrobial therapy, however, must be balanced against the risk of developing antimicrobial resistance.

Prevention

Evidence-based data on the efficacy of measures to prevent infections in patients with pacemakers and LVADs are lacking. Antibiotic prophylaxis recommendations for pacemakers and LVADs are modeled after those used to prevent surgical site infection. For LVAD drivelines, exit site care usually consists of daily sterile cleansing with povidone-iodine and isopropyl alcohol, dilute hydrogen peroxide, or chlorhexidine and placement of an occlusive dressing.[222] Although fungal LVAD infections are associated with a worse prognosis than bacterial infections, systemic antifungal prophylaxis does not appear to prevent fungal infection.[223]

INFECTIONS OF CENTRAL NERVOUS SYSTEM DEVICES

Epidemiology and Pathogenesis

Central nervous system (CNS) devices include cerebrospinal fluid (CSF) shunts, subarachnoid screws and bolts, and subdural catheters.[227] Infections usually are caused by skin flora introduced during surgical insertion. Skin-associated tract infections and ascending infection can occur postoperatively in patients with ventriculoperitoneal shunts.[228] The latter develops when the distal end of a ventriculoperitoneal shunt penetrates the bowel (or is surrounded by a collection of contaminated mesenteric/peritoneal fluid, i.e., "CSFoma") and are typically polymicrobial. Rarely, the ventriculoperitoneal catheter tip perforates the genitourinary system and becomes contaminated with local flora. Ventriculostomy catheters exit percutaneously to an external monitoring system and can become contaminated during placement or manipulation.[229,230] Moreover, skin flora can ascend from the exit site along the catheter and into the ventricle. Subcutaneous reservoirs can be contaminated during placement or subsequent access.

Infection rates for ventriculoperitoneal (VP) shunts range from 3% to 35%.[1,231–236] In general, rates are higher for second procedures (especially for replacement of an infected shunt, although the causative organisms may be dissimilar),[227] and for shunts placed for hydrocephalus due to intraventricular hemorrhage fluid shunt infections in children.[236] Infections rates generally are higher in children than adults.[237] Most infections occur within 2 months of shunt placement.[238] In a study from 41 children's hospitals, the rate of shunt infection at 24 months was 11.7% per patient and 7.2% per procedure, although rates varied widely across institutions.[239] A follow-up analysis revealed a reinfection rate of 14.8%, most of which occurred within the first 2 months post reinsertion.[240] One study found that rates of infection were highest in July, correlating with the arrival of new neurosurgical fellows in hospital programs.[233] As with other indwelling catheters, the rate of infection depends on the duration of catheterization.[241] Infection rates have been reported to be approximately 20% to 25% for subcutaneous reservoirs[241] and 10% for percutaneous ventriculostomies.

Clinical Manifestations and Laboratory Diagnosis

Catheter malfunction is the most common manifestation of infection. For shunts, malfunction produces signs of increased intracranial pressure (i.e., headache, vomiting, irritability, and/or mental status changes). Fever is usually but not always is present.[227,229] Abdominal symptoms can predominate when the gastrointestinal tract is the source of shunt infection or if primary ventricular infection causes clinical peritonitis. Seizure occasionally is a presenting sign. Shunt malfunction due to occlusion or disconnection is the major alternative diagnosis. A malfunctioning shunt should be considered infected until proven otherwise, even in the absence of systemic manifestations and CSF pleocytosis.[229] Up to 30% of malfunctioning shunts are ultimately proven infected.[233]

Most infections are caused by CoNS and other skin flora; gram-negative bacteria account for about 20%.[229-233,242,243] Skin flora, including *Corynebacterium* spp. and *Propionibacterium acnes,* can cause particularly indolent infections. Fungal infections most commonly are caused by *Candida* spp. and occur most commonly in prematurely born infants.[244]

Diagnosis requires examination and culture of ventricular fluid; lumbar CSF is not sufficient.[245] Pleocytosis is typical, but can range from zero to thousands of cells per mm.[5,231,236,245] Elevated ventricular fluid protein is more common than abnormal glucose concentration. Clinical and laboratory findings often are subtle in infections due to CoNS. Blood culture results usually are positive with ventriculoatrial shunt infection; likewise, pleural fluid culture can be positive in ventriculopleural shunt infections, and peritoneal fluid in VP shunt infections. Blood culture is rarely positive in VP shunt infection. Abdominal complications of VP shunts, including formation of pseudocyst (CSFoma), are best diagnosed with ultrasonography or computed tomography.[246,247] Lumbar puncture for CSF examination should be performed for a child with a lumbo-peritoneal shunt, or a VP shunt when the diagnosis of meningitis is suspected and ventricular shunt fluid is normal.

Management and Outcome

Treatment includes antimicrobial therapy and surgery.[227,229,233] Cure with systemic antimicrobial therapy alone is unusual. A common approach to treatment includes: (1) removing the ventriculostomy or shunt or externalizing the peritoneal end of the shunt; (2) beginning systemic antimicrobial therapy; and (3) sampling ventricular fluid daily. Empiric therapy consists of an antistaphylococcal agent with adequate cerebrospinal fluid penetration (nafcillin, oxacillin, or vancomycin); if abdominal signs are present or if a gram-negative infection is suspected, a broad-spectrum cephalosporin, such as cefotaxime, ceftriaxone, or ceftazidime, plus an aminoglycoside is added. Definitive therapy is based on susceptibility test results of isolate(s) and ability of the antimicrobial agent to penetrate the CSF. Rifampin may be useful in combination therapy for patients with infection due to CoNS. If the infection does not resolve promptly, antimicrobial agents also can be administered intraventricularly.[248,249]

Cultures should be repeated frequently to ensure that the infection is controlled and to use time-to-sterilization as a basis for

BOX 102-10. Complications of Central Nervous System Devices

ALL SHUNTS
Ventriculitis: loss of neurons

VENTRICULOPERITONEAL SHUNTS
Peritonitis: bowel obstruction, abdominal pseudocyst ("CSFoma"), loss of absorptive surface

VENTRICULOPLEURAL SHUNTS
Pleural effusion, empyema

VENTRICULOATRIAL SHUNTS
Bacteremia, endocarditis, nephritis

CSF, cerebrospinal fluid.

duration of therapy. The system is replaced after the infection is fully controlled and cultures are negative. Limited data inform duration of antimicrobial therapy or optimal timing for shunt replacement.[229,230,250] Some experts recommend 7 to 10 days of antimicrobial therapy after sterilizing CSF, with extension to 10 to 14 days for more virulent pathogens such as *S. aureus.*[251] Timing of shunt replacement must balance the risks of superinfection associated with prolonged externalization against the risk of premature internalization with contamination of a new system.

The major complication of ventriculitis is brain injury. Studies of children with myelomeningocele reveal that the number of shunt infections is a major determinant of low intelligence.[252] The prognosis for ventriculitis depends on the virulence of the pathogen and condition of the underlying host. Infections caused by slime-producing strains of CoNS may be more difficult to cure.[253] Infection in the immunocompromised host is more likely to result in morbidity or mortality. Complications of peritonitis include adhesions, bowel obstruction, and loss of fluid-absorptive capacity. Respiratory distress due to pleural effusion or infection can complicate infections of ventriculopleural shunts (Box 102-10). Ventriculoatrial infection can lead to endocarditis and immune complex-related glomerulonephritis.

Prevention

Prevention of infection depends on the appropriateness of antimicrobial prophylaxis as well as meticulous sterile technique during device placement and with each sampling of CSF. Shaving the scalp over the shunt button before CSF collection damages the skin and increases the risk of infection at subsequent samplings. Although some individual studies of antimicrobial prophylaxis have failed to show a significant impact on infection rate, a meta-analysis suggests that perioperative prophylaxis reduces the incidence of shunt infection.[254] The optimal antimicrobial regimen remains unclear.[232,255,256] Administration of antimicrobial agents for the duration of continuous intracranial pressure monitoring is not appropriate.[257]

Prophylaxis for CNS devices should be limited to the perioperative period. Catheters and shunts impregnated with antimicrobial agents, such as rifampin and clindamycin, have been shown in vitro and in animal models to inhibit bacterial colonization.[258,259] Small clinical trials in adults[260-262] and children[263] and a meta-analysis[254] also support the efficacy of antimicrobial catheters for infection prevention.

INFECTIONS ASSOCIATED WITH PERITONEAL CATHETERS

Epidemiology and Pathogenesis

Peritoneal catheters are most often inserted for continuing ambulatory peritoneal dialysis (CAPD). Peritoneal dialysis removes

PART II Clinical Syndromes and Cardinal Features of Infectious Diseases: Approach to Diagnosis and Initial Management

SECTION Q Infections Associated with Hospitalization and Medical Devices

complement and immunoglobulins and thus impairs host defenses.[264,265] In addition, the low pH of dialysate inhibits neutrophil function.[265] Peritoneal catheter-associated infections include catheter exit site and tunnel infections as well as peritonitis; the incidence of peritonitis in children is approximately 0.67 episodes per patient-year.[266] Longer duration of dialysis therapy, younger age, and decreased serum concentrations of immunoglobulin G are associated with a higher incidence of peritonitis.[267,268]

Organisms can enter the peritoneum during placement and subsequent manipulation of the catheter, with intrinsically or extrinsically contaminated peritoneal dialysis fluid, and after perforation of the bowel by the catheter tip.[269] Hematogenous seeding, ascending infection via the fallopian tubes, and transmural migration of bacteria across the bowel wall are less common routes of infection.[264] The most common organisms are those that colonize the skin around the catheter insertion site and that may enter the peritoneum via the catheter tract: *S. aureus* and CoNS are isolated in 50% to 60% of infections; gram-negative enteric bacilli in 20% to 30%; less frequently *Candida* spp., nontuberculous mycobacteria, molds, and *Nocardia* species.[264,268,270,271]

Clinical Manifestations and Laboratory Diagnosis

Clinical findings in peritonitis include fever, abdominal tenderness, and cloudy dialysate. Presentations range from subtle pain to sepsis syndrome.[269] The differential diagnosis includes chemical peritonitis, eosinophilic peritonitis, hemoperitoneum, chylous ascites, and (rarely) malignancy.[268] Examination of the dialysate fluid usually reveals pleocytosis. Cell counts vary, depending on fluid dwell time and the causal pathogen, but leukocyte counts >100 cells/mm^3 with neutrophil counts >50% suggest infection.[264,272] There is no consensus on the optimal method to culture fluid; methods include inoculation of a small sample or filtration of a large volume with inoculation of the filter disk on to solid media[264,272,273] Ultrasonography of the catheter tunnel can be useful in diagnosing tunnel site infection (particularly when exit site infection is apparent or in the setting of peritonitis) and after response to therapy.[274-276]

Management and Outcome

Exit site infections often respond to local therapy and oral antimicrobial therapy. Infections of the tunnel often require catheter removal.[264] Peritonitis is usually managed with intraperitoneal antimicrobial therapy and continuous dialysis.[269] Most patients with CAPD-associated peritonitis can be treated in the ambulatory setting. If the patient is systemically ill or if attempts to eradicate the bacteria fail, hospital admission and systemic antimicrobial therapy are warranted, and catheter removal should be considered. Catheter removal is essential for cure of fungal infection[271] and often is necessary for enterococcal and *Pseudomonas* infections.[270] Several reports indicate that simultaneous removal and replacement of the catheter is successful in selected instances,[277-279] particularly when infection is caused by staphylococci, the tunnel is involved, or in cases of recurrent peritonitis that clears intermittently with treatment. This approach is less likely to be effective in infections due to gram-negative organisms or fungi, or if there is ongoing inflammation between episodes of recurrent peritonitis.[279] There are no controlled studies on optimal duration of therapy; the recommended course for children is 2 weeks, and 3 weeks for *S. aureus*.[280] Complications include intra-abdominal abscess formation, adhesions with subsequent bowel obstruction, and impairment of the peritoneal surface available for dialysis.

Prevention

Staphylococcal carriage predisposes to peritonitis. Eradication of nasal or skin carriage with antistaphylococcal agents decreases the incidence of peritonitis due to *S. aureus*.[281-284] Systemic administration of rifampin (20 mg/kg once daily) combined with an antistaphylococcal agent for 7 days appears to be most effective.[281]

Topical application of mupirocin to the nose 2 to 4 times daily for 5 to 10 days can eliminate nasal carriage; elimination of nasal carriage was accompanied by elimination of hand carriage in one study.[282] None of these studies was related to community-associated methicillin-resistant *S. aureus*, eradication of which is difficult. Aseptic technique during catheter insertion and manipulation is essential.

INFECTIONS OF ORTHOPEDIC DEVICES

Epidemiology and Pathogenesis

Prosthetic joints are used less commonly in children than in adults, but pins, medullary nails, and rods are commonly placed in children for stabilization of fractures and during corrective surgery. Infection is a major complication of orthopedic devices;[285,286] incidence varies with type of procedure and patient population.[1] Prosthetic joint infections are the best studied; rates vary from 1% to 9%, depending on the joint involved.[285-287] Risk of infection is higher in the presence of underlying malignancy; in a surgical site infection not involving the prosthesis; with a National Nosocomial Infections Surveillance System surgical patient risk index of >1;[288] and after surgery related to a previously infected site.[289,290] Pin site infections are common, because the pin track creates a direct pathway for skin flora and contaminating organisms to reach soft tissues and bone. Infection risk depends on the mode and site of injury, amount of associated soft-tissue injury, and the time before pin removal. Solid medullary nails are associated with lower infection risk than hollow nails.[291]

Most infections are caused by CoNS and *S. aureus*. Other gram-positive cocci, such as group A streptococci, oral streptococci, and enterococci, as well as gram-negative enteric bacilli, are occasionally involved. Anaerobic bacteria account for <10% of infections. Organisms gain access to the joint and bone at the time of implantation, and later via spread from contiguous infections, or (less commonly) by hematogenous seeding.[285,286]

Clinical Manifestations and Laboratory Diagnosis

Clinical manifestations of implanted orthopedic device-associated infection frequently are subtle. Findings include pain, wound dehiscence, or loosening or malfunction of prosthetic joints. With pin-related infections, there is usually purulence at the skin exit site, but the depth of involvement is difficult to determine; infection can extend to the intramedullary cavity.[292] Toxic shock has been reported as a complication of pin site infection,[293] as has brain abscess secondary to a halo orthosis pin site infection.[294]

The diagnostic utility of most radiographic techniques in pin, nail, and joint infection is limited, because the appearance of infection mimics that of healing bone. For prosthetic joints, radiographs sometimes are helpful; periosteal reaction occurs with infection but also can occur with normal healing. An area of radiolucency surrounded by a sclerotic edge is suggestive of infection.[295] Radionuclide scans are sensitive but not specific and do not reliably differentiate infection from fracture and healing bone.[296,297] Computed tomography and magnetic resonance imaging are rarely helpful because the device often causes artifacts, obscuring the area of interest.[285] Assessment of inflammatory markers, including erythrocyte sedimentation rate and C-reactive protein, may help guide diagnosis and treatment.

Culture of superficial drainage from pin sites or draining sinuses can yield colonizing or contaminating organisms rather than the true etiologic agent. Direct sampling of the bone or joint for histologic examination and culture usually is required for definitive diagnosis.[286] Intraoperative specimens evaluated by frozen-section examination are useful in excluding active infection during surgery to revise loosened prostheses.[298]

Management and Outcome

The treatment of infections associated with surgical implants is challenging.[299] Therapy for superficial pin track infections involves pin removal and prolonged antimicrobial therapy. For infected rods and joints, removing the device offers the best chance of cure but is complicated by prolonged disability and deformity. Often, a two-step approach is used, in which the infection is first brought under control with systemic antimicrobial therapy and the device and all devitalized tissue and cement are removed. At a later date, the device is replaced.[300,301] There is no consensus regarding the ideal interval before replacement.

If removal of the device is not feasible, a combination of antimicrobial therapy and debridement can be attempted. This approach has a failure rate of 70% to 80%, however, and is best attempted only when the duration of symptoms before treatment is brief.[302,303] One study of adults with infected hip and knee prostheses demonstrated successful treatment with a combination of ciprofloxacin and rifampin for 3 to 6 months and retention of the prosthesis after initial debridement;[304] patients in this study had a short duration of symptoms before treatment.

Antimicrobial therapy for infected orthopedic devices typically is prolonged. For staphylococcal infections, the combination of a β-lactam or quinolone plus rifampin may be considered if the organism is susceptible and the device cannot be removed.[305] For cases in which the device is left in place, long-term suppressive therapy may be warranted. If there are large tissue defects over the involved area, skin and muscle flaps may help by providing a vascular source to enhance host defenses and improve antimicrobial delivery.[306]

Prevention

Methods designed to decrease contamination of the operative field during implantation of orthopedic devices have been studied, including increasing the number of operating room air exchanges as well as use of high-efficiency particulate air filters, laminar flow systems, and special barrier suits for surgeons.[307] A large prospective study involving >7000 patients showed no difference in rates of infection between the use of conventional operating suites and laminar flow rooms,[286] and more recent analyses suggest that laminar flow may increase the rate of surgical site infection following some orthopedic implants.[308]

Perioperative prophylaxis intravenously with antistaphylococcal agents is beneficial. Administration of prophylactic agents should be confined to the immediate perioperative period (i.e., from just before the procedure to 24 hours afterward). The appropriate drug, dose, and timing of antimicrobial prophylaxis prior to orthopedic implants is critical.[309] The clinical efficacy of dipping implants in antimicrobial solutions, antimicrobial coating of implants, or use of antimicrobial carriers (e.g., cements, beads) has not been established.[310,311] Debate exists about antimicrobial prophylaxis in persons with prostheses who undergo dental or surgical procedures.[312]

INFECTION OF URINARY CATHETERS

Epidemiology and Pathogenesis

The literature describing urinary catheter-associated urinary tract infections (CAUTIs) in children largely is limited by two factors: (1) Studies often fail to distinguish symptomatic from asymptomatic infections (i.e., catheter-associated bacteriuria from CAUTI), and (2) data describing epidemiology and strategies for the management and prevention of infections are sparse. Despite limitations, many principles of adult CAUTI are reasonably adapted to pediatrics.

Infection is the most common complication of urinary catheterization,[313] and catheter-associated bacteriuria is the most common healthcare-associated infection in adults worldwide.[314] Isolated cystitis occurs most commonly, but pyelonephritis and secondary BSI also can develop. Contamination can occur during catheter insertion, organisms can enter the bladder by ascending from the perineum on the outside of the catheter, or contamination can be introduced from the collection bag.[315,316]

Infection rates are approximately 1% for each catheterization episode.[317] The rate of infection of a catheter is 5% to 10% per day if a closed system is used.[1,316,317] Infection rates are higher with an open drainage system and when diarrhea is present,[102,318] there is diminished urine flow or urinary stasis (as occurs with ureteral reflux, bladder diverticula, and stenosis of the urethra).

The most common organisms that cause CAUTIs are members of the perineal flora. *Escherichia coli* is most common; other enteric gram-negative bacilli, *Enterococcus*, and *Candida* spp. also are frequent. Patients receiving antimicrobial agents are at high risk of infection due to resistant bacteria and fungi.[316,319]

Clinical Manifestations and Laboratory Diagnosis

CAUTIs often are asymptomatic.[320] Signs and symptoms of CAUTI include urgency, frequency, enuresis, dysuria, and cloudy or foul-smelling urine. Urinalysis and culture are useful to confirm infection. Urinalysis can reveal pyuria, but pyuria often is absent in bacteriuria associated with indwelling catheters. Diagnosis of CAUTI is established by isolation of organisms with colony counts of >10^2 CFU/mL from catheter urine.

Management and Outcome

Therapy for bacteriuria and infection should include removal of the catheter if possible. If the catheter remains in place, infection often persists despite appropriate antimicrobial treatment or recurs immediately after cessation of therapy. There is debate regarding the need for antimicrobial therapy for bacteriuria or cystitis, because these conditions often resolve spontaneously with removal of the catheter.[316] For complicating pyelonephritis and BSI, systemic therapy is necessary; the optimal duration is unclear.

The major complications of CAUTI are pyelonephritis and renal damage,[317] and BSI.[317,321] It is important to exclude UTI before major surgical interventions in catheterized patients. Prognosis is related to extent of the infection, the pathogen involved, and underlying host factors.

Prevention

Important strategies to prevent CAUTI are: (1) limiting catheterization to those for whom it is medically necessary; (2) attention to strict aseptic technique during catheter insertion; and (3) removal of the catheter as soon as possible. Catheters commonly are left in place for too long and "forgotten"; one study of adult medical inpatients revealed that clinicians were unaware that their patients had a catheter 28% of the time.[322]

Prophylactic antimicrobial therapy has been demonstrated to provide brief protection against bacteriuria;[323] however, few guidelines recommend this strategy because the risk of progression from asymptomatic bacteriuria to clinically significant UTI remains low for most patients.[314] In addition, prolonged antimicrobial therapy is not protective and often is harmful because of the increased risk of infection with resistant organisms.[315] Catheter care includes attention to handwashing, maintaining a closed system, minimizing entry to the system, and positioning the collecting system below the level of the bladder to avoid bladder urinary stasis or reflux.[23] In general, applying creams or attempting to wash the perineum raises the risk of UTI, probably because of movement of the catheter and an increase in introduction of perineal flora along the catheter and into the bladder.[324]

Clean intermittent catheterization is preferred to indwelling catheterization in children with neurogenic bladder.[325] The abdominal Credé method does not empty the bladder and may increase risk of infection.[19,315,326] Antiseptic-impregnated catheters have been shown to delay the onset of bacteriuria but few studies have examined cost-benefit and the associated risk of emerging resistant organisms associated with the use of these catheters.[327]

PART II Clinical Syndromes and Cardinal Features of Infectious Diseases: Approach to Diagnosis and Initial Management

SECTION R Infections in Patients with Deficient Defenses

SECTION R: Infections in Patients with Deficient Defenses

103 Evaluation of the Child with Suspected Immunodeficiency

E. Stephen Buescher

Although most primary immunodeficiency disorders are rare, referral for evaluation of these conditions is common in children with frequent infections. Epidemiologic studies show that children younger than 2 years normally have on average 5 to 6 acute respiratory tract illnesses per year (with a range up to 11 or 12 per year).[1,2] Infections such as otitis media and gastroenteritis occur with similar frequencies in children younger than 2 years of age, with up to 14 episodes per year at the far end of the normal spectrum.[3] Attendance at group childcare and exposure to secondhand smoke further increase frequency of these infections.[4] An approach that includes a carefully obtained history, a thorough physical examination, and selected laboratory tests often is required to differentiate the uncommon, immunologically abnormal child who requires more extensive evaluation from the common, "normal but unlucky" child.

IDENTIFICATION

The concept of the "normal but unlucky" child presumes that, in a group of normal children, the half who experience more than the average number of infections is "normal but unlucky."[5] Because "normal but unlucky" children can experience large numbers of infections, criteria other than the number of illnesses, as shown in Box 103-1, must be considered to identify the child who is "normal but unlucky." Further investigation is limited to those who lack these characteristics, and focuses on categorizing patients as to the likely cause for their recurrent infections.

Anatomic and Physiologic Abnormalities

A variety of anatomic abnormalities can alter natural host defenses, thus predisposing a child to recurrent infections (Table 103-1). Anatomy-related infections often localize at or near the site of the abnormality; thus, infections recur at the same site. In instances of congenital malformation, infections usually begin during infancy. Compared with the incidence of primary immunodeficiency disorders, congenital malformation as a cause of recurrent infections is common.

Underlying Conditions

The presence of underlying conditions, either natural or iatrogenic, can alter host defenses and predispose to recurrent infections or may be associated with an immunodeficiency (Box 103-2). In addition to the primary immunodeficiency syndromes, recurrent infections occur in more than 100 other syndromes,

which include growth deficiencies, specific organ system dysfunctions, inborn errors of metabolism, and miscellaneous and chromosomal anomalies.[6] Some underlying conditions only become serious considerations when specific data are obtained during a detailed history. Some conditions are suspected when constellations of noninfectious signs and symptoms are revealed by history and physical examination. Recurrent infections associated with

TABLE 103-1. Anatomic and Physiologic Abnormalities That Predispose to Recurrent Infections

Type of Infection	Predisposing Abnormality
Bloodstream infection	Asplenia
	Cardiac valve abnormality
	Intravascular cannula or thrombus
	Neutropenia
Bone infection	Foreign body
	Orthopedic device
Meningitis	Cochlear implant
	Dura mater (meningeal) defect
	Midline dermal sinus
	Mondini defect of inner ear
	Neurenteric fistula
	Occult skull fracture
	Ventricular cannula
Pneumonia	Abnormal cough reflex
	Atelectasis
	Bronchiectasis
	Endotracheal intubation
	Extrinsic airway compression
	Foreign body
	Gastroesophageal reflux
	Polyps
	Pulmonary cyst, fistula
	Pulmonary sequestration
	Tracheal web
	Tracheoesophageal fistula
	Tracheomalacia
	Tracheostomy
	Vascular ring
Soft-tissue infection	Diminished sensation
	Foreign body
	Lymphedema
	Thermal injury
Urinary tract infection	Genitourinary tract duplication, cyst, fistula, or obstruction
	Nephrostomy
	Urinary catheter
	Vesicostomy

BOX 103-1. History of a "Normal but Unlucky" Child

- Lack of documented, deep infections at multiple sites
- Normal growth and development
- Normal morphology and physiology between episodes of infection
- Lack of a family history of immunodeficiency

BOX 103-2. Underlying Conditions That Can Predispose to Recurrent Infections

Asplenia syndrome
Asthma
Bone marrow and solid-organ transplantation
Chemotherapy
Collagen vascular diseases
Congenital malformation
Corticosteroid therapy
Cystic fibrosis
Dermatologic syndrome with immunodeficiency
Diabetes mellitus
Down syndrome
Drug-induced cytopenia
Galactosemia
Gastrointestinal tract syndrome with immunodeficiency
Genetic/metabolic conditions
Glycogen storage disease type IB
Growth deficiency/immunodeficiency syndrome
Hematopoietic/immunologic conditions
Hemoglobinopathy
Ichthyosis
Immunosuppression
Isovaleric acidemia
Lymphohematopoietic malignancy
Malnutrition
α-Mannosidosis
Methylmalonic aciduria
Mucolipidosis II
Myelokathexis (WHIM syndrome)
Myotonic dystrophy
Nephrotic syndrome
Neurologic syndrome with immunodeficiency
Newborn state
Nutritional conditions
Orotic aciduria
Prematurity
Propionic acidemia
Protein-losing enteropathy
Radiation therapy
Renal conditions
Renal failure
Sarcoidosis
Tumor necrosis factor antagonist therapy
Werdnig–Hoffmann disease
WHIM (warts, hypogammaglobulinemia, infections, myelokathexis)

BOX 103-3. Characteristics of Children with Primary Immunodeficiency Disorders

- Infectious symptoms often begin in first days to weeks of life
- Therapeutic response is slow despite identification of a pathogen and administration of appropriate antimicrobial therapy
- Infection is suppressed rather than eradicated by appropriate therapy
- Common organisms cause severe manifestations or recurrent infection
- Unusual (sometimes sentinel) or "nonpathogenic" organisms cause infections
- Growth and development are delayed
- Multiple infections occur simultaneously
- Infection with common organisms leads to unexpected complications

underlying conditions either can be localized or disseminated and may or may not respond well even when appropriate treatment is given. Compared with the incidence of primary immunodeficiency disorders, this category of causes of recurrent infections also is common.

Primary Immunodeficiency Disorders

Recurrent infections due to primary immunodeficiency disease are rare in the general population (Table 103-2) and are relatively rare compared with other causes of recurrent infection. Common characteristics in children with primary immunodeficiency disorders are shown in Box 103-3.

The relative frequency of primary immunodeficiency disorders is shown in Table 103-3.[7,8] The component due to recognized disorders of the innate immune system, e.g., those affecting pattern recognition receptors or their associated signal transduction systems or both, probably is low, but is growing.[8] The list of recognized immunodeficiency conditions is long (Tables 103-4 to 103-6), and their degrees of characterization vary. More than 130 conditions presently are identified.[9,10] Some are well characterized, pathologic mechanisms are understood, and numerous affected patients have been described (chronic granulomatous disease,[11] X-linked severe combined immunodeficiency syndrome,[12] X-linked agammaglobulinemia,[13] leukocyte adhesive deficiency type I,[14] and adenosine deaminase deficiency[15]). Other conditions remain incompletely characterized, poorly understood, or have been observed in so few patients that they have not been studied extensively (lazy leukocyte syndrome,[16] common variable immunodeficiency,[17] reticular dysgenesis[18]).

TABLE 103-2. Estimated Frequencies of Selected Chronic Underlying Illnesses, Primary Immunodeficiency Disorders, and HIV Infection

Condition[a]	Frequency
Asthma[26]	1 in 26
IgA deficiency	1 in 500 to 1 in 700
Diabetes mellitus[26]	1 in 556
HIV infection	1 in 1000
Sickle-cell disease[26]	1 in 2200
Cystic fibrosis[27]	1 in 2500
Acute lymphocytic leukemia[26]	1 in 9000
Phenylketonuria[26]	1 in 10,000
Agammaglobulinemia[26]	1 in 50,000 to 1 in 100,000
Severe combined immunodeficiency	1 in 100,000 to 1 in 500,000
Chronic granulomatous disease[28]	1 in 255,000

HIV, human immunodeficiency virus; IgA, immunoglobulin A.

[a]Superscript numbers indicate references.

TABLE 103-3. Relative Frequency of Primary Immunodeficiency Disorders

Factors	Percentage
B lymphocytes	50–70
T lymphocytes	20–30
T and B lymphocytes	10–15
Phagocytic cells	15–20
Complement	2–5
Other innate immunity factors	<1

PART II Clinical Syndromes and Cardinal Features of Infectious Diseases: Approach to Diagnosis and Initial Management

SECTION R Infections in Patients with Deficient Defenses

TABLE 103-4. Characteristics of Primary Immunodeficiency Disorders Involving Immunoglobulins

Conditions	MIM[a]	Comment
CONDITIONS CAUSING DECREASES IN ALL IMMUNOGLOBULINS		
X-linked agammaglobulinemia	MIM +300300	XL inheritance, absent immunoglobulins, or low levels in "atypical" cases, absence or low blood levels of B lymphocytes; gene defect in *Btk* (Bruton thymidine kinase), gene location Xq21.3-q22
X-linked agammaglobulinemia with growth hormone deficiency	MIM #307200	XL inheritance, hypogammaglobulinemia, short stature, delayed puberty; mutation in *Btk* gene, gene location Xq21.3-q22
μ Heavy chain deficiency	MIM #601495 MIM *147020	AR inheritance, B lymphocytes low/absent, pro-B lymphocytes normal; mutations in μ heavy chain
λ5 deficiency	MIM #601495	AR inheritance, B lymphocytes low/absent, pro-B lymphocytes normal; mutations in IGLL1
Igα deficiency		AR inheritance, B lymphocytes low/absent, pro-B lymphocytes normal; mutations in Igα
Igβ deficiency		AR inheritance, B lymphocytes low/absent, pro-B lymphocytes normal; mutations in Igβ
BLNK deficiency	MIM +604515	AR inheritance, B lymphocytes low/absent, pro-B lymphocytes normal; mutations in BLNK, gene location 10q23.2
Thymoma with immunodeficiency		Heterogeneous findings: agammaglobulinemia, hypogammaglobulinemia, combined immunodeficiency; recurrent infections; usually adult onset
Antibody deficiency with transcobalamin II deficiency	MIM +275350	Early-onset megaloblastic anemia, low total immunoglobulin content; gene location 22q11.2-qter
CONDITIONS CAUSING DECREASES IN SELECTED IMMUNOGLOBULINS		
IgA deficiency 1 IgA deficiency 2	MIM %137100 MIM #609529	Deficiency of serum IgA, mucosal IgA or both, variable association with CVID, autoimmune disorders; IgAD1 gene location 6p21.3; IGAD2 associated with *TACI* defect, gene location 17p11.2
IgA deficiency with IgG subclass deficiency		Recurrent bacterial infections common
IgG subclass deficiencies		Usually asymptomatic, but can have recurrent viral/bacterial infections
IgG1		Total IgG usually low, frequent association with IgG3 deficiency
IgG2		Total IgG normal, often associated with IgG4 and IgA deficiency; poor responses to polysaccharide antigens
IgG3		Total IgG normal unless associated with IgG1 deficiency
IgG4		Total IgG normal, difficult to diagnose because IgG4 levels normally low
IgM deficiency	MIM 242850	Absence or low level of total IgM; association with intrahepatic sclerosing cholangitis
Immunodeficiency with hyper-IgM (type 1-5)	MIM *308230 MIM *300386 MIM #605258 MIM #606843 MIM 608184 MIM *191525	Type 1 (XL inheritance), gene location Xq26; type 2 (AR inheritance), gene location 12p13, lymph node hyperplasia due to giant germinal centers; type 3 (AR inheritance) gene location 20q12-q13.2; type 4, gene location unknown; type 5 (AR inheritance), defect in uracil DNA glycosylase, gene location 20q12-q13.2; all related to abnormalities in CD40-CD40 ligand signaling systems, low IgG, low IgA, normal or high IgM
AID deficiency	MIM *605257	Associated with immunodeficiency with hyper IgM, type 2; mutations in *AICDA* gene, gene location 12p13
Common, variable immunodeficiency	MIM #240500 MIM *604907	Heterogeneous group of disorders characterized by "acquired" hypogammaglobulinemia, antibody deficiency and recurrent bacterial infections, low-normal B-lymphocyte levels, poor antibody responses to immunization, occasionally IgG subclass "imbalances", associated with autoimmune, lymphoproliferative or granulomatous disorders
ICOS deficiency	MIM #607594	AR inheritance, clinically a CVID mimic; mutation in inducible costimulator (*ICOS*) gene, gene location 2q33
CD19 deficiency	MIM +107265	AR inheritance, hypogammaglobulinemia, recurrent infections, normal B-lymphocyte numbers; gene location 16p11.2
BAFF receptor deficiency		AR inheritance, low IgG and IgM, clinically a CVID mimic; mutations in *TNFRSF13C*
WHIM syndrome	MIM #193670	AD inheritance presumed, warts, hypogammaglobulinemia, infections and myelokathexis; defective CXC4 (chemokine) receptor signaling, gene location 2q21
Ectodermal dysplasia, hypohidrosis with immunodeficiency	MIM #300291 MIM *300248	Dysgammaglobulinemia, elevated IgM; susceptibility to mycobacterial infections; *IKK-γ* (NF-kB essential modulator, "NEMO") or *IKBKG* gene defects, gene location Xq28
Antibody deficiency with normal subclass deficiency, deficient antibody or high Ig levels		Normal total immunoglobulin levels, IgG responses to certain specific antigens (KLH, diphtheria toxoid, tetanus toxoid, pneumococcal polysaccharide)

AD, autosomal dominant; AR, autosomal recessive; XL, X-linked recessive; Ig, immunoglobulin; CVID, common variable immunodeficiency.

[a]*OMIM (Online Mendelian Inheritance in Man) access via WWW portal at http://www.ncbi.nlm.nih.gov/omim.*

TABLE 103-5. Characteristics of Primary Immunodeficiency Disorders Involving T Lymphocytes

Condition	MIM[a]	Comment
X-linked SCID (SCIDX1)	MIM #300400 MIM *308380	X-linked inheritance, defective IL-2 receptor γ-chain (also IL-4, IL-7, IL-9, IL-15, and IL-21 receptors), T lymphocytes absent, B lymphocytes present, peripheral blood lymphopenia; gene location Xq13
Autosomal SCID	MIM #601457	Multiple syndromes, all with autosomal inheritance, absent T lymphocytes, variable B lymphocytes, variable NK lymphocytes and deficient thymus, including:
	MIM #600802 MIM *600173	AR inheritance, T lymphocyte (–), B lymphocyte (+), NK lymphocyte (–): mutations in *JAK3* gene location 11q23, 5p13); *JAK3* functions in same signaling pathway as IL-2 receptor, so same immunologic phenotype as SCIDX1
	MIM *146661 MIM #608971	T lymphocyte (–), B lymphocyte (+), NK lymphocyte (+); defects in IL7R α-chain, gene location 5p13
	MIM #608971	T lymphocyte (–), B lymphocyte (+), NK lymphocyte (+); defects in CD45, gene location 1q31-q32
	MIM +186830 MIM *186790 MIM +186740	T lymphocyte (–), B lymphocyte (+), NK lymphocyte (+); defects in T-lymphocyte antigen receptor, in CD3D, CD3E, and CD3G chains, gene location 11q23
	MIM *608958 MIM #102700	AR inheritance, T lymphocyte (–), B lymphocyte (–), NK lymphocyte (–): mutations in ADA gene location 20q13.11; adenosine deaminase absent in erythrocytes, leukocytes, and fibroblasts; 50% of patients have radiographic abnormalities of vertebrae and ribs; SCID syndrome with early onset, delayed/late onset and partial ADA deficiency types patients have radiographic abnormalities of vertebrae and ribs; SCID syndrome with early onset, delayed/late onset and partial ADA deficiency types
	MIM +176947	ZAP 70 deficiency gene location 2q12, low CD8 cell numbers; deficient ZAP 70 expression. T lymphocyte (–), B lymphocyte (+), NK lymphocyte (+); "Coronin-1A deficiency"; failure of T-lymphocyte thymic egress; gene location 16p11.2
"Radiosensitive" SCID	MIM *605988	T lymphocyte (–), B lymphocyte (–), NK lymphocyte (+) with ionizing radiation sensitivity; mutation in Artemis gene producing V(D)J recombination and DNA repair defect, gene location 10p
	MIM #603554 MIM *175615	T lymphocyte (–), B lymphocyte (–), NK lymphocyte (+) with RAG1 or RAG2 defects; "Ommen syndrome"/ recombinase activating gene (RAG1 and RAG2) deficiency, gene location 11p13
	MIM *179616	T lymphocyte (–), B lymphocyte (+), NK lymphocyte (+); "DNA-dependent protein kinase catalytic subunit deficiency"; defective V(D)J recombination; increased sensitivity to ionizing radiation; erythroderma eosinophilia, chronic diarrhea; gene location 8q11
	MIM #606593 MIM *601837	"DNA ligase IV deficiency"; AR inheritance; growth failure, microcephaly, Fanconi-anemia-like syndromes, increased leukemia risk, increased sensitivity to ionizing radiation; impaired non-homologous end-joining in DNA repair; defective V(D)J recombination; gene location 13q22-q34
	MIM #611291	AR inheritance, T lymphocyte (–), B lymphocyte (+), NK lymphocyte (+); "Cernunnos deficiency"/"immunodeficiency with growth retardation and microcephaly"; microcephaly; impaired non-homologous end-joining in DNA repair; defective V(D)J recombination from NHEJ1 defect; gene location 2q35
Purine nucleoside phosphorylase deficiency	MIM +164050	Absent nucleoside phosphorylase in erythrocytes, leukocytes fibroblasts; carrier state with half normal levels; low uric acid, autoimmune hemolytic anemia, lymphopenia, phosphorylase deficiency; normal B lymphocyte numbers and Ig levels; neurologic impairment common; gene location 14q13.1
Nezelof syndrome	MIM %242700	Absent or low levels of T lymphocytes; thymic dysplasia present; Ig levels normal or near normal; low functional antibody; other characteristics heterogeneous
DiGeorge syndrome	MIM #188400 MIM *600594 MIM *601755 MIM %601362	Absence of T lymphocytes; congenital hypoparathyroidism, abnormal facies, congenital heart disease; type 1 gene location 22q112; type 2 gene location 10p14-p13
Calcium channel deficiency	MIM #612782 MIM *610277	Autoimmunity, anhydrotic ectodermal dysplasia, myopathy; defective T-cell proliferative responses; gene location 12q24
CD8 deficiency	MIM #608957 MIM *186910	AR inheritance, recurrent infections; T-lymphocyte, B-lymphocyte and NK lymphocyte numbers normal; CD8+ lymphocytes absent; defective CD8 α-chain, gene location 2p12
Reticular dysgenesis	MIM #267500	Early onset, severe leukopenia, severe lymphopenia; disruption of bone marrow differentiation; defect in mitochondrial adenylate kinase 2; gene location 1p34
Bare lymphocyte syndrome	MIM #209920 MIM *601962	Absence or deficiency of HLA antigen expression (MHC class I or II) on lymphocytes or platelets; multiple variants; MHC class II deficiency gene locations 16p13, 19p12, 13q14; MHC class I deficiency gene location 1q21.1-q21.3 (tapasin gene)
Short-limbed dwarfism/cartilage-hair hypoplasia	MIM #250250	Short stature, radiographic abnormalities in bone, short limbs, malabsorption, lax joints, redundant skin, sparse hair with absence of eyebrows and eyelashes, normal Ig levels; gene location 9p21-p12
Wiskott-Aldrich syndrome	MIM #301000 MIM #600903	XL (and rare AD) inheritance, petechiae and thrombocytopenia, eczematoid rashes; poor T- and B-lymphocyte function; poor antibody responses to polysaccharide antigens; elevated serum IgA and decreased serum IgM levels; predisposed to lymphoreticular malignancy; X-linked gene location Xp11.23-p11.22
Ataxia–telangiectasia syndrome	MIM *607585 MIM #208900	AR inheritance; recurrent sinopulmonary infections; progressive ataxia; progressive oculocutaneous telangiectasias; cutaneous anergy; IgA deficiency common; variable endocrinopathies; chromosomal breakages and cell sensitivity to ionizing radiation; gene location 11q22.3

Continued

Condition	MIM[a]	Comment
Biotin-dependent multiple carboxylase deficiency	MIM #253260	Multiple conditions, in vitro T-lymphocyte abnormalities in biotin-depleted culture media; nutritional biotin deficiency (e.g., excessive raw egg ingestion) indistinguishable; gene location 3p25
Chronic mucocutaneous candidiasis	MIM %212050 MIM %114580 MIM %607644	Heterogeneous disorder with at least 4 recognized groups; Candida sp. infection involving nails, skin, and mucous membranes; variable endocrinopathies; variable immunologic deficiencies (type 1 AD, gene location 2p22.3-p21; type 2 AR, gene location 9q34.3; type 3 finger and toe, nail familial candidiasis, gene location 11p13-q12; type 4 gene location 12p13.2-p12.3)
IPEX syndrome	MIM *300292 MIM #304790	immune dysregulation, polyendocrinopathy, enteropathy, x-linked; FOXP3 gene defective; gene location Xp11.23-q13.3.
APECED	MIM #240300 MIM *607358	Autoimmune polyendocrinopathy syndrome, type I; adrenal insufficiency, hypoparathyroidism, candidiasis; malabsorption/diarrhea prominent; AIRE gene dysfunction, gene location 21q22.3
ALPS	MIM #601859 MIM *134637 MIM #603909 MIM *601762	Autoimmune lymphoproliferative syndrome; massive lymphadenopathy, splenomegaly, hemolytic anemia, rash, thrombocytopenia; lymphocyte apoptosis defect due to CD95, Fas ligand, caspase 8, caspase 10, and unknown defects; AD and AR forms; gene locations 10q24.1, 2q33-q34
X-linked lymphoproliferative disease	MIM #308240 MIM *300490	XL inheritance; onset of immunodeficiency following viral infection (typically Epstein–Barr virus); multiple manifestations: agammaglobulinemia, combined immunodeficiency, B-lymphocyte lymphoproliferative disease; defect in SH2 domain protein 1A (SH2D1A); gene location Xq25
Itk deficiency	MIM #613011	AR inheritance, EBV-associated lymphoproliferation; gene location 5q32
Forkhead box N1 deficiency	MIM *600838	AR inheritance, T-lymphocyte immunodeficiency; congenital alopecia, nail dystrophy; winged-helix transcription factor defect; gene location 17q11-q12
IL-2 receptor α-chain deficiency	MIM #606367	AR inheritance, lymphoproliferation, recurrent infections, autoimmunity, impaired T-lymphocyte proliferation; CD25 deficiency; gene location 10p15.1
STAT5b deficiency	MIM *604260	AR inheritance, dwarfism (growth hormone insensitive), eczema, autoimmunity, lymphocytic interstitial pneumonitis; gene location 17q11.2
Hyper IgE syndrome	MIM #243700 MIM +611432	Extreme elevation of IgE; chronic eczema, recurrent staphylococcal infections, eosinophilia; AD and AR (DOCK8 defects) forms; AR gene location 9p24;AD gene location 17q21

AD, autosomal dominant; AR, autosomal recessive; XL, X-linked recessive; HLA, human leukocyte antigen; Ig, immunoglobulin; IL, interleukin; MHC, major histocompatibility complex; SCID, severe combined immunodeficiency.

[a]OMIM (Online Mendelian Inheritance in Man) access via WWW portal at http://www.ncbi.nlm.nih.gov/omim.

TABLE 103-6. Characteristics of Primary Disorders Involving Innate Immunity (Including Phagocytes and Complement) and Miscellaneous Conditions

Condition	MIM[a]	Comment
INNATE IMMUNITY DISORDERS		
IRAK4 deficiency	MIM #607676 MIM *606883	Recurrent pyogenic infections (particularly S. pneumoniae), poor inflammatory responses; normal Ig levels, normal T and B lymphocytes; normal phagocytes; pyogenic bacterial infections early in life, spontaneous amelioration with age; IL1-1R and toll R dysfunction; gene location 12q12
MyD88 deficiency	MIM #612260 MIM *602170	AR inheritance recurrent pyogenic infections (particularly S. pneumoniae), spontaneous amelioration with age, poor inflammatory responses; normal Ig levels, normal T and B lymphocytes; normal phagocytes; IL-1R and toll R adapter molecule defect, gene location 4q35
Toll-like receptor 3 (TLR3) deficiency	MIM *603029	Selective susceptibility to HSV-1 encephalitis; absent TLR3 signaling results in reduced IFN-α/β production in CNS; gene location 4q35
UNC93B protein mutation	MIM *610551	Selective susceptibility to HSV-1 encephalitis; mutation in adaptor protein for TLR3; reduced IFN-α/β and IFN-γ production in CNS; gene location 11q13
Mannose binding lectin deficiency	MIM +154545	Approximately 35% of normal population heterozygous for abnormal MBL alleles, while homozygosity for abnormal alleles is approximately 10 times more frequent in children referred for "immunodeficiency"; recurrent pyogenic infections and failure to thrive in small children; illnesses may ameliorate with age, individual cases of deficient adults with recurrent/severe infections; gene location 10q11.2-q21
MASP-2 deficiency	MIM +605102	Mannan binding lectin-associated serine protease-2 normally cleaves C2 and C4 to cause formation of C3; deficiency associated with pyogenic infections, inflammatory conditions, progressive pulmonary fibrosis; gene location 1p36.3-p36.2
IL-12 receptor deficiency	MIM *601604	Familial susceptibility to mycobacteria; deficiency of IL-12 receptor β1; gene location 19p13.1
IL-12 deficiency	MIM *161561 MIM *161560	Familial susceptibility to mycobacterial and Salmonella infection; deficiency of IL-12 production; β-chain deficiency gene location 5q31-q33.1; α-chain deficiency gene location 3p12-q13.2
Interferon-γ receptor deficiency	MIM *107470	Disseminated and/or recurrent mycobacterial infections and viral infections; gene location 6q23-q24
PHAGOCYTIC CELL DISORDERS		
Kostmann disease	MIM #202700 MIM *130130 MIM #610738 MIM #605998 MIM #613107 MIM *611045	Severe congenital neutropenia; multiple types: type 1 elastase mutations; type 2 GFI1 mutations; type 3 HAX-1 mutations (Kostmann disease); type 4 G6PCS3 mutations; some variants with abnormal G-CSF receptor; gene locations 19p13.3, 1p22, 1q213, 17q21, p35-p34.3

Condition	MIM[a]	Comment
Cyclic hematopoiesis (cyclic neutropenia)	MIM #162800	Recurrent episodes of neutropenia with 14–28 day cycle; duration of neutropenia shortened by G-CSF treatment inherited and acquired forms; elastase mutations; gene location 19p13.3
Chronic granulomatous disease	MIM #306400 MIM #233700 MIM #233710 MIM #233690 MIM 138990 MIM +608508	Multiple forms (AD, AR, XLR); absence of phagocyte superoxide production; abnormal nitroblue tetrazolium test/DHR 123 assay; gene locations Xp21.1, 7q11.23, 1q25, 16q24
Chédiak–Higashi syndrome	MIM #214500	Partial albinism, photophobia, nystagmus, giant leukocyte granules, malignant transformation LYST mutation; gene location 1q42.1-q42.2
Griscelli syndrome	MIM *603868 MIM #607624 MIM #214450	Hypomelanosis with primary neurologic impairment; type 1 no immunologic impairment; type 2 immune impairment, defect in RAB27A gene; type 3 no immunologic impairment, defect in melanophilin or MYO5A gene; development of hemophagocytic syndrome common
Hyper IgE/recurrent infection syndrome	MIM #147060 MIM #243700 MIM #611521	AD inheritance, recurrent sinopulmonary infections, eczematoid rashes, asymptomatic pneumatoceles, retained primary teeth, scoliosis and bone fractures; massively elevated IgE levels; STAT3 mutation; gene location 17q21; AR forms –DOCK8 (9p24) or TYK2 (19p13.2) mutations; some with susceptibility to intracellular bacterial infection
Myeloperoxidase deficiency	MIM #254600 MIM *606989	Absence of phagocyte peroxidase activity; gene location 17q23.1
Leukocyte adhesion deficiency	MIM #116920 MIM *600065 MIM #266265 MIM #612840	3 syndromes of defective leukocyte adhesion with different etiologies; type 1 leukocyte integrin deficiency, absent/low phagocyte CD11/CD18 surface expression, leukocytosis, periodontal disease; gene location 21q22.3; type 2 selectin dysfunction, Bombay erythrocyte phenotype, consanguinity, mental retardation, microcephaly, seizures, absence of sialyl-Lewis-X antigen on leukocytes, responsive to oral fucose administration; gene location 11p11.2; type 3 platelet and leukocyte defects, severe infection and bleeding tendency; defect in GDP fucose transporter (FERMT3); gene location 11q12
Secondary granule deficiency	MIM #245480	Absence of phagocyte lactoferrin, shortened respiratory burst; CEBPE (myeloid transcription factor) mutation; gene location 14q11.2
X-linked congenital neutropenia	MIM #300299	XL inheritance, present from birth, absolute neutrophil count repeatedly <1000/mm³; constitutively activating WAS mutation, gene location Xp11.23-p11.22
Neutrophil immunodeficiency syndrome	MIM #608203	Recurrent infections, leukocytosis (neutrophilia); diminished chemotaxis, cell polarization, granule secretion and superoxide production; RAC2 deficiency, gene location 22q12.3-13.2
COMPLEMENT DISORDERS		
Early (C1–C4) component deficiencies	MIM #216950 MIM +120700 MIM +120580 MIM +217000 MIM *120820 MIM +120550 MIM *217030 MIM #610984 MIM #609814 MIM +134370 MIM +120810	Recurrent infections, frequent autoimmune (SLE) and inflammatory (glomerulonephritis, proteinuria) manifestations
Individual component deficiencies		Variable deficiency of opsonic activity, absent or low levels of CH50
C5 deficiency	MIM #609536 MIM +120900	Seborrheic dermatitis, intractable diarrhea, recurrent local or systemic infections, marked wasting, disseminated gonococcal infection
C6–C8 deficiencies	MIM +120960 MIM *217050 MIM *217070 MIM +120950	Recurrent Neisseria spp. infections, absent or low levels of CH50
C9 deficiency	MIM +120940	CH50 level approximately 50% of normal; gene location 5p13
Factor D deficiency		Normal total hemolytic complement activity; deficiency of alternative complement activation pathway
Properdin deficiency	MIM #312060	XLR, normal hemolytic complement activity, deficiency of serum opsonic activity; fulminant meningococcal disease; gene location Xp11.4-11.23
MISCELLANEOUS DISORDERS		
Familial hemophagocytic lymphohistiocytosis	MIM #603552 MIM %267700 MIM #608898 MIM #613101 MIM *605014 MIM #603553	Massive infiltration of viscera with activated macrophages and lymphocytes; fever hepatosplenomegaly, cytopenias; 5 recognized types: type 1 unknown defect, gene location 9q21.3-q22; type 2 perforin defect (PRF1), gene location 10q22; type 3 UNC13D defect, gene location 17q25.1; type 4 syntaxin 11 defect (STX11), gene location 6q24; type 5 syntaxin binding protein defect (STXBP2), gene location 19p13.3-p13.2

AD, autosomal dominant; AR, autosomal recessive; XLR, X-linked recessive; CD, cluster designation (for antigens); CH50, 50% hemolyzing dose of complement; G-CSF, granulocyte colony-stimulating factor; hyper-IgE, hyperimmunoglobulin E; SLE, systemic lupus erythematosus; WAS, Wiskott–Aldrich syndrome protein.

[a]OMIM (Online Mendelian Inheritance in Man) access via WWW portal at http://www.ncbi.nlm.nih.gov/omim.

PART II Clinical Syndromes and Cardinal Features of Infectious Diseases: Approach to Diagnosis and Initial Management

SECTION R Infections in Patients with Deficient Defenses

EVALUATION OF A CHILD WITH RECURRENT INFECTIONS

History

A detailed history is the most powerful evaluation tool, and should gather information using all available sources, including medical records, parent or patient interviews, radiographs, and laboratory test results. Information is assembled into a chronology of data and events to determine whether episodes of illness have been characterized well enough to confirm that the patient truly has had recurrent infections. Additional important considerations are whether treatment of infectious episodes was appropriate, response to treatment was as expected, or other explanations for "infections" exist (e.g., fever from inflammatory rather than infectious disease).

Medical History

A description of each infectious episode is obtained, specifically: (1) date, duration, and site of infection; (2) how the diagnosis was established (i.e., specific cultures and diagnostic tests performed and their results); (3) severity of the episode (shock, tissue destruction, ventilator support, end-organ damage); (4) what treatment (need for parenteral or prolonged) was used and responses to specific treatments; (5) need for surgical intervention and quality of wound healing; and (6) temporal relationships to previous episodes. This level of detail often necessitates a prolonged interview, but is crucial for establishing whether an immunodeficiency is likely. Additional helpful details of the patient's history include immunizations administered and any clinical illnesses associated with them, pattern of growth and development, medications given (including long-term antibiotic use) and their effect on course of disease, compliance with treatments, presence of conditions that can predispose to or masquerade as infections, unusual blood phenotypes (e.g., McLeod phenotype in chronic granulomatous disease, Bombay phenotype in leukocyte adhesion deficiency type II), and healing pattern after skin and soft-tissue infection, injuries or surgery. If infections have been localized around an anatomic site, details should be obtained to focus on foreign-body aspiration, injuries or surgery at the site, medical problems involving the site, and timing of onset of infections relative to other events.

Historical details that decrease concern for a primary immunodeficiency are rapid responses to appropriate therapy, rapid resolution (versus suppression) of infected foci, healing without scarring, and inability to document infection. Details that are difficult to assess are poorly documented "infections," "infections" in the presence of allergic inflammation, and infections occurring in association with underlying conditions.

The category of microorganisms (and certain sentinel organisms) causing infections can suggest specific disorders (Table 103-7). Recurrent infections with extracellular, encapsulated microorganisms or chronic sinopulmonary infections frequently occur in people with asplenia, antibody deficiency conditions, or pattern recognition molecule (e.g., mannose-binding lectin or toll-like receptor) dysfunction. Deep fungal infections, multiple liver abscesses, or osteomyelitis suggest a phagocytic cell disorder. Recurrent infections accompanied by autoimmune symptoms or recurrent infections with *Neisseria meningitidis* suggest complement deficiencies. Recurrent infections due to opportunistic viral, protozoal, bacterial, mycobacterial, or fungal agents suggest T-lymphocyte deficiency. Unusual susceptibility to human papillomavirus infections occurs in WHIM (warts, hypogammaglobulinemia, infections, myelokathexis) syndrome and severe/disseminated mycobacterial infections are seen in defects related to interferon (IFN)-γ production/signaling.

Family History

Specific questions regarding the parents' ethnic heritage, the likelihood of parental consanguinity, early childhood deaths in the two previous generations, and gender bias in medical problems should be asked. Survival and significant illnesses and hospitalizations in all family members within two previous generations should be documented, as well as occurrence of peculiar infections or certain syndromes (particularly collagen vascular diseases and lymphoreticular malignancy) or both. Consanguinity or close ethnic heritage of the parents, occurrence of multiple early childhood deaths (particularly of male sex) in the family, serious infections in other family members, or presence of recognized syndromes in other family members (e.g., discoid lupus in heterozygous carriers for X-linked chronic granulomatous disease) heighten concern. Collagen vascular diseases in family members (associated with some complement deficiency states) and the presence of lymphoreticular malignancies (associated with a variety of immunodeficiency diseases[19]) are noteworthy.

Birth History

Both congenital anatomic malformations and primary immunodeficiency disorders can manifest within days to weeks of birth. History is sought about the mother's prenatal care, prenatal illnesses and exposures, and the infant's length of gestation and peripartum problems, delayed separation of the umbilical stump (leukocyte adhesion deficiency type I), requirement for blood transfusion (graft vs. host disease), and need for ventilator support.

TABLE 103-7. Sentinel Pathogens of Infections and Associated Conditions

Infectious Agent	Condition
Mucoid *Pseudomonas aeruginosa*	Cystic fibrosis
Nocardia spp., *Aspergillus* spp.	Chronic granulomatous disease
Burkholderia cepacia pneumonia	Chronic granulomatous disease, cystic fibrosis
Recurrent *Neisseria* spp. infections	Terminal complement component deficiency
Escherichia coli bloodstream infection	Galactosemia
Deep *Candida* spp. infection	Myeloperoxidase deficiency
Disseminated *Mycobacterium* spp. infection	T-lymphocyte deficiency, IFN-γ receptor deficiency, IL-12 defects
Pneumocystis jirovecii	T-lymphocyte deficiency
Recurrent/severe *Streptococcus pneumoniae* bloodstream infection	Asplenia, hemoglobinopathy, agammaglobulinemia, mannose-binding lectin deficiency, IRAK4 deficiency
Recurrent/severe *Staphylococcus aureus* infection	Chronic granulomatous disease, hyper-IgE/recurrent infection syndrome, Chédiak–Higashi syndrome, IRAK4 deficiency

IFN, interferon; IgE, immunoglobulin E.

Historical details of concern include lack of prenatal care, maternal drug use or multiple sexual partners (human immunodeficiency virus or other congenital infection), presence of congenital malformations, absence of a thymic shadow on a neonatal chest radiograph, perinatal blood transfusion, perinatal ventilator therapy (resulting in chronic lung disease), onset of infection in the first days of life, intracranial hemorrhage (resulting in dysfunction of hypothalamic temperature regulation), prenatal exposure to a teratogen, and the need for surgical removal of the umbilical stump. Separation of the umbilical stump normally occurs within 14 days, but assiduous umbilical cord care (aggressive application of triple dye and isopropyl alcohol to "keep the cord stump clean") can lead to its desiccation and failure to separate.

Social History

Because frequency of infection in small children mirrors frequency of exposure, details are sought of the patient's contacts with other children (e.g., siblings, classmates, playmates in childcare, nursery school, playgroups) that increase the frequency of exposures. In addition, exposure to tobacco smoke or other environmental pollutants affects infection rates and symptomatology, particularly in association with underlying atopy.

Review of the patient's dietary habits should include caloric intake and raw egg ingestion (excessive intake of avidin can lead to nutritional biotin deficiency). The length of time at the current residence, the type and duration of parental employment, and the child's daily activities or school performance can yield insights into the continuity of medical care. The impact that "recurrent infections" has had on the child and family gives a measure of their severity.

Review of Systems

The review of systems should focus on infection by organ systems involved. Skin, mouth, nasopharynx, lungs, and gastrointestinal tract are sites of constant contact with the microbially contaminated external environment and, therefore, are common sites of infection. The liver, spleen, and lungs provide defenses against systemic spread of infection and as a result can become sites of infection. The occurrence of cutaneous abscesses and extent of scarring when wounds heal, rashes (e.g., discoid lupus), rhinitis, dermatitis (generalized or localized, particularly behind the ears and in the diaper area), and paronychia provide clues to underlying disorders and the integrity of skin defenses. Questions about sinusitis, seasonal allergies, allergic shiners, snoring, and sleep disturbance (i.e., upper-airway obstruction) explore the possibility of an allergic diathesis. Gingivitis, periodontal disease, retained primary teeth, and aphthous stomatitis can be associated with specific primary immunodeficiency disorders. Focused questioning about pneumonia, diarrhea, perirectal or pararectal abscess, liver abscess, lymphadenitis, and bloodstream infections can reveal details sometimes missed in general review of systems.

Physical Examination

Points to be addressed by the physical examination are: (1) the physical status of the patient; (2) the presence of physical findings that confirm points of history; and (3) previously unrecognized but significant physiologic or anatomic abnormalities. Specific considerations during the physical examination are shown in Box 103-4.

Screening Laboratory Tests

If the history and physical findings are consistent with an anatomic cause of infection or the presence of an underlying condition, laboratory evaluation of the patient is directed at either defining the anatomic problem or diagnosing the underlying condition. If the history and physical findings do not point to a cause for recurrent, significant infections, a screening laboratory analysis (Table 103-8) provides a reasonable first evaluation.

BOX 103-4. Specific Considerations During the Physical Examination

- **Reconcile vital signs with historical details (e.g., normal pulse and respiratory rate despite significant lung disease infers physiologic compensation and, therefore, chronicity)**
- **Assess general habitus, growth, development (chronically ill versus robust; developmental delay; dysmorphism suggesting a genetic syndrome)**
- **Seek markers for atopy, nasopharyngeal lymphoid hyperplasia, or both**
- **Identify lymphoid tissue (absence of palpable or visible lymphoid tissue suggesting T-lymphocyte deficiency)**
- **Examine for midline defects in the head, neck, spine, or sacrum; or the presence of glucose-containing rhinorrhea**
- **Examine for scarring of tympanic membranes**
- **Examine for gingivitis, ulcerations, tooth loss, or periodontal disease (typical of immunodeficiency)**
- **Seek cutaneous stigmata:**
  Petechiae (suggesting Wiskott–Aldrich syndrome)
  Skin or conjunctival telangiectases (ataxia–telangiectasia syndrome)
  Eczematoid rash (Wiskott–Aldrich syndrome, hyperimmunoglobulinemia (hyper-Ig) E syndrome)
  Seborrhea-like dermatitis localized behind the ears (chronic granulomatous disease)
  Generalized seborrhea-like dermatitis (Langerhans histiocytosis, graft-versus-host disease, or T-lymphocyte deficiency)
  Nose-tip dermatitis (chronic granulomatous disease)
  Alopecia (graft-versus-host disease)
  Ectodermal dysplasia (anhidrotic ectodermal dysplasia with immunodeficiency)
  Cutaneous scars, with thin/poor formation at site of previous surgery or with tissue loss at site of previous infection (leukocyte defects)
- **Seek markers for chronic lung disease (pulmonary osteoarthropathy)**
- **Assess for acute or chronic sinus disease**
- **Identify the size of the liver and spleen**
- **Examine for pararectal inflammation, scarring from previous infections, or persistent inflammation**
- **Examine exhaustively any anatomic site where infections repeatedly localize, assessing normalcy of local anatomy and physiology**

Further Assessment

After the history, physical examination, and a screening laboratory evaluation have been completed, either the diagnosis will be clear and a plan of action can be proposed, or a diagnosis will be lacking and the decision must be made as to whether further, more detailed evaluation is appropriate. This decision is based on an overall impression of the severity, end-organ effects, documentation, and pathogens of the child's recurrent infections, family history, and physical findings. In the absence of repeated, documented infections in a patient in whom physical findings, growth and development, and appetite and activity are normal and the screening laboratory examination are unrevealing, the likelihood of a predisposing condition or immunodeficiency is remote and the child is assessed as "normal but unlucky." Prospective observation and documentation should be planned, and reassurance given.

Problems may resolve spontaneously or documentation of continuing problems may reveal their cause or lead to a need for specialized evaluation. If there are major incongruities between

PART II Clinical Syndromes and Cardinal Features of Infectious Diseases: Approach to Diagnosis and Initial Management

SECTION R Infections in Patients with Deficient Defenses

TABLE 103-8. Screening Laboratory Tests and Their Purposes in the Evaluation of Immunodeficiency Disorders

Test	Purposes
Complete blood count; differential and platelet counts	Assess numbers and morphology of cellular blood elements: leukopenia, leukocytosis, anemia, neutropenia, lymphopenia, Howell–Jolly bodies, bizarre erythrocyte forms, leukocyte morphology, thrombocytopenia
Total lymphocyte, T-lymphocyte and B-lymphocyte quantification	CD3 marker is used to estimate total lymphocyte number by flow cytometry; CD4 and CD8 markers are used to estimate T-lymphocyte subsets; B-lymphocyte numbers are estimated using surface Ig expression or CD19 or CD20 markers
Skin testing	Simple assessment of cell-mediated immunity (T-lymphocyte function)
Serum immunoglobulin quantification (IgA, IgG, IgM, IgE)	Assess for hypergammaglobulinemia, hypogammaglobulinemia, agammaglobulinemia
IgG subclass determinations	Assess for specific subclass deficiency
Specific antibody determinations	Assess production of antibody in responses to tetanus or diphtheria toxoid immunization as well as boosting; assess quantitative isohemagglutinin levels

Assess for Underlying Conditions	Test
Cystic fibrosis	Sweat test
HIV	HIV serology (and PCR testing, depending on patient age)
Sickle-cell disease, thalassemia	Hemoglobin electrophoresis
Posteroanterior and lateral chest radiograph	Assess for chronic lung disease, foreign body, presence of thymus, situs inversus, anatomic abnormality, or end-organ damage. If anatomic definition is inadequate, consider chest computed tomography
Total hemolytic complement activity (CH50)[a]	Absence or low activity in terminal complement component deficiencies

CD, cluster designation (for antigens); CH50, 50% hemolyzing dose of complement; HIV, human immunodeficiency virus; Ig, immunoglobulin; PCR, polymerase chain reaction.

[a]*Test is altered easily and unpredictably by inappropriate specimen handling and/or poor laboratory technique.*

TABLE 103-9. Specific Testing Approaches for Immunodeficiency Disorders

Disorder	Possible Testing Approaches
Cytopenia	Bone marrow examination/histochemistry
	Cytokine, colony-stimulating factor levels
Antibody deficiency	In vitro antibody production (Ig isotypes and subclasses)
	Cytokine levels
	In vitro specific antibody production
	Bruton thymidine kinase gene
T-lymphocyte deficiency	Adenosine deaminase activity
	Nucleoside phosphorylase activity
	In vitro proliferation responses (mitogens and specific antigens)
	Cytokine, growth factor levels
	Skin biopsy, intestinal biopsy (graft-versus-host disease)
Phagocytic cell dysfunction	Bactericidal activity
	Respiratory burst activity (nitroblue tetrazolium reduction, superoxide, dihydrorhodamine 123 oxidation test, or H_2O_2 production)
	Chemotaxis
Complement deficiency	CH50
	Individual complement component quantitation
	Serum opsonic activity

CH50, 50% hemolyzing dose of complement; Ig, immunoglobulin.

physical findings, historical details, and laboratory results, or when an unexplained lack of continuity in patient care is obvious, Munchausen syndrome or Munchausen by proxy should be considered.[20]

Specialized Testing

If anatomic problems or underlying conditions are suspected, appropriate testing/imaging is pursued. If immunodeficiency is suspected or is likely, specialized, targeted testing is planned. Because the range of specialized testing is broad, an all-inclusive testing approach is both labor- and time-intensive, extremely costly, and inappropriate in most circumstances. Focused testing should be performed in a stepwise fashion, pursuing abnormalities uncovered by history, physical examination, and screening laboratory tests (Table 103-9).

Genetic Testing

Genetic testing is a powerful diagnostic tool in primary immunodeficiency disorders. Current information on characteristics and genetics of most disorders is available at the Online Mendelian Inheritance in Man (OMIM) website, accessible through the National Center for Biotechnology Information portal (www.ncbi.nlm.nih.gov/omim). The genes responsible for all of the known X-linked and most of the known autosomal primary immunodeficiency disorders have been elucidated. For the X-linked disorders (see Tables 103-4 through 103-6), one-third of new cases are due to new mutations,[21] and two-thirds are inherited, that is, passed through female carriers. Carriers of some X-linked conditions (X-linked severe combined immunodeficiency,[22] X-linked agammaglobulinemia,[23] Wiskott–Aldrich syndrome[24]) sometimes can be identified through the use of X-chromosome inactivation analysis,[25] because cells expressing the normal X chromosome have a survival advantage over cells expressing the abnormal X chromosome. Carriers are recognized because of their homogeneous X-chromosome expression pattern (except in situations of "extreme" lyonization).

In classic autosomal-recessive conditions, recurrence risks follow Mendelian inheritance. More than 100 genes have now been associated with primary immunodeficiency diseases.[9] Although the availability of appropriate gene probes or diagnostic methods for most currently recognized primary immunodeficiency syndromes makes their diagnosis easier than in the past, clinical suspicion remains the fulcrum for testing. In some instances, the suspicion only arises after the death of an index patient; if specimens of tissues are appropriately preserved, genetic testing can be performed postmortem.

MANAGEMENT

When a child is identified with an anatomic abnormality, an underlying condition, or a recognizable primary immunodeficiency disorder, management is based on existing knowledge about the specific condition, as described in subsequent chapters. Management is more difficult for patients whose history or physical findings are suggestive of a defect but diagnostic testing is

104 Infectious Complications of Antibody Deficiency

Elisabeth E. Adderson

Antibodies play a central role in protective immunity against bacterial and certain viral infections. Immunoglobulin (Ig) molecules consist of two identical light chains and two identical heavy chains held together by disulfide bonds. The antigen-binding amino-terminal ends of the heavy (H) and light (L) chains are unique for each B-lymphocyte clone and are termed the variable regions. The carboxyl-terminal portions of these chains are the same for each of several classes (isotypes) or subclasses and are called constant regions. There are two types of light chains (κ and λ) and five classes of heavy chains (IgG, IgA, IgM, IgD, and IgE). There are also subclasses of IgG (IgG1, IgG2, IgG3, and IgG4) and of IgA (IgA1 and IgA2).

Antibodies bind to specific antigens on the surface of pathogens via the variable region of the Ig molecule. The constant region then performs an effector function, such as activation of complement, binding to a phagocytic cell, or antibody-dependent cell-mediated cytotoxicity. In some circumstances, the antigen-specific binding region functions alone by blocking the binding of a toxin or an infectious agent to the surface of a target cell.

B lymphocytes develop from a pluripotent precursor stem cell to IgM-expressing immature cell in the bone marrow, a process that does not require contact with antigen. Further maturation to an IgM/IgD-expressing mature B lymphocyte and to memory B or plasma cells takes place in peripheral lymphoid organs. Genes encoding Ig heavy-chain constant regions are arranged on chromosome 14 in the order: Cμ (IgM), Cγ3 (IgG3), Cγ1, (IgG1), Cα1 (IgA1), Cγ2 (IgG2), Cγ4 (IgG4), Cε (IgE), and Cα2 (IgA2). When naive B lymphocytes bind antigen, they are stimulated to differentiate. Beginning about a week after antigen stimulation, activated B lymphocytes can undergo a change in isotype expression from IgM to IgG, IgA, or IgE. Different antibody isotypes are more or less efficient at providing effector functions such as opsonization, complement activation, and antibody-dependent cell-mediated cytotoxicity. Simultaneously with isotype switching, genes encoding variable regions can undergo somatic hypermutation, a process that increases the affinity of antigen binding by antibody. Re-exposure to an antigen results in an accelerated memory (or secondary) immunologic response – this is the basis of "booster" vaccinations.

Antibody-mediated or humoral immunity is particularly important in the defense against infection caused by polysaccharide-encapsulated bacteria such as *Streptococcus pneumoniae* and *Haemophilus influenzae*, as well as some viral (poliovirus, non-polio enteroviruses) and protozoan (*Giardia lamblia*) pathogens. In some antibody deficiency disorders, such as X-linked agammaglobulinemia (XLA), immunodeficiency is present prenatally but transplacental transfer of maternal IgG in pregnancy protects against infection in the first several months of life. Children typically become symptomatic in the first 1 to 2 years of life after passive immunity wanes. The onset of other disorders, such as common variable immunodeficiency (CVID), can be delayed until adolescence or adulthood and immunodeficiency may be progressive.

unrevealing. Such patients often require management based more on skilled judgment and careful reassessment than on scientific knowledge. It is important to emphasize to parents that, although negative diagnostic test results cannot exclude all potential underlying conditions, they eliminate specific serious conditions; this

information can be comforting and helpful. In addition, delineating a specific plan for ongoing observation communicates a commitment to the child's wellbeing, which will help to ensure adherence to medically recommended interventions and continued contact with the patient.

The classification of primary antibody deficiencies was updated in 2009 by the International Union of Immunological Societies (Table 104-1) and diagnostic criteria for some of these disorders have been published.[1,2] Normal antibody synthesis and deficiencies are depicted in Figure 104-1.

APPROACH TO THE PATIENT WITH SUSPECTED ANTIBODY DEFICIENCY

A primary antibody deficiency should be considered in children with recurrent or chronic sinopulmonary infections, particularly in association with (1) poor growth, (2) unusual or unusually severe infections, (3) chronic or recurrent diarrhea, (4) a family history of recurrent and severe infections or of early childhood deaths, or (5) granulomatous or autoimmune disease (see Chapter 103, Evaluation of the Child with Suspected Immunodeficiency). Physical features suggesting humoral immunodeficiency include absent or small lymph nodes and tonsils, chronic lymphadenopathy, a dermatomyositis-like rash or hypertrophic osteoarthropathy.

Timely diagnosis of primary antibody deficiency and institution of immunoglobulin replacement therapy reduces the morbidity and mortality associated with these disorders.[3] Quantitative serum immunoglobulin concentrations should be compared with normal values for age and reduced levels of IgG, IgM, or IgA should prompt additional investigations. B lymphocytes are quantified by flow cytometry. The ability to generate a specific antibody response is assessed by measuring serum isohemagglutinins (naturally occurring antibodies to ABO blood group antigens) and antigen-specific serum antibody concentrations before and after vaccination. Quantifying IgG subclasses may be helpful in some cases but the wide range of normal values and an inconsistent correlation between low serum concentrations and clinical disease complicate the interpretation of results. A definitive diagnosis is possible for disorders caused by known genetic mutations. Carrier detection and prenatal diagnosis also is possible in some cases.

Patients with primary antibody deficiencies and severe symptoms should receive immunoglobulin replacement therapy, which reduces the rate and severity of infections. Ideally, trough serum IgG concentrations (immediately before the next administration of immunoglobulin) should be within the normal range of healthy persons.[4] Increasing use has been made of rapid subcutaneous infusion and home Ig infusion programs.[5] Immunoglobulin replacement therapy does not prevent all infections, perhaps due to quantitative and qualitative differences in IgG preparations.[5] Signs and symptoms of infection should be evaluated promptly and breakthrough infections treated aggressively. Some patients, particularly those with frequent or chronic respiratory infections, may benefit from prophylactic antibacterial therapy. Patients with CD40L deficiency (X-linked hyper-IgM syndrome, XHIM) have an increased susceptibility to *Pneumocystis jirovecii* infection and should receive trimethoprim-sulfamethoxazole or

TABLE 104-1. Immunodeficiencies Predominantly Involving Antibody Deficiency

Immunologic Finding	Serum Immunoglobulins	Circulating B Lymphocytes	Condition	Genetic Defect	Phenotype
All Ig isotypes severely reduced with low or absent B lymphocytes (agammaglobulinemias)	All isotypes decreased, no specific antibody responses	Low or absent	X-linked agammaglobulinemia Autosomal recessive agammaglobulinemia	*Btk* *Cμ, Igα, Igβ, CD179B(λ5), BLNK, LRRC8*	Recurrent and severe bacterial infections, chronic diarrhea, malabsorption, chronic enteroviral infection
Severe reduction in one or more Ig isotypes with normal or low numbers of B lymphocytes (common variable immunodeficiencies)	IgG decreased, IgA usually decreased, IgM variable, no or poor specific antibody responses	Normal or low	Common variable immunodeficiency	Most unknown, *TNFRSF13B(TACI), ICOS, CD19, TNFRSF13C(BAFF-R), Msh5*	Recurrent infections; autoimmune disorders; malignancy
Reduced IgG and IgA with variable IgM and normal numbers of B lymphocytes (hyper-IgM syndromes, class switch recombination defects)	IgG, IgA decreased; normal or elevated IgM No specific IgG response	Normal	CD40L deficiency CD40 deficiency	*CD40L* *CD40*	Recurrent and severe bacterial infections; *Pneumocystis jirovecii* infection; severe *Cryptosporidium* infection; parvovirus-induced aplastic anemia
			AID deficiency, UNG deficiency	*AICDA, UNG*	Opportunistic infections uncommon, lymphoid hyperplasia prominent; autoimmune disorders
Isotype or light chain deficiency with normal numbers of B lymphocytes	Variable	Variable	Ig heavy-chain deletions κ light-chain deficiency Isolated IgG subclass deficiency IgA with IgG subclass deficiency Selective IgA deficiency	*IgCH* *Cκ* Unknown Unknown Unknown	Usually asymptomatic Asymptomatic Most asymptomatic; recurrent infections Recurrent infections Most asymptomatic; recurrent infections; allergic and autoimmune disorders
Specific antibody deficiency with normal Ig concentrations and normal B lymphocyte numbers	IgG, IgM, IgA normal; IgG subclasses normal; impaired response to polysaccharide antigens	Normal	Specific antibody deficiency	Unknown	Recurrent or invasive bacterial infection
Transient hypogammaglobulinemia of infancy	IgG decreased, IgA and IgM variable	Usually normal		None	Recurrent infection; rarely, invasive bacterial infections

other effective prophylaxis. Vaccines composed of live-attenuated virus vaccines should not be administered to patients suspected of having a primary antibody deficiency.

ALL Ig ISOTYPES SEVERELY REDUCED WITH LOW OR ABSENT B CELLS (AGAMMAGLOBULINEMIAS)

The prototype of antibody deficiency syndromes is X-linked agammaglobulinemia (XLA), which has an incidence of approximately 1 in 200,000 persons and accounts for about 85% of cases of agammaglobulinemia (Table 104-2).[1-3] Passively transferred maternal antibody protects patients with XLA from infection in the first few months of life. Thereafter, serum IgG, IgA, and IgM levels are very low (>2 SD below the mean value for age), and patients have very poor or no specific antibody responses following infection or immunization.[2] Over half of patients are symptomatic by 1 year of age and almost all by 5 years of age.[6] Circulating CD19+ B lymphocytes are absent or present in very low numbers (generally <2%). This feature may distinguish patients with XLA from those with transient hypogammaglobulinemia. Plasma cells

are absent from lymph nodes and bone marrow and lymph nodes and tonsils are absent or small. T lymphocytes are normal in both number and function. Neutropenia can occur in association with acute infections.[7]

Children with XLA have recurrent bacterial infections in infancy or early childhood, including otitis media, sinusitis, and pneumonia. Other invasive bacterial infections, such as septicemia, meningitis, and osteoarticular infections, also are common. Most infections are caused by encapsulated bacteria, particularly *H. influenzae* type b (Hib), *S. pneumoniae*, *Staphylococcus aureus*, and *Pseudomonas* spp. Up to 50% of adults and a smaller proportion of children with XLA experience chronic diarrhea, steatorrhea, or malabsorption. In some cases, these symptoms have been associated with chronic rotavirus and *Giardia lamblia* infections.[8,9] Enteritis due to *Salmonella* spp. and *Campylobacter jejuni* is more common in patients with XLA than in healthy people.[10] Persistent *Mycoplasma* and *Ureaplasma* infections of the respiratory tract, joints, and urogenital tract also occur.

An exception to the general rule that antibody deficiencies lead primarily to greater susceptibility to bacterial, but not viral, infection is the occurrence of severe and chronic enteroviral infections

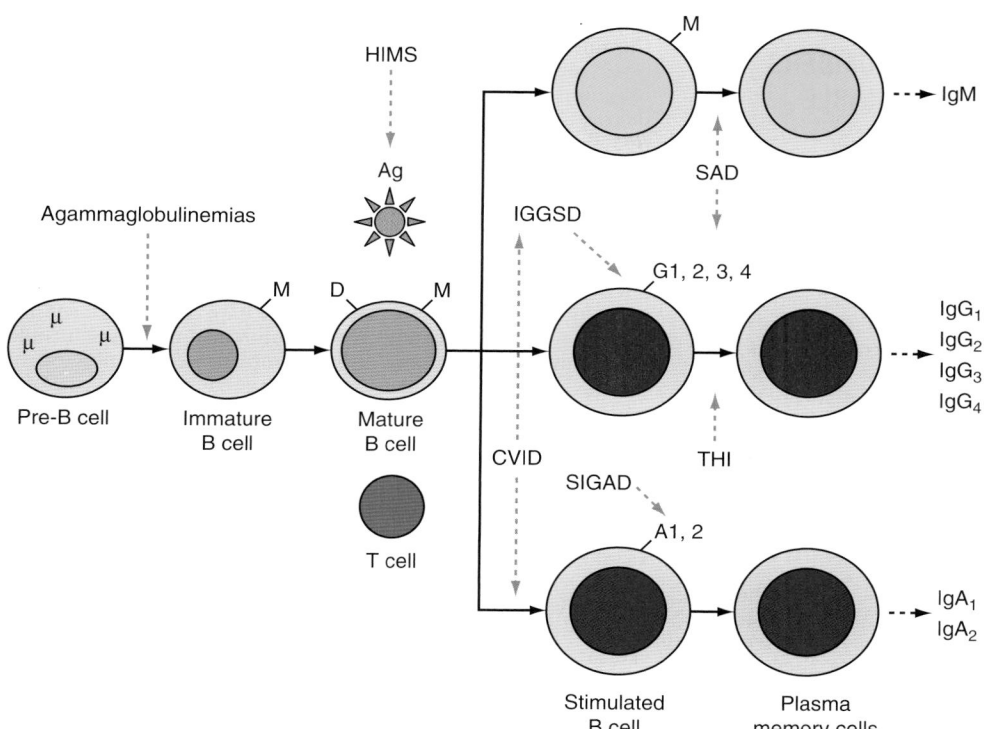

Figure 104-1. Normal antibody synthesis and primary deficiencies. μ, heavy chain of immunoglobulin (Ig) M; M, IgM; G, IgG; A, IgA; D, IgD; Ag, antigen; CVID, common variable immunodeficiency; IGGSD, IgG subclass deficiency; HIMS, hyper-IgM syndromes; SAD, specific antibody deficiency; SIGAD, selective IgA deficiency; THI, transient hypogammaglobulinemia of infancy.

in patients with XLA. Chronic enteroviral meningoencephalitis often has an insidious onset with ataxia, loss of cognitive skills, and paresthesias, or can manifest more acutely with fever, headache, and seizures.[11] Cerebrospinal fluid (CSF) pleocytosis with a lymphocytic predominance, increased protein levels and, frequently, decreased glucose levels is typical, although some children have normal or mildly abnormal findings. CSF abnormalities tend to worsen with clinical exacerbations. Enteroviral meningoencephalitis can be the initial manifestation of XLA and can occur despite intravenous IgG (IGIV) therapy. In regions of the world where wild-type or vaccine strain poliovirus strains circulate or live attenuated oral poliovirus vaccine is administered, patients

with XLA are at risk of paralytic disease.[12] Some individuals with chronic enteroviral infections develop a dermatomyositis-like syndrome characterized by muscle weakness, edema, and woody induration of the skin, and a violaceous rash over the extensor surfaces of joints.[11] The syndrome often is accompanied by hepatitis.

XLA is caused by mutations in the Bruton agammaglobulinemia tyrosine kinase (BTK) gene, *Btk*, which is required for the normal differentiation of pro-B cells to pre-B cells and mature B lymphocytes.[13,14] A family history of male relatives with recurrent infections is common; however, about half of patients represent new mutations. Over 600 distinct mutations have been described, some of which are associated with relatively mild clinical manifestations.[15] The severity of infectious complications also can differ among family members with the same mutation.

Approximately 10% to 15% of patients with a clinical history and laboratory findings consistent with XLA are females or males who do not have mutations in *Btk*.[1,16] As in XLA, these patients have low or absent serum Ig, poor specific antibody responses, and low or absent numbers of peripheral blood CD19+ B lymphocytes. Mutations in genes encoding the IgM heavy-chain constant region gene, *Cμ*, the surrogate light-chain complex *CD179B* (λ5), the Ig-associated alpha *CD79A* (*Igα*) and beta *CD79B* (*Igβ*), leucine-rich repeat-containing protein 8A (*LRRC8*), and the Ig-associated and B-lymphocyte linker protein (*BLNK*) have been reported to cause autosomal-recessive agammaglobulinemia.[17-22]

Patients with agammaglobulinemia and chronic enteroviral meningoencephalitis are treated with higher doses of IgG than other patients with agammaglobulinemia (to maintain trough levels of >1000 mg/dL) or with plasma or immune serum known to have high antibody titers to the enterovirus causing the infection.[11] Intrathecal IGIV also has been used. Aggressive and prolonged treatment of bacterial infections is critical. The prognosis of XLA has greatly improved with IGIV therapy, particularly when it is initiated at an early age. The most common causes of death remain chronic enteroviral and pulmonary infections. Prenatal diagnosis and carrier detection are possible if the mutation is known.

TABLE 104-2. Agammaglobulinemia

Onset	Infancy, early childhood
Clinical presentation	Recurrent respiratory and invasive infections, especially *Haemophilus influenzae* type b, *Streptococcus pneumoniae*
	Chronic diarrhea, malabsorption, chronic *Giardia* and rotavirus
	Chronic enteroviral meningoencephalitis, poliomyelitis, dermatomyositis-like syndrome
	Neutropenia with infection
	Lymph nodes and tonsils absent or small
Diagnosis	IgG, IgM and IgA more than 2 SD below mean for age
	Peripheral blood CD19+ B cells <2%
	Poor specific antibody responses, isohemagglutinins
	Mutation in *Btk*(X); rarely, mutations in *Cμ, Igα, Ig, CD179B(5), BLNK, LRRC8* (AR)
Treatment	Ig replacement

AR, autosomal recessive; Ig, immunoglobulin; SD, standard deviation; X, X-linked.

PART II Clinical Syndromes and Cardinal Features of Infectious Diseases: Approach to Diagnosis and Initial Management

SECTION R Infections in Patients with Deficient Defenses

SEVERE REDUCTION IN ONE OR MORE Ig ISOTYPES WITH NORMAL OR LOW NUMBERS OF B LYMPHOCYTES (COMMON VARIABLE IMMUNODEFICIENCY DISORDERS)

The common variable immunodeficiency (CVID) disorders are a heterogeneous group of disorders characterized by low serum Ig concentrations, defective production of specific antibodies, and an increased susceptibility to respiratory and gastrointestinal tract infections (Table 104-3).[2,23] CVID affects 1 in 25,000 to 1 in 75,000 persons and has an equal prevalence in males and females. Persons with CVID have serum total IgG concentration more than 2 SD below the mean for their age and impaired specific antibody responses.[2,23] Many also have IgA, IgM, or IgG subclass deficiencies. Numbers of peripheral B lymphocytes may be normal, reduced or even increased. The failure to produce antibodies in response to a known infection or vaccination is characteristic of CVID. Most patients fail to produce a fourfold increase in specific IgG to both protein and polysaccharide antigens. Immunodeficiency can be progressive.[23] CVID can develop in persons who initially manifest with clinical and laboratory findings suggestive of selective IgA or IgG subclass deficiencies.

Symptoms are unusual in children under 2 years of age, but bimodal peaks of incidence occur at ages 2 through 5 and 16 through 28 years.[24,25] Patients most commonly have recurrent sinopulmonary infection, chiefly due to bacteria such as *S. pneumoniae*, *Haemophilus influenzae*, *Moraxella catarrhalis*, and *Mycoplasma pneumoniae*.[24–26] Serious invasive bacterial infections occur in 10% to 25% of children.[25] Recurrent pneumonia sometimes progresses to bronchiectasis. Enteric infections caused by *Giardia*, *C. jejuni*, and *Salmonella* spp. also are frequent and can be more

severe and prolonged than in immunocompetent people.[24,27] Chronic genitourinary tract, joint, and systemic infections caused by *Mycoplasma* spp. have been described. Although most viral infections are not unusually severe in patients with CVID, an increased frequency or severity of hepatitis C virus, cytomegalovirus, measles, and varicella-zoster virus infection has been reported.[23–25,27] Complications of enteroviral infection, including chronic encephalomyelitis and dermatomyositis-like syndrome, have been reported in people with CVID, although less frequently than in XLA.[3]

Allergic symptoms are found in over 30% of children and adolescents with CVID.[25] Inflammatory or autoimmune diseases occur in 20% to 35% of patients and may cause more serious morbidity than infections. Lower respiratory disorders include granulomatous pulmonary disease, lymphocytic interstitial pneumonitis, and lymphadenopathy. Inflammatory bowel disease, lymphonodular hyperplasia, or nonspecific malabsorption affect up to 25% of patients and hematologic disorders such as autoimmune thrombocytopenia, hemolytic anemia, neutropenia, and pernicious anemia occur in 10%. About a quarter of patients have significant growth retardation.[25] The incidence of some cancers, particularly lymphomas and gastric carcinoma, is markedly elevated. Malignancies are uncommon in childhood.[25]

The genetic basis of most CVID is not known. Approximately 25% of cases are familial.[28] Relatives of patients with CVID may have decreased levels of total IgA, IgG subclasses, or both, or an increased incidence of autoimmune disease. Molecular defects described in patients with a CVID phenotype include mutations in genes encoding the transmembrane activator and CAML interactor (*TNFRSF13B/TACI*; autosomal-recessive inheritance, also observed in selective IgA deficiency), T-lymphocyte inducible costimulator (ICOS; autosomal-recessive inheritance), CD19, BAFF receptor (*TNFRSF13C*), and the DNA mismatch repair protein Msh5.[29–33] Other conditions causing antibody failure, including the X-linked and autosomal agammaglobulinemias, class switch recombination defects and X-linked lymphoproliferative disease, and "leaky" severe combined immunodeficiency syndromes, can manifest a CVID-like picture.[34–37] These, and secondary causes of hypogammaglobulinemia (drugs, chromosomal abnormalities, infection, malignancy, systemic illnesses), must be excluded. Current diagnostic criteria restrict CVID to children who are over 4 years of age in part due to the need to exclude other immunodeficiencies that manifest earlier in life.[2,23]

Most patients with CVID require antibody replacement using IGIV. Prophylactic antibiotics may benefit some patients, particularly those with recurrent respiratory infections and bronchiectasis. Patients require careful monitoring for autoimmune and lymphoproliferative complications.

TABLE 104-3. Common Variable Immunodeficiency

Onset	2 years to adult
Clinical presentation	Recurrent and severe sinopulmonary infections, especially *Streptococcus pneumoniae*, *Haemophilus influenzae*
	Gastrointestinal infections, especially *Giardia*, *Campylobacter jejuni*, *Salmonella* spp.
	Chronic *Mycoplasma* infection
	Severe infections due to hepatitis C, CMV, VZV, enteroviruses
	Autoimmune and inflammatory disorders (gastrointestinal lymphoid hyperplasia, inflammatory bowel disease, autoimmune cytopenias, arthritis, vasculitis)
	Lymphoid hyperplasia, splenomegaly, peripheral lymphadenopathy
	Increased risk of lymphoma, gastric carcinoma
Diagnosis	IgG usually more than 2 SD below mean for age; young children may present with progressive IgG subclass deficiency
	IgA usually >2 SD below mean for age, IgM normal or low
	Peripheral blood CD19+ B lymphocytess normal or reduced
	Poor specific antibody responses, absent isohemagglutinins
	Most genetic defects unknown, mutations in ICOS (AR), CD19 (AR), TNFRSF13B(TACI) (AD, AR, complex), TNFRSF13C(BAFFr) (AR), Msh5
Treatment	Ig replacement

AD, autosomal dominant; AR, autosomal recessive; CMV, cytomegalovirus; Ig, immunoglobulin; SD, standard deviation; VZV, varicella-zoster virus; X, X-linked.

REDUCED IgG AND IgA WITH VARIABLE IgM AND NORMAL NUMBERS OF B CELLS (HYPER-IgM SYNDROMES, CLASS SWITCH RECOMBINATION DEFECTS)

Children with hyper-IgM (HIM) syndromes have recurrent or serious infections in the first 5 years of life, absent or low levels of serum IgG, normal or elevated serum IgM, absent or poor specific immune responses, and normal or elevated numbers of B lymphocytes, but normal numbers of T lymphocytes (Table 104-4).[2]

Approximately 65% of cases are inherited in an X-linked recessive fashion, and are due to mutations of the gene encoding CD40L (*TNFSF5*).[38–40] Rare mutations of CD40 (*TNFRSF5*) cause a similar autosomal-recessive disorder.[41] B-lymphocyte signaling through CD40, which is required for isotype switching and the affinity maturation of antibody responses, are impaired in both CD40L and CD40 deficiency. A second autosomal-recessive disorder is caused by mutations of the activation-induced cytidine deaminase gene, *AICDA*.[42] A similar phenotype is caused by mutations of the gene encoding activation-induced cytidine deaminase,

TABLE 104-4. Class Switch Recombination Disorders (Hyper-IgM Syndromes)

Onset	Infancy, early childhood
Clinical presentation	Recurrent and severe sinopulmonary infections
	Severe or chronic *Cryptosporidium, Giardia*
	P. jirovecii infection in first year of life
	Neutropenia, parvovirus-induced aplastic anemia
	Autoimmune and lymphoproliferative disorders (sclerosing cholangitis, diabetes, arthritis, inflammatory bowel disease, uveitis)
Diagnosis	Serum IgG more than 2 SD below mean for age
	Absent specific IgG immune response, normal isohemagglutinins
	Normal or elevated B cells
	Normal T-cell numbers
	Absence of protein or mutation in *CD40L* (X), *CD40* (AR), *AICDA/UNG* (AR)
Treatment	Ig replacement, prophylaxis for *P. jirovecii* for patients with CD40L/CD40 deficiency, G-CSF for chronic neutropenia, hematopoietic stem cell transplant

AICDA, activation-induced cytosine deaminase; AR, autosomal recessive; G-CSF, granulocyte colony-stimulating factor; Ig, immunoglobulin; SD, standard deviation; UNG, uracil-DNA glycosylase; X, X-linked.

UNG. The protein products encoded by these genes are required for isotype switching from IgM to IgG and IgA. These disorders, therefore, are the result of a primary B-lymphocyte abnormality, rather than the defective interaction between B and T lymphocytes that is characteristic of CD40L and CD40 deficiency.

Patients with HIM have serum total IgG concentration greater than 2 SD below the mean for their age and impaired specific IgG responses, but most patients have normal isohemagglutinins, which are of the IgM isotype. Serum IgM levels are normal or increased. Circulating T- and B-lymphocyte numbers are within the normal range but T-lymphocyte proliferation is impaired in patients with CD40L and CD40 deficiency.

The median age at presentation of patients with CD40L and CD40 deficiency is 12 months.[43-45] That of AID deficiency is about 2 years, several years younger than patients with *UNG* deficiency. It is common for patients with *UNG* deficiency to have diagnosis delayed until adolescence or adulthood. Patients with CD40L/CD40 deficiency, who have both humoral and cellular immunodeficiencies, generally are more ill than patients with other antibody deficiency disorders.[43,46] Most patients have recurrent or severe bacterial infections, especially affecting the respiratory and gastrointestinal tracts. A predisposition to *P. jirovecii* pneumonia and to disseminated infections caused by *Cryptococcus*, cytomegalovirus, and herpes simplex virus infections distinguishes from other antibody deficiency disorders. Over half of patients have diarrhea, commonly associated with *Cryptosporidium, Salmonella*, or *Giardia*, and poor growth. Sclerosing cholangitis, sometimes progressing to cirrhosis, is common and can be idiopathic or a complication of *Cryptosporidium* infection. Neutropenia and anemia occur in 25% to 65% of patients; chronic anemia and pancytopenia occurs in association with human parvovirus B19 infection. Patients have a significantly increased risk of gastrointestinal and hepatic malignancies.

In contrast to CD40L and CD40 deficiency, opportunistic infections are uncommon in patients with *AICDA* and *UNG* deficiency. Lymphoid hyperplasia, especially of cervical lymph nodes and tonsils, is more pronounced than in CD40L/CD40 deficiency, especially in untreated patients. Autoimmune and inflammatory complications, including neutropenia, diabetes, arthritis, hepatitis, and inflammatory bowel disease, have been reported in approximately 20% of patients, including young children. Unlike CD40L/CD40 deficiency, there is no apparent increased risk of

malignancy; however, only small numbers of patients with these disorders have been identified and followed for long periods of time.

IgG replacement therapy is the mainstay for therapy of the class switch recombination defect disorders. Patients with CD40L and CD40 deficiency have an increased susceptibility to *P. jirovecii* infection and should receive trimethoprim-sulfamethoxazole or other effective prophylaxis. Patients should be counseled in regard to measures to prevent *Cryptosporidium* infections. Granulocyte colony-stimulating factor may be helpful in chronic neutropenia. Hematopoietic stem cell transplant may be curative – younger patients and those without liver disease appear to have the best outcomes.[47] Carrier detection and prenatal diagnosis are possible if the specific mutation is known.

ISOTYPE OR LIGHT CHAIN DEFICIENCIES WITH NORMAL NUMBERS OF B LYMPHOCYTES AND IMMUNOGLOBULIN HEAVY-CHAIN DELETION

Rarely, large deletions in the heavy-chain locus affect the expression of one or more heavy-chain constant regions.[48] Most affected people do not have significant problems with recurrent or severe infections and have relatively normal immune responses to vaccine antigens. Decreased serum concentrations of IgG1 or IgG2 and IgG4, with or without IgA1, IgA2, or IgE deficiency, are the most common abnormalities. Some subjects have elevated IgG1 or IgG3 levels, suggesting that this may compensate for the absence of other Ig isotypes.

IMMUNOGLOBULIN KAPPA-CHAIN DELETIONS

Individuals with partial or complete deficiencies of serum antibody containing kappa light chain have been described rarely.[49,50] Most patients are asymptomatic; lambda light chains appear to compensate for the absence of kappa light chains.

ISOLATED IgG SUBCLASS DEFICIENCY

Although the range of total IgG concentrations in serum from healthy adults is wide, the relative proportion of each of the IgG subclasses is constant. Normally, the composition of IgG is 60% to 65% IgG1, 20% to 25% IgG2, 5% to 10% IgG3, and 3% to 6% IgG4. Each IgG subclass rises to adult serum concentrations at a different rate, suggesting that they are regulated selectively during development. Differences in the various IgG subclass molecules are associated with functional differences in the ability to bind to receptors on phagocytic cells and activate complement.[51] Several biologic and technical problems have complicated the study of selective IgG subclass deficiencies and their clinical relevance. These include the wide range of normal values for each of the subclasses, marked differences among the subclasses in maturation to adult serum levels, and difficulties in the production of reliable reagents to quantify the different subclasses. IgG subclass deficiency (IgGSD) is defined as one or more serum IgG subclass levels greater than 2 SD below the mean for an individual's age but with normal total serum IgG and IgM levels (Table 104-5).[1] Absolute IgG subclass deficiency has been reported to result from mutations in individual genes in the IgG constant region. It is likely that defects in the regulation of expression of IgG subclasses are a more common cause.[52] Although some patients experience recurrent sinopulmonary infections or allergic or autoimmune disease, most are asymptomatic.[53-55] Some deficiencies resolve over time, suggesting that some children have a variant of transient hypogammaglobulinemia with delayed maturation of a particular IgG subclass. In some case series the risk of recurrent respiratory infections has correlated with impaired immune responses to polysaccharide antigens in children with IgG2 deficiency.[56]

Available evidence suggests that the ability to make specific antibody is most relevant to symptoms and prognosis in Ig subclass deficiency, and the evaluation should focus on this function. Patients must be managed according to their clinical status with

PART II Clinical Syndromes and Cardinal Features of Infectious Diseases: Approach to Diagnosis and Initial Management

SECTION R Infections in Patients with Deficient Defenses

TABLE 104-5. Isotype or Light Chain Deficiencies with Normal B-cell Numbers

Onset	Variable
Clinical presentation	Most asymptomatic
	Recurrent sinopulmonary infections (*Haemophilus influenzae* type b, *Streptococcus pneumoniae*) in patients with IgA + IgG subclass deficiency or, less frequently, with isolated IgG subclass deficiency
	Bacteremia (*H. influenzae* type b, *S. pneumoniae*) in patients with IgA + IgG subclass deficiency or, less frequently, with isolated IgG subclass deficiency
Diagnosis	≥1 IgG subclass more than 2 SD below mean for age
	Total IgG and IgM normal
	IgA normal or low
	Normal B-cell numbers
	Normal isohemagglutinins, antibody responses usually normal, impaired antipolysaccharide antibody responses may be present in IgG2 deficiency
	Most genetic defects unknown
Treatment	Usually none; may improve over time; Ig replacement in patients with recurrent or severe infections

Ig, immunoglobulin; SD, standard deviation.

TABLE 104-6. Specific Antibody Deficiency with Normal Ig Concentrations and Normal B-cell Numbers

Onset	Variable
Clinical presentation	Recurrent otitis media, sinopulmonary infections (*Haemophilus influenzae* type b, *Streptococcus pneumoniae*)
	Occasional serious invasive infection
	Allergic disease common
Diagnosis	Poor response to vaccination with polysaccharide antigen (<4-fold rise in serum specific IgG titer 4 weeks after vaccination or post-vaccination serum-specific IgG <1.3 g/mL)
	Normal serum total IgG, IgA, IgM
	B-cell numbers normal
Treatment	Prophylactic antibiotics, Ig replacement if severe or persistent

Ig replacement therapy reserved for patients with documented deficiencies of specific antibody responses and severe or recurrent infections.

SELECTIVE IgA DEFICIENCY

Selective IgA deficiency is defined as a serum IgA concentration of <0.07 g/L in the presence of normal total serum IgG and IgM levels (Table 104-5). Usually secretory IgA also is absent. Isolated IgA deficiency is the most common primary immunodeficiency, with an incidence ranging from 1 in 400 to 1 in 5000 persons in different ethnic populations. Young children may have a physiologic delay in IgA expression so the diagnosis of IgA deficiency should be deferred until age >4 years. Some cases of IgA deficiency are transient and may result from an exaggeration of this maturational delay. Secondary IgA deficiency has been reported as an adverse effect of anti-inflammatory and anticonvulsant drugs.

Most people with IgA deficiency have normal genes for the IgA heavy chain, and B lymphocytes expressing surface-positive IgA precursors usually are found in normal numbers. These B lymphocytes, however, have an immature phenotype and do not mature into plasma cells after antigen stimulation. Up to 20% of cases of selective IgA deficiency are hereditary. IgA deficiency, CVID, and IgG subclass deficiency have been reported in the same family, suggesting that these conditions may be part of a spectrum of abnormalities caused by the failure of appropriate signaling for B-lymphocyte maturation.[26]

Most people, even those with complete absence of IgA, do not have a recognizable increased susceptibility to infection. A third of patients, however, have recurrent infections, particularly of the respiratory tract. People with selective IgA deficiency have a higher incidence of autoimmune disorders than do the general population.[26,57]

As with IgG subclass deficiency, evaluation should focus on the patient's ability to generate specific antibody. Infections should be treated aggressively and some patients may benefit from prophylactic antibacterial therapy. Rare patients may benefit from Ig replacement therapy; however, minor amounts of IgA in IGIV preparations or other blood products can result in the development of anti-IgA antibodies and severe anaphylactic reactions in IgA-deficient patients.[58] Products low in IgA should be used if replacement therapy is necessary. In contrast to other primary antibody deficiency syndromes, routine vaccination with live attenuated viral vaccines is not contraindicated in selective IgA deficiency.

IgA DEFICIENCY WITH IgG SUBCLASS DEFICIENCY

Persons with IgA deficiency who also have associated deficiencies in IgG subclasses or specific antibody production have a greater predisposition to infection that those with selective IgA deficiency alone (Table 104-6). In addition to recurrent sinopulmonary infections, these patients have an increased risk of allergy, inflammatory gastrointestinal disease, and autoimmune disorders.[59,60] Deficiency of IgG2 is, in particular, associated with recurrent otitis media and sinopulmonary infections in children.[61] The most common associated defects associated with IgA deficiency are deficiencies of IgG4 (40%), IgG2 (28%), and IgG3 (17%). IgA, IgG4, and IgG2 deficiency sometimes are observed together. Patients should be evaluated and managed in the same manner as those with selective IgA deficiency.

SPECIFIC ANTIBODY DEFICIENCY WITH NORMAL IgG CONCENTRATIONS AND NORMAL B-LYMPHOCYTE NUMBERS

Patients with specific antibody deficiency (SAD) have poor responses to polysaccharide vaccines (specific serum IgG <1.3 µg/mL, or less than a fourfold rise in specific antibody levels 1 month after vaccination) with normal levels of serum Ig and IgG subclasses (Table 104-6). In children with allergic disease and recurrent respiratory infections, the incidence of SAD ranges from 0% to 10%; however, the incidence in the general population is not known.[62,63] The defect responsible for SAD has not been identified; some cases are familial.

Children with SAD typically present with recurrent bacterial infections. Otitis media and sinopulmonary infections are common and serious infections such as septicemia and meningitis can occur. Many children have associated allergic disease. The diagnosis of SAD in children is complicated by the physiologic delay in the development of specific immune responses to polysaccharide antigens and the poor standardization of laboratory testing for antipolysaccharide antibodies.[64] Responses of normal children younger than 2 years of age to polysaccharide antigens generally are poor, and responses to many of these antigens are unreliable until middle childhood. Serial testing over time often is required to conclude that a persistent deficiency exists. The natural history of the disorder is not well understood. Although antipolysaccharide antibody responses tend to improve with age, some patients progress to CVID.[65] Most children who fail to respond to immunization with polysaccharide vaccines have adequate responses to polysaccharide-protein conjugate formulations. Children with SAD and significant infections may benefit from a trial of prophylactic antibiotics. Ig replacement is considered if symptoms are severe and persistent.[66]

TRANSIENT HYPOGAMMAGLOBULINEMIA OF INFANCY

Passively transferred maternal IgG normally decreases with a half-life of 25 to 30 days, reaching a nadir at 3 to 6 months of age. After birth, a healthy infant actively begins making first IgM, then IgG, and last IgA. Sometimes the physiologic nadir of serum IgG concentrations is more persistent; this condition is called transient hypogammaglobulinemia of infancy (THI, Table 104-7). Because most transplacental transfer occurs during the third trimester, serum IgG in preterm infants can fall to very low concentrations and reach a nadir earlier than in infants born at term.

The incidence of THI has been estimated to be 20 to 60 per 100,000 live births,[67] and is slightly more common in males. Children come to attention with recurrent respiratory or gastrointestinal tract infections. Rare patients who have experienced invasive bacterial, fungal, or severe viral infections have been described. Infants with THI have normal numbers of circulating B lymphocytes and generally have normal specific immune responses. Low serum concentrations of IgA are present in up to 80% of patients and a smaller proportion of children has low serum IgM levels.

TABLE 104-7. Transient Hypogammaglobulinemia of Infancy

Onset	6 months to 3 years
Clinical presentation	Recurrent sinopulmonary and viral infections Rarely invasive bacterial infections
Diagnosis	IgG more than 2 SD below mean for age IgM usually normal, IgA variable B-lymphocyte numbers usually normal Usually normal specific antibody responses, isohemagglutinins Genetic defect unknown
Treatment	Usually none required, resolves by 2–4 years

SD, standard deviation.

The cause of the maturational delay in IgG production in THI is unknown. THI occurs with greater frequency in families with other immunodeficiency syndromes, but no specific genetic defects have been identified. THI is self-limited, with antibody concentrations normalizing by 2 to 4 years of age. The presence of invasive infections or poor specific anti-tetanus antibody responses at the time of presentation may identify children who will have more persistent immunodeficiency.[68] Most children with THI do not require specific treatment, but IGIV should be considered in children with frequent or severe infections. If initiated, the continued need for IGIV should be reassessed after 3 to 6 months.[27]

105 Infectious Complications of Complement Deficiencies

Michael M. Frank and Jerry A. Winkelstein

Complement, a part of the innate immune system, is comprised of over 30 plasma and cell membrane bound proteins that function cooperatively in antimicrobial and inflammatory reactions.[1-4] One of its most important roles is in the host's defense against infection.[4,5] These proteins are old in evolutionary terms and some of them were incorporated into the adaptive immune system as it developed to help promote a normal immune response.[6] This chapter reviews the biochemistry and biology of complement and its role in the host's defense against infection, and describes the infectious complications in individuals with inherited or acquired deficiencies of complement proteins.

BIOCHEMISTRY AND BIOLOGY OF COMPLEMENT

Most of the biologically significant effects of the complement system are mediated by the third component of complement (C3) and the late acting proteins (C5, C6, C7, C8, and C9). However, C3 and C5 through C9 must first be activated to generate their biologic activities. Three pathways are available by which C3 and C5 through C9 can be activated (Figure 105-1): the classical pathway, the alternative pathway, and the lectin pathway.[2,3]

The Classical Pathway

The classical pathway is so termed because it was the first pathway of activation studied. Activation of the classical pathway usually is initiated by antigen–antibody complexes.[7] Antibodies of the appropriate class (IgM or immunoglobulin G (IgG) subclass IgG1,

IgG2, IgG3) combine with microbial antigens to form an immune complex, which then binds and activates the first component of complement (C1). Only one molecule of pentameric IgM is needed for activation of C1. In contrast, two IgG molecules are necessary for C1 to bind and for activation to occur. The requirements for an IgG doublet greatly reduces the efficiency of IgG, compared with IgM, in activating C1 and the classical pathway, because thousands of IgG molecules may need to be deposited on a microbial surface in order for two of them to be aligned in close proximity.

C1 is a macromolecular complex composed of three biochemically distinct subcomponents, designated as C1q, C1r, and C1s. C1q binds to the immunoglobulin molecules in the immune complex.[2] This binding is followed by the cleavage of C1r and then cleavage of C1s. Activated C1s then cleaves both the fourth component of complement (C4) and the second component (C2), each into a smaller and a larger product. The larger fragment of C2 (C2a) remains complexed with the larger fragment of C4 (C4b) to form a bimolecular enzyme, C4b2a, which is responsible for activating C3 and initiating the assembly of the terminal components.

Because the classical pathway usually is activated by antibody, it is considered to be important especially in "acquired" immunity. However, some enveloped RNA viruses, some *Mycoplasma* species, and certain strains and species of both gram-negative and gram-positive bacteria bind C1q directly and activate the classical pathway.[5] Thus, under some circumstances, the classical pathway can be activated in an antibody-independent fashion and also functions in "natural" immunity.

PART II Clinical Syndromes and Cardinal Features of Infectious Diseases: Approach to Diagnosis and Initial Management

SECTION R Infections in Patients with Deficient Defenses

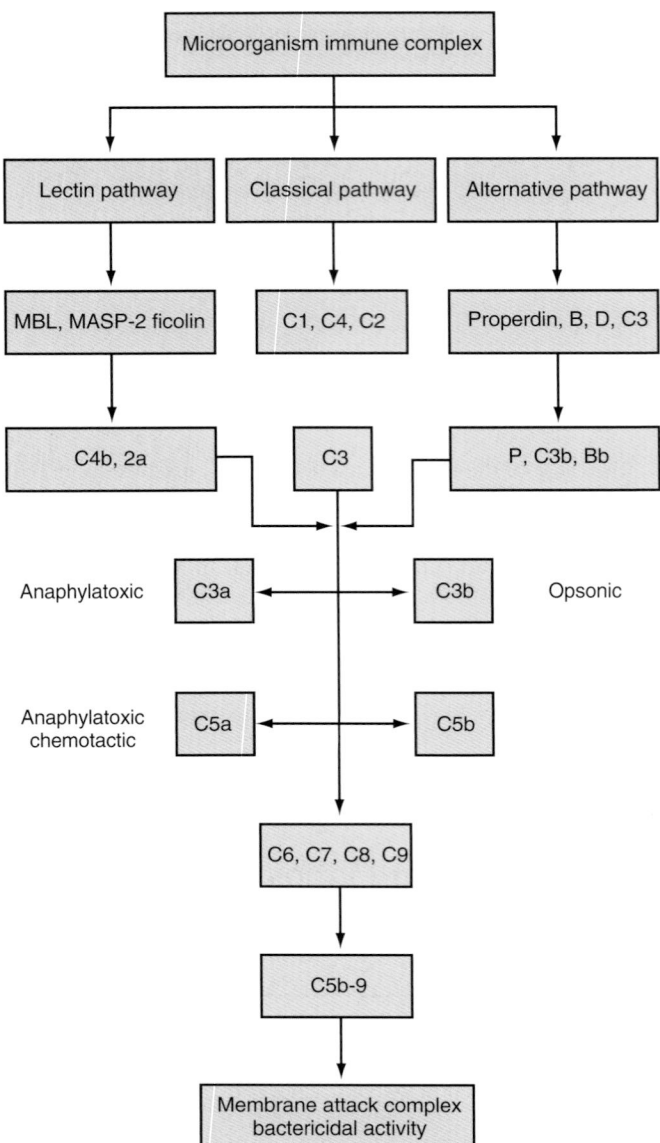

Figure 105-1. The complement system.

present on phagocytes and B cells, CD35 (sometimes termed complement receptor 1, CR1). Binding of microbes to CD35 markedly aids phagocytosis. The first step in C3b degradation leads to the decay fragment iC3b. This fragment with a cleaved α chain is recognized by the opsonization receptors CD11b/CD18 and CD11c/CD18, also termed CR3 and CR4. These receptors are deficient or abnormal in leukocyte adhesion deficiency (LAD). With the cleavage of the α chain this fragment no longer supports the continued activation of the complement cascade. This fragment is further degraded in several steps to the final fragment C3d recognized by CD21 (CR2), a receptor present on B cells and follicular dendritic cells and important in antigen processing and in immune response.

The Alternative Pathway

The alternative pathway provides an evolutionarily old and quite primitive innate immune defense mechanism.[6] Activation begins with the C3 molecule. Native C3 contains an internal thiol ester in its α chain that, under normal physiologic conditions, undergoes continuous low-grade hydrolysis to create a "C3b-like" molecule, $C3(H_2O)$.[2,3] $C3(H_2O)$ can bind a circulating alternative pathway protein factor B which allows its cleavage by a serine protease, factor D. Two cleavage products of factor B are generated, the larger Bb, and smaller Ba. The association of the hydrolyzed C3 with Bb creates a C3-cleaving enzyme, $C3(H_2O)Bb$ (termed the "priming" C3-convertase), which is responsible for a continuous, low-grade cleavage of C3 and hence, the generation of nascent C3b. If the nascent C3b binds covalently to a suitable surface, such as a bacterium, it can form a reversible complex with native factor B. This complex is cleaved by factor D to create a highly efficient C3-cleaving enzyme, C3bBb, termed the "amplification" C3-convertase.

Antibody is not required for the activation of the alternative pathway; however, antibody enhances activation.[2,7] Thus, the alternative pathway can participate in both innate and "acquired" antibody-mediated host defense.

Because C3b is both the product of the alternative pathway C3-cleaving enzyme and also forms part of it, the activation of C3 via the alternative pathway creates a positive-feedback amplification loop (see Figure 105-1). Moreover, activation of the classical pathway, by creating nascent C3b, can lead to activation of the alternative pathway. Thus, the alternative pathway can act to amplify the action of the classical pathway.

The Lectin Pathway

The lectin pathway is a third C3 activation pathway.[10] Mannose-binding lectin (MBL) is a naturally occurring member of the collectin family of proteins and is capable of binding to a number of sugars on the surface of a variety of microorganisms, including *Haemophilus influenzae, Neisseria meningitidis,* and streptococci. In the circulation MBL is associated with three serine proteases, mannose-binding lectin associated serine proteases (MASPs). The principal activation pathway involves MASP2, which, when activated, cleaves both C4 and C2 to create C4b2a with its C3 cleaving activity. Another less studied group of proteins of the lectin pathway, the ficolins, have similar structure, and presumably similar function, to MBL.

Activation of the Terminal Components

Activation of C5 by either the alternative or classical pathway by C5 convertases results in cleavage of the α chain of the native molecule to create a low-molecular-weight product, C5a, and a high-molecular-weight product, C5b. The smaller cleavage product, C5a, is released into the fluid phase where it, like C3a, acts as an anaphylatoxin.[8] In addition, C5a possesses potent chemotactic activity for neutrophils and monocytes.[11] The nascent C5b combines with native C6 to initiate formation of the membrane attack complex, a multimolecular assembly of C5b, C6, C7, C8, and C9, which is capable of cytolytic and bactericidal activity.[12]

Because C3 function and structure play a critical role in the activation of the alternative pathway, we describe C3 activation before we consider the alternative and lectin pathways.

Activation of C3

C3 is a two-chain molecule with the chains designated α and β.[2,3] One C3 activating enzyme (convertase) is formed by proteins of the classical pathway and a second is formed by the proteins of the alternative pathway. Hundreds of C3 molecules can be cleaved by each C3 convertase, allowing for amplification of the response. Cleavage releases a small peptide (C3a) from the α chain into the fluid phase, where it acts as an anaphylatoxin.[8] The remainder, C3b, is rapidly inactivated by hydrolysis. However, some C3b binds covalently to the microbial cell surface, where it acts as an opsonin.[5] The cell-bound C3b can be degraded by factor H and enzyme factor I as well as by other proteases, yielding a variety of products.[9] However, if it is not degraded, it joins the C3 convertases to continue the complement cascade. C3b degradation is complex and specific cellular membrane receptors recognize each of the degradation products and each appears to have a different biologic function. C3b itself is recognized by a specific receptor

Control of Complement Activation

Uncontrolled complement activation can result in widespread immunopathologic damage to the host and each step in the cascade is under complex control.[13] Each of these enzymes undergoes spontaneous decay under physiologic conditions. In addition, a number of control proteins inhibit the classical pathway (i.e., C1 esterase inhibitor, C4-binding protein, factor I, and decay-accelerating factor-CD55) and the alternative pathway (i.e., factors H and I and membrane cofactor protein, CD46). The membrane attack complex composed of C5b through C9 also is regulated by control proteins (i.e., CD59). Thus, the activation of complement proceeds in a highly controlled process and is limited to the immediate vicinity of the initiating substance (e.g., a microbial surface). Infectious agents have evolved proteins that control or prevent complement activation or binding or specifically bind complement control proteins from serum, allowing them to evade host immunity. Some well-studied examples involve staphylococci,[14] gonococci,[15] and vaccinia.[16]

ROLE OF COMPLEMENT IN HOST DEFENSE

The complement system is critical in the host's defense against infection caused by a wide variety of bacteria, viruses, and fungi. Animals that are pharmacologically depleted of complement or genetically deficient in individual complement components are more susceptible to infection with *Haemophilus influenzae*,[17] *Streptococcus pneumoniae*,[5] *Staphylococcus* spp.,[18] Sindbis virus,[19] influenza A virus,[14] and *Candida* spp.,[15] to name just a few.

The protective effects of complement appear to be most important in the first hours following the onset of infection. During this time complement helps to limit the spread of microorganisms from the initial site of infection.[20] Complement also plays a critical role in the clearance of pathogens from the bloodstream.[5] Different components of complement participate in different aspects of host defense. For example, in vivo studies have shown that the chemotactic cell activating activities associated with C5a are important in attracting neutrophils to the initial site of infection, whereas the opsonic activity of C3b is critical in the clearance of bacteria from the bloodstream.[5] Once the invading organism has established an infection, complement activation can contribute to further tissue damage.[20a]

GENETICALLY DETERMINED DEFICIENCIES OF COMPLEMENT

Most of the genetically determined deficiencies of the complement system are inherited as autosomal-recessive traits. However,

C1 esterase inhibitor deficiency is inherited as an autosomal-dominant trait and properdin deficiency is inherited as an X-linked recessive trait (Table 105-1). Heterozygous individuals with half normal levels of complement proteins usually do not have an increased incidence of infections, but susceptibility to infection is increased in many complete deficiencies. Many deficiencies are associated with rheumatic disorders and one, C1 esterase inhibitor deficiency, is associated with episodic attacks of angioedema.[21]

Patients with inherited deficiencies of complement develop certain types of infection depending on the function of the deficient protein in host defense. Patients with a deficiency in C3 dependent opsonization have increased susceptibility to organisms for which C3b-dependent opsonization plays an important role – organisms such as pneumococci, streptococci, and *H. influenzae* type b. Patients with deficiencies of C5, C6, C7, C8, or C9 are able to generate opsonically active C3b and thus have more limited increased susceptibility to these organisms.[22,23] However, because they lack the ability to generate C5 through C9-dependent bactericidal activity, they are especially susceptible to *Neisseria* species, for which bactericidal activity is a critical host defense mechanism.[18] Five to 15% of patients with systemic meningococcal infections have an inherited deficiency of one of the terminal components, C5 through C9.[24] The risk for having a complement deficiency is particularly high if the infection is caused by an uncommon serotype (i.e., X, Y, and W135) or if the individual or a first-degree relative had a previous meningococcal infection.

C1q Deficiency

Patients with C1q deficiency are unable to activate C3 and C5 through C9 via the classical pathway and thus have decreased C3b-dependent opsonizing activity and C5b through C9-dependent bactericidal activity.[22,23] Although their predominant clinical presentation is a lupus-like syndrome with 96% of the relatively rare C3-deficient individuals reported as having severe systemic lupus erythematosus, a few patients also have contracted septicemia or meningitis caused by encapsulated bacteria.

C1r or C1s Deficiency

Patients with C1r or C1s deficiency have markedly reduced concentrations of the deficient protein (<1% of normal) and levels of the related protein that are 20% to 50% of normal.[25] Similar to patients with C1q deficiency, C1r- or C1s-deficient patients are unable to activate C3 and C5 through C9 via the classical pathway and thus have decreased C3b-dependent opsonizing activity and C5 through C9-dependent bactericidal activity. Most C1r- or C1s-deficient patients have systemic lupus erythematosus or isolated glomerulonephritis rather than infection.

TABLE 105-1. Genetically Determined Deficiencies of Complement Associated with an Increased Susceptibility to Infection

Deficiency	Chromosomal Location	Inheritance	Major Clinical Manifestations
C1q	1p	Autosomal-recessive	Rheumatic disorders and pyogenic infections
C1r or C1s	12p	Autosomal-recessive	Rheumatic disorders and pyogenic infections
C4	6p	Autosomal-recessive	Rheumatic disorders and pyogenic infections
C2	6p	Autosomal-recessive	Rheumatic disorders and pyogenic infections
C3	19p	Autosomal-recessive	Pyogenic infections and rheumatic disorders
C5	9q	Autosomal-recessive	Meningococcal septicemia and meningitis
C6	5q	Autosomal-recessive	Meningococcal septicemia and meningitis
C7	5q	Autosomal-recessive	Meningococcal septicemia and meningitis
C8	1p(a,b,)	Autosomal-recessive	Meningococcal septicemia and meningitis
	9q(γ)	Autosomal-recessive	Meningococcal septicemia and meningitis
C9	5p	Autosomal-recessive	Meningococcal septicemia and meningitis
Factor I	4q	Autosomal-recessive	Pyogenic infections
Factor D	19p	Autosomal-recessive	Systemic meningococcal infections
Properdin	Xp	X-linked recessive	Meningococcal septicemia and meningitis
Mannose binding lectin	10q11	Autosomal dominant	Infection and increased rheumatic disease

PART II Clinical Syndromes and Cardinal Features of Infectious Diseases: Approach to Diagnosis and Initial Management

SECTION R Infections in Patients with Deficient Defenses

MBL Deficiency

MBL deficiency is believed to be the most common deficiency of a complement protein.[10] The normal serum level of MBL is low, 1–2 µg/mL. In about one-third of the population, mutations in either the chain coding or promoter regions of the gene lead to blood levels that are about one-tenth of normal. The literature suggests that individuals with MBL deficiency have a statistically increased frequency of infection, especially in the newborn period. Moreover patients with cystic fibrosis with low MBL levels are far more likely to have an early death from infection than are patients with normal levels, although the reasons for this are unclear.[26] Patients with MBL deficiency may have increased frequency of rheumatic diseases.

C4 and C2 Deficiency

C4 is encoded by two closely linked distinct loci (C4A and C4B) within the major histocompatibility complex (MHC) locus. Individuals with complete C4 deficiency are therefore deficient at both loci. As with other deficiencies of the classical pathway, C4-deficient patients do not generate C3b-dependent opsonizing activity or C5- through C9-dependent bactericidal activity through activation of the classical pathway. Their serum is able to generate these activities through microbial activation of the alternative pathway but not as quickly or to the same degree as serum containing C4.[23,27] Although the most common clinical manifestation of complete C4 deficiency has been a lupus-like syndrome, a substantial number of C4-deficient patients contract bacterial septicemia or meningitis. A number of studies have shown that homozygous C4B deficiency predisposes children to bacterial meningitis, presumably because they have to depend on the less functionally active C4A isotype to activate C3 through the classical pathway.[28]

C2 Deficiency

Although the ability of C2-deficient patients to generate complement-dependent opsonic and bactericidal activity via the classical pathway is reduced, activity is generated via the alternative pathway.[29] Affected individuals may be normal, but a subset of these patients have an increased susceptibility to infection and a number of rheumatic disorders.[30] Typical infections are septicemia or meningitis, and caused usual pathogens include encapsulated pyogenic bacteria such as the pneumococci and typable *H. influenzae*, and meningococci.

C3 Deficiency

C3 is central to the function of all activation pathways and C3-deficient individuals have deficient opsonic and bactericidal activity.[31] Affected patients typically manifest an increased susceptibility to infection and a variety of rheumatic diseases. Although septicemia and meningitis are most common, localized infections, such as recurrent otitis media, sinusitis, and pneumonia, also occur. The most common etiologic organisms are pneumococci, typable *H. influenzae*, and the meningococci.

iC3b interacts with CD11b/CD18 and CD11c/CD18; these receptors are deficient in patients with leukocyte adhesion deficiency.[32,33]

C5 Deficiency

Patients with C5 deficiency can generate opsonically active C3b through activation of the classical or alternative pathway, but cannot generate C5b through C9-dependent bactericidal activity.[22,23] They do not have an increased susceptibility to infection with encapsulated bacteria but, because normal host defense against *Neisseria* species depends on intact serum bactericidal activity, these patients have an increased susceptibility to systemic *Neisseria* species infections.[18] Patients with C5 deficiency fail to generate normal C5a, which is thought to contribute to infectious disease complications.

C6, C7, C8, C9, and Properdin Deficiency

Patients with C6, C7, or C8 deficiency can opsonize microbes but they are not able to generate complement-dependent bactericidal activity. Therefore, they have an increased risk for systemic meningococcal and gonococcal infections.[18,23]

Native C8 is composed of three distinct chains. The α and γ chains are covalently linked to form one subunit, which is non-covalently bound to the other subunit composed of the β chain.[34] There are two genetically distinct forms of C8 deficiency, one in which the α-γ subunit is deficient, and the other, in which the β subunit is deficient.[35] African Americans tend to have C8 α-γ chain deficiency and Caucasians tend to have deficiency of the β chain. In both forms, C8 functional activity and serum bactericidal activity are reduced markedly. The predominant clinical expression of C8 deficiency is an increased susceptibility to systemic *Neisseria* species infections.[18,36]

The assembly of C5b through C8 results in an unstable membrane attack complex that possesses limited bactericidal activity. Because the first patient described with C9 deficiency was asymptomatic, it was believed that C9 deficiency was not associated with increased infections. However, subsequently, an epidemiologic study has demonstrated the relationship between C9 deficiency and systemic meningococcal infections.[37]

Properdin acts to stabilize the alternative pathway C3-cleaving enzyme, C3bBb, thereby retarding its intrinsic decay. Deficiency of properdin increases susceptibility to bacterial infections, particularly those caused by *Neisseria* organisms.[38]

Deficiency of Factors H and I

Factor H deficiency is associated with atypical hemolytic uremic syndrome.[39] This protein is an important cofactor for C3 degradation and these diseases are thought to be associated with unregulated complement activation. It also is associated with age-related macular degeneration.[40] Multiple microbes have been found to bind factor H specifically in serum, thereby helping to down-regulate the ability of complement to destroy the organism.[18,41–43] Factor I is a cofactor for the cleavage of factor H bound C3b to iC3b. Factor I also functions with proteins that act as cofactors for the cleavage of C3b and iC3b to form C3d. These are the C3b receptor itself and CD46.[9] Patients with factor I deficiency have uncontrolled continuous activation of C3, with a resulting secondary serum C3 deficiency. These patients have an increased susceptibility to infection with the same encapsulated bacteria to which C3-deficient patients are susceptible.[44] Moreover, patients with mutations in factor I also have increased incidence of atypical hemolytic uremic syndrome.

Patients with factor D deficiency are unable to activate C3 via the alternative pathway. Rare families have been described in which patients with mutations of factor D have had systemic meningococcal infections.[45] Factor B is the protein in the alternative pathway that functions like C2 of the classical pathway; no deficiencies of factor B in humans have been reported.

SECONDARY DEFICIENCIES OF COMPLEMENT

Secondary deficiencies of complement can contribute to increased susceptibility to infection. For example, children with the idiopathic nephrotic syndrome who lose complement proteins in their urine have an increased susceptibility to pneumococcal peritonitis and sepsis.[46]

The Neonate

Serum concentrations of most of the individual complement proteins in term infants are reduced to between 50% and 80% of those found in adults. Even lower concentrations are found in premature infants.[47]

Sickle-Cell Disease

Patients with sickle-cell disease have a markedly increased susceptibility to systemic infections caused by *Streptococcus pneumoniae*.[48] Two defects in host defense contribute to this increased susceptibility; functional asplenia and a decrease in serum opsonizing activity. Deficient serum opsonizing activity is secondary to defective activation of the alternative pathway, although the exact basis for this defect is unknown.

DIAGNOSIS OF COMPLEMENT DEFICIENCIES

Screening for deficiencies of the early components of the classical pathway (C1, C4, and C2), C3, and the terminal components (C5–9) can be accomplished by measuring total serum hemolytic complement (CH50). Deficiency of any of these proteins leads to a reduction or absence of total hemolytic complement activity.[49]

Deficiencies of factors B, and D and properdin can be detected by a hemolytic assay that assesses lysis of rabbit erythrocytes mediated by the alternative pathway. This assay also is abnormal in patients with deficiencies of C3 or C5 through C9. Defects of MBL can be identified by enzyme immnoassays. The specific abnormality can be confirmed by sequencing the relevant genes.

In most cases the concentration of serum protein in question is a reliable test for a genetic defect. In some cases, however, such as in type 2 hereditary angioedema, the protein is present but nonfunctional; functional assays are needed for diagnosis. Patients with C8 deficiency lack either one (C8β) or two (C8α and γ) chains of the complete three-chain molecule. Therefore, C8 antigen is detected in the serum of such patients but their C8 function is reduced markedly. Individuals who are heterozygous for a deficiency of a single component usually have normal CH50 levels because this assay is not sufficiently sensitive to detect mild to moderate reductions in a single component.

Identification of the complement receptors or membrane-bound complement control proteins usually is established by flow cytometry.

MANAGEMENT

Replacement of specific components is usually not practical because of the short half-life of the complement proteins and the generation of an immune response to infused protein. Patients with complement deficiencies that predispose them to an increased susceptibility to infection may benefit from the administration of prophylactic antibiotics.

Immunization against vaccine-preventable infections in complement-deficient patients is critically important. Because antibody can act directly as an opsonin through engagement of Fc receptors on phagocytic cells, increasing concentrations of specific anticapsular antibody can provide increased opsonic activity, independent of complement. In addition, increased levels of specific antibody may increase activation of the classical pathway in patients with alternative pathway defects. Thus, complement-deficient individuals (see Chapter 6, Active Immunization) should be immunized, on a schedule similar to that of other immunodeficient hosts, against *S. pneumoniae*, *H. influenzae* type b, and *N. meningitidis*.

106 Infectious Complications of Dysfunction or Deficiency of Polymorphonuclear and Mononuclear Phagocytes

E. Stephen Buescher

Phagocytes perform critical roles in human host defense. Polymorphonuclear phagocytes (neutrophils, eosinophils, and basophils) defend against microbial invasion and contribute to various aspects of the inflammatory response. Mononuclear phagocytes (monocytes and macrophages) perform similar complementary functions in defense and inflammation. Despite their rarity, inherited disorders of these cell types provide insight into the critical role of phagocytes in human survival and health. One of the first phagocyte disorders to be recognized, chronic granulomatous disease (CGD), was described in 1957.[1,2] Despite its rare occurrence, CGD has been studied intensively and has become the paradigm for clinical management of infectious and inflammation-related problems common to disorders of phagocyte function.

TABLE 106-1. Characteristic Abnormalities of Disorders of Phagocytic Function

Disorder	Characteristics of Phagocytic Cells			
	Numbers	Chemotaxis	Adherence	Microbicidal Activity
Chronic granulomatous disease	NL	NL	NL	↓
Leukocyte adhesion deficiency	↑	↓	↓	NL
Chédiak–Higashi syndrome	↓[a]	↓	NL	↓
Myeloperoxidase deficiency	NL	NL	NL	NL[b]
Specific granule deficiency	↑/NL	↓	NL	↓
Hyper-IgE/recurrent infection syndrome	NL	↓/NL	NL	NL

Hyper-IgE, hyperimmunoglobulinemia E; NL, normal; ↑, increased; ↓, decreased.
[a]*Neutropenia is common during the accelerated phase.*
[b]*In vitro microbicidal activity against* Candida sp. *is deficient.*

PART II Clinical Syndromes and Cardinal Features of Infectious Diseases: Approach to Diagnosis and Initial Management

SECTION R Infections in Patients with Deficient Defenses

TABLE 106-2. Pathogens Associated with Disorders of Phagocytic Function

Organism	Chronic Granulomatous Disease	Leukocyte Adhesion Deficiency	Chédiak–Higashi Syndrome	Hyper-IgE/ Recurrent Infection Syndrome	Specific Granule Deficiency	Myeloperoxidase Deficiency
Staphylococcus aureus	++++	+++	++++	++++	+++	−
Streptococci	+	+	+++	+++	+++	−
Escherichia coli	++	+++	+	+	+	−
Burkholderia cepacia	+++	++	+	+	+	−
Serratia marcescens	+++	++	+	+	+	−
Candida spp.	++	++	+	++++	+	++++
Aspergillus spp.	+++	++	+	++	+	−
Nocardia spp.	+++	+	+	+	+	−
Pseudomonas aeruginosa	+	+++	+	+	++	−

Hyper-IgE, hyperimmunoglobulinemia E; ++++, most common or distinctive pathogen; +++, common pathogen; ++, less common pathogen; +, occasional pathogen; −, never associated.

ETIOLOGIC AGENTS

The major phagocyte function disorders and their abnormalities are outlined in Table 106-1. Because phagocytic cell responses are important both in normal host defense against extracellular microorganisms and in acute inflammatory responses, most of these conditions have the dual characteristics of recurrent infection plus deranged inflammatory responses. True pathogens or typically opportunistic agents cause infections in people with these disorders. Bacterial agents predominate in most conditions, but fungi are significant pathogens in many disorders (Table 106-2).

PATHOLOGIC FINDINGS

The systemic nature of these disorders explains their potential for infections at any anatomic site. However, interfaces between host and environment are the sites most commonly affected; skin and soft-tissue infections or abscesses, pneumonia, and infections of the upper airway or sinuses are typical (Table 106-3). Clinical manifestations depend on the nature of the underlying disorder. CGD phagocytes circulate in adequate numbers, move to tissues appropriately with normal locomotive and phagocytic function, and localize infection but fail to develop the respiratory burst required to kill certain pathogens. As a result, abscess formation

is common, but progressive, rapidly spreading cellulitis or septicemia is not. By contrast, disorders involving locomotive abnormalities (e.g., Chédiak–Higashi syndrome, leukocyte adhesion deficiency type I) demonstrate failure to localize infection, often resulting in rapid progression of infection or systemic spread, with a delayed appearance of inflammation.

Abnormal acute inflammatory responses contribute to ineffective wound healing that is characteristic of these conditions.[3] At sites of injury, histologic examination can show disordered inflammatory responses, such as combinations of acute and chronic inflammation (Figure 106-1) or poor accumulation of inflammatory cells.

CLINICAL MANIFESTATIONS

Manifestations of disorders of phagocyte function are highly variable. In some instances, inflammatory (rather than infectious) manifestations occur first.[4] Age at presentation varies from the first hours or days of life to adulthood,[5,6] but presentation early in life is more typical. Infectious agents can be recognized pathogens, opportunistic pathogens, or nonpathogens. Although few rules invariably apply, certain characteristics of infections raise concern for an underlying disorder (Table 106-4), and specific physical findings or infectious agents may suggest specific disorders (see Table 106-2).

TABLE 106-3. Infectious Complications of Disorders of Phagocytic Function

Infection	Chronic Granulomatous Disease	Leukocyte Adhesion Deficiency	Chédiak–Higashi Syndrome	Hyper-IgE/ Recurrent Infection Syndrome	Specific Granule Deficiency	Myeloperoxidase Deficiency
Lymphadenitis	++++	+	+	++	+	−
Septicemia	+	+++	++	++	+	++
Osteomyelitis	+++	+	+	++	++	++
Pneumonia	+++	++	+++	++++	++	+
Sinusitis	+	+	+	+++	+	−
Liver abscess	++	++	+	++++	+	++++
Meningitis	++	++	+	++	+	−
Poor healing	+++	+	+	+	+	−
Cellulitis	+	+++	+	+	++	−

Hyper-IgE, hyperimmunoglobulinemia E; ++++, most common; +++, common; ++, less common; +, occasional; −, rare.

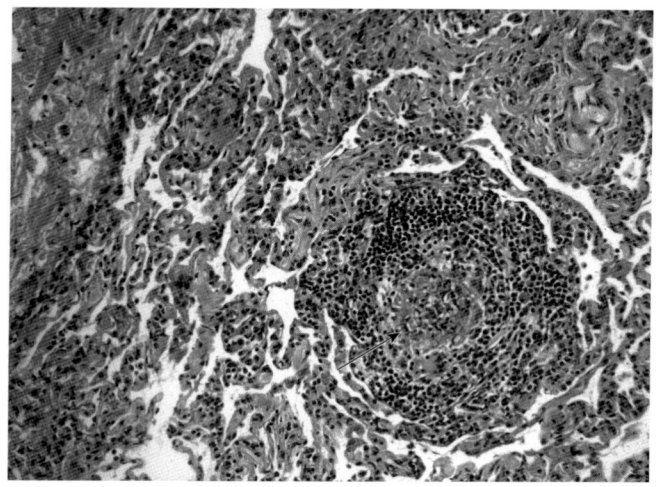

Figure 106-1. Pyogranuloma (acute inflammatory cells within granulomatous inflammatory response) (arrow) in lung of patient with chronic granulomatous disease and *Aspergillus* spp. pneumonia.

TABLE 106-4. Patterns of Clinical Illness Associated with Disorders of Phagocytic Function

Disorder	Clinical Illness
Chronic granulomatous disease	Liver abscess, aphthous stomatitis, discoid lupus erythematosus, McLeod blood phenotype, *Burkholderia cepacia* pneumonia, *Nocardia* spp. infections, *Aspergillus* spp. infections, retinitis pigmentosa, Duchenne muscular dystrophy, gastric or genitourinary tract wall thickening
Leukocyte adhesion deficiency type I	Failure of umbilical stump separation, early periodontal disease
Myeloperoxidase deficiency	Severe infections with *Candida* spp., often in presence of diabetes mellitus
Hyper-IgE/recurrent infection syndrome	Lung cysts or pneumatoceles, soft-tissue abscesses with minimal inflammation, retention of primary teeth, multiple bone fractures, scoliosis
Chédiak–Higashi syndrome	Recurrent cutaneous abscesses and cellulitis, invasive infections, progressive neuropathy, leukemia-like myeloproliferative process
Specific granule deficiency	Recurrent cutaneous and invasive infections

Hyper-IgE, hyperimmunoglobulinemia E.

CLINICAL APPROACH

The clinical approach to these patients centers around regular, repeated examination of target organ systems, preventive therapies, and prompt evaluation of acute clinical complaints. At the time of diagnosis, studies to define the anatomy of organ systems likely to be involved with future infection can provide baseline information for comparison. These studies include scintigraphy of the skeleton and computed tomography (CT) or magnetic resonance imaging (MRI) of the chest and abdomen (liver, spleen, para-aortic nodes, kidneys, and bladder). Regular examination of the hemogram, blood chemistry, coagulation, erythrocyte sedimentation rate, and C-reactive protein values aids in monitoring the patient's general state of health and provides data for comparison during illness.

Prompt evaluation of clinical complaints permits early recognition and treatment of conditions before serious complications or tissue damage occur. Local "dolor, rubor, calore, et tumor" of

a typical inflammatory response can be absent in these patients, and fever is variable. Simple problems, such as hangnail, insect bite, or minor injury, can become the source of progressive infection; expectant management, with attention to local care and administration of antibiotics, is required to prevent serious complications.

Any microorganism recovered from a normally sterile site, regardless of its nominal pathogenic potential, should be regarded as a likely infectious agent. This includes normal human flora or environmental organisms when the same organism is recovered repeatedly from the same site or from multiple sites. Recovery of multiple organisms from aspiration or biopsy materials should not be discounted, because polymicrobial infections including (bacteria or fungi) are well described in these patients.

MANAGEMENT

Identification of the Site of Infection

The ease with which sites of infection can be identified often varies from episode to episode. Skin, upper and lower respiratory tract, liver, bone, and lymph nodes are common sites of infection; spleen, gastrointestinal tract, central nervous system, and blood are less common. When the site of infection is accessible, material for culture and histology should be promptly obtained, preferably before administration of antimicrobial agents. When deep infections occur, clinical judgment must be used to decide whether antibiotic treatment can be delayed for 12 to 24 hours to acquire a surgical specimen. For patients with fever but no localizing signs or symptoms, a plan must be formulated early to define the length of clinical observation, while awaiting culture results or evolution of localizing findings, before initiating empiric antibiotic therapy. Anatomic sites previously infected should be carefully scrutinized because recurrent infections are common: technetium-99m bone scan and imaging studies of the chest and abdomen should be considered. Anatomic sites containing lymph nodes (hila of the lungs, paravertebral areas, mediastinum) should receive special attention because of the frequency of nodal suppuration in conditions such as CGD (see Table 106-3). Use of different imaging methods to examine the same anatomic areas (e.g., CT versus MRI) can be helpful (Figure 106-2). If, after 24 to 48 hours of close observation, the patient has no clinical change or has worsened, empiric antibiotic therapy should begin, usually with an antistaphylococcal agent plus an aminoglycoside or third-generation cephalosporin. In some instances, a previously unrecognized site of infection becomes evident after initiating empiric antibiotic therapy. If this occurs, appropriate surgical biopsy or drainage with culture of the specimen should be considered. Empiric antibiotic therapy alone rarely leads to resolution of unrecognized infection, which mandates repeated careful examinations of the patient and monitoring studies until the site of infection is identified.

Identification of the Infectious Agent

The importance of obtaining specimens for culture from sites of infection cannot be overemphasized; the variety of potential agents and the complicated nature of management require definitive knowledge for optimal treatment. Cultures of blood, urine, and cerebrospinal fluid (if appropriate) as well as cultures from all infected sites should be obtained before initiation of treatment. Surgical or imaging-guided biopsy is performed for deep infection (see Figure 106-2).

Delineation of Tissue Involvement and Debridement

For deep infections, meticulous and vigorous debridement of involved tissue should be performed at the time of biopsy; delayed control of infection, recurrence of infection, or slow healing all can result in excessive scarring and fibrosis. Tissue specimens (not swabs) should be sent for culture. For fungal infections, cure often requires surgical removal of the affected tissue. Close

PART II Clinical Syndromes and Cardinal Features of Infectious Diseases: Approach to Diagnosis and Initial Management

SECTION R Infections in Patients with Deficient Defenses

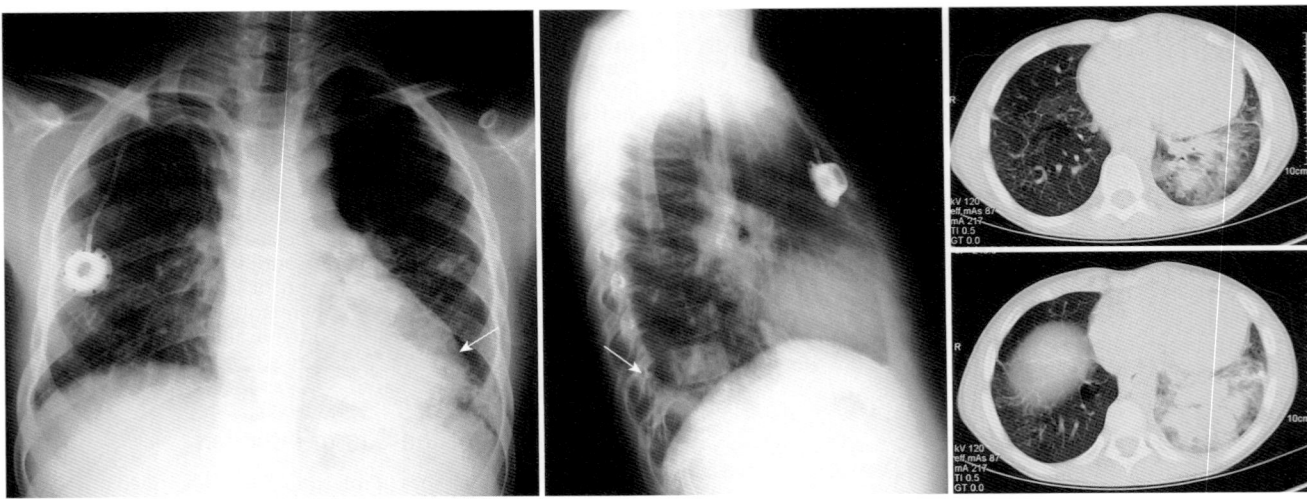

Figure 106-2. Chest radiograph and chest computed tomography (CT) scan of a 7-year-old child with chronic granulomatous disease with fever and dry cough. Plain films show a retrocardiac left-lower-lobe infiltrate (arrow), which appears small on the lateral view (arrow). CT (right) demonstrated more extensive disease throughout the left lower lobe. *Burkholderia cepacia* was isolated from the open-lung biopsy. Because this child had an episode of pneumonia caused by the same organism 12 months previously, the exposure history was more intensively examined, revealing that the child had a favorite outdoor activity of pulling up wild onions and playing with them.

collaboration with the surgeon, including the subspecialist's attendance at operative procedures, is required for optimal surgical intervention.

Initiation of Appropriate and Specific Treatment

When a surgical intervention is performed, prolonged postoperative drainage should be ensured, with slow advancement of drains, allowing perhaps twice the usual time for drainage to be achieved. Skin and soft-tissue sutures must be of maximal mechanical strength and left in place for a prolonged period because poor wound healing and weak scars in these patients lead to dehiscence. The duration of antimicrobial treatment typically is extended to approximately twice that required to treat an immunocompetent child with the same infection, with further tailoring of treatment

based on the extent of disease, antimicrobial susceptibility of microorganisms, effectiveness of surgery and therapy, and complications. Intravenous therapy is the standard for acute management, with oral treatment only used for chronic phases of therapy. Central venous catheters, if used, should be managed with meticulous aseptic technique because of associated risks of infection. Defervescence in patients receiving appropriate management typically is slow, but ineffective drainage, failure to identify and drain all foci, and iatrogenic causes, such as thrombophlebitis or drug fever, also must be considered when fever persists.

The frequency and severity of fungal infections, especially in patients with CGD (see Table 106-2), deserve specific comment.[7,8] Experience with CGD suggests that surgical resection of fungal infection offers the best chance of cure, but often, complete surgical resection is impossible. Amphotericin B, the mainstay of

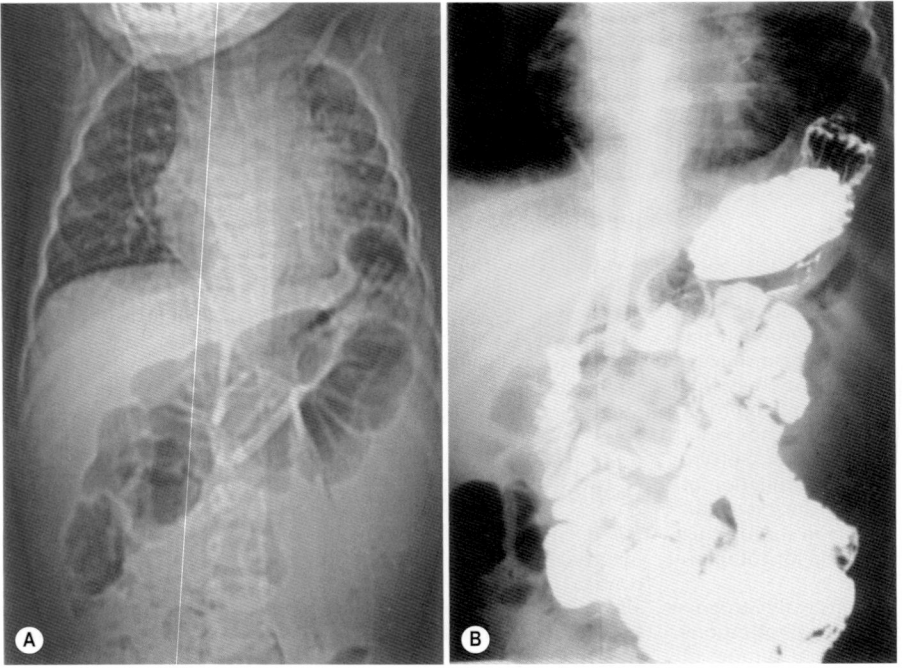

Figure 106-3. Plain radiograph **(A)** and barium study **(B)** illustrating herniation of the stomach through the incompetent left hemidiaphragm in a patient with chronic granulomatous disease. The left anterior chest wall, left lung, and, presumably, left hemidiaphragm had been infected with *Aspergillus fumigatus* 2 years previously, and had been effectively treated with white cell transfusions and parenteral antifungal treatment.

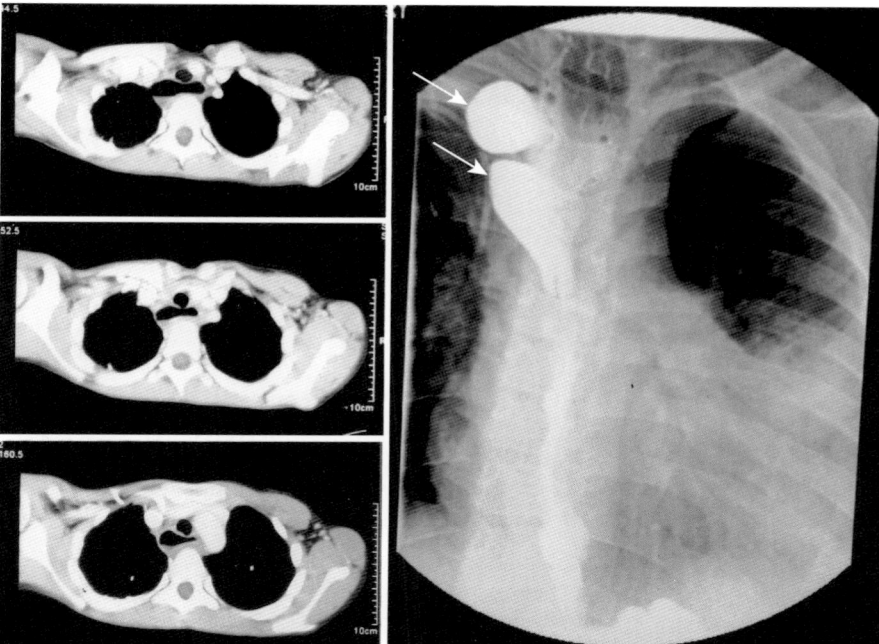

Figure 106-4. Barium swallow (right) and chest computed tomography (CT) images (left) of a 10-year-old patient with chronic granulomatous disease. Gastrointestinal granulomatosis was first diagnosed at 3 years of age and treated since with intermittent-pulse corticosteroid therapy for symptoms. Upper esophageal diverticulum (arrows) formed spontaneously over 4 years, during which time right-upper-lobe aspergillosis was diagnosed and treated. At age 7 years, right-upper-lobe resection was performed, with subsequent development of the lower diverticulum.

therapy in the past, remains effective against many fungi, but newer agents with less attendant toxicity, including itraconazole, voriconazole, caspofungin, and posaconazole, are supplanting its use.[8,9]

Under- rather than overtreatment of infectious episodes is common in these patients. When infection is suppressed instead of eradicated, smoldering infection and chronic inflammation lead to end-organ damage and scarring that eventually become insurmountable clinically, negatively affecting the patient's long-term prognosis.

Aggressive conventional approaches to treatment are not always successful. Unconventional adjunctive modalities must be considered in some situations, especially for fungal infections. Administration of functionally competent leukocytes via transfusion can be considered in situations of failure of aggressively applied conventional therapies, lack of localization of an infectious process, or life-threatening infection.[10] Most experience with leukocyte transfusions is based on care of patients with CGD,[11] often in the context of extensive, nonresectable fungal infection.[7,12,13] When used in this situation, it is prudent to separate leukocyte transfusion administration and infusion of amphotericin B by at least 6 hours to avoid acute pulmonary decompensation.[14] If used, it is important to understand that antileukocyte antibodies develop in approximately three-quarters of patients.[15]

COMPLICATIONS

Progressive tissue damage with associated loss of physiologic function or extension of infection (Figure 106-3) is the most serious consequence of ineffective treatment of infection. Progressive loss of pulmonary function, with parenchymal loss, bronchiectasis, and restrictive lung disease is a typical irreversible complication, which can be minimized or avoided by prompt definitive diagnosis and aggressive management.

Effects of inflammation-related masses, wound dehiscence, and mechanical failure of scar tissue are other major complications (Figure 106-4). In CGD, obstruction of the gastrointestinal or urinary tract by masses of granulomatous tissue, often without evidence of active infection, is a manifestation of the abnormal inflammatory response.[4,16,17] In some patients with CGD, gastric outlet obstruction is the first manifestation (Figure 106-5).[16] Corticosteroid therapy is used to re-establish normal function.[18] Inflammatory bowel disease-like colitis occurs in some patients

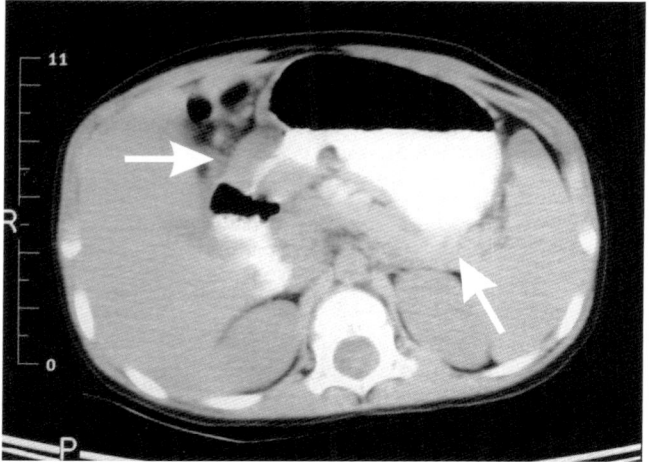

Figure 106-5. Abdominal computed tomography (CT) study of a 2-year-old boy with chronic granulomatous disease and persistent vomiting. Contrast material in the stomach forms an "apple-core" shadow as it passes through the pylorus (upper arrow), which is thickened by granulomatous inflammation. The posterior antral wall is also severely thickened (lower arrow). Vomiting resolved within 24 hours of starting oral prednisone treatment.

with CGD, and can be difficult to control. Complications of poor wound healing generally can be avoided by careful surgical technique and delayed removal of suture material.

PROGNOSIS AND SEQUELAE

The prognosis for patients with phagocyte functional disorders has improved steadily over time. With aggressive management of infections and careful follow up, 10-year survival in conditions such as CGD has improved from 15% to 25% previously[19] to 80% or greater.[6,20] Survival data for other conditions are not readily available. Rates of infection in patients with CGD can be reduced by prophylaxis with cotrimoxazole,[21,22] itraconazole,[23,24] and interferon-γ.[25] Patients with CGD and fungal pneumonia or disseminated fungal infection have mortality rates as high as 45%.[7]

PART II Clinical Syndromes and Cardinal Features of Infectious Diseases: Approach to Diagnosis and Initial Management

SECTION R Infections in Patients with Deficient Defenses

Bone marrow and stem cell transplantation have been performed in a limited number of patients, including some with CGD[26] and Chédiak–Higashi syndrome.[27] Gene insertion therapies have been successful in animal models of CGD,[28] but are not available for humans.

RECENT ADVANCES

Use of recombinant human hematopoietic growth factors has been examined in many phagocytic cell disorders and, in general, has not proven helpful, except in situations in which neutropenia accompanies abnormal function, as in glycogen storage disease Ib.[29] Use of cytokines in nonmalignant syndromes of cytopenia (congenital neutropenia, myelokathexis) also shows some promise.[30-32] Hematopoietic stem cell transplantation and gene therapy for CGD offer promise, but are still investigative.[33]

PREVENTION

Prevention of infections in people with phagocyte function disorders is based on prophylactic administration of antimicrobial agents, prompt attention and care of minor injuries, and avoidance of potentially harmful environments. Chronic administration of oral antibiotics daily has not been examined definitively in any of these conditions. Daily cotrimoxazole (Table 106-5) appears to prolong infection-free periods in CGD[21] but has less clear effects in other conditions. Prophylactic antibiotics should be administered before elective surgical and dental procedures (Table 106-6). Continuous prophylactic use of itraconazole to prevent fungal infections in patients with CGD results in significantly fewer invasive fungal infections.[24] Administration of ascorbic acid may be effective in reversing functional defects of phagocytes in Chédiak–Higashi syndrome[27,34] and CGD,[35] although beneficial effects have not been observed in all patients.[36] In several conditions, administration of recombinant interferon-γ appears to prolong infection-free periods. In a large randomized and placebo-controlled study, administration of subcutaneous interferon-γ (50 μg/m²) 3 times a week significantly prolonged periods between serious infections in patients with CGD,[25] and long-term treatment is safe.[37] In hyperimmunoglobulinemia E syndrome, in vitro interferon-γ exposure alters polymorphonuclear leukocyte locomotive responses, but clinical trials have not been performed.[38]

Minor wounds should be cleaned promptly and thoroughly and treated topically with an antiseptic or antibiotic agent (e.g., 1.5% to 3% solution of H_2O_2 or Neosporin ointment). To minimize gingivitis and periodontal disease, oral hygiene should include twice-daily brushing of teeth with 3% H_2O_2 and baking soda. Activities or environments that might predispose to infection should be avoided, including active and passive smoking; environments containing decaying plants, vegetables, or wood (e.g., hay, sawdust, compost, garden mulch) where *Burkholderia* species (see Figure 106-2), spores of *Aspergillus*, or other fungi might be aerosolized;[39] and situations in which medical care is inaccessible.

TABLE 106-5. Prophylactic Antibiotic Administration in Disorders of Phagocytic Function

| Drug | Dose/day[a] by Bodyweight | | Comments |
	<40 kg	>40 kg	
Trimethoprim-sulfamethoxazole	5 mg/kg	160 mg	Penetrates phagocytes
Dicloxacillin	12–25 mg/kg	500 mg	Remains extracellular
Clindamycin	10 mg/kg	300 mg	Penetrates phagocytes

[a]Divided into two equal doses.

TABLE 106-6. Antibiotics and Dosages for Surgical Prophylaxis

Drug	Dose	Schedule	Alternative Drug
Oxacillin	Child: 50 mg/kg IV	20–30 min before, every 3–4 hours during procedure[a] and 8 hours and 16 hours after procedure	Vancomycin: 10–20 mg/kg IV over 1 hour every 6 hours during procedure
	Adult: 2 g IV	20–30 min before, every 3–4 hours during procedure[a] and 8 hours and 16 hours after procedure	Adult: 0.5–1.0 g IV over 1 hour every 6 hours during procedure
Gentamicin	Child: 2.5 mg/kg IM or IV	30–60 min before, every 6 hours during procedure[a]	Cefotaxime: Child: 50 mg/kg IV every 6 hours during procedure[a]
	Adult: 1.5 mg/kg IM or IV	Every 6 hours during procedure[a]	Adult: 1 g IV every 6 hours during procedure[a]

[a]To maintain blood level above MIC of target organism throughout procedure.

SPECIFIC CONDITIONS

Chronic Granulomatous Disease

CGD is characterized by a defective or absent phagocyte respiratory burst in both polymorphonuclear and mononuclear phagocytes.[40] Absence of the respiratory burst results in failure to produce reactive oxygen metabolites and H_2O_2. Microbicidal activity against catalase-positive bacteria and fungi is defective; recurrent, life-threatening infections with these organisms result. CGD occurs in 1 : 250,000 births.[6] For initial screening, flow cytometric analysis of dihydrorhodamine 123 oxidation by blood leukocytes is used widely, but the nitroblue tetrazolium test remains rapid, relatively simple, and accurate. For confirmation, a quantitative test of the respiratory burst (superoxide assay or H_2O_2 assay)[41] or demonstration of an appropriate gene defect is necessary.

Both infectious and inflammatory syndromes are associated with CGD (see Table 106-2). Hepatic abscesses commonly cause fever, anorexia, and variable degrees of abdominal pain, often without abnormalities in serum transaminase levels. Abscesses can be multiple and variable in size (1 cm to >20 cm in diameter) (Figure 106-6). Surgical excision is the preferred management.[42,43] Suppurative adenitis can involve a single node, multiple contiguous nodes, or multiple geographically separate nodes. Surgical excision is preferred, followed by prolonged antibiotic therapy. Pneumonia, caused by either bacterial or fungal agents, requires aggressive, early diagnostic efforts (e.g., bronchoalveolar lavage, open-lung biopsy). Fungal pneumonia initially can be asymptomatic and is difficult to eradicate; excisional biopsy should be seriously considered if pneumonia is localized discretely to one lung area. Osteomyelitis can cause fever with or without initial bone pain. Hematogenous spread or local extension from a nearby nonosseous infection can occur. Bone scan usually is diagnostic and bone biopsy for identification of organisms should be performed. Concomitant antimicrobial prophylaxis may interfere with recovery of infectious agents, including fungi. Vertebral osteomyelitis caused by *Aspergillus* species is difficult to treat and is associated with a poor prognosis.[44] Inflammatory syndromes include granulomatous changes in viscera that produce mass effects (see Figure 106-5), poorly controlled inflammatory responses, poor scar formation, and slow wound healing.

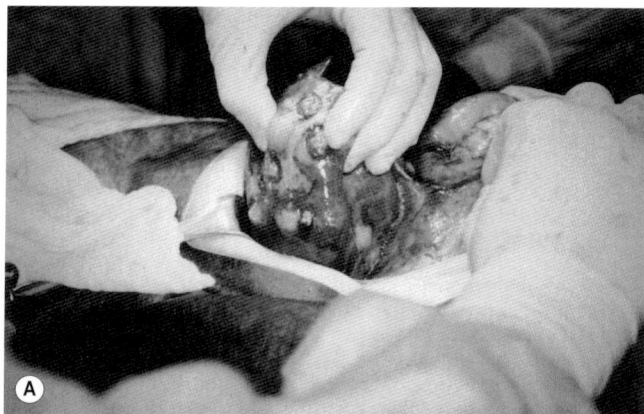

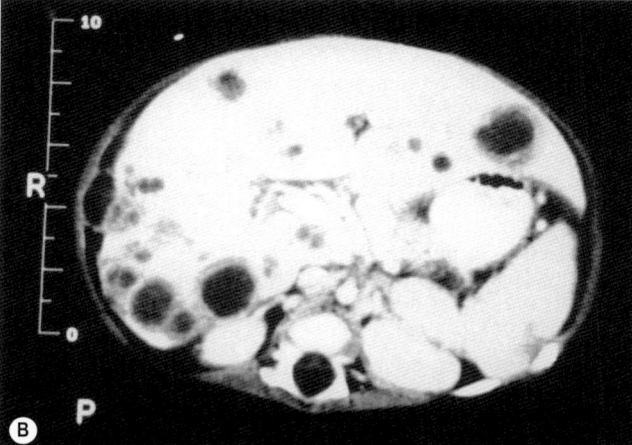

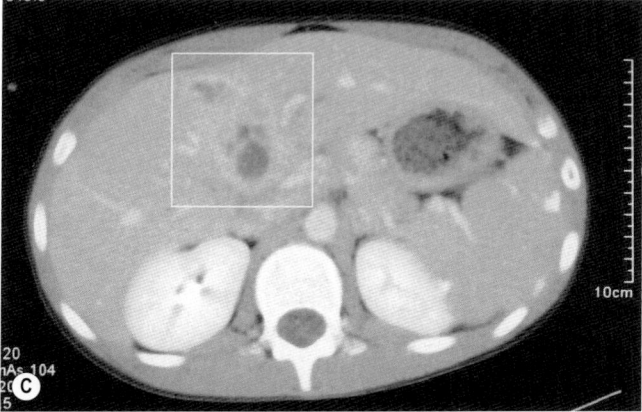

Figure 106-6. Intraoperative photograph **(A)** and abdominal computed tomography (CT) section **(B)** through the liver of a 3-month-old patient with chronic granulomatous disease, illustrating multiple liver abscesses, the number and location of which preclude resection en bloc. Abscesses were successfully drained using intraoperative, ultrasound-guided aspirations, followed by prolonged antibiotic therapy. **(C)** Single complex liver abscess (white box) in a 12-year-old patient with chronic granulomatous disease. Abscess is in the medial left lobe (box), in contact with the portal vein. Drainage was achieved by intraoperative ultrasound-guided needle aspiration, followed by prolonged antibiotic therapy.

Myeloperoxidase Deficiency

Myeloperoxidase (MPO) deficiency is the most common syndrome of phagocyte defect, occurring in approximately 1 in 2100 persons.[45-49] MPO deficiency affects both polymorphonuclear and mononuclear phagocytes, resulting in deficient conversion of chloride and H_2O_2 to hypochlorous acid and its microbicidal byproducts. The diagnosis of MPO deficiency relies on biochemical or histochemical determination of absence of peroxidase activity in blood polymorphonuclear leukocytes. In vitro, MPO-deficient cells have only minor (if any) microbicidal abnormalities against bacterial pathogens, but killing of *Candida* spp. is dramatically deficient[45,48] and may explain the severe candidal infections reported in some affected individuals.[45,48-50] Appropriate surgical debridement with antifungal treatment appears to be effective for these infections. MPO deficiency should be considered in any patient with unexplained (not caused by an indwelling device or cytopenia) severe candidal infection.

Hyperimmunoglobulinemia E/ Recurrent Infection Syndrome

Originally termed Job syndrome,[51,52] hyperimmunoglobulin E/ recurrent infection syndrome is a multisystem disorder of at least three different forms characterized by extreme elevations of serum immunoglobulin E (at least 10 times the upper limit of normal levels),[53,54] recurrent skin and sinopulmonary infections, and eczematoid rashes. Clinically, patients often have coarse facial features, retention of primary teeth, and candidiasis of the mouth, nails, or vagina. Recurrent sinopulmonary and cutaneous infections often begin in infancy; pneumonia frequently is severe and often is associated with pulmonary cyst or pneumatocele formation.[52,55,56] Bronchitis and sinusitis are common. Cutaneous infections typically are manifest as either abscesses (often with little associated evidence of inflammation) or cellulitis, but other types of cutaneous infections can occur.[57] When osteomyelitis occurs, it is often in proximity to a soft-tissue focus.[54] Expected infectious agents include *Staphylococcus aureus* (predominant), *Haemophilus influenzae*, *Candida albicans*, *Streptococcus pneumoniae*, and *S. pyogenes*,[53,54] but other organisms also are described.[56,58] Noninfectious manifestations include arthritis, arthralgia, multiple bone fractures,[52] hyperextensibility of joints, scoliosis, keratoconjunctivitis,[54] pulmonary cysts or pneumatocele,[55] and lymphoid cancer.[54,59] No single laboratory study establishes the diagnosis, but extreme elevation of serum IgE level and eosinophilia are common. The majority of cases are associated with mutations in STAT3 and its signaling systems.[52] Although originally proposed as a syndrome of primary phagocyte defect, it is now clear that the hyperimmunoglobulinemia E/recurrent infection syndrome is a multisystem disease involving dentition, bones, connective tissues, and defense systems; aberrant intracellular signaling causes the associated abnormalities of phagocyte function (i.e., chemotaxis).

Leukocyte Adhesion Deficiency Types I, II, and III

Three separate conditions involving abnormalities of leukocyte adhesion are identified as "leukocyte adhesion deficiency" type I, type II, or type III. The first descriptions of the condition now called leukocyte adhesion deficiency type I reported patients with recurrent infections, defective neutrophil mobility, and delayed separation of the umbilical cord.[60,61] Subsequently, the additional characteristics of severe periodontal disease, poor wound healing, and multiple adhesion-related abnormalities of phagocyte function, including poor adherence, spreading, chemotaxis, phagocytosis, and antibody-dependent cellular cytotoxicity responses, were described.[62] Partial ("moderate phenotype") or complete ("severe phenotype") absence of β_2 integrins ("leukocyte integrins," CD11/CD18) on mononuclear and polymorphonuclear phagocytic cells occur.[62,63] The result is slow mobilization and poor localization of phagocytic cells at inflammatory foci, resulting in severe, systemic, life-threatening infections, often resulting in death during infancy.[62] Infections involving cutaneous ulceration, delayed wound healing, pneumonia, and peritonitis are common.[62] Periodontal disease is common and can result in premature tooth loss. Leukocytosis without infection also is common, with marked leukocytosis often accompanying episodes of infection. Natural

PART II Clinical Syndromes and Cardinal Features of Infectious Diseases: Approach to Diagnosis and Initial Management

SECTION R Infections in Patients with Deficient Defenses

killer cell responses are diminished in vitro,[62] but whether this results in abnormal cell-mediated immunity is controversial. Spontaneous "regain of function" mutations in the defective β_2-integrin genes of 3 patients with LAD-1 have been documented.[63]

Leukocyte adhesion deficiency type II is an unrelated disorder in which absence of fucosylated ligands (sialyl-Lewis X antigen), which are the ligands for endothelial cell selectins on the surface of phagocytes, results in ineffective phagocyte-endothelial cell interactions.[64] Associated findings are severe mental retardation, short stature, and the Bombay erythrocyte phenotype. Dietary supplementation with oral fucose reverses the adhesive defect.[65]

Leukocyte adhesion deficiency type III is the most recently recognized LAD, involving failure of integrins to respond to activation signals. Multiple mutations in the *KINDLIN3* gene have been described, with resultant defects in leukocyte adhesion and platelet aggregation. Although it is unclear presently whether the type III condition is one or several distinct entities, all cases recognized to date have the common clinical characteristics of recurrent infection and severe bleeding tendencies.[66]

Chédiak–Higashi Syndrome

Chédiak–Higashi syndrome, consisting of recurrent pyogenic infections, partial oculocutaneous albinism with photophobia and nystagmus, and giant intracellular granules, is a rare, autosomal-recessive disorder of humans[67] and several types of animals.[68] Abnormal packaging of lysosomes is characteristic; all blood leukocytes show the diagnostic characteristic of abnormal, giant intracellular granules. In polymorphonuclear cells, these granules contain both primary and secondary granule markers[69] and are deficient in elastase and cathepsin G.[70] In vitro, microbial

killing is delayed, degranulation is abnormal, and chemotactic responsiveness is impaired.[71] Dysfunction of the lysosomal trafficking regulator gene (LYST) underlies the functional abnormalities of phagocytes in Chédiak–Higashi syndrome. Recurrent infections involving the respiratory tract and skin are most common, with *S. aureus* being the most common causative agent.[72] Progressive neuropathy is common, and a lymphoma-like "accelerated phase," accompanied by hepatosplenomegaly, lymphadenopathy, lymphohistiocytic proliferation or infiltration, anemia, neutropenia, and thrombocytopenia, develops in most patients during their first decade of life.[72] Limited studies addressing the use of prophylaxis with antibiotic agents in these patients have shown little effect.[71] In some patients, ascorbic acid treatment is reported to improve phagocytic cell function,[27,34] but this effect does not occur in all patients.[36] Ascorbic acid treatment does not alter progression to the accelerated phase, prompting investigation of bone marrow transplantation to correct this syndrome.[27]

Secondary Granule Deficiency

Secondary granule deficiency is a rare condition characterized by severe, recurrent infections and deficiency of the secondary granule marker lactoferrin[73,74] due to dysfunction of the myeloid-specific transcription factor CEBPE. These patients' phagocytes also lack all defensins, a class of phagocytic antimicrobial proteins.[70] Phagocytes from these patients have multiple functional abnormalities.[75,76] The diagnosis is made by demonstrating absence of antigenic lactoferrin in polymorphonuclear leukocytes. Clinically, patients manifest delayed localization of acute inflammatory cells at sites of injury, which leads to recurrent bacterial infections (both cutaneous and deep) and poor wound healing.[75]

107 Infectious Complications of Cell-Mediated Immunity Other than AIDS: Primary Immunodeficiencies

David B. Lewis

This chapter focuses on the infectious complications of primary immunodeficiencies in which lymphocyte-mediated immunity is compromised. Genetic disorders of cell-mediated immunity (CMI) that are mainly associated with hemophagocytic syndrome are discussed in Chapter 12 (Hemophagocytic Lymphohistiocytosis and Macrophage Activation Syndrome). Inherited immunodeficiencies that result in an autoimmune diathesis rather than compromised host defense, such as FoxP3 deficiency, are not included in this discussion.

OVERVIEW OF CELL-MEDIATED IMMUNITY AND ITS ROLE IN CONTROL OF INFECTIONS

Disorders of CMI that predispose to infection can be due to quantitative or qualitative deficiencies of thymus-derived lymphocytes (T cells) or natural killer lymphocytes (NK cells), as well as abnormalities in antigen-processing or presentation to T cells by antigen-presenting cells (APCs).[1,2] Limitations in cytokine production or cytokine responsiveness, e.g., deficiencies in cytokine receptors or downstream signaling molecules, also are important causes of genetic cell-mediated immunodeficiency.[1,2]

T lymphocytes play a critical role in the initiation and maintenance of antigen-specific immunity, and express heterodimeric

surface receptors for antigen, known as T-cell receptors (TCRs). T cells express heterodimeric TCRs that consist of either α and β chains (α/β T cells) or γ and δ chains (γ/δ T cells).[3] α/β T cells recognize antigens in the form of short peptides bound to histocompatibility leukocyte antigen (HLA) molecules on APCs. The CD4+ subset of α/β T cells recognize peptide antigens presented by major histocompatibility complex (MHC) class II molecules, which consist of HLA-DR, -DP, and -DQ proteins in humans. CD4+ T cells regulate the adaptive immune response by producing soluble cytokines, such as interleukin-2 (IL-2), IL-4, IL-13, IL-17, IL-21, interferon-gamma (IFN-γ), and tumor necrosis factor-alpha (TNF-α), and by expressing surface molecules, such as CD40-ligand (CD154), which interact with cognate ligands on other cells.[3] This CD4+ T-cell regulation includes promoting B-cell responses to protein antigens (by CD4+ T follicular helper (Tfh) cells secreting IL-21 and expressing CD40-ligand, which binds to CD40 on B cells), augmenting the microbicidal activity of mononuclear phagocytes (by CD4+ T helper 1 (Th1) cells secreting IFN-γ, IL-2, and TNF-α), enhancing the production of and tissue microbicidal activity of neutrophils (by CD4+ T-helper 17 (Th17) cells secreting IL-17A and IL-17F), and helping maintain CD8+ effector T cells that are involved in the control of persistent viral infections (by Th1 cells and less specialized CD4+ T cells secreting IL-2). Effector CD4+ T cells, especially Th1 cells, are important for the control of pathogens that infect cells for at least part of their life cycle, such as fungi (e.g., *Pneumocystis*, *Candida*, and *Aspergillus*), protozoa (e.g., *Toxoplasma* and *Leishmania*), some bacteria (e.g., *Listeria*, *Mycobacterium*, and *Salmonella*), and viruses (e.g., herpesviruses). Effector Th17 cells are important for the control of mucocutaneous candidal infection and also may help control pulmonary infection with bacteria that mainly have an extracellular life cycle, such as Enterobacteriaceae.

The human CD8 α/β T-cell subset recognizes peptide antigens presented by class I MHC molecules, which consists of HLA-A, -B, and -C molecules. CD8+ T cells are particularly important in killing infected host cells, such as those harboring viruses, by inducing them to undergo apoptosis (cell-mediated cytotoxicity).

Antigen-presenting cells (APCs) are not only involved in antigen presentation but also produce cytokines, such as IL-12p70 (a heterodimer of IL-12p40 and IL-12p35 chains), IL-23, and IL-27, that play an important role in directing the adaptive immune response. Dendritic cells are particularly important in initiating the immune response of naive CD4+ and CD8+ T cells to pathogens. Plasmacytoid dendritic cells are a type of APC that produces very high levels of type I interferon (multiple types of IFN-α and IFN-β) and are likely to be particularly important in the early response to viruses. NK cells are distinct from T cells in that they lack TCRs, and have the innate ability to lyse host cells (natural cytotoxicity) that are infected with intracellular pathogens, particularly herpesviruses. NK cells also secrete cytokines, such as IFN-γ, that contribute to the early cell-mediated immune response.

Most genetically defined primary lymphocyte-mediated immunodeficiency disorders are inherited as either autosomal-recessive (AR) or X-linked disorders, and compromise immunity from birth, e.g., severe combined immunodeficiency (SCID). Some inherited disorders typically require an infectious trigger for immunodeficiency to become manifest, e.g., Epstein–Barr virus (EBV) infection in the X-linked lymphoproliferative (XLP) syndrome. A few syndromes, such as selective absence of NK cells, are classified as idiopathic, since their inheritance or genetic defect has not yet been documented in most cases. Although primary lymphocyte-mediated immunodeficiencies collectively are rarer than acquired immunodeficiency disorders, they often present as unusual, severe, or recurrent infections, and frequently require more aggressive approaches for specific microbial diagnosis and therapy.

SEVERE COMBINED IMMUNODEFICIENCY SYNDROME

Definition

SCID is an inherited severe immunodeficiency of T- and B-cell function that occurs in about 1/50,000 live births. There is variable loss of NK-cell function, depending on the specific defect (Table 107-1).[4] The "combined" term in SCID reflects the fact that severe T-cell deficiency invariably compromises B-cell function, even if B cells are present in normal numbers. This is because CD4+ T-cell help for B-cell antibody production in the form of surface CD40 ligand and secreted cytokines, such as IL-21, is required for most antigens. In addition, as discussed below, in some forms of SCID the B cells that are present may have intrinsic functional defects.[5]

Specific Gene Defects and Their Inheritance Pattern

SCID can be due to single X-linked or AR gene defects[4] or, much less commonly, to chromosomal abnormalities, e.g., complete DiGeorge syndrome (DGS) secondary to interstitial deletions involving chromosomes 22 or 10. Peripheral T-cell dysfunction in most forms of SCID is due to perturbed intrathymic maturation of αβ-T cells;[4] an exception is coronin 1A deficiency, in which there is an intrathymic block of the release of mature thymocytes to the periphery.[6] X-linked SCID, which comprises about 50% of cases in most series, is due to deficiency of the common gamma

chain (γc) gene encoded in the Xq13.1 region. The γc protein (CD132) along with the IL-7Rα chain (CD127) comprises the specific receptor for the cytokine IL-7, and a lack of functional IL-7 receptors on developing thymocytes results in their arrested development.[4] Deficiency of the γc protein also results in the loss of functional surface receptors for IL-2, IL-4, IL-9, IL-15, and IL-21, and compromises the ability of γc-deficient B cells to receive IL-21-mediated help for immunoglobulin production.[7] Deficiency of the IL-7Rα chain or of Janus kinase-3 (JAK3), which is associated with the γc, result in a form of SCID similar to γc deficiency except that these have an AR rather than an X-linked inheritance pattern.[4] SCID with an AR inheritance pattern also can be due to defects in the ability of TCRs to transmit survival signals to the thymocyte (e.g., deficiencies of CD3-δ, TCR-zeta, zeta-associated protein of 70 kilodaltons (ZAP-70) kinase, CD45, or the Orai1 or Stim1 molecules that are involved in calcium signaling); defective thymocyte rearrangement of TCR genes (deficiencies of recombination activating gene (RAG)-1 and RAG-2 proteins, Artemis, Cernunos, DNA ligase IV, or DNA-dependent protein kinase catalytic subunit (DNA-PKcs)); increased thymocyte death from toxic effects of accumulated purine metabolites (deficiency of adenosine deaminase (ADA) or purine nucleoside phosphorylase (PNP)); a failure of the development of bone marrow precursors that normally colonize the thymus and give rise to thymocytes (reticular dysgenesis due to adenylate kinase 2 deficiency); impaired expression of MHC class II molecules (deficiency of the RFXAP, RFXANK, RFX5, or CTIIA transcription factors), which are required for the intrathymic development of CD4+ T cells from CD4+CD8+ thymocytes as well as antigen presentation to mature peripheral CD4 T cells; impaired development of thymic epithelium, which is required for thymocyte development (deficiency of the forkhead box N1 (FOXN1) transcription factor); or in proteins required for the egress of mature thymocytes to the periphery (deficiency of coronin 1A).[1,4,6,8,9] DGS results in SCID in less than 5% of cases, a form of the disorder that is referred to as complete DGS. Complete DGS may be more common, with interstitial deletion of the chromosome 10p14-13 region rather than the chromosome 22q11.2 region,[10] which is the more common cause of the disorder. CHARGE (coloboma, heart defect, atresia choanae, retarded growth and development, genital hypoplasia, ear anomalies/deafness) syndrome, which is due to heterozygous mutations of the *CHD7* gene, also can include a form of SCID with many clinical features that overlap with complete DGS.[11,12] AR SCID also can occur in some cases of the cartilage hair hypoplasia (CHH) syndrome (unpublished observations),[13] which is due to mutations in the RMRP RNA molecule[14] that has a poorly defined role in normal thymic development. ADA deficiency and RAG protein deficiencies have been estimated to comprise about 35%, and 5% respectively, of cases of AR SCID.[4]

Characteristic Infections

Even with the growing use of routine neonatal screening for SCID using Guthrie card blood spots, it remains important for the clinician to be aware of the frequent initial presentation of primary immunodeficiencies so that a specific diagnosis can be made rapidly and potentially life-saving therapies, such as immune reconstitution, can be considered. SCID disorders typically manifest early in infancy with infections caused by opportunistic organisms or with severe and/or protracted infections caused by common pathogens, especially viruses.[13,15–18] The infectious complications of SCID are similar regardless of the particular genetic defect. Infections with adenovirus, enterovirus, parainfluenza and influenza viruses, respiratory syncytial virus (RSV), and herpesviruses, such as cytomegalovirus (CMV), herpes simplex virus (HSV), or varicella-zoster virus (VZV), can be severe, e.g., with marked pulmonary, hepatic or central nervous system involvement.[13,15–18] This is due to a failure of adaptive immune mechanisms to control and ultimately eliminate intracellular viruses in these and other tissues. Failure to thrive is a prominent manifestation in most patients, and usually is due to persistent gastroenteritis from common pathogens, such as rotavirus, adenovirus,

TABLE 107-1. Clinical Characteristics of Some Well-Defined Forms of Severe Combined Immunodeficiency (SCID)

Syndrome/Gene Defect(s)/Mode of Inheritance	Gene Product Function	Mechanism of Immunodeficiency	Effect on Lymphocyte Numbers and Function	Characteristic Noninfection-Related Features
Common gamma chain (γc) deficiency/ CD132 gene/X-linked	Component of IL-2, IL-4, IL-7, IL-9, IL-15, and IL-21 receptors	Lack of IL-7 signaling leads to ↓↓ thymocyte development; lack of IL-15 signaling arrests NK-cell development	↓↓ T and NK; nl B but nonfunctional	None
JAK-3 deficiency/JAK-3 gene/AR	Signaling of cytokine receptors that use γc	Same as for γc chain deficiency	Same as for γc chain deficiency	None
IL-7 receptor α chain deficiency/CD127 gene/AR	Specific component of IL-7 receptor	Same as for γc, except that intact IL-15 function allows NK-cell development	↓↓ T; nl NK and B	None
RAG-1 or RAG-2 deficiency/RAG-1 or RAG-2 genes/AR	Enzymes required for TCR and Ig gene rearrangement	↓↓ T and B precursors	↓↓ T and B; nl NK	None
Artemis deficiency/ DCLRE1C gene/AR	Required for DNA repair process involved in TCR and Ig gene rearrangement	↓↓ T and B precursors	↓↓ T and B; nl NK	Radiation sensitivity
MHC class II deficiency/CTIIA, RFX5, RFXANK, or RFXAP genes/AR	Transcription of MHC class II (HLA-DR, -DP, and -DQ) genes	↓ Intrathymic maturation of CD4⁺ lineage cells and ↓↓ antigen presentation to peripheral CD4⁺ T cells	↓ or ↓↓ CD4⁺ T; nl or ↑ CD8⁺ T; nl NK and B	None
ZAP-70 kinase deficiency/ZAP-70 gene/ AR	TCR signaling of thymocytes and T lymphocytes	↓ Intrathymic development of CD8⁺ T cells; CD4⁺ T cells have ↓↓ function	↓↓ CD8⁺ T; nl or ↑ CD4⁺ T; nl B and NK	None
Cartilage hair hypoplasia (CHH) syndrome/RMRP gene/AR	RMRP encodes an RNA that is component of mitochondria	RMLP RNA/protein required for normal thymocyte growth	↓ to ↓↓ T – SCID only occurs with severe ↓↓	Absence of scalp and eyebrow hair, short-limb dwarfism
Adenosine deaminase deficiency/ADA gene/AR	Enzyme in purine salvage pathway	Thymocytes, immature B cells, and NK cells die from toxic effects of accumulated purine metabolites	↓↓ T and B in infantile-onset cases; ↓ NK cells	Rachitic flaring of costochondral junctions (50% of infantile-onset cases); renal mesangial sclerosis
Purine nucleoside phosphorylase deficiency/PNP gene/AR	Enzyme in purine salvage pathway	Purine metabolites that accumulate are less toxic to B than to T lymphocytes	↓↓ T; variable ↓ in B with poor function	Central nervous system disorders; autoimmune/allergic disorders
Reticular dysgenesis/ adenylate kinase 2 (AK2) gene/AR	Adenylate kinase 2 is an enzyme in the inner mitochondrial space required for hematopoietic stem cell development	Stem cell defect required for lymphocytes and granulocytes	↓↓ T, B, and NK ↓↓ PMNs	Bilateral sensorineural deafness
Omenn syndrome/partial RAG1 or RAG2 deficiency, some cases of IL-7Rα deficiency, CHH syndrome, or CHARGE syndrome	See RAG-1, RAG-2, IL-7Rα chain deficiencies, CHH syndrome	↓ T- and ↓↓ B-cell development; ↑ peripheral T cells with ↓↓ TCR repertoire	Nl or ↑ T cells with Th2 cytokine profile; ↓ regulatory T cells; ↓↓ B cells	Congenital/neonatal erythroderma, lymphadenopathy, hepatosplenomegaly; ↑↑ eosinophils and IgE

AR, autosomal recessive; B, B cell; HLA, human leukocyte antigen; Ig, immunoglobulin; IL, interleukin; MHC, major histocompatibility complex; NK, natural killer; nl, normal; ↓, moderately decreased; ↓↓, very decreased; ↑, moderately increased; PMN, polymorphonuclear leukocyte; T, T cell.

or enteroviruses. SCID patients also have increased risk for complications from live vaccines, such as paralytic disease from oral poliovirus vaccine or diarrhea due to persistent vaccine-acquired rotavirus infection.[19]

Fungal infections, which are suggestive of severe CD4⁺ T-cell immune deficiency, include persistent and severe mucocutaneous candidiasis, and *Pneumocystis jirovecii* pneumonia (PCP). *Pneumocystis* infection always should prompt a comprehensive search for SCID or another primary immunodeficiency involving CD4⁺ T cells.

Severe bacterial infections with pathogens that have a predominant intracellular presence, such as *Legionella*, *Listeria*, *Mycobacterium* (e.g., after vaccination with bacille Calmette-Guérin (BCG)), and *Salmonella* can occur and illustrate the requirement for CD4⁺ T-cell-mediated immunity in control of these pathogens. Other gram-negative bacteria, such as *Pseudomonas*, *Serratia*, *Klebsiella*, and *Escherichia coli*, also have been reported as causes of infection

even prior to hematopoietic cell transplantation,[15–18] and this may be explained by defects in Th17 cells.[3] Some cases of SCID can be complicated pretransplant by hemophagocytic syndrome,[20] which can include neutropenia that increases the risk of invasive bacterial disease, such as gram-negative bacteremia.[21] As maternally derived immunoglobulin G (IgG) level decreases over the first several months of life, patients develop marked and persistent hypogammaglobulinemia, and have increased risk for recurrent sinopulmonary infections from encapsulated bacteria, such as *Streptococcus pneumoniae* and *Haemophilus influenzae*.

In addition to infectious complications, some infants with SCID develop a skin rash and other organ dysfunction, such as hepatitis and gastrointestinal inflammation, from graft-versus-host-disease (GvHD). GvHD is mediated by T cells acquired transplacentally from the mother or from unirradiated blood transfusions, especially whole blood or platelets. Such maternally derived T cells also can cause hemophagocytic syndrome in untransplanted SCID patients.[21] Severe GvHD should also be distinguished from Omenn syndrome (OS), a form of SCID that classically is due to partial deficiency of one of the RAG proteins, but also can result from deficiency of Artemis, IL-7Rα chain, the CHH syndrome, or the CHARGE syndrome.[22,23] Patients with OS often have extensive erythroderma and failure to thrive. OS typically includes marked peripheral eosinophilia, highly elevated serum levels of IgE, increased levels of CD4[+] T cells producing Th2-type cytokines (IL-4, IL-5, and IL-13), and markedly reduced peripheral CD8[+] T cells and B cells.

Diagnosis

A history of other family members who experienced severe or recurrent infections in infancy or who died of unknown cause is suggestive of the diagnosis. However, a substantial number of cases of SCID, even cases of X-linked disease, result from new mutations, in which case the family history is not informative. Since SCID usually is due to severe thymic hypoplasia, there typically is a reduced or absent thymic shadow on imaging studies except in cases of coronin 1A deficiency. In cases of early-onset ADA deficiency, lateral chest radiograph can also reveal the rachitic-like flaring of the costochondral junctions. On physical examination, peripheral lymph node tissue is typically reduced, although there are exceptions, such as in OS, in which lymphadenopathy and hepatosplenomegaly are common. In a minority of cases, findings point to a specific disorder, e.g., the findings of short-limbed dwarfism and the absence of eyebrows and hair in the CHH syndrome, or the characteristic facies and congenital heart disease typical of complete DGS or velocardial facial syndrome (VCF syndrome: see Table 107-1).

In most cases of SCID, a complete blood count reveals a reduced absolute lymphocyte count (ALC) for age. This finding in early infancy never should be ignored, even in a well-appearing infant, as it can lead to an early diagnosis of immunodeficiency.[17] A severely reduced ALC is typical of forms of SCID that result in an arrest of both T- and B-cell development, such as complete RAG deficiency or ADA deficiency. A less severely decreased ALC is characteristic of forms of SCID due to defects in IL-7R signaling, since this spares human B-cell and NK-cell development (see Table 107-1). However, the ALC in some forms of SCID can be normal (e.g., some cases of X-linked SCID, MHC class II deficiency, and ZAP-70 deficiency) or even increased (e.g., some cases of ZAP-70 deficiency and most cases of OS). Normal or increased counts may reflect a compensatory increase in one lymphocyte population that masks the loss of another (e.g., the absolute increase in circulating numbers of CD4[+] T cells masking the absence of CD8[+] T cells in ZAP-70 deficiency) or a pathologic expansion (e.g., the marked expansion of a small population of activated CD4[+] T cells with a limited α/β TCR repertoire in OS). In some cases, maternal engraftment of T cells can partially offset the lymphopenia. Cases are described of X-linked SCID in which the numbers of CD4[+] and CD8[+] T cells are normal.[24] Therefore, regardless of the result of the ALC or T-cell subset analysis, if SCID is suspected clinically it is critical to enlist the help of a clinical immunologist so that appropriate tests can be performed to evaluate lymphocyte subpopulations (e.g., flow cytometry), and T-cell function (e.g., mitogen- and antigen-induced proliferation), specific gene sequencing, α/β TCR repertoire analysis, and determination of T-cell receptor excision circles (now in use in a number of states in the United States for neonatal screening using Guthrie card blood spots).[25]

Treatment

Once SCID is diagnosed and appropriate blood samples for total and antigen-specific immunoglobulin levels have been obtained, immune globulin intravenous (IGIV) usually is administered pending a definitive treatment plan. All live vaccines, including oral poliovirus vaccine, rotavirus vaccine, measles, mumps and rubella, varicella vaccine, vaccinia, BCG, and attenuated influenza vaccine and oral *Salmonella* Typhi vaccine, are contraindicated. IGIV therapy obviates the benefit of vaccination with "killed"

vaccines (e.g., inactivated poliovirus vaccine, inactivated influenza vaccine (TIV)) and antigen vaccines by providing passive antibody. Therefore, inactivated or protein/polysaccharide component vaccines, although safe in SCID and other immunodeficiencies, typically are not administered once IGIV therapy is begun. For ADA deficiency, either specific enzyme replacement with polyethylene glycol-associated ADA (Pegademase or Adagen) or gene therapy using retrovirally transduced patient-derived autologous hematopoietic stem cells to express an ADA gene segment (currently available as part of clinical research protocols at a number of centers)[26] are options for immune reconstitution. A similar retroviral-based gene therapy approach has also been used in X-linked SCID, and can result in significant T-cell and NK-cell immune reconstitution.[26] However, clinical trials of X-linked SCID gene therapy were halted after the development of T-cell leukemia in several treated patients, but recently have been restarted. For most SCID patients, the early transplantation of hematopoietic stem cells contained in bone marrow or peripheral blood, ideally from an HLA-matched relative, remains the standard treatment option for immune reconstitution.

Pneumonia in SCID

Pneumonia is often a presenting feature of SCID, as well as other serious disorders of T-cell immunity. Because virtually any microorganism can cause pneumonia in these hosts, it is imperative to establish a specific etiologic diagnosis, particularly if the patient shows signs of severe disease or deterioration. Although some etiologies of pneumonia in SCID patients can be established by bronchoalveolar lavage (BAL), lung biopsy should be strongly considered if there is not a prompt response to initial therapy.[27] Compared with lung biopsy BAL has a higher risk of both false-positive and false-negative results.[28] Open-lung biopsy poses a risk of morbidity and mortality, especially in patients with serious respiratory compromise. Therefore, depending on the location of the pneumonia, consideration should be given to using less invasive biopsy methods, such as thoracoscopically guided sampling.[28]

SELECTED NON-SCID DISORDERS OF T CELLS AND NK CELLS

Numerous non-SCID primary immunodeficiencies of T cells and/or NK cells can manifest with serious infections.[1,2] The genetic basis, clinical features, including infection predilection, diagnosis, and treatment of some of the better characterized disorders are discussed below and summarized in Table 107-2.

ADA and PNP Deficiency (late-onset)

ADA or PNP deficiency should be considered in HIV-negative patients of any age, including adults, in whom there is unexplained lymphopenia and recurrent infections. Notable infections include recurrent sinopulmonary disease, pneumonia, bacteremia, severe local papilloma infections, and recurrent herpes zoster. Late-onset infections associated with allergic or autoimmune hematologic disorders suggest partial enzyme defects.[29]

Ataxia-telangiectasia

Ataxia-telangiectasia (AT) is an AR progressive disorder with cerebellar degeneration and a high risk of cancer due to mutations of the *ATM* (ataxia telangiectasia mutated) gene. About two-thirds of patients also develop immunologic dysfunction, particularly those who have two null *ATM* alleles.[30] Immune dysfunction includes reduced antibody responses to polysaccharide antigens, such as in Pneumovax, absent IgA in serum, and progressive loss of T cells. Patients frequently have severe and recurrent bacterial sinopulmonary infections, which most likely is a reflection of markedly decreased antibody-mediated immunity. Infections typical of compromised T-cell immunity are not common, although reduced T-cell immunosurveillance may contribute to the high risk

PART II   Clinical Syndromes and Cardinal Features of Infectious Diseases: Approach to Diagnosis and Initial Management

SECTION R   Infections in Patients with Deficient Defenses

TABLE 107-2. Genetic and Clinical Features of Selected T-Cell and Natural Killer (NK)-Cell Immunodeficiencies

Syndrome/Gene Defect/ Mode of Inheritance	Gene Product Function and Mechanism of Immunodeficiency	Characteristic Noninfectious and Immune Features	Characteristic Infections
Ataxia telangiectasia/*ATM* gene/ AR	Protects from radiation-induced chromosomal damage by cell cycle arrest, allowing DNA repair; impaired V(D)J recombination and antibody isotype switching	Progressive cerebellar ataxia, bulbar and cutaneous telangiectasia; cellular hypersensitivity to radiation; ↓ IgA, IgM, T	Severe sinopulmonary infections and bronchiectasis; occasionally opportunistic infections if T-cell immunodeficiency is severe
Autoimmune polyendocrinopathy–candidiasis–ectodermal dysplasia (APECED) syndrome/*AIRE* gene/AR	Elimination of autoreactive thymocytes in thymic medulla, which if allowed to survive can contribute to autoimmunity	Autoimmune endocrinopathies, hepatitis, vitiligo, keratopathy; ↓ Th17 and Th22 immunity due to autoantibodies against IL-17A, IL-17F, and IL-22	Chronic mucocutaneous candidiasis
DiGeorge syndrome (DGS) and velocardiofacial (VCF) syndrome/interstitial deletion of chromosome 22q11.2/haploinsufficiency	Haploinsufficiency for the *TBX1* and *CRKL* genes result in hypoplasia of third and fourth branchial arch derivatives, including the thymus	Truncoconal congenital heart disease, characteristic facies, hypocalcemia; ↓ T (CD8 subset often ↓ more than CD4)	Usually asymptomatic if T cells >500/mm³; complete DiGeorge syndrome (naïve T cells <100/mm³) can manifest as SCID
Hyperimmunoglobulin E syndrome deficiency/*STAT3* gene/AD	STAT3 mutations that allow expression of mutated full-length protein inhibit the activity of STAT3 encoded by the normal allele	Eczema/dermatitis; osteoporosis, pathologic fractures, retention of deciduous teeth; coarse facies, joint hyper-extensibility, aneurysms; ↑↑ IgE; ↓↓ IL-17- and IL-22-producing CD4⁺ T cells	*S. aureus* skin boils (↓ IL-22); pneumonia and empyema due to *S. aureus* and other bacteria (↓ IL-17); pneumatoceles secondarily infected with *Aspergillus*, other fungi, nontuberculous *Mycobacterium*
Hyperimmunoglobulin M syndrome/CD40-ligand (*CD154*) gene/X-linked	Binds to CD40 and activates B cells and APCs; CD40 ligand/CD40 interaction required for generation of memory T and B cells, and isotype switching	Neutropenia and stomatitis common; normal or elevated IgM in 50% with ↓↓ serum IgG and IgA; poor specific antibody formation to protein antigens	Sinopulmonary infections and chronic parvovirus (↓ B-cell immunity); *Pneumocystis, Cryptococcus, Cryptosporidium, Toxoplasma*, CMV, PML (↓ T-cell immunity)
Hyperimmunoglobulin M syndrome/*CD40* gene/AR	Binds to CD40 ligand on B cells and APCs, which is required for generation of memory T and B cells, and immunoglobulin isotype switching	Neutropenia and stomatitis common; elevated or normal IgM; ↓↓ IgG and IgA; poor specific antibody formation to protein antigens	Sinopulmonary infections and T-cell immunodeficiency infections similar to X-linked hyperimmunoglobulin M syndrome
Interferon-gamma (IFN-γ) receptor deficiency/*IFN-γR1* or *IFN-γR2* genes/AR or, rarely, autosomal dominant	Specific cell surface receptor for IFN-γ, a potent activator of mononuclear phagocytes	Poor granuloma formation in response to mycobacterial infections; DTH response may be intact	Disseminated BCG and nontuberculous *Mycobacterium, Salmonella, Listeria*; recurrent oral and respiratory viral infections?
IL-12 or IL-12 receptor chain deficiency/*IL-12 p40* or *IL-12Rβ1* genes/AR	IL-12p40 is a component of IL-12p70 and IL-23, which respectively induce Th1 (IFN-γ) and Th17 (IL-17A and IL-17F) immunity by CD4 T cells	Granuloma formation in response to mycobacterial infection is normal	Nontuberculous mycobacteria, *Salmonella, Listeria*
NEMO mutation with immunodeficiency/*NEMO* gene/X-linked	Impaired activation of the NF-κB transcription factor impairs innate (e.g., NK cell function) and adaptive immunity by T and B cells	Hypohidrosis; conical/peg teeth, oligodontia, delayed tooth eruption; ↓ T-cell specific and ↓↓ specific antibody responses; ↓ NK-cell-mediated cytotoxicity	Disseminated nontuberculous *Mycobacterium*, gram-positive or gram-negative bloodstream infection, sinopulmonary infection; severe herpesviral infections; *Pneumocystis*
NK-cell deficiency/unknown/unknown	Unknown; lack of NK results in initially severe herpesvirus infections until T-cell immunity develops	? Myelodysplasia; ? malignancy; lack of NK cells based on CD16 and CD56 staining	Severe primary varicella, HSV, and CMV infection, but no ↑ in recurrent infection with these viruses
Wiskott–Aldrich syndrome/*WASP* gene/X-linked	Regulates leukocyte cytoskeletal function; required for normal function of T cells, B cells, and APCs, including dendritic cells	Thrombocytopenia with decreased mean platelet volume; eczema; IgA-mediated autoimmune disease; ↑ IgA and IgE, ↓ IgM and antigen-specific B cell responses	Recurrent sinopulmonary infections, herpesvirus infections, EBV lymphoproliferative disease; *Pneumocystis, Aspergillus*, mucocutaneous candidiasis
X-linked lymphoproliferative syndrome/*SAP/SH2D1A* gene/X-linked	Lymphocyte signal transduction molecule involved in T-cell and NK-cell function	Lymphoid neoplasm can occur in the absence of EBV infection (rare)	Primary EBV infection with fulminant hepatitis, hemophagocytic syndrome, neoplasm, or later hypogammaglobulinemia

APC, antigen-presenting cell; BCG, bacille Calmette-Guérin; CMV, cytomegalovirus; DTH, delayed-type hypersensitivity skin tests; EBV, Epstein–Barr virus; HSV, herpes simplex virus; IFN, interferon; Ig, immunoglobulin; IL, interleukin; MHC, major histocompatibility complex; PML, polymorphonuclear leukocyte; TCR, T-cell receptor; nl, normal; ↓, moderately decreased; ↓↓, very decreased; ↑, increased.

of EBV-related lymphoma. The *ATM* gene encodes a cytoplasmic molecule that helps arrest the progression of the cell cycle following radiation, allowing DNA repair to be completed prior to resumption of cycling. This accounts for the unusual sensitivity of AT patients to radiation-induced chromosomal breakage and the development of neoplasms. The *ATM* gene product is also required for normal rearrangement by V(D)J recombination of T-cell receptor and immunoglobulin genes. How *ATM* gene deficiency leads to neurologic abnormalities remains unclear. The serum concentration of α-fetoprotein usually is elevated and is a useful screening test for this disorder. Treatment of these patients is problematic, as the immunodeficiency and neurologic disease are progressive and the risk of developing cancer is high.

Autoimmune Polyendocrinopathy–Candidiasis–Ectodermal Dysplasia (APECED) Syndrome

Chronic mucocutaneous candidiasis is an invariable component of the APECED syndrome, also known as autoimmune polyglandular syndrome type I, an AR disorder.

The APECED syndrome can include autoimmune-mediated hypocortisolism, hypoparathyroidism, hypothyroidism, growth hormone abnormalities, hypogonadism, hepatitis, and vitiligo, as well as corneal and nail abnormalities. Chronic, intractable *Candida* infection of the oral mucosa, fingers, toes, and face is frequent,[31] and occasional patients have disseminated fungal infection. Prolonged antifungal therapy and prophylaxis is the mainstay of treatment. The APECED syndrome is due to a defect in the autoimmune regulator (AIRE) gene, and specific diagnosis is based on DNA sequence analysis. The *AIRE* gene is required for the optimal transcription by epithelial cells of the thymic medulla so that developing T cells reactive with these self-proteins can be eliminated by a process known as negative selection.[31] This may account for the frequent detection of T-cell-dependent autoantibodies against endocrine organ targets.[31] The increased susceptibility to candidal infection is explained, at least in part, by T-cell-dependent antibodies to self-proteins, in this case, to the cytokines IL-17A, IL-17F, and IL-22,[32] all of which provide important protection against fungal infection. The rest of immunologic function is usually normal.

DiGeorge Syndrome (DGS) and Velocardiofacial (VCF) Syndrome Due to Interstitial Deletions of Chromosome 22 (22q11.2 Deletion Syndrome)

Patients who are hemizygous for an interstitial deletion that includes the chromosomal 22q11.2 region may have features of either classic DGS or VCS. These include T-cell immunodeficiency due to thymic hypoplasia, transient postnatal hypocalcemia secondary to hypoparathyroidism, truncoconal cardiovascular anomalies, especially interrupted aortic arch, truncus arteriosus, and tetralogy of Fallot, and characteristic facial anomalies.[33] Haploinsufficiency of the *TBX1* and *CRKL* genes in the 22q11.2 region results in a developmental failure of the third and fourth pharyngeal pouches, accounting for the thymic hypoplasia and other characteristic features of DGS and VCS.[34] DGS also can result from other chromosomal abnormalities, such as deletion within the chromosome 10p14-13 region,[10] and this should be sought if screening for a 22q11.2 deletion or mutations in the *TBX1* gene are negative.

Peripheral α/β T cells in the 22q11.2 deletion syndrome appear to function normally in most respects. This probably accounts for the observation that patients with circulating T-cell counts in the range of 500 to 1500/mm³ do not usually show signs of immunodeficiency. In most moderately lymphopenic infants with this syndrome, the peripheral CD4⁺ and CD8⁺ T-cell counts normalize during the first year of life.[33] However, the assay of antigen-specific T-cell responses is particularly important, as peripheral T cells can undergo homeostatic expansion in a lymphopenic environment, giving the misleading impression that thymic function is relatively

intact when it is actually substantially reduced.[35] If such responses are normal, and the patient has a CD8⁺ T-cell count >400/mm³, live vaccines appear to be well tolerated. Moderately lymphopenic patients are at an increased risk for autoimmune hematologic disease in later childhood, suggesting that the thymic defect includes limitations in the induction of T-cell tolerance or its maintenance by regulatory T cells.

In a small fraction of cases (<5%), interstitial deletions of the chromosome 22q11.2 or, more commonly, chromosome 10p14-13, can result in severe thymic hypoplasia or aplasia, so that peripheral naive (CD45RA^high CD62-L^high) T-cell counts are persistently <100/mm³. These patients typically have SCID-like manifestations with severe infections (see Table 107-1). In this case, immune reconstitution by thymic transplantation[10] may be effective.

Hyperimmunoglobulin E (Hyper-IgE)–Autosomal Dominant (AD) Syndrome

Most cases of the hyper-IgE-AD syndrome are due to heterozygosity for mutations of the *STAT3* gene that allow protein expression.[36] These patients present with the triad of markedly elevated levels of IgE, recurrent pulmonary and skin infections, and eczema. Pneumonia due to *S. aureus* and other bacteria, such as *Streptococcus pneumoniae* and *Haemophilus influenzae*, often result in a striking amount of disease but a relative lack of symptoms, such as cough and fever. Pneumonias often are complicated by the development of empyema, pneumatoceles, and bronchiectasis. The pneumatoceles and bronchiectatic airways often serve as sites for secondary infection with fungi, such as *Aspergillus*, or with nontuberculous *Mycobacterium* species. The eczematous rash usually is present in the neonatal period, and skin furunculosis with *S. aureus* is invariably part of the syndrome. The predisposition to *S. aureus* pneumonia is likely due to impaired development of Th17 cells, and the predisposition to skin infections likely reflects a lack of CD4 T cells producing IL-22 (Th22 cells).[37] Children with hyper-IgE–AD syndrome frequently also have retention of their primary teeth beyond the usual age of exfoliation and joint hyperextensibility. They also develop coarse facies, osteoporosis, and pathologic fractures, particularly after childhood, and are at risk for a variety of vascular abnormalities, including aneurysms.

Hyperimmunoglobulin M (Hyper-IgM) Syndrome

The hyper-IgM syndrome is so named because of the frequent finding of an elevated serum level of IgM, and low levels of other immunoglobulin isotypes, particularly IgG.[38] The classic X-linked form of the disease is due to genetic deficiency in CD40 ligand, a surface protein that is expressed at high levels by activated CD4⁺ T cells. The interaction between CD40 ligand on the CD4⁺ T cells and the CD40 molecule on APCs, mononuclear phagocytes, and B cells, is essential for many adaptive immune responses, but this interaction is not required for normal T-cell or B-cell development. Patients have severe qualitative defects in B-cell function and a partial but important qualitative defect in T-cell function. Markedly reduced B-cell function frequently results in recurrent sinopulmonary infections with encapsulated bacteria and, rarely, in chronic parvovirus-induced anemia or enteroviral meningoencephalitis. These patients are extremely susceptible during infancy to PCP, an indication of the importance of CD40 ligand produced by CD4⁺ T cells in the normal control of this fungus. A variety of other infections indicative of T-cell immunodeficiency also have been reported,[39,40] including hepatobiliary infection with *Cryptosporidium*, cryptococcal meningitis, disseminated histoplasmosis, oral candidiasis, disseminated toxoplasmosis, severe CMV disease, and progressive multifocal leukoencephalopathy due to JC virus. Since the number of T and B cells and the ALC are normal, diagnosis requires assaying for functional CD40 ligand surface expression on activated CD4⁺ T cells using flow cytometry. Another frequent abnormality is neutropenia, the mechanism for which remains unclear. Oral ulcers often accompany neutropenia, but

PART II Clinical Syndromes and Cardinal Features of Infectious Diseases: Approach to Diagnosis and Initial Management

SECTION R Infections in Patients with Deficient Defenses

can occur independently. Patients should be treated with IGIV and should receive PCP prophylaxis. Some cases of severe neutropenia may respond to treatment with granulocyte colony-stimulating factor. Prognosis is poor even with these therapies; approximately 50% die by the fourth decade of life. Transplantation of hematopoietic stem cells from bone marrow, cord blood, or peripheral blood is curative of all features of the disease.

The hyper-IgM syndrome also can affect males and females in an AR inheritance pattern due to CD40 genetic deficiency. This is rare but clinically indistinguishable from its X-linked counterpart other than that girls and boys are equally affected.[41] The identical immunologic phenotype and clinical consequences for CD40 ligand and CD40 deficiency is consistent with CD40 being the only biologically important receptor for CD40 ligand. Other forms of AR hyper-IgM syndrome do not result in T-cell immunodeficiency but are associated with selective B-cell intrinsic defects in isotype switching and somatic hypermutation of immunoglobulin genes. These include defects in two enzymes, activation-induced cytidine deaminase (AID) and uracil N-glycolyase (UNG).[38] Patients with AID or UNG deficiency are predisposed to recurrent sinopulmonary and gastrointestinal infections associated with severe antibody deficiency, but are not susceptible to severe infections with intracellular pathogens, such as PCP.

Interferon-γ Receptor Deficiency

The IFN-γ receptor consists of two surface proteins, IFN-γR1 and IFN-γR2, which bind IFN-γ and mediate intracellular signaling. Complete genetic deficiency of either of these receptor components results in an AR disorder characterized by marked susceptibility to intracellular bacterial infections, particularly *Mycobacterium*, and *Salmonella* at extraintestinal sites, and occasionally, *Listeria*. Disseminated infection with BCG vaccine and environmental nontuberculous ("atypical") *Mycobacterium*, including species that do not cause disease in immunocompetent humans, such as *M. smegmatis*, is characteristic. These mycobacterial infections typically occur before 3 years of age and have a high mortality rate, with survivors requiring long-term multiple-drug antimycobacterial therapy.[42] Tissue that is infected with *Mycobacterium* characteristically lacks well-defined granulomas, demonstrating the importance of IFN-γ in the induction of this form of tissue reaction. Partial IFN-γR deficiency can occur, due to homozygous or compound heterozygous mutations that are hypomorphic, in which there is recovery from childhood infection with disseminated BCG, *M. tuberculosis*, and *Salmonella*, without specific chronic therapy.[42] Autosomal-dominant forms of IFN-γR deficiency also have been described. These forms tend to be less severe clinically than complete deficiency but more severe than partial deficiency.

Severe oral or respiratory tract viral infections, caused by CMV, HSV, VZV, parainfluenza virus, and RSV, can occur in patients with prior mycobacterial infection.[43] It remains unclear if IFN-γ receptor deficiency directly predisposes to such viral infections or if these viral infections occur mainly as a secondary complication of severe lung damage.

Diagnosis of IFN-γ receptor deficiency requires specialized tests to evaluate IFN-γ receptor expression and function, e.g., the production of TNF-α by monocytes after priming by exogenous IFN-γ, and confirmation of mutations using specific DNA gene sequencing. The differential diagnosis includes acquired autoantibodies to IFN-γ,[32] which is particularly a consideration when presentations with characteristic infections occur late in childhood or in adults. Treatment is problematic since patients with complete deficiency do not benefit from recombinant IFN-γ. Hematopoietic cell transplantation has been successful, but poses great risks for patients who are chronically infected with mycobacteria or who have sustained lung damage.

IL-12 p40 and IL-12 Receptor β1 Chain Deficiency

IL-12, a heterodimeric cytokine that consists of a p35 and a p40 chain, stimulates IFN-γ production by NK cells and T cells. IL-12

also promotes the differentiation of CD4+ T cells into a Th1 effector cells with a high capacity for IFN-γ production. Human genetic deficiencies of the IL-12 p40 chain, which is also a component of IL-23, and of one of the chains of the IL-12 receptor, the IL-12Rβ1 chain, which is also a component of the specific IL-23 receptor, have been identified.[2,37] Both deficiencies predispose to infections that are similar to those found in IFN-γ receptor deficiencies, except that extraintestinal infections with *Salmonella* are much more prominent than are disseminated infections with nontuberculous *Mycobacterium*. This high susceptibility to *Salmonella* infection most likely reflects the impairment of IL-12-mediated immunity, which is important for the generation of Th17 cells that limit gram-negative bacterial infection.[3,37] Granuloma formation in response to mycobacteria may occur normally, in contrast to patients with complete IFN-γ receptor deficiencies, most likely because IFN-γ production is only partially impaired. Treatment with recombinant IFN-γ should be considered in cases unresponsive to conventional antimicrobial therapy.

Natural Killer (NK)-Cell Deficiency

A few patients of both sexes have been identified with an apparent selective and complete deficiency of NK cells.[2] Most of these patients have presented after infancy with initially severe primary herpesvirus infections, including VZV (D. Lewis, unpublished observations), HSV, and CMV, requiring intravenous antiviral drug therapy. After recovery from a particular herpesvirus infection, the patients do not experience an increased frequency of recurrent infection, indicating the development of durable viral-specific T-cell immunity. There is a complete absence of circulating NK cells, based on flow cytometry using the CD16+ and CD56+ markers, and absent in vitro NK-cell activity in peripheral blood samples.[2] T-cell numbers and function appear to be normal in most cases. It is not clearly established that this is an inherited disorder, since, in most cases, families with more than one affected individual have not been described. IGIV has been used for therapy since this theoretically can increase antiviral function of cells other than NK cells, such as neutrophils and monocytes.

NF-κB Essential Modulator (NEMO) Mutation with Immunodeficiency

NEMO protein is encoded on the X chromosome and plays a critical role in the activation of the NF-κB protein by facilitating its release from the inhibitor of NF-κB (IκB) protein complex.[44,45] NEMO immunodeficiency occurs in boys with hypomorphic mutations of the NEMO gene; null mutations are lethal for the embryo. Ectodermal dysplasia, including hypohidrosis, sparse hair, conical or peg-shaped teeth, oligodontia, or delayed tooth eruption, occur in >90% of cases and reflect impaired function of the ectodysplasin A receptor, which utilizes NF-κB for signaling. NF-κB activation also plays a central role in both innate and adaptive immune responses, and the immunologic phenotype and predilection to infectious disease complications are therefore complex; these vary depending on the particular mutation and its location within the NEMO gene.[45] Decreased lipopolysaccharide-induced production of TNF-α by NEMO-deficient myeloid cells is observed, consistent with a central role for NEMO in the activation of toll-like receptors (TLRs) for NF-κB-dependent cytokine production (in this case, TLR4).[45] This block likely compromises the activation of mononuclear phagocytes and dendritic cells by pathogens and pathogen-derived products in vivo, which explains the susceptibility to sepsis caused by a variety of bacteria, including: *Listeria*, *Streptococcus pneumoniae*, *Klebsiella*, *Haemophilus influenzae*, and *Pseudomonas*. Severe and disseminated infections with nontuberculous mycobacteria also are frequent in this disorder, and may reflect both limitations in innate immunity as well as antigen-specific T-cell immune defects. PCP, CMV colitis, and severe herpesvirus infections also have been observed. NEMO-deficient NK cells have markedly impaired natural cytotoxic activity, which may contribute to the severity of herpesvirus infections.[45]

Finally, antibody response to both T-dependent and T-independent antigens often is decreased, and likely reflects the impact of impaired help to B cells from dendritic cells and CD4+ T cells, as well as intrinsic B-cell signaling defects, e.g., via CD40 engagement. Consistent with impaired CD40 signaling by B cells, some patients have a phenotype reminiscent of deficiency of CD40 ligand or of CD40, i.e., increased levels of IgM and low levels of IgG and IgA.[45] For unclear reasons, other patients can have markedly elevated levels of IgA or IgD.[45] Poor specific antibody responses in combination with limitations in neutrophil function likely contribute to the risk of bloodstream and other invasive infections caused by encapsulated organisms[45] and recurrent sinopulmonary infections.

Most patients will have abnormalities of TLR function, which can be screened using assays such as lipopolysaccharide-induced production of TNF-α, and decreased NK-cell-mediated cytotoxicity. Genetic sequencing is important for confirmation. IGIV replacement therapy is indicated because of the severity of humoral immunodeficiency. Hematopoietic cell transplantation is curative for the immunodeficiency component of this disorder, but may not correct enterocolitis, which most likely is a consequence of epithelial cell abnormalities of NF-κB signaling.

Wiskott–Aldrich Syndrome (WAS)

WAS is an X-linked disorder characterized by thrombocytopenia with small platelets, eczema of variable severity, and recurrent or severe infections due to mutations of the WAS protein gene (WASP). Immune abnormalities include severely depressed antibody response to unconjugated polysaccharide antigens, moderately depressed response to protein antigens, low serum IgM levels, and elevated serum IgA and IgE levels.[46] IgE elevation presumably is associated with the atopic diathesis of these patients.

WASP is widely expressed by hematopoietic cells and involved in the regulation of the cytoskeleton during cell signaling in the cytoplasm and also may regulate gene transcription in the nucleus.[47] WASP deficiency appears to substantially but selectively compromise the intrinsic function of T cells, B cells, and APCs.[47] In addition to recurrent pyogenic infections, especially otitis media, patients with WASP deficiency also are at increased risk for severe infection with certain viruses, especially VZV and HSV.[48] Patients with WASP deficiency, particularly those with mutations that result in undetectable levels of WASP, also can develop infections suggestive of severely compromised T-cell-mediated immunity, such as PCP, invasive Aspergillus infections, CMV encephalitis, and severe mucocutaneous candidiasis.[49] A substantial fraction of patients with WASP deficiency eventually develop autoimmune vasculitis associated with deposition of IgA-containing immune complexes that has many similarities to Henoch–Schönlein purpura. Autoimmune manifestations can include intussusception, arthritis, and nephritis. Bleeding can be severe or life-threatening in cases with profound thrombocytopenia. Splenectomy may be helpful in raising platelet counts, but this also increases the risk of life-threatening septicemia. Patients with WASP deficiency are at high risk for developing malignancy, especially lymphomas, starting after the second decade of life.

The diagnosis usually is evident, based upon the distinct features of the syndrome, and can be confirmed genetically by molecular analysis of the WASP gene. A determination of the precise WASP gene defect may not only allow screening of other potentially affected family members but also have prognostic value for the patient. Immune reconstitution by hematopoietic cell transplantation is curative of all disease manifestations, and appears to have the best outcome if performed early in life.

X-Linked Lymphoproliferative Disease

XLP disease is an X-linked immunodeficiency of males that affects T cells and B cells and is due to a mutation in the SH2D1A (SH2 domain protein 1A)/SAP gene.[50] The SH2D1A/SAP gene encodes SAP (SLAM-associated protein), a cytoplasmic protein associated with the SLAM receptor (CD150) that is involved in T-cell and NK-cell signal transduction. The immunodeficiency usually is silent clinically until primary infection with EBV results in a fatal infectious mononucleosis syndrome in about 50% to 60% of cases, a lymphoproliferative disorder, including malignant lymphoma in about 25 to 30% of cases, or a persistent dysgammaglobulinemia with decreased levels of IgG in about 30% of patients. Rarely, genetically affected individuals develop either lymphoma or dysgammaglobulinemia without prior EBV infection.

The mean age at development of infectious mononucleosis is about 5 years and infection usually is accompanied by severe hepatitis with periportal lymphocytic infiltration and bone marrow dysfunction with accompanying viral-associated hemophagocytic syndrome. In cases of hemophagocytosis, there are highly activated mononuclear phagocytes, many of which have internalized red blood cells in the bone marrow, lymph nodes, liver, and spleen (see Chapter 12, Hemophagocytic Lymphohistiocytosis and Macrophage Activation Syndrome). Meningoencephalitis also is common. Although there are no simple screening tests for diagnosis of this disorder, an absence of invariant NK T cells, a T-cell population that has some features of NK cells and a characteristic T-cell receptor, is suggestive but not pathognomonic of the disorder.[37,50] The diagnosis of XLP can be established definitively by analysis of SAP protein expression or the SH2D1A/SAP gene sequence. Patients with post-EBV hypogammaglobulinemia are treated with IGIV. The prognosis without definitive treatment, such as hematopoietic cell transplantation, is poor, with most patients dying before 40 years of age.

108 Infectious Complications in Special Hosts

Janet A. Englund and Jane L. Burns

SICKLE HEMOGLOBINOPATHY

The decrease in splenic function in young children with hemoglobin SS (Hb SS) disease results in increased susceptibility to fulminant bacterial infection, especially in early childhood. After recognition of excessive rates of septicemia and meningitis due to *Streptococcus pneumoniae* in patients with sickle-cell disease in the early 1970s,[1] mortality and morbidity due to pneumococcal disease have substantially decreased.[1,2] Retrospective studies reported rates of invasive infection in children 0 to 10 years of age with Hb SS disease prior to licensure of pneumococcal conjugate vaccine (PCV) to be 63.4 cases per 1000 person-years, a rate >10 times that in the general population. Mortality rates due to pneumococcal infections in United States children with Hb SS disease

PART II Clinical Syndromes and Cardinal Features of Infectious Diseases: Approach to Diagnosis and Initial Management

SECTION R Infections in Patients with Deficient Defenses

were reported to be as high as 2.8 per 1000 person-years, a rate 100 times that in the general population.[3] Patients with less severe hemoglobinopathies (sickle-cell hemoglobin C (Hb SC) disease, sickle-cell thalassemia (Hb S-thalassemia)) disease appear to have lower but increased risk for severe pneumococcal disease.[4,5] Bone and joint infections are relatively more common in patients with hemoglobinopathies, and the *Salmonella* spp. are isolated with greater frequency.[6,7]

Etiologic Agents

Encapsulated organisms, *S. pneumoniae, Haemophilus influenzae* type b, *Neisseria meningitidis*, and *Salmonella* spp. are the most common pathogens in patients with sickle-cell disease.[8,9] In African countries, infection with *Staphylococcus aureus, Escherichia coli, Salmonella*, and *Klebsiella* predominates, with *S. pneumoniae* responsible for fewer cases of infection than previously reported.[10] The incidence of *H. influenzae* type b (Hib) infections in the U.S. has dropped to very low levels since the introduction of Hib conjugate vaccines in infancy. Other microbes with special significance for patients with Hb SS disease are *Edwardsiella tarda, Yersinia enterocolitica, Mycoplasma* spp.,[8] *Chlamydophila* spp.,[11,12] and parvovirus B19.[13,14]

Epidemiology

Several studies of the natural history of Hb SS disease in the U.S., Saudi Arabia, and Jamaica have demonstrated increased mortality in young children: rates of pneumococcal infection have been 20-fold to 100-fold higher than in unaffected children in the first 5 years of life.[3,15] A study in Kenya reported an age-adjusted odds ratio for bloodstream infection (BSI) in children with Hb SS of 26 (95% CI, 14 to 48), with pneumococcus, *Salmonella*, and Hib disease documented most commonly.[16] Persistence of fetal hemoglobin is associated with fewer episodes of infection. Nasopharyngeal carriage rates and serotypes of pneumococci infecting children with Hb SS disease are the same as those infecting unaffected hosts.[2,17] Because of the frequent use of antimicrobial agents, close contact with many children in group childcare, and penicillin prophylaxis, up to 72% of the pneumococci colonizing children with Hb SS disease are penicillin nonsusceptible.[18-20]

Although infection was the major cause of death in a cohort of patients between the ages of 1 and 3 years with Hb SS who were monitored from 1979 to 1989, cerebrovascular accidents and trauma were more common causes in patients >10 years of age.[21] Other life expectancy studies suggest that at least 50% of patients with Hb SS currently followed survive beyond the fifth decade and that mortality most often is related to renal failure, chest syndrome, or stroke rather than infection.[22,23] Overall mortality associated with BSI in children with Hb SS has been documented as up to 23%,[20] with median survival estimated to be <5 years of age.[10]

The incidence of bacterial infection in Hb SC disease, although greater than that in healthy children, is less than that in Hb SS disease. Functional asplenia has been documented in adults with Hb SC by radionuclide liver-spleen scans, or by quantification of pitted erythrocytes. In one series, 4 of 51 children with Hb SC observed for 370 person-years were found to have 7 serious but nonfatal bacterial infections.[4] A second report describes 7 fatal episodes of pneumococcal septicemia in patients with Hb SC aged 1 to 15 years.[5]

Pathogenesis and Pathology

The increased incidence and morbidity of infections due to encapsulated microorganisms in patients with sickle hemoglobinopathies are attributable primarily to splenic dysfunction. The spleen is important as a reticuloendothelial filter and is involved in processing bacterial antigens and subsequent helper T-lymphocyte and B-lymphocyte responses. Encapsulated organisms cannot be phagocytosed efficiently without opsonization; thus, presence of type-specific antibody is critical to clearance of

organisms. The spleen and the liver (to a lesser extent) are important in clearing pneumococci from the blood. Additionally, the activation of complement by the alternative pathway, critical for phagocytosis in the absence of specific antibody, appears to be deficient in patients with Hb SS, although the specific defect has not been defined.

S. pneumoniae itself elicits a profound inflammatory response. Pneumococcal cell wall fragments trigger the expression of interleukin-1 and tumor necrosis factor, cytokines that in turn mediate systemic reactions associated with the clinical syndrome of septic shock. Thus, inability of the functionally asplenic, non-immune child with Hb SS to phagocytose and kill pneumococci efficiently results in bacteremia, multiple metastatic foci of infection, and unremitting upregulation of inflammatory mediators.

Clinical Manifestations

The clinical manifestations of infection (i.e., fever, pain, erythema, swelling) are no different from those in normal hosts without hemoglobinopathy. Differentiation of symptoms due to vaso-occlusive ischemia from those due to infection is problematic. Frequently, processes occur together. Children with Hb SS who appear "ill" should be treated aggressively for presumed septicemia while a specific diagnosis, including meningitis, is sought.

Pulmonary Symptoms

Bacterial pneumonia caused by *S. pneumoniae* is suspected in a patient with fever, cough, chest pain, sputum production (older patients), and abnormal chest film (lobar infiltrate or other parenchymal or pleural abnormalities). Patients often appear toxic. Laboratory findings include leukocytosis, frequently with an increase in immature forms. Causative agents include encapsulated bacteria, *Mycoplasma pneumoniae*[24] and *Chlamydophila pneumoniae*,[11] all of which have been shown to cause excessive morbidity in patients with sickle hemoglobinopathy.

Acute chest syndrome, described as fever and new pulmonary symptoms in a patient with Hb SS or Hb SC, commonly is precipitated by fat embolism and infection, usually community-acquired pneumonia.[25,26] Specific causes may be difficult to differentiate.[26,27] Patients have chest pain, rales on auscultation, and infiltrates caused by focal vaso-occlusive necrosis or frank pulmonary infarction, although the latter may be less frequent in children. Radiographic abnormalities may not be detected for several days after the onset of symptoms. Precipitating infections are bacteria, *Chlamydophila*,[11] viruses, and especially influenza.[28] Conversely, primary vaso-occlusive crisis involving ribs can cause splinting, diminished pulmonary toilet, and secondary bacterial pneumonia.

Laboratory data helpful in differentiating bacterial infection from vaso-occlusive processes are increased band count[9] and either extremely high or low white blood cell count (>30,000 or <5000 cells/mm[3]). Blood gas determinations from patients with acute pneumonia show oxygen desaturation, but patients with acute chest syndrome due to vaso-occlusion can have dramatic abnormalities as a result of ventilation-perfusion mismatch. Patients with significant vaso-occlusive pulmonary disease require prompt treatment with transfusion or exchange transfusion.

Central Nervous System Symptoms

In 1971, Barrett-Connor[1] calculated that children with Hb SS had a 300-fold higher risk of development of pneumococcal meningitis than unaffected children. Children with Hb SS in industrialized countries have a 6% to 8% chance of experiencing bacterial meningitis, with rates of 19% reported in Africa.[20] Of all children with Hb SS infected with *S. pneumoniae* in the modern era, meningitis develops in 20%, and 15% of patients die.[3] Factors associated with death in children with Hb SS and Hb SC include age >4 years, serotype 19F *S. pneumoniae*, and not being followed by a hematologist.[3] The rate of deafness after meningitis is increased in patients with Hb SS, with rates as high as 40%. A significant decline in the rate of pneumococcal meningitis was documented in the 1980s, and this rate has been reduced further in recent years by the prophylactic use of antimicrobial agents in young children with Hb SS, immunization with PCV, and prompt use of antimicrobial agents for febrile illnesses in these children.[2,8,9,21]

Lumbar puncture should be performed immediately in all febrile children with Hb SS who appear ill. This practice is particularly important in infants whose mental status can be difficult to evaluate or who have received oral antibiotics that can mask signs of infection. Central nervous system (CNS) vaso-occlusive disease (stroke) in young children with Hb SS is relatively uncommon, and typically, neurologic abnormalities are found in the absence of signs of infection. The management of pneumococcal meningitis includes consideration of early adjunctive corticosteroid therapy in an attempt to decrease the CNS inflammatory response.

Bone and Joint Infections

Bone and joint infection frequently is associated with ischemia and can manifest as dactylitis (in infants), pyogenic arthritis, or osteomyelitis with erythema, swelling, and pain.[6,7] An infectious cause may be suggested by the clinical presentation (e.g., as a complication of septicemia due to *S. pneumoniae* or a subacute presentation with less systemic illness due to *Salmonella*). Limp or refusal to bear weight may be the only clinical complaint. Bone and joint infections are associated with *S. aureus* in patients with Hb SS, as in unaffected children. *Salmonella* spp., particularly the serotypes associated with bone and joint infections *(S. choleraesuis, S. heidelberg)*, also are important because of splenic dysfunction and can manifest either as systemic infection or with localized signs and symptoms.[29] Blood and stool specimens as well as aspirates from infected sites should be obtained for culture before empirical antibiotic therapy is started. It is important to determine specific etiology and antimicrobial susceptibility, because prolonged therapy is generally required.

The differentiation between osteomyelitis and vaso-occlusive ischemia in the bone is difficult. Pain and tenderness out of proportion to physical findings, bilateral, symmetric involvement, and diffuse symptomatology over the metaphysis and shaft of long bones (or dorsum of the hands and fingers in infants) suggest infarction. Laboratory findings may be helpful. Elevated erythrocyte sedimentation rate (which is usually depressed in Hb SS) suggests bacterial infection. Bony destruction ("crumbling-bone disease") and periosteal new bone formation visualized on plain radiograph can occur with either condition. Imaging studies can be useful in establishing an etiology, but differentiation of infarction from infection is difficult (Figure 108-1). Radionuclide bone scanning is difficult to interpret. Magnetic resonance imaging may be useful for differentiating muscle and bone involvement. Bone aspiration or biopsy frequently is necessary to establish a bacterial cause. Prompt surgical decompression of infected joints often is diagnostic and also is critical for good outcome.

Management and Presumptive Therapy

Meningitis, Septicemia, and Pneumonia

Infants and young children with Hb SS and fever should be evaluated and treated for presumed bacterial infection. Initial evaluation usually includes a complete blood cell count, blood culture, and chest radiograph, particularly in young children in whom the physical examination may not be optimal. Patients who are at high risk for infection (i.e., who look ill and who have a body temperature >40°C or a white blood cell count >30,000 or <5000 cells/mm³) are likely to have pneumococcal infection and should be hospitalized for aggressive therapy.[9] Children who have had previous episodes of pneumococcal BSI are at increased risk for repeated infection and warrant special consideration.[30]

Patients who are febrile but do not appear ill have been managed successfully in a variety of ways, including: (1) observation in a short-stay area of the hospital for several hours after institution of antimicrobial therapy; or (2) parenteral administration of

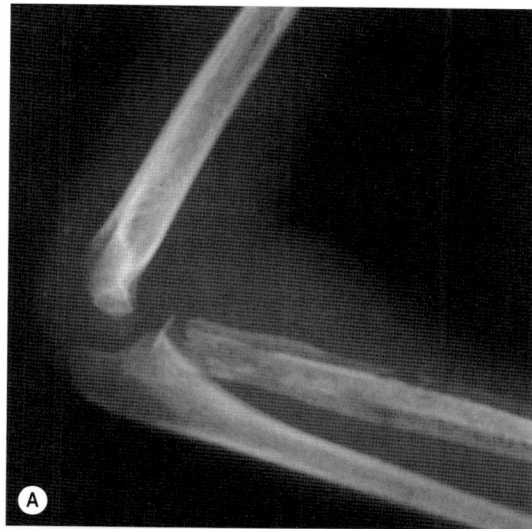

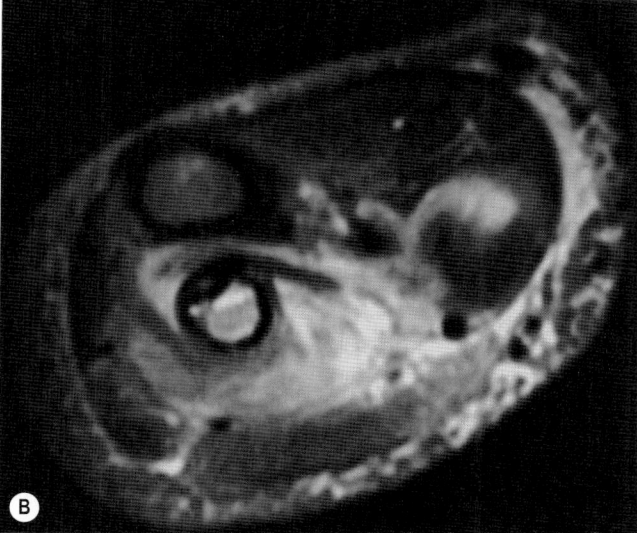

Figure 108-1. (A) Radiograph of elbow of 30-month-old patient with hemoglobin S (SS) disease and osteomyelitis due to *Salmonella* spp. There is joint effusion, marked destruction of bone, involucrum, and periosteal new bone formation. **(B)** Magnetic resonance imaging of elbow showing fat saturation fast T_2-weighted image in the axial plane. There is joint effusion, edema of the supinator muscle, and an active process within the radius more consistent with osteomyelitis than with infarction.

ceftriaxone and close observation on an outpatient basis.[9] Enthusiasm for the latter approach is tempered by case reports of severe and rapidly fatal immune-mediated hemolysis due to ceftriaxone in patients with Hb SS and other patients who have received multiple courses of the drug.[31,32] All febrile children with Hb SS should be given an antibiotic. In the case of disease highly likely to be a vaso-occlusive crisis, therapy could be given orally with close follow-up.

S. pneumoniae that is nonsusceptible to penicillin or cephalosporins poses a particular challenge,[19,33,34] especially for children <3 years of age who are receiving penicillin prophylaxis. Ampicillin-sulbactam plus gentamicin or a third-generation cephalosporin, plus vancomycin, are considered for presumptive therapy for BSI. Fluoroquinolones can be considered for therapy in developing countries where widespread antibiotic resistance is present.[20] For meningitis, particularly if corticosteroids are used, rifampin (20 mg/kg per day) plus vancomycin (60 mg/kg per day) plus cefotaxime or ceftriaxone are given empirically.

PART II Clinical Syndromes and Cardinal Features of Infectious Diseases: Approach to Diagnosis and Initial Management

SECTION R Infections in Patients with Deficient Defenses

Bone and Joint Infections

Empiric therapy for bone or joint infection includes agents effective against *S. aureus* (e.g., oxacillin, nafcillin, vancomycin, or clindamycin) and *Salmonella* (e.g., third-generation cephalosporin or fluoroquinolone). Extensive disease, particularly that due to *Salmonella* spp., usually requires debridement and prolonged antimicrobial therapy (e.g., 6 months or more) as for chronic osteomyelitis.

Prevention

The widespread use of pneumococcal vaccines has significantly decreased pneumococcal disease in children. A 13-valent pneumococcal conjugate vaccine (PCV) series is recommended for all children, beginning at 2 months of age (see Chapter 123, *Streptococcus pneumoniae*), including those with Hb SS.[35,36] PCV given in infancy decreases nasal colonization with *S. pneumoniae* as well as invasive disease.[37] For children who have received the 7-valent PCV vaccine, a dose of the 13-valent PCV vaccine (PCV13) now is recommended.[36] For children with Hb SS or other causes of functional asplenia, 23-valent pneumococcal polysaccharide vaccine (PPSV23) also is recommended following the PCV series beginning at 24 months of age.[35,36] A second immunization with PPSV23 is recommended 5 years after the first dose.[36] Opsonophagocytic activity has been documented in patients with Hb SS who have undergone immunization with the PCV followed by polysaccharide vaccine. Quadrivalent meningococcal conjugate vaccine (MCV4) also is indicated for children with Hb SS or Hb SC disease beginning at 2 years of age[38] with revaccination recommended every 5 years.[39]

Influenza vaccine should be targeted annually to children with Hb SS (as well as given to all children ≥6 months of age) because of the significant risk of complications due to influenza, including pneumococcal superinfection.

Substantial reduction in morbidity and mortality due to *S. pneumoniae* has been demonstrated in children <3 years of age with Hb SS through the use of prophylactic penicillin therapy.[2] The major placebo-controlled study (performed prior to routine use of PCV) demonstrated a decrease in the rate of pneumococcal infection from 9.8 to 1.5 per 100 patient-years.[8] Prophylactic penicillin is begun at 3 months of age. There is no consensus regarding the age at which prophylaxis should be stopped; studies do not support benefit of continuation beyond 5 years of age.[40,41] Adherence to an oral regimen may be erratic. Monthly injections of benzathine penicillin G are efficacious.

Special Considerations

Parvovirus B19 Infection

Transient aplastic crisis in Hb SS disease (worsening anemia and profound reticulocytopenia) has been associated with parvovirus B19 infection.[13] The cellular receptor for this virus is the blood group P antigen, explaining the tropism of the virus for erythroid progenitor cells; viral infection appears to trigger apoptosis.[14] Serologic studies of patients with Hb SS who have transient aplastic crisis demonstrate acute parvovirus B19 infection in 70%.[13] Patients have a high burden of virus, are highly contagious, and do not demonstrate the characteristic rash of erythema infectiosum. Neither chronic nor recurrent disease is reported in this patient group, and anti-B19 immunoglobulin (Ig) G antibodies remain detectable for several years following infection, suggesting protection.

ASPLENIA AND POLYSPLENIA

Asplenic patients have increased risk for overwhelming, life-threatening infections, most commonly due to *S. pneumoniae*.[42–45] The level of risk appears to correlate inversely with the amount of time a patient has had a functioning spleen. Adults who undergo splenectomy after trauma have a lower risk of serious infection than infants with congenital asplenia syndrome and children who undergo splenectomy after trauma. Children who undergo splenectomy as part of treatment for malignancy are at great risk. Overall, approximately 5% of children whose spleens are removed before the age of 4 years have significant infections, with a mortality rate of 30% to 60%. Risk of infection is greatest in the year after splenectomy (regardless of age) and continues to be significant for the next 7 to 10 years, after which time risk is low but never as low as for people with normal splenic function.

Children with congenital asplenia and polysplenia syndromes (e.g., Ivemark syndrome) are at increased risk of overwhelming septicemia.[46,47] Splenic function should be evaluated in children with congenital abnormalities of embryonic lateralization, such as heterotaxy syndromes involving a variety of abnormalities across the left–right axis of the body (situs inversus)[47], and a wide variety of cardiac defects including cono-truncal abnormalities, transposition of the great vessels, and endocardial cushion defects. Asplenia and polysplenia often are associated with other types of congenital abnormalities, including gastrointestinal malformations such as biliary atresia, neural tube anomalies, genitourinary defects, skeletal defects, and bronchopulmonary defects, including Kartagener syndrome, as well as bilobed and mirror-image lungs.

Because of the success of liver transplantation from living related donors in children with polysplenia syndrome, more such patients who have significant risks for infection are surviving. The polysplenia syndrome also has been reported as an incidental finding on computed tomography in adults, suggesting that some individuals may have immunologic impairment that is not as significant as that of asplenic patients.

Functional asplenia is confirmed by the presence of Howell–Jolly bodies in a peripheral blood smear (obtained after the first week of life), absence of splenic uptake on a technetium-99 sulfur colloid scan, or increased percentage (more than 3%) of pitted or pocked erythrocytes in peripheral blood. The last test is a useful means of monitoring splenic function after trauma and partial splenectomy.[48] Patients with severe or repeated pneumococcal infection should undergo evaluation of splenic function as well as tests for immunoglobulin deficiency and human immunodeficiency virus infection.

Etiologic Agents

Encapsulated organisms represent the greatest risk for asplenic patients. *S. pneumoniae* has been associated with 50% to 90% of the overwhelming infections occurring after splenectomy. Other pathogens are *H. influenzae* b and *N. meningitidis*. Fatal cases frequently are associated with meningitis.[43] It is not well documented that *N. meningitidis* infection is more fulminant in asplenic patients. Other streptococci, such as *Streptococcus agalactiae* (group B streptococcus) and *Enterococcus* spp., can cause fatal infection in asplenic hosts. Infections due to *Salmonella* spp. have been reported in asplenic patients, although the risk appears lower than with sickle hemoglobinopathy. Fulminant septicemia due to *Capnocytophaga canimorsus* (DF-2 bacillus), part of the mouth flora of dogs, occurs in asplenic patients, whose contact frequently is merely with pet's saliva.[49] The increased rates of gram-negative bacillary infections reported in asplenic hosts could be attributed to underlying malignancy, immunosuppression, and chemotherapy or to loss of splenic function.

Asplenic patients also have substantially higher risk for infection due to *Babesia microti*, an intraerythrocytic parasite endemic on islands off the coast of the eastern U.S. Whether asplenic patients are at greater risk of severe infection from *Plasmodium* species is not well established.[45]

Pathogenesis

The central roles of the spleen include: (1) mechanical clearance of antigen and foreign material; (2) synthesis of factors such as tuftsin that enhance phagocytosis; and (3) coordination of interactions of the T-lymphocyte and B-lymphocyte responses to organisms. The spleen is important in the *initial* response to a pathogen, perhaps as a result of its role in IgM production; the asplenic host is at a disadvantage when encountering a polysaccharide antigen for the first time. Asplenic patients are unduly affected by encapsulated organisms that require antibody and complement for opsonization and clearance. In the absence of preformed antibody, the spleen is critical in clearing the bloodstream. This may explain why adults who have developed a broad immunologic repertoire and older children who have been given pneumococcal vaccines have a lower risk than asplenic children for overwhelming infection after splenectomy.[45] Infants with congenital asplenia have profoundly impaired reticuloendothelial clearance mechanisms. Additionally, they have diminished T-lymphocyte responsiveness to a variety of antigens compared with age-matched controls.[50]

Management

Seemingly trivial febrile illnesses can herald life-threatening pneumococcal septicemia in the asplenic patient. Bacterial sepsis in a cohort of patients with visceral heterotaxy and asplenia has been reported to be 24% with a 44% mortality rate reported.[47] Clinical presentation of 26 episodes of BSI in children with asplenia included fever in 22, shock in 7, petechiae or purpura with respiratory distress in 5, and disseminated intravascular coagulopathy in 5 cases.[43] Febrile episodes require careful evaluation; empiric antibiotic therapy is begun urgently. Many physicians instruct patients to begin taking oral antibiotics at the earliest signs of infection, particularly if medical evaluation is not available immediately. For patients requiring parenteral antibiotics, empiric therapy is the same as for patients with Hb SS disease. Vancomycin and a third-generation cephalosporin usually are given.[51]

Prevention

Routinely recommended immunizations, especially PCV and PPSV23, should be given on schedule as for patients with Hb SS.[36] Hib conjugate vaccine, and varicella vaccine, are critically important for all asplenic children.[36,52] Meningococcal conjugate vaccine should be administered at 2 years of age and boosted every 5 years.[39] When splenectomy is elective, patients should be immunized at least 2 weeks before surgery.[27,53] Minimal side effects, chiefly induration and erythema at the injection site, are associated with revaccinations.[54]

It is less clear whether children with asplenia benefit from prophylactic antibiotics to the same extent as children with Hb SS. Most experts recommend penicillin prophylaxis for children who: (1) have congenital asplenia; (2) undergo splenectomy for hemolytic anemia, malignancy, or liver transplantation at any age; (3) undergo splenectomy before age 5 years; and (4) for persons of any age during the first years following splenectomy. There is no consensus as to when penicillin prophylaxis can be discontinued.[45] It is important to recognize that patients can experience fulminant infection while receiving antimicrobial prophylaxis or many years after splenectomy and, thus, require the same careful and urgent evaluation for febrile illness.

Isolated congenital asplenia (ICA) is more common than was thought previously with an autosomal dominant inheritance in at least some kindreds. Relatives of cases should be evaluated for ICA, as should children and young adults with severe invasive infections.[55]

RENAL DISEASE

Children with renal disease have increased risk for infection for a variety of reasons, including underlying disease and therapeutic modalities, such as immunosuppressive or corticosteroid therapy, and indwelling intravascular and peritoneal dialysis catheters. Children with nephrotic syndrome and accompanying hypogammaglobulinemia have increased risk for infection with encapsulated organisms, particularly *S. pneumoniae*, which require pre-formed IgG for efficient opsonization. A 1999 review of 452 admissions of 231 children with nephrotic syndrome described 10 episodes of septicemia (4 due to *S. pneumoniae*, 2 of which were fatal) and 8 episodes of peritonitis.[56] Gram-negative organisms, including *N. meningitidis* and *Salmonella* spp. as well as gut flora (*Escherichia coli, Klebsiella,* and *Enterobacter* spp.), accounted for 50% of the infections. Such patients require careful evaluation and empiric therapy effective against bowel flora as well as the encapsulated pathogens associated with BSI in patients with immunoglobulin deficiency. Patients with nephrotic syndrome also have an apparently higher frequency of urinary tract infections.

Children with nephrotic syndrome as well as other patients with chronic renal disease should be immunized with routine pediatric vaccines, including PCV13 and PPSV23.[57] Antibody levels in these patients are lower than in healthy children, but geometric mean antibody titers generally are within the protective range following immunization.[58] Duration of antibody protection may be reduced.[59] Higher doses of hepatitis B vaccine have proven more immunogenic than routine doses in children with renal failure.[60] The benefit of prophylactic penicillin in children with nephrotic syndrome is unclear because the risk of selection of multiple drug-resistant organisms is of concern. Some clinicians use prophylactic penicillin in children with nephrotic syndrome <2 or 3 years of age who have had an episode of *S. pneumoniae* BSI, as for children with sickle-cell disease.

Patients with end-stage renal disease who are undergoing ambulatory peritoneal dialysis or hemodialysis have additional risk of infection. Patients receiving chronic ambulatory peritoneal dialysis commonly experience low-grade peritonitis, which often is due to catheter-related coagulase-negative staphylococci (CoNS). Gram-negative organisms or fungi from the bowel can contaminate peritoneal fluid and cause frank peritonitis. The repeated use of vancomycin in these patients may predispose to multiple drug-resistant pathogens, such as vancomycin-resistant enterococci (VRE). Linezolid currently is considered the drug of choice for VRE infections in adults and often in children.[61] The use of indwelling arteriovenous shunts also can lead to infection, usually due to CoNS but also to *S. aureus* or other nosocomial pathogens.

Children with nephrotic syndrome who are being treated with corticosteroids (>2 mg/kg or >20 mg/day of prednisone) are at significant risk for severe varicella infection. A study of varicella vaccination in 20 children with corticosteroid-sensitive nephrotic syndrome found that anti-varicella antibodies remained high 2 years postvaccination, with only 3 subjects becoming mildly infected.[62] The use of varicella-zoster immune globulin (VariZIG) after known exposures is recommended, and some clinicians also treat exposed patients with acyclovir pre-emptively, although the oral dosages used may not achieve sufficient levels to be effective.

IRON OVERLOAD STATES

Patients with increased availability of free iron are at greater risk of serious infection due to *Yersinia enterocolitica*[63] and, less commonly, *Listeria monocytogenes, Vibrio vulnificus,* and *Klebsiella* spp.[64–67] Children at risk include those with: (1) β-thalassemia who require chronic transfusions and iron-aluminum chelation therapy with desferrioxamine;[68] (2) hemolysis due to glucose-6-phosphate dehydrogenase deficiency and other conditions; (3) idiopathic hemochromatosis; and (4) chronic renal failure managed with chronic transfusions and chelation.[69] The use of erythropoietin in chronic anemias should decrease the incidence of these infections.

Many in vitro studies demonstrate the importance of iron-scavenging systems in the virulence of bacteria and parasites as well as of free iron-depleting defense mechanisms of the host during acute infection.[64]

Most patients with iron overload syndromes have other deficiencies in immune function due to reticuloendothelial blockade and functional asplenia. However, increased free iron itself predisposes to *Yersinia* spp. infections and has been reported as a complication of acute iron ingestion.[70] In addition, a high rate of gram-negative BSI has been associated with the intramuscular injection of iron-dextran in neonates.[71] Acidosis, particularly

PART II Clinical Syndromes and Cardinal Features of Infectious Diseases: Approach to Diagnosis and Initial Management

SECTION R Infections in Patients with Deficient Defenses

diabetic ketoacidosis, leads to a greater availability of iron through a number of mechanisms and has been associated with infection due to Zygomycetes in patients with acidosis.[66]

Etiologic Agents and Pathogenesis

Y. enterocolitica has been associated with septicemia, mesenteric lymphadenitis, liver and splenic abscesses, and an acute appendicitis-like syndrome in patients with thalassemia and hemochromatosis.[68,72] Organisms can be found in blood, stool, and lymph nodes. *V. vulnificus* can cause severe and frequently fatal BSI in these patients, and also has been reported in necrotizing fasciitis in a child with congenital spherocytosis.[73] Infections caused by *L. monocytogenes*, *Salmonella* spp., *Klebsiella* spp., and Zygomycetes are reported in patients who are treated with desferrioxamine for iron overload associated with chronic transfusion.[67]

Yersinia spp., like other bacteria and fungi, require iron for growth. Unlike most other organisms, however, *Yersinia* spp. and the Zygomycetes are able to use iron complexed with the siderophore desferrioxamine and thrive under conditions of increased iron.[70] Several studies have demonstrated diminished immune function (decreased phagocytic function, impaired T-lymphocyte responsiveness) in the presence of elevated serum iron levels. Thus, both host and bacterial factors contribute to the greater susceptibility to infection.[71]

Clinical Manifestations and Management

The most common presentation of *Y. enterocolitica* infection in patients with thalassemia consists of fever, chills, and gastrointestinal complaints ranging from bloody diarrhea to frank peritonitis. Findings suggestive of acute appendicitis are associated with recovery of *Y. enterocolitica* from mesenteric lymph nodes. Normal hosts generally limit the organism to the intestinal mucosa, resulting in self-limited enteritis, appendicitis-like syndromes, and occasional extraintestinal infection.

Early recognition and specific treatment are important. Iron chelation therapy with desferrioxamine should be temporarily discontinued. Some *Y. enterocolitica* are susceptible to trimethoprim-sulfamethoxazole and aminoglycosides; most are susceptible to fluoroquinolones and third-generation cephalosporins. Parenteral therapy with a third-generation cephalosporin is appropriate for febrile, ill patients without focal signs of infection.

CILIARY DYSFUNCTION

Primary ciliary dyskinesia is an autosomal-recessive disease with an incidence of approximately 1 in 15,000 to 30,000 births. At least 11 distinct ultrastructural abnormalities of cilia have been associated with the immotile cilia syndrome.[74] Approximately one-half of patients with immotile cilia syndrome have situs inversus, which may be associated with Kartagener syndrome, dextrocardia, asplenia, or polysplenia. Lack of normal mucociliary clearance in the respiratory tract leads to a higher incidence of local infection. Patients with ciliary dysfunction have respiratory symptoms in the first month of life and often are colonized with *H. influenzae*.[74]

Recurrent mucopurulent rhinitis, otitis media, and bronchitis lead to bronchiectasis in as many as 85% of patients. Risk of invasive infection is not increased (unless there is an associated splenic abnormality), and pulmonary function usually is preserved until late in the course of disease. Longitudinal studies suggest that patients diagnosed early in life who are treated aggressively for infection have significantly better pulmonary function than those who are not treated for infection.[75] Bronchiectasis is the most significant complication, but young infants can have frequently acute otitis media (AOM), leading to hearing impairment.[76] The most common infecting organisms associated with bronchiectasis in primary ciliary dyskinesia are nontypable *H. influenzae* (47%), *S. pneumoniae* (32%), and *Pseudomonas aeruginosa* (16%).[77] In upper-airway infections, typical agents of AOM and sinusitis are common.

Bronchodilator therapy may be useful in some patients. Antimicrobial therapy is aimed at treating existent infection and decreasing inflammation. Physical therapy aids in clearance of secretions and prevention of atelectasis. Unlike cystic fibrosis, ciliary dysfunction does not reduce life expectancy significantly.

ASCITES

Patients with ascites due to either hepatic or renal dysfunction have increased risk for infection, particularly primary peritonitis. Historically, these infections were often due to group A streptococci or pneumococci. Although pneumococcal peritonitis remains a major problem in children with nephrotic syndrome, children with ascites due to hepatic disease also are at increased risk for peritonitis due to gram-negative bacteria. The close association of primary peritonitis and ascites due to hepatic disease suggests that the compromised reticuloendothelial function of the liver attributed to cirrhosis and portal hypertension allows organisms that would normally be cleared to contaminate hepatic lymph and pass into the peritoneal fluid. Because the liver is an important site for the clearance of bacteria from the bloodstream, significant compromise of this function leads to peritoneal infection, bloodstream infection, or both.[78,79] In studies of adults with peritonitis, up to 75% of patients have BSI. Experimental data suggest that bacteria also can traverse the intestinal wall to seed the peritoneal cavity. Thus, gram-negative bacilli can cause peritonitis. Although peritoneal fluid cultures are positive in the majority of patients with ascites and peritonitis, culture techniques inadequate for recovery of anaerobic organisms may explain some negative culture results.[80]

The composition of the ascitic fluid contributes significantly to the development of clinically significant peritonitis. Low levels of complement and immunoglobulins allow bacterial proliferation; a direct correlation exists between the amount of protein in ascitic fluid and susceptibility to infection.

The diagnosis and treatment of primary peritonitis in patients with ascites hinge on examination of peritoneal fluid and exclusion of other sources of infection, particularly intra-abdominal infection. Despite the presence of neutrophils, culture results can be negative; empiric treatment often is required. Choice of therapy is directed by Gram stain and likely sources of infection. A third-generation cephalosporin such as cefotaxime may be useful for activity against possible aerobic and facultative bowel flora and *S. pneumoniae*. In children repeatedly exposed to nosocomial pathogens who have received multiple courses of antibiotics, the use of a carbapenem plus metronidazole, for activity against *P. aeruginosa*, multiple-drug-resistant Enterobacteriaceae (*Enterobacter*, *Citrobacter*, *Serratia*, *Klebsiella* spp.), and anaerobic bacteria, may be warranted initially.

In adults with uncomplicated spontaneous bacterial peritonitis, a therapeutic course of a fluoroquinolone orally often is used.[79] In adults with cirrhosis, prophylactic use of a fluoroquinolone decreases the number of episodes of primary peritonitis, although it also raises the risk of selecting multiple drug-resistant pathogens and *C. difficile*.[81]

CYSTIC FIBROSIS

Cystic fibrosis (CF) is the most common lethal genetic disease of white people. It is caused by mutations in the CF transmembrane regulator (CFTR), an adenosine triphosphate-dependent chloride channel primarily expressed in the lung and exocrine glands.[82] Patients have chronic pulmonary infection with airway inflammation, and poor growth secondary to pancreatic exocrine insufficiency and malabsorption. Sinusitis secondary to abnormal secretions and nasal polyps as well as pancreatic endocrine insufficiency can cause significant morbidity. Aggressive medical management of the pulmonary and gastrointestinal manifestations of CF has more than doubled the life expectancy of affected patients from a median of 14 years in 1969 to a median of 37.4 years in 2005.[83,84]

TABLE 108-1. Age-Related Appearance of Pathogens in Cystic Fibrosis

Patient Age	Pathogens
Early infancy	*Staphylococcus aureus*
Early childhood	*Haemophilus influenzae*
Adolescence	*Pseudomonas aeruginosa*
Late in disease	*Burkholderia cepacia* complex *Stenotrophomonas maltophilia* *Achromobacter xylosoxidans* *Aspergillus fumigatus*

Etiologic Agents

The spectrum of bacterial pathogens colonizing and infecting the lungs of patients with CF is relatively limited (Table 108-1).[85] *S. aureus, H. influenzae* (mostly nontypable), and *P. aeruginosa* are the most commonly isolated bacterial pathogens, and several studies demonstrate bacterial lung infections within the first 3 years of life.[86,87] *P. aeruginosa* is the predominant pathogen in CF and is seen in between 45% and 62% of pediatric patients.[88] Although infection with both nonmucoid and mucoid phenotypes of *P. aeruginosa* is associated with a more rapid decline in lung function, mucoid isolates signal chronic infection and are very difficult to eradicate.[89,90] Later in the course of disease, multiple drug-resistant gram-negative organisms such as *Burkholderia cepacia* complex, *Stenotrophomonas maltophilia*, and *Achromobacter xylosoxidans* are isolated. Although *B. cepacia* complex organisms, particularly *B. cenocepacia* (genomovar III) and *B. multivorans* (genomovar II), have been associated with both fulminant pulmonary infection and chronic colonization,[91] the clinical significance of *S. maltophilia* and *A. xylosoxidans* is less well characterized.[92,93]

Fungi such as *Aspergillus* and *Fusarium* also cause disease in patients with CF. *A. fumigatus* can manifest as allergic bronchopulmonary aspergillosis,[94] lung transplantation, invasive dissemination (possibly related to corticosteroid use),[95] and as pulmonary or invasive disease.[96] In a multicenter study, nontuberculous mycobacteria were isolated from sputum in up to 13% of patients with CF, more commonly in older patients, those with a higher forced expiratory volume in 1 second, those with lower body mass, and those with *S. aureus*, but not *P. aeruginosa*, isolated from sputum. However, whether mycobacterial infection affects pulmonary decline remains unclear.[97] The role of infection with respiratory viruses and *Mycoplasma* spp. in patients with cystic fibrosis has been examined in several studies. There appears to be no difference in the numbers of upper respiratory tract viral infections between children with CF and unaffected controls. However, children with cystic fibrosis have significantly more episodes of lower respiratory tract disease.[98,99] Studies support a causative role for influenza in acute pulmonary exacerbations;[100] high morbidity and occasional fatality during acute influenza infection are recognized. During infancy, respiratory syncytial virus may be an important cause of early pulmonary morbidity, requiring hospitalization.[101] Rhinovirus and influenza are important viral pathogens of early childhood and adolescence.[102,103]

Epidemiology

The epidemiology of the acquisition of *P. aeruginosa* in CF increasingly is being examined. The majority of children with CF appear to have unique strains[104,105] and these early isolates share many phenotypic characteristics with environmental isolates.[106] Studies in siblings and at summer camps identify common strains in patients with close contact; it is uncertain whether these findings result from person-to-person spread or a common environmental source. Outbreaks of multiple drug-resistant *P. aeruginosa* in CF centers in Europe and Australia have identified epidemic strains that appear capable of person-to-person transmission.[107,108]

Epidemiologic studies also support the conclusion that *B. cepacia* complex can be spread from person to person. Molecular typing of *B. cepacia* complex has identified unique strains in each CF center, and studies of the epidemiology in summer camps attended by patients from different geographic areas have demonstrated cross-infection.[109] Social contact outside the hospital has also been implicated in the spread of *B. cepacia* complex.[110] Of the 9 named species in the complex, *B. cenocepacia* has specific clones, especially ET12, that have most clearly been associated with transmissibility.[111] A significant problem in understanding the epidemiology of *B. cepacia* complex is the demonstration that up to 2 years may elapse from the time of acquisition of the organism until it is detected by sputum culture.[112]

Pathogenesis

The molecular events responsible for the close association between *P. aeruginosa* and the lungs of patients with CF have not been defined fully. Inspissated secretions and dehydrated mucus decrease normal mucociliary clearance of organisms and facilitate chronic infection. Expression of increased numbers of asialylated glycolipid receptors for *Pseudomonas* pili on the epithelium of the lung in such patients may predispose them to colonization.[113] Some studies suggest that naturally occurring airway antimicrobial peptides are inhibited by the milieu in the lungs of patients with CF.[114] After colonization, *P. aeruginosa* grows in microcolonies, forming biofilms within the airway.[115,116] The environment within the lung in CF favors the proliferation of mucoid mutants of *P. aeruginosa* that produce large amounts of alginate exopolysaccharide, interfering with effective phagocytosis. Once a chronic infection is established, organisms are rarely, if ever, eradicated. Infection is endobronchial in location, with bacteria loosely enmeshed in a viscous layer of mucus that contains large amounts of cellular debris, neutrophil DNA, and actin. Histopathologic analysis shows that areas of focal infection surrounded by neutrophils. Eventually, chronic infection, fibrosis, and loss of the normal pulmonary parenchyma result. Much of the observed pathology is due to the inflammatory response to *P. aeruginosa*.

Clinical Manifestations

Because of their inability to eradicate bacterial pathogens from the lower airways, patients with CF have chronic pulmonary symptoms including chronic cough, expectoration of sputum, and progressive deterioration in pulmonary function. Acute episodes of clinical exacerbation are superimposed on chronic pulmonary symptoms. Because of wide variation in the severity of underlying manifestations, a pulmonary exacerbation is difficult to determine by clinical criteria alone.[117] Rather than new symptomatology, an exacerbation is more often heralded by a quantitative change in ongoing symptoms, for example, an increase in frequency and intensity of cough or in the quantity and purulence of sputum. The acute and chronic symptoms are the result of vigorous inflammatory responses to endobronchial infection. Increased airway disease manifests as tachypnea and increased work of breathing (retractions, use of accessory respiratory muscles, and wheezing). Systemic manifestations of pulmonary exacerbation include malaise, myalgia, anorexia, weight loss, and (rarely) low-grade fever.

Nonpulmonary symptoms of CF that can mimic infection include immune complex-mediated manifestations, such as vasculitic rashes[118] and arthritis.[119] In addition to pancreatic insufficiency, gastrointestinal manifestations include severe constipation, intestinal obstruction, and unrecognized or unusual presentations of acute appendicitis. Sinusitis secondary to nasal polyps is common.[120] Etiologic agents include the usual sinus pathogens plus organisms colonizing the lower airways in this population. In addition to causing acute and chronic disease, sinuses can serve as a reservoir for antibiotic-resistant organisms in patients undergoing lung transplantation.

PART II Clinical Syndromes and Cardinal Features of Infectious Diseases: Approach to Diagnosis and Initial Management

SECTION R Infections in Patients with Deficient Defenses

Laboratory Findings

Decline in results of pulmonary function studies is the most accurate and objective indicator of pulmonary exacerbation. Unfortunately, most patients <5 years of age cannot perform pulmonary function tests reproducibly, making the diagnosis of an exacerbation more difficult. The appearance of a new pulmonary infiltrate on a chest radiograph can be helpful; however, most pulmonary exacerbations, especially in patients with advanced disease, are unassociated with significant radiographic changes, probably because of the marked abnormalities present at baseline (Figure 108-2).

Sputum culture can accurately identify the bacterial pathogens colonizing lower-airway secretions.[121] Oropharyngeal culture (a suggested alternative in the nonexpectorating patient) is a relatively insensitive measure of lower-airway pathogens.[122] A technique combining the use of selective media and quantitative culture methods to identify infecting organisms in sputum also is used to evaluate therapeutic response.[123] This method circumvents the problem of rapidly growing mucoid strains of *P. aeruginosa*, which obscure the growth of more fastidious organisms such as *H. influenzae*.

Other laboratory studies helpful in defining a pulmonary exacerbation are white blood cell count with differential and measurements of acute-phase reactants, such as erythrocyte sedimentation rate and C-reactive protein level.[124] These tests are of limited value without baseline measurements for comparison. BSI rarely is seen[125] except in a subpopulation of patients infected with *B. cepacia* complex, with indwelling catheters, and immunosuppressed patients following lung transplantation. Blood cultures are not indicated routinely in patients with CF unless they have an indwelling central venous catheter, are colonized with *B. cepacia* complex, or have undergone lung transplantation.

Management

The goal of treatment is to prevent pulmonary damage from chronic infection and inflammation. Mainstays of therapy include nutritional support with pancreatic enzyme supplementation, chest physiotherapy to improve the drainage of pulmonary secretions, bronchodilator therapy to treat reactive airway disease, and antibiotic treatment to decrease bacterial density in the lungs. Antibiotic therapy in CF can take three forms: (1) early treatment of colonization (pre-emptive therapy); (2) suppression of chronic infection; and (3) treatment of acute pulmonary exacerbations.

Aggressive pre-emptive therapy for CF patients with their first *P. aeruginosa*-positive airway culture is the standard of care in several Scandinavian countries and is being implemented in other populations.[126–130] Since 1989, studies from Denmark in intermittently colonized CF patients have examined the clinical and microbiological efficacy of treatment with oral ciprofloxacin in combination with inhaled colistin and reported a decrease in acquisition of chronic *P. aeruginosa* infections as well as improvement in lung function.[130] Several other studies have demonstrated eradication of intermittent *P. aeruginosa* colonization with use of inhaled tobramycin.[126,128,129] In these studies, when *P. aeruginosa* reappeared, the organism most frequently was a new strain.[127,129]

The role of suppressive therapy in individuals with chronic *P. aeruginosa* infections has also been demonstrated, using antibiotics that have in vitro and in vivo antibacterial activity and those that demonstrate neither. Tobramycin has been used parenterally in pulmonary exacerbations for many years; most isolates of *P. aeruginosa* in patients with CF are susceptible. Use of high-dose inhaled tobramycin is associated with improvement in pulmonary function, decrease in the risk of hospitalization, and reduction in *P. aeruginosa* density in sputum without detectable ototoxicity or nephrotoxicity, and without a substantially higher rate of tobramycin resistance.[125–131] More recently, inhaled aztreonam lysinate has been shown to be safe and efficacious in CF.[132] Several randomized controlled trials of treatment with oral azithromycin, a macrolide agent with anti-inflammatory properties, to which *P. aeruginosa* routinely is resistant in vitro, also have demonstrated clinical improvement in lung function, body weight, number of exacerbations, and quality of life, but without a decrease in sputum bacterial density.[133–135]

Optimal antibiotic management of pulmonary exacerbations depends on knowledge of each patient's recent sputum bacteriology and susceptibility test results. Two drugs with antipseudomonal activity are normally given – usually a β-lactam agent or fluoroquinolone plus an aminoglycoside. Because of the potential for the induction of expression of the *Pseudomonas* chromosomal β-lactamase, combinations containing two β-lactam agents are avoided. Late in the course of disease, multiple-drug-resistant strains are frequently isolated, and synergy testing may identify combinations of antibiotics with potential efficacy. However, in a controlled clinical trial in subjects with clinical exacerbations, antibiotic therapy directed by combination susceptibility testing of *P. aeruginosa*, *B. cepacia* complex, *S. maltophilia*, and

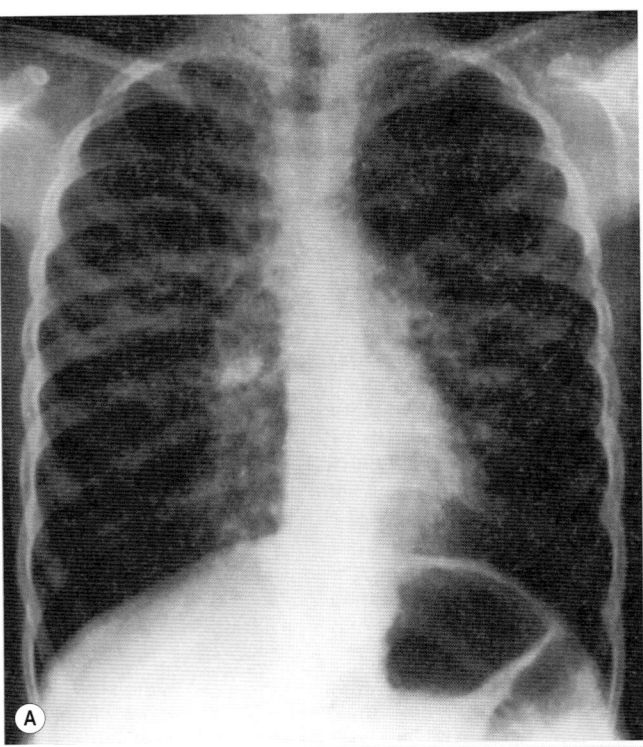

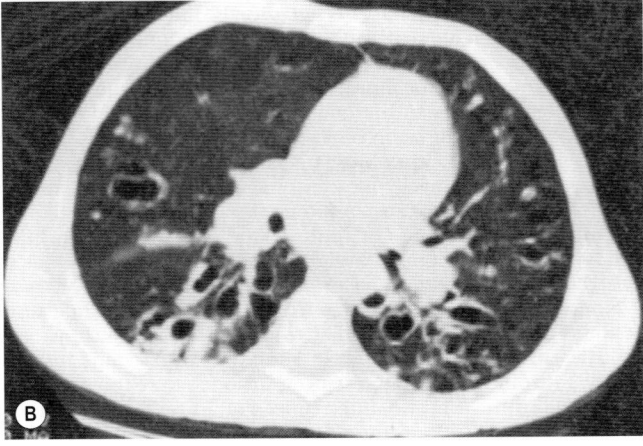

Figure 108-2. (A) Chest radiograph of a 14-year-old boy with cystic fibrosis demonstrating typical changes of hyperinflation, bronchial wall thickening, and areas of bronchiectasis and consolidation. **(B)** Computed tomography demonstrates the magnitude of changes and diffuse nature of the pulmonary involvement.

A. xylosoxidans did not result in better clinical or bacteriologic outcomes compared with therapy directed by standard testing.[136] Similar results have been reported for the use of biofilm susceptibility testing.[137]

Several problems are inherent to the selection and use of antibiotics in patients with CF. Chronic inflammation in the lung and localization of infection in the lumen of the airway make achievement of adequate levels of bioactive drug at the site of the infection difficult. The lack of a microbiologic endpoint for treating infections (organisms are never eradicated) makes definition of antibiotic resistance problematic. The differences in antibiotic pharmacokinetics identified in individuals with CF require the modification of drug dosing because the clearance of many drugs is higher compared with unaffected controls.[138–140]

Bilateral lung transplantation is a potential life-extending therapy for selected patients with end-stage pulmonary disease. However, infectious complications caused by multiple drug-resistant bacteria and fungi are a serious posttransplantation problem because of the immunosuppression required for transplantation.[141] Although infected lungs are removed, colonization of upper respiratory and gastrointestinal tracts persists. Bronchiolitis obliterans also is a potentially fatal complication of transplantation.

Recombinant human deoxyribonuclease has been demonstrated to improve pulmonary function and decrease the frequency of pulmonary exacerbations in patients with CF.[142] Improved mucociliary clearance results from lysis of the high concentrations of leukocyte DNA in the sputum of such patients.[143] Nebulized hypertonic saline, shown to improve mucociliary clearance, also has been demonstrated in short-term trials to improve mucociliary clearance, but is not recommended routinely in the management of individuals with CF.[144]

Recent Advances

Investigational efforts in CF have been divided between anti-infective–anti-inflammatory strategies and potentially curative therapies. Aerosol administration of other antimicrobial agents in addition to tobramycin and aztreonam[145] is potentially advantageous, because high concentrations of drug can be delivered directly to the site of infection and potential toxicity can be avoided.[129,132] The potential role of anti-inflammatory

medications, including corticosteroids and ibuprofen, has been demonstrated in well-controlled clinical trials, although treatment with systemic corticosteroids has unacceptable side effects.[146,147] Other anti-inflammatory strategies currently being examined include inhibitors of proinflammatory mediators, anti-inflammatory cytokines, modulators of proinflammatory signaling cascades, antioxidants, and protease inhibitors.[148]

Potentially curative therapies include gene therapy and pharmacologic approaches to correct the phenotype resulting from mutant CFTR. Although many CF-associated gene mutations have been identified and administration of CFTR cDNA to humans can complement the defect in vivo, the development of effective vectors to deliver the gene to the appropriate target cells and maintain its expression is challenging.[149,150] Another therapeutic strategy is the use of agents that restore activity of the mutant gene product such as CFTR potentiators, drugs that target protein folding and trafficking, and agents that induce translational read-through of stop codons and other nonsense mutations.[151] Pharmacologic agents that correct the ion transport defect in CF also are under development.[152]

Prevention

Approaches to the prevention of *P. aeruginosa* colonization have included the aggressive use of prophylactic antibiotics described above and the development of antipseudomonal vaccines for use in noncolonized patients. Preliminary studies demonstrated that a polyvalent *P. aeruginosa* conjugate vaccine was safe and immunogenic;[153] long-term follow-up of 26 young children demonstrated a longer time to *P. aeruginosa* infection and fewer chronic infections in the study group compared with matched controls.[154]

Patients with CF should receive all routine childhood and adolescent immunizations including PCV, varicella-zoster vaccine, and inactivated influenza vaccine.[155] In addition, their families should receive acellular pertussis and annual influenza vaccine because of the high rate of morbidity associated with infection in CF patients.[100,103] There is no specific recommendation for routine administration of PPSV23 in patients with CF; however, a single dose of PPSV23 is recommended at the age ≥2 years for any immunocompetent child with chronic illness (including chronic lung disease).[36]

---

109 Epidemiology and Prevention of HIV Infection in Children and Adolescents

Jennifer S. Read

The epidemiology of infection with human immunodeficiency virus type 1 (HIV) in children and adolescents has evolved dramatically since the first case of pediatric HIV infection was described almost three decades ago.[1] This evolution is a result of changes in the patterns of acquisition of HIV infection by children and adolescents, as well as improvements in the management of HIV infection, with resultant increased survival of individuals with HIV infection. This chapter addresses the epidemiology of HIV infection among children and adolescents, how HIV infection is acquired by and manifests itself in these populations, and prevention of HIV infection in children and adolescents.

EPIDEMIOLOGY

The epidemiology of HIV infection varies dramatically between resource-poor and resource-rich settings around the world. Estimates of the extent of the HIV epidemic, globally and in the United States, are updated regularly by the Joint United Nations Programme on HIV/AIDS and the World Health Organization (WHO)[2] and by the Centers for Disease Control and Prevention (CDC),[3] respectively. In the U.S., African American and other minority infants, children, and adolescents are disproportionately affected by HIV infection.[3] As among adults, HIV transmission to

PART II   Clinical Syndromes and Cardinal Features of Infectious Diseases: Approach to Diagnosis and Initial Management

SECTION S   Human Immunodeficiency Virus and the Acquired Immunodeficiency Syndrome

infants, children, and adolescents can occur through: sexual contact (vaginal, anal, or orogenital), percutaneous blood exposure (from contaminated needles or other sharp instruments), mucous membrane exposure to contaminated blood or other body fluids, and transfusion with contaminated blood products.[4] Unique to the pediatric population is the possibility of acquisition of HIV infection through mother-to-child transmission of infection.[4]

Of the estimated 33.4 million people living with HIV infection in 2008, 15.7 million were women and 2.1 million were children under 15 years of age, and most HIV-infected people (22.4 million) resided in sub-Saharan Africa.[2] An estimated 1.4 million HIV-infected individuals were in North America, and 850,000 in western and central Europe. Of the estimated 2.7 million new infections in 2008 (55,000 in North America and 30,000 in western and central Europe), 2.3 million were among adults and 430,000 among children.[2] Finally, among the estimated 2.0 million AIDS-related deaths in 2008 (25,000 in North America, 13,000 in western and central Europe), 1.7 million occurred in adults and 280,000 in children.[2] In 2007, the number of persons living with a diagnosis of HIV infection in 37 states and 5 U.S. dependent areas with confidential name-based HIV infection reporting included 9116 children (under age 13 years at diagnosis).[3]

Both in the U.S. and globally, mother-to-child transmission is the most common means of acquisition of HIV infection by children (Table 109-1). For example, of the 9116 children reported to be living with HIV infection in the 37 states and U.S. dependent areas in 2007,[3] 8019 (88%) were classified as having acquired infection through mother-to-child transmission.[3] While there has been a dramatic decrease in the rate of mother-to-child transmission of HIV and in the number of pediatric HIV infections and AIDS cases in the U.S., mother-to-child transmission has not been eradicated in the U.S. In 2006, there were an estimated 125,050 to 128,653 HIV-infected women in the U.S., and 8650 to 8900 infants were delivered of HIV-infected women.[5] The estimated number of cases of mother-to-child transmission of HIV in the U.S. peaked in 1991 (1650 infections).[6] By 2005, the number of cases of mother-to-child transmission in the U.S. had decreased to an estimated 215 to 370, representing a transmission rate of approximately 2.8%.[7]

Mother-to-child transmission of HIV can occur during pregnancy, around the time of labor and delivery, and postnatally (through breastfeeding).[8] Most transmission is estimated to occur during the intrapartum period (both in breastfeeding and non-breastfeeding populations).[9] Rates of mother-to-child transmission of HIV have been calculated in studies conducted in various countries prior to the development and implementation of interventions to decrease transmission.[10] Usually a transmission rate in the range of 25% to 30% was reported. Higher transmission rates were observed in resource-poor settings (13% to 42%) compared with rates in resource-rich settings (14% to 25%), in part attributed to the greater proportion of breastfeeding in resource-poor settings.

Various risk factors for mother-to-child transmission of HIV have been identified or are under investigation, and can be categorized as follows: (1) the amount of virus to which the child is exposed (e.g., maternal viral load[11-15]); (2) the duration of such exposure (e.g., the duration of ruptured membranes[16] or of breastfeeding,[17] vaginal versus cesarean delivery before labor and before ruptured membranes[18,19]); and (3) factors facilitating the transfer of virus from mother to child (e.g., mixed breastfeeding,[20,21] maternal breast pathology,[13,22-24] and infant oral candidiasis[23,24]). In addition to these risk factors, characteristics of the virus and the child's susceptibility to infection are important.

In 2007, the number of persons living with a diagnosis of HIV infection in 37 states and 5 U.S. dependent areas with confidential name-based HIV infection reporting included 7114 adolescents (13 to 19 years of age) and 17,922 young adults (20 to 24 years of age).[3] Improved estimation of HIV incidence is now possible with new assays that differentiate between recent versus chronic HIV infections.[25] The estimated incidence of HIV infection in the 50 states and the District of Columbia in 2006 was 19,200 among 13- to 29-year-old individuals.[25] Many cases of HIV infection in young adults represent infections that actually were acquired during adolescence, but not recognized until several years later. Among the estimated 430,892 male adults and adolescents living with HIV infection in 2007, 268,692 (62%) of these infections were acquired through male-to-male sexual contact, 74,692 (17%) were due to injection drug use, 31,036 (7%) were due to male-to-male sexual contact and injection drug use, and 53,687 (12%) were due to heterosexual contact[3] (Table 109-1). In contrast, among the estimated 159,808 female adults and adolescents living with HIV infection in 2007, 115,925 (72%) were acquired through heterosexual contact and 41,869 (26%) from injection drug use[3] (Table 109-1).

Aside from mother-to-child transmission, sexual transmission, and transmission related to intravenous drug use, other means of acquisition of HIV infection include transfusion of contaminated blood or blood products in settings in which routine and effective screening of blood is not available, percutaneous blood exposure (from contaminated needles or other sharp instruments), and mucous membrane exposure to contaminated blood or other body fluids (Table 109-1).[4] The first case of pediatric HIV infection in the U.S. was an infant who acquired HIV infection through a transfusion of contaminated blood,[1] and thousands of patients with hemophilia and other recipients of contaminated blood and blood products acquired HIV infection before screening of blood and blood products for HIV. Now, in the U.S. and many other countries, blood, blood components, and clotting factors undergo highly effective screening procedures. As a result, transmission of HIV through transfusion of blood or blood products in the U.S. has decreased substantially,[26-29] and virtually has been eliminated. The risk of transmission of HIV through blood transfusions in the U.S. in 2010 was estimated as 1:1,467,000.[29] In addition to intravenous drug use, other exposure to contaminated needles (e.g., with tattooing)[30] can result in HIV transmission. Possible transmission of HIV through receipt of food that has been pre-chewed by an HIV-infected caregiver with bleeding gums or open sores in the mouth has been reported.[31] There have been rare cases of household transmission of HIV between siblings,[32] but in these cases, there were opportunities for skin or mucous membrane exposure to HIV-infected blood. Thus, all caregivers of HIV-infected children should receive education regarding universal precautions.[33,34] Transmission of HIV rarely occurs in households or as a result of routine outpatient or inpatient care, and has not

TABLE 109-1. Modes of Acquisition of HIV Infection in Children and Adolescents

Children	Adolescents
MOST COMMON	**MOST COMMON**
Mother-to-child transmission	Sexual transmission: Males: male-to-male sexual transmission Females: heterosexual transmission Injection drug use
OTHER	**OTHER**
Transfusion of contaminated blood or blood products (if effective screening not available, e.g., among patients with hemophilia early in the HIV epidemic in the U.S.)	Percutaneous blood exposure (from contaminated needles or other sharp instruments, e.g., with tattooing)
Mucous membrane exposure to contaminated blood or other body fluids (e.g., through receipt of food that has been prechewed by an HIV-infected caregiver with bleeding gums or open sores in the mouth)	
Sexual abuse	

been described in schools or childcare settings in the U.S.[4,35-37] Finally, cases of HIV transmission to children through sexual abuse have been reported.[38-40]

CLINICAL MANIFESTATIONS AND PROGRESSION

Infection with HIV results in a myriad of clinical manifestations. Acquired immunodeficiency syndrome, or AIDS, refers to the most advanced disease stage of HIV infection. AIDS is defined by the development of life-threatening manifestations, including opportunistic infections and neoplasms, due to progressive immunosuppression induced by HIV infection. The CDC has developed and revised, most recently in 2008, the surveillance case definitions for HIV infection and AIDS.[41]

The CDC classifies HIV-infected children (below 13 years of age) according to their clinical status (ranging from N (not symptomatic), through A and B, to C (severely symptomatic; AIDS)) and immunologic status (Category 1 (CD4+ T-lymphocyte count or percentage indicating no evidence of immune suppression) to Category 3 (severe suppression)).[42] Thus, combining both the clinical and immunologic staging of children results in categories of N1 through C3. This classification system takes into account the age-related changes (<1 year, 1 to 5 years, 6 to 12 years) in the normal ranges of CD4+ lymphocyte counts. The classification system for adolescents and adults similarly classifies HIV-infected individuals according to their clinical and immunologic status, except that the clinical staging ranges from A to C (no category N).[43]

The natural history of HIV infection in infants who acquired HIV infection through mother-to-child transmission differs from that in adults. Plasma viral loads among untreated, infected infants increase rapidly after birth,[44] peaking at 1 to 2 months of age (median values of 318,000 and 256,000 copies/mL, respectively).[45] Untreated, viral loads decline slowly during the first 2 years of life,[45] reaching values observed in HIV-infected adults only at approximately 5 years of age.[46]

Early studies of disease progression among HIV-infected infants who acquired infection through mother-to-child transmission[47,48] were conducted in an era when pediatric antiretroviral treatment was much more limited than currently. In a study of 128 HIV-infected children in North America,[47] the median ages of progression to clinical classes A, B, and C were 5, 11, and 48 months, respectively. Among 392 HIV-infected children in Europe, an estimated 20% progressed to class C disease or death during the first year of life, and approximately 5% progressed per year thereafter.[48] The mortality rate at 6 years was 26%.[48] Early onset of clinical manifestations of HIV infection (lymphadenopathy, hepatomegaly, splenomegaly at 3 months of age or earlier) and positive HIV diagnostic testing within the first week of life were associated with more rapid disease progression.[47]

Since the late 1990s, with the introduction of more widespread antiretroviral treatment programs, and more effective antiretroviral regimens, the morbidity and mortality associated with HIV infection among infants, children, adolescents, and adults has decreased substantially.[49-61] Opportunistic and other infections were uncommon among HIV-infected children in 2000 to 2004,[62] and infection rates were lower than in those reported in earlier years.[63] Similarly, the incidence of certain noninfectious conditions (encephalopathy, pancreatitis, cardiac disorders) decreased between 2001 and 2006 among HIV-infected children and adolescents.[64]

Early diagnosis of HIV infection and early initiation of antiretroviral therapy reduced early infant mortality by 76% and HIV progression by 75% in a randomized trial conducted in South Africa.[65] Based on these data and the high risk of rapid progression in young infants, initiation of antiretroviral therapy for all infants is recommended, regardless of clinical, immunologic (CD4+ lymphocyte percentage), or viral load status.[66]

There is substantial variation in HIV disease progression among adolescents and adults; some individuals progress to AIDS in <5 years,[67] but some untreated individuals ("long-term non-progressors") do not deteriorate clinically or immunologically for many years.[68,69] Current guidelines for initiation of antiretroviral

therapy in HIV-infected adolescents and adults[70] recommend the initiation of antiretroviral therapy in individuals with a history of an AIDS-defining illness or with a CD4+ lymphocyte count of <350 cells/mm^3, in those with CD4+ lymphocyte counts between 350 and 500 cells/mm^3, in patients with HIV-associated nephropathy, and in those with hepatitis B virus co-infection when treatment of hepatitis B infection is indicated. Some experts recommend antiretroviral therapy in patients with CD4+ lymphocyte counts >500 cells/mm^3. Once antiretroviral therapy is initiated, therapy is generally continued for life.

PREVENTION

Mother-to-child transmission represents the means by which virtually all infants and young children acquire HIV infection. Most adults and adolescents acquire HIV infection through sexual transmission or percutaneous exposure (e.g., intravenous drug use). Discussion of prevention of HIV transmission to children and adolescents focuses on these routes of transmission.

Interventions to Prevent Mother-to-Child Transmission (Box 109-1)

Prevention of mother-to-child transmission of HIV is just one component of the overall management of HIV-infected women and their children. The WHO's Strategic Approach to Prevention of Pediatric HIV Infection[71] includes four components: primary prevention of HIV infection; prevention of unintended pregnancies among HIV-infected women; prevention of transmission of HIV infection from mothers to children; and provision of ongoing support, care, and treatment to HIV-infected women and their families. Ideally, primary prevention of HIV infection occurs, e.g., an HIV-uninfected woman does not acquire HIV infection either before or during pregnancy. To facilitate prevention of acquisition of HIV infection, individuals should know their own and their sexual partners' HIV infection status. This is accomplished through provision of and access to HIV counseling and testing. Prevention of unintended pregnancies is crucial for women who acquire HIV infection. Antiretroviral therapy for women who need treatment of their HIV infection, antiretroviral prophylaxis for women who do not yet meet criteria for treatment, antiretroviral prophylaxis for infants of HIV-infected mothers, and other interventions to prevent mother-to-child transmission of HIV, should be available. Finally, HIV-infected women and their children need ongoing support, care, and treatment, including infant feeding counseling and support.

Although different interventions to prevent mother-to-child transmission of HIV have been and are being investigated, efficacy has been demonstrated to date for only the following: antiretroviral prophylaxis,[72-78] cesarean delivery before labor and before ruptured membranes,[18] complete avoidance of breastfeeding,[79] and (in settings where complete avoidance of breastfeeding

---

BOX 109-1. Prevention of Mother-to-Child Transmission of HIV

- Antiretroviral therapy
  - Antiretroviral treatment for women (who meet criteria for treatment) or antiretroviral prophylaxis for women (who do not meet criteria for treatment or who do not want to use antiretroviral treatment) during the antepartum, intrapartum (and postpartum[a]) periods
  - For the non-breastfeeding infant (early postnatal period)
  - For the breastfeeding infant[a]
- Cesarean delivery before labor and before ruptured membranes
- Complete avoidance of breastfeeding
- Exclusive breastfeeding[a]

[a]When complete avoidance of breastfeeding is not feasible or safe.

PART II Clinical Syndromes and Cardinal Features of Infectious Diseases: Approach to Diagnosis and Initial Management

SECTION S Human Immunodeficiency Virus and the Acquired Immunodeficiency Syndrome

is not feasible) exclusive breastfeeding,[80] antiretroviral prophylaxis administered to the infant while breastfeeding,[81-83] and antiretroviral prophylaxis to the breastfeeding mother.[83,84] In addition to these interventions, observational data strongly suggest that maternal use of combination antiretroviral regimens, including highly active antiretroviral therapy (HAART), during pregnancy is associated with very low rates of transmission.[85]

Antiretroviral Management

Maternal use of antiretroviral agent(s) during pregnancy (whether for treatment of the woman's HIV disease itself or, for women who do not meet criteria for treatment, for prevention of mother-to-child transmission of HIV), and antiretroviral prophylaxis during the intrapartum and postnatal periods, are associated with significantly lower rates of mother-to-child transmission of HIV. In the first efficacy trial of antiretroviral prophylaxis, zidovudine alone was given to the mother during pregnancy and the intrapartum period and to the infant.[72] Subsequently, the U.S. Public Health Service issued guidelines regarding the use of zidovudine prophylaxis,[86] and such prophylaxis played a central role in the prevention of mother-to-child transmission in the U.S.[87] and other resource-rich settings. More recently, an increasing number of HIV-infected women have been using combination antiretroviral regimens, including HAART, during pregnancy.[85] Guidelines for initiation of antiretroviral therapy in adults and adolescents have been developed by the Department of Health and Human Services (DHHS) Panel on Antiretroviral Guidelines for Adults and Adolescents[70] and other groups. In addition, guidelines addressing the use of antiretroviral therapy, including combination antiretroviral regimens, in pregnant women have been developed by the DHHS Panel on Treatment of HIV-Infected Pregnant Women and Prevention of Perinatal Transmission,[88] the WHO,[89,90] and other groups. Use of antiretrovirals to prevent mother-to-child transmission of HIV in non-breastfeeding populations includes antiretroviral treatment of HIV-infected pregnant women who need antiretroviral therapy for their own health, antiretroviral prophylaxis for HIV-infected pregnant women who do not yet meet criteria for treatment, and antiretroviral prophylaxis for infants of HIV-infected mothers.

Antiretroviral therapies prevent mother-to-child transmission of HIV in three ways: decreasing the viral load in maternal blood and genital secretions,[12,91] and infant pre-exposure and postexposure chemoprophylaxis. Maternal viral load is an important risk factor for mother-to-child transmission.[91-93] However, the possibility of other mechanisms of action of antiretroviral therapy in preventing transmission besides simply lowering maternal viral load is suggested by several observations. First, there is no threshold maternal plasma viral load below which transmission does not occur; transmission has been observed at all levels of maternal viral load.[91,93,94] Secondly, among women with low plasma viral loads (below 1000 copies/mL), more intensive maternal antiretroviral regimens are associated with lower risks of transmission.[95] Also, maternal plasma load at delivery and antepartum antiretroviral use are each independent risk factors for transmission.[85] Pre-exposure infant prophylaxis can be accomplished through the maternal use of antiretroviral agents that cross the placenta and result in adequate systemic drug concentrations in the infant. Postexposure infant prophylaxis can be achieved through administration of antiretroviral agent(s) to the infant after birth. In this situation, the antiretroviral therapy can protect the infant from acquiring infection from virus transferred to the infant through maternal microtransfusions of blood during labor or from virus swallowed by the infant during delivery. The efficacy and effectiveness of intrapartum or neonatal antiretroviral regimens for prevention of mother-to-child transmission (i.e., initiated too late to prevent transmission by decreasing maternal viral load)[77,96-101] lend further support to the concepts of infant pre- and postexposure prophylaxis.

Guidelines for the use of antiretroviral management in HIV-infected pregnant women in the U.S. have been developed to address antiretroviral treatment for women who meet criteria for treatment, and antiretroviral prophylaxis for women who do not meet criteria for treatment.[88] Distinguishing between these two groups of women is accomplished by assessing the HIV disease stage (clinical manifestations, plasma viral load, CD4+ lymphocyte count) and has important implications with regard to when antiretroviral drugs are used during pregnancy, which drugs are used, and if antiretroviral agents are discontinued after delivery. Irrespective of whether antiretroviral agents are used during pregnancy or not, or whether antiretrovirals agents during pregnancy are used for treatment or prophylaxis, it is recommended that all infants of HIV-infected women should receive antiretroviral postexposure prophylaxis.

In general, indications for initiation of antiretroviral therapy in women of reproductive age or in pregnant women are the same as those delineated above for other HIV-infected adults and adolescents.[70] When an indication for antiretroviral treatment exists, therapy should be started as soon as possible (even during the first trimester) and continued through the intrapartum period and thereafter.

If an HIV-infected pregnant woman does not meet criteria for antiretroviral therapy, or chooses not to initiate antiretroviral therapy, use of antiretroviral agent(s) during pregnancy for prevention of mother-to-child transmission should be considered. Antiretroviral prophylaxis is recommended for all HIV-infected pregnant women, irrespective of plasma viral load. When used to prevent mother-to-child transmission, rather than to treat maternal infection, antiretroviral agents generally are initiated after the first trimester.

Antiretroviral resistance testing should be performed in all HIV-infected, pregnant women before initiation of antiretroviral prophylaxis. This testing is especially important if the woman received antiretrovirals previously for transmission prophylaxis (i.e., in a previous pregnancy).

Although it is argued that, for prophylaxis, combination antiretroviral regimens of at least three drugs should be offered to all HIV-infected women in the U.S.,[88] new clinical trial data indicate that the risk of transmission among women with CD4+ lymphocyte counts of 200 to 500 cells/mm^3 is indistinguishable whether a three-drug antiretroviral drug regimen or a simpler antiretroviral prophylaxis regimen is used.[84] Specifically, women in the Kesho Bora trial were randomized to receive: (1) zidovudine, lamivudine, and lopinavir/ritonavir; or (2) zidovudine (with a single dose of nevirapine at labor onset) beginning at 28 weeks' gestation. (Some women randomized to the latter regimen also received an antiretroviral "tail" therapy during the first week after delivery.) There was no statistically significant difference in transmission rates at birth: 1.8% among women receiving the triple drug prophylaxis and 2.2% among women randomized to zidovudine with single-dose nevirapine. Thus, although the standard of care for antiretroviral prophylaxis among U.S. women has been to use at least three antiretroviral agents (based on observational data), more complex antiretroviral regimens such as these do not appear to provide definitive additional benefit in transmission prevention. U.S. guidelines[88] suggest considering zidovudine alone if the plasma viral load is less than 1000 copies/mL. However, British guidelines for the management of HIV-infected women include zidovudine alone beginning at 28 weeks as a valid option for women with plasma viral loads below 10,000 copies/mL and with wild-type virus who do not require antiretroviral therapy for their own health or who do not want to use antiretroviral agent(s) during pregnancy, and who are willing to give birth by planned cesarean delivery.[102] In general, if antiretroviral agents during pregnancy are being used for transmission prophylaxis only, and not for treatment of the mother's own HIV disease, the drugs are discontinued after delivery.

Antiretroviral prophylaxis should be administered during the intrapartum period.[88] For women of unknown HIV infection status who present in labor, rapid HIV antibody testing should be performed. If the rapid test is positive, maternal and infant antiretroviral therapy should be initiated immediately, without waiting for the results of confirmatory HIV testing.

Infants of HIV-infected women in the U.S. should receive 6 weeks of oral zidovudine, irrespective of maternal use of antiretroviral agents during pregnancy. In the U.K., a 4-week infant prophylaxis regimen is recommended,[102] and this shorter regimen could be considered when there are concerns about adherence to the 6-week regimen or if significant toxicity is observed.

Among infants whose mothers did not receive any antiretroviral agents before the onset of labor, neonatal postexposure prophylaxis with a two- or three-drug antiretroviral regimen results in a lower rate of mother-to-child transmission of HIV than zidovudine alone.[102a] A two-drug regimen of zidovudine for 6 weeks with 3 doses of nevirapine during the first week of life (at birth and at 48 hours and 96 hours of life) is as effective but less toxic than a three-drug regimen of zidovudine, lamivudine, and nelfinavir.[102a] Therefore, current recommendations for infants of HIV-infected women who did not receive any antiretroviral drugs before the onset of labor are for administration of this two-drug neonatal prophylaxis regimen.[88]

The timing of initiation of zidovudine prophylaxis for the infant is very important. Zidovudine prophylaxis should begin as close as possible after birth and preferably within the first 12 hours of life.[103]

The effectiveness of antiretroviral therapy in improving maternal CD4+ lymphocyte counts and decreasing plasma viral load should be monitored carefully in any patient population, including HIV-infected pregnant women. Laboratory monitoring to assess antiretroviral drug-related toxicities is based upon the known adverse events related to the drugs being used by the HIV-infected pregnant woman.

In addition, the benefits of antiretroviral agents for HIV-infected women and their infants (treatment of the mother's own HIV infection, prevention of mother-to-child transmission of HIV) must be weighed against adverse events associated with these drugs. Potential adverse events related to in utero exposure to antiretroviral agents include congenital anomalies, malignancies, mitochondrial toxicity, and preterm birth. In addition, infant laboratory abnormalities have been associated with in utero or early postnatal exposure to antiretroviral agents. Studies to date evaluating in utero exposure to antiretroviral agents, especially first trimester exposure, generally have not demonstrated significant associations between exposure and infant congenital anomalies.[104-108] However, because of potential central nervous system abnormalities with first trimester exposure to efavirenz, use of this drug during the first trimester of pregnancy should be avoided. Findings to date regarding the short-term (e.g., within the first 2 to 4 years of life) risk of malignancies among infants with in utero antiretroviral exposure are reassuring.[109-112] However, the possibility that children with in utero exposure are at increased risk of cancer at older ages remains. In utero exposure to nucleoside and nucleotide analogue reverse transcriptase inhibitors has been linked to mitochondrial dysfunction in French infants.[113,114] But, other studies from the U.S. and Europe[109,115-120] have not corroborated the French studies. Therefore, in light of these conflicting data, further research in this area is needed. However, even if a clear association between in utero antiretroviral exposure and mitochondrial dysfunction is delineated, the absolute risk of severe mitochondrial dysfunction appears to be rare and generally is assessed to be outweighed by the benefit of antiretroviral therapy in reducing the risk of mother-to-child transmission of HIV. The possibility of an association between use of protease inhibitors during pregnancy (for treatment or prophylaxis) and infant preterm birth should be considered, although currently available data are conflicting.[121-133] In general, however, the benefits of antiretroviral use during pregnancy for therapy or for prophylaxis are felt to outweigh the small possible risk of preterm birth. Examples of laboratory abnormalities associated with in utero or early postnatal exposure to antiretroviral agents include anemia, and newborns with in utero or early postnatal exposure to zidovudine should have hematologic evaluation. Based on studies suggesting other laboratory abnormalities among infants with in utero or early postnatal exposure to antiretroviral agents,[113,115,134-139] some experts recommend more extensive laboratory assessments, such as a complete blood count with differential of white cells and hepatic transaminase assays.

The WHO recently revised its guidelines regarding use of antiretroviral drugs during pregnancy.[89,90] There were several key recommendations. The first set of recommendations addressed antiretroviral therapy for HIV-infected pregnant women and management of their infants. First, antiretroviral therapy is recommended for all HIV-infected pregnant women with CD4+ lymphocyte counts of 350 cells/mm³ or less, irrespective of WHO clinical stage, and for all HIV-infected pregnant women in WHO clinical stage 3 or 4, irrespective of CD4+ lymphocyte count. Second, antiretroviral therapy, if indicated, should be initiated as soon as possible (even during the first trimester) and, once initiated, should continue for life. Third, the preferred first-line therapeutic regimen and alternative regimens were delineated. Fourth, recommendations for infant antiretroviral prophylaxis were articulated. The second set of recommendations addressed antiretroviral prophylaxis for HIV-infected pregnant women. First, all HIV-infected pregnant women who do not meet criteria for antiretroviral therapy should receive antiretroviral prophylaxis. Such prophylaxis should be started as early as 14 weeks (second trimester), or as soon as possible if an HIV-infected woman first comes to attention late in pregnancy or in labor. Second, different options for antiretroviral prophylaxis for the HIV-infected woman and her infant were recommended.

Cesarean Delivery before Labor and before Ruptured Membranes

Cesarean delivery before labor and before ruptured membranes is effective in preventing mother-to-child transmission of HIV among HIV-infected women using no antiretroviral therapy during pregnancy,[18] and is associated with a lower risk of mother-to-child transmission of HIV among HIV-infected women using zidovudine alone during pregnancy.[19] In the late 1990s, results from a multicenter, randomized clinical trial conducted in Europe and a large individual patient meta-analysis of data from prospective cohort studies conducted in North America and Europe demonstrated the efficacy and effectiveness of cesarean delivery before labor and before ruptured membranes in reducing mother-to-child transmission of HIV.[18,19] In the clinical trial, the risk of mother-to-child transmission of HIV was 80% lower among women allocated to the group who underwent cesarean delivery before labor and before ruptured membranes. In analyses of the actual method of delivery, the risk of transmission was highest among women who delivered vaginally (10.2%), followed by those who had a cesarean delivery after onset of labor or ruptured membranes (8.8%), with the lowest risk among those who underwent cesarean delivery before labor and before ruptured membranes (2.4%).[18] The individual patient meta-analysis of data from 15 prospective cohort studies found that, after controlling for maternal age, use of antiretroviral agents during pregnancy (mostly zidovudine alone), and infant birthweight, cesarean delivery before labor and before ruptured membranes was associated with a lower risk of transmission of HIV (adjusted odds ratio 0.43; 95% confidence interval (CI), 0.33 to 0.56) compared with other modes of delivery.[19]

A large proportion of mother-to-child transmission of HIV occurs during the intrapartum period.[8,9] One potential mechanism of intrapartum HIV transmission is direct fetal exposure to infected maternal blood and cervicovaginal secretions in the maternal genital tract. An early study of twins born to HIV-infected women found that the firstborn twin was at higher risk of HIV transmission compared with the second twin.[140] This finding suggested that the first vaginally born infant may be at increased risk due to greater exposure to infected blood and secretions in the vagina since the first twin remains in the vagina for a longer period of time. In addition, a longer duration of ruptured membranes is associated with a greater risk of mother-to-child transmission of HIV.[141] For each hour increase in the duration of ruptured membranes, there is an approximate 2% increase in the risk of

PART II Clinical Syndromes and Cardinal Features of Infectious Diseases: Approach to Diagnosis and Initial Management

SECTION S Human Immunodeficiency Virus and the Acquired Immunodeficiency Syndrome

mother-to-child transmission of HIV.[141] This association suggests that intrapartum transmission results from ascending infection from the lower genital tract, once the integrity of the amniotic membranes is disrupted. Another potential mechanism for mother-to-child transmission of HIV is microtransfusions of maternal blood during uterine contractions. Placental microtransfusions occur when a small amount of maternal blood crosses the placenta to the fetus. Two studies assessing the levels of placental alkaline phosphatase found that the lowest cord placental alkaline phosphatase levels, and thus the lowest volumes of maternal-fetal transfusion, were among those undergoing cesarean delivery before labor and before ruptured membranes.[142,143]

Based on these studies, the American Congress of Obstetricians and Gynecologists (ACOG) and the DHHS Panel on Treatment of HIV-Infected Pregnant Women and Prevention of Perinatal Transmission recommend that: (1) HIV-infected women with plasma viral loads above 1000 copies/mL should be counseled on the benefits of cesarean delivery before labor and before ruptured membranes to prevent mother-to-child transmission; (2) cesarean delivery before labor and before ruptured membranes should be performed at 38 completed gestational weeks, based on the best clinical estimate, to minimize the odds of onset of labor and rupture of the membranes; (3) HIV-infected women should receive antiretroviral agents during pregnancy and these should not be interrupted before the cesarean delivery; and (4) women should receive intravenous zidovudine 3 hours prior to the cesarean delivery before labor and before ruptured membranes.[88,144] Following the release of data regarding mode of delivery and mother-to-child transmission of HIV,[18,19] and guidelines regarding mode of delivery for HIV-infected women,[88,144] cesarean delivery for HIV-infected women was performed with increasing frequency in clinical centers in the U.S.[145] However, cesarean delivery for prevention of mother-to-child transmission of HIV generally is not feasible in resource-poor settings because of the lack of a skilled attendant during labor and for other reasons.

Since a cesarean delivery is a major operative procedure, there are concerns about potential risks to the mothers, infants, and healthcare workers. In terms of maternal morbidity, there is an increased risk of intraoperative and postoperative complications associated with cesarean deliveries, particularly in emergency cesarean deliveries, compared with vaginal deliveries among HIV-uninfected women.[146–149] Several studies have compared postpartum morbidity according to mode of delivery among HIV-infected women.[18,150–153] The results of these studies, summarized in a Cochrane review,[154] indicate the risk of postpartum morbidity, primarily infectious (i.e., urinary tract infection, pneumonia, wound infection, toxoplasmosis, septicemia, and episiotomy infection), was highest with non-elective cesarean delivery, intermediate with elective cesarean delivery, and lowest with vaginal delivery. The DHHS Panel on Treatment of HIV-Infected Pregnant Women and Prevention of Perinatal Transmission[88] has concluded that the observed postpartum morbidity attendant to cesarean delivery before labor and before ruptured membranes among HIV-infected women is not of sufficient frequency or severity to outweigh the benefit of decreased transmission of HIV to the infant. Countries that have high HIV seroprevalence among pregnant women may not have adequate resources to perform cesarean deliveries for all HIV-infected women.

In terms of neonatal morbidity according to mode of delivery, studies among HIV-uninfected women have demonstrated that infants who are delivered before 39 weeks' gestation are at an increased risk for neonatal respiratory morbidity and other complications. In two recent analyses of data from prospective cohort studies,[155,156] respiratory morbidity among neonates of HIV-infected pregnant women was assessed according to mode of delivery. In an analysis of over 1000 mother–infant pairs in North America, the authors concluded that there was minimal neonatal respiratory morbidity risk in near-term infants born by cesarean delivery before labor and rupture of membranes.[155] In an analysis of over 1400 HIV-infected women and their infants in Latin America, few children who were born by cesarean delivery before labor and before ruptured membranes for prevention of

mother-to-child transmission of HIV had respiratory distress syndrome or transient tachypnea of the newborn, and only a minority required ventilator support.[156] At this point, the benefits of cesarean delivery for prevention of mother-to-child transmission of HIV outweigh the small risk of respiratory morbidity among near-term infants.[155,156]

In order to strike a balance between minimizing the risks of iatrogenic prematurity and ensuring that the cesarean delivery before labor and before ruptured membranes is performed prior to the onset of labor, the American College of Obstetricians and Gynecologists recommends that infants of HIV-infected women should be delivered a week earlier (at 38 completed weeks of gestation) than is customary among uninfected women (39 completed weeks of gestation).[144] Although the ACOG generally recommends testing amniotic fluid if elective delivery is being considered prior to 39 week to determine fetal pulmonary maturity,[157] amniocentesis should not be performed routinely in HIV-infected women. Therefore, clinicians generally should depend on the best clinical estimate of gestational age to determine when to deliver.[158]

Unresolved questions regarding mode of delivery and prevention of mother-to-child transmission of HIV include whether cesarean delivery before labor and before ruptured membranes is beneficial among HIV-infected, pregnant women with low plasma viral loads (less than 1000 copies/mL) and whether there is a benefit of cesarean delivery before labor and before ruptured membranes in women who are using combination antiretroviral regimens. In one recent study, the mother-to-child transmission rate in term births (including all modes of delivery) according to maternal viral load at delivery was 0.6% (less than 400 copies/mL).[159] A similarly low rate of transmission (0.8%) has been observed among women using combination antiretroviral regimens for at least the last 14 days of pregnancy, regardless of mode of delivery.[160] However, analyses of data from the European Collaborative Study[161] demonstrated an 80% lower risk of transmission with cesarean delivery before labor and before ruptured membranes when adjusting for use of combination antiretroviral regimens and preterm birth (adjusted odds ratio: 0.20; 95% CI, 0.05 to 0.65). Similarly, among 560 women with undetectable viral loads, cesarean delivery before labor and before ruptured membranes was associated with a 90% lower risk of transmission (odds ratio: 0.10; 95% CI, 0.03 to 0.33).[162]

Interventions to Prevent Breast Milk Transmission of HIV

Both the CDC[163] and the AAP[164] recommend that HIV-infected women in the U.S. not breastfeed their children. These recommendations are based in large part on the results of a randomized clinical trial conducted in Kenya, where the observed rate of mother-to-child transmission of HIV among mothers randomized to not breastfeed (i.e., they fed their children formula milk) was significantly lower than among mothers randomized to breastfeed (20.5% versus 36.7% at 2 years, P<0.001).[79]

The evidence for breast milk transmission of HIV and risk factors for such transmission have been summarized.[165] Risk factors for breast milk transmission of HIV include longer duration of breastfeeding, more advanced HIV disease in the mother, factors that facilitate transfer of HIV from mother to child, and the child's susceptibility to infection. A meta-analysis that included data from thousands of breastfeeding children of HIV-infected women in sub-Saharan Africa[17] demonstrated that breast milk transmission of HIV contributes substantially to overall mother-to-child transmission. After 4 to 6 weeks of age, the risk of breast milk transmission of HIV generally is constant; the longer breastfeeding continues, the greater the cumulative risk of HIV transmission. More advanced maternal disease stage, as manifested by low CD4+ lymphocyte counts, is a risk factor for breast milk transmission of HIV,[13,24] along with higher maternal peripheral blood or human milk viral load.[13–15] Certain factors that facilitate the transfer of the virus from mother to child, or otherwise facilitate mother-to-child transmission, including maternal breast abnormalities, infant candidiasis, and mixed feeding, are associated with breast milk transmission of HIV.[13–15,20,22–24]

If complete avoidance of breastfeeding is not safe or feasible, specific interventions to prevent breast milk transmission of HIV can be implemented. Some of these interventions have been evaluated in clinical trials, while others are currently under study.

First, since a longer duration of breastfeeding is associated with a greater risk of transmission,[17,79] early weaning was thought to be a reasonable intervention to decrease the risk of transmission. However, the morbidity associated with complete avoidance of breastfeeding (formula feeding) and with early weaning, due to contaminated water used in the preparation of replacement feeds, serves to counterbalance the benefits of such interventions to prevent mother-to-child transmission of HIV. For example, in the clinical trial of formula feeding versus breastfeeding, the two groups of children experienced similar mortality and malnutrition rates during the first 2 years of life.[166] Similarly, studies in Malawi and Uganda documented increased risks of severe gastroenteritis[167,168] and gastroenteritis-associated mortality[167] among HIV-exposed infants. In a randomized trial evaluating the safety and efficacy of early weaning,[169] there was no statistically significant difference in HIV-free survival between those children who ceased breastfeeding around 4 months of age and those who continued breastfeeding (P=0.27).

Secondly, since more advanced maternal disease (e.g., as manifest by a higher maternal viral load in breast milk) is associated with a greater risk of mother-to-child transmission of HIV, two types of interventions have been proposed to decrease the infectiousness of the breast milk of HIV-infected mothers: maternal use of antiretroviral agents while breastfeeding and treatment (chemical or heat) of breast milk. Two randomized clinical trials conducted in sub-Saharan Africa evaluated the use of antiretroviral prophylaxis by breastfeeding women and mother-to-child transmission of HIV.[83,84] In the BAN trial, HIV-infected, breastfeeding mothers with a CD4+ lymphocyte count of ≥250 cells/mm³ and their infants were randomized at 1 week of age to receive: maternal antiretroviral regimen for 28 weeks, infant nevirapine for 28 weeks, or no prophylaxis beyond the first week of age (control group). Prior to randomization, all mothers and infants had received standard perinatal prophylaxis, which included a single dose of oral nevirapine given to all mothers in labor and their newborn infants immediately after birth. In addition, all mothers had received zidovudine and lamivudine as a single tablet every 12 hours from the onset of labor to 7 days after birth and all infants received zidovudine until 7 days of age. Of 2369 mother–infant pairs who were randomized, 5% of infants were HIV-infected at 2 weeks of life. The estimated risk of mother-to-child transmission of HIV between 2 and 28 weeks was higher in the control group (5.7%) than in the other groups (maternal regimen group: 2.9%, P=0.009; infant regimen group: 1.7%, P<0.001). The estimated risk of infant HIV infection or death between 2 and 28 weeks was 7.0% in the control group, 4.1% in the maternal regimen group (P=0.02), and 2.6% in the infant regimen group (P<0.001).[83] In the Kesho Bora study, women with CD4+ lymphocyte counts between 200 and 500 cells/mm³ were randomized to either: (1) zidovudine with lamivudine and lopinavir/ritonavir (triple-ARV) at 28 to 36 weeks' gestation until 6 months postpartum; or (2) zidovudine at 28 to 36 weeks' gestation until the onset of labor, and then zidovudine with lamivudine and one dose of nevirapine at the onset of labor, followed by (in a later version of the protocol) zidovudine with lamivudine until one week after delivery (ZDV/sdNVP). All infants received one dose of nevirapine within 72 hours of birth along with one week of zidovudine. Among 882 enrolled women, 824 were randomized and delivered 805 singleton or first, liveborn infants. The cumulative risk of HIV transmission at 12 months was 5.4% in the triple-ARV arm and 9.5% in the ZDV/sdNVP arm (P=0.03), a 43% risk reduction.[84] Heat and chemical (e.g., sodium dodecyl sulfate) treatment of breast milk in order to decrease the amount of cell-free and cell-associated HIV have been evaluated in several studies.[170,171] In addition, a method of "flash-heating" of breast milk[172] will be evaluated further in East Africa.

Thirdly, because various factors facilitate the transfer of the virus from mother to child or otherwise facilitate mother-to-child transmission (e.g., maternal breast abnormalities, infant candidiasis, mixed breastfeeding), interventions to prevent or treat such factors have been developed. For example, programs have been developed to educate HIV-infected women who choose to breastfeed, addressing proper positioning during breastfeeding; prompt seeking of medical care if breast abnormalities develop or if the infant develops oral candidiasis or other lesions; and avoiding breastfeeding from a breast with mastitis or other abnormalities. Early findings from studies in Brazil and South Africa suggesting a lower risk of transmission with exclusive breastfeeding compared with mixed breastfeeding[20,173] prompted the development of additional studies in Zimbabwe,[21] South Africa,[80] and Zambia[169] which support the association of exclusive breastfeeding with a lower risk of mother-to-child transmission of HIV. For example, the transmission rate among infants who were still exclusively breastfeeding at 6 months of age was 15%, but was higher among those with mixed feeding at 6 months of age (27% among those who initiated mixed feeding before 14 weeks and 26% for those who initiated mixed breastfeeding after 14 weeks).[80] It is noteworthy that although mixed feeding has been hypothesized to damage the intestinal mucosa, thus facilitating HIV infection of the infant through increased permeability or intestinal immune activation, the evidence to date does not support this hypothesis.[173a] The exact mechanism by which mixed feeding is associated with a higher risk of transmission of HIV remains controversial.

Finally, interventions to decrease infant susceptibility to infection while breastfeeding (e.g., active and passive immunization of the infant, administration of antiretroviral prophylaxis to the infant while breastfeeding) have been or are being evaluated. Studies of the safety and immunogenicity of active immunization for prevention of mother-to-child transmission of HIV have been initiated.[174,175] Similarly, passive immunization with polyclonal immune globulin has been evaluated in clinical trials in the U.S. (formula-fed infants) and Uganda (predominantly breastfed infants).[174,175] Large studies of monoclonal antibody preparations with proven neutralizing activity have been proposed.

Several major studies have evaluated the efficacy of extended administration of antiretroviral prophylaxis to breastfeeding infants.[81–83,176] In a clinical trial in Botswana, infants were randomized to 6 months of breastfeeding along with zidovudine prophylaxis, or formula feeding with one month of zidovudine prophylaxis. HIV-free survival at 18 months was similar with both strategies.[176] However, in a combined analysis from three separate but coordinated randomized controlled trials in Ethiopia, India, and Uganda, extended (6-week) infant prophylaxis with nevirapine was compared with a single infant dose of nevirapine for outcomes of HIV-free survival at 6 weeks and 6 months of age among infants who were uninfected at birth. Although there was a reduction in the risk of HIV transmission by 6 weeks of age (P=0.009), there was no statistically significant reduction in the primary endpoint (HIV transmission at 6 months of age, P=0.16). These results suggested a longer course of daily infant nevirapine may be needed to prevent breast milk transmission of HIV.[81] A subsequent trial conducted in Malawi randomized infants after they had received one dose of nevirapine at birth followed by one week of zidovudine into three groups. Infants in one group received no additional prophylaxis, infants in a second group received nevirapine alone until 14 weeks of age, and infants in the third group were randomized to receive nevirapine and zidovudine until 14 weeks of age. HIV infection at 9 months of age was significantly lower in both of the extended prophylaxis groups, whether nevirapine alone (5.2%; P<0.001) or nevirapine plus zidovudine (6.4%; P=0.002), compared with the infection rate in the control group (10.6%).[82] As described above, extended infant prophylaxis with nevirapine until 28 weeks was highly efficacious in increasing HIV-free survival among infants of HIV-infected infants.[83] Finally, in a trial of daily infant nevirapine given to breastfeeding infants, extending daily infant nevirapine from 6 weeks to 6 months resulted in a lower risk of mother-to-child transmission of HIV, especially among infants whose mothers had a CD4 count of 350 cells/mm³ or more who were not using antiretroviral treatment.[176a]

Prevention of HIV Transmission in Adolescents

Essential components of the care of adolescents (Box 109-2) are counseling regarding behaviors that may put them at risk for acquisition of HIV infection and interventions to decrease the risk of transmission of HIV infection. In addition, adolescents should be educated regarding testing for HIV and postexposure prophylaxis.

Sexual transmission accounts for the majority of cases of HIV infection among adolescents and adults.[3] Although abstinence from sexual activity is the most effective means of avoiding acquisition of sexually transmitted infections (STIs), it is not possible to predict which adolescent will abstain. The AAP views provision of information regarding sex and STIs as an essential part of anticipatory guidance that pediatricians provide to their adolescent patients.[177] The AAP recommends that this information explicitly underscores the potential consequences of STIs, including HIV.[177] Adolescents with STIs, especially ulcerative diseases such as herpes simplex infection or syphilis, should be made aware of the association between such infections and transmission of HIV.[177] Screening for STIs in both public and private clinical settings represents an important component of prevention of HIV infection among adolescents and adults.[178]

Injection drug use or other percutaneous exposure to HIV is another important means of acquisition of HIV infection by adolescents and adults.[3] Adolescents should be informed about the dangers of injection drug use, as well as precautions to decrease the risk of transmission of HIV and other bloodborne viral pathogens due to contact with blood or open wounds (e.g., during contact sports).[177,179] In addition to injection drug use or other percutaneous exposures, the use of non-injection drugs (e.g., alcohol, cocaine, marijuana) is associated with an increased risk of acquisition of HIV infection due to impaired judgment associated with the use of these substances, which in turn may increase the likelihood of unsafe sexual practices.[177] Efforts to reduce the risk of adolescents initiating substance abuse, and to prevent acquisition of HIV infection among adolescents with a substance abuse problem, should be encouraged.[180]

The CDC recommends at least annual testing for sexually active men who have sex with men between the ages of 13 and 64 years.[181] HIV testing is treated as part of routine care, and it is performed unless the patient objects ("opts out"). General consent for medical care is considered to encompass consent for HIV testing, and no specific consent for HIV testing would be requested or required in order for the testing to be performed.[181] Testing for

---

BOX 109-2.   Prevention of HIV Transmission in Adolescents

- Counseling and education for adolescents regarding behaviors that put them at risk of acquisition of HIV infection and interventions to decrease that risk
  - Sexual transmission: counseling and education regarding safer sexual practices and about sexually transmitted infections
  - Substance abuse: counseling and education regarding prevention of initiation of substance abuse, and prevention of HIV acquisition among those with an existing substance abuse problem
- Screening for sexually transmitted infections
- HIV testing
- Postexposure prophylaxis

HIV infection is important in the prevention of HIV transmission since it provides the individual with knowledge of his or her HIV infection status, and, with this knowledge, most individuals reduce high-risk sexual behaviors.[182] In addition, testing is the first step in linking an HIV-infected person to appropriate care and treatment.

Recommendations for postexposure prophylaxis in children and adolescents for non-occupational exposure to HIV have been developed.[183] If postexposure prophylaxis is used, it should be initiated as soon as possible after exposure (no later than 72 hours) and continued for 28 days. Close follow-up is necessary to monitor adherence to and toxicity related to the prophylaxis, to provide psychological support, and to complete serial HIV testing.

SUMMARY

HIV infection among children and adolescents in the U.S. disproportionately affects minorities. Effective antiretroviral treatment and other care and support for HIV-infected children and adolescents have resulted in significantly decreased morbidity and mortality. Major successes have been achieved in prevention of mother-to-child transmission of HIV in the U.S. and other settings with the availability of effective interventions, but such transmission has not been eliminated. Acquisition of HIV infection among adolescents and adults continues at an alarming rate. Essential components of the care of adolescents include counseling and education regarding behaviors that put them at risk of acquisition of HIV infections and interventions to decrease that risk, and HIV testing.

---

110   Immunopathogenesis of HIV-1 Infection

Grace M. Aldrovandi and Chiara Cerini

In the absence of antiretroviral therapy (ART), most HIV-1 infections in children are due to mother-to-child transmission during pregnancy, birth, or breastfeeding. In settings where maternal HIV testing and treatment are available most infections occur during adolescence (see Chapter 109, Epidemiology and Prevention of HIV Infection in Children and Adolescents) as a result of sexual activity and/or injection drug use. In this chapter we review the main features of HIV-1 immunopathogenesis with an emphasis on the unique features of pediatric infection. We will also describe

how antiretroviral therapy (ART) allows preservation and reconstitution of immune function.

HIV REPLICATION

Activated CD4⁺ T lymphocytes represent the main cellular target of HIV-1 and the majority of these cells reside in the gastrointestinal tract. Once HIV establishes infection, high level replication results in CD4⁺ T-lymphocyte loss due to direct cytolytic activity and as a result of indirect effects described below. During acute infection, adolescents and adults frequently have nonspecific "viral" symptoms (see Chapter 111, Diagnosis and Clinical Manifestations of HIV Infection) but infants usually are asymptomatic.[1,2] In adolescents and adults, plasma viremia decreases and peripheral blood CD4+ T-cell counts increase after a few weeks even in the absence of ART. CD8+ cytotoxic T lymphocytes (CTLs) play a major role in this early control of viral replication.[3–5] Additional adaptive immune responses as well as innate immune responses increasingly are being recognized as important factors in the control of initial viral replication.[6–8] Following this acute period, adults and older children will have relatively constant levels of viremia, which is referred to as a "set point". This level of viremia is highly predictive of the later course of disease progression.[9,10]

In contrast to older children and adults, HIV-1-infected infants have high levels of plasma viremia and do not achieve a "set point" for several years.[11] These high and persistent levels of

---

BOX 110-1. Immunopathologic Consequences of HIV-1 Infection

T LYMPHOCYTES

Laboratory manifestations

Lymphopenia
Selective CD4+ T-lymphocyte depletion
Decreased CD4+/CD8+ T-lymphocyte ratio
Impairments in other T-lymphocyte subsets (Th17 and Treg depletion; switch Th1→Th2-type response) and gamma-delta cells

Impaired functions

Impaired delayed-type hypersensitivity (new and recall)
Impaired mitogen-antigen responses
Impaired alloantigen reactivity
Impaired T-lymphocyte cytotoxicity
Impaired cytokines production (IL-2, IFN-γ, others)

Clinical manifestations

Chronic active viral infections (i.e., varicella-zoster virus, cytomegalovirus, Epstein–Barr virus)
Neoplasms

B LYMPHOCYTES

Phenotypic perturbations

Over-representation of activated, exhausted, and terminally differentiated B lymphocytes
Over-representation of immature/transitional B lymphocytes
Reduced representation of CD27+ memory B lymphocytes

Impaired functions

Polyclonal B-lymphocyte activation
Hypergammaglobulinemia
Polyclonal immunoglobulin class switch recombination (switch from IgM to nonprotective IgG, IgA and IgE)
Impaired antibody responses (primary and secondary responses; T-lymphocyte-dependent and independent antigens)
Reduced proliferative capacity
Stunted immunoglobulin diversification
Increased circulating immune complexes
Loss of serological memory

Clinical manifestations

Impaired vaccine responses
B-cell malignancies
Autoimmune diseases

MONOCYTES AND MACROPHAGES

(including bone marrow precursors and microglial cells in the central nervous system)

Laboratory manifestations

Increased levels of circulating "pocked" red blood cells
Elevated levels of TNF
Impaired splenic clearance (antibody-coated red blood cells)

Impaired functions

Noncytopathic latent infection
Impaired delayed-type hypersensitivity
Impaired granuloma formation

Clinical manifestations

Opportunistic infections (mainly mycobacterial)
Pneumococcal bacteremia
HIV-associated encephalopathy

NATURAL KILLER (NK) LYMPHOCYTES

Laboratory manifestations

Reduced percentage of NK cells
Depletion of mature cytotoxic NK cell subsets (CD161+ CD56+ or CD16+)
Selective depletion of invariant natural killer T (NKT) lymphocytes

Impaired functions

Impaired cytolytic activity
Impaired immunoregulatory activity (DC-mediated helper function for Th1 and CTL responses)

Clinical manifestations

Chronic viral infection (i.e., herpesvirus)
Neoplasms

DENDRITIC CELLS (DCS)

Laboratory manifestations

Decreased numbers of both plasmacytoid and myeloid DCs in peripheral blood

Impaired functions

Impaired IFN-α production
Increased secretion of inflammatory cytokines and chemokines (including TNF and IL-6)

NEUTROPHILS

Laboratory manifestations

Neutropenia

Impaired functions

Impaired chemotaxis and expression of cellular adhesion molecules
Impaired phagocytosis
Impaired production of toxic oxygen species

Clinical manifestations

Opportunistic bacterial and fungal infections

CTL, cytotoxic T lymphocyte; IL, interleukin; IFN, interferon; Th, T helper; TNF, tumor necrosis factor; Treg, regulatory T lymphocyte.

PART II Clinical Syndromes and Cardinal Features of Infectious Diseases: Approach to Diagnosis and Initial Management

SECTION S Human Immunodeficiency Virus and the Acquired Immunodeficiency Syndrome

viremia are attributed to immunologic immaturity. HIV-specific CTL responses can be detected at birth in infants infected in utero, but these responses are insufficient to control infection.[12] Studies suggest that this failure is due to decreased functional capacity, lack of CD4+ T-lymphocyte help and targeting of epitopes that inhibit the virus less effectively.[12,13] The relatively high frequency of regulatory T cells also may contribute to the suppression of viral specific T-cell responses.[14,15] Other immune factors that may play a role include a decreased capacity of neonatal natural killer cells to mediate antibody-dependent, cell-mediated cytotoxicity (ADCC).

The availability of increased numbers of target cells also may contribute to the high level of viremia. The absolute number and relative percentage of CD4+ T lymphocytes are much higher in infants and children.[16] Relative to their body size, the mass of the thymus is increased and thymopoiesis is much more active during childhood.[17] Thus, a large renewable source of CD4+ T lymphocytes may serve as "fuel" for this infection and may account for the rapid tempo of disease progression observed in children.

IMMUNE CONSEQUENCES OF UNTREATED HIV-1 INFECTION

CD4+ T-lymphocyte depletion is the hallmark of HIV-1 infection. Although direct infection and activation are believed to account for most of this reduction, other mechanisms including decreased production of bone marrow precursors, thymic dysfunction, and immune-mediated destruction of infected CD4+ T lymphocytes may be involved. The effects on CD4+ T lymphocytes are not only quantitative. Their function and repertoire are also significantly perturbed. Moreover, CD4+ T lymphocytes are a heterogeneous and multifunctional population critical to steering immune responses such as B-cell antibody formation and the generation of effective CD8+ T-lymphocyte responses.[18–21] Other immune cells that are perturbed in HIV-1 infection are shown in Box 110-1.

Destruction of up to 60% of CD4+ T lymphocytes residing in the gastrointestinal tract has been identified as a critical early event in HIV-1 pathogenesis.[22–25] Unlike their counterparts in the blood, the numbers of these cells do not recover after the acute phase, and even with ART, their numbers infrequently are restored.[26–28] Most of the CD4+ T lymphocytes destroyed in the gut belong to the recently identified Th17 subset.[29–31] These cells regulate responses to bacterial and fungal pathogens at mucosal surfaces. This loss is associated with increased microbial translocation and immune activation, which contribute to enhanced HIV spread and CD4+ T-lymphocyte loss.[32,33]

The chronic phase of HIV-1 infection is characterized by a pathologic activation of the immune system. The extent of immune activation predicts disease progression better than either plasma viremia or CD4+ T-lymphocyte counts.[34,35] This activation is linked to immune exhaustion, impaired T-lymphocyte homeostasis, hypergammaglobulinemia and other perturbations that result in increased susceptibility to the opportunistic infections and cancers that characterize AIDS.[36]

EFFECTS OF ANTIVIRAL THERAPY ON IMMUNE FUNCTION

The advent of effective antiretroviral therapies has transformed HIV-1 infection into a chronic manageable disease. Higher levels of plasma viremia, variable pharmacokinetics, and poor adherence to therapy offer unique challenges to HIV-1 suppression in children. Nevertheless, with contemporary regimens, most children can achieve viral suppression with corresponding improvements in immune function. Normalization of both T- and B-lymphocyte numbers and function has been documented in many studies, particularly if therapy is initiated early in infection.[37–44] Increased thymic function also confers an advantage in HIV-infected adolescents.[45] Children who start therapy at low CD4+ T-lymphocyte levels may not experience full immunologic recovery.[29] Interestingly, some infants who achieve and maintain viral suppression in the first few months of life do not develop detectable HIV-specific responses (antibodies, CD4+, and CTL).[37,46] These infants mount appropriate responses to vaccines and other viral infections, suggesting that this defect is specific to HIV-1 infection. In contrast, adults who initiate effective therapy within a few months of infection have persistent HIV-1 specific immune responses.

However, at the initiation of ART, between 10 and 40% of individuals develop a pathologic immune response to antigens, especially latent or persistent mycobacterial and cryptococcal infection.[47–49] This acute inflammatory condition is referred to as "immune reconstitution inflammatory syndrome" (IRIS). It is similar to "paradoxical reactions" long recognized in *M. tuberculosis* infection. It is more common in individuals with low CD4+ T-lymphocyte levels, and recent data suggest that infants may be at greater risk.[50,51] Most individuals can be managed by the use of anti-inflammatory agents without interrupting ART.

111 Diagnosis and Clinical Manifestations of HIV Infection

Paul Krogstad, Heidi Schwarzwald, and Mark W. Kline

Most cases of HIV infection in infants and young children result from mother-to-child transmission. Most new cases of HIV in centers caring for children through 18 years of age in the United States currently are in youths, and can represent newly acquired or longstanding infection. Early diagnosis is a prerequisite to timely provision of potentially life-saving prophylactic medications and effective antiretroviral therapy. But the early clinical manifestations of HIV infection in children are varied and sometimes indistinct. Moreover, the diagnosis of human immunodeficiency virus (HIV) infection in children less than 18 months of age rests upon specialized laboratory testing. This chapter outlines diagnostic approaches for HIV infection in infants and children and focuses on the pathologic effects of HIV on various organ systems. Infectious complications of HIV infection are discussed in Chapter 112.

DIAGNOSIS

The detection of HIV infection in adults, adolescents, and children older than 18 months is based upon well-standardized antibody detection methods. HIV-specific antibodies are readily detected by screening tests, usually highly sensitive and specific enzyme immunoassays (EIAs). Infection is confirmed on the basis of repeated testing, using more specific assays. Transplacentally acquired maternal antibodies are present in children younger than 12 to 18 months who are born to HIV-infected women. In these

TABLE 111-1. Assays to Detect Human Immunodeficiency Virus Infection

Assay	Time	Advantages	Disadvantages
Antibody detection (rapid blood tests, enzyme immunoassay (EIAs), Western blot (WBs), immunofluorescence assays (IFAs))	Minutes (for rapid tests); hours for EIA, WB, IFA	Sensitive, suitable for screening	Transplacentally acquired maternal antibodies produce false-positive results in infants
Polymerase chain reaction (PCR) and other nucleic acid detection tests (NATs)	Days	Sensitivity very high	Small risk of false-positive results
p24 antigen detection assays	Hours	Inexpensive, quantitative	Less sensitive than NAT; false-positive results in the first week of life
Culture	Weeks	Sensitive, highly specific	Requires weeks to complete, technically complex; research use only

children, positive HIV antibody tests provide evidence of potential exposure to HIV infection in utero, at the time of delivery, or by breastfeeding, but do not confirm the presence of infection.[1] The critical determination of infection status in these infants is accomplished using virologic tests, usually assays to detect HIV RNA in plasma or HIV DNA within blood cells.[1-3] The characteristics of methods currently used for HIV diagnosis are discussed below and summarized in Table 111-1, and a schema for the diagnostic approach for pediatric patients is outlined in Table 111-2.

Screening Tests: Enzyme Immunoassay (EIA) and Rapid HIV tests

Two types of antibody tests are used to screen for the presence of antibodies to HIV. EIA tests use purified HIV proteins as antigens and detect antibodies in serum with high sensitivity (>99%). These assays also detect maternal antibodies present in an infant's blood for up to 18 months after birth. When used to screen for HIV infection in older children, adolescents, and adults, serum antibodies to HIV may not be present at detectable levels until 6 to 12 weeks after infection.

Several rapid tests also are available to detect HIV antibody in blood specimens collected by finger stick or by venipuncture.[4] In general terms, these tests are used like EIAs, and have similar limitations, including false positives in infants and children.[5,6] One currently approved rapid test also can be performed using oral fluid obtained with a special collection device. Since the results of rapid tests are available promptly, the effectiveness of posttest

counseling is increased.[7] Rapid tests also facilitate the determination of HIV status of pregnant women, allowing the timely administration of antiretroviral therapy to prevent mother-to-child transmission at the time of delivery.[8]

Confirmatory Antibody Tests

In the U.S., EIAs and rapid antibody tests are used only for screening. All positive results are confirmed by either a Western blot or immunofluorescence assays.[1] These confirmatory assays are more specific for HIV than EIA, but both are technically difficult to perform.

HIV Western blots demonstrate the presence of serum antibodies that bind to bands of HIV proteins immobilized to a solid substrate. If no bands are detected, the Western blot is negative. If most or all of the HIV protein bands specified by the manufacturer are seen, the Western blot is positive. Sequential EIA screening and Western blot confirmation is an accurate and proven strategy for the diagnosis of HIV infection. A survey of a low-prevalence population of U.S. Army recruits found a false-positive rate of 1 in 134,187 individuals.[9] An indeterminate Western blot, defined as the absence of one or more bands required by a test kit manufacturer for a positive test, may represent a transition to positive status and warrants repeating. A few individuals have persistently indeterminate Western blot results. If at low risk of HIV exposures, these patients usually are not infected.[10]

Immunofluorescence assays (IFAs) are used in some hospitals for confirmation of positive results of EIA or rapid HIV tests. An

TABLE 111-2. Schema for Evaluating Children at Risk for Human Immunodeficiency Virus (HIV) Infection

Age at Initial Evaluation	Stage of Evaluation	Test	Schedule	Comments
≤18 months	Maternal HIV status unknown	EIA or rapid test with Western blot (on mother or infant)	Immediate	If positive, warrants further evaluation
	Mother HIV-infected	Nucleic acid detection test (NAT)	Birth,[a] 2–3 weeks, 1–2 months, and 4–6 months	Two negative NATs at 1–2 months and >4 months of age provide definitive evidence that the child is not infected (in the absence of breastfeeding) Start PCP prophylaxis at 4–6 weeks of age pending results, unless two virologic tests have been performed (one at ≥4 weeks of age)
>18 months	Maternal HIV status unknown	EIA/rapid test on mother and infant	Immediate	If EIA/rapid test for either person is positive, proceed to next step
	Mother HIV-infected	Screening and confirmatory antibody testing or NAT	EIA/Western blot/IFA or NAT once immediately	EIA in uninfected children sereroverts to negative at a median age of 10 months Perform NAT initially to determine need for PCP prophylaxis or antiretroviral treatment If EIA/Western blot does not serorevert to negative by 15–18 months old, child usually is infected

EIA, enzyme immunoassay; PCP, Pneumocystis jirovecii pneumonia; PCR, polymerase chain reaction.
[a]*Recommended by some authorities so that prophylactic antiretroviral medications, if in use, may be stopped.*

IFA involves adding a patient's serum to a glass slide to which preservative-fixed HIV-infected cells are attached, followed by addition of fluorescent anti-human antibodies. Fluorescence of the infected cells provides evidence of the presence of antibodies to HIV in the serum specimen. False-positive IFA results are rare and usually are caused by the same conditions that produce persistently indeterminant Western blots.

In areas with a high prevalence of HIV, a second EIA or use of a rapid diagnostic test may be an acceptable approach for confirmation of an EIA or an initial rapid test result.[7,11,12]

Nucleic Acid Detection Tests

Antibody tests are not used for diagnosis of HIV in infants because of the persistence of transplacentally acquired maternal antibodies until up to 18 months of age. Virologic tests are used for these infants.[1-3] While HIV culture methods and EIA detection of HIV p24 antigen in serum have been used in research studies, the technical complexity of culture and the limited sensitivity and specificity of p24 detection assays in newborns limit their general use. PCR assays and other tests to detect HIV DNA or HIV RNA

BOX 111-1. Clinical Categories for Children with Human Immunodeficiency Virus (HIV)[a]

CATEGORY N: NOT SYMPTOMATIC

Children who have no signs or symptoms considered to be the result of HIV infection or who have only one of the conditions listed in category A

CATEGORY A: MILDLY SYMPTOMATIC

Children with two or more of the conditions listed below but none of the conditions listed in categories B and C:

- Lymphadenopathy (≥0.5 cm at more than two sites; bilateral, one site)
- Hepatomegaly
- Splenomegaly
- Dermatitis
- Parotitis
- Recurrent or persistent upper respiratory infection, sinusitis, or otitis media

CATEGORY B: MODERATELY SYMPTOMATIC

Children who have symptomatic conditions other than those listed for categories A or C that are attributed to HIV infection; examples of conditions in clinical category B include but are not limited to:

- Anemia (<8 g/dL), neutropenia (<1000/mm³), or thrombocytopenia (<100,000/mm³) persisting ≥30 days
- Bacterial meningitis, pneumonia, or sepsis (single episode)
- Oropharyngeal candidiasis, persisting >2 months in children >6 months of age
- Cardiomyopathy
- Cytomegalovirus infection, with onset before 1 month of age
- Diarrhea, recurrent or chronic
- Hepatitis
- HSV stomatitis, recurrent (>2 episodes within 1 year)
- HSV bronchitis, pneumonitis, or esophagitis with onset before 1 month of age
- Herpes zoster (shingles) involving ≥2 distinct episodes or >1 dermatome
- Leiomyosarcoma
- Lymphoid interstitial pneumonia (LIP) or pulmonary lymphoid hyperplasia complex
- Nephropathy
- Nocardiosis
- Fever persisting >1 month
- Toxoplasmosis, onset before 1 month of age
- Varicella, disseminated (complicated chickenpox)

CATEGORY C: SEVERELY SYMPTOMATIC

Children who have any condition listed in the 1987 surveillance case definition for AIDS, with the exception of LIP

- Serious bacterial infections, multiple or recurrent (i.e., any combination of ≥2 culture-confirmed infections within a 2-year period), of the following types: septicemia, pneumonia,

meningitis, bone or joint infection, or abscess of an internal organ or body cavity (excluding otitis media, superficial skin or mucosal abscesses, and indwelling catheter-related infections)
- Esophageal or pulmonary (bronchi, trachea, lungs) candidiasis
- Coccidioidomycosis, disseminated (at site other than or in addition to lungs or cervical or hilar lymph nodes)
- Extrapulmonary cryptococcosis
- Cryptosporidiosis isosporiasis with diarrhea persisting >1 month
- Cytomegalovirus disease with onset of symptoms at age >1 month (at a site other than liver, spleen, or lymph nodes)
- Encephalopathy (at least one of the following progressive findings present for at least 2 months in the absence of a concurrent illness other than HIV infection that could explain the findings): (1) failure to attain or loss of developmental milestones or loss of intellectual ability, verified by standard developmental scale or neuropsychological tests; (2) impaired brain growth or acquired microcephaly, demonstrated by head circumference measurements, or brain atrophy, demonstrated by CT or MRI (serial imaging is required for children <2 years of age); (3) acquired symmetric motor deficit manifested ≥2 of the following: paresis, pathologic reflexes, ataxia, or gait disturbance
- HSV infection causing a mucocutaneous ulcer that persists for >1 month; or bronchitis, pneumonitis, or esophagitis for any duration affecting a child >1 month of age
- Histoplasmosis, disseminated (at a site other than or in addition to lungs or cervical or hilar lymph nodes)
- Kaposi sarcoma
- Lymphoma, primary, in brain
- Lymphoma, small, noncleaved cell (Burkitt), or immunoblastic or large-cell lymphoma or B-cell or unknown immunologic phenotype
- *Mycobacterium tuberculosis,* disseminated or extrapulmonary
- *Mycobacterium avium* complex or *Mycobacterium kansasii,* disseminated (at site other than or in addition to lungs, skin, or cervical or hilar lymph nodes)
- *Pneumocystis jirovecii* pneumonia (previously known as *P. carinii* and *P. jirovecii*).
- Progressive multifocal leukoencephalopathy
- *Salmonella* (nontyphoid) septicemia, recurrent
- Toxoplasmosis of the brain with onset at >1 month of age
- Wasting syndrome in the absence of a concurrent illness other than HIV infection that could explain the following findings: (1) persistent weight loss >10% of baseline or (2) downward crossing of ≥2 of the following percentile lines on the weight-for-age chart (e.g., 95th, 75th, 50th, 25th, 5th) in a child ≥1 year of age or (3) <5th percentile on weight-for-height chart on two consecutive measurements ≥30 days apart, plus: (1) chronic diarrhea (i.e., at least two loose stools a day for ≥30 days) or (2) documented fever (for ≥30 days, intermittent or constant)

AIDS, acquired immunodeficiency syndrome; CT, computed tomography; HSV, herpes simplex virus; LIP, lymphoid interstitial pneumonia; MRI, magnetic resonance imaging.
[a]Centers for Disease Control. Classification system for human immunodeficiency virus in children under 13 years of age. MMWR 1987;36:225.
Adapted from Centers for Disease Control and Prevention. 1994 revised classification system for human immunodeficiency virus in children less than 13 years of age. MMWR 1994;43:1.

(also known as nucleic acid detection tests (NATs)) are now used throughout the world for early and accurate diagnosis of HIV infection in infants.

The sensitivity of DNA PCR detection of HIV is approximately 38% at 48 hours of life and 93% at 2 weeks of life.[13] By 1 month of age, DNA PCR tests have a sensitivity of 90% to 100% and a specificity of 95% to 100%.[14-16]

HIV RNA assays have equivalent or higher sensitivity than HIV DNA PCR for the diagnosis of neonatal HIV infection.[1-3,17] Since most infants have high plasma HIV-1 RNA concentrations, HIV RNA testing should be sensitive despite antiretroviral therapy.[18] For infants born to HIV-infected mothers, current U.S. Public Health Service recommendations include performance of HIV DNA PCR or an RNA detection test at 14 to 21 days, 1 to 2 months, and 4 to 6 months.[2] Some experts also recommend testing immediately after birth for infants whose mothers have poorly controlled HIV disease and other infants at higher risk of acquiring infection. An HIV RNA assay can be used as the confirmatory test for infants who have an initial positive HIV DNA PCR test. Cord blood specimens should not be used, due to the risk of contamination with maternal blood.[2]

HIV infection is presumptively excluded in non-breastfed infants who have had two or more negative virologic tests, with one test obtained at ≥14 days of age and one obtained at ≥1 month of age. Children with one negative virologic test result obtained at ≥2 months of age also are presumed to be uninfected. Definitive exclusion of HIV infection in a non-breastfed infant requires two or more negative virologic tests, with one obtained at ≥1 month of age and one at ≥4 months of age.

The worldwide genetic variability of HIV has an impact on the choice of NAT used. HIV exists in a variety of genetically distinct subtypes; subtype B is the predominate variant found in North America, South America, and Western Europe. Type C is the major subtype in sub-Saharan Africa and India. HIV DNA tests used in the U.S. will not detect all non-B subtypes of HIV.[19] HIV RNA assays appear to be more sensitive than HIV DNA PCR for detecting non-subtype B HIV as part of a diagnostic evaluation.[1,2]

Two or more negative HIV antibody tests from separate specimens obtained at ≥6 months of age also allow infection to be excluded, if an infant has not been breastfed. If breastfeeding has occurred, HIV infection cannot be definitively excluded until the infant has a negative diagnostic test ≥6 weeks after breastfeeding has ceased.[3]

EARLY SIGNS, SYMPTOMS, AND LABORATORY ABNORMALITIES FOLLOWING VERTICAL INFECTION

Infants with vertically acquired HIV infection usually are asymptomatic and have normal physical findings during the neonatal period. A purported congenital HIV syndrome, encompassing microcephaly and minor dysmorphic features, was reported early in the AIDS epidemic, but has not been seen consistently.[20]

Early manifestations of vertically acquired HIV infection are frequently nonspecific.[21] Lymphadenopathy, often associated with hepatosplenomegaly, is a commonly observed early sign of infection. Oral candidiasis, parotitis, failure to thrive, dermatitis, and developmental delay are other common presenting features. Before prophylactic therapy with trimethoprim-sulphamethoxazole and other agents became routine, *P. jirovecii* pneumonia (PCP) accounted for about half of all AIDS-defining conditions diagnosed during the first year of life in the U.S.[22]

Hyperimmunoglobulinemia G, A, E, or M is present in up to 90% of HIV-infected infants by 6 months of age.[23,24] By 1 or 2 months of age, HIV-infected infants have CD4+ lymphocyte counts that are significantly lower than those in HIV-exposed infants who are uninfected.[25] The U.S. Centers for Disease Control and Prevention (CDC) has outlined a classification scheme to characterize the severity of HIV infection in children (Box 111-1).[26]

The AIDS case definitions used for children are similar to those used for adults and individuals younger than 13 years,[27] with several exceptions.[28] Lymphoid interstitial pneumonitis (LIP) is a category B condition, while multiple or recurrent serious bacterial infections are only AIDS-defining conditions for children. Some infections, including cytomegalovirus and herpes simplex virus infections and central nervous system (CNS) toxoplasmosis, are only AIDS-defining conditions for children older than 1 month and adults.

ORGAN SYSTEM SPECIFIC MANIFESTATIONS OF HIV INFECTION

HIV infection has the potential to cause injury directly or indirectly to many organ systems. The following sections summarize the most common manifestations of HIV infection and AIDS in infants, children, and adolescents.

Neurologic

CNS abnormalities are extremely common in untreated HIV-infected children.[29-31] Prior to the availability of antiretroviral therapy, progressive HIV encephalopathy accounted for about 15% of all pediatric AIDS-defining conditions reported to the CDC.[32]

Clinical features of HIV-associated progressive encephalopathy are shown in Table 111-3. Characteristic computed tomographic findings are cerebral atrophy (in about 85% of cases) and bilateral symmetric calcification of the basal ganglia (in about 15% of cases)[29] (Figure 111-1). Results of cerebrospinal fluid (CSF) studies usually are normal; mild pleocytosis and elevated protein concentration are observed in some cases. A study from France suggests that the immature infant brain may be particularly sensitive to the effects of HIV.[33] This study found the rate of encephalopathy in HIV-infected infants younger than 1 year of age to be almost 30-fold that of adults. The rate decreased to 15-fold the adult rate in the second year of life, and thereafter the rates of development of encephalopathy were similar in children and adults. HIV-exposed infants are not different from unexposed controls with respect to neurologic function.[34] Encephalopathy is likely the result of direct HIV infection of the CNS rather than from complicating infection or malignancy. Evidence includes virus isolation from CSF, intrathecal synthesis of HIV antibody, and identification of HIV nucleotide sequences in brain tissue at autopsy.[35-38] Neuropathologic features noted in the brains of HIV-infected children include atrophy, subcortical inflammatory lesions, multinucleated giant cells, and vascular calcification.[35,37]

Blood-derived macrophages, resident microglia, their derivatives (including multinucleated giant cells), and astrocytes are the only cells that consistently have been shown to harbor HIV in the CNS.[34,35,39] It is hypothesized that activation of these cells by HIV results in overproduction of certain cytokines, arachidonic acid metabolites, nitric oxide, and quinolinic acid, which in turn may be responsible for some of the neuropathologic changes observed.[40-43] Elevated serum concentration of tumor necrosis factor (TNF) has been associated with progressive encephalopathy in HIV-infected children,[41-43] and TNF can produce white-matter destruction in vitro similar to that observed clinically and pathologically in children with encephalopathy.[44] Platelet-activating

TABLE 111-3. Features of Progressive Encephalopathy Associated with Human Immunodeficiency Virus

Clinical Features	Neuroimaging Features
Impaired brain growth	Cerebral atrophy
Developmental delay or regression	Symmetric calcifications in basal ganglia
Spastic weakness	
Pathologic reflexes	
Dystonia	
Gait disturbance	
Expressive language impairment	

PART II   Clinical Syndromes and Cardinal Features of Infectious Diseases: Approach to Diagnosis and Initial Management

SECTION S   Human Immunodeficiency Virus and the Acquired Immunodeficiency Syndrome

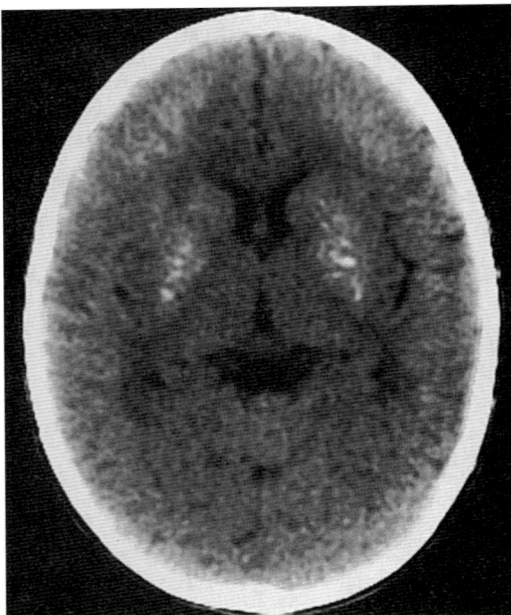

Figure 111-1. Computed tomography scan of the brain showing bilateral symmetric calcification of the basal ganglia in a 2-year-old boy with vertically acquired human immunodeficiency virus infection.

TABLE 111-4. Clinical Differentiation of LIP-PLH from PCP Pneumonia

Finding	LIP-PLH	PCP
CLINICAL		
Acute onset	No	Yes
Fever	No	Yes
Retractions	Late	Early
Crackles	No	Yes
Hypoxia	Late	Early
Clubbing	Yes	No
Salivary glands enlargement	Yes	No
BAL FLUID		
Lymphocyte predominance	Yes	No
Neutrophil predominance	No	Yes

BAL, bronchoalveolar lavage; LIP-PLH, lymphoid interstitial pneumonitis or pulmonary lymphoid hyperplasia; PCP, Pneumocystis pneumonia.

factor and products of arachidonic acid metabolism also may mediate CNS injury, possibly through upregulation of TNF or other cytokines.[42]

The rate of progression and severity of HIV encephalopathy vary tremendously and are modified by antiretroviral therapy. The effectiveness of antiretroviral therapy in preventing or reversing CNS abnormalities appears to depend upon the CNS penetration of the specific agents used and how early therapy is begun. Zidovudine attains therapeutic concentrations in CSF, and therapy with this agent alone has been shown to promote stabilization or reversal of encephalopathy in some cases.[45,46] CSF concentrations of stavudine are appreciable; CSF concentrations of didanosine are variable. However, treatment with all three of these nonnucleoside reverse transcriptase inhibitor agents (NRTIs) has been associated with improvement in neurodevelopmental testing.[47] HIV protease inhibitors, including ritonavir, saquinavir, and nelfinavir, do not penetrate the CSF and brain tissue well, and effective therapy with regimens that include these agents does not reverse neurocognitive abnormalities in all individuals.[48] Moreover, residual behavioral problems as well as neurologic, cognitive, and scholastic impairments still appear to be common with current antiretroviral therapy.[39,49] Frequent evaluation of developmental milestones and neuropsychological testing, as well as counseling and support for older children and adolescents, are critical components in the care of HIV-infected children.[2]

Pulmonary

Lymphoid Interstitial Pneumonia (LIP) and Pulmonary Lymphoid Hyperplasia (PLH)

Prior to the development of multidrug antiretroviral therapy, LIP and the clinically similar, but histologically distinct, PLH were second only to *P. jirovecii* pneumonia (PCP) among pulmonary diseases indicative of HIV infection and AIDS in children.[32] Although these conditions now are assigned to clinical category B because of their relatively benign course, one retrospective study showed more than twice the rate of hospitalization due to serious respiratory infections in patients with LIP-PLH than in controls with HIV but no LIP-PLH.[50]

Although the radiographic features of LIP-PLH and PCP can be similar, clinical features distinguish the two conditions (Table 111-4). The onset of LIP-PLH usually is insidious. Cough and tachypnea often are present. Examination of the chest generally reveals few auscultatory abnormalities. Marked generalized lymphadenopathy, hepatosplenomegaly, and salivary gland enlargement may be noted. Digital clubbing is observed in advanced cases of LIP-PLH. A chest radiograph typically reveals symmetric bilateral reticulonodular and interstitial infiltrates, sometimes in association with hilar adenopathy (Figure 111-2). Differentiation from miliary tuberculosis sometimes is difficult, although patients with LIP-PLH are more likely to be afebrile and relatively well-appearing; the chest radiograph shows less distinct (sometimes larger) lesions and more interstitial abnormality than in tuberculosis. There is no typical laboratory abnormality, but a marked increase in serum immunoglobulin concentrations often is present in patients with LIP-PLH, reflecting the presence of immunologic dysfunction.

Presumptive diagnosis of LIP-PLH can be made on the basis of characteristic radiographic features persisting for 2 months or longer; CT can enhance diagnostic evaluation.[51] A definitive

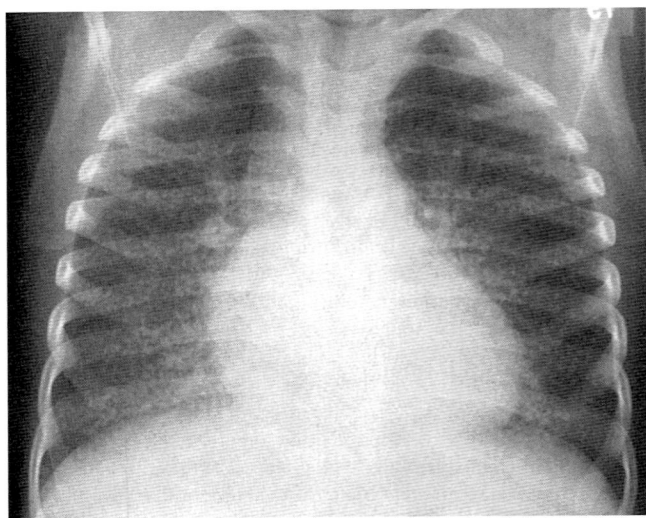

Figure 111-2. Chest radiograph demonstrating bilateral reticulonodular interstitial infiltrates of lymphoid interstitial pneumonitis/pulmonary lymphoid hyperplasia in a 4-year-old boy with vertically acquired human immunodeficiency virus infection.

diagnosis requires lung biopsy. Histopathologic and immunocytochemical analyses reveal a mononuclear interstitial infiltrate surrounding the airways composed of immunoblasts, plasma cells, and CD8[+] lymphocytes. The pathogenesis of LIP-PLH is poorly understood, although Epstein–Barr virus has been implicated as a cofactor.[52]

The clinical course of LIP-PLH is variable. Spontaneous clinical remission sometimes is observed. Exacerbation of clinical signs and symptoms can occur in association with intercurrent viral respiratory illnesses. In severe cases, there is progressive hypoxia and respiratory failure. The initial management of children with LIP-PLH is supportive. Some patients require supplemental oxygen, and anecdotal reports suggest that some cases with progressive hypoxemia may respond to corticosteroid therapy.[53] Antiretroviral treatment is associated with clinical improvement, including full resolution.[54]

Malignancy

Cancers are uncommon among HIV-infected children, but occur at much higher rates than in the general population.[32,55] The most common cancer is non-Hodgkin lymphoma (Burkitt or immunoblastic types).[56] Patients often manifest fever, weight loss, and evidence of "extranodal" disease (e.g., hepatomegaly and jaundice, abdominal distention, myelophthisis, or neurologic abnormalities). Children with CNS lymphoma can have delay or loss of developmental milestones, cranial nerve palsies, seizures, or hemiparesis.[57] Contrast-enhanced CT of the brain reveals hyperdense periventricular mass lesions similar to those seen in cerebral toxoplasmosis. CNS lymphoma more commonly causes an isolated brain mass in children than toxoplasmosis or other infectious agents. In addition to elevated protein and depressed glucose concentrations, examination of CSF can reveal malignant cells. Brain biopsy for definitive diagnosis is indicated for those children who have rapidly progressive disease or clinical or radiographic progression despite empiric therapy for toxoplasmosis.

The pathogenesis of AIDS-associated non-Hodgkin lymphoma is poorly defined; both Epstein–Barr virus[58] and mutations or rearrangements in the *c-myc* oncogene[59,60] have been implicated. Effective chemotherapeutic regimens are available.

Leiomyosarcoma, leiomyoma, and Kaposi sarcoma also occur with greater frequency in children with HIV infection than in the general pediatric population.[56] A strong association exists between Epstein–Barr virus and leiomyosarcoma or leiomyoma. Endobronchial leiomyosarcoma or leiomyoma can manifest with fever or cyanosis.[61] Multiple pulmonary parenchymal nodules can be visualized radiographically. Clinical manifestations of pulmonary Kaposi sarcoma, which is triggered by infection with human herpesvirus 8, include fever, cough, dyspnea, and hemoptysis. The radiographic features are diffuse reticulonodular infiltrates resembling those seen in LIP-PLH or PCP. Kaposi sarcoma also can present with involvement of lymph nodes, the oral cavity (hard palate or tonsils), or skin. Gastrointestinal lesions can occur with any of these malignancies, resulting in gastrointestinal bleeding, abdominal pain, or bowel obstruction.

Gastrointestinal

Wasting Syndrome

HIV infection was originally referred to as "slim disease" in African culture. Weight loss, or failure to gain appropriate weight, is a common presenting symptom in HIV-infected infants and children, and may appear within the first 2 to 3 months of life.[62] Several factors can contribute to wasting. HIV infection itself increases a child's nutritional requirements. In addition, opportunistic infections, especially those associated with fever, contribute to increased metabolic requirements. Oral lesions (e.g., thrush, herpes simplex infection, recurrent aphthous ulcers) can interfere with feeding. Chronic diarrhea and malabsorptive syndromes can inhibit caloric intake. Effective antiretroviral therapy and nutritional support are the primary approaches to treating wasting

---

BOX 111-2. Differential Diagnosis of Hepatitis in Children Infected with Human Immunodeficiency Virus (HIV)

INFECTION

Bacteria (e.g., *Mycobacterium avium* complex, *Mycobacterium tuberculosis*, or *Bartonella* spp.-induced bacillary peliosis hepatis)

Viruses (e.g., hepatitis A, B, or C; cytomegalovirus; Epstein–Barr virus; herpes simplex virus; adenovirus; or HIV)

Fungi (e.g., *Candida* spp., *Cryptococcus neoformans*, *Histoplasma capsulatum*, *Pneumocystis jirovecii*)

Protozoans (e.g., *Toxoplasma gondii*)

MALIGNANCY

Lymphoma

Sarcoma

DRUG-INDUCED

Sulfonamides

Antiretroviral agents (especially non-nucleoside reverse transcriptase inhibitors, tipranavir)

Antimycobacterial medications

Pentamidine

---

syndrome, and may include the use of nasogastric or gastrostomy tube feedings in some cases.

Hepatitis

Hepatomegaly, moderate increases in serum concentrations of hepatic enzymes (e.g., 5- to 10-fold increases in aspartate aminotransferase (AST) and/or alanine aminotransferase (ALT)), are common in HIV-infected children, but often are unaccompanied by clinical manifestations. The differential diagnosis of hepatitis in HIV-infected children is broad and includes a variety of infectious causes, neoplasms, and effects of medications (Box 111-2).[63] Elevation of transaminase values has been reported in association with the use of virtually all antiretroviral medications.[64] These elevations usually are clinically insignificant in children, but can necessitate discontinuation of antiretroviral medications in some cases. Coinfection with either hepatitis B or C and HIV can hasten the progression of liver disease.[65] The presence of hepatitis B (HBV) coinfection has an impact on the selection of antiretroviral medications, as flare in liver disease can occur with the removal of antiretroviral agents with activity against HBV. The clinical course of HIV-associated hepatitis is variable. Histopathologic studies of liver tissue obtained from HIV-infected children have identified giant-cell transformation of hepatocytes, fatty degeneration, and lymphoplasmacytic infiltration as prominent features.[66,67]

Cardiovascular Disease

Cardiac abnormalities are commonly observed in untreated HIV-infected children. Electrocardiographic abnormalities include conduction defects, unexplained sinus tachycardia, voltage abnormalities compatible with chamber enlargement, and dysrhythmias. Echocardiographic findings include ventricular dysfunction and pericardial effusion.[68] Many abnormalities are not apparent clinically but in one retrospective study of 81 HIV-infected children, serious dysrhythmia, congestive heart failure, and unexpected cardiac arrest occurred in 28 (35%), 8 (10%), and 7 (9%) patients, respectively.[68] The pathogenesis of cardiac disease in HIV-infected children is poorly understood, but epidemiologic associations between coinfection with Epstein–Barr virus and either bradycardia or congestive heart failure have been reported.[69] Adenovirus and cytomegalovirus sequences have been identified in a

PART II Clinical Syndromes and Cardinal Features of Infectious Diseases: Approach to Diagnosis and Initial Management

SECTION S Human Immunodeficiency Virus and the Acquired Immunodeficiency Syndrome

postmortem study of cardiac tissue from HIV-infected children with myocarditis, suggesting a possible etiologic role.[70] The relative importance of HIV-related and drug-related cardiac dysfunction, as well as value and timing of echocardiographic screening, is evolving with changing antiretroviral therapies.[71-73] Most HIV-infected children with cardiomyopathy and congestive heart failure demonstrate good response to antiretroviral therapy and specific management of the cardiac disease. Abnormalities of serum lipid concentrations and effect on electrocardiographic findings are well-known adverse effects of antiretroviral medications, especially the HIV protease inhibitors. When dyslipidemia is encountered, changes in diet and other lifestyle modifications, substitution of other medications, or pharmacologic treatment may be needed.[2]

Renal

Initially, nephropathy was found predominantly among children with advanced HIV disease.[74-76] Persistent proteinuria is a common finding. In one study, progressive renal disease with nephrotic syndrome and renal failure developed in 5 of 12 children with AIDS and proteinuria.[74] In a larger series of 556 HIV-infected children, 72 (12.9%) met the definition of HIV-associated nephropathy. Nineteen percent of those with nephropathy progressed to chronic renal insufficiency.[77] Histopathologic examination of the kidney has revealed a variety of lesions, including focal glomerulosclerosis, collapsing glomerulopathy, and mesangial hypercellularity. Immune complex deposition may be involved in the pathogenesis of HIV-associated nephropathy.[75,76] Antiretroviral therapy appears to be the most effective therapy, but addition of corticosteroids may improve renal function,[72,74,75] although corticosteroid therapy can be associated with additional risks of immune suppression and other complications.[78] Cyclosporine-induced remission of HIV-associated nephrotic syndrome also has been reported.[76,77]

Hematologic

Anemia, leukopenia, neutropenia, and thrombocytopenia are common manifestations of HIV infection in children. Many cases of normocytic or microcytic anemia are attributable to chronic disease; macrocytic anemia most often is secondary to zidovudine therapy. Other causes of anemia are iron deficiency, hemoglobinopathies, and red blood cell enzyme defects. Infectious diseases resulting in anemia in HIV-infected children include disseminated *Mycobacterium avium* complex infection, cytomegalovirus infection, and chronic parvovirus infection.[79]

The treatment of anemia in HIV depends on the etiology. Therapy with recombinant human erythropoietin facilitates continued use of zidovudine if alternative antiretroviral agents cannot be substituted.[2,80] Some patients with chronic parvovirus infection respond to high-dose immune globulin intravenous (IGIV) therapy.[79]

Leukopenia and neutropenia often result from medication-induced bone marrow depression caused by zidovudine, trimethoprim-sulfamethoxazole (TMP-SMX), ganciclovir, pentamidine, and other medications. Neutropenia also is observed during the course of various chronic and opportunistic infections, including parvovirus B19 and *Mycobacterium avium* complex. Granulocyte colony-stimulating factor therapy can be helpful in reversing drug- or disease-induced neutropenia and preventing infectious complications.[81]

Thrombocytopenia in HIV-infected children can occur as a result of either underproduction or shortened survival of platelets. Immune-mediated destruction is a common cause of thrombocytopenia, and antiplatelet antibodies are detectable in most patients. Antiretroviral therapy often leads to resolution of thrombocytopenia. Some children may exhibit an initial response to corticosteroid, IGIV therapy, or the use of intravenous anti-D antibody, but improvement often is short-lived and incomplete. Splenectomy may be indicated for the HIV-infected child with severe thrombocytopenia that is refractory to other measures.[82]

Rituximab also has been used in chronic, recurrent HIV-associated immune thrombocytopenia.[83]

Dermatologic Conditions

A wide variety of bacterial, fungal, viral, and parasitic infections of the skin occur in children with HIV infection. HIV-infected children also have a higher than expected incidence of noninfectious inflammatory, eczematoid, psoriatic, neoplastic, and drug hypersensitivity skin conditions.[84] Seborrheic dermatitis manifests as erythema and scaling of the face and scalp in HIV-infected infants or of the nasolabial folds, eyebrows, and postauricular areas in older children. Pruritic papular eruption (PPE) is a chronic eruption of papular lesions on the skin of unclear etiology. PPE may represent an overexuberant reaction to insect bites and has been associated with increased IgE.[85] PPE can cause substantial discomfort. Cutaneous eruptions occur with a variety of oral and parenteral medications, TMP-SMX and non-nucleoside reverse transcriptase inhibitors being the most commonly implicated. Cutaneous Kaposi sarcoma occurs in HIV-infected children internationally, but is rarely seen in the United States.

PROGNOSIS

In general, children with vertically acquired HIV infection have shorter clinical latent periods and more rapid disease progression than other individuals with HIV infection.[21,86] However, many children demonstrate late onset of symptoms with long-term survival.[86,87] Both the age at diagnosis of an AIDS-defining condition and clinical presentation are important determinants of prognosis. In one study, conducted before the advent of highly effective therapy, the overall median survival time for children with vertically acquired HIV infection was 30 months. But children who demonstrated AIDS in the first year of life had a median survival time of only about 7 months.[21] Presentation during infancy with opportunistic infection (especially PCP) or HIV encephalopathy[21,29,86] portends a poor prognosis, whereas slow decline of CD4+ lymphocyte count, late onset of signs and symptoms of HIV infection, and occurrence of LIP-PLH have been associated with a longer survival.[87]

The importance of weight growth velocity as a prognostic indicator for HIV-infected children has been highlighted in several studies.[62,88] In one study of HIV-infected children receiving zidovudine therapy, 9 of 28 (32%) children who gained weight at a rate lower than the 10th percentile during the first 6 months of therapy died within 24 months, whereas only 10 of 75 (13%) children with more normal growth velocity died during the same period of follow-up.[62]

Beyond infancy, CD4 T-lymphocyte counts and measurements of plasma HIV viral load have strong prognostic value. The HIV Paediatric Prognostic Markers Collaborative Study (HPPMCS) was a meta-analysis based upon data from 3941 children (with 7297 child-years of follow-up) who had received no antiretroviral agents, or zidovudine alone.[89] In the HPPMCS, CD4 percentage and HIV RNA levels were both independently predictive of the risk of clinical progression or death in children older than 12 months, although CD4 percentage was a stronger predictor of risk than HIV RNA concentrations (Figure 111-3).

The outlook for children with HIV continues to improve. Multidrug antiretroviral therapy (ART) is increasingly available throughout the world. ART is recommended for all infants by the World Health Organization, and is able to prevent, ameliorate, or reverse most of the clinical manifestations of HIV infection. Although adherence to medication regimens and tolerance of their side effects remain problematic, the number of pediatric deaths due to HIV/AIDS has been reduced markedly, wherever ART has been introduced. Hospitalizations have also decreased as a result of effective prophylaxis against opportunistic infections. Unfortunately, even with ART, the mortality rate for HIV-infected children and adolescents remains about 30-fold higher than that of other children in the U.S.[90]

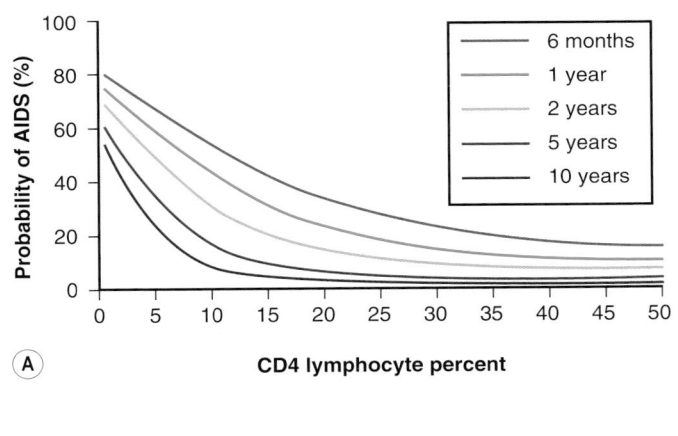

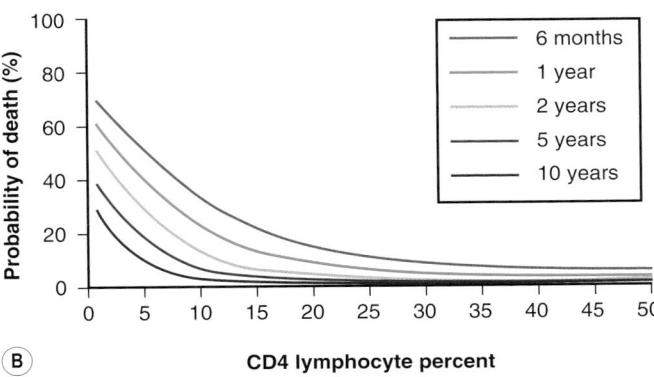

Figure 111-3. (A) Estimated probability of AIDS within 12 months by age and CD4 lymphocyte percentage in HIV-infected children receiving no therapy or zidovudine monotherapy. **(B)** Estimated probability of death within 12 months by age and CD4 lymphocyte percentage in HIV-infected children receiving no therapy or zidovudine monotherapy.[89]

NON-PERINATALLY ACQUIRED HIV

In the U.S. and throughout the world, adolescents and young adults are the fastest growing group of HIV-infected individuals, particularly youth of color. These youth most often are infected via high-risk behaviors including unprotected sex, sexual assault, and injection drug use. Numerous recent studies have shown a rise in coinfection of syphilis and HIV, particularly in young men who engage in sex with men.[90,91] One study in Louisiana found that of 141 newly infected adolescents, 75% of the women and 48% of the men presented with other sexually transmitted infections (STIs).[92] Hence, it is imperative that all patients newly diagnosed with HIV also be screened for syphilis and other STIs.

In one recent report, approximately 33% of adolescents and young adults newly diagnosed with HIV in the U.S. between the ages of 13 and 24 were infected recently.[93] The rest showed biologic markers of longer infection. This mixture of newly and chronically infected youth presenting for care correlates to the range of clinical presentations seen in adolescent care. A small number will present with findings consistent with acute retroviral syndrome (fever, sore throat, swollen lymph nodes or tonsils, and possibly rash). Youth presenting with these symptoms and history of high-risk behavior should be tested for HIV utilizing RNA or DNA PCR as any antibody-based test may be negative. Most adolescents are asymptomatic at the time of presentation, but obtain HIV testing through testing campaigns, partner notification, or provider-initiated testing in their primary care settings. Asymptomatic youths can be screened with an antibody-based test. For the asymptomatic, newly diagnosed adolescent, care should focus on education about HIV and prevention of transmission, obtaining psychosocial support as needed, and building a therapeutic relationship with the adolescent.

As not all newly diagnosed adolescents are newly infected, a small number will come to medical attention with severe opportunistic infections or AIDS-defining conditions. Clinical care will include starting treatment for opportunistic infections, prophylaxis based on CD4 lymphocyte count to prevent recurrences or new opportunistic infections, and assessing readiness for antiretroviral treatment. Most youth will respond robustly to antiretroviral therapy but psychological support is critical in caring for those youth who are infected because of behavioral risks, as high percentages have pre-existing mental health and substance abuse issues.[94,95]

112 Infectious Complications of HIV Infection

Russell B. Van Dyke and Mark W. Kline

Opportunistic infections are central to the definition of the acquired immunodeficiency syndrome (AIDS) and have been the major causes of human immunodeficiency virus (HIV)-associated morbidity and mortality. An unusual clustering of cases of *Pneumocystis jirovecii* (formally *P. carinii*) pneumonia (PCP) in the early 1980s led in part to the recognition of AIDS. Other AIDS-associated opportunistic infections, including disseminated mycobacterial disease, cryptococcal meningitis, cerebral toxoplasmosis, and cytomegalovirus (CMV) retinitis, were recognized soon thereafter. In the mid-1990s, improved treatment and prevention strategies and the introduction of highly active combination antiretroviral therapy (HAART) dramatically reduced the mortality from HIV and the incidence of opportunistic infections. Between 1994 and 2000, the mortality among HIV-infected children in the United States decreased from 7.2 to 0.8 deaths/100 person years[1]

(Table 112-1). Likewise, the incidence of most opportunistic infections fell dramatically.[2,3] Despite these advances, opportunistic infections continue to occur, and physicians must be familiar with the epidemiology and features of these infections to optimize early identification, prevention, and treatment.

PATHOGENESIS

The naivety of the developing immune system is invoked as a possible explanation for susceptibility of the infant or child infected with HIV to rapid HIV disease progression and complicating infections. The healthy neonate is at risk of serious infection because of immaturity of several components of the immune system, including B and T lymphocytes, phagocytes, and complement. As a consequence, defenses against primary HIV infection

TABLE 112-1. Incidence of Infections in Human Immunodeficiency Virus (HIV)-Infected Children Before and After the Advent of Highly Active Antiretroviral Therapy (HAART) (Cases/100 Patient-Years)

Condition	Pre-HAART 1986–1998[3,19]	Post-HAART 1997–2004[2,3]
OPPORTUNISTIC INFECTIONS		
Pneumocystis jirovecii pneumonia	1.3–5.8	0.09–0.3
Nontuberculous mycobacterial infection	1.3–1.8	0.2–0.14
Cytomegalovirus disease	0.7–1.5	0.03–0.1
Toxoplasmosis	0.06	NA
Progressive multifocal leukoencephalopathy	0.06	NA
Cryptosporidiosis	0.3–0.6	0–0.03
OTHER INFECTIONS		
Otitis media	57	NA
Upper respiratory infection	47	NA
Sinusitis	15	NA
Bacteremia	3.3	0.35
Bacterial pneumonia	11.1	2.1
Bacterial meningitis	0.1	0.05
Varicella	4.7	0.44
Herpes zoster	2.9	1.1
Candidiasis, esophageal or pulmonary	1.2–1.4	0.04–0.08
Urinary tract infection	1.6	0.35
Tuberculosis	0.4	<0.5

NA: not available.

From: references 2, 3, and 19.

and other opportunistic and nonopportunistic infections, as well as immune control of progression of HIV disease, are impaired.

HIV infection of the fetus or neonate can have profound effects on cellular immunity. Destruction of the thymus gland is observed in spontaneous abortuses from HIV-infected mothers. Surprisingly, depletion of CD4[+] lymphocytes is not recognized at the time of birth. However, as early as 1 or 2 months of age, HIV-infected infants have CD4[+] lymphocyte counts significantly lower than those of HIV-exposed but uninfected infants.[4] Suppression of cell-mediated immunity is responsible in large part for the susceptibility of HIV-infected individuals to PCP and opportunistic mycobacterial, fungal, and viral infections.

Despite the presence of hypergammaglobulinemia, humoral immune dysfunction is present in most children with symptomatic HIV infection. Humoral deficiency results from dysregulation of T-lymphocyte-mediated responses and polyclonal stimulation of B lymphocytes by poorly controlled infectious agents.[5-9] In vitro lymphoproliferative responses to B-lymphocyte mitogens and specific antigens often are poor. In vivo, there is impaired specific antibody production after immunization with either T-lymphocyte-independent antigens (e.g., capsular polysaccharide of Streptococcus pneumoniae), or T-lymphocyte-dependent antigens (e.g., bacteriophage OX174). Both primary humoral immune responses and recall responses (e.g., amplification and immunoglobulin class switch) are defective in children with HIV infection.

Phagocytic function also can be altered by HIV infection. Neutropenia and defects in neutrophil chemotaxis and bactericidal activity have been described.[10,11] Neutrophil superoxide production can be depressed in children with advanced HIV disease.[12,13] This combination of phagocyte abnormalities compromises the ability of an HIV-infected individual to kill bacterial and fungal pathogens. Although the precise pathogenesis of these abnormalities is unknown, studies suggest that neutropenia and neutrophil dysfunction are at least partly mediated by abnormal regulation by cytokines (e.g., granulocyte colony-stimulating factor

(G-CSF)).[14] Recombinant G-CSF administration in HIV-infected adults has been shown to reverse neutropenia and correct neutrophil-killing defects.[15]

IMMUNE RECONSTITUTION SYNDROME (IRIS)

Children with advanced immunosuppression who initiate HAART often have a rapid improvement in their immune competence, as reflected by an increase in their CD4[+] cell count. In the presence of an underlying infection, this can result in a worsening of the symptoms of the infection. The infection may be unrecognized prior to starting HAART and be "unmasked" by the resulting inflammatory response. In children, IRIS most often is seen with mycobacterial infections (Mycobacterium avium complex (MAC), M. tuberculosis, and the BCG vaccine), varicella-zoster virus (VZV), herpes simplex virus (HSV), and cryptococcal infections, but can be seen with PCP, CMV, hepatitis B and C, toxoplasmosis, and progressive multifocal encephalopathy (PML).[16,17] IRIS generally occurs within the first 2 to 3 months of initiating HAART and is associated with a low pre-treatment CD4[+] lymphocyte count. IRIS should not be interpreted as a failure of HAART. Children should be carefully evaluated for underlying occult infections prior to initiating HAART. The optimal time to start HAART in a child with an active opportunistic infection (OI) is unknown and should be individualized. For OIs without effective therapy (such as cryptosporidium, PML, and Kaposi sarcoma), HAART should be initiated promptly since immune reconstitution may clear the infection. For those with effective therapy (M. tuberculosis, MAC, PCP, and cryptococcal meningitis), treating the OI prior to starting HAART may prevent IRIS.[18] If symptoms of IRIS develop following HAART, the OI should be treated and HAART is generally continued.

EPIDEMIOLOGY AND ETIOLOGIC AGENTS

In children, as in adults, untreated HIV infection is characterized by an increased frequency of a specific group of serious opportunistic and nonopportunistic infections. There is also an increased frequency of common childhood infections of a less serious nature, which contribute to the overall morbidity of the disease. The frequency of the various opportunistic infections among HIV-infected children in the years preceding HAART varied by age, pathogen, and immunologic status.[19] The most common opportunistic infections among children in the U.S. included serious bacterial infections (SBIs, e.g., pneumonia and bacteremia), PCP, nontuberculous mycobacterial infections, and CMV disease (Table 112-1).[2,3,19,20] Despite a dramatic decrease in the rate of opportunistic infections due to HAART,[3,21,22] the types of infections observed have not changed.[23,24]

Before the advent of HAART and widespread use of P. jirovecii prophylaxis in early infancy, PCP was the most common AIDS-defining opportunistic infection in children (Table 112-2).[25] More than 50% of cases occurred between 3 and 6 months of age.[26] The disease accounted for about 60% of all AIDS-defining illness

TABLE 112-2. Common Acquired Immunodeficiency Syndrome (AIDS)-Defining Infections in Children Less than 13 Years of Age

AIDS-Defining Infection	AIDS-Defining Events (%)
Pneumocystis jirovecii pneumonia	35
Lymphoid interstitial pneumonitis	23
Recurrent bacterial infections	21
Esophageal or pulmonary candidiasis	21
Cytomegalovirus disease	11
Mycobacterium avium complex infection	9
Severe herpes simplex infection	5
Cryptosporidiosis	5

From CDC.[29]

occurring during the first year of life but only about 19% occurring subsequently. Between 7% and 20% of all HIV-infected infants manifested PCP. A low age-adjusted CD4+ lymphocyte count or percentage was the major determinant of risk. Although PCP still is observed in HIV-infected infants and children, the incidence has decreased dramatically in the U.S.[3]

Oral candidiasis occurs in approximately 15% to 40% of children with HIV infection and is more common among children with low CD4+ lymphocyte counts or symptomatic HIV disease than among those with normal counts or no symptoms.[27,28] Esophageal and pulmonary candidiasis account for approximately 17% and 4%, respectively, of all AIDS-defining illnesses in children.[29] Whereas oral candidiasis is common at all stages of HIV disease, esophageal and pulmonary candidiasis are far less common, and their occurrence is typically restricted to patients with advanced HIV disease.

Recognition of the frequently serious and recurrent nature of bacterial infections in HIV-infected children led to the designation of certain of these as indicator diseases for AIDS in children. A child <13 years of age with laboratory evidence of HIV infection is defined as having AIDS if any combination of the following bacterial infections occurs twice within 2 years: septicemia, pneumonia, meningitis, osteomyelitis or pyogenic arthritis, or abscess of an internal organ or body cavity. Recurrent bacterial infections accounted for 21% of all pediatric AIDS-defining illnesses reported to the Centers for Disease Control and Prevention (CDC) through 2007.[29]

Serious bacterial infections were reported in 40% to 60% of HIV-infected children prior to HAART.[30,31] Bloodstream infection (BSI) was common, with or without an identified localized infection such as pneumonia, urinary tract infection, meningitis, cellulitis, or lymphadenitis. In a multicenter placebo-controlled trial of immune globulin intravenous (IGIV) in the pre-HAART era, laboratory-proven (i.e., confirmed by bacterial culture or antigen assay) or clinically diagnosed (i.e., without a defined bacterial cause) serious bacterial infection (SBI) occurred in 38% of the children.[32] Minor infections (e.g., otitis media, urinary tract infection, or infections of skin or soft tissue) were 3-fold more common than serious infections (e.g., BSI, certain types of pneumonia or sinusitis, meningitis, osteomyelitis, septic arthritis, mastoiditis, or abscess of an internal organ). The most frequent laboratory-proven serious infections were BSI and pneumonia; pneumonia and sinusitis were the most common clinically diagnosed serious infections. The overall incidence of SBIs was 44 per 100 patient-years of follow-up. HAART has resulted in a dramatic drop in the incidence of SBI but rates remain higher than those of HIV-uninfected children (Table 112-1).

Risk factors for SBI in HIV-infected children have not been defined precisely, but studies have demonstrated that the incidence is highest in vertically infected children <1 year of age who have low CD4+ lymphocyte counts.[33] The Pediatric Spectrum of Disease Project evaluated 21,167 vertically infected children for SBI; 570 children had 1063 infections. Sixty-four percent were severely immunocompromised (CDC category 3) when the first SBI occurred. Of all children, 25% with SBIs had their first infection in the first 6 months of life, and 37% of infections occurred by 12 months of life. BSI, pneumonia, and urinary tract infection were the most common SBIs.[34]

Streptococcus pneumoniae is the single most common cause of SBI in HIV-infected children.[30–32,34,35] In a study of HIV-infected children <36 months of age, pneumococcal BSI occurred with an annualized rate of 11.3 episodes per 100 patient-years;[36] this rate is ≥3-fold that observed in children with sickle-cell anemia[37] and 12-fold that reported in one study of adults with AIDS.[38] Other bacteria commonly causing these infections include *Salmonella* species, *Staphylococcus aureus*, and *Neisseria meningitidis*. For children with indwelling venous catheters, *S. aureus* and coagulase-negative staphylococci, *Pseudomonas aeruginosa*, and enteric bacilli are likely.

CMV infection is common, but disseminated disease, chorioretinitis, and colitis caused by CMV are uncommon.[39] The role of CMV as a cause of pneumonia in HIV-infected children is controversial; CMV usually is found in association with another pathogen (often *P. jirovecii*). HSV commonly causes infection of the oral or genital mucous membranes;[40] esophageal or pulmonary disease occurs rarely. CMV disease, cryptosporidiosis,[41] and disseminated MAC[42,43] all occur predominantly among children with advanced HIV disease and severely depressed CD4+ lymphocyte counts. Without prophylaxis, up to 20% of HIV-infected children with CD4+ lymphocyte counts of <50 cells/mm³ have disseminated MAC infection; almost all children with MAC develop CD4+ lymphocyte counts <100 cells/mm³.

APPROACH TO THE HIV-INFECTED CHILD WITH SUSPECTED SYSTEMIC OR FOCAL INFECTION

Fever

Clinical manifestations and diagnostic considerations for HIV-infected children with fever are diverse. Febrile episodes can be acute or prolonged and may present with or without localizing signs. Prolonged fever (arbitrarily defined as more than 7 days) may be associated with a discernible cause, or a cause may not be evident even after careful physical examination and initial laboratory testing (i.e., fever of unknown origin).

Fever is a common reason for unscheduled outpatient clinic visits and hospital admission of HIV-infected children. At Texas Children's Hospital, 26 (11%) of 231 hospitalizations of HIV-infected children were because of fever without localizing signs, either acutely or with a duration >7 days. Fifty (31%) of 161 HIV-infected children had a total of 77 episodes of unexplained fever lasting ≥1 month.

Most HIV-infected children with acute febrile illnesses have mild, self-limited illnesses that appear to be caused by viral infection, however, some have BSI or other serious illnesses. Differentiation can be difficult (Box 112-1). Febrile HIV-infected children should be evaluated initially with a thorough medical history and physical examination. The character and duration of symptoms, HIV disease status including the most recent CD4+ lymphocyte count, use of prophylaxis, and history of recent exposures are particularly relevant. A careful search for evidence of focal infection or inflammation and a general assessment of severity of illness or "toxicity" should be performed. Clinical features of focal infection in HIV-infected children are similar to features observed in immunologically normal children. Fever and local signs of inflammation often are present. BSI should be suspected when certain serious focal infections (e.g., pneumonia, cellulitis, or osteomyelitis) are present or in the child who appears to be ill. Bacterial cultures of blood should be obtained from all such children.

The approach to the acutely febrile HIV-infected child without localizing signs is more problematic. Not all patients require

---

BOX 112-1. Causes of Fever of Unknown Origin in Human Immunodeficiency Virus (HIV)-Infected Children

Focal bacterial infection (e.g., sinusitis, pneumonia, or internal abscess)
Salmonellosis
Tuberculous or nontuberculous mycobacterial infection
Fungal infection (e.g., candidal esophagitis, cryptococcal meningitis, or pneumonia)
Pneumocystis jirovecii infection
Toxoplasmosis
Cytomegalovirus infection
Epstein–Barr virus infection
Herpes simplex virus infection
Hepatitis
Lymphoma and other types of malignancy
Drug fever

PART II   Clinical Syndromes and Cardinal Features of Infectious Diseases: Approach to Diagnosis and Initial Management

SECTION S   Human Immunodeficiency Virus and the Acquired Immunodeficiency Syndrome

diagnostic testing or antibiotic therapy, although both should be considered, especially in those with high-grade fever (>39.4°C) or advanced HIV disease. The white blood cell count, often used as a screening test for SBI in immunologically normal children, must be interpreted in the context of the patient's baseline values. Neutropenia commonly results from use of trimethoprim-sulfamethoxazole. Several other diagnostic studies, including blood culture, chest radiograph, lumbar puncture, urinalysis, and urine culture should be considered. Cultures for mycobacteria and fungi seldom have positive results (or are indicated) in the setting of acute fever without localizing signs except in children with very low CD4+ lymphocyte counts.

An individual approach to the therapy of acutely febrile, HIV-infected children with localizing signs is appropriate. The selection of antibiotic agents for expectant therapy is influenced by several factors, including the likely source of infection (e.g., community-acquired versus healthcare-associated infection), presence of a central venous catheter, immunization status, use of prophylactic antibiotics, and the child's HIV disease status. Expectant antibiotic therapy, when used, should be directed against a limited number of likely pathogens. Unless convincing clinical or laboratory evidence exists for serious opportunistic fungal, mycobacterial, or viral infection, therapy usually is directed against potential bacterial pathogens.

In general, antibiotic therapy for asymptomatic or mildly symptomatic HIV-infected children with fever should be similar to that used in the treatment of immunologically normal children with comparable clinical manifestations. Oral antibiotic therapy is appropriate in most cases. Children with more advanced HIV disease may require agents with broader activity, administered parenterally. Children with granulocytopenia resulting from HIV infection or from various medications should be given antibiotics similar to those given to children with granulocytopenia caused by other conditions (e.g., acute leukemia or chemotherapy).

Evaluation of fever of unknown origin (FUO) in children infected with HIV is informed by the degree of immunosuppression, as reflected in the child's CD4+ lymphocyte count. In a child with less advanced HIV disease who appears to be mildly ill, diagnostic studies are conducted in a stepwise manner with common causes of disease excluded first. With more advanced HIV disease or fulminant illness, immediate and extensive testing to address the full range of diagnostic possibilities is indicated. Opportunistic infections, such as disseminated MAC, *Cryptococcus neoformans*, or CMV retinitis, are more likely with advanced HIV disease.

Evaluation of FUO requires extensive diagnostic testing because of the many potential infectious and noninfectious causes (see Box 112-1). Such studies may include radiographs of the chest and sinuses; culture of blood for routine bacteria, mycobacteria, and fungi; culture of the throat, nasopharynx, urine, and blood for viruses (especially CMV); cryptococcal and other fungal antigen tests; Epstein–Barr virus serologic tests; hepatic enzyme measurements; and ophthalmologic examination for chorioretinitis. Cerebrospinal fluid (CSF) should be obtained for routine cell count; protein and glucose concentration; bacterial, fungal, and viral polymerase chain reaction (PCR) assays; cryptococcal antigen test; and cytologic tests. Bone marrow aspiration and biopsy occasionally are useful, particularly if hematologic abnormalities exist or if routine cultures and serologic test results are negative. Specimens should be obtained for Gram stain and bacterial culture, fungal stains and culture, stain for acid-fast bacteria, culture for mycobacteria and virus, histopathology, and cytology. As in immunologically normal children, expectant antibiotic therapy is rarely indicated in HIV-infected children with fever of unknown origin.

Pneumonia

More than 50% of all infants with vertically acquired HIV infection initially manifest signs and symptoms of a pulmonary disorder.[44] Many infectious and noninfectious pulmonary complications of HIV infection are recognized, but PCP, lymphocytic interstitial

pneumonitis/pulmonary lymphoid hyperplasia (LIP/PLH), and bacterial pneumonia are the most common. Predominant bacterial causes of pneumonia include *S. pneumoniae*, *S. aureus*, *Haemophilus influenzae* type b, *Klebsiella pneumoniae*, *P. aeruginosa*, and *M. tuberculosis*. There is an increased rate of tuberculosis among HIV-infected children and adults and, unlike other opportunistic infections, the CD4+ lymphocyte count is not a good indicator of risk of tuberculosis. Other infectious causes of pneumonia in HIV-infected children include common viruses (e.g., respiratory syncytial virus, parainfluenza virus, influenza virus, and adenovirus), CMV, HSV, and fungi (e.g., *Candida*, *C. neoformans*, and *Histoplasma capsulatum*).

Diagnostic evaluation is individualized on the basis of HIV disease status and clinical presentation. The likelihood of an unusual or opportunistic infectious agent increases as the patient's CD4+ lymphocyte count decreases. The usual manifestations of PCP include acute onset of fever, cough, tachypnea, and respiratory distress. Decreased breath sounds or rales may be present. The onset of LIP/PLH usually is insidious and the course is slowly progressive. Cough and wheezing may be present. Associated findings include generalized lymphadenopathy, hepatosplenomegaly, parotid enlargement, and digital clubbing. The clinical presentation of bacterial pneumonia in children with HIV infection is similar to that seen in immunologically normal children.

Radiographic features of pneumonia in HIV-infected children generally are nonspecific. The typical radiographic picture of PCP is diffuse interstitial and alveolar infiltrates, most prominent in the perihilar areas (Figure 112-1). Air bronchograms, focal infiltrates, pneumatoceles, or pneumothorax are seen in some cases. The chest radiograph can be normal at the time of presentation. The typical radiographic features of LIP/PLH include diffuse reticulo-nodular infiltration and hilar adenopathy (Figure 112-2). Bacterial pneumonia can be associated with focal or diffuse infiltration. The radiographic features of tuberculosis in HIV-infected children often are similar to those of HIV-uninfected children, although they are more likely to have atypical findings such as multilobar infiltrates and diffuse interstitial disease.

A tuberculin skin test (TST) or an interferon-γ release assay (IGRA) should be performed in every HIV-infected child with pneumonia. Annual TST is recommended for all HIV-infected children to diagnose latent infection. The use of control skin testing to identify anergy is not recommended; a negative TST (defined in the HIV-infected child as an induration of ≤5 mm) does not exclude tuberculosis regardless of the results of anergy testing.[45] IGRA test performance characteristics depend on

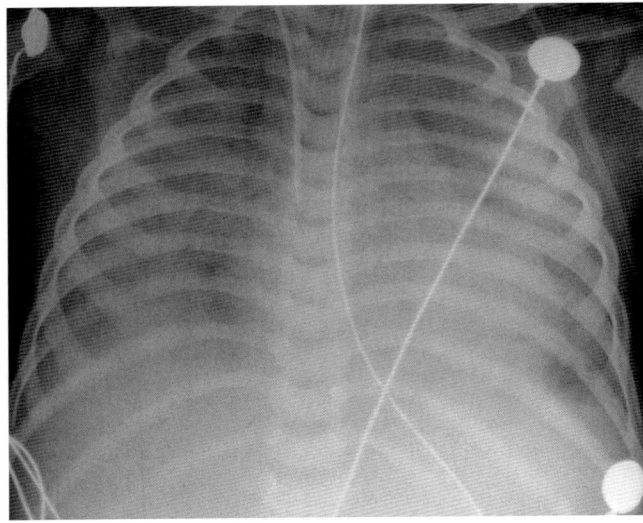

Figure 112-1. Chest radiograph showing *Pneumocystis jirovecii* pneumonia in a 2-year-old boy with vertically acquired human immunodeficiency virus infection. Note bilateral interstitial lung disease.

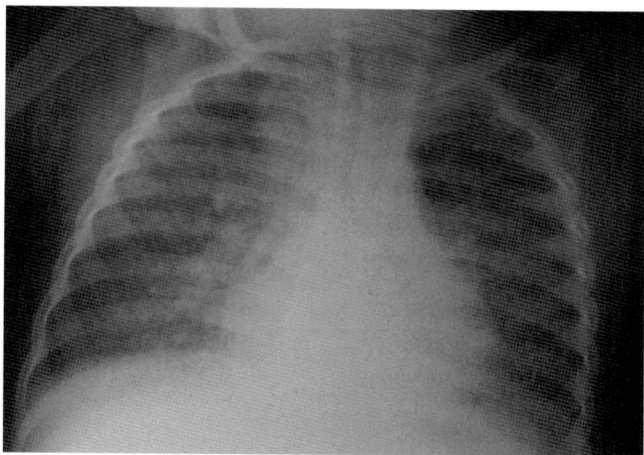

Figure 112-2. Typical lymphocytic interstitial pneumonitis/pulmonary lymphoid hyperplasia (LIP/PLH) as the presenting manifestation of vertically acquired HIV infection in a 23-month-old infant with slowly worsening "bronchiolitis" and hypoxia. Fungal, bacterial, and other viral causes were excluded. Plain radiograph shows diffuse reticulonodular infiltration and perihilar adenopathy. There was complete resolution 4 months after commencement of highly active antiretroviral therapy. (Courtesy of E.N. Faerber, J. Chen, and J. Foster, St. Christopher's Hospital for Children, Philadelphia, PA.)

immunologic capability, disease state, and age (not recommended <5 years of age). A complete blood cell count, measure of oxygen saturation, and routine blood cultures should be obtained in most cases. Most children with normal or unchanged results on chest radiograph and normal arterial oxygen saturation have self-limited (presumably viral) illness. A nasopharyngeal specimen for rapid diagnostic tests (e.g., fluorescent antibody test or enzyme immunoassay), nucleic acid testing, or culture for viruses may be helpful. Positive results of blood culture or evidence of a segmental or lobar infiltrate suggests bacterial pneumonia. A presumptive diagnosis of LIP/PLH can be made on the basis of characteristic clinical features and radiographic changes persisting for >2 months in the absence of another explanation. *P. jirovecii* is likely in a child with a low $CD4^+$ lymphocyte count and the acute onset of a diffuse reticular interstitial infiltrate associated with hypoxemia. Marked elevation of the serum lactate dehydrogenase concentration (>1000 IU/L) suggests PCP. Bronchoalveolar lavage is indicated for confirmation of suspected PCP and exclusion of other opportunistic infections in children with advanced HIV disease. If a high index of suspicion exists for tuberculosis in a child with a pulmonary infiltrate and negative results on TST, gastric or bronchoalveolar lavage is warranted. Atypical features of pneumonia may necessitate open-lung biopsy for histology and cultures to evaluate the wide array of diagnostic possibilities.

Empiric antibiotic therapy is indicated for HIV-infected children with characteristic features of bacterial pneumonia. A third-generation cephalosporin is appropriate for children with normal $CD4^+$ lymphocyte counts. The addition of vancomycin for possible methicillin-resistant *S. aureus* (MRSA) with or without an aminoglycoside should be considered for children with severe disease or profoundly depressed $CD4^+$ lymphocyte counts. Caution is warranted regarding repeated courses of ceftriaxone because rapidly fatal immune-mediated hemolysis has been described in HIV-infected children.[46]

Treatment of tuberculosis in HIV-infected children is complex since there are multiple drug interactions between antiretroviral drugs, other prophylactic agents such as the macrolides and azoles, and antimycobacterial drugs.[18] Advice should be obtained from an expert in the treatment of the two diseases. Tuberculosis treatment should be started immediately and the child's antiretroviral therapy altered as necessary. Directly observed therapy is essential. Specific considerations include the importance of rifampin in tuberculosis therapy and its potent induction of the hepatic CYP3A enzyme system that precludes use of all

protease inhibitors. Either rifabutin should be substituted, with appropriate dosage adjustments, or HAART should not include a protease inhibitor.

Central Nervous System Infections

Except for children with advanced HIV disease, the causative agents, clinical manifestations, and CSF findings of meningitis and encephalitis are similar to those observed in immunocompetent hosts. *C. neoformans* and JC virus are two opportunistic pathogens that can cause central nervous system (CNS) infection in HIV-infected children. *C. neoformans* is a common cause of meningitis in patients with advanced HIV disease and severely depressed $CD4^+$ lymphocyte counts. Cryptococcal meningitis often is characterized by an indolent course of illness. Complaints of fever, intermittent headache, and vomiting are common. Signs of meningeal inflammation can be absent. CSF complete cell count, glucose and protein levels can be normal. Important CSF diagnostic studies include India ink stain, cryptococcal antigen testing, and culture.

JC virus is a polyoma virus that causes progressive multifocal leukoencephalopathy (PML) in individuals with advanced immunosuppression. PML is a progressive demyelinating disease of the CNS, characterized by focal neurologic abnormalities (e.g., visual deficits and motor weakness), personality and cognitive changes, confusion, ataxia, and seizures. Neuroimaging reveals focal white-matter lesions without mass effect (Figure 112-3). Most cases of PML occur in individuals with advanced HIV disease. PML was uncommon in HIV-infected children prior to HAART and is now rare.[3,19] The usual clinical course is inexorable deterioration of CNS function, leading to death within a few months of diagnosis. The mainstay of therapy is to optimize ART since an improved immune status can result in clinical improvement. Antiviral agents directed against JC virus including cytosine arabinoside and cidofovir have no demonstrated efficacy.

CNS mass lesions in children with HIV infection pose special diagnostic considerations. Definitive diagnosis may require examination of tissue. Infectious causes include bacterial brain abscess, toxoplasmosis, cryptococcoma, and tuberculoma; noninfectious causes such as lymphoma also should be considered.

Cerebral toxoplasmosis occurs relatively frequently in patients with advanced HIV disease and severely depressed $CD4^+$ lymphocyte counts. Presenting features include fever, headache, seizures, focal neurologic abnormalities, and altered consciousness. Computed tomography or magnetic resonance imaging of the brain typically reveals multiple ring-enhancing lesions with surrounding edema. Toxoplasmosis almost invariably represents reactivated infection in HIV-infected individuals. The usefulness of serologic testing for *Toxoplasma* therefore is limited; patients who are found to be seronegative are unlikely to have cerebral toxoplasmosis. It is useful to document periodically the seronegative status of HIV-infected children. Brain biopsy, the definitive diagnostic procedure, usually is reserved for those patients who fail to respond clinically and radiographically to empiric therapy for toxoplasmosis. In addition to a variety of bacterial and fungal processes, the differential diagnosis of CNS toxoplasmosis includes CNS lymphoma.

Diarrhea

Many episodes of diarrhea in HIV-infected children are acute and self limited, with no apparent long-term effects. Persistent or recurrent diarrhea, however, can adversely affect quality of life and place the child at risk of malnutrition and further immunologic impairment.

Gastroenteritis can be caused by any of the usual pathogens including rotavirus, *Salmonella*, *Shigella*, enterotoxigenic *Escherichia coli*, *Campylobacter*, *Vibrio cholera*, *Clostridium difficile*, *Entamoeba histolytica*, enteric adenoviruses, and *Giardia intestinalis*, irrespective of the child's $CD4^+$ count. Opportunistic pathogens, such as CMV, MAC, *Cryptosporidium*, and *Cystisospora* spp., generally occur with advanced immunosuppression. Thus, the diagnostic

PART II Clinical Syndromes and Cardinal Features of Infectious Diseases: Approach to Diagnosis and Initial Management

SECTION S Human Immunodeficiency Virus and the Acquired Immunodeficiency Syndrome

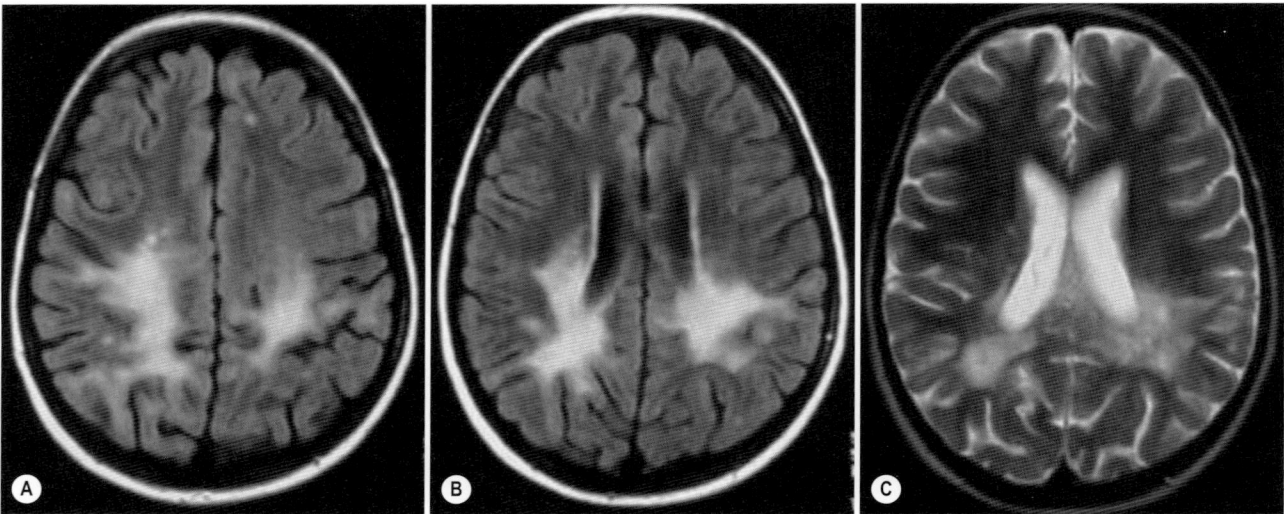

Figure 112-3. A 12-year-old boy, recently immigrated from Zambia, and newly diagnosed with acquired immunodeficiency syndrome (AIDS) had a 2- to 3-year history of severe headache and diarrhea. Magnetic resonance imaging showed predominantly right-sided white-matter lesions. Antimicrobial and highly active antiretroviral therapy (HAART) were begun; 9 weeks after starting HAART, human immunodeficiency virus (HIV) viral load was low but he was subdued, tearful, and had decreased strength and reflexes on the left. Imaging showed progression of previous abnormalities. Cerebrospinal fluid (CSF) was normal; CSF polymerase chain reaction was positive for JC virus. Note fluid-attenuated inversion recovery (FLAIR) **(A, B)** and T_2-weighted **(C)** magnetic resonance images showing increased signal within the periventricular white-matter tracts extending outward to the subcortical areas – involving parietal lobes, both hemispheres, the corpus callosum and brainstem – with no mass effect. (Courtesy of A.R. Feingold and D. Meislich, Cooper University Hospital, Camden, NJ.)

evaluation should be guided by the patient's HIV disease status and clinical presentation.

Many episodes of acute enteritis do not require diagnostic evaluation. However, if gastrointestinal symptoms are severe or persistent, a number of investigations should be considered. Examination of the stool for rotavirus (antigen or nucleic acid test), and ova and parasites (routine and acid-fast staining) for detection of *Cryptosporidium* and *Cystisospora* spp. should be considered. Stool cultures for bacterial enteric pathogens are obtained if the child has fever or stools containing blood or mucus. Blood culture is obtained to exclude *Salmonella* or *Shigella* BSI. Studies for *C. difficile* are performed if there is a history of recent antibiotic use. Documentation of active CMV replication by blood antigenemia, nucleic acid testing, or culture can be helpful. Stool cultures for CMV and MAC generally are not useful.

Upper endoscopy is reserved for the HIV-infected child with persistent diarrhea of unknown cause. Colonoscopy should be considered in patients with dysentery without an identified pathogen. Biopsies are obtained for evaluation of bowel histology and detection of *Giardia*, CMV, *Cryptosporidium*, and MAC.

Management of the HIV-infected child with diarrhea must include close attention to nutritional support. Empiric antibiotic therapy for *Salmonella* spp. should be considered for the child with dysentery and signs of toxicity. Other therapeutic interventions are guided by results of diagnostic studies.

Esophagitis

Esophagitis is common among individuals infected with AIDS. Affected children can have irritability, pain, difficulty swallowing, hiccups, or only fever. Esophagitis can be due to infectious and noninfectious causes. *Candida* species are the most common cause. Children with esophageal candidiasis do not always have concomitant oral candidiasis. Viral causes of esophagitis include CMV and HSV.[47] Esophageal disease caused by bacteria (including mycobacteria) is uncommon. Other causes of esophageal disease in HIV-infected children include lymphoma, acid reflux, and aphthous ulcers.

Empiric antifungal therapy is given when oral candidiasis and typical clinical features of esophagitis are present. Barium esophagography or endoscopy is considered if presentation is atypical or oral thrush is absent or if the patient fails to improve within 5

to 7 days. Radiographic differentiation of various types of esophageal ulcerative disease (e.g., candidiasis versus CMV disease) and recognition of dual infection are impossible. Therefore, if ulcerative or nodular lesions are identified radiographically, esophagoscopy and biopsy should be performed.

Oral Infections

Candidiasis is the most common oral infection of HIV-infected children.[40] Several clinical variants are recognized, including pseudomembranous, hyperplastic, and erythematous candidiasis and angular cheilitis. Although oral candidiasis may respond to oral nystatin or clotrimazole, oral fluconazole is more effective.

Oral ulcers also are common in HIV-infected children. CMV and HSV are common infectious causes. Aphthous ulcers also occur frequently, and are of three basic types: aphthous major (large ulcers persisting >3 weeks), aphthous minor (smaller ulcers that heal spontaneously within 5 to 10 days), and aphthous herpetiformis (multiple, discrete ulcers resembling those caused by HSV). Aphthous major is the most common form observed in HIV-infected individuals; concomitant pharyngeal and esophageal ulcers are present in some cases.

Diagnostic evaluation and management of HIV-infected children with oral ulcers are based on clinical presentation. A surface culture for HSV and empiric therapy with acyclovir may suffice for patients with lesions typical of herpetic stomatitis. Biopsy and cultures for viruses, mycobacteria, and fungi should be considered if initial diagnostic studies are negative, the ulcers are large or deep, or the ulcers fail to heal in an appropriate length of time, with or without empiric therapy.

PROPHYLAXIS AGAINST INFECTION

Separate guidelines for the prevention of opportunistic infections in HIV-infected children and adolescents/adults are published by the U.S. Public Health Service and the Infectious Diseases Society of America[18,48] and are updated regularly at http://aidsinfo.nih.gov/.

Routine Immunization

A modified immunization schedule for HIV-infected children and HIV-exposed infants with undefined HIV-infection status is available and should be consulted.[18] Children immunized prior to HAART generally have poor vaccine responses, associated with both a low CD4$^+$ count and high viral load at the time of immunization. With immune reconstitution following HAART, the response to immunization is much improved although protective immunity can wane over time.[49] Although it is likely that children with immune reconstitution following severe immunosuppression would benefit from reimmunization, data are not available to support specific recommendations. Reimmunization may be considered for children at increased risk of exposure to vaccine-preventable diseases.

The bacterial vaccines (diphtheria, tetanus, pertussis, *H. influenzae* type b, and peneumococcus) should be administered to all HIV-infected children according to the routine childhood schedule.[50,51] HIV-infected children should receive additional pneumococcal immunization according to the following recommendations[18]:

1. Pneumococcal conjugate vaccine (PCV) is recommended for all HIV-infected children <5 years of age. Administering PCV to HIV-infected children ≥5 years of age is not contraindicated.
2. For incompletely vaccinated children aged 24 to 59 months, administer 2 doses of PCV at least 8 weeks apart.
3. HIV-infected children who have received the PCV should receive a dose of the 23-valent pneumococcal polysaccharide (PPSV) vaccine at ≥24 months of age, at least 2 months after the last PCV dose.
4. If not previously vaccinated with PPSV, children and adolescents aged 7 to 18 years should receive 1 dose of PPSV.
5. If previously vaccinated with the PPSV, a single revaccination should be administered 5 years after the first dose.[50]

Beginning at 12 months of age, two doses of the live attenuated measles, mumps, rubella and varicella vaccines should be administered to HIV-infected children who are not severely immunosuppressed.[18] These live viral vaccines should not be administered to HIV-infected children who are severely immunosuppressed (i.e., CDC immunologic category 3; CD4$^+$ lymphocyte percentage <15%) because of the potential for dissemination of the vaccine virus. The quadrivalent measles-mumps-rubella-varicella (MMRV) vaccine should not be administered as a substitute for MMR and V vaccines administered at separate sites in HIV-infected children because immunogenicity and efficacy data for MMRV are lacking. Use of the rotavirus vaccine in HIV-infected children should be considered in accordance with guidelines by age.[18] Inactivated viral vaccines (hepatitis A, hepatitis B, and poliovirus) should be administered to all HIV-infected children according to the routine childhood immunization schedule. Inactivated influenza immunization is recommended annually for all HIV-infected children beginning at 6 months of age. In addition, it is important to immunize family members and other close contacts.

Passive immunization

VZV antibody (see Chapter 205, Varicella-Zoster Virus) should be administered as early as possible after exposure of a susceptible HIV-infected child to an individual with chickenpox or zoster.[18]

The beneficial effects of IGIV emerged from two National Institutes of Health-sponsored multicenter trials of IGIV for children with HIV infection.[32,52] The results of these trials formed the basis for U.S. Food and Drug Administration approval of IGIV for certain HIV-infected children. However, HAART and the widespread use of trimethoprim-sulfamethoxazole (TMP-SMX) prophylaxis has limited the benefits of IGIV. Current guidelines[18] recommend its use in HIV-infected children in the following situations: children with hypogammaglobulinemia (immunoglobulin G <400 mg/dL); or recurrent bacterial infections despite appropriate immunization and antibiotic prophylaxis.

Pneumocystis jirovecii Pneumonia (PCP) Prophylaxis

Identification of children at risk for PCP is complicated by two factors. First, some HIV-infected infants at greatest risk of PCP are

---

BOX 112-2. Classification of HIV Infection Status of Children Born to an HIV-Infected Mother

Definitive infection:
- Positive virologic results on two separate specimens at any age; OR
- Age >18 months and either a positive virologic test or a positive confirmed HIV-antibody test

Presumptive exclusion of infection in a non-breastfed infant:
- No clinical or laboratory evidence of HIV infection AND two negative virologic tests, both obtained at ≥2 weeks of age and one obtained at ≥4 weeks of age and no positive virologic tests; OR
- One negative virologic test at ≥8 weeks of age and no positive virologic test; OR
- One negative HIV antibody test at ≥6 months of age

Definitive exclusion of infection in non-breastfed infant:
- No clinical or laboratory evidence of HIV infection AND two negative virologic tests, both obtained at ≥4 weeks of age and one obtained at ≥4 months of age and no positive virologic tests; OR
- Two or more negative HIV antibody tests at ≥6 months of age

From reference 18.

---

either not known to be at risk for HIV infection (i.e., the mother is not known to be HIV-infected) or are known to be at risk but do not have confirmed infection (i.e., their HIV infection status is indeterminate). Second, because normal CD4$^+$ lymphocyte counts are age-specific, a single CD4$^+$ lymphocyte threshold cannot be used for defining the risk of PCP in all children. Guidelines for primary prophylaxis against PCP published by the CDC take these issues into consideration.[18] All HIV-infected infants should receive prophylaxis until they are 12 months of age, at which time the need for prophylaxis is determined by age-specific CD4$^+$ lymphocyte values. All HIV-infected children ≥12 months of age who meet criteria for CDC immunologic category 3 should receive prophylaxis. Prophylaxis should be considered for all HIV-exposed infants at 4 to 6 weeks of age. Infants with indeterminate infection status should receive prophylaxis until they are determined to be uninfected or presumptively uninfected (see Box 112-2). Prophylaxis is not recommend for children who meet the criteria for being uninfected or presumptively uninfected. Children 12 months of age and older who experience immune reconstitution following HAART can have primary prophylaxis stopped safely if they have received >6 months of HAART and CD4$^+$ cells exceeding CDC immunologic category 3 for >3 consecutive months. Children who have had an episode of PCP should receive secondary prophylaxis to prevent recurrence. Most children can have secondary prophylaxis safely stopped if they meet the criteria for stopping primary prophylaxis.

TMP-SMX is the drug of choice for PCP prophylaxis, given orally at 150 mg/m^2 body surface area of TMP per day (max 320 mg) in 2 divided doses on 3 consecutive days per week.[18] Alternative oral dosing schedules include a single dose on 3 consecutive days per week or 2 divided daily doses. TMP-SMX is also effective in preventing toxoplasmosis and some bacterial infections. Alternative regimens for children who are intolerant of TMP-SMX include oral dapsone, oral atovaquone, and aerosolized pentamidine.[18]

Mycobacterium avium Complex Infection

Clinical trials have demonstrated the effectiveness of clarithromycin and azithromycin as primary prophylaxis against MAC infection.[53,54] Although rifabutin also is effective for the prevention of

PART II   Clinical Syndromes and Cardinal Features of Infectious Diseases: Approach to Diagnosis and Initial Management

SECTION S   Human Immunodeficiency Virus and the Acquired Immunodeficiency Syndrome

MAC infection, it should be used as an alternative agent for patients who are unable to tolerate macrolide therapy. Current guidelines recommend that HIV-infected adults and adolescents receive prophylaxis if CD4$^+$ lymphocyte count is <50 cells/mm^3. Recommendations for starting MAC prophylaxis in children are based on the child's age and CD4$^+$ lymphocyte count: ≥6 years of age, <50 cells/mm^3; 2 to 6 years of age, <75 cells/mm^3; 1 to 2 years of age, <500 cells/mm^3; and <12 months, <750 cells/mm^3. Pediatric doses are clarithromycin, 7.5 mg/kg/dose (max 500 mg) orally twice a day; or azithromycin, 20 mg/kg/dose (max 1200 mg) orally once weekly.

Fungal Infections

Several trials of prophylaxis against *Candida* infections in adults using daily or weekly fluconazole indicate that clinical relapses can be prevented. Emergence of resistance to fluconazole, particularly among species of *Candida* other than *C. albicans,* is of concern.[55,56] Primary prophylaxis of candidiasis in HIV-infected infants and children is not recommended.[18] For children with infrequent recurrences, it is reasonable to treat each individual clinical episode. Children with frequent recurrences or a history

of esophageal candidiasis are candidates for prophylaxis with oral nystatin, clotrimazole, or fluconazole.

Specific circumstances dictate the use of antifungal agents for prophylaxis of systemic noncandidal fungal infections in HIV-infected patients.[18] Prospective controlled trials indicate that fluconazole and itraconazole are effective in the prevention of cryptococcosis in adults with advanced HIV disease (CD4$^+$ lymphocyte count <50 cells/mm^3).[48]

PROGNOSIS

Certain opportunistic and nonopportunistic infections can be important clinical indicators of HIV disease progression, immunologic deterioration, and early death. PCP, especially when it occurs during the first year of life, appears to portend a poor prognosis for long-term survival.[57,58] In one study, children with recurrent bacterial infections or LIP/PLH had at least a 4-fold longer survival time than those with PCP, disseminated MAC disease, CMV infection, tumors, or PML.[57] Pediatric HAART is associated with a marked reduction in rates of progression to AIDS, opportunistic infections, and hospitalizations, as well as improved survival.[1,59]

113   Management of HIV Infection

George Kelly Siberry and Rohan Hazra

The treatment and prognosis of pediatric HIV infection have changed dramatically since the start of the epidemic in the 1980s. The Department of Health and Human Services (DHHS) Panel on Antiretroviral Therapy and Medical Management of HIV-Infected Children has developed guidelines for the use of antiretroviral agents in pediatric HIV infection.[1] These guidelines are updated regularly to ensure that recommendations are based on the most recent evidence. Similarly, specialists in pediatric HIV infection periodically update guidelines for the prevention and treatment of opportunistic infections (OIs) in HIV-infected and HIV-exposed, uninfected children.[2] This chapter emphasizes the predominantly outpatient care-based approach to use of highly active antiretroviral therapy (HAART).

ANTIRETROVIRAL THERAPY

Therapeutic Agents

As of 2011, 23 different antiretroviral drugs are available for use in HIV-infected adults and adolescents; 17 have an approved pediatric treatment indication, and 15 are available as a pediatric formulation or capsule size (Table 113-1). These agents prevent viral entry (CCR5 antagonist and fusion inhibitor), block the early stage of viral replication (the nucleoside/nucleotide analogue reverse transcriptase inhibitors (NRTIs/NtRTIs) and nonnucleoside reverse transcriptase inhibitors (NNRTIs)), inhibit integration of the viral genome (integrase inhibitor), and interfere with the cleavage of HIV proteins by the viral protease (protease inhibitors (PIs)) (Figure 113-1).

Nucleoside and Nucleotide Analogue Reverse Transcriptase Inhibitors

The NRTIs were the first class of antiretroviral drugs available for the treatment of HIV infection. The NRTIs inhibit the HIV reverse transcriptase enzyme, responsible for the reverse transcription of

viral RNA into DNA. Like the NRTIs, the NtRTI tenofovir competitively inhibits viral reverse transcriptase, but because it already possesses a phosphate molecule, it bypasses the initial phosphorylation step required for activation of NRTIs.

NRTIs are the backbone of HAART. In general two of these agents are used with a PI or NNRTI as first-line therapy. Fixed-dose combinations of NRTIs/NtRTIs simplify dosing. With subsequent regimens, one or more of the NRTIs used in an earlier regimen often will be used again to take advantage of a favorable resistance profile.[3,4]

NRTIs/NtRTIs inhibit mitochondrial DNA (mtDNA) synthesis, leading to depletion of mtDNA and impaired mitochondrial function. This effect contributes to the toxicities associated with NRTIs/NtRTIs, such as peripheral neuropathy, pancreatitis, and myopathy. Unusual, but serious, toxicities that can occur with use of NRTIs/NtRTIs include lactic acidosis, hepatic steatosis, cardiomyopathy, and rapidly ascending muscular weakness. The order of potency of the NRTIs/NtRTIs in inhibiting mtDNA synthesis in vitro is didanosine (ddI) > stavudine (d4T) > zidovudine (ZDV) > lamivudine (3TC), abacavir (ABC), and tenofovir disoproxil fumarate (TDF).[5] Didanosine and stavudine are not used as first-line agents because of these toxicities. TDF appears to cause fewer mitochondrial toxicities but concerns about its deleterious effects on bone and kidneys limit use in children.

Non-Nucleoside Analogue Reverse Transcriptase Inhibitors

The NNRTIs have specific activity against HIV-1, but not HIV-2 or other retroviruses. They noncompetitively bind to and disrupt the catalytic site of reverse transcriptase.[6] Because drug resistance to NNRTIs requires a single mutation that does not appear to impact viral fitness, resistance can develop rapidly after initiation of NNRTI as part of a nonsuppressive regimen. Cross-resistance readily occurs between the NNRTIs efavirenz (EFV), nevirapine (NVP) and rilpivirine (RPV); cross-resistance is less common with

TABLE 113-1. Antiretroviral Drug Formulations and Pediatric Approval Status (as of September 2010)

Name (Abbreviation)	Formulations	Pediatric Approval
Nucleoside (NRTIs) and nucleotide (NtRTI) reverse transcriptase inhibitors		
Abacavir (ABC)	Solution, tablets	>3 months of age
Didanosine (ddI)	Powder for solution, capsules	>2 weeks of age
Emtricitabine (FTC)	Solution, capsules, FDCs	All ages
Lamivudine (3TC)	Solution, tablets, FDCs	All ages
Stavudine (d4T)	Solution, capsules	All ages
Tenofovir disoproxil fumarate (TDF)	Tablet, FDCs	>12 years of age and >35 kg
Zidovudine (ZDV)	Syrup, capsules, tablets, FDCs	All ages, including premature infants
Non-nucleoside reverse transcriptase inhibitors (NNRTIs)		
Efavirenz (EFV)	Capsules, tablets, FDC	> 3 years of age
Etravirine (ETR)	Tablets	No
Nevirapine (NVP)	Suspension, tablets	>15 days of age[a]
Rilpivirine (RPV)	Tablet, FDC	No
Protease inhibitors (PIs)		
Atazanavir (ATV)	Capsules	>6 years of age
Darunavir (DRV)	Tablets	>6 years of age
Fosamprenavir (FPV)	Suspension, tablets	>2 years of age
Indinavir (IDV)	Capsules	No
Lopinavir/ritonavir (LPV/r)	Solution, tablets	>14 days of age
Nelfinavir (NFV)	Powder for suspension, tablets	>2 years of age
Ritonavir (RTV)	Solution, capsules, tablets	>1 month of age[b]
Saquinavir (SQV)	Capsules, tablets	No
Tipranavir (TPV)	Solution, capsules	>2 years of age
Entry inhibitors		
Enfuvirtide (T-20)	Injection	>6 years of age
Maraviroc (MVC)	Tablets	No
Integrase inhibitors		
Raltegravir (RAL)	Tablets	No

FDC, fixed dose combinations.

[a]Approved for <14 days for use in prophylaxis against maternal–child transmission.

[b]RTV as part of LPV/r is approved for those >14 days of age.

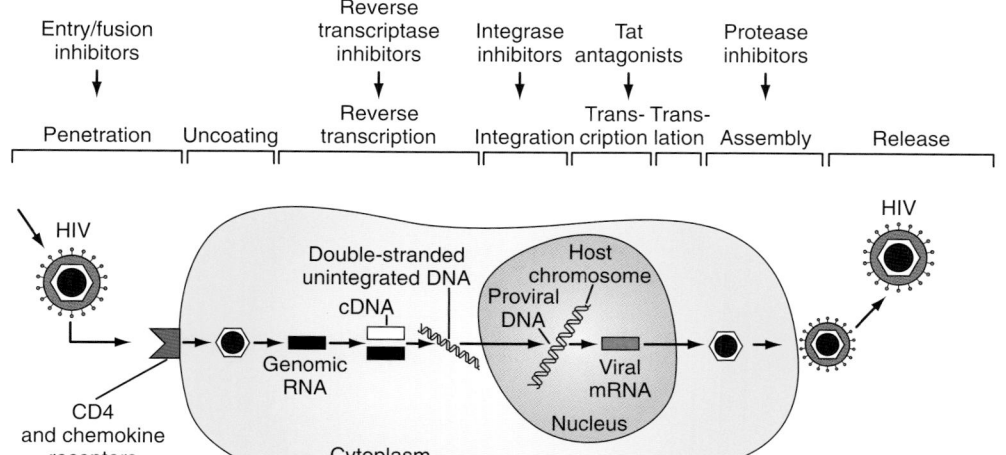

Figure 113-1. Human immunodeficiency virus (HIV) life cycle and location of action of various antiretroviral medications.

PART II Clinical Syndromes and Cardinal Features of Infectious Diseases: Approach to Diagnosis and Initial Management

SECTION S Human Immunodeficiency Virus and the Acquired Immunodeficiency Syndrome

etravirine (ETR). NNRTI-based HAART regimens are at least as effective as PI-based regimens in achieving durable viral suppression. In addition, NNRTIs appear to be associated with less long-term toxicity than PIs.[1]

NNRTIs are associated with several types of hepatic toxicity, including asymptomatic elevation in transaminases, clinical hepatitis, and hypersensitivity reactions with hepatitis. In HIV-infected adults, risk factors for NVP hepatic toxicity include elevated baseline serum transaminases, hepatitis B or C infection, female gender, and higher CD4+ lymphocyte counts. However, in contrast to what has been reported in adults, serious liver dysfunction appears much less common in children receiving NVP.[7]

Hypersensitivity reactions are reported more commonly with NNRTIs (especially NVP) than with other antiretroviral agents. EFV central nervous system (CNS) effects include confusion, hallucinations, and nightmares. EFV is classified as Food and Drug Administration (FDA) Pregnancy Class D (positive evidence of human fetal risk). Use of EFV in the first trimester of pregnancy should be avoided. ETR is not currently approved for use in children.

Protease Inhibitors

PIs inhibit the HIV protease enzyme, which is required to cleave viral polyprotein precursors and generate functional viral proteins. The protease enzyme is crucial for viral assembly.

PIs have potent antiretroviral effect, especially when used in combination with NRTIs and/or NNRTIs. Because resistance to PIs requires multiple mutations, some of which reduce viral fitness, PI resistance generally develops slowly. However, the PIs are associated with more toxicity than the NNRTIs, such as fat redistribution, lipodystrophy syndrome, hyperlipidemia, diabetes mellitus, and hyperglycemia. Most PIs require coadministration with a nontherapeutic dose of ritonavir (RTV) that inhibits CYP3A4 and increases the concentrations of other PIs. RTV is used almost exclusively in this pharmacokinetic "booster" role and seldom in therapeutic doses. The most commonly used PI in children is a co-formulation of lopinavir (LPV) and RTV. Other PIs boosted with RTV include: atazanavir (ATV), darunavir (DRV), fosamprenavir (FPV), and tipranavir (TPV).[1] All PIs are metabolized by and/or inhibit enzymes in the cytochrome P450 system; attention to potential drug–drug interactions is required.

Entry and Fusion Inhibitors

HIV enters target cells via a multistep process. First, HIV binds to the CD4 receptor, leading to conformational changes in the viral gp120 envelope protein that enable binding to chemokine co-receptors for HIV. Chemokine receptor engagement triggers conformational changes in the HIV gp41 envelope protein, leading to fusion of HIV and the target cell, resulting in delivery to the viral core.

Enfuvirtide (T-20) is the only FDA-approved fusion inhibitor; it requires twice daily subcutaneous injections. Maraviroc (MVC) binds to and alters the structure of the CCR5 chemokine receptor, preventing it from being used as a coreceptor by HIV. Since some strains of HIV also can infect cells by using the CXCR4 chemokine receptor molecule as a coreceptor, MVC is ineffective in individuals who harbor CXCR4 tropic or dual tropic (using both CCR5 and CXCR4) virus.

Integrase Inhibitors

Raltegravir (RAL) is the only available antiretroviral that acts by inhibiting the viral integrase-mediated integration of the viral genome into the host cell genome.

Indications for Initiation of Antiretroviral Therapy

The high mortality seen in HIV-infected infants under 12 months of age and the relatively poor ability of CD4 count and other factors to predict which infants will have rapid disease progression have led to a longstanding recommendation in the U.S. that all infected infants start HAART as soon as they are identified.[1] However, in resource-limited settings, adoption of this recommendation in the absence of clinical trial data was slow, given the resources necessary to treat all infected infants and concerns about toxicity related to such early initiation of therapy. The CHER trial provided clear evidence of the benefit to initiation of HAART in any infant below 12 months of age regardless of CD4+ lymphocyte count.[8] In this study, infected infants (6 to 12 weeks old) with CD4 percentage >25% were randomized either to initiate HAART or to delay until meeting defined criteria. The fourfold higher mortality rate in the delayed initiation arm led the World Health Organization (WHO) to recommend therapy for all infants. The increased mortality and poor predictive capacity of CD4 counts in those 1 to 2 years of age also led the WHO to recommend therapy in all 1- to 2-year-old children, though supporting clinical trial evidence is lacking.[9]

Unfortunately, limited virologic testing capabilities in many countries hinder timely diagnosis of perinatally infected children. Delayed presentation of children with HIV infection still occurs in the U.S., usually because of unrecognized perinatal HIV exposure.[10] In such cases, initiation of therapy is based upon clinical and immunologic criteria. Table 113-2 summarizes recommendations for initiating HAART.

TABLE 113-2. United States (U.S.) and World Health Organization (WHO) Recommendations for Criteria to Initiate HAART in HIV-infected Infants and Children

Age	U.S. Guidelines[1]	WHO Guidelines[10]
<12 months	Treat regardless of clinical symptoms, immune status, or viral load	Treat regardless of clinical symptoms or immune status
1 to <2 years	Treat if AIDS/CDC B[a] or C; CD4+ lymphocytes <25%; *OR* asymptomatic/mild symptoms, CD4+ lymphocytes >25% and VL >100,000 copies/mL. Consider if asymptomatic/mild symptoms, CD4+ lymphocytes >25% and VL <100,000 copies/mL	Treat regardless of clinical symptoms or immune status
2 to <5 years	Treat if AIDS/CDC B[a] or C; CD4+ lymphocytes <25%; *OR* asymptomatic/mild symptoms, CD4+ lymphocytes >25% and VL >100,000 copies/mL. Consider if asymptomatic/mild symptoms, CD4+ lymphocytes >25% and VL <100,000 copies/mL	Treat if CD4+ lymphocytes ≤750 cells/mm³; CD4+ lymphocytes ≤25%; *OR* WHO clinical stages 3 and 4, irrespective of CD4+ lymphocyte count
≥5 years	Treat if AIDS/CDC B[a] or C; CD4+ lymphocytes <500 cells/mm³; *OR* asymptomatic/mild symptoms, CD4+ lymphocytes >500 cells/mm³ and VL >100,000 copies/mL. Consider if asymptomatic/mild symptoms, CD4+ lymphocytes >500 cells/mm³ and VL <100,000 copies/mL	Treat if CD4+ lymphocytes ≤350 cells/mm³; *OR* WHO clinical stages 3 and 4, irrespective of CD4+ lymphocyte count

VL, viral load.

[a]Except for the following CDC category B conditions: single episode of serious bacterial infection or lymphoid interstitial pneumonitis (LIP).

Given the need to start multiple agents, comorbid conditions such as tuberculosis (TB) that require treatment with other medications that may interact with the ARVs, and many other complicating factors in the lives of families affected by HIV, treatment should not begin without intensive counseling and support. Families should be educated about the medications and the critical importance of adherence, and such counseling and support should continue at every visit.

Selection of ARV Drugs for Initial HAART Regimen

Guidelines for the treatment of pediatric HIV are published and updated regularly.[1,9] Initial therapy with three antiretroviral agents, usually consisting of two NRTIs and either a PI or NNRTI, is recommended. For infants who had perinatal exposure to nevirapine for failed prevention of maternal-to-children HIV transmission (PMTCT) as well as for infants who had no perinatal nevirapine exposure, the P1060 trial demonstrated that lopinavir/ritonavir-based HAART is superior to NVP-based HAART;[11,12] however, PENPACT-1 did not demonstrate an advantage of PI-based over NNRTI-based HAART in children without perinatal NVP exposure.[13] Factors to consider when deciding upon an initial HAART regimen for an infant or child include:[1]

- availability of appropriate (and palatable) drug formulations and pharmacokinetic information for the child's age group
- potency, dosing frequency, food and fluid requirements, and potential short- and long-term adverse effects of the antiretroviral regimen
- effect of initial regimen on later options
- presence of comorbidity, such as tuberculosis, hepatitis B or C virus infection, or chronic renal or liver disease

- potential antiretroviral drug interactions with other prescribed, over-the-counter, or complementary/alternative medications
- the ability of the caregiver and child to adhere to the regimen; and
- avoidance of efavirenz in adolescent females who may become pregnant.

CLINICAL AND LABORATORY MONITORING

Table 113-3 displays the schedule of clinical and laboratory evaluations for pediatric HIV management, based on HAART status.[1,14]

Once HIV infection has been diagnosed, it is important to stage disease, evaluate for coinfections and complications, assess need for opportunistic infection prevention, provide elements of routine primary health care, and address psychosocial needs. It is important to assess knowledge, attitudes, and potential barriers for taking antiretrovirals. Adherence counseling begins with readiness assessments prior to HAART initiation and monitoring at every clinical encounter once HAART has been prescribed. Clinical evaluations are recommended approximately every 3 months for HIV-infected children who have not yet met indications to initiate HAART.

Visit frequency, assessment, and counseling are intensified at the time HAART is initiated, allowing the provider to identify and intervene early in problems with adherence or adverse effects. Some patients require counseling every 1 to 2 weeks for several weeks to work through adherence and medication intolerance problems. By 4 weeks after initiation, a clinic visit should occur to allow for physical examination and laboratory testing for monitoring toxicity (Table 113-3). Additional monitoring may be indicated based on individual antiretroviral toxicity profiles. HIV viral

TABLE 113-3. Routine Monitoring Schedule for Management of Children with HIV-Infection

HAART Treatment Status	Visit Interval	Monitoring Treatment Efficacy and Adherence[a]	Toxicity Monitoring, Other Care and Monitoring[a,b]
Initial visit	N/A	Assess attitudes and readiness for potential HAART	History: complete clinical history, including pregnancy/delivery, opportunistic infections (OIs) and other HIV-related illnesses, ARV exposure/treatment, immunization record, comprehensive medical and family history
		HIV viral load	Psychosocial assessment; status of HIV disclosure to child and other family/contact
		CD4+ lymphocyte count/ percentage	Disclosure counseling; guardianship, permanency planning
			Complete physical examination
		HIV drug resistance genotype	Growth/nutritional assessment; pubertal and neurodevelopmental/educational assessment
			General laboratory: complete blood count and differential; chemistry panel (liver function, renal function, electrolytes, calcium, phosphate, amylase, lipase); lipid panel;[d] urinalysis (dipstick and microscopic); G6PD-deficiency screening; 25-OH vitamin D[e] level
			HBsAg, HBsAb, HBcAb; age-appropriate hepatitis C testing; Toxoplasma IgG, Varicella IgG
			TB assessment: exposure, symptoms, STS
			Sexually transmitted infection (STI) testing (syphilis, chlamydia, gonorrhea) based on maternal history (for infants); STI testing including cervical/anal Pap for sexually active youth; reproductive planning/risk reduction counseling for youth
Pre-HAART	3 months Shorter for infants or CD4+ lymphocyte values close to initiation threshold	Assess attitudes and readiness for potential HAART	History: interim clinical history
			Complete physical examination
		HIV viral load	General laboratory: complete blood count and differential; chemistry panel (liver function, renal function, electrolytes, calcium, phosphate)
		CD4+ lymphocyte count/ percentage	Immunization and OI prophylaxis assessment
			6–12 months:
			Growth/nutritional assessment; pubertal and neurodevelopmental/educational assessment
			Update of family and psychosocial history
			Disclosure counseling
			Amylase, lipase; urinalysis; lipid panel[d]
			HBsAb (annually); hepatitis C antibody testing (if at ongoing risk)
			TB assessment (annually)
			STI testing including cervical/anal Pap for sexually active youth; reproductive planning/risk reduction counseling for youth

Continued

PART II Clinical Syndromes and Cardinal Features of Infectious Diseases: Approach to Diagnosis and Initial Management

SECTION S Human Immunodeficiency Virus and the Acquired Immunodeficiency Syndrome

TABLE 113-3. Routine Monitoring Schedule for Management of Children with HIV-Infection—cont'd

HAART Treatment Status	Visit Interval	Monitoring Treatment Efficacy and Adherence[a]	Toxicity Monitoring, Other Care and Monitoring[a,b]
HAART initiation	1–2 weeks (in person or by phone), usually for at least initial 4 weeks	Adherence counseling and assessment Reinforce medication instructions Viral load (optional)	Adverse effects history Targeted physical examination Additional problem-based evaluations Interim clinical and psychosocial history
Early HAART	4–8 weeks	Adherence counseling and assessment Reinforce medication instructions Viral load CD4+ lymphocyte count (optional)	Adverse effects history Targeted physical examination Complete blood count with differential Chemistry panel (liver function, renal function, electrolytes) Additional problem-based evaluations Interim clinical and psychosocial history Intensive, interdisciplinary psychosocial support
Stable HAART	3 months	Adherence counseling and assessment Reinforce medication instructions Adjust ARV dosing for growth Consider ARV changes for convenience or tolerability, especially as child learns to swallow pills Viral load HIV viral load CD4 lymphocyte count/ percentage	Interim clinical history, including targeted history of drug adverse effects Targeted physical examination Additional problem-based evaluations Complete blood count and differential Chemistry panel (liver function, renal function, electrolytes, calcium) Drug specific toxicity monitoring[c] (e.g., phosphate for TDF; amylase, lipase for ddI) Interim psychosocial history Immunization and OI prophylaxis assessment **6–12 months:** Complete interim history and physical exam Growth/Nutrition assessment, pubertal and neurodevelopmental/educational assessment Update family and psychosocial history Disclosure counseling HBsAb (annually) Hepatitis C antibody testing (if at ongoing risk) TB assessment (yearly): history, STS STI testing including cervical/anal Pap for sexually active youth Reproductive planning/risk reduction counseling for youth. Optional/Selected patients: 25-OH vitamin D level;[e] bone mineral density assessment (by DXA[5])
Suspected treatment failure	24 weeks (in person and/or by phone)	Adherence counseling and assessment Reinforce medication instructions Confirm drug dosing, food and fasting requirements, interacting drugs Viral load HIV drug resistance genotype; also phenotype, if multidrug resistant (once at failure, ≥8–12 weeks if persistent failure and ready to start new HAART regimen)	Interim clinical history, including targeted history of drug adverse effects Targeted physical examination Complete blood count and differential Chemistry panel (liver function, renal function, electrolytes, calcium) Additional problem-based evaluations Interim clinical and psychosocial history Intensive, interdisciplinary psychosocial support

HB, hepatitis B; TB, tuberculosis; STS, skin test for tuberculosis.

[a]*Monitoring elements at each visit interval unless otherwise specified.* [b]*No toxicity monitoring before on HAART.* [c]*Individual ARV agent toxicitie and monitoring is covered elsewhere.* [d]*If lipid panel results abnormal on nonfasting specimen, obtain at least one fasting lipid panel per year.* [e]*Criteria for vitamin D and dual-energy X-ray absorptiometry (DXA) screening not well established.*

Adapted from DHHS Guidelines for the Use of Antiretroviral Agents in Pediatric HIV Infection.[1]

load should confirm the expected response to HAART. Clinical assessments should continue every 4 to 8 weeks or at shorter intervals if there are problems with adherence, intolerance, laboratory abnormalities, or lack of virologic response. In an uncomplicated case, encounters occur at 1 to 2 weeks, 4 weeks and then 12 weeks (or 3 months) after initiation. Successful HAART is expected to reduce viral load by at least one log from baseline at 8 to 12 weeks, attain viral load <400 copies/mL by 6 months, and reach undetectable viral load by ultrasensitive assays (e.g., <50 copies/mL) by 12 months.[1] Children whose pretreatment viral load is extremely high (>10[6] copies/mL) may take longer to achieve viral load suppression, but they should demonstrate nonetheless a one-log drop in viral load by 12 weeks and a consistent pattern of declining viral load measurements thereafter. For children who begin HAART with CD4+ lymphocyte >25% (or CD4 counts >500/mm³, for children at least 5 years old), successful HAART will result in maintaining those levels. For infants and children whose CD4+ lymphocyte percentages or counts are already depressed, successful HAART should generally result in gains of at least 5% or at least 50 cells/mm³ by the end of the first year of therapy.[1]

Once patients have a documented response to therapy on stable HAART, routine monitoring visits take place approximately every 3 months with the goals of assessing adherence; documenting ongoing treatment success (by viral load and CD4+ lymphocyte count/percentage); evaluating for toxicity; and ensuring that other aspects of comprehensive care are provided.

Illnesses in the initial 3 to 6 months of treatment do not always represent treatment failure, especially in the context of good virologic response; such illnesses may be the result of incomplete reversal of baseline immunosuppression or an immune-reconstitution inflammatory syndrome (IRIS) that occurs as an exaggerated or unmasked response to an infection in the context of an imbalanced, recovering immune system.[15] Mycobacterial infections, toxoplasmosis, cryptococcosis, and varicella zoster account for most IRIS events; in lower-resource settings, tuberculosis and bacille Calmette-Guérin (BCG) disease are especially common. Noninfectious IRIS syndromes, such as sarcoidosis and inflammatory response to Kaposi sarcoma, can occur. In addition to management of underlying infection or condition, IRIS may require treatment with nonsteroidal anti-inflammatory agents, and, when more severe, with systemic corticosteroids. HAART rarely is withheld and only in the most severe cases. Mortality is most often related to complications of CNS IRIS syndromes.

Treatment failure can manifest as lack of virologic suppression, decline or inadequate increase in CD4+ lymphocyte count/percentage, or new HIV-related clinical illness. The most common presentation of treatment failure is lack or loss of virologic suppression; the most common underlying reason is medication nonadherence. Drug resistance can be a primary cause of treatment failure or can emerge during periods of poor virologic control attributable to nonadherence. Any instance of deviation from expected viral load results merits prompt, reassessment. Isolated episodes of low-level viremia (<1000 copies/mL), or "blips", usually do not represent virologic failure.[16] However, repeated detection of even low-level viremia may signify failure.[16] If virologic failure is confirmed, assessment and counseling visits should: emphasize adherence improvement, evaluate for drug resistance with HIV genotypic testing, confirm ARV dosing and food and fasting requirements for individual ARVs, and exclude use of other drugs that interfere with ARV absorption, metabolism, or action (e.g., proton-pump inhibitors reduce atazanavir absorption). Switching to a new HAART regimen should only be undertaken once these issues – especially adherence – have been addressed.

INFECTION PREVENTION: IMMUNIZATIONS AND CHEMOPROPHYLAXIS

Chapter 112 (Infectious Complications of HIV Infection) provides a detailed discussion of management and prevention of infectious disease complications of HIV infection, and specific guidelines are published and updated periodically.[2] Indications for OI chemoprophylaxis and eligibility for vaccines should be reviewed at every clinical evaluation.

All HIV-infected infants require *Pneumocystis* pneumonia (PCP) prophylaxis, regardless of clinical, immunologic, or treatment status. Thereafter, indications for OI chemoprophylaxis should be based on CD4+ lymphocyte count and percentage obtained at the prior visit, interpreted according to normative values by age. Declines in CD4 values, resulting in new need for OI chemoprophylaxis, are most likely to occur in children who are not yet receiving HAART or who have not responded to HAART.

Primarily based on data from adults, primary and secondary OI chemoprophylaxis for PCP and for toxoplasmosis likely can be safely discontinued in children over one year old on stable HAART

with immune reconstitution.[2] Assessment at each HIV monitoring visit for the need to restart prophylaxis is important.

Specific recommendations for routine immunization have been developed for HIV-infected children,[2] because the safety, immunogenicity, efficacy, and protective durability of vaccines may be different in HIV-infected children than in otherwise healthy children.[17-19] These differences vary by specific vaccine as well as by demographic and clinical characteristics of vaccine recipients, including use of HAART and degree of immunosuppression.

The increase in HIV viral load and decline in CD4+ lymphocytes that can follow immunization are transient and without clinical consequences. Although increased mortality was reported after pneumococcal polysaccharide vaccine compared with placebo in a trial of HIV-infected African adults who were not receiving antiretroviral therapy,[20] there is no evidence of increased toxicity with use of pneumococcal or other non-live vaccines in adults receiving HAART or in HIV-infected children.[17-19] Thus, non-live vaccines generally are regarded as safe for use in HIV-infected children. Because severe and even fatal illnesses have occurred in severely immunocompromised HIV-infected children after receiving live virus vaccines, measles, mumps, rubella, and varicella vaccines are not recommended for HIV-infected children with severe immunosuppression but are used in those without severe immunosuppression. Increasing evidence suggests that rotavirus vaccines can be used safely in HIV-infected infants[21] and that cold-adapted live-attenuated intranasal influenza vaccine can be used safely in HIV-infected children.[22] BCG vaccine should not be given to infants with known HIV infection or to those with perinatal HIV exposure accompanied by symptoms suspicious for HIV infection. However, BCG vaccine can be given to infants who are asymptomatic, including those of undetermined HIV status born to HIV-infected mothers, in countries with high TB burden and established neonatal BCG vaccination programs.[23]

HIV-infected children demonstrate blunted humoral responses compared with uninfected children. Impaired response is particularly common with advanced HIV disease, lower CD4+ lymphocyte values, higher viral loads, and lack of HAART.[17,19] With effective HAART most HIV-infected children respond better to immunizations than their sicker predecessors, although still not as well as uninfected children. Potential strategies that have been explored to optimize protection of HIV-infected children include additional vaccine doses in primary series, higher-titer vaccine doses, more frequent booster doses, post-immunization confirmation of serologic response, and reimmunization after immune reconstitution. The majority of children who initiate HAART beyond infancy lack immunity related to vaccines they received prior to HAART.[24,25] Routine reimmunization may be indicated for such children, but further evidence is needed to confirm this recommendation.[24]

GROWTH AND NUTRITION

With effective HAART, HIV-infected U.S. children rarely suffer the AIDS-defining growth failure and severe malnutrition that were typical in the pre-HAART era. These manifestations now are restricted largely to those patients who are failing HAART and portend a poor prognosis. High-calorie supplementation orally or by gastrostomy tube and use of appetite stimulants can be used as adjunctive, supportive therapy, but the most important intervention is institution of effective HAART. While effective HAART routinely improves weight gain and linear growth, final height may not be attained, especially in children already stunted when HAART is begun.[26]

Growth failure that occurs in the setting of successful HAART merits a comprehensive evaluation, including for causes unrelated to HIV infection. There are no established associations of specific ARV agents and growth failure, but alterations in body appearance and fat distribution and metabolic derangements in HAART-treated children are common. Body mass index (BMI) should be monitored routinely and overweight children should be given nutrition and exercise counseling.

Evidence of delayed puberty in HIV-infected children is limited largely to the pre-HAART era. More recent data suggest that pubertal delay among children receiving HAART is uncommon and largely is confined to those with poor response to HAART.[27]

Vitamin D deficiency is common in HIV-infected children; ensuring vitamin D sufficiency and adequate intake of calcium should be emphasized.

DISCLOSURE

Developmentally appropriate disclosure of HIV infection status to children is strongly recommended.[28,29] Informing and educating a child about his or her HIV infection takes place in stages, often over years, beginning with general information about reasons for taking medicine and having an infection. Discussing HIV by name with the child requires the child to have an intellectual ability to understand the information and a capacity to understand the principle of keeping medical information private, usually at 8 to 10 years of age. A multidisciplinary team should provide ongoing counseling to parents and other caregivers about the purpose and process of disclosure; some parents prefer to have disclosure discussions with their children at home and others prefer to have staff present to participate in or even lead the disclosure discussions. Delaying disclosure until older ages increases the risk of inadvertent or unplanned disclosure and poor outcomes. Awareness of HIV status prior to onset of sexual activity is especially important for prevention of secondary transmission.

NEUROLOGIC FUNCTION

HIV infection commonly affects both the central and peripheral nervous systems. In the pre-HAART era, the impact of infection of the CNS was devastating in infants and children, with up to 50% of infected infants developing encephalopathy with substantial morbidity and mortality. Pathology included focal cerebral mass lesions, myelopathies, myopathies, seizures, cerebral vascular accidents, and peripheral neuropathies. With the advent of HAART, encephalopathy has almost disappeared.[30,31] However, with perinatally infected youth beginning to survive into young adulthood an emerging concern is more subtle CNS problems, such as cognitive deficits, problems with attention, and psychiatric disorders.[32,33] The etiology of these problems is not completely understood and likely is multifactorial. Potential causes include ongoing CNS infection or ongoing damage secondary to the initial CNS infection,[34] inflammatory changes,[35] ARV toxicities,[36] HIV- and ARV-related metabolic derangements, other exposures (e.g., in utero or current substance use), and social and demographic influences.

Many of the NRTIs can exacerbate or trigger peripheral neuropathy, though peripheral neuropathy can occur in HIV-infected children who are not being treated with ARVs. Efavirenz can cause impaired concentration, sleep disturbances, anxiety, vivid dreams, nightmares, and even psychosis. In most patients these symptoms are self-limited or manageable with nighttime administration of efavirenz, but efavirenz probably should not be used in children with psychiatric disorders.

CARDIOVASCULAR HEALTH

Cardiomyopathy caused by antiretroviral drugs (especially zidovudine) and HIV was a major cause of morbidity and mortality in the pre-HAART era.[37] In the HAART era, the proportion of deaths due to cardiomyopathy has remained relatively stable but the absolute number of cases has declined along with dramatic decreases in overall mortality.[38] An emerging concern, though, is the long-term effect of dyslipidemia and other metabolic derangements in children with well-controlled HIV disease. HIV itself is known to cause dyslipidemia, marked primarily by low high-density lipoprotein. A substantial proportion of perinatally infected children, especially those treated with NRTIs and PIs, have dyslipidemia (elevated cholesterol, triglycerides, or both), other metabolic derangements such as insulin resistance, and fat redistribution (with an overall appearance of peripheral wasting and central obesity that is associated with increased risk of cardiovascular disease).[39] Appropriate prevention and management

include standard recommendations about diet and exercise. The role of statins and other pharmacologic therapies that have been recommended in other high-risk pediatric groups[40] have not been evaluated fully. Substitution of lipodystrophy-promoting ARVs with ARVs associated with less lipid and metabolic derangement (e.g., unboosted fosamprenavir in place of coformulated lopinavir/ ritonavir) may be considered.

Another potential cardiac complication of the specific PIs atazanavir, lopinavir (coformulated with ritonavir), saquinavir, and ritonavir is prolongation of the PR interval and other conduction problems. Caution should be exercised when using these agents in patients known to have pre-existing conduction problems or in those receiving other drugs that also are associated with conduction problems.

HEPATIC FUNCTION

All perinatally HIV-infected children should be evaluated for hepatitis B virus (HBV) and hepatitis C virus (HCV) infections. The rate of HCV maternal–infant transmission is estimated to be 4% for HIV-uninfected women but rises to about 20% in HIV/HCV coinfected women.[41] It is not clear if the rate of HBV maternal–infant transmission is different if the mother also is HIV-infected. Infants of HBV/HIV coinfected women should receive the same HBV preventive management as infants of HBV monoinfected women. HBV surface antigen and HCV antibody testing also should be performed in older HIV-infected children in whom maternal information is lacking.

Several antiretroviral agents, including lamivudine, emtricitabine and tenofovir, have activity against HBV. For this reason, lamivudine or emtricitabine is routinely included in HAART regimens for HBV/HIV coinfected children. TDF also is used for coinfected older children; its use in younger children is limited by potential adverse effects.[1] Once HBV-active drugs are initiated, caution is advised against discontinuing these drugs, as flares of hepatic inflammation have been reported.

In children who have persistent, severe immunosuppression (CD4+ lymphocytes <50–100/mm³ or <15%), several opportunistic infections can involve the biliary system and produce a syndrome of right upper quadrant (RUQ) pain, fever, direct hyperbilirubinemia, and elevation of serum aminotransferase levels. Ultrasound or other imaging is indicated. Detection of the offending pathogen may require direct aspiration, biopsy, and/or ERCP-guided sphincterotomy and fluid sampling. Ascending bacterial cholangitis and obstructive conditions also should be considered. Such biliary problems are rare in children receiving HAART.

Tests of hepatic inflammation and function are part of routine monitoring. Jaundice due to indirect hyperbilirubinemia is commonly associated with atazanavir. This benign drug effect is thought to be related to inhibition of a uridine diphosphate glucuronyltransferase. At first occurrence, it is important to exclude elevated direct bilirubin or increased hepatic transaminases, as these abnormalities would suggest a different etiology. Even with continued use of the precipitating ARV, the indirect hyperbilirubinemia may abate. Hepatic transaminase elevation is common in HIV-infected children, and frequently no specific explanation is found; HIV infection itself, ARVs (especially NNRTIs – see Non-Nucleoside Analogue Reverse Transcriptase Inhibitors), non-ARV drugs, and hepatotropic viral infections should be considered. Persistent or moderate elevations deserve further evaluation. Intercurrent viral infections (e.g., EBV, enteroviruses) and effects of ARV and non-ARV drugs are the most common causes. HBV and HCV infection, withdrawal of HBV-active drugs in HBV-coinfected children, and HBV- or HCV-related IRIS are important to consider. There is concern that ongoing mild or subclinical liver inflammation may pose a long-term risk of progressive liver dysfunction, liver fibrosis, and cirrhosis.[42]

RENAL HEALTH

HIV infection frequently caused kidney disease in the pre-HAART era. HIV-associated renal disease has been classified into 4 groups:

(1) acute tubular disease, (2) immune-mediated glomerulopathies, (3) thrombotic microangiopathies, and (4) HIV-associated nephropathy. In the HAART era the proportion of deaths due to renal disease has increased relatively; cases probably represent end-stage HIV disease.[38] Rates of glomerular disease have decreased; rates of proteinuria as high as 33% in the pre-HAART era have fallen to less than 10% in the HAART era.[43,44] Specific ARVs, such as TDF and many of the PIs, are associated with renal disease. TDF-associated renal disease is a tubulopathy characterized by proteinuria, glycosuria, and renal phosphate wasting. Treatment with some PIs has been associated renal calculi.[45] In most cases, these toxic effects on the kidney are reversible with discontinuation of the offending ARV.

Appropriate monitoring for kidney disease includes measurements of serum creatinine and other electrolytes along with urinalysis prior to starting ARVs and then periodically during treatment. More intensive monitoring may be necessary for those receiving TDF.[46] Renal complications can develop as an insidious, progressive, chronic process exacerbated by nephrotoxic agents or other metabolic effects of longstanding HIV infection.[47] All of the NRTIs (except abacavir) and TDF are excreted by the kidney and require appropriate dose adjustments in the setting of impaired renal function.

BONE HEALTH

HIV infection in adults increases the risk of osteonecrosis (avascular necrosis), a condition resulting from ischemic death of cellular elements of bone.[48] The femoral head most commonly is affected but other involved areas include humeral heads and wrist bones. HIV-infected children also appear to be at increased risk, with an approximately 0.2% prevalence of avascular necrosis of the hip.[49] The most important osteonecrosis risk factor is corticosteroid use, which can be exacerbated by PI-mediated alterations in steroid metabolism. Other risk factors include alcohol use, hemoglobinopathies, hyperlipidemia, pancreatitis, low bone mineral density, and hypercoagulable states. Specific risk factors for HIV-infected children have not been determined. Limp, hip pain or periarticular pain and tenderness, and limited range of motion at the affected joint are typical. Imaging is used to confirm the diagnosis.[1] Less advanced osteonecrosis can be managed with avoidance of weight-bearing and use of analgesics, but surgical intervention often is required; consultation with an orthopedic specialist should be obtained early. Corticosteroid use and (in adolescents) alcohol intake should be minimized.

Decreased bone mineral density (BMD) is recognized as an emerging metabolic complication of HIV infection in adults and children.[50] Declining bone mass (osteopenia) frequently precedes osteoporosis. Dual energy X-ray absorptiometry (DXA) is the standardized method for measurement of BMD. Decreased BMD occurs in about 15% to 20% of HIV-infected adults and children in the HAART era; increased risk of fracture has been demonstrated in HIV-infected adults compared with uninfected adults,[51] but such findings have not been reported for children. The real impact on bone health of perinatally HIV-infected children will likely not be understood fully until these children reach adulthood, because of the normal maturational changes in BMD. The dual concern is that infected youth may not attain a normal peak bone mass in early adulthood and will continue to have high rates of ongoing bone loss, which would lead to high rates of osteoporosis and fractures as adults.

The causes of low BMD and osteoporosis in pediatric/adolescent HIV infection include low BMI, malnutrition, corticosteroid use, vitamin D insufficiency, and, in older adolescents, smoking, alcohol use and medroxyprogesterone injectable contraception, and HIV-specific factors, including effects of HIV infection and ARV use. Lower BMD was observed in HIV-infected patients in the pre-HAART era. Initiation of HAART has been associated repeatedly with loss of BMD. Specifically implicated ARVs include stavudine, tenofovir, and protease inhibitors.

There is no recommendation at the present time for routine assessment of BMD in children and youth by DXA or other measures.[1,50] BMD assessment by DXA (lumbar spine and whole body) should be obtained in any child who meets the general criteria for such screening.[52] In addition, current DHHS guidelines recommend considering DXA assessment at baseline and every 6 to 12 months for children in early puberty who are initiating treatment with TDF until more data are available about its long-term effects on bone mineral acquisition.[1] Given the high rates of vitamin D insufficiency in children with HIV infection, periodic assessment of vitamin D status is recommended.[53] Ensuring calcium and vitamin D sufficiency, encouraging weight-bearing exercise, and minimizing use of tobacco, alcohol, corticosteroids, and other drugs that compromise bone health are important interventions for maintenance and restoration of bone health. Consideration of substitution of tenofovir with a different ARV – balanced against feasibility of maintaining virologic suppression without tenofovir – may be warranted if very low BMD or osteoporosis is diagnosed.

PULMONARY CONDITIONS

Pulmonary infections in HIV-infected children were common before effective HAART became available. *Pneumocystis* pneumonia (PCP) was a common presentation for infants with unrecognized HIV infection. PCP and recurrent bacterial pneumonia are now uncommon in the U.S., and occur predominantly in children whose severe immunosuppression is a result of lack of effective HAART.

Tuberculosis (TB) commonly complicates HIV infection in children who live in TB-endemic areas. While much less of a problem for children in the U.S., HIV-infected children in the U.S. are at increased risk of exposure to *M. tuberculosis* because of living with HIV-infected, immunosuppressed adults with TB; having immigrated from TB-endemic areas; or having household contacts who immigrated from TB-endemic areas. HIV-infected children should have annual screening for TB risk and symptoms as well as tuberculin testing. Once infected with *M. tuberculosis*, HIV-infected children are at increased risk of developing TB disease, especially if CD4+ lymphocyte counts have not been preserved or restored by HAART.

Lymphocytic interstitial pneumonitis (LIP) is a chronic lymphoproliferative disorder observed in about one-third of HIV-infected children in the pre-HAART era (see Figure 111-2). Bronchiectasis and progressive pulmonary decompensation can ensue. Distinguishing the radiographic appearance of LIP from that of TB or PCP can be difficult. EBV has been implicated in the pathogenesis of LIP but the etiology is not definitively established. Episodic pulmonary exacerbations respond to systemic corticosteroids. LIP appears to be both treated and prevented by HAART.[54]

HEMATOLOGIC ABNORMALITIES

Anemia, thrombocytopenia, and neutropenia are commonly observed in HIV-infected children. These abnormalities can be related to HIV infection itself, toxicity of antiretroviral or other commonly used drugs, malnutrition or micronutrient deficiency, superinfections (e.g., parvovirus B19 or *M. avium* complex), or malignancy.

Anemia usually results from direct bone marrow suppression by HIV or from autoimmune hemolytic anemia. Both typically improve with HAART, though control of autoimmune hemolytic anemia may require use of corticosteroids. Anemia related to concomitant infection, malignancy, or other conditions improves with treatment of the underlying condition. Drug-related anemia usually is the result of marrow suppression (e.g., due to ZDV, cotrimoxazole) but also can be related to hemolysis in G6PD-deficient patients taking drugs such as dapsone or sulfonamides. ZDV-related anemia is common and usually is macrocytic. Erythropoietin injections have been used to mitigate severe nonhemolytic anemia and avoid transfusions in children without an alternative to ZDV or immediate option for treating an underlying condition.

PART II Clinical Syndromes and Cardinal Features of Infectious Diseases: Approach to Diagnosis and Initial Management

SECTION S Human Immunodeficiency Virus and the Acquired Immunodeficiency Syndrome

Neutropenia in HIV-infected children does not seem to carry the same risk of infection as neutropenia in children with malignancies. ZDV is the most common drug-related cause. Neutropenia also can be due to direct effects of untreated HIV infection, other drugs, intercurrent infections, and malignancy. Effective HIV treatment, substitution of offending drugs, and/or treatment of underlying conditions usually are sufficient. Granulocyte colony-stimulating factor (G-CSF) injections have been effective for severe or persistent neutropenia.[1]

Thrombocytopenia is more likely the result of HIV infection than the result of HIV treatment. Thrombocytopenia typically responds to HAART and is uncommon among children on effective HAART. Other causes include indinavir, non-ARV drugs (cotrimoxazole), opportunistic and non-opportunistic infections, recent live-virus immunizations, and malignancy. Severe thrombocytopenia has been managed successfully with the same therapeutic approaches as for HIV-unrelated immune thrombocytopenic purpura (ITP).[1]

LACTIC ACIDOSIS AND MITOCHONDRIAL DYSFUNCTION

NRTIs/NtRTIs inhibit mtDNA synthesis and impair mitochondrial function in vitro. HIV itself can also cause mitochondrial dysfunction. Clinical manifestations are broad, ranging from asymptomatic elevations in lactic acid (2.1–5.0 mmol/L) to a combination of symptoms and signs including fatigue, weakness, myalgia, abdominal pain, and dyspnea to severe multiorgan involvement (hepatic toxicity, pancreatitis, and respiratory failure), with elevated lactic acid concentrations. Mitochondrial toxicity can also play a role in peripheral neuropathy, cardiomyopathy, and CNS toxicity. Since asymptomatic elevations of lactic acid are quite common and of uncertain significance, routine assessment of lactic acid levels is not recommended. However, measurements should be performed whenever signs or symptoms of lactic acidosis are present.[1]

In the setting of symptomatic lactic acid elevations, all ARVs should be discontinued. After resolution of symptoms and normalization of lactic acid concentrations, a new ARV regimen that does not include the likely offending agents should be started. While in vitro data suggest that didanosine and stavudine are most likely to cause these problems and lamivudine and TDF less likely to do so, the clinical situation can be more complicated.[55,56] Therefore, NRTI/NtRTI-sparing regimens may be preferred in a patient who has experienced mitochondrial toxicity and lactic acidosis.

MALIGNANCIES

HIV-infected adults are at high risk for several cancers, including Kaposi sarcoma (KS) and non-Hodgkin lymphoma. In the HAART era, HIV-infected adults are much less likely to develop KS, but because of improved survival and other risk factors, a much broader array of malignancies are now seen. Cancer is a leading cause of death in adults infected with HIV in the U.S.[57] Cancer rates are low in infants and children infected with HIV but are still higher than the rates seen in the general pediatric population.[58]

REPRODUCTIVE HEALTH

By 19 years of age, 17% of perinatally infected girls in one cohort were pregnant at least once.[59] In this same cohort, 27% of 13-24-year-old girls were sexually active; those who were sexually active had higher viral loads and lower CD4[+] lymphocyte counts, factors that increase the risk of HIV transmission. In addition, less than 60% of sexually active girls had a Pap smear, but nearly half of those Pap smears were abnormal.

While cervical dysplasia screening (Pap smear) generally is deferred in adolescents until age 21 years, regardless of age of onset of sexual activity, sexually active HIV-infected adolescents should undergo cervical cytology screening twice in the first year after sexual activity onset and annually thereafter.[2,60] HPV vaccines are safe and immunogenic in perinatally HIV-infected children and youth;[61] HPV vaccine should be offered to all children, preferably by age 11 years but should not be withheld from older children, including those with evidence of HPV disease. Anal dysplasia screening (by anal Pap smear) also may be beneficial for HIV-infected women and men who have sex with men (MSM).[2]

Routine HIV care for perinatally infected adolescents should include regular reproductive health screening and counseling: discussion of current and planned sexual activity; prevention counseling for reducing risk of acquiring and transmitting sexually transmitted infections (STIs), including HIV infection; partner disclosure counseling; screening for STIs and for HPV-associated dysplasia; pregnancy planning and contraception. Condoms are recommended for prevention of HIV, HPV, and other STI transmission as well as for pregnancy prevention. Many forms of hormonal contraception can be used safely and effectively by HIV-infected women, but providers should be aware of potential drug interactions, especially between many protease inhibitors and oral contraceptives.[62] Most often, the infected youth's partner is not HIV-infected; periodic HIV testing for the partner is recommended and consultation with obstetric colleagues can be helpful for counseling about approaches to safe conception for the HIV-discordant couple.

INTERNATIONAL SETTINGS

In resource-limited countries HIV remains a devastating problem, but increased access to ARVs is expected to transform the pediatric HIV epidemic in those countries in a manner similar to that in the U.S. Numerous studies have shown that despite treatment being started in children at more advanced stages of disease, response to HAART in resource-limited settings is similar to results in the U.S. and Europe.[63] Nevertheless, many challenges remain, including the cost of treatment, limited medical care infrastructure, nutritional deficiencies and food insecurity, and comorbid conditions – especially TB and malaria – that are rarely seen in HIV-infected children in the U.S.

TRANSITION

The advent of effective combination antiretroviral therapy has transformed perinatal HIV from a progressive, fatal infection into a chronic disease. In addition to the possibility of cardiovascular and other long-term complications, survivors of perinatal HIV infection must also confront the same challenges of adolescence and adulthood faced by peers without HIV infection. Rather than focusing just on survival and avoidance of opportunistic illnesses, counseling of HIV-infected adolescents and young adults now must focus on school success and career choices, reproductive health and plans for marriage and families, and transition to adult medical care. Transition to the adult medical care model takes time and advance planning, as the pediatric and adult chronic care models are different. Awareness of patient and provider factors that facilitate or enhance transition can inform programs for perinatally HIV-infected young adults to enroll successfully in adult medical care.[64] Routine advance-care planning with youth and their families is as important as in any youth with chronic illness and has been shown to be well received and beneficial.

PART III

Etiologic Agents of Infectious Diseases

SECTION A: Bacteria

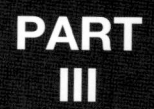

114 Classification of Bacteria

Joseph W. St. Geme III

The ability to discriminate between distinct groups of organisms and to communicate with a common language about organisms in the context of disease is essential for clinical microbiologists and physicians. The official taxonomic ranks for naming bacterial organisms are kingdom, division, class, order, family, genus, and species. A bacterial *species* is defined as a distinct group of organisms that share a constellation of properties. This definition is somewhat subjective, and as new data become available, reclassification is necessary occasionally.

IDENTIFICATION BY PHENOTYPIC CHARACTERISTICS

Historically, bacterial classification has been based on phenotypic characteristics. A useful first approach to classification was developed in 1884 by Christian Gram, who observed that some bacteria retain crystal violet dye after decoloration with ethanol and others do not. Organisms that retain crystal violet dye appear blue and are called *gram positive*. Bacteria that are decolorized appear red when counterstained with safranin and are referred to as *gram negative*. The staining characteristics of gram-positive and gram-negative bacteria reflect differences in cell wall structure. As shown in Figure 114-1, gram-positive cells have a relatively simple cell wall composed of an inner membrane and a surrounding peptidoglycan layer between 30 and 200 molecules thick. The gram-positive cell wall also contains teichoic acids and lipoteichoic acids, which are water-soluble polymers of polyol phosphates. Gram-negative organisms have a more complex cell wall, characterized by the presence of an inner membrane, a surrounding peptidoglycan layer one to two molecules thick, and an outer membrane (see Figure 114-1). The outer membrane contains lipopolysaccharide (endotoxin), which is unique to gram-negative organisms. The compartment between the inner and outer membranes is called the periplasm and contains a number of degradative enzymes and transport-related proteins.

Whereas most bacteria are gram-positive or gram-negative, some stain poorly or fail to stain at all with Gram reagents. Examples are mycobacteria, some actinomycetes, treponemes, rickettsiae, anaplasmae, chlamydiae, and mycoplasmas. Mycobacteria possess a complex cell wall that is rich in lipids and have been referred to as *acid fast* because of their resistance to decolorization with acid solutions. These organisms are best visualized microscopically with Ziehl–Neelsen or Kinyoun acid-fast stain. Most actinomycetes are gram positive, but *Nocardia* and *Rhodococcus* characteristically take up Gram stain irregularly. They have a cell wall structure similar to that of mycobacteria and, like the mycobacteria, are acid fast.

The family Treponemataceae contains five genera, namely *Treponema*, *Borrelia*, *Leptospira*, *Brachyspira*, and *Spirillum*. The treponemes generally do not stain with Gram reagents or other standard laboratory stains and usually are seen best with darkfield microscopy. Members of the family Rickettsiaceae and the family Anaplasmataceae (*Ehrlichia*, *Anaplasma*, *Wolbachia*, and

Neorickettsia) possess a cell wall typical of gram-negative bacilli but react weakly with Gram stain and are seen optimally with Giemsa or Gimenez stain. Members of the family Chlamydiaceae (*Chlamydia trachomatis*, *Chlamydophila psittaci*, and *Chlamydophila pneumoniae*) are obligate intracellular organisms that possess inner and outer membranes similar to those of gram-negative bacteria but lack a peptidoglycan layer and do not take up Gram stain. The two important members of the family Mycoplasmataceae are *Mycoplasma* and *Ureaplasma*. Mycoplasmas do not have a cell wall; their cytoplasmic contents are enclosed only by a well-developed plasma membrane.

Cellular morphology also plays an important role in classification. Bacteria can be separated into five major groups on the basis of morphology as viewed through the light microscope. Bacteria that are spherical or oval in appearance are described as *cocci*. Those that are rod-like or cylindrical are referred to as *bacilli*. Those with a comma-like or curved rod appearance are referred to as *vibrios*. Bacteria with a helical or more undulating appearance are called *spirochetes* if they are flexible and *spirilla* if they are rigid.

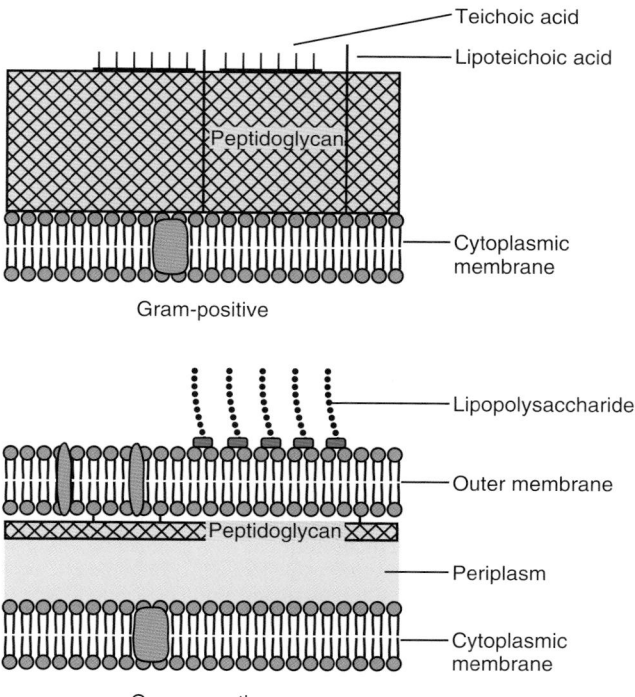

Figure 114-1. Schematic diagram of the cell wall structure of gram-positive and gram-negative bacteria.

After cell division, the cell wall between daughter cells in some species may not separate completely, giving rise to cell arrangements. These cell arrangements typically are distinctive and can be helpful in identifying related organisms. Common arrangements are cocci in pairs, cocci in chains, cocci in irregular clusters, cocci in packets of four or eight (called *sarcina*), bacilli in pairs, bacilli in chains, unusually short bacilli (called *coccobacilli*), and bacilli with tapered ends (called *fusiform* bacilli).

A wide range of other phenotypic characteristics also is employed commonly for the purpose of bacterial classification. For example, aerobic and facultative anaerobic organisms are distinguished from strictly anaerobic organisms, and spore-forming bacteria are distinguished from nonspore-forming species. Additional useful properties are carbohydrate fermentation abilities, susceptibilities to antibiotics and inorganic compounds, and reactivity with well-defined serologic reagents.

IDENTIFICATION BY MOLECULAR TECHNIQUES

Beyond phenotypic characteristics, molecular analysis also plays a major role in determining phylogenetic relationships among organisms and in classifying bacteria. The historical standard in this respect is DNA-DNA hybridization, which allows the total DNA from one organism to be compared with the total DNA of any other organism.[1] This technique involves incubating single-stranded DNA from one strain with single-stranded DNA from a second strain and assessing formation of a double-stranded DNA molecule. DNA reassociation is a specific, temperature-dependent reaction. The optimal temperature for DNA reassociation is 25°C to 30°C below the temperature at which native double-stranded DNA is denatured into single strands. Experience with several hundred species has led taxonomists to conclude that organisms with 70% or greater DNA-DNA relatedness belong to the same species. Occasionally, the 70% species-relatedness rule has been ignored when the existing nomenclature is both deeply ingrained and useful. One such example is *Escherichia coli* and the four species of *Shigella*. These organisms are all 70% or more related and should therefore be grouped into a single species instead of the present five species in two genera. However, to avoid confusion among members of the medical community, this change has not been made.

Mole percent guanine plus cytosine (G + C) content and genome size are two other measurements of DNA that often are helpful in classifying organisms.[2] The G + C content in bacterial DNA ranges from about 25% to about 75%. The G + C percentage is specific for a given species but is not unique for that species. Therefore, two strains with similar G + C contents may or may not belong to the same species. On the other hand, if the G + C contents are very different, the strains cannot be members of the same species. *Genome size*, or the molecular mass of bacterial DNA, ranges between 1×10^9 and 8×10^9 da. In certain circumstances, genome size determinations can distinguish between groups. Such determinations were used to distinguish *Legionella pneumophila* from *Bartonella* (formerly *Rochalimaea*) *quintana*. *L. pneumophila* has a genome size of 3×10^9 da, whereas the *B. quintana* genome is roughly 1×10^9 da.

In a number of cases, multilocus enzyme electrophoresis (MEE) has been applied for the purpose of classifying bacteria.[3] This method detects differences in the electrophoretic mobilities of individual soluble metabolic enzymes. The cellular proteins of an organism are separated by starch gel electrophoresis, and the individual enzymes are detected with the use of specific substrates. Variations in electrophoretic mobility of a given enzyme typically reflect amino acid substitutions that alter protein charge; these variations thus represent different alleles of the gene encoding the enzyme. Through the use of a relatively large number of enzymes, a positive correlation between estimates of relatedness obtained by MEE and by DNA hybridization of whole chromosomal DNA has been demonstrated. It is therefore possible to use MEE to determine the level of relatedness of two strains or a group of strains. This method has been useful particularly in yielding quantitative data about the relationships between organisms within a

given species. In addition, it has provided insights into bacterial evolution.

Two additional methods that are useful for determining genetic relatedness between strains and for characterizing the population structure of a given species are pulsed-field gel electrophoresis (PFGE) and amplified fragment length polymorphism (AFLP) analysis.[4,5] PFGE has been the accepted gold standard for many species and involves extraction of chromosomal DNA and then digestion of the DNA with a rare-cutting restriction enzyme, giving rise to a number of large (80 to 100 kb) fragments, which can be separated by applying an electrical field alternatively in two directions. The critical experimental variable is the *pulse time*, defined as the time a field is applied in one direction before it is abruptly switched to another direction. Each strain gives rise to a reproducible pattern of bands (a fingerprint), and the number of bands shared between strains provides a measure of relatedness. AFLP analysis involves extraction of genomic DNA and then digestion of this DNA with two restriction enzymes. Subsequently, two different double-stranded oligonucleotide adapters are added to the digested DNA, one compatible with the first restriction enzyme and the other compatible with the second enzyme. After ligation, an aliquot of the DNA sample is subjected to PCR amplification under highly stringent conditions with adapter-specific primers that have an extension of one to three bases at their 3-prime ends, running into the unknown chromosomal fragment. An extension of one base (e.g., adenine) in one primer results in amplification of one-fourth of the ligated fragments (e.g., those with a thymine, but not those with adenine, guanine, or cytidine at the complementary position), whereas an extension of two or three bases results in amplification of a smaller fraction of fragments. After polyacrylamide gel electrophoresis, a highly informative pattern of 40 to 200 bands is obtained.

The molecular technique that has taken on greatest importance for classifying bacteria is 16S (small subunit) ribosomal RNA (rRNA) gene sequencing. The 16S rRNA folds in a precise fashion with the large subunit rRNA to form ribosomes. *Ribosomes* are highly conserved structures found in all living cells that perform the crucial task of protein synthesis. Because the genes for 16S rRNA contain some sequences that have been highly conserved through the course of evolution and others that are highly variable, 16S rRNA gene sequence can be used to determine evolutionary and genetic relationships between organisms.[6] A further attribute of 16S rRNA gene sequencing is that cultivation of the organism is not required; for example, through the use of PCR and oligonucleotide primers that correspond to conserved regions of the bacterial 16S rRNA gene, a stretch of bacterial DNA can be

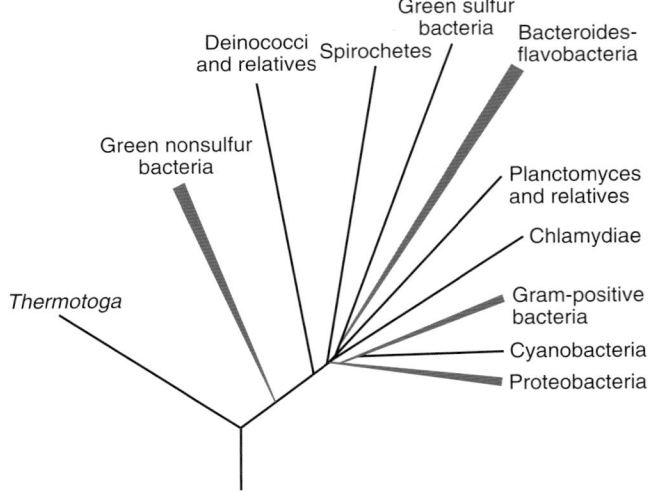

Figure 114-2. Phylogenic tree of the domain bacteria based on comparison of 16S ribosomal RNA sequences. Divisions that contain human pathogens are denoted by blue boldface branches. (Redrawn from Relman DA. The identification of uncultured microbial pathogens. J Infect Dis 1993;168:1–8.)

amplified directly from diseased tissue or any other relevant source.[7] The variable regions of the resultant DNA sequence form the basis for specific phylogenetic analysis. In general, consensus primers can be designed for any discrete group of organisms with common ancestry. On the basis of 16S rRNA sequence comparisons, the evolutionary relationships among all known extant bacterial species can be represented in a phylogenetic tree (Figure 114-2).[7]

Although 16S rRNA gene sequencing has clear strengths related to defining genetic relationships and classifying bacteria, using this technique alone has limitations. For example, isolates that have divergent 16S rRNA gene sequences are consistently unrelated, but isolates that have nearly identical 16S rRNA gene sequences may or may not belong to the same species, resulting in the need for another method to explore further whether isolates are sufficiently similar to be assigned to the same species. With this information in mind, multilocus sequence typing (MLST) is becoming more common, circumventing the potential effects of simple stochastic variation or recombination at a single locus. MLST uses profiles of alleles at multiple housekeeping genes (usually seven or so) to group isolates and determine relatedness between strains.[8,9] In recent years MLST has been especially useful in tracking the epidemiology of community-associated methicillin-resistant *Staphylococcus aureus* infection and the spread of virulent clones.[10,11]

Over the past decade there has been a steady increase in the number of completely sequenced bacterial genomes, reflecting advances in sequencing technology. The availability of this information has led to the development of DNA microarrays and has allowed comparison of the whole genomes of individual isolates. In the coming years, it is likely that whole genome information will be used increasingly to assist with bacterial classification in general terms and in clinical settings.[12,13]

Beyond nucleic acid based approaches to bacterial classification, whole-cell matrix-assisted laser desorption ionization-time of flight mass spectrometry (MALDI-TOF) has been demonstrated to be useful in classifying bacteria and comparing isolates for strain identity.[14,15]

Additional genetic and proteomic information continues to spur reclassifications.[16]

115 *Staphylococcus aureus*

Robert S. Daum

Staphylococcus aureus is the most common pathogen isolated among pediatric patients in North America, and is a major cause of morbidity and mortality. It is the most virulent species of the genus *Staphylococcus*. Its pathogenicity reflects its ability to acquire and integrate accessory genetic elements that confer virulence. *S. aureus* is responsible for community- and healthcare-associated infections and toxin-mediated diseases. The species is particularly adept at evolving strategies to elude antimicrobial therapy, leading to limited therapeutic options.

MICROBIOLOGY AND PATHOGENESIS

Staphylococci are aerobic or facultatively anaerobic gram-positive cocci that can persist in distressed environments such as acidic conditions, high sodium concentrations, and wide temperature variations. Staphylococci can survive on fomites, in dust, or on clothing for at least several days. The defining characteristics of *S. aureus* are the production of the extracellular enzyme coagulase and protein A (Figure 115-1). Clinical manifestations of *S. aureus*

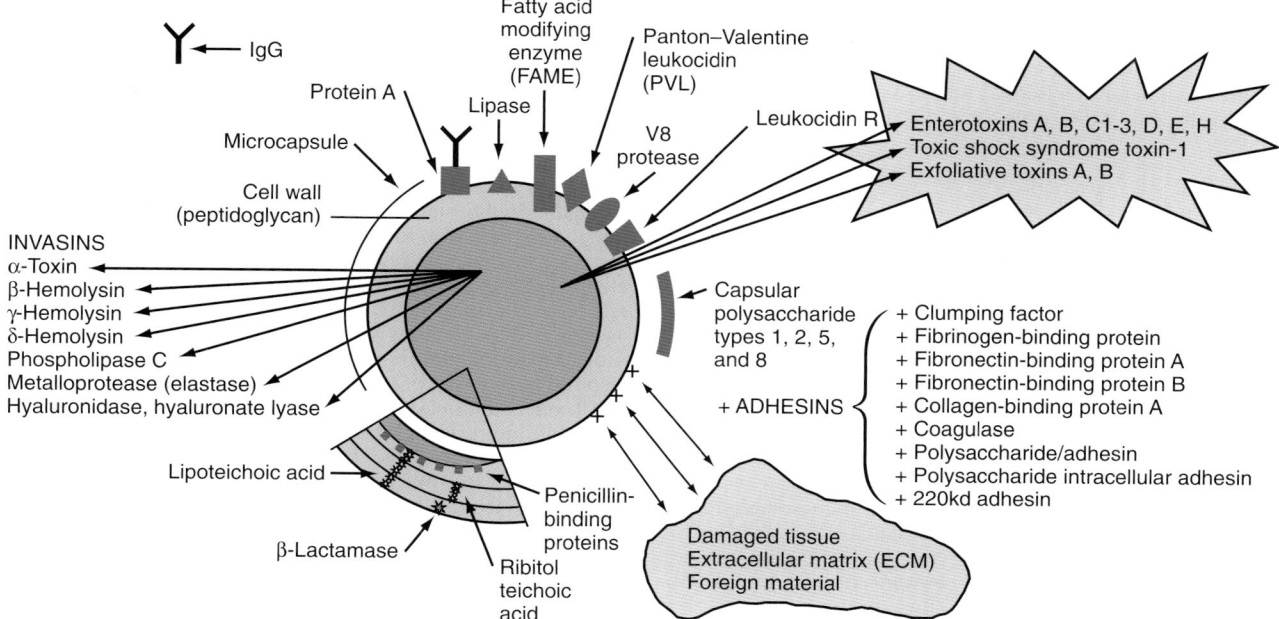

Figure 115-1. Virulence factors and relevant surface adhesins of *Staphylococcus aureus*. (Redrawn from Daum RS. *Staphylococcus aureus* vaccine. In: Plotkin SA, Orenstein WA (eds) Vaccines, 5th ed. Philadelphia, PA, Saunders Elsevier, 2008, pp 1307–1315.)

infection can result from tissue infection with inflammation, hematogenous dissemination, or toxin release inciting inflammatory cascades and tissue necrosis.

Capsule and Cell Wall

Many clinical *S. aureus* isolates have a polysaccharide capsule; 11 capsular serotypes have been described, but most experts believe that probably only 4 exist.[1] The high prevalence of two of the capsular polysaccharide types (5 and 8) in almost all collections of clinically important human and veterinary isolates suggests an important role for these polysaccharides in pathogenesis, but the mechanism is uncertain. Bloodstream infection (BSI) has also been caused by unencapsulated organisms, for example the so-called type 336 isolates and USA300.[2,3] Immunization with the type 5 and 8 polysaccharide conjugated to *Pseudomonas* exotoxoid A was the basis for two recent immunization trials, neither of which met its primary endpoints.[4–6]

The cell wall of *S. aureus* is composed of peptidoglycan, capsular polysaccharide when present, ribitol teichoic acid, lipoteichoic acid, and many surface proteins, including protein A, which binds to the Fc region of the immunoglobulin G (IgG) molecule.[7] IgG antibody binding to the staphylococcal cell surface in this non-physiologic manner decreases the efficiency by which *S. aureus* are opsonized and phagocytosed.[8–10]

Surface Proteins

Many proteins found on the surface of *S. aureus* isolates have been implicated in pathogenesis. Adherence of *S. aureus* to mammalian extracellular matrix components is mediated by a family of adhesins, the microbial surface components recognizing adhesive matrix molecules (MSCRAMMs).[11] Coagulase is found on the bacterial cell surface as well as in its environment. It binds to host prothrombin and forms staphylothrombin, an enzyme that catalyzes the formation of fibrin from fibrinogen.[12] The A and B clumping factors are cell surface proteins that bind to fibrinogen, producing the typical clusters of staphylococci when mixed with plasma.[13] Coagulase and the clumping factors breach host defenses by causing localized clotting; the clumping factors also may aid in adherence to traumatized skin, endothelial structures, and foreign surfaces. Recognition of this role for the *S. aureus* clumping factors has prompted investigation into their potential use as vaccine antigens.[14]

Iron is an essential component of cytochromes and other redox proteins. A cell wall-bound system of iron acquisition and importation has been identified in *S. aureus* and is under investigation to define an apparently essential role in pathogenesis.[15] An iron scavenging protein, isdB, currently is in a clinical trial as a vaccine candidate.[16]

Toxins

The virulence of *S. aureus* is due to a combination of variously elaborated virulence proteins that include extracellular products, such as α, β, γ, and δ hemolysins (also called toxins), leukocidins, proteases, lipase, deoxyribonuclease, a fatty acid-modifying enzyme, and hyaluronidase.[17–23] α-Hemolysin is the best studied of the exotoxins. It causes hemolysis of erythrocytes, necrosis of skin, and release of cytokines and eicosanoids that can produce shock. It is lethal when injected into animals, and *S. aureus* mutants lacking α-toxin are less virulent.[24] However, pathogenic *S. aureus* isolates that do not produce α-hemolysin have been identified. β-Hemolysin is a sphingomyelinase that can injure membranes that are rich in this lipid; most human isolates do not express β-toxin. The high prevalence of γ-leukocidin genes in isolates causing necrotizing skin infections suggests the importance of this toxin in the production of dermonecrosis. *S. aureus* possesses several leukocidins: synergohymenotropic toxins that damage membranes of certain cells as a result of the concerted action of two elaborated, secreted proteins. The Panton–Valentine leukocidin (PVL) is a pore-forming cytotoxin,[25] the toxic effect of which is said to result from the synergistic action of the proteins lukS-PV and lukF-PV.[26] PVL has been associated with severe inflammatory lesions, presumably through activation of granulocytes.[27] PVL-producing strains have been associated with severe skin infections and lung infections,[28] specifically necrotizing pneumonia.[29] The role of PVL in the pathogenesis of *S. aureus* infections has been controversial because of variation in susceptibility by species. Its importance in the pathogenesis of infections in humans was clarified recently.[30–32]

S. aureus causes a variety of so-called "toxin-mediated" diseases, including staphylococcal scalded-skin syndrome (SSSS), toxic shock syndrome (TSS), and staphylococcal food poisoning, which are caused by the action of exotoxins and enterotoxins. Exfoliative toxins A and B (ETA and ETB) cleave the glycoprotein desmoglein 1, promoting spread of *S. aureus* under the stratum corneum,[33,34] resulting in blistering of the superficial epidermis that is characteristic of SSSS and bullous impetigo. TSS toxin 1 (TSST-1) and staphylococcal enterotoxins B and C, SEB and SEC, have been implicated in most cases of TSS. These toxins have superantigen activity, i.e., stimulate T lymphocytes nonspecifically, and result in cytokine release and clinical toxic shock. At a skin or mucosal port of entry, TSST-1 can interfere with release of inflammatory mediators locally, which may be responsible for a surprisingly benign appearance at the local infective site. An expanding family of enterotoxins has been implicated in staphylococcal food poisoning; the most frequently implicated molecule is enterotoxin A, SEA.

Genetic Basis and Regulation of Pathogenicity Factors and Antimicrobial Resistance

The whole genome of *S. aureus* has been sequenced many times. It has a circular chromosome of about 2,800,000 basepairs.[35] Genes for many housekeeping functions are highly conserved. The genome also carries mobile genetic elements such as plasmids, transposons, prophages, and pathogenicity islands, many of which encode virulence factors or determinants of antibiotic resistance. These factors represent a subset of a large class of accessory gene products (including surface proteins, exotoxins, and other enzymes) that, although not required for growth and cell division, provide an advantage in particular environments.

S. aureus has evolved a remarkable network of regulatory mechanisms that control subsets of genes up- or downregulated under certain growth and environmental conditions. The best studied is the *agr* locus with its two-component signal transduction system and its effector RNAIII molecule. The *agr* locus upregulates genes encoding capsular polysaccharides, α-δ toxins, two-component synergohymenotropic toxins, enterotoxins, exfoliatins, and proteases, and downregulates others such as MSCRAMMS, other adhesins, and protein A. Other two-component signal transduction systems implicated in pathogenesis include *saeRS*, *srrAB*, *arlSR*, and *lytRS*. DNA-binding protein systems such as *sarA* and its regulatory homologs also regulate virulence factors. Additionally the sigma factor, σ^B, can combine with the RNA polymerase core enzyme to form a holoenzyme that can recognize promoter elements for at least 36 *S. aureus* genes involved in bacterial stress responses. Taken together, membrane sensing systems such as *agr* as well as DNA-binding regulatory systems afford *S. aureus* a versatile environmental response system and confer the capacity to respond to a myriad of environmental stimuli such as high or low NaCl concentrations, subinhibitory concentrations of protein synthesis inhibitors, low pH, low PO_2 or limitation of essential nutrients such as amino acids.

S. aureus can overcome environmental antibiotic pressure through the acquisition and transmission of resistance genes from other, usually less pathogenic, species and between isolates of the same species. Resistance to β-lactam antibiotics such as penicillins, cephalosporins, and carbepenems is one example. β-Lactam antibiotics bind to *S. aureus* penicillin-binding proteins (PBPs), thereby inhibiting cell wall synthesis.

Resistance to penicillin was documented almost immediately after its introduction into clinical practice in the 1940s and is mediated by the elaboration of a β-lactamase, encoded by a transposon borne on a plasmid. Almost all clinical isolates of *S. aureus* can elaborate this enzyme, rendering clinically ineffective antibiotics that are susceptible to β-lactamase hydrolysis.

The development of β-lactamase-resistant semisynthetic penicillins temporarily overcame the clinical problem created by the wide prevalence of β-lactamase-producing *S. aureus*. However, some strains became resistant to the semisynthetic compounds by acquiring *mecA*, a gene that elaborates PBP2a, a peptidoglycan-synthesizing enzyme that has decreased affinity for β-lactam antibiotics.[36,37] These resistant strains are termed methicillin-resistant *Staphylococcus aureus* (MRSA) and are responsible for nosocomial outbreaks and, more recently, a community-based MRSA epidemic. MRSA strains are resistant to all β-lactams with the exception of the recently licensed ceftaroline.

The *mecA* resistance gene is located on a mobile genetic element called the staphylococcal chromosome cassette *mec* (*SCCmec*),[38] which is present in all MRSA isolates with an occasional exception. *SCCmec* contains a *mec* complex, comprised of *mecA* and the variably present *mecI* and *mecRl* regulatory genes, and a *ccr* complex, comprised of genes that mediate insertion and excision of *SCCmec* from the genome. Insertion of *SCCmec* into the *S. aureus* genome is the genetic event that converts a methicillin-susceptible strain into a methicillin-resistant one. There currently are 8 *SCCmec* elements that have been sequenced or partially characterized (International Working Groups on the Classification of Staphylococcal Cassette Chromosome Elements (IWG-SCC) Classification of Staphylococcal Cassette Chromosomes mec (scc mec): Guideline for Replacing). Mobile elements *SCCmec* types I to III generally are found in healthcare-associated MRSA (HA-MRSA) isolates, whereas *SCCmec* types IV and V generally are found in community-associated MRSA (CA-MRSA) isolates, although these distinctions are blurring.[39]

Although the mechanism for the movement of *SCCmec* elements from strain to strain is unknown, the large size of types I to III is believed to limit easy transfer of the elements. Types IV and V, however, are smaller and probably, therefore, more mobile. Types IV and V have been found in multiple *S. aureus* genetic backgrounds, supporting the hypothesis that they are readily transferred from strain to strain.[40–42] Types VI through VIII have, to date, been identified in only a limited number of strains.

EPIDEMIOLOGY

Colonization

Humans and other mammals are the natural reservoirs for *S. aureus*. Asymptomatic colonization is frequent in humans and traditionally has been detected in the anterior nares. Other areas that can be colonized include the skin, nails, pharynx, axilla, perineum, throat, rectum, and vagina. Colonization rates range from 25% to 50%, with higher rates found in people with dermatologic conditions (e.g., eczema), frequent needle use (e.g., intravenous drug abusers), indwelling intravascular devices (e.g., dialysis patients), and healthcare personnel (HCP). Children have a higher colonization rate, possibly due to their frequent exposure to respiratory tract secretions. Three patterns of *S. aureus* colonization have been observed: about 20% of the population is persistently colonized, 60% is intermittently colonized, and 20% is almost never colonized.[43] Traditionally, nasal *S. aureus* carriage has been a risk factor for developing infection,[43–46] although most colonized individuals do not do so. Community-associated MRSA colonization affects more body sites, which correlates with increased risk of infection.

Healthcare-Associated Infections (HAIs)

S. aureus has demonstrated the ability to develop resistance to all classes of antimicrobial agents. Soon after the introduction of penicillin in the 1940s the acquisition by *S. aureus* of β-lactamase genes and their rapid dissemination resulted in widespread resistance among clinical isolates. Less than a year after the introduction of semisynthetic penicillins in the early 1960s that were active against so-called methicillin-susceptible *S. aureus* (MSSA), the first MRSA strain was reported. These multidrug-resistant, HA-MRSA strains spread worldwide within hospital settings. The National Healthcare Safety Network, NHSN (formerly the National Nosocomial Infections Surveillance System, NNIS) of the Centers for Disease Control and Prevention (CDC) reports *S. aureus* as a major pathogen among HAIs, with MRSA accounting for 64% of nosocomial *S. aureus* isolates in intensive care units (ICUs) in United States hospitals in 2003, an increase from 36% in 1992.[47] In January 2006 to October 2007, *S. aureus* was the second most common cause of HAIs, only exceeded by coagulase-negative staphylococci (CoNS).[48] In pediatric ICUs in the U.S., *S. aureus* is the major nosocomial pathogen in a variety of clinical situations, accounting for 9% of HA bloodstream infections (HA-BSIs), 17% of cases of HA pneumonia, and 20% of surgical site infections.[49] Current patterns of HA-MRSA isolates reveal decreasing rates of isolation[50] and decreasing resistance to non-β-lactam antibiotics, suggesting a shift in nosocomial MRSA epidemiology and probably reflecting the movement of "biologically fit" CA-MRSA isolates into the hospital.[39,51]

Additionally, at the University of Chicago, in recent years, there have been further reversals of roles. MSSA isolates have become healthcare-associated pathogens and patients with MRSA isolates no longer predominantly have exposure to a healthcare setting. Patients with MSSA were more likely than patients with an MRSA to have BSI. Such patients were also more likely to be transplant recipients, adults, or require intensive care.

Community-Associated MRSA Infections

The first report of prevalent MRSA infection outside of the healthcare setting was in 1982 in Detroit, MI, among intravenous drug users.[52] This and subsequent reports of CA-MRSA were associated with risk factors for infection similar to those known for HA-MRSA, including intravenous drug use, recent hospitalization or surgery, presence of indwelling catheters or devices, dialysis, or residence in a long-term care facility.[53–56] However, In the late 1990s, CA-MRSA infections began to emerge, occurring mostly in children with no identifiable predisposing MRSA risk factors.[57–61] Infections caused by these strains most commonly resulted in skin and soft-tissue infections, although some manifested as serious infections requiring hospitalization or resulted in death.[62] Recognition of CA-MRSA infections grew substantially in number and geographic distribution. Substantial evidence supports de novo rise of MRSA from MSSA in the community rather than movement of HA-MRSA into the community to explain most CA-MRSA disease, although both CA-MRSA and HA-MRSA can circulate in the community.[63,64]

A CA-MRSA infection has been defined as one occurring in an outpatient or within 72 hours of admission to the hospital in a patient without any of the following factors used to define risk for HA-MRSA: recent hospitalization or surgery, prolonged antibiotic therapy, underlying chronic disease, indwelling catheter or other device, healthcare contact, or residence in a long-term care facility.[65] Molecular definitions have also been used to distinguish HA- from CA-MRSA strains.[66] Outbreaks of CA-MRSA infections have been reported in group childcare centers,[56,67] sports teams,[68,69] correctional facilities,[70,71] and military units,[72,73] suggesting that close contact and suboptimal hygiene practices play a role in spread.

CA-MRSA isolates also can be distinguished from HA-MRSA by their lack of multidrug resistance. Most CA-MRSA isolates are susceptible to clindamycin, trimethoprim-sulfamethoxazole (TMP-SMX), and doxycycline, whereas HA-MRSA isolates more often are resistant to these agents. Genetic investigations such as multilocus sequence typing, *SCCmec* typing, and pulsed-field gel electrophoresis have elucidated important differences between HA-MRSA and CA-MRSA isolates. In the U.S., HA-MRSA usually contain *SCCmec* type II and genes that mediate resistance to several non-β-lactam antibiotics. In contrast, CA-MRSA isolates usually contain *SCCmec* types IV or V, and lack non-β-lactam antibiotic resistance genes.[38] Even among CA-MRSA isolates, however, non-β-lactam agent resistance determinants can be found elsewhere in the cell, e.g., on plasmids or in the chromosome. For example, erythromycin resistance is common among both HA- and CA-MRSA strains and can be mediated by a variety of phenotypic and genetic mechanisms. When the *erm* gene that commonly mediates erythromycin resistance is present, the constitutive or inducible MLS$_B$ phenotype is conferred (discussed below).[74,75]

Another difference between CA-MRSA and HA-MRSA isolates is their repertoire of toxin genes.[76] The most striking examples are the *lukS-PV* and *luk F-PV* genes that encode for PVL and are transferred from strain to strain by one of several bacteriophages.[77] They have been associated with MSSA and MRSA isolates causing SSTIs, necrotizing pneumonia, and empyema.[78–80] More severe infections, such as severe sepsis, thrombosis, and thromboembolism, also are caused by isolates containing the PVL genes.[29] Interestingly, while SCC*mec* IV or V and PVL together seem to confer a selective advantage for spread (i.e., transmission and colonization) and pathogenicity (i.e., excess rate of infection per colonized individual), the genes encoding PVL are transferred separately from the SCC*mec* element. The major circulating CA-MRSA genetic lineage in the U.S., called USA 300 by a nomenclature scheme based on its pulsed-field gel electrophoretic pattern, contains an island of foreign DNA called the ACME-encoded *arc* cluster. An important role for ACME in virulence of CA-MRSA has been postulated but is controversial.[81–83]

Vancomycin-Intermediate *S. aureus* (VISA) and Vancomycin-Resistant *S. aureus* (VRSA) Infections

S. aureus isolates with reduced susceptibility to vancomycin also emerged in the late 1990s. These strains, defined as having a minimum inhibitory concentration (MIC) of vancomycin >2 µg/mL typically have been isolated from patients with underlying medical conditions in whom vancomycin therapy has failed;[84,85] strains usually also are resistant to teicoplanin (a glycopeptide not licensed in the U.S.). Hence, the term glycopeptide-intermediately susceptible *S. aureus* (GISA) may be more appropriate. In 2002, the first high-level (MIC of vancomycin >16 µg/mL) vancomycin-resistant *S. aureus* (VRSA) strain was reported; this isolate apparently acquired the *vanA* vancomycin resistance genes from *Enterococcus*. To date, 11 VRSA isolates have been reported in the U.S. The strains evaluated to date all carry the *vanA* gene.[86–88]

CLINICAL MANIFESTATIONS

Skin and Soft-Tissue Infections

Impetigo

S. aureus is a major cause of several infections of the skin and its appendages. The most superficial is impetigo, which begins as a small, tender, erythematous papule. Often there is interruption of the integument by lesions such as an insect bite, a varicella vesicle, eczema, or a minor abrasion from trauma. Bullous impetigo is a specific *S. aureus* lesion in which transparent bullae rupture easily and expose a moist base surrounded by a thin rim of scale (see Figure 70-1). Bullous impetigo is mediated by the production of ETA and ETB.[89,90]

Several studies have demonstrated the superiority of topical or systemic antibiotics over simple cleansing for the treatment of impetigo. For uncomplicated impetigo outside the neonatal period, topical bacitracin or mupirocin can be appropriate and is associated with fewer side effects than systemic therapy. Bacitracin or mupirocin ointment should be applied 3 times daily for 7 to 10 days. Retapamulin recently was licensed for topical therapy for children 9 months of age or older with impetigo due to *S. pyogenes* or MSSA (but not MRSA).[91] Its place in the therapeutic armamentarium has yet to be determined. Many experts prefer systemic antimicrobial therapy for the treatment of bullous impetigo.[92]

Oral or parenteral antimicrobial therapy should be considered if impetigo is widespread. Because of the high prevalence of MRSA, in many areas a culture should be performed prior to the initiation of systemic therapy at least in patients with extensive involvement. Neonates with minor bullous impetigo (frequently near the umbilicus) who are afebrile and well, sometimes can be managed conservatively with oral empiric systemic antimicrobial therapy active against MRSA, but frequently are treated parenterally.

Abscess

S. aureus commonly causes superficial abscesses of the skin. Moist and hairy skin is particularly susceptible to furuncles, boils, folliculitis, and hidradenitis. When associated with a hair shaft, the term furuncle is often used (see Figure 70-6). Rupture yields a purulent discharge. A carbuncle is a larger lesion formed by the coalescence of furuncles. In most small skin abscesses, symptoms of pain and erythema are local, although fever can be present. Systemic signs can accompany larger lesions. In the neonate, a skin abscess or boil can progress rapidly to BSI and clinical sepsis.

S. aureus is the leading cause of breast abscess in infants, commonly occurring within the first 3 weeks of life when the breasts are enlarged physiologically. The abscess usually is unilateral, with erythema and induration. Occasionally, fever, leukocytosis, or BSI can occur. Isolation of the pathogen from discharge aids in management.[93]

Local cleansing and incision and drainage are essential components of the management of abscesses.[94,95] Sometimes small abscesses (e.g., <5 cm) can be treated without systemic antimicrobial therapy.[94,96] Neonates with skin abscesses and infants with a breast abscess should be treated. Additionally, any patient with the following should be treated with systemic antibiotic: severe or extensive disease, rapid progression of associated cellulitis, systemic illness, associated comorbidity or immunosuppression, abscess in an area difficult to drain (e.g., face, genitalia, hand), or associated phlebitis.[97]

Any abscess can heal with scarring. Some patients may suffer from recurrent furunculosis, which can be difficult to manage. Systemic and topical antimicrobial agents along with careful hand and nail hygiene may help to decrease recurrences.

Recurring MRSA skin and soft-tissue infection is common and poses a therapeutic challenge. Underlying skin conditions such as eczema should be managed aggressively. Attempts to decolonize with nasal mupirocin or applications of an antiseptic such as chlorhexidine often are unsuccessful. It is also unclear when to attempt such decolonization. Consideration of congenital or acquired immunodeficiency may be warranted in patients with recurrent disease, especially if response to therapy is slow or healing occurs with scarring.[98]

Cellulitis

Cellulitis is an infection of the subcutaneous tissues and the dermis, manifest as an area of erythema, warmth, edema, and tenderness. *S. aureus* is a major cause for all age groups and clinical sites. A blood culture should be performed before initiating antimicrobial therapy if systemic signs are present. Purulent material should be cultured when present. An aspirate or biopsy of a non-purulent cellulitis for culture can yield the infecting bacterium.[99]

Treatment is with oral or parenteral antimicrobial therapy, depending on the extent of disease and presence of systemic signs or toxicity.

Wound Infection

The likelihood of a postoperative or posttraumatic wound infection increases with the use of sutures, especially in poorly vascularized tissues. Infections often can be avoided by frequent dressing changes, meticulous daily wound care, and strict handwashing. *S. aureus* wound infections generally are recognized within a few days after trauma or surgery, with local signs of inflammation and, possibly, constitutional signs of illness. The exudate often is cloudy, hemorrhagic, and notably odorless. Extension of a wound infection to deeper tissues resulting in cellulitis, lymphadenitis, lymphangitis, or necrotizing fasciitis can occur. Bursitis usually is the complication of a contiguous skin infection, frequently with trauma, and must be differentiated from pyogenic arthritis.

Treatment of a wound infection includes exploration of the wound, drainage, removal of any foreign material, and optimization of skin hygiene. Topical or systemic antimicrobial therapy may be a useful adjunct for mild infections. Parenteral antimicrobial therapy should be considered for clinically serious or extensive infections or for wound infections on the head and neck.

Ocular Infections

S. aureus is an important cause of purulent conjunctivitis. The causative organism can be visualized by Gram stain or isolated from purulent discharge. Conjunctivitis usually resolves without treatment; topical ophthalmic antimicrobial agents frequently are used. *S. aureus* is the most frequently recognized cause of a stye or hordeolum, an infection of the sebaceous gland or eyelash follicle, respectively. Use of a topical antimicrobial agent may prevent spread of infection to adjacent hair follicles, but frequent application of warm compresses usually suffices for treatment.[100]

Preseptal (or periorbital) cellulitis is an infection of the tissues anterior to the orbital septum. It can result from extension of sinusitis or autoinoculation of skin flora following a break in the skin due to local trauma, an insect bite, an abscess, or impetigo.[101] *S. aureus* is the leading cause of skin lesion-related preseptal cellulitis. Because of the elasticity and thinness of the skin in and around the eyelid, the clinical presentation can be dramatic, with rapid onset of lid swelling, erythema, and tenderness.[102] Low-grade fever and leukocytosis can be present, although typically the child does not appear systemically ill. By definition, visual acuity is not affected in patients with preseptal cellulitis, and movement of the globe is not painful or limited. Treatment of preseptal cellulitis usually is initiated parenterally; oral therapy can be substituted after a demonstrated clinical response.

Orbital (or postseptal) cellulitis is an infection of the orbit proper. *S. aureus* is presumed to be the leading cause of orbital cellulitis following surgical or accidental trauma to the orbit, and can be responsible when orbital cellulitis complicates sinusitis.[103] Patients or parents note a red, swollen "eye"; physical examination reveals one or more of the following: decreased or painful movement of the globe, impaired visual acuity, chemosis, or proptosis.[102] Cavernous sinus thrombosis can complicate orbital infection, and should be suspected if the patient has abnormal neurologic findings.[104] Treatment of orbital cellulitis requires confirmation of the pathogen and antimicrobial susceptibility. Imaging by computed tomography (CT) helps distinguish between orbital phlegmon, subperiosteal abscess, and orbital abscess; staphylococci are more associated with abscesses. These diagnoses mandate assessment for surgical drainage in addition to intravenous antibiotics.[105] An extended course of antimicrobial therapy is given parenterally.

S. aureus endophthalmitis is an uncommon infection in children, and usually follows ocular surgery or penetrating trauma to the globe.[106] Symptoms include blurred vision, redness, pain, lid swelling, and the presence of a hypopyon. Systemic signs or fever and lethargy often are present. Treatment includes antibiotics both parenterally and instilled directly into the vitreal cavity, and vitrectomy. Visual outcomes are poor.[107]

Invasive Infections

Osteomyelitis

S. aureus is the major cause of hematogenous osteomyelitis, accounting for up to 90% of cases. The metaphyses of long, tubular bones are affected most frequently, although infection can occur in any bone.[108–111] Previous minor trauma may predispose to infection, probably as the result of subclinical minor vascular

injury, with a small area of bony necrosis acting as a nidus for seeding during what would otherwise have been asymptomatic bacteremia.[112] The classic clinical picture includes fever and point tenderness over the affected area of bone (usually at the metaphysis), decreased range of motion, and minor local signs of inflammation. Infants and toddlers can manifest only irritability, limp, or refusal to bear weight. Diagnosis requires a high degree of suspicion. The duration of symptoms prior to coming to medical attention usually is 1 week or less, but occasionally can be several weeks.[113]

Evaluation should include a blood culture as BSI is detectable in about 50% of patients.[114] At the time of clinical presentation, the erythrocyte sedimentation rate (ESR) and C-reactive protein (CRP) levels usually are increased, although normal values can be found, particularly among neonates or patients with sickle-cell disease, distal digital infection, or subacute cases (e.g., Brodie abscess). Other acute-phase reactants, such as a leukocyte count, may be normal.[115] A radiograph of the affected bone is likely to be normal in the first days after the onset of symptoms or show only deep soft-tissue swelling adjacent to the bony metaphysis; periosteal elevation or lucencies within the bone typically are not apparent until 10 to 21 days after the onset of infection. Technetium-99 methylene phosphonate scan performed in three phases identifies increases in regional perfusion and tracer uptake by inflamed bone (see Figures 78-3 and 78-4); scintigraphy is useful especially to detect multifocal infection. Although sensitive, scintigraphy can be normal in neonates and patients with sickle-cell disease with osteomyelitis. Magnetic resonance imaging (MRI) is the most accurate diagnostic test and can identify critical fascial and deep muscle phlegmon/abscess.[116]

Establishing the causative organism by needle aspiration or biopsy of the bone at the area of tenderness or imaging abnormality is important, especially if blood cultures are negative. Surgical intervention beyond a diagnostic needle aspiration is not usually required for simple acute osteomyelitis but can be indicated urgently in the presence of extensive subperiosteal or soft-tissue infection or ischemic compartment syndrome and frequently must be repeated. Surgery frequently is required for chronic infection to remove sequestra and debride affected bone.

Intravenous antibiotics should be initiated and subsequently modified according to microbiology test results. Most experts recommend a 4- to 6-week course of antimicrobial therapy for *S. aureus* osteomyelitis, using parenteral therapy initially. Deep-vein thrombosis adjacent to the bony site of infection and septic thromboembolism are increasingly recognized complications of *S. aureus* osteomyelitis, especially when caused by CA-MRSA or PVL-positive MSSA, and usually occurring in proximal long bones and vertebrae.[117] Total duration of the therapy and transition to oral therapy is individualized, depending on the extent of infection, susceptibility test results, the clinical setting, and course.[113,118,119]

Techniques to monitor therapeutic response vary, as few explicit data are available.[120] Most experts use rapid fall in CRP level as evidence of appropriate antibiotic choice and eventual fall in ESR as a guide to adequate duration of therapy. Generally, serial imaging of the infected bone does not provide useful information regarding the duration of therapy.

S. aureus can cause osteomyelitis secondary to an adjacent deep soft-tissue focus, by concurrent direct inoculation or by contiguous spread, such as by accidental puncture wound of the foot or the patella, a bite, trauma, an infected paronychia, or a surgical procedure.[121] Osteomyelitis following puncture wound frequently is termed "osteochondritis," partly to remind clinicians of the clinical and pathophysiologic features that distinguish it from hematogenous osteomyelitis. Symptoms and signs of acute hematogenous osteomyelitis usually are absent, although many patients have localized pain, fever, and erythema. The blood typically is sterile, and CRP levels can be minimally increased or normal. Surgical debridement is an important component of the therapeutic strategy in these nonhematogenous osteomyelitis/osteochondritis syndromes; antimicrobial therapy is adjunctive. The optimal duration of antimicrobial therapy for osteochondritis is uncertain, but frequently can be short (e.g., 7 to 14 days) following adequate surgical debridement in selected cases.[113]

Diskitis

Diskitis, or inflammation of an intervertebral disk, is uncommon and occurs primarily in children <5 years of age. Diskitis may be difficult to distinguish from vertebral osteomyelitis and probably the entities share a similar pathogenesis (see Chapter 78, Osteomyelitis, and Chapter 80, Diskitis). Children with diskitis usually are not febrile or ill, but refuse to walk, limp or, in the older child, have back pain. Among clinical findings, imaging studies (especially MRI) help distinguish diskitis from vertebral osteomyelitis. *S. aureus* is the most frequently identified organism in both entities, although specimens are collected more frequently and are positive more frequently in patients with vertebral osteomyelitis. Diskitis may resolve spontaneously without antimicrobial therapy; vertebral osteomyelitis does not.

Diskitis without adjacent vertebral involvement sometimes can be managed with observation alone. If the adjacent vertebrae are involved, it is impossible to exclude vertebral osteomyelitis, and these patients should receive a course of antimicrobial therapy appropriate for osteomyelitis. Follow-up imaging studies are appropriate in this circumstance.[122]

Pyogenic Arthritis

Hematogenous seeding of the synovium during *S. aureus* BSI is the most common pathogenesis of infectious arthritis in children. Pyogenic arthritis usually is heralded by warmth, tenderness, erythema, and limitation of range of motion of the involved joint. Manifestations of a hip infection, however, can be more subtle because of the depth of tissue surrounding the joint. In infants a subtle increase in resistance to movement or pain with movement may be the only clues. An imaging study, such as ultrasonography, is valuable.[123] Infants with osteomyelitis of the femur or humerus especially are prone to developing pyogenic arthritis of the adjacent joint due to the vascular and capsular anatomy in this region at this age[124] (see Figure 78-5).

If pyogenic arthritis is suspected, blood culture and aspiration of joint fluid are performed urgently; the hip usually is drained surgically. The fluid is evaluated by Gram stain and culture, total and differential cell counts, glucose and protein levels. In occasional cases of *S. aureus* arthritis, bacteria visualized on Gram stain are not isolated in culture because of the bacteriostatic nature of synovial fluid or prior antimicrobial therapy.

Treatment consists of surgical drainage and antimicrobial therapy. Antimicrobial therapy should be initiated when clinical suspicion is high and is continued for at least 3 weeks. Multiple aspiration procedures may be necessary. Open surgical drainage is employed when serial aspiration does not produce a rapid response, as an initial measure for involvement of the hip or the shoulder joint, or when establishing effective drainage by simple aspiration is technically difficult and the risk of long-term complications is high.[113] Poor outcome is associated with delay of appropriate treatment and concomitant osteomyelitis.[125]

Abscesses of Muscle and Viscera

S. aureus is the most common cause of pyomyositis (including iliopsoas and obturator internus abscess) and liver abscess, and is an important cause of renal, perinephric, splenic, and pancreatic abscess. These are all complications of BSI, which may have been asymptomatic, the patient coming to medical attention because of symptoms related to the focal infection or for fever of unknown origin (FUO), or associated with severe sepsis. Necrotizing fasciitis, especially due to CA-MRSA, usually occurs as a complication of skin infection but also can follow seeding of a deep site during BSI (see Figure 77-3A). Pyomyositis usually manifests with fever and an insidious or acute onset of cramping muscle pain, tenderness, and especially induration of a large muscle group such as those near the buttock, thigh, or hip. An obturator internus

abscess can cause a painful limp, pelvic girdle pain, or refusal to walk. An iliopsoas abscess can cause predominantly flank pain and tenderness. Visceral abscess and nephric abscesses are most likely to manifest as FUO, possibly accompanied by nonspecific abdominal or flank symptoms. A palpable mass is only present in approximately one-half of cases. A blood culture is positive in fewer than one-half of cases that present because of FUO or with localized complaints.

CT or MRI is highly likely to identify abnormalities. Management usually entails surgical decompression, debridement and drainage, and prolonged parenteral antibiotic therapy. Multiple, small visceral abscesses frequently can be treated with antibiotic therapy alone if the pathogen is identified and susceptibility test results are available. Necrotizing fasciitis is a surgical emergency and requires debridement of the involved tissue and antimicrobial therapy.

Upper Respiratory Tract Infections

Head and Neck Infections

S. aureus is an infrequent cause of acute otitis media or sinusitis but should be considered in the child who fails multiple courses

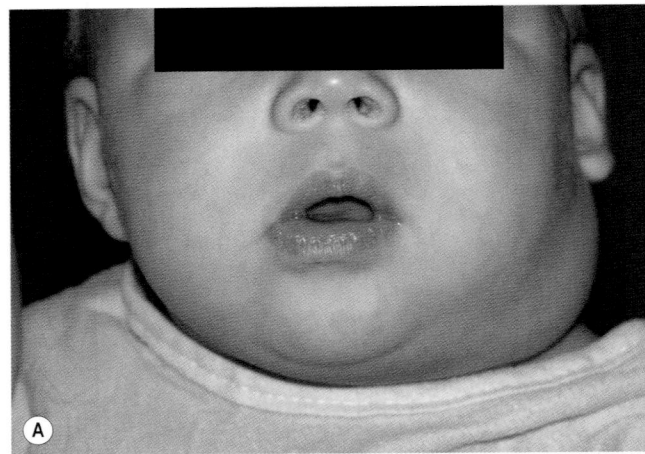

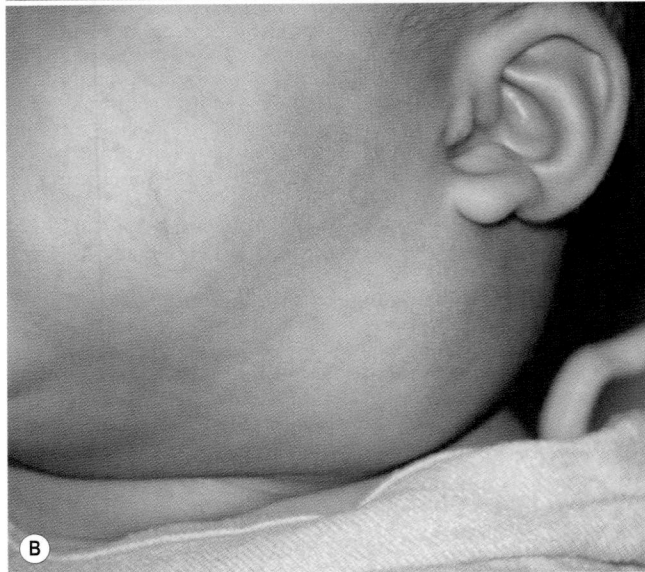

Figure 115-2. Necrotizing lymphadenitis in a 2-month-old infant. *Staphylococcus aureus* was isolated from specimen collected at the time of incision and drainage. There was no intraoral, skin, or middle-ear abnormality. Note location of mass **(A, B)** and elevation of the earlobe **(A)**. (Courtesy of J.H. Brien©.)

of empiric, oral antimicrobial therapy and in chronic or complicated disease. Both MSSA and MRSA increasingly have been isolated in cases of otorrhea following tympanostomy tube insertion and as complications of paranasal sinusitis.[103,126,127]

S. aureus is the leading cause of nasolacrimal duct abscess, suppurative parotitis, abscess of a lymph node below the angle of the jaw in very young infants (Figure 115-2) and retropharyngeal abscess in children <3 years of age (see Figure 28-1). Infection occurs presumably following nasopharyngeal or oropharyngeal colonization, sometimes in association with a viral infection. In older children and adolescents, *S. aureus* is the leading cause of peritonsillar and parapharyngeal abscess associated with recurrent pharyngeal infections and suppurative cervical lymphadenitis.

Tracheitis

Bacterial tracheitis caused by *S. aureus* can occur in an airway inflamed by a viral process or injured by medical manipulation. Affected patients manifest hoarseness and stridor (if the larynx is involved concomitantly) and can deteriorate suddenly, with respiratory distress and high fever. Diagnosis is made by visualization of thick, purulent secretions in the trachea and subglottic edema along with a positive Gram stain of secretions and recovery of *S. aureus* upon culture. Management includes establishment of an artificial airway and intravenous antibiotic therapy[128] (see Chapter 28, Infections Related to the Upper and Middle Airways).

Lower Respiratory Tract Infections

Pneumonia

S. aureus can cause rapidly progressive pneumonia following inhalation of the organism or seeding of the lungs during BSI. Clinical features include fever, cough, grunting, and tachypnea, which can evolve into rapidly progressive and severe respiratory distress. Chest radiograph demonstrates multiple patchy alveolar infiltrates that tend to coalesce to form large consolidations (Figure 115-3). Pleural effusion and empyema accompany ~90% of pulmonary infections; spontaneous pneumothorax occurs in 25% to 50%. A pneumatocele (an air- or fluid-filled cavitation resulting from dissolution of intra-alveolar septa) occurs in >50% of cases, and, if found radiologically, strongly suggests *S. aureus* as the etiologic agent of the pneumonia. The majority of cases occur in previously healthy children, although predisposing factors, such as young age (<1 year), chronic lung disease, immunosuppression, presence of a foreign body, skin infection, and concurrent use of antibiotics, may increase the likelihood of S. aureus community-associated and healthcare-associated pneumonia (CAP and HAP). A seasonal peak in *S. aureus* pneumonia is associated with viral respiratory tract infections such as influenza, presumably because viral illness transiently alters pulmonary defense mechanisms.[129]

The epidemiology of *S. aureus* pneumonia has changed dramatically with increasing frequency and geographic distribution of necrotizing CAP caused by both MSSA and MRSA strains, which usually contain the PVL genes.[28,130-133] Patients typically are young, immunocompetent hosts, often with a preceding viral illness who have acute worsening of respiratory symptoms, vital sign abnormalities, leukopenia, and rapidly progressive bilateral diffuse parenchymal pulmonary infiltrates.[29] This fulminant illness can progress to severe sepsis syndrome and has a high fatality rate. Histologic findings at autopsy reveal numerous *S. aureus* colonies throughout the lower respiratory tract with necrotic lesions extending from the tracheobronchial epithelium to the congested and hemorrhagic parenchyma of the lung[29,79] (Figure 115-4).

A high index of suspicion for *S. aureus* is critical in evaluating and aggressively treating possible cases. Diagnosis is made on clinical grounds and confirmed by recovery of the organism from pleural fluid, blood, or tracheobronchial aspirate. The duration of parenteral antimicrobial therapy is dependent upon the clinical course. Early intervention for empyema with video-assisted thoracoscopic surgery (VATS) or open surgical debridement decreases mortality and length of antimicrobial therapy compared with nonoperative treatment.[134]

Lung Abscess

Lung abscess can result as a complication of aspiration of infected material or a foreign body, can develop within a pre-existing infected site such as pneumonia, or can result from hematogenous seeding during *S. aureus* BSI and especially associated with thrombophlebitis. Lung abscess can be classified as primary or secondary, the latter referring to occurrence in children with an underlying condition. When bacteriology is proved for children with aspiration pneumonia, *S. aureus* can be recovered with or without facultative and anaerobic oral bacteria.[135,136]

Clinical features of *S. aureus* lung abscess include fever, cough, chest pain, dyspnea, anorexia, and weight loss.[135] CT helps determine the extent of disease and aids in following abscess resolution. Despite a dramatic appearance on radiograph, lung abscesses uncomplicated by pleural empyema usually can be treated adequately with intravenous antimicrobial therapy alone;[137] surgical drainage occasionally is required.[138] In these situations, percutaneous drainage is a well-established technique.[139-141]

Cardiovascular Infections

Endocarditis

S. aureus is the most common cause of infective endocarditis (IE).[142] IE develops when *S. aureus* BSI occurs in the setting of damaged cardiac endothelium, but also can affect previously normal valves and endothelium. IE occurs more frequently in patients with congenital heart disease, whether surgically repaired or not, compared with patients with structurally normal hearts.[143] Children whose cardiac lesions cause high-velocity blood flow or those with prosthetic valves or patches have increased risk of developing *S. aureus* IE.[144,145]

Fever, a new or changed heart murmur, and continuous BSI are the hallmarks of IE. Presentation can be indolent or acute; common complaints also include myalgia, arthralgia, general malaise, weight loss, and anorexia. Clinical progression can be rapid, with associated lethargy and cardiac failure, particularly when the aortic valve is involved. Right-sided endocarditis can be the source of emboli to the lungs, causing lung abscesses. Small-vessel embolic phenomena such as petechiae, splinter and conjunctival hemorrhages, and Janeway lesions are rarely manifest in children.[144]

The diagnosis is straightforward when echocardiography demonstrates a vegetation or abscess. However, this evidence may be lacking in children. A negative transthoracic or transesophageal echocardiogram does not exclude IE.[146,147] The modified Duke criteria have been used to identify children with IE based on major and minor clinical criteria (see Chapter 37, Endocarditis and Other Intravascular Infections).

Treatment requires 4 to 6 weeks of high-dose bactericidal antimicrobial therapy intravenously due to the relatively avascular nature of valves, high organism load, and decreased ability of polymorphonuclear leukocytes to function in endocarditis lesions. Guidelines for the therapy of *S. aureus* endocarditis, including consideration of combination therapy with aminoglycosides, can be found in Baddour et al.[148] and Chapter 37 (Endocarditis and Other Intravascular Infections). Fever may persist for about 1 week after antimicrobial therapy is initiated.[149] Sustained bacteremia spanning several days in usual. Serial blood cultures should be obtained until sterility is demonstrated. Occasionally, surgical intervention is necessary, particularly when embolic phenomena to major organs, intractable cardiac failure, or aortic insufficiency are documented, or when BSI persists despite appropriate antimicrobial therapy, particularly when a prosthetic valve or other foreign material is involved. Prosthetic valve endocarditis due to *S. aureus* has a high risk of mortality.[150,151]

Following cessation of therapy, close follow-up should be maintained because some patients can relapse and require definitive surgical intervention or removal of foreign material.

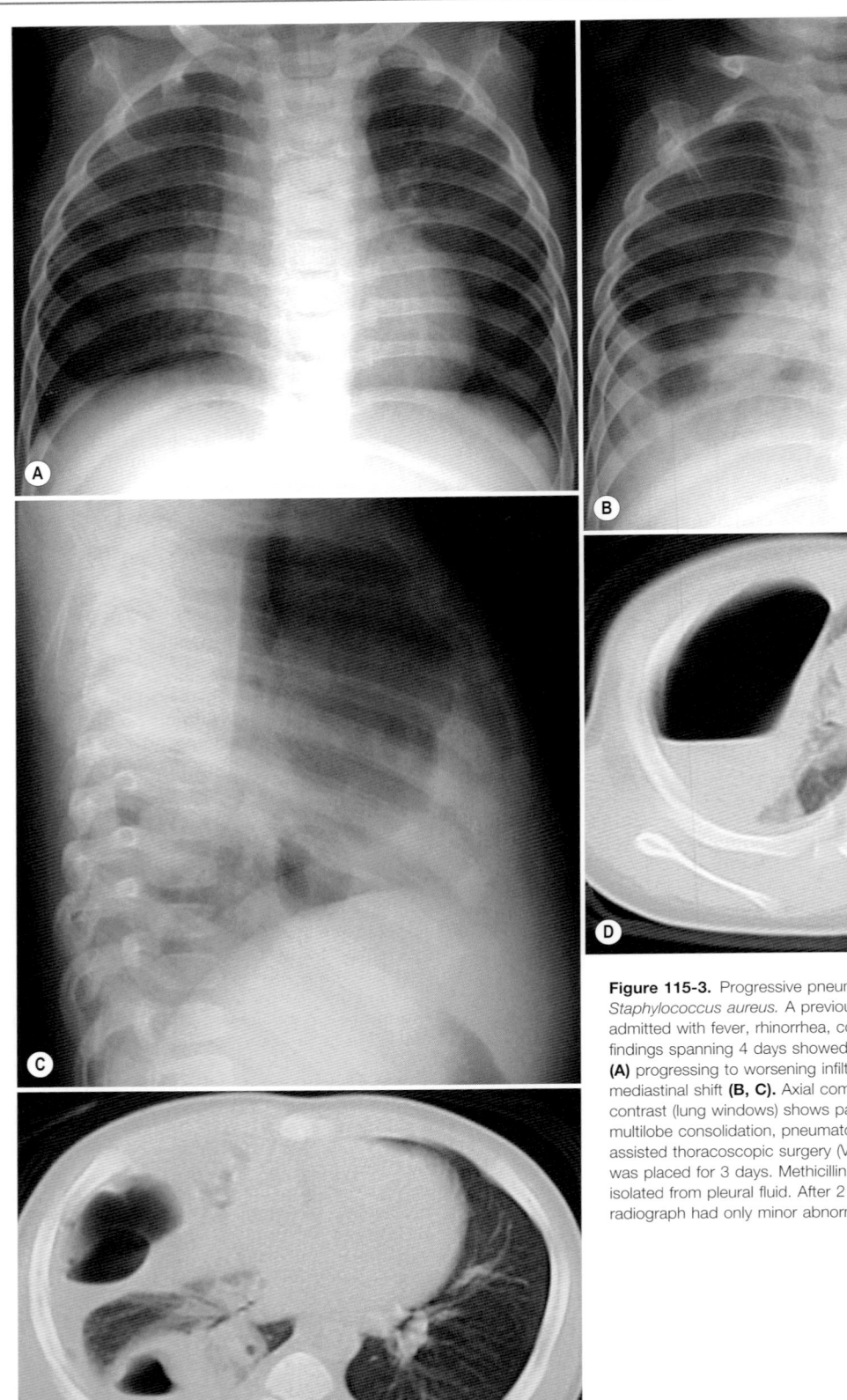

Figure 115-3. Progressive pneumonia with pneumatoceles due to *Staphylococcus aureus*. A previously healthy 9-month-old boy was admitted with fever, rhinorrhea, cough, and tachypnea. Chest radiographic findings spanning 4 days showed perihilar right lower lobe infiltrate **(A)** progressing to worsening infiltrate and large hydropneumothorax with mediastinal shift **(B, C)**. Axial computed tomography of the chest without contrast (lung windows) shows partial loculation of hydropneumothorax, multilobe consolidation, pneumatoceles, and atelectasis **(D, E)**. Video-assisted thoracoscopic surgery (VATS) was performed and a chest tube was placed for 3 days. Methicillin-resistant *Staphylococcus aureus* was isolated from pleural fluid. After 2 weeks of clindamycin therapy the chest radiograph had only minor abnormalities. (Courtesy of S.S. Long.)

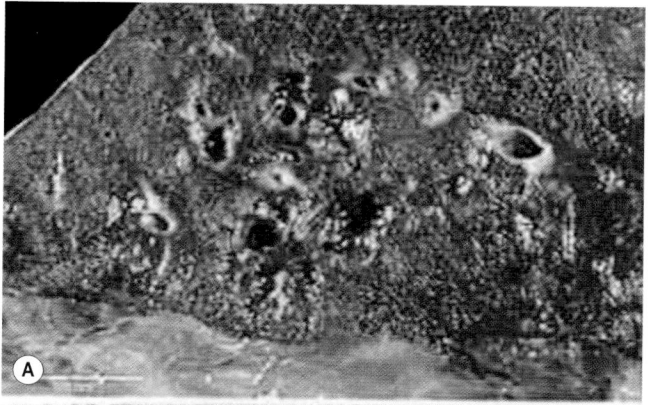

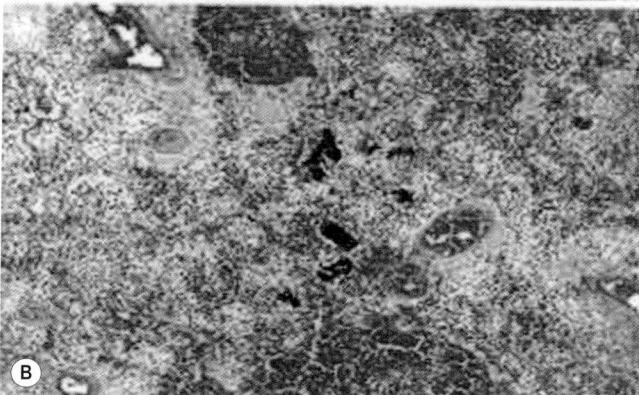

Figure 115-4. Pathology from a patient with fatal necrotizing pneumonia due to *Staphylococcus aureus* showing a gross specimen of lung with microabscesses **(A),** and histology of a section of lung with *S. aureus* colonies and hemorrhage **(B)** (hematoxylin and eosin). (From Adem PV et al. *Staphylococcus aureus* sepsis and the Waterhouse–Friderichsen syndrome in children. N Engl J Med 2005;353:1245–1251.)

Pericarditis

Bacterial pericarditis in children is a rare complication of *S. aureus* BSI or other focal, usually pleural, infection. Pericarditis should be suspected in any patient with BSI and cardiomegaly. Signs and symptoms of pericarditis include fever, dyspnea, cough, and precordial chest pain. The chest radiograph shows an enlarged heart; echocardiography demonstrates the presence of pericardial fluid. The diagnosis is made by examination of the pericardial fluid for the presence of inflammatory cells and bacteria. Management includes urgent pericardial decompression, closed or open pericardial drainage, and parenteral antimicrobial therapy.[152–154] Mortality is due to cardiac tamponade or the systemic inflammatory response syndrome; both complications are decreased by early medical and surgical treatment. Patients who develop constrictive pericarditis require pericardiectomy.

Suppurative Phlebitis and Septic Thrombophlebitis

Suppurative phlebitis and septic thrombophlebitis are serious endovascular infections that occur along a continuum of clinical severity, and most commonly are caused by *S. aureus*. Suppurative phlebitis usually occurs in a catheterized vessel wall and is characterized by a fluctuant, palpable vein that is warm, tender, and erythematous; pus may be expressed through the catheter or opening in the skin. Infection can progress to obstruction of the vessel or dissemination of infected thrombi to other sites or both. Treatment of suppurative phlebitis includes removal of a device, drainage or resection of the infected segment of the vessel, and intravenous antimicrobial therapy.

Septic thrombophlebitis also occurs in association with invasive *S. aureus* infection without catheterization of the infected vessel. The veins involved usually are major deep veins, especially pelvic or lower-extremity vessels, and commonly are adjacent to an area of osteomyelitis, pyogenic arthritis, or pyomyositis or other soft-tissue infection.[117] Long-term intravenous antibiotic therapy is warranted for this serious endovascular infection with attendant severe complications and mortality. Anticoagulant therapy and placement of an inferior vena cava filter have been considered when infected clots disperse septic emboli to the lungs.[155]

Central Nervous System Infections

Meningitis

S. aureus meningitis is increasing and can occur by several pathogenic mechanisms. Meningitis is an infrequent complication of BSI or endocarditis for reasons that are unknown. Meningitis can develop from extension of a parameningeal focus, including sinusitis, osteomyelitis of the skull bone, subdural empyema, epidural abscess, or rupture of a brain abscess into the lateral cerebral ventricles or the subarachnoid space. Congenital anomalies such as a dermal sinus or meningomyelocele can provide a portal of entry. Neurosurgical procedures are the most common cause of staphylococcal meningitis. Insertion of a cerebrospinal fluid (CSF) shunt is the most frequent predisposing procedure, although any neurosurgical procedure increases the risk for *S. aureus* meningitis.[156]

Treatment consists of parenteral antimicrobial therapy for 3 to 6 weeks, depending on the pathophysiology of the meningitis and removal of an indwelling device when present. Treatment of device-related infection is discussed below.

Brain Abscess

S. aureus brain abscess can result from direct extension of an adjacent infectious focus such as sinusitis,[103] mastoiditis, or otitis media, from inoculation of bacteria during a surgical procedure or as a consequence of trauma, or from seeding of the brain during bacteremia. Brain abscess more frequently complicates *S. aureus* BSI than BSI due to other pathogens[157,158] (see Chapter 46, Focal Suppurative Infections of the Nervous System). A *S. aureus* etiology should be considered especially when brain abscess complicates severe *S. aureus* BSI, a neurosurgical procedure or penetrating trauma. Cyanotic congenital heart disease also is a predisposing risk factor.[159]

Clinical features of brain abscess in children include headache, vomiting, irritability, focal neurologic defect, seizures, or other manifestations of increased intracranial pressure. The onset of symptoms can be insidious, depending on the pathophysiology; fever can be absent or low-grade. Findings on physical examination depend on the location of the abscess. Signs of meningitis are expected only if the abscess ruptures into a ventricle.

Radioimaging techniques are most often definitive in diagnosing brain abscess. Gadolinium-enhanced MRI is superior to CT, although both modalities are useful.[160] Principal advantages of MRI are discrimination of the central core of an abscess from a surrounding area of ring enhancement, identification of adjacent areas of cerebral edema, and for detection of abscesses in the posterior fossa.

Treatment consists of parenteral antimicrobial therapy and surgical drainage of the abscess, frequently by aspiration. Rarely, enucleation of the abscess is performed. Evolving abscesses in the non-necrotizing cerebritis stage and some small intracerebral abscesses can be treated with antimicrobial agents alone.[157] Corticosteroid therapy is limited to cases in which increased intracranial pressure is an important component. Patients typically are treated with antimicrobial agents parenterally for 6 weeks. Mortality associated with brain abscess is relatively low, but up to 60% of patients have neurologic sequelae, most commonly seizures.[161]

Spinal Epidural Abscess

S. aureus is the most common cause of spinal epidural abscess, which is a collection of purulent material external to the dura in the spinal canal, usually in the posterior aspect of the thoracic or lumbar vertebrae. Abscesses arise by seeding of the epidural space during BSI or by direct extension of an adjacent focus of infection such as pyomyositis or osteomyelitis. Complaints in children can be nonspecific and include fever, vomiting, lethargy, and irritability. With rare exception, spinal epidural abscess occurs among ambulatory children. There may be localized tenderness and refusal to lie prone. In older children, localized or radicular pain can be present. Paresis of limb muscles and loss of bowel or bladder control are specific and ominous signs as paralysis and loss of sensory modalities at levels below the affected area can ensue rapidly. History of a clinical illness compatible with bacteremia sometimes is elicited.[162]

Spinal epidural abscess must be distinguished from diskitis, extradural neoplasm, hematoma, disk herniation, and vertebral osteomyelitis. MRI is the diagnostic procedure of choice.[163] Lumbar puncture is deferred when this diagnosis is suspected. If performed, CSF findings are similar to those in other parameningeal infections, i.e., variable, modest pleocytosis, normal glucose, and modestly increased protein concentration.

Therapy includes immediate surgical decompression, debridement of the epidural space, and parenteral antimicrobial therapy, which generally is administered for 6 weeks.[164] Medical management alone is rarely considered in immunocompetent patients with a normal or stable neurologic examination, without signs of septicemia. Continuous reassessment is necessary to identify progressive pain or onset of any neurologic abnormality that necessitates urgent surgery.[165]

Device-Related Infections

Indwelling Vascular Catheters

Staphylococci are the most common causes of catheter-associated infections. For peripheral venous catheters, *S. aureus* is the most common infecting species, and for central venous catheters (CVCs), coagulase-negative staphylococci are recovered more commonly. Cutaneous colonization at the insertion site is the most important predictor of catheter-associated infections related to short-term, percutaneously inserted catheters. For surgically implanted CVCs, organisms introduced through the hub and lumen are the most important source of infection.

Local redness, pain, and warmth at the site of a simple peripheral catheter suggest local phlebitis, which is managed by removal of the device. Diagnosing central-line-associated BSI (CLABSI) can be more difficult. Fever and the presence of pain, fluctuance, erythema, purulence or soft-tissue infection at the site suggest CLABSI. Most often, however, the catheter entrance site appears normal.

Blood for culture is taken via the catheter; positive culture can represent CLABSI or BSI from another source. Isolation of *S. aureus* should not be regarded as a procedural contaminant. Repeated sampling and blood drawn simultaneously by venipuncture often helps to resolve the issue. Semiquantitative culture of the catheter tip following removal can implicate the catheter as the infectious nidus when the colony count is >15 colonies; a negative culture of the catheter tip does not exclude CLABSI.

S. aureus exit-site infections, whether in the presence of a tunnel track infection or BSI, are managed by removing the catheter and administering antimicrobial therapy. Because of the propensity of *S. aureus* BSI to persist and to cause clinical sepsis or to seed the endocardium, abdominal viscera, brain, lung, or bone, most experts recommend removal of an intravascular catheter when *S. aureus* infection is documented, even in the absence of an exit-site infection.

Vancomycin is the preferred empiric therapy for suspected *S. aureus* catheter-associated infection. Use of combination bactericidal therapy and an extended course of antimicrobial therapy (e.g., 4–6 weeks) frequently is recommended because of the known tendency of *S. aureus* BSI to seed and form abscesses at multiple sites. This point is controversial because of the lack of specific data (see Chapter 102, Clinical Syndromes of Device-Associated Infections). Careful, clean, and consistent techniques for handling catheters, such as skin disinfection, e.g., with chlorhexidine, aseptic technique of placement, and dedicated teams for ongoing catheter care, are among the measures shown to decrease the infection rate.

CSF Shunt Devices

A contaminated CSF shunt or subcutaneous reservoir device is the most common predisposing cause of staphylococcal meningitis.[156] Presumably *S. aureus* gains access to the catheter during surgical insertion, although the device and CSF can be seeded from subsequent adjacent primary SSTI, tract infection or during BSI – the presence of the catheter increasing the likelihood that the organism will survive and multiply.

Most CSF shunt infections occur within 2 months of shunt placement or revision. Low-grade fever and dysfunction of the shunt are variably present. For ventriculoperitoneal (VP) shunts, symptoms and signs attributable to peritonitis can be present commonly.[166,167] If surgery was recent, a wound infection may be evident. First-episode *S. aureus* shunt infection is positively predictive of a subsequent *S. aureus* shunt infection.[168]

Examination of the CSF (typically obtained by percutaneous puncture of the shunt reservoir/tubing) may reveal only mild abnormalities, e.g., modest pleocytosis, normal glucose, and normal or minimally elevated protein concentration. Microorganisms infrequently are visualized on Gram stain. Culture of CSF is the most sensitive test. CSF obtained by lumbar puncture frequently is not diagnostic of a VP shunt infection.

Most experts recommend combined medical and surgical treatment for CSF shunt infections. Typically, a temporary external ventricular drain is used while intravenous antimicrobial therapy is administered until the CSF is sterile and inflammation subsides, at which time a new CSF shunt can be placed.[169,170] Timing of this procedure is important. Insertion of the new catheter into an infected field must be avoided. However, maintaining an externalized catheter as a drainage device carries its own risk of infection, which accelerates after 5 to 7 days of use.

Toxin-Mediated Syndromes

Staphylococcal Food Poisoning

Staphylococcal food poisoning is caused by ingestion of *S. aureus* enterotoxins and accounts for up to one-third of foodborne gastrointestinal illnesses (see Chapter 61, Enteric Diseases Transmitted Through Food, Water, and Zoonotic Exposures). Protein-rich foods such as ham and chicken often are implicated as the outbreak source, as are dairy products, egg and potato salad. The individual who is responsible for inadvertently inoculating the food with *S. aureus* may have a clinical infection but usually is colonized asymptomatically.[171,172]

Illness begins shortly after consumption (at average, 4 hours) because ingestion of preformed toxin is responsible for the clinical manifestation. Classic symptoms are nausea, vomiting, abdominal pain, and diarrhea; headache and prostration ensue less commonly. Fever occurs in about 25% of patients. Hospitalization is required infrequently, and death occurs rarely.

S. aureus can be isolated from the vomitus or feces of ill people. Culture of the contaminated food may yield the offending organism. Therapy is supportive; antibiotics are not useful. The syndrome can be prevented by proper handling of food and careful hygiene practices of food handlers. When cases are recognized, the Department of Public Health must be notified.

Staphylococcal Scalded-Skin Syndrome (SSSS)

SSSS is an illness mediated by ETA and ETB.[89,90] Hematogenous spread of the toxins produces fever and widespread erythema of the skin that can be tender and quickly forms thin-walled, fluid-containing bullae that rupture, leaving a moist base of skin. Gentle friction applied to the skin produces Nikolsky sign, a sloughing of superficial sheets of skin (see Figure 13-2). Desquamation eventually follows.[173,174]

SSSS is diagnosed clinically or by isolation of *S. aureus* from a local site, ideally with demonstration by the isolate of toxin production or the toxin gene. Histologic evaluation of skin reveals separation of skin layers at the granular layer within the epidermis as opposed to the separation between the dermis and epidermis that is seen in drug-induced toxic epidermal necrolysis.[175]

Management of SSSS is primarily supportive with careful attention to electrolyte levels, as fluid shifts can occur across the denuded skin. Antiseptic measures should be taken to prevent infection of the unprotected, affected areas. Parenteral antimicrobial therapy is administered to decrease the staphylococcal burden. Topical antimicrobial agents are not helpful.[175]

Toxic Shock Syndrome

TSS is caused by *S. aureus* strains producing TSST-1 or certain enterotoxins (specifically SEB and SEC)[176] and is characterized by fever, rash, hypotension, and multisystem organ dysfunction[177]

BOX 115-1. Staphylococcal Toxic Shock Syndrome: Clinical Case Definition

An illness with the following clinical manifestations:
- Fever: temperature >38.9°C (102°F)
- Rash: diffuse macular erythroderma
- Desquamation: 1–2 weeks after onset of illness, particularly palms and soles
- Hypotension: systolic blood pressure ≥90 mmHg for adults or less than 5th percentile by age for children <16 years of age; orthostatic drop in diastolic blood pressure ≥15 mmHg from lying to sitting, orthostatic syncope, or orthostatic dizziness
- Multisystem involvement: ≥3 of the following:
  1. Gastrointestinal: vomiting or diarrhea at onset of illness
  2. Muscular: severe myalgia or creatine phosphokinase level ≥2× the upper limit of normal for laboratory
  3. Mucous membrane: vaginal, oropharyngeal, or conjunctival hyperemia
  4. Renal: blood urea nitrogen or creatinine ≥2× the upper limit of normal for laboratory or urinary sediment with pyuria (≥5 leukocytes per high-power field) in the absence of urinary tract infection
  5. Hepatic: total bilirubin, serum glutamic-oxaloacetic transaminase (SGOT), or serum alanine aminotransferase (ALT) or aspartate aminotransferase (AST) ≥2× the upper limit of normal for laboratory
  6. Hematologic: platelets <100,000/mm³
  7. Central nervous system: disorientation or alteration in consciousness without focal neurologic signs when fever and hypotension are absent
- Negative results on the following tests, if obtained:
  1. Blood, throat, or cerebrospinal fluid cultures (for all microorganisms except *Staphylococcus aureus*)
  2. Rise in antibody titer to *Rickettsia* or *Leptospira* species or rubeola

CASE CLASSIFICATION

Probable: a case with 5 of the 6 clinical findings described above
Confirmed: a case with all 6 clinical findings described above, including desquamation, unless the patient dies before desquamation could occur

Modified from Wharton M, Chorba TL, Vogt RL, et al. Case definitions for public health surveillance. MMWR Recomm Rep 1990;39:1–43.

(Box 115-1). The incidence of TSS peaked in the early 1980s; this was attributed to the use of superabsorbent tampons by menstruating women.[178] Subsequent public education and manufacturing regulations helped decrease the number of TSS cases, and now nonmenstrual TSS accounts for approximately half of all TSS cases.[179]

Risk factors for TSS include colonization of the skin with disruption of its integrity, colonization of mucous membranes, or any infection with a toxin-producing strain of *S. aureus*. TSS is often associated with surgery or trauma, manifesting several days after the event. The sudden onset of fever, chills, headache, vomiting, sore throat, myalgia, and diarrhea is followed by hypotension, respiratory distress, edema, and rash within 24 to 48 hours. Dizziness, listlessness, or disorientation are clues to hypotension; mental status changes can progress to coma.

The initial *S. aureus* focus can be without signs of inflammation or purulence. The rash can appear initially like that of scarlet fever, but classically is described as diffuse erythroderma, or "sunburn." The rash typically desquamates 1 to 2 weeks after onset of illness, most notably on the palms and soles.

Mucous membrane involvement includes conjunctival hyperemia, strawberry tongue, beefy red oropharyngeal membranes (sometimes with ulcerations), and lesions representing reactivation of herpes simplex virus.

A vaginal culture yields the organism in 85% of menstrual TSS cases. In nonmenstrual TSS cases, a nasopharyngeal or a wound culture may yield *S. aureus*; a blood culture should be obtained (to diagnose concurrent BSI) but is seldom positive.

Management consists of treating intravascular volume depletion, shock, and respiratory failure as well as the *S. aureus* infection. Any relevant focus of infection should be drained and any foreign body removed if possible. Intravenous antimicrobial therapy including an antibiotic that inhibits protein synthesis (such as clindamycin) may be preferable. The response to effective therapy can be rapid. When a patient does not respond to these interventions, immune globulin intravenous (IGIV) is recommended by most experts, based on presence of antibody to staphylococcal enterotoxins and TSST-1.[180,181] End-organ failure, particularly renal failure and the acute respiratory distress syndrome, can occur within the first few days of illness and is responsible for the attendant 3% mortality rate.

Severe Sepsis Syndrome

Severe sepsis syndrome (SSS) is defined as isolation of *S. aureus* from a clinically important site, hypotension (systolic blood pressure <5th percentile for age for children or less than 90 mmHg for adults), and respiratory distress syndrome or respiratory failure as well as involvement of the central nervous system, liver, kidneys, muscles, or skin or abnormal hemostasis, or the presence of leukopenia or thrombocytopenia. SSS is similar to TSS but does not fulfill all the clinical criteria and the *S. aureus* isolates do not produce TSST-1.[80]

S. aureus SSS classically occurs as an HAI, or as a community-associated infection in immunocompromised people with identifiable risk factors such as certain underlying medical conditions or intravenous drug abuse. Increasingly SSS occurs in children and adolescents with no underlying medical conditions or other identifiable risk factors.[80,182–184] Both MSSA and MRSA are implicated; genes encoding PVL frequently are identified in the infecting strain.

A primary infectious process such as pyogenic arthritis or pneumonia often is identified prior to clinical deterioration. However, patients can have overwhelming infection and subsequent rapid decline without a primary site of infection.[80,182,183] Skin lesions are common and manifest as erythroderma, pustules, petechiae, and/or purpura. *S. aureus* sepsis associated with the Waterhouse–Friderichsen syndrome,[185] staphylococcal purpura fulminans,[186] and necrotizing fasciitis has been reported.[187]

The diagnosis is made by isolation of *S. aureus* from a clinically important site such as the blood, a joint space, or respiratory secretions with concomitant systemic illness. A high index of suspicion is critical to instituting appropriate parenteral antimicrobial therapy and aggressive cardiopulmonary support. Mortality rates based on reviews of case reports approach 64%.[182]

MANAGEMENT

Invasive *S. aureus* infections have high mortality and morbidity. Treatment should be rapid and aggressive. Intravenous antimicrobial therapy should be initiated promptly to clear BSI and/or infected sites. The source of BSI and sites of possible metastatic infection should be sought aggressively. Drainage of abscesses and removal of CVCs or other foreign bodies should be performed when possible. Associated endocarditis or other endovascular infections always should be considered in patients with *S. aureus* BSI because this organism has a tropism for endothelial cells, and PVL-gene containing organisms have the propensity to cause thrombosis and thromboembolism.[117,188,189]

If rapid improvement does not occur or BSI continues after >24 hours of therapy, the therapeutic approach should be carefully re-evaluated because irreversible organ damage can progress rapidly. Once the antimicrobial susceptibility of the organism is known, therapy should be tailored to use the appropriate antimicrobial agent(s) with the narrowest appropriate spectrum of activity.

The CA-MRSA epidemic has refocused attention on the importance of adjunctive local treatments such as incision and drainage.[190] For many purulent skin and soft-tissue infections, incision and drainage may suffice. Guidelines for management using antibiotics and drainage are published.[97,191] Because susceptibility to β-lactam antibiotics cannot be assumed, obtaining a specimen for culture is essential in patients for whom antibiotic treatment is deemed necessary in order to further guide therapy.[190,192]

Antistaphylococcal Agents

The compounds below are considered further in Chapter 292 (Antimicrobial Agents).

β-Lactam Antibiotics

Previously, β-lactam antibiotics, particularly semisynthetic penicillins (nafcillin, oxacillin, cloxacillin, and dicloxacillin), were the gold standard for treatment of staphylococcal infections, particularly when the infection was acquired in the community. These agents inhibit cell wall synthesis and, thus, are bactericidal. They are relatively resistant to β-lactamase, well tolerated, and have a long record of therapeutic success. When an MSSA strain is isolated, β-lactams are drugs of choice for serious staphylococcal infections. Appropriate compounds are available for both intravenous and oral administration. Parenteral compounds in wide use in the U.S. include oxacillin and nafcillin; dicloxacillin is available for oral use although some children find the taste of the suspension unpleasant.

The β-lactam plus β-lactamase inhibitor combinations (ampicillin-sulbactam, amoxicillin-clavulanate, ticarcillin-clavulanate, and piperacillin-tazobactam) are active against MSSA but offer no advantage over the semisynthetic penicillins. The β-lactamase inhibitor is not a useful adjunct to the β-lactam compound against MRSA strains. So-called first-generation cephalosporins have antistaphylococcal activity superior to that of other generations of cephalosporin agents. Cefazolin for parenteral administration and cephalexin for oral administration are useful class compound examples, with similar efficacy to semisynthetic penicillins for treatment of non-life-threatening MSSA infections.

No currently available β-lactam antibiotic or cephalosporin has been useful for the therapy of MRSA infections until licensure of ceftaroline in 2010 for community-acquired pneumonia and complicated skin and soft-tissue infections. This compound, designated a fifth-generation cephalosporin, has activity against MRSA strains and broad-spectrum activity against many gram-positive and gram-negative bacteria. There is no reported evaluation for use in children.[193]

Clindamycin

Clindamycin is a lincosamide agent that inhibits protein synthesis at the chain elongation step by interfering with transpeptidation of the 50S ribosomal subunit. Most HA-MRSA isolates are resistant to clindamycin, but the majority of CA-MRSA isolates are susceptible,[190] particularly in children.[59,76,96,194,195] Despite its increasingly frequent use in treating CA-MRSA infections, clindamycin has not yet been licensed by the U.S. Food and Drug Administration for this purpose.

An important issue concerning clindamycin treatment is the risk of treatment failure if infection is caused by erythromycin-resistant *S. aureus* with the potential for selecting for clindamycin resistance. Erythromycin ribosomal methylase *(erm)* gene codes for the enzyme that modifies the binding site not only for macrolides but also for lincosamides and streptogramin B antibiotics. Thus, cross-resistance to these three classes of antibiotics, the so-called macrolide-lincosamide-streptogramin B (MLS$_B$) phenotype, is common among *S. aureus* isolates.[196] Phenotypic expression of the MLS$_B$ phenotype can be constitutive or inducible. When constitutive, the isolate tests as resistant to all MLS$_B$ antibiotics and the clinical microbiology laboratory will report the isolate as resistant to clindamycin. When inducible, however, the isolate will test as resistant to erythromycin and susceptible to clindamycin. Such an isolate can be induced to become resistant to lincosamides and streptogramin B antibiotics in the presence of a strong inducer of methylase synthesis, such as erythromycin. In this instance, the constitutive MLS$_B$ phenotype could be selected during clindamycin therapy.

The detection of erythromycin-inducible clindamycin resistance can be accomplished by the disk diffusion D-test[197] (see Chapter 290, Mechanisms and Detection of Antibiotic Resistance, and Figure 290-4). To date, although, the incidence of erythromycin resistance among CA-MRSA isolates is high, the incidence of clindamycin resistance is not.[190] If an MRSA isolate is D-test positive, clinicians should be aware that clindamycin treatment failure is possible, although it is unclear how frequently such failure occurs. The D-test should be performed on all CA-MRSA isolates with discordant erythromycin/clindamycin susceptibility, as recommended in 2004 by the Clinical and Laboratory Standards Institute.[197,198]

Clindamycin also is a potent suppressor of bacterial toxin synthesis. Clindamycin therapy may be clinically superior in toxin-mediated staphylococcal syndromes, although explicit data are lacking. When clindamycin is used in this setting, combination therapy with oxacillin or nafcillin (in areas with low prevalence of CA-MRSA infection) or with vancomycin is frequently used.

Clindamycin is bacteriostatic and does not cross the blood–brain barrier; clindamycin is not used alone in the treatment of endocarditis or other intravascular or CNS infections that can occur during *S. aureus* invasive infection. Poor taste of clindamycin can hamper adherence to oral therapy in children.

Clindamycin resistance rates among *S. aureus* isolates should be monitored locally. (In some areas rates of clindamycin resistance of MSSA can exceed those of MRSA). In areas where clindamycin resistance rates exceed 10% to 15% among *S. aureus* isolates, empiric therapy with this agent probably should be avoided. Several centers have documented increasing rates of resistance of CA-MRSA isolates to clindamycin.[199–201]

Vancomycin

Vancomycin is a glycopeptide that inhibits synthesis and assembly of the second stage of cell wall peptidoglycan of gram-positive bacteria. It is the therapeutic agent of choice for HA-MRSA infections. However, the emergence of VISA and VRSA isolates as well as decreased susceptibility (so-called MIC creep) has the potential to limit the effectiveness of vancomycin.[202–204] Some experts recommend use of higher doses to elicit higher serum trough levels of vancomycin but the effectiveness of these strategies is controversial.[97]

Vancomycin should be considered for children with suspected serious CA-MRSA infections, such as SSTIs with systemic manifestations requiring hospitalization, severe sepsis, TSS, central nervous system infection, necrotizing pneumonia, and necrotizing fasciitis. Considerations for empiric use for osteo-articular infections include the local prevalence of CA-MRSA, degree of illness, site of infection, and adequacy of culture specimens obtained to guide therapy.

Because vancomycin is less bactericidal than oxacillin or nafcillin for MSSA and can result in treatment failure or relapse, vancomycin should not be used for therapy of MSSA infection unless necessary, e.g., type 1 allergic reaction to β-lactam agents. In severely ill patients, semisynthetic penicillin frequently is given in addition to vancomycin pending culture and susceptibility test results. Vancomycin is only available in intravenous form for use in the therapy of *S. aureus* infections, and obtains poor concentration in the alveolar space. Oral vancomycin is not absorbed.

Linezolid

Linezolid is an oxazolidinone that inhibits protein synthesis by binding to the 50S ribosomal subunit during the formation of the initiation complex.[205] Linezolid has broad in vitro activity against MRSA, GISA, VISA, and VRSA isolates. Linezolid is well tolerated and is as effective as vancomycin in children with SSTIs and pneumonia caused by MRSA.[206–208] The oral bioavailability of linezolid is almost 100%, which facilitates transition from intravenous to oral therapy.

Linezolid is bacteriostatic against *S. aureus* and is not preferred for use in the treatment of endocarditis or other intravascular infections. Linezolid should be avoided if possible in patients taking adrenergic or serotonergic agents.[209] Linezolid is associated with development of thrombocytopenia (which can be idiosyncratic and severe), anemia, and neutropenia.[210] Complete blood count should be monitored in patients receiving therapy for longer than 2 weeks, those with underlying myelosuppression, or those taking other drugs that cause bone marrow suppression. A small number of cases of optic and peripheral neuropathy and lactic acidosis have been reported in adults during prolonged courses of therapy.

Resistance to linezolid has occurred in isolates from patients receiving long-term therapy with this agent. Resistant isolates have mutations in the 23S rRNA gene in the domain V region, of which *S. aureus* has five copies.[211,212] A mutation in ≥2 of the rRNA genes is required for the resistant phenotype.

More recently, additional resistance mechanisms have been identified in ribosomal proteins L4 and L3. More recently, plasmid-borne *cfr* genes have been identified that encode a methyltransferase that mediates linezolid resistance by methylatian of carbon-8 on the 23S rRNA base. *Cfr* genes confer cross-resistance to phenicols, lincosamides, pleuromutilins, and streptogramin A antibiotics.[213]

Linezolid is available in both intravenous and oral forms. There is a convenient pediatric suspension. The compound is extremely expensive, and negotiation with some third-party payers may be required for each use. Patients also can experience delays in procuring linezolid from private pharmacies as it often is not stocked routinely.

Trimethoprim-Sulfamethoxazole (TMP-SMX)

TMP-SMX interferes with the biosynthesis of tetrahydrofolic acid essential for microbial synthesis of proteins and nucleotides. Although most *S. aureus* isolates are susceptible in vitro, TMP-SMX was seldom used to treat *S. aureus* infections until the recent epidemic of CA-MRSA. There is minimal published clinical experience using TMP-SMX to treat CA-MRSA SSTIs (especially without surgical drainage of purulent lesions),[190] or more severe *S. aureus* infections. Moreover, if group A streptococcal infection is a possible etiology for the SSTI, TMP-SMX is a suboptimal choice. For ambulatory management of CA-MRSA infections, available data suggest that use of TMP-SMX requires careful follow-up as modified therapy may become necessary.[214] For treatment of invasive *S. aureus* infection, data show intravenous TMP-SMX to be inferior to vancomycin for MSSA and only equivalent to vancomycin for MRSA. (These data were obtained prior to the CA-MRSA era.[215]) The observation that thymidine can be released from injured tissue or bacteria has suggested a possible explanation for discordant in vitro and clinical outcomes.[216] Additional information is needed to establish the appropriate role for TMP-SMX in the anti-*S. aureus* armamentarium.

Tetracyclines (including Tigecycline)

Tetracyclines inhibit bacterial protein synthesis by binding to the 30S ribosomal subunit, thus blocking the attachment of the transfer RNA-amino acid to the ribosome. Tetracyclines have not been used widely for *S. aureus* infections, but with the advent of the CA-MRSA epidemic, tetracyclines such as doxycycline or minocycline have emerged as alternative oral antimicrobial agents for mildly to moderately ill patients with SSTIs. The majority of isolates are susceptible in vitro.[190,217] Tigecycline, a novel glycylcycline, recently licensed for parenteral use, has potent activity against *S. aureus* in vitro regardless of methicillin or vancomycin susceptibility.[218,219]

However, the U.S. Food and Drug Administration (FDA) issued a warning on September 1, 2010 linking tigecycline to increased mortality risk in patients being treated for HAP and CAP, complicated intra-abdominal infections, and complicated SSTIs, suggesting that tigecycline should be avoided for treatment of *S. aureus* infections.

All tetracyclines are bacteriostatic and should not be used for treatment of endocarditis, other intravascular or CNS infections. Tetracyclines also should be avoided when treating pregnant women or children <8 years of age because of concern regarding mottling of bones and teeth. Some tetracyclines are available in oral forms. Doxycycline and minocycline sometimes are recommended as useful oral agents for ambulatory management of CA-MRSA infections, although few explicit data are available to document efficacy.

Quinupristin-Dalfopristin

Synercid™ is a combination of two streptogramin antibiotics, one each from groups B (quinupristin) and A (dalfopristin) in a 30 : 70 ratio. Quinupristin-dalfopristin has good in vitro activity against *S. aureus*, including MRSA. The two streptogramins bind to sequential sites on the 50S ribosomal subunit, and have synergistic bactericidal effect resulting from inhibition of protein synthesis.[220] Recent trials have shown a lower bacteriologic success rate compared with standard therapy.[221] Quinupristin-dalfopristin is not cross-resistant to *S. aureus* isolates with MLS$_B$ resistance because the streptogramin A component remains active. Few data are available to ensure the clinical validity of this issue, however. Quinupristin-dalfopristin is available in an intravenous form only and has had minimal evaluation in children. Infusion site inflammation, thrombophlebitis, arthralgias, drug–drug interactions, myalgias, gastrointestinal toxic effects, and increased serum unconjugated bilirubin concentrations limit the widespread use of quinopristin-dalfopristin for the therapy of *S. aureus* infections.

Daptomycin

Daptomycin is a novel cyclic lipopeptide whose mechanism of action is not completely understood. It appears to bind to the gram-positive bacterial cell membrane, followed by calcium-dependent insertion[222] that results in a decrease in membrane potential, causing cell death by rapidly stopping DNA, RNA, and protein synthesis. It has potent bactericidal activity against MRSA.[223] Daptomycin was comparable with vancomycin in the treatment of complicated SSTIs,[224] but showed decreased effectiveness for treatment of CAP compared with standard treatment probably because of its propensity for binding surfactant.[225] Daptomycin is licensed by the U.S. FDA for the treatment of complicated SSTIs, BSI, and right-sided endocarditis; it is not, however, approved for the treatment of left-sided endocarditis.[226] Daptomycin is available in intravenous form only. Studies evaluating it for use in children are underway. Where the cell wall is thickened, e.g., in a VISA isolate or after exposure of a *S. aureus* isolate to vancomycin, resistance to daptomycin becomes evident, presumably because the compound cannot reach its cell membrane target.[227,228] Resistance to daptomycin can occur during therapy and was documented in 6 of 120 patients receiving daptomycin for endocarditis, or BSI.[229]

Telavancin

Telavancin is a lipoglycopeptide, licensed in 2009 for treatment of complicated SSTIs. The compound depolarizes bacterial membranes and also inhibits cell wall formation. It has received no formal evaluation in children. Drug is administered once daily. Telavancin can cause or worsen renal dysfunction and can be associated, like vancomycin, with the red man syndrome.

Rifampin

Rifampin is a bactericidal agent that blocks protein synthesis by inhibiting RNA polymerase, and is highly active against almost all *S. aureus* isolates. Resistance, however, emerges rapidly when rifampin is used as monotherapy. Combination regimens using rifampin with clindamycin, TMP-SMX, or doxycycline sometimes are recommended for the treatment of CA-MRSA infections, or for treating device- or prosthesis-associated *S. aureus* infections. It is unclear whether such combination regimens are more effective. Rifampin is available in both oral and intravenous forms, although a suspension suitable for use in young children is not available.

Aminoglycosides

Aminoglycosides such as gentamicin are potent bactericidal inhibitors of protein synthesis. Aminoglycosides alone are believed to be poorly efficacious against *S. aureus* infections. Aminoglycosides are synergistic with β-lactam antibiotics and vancomycin in vitro, and are commonly used in combination therapy for severe infections such as endocarditis. It is controversial whether such combination therapy offers a clinical advantage.

Empiric Therapy for Community-Associated Infections

It is impossible to distinguish between CA-MSSA and CA-MRSA infections on clinical grounds.[191] Clinicians must be aware of the frequency of CA-MRSA in their respective communities. In areas where the CA-MRSA disease burden is high (for example >10% of all *S. aureus* isolates), empiric β-lactam therapy is not appropriate. Figure 115-5 suggests an approach to the management of community-associated staphylococcal infections when CA-MRSA is among the likely etiologies. Therapy should be adjusted according to in vitro test results. A National Institutes of Health-sponsored study is underway that is addressing the optimal oral therapy of *S. aureus* skin and soft-tissue infections for outpatients.

Empiric Therapy for MRSA Infections Requiring Hospitalization

Vancomycin is indicated for empiric therapy of putative *S. aureus* infections when the patient is severely ill.[97,230] VISA isolates have been identified that are associated with vancomycin treatment

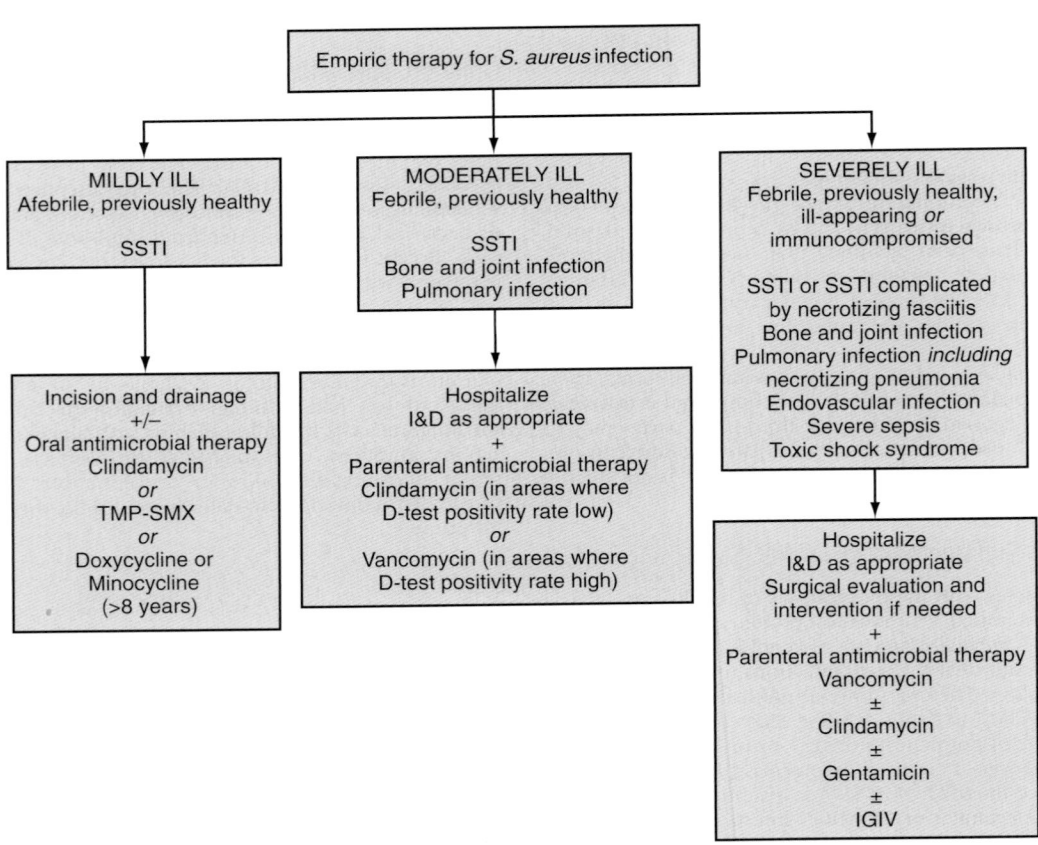

Figure 115-5. Schema for the empiric treatment of community-associated *Staphylococcus aureus* infections, determined by severity of illness. SSTI, skin and soft-tissue infection; I&D, incision and drainage; IGIV, immune globulin for intravenous use.

failure.[231,232] The Clinical and Laboratory Standards Institute defines VISA an MIC of vancomycin >2 μg/mL. In 2002, the CDC reported the first documented infection caused by *S. aureus* with high-level resistance (MIC >16 μg/mL) to vancomycin (VRSA); 10 additional VRSA strains have been isolated since.[86-88,233,234] VISA and VRSA isolates probably occur more frequently than documented because optimal tests to detect decreased vancomycin susceptibility often are not performed in clinical laboratories.[235]

Information about parenteral therapy with clindamycin, daptomycin, tigecycline, linezolid, telavancin and other agents useful in the therapy of MRSA infections in hospitalized children may be found in Chapter 292, Antimicrobial Agents. Guidelines from the Infectious Diseases Society of America also are available.[97]

PREVENTION

Efforts to prevent *S. aureus* HAIs have included general measures such as improved hand hygiene and attention to careful implementation of measures aimed at diminishing infections associated with intravascular catheters.[236] Other efforts specifically have been aimed at decreasing infections caused by *S. aureus*, usually focused on MRSA, and have included early identification of MRSA carriers, with isolation and cohorting of asymptomatically colonized patients. Patients presumed to have an MRSA infection often (but not universally) are cared for with contact precautions. Legislation in some states has mandated screening for MRSA transmission upon admission to the hospital or, in some cases, to an intensive care unit. Problems with such a screening approach have included the high cost of the program, concern about an overly intense focus on a single HA pathogen (thereby diminishing focus on other important pathogen), lack of agreement as to the best way to ascertain MRSA carriage, and lack of knowledge about the best approach to dealing with colonization when found. An additional concern is the relatively small impact of an effective institution-based strategy since most MRSA infections have onset in the community. Indeed, many institutions have achieved success at diminishing HA-*S. aureus* transmission only to find an increase in MRSA rate because of the impact of CA-MRSA disease.[236]

In the community setting, some sports teams have increased efforts to schedule equipment washing, discourage towel sharing, restrict infected members from play until lesions are healed, and encourage good hygiene among team members.[237,238] Several correctional facilities are increasing access to soap and water, improving laundry facilities, and improving attention to skin lesions to prevent the spread of CA-MRSA, as recommended by the Federal Bureau of Prisons.[71] The use of chlorhexidine-impregnated cloths to prevent skin and soft-tissue infections among military recruits was not successful.[239]

Attempted eradication of colonization by MRSA has been employed as a strategy to prevent recurrent disease and, possibly, to control outbreaks. MRSA decolonization has been attempted in outbreak situations but few randomized controlled trials have evaluated the efficacy of topical antibiotics and skin antisepsis in the eradication of *S. aureus* carriage.[98,240-243] Intranasal mupirocin ointment appears to have the most success in decreasing previous HA-MRSA nasal colonization with a subsequent decrease in carriage at other body sites. A 5-day application of intranasal mupirocin showed decreased short-term rates of colonization; however, recolonization occurred in at least one-half of the treated subjects, usually within a few months.[98] Unacceptably high recolonization rates, concern about mupirocin resistance,[244,245] and limited data regarding its effectiveness against CA-MRSA preclude recommendation for routine use.

Vaccine Development

It is controversial whether *S. aureus* infections can be prevented by vaccination and, if so, whether such a vaccine should be deployed universally or targeted to high-risk groups. A rigorous approach to vaccine development that considers the relevant vaccine antigens and the relevant immune responses and clinical endpoints will be required.

Much effort to date has been to identify the "protective" antigens. Many experts feel that more than one antigen will be required in the ideal vaccine because of the redundancy of many aspects of *S. aureus* pathogenicity. The traditional idea that production of opsonophagocytic antibody will be correlated with protection has been challenged with available data. In two vaccine trials of types 5 and 8 polysaccharide conjugate vaccine, immunization failed to provide protection against BSI.[246]

A protein vaccine containing an iron-scavenging, cell wall anchored protein, isdB, is currently in a phase II clinical trial. Potential enrollees are adults undergoing elective cardiac surgery that requires a sternotomy. The clinical endpoint is the occurrence of *S. aureus* mediastinitis. Enrollment is ongoing as of the spring of 2011.

Attempts to protect neonates passively with Veronate™, a high titer anti-clumping factor A polyclonal antibody product, appeared promising in an initial trial. However, a confirmatory trial suggested that this approach was not efficacious.[247] A clinical trial with a monoclonal antibody directed against lipoteichoic acid, pagibaximab, has been conducted among small premature infants aimed at preventing infections caused by *S. aureus* and coagulase-negative staphylococci. Enrollment was completed in November 2010 and data analysis is expected in 2011.

Recent attention has focused on the role of the Th17/IL-17 lymphocyte pathway.[248] One candidate vaccine, rAls3p-N, was derived from a *Candida* adhesin and protected mice against bacteremic challenge. Of great interest is that the efficacy of the vaccine was retained in B-cell deficient mice but not T-cell deficient mice. Further, adoptive transfer of CD4+ but not B220+ lymphocytes transferred immunity. The vaccine apparently stimulates proinflammatory Th1, Th17, and Th1/Th17 lymphocytes. These cytokines enhance neutrophil recruitment and activation.

116 *Staphylococcus epidermidis* and Other Coagulase-Negative Staphylococci

Philip Toltzis

Historically, *Staphylococcus epidermidis* and other coagulase-negative staphylococci (CoNS) have been considered nonpathogenic commensal organisms. It is now clear that these bacteria are true pathogens, particularly in hospitalized patients and those with indwelling foreign bodies. Indeed, multiple surveys conducted during the first decade of the 2000s have indicated that CoNS are the most frequent causes of nosocomial bloodstream infections (BSIs) across the globe.[1-7] The organisms are implicated particularly in bacteremic disease in patients in the intensive care unit[5,6,8–12] and patients with cancer;[13–20] 20% to 50% of all nosocomial BSIs in these patient groups are due to CoNS.

DESCRIPTION OF THE PATHOGEN

Staphylococci are members of the family Micrococcaceae and are nonmotile, nonspore-forming, catalase-positive bacteria.[21] They are gram-positive cocci that grow in irregular clusters. Staphylococci are among the hardiest of nonspore-forming bacteria and can survive many nonphysiologic environmental conditions. These organisms grow best under aerobic conditions but are capable of growth in an anaerobic environment as well. The optimal temperature for growth ranges between 30°C and 37°C, and the ideal pH ranges from 7.0 to 7.5. Although staphylococci grow readily on most routine laboratory media, sheep blood agar is recommended for primary isolation from clinical samples. Colonies are round, smooth, raised, and glistening and can be surrounded by a zone of hemolysis when grown on blood-containing media. Thioglycolate broth is the preferred liquid medium for primary isolation.

In the clinical microbiology laboratory, CoNS are distinguished from *Staphylococcus aureus* by their failure to produce coagulase, an enzyme that coagulates rabbit plasma. Originally, all CoNS were grouped together under the designation *Staphylococcus albus*; by 2010, however, over 40 species and numerous subspecies of CoNS were recognized, based upon biochemical and genetic differences (for the most current classifications, refer to http://www.bacterio.cict.fr/). Fifteen species are normal human flora: *S. epidermidis, S. haemolyticus, S. hominis, S. saccharolyticus, S. capitis, S. warneri, S. caprae, S. pasteuri, S. saprophyticus, S. cohnii, S. xylosus, S. simulans, S. auricularis, S. lugdunensis,* and *S. schleiferi.*[21] All CoNS primarily are skin commensals but can colonize the upper respiratory tract, gastrointestinal tract, genitourinary tract, and mammary glands. Some species exhibit niche preferences for certain areas of the skin, for example *S. capitis* for the sebaceous gland-rich scalp, *S. auricularis* for the external auditory canal, *S. hominis* and *S. haemolyticus* for the apocrine gland-rich axillae and pubis, and *S. saprophyticus* for the female genitourinary tract.

Many clinical microbiology laboratories continue to characterize isolates simply as CoNS. Commercially available kits, however, can rapidly distinguish CoNS species to an accuracy of 70% to >90%.[21] Most kits include a series of biochemical reactions, although systems based on high-resolution gas chromatography and PCR amplification of rRNA genes also have been developed.[21] Species identification of *S. lugdunensis* and *S. schleiferi* is particularly important in that they cause aggressive disease more typical

of *S. aureus* than other CoNS.[22] They can be distinguished in the laboratory from most other CoNS by yielding a positive rapid coagulase slide test (reflecting the presence of "clumping factor" rather than bound coagulase) but, like other CoNS, they test negative with the more definitive coagulase tube assay.[21] Both species are relatively uncommon on normal human skin but can colonize implanted materials such as catheters and drains. *S. lugdunensis* has been implicated in natural and prosthetic valve endocarditis, septicemia, brain abscess, peritonitis, soft-tissue infection, vascular graft infection, prosthetic joint infection, and catheter-related infection.[22–28] *S. schleiferi* has been reported rarely as a pathogen in the United States but in some European countries has caused brain empyema, wound infection, osteomyelitis, and BSI.[22,29,30]

PATHOGENESIS

Colonization is a prerequisite for CoNS disease. CoNS can be isolated from multiple skin surfaces, suggesting that the majority of infections originate from organisms on the skin.[31,32] Most patients in whom CoNS infection develops have an obvious disruption of the skin barrier caused by surgery, placement of a catheter, or insertion of a prosthesis. Systemic infection also can emanate from colonized mucous membranes of the pharynx and gastrointestinal tract when organisms enter the bloodstream either through breaks in the mucosa or by translocation through mesenteric lymph nodes.[33–35]

In distinction to *S. aureus*, CoNS typically do not elaborate virulent exotoxins. Consequently, infections caused by most CoNS characteristically are indolent and prolonged, even in compromised hosts. Their prominence as nosocomial pathogens stems largely from their propensity to adhere to the inanimate surfaces of catheters and prostheses, and in their ability, once established, to evade host defense mechanisms and antibiotic activity. Both characteristics are mediated by production of biofilm, a thick accumulation of bacteria arranged in multilayered clusters covered by an extracellular matrix. The importance of biofilm in CoNS pathogenesis has been confirmed repeatedly by demonstrations that mutants deficient in biofilm-related molecules are less disease-producing than their isogenic counterparts.[36,37]

Biofilm formation occurs in several stages, namely, attachment of the CoNS to unmodified polymer surfaces, further binding of the bacteria to host extracellular molecules that rapidly coat polymer surfaces, proliferation of organisms within the biofilm, and finally covering of the biofilm with bacteria-specific polysaccharide[38] (Figure 116-1). In the first stage, nonspecific factors, including long-range electromagnetic forces and surface hydrophobicity, promote initial attachment.[39] Several bacteria-specific

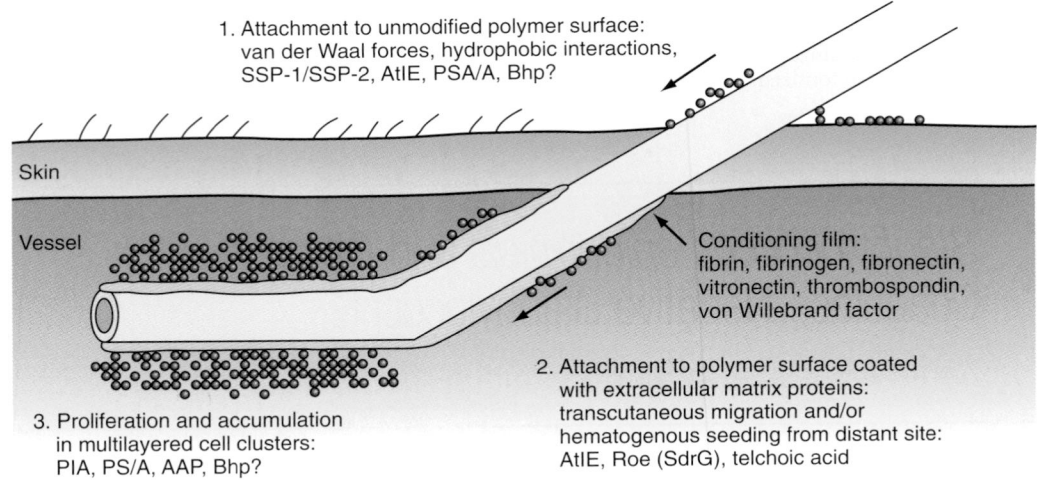

Figure 116-1. Schematic model of the phases involved in *Staphylococcus epidermidis* biofilm formation. AAP, accumulation-associated protein; AtlE, autolysin; Bhp, biofilm-associated (Bap)-homologous protein; Fbe, fibrinogen-binding protein; PIA, polysaccharide intercellular adhesin; PSA/A, polysaccharide/adhesin; SdrG, serine-aspartate-repeat-containing protein G; SSP-1/SSP-2, staphylococcal surface proteins. (Redrawn from von Eiff C, Peters G, Heilmann C. Pathogenesis of infections due to coagulase-negative staphylococci. Lancet Infect Dis 2002;2:677–685.)

products mediate the seminal stages of adherence. Chief among these is the polysaccharide capsular adhesin (PS/A),[40] which consists predominantly of galactose and glucosamine and promotes attachment to plastic polymers. A second attachment factor is the surface-associated autolysin AtlE, which shows significant homology to the major autolysin of *S. aureus*.[41] AtlE contains two biologically active domains generated by proteolytic processing, including a 60-kd amidase domain and a 52-kd glucosaminidase domain.[41] Two related staphylococci surface proteins, labeled SSP-1 and SSP-2, are fimbria-like polymers encoded by *S. epidermidis* that further mediate adherence to polymers.[42,43]

Once inserted into the body, plastic surfaces become coated with plasma and extracellular host proteins such as fibronectin, fibrinogen, vitronectin, thrombospondin, and von Willebrand factor. In the second stage of biofilm formation, bacterial molecules bind these host molecules as well (see Figure 116-1). AtlE and possibly other staphylococcal autolysins/adhesins have vitronectin-binding activity. Other CoNS products, particularly the 119-kd fibrinogen-binding protein Roe (also designated SdrG) and extracellular matrix-binding protein (Embp), as well as teichoic acid, may further mediate binding to plasma-coated plastic.[38,44,45]

After initial adherence, organisms multiply and form multilayered aggregates – the third and probably most critical stage of biofilm formation (see Figure 116-1). In 1994, Mack and coworkers found that a *S. epidermidis* transposon mutant lacking a polysaccharide antigen called polysaccharide intercellular adhesin (PIA) was unable to form multilayered cell clusters.[46] PIA has been confirmed as the central molecule in CoNS biofilm production.[45] Structural analysis revealed that PIA is a linear, β-1,6-linked glucosaminoglycan composed primarily of at least 130 2-deoxy-2-amino-D-glucopyranosyl residues, 80% to 85% of which are *N*-acetylated.[47,48] PIA is encoded by the *icaABCD* gene cluster, which is responsible for its synthesis and modification;[37,38,49] mutation of any of the four open reading frames in the *ica* gene complex interferes with maturation of CoNS biofilm.[45] The control of *ica* expression is incompletely understood but is influenced by several negative and positive regulators, presumably promoting the production of biofilm under specific environmental conditions.[45,50,51] Biofilm-producing *ica*-negative CoNS have been identified, however, indicating the existence of PIA-independent mechanisms of biofilm formation.[52–54] A second factor important for *S. epidermidis* intercellular adhesion and biofilm formation is a 140-kd extracellular protein called accumulation-associated protein (AAP).[55] Elimination of expression of AAP has no effect on initial adhesion to glass and polystyrene surfaces but disrupts bacterial accumulation.[56]

After adhesion and biofilm formation, most isolates elaborate copious amounts of a complex extracellular material generally referred to as slime.[57] In a hospital-wide survey, Ishak and associates[58] found slime production in 13 of 14 clinically significant bloodstream isolates of *S. epidermidis*, but in only 3 of 13 blood culture contaminants and 4 of 27 skin isolates. Studies of infants with CoNS infection have yielded similar results. In independent studies, slime production was noted in 82% of isolates from infants with invasive disease.[59]

Several biofilm-related molecules have been implicated in immune evasion.[49] PIA may render the organism more resistant to neutrophil clearance; *S. epidermidis* containing *ica* gene mutations and deficient PIA are phagocytosed more readily in vitro and are more susceptible to the toxic effects of neutrophil granules than their isogenic correlates.[37,60] PS/A may function as an antiphagocytic capsule by preventing C3 deposition and phagocytosis. These antiphagocytic properties may render the organism particularly pathogenic in premature infants who have depressed neutrophil function compared with that of term infants and adults.[61] Slime further functions as a nonspecific physical barrier to cellular and humoral defense mechanisms. In addition, slime inhibits neutrophil chemotaxis and phagocytosis, and suppresses lymphocyte blastogenesis.[62,63] Crude extracts of slime are capable of inhibiting the antimicrobial action of the glycopeptide antibiotics vancomycin and teicoplanin.[64] This effect appears to be limited

to the glycopeptide class of antibiotics inasmuch as slime extracts produce no change in the minimal inhibitory concentration (MIC) of cefazolin, clindamycin, or rifampin.

CoNS also elaborate a variety of exoproteins. Examples include urease, lipase/esterase, fibrinolysin, DNase, and a number of proteases. For the most part, the specific function of these bacterial products remains undetermined. In addition, some isolates produce δ-like toxin, an extracellular hemolysin that resembles the enteropathic δ-toxin of *S. aureus* in size, biologic properties, and antigenicity.[38] This δ-like toxin has cytotoxic effects on intestinal epithelium, and investigators have correlated free toxin in the stool of premature infants with the development of necrotizing enterocolitis (NEC).[65] *S. epidermidis* further produces a number of lantibiotics – antibiotic peptides containing the unusual amino acids lanthionine or methyllanthionine that can suppress growth of competing bacteria on skin and mucous membrane surfaces.[38]

S. saprophyticus elaborates a number of factors that may contribute to its ability to cause urinary tract infections (UTIs). A hemagglutinin/adhesin expressed on the surface of *S. saprophyticus* and the surface fibrillar protein Ssp both bind to uroepithelial cells and may explain the peculiar tropism of this species for the urinary tract. *S. saprophyticus* further elaborates a urease, which serves to damage bladder tissue once infection is established.[38,66–68]

EPIDEMIOLOGY

CoNS are acquired early in life, with virtually all infants carrying them at multiple sites by 2 to 4 days of age.[69] Beyond the newborn period, colonization among healthy persons remains ubiquitous. While in the past many community-associated CoNS were methicillin-susceptible, increasingly community strains are exhibiting resistance;[70,71] in one Japanese study, for example, nearly one-third of healthy children had nasal colonization with methicillin-resistant CoNS.[71] Community strains are of diverse lineage, but a substantial proportion carry the same cassette, labeled SCCmec IV, responsible for methicillin resistance in community-associated methicillin-resistant *S. aureus*.[70,71]

In distinction to the diversity of CoNS strains derived from the community, accumulating evidence suggests that one or more strain of CoNS can become predominant in a given hospital unit over a protracted period. This important epidemiologic finding was discovered using methods that enable strain identification by assessing similarities in bacteria DNA, including plasmid analysis, pulsed-field gel electrophoresis (PFGE), random amplification of polymorphic DNA (RAPD), and arbitrarily primed polymerase chain reaction.[72] Genetically identical or strongly related organisms have been isolated from multiple patients in an intensive care unit,[73–78] hematology-oncology unit,[79] and dialysis unit,[80] and even among multiple wards within a given hospital.[81–83] Dominant strains can circulate in affected units for many years.[75] The hands of nurses become colonized by hospital-associated strains of CoNS soon after employment,[84–86] suggesting their importance in patient-to-patient transmission. The biologic properties that confer strain predominance are not known, but interference with the growth of surrounding organisms or superior adherence to colonizing surfaces have been speculated to provide relative survival advantage.

CLINICAL MANIFESTATIONS

Bloodstream Infection and Intravascular Catheter-Related Infection Outside the Newborn Period

CoNS account for roughly one-third of all BSIs in children undergoing therapy for leukemia, lymphoma, or solid tumors.[87] In addition, CoNS are an important cause of septicemia in stem cell transplant recipients.[88] The strongest risk factors for CoNS BSI in these patients is the presence of a central venous catheter (CVC), although immunosuppressive therapy, neutropenia, and chemotherapy-induced gastrointestinal mucositis also are associated. Mortality from CoNS BSI in this group is reported to be as high as 11%.[87,89] Additionally, *S. epidermidis* is the most common species associated with CVC-related infections in patients in intensive care units with temporary, percutaneously inserted catheters.[90] Infection related to a CVC can occur at the exit site, along the catheter tunnel, or on the intravascular portion. Heavy skin colonization followed by tracking of the organisms along the external surface of the catheter is the principal mechanism of CoNS catheter-related BSI.[31,91] Additionally, the catheter hub can become contaminated and organisms can reach the intravascular portion along the inner surface.[31]

Although CoNS frequently are the cause of catheter-related BSI, CoNS also are the most common contaminants of blood cultures, and distinguishing true infection from contamination often is difficult. Some patients with a blood culture positive for CoNS experience systemic manifestations of infection, such as fever, tachycardia, tachypnea, and hypotension,[92] rendering the diagnosis of true infection relatively secure. In the patient with more subtle signs and symptoms, the most important evidence of true infection is a positive blood culture repeatedly from separate samplings spread 1 to 2 days apart.[93–97] The 2008 Centers for Disease Control and Prevention (CDC) diagnostic criteria for catheter-associated BSI caused by CoNS (and other skin commensals) require at least two positive blood cultures (www.cdc.gov/nhsn/PDFs/pscManual/4PSC/_CLABSIcurrent.pdf).

Several investigators have attempted to define additional diagnostic methods to confirm that the catheter is the source of bacteremia. Quantitative blood cultures are most useful in this regard;[98] specifically, the catheter is likely the source of the infection if the density of organisms in blood obtained through the catheter is at least 5- to 10-fold greater than that in blood drawn from a peripheral vessel.[90,99] When quantitative cultures are unavailable, relative concentrations of bacteria in central and peripheral blood can be estimated using the time-to-positivity of blood samples taken from the central line versus a peripheral site; a difference in time-to-positivity of >120 to 180 minutes suggests that the catheter is the source of infection (such comparison is only valid if samples are of equal volume).[100,101]

Culturing the intravascular portion of the catheter itself is the most reliable method of establishing the catheter as the source. Maki and associates[102] determined that catheter-related BSI can be confirmed by rolling the distal 5 to 7 cm of the removed catheter over an agar surface and finding growth of ≥15 colonies. This method requires catheter removal, however. Fortunately, most patients with CoNS exit site infection and roughly 75% with BSI from an operatively implanted tunneled catheter can be managed successfully without removing the catheter.[99] Although the risks of recurrent CoNS BSI are increased if the BSI is treated with the line in situ,[103,104] this practice did not contribute to increased mortality in one study.[103] Treatment typically is continued for 10 to 14 days after sterilization of the blood. Catheter removal is almost always necessary when tunnel infection is present. In nonoperatively placed, percutaneous catheters, particularly those commonly inserted in patients in the intensive care unit, catheter-related BSI generally requires catheter removal.

Neonatal Septicemia

Bacteremia and disseminated infection from CoNS are particularly prevalent in the neonatal intensive care unit (NICU), where they have been recognized as the most frequent cause of late-onset sepsis (occurring ≥7 days after hospitalization) in very-low-birth-weight infants.[9,105] CoNS have been implicated as principal pathogens in early-onset neonatal sepsis as well.[8,11,105,106] Unlike older patients, neonates with CoNS BSI often have focal complications, which are frequently heralded by persistent bacteremia.[107] In one series, skin abscess was present in more than 40% of cases.[108] Other sites of localized disease include the heart, intravenous thrombus, central nervous system, lungs, and bone and joints.[105] As in older children, CoNS BSI in the newborn is frequently, but not always, a consequence of CVC contamination. CVCs have been implicated in more than 50% of cases of neonatal CoNS BSI, especially catheters used to infuse parenteral nutrition,

particularly lipid emulsions.[109,110] Intralipid may provide an enriched medium for proliferation of CoNS.[110]

In a critically ill neonate, it is often impossible to perform more than a single blood culture before initiating antibiotic therapy. When CoNS is isolated from a single blood culture, assessment of the likelihood of true infection may be difficult. In one study that used quantitative cultures, peripheral blood yielding >50 colony-forming units (CFU)/mL occurred exclusively in infants with proven septicemia.[111] By contrast, low colony counts were observed with both septicemia and contamination. Infants with septicemia, including those with <50 CFU/mL, were significantly more likely to have a central catheter or an abnormal hematologic value (white blood cell count >20,000/mm^3 or <5000/mm^3, an immature-to-total neutrophil ratio >0.12, or a platelet count <150,000/mm^3). Infants who lacked these clinical features were more likely to have culture contamination. Several other studies have corroborated the utility of an elevated immature-to-total neutrophil ratio in identifying infants with true CoNS BSI.[107,112,113]

Neonatal Focal Intestinal Perforation and Necrotizing Enterocolitis

Gruskay and associates[114] described a series of newborn infants with *S. epidermidis* BSI and an associated syndrome of acute enterocolitis. By definition, all 19 infants had bloody stools in addition to signs and symptoms of enterocolitis and an abnormal abdominal radiograph. In this series, clinical courses were mild. Only 1 infant had pneumatosis intestinalis, and no child required surgical intervention or died. These findings are consistent with CoNS peritonitis due to focal intestinal perforation, which, in distinction to typical NEC, involves only a limited area of bowel.[115,116] By contrast, other authors have reported severe, even fatal cases of enterocolitis associated with *S. epidermidis* infection.[117,118]

Endocarditis

CoNS is an important cause of infective endocarditis. In older children and adults, CoNS account for approximately 5% of endocarditis involving previously normal valves.[119,120] Disease in this situation develops after a period of transient BSI with seeding of the valve. These organisms also have been implicated in native valve endocarditis in children with congenital heart disease, with the valves most often inoculated at the time of surgical repair. Finally, CoNS is the most common cause of prosthetic valve endocarditis and accounts for 25% to 40% of all cases;[121–125] pathogenesis is believed to involve contamination at the time of surgery, with subsequent formation of an abscess at the valvular ring.

Although some cases of CoNS endocarditis are caused by the intrinsically pathogenic *S. lugdunensis*, the majority are due to *S. epidermidis*.[119,121,126] Hence, the course of CoNS endocarditis typically is indolent, often evolving over a period of several months,[127] although acute onset with valvular destruction requiring surgical intervention also occurs.[119,121,126] Fever is the most common physical finding, present in approximately 90% of patients. Other findings include splenomegaly, petechiae, and a new or changed murmur. Classic manifestations of bacterial endocarditis, including Osler nodes, Roth spots, Janeway lesions, and splinter hemorrhages, are relatively uncommon. In practice, the initial blood culture isolation of CoNS in patients who later prove to have endocarditis frequently is dismissed;[126] timely diagnosis therefore requires a high level of suspicion. In the high-risk patient who has fever and multiple positive blood cultures, every effort should be made to detect valvular dysfunction. Evaluation should include two-dimensional transthoracic and, if necessary, transesophageal echocardiography.

In neonates, CoNS endocarditis usually is right-sided and tends to occur when the tip of an intravascular catheter is positioned in the right atrium.[105,128] Although the mortality associated with neonatal infective endocarditis caused by other pathogens is high, outcome of CoNS endocarditis is more favorable. An important diagnostic clue to the presence of endocarditis in the neonate is persistent bacteremia despite catheter removal and appropriate antibiotic therapy, especially in the presence of thrombocytopenia. It is sometimes difficult to distinguish endocarditis from an infected intravascular thrombus at an extracardiac site. The diagnosis is confirmed by echocardiography, which reveals intracardiac lesions associated with a valve or the endocardial wall. Removal of the catheter is fundamental to cure.

Cerebrospinal Fluid Shunt Infections and Meningitis

Infectious complications occur in approximately 10% of all cerebrospinal shunts placed in children within 24 months of their insertion,[129] and CoNS are the principal organisms implicated. *S. epidermidis* alone accounts for between 60% and 75% of CSF shunt infections. Seventy percent of shunt infections occur within 2 months of placement, which suggests that, in most cases, seeding occurs at the time of surgery.[130] Because infection is associated commonly with shunt or catheter obstruction, signs and symptoms frequently reflect increased intracranial pressure such as headache, vomiting, and depressed mental status. In addition, many patients have low-grade fever. Examination of CSF most often reveals modest pleocytosis, typically with elevated protein concentration and sometimes with slightly depressed glucose. Gram stain is variably positive. In some patients, CSF analysis is completely normal; in these cases, repeated isolation of the same strain is required to establish causation.

Few data guide the optimal approach to an infected CSF shunt, but most practitioners remove the contaminated apparatus and cure the infection with parenteral antibiotics while the CSF is drained through a temporary external ventriculostomy. A new internal shunt is then placed once the infection is cleared. Using mostly experiential data, a decision analysis concluded that this approach results in fewer deaths and treatment failures when compared with antibiotics plus immediate shunt replacement or with antibiotics alone.[122] In addition, some clinicians instill antibiotics directly into the ventricles through the drain,[131-133] but the benefits of this practice beyond those derived from systemic antibiotics and shunt removal alone are not known. In some circumstances removal of the infected shunt is not feasible surgically and the infection must be treated (usually including direct instillation of antibiotic) with the contaminated shunt left in place,[134] a strategy that is successful in approximately one-third of instances.[135] This approach is less likely to succeed if the infecting organism is slime-producing.[136,137]

In neonates, CoNS meningitis in the absence of an intraventricular foreign body has been reported, presumably as a result of BSI.[107,138] In one study, 10 infants were described who had *S. epidermidis* meningitis with unremarkable CSF white blood cell counts (mean, 6 cells/mm³; range, 0 to 14) and normal glucose and protein concentrations.[138] In this series, no deaths or cases of hydrocephalus secondary to meningitis were reported.[138] The possibility of more subtle, long-term sequelae was not assessed.[138]

Peritoneal Dialysis Catheter-Associated Peritonitis

Infection remains the most common complication of peritoneal dialysis.[139,140] According to several studies, the cumulative risk of peritonitis in patients undergoing continuous ambulatory peritoneal dialysis is approximately 60%.[140] *S. epidermidis* is the most common bacterial pathogen and accounts for roughly 40% of infections.[140] The most frequent symptoms of catheter-related peritonitis include abdominal pain, nausea, and vomiting. Fever is present in a minority of patients. Physical examination typically reveals abdominal tenderness, and in nearly all cases, cloudy peritoneal fluid is present.

Criteria for the diagnosis of catheter-related peritonitis are not uniform from one study to another, but generally they include some combination of abdominal pain, peritoneal fluid with >100 neutrophils/mm³, and a positive peritoneal fluid culture.[140] Gram stain of peritoneal fluid usually is negative. Routine cultures of small volumes of peritoneal fluid often fail to yield an organism, but inoculation of broth medium or culture of centrifugate of large volumes of peritoneal fluid improves the yield.[141] In the absence of CoNS tunnel infection, antibiotic treatment without removal of the catheter usually is successful.[141,142] Effective regimens have included intraperitoneal, parenteral, oral, or intraperitoneal plus oral administration of antibiotics. Treatment failures require retreatment or catheter removal.

Urinary Tract Infection

CoNS is an important cause of UTI, particularly in adolescent girls and young adult women.[143-146] *S. saprophyticus* is the species implicated most often and is identified readily in the clinical microbiology laboratory on the basis of its resistance to a 5 µg novobiocin disk.[147] *S. saprophyticus* UTI is almost always symptomatic and involves the upper urinary tract in approximately one-half of cases. Sexual intercourse is an important risk factor for infection, presumably by facilitating spread of bacteria from the urethra and periurethral area into the bladder. In one study, nearly 70% of females with *S. saprophyticus* UTI gave a history of sexual intercourse within the 24 hours preceding the onset of symptoms.[143]

Other species of CoNS occasionally cause UTI. Examples include *S. epidermidis* and *S. haemolyticus*. In contrast to *S. saprophyticus*, these species most commonly produce disease in hospitalized patients, generally those with an indwelling urinary catheter. On occasion, CoNS cause UTI in otherwise healthy children.[148]

Miscellaneous Infections

CoNS can cause a number of other infections. Most of these have been described primarily in neonates. Pneumonia from CoNS occurs almost exclusively in ill premature infants. In general, diagnosis is assigned when an infant with respiratory distress and a pulmonary infiltrate has CoNS isolated from blood. The series by Hall and coworkers[59] identified 12 infants with hospital-acquired pneumonia among 27 with CoNS BSI, 9 of whom were intubated at the time of the positive blood culture and pulmonary infiltrate, and 3 who had been intubated previously. Neonates can also experience omphalitis and abscesses due to CoNS.[149] Omphalitis is characterized by purulent discharge at the umbilical stump along with erythema, edema, and tenderness in the periumbilical area. Abscess formation secondary to CoNS can occur at a variety of sites, but the most frequent are the breast and the scalp. Breast abscess is encountered most often during the second or third week of life and occurs more frequently in females. Scalp abscess usually is a complication of a scalp electrode used for fetal monitoring. CoNS rarely can cause primary or secondary osteomyelitis in neonates, particularly in premature infants.[105,150] Recently CoNS has been implicated as a cause of hospital-acquired conjunctivitis in the NICU.[151]

In older children, CoNS is an important cause of endophthalmitis after intraocular trauma, and of mediastinitis after median sternotomy for open-heart surgery.[152-155] Additionally, central nervous system infection has been associated with a variety of other foreign bodies, including pacemaker wires, hemodialysis shunts, intravascular grafts, and prosthetic joints.[156,157]

ANTIBIOTIC TREATMENT

Resistance of CoNS to penicillin, methicillin, and gentamicin is common among hospital-associated isolates.[59,112,158] Full resistance to vancomycin is rare but has been reported in isolates of *S. haemolyticus*.[159,160] Higher, "creeping" MICs of vancomycin for CoNS are a concern. Intermediate resistance to vancomycin has been observed in *S. epidermidis*, and the percentage of all clinical isolates of CoNS with a vancomycin or teicoplanin MIC of 4 µg/mL has increased with continued use of glycopeptides.[161-164] Adequate area under the plasma drug-concentration time curve (AUC) is difficult to achieve when vancomycin MIC exceeds 1 µg/mL.

Vancomycin usually is initiated empirically when CoNS infection is suspected or proved. The treatment regimen is subsequently modified according to antibiotic susceptibility test results. When considering the results of susceptibility tests, several caveats are noteworthy. First, penicillin resistance in CoNS is frequently mediated by the production of β-lactamase, which is not always detected by microdilution methods.[165] Accordingly, all isolates that appear to be susceptible to penicillin or ampicillin should be tested specifically for the presence of β-lactamase.[165] Such testing should follow exposure to oxacillin, which induces β-lactamase expression. Second, although each organism in a population of CoNS may have the *mecA* genetic determinant for resistance to methicillin (and other penicillinase-resistant β-lactams), only a small fraction express this phenotype under testing conditions.[166] As a consequence, resistance to methicillin can be overlooked easily.[167] In vitro expression of resistance to methicillin is favored by testing a large inoculum and by incubation on salt-containing media at 30°C to 35°C. Third, routine susceptibility testing frequently indicates that isolates of CoNS resistant to methicillin are susceptible to cephalosporins; however, cross-resistance is extensive, and for clinical purposes, all staphylococci that are resistant to penicillinase-resistant penicillins should be considered resistant to cephalosporins as well.

Assuming rigorous testing, infections with penicillin-susceptible, β-lactamase-negative organisms can be treated with penicillin. For isolates that are resistant to penicillin but truly are susceptible to the penicillinase-resistant penicillins, therapy with oxacillin or nafcillin is preferred. Vancomycin is the preferred agent only for CoNS that are resistant to methicillin or for patients who are allergic to penicillin. The combination of rifampin and clindamycin (if CoNS is susceptible) might be an alternative regimen for patients allergic to penicillin.[168]

In some situations, such as endocarditis or infection related to an intraventricular CSF shunt, synergistic antibiotic therapy may be indicated. Synergy has been demonstrated in vitro for vancomycin or β-lactams in combination with rifampin and gentamicin (with isolates susceptible to each). For adult patients with CoNS endocarditis involving a prosthesis, therapy with three drugs (a cell-wall active agent, plus rifampin and an aminoglycoside) is recommended for the first 2 weeks, followed by an additional 4 weeks of the cell-wall active agent and rifampin.[169] Combination chemotherapy is commonly applied to CoNS native valve endocarditis, but it is uncertain if outcome is altered by therapy including agents in addition to a β-lactam or vancomycin alone.[121]

During the late 1990s and early 2000s, several agents were developed for the treatment of methicillin-resistant CoNS and other multidrug-resistant gram-positive pathogens. The semisynthetic lipoglycopeptides, dalbavancin and telavancin, possess more potent in vitro activity against CoNS compared with vancomycin.[170,171] Additionally, dalbavancin has a prolonged terminal half-life that allows once-a-week intravenous dosing.[172] Daptomycin, a parenteral lipopeptide, also has in vitro activity against almost all clinical isolates of CoNS tested to date,[173-175] but there is limited published experience of use in pediatrics. Linezolid, the first licensed agent of the oxazolidinone family of inhibitors of bacterial protein synthesis, also possesses activity against most isolates of CoNS and other gram-positive bacteria,[176,177] although epidemic clusters of clonally-related linezolid resistant CoNS infections have been reported.[178,179] Unlike other agents directed toward methicillin-resistant CoNS, linezolid is available in both a parenteral and oral preparation,[180] the latter allowing convenient, effective home therapy in the appropriate patient.

PREVENTION

Strict handwashing is of primary importance for minimizing horizontal spread of CoNS. In addition, meticulous skin preparation and surgical technique to limit intraoperative bacterial contamination has fundamental importance for minimizing infection related to foreign bodies.

Scanning and transmission electron microscopy shows that bacterial attachment is a dynamic process dependent on intrinsic properties of the catheter surface. Attempts to develop catheters that are inert and resistant to bacterial colonization, however, have been disappointing to date. More recent efforts have focused on

the possibility of preventing infection by using prosthetic materials impregnated with antibiotics.[181,182] Percutaneously inserted catheters impregnated with broad-spectrum antimicrobial agents, specifically silver sulfadiazine plus chlorhexidine or minocycline plus rifampin, have been tested in adults for their ability to reduce catheter-related BSIs due to CoNS and other pathogens. Although meta-analyses assessing their ability to prevent catheter infections have been positive,[43,183] controversy remains regarding their effectiveness.[184,185] Moreover, although pediatric-sized antibiotic-impregnated catheters are available, few data exist regarding their performance in children. Consensus opinion recommends their use only when other prevention measures fail.[33] Antibiotic-impregnated CSF shunts also are available, and some experiential data suggest effectiveness in reducing infection in children,[186,187] but use has not been embraced widely by pediatric neurosurgeons.[188]

The use of prophylactic antibiotics during the implantation of a foreign body has not been well studied, and the benefits of this practice remain uncertain. Studies of adding vancomycin to hyperalimentation fluid in neonates to reduce the incidence of CoNS CVC-associated BSI indicated efficacy,[189,190] but the risk of promoting vancomycin resistance outweighs the risk of CoNS BSI, even in very low birthweight infants. A stronger case has been made for the use of antibiotic lock to reduce the incidence of CVC-associated infections. Advantage is that a high concentration of antibiotic can be instilled and allowed to dwell in the catheter (permitting penetration of the biofilm) and then removed. A meta-analysis examining 11 randomized trials testing the effectiveness of antibiotic lock solutions, most of which employed gentamicin alone or with a second antibiotic, to reduce infection in hemodialysis catheters in adults and children indicated a significant reduction in catheter-associated BSIs compared with subjects who were infused only with anticoagulant.[191] Several studies have evaluated the effectiveness of lock solution composed of 70% ethanol, which possesses broad activity against gram-positive and gram-negative bacteria and fungi, in preventing catheter-associated infection.[192,193] Although mostly retrospective in design, these analyses report a statistically detectable reduction in incidence of infection.[192,193] Several important aspects of prophylactic antibiotic and ethanol lock strategies remain undefined, including the effects of prolonged exposure of the solutions on the integrity of the catheter,[194] and the ideal dwell time; when applied to infants, dwell time (even if short) can result in frequent episodes of hypoglycemia.[195] In older children, however, whose CVC is life-sustaining and who have experienced multiple central line infections despite other measures, lock strategies may be considered beneficial overall.

During the first decade of the 2000s several programs successfully promoted "best practices" to reduce central-line-associated BSIs (CLABSIs), with a consequent reduction of CoNS infections. "Bundles" of best practices were constructed based on published evidence and expert consensus. Most programs employed two sets of bundles, for line insertion and for line maintenance.[33,196-198] In many instances the results were dramatic. In the program adopted by 103 adult ICUs in Michigan, an 82% reduction of CLABSIs occurred within 3 months and was sustained over the subsequent year.[199] In 2009 alone, the CDC estimated that 25,000 fewer CLABSIs occurred in U.S. ICUs in people ≥1 year of age, a 58% reduction compared with 2001, with 6000 lives and >$400 million saved.[200] In the National Association of Children's Hospitals and Related Institutions collaborative intervention in pediatric ICUs, CLABSIs dropped from 5.4 per 1000 line-days to a sustained rate of 3.1 per 1000 line-days.[197] In the initial Vermont Oxford Network (VON) program implementing best practices in NICUs, incidence of CLABSI was reduced from 26.3% before intervention to 20.9% after intervention.[201] Subsequent VON collaborative groups have refined the methods to reduce CLABSIs and demonstrated further reductions.[202]

OTHER COAGULASE-NEGATIVE MICROCOCCACEAE

The family Micrococcaceae also includes *Micrococcus* species and *Rothia mucilaginosa*. Like other CoNS, these organisms are nonmotile, nonspore-forming, gram-positive cocci that grow as irregular clusters. Traditionally, micrococci and staphylococci have been grouped together based upon similar cellular morphology and positive catalase activity. The two genera differ considerably in amino acid content, however, and recently more complete genetic analyses confirm their distant relationship.[21] Organisms formerly belonging to the genus *Micrococcus* have been divided into six separate genera, including *Micrococcus* (which includes the species *M. luteus*), *Kocuria, Kytococcus, Nesterenkonia, Dermacoccus,* and *Arthrobacter*. The micrococci are normal residents of the skin and usually are not considered pathogenic. Occasionally micrococci, particularly those derived from the species *M. luteus*, can cause serious disease.[203] Generally, micrococci cause infections in people who have an indwelling medical device and an associated underlying condition such as catheter-related infection in leukemia, peritonitis in continuous ambulatory peritoneal dialysis, CSF shunt infections, and endocarditis in patients with prosthetic valves.[170] Micrococci also are common culture contaminants, and assessment of their significance can be difficult. Most isolates are susceptible to a wide range of antibiotics, including penicillin, methicillin, vancomycin, gentamicin, and erythromycin. However, because resistance to a variety of antibiotic classes has been reported, vancomycin is the preferred agent for empiric therapy.

R. mucilaginosa, formerly known as *Staphylococcus salivarius* and later as *Micrococcus mucilaginosus* and then *Stomatococcus mucilaginosus*, is differentiated from organisms in the genera *Micrococcus* and *Staphylococcus* by absent or weak catalase activity and failure to grow in a nutrient medium supplemented with 5% sodium chloride. *R. mucilaginosa* likely is underreported as a human pathogen because it can be mistaken for other microorganisms. When weakly catalase-positive, it can be confused with CoNS or micrococci, and when catalase-negative, it can be confused with streptococci. Traditionally believed to be an organism with low virulence, *R. mucilaginosa* is now recognized as an opportunistic pathogen that can cause BSI, meningitis, pneumonia, endocarditis, and peritonitis.[173,204–208] *R. mucilaginosa* also has been implicated in skin and soft-tissue infections in children.[208] Most affected children have leukemia or a solid tumor and profound neutropenia.[206,208] Other risk factors for infection include the presence of a CVC, valvular heart disease, continuous ambulatory peritoneal dialysis, and intravenous drug abuse.[204,205] *R. mucilaginosa* is a normal resident of the mouth and upper respiratory tract; oral mucositis, dental surgery, and head and neck surgery have been reported to predispose to infection.[203,206] The clinical course of *R. mucilaginosa* infection often is characterized by prolonged fever and a slow response to antibiotic therapy. On occasion, fulminant infection and fatality have occurred.[203,206,208] Based on the limited reported cases, *R. mucilaginosa* appears to be susceptible uniformly to vancomycin with most isolates also susceptible to penicillin, ampicillin, oxacillin, cefazolin, imipenem, clindamycin, tetracycline, erythromycin, and rifampin.[204]

Key Points. *Staphylococcus epidermidis* and Other Coagulase-Negative Staphylococci (CoNS)

MICROBIOLOGY

- Coagulase-negative gram-positive cocci that grow in irregular clusters
- Over 40 species identified, 15 of which are normal human flora
- Most reside on skin, but also are present on mucosa of the upper respiratory, gastrointestinal, and genitourinary tracts

PATHOGENESIS

- Gain entrance through a disruption in the skin or mucosal barrier, such as after placement of a device or a prosthesis, or performance of surgery
- Propensities to adhere to prosthetic surfaces and to form biofilm are principal pathogenic characteristics
- Do not produce exotoxins; infections usually are indolent

CLINICAL SYNDROMES

- Bloodstream infection, usually emanating from a contaminated intravascular catheter
- Endocarditis, especially in the presence of a prosthetic valve
- Infection related to cerebrospinal fluid shunt
- Infection related to peritoneal dialysis catheter
- Catheter-related urinary tract infection, although *S. saprophyticus* can cause community-associated infection in healthy young women
- Particularly prevalent in premature infants in whom infection is less commonly associated with instrumentation than in older children and adults

TREATMENT

- Many community-associated strains remain susceptible to semisynthetic penicillin and cephalosporins
- Most hospital-associated strains are methicillin-resistant and require use of vancomycin
- Need to remove infected prosthetic material depends on its location, composition, and clinical factors

---

117 Classification of Streptococci

David B. Haslam and Joseph W. St. Geme III

The genus *Streptococcus* is more diverse than any other bacterial genus and is the source of considerable confusion with respect to taxonomic classification.[1-3] The system for classifying streptococci was introduced at the beginning of the 20th century and is based on a series of external characteristics of the organisms. Classification based on pattern of hemolysis and serotype provides a useful framework for the clinician. Of note, a variety of gram-positive, catalase-negative cocci belonging to other genera often are erroneously referred to simply as "the streptococci" (Box 117-1).[4] Biochemical differentiation and clinical features of important species of *Streptococcus* and other genera of gram-positive catalase-negative cocci are discussed in subsequent chapters.

Streptococcus	*Gemella*
Enterococcus	*Lactococcus*
Leuconostoc	*Abiotrophia*
Pediococcus	*Granulicatella*
Aerococcus	

β-hemolytic organisms be classified as hemolytic and that all others (including the α-hemolytic streptococci) be considered nonhemolytic.

Beyond the broad classification of streptococci based on hemolysis, Lancefield[5] subdivided the streptococci on the basis of their reactivity with pools of antisera that now are known to recognize cell surface carbohydrates. Antigenically related strains are grouped alphabetically, A to H and K to V. Although the Lancefield grouping was utilized originally to distinguish among the β-hemolytic streptococci, it should be noted that hemolysis and Lancefield serogrouping are not mutually exclusive. For example, group C streptococci can be α-hemolytic, β-hemolytic, or nonhemolytic.

Colony morphology is used commonly to differentiate streptococci further. Indeed, in some circumstances colony size takes precedence over other features in the classification of an organism. Particularly notable in this regard are the "viridans streptococci," an extremely heterogeneous group that contains organisms within most Lancefield groups (excluding A, B, and D) and with all patterns of hemolysis. In general, a strain producing minute colonies on solid agar is grouped with the viridans streptococci regardless of its Lancefield reactivity or hemolysis.

When considered together, Lancefield group, hemolysis, and colony morphology enable a clinically useful subdivision of the genus (Table 117-1). For the most part, the Lancefield-grouped organisms are β-hemolytic and are associated with

The earliest subdivision of the genus *Streptococcus* was based on the ability to lyse sheep red blood cells. β-Hemolytic streptococci produce complete hemolysis on sheep blood agar and cause formation of a transparent ring around each colony. In contrast, α-hemolytic organisms produce partial red cell injury, due to bacterial release of hydrogen peroxide, resulting in a green or greyish zone surrounding colonies. When α-hemolytic organisms are grown under oxygen-depleted conditions, hydrogen peroxide is not formed, and colonies appear nonhemolytic. Nonhemolytic organisms are classified as γ-hemolytic and include most enterococci. In order to avoid confusion in the classification of partially hemolytic streptococci, some investigators prefer that only

TABLE 117-1. Classification of Streptococci Most Commonly Associated with Human Disease

Lancefield Group[a]	Species	Hemolysis	Most Common Human Diseases	Lancefield Group[a]	Species	Hemolysis	Most Common Human Diseases
A	*Streptococcus pyogenes*	β	Pharyngitis, skin infection, wound infection, pneumonia, conjunctivitis, postinfectious glomerulonephritis and rheumatic fever	G	*Streptococcus canis*	β	Puerperal infection, skin and wound infection, endocarditis, pyogenic arthritis
B	*Streptococcus agalactiae*	β	Neonatal septicemia, meningitis, osteomyelitis, pneumonia	Not groupable[d]	*Streptococcus pneumoniae*	α	Pneumonia, otitis media, sinusitis, meningitis
C[b]	*Streptococcus dysgalactiae* subsp. *equisimilis*[c]	β	Wound infection, cellulitis, endocarditis, epidemic pharyngitis, pyogenic arthritis		Other viridans streptococci *Streptococcus mitis* *Streptococcus salivarius* *Streptococcus anginosus* group *Streptococcus mutans* group *Streptococcus vestibularis* *Streptococcus parasanguinis*	α[e]	Endocarditis, septicemia, dental infections, intravascular catheter-related infection
	Streptococcus equi subsp. *zooepidemicus*	β	Septicemia, nephritis				
D	Enterococci *Enterococcus faecalis* *Enterococcus faecium* Nonenterococcal *Streptococcus bovis*	γ	Neonatal septicemia, intestinal and peritoneal infection, urinary tract infection, opportunistic infection				

[a]Serogroups E, F, H, and K through V are rarely associated with human infections.

[b]Other group C streptococci are unusual causes of human infections.

[c]Streptococcus equi subsp. equisimilis can possess other Lancefield antigens, including groups A, G, and L.

[d]Minute colony-forming Lancefield group C, D, and G organisms are included with the viridans streptococci.

[e]Occasional viridans streptococci are nonhemolytic, and others are β-hemolytic. Adapted from McMillan JA, Feigin RD. Group A streptococcal infections. In: McMillan JA, DeAngelis CD, Feigin RD, et al. (eds) Oski's Pediatrics: Principles and Practice, 4th ed. Philadelphia, Lippincott Williams & Wilkins, 2006, p 1130.

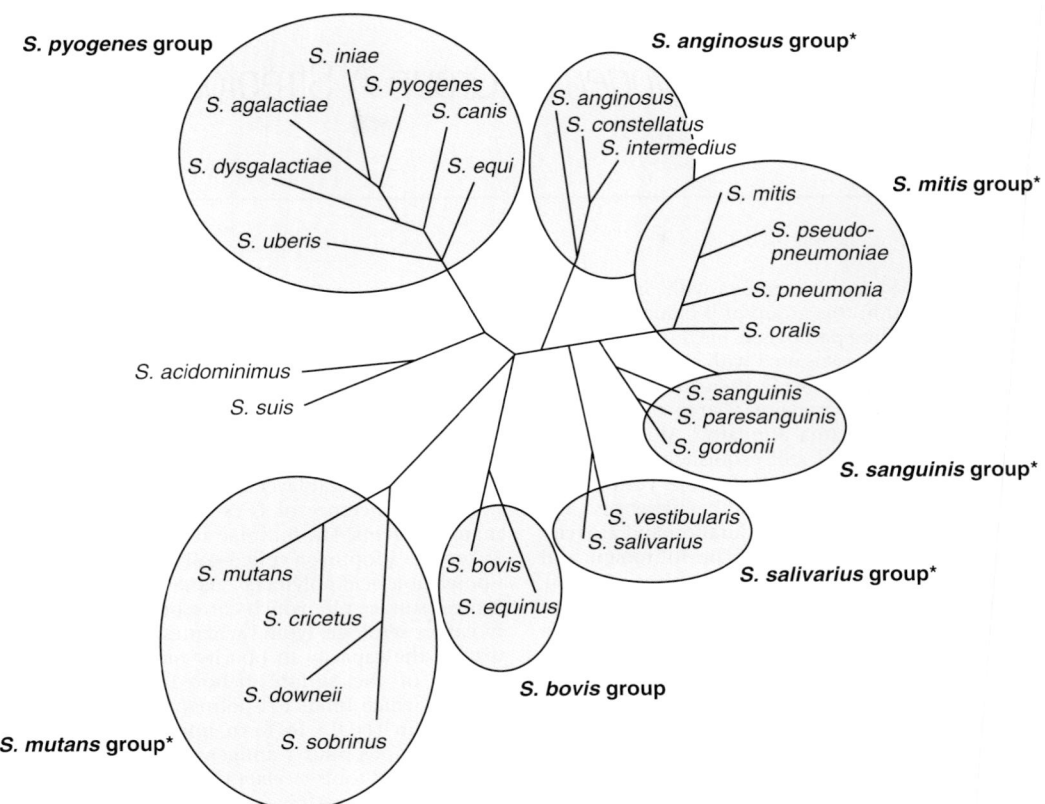

Figure 117-1. Schematic diagram of the phylogenetic relationship and classification of *Streptococcus* species. *Indicates the five groups constituting the viridans streptococci. Intraspecies distances are not to scale. (Originally adapted from Kawamura Y, Hou X, Sultana F, et al. Determination of 16S RNA sequences of *Streptococcus mitis* and *Streptococcus gordonii* and phylogenetic relationships among members of the genus *Streptococcus*. Int J Syst Bacteriol 1995;45:406.)

pyogenic infections. Nongroupable organisms usually belong in the viridans group and may be associated with bloodstream infection (BSI), endocarditis, and a variety of diseases in the compromised host. *S. pneumoniae* is now grouped among the viridans organisms based on its close genetic and phenotypic relatedness to the *Streptococcus mitis* group of organisms.

Other features commonly used to subdivide the streptococci are production of streptolysin O and streptokinase, susceptibility to bacitracin and optochin, production of acetoin upon metabolism of glucose (the Voges–Proskauer test), ability to grow in 6.5% NaCl, and ability to metabolize bile esculin or various carbohydrates.

With the advent of molecular techniques, the classification of streptococci has been subjected to reanalysis. On the basis of 16S rRNA gene sequences, the approximately 40 species constituting the genus *Streptococcus* have been subdivided into seven "species groups," which largely parallel phenotypic groupings (Figure 117-1 and Table 117-2).[6,7] Classification based on genetic relatedness is most useful for the viridans streptococci, because phenotypic classification of these organisms is particularly confusing and problematic (see Chapter 121, Viridans Streptococci, *Abiotrophia* and *Granulicatella* Species, and *Streptococcus bovis*).

Although no single scheme adequately differentiates all species, grouping of organisms on the basis of phenotypic, metabolic, and genetic criteria has provided a clinically useful framework for classifying the streptococci.

TABLE 117-2. Clinically Relevant Organisms Constituting Seven Species Groups in the Genus *Streptococcus*

Group	Species Included
S. pyogenes	*Streptococcus pyogenes*
	Streptococcus agalactiae
	Streptococcus canis
	Streptococcus dysgalactiae
	Streptococcus equi
S. mitis	*Streptococcus pneumoniae*
	Streptococcus pseudopneumoniae
	Streptococcus mitis
	Streptococcus oralis
S. sanguinis	*Streptococcus sanguinis*
	Streptococcus parasanguinis
	Streptococcus gordonii
S. salivarius	*Streptococcus salivarius*
	Streptococcus vestibularis
S. anginosus	*Streptococcus anginosus*
	Streptococcus constellatus
	Streptococcus intermedius
S. mutans	*Streptococcus mutans*
	Streptococcus cricetus
	Streptococcus downei
	Streptococcus sobrinus
S. bovis	*Streptococcus bovis*
	Streptococcus equinus

118 *Streptococcus pyogenes* (Group A Streptococcus)

Victor Nizet and John C. Arnold

Group A streptococcus (GAS) is synonymous with *Streptococcus pyogenes*, the only species within this group of β-hemolytic streptococci. GAS is one of the leading pathogenic bacteria that infects children and adolescents, and is associated with a wide spectrum of infections and disease states. Worldwide, there are estimated to be >600 million cases of GAS pharyngitis ("strep throat") and >100 million cases of GAS pyoderma annually.[1] Although uniformly susceptible to penicillin and still exquisitely susceptible to many other antimicrobial agents, GAS infections continue to present formidable clinical and public health challenges. The vast majority of GAS infections are of short duration and are relatively benign; however, invasive disease can be fulminant and life-threatening. In addition, GAS differs from other pyogenic bacteria in their potential to produce delayed, nonsuppurative sequelae (e.g., poststreptococcal acute glomerulonephritis (PSAGN) and acute rheumatic fever (ARF)) following uncomplicated infections. The importance of GAS infections in the United States was reinforced at the close of the 20th century by a resurgence of ARF[2] as well as by the appearance of severe invasive GAS infections (e.g., streptococcal toxic shock syndrome (STSS) and necrotizing fasciitis) with high morbidity and mortality.[3] On the global scale, GAS is an important cause of morbidity and mortality primarily in developing countries, with >500,000 deaths annually.[1]

DESCRIPTION OF PATHOGEN

Microbiology

GAS is a gram-positive coccoid-shaped bacterium that grows in chains. GAS produces small white to grey colonies with a clear zone of β-hemolysis on blood agar. Rare strains of GAS are not hemolytic.[4] GAS is distinguished from other groups of β-hemolytic streptococci by a group-specific polysaccharide (Lancefield carbohydrate C) located in the cell wall. Serologic grouping by the Lancefield method is precise, but group A organisms can be identified more readily by any one of a number of latex agglutination, co-agglutination, or enzyme immunoassay procedures.

GAS can be subdivided into >100 serotypes by the M-protein antigen that is located on the cell surface and by fimbriae (hairlike fuzz) that project from the outer edge of the cell. Classically, typing of the surface M protein relied upon available polyclonal antisera. This largely has been supplanted by a contemporary molecular approach that applies the polymerase chain reaction and DNA sequencing of the *emm* gene encoding the M protein. More than 130 distinct M genotypes have been identified using *emm* typing, and there has been a good correlation between known serotypes and *emm* types.[5,6]

M serotyping or genotyping has been valuable for epidemiologic studies; particular GAS diseases tend to be associated with certain M types. The M types commonly associated with pharyngitis rarely cause skin infections, and the M types commonly associated with skin infections rarely cause pharyngitis. A few of the "pharyngeal" strains (e.g., M type 12) have been associated with PSAGN, but far more of the "skin" strains (e.g., M types 49, 55, 57, and 60) have been considered nephritogenic. A few of the "pharyngeal" serotypes, but none of the "skin" strains, have been associated with ARF. However, recent evidence suggests that rheumatogenic potential is not solely dependent on the serotype, but rather is a characteristic of specific strains within several serotypes. Certain GAS M types are more strongly associated with invasive

disease, including M1, M3, M6, M12, M18, and M28. A globally disseminated clone of the M1 serotype has been the leading cause of severe invasive GAS infections such as necrotizing fasciitis and toxic shock syndrome over the past three decades.[7]

The GAS cell is a complex structure. In rapidly dividing strains (e.g., young cultures, epidemic strains), the cell is covered with a hyaluronic acid capsule that gives the colonies a mucoid or water drop appearance. Protruding from the cell surface and into the hyaluronic capsular layer are microscopic hairlike fimbriae, which promote adherence of GAS to epithelial cells and extracellular matrix proteins. The fimbriae are composed of a surface-anchored M protein adopting a coiled-coil structure, closely associated with lipoteichoic acid polymers.[8,9] GAS recently has been recognized to express surface pili, which correspond to the classical "T antigen" in earlier serologic typing schemes.[10] Roughly half of GAS strains display the capacity to opacify mammalian serum, through the activity of the surface-anchored serum opacity factor (SOF) protein, which binds to apolipoproteins to displace high-density lipoprotein (HDL) to form lipid droplets.[11] Serologic diversity among various pilus T antigens and SOF proteins can be helpful supplemental tools to *emm* typing in epidemiologic characterization of GAS strains.[12]

The group A carbohydrate, comprising 40% to 50% of the dry weight of the GAS cell wall, is a polymer of rhamnose units with side chains of *N*-acetyl-glucosamine and is responsible for its group (e.g., A) specificity.[13] Like other gram-positive species, a peptidoglycan polymer provides thickness and rigidity for the cell wall, consisting of glycan strands cross-linked by peptide bridges. M protein, pilus antigen, SOF, and other surface proteins are covalently attached to the GAS cell wall by recognition sequences on their C-terminal regions that interact with an anchoring enzyme called sortase.[14]

GAS produce and release into the surrounding medium a large number of biologically active extracellular products. Some of these are toxic for human and other mammalian cells. Streptolysin S (SLS) is a small oxygen-stabile toxin responsible for β-hemolysis of GAS on blood agar, while streptolysin O (SLO) is an oxygen-labile, cholesterol-dependent toxin related to staphylococcal α-hemolysin. Both SLS and SLO injure cell membranes, not only lysing red blood cells, but also damaging other eukaryotic cells and membranous subcellular organelles.[15] Streptolysin O is antigenic; streptolysin S is not. Streptococcal pyrogenic exotoxins (SPEs) are secreted factors with the capacity to act as superantigens and trigger T-cell proliferation and cytokine release.[16] GAS elaborates a broad-spectrum cysteine protease with multiple host targets, a variety of specific peptidases that cleave host chemokines and complement factors, and several nucleases. Finally, GAS produces bacteriocins, low-molecular-weight proteins that can kill a variety of other gram-positive bacteria, and thus may play a role in promoting infection or even persistence of colonization.[17]

The expression of GAS virulence genes is controlled by the interplay of several transcriptional regulatory systems.[18,19] These include the two-component "control of virulence" system (CovR/S) that regulates 10% to 15% of the GAS genome including its hyaluronic acid capsule synthesis operon, and the stand-alone Mga regulator controlling expression of M protein and nearby virulence factor genes. Genome sequencing has shown that bacteriophages have played an important role in the evolutionary genetics of GAS, including the transfer of genes encoding antibiotic resistance, SPEs and other virulence determinants.[20]

PATHOGENESIS AND VIRULENCE

GAS induces serious human disease by at least three mechanisms: suppuration, as in pharyngitis and pyoderma; toxin elaboration, as in STSS; and immune-mediated inflammation, as in ARF and PSAGN.[21] No complete explanation is available for the predilection of certain body sites for infection by GAS, nor for the ability of strains of certain M types to produce pharyngitis and of other M types to produce pyoderma.

The first step in GAS disease pathogenesis involves successful colonization of the upper respiratory mucosa or skin of human host. A large number of adherence factors for epithelial cells and extracellular GAS have been described, including lipoteichoic acid, M protein, pili, and fibronectin-binding proteins including Sfb1 and SOF.[22] GAS biofilm formation facilitates persistence within the human host.[23] Both M protein and fibronectin-binding proteins are important for subsequent endocytotic uptake of GAS into respiratory epithelial cells.[22] This process of intracellular invasion allows GAS access to a privileged intracellular niche, and represents a proximal step in the pathogenesis of systemic infection.[24]

The propensity of GAS to produce serious infection in otherwise healthy children and adults defines a capacity of the pathogen to resist host innate clearance mechanisms that normally function to prevent microbial dissemination.[25] For example, when GAS gains access to deeper tissues through cellular invasion or a break in epithelial integrity, it deploys specific peptidases that cleave and inactivate the neutrophil chemoattractants interleukin-8 and complement factor 5a. Likewise, the broad-spectrum secreted cysteine protease, streptococcal pyrogenic exotoxin (Spe) B, can degrade host immunoglobulins and cationic antimicrobial peptides.

M protein is a multifaceted immune resistance factor that promotes GAS resistance to opsonophagocytosis through multiple mechanisms, including the binding of fibrinogen, complement inhibitory factor H, and the Fc region of immunoglobulins.[26] M protein is essential to virulence in animal models, and immunization with M protein provides strong protection against infection with a type-specific GAS strain. During invasive infection, significant quantities of M protein are released from the cell surface by proteolysis, whereupon they can form a proinflammatory clot-like complex with human fibrinogen, leading to uncontrolled neutrophil activation, vascular leakage, and toxic shock symptomatology.[27,28] M protein also collaborates with the GAS virulence factor streptokinase to bind host plasminogen to the GAS surface, whereupon plasmin activity is generated, effectively coating the bacterial surface with a powerful protease to facilitate tissue spread.[29]

The pore-forming toxins SLS and SLO are toxic to multiple host cell types including macrophages and neutrophils, and thus promote GAS tissue damage and resistance to phagocytic clearance.[15] SLO in particular can induce the accelerated apoptosis of immune cells.[30] The GAS hyaluronic acid capsule is nonimmunogenic, mimicking a common human matrix component, and cloaks opsonic targets on the bacterial surface from phagocyte recognition.[31] In the case of the highly invasive globally disseminated M1T1 GAS clone, hyperinvasive forms bearing mutations in the *covR/S* two-component regulator gene arise in vivo under innate immune selection, leading to upregulation of capsule and other key virulence determinants.[32] Specific virulence determinants present in the hyperinvasive M1T1 clone include the phage-encoded DNAse Sda1, which allows GAS to escape killing within DNA-based neutrophil extracellular traps, and the serum inhibitor of complement (SIC), which binds and inactivates terminal complement components and host defense peptides.

The SPEs are a family of >15 bacterial superantigens, including the bacteriophage-encoded SPE A and SPE C.[33] These superantigens induce antigen-nonspecific T-lymphocyte activation, suppress antibody synthesis, potentiate endotoxic shock, induce fever, promote release of proinflammatory cytokines, produce reticuloendothelial blockade, and may contribute to multiorgan failure characteristic of STSS.[34] In the U.S., STSS commonly is associated with infections with SpeA-producing strains.[34] Susceptibility to STSS appears to be related to the absence of antibodies to both M protein and superantigens as well as the presence of specific human leukocyte antigen (HLA) haplotypes.[35] The SPEs share homology with staphylococcal enterotoxins but not with staphylococcal toxic shock syndrome toxin-1.[33] SpeA and SpeC are responsible for the rash of scarlet fever, stimulating the formation of specific antitoxin antibodies that provide immunity against future scarlatiniform rashes, but not against other GAS infections.

IMMUNOLOGIC RESPONSE

Although many GAS constituents and extracellular products are antigenic, protective immunity is type-specific, mediated by opsonic anti-M-protein antibodies. These antibodies protect against infection with a homologous M type but confer no immunity against other M types.[36] Therefore, multiple GAS infections attributable to different M types are common during childhood and adolescence. Anti-M antibodies persist for years, perhaps for life, protecting against invasive infection but not against pharyngeal carriage.[37] Type-specific antibody may be transferred across the placenta from mother to fetus.[38] Type-specific antibody against M protein is not usually detectable until 6 to 8 weeks after infection.[39] Therefore, its primary role may not be in the limitation or termination of active infection, but rather in the prevention of reinfection by the same serologic type. Opsonic type-specific antibodies do not appear after early and effective antimicrobial therapy.[40]

Humoral antibodies to specific streptococcal extracellular products such as antistreptolysin O (ASO) and anti-DNAse B can be demonstrated readily by neutralization assays. They have been particularly useful in allowing a more precise method of defining GAS infection in clinical and epidemiologic studies and in documenting the occurrence of a preceding GAS infection in patients with a suspected nonsuppurative complication. The ASO assay is the most commonly used streptococcal antibody test. Since SLO is also produced by group C or G streptococci, the test is not specific for GAS infections, and the response can be feeble in patients with streptococcal impetigo.[41] In contrast, the anti-DNAse B response is demonstrable after both skin and throat infections. Neutralizing antibody titers to SLO peak at 3 to 6 weeks and to DNAse B at 6 to 8 weeks. Antibody titers against GAS extracellular antigens reported by clinical immunology laboratories may vary. Upper limits of normal are higher for children than for adults and these values, even for the same age group, are higher in some populations than in others.[42]

SUPPURATIVE INFECTIONS

Epidemiology

GAS have a narrow host range, identified almost exclusively in humans and only rarely in other species.[43] GAS is highly communicable and can cause disease in individuals of all ages who do not have type-specific immunity. Disease in neonates is uncommon, probably because of placental transfer of maternal antibody. Significant differences exist between epidemiology of throat and skin infections due to GAS[44] (see Chapter 27, Pharyngitis, and Chapter 70, Superficial Bacterial Skin Infections and Cellulitis).

Severe invasive GAS infections had become uncommon in the U.S. and western Europe during the second half of the 20th century.[45] However, since the late 1980s, there has been a worldwide increase in severe invasive GAS infections.[46] The incidence of severe invasive GAS disease in industrialized societies (2 to 3 per 100,000 population) is similar in the geographically distinct regions of Europe, North America, and Australia.[47,48] This rate translates to ~10,000 cases of invasive GAS disease annually in the U.S.[49] However, rates of invasive disease in indigenous populations in Africa, the Asian subcontinent, and the Pacific Islands typically are much higher,[1] with rates as high as 82.5/100,000 reported in North Queensland, Australia.[50] Globally, it has been estimated that at least 663,000 cases of invasive GAS disease occur each year, resulting in 163,000 deaths.[1]

The stratified squamous epithelium of the oropharynx and skin is the principal barrier against invasive GAS disease. GAS can gain access to sterile sites via direct inoculation following an injury that breaches the mucous membranes or skin;[49] however, a substantial number of invasive streptococcal infections have no known site of entry.[51] Epidemiologic data suggest that the oropharynx is the primary site of origin for systemic GAS isolates; thus invasive disease is likely to occur as a result of transient bloodstream infection (BSI) originating from the oropharynx, possibly as a result of direct tissue penetration by GAS.[51] Varicella is a particularly important risk factor for severe invasive GAS infections in previously healthy children.[52] Other risk factors more common in adults include diabetes mellitus, human immunodeficiency virus infection, intravenous drug use, and chronic pulmonary or cardiac disease.

Clinical Manifestations or Clinical Syndromes

GAS is a common cause of acute pharyngitis (see Chapter 27, Pharyngitis) (Figure 118-1) and pyoderma (impetigo) (see Chapter 70, Superficial Bacterial Skin Infections and Cellulitis) in children and adolescents. GAS also produces a variety of other infections of the respiratory tract, including otitis media, retropharyngeal abscess, peritonsillar abscess, sinusitis, and mastoiditis; of the skin and soft tissues (Figures 118-2, 118-3, and 118-4), including cellulitis, erysipelas, perianal cellulitis, vaginitis, and blistering distal dactylitis (see Chapter 70, Superficial Bacterial Skin Infections and Cellulitis; Chapter 76, Subcutaneous Tissue Infections and Abscesses; and Chapter 77, Myositis, Pyomyositis, and Necrotizing Fasciitis); and invasive disease, including STSS (see Chapter 13, Mucocutaneous Symptom Complexes), necrotizing fasciitis, septicemia, meningitis, pneumonia, empyema, peritonitis, puerperal sepsis, neonatal sepsis, osteomyelitis, suppurative arthritis, myositis, and surgical wound infections. GAS also is the proven cause of two potentially serious nonsuppurative complications, acute rheumatic fever (ARF) and acute poststreptococcal glomerulonephritis (PSAGN), and the possible cause of two other potential nonsuppurative complications, poststreptococcal reactive arthritis (PSRA) and pediatric autoimmune neuropsychiatric disorders associated with streptococcal infections (PANDAS) (see below).

Severe invasive GAS infection is defined as the isolation of GAS from a normally sterile body site and includes three overlapping clinical syndromes. Cellulitis and BSI are the most common GAS invasive diseases, each accounting for ~20% to 40% of invasive GAS disease in published epidemiologic reports.[47,48] Clinically, cellulitis is characterized by acute onset of redness and inflammation of the skin, with associated fever, pain, and swelling. GAS BSI often triggers a rapid and robust proinflammatory cytokine response that results in high fever, nausea, and vomiting. While a serious health concern in their own right, cellulitis and BSI are

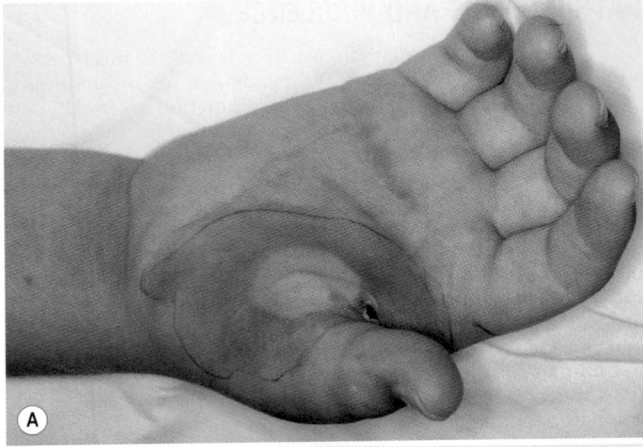
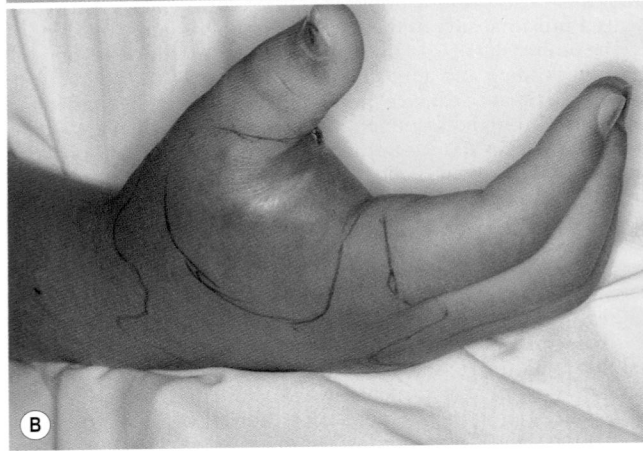

Figure 118-2. (A, B) Young girl with bullous, invasive local infection without trauma or foreign body due to group A streptococcus. (Courtesy of J.H. Brien©.)

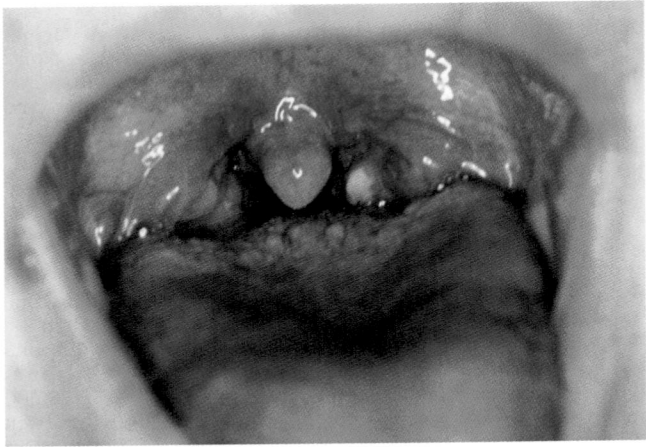

Figure 118-1. Typical group A streptococcal pharyngitis showing erythematous soft palate, uvula, and tonsils, with tonsillar exudate. (Courtesy of J.H. Brien©.)

commonly appreciated as preludes to the more serious invasive disease complications of necrotizing fasciitis and STSS.

The GAS "flesh-eating disease" necrotizing fasciitis is a devastating bacterial infection involving the skin, subcutaneous and deep soft tissue, and muscle. Necrotizing fasciitis involves rapid bacterial growth and spread along the fascial sheaths that separate adjacent muscle groups. As the infection progresses, the fascial sheaths are breached, resulting in necrosis of adjacent tissues.[53] Pathogenesis of necrotizing fasciitis is complex and incompletely understood at the molecular level. However, rapid tissue destruction and bacterial spread are thought to involve host and bacterial proteases (plasmin, SpeB), GAS pore-forming cytotoxins such as SLO and SLS, and tissue-damaging enzymes released by host neutrophils in response to GAS cell wall components and superantigens.[53] A major risk factor for the development of necrotizing fasciitis is prior blunt trauma, which is suggested to result in increased vimentin expression which tethers circulating GAS to the injured muscle.[54] Primary varicella (chickenpox) in unimmunized children also is a well-documented predisposing condition to GAS necrotizing fasciitis.[52,55]

Invasive GAS diseases also can result in STSS, a "cytokine storm," produced in response to GAS superantigens that substantially increases the risk of death.[47,48] GAS superantigens simultaneously engage MHC class II molecules and TCR β-chain variable regions, a molecular "bridging" that results in antigen-independent activation of large numbers of T lymphocytes. The resulting cytokine response by T lymphocytes (lymphotoxin α, interleukin (IL)-2, interferon (IFN)-γ) and antigen-presenting cells tumor necrosis factor (TNF)-α, IL-1β, IL-6) causes widespread organ dysfunction, disseminated intravascular thrombosis, and tissue injury.

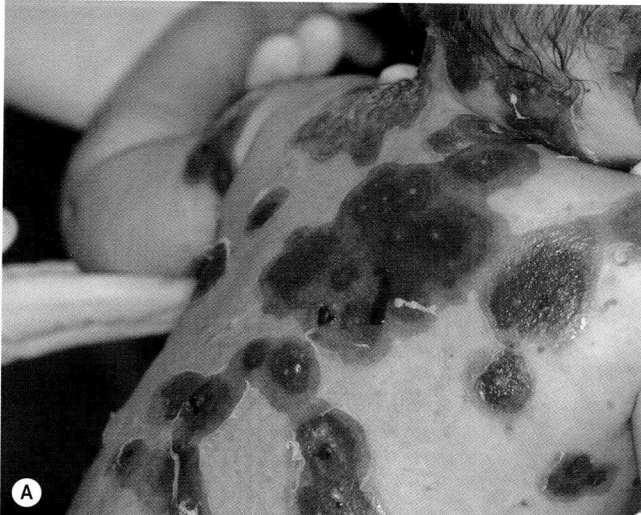

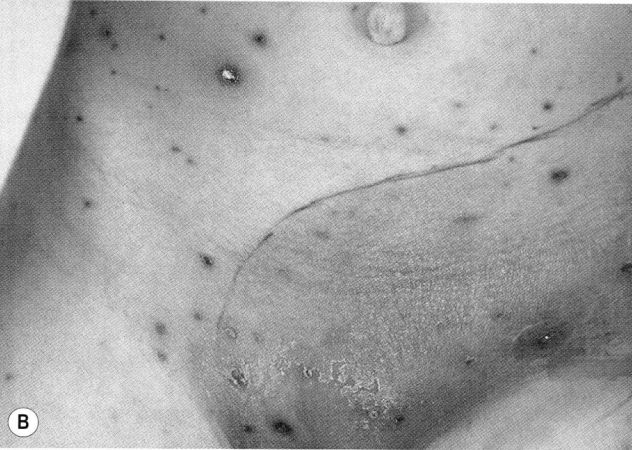

Figure 118-3. Toddler with *Staphylococcus aureus* and group A streptococcal infection complicating chickenpox **(A).** Necrotizing group A streptococcal cellulitis complicating chickenpox **(B).** (Courtesy of S.S. Long©.)

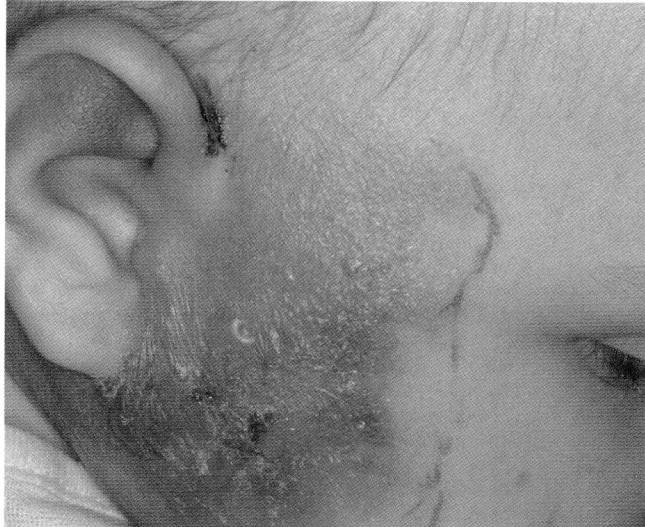

Figure 118-4. Toddler with erysipelas due to group A streptococcus. (Courtesy of J.H. Brien©.)

BOX 118-1. Definition of Streptococcal Toxic Shock Syndrome

CLINICAL CRITERIA
- Hypotension plus two or more of the following:
  - Renal impairment
  - Coagulopathy
  - Hepatic involvement
  - Adult respiratory distress syndrome
  - Generalized erythematous macular rash
  - Soft-tissue necrosis

DEFINITE CASE
- Clinical criteria plus isolation of group A *streptococcus* from a normally sterile site

PROBABLE CASE
- Clinical criteria plus isolation of group A *streptococcus* from a nonsterile site

The result is an acute, rapidly progressive illness typified by high fever, rapid-onset hypotension and accelerated multisystem failure.[56] The magnitude of the STSS inflammatory response is closely linked to disease severity. As the sites at which superantigens bind to HLA class II are polymorphic, there is strong epidemiologic and genetic evidence that host MHC class II haplotype influences susceptibility to STSS.[35,57] Specific criteria for diagnosis of STSS have been established (Box 118-1).[58]

Laboratory Findings and Diagnosis

The clinical course of severe invasive GAS infections often is precipitous, requiring rapid diagnosis and initiation of appropriate therapy. Although the initial clinical findings of STSS are nonspecific, a high index of suspicion is needed for this syndrome, particularly in patients at increased risk (e.g., those with varicella). Pain out of proportion to superficial signs of infection can be a clue to underlying necrotizing fasciitis. Hyper- or hypoesthesia, pallor, tenseness, duskiness or blistering (often hemorrhagic) at the site also are clues. Cultures of focal lesions are helpful in patients with skin or soft-tissue involvement. Results of blood cultures from patients with sepsis without an apparent focus of infection can also show GAS; a relatively normal total leukocyte count with a marked "left shift" of immature forms often is demonstrated on complete blood count. Blood pressure should be monitored frequently and carefully. Streptococcal toxic shock can be associated with multiorgan thromboses and multiorgan failure before or out of proportion to hypotension. If necrotizing fasciitis is suspected, magnetic resonance imaging may be helpful in confirming the diagnosis and determining degree of involvement of fascia and muscle.[39] Histologic examination of excised muscle/fascia tissue shows extensive necrosis, inflammation, and hemorrhage, with thrombosis of small vessels.

Treatment

Treatment of oropharyngeal, respiratory tract, and simple skin and soft-tissue infections is addressed by chapters specific to these clinical syndromes. Initial management of a child or adolescent with a severe invasive GAS infection includes hemodynamic stabilization and specific antimicrobial therapy to eradicate the GAS. When necrotizing fasciitis is suspected, prompt surgical drainage, debridement, fasciotomy, or amputation is often required. Patients with necrotizing fasciitis also need careful fluid and nutritional support and may require extensive skin grafting or other reconstructive surgery and physical therapy. Fluid resuscitation should be initiated as soon as possible for patients who are hypotensive, and frequently multiple boluses of fluid are required because of severe volume depletion and ongoing capillary leak. When fluid resuscitation alone is insufficient to maintain adequate tissue perfusion, inotropic agents (e.g., dobutamine, dopamine, norepinephrine) should be considered.

Parenteral antimicrobial therapy should include coverage for both GAS and *Staphylococcus aureus* until the results of bacteriologic studies are available. Once GAS has been identified, intravenously administered penicillin G (200,000 to 400,000 U/kg per day) in four to six divided doses is the drug of choice. However, a mouse model of streptococcal myositis suggests that clindamycin may be more effective than penicillin in eradicating GAS in severe, invasive infections.[41] In addition, clindamycin inhibits protein synthesis and the production of important virulence factors (e.g., M protein, SPEs). Therefore, many experts recommend intravenously administered clindamycin (25 to 40 mg/kg per day in three or four divided doses) in addition to penicillin. Fewer than 2% of GAS are resistant to clindamycin.

Several case reports have described the use of immune globulin intravenous (IGIV) therapy in patients with severe invasive GAS infections. An observational cohort study conducted in Canada reported significantly reduced mortality among patients treated with IGIV compared with those who were not treated.[59] However, this study had confounding factors that potentially affected mortality data, including use of historical controls and increased use of clindamycin among IGIV-treated patients. A European, multicenter, placebo-controlled trial was designed to evaluate the efficacy and safety of IGIV provided for 3 consecutive days (1 g/kg on day 1 and 0.5 g/kg on days 2 and 3) in the treatment of STSS, showing a slight trend (not statistically significant) toward a reduced mortality rate among the patients treated with IGIV.[60] Currently, IGIV should be reserved for those patients who do not respond to other therapeutic measures.

Prevention

The only specific indication for long-term use of antibiotics to prevent GAS infection is for patients with a history of ARF or rheumatic heart disease (RHD). Mass prophylaxis generally is not feasible except to reduce the number of infections during epidemics of impetigo and to control epidemics of pharyngitis in military populations and in schools.

Measures to prevent spread of GAS infections have variable effectiveness. Spread of throat or skin infection within a family unit often occurs before the index case is identified and isolated or treated. In epidemic situations, especially when there are cases of ARF or PSAGN, a culture survey with treatment of all individuals with positive cultures (mass prophylaxis) may be indicated. In families in which persistence or recurrence of streptococcal infection is a problem, simultaneous throat culture and/or culture of skin lesions of all members and treatment of all with positive results has been successful in eradicating the organism.

Clusters of invasive GAS infections have been reported within a chronic care facility or among members of a single household.[61] However, given the infrequency of these infections and the lack of a clearly effective chemoprophylactic regimen, available data currently do not support a recommendation for routine testing for GAS colonization or for routine administration of chemoprophylaxis to otherwise healthy household contacts of persons with invasive GAS disease. The Centers for Disease Control and Prevention recommend that healthcare providers inform household contacts of persons with invasive GAS about the clinical manifestation of pharyngeal and invasive GAS infections and emphasize the importance of seeking immediate medical attention if contacts develop such symptoms.[62]

Unfortunately, an effective vaccine to prevent GAS infection has yet to be developed. One major challenge derives from the great diversity of unique epitopes (>100) presented across GAS strains by the hypervariable N termini of the immunodominant surface M proteins. A second challenge is presented by data that suggests GAS components including the coiled-coil of the M protein or the GlcNac side chain on the cell wall group A carbohydrate antigen could elicit antibodies that cross-react with host muscle or neural tissues, thereby triggering ARF. Conserved, surface-associated GAS protein antigens such as pilus components, C5a peptidase, and

fibronectin-binding proteins have been explored as potential universal GAS vaccine candidates.[63] Two approaches have been taken to utilize the protective immunity of M protein without incurring the risks of molecular mimicry and autoimmune disease. One has used a conserved, noncross-reactive, C-repeat region of the M protein, found in the carboxy-terminal of the M protein proximal to the cell wall. In the other approach, molecular techniques have been used to genetically engineer highly complex multivalent M protein-based vaccines that appear to be free of potentially harmful tissue cross-reactive epitopes. A 26-valent vaccine has been shown to be well tolerated and immunogenic in adult volunteers and is now being considered for pediatric trials, which is the primary target group for the vaccine.[64]

Complications

Suppurative complications from the spread of GAS to adjacent structures were common before antibiotics were available. Cervical lymphadenitis, peritonsillar abscess, retropharyngeal abscess, otitis media, mastoiditis, and sinusitis still occur in children in whom the primary illness has gone unnoticed or in whom treatment of pharyngitis has been inadequate. GAS pneumonia occurs occasionally. Nonsuppurative complications are considered below.

ACUTE RHEUMATIC FEVER

ARF is an inflammatory disorder commonly involving joints and heart, and less commonly the brain and skin, which can develop as a complication of untreated GAS upper respiratory tract infection. The association of GAS and ARF was first postulated based on parallels in peak age (5 to 15 years) and seasonal (winter/spring) incidence, coupled with the observance that outbreaks of GAS pharyngitis in closed communities, such as boarding schools and military bases, could be followed by outbreaks of acute ARF. Subsequent serologic studies documenting anti-GAS antibodies in ARF patients provided further evidence. Finally, clinical studies showed that antimicrobial therapy that eliminates GAS from the pharynx also prevents initial attacks of ARF, and long-term, continuous prophylaxis that prevents GAS pharyngitis also prevents recurrences of ARF.

Epidemiology

While the incidence of ARF has declined substantially over the past eight decades in the U.S. and other developed countries (a decline that began even before the advent of penicillin), it still remains a major public health burden in much of the developing world. There are currently at least 15.6 million people worldwide with RHD, with 282,000 new cases and 233,000 deaths annually directly attributable to ARF or RHD.[1]

The incidence of ARF in some developing countries exceeds 50 per 100,000 children. Some of the highest incidence rates reported are in school-aged Pacific Islander children in New Zealand (80 to 100 per 100,000) and in aboriginal children in central and northern Australia (245 to 351 per 100,000). In contrast, the most recent ARF incidence data for an industrialized country come from the nonindigenous population of New Zealand (<100 per 100,000 children). The prevalence of RHD in children aged 5 to 14 years is highest in sub-Saharan Africa (570 per 100,000), the Pacific Islander and indigenous populations of New Zealand and Australia (350 per 100,000), and south central Asia (220 per 100,000). In contrast, the prevalence in developed countries usually is around 50 per 100,000.[65] A dramatic outbreak of acute ARF occurred in the Salt Lake City, Utah area beginning in 1985, with >200 cases in the first 4 years.[66] Other smaller U.S. outbreaks have been reported in various communities as well as among recruits in military training centers, but these resurgences have remained localized, not leading to a nationwide increase in cases.

The observation that only a small proportion of patients with GAS pharyngitis subsequently experience ARF suggests that specific characteristics of the organisms, the host, and the environment contribute to this complication. Although all risk factors have yet to be identified, certain potential factors have been described.

It has long been suspected, for example, that various strains of GAS differ in their ability to produce ARF, and a limited number of M serotypes have been linked epidemiologically with outbreaks of ARF. Strains of certain rheumatogenic serotypes (e.g., types 1, 3, 5, 6, and 18), which were isolated infrequently during the 1970s and early 1980s, reappeared dramatically as causes of pharyngitis during the localized outbreaks of ARF in the mid-1980s.[61] Additionally, mucoid strains of GAS had only rarely been isolated from throat cultures during the 1970s and early 1980s. However, during the focal outbreaks of ARF in the mid-1980s, mucoid strains of GAS (i.e., with high capsule expression) were commonly isolated from patients, family members, and residents in surrounding communities.

There appear to be genetic predispositions to ARF.[67] Studies in twins have shown a higher concordance rate of ARF in monozygotic than in dizygotic twin pairs. Associations between HLA class II alleles and the B-lymphocyte alloantigen D8/17 and susceptibility to ARF are under investigation; however, the association has not been consistent in various populations. In one highly defined group with mitral valve disease, collective data suggested that DRB1*0701, DR6, and DQB1*0201 confer susceptibility to ARF.[68]

Pathogenesis

The pathogenic link between a GAS infection of the upper respiratory tract and an episode of ARF still is not established definitively. Most attention has focused on the concept of autoimmunity based on molecular mimicry. This theory is supported by the latent period between GAS infection and ARF as well as by the observations of antigenic similarity between molecular constituents of GAS and several human tissues, including the heart, synovium, and basal ganglia. Sera of patients with ARF contain heart-reactive or myosin-reactive antibodies, frequently in high titers.[67] Studies of anti-GAS/anti-heart monoclonal antibodies from RHD have revealed that cardiac myosin, and GlcNac (the immunodominant epitope of the group A carbohydrate antigen), likely are cross-reactive antigens involved in antibody deposition on the valve.[68] Early work had demonstrated the persistence of increased levels of anti-group A carbohydrate antibody in RHD and their association with a poor prognosis.[69] More recently, human T-lymphocyte clones also have confirmed cross-reactivity between cardiac myosin sequences and GAS M proteins.[70] Strikingly, immunization of rats with recombinant GAS M6 protein induces autoimmune valvular heart disease.[71]

Clinical Features

Because no single clinical or laboratory finding is pathognomonic for ARF, T. Duckett Jones proposed guidelines in 1944 to aid in diagnosis and to limit overdiagnosis. The Jones criteria, as revised in 1992 by the American Heart Association (Box 118-2),[72] provide five major criteria and four minor criteria as well as the requirement for evidence (microbiologic or serologic) of recent GAS infection. The diagnosis of ARF is established according to the Jones criteria when a case fulfills two major criteria or one major plus two minor criteria and meets the absolute requirement for proof of antecedent GAS infection. ARF can be overdiagnosed even with strict application of the Jones criteria.

There are three circumstances in which the diagnosis of ARF can be made without strict adherence to the Jones criteria. Chorea can occur as the only clinical manifestation of ARF. Similarly, indolent carditis may be the only manifestation in patients who first come to medical attention months after onset.

Major Manifestations

Migratory Polyarthritis

Arthritis occurs in about 75% of patients with ARF and classically involves larger joints, particularly the knees, ankles, wrists, elbows, or hips. Rarely, the spine or small joints of the fingers or toes can be affected. Inflamed joints and periarticular tissues generally are hot,

---

BOX 118-2. Jones Criteria for Diagnosis of First Episode of Acute Rheumatic Fever (ARF)

DIAGNOSIS

Diagnosis of ARF requires two major criteria or one major and two minor criteria, with supporting evidence of antecedent group A streptococcal infection

MAJOR CRITERIA

Carditis
Polyarthritis
Chorea
Erythema marginatum
Subcutaneous nodules

MINOR CRITERIA

Clinical findings: fever; arthralgia
Laboratory finding: elevated acute-phase reactants (erythrocyte sedimentation rate or C-reactive protein); prolonged PR interval

SUPPORTING EVIDENCE OF ANTECEDENT GROUP A STREPTOCOCCAL INFECTION

Positive throat culture or rapid antigen test for GAS
or
Elevated or rising streptococcal antibody titer (ASO, anti-DNase B, etc.)

---

red, swollen and exquisitely tender; pain can precede and can appear disproportionate to other findings. The migratory nature is most characteristic; a severely involved joint can become normal within 1 to 3 days without treatment as one or more other large joints become similarly inflamed for up to 2 to 6 weeks. Another characteristic feature is a dramatic response to even small doses of nonsteroidal anti-inflammatory drugs (NSAIDs); lack of clear response should suggest an alternative diagnosis. Rheumatic arthritis almost never is deforming or associated with chronic changes.

Carditis

Carditis occurs in about 50% to 60% of ARF cases. Carditis and resultant chronic RHD are the most serious manifestations of ARF, accounting for essentially all associated morbidity and mortality. Rheumatic carditis is a pancarditis, with inflammation of myocardium, pericardium, and endocardium. Endocarditis (valvulitis), manifesting as one or more cardiac murmurs, is the hallmark feature of rheumatic carditis; myocarditis or pericarditis without evidence of endocarditis rarely is due to ARF or RHD. The vast majority of cases consist of isolated mitral valvular or aortic and mitral valvular disease. Valvular insufficiency is characteristic of acute and convalescent stages of ARF, whereas valvular stenosis develops over years or decades. In developing countries, systematic echocardiographic screening suggests the prevalence of chronic RHD may be as high as 2% to 3%, 10 times that previously estimated by clinical screening.[73]

Acute rheumatic carditis usually presents as tachycardia and cardiac murmurs with or without transient rhythm disturbances (reflecting myocardial involvement) or a friction rub (reflecting pericarditis). The characteristic murmur of mitral regurgitation is a high-pitched apical holosystolic murmur radiating to the axilla. Moderate to severe rheumatic carditis can result in cardiomegaly and congestive heart failure with hepatomegaly and peripheral and pulmonary edema. Currently, echocardiographic evidence of carditis without clinical support (i.e., auscultation of a new murmur) is neither a major nor minor Jones criterion.

Chorea

Sydenham chorea (St. Vitus dance) is a neurologic disorder that occurs in 10% to 15% of patients with ARF, often occurring much later (up to 6 months) than other manifestations. A frequently subtle disorder of behavior and movement, Sydenham chorea is characterized by emotional lability, incoordination, poor school performance, uncontrollable movements, and facial grimacing; symptoms are often exacerbated by stress and disappear during sleep. Onset can be insidious, with symptoms present for several months before recognition. Diagnosis of Sydenham chorea is based on clinical findings, with or without supportive evidence such as high serum levels of antistreptococcal antibodies. Although the acute illness is highly distressing, chorea rarely, if ever, has permanent neurologic sequelae.

Erythema Marginatum

Erythema marginatum is a rare but distinctive rash of ARF manifest by erythematous, serpiginous, macular lesions with pale centers that are not pruritic. It occurs primarily on the trunk and extremities, typically sparing the face, and is seen in fewer than 3% of patients with ARF.

Subcutaneous Nodules

Seen in less than 1% of ARF patients, firm nonpainful subcutaneous nodules approximately 1 cm in diameter can be palpated along the extensor surfaces of tendons near bony prominences. Subcutaneous nodules are often correlated with significant RHD.

Minor Manifestations

The two clinical minor manifestations included in the 1992 revised Jones criteria are: (1) arthralgia in the absence of the major criterion polyarthritis; and (2) fever, typically ≥38.9°C and occurring early in the course of illness. Two minor laboratory manifestations are: (1) elevations of acute-phase reactants, such as C-reactive protein and/or erythrocyte sedimentation rate (which is usually >50 mm/hour); and (2) demonstration of prolonged PR interval on electrocardiogram (first-degree heart block). Prospective studies have demonstrated that a prolonged PR interval alone does not constitute evidence of carditis nor predict long-term cardiac sequelae.

Recent Streptococcal Infection

Supporting evidence of a recent GAS infection is an absolute requirement for the diagnosis of ARF, except in isolated Sydenham chorea. Since ARF develops 2 to 4 weeks after acute GAS pharyngitis, clinical signs of pharyngitis are no longer present and throat culture or rapid GAS antigen test are positive in only 10% to 20% of cases; one-third of patients recall no history of antecedent pharyngitis. Elevated or rising serum antistreptococcal antibody titers thus provide the most reliable basis for diagnosis. If only ASO is measured, elevated titers (>500 Todd units) are found in 80% to 85% of patients who have ARF; 95% to 100% of such patients are identified if two additional antibody levels (e.g., anti-DNAse B, antistreptokinase or antihyaluronidase) are measured.

Differential Diagnosis

The differential diagnosis of ARF includes many infectious as well as noninfectious conditions associated with mono- or polyarticular arthritis (Table 118-1). Children with juvenile idiopathic arthritis (JIA) tend to be younger and usually have less joint pain relative to their clinical findings than those with ARF. Spiking fevers, lymphadenopathy, and splenomegaly are more suggestive of JIA than ARF. Response to salicylate therapy is much less dramatic with JIA than with ARF. Systemic lupus erythematosus (SLE) usually can be distinguished on the basis of the presence of antinuclear antibodies with SLE.

When carditis is the sole major manifestation of ARF, viral myocarditis, viral pericarditis, Kawasaki disease, and infective endocarditis should be considered. In general, the absence of a significant cardiac murmur excludes the diagnosis of ARF.

TABLE 118-1. Differential Diagnosis of Acute Rheumatic Fever

Arthritis	Carditis	Chorea
Juvenile idiopathic arthritis	Kawasaki disease	Huntington chorea
Systemic lupus erythematosus	Viral myocarditis	Wilson disease
	Viral pericarditis	Systemic lupus erythematosus
Serum sickness	Infective endocarditis	
Sickle-cell disease	Mitral valve prolapse	Cerebral palsy
Malignancy	Congenital heart disease	Tics
Gonococcal infection	Innocent murmur	Hyperactivity
Reactive arthritis (e.g., Shigella, Salmonella, Yersinia)		Encephalitis
Lyme arthritis		

Echocardiography can discriminate functional murmurs and murmurs caused by congenital heart defects. Patients with infective endocarditis can manifest both joint and cardiac manifestations; these patients usually can be distinguished on the basis of positive blood culture results or associated findings (e.g., hematuria, splenomegaly, splinter hemorrhages).

Treatment

Management of ARF involves antibiotic and anti-inflammatory therapy, symptomatic treatment, and interventions to prevent future GAS infections. Once the diagnosis of ARF has been established, the patient should receive either a single intramuscular injection of benzathine penicillin or 10 days of orally administered penicillin or amoxicillin (or a macrolide if penicillin allergic) to eradicate GAS from the upper respiratory tract, regardless of throat culture results. For patients who have definite arthritis and those who have carditis without cardiomegaly or congestive heart failure, salicylate therapy (50 to 75 mg/kg/day) should be initiated for 2 to 4 weeks, then tapered over the next 4 to 6 weeks. The response of the arthritis of ARF to salicylates is characteristically dramatic, and there is no evidence that other NSAIDs are superior. Patients with carditis and cardiomegaly or congestive heart failure should receive corticosteroid therapy (2 mg/kg/day) for 2 weeks with a slow taper over 4 to 6 weeks. Supportive therapies for patients with moderate to severe carditis include oxygen, fluid and salt restriction, diuretics, angiotensin-converting enzyme inhibitors, or digoxin. Bed rest for 2 weeks to 4 months, depending on the degree of carditis, is usually recommended. Because Sydenham chorea often occurs as an isolated manifestation after resolution of the acute phase of the disease, anti-inflammatory agents usually are not indicated. Patients may benefit from rest, limitation of external stimuli, and therapy with phenobarbital, haloperidol, or chlorpromazine as guided by a pediatric neurologist.

Secondary Prevention

Because ARF frequently recurs with subsequent GAS infections, secondary prevention is required to avoid recurrences that increase the likelihood and severity of RHD. Secondary prevention requires continuous antibiotic prophylaxis, which should begin immediately after the full course of antibiotic therapy has been completed. Patients who have had carditis with the initial episode of ARF should receive antibiotic prophylaxis well into adulthood and perhaps for life. Other patients have a relatively low risk of carditis with recurrences, and antibiotic prophylaxis can be discontinued in these patients after 5 years or when they reach the age of 21 years (whichever comes later). The decision to discontinue antibiotic prophylaxis should only be made after careful consideration of the potential risks and benefits and of epidemiologic factors, such as the risk of exposure to GAS infections.

Regimens for secondary prevention of ARF are shown in Table 118-2. A single injection of 1.2 million units of benzathine

TABLE 118-2. Secondary Prevention of Rheumatic Fever (Prevention of Recurrent Attacks)

Agent	Dose
Benzathine penicillin G	1,200,000 units IM every 4 weeks[a]
Penicillin V	250 mg PO twice daily
Sulfadiazine	0.5 g PO once daily for patients ≤27 kg; 1.0 g PO once daily for patients >27 kg
Erythromycin[b]	250 mg PO twice daily

IM, intramuscularly; PO, by mouth.

[a]*In high-risk situations, administration every 3 weeks is justified and recommended.*

[b]*For individuals allergic to penicillin and sulfadiazine.*

Adapted from Dajani A, Taubert Y, Ferrieri P, et al. Treatment of acute streptococcal pharyngitis and prevention of rheumatic fever: a statement for health professionals. Committee on Rheumatic Fever, Endocarditis, and Kawasaki Disease of the Council on Cardiovascular Disease in the Young, the American Heart Association. Pediatrics 1995;96:758.

penicillin G every 4 weeks is the regimen of choice. Continuous oral antimicrobial prophylaxis can be used in patients likely to adhere to the regimen. Penicillin given twice daily and sulfadiazine given once daily are equally effective when used in such patients. Although erythromycin resistance generally is ≤5%, frequency varies geographically, and clusters of cases with close contact can show higher resistance rates.

Prognosis

The prognosis for patients with ARF depends on the number and severity of clinical manifestations during the initial episode and whether recurrences were allowed to develop. In the absence of recurrent GAS infections, rheumatic fever does not reappear more than 8 weeks after the withdrawal of anti-inflammatory therapy. Approximately 70% of the patients with carditis during the initial episode of ARF recover with no residual heart disease if they are adherent to prophylaxis.

ACUTE GLOMERULONEPHRITIS

Epidemiology

PSAGN was described by Richard Bright in 1836 as hematuria after scarlet fever. Unlike ARF, PSAGN occurs as a consequence of either GAS pharyngitis or pyoderma. PSAGN is primarily a disease of preschool and school-aged children; approximately 60% of patients are between 2 and 12 years of age. Although the actual incidence of PSAGN is difficult to determine because many of cases are asymptomatic, PSAGN is by far the most common form of glomerulonephritis and acute renal insufficiency in children. Certain M types of GAS associated with pharyngitis, such as M1, M2, M3, M4, M12, and M15, as well as certain M types associated with pyoderma, such as M49, M52, M55, M59, M60, and M61, are commonly associated with PSAGN and, therefore, are considered nephritogenic.[74] However, not all strains of a given M type are nephritogenic. Although PSAGN is most often a sporadic disease, it also can occur in epidemic forms. Concomitant presence of ARF and PSAGN in a population is unusual and in a patient is rare.

Pathogenesis and Pathology

Although the pathogenic link between GAS infections and PSAGN is established clearly, the mechanisms of renal injury have not been defined clearly. There is considerable evidence, however, that PSAGN occurs when soluble immunoglobulin G immune complexes are deposited at the glomerular basement membrane, activating complement, with release of chemotactic factors leading to infiltration by inflammatory cells. Whether the antigen in these

complexes is a GAS antigen or a host-derived antigen that cross-reacts with antistreptococcal antibodies is not clear. Candidate GAS antigens for this process include glyceraldehyde-3-phosphate-dehydrogenase (GAPDH; also known as "nephritis-associated" streptococcal plasmin receptor) and the cysteine protease SpeB or its zymogen precursor.[75] Because these proteins are present in virtually all strains of GAS, additional host factors are suspected to influence susceptibility, but studies of HLA antigen distribution have failed to identify a specific association with PSAGN.[76]

Although renal biopsy is rarely indicated for patients with PSAGN, biopsy can be helpful if hypertension, hypocomplementemia, heavy proteinuria, or renal insufficiency persists. The glomerular lesions of PSAGN can be proliferative, exudative, or both; typically, all glomeruli are diffusely involved in the process. Electron microscopy reveals deposits consisting of immunoglobulin G and complement component C3, which usually are found in a subepithelial location during the first 3 to 6 weeks of the disease; the glomerular basement membrane usually appears normal.

Clinical Features

PSAGN typically occurs about 10 days after onset of acute GAS pharyngitis or 3 weeks after onset of GAS pyoderma. Edema (often periorbital) and hematuria most frequently bring patients with PSAGN to medical attention (Box 118-3). Approximately 30% to 50% of children with PSAGN have gross hematuria, which typically is described as "cola-colored" urine. Gross hematuria can persist for as little as a few hours or for as long as 2 weeks.

Approximately 50% to 90% of children with PSAGN have hypertension. The severity of hypertension is highly variable, but systolic pressures >200 mmHg and diastolic pressures >120 mmHg are not unusual. Most children with PSAGN also have evidence of circulatory congestion from the expansion of the intravascular fluid volume. Dyspnea, orthopnea, cough, or pulmonary rales may be present. Children with PSAGN also can have systemic symptoms such as lethargy, anorexia, fever, and abdominal pain, but they seldom appear extremely ill. Occasionally, a child with PSAGN can have a fulminant course, including severe oliguria congestive heart failure, or hypertensive encephalopathy. PSAGN typically is self-limited, however, with spontaneous diuresis, loss of edema, and improvement in hypertension occurring within 1 week.

Laboratory Findings

Virtually all children with PSAGN have microscopic hematuria, and 30% to 50% have gross hematuria. Pyuria and urinary hyaline, granular, or red blood cell casts also can be present. Most children with PSAGN also have proteinuria; approximately 30% have

---

BOX 118-3. Signs and Symptoms of Poststreptococcal Acute Glomerulonephritis (PSAGN)

COMMON FINDINGS

Hematuria (microscopic or macroscopic)
Edema
Hypertension
Oliguria

VARIABLE FINDINGS

Systemic symptoms (fever, nausea, anorexia, lethargy, abdominal pain)

UNCOMMON FINDINGS

Hypertensive encephalopathy (vomiting, headache, confusion, somnolence, seizures)
Anuria and renal failure
Congestive heart failure

proteinuria in the nephrotic range, with protein loss >2 g/m^2 per 24 hours.

During the initial 2 weeks of PSAGN, total hemolytic complement activity and C3 levels are depressed in almost all children. About one-third of patients have modest elevations of blood urea nitrogen and creatinine. During the first week of PSAGN, elevations of circulating immune complexes are seen in most patients, and the quantity of these immune complexes correlates with the severity of the PSAGN. Patients with moderate to severe impairment of renal function can demonstrate metabolic acidosis, hyperkalemia, hyperchloremia, hyponatremia, hypoalbuminemia, or dilutional anemia. In PSAGN, the best evidence of an antecedent streptococcal infection is a serologic response to GAS; 90% to 95% of patients have elevations of ASO and/or anti-DNAse B.

Treatment and Prognosis

Although antibiotic therapy does not affect the clinical course of PSAGN, therapy can eradicate the nephritogenic GAS strain that may still be present and thus reduce the risk of its transmission to others. Penicillin is the antibiotic of choice; a macrolide is the preferred agent for penicillin-allergic patients. No immunosuppressant or anti-inflammatory therapeutic agents have been shown to accelerate the resolution of the renal lesions in PSAGN. Therefore, treatment consists primarily of supportive measures directed at the complications of the disease. Children with PSAGN can occasionally have hypertension that is severe and is associated with encephalopathy. Circulatory congestion can also be severe and can lead to pulmonary edema and congestive heart failure. Although oliguria often is seen in children with PSAGN, anuria and renal failure are uncommon. Overall, the prognosis for children with PSAGN is favorable; >95% of children have spontaneous and complete resolution of symptoms, edema, and renal dysfunction. Urinalysis results are abnormal in <5% of individuals 15 years after the acute episode.[77]

Prevention

In contrast to ARF, which can be prevented with antibiotic therapy of the antecedent GAS infection, there is no evidence that PSAGN can be prevented once pharyngitis or pyoderma with a nephritogenic strain of GAS has occurred. However, antibiotic treatment of patients with PSAGN who are still harboring the nephritogenic strain can limit its transmission to others. During outbreaks of GAS pyoderma caused by nephritogenic strains, prophylactic administration of penicillin to children at risk may be beneficial.[78] Because recurrences of PSAGN are rare, long-term antibiotic prophylaxis after an episode is not indicated.

PEDIATRIC AUTOIMMUNE NEUROPSYCHIATRIC DISORDERS ASSOCIATED WITH STREPTOCOCCAL INFECTIONS (PANDAS)

In 1998, investigators described a series 50 patients with childhood-onset obsessive-compulsive disorder (OCD) and/or tics and

suggested these could arise as a result of a poststreptococcal autoimmune process.[79] The investigators coined the acronym PANDAS to denote pediatric autoimmune neuropsychiatric disorders associated with streptococcal infections. It was proposed that in response to GAS infection, this subset of patients with OCD and tic disorder produce autoimmune antibodies that cross-react with neuronal tissues in the basal ganglia and associated structures, reminiscent of the autoimmune response implicated in similar clinical manifestations of certain patients with ARF and Sydenham chorea. It was proposed that these patients could benefit from secondary antibiotic prophylaxis to prevent GAS infection and disease exacerbation, or in severe cases, immunoregulatory interventions such as plasma exchange or intravenous immunoglobulin therapy. Recently, two prospective blinded multicenter cohort studies of matched pairs have found no evidence for a temporal association between GAS infection and OCD/tic symptoms in children who met the published PANDAS diagnostic criteria.[80,81] In another study, no correlation was observed between clinical exacerbations in these patients and serum antibodies cross-reactive with brain tissues.[82] Inaccurate diagnosis and therapy of PANDAS is widespread in the pediatric medicine community;[83] new classification schemes will help delineate risks for this particular subtype of OCD or tic disorders. Current data indicate PANDAS remains an hypothesis, perhaps applicable to a very select subset of patients, but in which complicated interventions such as immune globulin or plasmapheresis may not be warranted.[81,84] Singer et al. propose a broader concept of childhood neuropsychiatric symptoms (CANS) and de-emphasis of tics and GAS.[85]

POSTSTREPTOCOCCAL REACTIVE ARTHRITIS

The term "poststreptococcal reactive arthritis" (PSRA) was first used in 1959 to describe an entity in patients who had arthritis following an episode of GAS pharyngitis but lacked other major criteria of ARF.[76] While ARF peaks in early childhood (4 to 9 years of age), PSRA has a bimodal distribution with a first peak at 8 to 14 years and a second peak in early adulthood.[86] The arthritis of ARF classically develops 14 to 21 days after an episode of GAS pharyngitis and responds rapidly to NSAID therapy, whereas PSRA does not respond readily to NSAIDs and occurs about 10 days following the GAS pharyngitis. In addition, the arthritis of PSRA is cumulative, persistent, and can involve large joints, small joints, or the axial skeleton, while the arthritis of ARF is migratory, transient, and usually involves only the large joints. All PSRA patients have serologic evidence of a recent GAS infection. A small proportion of such patients may go on to develop valvular heart disease; thus they should be monitored carefully for several months for carditis. In contrast to the arthritis of ARF, PSRA may have an extended duration (median 2 months) and can be recurrent. Some physicians administer secondary prophylaxis to these patients for a period of as short as 3 months and as long as 12 months. If carditis is not observed, prophylaxis can be discontinued. If carditis is detected, the patient should be classified as having ARF and should continue to receive secondary prophylaxis. Unfortunately, validated diagnostic criteria for PSRA have not been established.[86]

Key Points. Group A Streptococcus and Clinical Syndromes

EPIDEMIOLOGY, PATHOGENESIS, AND IMMUNITY

- >600 million cases of pharyngitis and >100 million cases of pyoderma annually worldwide
- 15.6 million people have rheumatic heart disease worldwide
- Infections can be nonsevere and of short duration or rapidly invasive and fulminant
- Unique among pyogenic bacteria in causing postinfectious, immunologically mediated diseases (acute rheumatic fever, acute glomerulonephritis)

- >130 distinct M-protein genotypes identified, which tend to be associated with infectious and nonsuppurative syndromes
- Genome sequencing shows that bacteriophages have been important in organism's evolutionary genetics (e.g., virulence determinants, toxins, etc.)
- Pathogenesis of serious disease can occur by 3 mechanisms: suppuration, toxin elaboration, and immune-mediated inflammation

Key Points. Group A Streptococcus and Clinical Syndromes—cont'd

- Expression of multiple specific virulence factors can lead to evasion of hosts innate clearance response, uncontrollable proinflammatory response, damage to phagocytic cells, accelerated apoptosis of immune cells, inactivation of terminal complement components, superantigen-induced T-lymphocyte activation, and more
- Opsonic anti-M-protein antibodies rise 6 to 8 weeks following infection and protect against M type-specific invasive infection

CLINICAL MANIFESTATIONS

- Causes wide spectrum of simple and complicated oropharyngeal and respiratory tract infections, skin and soft-tissue infections, invasive infections, and toxin-mediated syndromes
- Necrotizing cellulitis, myositis, fasciitis can be suspected when seemingly minor skin/soft-tissue infection is associated with disproportionate pain, hyper- or hypoesthenia, local pallor, tenseness, blistering lesion
- Proven cause of nonsuppurative acute rheumatic fever and acute glomerulonephritis (see text)
- Possible cause of nonsuppurative postinfectious reactive arthritis and neuropsychiatric disorders (see text)

TREATMENT OF SUPPURATIVE INFECTIONS

- Penicillin retains exquisite activity in vitro; no β-lactam antibiotic resistance exists
- Clindamycin usually is given in addition to a β-lactam agent for severe invasive or toxin-mediated disease to overcome the "Eagle effect" (loss of bactericidal capacity of β-lactam at high density of bacteria/stationary growth phase) and to inhibit protein synthesis/virulence factors
- Due to lack of compelling evidence of efficacy of IGIV therapy, use is reserved for severely affected patients under-responsive to other therapeutic measures

PREVENTION

- Vaccine development is thwarted by hypervariability and diversity of surface M proteins, and potential immunologic responses that might cross-react with cardiac or neural tissue
- Novel approaches explore the use of conserved or genetically engineered surface proteins

119 *Streptococcus agalactiae* (Group B Streptococcus)

Morven S. Edwards and Carol J. Baker

DESCRIPTION OF THE PATHOGEN

Microbiology

Streptococcus agalactiae is the species designation for Lancefield group B streptococcus (GBS). These gram-positive cocci appear on sheep blood agar as 3- to 4-mm, grey-white colonies with a narrow zone of β-hemolysis. The group B-specific cell wall carbohydrate antigen is common to all strains, and a surface capsular polysaccharide (CPS) allows classification into types Ia, Ib, II, III, IV, V, VI, VII, VIII, and provisional IX. A surface protein antigen, protein C, with α and β components, is common to all Ib strains, to 30% of type Ia, 60% of type II strains, and to some type IV, V, and VI strains.

Pathogenesis and Virulence

Pilus-like protein structures are found in all GBS strains of human origin. Antibodies to pili confer protection in experimental infection, suggesting an important role in mediating attachment and invasion.[1,2] The α C surface protein mediates translocation across epithelial barriers; GBS can also use a paracellular route by transiently opening cell junctions.[3,4] The β-hemolysin/cytolysin forms pores that compromise epithelial and endothelial barrier function.[5,6]

High-virulence clones of GBS have emerged.[7] Clonal complex ST-17 of type III has a tropism for meninges and typically is found among invasive but not colonizing neonatal isolates. CPSs allow the organism to evade ingestion by host phagocytic cells. GBS suppress phagocyte function and promote bacterial survival by engaging host CD33-related sialic acid-recognizing immunoglobulin superfamily inhibitory lectins.[8,9] Antibodies to CPSs are protective and risk for invasive infection correlates with low concentrations of antibodies to the infecting GBS CPS.[10]

TABLE 119-1. Pathogenesis of Early-Onset Group B Streptococcal Infection

Feature	Comment
Strain virulence	Clonal virulence; capsule type (e.g., III), amount of capsule, hemolysin production and certain surface components (e.g., sialic acid, β protein, among others) enhance virulence by facilitating invasion and down-regulating immune responsiveness
Genital inoculum	Risk of neonatal bacteremia correlates with high density of maternal genital colonization
Premature rupture of membranes	Risk of infection increases with rupture of membranes before onset of labor
Preterm delivery	Attack rate for early-onset disease correlates inversely with birthweight and gestational age
Prolonged rupture of membranes	Risk of early-onset disease increases significantly when membranes are ruptured >12 to 18 hours before delivery
Maternal bacteriuria due to group B streptococcus	Bacteriuria correlates with heavy maternal genital inoculum, premature rupture of placental membranes, and preterm delivery
Serum concentrations of immunoglobulin (Ig) G to colonizing serotype	Low levels of maternal IgG to capsular polysaccharide of colonizing strain increase risk

Immunity

The presence of GBS in the maternal genital tract at delivery is critical for early-onset neonatal infection. Early-onset infection occurs in ~1% of infants born to mothers with GBS vaginal or rectal colonization at delivery who do not receive intrapartum antibiotic prophylaxis (IAP). Replication of organisms in association with maternal chorioamnionitis further enhances fetal/infant risk. Early-onset disease incidence is influenced by a number of factors (Table 119-1). The higher the inoculum, the longer the duration of exposure and the greater the immaturity of the infant, the greater the risk of invasive neonatal infection.

As in early-onset infection, low concentrations of antibody to type III CPS are found uniformly in sera obtained during the acute phase of illness from infants with late- or late, late-onset infection. A viral infection preceding development may alter epithelial surfaces in a way that promotes entry of GBS into the bloodstream.[11] Extended hospitalization, as is required by very-low-birthweight infants, enhances risk of healthcare exposure to GBS, if hand hygiene is not optimal.[12]

EPIDEMIOLOGY

Depending on culture method employed and population studied, GBS can be isolated from the maternal genital or lower gastrointestinal tract in 15% to 40% of pregnant women. When specimens are obtained from the rectum and lower vagina, rather than the cervix, and when selective antibiotic-containing broth medium is employed rather than solid agar, colonization detection rates increase by 30% to 50%. Culture specimens obtained within 5 weeks of term gestation optimize the sensitivity to predict colonization at delivery.

Neonates acquire colonization with GBS vertically, either in utero by the ascending route or at delivery. Uninterrupted, the rate of vertical transmission of colonization from GBS-colonized mother to infant at delivery averages 50%. Infants born to mothers heavily colonized with GBS ($>10^5$ CFU/mL) or who have characteristics listed in Table 119-1 are at enhanced risk for invasive infection. Acquisition of colonization by infants can occur from mother or other household contacts after hospital discharge.

The incidence of early-onset GBS disease (within the first 6 days of life) has declined by 80% compared with the pre-prevention era baseline rate in 1993. In 2010, the provisional incidence was 0.25 cases per 1000 live births.[13] Attack rates for early-onset disease are related inversely to birthweight and can exceed 20 per 1000 live births in infants weighing less than 1000 grams. However, most (~70%) cases of early-onset infections still occur in term infants. The incidence of late-onset infection (7 to 89 days of age)

has not been reduced through maternal IAP; in 2010 this was provisionally 0.24 per 1000 live births.[13] GBS infections in infants aged ≥3 months occur primarily among those requiring prolonged hospitalization for complications of extreme prematurity.[14,15]

The CPS distribution of isolates causing early-onset disease parallels that of organisms colonizing the maternal genital tract.[16] Type V emerged in the 1990s.[17] The CPSs most commonly causing early-onset disease reported by the Centers for Disease Control and Prevention (CDC) are Ia (30% of cases), III (28%), V (18%), and II (13%).[18] In late-onset infections, CPS III accounts for one-half (51%), Ia for 24%, and V for 14% of cases. Infections occur occasionally in epidemic clusters; associated GBS types are similar to those causing late-onset disease.[19]

CLINICAL MANIFESTATIONS

Early-Onset Infection

Early-onset GBS infection is commonly associated with maternal obstetric complications (Table 119-2).[20] The presenting signs, such as lethargy, apnea, or bradycardia, and poor feeding, are not distinguishable from infections due to other bacteria. Irritability and hyperthermia are noted more often in term than preterm infants (Table 119-3), and bacteremia without signs of infection occurs almost exclusively in term infants.[21] Regardless of age of onset and focus of infection, respiratory distress often occurs in infants with early-onset infection. Radiographs can be consistent with pneumonia, respiratory distress syndrome, transient tachypnea of the neonate, or meconium aspiration.[15]

The clinical syndromes commonly associated with early-onset infection are bloodstream infection (BSI) without a focus (with shock in ~25%), pneumonia, and meningitis.[22,23] Payne and colleagues[24] identified six features that predict fatal outcome in early-onset disease: (1) birthweight <2500 g; (2) absolute neutrophil count <1500 cells/mm³; (3) hypotension; (4) apnea; (5) initial pH <7.25; and (6) demonstration of pleural effusion on initial chest radiograph. A clinical score was constructed that predicted outcome in 93% of patients.

Late-Onset Infection

The median age of onset for late-onset disease is 37 days.[18] Affected term infants usually have an unremarkable early neonatal course. BSI without a focus is the most common presentation, but meningitis occurs in ~30%. Characteristic features are fever, poor feeding, and irritability; infants usually recover uneventfully with antimicrobial and supportive therapy. Infants with meningitis can have similar presenting features, but some have fulminant onset

TABLE 119-2. Comparison of Early-Onset and Later-Onset Group B Streptococcal Infections

Feature	Early-Onset	Late-Onset	Late, Late–Onset
Age range	<7 days	7 to 89 days	>3 months
Median age at onset	1 day	37 days	Unknown
Maternal obstetric complications	Common	Preterm delivery	Varies
Frequency of gestation < 37 weeks	Frequent (~25%)	Frequent (~50%)	Typical
Usual clinical presentations	Septicemia (80–85%) Meningitis (5–10%) Respiratory diseases (10–15%)	Meningitis (25–35%) Bacteremia without focus (65%) Soft tissue, bone or joint Pneumonia (5–10%)	Bacteremia without focus (common) Bacteremia with a focus (occasional)[a]
Common capsular types	I (Ia, Ib), II, III, V	III (>50%), Ia, V	III, Ia, V
Mortality rate	3–10%[b]	1–6%	Low

[a]Includes peritoneum, urinary tract, skin and soft tissue, and central nervous system.

[b]<5% in term infants.

Modified from Edwards MS, Nizet V, Baker CJ. Group B streptococcal infections. In: Remington JS, Klein JO, Wilson CB, et al. (eds) Infectious Diseases of the Fetus and Newborn Infant, 7th ed. Philadelphia, Elsevier Saunders, 2011, p 419–469.

TABLE 119-3. Clinical Features of Early-Onset Group B Streptococcal Infection

Features	Term	Preterm
Respiratory distress	+++	++
Lethargy or poor tone	++	+++
Cyanosis	++	++
Poor feeding	++	++
Apnea or bradycardia	+	++
Poor perfusion	+	++
Hypotension	+	++
Irritability	+	–
Hyperthermia	+	–
Healthy-appearing	+	–

+++, Most common; ++, commonly observed (25–50%); +, occasionally observed (10–25%); –, rarely observed.

Modified from Weisman LE, Stoll BJ, Cruess DF, et al. Early-onset group B streptococcal sepsis: a current assessment. J Pediatr 1992;121:428–433.

and rapid progression. In these infants the presenting features can include poor color, grunting, altered level of consciousness, apnea, or seizures. A number of presenting clinical or laboratory findings are associated with a fatal outcome or abnormal neurologic examination at hospital discharge for infants with GBS meningitis (Table 119-4).[11,25,26] Seizures at admission remain a significant risk factor in multivariate analysis.[26]

Several other foci of infection can occur in late-onset disease, including osteomyelitis, arthritis, and cellulitis–adenitis syndrome. Osteomyelitis has an indolent presentation, with diminished mobility of an extremity or pain with motion that has been present for up to a month before diagnosis. Inflammatory signs are present occasionally but not reliably. The proximal humerus is the most frequent site in osteomyelitis; less frequently, long bones of the lower extremities and flat or small bones are involved.[27–29]

The mean age at diagnosis of pyogenic arthritis is 20 days. The duration of signs of infection is usually several days, and the hip and knee joints are common sites of involvement. GBS cellulitis–adenitis syndrome usually is unilateral, involving facial or submandibular sites, although inguinal, scrotal, and prepatellar sites have been described.[20,30,31] Presenting signs include poor feeding, irritability, and fever. Affected infants typically have BSI (>90% of

TABLE 119-4. Presenting Features that Predict an Adverse Early Outcome for Infants with Group B Streptococcal Meningitis[a]

Feature	Comment
Need for pressors	Indicates advanced or overwhelming infection
Coma or semicoma	Indicates advanced or overwhelming infection
Seizures	Indicates cerebritis
Pallor	Surrogate for shock
Low CSF glucose	<20 mg/dL
Elevated CSF protein	≥300 mg/dL
High antigen content in CSF	Concentration of type-specific antigen in CSF exceeding 3 µg/mL

CSF, cerebrospinal fluid.

[a]See reference 26.

cases), and aspiration of the involved soft tissue or lymph node often yields the organism. Abscesses can form, necessitating surgical drainage.

A number of less common or unusual foci of infection have been reported, including urinary tract infection with or without associated structural abnormalities, endocarditis, otitis media, and necrotizing fasciitis, and others.[20] Isolation of GBS from a normally sterile body site should be considered indicative of invasive infection.

Late, Late-Onset Infection

In one report of GBS disease, 20% of infants were older than 3 months.[15] For these infants, the terms *late, late-onset* or *very late-onset infection* are applicable. Most of these infections occur among very-low-birthweight infants who require protracted hospitalization. Immature immune function and continued mucous membrane colonization probably contribute to susceptibility. Among term infants with a very late presentation, immunodeficiency, including human immunodeficiency virus infection, should be considered. BSI, without a focus or with the foci described previously for late-onset infection, is the usual presentation (see Table 119-2). Among hospitalized infants, GBS infections associated with indwelling vascular catheters or necrotizing enterocolitis also have been observed.

LABORATORY FINDINGS AND DIAGNOSIS

The diagnosis of invasive GBS infection is established by isolation of the organism from a sterile body site. Lumbar puncture is critical to diagnose meningitis because as many as 30% of infants with meningitis have a sterile blood culture.[32] Cases of early-onset GBS infection occur among infants whose mothers have a negative culture for GBS colonization, so a negative maternal GBS screen should not discourage infant evaluation for septicemia.[33,34] The finding of GBS in gastric or tracheal aspirates or in maternal amniotic fluid contents indicates infant exposure but does not define clinical illness. Abnormalities in the white blood cell count, including leukopenia, neutropenia or an increased ratio of immature-to-total neutrophils, often are found but have poor sensitivity. Sensitivity in predicting early-onset GBS septicemia is improved if this testing is performed 6 to 12 hours after birth.[35,36]

Rapid antigen detection methods are not an appropriate substitute for cultures of blood or other normally sterile body fluids. With currently available radiometric blood culture technology, antigen detection is required or indicated uncommonly, and only serum or cerebrospinal fluid (CSF) is recommended for testing.[37] Repeating such tests during therapy is not recommended. Diagnostic imaging for infants with meningitis is not useful for diagnosis or managing the acute course of infection.

TREATMENT

Initial therapy for suspected GBS infection is ampicillin plus an aminoglycoside, typically gentamicin (Table 119-5). This regimen provides broad coverage for neonatal pathogens, and the combination is synergistic in vitro and in vivo for killing of GBS. When GBS has been confirmed as the causative pathogen, clinical response has been observed, *and* sterility of the bloodstream and CSF has been documented, treatment can be completed with penicillin G alone.

Penicillin is the drug of choice. The suggested dosages and expected duration of therapy are summarized in Table 119-5. These dosages have proved safe and effective, even in small premature infants. The rationale for use of the high doses recommended is that the minimal inhibitory concentration (MIC) of penicillin for GBS ranges from 0.01 to 0.6 µg/mL and MIC is affected directly by inoculum size, and inoculum at sites of infection can be high. Antibiotic levels achieved in the blood or CSF with the suggested doses will exceed the MIC even when infection is associated with a high inoculum of a strain with an MIC at the upper range of susceptibility.

TABLE 119-5. Antibiotic Therapy for Group B Streptococcal Infections

Type of Infection	Antibiotic (Dose)	Expected Duration of Therapy
Suspected meningitis (initial empiric therapy)	Ampicillin (300 mg/kg per day) *plus* Gentamicin (5–7 mg/kg per day)[a]	Until cerebrospinal fluid sterility *and* penicillin susceptibility documented
Suspected septicemia (initial empiric therapy)[b]	Ampicillin (150 mg/kg per day) *plus* Gentamicin (5–7 mg/kg per day)[a]	Until bloodstream sterility documented
Bacteremia	Ampicillin (150 mg/kg per day) *or* Penicillin G (200,000 U/kg per day)	Total of 10 days
Meningitis	Penicillin G (400,000–500,000 U/kg per day)	Total of 14–21 days
Arthritis	Penicillin G (200,000–300,000 U/kg per day)	Total of 2–3 weeks
Osteomyelitis	Penicillin G (200,000–300,000 U/kg per day)	Total of 3–4 weeks
Endocarditis	Penicillin G (200,000–300,000 U/kg per day)	Total of 4 weeks

[a]*Monitor serum concentration to maintain a peak level of 5–10 µg/mL and a trough of <2 µg/mL.*

[b]*Assumes that lumbar puncture to exclude meningitis has been performed and that cerebrospinal fluid has no detectable abnormalities.*

Reports from the United States and Japan describe point mutations in GBS penicillin-binding proteins conferring reduced susceptibility to penicillin and other β-lactam antibiotics.[38,39] Measured MICs are at the susceptibility threshold and clinical implications of these in vitro findings are unclear. In the usual circumstance, it is not necessary to determine MIC and minimal bactericidal concentration (MBC) of penicillin for the infecting GBS.[40] Determination of GBS MIC and MBC should be considered in the following circumstances: (1) a poor clinical or bacteriologic response to penicillin or ampicillin at the recommended doses; (2) unexplained relapse or recurrence of infection; and (3) infection in an infant with congenital or acquired immunodeficiency.

Provision of supportive care directed to treatment of shock, correction of metabolic abnormalities, assisted ventilation, and control of increased intracranial pressure is paramount for optimizing the outcome of GBS infections. Adjunctive use of human immune globulin intravenous (IGIV) remains investigational.[41,42] Administration of granulocyte colony-stimulating factor or an immunoglobulin preparation hyperimmune for GBS is clinically unproven.

Lumbar puncture should be considered before therapy for GBS meningitis is discontinued, usually at 14 days in uncomplicated cases. CSF findings that suggest inadequate therapy are a neutrophil value >30% of the total WBCs and a protein level >200 mg/dL. These findings are consistent with cerebritis or parenchymal destruction. It is our practice to continue therapy an additional week if CSF findings suggest inadequate resolution after 14 days of therapy, and to reassess the CSF at 21 days of therapy. It is rarely necessary to continue treatment for meningitis longer than 3 weeks.

Contrast-enhanced imaging of the brain should be obtained before antimicrobial therapy is discontinued for infants with GBS meningitis. Cranial imaging can reveal unresolved cerebritis or ventriculitis and can identify the rare infant with complications of subdural empyema or intracranial abscess. Imaging also identifies infarctions and other lesions that can affect prognosis. All infants recovering from GBS meningitis should undergo diagnostic auditory brainstem evoked audio-response testing.

SPECIAL CONSIDERATIONS

Prognosis

Case-fatality rates range from 3% to 10% for early-onset disease and 1% to 6% for late-onset disease. The risk of death for preterm infants is 8 times that for term infants for early-onset and 3 times that of term infants for late-onset disease.[18] Among survivors, premature infants with septic shock who demonstrate periventricular leukomalacia often have neurodevelopmental sequelae.[43]

Among 53 term and near-term infants with GBS meningitis in the past decade, infection was fatal in 6%, and 22% of survivors had neurologic impairment at hospital discharge, most commonly hypertonicity and persistent seizures.[26] Contemporary data suggest a 19% incidence of severe and a 25% incidence of mild-to-moderate neurologic sequelae among survivors of GBS meningitis.[44]

Recurrent Infection

The recurrence rate for early-onset disease is approximately 1%.[45–47] Green and colleagues[45] reported 9 episodes and reviewed 23 episodes of recurrent GBS disease. The mean age was 10 days at first episode and 42 days at recurrence. No common risk factors or underlying conditions predicted recurrence. The proposed causes included a persistent focus, inadequate dose or duration of therapy, reinfection with a second strain or type, and recurrent infection with the original strain in a non-immune patient. Two contemporary reviews provide evidence for the last hypothesis by documenting that 13 of 15 sets of isolates analyzed from first and second GBS episodes were genotypically identical.[45,47] In treating a recurrence, the following is suggested: (1) confirm penicillin susceptibility of the isolate by MIC testing; (2) assess serum immunoglobulin and human immunodeficiency virus status; (3) treat empirically for 1 week longer than the usual course; and (4) consider oral rifampin therapy after parenteral therapy is complete in an attempt to eradicate mucosal colonization. The suggested dose for rifampin is 20 mg/kg per day for 4 days; this intervention has a success rate of no more than 50%, probably because the drug is bacteriostatic rather than bactericidal against GBS.[48]

PREVENTION

Two approaches to prevention of GBS infections – chemoprophylaxis and immunoprophylaxis – are proposed. Both are achievable theoretically; intrapartum antibiotic prophylaxis (IAP) has proved efficacious for early-onset disease. In 1986, Boyer and Gotoff[49] demonstrated that IAP begun at 26 to 28 weeks of gestation to high-risk pregnant carriers of GBS significantly reduced vertical transmission to infants, early postpartum febrile morbidity in women, and early-onset sepsis. The American Academy of Pediatrics (AAP) published IAP guidelines in 1992.[50] A comprehensive approach was adopted in 1996 by AAP, the American College of Obstetricians and Gynecologists (ACOG), and the CDC.[51] Selection of women for IAP was based on antenatal cultures for GBS at 35 to 37 weeks of gestation or on the presence of a factor (without cultures) known to increase risk for neonatal GBS septicemia.

A large, population-based comparison demonstrated that culture-based screening was 50% more effective than risk-based intervention in preventing early-onset GBS disease.[52] In response, the 2002 revised guidelines from the CDC for prevention of perinatal GBS disease were endorsed by the AAP and the ACOG.[53,54] All pregnant women now are screened in each pregnancy for GBS carriage at 35 to 37 weeks of gestation (vaginal and rectal sites sampled and specimens processed in antibiotic-containing broth media). In women who previously delivered an infant with GBS disease or who experienced GBS bacteriuria during the current pregnancy screening is not needed; IAP should be given. At the time of labor or rupture of membranes, IAP should be given to all pregnant women identified as GBS carriers, with the exception of those undergoing a planned cesarean delivery before rupture of membranes and onset of labor (Table 119-6). The risk-based approach should be used only when culture results are not available at the time of delivery.

In 2010, CDC updated the guidelines to be more comprehensive, but reaffirmed the major prevention strategy—universal antenatal GBS screening and IAP for culture-positive and high-risk women—and included new recommendations for: (1) laboratory methods for identification of GBS colonization during pregnancy;

(2) algorithms for screening and IAP for women with preterm labor and premature rupture of membranes; (3) updated prophylaxis recommendations for women with a penicillin allergy; and (4) a revised algorithm for the care of newborns.[55] Options for GBS identification from vaginal/rectal swabs now include positive identifications from chromogenic media and identifications directly from antibiotic-containing broth. Nucleic acid amplification tests (NAATs), such as commercially-available PCR assays, are allowed for screening after enrichment if laboratories have validated their NAAT performance and use quality controls.

The maternal IAP regimen should consist of intravenous penicillin G (5 million units initially, then 3.0 million units every 4 hours) until delivery. Intravenous ampicillin (2 grams initially and 1 gram every 4 hours until delivery) is an acceptable alternative. Penicillin-allergic women who do *not* have a history of anaphylaxis, angioedema, respiratory distress or urticaria following administration of penicillin or a cephalosporin should receive cefazolin (2 grams initially and 1 gram every 8 hours until delivery). The definition of adequate IAP is receipt of antibiotic (penicillin, ampicillin, or cefazolin) at least 4 hours before delivery.[51,55,56] All other agents, doses or durations are considered inadequate for purposes of neonatal management. For high-risk penicillin-allergic women (anaphylaxis, angioedema, respiratory distress, or urticaria), clindamycin (900 mg every 8 hours until delivery) can be given if the colonizing GBS isolate has been documented to be clindamycin susceptible. Current data estimate that 30% of GBS isolates are clindamycin resistant. Early-onset GBS has been documented in an infant with a clindamycin-resistant organism whose mother received IAP with clindamycin.[57] Vancomycin (1 gram every 12 hours until delivery) is an alternative agent for women at high risk for penicillin allergy who have clindamycin-resistant GBS isolated from screening cultures. Clindamycin and vancomycin IAP have not been evaluated for efficacy in preventing early-onset GBS neonatal disease. In a pregnant woman with high-risk allergy to penicillin, susceptibility of her colonizing GBS isolate should be confirmed prior to use of IAP with clindamycin.

Management of infants depends on infant clinical status, presence or absence of maternal chorioamnionitis, duration of penicillin, ampicillin or cefazolin IAP before delivery, if indicated, duration of membrane rupture and gestational age. An algorithm of recommended infant management that applies to all newborns is summarized in Figure 119-1. If signs of sepsis are noted, full diagnostic evaluation and empiric antibiotic therapy are indicated. If a healthy-appearing infant is born to a mother with chorioamnionitis, a limited evaluation (blood culture at birth and complete blood count at birth and/or at age 6–12 hours) is recommended, based on the infant's exposure through established maternal infection. Healthy-appearing infants born to a mother who received appropriate doses of intravenous penicillin, ampicillin, or cefazolin 4 or more hours before delivery are observed in hospital for at least 48 hours before hospital discharge unless signs of sepsis develop that prompt full evaluation and initiation of antibiotic therapy. Infants with a gestational age of ≥37 weeks and membrane rupture <18 hours for whom the duration of IAP was <4 hours before delivery should have observation for 48 hours. Healthy-appearing infants whose gestational age is <37 weeks or membrane rupture is ≥18 hours before delivery and whose mothers received IAP ≥4 hours before delivery require a limited evaluation and observation for 48 hours. Exposure to antibiotics during labor does not change the clinical spectrum of disease or the age of onset of clinical signs of early-onset infection.[58]

With substantial reduction in early-onset GBS infection achieved through implementation of IAP policies, the current national projection is 1200 cases of early-onset and 1100 cases of late-onset GBS disease annually in the U.S.[13] Black infants remain at higher risk than white infants for GBS disease, possibly because of differences in access to prenatal care and rates of preterm births.[18] Further reduction in early-onset disease potentially could be realized by improving accuracy of culture screening methods and proper and timely IAP implementation.[33]

Whereas IAP is a desirable interim approach, IAP results in the administration of an antibiotic to approximately 30% of women

TABLE 119-6. Indications and Non-Indications for IAP to Prevent Early-Onset GBS Disease[55]

Intrapartum GBS Prophylaxis Indicated	Intrapartum GBS Prophylaxis Not Indicated
• Previous infant with invasive GBS disease	• Colonization with GBS during a previous pregnancy (unless an indication for GBS prophylaxis is present for current pregnancy)
• GBS bacteriuria during any trimester of the current pregnancy[a]	• GBS bacteriuria during previous pregnancy (unless an indication for GBS prophylaxis is present for current pregnancy)
• Positive GBS vaginal-rectal screening culture in late gestation[b] during current pregnancy[a]	• Negative vaginal and rectal GBS screening culture in late gestation[b] during the current pregnancy, regardless of intrapartum risk factors
• Unknown GBS status at the onset of labor (culture not done, incomplete, or results unknown) and any of the following: – Delivery at <37 weeks' gestation[c] – Amniotic membrane rupture ≥18 hours – Intrapartum temperature ≥100.4°F (≥38.0°C)[d] – Intrapartum NAAT[e] positive for GBS	• Cesarean delivery performed before onset of labor on a woman with intact amniotic membranes, regardless of GBS colonization status or gestational age

NAAT, nucleic acid amplification tests.

[a]Intrapartum antibiotic prophylaxis is not indicated in this circumstance if a cesarean delivery is performed before onset of labor on a woman with intact amniotic membranes.

[b]Optimal timing for prenatal GBS screening is at 35–37 weeks' gestation.

[c]Recommendations for the use of intrapartum antibiotics for prevention of early-onset GBS disease in the setting of threatened preterm delivery are discussed in reference 55.

[d]If amnionitis is suspected, broad-spectrum antibiotic therapy that includes an agent known to be active against GBS should replace GBS prophylaxis.

[e]NAAT testing for GBS is optional and might not be available in all settings. If intrapartum NAAT is negative for GBS but any other intrapartum risk factor (delivery at <37 weeks' gestation, amniotic membrane rupture at ≥18 hours, or temperature ≥100.4°F (≥38.0°C)) is present, then intrapartum antibiotic prophylaxis is indicated.

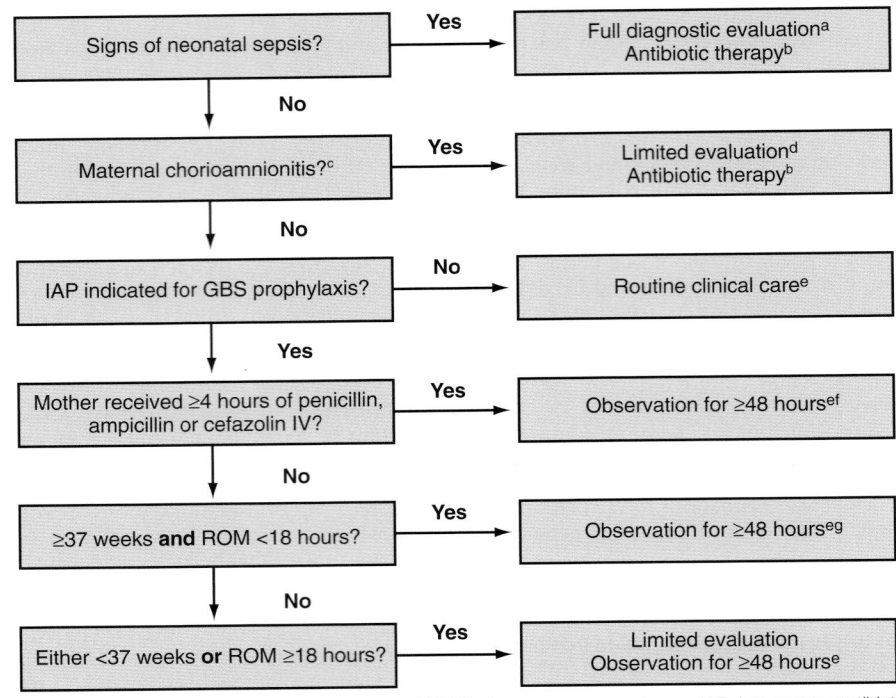

Figure 119-1. Algorithm for prevention of early-onset group b streptococcal (GBS) disease among newborns. IAP, intrapartum antibiotic prophylaxis; ROM, rupture of membranes.
[a]Full diagnostic evaluation includes a blood culture, a complete blood count (CBC) including white blood cell differential and platelet counts, chest radiograph (if respiratory abnormalities are present), and lumbar puncture (if patient is stable enough to tolerate procedure).
[b]Antibiotic therapy should be directed toward the most common causes of neonatal sepsis, including intravenous ampicillin for GBS and coverage for other organisms (including *Escherichia coli* and other gram-negative pathogens) and should take into account local antibiotic resistance patterns.
[c]Consultation with obstetric providers is important to determine the level of clinical suspicion for chorioamnionitis. Chorioamnionitis is diagnosed clinically and some of the signs are nonspecific.
[d]Limited evaluation includes blood culture (at birth) and CBC with differential and platelet counts (at birth and/or at 6 to 12 hours of life.
[e]If signs of sepsis develop, a full diagnostic evaluation should be conducted and antibiotic therapy initiated.
[f]If ≥37 weeks' gestation, observation may occur at home after 24 hours if other discharge criteria have been met, access to medical care is readily available, and a person who is able to comply fully with instructions for home observation will be present. If any of these conditions is not met, the infant should be observed in the hospital for at least 48 hours and until discharge criteria are achieved.
[g]Some experts recommend a CBC with differential and platelets at age 6 to 12 hours. (Adapted from Centers for Disease Control and Prevention. Prevention of perinatal group B streptococcal infection: revised guidelines from CDC, 2010. MMWR 2010;59(RR-10):1–31.)

at delivery, and emergence of antimicrobial resistance remains a concern.[23,59] Prevention of GBS invasive infections, irrespective of age of onset or presence of maternal risk factors, awaits development of suitable vaccines. Candidate CPS-protein conjugate vaccines are immunogenic and protective in experimental infection, and phase I and II clinical trials have been conducted. If efficacy is demonstrated, immunization of women of childbearing age to protect their neonates against GBS can be implemented. This model has been successful in prevention of tetanus, and it holds promise for application to perinatal GBS infection.[60]

120 *Enterococcus* Species

David B. Haslam and Joseph W. St. Geme III

Historically, enterococci, *Streptococcus bovis*, and *S. equinus* were grouped together as Lancefield group D streptococci. However, on the basis of DNA hybridization studies, these organisms have been reclassified, and enterococci are now recognized as a separate genus (Table 120-1). This chapter focuses on *Enterococcus* species; nonenterococcal group D streptococci are discussed in Chapter 121, Viridans Streptococci, *Abiotrophia* and *Granulicatella* Species, and *Streptococcus bovis*.

Enterococci were recognized as part of normal intestinal contents more than a century ago.[1] The improved ability to support critically ill patients, including extremely premature infants, and the widespread use of antimicrobial agents have led to the emergence of these organisms as an important cause of human disease. By contrast, other group D streptococci (*S. bovis* and *S. equinus*) remain less common causes of infection in children.

Species	Association with Disease in Children
ENTEROCOCCAL SPECIES	
Enterococcus faecalis	++
Enterococcus faecium	+
Other enterococcal species:	–
E. durans, E. avium,	
E. casseliflavus, E. dispar,	
E. flavescens, E. gallinarum,	
E. hirae, E. malodoratus,	
E. mundtii, E. pseudoavium,	
E. raffinosus, E. solitarius	
NONENTEROCOCCAL SPECIES	
Streptococcus bovis	+
Streptococcus equinus	–

++, Frequent; +, infrequent; –, rare.

DESCRIPTION OF THE PATHOGEN

Enterococcus species are gram-positive, facultatively anaerobic bacteria that grow as diplococci or in short chains. Most isolates are nonhemolytic on sheep blood agar, although some have α-hemolytic or β-hemolytic activity. Unlike other gram-positive, catalase-negative bacteria, group D organisms grow at 45°C and can withstand temperatures up to 60°C. They are capable of growth in bile, and they hydrolyze esculin, a feature not found in other Lancefield-groupable streptococci (5% of viridans streptococci and most lactococci, aerococci, pediococci, and leuconostocs share this property[2]). Clinical laboratories often distinguish *Enterococcus* species from nonenterococcal group D organisms on the basis of their ability to grow in 6.5% sodium chloride. The PYR reaction (hydrolysis of L-pyrrolidonyl-P-naphthylamide) also is a rapid means of distinguishing enterococci from *S. bovis* and *S. equinus*.[3] *S. pyogenes* is the only other PYR-positive *Streptococcus* and is distinguished easily from *Enterococcus* because of its positive reaction with group A antiserum and susceptibility to bacitracin. It is notable that occasional isolates of lactococci and aerococci also yield a positive PYR reaction. Within the *Enterococcus* genus, it is important to distinguish *E. faecalis* from *E. faecium*, two common human pathogens that are distinguished from each other on the basis of carbohydrate fermentation (Table 120-2).

Enterococci possess several important virulence factors, including adhesive factors called Esp, aggregation substance (AS), and

TABLE 120-2. Biochemical and Growth Characteristics of Clinically Important Enterococci and Group D Streptococci

	Enterococcus faecalis	*Enterococcus faecium*	*Streptococcus bovis*
Bile esculin	+	+	+
PYR reaction	+	+	–
Growth in 6.5% NaCl	+	+	–
Sorbitol	+	–	±
Mannitol	+	+	±
Lactose	+	+	+
Starch	–	–	+

+, Most isolates demonstrate the characteristic; ±, occasional isolates are positive for the characteristic; –, most isolates are negative.

Modified from Willett HP. Streptococcus. In: Joklik WK, Willett HP, Amos DB, et al. (eds) Zinser Microbiology, 22nd ed. Norwalk, CT, Appleton & Lange, 1992, p 417.

matrix binding proteins. Other virulence determinants include a cytolysin and degradative enzymes such as gelatinase, hyaluronidase, and a serine protease.[4] Many of these virulence factors are encoded on a pathogenicity island that is found more commonly among virulent than commensal isolates. The propensity of *E. faecalis* to cause endocarditis in adults may be related to surface carbohydrates that permit avid adherence to cardiac valves.[5] Once established on cardiac tissue, *E. faecalis* stimulates synthesis of fibrinogen, contributing to vegetation formation. Similarly, infection of the urinary tract may relate to the ability of the organism to adhere to renal epithelial cells.[6] *E. faecalis* cytolysin is encoded by the pathogenicity island and has lethal activity against a broad range of eukaryotic and prokaryotic cells. This factor contributes to virulence in experimental models of endocarditis, peritonitis, and endophthalmitis.[7] Antimicrobial resistance allows the persistence and proliferation of organisms in the setting of broad-spectrum antibiotic treatment. Enterococci have a remarkable propensity to exchange genetic material, both as donor and recipient. Sequencing of the *E. faecalis* strain V583 genome revealed that over 25% of its genetic material was comprised of mobile or exogenously acquired DNA. The ability to transfer DNA, including vancomycin resistance genes, to other species is a major concern.

EPIDEMIOLOGY

Enterococci are ubiquitous inhabitants of the gastrointestinal tract of humans and animals. *E. faecalis* is the predominant organism and is found in the feces of >90% of adults, usually at high density (approximately 10^7 colony-forming units per gram of stool). Nearly 50% of neonates are colonized with *E. faecalis* by 1 week of age.[8] Colonization with *E. faecium* is less common but appears to be increasing in frequency and is present in approximately 25% of adults. Although the gastrointestinal tract is the predominant habitat of enterococci, organisms also can be found in oral secretions and dental plaque, in the upper respiratory tract, on skin, and in the vagina.

E. faecalis accounts for 80% to 90% of enterococcal infections, which generally are presumed to arise from the patient's indigenous flora. Direct spread from person to person (i.e., via droplet or fecal–oral transmission) can occur, resulting in outbreaks of enterococcal septicemia in pediatric and neonatal intensive care units.[9,10] Epidemiologic investigations support the concept that outbreaks often are associated with clonal isolates that have greater potential to cause disease.

CLINICAL MANIFESTATIONS

Most enterococcal infections occur in individuals with breakdown of a normal physical barrier (such as the gastrointestinal tract, the tegument, or the urinary tract). Other factors associated with enterococcal infections in children are prolonged hospitalization, prior use of antibiotics, and compromise of the immune system. In neonates, enterococci are associated commonly with septicemia, whereas in older children and adults, they most often produce bacteremia, intra-abdominal abscess, or urinary tract infection (UTI). Among hospitalized adults, enterococci account for approximately 10% of BSIs, causing mortality in one-third of affected patients.[11]

Neonatal Infections

Enterococci account for up to 10% of all cases of neonatal BSI. The rate of enterococcal BSI fluctuates from year to year, possibly reflecting sporadic nosocomial spread of organisms. The incidence of enterococcal BSI appears to be increasing generally, concomitant with the longer survival of extremely premature infants. Most cases are due to *E. faecalis*. *E. faecium* is uncommon but has been reported as the cause of an outbreak of neonatal infection.[9]

Two apparently distinct syndromes of neonatal enterococcal BSI have been described. Early-onset BSI (within 7 days of birth) manifests similarly to early-onset group B streptococcal septicemia but tends to be milder. Early-onset infection most often occurs in full-term infants who are otherwise healthy. Late-onset infection (after 7 days of age) is associated with risk factors such as extreme prematurity, presence of an intravascular catheter, necrotizing enterocolitis, or a recent surgical procedure.[9,12] Symptoms in late-onset disease are more severe than those in early-onset disease and include apnea, bradycardia, and deteriorating respiratory function. In addition, focal infections such as scalp abscess and catheter-related infection are common. Mortality rates range from 6% in early-onset BSI to 15% in late-onset BSI associated with necrotizing enterocolitis.[12]

Enterococci are an occasional cause of meningitis. In neonates in particular, meningitis usually occurs as a complication of BSI. Alternatively, the organism gains access to the central nervous system via contiguous spread, such as through a neural tube defect, neurenteric cyst, intrathecal injection, or ventricular shunt placed for management of hydrocephalus.[13] Notably, enterococcal meningitis can be associated with minimal abnormality of the cerebrospinal fluid.

Infections in Older Children

Enterococci are the third most common organism causing BSI in hospitalized children.[14,15] Predisposing factors include an indwelling central venous catheter, gastrointestinal tract disease, immunodeficiency, cardiovascular abnormalities, and hematologic malignancy. Risk factors for vancomycin-resistant enterococcal BSI include prolonged mechanical ventilation, immunosuppression, and recent vancomycin exposure.[16] Genitourinary tract disease is a frequent predisposing factor in adults and is uncommon in children. Patients with community-acquired infections are younger than those with hospital-associated BSI, generally younger than 1 year. As in adults, polymicrobial BSI is common, probably reflecting the severity of underlying disease and the bowel as source.

Enterococci rarely cause UTIs in healthy children, but they account for approximately 15% of cases of hospital-associated UTI in both children and adults. Placement of an indwelling urinary catheter is the major risk factor for nosocomial UTI (CAUTI), and early removal of urinary catheters decreases the incidence of infection.[17] Enterococci also cause intra-abdominal abscesses after intestinal perforation. The significance of enterococci in these polymicrobial infections has been questioned, because use of an antimicrobial agent with poor activity against enterococci often is effective. In adults, enterococci cause up to 15% of cases of endocarditis, but in children these organisms rarely infect the heart.

Children colonized with vancomycin-resistant enterococci (VRE) are at highest risk of subsequent disease due to this organism. Approximately 15% of patients colonized with VRE will develop invasive infection, with the period of highest risk being the 3 months after initial colonization.[18]

BOX 120-1. Antimicrobial Resistance of Enterococci

INTRINSIC RESISTANCE (CHROMOSOMALLY ENCODED)

Aminoglycosides (low-level)
β-Lactams (especially semisynthetic penicillins and cephalosporins)
Clindamycin (low-level)

ACQUIRED RESISTANCE

Aminoglycosides (high-level)
Chloramphenicol
Erythromycin and high-level clindamycin
Fluoroquinolones
Penicillins (β-lactamase)
Tetracycline
Vancomycin

Adapted from Murray BE. Enterococci. In: Gorbach SL, Bartlett JG, Blacklow NR (eds) Infectious Diseases. Philadelphia, WB Saunders, 1992, p 1415.

TREATMENT

Enterococci demonstrate uniform resistance to cephalosporins and at least low-level resistance to other β-lactam agents. High-level resistance to aminoglycosides and vancomycin is increasingly prevalent. Antimicrobial resistance of *Enterococcus* spp. can be divided broadly into intrinsic and acquired forms.[19] In general, intrinsic resistance results from chromosomally encoded factors, whereas acquired resistance is carried on transposable elements (Box 120-1). In most cases of acquired resistance, plasmid-encoded factors are exchanged in a process mediated by sex pheromones. Receptive organisms respond to pheromones by aggregating, which facilitates subsequent conjugation and plasmid transfer.[20] On occasion, acquired resistance results from mutation of a chromosomal gene. Resistance is more common and generally is more significant in *E. faecium* than in *E. faecalis* (Table 120-3).

β-Lactam Resistance

Enterococci are highly resistant to cephalosporins and semisynthetic penicillins, such as nafcillin, oxacillin, and methicillin. Enterococci are moderately resistant to extended-spectrum penicillins, such as ticarcillin and carbenicillin. Ampicillin, imipenem, and penicillin are the most active β-lactam agents against enterococci, with minimal inhibitory concentrations (MICs) ranging from 1 to 8 µg/mL (see Table 120-3); however, the minimal bactericidal concentration (MBC) is often considerably higher, and

---

TABLE 120-3. Antimicrobial Susceptibility

Antimicrobial	*Enterococcus faecalis*			*Enterococcus faecium*		
	Range	MIC$_{50}$	MIC$_{90}$	Range	MIC$_{50}$	MIC$_{90}$
Penicillin	2 to >8	2	8	2 to >8	>8	>8
Ampicillin	0.25 to 8	2	2	0.25 to >128	128	128
Piperacillin	8 to 128	8	16	8 to 128	128	128
Imipenem	1 to >8	4	8	1 to >8	>8	>8
Chloramphenicol	8 to >16	8	16	8 to >16	8	>16
Levofloxacin	1 to >4	2	>4	1 to >4	>4	>4
Vancomycin	2 to >64	2	8	2 to >64	>64	>64
Linezolid	1 to 4	2	4	0.5 to 4	2	4

MIC, minimal inhibitory concentration; MIC$_{50}$, and MIC$_{90}$, required to inhibit 50% and 90% of isolates, respectively.

Data from Noskin GA, Siddiqui F, Stosor V, et al. In vitro activities of linezolid against important gram-positive bacterial pathogens including vancomycin-resistant enterococci. Antimicrob Agents Chemother 1999;43:2059.

tolerance to these antibiotics (defined as an MBC-to-MIC ratio >32) is common. Any active drug can be insufficient if used alone for serious infections in which high bactericidal activity is desired. Moreover, some strains of *E. faecalis* produce a plasmid-encoded β-lactamase similar to that found in staphylococci. These isolates are completely resistant to penicillins, necessitating the use of vancomycin, imipenem, or the combination of a penicillin plus a β-lactamase inhibitor. Penicillin- and imipenem-susceptible strains of *E. faecalis* generally are less susceptible, and can be resistant to meropenem, ertapenem, and doripenem; all *E. faecium* are resistant to all carbapenems.

Aminoglycoside Resistance

All enterococci have intrinsic low-level resistance to aminoglycosides (MIC, 8 to 250 µg/mL), probably reflecting poor transport of these antibiotics across the cell wall. Concomitant use of a cell wall-active agent such as a β-lactam or a glycopeptide antibiotic improves permeability of the cell wall for the aminoglycosides, resulting in synergistic killing.[21] High-level resistance is defined as an MIC >2000 µg/mL and is due to modification of aminoglycosides via adenylation, phosphorylation, or acetylation. Strains demonstrating high-level resistance (which usually are healthcare acquired) are increasingly recognized and are not affected by aminoglycosides plus cell wall-active antibiotics. Of note, some moderately resistant isolates also are not affected synergistically by aminoglycosides plus cell wall-active agents.

Vancomycin Resistance

For enterococci susceptible to both ampicillin and vancomycin, ampicillin has superior bactericidal activity. Traditionally vancomycin has been effective against multiple-drug-resistant enterococci. However, resistance to vancomycin emerged over the last decade and spread rapidly. The proportion of enterococcal infections caused by vancomycin-resistant organisms among hospitalized patients approaches 30%.[22] Resistance to vancomycin generally is accompanied by resistance to other glycopeptides, including teicoplanin and daptomycin. Both high-level resistance and moderate-level resistance are described for *E. faecalis* and *E. faecium*. High-level resistance (MIC ≥64 µg/mL) can be transferred via conjugation and usually is plasmid-mediated. The gene conferring high-level vancomycin resistance, *vanA*, encodes an inducible protein that creates a D-alanine:D-lactate ester rather than the normal D-alanine:D-alanine linkage in the cell wall. Vancomycin binds less avidly to the altered linkage and thus is unable to disrupt cell wall synthesis.[23] Moderate-level resistance (MICs 8 to 256 µg/mL) results from D-alanine:D-lactate activity expressed from a transposable homologue of *vanA* known as *vanB*.[24] Isolates that harbor the *vanB* gene are only moderately resistant to vancomycin because they possess residual D-alanine:D-alanine linkages. Although most *vanB* isolates are initially susceptible to teicoplanin, resistance can emerge during therapy. Other vancomycin phenotypes exist, encoded by *vanC*, *vanD*, *vanE*, and *vanG* genetic elements, but these are less prevalent and generally do not result in high-level resistance.

Other Antibiotics

Resistance to almost all classes of antibiotics, including tetracyclines, macrolides, and chloramphenicol, has been described among the enterococci, necessitating individual susceptibility testing for these antibiotics when their use is considered. Despite apparent in vitro susceptibility of organisms to trimethoprim-sulfamethoxazole, this combination agent has poor activity in vivo against enterococci; the organisms bypass the effect of this agent by efficiently scavenging thymidine and its precursors from blood and urine.

Antibiotics with activity against multiple-drug-resistant gram-positive organisms have been developed. Linezolid, an oxazolidone, inhibits bacterial protein synthesis. Linezolid is bacteriostatic against *E. faecium* and *E. faecalis*, demonstrating an

MIC90 of 4 µg/mL against both species, including vancomycin-resistant isolates.[25] Recent studies in children with VRE infection demonstrated a cure rate of approximately 70% with linezolid.[26] However, it is notable that resistance to linezolid among VRE isolates is described and can develop during prolonged therapy.

Daptomycin is the first lipopeptide antibiotic, and is approved for use in complicated skin infections. Daptomycin inserts into the bacterial membrane, resulting in depolarization and death of the organism without bacterial lysis. The agent has bacteriocidal activity against both *E. faecalis* and *E. faecium* and has been used as an adjunctive therapy in children with VRE infections with success, including a neonate with VRE BSI.[27,28] Daptomycin should not be used to treat pneumonia, as tissue levels are poor and the antibiotic is inactivated by pulmonary surfactants.

Quinupristin-dalfopristin (Synercid) is a combined streptogramin antibiotic that inhibits bacterial protein synthesis at two different stages. It has activity against many *E. faecium* strains, including those with high-level vancomycin resistance. Notably, it is inactive against *E. faecalis* and therefore should not be used as the sole agent for suspected gram-positive infection until culture results exclude the presence of *E. faecalis*. Recent reports suggest that only approximately 75% of VRE isolates are susceptible to quinupristin-dalfopristin in vitro. Experience in using quinupristin-dalfopristin in children infected with VRE is limited. One report documented microbiologic and clinical cure in 7 of 8 children infected with vancomycin-resistant *E. faecium*.[29] Emergence of resistance to quinupristin-dalfopristin during therapy is rare, occurring in <1% when isolates are examined before and after therapy.

Tigecycline is a tetracycline derivative that is approved for use in complicated intra-abdominal and skin and soft-tissue infections. Tigecycline is bacteriostatic against both vancomycin-resistant *E. faecalis* and vancomycin-resistant *E. faecium* and has been used with success in treatment of VRE infections in adults.[30]

Treatment Strategies

In the immunocompetent host, minor localized infections due to enterococci generally can be treated with ampicillin alone. Antibiotics containing β-lactamase inhibitors (clavulanate or sulbactam) only provide advantage for the few organisms that have high-level resistance due to production of β-lactamase. Most enterococci are susceptible to nitrofurantoin, and this agent is an alternative to penicillins for uncomplicated UTIs.

Systemic infections such as BSI, endocarditis, and meningitis usually are treated with a combination of penicillin or ampicillin and an aminoglycoside if the organism is susceptible to both. Vancomycin can be substituted for the penicillins if necessary but should not be used if penicillins can be used, and should be used with an aminoglycoside, because its action alone is only bacteriostatic. Infections due to strains possessing high-level resistance to aminoglycoside are problematic, because bactericidal activity usually cannot be achieved. As a result, endocarditis due to these strains can relapse even after prolonged therapy. High-dose or continuous-infusion penicillin has been proposed for treatment of these infections in adults.

In situations in which VRE are isolated, linezolid or daptomycin may be utilized. Quinupristin is an option for therapy of vancomycin-resistant *E. faecium* but not vancomycin-resistant *E. faecalis* infection. In patients with catheter-associated enterococcal BSI, the catheter should almost always be removed promptly. In one study of neonates, BSI persisted in all patients until the catheter was removed.[12] In patients with endocarditis due to aminoglycoside-resistant strains, valve replacement may be necessary.

PREVENTION

Strategies for preventing enterococcal infection include early removal of urinary and intravenous catheters and debridement of necrotic tissue. Contact isolation is suggested for hospitalized patients known to be colonized or infected with high-level aminoglycoside- and vancomycin-resistant organisms.[31] A number of trials have addressed the utility of using nonabsorbed antibiotics in attempts to eradicate intestinal colonization with VRE; however, decolonization has not gained wide acceptance. The Hospital Infection Control Practices Advisory Committee of

the Centers for Disease Control and Prevention (HICPAC) and the Society for Healthcare Epidemiology of America (SHEA) have published recommendations for education, infection control policy, and curtailment of use of vancomycin to prevent the spread of VRE.[32]

121 Viridans Streptococci, *Abiotrophia* and *Granulicatella* Species, and *Streptococcus bovis*

David B. Haslam and Joseph W. St. Geme III

The viridans streptococci are genetically diverse organisms that share the propensity to colonize humans and occasionally to penetrate local barriers to cause life-threatening disease. Their importance as the predominant cause of endocarditis in children and adults has been known for years. Improvements in identification and classification led to the recognition that these organisms are a significant cause of other infections, including septicemia and meningitis. In this chapter, *Abiotrophia* and *Granulicatella* (formerly nutritionally variant streptococci), and *Streptococcus bovis* are considered together with viridans streptococci. *S. bovis* is not uniformly classified within the viridans streptococci but shows significant clinical similarities to this group of organisms.

DESCRIPTION OF THE PATHOGEN

Like all streptococci, the viridans streptococci are gram-positive cocci that do not produce catalase. Most are facultatively anaerobic; however, some (including the *S. anginosus* group) are capnophilic, and others are microaerophilic. Viridans streptococci derive their name from the Latin word *viridis*, meaning green, reflecting the fact that most isolates cause α-hemolysis on sheep blood agar and produce a ring of greenish discoloration surrounding colonies. This pattern of hemolysis is predominantly due to red blood cell damage mediated by hydrogen peroxide, released from the organism when grown in the presence of oxygen. Many

viridans organisms are nonhemolytic when grown in oxygen and most are nonhemolytic when grown under anaerobic conditions. Although nucleotide sequence homology places *S. pneumoniae* among the viridans streptococci, *S. pneumoniae* generally is considered separately given its unique virulence potential. *S. pneumoniae* is differentiated from other viridans streptococci by its susceptibility to optochin and bile solubility. Whereas most viridans streptococci fail to react with the Lancefield antisera, there are a number of exceptions. For example, the *S. anginosus* group contains minute colony-forming, β-hemolytic organisms that may react with Lancefield group A, C, F, or G antisera.

SPECIATION

Speciation of the viridans streptococci has been the subject of considerable confusion. Nucleotide sequencing of the 16S ribosomal RNA (rRNA) genes has helped considerably in the classification of these organisms. Through the use of 16S rRNA sequences, the viridans streptococci now are classified into five groups, distinguished from *S. bovis* and the pyogenic streptococci (see Figure 117-1 in Chapter 117, Classification of Streptococci). In the clinical laboratory, viridans streptococcal species are differentiated on the basis of biochemical reactions and patterns of hemolysis (Table 121-1). The term "viridans streptococci" is preferred to "*Streptococcus viridans*" because it

TABLE 121-1. Biochemical Characteristics for Differentiation of Viridans Streptococci and *Streptococcus bovis*

Organism	Hemolysis	Voges–Proskauer Test Result	Hydrolysis of			Acid Production from					
			Esculin	Arginine	H₂O₂	Mannitol	Sorbitol	Lactose	Trehalose	Inulin	Raffinose
S. mutans	α, β, γ	+	+	–	–	+	+	+	+	+	+
S. mitis	α	–	–	–	+	–	–	+	v	–	v
S. oralis	α	–	–	–	+	–	–	+	v	–	v
S. sanguinis	α	–	v	+	+	–	v	+	+	+	v
S. gordonii	α	–	+	+	+	–	–	+	+	+	v
S. cristatus	α	–	–	v	+	–	–	v	+	–	–
S. salivarius	α	+	+	–	–	–	–	v	v	v	+
S. vestibularis	α	v	+	–	+	–	–	v	v	–	–
S. parasanguinis	α	–	v	+	+	–	–	+	v	–	+
S. anginosunis	α, β, γ	+	+	+	v	v	–	+	+	–	v
S. intermedius	α, γ	+	+	+	v	v	–	+	+	–	–
S. bovis	γ	NA	+	–	NA	+	–	+	+	+	+
G. morbillorum	α, γ	NA	–	–	NA	–	–	–	–	–	–

+, 85% or more of strains positive; –, 85% or more of strains are negative; G., Gemella; NA, not available; S., Streptococcus; v, variable.

Adapted from Sinner SW, Tunkel AR. Viridans streptococci and groups C and G streptococci. In: Mandell GL, Bennett JE, Dolin R (eds) Principles and Practice of Infectious Diseases, 7th Ed. New York, Churchill Livingstone, 2009.

avoids the misconception that these organisms belong to a single species or taxon.

Nutritionally variant streptococci (NVS) originally were believed to be mutant forms of *S. mitis*. Biochemical testing and genetic sequence analysis dispelled this notion, and these organisms are now classified as either *Abiotrophia* or *Granulicatella*. They are fastidious organisms that require pyridoxine (vitamin B_6) or thiol supplementation for growth. These requirements can be provided as metabolic byproducts from other bacteria; thus these organisms grow in culture as satellite colonies around other bacterial species, including *Staphylococcus aureus*.

Streptococcus bovis is a nonenterococcal group D organism and is an uncommon cause of disease in children. *S. bovis* resembles *Enterococcus* species (ability to hydrolyze esculin and grow in bile) but is differentiated by a negative PYR reaction (hydrolysis of L-pyrrolidonyl-P-naphthylamide) and failure to grow in 6.5% sodium chloride. Isolates of *S. bovis* can be further subdivided into biotypes I and II by detailed biochemical testing. Whereas biotype I strains cause most invasive *S. bovis* infections, occasional isolates are biotype II. *S. bovis* shares many biochemical characteristics with *S. salivarius*, necessitating careful testing to allow differentiation.

Automated biochemical identification systems commonly used in clinical microbiology laboratories can lead to incorrect species assignment of viridans streptococcal isolates. Advanced techniques such as 16S rRNA sequencing or MALDI-TOF mass spectrometry generally are more accurate, but still have difficulty distinguishing *S. pneumoniae* from *S. mitis* and *S. oralis*.[1]

Virulence Properties

Viridans streptococci lack classic virulence factors possessed by other streptococci, such as streptolysin O, streptolysin S, deoxyribonuclease B (DNAase B), adhesion-promoting M and F proteins, and pyrogenic exotoxins. The absence of such factors likely accounts for the low pathogenic potential of these organisms in the normal host. However, some viridans species have the predilection to cause endocarditis, a characteristic that appears to correlate with production of extracellular dextran. *S. mutans, S. sanguinis, S. mitis*, and, to some extent, *S. bovis* are most commonly implicated in endocarditis and all produce dextran. Dextran exopolysaccharide may have a dual role in the pathogenesis of endocarditis, mediating bacterial adherence to heart valves and also rendering organisms relatively resistant to penicillin. *S. mutans* also is known for its role in dental caries, a role that relates at least in part to adherence to dental enamel, mediated by glucan exopolysaccharides. *S. anginosus* organisms have a greater propensity to cause localized infections, such as dental and intra-abdominal abscesses. In contrast to other viridans streptococci, these organisms produce hydrolytic enzymes, such as hyaluronidase, DNAase, and chondroitin sulfatase, and can produce neuramidase. The role of these enzymes in pathogenesis remains to be elucidated. Finally, many viridans organisms produce an immunoglobulin (Ig) A protease that presumably attenuates the local immune response and allows organisms to persist in the mouth.

EPIDEMIOLOGY

Viridans streptococci are ubiquitous inhabitants of the mouth in both children and adults. Oral colonization occurs immediately after birth, and, by 8 hours of age, >30% of oral isolates are viridans streptococci.[2] Oral viridans organisms may confer protection for young infants by preventing overgrowth of more virulent organisms. Other sites of colonization are the upper respiratory, gastrointestinal, and female reproductive tracts.

Some viridans species occupy very well-defined niches. For example, *S. mitis* is localized predominantly to the buccal mucosa, whereas *S. mutans* and *S. sanguinis* are associated with the teeth, and *S. salivarius* is localized on the tongue. *S. bovis* is an inhabitant of the lower gastrointestinal tract.

CLINICAL MANIFESTATIONS

Endocarditis

Overall, viridans streptococci are the most common cause of bacterial endocarditis in children and adults.[3] In contrast, *S. bovis* is rarely isolated from children with endocarditis. The presentation of viridans endocarditis is insidious, usually with diagnosis delayed for several weeks. Fever is almost universally present. Malaise, anorexia, and weight loss can be prominent. Other classic signs of bacterial endocarditis, including splenomegaly, altered cardiac examination, petechiae, Osler nodes, Roth spots, Janeway lesions, and splinter hemorrhages, are found with varying frequency.

Major factors in the pathogenesis of bacterial endocarditis are turbulent flow within the heart and presence of bacteremia. Most children with viridans streptococcal endocarditis have either a ventricular septal defect or an abnormal heart valve (due to a congenital defect or rheumatic heart disease). Transient bloodstream infection (BSI) is common, particularly following dental trauma, which is an important risk factor for endocarditis. Up to 85% of children undergoing dental extraction are bacteremic, with viridans streptococci the most commonly isolated organisms.[4] Accordingly, children with certain heart lesions predisposing to severe outcomes from endocarditis should receive prophylactic antibiotics prior to dental procedures.

Abiotrophia and *Granulicatella* species (formerly NVS) account for approximately 5% of cases of endocarditis in adults. Although the frequency of endocarditis caused by these organisms appears to be lower in children, several pediatric cases have been described.[5] Historically, these organisms accounted for occasional cases of "culture-negative endocarditis"; however, most currently available blood culture media include L-cysteine or vitamin B_6 and thus support the growth of these fastidious organisms.

Bacteremia and Septicemia

The significance of recovery of viridans streptococci from blood cultures often is difficult to determine. Significance of isolation of these organisms increases if a single organism is isolated and when more than one blood culture is positive.

Viridans streptococci are a common cause of septicemia in children with cancer.[6] A particularly strong association between high-dose cytarabine and viridans streptococcal BSI has been reported. Mucositis and prolonged granulocytopenia are associated risk factors. Viridans streptococci typically are resistant to trimethoprim-sulfamethoxazole, and viridans streptococcal invasion may be enhanced by prophylaxis with this antibiotic.[7] Some patients with viridans streptococcal BSI have pulmonary complications, including acute respiratory distress syndrome (ARDS), or meningitis or both. Despite appropriate antimicrobial therapy patients with ARDS can deteriorate rapidly to septic shock. Fulminant cases generally are due to *S. mitis*, tend to occur after bone marrow transplantation, and are more common in children than adults.[8] A high proportion of these streptococci are resistant to penicillin and cephalosporins; vancomycin usually is added to the empiric treatment of neutropenic patients in whom viridans streptococcal infection is suspected.[9]

Approximately 3% to 5% of neonatal BSI are caused by viridans streptococci.[10] Risk factors are similar to those for BSI due to other organisms and include prematurity, low birthweight, and prolonged rupture of placental membranes. Clinical presentation resembles that of early-onset group B streptococcal infection, the predominant feature being respiratory distress. However, the onset tends to be later (mean age 3.5 days compared with <12 hours for group B streptococcus), and leukopenia, abnormal immature-to-total neutrophil ratio, and thrombocytopenia are less common. Associated localized infections are uncommon, although an infant with septicemia and meningitis associated with a viridans streptococcal scalp abscess has been described.[11]

Among immunocompetent older infants and children without underlying conditions, isolation of viridans streptococci from blood cultures generally represents contamination of blood

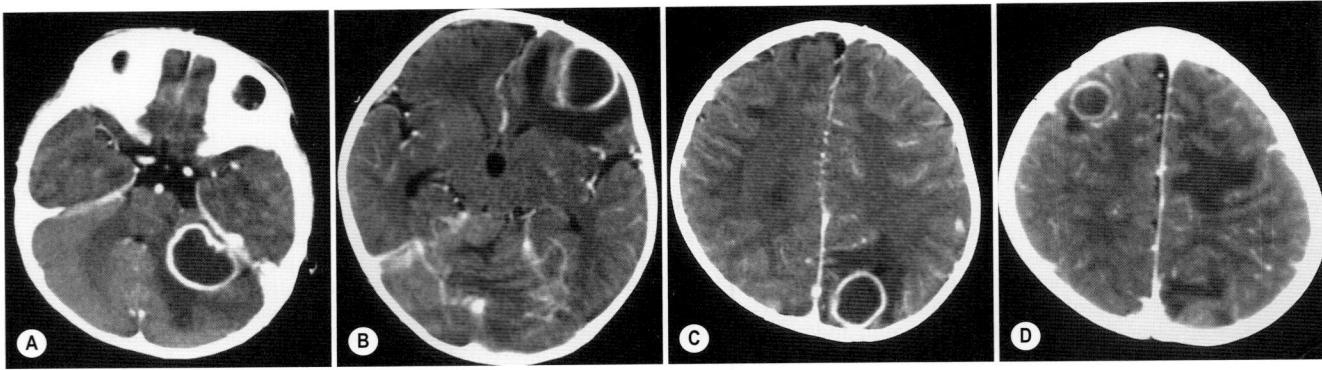

Figure 121-1. Multiple brain abscesses due to *Streptococcus intermedius* and *Eikenella corrodens* in an 11-month-old girl with tricuspid atresia, and pulmonary-to-systemic shunting of blood status post hemi-Fontan procedure. She had a 5-day history of fever, irritability, shaking chills, and then a right-sided seizure. She did not have a respiratory illness or pet exposure, pneumonia, or endocarditis. Axial contrast-enhanced computed tomography (CT) shows ring-enhancing brain abscesses with surrounding edema in the left cerebellar hemisphere **(A)**, frontal **(B)** and parietal lobes **(C)**, and right parietal lobe **(D)**, representing multifocal vascular territories. Note additional areas of cerebral edema in contralateral hemispheres **(D)** related to other abscesses. (Courtesy of E.N. Faerber and S.S. Long, St. Christopher's Hospital for Children, Philadelphia, PA.)

culture. In most cases, the patient remains asymptomatic despite lack of specific therapy.[12,13]

S. bovis occasionally is reported as a cause of neonatal BSI, often in association with a primary intestinal disorder.[14] The true incidence of *S. bovis* BSI is difficult to determine because the organism can be classified among enterococci (as a group D streptococcus) in some studies and viridans streptococci in others. No clinical features distinguish neonatal BSI due to *S. bovis* from BSI caused by more typical neonatal pathogens. Rarely, *S. bovis* BSI is complicated by meningitis, even in otherwise healthy infants born at term.[15]

Other Infections

Viridans streptococci are a rare cause of meningitis, accounting for approximately 0.3% to 3% of cases in adults. Few data exist for children, although one study implicated these organisms in approximately 1% of pediatric cases.[16] Most children are younger than 1 year and have concomitant BSI. Predisposing factors in older children include endocarditis and trauma, surgery or anomaly involving the central nervous system.

Dental infections, including dental caries, abscesses, and periodontal disease, often are due to viridans streptococci, most commonly *S. mutans* and the *S. anginosus* organisms. Infections usually are polymicrobial, but viridans streptococci sometimes are isolated as sole pathogens.

Pneumonia, empyema, sinusitis, and otitis media occasionally are ascribed to viridans streptococci. Because these organisms colonize the mouth in such high numbers, implication as the cause of respiratory tract infection is confirmed only when isolated from percutaneously aspirated specimens. Pure growth of a viridans organism has been obtained from bronchoscopy material and from aspirated pleural fluid.[17] Growing evidence supports a role for *S. anginosus* organisms as a contributor to pulmonary disease in some patients with cystic fibrosis.

Viridans streptococci can be associated with brain abscess and intra-abdominal infections, including hepatic and subphrenic abscesses. Among the viridans streptococci, the *S. anginosas* group accounts for most such infections, reflecting the proclivity of these organisms to cause localized pyogenic infections, frequently in association with other organisms (Figure 121-1).

TREATMENT

In previous decades, >80% of viridans streptococci were susceptible to penicillin (minimal inhibitory concentration (MIC) ≤0.1 µg/mL). However, resistance has increased, perhaps as a consequence of the widespread use of β-lactam antibiotics.[18] Strains with an MIC >0.12 µg/mL and <0.5 µg/mL are classified by the American Heart Association as relatively resistant, whereas those

with an MIC ≥0.5 µg/mL are considered resistant. Tolerance (ratio of minimal bactericidal concentration to MIC >32) is uncommon among viridans streptococci and is of unclear clinical significance. High-level penicillin resistance (MIC >4.0 µg/mL) is described but remains rare in North America. Penicillin nonsusceptible viridans streptococci appear to have altered penicillin-binding proteins (PBPs). The nucleotide sequence of the *PBP 2B* gene from highly resistant *S. pneumoniae* demonstrates striking homology with the *PBP 2B* gene from resistant *S. oralis* isolates, suggesting transfer of the mutated gene between the two species.[19]

Viridans streptococci are resistant to aminoglycosides used as single agents. However, aminoglycosides are synergistically bactericidal when used in combination with penicillin. Other antibiotics with good activity against the viridans streptococci are cephalosporins (especially ceftriaxone), vancomycin, teicoplanin, meropenem, and chloramphenicol. Susceptibility to tetracycline, clindamycin, and erythromycin is variable, and most isolates are resistant to trimethoprim-sulfamethoxazole. Newer antibiotics with activity against β-lactam-resistant viridans streptococci include linezolid, tigecycline, and daptomycin, although clinical experience with these agents for viridans streptococcal infection is limited.

Approximately one-half of the *Abiotrophia* and *Granulicatella* species are nonsusceptible to penicillin, and occasional isolates demonstrate high-level resistance.[20] Furthermore, strains with apparent susceptibility to penicillin often are tolerant to bactericidal activity. Relative resistance of these organisms to aminoglycosides also is common, although high-level resistance (MIC >500 µg/mL) is not described. Combination therapy with a cell wall-active agent, such as penicillin or vancomycin, and an aminoglycoside results in synergistic bactericidal activity.

The therapeutic recommendations of the American Heart Association for viridans streptococcal endocarditis involving native valves are listed in Table 121-2. Patients with endocarditis due to penicillin-susceptible isolates can be treated with penicillin alone for 4 weeks. Alternative therapy is the combination of penicillin plus an aminoglycoside for 2 weeks, with or without 2 additional weeks of penicillin alone. Relatively resistant isolates are treated with penicillin plus an aminoglycoside for 2 weeks, followed by 2 weeks of penicillin alone. Isolates with a penicillin MIC >0.5 µg/mL are treated for 4 to 6 weeks with both penicillin and an aminoglycoside. For endocarditis involving prosthetic valves or due to organisms other than viridans streptococci, the reader is referred to the American Heart Recommendations[21] and Chapter 37 (Endocarditis and Other Intravascular Infections).

Vancomycin can be substituted for penicillin in patients who have immediate-type hypersensitivity to penicillin. A 4-week course of vancomycin is recommended if the isolate has a penicillin MIC <5 µg/mL. If the isolate has an MIC ≥0.5 µg/mL, the

TABLE 121-2. Suggested Therapy for Native Valve Endocarditis Due to Viridans Streptococci According to Penicillin Minimum Inhibitory Concentration (MIC)[a,b]

Isolates with Penicillin MIC ≤0.12 µg/mL		Isolates with Penicillin MIC >0.12 µg/mL and <0.5 µg/mL		Isolates with Penicillin MIC ≥0.5 µg/mL	
Antibiotic	**Duration (Weeks)**	**Antibiotic**	**Duration (Weeks)**	**Antibiotic**	**Duration (Weeks)**
1. Penicillin G	4	1. Penicillin G	4	1. Penicillin G	4–6
or		or		plus	
Ceftriaxone	4	Ceftriaxone	4	Gentamicin[c]	4–6
2. Penicillin G	2	plus		2. Ampicillin	4–6
or		Gentamicin[c]	2	plus	
Ceftriaxone		2. Vancomycin	4	Gentamicin[c]	4–6
plus				3. Vancomycin	4–6
Gentamicin[c]	2			plus	
3. Vancomycin[d]	4			Gentamicin[c]	4–6

[a]Numbers indicate alternate, independent regimens.

[b]Suggested dosages: penicillin G, 150,000–200,000 U/kg per day (not to exceed 20 million U/day) intravenously either continuously or in six equally divided doses; gentamicin, 2.0–2.5 mg/kg per dose intravenously or intramuscularly q8 hours; streptomycin, 15 mg/kg/dose (not to exceed 500 mg) q12 hours; vancomycin, 30–40 mg/kg per day divided q8–12 hours; ceftriaxone, 75 mg/kg per day divided q12 hours. Aminoglycoside and vancomycin serum levels should be monitored and the dose adjusted accordingly.

[c]Streptomycin is a suitable alternative to gentamicin.

[d]Vancomycin therapy is suggested for penicillin-allergic patients.

Table derived from data in Baddour et al.[21]

patient should be treated with 4 to 6 weeks of vancomycin plus an aminoglycoside.[21]

Some cases of endocarditis in children do not respond to antimicrobial treatment alone and require operative therapy. Relative indications for surgical intervention include persistent infection, embolic phenomena, and worsening of congestive heart failure.

Septicemia, meningitis, and other serious infections due to penicillin-susceptible viridans streptococci can be treated with penicillin alone or in combination with an aminoglycoside. Vancomycin is the drug of choice in penicillin-allergic patients or when penicillin-highly resistant organisms are isolated. Empiric therapy for viridans streptococcal sepsis in pediatric oncology patients should include vancomycin, linezolid, or daptomycin as resistance to these agents remains rare among the S. mitis group.

Penicillin is the treatment of choice for infections caused by S. bovis, because virtually all isolates are susceptible, with an MIC <0.1 µg/mL. A single S. bovis isolate demonstrating the vanB pattern of vancomycin resistance has been described.[22]

PREVENTION

Nonspecific measures to prevent viridans streptococcal BSI in children with cancer include assiduous mouth care and maintenance of oral hygiene, particularly when mucositis is present. Studies suggest that penicillin prophylaxis in neutropenic patients may decrease the incidence of viridans streptococcal septicemia; however, this practice can lead to a greater prevalence of penicillin-resistant organisms and is not widespread currently.

Updated recommendations from the American Heart Association for prevention of endocarditis suggest antimicrobial prophylaxis for: patients with prosthetic cardiac valves, those with previous infectious endocarditis, cardiac transplant recipients with cardiac valvulopathy, and specific patients with congenital heart disease.[23] In such patients prophylactic antimicrobial therapy is recommended for tonsillectomy, adenoidectomy, and for dental procedures that involve manipulation of gingival tissue or the periapical region of teeth or perforation of the oral mucosa. Ampicillin remains the mainstay of prophylactic therapy for these situations. Recommendations differ for those with penicillin allergy, inability to take oral medications, chronic antibiotic prophylaxis, or for patients undergoing procedures such as drainage of focal respiratory infection or procedure involving infected skin or musculoskeletal tissue. Detailed guidelines for prophylaxis against endocarditis can be found in recommendations from the American Heart Association[23] and in Chapter 7 (Chemoprophylaxis).

122 Groups C and G Streptococci

David B. Haslam and Joseph W. St. Geme III

The β-hemolytic streptococci can be subdivided on the basis of whether they form large colonies or minute colonies on solid agar. Most notable among those that form large colonies are *Streptococcus pyogenes* (group A) and *S. agalactiae* (group B). Among the remaining Lancefield-reactive β-hemolytic streptococci, groups C and G organisms are most commonly associated with human disease. In this chapter, groups C and G streptococci refer exclusively to the large colony-forming organisms, often called "*S. pyogenes*-like" as their microbiologic and clinical features can mimic those of group A streptococcus. Minute colony-forming species belonging to groups C and G are placed in the *S. anginosus* group (see Chapter 121, Viridans Streptococci, *Abiotrophia* and *Granulicatella* species, and *Streptococcus bovis*). In some series of hospitalized cases of invasive bacterial infections, group G

TABLE 122-1. Differentiation of β-Hemolytic Group C and G Isolates from *Streptococcus pyogenes* and *Streptococcus anginosus*

Organism	Lancefield Group	Bacitracin	PYR Test Result	VP Test Result
Streptococcus pyogenes-like groups C and G (large colony-forming)	C or G	Resistant[a]	–	–
Streptococcus pyogenes	A	Sensitive	+	–
Minute colony-forming groups C and G (*Streptococcus anginosus* group)	C or G	NA	NA	+

+, The majority of isolates produce a positive reaction; –, most isolates produce a negative reaction; NA, data not available; PYR, L-pyrrolidonyl-β-naphthylamide; VP, Voges–Pruskauer.

[a]Occasional isolates are susceptible to bacitracin.

streptococci cause more cases than *S. pyogenes*,[1] perhaps because group G streptococci are more commonly associated with infection in immunocompromised hosts.

DESCRIPTION OF THE PATHOGENS

Groups C and G organisms are catalase-negative, gram-positive cocci. Human isolates are almost always β-hemolytic on sheep blood agar culture, although rare isolates are α-hemolytic or non-hemolytic. Groups C and G organisms resemble *S. pyogenes* on blood agar, necessitating biochemical testing and serologic analysis for definitive identification. Latex agglutination typically is used in clinical microbiology laboratories to determine the Lancefield grouping of large-colony β-hemolytic streptococci. Although most groups C and G isolates are resistant to bacitracin, an important fraction is susceptible, making this test alone unreliable in distinction from *S. pyogenes*. Hydrolysis of L-pyrrolidonyl-β-naphthylamide (PYR reaction) is a useful adjunctive test, because groups C and G streptococci are PYR negative while *S. pyogenes* is PYR positive. Colony morphology and lack of acetoin production (negative results on the Voges–Proskauer (VP) test) differentiate large-colony groups C and G streptococci from the *S. anginosus* group (Table 122-1).

Speciation

Large-colony group C and G human isolates now are grouped together as *S. dysgalactiae* subspecies *equisimilis*.[2] The remaining large-colony group C streptococci, which predominantly are animal pathogens, are grouped as *S. dysgalactiae* subspecies *dysgalactiae*. Non-human group G isolates often are considered part of a single species designated as *S. canis* and are genetically distinct from the *S. dysgalactiae* subsp. *equisimilis* group G organisms.

Virulence Properties

The groups C and G streptococci share a number of virulence factors with *S. pyogenes*. Both group C and group G isolates produce streptolysin O and can stimulate an increase in the antistreptolysin O (ASO) titer. In addition, both produce degradative enzymes, including hyaluronidase.

Group G isolates also produce streptolysin S and often produce a DNAase that is antigenically similar to *S. pyogenes* DNAase B. Moreover, group G streptococci produce an M protein that is similar immunologically to that of *S. pyogenes* and may be responsible for the occasional association of group G isolates with postinfectious glomerulonephritis. Glomerulonephritis after group C streptococcal infection also is well described. Whereas these isolates fail to produce an M protein, they can produce endostreptosin, which is felt to be involved in the pathogenesis of *S. pyogenes*-induced glomerulonephritis.

A toxic-shock-like syndrome associated with group C and G streptococcal infection has been reported. Some of these cases have been associated with a strain that possesses genes homologous to the *S. pyogenes* genes encoding streptococcal pyogenic exotoxins or that elaborates an unidentified substance with super-antigen activity.[3]

EPIDEMIOLOGY

Asymptomatic pharyngeal carriage of groups C and G streptococci is detected in up to 5% of children. In tropical climates, the pharyngeal carriage rate is much higher. The skin, gastrointestinal tract, and vagina also are frequent sites of groups C and G streptococci colonization. *S. dysgalactiae* subsp. *equisimilis* can be isolated from the umbilicus of healthy neonates but rarely causes invasive disease.

CLINICAL MANIFESTATIONS

Groups C and G streptococci are associated with the same spectrum of illnesses caused by *S. pyogenes*. In children, these organisms are implicated most commonly in respiratory tract infections, particularly pharyngitis. The true incidence of groups C and G streptococcal pharyngitis is difficult to determine, because asymptomatic colonization occurs.[4] Nevertheless, there is compelling evidence for group C and G streptococci as a true cause of pharyngitis. For example, several epidemics of group C and group G streptococcal pharyngitis have been reported. Foodborne outbreaks provide even more convincing evidence. The clinical presentation of pharyngitis due to groups C and G streptococci is indistinguishable from pharyngitis caused by *S. pyogenes*.[5]

Isolated case reports have described group C streptococcal pneumonia in children. Similar to group A streptococcal infection, tissue destruction is considerable. Abscess formation, empyema, and bacteremia are common. Despite effective antimicrobial therapy, these infections typically respond slowly, with persistent fever for >7 days.[6] Other respiratory tract infections reported include epiglottitis[7] and sinusitis.

Groups C and G streptococci also cause skin and soft-tissue infections. These organisms can colonize the skin and gain access to subcutaneous tissues after a break in skin integrity. As with *S. pyogenes*, lymphangitis can complicate superficial infections caused by groups C and G organisms. Musculoskeletal infections, particularly pyogenic arthritis, occasionally are caused by groups C and G streptococci infection. Most cases involve adults with underlying disease.[8] Pediatric cases are uncommon, although at least three well-documented cases resulting from group C streptococci have been described.[9]

Rarely, these organisms cause neonatal septicemia, accounting for up to 2% of cases in some series. Risk factors are similar to those for early-onset group B streptococcus and septicemia, include prematurity and prolonged rupture of membranes. Clinical courses may be indistinguishable and include respiratory distress, hypotension, apnea, bradycardia, and disseminated intravascular coagulation. Associated maternal infections are found commonly. Neonatal streptococcal toxic shock syndrome caused by *Streptococcus dysgalactiae* subsp. *equisimilis* has been described.[10]

Endocarditis, bacteremia, central nervous system infections (particularly brain abscess), and toxic shock caused by groups C and G streptococcal infection have been described but are uncommon in children. These infections generally occur in children with immune deficits or in adolescents after delayed recognition of sinusitis.[11]

In addition to postinfectious glomerulonephritis associated with groups C and G streptococcal infection, reactive arthritis has been described after group C streptococcal infection. There has been no convincing evidence of acute rheumatic fever after group C or G streptococcal infection, thus contrasting with group A streptococcal infection and arguing against the need for antibiotic treatment of pharyngitis to prevent this complication.[12]

THERAPY

Groups C and G streptococcus are highly susceptible to penicillin (mean minimum inhibitory concentration (MIC) <0.2 mg/mL), and penicillin is the drug of choice in most circumstances. However, some isolates demonstrate tolerance to penicillin, with a minimal bactericidal concentration-to-MIC ratio as high as 512:1. Although the clinical significance of tolerance is unclear, one study demonstrated that in adults with endocarditis resulting from tolerant group C streptococci infection, treatment with penicillin plus an aminoglycoside resulted in improved outcome.[13]

Other antibiotics with activity against groups C and G streptococci include other β-lactam agents, carbapenems, linezolid, quinupristin-dalfopristin, and vancomycin.[14] Occasional isolates demonstrate tolerance to vancomycin. Chloramphenicol, clindamycin, and erythromycin have poor bactericidal activity, particularly against group G streptococci. Up to 70% of group C streptococci produce a chromosomally encoded factor that mediates resistance to tetracycline.

123 *Streptococcus pneumoniae*

Krow Ampofo and Carrie L. Byington

In the introduction to his classic 1938 monograph *The Biology of the Pneumococcus,* Benjamin White wrote that the "pneumococcus is altogether an amazing cell. Tiny in size, simple in structure, frail in make-up, it possesses physiological functions of great variety, performs biochemical feats of extraordinary intricacy and, attacking man, sets up a stormy disease so often fatal that it must be reckoned as one of the foremost causes of human death."[1] More than 70 years later, the pneumococcus remains a major cause of respiratory tract and invasive diseases, and contributes significantly to mortality in children younger than 5 years.[2,3]

DESCRIPTION OF THE PATHOGEN

Microbiology

Streptococcus pneumoniae is a gram-positive, catalase-negative, facultative anaerobic organism that grows as lancet-shaped diplococci and in short chains. Growth is enhanced in 5% carbon dioxide or anaerobic conditions. Autolysis may be responsible for failure of the organism to grow in subculture despite a positive Gram stain reaction. On blood agar, colonies are α-hemolytic and can be identified presumptively from their susceptibility to optochin or the latex agglutination test. The specific pneumococcal type based on polysaccharide capsule can be identified using pooled typing sera and microscopy or by molecular techniques.

Ninety immunologically distinct capsular polysaccharides within 45 serogroups have been identified.[4] In the widely accepted Danish system, serotypes are grouped according to antigenic similarities. For example, serogroup 9 includes types 9A, 9L, 9N, and 9V. Immunologic cross-reactivity among serotypes in the same serogroup can result in some cross-protection but no cross-reactivity exists among different serogroups.[5]

Nucleic acid amplification tests (NAATs) such as real-time polymerase chain reaction (rPCR) have been used for *S. pneumoniae* identification, and have improved pneumococcal diagnosis. These assays rely on amplification of a number of gene sequences such as autolysin (*lytA*), pneumolysin (*ply*) and pneumococcal surface adhesin (*psa A*) to identify *S. pneumoniae*.[6-8] While useful in the rapid identification of *S. pneumoniae* from bacterial colonies,[6] these assays also have been used to detect *S. pneumoniae* in a variety of clinical specimens including blood, middle-ear fluid,[6] tissue,[9] cerebrospinal fluid,[10] and pleural fluid.[11-13] PCR-based techniques also have been used for *S. pneumoniae* serotyping.

Assays interrogate the *S. pneumoniae* gene responsible for capsular polysaccharide synthesis located at the *cps* locus. Serotype is determined by amplification of the entire *cps* locus followed by restriction fragment length polymorphism analysis[14] or by a sequence-based system using multiplex PCR.[15] The advantage of the PCR-based assay is that it can be used for *S. pneumoniae* serotyping of either living bacterial colonies or in the absence of viable isolates, and for detection of tissue or body fluids.[10,13]

Prior to 2000 and the licensure of the 7-valent conjugate pneumococcal vaccine (PCV7) in the United States, most pneumococcal disease was caused by relatively few serotypes. The most frequent types responsible for acute otitis media (AOM) in children were 23F, 19F, 6B, 6A, 14, 19A, 11, 15, 18C, 3, and 9V, although rank order varied by geographic location as exemplified by data from Finland,[5] Alabama,[16] and the Czech Republic and Slovakia.[17] Serotypes responsible for invasive pneumococcal disease (IPD) such as bacteremia or meningitis also were limited, with infection by types 14, 6B, 19F, 18C, 23F, 4, and 9V reported most commonly.[18] There have been shifts in AOM and IPD serotype distribution coincident with PCV7 licensure. Emerging AOM types include the non-PCV7 serotypes 3, 6A, 6C, and 19A.[19-22] Similarly, serotypes responsible for IPD reflect increases in non-PCV7 types including 3, 15, 19A, 22F, and 33F, with serotype 19A reported as the predominant cause of culture-confirmed IPD in U.S. children.[23-26] Genetic transformation, whereby the polysaccharide capsule switches to a different type is a well-documented mechanism for the pneumococcus to evade the host immune response.[27-29] Strain replacement (in part facilitated by capsular switching) in response to the selective pressure exerted by a successful pneumococcal vaccine program that targets a limited number of serotypes could limit the utility of pneumococcal conjugate vaccines.

Pathogenesis and Virulence

The most important factors in the development of pneumococcal disease are the virulence of the serotype, the absence of type-specific humoral immunity, and the presence of viral respiratory tract disease. *S. pneumoniae* colonizes the nasopharynx of healthy children. *S. pneumoniae* can infect the middle ear, sinuses, and lungs by contiguous spread or can invade the bloodstream and establish foci in the meninges and other sites. Pneumococcal AOM is associated with recent nasopharyngeal acquisition of a serotype rather than with prolonged colonization (carriage).[30,31] Recent acquisition also is associated with IPD. Not all pneumococcal types are equally invasive. The composition and quantity of capsular polysaccharide have major roles in virulence and invasive potential. Thus while certain serotypes are infrequently isolated from the nasopharynx, they may contribute disproportionately to IPD. In large studies, serotypes 1, 2, 7F, 9, 14, and 16 are among the most invasive, while serotypes 3, 6, 15, 19, and 23 are among the least invasive.[32,33]

Once pneumococcus enters the bloodstream, encapsulation provides protection from host defense mechanisms by inhibiting neutrophil phagocytosis and classic complement-mediated bactericidal activity. Several protein virulence factors, such as *ply* and *psa A*, also have been identified from studies in experimental animals.[34]

In the healthy host, bacteria reaching the lung usually are cleared rapidly by alveolar macrophages or migrating neutrophils. Pneumonia results when disruption of the integrity of the epithelium of the lower respiratory tract is caused by microbiologic (e.g., viral infection), chemical (e.g., alcohol), or mechanical (e.g., aspiration) factors. Bacterial clearance is delayed, resulting in proliferation of *S. pneumoniae*. The role of respiratory tract viral infection as an antecedent or co-pathogen with *S. pneumoniae* is suggested by the seasonality of IPD and correlation with respiratory viral activity.[35–37] Further, in pneumococcal conjugate vaccine trials, the 9-valent vaccine prevented 31% of cases of pneumonia associated with respiratory viruses in children.[38,39]

Immunity

The polysaccharide capsules of pneumococci are chemically distinct and have immunologically specific features that form the basis of vaccine development. Type-specific, protective antibodies against capsular polysaccharide develop after pneumococcal disease or immunization. Children <2 years of age require immunization with protein conjugate vaccine to produce type-specific antibody. Antibody facilitates destruction of the pneumococcus by complement-mediated lysis and protects against both local and invasive disease.

Carriage of a particular serotype usually does not produce immunity sufficient to prevent reacquisition of that serotype. Human breast milk may protect infants from pneumococcal infection,[40,41] but specific protective factors provided by human milk against pneumococcal infections have not been identified.

EPIDEMIOLOGY

Initial acquisition of pneumococci occurs in the first months of life with a mean age of 6 months.[42] In developing countries, cumulative acquisition in several studies has exceeded 90% before 6 months of age. Nasopharyngeal carriage rates have been reported to range from 11% to 93% and vary by age, geographic region, and population.[42–45] In a study of healthy families in Charlottesville, VA, carriage rates were as high as 35% in preschool- and school-aged children, with lower rates in adolescents (9%). Adults with preschool-aged children had higher rates of carriage (18%) than those without (9%).[46] Duration of carriage varies with serotype, is inversely correlated with age, and most commonly is 2 to 4 months but may be longer.[30,47,48]

Nasopharyngeal carriage of PCV7 serotypes decreases in children who have received vaccine, but carriage of non-PCV7 serotypes increases.[49,50] Factors associated with higher carriage rates include age <2 years, attendance at out-of-home childcare, crowding, winter, and parental smoking.[42]

Pneumococci are transmitted from person to person by respiratory droplets. Most disease is episodic, but epidemic disease has occurred in closed populations, such as military recruits,[51] and clusters of cases of IPD have been reported in children attending childcare facilities.[52]

Although type-specific immunity results from prior infection, recurrent infections by the same pneumococcal type can occur in immunocompromised hosts. Recurrent episodes of IPD occur in

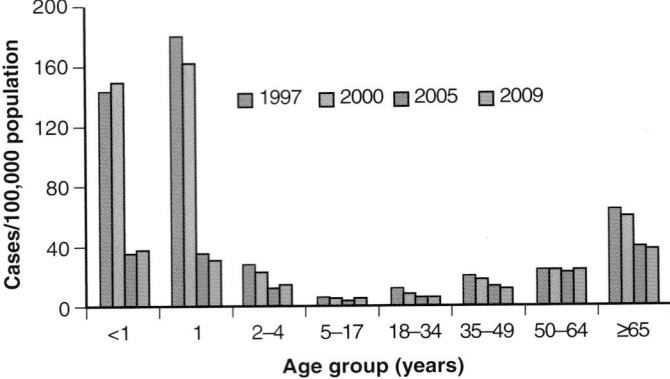

Figure 123-1. Rates of invasive pneumococcal disease by age group – United States, 1997, 2000, 2005 and 2009. Redrawn from Centers for Disease Control and Prevention. Active Bacterial Core Surveillance (ABCs)/ Emerging Infectious Program (EIP) network, 2009 (www.cdc.gov/ncidod/ dbmd/abcs).

~2.5% of patients who survive their initial episode.[53,54] The risk of recurrence is higher in persons with HIV infection and children <5 years of age with chronic illness. Recurrent pneumococcal meningitis is associated with congenital or acquired disruption of the integrity of the skull, such as fractures of the cribriform plate and nasal, otic, or neurosurgical procedures.

The highest age-specific attack rate of IPD occurs in the first 2 years of life, with a peak between 6 and 11 months of age. This pattern continued during the PCV7 era (Figure 123-1).[26] Males are more commonly affected than females in most studies. Type-specific antibody is passively transferred from the mother to the newborn and protects infants in the first several months. Accordingly, pneumococcal septicemia is rare in newborns, neonates accounting for only 20 cases in a review of 4428 episodes of IPD from 1993 to 2001.[55] In neonatal infection, the organism usually is acquired from the maternal genital tract and both early-onset and late-onset disease has been reported.[55,56]

Certain groups of children are at higher risk of IPD (Table 123-1). In the U.S. prior to introduction of PCV7, African Americans, Alaska Natives, and members of specific American Indian groups had higher rates of IPD compared with white people.[49,57] Following introduction of PCV7 the racial disparity for IPD diminished, although African Americans, Alaska Native, and some American Indian populations continue to have increased incidence of IPD compared with white people.[25,58–60] The extent to which increased risks are attributable to factors other than race or ethnicity is not clear. The increased risk of race persists despite controlling for income.[49] However, a number of case-control studies have demonstrated the strong association of IPD with underlying disease, larger family size,[41] and with attendance at out-of-home childcare in the preceding 3 months, suggesting that nonracial factors also contribute to higher risk.[40] During the PCV7 era, children with either underlying illness or no insurance coverage were at increased risk for IPD with PCV7 serotypes. Conversely, infections with non-PCV7 serotypes were more likely to occur in children who attended group childcare, lived in low-income households, or had asthma. Immunization with PCV7 did not influence the risk for nonvaccine-type IPD.[26]

Children with sickle-cell disease (SCD) or with human immunodeficiency virus (HIV) infection, especially those <3 years of age, have a markedly higher incidence of IPD.[49,61] The risk also is increased in children with other hemoglobinopathies, asplenia, nephrotic syndrome, immunodeficiency other than HIV and in children who are receiving immunosuppressive therapy or have cerebrospinal fluid leak (Table 123-1).[49,61,62] Children with a cochlear implant, in particular those who received an implant with a positioner, also have an increased risk for pneumococcal meningitis.[63]

TABLE 123-1. Underlying Medical Conditions That Are Indications for 23-Valent Pneumococcal Polysaccharide Vaccination (PPSV23) Among Children, by Risk Group[a]

Risk Group	Condition
Immunocompetent children	Chronic heart disease[b]
	Chronic lung disease[c]
	Diabetes mellitus
	Cerebrospinal fluid leaks
	Cochlear implant
Children with functional or anatomic asplenia	Sickle-cell disease and other hemoglobinopathies
	Congenital or acquired asplenia, or splenic dysfunction
Children with immunocompromising conditions	HIV infection
	Chronic renal failure and nephrotic syndrome
	Diseases associated with treatment with immunosuppressive drugs or radiation therapy, including malignant neoplasms, leukemias, lymphomas and Hodgkin disease; or solid organ transplantation
	Congenital immunodeficiency[d]

[a]*PPSV23 is given in addition to pneumococcal conjugate vaccines. Advisory Committee on Immunization Practices, Centers for Disease Control and Prevention 2010.[177]*

[b]*Particularly cyanotic congenital heart disease and cardiac failure.*

[c]*Including asthma if treated with high-dose oral corticosteroid therapy.*

[d]*Includes B- (humoral) or T-lymphocyte deficiency; complement deficiencies, particularly C1, C2, C3, and C4 deficiency; and phagocytic disorders (excluding chronic granulomatous disease).*

CLINICAL MANIFESTATIONS

The manifestations of pneumococcal infection are not distinctive from those caused by other bacteria. The major exception is the classic syndrome of pneumococcal pneumonia described below that occurs in older children and adults.

In the pre-PCV7 era, the most common infections were AOM, pneumonia, and bacteremia with or without a focus, also termed "occult bacteremia."[49] In infants and young children with occult bacteremia, *S. pneumoniae* was the predominant isolate, accounting for 83% and 92% of cases in two studies in the post-Hib and pre-PCV7 era.[64,65] In the PCV7 era, occult bacteremia in febrile children is uncommon in the U.S.[66–72] However when present, occult pneumococcal bacteremia can be caused by non-PCV7 serotypes.[73–75] Pneumococcal bloodstream infection in patients with SCD or asplenia can have a rapidly progressive course marked by abrupt onset, purpura, disseminated intravascular coagulation, and death in 24 to 48 hours; the spectrum resembles that of Waterhouse–Friderichsen syndrome.

In the U.S., *S. pneumoniae* remains the leading bacterial cause of pneumonia, although ~70% of pneumonia occurring beyond the neonatal period is caused by respiratory viruses. Data from the PCV7 trials indicated that *S. pneumoniae* was responsible for approximately one-third of radiographically diagnosed cases of pneumonia in infants.[76]

The classic presentation of pneumococcal pneumonia in older children includes a prodrome of viral respiratory tract infection typically followed by the abrupt onset of shaking chills, high fever, pleural pain, dyspnea, prostration, rust-colored sputum, and radiographic and physical findings indicating lobar consolidation. The spectrum of manifestations of pneumococcal pneumonia in infants and young children is broad and includes mild, nonspecific respiratory symptoms; cough can be absent, at least initially. In infants and toddlers, fever, vomiting, abdominal distention, and pain can be predominant and can suggest appendicitis.

Patients with right upper lobe pneumonia can have nuchal rigidity suggestive of meningitis.[77]

The characteristic radiographic finding in pneumococcal pneumonia in adolescents and adults is lobar consolidation, but in infants and young children, bronchopneumonia with scattered distribution of alveolar and parenchymal consolidation is common. Other radiographic findings are pleural fluid, lung abscess resulting from necrotizing lobar pneumonia, and, infrequently, pneumatoceles.

Although *S. pneumoniae* continues to be the leading cause of bacterial pneumonia in children, the overall incidence of pneumonia has declined significantly.[26,76,78–80] In contrast to pneumonia, parapneumonic empyema and hospitalizations due to complicated pneumonia, empyema, lung abscess and necrosis caused by *S. pneumoniae* have increased in regions of the world with widespread use of PCV7.[11,81–83] In children with pleural empyema, *S. pneumoniae* continues to be the leading cause in the U.S. and worldwide, although pleural empyema due to methicillin-resistant *S. aureus* (MRSA) is increasing.[13,83,84] An increased incidence of empyema has been associated with *S. pneumoniae* serotype 1[85,86] and necrotizing pneumonia associated with serotype 3.[87]

Among children with pneumococcal meningitis, approximately one-half manifest the classic triad of fever, nuchal rigidity, and change in mental status, and the remaining have at least one of these findings.[88] Common manifestations vary by age in children: seizures, irritability, diarrhea, and a bulging fontanel <6 months of age; vomiting, altered mental status, and poor feeding between 6 months and 2 years; neck stiffness, vomiting, and drowsiness between 2 and 10 years; neck stiffness, focal neurologic sign, headache, and vomiting >10 years of age.[89] Cerebrospinal fluid (CSF) often demonstrates typical lancet-shaped gram-positive cocci in pairs with accompanying pleocytosis (predominantly neutrophils), a low CSF-to-serum glucose ratio (<0.6) and high CSF protein concentration. In children with confirmed pneumococcal meningitis, CSF culture is positive in >90% and blood culture is positive in ~75%.[88,90] Common complications associated with pneumococcal meningitis include shock, respiratory failure, and residual neurologic sequelae, including hearing loss, seizures, and motor and behavioral deficits.[91–93] Features associated with increased morbidity and mortality include altered mental status and shock at admission as well as low CSF white cell count and glucose.[88,94]

Pneumococcal diseases also include conjunctivitis,[95–97] sinusitis,[98] soft-tissue infections, such as buccal and periorbital cellulitis, erysipelas, cystic gingival lesions, and glossitis,[99,100] and invasive infections, including peritonitis,[101] pyogenic arthritis and osteomyelitis,[102] tubo-ovarian abscess and salpingitis,[103] and endocarditis.[104,105] Rare complications of pneumococcal infection include hemorrhage and shock,[106] hemolytic-uremic syndrome,[107–109] and rhabdomyolysis.[110]

LABORATORY FINDINGS AND DIAGNOSIS

The diagnosis of pneumococcal infection can be made by isolation of the organism from culture of blood or other normally sterile site, such as CSF, middle-ear, pleural, or synovial fluid. In suspected IPD, specimens for culture should be obtained, whenever possible, before antimicrobial therapy is initiated. Specimens should be inoculated into culture media immediately or, if delay in processing is unavoidable, stored in nutrient media at 4°C. Blood culture results usually are positive within 18 hours of incubation.[65]

Gram stain of infected body fluids also should be performed, because the finding of gram-positive diplococci suggests pneumococcal etiology. In patients with fulminant infection, organisms may be seen on microscopic examination of a stained smear of buffy coat of peripheral blood, reflecting the high concentration of circulating organisms.

Early in-vitro studies of PCR demonstrated lack of sufficient sensitivity or specificity to be useful clinically.[111–113] More recently, sensitive rPCR-based assays have been developed that allow for the accurate detection of *S. pneumoniae*. In one study of children with community-acquired pneumonia (CAP), rPCR was significantly more sensitive than culture in revealing bacteremic pneumonia.[114] In another study of adult CAP, rPCR was more sensitive than routine blood culture in identifying pneumococcal pneumonia and a positive blood rPCR was associated with higher mortality, risk for shock, and the need for mechanical ventilation in adults.[115] Recent studies also have demonstrated the utility of PCR for identifying pneumococci in pleural fluid.[12,13,116]

In the absence of a positive culture or PCR assay, definitive diagnosis of pneumococcal pneumonia is difficult. In adults and older children, culture and Gram stain of expectorated sputum may be useful. Lower respiratory tract secretions can be obtained by tracheal aspiration through a catheter, protected brush, or by bronchoalveolar lavage. Lavage is warranted in children in whom microbiologic diagnosis is essential for management. The most accurate test is needle aspiration and culture of infected lung parenchyma, but the procedure is not justified in most children with uncomplicated pneumonia.

Rapid antigen tests for pneumococcal capsular polysaccharide have limited value in the diagnosis of pneumococcal infection. A urine antigen assay used in children demonstrated high sensitivity for pneumococcal bacteremia and focal pneumonia. However, the rate of false-positive tests among febrile children without identified pneumococcal infection was 15%.[117] In children with suspected bacterial meningitis, rapid antigen tests of CSF have approximately the same yield as that of Gram stain,[118] but recent findings with an immunochromatic test demonstrated better performance using CSF.[119] In children with pleural empyema, the confirmation of pneumococcal etiology can be enhanced by use of latex agglutination and PCR assays performed on pleural fluid.[13,120]

TREATMENT

Antimicrobial Susceptibility

Historically, pneumococci were susceptible in vitro to penicillins, cephalosporins, macrolides (including erythromycin, clarithromycin, and azithromycin), clindamycin, rifampin, vancomycin, and trimethoprim-sulfamethoxazole. Chloramphenicol and sulfonamides had moderate activity. In the early 1990s, pneumococcal strains resistant to penicillin and other antimicrobial agents emerged and increased. Associated with the introduction of PCV7 in 2000, and a change in definition of nonsusceptibility, antimicrobial resistance decreased during the first decade of the 21st century.

Isolates of *S. pneumoniae* are tested by broth dilution assays or the E test (AB Biodisk NA), which provide specific susceptibility data. Interpretive definitions are recommended by the Clinical Laboratory Standards Institute (CLSI).[121] Nonsusceptible isolates are subdivided into intermediate and resistant strains. Most strains of penicillin-nonsusceptible pneumococci have a minimum inhibitory concentration (MIC) of <2 μg/mL. However, in the late 1990s strains of *S. pneumoniae* with MIC of >8 μg/mL emerged.[122] In 2002, definitions of susceptibility and nonsusceptibility for penicillin, cefotaxime and ceftriaxone were revised and resulted in a decrease in nonsusceptibility rates (Table 123-2).[121]

The mechanism of penicillin resistance in pneumococci is alteration in the penicillin-binding cell wall proteins, which results in decreased drug affinity (Table 123-3). Most strains of penicillin-resistant pneumococci also are resistant to other antimicrobial agents. Penicillin resistance correlates directly with resistance to broad-spectrum cephalosporins. Strains that are more resistant to cefotaxime or ceftriaxone than to penicillin are rare.[123] The mechanisms of resistance of pneumococci are determined genetically. In addition to changes in antibiotic-binding proteins (for penicillins and cephalosporins), resistance mechanisms include induction of enzymes that inactivate the drug (e.g., chloramphenicol) and decreased drug permeability, such as with the fluoroquinolones.[124] Macrolide resistance is expressed as two phenotypes. The more common M phenotype is an efflux pump mechanism associated with the *mefE* gene and does not affect clindamycin susceptibility.

The MLS$_a$ phenotype is a result of the *ermAM* gene encoding erythromycin-ribosomal methylase, which blocks the binding of macrolide, clindamycin, and quinupristin-dalfopristin antibiotics (Table 123-3).[125] In the past decade, newly developed antimicrobial agents such as the oxazolidinones (e.g. linezolid) and

TABLE 123-2. Comparison of Former and New Antimicrobial Agents Breakpoints (Minimum Inhibitory Concentrations) for *Streptococcus pneumoniae*, by Susceptibility Category – Clinical and Laboratory Standards Institute (CLSI), 2008

Standard	Susceptibility Category MIC (μg/mL)		
	Susceptible	Intermediate	Resistant
PENICILLIN			
Former (all clinical syndromes and administered routes)	<0.06	0.12–1	≥2
New (by clinical syndrome and administered route)			
Meningitis, IV penicillin	<0.06	—[a]	≥0.12
Nonmeningitis, IV penicillin	<2	4	≥8
Nonmeningitis, oral penicillin	<0.06	0.12–1	≥2
CEFOTAXIME OR CEFTRIAXONE			
Former (all clinical syndromes and administered routes)	<0.5	1.0	≥2.0
New (by clinical syndrome and administered route)			
Meningitis	<0.5	1.0	≥2.0
Nonmeningitis	≤1.0	2.0	≥4.0

MIC, minimum inhibitory concentration; IV, intravenous.

[a]*No intermediate category for meningitis under new penicillin breakpoints.*

TABLE 123-3. Mechanisms of Antimicrobial Resistance in *Streptococcus pneumoniae*[a]

Agent	Mechanism of Resistance (Proven or Suspected)
Penicillins and cephalosporins	Alterations in penicillin-binding enzymes lead to a decreased affinity between penicillin-binding protein and the beta-lactam drugs
Chloramphenicol	Acetyltransferase
Macrolides	Expression of a ribosomal methylase encoded by *ermB* gene is responsible for high-level macrolide resistance and complete cross-resistance to clindamycin
	Efflux of macrolide from cell encoded by the *mefE* gene is responsible for low-level resistance but no effect on susceptibility to clindamycin
Trimethoprim	Reduced affinity of trimethoprim for its target enzyme dihydrofolate reductase
Quinolones	Reduced affinity of DNA gyrase (increased drug concentrations needed to obtain the same degree of enzyme inhibition) or active efflux of drug out of the bacterial cell

[a]*Data from Jacoby GA. Prevalence and resistance mechanisms of common bacterial respiratory pathogens. Clin Infect Dis 1994;18:951–957; Hyde TB, Gay K, Stephens DS, et al. Macrolide resistance among invasive Streptococcus pneumoniae isolates. JAMA 2001;286:1857–1862; Applebaum PC. Resistance among Streptococcus pneumoniae: implications for drug selection. Clin Infect Dis 2002;34:1613–1620.*

TABLE 123-4. Antibiotic Susceptibility Patterns for Invasive Pneumococcal Strains in 2000, 2005, and 2009,[a] Based on the Clinical and Laboratory Standards Institute (CLSI) Laboratory Testing Definitions

	S (%)			I (%)			R (%)		
	2000	2005	2009	2000	2005	2009	2000	2005	2009
Penicillin	72.6	76.4	89.8	9.8	13.7	5.2	17.6	9.9	5
Cefotaxime	82.3	94.7	91.9	9.8	4.1	6.2	8.0	1.2	1.9
Erythromycin	78.4	79.8	74.9	0.2	0.1	0.21	21.5	20.1	24.9
Trimethoprim-sulfamethoxazole	67.9	78.1	77	6.1	6.9	7.3	26.1	15	15.7
Levofloxacin	99.7	99.4	99.7	0	0.03	0	0.3	0.6	0.35
Vancomycin	100	100	100	0	0	0	0	0	0

S, susceptible; I, intermediate; R, resistant based on 3691 isolates in 2000, 3499 isolates in 2005, and 3743 isolates in 2009 using the Clinical and Laboratory Standards Institute (CLSI) definitions.

[a]*From the Active Bacterial Core Surveillance Report: Emerging Infections Program Network* Streptococcus pneumoniae *(www.cdc.gov/ncidod/dbmd/abcs).*

lipopeptides (e.g. daptomycin) have demonstrated in vitro activity and clinical efficacy against resistant *S. pneumoniae* isolates and infection.[126,127] No clinical isolates resistant to linezolid have been reported.

The Centers for Disease Control and Prevention (CDC) conducts population-based surveillance through the Active Bacterial Core Surveillance (ABCs), to monitor drug resistance and study the epidemiology of IPD in the U.S. Current and past data for drug resistance for various bacterial pathogens, including the pneumococcus, are available at the ABCs CDC website (http://www.cdc.gov/abcs/index.html). In 1998, 14% to 16%[128,129] of *S. pneumoniae* isolates were nonsusceptible to one or more antimicrobial agents tested, and increased to 22% by 2002 and 2003.[130,131] Following the introduction of PCV7 in 2000, the incidence of drug-resistant pneumococci decreased (Table 123-4). The reduction in single and multidrug resistance is likely due to both the reduction in pneumococcal disease resulting from the universal usage in the U.S. of PCV7 and the education of physicians and parents to restrict use of antimicrobial agents to appropriate indications.[132,133]

Prior to PCV7 licensure, risk factors associated with multidrug-resistant pneumococcal nasopharyngeal carriage and disease were age <5 years, white race,[129,134] out-of-home childcare in the previous 3 months,[40] recent antimicrobial treatment,[40,135] and residence in a community with high utilization of antibiotics.[136] With widespread use of PCV7, antimicrobial resistance of emerging non-PCV7 serotypes to penicillin has increased, with childcare attendance, upper respiratory tract infection, and the presence of young siblings important predictors.[132,137,138]

Antimicrobial Therapy

Acute Otitis Media

In guidelines published by the American Academy of Pediatrics (AAP) and the American Academy of Family Physicians in 2004, amoxicillin at a dose of 80 to 90 mg/kg per day in 2 divided doses is the first choice in uncomplicated AOM.[139] This dosing results in concentrations of drug in the middle ear sufficient to eliminate most penicillin-nonsusceptible (resistant) strains.[140] When amoxicillin fails, alternatives include amoxicillin-clavulanate (14 : 1 formulation) in a dosage of 80 to 90 mg/kg per day of the amoxicillin component in 2 divided doses. This regimen (which has activity against β-lactamase-producing organisms, but not enhanced activity against pneumococcus) has been demonstrated to be superior to placebo for children 6 through 23 months of age with AOM.[141] Cefuroxime axetil and intramuscular ceftriaxone are alternatives. Clindamycin, azithromycin, or clarithromycin are the preferred agents for AOM in children who are allergic to β-lactam antimicrobial agents, although substantial number of pneumococci are resistant to macrolides (azithromycin and erythromycin). The recommended duration for therapy for children <2 years of age with

uncomplicated infection is 10 days, while children >2 years of age can be treated for 5 days.[62] Tympanocentesis and myringotomy should be considered in the child who is toxic and in whom AOM has shown poor response to initial therapy in order to determine bacteriology and antimicrobial susceptibility.

Meningitis

The preferred regimen for initial therapy of infants and children with presumed bacterial meningitis is vancomycin (60 mg/kg per day in four divided doses) plus ceftriaxone (100 mg/kg per day in one or two doses) or cefotaxime (300 mg/kg per day in three doses).[62] Specific susceptibility breakpoints for penicillin for pneumococcal meningitis must be applied (Table 123-2). If *S. pneumoniae* is identified as the etiologic agent and is susceptible to penicillin, vancomycin should be discontinued, and penicillin G (250,000 to 400,000 units/kg per day in four or six divided doses), ceftriaxone (100 mg/kg per day in one or two divided doses), or cefotaxime (300 mg/kg per day in three or four divided doses) should be given.[142] If the pneumococcal isolate is not susceptible to penicillin (intermediate or resistant) but susceptible to ceftriaxone and cefotaxime, vancomycin can be discontinued, and ceftriaxone or cefotaxime continued. If the isolate is nonsusceptible to penicillin, ceftriaxone, and cefotaxime (intermediate or resistant), vancomycin plus ceftriaxone or cefotaxime are continued, and rifampin (20 mg/kg per day in two divided doses) may be added.[143] No human data are available to determine the treatment of ceftriaxone-resistant pneumococcal meningitis, but results from a rabbit model indicate more rapid elimination of organisms with vancomycin plus ceftriaxone than with vancomycin alone.[144] The duration of therapy in uncomplicated cases of pneumococcal meningitis is 10 days.

Adjunctive therapy with dexamethasone has been demonstrated to decrease the incidence of neurologic and audiologic sequelae in children with meningitis due to *H. influenzae* type b. Its efficacy in this respect in patients with pneumococcal meningitis is controversial.[145-147] However, a meta-analysis of randomized clinical trials indicates that dexamethasone significantly reduces the incidence of severe hearing loss in pneumococcal meningitis and also might be effective in preventing hearing or neurologic deficit, provided that dexamethasone is initiated with or before antibiotic therapy.[148] In a recent Cochrane review, the use of corticosteroids (dexamethasone at 0.6 mg/kg daily given before or with the first dose of antibiotics) in children with acute bacterial meningitis including *S. pneumoniae* in high-income countries was beneficial by decreasing mortality, although the strength of the evidence was not optimal.[147] As a result, the AAP recommends consideration of use of dexamethasone in the initial therapeutic regimen for infants and children ≥6 weeks of age with possible pneumococcal meningitis.[62] Duration of dexamethasone is 48 hours, in a regimen of 0.15 mg/kg per dose every 6 hours. A repeat lumbar puncture should be considered at 24 to 48 hours of therapy to help guide further therapy if the organism is penicillin nonsusceptible, dexamethasone has been used, or the clinical response is not optimal.

Pneumonia

In 2011, the Infectious Disease Society of America and the Pediatric Infectious Disease Society issued guidelines for the management of pediatric community acquired pneumonia (CAP).[149] *S. pneumoniae* was recognized as the most common cause of bacterial CAP in children. The guidelines recommend that amoxicillin be used as first-line therapy for outpatient treatment of previously healthy, appropriately immunized infants, preschool, and school-aged children with mild to moderate CAP suspected to be of bacterial origin. Providing a daily dose of amoxicillin of 90 mg/kg/day divided into 3 equal doses is predicted to achieve clinical and microbiologic cure in 90% of children compared with 65% treated with the same daily dose divided into 2 doses.[149] The guidelines recommend the addition of a macrolide antibiotic primarily in school-aged children and adolescents evaluated in an outpatient setting with findings compatible with CAP caused by atypical pathogens.

For hospitalized children, the guidelines recommend penicillin G (up to 300,000 units/kg/day divided every 4 hours) or ampicillin (up to 400 mg/kg/day divided every 6 hours) be administered to the fully immunized infant or school-aged child admitted to a general medical unit with CAP when local epidemiologic data document lack of substantial high-level penicillin resistance for invasive *S. pneumoniae*. Empiric therapy with a third-generation parenteral cephalosporin (ceftriaxone or cefotaxime) should be prescribed for hospitalized infants and children who are not fully immunized, or in regions where local epidemiology of invasive pneumococcal strains documents high-level penicillin resistance, or for infants and children with life-threatening infection, including those with empyema.[149]

PROGNOSIS

Mortality in pneumococcal infection occurs most commonly in immunocompromised hosts, such as those with SCD, asplenia, congenital or acquired immunodeficiency, and in children from developing countries with limited access to medical facilities. With current antimicrobial therapies, mortality from bacterial meningitis in children beyond the neonatal period is <10%, but neurologic sequelae, including hearing loss and mild to severe motor and intellectual deficits, remain relatively common. In one multicenter study of pneumococcal meningitis, 7.7% of children died, 32% had hearing loss at discharge, and 25% experienced neurologic sequelae.[150] In another study, pneumococcal meningitis was associated with hearing loss in 36%.[93]

Children with pneumococcal otitis media uncommonly suffer suppurative complications, such as chronic suppurative otitis media, mastoiditis, petrositis, labyrinthitis or brain abscess, and meningitis. However, since the introduction of PCV7, one large children's hospital has reported an increase in pneumococcal mastoiditis due to multidrug-resistant serotype 19A.[151]

PREVENTION

Vaccine

The morbidity and mortality of pneumococcal infection in the antibiotic era led to the development and licensure in 1977 of a polyvalent polysaccharide vaccine in the U.S. The currently available 23-valent pneumococcal polysaccharide vaccine (PPSV23) is composed of purified capsular polysaccharide antigens of 23 serotypes that offered some protection against ~90% of the serotypes causing IPD in the U.S. between 1998 and 1999 and up to 84% by 2006 and 2007 in children <5 years of age.[26,49] Whereas PPSV23 elicits type-specific antibody responses in most healthy adults and children older than 5 years, the serologic response to the polysaccharide antigens is generally poor in children <2 years of age.[152]

To increase the immunogenicity of pneumococcal vaccine in infants, the age groups with the highest incidence of IPD, vaccines were developed in which the purified capsular polysaccharides of different pneumococcal serotypes were covalently bound to a protein carrier. The conjugate vaccines are immunogenic for infants as young as 2 months of age, induce B-lymphocyte memory cells resulting in an anamnestic response with subsequent doses, and reduce carriage of vaccine serotypes.

The PCV7 (Prevnar, Wyeth Lederle Vaccines) was approved in 2000 for universal infant immunization in a four-dose schedule in the U.S.[49,61] PCV7 contains the polysaccharides of serotypes 4, 6B, 9V, 14, 18C, 19F, and 23F. These serotypes accounted for the majority of cases of bacteremia, meningitis, pneumonia, and AOM in U.S. children <6 years of age during the period 1978 to 1994.[49] Infants respond to each conjugate polysaccharide type with substantial concentrations of serum antibody believed to be protective against invasive disease.[153] Protective titers are achieved after doses administered at ages 2, 4, and 6 months but wane during the following 6 months, requiring a booster dose between the ages of 12 and 15 months.

The efficacy of PCV7 initially was demonstrated in prospective, randomized clinical trials in northern California[153] and Finland.[5] In the large randomized study involving 38,000 children <2 years of age in northern California, PCV7 was somewhat efficacious against placement of tympanostomy tubes, AOM episodes and related office visits, moderately efficacious against pneumonia, and highly efficacious in preventing IPD.[153,154] Adverse events were limited to mild erythema, induration, and tenderness at the injection site, and fever (39°C or greater) in approximately 1% to 2% of recipients.[153]

On the basis of safety and efficacy data, PCV7 was recommended by the AAP and CDC in 2000 for all infants in a four-dose schedule at ages 2, 4, 6, and 12 to 15 months.[49,61] The recommendations also included PCV7 immunization of children at high risk for IPD as well as PPSV23 immunization (Table 123-1). Children who have been given PPSV23 should receive a booster dose once 5 years after the first dose. In 2003, the CDC recommended that all children with cochlear implants receive the age-appropriate pneumococcal vaccination and those persons planning to receive a cochlear implant be vaccinated at least 2 weeks prior to surgery.[155] In 2007, the ACIP further revised its recommendation for routine use in all children aged 2 through 59 months of age.[156] The CDC's national immunization survey data indicate that in 2009, PCV7 coverage among U.S. children 19 through 35 months of age was 93% for ≥3 doses and 80% for ≥4 doses.[157] Studies have demonstrated that PCV7 also is effective when given in different and abbreviated schedules from that of the 4 doses recommended in the U.S.[158,159] Surveillance through the Vaccine Adverse Event Reporting System (VAERS), a U.S. passive database, has confirmed the safety of PCV7.[160]

By December 2010, over 300 million doses of PCV7 had been distributed worldwide; the majority of the doses were distributed in the U.S. (P. Paradiso, personal communication March 1, 2011). PCV7 post-licensure surveillance and ecologic studies have demonstrated significant changes in epidemiology of IPD in the U.S. Overall, there have been significant declines in the burden of IPD, pneumonia, meningitis and AOM, and decreasing incidence of penicillin resistance among pneumococci.[161-165] The CDC ABCs report that the incidence of all serotypes of IPD in children <5 years of age decreased from 95 cases per 100,000 in 1999 to 22 to 25 cases per 100,000 annually from 2002 through 2007, a decrease of more than 70%.[131] The indirect effects of PCV7 are demonstrated by declines in IPD in other age groups in whom the PCV7 was not indicated (Table 123-5).[23,26] Comparable decreases in IPD also have been reported in other countries where PCV7 is used widely.[166,167] The decreases in IPD were greatest among children <12 months and those 12 through 23 months of age (Figure 123-2).[26]

Some regions in the U.S. (including Alaska and Utah) and other regions of the world reported a less dramatic decrease in IPD and the early emergence of IPD due to non-PCV7 serotypes.[24,25,69,84,116] Ongoing surveillance of IPD at the CDC's ABCs sites through 2007

TABLE 123-5. Changes in Incidence of Invasive Pneumococcal Disease, by Age Group and Serotype, 1998–1999 Average (Baseline) versus 2007[26]

| Age Group (Years) | Serotype | Incidence, Cases per 100,000 Population | | Change in Rate (2007 vs. Baseline) |
		1998–1999 (n = 4048)	2007 (n = 2576)	Change, % (95% CI)
<5	All types	98.7	23.6	−76 (−79 to −73)
	Vaccine[a]	81.9	0.4	−100 (−100 to −99)
	Vaccine-related	7.3	1.7	−77 (−85 to −64)
	Nonvaccine	6.8	10.3	+51 (+20 to +90)
5–17	All types	4.2	2.4	−43 (−55 to −26)
	Vaccine[a]	2.4	0.2	−94 (−97 to −85)
	Vaccine-related	0.2	0.2	+4 (−59 to +164)
	Nonvaccine	1.5	1.4	−2 (−31 to +40)
18–49	All types	13.3	8.0	−40 (−45 to −35)
	Vaccine[a]	7.6	0.7	−91 (−93 to −88)
	Vaccine-related	1.1	1.1	+1 (−22 to +29)
	Nonvaccine	4.2	4.8	+14 (+1 to +29)
50–64	All types	24.0	19.8	−18 (−25 to −9)
	Vaccine[a]	12.8	1.7	−87 (−90 to −83)
	Vaccine-related	1.9	2.6	+35 (+1 to +80)
	Nonvaccine	8.6	12.3	+43 (+25 to +64)
≥65	All types	60.1	37.9	−37 (−42 to −32)
	Vaccine[a]	33.7	2.7	−92 (−94 to −89)
	Vaccine-related	5.8	7.2	+25 (+1 to +54)
	Nonvaccine	18.3	22.5	+23 (+9 to +38)

[a]*PCV7 vaccine.*

also demonstrated relative increases in non-PCV7 serotypes from 17% in 1998–1999 to 98% in 2006–2007 (Table 123-5). By 2007, serotypes 3, 15B/C, 19A, 22F, and 33F were the most common serotypes causing IPD among children <5 years of age in the U.S.[24,26,168,169] In many regions in the U.S., serotype 19A emerged as the leading cause of IPD during the PCV7 era. A retrospective review of IPD in 8 children's hospitals from 1994 through 2008 showed significant increases in IPD caused by non-PCV7 serotypes. By 2007–2008, serotype 19A accounted for 46% of 369

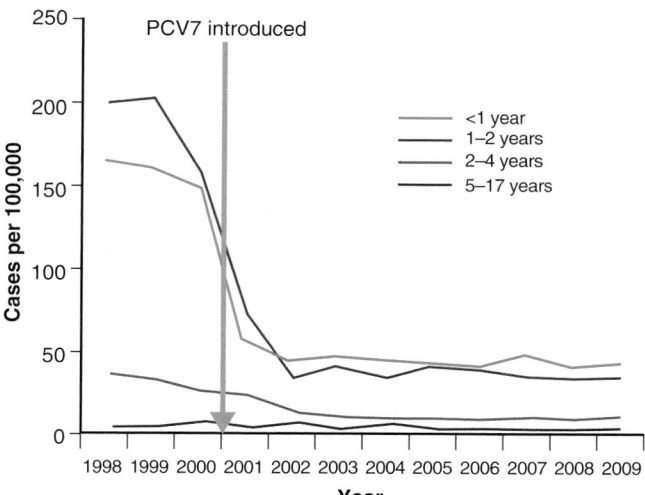

Figure 123-2. Rates of invasive pneumococcal disease among children under 18 years old, according to age and year. Data are from the Active Bacterial Core Surveillance from 1998 through 2009 (http://www.cdc.gov/abcs/index.html).

non-PCV7 IPD isolates while serotypes 1, 3, and 7F combined accounted for 22%.[75] In Massachusetts, serotype 19A increased from 10% of IPD cases in 2002 to 41% in 2006.[170] A similar trend also was noted in Texas, where significant increase in infections due to serotype 19A were noted between 1999 and 2008.[171]

Clinical syndromes associated with IPD changed in regions of the world where PCV7 is used widely. *S. pneumoniae* bacteremia without focus is now uncommon, accounting for <1% of bacteremia in febrile infants and children up to 36 months.[66,172] There also have been significant declines in pneumococcal pneumonia following PCV7 licensure. Data from the Nationwide Inpatient Sample database demonstrated a sustained 33% decrease in hospitalized children with pneumonia <2 years of age in the PCV7 era (2001–2007), compared with 1996–1999.[173] Similarly, pneumococcal meningitis decreased with the widespread use of PCV7. Data from the CDC's ABCs sites have showed a 30% decrease in incidence from 1.13 cases to 0.79 case per 100,000 persons between 1998–1999 and 2004–2005, respectively. The largest decline in meningitis (65%) was among children <2 years of age.[168] Similar decreases were noted in national trends in rates of hospitalization for pneumococcal meningitis, using data from the Nationwide Inpatient Sample.[174] However, many sites in the U.S. and Europe have reported significant increases in pneumococcal empyema.[11,81-85,175] Li and Tancredi showed a 70% increase in pneumococcal empyema hospitalization in the U.S. from 2.2 per 100,000 in 1997 to 3.7 per 100,000 in 2006 in children <18 years of age. The largest increase was among children <5 years of age.[82] Similarly Grijalva et al. noted a 2-fold increase in hospitalizations of pneumonia complicated by empyema from 3.5 cases per 100,000 children in 1996–1998 to 7.0 cases per 100,000 children in 2005–2007.[83]

As a result of the changing serotype distribution and epidemiology of IPD in U.S. children, a new 13-valent pneumococcal polysaccharide-protein conjugate vaccine (PCV13 (Prevnar13), Wyeth Pharmaceuticals, Inc., marketed by Pfizer, Inc.) was approved by the U.S. Food and Drug Administration (FDA) in 2010 for prevention of IPD in infants and young children aged 6 weeks through 71 months of age. PCV13 contains the 7 serotypes included in PCV7 and 6 additional serotypes (1, 3, 5, 6A, 7F, and 19A). PCV13 replaces PCV7.[176,177] PCV13 also is approved for the prevention of AOM caused by the 7 serotypes also covered by PCV7. PCV13 is formulated and manufactured using the same processes as PCV7 and was licensed by the FDA on the basis of studies demonstrating safety and an ability to elicit antibodies protective against IPD comparable with those of PCV7.

The safety and adverse reactions after administration of PCV13 in clinical trials was assessed in three clinical trials in the U.S. Injection-site reactions, fever, decreased appetite, irritability, and increased or decreased sleep were solicited adverse reactions reported in ≥20% of subjects. The incidence and severity of solicited local reactions at the injection site (pain, tenderness, erythema, and induration/swelling) and solicited systemic reactions (irritability, drowsiness/increased sleep, decreased appetite, fever, and restless or decreased sleep) were similar in the PCV13 and PCV7 groups.[178]

Based on the 2007 rate of IPD in children <5 years of age, an estimated 4600 cases of IPD occurred in the U.S. Among those cases, an estimated 70 were caused by serotypes covered in PCV7 and 2900 were caused by serotypes covered in PCV13.[178] Although the incidence of IPD is expected to decline further with the introduction of PCV13, cases of disease will continue to occur. Some children will be unimmunized or incompletely immunized, children who have immune deficits may not respond with protective titers to the vaccine, and cases of disease due to nonvaccine serotypes will persist. Ongoing surveillance of pneumococcal serotypes, clinical syndromes and age distribution of children with IPD post licensure of the PCV13 will be critical in determining national vaccine policy.

Passive Immunoprophylaxis

Immune globulin reduces the incidence of pneumococcal and other bacterial infections in several circumstances. In a placebo-controlled trial in HIV-infected children with clinical or immunologic evidence of disease, children given immune globulin intravenous (IGIV) (400 mg/kg given every 28 days) had a longer time before serious bacterial infection and a smaller number of infections compared with the control group.[179] Benefit in preventing serious infections primarily was against IPD and clinically diagnosed acute pneumonia. As a result of this study, the Working Group on Antiretroviral Therapy and Medical Management of Infants, Children and Adolescents with HIV Infections recommended IGIV therapy for HIV-infected children who have recurrent serious bacterial infections despite appropriate antimicrobial prophylaxis and in whom humoral immunodeficiency is present.[180]

Chemoprophylaxis

For prevention of IPD in children with functional or anatomic asplenia, particularly SCD, daily antimicrobial prophylaxis with oral penicillin V or G (125 mg twice daily for children <5 years of age; 250 mg twice daily for children ≥5 years of age) is recommended.[61] A chemoprophylactic regimen of penicillin reduced the incidence of IPD by 84% in a randomized, placebo-controlled trial in children with SCD.[181] These data are the basis for the recommendation to give daily penicillin prophylaxis to these patients beginning before 2 months of age or as soon as the diagnosis is made.[61] Prophylactic penicillin may be discontinued in children with SCD after 5 years if they have not experienced IPD and they have received the recommended pneumococcal immunizations.[182] The duration of prophylaxis for children with asplenia due to other causes is unknown. Some experts continue prophylaxis throughout childhood.[62]

Prevention of Disease in Contacts

Because secondary cases of IPD are uncommon, chemoprophylaxis is not indicated for contacts of patients with such infection.[62] Universal precautions are recommended for hospitalized patients with IPD and droplet precautions are recommended for infants and children with presumed bacterial meningitis for the first 24 hours of therapy because of the possibility of infection with pathogens other than *S. pneumoniae* such as *Neisseria meningitidis* or Hib.

Acknowledgment

KKA and CLB gratefully acknowledge the contributions of Georges Peter, MD and Jerome O. Klein, MD for their work on this chapter in the previous edition.

Key Points. Diagnosis and Management of *Streptococcus pneumoniae* Infection

MICROBIOLOGY

- Catalase-negative, gram-positive lancet-shaped cocci
- Facultative anaerobe, enhanced growth in 5% CO_2, α-hemolysis on blood agar and susceptible to optochin
- Based on *S. pneumoniae* polysaccharide capsule, there are over 90 serotypes

EPIDEMIOLOGY

- Normal oropharyngeal flora, with some serotypes more invasive than others
- High prevalence of invasive pneumococcal disease among children <5 years of age
- *S. pneumoniae* serotype distribution has changed since the introduction of 7-valent conjugate pneumococcal vaccine (PCV7), with the emergence of serotypes 19A, 3, 1, 7F, and 22F responsible for infection during the PCV7 era
- There have been decreases in *S. pneumoniae* otitis media, bloodstream infection, pneumonia, meningitis, but increases in complicated pneumonias and empyema coincident with the licensure of PCV7 in the U.S.
- PCV13 provides coverage for 6 additional serotypes (including 19A), has been licensed for use in U.S. children, and will replace PCV7

DIAGNOSIS

- Lancet-shaped gram-positive cocci in cerebrospinal fluid (CSF) and other sterile body fluid suggest *S. pneumoniae*
- PCR can detect *S. pneumoniae* DNA in pleural fluid, CSF and other sterile body fluids

TREATMENT

- Choice of antibiotic and route of antibiotic for treatment depends on site of *S. pneumoniae* infection/isolation, i.e., CSF or blood, as *S. pneumoniae* minimum inhibitory concentration (MIC) differs by site
- Penicillin is drug of choice for infections caused by penicillin-susceptible *S. pneumoniae*
- Generally susceptible (>90%) to cephalosporins, and fluoroquinolones, and less (<80%) to the erythromycins and trimethoprim-sulfamethoxazole
- All *S. pneumoniae* isolates are susceptible to vancomycin and linezolid

DURATION OF THERAPY

- Response to therapy usually is rapid
- Duration of therapy depends on site of infection

Other Gram-Positive, Catalase-Negative Cocci

David B. Haslam and Joseph W. St. Geme III

DESCRIPTION OF PATHOGENS

Among the gram-positive, catalase-negative cocci, streptococci and enterococci cause most human infections. The remaining organisms belong to five genera that can be identified according to the criteria proposed by Facklam and colleagues[1] (Table 124-1) and form colonies that are α-hemolytic or nonhemolytic on sheep blood agar and are easily confused with *Streptococcus pneumoniae* or viridans streptococci. These organisms appear to lack typical virulence determinants and consequently are uncommon pathogens.

Of these genera, *Leuconostoc* and *Pediococcus* account for most human infections and are notable for their intrinsic high-level resistance to vancomycin. The genus *Leuconostoc* consists of six species, of which *L. mesenteroides* and *L. paramesenteroides* are most commonly associated with pediatric infections.[2] The genus *Pediococcus* consists of eight species, but only *P. acidilactici* and *P. pentosaceus* are recognized as potential pathogens.[3]

EPIDEMIOLOGY

Leuconostoc and *Pediococcus* species are found on a number of foods, including vegetables, dairy products, and processed meats. Occasionally they can be isolated from culture of vaginal and gastrointestinal tract specimens. *Leuconostoc* can colonize other mucosal surfaces as well, including gastrostomy and tracheostomy sites.

CLINICAL MANIFESTATIONS

Leuconostoc Species

Invasive disease due to *Leuconostoc* is unusual, with approximately 20 cases reported in children. Most infants with systemic infection have an underlying disorder, such as prematurity or a gastrointestinal tract abnormality.[4] Rarely, however, bloodstream infection (BSI) can occur in infants without underlying conditions. Older children with *Leuconostoc* infection typically have an immunodeficiency. In patients of all ages, additional risk factors appear to include previous therapy with vancomycin and the presence of an indwelling catheter. Contaminated enteral feedings, including infant formula, have been implicated as the source of BSI in isolated cases. There is an association between *Leuconostoc* infection and enteral feeding in patients with short-gut syndrome. In many children with underlying gastrointestinal disease, BSI is polymicrobial and involves *Leuconostoc* plus enteric organisms.

Leuconostoc meningitis, pneumonia, and osteomyelitis have been reported in children, almost always in association with an underlying condition such as gastrointestinal disease, immunodeficiency, or an indwelling ventricular shunt. Other reported infections include peritonitis in a child with an indwelling peritoneal dialysis catheter.

Pediococcus Species

Few pediatric cases of invasive pediococcal disease have been described.[3] Reported patients have been younger than 1 year, have recently undergone surgery for gastrointestinal abnormalities, and have shown response to antibiotic regimens that contained a β-lactam and an aminoglycoside.

Other Genera

Aerococcus viridans is a rare cause of invasive disease in children and has been associated with fewer than 10 cases of meningitis or BSI reported.[5] *Gemella* spp. are also an uncommon cause of pediatric disease. However, endocarditis and BSI due to *Gemella* spp. have occurred in children without underlying conditions[6] or as a

TABLE 124-1. Biochemical Differentiation of Catalase-Negative Gram-Positive Cocci

Test	*Streptococcus*	*Enterococcus*	*Pediococcus*	*Leuconostoc*	*Aerococcus*	*Gemella*	*Lactococcus*
Arrangement of cells	Chains, pairs	Pairs, chains	Tetrads, some pairs	Pairs, chains	Tetrads, pairs	Pairs, short chains	Pairs, short chains
Gas from glucose	−	−	−	+	−	−	−
Vancomycin	S	S[a]	R	R	S	S	S
Streptococcal group antigen	v	+	+	+[a]	−	−	−
Growth in bile-hydrolysis of esculin	v	+	+	+[a]	v	−	v
PYRase[b]	−[c]	+	−	−	+	+	v
Leucine aminopeptidase	+	+	+	−	−	+	+
Growth in:							
65% NaCl	−	+	v	v	+	−	v
45°C	v	+	+[a]	−	−	−	−[a]
10°C	−	+[a]	−	+	−	−	+

R, resistant to vancomycin (absence of a zone of inhibition); S, susceptible to vancomycin; v, variable reaction.

[a]*Occasional exceptions exist.*

[b]*Hydrolysis of L-pyrrolidonyl-β-naphthlyamide.*

[c]*Except Streptococcus pyogenes, which is PYR-positive.*

Adapted from Facklam R, Hollis D, Collins D. Identification of gram-positive coccal and coccobacillary vancomycin-resistant bacteria. J Clin Microbiol 1989;27:724.

complication of tongue piercing.[7] Invasive *Lactococcus* infections in children are extremely rare, although a case of catheter-associated BSI in a young infant was reported.[8]

THERAPY

Leuconostoc and *Pediococcus* genera have intrinsic high-level resistance to vancomycin (minimum inhibitory concentration (MIC) ≥64 µg/mL). The mechanism of resistance in both genera is unknown but appears to be chromosomally mediated and is distinct from the mechanism demonstrated by vancomycin-resistant enterococci.

Leuconostoc and *Pediococcus* species are moderately resistant to penicillin, with MICs ranging from 0.03 to 2 µg/mL; 90% of isolates have an MIC <1 µg/mL.[2] Many isolates are tolerant to

penicillin (minimum bactericidal concentration to MIC ratio >32), although the clinical significance of this finding is unclear. Penicillin, either alone or in combination with an aminoglycoside, is the treatment of choice for *Pediococcus* and *Leuconostoc* infections. Chloramphenicol, aminoglycosides, and imipenem also are active against these organisms, but the activity of clindamycin, trimethoprim-sulfamethoxazole, and third-generation cephalosporins is unreliable.[9] Antibiotics belonging to the ketolide family, such as telithromycin, demonstrate excellent activity against *Pediococcus* and *Leuconostoc*. Daptomycin has been successfully used to clear persistent *Pediococcus* BSI.[10] *Aerococcus* and *Gemella* spp. are susceptible to penicillin, cephalosporins, erythromycin, and vancomycin; penicillin alone or in combination with an aminoglycoside is the treatment of choice for invasive disease due to these organisms.

125 *Neisseria meningitidis*

Andrew J. Pollard and Adam Finn

Neisseria meningitidis (meningococcus) is one of the leading causes of serious bacterial infections in children, most commonly presenting as purulent meningitis or septicemia. However, asymptomatic nasopharyngeal colonization is a far more common association of the organism with humans, who are the only reservoir.[1] Gaspard Vieusseux provided the first clinical description of meningococcal disease during an outbreak in Geneva, Switzerland, as recently as 1805,[2] which was followed by epidemics across Europe for the next 50 years. The first description in North America was in Medfield, Massachusetts, in 1806.[3] Further cases appeared in New England and Canada during the following decade. In 1887 Anton Weichselbaum described paired cocci inside white blood cells in cerebrospinal fluid (CSF) and named the organism *Diplococcus intracellularis*[4] and the organism was later reclassified as *Neisseria meningitidis*.

MICROBIOLOGY

N. meningitidis is a nonmotile, gram-negative coccus, usually appearing in pairs with abutting sides flattened. The genus *Neisseria* also includes *N. gonorrhoeae* and several commensal organisms, including *N. flavescens*, *N. lactamica*, *N. mucosa*, *N. sicca*, and *N. subflava*.

N. meningitidis has complex nutritional requirements but grows well on chocolate, blood, Mueller–Hinton, trypticase soy and GC agar in a humidified environment at 35°C to 37°C. *N. meningitidis* like *N. gonorrhoeae* require additional carbon dioxide for growth. The organism is highly susceptible to drying, cold, sunlight, and either high or low pH. *Neisseria* species are differentiated initially by biochemical characteristics. *N. meningitidis* can produce acid from glucose and maltose, but *N. gonorrhoeae* utilizes maltose alone. All *Neisseria* produce catalase and are oxidase-positive.

The cell envelope of *N. meningitidis* has three layers (Figure 125-1): a cytoplasmic membrane, a peptidoglycan cell wall, and an outer membrane, which contains lipopolysaccharide (LPS), phospholipid, and outer membrane proteins (OMPs). Invasive meningococci also have a polysaccharide capsule surrounding the cell envelope which confers the serogroup. The recent appearance of invasive meningococcal disease in 1805 might indicate the acquisition of capsule genes in the last 200 years which have conferred virulence potential on an organism that previously was only a commensal.

The antigen responsible for serogroup specificity is the capsular polysaccharide. Thirteen different serogroups of meningococci have been identified – A, B, C, D, X, Y, Z, 29E, W135, H, I, J, and L – each with different saccharide subunits, but only five are commonly associated with disease: A, B, C, Y, and W135 (Table 125-1).[5] The other serogroups are responsible for occasional sporadic cases and there have been recent epidemics in West Africa caused by serogroup X, but are isolated more commonly from asymptomatic carriers than from people with disease.

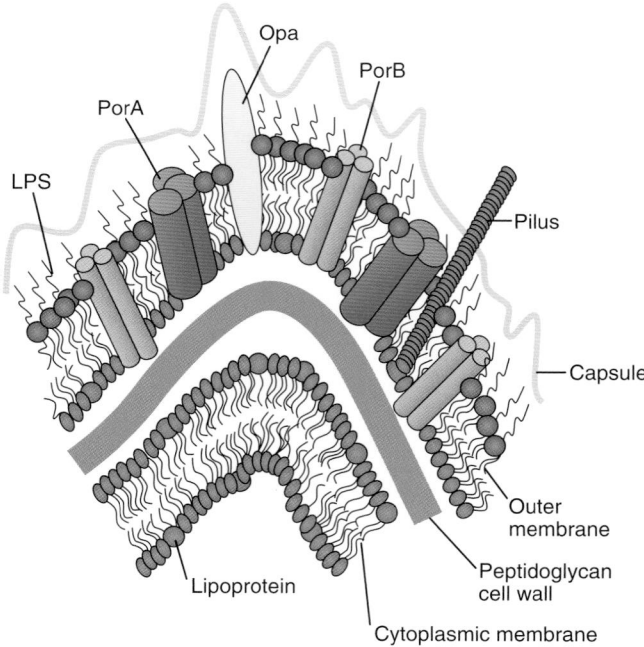

Figure 125-1. Drawing of the surface structures of *Neisseria meningitidis*. LPS, lipopolysaccharide. (From Pollard AJ, Levin M. Vaccines for prevention of meningococcal disease. Pediatr Infect Dis J 2000;19:333–345, with permission.)

TABLE 125-1. Chemical Structure of Meningococcal Polysaccharide Capsules

Serogroup	Chemical Structure
A	N-acetyl mannosamine-1-phosphate
B	α2-8 N-acetyl neuraminic acid (a2-8 NANA)
C	α2-9 N-acetyl neuraminic acid (a2-9 NANA)
29E	3-deoxy-D-manno-octulosonic acid
X	α1-4 N-acetyl-D-glucosamine 1-phosphate
Y	Copolymer of NANA with glucose
W135	Copolymer of NANA with galactose

Within each serogroup, serotypes and subtypes can be identified on the basis of differences in two OMPs, PorB and PorA respectively, while the immunotype is defined by the LPS structure.[6] More recently, sero(subtyping) has been undertaken by molecular methods in view of the limited availability of serologic reagents[7] and with the advent of novel vaccines based on surface proteins antigen-gene sequence-typing is growing in importance to describe diversity and predict potential vaccine coverage. In addition to serologic differentiation based on surface antigens, related meningococcal isolates previously have been described by differences in the electrophoretic mobility of cytoplasmic enzymes (multilocus enzyme electrophoresis, MLEE). However, genetic relatedness between strains now is best described using multilocus sequence typing (MLST)[8] that defines meningococci using sequence data from seven housekeeping genes. Using this method, seven hyperinvasive lineages have been described that cause the majority of invasive meningococcal disease worldwide. With the recent availability of low-cost, high-throughput sequencing, routine whole-genome sequencing likely will replace other typing methods in the decade to come.

Complete genome sequences were determined for several meningococcal isolates a decade ago[9,10] and shown to contain a large number of repeating sequences. In addition, the meningococcal genomes contain multiple insertion sequences, responsible for the uptake of DNA from the microbial environment,[11] thus allowing the addition of new genes. For example, meningococci can acquire the capsular operon from another serogroup and switch to expression of the donor gene product (e.g., switch from serogroup B to serogroup C and vice versa).[11,12] Meningococci also import DNA at high rates from other commensal *Neisseria* spp. during mixed colonization in the nasopharynx.[13] Phase variation of surface structures during colonization and invasion can augment the above mechanisms in helping evade host responses. Variability in the expression of immunogenic proteins may be important for persistence of the organism but hampers vaccine development.

Sequence data from the meningococcal genome have been used to identify genes encoding potential vaccine candidates that are being tested in new-generation vaccines.[14,15]

VIRULENCE AND PATHOGENESIS

The rare episodes of invasive meningococcal disease that occur probably do not provide any survival advantage for the meningococcus. It seems likely that the virulence factors that have been associated with the pathogenic meningococci have evolved as a result of a fitness advantage that they confer in the transmission–colonization cycle that describes the organism's normal lifestyle and in the polymicrobial environment of the human nasopharynx. The polysaccharide capsule enhances invasiveness by inhibiting phagocytosis but may also be important, for example, for avoiding desiccation during transmission. Immunoglobulin (Ig) A1 protease, a neutral endopeptidase with specific enzymatic activity against human IgA1, appears to enhance the ability of pathogenic *Neisseria* to colonize mucosal surfaces. The ability of pathogenic *N. meningitidis* to survive and multiply within the human host is facilitated by the organism's ability to extract iron

from high-affinity iron-binding proteins by means of a non-energy-requiring cell surface mechanism.

Colonization involves a series of interactions between meningococcal surface structures (including pili and Opa) and specific ligands on the surface of cells in the nasopharyngeal mucosa of the human[16-18] and must precede invasive infection. Invasion of *N. meningitidis* through the nasopharyngeal mucosa into the bloodstream is incompletely understood but appears to be dependent on phase variation of meningococcal surface structures, including the capsule, and results in the release of endotoxin (LPS), contained in blebs formed from the outer membrane during bacterial growth. A cascade of mediators is triggered in an inflammatory storm at the core of which are the interactions between LPS and CD14 and toll-like receptor 4 and between lipoprotein or peptidoglycan and toll-like receptor 2. The subsequent cytokine release (rather than direct tissue injury by microbial products) is thought ultimately to produce the features of septic shock in susceptible individuals. High levels of meningococcal LPS are found in severe meningococcal disease and these correlate strongly with mortality.[19] A wide variety of genes are involved in these responses and various human gene polymorphisms have been associated with susceptibility to meningococcal infection or severity of disease.[20] Early in meningococcal disease high levels of tumor necrosis factor (TNF)-α, soluble TNF-α receptor (sTNFR), interleukin-1 (IL-1), IL-1ra, IL-1β, IL-6, IL-8, IL-10, plasminogen activator inhibitor (PAI-1), and leukemia-inhibitory factor are detectable in blood and elevated levels of many of these cytokines have also been associated with disease severity or fatality.[21] Indeed, the balance between these cytokines and their antagonists may influence the outcome of meningococcal disease.[22]

Although during meningococcal meningitis, an inflammatory cascade of cytokines also is released in the subarachnoid space, their levels are not obviously associated with death.[23] Nevertheless, the inflammatory response is thought to mediate neurologic injury in meningococcal meningitis and might be suppressed by use of corticosteroids, although clinical data to support this adjunctive treatment for meningococcal meningitis are limited.[24,25]

IMMUNITY

In 1918, Matsunami and Kolmer demonstrated that the bactericidal activity of clotted whole blood from various laboratory animals was related to the resistance of these animals to infection with *N. meningitidis*.[26] They also demonstrated that the bactericidal activity of serum from adults was greater than the activity of serum from children, providing the first link between serum bactericidal activity and the susceptibility of young children to meningococcal disease. Soon afterwards, Heist et al. found that there was individual variation in the bactericidal activity of sera and individual susceptibility to infection.[27] Unfortunately Heist's own serum contained inadequate bactericidal activity against meningococcus to protect him and he died from invasive meningococcal disease before the publication of these observations.

Goldschneider et al. are credited with firmly establishing the importance of the relationship between serum bactericidal activity (defined as killing of meningococci after mixing with serum and exogenous complement in vitro) and susceptibility to infection. They showed in 1969 that susceptibility to invasion by a newly acquired strain of *N. meningitidis* was associated with the absence of bactericidal antibody against that strain,[28,29] an observation reconfirmed in 2000 during an outbreak in the United Kingdom.[30] This is further supported by the age-specific incidence of meningococcal disease caused by serogroups A, B, and C, which correlates inversely with the age-specific prevalence of protective bactericidal antibody (Figure 125-2).[29,31,32] Titers of antimeningococcal bactericidal antibody in a newborn infant are similar to those in the mother but decline after birth, reaching a nadir at about 6 months of age, which correlates with the peak incidence of meningococcal disease at 5 to 9 months of age.

Individuals with hypogammaglobulinaemia may have a moderately increased rate of meningococcal infection.[33,34] Conversely, serum therapy was successfully used in the treatment of

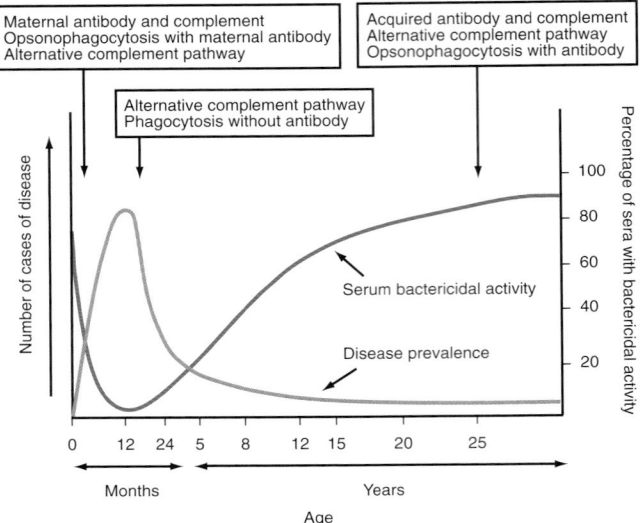

Figure 125-2. Age-specific incidence of meningococcal disease contrasted with serum bactericidal activity. (After Goldschneider I, Gotschlich E, Artenstein M. Human immunity to the meningococcus. I: The role of humoral antibodies. J Exp Med 1969;129:1307.)

meningococcal disease before the advent of antibiotics. The mortality rate from untreated meningococcal disease fell from between 60% and 80% following the introduction of therapy using horse serum shortly after 1900 to between 13% and 30% in treated patients, depending upon how promptly it was initiated.[35]

The bactericidal activity of immune sera requires the presence of both antibody and complement. Approximately 0.3% of individuals with meningococcal disease have complement deficiency.[36] Fifty percent of individuals with a late complement component deficiency (C5 to C9) will develop meningococcal disease and half of these will have recurrent attacks, highlighting the importance of complement in defense against this infection.[37,38] These episodes are usually in older age groups and are often associated with the less common serogroups and rarely with serogroup B disease.[36,39,40] There is a relative deficiency of late complement components in infancy,[41] which may add to the susceptibility to meningococcal infection in this age group. In contrast to those with terminal complement component deficiency, susceptible complement-deficient individuals who have either properdin or factor D deficiency have a case fatality of over 50% while recurrence is rare in survivors.[38,42,43]

In vitro opsonophagocytosis plays a greater role in killing serogroup B meningococci than A, C, Y, or W135 meningococci despite equivalent C3 binding to the surface of the serogroup B and Y organisms[44] and may explain the relative resistance of complement-deficient individuals to serogroup B infection and their susceptibility to serogroup Y infection.

Some further data suggest that phagocytic function may be important in immunity against meningococci. Congenital impairment of binding by phagocytes of IgG2 also can predispose to invasive meningococcal disease. In one study, children with fulminant meningococcal disease were more likely than healthy controls to have poor IgG2-binding by the opsonic Fc-γ receptor IIa, which is expressed by phagocytes.[45] The decreased binding results in marked reduction in phagocytosis of meningococci opsonized with IgG2, but not of those opsonized with IgG1.

During the first two decades of life, the majority of individuals develop bactericidal antibody directed against the capsular polysaccharides and subcapsular structures such as OMP, and LPS and these antibodies are thought to mediate naturally acquired immunity.[46] Of the known surface proteins that are important in anti-meningococcal immunity, PorA appears to be the dominant immunogen (with short surface exposed segments of loop 1 and 4 of the protein containing the immunogenic epitopes) but

bactericidal activity mediated by these antibodies is largely strain specific.[47] Within 2 weeks of asymptomatic acquisition of a meningococcus, the titer of bactericidal antibody against the colonizing strain increases. Cross-reacting (i.e., non-strain-specific) antibodies are primarily directed against OMP and LPS antigens.

Natural immunity can develop as a result of asymptomatic colonization with meningococci or colonization with unrelated organisms bearing cross-reactive antigenic structures.[29,48] Carriage of pathogenic meningococci in early childhood is uncommon and therefore unlikely to be responsible for the induction of early natural immunity.[48] However, carriage of *N. lactamica* and of nontypable *N. meningitidis* is common and does induce cross-reacting bactericidal antibodies against other strains of meningococci.[49] Enteric bacteria bear many similar surface structures that also can cross-react with meningococci. The *Escherichia coli* K1 capsular polysaccharide cross-reacts antigenically with serogroup B meningococci,[50] and the *E. coli* K92, with serogroup C polysaccharide.[51]

The role of T lymphocytes in immunity to meningococcus is unclear. Lymphoproliferative responses to Opa, Opc, and PorA proteins of the bacterial outer membrane have been described[52] and age-dependent differences in the cytokine response of peripheral blood mononuclear cells following disease have been observed.[53] The age-dependent emergence of specific mucosal T-lymphocyte immunity to meningococcus also has been demonstrated recently and may be important in the development of local immunity to colonization and invasion.[54]

EPIDEMIOLOGY

There are two largely distinct epidemiologic patterns of meningococcal disease observed, endemic and epidemic disease.

Endemic disease consists of isolated sporadic cases and occasional small clusters of cases that are associated temporally and geographically. This pattern appears to occur everywhere that disease surveillance is carried out, although baseline incidence rates vary markedly between different geographic areas within the approximate range 0.3 to 7 cases per 100,000 population per year.[55] Over the past 20 years, disease rates in the U.S. remained at around 1/100,000,[56] falling recently to 0.3/100,000. The exception was in the Pacific Northwest,[57] where higher rates were reported in the late 1990s due to an increase in cases caused by hyperinvasive serogroup B strains. By contrast, during the 1990s disease rates increased in the British Isles to over 5/100,000, higher than other regions of Europe,[58] largely due to a highly virulent clone bearing the serogroup C capsule[59] until controlled by vaccination from 1999 onwards. Most cases of endemic disease occur during the winter season in temperate climates, which may reflect an association with respiratory viral infections.

Serogroup distribution varies with time and place. During the late 1990s there was a rising incidence of serogroup C disease in Europe and of serogroup Y in North America.[60] Until recently, serogroups B and C were the most prevalent serogroups in most industrialized nations, but rates of serogroup C disease have recently fallen following the introduction of serogroup C meningococcal vaccines in many countries in Europe and in Canada and Australia,[61] and serogroup B meningococci are now the predominant cause of disease in these regions. Serogroups A and W135 cause only a minority of the cases of meningococcal disease in Europe and North America today. However, serogroup A was the most commonly isolated organism on both sides of the Atlantic during the periods after World Wars I and II and in various parts of Europe, including Finland, and in North America during the 1970s.[62] Serogroup A meningococci caused a significant amount of disease in New Zealand during the 1980s[63] but were replaced by high rates of serogroup B disease from the early 1990s,[64] leading to a vaccine intervention program in 2005. Outbreaks of serogroup A meningococcal disease in Russia[65] and Poland[66] highlight the proximity of areas with a high disease prevalence to western Europe.

Epidemic meningococcal disease in Africa has occurred predominantly during the dry season in an east–west belt from The Gambia to Ethiopia below the Sahara desert, with cases declining at the onset of the rainy season.[67] Epidemics also have been reported in other developing countries, including China, Nepal, Mongolia, India, and Pakistan. Rates are far higher than endemic disease. For example, in a very severe epidemic in Africa in 1996, attack rates of up to 1 in 100 people were recorded. The predominant serogroup is A, although epidemics of serogroup C, W135, and X have been recorded.[68–70] Significant epidemics of disease also have occurred in conditions of overcrowding,[71] and epidemics of serogroups A and W135 have been associated with the Hajj pilgrimage to Saudi Arabia, leading to a requirement for immunization prior to travel.[72]

Factors Influencing Disease Susceptibility and Severity

Susceptibility

Host and pathogen factors that determine susceptibility to meningococcal disease are summarized in Box 125-1. The most important host factor is age. The peak incidence of endemic meningococcal disease occurs in the first year of life, with 35% to 40% of cases occurring in children younger than 5 years.[1,56,73] A review of 807 cases of meningococcal disease occurring between 1992 and 1996 in the U.S. found that infants younger than 1 year had the highest incidence of disease, regardless of serogroup.[56] The median ages for patients with disease due to serogroups B, C, Y, and W135 in this report were 6, 17, 24, and 33 years, respectively – an observation that may be important for vaccine programs. Thirty percent of cases of group B meningococcal disease occurred in infants younger than 1 year, compared with 14% of cases of disease due to other serogroups. Median age increases during epidemics.

Other factors predisposing to meningococcal disease are overcrowding, poverty, cigarette smoking or exposure to cigarette smoke, prior viral respiratory tract infection, winter or dry season,[74] moving into new communities,[75,76] and certain immunodeficiencies.[77–84] In a case-control study, household smoking had an odds ratio for meningococcal disease of 4.1 (95% confidence interval (CI), 1.6 and 10.7).[78] In a study of military recruits, active or passive smoking raised the risk of carriage of *N. meningitidis*.[85] Coexistent colonization or infection with respiratory viruses and *Mycoplasma* species was associated with meningococcal disease in a study from Chad[86] and previous studies have implicated influenza A as a predisposing factor.[87] Individuals with a low socioeconomic status also are more likely to be carriers and to develop disease.[88]

Deficiency of either antibody or complement increase risk of meningococcal disease. Compared with the general population, inherited deficiency of properdin or of a terminal component of complement (C5 to C8) increases the risk of invasive meningococcal disease by 250-fold or 600-fold, respectively,[89,90] as a result of impaired bacteriolysis even in the presence of specific antibody.[91] However, the proportion of all cases of meningococcal disease that are associated with complement deficiency is small.

BOX 125-1. Risk Factors for Invasive Meningococcal Disease

- Lack of bactericidal antibody to acquired strain
- Age <1 year or 15–24 years of age
- Crowded living conditions/close contact (poor housing, military barracks, students in dormitories)
- Cigarette smoking, active or passive
- Prior viral respiratory infection (especially influenza)
- Inherited properdin or factor D deficiency
- Inherited terminal complement component deficiency (C5-C9)
- Family/household contact of person with meningococcal disease

---

Indications for screening for complement deficiency by performance of total hemolytic complement activity assay are: recurrence of meningococcal disease, chronic meningococcemia, endemic disease due to serogroups other than A, B, and C, and history of a sibling with recurrent meningococcal disease. Routine screening of all patients with meningococcal disease for complement deficiencies probably is not indicated.[92]

Patients with terminal complement component deficiency should be vaccinated with the conjugated quadrivalent meningococcal vaccine (A/C/Y/W135), which reduces the risk of recurrent disease.[93] In addition, both the patients and their families should be aware of the patient's need for prompt care for acute febrile illnesses.

Studies of human single nucleotide polymorphisms have indicated various host factors that may be associated with susceptibility to invasive meningococcal infection and are reviewed by Emonts and coworkers.[20] Polymorphisms in Fc-gamma receptor II and III (CD32 and CD16) are more common in children with meningococcal disease presumably as a result of reduced binding of IgG2 on the surface of phagocytes.[94] A multinational European study showed excess of structural variants in mannose-binding lectin exon 1 in cases of meningococcal infection compared with controls,[95] and a recent study found that SNPs in factor H binding protein were associated with increased risk of disease.[96]

Seven families of genetically related meningococci have been described – the hyperinvasive lineages – that account for a majority of the invasive infections.[8] These organisms appear to be genetically stable over time and across all geographic regions, indicating that they have adapted well to a particular life cycle of colonization and transmission that maintains the persistence of the clonal group. Acquisition of a hyperinvasive meningococcus increases the risk of disease.

Severity

Severity of meningococcal disease is related to host, pathogen, and other environmental factors. A large number of polymorphisms in human genes involved in inflammation, coagulation, and the immune response have been studied and several associations reported (reviewed by Emonts et al.[20] and Texereau et al.[97]). Furthermore, some meningococcal clones have been associated with higher case fatality and more severe disease.

The delivery of early and optimal medical care to patients with meningococcal disease has been shown to be an important factor in outcome in a recent study of deaths in the U.K. Late diagnosis and suboptimal medical care were associated with a worse outcome. Although there has been an emphasis on early administration of antibiotics in the past, observations on changing case management in the U.K. suggest that early and rapid cardiovascular resuscitation (particularly volume replacement) may be the most important intervention.[98–101]

Transmission and Colonization

Transmission of *N. meningitidis* occurs by means of respiratory droplets and requires close, direct contact. In a recent systematic review and meta-analysis, carriage prevalence of *N. meningitidis* increased through childhood from 4.5% in infants to a peak of 23.7% in 19-year-olds and subsequently decreased in adults to 7.8% in 50-year-olds.[102] Most strains recovered from carriers younger than 5 years are not encapsulated; carriage of encapsulated strains is uncommon until adolescence.[102,103] Serogroup B is the most frequently isolated capsular type in carriage studies from Europe (30% to 40%), followed by serogroup Y (10% to 15%), C (5% to 7%), W135 (3% to 4%), and A (2%).[104,105]

Asymptomatic carriers are the most common source of transmission and evaluation of herd immune effects following introduction of serogroup C meningococcal vaccines suggests that adolescents and young adults are the main vehicle of transmission for this serogroup in the population. Close contacts are the source of acquisition in most individual cases. Disease is more correctly associated with acquisition than carriage since the incubation period is very short in most cases. Studies in military recruits show that illness often occurs within 48 to 72 hours of colonization.[106] During outbreaks of disease in military recruits, intense transmission occurs, so that 60% to 80% of recruits become carriers of outbreak strains within 6 to 8 weeks of starting basic training. High colonization rates have not been associated with disease outbreaks in semiclosed civilian populations, such as colleges and universities.[107,108] The highest carriage rates are detected at the beginning of the first term in the first year of higher education.[109]

When members of the households of individuals with serogroup B or C disease are studied, 20% to 40% of contacts are found to carry the disease strain and secondary cases occur among close contacts at rates up to 1000 times higher than that of the general population.[110]

With the introduction of the serogroup C meningoccoccal conjugate vaccine in the U.K., which included a catch-up program in children and young adults as well as a rolling program for infants, carriage rates of serogroups A, B, Y, and W135 remained unaffected, whereas those of serogroup C decreased from 0.45% to 0.15% in 15- to 17-year-olds.[111] This study highlights the fact that colonization rates of disease-associated meningococci in the general population usually are <5%[112,113] even during outbreaks in a college or school population.[114,115]

There are few longitudinal studies that have attempted to address duration of carriage. A study of serogroup A stains in Africa suggested that the organism might persist in the nasopharynx for 3 months.[116] By contrast, the median duration of carriage of serogroup B in another study was 9 months.[117]

Outbreaks

School-related outbreaks have been associated with serogroup B,[118] but most have been due to serogroup C strains.[119-122] The first described outbreaks occurred in Canada in the late 1980s, but subsequent outbreaks related to schools, colleges, and universities have been reported from the U.S.,[56,82] the U.K.,[114] Sweden,[123] Germany,[124] Spain,[125] Argentina,[126] and Australia.[127] The number of cases in each outbreak is small (<10), but in most outbreaks, there is a high proportion among cases of fatal meningococcemia in 15- to 24-year-old patients.[82]

Risk factors for college and university outbreaks are summarized in Box 125-2. As in outbreaks of meningococcal disease among military recruits, risk of disease is greatest in first-year college students, especially those living in dormitories.[114,128-130] Meningococcal carrier rates rise rapidly in the first few months after students arrive at college.[84] The highest carriage rates among first-year university students in the U.K. are during the first week of their first term.[109] These data and the higher age-specific incidence of disease in people 15 to 19 years old,[131] as well as the overrepresentation of people between 12 and 19 years of age in cases occurring in the school-related clusters in Canada and among freshman college dormitory residents in the U.S., suggest that adolescents transmit meningococci to one another.[82,119] Behaviors such as kissing, smoking, and prolonged duration of close contact in relatively small groups (at dances, parties, and bars as well as in dormitories) may facilitate transmission of meningococci.[109,132,133]

Although cases arising in college-related outbreaks account for only 3% of all cases in the U.S., the resulting disruption of college

---

BOX 125-2. Risk Factors Associated with Meningococcal Disease in College and University Outbreaks

- Being a first-year student
- Living in a dormitory
- Attending a bar, nightclub, disco, or social function within 10 days prior to onset of index case
- Smoking
- Intimate kissing

---

activities and the costs of outbreak management led the American College Health Association to recommend in 1997 that college health services alert students and parents about the risks of meningococcal disease and the benefits of vaccination. Following earlier recommendations concerning polysaccharide vaccine and following licensure in 2005, the U.S. Centers for Disease Control and Prevention (CDC) and American Academy of Pediatrics recommended universal administration of quadrivalent conjugate meningococcal vaccine (MCV4) to young adolescents (at 11 to 12 years), with catch-up immunization of students entering high school or 15-year-olds, and college freshmen who will be living in dormitories.[133] In 2010, the CDC and AAP recommended a booster dose of MC4 at 16 years for persons immunized at age 11 or 12 years to assure persistence of protective levels of bactericidal antibody.[134]

CLINICAL MANIFESTATIONS

The spectrum of clinical manifestations of infection with *N. meningitidis* ranges from asymptomatic carriage, the most common form of infection, to death within hours with fulminant meningococcal septicemia (meningococcemia). Meningococcal meningitis and septicemia are the most frequently reported clinical syndromes associated with *N. meningitidis*.

"Benign or unsuspected meningococcemia" has been observed in infants and young adults[135] in whom the clinical presentation is fever and signs of upper respiratory tract infection without toxicity, meningismus, or rash. Neither clinical features nor laboratory tests reliably distinguish febrile children with unsuspected meningococcemia (i.e., with fever but with no characteristic rash) from those without bacteremia.[136] Although some infants eliminate unsuspected meningococcemia without antibiotic treatment, two-thirds of untreated cases progress to meningitis, fulminant meningococcemia, or other complications.[137]

Several clinical algorithms for assisting in the diagnosis and management of the child presenting with a fever and a nonblanching rash have been described[138-141] but none has been fully, independently validated. These algorithms may enable the clinician to improve the specificity of the diagnosis but loss of sensitivity for diagnosis of meningococcal disease could obviously have serious consequences.

The rash in all forms of meningococcal disease begins as macules, maculopapules, or urticaria but usually becomes petechial within hours of onset. Large purpuric lesions evolve in severe cases but some children who die from overwhelming sepsis may have no rash at all.

However, the more frequent clinical problem is the child with fever and a petechial rash (Figure 125-3). Only 2% to 11% of children with fever and a petechial rash have meningococcal disease; most of the remainder have a viral illness, predominantly due to enterovirus. Other viruses associated with petechiae include influenza and other respiratory viruses, parvovirus, Epstein–Barr virus, cytomegalovirus, and measles.[142-144] Petechiae or purpura also can occur with coagulation disorders such as congenital or acquired (after varicella infection) protein S or C deficiency.[145,146] Other disorders associated with petechial rash include platelet disorders (such as idiopathic thrombocytopenic purpura, drug effects, and bone marrow infiltration), Henoch–Schönlein purpura, connective tissue disorders, and trauma (including non-accidental injury in children). Differential diagnosis of other invasive infection includes septicemia due to pneumococci, streptococci, staphylococci, gram-negative bacilli, or rickettsia.[147,148] In the case of pneumococcal purpura fulminans, hyposplenism is an important association.

Histologic analysis of skin lesions shows widespread endothelial necrosis of small veins and capillaries in the dermis and subcutaneous tissue, infiltration of neutrophils, and occlusion of damaged vessels with platelets, white blood cells, fibrin thrombi, and hemorrhage.[149] Meningococci are present within the endothelium and thrombi.

Meningitis is the most common form of invasive meningococcal disease and is associated with a petechial rash in two-thirds of

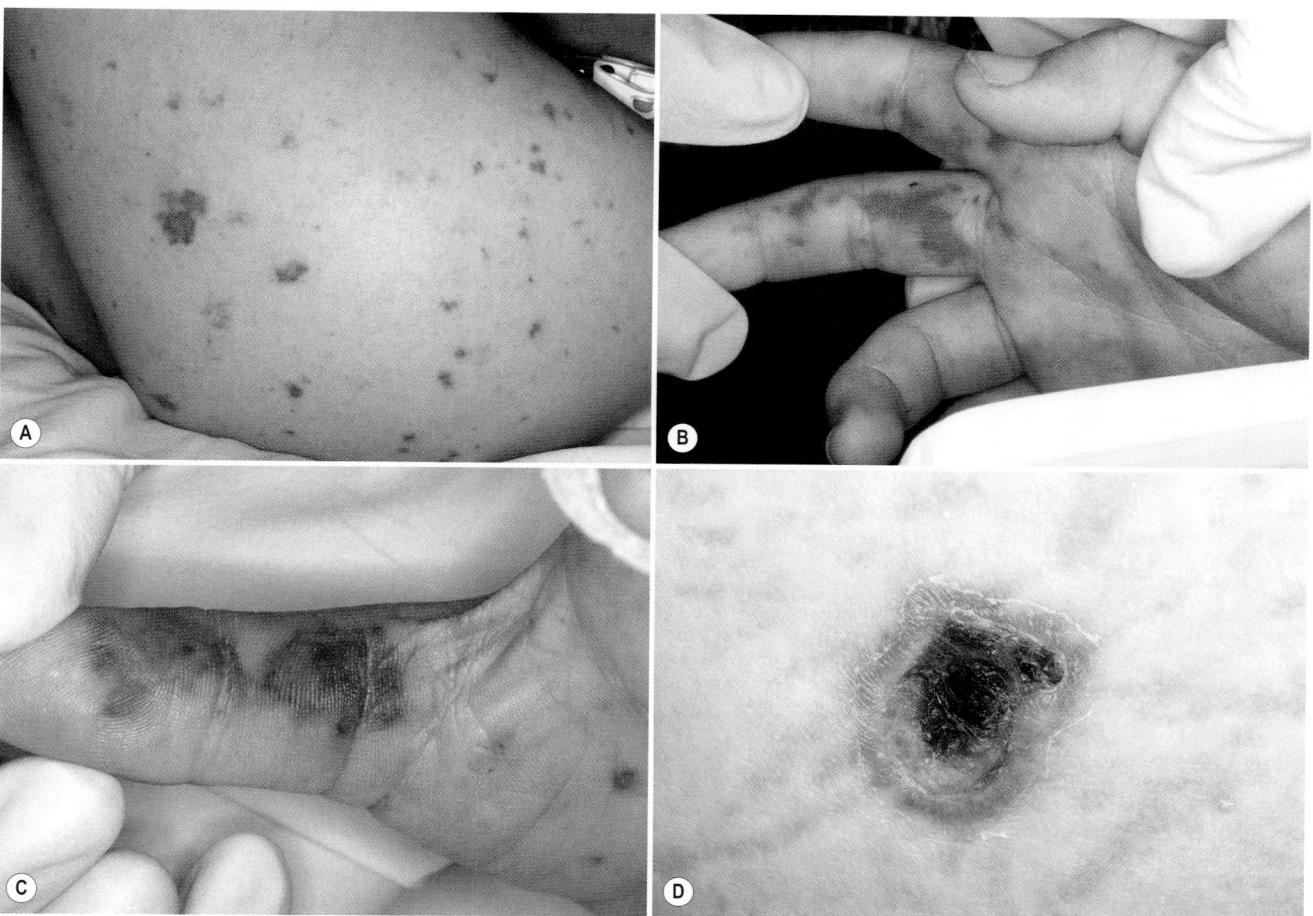

Figure 125-3. An 8-year-old boy had acute onset of fever, purpuric rash and shock. *Neisseria meningitidis* was isolated from blood culture. He recovered. Typically, petechiae and purpura are most dense on buttocks, lower extremities (**A,** day 1) and peripherally (**B,** day 1). Tissue damage and necrosis can ensue (**C,** day 4, **D,** day 10). (Courtesy of J.H. Brien©.)

patients.[1] Headache, fever, vomiting, irritability, photophobia, lethargy, and neck stiffness can be present and Kernig sign can be positive in advanced cases in older children. Seizures occur in as many as 20% of cases and mental state is altered as disease progresses. Many of the features of meningitis are not reported by younger children and misery can be the dominant clinical feature. Infants can present with poor feeding, unconsolable irritability, a high-pitched cry, and a bulging fontanel.

Meningococcal septicemia is a fulminant illness characterized by the onset of a nonspecific febrile illness followed within a few hours by rapid deterioration. Many deaths occur within 12 hours, and almost all within 48 hours, of onset. Initial symptoms include fever, headache, myalgia, shivering, cold hands and feet, and influenza-like symptoms and may be associated with vomiting and abdominal pain. Limb pain is a feature in some patients. Features of shock include tachycardia, poor peripheral perfusion, tachypnea, and oliguria. As shock progresses there is decreased cerebral perfusion resulting in alteration in mental status (confusion, agitation, or decreasing consciousness), multiorgan failure and, as a preterminal event, hypotension can be present.[120-153] A petechial rash can progress rapidly to purpura and ecchymoses.

Meningococcal septicemia accounts for 15% to 20% of all cases of invasive meningococcal disease but some patients also have a mixed picture of meningitis and septicemia. Septicemia is more common in infants and young children.[154,155] The case-fatality rate exceeds 40% in older case series, although more recent reports from specialist pediatric intensive care units in the U.K. show improved survival; mortality was under 5%, with an emphasis on early correction of shock with volume replacement.[99] Many

survivors lose extremities or extensive areas of skin as a result of vascular damage and peripheral ischemia and infarction.[156-158] Predictors of mortality and poor outcome include young age, the absence of meningitis, the presence of coma, temperature <38 °C, hypotension (mean arterial blood pressure <2 SD below mean for age) leukopenia (white cell count <10,000/mm^3), and thrombocytopenia (platelet count <100,000/mm^3).[159,160]

Less common manifestations of invasive meningococcal disease are pneumonia, pyogenic arthritis, purulent pericarditis, myocarditis, endophthalmitis, conjunctivitis, primary peritonitis, and osteomyelitis. The incidence of meningococcal pneumonia is not known because it is only confirmed if blood or pleural fluid culture results are positive. Compared with patients who have meningitis or bacteremia due to *N. meningitidis*, patients with pneumonia tend to be older (94.4% >10 years old) and are more likely to be infected with less common serogroups, such as Y, W135, and Z.[161,162] Meningococcal conjunctivitis should be managed as for invasive disease since topical therapy does not prevent invasion and secondary cases can occur.

Chronic meningococcemia, first described in the early 1900s,[163] is a rare form of meningococcal infection, characterized by recurrent episodes of fever, rash, and arthralgia or arthritis and headache over weeks to months in association with bacteremia that often clears without treatment. The same strain is usually responsible for recurrent episodes and the patient is well between attacks.[164,165] A recent study indicated that chronic meningococcemia was associated with the LpxL1 mutant strain that has a less toxic pentacylated LPS molecule.[166] Chronic meningococcemia can mimic acute rheumatic fever, bacterial endocarditis, anaphylactoid (Henoch–Schönlein) purpura, infectious mononucleosis, disseminated gonococcal infection, and immune-mediated vasculitis. The diagnosis is difficult because blood culture results are only positive if the specimen is obtained during a febrile episode. If not recognized and treated, chronic meningococcemia can progress to meningitis or acute meningococcemia. The pathogenesis of chronic meningococcemia is unknown but inherited deficiencies of terminal components of complement have been found in some cases.[167]

DIAGNOSIS

Diagnosis of meningococcal disease should be made clinically and appropriate therapy instituted immediately. However, microbiologic confirmation is important for public health control and to exclude an alternative diagnosis. Specimens from normally sterile sites (most commonly CSF and scraping from skin lesion) are inoculated onto chocolate agar and incubated in 3% to 5% carbon dioxide. Specimens from mucosal sites are inoculated on selective media (e.g., Thayer–Martin chocolate agar) to which vancomycin, colistin, and nystatin have been added to inhibit growth of competing microbes. Visualization of intracellular or extracellular diplococci on Gram staining of CSF, fluid from skin lesions, or the buffy coat of blood can provide positive results immediately.

Blood culture results may be positive in 40% to 75%, and CSF culture results positive in 90%, of patients with meningococcal meningitis who have not received antibiotics. Some blood culture media contain sodium polyanethol sulfate, which can inhibit *Neisseria* spp., and these organisms are very sensitive to a delay in transport to the microbiology laboratory or inoculation of CSF samples onto agar. Results of Gram stain of CSF are positive in 75% to 80% of untreated cases of meningitis, and the test has a specificity of 97%. Combining results of blood and CSF cultures with those of the CSF Gram stain identifies 94% of cases of meningitis. Culture of blood, CSF, and skin lesions improves laboratory confirmation of disease. However, administration of oral or parenteral antibiotics before specimens are obtained reduces the rate of positive results of blood cultures to <10% and of CSF cultures to approximately 50% in patients who have meningitis.[155]

Detection of meningococcal antigen in CSF, by latex agglutination, can be useful in patients who previously received antibiotics but the test has poor sensitivity and specificity, particularly for serogroup B, the predominant cause of the disease in most industrialized countries and is not recommended routinely if PCR is available as an adjunct to culture.[168] PCR assays can detect meningococcal DNA in CSF, plasma, and serum.[169-171] PCR assays may use different amplification methods and gene targets;[169,172] better PCR systems are reported to have sensitivity and specificity of >90% and to permit diagnosis within 4 to 8 hours.[172,173] PCR is more sensitive than blood culture and the proportion of laboratory-confirmed cases of meningococcal disease is increased by 30% to 40% when this assay is included in the investigation of suspected meningococcal disease, since the assay is relatively unaffected by prior antibiotic therapy.[174]

Lumbar puncture can be associated temporally with deterioration in some patients with meningococcal disease and in patients with shock the procedure can compromise cardiovascular function.[175-177] Lumbar puncture is contraindicated where there is cardiorespiratory insufficiency, raised intracranial pressure, coagulopathy, extensive or spreading purpura, and after convulsions until stabilized. Lumbar puncture can be deferred until the patient is stabilized, when abnormal CSF can confirm meningitis and PCR can be used to confirm etiology.

Some patients come to medical attention in coma and computed tomography (CT) brain imaging may be helpful to exclude intracranial hemorrhage in patients for whom diagnosis is unclear. However, clinically significant raised intracranial pressure or cerebral edema may not be evident on CT and the decision to perform a lumbar puncture should be made on clinical assessment.[178,179]

METABOLIC AND HEMATOLOGIC ABNORMALITIES

In bacterial meningitis caused by *N. meningitidis*, the CSF white blood cell (WBC) count, the peripheral blood WBC count, and inflammatory markers (C-reactive protein,. procalcitonin and erythrocyte sedimentation rate) typically are elevated. Biochemical tests and coagulation are usually normal but inappropriate antidiuretic hormone (ADH) secretion can occur and lower the plasma sodium. The CSF shows pleocytosis with raised protein, low glucose, and presence of gram-negative diplococci.

In meningococcal septicemia, metabolic derangements are common and contribute to depressed myocardial function. Hypoglycemia, hypokalemia, hypocalcemia, hypomagnesemia, hypophosphatemia, and metabolic acidosis frequently are present in severely affected children and should be corrected.[101,180] Renal failure, anemia and coagulopathy also can occur and there may be spontaneous pulmonary, gastric, or cerebral hemorrhage, particularly in the presence of thrombocytopenia. Protein C, fibrinogen, prothrombin, coagulation factors (V, VII, and X), and antithrombin levels typically are depressed. Tissue factor pathway inhibitor is raised. Coagulopathy can be corrected with fresh frozen plasma, platelets, and, in severe cases, cryoprecipitate, to prevent life-threatening hemorrhage.

TREATMENT

Antimicrobial Agents

Use of a third-generation cephalosporin, such as ceftriaxone or cefotaxime, for initial therapy of suspected meningococcal disease seems prudent, because meningococcal strains that are relatively resistant to penicillin appear to be susceptible to these antibiotics (discussed below) and because third-generation cephalosporins also provide coverage for *Haemophilus influenzae* and penicillin-resistant *Streptococcus pneumoniae*. Where penicillin/cephalosporin resistant pneumococci are prevalent addition of vancomycin is recommended.

Pre-hospital antibiotic therapy is recommended in some countries, especially where there is likely to be any delay in transfer to hospital. However, there are no high quality studies that have addressed the benefit of such an approach and the available observational data have conflicting results. Urgent transfer to hospital may improve outcome among those with septicemia since fluid resuscitation appears to be the clinical priority.

For confirmed disease, ceftriaxone (75 to 100 mg/kg per day, maximum 4 g/day, in 1 to 2 divided doses, intravenously), cefotaxime (200 mg/kg per day, maximum 8 g/day, in 4 divided doses, intravenously), penicillin G (250,000 U/kg per day, maximum 12 million U/day, in 4 divided doses, intravenously; or 50 mg/kg per day, maximum 2–4 g/day in 6 divided doses), and chloramphenicol (75 to 100 mg/kg per day, maximum 2 g/day, in 4 divided doses orally or intravenously) are all effective alternatives for treatment.[181] However, ceftriaxone sterilizes the CSF more rapidly than cefotaxime, ampicillin, or chloramphenicol ($P<0.01$), although the clinical significance of this is unknown.[182] Many countries recommend penicillin for confirmed disease in view of its low cost and narrow spectrum. Chloramphenicol is widely used and effective in resource-poor settings and is used elsewhere in patients with severe β-lactam allergy. One randomized controlled trial in Turkey found that necrotic skin lesions occurred more frequently with penicillin G than ceftriaxone ($P<0.05$).[183] In the U.K., ceftriaxone is recommended as definitive therapy for penicillin-susceptible organisms as it appears to be cheaper when administration costs are considered, and the long half-life and dose interval also permit children who have made a good recovery to complete treatment as outpatients.[36]

Emergence of strains with increased resistance to penicillin (i.e., with a minimum inhibitory concentration between 0.12 and 1.0 μg/mL) has been reported from Africa, the U.K., Spain, Argentina, the U.S., and Canada.[184] Failure of penicillin therapy for meningitis due to such strains is reported but these strains remain susceptible to third-generation cephalosporins.[185] Resistance is due to a genetic mutation that appears to have been acquired from avirulent *N. lactamica* or other *Neisseria* spp. through DNA transformation and causes alteration in penicillin-binding protein 2. The highest prevalence of penicillin resistance has been reported from Spain, where rates exceed 40%.[186] Although the frequency of penicillin-resistant *N. meningitidis* has increased in many parts of the world, the prevalence in the U.S. remained unchanged at 3% between 1991 and 1997.[187]

Although the recommended duration of therapy for meningitis and meningococcemia is 7 days, there are no high quality studies to support any specific duration of therapy in meningococcal disease. In some studies treatment with penicillin, chloramphenicol, or ceftriaxone for 4 to 5 days appeared to be effective. Treatment with 1 or 2 doses of ceftriaxone or long-acting oily suspension of chloramphenicol were shown to be as effective as more prolonged therapy.[188–195]

The appropriate duration of therapy for meningococcal infections at other sites (bone, joint, heart, lung) has not been established; patients with such infections should be treated at least until all clinical and laboratory signs of infection have resolved.

Adjunctive Therapy

The use of corticosteroid therapy for presumed meningococcal meningitis is controversial since no pediatric studies have had an adequate sample size to assess benefit, although benefit has been shown for other bacterial causes of meningitis.[196] Studies in developing countries do not show any benefit from corticosteroid therapy in bacterial meningitis.[197] However, adult studies have shown benefit in all-cause meningitis and a trend towards benefit in meningococcal meningitis.[198] If used, dexamethasone can be administered in a dose of 0.15 mg/kg four times daily for 4 days.

There are no studies of high-dose corticosteroid treatment in children with meningococcemia or other types of shock but data from adult studies showed no benefit and the potential for harm. Studies of low ("physiologic") doses in adults showed conflicting results but some authorities believe that replacement doses (25 mg/m^2 hydrocortisone four times daily) may be useful in children who have refractory shock in association with impaired adrenal gland responsiveness; there is ongoing investigation in Europe.[199,200]

Reduced concentrations of protein C have been found in the plasma of patients with meningococcal sepsis and low levels are associated with increased risk of death. Activated protein C inhibits both inflammatory and procoagulant pathways that are activated by the proinflammatory cytokines released in response to sepsis and reduces mortality in adults with sepsis.[201] Small controlled trials have shown a reduction in mortality in treated patients.[202–204] However, a randomized, placebo-controlled study of the use of activated protein C in children with severe sepsis failed to demonstrate any obvious benefit in children with septic shock, and serious bleeding was a complication.[205] Protein C is not recommended.

Recombinant bactericidal permeability-increasing protein (rBPI), which binds to endotoxin and blocks the inflammatory cascade, was studied in a randomized multicenter placebo-controlled trial, but the study was not sufficiently powered to assess adequately a reduction in mortality.[206,207] However, children who received rBPI had fewer amputations, decreased blood product transfusions, and improved functional outcome and fewer children died who received a full 24-hour infusion of rBPI (2% rBPI vs. 6% placebo, P = 0.07).

Various other agents and other adjunctive therapies have been used or considered in the management of septicemia including fibrinolysis, extracorporeal membrane oxygenation, plasmapheresis, and anti-mediator therapy, but only the antiendotoxin antibody, HA1A, has been subjected to rigorous clinical trials and was not found to have benefit.[208] None of these adjunctive therapies can be recommended.

EMERGENCY MANAGEMENT

Pulmonary edema or poor pulmonary perfusion and hypoxia can be present in meningococcal septicemia and requires elective endotracheal intubation during volume resuscitation. Intubation also is recommended if the patient is still in shock after 40 to 60 mL/kg of volume resuscitation as pulmonary edema is common during ongoing resuscitation. After securing the airway there are two clinical management priorities in children with meningococcal disease: correction of cardiovascular shock and control of raised intracranial pressure. Most patients die from decompensated shock and a small proportion from raised intracranial pressure. Aggressive volume resuscitation and inotropic support to maintain tissue perfusion are critical to improving survival and minimizing sequelae in patients with fulminant disease and shock. Children with meningococcal septicemia may require fluid replacement volumes equivalent or several times greater than their circulating blood volume. Fluid replacement should be administered initially as 0.9% sodium chloride solution in a volume of 20 mL/kg over 5 to 10 minutes and repeated until shock improves (reduction in heart rate and increased tissue perfusion). Human albumin solution (4.5%) is recommended as an alternative by many intensivists but there are currently no data to support the type of fluid. If the child is still in shock after receiving 40 to 60 mL/kg of fluid, vasoactive therapy is required. Metabolic derangements, anemia, and coagulopathy should be monitored and corrected as appropriate. Renal support may be necessary. For the child with raised intracranial pressure, management should be directed at ensuring adequate cerebral perfusion by correcting coexistent shock and by providing neurointensive care. In bacterial meningitis caused by *N. meningitidis* without raised intracranial pressure or inappropriate secretion of ADH, volume resuscitation should be aggressive. There is no evidence to support the historical practice of fluid restriction in such cases and one study found increased rates of neurologic sequelae among those who received fluid restriction.[209]

An algorithm has been developed to assist direction of early management in both children and adults[102,210] and updated versions are available from the Meningitis Research Foundation website (www.meningitis.org).

OUTCOME

Mortality

The overall case-fatality rate for invasive meningococcal disease is approximately 10%.[56,172,211,212] In a case series from the Netherlands,[213] the risk of death was higher in infants younger than 6 months, adolescents, and adults older than 50 years (odds ratio 5.1, 3.4, and 9.8, respectively) than in children 1 to 9 years old. The risk of death was greater among females (odds ratio 2.3; 95% CI, 1.2 and 4.7).

Death or severe ischemic damage with extremity loss or extensive skin gangrene occurs much more commonly in fulminant meningococcemia than in meningitis. Optimized initial management and aggressive supportive care in the pediatric intensive care unit of the most severely affected patients have been associated with a reduction in mortality in this group of patients from a predicted risk of death of 25% to less than 5%.[130] With prompt and appropriate antibiotic and support therapy, uncomplicated cases of meningococcal disease improve rapidly. Most patients with meningitis return to a normal state of consciousness within 2 days, are afebrile within 3 to 4 days, and show resolution of meningismus within 4 to 5 days.

Prognostic scoring systems have been developed that use presenting clinical signs and laboratory findings.[214–216] The first of these demonstrated that the combination of 3 or more of the following features was associated with a poor prognosis: (a) petechiae for less than 12 hours before presentation; (b) hypotension; (c) absence of meningismus; (d) peripheral blood white cell count below 10,000 cells/mm^3 and an erythrocyte sedimentation rate less than 10 mm/h.[217] The Glasgow meningococcal septicemia prognostic score[218] has been widely used as a research tool but tends to overestimate mortality. The clinical utility of scoring systems has not been fully established.

Postinfectious Inflammatory Syndromes

A variety of immunologic or reactive complications, such as arthritis, cutaneous vasculitis, iritis, and pericarditis, can occur in patients with meningococcal disease from 4 days after the onset of invasive disease (after bacteriologic eradication). The mechanism is focal deposition of immune complexes containing meningococcal polysaccharide antigen, IgG, and C3, which results in acute inflammation.[219] All of these forms of reactive disease resolve spontaneously. Symptoms usually can be relieved by administration of acetylsalicylic acid or other nonsteroidal anti-inflammatory agents.

The rate of reactive arthritis is 5% to 8%.[220] This complication is more often reported in adults than children and affects medium-sized joints preferentially. Fever occurs at the time of onset of joint pain; arthritis resolves within 6 to 10 days without residual damage. The onset of arthritis is associated with disappearance of meningococcal antigen from the serum, a rise in antibody titer, and a drop in serum C3 concentration.[221]

Cutaneous vasculitis occurs in approximately 2% of patients, with onset 5 to 9 days after appearance of disease.[204] Small numbers of warm, red papules appear, mainly on the extremities, and often progress to form bullae that rupture, leaving a shallow ulcer. Several crops of papules can appear over 2 to 3 days. Healing occurs without scarring in 4 to 8 days.

Inflammation of the iris or sclera occurs in approximately 1% of patients, often in association with reactive arthritis or vasculitis.[220] Reactive pericarditis, characterized by chest pain, pericardial friction rub, recurrence of fever, and sterile, non-purulent pericardial exudate, can also occur.[222] Concurrent presence of polyarthritis and polyserositis is common. Pericardial effusion rarely leads to tamponade or requires drainage.

Sequelae

Rates of severe and moderate neurologic sequelae after 5 years are lower after meningitis due to *N. meningitidis* (2.9% and 6.5%, respectively) than those following *Haemophilus influenzae* (3.4% and 7.3%, respectively) or *S. pneumoniae* (9.7% and 13.9%, respectively) meningitis.[223] In 562 cases of meningococcal disease in the Netherlands, 8.5% of survivors had one or more sequelae, including deafness in 3.1%, motor dysfunction in 1.2%, and other neurologic deficits in 1.2%.[214] The frequency of sequelae did not vary significantly with the serogroup or serotype of the pathogen or with the sex or age of the patient. A review of 471 cases of invasive meningococcal disease in Quebec, Canada, between 1990 and 1994 demonstrated significantly higher rates of death and major complications (skin scars, amputations) in patients infected with serogroup C than in those with serogroup B meningococci (Table 125-2).[211]

Psychological problems are frequently reported and neurologic deficits are found in 7% of cases.[36] It is important to perform follow-up of auditory testing in all cases of meningococcal disease to identify hearing loss (rate of occurrence 2% to 15% of cases in various studies),[224] and to provide hearing aids and plan cochlear implantation as necessary, in a timely manner.

Perfusion of the skin and muscle can be severely compromised in meningococcal shock and areas affected by purpura and pressure areas can be necrotic and at risk of secondary infection. In one study, ischemic infarction of skin and soft tissues resulted in significant scarring or extremity loss in 3.9% of survivors, most often after fulminant meningococcemia.[214] Multiple areas are involved in most patients. The limbs are the predominant sites of damage. In one study of 21 patients with skin infarction, the lower limbs were involved in 20, the arms in 9, the trunk in 8, the face in 4, and the scalp and ear in 1 each.[225] The mean area of skin necrosis was 13% of total body surface area. Skin damage or scarring across several studies was noted in 13% of cases.[36]

Limb compartment syndromes often are observed during the course of disease and fasciotomy has been used in management

TABLE 125-2. Outcome of Invasive Meningococcal Disease in Quebec, Canada, 1990–1994

Outcome	Outcomes in Indicated Serogroup (%)		
	B (*n* = 167)	C (*n* = 304)	P[a]
Death	7.2	13.8	<0.05
One or more major complications[b]	3.2	15.3	<0.0005
Skin scars	1.3	11.5	<0.0005
Amputations	0.6	4.6	<0.05
Deafness[c]	1.9	1.9	NS
Renal failure	0.0	1.1	NS
Other	2.5	3.3	NS

[a]*P value of chi-square analysis; NS, not significant.*

[b]*Some cases had multiple sequelae.*

[c]*Deafness in survivors with meningitis due to serogroups B and C: 3.2% and 2.9%, respectively.*

Adapted from Erickson L, DeWals P. Complications and sequelae of meningococcal disease in Quebec, Canada, 1990–1994. Clin Infect Dis 1998;26:1159.

in some circumstances but its role is not established clearly.[226] Except in the presence of infection, amputations of ischemic limbs should be undertaken late in order to allow maximum limb recovery before lines of viability are finalized. Amputations are necessary in approximately 3% of cases, with a further 3% suffering other orthopedic complications.

Impaired organ perfusion results from hypovolemia, vasoconstriction, and myocardial depression resulting in prerenal failure in some patients, with oliguria or anuria or acute tubular necrosis. Most patients recover without any renal support, some require hemofiltration, and rarely permanent renal failure ensues.

PREVENTION

Management of Contacts

Household and kissing contacts of a patient with meningococcal disease are at significantly increased risk of meningococcal disease (Box 125-3).[82,227,228] The incidence of disease in household contacts, although still low, is 500 to 1000 times that in the general population.[229] In sporadic cases of disease, 1% to 3% of households have one or more secondary cases of disease within 30 days of onset of the index case, if there is no intervention.[230]

BOX 125-3. Contacts of a Patient with Meningococcal Disease Who Are at Increased Risk of Disease

- Household members
- Childcare center and nursery school contacts
- School or college contacts during outbreak
- Anyone directly exposed to a patient's oral secretions through mouth-kissing or the sharing of food, drinks, utensils, glasses, water bottles, or anything that has been in the mouth of the patient
- Healthcare personnel exposed directly to patient's oral secretions through mouth-to-mouth resuscitation, or endotracheal intubation or tube management in the first 2 days of therapy without wearing a surgical mask[a]

[a]Healthcare workers without such exposure are *not* at increased risk. Adapted from Advisory Committee on Immunization Practices. Prevention and control of meningococcal disease: recommendations of the Advisory Committee on Immunization Practices (ACIP). MMWR 2000;49:1; and Pollard A, Begg N. Meningococcal disease and healthcare workers. Br Med J 1999;319:1147.

TABLE 125-3. Chemoprophylaxis Regimens for Contacts of Patients of Meningococcal Disease

Antibiotic	Dose
Rifampin	10 mg/kg per dose (maximum dose 600 mg) PO every 12 hours for 4 doses (for infants <1 month of age, 5 mg/kg per dose)
Ceftriaxone	Single injection of 125 mg IM for children <12 years; 250 mg IM for children ≥12 years and adults
Ciprofloxacin	Single dose 500 mg PO for adults

IM, intramuscularly; PO, by mouth.

Approximately 20% of secondary cases are coprimary infections (i.e., occurring on the same day as the index case); 30% of secondary cases occur in the first week, 20% in the second week, and 30% in weeks 3 to 8 after the index case. Because of the rapid onset of 50% of related cases, early antibiotic prophylaxis when indicated, education, and close follow-up of contacts to ensure rapid intervention if they experience febrile illness are important. Culture of specimens from contacts to aid management is of no value.

Trials of mass prophylaxis with sulfadiazine in military recruit camps during World War II suggested the efficacy of this approach for eradication of carriage and interruption of epidemics. However, mass prophylaxis has not been effective in other situations[231] and usually is avoided. The emergence of worldwide resistance of serogroups A, B, and C to sulfa drugs after 1963 led to the investigation of other agents for use in eradication of meningococcal carriage as a means of prophylaxis. Efficacy against all serogroups has been noted for rifampin, minocycline, ceftriaxone, ciprofloxacin, and ofloxacin. Minocycline is rarely used for prophylaxis because of its high rate of adverse effects (dizziness, nausea, and vomiting).

Rifampin is the only agent that has been studied widely, but it has the following disadvantages: (1) eradication rate is only 80% to 85%; (2) adverse effects occur in 25% of patients; (3) four doses are required; (4) it is expensive and not readily available; and (5) a liquid suspension is not always available for children.[229] Moreover, emergence of resistance to rifampin can occur rapidly. Ceftriaxone, administered as a single intramuscular injection, has been shown to be >97% effective in eradicating carriage;[232] Additional advantages are single-dose therapy and its safety during pregnancy. Disadvantages are the pain associated with intramuscular injection and the potential adverse effects on mucosal flora. Ciprofloxacin and ofloxacin effectively eradicate meningococcal carriage after a single oral dose.[233–236] However, fluoroquinolones are not approved for use in pregnant women and their use is limited in children in some countries.

It is essential that all contacts be treated immediately and concurrently, otherwise disease can not be prevented, and untreated carriers could infect contacts who have already completed prophylaxis. Treatment of index cases with ceftriaxone eradicates carriage. Patients who are treated with other antibiotics should receive appropriate prophylaxis before hospital discharge to prevent reintroduction of meningococcus into the household or community.

Details of prophylactic regimens are given in Table 125-3. Prophylaxis is not routinely recommended for: (1) school, church, or community contacts; or (2) medical personnel caring for the patient, except for those who have unusual, direct exposure to respiratory secretions through mouth-to-mouth resuscitation, or intubation or suctioning without wearing a mask.[237] Prophylaxis is recommended for infants and young children in close contact in daycare centers.

Immunization

Polysaccharide Vaccines

Vaccines composed of purified capsular polysaccharide of large molecular size have been developed against serogroups A, C, Y, and W135 and have been formulated as monovalent A and C, bivalent A/C, and quadrivalent A/C/Y/W135 vaccines. The major vaccine-related determinants of immunogenicity are the molecular size and dose of the vaccine, and the major host factor is age.[238,239] A dose–response effect has been observed in the dose range 10 to 200 µg, but in the range 25 to 100 µg there is little difference in peak antibody responses.[238] Currently licensed vaccines contain 50 µg of each serogroup polysaccharide per dose. Vaccines are safe, with rare reports of serious systemic events.[239–242] Benign febrile seizures have been reported rarely in young children who have undergone vaccination with bivalent group A and group C vaccine.[243] Transient local reactions, such as erythema and tenderness, can occur at the site of injection. These reactions are more common after quadrivalent vaccine (30% to 40%) than after monovalent group A or C vaccines (8% to 10%).

In U.S. adults vaccinated with quadrivalent A/C/Y/W135 vaccine, bactericidal antibodies directed at group A and C polysaccharides peak at 1 month, decline after 2 years, but remain higher than baseline for 10 years after vaccination.[244] In rural Nigeria, however, one study found that antibody to group A polysaccharide was not sustained 2 years after vaccination.[245]

Protection induced by meningococcal vaccine is serogroup specific. Group A vaccine is effective in preventing disease in all age groups (Box 125-4). Two doses administered 2 to 3 months apart

BOX 125-4. Recommended Uses of Meningococcal Conjugate Vaccines[a]

RECOMMENDED USES

Routine immunization of infants or toddlers with monovalent serogroup C meningococcal conjugate vaccine (MCC) is recommended in some countries (currently not available in the U.S.)

Routine immunization of children at 11 or 12 years of age and with catch-up immunization of those through 18 years of age, using a quadrivalent conjugate serogroup ACYW vaccine (MCV4) is recommended in the U.S.

Immunization of at-risk populations for control of outbreaks caused by serogroups contained in vaccine[b]

Immunization of travelers to an epidemic area[b]

Routine immunization in high-risk setting (e.g., military recruits, laboratory personnel)

Immunization of children with persistent complement deficiencies at 9 months of age and those with other high-risk conditions such as asplenia at 2 years of age, using MCV4 in a 2-dose series 3 months apart

REVACCINATION

Routine booster immunization of persons at 16 years of age who received MCV4 at 11 or 12 years of age, or at 18 years of age for those who received MCV4 at 13 or 14 years of age. No booster is recommended routinely for persons who received MCV4 ≥15 years of age

Booster immunization of persons in high risk groups every 5 years (with first booster after 3 years in those immunized under 2 years of age who continue to be at high risk of disease)

CONTRAINDICATIONS[c]

Severe reaction (anaphylaxis) to previous dose of vaccine

[a]Recommendations except for MCC are those of the U.S. Centers for Disease Control and Prevention for use of MCV4.[134]
[b]MCV4 can be given at 9 months of age, with second dose at interval of 3 months (or 2 months if in epidemic outbreak or time of travel does not permit longer interval).[134a]
[c]Pregnancy is not a contraindication to vaccination.

in infants 3 to 18 months (or 1 dose in older children and adults) have a protective efficacy >95%.[62,63] Group A vaccine has been effective in terminating epidemic group A disease. However, because duration of protection against invasive disease in adults does not appear to last more than 3 to 5 years, vaccine is not recommended for routine use.

Immunization with the group C vaccine has been >90% effective in preventing disease in young adults, and its routine use in the military eliminated outbreaks of group C disease.[246,247] However, group C vaccine is poorly immunogenic in infants. Repeated doses of group C vaccine, unlike group A vaccine, do not cause an anamnestic response at any age. Indeed, one dose of group C polysaccharide vaccine has been shown to induce immunologic hyporesponsiveness to subsequent doses in infants, toddlers, and adults.[239,248-250] The duration and clinical relevance of such hyporesponsiveness are uncertain but the phenomenon may be several years in duration.[237,251]

Group Y and group W135 polysaccharide vaccines are immunogenic in children older than 12 to 24 months. Proof of efficacy cannot be obtained because of the absence of epidemics due to these serogroups.

The polysaccharide vaccines have now largely been superseded by the glycoconjugate vaccines.

Conjugate Vaccines

Conjugation of groups A, C, Y, and W135 polysaccharides to proteins (MCV4), such as CRM197, tetanus toxoid, and diphtheria toxoid, achieves similar or greater immunogenicity and duration of protection in infants, children, adolescents, and adults without any increase in reactogenicity, compared with plain polysaccharide vaccine.[248-254] Moreover, the conjugated vaccines induce immunologic memory,[249,251] unlike the polysaccharide vaccines, and can overcome the hyporesponsiveness induced by previous doses of polysaccharide vaccine.[250,255] Conjugated group C vaccines have also been shown to induce salivary IgG and IgA antibodies in infants vaccinated at 2, 3, and 4 months of age,[256] adolescents,[257] and young adults,[258] and general use of the vaccine is associated with reduction in carriage rates.[111]

Because of a significant rise in the incidence of group C disease, a mass immunization program was started in November 1999 in the U.K. with meningococcal conjugate C (MCC) vaccines from three manufacturers.[259] Vaccination was offered first to infants younger than 1 year and adolescents 15 to 17 years old, the age groups at highest risk. Subsequently, vaccine was offered to all children and young adults under 24 years. The campaign proved to be highly effective both as a result of direct protection of the individual and as a result of herd immunity through reduction in transmission of the organism.[111,260,261]

MCC vaccines have been licensed and used in many other countries on the basis of the efficacy demonstrated in the U.K., using either a three-dose infant schedule or a single-dose toddler schedule with a catch-up campaign.[61,262] Data from the U.K. have shown that persistence of antibody after primary infant immunization is poor, and effectiveness data indicate that protection wanes to zero by 1 year after completion of the three-dose infant schedule.[260] In response to this, the U.K. Department of Health announced the addition of a booster dose of MCC vaccine in 2006 to be administered in the second year of life. However, recent studies suggest that persistence of functional antibody is poor even after this booster dose given at 1 year of age.[263] By contrast, persistence of antibody is more sustained after primary immunization of children over 10 years of age.[264] Furthermore, there is a marked response to a booster and persistence of antibody for at least 1 year if the booster is administered beyond 6 years of age.[265] Booster doses in adolescents are now implemented or being considered in several countries with an infant MCC program. In a study of 53 people who developed invasive group C meningococcal disease despite receipt of MCC vaccine, antibody response to disease was consistent with an anamnestic response, indicating that persistence of antibody may be a better correlate of long-term protection than priming for immune memory.[266]

In 2005, MCV4 containing A, C, Y, and W135 polysaccharides was licensed and recommended for universal use in the U.S. at the age of 11 years.[133] Preliminary data from the U.S. CDC in 2010 indicated a vaccine effectiveness of 75% (95% CI, 17 to 93).[267] Cases of Guillain–Barré syndrome occurring within 6 weeks of receipt were reported soon after implementation of MCV4 for adolescents in 2005; ongoing investigations since then in the U.S. as well as surveillance in Canada describe no excess cases or rare excess cases over that predicted.[268,269] A CRM197 ACYW meningococcal conjugate and similar combination conjugates from other manufacturers are expected to be available within a few years. In view of their immunologic advantages, the MCV4 vaccines should replace the plain polysaccharide vaccines for all indications in children and adults through 54 years of age. MCV4 vaccines are licensed in the U.S. down to 2 years of age, and are recommended for people at high risk of meningococcal disease (see Box 125-4).[134]

Waning of bactericidal antibody following MCV4 immunization given at 11 or 12 years of age led to the U.S. recommendation in 2010 for a second dose at 16 years of age, or at 18 years of age if the primary dose was given at 13 through 15 years of age.[134] In countries with established monovalent C conjugate programs in early childhood the quadrivalent vaccines are set to be used for adolescent boosters to overcome waning immunity.

Prospects for control of epidemic group A meningococcal disease in the meningitis belt of Africa have been enhanced by an alliance between the World Health Organization (WHO) and the Program for Appropriate Technology in Health (PATH) to develop a monovalent serogroup A meningococcal vaccine for Africa, funded by the Bill & Melinda Gates Foundation. Vaccine program implementation began across the meningitis belt of Africa during 2010 and early results indicate a decline in disease among vaccinated populations.[270]

Development of polysaccharide vaccine against group B meningococci, a major cause of endemic disease, is thwarted by lack of immunogenicity in humans.[271] The group B polysaccharide has structural and immunologic similarity to neural cell adhesion molecule, a membrane glycoprotein on human brain cells.[272] Protein vaccines prepared from PorA proteins induce bactericidal antibody but have been of limited success.[273] However, field trials of an OMP vaccine containing outer membrane vesicles (OMVs) from a Norwegian outbreak strain reduced the incidence of group B disease among schoolchildren aged 14 to 16 years by 53%.[274] A Cuban OMV vaccine from a local outbreak strain may have had somewhat greater efficacy in Cuba[275] but did not perform so well when tested in other settings. OMP vaccines may have limited utility because the bactericidal antibody elicited appears to be limited largely to the strain from which they are derived. However, this makes them ideal for control of an outbreak due to a single clone of meningococci such as the situation in New Zealand in which a single serogroup B clone caused a prolonged epidemic of disease starting in the early 1990s. An OMV vaccine based on the outbreak strain was launched during 2005 and had high effectiveness.[276]

Development of a comprehensive serogroup B vaccine continues to be an important public health goal and a large number of vaccine candidates have been considered over the past 2 decades (reviewed in Sadarangani and Pollard).[277] Data from the genome-sequencing projects have provided information about novel vaccine candidates[14] and two vaccines are now advancing through clinical trials: a 4-component vaccine containing meningococcal factor H binding protein, neisserial adhesion A, neisserial heparin binding antigen, and PorA; and a 2-component vaccine containing 2 variants of meningococcal factor H binding protein. Data from studies of these candidate vaccines in adults and children indicate that the vaccines induce bactericidal antibody against strains bearing the antigens contained in the vaccine. Results of larger clinical trials of candidate vaccines should determine their potential to provide cross-protection to other non-vaccine strains.

Key Points. Diagnosis and Management of *Neisseria meningitidis* Infection

MICROBIOLOGY

- Catalase-positive, oxidase-positive, piliated gram-negative coccus that oxidizes glucose and maltose
- Outer phospholipid membrane contains endotoxin and various outer membrane proteins that are subject to phase variation
- Can be surrounded by a polysaccharide capsule or acapsulate; 5 capsule "serogroups" associated with most global disease: A, B, C, Y, and W135
- Grows well on chocolate or blood agar; enhanced growth in humidified CO_2 environment

EPIDEMIOLOGY

- Highest rate of colonization (up to 40%) in adolescents and young adults; colonization rare in children <10 years
- Respiratory route of transmission
- Peak of disease in children under 2 years of age and smaller peak in adolescence
- Risk of disease increased by smoking (active and passive), overcrowding, prior viral respiratory tract infection, winter or dry season, moving into new communities, complement deficiency, and various human single nucleotide polymorphisms
- Serogroup distribution varies over time and with geographical location: B and C account for most disease in Europe; B, C, and Y in North America; and serogroup A in Africa and Asia
- In developed countries most cases are sporadic but small clusters can occur (mostly serogroup C strains). Epidemics of disease can occur (mainly serogroup A, with some X or W135) in developing countries, especially the meningitis belt of Africa

CLINICAL FEATURES

- Four presentations all of which are most often associated with a non-blanching (petechial or purpuric) rash:
  - Meningitis with mortality under 5%
  - Septic shock (meningococcaemia/meningococcal septicaemia) with high mortality
  - A mixed picture of meningitis and shock
  - Bloodstream infection without shock or meningitis
- Death usually is caused by cardiovascular collapse in septic shock cases or, rarely, by raised intracranial pressure in meningitis cases
- Complications include a self-limiting inflammatory reactive syndrome; neurologic sequelae (including deafness) following

meningitis; and limb, digit and skin scarring/loss after septic shock

DIAGNOSIS

- Microbiologic diagnosis usually is made by Gram stain of CSF and/or culture of blood (automated culture system) or CSF
- PCR of blood or CSF can yield higher rate of identification (especially with receipt of antibiotic prior to sampling)

TREATMENT

- Ceftriaxone is recommended as empiric therapy for suspected cases
- Urgent management of shock includes volume replacement therapy and supportive care (mechanical ventilation and inotropic drugs)
- Meningococcal meningitis should be managed with antibiotics and maintenance fluids with careful assessment for coexistent shock or raised intracranial pressure

DURATION OF THERAPY

- Duration of therapy should be 5–7 days but some studies suggest that as little as one dose of an appropriate antibiotic may be sufficient
- Response to therapy usually is rapid

VACCINE PREVENTION

- Monovalent serogroup C meningococcal conjugate vaccines (MCC) are widely used in Europe, Australia, and Canada for routine immunization of infants/toddlers and are highly effective, though optimal timing of booster doses is still unclear
- Quadrivalent meningococcal A, C, Y, W135 conjugate vaccines (MCV4) are used routinely in North America for adolescent immunization and are now recommended in many countries for high-risk groups and travelers (as young as 9 months of age)
- Booster dose(s) of MCV4 are recommended in the U.S. for high-risk children and persons immunized at <15 years of age
- Serogroup B vaccines have been used successfully for outbreaks involving single clones but are not suitable for endemic, polyclonal disease
- Novel serogroup B vaccines aimed at broad serogroup B coverage are in an advanced stage of development but there are no currently licensed vaccines for widespread use

126 *Neisseria gonorrhoeae*

Katherine K. Hsu, Peter A. Rice, and Jay M. Lieberman

Neisseria gonorrhoeae is a pathogen only of humans. Gonorrhea, one of the oldest known human illnesses, continues to result in significant morbidity – an estimated 62 million cases occur worldwide each year.[1] In the United States, gonorrhea is the second most frequently reported communicable disease, after *Chlamydia trachomatis*.[2] The reader is referred to organ- or syndrome-specific chapters for the overall approach to genital tract infections.

Gonorrhea is primarily a sexually transmitted infection (STI), although vertical transmission from infected mothers to their infants also occurs. The major public health impact of gonorrhea is as a cause of acute salpingitis, which is a leading cause

of infertility in women worldwide. Gonorrhea also is a potent amplifier of the spread of human immunodeficiency virus (HIV), increasing rates of HIV sexual transmission up to 5-fold.[3]

MICROBIOLOGY, IMMUNOLOGY AND PATHOGENESIS

N. gonorrhoeae, an oxidase-positive, gram-negative diplococcus, primarily infects columnar or transitional epithelial cells in the human genital tract. Transmission results almost exclusively from

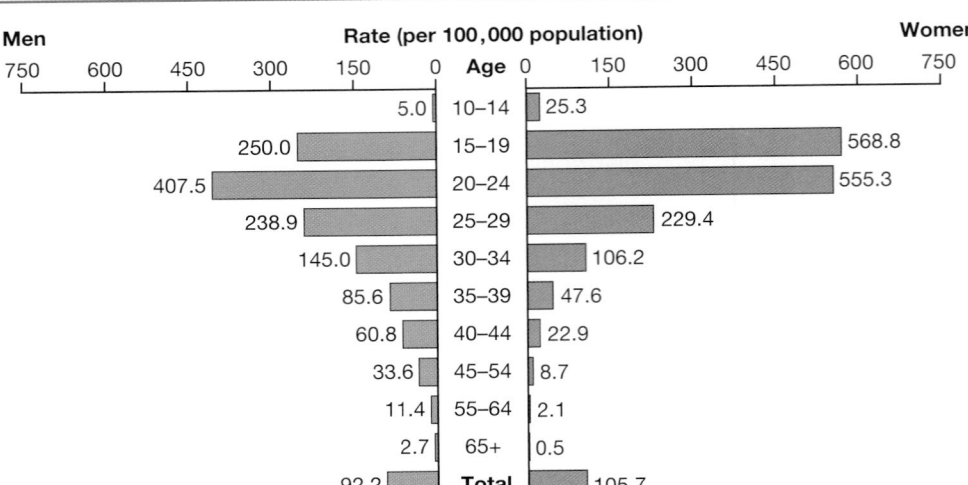

Figure 126-1. Age- and sex-specific rates for gonorrhea, United States, 2009. (Reprinted from Centers for Disease Control and Prevention. Sexually Transmitted Disease Surveillance. Atlanta, GA, United States Department of Health and Human Services, 2010.)

intimate contact, such as sexual activity or parturition. Adherence to mucosal epithelium is mediated by numerous gonococcal surface structures including pili, opacity-associated outer membrane (Opa) proteins, and lipo-oligosaccharides (LOS), which is followed by penetration of organisms between and through epithelial cells to submucosal tissue.[4] Cytokine release, which usually occurs in the process of invasion of male urethral cells, contributes to the symptomatic nature of gonococcal disease in men.[5] A neutrophil response follows, with subsequent sloughing of the epithelium, pus formation, and development of submucosal microabscesses. If infection is untreated, macrophages and lymphocytes eventually replace neutrophils. In contrast, subversion of host immune function can occur in women with uncomplicated cervical infection, resulting in lack of antibody and interleukin production.[5] However, in a model of upper genital disease using organ explant culture of fallopian tubes, gonococcal endotoxin (lipopolysaccharide) impairs ciliary motility and contributes to the destruction of surrounding ciliated cells.[6] Both humoral and local secretory antibodies to N. gonorrhoeae are induced during some uncomplicated gonococcal infections, and a cellular immune response is detectable in persons with recurrent infections. The exact role of host defense mechanisms in modulating infection or conferring immunity to reinfection is unclear.

N. gonorrhoeae has evolved multiple mechanisms to evade or thwart the host's immune response; repeated infections are common. Gonococcal virulence factors (e.g., pili, Opa proteins, and LOS) undergo phase and antigenic variation in response to selective environmental pressures, resulting in successful adaptation to variable microenvironments (such as the male urogenital tract, the female lower and upper genital tracts that also vary throughout the menstrual cycle, and the human bloodstream).[5] For example, the organism can: (1) turn on or off the synthesis or shift the expression of pili, Opa proteins, and LOS; (2) vary surface immunoaccessibility of porin (Por) and LOS antigens; (3) elicit antibody responses that are not protective (e.g., antibodies to the reduction-modifiable protein (Rmp) that block bactericidal activity of other antibodies against Por and LOS); and (4) alter LOS enzymatically by sialylation, causing loss of serum bactericidal activity.[7]

EPIDEMIOLOGY

Approximately 700,000 new N. gonorrhoeae infections occur annually in the U.S.[8] In 2009, 301,174 U.S. cases were reported; the incidence of reported disease was 99.1 cases per 100,000 population, which has remained relatively stable over the past 15 years.[2] Before 1996, men had higher rates of infection than women, but reported incidence now is higher in women. The highest incidence

is among women 15 to 19 years of age and among men 20 to 24 years of age (Figure 126-1).[2] When data are examined by single-year age groups, in California, rates of infection are much higher in women 18 and 19 years of age than women 15, 16, or 17 years of age, indicating potential for more targeted prevention and treatment efforts in settings serving older adolescents and young adults.[9] Prevalence continues to be highest in females, age group of 14- to 19-year-olds, non-Hispanic blacks, and residents of inner cities.[10,11] Risk of adolescents and young adults is multifactorial, including increased likelihood of multiple sex partners, unprotected sex, and susceptibility to infection due to cervical ectopy (in adolescent women), as well as less access to STI prevention services (lack of insurance or other ability to pay, lack of transportation, discomfort with facilities designed for adults, and concerns about confidentiality).[2,12] Additional risk factors include older sexual partners and substance abuse, particularly alcohol and marijuana.[13,14]

The likelihood of transmission depends on the anatomic site exposed and the number of exposures. A man's risk of acquiring urethral N. gonorrhoeae after a single episode of vaginal intercourse with an infected woman is about 20%; the risk increases to 60% to 80% after 4 exposures.[15-17] The risk of male-to-female transmission has not been evaluated as thoroughly but probably is ~50% to 70% after a single contact, with little evidence that risk increases with multiple exposures.[17,18] The risk of transmission via rectal or oral contact is less well defined, but is thought to be relatively efficient for insertive or receptive rectal intercourse. Pharyngeal gonorrhea can be acquired easily through fellatio; fellatio may account for 26% of urethral gonorrhea in men who have sex with men (MSM).[17] Oral sex is a highly prevalent practice among heterosexual young people, regardless of whether they have engaged in penetrative intercourse. As a result, pharyngeal gonorrhea has become increasingly prevalent, particularly among adolescents. In two Los Angeles STI clinics, 65% of patients between 15 and 24 years of age reported having oral sex; in this group, the prevalence of pharyngeal gonorrhea was 6% compared with 7% for urogenital gonorrhea.[19]

Prevalence in a community is sustained through continued transmission by asymptomatically infected individuals and also by a "core group" of transmitters who are more likely than the general population to become infected and to transmit N. gonorrhoeae to their sex partners.[20] Characteristics of core groups include demography (e.g., low socioeconomic status, geographic clustering in innercities) and unique behavior (e.g., history of repeated gonococcal infections, drug use, multiple sex partners, prostitution, and failure to abstain from sex despite symptoms or knowledge of recent exposure).[21-24] Effective control efforts for gonorrhea must target both asymptomatically infected individuals and infected core group members.

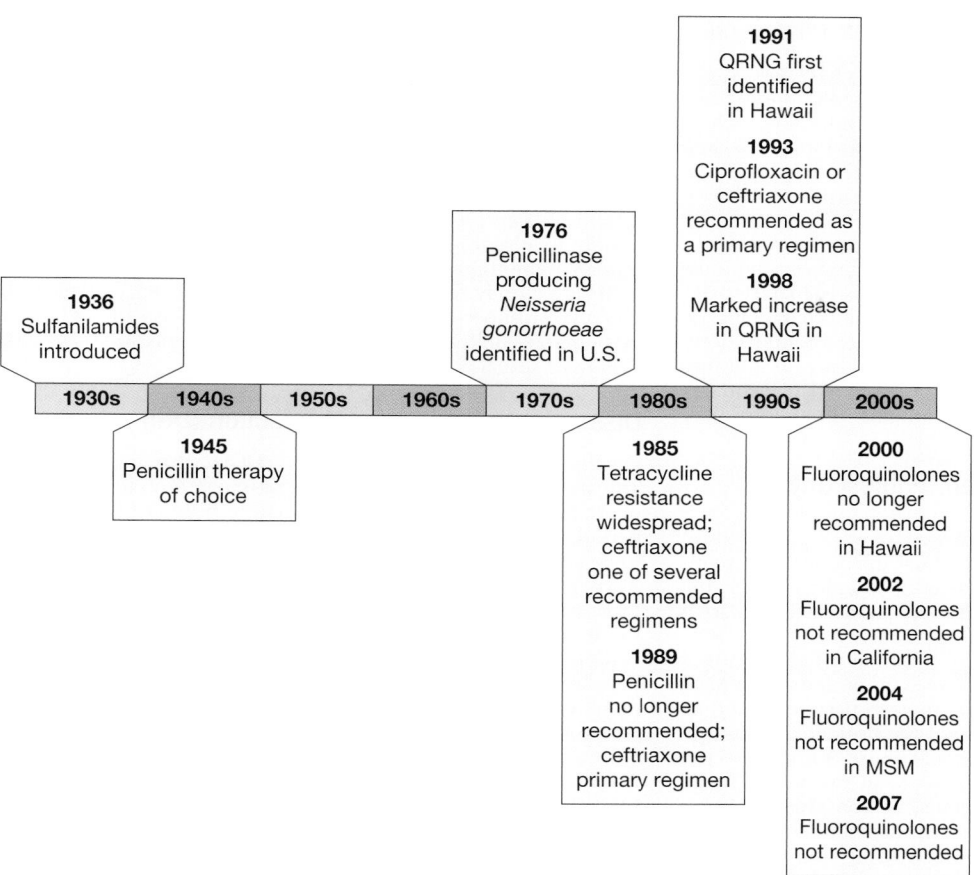

Figure 126-2. Historical perspective on gonococcal antimicrobial resistance in the United States. QRNG, fluoroquinolone-resistant *Neisseria gonorrhoeae*; MSM, men who have sex with men. (Redrawn from Workowski KA et al., Emerging Antimicrobial Resistance to *Neisseria gonorrhoeae:* Urgent Need to Strengthen Prevention Strategies, Ann Intern Med 2008;148:606–613.)

ANTIBIOTIC RESISTANCE

N. gonorrhoeae is facile at developing resistance to commonly used antimicrobial agents. The epidemiology, genetics, and mechanisms of resistance have been described.[17,25–28] Risk factors for antibiotic resistance include travel outside the community, high-risk behaviors, and recent antibiotic use, but are not always identified in individuals infected with resistant *N. gonorrhoeae*.[21–24,29,30]

The history of recommended antimicrobial therapy and development of resistance has been well described (Figure 126-2).[31] Although fluoroquinolone antibiotics were among agents primarily recommended for uncomplicated gonorrhea, their use is no longer recommended by the U.S. Centers for Disease Control and Prevention (CDC).[32]

Cephalosporin resistance is not reported in the U.S., although a few isolates with reduced susceptibility to ceftriaxone and cefixime have been identified.[33,34] Although most definitions of cephalosporin resistance are based on ceftriaxone, there may be important differences in susceptibility across cephalosporins, making cephalosporin susceptibility monikers not generalizable. Resistance mechanisms include altered penicillin binding proteins, reduction of antimicrobial entry into cells or active efflux. β-Lactamase has not been found in strains of *N. gonorrhoeae* that express relative cephalosporin resistance. Currently the only reliable method to detect resistance to cephalosporins is isolation and susceptibility testing. Limitations of direct specimen testing using nucleic acid amplification tests (NAATs) are incomplete correlations between identification of specific mutations, mean inhibitory concentrations (MICs), and clinical outcomes.[34]

CLINICAL MANIFESTATIONS

N. gonorrhoeae typically infects susceptible columnar or transitional epithelial cells (e.g., mucous membranes of the conjunctiva, pharynx, urethra, endocervix, and rectum). Infection often remains localized to the site of inoculation but can disseminate.

Perinatal Infections

Perinatal infection generally is acquired during passage through an infected birth canal, although transmission can occur after cesarean delivery, especially following premature rupture of membranes. Infant risks for infection include lack of appropriate ophthalmic prophylaxis, lack of maternal prenatal care, and maternal history of STI or substance abuse. An infant born to a woman with cervical gonococcal infection has an approximate 30% risk of acquiring ophthalmic infection,[35] versus <5% if ocular prophylaxis is given.[36]

Ophthalmia Neonatorum

The usual incubation period for gonococcal ophthalmia neonatorum is 2 to 5 days, but onset can be as early as several hours after birth (following prolonged rupture of membranes) or as late as several weeks.[37] Prematurity and premature rupture of membranes are significant risk factors for gonococcal ophthalmia. The time of onset and clinical findings do not reliably distinguish *N. gonorrhoeae* from *Chlamydia trachomatis* conjunctivitis.

Typical findings of gonococcal conjunctivitis are marked bilateral eyelid edema, chemosis, and copious purulent discharge. Asymptomatic infection or mild chronic infection with intermittent symptomatology lasting for several months also has been reported.[38] Although gonococcal conjunctivitis generally is less severe in neonates than in adults, corneal complications, such as ulceration and perforation of the globe (rarely), panophthalmitis, and blindness, can occur.[8]

Other Perinatal Infections Including Systemic Infection

N. gonorrhoeae can be isolated from culture of pharyngeal swabs or orogastric fluid in about one-third of infants with ophthalmia neonatorum.[39,40] Examples of neonatal mucosal infections include vaginitis (uncommon because neonatal vaginal mucosa is well estrogenized by circulating maternal hormone), urethritis, rhinitis, anorectal infection, and funisitis. *N. gonorrhoeae* scalp abscess can follow fetal electrode monitoring.[41,42]

Disseminated disease is rare in neonates; pyogenic arthritis is the most common manifestation.[43,44] Clinical symptoms typically develop at 1 to 4 weeks of age; pseudoparalysis is characteristic. Multiple joint involvement is common.[43] Most affected infants do not have/have not had conjunctivitis or other mucosal infections. Skin lesions representing septic emboli of bloodstream infection (BSI), commonly seen in adults, are not described in neonates. Rarely, neonatal infection results in meningitis[45] or endocarditis.

Mucosal Infections in Children, Adolescents, and Adults

N. gonorrhoeae causes a variety of mucosal infections in sexually active adolescents and adults as well as in sexually abused children. Transmission by fomites or through nonsexual contact is extremely rare.

In prepubertal children, gonococcal infection usually occurs in the genital tract, and vaginitis is the most common manifestation (the nonestrogenized alkaline vaginal mucosa permitting colonization). *N. gonorrhoeae* infection should be considered in any girl with vaginal discharge, even when sexual abuse is not suspected. In one study of 43 girls <12 years of age with vaginal discharge, 9% had gonorrhea.[46] Sexual abuse must be considered strongly when gonococcal infection is diagnosed in prepubertal children (beyond the newborn period).[47] Among sexually abused children, pharyngeal and anorectal gonococcal infections are common and often are asymptomatic.[47,48] Gonococcal urethritis, perihepatitis, and pelvic inflammatory disease (PID) are uncommon but possible in prepubertal children.

The majority of men who come to medical attention with *N. gonorrhoeae* infection are symptomatic; asymptomatic or minimally symptomatic infections may be more common than appreciated but usually are recognized only through screening programs or after symptomatic infection in a contact.[49] In a cohort of men whose time of acquisition was defined, only 2.5% remained asymptomatic for 2 weeks.[17] However, certain phenotypes of gonococci have been more frequently associated with asymptomatic infection.[50] Acute urethritis is the major clinical manifestation in men, who complain of dysuria or note a mucoid or mucopurulent discharge 2 to 5 days after infection. Discharge often becomes profuse and purulent within 24 to 48 hours of onset.

Women are more likely than men to have asymptomatic infection or mild, sometimes unappreciated, symptoms. The endocervical canal is the predominant site of urogenital infection; urethral colonization also occurs in most cases in which the cervix is involved. The incubation period for urogenital infections in women is less certain and more variable, but in most symptomatic women, the symptoms develop within 10 days of infection.[51,52] Symptomatic females can have vaginal discharge, dysuria, abdominal pain, and intermenstrual bleeding; symptoms and signs range from mild to severe. The cervix can appear normal or can exhibit edema, erythema, or friability as well as purulent or mucopurulent discharge.[53]

Pharyngeal infection occurs in about 3% to 7% of *N. gonorrhoeae* infection in heterosexual men and 10% to 20% in heterosexual women or MSM.[54-56] However, pharyngitis is the sole site in <5% of infections. Most pharyngeal infections are asymptomatic; rarely, acute tonsillopharyngitis or cervical lymphadenopathy occurs.[54,55]

Asymptomatic rectal infection is present in 26% to 68% of women with gonococcal cervicitis; translocation of infected secretions is thought to be the mechanism, because rectal positivity correlates with duration of infection.[57,58] The rectum is the sole site of infection in <5% of women. In MSM, rectal mucosa can become infected after receptive anal intercourse.[57] Anorectal infection often is asymptomatic. Symptomatic infections range from painless mucopurulent discharge and scant rectal bleeding to overt proctitis with associated rectal pain and tenesmus.[57,58]

Gonococcal conjunctivitis is rare in adults, usually results from autoinoculation, and occurs most often in people with anogenital infection. Untreated gonococcal conjunctivitis can progress rapidly to ulcerative keratitis and corneal perforation; however, mild or asymptomatic conjunctival infection also occurs. Outcome correlates closely with the severity of disease at the initiation of therapy.[59] Gonococcal conjunctivitis also has been described in prepubertal children without laboratory evidence or suggestive history of sexual abuse.[60]

Disseminated Gonococcal Infection (DGI)

Disseminated gonococcal infection (DGI), also known as the arthritis–dermatitis syndrome, is the most common manifestation of acute systemic gonococcal infection beyond the neonatal period; in the 1970s when gonococcal strains with a propensity to disseminate (see below) were common, DGI occurred in up to 3% of people with untreated mucosal gonorrhea;[61-63] DGI is much less common currently. The characteristic findings of acute arthritis, tenosynovitis, dermatitis (alone or in combination) result from intermittent BSI. Fewer than one-half of patients with DGI have *N. gonorrhoeae* isolated from blood, joint fluid, skin lesions, or other sterile sites, but *N. gonorrhoeae* can be isolated from a mucosal site or from a sex partner in about 80% of cases.[61-64]

Dermatitis occurs in about 75% of patients with DGI. The classic skin lesions are discrete, tender necrotic pustules on erythematous bases located distally on an upper extremity; macules, papules, petechiae, bullae, or ecchymoses also have been described. Results of culture or Gram stain of lesions are positive for *N. gonorrhoeae* in only about 10% to 15% of cases. Migratory polyarthralgia or tenosynovitis (especially in the flexor and extensor tendon sheaths) affecting smaller joints is an early finding. Pyogenic monoarticular or polyarticular arthritis develops later in about one-third of patients; the wrist, metacarpophalangeal, ankle, or knee joints are involved most commonly.[61-64]

Gonococcal endocarditis is a rare complication, occurring in about 1% to 3% of patients with DGI.[61,62,65] The aortic valve is affected most often; valvular damage can progress rapidly if untreated. Hepatitis and meningitis also are uncommon complications of DGI.

DGI is more common in women, with onset within 7 days of the start of menstruation in about one-half of cases.[61-63] Certain strains of *N. gonorrhoeae* (uncommon in the U.S. currently) are associated with disseminated infection. DGI strains often cause asymptomatic urogenital infection and typically, although not always, are penicillin G-susceptible, and resistant to the complement-mediated bactericidal activity of human serum.[62,63] Complement deficiency, which predisposes to gonococcal or meningococcal BSI, is found in up to 13% of patients with DGI.[66,67]

LABORATORY FINDINGS AND DIAGNOSIS

Laboratory confirmation of *N. gonorrhoeae* infection is essential in children because of the legal implications of potential sexual abuse. Confirmation also is important in adolescents and adults to improve adherence to therapy and referral of sex partners.

Gram Stain

Gram-stained smears of exudate from the conjunctivae, endocervix of postpubertal females, vagina of prepubertal girls, male urethra, skin lesions, synovial fluid, and cerebrospinal fluid may be useful, if positive, in the initial evaluation of individuals with suspected gonococcal infection. Visualization of intracellular gram-negative diplococci (most often as multiple kidney bean-shaped diplococci within a relatively few neutrophils in the specimen) is presumptive evidence of *N. gonorrhoeae* infection; identifying only extracellular organisms is less specific in mucosal specimens. Compared with culture, Gram stain is 90% to 95% sensitive in urethral specimens from men with symptomatic urethritis, but only 50% to 70% sensitive in endocervical specimens from women with uncomplicated gonorrhea.[17,68-70] Gram stain of pharyngeal or rectal specimens is not recommended due to lack of specificity.

Culture

Isolation of *N. gonorrhoeae* by culture is critical to monitoring development of resistance to current antimicrobial treatment regimens.[71] *N. gonorrhoeae* does not tolerate drying; clinical specimens should be inoculated immediately onto appropriate culture media and incubated at 35°C to 37°C in an atmosphere of high humidity and 4% to 6% carbon dioxide. "Bedside" inoculation in a nutritive transport system (e.g., a polystyrene dish containing selective gonococcal media and an inner well containing a carbon dioxide-generating tablet is an acceptable alternative). *N. gonorrhoeae* only grows well on chocolate agar or similarly enriched media; media used for specimens from the urogenital tract or pharynx should contain antimicrobial agents (e.g., vancomycin, colistin, plus an antifungal agent) to inhibit growth of saprophytic organisms. Thayer–Martin and Martin–Lewis are the most commonly used enriched antimicrobial media. Sterile body fluids (e.g., blood, synovial fluid, cerebrospinal fluid) should be inoculated onto antibiotic-free, enriched media such as chocolate agar.

N. gonorrhoeae are oxidase-positive, gram-negative diplococci that utilize glucose but not maltose, sucrose, fructose, or lactose. *N. gonorrhoeae* can be distinguished from other *Neisseria* species and from *Moraxella catarrhalis* by carbohydrate utilization or by a nucleic acid confirmation test. Although specimens from urogenital infections generally give straightforward results, confirmation at a reference laboratory occasionally is necessary. Presumptive identification of *N. gonorrhoeae* from extragenital mucosal sites such as the pharynx should be interpreted with caution because of the expected presence of nonpathogenic *Neisseria* species; at least two confirmatory bacteriologic tests using different methodologies (e.g., biochemical and enzyme substrate) should be performed.[72,73]

The sensitivity of a single, properly obtained specimen inoculated onto selective media is >95% for males with symptomatic urethritis, and 80% to 90% for women with endocervical infections. Obtaining a second endocervical specimen improves culture sensitivity in women.

Advantages of culture include low cost and availability of an isolate for further studies, e.g., antibiotic susceptibility testing or subtyping. Disadvantages include transport and growth requirements and time-delay of 24 to 72 hours from specimen collection to presumptive result.[74]

Nonculture Tests

The sensitivity of NAATs for the detection of *N. gonorrhoeae* at genital and nongenital anatomic sites is superior to culture but varies by NAAT type.[8] Product information inserts for each NAAT test must be read carefully because specimen types approved by the Food and Drug Administration (FDA) vary by test. NAATs are not FDA-approved for use on specimens from the rectum, pharynx, conjunctiva, joint fluid, blood, or CSF. Despite lack of FDA approval, and to facilitate patient management, some commercial and public health laboratories have established performance specifications to satisfy Centers for Medicare and Medicaid Services (CMS) regulations for FDA Clinical Laboratory Improvement Amendment (CLIA) compliance in testing and reporting results for nongenital specimens. Specificity is the key factor for performance due to cross-reaction with nongonococcal *Neisseria* species. Advantages of NAATs include flexibility in sampling source, and utility when transport problems preclude the use of culture.[71,74]

Use of NAATs performed on urine or other easily obtained genital specimens offers several advantages for detection of reproductive tract infection. Advantages include patient preference (compared with speculum examinations of women and urethral swabs of men) and the feasibility of testing in settings where traditional genitourinary examinations are not performed, such as schools. For men, urine is the preferred sample for testing or screening because testing specimen of urine is more sensitive than urethral swab and has equivalent specificity.[71] However, NAATs may be less sensitive in women when performed on urine compared with genital swab samples (vaginal or endocervical).[71] For women, vaginal swab samples are preferable to endocervical swabs for screening for *N. gonorrhoeae* by NAATs because of convenience and equivalent sensitivity and specificity compared with endocervical swabs. Endocervical swabs are acceptable when pelvic exams are done, but vaginal swab specimens are an appropriate sample type even when a full pelvic examination is being performed.[71]

For detection of rectal and pharyngeal infections, NAATs are superior to culture.[75-77] However, not all commercially available NAATs are equivalently specific (particularly polymerase chain reaction tests) for pharyngeal specimens or FDA-approved, and results must be interpreted cautiously (see above).[71,75,76]

Data on the use of NAATs are limited in children and performance is both sample-site and test dependent. In a multicenter study of testing using strand displacement amplification or transcription-mediated amplification in children being evaluated for sexual abuse, sufficient data were collected from prepubertal girls to conclude that testing of urine samples using these 2 commercially available NAATs is a reliable alternative to vaginal culture for detection of *N. gonorrhoeae*.[78] However, culture still remains the recommended method for detection of *N. gonorrhoeae* in urethral specimens from boys and for extragenital specimens (conjunctiva, pharynx and rectum) from all children because NAATs have not yet been sufficiently evaluated for these populations and sample sites.[8]

Because accurate diagnosis is the goal, there is no justification for the routine use of less sensitive non-amplified technologies such as enzyme immunoassays (EIA) or DNA probe assays except perhaps when an immediate positive diagnosis provides a therapeutic advantage.[71] Serologic assays for diagnosis or screening for gonococcal infection are neither recommended nor available.

TREATMENT

Management Considerations

The goals of antibiotic therapy are to relieve symptoms, reduce the risk of sequelae, eradicate infection, and halt transmission. Persons with suspected gonococcal infections should be treated empirically, before susceptibility test results of the isolate are known. Selection of an appropriate regimen requires consideration of local and national resistance patterns, anatomic site(s) of infection, likelihood of concurrent infections with *C. trachomatis* or another STI, side effects, and relative cost. Generally, ceftriaxone or another third-generation cephalosporin is the drug of choice for all gonococcal infections in the U.S., with dosing dependent upon age and weight, and length of therapy varying by site and severity of infection (Table 126-1). Coinfection with *C. trachomatis* is common (up to 46% in some studies)[10,79] so persons treated presumptively for gonorrhea should be treated routinely with a dual regimen that is effective against both pathogens (see Chapter 167, *Chlamydia trachomatis*). All persons treated for *N. gonorrhoeae* also should be evaluated for *Chlamydia*, syphilis, HIV, and other STIs.[8]

Return visits for test-of-cure cultures are not recommended for persons with uncomplicated gonorrhea who become/remain asymptomatic following treatment with a recommended regimen. If symptoms persist after therapy, a culture for *N. gonorrhoeae* should be obtained, and antimicrobial susceptibility testing performed. Symptoms of persistent urethritis, cervicitis, or proctitis also can be caused by *C. trachomatis, Mycoplasma hominis,*

TABLE 126-1. Treatment of Gonococcal Infections

	Infection	Treatment Regimen	Length of Therapy
Neonates	Ophthalmia neonatorum	Ceftriaxone[a] 25–50 mg/kg IV or IM once (max. 125 mg) plus lavage infected eye frequently until discharge eliminated	Once
	Disseminated infection Scalp abscess Septic arthritis	Ceftriaxone[a] 25–50 mg/kg IV or IM qd *Or* Cefotaxime 50 mg/kg IV or IM q8–12h[b]	7 days
	Meningitis	Ceftriaxone[a] 25–50 mg/kg IV or IM qd *Or* Cefotaxime 50 mg/kg IV or IM q12h[b]	10–14 days
	Endocarditis	Ceftriaxone[a] 25–50 mg/kg IV or IM qd *Or* Cefotaxime 50 mg/kg IV or IM q12h[b]	Minimum 28 days
Children <45 kg	Pharyngeal infection Anorectal infection Urogenital infection	Ceftriaxone 125 mg IM	Once
	Conjunctivitis	Ceftriaxone 50 mg/kg IM (max. 1 g) plus lavage infected eye with saline solution	Once
	Disseminated infection Septic arthritis	Ceftriaxone 50 mg/kg IV or IM qd (max. 1 g daily)	7 days
	Meningitis	Ceftriaxone 50 mg/kg IV or IM q12h (max. 2 g daily)	10–14 days
	Endocarditis	Ceftriaxone 50 mg/kg IV or IM q12h (max. 2 g daily)	Minimum 28 days
Adults, adolescents, and children ≥45 kg	Anorectal infection Urogenital infection	Ceftriaxone 250 mg IM *Or, if not an option* Cefixime 400 mg PO[c] *Or* Other single-dose injectable cephalosporin[d]	Once
	Pharyngeal infection	Ceftriaxone 250 mg IM	Once
	Conjunctivitis	Ceftriaxone 1 g IM plus lavage infected eye with saline solution	Once
	Disseminated infection Septic arthritis	Ceftriaxone 1 g IV or IM qd[e]	7 days
	Meningitis	Ceftriaxone 1 g IV or IM q12h	10–14 days
	Endocarditis	Ceftriaxone 1 g IV or IM q12h	Minimum 28 days

[a]*Ceftriaxone should not be administered to neonates with hyperbilirubinemia.*

[b]*Dose and/or dosing frequency change after postnatal age >7 days of life – consult neonatal dosing references.*

[c]*Cefixime should not be used if pharyngeal infection is suspected.*

[d]*See text for details.*

[e]*Continue for 24–48 hours after improvement occurs, at which time therapy can be changed to cefixime 400 mg PO every 12 hours to complete at least 7 days of therapy.*

Ureaplasma urealyticum, and other organisms. Gonococcal infection detected after an appropriate course of therapy usually represents reinfection rather than treatment failure. Because infection occurs most commonly in patients who have been diagnosed and treated for gonorrhea in the preceding several months, patients with gonorrhea should be retested 3 months after treatment or whenever they seek medical care within the following 12 months.[8]

Gonorrhea is a reportable disease, and partner notification for evaluation and treatment is imperative to prevent reinfection of the index case patient, to eradicate large numbers of asymptomatic infections, and to interrupt transmission. In heterosexual adolescents and adults, expedited partner therapy (detailed below) should be considered.

Perinatal Infections

Infants born to mothers who have untreated gonorrhea are at high risk for infection and should be given a single intravenous (IV) or intramuscular (IM) dose of ceftriaxone, even in the absence of signs or symptoms.[8] Neither ocular silver nitrate nor topical antibiotic ointment (e.g., erythromycin, tetracycline) is adequate therapy for established gonococcal ophthalmia.[37] Infants with

gonococcal ophthalmia should be hospitalized and disseminated infection excluded; considering the rarity of gonococcal meningitis most experts would not perform a lumbar puncture in a well-appearing, afebrile infant. Infants with uncomplicated ophthalmia neonatorum should be treated with ceftriaxone; additional topical therapy is unnecessary, but frequent saline irrigations are important.[8,39]

Some physicians elect to continue ceftriaxone once daily until blood, joint, and cerebrospinal fluid (if obtained) culture results are negative at 48 to 72 hours. Ceftriaxone should be administered cautiously to infants with hyperbilirubinemia, especially preterm infants; cefotaxime is an alternative in these cases.[73] The mother of an infant diagnosed with a gonococcal infection (and her sex partner) also should receive appropriate evaluation and treatment, and the infant should be evaluated for *Chlamydia trachomatis*, syphilis, and HIV.

Mucosal Infections in Adolescents and Adults

Single-dose ceftriaxone 250 mg IM cures >99% of uncomplicated anorectal and urogenital infections and 99% of pharyngeal infections. Gonococci are eradicated from the urine, urethra, and semen of symptomatic men within 24 hours of therapy.[80] Azithromycin given orally in a single dose, or doxycycline orally twice daily for 7 days, also should be given routinely to treat *C. trachomatis*.

If ceftriaxone is not available, oral cefixime or other single-dose injectable cephalosporin regimens (ceftizoxime 500 mg IM, cefoxitin 2 g IM administered with probenecid 1 g orally, or cefotaxime 500 mg IM) can be used to treat uncomplicated anorectal and urogenital infection. Although oral therapy avoids the cost and inconvenience of injections and decreases the risk of accidental needlestick injuries to medical personnel who may be treating a population at high risk of HIV infection,[80] the recommended 400 mg oral dose of cefixime does not provide as high nor as sustained a bactericidal level as that provided by the 250 mg IM dose of ceftriaxone. In published clinical trials, cefixime 400 mg orally cured 98% of uncomplicated anorectal and urogenital infections, but only 92% of pharyngeal infections. None of the other injectable cephalosporins offers any advantage over ceftriaxone for urogenital infection, and efficacy for pharyngeal infection is less certain.[8]

Gonococcal conjunctivitis should be treated with a single dose of ceftriaxone 1 g IM; lavage with saline solution (once) should be considered. Presumptive treatment for concurrent *C. trachomatis* infection also should be given.[8]

Alternative Regimens

Although cefpodoxime 400 mg orally, cefpodoxime-proaxetil 200 mg orally, and cefuroxime-axetil 1 g orally all meet minimum efficacy criteria for alternative regimens for urogenital infections, efficacy in treating pharyngeal infections is unsatisfactory (estimated to be 70%, 79%, and 57%, respectively) and there are concerns about the pharmacodynamics of both the lower dose of cefpodoxime and the 1 g dose of cefuroxime-axetil.

Spectinomycin in a single 2 g IM dose might be useful in persons who cannot tolerate cephalosporins (estimated efficacy 98% for uncomplicated urogenital and anorectal infections), but the drug is relatively expensive, must be injected, is not effective against pharyngeal gonococcal infection (estimated efficacy 52%) or incubating syphilis, and is not available currently in the U.S.[8,81,82]

Azithromycin, approved for the treatment of nongonococcal infections, has been evaluated for treating gonococcal infections. Azithromycin 2 g orally is effective (estimated efficacy 99%) for uncomplicated urogenital, anorectal, and pharyngeal gonococcal infections,[83] and this dose is approved by the FDA for therapy of gonorrhea. Azithromycin 1 g orally, the dose approved to treat *C. trachomatis* infections, meets alternative regimen criteria (estimated efficacy 98%), but it is not recommended because of documented treatment failures and reports of strains of *N. gonorrhoeae* with decreased susceptibility to azithromycin.[84,85] Although a single oral-dose regimen of azithromycin to eradicate both *N. gonorrhoeae* and *C. trachomatis* is appealing, concerns about possible rapid emergence of macrolide resistance as well as the high rate of gastrointestinal symptoms associated with the 2 g dose limit its usefulness.[8]

Disseminated Infection Including Meningitis and Endocarditis in Adolescents and Adults

Hospitalization usually is recommended for initial therapy of DGI to establish the correct diagnosis and especially when purulent synovitis or another major complication is present. Daily parenteral ceftriaxone should be administered until at least 24 to 48 hours after clinical improvement begins. Alternative agents include cefotaxime 1 g IV every 8 hours or ceftizoxime 1 g IV every 8 hours. Following the parenteral regimen, the patient can be given cefixime orally to complete at least 1 week of therapy. Persons treated for DGI should be treated presumptively for concurrent *C. trachomatis* infection.[8] Patients with gonococcal meningitis or endocarditis should be treated with parenteral ceftriaxone *twice* daily, for longer (Table 126-1).[8]

Childhood Infections

Treatment regimens for children weighing ≥45 kg are the same as for adolescents and adults. In children <45 kg, single-dose ceftriaxone 125 mg IM is recommended for treatment of uncomplicated vulvovaginitis, cervicitis, urethritis, proctitis, or pharyngitis; weight-based dosing is used to treat conjunctivitis or disseminated infections including arthritis, meningitis, and endocarditis (Table 126-1).[8]

SPECIAL CONSIDERATIONS

Pelvic inflammatory disease, a spectrum of inflammatory disorders of the female upper genital tract, can be any combination of endometritis, salpingitis, tubo-ovarian abscess, and pelvic peritonitis. Women who have gonococcal versus nongonococcal salpingitis are more likely to be febrile, to appear acutely ill, and to seek medical attention during the first 3 days of symptoms, although laparoscopic studies have shown that the severity of tubal disease is similar in gonococcal versus nongonococcal disease.[86] In PID, isolation of *N. gonorrhoeae* from the cervix does not necessarily mean that it is the sole pathogen. Acute perihepatitis (Fitz-Hugh–Curtis syndrome) can occur with gonococcal or chlamydial infections. PID is the most common complication of gonorrhea in women, occurring in about 10% to 20% of women with infection.[87,88] Even asymptomatic infections can progress to PID. Prevention of PID is critical because of potential long-term consequences – tubal infertility, ectopic pregnancy, and chronic pelvic pain.

Without treatment, gonococcal urethritis usually resolves spontaneously over several weeks, and >95% of untreated patients become asymptomatic within 6 months.[17] Most men with gonococcal epididymitis also have overt urethritis.[17] Epididymitis currently is an uncommon complication, and acute or chronic gonococcal prostatitis occurs rarely. Other unusual local complications of gonococcal urethritis include edema of the penis due to dorsal lymphangitis or thrombophlebitis, periurethral abscess or fistulae, seminal vesiculitis, and balanitis in uncircumcised men.

The manifestations of gonorrhea during pregnancy are not distinctive, except that pharyngeal infections appear to be more prevalent and PID probably is less common.[17,89] Reported complications in pregnancy include spontaneous abortion, premature rupture of membranes, premature delivery, intrauterine growth retardation, and acute chorioamnionitis, in addition to infection in the neonate.[17,89]

In immunocompromised people such as HIV-infected patients, the manifestations and sequelae of gonococcal infections are not different or more common than in HIV-uninfected patients. However, nonulcerative STIs enhance HIV transmission by 3- to 5-fold, in part because of increased viral shedding by persons with urethritis or cervicitis. Gonococcal infection also may increase an individual's risk for acquisition of HIV, with the presence of significantly increased numbers of HIV-susceptible CD4+ T lymphocytes and dendritic cells the hypothesized mechanism.[90]

Complement deficiencies, particularly of components involved in the assembly of the membrane attack complex (C5 through C9), predispose to *Neisseria* BSI generally, and are found in up to 13% of patients with DGI.[66,67]

PREVENTION AND CONTROL

Ocular Prophylaxis

Ocular prophylaxis with topical silver nitrate (1% aqueous solution), erythromycin (0.5%), or tetracycline (1%) ophthalmic ointment reduces the incidence of gonococcal ophthalmia neonatorum with equivalent efficacy.[73,91] Insufficient data exist to recommend 2.5% povidone-iodine for standard prophylaxis in the U.S.[8,92] Topically applied antibiotics are less irritating than silver nitrate but are slightly more expensive, and have been associated with emergence of gonococcal resistance.[93] Silver nitrate and tetracycline ophthalmic ointment are no longer manufactured in the

U.S., leaving erythromycin ophthalmic ointment as the only recommended agent for ocular prophylaxis.[88] Single-use tubes or ampules are recommended, and prophylaxis should be administered as soon as possible to all newborn infants after delivery.[8,73] If erythromycin ointment is not available, infants at risk for *N. gonorrhoeae* (especially those born to a mother with untreated gonococcal infection or who has not received prenatal care) can be given ceftriaxone 25 to 50 mg/kg IV or IM, not to exceed 125 mg, in a single dose. Properly administered ocular prophylaxis can fail to prevent infection acquired before delivery as a result of prolonged rupture of membranes, or after administration of prophylaxis.

Partner and Expedited Partner Therapy for STI

All sex partners within 60 days (or, if none, the last partner >60 days) of the patient's diagnosis of any gonococcal infection should be examined and treated presumptively.[88] Delivery of antibiotic therapy or a certified prescription for antibiotic therapy for gonorrhea (forms of expedited partner therapy or EPT) by heterosexual patients to their partners should be considered in states where EPT is permissible.[94] Randomized controlled trials demonstrate safety and noninferiority of EPT versus traditional care in heterosexual patients.[95] The American Medical Association,[96] the American Academy of Pediatrics, and the Society of Adolescent Health and Medicine[97] endorse EPT for heterosexual patients when in-person evaluation and treatment are impractical or unsuccessful. Partners, however, should be encouraged to seek clinical evaluation to optimize management of STIs. Because of the high risk for coexisting undiagnosed STIs including HIV, EPT is not considered a routine partner management strategy in MSM.[8]

Screening as Prevention

Because gonococcal infections may not be associated with overt symptoms, particularly in women, annual screening of individuals at risk or living in an area with high prevalence of gonococcal infection is important to prevent disease and sequelae.[8,98] Active gonococcal screening programs decrease prevalence of *N. gonorrhoeae* infections. Although the U.S. Preventive Services Task Force has not defined high prevalence area, a threshold of 4.75% has been cited as a level for cost-effectiveness for screening of women aged <25 years with risk factors (previous gonococcal infection, other STIs, new or multiple sex partners, inconsistent condom use, commercial sex work, and drug use).[98,99] Frequent re-screening in previously infected people is important; reinfection rate is high (median, 7% in males and 12% in females).[100,101] Sexually active MSM should be screened at least annually, preferably using NAAT of all sites involved in intercourse (urine, rectal swab, and/or pharyngeal swab).[8] Pregnant women at risk or living in an area with high prevalence should be screened for *N. gonorrhoeae* at the initial antenatal visit, and at-risk patients (including those found to have gonococcal infection) should be screened again during the third trimester.[98]

Vaccination

Although understanding of the pathobiology and immunology of gonorrhea has advanced, limits to knowledge about what constitutes protective immunity and lack of a suitable animal model that mirrors human disease have hampered vaccine development.[7,102] It is likely that multiple immunogens will be required in any *N. gonorrhoeae* vaccine to protect against diverse strains.[7,102,103]

Key Points. Diagnosis and Management of *Neisseria gonorrhoeae* Infections

MICROBIOLOGY

- Oxidase-positive, gram-negative diplococcus
- Requires chocolate agar or other enriched media and CO_2 for initial growth in vitro
- Penicillin, tetracycline, and fluoroquinolone resistance well described

EPIDEMIOLOGY

- Highest prevalence in adolescents and young adults 15 to 24 years of age
- Prevalence of gonorrhea in a community is sustained via continued transmission by asymptomatically infected individuals and by "core group" transmitters
- Transmission is primarily sexual (oral, rectal, genital contact) or perinatal during delivery
- Infection often is localized to the site of inoculation but can disseminate

DIAGNOSIS

- Majority of diagnoses are made by nucleic acid amplification testing (NAAT) of urine, or urethral, vaginal, cervical, rectal, or pharyngeal swab
- Maintaining culture capability to isolate *N. gonorrhoeae* remains critical as the only method to monitor development of resistance to current antimicrobial treatment regimens

TREATMENT

- Ceftriaxone is drug of choice for most infections
- Variable susceptibility to other cephalosporins (heterogeneous mechanisms of resistance)
- Co-treatment for *Chlamydia* is advised because of high incidence (~45%) of coinfection
- Sex partners within 60 days of onset of patient's symptoms should be examined and *treated presumptively*

---

127 Other *Neisseria* Species

Katherine K. Hsu and Jay M. Lieberman

Neisseria meningitidis and *N. gonorrhoeae* are the two pathogenic *Neisseria* species. Other *Neisseria* species are common inhabitants of the upper respiratory tract and oral cavity of humans. Often considered nonpathogenic, these species rarely can cause clinical disease.[1–3]

MICROBIOLOGY AND LABORATORY DIAGNOSIS

Neisseria species are gram-negative, oxidase-positive bacteria. All are catalase-positive, except *N. bacilliformis* and *N. elongata*. All are diplococci, except *N. bacilliformis*, *N. elongata*, and *N. weaveri*.

TABLE 127-1. Selected Characteristics of *Neisseria* Species

Species	Pigment	Polysaccharide Synthesis	Acid Produced From				Reduction of NO₃
			Glucose	Maltose	Sucrose	Lactose	
Neisseria gonorrhoeae	−	−	+	−	−	−	−
Neisseria meningitidis	−	−	+	+	−	−	−
Neisseria bacilliformis	+	−	−	−	−	−	±
Neisseria cinerea	−	−	−	−	−	−	−
Neisseria elongata	+	−	±	−	−	−	−
Neisseria flavescens	+	+	−	−	−	−	−
Neisseria lactamica	−	−	+	+	−	+	−
Neisseria mucosa	+	+	+	+	+	−	+
Neisseria polysaccharea	−	+	+	+	−	−	−
Neisseria sicca	±	+	+	+	+	−	−
Neisseria subflava	+	±	+	+	±	−	−
Neisseria weaveri	±	−	−	−	−	−	−

+, strains are typically positive, but mutations lacking the specific enzyme activity are occasionally found; −, most strains are negative; ±, strains are variable.

Whereas meningococci and gonococci require additional carbon dioxide for optimal growth and grow only at temperatures of 30°C to 37°C, the other species are less fastidious; they do not require extra carbon dioxide and can grow at 22°C to 25°C. Unlike *N. meningitidis* and *N. gonorrhoeae*, the other *Neisseria* species (except *N. lactamica*) generally do not grow on selective media such as Thayer–Martin agar. The commensal species can be distinguished from *N. meningitidis* and *N. gonorrhoeae* by biochemical and serologic tests. Carbohydrate utilization reactions, production of polysaccharide from sucrose, and reduction of nitrate are commonly used for identification (Table 127-1).[2–5] Difficulties in accurate identification of certain species resulted in some confusion and incorrect identifications in earlier literature.[2]

EPIDEMIOLOGY

Neisseria species commonly colonize the upper respiratory tract and occasionally the genital tract. In a study evaluating carriage rates of two *Neisseria* species in healthy infants and children, the prevalence of *N. lactamica* carriage was 3.8% at 3 months of age, peaked at 21% at 18 months of age, and declined to 1.8% by early adolescence.[6] In contrast, the rate of *N. meningitidis* carriage was 0.7% in the first 4 years of life and increased to 5.4% by early adolescence. Similarly, among 1400 healthy children 0 to 10 years of age in Turkey, 17.7% were colonized with *N. lactamica*, whereas only 1.2% were colonized with *N. meningitidis*.[7]

Carriage of nonpathogenic strains may be important, because *N. meningitidis* and *N. lactamica* share cross-reactive carbohydrate antigens; carriage of *N. lactamica* is likely associated with the development of "natural" immunity against *N. meningitidis*.[8] Cross-reacting antibodies to *N. meningitidis* were found in 66% of children who had asymptomatic colonization with *N. lactamica*, compared with 5% of children who were not colonized.[6] *N. lactamica*-based vaccines are being evaluated as a potential strategy to prevent meningococcal disease.[9–11]

Most adults are colonized, either densely or sparsely, by two or three *Neisseria* strains. For example, oropharyngeal cultures from individuals cared for in a clinic for sexually transmitted infections revealed *N. perflava* in >95%; *N. cinerea*, *N. mucosa*, and *N. flava* in 25%; and *N. lactamica* in 1%.[12]

CLINICAL MANIFESTATIONS

Information on clinical disease caused by commensal *Neisseria* species is accrued primarily through case reports. Characteristics of various species and some infections caused by the organisms are briefly described here. Antibiotic susceptibility testing should be performed on all clinically relevant isolates, because some organisms are penicillin resistant due to β-lactamase production or altered penicillin-binding proteins.

Neisseria bacilliformis. Strains of *N. bacilliformis* grow as light grey colonies that resemble *N. elongata* on sheep blood agar or chocolate agar at 35°C with 5% carbon dioxide. *N. elongata* and *N. bacilliformis* are the only bacillary *Neisseria* species isolated from humans. Biochemically *N. bacilliformis* is negative for indole production and reactions in catalase, nitrate reduction, and tributilin tests vary by strain. Sequencing of the 16S rRNA gene is the most reliable way to identify *N. bacilliformis*.[5]

N. bacilliformis predominantly causes infections of the oral cavity and respiratory tract in immunocompromised individuals, but one case of bicuspid aortic valve endocarditis was reported in a previously healthy adult male.[13]

Neisseria cinerea. *N. cinerea* grows as translucent colonies that closely resemble *N. gonorrhoeae* on isolation media. Misidentification as *N. gonorrhoeae* also can occur when these strains are grown on gonococcus-selective media (e.g., Martin–Lewis medium)[14] or when the Bactec radiometric system is used for detection of glucose utilization.[15] However, susceptibility to colistin and ability to grow in trypticase soy broth or Mueller–Hinton agar are characteristics of *N. cinerea* and not *N. gonorrhoeae*.

N. cinerea has been isolated from the oropharynx and nasopharynx and, rarely, from the genital tract. The spectrum of disease attributed to this species includes hospital-associated pneumonia in a patient with human immunodeficiency virus infection,[16] pulmonary cavitation in a renal transplant patient,[17] chronic cervical lymphadenitis in a child with dysgammaglobulinemia,[18] bacterial peritonitis associated with chronic ambulatory peritoneal dialysis,[19] bloodstream infection (BSI),[20] endocarditis,[21] proctitis,[22] orbital cellulitis, and conjunctivitis.[23] In some cases, the isolate was initially misidentified as *N. gonorrhoeae*.

Neisseria elongata. *N. elongata* are rod-shaped and elongate into filaments when exposed to sublethal concentrations of penicillin. Despite its shape, *N. elongata* is considered to be a member of the genus *Neisseria* because of similarities in genetic makeup, glycolytic enzymes, and lipid and carbohydrate composition. There are multiple reports of *N. elongata*, particularly subsp. *nitroreducens* (formerly known as Centers for Disease Control and Prevention (CDC) group M-6), as a cause of endocarditis.[24–29] One case of endocarditis was associated with septic embolization and brain abscess formation.[30] Many of these infections followed dental procedures and occurred in people with pre-existing heart disease; the infection frequently caused valvular damage that required surgical intervention. Other infections associated with *N. elongata* include bloodstream infection and osteomyelitis.[25]

Neisseria flavescens. *N. flavescens*, a yellow-green-pigmented strain, does not utilize carbohydrates. This species has been recovered in cases of meningitis[31] and endocarditis.[32]

Neisseria lactamica. *N. lactamica* resembles *N. meningitidis* in colony morphology, in growth on selective media containing vancomycin, colistin, and trimethoprim, and in production of acid from glucose and maltose. However, *N. lactamica* is differentiated by its ability to produce β-galactosidase, which can cleave lactose to glucose; this causes a color change when *o*-nitrophenyl-β-D-galactopyranoside medium is used.

N. lactamica colonizes the nasopharynx, especially of infants and children,[6,7] and rarely the genital tract.[33] *N. lactamica* has been isolated from several infants and children with meningitis[34,35] and from adults, including one who developed meningitis secondary to traumatic fracture of the cribriform plate with cerebrospinal fluid leak,[36] an organ transplant recipient with cavitary lung disease,[37] a patient with liver cirrhosis who developed bacteremic pneumonia,[38] and a patient with myeloma receiving corticosteroids who developed arthritis and septicemia.[39]

Neisseria mucosa. On blood and chocolate agar, *N. mucosa* forms large, colorless, moist, mucoid colonies but can be differentiated from other species by its ability to reduce nitrate to nitrite and gaseous nitrogen. Clinical manifestations attributed to this encapsulated organism include post-pneumonectomy empyema,[40] endocarditis,[41–43] purulent pericarditis,[44] meningitis,[45] peritonitis,[46] and neonatal conjunctivitis.[47] In patients with chronic granulomatous disease, *N. mucosa* has caused pneumonia (a pulmonary coin lesion[48]) and visceral botryomycosis.[49]

Neisseria polysaccharea. *Neisseria polysaccharea*, a nonencapsulated *Neisseria* species, is so named because of its ability to produce polysaccharide from sucrose, and acid from glucose and maltose. Although the biochemical reactions of *N. polysaccharea* strains are similar to those of *N. lactamica* and *N. meningitidis*, it can be distinguished by its unique production of polysaccharide. Some *N. polysaccharea* strains can also grow on colistin-containing selective media (i.e., Thayer–Martin).[50] The organism has not been implicated in disease.

Neisseria sicca. *N. sicca*, a variably pigmented species, grows on agar in dry, wrinkled colonies but rarely grows on gonococcus-specific media because it is susceptible to colistin. *N. sicca* colonizes the upper respiratory tract and may be responsible for inflammation of the oral mucous membranes.[51] Ascribed infections include meningitis,[52] meningitis as a complication of ventriculostomy placement for subarachnoid hemorrhage,[53] cerebrospinal fluid shunt infection,[54] endocarditis,[55–57]

pneumonia,[58] peritonitis,[59] liver abscess after repeated transcatheter arterial embolization,[60] and vertebral osteomyelitis.[61]

Neisseria subflava. *N. subflava*, a yellow-pigmented species, is a common inhabitant of the respiratory and genitourinary tracts; the former species *N. subflava*, *N. flava*, and *N. perflava* have been reclassified as one species, *N. subflava*.[2] This organism is reported as a rare but serious cause of BSI,[62,63] meningitis,[64,65] endocarditis,[66,67] epidural abscess–diskitis–vertebral osteomyelitis,[68] and endophthalmitis.[69] In children, *N. subflava* can cause fulminant infection associated with a petechial or purpuric rash, resulting in death in about a third of cases. Thus, infection with *N. subflava* can be clinically indistinguishable from that due to *N. meningitidis*, and because the strains have similar fermentative patterns, they can be confused without additional testing.[62]

Neisseria weaveri. *Neisseria weaveri* (formerly known as CDC group M-5) is a common inhabitant of the oropharyngeal flora of dogs. Like *N. elongata*, it is rod-shaped and sometimes occurs in pairs or short chains. It can be an important pathogen associated with dog bite wound infections of humans[70] and has caused BSI.[71]

SPECIAL CONSIDERATIONS AND PREVENTION

Disease caused by the commensal species of *Neisseria* occurs infrequently, and there are no reports of secondary cases in contacts. Accordingly, there are no recommendations to administer antibiotic prophylaxis to close contacts. Misidentification of these species as *N. meningitidis*, however, can result in the unnecessary administration of antibiotic prophylaxis and unwarranted concern in the community regarding potential spread of meningococcal infection. Their misidentification as *N. gonorrhoeae* can have important social and medicolegal ramifications, particularly in children.

Several studies have examined the potential role of commensal *Neisseria* as a reservoir for transferring β-lactam antibiotic resistance to pathogenic *Neisseria* strains.[72,73] A 25.2-Md conjugative plasmid, similar to that isolated from *N. gonorrhoeae*, has been found in some tetracycline-resistant isolates of *N. meningitidis*. By contrast, some tetracycline-resistant strains of *N. subflava* and *N. mucosa* appear to carry the *TetM* determinant in the chromosome.[74] The role of commensal *Neisseria* in the emergence of antibiotic-resistant pathogenic strains requires further study. Surveillance for changes in resistance patterns is important.

128 *Arcanobacterium haemolyticum*

Denise F. Bratcher

Arcanobacterium haemolyticum was first identified as *Corynebacterium haemolyticum* in 1946 in pharyngeal cultures of World War II soldiers and Pacific Islanders with pharyngitis that was indistinguishable clinically from infection caused by group A streptococcus.

EPIDEMIOLOGY

Humans are the primary reservoir of *A. haemolyticum* where the organism is found in the pharynx and on the skin. Although many studies reporting an association of *A. haemolyticum* with pharyngitis fail to exclude viral pathogens and *Mycoplasma pneumoniae*, *A. haemolyticum* has been implicated increasingly in association with pharyngitis (reported incidence of 0.3% to 9.3%) and rash in older children and young adults, with an increased incidence reported among adolescents aged 15 to 18.[1] Multiple single case

reports document infection at pulmonary and extrapulmonary sites.[2–4] A slight predominance in females is noted among reported pharyngitis series, but a male predilection is noted in systemic *A. haemolyticum* infections.[5] Transmission occurs from person to person purportedly by droplet transfer;[6] the incubation period is uncertain.

MICROBIOLOGY

A. haemolyticum is a gram-positive or gram-variable, pleomorphic, nonmotile, nonsporulating bacillus. It appears strongly gram-positive in young cultures, becoming gram-variable after 24 hours. Optimum growth occurs on human or rabbit blood agar and is enhanced in carbon dioxide; after 48 hours of incubation, colonies on horse or sheep blood agar (the preferred medium for throat cultures) are small (0.1 to 0.5 mm), with a narrow zone

(1 mm) of hemolysis. A black, opaque dot appears at the center of each colony and a tiny dark pit is noted if the colony is scraped aside. Smooth and rough colonies, associated respectively with wound and respiratory isolates, have been noted.[7] *A. haemolyticum* resembles *Corynebacterium diphtheriae* on Loeffler medium, whereas growth of *A. haemolyticum* on tellurite medium is poor. A mupirocin-containing selective medium for *A. haemolyticum* isolation has been developed.[8] The organism is catalase-negative and ferments glucose and maltose, usually within 4 days. Production of a dermonecrotic toxin has been demonstrated. Kits are available to identify *A. haemolyticum*.[9]

Many cases of *A. haemolyticum* pharyngitis may go undetected because of the slow growth of the organism in culture (requiring at least 72 hours of incubation) and if streptococcal antigen testing is performed without a backup throat culture.

CLINICAL MANIFESTATIONS

A. haemolyticum is reported most frequently in association with pharyngitis in individuals 10 to 30 years old. Most patients complain of mild fever and sore throat. Some have persistent or recurrent pharyngeal symptoms for weeks before diagnosis. Pharyngeal erythema is present universally, and tonsillar exudate is common, occurring in up to 70% of cases. Membranous pharyngitis mimics diphtheria[10] and peritonsillar abscess. Lymphadenopathy occurs in 26% to 81% of reported patients, primarily involving the anterior cervical or submandibular lymph nodes bilaterally.

An associated rash was noted in 23% to 75% of cases reported, most frequently involving the extensor surfaces of the extremities, the neck, and trunk; face, palms, and soles typically are spared, although a single case report of vesicular lesions of the palms and soles exists.[6] The exanthem, commonly described as a scarlatiniform rash (erythematous, blanching fine papules), usually develops 1 to 4 days after the onset of sore throat, although rash has been noted before the development of pharyngitis.[10] Mild desquamation of the skin on the hands and feet follows. The rash appears to occur only in association with pharyngeal infection. Pruritus occurs in approximately 50% of patients, and urticaria and erythema multiforme have been described.[10]

In both normal and immunocompromised hosts, *A. haemolyticum* is the cause of sporadic invasive infections, including septicemia, endocarditis, meningitis, brain abscess, pneumonia, pleural effusion, sinusitis, urinary tract infections, pelvic abscess, spontaneous bacterial peritonitis, and bone and joint infections.[2-4,11-24] Cellulitis, cutaneous abscesses, skin ulcers, wound infections, a paravertebral abscess, and paronychia also have been reported.[4,19-22,25-30]

Similar to the most common clinical manifestation of pharyngitis, most invasive *A. haemolyticum* infections that are reported among children occur in adolescents. These include septicemia, brain abscess, pneumonia, empyema, peritonsillar abscess, sinusitis associated with orbital cellulitis, and membranous pharyngitis.[3,11,14,16,19,20,31-34] Septicemia has been reported rarely in adolescents with Epstein–Barr virus infections.[11,35] Coinfection of

A. haemolyticum with *Fusobacterium necrophorum, Streptococcus agalactiae, Streptococcus milleri, Staphylococcus aureus, Bacteroides* species, *Veillonella* species, *Mycobacterium tuberculosis*, and *Mycoplasma pneumoniae* has been reported.[9,14,18,20,27,35–37]

DIAGNOSIS

Diagnosis is made when *A. haemolyticum* is isolated from clinical specimens. Pharyngeal isolates of *A. haemolyticum* can be confused with streptococci or *C. diphtheriae* or may be disregarded because colonies are confused with normal oral flora. Group A streptococcus and other streptococci have been isolated concomitantly with *A. haemolyticum* from pharyngeal specimens. If *A. haemolyticum* infection is suspected, particularly in an adolescent or young adult with pharyngitis and exanthem, consideration should be given to inoculating agar containing human or rabbit blood, or to holding cultures on sheep blood agar for at least 72 hours, in an effort to identify the small α-hemolytic colonies of *A. haemolyticum*. Mild leukocytosis with neutrophilia is common. Biopsy of skin lesions shows only mild lymphohistiocytic perivascular infiltrate.

TREATMENT

No prospective, randomized clinical trial has established the benefit of antimicrobial treatment of *A. haemolyticum* pharyngitis or compared the efficacy of therapeutic agents. In case reports, *A. haemolyticum* isolates are susceptible in vitro to penicillin, erythromycin, cefotaxime, cephalothin, chloramphenicol, clindamycin, and tetracycline.[38,39] Bacteriologic failure has been reported after penicillin treatment of pharyngitis, although the significance of persistent colonization is uncertain. *A. haemolyticum* can invade respiratory epithelial cells, potentially creating an intracellular reservoir; in the laboratory, erythromycin kills intracellular bacteria more efficiently than penicillin.[40] Empiric therapy for pharyngitis with erythromycin or other macrolides is effective against *A. haemolyticum*.[41]

Anecdotal experiences with extrapharyngeal infections due to *A. haemolyticum* report resolution with intravenous therapy with penicillin G. Penicillin tolerance of *A. haemolyticum* among pharyngeal isolates has been demonstrated in vitro,[38] and clinically significant tolerance to ampicillin and penicillin has been described in an *A. haemolyticum* strain that causes endocarditis.[13] Minimum inhibitory concentrations by E-test of 10 invasive *A. haemolyticum* strains determined all isolates to be susceptible to penicillin, cephalosporins, macrolides, clindamycin, ciprofloxacin, and vancomycin but resistant to trimethoprim-sulfamethoxazole.[42] One case report notes resistance to ciprofloxacin in an *A. haemolyticum* isolate from a brain abscess.[17] Suggested treatment options for pharyngitis include high-dose penicillin plus an aminoglycoside,[13] broad-spectrum β-lactam antibiotics, clindamycin, and macrolides.[12] Antimicrobial treatment of extrapharyngeal infections caused by *A. haemolyticum* is based on the susceptibility pattern of a specific isolate and testing for penicillin tolerance.

129 *Bacillus* Species (Anthrax)

Denise F. Bratcher

Bacillus species, ubiquitous in the environment, are found in soil, water, dust, and air. With the exception of *B. anthracis*, which causes anthrax, the *Bacillus* spp. previously have been considered nonpathogenic when isolated from clinical specimens. However, non-anthrax species are increasingly recognized as pathogens in

immunosuppressed individuals and patients with indwelling devices. Isolates are more likely to be significant if the organism is present on direct smear of the original specimen or is isolated repeatedly from blood cultures.[1] In addition, *B. anthracis* has long been recognized as a potential biologic weapon.[2] In the fall of

2001, the deliberate release of *B. anthracis* through the United States Postal System provided experience in the clinical presentation, diagnosis, prophylaxis, and treatment of anthrax disease following a bioterrorism-related outbreak.

Immediate notification of the local hospital epidemiologist, the local or state health department, and local or state health laboratories should occur at the first suspicion of an anthrax illness. When bioterrorism alleging the use of anthrax or other agents occurs, the local emergency response system should be activated or local law enforcement agents should be notified.[3]

Bacillus spp. are aerobic or facultatively anaerobic, gram-positive or gram-variable, encapsulated, spore-forming rods that usually are motile. *Bacillus* spp. produce a number of toxins, including enterotoxin, emetic toxin, phospholipases, proteases, and hemolysins.[4] The species are differentiated by a variety of laboratory observations involving colony morphology, growth on selective media, agglutination reactions, and penicillin susceptibility. *B. anthracis* grows well on blood agar as large, opaque, irregular "curled-hair" colonies.[5]

BACILLUS ANTHRACIS

B. anthracis, a large, gram-positive, encapsulated, spore-forming, nonmotile rod, is the cause of anthrax. Anthrax, a disease of herbivores who acquire *B. anthracis* while grazing in areas where soil is contaminated by spores, is a zoonotic disease of worldwide occurrence. Disease tends to occur in animals in summer and fall;[6] insects can serve as vectors.[7] Humans typically become infected as they contact infected domestic or wild animals or their products.[6] *B. anthracis* spores can survive for prolonged periods, permitting relapsing infection. Human infections have resulted from contact with contaminated products, such as hides, wool, bone meal, and imported dolls, drums, and toys.[8,9] Discharge from cutaneous lesions potentially is infectious, and possibility of person-to-person transmission is possible. The incubation period is 1 to 7 days but can be up to 60 days depending on host factors, exposure dose, and chemoprophylaxis. Naturally occurring human disease is rarely reported in the U.S.[10] Before the bioterrorism-related anthrax outbreak of 2001, only 18 cases of inhalational anthrax had been reported in the U.S. in the 20th century.[10] A series of recently reported US cases have involved exposure to imported animal hides associated with drumming or drum making.[9,11,12]

Three forms of human disease occur:

1. *Cutaneous anthrax*[13] accounts for most anthrax seen in the U.S. and worldwide; infection follows inoculation of existing skin lesions with *B. anthracis* spores. A painless lesion develops as a pruritic papule (malignant papule) that evolves to a vesicular lesion and eventually forms an eschar (Figure 129-1). Striking local edema occurs as a result of release of extracellular toxin, and regional lymphadenopathy and lymphangitis also are noted. Although antibiotic treatment does not alter progression of an anthrax lesion itself, mortality approaches 20% in untreated cases.

2. *Inhalational anthrax* (woolsorters' disease) results from inhalation of aerosolized spores. A biphasic disease, when it occurs naturally, begins with mild upper respiratory tract symptoms that progress to dyspnea, cyanosis, tachycardia, fever, hypoxemia, shock, and usually death. Bacteremia and hemorrhagic meningitis are common.[14] A chest radiograph typically shows a widened mediastinum consistent with massive lymphadenopathy. This finding in a previously healthy patient with evidence of overwhelming flulike illness essentially is pathognomonic of advanced inhalation anthrax; pleural effusions also are common. Mortality is reported to approach 90%;[2] the case-fatality rate among individuals who received intensive care in the 2001 attacks was 45%.[15] The first case of naturally acquired inhalation anthrax in the U.S. since 1976 was reported in 2006 in an adult male who made African drums from imported animal hides.[11]

3. *Gastrointestinal disease,* is a result of ingestion of contaminated, undercooked meat, with deposition of spores in the lower gastrointestinal tract. Disease manifests as abdominal pain and distention, with vomiting and diarrhea, followed by ascites, hemorrhagic lymphadenitis, and septicemia. An anthrax case involving the gastrointestinal form of disease was reported following animal-hide drum exposure.[9] *Pharyngeal anthrax* can follow upper gastrointestinal mucous membrane infection acquired from consumption of contaminated meat and manifests as lesions at the base of the tongue or tonsils, profound swelling of the neck, lymphadenopathy, and systemic symptoms.[16]

All forms of anthrax can progress to septicemia and meningitis.[1] Multiple cases of anthrax have been reported in children, including meningitis, hemorrhagic meningoencephalitis, periorbital cellulitis, neonatal septicemia and meningitis, and intestinal and cutaneous anthrax.[6,12,17–23] During the 2001 Postal Service anthrax outbreak, a 7-month-old infant developed cutaneous anthrax with microangiopathic hemolytic anemia; anthrax spores were identified at his mother's workplace, a national television news office.[24]

B. anthracis can be isolated from ordinary nutrient broth and on blood agar.[5] Gram stain and culture of vesicular fluid confirm the diagnosis of cutaneous anthrax. Peripheral blood smears can show visible bacilli on Gram stain, and blood culture shows growth of the bacillus within 24 hours in inhalational and gastrointestinal anthrax. Laboratory diagnosis of anthrax is suspected when characteristic large, gram-positive, sporulating bacilli are seen on Gram stain of an isolate. A direct fluorescent antibody test is available for analysis of a smear of vesicular fluid. Enzyme immunoassay, immunohistochemistry, and polymerase chain reaction tests are available at national reference laboratories. The microbiology laboratory should be alerted if anthrax is suspected.

Successful management depends on a high index of suspicion and early effective antibiotic administration. Although no controlled clinical studies of the treatment of human anthrax exist, high-dose intravenous penicillin therapy historically has been the drug

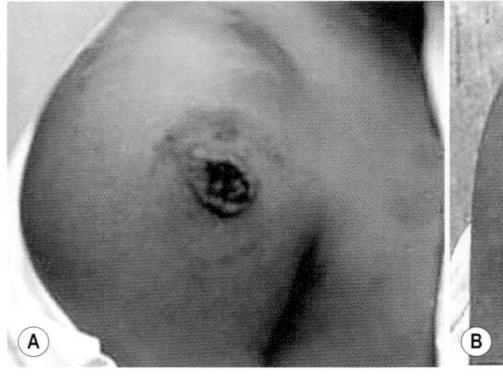
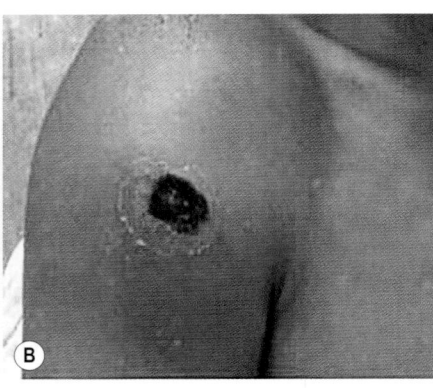

Figure 129-1. Sequential lesion of cutaneous anthrax, progressing from a painless ulcerative vesicle with surrounding erythema **(A)** to black eschar with persisting erythema **(B).** (From Centers for Disease Control and Prevention: http://www.bt.cdc.gov/agent/anthrax/anthrax-images/cutaneous.asp. Accessed January 10, 2011.)

of choice for all forms of anthrax. Based on more recent data indicating the presence of constitutive and inducible β-lactamases in *B. anthracis* isolates, the use of a penicillin alone for treatment of systemic *B. anthracis* infection is not recommended.[25] *B. anthracis* also produces a cephalosporinase, inhibiting the use of cephalosporins in treatment.[26] Because of concerns regarding genetically engineered *B. anthracis*, the Working Group on Civilian Biodefense recommends that antibiotic resistance to penicillin and tetracycline antibiotics be assumed after a terrorist attack until laboratory testing demonstrates otherwise.[2] Due to the high mortality associated with inhalational anthrax, initial intravenous therapy with two or more antimicrobial agents, including either ciprofloxacin (approved by Food and Drug Administration) or doxycycline, is recommended for infants, children, or adults.

Other agents with in vitro activity against *B. anthracis* that are suggested for use in conjunction with ciprofloxacin or doxycycline include rifampin, vancomycin, imipenem, chloramphenicol, penicillin, ampicillin, clindamycin, or clarithromycin. If meningitis is suspected, ciprofloxacin is preferred, owing to doxycycline's poor central nervous system penetration. Anthrax immunoglobulin has been utilized in recent inhalational and gastrointestinal anthrax cases.[27,28] A human monoclonal antibody, raxibacumab, directed against a component of the anthrax toxin has shown improved survival in animal studies of inhalational anthrax.[29]

For cutaneous anthrax, oral ciprofloxacin or doxycycline is considered first-line therapy. If signs of systemic involvement, extensive edema, or head and neck lesions are noted, a multidrug intravenous therapy regimen, as for inhalational disease, is recommended. When disease is thought to result from aerosol exposure, antimicrobial therapy is continued for 60 days due to the potential persistence of spores in the respiratory tract. Oral antimicrobial agents can be used for completion of therapy. Corticosteroid therapy has been suggested for extensive edema, respiratory compromise, and meningitis associated with inhalational anthrax, and for extensive edema of the head and neck region associated with cutaneous anthrax.[25]

Initial antimicrobial treatment recommendations for children with inhalational or cutaneous anthrax are essentially the same as for adults, i.e., intravenous ciprofloxacin (10 mg/kg per dose every 12 hours, maximum 400 mg dose) or doxycycline (2.2 mg/kg every 12 hours, maximum 100 mg/dose) plus one or two additional agents. When *B. anthracis* is known to be penicillin-susceptible, amoxicillin (80 mg/kg per day orally divided every 8 hours, maximum 500 mg/dose) is an option for completion of lengthy treatment courses in children to avoid potential adverse effects of prolonged use of doxycycline (oral dose same as intravenous) or ciprofloxacin (oral dose 15 mg/kg per dose every 12 hours, maximum 500 mg dose).[30]

Following a confirmed or suspected aerosol exposure, postexposure prophylaxis is indicated to prevent inhalational anthrax.[31] Initial therapy with ciprofloxacin or doxycycline is recommended for adults and children until antimicrobial susceptibilities of the implicated *B. anthracis* isolate are known. If penicillin susceptibility is confirmed, oral amoxicillin is appropriate prophylactic therapy for children (80 mg/kg per day divided every 8 hours; maximum dose, 500 mg every 8 hours).[30,32] Oral amoxicillin (when susceptible) also is an option for antimicrobial prophylaxis in breastfeeding mothers. Ciprofloxacin and doxycycline are considered to be compatible with breastfeeding, but little is known about the safety of long-term use. The most current information related to the treatment of anthrax is available through the Centers for Disease Control and Prevention website at www.cdc.gov.

As a result of the intentional delivery of *B. anthracis* spores through the mail, 22 cases of bioterrorism-related anthrax were identified in October and November 2001 in the U.S. Eleven cases were confirmed as inhalational anthrax, and 11 cases were cutaneous.[33] All but two of the inhalational anthrax cases had likely direct exposure to a *B. anthracis*-containing envelope. Five patients exhibited fulminant signs of inhalational illness at presentation and subsequently died. Patients who were ill but came to medical attention and received antibiotics with activity against *B. anthracis* in the initial phase of illness all survived (~55% overall survival).

Fever, chills, fatigue, malaise, and lethargy with minimal or nonproductive cough and nausea or vomiting were common symptoms in inhalational anthrax. A biphasic illness was not noted, but profuse, drenching sweating was a prominent feature. No initial chest radiograph was normal, and pleural effusions were common. All patients received combination antimicrobial therapy with activity against *B. anthracis*, which, in combination with better supportive care and potentially other factors, likely contributed to improvement in survival compared with previous reports.[26]

Prevention of naturally occurring human disease depends on control of animal disease and industrial contamination. Precautions to prevent transmission from draining wounds and secretions are advised for medical personnel during the first 72 hours of treatment[34] of patients with cutaneous or inhalational anthrax.

Animal and human vaccines are available.[35] The human anthrax vaccine available in the U.S. is made from the cell-free filtrate of a nonencapsulated, attenuated strain of *B. anthracis* (Emergent BioSolutions, Lansing, MI).[10] Anthrax vaccine is indicated for workers who contact imported animal hides, hair, or textiles in the workplace and for those involved with diagnostic or investigational work; vaccine is not licensed for use in children. The current pre-exposure vaccine series consists of two intramuscular (IM) injections administered 4 weeks apart, followed by three subsequent injections at 6, 12, and 18 months, plus annual booster doses; administration in the deltoid muscle is recommended.[15] Local reactions, including edema, erythema, warmth, tenderness, and pruritus, are substantially reduced by IM versus subcutaneous injections. Systemic reactions are rare.

Due to the threat of anthrax as a potential biologic weapon, U.S. military personnel with a calculated risk for anthrax exposure are given pre-exposure anthrax vaccination.[36] After a biologic attack, postexposure vaccination (three-dose subcutaneous injection series) with antibiotic prophylaxis is recommended and may also be recommended for children.[2] Antibiotic postexposure prophylaxis depends on antibiotic susceptibility of the *B. anthracis* strain of the index case and should be continued for 30 days (previously vaccinated) to 60 days (not vaccinated previously).[2,6] Recommendations for the use of anthrax vaccine in the U.S. are limited.[10] Newer vaccine technologies offer the potential for improved anthrax vaccines, and alternate treatment and prophylactic modalities are under investigation.

BACILLUS CEREUS

Bacillus cereus is a significant cause of toxin-induced food poisoning characterized by emesis and diarrhea.[37] Although a variety of foods have been implicated, including infant cereal, contaminated fried rice most frequently is associated with the emetic form of disease, which is caused by heat-resistant, preformed toxin, cereulide, or *B. cereus* spores that germinate when boiled rice is left unrefrigerated.[38,39] Nausea, vomiting, and diarrhea with abdominal cramping can occur within 1 to 6 hours of ingestion of contaminated food. The isolated diarrheal form, which is associated with profuse diarrhea produced by an enterotoxin similar to *Clostridium perfringens*, has a longer incubation period of 6 to 24 hours. *B. cereus* can be isolated from stools of asymptomatic individuals, but person-to-person transmission does not occur.[36] Confirmation of food poisoning requires the isolation of *B. cereus* from a stool or emesis in addition to the isolation of *B. cereus* (10^5 colony-forming units/g) in contaminated food. *B. cereus* food poisoning typically is brief and self-limited, requiring no antimicrobial therapy. A few fatal cases due to *B. cereus* emetic toxin have been reported, including fulminant hepatic failure and rhabdomyolysis in an adolescent following consumption of contaminated pasta;[40] hepatic failure and pulmonary hemorrhage in a 7-year old following consumption of contaminated pasta salad;[41] and acute encephalopathy in a 1-year-old 6 hours after eating reheated fried rice.[42] This patient and his 2-year old sibling had cereulide detected in serum at presentation; the sibling recovered after plasma exchange and hemodialysis. Another child developed fulminant hepatitis, shock, and prolonged seizures associated with *B. cereus* food poisoning.[43]

Multiple other human infections due to *B. cereus* have been reported.[4] *B. cereus* ranks as the second most common pathogen of posttraumatic ophthalmitis, after *Staphylococcus epidermidis*.[44,45] The organism typically is introduced by a projectile foreign body or open globe injury, producing a rapidly severe infection that frequently results in enucleation or poor visual outcome. A postsurgical endophthalmitis outbreak has been described, but *B. cereus* is an uncommon cause of postoperative endophthalmitis.[46] Management is aggressive, including surgical intervention and parenteral, intravitreal, and topical antimicrobial treatment.

B. cereus is a cause of clinically significant bloodstream infection and, occasionally, fulminant septicemia in neonates, intravenous drug abusers, and immunocompromised patients, including children with cancer and those with an indwelling catheter or prosthetic device.[4,47–57] Septicemia has followed transfusion of *B. cereus*-contaminated platelets and dietary tea consumption in children with cancer.[58,59] Endocarditis, typically involving a prosthetic valve or the tricuspid valve in intravenous drug abusers, also has been described.[60–63] Pneumonia was reported in immunosuppressed patients and neonates[4,62,64] and was associated with fulminant septicemia in two previously healthy welders.[65] *B. cereus* was isolated from ventilated pediatric patients in association with inadequate disinfection of reusable ventilator air-flow sensors.[66] Meningitis, hemorrhagic meningoencephalitis, and brain abscess caused by *B. cereus* have been reported, often affecting neonates, immunocompromised children, or children with ventriculoperitoneal shunts.[4,50,62,67–75] Lequin et al. describe serial ultrasonography and magnetic resonance imaging findings of hemorrhagic and early, cavitating, selective white matter destruction as typical of neonatal *B. cereus* meningoencephalitis.[76] Although isolation from wounds is difficult to interpret, *B. cereus* has caused local infection after burns, trauma, or surgery.[77,78] Primary cutaneous infections in neutropenic children[79] and necrotizing cellulitis due to *B. cereus* have been reported.[80] Osteomyelitis, usually associated with accidental or surgical trauma or intravenous drug abuse, is described.[81]

B. cereus also has been associated with urinary tract infection in a patient with invasive bladder cancer and with peritonitis in patients undergoing peritoneal dialysis.[82–84]

B. cereus is resistant uniformly to β-lactam antibiotics. Antibiotic therapy is indicated in invasive *B. cereus* infections; vancomycin or clindamycin in combination with an aminoglycoside is recommended most commonly. Removal of the prosthetic device usually is necessary for cure, and was associated with significantly lower recurrence rate in one study.[49,84,85] Surgical intervention typically is required in ophthalmic and soft-tissue infections. Endophthalmitis typically is treated with intravitreal vancomycin, vitrectomy, and topical and systemic fluoroquinolone therapy.

BACILLUS SUBTILIS AND OTHER BACILLUS SPECIES

Other *Bacillus* spp. implicated in human infections include *B. alvei*, *B. brevis*, *B. circulans*, *B. coagulans*, *B. infantis*, *B. idriensis*, *B. laterosporus*, *B. licheniformis*, *B. macerans*, *B. pumilus*, *B. sphaericus*, *B. subtilis*, and *B. thuringiensis*.[4,45,49,54,62,86–93] Non-anthrax *Bacillus* species have been associated with bloodstream infection (including catheter-related), brain abscess, meningitis, pneumonia, pleuritis, endocarditis, pericarditis, urinary tract infection, peritonitis, periorbital cellulitis, and ocular infections. *B. thuringiensis* has been associated with foodborne gastrointestinal illnesses.[37] Case reports of infections due to *Bacillus* species are sometimes difficult to interpret, because the species frequently is identified incorrectly or may represent a contaminant of the culture.

B. subtilis specifically is described in association with BSI, cholangitis, meningitis, chronic osteomyelitis, panophthalmitis, pneumonia, and ventriculoperitoneal shunt infections.[4,62,94] Unlike *B. cereus*, *B. subtilis* is susceptible to penicillins in addition to vancomycin, clindamycin, aminoglycosides, and third-generation cephalosporin agents.

130 *Corynebacterium diphtheriae*

Irini Daskalaki

Diphtheria is a toxicosis caused by infection with *Corynebacterium diphtheriae*. Genus and species are derived from Greek roots: *korynee* ("club") after the microscopic appearance of the organisms and *diphtheria* ("leather hide") for the pseudomembrane that is the hallmark of respiratory tract infection. Once a major cause of childhood death, diphtheria was among the first infectious diseases to be controlled employing modern principles of microbiology, immunology, and public health. Increased immunization rates, rare circulation of toxigenic strains, and improved living conditions have controlled diphtheria in developed countries. The rare importation of diphtheria into the United States from developing countries and recent outbreaks in developed countries have underscored the continuing need for diphtheria immunization.

ETIOLOGY

Corynebacterium species are aerobic, nonencapsulated, nonspore-forming, mostly nonmotile, pleomorphic gram-positive bacilli. Isolation is enhanced by the use of selective media such as cystine-tellurite blood agar that inhibits the growth of competing organisms and, when reduced by *C. diphtheriae*, colonies are grey to black. Modified Tinsdale medium and Löffler or Pai slants are

additional effective enrichment media. Growth occurs within 48 hours; Gram stain of typical colonies from Löffler or Pai media can confirm a presumptive identification. Three phenotypes (*mitis*, *gravis*, and *intermedius*), each capable of causing diphtheria, are distinguished by colonial morphology, hemolysis, and fermentation reactions. A lysogenic bacteriophage encoding for production of exotoxin confers no essential protein to the bacterium, but factors other than toxin production also can provide virulence and facilitate the spread of infection.[1]

Production of diphtheria toxin can be demonstrated in vitro by use of an agar well or antitoxin membrane immunoprecipitin technique (Elek test) or by in vivo toxin neutralization tests in the guinea pig.[2,3] Investigational polymerase chain reaction (PCR) tests detect the presence of genes for both A and B toxin subunits but do not prove toxin production directly.[4] Toxigenic strains are indistinguishable by colony type, microscopy, or biochemical tests. Expression of toxin is enhanced in vitro by nutrient or iron depletion or exposure to ultraviolet light. Nontoxigenic *C. diphtheriae* can be converted to toxigenic strains by lysogenic infection. Studies of outbreaks in which molecular techniques were used suggest that indigenous nontoxigenic *C. diphtheriae* strains can be rendered toxigenic, producing clinical diphtheria after importation of single cases of toxigenic *C. diphtheriae*.[5] Non-diphtheria strains of *Corynebacterium* such as *C. ulcerans* can produce diphtheria toxin and cause a respiratory diphtheria-like illness.[6]

EPIDEMIOLOGY

Coryneform bacteria ("diphtheroids") are ubiquitous in nature, found on human skin and mucous membranes, as well as on plants, and in soil, fresh water, and salt water. Humans are the only known reservoir of *C. diphtheriae*. The primary modes of spread are by airborne respiratory droplets, direct contact with respiratory secretions, or exudate from skin lesions. Asymptomatic or convalescent respiratory carriers are important reservoirs for transmission. In endemic areas, 3% to 5% of healthy individuals harbor toxigenic organisms, but pharyngeal carriage of these strains is very uncommon if clinical diphtheria is rare. Skin infection, or carriage, can be the silent reservoir of toxigenic diphtheria. Viability in dust and on fomites for up to 6 months has unknown epidemiologic significance. Transmission via animals, contaminated milk, and an infected food handler has been proved or suspected.[7]

Diphtheria occurs worldwide and remains endemic in many developing countries. Incidence is higher in temperate climates, occurring predominantly in poor socioeconomic conditions, crowded areas, and in countries with inadequate rates of immunization. The risk of diphtheria can be increased during travel to endemic areas. The main risk factor for acquisition of toxigenic *C. diphtheriae* in a study from the United Kingdom was travel to the Indian subcontinent, Africa or Southeast Asia, or laboratory acquisition.[8] A complete list of diphtheria endemic areas is available from the U.S. Centers for Disease Control and Prevention (CDC).[9]

Before 1930, more than 125,000 cases and 10,000 deaths due to diphtheria were reported annually in the U.S. (incidence, 100 to 200 cases per 100,000). Highest fatality rates occurred in very young and in elderly persons. From 1921 to 1924, diphtheria was the leading cause of death among Canadian children aged 2 to 14 years. With widespread use of diphtheria toxoid vaccine in the U.S. after World War II, the incidence declined steadily. Since 1980, 5 or fewer cases of respiratory tract diphtheria have been reported yearly, with incidence rates of 0.001 per 100,000 population; no case has been reported from 2004 to 2007.[10] Since 1988, all U.S. cases have been imported. Although immunization does not prevent respiratory or cutaneous carriage or infection with toxigenic *C. diphtheriae*, neutralization of toxin diminishes local tissue spread, necrosis, multiplication, and transmission, thus providing herd immunity. It is estimated that 70% to 80% of a population must be immunized to prevent epidemic spread.[11]

Despite a low rate of circulating toxigenic *C. diphtheriae* in most industrialized countries, subgroups of individuals at risk have been identified if the organism were introduced due to underimmunization. In a multicenter European study, screening of upper respiratory specimen cultures revealed both toxigenic and nontoxigenic strains of *C. diphtheriae* representing carriage in highly vaccinated populations.[12] The National Immunization Survey in the U.S. has demonstrated that greater than 95% of children 19 to 35 months old have received at least three doses of diphtheria toxoid.[13] Immunization requirements for school entry have assured protection for most U.S. children. However, during the 1990s, 20% of 396 children younger than 5 years surveyed in Dade county, Florida, lacked protective serum immunity (antitoxin level >0.01 IU/mL).[14] In serosurveys in the U.S. and western European countries, where there is universal immunization in childhood, 25% to more than 60% of adults were found to lack protective antitoxin levels. The elderly had particularly low levels.[11,15–17]

Low levels of antitoxin in some populations may reflect relatively poor booster administration rates of diphtheria vaccines following primary immunization in childhood. The recent epidemiology of diphtheria demonstrates a shift from endemic disease in childhood to outbreaks in adults. In 27 sporadic cases of respiratory tract diphtheria in the U.S. in the 1980s, 70% occurred in persons older than 25 years.[16]

From 1990 to 1996, a massive outbreak of diphtheria occurred in the Newly Independent States of the former Soviet Union. Beginning in 1990 in the Russian Federation state, more than 150,000 cases occurred by the end of 1996 in 14 of 15 of the states.[18] Case-fatality rates ranged from 3% to 23% by state, and >60% of cases occurred among persons older than 14 years. Factors contributing to the epidemic included a large population of susceptible (i.e., underimmunized) adults, decreased childhood immunization, population migration, crowding, and a failure to respond aggressively during early phases of the epidemic. Attempts to control the epidemic with childhood immunization alone failed, whereas mass immunization of both children and adults was successful. Cases of diphtheria among travelers were transported to many countries in Europe. Molecular characterization of the Russian *C. diphtheriae* isolates by ribotyping and multilocus enzyme electrophoresis demonstrated that a distinct clonal group emerged in Russia in 1990 as the epidemic began and was responsible for the wider epidemic.[19]

Cutaneous diphtheria may be central to the changing epidemiology of diphtheria. Cutaneous diphtheria has accounted for more than 50% of *C. diphtheriae* isolates reported in the U.S. since 1975. Cutaneous infection is infrequently associated with toxic complications, and is caused by toxigenic and nontoxigenic strains, often in association with other bacteria. In contrast to respiratory tract infection, cutaneous diphtheria is associated with prolonged bacterial shedding, increased environmental contamination, and increased transmission to close contacts. Previously a disease of tropical countries and U.S. below the 37th parallel, recent outbreaks of cutaneous diphtheria have occurred in the Pacific northwest and sporadically throughout the country. Such outbreaks have been associated with homelessness, crowding, poverty, alcoholism, poor hygiene, contaminated fomites, underlying dermatosis, and introduction of new strains from exogenous sources. From 1971 through 1982, a total of 1100 *C. diphtheriae* infections were documented in Seattle; 86% were cutaneous, and 40% involved toxigenic strains.[20] Currently, cutaneous diphtheria is a reservoir for toxigenic *C. diphtheriae* in the U.S. and has been a frequent mode of importation of source cases for sporadic respiratory tract diphtheria. In an attempt to focus attention on respiratory tract diphtheria, however, which is much more likely to cause complications and toxic manifestations, cutaneous diphtheria has not been a nationally reportable disease since 1980.

PATHOGENESIS

Both toxigenic and nontoxigenic *C. diphtheriae* organisms cause skin and mucosal infection as well as rare distant infection after bacteremia. Organisms remain confined to superficial layers of skin lesions or respiratory mucosa and induce a local inflammatory reaction. The major virulence factor is a potent 62-kd polypeptide exotoxin that consists of a binding segment A and an active segment B, which, when cleaved, is internalized and inactivates transfer RNA translocase, preventing addition of amino acids during protein synthesis. Within the first few days of respiratory tract infection, a dense, necrotic "pseudomembrane" forms. The pseudomembrane, which advances and becomes adherent, consists of organisms, epithelial cells, fibrin, leukocytes, and erythrocytes. Removal is difficult and reveals a bleeding edematous submucosa. Paralysis of the palate and hypopharynx are early local effects of the toxin. Absorption and hematogenous dissemination of toxin can lead to necrosis of kidney tubules, hepatic parenchyma, amegakaryocytic thrombocytopenia, myocardiopathy, and demyelinating neuropathy. Cardiomyopathy and neuropathy occur 2 to 10 weeks after initial mucocutaneous infection and may involve an immune-mediated pathophysiology as well as a delayed appearance of toxic tissue damage.

CLINICAL MANIFESTATIONS

Respiratory Tract Diphtheria

In a classic description of 1400 cases of diphtheria, infection involved the tonsils or pharynx in 94%; the nose and larynx were the next two most common sites.[21] After an average incubation

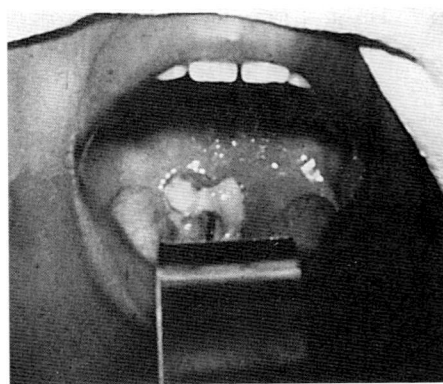

Figure 130-1. Four-year-old girl with faucial diphtheria.

period of 2 to 4 days, local signs and symptoms of inflammation develop. Fever is low-grade or absent. Infection of the anterior nares (more common in infants) causes serosanguineous, erosive rhinitis with membrane formation. Shallow ulceration of the external nares and upper lip is characteristic. Sore throat is a universal early symptom of tonsillar or pharyngeal diphtheria, but only 50% of patients have fever, and fewer than 50% of patients have dysphagia, hoarseness, malaise, or headache. Mild pharyngeal injection is followed by unilateral or bilateral tonsillar membrane formation, which extends off tonsillar tissues to variably affect the uvula, soft palate, posterior oropharynx, hypopharynx, and glottic areas (Figure 130-1). Underlying soft-tissue edema and enlarged lymph nodes can cause cervical swelling (e.g., "bull-neck"), characterized by obliteration of borders of the mandible, sternocleidomastoid muscle, and clavicle by brawny, pitting, warm, tender, but nonerythematous, edema. The degree of toxin extension correlates directly with symptoms of prostration, "bull-neck," airway compromise, and subsequent toxin-mediated complications of distant organs. A patient with laryngeal diphtheria is highly prone to acute airway compromise due to local edema and formation of the pseudomembrane. Establishment of an artificial airway and resection of pseudomembrane may be life-saving.

Appearance of a leather-like adherent pseudomembrane extending beyond the faucial tonsillar area, and a relative lack of fever and dysphagia, help distinguish diphtheria from exudative pharyngitis due to *Streptococcus pyogenes*, adenovirus, and Epstein–Barr virus. Absence of exanthem or ulcers elsewhere on the oral mucosa and tongue distinguishes diphtheria from other viral causes. Vincent angina and Lemierre disease, phlebitis and thrombosis of jugular veins, mucositis in patients undergoing cancer chemotherapy, and faucial membrane after tonsillectomy usually are distinguished by the clinical setting. Diphtheritic infection of the larynx, trachea, or bronchi can be primary or from secondary extension after pharyngeal infection; hoarseness, stridor, dyspnea, and "croupy" cough are clues to infection of these sites. Differentiation from bacterial epiglottitis, severe viral laryngotracheobronchitis, and staphylococcal or streptococcal tracheitis hinges partially on relative paucity of other signs and symptoms in a patient with diphtheria and primarily on visualization of an adherent pseudomembrane at the time of laryngobronchoscopy and intubation.

Cutaneous Diphtheria

Cutaneous diphtheria usually is an indolent, nonprogressive infection characterized by a superficial ecthymic nonhealing ulcer with a grey-brown membrane. Often, diphtheritic skin infection cannot be distinguished from streptococcal or staphylococcal impetigo, and the conditions frequently coexist. In the Seattle outbreak,[20] *Streptococcus pyogenes* was isolated in 73% of diphtheritic skin lesions. The role of *C. diphtheriae* as the cause of localized findings is not clear. Ulcers do not respond to antitoxin therapy, but infection elicits high antitoxin levels. In most cases, underlying dermatoses, lacerations, burns, bites, or impetigo have become secondarily

contaminated. Extremities are affected more often than the trunk or head. Pain, tenderness, erythema, and exudate are typical. Local hyperesthesia or hypoesthesia can occur. Respiratory tract colonization or symptomatic infection, as well as toxic complications, occur in a minority of patients with cutaneous diphtheria. Among infected Seattle adults, 3% with cutaneous infections versus 21% with symptomatic nasopharyngeal infection with or without skin involvement had toxic myocarditis, neuropathy, or obstructive respiratory tract complications.[20] All had received at least 20,000 units of equine antitoxin at the time of hospitalization.

Infection at Other Sites

C. diphtheriae occasionally causes infections at other mucocutaneous sites such as the ear (otitis externa), eye (purulent and ulcerative conjunctivitis involving primarily palpebral areas), and genital tract (purulent and ulcerative vulvovaginitis). Clinical setting, ulceration, pseudomembrane formation, and submucosal bleeding help distinguish among other bacterial and viral causes.

Rare cases of septicemia with *C. diptheriae* have been described and such cases often are fatal. Sporadic cases of endocarditis occur, and clusters among intravenous drug users have been reported,[22,23] as have occasional cases in children living in endemic areas.[24,25] Notable clinical features are aggressive valvular destruction, with associated pyogenic arthritis and major vascular complications (emboli and aneurysms) due to large size of vegetations; most complications have been caused by nontoxigenic strains. Most patients did not have respiratory tract symptoms. Although skin lesions were not described, skin is likely to have been the portal of entry. Sporadic cases of pyogenic arthritis, mainly due to nontoxigenic strains, have been reported in adults and children.[26] "Diphtheroids" isolated from sterile body sites should not be dismissed as contaminants without careful consideration of the clinical setting and should be identified to the species level if validly associated with invasive disease. If *C. diphtheriae* is isolated, toxigenicity studies of the isolate should be completed and prophylaxis for contacts should be considered.

Toxic Myocardiopathy

Toxic myocardiopathy occurs in approximately 10% to 25% of patients with diphtheria and is responsible for 50% to 60% of deaths. Subtle signs of myocarditis may be detectable in many patients, especially in the elderly, but the risk of significant complications for an individual correlates directly with the extent and severity of exudative oropharyngeal disease and delays in administration of antitoxin.[20-22]

Most often, first evidence of cardiomyopathy is recognized in the second to third week of illness, as pharyngeal disease improves, but cardiomyopathy can appear as early as the first week (when fatal outcome is high) or insidiously as late as the sixth week of illness. Tachycardia out of proportion to fever is common evidence of cardiac toxicity or autonomic nervous system dysfunction. Prolonged P-R interval or ST-segment and T-wave changes are relatively frequent findings on electrocardiogram, and dilated or hypertrophic cardiomyopathy is frequently observed on echocardiogram. Single or progressive cardiac arrhythmias can occur, such as first-, second-, and third-degree heart block, atrioventricular dissociation, and ventricular tachycardia. Clinical congestive heart failure can have insidious or acute onset. Elevation of serum aspartate aminotransferase concentration closely parallels the severity of cardiac myonecrosis. Severe arrhythmia portends death.[14,21,27] Histologic postmortem findings can show minor abnormality or diffuse myonecrosis with acute inflammatory response. Except for survivors of more severe arrhythmias, who may have permanent conduction defects, recovery from toxic myocardiopathy usually is complete.

Toxic Neuropathy

Neurologic complications also parallel the extent of primary infection and are multiphasic in onset.[20,21,27] Two to 3 weeks after onset of oropharyngeal inflammation, hypoesthesia and local paralysis of soft palate commonly occur. Weakness of posterior pharyngeal, laryngeal, and facial nerves may follow, causing a nasal quality in voice, difficulty in swallowing, and risk of death from aspiration. Cranial neuropathies usually occur in the fifth week, leading to oculomotor and ciliary paralysis, manifest as strabismus, blurred vision, or difficulty with accommodation. Symmetric polyneuropathy can have its onset 10 days to 3 months after onset of oropharyngeal infection and principally causes motor defect and diminished deep tendon reflexes.

Both proximal muscle weakness of extremities progressing distally and, more commonly, distal weakness progressing proximally, have been described. Clinical and cerebrospinal fluid findings are indistinguishable from that of the polyneuropathy of Guillain–Barré syndrome. Paralysis of the diaphragm can ensue. Complete recovery is likely. Rarely, 2 or 3 weeks after onset of illness, dysfunction of vasomotor centers can cause hypotension or cardiac failure.

MANAGEMENT

Patients

Diagnostic Tests

Specimens for culture should be obtained from nose and throat and from any affected mucocutaneous site. A portion of membrane as well as underlying exudate should be removed and submitted for testing. Growth from slants are stained with Neisser or Löffler methylene blue and examined for metachromatic granules. At the time of submission of specimens, the laboratory must be notified to use selective media for isolation. *C. diphtheriae* survives drying, but if transport to a laboratory will require more than 24 hours, a transport media should be used. In remote areas, a swab specimen can be placed in a silica gel pack and sent to a reference laboratory. Evaluation of direct smears using Gram stain or specific fluorescent antibody is unreliable. When coryneform bacteria are isolated from sterile body sites or from mucocutaneous sites in suspected cases or contacts, organisms should be identified to species level and toxigenicity and antimicrobial susceptibility tests performed on *C. diphtheriae* isolates. While the only commercially available methods to diagnose *C. diphtheria* infection are culture and toxigenicity tests, the CDC performs a PCR assay that allows detection of the regulatory gene for toxin production (*dtxR*) and the diphtheria toxin gene (*tox*). This assay provides supportive evidence for the diagnosis and is not sufficient for confirmation but can be particularly useful if nonviable organisms are present in clinical specimens.[28] Measurement of serum antibodies to the toxin is performed by few laboratories, but, if performed before administration of antitoxin, could be helpful in assessing the probability of the diagnosis.

Antitoxin

Specific antitoxin neutralizes free toxin only; therefore, if the clinical findings and epidemiology support the diagnosis, antitoxin should be administered promptly, before culture confirmation. Mortality is less than 1% if antitoxin is administered on the first day of disease and increases 20-fold if treatment is delayed until the fourth day.

Antitoxin of human origin is available in some countries, but only an equine preparation is available in the U.S. Currently the U.S. supply of equine diphtheria antitoxin (DAT) is available from the CDC through an investigational new drug (CDC Emergency Operations Center, 24-hour telephone 770-488-7100).[29] Antitoxin is administered once at an empiric dosage based on the degree of toxicity, site and size of the membrane, and duration of illness.[29] The intravenous route is preferred. Antitoxin is probably of no value for local manifestations of cutaneous diphtheria but is recommended because toxic sequelae can occur.

Approximately 8% of patients given equine antitoxins develop serum sickness. Up to 10% of individuals have pre-existing hypersensitivity to horse protein. Even very sick patients must be tested before infusion, with desensitization by protocol performed in those showing immediate reactions.[29]

Commercially available immune globulin preparations for intravenous use contain antibodies to diphtheria toxin, but the amounts likely vary from lot to lot. Their use for therapy of diphtheria is not proved or recommended. Antitoxin is not recommended for asymptomatic carriers.

Antimicrobial Therapy

Antimicrobial therapy is indicated to limit further presumed continuing toxin production, treat localized infection, and prevent transmission of organism to contacts, but antibiotic therapy is not a substitute for antitoxin therapy. *C. diphtheriae* usually is susceptible in vitro to penicillins, erythromycin, newer macrolides (clarithromycin, azithromycin), clindamycin, rifampin, fluoroquinolines, and tetracycline. Resistance to erythromycin has been documented in cutaneous diphtheria outbreaks in the U.S.[20] Only penicillin and erythromycin have been evaluated in prospective trials and are the sole agents recommended. Erythromycin is marginally superior to penicillin for eradication of nasopharyngeal carriage. Appropriate therapy is erythromycin given orally or parenterally (40 to 50 mg/kg per day, maximum 2 g/day); or aqueous crystalline penicillin G intramuscularly or intravenously (100,000 to 150,000 U/kg per day divided into 4 doses) or procaine penicillin intramuscularly (25,000 to 50,000 U/kg per day divided into 2 doses). Therapy is given for 14 days. Some patients with cutaneous diphtheria have been treated for 7 to 10 days. Elimination of the organism should be documented by two successive cultures from the nose, throat, and skin (when appropriate) at least 24 hours apart after completion of therapy. Treatment with erythromycin is repeated if culture is positive.

Other Measures

Droplet isolation is recommended for patients with pharyngeal diphtheria; contact isolation is sufficient for patients with cutaneous diphtheria. Isolation is continued until at least two cultures from the nose and throat (and skin lesions, if present) taken after cessation of therapy are negative. Cutaneous wounds should be thoroughly cleansed with soap and water. Bedrest is recommended during the acute phase of disease. Return to physical activity should be guided by degree of toxicity and cardiac involvement. Complications of airway obstruction and aspiration should be anticipated with careful observation of oropharyngeal and laryngeal diphtheria, and an artificial airway should be established pre-emptively. Congestive heart failure and malnutrition should be anticipated and prevented when possible.

Corticosteroid therapy is not recommended. In a study of 66 children with respiratory tract diphtheria alternately treated with prednisone or no steroid therapy for 14 days from the time of diagnosis, toxic myocarditis occurred in 26%, neuritis in 17%, and bullneck diphtheria in 10%, with no difference in occurrence or death in those who received steroids.[27] Use of digitalis for treatment of myocarditis is associated with excess occurrence of arrhythmia.

Prognosis of diphtheria is dependent on the virulence of the organism, age, immunization status, site of infection, the presence and severity of complications, and speed of administration of antitoxin. Mechanical obstruction from laryngeal or bullneck diphtheria and complications of myocarditis account for most deaths.[30] Ventricular ectopy with or without evident clinical myocarditis at the time of initiation of therapy predicted fatal outcome with 100% sensitivity and specificity in children with severe diphtheria. A minimum case-fatality rate of 10% for respiratory tract diphtheria has not changed in 50 years,[11] and mortality was 18% and 23% in outbreaks that occurred in the 1980s and 1990s in Sweden[1] and states of the former Soviet Union,[18] respectively, and 33% in a retrospective study from the U.K. where deaths were observed only in nonimmunized individuals.[8]

Because sustained immunity does not develop in all patients after infection, administration of diphtheria toxoid is indicated at recovery to complete the primary series or booster doses of immunization.

Exposed Persons

Public health officials should be notified promptly when a diagnosis of diphtheria is suspected or proved. Investigation is aimed at preventing secondary cases in exposed individuals and at determining the source case and carriers to halt spread to unexposed individuals. Reported rates of carriage in household contacts of case-patients have ranged from 0% to 25%.[7,14,31] The risk of developing diphtheria after household exposure to a case is approximately 2%; it is 0.3% after similar exposure to a carrier.

Asymptomatic Case Contacts

Prompt identification and investigation of close contacts (defined as all household contacts and those who have had intimate respiratory or habitual physical contact with the patient) are the highest priorities. The following steps should be taken in these individuals:

- Monitor closely for illness through the 7-day incubation period.
- Perform cultures of the nose, throat, and any cutaneous lesion.
- Give antimicrobial prophylaxis, regardless of immunization status, with oral erythromycin (40 to 50 mg/kg per day for 7 to 10 days, maximum 2 g/day). If the individual is intolerant to erythromycin or if complete adherence is not assured, intramuscular benzathine penicillin should be administered (600,000 U for those <30 kg or 1,200,000 U for those ≥30 kg). The efficacy of antimicrobial prophylaxis is presumed but not proved, and the newer macrolides, such as clarithromycin and azithromycin, have not been evaluated for their ability to eliminate carriage of C. diphtheriae.
- Give diphtheria toxoid vaccine doses or other suitable combination vaccine (e.g., childhood diphtheria and tetanus toxoids (DT); childhood diphtheria and tetanus toxoids, and acellular pertussis (DTaP) vaccine; adult or childhood diphtheria and tetanus toxoids, and acellular pertussis (Tdap) vaccine; or adult tetanus and diphtheria toxoids (Td)), appropriate for age, to immunized individuals who have not received a booster dose within 5 years. Some experts suggest that the duration of protective antibody is variable and recommend a booster be given to close contacts if 1 year has elapsed since immunization.[32,33] Tdap adolescent and adult vaccines have not been evaluated in control of outbreaks, but should be reliable based on the immune responses to these vaccines which produce high antibody levels when given to subjects who have received a primary series of DTaP. Children who have not received their fourth or fifth dose of DTaP should be vaccinated. Those who have received fewer than three doses of diphtheria toxoid or for whom knowledge of immunization status is lacking should be immunized with an age-appropriate preparation on a primary schedule. The use of the Schick test (intradermal injection of diphtheria toxin) to determine immunity in contacts is no longer recommended, and the reagents for testing are generally no longer available.

Asymptomatic Carriers

When an asymptomatic carrier is identified, the following steps should be taken:

- Give antimicrobial prophylaxis for 7 to 10 days.
- Give age-appropriate preparation of diphtheria toxoid immediately if the individual has not received a booster within 1 year.
- Place individuals in droplet isolation (respiratory tract colonization) or contact isolation (cutaneous colonization only) until at least two subsequent cultures taken at least 24 hours apart after cessation of therapy are negative for C. diphtheriae.
- Perform repeat cultures at a minimum of 2 weeks after completion of therapy in cases and carriers, and, if cultures are positive,

an additional 10-day course of oral erythromycin should be given and follow-up cultures performed.

Neither antimicrobial agent eradicates carriage in 100% of individuals. In one report,[34] eradication failed in 21% of carriers after a single course of therapy. Antitoxin is not recommended for close contacts or asymptomatic carriers even if they are inadequately immunized because of the adverse effects of horse serum and no demonstrable evidence of benefit above antimicrobial prophylaxis. Booster immunization elicits rapid rise in antitoxin levels.

Transmission of diphtheria in modern hospitals is rare.[35] Meticulous handwashing and handling of secretions are mandatory. Only those who have had unusual contact with respiratory or oral secretions should be managed as contacts. Investigation of casual contacts of patients and carriers, or persons in the community without known exposure, has generally yielded extremely low carriage rates and is not recommended routinely.

PREVENTION

Universal immunization with vaccines containing diphtheria toxoid to provide constant protective antitoxin levels and to reduce indigenous C. diphtheriae is the only effective control measure. This requires multiple injections in childhood and adulthood. Serum antitoxin levels, measured by toxin neutralization tests in Vero cell culture or rabbit skin or measured by hemagglutination, are roughly equivalent. Concentration of 0.01 to 0.1 IU/mL is conventionally accepted as the minimum protective level although the protective limit of antibody has not been precisely defined. In outbreaks, 90% of individuals with clinical disease have had antitoxin levels <0.01 IU/mL and 92% of asymptomatic carriers have had titers >0.1 IU/mL.[29]

Vaccine Preparations

Diphtheria toxoid is prepared by formaldehyde treatment of toxin and is standardized for potency according to the U.S. Food and Drug Administration. Toxoid is adsorbed to aluminum salts, which enhances immunogenicity. Two preparations of diphtheria toxoids are formulated according to limit of flocculation (Lf) content, a measure of quantity of toxoid. Pediatric preparations (DTP, DT, DTaP) contain ≥6.7 Lf units of diphtheria toxoid/0.5 mL dose whereas adult preparations of combination vaccines of diphtheria–tetanus (Td) or tetanus–dipththeria–acellular pertussis (Tdap) contain no more than 2 Lf units of toxoid/0.5 mL dose. The higher potency (D) formulation of toxoid is used for the primary series and booster doses for children through 6 years of age because of superior immunogenicity and minimal reactogenicity. For individuals 7 years of age and older, Td or Tdap (for one dose only) is recommended for primary series and booster doses because the lower concentration of diphtheria toxoid is adequately immunogenic and because increasing content of diphtheria toxoid heightens reactogenicity with increasing age.

Schedules

Children from 6 Weeks through 6 Years of Age

Five 0.5 mL doses of diphtheria-containing (D) vaccine should be given. The adult preparations (d) should not be used in children younger than 7 years because of reduced immunogenicity. The primary series includes doses at approximately 2, 4, and 6 months of age. The fourth dose is an integral part of the primary series and is given approximately 6 to 12 months after the third dose to maintain adequate immunity during preschool years. A booster dose is given at 4 to 6 years (unless the fourth primary dose was administered after the fourth birthday).

Persons 7 Years of Age or Older

Three 0.5 mL doses of diphtheria containing (Td, or Tdap for one dose) vaccine are recommended as a primary series; this primary series includes two doses 4 to 8 weeks apart and a third dose 6 to 12 months after the second dose; the preferred schedule is Tdap followed by Td but Tdap can replace any single dose of Td. The only contraindication to diphtheria toxoid is a history of neurologic or severe hypersensitivity reaction after a previous dose.

Children in Whom Pertussis Immunization is Contraindicated

D or d toxoids (DT or Td) are used as follows: those who began with either diphtheria–tetanus–pertussis or DT at age <1 year should have a total of five 0.5 mL doses of D-containing vaccine by 6 years. For those beginning at or after 1 year of age, the primary series is two 0.5 mL doses of D vaccine, with a third dose 6 to 12 months later, and a booster given at 4 to 6 years unless the third dose was given after the fourth birthday.[32,36]

Further reduction in the number of cases of diphtheria in industrialized countries will require universal booster immunization throughout life. Booster doses of 0.5 mL Td should be given every 10 years (most conveniently given to most persons at 15 years, 25 years, 35 years of age, and so forth). Tdap should be given to replace one dose of Td for routine administration. Vaccination with diphtheria toxoid should be used whenever tetanus toxoid is indicated to ensure continuing diphtheria immunity. There is no known association of DT or Td with increased risk of convulsions. Local side effects alone do not preclude continued use. Persons who experience severe Arthus-type hypersensitivity reactions after a dose of Td usually have high serum tetanus antitoxin levels and should not be given Td more frequently than every 10 years, even if significant tetanus-prone injury is sustained. DT or Td can be given concurrently with other vaccines. *Haemophilus influenzae* conjugate vaccines containing diphtheria toxoid (PRP-D) or the variant of diphtheria toxin, CRM1$_{97}$ protein (HbOC), are not substitutes for diphtheria toxoid immunization.

Acknowledgment

The author acknowledges substantial use of content contributed to prior editions by G.D. Overturf.

Key Points. Diagnosis and Management of *Corynebacterium diphtheriae* Infection

MICROBIOLOGY

- Pleomorphic gram-positive bacilli
- Selective or enrichment media are required for growth
- Infection of the bacteria with a lysogenic bacteriophage is responsible for exotoxin production

EPIDEMIOLOGY

- Humans are the only reservoir
- Infection spreads by respiratory droplets or direct contact with respiratory or skin secretions
- Due to universal childhood immunization in the U.S. diphtheria cases are imported but diphtheria is still endemic in many developing countries
- Classic presentations include pharyngitis and cutaneous diphtheria, but endocarditis or arthritis cases have been documented
- Complications include toxic cardiomyopathy and neuropathy

DIAGNOSIS

- Isolation from the nasopharynx, or skin lesions
- Coryneform bacteria isolated from blood in patients with suspicion of diphtheria should not be discounted as contaminants before identification to the species level

- PCR (not commercially available) allows detection of toxin production regulatory genes

TREATMENT

- Specific antitoxin is life-saving if administered in first 24 hours of symptom onset
- Equine antitoxin is available in the U.S. only through CDC Emergency Operations Center
- Antimicrobial therapy is indicated to limit toxin production and prevent transmission
- Strains usually are susceptible to penicillins and macrolides
- Administration of diphtheria toxoid vaccine is indicated at recovery since sustained immunity does not develop in all patients after infection

INFECTION CONTROL/PREVENTION

- Droplet isolation is indicated for pharyngeal and contact isolation for cutaneous diphtheria cases
- Universal immunization with vaccines containing diphtheria toxoid and booster doses throughout life is the only effective control measure

---

131 Other Corynebacteria

Denise F. Bratcher

Corynebacterium species are recognized as members of the normal human flora, and are isolated from the skin, mucous membranes, and gastrointestinal tract. Although frequently they are dismissed as contaminants in clinical specimens, they have become recognized more often as pathogens, particularly among immunocompromised hosts.[1,2] In addition, infections due to *Corynebacterium* species have occurred predominantly among those with prosthetic devices, and other medical devices. Further definition of the pathogenic role of *Corynebacterium* species in human infections and of

the mechanisms of pathogenesis remains to be elucidated. Many case reports are questioned due to the limitations of commercial identification systems and inappropriate identification methods, significant changes in the taxonomy of coryneform bacteria, and lack of distinction between colonization and infection.[1] Identification of significant clinical isolates of *Corynebacterium* spp. and antimicrobial susceptibility and synergy testing are warranted. Characteristics of reported infections due to *Corynebacterium* species are outlined in Table 131-1. *Corynebacterium*

TABLE 131-1. Characteristics of Infection and Habitat of *Corynebacterium* Species

Species	Normal Flora	Infection				Unusual Features	References
		Normal Host	Compromised Host[a]	Children	Antibiotic Susceptibility[b]		
C. afermentans	Human Animal	Brain abscess Hepatic abscess	Bacteremia Endocarditis Pulmonary infections				22–26
C. amycolatum		Septic arthritis Endocarditis	Bacteremia Endocarditis Peritonitis	Bacteremia	S: Vanc, Teico, Tet R: Multiple drugs	Often nosocomial	1, 3, 18–20, 27–29
Former *C. aquaticum* (*Leifsonia aquatica*)		Skin infection	Bacteremia/Sepsis Peritonitis Skin infection	Bacteremia Endocarditis Meningitis Peritonitis Urinary tract infection	S: Vanc, Amg, Clin V: Pcn, 1G and 3G Ceph, Dapto	Habitat natural fresh water; resembles *Listeria* spp.	30–36
C. bovis	Animal	Skin infection Meningitis Mastoiditis	Bacteremia Endocarditis Glomerulonephritis Meningitis		S: Ery, Rif V: Pcn	Causes rancidity of milk	1, 37
C. coyleae			Ascites Sepsis Skin/soft tissue infection	Bacteremia	S: Pcn, Cephs, Vanc, Tet, Rif, Lin V: Ery R: Clin	Diagnostic procedures main risk; commercial identification challenging	38
C. jeikeium	Human	Bacteremia Otitis media Septic arthritis	Absces Bacteremia Endocarditis Enteritis Meningitis Osteomyelitis Peritonitis Pneumonia Pyelonephritis Skin infections Transverse myelitis Urinary tract infection Ventriculitis	Abscess Bacteremia Endocarditis Meningitis	S: Vanc, Tig R: Multiple drugs	Most common cause of diphtheroid endocarditis; removal of prosthetic device usually required for cure; major nosocomial pathogen	1, 3, 4–15, 39–46
C. kutscheri[c]	Animal		Chorioamnionitis Septic arthritis	Pneumonia Soft tissue (after rat bite)	S: Vanc, 1G Ceph	Causes visceral lesions in rodents; pathogenicity questioned in humans	1, 47–49
C. macginleyi			Catheter-related infection Conjunctivitis Endocarditis Endophthalmitis Keratitis Sepsis Urinary tract infection		S: Multiple V: Fq R: Ery	Almost exclusively from eye specimens	50–57
C. minutissimum[c]	Human	Bacteremia Cellulitis Erythrasma (polymicrobial) Meningitis	Abscess Bacteremia Endocarditis Erythrasma Peritonitis	Erythrasma Pyelonephritis	S: Ery, Tet, T/S, Vanc V: Ceph, Chloro, Pcn	Involved skin fluoresces coral red with Wood light	1, 58–65
C. pilosum[c]	Animal		Abscess Endocarditis		S: 3G Ceph, Pcn, Tet, Vanc	Infections associated with animal contact	1, 66

Continued

TABLE 131-1. Characteristics of Infection and Habitat of *Corynebacterium* Species—cont'd

Species	Normal Flora	Infection Normal Host	Infection Compromised Host[a]	Infection Children	Antibiotic Susceptibility[b]	Unusual Features	References
C. pseudodiphtheriticum (*Corynebacterium hofmannii*)	Human	Conjunctivitis/ keratitis Discitis Endocarditis Lymphadenitis Pharyngitis (membranous) Pulmonary infections Skin infections	Endocarditis Pulmonary infections Septic arthritis Urinary tract infection[c]	Endocarditis Lymphadenitis Otitis media Pharyngitis (membranous) Pulmonary infections	S: Amg, Vanc, Fq, Rif, Tet V: 1G & 2G Ceph, Pcn, Chloro, Clin R: Ery	Commensal of human nasopharynx; Gram stain parallel rows of bacilli	1, 67–78
C. pseudotuberculosis (*Corynebacterium ovis*)	Animal	Lymphadenitis Pneumonia	Abscess Lymphadenitis Pneumonia	Lymphadenitis Septic arthritis	S: Amg, Ery, Clin, Pcn, Tet, Vanc,[d] Chloro, Rif	Produces dermonecrotic toxin; usually associated with animal contact	1, 79, 80
C. striatum[c,e]	Human		Endocarditis Bacteremia Central line infection Chorioamnionitis Meningitis Osteomyelitis Peritonitis Pulmonary infections Septic arthritis Skin/soft tissue infection	Ventriculitis	S: Vanc, Teico, Imip, Dapto V: Clin, Ery, Lin, Pcn, Amg, Tet R: FQ, Rif	Nosocomial infections	1, 3, 12, 81–96
C. ulcerans	Animal	Pharyngitis (membranous) Sinusitis Skin ulcers	Pharyngitis Pneumonia Pulmonary nodules	Pharyngitis (membranous) Otitis media	S: multiple drugs; Ery: drug of choice	Produces exotoxins of *C. diphtheriae* and *C. pseudotuberculosis*; treatment includes antitoxin; associated with raw milk	1, 97–105
C. urealyticum (group D2)	Human		Bacteremia Endocarditis Osteomyelitis Pericarditis Pneumonia Urinary tract infection Wound infection	Soft-tissue infection Urinary tract infection	S: Teico, Vanc V: Fq, Rif, Ery, Tet R: Multiple drugs	Urease activity produces alkaline urine; leads to crystal formation	1, 106–112
C. xerosis[c]	Human	Endocarditis	Bacteremia Central nervous system Infections Endocarditis Osteomyelitis Peritonitis Pulmonary infections Septic arthritis	Bacteremia Endocarditis Meningitis Pericarditis Ventriculitis	S: Vanc, 3G Ceph, Fq V: Amg, Clin, Ery, Pcn	Nosocomial infections	1, 113–119

Amg, aminoglycosides; 1G Ceph, first-generation cephalosporins; 3G Ceph, third-generation cephalosporins; Chloro, chloramphenicol; Clin, clindamycin; Dapto, daptomycin; Ery, erythromycin; Imip, imipenem; Lin, linezolid; Pcn, penicillin; Fq, fluoroquinolones; Rif, rifampin; Teico, teicoplanin; Tet, tetracyclines; Tig, tigecycline; T/S, trimethoprim-sulfamethoxazole; Vanc, vancomycin.

[a]*Compromised hosts include immunodeficient patients, neutropenic patients, those with indwelling devices, and postsurgery and trauma patients.*

[b]*There are no reports of controlled clinical trials using different antimicrobial agents in the treatment of infections with Corynebacterium species. Notation is based on antimicrobial susceptibilities reported in cases and laboratory evaluations. S, susceptible; R, resistant; V, variable.*

[c]*Some reports likely represent misidentification of Corynebacterium amycolatum or another Corynebacterium strain.[1]*

[d]*Surgical excision following parenteral antibiotic therapy is necessary for cure.*

[e]*Multidrug resistance is reported; only drugs active against these strains are glycopeptides, linezolid, quinopristin/dalfopristin, daptomycin, and tigecycline.*

infections among children rarely cause severe symptoms or mortality.[3]

CORYNEBACTERIUM JEIKEIUM

Corynebacterium jeikeium, formerly known as Centers for Disease Control and Prevention (CDC) group JK, was first identified as a distinct group in 1976; a pathogenic role in endocarditis after cardiovascular surgery has been noted since 1963. Over the subsequent decades, *C. jeikeium* has been identified increasingly in association with a variety of clinical entities, predominantly in immunocompromised hosts, and has become recognized as a significant nosocomial pathogen.

Only pathogenic for humans, *C. jeikeium* is found in soil and water and is part of normal human skin flora. Colonization rate increases with hospitalization; it has been reported in hospital personnel and up to 40% of hospitalized patients, especially on the skin of the perirectal area, groin, and axilla.[4] Infection is thought to occur when *C. jeikeium* invades through mucosal breaks and colonizes prosthetic devices. Risk factors for *C. jeikeium* infection include: prolonged hospitalization; profound, extended granulocytopenia; multiple or prolonged course(s) of antibiotic therapy; disruption of mucocutaneous barriers; and presence of a medical device.

C. jeikeium was recognized as the most frequent cause of bloodstream infection (BSI) among bone marrow transplant patients in one study;[4] BSI also has been reported among immunocompetent and immunosuppressed patients. *C. jeikeium* is the most common cause of diphtheroid endocarditis of prosthetic valves[5] but also can infect native valves. Other infections attributed to *C. jeikeium* include skin and wound infections, catheter-related infections, enteritis, meningitis, osteomyelitis, peritonitis, pneumonia, prosthetic joint infections, pyelonephritis, and liver abscess in a patient with acquired immunodeficiency syndrome (AIDS).[6–12] Several infections due to *C. jeikeium* have been reported in children, including meningitis associated with ventriculoperitoneal shunt, BSI endocarditis, and a localized skin abscess at a puncture site.[13–15] Most cases were associated with immunosuppression, a medical device, or trauma.

C. jeikeium is a nonmotile, gram-positive bacillus that can appear to be coccobacillary. Growth appears as discrete, pinpoint, smooth, white colonies that take on a characteristic metallic sheen after 24 to 48 hours of incubation. Identification is frequently confirmed on the basis of its resistance to many antibiotics, including β-lactams, aminoglycosides, erythromycin, and tetracycline. Vancomycin generally is the most active antibiotic agent and is the drug of choice in *C. jeikeium* infections. Telithromycin, linezolid, and quinopristin/dalfopristin have good in vitro activity.[16] While it has been suggested that removal of a central venous catheter may not be necessary, removal of involved prosthetic devices usually is required for cure.[4,17] Prevention of nosocomial transmission of *C. jeikeium* depends on meticulous handwashing and aseptic techniques. Greater elucidation of the modes of transfer of *C. jeikeium* in hospital settings may suggest further methods of infection control.

OTHER *CORYNEBACTERIUM* SPECIES

In addition to the increasing frequency of infections over the past 20 years, many new *Corynebacterium* species have been established; further new identifications are expected.[1] Corynebacteria are diverse morphologically, metabolically, and structurally. Multiple changes and improvements in the taxonomic framework for coryneform bacteria have facilitated associations.

C. amycolatum, a newly established species in 1988, probably accounts for many previously reported infections misidentified as *C. kutscheri*, *C. minutissimum*, *C. striatum*, and *C. xerosis*.[1] *C. amycolatum* is one of the species most commonly isolated from clinical specimens[1] and has been reported as a cause of septicemia in a diabetic patient[18] and a premature infant[19] and of pyogenic arthritis.[20] *C. amycolatum* typically is resistant to multiple antibiotics and is susceptible to vancomycin and teicoplanin.

Other newly identified *Corynebacterium* spp. that have been reported rarely in association with human disease include *C. accolens*, *C. afermentans*, *C. argentoratense*, *C. auris*, *C. falsenii*, *C. glucuronolyticum*, *C. macginleyi*, and *C. propinquum*.

Current methods for identification of *Corynebacterium* species, especially those relying on commercial identification systems, may be inadequate because a limited number of species are represented. Similarly, numerous differences within reference strains of *Corynebacterium* species have been noted.[1] Referral of isolates to a reference laboratory may be necessary. Standardized guidelines for susceptibility testing of *Corynebacterium* species were published in 2006.[21] Variable susceptibility to antimicrobial agents mandates specific testing of each clinical isolate.

132   *Listeria monocytogenes*

Bennett Lorber

The bacterium *Listeria monocytogenes* is an uncommon cause of illness in the general population. In some groups, however, including neonates, pregnant women, elderly persons, and those with impaired cell-mediated immunity, it is an important cause of life-threatening bacteremia and meningoencephalitis.[1,2] Growing interest in this organism has resulted from foodborne outbreaks, concerns about food safety, and the recognition that foodborne infection can result in self-limited febrile gastroenteritis as well as invasive disease.

DESCRIPTION OF THE PATHOGEN

L. monocytogenes is a facultatively anaerobic, nonsporulating, catalase-positive, oxidase-negative, short, nonbranching gram-positive bacillus that grows readily on blood agar, producing incomplete β-hemolysis.[3,4] The bacterium possesses polar flagellae and exhibits a characteristic tumbling motility at 25°C. Unlike most bacteria, *L. monocytogenes* grows well at refrigerator temperature (4°C to 10°C), and, by so-called cold enrichment, it can be separated from other contaminating bacteria by long incubation in this temperature range. Selective media have been developed to isolate the organism from specimens containing multiple species (food, stool) and appear to be superior to cold enrichment.[3,5]

In clinical specimens, the organisms can be gram-variable and can resemble diphtheroids, cocci, or diplococci. Media typically used to isolate diarrhea-causing bacteria from stool cultures inhibit listerial growth. Laboratory misidentification as diphtheroids, streptococci, or enterococci is not uncommon, and the isolation of a "diphtheroid" from blood or cerebrospinal fluid (CSF) should always alert one to the possibility that the organism is really *L. monocytogenes*.[6,7]

Of the six listerial species (*L. monocytogenes*, *L. seeligeri*, *L. welshimeri*, *L. innocua*, *L. ivanovii*, and *L. grayi*), only *L. monocytogenes* is pathogenic for humans. There are at least 13 serovars of *L. monocytogenes*, but almost all disease is due to types 4b, 1/2a, and 1/2b.[2,8] A number of molecular techniques, including pulsed-field gel electrophoresis, ribotyping, and multilocus enzyme electrophoresis, have been employed to separate isolates into distinct groups and have proved useful for investigating epidemics.[9–12]

EPIDEMIOLOGY

L. monocytogenes is an important cause of zoonoses, especially in herd animals. It is widespread in nature, being commonly found in soil, decaying vegetation, and as part of the fecal flora of many mammals.[3,8] The organism has been isolated from the stool of approximately 5% of healthy adults,[8,13] with higher rates of recovery reported from household contacts of patients with clinical infection.[14] In three healthy, asymptomatic adults followed for one year, *L. monocytogenes* was present transiently in 3.5% of stool specimens.[15] Many foods are contaminated with *L. monocytogenes*, and recovery rates of 15% to 70% or more are common from raw vegetables, raw milk, fish, poultry, and meats, including fresh or processed chicken and beef available at supermarkets or delicatessen (deli) counters.[4] Ingestion of *L. monocytogenes* must be a common occurrence.

Listeriosis became a nationally reportable disease in 2000. Two active surveillance studies performed in the 1980s by the Centers for Disease Control and Prevention (CDC) indicated annual infection rates of 7.4 in 1 million population, accounting for approximately 1850 cases a year in the United States, with 425 deaths.[16] By 1993, after food industry regulations were instituted to minimize the risk of foodborne listeriosis, the annual incidence had declined to 4.4 cases per million, or 1092 cases, with 248 deaths.[17] From 1996 through 2003 the incidence decreased 26% and estimated cases dropped from 2228 to 1803 and deaths from 462 to 378.[18] The highest infection rates are seen in infants <1 month and in adults >60 years of age (Figure 132-1).[11,16] Pregnant women account for about 30% of all cases and 60% of cases in the 10- to 40-year age group. Almost 70% of nonperinatal infections occur in those with hematologic malignancy, the acquired immunodeficiency syndrome (AIDS) or organ transplant recipients, or in those receiving corticosteroid therapies.

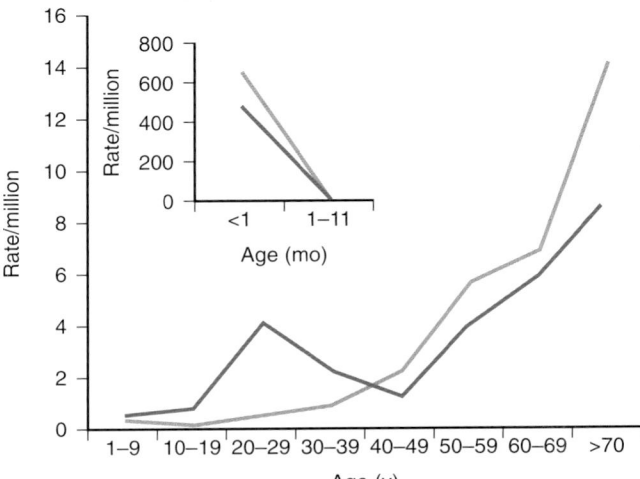

Figure 132-1. Age-specific incidence of listeriosis, by sex. Orange line indicates male patients; blue line, female patients. (Redrawn from Ciesielski CA, Hightower AW, Parsons SK, et al. Listeriosis in the United States: 1980–1982. Arch Intern Med 1988;148:1416–1419.)

Subsequent to a 1983 report[13] of a foodborne outbreak of human listerial infection due to contaminated coleslaw, a number of other foodborne outbreaks resulting in invasive disease (bloodstream infection, meningitis) have been documented,[11] with vehicles including milk,[19] soft cheeses,[20,21] ready-to-eat pork products,[22] hot dogs, and deli-ready turkey.[23] A 2002 outbreak traced to deli-style turkey produced illness in 54 people in nine states, and led to the largest recall of meat in U.S. history (>30 million pounds of food products).[24] Sporadic cases have been traced to contaminated cheese,[25] turkey franks,[26] and alfalfa tablets.[27] The importance of food as a source of sporadic listeriosis is illustrated by two CDC studies in which 11% of all refrigerator food samples were contaminated, 64% of infected patients had at least one contaminated food, and, in 33% of instances, the patient and food isolates had identical strains.[28,29] Deli-style ready-to-eat meats, especially chicken, had the highest rates of contamination. Cases were more likely than were controls to have eaten soft cheeses or deli meats, and 32% of sporadic cases could be attributed to these foods.

Although most human listeriosis appears to be foodborne, other modes of transmission occur. These include transmission from mother to child transplacentally or through an infected birth canal and cross-infection in neonatal nurseries.[30,31] One common source outbreak was traced to contaminated mineral oil used for bathing infants.[32] Localized cutaneous infections have occurred in veterinarians and farmers after direct contact with aborted calves and infected poultry.

In 1998, the CDC added *L. monocytogenes* to PulseNet (http://www.cdc.gov/pulsenet/), a network of public health and food regulatory laboratories that use pulsed-field gel electrophoresis to subtype foodborne pathogens in order to speed detection of disease clusters that may have a common source.[33] This system has proved effective in the early detection of outbreaks of listeriosis.[11,34]

PATHOGENESIS

Except for vertical transmission from mother to fetus and rare instances of cross-contamination in the delivery suite or neonatal nursery, human-to-human infection has not been documented.

Most often, listeriae are acquired via the ingestion of contaminated food.[2,4,11] The oral inoculum required to produce clinical infection is unknown; experiments in healthy mammals indicate that 10^9 organisms are required.[35] Alkalinization of the stomach by antacids, H_2-blocking agents, proton pump inhibitors, or ulcer surgery may promote infection.[36,37] The incubation period for invasive infection is not well established, but evidence from a few cases related to specific ingestions points to a mean incubation period of 31 days, with a range from 11 to 70 days. Virulent *L. monocytogenes* organisms can cause disease without promoter organisms, but a 1987 outbreak in Philadelphia for which no particular source was found suggested that intercurrent gastrointestinal infection with another pathogen may enhance invasion in individuals colonized with *L. monocytogenes*.[25] Evidence for this hypothesis is found in the common history of antecedent gastrointestinal symptoms in patients and household contacts, the long incubation period from ingestion to clinical illness, and two instances in which clinical listeriosis closely followed shigellosis.[38,39] Both listerial meningitis and bacteremia have occurred shortly after colonoscopy or sigmoidoscopy.[40,41]

In the intestine, *L. monocytogenes* crosses the mucosal barrier aided by active endocytosis of organisms by endothelial cells.[4,42] Once in the bloodstream, dissemination can occur to any site; *L. monocytogenes* has a particular predilection for the central nervous system (CNS) and the placenta. It is generally believed that listeriae reach the CNS by a bacteremic route, but animal experiments suggest that rhombencephalitis can develop by intra-axonal spread of bacteria from peripheral sites to the CNS.[43]

The intracellular, molecular pathogenesis of listeriosis has been reviewed in detail.[44–46] Several virulence factors enable *L. monocytogenes* to function as an intracellular organism. A specific surface protein, LPXTG, aids adherence to mucosal surfaces.[47] Another cell

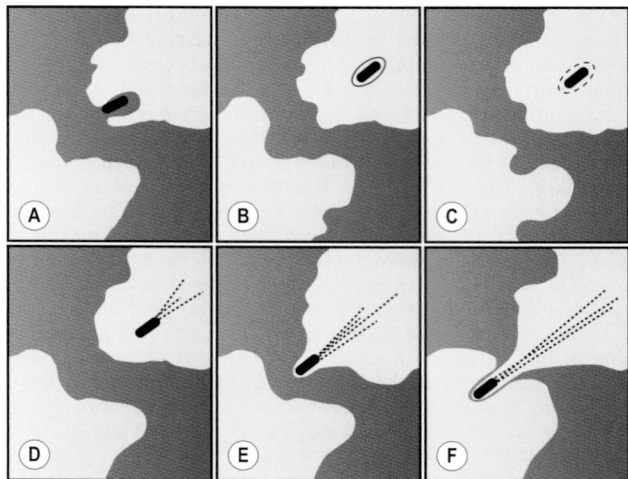

Figure 132-2. Steps in the engulfment of *Listeria monocytogenes* with subsequent transfer of the bacterium from one macrophage to another. **(A)** Adjacent macrophages, one of which has been induced to phagocytose *L. monocytogenes*. **(B)** After ingestion, the organism is held in a single membrane phagosome. **(C)** Through the action of listeriolysin O, the bacterium escapes from the phagocytic vacuole before it is damaged and replication occurs. **(D)** Host cell actin is induced by the organism, now free in the cytoplasm. **(E)** Polymerized actin forms an elongating lattice that propels the bacterium to the host cell membrane, forming a pseudopod-like extension. **(F)** The pseudopod-like extension containing a bacterium is engulfed by an adjacent macrophage, resulting in a double-membrane vacuole.

surface protein, internalin, interacts with E-cadherin, a receptor on macrophages and intestinal lining cells, to induce its own ingestion;[48] the major virulence factor, listeriolysin O, along with phospholipases, enables listeriae to escape from the phagosome and avoid intracellular killing.[49] Once free in the cytoplasm, the bacterium can divide and, by inducing host cell actin polymerization, propel itself to the cell membrane[50] where pseudopod-like projections enable invasion of adjacent macrophages (Figure 132-2). The bacterial surface protein Act A is necessary for the induction of actin filament assembly and cell-to-cell spread and, therefore, is a major virulence factor. Thus, through this novel life cycle, *L. monocytogenes* moves from cell to cell, evading exposure to antibodies, complement, or neutrophils. Siderophores are important virulence factors of *L. monocytogenes*, enabling scavenging of iron from transferrin.[4] In vitro, iron enhances organism growth, and, in animal models of listerial infection, iron overload is associated with enhanced susceptibility to infection and iron supplementation with enhanced lethality, whereas iron depletion results in prolonged survival.[51] The clinical associations of sporadic listerial infection with hemochromatosis[7] and of outbreaks with transfusion-induced iron overload in patients receiving dialysis[52] attest to the importance of iron acquisition as a virulence factor in humans.

IMMUNITY

Resistance to listerial infection involves both innate and adaptive immune responses.[53] The adaptive response primarily is cell-mediated as evidenced by experiments[54] showing that immunity can be transferred by sensitized lymphocytes but not by antibodies. Further evidence is provided by the overwhelming clinical association between listerial infection and conditions of impaired cellular immunity, including lymphoma, pregnancy, AIDS, and corticosteroid immunosuppression.[1,2,6,7,55–57] Invasive listeriosis has complicated the use of tumor necrosis factor (TNF)-α–neutralizing agents (e.g., infliximab) in a variety of conditions.[58–62] In a murine model, TNF was found to play a critical role in the intracerebral control of *L. monocytogenes* infection.[63] Toll-like

receptor 2 contributes to the recognition and control of listeriosis.[64] The role of humoral immunity is unknown, although both immunoglobulin M (absent in neonates) and classical complement activity (low in neonates) have been shown to be necessary for efficient opsonization of *L. monocytogenes*.[65]

Although listeriosis is 100 to 1000 times more common in patients with AIDS compared with the general population,[66,67] it is somewhat surprising that it is not seen more commonly, given the ubiquity of the organism.[68–71] Use of trimethoprim-sulfamethoxazole (TMP-SMX) for prophylaxis against *Pneumocystis jirovecii* pneumonia (PCP) provides protection against listeriosis.[66] Frequency of listeriosis is not increased in those with deficiencies in neutrophil numbers or function, splenectomy, persistent complement deficiency, or immunoglobulin disorders; the latter finding is not surprising, because *L. monocytogenes* can pass from cell to cell without being exposed to antibody.

CLINICAL SYNDROMES

The species name derives from the fact that an extract of the *L. monocytogenes* cell membrane has potent monocytosis-producing activity in rabbits, but monocytosis is an uncommon feature of human infection.[72,73]

Infection in Pregnancy

During gestation, mild impairment of cell-mediated immunity occurs, and pregnant women are prone to developing listerial bloodstream infection (BSI) with an estimated 17-fold increase in risk.[74,75] Listeriae proliferate in the placenta in areas that appear to be unreachable by usual defense mechanisms, and cell-to-cell spread facilitates maternal–fetal transmission.[76,77] For unexplained reasons, CNS infection, the most commonly recognized form of listeriosis in other groups, is extremely rare during pregnancy in the absence of other risk factors.[1,13,16] BSI manifests clinically as an acute febrile illness, often accompanied by myalgia, arthralgia, headache, and backache. Illness usually occurs in the third trimester, probably related to the major decline in cell-mediated immunity seen at 26 to 30 weeks of gestation.[74] Twenty-two percent of perinatal infections result in stillbirth or neonatal death; premature labor and spontaneous abortion are common.[1] Untreated BSI generally is self-limited, although if there is a complicating amnionitis, fever can persist in the mother until the fetus is aborted. Early diagnosis and antimicrobial therapy can result in the birth of a healthy infant.[78,79]

There is no convincing evidence that listeriosis is a cause of habitual abortion in humans.

Neonatal Infection

In a pregnant primate model, oral administration of *L. monocytogenes* resulted in stillbirth with isolation of the bacterium from placental and fetal tissues.[80] Infection in utero can precipitate spontaneous abortion in humans. The fetus may be stillborn or die within hours of a disseminated form of listerial infection known as granulomatosis infantiseptica, which is characterized by widespread microabscesses and granulomas that are particularly prevalent in the liver and spleen. In this entity, abundant bacteria often are visible on Gram stain of meconium.[81,82]

More commonly, neonatal infection manifests similarly to group B streptococcal disease in one of two forms[2]: (1) early-onset sepsis syndrome, usually associated with prematurity and probably acquired in utero; or (2) late-onset meningitis, occurring at about 2 weeks of age in term infants, who most likely acquired organisms from the maternal vagina at parturition. Cases have occurred after cesarean delivery, however, and nosocomial transmission also has been suggested.

In early-onset disease, *L. monocytogenes* can be isolated from the conjunctivae, external ear, nose, throat, meconium, amniotic fluid, placenta, blood, and, sometimes, CSF. Gram stain of meconium may show gram-positive rods and provide early diagnosis. The highest concentrations of bacteria are found in the neonatal lung and gut, which suggests that infection is acquired in utero from infected amniotic fluid, rather than via a hematogenous route.[83] Purulent conjunctivitis and a disseminated papular rash have been described rarely in neonates with early-onset disease, but clinical infection is otherwise similar to that due to other bacterial pathogens.

Bacteremia

Bacteremia without an evident focus is the most common manifestation of listeriosis after the neonatal period.[1,2,11] Clinical manifestations typically include fever and myalgias; a prodromal illness with nausea and diarrhea can occur.

Central Nervous System Infection

Organisms that cause bacterial meningitis most frequently *(Streptococcus pneumoniae, Neisseria meningitidis,* and *Haemophilus influenzae)* rarely cause parenchymal brain infections such as cerebritis and brain abscess. By contrast, *L. monocytogenes* has tropism for the brain itself (particularly the brainstem), as well as for the meninges.[2,7] Many patients with meningitis experience altered consciousness, seizures, or movement disorders and truly have meningoencephalitis.

Meningitis

A 1995 active surveillance study of bacterial meningitis showed that *L. monocytogenes* accounted for 20% of cases in neonates and 20% in those >60 years of age.[84] Worldwide, *L. monocytogenes* is one of the three major causes of neonatal meningitis, is second only to pneumococcus as a cause of bacterial meningitis in adults >50 years, and is the most common cause of bacterial meningitis in patients with lymphoma, organ transplants, or those receiving corticosteroid immunosuppressive therapy for any reason.[2,85-87]

Clinically, meningitis due to *L. monocytogenes* usually is similar to that due to more common causes;[88] features particular to listerial meningitis are summarized in Table 132-1.

The first prospective study of meningitis due to *L. monocytogenes* was reported in 2006.[89] In this nationwide cohort study from the Netherlands, notable clinical features of 30 cases of listerial meningitis included headache in 88%, nausea in 83%, and fever in 90%; but only 75% of patients had a stiff neck at the time of presentation. A focal neurologic deficit was present in 37% (likely reflective of propensity for brain parenchymal involvement). Only 43% had the classic meningitis triad of fever, neck stiffness, and change in mental status. At the time of presentation, 19 out of 30 patients had symptoms persisting for greater than 24 hours and 8 had symptoms for ≥4 days. Remarkable CSF findings included a median white blood cell count of 620 (range 24–16,003) and protein of 252 mg/dL. Gram stain of CSF revealed a gram-positive rod in only 28% of patients, and blood cultures were positive in only 46% of patients. Sequelae in survivors included hemiparesis in two patients and cranial nerve palsies in two others; mortality was 15%.

Brainstem Encephalitis (Rhombencephalitis)

An unusual form of listerial encephalitis involves the brainstem[90] and is similar to the unique zoonotic listerial infection known as circling disease of sheep.[91] In contrast to other listerial CNS infections, this illness usually occurs in healthy older children and adults; neonatal cases have not been reported. The typical clinical picture is one of a biphasic illness with a prodrome of fever, headache, nausea, and vomiting lasting about 4 days, followed by the abrupt onset of asymmetric cranial nerve deficits, cerebellar signs, and hemiparesis or hemisensory deficits, or both. Respiratory failure develops in about 40% of cases. Nuchal rigidity is present in about 50%. CSF is only mildly abnormal, and CSF culture is positive in about one-third; almost two-thirds are bacteremic. Magnetic resonance imaging is superior to computed tomography for demonstrating rhombencephalitis.[90,92] Mortality is high, and serious sequelae are common in survivors.

Brain Abscess

Macroscopic brain abscesses account for about 10% of CNS listerial infections. Bacteremia is almost always present, and concomitant meningitis with isolation of *L. monocytogenes* from the CSF is found in 25%; both of these features are rare in other forms of bacterial brain abscess.[93] About 50% of cases occur in known risk groups for listerial infection. Subcortical abscesses located in the thalamus, pons, and medulla are common; these sites are exceedingly rare when abscesses are due to other bacteria. Mortality is high, and survivors usually have serious sequelae.[94]

Endocarditis

Listerial endocarditis accounts for about 7.5% of adult listerial infections,[7] affects the population at risk for viridans streptococcal endocarditis, produces both native valve and prosthetic valve disease, and has a high rate of septic complications and a mortality of 48%.[95] Cases in children are rare.

Localized Infection

Rare reports of focal infections from which *L. monocytogenes* has been isolated include direct inoculation resulting in conjunctivitis,[25] skin infection,[96] and lymphadenitis.[7] BSI can lead to hepatic infection,[97,98] cholecystitis,[99] peritonitis,[100,101] splenic abscess,[8] pleuropulmonary infection,[102-104] pyogenic arthritis,[105] osteomyelitis,[106] pericarditis,[107] myocarditis,[108] arteritis,[109] and endophthalmitis.[7] Complications, including disseminated intravascular coagulation,[110] adult respiratory distress syndrome,[111] and rhabdomyolysis with acute renal failure,[112] have been documented. There is nothing clinically unique about these localized infections; many, but not all, have occurred in those known to be at risk for listeriosis.

Febrile Gastroenteritis

Many patients with invasive listeriosis have a history of antecedent gastrointestinal illness, often accompanied by fever. Although isolated cases of gastrointestinal illness due to *L. monocytogenes*

TABLE 132-1. Distinctive Features of Listerial Meningitis Compared with More Common Bacterial Etiologies

Feature	Rate of Occurrence (%)
CLINICAL AND LABORATORY	
Subacute presentation is more common (>24 hours)	~60
Unimpaired neck movement is more common	25
Movement disorders (ataxia, tremors, myoclonus) are more common	15–20
Seizures are more common	~25
Fluctuating mental status is common	~75
Focal neurologic findings are more common	35–40
Positive blood culture is more common	75
CEREBROSPINAL FLUID (CSF)	
Positive Gram stain is less common	40
Normal CSF glucose is more common	>60
Mononuclear cell predominance is more common	~30

BOX 132-1. Clinical Settings in Which Listeriosis Should Be Considered

- Septicemia or meningitis in infants <2 months of age
- Meningitis or parenchymal brain infection in a patient with:
  (a) hematologic malignancy, acquired immunodeficiency syndrome, organ transplantation, corticosteroid or antitumor-necrosis factor immunosuppression;
  (b) subacute presentation;
  (c) adult >50 years; and
  (d) cerebrospinal fluid (CSF) shows gram-positive bacilli
- Simultaneous infection of the meninges and brain parenchyma
- Subcortical brain abscess
- Fever during pregnancy
- Blood, CSF, or other normally sterile specimen reported to have "diphtheroids" on Gram stain or culture
- Foodborne outbreak of febrile gastroenteritis when routine cultures fail to identify a pathogen

appear to be quite rare,[113] at least seven outbreaks of foodborne gastroenteritis due to *L. monocytogenes* have been documented.[114] In the largest outbreak to date, 1566 individuals, most of them children between the ages of 6 and 10, became ill after eating caterer-provided cafeteria food at two schools, and 19% were hospitalized.[115] Illness typically occurs 24 hours (range 6 hours to 10 days) after ingestion of a large inoculum of bacteria and usually lasts 1 to 3 days (range 1 to 7 days); attack rates are high (52% to 100%). Common symptoms include fever, watery diarrhea, nausea, headache, and pains in joints and muscles. Vehicles of infection have included chocolate milk, cold corn and tuna salad, cold smoked trout, and deli meat. *L. monocytogenes* should be considered to be a possible etiology in outbreaks of febrile gastroenteritis when routine cultures fail to yield a pathogen.

DIAGNOSIS

Listeriosis should be considered strongly as part of the differential diagnosis in any of the clinical settings shown in Box 132-1. Diagnosis requires isolation of *L. monocytogenes* from clinical specimens (e.g., CSF, blood) and identification through standard microbiologic techniques. Antibodies to listeriolysin O have not proved useful in invasive disease,[116] nor have polymerase chain reaction probes.[117] Antibodies to listeriolysin O may be useful during investigations of outbreaks of febrile gastroenteritis.[118] MRI is superior to CT for demonstrating parenchymal brain involvement, especially in the brainstem.[90,92]

TREATMENT

Comprehensive reviews of treatment are available.[119,120] No controlled trials have established drug of choice or duration of therapy for listerial infection. Ampicillin generally is considered the preferred agent.[7,120–122] Based on synergy in vitro and in animal models,[123] most authorities suggest adding gentamicin to ampicillin for treatment of BSI in those with severely impaired T-lymphocyte function and in all cases of meningitis and endocarditis.[120] In one non-randomized study,[124] the combination of TMP-SMX plus ampicillin was associated with a lower failure rate and fewer neurologic sequelae than ampicillin combined with an aminoglycoside.

For those intolerant of penicillins, TMP-SMX is the best alternative.[120,125–127] In rare instances, oral TMP-SMX has been used effectively.[128] No currently available cephalosporin should be used; none has adequate activity,[120,129] and meningitis has developed in patients receiving cephalosporins.[130] For this reason, ampicillin is always included in empiric therapy for septicemia or meningitis in infants <2 months of age.

Vancomycin has been used successfully in a few patients with penicillin allergy,[131,132] but other patients have developed listerial meningitis while receiving the drug.[133] Rifampin is active in vitro; clinical experience is minimal, however, and in animal models the addition of rifampin to ampicillin was not more effective than was ampicillin used alone.[121] While fluoroquinolones and linezolid show good in vitro activity, clinical experience is mixed,[134–136] and, to date, too limited to support recommending these agents for therapy.

Initial dosing of antibiotics as for meningitis is prudent for all patients, even in the absence of CNS or CSF abnormalities, because of the high affinity of this organism for the CNS. Patients with meningitis should be treated for no fewer than 3 weeks; bacteremic patients without CSF abnormalities can be treated for 2 weeks.

No data exist concerning antimicrobial efficacy in listerial gastroenteritis; the illness is self-limited, and treatment is not warranted.

In patients with iron deficiency, it seems prudent to withhold iron replacement until infection resolves.

Nine neonates with septicemia, pneumonia, and severe respiratory failure due to *L. monocytogenes* who were supported by venoarterial bypass have been reported, with recovery in 6 infants. The duration of extracorporeal membrane oxygenation was comparatively prolonged (median, 9 days), probably because of the necrotizing nature of listerial lung infection.[137]

PREVENTION

Recommendations for prevention of listeriosis from a foodborne source are presented in Box 132-2.[138,139]

Neonatal listerial infection complicating successive pregnancies is virtually unheard of, and intrapartum antibiotic therapy is not recommended for mothers with a history of perinatal listeriosis. There is no vaccine. Listerial infections are effectively prevented by TMP-SMX given as PCP prophylaxis to recipients of organ transplants or to individuals with the human immunodeficiency virus.[140]

BOX 132-2. Dietary Recommendations for Preventing Foodborne Listeriosis

FOR ALL PERSONS

1. Cook raw food from animal sources (e.g., beef, pork, and poultry) thoroughly
2. Wash raw vegetables thoroughly before eating
3. Keep uncooked meats separate from vegetables, cooked foods, and ready-to-eat foods
4. Avoid consumption of raw (unpasteurized) milk or foods made from raw milk
5. Wash hands, knives, and cutting boards after handling uncooked foods

ADDITIONAL RECOMMENDATIONS FOR PERSONS AT HIGH RISK[a]

1. Avoid soft cheeses (e.g., Mexican-style, feta, Brie, Camembert) and blue-veined cheese; there is no need to avoid hard cheeses, cream cheese, cottage cheese, or yogurt
2. Reheat until steaming hot leftover foods or ready-to-eat foods (e.g., hot dogs) before eating
3. Consider avoidance of foods in delicatessen counters[b]

[a] Those immunocompromised by illness or medications, pregnant women, and the elderly.
[b] Although the risk for listeriosis associated with foods from delicatessen counters is relatively low, pregnant women and immunosuppressed persons may choose to avoid these foods or to reheat cold cuts thoroughly before consumption.

MICROBIOLOGY

- Gram-positive rod; often mistaken for diphtheroids, streptococci or enterococci
- Isolation of a "diphtheroid" from a normally sterile body fluid, particularly CSF, should alert the clinician to possibility of listeriosis

EPIDEMIOLOGY

- Zoonotic illness, particularly in herd animals
- Mother-to-fetus/neonate transmission in utero or a time of birth in humans
- After neonatal period infection typically foodborne illness; highest risk with deli-style ready-to-eat meats and unpasteurized cheeses
- At-risk populations include neonates, pregnant women, and those with impaired cell-mediated immunity due to disease (e.g. lymphoma, AIDS) or therapy (corticosteroids, anti-TNF agents)

CLINICAL FEATURES

- Bloodstream and meningoencephalitis most common invasive infections

- Meningitis can be subacute
- Neonatal infection occurs as both early- and late-onset similar disease, similar to group B streptococcus
- Can cause acute febrile gastroenteritis; consider especially in foodborne outbreak with negative routine stool cultures

DIAGNOSIS

- Consider listeriosis especially in the following: sepsis or meningitis in infants <2 months of age; meningitis or parenchymal brain infection in those with impaired cell-mediated immunity; fever during pregnancy; subcortical brain abscess or brainstem infection

TREATMENT

- Ampicillin plus gentamicin is recommended for CNS infection
- Cephalosporins are not adequate therapy
- Trimethoprim-sulfamethoxazole is recommended for penicillin allergic patients

133 Other Gram-Positive Bacilli

Denise F. Bratcher

Many pleomorphic, nonsporulating gram-positive bacilli have long been identified as "diphtheroids" and dismissed as contaminants. Because many can cause endocarditis and other serious diseases, especially in immunosuppressed patients, coryneform bacteria isolated from clinical specimens should be identified routinely, particularly if they are found in pure culture or are from multiple specimens or immunocompromised patients.

ERYSIPELOTHRIX RHUSIOPATHIAE

Erysipelothrix rhusiopathiae, first isolated in 1878 from mice by Koch, was later identified as the cause of swine erysipelas and as a human pathogen. In recent years, *E. rhusiopathiae* has been more commonly recognized as a cause of serious human diseases.[1]

Microbiology

E. rhusiopathiae is a gram-positive, pleomorphic, nonspore-forming, nonmotile, encapsulated, aerobic, or facultatively anaerobic bacillus. Due to the propensity for older colonies to lose cell wall integrity, the bacillus also can appear to be gram-negative or gram-variable. The organism grows readily on standard media and in conventional blood culture systems. Both rough and smooth colonies are noted on blood agar. Smears from rough colonies can show granular, nonbranching filaments. Some strains produce α-hemolysis in 48 to 72 hours. *E. rhusiopathiae* is readily distinguished from other morphologically similar gram-positive bacteria (*Listeria* species and diphtheroids) by absence of motility, negative catalase reaction, and production of hydrogen sulfide (H₂S). *E. rhusiopathiae* also is oxidase- and urease-negative and produces acid from glucose and lactose. A "test-tube brush" or "pipe cleaner" pattern of growth in gelatin stab cultures is highly characteristic.

Epidemiology

E. rhusiopathiae is a ubiquitous organism that primarily is a pathogen of animals. It has been isolated from wild mammals, various fowl, fish, shellfish, and domestic animals, such as pigs, sheep, cattle, and horses.[1,2] Contaminated soil is thought to be a source. Human infections often are due to occupational exposure to infected animals or contaminated animal products. Persons at risk include slaughterhouse workers, butchers, poultry workers, fishermen, fish marketers, veterinarians, farmers, and housewives.[2] There is a greater incidence of human infections in summer months. A 4:1 male preponderance may reflect male occupational exposure.

Clinical Manifestations

There are three major forms of clinical disease: (1) the most common, *localized*, self-limited, *cutaneous* form known as erysipeloid (because it resembles streptococcal erysipelas); (2) a *diffuse cutaneous* form with multiple skin lesions and systemic symptoms; and (3) a *systemic* form including septicemia and endocarditis. Erysipeloid is a painful, inflammatory lesion of the skin that usually involves the hands and fingers and commonly occurs at the site of a scratch that has become contaminated by contact with animals or other infectious material. The incubation period is 1 to 7 days after inoculation and usually is <4 days. The lesion appears with a characteristic purplish-red hue and irregular, raised borders that spread peripherally as central clearing occurs. The lesion can spread proximally to involve an adjacent joint. Although characterized by recurrences, erysipeloid usually is self-limiting, with spontaneous recovery in 1 to 4 weeks.

The rarely reported diffuse cutaneous form of *E. rhusiopathiae* infection, with progression of violaceous lesions remote from the initial site, is associated more frequently with systemic symptoms. These include fever, malaise, arthralgia, myalgia, and severe headache. Although not accompanied by bacteremia, the clinical course of this form is more protracted and often is complicated by recurrences.[2-4]

Septicemia and endocarditis are rare complications of *E. rhusiopathiae* infections, including occupationally acquired diseases.[1] In >50 reported cases of bloodstream infection (BSI) due to *E. rhusiopathiae*, approximately 90% were associated with endocarditis, which manifests as an acute or subacute process and is predated by erysipeloid lesions in only 36% of cases. Infection commonly affects normal hosts and native valves and involves the aortic valve in 70% of reported cases; approximately 40% of patients have previous heart disease. Intracranial complications are reported.[5-8]

A variety of other infections associated with *E. rhusiopathiae* have been reported: BSI resulting from colonic perforation by a toothpick, BSI in a patient with lupus nephritis and another with human immunodeficiency virus (HIV) infection, chronic meningitis, pyogenic arthritis, infected arthroplasty, peritonitis associated with peritoneal dialysis, intra-abdominal abscess, necrotizing fasciitis, and infection following cat bites.[4,9-19]

Reported infections in children include endocarditis; BSI in the settings of acute leukemia, systemic lupus erythematosus, and HIV infection; systemic disease and pleural effusions; and localized infection of the knee.[3,6,20,21]

Diagnosis

The diagnosis of erysipeloid predominantly relies on clinical recognition and an epidemiologic link to animal exposure. Because the organism is located deep in the reticular layer of the dermis, successful isolation of the organism from a skin lesion requires full-thickness biopsy obtained from the peripheral quadrant of the lesion.[4] *E. rhusiopathiae* is isolated from blood in patients with septicemia or endocarditis. A high index of suspicion is necessary, as these isolates occasionally are misidentified as streptococci or considered insignificant diphtheroids.[2,11] Serologic diagnostic methods are unreliable, but polymerase chain reaction methods may improve diagnostic accuracy in the future.[3]

Treatment

Penicillin is considered the drug of choice for *E. rhusiopathiae* infections, based on exquisite susceptibility in vitro and limited clinical experience. The most active antibiotics against *E. rhusiopathiae* in vitro are penicillin and imipenem, followed by cefotaxime, clindamycin, tetracycline, and chloramphenicol. The organism consistently is resistant to aminoglycosides, vancomycin, teicoplanin and trimethoprim-sulfamethoxazole.[19] Vancomycin resistance is noteworthy, since it frequently is used as empiric therapy for endocarditis, especially in patients allergic to penicillin. Oral penicillin therapy usually is adequate for erysipeloid; BSI and endocarditis caused by *E. rhusiopathiae* are best treated with aqueous penicillin G, 12 to 20 million units daily, given intravenously in divided doses every 4 hours for 4 to 6 weeks.[1,2] No data exist to evaluate in vitro synergy with an aminoglycoside. Considerations for penicillin-allergic patients include cephalosporins, imipenem, and fluoroquinolones.[22]

ROTHIA DENTOCARIOSA

Microbiology

Rothia dentocariosa is a nonmotile, nonspore-forming, nonacid-fast, gram-positive bacillus with variable morphology – from coccoid to branching filamentous forms. Preferring aerobic conditions, *R. dentocariosa* grows less well in microaerophilic environments. The organism is slow-growing and occasionally is isolated from anaerobic cultures that have been held longer than aerobic cultures. Colonies are either smooth and convex or rough with a "spoke-wheel" surface with scalloped edges.[23] *R. dentocariosa* produces acid from glucose, sucrose, maltose, and glycerol, is

catalase-positive and oxidase-, indole-, and urease-negative (although urease-positive and catalase-negative strains have been identified). *R. dentocariosa* hydrolyzes esculin, reduces nitrate, produces hydrogen sulfide, and typically is identified correctly by commercial identification systems.

Epidemiology

R. dentocariosa was first isolated from dental caries in 1949 and currently remains a constituent of carious teeth.[24] Considered normal flora of the human mouth, this organism's pathogenic potential has been confirmed by a growing body of case reports, predominantly involving infective endocarditis.

Clinical Manifestations

The first human infection involving *R. dentocariosa*, a periappendiceal abscess, was reported in 1975. Since then, rare *R. dentocariosa* infections have been reported in normal hosts: BSI, periodontitis, and pericoronitis, maxillary cyst, pilonidal cyst, and endocarditis.[25-34] Endocarditis associated with *R. dentocariosa* is reported most commonly, and typically involves native valves with pre-existing cardiac abnormalities in patients with carious dentition, periodontitis, or dental manipulation; prosthetic valves are involved occasionally.[28-38] Complications of endocarditis include brain abscess, multiple intracranial hemorrhages, mycotic aneurysms, and subarachnoid hemorrhages and aneurysm.[29-33] Two reported patients also had an underlying malignancy.[28,36] Additionally, *R. dentocariosa* has caused pneumonia in patients with underlying lung cancer and leukemia, BSI associated with leukemia, peritonitis associated with peritoneal dialysis, and arteriovenous fistula infection in a diabetic patient who was undergoing hemodialysis.[39-43] A proposed etiologic association with cat-scratch disease was not verified.

Few *R. dentocariosa* infections have involved children.[34] Reported cases include BSI without endocarditis (in a neonate); and complicating lymphoproliferative disease following renal transplantation, congenital heart disease, and herpangina. Case reports also include a case of severe exudative tonsillitis in a healthy 4-year-old child and corneal abscess in an 11-year-old boy who wet his fingertip with saliva before rubbing his eye.[44-48]

Treatment

Penicillin appears to be the drug of choice for *R. dentocariosa* infections, based on clinical experience of cure in patients with endocarditis.[28-31,33,35-38] Most treatments also included an aminoglycoside. Although data are limited, the organism consistently is susceptible in vitro to penicillin, ampicillin, cephalothin, third-generation cephalosporins, erythromycin, rifampin, and vancomycin and is variably susceptible to clindamycin, aminoglycosides, tetracycline, and trimethoprim-sulfamethoxazole. Determination of in vitro susceptibilities is advisable because individual instances of β-lactam resistance and other variable resistance patterns have been described. Treatment failure has been observed in a few cases of endocarditis initially treated with vancomycin.

RHODOCOCCUS (CORYNEBACTERIUM) EQUI

Microbiology

Rhodococcus (Corynebacterium) equi is a gram-positive, encapsulated, intracellular bacillus, varying from coccoid to long and club-shaped. *R. equi* produces small, white, mucoid colonies initially, which become large, salmon-colored colonies on standard media in approximately 4 days. The bacillus can demonstrate a weak acid-fast reaction due to the presence of mycolic acids in its cell walls, and does not ferment carbohydrates or liquefy gelatin. It is catalase-positive and oxidase-negative. *R. equi* strains have been categorized as virulent, of intermediate virulence, and avirulent on the basis of virulence-associated antigens and plasmids.[49]

Epidemiology

R. equi is a well-established pathogen in animals. The first human infection, a lung abscess, was described in 1967. A continually increasing number of *R. equi* infections have been reported subsequently, occurring predominantly among immunocompromised patients.[50] The natural habitat of *R. equi* is soil; infections are believed to be acquired through the respiratory route. *R. equi* is an intracellular organism, surviving and replicating in macrophages by preventing fusion of phagolysosomes.[51] Many infected patients have had contact with animals.

Clinical Manifestations

The majority of *R. equi* reports involve patients infected with HIV in whom the associated mortality rate is >50% (versus 20% in non-HIV-infected patients).[52] The lung is the most commonly reported site among both immunocompetent and immunocompromised populations, with increasing reports among solid-organ transplant recipients.[53] The clinical course of pneumonia mimics mycobacterial disease, with necrotizing, cavitary lesions and common involvement of the upper lobe.[54] Empyema, lung abscess, mediastinitis, malakoplakia, and other pulmonary manifestations have been described.[54–59] Other reported clinical associations among immunocompetent and immunocompromised hosts include BSI; diarrhea; meningitis; abscesses of the brain, thyroid, adrenal glands, liver, spleen, and paravertebral area; skin and soft-tissue infections; lymphadenitis; mastoiditis; peritonitis; granulomatous hepatitis; colonic polyps; pericarditis; osteomyelitis; mandibular osteitis; foot mycetoma and disseminated infection; endophthalmitis; orbital implant infection and peritonitis complicating chronic ambulatory peritoneal dialysis.[60–86]

R. equi infections occasionally have been reported in children, often involving extrapulmonary sites. These include pneumonia (complicated by brain abscesses, and cavitary lesion in patients with acquired immunodeficiency syndrome (AIDS)), BSI (alone or associated with pneumonia and lymphadenitis), malakoplakia, eye infections, meningitis resulting from orbital trauma, osteomyelitis following trauma, and wound infection resulting in pyogenic arthritis.[76,87–95] *R. equi* infections are reported less commonly among immunocompromised children than adults; infections have been reported in children with HIV, leukemia, ependymoma; toxic epidermal necrolysis, and congenital hepatic fibrosis with polycystic kidney disease.[77,87–94]

Treatment

The optimal treatment of *R. equi* infections is unknown and many different methods of susceptibility testing have been applied in case reports. Widespread resistance and tolerance to β-lactam agents, tetracyclines, macrolides, chloramphenicol, and rifampin have been noted. *R. equi* is resistant to intracellular killing by macrophages; therefore treatment requires use of an antibiotic with intracellular activity. Combinations of antibiotics with bactericidal activity are recommended strongly because antibiotic-resistant mutants can easily be selected using monotherapy.[56] Choice is based on antimicrobial susceptibility and intracellular penetration. Some experts suggest initial treatment with vancomycin plus imipenem, rifampin, erythromycin, teicoplanin, ciprofloxacin, or aminoglycoside followed by oral therapy with a combination of erythromycin plus rifampin, erythromycin plus ciprofloxacin, or rifampin plus ciprofloxacin. Others suggest initial intravenous combination therapy including imipenem as optimal. Azithromycin in combination with others appears appropriate due to high tissue levels.[96] Levofloxacin also has been used with rifampin.[97,98] Because of the high incidence of relapse among immunocompromised patients, especially those with HIV infection, treatment is recommended for at least 2 months, and possibly up to 6 months.[56,99] Surgical drainage or resection of lesions often is required.

GARDNERELLA VAGINALIS

Gardnerella vaginalis, formerly known as *Haemophilus vaginalis* and *Corynebacterium vaginale*, has been implicated as the cause of bacterial vaginosis (BV) since 1955. *G. vaginalis* is consistently isolated as the predominant organism in women with BV, but its role in the pathogenesis of this syndrome is confounded by isolation rates of up to 69% from vaginal specimens from healthy women.[100]

Microbiology and Pathogenesis

G. vaginalis is a facultatively anaerobic, nonmotile, pleomorphic, gram-negative or gram-variable bacillus that is oxidase-and catalase-negative. Electron microscopic studies demonstrate a cell wall consistent with gram-positive and gram-negative organisms and a laminated cell wall typical of neither. *G. vaginalis* ferments a wide variety of carbohydrates, producing acetic acid as an end product. *G. vaginalis* does not reduce nitrate or hydrolyze urea. Colonies on blood agar are 0.3 to 0.5 mm in diameter after 48 hours of incubation, demonstrating a distinct β-hemolysis on human and rabbit blood agar but not on sheep agar.

The ability of *G. vaginalis* to adhere to vaginal and urinary epithelial cells at a pH of 5 to 6 is thought to contribute to its role in the pathogenesis of BV and urinary tract infections.[101] It is hypothesized that other undefined factors disturb the ecologic balance between *G. vaginalis* and *Lactobacillus* species in the female genital tract, allowing *G. vaginalis* and anaerobic organisms to proliferate, which leads to BV.[102]

G. vaginalis also produces phospholipase, which breaks down phospholipids to arachidonic acid, producing a cascade of prostaglandins that may explain the relationship between BV and the onset of preterm labor.[103]

Epidemiology

The incidence of bacterial vaginosis due to *G. vaginalis* is difficult to define because of prominence in normal flora. Sexual transmission is proposed as the main mode of transmission, supported by isolation of *G. vaginalis* of the same biotype from urethral cultures of men and their partners with BV.[104] Colonization of the genital tract also may result from transfer from an endogenous intestinal site.[105]

G. vaginalis is rare among prepubertal females but has been found in vaginal cultures of children with and without a history of sexual contact.[106–110] In a study of prepubertal males with no history of suspected or known sexual abuse, *G. vaginalis* colonization of the urethra, glans, or rectum was not found.[111] The presence of *G. vaginalis* in a vaginal specimen from a prepubertal female or isolation from a symptomatic prepubertal boy should heighten suspicion of sexual abuse but is not incontrovertible evidence of sexual abuse (see Chapter 56, Infectious Diseases in Child Abuse).[108,111]

Clinical Manifestations

Clinical features of BV are addressed in Chapter 53, Urethritis, Vulvovaginitis, and Cervicitis. *G. vaginalis* also is a cause of postpartum or postabortion septicemia and is associated with fever, vaginal discharge, abdominal tenderness, and leukocytosis.[112] BSI has been described rarely in women undergoing gynecologic procedures and in men following urologic surgery. *G. vaginalis* infection has been associated with endometritis, chorioamnionitis, episiotomy and hysterectomy wound infections, intra-uterine infections, and vaginal abscess.[112,113] Urinary tract infections (UTIs) have occurred in both sexes, especially in pregnant women and renal transplant recipients.[114] Balanoposthitis, nonspecific urethritis, cystitis, and prostatitis in males have been associated with *G. vaginalis*.[113,115] Lung abscess, empyema, and BSI resulting from inhalation pneumonia were reported in an individual with alcoholism.[116]

Neonates have been reported with *G. vaginalis* septicemia, meningitis, cellulitis, conjunctivitis, and pneumonia.[117–121] *G. vaginalis* also has been the presumed cause of osteomyelitis complicating a cephalhematoma following use of an internal scalp electrode, and early-onset infection of a scalp hematoma.[122,123] *G. vaginalis* grew from the purulent exudate of a 20-month-old boy with balanitis; no evidence of sexual abuse was found.[111] The only other reports of *G. vaginalis* infection among pediatric patients are UTIs.[124]

Diagnosis

Culture of vaginal secretions is not recommended for diagnosis of BV.[125] Direct smear, especially Gram stain, is the preferred diagnostic test (to assess relative numbers of *G. vaginalis* and *Lactobacillus* species). On direct examination of vaginal secretions from patients with BV, clue cells (epithelial cells coated peripherally with *G. vaginalis*) are observed (see Figure 53-1).[125] Addition of 10% potassium hydroxide to specimen results in a fishy, amine-like odor (known as the amine, or whiff, test). Clinical criteria for diagnosis of BV include the following: (1) vaginal pH >4.5; (2) positive results on the whiff test; (3) presence of clue cells; and (4) homogeneous vaginal discharge. The indirect fluorescent antibody method also is available to detect *G. vaginalis* in specimens of vaginal secretions. Identification of the organism from culture is based on the demonstration of thin gram-variable rods that are catalase-negative, growing with a narrow zone of β-hemolysis after 48 hours of incubation.

Treatment

Metronidazole (1 g/day orally in two divided doses for 7 days) is the drug of choice for treatment of BV: initial cure rates are ≥90%.[113] Other options include orally administered clindamycin (600 mg/day in two divided doses for 7 days), intravaginally applied metronidazole gel (0.75%, 5 g or one applicator once daily for 5 days) or clindamycin cream (2%, 5 g or one applicator at bedtime for 7 days). Treatment of sexual partners has not been shown to alter the clinical course of BV or to prevent relapsing or recurrent infections.[126,127] Development of metronidazole resistance after treatment has been noted.[128] *G. vaginalis* isolates are susceptible in vitro to penicillin, ampicillin, erythromycin, clindamycin, chloramphenicol, and trimethoprim, which provides several options for treatment of extragenital infections.[129]

LACTOBACILLUS SPECIES

Epidemiology and Microbiology

Lactobacillus species are normal flora of the mouth, gastrointestinal tract, and female genital tract, where they produce lactic acid (affecting a low pH) and competitively inhibit pathogenic organisms. *Lactobacillus* species are associated with dental caries.[130,131] Lactobacilli are small, slender, nonmotile, gram-positive bacilli in chains. Immature colonies appear smooth, convex, and translucent. Organisms are microaerophilic or anaerobic and oxidase- and catalase-negative; they hydrolyze esculin and ferment carbohydrates.

Clinical Manifestations

Usually regarded as commensals or contaminants in clinical specimens, lactobacilli increasingly are identified as pathogens. Endocarditis is the most common infection, frequently associated with a structural heart defect or an immunocompromised state, including cardiac transplant.[132–134] Previous dental manipulation or parturition is a common factor in the patient history. Endocarditis usually affects the left side of the heart and rarely involves prosthetic valves; pulmonic and tricuspid valve involvement has been reported.[135,136] Species associated with endocarditis include *L. acidophilus*, *L. casei* (subspecies *alactosus*, *casei*, and *rhamnosus*), *L. fermentum*, *L. jensenii*, *L. plantarian*, and *L. salivarius*. Failure of antibiotic treatment of endocarditis has been described; and typically is associated with use of single-drug regimens.

Cases of *Lactobacillus* endocarditis have been noted in children.[137] Other infections reported in pediatric patients include *L. acidophilus* BSI in an infant,[138] *L. casei* BSI in a child with congenital HIV infection,[139] *L. rhamnosus* BSI and pericarditis in bone marrow transplant recipient,[140] and fatal pneumonia due to *L. rhamnosus* in a child with aplastic anemia.[141] Four children with *Lactobacillus* BSI were reported in a case series including *L. rhamnosus* in an infant with necrotic bowel, *L. sakei* ssp. *carnosus* in a neutropenic patient with an ependymoma, *L. curvatus* following trauma, and *L. paracasei* ssp. *paracasei* following a burn.[142] A retrospective review of clinical isolates identified 41 *Lactobacillus* species isolated from 40 children, including *l. acidophilus*, *L. fermentum*, *L. jensenii*, *L. catenaforme*, and others.[143] Sources for these isolates included abscesses (dental, subcutaneous, vulvovaginal, abdominal, subdiaphragmatic, lung, and tonsillar), pneumonia, ear infection, catheter-related BSI, and conjunctivitis. Infections were polymicrobial in 90% of patients.

Rarely reported clinical infections due to *Lactobacillus* species, typically among immunocompromised hosts, include BSI, pneumonia, empyema, abscesses (liver, spleen, pelvic, peritonsillar and retropharyngeal, and abdominal wall), peritonitis, endometritis, endophthalmitis, UTI, and empyema of the gallbladder.[144–160] Little is known about the pathogenesis of infection. The most common *Lactobacillus* species reported as pathogenic are *L. casei*, *L. fermentum*, and *L. acidophilus*, although species often are not identified completely. Infections are frequently polymicrobial.

Probiotic agent-related invasive disease attributable to *L. rhamnosus* GG is reported rarely in children. Short bowel syndrome appears to be the most common clinical association in children presenting with *L. rhamnosus* GG BSI after enteral *L. rhamnosus* GG therapy. Another child with congenital heart disease developed an atrial wall thrombus in association with *L. rhamnosus* GG BSI.[161–164]

Treatment

Lactobacillus species demonstrate intrinsic resistance to vancomycin and many cephalosporins.[165] High-dose penicillin and gentamicin are synergistic, and combination therapy is considered the standard of care in endocarditis and other serious or deep-seated infections. Because reported *Lactobacillus* isolates have had unusual and varied antimicrobial susceptibility, decisions regarding antibiotic therapy are best guided by clinical presentation and susceptibility testing of the specific isolate.

TSUKAMURELLA SPECIES

Epidemiology and Microbiology

Tsukamurella species were first isolated from the ovaries of bed bugs in 1941 and also have been found in soil and sludge. The first human isolate, then known as *Gordona aurantiaca*, was described in 1971 from sputum samples of patients with chronic pulmonary disorders.[166] On the basis of analysis of gene sequences, *Tsukamurella* was first proposed as a genus in 1988. Seven *Tsukamurella* species have been identified; five have been reported to cause infections in humans, including *T. inchonensis*, *T. paurometabola*, *T. pulmonis*, *T. strandjordae*, and *T. tyrosinoslovens*.[167]

Tsukamurella species are gram-positive, aerobic, nonmotile, nonspore-forming bacilli. They are partially acid fast due to mycolic acid in the cell envelope. They demonstrate rapid growth on MacConkey agar and appear as yellow, rough, irregular, flat, dry colonies. *Tsukamurella* species can be misidentified due to characteristics similar to *Rhodococcus*, *Nocardia*, and rapidly growing mycobacteria.[166] High-performance liquid chromatography or DNA sequence methods can identify organisms appropriately.

Clinical Manifestations

Rare reported *Tsukamurella* infections in humans are related to medical devices, including catheter-related BSI, peritoneal dialysis catheter-related peritonitis, infection related to an implantable cardioverter-defibrillator, knee prosthesis, and keratitis following trauma or corneal grafting.[166–175] *Tsukamurella* pulmonary infections have occurred in patients with underlying pulmonary disease, in an AIDS patient (with cavitary lesion), and as a cause of community-acquired pneumonia.[176–179] Local skin infection, subcutaneous abscess with necrotizing fasciitis, conjunctivitis, cerebellar abscess complicating chronic otitis media, and fatal meningitis in a leukemic patient have also been associated with *Tsukamurella* species.[166,167,180–182]

Among children, three cases of *Tsukamurella* BSI have been reported in immunosuppressed patients with central venous catheters: *T. strandjordae* in a patient with acute myelogenous leukemia;[183] *T. pulmonis* in a patient who underwent bone marrow transplant for severe combined immunodeficiency; and an untyped *Tsukamurella* species in an infant with myelodysplastic syndrome.[166]

Treatment

Limited data regarding antimicrobial susceptibility testing of *Tsukamurella* isolates are available, but reported susceptibility patterns are similar among different *Tsukamurella* species. *Tsukamurella* typically are resistant to penicillins, cephalosporins (including cefoxitin, which often is used empirically for nontuberculosis mycobacterial infections – one of a number of species for which *Tsukamurella* is easily confused). Susceptibility to amikacin, ciprofloxacin, clarithromycin, imipenem, and sulfamethoxazole is reported.[166] *T. paurometabola* demonstrates high-level resistance to imipenem.[184] Combination therapy has been suggested to treat *Tsukamurella* infections.[166,177] Catheter removal is indicated in catheter-related infections.

CELLULOSIMICROBIUM (FORMERLY *OERSKOVIA*) SPECIES

Epidemiology and Microbiology

Human infections caused by *Nocardia*-like, diphtheroid-like organisms of the *Cellulosimicrobium* (formerly *Oerskovia*) genus have been described rarely. The genus consists of two species, *C. cellulans* and *C. funkei*, formerly *O. xanthineolytica* and *O. turbata*, respectively, which are found in grass cuttings, aluminum hydroxide gel, and soil in many parts of the world. *Cellulosimicrobium* are gram-positive, branched, filamentous, nonacid-fast bacilli that fragment into motile rods. The bright yellow pigment of colonies is characteristic. Organisms produce acid from glucose, lactose, maltose, sucrose, and xylose, hydrolyze esculin, and reduce nitrate. They are catalase-positive and oxidase- and urease-negative.

Clinical Manifestations

Rare *Cellulosimicrobium* infections in human hosts usually involve immunocompromised hosts with indwelling foreign devices.

Individual case reports of *C. cellulans* BSI include patients with alcoholic cirrhosis, short bowel syndrome, colon cancer, and breast cancer.[185–188] Endocarditis was reported in bone marrow and renal transplant recipients.[189,190] *C. cellulans* has caused peritoneal dialysis-related peritonitis[191–193] (including in a 13-year-old with recurrent and culture-negative peritonitis),[193] ventriculoperitoneal shunt-associated meningitis,[194] a prosthetic knee joint infection,[195] endophthalmitis after penetrating foreign body,[196] flexor sheath tenosynovitis following multiple splinters,[197] keratitis in a contact-lens wearer,[198] and chronic tongue ulcerations in an HIV-infected patient.[199]

C. funkei was responsible for two cases of BSI (one in a patient with AIDS,[200] the other in a 3-year old child with leukemia[201]), endocarditis in a patient with Crohn disease associated with ankylosing spondylitis and aortic insufficiency,[202] and an axillary abscess in another patient with AIDS.[203] Individual cases of pyonephrosis[204] and BSI related to contaminated parenteral nutrition solution[205] were caused by unspecified *Cellulosimicrobium* species.

Treatment

Although antimicrobial susceptibility varies among isolates reported, *Cellulosimicrobium* species consistently are susceptible to vancomycin and imipenem (only three isolates reported); variably susceptible to amikacin, ampicillin, cephalosporins, ciprofloxacin, penicillin, tetracyclines, and trimethoprim-sulfamethoxazole; and resistant to clindamycin, erythromycin, gentamicin, and tobramycin. Optimal therapy generally involves removal of hardware.

KURTHIA SPECIES

Microbiology

Kurthia species are coryneform organisms identified as short, plump, nonspore-forming, aerobic gram-positive bacilli. Organisms grow poorly in anaerobic environments, demonstrate motility at 36°C but not at 21°C, are catalase-positive, oxidase-negative, and urease-positive after 24 hours and do not ferment carbohydrates or reduce nitrate.

Clinical Manifestations

Kurthia species have been isolated from clinical specimens, including feces, sputum, pilonidal cyst, and conjunctiva, although they were not considered significant clinically. The course of a 31-year-old narcotic user with *K. bessonii* native aortic valve endocarditis was complicated by cusp abscess and fistula.[206]

Treatment

Typically, organisms are susceptible to penicillin, ampicillin, carbenicillin, cephalothin, gentamicin, amikacin, erythromycin, chloramphenicol, and trimethoprim-sulfamethoxazole and resistant to oxacillin, clindamycin, and kanamycin.

134 *Mycobacterium tuberculosis*

Jeffrey R. Starke

The genus *Mycobacterium* consists of a diverse group of acid-fast bacilli (AFB) with a cell wall high in lipid content. The bacilli are aerobic, nonspore-forming, nonmotile, and slightly curved or straight, ranging in length from 1 to 10 μm and in width from 0.2 to 0.6 μm. Mycobacteria take up stain poorly but retain specific dyes despite treatment with acid-alcohol solutions. This property is demonstrated with fuchsin stain techniques (acid-fastness), such as the Ziehl–Neelsen and Kinyoun methods, or the fluorochrome method using auramine and rhodamine stains. The *M. tuberculosis* complex consists of *M. tuberculosis, M. bovis, M. africanum* (causing one-half of pulmonary tuberculosis in West Africa), *M. canetti* (may be an ancestral strain of *M. tuberculosis*), and several species that cause tuberculosis primarily in animals, and occasionally through animal exposure, in humans: *M. microti* (rodents), *M. pinnipedii* (acquatic mammals), and *M. capral* (animals in Europe).

IMMUNOLOGY

Clinical manifestations of *M. tuberculosis* infection in humans reflect the spectrum of immunologic responses, from asymptomatic infection and positive tuberculin skin test result to hematogenous dissemination with severe or fatal disease.[1-5] Dissemination is associated with a high frequency of a negative tuberculin skin test reaction and failure of T lymphocytes to proliferate in response to *M. tuberculosis* antigens. Progressive primary pulmonary tuberculosis represents an ineffective immune response and can be fulminant or life-threatening, with negative tuberculin skin test results in 20% to 30% of patients. By contrast, patients with tuberculous pleuritis have an effective immune response; few bacilli are present in the pleural fluid and tissue, the tuberculin skin test result is positive in 90% of cases, and resolution without therapy is common.[3,4] Immunologic defenses against mycobacteria are primarily mediated by T lymphocytes and macrophages. The central role of tumor necrosis factor (TNF) is evident by the greatly increased risk of tuberculosis among patients treated with anti-TNF monoclonal antibodies.[6,7] Although neutrophils and natural killer cells manifest mycobacteriostatic effects in vitro[5,8] and B-lymphocyte responses and antibodies can be demonstrated, their significance is unproved. Several recent reviews provide excellent descriptions of the full immune response to *M. tuberculosis*.[1-5]

EPIDEMIOLOGY

Transmission

Transmission of *M. tuberculosis* usually is person to person, by mucous droplets that become airborne when an individual with pulmonary tuberculosis coughs or sneezes.[9] Droplets containing tubercle bacilli dry, becoming droplet nuclei that can remain suspended in the air for hours. Only small droplet nuclei (<10 μm in diameter) reach alveoli. Transmission rarely occurs by direct contact with infected body fluids such as urine or wound drainage, or fomites such as syringes or gastric lavage tubes; improperly cleaned bronchoscopes have transmitted infection.

The most important marker of contagiousness is the presence of organisms on a smear of sputum.[10,11] Children with primary pulmonary tuberculosis have sparse bacilli in endobronchial secretions, little cough, and diminished force of cough; they rarely infect others.[12,13] Adolescents with reactivation pulmonary tuberculosis are potentially infectious.[14] For all patients with tuberculosis, caution must be used within medical facilities to avoid infection of healthcare personnel (HCP) and others.[15] Children with extensive disease, especially with attributes similar to adult-type tuberculosis (cavities, extensive upper-lobe infiltrates, productive cough, positive acid-fast smear of sputum), should be treated with the same infection control measures as used for adults.[15-17] Most outbreaks of tuberculosis in children's healthcare facilities have been linked to a parent or adult visitor.[18,19] Adult and adolescent hospital visitors to children with suspected tuberculosis should undergo screening for cough illness (and subsequent chest radiography) promptly to exclude them as transmissible sources of infection.[12,13]

The decision that a patient is no longer contagious usually is based on improvement in symptoms, decreased number of AFB in the sputum smear, changes in radiographic findings, and adherence to an effective treatment regimen.[15] Retrospective epidemiologic studies and studies of transmission to animals indicate that most infectious patients with drug-susceptible tuberculosis become noninfectious within 2 weeks of starting effective treatment. However, many patients become noninfectious within several days, and occasional patients (especially those with multiple-drug-resistant (MDR) organisms) remain infectious for weeks to months.

Mycobacterium tuberculosis Infection

It is estimated that one-third of the world's population is infected with the tubercle bacillus. In many areas of Africa and Asia, new infection rates for all ages are 2% to 5% annually. Specific data in children are lacking.[20] All countries except two (the United States and the Netherlands) have used Calmette–Guérin bacillus (formerly *bacille Calmette–Guérin* (BCG)) vaccine extensively, limiting population surveys for infection using the tuberculin skin test. Historical data also are lacking in the U.S., because *M. tuberculosis* infection was a reportable condition in only several states and because national surveys of infection rates in children were discontinued in 1971.

In the U.S., the estimated total risk of acquiring *M. tuberculosis* is <1% for children.[21] In some urban populations, the risk is substantially higher.[22] A 2003 study of New York City public schools showed that 9.7% of high-school students had positive tuberculin skin test (TST).[23] Although Los Angeles[24] and Houston[25] have had infection rates between 2% and 10% in elementary and high-school children, other large cities have an infection rate <1% in school-aged children. Many of these children are foreign born; testing for tuberculosis infection in children immigrating to the U.S. was begun only in 2007. The most efficient method of finding children infected with *M. tuberculosis* is through contact investigations of adults with contagious pulmonary tuberculosis.[26] On average, 30% to 50% of household contacts of a case have a reactive TST.

Mycobacterium tuberculosis Disease

The World Health Organization (WHO) estimates that 8 to 10 million people develop tuberculosis in the world every year and 2 to 3 million die from tuberculosis. Approximately 1.3 million cases of tuberculosis and 400,000 tuberculosis-related deaths occur annually among children <15 years of age.[27] There is no indication that tuberculosis case rates among adults or children in developing nations are declining; infection and disease rates are increasing, especially where HIV infection is prevalent. In many high-burden countries, children represent 40% to 50% of the population and tuberculosis case rates in children are underreported.

Because children acquire *M. tuberculosis* from adults, understanding the epidemiology of childhood tuberculosis requires thorough knowledge of the disease's epidemiology in adults. In the U.S., from 1953 to 1984, the incidence of tuberculosis declined an average of about 6% per year. Beginning in 1985, this downward trend was reversed for both adults and children. In 1993, 25,287 cases of tuberculosis were reported in the U.S., an 18% increase since 1985.[28] From 1985 through 1998, >85,000 additional cases of tuberculosis were reported than would have been expected if the previous decline had continued. Although there are multiple reasons for the resurgence, the most important causes were the epidemic of HIV infection, immigration of people to the U.S. from countries with high prevalence, and inadequate implementation of public health policy. Fortunately, with the invigoration of tuberculosis control efforts in the U.S. in the 1990s, the annual number of tuberculosis cases dropped to 11,545 in 2009.[28] Strategies to reduce tuberculosis among foreign-born persons should be directed toward early detection of disease and treatment of latent infection (Figure 134-1).[29-31]

When tuberculosis was more prevalent in the U.S., risk of exposure to a contagious adult was high and uniform throughout the population. At present, high risk of exposure is more confined to well-defined groups (Box 134-1). Among young adults in the U.S., tuberculosis is predominantly a disease of racial or ethnic minorities who are socially and economically disadvantaged. Approximately 58% of persons with tuberculosis are foreign-born, with

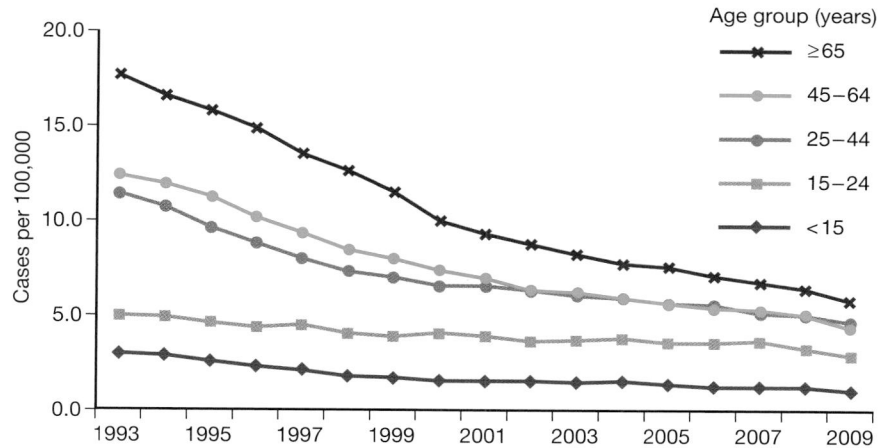

Figure 134-1. Reported tuberculosis cases per 100,000 people by age group in the United States, 1993 to 2009. (Data from the Centers for Disease Control and Prevention, Reported Tuberculosis in the United States, 2009. Atlanta, GA: U.S. Department of Health and Human Services, CDC, 2010.)

six countries (Mexico, Philippines, India, Vietnam, China, and Guatemala) accounting for 59% of the cases.[28] About 18% of persons bringing tuberculosis from other countries are identified within 5 years of immigration, suggesting either rapid development of disease after immigration or undetected tuberculosis disease during immigration.[28]

Residence in jails, prisons, or homeless shelters, use of illicit intravenous drugs, and social and economic disadvantage historically have been associated with increased risk of tuberculosis infection, especially in large urban sites. Metropolitan areas with >500,000 people accounted for 63% of the U.S. population and for 79% of tuberculosis cases in 2009.[28]

Between 1953 and 1980, the number of cases of childhood tuberculosis in the U.S. also declined to approximately 6% per year. From 1980 to 1987, case rates remained relatively flat, but they began a steady increase in 1988. In 1993, 1721 cases of tuberculosis were reported in children <15 years of age, a 40% increase over 1987. By 2009, the number of cases of tuberculosis in children <15 years of age had declined to 646, a reduction of 62% since 1993.[28]

Although there is no evidence that age or sex influences the likelihood of infection with *M. tuberculosis*, both factors probably influence the risk of development of disease.[32] Almost 60% of the U.S. childhood cases of tuberculosis occur in children <5 years of age.[33] Those >14 years of age also have higher risk of clinical disease, with the lowest risk during the interval between the ages 5 and 14 years. Age also affects the clinical site of infection.[34] Infants and younger children are more likely to have meningeal, disseminated, and lymphatic tuberculosis. Adolescents more commonly have pleural, genitourinary, or peritoneal disease. Among younger children, the sex ratio for clinical tuberculosis is equivalent, but girls may have a slightly higher incidence during adolescence.

In the U.S., eight states (Arizona, California, Florida, Georgia, Illinois, New York, Texas, and Washington) account for 61% of reported cases among children <5 years of age.[28] Childhood case rates are significantly higher among foreign-born and ethnic and racial minorities.[22] Most children are infected at home, but outbreaks also have occurred in elementary and high schools, nursery schools, daycare homes, and churches, and on school buses. In most cases, a highly contagious adult working in the area was the source case. During a 1994 outbreak in a St. Louis elementary school, in which a teacher had extensive, long-standing, unrecognized pulmonary tuberculosis, almost 50% of the students had *M. tuberculosis* infection and 11% had radiographic evidence of disease.[35]

Tuberculosis in Immunocompromised Children

Epidemiology of tuberculosis among children has been affected profoundly by the epidemic of HIV infection.[36-39] HIV-infected adults are more likely to have tuberculosis infection, pulmonary disease, lack of classic features allowing prompt diagnosis, and failure to respond rapidly to therapy. Children with HIV infection have higher risk of progressing from tuberculosis infection to disease after acquiring the organism.

Pulmonary tuberculosis is a defining condition for the diagnosis of acquired immunodeficiency syndrome (AIDS) for both adults and children. HIV-infected adults with pulmonary tuberculosis may be slightly less likely to have a positive acid-fast sputum smear than non-HIV-infected adults. Studies from Africa and New York City have suggested that HIV-seronegative and HIV-seropositive adults with smear-positive pulmonary tuberculosis are equally infectious. A retrospective study in Florida showed that an observed increase in childhood tuberculosis was linked to an increase in pulmonary tuberculosis among HIV-infected adults in the community.[40] Across the U.S., the highest rates in childhood tuberculosis over the past two decades have been in cities with high rates of HIV infection in the adult population.

Both clinical and autopsy studies in countries with high burdens of tuberculosis have demonstrated excessive risk of development of tuberculosis in most HIV-infected cohorts of children.[41-44] In both economically developing and developed nations, tuberculosis probably is underdiagnosed in HIV-infected children because

---

BOX 134-1. Positive Interpretation of Mantoux Tuberculin Test According to Diameter of Induration and Risk Category

INDURATION ≥5 MM IN DIAMETER

Contact with infectious case
Abnormal chest radiograph
Human immunodeficiency virus infection
Other immunosuppression

INDURATION ≥10 MM IN DIAMETER

Foreign-born individual from high-prevalence country
Frequently exposed to high-risk adults[a]
User of illicit intravenous drug(s)
Other medical risk factor(s)[b]
Healthcare worker
Member of locally identified high-risk population
Age ≤4 years

INDURATION ≥15 MM IN DIAMETER

Regardless of age or risk factors

[a]Such as HIV-infected, homeless, users of illicit drugs, residents of nursing homes, incarcerated or institutionalized, or migrant farm workers.
[b]Such as Hodgkin disease, lymphoma, diabetes mellitus, chronic renal failure, malnutrition.

---

clinical presentations are similar to those of opportunistic infections, skin test anergy is frequent, and culture confirmation is difficult. All children with suspected tuberculosis should have serologic testing for HIV, because the two infections are linked epidemiologically.

Adults and children with HIV infection and tuberculosis are prone to developing immune reconstitution inflammatory syndrome (IRIS) if antiretroviral drugs are started with or shortly after the initiation of antituberculosis therapy.[45,46] In IRIS, as the HIV load drops and the CD4+ lymphocyte count rises rapidly, tuberculosis disease appears to worsen or new foci of infection (tuberculoma of the brain, abdominal lesions) appear despite the use of effective chemotherapy. IRIS is an immunologically mediated phenomenon and does not indicate inadequate treatment for tuberculosis. The addition of corticosteroids to the treatment regimen usually hastens resolution of new lesions.

Other causes of immune suppression – including malignancies and their therapy, and use of high-dose corticosteroids – have been associated with higher rates of tuberculosis disease. Anti-TNF drugs used to control inflammatory bowel disease and several rheumatologic diseases greatly increase the risk of tuberculosis infection progressing rapidly to tuberculosis disease in adults.[47,48]

CLINICAL MANIFESTATIONS

Intrathoracic Disease

Pulmonary Disease

The vast majority of children with *M. tuberculosis* infection develop *silent pulmonary infection* weeks after acquisition, with no signs, symptoms, or radiographic abnormality.[49] The initiation of infection occasionally is marked by several days of low-grade fever and mild cough. Some children have fever and mild systemic symptoms at the onset of tissue hypersensitivity several weeks after infection; symptoms resolve over 1 to 3 weeks. The likelihood of symptom development at primary infection depends on the child's age. Between 80% and 90% of newly infected older children have completely asymptomatic infection, whereas 40% to 50% of infected infants develop symptoms or radiographic abnormalities.[50]

The primary pulmonary complex includes infection of the lung parenchyma and infection and hyperplasia of regional lymph nodes. Approximately 70% of primary foci are subpleural, and localized pleural reaction is a common part of the primary complex. Lobes of the lung are affected equally, and 25% of cases have multiple parenchymal foci.[51] Initial inflammatory response

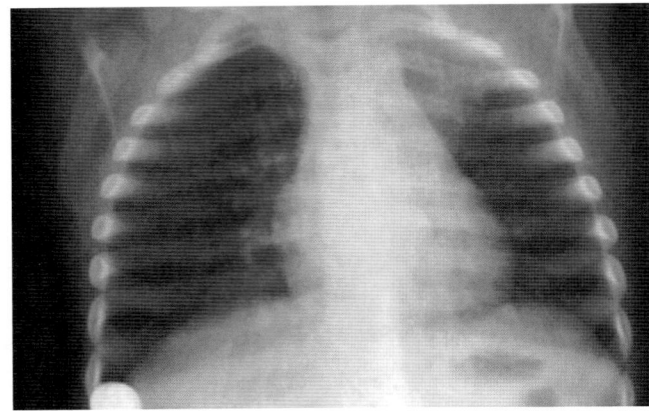

Figure 134-3. Mediastinal adenopathy and left upper-lobe segmental lesion in a child with primary pulmonary tuberculosis.

is not usually visible radiographically, but a localized, nonspecific infiltrate can be seen. Within days, infection spreads to regional lymph nodes. As tissue sensitivity develops, inflammatory reaction in lung tissue and lymph nodes intensifies. The hallmark of primary tuberculosis is disproportionately enlarged regional lymph nodes compared with a relatively minor parenchymal focus (Figure 134-2).

In most children, infiltrate and adenopathy resolve quickly, often by the time the chest radiograph is obtained. In some children, particularly infants, lymph nodes continue to enlarge. External compression can cause partial or complete bronchial obstruction.[51] The inflammatory response can erode the bronchial wall, leading to luminal infection. This process usually results in partial or complete obstruction of the bronchus. A common radiographic sequence is adenopathy followed by localized hyperinflation and then atelectasis of contiguous parenchyma, referred to as *segmental lesions* (Figure 134-3). This radiographic picture is unlike that of other bacterial pneumonias but mimics foreign-body aspiration and other obstructive disorders.

Obstructive emphysema of a lobar segment occurs rarely but most often is found in children <2 years of age. Resolution of obstruction usually occurs spontaneously and may be hastened with the use of corticosteroids; however, complete resolution often takes several months. Up to 40% of children <1 year of age who are infected with *M. tuberculosis* develop a segmental lesion,

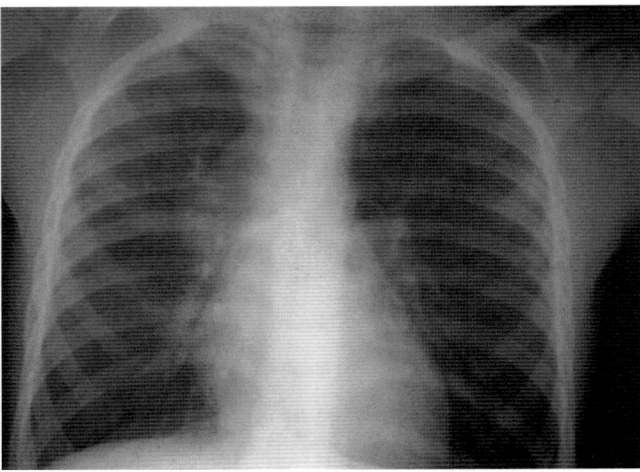

Figure 134-2. Right-sided hilar lymphadenopathy with minor parenchymal infiltrate in a 3-year-old boy with primary pulmonary tuberculosis. (Courtesy of S.S. Long.)

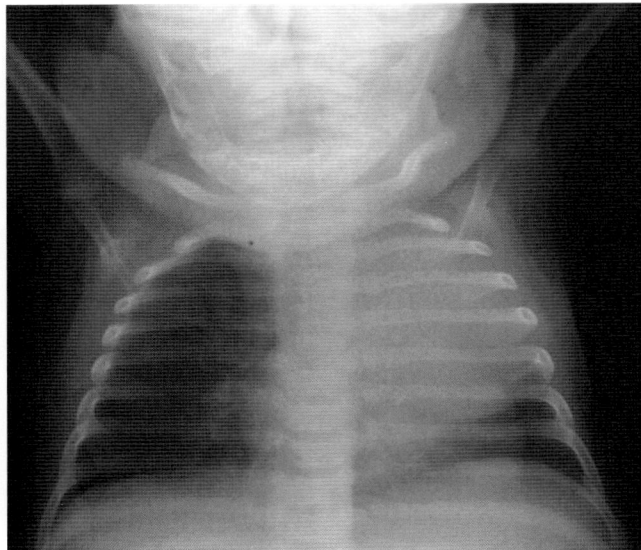

Figure 134-4. Left upper-lobe consolidation in a 16-month-old toddler with primary pulmonary tuberculosis. (Courtesy of S.S. Long.)

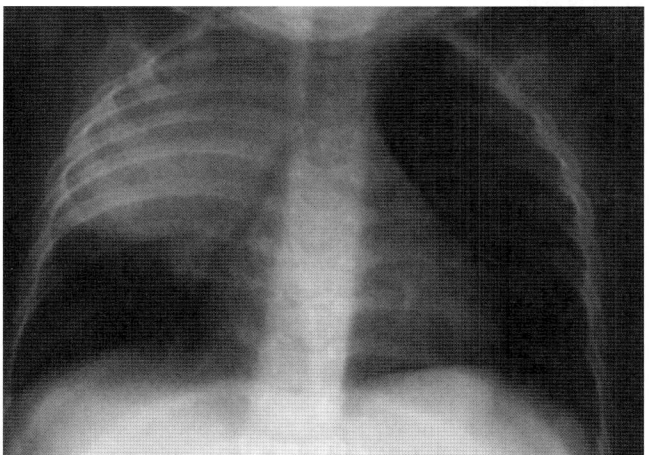

Figure 134-5. Lobar pneumonia with bulging of the horizontal fissure in a child with primary pulmonary tuberculosis.

compared with 15% of children 11 to 15 years of age. Occasionally, the radiographic abnormality is lobar pneumonia (Figures 134-4 and 134-5). Enlarged subcarinal nodes can impinge on the esophagus, causing swallowing difficulty or the development of a bronchoesophageal fistula; other enlarged nodes can compress the

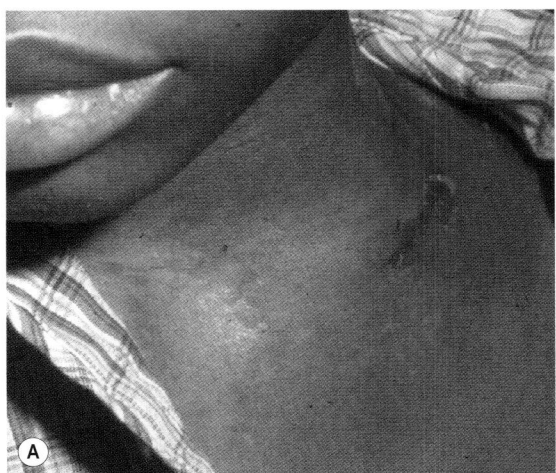

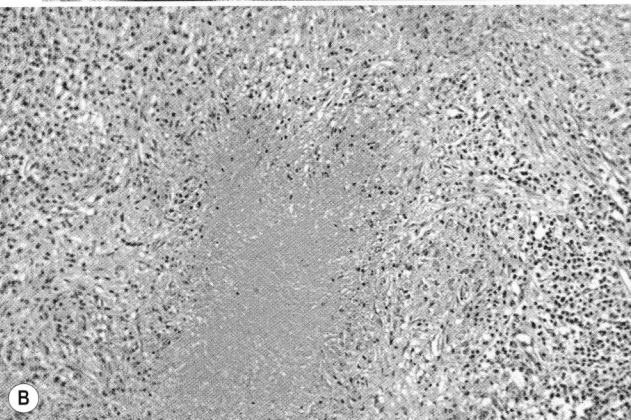

Figure 134-6. An adolescent girl had biopsy performed of a supraclavicular mass **(A)** to exclude lymphoma because of a 1-month history of fever and weight loss, and a chest radiograph showing a mediastinal mass. Histology **(B)** revealed caseous necrosis and granulomatous reaction. 400×, hematoxylin & eosin stain. (Courtesy of S.S. Long.)

subclavian vein, causing edema of the hand or arm. Occasionally, nodes rupture into the mediastinum, leading to supraclavicular adenitis (Figure 134-6).

The symptoms and signs of pulmonary tuberculosis in children usually are minor and are more commonly present in infants and young children.[52,53] Nonproductive cough and mild dyspnea are the most common symptoms in infants. Fever, night sweats, anorexia, and irritability are less common. Some infants have failure to thrive, which may not improve for months after appropriate chemotherapy is begun. Tachypnea, localized wheezing, or decreased breath sounds can occur with bronchial obstruction, but respiratory distress is rare.[54,55] Nonspecific signs and symptoms occasionally resolve after routine antibiotic therapy, suggesting bacterial superinfection distal to nodal obstruction.

A rare but serious complication of primary pulmonary tuberculosis occurs when the parenchymal focus enlarges and develops a large caseous center. The clinical course and radiographic appearance (progressive primary tuberculosis) can resemble those of

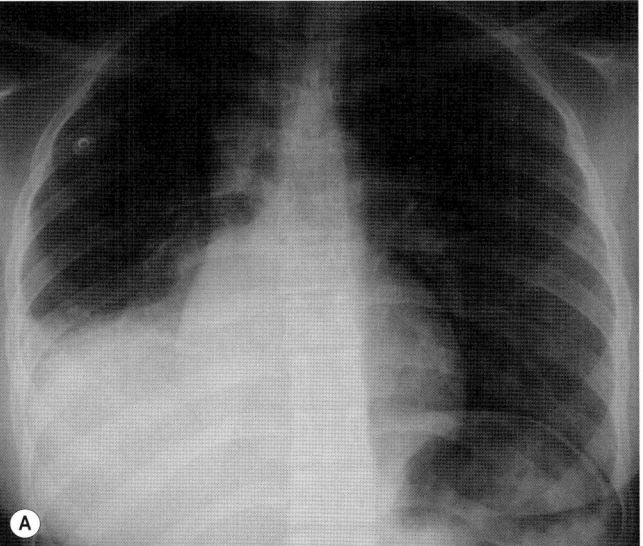

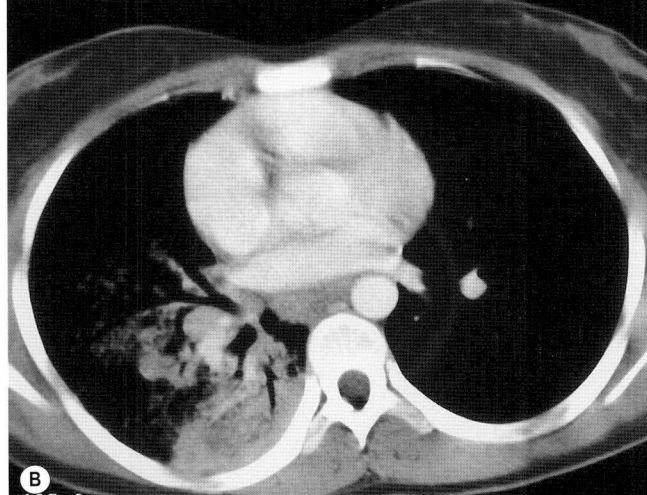

Figure 134-7. Progressive primary pulmonary tuberculosis with hemoptysis. **(A)** Chest radiograph shows right lower-lobe consolidation. Bronchoscopy revealed hemorrhage and a large clot obscuring lumen to the right lower lobe. Computed tomography showed multiple nodes abutting airways, and consolidation and atelectasis of the right lower lobe. A hilar node and the most rostral lower lobe infiltrate are shown **(B).** Bronchoalveolar lavage was smear-negative but culture-positive for *Mycobacterium tuberculosis.* (Courtesy of S.S. Long.)

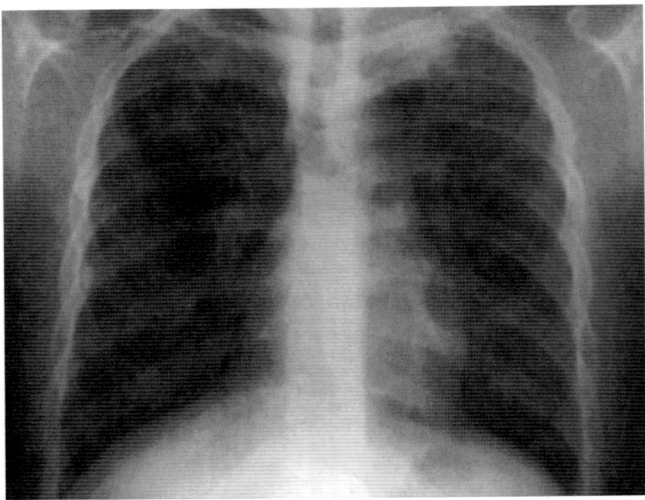

Figure 134-8. Bilateral upper-lobe infiltrates caused by reactivation tuberculosis in an adolescent. The calcified primary focus can be seen at the periphery of the right lung.

bacterial pneumonia.[56-58] Hyperpyrexia, moderate to severe cough, night sweats, dullness on chest percussion, rales, and decreased breath sounds over the affected area are common. Central liquefaction can result in formation of a thin-walled cavity; by producing a ball-valve mechanism, such a cavity can cause rupture into either the pleural space (leading to a bronchopleural fistula or pyopneumothorax) or the pericardium (causing acute pericarditis with constriction). Before the advent of antituberculosis chemotherapy, the mortality of progressive primary tuberculosis in children was 30% to 50%. With current treatment, the prognosis is excellent for full recovery.

Older children can have reactivation pulmonary tuberculosis that resembles disease in adults.[59-61] This form of tuberculosis is more common when infection is acquired after 7 years of age, especially at the onset of puberty (Figure 134-7).[60] Fever, anorexia, weight loss, night sweats, productive cough, chest pain, and hemoptysis are typical. Findings on physical examination usually are minor or absent, but the radiographic appearance is disproportionately abnormal. Extensive upper-lobe infiltrates (Figure 134-8) or upper-lobe cavities (Figure 134-9) are typical. Infection usually remains localized to the lungs, because the immune response induced by the initial infection prevents further lymphohematogenous spread. Most signs and symptoms improve within several weeks of the start of effective treatment, although cough can persist for several months.

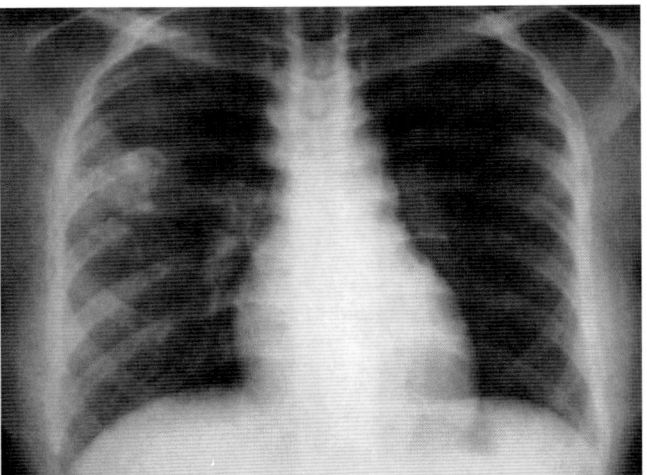

Figure 134-9. Multiloculated cavity due to reactivation tuberculosis.

Pleural Disease

Pleural tuberculosis is caused by the hypersensitivity response to the discharge of a few bacilli from a subpleural focus into the pleural space.[62] Occasionally, a larger discharge causes a generalized pleural effusion, which is unilateral and usually occurs within 6 to 9 months of initial infection.[63] Pleural tuberculosis is not associated with segmental pulmonary lesions, and only rarely with miliary tuberculosis. Onset usually is abrupt, consisting of fever, chest pain, and shortness of breath, with dullness to percussion and diminished breath sounds on the affected side. Fever often is high and can persist for several weeks during treatment.[64]

Stain of pleural fluid for AFB usually is negative, but culture results are positive in 30% to 50% of cases. Biopsy of the pleural membrane demonstrates caseating granulomas in up to 90% of cases, and culture of tissue is positive in up to 70% of cases. Pleural fluid typically is yellow and occasionally is blood-tinged, with specific gravity 1.012 to 1.025, protein 2 to 4 g/dL, glucose 20 to 40 mg/dL, and white blood cell count ranging from 100 to 1000 cells/mm^3, with predominance of neutrophils early, followed by a high proportion of lymphocytes.

Cardiac Disease

Pericarditis is the most common form of cardiac tuberculosis, occurring in 1% to 4% of tuberculosis cases in children.[65] Pericardial fluid is serofibrinous or slightly hemorrhagic initially and tuberculosis can be suggested by detecting stranding on echocardiography.[66] In approximately 10% to 20% of cases, fibrosis leads to constrictive pericarditis over a period of months to years. Early symptoms of serofibrinous pericarditis are nonspecific and usually consist of low-grade fever, malaise, weight loss, and cough; in children, chest pain is unusual. Signs of a pericardial friction rub, distant heart sounds, and pulsus paradoxus can follow, especially with constriction. Smear of pericardial fluid for AFB rarely is positive, but culture of fluid is positive in 30% to 70% of cases. Pericardial biopsy shows caseating granulomas in 50% to 75% of cases, and culture usually is positive. The TST is positive in 75% of cases.

Extrathoracic Disease

Lymphohematogenous Disease

Tubercle bacilli disseminate to distant anatomic sites in all asymptomatic and symptomatic *M. tuberculosis* infections of the lung. Clinical manifestations of dissemination depend on the burden of organisms and the host immune response. Infants and HIV-infected children are more likely to have severe forms of disseminated disease.[67] Dissemination during initial infection usually is occult but can result in extrapulmonary disease that becomes clinically evident months to years later.

Intermittent release of bacilli from erosion of a caseous focus into a pulmonary vessel rarely causes protracted bloodstream infection (BSI). There may be acute onset of spiking fever, but an indolent and prolonged intermittent fever is common. Involvement of multiple organs is common, with hepatosplenomegaly, lymphadenitis of superficial or deep nodes, and appearance of papulonecrotic tuberculids in crops on the skin. Meningitis, which occurs late in the course, was often the cause of death in the prechemotherapy era. Initial mild pulmonary involvement becomes diffuse after several weeks. Culture of gastric aspirate often is negative; blood or urine culture can be positive, and biopsy of bone marrow or liver yields a high rate of positive stain and culture results.

The most common clinically significant form of disseminated tuberculosis is *miliary disease*, which occurs when massive BSI causes disease in ≥2 organs.[67-69] Miliary tuberculosis occurs as an early complication of the primary infection (i.e., within 2 to 6 months). Miliary tuberculosis usually is a disease of infants and young children, but breakdown of a healed primary pulmonary lesion can cause miliary spread in older individuals. Clinical manifestations are protean, depending on the number and final location of disseminated organisms.[69] Lesions usually are largest and most numerous in the lungs, spleen, liver, and bone marrow.

The clinical onset of miliary tuberculosis can be explosive over several days but more often is indolent. Early manifestations are malaise, anorexia, listlessness, weight loss, and low-grade fever with normal physical findings. Higher fever, hepatosplenomegaly, and generalized lymphadenopathy develop within several weeks in approximately 50% of children. Respiratory symptoms are few, and the chest radiographic findings can be normal. Within the next several weeks, respiratory distress, cough, rales, or wheezing occurs as lungs often become filled with tubercles, and characteristic radiographic findings appear.[69] If pulmonary disease progresses, alveolar-capillary block can result in respiratory distress, hypoxia, and pneumothorax. Differential diagnosis of miliary parenchymal disease includes lymphocytic interstitial pneumonia in HIV-infected children, histoplasmosis, disseminated neuroblastoma or thyroid carcinoma, and histiocytosis. Headache usually indicates meningitis, whereas abdominal pain or tenderness often heralds tuberculous peritonitis.[68,70] Choroid tubercles have been detected on ophthalmologic examination in 13% to 87% of children in various studies.

Timely diagnosis of miliary tuberculosis requires a high index of suspicion. Eliciting a history of exposure to an adult with contagious tuberculosis is most important. At least 30% of children with miliary tuberculosis have a negative TST before treatment. Biopsy of the liver or bone marrow facilitates rapid diagnosis. In one review, the premortem diagnosis could be confirmed microbiologically in only 33% of cases in children.[67] With timely treatment, the prognosis of miliary tuberculosis in children is excellent. The general sense of wellbeing improves within 2 weeks of beginning therapy, but resolution of other signs and symptoms may take several weeks, weight gain may be delayed by weeks to months, and abnormalities on chest radiograph often persist for months.

Lymphatic Disease

Tuberculosis of the superficial lymph nodes (scrofula) is the most common form of extrapulmonary tuberculosis among children, accounting for approximately 67% of cases. Historically, scrofula often was caused by drinking unpasteurized cow milk laden with *M. bovis.* Most current cases are due to primary pulmonary infection with *M. tuberculosis* acquired by aerosol or droplet nuclei. The supraclavicular, anterior cervical, tonsillar, and submandibular nodes most often are involved secondary to extension of a primary lesion of the upper lung fields or abdomen. Tuberculous inguinal, epitrochlear, or axillary lymphadenopathy usually results from tuberculosis of the skin or skeletal system and is rare in children.[71]

Infected lymph nodes usually enlarge gradually in the early stages, are discrete and firm but not hard or tender. Nodes often feel fixed to underlying or overlying tissues.[71-73] Involvement usually is unilateral but can be bilateral because of crossover drainage of lymphatic vessels in the chest and lower neck. Infection can progress to affect several nodes, resulting in a matted mass. Other than low-grade fever, systemic signs and symptoms usually are absent. The TST usually is reactive. A primary pulmonary focus almost always is present but is visible radiographically in only 30% to 70% of cases, and usually is asymptomatic. Occasionally, lymphadenitis is more acute, with rapid enlargement associated with high fever, tenderness, and fluctuation. The initial presentation rarely is a fluctuant mass with overlying cellulitis.

Untreated lymphadenitis can resolve but more often progresses to caseating necrosis, capsular rupture, and spread to adjacent nodes as well as overlying skin, which becomes effaced, shiny, and erythematous (see Figure 134-6). Rupture through the skin results in a draining sinus tract that may require surgical removal.[73] Distinguishing lymphadenitis due to *M. tuberculosis* from nontuberculous mycobacterial (NTM) infection is challenging.[72] Both conditions cause chronic, nontender adenopathy with tissue breakdown or sinus tracts or both. Chest radiographic findings usually are normal in both infections. The TST reaction almost always is positive in *M. tuberculosis* disease and can be moderately positive or negative in NTM infections. Identification of an adult source case is important in cases of tuberculosis. Excisional biopsy with culture of the lymph nodes often is required to establish etiology.

Central Nervous System Disease

Central nervous system (CNS) disease usually is fatal without treatment. CNS disease arises from either the renewed activity in a caseous lesion in the cerebral cortex or meninges that was established during early occult lymphohematogenous dissemination,[74] or rapidly from direct invasion during uncontrolled dissemination.[75,76] Lesions enlarge and discharge small numbers of bacilli into the subarachnoid space. The resulting exudate infiltrates the cortical or meningeal blood vessels, producing inflammation, obstruction, and subsequent infarction of the cerebral cortex. The base of the brain is affected most commonly, accounting for frequent involvement of cranial nerves III, VI, and VII. Exudate can interfere with flow of cerebrospinal fluid (CSF) at basilar cisterns, leading to communicating hydrocephalus.[77] The combination of vasculitis, infarction, cerebral edema, and hydrocephalus results in severe damage that can occur gradually or rapidly. Hyponatremia and volume expansion, caused by the inappropriate secretion of antidiuretic hormone, are common and contribute to the pathophysiology.[78]

Tuberculous meningitis complicates approximately 0.5% of untreated primary infections in children. It is extremely rare in infants <4 months of age, and is most common in children between 6 months and 4 years of age. Meningitis often occurs within 2 to 6 months of initial infection.

The clinical onset of tuberculous meningitis can be rapid or gradual.[79-81] Rapid progression occurs more often among infants and young children, who may have symptoms for only several days before the onset of hydrocephalus, seizures, or cerebral edema. More often, signs and symptoms progress over several weeks and can be divided into three stages.[82] Stage I typically lasts 1 to 2 weeks and is characterized by nonspecific symptoms such as fever, headache, irritability, and drowsiness. Focal neurologic signs are absent, but infants can lose developmental milestones. This stage can be recognized as early tuberculous meningitis only in retrospect. Stage II usually begins more abruptly, with lethargy, nuchal rigidity, presence of Kernig or Brudzinski sign, seizures, hypertonia, vomiting, cranial nerve abnormalities, and other focal neurologic signs. If significant hydrocephalus is present, early placement of a ventriculoperitoneal shunt or extraventricular device can relieve the symptoms.[83] Some children have signs only of encephalitis, such as disorientation, abnormal movements, and speech impairment. Stage III is marked by coma, hemiplegia or paraplegia, hypertension, decerebrate or decorticate posturing, progressive abnormalities of vital signs, and eventual death.

The prognosis of tuberculous meningitis correlates closely with the clinical stage of illness at the time effective treatment is begun.[82,84,85] Most patients whose treatment begins at stage I have an excellent outcome, whereas most survivors of stage III have permanent disabilities that include blindness, deafness, paraplegia, diabetes insipidus, and mental retardation. Antituberculosis treatment should be instituted empirically (while the diagnosis is being established) for any child with basilar meningitis and hydrocephalus, infarction, or cranial nerve involvement that has no other apparent cause. The key to the diagnosis in children often is identification of the adult source case.

Rapid confirmation of tuberculous meningitis can be extremely difficult. The tuberculin skin test result is nonreactive in up to 40% of cases, and chest radiographic findings are normal in up to 50% of cases. The lumbar CSF leukocyte cell count ranges from 10 to 500 cells/mm³. Neutrophils can predominate early, but lymphocytic predominance is more typical. The CSF glucose level is usually between 20 and 40 mg/dL (but can be <10 mg/dL); CSF protein concentration is elevated, sometimes markedly (>400 mg/dL). Positivity of CSF stain or culture results is directly related to

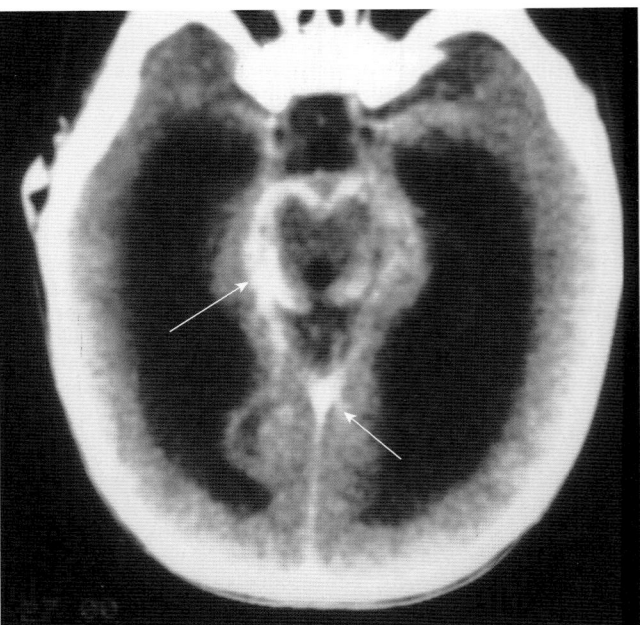

Figure 134-10. Tuberculous meningitis in a 6-month-old infant, with a 2-week history of lethargy, and acute onset of seizures, right facial paralysis, and right-sided hemiparesis. Contrast-enhanced axial computed tomography shows enlarged ventricles and prominent basilar cisternal enhancement (arrows). *Mycobacterium tuberculosis* was isolated from gastric aspirates. (Courtesy of S.S. Long.)

the quantity of CSF sampled. When 10 mL of lumbar CSF is sampled, the acid-fast stain yields a positive result in up to 30% of cases, and the culture result is positive in up to 70% of cases. Ventricular CSF often is normal as the pathology occurs distal to the lateral ventricles. Cranial computed tomography (CT) and magnetic resonance imaging can be helpful in the diagnosis of tuberculous meningitis. Although CT findings can be normal during early stages of the disease, basilar enhancement with communicating hydrocephalus and signs of cerebral edema or focal ischemia are helpful clues (Figure 134-10).

Tuberculoma, another manifestation of CNS infection, usually manifests as a space-occupying lesion and occurs most often in children <10 years of age. A typical lesion is singular and infratentorial, usually located at the base of the brain near the cerebellum.[86] Tuberculoma and tuberculous meningitis were once considered to be distinct entities, but neuroimaging has demonstrated that many small children with CNS tuberculosis develop both. The most common symptoms are headache, fever, and convulsions. Usually the TST result is positive, and chest radiographic findings are normal. Although surgical excision is not necessary, biopsy often is performed for diagnosis.

Paradoxical appearance of a tuberculoma during effective therapy of tuberculous meningitis can occur.[87,88] Probably an immunologic or inflammatory reaction, its appearance does not signify drug failure or need for change, and usually responds to corticosteroid therapy. The condition should be suspected if focal neurologic abnormality arises during treatment of meningitis. Tuberculomas can resolve slowly, over months to years. The necessary duration of antituberculosis or corticosteroid treatment is unclear.

Osteoarticular Disease

Bone and joint infections can originate from direct lymphohematogenous seeding, extension of a caseous regional lymph node, or extension from adjacent infected bone. The interval between infection and clinical manifestations can be 1 month (tuberculous dactylitis) to years (osteoarthritis of the hip). Infection usually begins in the metaphysis of the bone, causing necrosis by infection

or pressure of granulation tissue and caseation. Soft-tissue abscess and extension of the infection through the epiphysis into the nearby joint complicates bone infection. The disease often becomes clinically apparent when the joint becomes involved.

Weight-bearing bones and joints are affected most commonly, especially vertebrae, when such an infection is called *Pott disease*.[89] Any or multiple vertebral bodies can be involved, but there is a predilection for the lower thoracic or upper lumbar vertebrae. Multiply affected vertebrae usually are contiguous, but there can be skip areas between lesions.[90] Infection in the body of the vertebra leads to bone destruction and collapse, spondylitis of one or several disk spaces, collapse and wedging of the vertebral body with subsequent angulation of the spine (gibbus), or kyphosis. Infection can rupture into soft tissue, causing paraspinal abscess (Pott disease), psoas abscess, or retropharyngeal abscess. The most common manifestations of Pott disease in children are low-grade fever, irritability, and restlessness; back pain (usually without significant tenderness); and abnormal positioning or refusal to walk. Rigidity of the spine results from involuntary immobilization and muscle spasm.

Other common sites of skeletal tuberculosis are the knee, hip, elbow, and ankle.[91-93] The extent of involvement ranges from mild joint effusion without bone destruction to frank destruction of bone and restriction of the joint caused by chronic fibrosis of the synovial membrane. The process usually evolves over months to years, most commonly causing mild pain, stiffness, limping, and restrictive movement. The TST is reactive in 80% to 90% of cases. Culture of joint fluid or bone biopsy usually yields the organism. One form of bony tuberculosis peculiar to infants is tuberculous dactylitis. Affected children have distal endarteritis followed by painless swelling of hands or feet and cystic bone lesions. Abscesses are rare, but the TST result usually is positive.

Abdominal and Gastrointestinal Disease

Tuberculous enteritis can be caused by hematogenous dissemination or swallowing of tubercle bacilli discharged from the patient's lungs. The jejunum and ileum near Peyer patches and the appendix are the most common sites of involvement.[94-96] Shallow ulcers that cause pain, diarrhea or constipation, and weight loss are the usual findings. Mesenteric lymphadenitis usually complicates the infection. Nodes can obstruct the intestines or erode through the omentum to cause generalized peritonitis. Tuberculous enteritis should be considered for any child with chronic gastrointestinal complaints who has a positive TST result.[97] Biopsy, stain, and culture of lesions usually are necessary to confirm the diagnosis.

Tuberculous peritonitis is uncommon in adolescents and rare in young children. Generalized peritonitis can result from subclinical or miliary hematogenous dissemination. Localized peritonitis is caused by direct extension from an infected abdominal lymph node, an intestinal focus, or tuberculous salpingitis.[98] Pain and tenderness usually are mild initially. Rarely, lymph nodes, omentum, and peritoneum become matted and can be palpated as a doughy, irregular, nontender mass. Ascites and low-grade fever are common. The TST result is almost always positive. Diagnosis is confirmed by paracentesis or biopsy with appropriate stains and cultures, but the procedure must be performed extremely carefully to avoid entering fixed bowel intertwined with the matted omentum.

Genitourinary Disease

Renal tuberculosis is rare in children because the incubation period is at least several years.[99] Tubercle bacilli reach the kidney during lymphohematogenous dissemination, as documented by their transient recovery from urine in many cases of miliary or primary pulmonary tuberculosis. Small caseous tubercles develop in the renal parenchyma and release *M. tuberculosis* into the tubules. A large mass can develop near the renal cortex that discharges large numbers of bacteria through a fistula into the renal pelvis. Infection spreads locally to the ureters, prostate, or epididymis. Renal tuberculosis often is silent clinically in the early stages, the only signs being sterile pyuria and microscopic hematuria.[100] As disease progresses, dysuria, flank or abdominal pain, and gross hematuria can develop. Superinfection frequently occurs and can delay recognition of underlying tuberculosis. Ureteral stricture or hydronephrosis complicates the disease.[101] Urine culture results are positive in 80% to 90% of cases. Results of acid-fast stains of large volumes of urine (sedimented) are less frequently positive. The TST result usually is positive.

Tuberculosis of the genital tract is uncommon in both sexes before puberty. Infection usually originates from lymphohematogenous seeding, although it can be spread directly from the intestinal tract or bone. Adolescent girls can have hematogenous genital tract tuberculosis during the primary infection. The fallopian tubes most often are involved, followed by the endometrium, ovaries, and cervix. Usual symptoms are lower abdominal pain and dysmenorrhea or amenorrhea. Epididymitis or orchitis can occur in adolescent males, manifesting as a unilateral, nodular, painless swelling of the scrotum. Involvement of the glans penis is rare. For both girls and boys, systemic manifestations are usually absent, and chest radiographic appearance is normal. The TST result is usually positive. Because unrecognized genital tract tuberculosis can lead to infertility in women, and in vitro fertilization (IVF) has been associated with congenital tuberculosis, women from endemic regions should have TST testing prior to IVF.[102]

Cutaneous Disease

Tuberculosis of the skin, more common decades ago, arises as a primary infection, hematogenous dissemination, or hypersensitivity to the tubercle bacillus.[103] Direct inoculation of the skin through an abrasion, cut, or insect bite leads to the primary complex. Regional lymphadenitis is striking, but systemic symptoms usually are lacking. The most common form of hypersensitivity lesion is *erythema nodosum*, characterized by large, painful, purple-brown nodules on shins and extensor forearms. *Scrofuloderma* occurs when a caseous lymph node ruptures through the skin and leaves an ulcer or sinus tract. *Papulonecrotic tuberculids* are miliary lesions of the skin appearing most frequently on the face, trunk, and upper thighs. The characteristic "apple-jelly" center of such a lesion is best demonstrated by placing a glass slide over it. *Verrucosa cutis* is a tuberculous wart-like lesion, most common on the arms or legs that represents autoinoculation of tubercle bacilli in a person already sensitized to the organism.[104]

Congenital Disease

Congenital tuberculosis is rare, with fewer than 400 cases reported in the English language literature.[105] The affected infant's mother can have tuberculous pleuritis, meningitis, genital tract infection or disseminated disease during pregnancy, but in some series of congenital tuberculosis, diagnosis of tuberculosis was made in the mother at or after delivery in <50% of cases.[106] Occurrence and intensity of hematogenous dissemination during pregnancy determine congenital infection. Placental infection is probably required to transmit infection to the fetus by blood or aspiration of amniotic fluid. However, even massive tuberculous placentitis does not always give rise to congenital infection.

In hematogenous congenital tuberculosis, *M. tuberculosis* reaches the fetus via the umbilical vein and disseminates widely. If bacilli infect the liver, a primary focus develops, with involvement of periportal lymph nodes.[107] Hematogenous primary focus in the fetal lung usually remains dormant until after birth, when oxygenation and circulation increase significantly. Congenital infection of the infant also occurs via aspiration or ingestion of infected amniotic fluid.[108]

Symptoms of hematogenous congenital tuberculosis can be present at birth but more commonly appear by the second or third week of life.[105,106] The most common manifestations are respiratory distress, fever, hepatosplenomegaly, poor feeding, lethargy or irritability, lymphadenopathy, abdominal distention, ear drainage, and skin lesions. Clinical manifestations vary in relation to the site and size of lesions. Some infants have a normal chest

radiograph early in the course but most have diffuse radiographic abnormalities as disease progresses. The most common early findings on chest radiograph are hilar lymphadenopathy and parenchymal infiltrates; approximately 50% have a miliary pattern.

Clinical presentation of tuberculosis in the young infant mimics septicemia and other congenital infections. Congenital tuberculosis should be suspected in any infant who has compatible signs and symptoms with no response to antibiotic therapy and an unrevealing evaluation for other congenital infections. Suspicion also is high if the mother has risk for, has, or has had tuberculosis.

Timely diagnosis of congenital or neonatal tuberculosis often is difficult. The TST result usually is negative, frequently becoming reactive after 1 to 3 months of therapy. Diagnosis is established by positive results of acid-fast stains or culture of body fluids or tissues. A positive result of an acid-fast smear of gastric or tracheal aspirates in a neonate is almost diagnostic, because false-positive smear results are rare. Diagnosis by direct acid-fast smears from middle-ear fluid, bone marrow, tracheal aspirate, or tissue biopsy are useful and should be attempted.[105] Examination and culture of CSF should be performed, although the yield of such tests is low because only 20% of affected children have meningeal involvement. The mother should be examined; endometrial specimens almost always yield positive culture results.

DIAGNOSIS

Tuberculin Skin Test

The definitive TST uses 5 tuberculin units (TU) of purified protein derivative (PPD) stabilized in Tween 80, injected intradermally with the Mantoux technique, with use of a 27-gauge needle and tuberculin syringe, on the volar surface of the forearm.[109] Older, prong-type Tine test is no longer available in the U.S. because of inferior test performance. Delayed hypersensitivity reaction to TST usually peaks at 48 to 72 hours. In some individuals, reaction occurs after 72 hours and should be considered a positive result. The diameter of induration is measured and recorded in millimeters. For accuracy, the TST should be interpreted by trained HCP, not by a parent or relative. An allergic or Arthus-like reaction to TST components occasionally causes erythema and induration beginning within hours after application, peaking as late as 24 hours (for the Arthus reaction), and waning at 48 hours; these are not indications of *M. tuberculosis* infection.

A nonreactive TST result does not exclude *M. tuberculosis* infection or disease. A variety of factors can lower tuberculin reactivity (Box 134-2).[110] Approximately 10% of immunocompetent children with culture-documented tuberculosis do not react initially to 5 TU of PPD (TST).[16,111] Most of these children have a positive test result after several months of treatment, suggesting that tuberculosis was acquired recently or that untreated disease depressed specific immune responses. Additionally, many adults and children with disseminated tuberculosis and many with advanced, untreated HIV infection and *M. tuberculosis* infection are anergic.[112]

False-positive reactions to tuberculin also occur. Recent infection with NTM can result in cross-sensitization and a false-positive TST. Exposure to NTM varies geographically and is greater nearer the equator. Cross-reactions usually are ≤10 mm (but can be larger) and transient, lasting for several months.

A second cause of false-positive TST result is prior receipt of BCG vaccine.[113–117] Tuberculin reactions caused by BCG vaccination cannot be distinguished with certainty from infection with *M. tuberculosis* by the TST alone. Countries using BCG vaccine frequently have high rates of endemic tuberculosis. In most studies of newborn infants vaccinated with BCG, only about 50% have a positive TST result, and 80% to 90% lose such reactivity within 5 years. Older children or adults have higher initial and longer responses to BCG, but most lose tuberculin reactivity within 10 years of vaccination.[113] Degree of reactivity also is affected by BCG product and nutritional status.[114,115] TST reactivity after BCG vaccination is expected to measure <10 mm of induration at 48 to 72 hours (although reactions of 10 to 15 mm can occur). Prior receipt of BCG vaccine is not a contraindication to tuberculin testing. In general, in the U.S., the TST result is interpreted similarly for persons with and without a history of vaccination.[16] However, the interferon-gamma (IFN-γ) release assays may help distinguish between *M. tuberculosis* infection and a positive test due to BCG or NTM (see below). Several studies have demonstrated that a positive TST in a previously BCG-vaccinated child who is a close contact with an active case of tuberculosis is likely to represent *M. tuberculosis* infection, and the child should be evaluated and treated.[116,117]

During the past decade, the approach to interpretation of the TST result has changed with the epidemiology of tuberculosis.[16] Size of induration interpreted as a positive result is a statistical attempt to minimize false-positive or false-negative readings, and

thus varies according to individual and epidemiologic factors, with possible exposure to *M. tuberculosis* the most heavily weighted factor (see Box 134-1). For children at highest risk for infection progressing to disease, induration diameter ≥5 mm is classified as a positive result, likely indicating *M. tuberculosis* infection. For other high-risk groups, an induration diameter ≥10 mm is a positive result. For children at low risk, an induration diameter ≥15 mm is a positive result.

In the U.S., it is preferable to screen children for *M. tuberculosis* infection risk factors with a questionnaire;[110] the TST should be performed when risk factors are discovered through the questionnaire. Local public health authorities should help determine interpretation of TST reactivity for each community. Age and intervals for TST are based on personal and epidemiologic risk factors.

Interferon-γ Release Assays

Interferon-γ release assays (IGRAs) are blood tests that detect the secretion of IFN-γ ex vivo by sampled lymphocytes after stimulation with 2 or 3 proteins that are fairly specific for *M. tuberculosis*. There are two commercially available IGRAs: one measures the total amount of IFN-γ produced by the lymphocytes while the other determines the number of lymphocytes producing IFN-γ.[118] Both tests are performed with positive and negative controls; threshold values that determine test positivity were determined using samples from adults with culture-confirmed *M. tuberculosis* disease. Like the TST, IGRAs cannot distinguish between tuberculosis infection and disease. Although the proteins in the tests are found on several rare species of NTM, they are not found on *M. avium* complex (MAC) or the BCG organisms. The IGRAs have been tested extensively in a variety of adult populations.[119–121] As expected, IGRAs are more specific than the TST; however, the difference in sensitivity is small. Data available from fewer studies in children demonstrate increased specificity of IGRAs but not increased sensitivity compared with the TST.[122–126] Indeterminate results also are problematic. IGRAs are particularly useful for testing individuals in low-burden settings who have received one or more BCG vaccinations; IGRA is the preferred test for these individuals.[127] However, usefulness of IGRA is limited in high-burden countries because of their cost, the need for laboratory equipment, the need to draw blood, and their lack of advantage in sensitivity over the TST.

Laboratory Diagnosis

Diagnostic tests for tuberculosis are based either on detection of *M. tuberculosis* in a clinical sample or recognition of the host response to the organism.[128–132] Methods of laboratory diagnosis are summarized in Table 134-1. Acid-fast staining and microscopic examination followed by culture confirmation is the standard, but this method can be slow, expensive, and insensitive for clinical samples from children.

TABLE 134-1. Summary of Laboratory Methods for Diagnosis of Tuberculosis

Identification Method	Test System	Use
CULTURE		
Conventional media	Colony morphology (3–5 weeks)	Preliminary identification
	Biochemical tests	Species identification
Radiometric methods	Positive growth index (5–14 days)	Differentiates *Mycobacterium tuberculosis* from nontuberculous mycobacteria species
Chromatography	HPLC mycolic acid profile	Speciates all common mycobacteria
	Gas chromatography-fatty acid profile	Speciates all common mycobacteria
RAPID DIRECT TESTS		
Direct smear	Acid-fast or fluorochrome stains	Easy, inexpensive, moderately sensitive
Nucleic acid detection	PCR amplification	Moderately sensitive, highly specific, technically complex

HPLC, high-performance liquid chromatography; PCR, polymerase chain reaction.

Strains of *M. tuberculosis* traditionally have been distinguished by drug susceptibility testing and phage typing, tests that are limited because of similarities of >90% and >50%, respectively, among strains in the U.S. Genotyping, spoligotyping and restriction fragment-length polymorphism are powerful tools allowing differentiation of strains for epidemiologic study.[133-135] Currently, the insertion sequence IS6110 is a strain-specific marker employed in many laboratories in the U.S. and worldwide.

Culture

Culture is the most important laboratory test for the diagnosis and management of tuberculosis. Unfortunately, positivity of cultures from early-morning gastric aspirates from children with pulmonary tuberculosis is <40%.[131] Yields of culture from sites of extrapulmonary tuberculosis often are far lower. Culture is most important when the source case is unknown or is known to have drug-resistant tuberculosis.[134,135] Two studies evaluating the role of bronchoscopy document culture yield of 13% to 62% in children with pulmonary tuberculosis.[136,137] In both studies, the yield from gastric aspirate was superior to that from bronchoalveolar lavage. A new technique (which can be used in an outpatient setting) of inducing sputum with warm saline and salbutamol has yielded positive cultures even from infants with pulmonary tuberculosis at a rate comparable with gastric aspirate sampling performed in the hospital.[138,139]

Traditional culture methods using Löwenstein–Jensen and Middlebrook solid media often require 4 to 6 weeks until positivity, followed by an additional 2 to 4 weeks for susceptibility testing. Radiometric techniques using liquid media provide more rapid detection, identification, and drug susceptibility testing of mycobacteria.[140] The recovery rate of *M. tuberculosis* using liquid media is substantially higher and faster compared with any single solid medium. The presence of mycobacteria in broth is confirmed by acid-fast stain, with speciation by traditional testing or high-pressure liquid chromatography.[141,142] Using these techniques, total time to isolation and speciation results averages 17 days for *M. tuberculosis*. With use of more sensitive culture assays, blood or urine samples from children and adolescents with mild or asymptomatic primary pulmonary tuberculosis occasionally can yield positive results.

Nucleic Acid Amplification Methodology

Serology has not performed well for diagnosis of tuberculosis.[143] However, several newer technologies have been somewhat successful. A number of nucleic acid amplification-based assays for mycobacteria have been developed with varied target sequences, assay formats, and specimen-processing procedures.[144-154]

The DNA sequence most frequently used to detect *M. tuberculosis* is the insertion element IS6110.[150] Test performance has varied among reference laboratories, but for adults, sensitivity and specificity of the polymerase chain reaction (PCR) test of sputum samples are >90% compared with culture.[151] Study of PCR tests in children is limited. Compared with a clinical diagnosis of pulmonary tuberculosis in children, the sensitivity of PCR has ranged from 25% to 83%, and specificity from 80% to 100%.[152-154] The PCR test on gastric contents can be positive in a recently infected child with a normal chest radiograph, but the clinical implications of such a finding are unclear. A negative PCR result does not exclude tuberculosis, nor does a positive result completely confirm the disease. PCR testing may be useful in evaluating immunocompromised children with pulmonary disease (especially children with HIV infection) and for confirming the diagnosis of extrapulmonary tuberculosis, although published information also is limited in this area.[144,155]

THERAPY

Antituberculosis Agents

Antituberculosis drugs are either bacteriostatic or bactericidal (Table 134-2).[156,157] Traditionally, antituberculosis regimens consisted of combinations of bactericidal and bacteriostatic agents, such as isoniazid and ethambutol. With such treatment regimens, microbiologic cure could be achieved in 18 to 24 months. In one study, the addition of rifampin to regimens containing isoniazid and streptomycin led to cure rates approaching 100% in patients with pulmonary tuberculosis after only 9 months of therapy.[135] Pyrazinamide used in combination with isoniazid and rifampin achieves cure rates of 98% in 6 months.[158]

Isoniazid, rifampin, pyrazinamide, and ethambutol are mainstays of antituberculosis treatment in adults and children. Successful treatment regimens use multiple drugs to which the patient's organism is susceptible plus regular administration for an extended period. The total duration of treatment is dictated by the extent of tuberculosis disease, adherence to treatment, adverse reactions to drugs, and clinical and bacteriologic response.[159,160]

Isoniazid

Isoniazid is the most widely used antituberculosis medication. Isoniazid is an ideal agent because it is bactericidal, easily administered, inexpensive, and relatively nontoxic in children. Isoniazid is almost completely absorbed from the gastrointestinal tract and penetrates all body fluid cavities, in which drug levels are similar to serum levels. Isoniazid has been associated with symptomatic pyridoxine deficiency in adults (e.g., pregnant women and persons with seizure disorders), but mainly only in children who are malnourished or have HIV infection.[160] Simultaneous administration of pyridoxine is not necessary in otherwise healthy children. The major toxicity of isoniazid is hepatic inflammation.[160] Almost 10% of children develop transiently elevated serum alanine aminotransferase (ALT) levels while taking isoniazid, but clinical toxicity is exceedingly rare. Most children are followed clinically, without serum biochemical monitoring. Isoniazid interferes with the metabolism of phenytoin, leading to high levels of phenytoin. A dose of isoniazid exceeding 15 mg/kg per day, or in combination with rifampin, enhances toxicity.

Rifampin

Rifampin is bactericidal for *M. tuberculosis*, is relatively nontoxic, and generally is well tolerated at a dose of 15 mg/kg per day. Although approximately 75% of drug is protein-bound, rifampin penetrates well into most tissues and fluids. Rifampin penetrates meninges only in the presence of inflammation. Gastrointestinal upset is the most common side effect. Other reactions are skin eruptions, hepatitis, and occasional thrombocytopenia or cholestatic jaundice.[160] Rifampin is excreted in urine, tears, sweat, and other body fluids. In 80% of recipients, body fluids and contact lenses are discolored orange during consumption of rifampin. Discoloration of body fluids can be a useful indicator of adherence to therapy. Rifampin can lower the effectiveness of oral contraceptive drugs and accelerate excretion of other drugs that undergo hepatic metabolism.

Pyrazinamide

Pyrazinamide is bactericidal for *M. tuberculosis* when organisms are located in an acid environment such as the macrophage. Pyrazinamide exerts maximum effect during the early phase (2 months) of therapy. Pyrazinamide is well absorbed from the gastrointestinal tract and penetrates most tissues, including CSF.[161,162] The optimal dose in children has not been established because of a lack of pharmacokinetic data. Doses of 30 mg/kg per day produce little toxicity in adults and are well tolerated in children.[163] Hepatic dysfunction, gastrointestinal upset, and skin rashes can be associated with pyrazinamide administration.[160] Adults taking pyrazinamide can experience symptomatic hyperuricemia with arthralgia or arthritis.

Ethambutol

Ethambutol generally is considered to have a bacteriostatic effect on *M. tuberculosis*, especially at lower dosages. Easily administered

TABLE 134-2. Antituberculous Drugs Used for Children

Drugs	Dosage Forms	Daily Dosage (mg/kg per day)	Twice-Weekly Dosage (mg/kg per dose)	Maximum Dose
Isoniazid[a]	Scored tablets 100 mg 300 mg Syrup 10 mg/mg[b]	10–15	20–40	Daily: 300 mg Twice weekly: 900 mg/dose
Rifampin	Capsules 150 mg 300 mg Syrup Formulated from capsules[c]	10–20	10–20	Daily: 600 mg Twice weekly: 600 mg/dose
Pyrazinamide	Scored tablets 500 mg	20–40	50–70	2 g
Streptomycin	Vials 1 g 4 g	20–40 (IM)[d]	20–40 (IM)[d]	1 g
Ethambutol	Scored tablets 100 mg 400 mg	20	50	2.5 g
Ethionamide	Tablets 250 mg	10–20	–	1 g
Amikacin	Vials 1 g	15 (IM or IV)[d]	15–25 (IM or IV)[d]	1 g
Cycloserine	Capsules 250 mg	10–20	–	1 g
Levofloxacin	Tablets 250 mg 500 mg Vials 25 mg/mL	Adults: 500 total dose per day Children: 5–10 total dose per day	1 g[e] total dose per day	1 g
Ciprofloxacin	Tablets 250 mg 500 mg 750 mg	500–1500 mg divided bid[e]	1.5 g[e] total dose per day	1.5 g

[a]Rifamate is a capsule containing 150 mg of isoniazid and 300 mg of rifampin. Two capsules provide the usual adult (≥50 kg) daily dose of each drug. Rifater is a tablet containing 50 mg isoniazid, 120 mg rifampin, and 300 mg pyrazinamide. Neither combination has been studied in children nor is either available in pediatric formulation.

[b]Many experts recommend avoidance of isoniazid syrup, because it is unstable and is associated with frequent gastrointestinal complaints, especially diarrhea.

[c]Merrell Dow Pharmaceuticals (Cincinnati, OH) issues directions for preparation of this "extemporaneous" syrup.

[d]IM, intramuscular: possibly intravenous.

[e]Total adult daily dosage. Fluoroquinolones can cause gastrointestinal disturbance, rash, and headache. They could theoretically affect growing cartilage.

and well absorbed, ethambutol penetrates poorly into CSF even in the presence of inflammation.[164,165] Ethambutol primarily is used when there is a possibility of initial drug resistance to other first-line drugs. Retrobulbar neuritis is the most serious adverse effect;[160] symptoms are blurred vision, central scotoma, and red-green color blindness. Neuritis is exceedingly rare in children and all persons with normal renal function.[166] Complications appear to be dose-related and rarely occur with a daily dose of 20 mg/kg per day.

Other Agents

Para-aminosalicylic acid, ethionamide, linezolid, cycloserine, capreomycin, kanamycin, and streptomycin occasionally are used for the treatment of tuberculosis in children. Ethionamide crosses the blood–brain barrier especially well and is a useful drug for tuberculous meningitis and tuberculoma. A number of additional drugs have been evaluated in children or adults with M.

tuberculosis infections, including amikacin, fluoroquinolones, rifamycin derivatives, clofazimine, and β-lactams. Rifabutin induces the cytochrome P450 enzyme system less than does rifampin, which may make rifabutin the better choice in HIV-coinfected children receiving protease-inhibitor therapy. In vitro, levofloxacin has better activity than ciprofloxacin (and ciprofloxacin than ofloxacin) against M. tuberculosis. None of these drugs has been evaluated in well-designed, randomized trials for the treatment of tuberculosis in children. Optimal doses and dosage intervals for use to treat tuberculosis in children have not been established. Their use should be restricted to specific instances of multidrug resistance or medication intolerance and after consultation with an expert in tuberculosis.

Latent *Mycobacterium tuberculosis* Infection

One study of 2750 children with latent M. tuberculosis infection (LTBI: positive TST result, normal chest radiograph) showed that isoniazid therapy produced a 94% reduction in tuberculosis disease during the first year after treatment and a 70% reduction over the subsequent 9-year period.[167] Placebo-controlled trials of isoniazid preventive therapy involving more than 125,000 subjects have been reported; the largest of these studies was undertaken by the U.S. Public Health Service in the 1950s.[168] Data combined from several studies showed the median risk reduction for tuberculosis in adults after 1 year of isoniazid therapy and follow-up to be 60% in the treated group. When analysis was limited to subjects with good adherence to medication, effectiveness approached 90%.

Guidelines and recommendations for the treatment of LTBI have been published.[32,110] The following aspects of the natural history and treatment of LTBI in children must be considered in the formulation of recommendations about therapy: (1) infants and children <5 years of age with LTBI have been infected recently; (2) the risk for progression to disease is high; (3) untreated infants with LTBI have up to a 40% chance of development of tuberculosis disease; (4) the risk for progression decreases gradually through childhood; (5) infants and young children are more likely to have life-threatening tuberculosis disease, including meningitis and disseminated disease; and (6) children with LTBI have more years at risk than adults for development of disease.

Isoniazid therapy for LTBI appears to be more effective for children than adults, with several large clinical trials demonstrating risk reduction of 70% to 90%.[169,170] Also, the risk of isoniazid-related hepatitis is minimal in infants, children, and adolescents, who generally tolerate the drug better than adults.[171,172]

The recommended regimen for treatment of LTBI in children is a 9-month course of isoniazid as self-administered daily therapy or by twice- or thrice-weekly directly observed therapy (DOT).[110] Isoniazid given twice weekly has been used extensively to treat LTBI in children, especially schoolchildren and close contacts of case patients.[173,174] However, no controlled clinical trials of intermittent isoniazid therapy of tuberculosis infection have been undertaken. In a community-based study conducted in Bethel, Alaska,[175] persons who took <25% of the prescribed regimen (daily isoniazid for 1 year) had a 3-fold higher risk for tuberculosis disease than those who took >50% of the regimen.

Rifampin alone has been used for the treatment of LTBI in infants, children, and adolescents when isoniazid could not be tolerated or the child has had contact with a source case infected with an isoniazid-resistant but rifamycin-susceptible organism.[176] However, no controlled clinical trials have been conducted. The optimal duration of rifampin therapy in children with LTBI is not known, but many experts recommend at least a 6-month course.[110] A 3-month regimen of rifampin and isoniazid has been used in Europe, with programmatic and case-control data suggesting that the regimen is effective.[177-181]

No controlled studies have been published regarding the efficacy of any form of treatment for LTBI in HIV-infected children. A 9-month course of isoniazid is recommended.[110] Most experts recommend that routine monitoring of serum hepatic enzyme concentrations be performed and pyridoxine be given when HIV-infected children are treated with isoniazid.

Isoniazid should be given to young children who have negative TST results but who have known or suspected exposure to an adult with contagious tuberculosis disease (so-called window prophylaxis). By the time delayed hypersensitivity develops (2 to 3 months), an untreated child can develop severe tuberculosis. For these children, TST is repeated 3 months after contact with the source case for tuberculosis has been broken (*broken contact* defined as physical separation or adequate initial treatment of the source case). If the second TST is positive, isoniazid therapy is continued for the full duration, but if the result of the second test is negative, treatment can be stopped.[182]

Pulmonary Tuberculosis

Regimens of treatment of pulmonary tuberculosis for 12 to 18 months, recommended in the 1970s, were effective, but failure

rates were high because of poor adherence. Extensive studies in children and adults show that 6 months of treatment with certain regimens is successful for most forms of tuberculosis. The critical factors in this new approach, called *short-course chemotherapy,* are (1) intensive initial therapy with multiple bactericidal drugs and (2) monitored adherence with DOT.[183]

Principles of Antimicrobial Approach

Success of antimicrobial therapy against *M. tuberculosis* depends on number, activity, primary or secondary resistance, and site (open cavities, closed caseous lesions, within macrophages) of organisms. At the high oxygen tension and lower pH in open cavities, *M. tuberculosis* can grow to a density of $>10^9$ organisms. Reactivation tuberculosis is associated with high density of organisms at all three sites. Most children with primary pulmonary tuberculosis are infected with a smaller number of organisms because there is no cavitary population.

Although an entire population of bacilli may be considered susceptible to one or more drugs, a subpopulation of drug-resistant organisms is found predictably before initiation of therapy.[156] Primary drug-specific resistance mutations occur at predictable frequency: for streptomycin, resistance mutations per organism occur at a density of 10^{-6}; for ethambutol, 10^{-7}; for isoniazid, 10^{-6} to 10^{-7}; and for rifampin, 10^{-8}. A cavity containing 10^9 tubercle bacilli has thousands of drug-resistant organisms; a closed caseous lesion with 10^6 bacilli has few or none. Fortunately, because the genetic loci for resistance are unlinked on the mycobacterial chromosome, the chance occurrence of resistance to one drug is unrelated to that for any other drug. For an organism to be "naturally" resistant (primary drug resistance) to two drugs, it would have to have a density of 10^{11} to 10^{16}, which is rarely, if ever, achieved clinically.

In adults with pulmonary cavities and children with extensive pulmonary infiltrates, bacterial density dictates the presence of many bacilli that are resistant to a single drug; treatment requires the use of at least two antituberculosis drugs. A single effective drug would select for emergence of a dominantly resistant population and produce secondary drug-resistant tuberculosis. Conversely, in children with latent *M. tuberculosis* infection, bacterial density is low, and a single drug is used; in children with limited primary pulmonary tuberculosis or moderate extrapulmonary disease, bacterial density is moderate, and effective therapy requires at least two bactericidal drugs.

Regimens

The earliest treatment regimens combined a bactericidal drug (such as isoniazid) with a bacteriostatic drug, to prevent development of isoniazid resistance. Because a few drug-susceptible organisms persist, treatment was given for 18 to 24 months to permit their elimination by the host. Despite prolonged treatment, relapse rate among adults was 5% to 10%. Use of bactericidal rifampin with isoniazid in adults led to cure in almost 100% of patients treated for 9 months.[184] Addition of pyrazinamide to isoniazid and rifampin during the first 2 months of treatment of pulmonary tuberculosis in adults led to cure rates >98% and relapse rates <3% after a total of 6 months of treatment.[158] The addition of streptomycin added little to effectiveness. Regimens of <6 months' duration were less effective even when four or five drugs were used initially.

During the past three decades, many therapeutic trials for tuberculosis in children have been reported. In 1983, Abernathy and colleagues[185] reported successful treatment of 50 children with pulmonary tuberculosis in an area with low rates of drug resistance using isoniazid (10 to 15 mg/kg) and rifampin (10 to 20 mg/kg) daily for 1 month, followed by isoniazid (20 to 40 mg/kg per dose) and rifampin (10 to 20 mg/kg per dose) twice weekly for 8 months, a total treatment course of two drugs for 9 months. Some patients with hilar lymphadenopathy alone were successfully treated with two drugs given for 6 months.[185,186] Although a study from Brazil reported successful treatment of 117 children with pulmonary tuberculosis using isoniazid and rifampin daily for 6 months, this regimen has not been adopted because of limited data and the concern for drug resistance.[187] The Brazilian study also highlighted difficulties with adherence in taking medications long term; even with this relatively simple regimen, 17% of children did not complete treatment.

Several studies of 6-month regimens (using at least three drugs) for drug-susceptible pulmonary tuberculosis in children have been reviewed.[159,188-192] The most common regimen was a 6-month period of administration of isoniazid and rifampin, supplemented during the first 2 months with pyrazinamide. Most trials used daily therapy for the first 2 months, with the exception of recent trials in which daily therapy was given for only 0 to 2 weeks, followed by twice- or thrice-weekly therapy to complete 6 months.[188,189] Regimens using intermittent therapy were as safe and effective as those using daily therapy. In all these trials, the overall success rate was >95% for cure and >99% for significant improvement during a 2-year follow-up.

Current Recommendations for Suspected Isoniazid-Susceptible Tuberculosis

The American Academy of Pediatrics (AAP) and the American Thoracic Society endorse the standard therapy for intrathoracic tuberculosis in children of 6 months of isoniazid and rifampin supplemented during the first 2 months by pyrazinamide and ethambutol (so called "RIPE" therapy).[193] Ethambutol is recommended routinely because it is safe in children and helps to prevent the emergence of rifampin resistance if isoniazid resistance already is present.[194] If the isolate from the child or the likely source case is fully drug-susceptible, ethambutol can be stopped. Daily administration of drugs is desirable for the first 2 weeks to 2 months; subsequently, drugs can be administered daily or twice- or thrice-weekly under directly observed therapy (DOT). When adherence to a regimen is likely to be unreliable, drugs have been given 2 or 3 times a week by DOT from initiation of therapy. Usual doses of antituberculosis medications are listed in Table 134-2.

Treatment for Children with HIV Infection

The optimal treatment of tuberculosis in children with HIV infection has not been established.[195,196] Adults with HIV and tuberculosis usually can be treated successfully with standard regimens if the total duration of therapy is extended to 9 months, or to 6 months after results of sputum smears and cultures become negative, whichever is longer.[197] Data for children are limited to isolated small series. Children with drug-susceptible tuberculosis and HIV usually are given isoniazid and rifampin for 9 months, with pyrazinamide and ethambutol (RIPE) for the first 2 months.[38,196] Rifabutin can be substituted for rifampin, especially in patients undergoing protease-inhibitor antiretroviral therapy.[198-200] Treatment of latent tuberculosis infection for HIV-infected children consists of 9 months of isoniazid. For an anergic child with HIV who is exposed to an adult with tuberculosis, the safest course of action is administration of isoniazid for 9 months.

Extrapulmonary Tuberculosis

Clinical trials for treatment of extrapulmonary tuberculosis in children have not been conducted. Several trials in children of 6-month, 3-drug regimens included cases of lymph node and disseminated tuberculosis; both types of disease responded favorably.[192,201] Most data come from series of cases of extrapulmonary tuberculosis in adults.[11,58,202,203] Most non-life-threatening forms have responded well to a 6-month regimen using 3 or 4 drugs in the initial phase of therapy. In general, treatment for most extrapulmonary tuberculosis is the same as that for pulmonary tuberculosis. One exception is bone and joint tuberculosis, for which 6-month regimens (especially without surgical intervention) have been associated with a higher failure rate.[203,204] For bone and joint tuberculosis, 9 to 12 months of chemotherapy is recommended.

Meningitis usually has not been included in trials for extrapulmonary tuberculosis because of its serious nature and low incidence. For drug-susceptible infection, treatment with isoniazid and rifampin for 12 months generally has been effective.[205] A study from Thailand has demonstrated better survival and less morbidity when pyrazinamide (which crosses the blood–brain barrier well) is added to the initial 2 months of treatment.[206] The AAP recommends 9 to 12 months of therapy with the use of at least isoniazid, rifampin, and pyrazinamide. Many experts believe that a treatment duration of 6 to 9 months is adequate if pyrazinamide is included in the initial phase, with a fourth drug added initially (streptomycin, ethionomide, or another aminoglycoside) if antibiotic susceptibility of the particular case is not known. However, some experts continue to recommend 12 months of treatment.[207]

Newborn or Infant with a Contagious Household Contact

A newborn infant or young infant whose mother (or other household contact) is suspected of having tuberculosis is at high risk of infection and disease. If possible, separation of the mother (or contact) and infant should be minimized. Recommendations in a variety of settings follow.[110]

Mother (or other household contact) has positive TST reaction and no evidence of active disease. Investigation of other members of the household or extended family (to whom the infant could be exposed) is recommended. If no evidence of disease is found, the infant does not need further evaluation. Isoniazid therapy should also be considered for the mother.

Mother has noncontagious disease that is untreated, or has been treated for 2 weeks or longer and is judged to be noncontagious at delivery. For the infant of a woman who is newly diagnosed as having tuberculosis (e.g., hilar lymphadenopathy, apical scarring) or whose tuberculosis has been treated for at least 2 weeks, careful contact investigation of household members and extended family is mandatory. A chest radiograph and TST should be performed on the infant at 3 months and again at 6 months of age. Separation of the mother and infant is not necessary if treatment/follow-up of both is ensured. The infant can breastfeed.

The infant should receive isoniazid regardless of the infant's TST result because of the high risk for disseminated disease and the delayed manifestations of a positive skin test result as late as 6 months of age if the infant was infected at birth. Isoniazid therapy can be discontinued if the infant's TST result and chest radiograph and physical findings are normal at 3 to 4 months of age, the mother is adherent to therapy and shows a satisfactory clinical response to treatment, and no other family members have infectious tuberculosis.

Mother has active disease and is suspected to be contagious at delivery. Management is the same as for the infant of a mother judged to be noncontagious at delivery (above). Additionally, the mother and infant should be separated until the infant is receiving therapy with adherence ensured and the mother is confirmed to be noninfectious.

Mother has hematogenously spread tuberculosis. The infant of a mother with hematogenously spread tuberculosis (e.g., meningitis, miliary disease, or bone or joint involvement) should be evaluated for congenital tuberculosis and treated accordingly. Evaluation of the placenta for *M. tuberculosis* should be conducted. If clinical and radiographic findings do not suggest congenital tuberculosis, the infant is separated from the mother until she is judged to be noncontagious, the infant is given isoniazid until 3 or 4 months of age at which time the TST is performed. If the TST result is positive, isoniazid should be continued for a total of 9 months. If the TST result and chest radiograph findings are normal, isoniazid can be discontinued, depending on the status of the mother and household contacts.

Adjunctive Measures and Monitoring

Corticosteroid Therapy

Corticosteroid agents are beneficial in the management of tuberculosis in children when the host inflammatory reaction contributes significantly to tissue damage or impaired function.[208] Corticosteroids decrease mortality rates and long-term neurologic sequelae in patients with tuberculous meningitis by reducing vasculitis, inflammation, and increased intracranial pressure.[209] A CNS inflammatory mass that arises during therapy of tuberculous meningitis usually responds to corticosteroid therapy. Children with enlarged hilar lymph nodes that compress the tracheobronchial tree, causing respiratory distress, localized emphysema, or collapse-consolidation lesions, frequently benefit from corticosteroid therapy.[210] Corticosteroids may benefit the course of miliary disease associated with alveolar-capillary block, pleural effusion, or pericardial effusion. Prednisone is used most commonly at the dose of 1 to 2 mg/kg per day for 4 to 6 weeks.

Follow-Up During Antituberculosis Therapy and Directly Observed Therapy

Major goals of following children during treatment, in order of importance, are: (1) to ensure adherence; (2) to monitor for toxic or other side effects of the medications; and (3) to assess clinical response. Patients are evaluated periodically and should be given only enough medicine for the interval between evaluations. Suspected cases of tuberculosis must be reported so that the local public health department can compile accurate statistics, perform necessary contact investigations, and help patients and HCP overcome barriers to adherence to therapy. Nonadherence and missed appointments should be quickly brought to the attention of responsible public health officials, who may be able to use various incentives or behavior modification. In extreme cases, a child may have to be removed from the home to ensure adherence to therapy. The use of DOT in a population of patients with increased risk factors for nonadherence (homelessness, intravenous drug use, HIV infection, and lower socioeconomic status) demonstrated reductions in primary drug resistance, secondary drug resistance, relapse rates, and relapses with MDR organisms.[211] Most children and adolescents with tuberculosis should be managed with DOT.[212,213]

Monitoring for Adverse Effects of Treatment

Rates of adverse reactions to antituberculosis medications among children are low.[110,160] Asymptomatic elevations (<3 times normal) of serum ALT occur frequently during isoniazid or rifampin treatment, do not predict hepatotoxicity, and are not indications for discontinuing drugs. Routine biochemical monitoring usually is not indicated. Education of caregivers regarding signs and symptoms of potential adverse events is preferable. Anorexia or vomiting (beyond 1 to 2 days of presumed intercurrent illness), abdominal pain, or jaundice should elicit discontinuation of medications and evaluation by a physician. Children taking ethambutol require regular monitoring of visual acuity and color discrimination, if possible. Biochemical monitoring is recommended for pregnant or postpartum adolescents because of possible excessive hepatotoxicity.[110]

Frequent radiographic monitoring usually is not necessary. Improvement of intrathoracic tuberculosis in children occurs slowly. Chest radiographs usually are obtained at diagnosis, 1 or 2 months into therapy, and at the conclusion of therapy. Normal chest radiograph appearance is not a necessary criterion for completion of therapy. After the end of chemotherapy, resolution of hilar lymphadenopathy commonly continues for 2 to 3 years.

DRUG-RESISTANT TUBERCULOSIS

Factors contributing to the increase in drug resistance in tuberculosis have been: (1) the deterioration of the public health service infrastructure; (2) inadequate training of HCP regarding the epidemiology, treatment, and control of tuberculosis; (3) a switch to predominantly unmonitored outpatient therapy for tuberculosis; (4) a rise in the incidence of tuberculosis in populations with easy access to antituberculosis medications; (5) an increase in the number of individuals at high risk for the acquisition of tuberculosis and for potentially serious forms of the disease, with subsequent inadequate treatment; and (6) the epidemic of HIV infection.[17,214] Factors contributing to recent outbreaks and the continued spread of drug-resistant tuberculosis are: (1) the increased number of patients coinfected with *M. tuberculosis* and HIV; (2) inefficient infection control procedures and facilities; (3) laboratory delays in identification and susceptibility testing of *M. tuberculosis* isolates; and (4) failure to recognize the ongoing infectiousness of patients.[17]

The prevalence of drug-resistant organisms among patients with pulmonary tuberculosis in the U.S. has risen steadily from about 2% to 9% in the past 3 decades. The consideration of drug-resistant tuberculosis and of local epidemiologic circumstances has led to major changes in recommendations for initial treatment, retreatment, control, and prevention of tuberculosis throughout the world.[17,215]

MDR tuberculosis is defined as infection caused by a strain of *M. tuberculosis* that is resistant at least to isoniazid and rifampin. *XDR tuberculosis* refers to infection due to organisms that are resistant to isoniazid and rifampin, fluoroquinolones, and at least one aminoglycoside. The importance of prior exposure to antituberculosis drugs in this situation is highlighted by the finding that 100% of the organisms in an initially mixed population of susceptible and resistant organisms can become resistant if exposure to that specific drug persists.

Treatment

For treatment of tuberculosis in adults and children, an initial regimen of 4 drugs, usually RIPE, when resistance is a risk, is used empirically.[193] This regimen usually will prevent emergence of resistance to rifampin if isoniazid resistance is already present but not yet verified. It is difficult for the clinician to anticipate other patterns of drug resistance before drug susceptibility results are known. The selection of antituberculosis treatment regimens requires knowledge of local epidemiology, assessment of the patient's history of treatment and contact with drug-resistant tuberculosis, and performance of complete laboratory studies to characterize the susceptibility of *M. tuberculosis*.

Most recommendations about treatment of drug-resistant tuberculosis in children have been based on case reports and extrapolation from adult series.[216–221] Several recent series of management of drug-resistant tuberculosis in children have shown that[222–225]: (1) children generally tolerate second-line therapy well, despite the lack of pediatric dosage forms; (2) children with intrathoracic tuberculosis generally respond well when at least 3 to 4 drugs to which the isolate is susceptible are used; (3) prognosis is poorer for children with tuberculous meningitis, HIV coinfection, or poor access to health resources; and (4) treatment can be community-based for all or most of the course in most children. The specific regimen to be used depends on drug susceptibility test results; if drug resistance is confirmed, an expert in managing drug-resistant tuberculosis should be involved in designing the treatment regimen.

CALMETTE–GUÉRIN BACILLUS (BCG) VACCINE

Although BCG vaccines have been administered to over 4 billion people and have been used routinely in every country except the Netherlands and the U.S., tuberculosis remains a major cause of morbidity and mortality throughout the world.[226] A major hindrance to evaluation of BCG is the lack of known in vitro correlates for immunity to *M. tuberculosis*. Immune response to BCG vaccine and its mechanism of action are not well understood. BCG does not appear to prevent primary pulmonary infection. Clinical trials and case-control studies show higher levels of protection against the more serious forms of disease, such as meningitis and miliary tuberculosis.[227,228]

Eight clinical efficacy trials conducted from the 1930s through the 1970s demonstrated wide-ranging and conflicting results, with efficacy in prevention of disease ranging from 0% to 80%. Trials differed in eligibility criteria, methods of disease surveillance, diagnostic criteria, vaccine strain and administration, and environmental factors. Heterogeneity among these trials is not unexpected because they were conducted over 4 decades in 9 different geographic areas in 3 different countries and involved myriad investigators and organizations. Meta-analyses of published trials and case-control series suggest that BCG vaccination prevents about 50% of all cases of tuberculosis disease in children, 60% to 80% of severe cases (meningitis, military), and 60% to 80% of deaths from tuberculosis.[229-232]

The low risk of *M. tuberculosis* infection in the general population of the U.S. and the unknown vaccine efficacy make a national BCG vaccination policy inappropriate. BCG vaccination is recommended for infants and children with negative TST results who: (1) are at high risk of intimate and prolonged exposure to persistently untreated or ineffectively treated individuals with infectious pulmonary tuberculosis, cannot be removed from the source of exposure, and cannot be given appropriate preventive therapy; or (2) are continuously exposed to people with tuberculosis who have bacilli resistant to isoniazid and rifampin.[233] In healthcare settings with a high risk of transmission of drug-resistant *M. tuberculosis* where aggressive infection control measures have failed, BCG vaccination for HCP might be considered.

BCG vaccine is contraindicated in: (1) individuals whose immunologic responses are impaired because of HIV infection, congenital immunodeficiency, leukemia, lymphoma, or generalized malignancy; (2) persons receiving corticosteroids, alkylating agents, antimetabolites, or irradiation; and (3) pregnant women.[233] Patients who are undergoing treatment for tuberculosis or who receive BCG vaccine can be given measles vaccine or other live-virus vaccines as otherwise indicated, unless they are taking corticosteroids, are severely ill, or have specific vaccine contraindications.

Complications of BCG vaccine include BCG lymphadenitis and abscesses; in immunosuppressed individuals and occasionally in normal hosts (especially infants and toddlers), infection can occur at disseminated sites, such as bone, brain, liver, and lung.[234-243] Standard antituberculosis therapy (except for pyrazinamide) is recommended to treat osteitis and disseminated disease caused by BCG and could be considered for treatment of chronic suppurative lymphadenitis when surgical excision cannot be performed.

TUBERCULOSIS CONTROL IN CHILDREN

Considering that tuberculosis disease can be cured with a drug cost of $50, and most cases should be prevented with effective treatment of LTBI, the failure to control tuberculosis in adults and children is a tragedy – a failure of public health policy.[244] The number of childhood cases of tuberculosis occurring even in the poorest countries can be reduced drastically if children who live with adults with pulmonary tuberculosis are appropriately evaluated and treated in a timely fashion.[245-248] Because most childhood tuberculosis cases occur 2 to 9 months after infection, early intervention is highly effective and highly cost-beneficial.[249] Children should be a major focus of all tuberculosis control programs.[250]

135 *Mycobacterium* Species Non-*tuberculosis*

Marc Tebruegge and Nigel Curtis

More sophisticated microbiologic techniques in the recent two decades have enabled more rapid and more accurate identification of "older" species of nontuberculous mycobacteria (NTM) as well as identification of multiple "new" species that are emerging as human pathogens.[1,2] Newer technologies include high-performance liquid chromatography (HPLC), commercial DNA probes, automated broth culture techniques, and sequencing or restriction fragment length polymorphism (RFLP) analysis of DNA sequences.[3] Most laboratories use a variety of traditional morphological and biochemical characteristics in addition to newer techniques. More than 140 species of mycobacteria are recognized currently.

EPIDEMIOLOGY

NTM species are ubiquitous in soil, water, foodstuffs, and domestic and wild animals.[4,5] Human strains of *Mycobacterium avium* and *M. intracellulare* (*M. avium* complex or MAC) are found in fresh and brackish waters in warm climates as well as in some animals, particularly swine. Despite earlier impressions, bird strains of *M. avium* differ on a molecular level from human strains.[6] Tap water has emerged as the major reservoir for a number of NTM species, including *M. kansasii*, *M. xenopi*, *M. gordonae*, *M. simiae*, and *M. mucogenicum*,[7] and also *M. fortuitum*, *M. chelonae*, and *M. abscessus*.[4] Fish and fishtank water are a major reservoir for *M. marinum*.[8-12] Rapidly growing mycobacteria (*M. fortuitum*, *M. mucogenicum*, *M. immunogenum*, and *M. abscessus*) have been associated with healthcare-associated infection (HAI) presumably from environmental sources.[13-17] When identical methods are used, isolation rates of NTM are remarkably similar in diverse geographic areas.[18]

There are particular geographic regions in which pathogenic species are found more commonly in the local environment and as etiologic agents of disease.[19] These include *M. simiae* (southwestern United States, Europe, Israel), *M. malmoense* (northern and central Europe), *M. xenopi* (Canada, U.S., Europe), *M. ulcerans* (Australia, Africa), and *M. kansasii* (Europe, selected areas of the central and southern U.S.).[18-36]

The incidence of human disease due to NTM increased significantly in the 1980s and 1990s in parallel with increasing numbers of AIDS cases.[37] Additionally, epidemiologic data suggest that the incidence of NTM infections in seemingly immunocompetent individuals also has risen in the last few decades.[19,20,34,35,38-40] However, it is uncertain whether the increase is real or reflects increased awareness and enhanced laboratory detection.[19,35]

PATHOGENESIS

Knowledge of pathogenesis of NTM infection in humans is limited. Humans are thought to acquire these organisms from environmental sources. There is no evidence of human-to-human transmission.[18,40-44] Pulmonary NTM infection results from inhalation of airborne particles containing organisms, whereas skin and soft-tissue infections result from direct inoculation. Ingestion of NTM can lead to gastrointestinal disease or to cervical lymphadenitis. The pathogenesis of disseminated disease,

TABLE 135-1. Clinical Manifestations of Infection Caused by Nontuberculous Mycobacteria

Infection Site	Predominant Species	Typical Lesions	Setting
Skin and soft tissue	*Mycobacterium marinum*	Papular, nodular or plaque-like; less commonly ulcerative	Usually associated with aquatic trauma (aquarium granuloma, swimmer's granuloma)
	M. fortuitum	Granuloma	Postsurgical, CVC-associated, following trauma/penetrating injury
	M. abscessus	Granuloma	Following local trauma
	M. chelonae	Granuloma	Following local trauma
	M. ulcerans	Ulcer	Mode of transmission is uncertain
Lymphadenitis	*M. avium* complex	Submandibular or anterior cervical mass	Typically unilateral; subacute; age 1–5 years
	M. haemophilum		
	M. malmoense[a]		
Otitis media/mastoiditis	*M. abscessus*	Chronic otorrhea; unresponsive to conventional antibiotics	Almost exclusively in patients with tympanostomy tubes in situ
	M. avium complex		
Pulmonary infection	*M. avium* complex	Cavitation or nodular; bronchiectasis	Typically patients with pre-existing lung disease; in children and adolescents: cystic fibrosis and bronchiectasis; in adults: chronic obstructive pulmonary disease
	M. kansasii		
	M. abscessus		
	M. fortuitum		
	M. simiae[a]		
Disseminated infection	*M. avium* complex	Organism recovered from blood, bone marrow, liver, lymph nodes	Immunocompromised host (malignancy, impaired cell-mediated immunity, HIV infection, immunosuppressive treatment or chemotherapy)
	M. kansasii		
	M. abscessus		
	M. chelonae		
	M. haemophilum		

[a]*Only common in certain geographic areas (see text).*

especially for rapidly growing mycobacteria, usually is not apparent,[45] although central venous catheters (CVCs) may be important. Multiple host factors that increase the risk of NTM infection have been identified.[18] Each species has a characteristic level of virulence and propensity to cause infection in particular organs/settings (Table 135-1). This includes contaminated wounds and open fractures (*M. fortuitum, M. goodii*), prosthetic devices such as indwelling CVCs (*M. fortuitum, M. mucogenicum*) and prosthetic heart valves (*M. fortuitum, M. abscessus*),[45–47] tympanostomy tubes (*M. abscessus*, MAC),[14,17] immune suppression with organ transplantation (*M. chelonae, M. abscessus*),[48] and bronchiectasis in the setting of cystic fibrosis (CF) (MAC, *M. abscessus*).[49–51] A further iatrogenic factor predisposing to mycobacterial disease is treatment with tumor necrosis factor (TNF)-α inhibiting agents (e.g., infliximab and etanercept), usually in the context of rheumatoid arthritis or inflammatory bowel disease.[52–55] Investigation of genetic polymorphisms that enhance host susceptibility to NTM is ongoing. There is increasing recognition of the importance of the interferon (IFN)-γ, TNF-α, and interleukin (IL)-12 pathways in the host immune response to mycobacteria. Isolated immune defects identified in patients with disseminated mycobacterial infections include mutations in the IFN-γ receptor gene and IL-12 receptor deficiency.[56–62]

Virulence factors that enhance invasiveness of NTM largely are unknown, in part because only a few NTM species have undergone genomic sequencing. The complete genome of *M. ulcerans* was published in 2007, followed by the genomes of *M. avium, M. marinum*, and *M. abscessus*.[63–68] *M. ulcerans* has been shown to produce mycolactone, a polyketide toxin that induces tissue necrosis and has immunosuppressive properties.[69] The genes required for mycolactone production are plasmid encoded.[70]

LABORATORY DIAGNOSIS

Mycobacterial species, the site of specimen origin, and quantity of growth in culture are important in assessing the potential pathogenic role of an NTM isolate.[18] Heavy growth of a single organism usually indicates infection, whereas light growth from a single sputum sample may indicate colonization/contamination.[18] Isolation of NTM from normally sterile body fluids or bronchoalveolar lavage (BAL) fluid, confirms infection.[18] Recommendations for isolation and interpretation of culture results are published.[18]

Because some NTM have unusual requirements for nutrition and incubation (e.g., *M. haemophilum, M. ulcerans, M. genavense, M. marinum*),[2,9,18,71] laboratory personnel should be consulted, to optimize specimen collection and culture.

Conventional methods used for *M. tuberculosis* remain useful for processing and staining specimens for NTM. Typically, *N*-acetyl-L-cysteine is used as a mucolytic agent to free acid-fast bacilli from proteinaceous material, followed by 2% sodium hydroxide to kill non-acid-fast organisms. Some NTM species, especially rapidly growing mycobacteria such as *M. abscessus*, are highly susceptible to sodium hydroxide procedures and lose viability.[72] Chlorhexidine decontamination may be preferable when *M. abscessus* is suspected.[72] For tissue samples and fluids from normally sterile sites, decontamination procedures are not required.[18]

Fluorochrome, Kinyoun, and Ziehl–Neelsen stains are used for direct staining.[3,18] The appearance of mycobacteria in stained specimens is variable, requiring experience for accurate interpretation. Colony morphology, growth rates, and pigmentation are superior to microscopic morphology as an indication of mycobacterial group; however, neither should be used to identify species.

Standard culture methods involve a combination of broth and solid media. Although most NTM species grow well with standard incubation at 37°C, some, including *M. ulcerans* and *M. marinum*, grow poorly or not at all at 37°C. If these organisms are suspected, additional cultures should be incubated in parallel at 30 to 32°C.[9,73,74]

Historically, isolation of mycobacteria on solid media required 2 to 4 weeks, and identification based on biochemical tests took another 4 to 6 weeks. However, the use of broth culture incubation systems, such as the BioFM (Bio-Rad) and the Bactec MGIT 960 (Becton Dickinson), has reduced the time for detection of growth to an average of 1 to 2 weeks, depending on species and positivity of direct smear.[3,75–77] A more rapid method for species identification is cell wall mycolic acid analysis by thin-layer chromatography, gas–liquid chromatography, or high-performance liquid chromatography (HPLC).[1,78–81] A variety of molecular methods also can be used for species identification, including commercial DNA probes (*M. tuberculosis* complex, MAC, *M. gordonae*, and *M. kansasii*) (AccuProbe, Gen-Probe), and a commercial hybridization strip for multiple species (INNO-LiPA, InnoGenetics).[18,82–86] Other methods include a commercial 16S rRNA gene sequencing kit (MicroSeq, Applied Biosystems),[87,88] noncommercial (in-house) sequencing and polymerase chain reaction (PCR) plus RFLP analysis (PRA) of the *hsp*65 gene.[89–92]

DNA probes, target amplification methods (e.g., PCR), signal amplification methods, and gene amplification are being studied to detect and identify NTM directly from clinical specimens.[3,93] The most effective method has been amplification followed by identification of the 16S rRNA or the *hsp*65 gene.[3,93] None of these is available commercially, and both gene targets unfortunately are single-copy genes, which greatly reduces detection sensitivity. Recent publications have reported the identification of NTM by means of pyrosequencing of the hypervariable regions of the 16S rRNA gene.[94–96] This method allows higher throughput and is generally less expensive than "traditional" chain-termination ("Sanger") sequencing, and has a high level of accuracy for distinguishing between different mycobacterial species. The automated PCR-based GeneXpert system (Cepheid) permits concurrent rapid detection of *M. tuberculosis* and rifampin resistance, but has not been developed for NTM.[97]

In 2003, the Clinical Laboratory Standards Institute published standardized procedures for susceptibility testing of NTM.[98] Generally, both slowly and rapidly growing pathogenic mycobacteria are tested using broth systems. Susceptibility or resistance of NTM species in vitro often does not correlate well with clinical efficacy, with the exception of clarithromycin resistance for treatment of disseminated or pulmonary MAC, clarithromycin resistance for *M. chelonae* and *M. abscessus* infections, and rifampin resistance for pulmonary *M. kansasii*.[99–102]

Immunoassays in the Diagnosis of Nontuberculous Mycobacterial Infections

IFN-γ release assays (IGRA) have emerged as a novel tool for the diagnosis of tuberculosis. The common principle of IGRA is the detection of IFN-γ produced by sensitized T lymphocytes upon exposure to mycobacterial antigens.[103,104] Two commercial assays are available currently: the QuantiFERON-TB Gold assay (Cellestis; currently in second- and third-generation versions) and the T-SPOT.*TB* assay (Oxford Immunotech). The former is a whole-blood assay, the latter an ELISPOT assay, which uses peripheral blood mononuclear cells. The second-generation QuantiFERON-TB Gold assay and the T-SPOT.*TB* assay incorporate early secretory antigenic target 6 (ESAT-6) and culture filtrate protein 10 (CFP-10) as stimulatory antigens; the third-generation QuantiFERON-TB Gold assay (QuantiFERON-TB Gold In Tube) incorporates TB7.7 as an additional antigen. Both ESAT-6 and CFP-10 are encoded in the RD1 region of the *M. tuberculosis* genome, and are absent from most nontuberculous mycobacteria, with the notable exceptions of *M. kansasii*, *M. marinum*, and *M. szulgai*.[103–105] Consequently, IGRAs have overall greater specificity for tuberculous infections compared with the Mantoux tuberculin skin test (TST). However, IGRAs have several limitations, particularly in children: (a) evidence that their performance is less robust in young children,[106–109] (b) high proportions of indeterminate (i.e., uninterpretable) results are reported in some pediatric studies,[106,109,110] and (c) the mechanisms underlying discordance with TST results, which frequently is attributed (without definitive evidence) to prior BCG vaccination or exposure to NTM, are understood incompletely.[106,111–113]

IGRAs, however, may be useful adjunctively to help differentiate between tuberculous and NTM disease. One study that included a subgroup of children with mycobacterial lymphadenitis (mainly caused by *M. avium*) showed that both the QuantiFERON-TB Gold

assay and the T-SPOT.*TB* assay have a greater ability than TST to discriminate between tuberculous and NTM lymphadenitis.[114] Other studies illustrate that both commercial IGRAs can be useful to distinguish between lung disease due to *M. tuberculosis* and certain NTM, including MAC, *M. malmoense*, *M. ganavense*, and *M. gordonae*.[115–120] A recent meta-analysis of published studies, however, shows that the pooled sensitivity of the QuantiFERON-TB Gold In Tube assay and the T-SPOT.*TB* assay in patients with active tuberculosis is only 81% and 88%, respectively.[121] Additionally, a positive IGRA result does not prove *M. tuberculosis* infection; the majority of patients with NTM disease caused by *M. kansasii*, *M. marinum*, or *M. szulgai* have positive IGRA results.[116,117,120,122,123] Case reports suggest that these tests can be useful to support a suspected diagnosis of *M. marinum* skin infection while PCR and culture results are pending.[124,125]

CLINICAL MANIFESTATIONS

Localized Skin, Soft-Tissue, and Bone Infections

The NTM responsible for most posttraumatic or postsurgical skin and soft-tissue infections are *M. marinum*, *M. ulcerans*, *M. fortuitum*, and *M. chelonae*, as well as the more recently recognized *M. goodii*.[18,45,126–129] Diagnosis requires demonstration of the organism in a biopsy specimen or culture of aspirated fluid from a skin nodule, wound, or abscess. In immunocompetent hosts, cutaneous NTM infection usually represents the primary site of infection following local trauma.[45] In immunocompromised hosts, cutaneous lesions can be a manifestation of disseminated disease.[18,130–132]

Infection with *M. marinum* usually follows cutaneous trauma in non-chlorinated swimming pools, aquariums, or natural bodies of water.[8,9,124,133,134] Infection is acquired most commonly from home aquariums.[8,9,12] Less frequently, *M. marinum* infection results from injuries inflicted by marine life (i.e., fish spine or bite injuries). Lesions typically are nontender and papular, nodular or plaque-like. The hands and arms are affected most commonly, followed by the legs; truncal lesions are rare. A sporotrichoid distribution (i.e., a linear distribution along lymphatic vessels) of multiple lesions is seen in about one-quarter to one-third of cases.[12,135–137] Regional lymphadenitis or systemic symptoms are very rare.[12] Locally invasive disease, including tenosynovitis, arthritis, and osteomyelitis, is uncommon.[138] Disseminated infection is rare, and almost exclusively occurs in immunocompromised hosts.[8,132,139,140]

M. ulcerans infection mainly occurs in sub-Saharan Africa and Australia, where it is referred to as Buruli ulcer and Bairnsdale ulcer, respectively.[18,24,25,92,126,141–143] However, cases are also reported from some Asian countries and Latin America.[141,142,144–148] The infection is most commonly acquired in riverine and coastal areas. Although the mode of transmission currently is unknown, some data suggest a role of aquatic insects or mosquitoes.[142,149,150] The initial lesion is a single subcutaneous nodule, which evolves into a painless, undermined ulcer, typically located on the extensor surface of the lower extremities. Local necrosis and, occasionally, widespread secondary necrosis occur with or without satellite lesions. Infection can spread to deep tissue planes. Healing may occur slowly over a period of 6 to 9 months, often resulting in severe limb deformity.[143] Lymph node enlargement and systemic symptoms are rare.

M. fortuitum, *M. abscessus*, and *M. chelonae* are rapidly growing mycobacteria that cause a wide spectrum of cutaneous infections.[45] Primary cutaneous disease often follows penetrating injury and usually manifests as localized cellulitis, a draining abscess, or individual nodule with minimal tenderness.[18,36,45,127,133] Outbreaks of cutaneous abscesses following injections have been associated with use of contaminated multiple-dose vials.[15,16] Outbreaks of postoperative wound infections have been reported after median sternotomy,[45,151,152] plastic surgery using contaminated gentian violet,[153] and plastic surgery procedures such as liposuction and mammoplasty.[13,45] Sporadic infections have been described in association with a wide variety of surgical procedures. In contrast

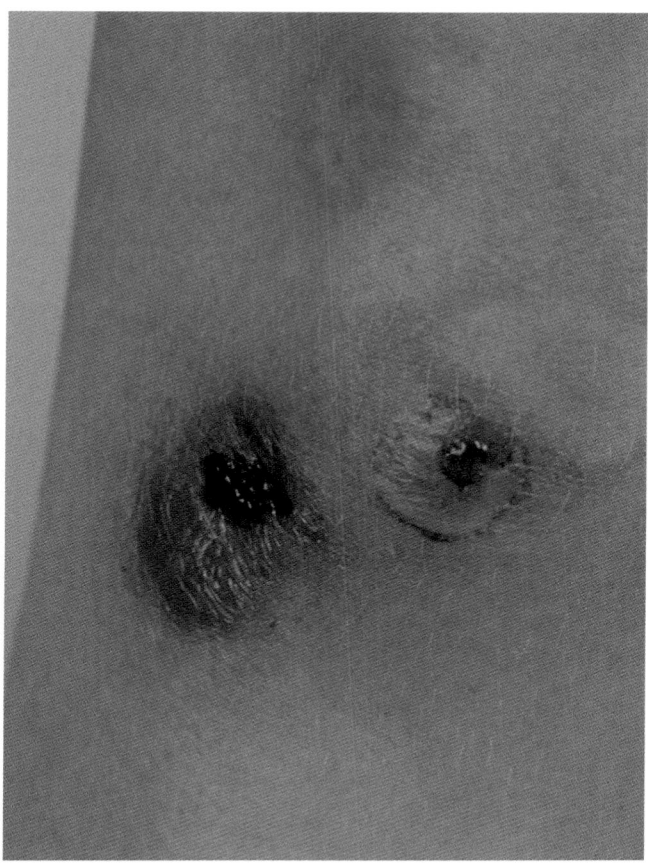

Figure 135-1. Lesion on the right knee of a previously well 5-year-old girl that developed over a 1- to 2-month period and did not respond to conventional antibiotics. Biopsy of the lesion showed granulomatous inflammation and acid-fast bacilli; *Mycobacterium avium* complex was identified by culture. Immunologic testing, including investigation of the interferon-γ/IL-12 pathway, did not reveal evidence of immunodeficiency. The lesion resolved almost completely within 3 months of starting a combination of rifampin and clarithromycin.

with a high prevalence in the southeastern U.S.[18,20,36,38,133,154–160] In contrast, children >12 years with mycobacterial adenitis generally have tuberculous infection.[156,159] In industrialized nations with low TB prevalence, NTM infections account for most cases of chronic cervical lymphadenitis.[157] MAC now accounts for 70% to 90% of cases of culture-positive NTM lymphadenitis, although *M. scrofulaceum* (now rare) was the predominant etiologic agent when the disease was first recognized.[18,20,21,36,38,133,154–161] In northern and central Europe, a significant proportion of NTM lymphadenitis is caused by *M. malmoense*.[20,161] The importance of *M. haemophilum* as a cause of cervical lymphadenitis previously was underestimated because of its unusual growth requirements (iron supplementation and optimal incubation temperature of 30°C).[71,160,162,163] Incidence of *M. haemophilum* in some series approaches 25%.[157] Other relatively uncommon causes of lymphadenitis are *M. kansasii*, *M. simiae*, *M. chelonae*, and *M. fortuitum*.[21,22,36,155,157–159]

Lymphadenitis due to NTM usually is unilateral and most commonly involves the anterior cervical or submandibular lymph nodes (Figure 135-2); the preauricular lymph nodes are

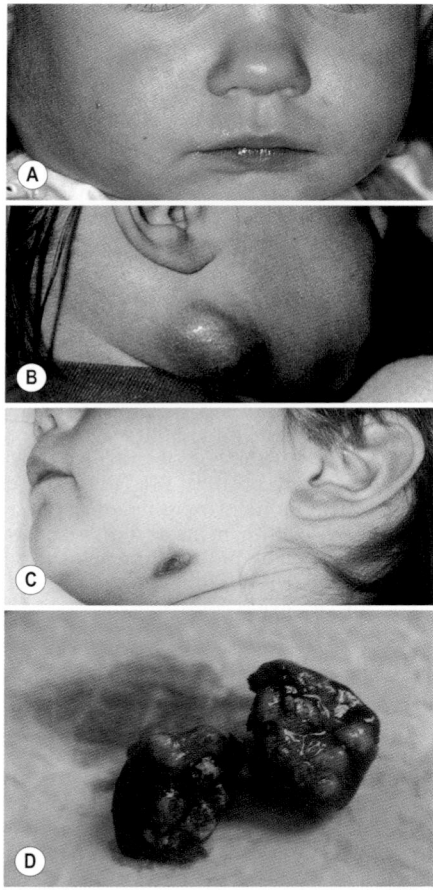

Figure 135-2. Three toddlers with characteristic ages, sites, appearances, and courses of nontuberculous lymphadenitis. Patient **A** had a 9 mm reactive tuberculin skin test (TST), was treated with clarithromycin, and the node regressed without suppuration. Patient **B** had typical erythematous, effaced skin overlying a *Mycobacterium avium* complex abscess; management included aspiration, antimycobacterial therapy, and then surgical excision. Photograph of patient **C** was taken 7 months after incision and drainage were performed (misdiagnosed as acute lymphadenitis), and 6 months after beginning clarithromycin and rifampin therapy; eventually intermittent drainage ceased and the scar lightened. Nine years after treatment, a mass recurred at the edge of the surgical scar. Two masses were excised measuring 0.7 and 1 cm in diameter **(D).** Microscopy confirmed noncaseating granulomas; mycobacterial culture was negative. (Courtesy of S.S. Long and B. Burkey, St. Christopher's Hospital for Children, Philadelphia, PA.)

to pyogenic infections, there is often a considerable gap between the surgical procedure and the onset of symptoms (typically 1 to 5 weeks).[151] Patients have poor wound healing or breakdown of a healed wound, with drainage of serous fluid. *M. fortuitum* has been associated with infections of the foot after puncture wound; such infections can be indistinguishable clinically from pseudomonal or staphylococcal infection.[36,45,129] The most common healthcare-associated NTM infections are CVC-associated infections due to *M. fortuitum*.[18,46,47]

Synovial infections are seen with MAC, and usually manifest as tenosynovitis of the hands or upper extremity. Usually they are localized and occur as a result of local trauma. Skin lesions due to MAC are rare and usually are the manifestation of disseminated disease (Figure 135-1).[131]

Infection of bones, bursa, and tendon sheaths can follow penetrating trauma or surgical procedures. *M. fortuitum* is most common in this setting; less commonly, *M. terrae* complex, MAC, and *M. goodii* are implicated.[18] Rare cases of disseminated osteomyelitis in children have been reported. The clinical presentation of skeletal infection (especially vertebral osteomyelitis) resembles that of *M. tuberculosis* and has an indolent, chronic course.[154]

Lymphadenitis

Lymphadenitis is the most common manifestation of NTM infection in children, generally occurring in otherwise healthy children <12 years of age (peak incidence 1 to 5 years of age), less commonly affected.[38,155–158,160,161,164] In about 5% of patients, infection involves intrathoracic (paratracheal or mediastinal) nodes.[156,165] Patients generally are well, without constitutional signs or symptoms, and have no or only mild local tenderness.[161] The lesion can be fluctuant or non-fluctuant.[156–158] If untreated, the overlying skin often becomes violaceous and effaced as the lymph nodes enlarge and soften.[157,166] Nodes then can rupture, and drain for prolonged periods of time through a sinus tract to the skin (Figure 135-2C). Infection sometimes resolves spontaneously or lymph nodes do not rupture but heal, leading to fibrosis and calcification that can be disfiguring.[156,167] Remote recrudescence also can occur (Figure 135-2D).

In the vast majority of patients the complete blood count is unremarkable; only a small proportion of patients have leukocytosis.[156,157,161] Some patients have an elevated erythrocyte sedimentation rate.[156,157,161] Chest radiography is unremarkable in approximately 90% to 95% of cases.[155,156,161] Some studies reported Mantoux TST yields a negative result in the majority of patients;[38,161] others suggest that approximately one-half of cases have a positive test result (induration >6 mm[158] or >10 mm[159] at 48 to 72 hours). Skin testing with mycobacterial sensitins (i.e., purified proteins) derived from NTM (e.g., *M. avium*, *M. scrofulaceum*, *M. kansasii*) is more sensitive than TST;[168] however, sensitins for clinical use are not available currently, and their potential usefulness is limited by their poor ability to distinguish between different causative NTM.

The differential diagnosis of NTM lymphadenitis is extensive and includes infection due to *M. tuberculosis*, *Bartonella henselae*, Epstein–Barr virus, *Toxoplasma gondii*, malignancy, and cystic hygroma (see Chapter 17, Cervical Lymphadenitis and Neck Infections). The diagnosis is supported by the histopathologic appearance of the lymph node, which shows caseating or noncaseating granulomas.[133,156,161,163] Acid-fast bacilli are detected only in approximately one-half to two-thirds of cases.[155,156,161] Although TST frequently is reactive, a negative result does not exclude NTM. Diagnosis is confirmed by isolating NTM from a lymph node or by molecular detection. In most series (using older, conventional culture media), organisms were isolated from only about 50% of infected lymph nodes.[155,156]

Bilateral lymphadenitis and involvement of posterior cervical, supraclavicular, axillary, or inguinal nodes suggest TB rather than NTM (see Figure 134-6). Tuberculous lymphadenitis is more often associated with a strongly positive TST, abnormal chest radiograph, history of constitutional symptoms, and contact with a case of active tuberculosis. Nodes in acute bacterial lymphadenitis often are larger, evolve rapidly, and are more tender and erythematous; fever is prominent and white cell count and C-reactive protein are typically elevated.[156,167,169]

Pulmonary Infection

Until recently, pulmonary infection with NTM was rare in children.[5,127] The recognition that NTM lung infections occur in the setting of bronchiectasis, especially in patients with cystic fibrosis (CF), has dramatically changed this perception.[49–51,170–172] Typically NTM lung infection in CF occurs in an adolescent or young adult with relatively mild disease. Some infections are difficult to distinguish from symptoms of CF, whereas other patients have fever, weight loss, and fatigue that does not respond to antipseudomonal therapy.[172] The disease appears to be more common in the south and southeastern U.S., where up to 20% of adolescents are infected. The most common reported species affecting the lung in CF patients are MAC, *M. abscessus*, *M. chelonae*, and *M. fortuitum*.[50,172–174] NTM organisms should be considered as possible pathogens when recovered repeatedly from sputum in patients with CF and severe lung disease or pulmonary exacerbation is unresponsive to broad-spectrum antibiotics.[167,171,172]

Most children with non-CF-associated, isolated pulmonary infection due to NTM are immunocompetent and have no underlying pulmonary disease.[154,175] Reported cases in children have been due to MAC, or other NTM (*M. kansasii*, *M. abscessus*, *M. chelonae*, and *M. fortuitum*).[36,175–179] Signs and symptoms are variable and nonspecific, including fever, cough, dyspnea,

hemoptysis, malaise, and fatigue. Weight loss and night sweats are relatively uncommon.[27,177] Enlargement of mediastinal and hilar lymph nodes is common.[175,177] Endobronchial obstruction can occur (either due to external compression or endobronchial granulation tissue), which can cause reduced air entry and persistent wheezing, thereby mimicking foreign body aspiration.[175,177] The diagnosis of pulmonary NTM should be suspected in a child who has a pulmonary illness consistent with tuberculosis who is not responding well to usual antituberculous medications.

NTM are recognized increasingly as causes of graft dysfunction in lung transplant recipients.[180]

Physical examination and routine laboratory tests seldom provide etiologic clues. Chest radiographic findings are nonspecific and cannot be differentiated easily from those of tuberculosis or fungal infection. However, cavitating lesions are less common in pulmonary NTM disease compared with tuberculosis.[27] Involvement of multiple pulmonary segments is common.[181] Chest computed tomography, including high-resolution studies, is used increasingly for diagnosis and follow-up.[182] Imaging features depend on whether lung disease primarily is fibrocavitary (similar to tuberculosis) or is characterized by nodules and bronchiectasis.[18,181,182] Isolation of NTM is essential for diagnosis. The interpretation of positive sputum or gastric aspirate culture results is confounded by ubiquity of NTM in the environment. A single positive culture does not establish NTM disease.[18] Diagnosis requires growth of the same NTM organism from multiple sputum samples or a BAL specimen after the exclusion of other causes for the clinical symptoms. Certain NTM that are generally nonpathogenic – including *M. gordonae*, *M. terrae* complex, and *M. mucogenicum* – are likely to be contaminants.[18] The American Thoracic Society (ATS) has established diagnostic criteria for NTM pulmonary infection in adults, but their validity for children is not established.[18] The role and importance of BAL cultures in CF also have not been established, nor have the sensitivity or specificity of sputum cultures versus BAL cultures. In cases where the underlying etiology remains uncertain, lung biopsy should be considered to exclude other causes, to demonstrate histopathologic changes consistent with mycobacterial disease (e.g., granulomatous inflammation with or without acid-fast bacilli), and to obtain specimens for culture.[18]

Otitis Media

Otitis media with or without mastoiditis due to NTM occurs almost exclusively in children with tympanostomy tubes.[183–191] Outbreak[17] and sporadic[14] infections are described. The most commonly implicated NTM are *M. abscessus*, although cases caused by MAC are described. Patients usually present with persistent drainage unresponsive to standard antibiotic therapy.

Disseminated Infection

Disseminated disease due to NTM is rare in healthy persons, generally occurring in immunocompromised hosts, such as in patients with underlying malignancy or congenital or acquired defects of cell-mediated immunity,[8,18,45,48,132,139,140,192] isolated defects in the IFN-γ/IL-12 pathway,[60,62] solid-organ and stem cell transplant recipients,[192–198] and long-term corticosteroid therapy or cytotoxic chemotherapy.[192,199] Often, patients exhibit skin lesions as the earliest manifestation of disseminated disease, sometimes related to an indwelling CVC. The most common pathogens in these settings are *M. chelonae* and *M. abscessus*.[45,199] Other pathogens include MAC, *M. haemophilum*, *M. kansasii*, *M. fortuitum*, and *M. simiae*.[18,45,192,196,200] Skin or soft-tissue manifestations of *M. kansasii* infection are rare compared with rapidly growing mycobacteria and include verrucous or granulomatous papules, cellulitis, sporotrichoid eruptions, ulcers, and necrotic papulopustules.[130,192] Multiple skin nodules occurring in clusters or without a definite pattern can be associated with *M. haemophilum* infection, usually in an immunocompromised host.[18]

Disseminated disease with NTM, primarily MAC, has long been recognized in patients with AIDS, as well as in patients with congenital immunodeficiencies, including severe combined immunodeficiency (SCID).[20,201-203] MAC infection is reported to occur in 6% to 14% of children infected with human immunodeficiency virus (HIV), increasing to 24% in those with severe depletion of CD4⁺ T lymphocytes (<100 cells/mm³).[204-206] As in the adult population,[37] disseminated MAC infection generally occurs late in the course of symptomatic HIV infection.

Disseminated MAC infection in children with AIDS is associated with systemic symptoms, including fever, weight loss, night sweats, and gastrointestinal complaints, often accompanied by neutropenia, anemia, or both. Although directly attributable mortality is difficult to establish, morbidity can be significant.[205,206] Early autopsy studies suggested that MAC infection is rarely a cause of death; later studies found disseminated MAC infection to be associated with shortened survival.[37]

Clinicians should have a high index of suspicion for disseminated MAC infection in HIV-infected children with low CD4⁺ T-lymphocyte counts. Definitive diagnosis rests on recovery of MAC from blood, bone marrow, liver, visceral lymph nodes, or other normally sterile body sites.[201] MAC bacteremia can be intermittent and low-grade; multiple blood specimens must be collected to detect infection.[206] A positive stool culture in the absence of symptoms is not uncommon and most likely represents gastrointestinal colonization or localized disease.

Immune reconstitution inflammatory syndrome (IRIS) related to NTM infection has been described repeatedly in HIV-infected patients with a good response (i.e., increasing CD4⁺ T lymphocyte counts) to antiretroviral therapy.[207-210] Typically, IRIS manifests as localized disease, e.g., peripheral lymphadenitis, pulmonary disease, or abdominal disease. The long-term prognosis generally is good, although the role of corticosteroid therapy or antimycobacterial therapy has not been established.[207]

TREATMENT

Many NTM species are resistant to traditional, first-line drugs used to treat *M. tuberculosis*. Antimicrobial susceptibility testing is essential for appropriate selection of an effective treatment regimen.

Localized Skin, Soft-Tissue, and Bone Infections

The optimal treatment for *M. marinum* infection remains uncertain due to the absence of controlled trials. The latest ATS/Infectious Diseases Society of America (IDSA) guidelines recommend combination therapy comprising clarithromycin plus ethambutol or rifampicin (international nonproprietary name; rifampin, U.S. adopted name).[18] However, the largest published study on *M. marinum* infections reported that 18% of the patients receiving clarithromycin (alone or in combination with other antimycobacterial antibiotics) failed to respond, or relapsed.[12] Some experts suggest adding rifampin as a third agent in patients with bone or joint involvement.[8,9,18,211] Cases with extensive locally-invasive disease may require surgical debridement. Antibiotic treatment should be continued for 1 to 2 months after resolution of all lesions.[8,9,211,212]

Traditionally, lesions due to *M. ulcerans* were treated by surgical excision with or without skin grafting;[141] circumstantial evidence suggests that radical excision with a wide safety margin is more effective than more limited surgery.[213] However, incomplete cure and recurrence are not uncommon with surgery alone, even with radical excision.[143,213-215] Systemic therapy with trimethoprim-sulfamethoxazole, minocycline, dapsone, or clofazimine has been used, but clinical response in long-standing ulcerative lesions is poor.[25,141,142,216] However, anecdotal reports and data from observational studies suggest that treatment with rifampin-containing combination therapy can be curative without surgery.[217,218] Data from a randomized controlled trial in patients with early, limited *M. ulcerans* infection support efficacy of antimycobacterial treatment alone.[219] Patients in this study received either rifampin plus streptomycin for 8 weeks, or the same combination for 4 weeks followed by 4 weeks of rifampin plus clarithromycin; cure rates were >90% in both groups. In a recent pilot study including 15

patients, an 8-week course of oral rifampin plus clarithromycin was curative without surgery.[220]

Primary cutaneous lesions due to *M. fortuitum*, *M. chelonae*, and *M. abscessus* require drainage of localized abscesses and removal of any foreign body.[18] With currently available antimicrobial agents, surgical excision of infected tissue is not required routinely. Susceptibility testing is essential because susceptibilities vary between and within species.[18,221] *M. fortuitum* isolates usually are susceptible to several oral antibiotics, including clarithromycin, doxycycline and minocycline, sulfonamides, and fluoroquinolones.[18] However, *M. fortuitum* can contain an inducible *erm* gene that confers resistance to macrolides;[222] hence these drugs should be used with caution.[18] Limited data suggest that clarithromycin monotherapy usually is effective for *M. chelonae* skin infections.[18,199] Serious skin and soft-tissue infections with *M. abscessus* should be treated empirically with a macrolide (clarithromycin or azithromycin) plus a parenteral agent (amikacin, cefoxitin, or imipenem).[18] The duration of therapy must be individualized according to host factors, clinical response to treatment, and extent of infection. However, standard recommended duration of therapy for severe disease, including osteomyelitis, is 6 months.[18]

Lymphadenitis

Standard therapy for NTM lymphadenitis is surgical excision with removal of all visibly affected nodes.[18,127,155,167,169] A single published randomized controlled trial investigated the efficacy of surgery compared with antimycobacterial antibiotics (clarithromycin plus rifabutin) in children with NTM cervical lymphadenitis.[160] Cure rate was significantly higher in the group allocated to surgery (96%) versus antibiotics (66%). However, 6 patients (12%) in the surgery group developed postsurgical wound infections, and 7 (14%) had facial nerve dysfunction postoperatively, which was permanent in 1 patient (2%). Adverse events in the antibiotic group were mild and transient. Importantly, outcome is highly dependent on surgical expertise and these data can be generalized. Subsequently published data from the same study suggest that the aesthetic outcome is better with primary surgery compared with antimycobacterial management.[166] When complete excision is not possible (e.g., submandibular lymphadenitis with extensive facial nerve involvement) partial excision, thorough curettage, or treatment with antimycobacterial antibiotics alone, are options. Since MAC is by far the most common causative agent of NTM lymphadenitis, empiric treatment with clarithromycin and rifabutin with or without ethambutol is suitable.[18,160,169,223-226] Incisional drainage is not advisable, as a high proportion of cases develop a draining sinus tract as a result, and recurrent disease is not uncommon (see Figure 135-2C and D).[155,156,164] Drainage by needle aspiration remains controversial; sinus tract formation can occur with this approach.[161]

Pulmonary Infection

Treatment regimens for NTM pulmonary disease in children are not well established. Patients with minimal symptoms potentially can be observed without treatment, although increasing recognition of the pathogenicity of NTM makes this approach increasingly uncertain. Patients with more severe clinical symptoms, radiographic findings, and/or persistently positive culture results require treatment.[18] The ATS/IDSA guidelines suggest a 3-drug regimen comprising clarithromycin or azithromycin, plus ethambutol, plus rifampin or rifabutin for adults with MAC lung disease, with the addition of an aminoglycoside intravenously for severe disease.[18] The same guidelines recommend a combination of rifampin, isoniazid, and ethambutol for pulmonary *M. kansasii* infection. Notably, a study in adults with *M. kansasii* lung disease showed a regimen of clarithromycin, rifampin, and ethambutol to be effective.[227] In adults, the guidelines recommend a duration of therapy for MAC or *M. kansasii* disease of 12 months after the sputum culture result is negative.[18] Some adults with disease confined to one lobe of the lung have benefited from surgical lobectomy, particularly if response to medical therapy was poor.[18] However, currently there are no uniform criteria for the selection of patients with NTM lung disease for surgical therapy.[18] Doses, drugs, and endpoints of therapy have not been established for CF patients with MAC or *M. abscessus*. *M. abscessus* lung disease in the setting of CF generally is treatable but incurable. Long-term intravenous therapy with amikacin combined with cefoxitin or imipenem is suggested in the ATS/IDSA guidelines.[18] Clinical and microbiologic response of *M. abscessus* lung disease to clarithromycin has been poor despite in vitro susceptibility.[18] Adolescents with CF who are being considered for macrolide monotherapy or immunotherapy for CF should have sputum cultured for NTM before therapy, and periodically thereafter. Those with repeated isolation of NTM should not receive macrolide monotherapy.[18]

Disseminated Infection

Empiric treatment of disseminated NTM infection in patients with AIDS is a multiple-drug regimen consisting of at least two agents: clarithromycin or azithromycin plus ethambutol. A third drug, such as rifabutin or amikacin, often is added.[18] In vitro susceptibilities to drugs other than macrolides do not predict clinical outcome, and should not be used to direct therapy.[18,221] Symptomatic improvement may take from 2 or 3 weeks to 2 months; repeated blood cultures are useful to assess reduction of bacterial load. Neither a durable response nor an extension of survival has been demonstrated definitively in prospective clinical trials (in the absence of immune reconstitution). However, when clinical improvement is observed, therapy should be continued for the patient's lifetime or until sufficient immune reconstitution has occurred.

For patients with CVC-related infection (or infection related to prosthetic devices, such as ventriculoperitoneal shunts and peritoneal dialysis catheters), removal of the device is essential. Choice of agents for and duration of antimicrobial therapy are based on causative species, results of in vitro susceptibility tests, and the degree of immunocompromise. It is not unusual for new skin lesions to appear during successful therapy of disseminated disease; these may be immunologically mediated. After 4 to 6 weeks of therapy for *M. chelonae*, culture of a biopsy specimen from a new lesion is expected to be sterile.[199] *M. abscessus* often requires 3 to 4 months of treatment to become culture negative. In children with cancer, *M. chelonae* and *M. fortuitum* have caused infections related to venous or implanted catheters in which blood cultures were transiently positive and disseminated skin lesions persisted despite removal of the device and therapy. Treatment of bone infections (especially with open fractures and the presence of foreign material) often requires surgical debridement and prolonged multidrug therapy.[18]

Prophylaxis against disseminated MAC in adults with AIDS has been studied extensively. Clarithromycin or azithromycin prophylaxis now is recommended by the U.S. Public Health Service for HIV-infected adults and adolescents whose CD4$^+$ T lymphocyte counts are <50 cells/mm^3.[228] Before the initiation of prophylaxis, patients must be evaluated to exclude active disease due to disseminated MAC, *M. tuberculosis*, or other mycobacterial species. Similarly robust data do not exist in children. However, prophylaxis consisting of daily clarithromycin (15 mg/kg per day divided into 2 doses, maximum 500 mg/day) or once-weekly azithromycin (20 mg/kg, maximum 1200 mg) is recommended in the U.S. guidelines for HIV-infected children with profound CD4$^+$ lymphocytopenia.[229]

Acknowledgments

The authors wish to acknowledge significant use of the work of Richard J. Wallace, Jr from the 3rd edition.

136 *Nocardia* Species

Ellen Gould Chadwick and Richard B. Thomson, Jr

Since the first reported case of human nocardiosis in 1890, *Nocardia* spp. increasingly have been recognized as serious human pathogens. Recent molecular analyses have shown that more than 80 species comprise the *Nocardia* genus, necessitating ongoing evolution in the understanding of *Nocardia* taxonomy.[1,2] Although identification of *Nocardia* isolates to the species level is challenging, it is nevertheless important, in order to determine pathogenicity and predict antimicrobial susceptibility.[1] The more common clinical isolates reported by laboratories in past decades as *N. asteroides* have been divided into six different groups based on unique antimicrobial susceptibility patterns. These six groups were initially referred to as *N. asteroides* complex groups I to VI; subsequently all six groups were shown to be valid taxonomic clusters by gene sequencing and given species or "complex" names. *Nocardia asteroides* complex is not a recognized taxonomic designation but is used for convenience, referring to all six groups in place of or until full identification is available. The term "complex", when used with one of the six species groups, refers to a cluster of multiple but similar strains that have not been studied adequately to name all as individual species (Table 136-1). Current designations for the six groups, collectively referred to as the *N. asteroides* complex, are *N. abscessus* complex, *N. brevicatena* complex, *N. nova* complex, *N. transvalensis* complex, *N. farcinica*, and *N. cyriacigeorgica*.[2-4] The *N. farcinica* and *N. cyriacigeorgica* groups each contain closely related strains that represent a single species. Using the new taxonomy, nearly all of the clinically significant *Nocardia asteroides* complex isolates identify as *N. cyriacigeorgica*, *N. farcinica*, *N. abscessus* complex, or *N. nova* complex.[2,5] Human pathogens belonging to the *Nocardia* genus not identified as belonging to the *N. asteroides* complex usually are *N. brasiliensis* or *N. otitidiscaviarum* complex (formerly *N. caviae*). *N. brasiliensis* has been subdivided into *N. brasiliensis* and *N. pseudobrasiliensis*. Whereas *N. brasiliensis* infections often are limited to skin and subcutaneous tissue in healthy individuals, all species have been reported in pulmonary and systemic infections.[3,6-10]

MICROBIOLOGY

The family Nocardiaceae is composed of aerobic actinomycetes and characterized by filamentous growth with true branching. *Nocardia* spp. are catalase- and urease-positive and grow on multiple media, including Sabouraud dextrose agar, Löwenstein–Jensen medium, brain–heart infusion agar, and simple blood agar. Although growth occurs over a wide temperature range, *Nocardia* spp. grow best at 37°C in the presence of 10% carbon dioxide. Unlike most other *Nocardia* spp., *N. farcinica* grows as well at 45°C as it does at 35°C, and this property can be used to differentiate this species.[11] Many selective (i.e., inhibitory) media used for isolation of pathogenic fungi do not support the growth of *Nocardia* spp. Colonies can appear within 48 hours when present in pure

TABLE 136-1. Changing Classification of Medically Relevant *Nocardia* Species

Current Classification	Classification Circa 1990–2000	Classification Before 1990
Nocardia abscessus complex[a]	*Nocardia asteroides* complex group I	*Nocardia asteroides*
Nocardia brevicatena complex[a]	*Nocardia asteroides* complex group II	*Nocardia asteroides*
Nocardia nova complex[a]	*Nocardia nova* (group III)	*Nocardia asteroides*
Nocardia transvalensis complex[a]	*Nocardia asteroides* complex group IV	*Nocardia asteroides*
Nocardia farcinica	*Nocardia farcinica* (group V)	*Nocardia asteroides*
Nocardia cyriacigeorgica	*Nocardia asteroides* complex group VI	*Nocardia asteroides*
Nocardia otitidiscaviarum complex[a]	*Nocardia otitidiscaviarum*	*Nocardia caviae*
Nocardia brasiliensis	*Nocardia brasiliensis*	*Nocardia brasiliensis*
Nocardia pseudobrasiliensis	*Nocardia pseudobrasiliensis*	*Nocardia brasiliensis*

[a]These taxa include diverse strains within the species groups. It is recommended that the term "complex" be used with the species names indicating their heterogeneity and that the taxonomy will eventually be more clearly defined.[2]

Based on references 1, 2, 40, and 56.

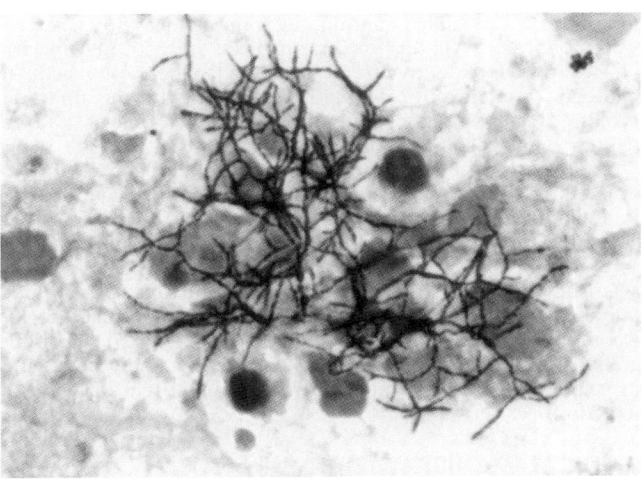

Figure 136-2. Modified acid-fast stained smear (oil immersion objective, 1000×) *of Nocardia* sp. in the same purulent sputum specimen shown in Figure 136-1.

irregular staining that creates a beaded appearance. Many *Nocardia* spp. are acid-fast but retain fuchsin less avidly than *Mycobacterium* spp. Organisms from initial isolation are most reliably acid-fast but become progressively less so on repeated subculture. A modified Ziehl–Neelsen or Kinyoun stain, with the use of 1% sulfuric acid instead of acid alcohol for decoloration, is best for demonstrating acid-fast *Nocardia* in clinical specimens (Figure 136-2).

EPIDEMIOLOGY

Nocardia are ubiquitous saprophytic soil organisms which are easily aerosolized, having been identified in house dust, garden soil, decaying vegetation, beach sand, fresh and salt water, and swimming pools. The lung is the primary portal of entry, and underlying pulmonary dysfunction with decreased bronchociliary clearance mechanisms (e.g., cystic fibrosis, asthma, or bronchiectasis) predisposes to sporadic colonization, although infection only rarely occurs in the absence of corticosteroid therapy in patients with such dysfunction.[5,12,13]

PATHOGENESIS

Inhalation of *Nocardia* spp. can lead to primary pulmonary disease that either resolves spontaneously or progresses to pneumonia; disseminated infection occurs via hematogenous spread from the respiratory tract, especially in immunocompromised hosts. Primary cutaneous infections usually are the result of trauma with soil contamination of the wound, resulting in infection localized to the skin and subcutaneous tissue. Keratitis, either posttraumatic or associated with contact lens use, and endophthalmitis have been reported.[14–16] A few case clusters have been described, and person-to-person transmission has been documented on rare occasions.[17,18]

Patients with deficient host defenses, such as those with lymphoreticular malignancy, chronic obstructive pulmonary disease, chronic granulomatous disease, dysgammaglobulinemia, human immunodeficiency virus infection, and patients receiving corticosteroid therapy are at high risk of invasive nocardiosis.[5,7,9,13,19–21] Recipients of bone marrow or solid-organ transplants are reported to be at particularly high risk; in the latter group, high-dose corticosteroid therapy, a history of cytomegalovirus disease, and high levels of calcineurin inhibitors have been found to be independent risk factors for *Nocardia* infections.[22] There are multiple reports of *Nocardia* infections developing in adults treated with tumor necrosis factor inhibitors, especially infliximab.[23] Host response to *Nocardia* consists of early neutrophil mobilization to localize

culture; in mixed culture from clinical specimens such as sputum, other organisms often obscure small *Nocardia* colonies, making it difficult to recognize the typical morphologic characteristics until 2 to 4 weeks of growth have occurred. Laboratory personnel should be notified to observe cultures for 4 weeks when nocardiosis is being considered. Colonies can be smooth and moist or waxy; with further incubation, development of aerial hyphae causes a velvety or chalky appearance. Primary isolates generally are light orange, but color can vary from cream to brick-red. Microscopically, *Nocardia* spp. often are detected first on Gram stain, where they appear as delicately branched, weakly gram-positive organisms that tend to fragment into coccoid and bacillary elements (Figure 136-1). Filaments show true branching, with

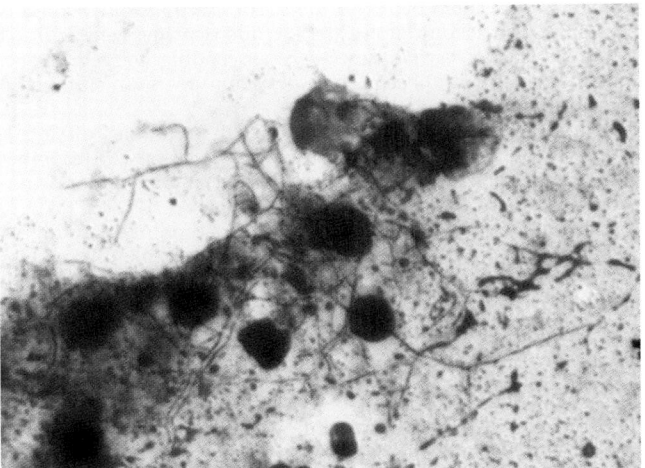

Figure 136-1. Gram-stained smear (oil immersion objective, 1000×) of *Nocardia* sp. in purulent sputum specimen. Note filamentous, branching, beaded, or stippled gram-positive rods.

infection; cell-mediated immunologic mechanisms then supervene, followed by killing of the organism via activated macrophages and cytotoxic T lymphocytes.[24] As a facultative intracellular pathogen, virulence of *Nocardia* is associated with the ability to inhibit phagosome–lysosome fusion in macrophages and to neutralize phagosomal acidification.[9]

Nocardiosis produces suppurative necrosis and abscess formation similar to that seen in pyogenic infection. Although tuberculoid granulomas and giant cells have been reported, lesions generally do not demonstrate granulomatous inflammation or tissue fibrosis. Confluent abscesses without capsules are characteristic of nocardial infection; this feature may explain the frequency of dissemination from the primary pulmonary focus. *Nocardia* "granules" or "grains," which are similar to the sulfur granules characteristic of actinomycosis, occasionally are found in superficial *Nocardia* infections but are absent in visceral infections.

CLINICAL MANIFESTATIONS

The most common clinical manifestation of nocardiosis is pulmonary disease, occurring in more than two-thirds of cases. Infection causes acute, subacute, or chronic suppurative disease, which tends to remit and relapse. Acute onset with fever and systemic symptomatology is uncommon. Pulmonary infection can manifest with cough or dyspnea as well as with nonspecific symptoms such as anorexia and weight loss; hemoptysis occasionally occurs in the presence of cavitary disease. Untreated pulmonary nocardiosis is much like tuberculosis, with a chronic course that can resolve spontaneously, obscuring the source of subsequent metastatic infection. Chest radiographic findings are variable, including bronchopneumonia, alveolar infiltrates, single or scattered nodules or abscesses, and interstitial reticular infiltrates. Cavitation or pleural involvement or both is not uncommon.

Widespread dissemination can occur, especially in solid-organ transplant recipients and other immunocompromised hosts. The central nervous system is the most common secondary site, where disease manifests as single or multiple brain abscesses. *N. farcinica* and *N. otitidiscaviarum* have been reported in brain abscesses with increasing frequency, which may have implications for treatment due to their antibiotic resistance patterns.[25–27] *Nocardia* also has been recognized as a cause of persistent neutrophilic meningitis, despite negative routine cultures. Neurologic symptomatology ranges from headache to coma, with a subacute to acute presentation. Neurotropism is so prominent a feature of nocardiosis that cranial imaging should be performed in patients with pulmonary infection even without symptoms of central nervous system disease. Computed tomography (CT) or magnetic resonance imaging (MRI) typically shows a necrotic cavity surrounded by a contrast-enhancing smooth capsule of uniform thickness and surrounding edema, in contrast to the more irregular capsule seen in malignant tumors.[25] T_2-weighted MRI can show multiple concentric rings with varying signal intensities.[28]

Skin manifestations of disseminated disease can be indistinguishable from primary cutaneous nocardiosis. Cutaneous lesions include cellulitis, pustules, ulcerations, pyoderma, subcutaneous abscesses, and mycetoma, which is a slowly progressive, often painless granulomatous mass associated with nodules, sinuses, and granules, usually involving the foot. Patients manifesting skin involvement should be evaluated thoroughly to exclude disseminated disease. Subcutaneous "abscesses," which are more nodular than fluctuant, do not have the same propensity for fistulous drainage as those caused by *Actinomyces*.[8,29] A cervicofacial syndrome with cervical adenitis due to *Nocardia* has been described in children.[30]

Lymphocutaneous infection caused by *N. brasiliensis* can be indistinguishable from sporotrichosis, manifesting as a primary ulcerative lesion at the site of injury, often on the lower extremity, with nodular lymphangitis, sometimes associated with regional adenopathy and mild systemic symptoms;[6,8,29] this syndrome also has been described at the site of a cat scratch.[31]

Nocardia can disseminate to almost any organ, including kidneys, intestine, pancreas, heart, spleen, liver, joints, bones, eye, spinal cord, thyroid, and adrenal glands.[7,16,20,32,33] Organ infection with *Nocardia* spp. consists of single or multiple nodules or abscesses. Renal infection can cause dysuria, hematuria, or pyuria. Nocardia bacteremia is rare, but infections associated with central venous catheters (CVCs) and peritoneal dialysis catheters have been reported; removal of the CVC followed by 3 months of antibiotic treatment has been successful in these cases.[19,34] Limited case reports of nocardiosis in children suggest that clinical presentations are similar to those in adults.

LABORATORY FINDINGS AND DIAGNOSIS

Nocardia spp. in tissue appear as branching, beaded gram-positive filaments when stained by the Brown–Brenn modification of the Gram stain or other standard tissue Gram stain as well as Gomori methenamine–silver stain. *Nocardia* are not visible when stained with hematoxylin and eosin or periodic acid–Schiff. Identification in tissue can be confirmed using a modified acid-fast stain, since *Nocardia* spp. are acid-fast while other branching gram-positive rods are not.

Although growth of *Nocardia* is best on antibiotic-free media, the rate of recovery can be improved with the use of selective techniques to prevent overgrowth of more rapidly growing organisms in specimens from skin or mucosal sites. A method in which secretions are pretreated with an acid wash and inoculated onto selective buffered charcoal–yeast extract agar, as formulated for the detection of *Legionella* spp., has been reported to increase the recovery of *Nocardia* from respiratory specimens.[35] Although uncommon, *N. asteroides* complex strains can be isolated from blood cultures, especially from specimens in patients receiving immunosuppressive therapy. The organism can be recovered using automated blood culture systems; however, performing blind subcultures on day 5 of incubation on "negative" specimens can increase the recovery.[36] Notably, when *Nocardia* infection is not suspected, cultures generally are discarded without terminal subculture or too early to allow growth of the organism.

Usual laboratory biochemical methods can be used to differentiate *N. asteroides* complex, *N. otitidiscaviarum* complex, and *N. brasiliensis*; however, phenotypic testing does not identify the many species within the *N. asteroides* complex or the less common human pathogens within the genus.[4,11,37] Definitive identification requires analysis of gene sequences by molecular methods (16s rRNA gene; multilocus sequence analysis of 5–7 housekeeping genes have been most successful) and may be necessary for some patients with serious disease.[1,2,4,38–40] Presumptive identification of a limited number of *N. asteroides* complex isolates can be provided using an abbreviated battery of tests. For example, *N. farcinica* is resistant to ceftriaxone, grows at 45°C and opacifies Middlebrook agar, whereas *N. cyriacigeorgica* is susceptible to ceftriaxone, imipenem, and amikacin but resistant to ampicillin and erythromycin.[1,41,42]

Performance of bronchoalveolar lavage in pulmonary disease or biopsy of an affected tissue site may be necessary when other clinical specimens are nondiagnostic, especially in immunocompromised hosts.

Clinical laboratory methods for the susceptibility testing of *Nocardia* spp. have been standardized, with breakpoints established for interpretation of susceptibility and resistance.[43] Initial selection of antimicrobial therapy must be empiric, as isolation and susceptibility testing can require days to weeks.[42,44]

TREATMENT

On the basis of accumulated clinical experience, a sulfonamide always has been considered the treatment of choice for nocardiosis in conjunction with appropriate surgical drainage or excision of empyema or large abscesses. Trimethoprim-sulfamethoxazole (TMP-SMX) has been reported to be effective in many clinical series, supplanting sulfonamides as the treatment of choice of many experts.[45] Increasing reports of sulfonamide resistance or lack of effectiveness in immunosuppressed patients has led most clinicians to use additional agents in combination with a sulfonamide, at least initially. Nephrotoxic interaction between TMP-SMX and cyclosporine may necessitate the use of alternative agents in organ transplant recipients.[20] Importantly, thrice-weekly TMP-SMX used for prophylaxis against *P. jirovecii* infections is frequently ineffective in preventing nocardiosis.[19,22]

Primary drug resistance exists among *Nocardia*, necessitating in vitro susceptibility studies for all clinically significant isolates; however, because performance and interpretation of susceptibility testing of *Nocardia* is complex, laboratories with limited experience should consider sending isolates to reference laboratories for testing.[3] A retrospective study of >750 *Nocardia* isolates sent to the Centers for Disease Control and Prevention from 1995 to 2004 found increasing resistance over time.[46] Among the four most prevalent *Nocardia* species, TMP-SMX resistance ranged from 20% for *N. brasiliensis* to 80% for *N. farcinica*. Linezolid was the only antibiotic to which 100% of the isolates were susceptible. Resistance among all strains tested was lowest for amikacin (5%), imipenem (30%), and ceftriaxone (52%), although *N. farcinica* virtually always is resistant to the cephalosporins.[3,47] In vitro studies have shown that meropenem is more active than imipenem against most *Nocardia* spp. but less active against *N. farcinica* and *N. nova*; in contrast, most *Nocardia* spp. are resistant to ertapenem.[5,13,48] Amoxicillin-clavulanate is active against many strains of *Nocardia*, except *N. nova*, *N. otitidiscaviarum*, and *N. cyriacigeorgica*, which are resistant.[46,47,49] Moxifloxacin generally is more active than ciprofloxacin, and was shown in one report to be successful in treating a *N. farcinica* brain abscess in an immunosuppressed patient.[50] Because of linezolid's excellent in vitro activity, with minimum inhibitory concentrations <8 μg/mL against all strains of *Nocardia*, linezolid may be useful as initial therapy until speciation and/or susceptibility of the isolate is available.[51] Although linezolid is approved only for short courses at this time, it has been used for longer-term therapy when there were no alternative active agents, remembering that data about adverse effects of long-term use are incomplete and its high cost often is prohibitive. Although clinical improvement can occur

with single-drug therapy, two or three drugs with activity in vitro (preferably a combination demonstrating synergy, such as TMP-SMX with amikacin or a carbapenem) should be used for progressive disease, especially in immunocompromised hosts.

Duration of therapy for nocardial infection depends on the site of infection and the immune status of the host. For primary cutaneous nocardiosis, a course of 6 to 12 weeks of sulfonamide therapy is appropriate, although spontaneous resolution of disease without therapy has been reported. For individuals with isolated pulmonary disease, 6 to 12 months of therapy is preferred.[52] Brain abscess or meningitis requires longer therapy, at least 12 months in most cases; a second or third drug with proven activity in vitro, such as amikacin and ceftriaxone, usually is given for the first 4 to 12 weeks of treatment or until clinical and radiographic improvement is observed.[5,13,52] Parenteral therapy should be used for the first 3 to 6 weeks, until a response to therapy has been documented and the species and its antibiotic susceptibilities have been determined; thereafter, oral therapy can be used to complete the course of treatment.

Relapses after prolonged therapy occur but are uncommon. Lifelong suppressive therapy for nocardiosis is probably prudent in patients with acquired immunodeficiency syndrome and persistent, severe CD4+ T-lymphocyte depletion.[47] Delayed appearance of metastatic abscesses, even during effective therapy, often represents the evolution of a previously seeded focus. Because infection by *Nocardia* can present concurrently with infection due to other opportunistic pathogens in immunocompromised patients, poor response to therapy or the development of new lesions should raise the possibility of a concomitant pathogen, such as *Mycobacterium tuberculosis*, *Pneumocystis jirovecii*, or *Aspergillus*.

Although older series report mortality from 44% to 85%, more recently published mortality rates range from 15% to 26%.[5,12,20,53-55] Mortality among patients with cancer may be as high as 60%; factors that increase mortality include concurrent corticosteroid or antineoplastic therapy and coinfection with cytomegalovirus.[19] Consideration of nocardial infection in the differential diagnosis of immunocompromised or debilitated patients and aggressive diagnostic pursuit can lead to earlier diagnosis and improved outcome.

Key Points. Epidemiology, Clinical Syndromes, Diagnosis and Treatment of *Nocardia* Infections

EPIDEMIOLOGY
- Ubiquitous soil organisms
- Lung is the primary portal of entry into the body
- Most infections occur in children with immunodeficiency, i.e., chronic granulomatous disease, HIV infection, chronic high-dose corticosteroid therapy, lymphoreticular malignancies, bone marrow and solid-organ transplantation, and dysgammaglobulinemia

CLINICAL SYNDROMES
- Pulmonary infiltrates or abscess(es) ± pleural effusion
- Disseminated disease usually includes pulmonary infection and central nervous system involvement; however, any organ can be affected
- Primary cutaneous or lymphocutaneous due to direct inoculation

DIAGNOSIS
- Tissue diagnosis (e.g., bronchoalveolar lavage, tissue biopsy) often necessary
- Branching, beaded gram-positive filaments using standard Gram staining procedures for tissue or smears

- Modified acid-fast stain confirms identification, since *Nocardia* spp. are weakly or partially acid-fast while other branching gram-positive rods are not
- Selective media (e.g., selective buffered charcoal-yeast extract agar) may be necessary to prevent overgrowth of more rapidly growing organisms in specimens from skin or mucosal sites
- Laboratory personnel should be notified to hold cultures for at least 2 weeks to allow for slow growth of *Nocardia*
- Definitive species identification requires gene sequencing

TREATMENT
- Trimethoprim-sulfamethoxazole (TMP-SMX) is the historical treatment of choice
  - Emergence of resistant strains dictates broader coverage
- Empiric combination therapy for pulmonary or disseminated disease, especially in immunocompromised hosts
  - 2–3 active agents including TMP-SMX, linezolid, amikacin, carbapenem or ceftriaxone; definitive therapy guided by in vitro susceptibility tests
- Surgical debridement as adjunctive therapy often required
- Duration of therapy for invasive disease is 6 to 12 months or longer

137 *Escherichia coli*

James P. Nataro and Jorge J. Velarde

Escherichia coli comprise the predominant facultative anaerobic flora of the human gastrointestinal tract and as such serve useful homeostatic functions in the human large intestine.[1] However, *E. coli* also are among the most versatile bacteria known, and certain strains have adapted to niches of human and animal virulence.

E. coli are gram-negative, motile bacilli of the family Enterobacteriaceae. Approximately 90% ferment lactose, although often slowly, and produce indole and cadaverine, via lysine decarboxylase.[2] There are over 170 somatic (O) and 56 flagellar (H) antigens recognized. Pathogenic *E. coli* have evolved various pathotypes, each with distinct pathogenetic, epidemiologic, and clinical features.[3] Patho-adapted *E. coli* cause three main types of human disease: urinary tract infection; enteric infection; and systemic infection, including bloodstream infection (BSI) and pneumonia.[3] Specific virulence traits have been described for each pathotype; these virulence factors usually are encoded by large virulence-related plasmids and/or chromosomal pathogenicity islands.[3] In addition to these virulence factors, each pathotype features characteristic O and H antigen combinations (i.e., serotypes).[1] *E. coli* lacking specific virulence factors can be opportunistic pathogens of compromised hosts.

PATHOGENESIS

Uropathogenic *E. coli*

The pathogenesis of *E. coli* urinary tract infection (UTI) is complex. Uropathogenic *E. coli* (UPEC) colonize the kidney and bladder epithelium by virtue of specially adapted surface fimbriae.[4,5] Best characterized are the P fimbriae, which are hollow proteinaceous rods 7 nm in diameter.[5] P fimbriae mediate binding to renal epithelium and are associated with pyelonephritis. Other fimbriae, including type 1 fimbriae, have been shown to facilitate colonization of the renal or bladder epithelium.[4] Following successful colonization, UPEC must evade host defense mechanisms, a function mediated in part by fimbrial adherence,[4] by resistance to the killing power of serum, and by the ability to scavenge iron via siderophore aerobactin.[4,6,7] The pathogenesis of renal damage by *E. coli* is not elucidated completely, but two possible mechanisms have been suggested: (1) *E. coli* hemolysin has been shown to cause direct cellular damage, in part by forming pores in the eukaryotic cell wall;[4,7] and (2) cell culture experiments suggest that some UPEC directly invade renal epithelial cells.[8]

Some investigators have suggested that UPEC form intracellular biofilms called pods, which may promote persistence and relative antibiotic resistance.[9]

Diarrheagenic *E. coli*

Diarrheagenic *E. coli* are subdivided into five recognized pathotypes, each with a distinct clinical presentation, epidemiology, and pathogenesis[1,3] (Table 137-1). Enterotoxigenic *E. coli* (ETEC) adhere to the small bowel mucosa using one of several different fimbrial colonization factor antigens (CFAs).[1] Following colonization, ETEC elaborate one or two enterotoxins, which increase secretion of fluid and electrolytes from the small bowel mucosa.[1,10,11] The heat-labile toxin (LT) is an A-B subunit ADP-ribosylating toxin with genetic and mechanistic similarity to cholera toxin, which acts by inducing adenylate cyclase.[10] The second toxin, heat-stable toxin (ST), acts through a cGMP-dependent mechanism that is only partially understood.[11] Epidemiologic studies suggest that ST is the more important virulence factor.[12]

Enterohemorrhagic *E. coli* (EHEC) adhere to luminal enterocytes and disrupt the apical cytoskeleton, giving rise to the characteristic "attaching and effacing" lesion (Figure 137-1).[13] An outer membrane protein, termed intimin (the *eae* gene product), is necessary to induce this lesion in animal models.[13] Remarkably, the intimin receptor is of bacterial origin, and is injected into the epithelial cell early in the infectious process. Once established in the colon, EHEC release one or more toxins related to the Shiga toxin of *Shigella dysenteriae* (designated Shiga-like toxin or Stx); Stx is cytotoxic to the vascular endothelium.[14] Stx also is referred to as verotoxin because of its ability to kill Vero cells in vitro. Stx circulates systemically in persons with EHEC disease. Its propensity to induce necrosis of cerebrovascular and renal endothelium gives rise to the characteristic sequelae of EHEC infection, most notably the hemolytic uremic syndrome (HUS).[15] Stx contributes to but is not required for EHEC diarrhea.[15]

Enteropathogenic *E. coli* (EPEC) are pathogens of the small intestine, where they induce an attaching and effacing lesion similar to that caused by EHEC.[16] The proposed three-stage model of EPEC infection includes: (1) intestinal colonization mediated by the bundle-forming pilus (BFP), (2) induction of the attaching and effacing lesion via intimin and other secreted proteins, and finally (3) signal transduction, resulting in induction of a net secretory state.[17]

The pathogenic mechanisms of enteroinvasive *E. coli* (EIEC) are virtually identical to those of *Shigella* spp.[1,18] EIEC invade colonic enterocytes and spread laterally through the mucosa and lamina propria; genes essential to invasion are encoded on 140-Md plasmids. In addition, EIEC elaborate secretogenic enterotoxins that may account for the watery diarrheal phase of disease that occur in most cases.[19]

TABLE 137-1. Pathogenesis and Manisfestations of Diarrheagenic *E. coli* Infection

Category	Adherence Factors	Toxins	Invasiveness	Type of Diarrhea
ETEC	CFAs, other fimbriae	ST, LT	No	Watery
EHEC	Fimbriae, intimin	Stx 1, Stx 2	AE lesion	Afebrile, bloody colitis
EPEC	BFP, intimin	None	AE lesion	Watery
EIEC	Membrane proteins	EIET	Shigella-like	Watery, dysentery
EAEC	AAFs	EAST, Pet ShET1	No	Persistent watery

AAF, aggregative adherence fimbriae; AE, attaching and effacing; BFP, bundle-forming pilus; CFA, colonization factor antigen; EAEC, enteroaggregative E. coli; *EHEC, enterohemorrhagic* E. coli; *EIEC, enteroinvasive* E. coli; *EIET, EIEC enterotoxin; EPEC, enteropathogenic* E. coli; *ETEC, enterotoxigenic* E. coli; *LT, heat-labile toxin; Pet, plasmid encoded toxin; ShET1, Shigella enterotoxin 1; ST, heat-stable toxin; Stx, Shiga-like toxin.*

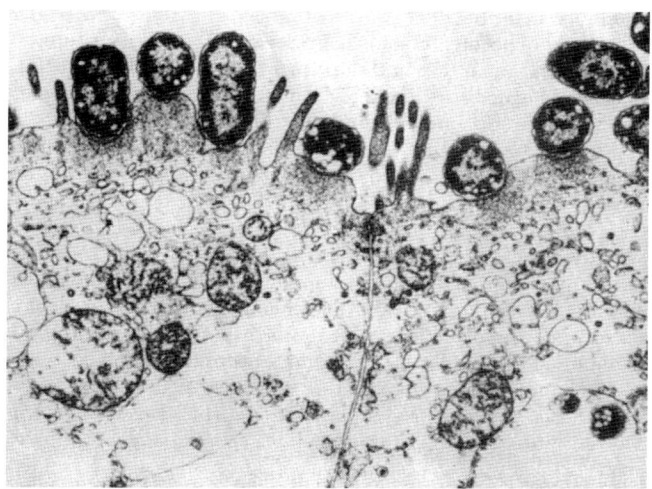

Figure 137-1. Electron photomicrograph of the attaching and effacing lesion induced in the gnotobiotic piglet ileum after oral administration of a human EPEC strain. Bacteria are seen intimately attached to the epithelial cells, which respond by forming cup-like pedestals composed of cytoskeletal protein. An identical lesion can be induced by human EHEC strains. (From Baldini MM, Kaper JB, Levine MM, et al. Plasmid-mediated adhesion in enteropathogenic *Escherichia coli*. J Pediatr Gastroenterol Nutr 1983;2:543, with permission.)

Enteroaggregative *E. coli* (EAEC) adhere tenaciously to the intestinal mucosa in a characteristic biofilm.[20] Adherence is mediated by fimbrial organelles called aggregative adherence fimbriae (AAFs). Once colonization is achieved, EAEC secretes a series of cytotoxic, secretogenic, and proinflammatory proteins.[20]

Other categories of diarrheagenic *E. coli* have been proposed, including diffusely adherent *E. coli*,[21] and strains elaborating the cytolethal distending toxin[22] or cytotoxic necrotizing toxin.[23] Definitive roles for these strains in human disease have yet to be established.

E. coli Causing Disseminated Infection

E. coli isolated from neonates with septicemia and/or meningitis belong to certain characteristic serotypes, with organisms displaying the K1 antigen accounting for approximately 40% of cases.[24,25] Pathogenic *E. coli* acquired by infants, either vertically or horizontally, are capable of translocating through intestinal or nasopharyngeal mucosa to cause systemic disease.[26]

K1 antigen is an acidic polysaccharide, colominic acid, which is a homopolymer of *N*-acetylneuraminic (sialic) acid.[27] Sialic acid is a common constituent of human tissues. K1 is identical in chemical and immunologic structure to the group B acidic polysaccharide of *Neisseria meningitidis*. The virulence of K1-encapsulated *E. coli* is thought to be related in part to the ability of the K1 capsule to mimic host antigens and to mask underlying structures of the bacterial cell surface, preventing development of specific antibody responses and activation of the alternative complement system.[24,27] Possession of K1 antigen alone, however, does not confer invasiveness to *E. coli*[27] through either the gastrointestinal tract or the meninges, and several additional virulence factors have been described.[28,29]

Many *E. coli* isolated from patients with central nervous system (CNS) infection express S fimbriae that mediate adherence to vascular epithelium, brain cells, and laminin.[30,31] S fimbriae also promote conversion of plasminogen to plasmin, which activates the fibrinolytic process and may facilitate spread of the bacterium within the CNS.[31] Presence of S fimbriae correlates with increased virulence of *E. coli* in animal models. Penetration of the meninges may be mediated by specific bacterial outer membrane proteins.[28]

EPIDEMIOLOGY

Each pathotype of diarrheagenic *E. coli* (i.e., EHEC, ETEC, EIEC, EPEC, and EAEC) has distinct epidemiologic features. All pathotypes, however, have been associated with widespread diarrheal disease, predominantly affecting infants or children and occurring most commonly in warmer months.[1]

Most EHEC disease has been reported from North and South America, Europe, Australia, and parts of Asia.[32] In the United States, both endemic and epidemic disease occurs. Outbreaks have been associated mainly with consumption of undercooked contaminated beef, but many other vehicles, including water, milk, apple cider, yogurt, and vegetables including sprouts have been implicated;[32,33] these alternative sources usually are contaminated by bovine manure. Although most EHEC infections are contracted via the fecal–oral route, person-to-person transmission is common in outbreaks.[32–34]

ETEC are ubiquitous in developing countries and frequently are transmitted via contaminated food or water.[35] Infants typically experience ETEC diarrhea upon introduction of foods to supplement human milk. ETEC are the leading cause of bacterial gastroenteritis in travelers to developing countries.[1,12,36]

EIEC is a relatively uncommon cause of diarrhea globally. In the U.S., transmission of EIEC is most notably via outbreaks of foodborne disease.[37] In the developing world, person-to-person transmission also is thought to occur,[18] although the infectious dose is higher than that required for transmission of *Shigella* species.[38]

EPEC was associated classically with severe outbreaks of infantile diarrhea in the developed world in the 1940s to 1960s.[1,17,39] After this period, infection all but disappeared, only to resurface as one of the most prevalent causes of diarrheal infection among infants in developing countries.[17,39] There is predilection for infants <6 months of age who are not fed human milk exclusively.[39] No animal host has been identified for EPEC; it is thought that older infants and children who excrete organisms asymptomatically are an important reservoir. The vehicle by which EPEC are transmitted to infants is not known, although in outbreaks heavy environmental contamination has been documented.[39]

EAEC is a highly versatile pathogen of all ages, occurring in both industrialized and developing countries.[40] EAEC particularly is prevalent in patients with HIV/AIDS, where it is an important cause of persistent diarrhea.[41] EAEC may be a common cause of traveler's diarrhea.[40]

E. coli that causes systemic infection can be acquired from the mother during delivery or horizontally after birth. Why only a small percentage of colonized infants develop invasive disease is unclear, but epidemiologic clues suggest that susceptibility to *E. coli* K1 disease is due to host factors as well as bacterial virulence.[25]

CLINICAL MANIFESTATIONS

Clinical manifestations of *E. coli* UTI are similar to those caused by other pathogens, as are manifestations of systemic *E. coli* infections in the neonate or older child. The clinical setting in older children with *E. coli* bacteremia or septicemia characteristically begins with primary pathology in the gastrointestinal tract (e.g., ruptured appendicitis, shigellosis, short bowel syndrome) or genitourinary tract (e.g., pyelonephritis, obstructive uropathy). Endotoxemia and induction of inflammatory mediators are responsible for profound clinical derangements (Chapter 11. The Systemic Inflammatory Response Syndrome (SIRS), Sepsis. and Septic Shock).

ETEC, EPEC, and EAEC generally cause a self-limited watery diarrheal syndrome with a short incubation period (6 to 48 hours).[1] Patients can have nausea, abdominal cramps, and low-grade fever. Persistent diarrhea (>14 days) has been reported with EPEC[42] and especially with EAEC.[40] EIEC causes diarrhea that usually is watery, but dysentery develops in a minority of cases.[1] Hemorrhagic colitis without fever, characteristic of EHEC infection, often is confused with intussusception, inflammatory bowel disease, or ischemic colitis.[33,43] Patients can develop CNS disease (ischemia, hemorrhage) and/or HUS.

DIAGNOSIS

Diagnosis of *E. coli* septicemia, meningitis, and UTI is made when *E. coli* is isolated from normally sterile body fluids. Diagnosis of diarrheagenic *E. coli* infection relies on isolation of the offending bacterium from stool and its subsequent differentiation from non-pathogenic stool flora using methods described in Table 137-2. Genetic probes are available that correspond to each phenotype. Use of these probes generally is preferred to assays that identify phenotype directly.[1]

Although multiple EHEC serotypes are encountered frequently in other countries, EHEC isolated in the U.S. are almost entirely serotype O157:H7.[32,33] Strains of this serotype have the unusual biochemical trait of inability to ferment sorbitol, yielding colorless colonies following incubation on MacConkey agar base with added sorbitol.[1,32] Definitive identification is confirmed by agglutination with O and H antisera. The yield of O157:H7 is substantially higher when stool culture is performed within the first 6 days of diarrheal illness.[45] Several other assays have been proposed to assist in the identification of EHEC disease,[1,46] including detection of Stx in stool specimens or colony lysates, and seroconversion to O157 lipopolysaccharide following recovery. Several chromogenic agars have been developed to facilitate laboratory identification of the O157:H7 serotype.[2]

TREATMENT

Management of diarrhea due to *E. coli* is summarized in Table 137-2. Support of fluid and electrolyte status is the first therapeutic priority. Antimotility agents may be useful in controlling ETEC diarrhea,[47] but these agents are contraindicated in EHEC[33] and EIEC infections unless administered concurrently with antibiotics[47] and can be dangerous if given to infants and young children.

Administration of oral antibiotics for 5 days is considered adequate therapy for ETEC, EIEC, EAEC, and EPEC infections.[47] Antimicrobial therapy of ETEC disease is limited, by frequent resistance to commonly used antibiotics. In adults, fluoroquinolones are effective against most ETEC isolates. Since these agents are not approved for use in children, an alternative agent should be selected, based on antibiotic susceptibility patterns of the isolated agent or known local resistance patterns. Cefixime and azithromycin may be effective alternatives to fluoroquinolones. Antibiotic therapy for EHEC has not been shown to impact favorably on the course of diarrheal illness or to prevent development of HUS;[33] some clinical data suggest that antibiotics may increase the likelihood of subsequent HUS[48] (most likely by promoting release of Stx) although this remains controversial.[49] Therefore, antibiotics should be withheld in patients who are likely to have EHEC hemorrhagic colitis.

Antimicrobial therapy of neonates with septicemia and/or meningitis initially must include agents effective against group B streptococcus, *Listeria monocytogenes*, and gram-negative bacilli including *E. coli*. Initial therapy generally is ampicillin plus an aminoglycoside or ampicillin plus cefotaxime. Due to rapid emergence of cephalosporin-resistant strains, especially *Enterobacter cloacae* and *Serratia* species, routine use of third-generation cephalosporins in neonatal intensive care units (NICUs) for empiric treatment of infections is not recommended, unless gram-negative bacillary meningitis is suspected. Meropenem may need to be used empirically for suspected gram-negative bacillary meningitis in an infant who has been heavily exposed to cephalosporins. Definitive therapy of septicemia and/or meningitis due to *E. coli* should be based on in vitro susceptibility tests. Repeat lumbar puncture is recommended to document eradication of the infecting pathogen. Duration of therapy is based on response and usually is 10 to 14 days in neonates with uncomplicated septicemia, and a minimum of 21 days (and at least 14 days after sterilization of cerebrospinal fluid) for meningitis. All infants should be monitored to detect neurologic sequelae, including hearing loss.

HEMOLYTIC UREMIC SYNDROME

HUS is defined by the triad of microangiopathic hemolytic anemia, thrombocytopenia, and acute renal dysfunction. Two principal subgroups are defined in children: diarrheal and non-diarrheal HUS.[1,33] The first includes typical cases, which manifest with a diarrheal prodrome of sudden onset. This typical form most often is associated with Stx-producing *E. coli* or *Shigella dysenteriae* type 1. *E. coli* O157:H7 traditionally had been the most associated Stx-producing bacteria, but an outbreak due to previously rare *E. coli* O104:H4 began in Germany in May, 2011 and extended rapidly to 14 European countries and to the U.S. and Canada.[50] The second nondiarrheal (formerly atypical) group of HUS cases is heterogeneous in cause, may include a genetic predisposition, lacks antecedent diarrhea, has a tendency to relapse, and has a worse prognosis.[51,52] This nondiarrheal form is not associated with Stx of EHEC or *S. dysenteriae* type 1, has been reported with a variety of infections and notably with complicated pneumococcal pneumonia.[53] Neuraminidase produced by *S. pneumoniae* is important pathogenically.

Much attention has been devoted to EHEC and the mechanisms underlying HUS.[54-56] EHEC colonize the large intestine, where development of the attaching and effacing lesion elicits diarrhea.[13]

TABLE 137-2. Diagnosis and Treatment of Diarrheagenic *E. coli* Infections[a]

Category	Distinguishing Phenotype or Property	Non-Nucleic Acid Detection of Choice	Antimicrobial Agent
ETEC	Heat-labile toxin	GM1 EIA	TMP-SMX, cefixime, azithromycin, fluoroquinolones
	Heat-labile toxin	Suckling mouse	
EHEC	Shiga-like toxins	Vero cytotoxicity	Not indicated
	60-Md[b] plasmid	None	
EIEC	140-Md plasmid	Guinea pig	TMP-SMX
		Keratoconjunctivitis	
EPEC	60-Md[b] plasmid	LA adherence[44]	Neomycin, colistin sulfate
	Bundle-forming pilus	LA adherence	TMP-SMX fluoroquinolone
EAEC	60-Md[b] plasmid	AA adherence[44]	

AA, aggregative adherence to HEp-2 cells in culture; EIA, enzyme immunoassay; LA, localized adherence to HEp-2 cells in culture; TMP-SMX, trimethoprim-sulfamethoxazole. For other abbreviations, see Table 137-1.

[a]*In age-appropriate patients.*

[b]*The 60-Md plasmids of EHEC, EPEC, and EAggEC share minimal homology.*

The bloody nature of the diarrhea is thought to be caused by mucosal necrosis resulting from Stx production.[15] Stx acts by depurination of residue 4324 of the eukaryotic 28S rRNA;[14,55] this effect abolishes protein synthesis in the eukaryotic cell, resulting in cell death. Absorption of Stx to the circulation gives rise to the systemic complications of EHEC infection. Not all cells express receptors for Stx, which determines the organ specificity of clinical manifestations. Cells of the gastrointestinal tract and CNS vascular endothelium and that of the glomerulus are most affected.[33,56] Classically, patients manifest the clinical triad of HUS within a week after developing bloody diarrhea. Incomplete forms and atypical presentations are described.[33,52,54] The proportion of patients who develop HUS after EHEC infection ranges from 2% to over 20%.[33] Around 4% to 10% of children with HUS develop chronic renal failure; a larger percentage develop milder renal sequelae.[33] The overall fatality rate has been reported to be 5% to 10% in children, but improved management strategies have reduced mortality. Complicated hospital course and mortality are higher in adults and children with nondiarrheal HUS. Renal failure as well as cerebral, myocardial, and intestinal infarctions contribute to fatality.[32,33,43]

MANAGEMENT

Fluid and electrolyte balance should be corrected and maintained before and after HUS develops. Prompt recognition of acute renal failure may prevent fluid overload and lessen hypertension. Antimotility agents should not be administered to anyone with inflammatory or bloody stools or to any child with diarrhea exposed to a person with HUS or hemorrhagic colitis. Antimotility agents have been shown to be a risk factor for progression of diarrhea caused by *E. coli* O157:H7[57,58] and have been associated with an increased risk of neurologic manifestations.[59] One study suggested that early volume expansion may mitigate the risk of developing oligoanuric HUS.[60]

Several studies have shown that patients who receive antibiotics are at increased risk of diarrhea-associated HUS.[48,57] In vitro studies add support to this hypothesis, as cephalosporins and fluoroquinolones induce expression of STx encoded on the Shiga phage.[61] However, a meta-analysis of all available studies did not reveal a consistent association of antibiotic administration with increased risk of HUS.[48] Although controversy persists, it is clear that antibiotics routinely prescribed for bacterial gastroenteritis do not mitigate either the signs and symptoms of EHEC colitis or the risk of sequelae.

Many therapeutic interventions have been proposed for patients with HUS,[1,33,62] including plasma infusions, plasma exchange, intravenous immunoglobulin, Stx inhibitors, prostacyclin, antithrombotic therapy, vitamin E, recombinant tissue-type plasminogen activator, transfusion with PI-antigen positive erythrocytes, aurintricarboxylic acid (to bind von Willebrand factor multimers), or recombinant fragment of von Willebrand factor monomer. These nonconventional therapies primarily have been tried in small numbers of patients with nondiarrheal HUS. Additional data supporting their effectiveness are needed.

PREVENTION

Prevention of diarrheagenic *E. coli* infection is based on avoidance of contaminated vehicles. Travelers should consume only cooked food and boiled or bottled beverages when visiting developing areas. Prevention of EPEC and EIEC in indigenous populations is best accomplished by improvements in sanitation, food storage, and personal hygiene. The prevention of EHEC infection has centered around protection of the food supply, especially beef products. All commercially prepared hamburgers are required to reach an internal temperature of 68°C (155°F), a temperature shown to kill *E. coli*.[63] Hamburgers should be cooked until no pink remains and until juices are clear.

Development of vaccines against diarrheagenic *E. coli*, especially ETEC and EHEC, has received a great deal of attention.[1,64] Purified ETEC fimbriae fed to human volunteers in biodegradable microspheres (to enable protection from gastric acidity) have been shown to be immunogenic and partially protective. Killed ETEC vaccines have induced partial protection for short periods, and may be attractive for travelers.

Vaccines have been prepared against the K1 capsule, associated with the virulence of invasive *E. coli*. Thus far, these vaccines have not been shown to be protective; in fact, the similarity of the capsular antigen to host sialic acid has raised the possibility of serious autoimmune reactions as a result of vaccination.[65] Vaccines against *E. coli* associated with UTI have not proved effective.

---

138 *Klebsiella* and *Raoultella* Species

William J. Barson and Mario J. Marcon

MICROBIOLOGY AND EPIDEMIOLOGY

The Klebsiellae, family Enterobacteriaceae, contains at least five *Klebsiella* spp. and three *Raoultella* spp.: *K. pneumoniae, K. oxytoca, K. granulomatis, K. variicola, K. singaporensis, R. terrigena, R. ornithinolytica,* and *R. planticola*.[1-6] The two most important human pathogens in terms of frequency and disease severity are *K. pneumoniae* and *K. oxytoca*. *K. pneumoniae* has been divided further into subspecies *pneumoniae, ozaenae,* and *rhinoscleromatis*. The latter two *K. pneumoniae* subspecies are associated with chronic respiratory tract infections with somewhat unique clinical presentations, namely an atrophic rhinitis called ozena or other nasal infections and rhinoscleroma, and a chronic granulomatous infection of the nose, respectively; these diseases occur most frequently in the tropics. These subspecies may be difficult to separate from each other and from biochemically inactive strains of *K. pneumoniae* subsp. *pneumoniae*. *K. granulomatis*, formerly known as *Calymmatobacterium granulomatis*, is the agent of granuloma inguinale or donovanosis, a sexually transmitted ulcerative disease of skin and subcutaneous tissues of the genital region (see Chapter 139, *Klebsiella (Calymmatobacterium) granulomatis* (Granuloma Inguinale)). It is noncultivable on standard laboratory agar media.

Most *Klebsiella* and *Raoultella* spp. are ubiquitous in nature, being found both in environmental sources such as surface and drinking waters, soil, vegetation, sewage, and industrial waste, as well as in association with mucosal surfaces and disease states of humans, other mammals, birds, and reptiles.[5,7] *K. variicola* is a newly described species that has been isolated from both plants and human sources including the bloodstream. In contradistinction, *K. ozanae, K. rhinoscleromatis,* and *K. granulomatis* have been recovered only from human clinical specimens. *Raoultella* spp. are isolated infrequently from human sources. *Raoultella ornithinolytica* and *R. planticola* produce histidine decarboxylase and have been implicated in causing scombroid fish poisoning.[8]

Members of the genera *Klebsiella* and *Raoultella*, like most other Enterobacteriaceae, are facultative, gram-negative bacilli, catalase-positive, and oxidase-negative, reduce nitrate to nitrite and use glucose and other carbohydrates fermentatively. In addition, they are nonmotile, usually encapsulated, and generally produce lysine but not ornithine decarboxylase, except for *R. ornithinolytica* which produces ornithine decarboxylase. *Klebsiella* spp. generally utilize citrate as a sole carbon source, often produce urease, and are positive in the Voges–Proskauer test.[1-6] They are H_2S- and indole-negative except for *K. oxytoca* which is indole-positive.

K. pneumoniae subsp. *pneumoniae* and *K. oxytoca* generally appear as large, mucoid, lactose-fermenting colonies on MacConkey agar. Commercial or conventional biochemical identification systems perform well for identifying and differentiating these two species; however, the lack of indole production by *K. pneumoniae* is the single main differentiating feature. *K. pneumoniae* is difficult to differentiate from *R. planticola* and *R. terrigena* using basic biochemical tests and commercial identification systems. Studies conducted in Europe have suggested that a significant percentage of organisms identified as *Klebsiella* spp. may by *R. planticola*; however, similar studies conducted in the United States suggest that *R. planticola* isolates are rare.[9,10] Thus prevalence of these organisms in human disease may vary by geographic location.

The role of specific virulence factors in the pathogenesis of infection due to *Klebsiella* spp. is unclear, and the importance of the various factors may vary by site of infection. Specific virulence factors identified include: (1) cell surface adhesins that may mediate attachment to mucosal surfaces; (2) cell surface capsular polysaccharides and lipopolysaccharide that may inhibit phagocytosis and serum bactericidal activity; and (3) a variety of other factors, including siderophores (iron-chelating compounds), cytotoxins, enterotoxins, and hemolysins.[4,5] Adhesins produced by *K. pneumoniae* include both fimbrial and nonfimbrial proteins. Type I fimbriae have been shown to be important in adherence to epithelial cells of the urinary tract in animal models. Strains of both *K. pneumoniae* and *K. oxytoca* that produce enterotoxins and cytotoxins have biologic effect in various animal models of gastrointestinal pathology. It is postulated that overgrowth of these organisms in the gut of patients receiving antibiotics may lead to gastrointestinal syndromes including antibiotic-associated colitis.[11]

K. pneumoniae subsp. *pneumoniae* and *K. oxytoca* may be carried in the nasopharynx (1% to 6%) and in the intestinal tract (5% to 40%) of the general population.[4] Carriage in hospitalized patients and healthcare personnel can be dramatically higher, particularly carriage in the respiratory tract. Airway colonization with *Klebsiella* spp. and other gram-negative bacilli in the mechanically ventilated neonate is a moderate risk factor for bloodstream infection (BSI) and is associated with severe bronchopulmonary dysplasia.[12]

CLINICAL MANIFESTATIONS

Klebsiella spp. are important opportunistic pathogens of children, causing a wide variety of infections including healthcare- and community-associated BSI, infections of the central nervous system, respiratory tract, urinary tract, and peritoneal cavity, as well as deep abscesses and postsurgical, trauma, and burn wound infections; approximately 75% of cases of BSIs are healthcare-associated (HA-BSI).[13-21] Outbreaks in neonatal units are of major concern.[22] Neonatal infections include BSI, meningitis, brain abscess, conjunctivitis, hepatic abscess, endocarditis, pneumonia, necrotizing fasciitis, arthritis, osteomyelitis, urinary tract infection (UTI), and necrotizing enterocolitis (NEC).[23-29] The clinical manifestations of infection are not different from those of other gram-negative bacilli. Although *Escherichia coli* is the most frequent etiology of UTI, *Klebsiella* and *Proteus* spp. are the other more common Enterobacteriaceae associated with UTI.[30]

Gram-negative organisms account for more than 50% of all BSIs reported in children. During a 6-year prospective study of gram-negative BSI in a pediatric tertiary care medical center in Israel, *K. pneumoniae* was the most commonly identified pathogen, comprising 26% (109 of 419) of isolates.[16] In a review of 57 cases of pediatric BSI caused by *K. pneumoniae*, 67% were <12 months of age, and almost all had at least one underlying condition including gastrointestinal tract abnormality in 56%, central venous catheter in 35%, neutropenia in 25%, and urinary tract abnormality in 16%.[31] The Surveillance and Control of Pathogens of Epidemiologic Importance project based at Virginia Commonwealth University in Richmond has provided important data identifying the predominant pathogens responsible for HA-BSI in children.[32] While gram-positive organisms especially coagulase-negative *Staphylococcus* spp. accounted for >50% of isolates, *Candida* spp. accounted for 9.3%; and *Klebsiella* spp., *Enterobacter* spp., and *Escherichia coli* for 5.8%, 5%, and 5% of isolates, respectively. Other conditions associated with *Klebsiella* spp. BSI in childhood include: prematurity, prior antibiotic exposure, preceding rotavirus gastroenteritis, Kasai procedure for biliary atresia, malignancy, postoperative status, burns, multiple trauma, acquired immunodeficiency syndrome, granulocyte disorders, homozygous sickle-cell disease, solid-organ transplantation, the postoperative period following splenectomy, systemic lupus erythematosus, and interleukin-12 receptor β1 deficiency.[16,32-38] Contaminated intravenous solutions also have been identified as a source of *Klebsiella* spp. BSI.[39]

The overall mortality rate for *Klebsiella* spp. BSI is approximately 11%, with a rate of 14.5% for HA-BSI.[16,32] Increased mortality is significantly associated with acute leukemia, neutropenia, HA infections, and previous corticosteroid therapy.

Cytotoxin-producing strains of *K. oxytoca* have been implicated in antibiotic-associated hemorrhagic colitis.[11,40,41] The clinical manifestations of abdominal pain and bloody diarrhea usually are preceded by antibiotic treatment with a β-lactam agent. Colitis usually is segmental and located predominantly in the right colon. Cessation of the offending antimicrobial agent and supportive care typically result in clinical resolution. Enterotoxigenic and enteroaggregative strains of *K. pneumoniae* also have been implicated as potential causes of childhood gastroenteritis.[42]

Raoultella spp. have been reported inconsistently as colonizing bacteria of the gastrointestinal tract of hospitalized neonates, and as agents of BSI and adult pneumonia.[43,44] *R. planticola* has been isolated from adult urine, wounds including an intra-abdominal abscess associated with pancreatitis, and contaminated infant formulas.[45-47] *R. ornithinolytica* has been recovered from the blood of a neonate with visceral heterotaxy, functional asplenia, and complex congenital heart disease experiencing NEC, and from one adult with a giant renal cyst and from another with an enteric fever-like syndrome.[48-50] Both *R. ornithinolytica* and *R. planticola* appear to be the cause of scombroid (histamine) fish poisoning.[8] This condition follows ingestion of improperly stored (>20°C) scombroid fish (tuna, mahi-mahi, bonito, mackerel, and sardine), and results from the breakdown of high concentrations of histidine into histamine by the action of bacterial histidine decarboxylase.[48,50] The incubation period can be as short as 1 minute to 3 hours; clinical manifestations can include marked skin flushing (especially of the face, upper trunk, and arms), headache, dizziness, abdominal cramps, vomiting, diarrhea, burning of the mouth, urticaria, generalized pruritus, and rarely hypotension and bronchospasm.

THERAPY

K. pneumoniae and *K oxytoca* frequently are susceptible to the aminoglycosides, carbapenems, third- and fourth-generation cephalosporins, extended-spectrum penicillin/β-lactamase inhibitor combinations, trimethoprim-sulfamethoxazole, and fluoroquinolones; *K. pneumoniae* also is susceptible commonly to cefazolin.[51] Both organisms are routinely resistant to ampicillin due to the presence of plasmid-mediated β-lactamases such as TEM-1, TEM-2, and SHV-1.[30,52,53] Additionally, HA infections due to extended-spectrum β-lactamase (ESBL)-producing isolates of *K. pneumoniae* and *K. oxytoca* have emerged.[19,31,32] The ESBLs are a group of diverse enzymes derived primarily from genes coding for TEM- or SHV-type enzymes by single or multiple amino acid substitutions near the active site of the enzyme.[4,54,55] ESBLs can hydrolyze third- and fourth generation cephalosporins and monobactams, rendering organisms harboring such enzymes clinically resistant to these agents; however, in vitro ESBL activity may be variable against different β-lactam agents and resistance not always detected. β-Lactamase inhibitor combination antibiotics, such as piperacillin-tazobactam or ticarcillin-clavulanate, can retain some activity in vitro due to inhibition of ESBL by the β-lactamase inhibitor; however, reduced susceptibility is typical. Susceptibility to the cephamycins and carbapenems is maintained.

Genes coding for ESBLs generally are located on transferable plasmids that also can harbor resistance determinants to other antimicrobial agents, including the fluoroquinolones and aminoglycosides.[54,55] In 1998, the incidence of ESBL-producing isolates of *K. pneumoniae* in the U.S. was reported to be about 5% in the National Nosocomial Infection Study system.[4] In another U.S. surveillance network study conducted from 1996 to 2000, the ESBL rates for *K. pneumoniae* and *K. oxytoca* rose from 7% to 9% and 3% to 6%, respectively.[56] Fortunately, ESBL prevalence among organisms isolated from children is considerably lower. The SENTRY Antimicrobial Surveillance Program reported 1.9% of *E. coli* and 1.1% to 3.2% of *Klebsiella* spp. as ESBL producers.[57] Although TEM-type ESBLs have been prevalent in the U.S., CTX-M-type ESBLs have emerged as the predominant ESBL type in many regions of the world and are also common in the U.S.[58,59] These enzymes preferentially hydrolyze cefotaxime over ceftazidime.

The incidence of ESBLs in *Klebsiella* spp. in the U.S. varies by institution, due mainly to the isolation of ESBL-positive *K. pneumoniae* in intensive care units and in immunocompromised hosts in tertiary care institutions.[30,52,53] Among 296 pediatric BSI isolates of *E. coli* and *Klebsiella* spp. from hospitalized U.S. children in 1999 to 2003, 35 (12%) were ESBL-producing: 17 *K. pneumoniae*, 10 *K. oxytoca*, and 8 *E. coli* isolates; ESBL-positive *Klebsiella* spp. represented 18% of all BSI isolates of *Klebsiella* spp.[60] In this population, exposure to third-generation cephalosporins in the 30 days before infection, female gender, infection with a *Klebsiella* sp., and corticosteroid use in the 2 weeks before infection were significant risk factors for BSI due to an ESBL-producing *E. coli* or *Klebsiella* spp. Children with these infections tended to experience high rates of mortality and longer lengths of hospitalization after infection compared with children with BSI due to similar non-ESBL-producing isolates. During 2003 to 2007, rates of ESBL-positive isolates in one children's hospital increased from 0.53% to 1.4%, an increase in incidence from 0.14% to 0.3% infections per 10,000 encounters.[61]

Bacterial strains producing ESBLs may be underdetected as generally they do not demonstrate overt resistance to all third- and fourth-generation cephalosporins and monobactams by standard in vitro laboratory test methods. Detection can be better accomplished by using screening and confirmatory tests recommended by the Clinical Laboratory and Standards Institute (CLSI).[62] In vitro screening tests are designed to detect possible ESBL-producing strains of *K. pneumoniae*, *K. oxytoca*, *E. coli*, and *Proteus mirabilis* based on an elevated minimum inhibitory concentration (MIC) or a reduced zone of inhibition by disk diffusion testing to select cephalosporins while still falling within traditional "susceptible" interpretative categories. Multiple antimicrobial agents are used in screening tests because in vitro activity of ESBL enzymes against different β-lactam agents varies. Failure to identify such a strain may lead to a report of false susceptibility to third- and fourth-generation cephalosporins, selection of inappropriate therapy, and possible treatment failure.

If a screening test suggests the presence of an ESBL, confirmation depends upon demonstrating that the activity of one or more antimicrobial agents, commonly both ceftazidime and cefotaxime, is enhanced by the addition of clavulanic acid. A ≥8-fold decrease in the MIC, or a minimum of a 5 mm increase in zone diameter of inhibition by disk diffusion, for either test agent confirms the presence of an ESBL because β-lactamase-inhibiting agents have activity against ESBLs. If confirmed, such an isolate is reported as resistant to all penicillin, cephalosporin, and monobactam agents, with comment that the organism has been confirmed to produce an ESBL. Although the fourth-generation cephalosporins have greater in vitro activity against these isolates, their clinical efficacy is unclear; thus, these compounds also should be reported as resistant.[51-55] Although the CLSI recommendation is to report activity of extended-spectrum penicillin/β-lactamase inhibitor combination agents, some consider the use of these agents in treatment of ESBL-positive organisms as ill-advised. Until these controversies are resolved, it would be prudent not to use these agents as monotherapy for serious infections due to ESBL-producing organisms.

CLSI also has published an alternative method for detecting and reporting possible ESBL producers among the Enterobacteriaceae.[62] This method uses revised MIC and disk diffusion breakpoints for reporting several antibiotics including cefotaxime, ceftriaxone, ceftazidime, and aztreonam. The lower MIC and larger disk diffusion breakpoints required to categorize an isolate as susceptible allow for reporting of susceptibility test results for these agents without the use of screening and confirmatory tests for ESBLs, a significant advantage for many laboratories. The conventional screening and confirmation method, as well as the newer method using revised breakpoint, are both appropriate for laboratory detection of ESBLs and some laboratories in the U.S. have adopted the newer approach. An additional advantage of the revised breakpoint approach is that it is applicable for detection of ESBLs in all Enterobacteriaceae compared with the traditional screening and confirmation test approach applicable only to *Klebsiella* spp., *E. coli*, and *P. mirabilis*. One of the difficulties in adopting the newer approach is that FDA-cleared commercial antimicrobial test systems currently use the traditional breakpoints. Thus, laboratories desiring to adopt the newer breakpoints must verify the newer breakpoints and devise approaches to reinterpret MIC results from the test systems before reporting. In addition, some commercial systems do not have adequate low-end antimicrobial concentrations to allow for interpretation with the revised lower-susceptibility breakpoints. Whatever system is used, it is imperative that laboratories clearly communicate and physicians understand how susceptibility test results are being interpreted and reported.

Fluoroquinolones, aminoglycosides, and carbapenems generally maintain activity against ESBL-producing Enterobacteriaceae.[60-65] Amikacin may be the most active aminoglycoside, with susceptibility of 89% of ESBL-producing *E. coli* and *Klebsiella* spp.[60] Fluoroquinolone resistance among *Klebsiella* spp. causing UTI ranges from 4.2% to 7.8%, with 80% of ESBL-producing *E. coli* and *Klebsiella* spp. susceptible to ciprofloxacin.[60,65] The carbapenems retain full activity against ESBL-producing isolates and should be used for treatment of serious infections.[63,64]

Klebsiella spp. also can harbor other plasmid-mediated β-lactamases, including AmpC β-lactamases, similar to those chromosomal enzymes commonly found in *Enterobacter* spp., inhibitor-resistant TEMs, and carbapenemases. The AmpC β-lactamases are not inhibited by clavulanic acid and other β-lactamase inhibitors, and thus extended-spectrum penicillin/β-lactamase inhibitor combination antibiotics, as well as the cephamycins, are generally ineffective; the fourth-generation cephalosporins and carbapenems retain activity.[4,54-57,66] Perhaps most alarming is the emergence of carbapenem resistance due to the presence of carbapenemases among Enterobacteriaceae. Organisms harboring these enzymes have been responsible for many HA infections worldwide.[67-69] The most common carbapenemases in the Enterobacteriaceae are the *K. pneumoniae* carbapenemases (KPCs), first identified in the U.S. in a *K. pneumoniae* isolate in North Carolina.[70] The majority of reports of infections due to KPC-positive organisms are from metropolitan centers in the northeast, but increasingly they are reported throughout the U.S. The KPCs constitute a group of similar enzymes (serine carbapenemases) that can be found in *K. pneumoniae*, *K. oxytoca*, *E. coli*, *Citrobacter freundii*, *Enterobacter* spp., and other gram-negative bacilli; however, the enzymes occur most frequently in isolates of *K. pneumoniae*. They confer resistance to all of the carbapenems as well as all third- and fourth-generation cephalosporins. Although β-lactamase inhibitors such as clavulanic acid and tazobactam demonstrate some inhibition of KPCs, inhibition generally is not sufficient to render β-lactam/β-lactamase inhibitor combination antibiotics active against these organisms. There have been recent reports in the U.S. of carbapenem-resistant Enterobacteriaceae harboring metallocarbapenemases, including Verona integron-encoded (VIM) and New Delhi type-1 (NDM-1) metallocarbapenemases.[71,72] The three U.S. cases of infections due to organisms harboring the NDM-1 enzyme included an *E. coli*, *K. pneumoniae*, and *E. clocacae* isolate. All three patients had received recent medical care in India. A single patient with infection due to a strain of *K. pneumoniae* producing a VIM-type enzyme was previously hospitalized in Greece. Laboratories and physicians alike must be alert to the possibility of infections due to such organisms, particularly when patients have traveled to areas where these organisms are prevalent.

CLSI recently has published updated susceptibility test interpretive criteria for the Enterobacteriaceae with lower MIC and higher disk diffusion breakpoints to define isolates susceptible to the carbapenem antibiotics including ertapenem, meropenem, imipenem-cilastatin and doripenem.[73] The revised breakpoints are designed to better identify organisms that may be harboring carbapenemases but would not be reported as intermediate or resistant with the older breakpoints. Laboratories either can implement newer breakpoints or can continue to use screening and confirmatory tests with the older breakpoints to identify carbapenemase-producing Enterobacteriaceae in much the same way as using screening and confirmatory tests for detection of ESBLs. The recommended confirmatory test for carbapenemase production is the modified Hodge test.[73] In this test, performed on an agar plate, the presence of carbapenemase activity in a test organism is demonstrated by the ability of the enzyme to inactivate the activity of a carbapenem antibiotic, thus allowing a carbapenem-susceptible indicator *E. coli* organism to show enhanced growth in the presence of the antibiotic.

Raoultella spp. exhibit similar antibiotic susceptibility patterns to *Klebsiella* spp.[45]

Empiric treatment of the seriously ill patient with suspected HA infection due to a *Klebsiella* spp. or other gram-negative bacillus should include the combination of meropenem and amikacin. For patients with BSI (including those with granulocytopenia or hypotension) or other serious infections due to such organisms, combination therapy with a β-lactam antibiotic plus an aminoglycoside

to which the organism is susceptible is reasonable.[74,75] Fluoroquinolones and piperacillin-tazobactam have been used to treat serious infections caused by *Klebsiella* spp. that were resistant to the aminoglycosides and cephalosporins.[76,77] Unfortunately, resistance to these agents also is reported and definitive antimicrobial therapy must be guided by the results of susceptibility testing.

For meningitis due to antibiotic-susceptible *Klebsiella* spp., a third-generation cephalosporin and aminoglycoside administered intravenously is currently the regimen of choice. In one study of children 4 days to 7 months old who were receiving cefotaxime and amikacin parenterally, the mean duration of positive cerebrospinal fluid (CSF) cultures was 5.8 ± 4.7 days (range, 2 to 15 days).[74] Five of these patients also received from 1 to 25 doses of intraventricular amikacin; however, intraventricular instillation is not recommended in children who do not have a central nervous system device in place. The efficacy of treatment in children with gram-negative bacillary meningitis should be monitored by repeated examinations and cultures of CSF. Patients with prolonged positive cultures may be candidates for meropenem, if supported by susceptibility testing. Therapy should be continued for at least 2 weeks after the first sterile CSF culture, or for a total course of 21 days, whichever is longer.

Management recommendations for infections associated with intravascular devices due to *Klebsiella* spp. and other members of the Enterobacteriaceae family generally have included the removal of the foreign body. For device-associated BSI due to gram-negative bacilli, attempt to treat with antibiotics without device removal is reasonable if the patient is stable clinically and the bloodstream is sterilized quickly.[78] Oral cephalosporins, trimethoprim-sulfamethoxazole, or fluoroquinolones can be considered for treatment of UTIs due to susceptible organisms.

Treatment of infections due to carbapenem-resistant Enterobacteriaceae may be problematic because these organisms are resistant to all β-lactam class antibiotics and also can be resistant to the aminoglycosides and fluoroquinolones. The newer agent tigecycline, and the revived agent colistin, may offer therapeutic options.[79]

A 24-valent *K. pneumoniae* capsular polysaccharide vaccine has been shown to be immunogenic in patients who have sustained trauma, a group known to be at risk for serious infection due to gram-negative bacteria.[80] In the future, active immunoprophylaxis may be a consideration for individuals at risk for infections caused by *Klebsiella* spp. and other gram-negative bacilli.

139 *Klebsiella (Calymmatobacterium) granulomatis* (Granuloma Inguinale)

Bradley P. Stoner

Granuloma inguinale, or donovanosis, is a chronic, slowly destructive, ulcerative disease of skin and subcutaneous tissues caused by *Klebsiella* (formerly *Calymmatobacterium*) *granulomatis*.[1,2] Uncommon in industrialized countries, donovanosis historically has been seen among adolescents and adults in some tropical and developing regions, including Papua New Guinea, central Australia, South Africa, Brazil, and regions of India.[3-7] Sporadic cases also have been reported in the West Indies, South America, and other areas of southern Africa. Children rarely are diagnosed with donovanosis.[8,9] In recent years, several endemic regions have

reported substantial declines in prevalence.[10-12] The published literature on donovanosis represents few geographic locations, reflects limited microbiologic testing, and relies on syndromic genital ulcer disease (GUD) surveillance in areas where donovanosis is thought to be most common.[13] Increased awareness of the role of GUD in human immunodeficiency virus (HIV) transmission may raise public health interest in donovanosis.[14,15]

The sexual transmission of donovanosis has been controversial, but there is substantial evidence that *K. granulomatis* is transmitted sexually.[13,16] Transmission rates of up to 52% have been reported

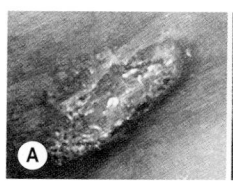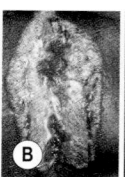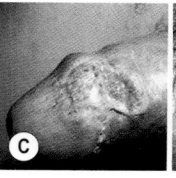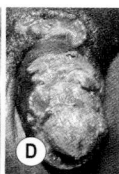

Figure 139-1. Lesions in patients with donovanosis. **(A)** Healing inguinal ulcer. **(B)** Perianal skin ulcer. **(C)** penile ulcer. **(D)** Penile ulcer with extensive tissue damage. (Photos from the Centers for Disease Control and Prevention's Public Health Image Library for public use: http://phil.cdc.gov/phil/home.asp.)

among steady sexual partners of persons with donovanosis.[8] Although rare, vertical transmission of donovanosis has been reported.[17] There also is evidence that transmission can occur through fecal contamination.[18]

CLINICAL MANIFESTATIONS

Donovanosis lesions involve the genitalia (typically the prepuce or glans in men and the vagina or labia minora in women) in 80% to 90% of cases, but also can involve the inguinal and anal regions (Figure 139-1A, B). Beginning as a small papule (or multiple papules) at the site of inoculation, donovanosis typically manifests with painless, easily bleeding ulcers or vegetative lesions (Figure 139-1C), which can be ulcerogranulomatous, hypertrophic, necrotic, or sclerotic.[19] Ulcerative lesions expand slowly and become clean, shallow, well-demarcated ulcer(s) with a beefy red granular base (Figure 139-1D). Prominent lymphadenopathy often develops, leading to further ulceration of overlying skin.[20] In most cases, clinical findings are suggestive of donovanosis, but are not highly specific.[8,16,21]

Untreated lesions can cause extensive local tissue damage, including pelvic and perianal fistulas, urethral obstruction, and lymphedema.[16] Although uncommon, lesions can develop secondary bacterial infection and cellulitis. Systemic infections can cause fever, weight loss, and anemia. Involvement of the bone, joint, and liver can occur infrequently and is thought to be more common in pregnant women. Involvement of the head and neck also has been described.[22]

The differential diagnosis of donovanosis includes syphilis, lymphogranuloma venereum, chancroid, lymphoma, carcinoma, tuberculosis, blastomycosis, and other granulomatous diseases. People suspected of having donovanosis should have a careful complete examination, and should be tested for syphilis and other sexually transmitted infections (STI), including HIV, which can coexist with donovanosis.[16,23] The increased risk of HIV transmission associated with GUD (such as due to syphilis, herpes simplex virus infection and donovanosis), further underscores the importance of prompt recognition and treatment.[14]

LABORATORY DIAGNOSIS

K. granulomatis is a pleomorphic, intracellular, gram-negative bacterium. Difficult to grow on artificial media, *K. granulomatis* can be identified using tissue "crush" or biopsy specimens. For tissue crush specimens, granulation tissue is collected from a lesion and crushed between two microscopic slides. Once excess material has been removed from the ulcer base with a cotton swab, the first swab collection is most sensitive.[13,19] "Donovan bodies," which look like safety pins clustered in macrophages when stained with Wright or Giemsa stain, are diagnostic of *K. granulomatis*. A polymerase chain reaction test for *K. granulomatis* is available for use in some research settings,[24,25] but this is not available commercially. Light microscopy is a less reliable diagnostic technique for donovanosis.[8,21,26]

TREATMENT AND MANAGEMENT

Prompt identification and treatment are important in optimal management.[27] However, in most donovanosis-endemic areas,

diagnostic testing is limited, and treatment is determined by syndromic algorithm. Syndromic algorithm for GUD should be evaluated routinely to determine whether donovanosis therapy should be included in the GUD treatment provided.

Initiation of antibiotic therapy slows progression of lesions, but prolonged therapy usually is required for effective treatment. Several antimicrobial regimens are effective, but few controlled trials have been published. The recommended first-line therapy for adults according to the Centers for Disease Control and Prevention (CDC) STI treatment guidelines is doxycycline (100 mg dose orally twice daily) (http://www.cdc.gov/std/treatment/2010/default.htm).[28] Alternative regimens include: azithromycin (1 g dose orally once per week), ciprofloxacin (750 mg dose orally twice daily), erythromycin base (500 mg dose orally four times a day), trimethoprim-sulfamethoxazole (one double strength (800 mg/160 mg) tablet orally twice daily).

Studies of azithromycin for treatment of donovanosis have involved few cases to date, and treatment regimens have not been standardized.[29,30] Nevertheless, results with azithromycin have been promising, and recently-published European guidelines now recommend azithromycin as first-line treatment for donovanosis (1 g dose weekly or 500 mg dose daily for adults, and 20 mg/kg once daily for children).[19] The World Health Organization 2003 STI management guidelines recommend either azithromycin (1 g for 1 day, followed by 500 mg daily) or doxycycline (100 mg dose twice daily).[31]

Recommendations for duration of antimicrobial therapy vary. The CDC recommends treatment for at least 3 weeks and until all lesions have healed completely. Some specialists recommend addition of an aminoglycoside (e.g., gentamicin 1 mg/kg intravenously every 8 hours) if clinical improvement is not evident within the first few days of antibiotic therapy.[28]

Clinical studies suggest a variable incubation period for donovanosis of approximately 1 to 8 weeks or longer.[8,19] Contact intervals are not standardized. CDC STI treatment guidelines recommend that sex partners within 60 days before the onset of the patient's symptoms be examined and offered therapy. However, the value of empiric therapy in the absence of clinical signs and symptoms has not been established.[18,28]

Because doxycycline and ciprofloxacin are contraindicated in pregnant women (and pregnancy is a relative contraindication to the use of sulfonamides), pregnant and lactating women should be treated with the erythromycin regimen, and consideration should be given to the addition of an aminoglycoside. Azithromycin may be effective and useful for treating donovanosis in pregnancy, but published data are lacking.[28]

Few data exist regarding the clinical presentation and treatment of HIV-infected people. However, one study found no difference in duration of ulcer healing and rate of recurrence between HIV-infected and uninfected pregnant women.[32] The CDC STI treatment guidelines recommend that people with both granuloma inguinale and HIV infection should receive the same regimens as people who are HIV uninfected; however, patients should be monitored closely for relapse or treatment failure, and if failing the initial antimicrobial therapy, an aminoglycoside (e.g., gentamicin) can be added.

The risk of complications, such as complete genital erosion and urethral obstruction, can be minimized with early therapy. If extensive tissue destruction has occurred, surgery may be required.[33] Relapse is common, especially if duration of treatment is inadequate, and can occur 6 to 18 months after apparently effective therapy.

PREVENTION AND CONTROL

Few data exist regarding effective prevention and control. Prevention should be part of a broad STI prevention and control program, with emphasis on providing information about risks and complications of STIs (including HIV), safer sex practices, early recognition and treatment of STIs, and sex partner evaluation and treatment.[6,20,28]

140 *Enterobacter, Cronobacter,* and *Pantoea* Species

Dennis J. Cunningham and Mario J. Marcon

MICROBIOLOGY AND EPIDEMIOLOGY

The genus *Enterobacter* has undergone significant taxonomic revision based on DNA-DNA hybridization and 16S ribosomal RNA sequencing studies and now contains upwards of 15 named species.[1-5] Many former members of this genus have been transferred to other genera in the family Enterobacteriaceae, including the genera *Klebsiella, Serratia, Hafnia,* and *Pantoea*. In fact, there is significant current genetic evidence to support the transfer of *Enterobacter aerogenes* to the genus *Klebsiella* and to reclassify a number of genospecies in the *E. cloacae* complex of organisms into different named species. Similarly, some organisms formerly assigned to the genus *Erwinia* or given Centers for Disease Control and Prevention "enteric group" designations have been reclassified within the genus *Enterobacter*.

The genus *Pantoea* has been proposed to accommodate several isolates with significant biochemical and nucleic acid diversity that were formerly included in the heterogeneous taxon referred to as the "*Enterobacter agglomerans*" group.[6] Two species recovered from human and other sources are included in the genus – *P. dispersa* and *P. agglomerans*. Some have suggested that until the proper taxonomic relationship and biochemical identification of these organisms have been clarified, they should be referred to as members of the *E. agglomerans* group. Notwithstanding, some commercial biochemical identification systems include *P. agglomerans* or *P. agglomerans* group in their databases.

The *Enterobacter* spp. most commonly recovered from human sources include *E. cloacae, E. aerogenes,* and to a lesser extent *Pantoea (Enterobacter) agglomerans* group, *Cronobacter* spp. (formerly *E. sakazakii*), *E. gergoviae,* and *E. asburiae; Enterobacter cloacae* is by far the most common clinical isolate. A number of newly named species were formerly included in the *E. cloacae* group and are difficult to differentiate by biochemical test methods.[1-5] Similarly, organisms formerly classified as *E. sakazakii* comprised a diverse group but were lumped together as a single species. They have now been renamed as *Cronobacter* spp., which comprise at least five named distinct species including *C. sakazakii*. Some commercial biochemical identification systems use the terms *E. cloacae* group and *C. Sakazakii* group to describe these closely related organisms that are difficult to distinguish by biochemical testing methods.

Enterobacter, Cronobacter, and *Pantoea* spp. are nonfastidious in nature and grow on enriched media such as blood and chocolate agar, as well as selective media for enteric bacteria. On MacConkey agar, *E. cloacae* and *E. aerogenes* commonly appear as pink, lactose-positive, mucoid colonies similar in appearance to *Klebsiella pneumoniae* and *K. oxytoca*. Most isolates of *Cronobacter* spp. and *P. agglomerans* group organisms produce a nondiffusible yellow pigment which often is more intense on enriched media at 25°C versus 35°C. Colonies of *Cronobacter* can appear as dry, wrinkled, and leathery on some media. Most isolates of *Enterobacter* spp. are motile, utilize citrate as a sole carbon source, and give a positive Voges–Proskauer test but do not produce indole or H_2S. With the exception of the *P. agglomerans* group organisms, most isolates have ornithine decarboxylase activity. Motility and ornithine reactions help differentiate *Enterobacter* spp. from the common human isolates of *Klebsiella* spp. Commercial or conventional biochemical identification systems generally perform well for identifying and differentiating *E. cloacae, E. aerogenes, P. agglomerans* and *Cronobacter* spp.; however, the other species present a greater challenge and are not all represented in the databases of commercial systems. In general, a report of *Enterobacter* spp. or

Cronobacter spp. may be sufficient for most patient care decisions, although knowledge of the specific species would be important in the setting of a potential nosocomial outbreak or when the clinical significance of the isolate is questioned.

Enterobacter spp. and *Pantoea* spp. are common inhabitants of the gastrointestinal tract of humans and other mammals, and also can be found in water, sewage, soil, and in association with plant material and foods. Even the more common human isolates, *E. cloacae* and *E. aerogenes,* have been described as ubiquitous in animal and environmental distribution. A number of *Pantoea* spp. are well-known agents of disease in plants. In humans, *Enterobacter* spp. and *Pantoea* spp. are opportunistic pathogens and are among the most common organisms causing nosocomial infections such as pneumonia, urinary tract infection, surgical wound infection, and catheter-related bloodstream infection. These organisms frequently colonize the skin, respiratory, urinary, and gastrointestinal tracts of hospitalized patients; these sites act as portals of entry for localized or invasive disease.[1-5] *Enterobacter* spp. and *Pantoea* spp. also cause community-acquired infections including urinary tract, skin and soft-tissue and other infections, although at much lower rates than other gram-negative rods such as *E. coli, Proteus* spp., and *Klebsiella* spp. Community-acquired infections due to *P. agglomerans* have been associated with plant thorn and wood splinter injuries.

Enterobacter spp. accounted for 4.7% of all bacterial pathogens and 9.4% of gram-negative rods in >4000 episodes of nosocomial or community-acquired bloodstream infection (BSI) in North America and Latin American in 1997.[7] Of nearly 75,000 gram-negative bacilli recovered from BSIs in patients in intensive care units (ICUs) in the United States between 1993 and 2004, *Enterobacter* spp. accounted for 13.5% of isolates.[8] Two U.S. studies indicate that *Enterobacter* spp. are the fourth and seventh most common pathogens causing BSI in pediatric ICUs and neonatal ICUs, respectively.[9,10] An additional 2003 U.S. study of ICU nosocomial bacterial infections reported that *Enterobacter* spp. accounted for 10%, 4.4%, 9.0%, and 6.9% of pneumonia, BSI, surgical-site, and urinary tract infections due to gram-negative rods.[11] *Enterobacter* spp. also accounted for 15% of all gram-negative childhood BSIs in Israel.[12]

An endogenous source of *Enterobacter* spp. is most common in nosocomial infections. Approximately 40% of infants are fecal carriers of either *Klebsiella* or *Enterobacter* spp. upon discharge from neonatal ICUs. Colonization in nursery settings has been associated with overcrowding, inadequate handwashing, low birthweight, prematurity, endotracheal intubation, prolonged hospitalization, contaminated infant formula or parenteral nutrition, and the use of antibiotics or central venous catheters (CVCs). Risk factors for infection include immunosuppression from any cause, prematurity, the use of a foreign device such as a CVC, endotracheal tube, or urinary catheter, and the prior use of antibiotics. The role of microbial virulence factors in pathogenicity of these organisms has been reviewed.[5]

CLINICAL MANIFESTATIONS

Bloodstream infection is the most common form of invasive infection due to *Enterobacter* spp;[13-18] signs and symptoms are similar to those due to other gram-negative enteric bacteria. Fever occurs in 83% to 87% of children, whereas hypotension or shock occurs in 8% to 28%. Leukocytosis or leukopenia can develop and mortality rates in children range from 6% to 24%.[13-17]

Lower respiratory tract infection including pneumonia with BSI is the second most common pediatric infection due to *Enterobacter* spp. In the pediatric national nosocomial surveillance studies, *Enterobacter* spp. were the third and fourth leading causes of nosocomial pneumonia in pediatric and neonatal ICUs, respectively.[9,10] Pneumonia due to *Enterobacter* spp. occurs more often in infants younger than 2 months than in older infants and children. The relative frequency of *Enterobacter* spp. as a cause of nosocomial pneumonia in pediatric ICUs rose from 7.4% in 1992 to 13% in 1997.[10]

Other *Enterobacter* spp. infections in infants and children include meningitis, brain abscess, endocarditis, pyogenic arthritis, and peritonitis. *Klebsiella* or *Enterobacter* spp. accounted for 16% of all cases of meningitis due to gram-negative enteric bacteria during a 21-year period in Dallas.[19] *Enterobacter* spp. also are associated with nosocomial gastrointestinal, urinary tract, surgical site, eye, ear, nose, and throat infections (Table 140-1).[9,10]

Cronobacter spp. (also *Cronobacter sakazakii* group; formerly *Enterobacter sakazakii*) have particular importance in young infants because of association with powdered infant formula feeding[20] and because of its propensity for causing meningitis in a similar fashion to *Citrobacter koseri* (see Chapter 141, *Citrobacter* Species). Neonatal meningitis due to *Cronobacter* is associated with a high prevalence of brain abscess or cyst formation, a high mortality rate (40% to 80%), and long-term neurologic sequelae in survivors. There is controversy as to whether the cystic lesions visualized on brain computed tomography (CT) in neonates with *Cronobacter* meningitis result from infarction leading to sterile liquefaction cysts or from abscess formation. *Cronobacter* has been isolated from brain "cysts," suggesting a need to obtain cyst aspirates for Gram stain and culture whenever possible. Whenever *Cronobacter* is recovered from neonatal blood or cerebrospinal fluid cultures, serial CT or magnetic resonance imaging studies should be performed to evaluate for brain cyst and abscess formation to guide optimal management.[21] The World Health Organization has recommended preparation guidelines and continued improvement of powdered infant formula manufacturing processes to reduce this mode of acquisition of *Cronobacter* spp.[20]

Pantoea agglomerans is an uncommon human pathogen and has been reported to cause BSI, including neonatal BSI related to administration of contaminated IV solutions or associated with contamination of indwelling catheters. Septic shock, respiratory failure, and mortality occurred in 7 of 8 patients in one outbreak related to contaminated parenteral fluid.[22] Another study reported 5 sporadic cases of *Pantoea agglomerans* bacteremia in preterm neonates over a 2-year period at one hospital; no source was identified.[23] Additional reports include peritonitis during chronic ambulatory peritoneal dialysis, suppurative arthritis, or skin and soft-tissue infections presumably resulting from catheter contamination or from plant thorn injury during rose gardening.[24,25]

Pantoea spp. endophthalmitis developed in a patient after ocular trauma while using a lawn mower; a metal fragment was found lodged in the lens of the eye.[26]

TREATMENT

Antibiotic susceptibility patterns for *Enterobacter* spp. vary among facilities and among species, making careful monitoring of antimicrobial susceptibility patterns critical. *Cronobacter* spp. and *E. gergoviae* may be susceptible to ampicillin, cefazolin, and other narrow-spectrum cephalosporins; however, *E. cloacae, E. aerogenes,* and several other *Enterobacter* spp. uniformly are resistant to these agents.[27]

Both *E. cloacae* and *E. aerogenes,* along with other select Enterobacteriaceae, including *Citrobacter freundii, Proteus vulgaris, Morganella morganii, Serratia* spp., and *Providencia* spp., harbor a chromosomal gene (*ampC*) coding for AmpC-type β-lactamase.[28] This enzyme, which may be produced at low levels on initial laboratory isolation of the organism, can be induced to high-level production following in vitro or in vivo exposure to select β-lactam antibiotics, particularly compounds like ampicillin, first- or second-generation cephalosporins, and clavulanic acid. Initial isolates of these organisms can show susceptibility to extended spectrum β-lactam agents by in vitro test methods, particularly rapid susceptibility test methods. Additionally, AmpC β-lactamase production can be stably de-repressed in these organisms due to a chromosomal mutation of the *ampD* gene that normally plays a role in repressing *ampC* gene transcription and attendant high-level β-lactamase production. These strains, referred to as "stably de-repressed mutants," can emerge during selective antimicrobial pressure within days of starting a course of β-lactam therapy, and produce high levels of AmpC β-lactamase constitutively.[27–29] Emergence of resistance appears to occur more often in *Enterobacter* spp. than in other enteric bacteria known to harbor *ampC* genes.[29] High level AmpC production renders the organism resistant to many β-lactam antibiotics including third-generation cephalosporins and extended-spectrum penicillin/β-lactamase inhibitor combination drugs; susceptibility to fourth-generation cephalosporins and carbapenems is retained.

Currently, there are no routine procedures recommended by the Clinical Laboratory and Standards Institute (CLSI) for laboratory detection of inducible AmpC-mediated resistance in *Enterobacter* spp. and related organisms. A "double-disk" approximation test can be used, in which a known AmpC inducer antibiotic disk and an indicator antibiotic disk are placed in adjacent positions on a lawn of a test organism. A measurable reduction or "flattening" in the zone of inhibition on the side of the indicator antibiotic disk adjacent to the inducer antibiotic disk suggest AmpC production.[30] An alternative approach for the detection uses AmpC inhibitor compounds in a disk diffusion test format similar to the CLSI disk test for extended spectrum β-lactamase (ESBL) confirmation (see Chapter 138, *Klebsiella* and *Raoultella* Species).[31]

In areas where inducible AmpC resistance is common, it seems prudent to report *Enterobacter cloacae* and other known AmpC-producers as resistant to third-generation cephalosporins and extended-spectrum penicillin/beta-lactamase inhibitor combination drugs or, at the very least, to caution against their use as monotherapy for serious infections.[32] It is equally important to repeat testing of secondary isolates of *Enterobacter* spp. and other gram-negative bacilli recovered from normally sterile body sites when recovered after 24 or 48 hours of appropriate antibiotic therapy.

Enterobacter spp. also can contain plasmids encoding for ESBLs and other genes coding for resistance to other classes of antibiotics.[33]

In a North American and Latin American survey of gram-negative BSI in which 399 *Enterobacter* spp. isolates were tested, meropenem, imipenem, and cefepime were the most active antimicrobial agents with >99% of isolates susceptible. The fluoroquinolones and aminoglycosides also had good activity, with 90% to 96% of isolates susceptible. No other antibiotic demonstrated activity for >78% of isolates.[7]

TABLE 140-1. Percentage of All Pediatric Infections Caused by *Enterobacter* spp. Reported by the National Nosocomial Infections Surveillance System[a]

Infection	Percentage of Cases by Intensive Care Unit (ICU)	
	Neonatal ICU	Pediatric ICU
Bloodstream	2.9	6.2
Gastrointestinal tract	5.5	ND
Pneumonia	8.2	9.3
Lower respiratory tract other than pneumonia	ND	12.2
Urinary tract	ND	10.3
Surgical site	7.6	8.1
Eye, ear, nose, throat	4.5	ND

Abbreviation: ND, no data.
[a]Data collated from references 9 and 10.

Optimal antibiotic therapy for infections due to *Enterobacter* spp. is unclear. In serious infection, it may be prudent to avoid use of single-agent, extended-spectrum cephalosporin or penicillin/β-lactamase inhibitor combination drug therapy other than a fourth-generation cephalosporin because of the possibility of rapid selection of resistance. A combination of an extended-spectrum cephalosporin or penicillin/β-lactamase inhibitor combination drug and an aminoglycoside is reasonable for infections outside the central nervous system. For treatment of meningitis, meropenem may be the optimal choice.[34,35] Many experts would use meropenem and an aminoglycoside in this setting. For patients with type I hypersensitivity reactions to β-lactams, use of a fluoroquinolone with an aminoglycoside may be effective.

Careful monitoring of the patient's clinical course, particularly for occurrence of central nervous system complications, is essential, especially with *Cronobacter* infection. Appropriate specimens must be obtained sequentially to demonstrate sustained bacteriologic response. Prompt removal of contaminated prosthetic devices is essential to eradicate the organism and effect cure; failure to remove such devices compromises rapid bacteriologic response and increases the likelihood that resistant organisms will emerge. The use of broad-spectrum antimicrobial agents should be limited and unnecessary antimicrobial therapy should be avoided. Good handwashing technique and other infection control practices must be followed.

141 *Citrobacter* Species

Dwight A. Powell and Mario J. Marcon

MICROBIOLOGY AND EPIDEMIOLOGY

The genus *Citrobacter* has undergone significant taxonomic revision through the use of newer techniques based on DNA relatedness. The genus now contains 11 named species: *Citrobacter freundii, C. koseri, C. amalonaticus, C. youngae, C. farmeri, C. braakii, C. werkmanii, C. sedlakii, C. gillenii, C. murliniae,* and *C. rodentium*.[1-5] *Citrobacter koseri* has replaced the taxon formerly known as *Citrobacter diversus,* and *Citrobacter farmeri* is the new taxon assigned to the former *Citrobacter amalonaticus* biogroup 1. All species except *C. rodentium* have been recovered from human clinical sources (some rarely) including blood and other normally sterile body sites, wounds, respiratory and urinary tract; however, *C. freundii* and *C. koseri* are the most important human pathogens. *C. freundii, C. koseri,* and *C. amalonaticus* appear to be distinct organisms; however, only *C. koseri* appears to be genetically homogeneous. Several other named species form a closely related group and are difficult to differentiate biochemically; they are sometimes referred to as *C. freundii*-complex organisms.

Members of the genus *Citrobacter* share all the general properties and biochemical characteristics of the family Enterobacteriaceae, including the following: gram-negative rod, catalase-positive and oxidase-negative, growth on MacConkey agar, reduction of nitrate to nitrite, growth both aerobically and anaerobically, and fermentation of glucose and other carbohydrates. Most isolates are motile and utilize citrate as a sole carbon source, but lack urease and lysine decarboxylase activity; production of hydrogen sulfide is variable, occurring with *C. freundii* and a few other species. On salmonella-shigella agar, lactose-negative/hydrogen-sulfide positive isolates of *Citrobacter* spp. produce black colonies resembling *Salmonella* spp. The lysine decarboxylase reaction allows for separation of the hydrogen sulfide-producing isolates of *Citrobacter* spp. from *Salmonella* spp.[1-5] Select isolates of *C. freundii* have "O" (somatic) cell wall antigens closely related to the O antigens of *Salmonella* spp. and thus cross-react with *Salmonella* typing antisera.[5] In addition, rare isolates of *C. freundii* and *C. braakii* cross-react with some commercial *Escherichia coli* O157 typing antisera.[5] For this reason, it is always prudent to confirm the identification of suspected *Salmonella* spp. and *E. coli* O157 by the use of both biochemical and serologic methods. Although biochemical identification of the newer species can be accomplished through the use of conventional tests, most commercial identification systems do not include all species in their databases. This limitation hampers the correlation of the newer species with human disease.

Citrobacter spp. are primarily inhabitants of the intestinal tract of mammals and other vertebrates. Their isolation from environmental sources such as water and soil likely is the result of fecal excretion. *Citrobacter* spp. are not common agents of human disease, and are most often recovered from stool as colonizing flora of the gastrointestinal tract. When associated with significant human infection, *Citrobacter* can be recovered from blood, cerebrospinal fluid (CSF), urine, respiratory tract secretions, and wounds. The most common *Citrobacter* spp. isolated from human sources are *C. freundii* (all sites listed above), *C. koseri* (all sites but CSF and brain most commonly), *C. amalonaticus* (all sites except CSF), *C. braakii* (primarily stool), and *C. youngae* (primarily stool).

The pathogenesis of *Citrobacter* infections has not been characterized fully. Most *C. koseri* isolates produce hemolysins, are piliated, and are resistant to killing by pooled human sera. Tropism for the central nervous system may be due to specific outer membrane proteins. In one study, 79% of strains of *C. koseri* isolated from CSF had a unique 32-kd outer-membrane protein, which was found in only 9% of isolates from other kinds of specimens.[6] *Citrobacter koseri* also has the ability to enter macrophages, survive phago-lysosomal fusion, and replicate intracellularly. These infected macrophages then infiltrate blood vessels in the brain, which may be one of the main mechanisms of infecting brain microvascular endothelial cells, thus starting the process leading to brain abscess.[5,7,8]

In the pediatric population, infections due to *Citrobacter* spp. occur most commonly in neonates.[9,10] Organisms can be transmitted by vertical transmission from mothers or by nosocomial spread. Direct mother-to-infant transmission has been confirmed by ribotyping and DNA fingerprinting.[11,12] It is likely that individual strains of *Citrobacter* spp. circulating in the community periodically gain access to a hospital nursery from the hands of nursery personnel and visitors.[13] One nursery outbreak of *C. freundii* was traced to contaminated infant formula.[14] Outbreaks in nursery settings can last for months or years and appear to be best controlled by cohorting of patients and personnel.

CLINICAL MANIFESTATIONS

Neonatal septicemia and meningitis are the most common infections due to *Citrobacter* spp. in infants.[9,10] Septicemia is associated with meningitis in about one-half of cases. From 1969 to 1989 in Dallas, TX, *Citrobacter* spp. accounted for 9% of 91 cases of gram-negative enteric meningitis in infants aged 1 day to 2 years.[15] *C.*

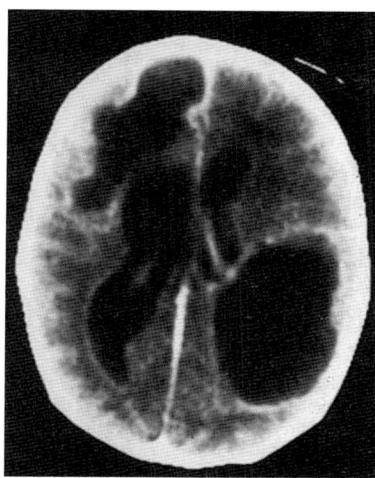

Figure 141-1. Computed tomographic scan of a neonate with multiple brain abscesses caused by *Citrobacter koseri*.

koseri was responsible for 90% of cases and *C. freundii* caused most of the remaining cases. Neonatal sepsis and meningitis can manifest as early-onset (<1 week of life) or late-onset (>1 week of life) disease. In 2002–2003, *Citrobacter* spp. caused 2.9% of early-onset sepsis in very-low-birthweight infants.[16] The illness can be fulminant or insidious. No early features distinguish meningitis due to *Citrobacter* spp. from meningitis due to other gram-negative rods; however, approximately 80% of infants with meningitis due to *Citrobacter* spp. develop ≥1 intracerebral abscesses (Figure 141-1). In contrast, <10% of cases of infants with meningitis due to other gram-negative organisms have associated abscess(es).[9,10] Brain abscesses can occur at any time during the acute course, including several weeks after the start of treatment. In a review of brain abscesses in neonates <1 month of age, 3 of 5 were due to *Citrobacter* spp.[17] A similar clinical presentation of neonatal brain abscess occurs with *Cronobacter* (formerly *Enterobacter*) *sakazakii* and *Serratia marcescens*.

The prognosis for meningitis due to *Citrobacter* spp. in neonates generally is poor. Approximately 30% to 35% of infected infants die, and only 15% to 20% survive with a structurally normal brain at completion of therapy; however, data on long-term prognosis are limited.[9] Although at least 40% of survivors show some form of developmental delay, physical impairment, or both, there are reports of infants with brain abscesses due to *Citrobacter* spp. who develop normally.[18]

Citrobacter spp. are the cause of urinary tract infection (UTI) in <3% of adults and children.[19,20] In a review of 37 pediatric cases, the mean age was 6.9 years, with a range of 1 month to 18 years.[20] Females predominated, and 56% of patients had underlying urinary tract or renal anomalies or neurologic impairment. Presenting symptoms were similar to those of UTI from other causes, with dysuria, fever, incontinence, frequency, flank pain, or hematuria. *C. freundii* accounted for 71% of cases, and *C. koseri* for the remainder. Mixed UTI involving other enteric bacilli occurred in about 25% of patients.

Other illnesses in infants due to *Citrobacter* spp. occur rarely and include gastroenteritis, osteomyelitis, pyogenic arthritis, pulmonary infections, pneumatosis intestinalis, and sepsis.[10] In older children and adults, *Citrobacter* spp. is associated most commonly with urinary tract, bloodstream, intra-abdominal, skin and soft-tissue, and respiratory tract infections.[21] *C. freundii* caused 2.3% of bloodstream infections in the first year following lung

transplantation in 190 pediatric patients.[22] An outbreak of severe gastroenteritis associated with several cases of hemolytic-uremic syndrome occurred in a nursery school.[23] The source of this outbreak was sandwiches prepared with green butter containing a toxigenic strain of *C. freundii*. The butter had been made with contaminated parsley grown in an organically fertilized garden.

TREATMENT

Most data on in vitro antimicrobial susceptibility and therapeutic management are for infections due to *C. freundii* and *C. koseri*. These organisms can harbor a wide variety of β-lactamases. Both species are resistant uniformly to ampicillin and *C. freundii* is also resistant to first-generation cephalosporins. *C. freundii* and some other *Citrobacter* spp. harbor chromosomal AmpC-type β-lactamases that can inactivate third-generation cephalosporins (see Chapter 140, *Enterobacter, Cronobacter,* and *Pantoea* Species).[24] This enzyme is not inhibited by β-lactamase inhibitors such as tazobactam or clavulanate, thus isolates can be resistant to agents such as ticarcillin/clavulanate and piperacillin/tazobactam. Some strains of *C. freundii* also harbor extended spectrum β-lactamases and *Klebsiella pneumoniae*-type carbapenemases (KPCs) that are found more commonly in *Klebsiella* spp. (see Chapter 138, *Klebsiella* and *Raoultella* Species). These plasmid-mediated enzymes are problematic in that they are readily transferred from one strain to another in a healthcare environment.[25,26]

Citrobacter spp. are more susceptible to fourth-generation cephalosporins such as cefepime (compared with third-generation cephalosporins such as ceftriaxone or ceftazidime) due to relative stability to inactivation by AmpC enzymes; carbapenems are almost always active. Susceptibility for *C. koseri* to trimethoprim-sulfamethoxazole and the aminoglycosides is variable but is much more likely than for *C. freundii*. Among 117 *Citrobacter* spp. from U.S. hospitals in 2007, the rates of susceptibility to the agents listed were: meropenem and imipenem 100%, cefepime 98%, ceftriaxone 95%, ceftazidime 86%, piperacillin/tazobactam 94%, gentamicin 96%, tobramycin 95%, and ciprofloxacin and levofloxacin 97%.[27]

Optimal therapy of *C. koseri* meningitis has not been established, but a combination of a third-generation cephalosporin and an aminoglycoside to which the organism is susceptible is reasonable.[10] Imipenem-cilastatin or high-dose cefotaxime or ceftriaxone alone has also been reported to be successful.[28,29] Meropenem would seem to be the more logical carbapenem of choice due to less potential for neurotoxicity. For patients with accessible brain abscess, neurosurgical drainage is recommended, and for children who have progressive hydrocephalus and fibrous compartmentalization of the ventricular space, instillation of intraventricular urokinase has been performed.[30] With recognition of the possible role of intracellular *C. koseri* in the pathogenesis of cerebral abscesses, treatment with a third-generation cephalosporin in combination with ciprofloxacin has been suggested.[31] Cultures of CSF should be performed on a regular basis until sterility is documented, while understanding that abscesses can remain culture positive for weeks. Results of sequential cultures of material aspirated from the abscesses aids in determining length of therapy. An aminoglycoside has been administered directly into the abscess in some cases.[29] Meningitis without abscess formation is treated for a minimum of 21 days, or 2 weeks after the first sterile CSF culture, whichever is longer. When abscesses are present, a 4- to 6-week course is the minimum duration generally recommended.[8,9]

Prevention of infections due to *Citrobacter* spp. is related predominantly to preventing healthcare-associated infections. Strict cohorting of infected or colonized neonates may not effectively control nursery outbreaks; meticulous handwashing is mandatory.

142 Less Commonly Encountered Enterobacteriaceae

Katalin I. Koranyi and Mario J. Marcon

MICROBIOLOGY, EPIDEMIOLOGY, CLINICAL MANIFESTATIONS, AND TREATMENT

More than 99% of Enterobacteriaceae recovered in clinical laboratories belong to a few dozen species; three species, *Escherichia coli*, *Proteus mirabilis*, and *Klebsiella pneumoniae*, make up more than 90% of isolates and several other well-recognized species account for most of the remaining clinical isolates.[1] Of the remaining Enterobacteriaceae, some genera have clinically important member species that have been well described, whereas others are newly described genera with species that have rarely been reported to cause human infections.[1-6] Many of these newly described species were formerly classified as "atypical" members of recognized species or by various group designations, such as "enteric group" organisms, with a numerical designation. DNA relatedness and 16S ribosomal RNA gene sequencing studies have allowed the placement of these organisms into new genera. No single commercial identification system includes all these species in its database, and it may be appropriate for laboratories to report such organisms with questionable identities as "*Escherichia coli*-like" or "*Enterobacter*-like" and to refer the isolate to a reference laboratory for definitive identification when clinically warranted. Antibiotic susceptibility testing of these organisms should produce reliable in vitro results given that they are members of the family Enterobacteriaceae for which standardized test methods are available. The taxonomic classification of these newly described organisms will evolve as additional genetic relationships among the Enterobacteriaceae are discovered. Similarly, our understanding of their true clinical significance will evolve as better laboratory identification methods become available.

Cedecea Species

The genus *Cedecea* includes three named species, *C. davisae*, *C. lapagei*, *C. neteri*, and several unnamed species. Strains of *Cedecea* spp. have biochemical reactions similar to those of the genus *Serratia* including lipase positivity and resistance to polymixin B, but lack deoxyribonuclease and gelatinase activity. *Cedecea* spp. are rare human pathogens and the clinical significance of these organisms is unclear. Most isolates have been reported from the respiratory tract or in association with soft-tissue infections. There are at least three cases of bloodstream infection (BSI) due to *C. davisae* or *C. neteri* reported in the literature and a case of BSI and wound infection due to *C. lapagei* in a patient with a cement-related chemical burn.[6-10] Antibiotic susceptibility data for *Cedecea* spp. are limited, but some isolates have been reported to be resistant to extended-spectrum cephalosporins and the aminoglycosides.[6-10]

Edwardsiella Species

Organisms of the genus *Edwardsiella* are found in freshwater environments and cold-blooded animals, including fish, reptiles, and amphibians, but occasionally also in birds and mammals. *E. tarda*, *E. hoshinae*, and *E. ictaluri* are the three recognized species of this genus, but only *E. tarda* has been associated with human disease.[1-6] *Edwardsiella* generally are positive for both lysine and ornithine decarboxylase activity, but yield a negative Voges–Proskauer test result and do not use citrate as a sole carbon source. Most clinical isolates of *E. tarda* produce indole and hydrogen sulfide, but do not ferment lactose so appear as colorless colonies

on MacConkey agar. This characteristic, along with the production of hydrogen sulfide on salmonella-shigella agar, necessitates further testing of such isolates to exclude *Salmonella* spp.[1-6] *E. tarda* is not considered to be part of the normal human intestinal flora, being recovered in <1% of stool samples in studies of carriage. Thus human infections generally result from exposure to the organism from its natural environments.

A variety of human infections due to *E. tarda* are described, but none has been associated with outbreaks or epidemics of disease.[11-19] Infections due to *E. tarda* can be divided into intestinal and extraintestinal. The pathogenesis of gastroenteritis due to *E. tarda* is not well established. The organism is negative for Shiga-like enterotoxin and in the Sereny test of entero-invasiveness, but it does produce cell-associated hemolysins and siderophores and can penetrate HeLa and HEp-2 cells in culture.[17] Intestinal infections usually manifest as self-limiting gastroenteritis associated with consumption of raw seafood or snake flesh or other exposure from aquatic environments. Evidence supporting the association of *E. tarda* with gastroenteritis is largely circumstantial. *E. tarda* is isolated from stool cultures significantly more frequently in individuals with diarrhea than in asymptomatic individuals.[1,2] The gastroenteritis typically is an acute secretory diarrheal illness, although serious cases of dysentery can also occur. Intestinal infections in immunocompromised patients including transplant patients can be severe.[19] Reported extraintestinal infections include: wound infections such as cellulitis and gas gangrene associated with trauma; septicemia and meningitis; and focal infections, including cholecystitis, prosthetic valve endocarditis, hepatic abscesses, tubo-ovarian abscess, pyogenic arthritis, and osteomyelitis.[1,11-15]

Wound infections are perhaps the most important infections caused by *E. tarda*. They usually occur after local trauma, such as abrasion, laceration, or penetrating injury. Many infections have been associated with aquatic injuries and represent combined infection due to *E. tarda* and *Aeromonas hydrophila*.[1] Pyogenic arthritis caused by *E. tarda* after catfish puncture wound has been reported.[15] *E. tarda* BSI is most commonly associated with an underlying condition. In adults, liver disease is a common predisposing factor. In children, sickle-cell anemia has been linked to serious infections due to *E. tarda*, as it has been with *Salmonella* spp.[11] Osteomyelitis and meningitis have occurred in individuals with hemoglobinopathies. The gastrointestinal tract is presumably the site of *E. tarda* colonization in these patients, with invasion leading to BSI and subsequent focal infection. Neonatal septicemia and meningitis due to *E. tarda* has been reported in association with acquisition from mother.[13]

Typically, *E. tarda* is susceptible to ampicillin, cefazolin, third-generation cephalosporins, extended-spectrum penicillin/inhibitor combination antibiotics, aminoglycosides, fluoroquinolones, and trimethoprim-sulfamethoxazole. In serious invasive infections, combination therapy with an extended-spectrum cephalosporin and an aminoglycoside has been successful. Antibiotic therapy of individuals with gastroenteritis due to *E. tarda* probably is not indicated.

Ewingella Species

Ewingella americana is the only species in the genus *Ewingella*. Biochemically, this organism is similar to *Pantoea agglomerans* but does not utilize arabinose. *E. americana* has been recovered rarely from miscellaneous specimens such as wounds, urine, stool, and sputum, but the clinical significance of these isolates is unclear. In adults, *E. americana* has caused postoperative infection, and peritonitis during peritoneal dialysis.[6,20–22] A contaminated ice bath in which surgical equipment was cooled appeared to be the source of the postoperative infections. *E. americana* caused a number of cases of pseudo-BSI due to contamination of blood culture bottles by the use of nonsterile citrated blood collection tubes in a children's hospital. Exacerbation of chronic obstructive pulmonary disease and keratoconjunctivitis also have been reported.[22–24] An elderly woman died from overwhelming sepsis caused by *E. americana*.[25] Most clinical isolates are susceptible to a wide variety of antibiotics, but multidrug resistance has been reported to include the aminoglycosides, carbapenems, and fluroquinolones.[22]

Hafnia Species

Hafnia alvei is the only named species of the genus *Hafnia*, although organisms presently classified as *H. alvei* can be separated into three distinct genospecies.[26] Unlike *E. tarda*, *H. alvei* is commonly found in feces of humans and animals, as well as in sewage and soil. In fact, several reports suggest that *H. alvei* is one of the most frequently recovered members of the family Enterobacteriaceae in the gastrointestinal tract of humans. Organisms can be recovered on routine laboratory enteric media such as Mac-Conkey agar, appearing as colorless colonies similar in appearance to *Salmonella* or *Shigella* spp. In addition, *H. alvei* appears similar to *Escherichia coli* O157 on sorbitol–MacConkey agar because both of these organisms commonly are D-sorbitol negative. *H. alvei* is lysine- and ornithine decarboxylase-positive and also positive in the Voges–Proskauer test.

H. alvei is an uncommon cause of infection, having been implicated as a cause of diarrhea, BSI, meningitis, urinary tract infection (UTI), wound infection, intra-abdominal abscess, and empyema in immunocompetent and immunocompromised individuals.[27–34] Most infections in adults are healthcare-associated. A few cases of extraintestinal infections are described in pediatrics including an 8-day-old infant with septicemia.[32] Four cases of BSI were reported in a pediatric surgical cardiac unit.[34] The antibiotic susceptibility pattern of *H. alvei* appears to be similar to that of *Enterobacter* spp., with resistance to both ampicillin and cefazolin. A number of isolates also produce broad-spectrum β-lactamases; in one report, strains resistant to ceftazidime, cefotaxime, and ceftriaxone due to an ampC-type β-lactamase were isolated from 13 patients in the same intensive care unit.[29]

Kluyvera Species

The genus *Kluyvera* includes four species, *K. cryocrescens*, *K. ascorbata*, *K. georgiana*, and *K. cochleae*. *Kluyvera* spp. are phenotypically similar to *Escherichia coli* but are citrate-positive. Found in water, soil, and sewage and in healthcare environments, most human infections are due to *K. ascorbata*. Soft-tissue infection, catheter-associated BSI, UTI, mediastinitis, sepsis, and peritonitis have been reported.[6,35–38] *Kluyvera* spp. also have been implicated in opportunistic infections of immunocompromised patients and have been recovered from stool cultures in adults with diarrhea associated with neutropenia and cancer. Most isolates are susceptible to aminoglycosides, extended-spectrum cephalosporins, and trimethoprim-sulfamethoxazole, but one case of multidrug-resistant *K. ascorbata* causing septicemia has been reported.[38]

Leclercia Species

The genus *Leclercia* is composed of a single species, *L. adecarboxylata*. This organism was previously known as *Escherichia adecarboxylata* on the basis of its similarity to *E. coli* but with negative decarboxylase reactions. *Leclercia* have been isolated from environmental sources including food and water, but also rarely from clinical specimens including sputum, blood, peritoneal fluid,

synovial fluid, wounds, and stool.[6,39–44] In some cases, the clinical significance of isolation from human sources could not be established and most often *Leclercia* have been isolated as part of mixed bacterial growth. Most clinical isolates of *L. adecarboxylata* are susceptible to antibiotics active against *E. coli*, but an extended-spectrum β-lactamase producing BSI isolate has been reported.[44]

Leminorella Species

The genus *Leminorella* contains at least two named species, *L. grimontii* and *L. richardii*, and possibly a third unnamed species. Most human isolates have been recovered from feces and urine. The role of these organisms as primary human pathogens is unclear, but a number of healthcare-associated infections have been reported including urinary tract, soft-tissue, and surgical site infections, as well as BSI and peritonitis.[6,45,46] *Leminorella* spp. isolates have shown variable susceptibility to a variety of antimicrobial agents including the extended-spectrum cephalosporins and penicillin/β-lactamase inhibitor combinations; imipenem and amikacin showed the most activity.[45]

Moellerella Species

The genus *Moellerella* contains one species, *M. wisconsensis*. Isolates have been recovered primarily from stool, mainly from individuals in the state of Wisconsin, but have not been shown to cause diarrhea. The organism was also isolated from the gallbladder and bronchial aspirate in one adult patient.[6] The first case of *M. wisconsensis* BSI was described recently in an adult.[47] The few clinical isolates tested generally have been susceptible to most antibiotics effective against *E. coli*.

Photorhabdus Species

The genus *Photorhabdus* consists of at least three species, but only *P. asymbiotica* has been isolated from humans. Organisms in this genus are noteworthy in that they are luminescent and live symbiotically in the intestinal lumen of various nematodes and are infective for insects. *Photorhabdus* spp. are nonfastidious and can be recovered in the laboratory on blood and MacConkey agars. Colonies can have yellow pigment and are bioluminescent when viewed in a darkened room. *P. asymbiotica* has been recovered from cutaneous lesions, wounds, sputum, and blood; some infections have relapsed and required prolonged antimicrobial therapy.[6,48,49] The antimicrobial susceptibility pattern is reported for only a few isolates. Most were susceptible to the aminoglycosides, fluoroquinolones, extended-spectrum cephalosporins, and trimethoprim-sulfamethoxazole, but resistant to ampicillin and cefazolin.[6]

Rahnella Species

The genus *Rahnella* consists of one primary species, *R. aquatilis*, and at least two additional genospecies. Most isolations of *R. aquatilis* are from water, but the organism also has been recovered from burn wounds and from immunocompromised patients with urinary tract infection, BSIs including catheter-related infections, and from bronchial washings in an adult with acquired immunodeficiency syndrome.[6,50,51] One case of BSI due to *R. aquatilis* occurred in an immunocompetent adult who received a contaminated intravenous infusion.[51] *R. aquatilis* is reported to be susceptible to aminoglycosides, extended-spectrum cephalosporins, and fluoroquinolones.

Tatumella Species

The genus *Tatumella* contains one species, *T. ptyseos*. Most human isolates are from the respiratory tract, but a few have been from BSIs. A unique property differentiating this organism from other Enterobacteriaceae is its exquisite susceptibility to penicillin in vitro. Association of this organism with human disease is unknown.[6]

Trabulsiella Species

The genus *Trabulsiella* contains one species, *T. guamensis*. This organism resembles *Salmonella* spp. biochemically, because it is positive for hydrogen sulfide production and lysine and ornithine decarboxylase activity (arginine is variable); it has been recovered from soil and human stool, but its clinical significance is unknown.[6]

Yokenella Species

The genus *Yokenella* contains one species, *Y. regensburgei*, formerly called *Koserella trabulsii*. This organism is biochemically similar to *Hafnia alvei* but is citrate positive; it has been isolated from respiratory tract, wounds, feces, and urine specimens. *Y. regensburgei* also has been isolated from an adult with pyogenic arthritis and an immunocompromised adult with transient BSIs.[6,52]

143 *Plesiomonas shigelloides*

Shai Ashkenazi

Plesiomonas shigelloides, common inhabitants of surface water and fish, are a cause of acute gastroenteritis and an uncommon cause of extraintestinal infections in children.[1-5]

DESCRIPTION OF THE PATHOGEN

P. shigelloides is a single species in the genus *Plesiomonas*. Based on phenotypic characteristics, *P. shigelloides* was classified in the Vibrionaceae family.[1] However, analysis of the sequence of 5S rRNA, 16S rRNA, and 16s rDNA indicates that phylogenetic ancestry of *P. shigelloides* is aligned more closely with the tribe Proteaceae in the Enterobacteriaceae family.[6]

P. shigelloides are facultative anaerobic, gram-negative rods, which are motile via a polar flagellum. Some isolates of *P. shigelloides* share the capsular O-antigen with that of *Shigella sonnei*. *P. shigelloides* are oxidase-, indole- and catalase-positive. They also are ornithine-, lysine- and arginine decarboxylase-positive. *P. shigelloides* grow well on traditional enteric media, including MacConkey, Hektoen enteric deoxycholate citrate (Leifson), and salmonella-shigella (SS) agars,[1] with growth enhanced when inoculated on selective media, such as trypticase soy broth with ampicillin. Organisms do not grow on thiosulfate citrate bile salts sucrose agar. *P. shigelloides* growth produces grey nonhemolytic colonies after 18 to 24 hours of incubation at 37°C;[1] optimal growth occurs at temperatures of 40°C to 44°C.

PATHOGENESIS

Although there is a strong epidemiologic association with gastroenteritis, particularly in the first 2 years of life,[7,8] when fed to adult human volunteers, *P. shigelloides* does not cause diarrhea. In vitro and in vivo studies of pathogenicity suggest low pathogenic potential.[9] Clinical manifestations of gastroenteritis suggest enteroinvasion as a possible mechanism of disease. However, *P. shigelloides* yields negative or variable results by most standard assays of invasiveness.[1,8-10] DNA probes for virulence genes of *Shigella* spp. and enteroinvasive *Escherichia coli* also are negative.[8,10] *Plesiomonas* does not produce an enterotoxin; cytotoxin production has been demonstrated in some strains.[8,10,11] A high-molecular-weight plasmid (>120 megadaltons) has been identified in most strains of *P. shigelloides*, but the role of this plasmid in the pathogenesis of diarrhea has not been elucidated.[9] Investigations have demonstrated pronounced cell adhesion of clinical isolates of *P. shigelloides*, a characteristic not observed in environmental isolates.[12] It is unclear whether some strains are virulent whereas others are nonpathogenic, or whether there is age- and immunity-related susceptibility. In a case-control study of childhood diarrhea in Dhaka, Bangladesh, *P. shigelloides* was isolated with similar frequency from stool specimens in cases and controls.[13]

EPIDEMIOLOGY

Humans are infected with *P. shigelloides* after ingestion of contaminated food or water, or by contact with colonized animals. *P. shigelloides* can cause foodborne outbreaks[14] and the organism has been recovered from fresh water and estuaries in temperate and tropical regions and occasionally from seawater during summer months. *Plesiomonas* colonizes the gut of cold- and warm-blooded animals and has been isolated from cats, dogs, pigs, cows, snakes, newts, fish, shellfish, monkeys, and vultures. Occupations associated with an increased risk of *P. shigelloides* infection include veterinarians, aquaculturists, fish handlers, and zoo keepers.[1] *P. shigelloides* can be isolated from stools of patients with gastroenteritis who reside in tropical and subtropical regions of Africa, Asia, and Australia.[1] Asymptomatic carriage of *P. shigelloides* in humans living in developed countries is uncommon, but in Asia asymptomatic colonization is common. The organism has been isolated from coastal waters of the Gulf of Mexico and has been implicated as a cause of diarrhea in travelers to Mexico and the Caribbean.[2] Although *Plesiomonas* has been identified in about 1% of tropical fish tanks, aquarium-associated illness is rare. In the United States and Europe, most cases of gastroenteritis are associated with travel to tropical areas or with consumption of raw oysters or shellfish.[1,2]

CLINICAL MANIFESTATIONS

About 70% of cases of *P. shigelloides*-gastroenteritis are associated with either an underlying illness or an identifiable risk factor, such as travel or consumption of raw seafood.[1,3] The clinical presentation is variable; symptoms include abdominal cramps, dehydration, fever, headache, vomiting, and diarrhea, which usually last for a few days.[1,2] A study from Bangladesh suggests that diarrhea primarily occurs in the first 2 years of life. Most illness is manifest by acute watery diarrhea (84%), although dysenteric disease (16%) and persistent diarrhea lasting more than 2 weeks (13%) also occur. A Canadian study documented persistent symptoms (>2 weeks in 76%, >4 weeks in 32%), mostly in people who recently had traveled, been exposed to seafood, or had contact with contaminated water in the previous week. This high frequency of persistent symptoms may reflect selection biases.

Extraintestinal manifestations are rare and include bacteremia, meningitis, osteomyelitis, septic arthritis, cellulitis, endophthalmitis, proctitis, peritonitis, pseudoappendicitis, pancreatitis, and cholecystitis.[1,4,5,15-19] Underlying illnesses associated with extraintestinal infections include immunodeficiency, sickle-cell disease, and cirrhosis.[1] There are reported cases of early-onset neonatal septicemia and meningitis.[4,15,17] Mortality is high when extraintestinal infection occurs; in neonates, the mortality rate can be >80%.

DIAGNOSIS

Isolation of the organism after growth in appropriate medium is essential for diagnosis of *P. shigelloides*. Clinical laboratories sometimes underrecognize the organism because up to 30% of the clinically significant isolates ferment lactose. Thus, if an oxidase test is not performed, these lactose-fermenting isolates can be misidentified as normal enteric flora.[2] Therefore, when *P. shigelloides* is considered either on the basis of a history of foreign travel or of ingestion of raw seafood or untreated water, oxidase test should be performed. Selective media also can be used. *P. shigelloides* is isolated readily from normally sterile body fluids when extraintestinal infection is present.

TREATMENT

Acute Gastroenteritis

Because *P. shigelloides*-associated gastroenteritis usually is self-limited, use of antimicrobial therapy for diarrhea due to this pathogen is controversial. In some studies, antimicrobial therapy appears to shorten the duration of illness. However, a case-controlled study in Thai children found no difference in duration of diarrhea in the treated versus untreated groups.[20] Antimicrobial therapy is recommended for gastroenteritis in children with underlying conditions. *P. shigelloides* is susceptible to trimethoprim-sulfamethoxazole and fluoroquinolones. Many isolates produce β-lactamase and are therefore resistant to ampicillin and other penicillins, but usually are susceptible to most cephalosporins, carbapenems, and tetracycline and variably susceptible to aminoglycosides.[3,21,22]

Extraintestinal Infections

Antimicrobial therapy is essential for children with extraintestinal infections. For these infections, antimicrobial therapy should be given intravenously and guided by susceptibility of the individual isolate, since there is considerable variability in antimicrobial susceptibility from strain to strain. Empiric therapy with an extended-spectrum cephalosporin is reasonable, because isolates typically are susceptible in vitro and because of good penetration into the cerebrospinal fluid.[3,21,22]

144 *Proteus, Providencia,* and *Morganella* Species

William J. Barson and Mario J. Marcon

MICROBIOLOGY AND EPIDEMIOLOGY

Organisms belonging to the genera *Proteus, Providencia,* and *Morganella* are phylogenetically related members of the family Enterobacteriaceae and often referred to as the Proteeae. All members of these genera have phenylalanine deaminase activity, and most also have urease activity and motility. Organisms can be isolated readily in the laboratory on enriched media, such as blood and chocolate agars, and on gram-negative selective media, such as MacConkey agar, on which they appear as "colorless colonies" because they do not utilize lactose.[1-5]

There are at least five named *Proteus* spp. and several unnamed genospecies. The named species include *P. mirabilis, P. vulgaris, P. penneri, P. hauseri,* and *P. myxofaciens.* The two species of primary human clinical significance are *P. mirabilis* and *P. vulgaris.* Both species generally produce hydrogen sulfide and swarm on non-inhibitory agar medium. *P. mirabilis* is positive for ornithine and negative for indole, whereas *P. vulgaris* is negative for ornithine but positive for indole. *P. penneri* is a species that accommodates indole-negative, genetically distinct variants of *P. vulgaris.*

There are also five named *Providencia* spp. including four that are positive for indole production; these four are *P. stuartii, P. rettgeri, P. alcalifaciens,* and *P. rustigianii. P. stuarti* and to a lesser extent *P. rettgeri* are the two species of primary human significance. *Providencia* spp. can be differentiated from *Proteus* spp. and *M. morganii* based on their ability to use citrate as the sole carbon source and to ferment D-mannitol. Currently, there is only one named *Morganella* species, *M. morganii,* with subspecies *morganii* and *sibonii. Morganella morganii* generally is positive for indole, urea, and ornithine.[1-5]

Proteus, Providencia, and *M. morganii* are found in the natural environment in soil and water and in environmental sources in healthcare facilities. They are normal flora in the gastrointestinal tract of humans and other mammals and birds.[1,5] These organisms can colonize the skin and respiratory mucosa of hospitalized patients and healthcare personnel (HCP) and can be transmitted to other patients. Members of all three genera also commonly colonize reptiles and fish.

Investigations of pathogenic mechanisms of these organisms have focused on *P. mirabilis* as an agent of urinary tract infection (UTI). Virulence factors that appear to contribute to pathogenicity include motility and production of fimbrial proteins and other factors that facilitate attachment to uroepithelial cells.[5] Once attached, proteases, hemolysins, and potent urease enzymes that hydrolyze urea and alkalinize the urine contribute to tissue invasion and pathology. Other studies have demonstrated the ability of *Providencia* spp. to attach and invade human cells in tissue culture and implicated these organisms as agents of gastroenteritis including travelers' diarrhea.[5]

P. mirabilis causes the majority of cases of infection due to members of these three genera and is considered primarily, but not exclusively, a community-associated pathogen. Other members of these genera often are isolated in healthcare-associated infections (HAIs), such as UTI, burn wounds, and bloodstream infection (BSI). *P. mirabilis* was the cause in 4% of HAIs at major centres in the National Nosocomial Infections Surveillance System during the period from 1986 to 1989. *Proteus* spp. accounted for 3% of HA-UTI in children, frequently associated with indwelling bladder catheters.[6] Wound infections due to *Proteus* spp. have occurred after surgical procedures (e.g., spinal fusions, myocutaneous flap surgery in patients with spinal injury), animal bites, burns, and with decubitus ulcers.[5,7-10]

CLINICAL MANIFESTATIONS

P. mirabilis is the third most frequent agent of UTI in childhood after *Escherichia coli* and *Klebsiella* spp.[11,12] In one series of primary

UTI in males, *P. mirabilis* replaced *E. coli* as the most prevalent pathogen.[13] *Proteus* spp. also are found frequently as a cause of recurrent UTI. The urease enzyme produced by *P. mirabilis* and other related bacteria hydrolyzes urea in the urine, forming ammonium hydroxide. This reaction increases urinary pH, resulting in toxicity to renal cells and promoting precipitation of inorganic and organic compounds leading to the formation of struvite stones.[14] These stones can act as foreign bodies, rendering infections difficult to eradicate and promoting reinfection. Recovery of *Proteus* spp. from urine should alert the physician to the possibility of urolithiasis. Toxic encephalopathy due to a high concentration of ammonia has been reported as a complication of *P. mirabilis* and *P. rettgeri* UTI in children with prune-belly syndrome.[15,16] *P. mirabilis* also is associated with infections in males with urinary tract anomalies.[17] Xanthogranulomatous pyelonephritis, most commonly due to *E. coli* and *P. mirabilis*, is a rare type of chronic pyelonephritis that can be mistaken for Wilms tumor.[18] This diagnosis should be considered in a child presenting with a renal mass, hematuria, anemia, and leukocytosis, and can be associated with urinary tract obstruction and nephrolithiasis.

Proteus, *Providencia*, and *Morganella* spp. have been recovered from children with a variety of infections other than UTI, including chronic suppurative otitis media.[19] *P. mirabilis* is the third most common organism recovered from cultures of ear drainage in children with tympanostomy tubes; *Pseudomonas aeruginosa* and *Staphylococcus aureus* are recovered more commonly.[20] Intracranial and extracranial complications due to *P. mirabilis* have been reported in association with mastoiditis and chronic otitis media.[21,22] *Proteus* spp. have been reported as a cause of folliculitis, pneumonia, BSI, and meningitis; hepatic, pulmonary, and splenic abscesses; osteomyelitis in patients with sickle-cell anemia; sinusitis in neurologically impaired children; necrotizing fasciitis associated with omphalitis; and brain abscess as a complication of neonatal meningitis and following neurosurgical procedures.[5] Many of these infections occur in neonates and immunocompromised hosts.

In a 21-year review from Dallas, *P. mirabilis* was the cause of gram-negative meningitis in 3 of 49 (6%) term infants and in 1 of 18 (6%) infants who were 1 to 3 months old.[23] *Proteus* spp. also have been associated with "pump pocket" infections in patients receiving intrathecal baclofen for spasticity.[24] Neonatal infections, including early- and late-onset septicemia and brain abscess, also have been reported due to *M. morganii*.[5,25,26] *M. morganii* also has been recovered from the following infections: middle-ear infections in pediatric cardiac transplant patients, deep-neck space infections, tubo-ovarian abscesses associated with relapsing Henoch–Schönlein purpura, pericarditis associated with X-linked agammaglobulinemia, and necrotizing fasciitis following a chicken scratch.[27–31] *Proteus* spp. and *M. morganii* can secrete the enzyme L-histidine decarboxylase which can convert the free amino acid histidine, found in muscle tissue of certain fish (tuna and mackerel), into histamine. This occurs in improperly stored fish and can lead to scombroid poisoning with an anaphylactic-like syndrome following human consumption.[5] One study in Brazil reported on the microbiology of abscesses secondary to *Bothrops* spp. snake bites and found *M. morganii* in 23 of 40 (58%) and *P. rettgeri* in 7 of 40 (18%) abscesses; 16 of 40 (40%) cases were polymicrobial.[32] *Providencia* spp. are recovered occasionally from patients with chronic otitis media, infected burn wounds, and also can be responsible for diarrhea (especially *P. alcalifaciens*).[33–35] *P. alcalifaciens* was implicated in a large outbreak of foodborne diarrhea in Japan in multiple schools and affecting teachers and students.[33] When recovered from the urinary tract, *Providencia* spp. typically are found in the setting of an underlying structural, physiologic, or neurologic abnormality (e.g., neurogenic bladder).[5]

TREATMENT

Treatment of infections due to these organisms can be difficult because of frequent antimicrobial resistance. The majority of isolates of *P. mirabilis* remain susceptible to ampicillin and first-generation cephalosporins, but plasmid-mediated resistance to penicillins and cephalosporins due to β-lactamases is becoming more common.[36] *P. mirabilis* is resistant intrinsically to nitrofurantoin, a characteristic useful for identification. The indole-positive members of the Proteeae, including *Proteus vulgaris*, *Providencia* spp., and *M. morganii*, typically are resistant to ampicillin and cefazolin, as is the indole-negative species *Proteus penneri*. Historically, third- and fourth-generation cephalosporins, aztreonam, piperacillin-tazobactam, carbapenems, fluoroquinolones (FQs), and trimethoprim-sulfamethoxazole (FMP-SMX) usually were active.[5,37–39]

There are increasing recent reports of resistance to TMP-SMX and FQs among *P. mirabilis* and *M. morganii* with resistance rates for *P. mirabilis* of 16% to TMP-SMX and 15% to FQs, and for *M. morganii* of 25% to TMP-SMX and 22% to FQs; higher resistance rates were associated with overuse of these agents.[5,39]

There also are reports of extended-spectrum β-lactamase (ESBL)-producing strains of *P. mirabilis* and other species of the Proteeae causing infections in children.[40–42] Isolates harboring these enzymes can be resistant to a wide range of β-lactam antibiotics and may not be detected readily by laboratory testing unless appropriate in vitro procedures are utilized.[43] Healthcare-associated outbreaks have occurred due to strains of *P. mirabilis* that have acquired plasmid AmpC-type β-lactamases similar to the chromosomal AmpC enzymes found in *Enterobacter cloacae* and other Enterobacteriaceae.[44] Most isolates of *M. morganii* carry genes coding for AmpC-type β-lactamase enzymes. Stable derepression of such genes leads to high-level enzyme production and can be associated with emergence of resistant subpopulations during monotherapy with β-lactam antibiotics.[5,45] A neonate with early-onset *M. morganii* sepsis developed persistent ventriculitis due to emergence of a cefotaxime-resistant variant as a result of derepression of its AmpC β-lactamase.[45] Combination therapy with meropenem, ciprofloxacin, and gentamicin resulted in a microbiologic cure. Use of third-generation cephalosporins as monotherapy should be reconsidered when treating serious infections due to organisms known to harbor AmpC β-lactamases. (See Chapter 138, *Klebsiella* and *Raoultella* Species, for a more complete discussion of ESBL enzymes including laboratory detection and Chapter 140, *Enterobacter*, *Cronobacter*, and *Pantoea* Species, for a more complete discussion of Amp-C β-lactamases).

The activity of the aminoglycosides against the Proteeae is variable, with amikacin tending to have the most reliable activity. When infection with one of these organisms is suspected, initial empiric treatment regimen for serious infection should include both meropenem and amikacin. For infection of the central nervous system, a minimum of 2 weeks of antibiotic therapy after documented bacteriologic cure is recommended. Drainage of brain abscesses may be required, but resolution of smaller abscesses following antibiotic therapy alone has been reported. Specific therapy should be guided by the results of definitive identification and susceptibility testing. (See Chapter 46, Focal Suppurative Infections of the Nervous System, for a more complete discussion of management of such infections.)

Gram-negative bacillary otitis externa can be treated effectively with topical ofloxacin otic solution.[46,47] A 7- to 10-day course of antibiotics usually is adequate for treatment of uncomplicated UTI; removal of a urinary catheter, if present, hastens eradication. Otherwise, failure to eradicate the bacteria should alert the physician to the possibility of urolithiasis or a structural anomaly. Removal of stone(s) or surgical correction of obstruction often is required for cure.

145 *Serratia* Species

Dwight A. Powell and Mario J. Marcon

MICROBIOLOGY AND EPIDEMIOLOGY

The genus *Serratia*, family Enterobacteriaceae, contains at least 10 separately named species. *Serratia marcescens* is the primary pathogen in this genus, but occasional or rare cases of human infections have been described for *S. liquefaciens*, *S. rubidaea*, *S. plymuthica*, *S. odorifera*, *S. ficaria*, and *S. fonticola*. *S. marcescens*, *S. liquefaciens*, and *S. odorifera* are diverse groups with several subspecies or biogroups based on DNA hybridization analyses.[1-4]

Like other enteric bacteria, *Serratia* spp. are readily recovered in the laboratory on enriched, nonselective agars including blood and chocolate agars, as well as selective enteric agars such as Mac-Conkey or salmonella-shigella agar. Most human isolates of *Serratia* spp. do not ferment lactose (and thus appear as colorless colonies on the enteric agars), reduce nitrate to nitrite, are catalase positive, cytochrome oxidase-negative, and ferment glucose and a number of other sugars. Most isolates react positively in the Voges–Proskauer test and utilize citrate as a sole carbon source, but do not produce hydrogen sulfide or indole. Hydrolytic enzymes, including gelatinase, lipase, and DNAse, are produced commonly, a property somewhat unique among the Enterobacteriaceae. These and other extracellular enzymes, including esterase, caseinase, and lecithinase, may be potential virulence factors that promote tissue invasion. Strains of *S. rubidaea* and *S. plymuthica* commonly produce the red pigment prodigiosin; *S. marcescens* also can produce prodigiosin. The most important biochemical tests for differentiating among *Serratia* spp. are pressure of lysine and ornithine decarboxylase and acid production from a number of sugars.[1-4]

Serratia spp., especially *S. marcescens*, are almost exclusively nosocomial pathogens and associated with rapidly spreading outbreaks in intensive care settings. In a national surveillance of pediatric intensive care units (PICUs) for nosocomial infections, *Serratia* spp. accounted for 2% of bloodstream infections (BSIs), 3.6% of pneumonias, 3.6% of lower respiratory infections other than pneumonia, 1.2% of urinary tract infections, and 2.8% of surgical site infections.[5] In two U.S. neonatal intensive care units (NICUs), *S. marcescens* accounted for 11% and 16% of gram-negative BSIs.[6,7] In a review of 239 *S. marcescens* infections reported from 27 NICUs and PICUs, the most common sites of infection were BSIs (47%), conjunctivitis (26%), pneumonia (13%), urinary tract infection (8%), meningitis with or without brain abscess (7%), and surgical site infections (3%). Other less common infections were otitis externa, gastroenteritis, omphalitis, septic arthritis, and intraperitoneal infections.[8]

Although *Serratia* spp. have been isolated from a large number of environmental sources, point source outbreaks are rare. *Serratia* spp. are more commonly spread from person to person on the hands of healthcare personnel.[8,9] The most common sites for colonization are the respiratory and gastrointestinal tracts of infants and the respiratory tract of adults. Prolonged colonization can occur, particularly in immunocompromised hosts.[10] Control of outbreaks depends on stringent cohorting of cases and aggressive education regarding handwashing by healthcare professionals. Additional risk factors for acquiring infection include exposure to contaminated instruments and fluids, use of intravenous or urinary catheters, long duration of hospitalization, previous antibiotic therapy, and underlying diseases such as prematurity, diabetes mellitus, and altered host defenses.[8] A recent outbreak of *S. marcescens* (BSI) at an outpatient infusion therapy center implicated contamination of syringes prefilled with heparin and saline.[11]

CLINICAL MANIFESTATIONS

The symptoms and signs of neonatal septicemia and meningitis due to *S. marcescens* are not unique and can include apnea and bradycardia, hypo- or hyperthermia, hypo- or hyperglycemia, and shock; mortality rate can be as high as 24 to 44%.[12,13] Neonatal meningitis can be present in about 25% of infants with *S. marcescens* BSI but cerebrospinal fluid can have normal cell count and glucose concentration in up to 50% of patients; protein concentrations usually are elevated.[13,14] Additionally, meningitis can develop during therapy for septicemia and can be associated with ventriculitis, hydrocephalus, or striking destruction of brain parenchyma. These processes can lead to loculated areas of infection or cyst formation, similar to infections due to *Cronobacter* species (formerly *Enterobacter sakazakii*) and *Citrobacter* spp. Serial neuroimaging studies should be performed during therapy.[15] Mortality exceeds 40%, and most survivors are neurologically impaired.[16] BSI due to *Serratia* spp. in pediatric and adult cancer patients usually manifests as fever. Shock and disseminated intravascular coagulopathy appear less commonly than in infection with other gram-negative bacteria including *Pseudomonas* spp. Survival rates may be >75%.[17]

Urinary tract infections are almost always associated with an indwelling urinary bladder catheter. Nosocomial pneumonia due to *Serratia* spp. occurs in children less frequently than in adults and can result in empyema.[18] *Serratia marcescens* has been implicated in endophthalmitis, keratoconjunctivitis, contact lens and non-contact lens-related keratitis, and contact lens-induced acute red eye. These infections are associated with corneal grafts, use of topical medications such as corticosteroids and anti-glaucoma drops, and contamination of water or solutions used to clean or moisturize contact lenses.[19,20] Rare cases of necrotizing fasciitis in adults with diabetes or malignancies have been reported.[21]

Community-acquired *Serratia* infections are not uncommon in children with chronic granulomatous disease (CGD), and are sentinel infections for the disorder. In a national registry of 368 patients with CGD, *Serratia* was the leading bacterial cause of osteomyelitis (29%) and the second most frequent cause of suppurative lymphadenitis (9%).[22] *Serratia* spp. also were isolated frequently from CGD patients with subcutaneous abscesses (15%), BSI (6%), and pneumonia (5%); however, they were uncommonly associated with deep tissue abscesses (<1%). Any child with a community-acquired infection due to a *Serratia* spp., particularly infections of bone or lymph nodes, should be evaluated for CGD.

TREATMENT

Serratia spp., especially *S. marcescens*, harbor an intrinsic, chromosomal AmpC-type β-lactamase (see Chapter 140, *Enterobacter*, *Cronobacter*, and *Pantoea* Species).

The AmpC β-lactamases can be expressed at low level and go undetected in standard laboratory susceptibility tests; however, the genes coding for these enzymes can be induced or stably de-repressed, leading to high-level enzyme production. Treatment failure during monotherapy with a third-generation β-lactam antibiotic can follow. *Serratia* spp. also can carry other β-lactamases including extended-spectrum β-lactamases (ESBLs)[23,24] and to a lesser extent carbapenemases. There are no Clinical and Laboratory Standards Institute (CLSI) recommended screening and confirmation tests for detection of AmpC and ESBL enzymes in *Serratia* spp; however, CLSI recently recommended the adoption of revised susceptibility test breakpoints for the Enterobacteriaceae to more accurately categorize the susceptibility of beta-lactamase-producing isolates to the β-lactam agents.[25] Carbapenemases found in various strains of *S. marcescens* include serine carbapenemases such as plasmid-borne KPC-type enzymes and chromosomal SME-type enzymes, as well as plasmid-borne metallo-carbapenemases including IMP- and VIM-type enzymes.[26,27] There are also recent data suggesting that carbapenem resistance in *S. marcescens* can be mediated by hyperproduction of AmpC β-lactamase along with mutation of outer membrane porin proteins.[28] Fortunately, these enzymes are uncommon in U.S. strains of *S. marcescens,* and susceptibility to carbapenem antibiotics including meropenem and imipenem currently is >99%.

The following were the percentage susceptible of >4000 isolates of *Serratia* spp. from hospitalized patients in the U.S.: imipenem (99%), amikacin (98%), cefepime (95%), ceftazidime (96%), ceftriaxone (90%), piperacillin-tazobactam (87%), and ciprofloxacin (90%).[29]

Treatment of serious infections due to *Serratia* spp. should consist of a carbapenem, an extended-spectrum cephalosporin, or an extended-spectrum penicillin/β-lactamase inhibitor combination antibiotic plus an aminoglycoside pending results of in vitro susceptibility testing. Antibiotic susceptibility test results should direct subsequent therapy. Duration of treatment is dictated by the condition and rate of clinical response. In management of neonatal meningitis due to *Serratia* spp., cerebrospinal fluid cultures should be performed repeatedly until sterility is confirmed.[16] Therapy should be continued for a minimum of 21 days or 10 to 14 days after cerebrospinal fluid sterility has been documented, whichever is longer. Imaging studies also should guide medical and surgical management; 4 to 8 weeks of antibiotic therapy may be required for infants with ventriculitis, abscesses, encephalitis, or infarction.

146 *Salmonella* Species

Megan E. Reller

Nontyphoidal *Salmonella* organisms are found widely in animals and cause a broad spectrum of clinical infections that include asymptomatic carriage, gastroenteritis, bloodstream infection (BSI), and metastatic focal infections. In contrast, *Salmonella* serotypes Typhi and Paratyphi A are human-specific pathogens that cause typhoid or enteric fever, a protracted febrile illness with myriad manifestations.

DESCRIPTION OF THE PATHOGEN

Salmonella species are gram-negative bacilli that belong to the family Enterobacteriaceae and as such ferment glucose, reduce nitrate to nitrite, and are oxidase-negative. Almost all *Salmonella* species are motile, indole-negative, and do not ferment lactose. Clinical microbiology laboratories further characterize *Salmonella* isolates by biochemical criteria; complete serotyping is performed in public health laboratories.

All *Salmonella* organisms are so closely related by DNA-DNA hybridization studies as to be considered a single species, namely, *Salmonella enterica*.[1] Serologic studies of *Salmonella* have enabled delineation of at least 2463 serotypes, which has proved enormously useful as an epidemiologic tool. Reactions of *Salmonella* with antisera to specific O (somatic) antigens determine the serogroups A, B, C_1, C_2, D, and E and further O, H (flagellar), and Vi (capsular) antigenic characterization results in a unique serotype that traditionally has served as a surrogate species designation, e.g., *S. typhi* (*S.* Typhi now recommended). To clarify this complex *Salmonella* nomenclature, the Centers for Disease Control and Prevention (CDC) has published guidelines for the modern, consistent terminology (Table 146-1) that is used herein.[1] Some clinical laboratories perform preliminary serogrouping; examples of serotypes are: A (*S.* Paratyphi A), B (*S.* Typhimurim, *S.* Heidelberg, *S.* Paratyphi B), C_1 (*S.* Choleraesuis, *S.* Infantis), C_2 (*S.* Newport), and D (*S.* Enteritidis, *S.* Typhi).

PATHOLOGY

Enterocolitis with diffuse mucosal inflammation, edema, and microabscesses is the typical intestinal tract disease caused by nontyphoidal serotypes of *Salmonella*. Destruction of epithelial cells and production of ulcers are not common. Intestinal lymphoid tissue and mesenteric lymph nodes hypertrophy and can develop small areas of necrosis; in the case of *S.* Typhi, these areas can ulcerate, causing intestinal perforation.[2,3]

PATHOGENESIS

The pathogenesis of *Salmonella* infections is complex, but is being unraveled now that genome sequencing has provided a complete blueprint of the genetic repertoire for several species of *S. enterica*, including *S.* Typhimurium, *S.* Typhi, and *S.* Paratyphi.[4] Examination of the *S.* Typhi genome has identified up to 10 pathogenicity islands and comparisons with the *S.* Typhimurium genome have disclosed other smaller *S.* Typhi-specific gene clusters or

TABLE 146-1. *Salmonella* Nomenclature

Complete Name	CDC Designation	Common Clinical Usage (Recommended)
Salmonella enterica subsp. *enterica* ser. Typhi	*Salmonella* ser. Typhi	*Salmonella typhi* (Typhi)
Salmonella enterica subsp. *enterica* ser. Paratyphi A	*Salmonella* ser. Paratyphi A	*Salmonella paratyphi* A (Paratyphi A)
Salmonella enterica subsp. *enterica* ser. Typhimurium	*Salmonella* ser. Typhimurium	*Salmonella typhimurium* (Typhimurium)
Salmonella enterica subsp. *enterica* ser. Enteritidis	*Salmonella* ser. Enteritidis	*Salmonella enteritidis* (Enteritidis)
Salmonella enterica subsp. *enterica* ser. Dublin	*Salmonella* ser. Dublin	*Salmonella dublin* (Dublin)

CDC, Centers for Disease Control and Prevention; ser., serotype; subsp., subspecies.

Adapted from Brenner FW, Villar RG, Angulo FJ, et al. Salmonella nomenclature. J Clin Microbiol 2000;38:2465.

individual genes. Further studies of virulence genes should enable an understanding, for example, of why *S.* Typhi infects only human beings and why the rare animal serotype *S.* Dublin is nearly 80-fold more likely to invade the bloodstream than is *S.* Typhimurium.[5]

Most nontyphoidal *Salmonella* do not extend beyond the lamina propria and local lymphatics of the gut, whereas *S.* Choleraesuis and *S.* Dublin rapidly cause bacteremia with little or no intestinal involvement. The quintessential invasive serotype is *S.* Typhi, the pathogenesis of which is best known.[4,6] Upon reaching the small intestine, *S.* Typhi adheres to the specialized epithelial M cells overlying Peyer patches. Penetration of the mucosa includes cytokine secretion (interleukin-8, interleukin-6), uptake by macrophages, and translocation to lymphoid follicles in the gut and the draining lymph nodes. An ensuing silent bacteremia disseminates *S.* Typhi throughout the body, where the bacteria survive and multiply within mononuclear cells of the liver, spleen, and bone marrow. Seven to 14 days later (incubation period), a sustained secondary BSI heralds the onset of symptoms.

Multiple factors predispose to *Salmonella* infection (Table 146-2). The dose of organisms ingested is an important determinant of the incubation period, symptoms, and severity of acute salmonellosis. Gastric acidity is an important barrier to infection. Achlorhydria, antacid use, and rapid gastric emptying (after gastrectomy and gastro-enterostomy) favor survival of ingested organisms.[6] The hypochlorhydria and rapid gastric emptying time of neonates and young infants explain, at least in part, their vulnerability to symptomatic salmonellosis.[7]

Impaired reticuloendothelial or cellular immune response (which occurs in people with chronic granulomatous disease, post transplantation, hemoglobinopathy, schistosomiasis, malaria, the acquired immunodeficiency syndrome (AIDS), cancer, *Bartonella bacilliformis* infection (Oroya fever), and systemic lupus erythematosus) raise the risk for severe, complicated infection.[7,8] Children

with sickle-cell disease are prone to septicemia and osteomyelitis when infected with nontyphoidal *Salmonella*. Decreases in phagocytic and opsonizing capacity of patients with sickle-cell disease, along with infarcts in the gastrointestinal tract, bones, and reticuloendothelial system (RES), contribute to the high infection rate.

EPIDEMIOLOGY

Nontyphoidal *Salmonella*

Since 2005 a range of 45,000 to 51,000 cases of culture-proven nontyphoidal salmonellosis have been reported each year in the United States; however, an estimated ~1.4 million diarrheal illnesses and 600 deaths annually are attributed to *Salmonella*.[8-12] About one-third of cases occur in children <4 years of age, and children in the first few months of life have the highest incidence. Nontyphoidal *Salmonella* infections have worldwide distribution, with a prevalence that varies according to public health standards, water treatment, sewage disposal, animal exposures, and food-handling practices. *Salmonella* infections occur particularly during warm summer months in temperate climates. The frequency of *Salmonella* infection has risen over the last several decades. *Salmonella* serotypes most often encountered in the U.S. since 1996 are Typhimurium and Enteritidis (www.cdc.gov/narms).

The Foodborne Surveillance Network (FoodNet), a collaborative program among state health departments, United States Department of Agriculture, U.S. Food and Drug Administration, and CDC, was established in 1996 and has enhanced outbreak recognition by adding pulsed-field gel electrophoresis analyses to traditional serotyping.[10-12]

The major reservoir of nontyphoidal *Salmonella* is the gastrointestinal tract of infected, often asymptomatic, birds, mammals, and reptiles; chickens, turkeys, ducks, sheep, cows, pigs, and various pets, especially turtles, snakes, lizards, iguanas, and hedgehogs, commonly are infected.[13-17] Some serotypes can be isolated from a variety of warm- and cold-blooded animals; others are relatively restricted (Table 146-3). Isolation of an uncommon serotype can suggest a likely source of infection. Illness can result from exposure to pets and to animals in public settings[18,19] and from environmental contamination even without direct contact with an infected animal, as was demonstrated in an outbreak of *S.* Enteritidis related to a Komodo dragon exhibit in a zoo.[20] Even handling pet food treats containing dried beef has caused infections.[21]

TABLE 146-2. Factors Predisposing to *Salmonella* Infection or Dissemination

Site of Defect	Mechanism and Clinical Setting
Gastric acid barrier	Achlorhydria
	Anatomic: gastrectomy, gastroenterostomy
	Functional: ingestion of buffers, vagotomy
	Rapid emptying (neonates, postgastrectomy)
Intestinal mucosal barrier	Inflammatory bowel disease
	Tissue ischemia/infarction (sickle-cell anemia, trauma)
Gut flora	Prior antimicrobial therapy (results in increased infection and prolonged carriage)
Opsonins	Sickle-cell anemia (defect in alternate complement pathway)
Neutrophils	Chronic granulomatous disease
Cell-mediated immunity	After organ transplantation or with defects associated with acquired immunodeficiency syndrome, infancy, malnutrition, or corticosteroid therapy
	Defects in type 1 helper T-lymphocyte (Th1) functions (interleukin-12/interferon-gamma axis), including mutations in the genes for interleukin-12Rβ1 and interleukin-12
Sequestered organisms	Schistosomiasis
	Reticuloendothelial cells (typhoid fever)
	Solid tumors
	Gallbladder disease
Reticuloendothelial system	Overload with hemoglobin or iron (hemolytic anemia, such as sickle-cell disease, thalassemia, bartonellosis, malaria) or impaired function due to malignancy, such as leukemia or lymphoma

TABLE 146-3. Examples of *Salmonella* Serotypes Associated with Warm-Blooded and Cold-Blooded Animals

Animal Reservoir	Serotypes Isolated
Snake	Arizonae, Montevideo, Eingedi
Iguana	Marina, Montevideo, Poona
Lizard	Poona
Komodo dragon	Enteritidis
Terrapin	Tel-el-kebir
Turtle	Pomona, Chester, Typhimurium, Muenchen, Java
Gecko	Weltevreden, Typhimurium, Enteritidis, Saintpaul, Agama
Crocodile	Typhimurium, Tsevie, Duval, Schwerin, Tinda, Tallahassee
Chicken	Typhimurium, Enteritidis, Heidelberg, Hadar, Montevideo, Thompson, Berta, Livingstone, Virchow
Turkey	Kentucky, Anatum, Heidelberg, Reading, Senftenberg, Saintpaul
Pig	Infantis, Choleraesuis, Typhimurium
Cattle	Dublin, Typhimurium
Hedgehog	Tilene

Salmonella serotypes have been isolated from up to 20% to 75% of fresh or thawed retail poultry samples, but also are found in pork, beef, and frozen egg products. Foods containing raw or undercooked eggs (e.g., Caesar salad, egg-dipped bread, and homemade eggnog) can be contaminated. Eggs become contaminated by organisms on the shell surface that penetrate the egg or from direct transovarian inoculation to the egg yolk. Other dairy products, such as ice cream, cream cakes, and mayonnaise, also have been incriminated as sources of human infections. *Salmonella* can be killed by heating to 54.4°C for 1 hour or 60°C for 15 minutes, but remain viable at ambient or reduced temperatures for days to weeks.

The number of bacteria that must be ingested to cause symptomatic disease in healthy adults is 10^6 to 10^8 nontyphoidal *Salmonella* organisms.[22] In infants and in other people with certain underlying conditions, a smaller inoculum can produce disease, so direct person-to-person transmission sometimes occurs. Nursery outbreaks are a result of several factors including neonatal susceptibility to low numbers of *Salmonella*. Both transplacental infection and perinatal transmission during vaginal delivery have been reported.[23] Healthcare-associated infections also have been related to contaminated medical equipment (e.g., endoscopes) and diagnostic or pharmacologic preparations, particularly those of animal origin (e.g., pituitary extracts, bile salts, pancreatic extracts, pepsin, and vitamins).

After infection, nontyphoidal salmonellae are excreted in feces for a median of 5 weeks. In infected children younger than 5 years of age, excretion is prolonged; approximately 40% of these children excrete organisms for 20 weeks after illness. In older children and adults, *Salmonella* excretion lasting more than 8 weeks after infection is uncommon, but unnecessary antimicrobial therapy may prolong excretion.

Emerging antimicrobial resistance in animal-associated serotypes of *Salmonella* has become an international public health problem, especially of industrialized countries.[24] A zoonotic strain of *S.* Enteritidis known as definitive phage type 104 (DT104) with chromosomal resistance to ampicillin, chloramphenicol, streptomycin, sulfonamides, and tetracycline was recognized in the 1990s in several countries in Europe and in the U.S.[8] Subsequently, clonal spread of fluoroquinolone-resistant DT104 strains from food animals to humans has been documented in Denmark.[24] In 2000 in the U.S. and 2002 in Canada, cattle-associated multidrug-resistant (MDR) strains of *S.* Newport with plasmid-encoded AmpC β-lactamase were isolated from ill children.[21] These ceftriaxone-resistant Newport-MDR AmpC strains were estimated by CDC to cause over 20,000 *Salmonella* infections in 2001 alone.[25] Although most extended-spectrum cephalosporin resistance is due to plasmid-encoded AmpC β-lactamases, extended-spectrum β-lactamases have been reported.[26] Fluoroquinolone-resistant invasive *S.* Choleraesuis strains in Taiwan have spread to humans from pigs and life-threatening infantile diarrhea from highly resistant *S.* Typhimurium with mutations in both *gyrA* and *parC* genes has been reported.[27,28] In aggregate, these epidemiologic realities have led to restriction and/or prohibition in food animals of fluoroquinolones and other antimicrobial agents used for treating human disease.[24–28]

The scourge of MDR nontyphoidal *Salmonella* has not spared Africa, where unregulated over-the-counter sale of antimicrobial agents rather than use in animals has fueled resistance.[29,30] Over the past decade, increasing resistance encoded on large, self-transferable plasmids of a few clones has been documented in 30% to 80% of the serotypes Typhimurium and Enteritidis, which account for nearly 80% of the nontyphoidal *Salmonella* isolated from blood, feces, and cerebrospinal fluid in Kenyan studies.[29,30]

Salmonella Typhi

The worldwide disease burden of typhoid and paratyphoid fever is estimated to approach 20 million illnesses, with up to 600,000 deaths yearly.[6] The impoverished and children suffer disproportionately, especially in south-central and southeast Asia and southern Africa.[31] About 300 cases of typhoid fever are reported annually in the U.S.; most (nearly 80%) occur in travelers to or visitors from highly endemic areas, especially the Indian subcontinent, and children account for about 40% of cases.[32] Since *S.* Typhi and Paratyphi A have no animal reservoir, fecal contamination of food or drink by ill, convalescing, or asymptomatically infected people accounts for most cases of enteric fever. Infection by person-to-person contact is thought to be rare, but sexual transmission has been documented.[33] The inoculum required for *S.* Typhi varies between 1000 and 1 million organisms, which is about 1000-fold lower than that customarily associated with other *Salmonella*.[6,22] Systemic and local humoral and cellular immune responses result from typhoid infection, but immunity is not robust and confers incomplete protection from relapse and reinfection.[6]

Antimicrobial resistance of *S.* Typhi to chloramphenicol became widely recognized in the 1970s and plasmid-mediated, multidrug resistance emerged in the 1990s. These MDR strains commonly were resistant to all drugs used for front-line treatment of enteric fever (ampicillin, chloramphenicol, and trimethoprim-sulfamethoxazole).[6] Resistance to fluoroquinolones has become widespread and ceftriaxone resistance is emerging. Reports buttressed by elegant molecular studies have documented MDR clones of *S.* Typhi in Africa and Asia that now account for many (85% to 100% of outbreak strains in Kenya) isolates.[34–36] These patterns of resistance appear to be shifting with changing pressures in antimicrobial use. Fluoroquinolone-resistant *S.* Paratyphi A is an emerging problem in India and Nepal as fluoroquinolone use has flourished.[37–39] Despite a steady rise in resistance in most studies, re-emergence of strains susceptible to first-line antimicrobial agents, including ampicillin, chloramphenicol, and co-trimoxazole, has been reported.[40]

CLINICAL MANIFESTATIONS

Several distinct clinical syndromes can develop in children infected with *Salmonella*, depending on both host factors and the specific serotype involved.

Gastroenteritis

Gastroenteritis is the most common clinical presentation of nontyphoidal *Salmonella* infection. After an incubation period of 6 to 72 hours (mean, 24 hours), abrupt onset of nausea, vomiting, and crampy abdominal pain in the periumbilical area and right lower quadrant is followed by watery or dysenteric diarrhea (containing blood and mucus). Fever (38.5°C to 39°C) is present in approximately 70% of cases, and the abdomen can be tender. Feces may contain neutrophils and occult blood. Mild peripheral blood leukocytosis with left shift commonly is present. Symptoms subside in <1 week in most healthy children. In neonates, young infants, and children with immunodeficiency, symptoms can persist for weeks. In patients with AIDS, the infection can disseminate, with multisystem involvement, shock, and death. In patients with inflammatory bowel disease, especially active ulcerative colitis, *Salmonella* gastroenteritis can be associated with invasion of the bowel wall and rapid development of toxic megacolon, systemic toxicity, and death. Reactive arthritis without clinical joint infection follows *Salmonella* gastroenteritis in 2% of cases, usually in adolescents or adults with the human leukocyte antigen (HLA)-B27 antigen. The duration of fecal shedding after symptoms subside can be prolonged in children <5 years of age (median, 7 weeks).[6]

Bloodstream Infection

Nontyphoidal *Salmonella* gastroenteritis is complicated by transient BSI, usually associated with fever, chills, and toxicity, in 1% to 5% of patients overall, and more frequently in infants and malnourished children.[41,42] Typhimurium and Enteritidis are the most common serotypes of *Salmonella* associated with BSI in the U.S., Greece, and tropical Africa.[7,30,42,43] Certain serotypes (e.g., Choleraesuis and Dublin) cause BSI more often than they cause gastroenteritis.[5,27] Children, especially neonates, may be afebrile and nontoxic despite BSI.

The occurrence, morbidity, and mortality of nontyphoidal *Salmonella* BSI are related to age and presence of underlying conditions. Infants with BSI uncommonly (~20% of cases) have immunocompromising conditions, whereas older children with BSI usually (~75% of cases) have a predisposing condition.[44] Death is more common if the patient has an underlying condition. Metastatic foci of infection and death are more common in the first year of life.[7,45]

Nontyphoidal *Salmonella* BSI commonly persists when treated with oral antibiotics or single-dose parenteral antibiotics. Laboratory and clinical findings do not predict adequately which children will experience persistence of BSI. Children with underlying medical conditions, particularly immunocompromising conditions, are at risk (~35%) for development of serious focal infections (meningitis, osteomyelitis, pyogenic arthritis, or pneumonia) during BSI, whereas previously healthy children are at relatively low risk (3%).[46–48]

Recurrent *Salmonella* septicemia without an obvious focus sometimes complicates infection in people with AIDS and occurs despite antibiotic therapy.[7,8] Prolonged or recurrent bacteremia also occurs in patients with schistosomiasis, who exhibit persistence of infection unless the schistosomiasis also is treated. *Salmonella* organisms are able to multiply within the schistosomes, where they are protected from antimicrobial agents. Hemolytic anemia, such as that occurring with sickle-cell disease, malaria, and *Bartonella bacilliformis* infection, is associated with a higher risk of BSI, presumably because of blockade of the reticuloendothelial system. Invasive nontyphoidal salmonellosis during pregnancy in otherwise healthy women is rare and prognosis for the mother is favorable, but transplacental infection is usually lethal for the fetus.[23]

Extraintestinal Focal Infections

Salmonella can cause metastatic infection in almost any organ. Sites with pre-existing anatomic abnormalities typically are involved (e.g., polycystic kidney or liver, hyperplastic lymph nodes, tumor). Bone infections due to *Salmonella* occur in infarcted bone of children with sickle-cell disease. Both osteomyelitis and suppurative arthritis can develop at sites of previous trauma, in skeletal prostheses, and occasionally without any predisposing factor.[8] Infants <2 months of age with *Salmonella* gastroenteritis have increased risk of BSI, meningitis, and other foci of infection. Meningitis is primarily a disease of infants; neonates may have little or no fever initially but show rapid deterioration, high mortality (approximately 50%), and neurologic sequelae if they survive the disease.[7,30,49–52] *Salmonella* meningitis and brain abscess also can complicate infection in people with AIDS. Persistent BSI can occur in patients with endocarditis, arteritis, or infected aneurysm. Rarely, other focal infections, such as urinary tract infection, pericarditis, peritonitis, pneumonia, and empyema, complicate *Salmonella* bacteremia.[53]

Enteric Fever (Typhoid Fever)

Although enteric fever classically is associated with *S.* Typhi and Paratyphi, other *Salmonella* occasionally cause disease mimicking this syndrome.[6,31,54–57] The clinical features of enteric fever with *S.* Typhi and Paratyphi are indistinguishable.[38] During the first week of illness, there is a stepwise, insidious increase in fever, which eventually becomes unremitting and is associated with systemic symptoms such as headache, lethargy, malaise, myalgia, and abdominal pain. In the second week, hepatosplenomegaly occurs and rose spots may be seen; headache is replaced by stupor. Relative bradycardia is not a feature of typhoid fever in children.[58] During the third to fourth week of fever, intestinal hemorrhage

and perforation are common; fever begins to show morning remissions, and there is a gradual decline in fever spikes. Myocarditis, shock, meningitis, and pneumonia can complicate the course.[59]

Diarrhea with blood and fecal leukocytes often is present in children during the first several weeks of illness, although in a few patients diarrhea does not begin until the third week. Occasionally, resolution does not occur until 6 weeks after onset. Even in the preantibiotic era, recurrences were sometimes seen after apparent resolution. Death related to central nervous system involvement, intestinal hemorrhage, or perforation generally does not occur until after the first week of illness. In infants and young children, *S.* Typhi can cause less impressive fever and toxicity the resultant nonspecific syndrome can be misinterpreted as a viral infection.

Asymptomatic Infection

After clinical recovery from nontyphoidal *Salmonella* gastroenteritis, asymptomatic fecal excretion of *Salmonella* continues for weeks and can be a source for contamination of food or drink and transmission to others.[8] Excretion of *Salmonella* for several months is typical in infants infected very early in life. Asymptomatic fecal excretion for weeks is also seen after typhoid fever in all ages. The role of convalescing excretors of *S.* Typhi among children in endemic areas is more important than chronic carriage in perpetuating transmission. Convalescent (up to 1 year) and chronic (over 1 year) carriage in adults is a consequence of biliary tract disease, especially gallstones, which usually are asymptomatic.[33]

DIAGNOSIS

Gastroenteritis is best diagnosed by cultures of stool specimens rather than rectal swab specimens. Selective media that inhibit the growth of normal flora, such as MacConkey, Hektoen enteric, or xylose-lysine-deoxycholate (XLD) agar, should be used. Enrichment broth, e.g., selenite F, can be used to enhance isolation when low numbers of *Salmonella* are present in stools. Rare lactose-fermenting *Salmonella* may pose a diagnostic problem, but other biochemical features enable accurate identification.[60]

Blood cultures are the best method for diagnosing typhoid fever and BSIs that can complicate other *Salmonella* infections.[6,31,55–59] The sensitivity of blood cultures (60% to 80%) depends principally on the volume of blood sampled in children as well as adults.[6] Quantitative studies of blood and bone marrow have shown a median of 0.3 (interquartile range (IQR), 0.1 to 10) organisms per mL versus 9 organisms per mL (IQR, 1.0 to 85) in bone marrow (which matches the pathophysiology of typhoid fever).[61] Consequently, a minimum of 1 to 15 mL of blood, depending on the age and weight of the child, should be cultured.[6] Culture of bone marrow is more sensitive (80% to 95%), but is done less often now that most children in endemic areas are treated outside hospital. Bone marrow cultures may be useful when the diagnosis is elusive in persistently febrile patients. Metastatic focal infections that can complicate infection due to many *Salmonella* serotypes are best diagnosed by cultures of aspirates of pus, biopsy specimens, or cerebrospinal fluid.[8,31]

Given the worldwide prevalence of MDR in *Salmonella*, accurate antimicrobial susceptibility testing in accord with Clinical Laboratory Standards Institute methods and interpretive criteria is imperative and results should guide or refine therapy.[62] For fecal isolates of *Salmonella*, only ampicillin, a fluoroquinolone, and trimethoprim-sulfamethoxazole should be tested and reported routinely; chloramphenicol and an extended-spectrum cephalosporin should be tested for extraintestinal isolates. Resistance to nalidixic acid is a practical surrogate test for gyrase (*gyrA* and *gyrB*) and topoisomerase IV (*parA* and *parC*) mutations that render isolates less responsive or refractory to fluoroquinolone therapy. Validated interpretive criteria for susceptibility to azithromycin do not exist currently.

DIFFERENTIAL DIAGNOSIS

Clinically, *Salmonella* gastroenteritis cannot be distinguished easily from other bacterial causes of bloody diarrhea, although age, exposures, presence of fever, associated enteritis symptoms, and various epidemiologic features sometimes suggest an etiologic agent. The presentation of inflammatory diarrhea with fever also is consistent with *Shigella*, enteroinvasive *Escherichia coli*, entero-hemorrhagic *E. coli*, *Campylobacter jejuni*, *Yersinia enterocolitica*, and *Clostridium difficile* infections. *Trichuris trichiura*, *Balantidium coli*, and *Entamoeba histolytica* are important possible parasitic causes of bloody mucoid diarrhea. When abdominal pain and tenderness are severe, alternative diagnoses such as appendicitis, perforated viscus, and ulcerative colitis merit consideration. Typhoid fever can mimic other infections of the reticuloendothelial system, including Epstein–Barr virus infection, disseminated tuberculosis or histoplasmosis, ehrlichiosis, anaplasmosis, brucellosis, tularemia, plague, and murine typhus.

TREATMENT

For people with gastroenteritis, initial therapy is focused on rehydration, correction of electrolyte disturbances, and general supportive care. Antimicrobial agents usually are not indicated for uncomplicated gastroenteritis, because they do not speed resolution of symptoms. Rather than eliminating fecal excretion, antimicrobial agents can prolong colonization. Antimicrobial therapy may be appropriate for patients with gastroenteritis who are at high risk of complications, although the efficacy of this measure is unproven.

Suspected or proven BSI and extraintestinal focal *Salmonella* infections should be treated with a third-generation cephalosporin unless susceptibility data demonstrate that the organism is susceptible to ampicillin, trimethoprim-sulfamethoxazole (TMP-SMX), or chloramphenicol; usual doses are listed in Table 146-4. Considering the intracellular site of *Salmonella* in the RES, TMP-SMX or fluoroquinolones may have a theoretical advantage over ampicillin for treatment of enteric fever. About 40% of nontyphoidal *Salmonella* isolates in the U.S. are resistant to one or more antimicrobial agents; worldwide MDR of all *Salmonella* is increasing.[5,6,21,24-30,34-39] Fluoroquinolones are best avoided in children under 18 years of age, unless alternative agents are not available.[6]

Duration of therapy depends on serotype and site of infection. Therapy usually is continued for 10 to 14 days in children with BSI, for 4 to 6 weeks for acute osteomyelitis, and for 4 weeks for meningitis.[8,59] Meningitis can recur even after 4 weeks of therapy, although most patients who experience relapse have received <3 weeks of antimicrobial therapy. Surgical drainage of focal purulent collections is indicated.[59] In the developing world, *Salmonella* infection associated with schistosomiasis requires treatment of both infections to achieve resolution.

S. Typhi infection usually is treated with a minimum of 10 to 14 days of therapy. Ceftriaxone is the best initial parenteral choice because of widespread resistance to other agents. For susceptible strains, ampicillin, trimethoprim-sulfamethoxazole, and chloramphenicol have all been used successfully, and fluoroquinolones

have been used extensively, even in children in endemic areas.[6,31] Defervescence in typhoid fever usually requires at least 36 hours of therapy and fever can persist for 5 to 7 days, even with ultimately effective therapy. Azithromycin has been effective in children with strains resistant to first-line agents.[63,64] Corticosteroids are used as adjunctive therapy in the presence of delirium, obtundation, stupor, coma, or shock in children with typhoid fever; a dose of 3 mg/kg dexamethasone initially, followed by 1 mg/kg every 6 hours for 48 hours, was associated with reduction of mortality from between 35% and 55% to 10%.[65] For patients in whom intestinal perforation develops, surgery coupled with broad-spectrum antimicrobial therapy directed at anaerobic and gram-negative enteric bacteria is indicated. The mortality after perforation can be as high as 10% to 30%.[6]

PROGNOSIS

An uneventful recovery without antimicrobial therapy usually occurs in immunocompetent children with *Salmonella* gastroenteritis. Young infants and immunocompromised patients, particularly patients with focal infection after BSI, can have prolonged, complicated courses. *Salmonella* meningitis has a poor prognosis and high relapse rate, particularly if treated with too short a course of therapy. Antimicrobial-resistant nontyphoidal *Salmonella* is associated with excess BSIs, hospitalization, and mortality.[5,66]

Even with appropriate therapy, patients can have recurrence of typhoid fever after completion of therapy (5% to 20% relapse rate). Relapses of *Salmonella* infections presumably reflect the difficulty in killing intracellular organisms. Because relapse is sometimes due to resistant bacteria, an agent different from the initial drug should be used empirically while awaiting culture and susceptibility test results. Antibiotic-resistant strains of *S.* Typhi are independently associated with increased virulence and adverse outcomes.[67,68]

PREVENTION

Chlorination of water, proper sewage disposal, and appropriate food-handling practices are necessary to prevent salmonellosis. Hand hygiene is critical to the prevention of person-to-person transmission via food. People who excrete *S.* Typhi should be excluded from occupations in food preparation and childcare until results of repeated stool cultures are negative; infected children <5 years of age also are excluded until repeated stool cultures are negative. For nontyphi salmonellosis, recovery from symptomatic disease but not stool culture negativity is required for return to group childcare.[69] In hospitalized infants and children, enteric precautions are recommended, because low inocula are capable of causing infection in children. Prolonged breastfeeding reduces the infection rate.[70]

No vaccine against nontyphoidal *Salmonella* or *S.* Paratyphi infections is available, although two vaccines are available for *S.* Typhi (Table 146-5).[71-74] These vaccines have similar efficacy, generally in the range of 50% to 75% for reducing the number of laboratory-confirmed cases within 2 to 3 years. Seven-year follow-up data with enteric-coated capsules containing Ty21a live vaccine suggest greater than 60% long-term protection. The live-attenuated vaccine should not be used in immunocompromised hosts or in people receiving antimicrobial agents at the time of immunization. Pediatric use of typhoid vaccines has been limited to children who: (1) will travel in areas where prolonged exposure to *S.* Typhi is likely; (2) live where MDR strains are prevalent; or (3) are members of households of documented carriers.

Mass vaccination of children to prevent typhoid fever in endemic areas is desirable. Neither of the two FDA-licensed vaccines is effective against *S.* Paratyphi A, which is an emerging, often antibiotic-resistant cause of enteric fever.[37,38] The *S.* Typhi Vi conjugate vaccine (Vi-rEPA) appears effective.[75] A substantial proportion of typhoid occurs in children <5 years of age for whom the oral vaccine is not approved.[54] WHO has recommended widespread use of the Vi vaccine in developing countries in which typhoid fever is endemic; a recent cluster-randomized trial suggests efficacy in preschool children.[54,74]

TABLE 146-4. Antimicrobial Agents Useful in Extraintestinal *Salmonella* Infections[a]

Drug	Dosage
Ampicillin	200 mg/kg per day in 4 divided doses
Trimethoprim-sulfamethoxazole	10 mg/kg per day trimethoprim in 2 divided doses
Cefotaxime	150–200 mg/kg per day in 3–4 divided doses
Ceftriaxone	100 mg/kg per day in 1–2 divided doses
Chloramphenicol	50–75 mg/kg per day in 4 divided doses

[a]*Serotype, site infected, and susceptibility determine optimal agent and duration of therapy.*

TABLE 146-5. Vaccines for Prevention of *Salmonella* Typhi

Vaccine	Age Indicated	Dose and Route	Adverse Reactions
Oral live-attenuated Ty21a vaccine (Vivotif)	≥6 years		0–5% fever or headache
Primary series		1 enteric-coated capsule every 2 days for 4 doses	
Booster (every 5 years)		1 enteric-coated capsule every 2 days for 4 doses	
Vi capsular polysaccharide vaccine (Typhim Vi)	>2 years		0–1% fever, 1.5–3% headache, 7% redness or induration at injection site
Primary series		A single dose of 0.5 mL (25 µg) IM	
Booster (every 2 years)		A single dose of 0.5 mL (25 µg) IM	

IM, intramuscular.

Key Points. Diagnosis and Management of *Salmonella* Infection

MICROBIOLOGY

- Gram-negative bacillus, usually nonlactose-fermenting
- Characterization based on O (somatic), H (flagellar), and Vi (capsular) antigens
- Chromosomal and plasmid-mediated antimicrobial resistance to ampicillin, chloramphenicol, and sulfonamides; emerging resistance to fluoroquinolones and extended-spectrum cephalosporins

EPIDEMIOLOGY

- Flora of birds, mammals, and reptiles, except Typhi and Paratyphi, which are uniquely human pathogens
- Highest prevalence in children <5 years of age, in whom excretion is prolonged
- Person-to-person transmission is rare, especially for Typhi and Paratyphi
- Host factors and serotype contribute to clinical manifestations
- Enteric fever classically with Typhi and Paratyphi, gastroenteritis more common with others
- Children with compromised immune systems are at increased risk for serious focal infections

DIAGNOSIS

- Recovery from blood (typhoidal, infants and malnourished) or stool (nontyphoidal > typhoidal)
- Stool cultures require selective and inhibitory media to suppress normal flora; enrichment broth enhances isolation
- Antimicrobial susceptibility testing is imperative with extended testing for extraintestinal isolates

TREATMENT

- Antimicrobial agents prolong colonization and are not recommended for uncomplicated gastroenteritis
- Third-generation cephalosporin is empiric choice for bloodstream infection and extraintestinal focal infections
- Azithromycin has been effective for typhoidal strains resistant to first-line agents
- Salmonellae are resistant to first- and second-generation cephalosporins

DURATION OF THERAPY

- Length of therapy required depends on serotype and site of infection
- Usual treatment 10 to 14 days for bacteremia, 4 to 6 weeks for acute osteomyelitis, and 4 weeks for meningitis

---

147 *Shigella* Species

Shai Ashkenazi and Thomas G. Cleary

Shigella spp. cause acute gastrointestinal tract infections, sometimes with extraintestinal manifestations. These infections are of major public health relevance, especially in developing countries, where they cause substantial pediatric morbidity and mortality. It has been estimated that 1.1 million deaths result from the 164.7 million annual cases worldwide.[1] The term *dysentery* denotes the presence of colitis manifest as frequent painful passage of stools containing blood or mucus. Bacillary dysentery is caused by bacteria, including shigellae and enteroinvasive *Escherichia coli*, which possess *Shigella* virulence genes.[2,3]

DESCRIPTION OF THE PATHOGEN

Shigella are nonmotile, nonencapsulated, gram-negative bacilli in the family Enterobacteriaceae. They do not ferment lactose, and lack urease activity. When grown on triple-sugar iron agar and lysine iron agar slants, shigellae characteristically show an alkaline slant and acid butt and no gas production. Nearly fifty serotypes, belonging to four serogroups (or species), have been identified: group A *(Shigella dysenteriae)*, group B *(S. flexneri)*, group C *(S. boydii)*, and group D *(S. sonnei)*.

PATHOGENESIS AND IMMUNITY

Shigellosis is one of the most communicable forms of diarrhea caused by bacteria. As few as 10 organisms have caused diarrhea in some adult volunteers. The low dose required to cause disease helps explain the ease of person-to-person spread.

The central event in pathogenesis is invasion of colonic mucosa.[4] The current model of this process involves multiple steps.[5,6] First, ingested Shigella cross the colonic epithelium via transcytosis through M cells, the specialized cells that cover the lymphoid follicles of the intestinal mucosa. At the dome area of the lymphoid follicle, the bacteria are phagocytosed by macrophages, which the bacteria kill by inducing apoptosis.[6] With this strategy, Shigella reach the subepithelial tissue and invade colonic epithelial cells through their basolateral surface. During the initial step of cellular entry, Shigella induce actin polymerization in epithelial cells with formation of filopodes. After entry, the bacteria free themselves from membrane-bound vacuoles, proliferate in cytoplasm, and spread via actin-based motility. This enables infection of neighboring cells by formation of finger-like protrusions. Intracellular Shigella also reprogram host cells to express proinflammatory cytokines, such as interleukin (IL)-1, IL-6, and IL-8, which augment local inflammation and attract neutrophils. Leukocytes transmigrate the epithelium into the lumen of the colon. Shigella kills neutrophils by inducing necrosis; release of granular proteins can further contribute to epithelial disruption.[6] Extensive destruction of the epithelial layer is followed by more inflammation.

These events have been elucidated at the molecular level: plasmid and chromosomal virulence genes have been defined in Shigella and invasive E. coli. Specific chromosomal genes enhance replication (e.g., the siderophore aerobactin facilitates multiplication of Shigella within tissues), increase bacterial resistance to nonspecific defense mechanisms (e.g., somatic antigens), or prevent killing by phagocytic cells (e.g., superoxide dismutase).[6] S. dysenteriae serotype 1 can increase severity of illness further via expression of Shiga toxin.[7] This toxin belongs to the family of toxins that contain an enzymatically active (A) subunit and five cell-binding (B) subunits. The A subunit irreversibly inhibits mammalian protein synthesis by cleaving an N-glycosidic bond at adenine 4324 in the 28S ribosomal RNA, blocking elongation factor 1-dependent binding of aminoacyl transfer RNA to the ribosome. Five identical copies of subunit B bind to the cell receptor glycolipid, globotriosyl ceramide. Chromosomal genes also act by regulating expression of genes on the Shigella virulence plasmid. The malA gene product functions in the inner membrane as a sensor for the high osmolarity of the colonic contents in the primate intestine, inducing expression of plasmid invasion genes. The chromosomal keratoconjunctivitis provocation gene (kcpA) is responsible for movement of Shigella in the cytoplasm. The virR regulatory loop gene responds to conditions outside the bacteria by inhibiting expression of the invasive phenotype at 30°C.

All virulent Shigella contain a 120- to 140-megadalton (200- to 220-kilobase) plasmid.[8] As with the chromosomal genes, plasmid genes can be involved in regulatory functions, invasion, or intercellular spread; virF governs the plasmid virulence regulon by directly activating transcription of two other gene loci, virG and virB. This latter locus then activates invasion plasmid antigens ipaABCD. The ipaABCD genes are highly conserved in Shigella invasion plasmids.[2] These proteins are the dominant virulence plasmid antigens recognized during the humoral immune response to Shigella. Intracellular and intercellular bacterial spread is encoded by virG, which has a sequence of repeating motifs in its amino terminus that is involved in polymerization of actin monomers to provide the force to propel Shigella within the cytoplasm and into adjacent cells.

This model explains the histologic observations of early neutrophil efflux in colonic crypts and bacterial invasion. The desquamation, ulceration, and formation of microabscesses in the colonic mucosa inhibit absorption of water, with production of stools that are frequent, scanty, and contain blood, inflammatory cells, and mucus. Invasion beyond the mucosa to the bloodstream seldom occurs.

Although mucosal secretory immunoglobulin (Ig) A antibodies develop against the virulence plasmid invasion antigens (ipaABCD) after natural infection, immunity has been shown to be serotype (lipopolysaccharide)-specific. It is unclear why occasional children and adults can be infected with Shigella and remain asymptomatic.[9] Cellular immunity and cytokine production develop during acute illness. IL-1α, IL-1β, tumor necrosis factors (TNFs) α and β, IL-4, IL-8, IL-6, and transforming growth factor β are induced, whereas interferon-γ is suppressed.[10,11]

PATHOLOGY

Shigella primarily affects the colon.[12] Macroscopically, the affected mucosal surface is edematous and erythematous, covered by a layer of grey mucopurulent exudate with varying severity of ulceration and hemorrhage. Microscopic examination typically reveals hyperemia, edema, and neutrophil infiltration of the colonic mucosa. In early stages, the surface epithelium can be reduced in height and infiltrated with neutrophils; as disease progresses, epithelial cells detach from the edematous lamina propria, leaving microulcerations. With advanced disease, large numbers of lymphocytes and plasma cells can be seen in the lamina propria. At the base of deep necrotic ulcerated mucosa, a thick pseudomembrane forms, composed of neutrophils, erythrocytes, fibrin, and desquamated epithelial cells. Crypt abnormalities include a marked reduction of goblet cells and hyperplasia of epithelial cells, crypt abscesses, and distention due to exudates. Aphthoid ulcers form over lymphoid aggregates. Shigellosis produces striking proliferation of crypt epithelial cells, even at sites distant from ulcers.

In small blood vessels near the lamina propria, pathologic changes include hyperemia, edema, focal hemorrhage, and swelling of endothelial cells. In some cases, thrombosis of blood vessels in the lamina propria and submucosa is associated with widespread necrosis of colonic mucosa. The pathophysiologic basis for the initial watery diarrheal presentation has not been fully elucidated.

EPIDEMIOLOGY

The number of annual cases of shigellosis reported in the United States to the Centers for Disease Control and Prevention (CDC) varies considerably, from 22,625 in 2008 to 14,786 in 2010.[13,14] Shigella sonnei infections account for over 75% of cases in the U.S.[13] The calculated reported incidence is about 4 to 10 per 100,000 people, with highest rates reported from western states (10 cases per 100,000).[13,15] Because of underreporting, the actual numbers are estimated to be approximately 20 times higher. The highest risk is in children between 1 and 4 years of age (particularly children 12 to 36 months), followed by children between 5 and 9 years of age.[15] Large childcare-associated outbreaks are common and are difficult to control (see Chapter 3, Infections Associated with Group Childcare). In the U.S., seasonality of shigellosis has changed from a peak in summer to a higher incidence in the second half of the year. In developing countries with tropical climates, Shigella infection is common throughout the year, but higher isolation rates occur during the summer and rainy seasons.

Shigella are hardy organisms that can be recovered for up to 6 months from contaminated water samples maintained at room temperature. Organisms can survive for up to 30 days in foods such as milk, whole eggs, oysters, shrimp, and flour. Shigella can be isolated from toilet surfaces in homes of patients with dysentery, and from fingers of patients who use toilet paper. The ability to survive, coupled with a low infectious dose, explains contagion. Most cases of shigellosis probably result from person-to-person transmission of small inocula through the fecal–oral route. There is a high risk of spread within families, in childcare centers, custodial care institutions, prisoner-of-war camps, Indian reservations, and among men who have sex with men. Water and food are responsible for large outbreaks of shigellosis in closed populations, such as military camps, cruise ships, community gatherings, and restaurants. Water plays a major role in transmission in developing countries, as does poverty, overcrowding, and unsanitary conditions.

Healthy people who become infected with *Shigella* can shed organisms for up to a month; antibiotic treatment reduces the period of excretion to a few days. Malnourished children shed the organism for prolonged periods as a result of their inability to eliminate the organism or to prevent reinfection. In patients with acquired immunodeficiency syndrome (AIDS), prolonged, relapsing symptomatic shigellosis and lengthy carrier states have been described despite proper treatment.

The prevalence of *Shigella* serotypes varies over time and geography. *Shigella sonnei* account for about 80% of *Shigella* isolates in developed countries, with an increasing relative prevalence in the last decades.[13,15] By contrast, in developing countries, *S. flexneri* is most common, with occasional outbreaks caused by *S. dysenteriae* serotype 1.[16]

CLINICAL MANIFESTATIONS

Uncomplicated Shigellosis

Studies conducted on adult volunteers have established that the first symptoms of shigellosis usually occur within 12 to 48 hours of exposure, but symptoms can be delayed for up to 1 week. In mild infections, the only complaints may be development of watery or loose stools for a few days with minimal or no constitutional symptoms. In contrast, typical disease in children includes acute onset of high fever, malaise, abdominal cramps, and copious watery diarrhea followed by resolution or by heightened toxicity, appearance of nausea and vomiting, and passage of frequent, scanty, mucoid, bloody stools associated with pain and tenesmus. Some children have bloody mucoid diarrhea from onset of illness. Physical findings include body temperature of 38.5° C or higher, general toxicity, mild dehydration (because <30 mL/kg per day of diarrheal fluid usually is lost in the dysenteric phase), lower abdomen tenderness, and increased bowel sounds. Rectal examination elicits severe pain. In most cases, symptoms resolve without antimicrobial therapy within one week; however, therapy shortens clinical illness and fecal excretion of organisms.

Complications of Shigellosis

The main complications of shigellosis include dehydration due to fluid loss through diarrhea and vomiting, electrolyte imbalance (including hyponatremia and hypokalemia, commonly observed with *S. dysenteriae*), and, less commonly, hypoglycemia due to failure of glycogenolysis and gluconeogenesis. Hypoglycemia and hyponatremia have been associated with a higher risk of death. Protein-losing enteropathy can contribute to poor nutrition. In malnourished children with chronic diarrhea or frequent relapses, rectal prolapse can be observed. Hemolytic-uremic syndrome is a major complication of infections due to *S. dysenteriae* serotype 1, being associated with production of Shiga toxin and damage to vascular endothelium.

Bloodstream Infection

Severe colitis and ulceration can result in loss of the mucosal protective barrier, with entry into the circulation of bacteria or bacterial lipopolysaccharide.[17,18] However, bloodstream infection (BSI) during shigellosis is rare in developed countries.[17] In contrast, one study from Bangladesh found that 4% of patients with shigellosis had *Shigella* bacteremia.[17] In this setting, BSI was more common in malnourished infants and was associated with significant mortality. BSI with disseminated intravascular coagulation, endotoxic shock, and death, is more commonly associated with *S. dysenteriae* than with other *Shigella* species. A study from southern Israel described 15 children with *Shigella* BSI.[19] Most patients were infants and 13 (87%) had failure to thrive. Most (87%) of the isolates were *S. flexneri*, with no isolates of *S. dysenteriae* serotype 1 and no deaths. In patients with AIDS, shigellosis is more common, more severe, and is more often associated with BSI. In addition to *Shigella* BSI, enteric gram-negative bacilli can cross the damaged mucosa and cause secondary BSI.[20,21]

Surgical Complications

A review of 57 published cases of surgical complications of shigellosis in children over a 40-year period categorized complications into four groups: (1) intestinal obstruction (53%); (2) appendicitis with or without perforation (28%); (3) colonic perforation (17%); and (4) intra-abdominal abscesses (2%). Thirteen children (23%) died, often despite antimicrobial therapy.[22]

Extraintestinal Infections

Extraintestinal infections caused by *Shigella* spp. are rare. Of these, urogenital infections are relatively common. Vulvovaginitis with vaginal discharge and urinary tract infections (mainly cystitis) caused by *Shigella* spp. are well documented.[23,24] Publications from developed countries highlight the problems of delayed diagnosis and inappropriate treatment of people with these infections.[25,26] Eye infections include keratitis, conjunctivitis, iritis, and iridocyclitis.[26]

Neurologic Symptoms

In series of hospitalized children, 10% to 45% have neurologic symptoms, including brief generalized seizures, lethargy, confusion, hallucinations, and severe headache.[26] Neurologic symptoms are overrepresented in series based on hospitalized patients, because seizures often are the indication for admission. In longitudinal outpatient-based studies, convulsions are uncommon. Neurologic symptoms can precede the onset of diarrhea and can suggest a central nervous system intoxication or infection. Cerebrospinal fluid usually is normal; mild lymphocytic pleocytosis (up to 12 cells/mm³) has been observed.[27]

The pathogenesis of *Shigella*-induced neurologic symptoms is not understood fully; clinical and complementary studies in a murine model documented the role of bacterial components, host inflammatory mediators, such as TNF-α, IL-1β, and nitric oxide, and early development of brain edema.[26,28] Most children recover completely with no residual neurologic deficit, although studies conducted in Bangladesh found altered consciousness, seizures following stopping of breastfeeding in the neonatal period, and dehydration to be unfavorable prognostic signs.[29,30] Fatalities sometimes occur early in the course of illness in children who lack significant dehydration or septicemia but demonstrate stupor, coma, hyperpyrexia, shock, convulsions, and decorticate or decerebrate posturing (related to cerebral edema). This Reye-like syndrome may be the most common cause of death from shigellosis in developed countries.[31] *S. flexneri* and *S. sonnei* are the most frequently associated species. This fulminant toxic encephalopathy (called Ekiri syndrome in Japan) has a poor prognosis.[31,32] Hypocalcemia may play a role in pathogenesis.[31]

Musculoskeletal Symptoms

A nationwide study of 278 consecutive patients with shigellosis and 597 controls found that 7% of the patients had reactive arthritis.[33] An additional 2% had other musculoskeletal symptoms, including tendinitis, enthesopathy, or bursitis. Only a single control subject had reactive arthritis. Human leukocyte antigen (HLA) B27 was positive in 36% of the patients with reactive arthritis.[33] Reiter syndrome (arthritis, urethritis, and conjunctivitis) was reported mainly in adults.

Neonatal Shigellosis

Shigellosis in neonates and young infants has several unique features. Neonatal shigellosis is relatively rare, accounting for only 0.6% of all cases in children less than 10 years of age.[34] This finding may be explained by the presence of maternal protective factors that pass through the placenta or by breastfeeding.

Conversely, complications – including dehydration, hypothermia, septicemia, meningitis, rectal prolapse, toxic megacolon, and colonic perforation – are more common in infants than in older children; paradoxically neonates often have a shorter duration of diarrhea.[35-38] The mortality rate for infants 3 months of age or younger who were hospitalized with shigellosis was at least double that of older children. Risk factors associated with poor outcome include ileus, hypoproteinemia, gram-negative BSI, and hyponatremia.[38]

LABORATORY FINDINGS AND DIAGNOSIS

The differential diagnosis for watery diarrhea associated with fever due to *Shigella* includes viral agents (rotavirus, enteric adenovirus, norovirus, astrovirus) as well as bacterial agents (*Salmonella, Campylobacter, Yersinia enterocolitica, Clostridium difficile,* diarrheagenic *E. coli, Aeromonas, Plesiomonas*). For patients with clinical dysentery, *Entamoeba histolytica, Balantidium coli,* and noninfectious diseases (e.g., inflammatory bowel disease, allergic proctitis in infancy) also are considered.

The peripheral white blood cell count in bacillary dysentery can show a dramatic left shift, but this finding is not present consistently. Microscopic (or macroscopic) fecal blood and fecal leukocytes are each present in approximately 70% of cases of *Shigella* infection; both are present in 50%.[39] Although seen more commonly in shigellosis than in other types of bacterial enteritis, findings of fecal blood and leukocytes are signs of colitis due to any etiology.

Stool culture to isolate *Shigella* is the basis for diagnosis. Culture, however, has some limitations: a few days of incubation is required; the sensitivity is only 72% to 80%, the organism may not survive transportation to the laboratory, and the culture can be negative in children who have received antimicrobial therapy. Additional diagnostic methods hold promise. Studies showed that polymerase chain reaction (PCR) testing of stool specimens increased diagnosis by 50% compared with culture.[40,41] Diagnosis by microarrays using the *gyrB* genes was sensitive and also enables simultaneous identification of other enteric pathogens, such as *Salmonella* spp. and diarrheagenic *E. coli*.[42] Immune assay with monoclonal antibodies to the IpaC protein detected *Shigella* spp. and enteroinvasive *E. coli* with high sensitivity and specificity.[26] Serology has little value in the diagnosis of acute infection.

TREATMENT

Rapid correction of fluid and electrolyte deficits, early reinstitution of feeding (<12 hours after initiation of treatment), and continual replacement of ongoing losses are key elements of therapy.[26] Oral rehydration is the treatment of choice, although patients in shock or coma, as well as patients with ileus, should be treated with intravenous replacement of fluids and electrolytes.

Appropriate antimicrobial therapy of shigellosis shortens the duration of fever, diarrhea, and fecal excretion of the pathogen (thereby reducing infectivity) and apparently also reduces the risk of complications.[26,43] Empiric antimicrobial treatment generally is recommended for people with colitis or dysentery until results of culture and clinical response are known. Because *Shigella* is not always isolated from stool when it is the cause of illness, response to an antimicrobial agent in <24 hours after initiation of therapy (the typical course of treated shigellosis) can be an appropriate basis for continuing therapy despite negative fecal culture results. Lack of response to therapy or inability to confirm infection should prompt collection of stool specimens for a second culture and consideration of other possible diagnoses. Identification of a pathogen other than *Shigella* should refocus therapy when appropriate.

Empiric therapies used in the past (e.g., trimethoprim-sulfamethoxazole (TMP-SMX) and ampicillin) often are inappropriate because of bacterial resistance.[16,44] Most resistance is plasmid-mediated and easily transferable among bacteria. Parenteral therapy with a third-generation cephalosporin may represent optimal empiric therapy for hospitalized or severe cases

TABLE 147-1. Antibiotic Therapy for Children with Suspected or Proven Shigellosis[a]

Drug[b]	Dosage
Cefixime[c]	8 mg/kg per day PO once daily
Ceftriaxone	50 mg/kg per day IV or IM in one dose daily (maximum 1.5 g/day)
Trimethoprim-sulfamethoxazole[d]	10 mg/kg per day (TMP) PO in two divided doses (maximum 320 mg TMP/day)
Ampicillin[d]	100 mg/kg per day IV or PO in four divided doses
Azithromycin	12 mg/kg (maximum 500 mg) on the first day, then 6 mg/kg (maximum 250 mg) for 4 days

IM, intramuscular; IV, intravenous; PO, by mouth; TMP, trimethoprim.

[a]Therapy is given for a total of 5 days. Susceptibility test results are used to tailor therapy.

[b]Ciprofloxacin or other fluroquinolones may be appropriate (see text).

[c]Cefixime is not available in some locations.

[d]Resistance is common.

because of the excellent clinical and microbiologic response and rare resistance[45,46] (Table 147-1). A single dose of ceftriaxone showed bacteriologic failures, but a 2-day course was as effective as a 5-day course in one study[46] and can be used when there is a good clinical response and no extraintestinal infection.

Because of the worldwide high resistance rates, the choice of the empiric oral antimicrobial treatment is problematic. TMP-SMX is appropriate for patients who are infected with a susceptible organism or persons who have acquired infection in a locale with low resistance. For patients infected with an ampicillin-susceptible, TMP-SMX-resistant organism, ampicillin can be given (see Table 147-1). Cefixime, an oral third-generation cephalosporin, was clinically effective in children infected mostly with *S. sonnei* but showed a relatively high bacteriologic failure rate in children[47] and was less effective in adults with severe shigellosis caused mostly by *S. dysenteriae* and *S. flexneri*.[48] A 2-day course of cefixime was less effective than 5 days.[49] Azithromycin was effective in adults with shigellosis.[50] In an open randomized study in children, azithromycin and cefixime had similar clinical efficacy, but azithromycin had a better bacteriologic response.[51] Azithromycin was superior clinically and microbiologically to nalidixic acid in an outbreak setting of shigellosis in children.[52] In some settings, antimicrobial resistance patterns leave only fluoroquinolones, such as ciprofloxacin or ofloxacin, as therapeutic options.[53] Ciprofloxacin (10 mg/kg every 12 hours for 5 days, maximum single dose 500 mg) is effective treatment.[54] If the patient shows no improvement by 72 hours of therapy with one of these agents, use of an alternative drug should be considered. Resistance of *Shigella* to azithromycin and fluoroquinolones has been reported.[44,55]

Antimicrobial resistance patterns of *Shigella* strains in the U.S. are monitored by the CDC (www.cdc.gov/narms).

Antimotility agents should be avoided in shigellosis as well as in other infectious causes of colitis.[56] Data suggest that such drugs prolong symptoms (diarrhea and fever) and shedding of the organism. In countries where vitamin A deficiency is common, a single oral dose of vitamin A (200,000 IU) in addition to antimicrobial therapy reduces severity of illness.[57] Zinc supplementation (20 mg/day, elemental) in Bangladeshi children shortened the duration of the acute disease,[58] promoted weight gain[58] and also improved the immune response.[59] In addition, a high-protein diet rich in animal proteins (milk, eggs, chicken) given for 21 days after completion of antimicrobial therapy for shigellosis resulted in significantly greater height gains in Bangladeshi children.[60]

PREVENTION

The best strategy to prevent shigellosis in young children is prolonged breastfeeding.[61,62] Specific protective antibodies present in milk of women living in endemic areas decrease the severity of infection in infants.[63,64] Clean running water and appropriate sanitation are crucial. For toddlers and older children, good hygiene practices are helpful but are difficult to implement. Adults involved in food preparation should be instructed in proper hand hygiene technique.[65,66] Fly control also has been suggested to aid control of spread.

Despite continuing efforts and substantial progress, a *Shigella* vaccine is not available commercially. Several strategies for vaccine development are under study. Lipopolysaccharide-based conjugate vaccines showed minor adverse reactions and a good homologous immune response in children 4 to 7 years[67] and 1 to 4 years of age,[68] and promising efficacy.[69]

Antibiotic prophylaxis against shigellosis generally is not recommended for children, although for certain brief, high-risk exposures, such prophylaxis may be reasonable. Treatment of symptomatic people shortens duration of excretion and thereby decreases secondary spread to close contacts, especially in settings where close contact occurs, such as group childcare.

Key Points. Epidemiology, Clinical Manifestations, and Management of *Shigella* Infections

EPIDEMIOLOGY

- Peak incidence is in children 1 to 4 years of age
- Because of the low infectious dose, direct person-to-person transmission through the fecal–oral route is most common, especially in young children and in childcare settings
- Transmission can occur by contact with contaminated environmental surfaces and by consumption of contaminated food or water used for drinking or recreational purposes

CLINICAL FEATURES

- Incubation period of 24 to 48 hours, but can be as long as 1 week
- Acute onset of diarrhea (often with blood or mucus), with fever, nausea, vomiting, and abdominal cramps
- Dehydration and electrolyte imbalance are the most common complications, especially in very young children

- Extraintestinal complications are uncommon, and occur more frequently in neonates or immunocompromised children

MANAGEMENT

- Mainstay is replacement of fluid and electrolyte losses, preferably by oral rehydration solutions
- Antimicrobial therapy shortens duration of diarrhea, fever, and fecal shedding (thereby reducing infectivity) and apparently reduces risk of complications
- Empiric antibiotic therapy should be based on local resistance patterns
- In most locations, the preferred oral and parenteral antimicrobial agents are azithromycin and a third-generation cephalosporin, respectively
- No vaccine is available

---

148 *Yersinia* Species

Theresa J. Ochoa and Miguel O'Ryan

Bacteria of the genus *Yersinia* belong to the family Enterobacteriaceae. There are 15 species of *Yersinia*; among them, only *Yersinia enterocolitica*, *Y. pseudotuberculosis*, and *Y. pestis* are human pathogens. The most infamous of the three is the black death-associated agent *Y. pestis*, which causes *bubonic plague* when transmitted by a flea bite and *pneumonic plague* when acquired by an aerosol. *Y. enterocolitica* and *Y. pseudotuberculosis* are enteropathogens transmitted by consumption of contaminated food or water and cause gastrointestinal syndromes that can develop into fatal septicemia in immunocompromised people.

Yersinia are gram-negative, aerobic and facultatively anaerobic, rod-shaped nonspore-forming bacteria; these microorganisms ferment glucose, are oxidase-negative, and reduce nitrates to nitrites. *Yersinia* do not react with hydrogen sulfide, citrate, potassium cyanide (KCN), lysine decarboxylase (LDC), and arginine dihydrolase, but do react with methyl red and indole. *Yersinia* species are nonpigmented, are nonlactose-fermenting, and produce acid from glucose. Species are differentiated by a variety of traits, such as urease (*Y. pestis* is negative), motility (*Y. pestis* is nonmotile at both 25°C and 37°C), ornithine decarboxylase (*Y. enterocolitica* is positive), and rhamnose (*Y. pseudotuberculosis* is positive), as well as several carbohydrate fermentation reactions for which *Y. enterocolitica* is positive.

Despite differences in their mode of entry into the host, clinical manifestations, and disease severity, all three pathogenic *Yersinia* have in common a tropism for lymphoid tissue. Virulence factors shared by all three species include factors that promote serum resistance, coordinate gene expression, and iron acquisition, and presence of a 70-kb virulence plasmid (pYV) encoding for a type III secretion system (TTSS) essential for sustained bacterial replication in host tissue.[1–4] Although it is clear that the bulk of bacterial multiplication occurs in the extracellular space, there is evidence that all three pathogenic *Yersinia* survive and multiply within macrophages, especially during the early stages of colonization.[5]

Virulence genes unique to single species also are present. For example, *Y. enterocolitica* has a chromosomal gene that encodes for a guanylate cyclase-stimulating enterotoxin structurally related to the heat-stable enterotoxin produced by enterotoxigenic *Escherichia coli*.[6] Enteropathogenic *Yersinia* harbor three adhesins/invasins that facilitate invasion: *Yersinia* adhesin A, invasin, and an attachment and invasion locus (Ail). Virulence of this species also is associated with an iron-repressible outer membrane polypeptide. *Y. pestis* has two additional specific plasmids: *pPCP1* encoding for a plasminogen activator and *pPMT1* for a toxin that affects intestinal blockade and survival in fleas, and the F1 capsule that has the ability to block phagocytosis.[7,8]

YERSINIA ENTEROCOLITICA

Epidemiology

Yersiniosis due to infection with *Y. enterocolitica* is a zoonotic gastrointestinal disease in humans. *Y. enterocolitica* can be isolated from a variety of domestic and wildlife animals, e.g., pigs, cattle, sheep, goat, rabbits, dogs, cats, wild boars, and small rodents. Pigs are considered to be the main reservoir of human pathogenic strains. Individuals who eat or handle pork are at risk of illness. Pork intestines (chitterlings) are a documented source of infection.[9] Eating food prepared from raw products or treated sausage, and contact with domestic animals, are the main risk factors for domestic sporadic yersiniosis in children.[10] Milk and other dairy products, even if pasteurized, can sometimes be the source of outbreaks, because organisms proliferate at refrigerator temperatures; thus, low levels of contamination can lead to significant risk. Refrigerated stored blood is a source of transfusion-acquired illness.[11] Contaminated water also can be a source of infection. Familial and nosocomial spread of *Y. enterocolitica* suggest that person-to-person transmission occurs.

Human infections are more common in cooler climates and tend to cluster in winter months. Most reported cases have been from Canada, Europe, and the United States. The average annual incidence of *Y. enterocolotica* infection in the U.S. (FoodNet) during 1996–2007 was 3.5 cases per million people.[12] In comparison, the average annual incidence of *Y. enterocolotica* infection in Germany (SurvNet) during 2001–2008 was 7.2 per 100,000 people, with the highest incidence in children <5 years of age (58/100,000 population), specifically in the subset <1 year of age (108/100,000 population).[13] Black infants have the highest incidence of *Y. enterocolitica* infection in the U.S.[14] In general, after campylobacteriosis and salmonellosis, yersiniosis ranks third among notified bacterial zoonosis in the European Union.

Clinical Manifestations

Enteric Disease

The most common clinical syndrome is enterocolitis associated with fever, abdominal pain, vomiting, and diarrhea that contains mucus and gross blood. This presentation occurs most frequently in children <5 years of age. During the first 3 months of life, enteritis is complicated by bloodstream infection (BSI) in up to 28% of cases.[15–18] The relative frequency of specific symptoms may vary by strain biotype/serotype.[13,19] Diarrhea commonly persists for >2 weeks, and occasionally for several months. Untreated people shed organisms for several weeks. Abdominal complications of enteric infection include intestinal perforation, peritonitis, intussusception, toxic megacolon, mesenteric vein thrombosis, chronic ileitis, and gangrene of the bowel wall. Less than 10% of adolescents and adults have bloody diarrhea associated with *Y. enterocolitica*. In older children, mesenteric lymphadenitis (pseudoappendicitis) or, less commonly, terminal ileitis is the major clinical manifestation, accompanied by one or more of the following: fever, abdominal pain, right lower quadrant tenderness, and leukocytosis. *Y. enterocolitica* enteritis sometimes can mimic appendicitis or other surgical conditions and should be considered in the differential diagnosis of children presenting with an "acute abdomen".

Extraintestinal Manifestations

The major complication of *Yersinia*-associated enteric infection is BSI in the very young child and in individuals with iron overload syndromes, including those undergoing frequent transfusion due to sickle-cell anemia, β-thalassemia, aplastic anemia, cirrhosis with hemochromatosis, or malignancy, as well as those undergoing long-term hemodialysis and receiving oral iron supplementation.[9,20–23] Clinical presentations in patients with iron overload most commonly include enteritis or a pseudoappendicitis syndrome.[24]

Other occasional manifestations and complications are chronic infection with prolonged fever, granulomatous hepatitis, multiple liver and spleen abscesses, acute and chronic pancreatitis, acute pharyngitis, meningitis, osteomyelitis, pyomyositis, myocarditis, endocarditis, conjunctivitis, pneumonia and pleural empyema, urinary tract infection, and renal abscess. Dermatologic manifestations include primary cutaneous infections (cellulitis, abscess), erythema nodosum, erythema multiforme, and cutaneous vasculitis. *Yersinia* infection rarely has been associated with Sweet syndrome.

In adults, postinfectious sequelae such as erythema nodosum, arthralgia or arthritis, and uveitis are the most common complications; polyarthritis occurs particularly in individuals with major histocompatibility class (MHC) 1 antigen HLA-B27.[25] Although swelling of several joints can persist for >4 months, the long-term prognosis of this form of arthritis is usually good.[26] Chronic inflammatory bowel disease also has been associated with *Y. enterocolitica* infection.[27]

Laboratory Findings and Diagnosis

Fecal leukocytes are common although non-pathognomonic in patients with colitis. *Y. enterocolitica* can be isolated from culture of stool and sometimes from mesenteric lymph nodes or peritoneal fluid specimens from children who have undergone appendectomy. *Y. enterocolitica* grows on all commonly used enteric media. Cold enrichment in phosphate-buffered saline or phosphate-buffered saline with sorbitol and bile salts, and several other selective enrichment media, are useful for recovery of *Y. enterocolitica*. Cefsulodin–irgasan–novobiocin (CIN) agar, selective for growth of *Yersinia*, is preferred for isolation from fecal samples. Growth of pathogenic *Yersinia* can require up to 4 weeks of incubation.[28]

Yersinia are coccobacillary and exhibit bipolar staining in blood agar. Old cultures or cultures grown on more restrictive media show morphologic variability with Gram stain. Avirulent strains are pyrazinamidase-positive and fail to autoagglutinate; virulent strains yield positivity with crystal violet and Congo red binding assays.[29] Several organisms previously classified as *Y. enterocolitica*-like now are classified as separate species, including *Y. intermedia*, *Y. kristensenii*, and *Y. frederiksenii*.[30] These organisms infrequently cause illness in immunocompetent individuals.

Y. enterocolitica species is divided into six biotypes (1A, 1B, 2–5), which include several serotypes. Most human pathogenic *Y. enterocolitica* strains are classified as biotype 4, serotype O:3. Serotypes most commonly associated with disease in North America are different from those identified in Europe. Serologic responses can be used as evidence of infection when culture results are negative and a compatible syndrome is present. Titer determinations are available through commercial laboratories for the most common serotypes, but results should be interpreted with caution. Children <1 year of age are less likely to develop a serologic response compared with older children.[31] Cross-reactions with *Brucella abortus*, *Morganella morganii*, *Salmonella*, *Bartonella henselae*, *Chlamydophila pneumoniae*, *Rickettsia rickettsii*, and *Borrelia burgdorferi*, as well as persistence of titers for several years after *Y. enterocolitica* infection limit the usefulness of serodiagnosis. Using antibodies raised against the recombinant attachment-invasion locus protein (Ail), detected by indirect enzyme immunoassay (EIA) and Western blot immunoassay, could aid in identifying pathogenic *Y. enterocolitica* strains.[32]

Several different DNA-based methods have been developed to characterize *Y. enterocolitica* strains (conventional PCR, real-time PCR, oligonucleotide-based DNA microarray) in clinical, food, and environmental samples. Many of these assays use primers targeting plasmid (*yadA* or *virF*) and/or chromosomal-encoded virulence genes (*ail*, *inv*, and *yst*). In addition, PCR assays using the *Yersinia*-specific region of the 16S rRNA gene have been designed to detect *Yersinia* spp., especially in blood samples.[33] Detection rate of pathogenic *Y. enterocolitica* in clinical specimens is clearly higher using PCR assay than culture. Results must be interpreted with caution, however, when the sample is from a nonsterile site.

Treatment

The benefit of antibiotics for management of immunocompetent individuals with *Yersinia* enterocolitis has not been established conclusively. Patients who are immunocompromised and patients with extraintestinal dissemination should be treated with antibiotics. *Y. enterocolitica* generally are susceptible in vitro to trimethoprim-sulfamethoxazole, chloramphenicol, fluoroquinolones, aminoglycosides, tetracycline, piperacillin, and extended-spectrum cephalosporins, and are resistant to most penicillins and first-generation cephalosporins. If septicemia develops during desferrioxamine treatment in patients with iron overload states, chelation should be stopped temporarily. Antibiotic therapy has no beneficial effect on postinfectious syndromes.

Prevention

Outbreaks of illness due to *Y. enterocolitica* often are foodborne and should receive prompt and thorough investigation. Recall of suspect contaminated items can abort an outbreak. Careful attention to appropriate cooking practices in handling of pig products, especially intestines, should decrease the risk associated with these food products. Consumption of uncooked meats should be avoided, and meat should not be refrigerated for prolonged periods before consumption because *Y. enterocolitica* growth can be enhanced at refrigerator temperatures. There is no vaccine currently available against *Y. enterocolitica* although several candidates are under evaluation.

YERSINIA PSEUDOTUBERCULOSIS

Epidemiology

Y. pseudotuberculosis is distributed worldwide in animals, including rodents, birds (turkey, duck, geese, pigeons, and canaries), rabbits, deer, and farm animals. Infection can follow exposure to well and mountain water. This organism was originally described as causing tuberculosis-like lesions in guinea pigs. Household pets often are the source of infection for children. *Y. pseudotuberculosis* also can be transmitted through food products and outbreaks have been linked to pasteurized milk, lettuce, and carrots.[34-36] As with *Y. enterocolitica*, infections in humans cluster in cold weather months. Human infections are most common among individuals 5 to 15 years of age, with a 3-fold male predominance. Most cases have been reported from Europe, although the organism has a worldwide distribution. The average annual incidence of *Y. pseudotuberculosis* infection in the U.S. (FoodNet) during 1996–2007 was 0.04 cases per million people.[12] Compared with *Y. enterocolitica*, *Y. pseudotuberculosis* infects older individuals, who are more likely to require hospitalization for invasive infection. Patients with iron overload are at increased risk for infection although this seems to be a less common risk factor compared with *Y. enterocolitica* infections.

Clinical Manifestations

Y. pseudotuberculosis causes acute gastroenteritis and mesenteric lymphadenitis, often accompanied by fever and abdominal pain. The most common clinical syndrome is "pseudoappendicitis" (mesenteric lymphadenitis, occasionally with associated terminal ileitis) characterized by abdominal pain, right lower quadrant tenderness, fever, and leukocytosis. Less commonly, *Y. pseudotuberculosis* can mimic Kawasaki disease and has been implicated as a possible cause of Kawasaki disease.[37-40] Septicemia or extraintestinal spread of *Y. pseudotuberculosis* is uncommon and has been reported in patients with underlying conditions such as cirrhosis, malignancy, diabetes, aplastic anemia, thalassemia, iron overload, and HIV infection. Acute renal failure with tubulointerstitial nephritis complicates *Y. pseudotuberculosis* infection in up to 14% of patients although prognosis of these patients generally is good.[41] *Y. pseudotuberculosis* infection occasionally leads to postinfectious sequelae such as reactive arthritis and erythema nodosum. *Y. pseudotuberculosis* serotype O:3 has been associated particularly with reactive arthritis and a severe clinical outcome.[42]

Laboratory Findings and Diagnosis

Stool cultures of individuals with *Y. pseudotuberculosis*-associated pseudoappendicitis commonly are negative even though intestinal infection must have preceded spread to mesenteric nodes. Culture of mesenteric nodes removed at appendectomy can be positive. Cold enrichment of stool cultures appears to enhance recovery of *Y. pseudotuberculosis*, as does culture use of CIN agar. Identification of *Y. pseudotuberculosis* from food products and environmental sources using solely biochemical reactions can be misleading and serotyping or molecular methods for virulence determinants should be used.[43] Although 21 serotypes of *Y. pseudotuberculosis* have been identified, 80% of human cases are due to O-group I. Several PCR assays have been developed to characterize *Y. pseudotuberculosis* in clinical, food, and environmental samples, alone or in conjunction with genes for *Y. enterocolitica* or *Y. pestis*.

Treatment

Recovery from *Y. pseudotuberculosis* infection can occur without specific therapy. *Y. pseudotuberculosis* generally is susceptible to ampicillin, aminoglycosides, cephalosporins, trimethoprim-sulfamethoxazole, tetracycline, and chloramphenicol. Optimal antibiotic treatment of the rare patient with septicemia is unclear. Mortality from *Y. pseudotuberculosis* septicemia is 75% despite the use of an antimicrobial agent effective in vitro.

Prevention

There is no practical way to prevent sporadic cases of this rare disease; outbreaks can be managed through careful epidemiologic

---

Key Points. Epidemiology, Clinical Manifestations, Diagnosis, and Management of *Yersinia enterocolitica* and *Yersinia pseudotuberculosis* Infections

EPIDEMIOLOGY

- Yersiniosis is a zoonotic gastrointestinal disease
- Contact with pork is a risk factor
- Infections tend to cluster during winter months
- Highest incidence:
  - *Y. enterocolitica:* children <5 years of age
  - *Y. pseudotuberculosis:* children 5 to 15 years of age

CLINICAL MANIFESTATIONS

- Most commonly:
  - *Y. enterocolitica:* febrile enterocolitis
  - *Y. pseudotuberculosis:* "pseudoappendicitis" and less commonly Kawasaki-like illness
- Most serious complication: bacteremia mainly in infants and immunocompromised individuals

DIAGNOSIS

- Stool culture using selective enrichment media
- Mesenteric lymph node/peritoneal fluid culture in children undergoing surgery
- PCR assays available for clinical samples, food products, and environmental samples

TREATMENT

- Benefit of antimicrobial treatment not established conclusively for immunocompetent children
- Antimicrobial therapy should be used in immunocompromised patients with enterocolitis, and patients with extraintestinal infection
- Trimethoprim-sulfamethoxazole, chloramphenicol, fluoroquinolones, aminoglycosides, tetracycline, piperacillin, and extended-spectrum cephalosporins generally are active in vitro
- Mortality from *Y. pseudotuberculosis* septicemia is 75% irrespective of antimicrobial use

investigation and intervention. Case contacts generally are at low risk and should not receive prophylactic antibiotics. Several candidate vaccines are under evaluation.

YERSINIA PESTIS

Y. pestis represents a clone that evolved from *Y. pseudotuberculosis* sometime during the past 20,000 years.[44] Three documented plague pandemics have occurred: during the 6th century, the 14th century, and the current pandemic which began in the mid-19th century. In the early decades of this pandemic, millions died in China and India.[45] Devastation of this magnitude no longer occurs, because of improved microbiologic and epidemiologic understanding, sanitation, and the development of antibiotics. Nevertheless, plague persists, mainly in underdeveloped regions.

Epidemiology

Plague, or *black death* (so-called because of the purpuric lesions associated with disseminated intravascular coagulation), has been known for centuries. Fleas transmit *Y. pestis* from domestic rats (murine plague) to humans causing bubonic plague. Plague also occurs in wild animals (sylvatic plague), such as rabbits, prairie dogs, bobcats, coyotes, ground squirrels, rock squirrels, and wild mice, representing an additional reservoir for infection.

The oriental rat flea (*Xenopsylla cheopis*) is the most efficient vector among many fleas capable of transmitting plague. A blood meal containing the bacillus clots in the flea's gut and causes intestinal obstruction. When the flea continues to feed, it regurgitates organisms into the victim's skin. Cases of human infection often occur after large numbers of infected rats have died, forcing fleas to seek other hosts. *Y. pestis* also can be transmitted via secretions leading to pneumonic plague. Primary pulmonary plague follows contact with a sick pet or another human with pulmonary infection. Because of potential infectivity by aerosol, *Y. pestis* is considered a Category A agent of bioterrorism.

Currently, plague is a disease of people living in unsanitary conditions. Although predominantly rural, there have been outbreaks among urban populations, mainly in Madagascar and Tanzania. The World Health Organization reported 12,503 human cases of plague, including 843 deaths, in 16 countries from Africa, Asia, and the Americas between 2004 and 2009. The global case-fatality rate was 6.7%. Only 4 countries reported cases of human plague every year during the period: The Demographic Republic of Congo, Madagascar, Peru and the U.S. An upward trend in the incidence of human plague has been observed starting in 2005, with a global average incidence of 2083 cases annually.[46] Human plague has seasonal variations with a peak coinciding with epizootics in which a high mortality of susceptible rodents occurs.[47] In the U.S., most cases of plague occur in New Mexico, Arizona, Colorado, Utah, and California and are associated with a sylvatic rather than murine reservoir.[48] Plague has been increasing in frequency in the U.S., mostly between May and September and among individuals <20 years of age, and associated with outdoor activities likely to bring people into contact with rodents and fleas. Off-season cases often are associated with rabbit hunting. High-risk behavior for plague includes handling and skinning of wild animals. Occasionally, fleas of a pet dog or cat are the source of infection. Cats also can develop symptomatic plague and spread infection through biting, scratching, or coughing. From 1947 to 2001, 421 cases of plague were reported to the U.S. Centers for Disease Control and Prevention (CDC); 183 (44%) were in people ≤18 years of age. Pediatric patients mainly were white non-Hispanic (51%) and Native American (35%). Most likely infective sources identified were flea bites (67%), direct contact (9%), airborne from a sick cat (<1%), and unknown (23%).[49] In 2006 in the U.S., 13 cases, with 2 deaths, were reported in the states of New Mexico, Colorado, California and Texas; the age range was 13 to 79 years, and 8 of the 13 cases occurred in females.[50]

Clinical Manifestations

Clinical syndromes associated with *Y. pestis* infection are bubonic, pneumonic, septicemic, and meningeal plague. Asymptomatic infections also occur.

Bubonic plague. Bubonic plague is the most common form of plague. Symptoms appear 2 to 10 days after a flea bite and are characterized by exquisitely tender, non-fluctuating lymphadenitis (bubo) within regional lymph nodes draining the bite area. A papule, vesicle, or ulcer at the inoculation site develops in ~25% of cases. Tenderness of the involved node is remarkable; suppuration, sometimes with drainage, occurs in ~20%. In 90% of cases, the bubo is unilateral and can be up to 10 cm in diameter. Although the onset of fever usually coincides with the lymphadenitis, fever can precede the bubo by several days. Fever occurs during BSI, is high (up to a mean 103°F/39°C) and is accompanied by chills, headache, malaise, anorexia, vomiting, myalgia, and prostration. The skin may show insect bites and scratch marks, but there is no associated ascending lymphangitis. Localized cellulitis or abscess at the flea bite site is rare. Complications include endotoxic shock and purpura/gangrene of extremities due to disseminated intravascular coagulopathy (DIC). Untreated plague has a mortality of approximately 50%.

Pneumonia. Pneumonia occurs in <16% of cases due to inhalation (primary plague pneumonia) or to hematogenous seeding associated with bubonic or septicemic plague (secondary pneumonia). Symptoms include chest pain, progressive tachypnea, dyspnea, hypoxia, and productive cough (sputum can be watery, frothy, bloody-tinged, hemorrhagic or purulent). Chest radiograph characteristically shows alveolar infiltrations and extensive bronchopneumonia; cavitation can be present. Primary plague pneumonia is characterized by a short incubation period lasting from a few hours to 2 to 3 days, with death occurring as early as the first day of symptoms. Plague pneumonia is more common and severe in patients with septicemia than in those with bubonic plague (57% versus 6%, with 71% versus 3% mortality). Rarely, pharyngeal plague can follow direct contact with infectious materials. A case of pneumonic plague can be the source of an outbreak occurring in large families. The association of aerosol transmission and severe disease of pneumonic plague provide a basis for considering *Y. pestis* a potential biological weapon.[45]

Septicemia. From 10% to 25% of plague cases manifest as primary septicemia (severe endotoxemia, hypotension, shock, and multiorgan system failure) without obvious lymph node involvement. These patients have a high mortality rate, exceeding 30% despite appropriate antimicrobial treatment.[45,49] Abdominal pain, nausea, vomiting and diarrhea can occur and confuse the initial diagnostic approach.

Meningitis. Altered mental status including lethargy, stupor, or delirium is common in bubonic plague, but meningitis tends to be a late complication, in patients receiving inadequate treatment. Meningitis is more common in children than in adults occurring in about 10% of children with plague in the U.S.[49,51]

Pediatric considerations. Most cases of plague in recent years have occurred in children (with a mild male predominance) in whom diagnosis often has been delayed. Among 183 U.S. pediatric cases from 1947 to 2001, primary clinical presentations were bubonic (91%) and septicemic plague (7%). One-third of the bubonic cases developed secondary complications (BSI, meningitis, pneumonia). In this series children were somewhat more likely than adults to manifest as bubonic plague (91% vs. 79%), develop complications (32% vs. 27%), and to die (17% vs. 14%).[49]

Laboratory Findings and Diagnosis

Rapid diagnosis can be made by staining of clinical specimens (bubo needle aspirate, cerebrospinal fluid, or sputum) with Gram, Wayson or other polychromatic or fluorescent antibody methods, by antigen detection or by PCR; confirmation is made by culture and serology. Wright–Giemsa staining of a routine blood smear can reveal the organism and is a poor prognostic sign. White blood cell count usually ranges from 10,000 to 20,000 cells/mm³. Evidence of DIC is common and renal function becomes impaired in patients developing hypotension.[52]

Y. pestis grows in routine culture media, including blood agar, within 48 hours. In children, blood cultures are positive in approximately 60% with bubonic plague and in 100% with septicemic plague. Quantitative blood culture data suggest that a bacterial density >10² organisms/mL is associated with a greater risk of hypotension and death. Cerebrospinal fluid in meningitic plague has features common to all bacterial meningitis, such as neutrophilic pleocytosis and a positive Gram stain. *Y. pestis* can be confused in the laboratory with *Enterobacter agglomerans*; not all automated test systems are programmed to identify *Y. pestis*, leading to misidentification. Clinical suspicion of plague should lead to microbiologic re-evaluation.

Rapid diagnosis is possible by detection of *Y. pestis* F1 antigen by immunofluorescence and dipstick test.[53] PCR tests that use structural genes for F1 antigen, plasminogen activator, and murine toxin have been developed.[47]

In the absence of a definite *Y. pestis* isolate, a diagnosis can be made by seroconversion (≥4-fold rise in titer) to *Y. pestis* F1 antigen by passive hemagglutination or EIA testing of paired serum specimens. Seroconversion can occur as early as 5 days but more commonly between 1 and 2 weeks after disease onset.[45]

Y. pestis is dangerous for laboratory workers (considered a hazard group 3 or P3 pathogen); laboratory personnel should be notified and all samples sent from suspected cases should be labeled as high risk and handled in a biosafety cabinet.[45]

Differential Diagnosis

The differential diagnosis of bubonic plague includes streptococcal and staphylococcal lymphadenitis, tularemia, and cat-scratch disease. Common causes of community-acquired pneumonia, as well as tularemia and hantavirus infection, should be considered in the differential diagnosis of pneumonic plague. Septicemic plague, especially in patients with purpura and peripheral gangrene, can be confused with meningococcemia or with sepsis due to other gram-negative pathogens.[49]

Treatment

Y. pestis from human cases have been susceptible universally to β-lactams, tetracycline, aminoglycosides, chloramphenicol, and fluoroquinolones. Most isolates are resistant to colistin, polymyxin B, and macrolides, including clarithromycin.[47] Plasmid-mediated multidrug resistance has been documented only in 2 human isolates.[54] The drug of choice in many countries is intramuscular streptomycin (20 to 30 mg/kg/day in 2 doses for 7 to 10 days). Gentamicin, alone or in combination with tetracycline, or doxycycline are alternative drugs of choice.[55,56] Fever resolves within 1 to 15 days (average, 6 days) after initiation of effective antimicrobial therapy. For patients in shock (for whom absorption of intramuscular streptomycin can be erratic) and for individuals with meningitis, chloramphenicol (75 to 100 mg/kg/day) is appropriate; drug levels should be monitored to avoid cardiac toxicity. In the rare older child or adult who is well enough to be managed as an outpatient, oral tetracycline is appropriate. Relapse after completion of therapy is rare despite the fact that organisms occasionally can be recovered from buboes late in therapy. Patients with pneumonic plague who do not receive therapy within 18 hours of onset of respiratory symptoms are unlikely to survive. Mortality ranges from 50% to 90% for untreated bubonic plague, and approaches 100% for untreated pneumonic and septicemic plague. With effective antibiotic therapy, the case-fatality rate can be as low as 5% for bubonic plague but is ≥30% for septicemic plague.[57] Intravenous fluids for correction of shock and dehydration usually are required as part of initial management of plague. Corticosteroid therapy is not indicated, and heparin has been of no proven value for treatment of associated DIC.

Because plague is highly contagious, *Y. pestis* is considered a Category A agent of biologic warfare.[58] Children exposed to individuals with symptoms suggesting plague (particularly plague pneumonia) can be given prophylaxis with doxycycline (2.2 mg/kg twice daily), trimethoprim-sulfamethoxazole (8 to 12 mg/kg of the trimethoprim component twice daily), ciprofloxacin (15 to 20 mg/kg twice daily), or, if necessary, chloramphenicol (25 mg/kg every 6 hours) for 7 days.[59,60] Doxycycline or ciprofloxacin is recommended for mass treatment of prophylaxis after a potential bioterrorism event.[58]

Prevention

People living in plague-endemic areas should take measures to decrease rat and flea exposures. Use of an insect repellent containing *N,N*-dietheylmethyltoluamide applied to the legs and ankles is helpful if exposure is likely. Care in handling of dead animals is important. Insecticides and rat control are useful in prevention of murine plague. Flea control for pet dogs and cats is important. Public health officials should be notified when a case of plague is diagnosed in order to assist in managing environmental reservoirs and vectors.

Spread of plague pneumonia is best prevented by early diagnosis and initiation of appropriate therapy, and strict isolation (including droplet precautions) for patients in whom plague is suspected for several days after initiation of appropriate therapy. Contacts of individuals with plague pneumonia should receive tetracycline prophylactically for 7 days. Microbiology laboratory personnel should be alerted when receiving samples possibly containing plague bacillus in order to exercise extreme caution in handling.

Live attenuated and killed whole cell vaccines against *Y. pestis* have been available for many years, but they have a number of shortcomings including unproven effectiveness. New candidate vaccines are being evaluated, mainly subunit vaccines based on the F1 and LcrV antigens.[61] The potential use of *Y. pestis* for bioterrorism emphasizes the need to develop more effective vaccines against airborne infection.

Key Points. Epidemiology, Clinical Manifestations, Diagnosis, and Management of *Yersinia pestis* Infection

EPIDEMIOLOGY

- *Y. pestis* causes *bubonic plague* or *pneumonic plague* when acquired through a flea bite or aerosol aspiration, respectively
- Plague is a disease especially in poor people in contact with rodents particularly in endemic countries in Africa, Asia, and the Americas

CLINICAL MANIFESTATIONS

- Bubonic plague
  - The most common form of plague; symptoms appear 2 to 10 days after a flea bite
  - Symptoms: bubo (exquisitely tender, non-fluctuating lymphadenitis), high fever, headache, malaise, anorexia, vomiting, myalgia, and prostration
  - Complications: endotoxic shock and purpura/gangrene of extremities
- Pneumonic plague
  - Primary or secondary pneumonia occurs through inhalation or hematogenous seeding, respectively
  - Symptoms: chest pain, progressive tachypnea, dyspnea, hypoxia and productive cough (sputum can be watery, frothy, bloody-tinged, hemorrhagic or purulent)

Key Points. Epidemiology, Clinical Manifestations, Diagnosis, and Management of *Yersinia pestis* Infection—cont'd

– Chest radiograph: alveolar infiltrates and extensive bronchopneumonia with cavities
– Aerosol transmission combined with a high potential for severe disease make *Y. pestis* a potential biologic weapon
• Septicemic plague
  – The sole clinical manifestation in 10% of plague cases
  – Symptoms: hypotension, shock, and multiorgan system failure. Abdominal pain, nausea, vomiting and diarrhea
• Meningitic plague
  – Late complication in patients receiving inadequate treatment for bubonic plague
  – More common in children compared with adults
  – Symptoms: altered mental status including lethargy, stupor, or delirium

DIAGNOSIS

• Characteristic bipolar-staining coccobacilli in bubo aspirate, cerebrospinal fluid or sputum using Wright–Giemsa or Wayson stain
• Rapid diagnosis: antigen detection tests and PCR

TREATMENT

• Susceptible in vitro to β-lactams, tetracycline, aminoglycosides, chloramphenicol, and fluoroquinolones
• Drugs of choice: intramuscular streptomycin; gentamicin, alone or in combination with tetracycline; doxycycline
• Chloramphenicol should be considered for patients in shock or with meningitis
• Mortality ranges from 50% to 100% for untreated plague, 5% for treated bubonic plague, and ≥30% for treated septicemic plague

---

149 *Acinetobacter* Species

Dwight A. Powell and Mario J. Marcon

MICROBIOLOGY AND EPIDEMIOLOGY

Acinetobacter spp. are nonmotile, oxidase-negative, catalase-positive, strictly aerobic, gram-negative coccobacilli. Their inability to ferment glucose or to reduce nitrate clearly separates these organisms from the family Enterobacteriaceae. The genus *Acinetobacter* was formerly placed within the family Neisseriaceae, but it is now located in the family Moraxellaceae along with the *Moraxella*, *Psychrobacter*, and other genera.[1–5]

There are currently at least 25 DNA homology groups or genospecies in the genus *Acinetobacter* with species names assigned to 11, and differential biochemical and growth tests published for at least 19. These include *Acinetobacter calcoaceticus* (genospecies 1), *A. baumannii* (genospecies 2), *A. haemolyticus* (genospecies 4), *A. junii* (genospecies 5), *A. johnsonii* (genospecies 7), *A. lwoffii* (genospecies 8), and *A. radioresistens* (genospecies 12).[1–5] Most of the other genospecies cannot be separated easily with conventional biochemical tests or commercial identification systems. Isolates of *A. calcoaceticus, A. baumannii,* and genospecies 3 and 13 strains are capable of utilizing glucose oxidatively. It has been suggested that these biochemically similar, saccharolytic species should be reported as "*Acinetobacter calcoaceticus–A. baumannii* group" organisms; however, this classification is not totally satisfactory due to the increased clinical significance of *A. baumannii* in a variety of human infections. Indeed it has been suggested that *A. calcoaceticus* is unlikely to be a significant human pathogen. Thus it is probably best to use the term "*A. baumannii* group" to refer to this organism and related genospecies 3 and 13 strains only. Similarly, nonglucose-oxidizing isolates of *A. lwoffii, A. johnsonii,* and *A. junii* may be reported as "nonsaccharolytic *Acinetobacter* spp." Most nonhemolytic, glucose-oxidizing clinical isolates are *A. baumannii,* and most nonhemolytic, glucose-nonoxidizing clinical isolates are *A. lwoffii.* Most hemolytic isolates of *Acinetobacter* spp. are *A. haemolyticus.*[1–5] Older literature includes references to two subspecies of *Acinetobacter calcoaceticus* – subsp. *anitratus* and subsp. *lwoffi* – but these names have no official standing in bacterial nomenclature. More definitive identification methods based on DNA relatedness will help to further clarify the importance of the various *Acinetobacter* spp. in human disease.

Acinetobacter spp. can be isolated readily from clinical material on blood, chocolate, and usually MacConkey agar; however, some fastidious strains grow poorly or not at all on the latter medium. Colonies first appear as small and nonpigmented on blood and chocolate agars, and as colorless, light-pink or purplish colonies on MacConkey agar. On Gram stain, *Acinetobacter* are short, plump coccobacilli or rods, sometimes resembling *Moraxella* or *Neisseria* spp. but distinguished easily by their lack of cytochrome oxidase activity. In addition, some cells can hold the crystal violet of Gram staining and appear as "staphylococcal-like" gram-positive cocci. This latter characteristic also can be seen in smears prepared directly from clinical material or from positive blood culture bottles.

There are limited data on virulence factors associated with *A. baumannii* and other *Acinetobacter* spp.; virulence factors that have been described are not unique to this genus. Factors include capsular polysaccharides, protein adhesins, proteolytic and lipolytic enzymes, factors associated with boil formation, and lipopolytic lipopolysaccharide.[1,5] *A. baumannii* has limited virulence in animal models of peritonitis and pneumonia; virulence is potentiated in models of mixed infection.[1] Notwithstanding, *A. baumannii* has emerged as an important pathogen of healthcare-associated infections (HAIs) worldwide, partly due to its ability to (1) survive for prolonged periods in the hospital environment, (2) resist inactivation by disinfectants, and (3) acquire resistance to a wide variety of antibiotics.

Acinetobacter spp. are found in a wide variety of environmental sources, including water, soil, foods, and arthropods, and can survive on dry surfaces much longer than other bacteria associated with HAIs.[6,7] Unlike most other gram-negative bacilli, *Acinetobacter* also are capable of colonizing both dry and moist areas of healthy human skin. In one study of skin and mucous membranes, up to 43% of nonhospitalized individuals were colonized with *Acinetobacter* spp., with *A. lwoffii, A. johnsonii,* and *A. junii* being the most common species detected.[8] Interestingly, *A. baumannii* uncommonly colonized healthy human skin and it was recovered infrequently from environmental sources outside the hospital; its natural habitat has yet to be determined.[5]

Acinetobacter spp. often are associated with opportunistic HAIs, in hospital and home care settings. In one large North American study including pediatric and adult patients, *A. baumannii* (54%), "*A. anitratus*" (15%), and *A. calcoaceticus* (15%) were the species most often isolated.[9] In a study of *Acinetobacter* spp. bloodstream infection (BSI) in a children's hospital, the most common species recovered were *A. baumannii* (44%) and *A. lwoffii* (39%).[10] While many pediatric infections due to *Acinetobacter* spp. are nosocomial in origin, this study found that children with *Acinetobacter* spp. BSIs were significantly more likely to develop their infection in the home setting. Most patients had indwelling central venous catheters, and exposure to water or soil was thought to be the major risk factor for infection.[10]

Following admission to the hospital and particularly to an intensive care unit (ICU), the rate of colonization with *Acinetobacter* spp. of the skin, oral mucosa, and gastrointestinal tract increases rapidly. Hospital reservoirs include tap water, sinks, room humidifiers, water baths, air conditioners, tap water aerators, respiratory care equipment, dusty filters, and the skin of hospital personnel. All these sources have been implicated as reservoirs in specific nosocomial outbreaks.[11-13] Contaminated parenteral solutions have been identified as the clear source point for infection in other cases.[14] Patient-to-patient transmission of *A. baumannii* probably occurs via transient colonization and spread from the hands of healthcare personnel (HCP).

Acinetobacter spp. are considered pathogens of low virulence, causing opportunistic infections only in individuals with compromised immune status or with an indwelling device or both. Of the top 10 organisms causing HA-BSI in U.S. hospitals from 1995 to 2002, *Acinetobacter* spp. ranked tenth in incidence (0.6/10,000 admissions) but second in crude mortality (34%).[15] In two SENTRY surveillance studies of pediatric blood, urine, pulmonary or wound infections covering the periods 1998–2003 and 2004, *Acinetobacter* spp. accounted for 1.8% of all pathogenic isolates.[16,17] Risk factors for *Acinetobacter* infection included the use of intravenous devices and urinary tract catheters, immunosuppression, admission to an ICU or burn unit, respiratory failure at ICU admission, previous antimicrobial therapy, diabetes mellitus, and chronic lung disease.[18-20] In a report of the National Nosocomial Infections Surveillance System of the Centers for Disease Control and Prevention (CDC) between 1992 and 1997, *Acinetobacter* spp. accounted for the following percentages of total infections among patients in pediatric ICUs: 2% of BSIs, 3% of pneumonia, 3% of lower respiratory infections other than pneumonia, and <1% of urinary tract or surgical site infections.[21] Other pediatric infections cited during this reporting period included endocarditis, meningitis after neurosurgical infections, and peritonitis.

Because of the widespread distribution of these organisms in nature and on human skin, *Acinetobacter* spp. can be recovered in culture from blood or other specimen types as contaminating or colonizing organisms, thus complicating the interpretation of such positive cultures.

CLINICAL MANIFESTATIONS

The clinical manifestations of *Acinetobacter* BSI are not unique. In infants, temperature instability, central apnea, and thrombocytopenia can occur.[14] In a study of 29 episodes of *Acinetobacter* spp. BSI in children with cancer, 11 episodes were polymicrobial and only 3 occurred in children with an absolute neutrophil count <500/mm³. Risk of infection was associated with osteosarcoma, presence of an intravascular catheter, and recent chemotherapy treatments. There were few manifestations of gram-negative septicemia other than fever and malaise, and none of the children developed septic shock.[22]

In a review of 25 patients including 5 children with nosocomial meningitis due to *Acinetobacter* spp. after neurosurgery, fever and signs or symptoms of central nervous system infection were noted in most patients.[23] The average cerebrospinal fluid white blood cell count was 5700/mm³ with 90% neutrophils. *A. lwoffii* was more commonly associated with meningitis that other *Acinetobacter* spp. Risk factors for *Acinetobacter* spp. meningitis in infants included presence of ventriculoperitoneal shunt, previous neurosurgery, and central nervous system abnormalities.[24]

Most cases of suspected or confirmed pediatric pneumonia due to *Acinetobacter* spp. are HAIs in intubated children. Clinical manifestations are indistinguishable from pneumonia due to other gram-negative organisms. It is often difficult to determine the precise pathologic role of *Acinetobacter* spp. in such cases because colonization of the upper respiratory tract with *Acinetobacter* spp. and other gram-negative bacilli is not uncommon in such intubated patients and tracheal aspirates often submitted for culture may be contaminated with organisms colonizing the upper respiratory tract. Quantified recovery of *Acinetobacter* spp. from specimens collected by bronchoalveolar lavage is more meaningful in defining infection versus colonization. Mortality from pneumonia due to *Acinetobacter* spp. in ventilated patients may be as high as 23% to 73%.[25]

Urinary tract and wound infections due to *Acinetobacter* spp. are relatively uncommon in children and usually occur in patients with hematologic malignancies, neonates, or those with neurologic disorders and bladder dysfunction.[26] *Acinetobacter junii* has been reported to be a rare cause of BSI and ocular infection in pediatric patients.[27,28]

TREATMENT

Antimicrobial susceptibility of *Acinetobacter* spp. varies widely among institutions and countries; however, the emergence of multidrug-resistant strains of *A. baumannii* is a worldwide problem.[29,30] Mechanisms of resistance include production of inactivating enzymes, including broad-spectrum β-lactamases and aminoglycoside-modifying enzymes; alteration of penicillin-binding proteins; alterations of DNA gyrase and topoisomerase IV, the target sites for quinolone antibiotics; decreased permeability of the outer membrane to β-lactam antibiotics; and overexpression of efflux pumps.[30]

All strains of *A. baumannii* harbor chromosomally encoded AmpC-type enzymes, referred to as *Acinetobacter*-derived cephalosporinases, somewhat analogous to AmpC enzymes found in *Enterobacter* spp. and other Enterobacteriaceae.[5] Overexpression of these enzymes results in resistance to extended-spectrum cephalosporins, but cefepime and carbapenem antibiotics retain activity. A wide variety of extended spectrum β-lactamases (ESBLs) also can be found in *Acinetobacter* spp.; these enzymes appear to be similar to ESBLs found in *Klebsiella* spp. and other Enterobacteriaceae and also in *Pseudomonas aeruginosa*. Perhaps most importantly, *A. baumannii* can carry OXA-type serine carbapenemases and metallo-carbapenemases, but KPC-type serine carbapenemases such as are found in *Klebsiella* spp. and other Enterobacteriaceae have not been found in *A. baumannii*.[5]

In a U.S. report on pediatric BSIs, *Acinetobacter* spp. in vitro susceptibility to the following agents was: 53% to cefotaxime, 71% to ceftazidime, 97% to imipenem, 90% to ticarcillin-clavulanate, 93% to trimethoprim-sulfamethoxazole, and 97% to ciprofloxacin.[10] A similar percentage of susceptible isolates was found for 84 *Acinetobacter* spp. from a North American SENTRY study of infections in children <7 years old.[16] However, healthcare outbreaks due to carbapenem-resistant strains of *Acinetobacter* spp. are reported increasingly.[30,31] In two pediatric ICUs in Thailand and Greece, 64% and 62% of *Acinetobacter* spp. were carbapenem resistant.[32,33]

Because few antibiotics remain effective in treatment of infections due to such multidrug-resistant strains, the search for new drugs and the re-evaluation of older agents has become a priority. The β-lactamase inhibitor agent sulbactam and the polymyxin antibiotic colistin have been used with some success in a limited number of nonrandomized clinical trials.[34-38] Sulbactam has both β-lactamase inhibitor activity and direct antibacterial activity against *Acinetobacter* spp. by irreversibly binding to penicillin-binding protein 2. Sulbactam has been shown to have excellent in vitro activity against *Acinetobacter* spp. and to be effective in treating *Acinetobacter* infections. In vitro synergy with meropenem has also been demonstrated.[36] Ampicillin-sulbactam is more active than ticarcillin-clavulanate or piperacillin-tazobactam and was more effective than polymyxins for the treatment of infections due to multidrug-resistant (including carbapenem-resistant) *Acinetobacter* spp.[34,35] Several uncontrolled studies of intravenous colistin for treatment of multidrug-resistant *Acinetobacter* spp. infections appear to demonstrate effectiveness and safety.[37,38] Both minocycline and tigecycline, a new semisynthetic derivative of minocycline, have in vitro activity against *A. baumannii*, but clinical efficacy data are limited, particularly in pediatrics.[39]

Although both disk diffusion and dilution minimum inhibitory concentration (MIC) methods of susceptibility testing are recommended for *Acinetobacter* spp. by the Clinical and Laboratory Standards Institute (CLSI), differences between the categorical interpretations of these two methods against select β-lactam agents have been reported.[40,41] There also are differences between gradient agar diffusion E-test MIC versus broth microdilution MIC for *Acinetobacter* spp. against the polymyxins. Furthermore, there are no CLSI disk diffusion or MIC breakpoints for tigecycline against *Acinetobacter* spp. It is also important to note that discordance in susceptibilities between carbapenems is increasingly described; thus one cannot equate susceptibilities of imipenem, meropenem, and doripenem.[42]

The current approach to treating serious, deep-seated infection involving *Acinetobacter* spp. should include an effective cephalosporin, carbapenem, or penicillin/β-lactamase inhibitor combination agent with the addition of an aminoglycoside. Contaminated indwelling devices should be removed. The use of prolonged infusion times, increased drug doses, and altered routes of administration such as nebulized therapy for pulmonary infections may be helpful in treatment of infections due to *Acinetobacter* spp. resistant to all available antibiotics.[30,41] Prevention of *Acinetobacter* spp. infections requires judicious use of medical devices and antimicrobial agents and meticulous adherence of HCP to infection control practices.

150 *Aeromonas* Species

Miguel O'Ryan and Yalda C. Lucero Alvarez

DESCRIPTION OF THE PATHOGEN

The genus *Aeromonas* consists of environmental, facultatively anaerobic, mesophilic, gram-negative bacilli that are predominantly motile due to a single polar flagellum, and which produce oxidase, catalase, nitrate reductase, and an array of exoenzymes. Although there are at least 21 species described in this genus, only *A. hydrophila*, *A. caviae*, *A. veronii* biovar *sobria*, and *A. trota* are important human pathogens.[1,2]

Aeromonads can produce a variety of potential virulence factors, including heat-stable and heat-labile enterotoxins, hemolysins, proteases, leukocidin, elastase, fibrinolysin, DNase, lecithinase, lipases, amylase, adhesins, agglutinins, pili, and an array of outer membrane proteins.[1,3,4] Reports of endemic diarrhea associated with *Aeromonas* suggest that clinical severity is related to expression of a specific combination of enterotoxins.[1,5]

EPIDEMIOLOGY

Aeromonas spp. are ubiquitous organisms that can be isolated from almost any environmental niche. Most environmental isolates come from fresh or brackish water sources; contamination of chlorinated tap water has been reported. *Aeromonas* spp. colonize and can cause disease in cold-blooded animals, including fish, amphibians, and reptiles, which may act as reservoirs.[1,6,7] Humans acquire infection most frequently during warm weather months, through contaminated food or water, unpasteurized milk, red meats, poultry, vegetables, fish, or other seafoods, or by swimming/bathing in contaminated bodies of water.[1,6–8]

Aeromonas disease burden is difficult to determine due to underreporting and lack of routine diagnosis. Specific diagnostic tests are required to differentiate pathogenic species from normal flora and other pathogenic gram-negative bacilli such as *Vibrio* spp. and *Plesiomona* spp.[1,2,8] Asymptomatic fecal carriage is observed in approximately 1% to 2% of healthy people residing in nontropical regions and in up to 27% of healthy adults residing in tropical areas of Asia.[5,9,10]

The first report of a human *Aeromonas* infection occurred in 1954 in a woman from Jamaica with myositis. In 1961, *Aeromonas* spp. were first isolated from human feces. Since then *Aeromonas* spp. have been incriminated as agents of diarrhea although unequivocal evidence of their pathogenic role in the intestine remains controversial.[5,11] *Aeromonas* have been implicated in 1% to 13% and 2% to 7% of endemic diarrhea in children and adults,

respectively. These pathogens also have been associated with 1% to 4% of travelers' diarrhea, especially in people traveling to Southeast Asia.[1]

A prospective multicenter, 6-month hospital surveillance study in France reported 78 *Aeromonas* spp. associated infections of which 44% were skin and soft-tissue infections, 26% bacteremia, 19% gastroenteritis, 6% respiratory tract infection, and 5% miscellaneous.[7]

CLINICAL MANIFESTATIONS

Gastroenteritis

Gastroenteritis is the most common clinical illness attributed to *Aeromonas* infection in humans.[5,7] Both the small and large intestine can be compromised by infection. A self-limited watery diarrhea is the most common clinical manifestation of enteritis although a cholera-like illness has been reported.[1,12–15] Fever and vomiting are common in children. One-third of patients have a dysentery-like syndrome with bloody mucoid diarrhea associated with colitis;[16] malaise and fever are more common in this presentation. In contrast to other causes of dysenteric bacterial gastroenteritis, stool leukocytes are uncommon. Chronic or intermittent diarrhea lasting for weeks has been described in one-third of patients infected by *A. caviae*.[1,16] Reported complications include bacteremia, intussusception, failure to thrive, hemolytic-uremic syndrome, and strangulated intestinal hernia.[1,17]

Skin and Soft-Tissue Infections

Skin and deep soft tissue are the second most common anatomic sites associated with *Aeromonas* infections. *A. hydrophila* is the most common species associated with tissue infections, with an incidence peaking during the warmer months. Major predisposing factors are local trauma occurring in people during recreational swimming, exposure to contaminated water in occupational or recreational activities, and shark or reptile bites. Soft-tissue infection also has been reported in patients immersed in water immediately after being burned, and more rarely after folk or standard medical procedures such as medicinal leech therapy and gastrointestinal tract surgery.[1,7,15]

Cellulitis develops 8 to 48 hours after trauma, followed by a rapid spread to deep tissues. The clinical spectrum includes localized skin nodules, soft-tissue abscess, furunculosis, ecthyma gangrenosum, bullous cellulitis with crepitance, synergistic necrotizing cellulitis, and myonecrosis. *Aeromonas* soft-tissue infection can mimic cellulitis caused by group A streptococcus, *Clostridium* species, and ecthyma gangrenosum caused by *Pseudomonas aeruginosa*.[1,18,19]

Septicemia

Septicemia is the most serious and life-threatening complication of *Aeromonas* infection. Septicemia occurs primarily in immunocompromised patients, especially people with hematologic malignancies, hepatobiliary conditions, and malnutrition.[20–22] Cases are reported increasingly in immunocompetent hosts, and associated with burns, penetrating trauma, and recreational or professional activities with exposure to contaminated water.[1,7]

A. hydrophila is the predominant species in patients with mild to moderate underlying illness while *A. caviae* is more commonly isolated in patients with severe underlying illness, often associated with polymicrobial septicemia. Although most cases are community acquired, nosocomial bloodstream infection (BSI) occurs in patients with cancer.

Aeromonas bloodstream infection (BSI) occurs throughout the year, with a higher incidence in warmer months. Clinical presentation is similar to that caused by other gram-negative bacilli, including fever (74% to 89%), jaundice (57%), abdominal pain (16% to 45%), septic shock (40% to 45%), and dyspnea (12% to 24%). Diarrhea immediately preceding or concurrent with the onset of BSI is uncommon (9% to 14%). Most infections are monomicrobic (60% to 76% of cases), but BSI can occur in association with *Escherichia coli*, *Klebsiella pneumoniae*, and *Staphylococcus aureus*. A secondary focus of infection in ascitic fluid, bile, wounds, or urine can be found in up to 25% of patients.[1,7,8,20–22]

BSI-associated mortality is high, ranging from 5% to 60%, depending on the underlying condition. Poor prognosis has been associated with altered consciousness, septic shock, underlying liver cirrhosis and cancer, persistent BSI, community-acquired focal infection, or secondary bacteremia.

Uncommon Clinical Presentations

Aeromonas spp. rarely have been associated with a variety of other systemic and local infections including intra-abdominal infections (peritonitis, pancreatitis, cholangitis, hepatic abscesses), pneumonia (aspiration associated with a near-drowning episode), lung abscess, endophthalmitis, tonsillitis, otitis media, urinary tract infection, endocarditis, meningitis, osteomyelitis, pyogenic arthritis, and suppurative thrombophlebitis.[1,7,15,23]

LABORATORY FINDINGS AND DIAGNOSIS

Gastroenteritis can be associated with abnormalities of acid–base and renal function; white blood cell count and serum C-reactive protein level can be mildly elevated.[1,7] In skin and soft-tissue infections, other invasive infections, and BSI, moderate increase of leukocytes (up to 16,000 cells/mm³) and high serum C-reactive protein value (up to 15 mg/dL) is expected.[21]

Bacterial isolation is essential to support the diagnosis. Although a variety of transport media can be used for stool, specimens, Cary–Blair media is used most commonly. Samples should be transported at room temperature. *Aeromonas* grows easily on routine enteric isolation media such as MacConkey, XLD, HE, SS, and DC. Because *Aeromonas* are non-lactose fermenting, colonies can be misclassified as normal enteric flora. Use of a selective media such as sheep blood agar containing ampicillin is recommended. DNase-toluidine blue agar can be used to detect nonhemolytic and ampicillin-susceptible strains that represent <10% of pathogenic strains. Cefsulodin-irgasan-novobiocin (CIN) agar is more cost-effective, because it allows concomitant isolation of

Yersinia and *Plesiomonas* species. *Aeromonas* agar is a highly selective media that contains irgasan, and D-xylose.[1]

Aeromonas can be differentiated from other gram-negative bacilli by biochemical testing. *Aeromonas* are oxidase positive, indole positive, and urease negative. Oxidase activity helps differentiate *Aeromonas* from Enterobacteriaceae.

DNA probes have been developed for species identification, and are useful epidemiologic and environmental surveillances. Commercial PCR assays designed for detection of gram-negative bacilli have been used for *Aeromonas* characterization but major errors in genus and species identification have been reported.[24] 16S rRNA sequencing has not been useful for species discrimination, but partial sequence analysis of house-keeping genes such as *gyrB* and *rpoD* is promising for use in epidemiologic studies.[25,26]

TREATMENT

Most cases of *Aeromonas*-associated gastroenteritis are self-limited; appropriate rehydration strategies should be implemented. Antimicrobial therapy has not been proven to be useful consistently although data from uncontrolled studies suggest benefit in shortening the duration of disease.[13] Antibiotics can be recommended in patients with dysenteric illness, prolonged diarrhea (>7 days), and in immunocompromised patients. For skin and soft-tissue infections an early diagnosis, aggressive surgical debridement, and parenteral antibiotics are of utmost importance.[15,18,27] BSI must be treated with parenteral antimicrobial therapy and a thorough search for focal infections is required.

In vitro antimicrobial susceptibility testing of clinical isolates is important. Most *Aeromonas* are resistant to penicillin, ampicillin, cephalothin, vancomycin, clarithromycin, clindamycin, and carbenicillin.[1,13,14] Susceptibility to first- and second-generation cephalosporins varies among species. At least four different types of β-lactamases have been reported in *Aeromonas* species; inducible chromosomal β-lactamase is predominant. Isolates producing expanded spectrum β-lactamases have been described sporadically. Individual strains can harbor up to three different β-lactamases coordinated by a single mechanism of expression.

Most isolates are susceptible to trimethoprim-sulfamethoxazole, fluoroquinolones, aminoglycosides, tetracycline, chloramphenicol, aztreonam, imipenem, meropenem, and extended-spectrum cephalosporins including ceftriaxone, ceftazidime, and cefepime. Isolates from Asia can be resistant to tetracyclines, piperacillin, imipenem, third-generation cepholosporins, and trimethoprim-sulfamethoxazole.[1,13,14]

A 3-day treatment with TMP-SMX, azithromycin, or ceftriaxone in children and TMP-SMX, ciprofloxacin, or azithromycin in adults is recommended for treatment of *Aeromonas* gastroenteritis, but benefits of therapy are unknown. Expanded spectrum cephalosporins, carbapenem, TMP-SMX, tetracycline, or ciprofloxacin are reasonable empiric therapies for skin and soft-tissue infections and BSI. Although induction of β-lactamases in the clinical setting is rare, clinicians should monitor the patient closely for a potential relapse when using a cephalosporin for a serious *Aeromonas* infection.

PREVENTION

Aeromonas are present in fresh and brackish nonprocessed water, in fish, shellfish, meat, and fresh vegetables. Avoiding ingestion of natural source water and contaminated food especially by infants and immunocompromised patients is important. Cooking and smoking food products eliminates these organisms. Cross-contamination after processing should be avoided. Food products should be handled appropriately, i.e., storing raw and processed products separately and chilling until consumption.

Aeromonas should be considered in the management of traumatic wounds sustained in or exposed to aquatic natural environments.

151 Less Commonly Encountered Nonenteric Gram-Negative Bacilli

Michael T. Brady and Mario J. Marcon

MICROBIOLOGY AND EPIDEMIOLOGY

A number of genera of nonglucose-fermenting gram-negative rods are infrequent opportunistic human pathogens. As a group, most are nonfastidious, aerobic, catalase-positive organisms; motility, oxidase activity, and growth on MacConkey agar are variable. Those that grow on MacConkey agar typically produce colorless colonies. The organisms are widely distributed in natural environments including plant material, soil and water, as well as in the environment in healthcare facilities. Some species can colonize mammalian mucosal surfaces.[1-4] In many ways, these organisms resemble more commonly isolated *Pseudomonas* spp. including *Pseudomonas aeruginosa*. The taxonomy of these organisms continues to undergo significant change based on DNA homology studies and 16S ribosomal RNA gene sequencing. This chapter focuses on select taxonomic family groups of nonenteric gram-negative bacteria not discussed in other chapters.

Pseudomonadaceae. A number of organisms in the family Pseudomonadaceae have been reclassified. An earlier classification scheme grouped the pseudomonads into five homology groups based on similarities in 16S ribosomal RNA gene sequence. At present, only the former members of rRNA homology group I are retained in the amended genus *Pseudomonas*. The most common *Pseudomonas* spp. isolated from human clinical specimens are the fluorescent pseudomonad group organisms, *P. aeruginosa*, *P. putida*, and *P. fluorescens*. *P. stutzeri*, *P. mendocina*, *P. alcaligenes*, *P. pseudoalcaligenes*, *P. luteola*, and *P. orzyhabitans* are isolated much less frequently (see Chapter 154, *Pseudomonas* Species and Related Organisms). Both *Pseudomonas luteola* (formerly *Chryseomonas luteola*) and *P. oryzihabitans* (formerly *Flavimonas oryzihabitans*) are catalase-positive, oxidase-negative, motile, gram-negative bacilli that form yellow pigmented, often wrinkled colonies on blood and MacConkey agar. The negative oxidase reaction of these organisms is somewhat unique among *Pseudomonas* spp. *Pseudomonas luteola* can be differentiated from *P. oryzihabitans* on the basis of its ability to hydrolyze esculin and orthonitrophenyl-β-D-galactopyranoside.[3]

Ribosomal RNA homology group II organisms now are designated as *Burkholderia* spp., *Ralstonia* spp., *Cupriavidus* spp., *Pandoraea* spp., and related organisms in the family Burkholderiaceae; rRNA homology group III contains *Comamonas* spp., *Delftia* spp., and *Acidovorax* spp. in the family Comamonadaceae; rRNA homology group IV pseudomonads now are classified as *Brevundimonas* spp. in the family Caulobacteraceae; and rRNA homology group V pseudomonads are now *Stenotrophomonas* spp.[1]

Alcaligenaceae. Both *Achromobacter* and *Alcaligenes* spp., along with the closely related *Bordetella* spp., currently are grouped together within the family Alcaligenaceae. The clinically relevant *Achromobacter* and *Alcaligenes* spp. include: *Alcaligenes faecalis*, *Achromobacter piechaudii*, *Achromobacter denitrificans*, and *Achromobacter xylosoxidans*.[2,5] The first three organisms listed are asaccharolytic and biochemically similar to the *Bordetella* spp. and *Oligella ureolytica*, also members of this family.[6] *Achromobacter xylosoxidans* is saccharolytic and biochemically similar to several organisms of uncertain taxonomic position, including *Achromobacter* groups B, E, and F and *Ochrobactrum anthropi*; the former *Achromobacter* groups A, C, and D are biovars of *O. anthropi*.[7] *Ochrobactrum* spp. have been placed in the family Brucellaceae. The genus *Oligella* contains two species of clinical significance,

O. urethralis and *O. urealytica*.[6] *O. urethralis* (formerly *Moraxella urethralis*) is nonmotile and shares several characteristics with *Moraxella* spp.; it is thought to be a commensal organism of the genitourinary tract. *Oligella urealytica* is motile and biochemically similar to *Bordetella bronchiseptica*, including the property of rapid hydrolysis of urea.

Caulobacteraceae. There are a number of named *Brevundimonas* species, but only *B. diminuta* and *B. vesicularis* are of human clinical significance. These species currently are placed in the family Caulobacteraceae. All these organisms are aerobic, oxidase-positive, motile, gram-negative bacilli that can be isolated in the laboratory on blood or chocolate agar; most but not all strains also grow on MacConkey agar. Some isolates produce a yellow or tan-brown pigment.

Comamonadaceae. Current members of the family Comamonadaceae include *Comamonas testosteroni* and *C. terrigena*; *Delftia acidovorans* (formerly *Comamonas acidovorans*) and *D. tsuruhatensis*; and three Acidovorax spp. – *A. facilis*, *A. delafieldii*, and *A. temperans*.

Flavobacteriaceae. The family Flavobacteriaceae has undergone extensive revision and now contains many genera including *Chryseobacterium*, *Elizabethkingia*, *Flavobacterium*, *Weeksella*, *Bergeyella*, *Empedobacter*, and *Myroides*. *Elizabethkingia meningoseptica* (formerly *Chryseobacterium meningosepticum*; *Flavobacterium meningosepticum*), an important opportunistic pathogen of children, and *Chryseobacterium indologenes*, are the most common human isolates of this group.[1-5] *Elizabethkingia meningosepticum* produces large, smooth colonies on blood and chocolate agars within 24 hours, but most isolates of do not grow on MacConkey agar. Gram stain of growth on agar reveals long, thin rods that can be filamentous. Isolates are encapsulated and produce proteolytic enzymes including elastase, a potential virulence factor. Ribotyping has been used to demonstrate heterogenicity among strains of *E. meningoseptica*.[3] Other *Chryseobacterium* spp. produce colonies of similar appearance; some produce yellow-pigmented colonies on blood agar, but pigment production may be negative or weak, except for the deep-yellow pigment produced by *C. indologenes*.[1]

Flavobacterium breve has been reclassified as *Empedobacter brevis*. Organisms formerly classified as *F. odoratum* are now classified as two distinct species, *Myroides odoratus* and *M. odoratimimus*. *Weeksella zoohelcum* has been reclassified as *Bergeyella zoohelcum*, and *Weeksella virosa* remains as the single species in the genus. Unlike the other flavobacteria, which are environmental organisms, *W. virosa* and *B. zoohelcum* are found on mucosal surfaces of humans or other mammals.[1-5] Colonies of *W. virosa* are mucoid, adherent to agar, and may develop a tan appearance, whereas colonies of *B. zoohelcum* may be sticky and tan in appearance. Useful tests to differentiate these organisms include hydrolysis of gelatin, starch, and esculin; DNase and urease production; nitrate reduction; and susceptibility to penicillin and polymyxin B.[1-5]

Methylobacteriaceae. *Methylobacterium* spp. and *Roseomonas* spp., members of the family Methylobacteriaceae, are oxidase-positive and produce characteristic pink or coral pigmented colonies on a variety of media, including blood, Sabouraud, Thayer–Martin, and buffered charcoal–yeast extract agar. These are environmental organisms that also can be found in the healthcare environment. Colonies of *Methylobacterium* spp. generally are dry in appearance and Gram stain shows large, highly vacuolated, pleomorphic bacilli; growth on MacConkey agar above 40°C usually is negative. In contrast, colonies of *Roseomonas* spp. are mucoid in culture and show non-vacuolated, coccoid bacilli on Gram stain; these organisms usually grow on MacConkey agar at temperatures up to 42°C.[3]

Rhizobiaceae. *Rhizobium* spp. *and Agrobacterium* spp. are members of the family Rhizobiaceae and are natural inhabitants of soil and are well-known pathogens of plants. *Rhizobium radiobacter* (formerly *Agrobacterium radiobacter; A. tumefaciens*) is the only medically important species in the family.[8] Colonies of the organism can appear mucoid and pink on MacConkey agar, resembling colonies of *Klebsiella* spp.

Sphingomonadaceae. The family Sphingomonadaceae contains a number of species but only two species are considered of human clinical significance, *Sphingomonas paucimobilis* (formerly *Pseudomonas paucimobilis*) and *S. parapaucimobilis. S. paucimobilis* is slow-growing and produces yellow colonies; however, in contrast to *Sphingobacterium* spp., most isolates of *S. paucimobilis* are urease-negative and susceptible to polymyxin B.[2]

Sphingobacteriaceae. The family Sphingobacteriaceae contains a number of former *Flavobacterium* spp., but only two species are considered of human clinical significance, *Sphingobacterium multivorum* and *S. spiritivorum. Sphingobacterium* spp. generally are yellow pigmented, urease-positive, and resistant to polymyxin B; this latter property is shared with *Burkholderia* spp., *Chryseobacterium* spp., and a few other genera of nonfermentative gram-negative bacilli.[2]

Shewanellaceae. There are over 20 species in the genus *Shewanella*, family Shewanellaceae, but only *S. putrefaciens* and *S. algae* are thought to be of clinical importance. *S. algae* is a halophilic and asaccharolytic organism and thought to be the more common human isolate, while *S. putrefaciens* is non-halophilic and saccharolytic and more commonly isolated from the environment. Among nonfermentative gram-negative bacilli, these organisms have the unique property of producing hydrogen sulfide in Kligler or triple sugar iron agar.[2]

CLINICAL MANIFESTATIONS AND TREATMENT

As a group, these organisms are opportunistic pathogens that cause relatively few human infections. Most infections occur in individuals with underlying medical conditions and/or with indwelling medical devices. In addition, for many organisms, there are no standardized and recommended methods for in vitro antimicrobial susceptibility testing. Thus, patient management should rest on clinical experience and published literature. If in vitro testing is performed as an aid to guide patient management, it should be done by a dilution method to establish a minimum inhibitory concentration. An in vitro test result of "resistant" indicates likely treatment failure, but a result of "susceptible" may not predict treatment success.

Acidovorax, Brevundimonas, Comamonas, and *Delftia* spp.

Acidovorax spp. typically are plant pathogens and infections are extremely rare in humans. Single cases of bloodstream infection (BSI) and implanted port/catheter-related infections have been reported.[9,10] *Brevundimonas vesicularis* BSI has been reported in a patient undergoing hemodialysis and in a patient with sickle-cell disease; *B. diminuta* also has been associated with BSI and vascular catheter infections primarily in patients with cancer[11] as well as peritonitis in patients undergoing chronic ambulatory peritoneal dialysis (CAPD),[12] septic arthritis,[13] and cutaneous infections[14] in immunocompetent individuals. *Comomonas testosteroni* infections commonly are polymicrobial and occur most often in the abdomen including following perforation of the appendix.[15] *C. testosteroni* has been reported to cause catheter-associated BSI,[16,17] endocarditis,[18,19] and meningitis in a patient with recurrent cholesteatoma.[20] *Delftia acidovorans* has caused catheter-associated BSI, endocarditis associated with intravenous drug

use, conjunctivitis, and otitis externa.[21-24] *Delftia tsuruhatensis* has caused catheter-associated BSI.[25] Antibiotic susceptibility of this group of organisms is variable, but most isolates are susceptible to broad-spectrum cephalosporins, carbapenems, and fluoroquinolones; however, *B. diminuta* is intrinsically resistant to fluoroquinolones[11] and susceptibility to aminoglycosides is variable.

Achromobacter and *Alcaligenes* spp.

Achromobacter and *Alcaligenes* spp. are opportunistic human pathogens causing sporadic cases of pneumonia, septicemia, peritonitis, urinary tract and other infections.[26-29] *Achromobacter xylosoxidans* and *Alcaligenes faecalis* are the most common isolates and agents of human disease in these genera, but little is known about factors promoting virulence. BSI, meningitis, and pneumonia are among the most common forms of infection, although these organisms have been recovered from many other sites including peritoneal fluid in CAPD, joint fluid, bone, and urine.[26-30] Infections have been associated with contaminated medical supplies and devices, such as transducers, topical medications, nuclear medicine tracers, deionized water used for hemodialysis, and fluids from incubators and humidifiers.[28,29] In individuals with cancer, the gastrointestinal tract can be the source of infection.[27] *Achromobacter xylosoxidans*, which has been isolated from blood and cerebrospinal fluid of neonates with nosocomial infection, rarely has been associated with maternal BSI.[28,31] *A. xylosoxidans* has been recovered from bone cultures after penetrating nail injury in older children.[26] Clinical illness due to *A. xylosoxidans* BSI is indistinguishable from that of other gram-negative bacilli.[32] Intravascular catheters frequently are a predisposing factor to infection, but neutropenia is not a major risk factor.[27]

Achromobacter xylosoxidans and *Alcaligenes faecalis* have been shown to colonize the respiratory tract of intubated children and patients with cystic fibrosis.[30] *A. xylosoxidans* can be isolated as a "late colonizer" in up to 8.7% of patients with cystic fibrosis and can contribute to exacerbation of pulmonary disease,[33,34] and has been reported as a cause of lymphadenitis in patients with chronic granulomatous disease[35] and hyper-immunoglobulin M syndrome.[36]

The antimicrobial susceptibility pattern of these organisms is variable.[27,37] Isolates of *Achromobacter xylosoxidans* and *Alcaligenes faecalis* produce several types of β-lactamases that hydrolyze a variety of the penicillins and cephalosporins. Ceftazidime generally retains good in vitro activity against *A. xylosoxidans*; meropenem and trimethoprim-sulfamethoxazole typically also are active. Resistance to the aminoglycosides and aztreonam is expected; activity of ureidopenicillins, ticarcillin-clavulanic acid, and the fluoroquinolones is variable. Monotherapy is probably sufficient in most cases of infection, but two agents may be required to eradicate the organism in severe, deep-seated infections such as endocarditis. Removal of contaminated venous catheter or other device often is necessary to clear infections.

Rhizobium radiobacter

Virtually all reported cases of human infections due to members of the Rhizobiaceae family are of *Rhizobium radiobacter* and have occurred in immunocompromised hosts or in patients with medical devices, especially central venous catheters (CVCs), CAPD catheters, or implanted biomedical prostheses.[38-46] The ability of this organism to adhere to silicone and other inert surfaces may explain the associations. About 20% of cases of human infections have occurred in individuals 16 years of age or younger. More than 50% of these cases required antibiotic therapy and removal of the device for resolution. In addition to infections associated with medical devices, *Rhizobium radiobacter* has caused native valve endocarditis and urinary tract infection.[38-46]

The antimicrobial susceptibility pattern of *R. radiobacter* is variable. Many isolates are multiply resistant to various classes of antimicrobial agents because of production of antibiotic-inactivating enzymes. Most strains are inhibited by broad-spectrum cephalosporins including ceftriaxone but not ceftazidime, gentamicin but not tobramycin, and trimethoprim-sulfamethoxazole; piperacillin-tazobactam, ciprofloxacin, and carbapenems usually also have activity. While *R. radiobacter* infections are typically of low virulence, the variable antibiotic susceptibility and lack of optimal therapeutic regimens makes them difficult to treat.[38–40]

Chryseobacterium, Elizabethkingia, Bergeyella, Weeksella, Myroides, and *Empedobacter* spp.

Members of the genera *Chryseobacterium, Elizabethkingia, Bergeyella, Weeksella, Myroides,* and *Empedobacter* spp., all once classified as *Flavobacterium* spp., have been responsible for infrequent human infections. *Elizabethkingia* (formerly *Flavobacterium*) *meningoseptica* is the species of greatest medical importance among these organisms. Although this organism has been recovered from patients with community-acquired infections, it is most frequently an opportunistic nosocomial pathogen of infants 3 months of age or younger. Infection in this age group accounts for >75% of reported cases.[47,48] *Elizabethkingia meningoseptica* has caused numerous outbreaks of neonatal infection, especially BSI and meningitis.[49] Approximately one-half of reported cases of meningitis due to *E. meningoseptica* in neonates have occurred in nursery outbreaks.[50] Outbreaks have been associated with contamination of solutions and equipment in the hospital environment, including containers of antiseptic solutions, vials of intravenous drugs, chlorinated water sources, and respiratory care equipment.[50]

Infants become colonized with *E. meningoseptica* in the nose, throat, or gastrointestinal tract before development of invasive infection. The clinical course of BSI or meningitis is similar to that of other gram-negative bacilli; meningitis can have either an early or late onset. The onset of disease can be insidious, and cerebrospinal fluid (CSF) evaluation can be unremarkable initially.[49] Morbidity and mortality rates from neonatal meningitis due to *E. meningoseptica* are high; the mortality rate is more than 50%, and survivors frequently have severe neurologic sequelae, including hydrocephalus. A significant association exists between the development of hydrocephalus and administration of intrathecal antibiotics or positive results of CSF cultures for greater than 10 days.[49]

Elizabethkingia meningoseptica rarely causes infection beyond the neonatal period in an immunocompetent host, but infections in immunocompromised individuals occur as outbreaks in intensive care units or as isolated cases.[48] In contrast to infection in neonates, pneumonia is the most common presentation outside of the neonatal period, accounting for 40% of reported cases. Nosocomial infections account for >90% of cases. The mortality rate in immunocompromised patients is more than 60%. Other reported *E. meningoseptica* infections include endocarditis, ophthalmologic infections, cellulitis, pyogenic arthritis related to an elbow joint prosthesis, abdominal abscesses, and burn wound sepsis.[51] Prolonged antibiotic therapy may predispose the infection.

Although *Chryseobacterium indologenes* is the most common human isolate within this group, recovery of the organism is not always associated with infection. *C. indologenes* has been reported to cause BSI in immunocompromised patients and in those with indwelling intravascular devices.[52] *C. indologenes* also has been implicated in cases of cellulitis, bacteremia, pneumonia, meningitis, pyomyositis, and keratitis.[52–56]

Weeksella virosa has been recovered primarily from urine and urogenital tract specimens, but its clinical significance has been questioned. *Bergeyella zoohelcum* is an inhabitant of the oropharynx of dogs and cats and has been recovered in bite wound infections and in a case of meningitis that followed multiple bites.[57–60] *Bergeyella* sp. was recovered from amniotic fluid of a mother delivering a preterm infant but its significance was unclear.[61] The two current *Myroides* spp., *M. odoratus* and *M. odoratimimus*, are uncommon human isolates from urine, respiratory tract, and rarely blood. *Empedobacter brevis* also is reported rarely as an agent of human disease.

Elizabethkingia meningoseptica and other related species can be resistant to antimicrobial agents routinely prescribed for gram-negative infections including third- and fourth-generation cephalosporins, carbapenems, aztreonam, and the aminoglycosides; however, *E. meningoseptica* may test as susceptible in vitro to antimicrobial agents generally used to treat infections due to gram-positive organisms including rifampin, vancomycin, clindamycin, and erythromycin. Moreover, in vitro susceptibility test results may not correlate with clinical efficacy for this organism. Antibiotics with the most consistent in vitro activity against both *E. meningoseptica* and *C. indologenes* are minocycline, rifampin, and levofloxacin. Ciprofloxacin, trimethoprim-sulfamethoxazole, and piperacillin or piperacillin-tazobactam are less active.[48,49,62–64] Both *W. virosa* and *B. zoohelcum* are susceptible to a wide variety of antimicrobial agents. Susceptibility testing must be performed for each clinically significant isolate to guide therapy. A dilution method should be used to establish specific minimal inhibitory concentrations of potential therapeutic agents; disk diffusion susceptibility testing of *Chryseobacterium* spp. and other related agents can be unreliable.[62,63]

Optimal therapy for serious infections, including meningitis, due to *E. meningoseptica* is not well established. Several authors have identified vancomycin as the drug of choice for neonatal meningitis, although others have pointed out that vancomycin MICs are high for nearly all isolates. A study of four *E. meningoseptica* isolates recovered from neonatal CSF demonstrated synergy in vitro between vancomycin and rifampin in three of four isolates; and additive interaction between vancomycin and ciprofloxacin and antagonism between vancomycin and meropenem in all four isolates.[65] These data and several clinical cases suggest that intravenous therapy with high-dose vancomycin and rifampin may be optimal therapy for management of these infections.[65] Rifampin should not be used as monotherapy because of the potential for rapid emergence of resistance. Outside the central nervous system, minocycline for patients ≥8 years of age, trimethoprim-sulfamethoxazole, or a quinolone could be considered as treatment options, based on susceptibility testing.

Methylobacterium and *Roseomonas* spp.

Methylobacterium mesophilica and *Roseomonas gilardi* are the species most frequently isolated from humans. Both have been reported as agents of BSI, primarily in association with indwelling CVCs, hemodialysis catheters, and contaminated endoscopes. Other infections associated with these organisms include peritonitis related to CAPD, septic arthritis, endopthalmitis, cellulitis, bacteremia, keratitis, ventilator-associated pneumonia, and urinary tract infections.[66–76] These organisms generally are susceptible to carbapenems, aminoglycosides, tetracycline, and fluoroquinolones.[77–79] *Rosemonas mucosa* strains typically are more resistant than strains of *R. gilardii*.

Ochrobactrum spp.

Ochrobactrum anthropi is the most common *Ochrobactrum* sp. resulting in human disease. This organism may colonize the respiratory tract or wounds and subsequently cause a variety of opportunistic infections including primarily CVC-associated BSI, prosthetic valve endocarditis, septic arthritis, osteomyelitis, peritonitis, BSI, and meningitis.[40,80–96] Other *Ochrobactrum* spp. including *O. haematophilum* and *O. pseudogrignonense* have been isolated rarely from human clinical specimens.[97] The closely related *Achromobacter*-like groups B, E, and F organisms have been recovered most commonly from blood cultures of patients with deep CVCs.[98] Most isolates of these *Achromobacter*-like groups and *O. anthropi* are susceptible to aminoglycosides, carbapenems, fluoroquinolones, and trimethoprim-sulfamethoxazole.[99]

Oligella spp.

The two *Oligella* spp. of clinical significance, *O. urethralis* and *O. urealytica*, have been recovered primarily from the urogenital tract and rarely as agents of urosepsis or pyogenic arthritis.[100,101] *O. urethralis* has an antibiotic susceptibility pattern similar to *Moraxella* spp., including susceptibility to penicillin; the antibiotic susceptibility pattern of *O. urealytica* is variable.

Pseudomonas luteola and Pseudomonas oryzihabitans

Both *Pseudomonas luteola* and *P. oryzihabitans* are found in natural environments such as soil, water, and damp environments including rice paddies, as well as in the hospital environment in sinks and respiratory therapy equipment. Both organisms have been isolated most commonly in patients with medical devices and in people with immunosuppressive conditions.[102-107] Osteomyelitis, peritonitis, endocarditis, meningitis after a neurologic procedure, leg ulcer in a patient with sickle-cell disease, polymicrobial BSI, cellulitis, abscesses, and wound infections have also been reported.[108-113] Both *P. luteola* and *P. oryzihabitans* have caused postoperative endophthalmitis following cataract surgery.[114,115]

There are insufficient published data to recommend a treatment regimen for infections due to these organisms. *P. luteola* and *P. oryzihabitans* are susceptible to most extended-spectrum penicillins, third-generation cephalosporins, fluoroquinolones, and aminoglycosides, but usually are resistant to ampicillin and first- and second-generation cephalosporins.[102-105] Antimicrobial susceptibility testing is required for all isolates to select the most appropriate agent. Because of the low virulence of *P. oryzihabitans*, patients can recover spontaneously from infection after removal of foreign material.[107]

Sphingobacterium, Sphingomonas, and Shewanella spp.

Sphingobacterium multivorum and *S. spritivorum* are the species most commonly recovered from human clinical specimens. Most human isolates have been from blood and urine. Isolates are generally resistant to the aminoglycosides and polymyxins, susceptible to fluoroquinolones and trimethoprim-sulfamethoxazole, and variably susceptible to the β-lactam agents.[116-118]

Sphingomonas paucimobilis and other *Sphingomonas* spp. have been recovered from blood, cerebrospinal fluid, urine and urogenital sites, and wounds.[119-125] These organisms can cause sporadic or community-acquired infections including BSI, osteomyelitis, pyogenic arthritis, meningitis, urinary tract infection, and wound infection. Infections follow acquisition from the environment or nosocomially from contaminated fluids orequipment.[115-117] There is a single report of BSI due to *S. mucosissima* in a patient with sickle-cell disease.[125] Most isolates are susceptible to the aminoglycosides, fluoroquinolones, and trimethoprim-sulfamethoxazole; susceptibility to β-lactam agents is variable.[120]

Shewanella algae and *S. putrefaciens* have human clinical importance. *Shewanella* spp. have been recovered in association with BSI, CVC-associated BSI, ventilator-associated pneumonia, exudative tonsillitis, cerebellar abscess, ventriculoperitoneal shunt infection, peritonitis, osteomyelitis, pyogenic arthritis, and external ear and skin and soft-tissue infections following trauma.[126-137] These organisms are generally susceptible to a wide variety of antimicrobial agents, except for first-generation penicillins and cephalosporins.[126-137]

---

152 | Eikenella, Pasteurella, and Chromobacterium Species

Michael T. Brady and Mario J. Marcon

MICROBIOLOGY AND EPIDEMIOLOGY

Eikenella, Pasteurella, and *Chromobacterium* species display both common and contrasting characteristics of laboratory properties, epidemiology, and clinical presentations. The genus *Eikenella* contains only one species, *Eikenella corrodens,* which belongs to the family Neisseriaceae along with the genera *Neisseria* and *Kingella.*[1-4] The genus *Pasteurella* contains a number of species of clinical significance and belongs to the family Pasteurellaceae along with the genera *Aggregatibacter, Actinobacillus,* and *Haemophilus.* The genus *Chromobacterium* contains only one species of human significance, *C. violaceum,* and also is currently placed in the family Neisseriaceae; a number of other *Chromobacterium* spp. recovered from environmental sources have been proposed. Most of these organisms are microaerophilic, facultatively anaerobic, somewhat fastidious, gram-negative bacilli that can appear pleomorphic or coccobacillary in direct smears or smears prepared from culture. *Eikenella* and *Pasteurella* spp. are nonmotile, while *C. violaceum* is motile and less fastidious than the others.

Eikenella corrodens is a small straight rod that can appear coccobacillary. The organism is oxidase-positive and ornithine decarboxylase-positive, reduces nitrates to nitrites, but does not produce catalase, urease, or indole.[1-4] *E. corrodens* originally was thought to be related to the strictly anaerobic bacterium *Bacteroides urealyticus* (formerly *Bacteroides corrodens*) because of the characteristic "corroding" or "pitting" of the surface of blood or chocolate agar by some isolates, suggesting a preference for anaerobic growth.

Most *Pasteurella* spp. are oxidase- and catalase-positive, reduce nitrates, and utilize glucose and a variety of other carbohydrates. The most important species of human significance include *P. multocida* subsp. *multocida, P. multocida* subsp. *septica, P. canis, P. dagmatis,* and *P. stomatis.*[1,2,5-7] A number of other *Pasteurella* spp. are rarely if at all associated with human disease.[1,2,5-7] The classification of *Pasteurella* spp. is undergoing revision based on DNA-DNA hybridization studies and ribosomal RNA sequence analysis and several species, including *P. pneumotropica, P.aerogenes,* and *P. bettyae,* may be reclassified as members of the genus *Actinobacillus* or other genera in the family Pasteurallaceae.[7-9] Organisms formerly classified as *P. gallinarum* now are *Avibacterium gallinarum* and some formerly classified as *P. haemolytica* now are *Mannheimia haemolytica.*

Chromobacterium violaceum is a long gram-negative, slightly curved bacillus. *C. violaceum* is positive for catalase, nitrate reductase, and arginine dihydrolase; grows on sheep blood, MacConkey, chocolate and Mueller–Hinton agar; and produces a deep purple pigment (violacein) that can result in black-appearing colonies. The pigment also can be produced during infection, resulting in a violaceous cellulitis.

Eikenella corrodens is part of the normal flora of the oral cavity, upper respiratory tract, and mucosal surfaces of the gastrointestinal and genitourinary tracts of humans and some mammals.[10,11] From both a clinical and laboratory diagnostic perspective, it is useful to discuss *E. corrodens* in the context of the so-called "AACEK" (formerly "HACEK") group organisms. This mnemonic stands for *Aggregatibacter aphrophilus* (formerly *Haemophilus aphrophilus* and *H. paraprophilus*), *Aggregatibacter* (formerly *Actinobacillus*) *actinomycetemcomitans*, *Cardiobacterium hominis*, *E. corrodens*, and *Kingella kingae* and other *Kingella* spp. As a group, these are slow-growing organisms of the normal flora of the upper respiratory tract, often requiring elevated carbon dioxide concentrations and hemin in the culture medium for optimum growth.[10] AACEK organisms are clinically important in specific disease syndromes, including disseminated diseases, such as subacute bacterial endocarditis and pyogenic arthritis, and localized pyogenic diseases of the oral cavity, head, and neck.[11] Compared with the other organisms in the AACEK group, *E. corrodens* is less fastidious and generally is recoverable within 24 to 48 hours on routine blood and chocolate agar media. Because of improvements in composition of broth media and detection techniques, blood cultures from patients with suspected endocarditis due to *E. corrodens* or other AACEK group organisms generally need not be incubated beyond the routine 5 days used in most laboratories.[1–3,12]

There are limited data on potential virulence factors produced by *E. corrodens* that may contribute to invasion or pathogenic processes. A lectin-like protein and multiple pilus proteins are found on the bacterial cell surface and may contribute to adherence to mucosal epithelial cells. Some genes coding for pilus proteins share nucleotide homology, and the pilus proteins show amino acid sequence homology, with pilin genes and proteins from *Moraxella* spp. and *Neisseria gonorrhoeae*. Other cell surface proteins have the ability to agglutinate red blood cells. Like other gram-negative bacteria, the outer cell membrane of *E. corrodens* contains unique proteins, the cell wall possesses lipopolysaccharide, and the organism can synthesize an extracellular polysaccharide or slime layer. It is difficult to determine the specific contribution of each of these factors to virulence, but they may play a role in inhibiting phagocytosis or modulating macrophage activity.[2]

Pasteurella spp. are commensals of the upper respiratory tract of many animal species. Oropharyngeal carriage of *P. multocida* occurs in most dogs and cats, including large cats (lions, tigers, panthers), as well as in swine, rats, opossums, rabbits, fowl, and possibly humans.[13] *Pasteurella* spp. are primary pathogens of a variety of animals and several species can cause a variety of human infections, most commonly associated with animal bites or scratches. In one study of 159 human isolates of *Pasteurella* spp. recovered from dog or cat bites, *P. multocida* subsp. *multocida* accounted for 60% of isolates, *P. canis* for 18%, *P. multocida* subsp. *septica* for 13%, *P. stomatis* for 5%, and *P. dogmatis* for 3%.[6] *Pasteurella* also can be acquired through aerosol inhalation, and there may be differences in the propensity of the two *P. multocida* subspecies to cause respiratory tract disease.[14] Although an animal source is present in most human *P. multocida* infections, there is no known animal exposure in 5% to 15% of cases. *Pasteurella* spp. generally can be isolated from culture on blood or chocolate agar within 24 to 48 hours of incubation; most strains do not grow on MacConkey agar. Gram-stain smears of growth on agar reveal small gram-negative coccobacilli. Biochemical identification of *P. multocida* is straightforward, particularly when a clinical history is provided; however, identification of some other *Pasteurella* species may be more difficult.[7–9]

Studies of virulence factors of *Pasteurella* spp. have been focused on *P. multocida*. Virulence of *P. multocida* may be associated with production of neuraminidase and lipopolysaccharide endotoxin. A dermonecrotic toxin, a known virulence factor in animals, may be detected more commonly in strains isolated from adults with chronic bronchitis than from other sources. In addition, certain strains have been reported to produce a cytotoxin.[15]

Chromobacterium violaceum is a common saprophyte of soil and water, especially in tropical and subtropical areas.[16,17] The organism usually gains entry through the skin to cause localized wound infection, but bloodstream and disseminated infection can occur in patients with select immune dysfunction. *C. violaceum* can be isolated readily from blood, abscess fluid, or purulent drainage. Factors promoting virulence have not been identified.

CLINICAL MANIFESTATIONS

Most infections due to *E. corrodens* involve the head, neck, or respiratory tract or are related to human bites or fist-fight injuries.[11,18–21] Localized infections generally are indolent and follow a slowly progressing course, often becoming manifest no earlier than one week after injury. *E. corrodens* is a cause in about 25% of infections resulting from clenched fist injuries. These slowly evolving infections can lead to complications such as a stiff joint or, rarely, even amputation.[18] Oral contamination can lead to infection of surgical wounds, such as after craniofacial or esophageal reconstruction. *E. corrodens* is prevalent in subgingival plaque of adults with periodontitis.[22] Pleuropulmonary infections also can occur, presumably as a result of aspiration of oral contents or leaking of oral secretions into the pleural space after surgery. In these cases, pneumonia, empyema, or pulmonary cavitation can result.[21–23] *E. corrodens* often is part of a polymicrobial infection, especially with viridans or β-hemolytic streptococci, staphylococci, and oral anaerobic bacteria in human bites, head and neck infections, respiratory tract infections, and hepatic abscesses.[1–3,24–26] *E. corrodens* infections occur in immunocompromised individuals as well as in individuals with normal immune function.[27] *E. corrodens* can be found concurrently with *Actinomyces* spp. and may contribute to the pathogenesis of actinomycosis,[1,28] and has been implicated with *Actinomyces* spp. in a distinctive clinical infection known as chronic diffuse sclerosing osteomyelitis of the mandible.[28]

E. corrodens also can be recovered from peritoneal cultures after ruptured appendix, gastric surgery, traumatic duodenal rupture, gastric cancer, and abscesses of the spleen, liver and pancreas.[29–31] Other serious *E. corrodens* infections include bloodstream infection (BSI), endocarditis, pyogenic arthritis, chorioamnionitis, neonatal sepsis, neonatal conjunctivitis, meningitis, sinusitis, submandibular abscess, thyroid abscess, renal abscess, and brain abscess.[20,32–41] Invasion of the central nervous system (CNS) can occur by extension from periodontal, middle ear, or sinus infections (Figure 152-1). BSI and endocarditis most often occur in immunocompromised hosts, intravenous drug abusers, and individuals with previous cardiac valve damage. Osteomyelitis of the calcaneus has been reported subsequent to penetration of the heel by a toothpick.[19] Injection and fingerstick site abscesses due to *E. corrodens* have been reported in adolescents with insulin-dependent diabetes mellitus; licking or biting skin or nails might

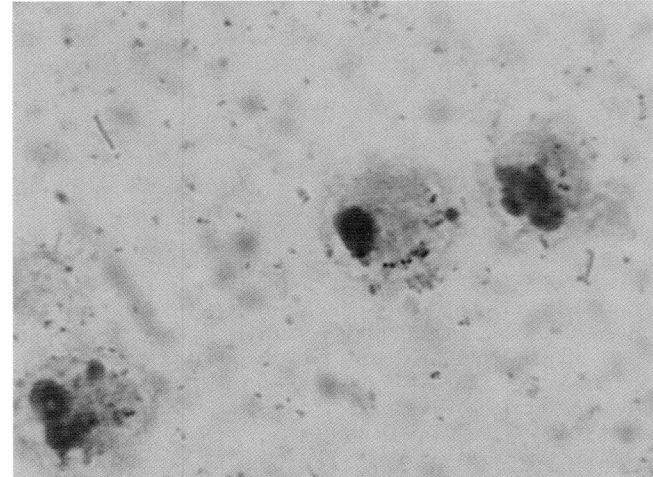

Figure 152-1. Gram stain of epidural fluid from 6-year-old boy with acute onset of fever, sinusitis, mental status change, and hemiparesis. *Eikenella corrodens* and group C streptococcus were isolated. (Courtesy of E.D. Thompson and K.D. Herzog, St. Christopher's Hospital for Children, Philadelphia, PA.)

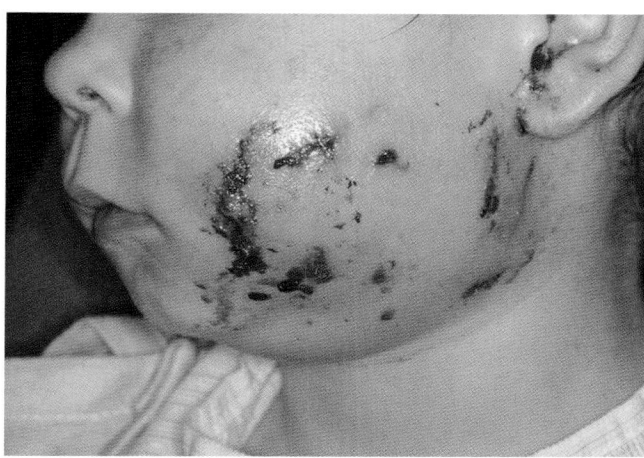

Figure 152-2. A toddler with facial cellulitis due to *Pasteurella multocida* following a dog bite. (Courtesy of J.H. Brien©.)

provide opportunity for the organism to contaminate traumatized skin.[42]

Infection caused by *Pasteurella* spp., most commonly *P. multocida,* generally occurs after an animal bite.[43-45] *P. multocida* is the pathogen in >50% to 75% of infections following a cat bite and up to 50% of those following a dog bite[44] (Figure 152-2). Cat scratches also can be complicated by *P. multocida* infection. Infection can occur after bite injuries from lions, tigers, or other large cats as well as rats, rabbits, and other animals. Wound infections due to *P. multocida* typically develop rapidly, within 12 to 24 hours after injury, and manifest with warmth, swelling, redness, and tenderness and with serosanguineous-to-purulent discharge at the site.[43] Regional lymphadenopathy, chills, and fever are common. In one review spanning 10 years, the highest rate of infection occurred in children <5 years of age and in adults >55 years of age.[43] Tenosynovitis and tendon sheath abscess formation, osteomyelitis, and pyogenic arthritis are complications related to deep penetration by the teeth or claws of the animal.[44] Pre-existing joint disease may predispose patients to pyogenic arthritis.

Some cases of infection due to *Pasteurella* spp. occur in individuals with frequent animal exposure but without a bite or scratch injury. These cases include infections of the upper respiratory tract, soft-tissue infection secondary to accidental injury, intra-abdominal infections, meningitis, and bone and joint infections.[44] Pneumonia with or without empyema is rare and occurs chiefly in adults with underlying chronic bronchopulmonary disease. *P. multocida* can cause BSI and meningitis in infants and children, with most cases occurring in infants <12 months of age.[46-49] Exposure to animals was frequently nontraumatic and typically subsequent to a pet dog or cat licking the infant's face. The symptoms of CNS infection and abnormalities of cerebrospinal fluid (CSF) in infected children are typical of bacterial meningitis; however, a CSF mononuclear cell predominance has been reported.[47,48,50,51] BSI is documented in about 50% of patients with meningitis. Neurologic sequelae are uncommon. Other *P. multocida* CNS infections include brain abscess secondary to direct penetration of the brain parenchyma after a dog bite, subdural empyema, and ventriculoperitoneal shunt infections.[50,51]

P. multocida is a rare cause of fetal infection secondary to maternal BSI and invasion via the placenta.[52] Ascending infection due to *P. multocida* also has been postulated.[53,54] This is in contrast to fetal infections in animals, in which *Pasteurella* spp. are well-documented causes of septic abortion. Neonatal systemic infection with *P. multocida* has been reported only rarely. The presentation is similar to early-onset group B streptococcal disease and is characterized by fulminant septicemia with or without meningitis. Neonatal infection usually occurs in the setting of maternal obstetric complication, including chorioamnionitis, premature onset of labor, prolonged rupture of membranes, postpartum fever, or premature delivery.[55,56] The mortality rate is high, particularly in infants who acquire infection in utero and who are symptomatic at birth. The maternal genital tract is the source of the infection for both infant and mother. Genital colonization is thought to occur as a result of hand inoculation after animal contact.[56] Late-onset meningitis and cervical spine osteomyelitis has been reported in a 20-day-old infant from a household with two pet cats.[57] The infection occurred without an obvious history of cat bites, scratches, or licks.

Individuals with underlying abnormalities of host defense, especially liver disease, are predisposed to BSI due to *P. multocida* infection.[43] Direct trauma due to an animal bite or scratch has occurred in some patients, but oropharyngeal colonization secondary to contact with secretions of a pet also may be the source of invasive infection. Septic shock develops in approximately 50% of patients, and the mortality rate approaches 40%. Contiguous spread of infection from liver to lung with involvement of the diaphragm has been reported.[58] *P. multocida* also has been associated with peritonitis secondary to a ruptured appendix or peritoneal dialysis, endophthalmitis after a cat scratch, prosthetic vascular graft infection, and granulomatous hepatitis.[59-61] Urinary tract infection (UTI) due to *P. multocida* is rare but has been reported in children with underlying renal disease.[62,63] Repeated catheterization and skin contamination with *P. multocida* may contribute to introduction of the organism into the urinary tract.[62] A case of *P. multocida* BSI in a patient with Kikuchi disease has been reported, but relationship between Kikuchi disease and *P. multocida* infection could not be established.[64] The authors conjectured that *P. multocida* infection might have served as an antigenic stimulus for the development of Kikuchi disease.

Several other *Pasteurella* spp. have been reported as human pathogens. *Pasteurella canis, P. dagmatis,* and *P. stomatis* have been associated with wound infections and osteomyelitis after cat or dog bites, as well as with endocarditis, peritonitis, and sepsis in a patient with cirrhosis, and septicemia in a diabetic patient.[65-68] The reservoir of *P. canis* is the oral cavity of dogs, while the latter two species have been recovered from the oral cavity of both dogs and cats. *P. aerogenes* has been associated with animal bite wounds, UTI, and peritonitis in humans.[9,69] *P. bettyae* has been recovered from amniotic fluid, blood (usually in the neonatal period), finger lesions, abscesses, wounds following rectal surgery, and genitourinary lesions, particularly Bartholin gland abscesses.[9,70] *P. aerogenes* and *P. pneumotropica* peritonitis have been reported in a patient undergoing peritoneal dialysis following bites of hamsters.[71,72]

C. violaceum is a rare human pathogen but is a common soil and water inhabitant in tropical and subtropical areas; most infections are reported from Southeast Asia.[1,16,17] All cases of infection reported in the United States have been in the southeast, especially Florida, Georgia, Louisiana, and South Carolina. Infections occur primarily in males during the summer months and usually involve injury to the skin in association with exposure to soil or water. Initial symptoms typically are pain at the wound site. Infection may be localized and limited to the wound, or disseminate rapidly, causing overwhelming septicemia with a high mortality rate.[16,73] Fever, nausea, vomiting, abdominal pain, and diarrhea frequently are noted. Septic shock, pneumonia, osteomyelitis, lymphadenitis, diarrhea, UTI, conjunctivitis, orbital cellulitis, and abscesses of spleen, lung, brain and liver have been described.[74-81] Pneumonia after aspiration of fresh warm water has been reported in two cases of near drowning.[77] Multiple sites of abscess formation also tend to occur, especially in the liver, spleen, and lungs. Although most *C. violaceum* infections have occurred in individuals presumed to be immunologically competent, chronic granulomatous disease predisposes to *C. violaceum* infection.[81] There are similarities in clinical presentations of *C. violaceum* infection and the septicemic form of melioidosis due to *Burkholderia pseudomallei.*[74] Diagnosis is made by culture of wound exudate, biopsy specimen, blood, or abscess fluid.

Key Points. Diagnosis and Management of *Eikenella corrodens* Infections

MICROBIOLOGY

- Catalase-negative, oxidase-positive, small gram-negative, straight bacilli
- Good growth on blood and chocolate agars but not MacConkey agar; enhanced growth in CO_2
- Colonies often show a fringe of spreading growth and can pit the agar
- Generally susceptible to penicillin, but β-lactamase-producing strains occur (susceptible to penicillin/β-lactamase inhibitor compounds)

EPIDEMIOLOGY

- Normal oropharyngeal and transient gastrointestinal tract flora
- Associated with juvenile and adult periodontitis
- Oral, pleuropneumonic, and abdominal infections; often polymicrobial
- Wound infection associated with human bites and fist-fight injuries
- Can cause bone and joint infection
- Agent of subacute bacterial endocarditis, especially subsequent to dental manipulation or IV drug abuse

DIAGNOSIS

- Recovery in culture using standard laboratory procedures
- PCR and 16S rRNA gene sequencing have been used for diagnosis but are not available widely
- *E. corrodens*-specific DNA probes have been used to analyze the microbial flora associated with periodontal disease

TREATMENT

- Penicillin is drug of choice for infection due to β-lactamase-negative organism
- Susceptible generally to ampicillin and amoxicillin (if β-lactamase negative), amoxicllin-clavulanate, extended-spectrum cephalosporins, ciprofloxacin, doxycycline; generally resistant to clindamycin and the macrolides

DURATION OF THERAPY

- Response to therapy usually is rapid
- Duration of therapy for systemic infection including osteoarticular infections or endocarditis is similar to that for other infectious agents

---

TREATMENT AND PREVENTION

E. corrodens generally is susceptible in vitro to penicillin, ampicillin, or amoxicillin; amoxicillin-clavulanate and ampicillin-sulbactam; most second- and third-generation cephalosporins; carbapenems; ureidopenicillins; tetracyclines; and newer fluoroquinolones.[26,82,83] Clindamycin, antistaphylococcal penicillins, macrolides, metronidazole, and aminoglycosides generally are inactive and first-generation cephalosporins have variable activity with that of cefazolin greater than cephalothin. First-generation cephalosporins should not be given for suspected *E. corrodens* infections.[27] β-Lactamase-producing stains have been reported rarely; these strains were highly susceptible to amoxicillin-clavulanate and ampicillin-sulbactam.[84] Because many infections involving *E. corrodens* are polymicrobial and can include anaerobic bacteria, selection of therapy should take into account other potential pathogens. Parenteral therapy is appropriate for initial therapy of severe infection, while amoxicillin or amoxicillin-clavulanate administered orally can be used to complete treatment in most instances. Surgical drainage of abscesses may be required. Standardized methods for in vitro antimicrobial susceptibility testing are published.[85]

P. multocida is susceptible to penicillin, which is the drug of choice for treatment of these infections. Other active agents include ampicillin, amoxicillin-clavulanate, cefuroxime, cefoxitin, fluoroquinolones, tetracyclines, and trimethoprim-sulfamethoxazole.[82,86] Erythromycin, clindamycin, cephalexin, cefadroxil, cefaclor, and dicloxacillin have poor activity against *P. multocida* and should not be used to treat infection.[46,86,87] β-Lactamase-producing strains of *P. multocida* have been isolated from human infections. In one case, the strain was resistant to penicillin, ampicillin, ticarcillin, sulfonamides, and tetracycline. The addition of any of the β-lactamase-inhibiting compounds reduced the minimal inhibitory concentration of this organism at least 64-fold.[87] In another report of a lung abscess due to a β-lactamase-producing strain, investigators speculated that the resistance gene may have been acquired from *Haemophilus influenzae*. Testing for β-lactamase using a chromogenic cephalosporin (nitrocefin test) is recommended for isolates from normally sterile body sites. Other susceptibility testing usually is not necessary. Standardized methods for in vitro testing of *Pasteurella* spp. are published.[85,88]

Although most wound infections due to *P. multocida* typically respond well to appropriate oral antibiotic therapy, worsening of disease during the first 24 hours of treatment is not unusual. When polymicrobial wound infection is suspected, amoxicillin-clavulanate or cefuroxime is recommended. The duration of oral antibiotic therapy for localized infections typically is 7 to 10 days.

Hospitalization should be considered for certain *P. multocida* infections: systemic infections, infections in individuals with diabetes mellitus or immunocompromising conditions, and for serious infections of the head, hands, joint spaces, or tendons. Parenteral antimicrobial agents active against *Pasteurella* spp. include penicillin, ampicillin, ampicillin-sulbactam, piperacillin, cefuroxime, and cefotaxime.[46,86] The duration of parenteral therapy for severe or disseminated infections should be 10 to 14 days. When mixed infection is considered, ticarcillin-clavulanate, cefuroxime, ampicillin-sulbactam, or meropenem should be effective. Because *P. multocida* is susceptible to penicillin or ampicillin, current regimens for empiric therapy for presumed septicemia or meningitis in the neonate would be effective.

Parents should be discouraged from allowing pets to lick infants and children on the face or on wounds. Handwashing after pet contact is prudent. Limiting contact with wild and domestic animals probably is the only way to prevent human infections due to *Pasteurella* spp. Animal bites and scratches should be vigorously cleaned, irrigated, and debrided promptly. The use of antibiotic prophylaxis to prevent wound infection secondary to animal bites is controversial. Some experts recommend prophylactic antibiotic therapy in persons with the following: (1) cat bite; (2) severe bite wound accompanied by edema, crush injury, or involvement of bone, joint, or tendon sheath; (3) immunocompromising condition, asplenia, or diabetes mellitus; (4) injury sustained ≥8 hours before medical assistance is sought; and (5) bite on the hands, feet, or genital area.[46] Amoxicillin-clavulanate is a good choice when antimicrobial prophylaxis or pre-emptive therapy of a bite wound is indicated. For the penicillin-allergic child, trimethoprim-sulfamethoxazole or cefuroxime axetil can be considered. Minimal data exist about the role of suturing bite wounds and risk of infection.[46]

C. violaceum usually is susceptible to chloramphenicol, aminoglycosides, tetracyclines, meropenem, fluoroquinolones, and trimethoprim-sulfamethoxazole but is resistant to penicillin, ampicillin, and first-generation cephalosporins.[16,17,74] Trimethoprim-sulfamethoxazole plus ciprofloxacin is the treatment of choice for initial therapy, but chloramphenicol plus an aminoglycoside, or a carbapenem, may be effective alternate

---

Key Points. Diagnosis and Management of *Pasteurella multocida* Infections

MICROBIOLOGY

- Catalase- and slow oxidase-positive, small gram-negative, coccoid to short bacilli
- Good growth on blood and chocolate agar but not MacConkey agar; does not require CO_2
- Colonies can be mucoid, particularly those recovered from the respiratory tract
- Generally susceptible to penicillin, but β-lactamase-positive strains causing penicillin and ampicillin resistance occur (susceptible to penicillin/β-lactamase inhibitor compounds)

EPIDEMIOLOGY

- Normal inhabitants of the nasopharynx, gingival, and oral cavity of a wide variety of wild and domestic mammals including cats and dogs; also found in the respiratory tract of birds
- Associated with wound infections following animal bites, scratches, or other exposures (licking of open skin lesions)
- Infected cat bites more likely than infected dog bites to contain *P. multocida*
- Causes respiratory tract infection including sinusitis and bronchitis, pneumonia, and empyema, primarily in people with underlying disease
- Two subspecies, *P. multocida* subsp. *multocida* and subsp. *septica*; the former is responsible for the majority of infections

- Can cause bloodstream and disseminated infection, including meningitis, endocarditis, peritonitis, bone and joint infection

DIAGNOSIS

- Recovery in culture from most body sites using standard laboratory procedures
- PCR and 16S rRNA gene sequencing have been used for diagnosis but are not available widely

TREATMENT

- Penicillin is drug of choice for β-lactamase-negative infections
- Susceptible generally to ampicillin and amoxicillin (if β-lactamase negative), amoxicillin-clavulanate, extended-spectrum cephalosporins, ciprofloxacin, TMP-SMX; generally resistant to clindamycin while macrolides and aminoglycosides have reduced activity

DURATION OF THERAPY

- Response to therapy usually is rapid, particularly with administration of antibiotic parenterally; however, disease can progress initially after starting an appropriate antibiotic, particularly an oral agent
- Duration of therapy for systemic infection including osteoarticular infections or endocarditis is similar to that for other infectious agents

---

therapies.[83] Erythromycin is not effective for treatment, regardless of susceptibility test results, and resistance to the aminoglycosides and broad-spectrum β-lactam agents has been documented.[77,89] Antimicrobial susceptibility testing may be helpful in guiding management; however, there are currently no standardized methods for in vitro testing of *C. violaceum* and test results should be interpreted cautiously. Antimicrobial therapy for infections due to *C. violaceum* should be initiated with parenteral antibiotics until the patient is stable and improving, followed by oral therapy (trimethoprim-sulfamethoxazole or tetracycline), for at least an additional 4 weeks for disseminated infection. Necrotizing skin lesions should be debrided and abscesses drained aggressively at initiation of antimicrobial therapy. Disseminated infection requires aggressive supportive care. Relapse of BSI is a documented complication, occurring about 2 weeks after completion of therapy. *C. violaceum*, along with the more common *Aeromonas hydrophila*, should be considered when choosing empiric antibiotic therapy for cellulitis or rapidly progressive illness following exposure to soil or water, particularly stagnant water in the southeastern U.S.[76]

---

153 *Moraxella* and *Psychrobacter* Species

Eugene Leibovitz and David Greenberg

MICROBIOLOGY, PATHOGENESIS, AND EPIDEMIOLOGY

Discovered at the end of the 19th century, *Moraxella catarrhalis* (formerly *Micrococcus catarrhalis*, *Neisseria catarrhalis*, and *Branhamella catarrhalis*) has undergone several changes of nomenclature and changes in status as either a commensal of the upper respiratory tract or a true pathogen of both the upper and lower respiratory tract.[1-4] *M. catarrhalis* is morphologically and phenotypically similar to *Neisseria* spp., leading to its misidentification in the past as a *Neisseria* species particularly as *N. cinerva* (a commensal of the adult pharynx).[3,4] Later DNA-DNA and rRNA-DNA hybridization techniques studies showed little homology between *M. catarrhalis* and Neisseriaceae species and demonstrated that *M. catarrhalis* is more closely related to the *Moraxella* than to *Branhamella* species.[3-7]

M. catarrhalis is a cause of acute otitis media (AOM), being responsible for up to 20% of the cases (the third most common etiologic agent after nontypable *Haemophilus influenzae* and *Streptococcus pneumoniae*).[8,9] *M. catarrhalis* also is the second (after *H. influenzae*) most common cause of exacerbations of chronic obstructive pulmonary disease (COPD) in adults, being responsible for 2–4 million episodes of the syndrome in the United States.[10]

Members of the genus *Moraxella* are nonmotile, oxidase-positive, catalase-positive, aerobic, asaccharolytic, gram-negative coccobacilli or diplococci that tend to resist decolorization on Gram stain.[1] *M. catarrhalis*, *M. osloensis*, *M. nonliquefaciens* (the second most frequently isolated species after *M. catarrhalis*), and *M. lincolnii* are part of the normal flora of the respiratory tract while *M. canis* has been recovered in the upper respiratory tract of cats and dogs. Other pathogens include *Psychrobacter phenylpiruvicus*, whose differential diagnosis from *Brucella* spp. is important and requires microscopy and tests for acidification of xylose and glucose. Because of their similar pathogenic significance and possibility of equivocal biochemical reactions, most laboratories do not perform species identification of these organisms except for *M. catarrhalis*. Colonies of *M. catarrhalis* grow well on both blood and chocolate agar, and some strains also grow well on modified Thayer–Martin and other selective media. Colonies are grey-white, opaque and smooth. Another useful feature for identification of *M. catarrhalis* is the observation that colonies can be pushed over the surface of a blood agar plate much like an ice-hockey puck is pushed over ice.[1] *M. catarrhalis* may be distinguished easily from *Neisseria* spp. by its ability to hydrolyze ester-linked butyrate groups. Almost all *M. catarrhalis* isolates produce β-lactamases today.[11,12]

M. catarrhalis colonizes the mucosal surfaces of upper and lower respiratory tract by a process requiring the expression of adhesins and the activation of metabolic pathways to overcome specific nutrient limitations. The *M. catarrhalis* adhesion is a multifactorial event mediated by several adhesin macromolecules. A number of *Moraxella* adhesins and their corresponding receptors have been identified and characterized.[13] The family of ubiquitous surface proteins (Usps), consisting of at least three proteins (UspA1, UspA2 and UspA2H), are the most extensively studied outer membrane proteins (OMPs) of *M. catarrhalis* and were found to have major roles in adhesion, invasion, and protection against the complement system. The *Moraxella* immunoglobulin D-binding protein (MID, also named hemagglutinin) is another extensively studied and highly conserved OMP that has a unique ability to bind immunoglobulin D and also type II alveolar epithelial cells.[13,14] The pathogen also possesses several mechanisms of evasion of the host immune system, such as the ability to withstand the action of human complement system as demonstrated in clinical isolates obtained from patients with otitis media or COPD.[13,15,16] UspAs are the most important OMPs involved in *M. catarrhalis* resistance to complement, interfering with both the classical and the alternative complement pathway. *M. catarrhalis* can be divided, by molecular typing methods, into two distinct phylogenetic lineages, serosensitive and seroresistant.[17] The seroresistant lineage is more virulent and is represented predominantly by strains resistant to complement-mediated killing and able to adhere to epithelial cells.[13,18] The membrane lipooligosaccharides (LOS) also are considered important for *M. catarrhalis* adhesion and virulence.[13,19]

The capacity of *M. catarrhalis* to form biofilms has been confirmed in vitro and the pathogen has been detected in biofilms in vivo in the middle ears of patients with chronic otitis media.[20,21] The presence of UspA1 and UspA2H affects biofilm formation positively.

At the respiratory tract mucosal level, *M. catarrhalis* activates an inflammatory response that is mainly dependent on toll-like receptor 2 (TLR2). Following infection with *M. catarrhalis*, the activation of TLR2 initiates a cascade of reactions resulting in the transcription of proinflammatory genes, such as those encoding interleukin-8 and the granulocyte-macrophage colony-stimulating factor.[13,22] On the other hand, despite the activation of TLR2 cascade, *M. catarrhalis* was found to be able to inhibit the proinflammatory cascade and to evade human immune responses, leading to persistent mucosal surface colonization.[23]

The replacement phenomenon in AOM related to the introduction of pneumococcal conjugate vaccines (by which pathogens not targeted in the vaccine take the place of the eradicated vaccine strains) and potential future use of vaccines against nontypable *H. influenzae*, as well as the increasing resistance rates of *M. catarrhalis* to antimicrobial agents, make the development of a vaccine for *M. catarrhalis* a real scientific challenge.[11,12,24,25] Several adhesin molecules with different specificities for host cell receptors have been identified and their immunogenicity and generation of a protective immune response evaluated in animal studies. At the present time UspA1, UspA2, and MID/hemagglutinin are considered important OMP adhesin candidates for the development of a *Moraxella catarrhalis* vaccine.[26–28]

Colonization rates with *M. catarrhalis* in the upper respiratory tract vary greatly with age, with rates highest in the first year of life (28% to 100% of infants) and comparable with those of more traditionally recognized pathogens such as *S. pneumoniae*.[28,29] At this age, *M. catarrhalis* strains may persist for several months and earlier colonization was associated with higher risks of AOM and recurrent disease.[29] At any one time, 5% to 32% of the elderly adults with COPD may have, *M. catarrhalis* colonizing the respiratory tract, with a median carriage duration of 30 to 40 days.[30]

CLINICAL MANIFESTATIONS

AOM, sinusitis, bronchitis, and pneumonia are the most common infections due to *M. catarrhalis*. Most cases of *M. catarrhalis* AOM resolve spontaneously, unlike AOM caused by *S. pneumoniae*. Compared with AOM caused by other pathogens, *M. catarrhalis* AOM most frequently is part of a mixed-infection AOM, and is less often associated with spontaneous perforation and mastoiditis.[31] Other suppurative complications of AOM, such as osteomyelitis, meningitis or brain abscess, are almost never caused by this organism.

M. catarrhalis represents a major diagnostic challenge in children with community-acquired pneumonia; the yield of diagnostic tests for *M. catarrhalis* is low and growth of the pathogen from upper respiratory tract secretions is weak evidence that the organism is the true cause of pneumonia.[32,33] *M. catarrhalis* bacteremia is reported to occur mainly in children <2 years old, mainly in immunocompetent hosts, associated with community-acquired pneumonia. Characteristic clinical features of pneumonia include low-grade fever, lack of leukocytosis at presentation, prolonged hospitalizations in several cases, and a favorable overall prognosis.[34]

M. catarrhalis can cause purulent conjunctivitis, periorbital cellulitis, endophthalmitis, septic arthritis, pancreatitis, pericarditis, and endocarditis.[35–41] *M. catarrhalis* septicemia has been reported in immunocompromised patients with leukemia, AIDS, and agammaglobulinemia.[42–44]

Meningitis caused by *Psychrobacter immobilis* in a 2-day-old infant was initially thought to be caused by *N. gonorrhoeae*.[45] Septicemia associated with diarrhea in children caused by *M. osloensis*, *M. nonliquefaciens*, and *M. lacunata* has been reported.[46] Septicemia, endocarditis, and pyogenic arthritis caused by *M. liquefaciens* and *M. nonliquefaciens* also have been reported.[47–50] *M. osloensis* has been associated with osteomyelitis, peritonitis, catheter-related bloodstream infection, and other deep-seated infections.[51] *M. canis* has been associated with rare cases of bloodstream infection and wound infections following dog bites, and infection of a skin-ulcerating malignant lymph node.[52,53]

TREATMENT

Most *Moraxella* and *Psychrobacter* spp. other than *M. catarrhalis* are susceptible to penicillin and ampicillin, cephalosporins, tetracyclines, macrolides, aminoglycosides, and fluoroquinolones; however, β-lactamase-producing strains have been identified in some species, including strains of *M. osloensis* and *P. phenylpyruvicus*.[1,54,55] It is therefore prudent to test clinically significant isolates for β-lactamase production.

M. catarrhalis is almost uniformly resistant to penicillin, ampicillin, and amoxicillin due to the production of a *Branhamella/Moraxella* (BRO)-1 or BRO-2 β-lactamase.[1,56] The drug of choice to treat *M. catarrhalis* infections is amoxicillin-clavulanate. Second- or third-generation cephalosporin drugs are alternative therapeutic agents. With a wide variety of antimicrobial agents (including fluoroquinolones and carbapenems) uniformly active against this organism, there is rarely a need for susceptibility testing other than testing for β-lactamase, which may be used as an aid in identification.[1,56]

154 *Pseudomonas* Species and Related Organisms

Jane L. Burns

Pseudomonas species primarily are water and soil organisms of relatively low virulence that are catalase-producing, nonglucose-fermenting gram-negative bacilli that grow well on routine microbiologic culture media at 37°C. Pseudomonads are motile and both indophenol- and oxidase-positive; many produce pyoverdins or other visible or fluorescent pigments. Speciation is based primarily on physical characteristics (pigment production, odor, colonial morphology, and flagellar structure) and biochemical profiles (including carbohydrate fermentation patterns and production of arginine dihydrolase and lysine decarboxylase). There are several related genera, many of which used to be species within the genus *Pseudomonas* (Box 154-1). Still remaining within the genus are *Pseudomonas aeruginosa*, *P. stutzeri*, *P. putida*, and *P. fluorescens*. In addition, *P. oryzihabitans* (formerly *Flavimonas*) and *P. luteola* (formerly *Chryseomonas*) have been returned to the genus (Table 154-1).[1]

As a group, pseudomonads and closely related species are nutritionally diverse, and many are used in industry because of their unique ability to catabolize toxins. Although *P. aeruginosa* is the most important human pathogen within this group, other species have been reported to cause nosocomial infections in immunocompromised and postoperative patients and those with indwelling catheters, and to cause sporadic infections in previously healthy individuals. In addition, some organisms occupy specific environmental niches. Several of these species, including *P. fluorescens* and *Ralstonia* spp., are isolated commonly from the sputum of patients with cystic fibrosis, but are of unknown clinical significance. *R. mannitolilytica* is the most commonly isolated *Ralstonia* species from patients with cystic fibrosis (46% of positive individuals), followed by *R. respiraculi* and *R. pickettii* (19% and 18%, respectively).[2] Other pediatric isolates of *Ralstonia* occur mainly in nosocomial infections and infections among young patients with malignancy.[3] In 2005, *Ralstonia* spp. was found contaminating a high heat/humidity/delivery respiratory gas administration device.[4] Related cases of colonization and infection were found in neonates and children. *Sphingomonas paucimobilis* can cause nosocomial infections, most commonly in immunocompromised individuals; contaminated solutions often are the cause.[5] Bloodstream infection (BSI) in the presence of a central venous catheter has been reported in children with neonatal sepsis, malignancy, and aplastic anemia; patients undergoing continuous peritoneal dialysis also are at risk for catheter-associated peritonitis.[6]

The fluorescent group of *Pseudomonas* includes *P. aeruginosa*, *P. fluorescens*, *P. putida*, *P. veronii*, and *P. monteilii*. *P. fluorescens* and *P. putida* are difficult to differentiate in the laboratory and often are reported as *P. fluorescens/putida*. These organisms have been described in both nosocomial and community-associated infections in children, including BSI, pneumonia, urinary tract infection and postoperative wound infection.[7] In 2008, a multistate outbreak of *P. fluorescens* BSI was reported, associated with exposure to contaminated heparinized saline flushes.[8] Isolated case reports include *P. putida* septicemia in a neonate with staphylococcal scalded skin-like syndrome and in a hypothermic child with panhypopituitarism.[9,10] There are few studies of susceptibility of these organisms because they are uncommon human pathogens; in vitro susceptibility testing should guide therapy.

P. oryzihabitans, *P. luteola*, and *P. stutzeri* are members of the nonfluorescent group. Although rare human pathogens, they are reported occasionally as nosocomial pathogens in both previously healthy and immunocompromised individuals. *P. oryzihabitans* has been described as an etiologic agent of BSI in premature neonates and children with malignancy, postoperative infections and catheter-associated infections.[11,12] There are case reports of *P. luteola* causing brain abscess, meningitis, and endocarditis.[13,14] *P. stutzeri* has been reported to cause posttraumatic pyogenic arthritis and postoperative brain abscess.[15,16] Other pseudomonads, including *Brevundimonas vesicularis*, *Comamonas acidovorans*, *C. testosteroni*, *Acidovorax avenae*, and *Shewanella putrefaciens*, can cause sporadic infections or nosocomial outbreaks in immunocompromised individuals but have not been identified as significant human pathogens.[17-20]

BOX 154-1. Closely Related Genera Formerly Included with *Pseudomonas*

Burkholderia
Stenotrophomonas
Comamonas
Shewanella
Ralstonia
Methylobacterium
Sphingomonas
Acidovorax
Brevundimonas

TABLE 154-1. Human Pathogens Included within the Genus *Pseudomonas* (non-*aeruginosa*)

Species	Subspecies
Pseudomonas stutzeri	18 genomovars
Pseudomonas putida	2 biovars
Pseudomonas fluorescens	5 biovars
Pseudomonas veronii	(closely related to *Pseudomonas fluorescens*)
Pseudomonas monteilii	(closely related to *Pseudomonas putida*)
Pseudomonas oryzihabitans	(formerly *Flavimonas oryzihabitans*)
Pseudomonas luteola	(formerly *Chryseomonas luteola*)

155 *Pseudomonas aeruginosa*

Alice S. Prince

MICROBIOLOGY

Pseudomonas aeruginosa is a gram-negative bacillus found widely in nature, in soil and water. Classified as an opportunistic pathogen, *P. aeruginosa* causes disease infrequently in normal hosts but is a major cause of infection in patients with underlying conditions. The sequencing of the genome of several strains including the prototypic laboratory strain PAO1 (www.pseudomonas.com), which is especially large for a prokaryote, has provided an understanding of the metabolic and pathogenic mechanisms that underlie the success of this versatile pathogen. This large genome endows the organism with tremendous genetic flexibility. *P. aeruginosa* has few nutritional requirements and can adapt to conditions not tolerated by other organisms. It does not ferment lactose or other carbohydrates but oxidizes glucose and xylose. Organisms grow aerobically or anaerobically if nitrate is available as an inorganic electron acceptor, as is the case in the lungs of individuals with cystic fibrosis (CF).[1] *P. aeruginosa* gene expression responds to environmental conditions – with discrete patterns typical of environmental isolates, which are motility, piliation, and expression of numerous exoproducts. In subacute and chronic infections, the accumulation of intracellular dinucleotides (c-di-GMP) favors a biofilm mode of growth, with the formation of an extracellular polysaccharide matrix[2] enabling the organisms to avoid innate immune clearance mechanisms and persist in human airways.[3]

The organism produces fluorescent siderophores pyoverdin and pyochelin, which function to scavenge iron, and pyocyanin, a pigment with oxidant activity that gives *P. aeruginosa* its characteristic blue color.[4] *P. aeruginosa* can be identified biochemically as having indophenol oxidase-positive, citrate-positive, and L-arginine dehydrolase-positive activity. Differentiation of *P. aeruginosa* from the non-*aeruginosa* pseudomonads or organisms such as *Burkholderia* species, *Stenotrophomonas maltophilia*, and *Achromobacter* spp. occasionally can require testing for DNAse activity, growth at 42°C, and differential carbohydrate metabolism or molecular methods.

VIRULENCE FACTORS AND PATHOGENESIS

Multiple virulence factors and their purported roles in pathogenesis are shown in Table 155-1. *P. aeruginosa* is a typical "opportunist" and thrives under conditions that would be adverse to many other bacteria, requiring only a minimal carbon source and a moist environment. Because of intrinsic resistance to many classes of antimicrobial agents and acquisition of additional antibiotic resistance genes from other organisms, *P. aeruginosa* flourishes under the selective pressures that eliminate competing flora. Depending on specific environmental conditions (e.g., availability of nutrients, iron) and immune responses, specific virulence factors are expressed in a highly regulated manner. Hosts without underlying conditions occasionally experience serious *P. aeruginosa* infections if there is a break in normal barrier defenses through puncture wounds,[5] skin trauma or burns.[6] More commonly, *P. aeruginosa* acts as an opportunist, infecting the patient with defective mucosal immunity, pulmonary clearance as in CF, or disease-induced or iatrogenic neutropenia.[7,8]

P. aeruginosa expresses numerous virulence factors that stimulate both airway epithelial cells and professional immune cells to produce proinflammatory cytokines and chemokines, such as interleukin-8,[9] IL-17A/F,[10] granulocyte-macrophage colony-stimulating factor,[11] and mucin.[12] Secreted exoenzymes interact with specific eukaryotic targets to affect cytoskeletal components,

TABLE 155-1. Virulence Factors of *Pseudomonas aeruginosa*

Component	Mechanism	Role in Pathogenesis
Pilus	Adhesin: recognizes the GalNAcbeta1-4Gal receptor in asialoglycolipids	Mediates attachment to epithelial surfaces, required for secretion of type III virulence factors, provides twitching motility – essential for biofilm formation, activates inflammation
Flagella	Motility, chemotaxis, mucin-binding, major immunostimulant through toll-like receptor 5 recognition	Facilitates tissue invasion, activates inflammation
Alginate mucoexopolysaccharide	Antiphagocytic	Characterizes chronic infections in cystic fibrosis
Elastase	Cleaves elastin, proteins including IgA	Destroys extracellular matrix components
Alkaline protease	Cleaves proteins	Causes tissue destruction
Phospholipase C (hemolytic and nonhemolytic)	Cleaves phosphatidylcholine and sphingomyelin	Degrades pulmonary surfactant, facilitates infection in the lung
Neuraminidase	Releases sialic acid from glycoconjugates	Facilitates colonization
Cytotoxin	Forms pores in membranes	Causes tissue destruction
Pseudomonas autoinducer (PAI)	Homoserine lactone derivative, a secreted cofactor necessary for the expression of elastase, alkaline protease, neuraminidase, and biofilm formation	Coordinates gene expression within a population of organisms
Exotoxin A	ADP ribosylating enzyme, which inactivates EF-2, inhibiting protein synthesis	Causes tissue destruction
Exoenzyme S, T, U (type III secreted toxins)	ADP ribosylating enzymes (S and T) and toxins with specific eukaryotic targets, including GTPases; phospholipase A2	Facilitates invasion, cytotoxicity, interferes with cytoskeletal integrity
Siderophores (pyochelin, pyoverdin)	High-affinity iron-binding capacity	Facilitates iron acquisition for bacterial metabolism
Pyocyanin	Blue-green pigment – oxidant activity	Destroys ciliary activity, toxic to airway cells

ADP, adenosine diphosphate; EF-2, elongation factor-2; GTPases, guanosine triphosphatases; IgA, immunoglobulin A.

disrupting the integrity of the epithelial tight junctions and inducing inflammation.[11] Products of type III secretion systems (TTSS) are expressed commonly in acute infection often in the setting of hospital-acquired pneumonias, causing cytotoxicity and facilitating invasion.[13] The TTSS effector proteins include ExoU, a potent phospholipase A2 which requires host superoxide dismutase for activation and is often associated with severe pneumonia;[14] ExoS or ExoT, closely related toxins with both adenosine diphosphate (ADP) ribosyltransferase activity and Rho GTPase activating protein activity,[13] are expressed commonly in clinical isolates from acute infections. The type III secreted virulence factors have been associated with severe *P. aeruginosa* pneumonia in hospitalized patients[15] and have been targeted as potential antigens in *Pseudomonas* vaccines and immunotherapy.

Whereas lipopolysaccharide (LPS) often is considered the major immunostimulatory factor in gram-negative bacteria, *P. aeruginosa* LPS does not activate proinflammatory signaling as potently as does LPS of other organisms.[16] *P. aeruginosa* flagella are important in pathogenesis signaling primarily through toll-like receptor 5 (TLR5) to initiate the host proinflammatory responses to the organisms.[17] Genetically engineered mice have been used extensively to define the critical components of the host immune response to *P. aeruginosa* infection. In addition to the TLRs, additional host factors such as the shedding of syndecan-1,[18] activation of matrilysins,[19] and signaling through purinergic receptors[20] all contribute to host defenses against this pathogen.

Initial pulmonary infections in CF are caused by environmental strains of *P. aeruginosa* that may be cleared intermittently in the course of disease. Distinct patterns of host gene expression are activated by the initial colonizing bacteria that are motile compared with those expressed by the organisms associated with chronic infection.[21] Once a sufficient density of organisms is resident in the airways, bacterial gene expression is regulated by a quorum sensing system – the secretion of freely diffusable homoserine lactones that act along with transcriptional activators to coordinate the gene expression of the entire population of bacteria. This facilitates a biofilm mode of growth, turning off expression of the more immunostimulatory gene products such as

exoenzymes and flagella while favoring secretion of exopolysaccharides.[22] Although few organisms are directly adherent to the epithelial surface, huge numbers of organisms persist in the airways due to reduced mucociliary clearance and loss of airway surface hydration.[23] The shedding of immunostimulatory components from the bacteria activates cytokine and chemokine production by both the airway epithelial cells and recruited immune cells. The milieu within the CF airways is relatively anaerobic, which affects both bacterial gene expression as well as antimicrobial susceptibility.[24] Because organisms within biofilms are relatively less susceptible to antimicrobial agents and phagocytosis, the ability to persist in biofilms provides a major selective advantage to the species.[25]

From this population of bacteria in the CF lung, phenotypically mucoid organisms, *muc* mutants, often are selected. These mutants, virtually pathognomonic for CF isolates, express copious amounts of alginate, a polymer of mannuronic and guluronic acids.[26] Although resistant to phagocytosis, these organisms are not invasive, but chronically infect the airways. The *muc* mutants and wild-type bacteria persist in equilibrium. The planktonically growing bacteria that break off from the biofilm surface are more immunostimulatory and more susceptible to antimicrobial therapy.

EPIDEMIOLOGY AND CLINICAL MANIFESTATIONS

P. aeruginosa is associated with a wide variety of infections, depending on the nature of the host and severity of underlying disease, ranging from self-limited folliculitis[27] to overwhelming septic shock.[28] Due to its exceptional genetic plasticity, *P. aeruginosa* adapts readily to healthcare settings and has become a major cause of healthcare-associated infections[29] including ventilator-associated pneumonia and infections of indwelling catheters.[30] Genomic sequencing studies suggest that a relatively limited number of clones may be responsible for these infections, but with extensive phenotypic diversity within the clones.[31] In CF patients, there is usually clonal expansion of a single *P. aeruginosa* strain over time, with reduced virulence.[32] Tables 155-2 and 155-3

TABLE 155-2. Epidemiology and Clinical Manifestations of Community-Acquired and Nosocomial *Pseudomonas aeruginosa* Infection in the Normal Host

Infection	Clinical Characteristics
COMMUNITY-ACQUIRED	
Ocular	Keratitis is common after minor eye trauma (as in wearers of contact lenses) or penetrating eye trauma; treatment often involves subtenon or intravitreal injections
Otitis externa	"Swimmer's ear" is associated with excessive moisture, or otitis externa results from chronic suppurative otitis media; topical treatment is sufficient; malignant otitis externa is a severe systemic infection usually limited to diabetic patients and other compromised hosts; parenteral therapy and debridement are required
Endocarditis	Intravenous drug abusers can develop *Pseudomonas aeruginosa* endocarditis, usually of the tricuspid valve; injected foreign materials may damage endothelium and create a niche for injected organisms to adhere; septic emboli cause pneumonia; therapy may require surgery
Bone and soft tissue	Puncture wounds of the foot are complicated especially by *P. aeruginosa* infection, because the organisms are found in the moist environment within the soles of sneakers; biopsy of bone may be necessary to differentiate osteomyelitis from a contaminated drainage tract and exploration to remove a retained foreign object
Folliculitis	Immersion in contaminated bathtubs, hot tubs, and pools has been associated with superficial, self-limited infection, commonly confined to abraded areas and those areas covered by bathing suits; infants or patients who experience cellulitis may have severe systemic signs of infection and require anti-*Pseudomonas* treatments
NOSOCOMIAL	
Respiratory tract	Ventilator-associated pneumonia, intubation and use of broad-spectrum antibiotics predispose to pneumonia; *P. aeruginosa* pneumonia (fever, purulent secretions, necrotizing pneumonia, and respiratory deterioration) must be differentiated from colonization; outbreaks of *P. aeruginosa* respiratory infection in intensive care units suggest contamination of a common source, such as respiratory equipment, sinks, blood pressure transducers, or common intravenous flush vials
Urinary tract	Use of prophylactic or broad-spectrum antibiotics, indwelling urinary catheter, another foreign body, or obstruction are predisposing factors; successful treatment almost always requires removal of the foreign body
Surgical	Wound infection can follow neurosurgery, urologic surgery, or orthopedic surgery; osteomyelitis is an infrequent complication that often requires debridement to effect a cure; antimicrobial therapy is prolonged, with few clinical endpoints; neurosurgical infections involving shunts require removal of the foreign material

TABLE 155-3. Epidemiology and Clinical Manifestations of *Pseudomonas aeroginosa* Infections in Special Hosts

Infection	Clinical Characteristics
NEUTROPENIA OR NEUTROPHIL DYSFUNCTION	
Septicemia	Healthcare-associated infection and complication of chemotherapy that causes profound neutropenia, associated with higher mortality and morbidity than from other pathogens; successful outcomes associated with recovery or engraftment of bone marrow, recovery of neutrophils; immunodeficiency patients, extremely small birthweight infants
	Central venous access devices are a source
Ecthyma gangrenosum	These erythematous tender lesions with an area of central necrosis are usually manifestations of or are associated with septicemia; perianal lesions portend poor outcome (Figures 155-1 to 155-3)
Central nervous system	Infection occurs by direct extension from sinuses, bacteremic spread, or secondary to contamination of shunts or reservoirs; in immunosuppressed patients, CNS infections can be insidious
HIV INFECTION	
Pneumonia/bacteremia	*Pseudomonas aeruginosa* is a rare cause of community-acquired pneumonia in HIV-infected adults and children, usually those NOT on effective antiretroviral therapy
Burns	Burn wound sepsis is a complication accompanied by high mortality; meticulous debridement, grafting, and judicious use of antibiotics can help to decrease the incidence of most such infections
Cystic fibrosis	Infection usually occurs early in infancy and childhood, leading to neutrophil-dominated inflammation of the airway, chronic inflammation, fibrosis, and loss of pulmonary function; aggressive anti-*Pseudomonas* therapy and control of inflammatory response are mainstays of therapy

CNS, central nervous system; HIV, human immunodeficiency virus.

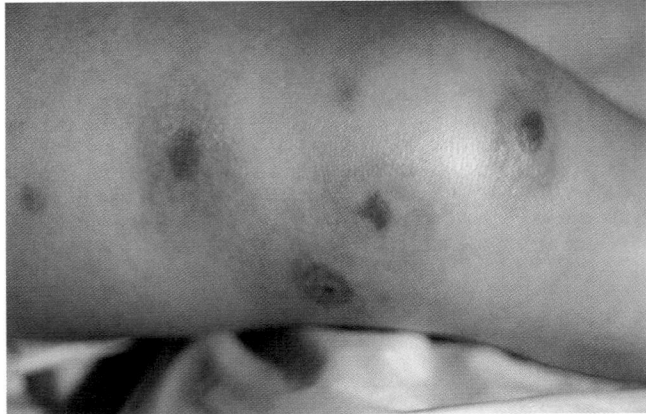

Figure 155-1. Multiple early skin lesions of *Pseudomonas aeruginosa* septicemia in an infant as the initial manifestation of congenital neutropenia. (Courtesy of S.S. Long.)

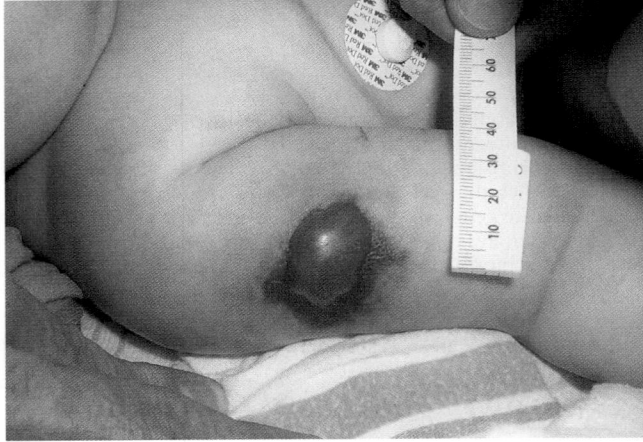

Figure 155-2. Ecthyma gangrenosum lesion as the initial manifestation of chronic granulomatous disease in an infant boy. (Courtesy of S.S. Long.)

show the epidemiology and clinical manifestations of *P. aeruginosa* infection in normal and special hosts.

Antibiotic Resistance

Epidemiologic Trends

Much of the reputation of *P. aeruginosa* as a feared pathogen is due to the combined effects of its many intrinsic virulence factors and readily acquired resistance to antimicrobial agents. By virtue of its large genome, numerous virulence factors, and prodigious ability to mutate in response to immune and chemotherapeutic pressure, numerous reports of human clinical isolates resistant to all available antimicrobial agents including polymyxins are not surprising.[33] Moreover, particularly in patients harboring large numbers of organisms, as in CF, hypermutable strains are recovered that have increased rates of spontaneous mutations due to alterations in the DNA mismatch repair systems.[34] Such hypermutable strains rapidly acquire resistance to multiple antimicrobial agents. National surveillance of antimicrobial resistance rates for *P. aeruginosa* suggest relatively stable resistance trends[35] but with important geographic differences in resistance patterns across the United

States. As might be expected, multidrug-resistant isolates often are associated with healthcare facilities and are more frequent in the CF population.

Mechanisms of Antibiotic Resistance

Permeability factors and efflux systems. Analysis of the *P. aeruginosa* genome has demonstrated that the organism has multiple redundant mechanisms to deal with the potential threat of antimicrobial agents, a likely consequence of its origin in the soil along with fungi that produce common antimicrobial agents. Perhaps the most critical resistance mechanism is the organism's ability to limit permeability through a number of efflux pumps. These efflux pumps have been shown to be important in the export of the quorum sensors that regulate biofilm production, in invasiveness, as well as in antimicrobial susceptibility.[36] The *mexAB* operon is thought to be the major cause of the "intrinsic" resistance of *P. aeruginosa* to many classes of antibiotics, including tetracyclines, fluoroquinolones, chloramphenicol, macrolides, and trimethoprim, as well as β-lactams and β-lactamase inhibitors. Genome analysis has revealed the presence of at least 20 homologues of the mexAB system in *P. aeruginosa*. The combination of limited permeability (increased efflux) and strategically

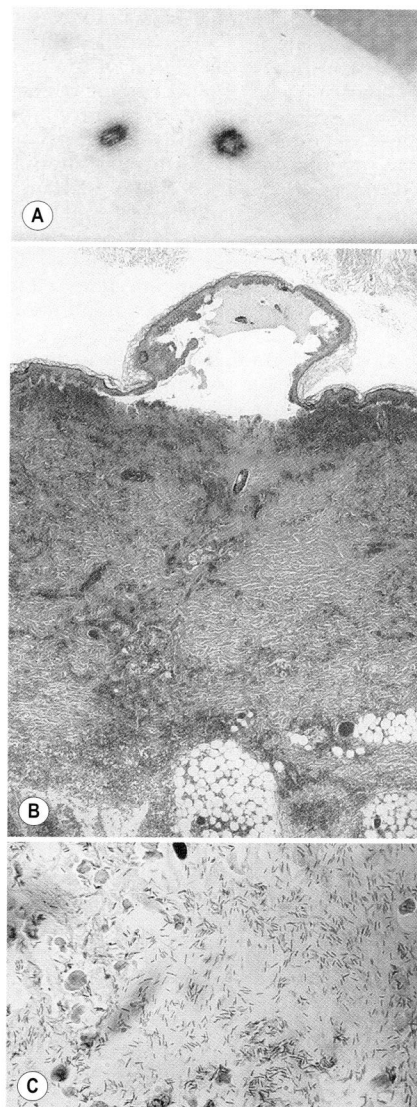

Figure 155-3. (A) Early skin lesions of *Pseudomonas aeruginosa* septicemia in an infant with leukemia. **(B)** Hematoxylin & eosin stain of biopsy of lesion (200×) showing characteristic ischemic necrosis and vesicle formation. **(C)** Tissue Gram stain of fluid from biopsy specimen (1000×). (Courtesy of J.H. Brien©.)

placed enzymes such as β-lactamases within the periplasmic space accounts for much of the antimicrobial resistance of the species.

β-Lactamase production. *P. aeruginosa* expresses both chromosomally mediated as well as plasmid-associated enzymes that degrade β-lactam antibiotics. Chromosomal expression of ampC, an inducible enzyme that preferentially cleaves the 6-membered nucleus of the cepahalosporin family, is a conserved gene in this species. Although normally repressed, the chromosomal enzyme can be induced, particularly by cephalosporin compounds, resulting in clinically significant antibiotic resistance. This chromosomal enzyme is not inhibited by the β-lactamase inhibitors currently in clinical use – tazobactam (as in piperacillin-tazobactam) or clavulanate.[37] In addition, *P. aeruginosa* proficiently accepts plasmid-mediated β-lactamases of many different types. These constitutively expressed enzymes readily cleave most penicillins. β-Lactamase enzymes with inhibition of extended-spectrum β-lactam agents (ESBLs) are increasingly common and have significant activity against a variety of β-lactam and carbapenem structures. Whereas the most common TEM-type plasmid-mediated β-lactamases are susceptible to clavulanate

and tazobactam, many of the more recently identified ESBLs are resistant. Large numbers of bacteria, frequently associated with pulmonary infections such as in patients with CF or in burn wounds, facilitate the selection of mutants resistant to entire classes of antimicrobial agents.

Aminoglycoside-modifying enzymes. Plasmid-encoded or transposon-associated enzymes that can acetylate, phosphorylate, or adenylate specific sites on aminoglycosides can be associated with clinically significant aminoglycoside resistance. The prevalence of these genes varies widely among healthcare facilities. In general, amikacin is less susceptible to modification by these enzymes than is tobramycin or gentamicin, and rates of resistance to amikacin have been lower than to other aminoglycosides. Most aminoglycoside resistance, however, is due to efflux systems resulting in limited uptake of the drug, either alone or in combination with these enzymes.

TREATMENT

Uncomplicated Infections in a Normal Host

The major clinical decisions in treating *P. aeruginosa* infections involve the quality of the host, whether the immune system is normal, the site of infection, the size of the bacterial inoculum and the potential for antimicrobial resistance. There is ongoing debate as to whether the organism requires treatment with two, potentially synergistic antibiotics, or if one drug could suffice in specific clinical settings. Thus, in a *P. aeruginosa* osteomyelitis associated with a puncture wound in a healthy adolescent, or folliculitis acquired in a hot tub, a single drug with high activity against the isolate would be sufficient, and the patient could be treated orally. Similarly, otitis externa (swimmer's ear) in a healthy child, commonly caused by *P. aeruginosa*, often can be treated topically, whereas otitis externa in a person with diabetes requires systemic and usually parenteral therapy. Systemic illness due to *P. aeruginosa* is usually treated with two drugs likely to have synergistic activity against the organism. Outcome of *P. aeruginosa* bloodstream infection is significantly improved if the empiric regimen includes at least one antibiotic with activity against the *P. aeruginosa* isolated.[38] Recent surveys across the U.S. indicate the following rates of *P. aeruginosa* susceptibility: piperacillin-tazobactam, 86%; ceftazidime, 80%; ciprofloxacin, 67%; and levofloxacin, 67%.[35] Isolates from patients with CF generally are more resistant than isolates from individuals without CF.

Infection in Immunocompromised Hosts

Despite the lack of well-controlled blinded studies, most clinicians would treat a "serious" *P. aeruginosa* infection such as bloodstream infection in a neutropenic host or sepsis in a premature infant – with two antipseudomonal agents and preferably with drugs likely to have synergistic activity. As oncology patients and particularly patients with stem cell transplantation often have prolonged periods of neutropenia and frequent febrile episodes, empiric antimicrobial regimens in such patients always include agents with activity against *P. aeruginosa*. Fluoroquinolones or β-lactam agents are commonly used often combined with an aminoglycoside despite the potential for renal toxicity, especially in this patient population. It is noteworthy that the frequency of *P. aeruginosa* infection in these patients has decreased substantially whereas the isolation of gram-positive pathogens and fungi has increased. Most CF patients are managed with chronic inhaled tobramycin and several other antimicrobial agents (e.g., aztreonam and amikacin), some of which will be available for aerosol delivery in this patient population within the near future. Exacerbations in CF often are treated in the outpatient setting and may include parenteral therapy.

Renal Infection

Because extremely high concentrations of most of the antipseudomonal antibiotics are achieved in the urine of patients with normal renal function, most urinary tract infections due to this organism can be treated with a single agent. Patients with obstruction, renal stones, or foreign bodies often fail antimicrobial therapy alone or relapse, as the organisms commonly form biofilms in this setting and are substantially less susceptible to antimicrobial agents.

Central Nervous System Infections

P. aeruginosa shunt infections are generally treated with removal of the contaminated shunt. Agents that cross the blood–brain barrier and have high anti-*P. aeruginosa* activity, such as the carbapenems[39] or fluoroquinolones,[40] usually are effective. As aminoglycosides do not accumulate in the central nervous system, they are of questionable value.

Ocular Infections

Usually associated with accidental or surgical trauma, ocular infection requires urgent and careful ophthalmologic examination to define the extent of the infection and guide the aggressiveness of antipseudomonal therapy. Superficial infections may respond to topical therapy; superfortified aminoglycoside and fluoroquinolone preparations for ocular administration are available. More invasive infections require intraocular treatment to achieve high local levels of drug. Ciprofloxacin and imipenem have some ocular penetration.[41] Infection of the vitreous or anterior chamber usually requires intravitreal or subtenon administration of the antibiotic, chosen according to results of specific susceptibility tests, and vitrectomy may be required.

Pulmonary Infections

Because pneumonia usually involves a high inoculum, treatment conventionally includes two antipseudomonal agents that are likely to be synergistic. This usually includes a β-lactam agent such as piperacillin/tazobactam, a fluoroquinolone, and/or an aminoglycoside. Antipseudomonal cephalosporins (ceftazidime or cefepime) also are effective, although these drugs can select for mutants with constitutive expression of the *ampC* chromosomal enzyme. Carbapenems (imipenem, meropenem, or ertapenem) are often used for isolates resistant to other agents, particularly those that express extended-spectrum β-lactamases. In CF patients who require parenteral therapy, an aminoglycoside (often inhaled tobramycin) is used with a β-lactam or a fluoroquinolone. Fluoroquinolones (ciprofloxacin and levofloxacin) are used widely, both as single agents and in combination with other classes of drugs. Aminoglycosides can be given in large doses by the aerosol route for these pulmonary infections without systemic side effects (see Chapter 108, Infectious Complications in Special Hosts).

Single daily dosing of aminoglycosides is frequently used and appears effective on the basis of studies performed in neonates, children with CF, and neutropenic hosts.[42] The carbapenems and monobactam-aztreonam regimens generally are reserved for infections caused by organisms resistant to the other β-lactams, or for patients with renal disease who are at risk of aminoglycoside-related nephrotoxicity. Multidrug-resistant isolates have been treated successfully with colistin (polymyxin)[43] and polymyxins that can be delivered by aerosol.[44]

PREVENTION

Nosocomial acquisition of the organism is prevented through handwashing, prevention of exposure to high-density organisms from water sources, and adherence to general principles of infection control. Avoidance of uncooked foods, raw fruits, and vegetables in neutropenic patients may decrease ingestion of *P. aeruginosa*. Despite decades of interest in the development of an antipseudomonal vaccine for patients known to be at high risk, there are no vaccines currently available for use. A flagellin-based vaccine has been developed for use in patients with CF, but has been difficult to evaluate due to the efficacy of routine prophylactic antimicrobial therapy for *P. aeruginosa*.[45]

156 *Burkholderia cepacia* Complex and Other *Burkholderia* Species

Jane L. Burns

The genus *Burkholderia* was proposed in 1992 for seven species that previously were in *Pseudomonas* homology group II.[1] All are animal or plant pathogens but are not significant pathogens in healthy humans. Like the pseudomonads, *Burkholderia* are nutritionally diverse water- and soil-organisms; they are catalase-producing and nonglucose-fermenting. Species are distinguished primarily on the basis of phenotype (pigment production, colony morphology, motility, and flagellar structure) and biochemical characteristics (including carbohydrate fermentation patterns and production of indophenol oxidase, arginine dihydrolase, and lysine decarboxylase). All are resistant to polymyxin.

Infections associated with *Burkholderia* species are shown in Table 156-1. *B. cepacia* complex, including both named and unnamed species, has been associated with severe pulmonary infections in patients with cystic fibrosis (CF) and with fatal bloodstream infection (BSI) in patients with chronic granulomatous disease (CGD). *B. pseudomallei* is the cause of melioidosis, an endemic disease in Southeast Asia and northern Australia, and *B. mallei* is the organism that causes glanders, an equine infection seen in Asia and Africa that can be transmitted to humans. *B. gladioli* has been isolated from patients with CF and from immunocompromised individuals. Other *Burkholderia* species can cause sporadic infections or nosocomial outbreaks in immunocompromised individuals but have not been associated with specific syndromes.

BURKHOLDERIA CEPACIA COMPLEX

B. cepacia has recently been recognized as a complex of at least 17 subspecies (genomovars), some of which can be distinguished phenotypically and others that require genotypic identification.[2] Nine of these genomovars have been given species names (Table 156-2)[3] although additional novel species recently have been proposed including *B. latens* sp. nov., *B. diffusa* sp. nov., *B. seminalis*

TABLE 156-1. Infections Caused by *Burkholderia* Species

Organism	Underlying Disease	Disease Caused	Site of Infection
Burkholderia cepacia complex	Cystic fibrosis Chronic granulomatous disease		Lungs Lungs and pleura Lymph nodes Skin and soft tissue Bloodstream Septicemia
Burkholderia pseudomallei	Immunocompromised state Diabetes mellitus Renal insufficiency	Melioidosis	Septicemia Lungs Skin and soft tissue Bone
Burkholderia mallei		Glanders	Septicemia Skin Peritoneum Lymph nodes
Burkholderia gladioli	Cystic fibrosis Chronic granulomatous disease		Lungs Lungs and pleura Lymph nodes Skin and soft tissue Bloodstream Septicemia

TABLE 156-2. Named Species (Genomovars) *Burkholderia cepacia* Complex

Genomovar	Species Name[a]
I	*Burkholderia cepacia*
II	*Burkholderia multivorans*
III	*Burkholderia cenocepacia*
IV	*Burkholderia stabilis*
V	*Burkholderia vietnamiensis*
VI	*Burkholderia dolosa*
VII	*Burkholderia ambifaria*
VIII	*Burkholderia anthina*
IX	*Burkholderia pyrrocinia*

[a]*Only those species that can be distinguished phenotypically have been named.*

sp. nov., and *B. metallica* sp. nov. It has also been suggested that *B. ubonensis* should be considered a member of the complex.[4] *B. cepacia* complex primarily is a nosocomial pathogen and is relatively avirulent in the healthy host. In fact, multiple outbreaks of *B. cepacia* complex infection associated with the contamination of intravenous solutions, intravascular devices, bronchoscopy equipment, and urinary catheters have resulted in minimal morbidity.[5–9] Because *B. cepacia* complex is able to grow in many commonly used disinfectants, such outbreaks are frequently associated with contaminated cleaning solutions.[7,9] Endemic *B. cepacia* complex infections in a large pediatric hospital were associated with contamination of ultrasound gel.[10] *B. cepacia* complex BSI also has been reported in children with hemoglobinopathies[11] and cancer.[12] Patients with CF[13–15] and CGD[16,17] appear to be specifically susceptible to infection by *B. cepacia* complex; such infections can be fatal.

Virulence and Pathogenesis

Despite its virulence in certain subpopulations of patients, specific virulence factors have only recently been identified in *B. cepacia* complex.[18,19] Known *Pseudomonas aeruginosa* cytotoxins, exotoxin

A and exoenzyme S, have not been detected in *B. cepacia* complex.[20] However, the abilities to acquire mobile DNA elements, including genomic islands and insertion sequences, and to use quorum sensing to regulate gene expression are clearly components of virulence. Gene expression changes observed when *B. cenocepacia* is grown in CF sputum are linked to antibiotic resistance, oxidative stress, iron depletion, and motility.[21] In addition, *B. cepacia* complex has an outer membrane that limits antibiotic entry, primarily through limited porin size and efflux pumps,[22] and lipopolysaccharide that is proinflammatory.[23]

Epidemiology

Like many pseudomonads, *B. cepacia* complex is a ubiquitous organism found in soil and water. It was originally described as the cause of onion rot, and *B. cepacia* complex generally is considered a plant pathogen.[24] However, because of its antifungal activity and nutritional diversity, it has become an important organism for biologic control and bioremediation.[25] Nosocomial spread of *B. cepacia* complex most frequently occurs because of the contamination of disinfectant solutions used to clean reusable patient equipment, such as bronchoscopes and pressure transducers, or to disinfect skin.[9,26] The source for acquisition of *B. cepacia* complex by patients with CGD has not been identified.

The epidemiology of *B. cepacia* complex in CF has been well characterized using restriction fragment length polymorphisms, pulse-field gel electrophoresis, and typing strategies based on polymerase chain reaction (PCR). There appears to be a predominant *B. cepacia* strain at each CF center, and epidemiologic studies of movement of patients between centers, CF summer camps, and other social events attended by patients from different geographic areas have demonstrated person-to-person transmission.[3]

In *B. cenocepacia*, one of the pathogenicity islands encodes the *B. cepacia* epidemic strain marker (BCESM), a transcriptional activator that has been associated with transmissibility as well as virulence.[27] The surface cable (Cbl) pilus, which binds CF mucin and is expressed by many *B. cenocepacia* strains, also has been associated with person-to-person transmission in CF.[28]

Recent investigation of the epidemiology of *Burkholderia* in CGD found that, unlike CF, patients are repeatedly infected with distinct strains. *B. cepacia* complex infections in CGD also involve multiple species including *B. ambifaria* and *B. metallica*.[16]

Clinical Manifestations

The expression of nosocomial infections with *B. cepacia* complex is most frequently BSI,[29] although wound infections, urinary tract infections, and pneumonia can occur when those sites are contaminated.[10] BSI is the most frequently occurring infection in immunocompromised patients;[11,12] even in this population, patients rarely succumb to *B. cepacia* complex BSI.

Pulmonary infection in patients with CF usually does not have a discrete onset. Patients become culture positive for the organism late in the course of their disease, virtually always after infection with *P. aeruginosa* has been established. Patients with positive-culture results for *B. cepacia* complex experience one of the following three clinical patterns: (1) transient colonization and no change in the rate of pulmonary decompensation; (2) chronic colonization and a more rapid pulmonary deterioration; or (3) an unexpectedly rapid decline in clinical status that results in death.[13] Epidemiologic studies suggest that specific genomovars, including *B. cenocepacia* and *B. dolosa*, can cause more severe disease in patients with CF,[14,30] although other genomovars cannot be considered nonpathogenic.

In CGD, pneumonia is the most common infection caused by *Burkholderia*;[17,31] lymphadenitis and bacteremic soft-tissue infections also occurred. A tuberculosis-like illness with hemophagocytic syndrome and splenic microabscesses has been reported.[32] The onset of disease is insidious, with low-grade fever and malaise early in the course of disease and signs of systemic toxicity 3 to 4 weeks later. Pleural effusion was seen in 50% of reported cases, and several patients with cavitary lesions have been described.[31,32] The organism is rarely isolated from sputum in these patients; cultures of blood, pleural fluid, bronchoscopy, and lung biopsy specimens have yielded *B. cepacia* complex.

Treatment

B. cepacia complex organisms are difficult to eradicate because they are highly resistant to antibiotics. Organisms are resistant uniformly to the aminoglycosides and polymyxin because of the intrinsic structure of the bacterial cell wall.[33] The outer-membrane porins of *B. cepacia* complex, which serve as channels for the entry of water-soluble antibiotics (such as the β-lactam antibiotics), are relatively impermeable[34] and this, combined with the induction of chromosomal β-lactamases,[35] results in nearly uniform resistance to the β-lactam antibiotics. Multiple antibiotic efflux mechanisms also have been reported in *B. cepacia* complex organisms.[22] The agents with the greatest in vitro activity against *B. cepacia* complex include minocycline, meropenem, ceftazidime, and doxycycline; however, in vitro synergy studies find very few synergistic two-drug combinations.[36] Multiple-combination bactericidal testing suggests that two- and three-drug combinations that include meropenem have the best in vitro activity against *B. cepacia* complex isolates.[37] However, a randomized trial in CF patients comparing clinical outcomes demonstrated no difference between the group receiving standard antibiotic therapy and the group receiving therapy directed by multiple-combination bactericidal testing.[38]

BURKHOLDERIA PSEUDOMALLEI

B. pseudomallei is a major cause of community-acquired septicemia in Southeast Asia and infection is no longer confined to Southeast Asia. Melioidosis, the disease it causes, has been reported in northern Australia, India, and Central America and in travelers returning from endemic areas. Melioidosis occurs in rural populations and is associated with underlying risk factors, including diabetes mellitus and renal insufficiency. Risk factors for melioidosis are rare in pediatric patients and the disease itself is much less common in children than in adults (0.68/100,000 population per year).[39]

However, seroconversion between the ages of 6 and 42 months is estimated to be 24% of the population per year, and symptomatic infection can occur in children as young as 12 months.[40]

Melioidosis can manifest as a localized infection or fulminant septicemia. In pediatric melioidosis, localized infection is the most common presentation (46.2%), followed by septic shock (38.4%) with or without lung involvement.[39] Localized infection in children is most commonly skin and soft-tissue infection of the head and neck, including cervical and submandibular abscesses and suppurative parotitis.[41] Children presenting with melioidosis with septic shock frequently have pneumonia and multiorgan failure can occur. In a small pediatric study, mortality in melioidosis with septic shock was 80%,[39] and in adults the mortality rate in septicemic melioidosis ranges from 17% to 40%, even with antimicrobial therapy.[42,43] Diagnosis can be made by isolation of the organism from the blood or infected site; however, because of the high mortality in septicemia, rapid tests are desirable. Culture remains the gold standard for diagnosis in the absence of other commercially available tests. The indirect hemagglutination antibody assay has been the serologic test used most often. It is more specific in young children than in older children and adults because of the background seroprevalence in older age groups.[40] Immunochromatographic IgM and IgG assays have a sensitivity and specificity of 95% when both tests are used and can have results available in less than 10 minutes.[44] PCR detection of the *B. pseudomallei* type 3 secretion system in DNA extracted from clinical samples, including blood, sputum, urine, body fluids, and swabs of affected areas, has been reported to have a sensitivity of 65% and a specificity of 100%, with no PCR-positive results in specimens from patients without melioidosis.[45]

Treatment of *B. pseudomallei* is difficult. Agents demonstrating in vitro activity include ceftazidime, piperacillin, doxycycline, chloramphenicol, and trimethoprim-sulfamethoxazole.[46] The antibiotic of choice for severe infections is ceftazidime, frequently in combination with trimethoprim-sulfamethoxazole, although there is no demonstrated decrease in acute mortality with the addition of trimethoprim-sulfamethoxazole.[47] Antibiotic resistance testing in *B. pseudomallei* is difficult because of inaccuracy of the disk diffusion method.[48] Because of the high relapse rate in melioidosis,[49] prolonged therapy (up to 6 months) is recommended.

BURKHOLDERIA MALLEI

B. mallei is the cause of glanders, an equine infection seen primarily in the Far East and only rarely spread to humans. The organism is present in the nasal secretions and pustular drainage of infected horses and can be spread by contact with these infected materials. The disease in humans is a severe systemic infection with ulcerative necrosis of the upper respiratory tract, cervical and mediastinal lymphadenopathy, pustular skin lesions and pneumonia, with subsequent septicemia.[50] Infection can be acute or chronic. *B. mallei* infections have been treated successfully with the sulfonamides. Tetracyclines, aminoglycosides, ceftazidime, β-lactam/β-lactamase inhibitor combinations, carbapenems, and fluoroquinolones demonstrate activity in vitro.[46]

BURKHOLDERIA GLADIOLI

Because of its pigmentation and ability to grow on selective agars, *B. gladioli* frequently is misidentified as *B. cepacia* complex. *B. gladioli* can be distinguished biochemically because it is usually indophenol oxidase-negative and does not produce an acid reaction on lactose- and maltose-containing media. *B. gladioli* has been isolated from the sputum of patients with CF with variable clinical impact,[51] but sometimes associated with severe lung disease. *B. gladioli* infections in immunocompromised children and adults also have been reported.[52]

157 *Stenotrophomonas maltophilia*
Jane L. Burns

Stenotrophomonas maltophilia originally was classified as a *Pseudomonas,* transferred to the genus *Xanthomonas* because of common biochemical reactions,[1] and then transferred to its own genus, *Stenotrophomonas,* primarily because it differs markedly in appearance from the other xanthomonads and is not a phytopathogen.[2] The biochemical reactions this organism has in common with *Xanthomonas* include a negative indophenol oxidase reaction and a shared pattern of carbohydrate metabolism. Many strains require methionine for growth. A unique feature of *S. maltophilia* that can aid in its identification is a positive reaction on deoxyribonuclease (DNase) test agar.

VIRULENCE FACTORS

Potential virulence factors identified in *S. maltophilia* include protease, elastase, lipase, mucinase, hyaluronidase, deoxyribonuclease, ribonuclease, and hemolysin. Clinical correlation of these factors with disease has not been reported. However, in a single immunocompromised patient with ecthyma gangrenosum caused by *S. maltophilia,* intense production of protease and elastase by the organism was identified.[3]

EPIDEMIOLOGY

S. maltophilia is similar to the pseudomonads in two important features: ubiquity (frequently being isolated from soil and water), and association with healthcare-related infections in patients with comorbidities.[4] In some patients, it can be difficult to distinguish colonization from true infection. Bloodstream infection (BSI) and pneumonia are the most common infections, but *S. maltophilia* also has been reported to cause ecthyma gangrenosum, endocarditis, ocular infection, urinary infection, wound infection, and other nosocomial infections.[4-8] In a study of pediatric BSI caused by glucose nonfermenting gram-negative bacilli other than *Pseudomonas aeruginosa, S. maltophilia* was the most common, occurring in 67% of patients.[9] Like *Burkholderia cepacia, S. maltophilia* can persist in commonly used disinfectant solutions, resulting in both true infections and pseudoinfections.[10,11] Risk factors associated with pediatric *S. maltophilia* BSI are listed in Box 157-1.[7] Unlike many other gram-negative pathogens, community-associated infections are not uncommon[4] and polymicrobial infections are typical in children.[7] In children with human immunodeficiency virus infection or malignancy, *S. maltophilia* has been reported as an important cause of central venous catheter-associated BSIs.[12] Risk factors associated with *S. maltophilia* BSI in oncology patients include severe mucositis, diarrhea, and use of

BOX 157-1. Risk Factors Associated with *Stenotrophomonas maltophilia* Bloodstream Infections in Children

- Malignancy
- Acquisition of infection in the community
- Trimethoprim-sulfamethoxazole exposure in previous 30 days
- Receipt of corticosteroids or other immunosuppressive therapy
- African American race

metronidazole. There have been several reports of cross-infections in neonatal nurseries.[13,14]

S. maltophilia is an emerging pathogen in cystic fibrosis (CF). *S. maltophilia* was isolated from respiratory tract specimens of 12.5% of CF patients in one study,[15] with prevalence doubling in the last decade.[16] In one study, isolation of *S. maltophilia* from the respiratory tract was associated with oral fluoroquinolone use.[17] Although *S. maltophilia* is more frequently isolated from patients with more severely impaired pulmonary function, an association with increased rate of decline has not been demonstrated clearly.[18,19] However, a recent study found that *S. maltophilia* was an independent risk factor for pulmonary exacerbations in CF.[20]

CLINICAL MANIFESTATIONS AND TREATMENT

Infections caused by *S. maltophilia* are not distinct from nosocomial infections caused by other gram-negative organisms, with the possible exception of ecthyma gangrenosum. This manifestation appears more commonly during *S. maltophilia* BSI than during other non-*Pseudomonas aeruginosa* gram-negative infections.

S. maltophilia is highly resistant to antibiotics, making treatment difficult. The organism virtually is always resistant to the carbapenem antibiotics and aminoglycosides and is variably susceptible to cephalosporins and penicillins.[21,22] The most active agents in vitro continue to include the newer fluoroquinolones, minocycline, and doxycycline, but resistance to trimethoprim-sulfamethoxazole and ciprofloxacin is increasing.[13,21-23] Unlike many multidrug-resistant gram-negative non-Enterobacteriaceae, *S. maltophilia* appears to be susceptible to the β-lactamase inhibitor clavulanic acid. Both ticarcillin-clavulanate and aztreonam-clavulanate demonstrate some activity in vitro.[24] With the exception of trimethoprim-sulfamethoxazole, isolates from individuals with CF are more resistant than isolates from individuals without CF.[21]

158 *Vibrio cholerae* (Cholera)
Anagha R. Loharikar, Manoj P. Menon, Robert V. Tauxe, and Eric D. Mintz

Cholera is an acute diarrheal disease with great potential for epidemic spread. For centuries cholera has caused considerable morbidity and mortality, particularly in the most impoverished areas of the world, where it remains a major public health challenge.

Cholera is caused by two toxin-producing serogroups of the bacterium *Vibrio cholerae,* O1 and O139. When severe, cholera causes rapid loss of fluid and electrolytes; unless volume resuscitation is prompt, death can result.

DESCRIPTION OF THE PATHOGEN

V. cholerae is a gram-negative bacterium of the family Vibrionaceae. Measuring 1.4 to 2.6 μm in length, *V. cholerae* is a curved bacillus with a single polar flagellum. Somatic (O) antigens differentiate the serogroups. Epidemic cholera is caused by toxin-producing strains of serogroup O1 or O139. Nontoxigenic and non-O1, non-O139 strains can cause diarrhea and septicemia, but only O1 and O139 have caused epidemics (see Chapter 159, Other *Vibrio* Species). *V. cholerae* O1 is further divided into two major serotypes (Inaba and Ogawa) and two biotypes, classic and El Tor. During epidemics, a shift from one serotype to another can occur.[1,2] *V. cholerae* O139 closely resembles the El Tor biotype but, unlike *V. cholerae* O1, possesses both a capsule and a distinct lipopolysaccharide and does not agglutinate with O1 antisera.[3,4]

The complete genome of *V. cholerae* O1 has been sequenced, and consists of two circular chromosomes. The larger chromosome I, comprising some 2.96 million basepairs, contains most of the essential genes as well as loci determining virulence.[5] The toxin-associated genes reside within a lysogenized filamentous phage, which suggests that these genes came from another organism via horizontal transfer.[6] Chromosome II, which consists of roughly 1.07 megabases,[5] may have been acquired as a plasmid or by excision from a single large genome. Chromosome II harbors unique copies of critical genes, including a large cluster of integrons (mobile DNA elements capable of gene acquisition).[5]

MICROBIOLOGY

V. cholerae ferments glucose and sucrose, is oxidase-positive, and is exquisitely sensitive to acid and to drying. Although *V. cholerae* can be grown on commonly used media, a selective medium such as thiosulfate citrate bile salts sucrose (TCBS) agar facilitates isolation. On TCBS agar, *V. cholerae* colonies are large (2 to 4 mm in diameter) and yellow with opaque centers and translucent edges. Presumptive identification is based on slide agglutination with O1 or O139 antiserum. Two biotypes of *V. cholerae* serogroup O1 – classic and El Tor – and have been described on the basis of biochemical and other phenotypic markers. The classic biotype was predominant until the 1960s, when the El Tor biotype spread around the world as the seventh pandemic. More recently, "variant" or "hybrid" strains that possess all of the properties of El Tor biotype strains but include cholera toxin genes that more closely resemble those typically found in classic biotype strains have been described.[7] Serogroup O1 isolates react with Inaba or Ogawa antiserum; both serotypes are found among classic and El Tor biotype strains. Confirmation of O139 isolates involves demonstration of either cholera toxin production or the presence of cholera toxin gene sequences.[8]

VIRULENCE AND PATHOGENESIS

Infection with toxigenic strains of *V. cholerae* O1 and O139 causes a spectrum of illness. A study in Bangladesh found that 59% of people infected with the classic biotype of *V. cholerae* O1 were asymptomatic compared with 75% of those infected with the El Tor biotype. Among those with symptomatic infection, 11% of those infected with the classic biotype compared with only 2% to 5% of those with El Tor infections were hospitalized for severe cholera. The remainder had mild or moderate illness.[9,10] Mortality in severe cases can reach 50% in remote regions or among populations for whom treatment is not readily available. However, with prompt and appropriate volume resuscitation, mortality should be <1%.

V. cholerae O1 and O139 remain in the gastrointestinal tract and typically do not invade the bloodstream; however, there are some reports of cholera bacteremia resulting from *V. cholerae* O139.[11,12] The voluminous secretory diarrhea of cholera results from the action of cholera toxin on the small intestinal mucosa and the effect of a pilus colonization factor, toxin coregulated pilus (TCP).[13] Cholera toxin, like the heat-labile (LT) *Escherichia coli* toxin, is a protein enterotoxin. The toxin is composed of an A

subunit and five B subunits arranged in circular form. After the B subunits bind to intestinal epithelial cells, the A subunit activates adenylate cyclase in the mucosa. As a result, increased intracellular concentrations of cyclic adenosine monophosphate (cAMP) fuel secretion of sodium and chloride into the gut lumen; water follows passively. Isotonic fluid is secreted at a rate that exceeds the absorptive capacity of the colon.[14] The mechanism of TCP remains unclear. Three additional enterotoxins, the zona occludens toxin (ZOT),[15] accessory cholera enterotoxin (ACE),[16] and WO7 toxin[17] produced by *V. cholerae* O1, have been described. Although the mechanism of these toxins differs, they each appear to increase mucosal permeability.

IMMUNITY

Immunity to cholera is incompletely understood. Nonspecific defense mechanisms include gastric acidity and intestinal peristalsis. People with blood group O are particularly likely to experience severe cholera; the reason is unknown.[18,19] A study in Bangladesh found that although people with blood group O were more likely to develop severe disease once they were infected, they were less likely to become infected with *V. cholerae* O1 in the first place, a finding consistent with the hypothesis of adaptive immunity.[20] Incubation period varies with the ingested dose and gastric pH but averages 1 to 3 days, with a range of a few hours to 5 days.

Antimicrobial therapy decreases volume and duration of diarrhea, and shortens the duration for which *V. cholerae* is detectable in stool.[21,22] Without antimicrobial therapy, *V. cholerae* is detectable in stools for approximately 1 to 2 weeks. Prolonged carriage is rare but does occur.[23] Infection with *V. cholerae* O1 induces development of serum antibacterial (vibriocidal) and antitoxin antibodies. As with other noninvasive enteric infections, specific immunity is provided primarily by secretory immunoglobulin (IgA), which, in the case of cholera, lasts but a few months. However, cholera infection can induce long-lasting immunologic memory.[24]

A study comparing the immune response of patients infected with *V. cholerae* O1 and O139 revealed that both serogroups can elicit vibriocidal and cholera toxin-specific responses. However, previous infection with serogroup O1 does not offer protection against infection with serogroup O139.[25,26] Where cholera is prevalent, children who are not breastfed are infected more often than breastfed children. A mother who breastfeeds not only protects her infant from unsafe alternative food sources[27] but also, if previously exposed to *V. cholerae*, may transfer specific IgA antibodies in her milk.[28]

EPIDEMIOLOGY

Cholera can be endemic, epidemic, or pandemic. For centuries, cholera has remained endemic in countries bordering the Bay of Bengal and has spread in periodic pandemic waves. Worldwide, epidemics tend to occur during warm seasons.

The modern era of cholera comprises seven pandemics; the first six occurred between 1817 and 1923. Most originated in Asia, usually the Indian subcontinent, and subsequently extended to Europe and the Americas.[29] During the second pandemic, the English physician John Snow traced cholera in London to the Broad Street pump and documented waterborne disease transmission before the etiology of the disease was known. During the fifth pandemic, Robert Koch isolated *V. cholerae* from patients with diarrhea, thereby establishing the etiology of cholera. Strains of the fifth and sixth pandemics were classic biotype.

The ongoing seventh pandemic, already the longest and most widespread, began in 1961, when *V. cholerae* O1, biotype El Tor, spread from a focus in Sulawesi (formerly Celebes), Indonesia. In 1971, it reached both East and West Africa, where it remains endemic. After more than 100 years without epidemic cholera, the pandemic reached the Americas, in January 1991, when *V. cholerae* O1 appeared in Peru and spread swiftly through much of South and Central America.[30,31] Compared with epidemics of the 19th century, attack rates were higher but mortality rates were lower.[32,33]

From 1991 through 1996, more than 1.3 million cases of cholera, and nearly 12,000 associated deaths, were reported from 20 countries in Latin America, sparing the Caribbean.[34] In stark contrast to Africa, cholera was nearly eliminated from Latin America within a decade, due to investments in water and sanitation infrastructure that brought additional benefits, such as decreased infant mortality.[35,36] Cholera incidence during the Latin American epidemic correlated with infant mortality, suggesting that they share a common denominator of unsafe drinking water and poor sanitation.[37] Cholera remains endemic in sub-Saharan Africa, the region with the lowest population coverage for improved water sources and sanitation, with recurrent outbreaks in several countries.[38–48] Currently, Africa reports the "lion's share" of cholera to the World Health Organization (WHO); from 2000 through 2009, more than 1.5 million cases of cholera and over 38,000 associated deaths, were reported from 36 countries in Africa.[39–49]

In 2009, the latest year for which data were available, 45 countries notified WHO of a total of 221,226 cholera cases and 4946 deaths (case-fatality rate 2.2%), an increase of 16% in reported cases compared with 2008.[39] Thirty (67%) countries reporting cholera to WHO were from sub-Saharan Africa, and, as has been the trend in recent years, Africa reported the largest percentage of cases (98%) and deaths (99%).[38] Underreporting, which results from concern about the political and economic ramifications of reporting cholera cases, has been and remains a problem; however, although differences in reporting may account for some of the disparity, issues regarding water, sanitation and hygiene infrastructure and access to basic medical care clearly play a role. In 2009, countries most affected by cholera, with over 10,000 reported cases each, included Democratic Republic of Congo, Ethiopia, Kenya, Mozambique, Nigeria, Sudan, South Africa, and Zimbabwe. Zimbabwe faced a large outbreak of cholera causing over 68,000 cases and 2700 deaths in 2009, on top of 60,000 cases and nearly 3000 deaths in late 2008.

Haiti has long had the lowest population coverage with improved water sources and sanitation in the western hemisphere. Tragically, 9 months after the devastating earthquake in January, 2010, Haiti experienced its first outbreak of cholera in over a century.[50,51] Within 1 month of the first recognized cases in late October 2010, cholera had reached all 10 Departments in Haiti and related cases had been recognized in the neighboring Dominican Republic and the United States.[52,53] As of December 31, 2011, Haiti had reported 523,904 cases, 282,441 hospitalizations, and 7018 deaths due to cholera (case fatality rate CFR 1.3%).

In October 1992, a new strain of *V. cholerae* was identified in Chennai (formerly Madras), India. The strain did not agglutinate with O1 antiserum nor with antisera to any of the other 137 previously known serogroups, and spread rapidly to 11 countries in South Asia.[11,54] Designated *V. cholerae* O139 Bengal, it was the first non-O1 *Vibrio* to cause epidemic disease. Because immunity to *V. cholerae* O1 was not protective against this strain, the proportion of adults affected was unusually high. Given the potential evolutionary advantage of this relatively new bacterial serotype, concern was expressed that the advent of *V. cholerae* serogroup O139 marked the beginning of the eighth pandemic of cholera.[37] Thus far, however, O139 has remained confined to South and Southeast Asia and only transiently displaced O1 as the dominant serogroup.[55]

Brackish aquatic environments are the natural reservoirs of both O1 and non-O1 strains of *V. cholerae*. When conditions are favorable, *V. cholerae* multiplies and can survive for years, independent of human fecal contamination, in brackish waters in association with invertebrates such as copepods, crabs, shrimp, and oysters. Endemic foci of *V. cholerae* O1 persist in several areas of the developed world, including the Gulf Coast waters of the U.S. where a unique O1 strain was first identified in 1973.[56] In the developed world, rare sporadic human cases may follow ingestion of water or undercooked shellfish[57] from such reservoirs; more commonly, they occur in travelers returning from areas where disease is epidemic.[58]

Introduction of cholera into a developing area, where the drinking water supply is not protected from human fecal contamination, can cause explosive epidemics. Infection typically follows

drinking contaminated water or consumption of food washed with, or seafood harvested from, contaminated water, or food prepared by an individual who is excreting *V. cholerae*.[59] Waterborne transmission of *V. cholerae* was identified in multiple investigations during the epidemics in Latin America, from contamination of municipal source water as well as stored water in the home.[60] Foodborne transmission can occur through foods and beverages in the market or the home, including foods from street vendors, leftover rice, and unwashed fruits and vegetables. Foods and drinks sold by street vendors are often prepared in unhygienic ways. Foods may be held at ambient temperatures for long periods of time, and beverages may use unsafe ice. Drinking water from wide-mouthed household storage containers raises the risk of illness.[37,61] However, direct person-to-person spread of cholera has not been documented convincingly.[62]

CLINICAL MANIFESTATIONS

The hallmark of cholera is watery diarrhea leading to varying severity of volume depletion and dehydration. Mild or moderate disease may be difficult to distinguish from disease caused by several other enteric pathogens, including enterotoxigenic *E. coli* (ETEC) or rotavirus; however, severe cholera is distinctive. No other diarrheal illness produces volume depletion as rapidly as cholera. Cholera usually begins with watery colorless diarrhea flecked with mucus – "rice-water stools" – without abdominal cramps or fever. Stools can have a mild fishy odor. Vomiting is common, can be severe, and can precede or follow diarrhea. Patients with cholera typically do not have fever.

In untreated severe cholera, diarrhea and vomiting usually result in volume depletion with shock in 4 to 12 hours and death in 18 hours to several days. When the disease is most severe, patients lose 1 liter of fluid per hour and die within hours. The early signs of dehydration – thirst, tachycardia, dry mucous membranes, loss of skin turgor, and sunken eyes – are followed quickly by hypotension and anuria. Renal failure secondary to hypovolemia is reversible with volume resuscitation. Altered mental status is common but usually is mild and can consist of somnolence, restlessness, or lethargy. Rarely, patients have abdominal distention and ileus without diarrhea; this has been called "cholera sicca," or dry cholera.[63]

Other clinical manifestations result from electrolyte imbalances. Profuse watery diarrhea rich in potassium and bicarbonate (Table 158-1) leads to hypokalemia with arm and leg cramps

TABLE 158-1. Electrolyte Composition of Diarrheal Stools from People with Cholera and Composition of Rehydration Solutions

	Sodium (mEq/L)	Potassium (mEq/L)	Chloride (mEq/L)	Base[a] (mEq/L)	Carbohydrate (mmol/L)
CHOLERA STOOLS					
Adults	135	15	100	45	
Children	105	25	90	30	
ORAL SOLUTIONS					
WHO-ORS	90	20	80	30	111
WHO-ORS (reduced osmolarity)	75	20	65	10	75
Ceralyte 70 (rice-based)	70	20	60	30	40 g/L
Ceralyte 90 (rice-based)	90	20	80	30	40 g/L
RINGER LACTATE	130	4	109	28	

WHO-ORS, World Health Organization oral rehydration solution.

[a]*Consists of bicarbonate, or citrate.*

Modified from Swerdlow DL, Ries A. Cholera in the Americas: guidelines for the clinician. JAMA 1992;267:1495–1499.

and metabolic acidosis, which can increase the frequency of vomiting. Hyperglycemia, resulting from high concentrations of epinephrine, glucagon, and cortisol, is more common overall than hypoglycemia, which can occur when glycogen stores are depleted and gluconeogenesis is impaired.[64] However, children with cholera are especially prone to hypoglycemia, which can lead to convulsions and poor outcomes.[65] Fever and obtundation also are more common in children.[66] Sequelae related to fluid and electrolyte derangements, followed by hypoglycemia, are the most important life-threatening consequences of cholera. During pregnancy, cholera can be particularly severe; despite prompt resuscitation the fetal death rate may be as high as 50% for women in the third trimester who experience severe volume depletion.[67]

LABORATORY FINDINGS AND DIAGNOSIS

Cholera is a clinical diagnosis. Once cholera is suspected, treatment must be begun before laboratory confirmation is obtained. Cholera should be considered in any patient with profuse watery diarrhea, often described as "rice-water stools," and vomiting. Clinical suspicion should increase if these symptoms are severe in any patient who has returned from an area with epidemic cholera or who has eaten undercooked shellfish in the 5 days before onset of illness.

Cholera is diagnosed definitively by isolation of toxigenic *V. cholerae* O1 or O139 from a stool specimen or rectal swab, which should be collected before antibiotics are given.[68] Rectal swabs should be placed in a transport medium such as Cary–Blair medium at room temperature; buffered glycerol saline is not acceptable. Because *V. cholerae* rarely is isolated routinely by laboratories in the U.S., clinicians should alert the laboratory if cholera is suspected so that specimens can be inoculated on TCBS agar or other appropriate media. Isolates of *V. cholerae* should be sent to the state public health laboratory for testing with O1 and O139 antisera, and then to the Centers for Disease Control and Prevention (CDC) for confirmation of serogroup and serotype and detection of toxin production.

Antimicrobial susceptibility can be determined by disk diffusion or broth microdilution testing. Interpretive criteria have been established for ampicillin, chloramphenicol, sulfonamides, tetracycline, and trimethoprim-sulfamethoxazole.[69] Susceptibility results for tetracycline by disk diffusion are used to predict susceptibility to doxycycline. There are no available cutpoint values for disk diffusion testing for ciprofloxacin or azithromycin. Increases in serum vibriocidal antibody titers can confirm infection retrospectively in clinically compatible cases; however, this test is not used routinely for diagnosis of cholera. Rapid immunoassays for presumptive detection of *V. cholerae* O1 or O139 in stool in field

settings have been developed[70–73] but do not replace culture for definitive diagnosis.

Nonspecific abnormalities in laboratory test results include hypoglycemia or hyperglycemia, hypercalcemia, hypermagnesemia, and hyperphosphatemia. Potassium deficit may not become apparent until the patient's metabolic acidosis is corrected. Serum sodium and chloride concentrations usually are normal or slightly decreased. The white blood cell count can be elevated. Volume depletion often results in increases in hematocrit and total serum protein concentration, and can cause elevated blood urea nitrogen and serum creatinine values.

TREATMENT

Volume Replacement

Steps in management of people with suspected cholera are listed in Box 158-1. Rapid volume resuscitation is the cornerstone of therapy. Treatment options depend on available resources and training of healthcare providers. A simple scheme can be used to determine the severity of volume depletion (Table 158-2) and to guide fluid resuscitation after acute diarrhea of any cause.

Oral rehydration therapy is as effective as intravenous rehydration;[74,75] patients with mild to moderate volume depletion can be treated with oral solutions alone, administered in small sips to patients who are vomiting.[76] In the U.S., WHO oral rehydration solution (ORS) is available in salt packets by the case or carton (Jianas Brothers, St. Louis, MO; 816-421-2880; http://rehydrate.org/resources/jianas.htm). When mixed with 1 liter of clean water per

---

BOX 158-1. Steps in Management of People with Suspected Cholera

1. Assess for volume depletion
2. Rehydrate with oral and/or intravenous fluids and monitor frequently
3. Maintain hydration: replace continuing fluid losses until diarrhea and vomiting ceases
4. Consider zinc supplementation in addition to rehydration
5. Give oral antibiotics to patients with moderate or severe volume depletion
6. Resume feeding with a normal diet; continue breastfeeding infants and young children

Modified from World Health Organization. Guidelines for Cholera Control. Geneva, World Health Organization, 1993.

TABLE 158-2. Signs and Symptoms of Dehydration in Patients with Watery Diarrhea

	Degree of Dehydration		
	Mild (3–5%)	**Moderate (6–9%)**	**Severe (≥10%)**
OBSERVATIONS			
Mental status	Alert	Restless, irritable	Lethargic or unconscious
Thirst	Slightly increased	Moderately increased	Very thirsty or too lethargic to drink
Mucous membranes	Slightly dry	Dry	Very dry
Tears	Present	Absent	Absent
Eyes	Normal	Sunken	Very sunken and dry
EXAMINATION			
Pulse	Normal	Faster than normal	Very fast, weak, or nonpalpable
Pinched skin	Retracts rapidly	Retracts slowly	Retracts very slowly
Extremities	Warm; normal capillary refill	Delayed capillary refill	Cool, mottled
Fontanel	Normal	Sunken	Very sunken
THERAPY	Oral rehydration	Oral or intravenous rehydration	Intravenous rehydration

Modified from World Health Organization. Guidelines for Cholera Control. Geneva, World Health Organization, 1993; and Centers for Disease Control and Prevention. The management of acute diarrhea in children: oral rehydration, maintenance, and nutritional therapy. MMWR 1992;41:1–20.

packet, the resulting solution can be used to restore fluid and electrolyte balance in patients with cholera (see Table 158-1). A systematic review of ORS among a pediatric population found that a solution with 75 mEq/L of sodium compared with the standard solution of 90 mmol/L of sodium was associated with reduction in stool output, vomiting, and intravenous fluid use.[77] Based in part on these findings, WHO advocated for a solution with reduced osmolarity in the year 2002. The current recommended solution contains 75 mEq/L of sodium with an osmolarity of 245 mOsm/L. Ceralyte (Cera Products, Columbia, MD; 1-888-237-2598; http://www.ceraproductsinc.com/productline/ceralyte.html). A rice-based product also is available. This glucose polymer-based ORS has been shown to result in a greater reduction of stool output than glucose-based ORS.[78] Oral solutions with sodium concentrations <75 mEq/L should not be used in the treatment of cholera. For alert patients unable to drink sufficient quantities of ORS, use of an orogastric or nasogastric tube should be considered.[79] If ORS is not available, volume resuscitation should be started immediately with intravenous fluids.

Zinc supplementation, in addition to rehydration, can reduce duration and severity of cholera diarrhea, particularly in children.[80] Treatment with antibiotics also has been shown to reduce duration of diarrhea, and improve fluid losses (see Antimicrobial Agents below).

Patients without Volume Depletion

Patients without signs of volume depletion can be treated at home with ORS. Using a teaspoon, syringe, or medicine dropper, the caregiver initially should provide small volumes of fluid (e.g., one teaspoon) and then gradually increase the amount as tolerated.[81] Ongoing fluid losses are replaced as described later. The caregiver should be given a 2-day supply of ORS and instructed to seek medical attention immediately if the patient's intake cannot keep pace with vomiting or diarrhea losses.

Patients with Mild to Moderate Volume Depletion

ORS (50 mL/kg) should be given initially to people with mild volume depletion (loss of 3% to 5% of body weight) in the first 2 to 4 hours of therapy, and 100 mL/kg to people with moderate volume depletion (loss of 6% to 9% of body weight). In both cases, volume status is reassessed at 4 hours. If volume depletion is corrected, treatment enters the maintenance phase. If losses continue, fluid deficit is re-estimated, and fluid administration is resumed.[81] Ongoing losses can be replaced at home with ORS after initial observed volume resuscitation. Additional ORS always can be administered coincident with thirst.

Patients with Severe Volume Depletion

If volume depletion is severe (loss of ≥10% of body weight), or if patients are unable to tolerate oral rehydration because of mental status changes or intractable vomiting, intravenous therapy should be started immediately. Rapid volume resuscitation can even save patients whose pulse is not initially detectable. Ringer lactate is the appropriate fluid in the U.S. (see Table 158-1); normal saline is far less effective because it lacks potassium and bicarbonate. Dextrose–water solutions should not be used, as they do not effectively replete volume. Ringer lactate is infused rapidly until pulse, perfusion, and mental status return to normal. Volume status is reassessed frequently. ORS (about 5 mL/kg per h) should be added as soon as the patient is able to drink. Oral fluids should replace intravenous fluids as early as is practical.

ORS can be administered through the nasogastric route if the patient has mild to moderate volume depletion and cannot drink or if volume depletion is severe and intravenous therapy is not possible. Urine output usually resumes within 6 to 8 hours. Regular urinary output, 1 mL/kg per h or more every 3 to 4 hours, signifies adequate fluid administration. Volume status is reassessed frequently, and ongoing fluid losses are replaced. Infants and young children should continue breastfeeding, and other

TABLE 158-3. Antibiotics for Treatment of Cholera[a]

Antibiotic	Dose	
	Children (mg/kg)	Adults (mg)
Drug of choice:		
Doxycycline (a single dose)	6	300
Alternative for children <8 years:		
Azithromycin (single dose)	20	1000
Alternative for pregnant women:		
Azithromycin (single dose)	N/A	1000

[a]*See text.*

older children should resume a normal diet, as soon as they are able.

Replacement of Ongoing Fluid Losses

During both initial volume resuscitation and maintenance, ongoing fluid losses from stool and vomit should be replaced, initially by 10 mL/kg of ORS for each watery stool passed and 2 mL/kg for each episode of emesis. Ongoing fluid losses during maintenance therapy can be replaced with either low-sodium ORS or ORS containing 75 to 90 mEq/L of sodium accompanied by another source of low-sodium fluid (e.g., human milk, formula, or water; see Table 158-1).[81]

Antimicrobial Agents

Although the cornerstone of treatment for cholera is replacement of fluid volume and electrolytes, treatment with antimicrobial agents decreases duration of illness, volume of stool output, and period of excretion of *V. cholerae*. Single-dose doxycycline orally is recommended as the first-line treatment in adults;[82] single-dose azithromycin or ciprofloxacin can be used as effective alternatives (Table 158-3).[83] Azithromycin, as a single dose, is recommended as the first-line treatment in children and pregnant women.[84] Antibiotic susceptibility patterns should be determined, particularly in outbreak settings, because antibiotic-resistant strains of *V. cholerae* are common, and antibiotic choices should be informed by local susceptibility patterns.[56–58] Antibiotics should not be used routinely for prophylaxis, but may be considered for outbreaks occurring in institutionalized populations.[85] Antidiarrheal and antispasmodic agents should not be used.

PREVENTION
Public Health Measures

In the developed world, water and sewage treatment makes epidemic spread of cholera extremely unlikely, although some underserved populations may be at risk.[86] In the developing world, however, contaminated drinking water and food set the stage for epidemic cholera. Prophylaxis is not recommended in the U.S. In the developing world, prophylaxis can be considered during outbreaks occurring in institutionalized settings, such as prisons. Chemoprophylaxis of household contacts in the developing world has been suggested.[87] However, this measure may promote development of antibiotic resistance and is not recommended routinely.[88,89] Education about protecting drinking water and about washing hands with soap and water after defecation and before preparation or eating of food may help control the epidemic. A strategy that empowers families to disinfect drinking water with chlorine and safely store drinking water in closed, narrow-mouth vessels to prevent re-contamination (see www.cdc.gov/safewater/) was developed in the course of the cholera epidemic in Latin America.[90] This approach may reduce the introduction as well as spread of cholera in households and has been used widely in Africa.[91,92] Breastfeeding protects infants, whether or not the mother has immunity to *V. cholerae*.[27,28] Quarantine of patients, mass chemoprophylaxis, and mass vaccination have not halted epidemic cholera, and are not recommended as epidemic control measures.

Vaccination

The search for an inexpensive and effective vaccine has been ongoing for over a century. Historically parenteral vaccines have not been favored given the low efficacy and high rate of side effects. However, in the past two decades, considerable progress has been made in development of both live and killed oral cholera vaccines.

Currently two types of oral vaccines are available in some countries, although none is licensed in the U.S. These include: (1) Dukoral, manufactured by Crucell/SBL Vaccine, Sweden, and containing a mixture of heat- and formalin-killed classic and El Tor *V. cholerae* strains and a recombinant B subunit of cholera toxin (WC/rBS);[39] and (2) ShanChol (manufactured by Shantha Biotechnics, India) and mORCVAX (manufactured by VABIO-TECH, Vietnam), which contain different mixtures of killed strains without a cholera toxin subunit.[93,94]

A previously marketed oral live attenuated single-dose vaccine, CVD 103-HgR, is no longer available.[94] An injectable vaccine prepared from phenol-inactivated strains is no longer manufactured or available, due to its limited efficacy and short duration of protection.[95]

When WC/rBS was tested extensively in a field trial in Bangladesh in a location where both El Tor and classic strains were present, vaccine yielded protective efficacy of 62% in the first year of the trial.[96] Efficacy waned after 2 years, and was substantially lower among people of blood group O,[97] among children, and against infection with El Tor biotype as opposed to classic biotype.[98] In this cluster randomized trial in an endemic area, although vaccine coverage rates varied, herd protection was observed.[99]

Given concern about the effectiveness of a vaccine in an area with a high prevalence of HIV, a case-control study was conducted in a city in Mozambique with an HIV-seroprevalence rate of >20%. The WC/rBS vaccine was found to be effective, with vaccination providing 78% protection.[100] In a trial in Kolkata, Shanchol, a modified killed-whole cell oral vaccine, provided safe and efficacious protection against clinically significant cholera, while being easier to administer and less costly; Shanchol is pending prequalification by WHO.

These cholera vaccines have not been shown to prevent epidemic cholera transmission and are not recommended for the general population. Given the extremely low risk of cholera for travelers in areas with epidemic or endemic disease, counseling about risk avoidance is more cost-effective than vaccination. Even in stable refugee populations at risk for epidemic cholera, vaccination generally is a less cost-effective intervention than improvements in water sanitation and treatment.[101]

Vaccination should be considered in areas where cholera is endemic.[94] However, it should always be done in conjunction with

---

BOX 158-2. Advice for Travelers to Areas Affected by Epidemic Cholera

USUALLY SAFE
Cooked foods that are still hot
Fruits peeled by the traveler
Carbonated bottled water without ice
Other carbonated beverages
Beverages made with boiled water

UNSAFE. AVOID
Cooked food stored at ambient temperature
Salads and raw vegetables
Raw or undercooked fish and shellfish
Food and beverages from street vendors
Unboiled or untreated water or ice

Modified from Swerdlow DL, Ries A. Cholera in the Americas: guidelines for the clinician. JAMA 1992;267:1495–1499.

---

the implementation of safe water, sanitation and hygiene promotion programs. In resource-poor areas, vaccination should be targeted at children aged ≥2 years. After taking into account herd immunity, cholera vaccination may be a cost-effective measure in some endemic mid-low resource settings.[94]

Cholera vaccine has not been recommended in outbreak settings or complex humanitarian emergencies because of the logistical challenges of administering a 2-dose vaccine, and the concern that large-scale vaccination would divert limited resources from higher priority measures, including treatment, and could provide a false sense of security.[102]

Epidemiologic Investigations

Because of the potential for epidemic spread in the developing world, even a single case of cholera has important public health implications. Because many *V. cholerae* infections are mild or asymptomatic, a single recognized case portends a larger outbreak. If a case is suspected, local public health authorities should be notified, and a search begun immediately to identify the source. CDC can assist state and local health departments and other countries with these epidemiologic investigations.

Advice For Travelers[103,104]

Travelers to areas where epidemic cholera occurs can prevent infection by following the precautions described for prevention of travelers' diarrhea (Box 158-2). When simple precautions are followed, the risk of cholera is low.[34] Nonetheless, travelers to areas with cholera who experience profuse watery diarrhea, especially if it is accompanied by vomiting, should seek medical attention immediately, because prompt volume resuscitation can be life-saving.

---

159 Other *Vibrio* Species

Emily J. Cartwright and Patricia M. Griffin

In addition to organisms that cause cholera (see Chapter 158 on *Vibrio cholerae* (Cholera)), several other *Vibrio* species cause clinical illness. These organisms, with the exception of *V. parahaemolyticus* and *V. vulnificus* biogroup 3, rarely cause outbreaks.

Organisms that do not cause cholera are referred to collectively as nontoxigenic vibrios and include serogroups of *V. cholerae* other than O1 and O139, nontoxigenic strains of *V. cholerae* O1, and several other *Vibrio* species associated with human disease

TABLE 159-1. Nontoxigenic *Vibrio* Species Most Commonly Associated with Human Disease in the United States, 2007–2008

Vibrio Species	Site of Isolation			Percentage of All Reported *Vibrio* Species[a]
	Blood	**Stool**	**Wound**	
V. parahaemolyticus	+	+++	++	47
V. vulnificus	+++	+	++	17
V. cholerae nontoxigenic[b]	++	+++	++	9
V. alginolyticus	+	+	+++	18
V. fluvialis	+	+++	++	4
Grimontia (Vibrio) hollisae	+/–	+++	++	1
V. mimicus	+	+++	+	4

+++, *common (51% to 100% of isolates); ++, occasional (10% to 50% of isolates); +, infrequent (1% to 9% of isolates); +/–, rare (<1% of isolates).*

[a]*Based on 1080 nontoxigenic* Vibrio *illnesses reported to the Centers for Disease Control and Prevention's Cholera and Other* Vibrio *Illness Surveillance System, 2007–2008.[3] Species constituting ≥1% of all reported* Vibrio *species are listed.*

[b]*Includes nontoxigenic* V. cholerae *O1 (8 isolates), and other nontoxigenic* V. cholerae *non-O1 non-O139 (293 isolates).*

BOX 159-1. Guidance[11]

- Persons should be informed that consumption of raw or undercooked seafood and open-wound contact with warm seawater increases the risk of *Vibrio* infection
- Persons who are immunocompromised, especially those with chronic liver disease, are at highest risk for severe *Vibrio* infection
- To ensure appropriate diagnosis of infection, clinicians should request microbiologic culture with selective media when *Vibrio* is suspected
- Clinical laboratories should send all *Vibrio* isolates to their state public health laboratory for confirmation and species identification

(Table 159-1). The nontoxigenic *Vibrio* species can be divided into two groups: (1) invasive species primarily associated with septicemia and wound infections (of which *V. vulnificus* is the prototype); and (2) species that typically cause gastroenteritis (e.g., *V. parahaemolyticus*).

DESCRIPTION OF THE PATHOGENS

Vibrios are gram-negative bacteria of the family Vibrionaceae. They are fermentative, facultatively anaerobic, gram-negative bacilli with a single polar flagellum. Except for *V. cholerae* and *V. mimicus*, all *Vibrio* species are halophilic (salt-requiring).

Several possible virulence factors have been described for the nontoxigenic *Vibrio* species, including cell-associated adhesins, extracellular toxins, and various proteases.[1] However, the actual role of these factors in disease is unknown. Some *V. cholerae* non-O1, non-O139 strains[2] and *V. mimicus* strains can produce cholera toxin. Little is known about the mechanisms of immunity against nontoxigenic vibrios.

Vibrios are free-living inhabitants of marine coastal waters and, occasionally, brackish inland lakes and streams; their presence does not indicate fecal contamination of the water. Environmental factors, specifically water surface temperatures and salinity, affect the concentrations of most *Vibrio* species. Accordingly, most *Vibrio* infections occur during the summer and fall months, when surface waters tend to be relatively warm.

EPIDEMIOLOGY

Vibrio infections are reported more commonly from coastal than inland states.[3] Estuarine filter feeders (such as oysters, clams, mussels, shrimp, and crabs) can sequester and concentrate vibrios, and *Vibrio* infections often occur in people who have consumed raw or undercooked seafood, especially shellfish.[3] *Vibrio* infections also can occur after exposure of a wound to seawater.[4] The incidence of *Vibrio* infections other than toxigenic *V. cholerae* in the United States is estimated to be almost 80,000 cases per year, with most infections occurring in adults.[5] Not all cases are detected, partly because most laboratories do not routinely use media that are selective for vibrios.[6,7] Historically, only infections with toxigenic *V. cholerae* serogroups O1 and O139 were notifiable nationally, but, in 2007, infection caused by any *Vibrio* species became notifiable nationally.[3]

Vibrio vulnificus

V. vulnificus was first described by the Centers for Disease Control and Prevention (CDC) in 1979. It is the *Vibrio* species most commonly associated with life-threatening illness in the U.S.[3,8] *V. vulnificus* causes an estimated 207 cases of illness each year, with 202 hospitalizations and 77 deaths.[5] The organism is responsible for two major syndromes: primary septicemia and wound infection.

Infections are classified as primary bloodstream infection (BSI)/septicemia when *V. vulnificus* is isolated from a normally sterile site, and the patient had no evidence of a preceding wound infection. A review of *V. vulnificus* infections in the U.S. occurring between 1988 and 1996 found that 96% of patients with primary BSI had consumed raw oysters in the 7 days before symptoms.[9] Almost all patients with primary BSI have an underlying condition, such as liver disease, malignancy, hemochromatosis, or are immunocompromised.[3,9] CDC has issued guidance regarding the risks of consuming raw or undercooked seafood, particularly in people with underlying conditions (Box 159-1).[10,11]

The second important clinical syndrome caused by *V. vulnificus* is wound infection. Wound infection occurs most commonly in adults with an underlying condition.[8,12,13] Infection typically occurs through exposure of an open wound to warm seawater.[14,15] Severe wound infections with *V. vulnificus* biogroup 3 have been reported from Israel among previously healthy persons handling live tilapia fish.[16]

Gastroenteritis is a rare presentation of *V. vulnificus* infection, accounting for approximately 5% of reported cases, and typically occurs in healthy persons who have recently consumed raw oysters.[11]

Vibrio parahaemolyticus

V. parahaemolyticus is the most frequently reported cause of *Vibrio* illness in the U.S.,[3] where it causes both sporadic cases and outbreaks of gastroenteritis.[17,18] Patients frequently report eating raw oysters in the week before onset of the illness.

Other *Vibrio* Species

Non-O1, non-O139 *V. cholerae* strains are common inhabitants of coastal and estuarine saltwater areas, although infections also have occurred after exposure to freshwater inland lakes.[19] These organisms are isolated commonly from oysters and other shellfish, especially during the warmer months. Gastroenteritis is the most common presentation, although septicemia and wound infections also occur. Non-O1 strains of *V. cholerae* can produce a polysaccharide capsule, a feature that may explain their ability to cause invasive disease.

V. alginolyticus and *Photobacterium (Vibrio) damselae* usually are associated with external ear and wound infections, respectively, in persons exposed to saltwater, whereas *Grimontia (Vibrio) hollisae*, *V. fluvialis*, *V. mimicus*, and nontoxigenic strains of *V. cholerae* O1 typically cause gastrointestinal tract infection.[1] Cases of wound infection with *V. carchariae*[20] and meningitis-bacteremia caused by *V. cincinnatiensis*[21] have been reported. Human isolates of two other *Vibrio* species, *V. furnissii* (from stool and wounds) and *V. metschnikovii* (from blood, stool, urine, and wounds) have been reported.[22,23] Isolation of an uncommon *Vibrio* species does not prove that it is the cause of clinical symptoms; the pathogenicity of some vibrios is not established clearly.

CLINICAL MANIFESTATIONS

Vibrio vulnificus

Primary BSI caused by *V. vulnificus* is often fulminant and rapidly fatal. One-third of patients come to medical attention in shock, and 90% of these people die, usually within 48 hours of hospitalization.[14] Most patients have characteristic bullous skin lesions. Necrotic ulcers can progress to necrotizing fasciitis. Thrombocytopenia is common, and disseminated intravascular coagulation can occur. Initial hypotension, leukopenia, thrombocytopenia, and low serum albumin levels predict a fatal outcome.[14,24] The case-fatality rate in primary *V. vulnificus* BSI is 61%.[9] Patients with *V. vulnificus* wound infections typically have fever and cellulitis, swelling, and intense pain at the wound site. In severe cases, fasciitis, myositis, or secondary BSI can ensue. In one series, 17% of persons presenting with a *V. vulnificus* wound infection died, and patients with underlying liver disease were significantly more likely to die than others.[4] For any of the syndromes caused by *V. vulnificus*, the typical incubation period is about 18 hours but ranges from 12 hours to 4 days.

Vibrio parahaemolyticus

Gastroenteritis due to *V. parahaemolyticus* usually causes stools that are watery but can contain mucus or blood. Patients typically experience diarrhea 24 hours (range, 4 to 96 hours) after consumption of contaminated raw or undercooked seafood. Diarrhea can be accompanied by abdominal cramps, nausea, vomiting, and headache. Fever is absent or low grade, dehydration rarely occurs, and illness usually is self-limited, with a median duration of 2.5 days.[1]

Other *Vibrio* Species

Diarrhea associated with *V. cholerae* non-O1, non-O139 strains ranges from mild to profuse and watery, similar to that of patients with cholera.[2,25] Abdominal cramps, fever, visible blood in stool, and vomiting also can occur. *V. cholerae* non-O1, non-O139 also can cause primary BSI, usually in patients with underlying immunodeficiency, hematologic malignancy, or cirrhosis.[25,26] Symptoms resemble those of BSI caused by *V. vulnificus* but usually without bullous skin lesions. The case-fatality rate of BSI is >50%.[26] Nontoxigenic vibrios occasionally are isolated from other body sites.

Infections attributed to *Vibrio* species include otitis media, otitis externa, meningitis, pneumonia, peritonitis, cholecystitis, and panophthalmitis.[27]

LABORATORY FINDINGS AND DIAGNOSIS

Vibrio infection should be suspected in any patient with septicemia, wound infection, or gastroenteritis who has a history of shellfish consumption or exposure to saltwater or brackish water. *Vibrio* species are isolated readily from blood on sheep blood agar. However, isolation from stool or wounds is best accomplished using selective media, such as thiosulfate-citrate bile salts sucrose (TCBS) agar,[28] which are not typically included in routine microbiologic testing of stool.[6] All pathogenic *Vibrio* species (with the exception of *Grimontia* (*Vibrio*) *hollisae*) grow on TCBS agar. Final identification is made by standard biochemical tests.[29]

TREATMENT

Patients with primary septicemia require prompt supportive care, including monitoring of hemodynamic status and fluid management. Early antimicrobial therapy for *V. vulnificus* septicemia can decrease the case-fatality rate.[14] Recommended therapy has been trimethoprim-sulfamethoxazole plus an aminoglycoside for children (although organisms are not susceptible uniformly to either agent), and doxycycline plus a third-generation cephalosporin or fluoroquinolone for adults.[30] A single-agent regimen with a fluoroquinolone such as levofloxacin, ciprofloxacin, or gatifloxacin has been reported to be at least as effective in an animal model as combination drug regimens with doxycycline and a cephalosporin.[31] This would be an appropriate use for a fluoroquinolone in children. For patients with wound infections or necrotizing fasciitis, prompt debridement is often necessary.[32,33] In one retrospective analysis of critically ill patients with *V. vulnificus* wound infections, prompt surgical intervention was associated with improved survival.[34] Most gastrointestinal tract infections are mild and self-limited and do not require treatment other than oral rehydration (see Chapter 158, *Vibrio cholerae* (Cholera)).

PREVENTION

Although the risk of *Vibrio* infection in consumers of raw oysters is greatest during the summer and fall, cases occur throughout the year. Guidelines for prevention of *Vibrio* infections have been developed for high-risk groups, with particular focus on persons with liver disease.[11] However, because most cases of *Vibrio* gastroenteritis and wound infections occur among healthy persons, such guidelines are appropriate for everyone. Effective preventive measures are: (1) thoroughly cooking shellfish; (2) refrigerating cooked seafood if it is not eaten immediately; (3) preventing cross-contamination of other foods with raw seafood; and (4) avoiding exposure of open wounds or broken skin to warm saltwater or brackish water or to raw shellfish harvested from such waters.

160 *Bartonella* Species (Cat-Scratch Disease)

Gordon E. Schutze and Richard F. Jacobs

The genus *Bartonella* consists of more than 20 species, of which the best known is *B. henselae*. The role of *B. henselae* in most cases of cat-scratch disease has been established through serologic analysis of patients and their cats, polymerase chain reaction (PCR) tests on lymph nodes and skin test antigen, and isolation of the organism from lymph nodes and cats.[1-6] *B. quintana*, the cause of louse-borne trench fever, and *B. henselae* have both been identified as the causes of bacillary angiomatosis, bacillary peliosis, bacteremia, and endocarditis in the immunocompromised host. *B. bacilliformis* is the cause of bartonellosis (also known as Carrión disease), and other *Bartonella* species (e.g., *B. elizabethae*, *B. alsatica*) have been described to cause endocarditis.

DESCRIPTION OF THE PATHOGEN

Bartonella spp. are small, curved, pleomorphic, gram-negative bacilli with fastidious growth requirements. Lysis centrifugation tubes can be used to isolate *Bartonella* spp. from blood. Recovery on solid agar is best achieved through inoculation of tissue homogenate onto fresh chocolate agar or heart infusion agar plates with 5% rabbit blood. Inoculated agar plates are incubated in 5% carbon dioxide at 35°C for 2 to 6 weeks.

EPIDEMIOLOGY

The true incidence of cat-scratch disease in the United States is unknown, although an estimated 22,000 ambulatory patients are diagnosed annually, with a national hospitalization rate of 0.42/100,000 to 0.86/100,000.[7,8] A slightly larger proportion of cases occurs in males than in females. Although children are more likely to be affected than adults, the disease is rare in infancy.[9] Incidence is highest in southern states and lowest in arid, western states.

The domestic cat is a major reservoir for *B. henselae* as well as a major vector for the transmission of *B. henselae* to humans. *B. henselae* bacteremia in otherwise well-appearing cats is common and can be prolonged.[10] Recent studies have demonstrated that 41% of pet and impounded cats have bacteremia with *B. henselae*,[6] whereas 93% of feral cats and 75% of pet cats have been found to be seropositive.[11] Although flea-borne (*Ctenocephalides felis*) transmission of *B. henselae* from cat to cat appears to be efficient, epidemiologic data do not support the efficient transmission from cats to humans by cat fleas.[12]

More than 90% of patients with cat-scratch disease have a history of recent contact with a cat, often a kitten, and 50% to 87% of these patients have been scratched. The incubation time from the cat scratch until the appearance of lymphadenopathy is from 5 to 50 days (median, 12 days). There are anecdotal reports of transmission by other animals, such as dogs and monkeys, as well as by inanimate objects, such as pins and splinters.

Cat-scratch disease is a sporadic illness with no evidence of person-to-person transmission. Even if asymptomatic, persons in households in which a case has been diagnosed are more likely to be seropositive than the general population.[2] Multiple cases have occurred in families, presumably resulting from contact with the same animal. Several widespread outbreaks also have been described. A survey of 33 geographic regions throughout North America showed that increasing prevalence of antibody to *B. henselae* in cats paralleled increasing climatic warmth and annual precipitation.[13] Seroprevalence was highest in regions with warm, humid climates, which also have a higher incidence and severity of flea infestation of cats.

Most cases of cat-scratch disease occur in fall and winter; 71% to 93% are reported from August through January.[2,7,9] Seasonality may be related to feline reproductive cycles, in combination with flea activity; that is, a cohort of kittens is born midsummer (while flea activity is high) and is weaned in early fall. Kittens are more commonly implicated as sources of infection than adult cats, possibly because kittens are more likely to scratch. However, a recent survey of cats indicated that seroconversion occurred during the first year of life, suggesting that young cats are more likely to have active infection than older ones.[14]

The arthropod vector for *B. bacilliformis* is the sandfly.[15] The vector involved in transmission of *B. quintana* is unknown but is suspected to be the body louse, because of the association of body lice and trench fever during World War I. Humans are the only known vertebrate hosts for *B. quintana* and *B. bacilliformis*. Both of these species can produce prolonged periods of asymptomatic bacteremia, providing a reservoir from which the body louse and sandfly, respectively, can transmit the organisms to another human host.

Bacillary angiomatosis is a rare vasoproliferative disorder that occurs almost exclusively in severely immunocompromised persons.[16,17] It also has been reported in a few apparently immunocompetent individuals. In patients with bacillary angiomatosis, those infected with *B. henselae* often have a history of cat exposure, but those infected with *B. quintana* do not. Bacillary peliosis occurs primarily in terminally ill patients with acquired immunodeficiency syndrome, but also has occurred in other chronic debilitating diseases, such as tuberculosis and malignancy. Persistent or relapsing fever with bacteremia due to *B. henselae* or *B. quintana* occurs primarily in immunocompromised persons but also has been reported in immunocompetent persons.[18]

B. bacilliformis infection (bartonellosis, Carrión disease) has not been reported to occur outside a very restricted geographic region in the Andes mountains in western South America. There are two different forms of this disease. The acute form, known as Oroya fever, is a severe febrile illness with a high mortality rate. The chronic phase, known as verruca peruana, is characterized by red, warty, vascular cutaneous lesions that resemble bacillary angiomatosis.[19]

CLINICAL MANIFESTATIONS

Cat-Scratch Disease

Human infections due to *B. henselae* can be asymptomatic or symptomatic (Figure 160-1A to J). For symptomatic patients, regional lymphadenopathy, fever, and mild constitutional symptoms are common. Cat-scratch disease is the most common cause of chronic unilateral regional lymphadenitis in children in the United States.[9,18–20] After an incubation period of 7 to 12 days, one or more erythematous papules 2 to 5 mm in diameter appear at the inoculation site. This primary lesion persists for 1 to 4 weeks and then regresses spontaneously with the appearance of lymphadenitis, the hallmark of cat-scratch disease.

Lymphadenitis usually involves nodes that drain the site of inoculation; however, in as many as 20% of cases, additional lymph node groups are affected. At any particular site of lymphadenitis, a single lymph node is involved in approximately half of cases, whereas in the remainder, multiple nodes are involved. The site most commonly involved is the axilla, followed by the cervical, submandibular, and inguinal areas. The area around an affected lymph node typically is tender, warm, erythematous, and indurated. In as many as 30% of cases, the affected node suppurates spontaneously. Lymphadenitis usually regresses over 4 to 6 weeks.

The majority of patients with cat-scratch disease are afebrile and lack constitutional symptoms. When present, constitutional symptoms typically are low-grade fever, malaise, anorexia, fatigue, and headache. Parinaud oculoglandular syndrome is a distinctive presentation of cat-scratch disease in which the site of inoculation is the eyelid or conjunctiva, and a papular lesion and conjunctivitis develop at the inoculation site accompanied by ipsilateral preauricular lymphadenitis (Figure 160-1).

Systemic cat-scratch disease occurs in a small proportion of cases, but there has been an apparent increase in incidence over the last decade that may be due to greater recognition.[18,21,22] Patients with systemic cat-scratch disease typically come to medical attention for prolonged fever (1 to 3 weeks), malaise, listlessness, myalgia, and arthralgia; some have skin eruptions, weight loss, abdominal pain (which can be severe), peripheral lymphadenopathy, hepatomegaly, and splenomegaly. In two case series in which presentation was fever of unknown origin, abdominal pain was present in more than half of patients and lymphadenopathy in less than half.[23,24] On ultrasonography (US) and computed tomography (CT), multiple microabscesses or granulomas of the liver or spleen can be identified in some cases. Other less common manifestations include encephalitis, aseptic meningitis, neuroretinitis, osteolytic lesions, bone marrow granulomas, granulomatous hepatitis, pneumonia, thrombocytopenic purpura, and erythema nodosum. Anecdotal cases (Figure 160-1), magnetic resonance imaging, and technetium-99 bone scan have demonstrated bony involvement, without osteolytic lesions on plain film.

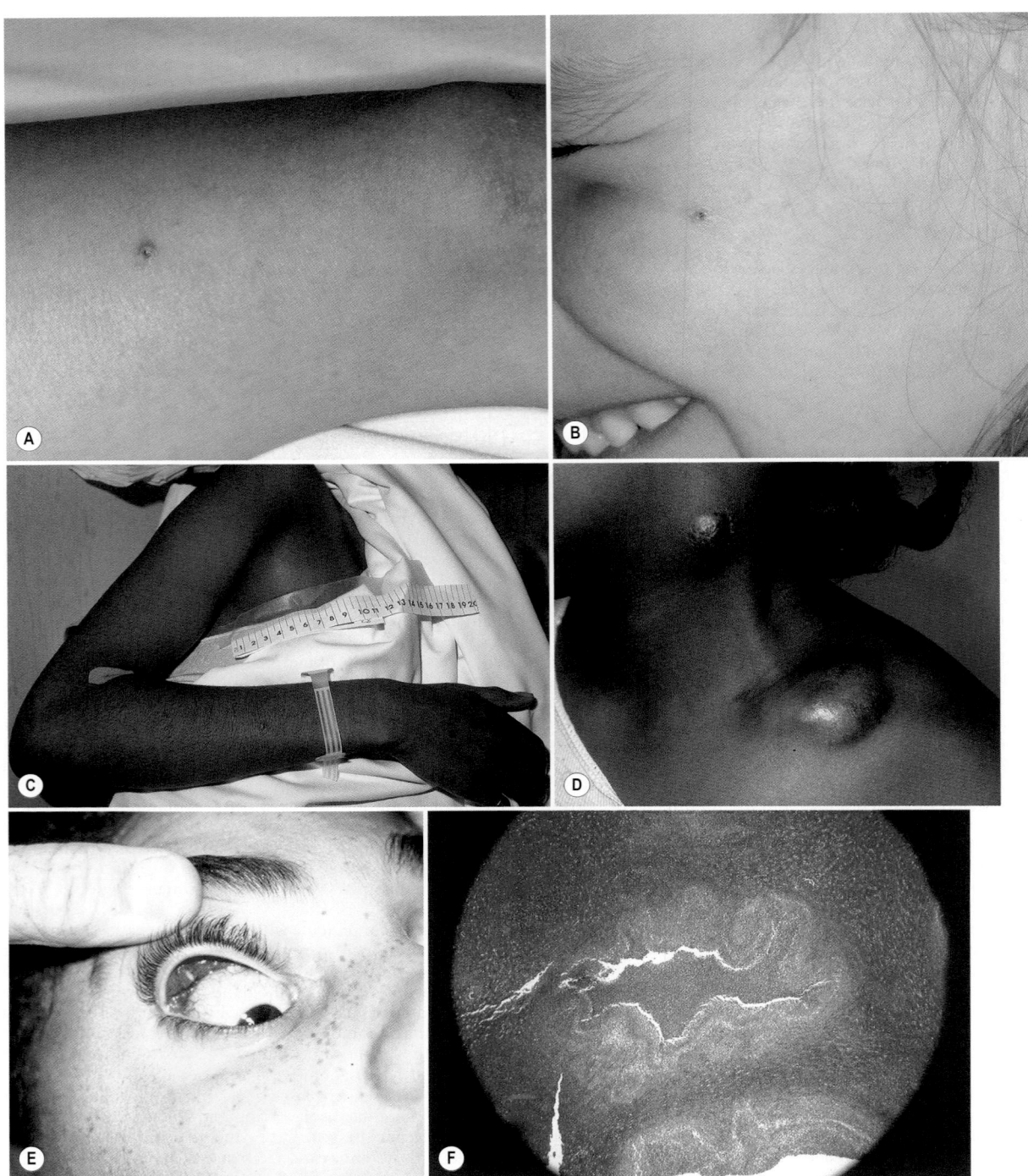

Figure 160-1. Typical clinical findings of *Bartonella henselae* infection (cat-scratch disease). Simple papule at the scratch site on the leg **(A)** of a young boy, and the face of a young girl **(B)**. Papular lesion on the arm and axillary lymphadenopathy in an adolescent **(C)**. Papular lesion and fluctuant, enlarged lymph nodes in the supraclavicular and neck areas of an adolescent girl who frequently cuddled her kitten over her chest and shoulder **(D)**. Granulomatous conjunctivitis and preauricular lymphadenopathy in a 12-year-old boy **(E)**. Histologic specimen of an excised neck mass showing a lymph node with granuloma and stellate microabscess (hematoxylin & eosin, 200×) **(F)**.

Other *Bartonella henselae* and *Bartonella quintana* Infections

Bacillary angiomatosis is characterized by the gradual appearance of vascular proliferative lesions of the skin and subcutaneous tissues.[18,21] These lesions can be verrucous, papular, or pedunculated, and although they usually have an erythematous base and a vascular appearance, the lesions are occasionally dry, scaly, hyperkeratotic, or plaque-like. The lesions can occur singly or in large numbers so as to cover the entire body; they usually enlarge if untreated. Bacillary angiomatosis also can manifest either as subcutaneous nodules with or without overlying tenderness and erythema or as deep soft-tissue masses.

Bacillary peliosis is characterized by the appearance of reticuloendothelial lesions in visceral organs, primarily the liver (peliosis hepatis); however, the spleen, abdominal lymph nodes, and

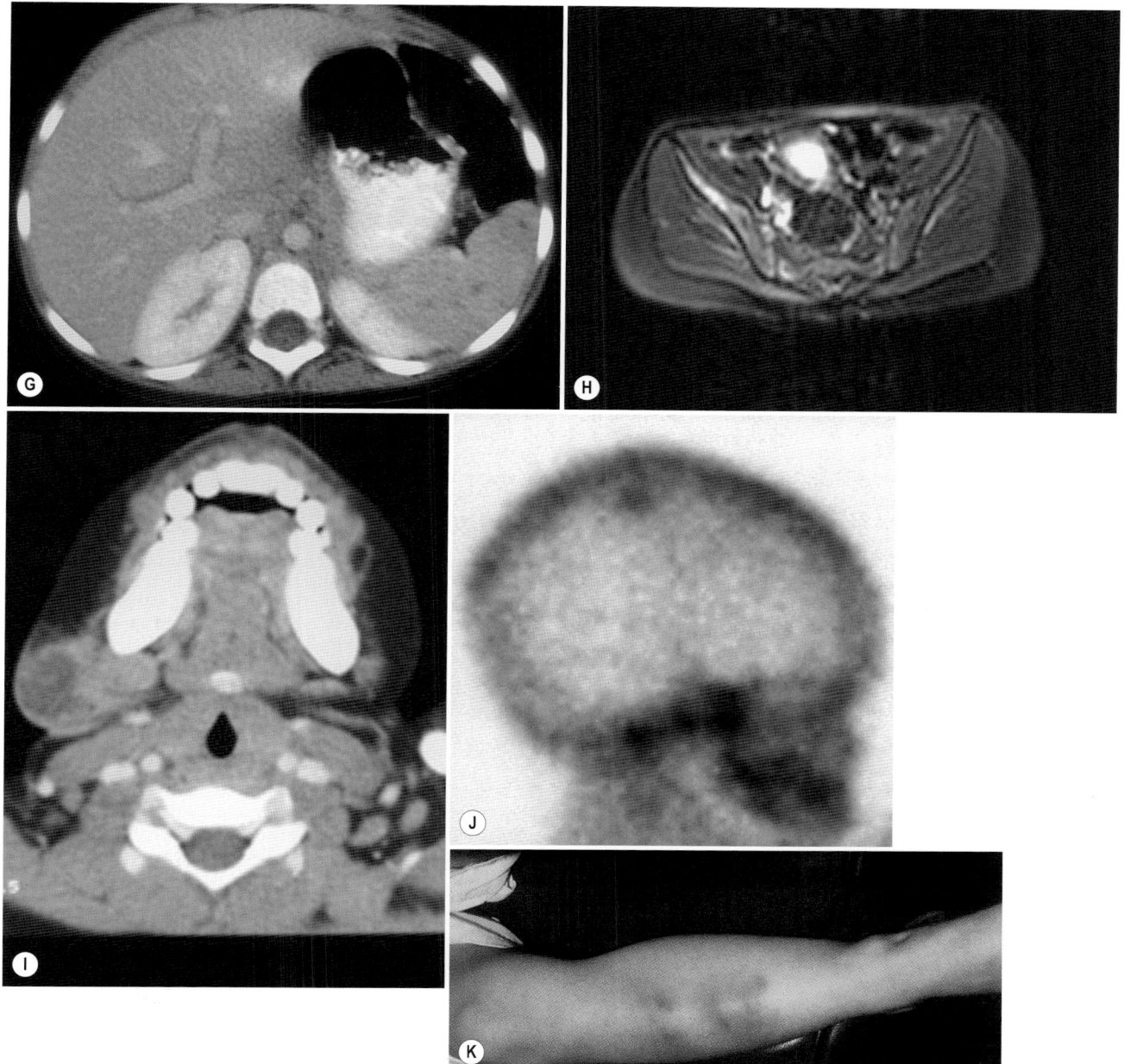

Figure 160-1, cont'd Computed tomography of the abdomen without contrast in a young girl with fever of unknown origin showing multiple hypodense areas in the spleen **(G),** which changed minimally following administration of contrast. Gadolinium-enhanced axial magnetic resonance imaging showing bone marrow enhancement of the ilium in a 6-year-old girl who came to attention for fever of unknown origin and right hip pain; no osteolytic lesion was evident on plain film **(H).** Computed tomography of the neck showing superficial necrotizing mass **(I),** and delayed phase of technetium-99 bone scan showing increased uptake in the skull **(J)** (and ilium: not shown) in a 5-year-old with persistent fever and hip pain while being treated with amoxicillin for lymphadenitis; she had no signs or symptoms referable to the skull finding. **(K)** Erythema nodosum in a 7-year-old girl with axillary lymphadenopathy. (Courtesy of J.H. Brien© (A, B, E, H), Scott & White Memorial Hospital, Temple, TX; S.S. Long (C, D, F, K) and E.D. Thompson (G, I, J), St. Christopher's Hospital for Children, Philadelphia, PA.)

bone marrow also can be involved. The visceral lesions of bacillary peliosis can be accompanied by the cutaneous lesions seen in bacillary angiomatosis.

Immunocompromised patients who are infected with *B. henselae* or *B. quintana* can manifest persistent or relapsing fever with bacteremia, frequently accompanied by weight loss and other constitutional symptoms. Bacteremia can be complicated by subacute endocarditis.

LABORATORY FINDINGS AND DIAGNOSIS

Results of routine laboratory evaluation of patients with cat-scratch disease usually are unremarkable. The most consistently reported abnormality is an elevated erythrocyte sedimentation rate and C-reactive protein.[18,21] In disseminated disease, hepatic transaminase concentrations can be elevated if the liver is involved (but not in all cases of hepatic infection), and occasionally, a biliary obstructive pattern of abnormalities can be seen. US or CT can reveal multiple round, oval, or irregular lesions from 3 to 30 mm in diameter.

Several serologic tests for cat-scratch disease have been developed. Using strict clinical case criteria, immunoglobuoin M (IgM) and IgG indirect immunofluorescence antibody (IFA) assays show sensitivity of 88% and specificity of 98%).[3,25] An enzyme immunoassay (EIA) has excellent specificity (IgM 99%; IgG 98%).[1,2,18,26] Rates of background seropositivity (titer ≥1:64) with the IFA test are low (2% to 6%) but may be higher in cat owners. Demonstration of a rising IgG titer provides the best evidence of infection; however, most patients with cat-scratch disease already have high titers at the time of presentation, and titers may not fall for 2 to 6 months. In a prospective trial of antibody kinetics, EIA (IgM) remained positive for 3 months and indicated acute infection. EIA (IgG) antibody decreased over time, with 25% of patients remaining positive for 1 year after the onset of cat-scratch disease. No association was found between height of antibody titers or their kinetics and the clinical manifestations or duration of disease.[26] Cross-reactivity among *Bartonella* spp. is common, and serologic tests do not yet accurately distinguish between species.

If tissue specimens are obtained from patients with cat-scratch disease, attempts to isolate *Bartonella* species usually are not helpful because in vitro incubation is 2 to 4 weeks, and for poorly understood reasons, live organisms are rarely isolated from such patients. The histologic findings of lymph nodes or other affected tissues are characteristic, but not pathognomonic. Early histologic changes consist of lymphocytic infiltrates with epithelioid granuloma formation. Later histologic changes consist of neutrophilic infiltrates within granulomas that have begun to fuse and become necrotic (stellate microabscesses) (Figure 160-1), followed by large pus-filled sinuses that eventually rupture through the node capsule into surrounding tissue. Organisms can be visualized using a Warthin–Starry silver impregnation stain; however, this test is not specific for *B. henselae*.

In cases of bacillary angiomatosis and bacillary peliosis, diagnosis usually is made by biopsy. The histologic appearance of each of these lesions is characteristic, and clusters of organisms can be demonstrated with Warthin–Starry staining. Attempts to culture *Bartonella* have been more successful in specimens collected from patients with these manifestations than in those collected from patients with typical cat-scratch disease.[22] Serologic tests have proved useful, even in patients with human immunodeficiency virus infection.

The most sensitive method of diagnosing a *B. henselae* or *B. quintana* infection is by PCR testing performed on various clinical specimens. Several different procedures have been developed that are accurate and can discriminate among different species of *Bartonella*.[27-30] Although many PCR assays use different gene products, a recent description of the htrA gene from *B. henselae* demonstrated a 76% positivity rate in 29 definite cases of cat-scratch disease utilizing tissue or fine-needle aspirates.[30] A skin test that was widely used in the past was never licensed or known to be free of transmissible agents, however, and should not be used.

TREATMENT

The management of typical cat-scratch disease primarily is supportive; the disease usually is self-limited, resolving spontaneously in 2 to 4 months. Painful suppurative nodes can be treated with needle aspiration for relief of symptoms; surgical excision generally is unnecessary. *B. henselae* is susceptible in vitro to a wide range of antimicrobial agents, including penicillins, tetracyclines, macrolides, trimethoprim-sulfamethoxazole, rifampin, fluoroquinolones, aminoglycosides, and later but not first-generation cephalosporins. Anecdotal reports of patients with systemic infection[22,23,31] and typical cat-scratch disease[32,33] suggest a clinical response to a number of antimicrobial agents, including trimethoprim-sulfamethoxazole, rifampin, ciprofloxacin, and gentamicin. A prospective, randomized, double-blind, placebo-controlled investigation of 5 days of oral azithromycin therapy for patients with laboratory-confirmed typical cat-scratch lymphadenitis demonstrated a modest clinical benefit.[34] Patients who received azithromycin compared with placebo recipients had a significantly greater decrease in lymph node volume during the first month of treatment, as determined by serial US evaluation. In the absence of data from controlled trials demonstrating a substantial clinical benefit, the value of antimicrobial therapy for patients with any form of cat-scratch disease remains uncertain.

Although the benefit of antimicrobial therapy for patients with bacillary angiomatosis or bacillary peliosis has not been studied systematically, experience suggests that such therapy is beneficial and clearly is indicated.[21] The lesions and symptoms of these diseases respond rapidly to erythromycin or doxycycline therapy.[35] Tetracycline, minocycline, and azithromycin also have been shown to be effective.[36] Rifampin also may be effective but usually is recommended as a second drug in combination with either erythromycin or doxycycline. Patients who have only cutaneous lesions should be treated for at least 2 weeks, and those who have visceral lesions should be treated for at least 4 weeks.

The observation that cat-scratch disease does not respond as rapidly and as consistently to antimicrobial therapy as bacillary angiomatosis has several possible explanations. One is that immunocompetent patients sequester infectious organisms beyond the reach of antimicrobial agents, whereas immunocompromised patients do not. This is supported by results of PCR testing on lymph nodes, liver, or skin biopsies compared with blood. Another explanation is that many of the clinical findings in cat-scratch disease may be immunologically mediated. Therefore, antimicrobial therapy may have limited ability to modify these findings in patients with intact immune responses but has impact on the infectious disease in immunocompromised patients.[10]

COMPLICATIONS, SEQUELAE, PROGNOSIS

Complications of cat-scratch disease are unusual. Encephalopathy is the most serious complication of cat-scratch disease, occurring in up to 5% of patients.[2,37] Typically, 1 to 3 weeks after the onset of adenopathy, the patient experiences sudden appearance of neurologic symptoms, which can include seizures, combative or bizarre behavior, lethargy, and coma. Neurologic imaging findings generally are normal, and lumbar puncture results are normal or show only a slight lymphocytic pleocytosis or elevation of protein. Fever usually is absent or low-grade, and systemic symptoms are minimal. The patient usually improves rapidly, sometimes returning to normal within a few days. In a series of 61 patients with cat-scratch encephalopathy, two-thirds had fully recovered by 4 weeks, and none showed any residual encephalopathy after 1 year.[38] Data also suggest that cat-scratch encephalopathy should be included in the differential diagnosis of new-onset status epilepticus in previously healthy school-aged children.[39]

Optic neuritis or neuroretinitis, with painless unilateral visual loss, also can occur as a complication of cat-scratch disease several weeks after the onset of adenopathy. Although visual loss can be profound, patients usually recover completely over a period of months. A report of 3 cases of acute sight impairment with papillary edema and stellate neuroretinitis documented prolonged visual impairment in 1 patient.[40] Peripheral neuralgia and paresthesia as well as facial nerve palsies also have been reported.[38] Other complications of cat-scratch disease are erythema nodosum (Figure 160-1K), osteolytic lesions, endocarditis, thrombocytopenic and nonthrombocytopenic purpura, nonimmune hemolytic anemia, atypical pneumonia, and glomerulonephritis.[41-49] Osteolytic lesions frequently are associated with a soft-tissue phlegmon, can be multiple, and frequently involve unusual sites such as the spine, cranium, sternum, or fibula[46] (Figure 160-1).

Although acute illness due to cat-scratch disease can be dramatic, the prognosis for all forms of this illness is excellent. Even in the absence of treatment, almost all immunocompetent patients recover fully. Reinfection appears to be extremely rare.

Bacillary angiomatosis and bacillary peliosis, even in severely immunocompromised patients, usually respond to antimicrobial therapy. However, relapses are common.

PREVENTION

Avoiding cats is a simple, although not popular, method of preventing infections with *B. henselae*. Removing a family pet to which a case of cat-scratch disease has been attributed is unnecessary because the capacity for disease transmission appears to be transient. However, declawing such a pet might be considered. Persons with immunodeficiency should avoid contact with cats that scratch or bite, and, if obtaining a new pet, they should avoid cats younger than 1 year. People should immediately wash sites of cat scratches or bites, and they should not allow a cat to lick their open cuts or wounds. Control of flea infestation has the potential for limiting transmission of *B. henselae* among cats. At present, recommendations for prevention of *B. quintana* infection are limited to avoiding contact with lice and promptly eradicating lice infestation.[19]

Key Points. Diagnosis and Management of *Bartonella henselae* Infection

MICROBIOLOGY

- Small, slow growing, pleomorphic, gram-negative bacilli
- Fastidious growth requirements

EPIDEMIOLOGY

- True incidence of human disease is unknown
- Sporadic and asymptomatic human disease is common
- There is no person-to-person transmission
- Domestic cats are the natural reservoir
- Incidence of disease is highest in fall and winter of each year

DIAGNOSIS

- Routine laboratory tests usually are not helpful
- Serology is used to establish most diagnoses
- Polymerase chain reaction is the most sensitive method for establishing the diagnosis

TREATMENT

- The management of most infections is supportive
- *B. henselae* is susceptible in vitro to penicillins, tetracyclines, macrolides, trimethoprim-sulfamethoxazole, rifampin, fluoroquinolones, and aminoglycosides
- Only azithromycin has been evaluated in a prospective, randomized, double-blind, placebo-controlled investigation; modest clinical benefit was shown for reduction in size of lymph node
- Azithromycin therapy for cat-scratch lymphadenitis typically is 5 days
- There is only anecdotal guidance for treatment of systemic forms of *B. henselae* infection
- Optimal agent(s) and duration of therapy for systemic forms of disease is unknown

---

161 *Brucella* Species (Brucellosis)

Edward J. Young

Brucellosis is an infection of animals (zoonosis) that is transmissible to humans.[1] The genus *Brucella* consists of six named (nomen) species classified according to their preferred natural hosts (Table 161-1). Nucleic acid homology studies and genome sequencing indicate a high degree of relatedness among *Brucella* spp., suggesting a single species with multiple biovars.[2] *Brucella* spp. also have been isolated from a variety of marine mammals, but their taxonomy is undecided and they rarely cause human infection.[3,4]

TABLE 161-1. Genus *Brucella*

Nomen Species	Biovars	Preferred Hosts	Human Pathogen
Brucella abortus	1–6, 9	Cattle	Yes
Brucella melitensis	1–3	Goats, sheep	Yes
Brucella suis	1–3	Swine	Yes
	4	Caribou, reindeer	Yes
	5	Rodents	Yes
Brucella canis[a]	None	Dogs	Yes
Brucella ovis[a]	None	Sheep	No
Brucella neotomae	None	Desert wood rats	No

[a]Signifies naturally rough strains (lacking O-polysaccharide).

PATHOGEN AND PATHOGENESIS

Brucellae are small, gram-negative coccobacilli that lack endospores, capsules, or native plasmids. Their metabolism is oxidative, and all strains are aerobic (some strains may require added CO_2 for primary isolation). A variety of media support the growth of brucellae in vitro; however, prolonged incubation ($\geq$21 days) may be required. Rapid isolation techniques, such as Bactec systems, have shortened the time to isolation. Cultures of bone marrow may have a higher yield than routine cultures of blood.

Brucella strains are always catalase-positive, but production of oxidase, urease, and hydrogen sulfide is variable. Rapid identification systems have misidentified *Brucella* as *Moraxella*, *Haemophilus*, and *Ochrobactrum* species.[5] Owing to the risk of laboratory-acquired infection, biosafety level 3 (BSL-3) practices, containment equipment and facilities are recommended for handling cultures when *Brucella* is suspected.[6,7]

A major virulence factor of brucellae is cell wall lipopolysaccharide that is similar in many ways to the endotoxins of other gram-negative bacteria.[8] For reasons that are not entirely clear, *B. melitensis* and *B. suis* are more virulent than *B. abortus*.[9]

Brucella spp. are facultative intracellular pathogens that can survive and replicate within phagocytic cells of the host. Innate and acquired humoral immunity play some role in resistance to infection. However, cell-mediated immunity is the major mechanism for recovery from brucellosis. Coincident with acquired cellular resistance, hypersensitivity to *Brucella* antigens develops,

TABLE 161-2. Routes of Acquisition of Brucellosis

Nomen Species	Route	Common Settings
Brucella abortus	Intracutaneous	Delivering aborting cattle or slaughtering infected animals
	Oral	Ingestion of unpasteurized milk
Brucella abortus (strain 19)	Intracutaneous	Accidental needlestick with vaccine
	Conjunctival	Accidental splash with vaccine
Brucella melitensis	Oral	Ingestion of unpasteurized milk or cheese
Brucella melitensis (strain Rev-1)	Intracutaneous	Accidental needlestick with vaccine
	Conjunctival	Accidental splash with vaccine
Brucella suis	Respiratory	Inhalation of aerosol in abattoir
	Conjunctival	Inoculation of infected blood
	Oral	Ingestion of undercooked meat, blood, or bone marrow (traditional foods)
	Intracutaneous	Slaughtering and dressing feral swine
Brucella canis	Intracutaneous	Attending aborting dogs
		Accidental needlestick in laboratory
	Oral	Accidental ingestion while pipetting blood or serum in laboratory

which may contribute to some of the clinical manifestations of disease.

EPIDEMIOLOGY

Brucellosis exists worldwide but is prevalent especially in the Mediterranean basin, Arabian peninsula, the Indian subcontinent, and in parts of Mexico, Central, and South America. Brucellosis also has re-emerged in eastern Europe where the collapse of the former Soviet Union has led to social and economic upheaval with a decline in veterinary and human health services.[10,11] Although once common in the United States, eradication of bovine brucellosis has reduced the incidence of human infection to less than 0.5 cases per 100,000 population. In states bordering Mexico, where *B. melitensis* is widespread in goats, brucellosis is 8 times more prevalent than elsewhere in the U.S.[12]

Humans are accidental hosts, contracting the disease by direct contact with infected animals, their carcasses, or their milk. Hence, farmers, veterinarians, abattoir workers, and laboratory personnel are at increased risk of infection. Increasingly, cases of brucellosis

are linked to ingestion of fresh goat-milk cheese imported from countries where the disease is enzootic.[13] Consequently, people of all ages can be affected, and there may be no history of direct animal contact. In the evaluation of patients with unexplained fever, clinicians should obtain a thorough history of travel (e.g., to enzootic areas), food consumption, occupation, and avocations (e.g., hunting feral swine).[14]

The usual routes of transmission of brucellosis from animals to humans are listed in Table 161-2. Human-to-human transmission is rare, but isolation of brucellae from banked sperm raises the possibility of venereal disease.[15,16] Brucellosis during pregnancy poses a risk of spontaneous abortion[17] and cases of neonatal infection suggest the possibility of transplacental passage.[18,19] Moreover, brucellosis has been transmitted from mother to child via human milk.[20]

Once considered rare, brucellosis in children is now recognized to be common in countries where *B. melitensis* is endemic.[21] In such areas, fresh milk from goats and camels is fed to children, and newborn animals often share the family's living space, providing conditions favorable to transmission.[22,23] In countries where

TABLE 161-3. Clinical Findings in Childhood Brucellosis from Selected Series[a]

Symptoms (%)	Series I[24] (102 Cases)	Series II[25] (157 Cases)	Series III[26] (200 Cases)	Series IV[27] (48 Cases)	Series V[28] (52 Cases)
Fever	91	80	70	88	88
Chills	20	NR	NR	75	NR
Sweats	19	NR	22	79	19
Fatigue/malaise	60	91	67	77	29
Anorexia	40	68	NR	NR	NR
Weight loss	48	68	67	56	NR
Arthralgia	73	25	74	32	62
Headache	11	NR	NR	47	21
Backache	16	NR	NR	73	NR
Abdominal pain	11	20	22	44	19
Cough	NR	20	NR	21	12
Arthritis	37	NR	30	11	NR
Lymphadenopathy	16	18	NR	67	23
Splenomegaly	35	55	23	38	52
Hepatomegaly	28	31	23	25	33

NR, not reported.

[a]*Superscript numbers indicate references.*

brucellosis is no longer common, failure to consider the diagnosis may contribute to the low reported incidence of childhood infection.

CLINICAL MANIFESTATIONS

In children or adults, brucellosis is a systemic illness characterized by a multitude of nonspecific complaints and a paucity of abnormal physical findings. The onset can be insidious or acute, with symptoms generally beginning 2 to 4 weeks after exposure. Series of childhood brucellosis caused by *B. melitensis* indicate that fever, sweating, malaise, lethargy, anorexia, and joint pains are the most common complaints.[24-30] A common constellation in young children is lassitude, refusal to bear weight on an extremity, and failure to thrive.

In contrast to the multiple somatic complaints, physical abnormalities can be few – notably, fever, arthritis, and, occasionally, hepatosplenomegaly (Table 161-3). The fever pattern can vary widely over time, referred to as *undulant fever*. Any organ or tissue can be involved, and morbidity is significant, but mortality is rare and usually results from infection of the heart or brain.

ORGAN SYSTEMS OF INVOLVEMENT

Skeletal System

Osteoarticular involvement is common and often is the predominant manifestation in children.[31,32] In contrast to adults, in whom sacroiliitis predominates, childhood brucellosis most often affects large peripheral joints (knees, hips, and ankles). Arthritis usually is accompanied by fever, malaise, weight loss, and other systemic symptoms and must be distinguished from juvenile idiopathic arthritis. In one series of 50 children with brucellosis, monoarthritis was reported in 35 cases, polyarthritis involving two joints in 11 cases, and three or more joints in 4 cases.[33] Limitation of movement with swelling and tenderness of the affected joints is prominent, similar to observations in pyogenic arthritis caused by other organisms.[34] Osteomyelitis involving the vertebrae and long bones also is reported.[35-37] *Brucella* sacroiliitis is rare in children and is difficult to diagnose because plain radiographic findings usually are normal.[38] Most authorities agree that treatment of spinal brucellosis should continue for at least 3 months.[39-41]

Central Nervous System

Although headache, mental inattention, and depression are common complaints in brucellosis in humans, invasion of the nervous system is rare. In one study of 1100 children with brucellosis, only 9 experienced neurologic complications.[42] Meningitis is the most common neurologic manifestation, and fever, headache, confusion, and gait disorders are frequent.[43,44] Cerebrospinal fluid (CSF) reveals lymphocytic pleocytosis, elevated protein, and often hypoglycorrhachia; tuberculous meningitis must be differentiated. Cultures of CSF are positive in less than half of cases, but confirmation of neurobrucellosis is made by demonstrating *Brucella* antibodies or antigen in the CSF.[45-47] Other neurologic complications include encephalitis, myelitis, neuritis, radiculopathy, mycotic aneurysms, and brain abscess.[48,49]

Alimentary Tract

Nausea, vomiting, anorexia, weight loss, and abdominal discomfort occur in two-thirds of cases of acute brucellosis.[50] Rare cases of cholecystitis, ileitis, colitis, and pancreatitis have been reported in patients infected with *B. melitensis*.

Reticuloendothelial System (RES)

As the largest organ of the RES the liver probably always is involved in brucellosis; however, hepatic enzymes are only mildly elevated and can be normal. Histologically, infection with *B. abortus* shows

noncaseating granulomas, whereas *B. suis* generally causes suppurative abscesses. *B. melitensis* can result in a variety of hepatic lesions, including nonspecific reactive hepatitis, granulomas, and acute hepatitis with focal necrosis.[51,52] Rarely, chronic hepatosplenic abscesses caused by *B. suis* or *B. melitensis* may require surgical intervention for cure.[53]

Cardiovascular System

Infective endocarditis in brucellosis occurs rarely in children (0.5%),[54] but it was once considered the principal cause of death from the disease. Advances in diagnosis and combined medical and surgical treatments have improved dramatically the prognosis of *Brucella* endocarditis.[55-57] Myocarditis and pericarditis can occur with or without endocarditis.[58]

Genitourinary Tract

Orchitis or epididymitis has been reported in 2% to 20% of patients with brucellosis.[59,60] Although *Brucella* can be recovered from urine using appropriate techniques, infection generally does not compromise renal function.[61] Nephritis or glomerulonephritis usually occurs in conjunction with endocarditis.[62]

Respiratory Tract

Although cough is common in brucellosis, respiratory tract lesions are documented in <5% of cases in most series.[63] Only rarely are brucellae seen on stains or grown from expectorated sputum; therefore, diagnosis depends on isolating the organism from other sites. The spectrum of pulmonary involvement is wide, including pneumonia, pulmonary nodules, and empyema.[64,65]

LABORATORY FINDINGS AND DIAGNOSIS

A definitive diagnosis is made by recovering *Brucella* organisms from blood, bone marrow, or other tissue. In the absence of bacteriologic confirmation, a presumptive diagnosis is made by demonstrating high or rising titers of specific antibodies in serum.[66] Routine laboratory tests are not particularly helpful, except that the white blood cell count is often normal or low. Anemia and thrombocytopenia are common and some patients present with epistaxis. Rarely, thrombocytopenic purpura can be associated with hypersplenism, bone marrow hemophagocytosis, immunologic reactions, or a combination of such factors.[67,68]

The most widely used test for serodiagnosis is the serum agglutination test (SAT). Using antigen from *B. abortus* strain 1119, this test can detect antibodies against all brucellae containing smooth lipopolysaccharide (LPS). For detection of antibodies to *B. canis*, a rough-LPS antigen is required.[69] The immunologic response in brucellosis is characterized by an initial rise in immunoglobulin M (IgM) antibodies followed by a switch to IgG synthesis. With treatment, both antibody isotypes decline over time. The SAT measures the total quantity of agglutinating antibodies; therefore, to differentiate IgM from IgG, serum samples are run in parallel with and without addition of disulfide-reducing agents, such as 2-mercaptoethanol or dithiothreitol, either of which destroys the agglutinability of IgM.[70] Although low levels of IgM antibodies can persist for years, persistence of IgG agglutinins is suggestive of unresolved infection.[62]

Among other tests, enzyme immunoassay (EIA) appears to be the most sensitive method to detect antibodies to *Brucella*. However, there may be variability in results from commercial laboratories.[71,72] A convenient and rapid flow assay for *Brucella* IgM/IgG is reported to have good correlation with agglutination test results.[73] No single antibody titer is always diagnostic; however, the majority of patients with active infection have titers ≥1:160. Cross-reactions can occur with any assay so it is important to understand the limitations of each test.[66,72] Moreover, it is imperative to interpret serologic test results in the context of epidemiologic and clinical findings. There also are a number of antigen

TABLE 161-4. Recommended Therapies for Human Brucellosis

Condition	Antimicrobial Agents	Adult Dose	Route	Duration of Therapy
ADULTS				
Acute brucellosis or relapse	Doxycycline	200 mg/day	PO	6 week
	Plus			
	Streptomycin	1 g/day	IM	2 week
	Or			
	Gentamicin	3–5 mg/kg per day	IM or IV	1 week
Alternative	Doxycycline	200 mg/day	PO	6 week
	Plus			
	Rifampin	15–20 mg/kg per day	PO	6 weeks
CHILDREN				
>8 years	Same as adults			
<8 years	TMP-SMX[a]	2 DS tablets/day	PO	45 days
	Plus			
	Rifampin	15–20 mg/kg per day	PO	45 days
COMPLICATIONS[b]				
Meningitis	Doxycycline	200 mg/day	PO	4–6 months
	Plus			
	Rifampin;	900 mg/day	PO	4–6 months
	Or			
	TMP-SMX[a]	2 DS tablets/day	PO	4–6 months
	Plus			
	Rifampin	900 mg/day	PO	4–6 months
Endocarditis	Same as meningitis[c]			
Pregnancy	Rifampin	900 mg/day	PO	6 weeks

DS, double-strength; IM, intramuscular; IV, intravenous; PO, by mouth; TMP-SMX, trimethoprim-sulfamethoxazole.

[a]*TMP-SMX standard formulation (80 mg trimethoprim/400 mg sulfamethoxazole) is given as four standard tablets or two double-strength tablets per day.*

[b]*See text.*

[c]*Valve replacement surgery may be necessary.*

detection assays including polymerase chain reaction (PCR) using a variety of gene sequences as targets, but these generally are not available in most clinical laboratories.[74–76]

TREATMENT AND OUTCOME

Many drugs are active in vitro against *Brucella* spp., but clinical efficacy is not always predicted by in vitro results.[77,78] General recommendations for treatment of brucellosis are shown in Table 161-4. The tetracyclines (especially doxycycline) remain the most useful drugs, and, when used in combination with an aminoglycoside, are associated with the fewest relapses.[79–81] In an attempt to find a completely oral treatment regimen, in 1986 the WHO recommended the combination of doxycycline plus rifampin administered for 45 days. While this combination has been used successfully for uncomplicated cases, it is less effective than doxycycline plus an aminoglycoside for focal complications such as spondylitis.[82,83] A meta-analysis (based on results of two trials) recommended doxycycline plus aminoglycoside plus rifampin for the first 7 to 14 days and then doxycycline plus rifampin for 6 to 8 weeks.[84] For children younger than 8 years of age, TMP-SMX (fixed combination of 80 mg trimethoprim, 400 mg sulfamethoxazole) once was considered satisfactory. Subsequently, controlled studies indicated a high rate of relapse when TMP-SMX was used alone.[85] Consequently, TMP-SMX is used in combination with rifampin for childhood brucellosis.[86,87] Many fluoroquinolones have in vitro activity against *Brucella*[88] but they too are most effective when used in combination with other drugs such as rifampin.[89,90]

Osteoarticular complications rarely present special problems in treatment but may require a longer course of therapy depending on the clinical evolution.[91] Surgical intervention may be required to drain pyogenic joint effusions, rare paraspinal abscesses, or chronic hepatic/splenic abscesses.

Neurobrucellosis requires a prolonged course of therapy, usually with multiple-drug regimens. Extended-spectrum cephalosporins, with excellent penetration of the blood–brain barrier, have been disappointing when used as monotherapy for brucellosis.[92] The use of corticosteroids as an adjunct to antibiotics may be of benefit in children with confirmed *Brucella* meningitis.

There is no established optimal therapy for *Brucella* endocarditis. However, combinations of drugs, including bactericidal agents such as rifampin and TMP-SMX, have been used with success. Valve replacement surgery often is required in addition to prolonged antibiotic therapy.

Pregnancy with concomitant brucellosis can lead to spontaneous abortion. However, early diagnosis and treatment can result in a successful outcome for mother and child.[93] Rifampin (900 mg once daily for 6 weeks) is the treatment of choice; while TMP-SMX is an alternative after 13 weeks of gestation.

PREVENTION

Live-attenuated vaccine strains of *B. abortus* (strain 19) and *B. melitensis* (strain Rev-1) provide protection in animals but are too virulent for use in humans. Another strain of *B. abortus* (RB51) appears less pathogenic for humans but is used only for immunization of animals. No vaccines are available for use against *B. suis* or *B. canis*. Children and adults can be protected against foodborne infection with brucellae by ensuring pasteurization of milk and milk-containing products including cheese, and thorough cooking of meat from susceptible animals.

162 *Bordetella pertussis* (Pertussis) and Other *Bordetella* Species

Sarah S. Long, Kathryn M. Edwards, and Jussi Mertsola

Pertussis is an acute respiratory tract infection that was well described in the 1500s and endemic in Europe by the 1600s; its current worldwide prevalence is dampened only by continuous use of active immunization since the 1940s. Sydenham first used the term *pertussis* (intense cough) in 1670. Inexorable spasms of coughing and a protracted course characterize pertussis, as attested to by names given to the disease in many languages: *tos ferina* and *tosse canina* (dog's bark) in Spanish and Italian, respectively, *chincough* (gasping cough) in old English, *coqueluche* (cock's crow) in French, and the "cough of 100 days" in Chinese.

ETIOLOGY

Bordetella pertussis is the sole cause of epidemic pertussis and the usual cause of sporadic pertussis. *B. parapertussis* accounts for 5% of isolates of *Bordetella* spp. in the United States[1,2] and characteristically causes a less protracted illness.[3] *B. parapertussis* contributes more significantly to total cases of pertussis and bronchitis in Europe.[4-6] *B. pertussis* is exclusively a human pathogen. *B. parapertussis* also has been found in lambs, but ovine and human strains are genetically distinct. *B. bronchiseptica* is a common animal pathogen causing kennel cough in dogs and cats, snuffles in rabbits, and atrophic rhinitis in swine. Occasionally, *B. bronchiseptica* infects humans causing upper and lower respiratory tract infections, endocarditis, septicemia, posttraumatic and postsurgical meningitis, and peritonitis. Typically, cases occur in immunocompromised people, patients with cystic fibrosis, or young children with exposure to infected farm animals or companion pets.[7-9] Recently, *B. hinzii* has been recovered from blood of patients with immunodeficiency states without a respiratory illness, and from sputum of patients with cystic fibrosis.[9] *B. holmesii* and *B. holmesii*-like organisms have been associated with cases of bronchitis, suspected pertussis, septicemia and endocarditis, predominantly in asplenic or immunosuppressed individuals and possibly acquired from dogs.[10-14]

Protracted coughing can be caused by *Mycoplasma* spp., adenoviruses, parainfluenza or influenza viruses, enteroviruses, and respiratory syncytial virus.[15] However, none of these pathogens is responsible for as much paroxysmal cough as pertussis. Prolonged coughing episodes due to *Mycoplasma pneumoniae* or *B. pertussis* in adolescents can be difficult to distinguish.[16] Dual infections are not uncommon. An outbreak of pertussis-like illnesses has been ascribed to *Chlamydophila pneumoniae*.[17]

EPIDEMIOLOGY

Worldwide, there continue to be 50 million cases of pertussis annually, causing 300,000 deaths. During the prevaccine era in the United States, pertussis was the leading cause of death from communicable disease among children younger than 14 years. A peak of 9000 deaths and 260,000 cases occurred in 1923 and 1934, respectively. Widespread use of pertussis vaccine since the late 1940s was responsible for the more than 100-fold decline in incidence per 100,000 from 110 (1922 to 1948) to 0.5 (1981). The 1010 cases and 7 deaths reported in 1976 are the all-time lowest ever recorded. There is a high incidence of disease in developing and certain developed countries related to low vaccine coverage[18,19] or use of less potent vaccines.[20] The dramatic resurgence of disease in developed countries when the immunization policy was rescinded[21] attests to the pivotal role of vaccination. Despite high immunization rates in children <7 years of age in the U.S., pertussis was increasingly recognized in the mid-1980s to 1990s, first cyclically every 3 to 4 years and then more steadily until 2004, when the 25,827 cases in the U.S. were the highest number reported since 1959 (Figure 162-1).[22]

During the prevaccine era in the U.S. and currently in countries with low immunization rates the peak incidence of pertussis is in children 1 to 5 years of age, with infants younger than 1 year and individuals older than 10 years each accounting for less than 15% of cases.[18,20,21] However, by 1993, 44% of the almost 6400 cases of

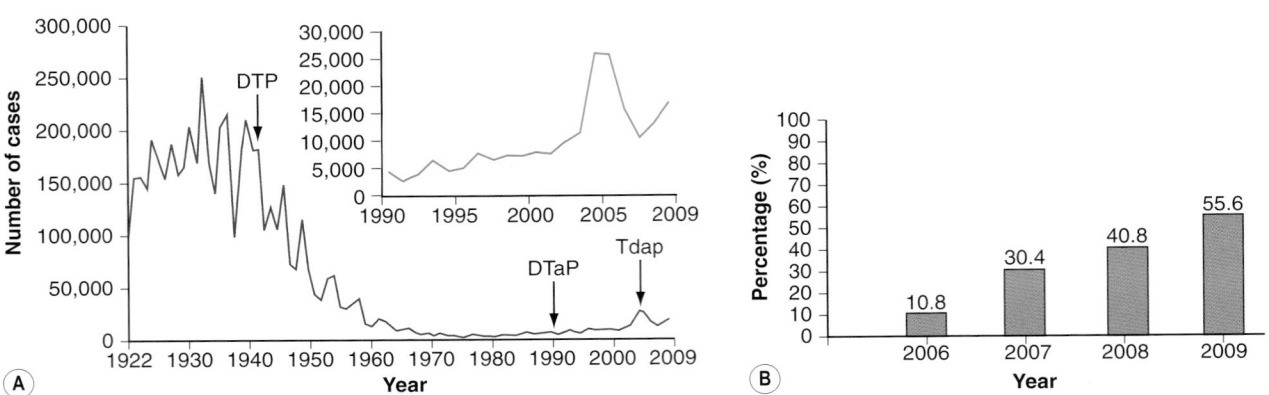

Figure 162-1. Annual reported cases of pertussis in the United States, 1922 through 2009. Data from National Notifiable Diseases Surveillance System for 1950 to 2009, and from passive reports to the Public Health Service for 1922 to 1949. (Redrawn from Centers for Disease Control and Prevention data.)

pertussis reported to the Centers for Disease Control and Prevention (CDC) for which patient age was known occurred in children younger than 1 year. The incidence in young infants has continued to rise (Figure 162-2).[22,23] Currently, infants under 2 months of age have the highest age-related risk of pertussis (incidence ~200 per 100,000 in 2004 (Figure 162-2). Infants <6 months of age are at highest risk for pertussis-related hospitalizations and complications and from 1980 to 2004, 235 pertussis-related deaths in infants <6 months of age were reported to the CDC.[24]

While young unimmunized infants have the highest risk of pertussis, their proportionate number of cases was eclipsed by cases diagnosed in adolescents and adults in the last decade. By 2004, 34% of all reported cases of pertussis occurred in adolescents 11 to 18 years of age (incidence ~30 per 100,000).[22] In studies where enhanced surveillance was employed, it was estimated that reported cases represent less than 10% of actual cases.[20,25,26] This is especially true for cases in previously immunized individuals. From 2001 to 2003, Massachusetts, which uses enhanced serologic surveillance, had an annual reported incidence of pertussis in 10- to 19-year-olds of 78.8 per 100,000 while the median average annual incidence in this age group in other states was only 3.7 per 100,000 population, a 20-fold difference.[26] In two prospective studies using extensive methods for evaluation and diagnosis, annual incidence of cough illness due to pertussis in adolescents and adults was estimated to be 370 and 450 per 100,000 population, respectively.[27,28] Studies of prolonged cough illnesses in adolescents and adults in the 1990s indicated that

between 12% and 32% of adolescents and young adults with prolonged cough illnesses have pertussis.[29,30]

Schools are a major source of contagion for pertussis in the community. In Massachusetts in 1996,[29] Arizona in 2002 to 2003,[31] and Wisconsin in 2003 to 2004,[32] the highest attack rates and numbers of cases in community outbreaks occurred among 10- to 19-year old people. Pertussis outbreaks have occurred even in elementary schools with high vaccination coverage and despite vaccination effectiveness of 80%.[33] Exemptions from pertussis immunization have been linked to increased personal risk and school and community outbreaks.[34,35] Imperfect vaccines and incomplete implementation of vaccine policy, waning immunity, and lower transplacental protection for infants[36,37] all play a role in the current epidemiology of pertussis. Neonates with pertussis are more likely to have been born prematurely or have young mothers with a cough illness.[38–40] Taken together, data are compelling evidence that older individuals are a major reservoir for *B. pertussis* and sources of infection for susceptible peers and infants.[40-44] In 2006 in the U.S., universal vaccination at 11 to 12 years was recommended using tetanus toxoid, reduced content diphtheria toxoid and pertussis antigen vaccine (Tdap).[44] With 53% of U.S. 13- to 18-year-olds vaccinated by 2009, there was approximately 50% reduction in pertussis in 11- to 19-year-olds (Figure 162-3). An epidemic of pertussis began in California in

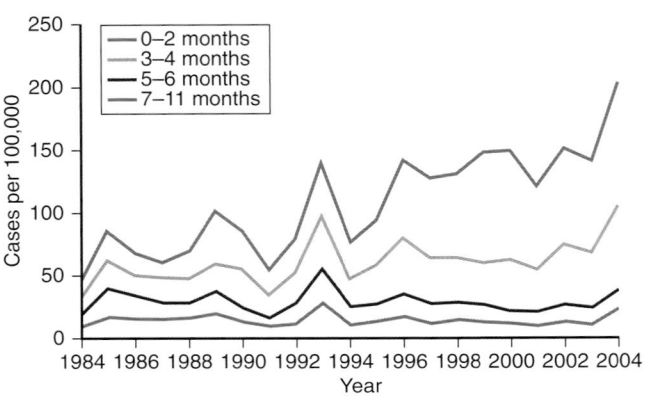

Figure 162-2. Incidence of reported cases of pertussis per 100,000 in infants in the United States by month of age, 1984 to 2004. (Centers for Disease Control and Prevention, unpublished data, 2005.[22,23])

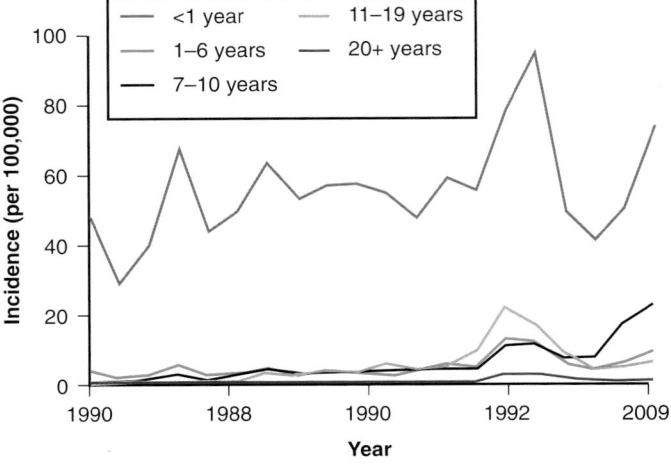

Figure 162-3. Age-related incidence per 100,000 of pertussis in the United States, 1990 through 2009. (Data from National Notifiable Diseases Surveillance System. Redrawn from Centers for Disease Control and Prevention data.)

2009 and escalated to more than 8000 cases and 10 infant deaths in 2010; the peak age group affected was 10-year-olds.[45]

Transmission

Pertussis is highly contagious, with attack rates as high as 100% in susceptible individuals exposed to aerosol droplets at close range. Chronic carriage by humans is not documented. After intense exposure, as in households and childcare centers, the rate of subclinical infection or mild disease exceeds 50% in fully immunized or naturally immune individuals.[46,47] When carefully sought, a symptomatic source case can be found for most patients.[39,47] Vaccination reduces transmissibility of *B. pertussis* even when vaccinated individuals become symptomatically infected.[48]

Immunity

B. pertussis causes mucosal infection and produces toxins with local and systemic effects. Natural disease and vaccination elicit broad antibody and cell-mediated immune responses. Neither disease nor vaccination provides complete or lifelong immunity against reinfection or disease. There is no generally accepted laboratory correlate of protective immunity. Taken together, data suggest that high levels of antibody against pertussis toxin (PT), combinations of antibodies against multiple *B. pertussis* antigens, and cell-mediated immunity play important roles.[49,50] Cell-mediated immune response may last longer,[50] while antibody levels fall to preinfection levels within 5 years after natural pertussis,[51] and protection against typical disease begins to wane 3 to 5 years after vaccination[52] and rapidly thereafter.[53] Subclinical reinfection as well as mild recurrent disease, which was common when pertussis was circulating widely, undoubtedly contributed significantly to protection against disease. Natural opportunities to boost pertussis immunity continue to occur, with the annual incidences of silent reinfection as high as 8% to 12% in studies of urban infants and adolescents, respectively.[52,54] However, such opportunities are not universal. Young adolescents and adults in the United States who have not received pertussis immunization since preschool age have inadequate protection against *B. pertussis*.[55,56] Outbreaks of pertussis also have occurred in the elderly, in nursing homes and in residential facilities with limited exposure to *B. pertussis*, as a result of waning immunity.

PATHOGEN AND PATHOPHYSIOLOGY

Microbiology

Bordetella are tiny, gram-negative coccobacilli that grow aerobically on starch-blood agar or completely synthetic media with nicotinamide supplemented for growth, amino acids for energy, and charcoal or cyclodextrin resin to absorb fatty acids and other inhibitory substances. *Bordetella* do not ferment carbohydrates. *B. pertussis* and *B. parapertussis* are nonmotile and all *Bordetella* spp. share a high degree of DNA homology among virulence genes. Only *B. pertussis* expresses PT, the major virulence protein. Electrophoretic mobility patterns of nonvirulence-related enzymes align *B. parapertussis* closely with *B. bronchiseptica*. *Bordetella* spp. possess a common O antigen.

Speciation of clinical isolates is based on phenotypic characterization and direct fluorescent antibody (DFA) testing using specific antisera. Serotyping depends on heat-labile K agglutinogens. Of 14 agglutinogens, 6 are specific to *B. pertussis*. Two principal agglutinogens are fimbrial proteins (FIM2, FIM3). Currently, there is discrepancy in nomenclature among countries because of slightly different serotyping systems. Serotypes vary geographically and with time. Pulsed-field gel electrophoresis of chromosomal DNA and multilocus variable number tandem repeat analysis of *B. pertussis* isolates from epidemiologic studies show dominance of certain strains, as well as diversity of strains geographically, over time, and between endemic and epidemic pertussis, as well as relatedness of epidemiologically linked cases.[57-60]

Virulence

B. pertussis is uniquely an infection of humans, with little information provided by animal models. *Bordetella* organisms elaborate a number of biologically active substances; their role in pathogenesis and protection has been reviewed by Hewlett[61] (Table 162-1). *B. pertussis* organisms are acquired by inhalation and have a strict tropism for ciliated epithelium of the respiratory tract to which infection is limited. Attachment to ciliated cells is mediated by several surface molecules, including PT and filamentous hemagglutinin (FHA). Bacterial survival is aided by ciliostasis related to tracheal cytotoxin (TCT) and impaired leukocyte function due to PT and adenylate cyclase (AC) toxin. Local epithelial damage and respiratory tract symptomatology are postulated to be mediated by TCT and AC toxin.

TABLE 162-1. Components of *Bordetella pertussis* and Possible Roles in Pathogenesis and Immunity

Component	Cellular Site	Biologic Activity
Pertussis toxin (PT)	Extracellular	Promotes attachment to respiratory epithelium
		Sensitizes to histamine
		Elicits lymphocytosis
		Enhances insulin secretion
		Causes T-lymphocyte mitogenesis
		Stimulates production of interleukin-4 and immunoglobulin E
		Inhibits phagocytic function of leukocytes
		Causes cytopathic effect on Chinese hamster ovary cell
Filamentous hemagglutinin (FHA)	Cell surface	Promotes attachment to respiratory epithelium
		Agglutinates erythrocytes in vivo
Pertactin (PRN)	Cell outer membrane	Promotes attachment to respiratory epithelium
Agglutinogen (FIM)	Cell surface Fimbriae-associated	Promotes attachment to respiratory epithelium
Adenylate cyclase (AC) toxin	Extracytoplasmic	Inhibits phagocytic function of leukocytes
		Induces apoptosis in macrophages; catalyzes supraphysiologic production of cyclic adenosine monophosphate
		Causes hemolysis in vitro
Tracheal cytotoxin (TCT)	Extracellular	Elicits interleukin-1 and nitric oxide synthase
	Peptidoglycan-like	Causes ciliary stasis, cytopathic effect on tracheal mucosa in mice, necrosis of mouse tracheal explants

PT has multiple proven biologic activities, some of which account for systemic manifestations of disease. PT is a complex bacterial toxin, composed of six subunits with an A protomer responsible for biologic activities and a B pentamer directing binding and entry of the A subunit into the cytoplasm. PT causes immediate lymphocytosis in experimental animals by preventing their migration from the circulating blood pool. Severe or fatal pertussis has been correlated with degree of lymphocytosis, a manifestation of PT.[62,63] Although a hydrogen peroxide-detoxified PT vaccine protects children in the short term against severe disease,[49] multiple lines of evidence support a central but not singular role for PT. There is no evidence of neurotoxic effects of *B. pertussis*. Parenchymal brain hemorrhage with hypoxic-ischemic necrosis is seen in fatal cases of pertussis, suggesting hypoxia from cough illness as causative.

There is evidence of ongoing evolution of *B. pertussis* virulence in vaccinated populations.[60,64] These virulence factor proteins are included in current vaccines. A dramatic increase in pertussis in the Netherlands was temporally associated with emergence of *B. pertussis* strains carrying a novel allele for PT promoter, which confers increased PT production.[65] In an animal model testing the effect of vaccines against different strains of *B. pertussis*, strains expressing a new type of PT (ptxA1) and pertactin (prn2) conferred a survival advantage over other strains. These results suggest that an allelic shift may play a role in emergence of pertussis in vaccinated populations.[66] "Shifted" strains of *B. pertussis* have caused outbreaks of pertussis in Finland exclusive of recently vaccinated individuals, suggesting that changes in virulence genes do not cause "vaccine resistance." Major increase in cases in outbreaks occurred in adolescents and young adults, leading to the speculation that genetic adaptation (i.e., increased PT production and colonizing ability) might play a substantial role during the waning phase of immunity.[67]

CLINICAL MANIFESTATIONS

Cadence of Symptoms

Pertussis is a lengthy disease classically divided into catarrhal, paroxysmal, and convalescent stages, each of which lasts 2 weeks (Figure 162-4). These three stages provide useful markers for progression of disease and timing of potential complications; the duration of each, however, depends on the patient's age and immunization status. Classic pertussis is seen in unimmunized toddlers and children. In infants younger than 3 months, the catarrhal phase usually lasts a few days or is unrecognized, and paroxysmal and convalescent stages are protracted, with periods of spasmodic cough throughout the first year of life. In immunized children, all stages of pertussis are foreshortened. Adults with the disease do not demonstrate distinct stages.

In classic pertussis, an incubation period of 3 to 12 days is followed by the occurrence of nondistinctive catarrhal symptoms. Coughing then begins as a dry, intermittent, irritative hack and evolves into paroxysms that are the hallmark of pertussis. With insignificant provocation, the well-appearing playful toddler suddenly expresses an anxious aura and commences a machine-gun burst of uninterrupted coughs (tongue protruding, eyes bulging and watering, face reddened) on a single breath, followed by a loud whoop as inspired air traverses the still partially closed glottis. The episode may end with expulsion of a thick mucus plug. In infants younger than 3 months, gagging, gasping, choking, cyanosis, apnea, or an "apparent life-threatening event" are frequently the presenting features rather than paroxysmal cough, and the whoop is absent.[23,68–70] Adults describe a sudden feeling of strangulating suffocation as spasms of coughing begin.

Post-tussive emesis is common in pertussis at all ages and is a clue to the diagnosis in adolescents and adults. Post-tussive

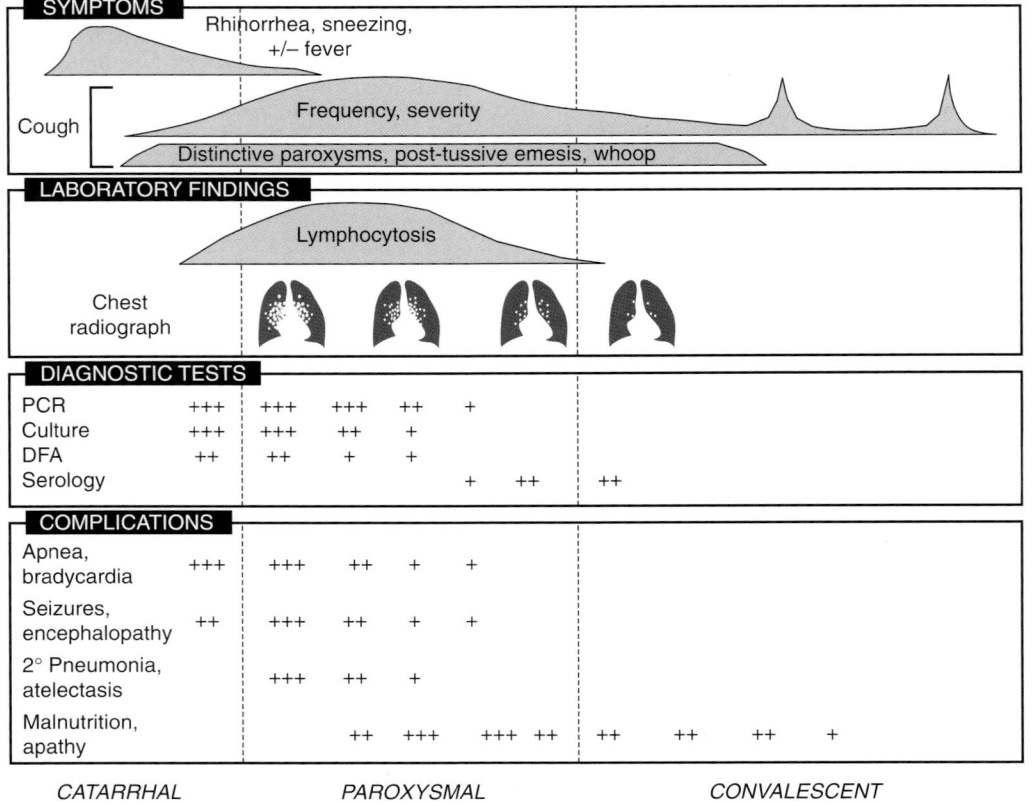

Figure 162-4. Manifestations and complications of pertussis. Duration of stages depends on patient's age and immunization status. +++, most likely to be positive or to occur; ++, can be positive or can occur; +, occasionally positive or occurring. DFA, direct fluorescent antibody; PCR, polymerase chain reaction. (Redrawn from Cherry JD, Brunell PA, Golden GS, et al. Report of the task force on pertussis and pertussis immunization-1988. Pediatrics 1988;81(Suppl):939–984.)

TABLE 162-2. Predictive Factors for Uncomplicated Pertussis

Positive Factors	Negative Factors
Coughing contact	Fever
Incomplete immunization	Diarrhea
Years since immunization	Exanthem
Pure or predominant cough	Enanthem
Paroxysmal cough	Tachypnea
Well between paroxysms	Wheezes
Whoop	Rales
Post-tussive vomiting	Lymphadenopathy
Apnea, bradycardia (infant)	Neutrophilia
Choking, gasping spells	Neutropenia
Petechiae above the clavicles	Lymphocytosis (atypical cells)
Lymphocytosis (normal cells)	

exhaustion is universal. Paroxysms progress in number and severity over days to a week and remain at peak for days to weeks, sometimes with multiple episodes hourly, before fading into convalescence, when the number, severity, and duration of episodes diminish. In young infants whoop may become louder and more classic in convalescence. With subsequent respiratory illnesses over several months, paroxysmal coughing can recur; this is not due to recurrence or reactivation of *B. pertussis* infection and the pathogenesis is unclear.

The physical examination between paroxysms is normal; this finding supports the diagnosis of pertussis. Fever and signs of lower respiratory tract disease are not seen. Conjunctival hemorrhages and petechiae on the upper body are common.

Spectrum of Symptoms

Pertussis should be suspected in any individual who has a pure or predominant complaint of paroxysmal cough that is escalating in the second week of illness. In prospective studies, nonspecific, protracted cough illness is the most frequent manifestation in adolescents and adults. Symptoms differ according to method of case ascertainment, age, immunization status, and prior exposures. In four series of reported cases of pertussis that included an adolescent age group,[37,41,71,72] the following symptoms were reported in adolescents: cough for >28 days, 41% to 76%; paroxysms, 82% to 100%; vomiting, 45% to 71%; whoop, 30% to 67%; cyanosis, 6% to 15%; and apnea 19% to 86%. Findings with predictive value are listed in Table 162-2. Clinical case definitions for pertussis have been developed for purposes of epidemiology and evaluation of vaccines. The Council for State and Territorial Epidemiologists (CSTE) defines a sporadic clinical case as a cough illness lasting 14 or more days with at least one associated symptom of paroxysms, whoop, or post-tussive vomiting with no other apparent cause. This definition had a sensitivity of 81% and specificity of 58% using culture confirmation (see comments below) as the standard in one study.[73] In Canadian adults, prolonged duration of violent cough (median 43 days) and post-tussive vomiting distinguished those with pertussis from others.[74]

Sudden infant death syndrome (SIDS) can be the manifestation of pertussis in young infants. Postmortem evidence of *B. pertussis* was found in 3 of 12 infants with SIDS studied in Syracuse, New York.[75] During pertussis outbreaks in the United Kingdom in the 1980s and Norway and Sweden in 1997, 3% to 5% of sudden infant deaths were associated with *B. pertussis* infections.[76,77] In a prospective study of 254 German infants with SIDS, respiratory tract specimens were positive by polymerase chain reaction (PCR) testing for *B. pertussis* in 5% of cases.[78]

DIFFERENTIAL DIAGNOSIS

Adenovirus infections frequently can be distinguished on the basis of associated features, such as fever, sore throat and conjunctivitis. In one study, median days of cough was 18 for adenovirus infection, compared with 35 days for pertussis. However, almost 50% of children with adenovirus had paroxysmal cough for >21 days and 53% had post-tussive vomiting; fewer (20%) had whooping.[15] *Mycoplasma* infection is difficult to distinguish from pertussis clinically,[15] although a history of fever, headache, and systemic symptoms at the onset of disease as well as the frequent finding of rales on auscultation, if present, differentiate *Mycoplasma*. *Chlamydia trachomatis* in young infants can be distinguished by the typical staccato cough (breath with every cough), purulent conjunctivitis, tachypnea, and rales; and respiratory syncytial virus (RSV) by wheezing. Unless the infant with pertussis has developed a secondary bacterial pneumonia, or has a dual infection with a virus, such as RSV, the physical findings between paroxysms generally are normal. A young infant who is being evaluated because of a history of paroxysmal cough who appears completely well should have a paroxysm witnessed by medical personnel before disposition is planned.

LABORATORY FINDINGS AND DIAGNOSIS

Leukocytosis (leukocyte counts of 15,000 to 100,000 cells/mm^3) due to an absolute lymphocytosis is characteristic in late catarrhal and paroxysmal stages of pertussis, being present in at least 75% of unvaccinated children.[38] Lymphocytes are both T and B cells and are normal small cells rather than the large atypical lymphocytes classically found in some viral infections. Lymphocytosis is not common in adolescents, adults, and partially immunized children with pertussis. Absolute increase in neutrophils or shift to immature forms suggests a secondary bacterial infection. Eosinophilia is not a feature of pertussis, even in young infants.

Lymphocytosis and thrombocytosis parallel the severity of illness. Lymphocytic leukemoid reactions and extreme thrombocytosis in infants are associated with fatal outcome.[59,60] Hypoglycemia (a PT effect) is reported only occasionally. The chest radiograph is abnormal in most hospitalized infants, showing perihilar infiltrate or interstitial edema (sometimes with a butterfly appearance) and variable atelectasis. Parenchymal consolidation suggests secondary bacterial infection. Pneumothorax, pneumomediastinum, and soft-tissue air can be seen occasionally.

All current methods for confirmation of *B. pertussis* infection have limitations in sensitivity, specificity, or practicality. Culture remains the diagnostic standard[1,73] and frequently is positive during the catarrhal stage and escalating paroxysmal stage in unimmunized children when proper specimen collection, transport, and isolation techniques are used. However, culture is positive in fewer than 20% of immunized individuals, in individuals who have received macrolides or trimethoprim-sulfamethoxazole, or in those who come to attention late in illness.

The best culture specimens are obtained by deep nasopharyngeal aspiration, nasal wash, or by placing a flexible swab in the posterior nasopharynx for 30 seconds. A calcium alginate- or Dacron-tipped swab is preferable to a rayon- or cotton-tipped one. Throat swabs are not adequate specimens.[79] If the specimen cannot be inoculated immediately onto solid media, 1% casamino acid liquid medium is acceptable for holding up to 2 hours. Otherwise, Stainer–Scholte broth with cyclodextrin or Regan–Lowe semisolid transport medium is used and allows adequate recovery of organisms for up to 4 days.[73] Regan–Lowe charcoal agar with 10% horse blood and 5 to 40 μg/mL cephalexin, or Stainer–Scholte medium with cyclodextrin resins are preferred media for culture. Cultures should be incubated at 35°C to 37°C in a humid environment (with or without 5% carbon dioxide) and should be examined with a stereoscopic microscope daily for 7 days to detect tiny glistening colonies. Culture detection is optimized by DFA testing of colonies using specific antibody for *B. pertussis* to *B. parapertussis*.

DFA testing of nasopharyngeal secretions is reliable only if performed by laboratory technologists who have extensive experience. PCR tests for nasopharyngeal specimens have been developed, using target regions of the repeated insertion sequence 481, the PT promoter region, or the porin gene.[80,81] Use of multiple targets may improve specificity; the CDC has published best practices for PCR testing for pertussis (www.cdc.gov/pertussis/clinical/diagnostic-testing/diagnosis-pcr-bestpractices.html). PCR testing is more sensitive than culture, especially in mildly symptomatic cases.[53,82,83] However, in adolescents and adults with pertussis, culture or PCR test results are positive in <10% of cases confirmed by serology, especially when PCR is performed >2 weeks after onset of cough.[40,83,84] False positive interpretation of PCR tests is problematic[85] and led to massive interventions in one pseudo-outbreak of pertussis among healthcare workers.[86]

Serologic tests using enzyme immunoassay (EIA) for detection of antibodies to components of *B. pertussis* are the most sensitive tests for diagnosis in distantly immunized individuals and those evaluated after the second week of cough, particularly adolescents and adults.[87] Currently, these tests are not standardized and may be difficult to interpret in immunized individuals. Tests for immunoglobulin A (IgA) and IgM antibodies to nonpurified and purified pertussis antigens lack sensitivity, specificity, and reproducibility. When standardized and available, anti-PT IgG antibody appears to be the most reliable serologic test. An anti-PT IgG level of >94 EU/mL in a standardized assay has been proposed as a diagnostic cutoff point (with sensitivity of 80% and specificity of 93% in culture-confirmed cases).[87] Anti-PT IgG level >50 EU/mL ≥5 years after immunization is highly unusual, and is supportive when the clinical diagnosis is suggestive evidence (personal experience of authors). Antibody to PT is specific for *B. pertussis*, whereas antibody to FHA, pertactin, and FIM can cross-react with organisms such as *B. parapertussis*, *B. bronchiseptica*, and nontypable *Haemophilus influenzae*.[41,52,83,87]

COMPLICATIONS AND OUTCOME

The principal complications of pertussis are apnea, secondary bacterial infections (such as pneumonia and otitis media), respiratory failure (from apnea, pneumonia, or pulmonary hypertension) and physical sequelae of forceful coughing. Reported rates of complications of pertussis are affected by age, immunization status, and completeness of diagnosis and reporting.[25,37,38,55] Infants younger than 6 months have high morbidity and mortality,[18,20,25,84] especially those younger than 2 months,[24,62,68,69] with the highest reported rates of pertussis-associated hospitalization (>90%), pneumonia (13% to 25%), seizures (2% to 4%), encephalopathy (0.4% to 1%), and death (0.5% to 1%).[23,37,88] Of 23 infants with fatal pertussis in the U.S. reported during 1992 and 1993, 96% had pneumonia, 17% had seizures, and 13% had encephalopathy.[38] In a Canadian study, infants intubated because of respiratory failure had a worse prognosis than those intubated because of apnea.[63]

Pertussis-related deaths are increasingly clustered among very young infants; 64% of deaths reported to CDC during the 1980s, 82% in the 1990s, and all 17 deaths in 2000 were in infants younger than 4 months.[68,89] With striking similarity, 94% to 100% of pertussis-related deaths reported from the United Kingdom,[90] Canada,[63] and Australia[91] in the last decade were seen in children <2 months of age. Other risk factors associated with death include Hispanic ethnicity, multiple births, premature birth, and household source of infection.[62,63,68,89,90] Pulmonary hypertension is an increasingly recognized complication of pertussis in young infants leading to dilatation of the right ventricle and respiratory failure.[69,92] It can be misdiagnosed as pneumonia. Infants with pulmonary hypertension generally are younger than 4 weeks of age and frequently born at <39 weeks of gestation. Pathologic findings identified in the respiratory tract of fatal cases, and the known physiologic responses of the infant's lung to hypoxia, suggest that *B. pertussis* triggers a cascade of events that includes pulmonary vasoconstriction, luminal aggregation of abundant leukocytes in pulmonary vessels, and compromised pulmonary blood flow; hypoxemia is exacerbated and refractory pulmonary hypertension ensues.[92] Progressive respiratory failure in the absence of distinct manifestations of pneumonia in young infants should prompt evaluation for pulmonary hypertension, including an echocardiogram. In older children and adolescents, only 1%

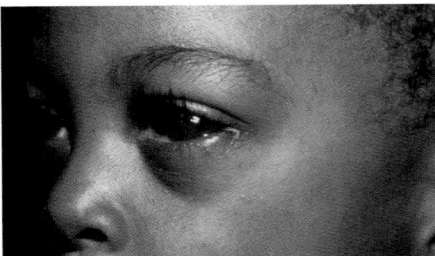

Figure 162-5. Bilateral scleral hemorrhages and periorbital edema in a young boy with pertussis.

to 7% are hospitalized and complications occur in only 5%, with pneumonia and otitis media most common.[37,41,71,72,74] Individuals with underlying cardiac, pulmonary, muscular, or neurologic disorders have high risk for severe disease. Patients with acquired immunodeficiency syndrome have unusually prolonged cough with prolonged recovery of *B. pertussis* from respiratory tract secretions.

Fever, tachypnea, and respiratory distress between paroxysms and absolute neutrophilia are clues to secondary bacterial pneumonia. Expected pathogens include *Staphylococcus aureus*, *Streptococcus pneumoniae*, and bacteria of oropharyngeal flora.

Increased intrathoracic and intra-abdominal pressure during coughing can result in conjunctival and scleral hemorrhages (Figure 162-5), petechiae on the upper body, epistaxis, central nervous system and retinal hemorrhages, pneumothorax and subcutaneous emphysema, umbilical and inguinal hernias, rib fracture, and urinary incontinence. Laceration of the lingual frenulum is not uncommon.

Central nervous system abnormalities are almost always the result of hypoxemia or hemorrhage associated with coughing or apnea in young infants. Apnea or bradycardia or both can occur from apparent vagal stimulation or laryngospasm just before a coughing episode, from obstruction during an episode, or hypoxemia after an episode. Occasionally, apnea or bradycardia occurs without coughing. Seizures usually are the result of hypoxemia, but hyponatremia from inappropriate secretion of antidiuretic hormone in the setting of pneumonia also should be considered.

MANAGEMENT

Assessment and Supportive Care

The goals of management are to limit the number of paroxysms, to observe the severity of cough and provide assistance when necessary, and to maximize nutrition, rest, and recovery without sequelae. Infants younger than 3 months are admitted to the hospital almost without exception, as are many between 3 and 6 months old unless their witnessed paroxysms are not severe.

The specific, limited goals of hospitalization are to: (1) assess progression of disease and likelihood of life-threatening events; (2) prevent or treat complications; and (3) educate parents about the natural history of the disease and the care that will be needed at home. For most infants older than 2 months without complications, these goals usually are accomplished within a 48- to 72-hour hospitalization. Feeding, vomiting, and daily weight gain are documented. Continuous electronic monitoring is performed, with alarm settings so that each paroxysm is witnessed by healthcare personnel. A detailed cough record is constructed to quantify episodes, to interpret risks and trajectory of the clinical course, and to assess safety/timing of discharge (Table 162-3). Infants whose paroxysms repeatedly lead to life-threatening events require intubation, paralysis, and ventilation. Subsequent management is challenging, with frequent intervention required because of airway obstruction, bradycardia, or cardiopulmonary complications.

Mist by tent is useful for some infants with thick tenacious secretions and extremely irritable airways. The benefit of a quiet, low-lit, undisturbed, and comforting environment cannot be

TABLE 162-3. Assessment of Severity of Paroxysms During Pertussis

Clinical Assessments	Expected	Worrisome
Duration of paroxysm	<45 seconds	>60 seconds
Demeanor during paroxysm	Anxious, unconsolable, nondistractable; rigid; eyes bulging; tearing	Limp
Character of cough	Loud, forceful uninterrupted bursts until all air expelled	Gagging/choking/gasping > coughing
Color change	Red	Blue
Tachycardia	Resolves <30 seconds after end of paroxysm	Persists
Bradycardia (<60 in infant <3 months)	Resolves at end of paroxysm without stimulation	Persists, requires stimulation
Oxygen desaturation	Resolves <30 seconds after end of paroxysm	Persists
Mucus plug	Self-expectorated	Obstructive, requires suctioning
Self-rescue breath	Immediate, large volume	Apnea or feeble attempt
Whoop	Strong	None
Post-tussive state	Exhausted	Unresponsive

overestimated or forfeited by the desire to monitor and intervene. Feeding children with pertussis is challenging. The risk of precipitating cough by nipple feeding does not warrant the use of nasoenteral or parenteral alimentation in most infants. However, large-volume feedings should be avoided.

Therapeutic Agents

Antimicrobial Agents

In vitro, *B. pertussis* is susceptible to erythromycin, newer macrolides, fluorquinolones, third-generation cephalosporins, and meropenem.[93] Ampicillin, rifampin, and trimethoprim-sulfamethoxazole are modestly active, but first- and second-generation cephalosporins are not. Rare isolates of erythromycin-resistant *B. pertussis* have been identified in children who had prolonged symptoms despite erythromycin therapy.[94–96] *B. parapertussis* is less susceptible in vitro to all agents except macrolides. In vitro, *B. bronchiseptica* is most susceptible to antipseudomonal penicillins, aminoglycosides, fluoroquinolones, and tetracycline (with antagonism demonstrated between the last two drugs); erythromycin resistance is not uncommon.[7] *B. holmesii* isolates are most susceptible to fluoroquinolones and carbapenems.[14] Use of agents with proven activity in vitro does not necessarily correlate with observable clinical benefit.

An antimicrobial agent should always be given when pertussis is suspected or confirmed in infants <1 year of age within 6 weeks of cough onset, and in persons >1 year of age within 3 weeks of cough onset[97,98] (Table 162-4). Erythromycin, clarithromycin, or azithromycin can be used in persons aged ≥1 month. However,

because of the association of erythromycin use and infantile hypertrophic pyloric stenosis (IHPS), infants aged <1 month should receive azithromycin. The association between erythromycin and IHPS was shown in infants younger than 6 weeks, with a 7- to 10-fold relative risk.[99,100] The highest risk appears to be in the first 2 weeks of life in term infants, and with courses of 14 days or more. In one reported experience of azithromycin use in 58 neonates, IHPS did not occur.[101] However, in another report, 2 of 3 triplets born at 32 weeks of gestation who were given azithromycin for 5 days at 7 weeks of age developed IPHS at 12 and 13 weeks of age, respectively.[102] Neonates with pertussis disease or exposure should always be treated and monitored clinically for IPHS.

Antimicrobial clinical efficacy is most evident in young infants and others who come to clinical attention quickly; otherwise the purpose of therapy is to eliminate contagiousness. Infants under 6 months of age (and other incompletely immunized children) have higher density and duration of colonization; azithromycin dose is 10 mg/kg per day for 5 days. In clinical studies, macrolides are superior to amoxicillin for eradication of *B. pertussis*. In those ≥2 months of age who are intolerant of macrolides, trimethoprim-sulfamethoxazole is the alternative agent.[97] However, alternative therapies are not well studied. Patients with pertussis and pneumonia should be treated with antibiotic(s) in addition to a macrolide.

Other Therapies

No randomized, blinded clinical trial of sufficient size has been performed to evaluate the usefulness of corticosteroids in the

TABLE 162-4. Recommended Antimicrobial Agents for Treatment and Postexposure Prophylaxis of Pertussis[a]

Agents	<1 month	1–5 months	≥6 months and Children	Adults
Age Group				
PRIMARY AGENTS				
Azithromycin	Recommended agent 10 mg/kg, once daily × 5 days	10 mg/kg once daily × 5 days	10 mg/kg (max 500 mg) once on day 1; then 5 mg/kg (max 250 mg) once on days 2–5	500 mg once on day 1; then 250 mg once on days 2–5
Clarithromycin	Not recommended	15 mg/kg/day divided bid × 7 days	15 mg/kg/day (max 1 g/day) divided bid × 7 days	1 g/day divided bid × 7 days
Erythromycin	Not preferred	40–50 mg/kg/day divided qid × 14 days	40–50 mg/kg/day (max 2 g/day) divided qid × 14 days	2 g/day divided qid × 14 days
ALTERNATE AGENT				
TMP-SMX	Contraindicated	Contraindicated at age <2 months. At ≥2 months, TMP 8 mg/kg/day-SMX 40 mg/kg/day divided bid × 14 days	TMP 8 mg/kg/day-SMX 40 mg/kg/day (max TMP 320 mg/day) divided bid × 14 days	TMP 320 mg-SMX 1600 mg/day divided bid × 14 days

TMP-SMX, trimethoprim-sulfamethoxazole.

[a]Modified from Tiwari T, Murphy TV, Moran J, et al. National Immunization Program. Centers for Disease Control and Prevention. Recommended antimicrobial agents for treatment and postexposure prophylaxis of pertussis. *MMWR Recomm Rep* 2005;54(RR-14):1–13.

management of pertussis and use of these agents is not warranted. A handful of small clinical trials suggest a modest reduction in symptoms with the use of aerosolized albuterol. However, one small study showed no effect,[103] and use can trigger paroxysms of coughing.

Hyperimmune serum (raised by immunization of adults with acellular pertussis vaccines) given intramuscularly reduced whooping significantly in infants treated in the first week of disease in a double-blind study in Sweden.[104] Pertussis immune globulin, intravenous (P-IGIV), prepared from plasma of adults immunized with pertussis toxoid was evaluated in a prospective, placebo-controlled clinical trial in the U.S. and Canada but was terminated prematurely because of expiration of P-IGIV lots. No benefit was noted in these studies[105] and P-IGIV product is no longer available. Commercial IGIV is not indicated.

Several reports show that infants with pertussis who fail artificial ventilation and are managed using extracorporeal membrane oxygenation have extremely high death rates (>80% in infants <6 weeks of age).[63,69,89] Several single cases and small series of young infants with extreme leukocytosis, respiratory insufficiency despite ventilator therapy, and pulmonary hypertension have been reported to survive after rapid leukoreduction by leukopheresis or exchange transfusion.[106-110] In a single case report, an infant with severe pulmonary hypertension treated with sildenafil and inhaled nitric oxide survived.[111]

CONTROL MEASURES

Isolation

In addition to standard precautions, droplet precautions are recommended for at least 5 days after initiation of macrolide therapy. For infants who require longer hospitalization, isolation frequently is continued to avoid any possibility of spread, to reduce noxious stimuli, and to avoid the protective concern of other families.

Care of Household and Other Close Contacts

Postexposure prophylaxis (PEP) with a macrolide agent should be given promptly to all household contacts and other close contacts (such as those in childcare facilities) regardless of age, history of immunization, or symptomatology.[97,98] PEP may not be necessary for out-of-home exposures in adolescents, and when healthcare personnel (HCP) who have received Tdap and will not likely expose patients at risk of severe pertussis (e.g., hospitalized neonates and pregnant women) can be monitored for symptoms for 21 days.[112,112a] In some European countries, PEP is limited to families with infants under 6 months of age or with older children who are underimmunized. Choice of agents, dosage, and duration for PEP is the same as for treatment (see Table 162-4). Repeatedly, studies have shown high transmission rates and efficacy of macrolide chemoprophylaxis for maternal–neonatal exposure,[113] as well as in households[114,115] when prophylaxis is given before onset of a secondary case,[116] in residential facilities,[56] and hospitals.[117] Visitation of coughing family members to the hospital must be controlled until they have taken a macrolide for 5 days. For outbreaks in childcare facilities and schools, all children, students, and staff who have cough illness compatible with pertussis should be excluded for 5 days after they begin therapy or for 21 days after onset of cough if they are not treated.

Immunization status of close contacts also should be considered. Children <7 years of age who have received fewer than four doses of a pediatric pertussis-containing vaccine (DTP/DTaP) should be given further dose(s) to complete the recommended series; children who received a third dose 6 months or more before exposure, or a fourth dose 3 years or more before exposure, should be given a booster DTaP dose. Adolescents 10 years of age or older and adults who have not received Tdap, and DTaP underimmunized children 7 through 10 years of age, should be given a single dose of Tdap.

Multiple outbreaks of pertussis have been described in a variety of inpatient and ambulatory healthcare settings, affecting HCWs, with subsequent transmission from HCWs to patients.[70,117-120] Guidance for management is available at http://www.cdc.gov.nip/publications/pertussis/guide.htm. Postexposure strategies are resource-intensive and include contact identification, PEP, surveillance, and furlough of coughing HCWs.[121] PEP strategy has limited impact as many cases and exposures are unrecognized.[65] Preexposure vaccination is a better strategy. Brisk response (by 2 weeks) of adults to Tdap also supports a role for vaccination in outbreak control.[122] Even when *B. pertussis* infection is documented, the individual should complete the recommended immunization series, i.e., DTaP for those <7 years, and Tdap booster for adolescents and adults.[22,44]

Even when *B. pertussis* infection is documented, the individual should complete the recommended immunization series, i.e., DTaP for those <7 years, and Tdap booster for adolescents and adults.[22,44]

PREVENTION

Purified component (acellular) pertussis vaccines (DTaP) that are less reactogenic than whole-cell pertussis vaccines (DTP) have been used exclusively in the U.S. since 1997. DTaP is given in a 5-dose series in children 6 weeks through 6 years of age. Tetanus toxoid reduced-content diphtheria toxoid and reduced-content pertussis antigen vaccine (Tdap) was recommended in 2006 for routine booster immunization to replace Td at 11 or 12 years of age, with catch-up for older adolescents;[22,44] for healthcare workers;[112] for all adults <65 years of age to replace one decennial dose of Td, and for wound prophylaxis. In 2010, a single dose of Tdap was recommended for children 7 through 10 years of age who previously were not fully immunized against pertussis.[123,124]

The compositions of diphtheria and tetanus toxoids and acellular pertussis vaccines available in the U.S. are shown in Table 162-5. Vaccine efficacies for DTaPs range from 75% to 90% after the primary series, depending on the definition of disease, the vaccination schedule, and the rates of immunization in the population. Licensure of Tdap vaccine is based on comparable immunogenicity in adolescents and adults to that seen in infants who were enrolled in previous clinical efficacy trials of the primary series of matched pediatric DTaPs.[22,125,126] Additionally, a multicenter randomized blinded efficacy study of acellular pertussis (aP) vaccine in U.S. adolescents and adults revealed a vaccine efficacy of 92%.[28] Effectiveness of adolescent Tdap during outbreaks in two early studies in Australia and the U.S. Virgin Islands was 66% and 85%.[127,128]

Goals of adolescent and adult immunization are to protect the individual from a significant cough illness, to control endemic and epidemic disease, and to decrease contagion for young infants. Two U.S. economic studies of Tdap booster strategies identified universal immunization of adolescents as the most cost-effective strategy, being cost-acceptable (~$21,000 per quality-adjusted life-year gained) or cost-saving depending on the true incidence of pertussis.[129,130]

Many studies have shown that household contacts are sources for pertussis in neonates.[43,131-133] The American Academy of Pediatrics (AAP), the CDC, the American College of Obstetricians and Gynecologists, and many European countries recommend a cocoon strategy to increase protection of young infants.[44,131,134] The cocoon strategy consists of pertussis immunization of women, families, and contacts. The AAP[44] and CDC[134a] recommend universal Tdap for all pregnant women (who previously have not received Tdap) after 20 weeks' gestation. If not administered during pregnancy, Tdap should be administered immediately postpartum. The cocoon strategy also includes catch-up immunization for underimmunized siblings (DTaP for those <7 years of age and Tdap for those 7 through 10 years of age) and for adolescents and adults of all ages.[123,124] The CDC further expanded Tdap recommendation to all adults 19 years of age and older (i.e., beyond 64 years of age) who previously did not receive Tdap who have or anticipate having contact with children under 12 months

TABLE 162-5. Diphtheria and Tetanus Toxoid and Acellular Pertussis Antigen Content of U.S. Vaccines (0.5 mL dose)

Age Group of Licensure Doses	Tripedia[a] 6 wks–6 yrs 5	Daptacel 6 wks–6 yrs 5	Pentacel[b] 6 wks–4 yrs 4	Infanrix[c] 6 wks–6 yrs 5	Adacel 11 yrs–64 yrs 1	Boostrix 10 yrs and Older 1
PT (µg)	23.4	10	20	25	2.5	8
FHA (µg)	23.4	5	20	25	5	8
PRN (µg)	–	3	3	8	3	2.5
FIM 2+3 (µg)	–	5	5	–	5	–
D (Lf)	6.7	15	15	25	2	2.5
T (Lf)	5	5	5	10	5	5

PT, pertussis toxoid; FHA, filamentous hemagglutinin; PRN, pertactin; FIM, fimbrial agglutinogens; D, diphtheria toxoid; T, tetanus toxoid; Lf, limits of flocculation; "–" in age range denotes "through."

[a]*TriHIBit also contains these DTaP components.*

[b]*Pentacel also contains IPV types 1, 2, 3 and is reconstituted with* Haemophilus influenzae *b PRP-T 10 µg.*

[c]*Pediarix and Kinrix also contain these DTaP components.*

of age.[123] In 2011, one Tdap product (Boostrix) was FDA licensed for use in people 65 years of age and older. In 2009, the German Standing Committee on Vaccination (STIKO) extended previous recommendations to include a decennial Tdap booster for all HCP and all persons who are employed in the care of children and in schools or in other institutions caring for older children.[135] In a Finnish study, a decennial second dose of Tdap in adults was immunogenic and well tolerated.[136] U.S. recommendations for decennial Tdap boosters throughout life depend on further study and licensure of a product.

The cocoon strategy in the U.S. has been implemented poorly.[131] A few studies show feasibility but requirement for intensive resources.[137–139] Pertussis vaccination of neonates has been studied and is associated with interference with responses to other infant vaccines.[140–143] The effect of Tdap immunization during pregnancy on subsequent infant/toddler responses to DTaP and other vaccines is under prospective study. Follow-up data on 16 infants' pertussis antibodies and responses to vaccines following maternal receipt of Tdap in pregnancy during a mass vaccination campaign of HCP appear to be reassuring.[144]

Rates of local and systemic adverse reactions after vaccination are lower following DTaP than DTP vaccine, as are hypotonic-hyporesponsive episodes and febrile seizures. In a study of 14 children who had alleged, temporally associated, pertussis-containing vaccine encephalopathy with seizure onset within 72 hours of vaccination, 11 patients were found to have genetic epileptic encephalopathy due to mutations in a neuronal sodium channel gene, *SCN1A*,[145] with fever likely unmasking the condition. Rates of local reactions are increased with the fourth and fifth doses of an all-DTaP regimen although they still are less than for DTP. In individuals who have received 5 consecutive doses of DTaP, the sixth Tdap booster does not appear to be more reactive than the fifth dose.[146] Data from several reported studies show local and systemic events following administration of Tdap similar to those following Td,[147–149] with no increase in reactogenicity if there is a short interval (1 month to 2 years) between receipt of DT/Td-containing vaccines and Tdap.[150–154] In 2010, the CDC and AAP recommended administration of Tdap when indicated regardless of interval since receipt of diphtheria- or tetanus-toxoid containing vaccines.[123,124]

Extensive limb swelling (ELS) of the injected extremity has been reported in 2% to 6% of children receiving the fourth or fifth doses of DTaP.[155–157] ELS is self-limited; the pathogenesis is not fully understood, and the reaction is not consistently related to diphtheria or tetanus content, pertussis proteins, or aluminum content of vaccines.[158,159] ELS has been reported almost as frequently following Td and hepatitis B vaccination in adolescents.[157] In a study of 20 children who had ELS after dose 4 of DTaP, 5 again had ELS and 7 had swelling >5 cm after dose 5, but all events were well tolerated and resolved rapidly.[160] ELS is not a contraindication to further recommended doses of DTaP, or to Tdap.[22,44,98]

163 *Campylobacter jejuni* and *Campylobacter coli*

Manuel R. Amieva

Campylobacter strains are among the most common pathogens in humans and are commensals in cattle, swine, and birds. They are the most common cause of culture-proven bacterial gastroenteritis in developed and developing countries, responsible for 400 to 500 million cases of diarrhea each year. In North America, >1% of the population acquires the infection yearly, with the highest incidence in children <5 years of age. Although diarrhea is the most frequent clinical manifestation, a broad clinical spectrum is associated with *Campylobacter* infection, from asymptomatic carriage to systemic illness and bloodstream infection (BSI) to localized infection. Also *Campylobacter* increasingly is associated with a variety of inflammatory and autoimmune sequelae including Guillain–Barré syndrome (GBS).

DESCRIPTION OF THE PATHOGEN

Campylobacters belong to the class epsilon-Proteobacteria and the order Campylobacteriales. This order contains the family Helicobacteraceae, which includes the human gastric pathogen *Helicobacter pylori*, as well as the Campylobacteraceae, which includes

TABLE 163-1. Taxonomy, Clinical Syndromes, and Common Sources of Campylobacteriaceae That Are Pathogenic to Humans

Organism	Associated Illness	Reservoir
CAMPYLOBACTER SPECIES		
Campylobacter jejuni subsp. jejuni	Diarrhea, bacteremia, meningitis, Guillain–Barré syndrome, reactive arthritis	Poultry, cattle, dog, cat, sheep, monkey
Campylobacter jejuni subsp. doylei	Diarrhea	Pig
Campylobacter coli	Diarrhea	Pig, poultry
Campylobacter upsaliensis	Diarrhea, bacteremia	Dog, cat
Campylobacter lari	Diarrhea, bacteremia	Seagull, dog, cat, poultry, monkey
Campylobacter fetus subsp. fetus	Bacteremia, endocarditis, abscess, meningitis	Cattle, sheep
Campylobacter hyointestinalis	Diarrhea	Pig, cattle, hamster
Campylobacter concisus	Periodontal diseases, diarrhea, bacteremia	Human oral cavities and gastrointestinal tract
Campylobacter sputorum subsp. sputorum	Lung, scrotal, and axillary abscess	Human oral cavity
Campylobacter curvus	Alveolar abscess	Human oral cavity
Campylobacter rectus	Periodontitis	Human oral cavity
ARCOBACTER SPECIES		
Arcobacter skirrowii	Bacteremia	Cattle, sheep
Arcobacter butzleri	Abdominal cramps, diarrhea	Pig, cattle, primates

the genera *Campylobacter, Arcobacter, Sulfurospirillum,* and *Thiovulum*. The genus *Campylobacter* (from the Greek and Latin meaning "curved rod") comprises gram-negative, mostly microaerophilic bacteria. These curved, spiral, or S-shaped cells are 0.2 to 0.5 μm wide and 1 to 5 μm long and possess rapid and darting motility in corkscrew fashion by means of a single, unsheathed flagellum in one (monotrichous) or both (amphitrichous) ends. Campylobacters are commensal organisms living in the gastrointestinal tract of birds and mammals for prolonged periods, mostly asymptomatically. *Campylobacter* genomes are relatively small (approximately 1600 to 1900 genes). The complete genomes of several *Campylobacter* strains have now been sequenced and revealed an unexpected variety of genes involved in biosynthesis and modification of carbohydrate surface structures that may be involved in antigenic variation and molecular mimicry.[1–4]

More than 20 species have been recognized within the family Campylobacteraceae, although only 13 are considered pathogenic in humans (Table 163-1). The genus *Campylobacter* comprises 15 species and 6 subspecies although human illness is mostly due to *C. jejuni* and *C. coli* and less frequently to *C. upsaliensis, C. lari,* and *C. fetus*.

All species associated with human diseases grow better in a microaerophilic atmosphere containing 5% to 10% oxygen, and 3% to 5% CO_2, and all are thermotolerant and can grow at 37°C. *C. jejuni* and *C. coli*, which account for almost all cases of enteritis,[5] grow best at 42°C. This likely represents an adaptation for life in the intestine of birds, the natural hosts of thermophilic campylobacters, since normal avian body temperature is in that range (38 to 42°C). Species that are pathogenic for humans can be commensals and nonpathogenic in animals and can be distinguished by their host range. *C. jejuni* is predominant in poultry and *C. coli* in swine, and both also colonize cattle.

Isolation from stool culture is the gold standard for establishing the diagnosis of *Campylobacter* enteritis. Several methods are available for isolation of campylobacters from stool, food, and environmental samples that take advantage of their innate antibiotic resistance, slender morphology, and tolerance to high temperatures.[6–8] Use of blood or charcoal agar containing selective antibiotics that suppress the growth of the normal human colonic microflora permit growth as non-pigmented colonies that have oxidase activity.[9] Many *Campylobacter* species other than *C. jejuni* and *C. coli*, however, can be susceptible to the selective antibiotics. To avoid selective antibiotics some methods use filtration enrichment through cellulose membranes that trap most colonic organisms but allow slender campylobacters to pass through.[10]

Campylobacters grow best in microaerophilic conditions, and *C. jejuni* and *C. coli* can be selectively enriched by growth at higher temperature. For optimal recovery of all *Campylobacter*, filtration and enrichment is used.[11]

Molecular detection techniques, such as polymerase chain reaction (PCR)-based methods, and enzyme immunoassays (EIAs) are available for diagnosis and speciation directly from stool.[12,13] In some conditions these are more sensitive than culture.[14] *Campylobacter* can be isolated from normally sterile body fluids without using selective media, using any enrichment medium incubated under microaerophilic conditions.

C. jejuni is the most common species of *Campylobacter* isolated from patients with diarrhea.[5,15–21] *C. jejuni* is differentiated from other members of the genus by its ability to hydrolyze hippurate, although a few hippurate-negative strains have been isolated. For practical purposes, *C. jejuni* and *C. coli* are discussed together because they have similarities in epidemiology and clinical features, and they belong to the same cluster phylogenetically.

EPIDEMIOLOGY

Enteric *Campylobacter* infections are common worldwide. *C. jejuni* is a major cause of diarrhea of bacterial origin in both developed and developing countries. The rate of isolation of *C. jejuni* from children with diarrhea in industrialized countries ranges from 5% to 16%, with a prevalence of infection in healthy individuals of 0% to 1.5%.[19] In the United States, an estimated 2 million cases of campylobacteriosis occur each year.[22] *Campylobacter* fluctuates with *Salmonella* as the most common bacterial cause of foodborne illness in the U.S.[19,23] The overall incidence of laboratory-confirmed *Campylobacter* infections is 13 per 100,000 population.[23] There has been a 30% decline in the incidence of culture-confirmed *Campylobacter* infection from the 1996 baseline. However, no further decrease has occurred since 2006.[23,24] Age-specific rates of *C. jejuni* isolation in patients with diarrhea differ among countries. Population-based studies in England, the U.S., and Sweden have shown a bimodal distribution, with a peak of illness in children <5 years of age and in people 15 to 29 years of age.[16,20,21,23] The highest isolation rate of 15 per 100,000 occurs in the first year of life. Infection occurs more often during the summer.

In rural populations where raw milk is often consumed, the incidence is 5- or 6-fold higher than in urban settings.[25] In the United Kingdom, approximately 54,000 laboratory-confirmed cases are reported each year, with an estimated annual incidence of 870 to 1010 cases and 600 hospitalizations per 100,000 people.[21]

In the Netherlands, intestinal infection in general accounts for 3000 to 10,000 disability-adjusted life years (DALYs) per year, and *Campylobacter* infections account for 1400 DALYs per year, that is, at least one-third of the disease burden of all intestinal infections.[26] *Campylobacter* infection generally is associated with mild illness although up to 17% of culture-confirmed cases are hospitalized.[27] The mortality rate of symptomatic, confirmed *Campylobacter* infection is estimated to be 0.1% or 120 deaths annually in the U.S.[27]

In endemic areas in developing countries, the isolation rate in children with diarrhea is 8% to 45%, with a similar rate of isolation in asymptomatic children.[28–33] The highest proportion of *C. jejuni* isolations are in children <5 years of age.[28,32] The annual incidence of *Campylobacter* infections can be as high as 2.1 episodes per child. Infections acquired under 5 years of age are more likely to be associated with diarrhea, whereas those occurring later, although relatively common, are mostly asymptomatic.

Enteric *Campylobacter* infection has several well-defined modes of transmission. The most important is the ingestion of contaminated food such as undercooked poultry and meat, and unpasteurized milk.[19,25,34–40] Ingestion of contaminated water[41,42] and direct contact with animals, including pets and animals on farms and in slaughterhouses, has also been documented.[34,36,43,44] Wild birds (e.g., magpies) also have been implicated in directly contaminating milk bottles, resulting in *Campylobacter* outbreaks.[45,46] Person-to-person transmission is rare, but does occur in childcare centers and in families,[47,48] as does perinatal transmission through contact with a contaminated birth canal,[49] sexual contact among homosexuals,[50,51] and acquisition during travel to developing countries.[52,53]

Pasteurization and chlorination of water kill *C. jejuni*, but organisms survive in milk or other foods kept at 4°C. Although many milkborne outbreaks have been reported as a result of the consumption of unpasteurized or ineffectively pasteurized milk[36,38,40] and a few waterborne outbreaks have occurred,[54,55] together they account for <10% of all reported cases. Since campylobacters have relatively high temperature requirements, they tend not to multiply in foods (in contrast to *Salmonella*) and therefore most cases are sporadic rather than occurring in large outbreaks.

Modes of transmission of *Campylobacter* differ in developed and developing countries. In industrialized regions, most sporadic cases can be attributed to the handling, preparation, and consumption of contaminated raw or undercooked poultry.[15,17,19,36,37] Among college students in the U.S., 70% of *Campylobacter* infections were caused by eating undercooked chicken, and in 30% of cases, contact with cats was reported.[35] Poor kitchen hygiene also can play a role, since the risk of infection is inversely associated with the frequency of using soap to clean the cutting board.[17] *Campylobacter* can be isolated from 50% to 90% of raw chicken meat purchased in supermarkets from different countries in the developed world.[56–61] For infants, riding in shopping carts has been a risk factor, through contact with leaky packages of uncooked meat products.[62,63]

In developing countries, the main factors involved in transmission are free-roaming poultry in the household, toddlers in the family, a limited water supply, and lack of adequate disposal of sewage. Transmission can be reduced substantially by education regarding personal and domestic hygiene, penning of chickens outside the house, avoidance of contact with their feces, piped water, flush toilets, and handwashing.[28,34] *C. coli* has been isolated more frequently in populations with intimate contact with swine. *C. jejuni* subsp. *doylei* is isolated more often in socially deprived communities and in persons who have contact with cats and dogs. The incubation period of *C. jejuni* is 2 to 4 days (range 2 to 7 days).

PATHOGENESIS

In susceptible individuals, as few as 500 organisms are required to induce diarrhea.[64] Although *C. jejuni* is killed by hydrochloric acid at pH 2.3, it can survive in milk or water for several weeks. The mechanisms by which *C. jejuni* induces disease are not well understood, but the process involves bacterial virulence and colonization factors involved in surviving passage through the stomach and small intestine, and subsequent colonization and growth in the distal ileum and colon.[65,66]

Studies of *Campylobacter* genome sequences[3,67] have failed to identify classical virulence factors found in other bacteria that cause diarrhea, like enterotoxins and pili. The only toxin genes present are for cytolethal distending toxins (CDTs). Genes involved in biosynthesis of surface carbohydrates comprise up to one-tenth of the genome. These genes influence glycosylation of several bacterial surface structures, including the capsule, lipooligosaccharides, and the flagella.[68] Modifications are highly variable and give campylobacters increased diversity that avoids host immune responses. Some lipooligosaccharides, for example, resemble human neuronal gangliosides and molecular mimicry is thought to be responsible for autoimmune sequelae like GBS.[69] Much of the "virulence" of campylobacters may be due to aberrant immune responses by the host, including some serious postinfectious sequelae. Three general stages during *Campylobacter* infection have been postulated to lead to different clinical syndromes:[65,70,71] (1) colonization and adherence to the epithelium of the distal ileum and colon may result in non-inflammatory diarrhea through unknown mechanisms; (2) invasion and proliferation within the intestinal epithelium causes cell damage and an inflammatory response clinically manifest as dysentery with fecal leukocytes;[72–75] and (3) translocation across the intestinal epithelium and into the lamina propria potentially can spread to mesenteric lymph nodes causing mesenteric adenitis, and also to deeper sites causing extraintestinal infections such as meningitis, cholecystitis, and urinary tract infection. The ability of some clinical strains to invade has been demonstrated in in vitro assays[76] and animal models.[75,77] Prior to attachment and invasion, the bacteria must navigate to the epithelial surface, and both motility and chemotaxis have been shown to be important in colonization and disease.[78] Studies in experimental animals and in volunteers have shown that nonmotile variants of *C. jejuni* fail to colonize or induce disease.[79] Flagella are postulated to be involved directly in attachment to the cell surface and to serve as a secretion apparatus involved in adhesion.[80–84] Several other putative adhesins have been identified that either bind specific protein receptors on the cell surface[85–87] and fucosylated residues on glycoproteins,[88] or bind extracellular matrix components such as fibronectin found in the basolateral side of the epithelium.[89] *Campylobacter* also produce a multi-subunit protein toxin, CDTs, that causes DNA damage and cell death. CDT is not unique to *Campylobacter*, having homologues in several other gram-negative bacterial pathogens.[90,91] CDTs also are involved in the inflammatory response, inducing release of interleukin-8 (IL-8) from intestinal epithelial cells and promoting proinflammatory response in animal models.[92] The clinical relevance of CDTs requires further study.[93]

Invasion of epithelial cells in the intestine is considered an important virulence factor of *Campylobacter* infection, since intracellular *Campylobacter* are found during invasive enterocolitis in humans and in animal models,[94,95] and also invade a number of epithelial cell types in vitro.[76,96–100] The ability to penetrate epithelial cells involves attachment followed by manipulation of the host cytoskeletal machinery. Campylobacters seem to utilize both microfilament- and microtubule-mediated entry mechanisms.[101,102] After internalization, campylobacters are found within vacuoles of the epithelial cell and do not exit into the cytosol. Whether the bacteria can replicate intracellularly remains controversial. Survival mechanisms inside the cells require genes involved in bacterial stress responses.[103,104] *Campylobacter* also can survive within macrophages and monocytes in cell culture conditions, suggesting a mechanism to prolong infection within the lamina propria.[105] An important feature of *C. jejuni* enterocolitis is activation of a proinflammatory response in colonic epithelium,[106,107] which likely contributes to the inflammatory diarrhea seen in some patients.

C. jejuni BSI or extraintestinal infection is rare, occurring mainly in neonates, the elderly, and immunocompromised hosts (especially those with humoral immunodeficiency such as agammaglobulinemia), patients with malignancies treated with chemotherapy, and patients with acquired immunodeficiency syndrome (AIDS).[108,109]

IMMUNITY

Immunity to *C. jejuni* develops after one or more infections.[110-114] Children living in endemic areas have a progressive decrease in the illness-to-infection ratio with increasing age.[19] Cohort studies also demonstrate that *Campylobacter* diarrhea occurring in young children protects against subsequent infections; however, no protection seems to occur after a symptom-free infection.[19] Serum antibodies to specific antigens of *Campylobacter* increase after natural infection,[110,112,115] and in children from some developing countries, an inverse relationship is seen between levels of antibodies and the incidence of diarrhea. Further evidence of the importance of antibodies in protecting against *C. jejuni* is the prolonged, severe, and recurrent *C. jejuni* infection in immunodeficient patients[108,116] and the failure of patients with AIDS to respond to therapy or mount a humoral immune response to infection.[117] Experimental studies in volunteers have further substantiated the acquisition of antibodies after symptomatic infection and protection from subsequent illness after rechallenge.[64,114]

Production of serum and gut mucosal antibodies mainly is responsible for elimination of the organism. A rapid and intense serum response involving both monomeric and polymeric IgA occurs in the first week, reaches a peak after the second week, and declines to low levels within 30 days after the onset of symptoms. Patients infected with *C. jejuni* O:19, the serotype most frequently associated with GBS, had a significantly higher IgA antibody response than did patients infected with other serotypes.[112] A local secretory IgA response also occurs after *Campylobacter* enteritis.[118] Isotype-specific IgG and IgM antibodies peak on days 15 to 21 and decrease to low levels within 3 months after onset of symptoms.[110,112] In persons who are chronically exposed in hyperendemic areas, serum-specific IgA antibodies increase progressively through life.[110] *Campylobacter* antibody levels in populations in developed compared with developing countries are significantly lower.[70] Studies in breastfed Mexican children have demonstrated protection against *Campylobacter* diarrhea conferred by specific secretory IgA antibodies present in human milk.[115,119] Human and mouse[120] experimental infections also suggest that cell-mediated immune responses are important and correlate with protection against *Campylobacter* enteric infections. For example, antigen-dependent production of interferon-γ by monocytes of volunteers correlated strongly with protection from experimental campylobacteriosis.[114]

CLINICAL MANIFESTATIONS

Campylobacter infections produce a broad range of clinical manifestations that are associated with the species involved and some characteristics of the host, such as age, immunosuppression, and underlying chronic and debilitating illnesses (see Table 163-1). The most common clinical finding is enteritis, for which >95% of cases are caused by *C. jejuni*.[5,21] BSI, extraintestinal, and perinatal infections are rare and are caused by other *Campylobacter* species.

Enteritis

Several clinical manifestations of *Campylobacter* enteritis occur in children:[19,121] mild episodes of loose stools; watery, secretory-type diarrhea; and inflammatory diarrhea, which occasionally is severe. Substantial differences in the clinical characteristics of diarrhea occur in children in developed and developing countries. Inflammatory diarrhea is more common in developed countries, while secretory diarrhea seems to prevail in underdeveloped areas. In general, episodes are mild and self-limited; 60% to 70% subside within 1 week, 20% to 30% subside in 2 weeks, and 5% to 10% persist for several weeks. Relapses can occur. In one-third to one-half of patients, the onset of diarrhea is preceded by intense abdominal pain, malaise, myalgia, and headache.[122] Vomiting

occurs frequently. Pain generally is periumbilical and cramping and when present can be severe in 20% of patients, sometimes mimicking appendicitis.[123] When laparotomy is performed in these patients, mesenteric lymphadenitis or signs of ileocolitis are found. Pain usually subsides within a week. Secretory diarrhea is more common in younger children, who have 10 or more profuse watery stools per day. Dehydration occurs in about 10% of children.

The clinical features of inflammatory diarrhea are indistinguishable from those caused by *Shigella* and are characterized by generalized malaise, fever, abdominal cramps, tenesmus, bloody stools, and the presence of fecal leukocytes by light microscopy. Severe cases, which are rare, can occur in adolescents and young adults and can be mistaken for ulcerative colitis, Crohn disease, or pseudomembranous colitis; occasionally, disease progresses to toxic megacolon, massive bleeding, or colonic perforation.[124-126] In neonates, blood-streaking of formed stool (hematochezia) is associated with *C. jejuni*.[127,128] Abdominal examination reveals tenderness to deep palpation, especially in the right lower quadrant. Splenomegaly has been reported rarely.

In patients who have undergone proctoscopy or colonoscopy because of a protracted course of illness, normal mucosa is found in approximately 50%. In the rest, mucosal edema, congestion, friability, and granularity are seen. The spectrum of histologic changes ranges from minimal edema with acute and chronic inflammatory cells without vascular congestion, to moderate inflammation and cryptitis, to crypt abscess formation.[129]

The peripheral white blood cell count usually is normal, although a shift to the left is common. Mild elevations in serum alanine aminotransferase, alkaline phosphatase, and the sedimentation rate are observed in up to 25% of patients. If specific treatment is not given, fecal shedding of *Campylobacter* persists for a median of 2 to 3 weeks, with a range of 3 days to several months.[19,127,130] Younger children tend to shed the organism for longer periods.[131] Severe, persistent, and recurrent *C. jejuni* infections and emergence of erythromycin resistance during therapy have been reported in patients with immunodeficiencies, including congenital or acquired hypogammaglobulinemia and AIDS.[108,116,117,130]

Bloodstream Infections

Campylobacter BSI is uncommon (approximately 1.5 per 1000 cases of enteritis) and occurs mostly in malnourished children or patients with chronic debilitating illnesses or immunodeficiency. BSI can be transient and asymptomatic in normal hosts, but severe in immunosuppressed hosts.[108] *C. fetus* infections, although rare, usually are associated with BSI and systemic infections.[117,132] *C. fetus* rarely causes diarrhea, except in debilitated or immunocompromised hosts. Three clinical manifestations of BSI are described: (1) cryptogenic BSI, which occurs as an isolated event that is self-limited or readily responds to antibiotics; (2) secondary BSI, the most common manifestation, which is associated with focal infections such as meningitis, pneumonia, endocarditis, and thrombophlebitis; and (3) chronic BSI with relapses that can persist for several months (mostly in immunosuppressed patients). Contrary to the age-specific distribution of *Campylobacter* enteritis, BSI peaks in patients >65 years of age. BSI occurs in approximately 1 in 3000 intestinal infections in children <14 years of age, and in 1 in 170 intestinal infections in people >65 years of age.[132,133] *C. jejuni* or *C. coli* account for 60% to 90% of blood isolates, followed by *C. fetus* in 8% to 15%. Most episodes of BSI occur in patients with diarrhea. BSI appears to be more common in children in developing countries, with a rate as high as 45 per 1000 intestinal infections, with *C. jejuni* subsp. *jejuni* (41%), *C. jejuni* subsp. *doylei* (24%), and *C. upsaliensis* (5.6%) the most common blood isolates.

Localized Extraintestinal Infections

A focal lesion can be the first manifestation of *C. jejuni* infection, or can occur after or simultaneously with BSI. Extraintestinal infections caused by *C. jejuni* include cholecystitis,[134] urinary tract infection,[135] spontaneous splenic rupture, pancreatitis,[136] septic arthritis[137] and osteomyelitis,[138] and meningitis.[109,139] These manifestations are uncommon and generally occur in patients who are immunosuppressed or at the extremes of age.[133]

Perinatal Infections

Perinatal infections have been associated with *C. fetus* and rarely with *C. jejuni*.[140] *C. fetus* has tropism for the genital tract and fetal tissue. Three clinical manifestations of perinatal infection have been described: abortion and stillbirth, premature labor, and neonatal septicemia and meningitis.[109,139-146] Perinatal infections with BSI and meningitis associated with *C. jejuni* are rare.[109,139,140] Infected infants often are premature, and in most cases, maternal infection has been implicated. Symptomatic gastroenteritis and asymptomatic bloody diarrhea attributable to *C. jejuni* are reported in neonates,[127] with the mother (who can be symptomatic or asymptomatic at the time of delivery) generally being the source.[140] In general, perinatal infections caused by *C. jejuni* are less severe than those caused by *C. fetus*.

Immunoreactive Complications

Immunoreactive complications such as GBS,[147-150] Reiter syndrome,[151,152] reactive arthritis,[137] and erythema nodosum[153] occur occasionally after *C. jejuni* diarrhea. *Campylobacter* is the single most common cause of GBS, as suggested by case-control and cohort studies; GBS is rare in children.[154,155] It is estimated that a *Campylobacter* infection occurred in the previous 2 weeks in 30% to 40% of cases of GBS. A cohort study reported a rate of 30.4 cases of GBS for every 100,000 laboratory-confirmed *Campylobacter* infections.[156] The risk of GBS within 2 months of a symptomatic *Campylobacter* infection is 100-fold that in the general population. People ≥60 years of age are at highest risk for GBS (248 cases in 100,000 *Campylobacter* infections). *Campylobacter*-associated GBS is more frequent during the summer. The mean interval between diarrhea and the onset of symptoms is 10 days (range 6 to 21 days).[157] Patients with *C. jejuni*-associated GBS are more likely than other GBS patients to have more neurophysiologic features of axonal neuropathy, antibodies to ganglioside GM_1, pure motor GBS, a less elevated cerebrospinal fluid protein concentration, and a worse outcome.[148,149,158] Cranial nerve involvement occurs in one-third of cases, and recovery is complete in most patients. Miller Fisher syndrome, a polyneuritis variant characterized by ophthalmoplegia, areflexia, ataxia, and high levels of IgG antibodies to ganglioside GQ_{1b}, also has been associated with preceding *Campylobacter* infection.[157,159-161] A third variant is acute motor axonal neuropathy, or Chinese paralytic syndrome, which is characterized by an explosive onset with rapid progression to tetraplegia and respiratory failure.[162,163] The illness is a reversible lesion of the motor nerve terminal or anterior horn cell. Epidemics of acute motor axonal neuropathy have occurred in northern China for >20 years, taking place in the summer and fall, in rural areas and involving children mainly. Studies using serology and culture have found a strong association with *Campylobacter* infection.[164,165] The pathogenesis of *Campylobacter*-induced GBS is not completely understood, but experiments in rabbits show that molecular mimicry between *Campylobacter* lipooligosaccharides and human gangliosides GM_1 are sufficient to reproduce a clinical syndrome like GBS.[69] These data suggest that infection with *C. jejuni* carrying GM_1-like lipooligosaccharides may result in autoantibodies that bind to GM1 on the motor nerve axons in the spinal roots. Deposited IgG recruits macrophages into the periaxonal space where they attack the axon, causing Wallerian-like degeneration. Molecular mimicry between the lipooligosaccharide of some *Campylobacter* serotypes (O:19, O:41) and gangliosides GM_1, GD_{1a}, GD_3, GT_{1a}, and GQ_{1b} of peripheral nerve glycolipids or myelin[166-170] may play a role in the pathogenesis of *Campylobacter*-related GBS, where the immune response to *Campylobacter* infection could generate antibodies cross-reactive with neural antigens. Possible host susceptibility to GBS is suggested by the observations that antibodies to GM_1 ganglioside do not develop in all patients with *C. jejuni*-induced GBS and GBS does not develop in many patients who have enteritis caused by the predominant serotypes O:19 and O:41 (which have GM_1 epitopes). Although the association of GBS with histocompatibility antigens is unclear, studies suggest a link with HLA-DQB1*03, HLA-B35, and HLA-DRB1*1312.[158]

Reactive arthritis can be associated with *Campylobacter* enteritis as well as with *Salmonella*, *Shigella*, and *Yersinia* enteritis.[137,151,152] It is relatively more common in young male adults. Arthritis begins 3 to 40 days (mean 11 days) after the onset of diarrhea, usually is oligoarticular and asymmetric (affecting mainly the knees), is of short duration (range 1 to 21 days), and has no sequelae. Arthralgias are reported in up to 20% of infected patients, but symptoms of arthritis occur in 2% to 9%. Synovial fluid is sterile and fever and leukocytosis are absent, but the sedimentation rate is elevated. The histocompatibility antigen HLA-B27 has been associated with more severe or prolonged illness in some but not all studies.[171]

Some studies also suggest an association between *Campylobacter* infection and postinfectious irritable bowel syndrome, especially in those having diarrhea for >7 days.[172] Other potential host predisposing factors for postinfectious irritable bowel syndrome include younger age, female sex, prior anxiety/depression, and fever and weight loss during the acute enteric illness.[173,174]

DIAGNOSIS

The diagnosis can be suspected clinically by the occurrence of watery diarrhea sometimes followed by blood-streaked stools and preceded or accompanied by abdominal pain. Microbiologic confirmation is required. A rapid diagnosis of *Campylobacter* enteritis can be made tentatively by direct examination of stool with carbolfuchsin stain, the indirect fluorescent antibody test, or darkfield microscopy. PCR techniques using oligonucleotide primers encoding for 16S ribosomal RNA have been designed for specific detection of *C. jejuni*, *C. coli*, and other species.[175] In a large-scale survey of *Campylobacter* species in diarrheal cases, this method was as sensitive as culture methods, and it was excellent for diagnosing mixed infections with more than one *Campylobacter* species, including non-*C. jejuni* and non-*C. coli* infections.[176] Rapid EIA antigen testing of stool may be as sensitive and specific as culture methods, but false-positive results can occur (possibly related to blood) that misdirect management.[13,177]

TREATMENT

Rehydration and correction of electrolyte abnormalities are the mainstay of treatment for enteritis. Need for antibiotic treatment is debated but should be considered for *C. jejuni*-infected patients who have bloody or severe diarrhea, fever, or worsening of symptoms, and in those who are immunosuppressed. Antimotility agents have been associated with prolongation of symptoms and fatalities and should not be used.

Campylobacter species often are resistant to penicillin, ampicillin, and cephalosporins, with an alarming increase in fluoroquinolone resistance in the past two decades in most countries.[178] Rise in resistance coincides with the licensure of fluoroquinolones for use in poultry and veterinary medicine.[179,180] In some countries like Spain, Thailand, Taiwan, and Hong Kong, fluoroquinolone resistance is ≥80%.[181,182] Most strains of *C. jejuni* and *C. coli* are susceptible to erythromycin, azithromycin, gentamicin, carbapenems, and chloramphenicol.[183-186] When antibiotic therapy is indicated for gastroenteritis, erythromycin or azithromycin are the drugs of choice.[187-189] Erythromycin shows little propensity to select for plasmid-mediated resistance, which mainly is selected by point mutations. Although erythromycin resistance is low currently, it is an emerging health concern especially in countries that use erythromycin in food-producing animals.[190,191] *C. coli* harbors higher rates of erythromycin resistance than *C. jejuni*.[181] Macrolide-resistant isolates tend to be multidrug resistant.[192] Studies have shown no clinical benefit of erythromycin therapy versus placebo if given late in the course of disease.[186,187,193] If antibiotic therapy was initiated within the first 4 days of illness, a reduction in fecal excretion also occurred, but conflicting results were reported with regard to resolution of symptoms.[190,194,195]

PROGNOSIS

Campylobacter BSI in immunocompromised hosts or neonates is associated with high mortality.[109,196] The few cases reported preclude providing an estimate of the mortality rate, particularly when early or effective antimicrobial therapy is administered. The prognosis of patients with *C. jejuni* or *C. coli* enteritis appears to be good in immunocompetent hosts, but enteritis can be severe, prolonged, and recurrent in individuals who are immunocompromised.

Key Points. *Campylobacter jejuni* and *C. coli*

EPIDEMIOLOGY

- Major cause of culture-proven bacterial gastroenteritis worldwide
- Highest incidence occurs in children <5 years of age
- Well-defined modes of transmission are undercooked poultry and meat and unpasteurized milk

CLINICAL FEATURES

- Generally a mild illness but inflammatory diarrhea and hospitalization can occur; extraintestinal infections and death are rare
- Most common cause of Guillain–Barré syndrome
- Most perinatal infections are caused by *C. fetus*

DIAGNOSIS

- Stool samples cultured on selective media is the gold standard

- Selective media is not necessary for isolation from normally sterile body fluids

TREATMENT AND PREVENTION

- Rehydration and correction of electrolyte abnormalities are the mainstays of therapy
- Consider antimicrobial therapy in patients with bloody or severe diarrhea, fever, worsening of symptoms, or patients who are immunosuppressed
- Drugs of choice are azithromycin or erythromycin if given within the first 4 days of illness
- Antimotility agents should not be used
- Pasteurization and chlorination of water kill *C. jejuni*

---

164 Other *Campylobacter* Species

Manuel R. Amieva and Guillermo M. Ruiz-Palacios

The genus *Campylobacter* includes approximately 18 species and subspecies. Of the *Campylobacter* species that are associated with human disease, *C. jejuni* is the prototype for enteric infections, and *C. fetus* is the prototype for extraintestinal infections. *Helicobacter cinaedi* and *H. fennelliae* originally were identified as *Campylobacter* species but have been reclassified (see Chapter 175, Other Gastric and Enterohepatic *Helicobacter* Species). Refinement of microbiologic techniques for isolation of *Campylobacter* spp. and use of molecular assays have expanded our knowledge of the extent of human infections with these organisms.[1-4] However, *Campylobacter* species other than *C. jejuni* and *C. coli* may be significantly underdiagnosed as causes of gastrointestinal tract disease as a consequence of: (1) use of selective *Campylobacter* media that may inhibit their growth; (2) lack of use of stool filtration techniques; and (3) lack of speciation of *Campylobacter* isolates, because of growth requirements and indistinguishable biochemical characteristics.[5]

Phylogenetic trees have been established for *Campylobacter* on the basis of 16S ribosomal DNA sequences. These trees contain three distinct clades (species groups) (Table 164-1). The first clade consists of *C. fetus*, *C. hyointestinalis*, and *C. mucosalis*, generally associated with disease in farm animals. The second clade consists of *C. coli*, *C. jejuni*, *C. helveticus*, *C. lari*, and *C. upsaliensis* species; all (except *C. helveticus*) have been associated with gastroenteritis in humans. The third contains *C. curvus*, *C. concisus*, *C. gracilis*, *C. rectus*, *C. showae*, and *C. sputorum*, organisms generally associated with the periodontal cavity of humans and animals. *C. jejuni* and

TABLE 164-1. Location of and Disease Associated with *Campylobacter* Species

Association or Disease	*Campylobacter* Species
Disease in farm animals	Campylobacter fetus[a]
	Campylobacter hyointestinalis[a]
	Campylobacter mucosalis
Gastroenteritis and, occasional, bacteremia	Campylobacter coli[a]
	Campylobacter jejuni[a]
	Campylobacter helveticus
	Campylobacter lari[a]
	Campylobacter upsaliensis[a]
Periodontal cavities of humans and animals	Campylobacter curvus
	Campylobacter concisus
	Campylobacter gracilis
	Campylobacter rectus
	Campylobacter showae
	Campylobacter sputorum

[a]Associated with human disease.

C. coli are described in Chapter 163, *Campylobacter jejuni* and *Campylobacter coli*.

CAMPYLOBACTER FETUS

Two subspecies of *C. fetus* have been recognized, *C. fetus* subsp. *fetus* and *C. fetus* subsp. *venerealis*. These organisms cause infection of the genitourinary tract of cattle and sheep, and only *C. fetus* subsp. *fetus* is considered a human pathogen, causing perinatal infections, and bloodstream infection (BSI) in the immunocompromised host. In 1913, McFadyean and Stockman[6] found a *Vibrio*-like organism in aborted ovine fetuses and proposed the name *Vibrio fetus ovis*. The same organism later was implicated as a cause of abortion and infertility in other domestic animals, and the name was shortened to *V. fetus*.[7] A second type of infection in cattle and sheep, causing sporadic abortion, but not infertility, was recognized; the causal agent was named *V. fetus* subsp. *venerealis*, which has not been found to be a human pathogen.[8] In 1947, Vincent and colleagues[9] reported the first human infection by *C. fetus* in a pregnant woman with BSI who aborted at 6 months of gestation.

Microbiology and Epidemiology

C. fetus subsp. *fetus* are curved, gram-negative, microaerophilic bacteria that are oxidase-, catalase-, and nitrate-positive; they grow at 25°C and 37°C but not at 42°C. They are susceptible to cephalothin and resistant to nalidixic acid. In national surveillance in the United States, *C. fetus* represented only 0.3% of all *Campylobacter* species reported; most isolates of *C. fetus* were from blood, with isolation rates peaking in children <1 year of age and among elderly people.[10] In the adult population, the male-to-female ratio was 3:1; among children there is no sex predominance. Most cases occur in patients with underlying diseases.[11,12] A source of *C. fetus* infection seldom is identified, although a few cases have been reported after ingestion of raw milk[13,14] or contaminated food[15] or water, by sexual and transplacental transmission,[16] and in neonates after vaginal delivery.[17] Unlike *C. jejuni*, broiler chickens are not likely to be contaminated by *C. fetus* probably because of the higher body temperature,[18] but sheep and cattle are common carriers and may be a source of infection.[19]

C. fetus infections in pregnant women occur predominantly during the third trimester of pregnancy. In other adults infected with *C. fetus* there is often a history of farm or animal exposure.[20,21] An infected woman, with or without symptoms, can have recurrent abortions or premature deliveries or can serve as a source of life-threatening perinatal infection.[16,22-28] In several cases of neonatal septicemia and meningitis, *C. fetus* was isolated from the maternal cervix or vagina.[24,28,29] Cervical cultures remained positive in women who had recurrent abortions and whose husbands had high antibody titers to the organism.[30]

Clinical Manifestations and Management

In humans, *C. fetus* infection generally causes a systemic illness manifesting as enteric fever, and can be associated with translocation of the organism through a relatively intact intestinal mucosa to the reticuloendothelial system and the bloodstream.[31] BSI principally occurs in children with acquired or primary immunodeficiency or in the very young. A paracrystalline protein structure composed of S-layer proteins surrounding the bacterial outer-membrane is a unique virulence factor of *C. fetus* and *C. rectus*. This structure is implicated in invasion, resistance to phagocytosis, resistance to complement-mediated killing, and immune evasion by antigenic variation.[32-36] The pathology of perinatal *C. fetus* infection consists of placental necrosis, and of widespread endothelial proliferation, intravascular fibrin deposition, perivascular inflammation, and hemorrhagic necrosis in the brain of the neonate.[37] *C. fetus* rarely causes diarrhea but can do so in debilitated or immunodeficient hosts.[38]

BSI is the most common manifestation of *C. fetus* infection; this organism appears to have a predilection for vascular endothelium, with manifestations such as thrombophlebitis, pericarditis, mycotic aneurysms, and endocarditis.[39-44] Patients with BSI due to *C. fetus* should be evaluated for localized vascular infection. Confusion and lethargy are common, although focal neurologic signs are unusual except when meningitis or cerebral abscesses are present. The following three clinical presentations of BSI have been described: (1) cryptogenic BSI occurring as an isolated event that is self-limited or readily responds to antimicrobial therapy; (2) secondary BSI, the most common presentation, associated with focal infections such as meningitis, pneumonia, endocarditis, and thrombophlebitis; and (3) chronic BSI with relapses that can persist for several months, occurring mostly in immunosuppressed patients.

Mortality from *C. fetus* BSI has been estimated at 30% to 40%, with higher rates among patients who have secondary BSI with a distant focal infection. In children with agammaglobulinemia, severe septicemia and hepatitis have been described.[45] Systemic infections generally occur in patients with predisposing conditions such as chronic alcoholism, liver disease, diabetes mellitus, human immunodeficiency virus infection, and malignancies,[11,46-50] or in women during pregnancy.[51] *C. fetus* infections in children usually are confined to the neonatal period and occur in association with maternal infections.[52]

A focal lesion can be the first manifestation of *C. fetus* infection, or can occur following or simultaneously with BSI. Meningitis, cholecystitis, pancreatitis, cellulitis, urinary tract infection, lung and gluteal abscesses, pericarditis, endocarditis, thrombophlebitis, septic arthritis, and salpingitis have been reported.[29,53-59] Perinatal infections are associated with *C. fetus*.[17]

Infections with *C. fetus* usually are systemic and therefore require parenteral antibiotic therapy. *C. fetus* organisms often are susceptible to ampicillin and gentamicin, but imipenem or meropenem is preferred for treatment pending results of in vitro susceptibility tests.[60,61] Duration of therapy is empiric. Central nervous system infections should be treated for several weeks.

CAMPYLOBACTER UPSALIENSIS

Microbiology

A species of thermotolerant, catalase-negative or weakly catalase-positive, cephalothin-susceptible *Campylobacter* was isolated from dogs with diarrhea in 1982.[62] DNA hybridization and phylogenetic studies with comparison of the 16S rRNA sequence demonstrated that this organism belongs to a new species, *C. upsaliensis*, named after the Swedish city in which it was first isolated.[63,64] Although initially isolated from dogs and cats,[65] *C. upsaliensis* now is considered a relatively common enteric pathogen of humans[66,67] and also is a cause of BSI in malnourished children and immunocompromised adults.[68-70]

C. upsaliensis can be differentiated from other *Campylobacter* species on the basis of several phenotypic characteristics.[63] Most strains are thermotolerant, which means that they grow well at 42°C, but not at 25°C. *C. upsaliensis* is weakly positive or negative for catalase production and does not produce hydrogen sulfide in triple sugar medium or hydrolyze hippurate. A high proportion of isolates possess multiple plasmids. All strains are susceptible to cephalothin and nalidixic acid. *C. upsaliensis* is susceptible to the antimicrobial agents used in *Campylobacter*-selective media and therefore is not detected in cultures using these media.[71]

Epidemiology, Clinical Manifestations, and Treatment

C. upsaliensis is under-identified in routine clinical laboratories, making the true prevalence of infection with this pathogen difficult to estimate.[72,73] *C. upsaliensis* is the second most common *Campylobacter* species isolated after *C. jejuni* subsp. *jejuni*.[66,67] *C. upsaliensis* is isolated more frequently from populations with poor sanitation and overcrowded conditions, and frequently is isolated from dogs and cats with diarrhea.[72,74,75] An outbreak of *C. upsaliensis* diarrhea was described in childcare centers in Brussels, with attack rates of 21% to 77%. Infection was associated with chronic or relapsing diarrhea in which fecal–oral transmission was likely.[76] Infections in humans sometimes are associated with close contact with infected dogs.[74,77–79] Although no studies are available to define associated risk factors, *C. upsaliensis* is isolated more commonly from October through December.[66] Children are affected more often than adults. Diarrhea of short duration is the most common clinical presentation; 25% of patients have gross or occult blood in stools, one-fourth have fecal leukocytes, and vomiting occurs occasionally but the disease appears to be milder than that caused by *C. jejuni*.[67]

In immunocompromised children and in malnourished children with diarrhea the infection can progress to septicemia.[68–70,80] *C. upsaliensis* infection has been associated with abortion, and BSI was described in a patient with ruptured ectopic pregnancy.[81]

Experience with antimicrobial treatment of *C. upsaliensis* is limited and clinical studies are needed. Most isolates are resistant to vancomycin, methicillin, trimethoprim, and piperacillin, but susceptible to cephalosporins, fluoroquinolones, tetracycline, and aminoglycosides.[63,82,83] Diarrhea generally has been treated with erythromycin but no controlled trials have been conducted and in some studies up to 13% to 15% of *C. upsaliensis* strains are resistant to macrolides in vitro.[83]

CAMPYLOBACTER LARI

In the early 1980s, Skirrow and Benjamin[84] isolated nalidixic acid-resistant, thermophilic campylobacters in seagulls (*Larus argentus*) as well as in feces of domestic animals, seals, and ducks. Although *C. lari* has been isolated in up to 10% of cloacal swabs from chickens, transmission to humans is rare. *C. lari* accounts for 1% of all diarrhea-associated *Campylobacter* isolates.[85] *C. lari* BSI has been described in immunocompromised patients and neonates.[86–88] An outbreak of diarrhea occurred among construction workers who drank water contaminated by surface water from Lake Ontario.[89]

OTHER *CAMPYLOBACTER* SPECIES

C. curvus, *C. concisus*, *C. gracilis*, *C. rectus*, *C. showae*, and *C. sputorum* generally are associated with the periodontal cavities of humans and animals and have no definitive association with human gastroenteritis. However, *C. curvus* has been isolated from patients with bloody and chronic diarrhea[90] and *C. curvus* and *C. rectus* have been reported as the cause of extraoral abscesses in humans.[91,92] Reports of the isolation of *C. concisus* from nonoral human clinical specimens (from blood and stool of patients with diarrhea, and from the foot of a diabetic patient with osteomyelitis) suggest that this organism can be a true pathogen in humans.[93] *C. concisus* was found in stools of control children and adults as often as in children and adults with diarrhea,[94] although it may be an opportunistic pathogen causing diarrhea in immunocompromised patients.[95]

C. hyointestinalis has been associated with human disease. In two studies, the rates of diarrhea due to *C. hyointestinalis* were 0.01% and 0.08% of all *Campylobacter*-associated episodes.[2,66] Other reports have described this organism as an uncommon cause of diarrhea in humans[96–98] and BSI.[99]

165 *Capnocytophaga* Species

Lorry G. Rubin

Capnocytophaga is a genus encompassing a group of slow-growing, capnophilic (carbon dioxide-loving), facultative anaerobic, gram-negative fusiform bacilli. Their recovery in culture requires incubation in an environment with enhanced carbon dioxide concentration under aerobic or anaerobic conditions. Colonies are detectable after 2 to 4 days or longer on several media; growth does not occur on MacConkey agar. Generally, species in this genus ferment carbohydrates except mannitol and xylose. The seven species were formerly classified as Centers for Diseases Control and Prevention (CDC) biogroups DF-1 and DF-2, five in the DF-1 group and two in the DF-2 group.[1] Species can be distinguished by means of DNA hybridization or 16S rRNA analysis.[2] These two groups are considered separately because the patient population, epidemiology, and antimicrobial treatment are distinct.

HUMAN (DF-1 GROUP) *CAPNOCYTOPHAGA*

Microbiology and Epidemiology

The DF-1 *Capnocytophaga* species *C. ochracea*, *C. gingivalis*, *C. sputigena*, *C. haemolytica*, and *C. granulosa* ("human" *Capnocytophaga*) are normal flora of the gingival sulci of humans.[1,3] They are closely related to both *Fusobacterium* and *Bacteroides/Prevotella* spp. Colonies tend to glide along the agar. Identification by conventional tests is not always successful. DF-1 organisms are responsible for invasive infection in the presence of neutropenia and oral mucosal ulceration, often cancer chemotherapy-induced, implicating the neutrophil as specifically important in host defense. Possible virulence factors include a serum-resistant phenotype, production of immunoglobulin A protease, and bacterial factors that interfere with host responses to infection, such as neutrophil migration.[3]

Clinical Manifestations and Treatment

The most significant infections are bloodstream infections (BSIs) at times polymicrobial, in children or adults with malignancies, including recipients of stem cell transplantation.[3] These patients generally are neutropenic and have oral lesions such as mucositis or aphthous stomatitis.[4] Based on series of cases reported from France[4] and Spain,[5] the mortality rate associated with BSI in these patients is <2%. *Capnocytophaga* spp. have been recovered from blood and infected sites such as the lung, pleural space, eye, brain, wounds, heart, bone, and joints in immunocompetent patients, commonly but not always in association with other bacteria.[6] These organisms occasionally are documented as a cause of chorioamnionitis and early-onset sepsis in premature neonates[7] and are important pathogens in juvenile periodontitis.

Although many isolates are susceptible to penicillin, strains resistant to penicillin and cephalosporins due to β-lactamase production including a strain with an extended spectrum β-lactamase,[8] and resistant to other antimicrobial agents, have been reported.[4,9,10] Imipenem or a β-lactam–β-lactamase inhibitor combination is highly active against *Capnocytophaga;* either can be considered a drug of first choice until results of antibiotic susceptibility testing, including a test for β-lactamase production, are available.[11] Clindamycin, chloramphenicol, and tetracycline show good activity and linezolid has been used successfully.[12,13] Cephalosporins, ciprofloxacin, and trimethoprim-sulfamethoxazole have variable activity. Aminoglycosides, metronidazole, and vancomycin have no activity.

CANINE (DF-2 GROUP) *CAPNOCYTOPHAGA*

Microbiology and Epidemiology

In 1989, Brenner and associates[14] classified DF-2 organisms as *C. canimorsus.* "DF-2-like" organisms are now classified as *C. cynodegmi.* Both of these species are found commonly in the oral flora of dogs[15] and cats.[16] They differ biochemically and by DNA-relatedness from the *Capnocytophaga* spp. of human oral origin (DF-1). *C. canimorsus,* the predominant pathogen, resists phagocytosis by human polymorphonuclear leukocytes[17] and causes invasive disease in asplenic hosts and patients with alcoholic cirrhosis, implicating the spleen as important for protection against invasive infection. Infections with *C. canimorsus* are zoonotic; patients with septicemia or meningitis report a dog bite or scratch or at least dog exposure (or cat exposure) before the onset of infection.[18,19] The vast majority of cases have occurred in adults, although infections have been reported in children, including neonates.

Clinical Manifestations and Treatment

Septicemia with or without cellulitis is the most common clinical infection due to *C. canimorsus,* occurring ~5 days (range, 1 to 8 days) after a dog (or less commonly cat) bite or exposure to saliva.[18,19] Meningitis also occurs and has a lower case-fatality rate than cases of septicemia.[20] Localized cellulitis following a dog-bite wound also can occur, and there have been reports of endocarditis and pneumonia. *C. cynodegmi* causes localized wound infection but rarely causes BSI. Although septicemia due to *C. canimorsus* can occur in immunologically normal hosts, many patients have an underlying condition, such as asplenia, alcohol abuse, or corticosteroid therapy.[19] Infection is fulminant in more than one-half of asplenic patients.[14] Case reports include cases of vertebral osteomyelitis and brain abscess. Several case reports have described an acute febrile illness in adults due to *C. canimorsus* and a syndrome in which septicemia is accompanied by thrombotic thrombocytopenic purpura with hemolytic uremic syndrome.[21]

Diagnosis is made through culture of blood or cerebrospinal fluid. Gram stain of a buffy coat smear of blood can reveal organisms in asplenic patients. Strains are susceptible to penicillin, the antibiotic of choice, as well as to newer cephalosporins, chloramphenicol, clindamycin, erythromycin, and tetracycline.[11] Susceptibility to aminoglycosides and trimethoprim-sulfamethoxazole is variable. Strains are resistant to aztreonam. Asplenic patients should be given penicillin prophylactically after a dog bite in an attempt to prevent this life-threatening infection (see Chapter 90, Infection Following Bites).

166 *Chlamydophila (Chlamydia) pneumoniae*

Samir S. Shah

THE PATHOGEN

Chlamydiae are obligate intracellular pathogens that had been classified under the order Chlamydiales with their own family (Chlamydiaceae) and genus *(Chlamydia)* on the basis of phenotypic, morphologic, and limited genetic criteria. Genome sequencing and comparative analysis of the ribosomal operon have led to a new, albeit controversial,[1] proposed taxonomic classification in which the genus *Chlamydia pneumoniae* would be replaced with a new genus name, *Chlamydophila pneumoniae,* with three biovars – human (TWAR), koala, and equine.[2] In this chapter, the term *C. pneumoniae* will refer to *Chlamydophila pneumoniae,* biovar TWAR, the agent causing infection in humans.

C. pneumoniae was first described as a human respiratory tract pathogen in the mid-1980s.[3,4] This obligate intracellular pathogen causes atypical pneumonia and upper respiratory tract disease and has been associated with a number of nonrespiratory conditions. *Chlamydia* spp. are classified as bacteria because of the ability to reproduce by binary division. Like *Chlamydia trachomatis* and *Chlamydophila psittaci, C. pneumoniae* has a biphasic developmental cycle of replication. The infectious bacterial form, known as the elementary body, enters the eukaryotic cell by endocytosis, resides within a cytoplasmic inclusion, and then transforms into a vegetative form (the reticulate body) to replicate by binary fission. As the inclusion fills with progeny, chlamydiae transform back into the metabolically inactive but infectious elementary body and are released through host cell rupture or fusion of the inclusion with the host cell plasma membrane.

EPIDEMIOLOGY

C. pneumoniae is a common infection worldwide.[5–10] Variable quality of diagnostic assays and lack of standardization remain important challenges to a precise description of the epidemiology, but many retrospective serologic studies as well as prospective studies using culture and polymerase chain reaction (PCR) testing have identified the mode of transmission, incidence of disease, and clinical characteristics of infection.[3,5,11–15]

Infection occurs most commonly in late winter or early spring.[16] The age at which primary infection apparently occurs differs according to the diagnostic test used. Population-based serologic studies indicate that acquisition of specific antibody occurs most often in children between 5 and 15 years of age;[17] the seroprevalence in this age group is approximately 30%.[18] New or repeat infections continue through adolescence and adulthood, culminating in 70% to 80% seropositivity in the elderly.[19] Acute infections (either primary infection or reinfection) are most common in school-age children. In a prospective population-based study in Seattle, the incidence of acute infection by age groups per 100 person-years was as follows: 0 to 4 years (no cases); 5 to 9 (9.2); 10 to 14 (6.2); 15 to 19 years (2.2); and >20 years (1.5).[17] In contrast, a population-based study in Thailand identified rates of *C. pneumoniae* pneumonia of 2 to 20 per 100,000 population with the highest rates occurring in those <1 year and >65 years of age.[20] If culture or PCR testing is used for such studies, colonization (or possibly infection) in younger children also is identified commonly in the absence of a detectable antibody response.[12,15,21,22]

Whether the absence of a serologic response in young children results from an insensitive test or from the absence of invasion remains unresolved. *C. pneumoniae* was isolated from the nasopharynx or throat of 1% to 10% of asymptomatic children and has been identified by PCR testing in 5% to 25% of children who attend childcare centers; those with respiratory tract symptoms and those from large families had the highest rates of identification of *C. pneumoniae*.[11,12,14,23-26]

C. pneumoniae is shed from the respiratory tract during the acute clinical illness and for up to 1 year later.[24] Asymptomatic infection with antibody response also is common.[17,23,24,27-29] It is not known whether the presence of symptoms increases the likelihood of transmission. Animal experiments suggest that aerosolized particles are an inefficient means of spreading *C. pneumoniae*. Although the organism remains viable only briefly on skin, it survives for 20 to 30 hours on environmental surfaces, suggesting that direct inoculation may be the predominant mode of transmission in clinical settings.[13]

Among military trainees in Finland, attack rates during a *C. pneumoniae* epidemic ranged from 60 to 84 per 1000 exposed men.[29] Attack rates were higher during institutional outbreaks, ranging from 44% to 68% among nursing home residents and 22% to 34% among nursing home staff.[30,31] The incubation period is 2 to 4 weeks as determined by the temporal clustering of cases during institutional[31] and military[29] outbreaks. Protracted epidemics of *C. pneumoniae* infection may occur in some settings. Epidemics among military trainees in Finland lasted approximately 6 months.[29] Some evidence points to epidemic periods occurring every 6 months to 3 years, superimposed upon low levels of endemic *C. pneumoniae* infection.[4,27,29]

CLINICAL MANIFESTATIONS

C. pneumoniae infects the upper respiratory tract epithelium of young children, where it occasionally causes or contributes to acute otitis media and sinusitis, as well as prolonged cough illness and community-acquired pneumonia. *C. pneumoniae* has been identified by culture and PCR testing of middle-ear fluid specimens from approximately 5% of children with acute otitis media.[11,12,32] Most often, the organism is found in addition to other bacterial pathogens and infection resolves in the absence of therapy directed at *C. pneumoniae*. The organism has not been detected in individuals with chronic middle-ear effusions.[33] *C. pneumoniae* may be a cause of prolonged cough illness. The organism has been detected in 5% to 17% of individuals with prolonged cough; the clinical features resemble those of pertussis.[14,34] In patients with prolonged cough during outbreaks of pertussis-like illness, the mean duration of cough associated with *C. pneumoniae* infection has been 25 to 30 days, compared with 50 days for cough associated with *Bordetella pertussis*.[14,35,36] *C. pneumoniae* associated fever and upper respiratory tract symptoms, including sore throat and hoarseness, can be self-limited or can progress to coughing and lower respiratory tract involvement.[15,21,37]

C. pneumoniae has been implicated in 5% to 14% of cases of pediatric community-acquired pneumonia.[5,10,15,25,38-45] The illness tends to have a subacute onset, indistinguishable from that due to *Mycoplasma pneumoniae* or influenza. More than half of infected patients have fever, cough, shortness of breath, chills, nausea, headache, and myalgia.[37,46] Crackles, wheezing, and rhonchi often are detected on physical examination. Physical examination and chest radiograph can indicate pneumonia even when respiratory tract symptoms are mild. Because of the prolonged and relatively mild nature of initial symptoms, the patient may seek medical attention more than 1 week after the illness onset, at which time fever and signs of systemic illness may have resolved.[37] Studies have not identified findings that reliably differentiate *C. pneumoniae* from other causes of pneumonia in children. Among adults requiring hospitalization for community-acquired pneumonia, patients with *C. pneumoniae* were more likely than those with pneumonia due to a typical bacterial etiology to have a duration of illness >7 days (odds ratio, 3.5; 95% confidence interval: 1.3 to 9.4) and less likely to have a productive cough (odds ratio, 0.3; 95% confidence interval: 0.1 to 0.7).[38]

TABLE 166-1. Diseases Associated with *Chlamydophila (Chlamydia) pneumoniae* Infection

Pathologic Role Established	Association Supported by Several Lines of Evidence
Pneumonia	Otitis media
Prolonged cough illness	Cardiovascular disese
Acute bronchitis	Asthma
Speculative Association	
Meningoencephalitis	Multiple sclerosis
Alzheimer disease	Myalgia
Kawasaki disease	Conjunctivitis
Lung cancer	Arthritis
Hypertension	Adult respiratory distress syndrome
Erythema nodosum	Chronic fatigue syndrome
Chronic bronchitis	Ischemic stroke

Modified from Sanchez F, Dowell S. Chlamydia pneumoniae infection in children: a pediatric infection with possible consequences in adults? Pediatr Infect Dis J 1999;19:367–373.

C. pneumoniae pneumonia has been associated with severe illness. The organism was isolated from culture of the respiratory tract and pleural fluid of a previously healthy adolescent boy with severe pneumonia complicated by respiratory failure and parapneumonic effusions.[47] A 13-year-old girl developed pneumonia and hemorrhagic pericarditis; *C. pneumoniae* was detected in the pericardial fluid by PCR.[48]

Most studies that include appropriate control groups fail to demonstrate an association between asthma and acute or chronic *C. pneumoniae* infection.[49-53] For example, *C. pneumoniae* was identified in 3.4% of children during an asthma exacerbation, in 6% of children during an initial episode of wheezing, and in 2.5% of patients with stable asthma or allergic rhinitis.[49] However, Teig et al. detected *C. pneumoniae* by PCR from 24% of children with stable asthma but from 0% of healthy nonasthmatic children;[54] it is not clear why *C. pneumoniae* was detected less frequently in the control population in this study compared with previous studies.

Nonstandardized laboratory testing has resulted in widely varying and often unconfirmed reports of new clinical manifestations of *C. pneumoniae*, including Alzheimer disease, atherosclerotic cardiovascular disease, multiple sclerosis, meningoencephalitis,[55-57] pyoderma gangrenosum,[58] and a variety of other diseases in children and adults (Table 166-1). *C. pneumoniae* was identified by immunohistochemistry in cardiovascular tissue of sporadic cases of Kawasaki disease.[59] However, this association was not confirmed in a case-control study.[60]

LABORATORY DIAGNOSIS

None of the many diagnostic assays used worldwide to identify *C. pneumoniae* has received approval by the United States Food and Drug Administration for clinical use. Recommendations for standardized approaches to culture, PCR testing, serology, and immunohistochemistry were published in 2001 by the U.S. Centers for Disease Control and Prevention (CDC) and the Canadian Laboratory Centres for Disease Control (LCDC).[61] The lack of standardization has resulted in substantial variation in interlaboratory test performance, even when using the same test and diagnostic criteria.[62]

Serology has been the primary means of clinical diagnostic testing for *C. pneumoniae* because of its widespread availability and relative simplicity. However, many of the available assays, including complement fixation, whole-inclusion fluorescence, and various enzyme immunoassays, perform poorly or have not been adequately validated; microimmunofluorescence testing remains the only endorsed approach, despite its limitations.[61] During primary infection, immunoglobulin M (IgM) antibody appears 2 to 3 weeks after illness onset. IgG antibody may not reach high titer until 6 to 8 weeks after the onset of illness. Therefore, confirmation of primary acute infection requires documenting an IgM titer of ≥1:16 or a 4-fold rise in IgG titer between acute and convalescent serum specimens. In case of reinfection, IgM antibody may not appear and the level of IgG antibody titer may rise quickly within 1 to 2 weeks of infection.[61] Criteria proposed in the past, including a single IgG titer >1:512 and elevated IgA titers, are no longer endorsed because of their low specificity. IgG titers of ≥1:16 are consistent with previous exposure and are found in approximately one-half of adults. Therefore, a single elevated IgG titer does not confirm the diagnosis *C. pneumoniae* infection.

The organism or its DNA can be identified directly in specimens from nasopharyngeal or throat swabs, sputum, blood, or tissue by culture or PCR testing. Culture traditionally has been considered the reference-standard diagnostic method. For culture, a specimen can be collected on a Dacron-tipped, wire- or plastic-shafted swab. The specimen, transported in appropriate media at 4°C, is then centrifuged onto HEp-2 (human epithelial cell line type 2) or HL (heteroploid line with a slow life cycle) cell lines, passaged twice, and examined at 3 to 7 days after staining with monoclonal antibodies to identify the *C. pneumoniae* inclusions. Observation of inclusions constitutes a presumptive positive result; confirmation requires either successful passage of the isolate or confirmation with PCR. Swabs with calcium alginate or cotton tips and wooden shafts can inhibit the growth of the organisms, depending on the adhesive used. Specimens that cannot be processed within 24 hours should be frozen and held at −70°C.

Only 4 of >30 published PCR assays met validation criteria proposed by CDC/LCDC.[61,62] Validation in these 4 studies was primarily analytical; extensive validation on clinical specimens has not yet been performed. No assay has yet received approval by the FDA for detection of *C. pneumoniae* in respiratory or other specimens. Reports of the identification of the organism by PCR in clinical specimens as well as in research studies on atherosclerotic plaques, peripheral blood mononuclear cells, brain, lung, and other tissues should be interpreted in the context of other confirmatory information. Identification of *C. pneumoniae* in the respiratory tract by culture or PCR testing does not necessarily establish the organism as the cause of disease, because prolonged asymptomatic shedding of *C. pneumoniae* has been documented.[24,28,63] Despite CDC recommendations, there remains a high degree of heterogeneity in serologic methods and diagnostic criteria among studies of *C. pneumoniae* respiratory tract infections.[62]

Identification of the organism in tissue specimens can be performed using PCR testing or in situ hybridization, but immunohistochemical techniques have been used most commonly. The prevalence of the organism in arterial plaques has varied in reports from 0% to more than 50%, highlighting the importance of appropriate selection of the monoclonal antibody, use of appropriate controls in the staining procedures, and careful interpretation to exclude false-positive staining responses.[61,64]

Routine laboratory studies do not distinguish *C. pneumoniae* from other causes of acute respiratory tract infection.[15,21,37] The erythrocyte sedimentation rate typically is elevated (range 21 to 75 mm/hour). Peripheral white blood cell count can be normal or elevated although usually with neutrophil predominance.[46] On radiographic evaluation, pneumonia usually is associated with bilateral ground-glass or nodular infiltrates although unilateral parenchymal infiltrate and pleural effusion have been reported in more than one-quarter of patients.[46,47,63,65]

TREATMENT

Standards for in vitro susceptibility testing have not been established but *C. pneumoniae* appears to be susceptible to the tetracyclines, macrolides, ketolides, and most fluoroquinolones (e.g., levofloxacin and moxifloxacin but not ciprofloxacin), and resistant to sulfa drugs.[63,66–69] Microbiologic eradication of the organism from the nasopharynx occurs in 70% to 90% of children with *C. pneumoniae* pneumonia after a 10-day course of erythromycin or clarithromycin, or a 5-day course of azithromycin.[21,70,71] Clinical resolution occurs in a high percentage of children who are not treated[72] or are treated with a β-lactam agent predicted to be ineffective.[11,70] Typical treatment regimens, when prescribed, are 14 to 21 days for tetracycline or doxycycline, 14 days for erythromycin, 7 to 14 days for fluoroquinolones or clarithromycin, and 5 days for azithromycin. In some patients, clinical symptoms and persistent isolation of the organism occur despite 10- to 30-day courses of appropriate therapy.[28,73] The role of prolonged therapy in patients with persistent or relapsing symptoms, while possibly beneficial, also is not clear.

COMPLICATIONS

Complications associated with acute *C. pneumoniae* infection are rare. The possibility that *C. pneumoniae*, like *C. trachomatis*, can establish a state of persistent infection has lent plausibility to a number of associations with chronic diseases. The association between *C. pneumoniae* and atherosclerotic cardiovascular disease is based on higher prevalence of serum antibodies in patients with coronary heart disease than in controls,[64] detection and culture of the organism in atheromatous plaques,[64,74,75] and animal studies and small human trials suggesting a benefit of treatment with macrolides.[76–78] A meta-analysis has failed to support a significant serologic association,[79] and large, prospective, randomized trials thus far have not found evidence of a treatment benefit of the magnitude suggested by the earlier studies.[80] A longitudinal study of children found no association between recurrent anti-*Chlamydophila* treatments in childhood and early vascular changes, suggesting that antimicrobial therapy does not prevent atherogenicity potentially associated with repeated infectious insults.[81] Although fewer investigators have pursued other disease associations, similarly conflicting evidence exists for *C. pneumoniae* as a causative agent in Alzheimer disease,[82–84] ischemic stroke,[85,86] asthma,[51,52,87,88] multiple sclerosis,[89–92] Kawasaki disease,[59,60] and other conditions (see Table 166-1).[55,58,93]

167 *Chlamydia trachomatis*

Toni Darville and G. Ingrid J.G. Rours

THE PATHOGEN

Chlamydiae are obligate, intracellular, nonmotile, gram-negative bacteria with a unique biphasic developmental cycle consisting of extra- and intracellular forms. Chlamydiae have an outer membrane that contains lipopolysaccharide (LPS) and membrane proteins but their outer membrane contains no detectable peptidoglycan. Although chlamydiae contain DNA, RNA, and ribosomes, they obtain high-energy phosphate compounds from the host cell. *Chlamydia trachomatis* encodes an abundant protein called the major outer membrane protein (MOMP or OmpA) that is surface exposed and is the major determinant of serologic classification.

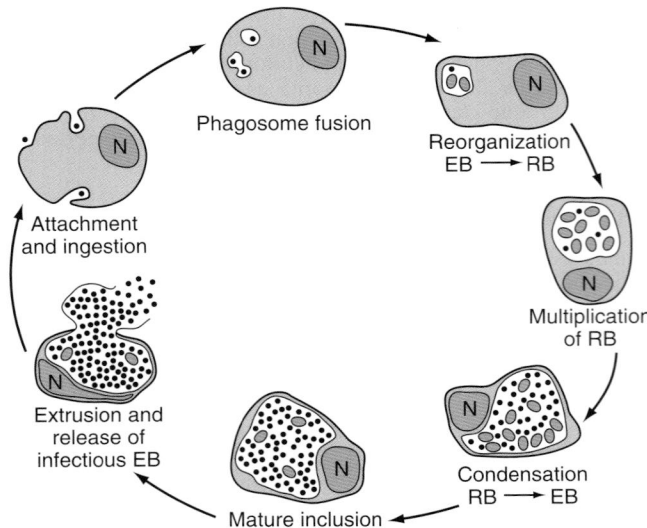

Figure 167-1. Life cycle of *C. trachomatis* in tissue culture. N, nucleus; EB, elementary bodies; RB, reticulate bodies. (Redrawn from Jones RB. *Chlamydia trachomatis* (trachoma, perinatal infections, lymphogranuloma venereum, and other genital infections). In: Mandell GL, Bennett JE, Dolin R (eds) Principles and Practice of Infectious Diseases, 5th ed. New York, Churchill Livingstone, 2000, p 1990.)

LIFE CYCLE

The biphasic developmental cycle of chlamydiae is unique among microorganisms and involves two highly specialized characteristic morphologic forms, as shown in Figure 167-1. The extracellular form or *elementary body* (EB) has a rigid, thick outer membrane that contains extensive disulfide cross-links both within and between OMPs and is stable outside of the cell. The small (350 nm in diameter) EB is infectious but inactive metabolically.

The developmental cycle is initiated when an EB attaches to a mucosal epithelial cell. A number of candidate adhesins have been proposed, but their identity and that of associated epithelial cell receptors remain uncertain. Once inside the cell, the EB resides within a membrane-limited endosome and prevents fusion of the endosome with lysosomes, protecting itself from enzymatic destruction. Escaping from host attack by antibody or cell-mediated defenses, the EB enlarges and reorganizes into the replicative and metabolically active form, the *reticulate body* (RB). Chlamydiae hijack certain host cell signaling pathways to protect the cell from recognition and attack while preventing apoptosis and maintaining integrity of their host cells.[1]

RBs remain strictly intracellular, successfully parasitizing the host cell, synthesizing mRNA, dividing and multiplying. As the RB divides by binary fission it fills the endosome, now a cytoplasmic *inclusion*, with its progeny. After 48 to 72 hours, multiplication ceases and nucleoid condensation occurs as the RBs reorganize and transform again to new infectious EBs. Eventually, the host cell's nutrients are expended and EBs are released from the cell by cytolysis,[2] exocytosis, or extrusion of the whole inclusion,[3] leaving the host cell intact. The last fact may explain the frequency of asymptomatic or subclinical chlamydial infections. The release of the infectious EBs allows infection of new host cells to occur.

CLASSIFICATION

Based on analysis of signature sequences in the 16S and 23S ribosomal genes, a proposal has been made to add a new genus, *Chlamydophila*, to the family of Chlamydiaceae that previously contained the single genus, *Chlamydia*.[4] The mouse and porcine strains of *C. trachomatis* are contained in the *Chlamydia* genus, whereas *C. pneumoniae* and *C. psittaci* species may be classified as *Chlamydophila* spp. The scientific community has not accepted this split of the genus.[5] *C. trachomatis* is divided into subgroups based on antigenic variation in the major OMPs (serovars) and clinical expression. Microimmunofluorescence and monoclonal antibody testing have shown that there are more than 18 serovars of *C. trachomatis* with several distinctive clinical patterns of disease:[6–8] trachoma is caused by serovars A, B, Ba, and C; oculogenital and neonatal disease by serovars B, Da, Ga, Ia, and D-K; and lymphogranuloma venereum (LGV) by serovars L1, L2, L2a, and L3.

PATHOGENESIS

LGV serovars can replicate in lymph nodes and macrophages, whereas replication of the other serovars of *C. trachomatis* is confined to mucosal epithelial cells. After an incubation period of 10 days (between 7 and 21 days) a variety of clinical manifestations can result from the host inflammatory response and tissue destruction. Primary infection is characterized by a marked influx of neutrophils, especially early in infection.[9–12] Lymphocytes and plasma cells also participate in the primary response, but they appear later, concurrently with resolution of infection.[13] In ocular and genital infections, plasma cells can be present in large numbers,[14–16] whereas in infants with pneumonia, eosinophils and neutrophils predominate.[17] In animal models, inflammation associated with a single infection can lead to genital tract tubal dilatation.[12,18]

The host is assumed to develop some sort of protective immune response since chlamydial infections can be self-limiting,[19,20] and asymptomatic infection can be chronic, lasting for months or even years.[21–23] However, natural infection with *C. trachomatis* appears to confer little protection against reinfection and that which is conferred is short-lived. The potential for chronic, untreated infections is great, because most chlamydial genital tract infections are asymptomatic. The potential importance of reinfection was first recognized during human trachoma vaccine trials, in which low-dose immunization resulted in more severe disease when vaccinees became infected with heterologous strains.[24]

EPIDEMIOLOGY

C. trachomatis strains exhibit tissue tropism with different strains infecting either the mucosa of the genital tract or the eye. *C. trachomatis* is the leading cause of bacterial sexually transmitted infection (STI) in the world. However, in endemic areas, mostly in Africa and the Middle East, *C. trachomatis* causes trachoma, the leading cause of preventable blindness worldwide.

The World Health Organization estimated that 92 million new cases of *C. trachomatis* infection occur annually worldwide.[25] It is estimated that >4 million chlamydial infections occur annually in sexually active adolescents and adults in the United States.[26] Most infected men and women are either asymptomatic or minimally symptomatic and diagnosis is a result of screening or because a contact is symptomatic. In 2007, 1,108,374 chlamydial infections were reported to the U.S. Centers for Disease Control and Prevention (CDC), the highest rate ever reported. The reported number of cases of chlamydial infection was >3 times that of reported cases of gonorrhea. From 1988 through 2007, the reported rate of chlamydial infection in women increased ~5-fold.[27] Possible reasons for the increase are increased screening, increased use of nucleic acid amplification tests (NAATS), and improved reporting, as well as continuing high burden of disease. Table 167-1 outlines prevalence estimates reported for selected patient groups and conditions.[27–34]

Young age (<20 years) is the sociodemographic factor most strongly associated with chlamydial infection. A study in Louisiana public high schools revealed an overall prevalence of *C. trachomatis* of 6.5%, with rates among girls more than twice that of boys (9.7% versus 4.0%).[35] In a study of over 3000 sexually active adolescent females attending middle school health centers in Baltimore, MD, chlamydial infection was found in ~24% at the first visit and 14% at repeat visits; 14-year-old females had the highest age-specific prevalence rate (28%).[31] Unfortunately, independent predictors of chlamydial infection failed to identify a subset of adolescent females with the majority of infections.

TABLE 167-1. Prevalence of Chlamydial Genital Infection in Selected Patient Groups and Conditions

Subject Group or Condition	Females (%)	Males (%)
Adolescents	8–37	13–15
Adults (asymptomatic)	4–8	3–5
Adults (STD clinic)	>20	15–20
Gonorrhea	25–50	5–30
Mucopurulent cervicitis or nongonococcal urethritis	9–15	30–40
Pelvic inflammatory disease or epididymitis	8–54	50

Data collated from Turner CF, Rogers SM, Miller HG, et al. Untreated gonococcal and chlamydial infection in a probability sample of adults. JAMA 2002;287:726–733; and Centers for Disease Control and Prevention. Recommendations for the prevention and management of Chlamydia trachomatis infections, 1993. MMWR Recomm Rep 1993;42:1–39.

Substantial racial/ethnic differences exist in the prevalence of both chlamydial and gonococcal infections in the U.S. A cross-sectional analysis in a prospective cohort study of a nationally representative sample of 14,322 young adults aged 18 to 26 years revealed the overall prevalence of chlamydial infection to be 4.2%.[36] Women (4.7%) were more likely to be infected than men (3.7%). The prevalence of chlamydial infection was highest among black women (14%) and black men (11%), and lowest among white women (2.5%), white men (1.4%), and Asian men (1.1%). Prevalence of chlamydial infection was highest in the south (5.4%) and lowest in the northeast U.S. (2.4%).

In a study of adolescents, oral contraceptives had no effect on risk of chlamydial infection, but use of depot medroxyprogesterone acetate injections increased the risk for infection 5-fold compared with nonhormone users.[37] A recent prospective study in 948 Kenyan prostitutes revealed that users of oral contraceptives were at increased risk for acquisition of *Chlamydia* (hazard ratio, 1.8; 95% confidence interval, 1.1 to 2.9). Women using depot medroxyprogesterone acetate also had a significantly increased risk of *Chlamydia* infection (hazard ratio, 1.6; 95% confidence interval, 1.1 to 2.4), but a significantly decreased risk of pelvic inflammatory disease (PID) (hazard ratio, 0.4; 95% confidence interval, 0.2 to 0.7).[38]

Partner transmission rates have been found to be approximately 65% and appear to be similar for female–male and male–female transmission.[31,39,40] The number of exposures or coinfection with *Neisseria gonorrhoeae* did not affect the transmission rate.

CLINICAL MANIFESTATIONS

C. trachomatis infects susceptible nonciliated squamocolumnar or transitional epithelial cells (e.g., mucous membranes of the conjunctivae, posterior nasopharynx, urethra, endocervix, and rectum).

Perinatal Infection

Neonatal infection generally is acquired during passage through an infected birth canal. In a recent Chinese study, the vertical transmission rate was found to be 67% after vaginal delivery and 8% after cesarean delivery.[41] Prospective studies of infants born to women with a chlamydial infection of the cervix have shown a 50% to 75% risk that the infant will acquire *C. trachomatis* at ≥1 anatomic sites.[42–47] In infants exposed to *C. trachomatis*, risk of conjunctivitis is 20% to 50% and risk of pneumonia is 5% to 20%.

In ~14% of infants born to women with chlamydial infection, asymptomatic rectal or vaginal *C. trachomatis* can be detected, which can persist for ≥18 months.[48] Persistence of *C. trachomatis* in the genital tract can confound evaluation for possible sexual abuse and requires thorough and appropriate investigation.[49,50]

Inclusion Conjunctivitis

C. trachomatis is the most common cause of ophthalmia neonatorum, the major clinical manifestation of neonatal chlamydial infection.[51] The usual incubation period is 5 to 14 days after birth, but symptoms can occur earlier after premature rupture of membranes or as late as 6 weeks after birth.[42] At least 50% of infants with chlamydial conjunctivitis have concurrent infection in the nasopharynx.

The most common presenting symptom is watery ocular discharge that progressively becomes more purulent (95%), followed by swelling of the eyelids (73%) and conjunctival erythema (65%)[51] (Figure 167-2). The majority of chlamydial conjunctivitis resolves spontaneously during the first few months of life. However, if the condition is untreated, chronic conjunctivitis can develop. Although conjunctivitis can be quite severe, corneal ulceration, scars, and pannus formation are rare and recovery is expected without visual impairment.[52]

Chlamydial conjunctivitis must be distinguished from that produced by pyogenic bacteria, particularly *N. gonorrhoeae*. Gonococcal ophthalmia usually occurs earlier (around 2 to 5 days after birth) and usually progresses more rapidly. On the basis of clinical

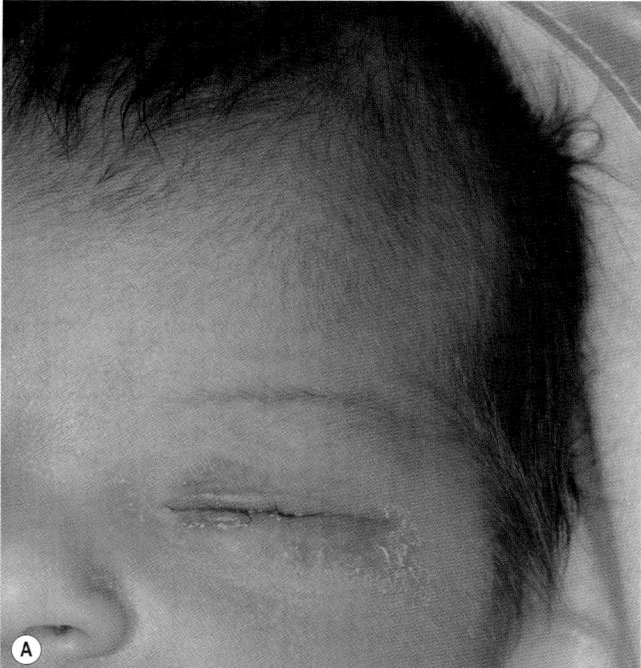

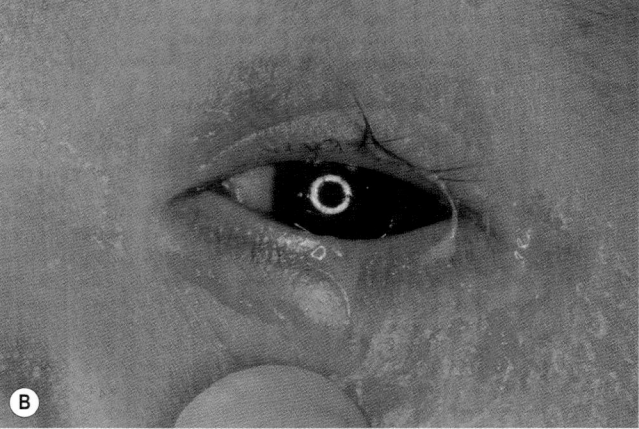

Figure 167-2. (A and **B)** A neonate with chlamydial conjunctivitis. (Courtesy of J.H. Brien©.)

findings, neonatal conjunctivitis caused by *N. gonorrhoeae* or other pathogens can be indistinguishable from that due to *C. trachomatis*.[23]

Pneumonia in Infancy

Pneumonia caused by *C. trachomatis* in infancy occurs characteristically between 3 and 12 weeks of age, but sometimes can manifest later.[53-57] Characteristically, the infant has been symptomatic for 3 or more weeks before presentation. Most infants are only modestly ill and are afebrile. Symptoms of nasal obstruction and a pertussis-like (but nonproductive staccato) cough gradually worsen over ≥1 week. Physical findings include tachypnea and rales but not wheezing. About 50% of the affected infants have a history or evidence of conjunctivitis.[55] Laboratory findings include hyperinflation with symmetric interstitial infiltrates on chest radiography, peripheral eosinophilia (>400 cells/mm^3), and increased levels of serum immunoglobulins. Pneumonia in preterm neonates has been described to manifest differently. Symptoms occurred as early as 48 hours after birth, presenting as idiopathic respiratory distress syndrome that initially improved but was complicated by apneic spells and feeding problems.[58-63]

Oculogenital Infections

C. trachomatis causes a variety of oculogenital infections in sexually active adolescents and adults, as well as in children who have been sexually abused (see Table 167-1).[64] The majority of infected persons are asymptomatic. In the National Longitudinal Study of Adolescent Health, 95% of *C. trachomatis*-infected people did not report symptoms in the 24 hours preceding specimen collection.[36] Among infected men, urethral discharge and dysuria were present only in 3% and 2%, respectively. Among infected women, vaginal discharge and dysuria were presently only in 0.3% and 4%, respectively. Among men reporting urethral discharge, the prevalence of chlamydial infection was high (38%), whereas the prevalence of chlamydial infection was only 1% among the women reporting vaginal discharge. Of note, 6% of the women reporting dysuria had chlamydial infection.

The incubation period for symptomatic males is 7 to 14 days. They may complain of dysuria, a slight, clear or mucopurulent urethral discharge, stained underwear in the morning, or discharge that may be detected only after penile stripping during genital examination by a healthcare provider.[65] The primary complications of chlamydial urethritis in men are: epididymitis, reactive arthritis (including Reiter syndrome), and transmission to women. *C. trachomatis* and *N. gonorrhoeae* are the most frequent causes of epididymitis in men <35 years of age; urethritis also usually is present.

Although asymptomatic rectal carriage of *C. trachomatis* occurs in both infants[66] and adults,[67] *C. trachomatis* is a fairly common cause of proctitis and proctocolitis in men who have sex with men (MSM).[68] Approximately 1% of men with nongonococcal urethritis develop acute aseptic arthritis of presumed immune-mediated etiology.[69] One-third of patients have the full complex of Reiter syndrome (arthritis, nonbacterial urethritis, and conjunctivitis); most such patients carry the histocompatibility antigen HLA-B27.[70]

The natural course of *C. trachomatis* infection in women was described in a study of Colombian women followed for a 5-year period using serotyping and polymerase chain reaction (PCR) on cervical-scrape samples.[23] Approximately 46% of infections, if not treated, were persistent at 1 year, 18% at 2 years, and 6% at 4 years of follow-up. Symptoms of *C. trachomatis* infection in women include a dysuria/pyuria syndrome, vaginal discharge, intermittent bleeding, and mild abdominal pain. The cervix can appear normal or can exhibit edema, erythema, friability, or mucopurulent discharge. In prepubertal girls, vaginitis can occur secondary to *C. trachomatis* infection of transitional cell epithelium. In contrast, the squamous epithelium of the adult vagina is not susceptible, and vaginal discharge generally reflects endocervical infection.

In some women, ascending infection of the genital tract develops, resulting in endometritis and salpingitis (Figure 167-3).

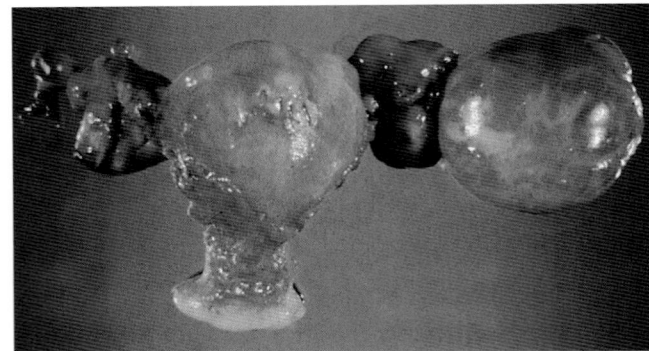

Figure 167-3. Pathologic specimen of uterus and salpinx from a patient with involuntary infertility and a history of repeated chlamydial infections.

Eighteen (16%) of the infected asymptomatic adolescent women in one study who were monitored for 2 months or more became symptomatic, but <2% developed clinical PID.[71] A recent review of 24 studies examined PID diagnosis and sequelae after untreated chlamydial infection.[72] On average in high-risk settings, 2% to 5% of untreated females developed PID within the ~2-week period between testing positive for *C. trachomatis* and returning for treatment.[73,74] In several studies, repeated chlamydial infection was associated with PID and other reproductive sequelae, although it was difficult to determine whether the risk per infection increased with each recurrent episode.[75,76] No prospective study has directly assessed the risk of infertility after untreated *C. trachomatis* infection. However, according to the largest studies, after symptomatic PID of any cause has occurred, up to 18% of women may develop infertility.[77]

C. trachomatis and *N. gonorrhoeae* are the most common causes of PID, with more than half of cases due to one or both organisms. The spectrum of PID associated with *C. trachomatis* infection ranges from asymptomatic to acute, severe disease with perihepatitis and ascites (Fitz-Hugh–Curtis syndrome). Compared with women who have gonococcal or nongonococcal-nonchlamydial salpingitis, women with chlamydial salpingitis are more likely to experience a chronic, subacute course with a longer duration of abdominal pain before they seek medical care. Yet, they have as much or more tubal inflammation at laparoscopy.[78] Chronic infections, even if subclinical, can lead to infertility and ectopic pregnancy.[79]

Adolescents and adults with genital tract disease presumably can auto-inoculate their eyes, leading to inclusion conjunctivitis.[80,81] Additionally, infection can follow exposure to infected eye secretions without sexual contact or can occur in conjunction with unrecognized genital infection that has resolved. Acute follicular conjunctivitis is typical. Symptoms are those of a foreign body sensation in the eye. The infection usually resolves without complications, but, if untreated, can persist for months and scarring can occur.

Pregnancy

C. trachomatis infection can negatively influence pregnancy.[82] Previous chlamydial infection has been associated with increased risk for ectopic pregnancy as evidenced by serologic studies, isolation of *C. trachomatis* from fallopian tubes, and chlamydial DNA detection from cervical, endometrial, or salpingectomy tissues.[83,84] In addition, *C. trachomatis* infection has been associated with spontaneous abortion and stillbirth. Spontaneous abortion has been proposed to be due either to direct zygote infection or to an immune response to heat shock proteins expressed by the zygote which is triggered by previous chlamydial infection, reactivation of latent chlamydial infection, or endometrial damage from past chlamydial infection.[85-87] Stillbirth is related to fetal chlamydial infection as can be detected by testing for chlamydial IgM antibodies in cord blood.[86,88,89] Furthermore, *C. trachomatis* infection has been associated with chorioamnionitis, premature rupture of membranes, and preterm delivery. A 2.6- and 3-fold increased risk of preterm delivery were determined in women with positive serology detected at 17 weeks' gestation or diagnosed with cervical infection at 24 weeks' gestation, respectively.[88,90] Although earlier studies based on serology and cultures were at variance regarding preterm delivery, evidence grows with the use of NAAT that preterm delivery is associated with *C. trachomatis* infection.[91-93]

Lymphogranuloma Venereum

LGV is an STI caused by the L1 to L3 serovars of *C. trachomatis*. The bubonic form is endemic in tropical and subtropical areas but its description is rare in the U.S. Classically, LGV is a disease of the lymphatic tissue with acute and chronic manifestations.[94] The primary lesion of LGV is a small, inconspicuous, asymptomatic genital papule or ulcer that heals without a scar. Days to weeks later, unilateral acute lymphadenitis with bubo formation occurs at the site of lymphatic drainage of the primary lesion; acute hemorrhagic proctitis develops after a rectal lesion. Systemic symptoms can include fever, myalgia, or headache. About one-third of inguinal buboes become fluctuant and rupture; the remainder involute slowly. Although most patients recover from LGV following this secondary stage, a small number develop a chronic inflammatory response with fibrosis (due to the persistence of chlamydiae in anogenital tissues) that can result in chronic genital ulcers or fistulas, rectal strictures, or genital elephantiasis.

Rare in the western world prior to 2003, outbreaks of LGV proctitis have been reported in the Netherlands,[95] Europe, North America, and Australia among MSM.[96] The majority were HIV-infected with high-risk sexual behavior and a high rate of concomitant STIs, including hepatitis C.[97]

Ocular Trachoma

Trachoma is still one of the world's leading causes of blindness; approximately 30% of the children in a holoendemic area are at risk for blindness due to severe trachoma.[98] Extensive studies in Taiwan have revealed the importance of reinfection in the pathogenesis of trachoma.[99] Both pannus formation (the superficial vascularization that is pathognomonic of trachoma) and progressive disease with scarring are believed to be due to a cycle of active infection and resolution repeated over many years.

In areas that are endemic for trachoma, infections occur early in life, and active disease persists for several years. Poor hygiene and presence of eye-seeking flies enhance transmission. Initially, chronic follicular conjunctivitis typical of inclusion conjunctivitis develops, followed by more intense inflammation of the conjunctivae and then by scarring of the tarsal conjunctiva. Following severe scarring of the inner surface of the lids, trichiasis (inturning of the eyelashes) often develops. This results in further corneal ulceration, scarring, opacification, and loss of vision. *C. trachomatis* can be isolated from conjunctival scrapings and nasopharyngeal cultures obtained from young children with active trachoma. The clinical spectrum of trachoma can vary from mild to severe; a simplified World Health Organization (WHO) grading scheme can be used for standardized clinical assessment.[100] Young preschool children who have persistent or severe disease and chronically shed *C. trachomatis* act as an important reservoir of infection within a family unit.[99,101]

LABORATORY DIAGNOSIS

The diagnosis of trachoma in endemic areas can be based on clinical findings. Other chlamydial infections generally require laboratory confirmation to distinguish them from other conditions. A positive laboratory test for *C. trachomatis* can be utilized for patient education and to both improve adherence to treatment regimens and increase the likelihood of referral of sexual partners. The development of tissue cell culture methods in the 1960s was a major advance, but has been replaced by NAATs as methods of diagnostic choice.

Definitive diagnosis of chlamydial infection, as would be required in a medico-legal setting (i.e., suspected sexual abuse or rape), still requires isolation of *C. trachomatis* in cell culture or a positive NAAT confirmed by a second NAAT that targets a different gene sequence.[102]

Diagnostic Specimens

Many screening tests for *C. trachomatis* require appropriately handled samples containing columnar epithelium from mucosal sites rather than exudate.

The discomfort caused by obtaining a urethral swab in males has precluded its widespread use in asymptomatic men. A dipstick test for leukocyte esterase (LE) performed on the first portion of voided urine is a cost-effective and relatively sensitive screen (72% to 95%) in asymptomatic young men.[103] Sediment from LE-positive urine is then used for a nonculture diagnostic test and, in members of low-risk populations, as a second confirmatory test. When feasible, urine NAAT provides a more sensitive and equally noninvasive method of detection.

Diagnostic Methods

Cell Culture

Use of chlamydial transport media containing antibiotics maximizes recovery. Swabs used to obtain a specimen should have plastic or metal shaft, and a tip made of cotton or Dacron as this causes less inhibition than nylon or alginate. Storage at 4°C or maintenance at −70°C is required if inoculation within 24 hours is not possible. Cycloheximide-treated McCoy or HeLa cell lines are used most frequently to isolate *C. trachomatis*. Centrifugation techniques enhance absorption of chlamydiae to cells. Intracytoplasmic inclusions can be detected at 48 to 72 hours with species-specific immunofluorescent monoclonal antibodies or Giemsa or iodine staining.

Nonculture Tests

NAATs have a higher sensitivity than all other tests, while retaining high specificity when cross-contamination is avoided.[104] NAATs have Food and Drug Administration (FDA) approval for testing cervical swabs from women, urethral swabs from men, and urine from men and women.[105,106] NAATs detect *C. trachomatis* in urine or in self-administered vaginal swab specimens with sensitivity comparable with clinician-obtained urogenital swab specimens, which makes noninvasive testing possible.[103,107] Data suggest that NAATs are equivalent to or better than culture for the detection of *C. trachomatis* in the conjunctiva and nasopharynx of infants,[108] and are being used currently in evaluation of newborns with conjunctivitis or pneumonia.

Direct fluorescent antibody assays (DFAs) use fluorescein-conjugated monoclonal antibodies to stain chlamydial antigens in smears. DFAs are FDA-cleared for use with pharyngeal specimens, and potentially have high specificity if a *C. trachomatis*-specific stain is used. The tests also perform well on conjunctival specimens, with sensitivities >90%, and specificities ≥95% compared with culture.[109,110] DFAs that use antibodies specific for chlamydial MOMP are highly specific, but certain commercial kits use anti-LPS antibodies, which can lead to false-positive results.

Enzyme immunoassays (EIAs) detect chlamydial LPS but are less sensitive than culture and NAATs, and there is a potential for false-positive results caused by cross-reaction with LPS of other microorganisms, including other *Chlamydia* species.[111] Serologic tests are of limited value in individual cases and are used primarily for population studies. However, serology can be used to detect *C. trachomatis* in women with tubal-factor infertility and in newborns. The detection of specific serum IgM or tear IgA antibodies in an individual is suggestive of current infection. In infants IgM levels often are elevated with neonatal pneumonia, but not with conjunctivitis.[112] Cytology is used mainly to diagnose conjunctivitis. Glycogen accumulates only in inclusions of *C.*

trachomatis, which permits its specific staining in cell culture. Characteristic intracytoplasmic inclusions can be identified in Giemsa-stained conjunctival scrapings from up to 90% of infants and 50% of adults who have inclusion conjunctivitis but from only 10% to 30% of patients who have active trachoma.[113] This method allows for visualization of *C. trachomatis* and other bacteria, such as gonococci, and of cytologic findings suggesting viral infection. Glycogen staining does not exclude other pathogens, is not helpful in patients with mild disease, and is not recommended for evaluation of endocervical specimens.

TREATMENT

Antibiotics against *C. trachomatis* act by inhibiting protein synthesis, growth and division of RBs, DNA-gyrase activity, or cell wall biosynthesis. Antibiotics used should be able to gain access to and exhibit activity in intracellular sites. The 72-hour life cycle and the asynchronous nature of chlamydial infection further require the maintenance of adequate antibiotic concentration in tissues. Table 167-2 summarizes treatment regimens for chlamydial infections. Antibiotic resistance has been described only rarely for chlamydial infection.

Perinatal Infection

Topical treatment of inclusion conjunctivitis is not recommended, because local therapy does not eliminate nasopharyngeal carriage and subsequent risk of pneumonia or recurrent conjunctivitis.[114] Conjunctivitis or pneumonia caused by *C. trachomatis* in young infants is treated with a macrolide orally.[110,112] The efficacy of erythromycin therapy is approximately 80%; a second course may be required in some cases.[115] Erythromycin can have gastrointestinal side effects and interact with other drugs, and has been associated with infantile hypertrophic pyloric stenosis (IHPS) in infants <6

weeks of age who were given the drug for prophylaxis after nursery exposure to pertussis.[116] The risk of IHPS after treatment with other macrolides is unknown. Azithromycin use in 58 neonates for prophylaxis against pertussis was not associated with IHPS in one study[117] but cases have been reported.[118] Azithromycin suspension was shown to be safe and effective for neonatal chlamydial conjunctivitis in one study.[119] The recommended dosage was 20 mg/kg/day for 3 days. Mothers of infants diagnosed with chlamydial infection (and their sex partners) also should receive appropriate evaluation and treatment.

Prophylactic therapy of infants born to women known to have untreated chlamydial infection is not indicated, because the efficacy of such prophylaxis is limited. Such infants should be monitored for signs of infection and to insure appropriate treatment if infection develops.

Oculogenital Infection

Treatment for uncomplicated oculogenital infections in nonpregnant adolescents and adults is doxycycline for 7 days or azithromycin in a single dose.[120] Erythromycin is less efficacious than both azithromycin and doxycycline, and gastrointestinal side effects discourage adherence to treatment.

Sex partners should be evaluated, tested, and treated if they had sexual contact with the patient during the 60 days preceding either onset of the patient's symptoms or diagnosis of *Chlamydia.* The most recent sex partner should be treated even if the time of the last sexual contact was >60 days before diagnosis of the index case. Patients do not need to be retested for *Chlamydia* after completing treatment with doxycycline or azithromycin unless symptoms persist or reinfection is suspected. A test of cure may be considered 3 weeks after completion of treatment with erythromycin. Testing at <3 weeks after completion of therapy to identify cases that did not respond to therapy may not be valid.[121]

TABLE 167-2. Recommended Oral Treatment Regimens for *Chlamydia trachomatis* Infections[124,137]

Condition	Treatment
PERINATAL INFECTIONS	
Inclusion conjunctivitis *or* Pneumonia of infancy	Erythromycin (50 mg/kg/day in 4 doses) for 10–14 days *or* Azithromycin (10 mg/kg/day) for 5 days[a]
OCULOGENITAL INFECTIONS	
Children: <45 kg	Erythromycin (50 mg/kg/day in 4 doses) for 10–14 days
Children: >45 kg but <8 years old	Azithromycin (1 g in a single dose)
Children: >8 years old	Azithromycin (1 g) single dose Doxycycline (100 mg twice daily) for 7 days
Nonpregnant adolescents or adults	Doxycycline (100 mg twice daily) for 7 days *or* Azithromycin (1.0 g) single dose *or* Ofloxacin (300 mg twice daily) for 7 days *Alternative regimen:* Erythromycin base (500 mg 4 times daily) for 7 days *or* Erythromycin ethylsuccinate (800 mg 4 times daily) for 7 days
Pregnant adolescents or adults	Azithromycin (1 g) single dose *or* amoxicillin (500 mg 3 times daily) for 7 days *Alternative regimen:* Erythromycin base (500 mg 4 times a day) for 7 days *or* Erythromycin base (250 mg 4 times daily) for 14 days *or* Erythromycin ethylsuccinate (800 mg 4 times daily) for 7 days *or* Erythromycin ethylsuccinate (400 mg 4 times daily) for 14 days
LYMPHOGRANULOMA VENEREUM	Aspiration of fluctuant buboes plus doxycycline (100 mg twice daily) for 21 days *plus* erythromycin base (500 mg 4 times daily) for 21 days
TRACHOMA	Topical erythromycin, tetracycline, or sulfacetamide ointment twice daily either for 2 months or the first 5 days of 6 consecutive months, *or* Doxycycline or erythromycin for 40 days if severe, *or* Azithromycin (20 mg/kg to max of 1 g once per week) for 3 weeks

[a]*Azithromycin therapy has limited evaluation for treatment of* C. trachomatis *infections in infants.*[119] *It is an accepted agent for treatment or prophylaxis of pertussis in neonates.*[138]

Azithromycin is the recommended first choice for treatment of pregnant women, with amoxicillin as alternative.[122] Doxycycline and ofloxacin are contraindicated in pregnant women. Azithromycin is widely prescribed during pregnancy and lactation and is excreted minimally in breast milk. The benefits of human milk feeding outweigh the risks of infant exposure to small amounts of azithromycin.[123]

Lymphogranuloma Venereum

Recommended oral treatment for LGV is doxycycline for 21 days or erythromycin base for 21 days.[116,124] Fluctuant buboes should be aspirated through intact skin to prevent bubo rupture with formation of sinus tracts.

Trachoma

It is estimated that half the cases of blindness can be prevented with topical treatment of trachoma. Current treatment recommendations vary, but the most widely used include topical treatment with erythromycin, tetracycline, or sulfacetamide ointment twice daily for 2 months, or for the first 5 days of each month for 6 months.[125,126] The latter schedule is recommended by the WHO for mass treatment, in which topical therapy is applied concurrently to all the children in a given area with endemic trachoma. Oral erythromycin or doxycycline for 40 days also is given in severe cases; cycles of weekly or monthly courses can minimize dental staining associated with doxycycline, as most treated children are <7 years of age. Preliminary results of trials of mass treatment with single doses of azithromycin at the village level indicate that both infection and clinical disease are markedly decreased at 6 and 12 months after such treatment.[127–129]

COMPLICATIONS AND SEQUELAE

Chlamydiae can persist in host cells in a quiescent state for extended periods. *C. trachomatis* has been implicated as a pathogen in 8% to 54% of women who have PID and has been associated with the long-term consequences of tubal infertility (17%), ectopic pregnancy (10%), or chronic pelvic pain (17%).[130] Untreated pregnant women with chlamydial infection are at risk for endometritis following delivery or induced abortions,[130,131] and can experience adverse pregnancy outcomes such as premature rupture of membranes, prematurity, low birthweight, and stillbirth.

C. trachomatis infection and its complications account for serious morbidity and economic cost. In males, epididymitis, prostatitis, and reactive arthritis are the most common sequelae. Furthermore, untreated or incorrectly treated chlamydial conjunctivitis can result in chronic conjunctivitis that can develop alone or as part of Reiter syndrome, which includes urethritis, conjunctivitis, mucosal lesions, and reactive arthritis.

PREVENTION

Screening of asymptomatic high-risk patients for *C. trachomatis* infection is the most effective means of preventing disease and sequelae. Behavioral interventions (e.g., delaying intercourse, decreasing the number of sex partners, and using barrier contraception) should be pursued aggressively. Women with any of the following risk factors should be tested routinely for *Chlamydia*: mucopurulent cervicitis, sexually active and <20 years of age, >1 sex partner during the last 3 months, or inconsistent use of barrier contraception while in a nonmonogamous relationship.[102] Because of the frequency of repeated chlamydial infections within the first several months following treatment of an initial infection, more frequent (e.g., every 6 months) screening of asymptomatic sexually active adolescents may be necessary.[31] A cost-effectiveness study in women attending family planning clinics revealed that a strategy that combined use of PCR on cervical specimens in women receiving pelvic examinations, and PCR on urine of women with no medical indication for a pelvic examination prevented the most cases of PID and provided the highest cost savings.[132]

Pregnant women should be screened and treated for *C. trachomatis* to prevent adverse pregnancy outcomes, chlamydial infection among infants, and maternal postnatal complications. In neonates, ocular prophylaxis with topical erythromycin or tetracycline has reduced the incidence of gonococcal ophthalmia but does not appear to be effective against *C. trachomatis* while masking infection at other sites.[133]

To combat trachoma, the WHO has endorsed an integrated strategy known as SAFE: Surgery for people at immediate risk of blindness, Antibiotic therapy to treat individual active cases and reduce the community reservoir of infection, Facial cleanliness and improved hygiene to reduce transmission, and Environmental improvements to make living conditions better so that the environment no longer facilitates the maintenance and transmission of trachoma. In many areas, the life-changing benefits of the SAFE program are being observed due to efforts of the International Trachoma Initiative.[128]

During the extracellular EB stage, antibodies can act to inhibit infection. However, since the replicating RB form resides within the intracellular inclusion, bacterial killing at this stage requires a cell-mediated immune response with the primary effectors being interferon-γ secreting Th1 cells. Thus, an ideal *C. trachomatis* vaccine should induce both local antibodies to prevent infection by EBs, and a strong Th1 response to limit infection once initiated. Efforts to develop a *C. trachomatis* vaccine have concentrated primarily on the use of recombinant *Chlamydia* antigens with immune adjuvants.[134,135] The use of a purified native preparation of MOMP combined with Th1-inducing adjuvants induced significant resistance in mice, but sterilizing immunity was not achieved.[136] Future work may incorporate molecular technology and our increasing understanding of the host response to chlamydiae to develop new vaccine candidates.

168 *Chlamydophila (Chlamydia) psittaci* (Psittacosis)

Laura M. Conklin

THE PATHOGEN

Chlamydophila psittaci is a gram-negative obligate intracellular bacterium that causes both systemic infection and pneumonia, often referred to as psittacosis or ornithosis. Formerly classified under the genus *Chlamydia*, *C. psittaci* is now grouped with *C. pneumoniae*, *C. pecorum*, *C. abortus*, *C. caviae*, and *C. felis* in the genus *Chlamydophila* of the family Chlamydiaceae.[1] There now is considerable debate as to whether *C. psittaci* should be returned to its previous genus, *Chlamydia*. Although psittacosis originally

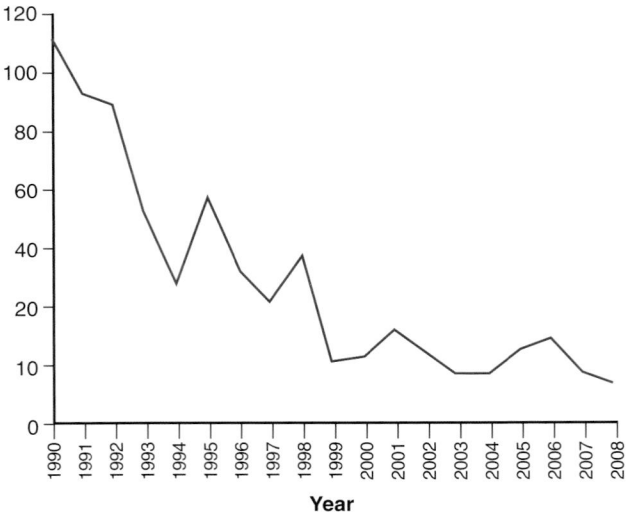

Figure 168-1. Cases of psittacosis reported to the Centers for Disease Control and Prevention, 1990 to 2008.

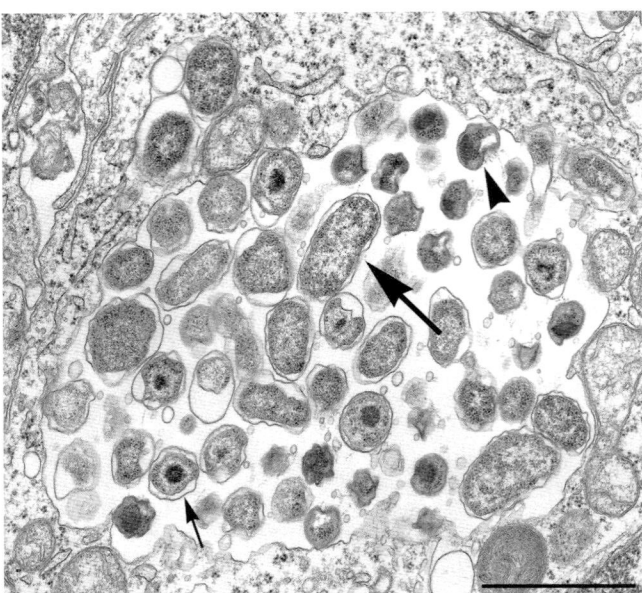

Figure 168-2. Electron micrograph of *Chlamydophila psittaci*. The large arrow indicates a reticulate body, the small arrow an intermediate body, and the arrowhead an elementary body. (Courtesy of C. Goldsmith and B. Wolff, Centers for Disease Control and Prevention.)

was named parrot fever because of its association with psittacines (e.g., parrots, parakeets), psittacosis can be transmitted through virtually all domestic and wild birds.[2,3]

EPIDEMIOLOGY

From 1990 through 2008, the Centers for Disease Control and Prevention (CDC) received 756 reports of psittacosis, of which 9% occurred in people under 20 years of age.[4] Improved sensitivity of testing methods in the 1990s corresponded to a substantial decline in the number of cases reported, which has since remained relatively stable (Figure 168-1). The low number of reported cases, especially pediatric cases, is likely an underestimate of the actual number of cases because of: (1) lack of recognition by clinicians; (2) difficulties in diagnosis of infection; and (3) underreporting. As of 2008, psittacosis was reportable in all states except for Connecticut and Texas (http://www.cste.org/nndssmainmenu2005.htm). Disease incidence does not vary by season.

C. psittaci is transmitted through inhaled aerosols from the respiratory tract secretions, eye secretions, urine, or feces of infected birds. Mouth-to-beak contact, handling of plumage, and lawn-mowing have been reported modes of exposure.[5] Illness can occur after even brief exposure to infected birds or their droppings. Most reported psittacosis cases have a known exposure to pet birds. However, outbreaks associated with wild birds, poultry processing, veterinary clinics, and aviaries have been described.[6-10] Infected birds can be asymptomatic or only mildly ill and can shed the organism for prolonged periods after recovery. Because *C. psittaci* resists drying and can remain infectious in the environment for months, bird exposure may not be reported in some cases. Although biologically plausible, reports of person-to-person transmission are rare.[11,12] Confirmed and probable cases of psittacosis should be reported to the local or state health department to prevent further transmission.[13]

CLINICAL MANIFESTATIONS

Psittacosis classically causes an "atypical" pneumonia (Figure 168-2). However, disease manifestations can range from a mild, influenza-like illness to severe systemic disease (Box 168-1). Symptoms generally develop after an incubation period of approximately 5 to 14 days but can occur up to one month after exposure.[10] Because signs and symptoms of *C. psittaci* infection are similar to those caused by other community-acquired pneumonia

BOX 168-1. Clinical Manifestations of Psittacosis

COMMON

Fever
Chills
Weakness
Fatigue
Myalgia
Headache
Cough

LESS COMMON

Pulse-temperature dissociation (fever without elevated pulse)
Splenomegaly
Rash

RARE

Myocarditis
Hepatitis
Arthritis
Keratoconjunctivitis
Encephalitis
Placental infection and fetal compromise (gestational psittacosis)

pathogens (including *Mycoplasma pneumoniae*, *C. pneumoniae*, *Coxiella burnetii*, and influenza virus), psittacosis should be considered in any child with pneumonia who has had close exposure to birds.[14,15]

DIAGNOSIS

Culture and isolation of *C. psittaci* rarely is undertaken outside research laboratories, largely due to technical difficulties. Diagnosis usually is made by observing a fourfold increase in antibody to a reciprocal titer of >32 between acute and convalescent sera. In the absence of a clear exposure to birds, serologic testing should be interpreted cautiously because of the potential for cross-reactivity with other *Chlamydia* spp. Use of complement fixation is discouraged due to its poor specificity. Microimmunofluorescence is the preferred assay because it more reliably discriminates between *C. psittaci* and *C. pneumoniae*. Acute serum collection should occur as soon as possible after onset of clinical illness, with convalescent serum collection 2 to 4 weeks later. A real-time polymerase chain reaction assay for *C. psittaci* has been developed and validated in avian specimens but is not yet available commercially for use in humans.[16] Information on availability of laboratory testing can be obtained from most state public health laboratories.[2]

TREATMENT

Tetracyclines are the drugs of choice for treating *C. psittaci* infections. In groups for whom tetracyclines are contraindicated, i.e., pregnant women and children less than 8 years of age, macrolide antibiotics are considered the best alternative, although in vivo efficacy has not been determined.[17] Clinical response to therapy usually occurs within 48 to 72 hours; however, treatment should continue for 10 to 14 days after fever ceases in order to avoid relapse.[2] Tetracycline resistance has not been reported in *C. psittaci* but has been documented in other *Chlamydophila* spp.[18]

169 *Coxiella burnetii* (Q Fever)

Gilbert J. Kersh, Alicia D. Anderson, and Herbert A. Thompson

THE PATHOGEN

Q fever (or "query" fever) is caused by the intracellular bacterium *Coxiella burnetii,* which belongs to the order Legionellales, family Coxiellaceae. *C. burnetii* is primarily a zoonotic pathogen. The organism can be present in high concentrations in the placenta and amniotic fluid of parturient animals, and can be transmitted to humans via inhalation or direct contact.[1,2] *C. burnetii* is highly infectious to humans, and as little as a single inhaled organism can be sufficient to initiate infection.[1,2] The organism survives and replicates in eukaryotic cells, but also is remarkably long-lived in the environment, where it is resistant to environmental extremes and desiccation.[1,2] The organism is thus classified as a Category B bioterrorism agent. Human Q fever was made nationally reportable in 1999.[3]

Variation in the outer lipopolysaccharide of *C. burnetii* causes two antigenic phases; people with acute infection show antibodies primarily directed against phase II antigen, whereas people with chronic Q fever infections show a predominantly phase I antibody response.[4]

EPIDEMIOLOGY

Q fever is enzootic in domestic ruminants throughout the world, and human cases have a similar worldwide distribution.[1] Large outbreaks of Q fever have been reported from numerous geographic locations, including the United States, Australia, and Europe.[1] A particularly large outbreak has recently occurred in the Netherlands with >3500 cases of Q fever documented in 2007–2009.[5] Classically, outbreaks are linked to occupational exposure (farm or slaughterhouse workers) or research institutions that use pregnant livestock in research. Several outbreaks of Q fever have been documented among people living downwind from infected livestock, strongly implicating windborne transmission.[6,7] Although sheep, cattle, and goats are implicated most commonly in transmission of Q fever to humans, outbreaks also have been associated with other parturient animal species, including dogs and cats.[8,9] Ticks are known to harbor *C burnetii,* and can transmit infection in rare circumstances.[10,11] Consumption of unpasteurized dairy products also has been suggested as a possible means of transmission.[12]

In the U.S., Q fever is widespread in cattle, sheep, and goats, with antibodies to *C. burnetii* detected in 3%, 16%, and 42% of individual animals, respectively.[13] In disease-endemic areas, sporadic cases or localized outbreaks of Q fever occur in humans from contact with infected animals. From 1999 through 2004, the average annual reported incidence was 0.28 per million persons

in the U.S.[14] Although the disease is reported rarely, the true incidence of infection likely is much higher due to difficulties in recognizing infection and establishing a diagnosis. Seroprevalence surveys suggest that 3.1% of the general U.S. population has antibodies to *C. burnetii.*[15] This is likely to be higher among persons with livestock contact; a survey of veterinarians found a seroprevalence of 22%.[16]

Q fever is considered to be a disease primarily of middle-aged adults rather than children, probably because of its strong occupational associations. The reported annual incidence of Q fever in children in the U.S. is <0.05 cases per million persons (Figure 169-1), and from 1999 though 2003, only 7 cases of Q fever were reported in children <18 years of age.[14] Studies examining age distribution in large outbreaks have shown that children less frequently develop symptomatic illness, even when exposures and seroconversion rates are similar to those observed in adults.[17] However, pediatric cases of Q fever have been recognized, especially in countries where Q fever is reported frequently.[18,19] A report of Q fever infections among children in Greece suggests that specific pediatric age groups (11 to 14 years of age) and risk factors (livestock contact, consumption of unpasteurized dairy products) may be associated with infection.[19]

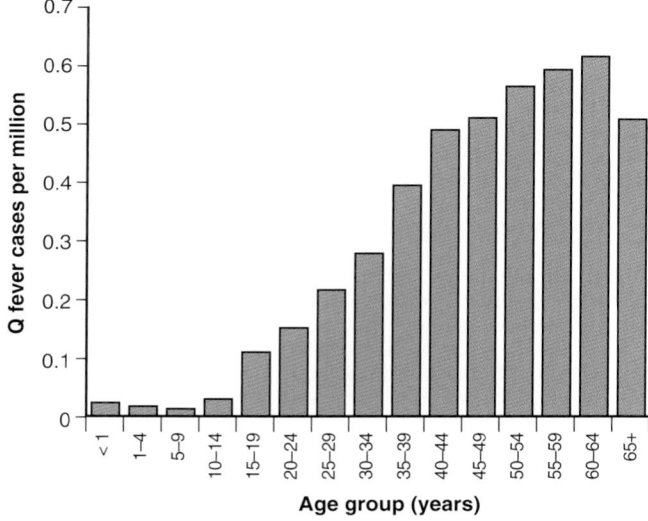

Figure 169-1. Annual incidence of Q fever by age, United States, 2000–2008. (Data from U.S. Centers for Disease Control and Prevention.)

CLINICAL MANIFESTATIONS

Outbreak investigations have suggested that >50% of adults, and >80% of children exposed to *C. burnetii* have asymptomatic infections.[17,20] Apparent infections can result in signs and symptoms ranging from mild to severe. Although acute infection can be self-limiting, all recognized cases should be treated. Chronic forms of infection are more severe, can be life-threatening, and require long-term treatment.[1,2] Classic symptoms of acute, respiratory Q fever in North America include sudden onset with fever, headache (often frontal), chills, general malaise, cough, anorexia, and myalgia. These symptoms should prompt inclusion of Q fever in the differential diagnosis particularly in patients with a history of exposure to ruminants. However, the lack of direct animal contact should not preclude a clinical suspicion because airborne transmission can occur. It is important to note that severity of acute disease and length of incubation period often are related to dose size,[21] and that specific symptoms and direction of disease progression may often be dependent upon route of infection.[22]

Acute Q fever infection follows 1 to 3 weeks after the initial exposure, and symptoms in children usually are similar to those recognized in adults. Acute infection typically is a self-limited febrile illness or pneumonia.[1,2,23] In children, Q fever pneumonia can be characterized by a cough (up to 90% of cases), and radiographic changes that include bilateral infiltrates, atelectasis, and pleural effusion.[23] Respiratory failure and death is uncommon, but can occur in patients with underlying conditions.[24] Gastrointestinal tract symptoms, such as abdominal pain, vomiting, or diarrhea may be present.[25] A review of 18 cases of Q fever in infancy listed fever of unknown origin as the most frequent clinical manifestation; pneumonia, convulsions, and malaise also were reported.[26] Common clinical signs among infants in the series included anorexia, cough, and diarrhea.[26] In a review of hospitalized children with Q fever in Spain, common symptoms included fever (92%), gastrointestinal tract symptoms (83%), hepatomegaly (67%), fatigue (50%), cough (50%), headache (42%), splenomegaly (25%, arthralgia (17%), and nuchal rigidity (8%).[17,25] In a review of pediatric Q fever cases in Australia, most experienced a clinical illness similar to illness observed in adults, and 14% reportedly experienced protracted symptoms of fatigue >3 months after acute infection.[18] More severe manifestations of acute disease include severe atypical pneumonia, hepatitis, myocarditis, pericarditis, rhabdomyolysis, or meningoencephalitis.[1,2,17,19,25,27–29] A case of hemolytic-uremic syndrome also has been reported.[30]

Chronic Q fever occurs months or years after the initial acute infection, and can be difficult to diagnose because of its lack of a temporal association with specific exposures. Chronic infection is characterized by development of chronic hepatitis, osteomyelitis, or infective endocarditis.[1,2,17,27,31] Children with Q fever osteomyelitis may not show systemic illness, but often experience recurrent, multisite episodes that are poorly responsive to traditional treatment.[31] Children with a history of underlying valvular heart defect or immunocompromising conditions may be at increased risk for developing chronic Q fever endocarditis, which manifests as a culture-negative endocarditis.[17] Chronic Q fever endocarditis can be fatal, especially if it is not recognized and treated.

LABORATORY FINDINGS AND DIAGNOSIS

Abnormal laboratory findings in children with Q fever include elevation of serum hepatic enzymes, leukopenia or leukocytosis, and thrombocytopenia.[2,25] Because of the vague clinical signs associated with Q fever, most physicians rely on serologic tests for confirmation. Indirect immunofluorescent antibody assays (IFAs) are used most commonly. These tests can detect either phase II or phase I antibodies, which can help differentiate between acute and chronic infection.[4] In general, chronic infections are associated with a higher ratio of phase I to phase II antibodies than acute infections.[4]

Although considered the gold standard for diagnosis, serologic confirmation of Q fever infection can be difficult. Most serologic tests are based on detection of IgG, which usually appears 9 to 14 days after onset of clinical signs.[4] However, some patients may not have detectable IgG titers for several weeks after onset. Laboratory confirmation is further complicated by the fact that patients may have elevated IgG titers for years following an initial exposure to Q fever, so a single elevated IgG titer may not be strong evidence of recent infection. The presence of specific IgM antibodies provides stronger evidence for recent infection, and IgM antibodies can appear as early as 4 days after symptom onset.

The most reliable method for diagnosis of Q fever is the laboratory examination of paired acute- and convalescent-phase serum samples. Paired serum samples that show a 4-fold change in phase II IgM or IgG titer should be considered indicative of confirmed cases of Q fever for reporting purposes.[3] Patients with a clinically compatible illness that show a single elevated titer should be considered probable cases of Q fever.[3]

Demonstration of *C. burnetii* in blood or tissue samples via polymerase chain reaction (PCR), immunohistochemistry, or culture also can be used for diagnosis.[4] PCR on blood or serum is considered essential for diagnosis in the early stages of infection before antibody titers are detectable.[32] Immunohistochemistry and culture are useful on excised heart valve tissue for patients with endocarditis undergoing valve replacement surgery. However, because *C. burnetii* is highly infectious to humans, only biosafety-level 3 laboratories should attempt isolation and culture of the organism.

TREATMENT

Because a definitive diagnosis of Q fever can be delayed due to slow development of antibodies and the lack of routine PCR testing, clinicians should provide empiric treatment based on a suspicion of Q fever. Although most cases of acute Q fever resolve without treatment, treatment with rickettsiostatic antibiotics may shorten the length of clinical illness.[1,2,17] Furthermore, although no long-term studies have been conducted, antibiotic treatment may prevent severe disease and help prevent chronic infection. For treatment of acute Q fever in children, doxycycline (2.2 mg/kg twice daily, with a maximum of 200 mg/day) should be administered to patients for 14 days.[17,33] The highly effective action of doxycycline against *C. burnetii* warrants its use in children, especially in patients with severe illness. Studies suggest that the dosage and duration of doxycycline suggested here will have minimal effects on tooth color.[34,35] Alternative antibiotics that might be considered in milder cases include cotrimoxazole or rifampin.[17]

Treatment of chronic Q fever requires aggressive, long-term antibiotic therapy. Combination therapy consisting of oral doxycycline and hydroxychloroquine for at least 18 months usually is required.[17,36] The patient's serologic response should be monitored during treatment, and therapy should be extended beyond 18 months if the patient's phase I IgG antibody titer remains ≥1 : 800.[36] Even with long-term therapy, relapse can occur following cessation of antibiotic treatment. Surgical excision of affected heart valves also may be necessary. Routine (twice yearly) ophthalmologic examination for chloroquine accumulation should accompany hydroxychloroquine use.[36]

SPECIAL CONSIDERATIONS

Children with chronic immunosuppressive conditions may be at increased risk for *C. burnetii* infection. There is a case report describing fatal Q fever pneumonia in a child with chronic granulomatous disease,[24] and patients with congenital heart defects or chronic immunosuppressive conditions may be predisposed to develop Q fever endocarditis.[17] Up to 75% of patients with preexisting valvular heart disease who experience acute Q fever develop endocarditis within 2 years.[17,37] Such patients should have careful serologic monitoring to allow early detection and rapid treatment of chronic infection.

Case reports suggest women infected with *C. burnetii* during pregnancy can experience abortion or premature delivery, and *C. burnetii* has been isolated from the placenta and milk of infected mothers.[17,38,39] Infected women may pose a risk for infection to healthcare providers during delivery because of aerosolization of infectious material.[39] Pregnant women who are diagnosed with Q fever should be treated with cotrimoxazole during their entire pregnancy, and followed serologically to evaluate possible progression to chronic infection.[17,40]

PREVENTION

Children can be protected by minimizing their contact with parturient and newborn animals, especially livestock including sheep, goats, and cattle, but also dogs and cats. Adults who come in contact with parturient or newborn animals should take care to minimize their own contact with children until they can shower and wash potentially contaminated clothing.[9] Because dairy products have sometimes been implicated as a means of transmission, children should be allowed to consume only milk and dairy products that have been boiled or pasteurized. A Q fever vaccine is not currently licensed for use in the U.S., but a licensed vaccine is available in Australia. Its use is generally limited to persons with high-risk occupations, such as abattoir workers and laboratory technologists who work with *C. burnettii*.[1,2,41]

Key Points. Diagnosis and Management of *Coxiella burnetii* Infection (Q Fever)

MICROBIOLOGY

- Obligate intracellular, gram-negative gamma-proteobacterium
- Can be grown in embryonated eggs, mice, guinea pigs, or tissue culture of host cells
- Has been grown in host cell-free liquid culture in the laboratory

EPIDEMIOLOGY

- A zoonotic pathogen with worldwide distribution
- Cases and outbreaks usually are associated with exposure to domestic ruminants
- Occupational exposure to infected animals is a significant risk factor
- Seroprevalence in U.S. is 3.1%
- Very likely that disease is underreported due to nonspecific flu-like symptoms

DIAGNOSIS

- Acute form of Q fever usually manifests 1 to 3 weeks after exposure with flu-like symptoms, sometimes also with pneumonia and/or hepatitis

- Chronic Q fever can develop many months after initial infection
- Serologic detection of 4-fold rise in phase II IgG antibody titer is the most common method of diagnosis
- Antibody titers usually do not increase until at least 2 weeks after symptom onset
- PCR detection of *C. burnetii* can be used on blood or serum samples during first 2 weeks of symptoms and prior to antibiotic administration

TREATMENT

- Doxycycline (2.2 mg/kg twice a day, maximum 200 mg/day) is the optimum treatment
- No significant drug resistance is reported
- Chronic cases can result in culture-negative osteomyelitis or endocarditis (possibly requiring valve replacement)

DURATION OF THERAPY

- 14-day course of antibiotic for acute infections
- Treatment may need to be ≥18 months for chronic infections

---

170 *Ehrlichia* and *Anaplasma* Species (Ehrlichiosis and Anaplasmosis)

Joanna J. Regan and William L. Nicholson

DESCRIPTION OF THE PATHOGENS

The family Anaplasmataceae is in the order Rickettsiales and contains six genera of obligate intracellular bacteria. Three of the genera contain members that can infect humans. These zoonotic agents are transmitted by invertebrate vectors and cause potentially life-threatening diseases in humans and animals. As of 2010, four species in the genus *Ehrlichia* and one species in the genus *Anaplasma* have been documented causes of human disease (Table 170-1). Four species responsible for disease in the United States, *Ehrlichia chaffeensis*, *E. ewingii*, *E. muris*-like, and *Anaplasma phagocytophilum*, are all transmitted by ticks and have been described since 1987. In addition to these species, an *Ehrlichia canis*-like agent has been identified from blood of an asymptomatic patient in South America.[1] It is possible that additional *Ehrlichia* and *Anaplasma* species capable of causing human disease will be described in the U.S. and worldwide.

Ehrlichia and *Anaplasma* are small (0.5 to 1.5 μm) gram-negative cocci.[2] The genomes of these organisms are relatively small with a size of 1.18 Mb for *E. chaffeensis* and 1.47 Mb for *A. phagocytophilum*.[3] *Ehrlichia* and *Anaplasma* species that infect humans are specialized for infecting leukocytes. After attachment to membrane receptors and subsequent induction of phagocytosis,[4] the organisms multiply in early endosomes that fail to develop into mature phagocytic or lysosomal vacuoles. Although the complete repertoire of cell receptors used is not known, *A. phagocytophilum* binds to the P-selectin binding domain of the P-selectin glycoprotein ligand PSGL-1 on human granulocytes before cell internalization.[5] Within the cell cytoplasm of infected leukocytes, organisms replicate within membrane-bound vesicles, developing into microcolonies called morulae. The morphologic features of morulae vary among the species in size, number of individual organisms, and the presence of a fibrillar matrix.[6] Individual morulae can contain more than 50 bacteria, which are released into the extracellular space after cell lysis or by exocytosis after fusion of the vacuole membrane with the plasma membrane.[2] Ehrlichiae in morulae stain with eosin-azure-type stains and occasionally are observed in circulating leukocytes of acutely ill patients.

How *Ehrlichia* and *Anaplasma* cause disease in humans is incompletely understood, although they may kill infected leukocytes directly.[2] Perivascular inflammatory infiltrates become apparent in many organs, and morulae can be visualized within the leukocyte populations present in these infiltrates.[7] However, factors leading to the inflammatory response are not known. Mechanisms of

TABLE 170-1. Disease and Distribution of *Ehrlichia* and *Anaplasma* Species that Cause Disease in Humans

Ehrlichia Species	Disease (Date of First Description)	Distribution[a]
Ehrlichia chaffeensis	Monocytic ehrlichiosis (1987)	United States
Ehrlichia ewingii	Granulocytic ehrlichiosis (1999)	United States
Ehrlichia muris-like	Monocytic ehrlichiosis (2009)	United States
Ehrlichia canis	Monocytic ehrlichiosis (1996)[b]	Venezuela
Neorickettsia sennetsu	Sennetsu fever (1953)	Japan, Malaysia
Anaplasma phagocytophilum	Granulocytic anaplasmosis (1994)	United States, Europe

[a]*Organism isolated or identified in humans by molecular characterization.*
[b]*Single report.*

many of the hematologic and biochemical perturbations (e.g., cytopenia and abnormal serum hepatic enzyme levels) are not clear. Infections do not cause the vasculitis or endothelial damage characteristic of other rickettsial diseases (e.g., Rocky Mountain spotted fever (RMSF) caused by *Rickettsia rickettsii*).

EPIDEMIOLOGY

Although these infections can result in life-threatening disease in children, this outcome has been reported relatively infrequently in the pediatric population. Among the first 250 cases described (mostly human monocytic ehrlichiosis (HME) caused by *E. chaffeensis*), less than 10% were in people 2 to 13 years of age.[8] Active surveillance for *A. phagocytophilum* (also called human granulocytic anaplasmosis; HGA) indicates that the age-specific incidence of HGA also is notably low in people <18 years of age and is highest in adults >50 years of age.[9] The reasons for the low number of cases reported in younger patients remain unclear, and the frequency of asymptomatic infection in children is unknown.

Documentation of infection by isolation or molecular characterization of the etiologic agent from humans has occurred in some locations (see Table 170-1). However, serologic studies indicate that *Ehrlichia* and *Anaplasma* species (listed in Table 170-1), or antigenically related species, cause human infections throughout Europe and Scandanavia,[10] South and Central America,[11,12] Africa,[13] and China.[14] In the U.S., the number of cases of ehrlichiosis due to *E. chaffeensis* that have been reported to the Centers for Disease Control and Protection (CDC) has increased from 200 cases in 2000, to 740 cases in 2010. The number of anaplasmosis cases reported in the U.S. also has increased, from 348 in 2000, to 1761 cases in 2010.[15] The estimated incidence of hospitalized cases of *E. chaffeensis* infection is 5.5 per 100,000 people in southeastern Georgia, which was higher than the incidence of RMSF in the same population during the study period.[16] Active surveillance for HGA in Connecticut estimated an incidence of between 24 and 51 cases per 100,000 residents living in counties where the disease is endemic.[9]

Human ehrlichioses and anaplasmosis share certain epidemiologic features. In addition to being reported most commonly in adults, these diseases have been reported most frequently in males.[17] Approximately 60% of the recorded pediatric cases have occurred in boys.[8,18,19] Although it is possible for cases to occur year round, the peak incidence of disease occurs in May through August.[15,17,19,20] While generally a sporadic disease, clusters of cases have occurred during recreational activities (e.g., golf)[21] and occupational exposure (e.g., military maneuvers).[22]

The endemic region for specific diseases can be approximated by the geographic distribution of each agent's primary tick vector. Infections caused by *E. chaffeensis* and *E. ewingii* are associated with the bite of the lone star tick, *Amblyomma americanum*.[23,24] This tick is distributed primarily across central Texas and eastern Oklahoma, eastward throughout the southeastern U.S., and north along the Atlantic coastal plain into New England. The greatest number of

cases of *E. chaffeensis* ehrlichiosis and all those caused by *E. ewingii* have been reported from the southeastern and south central U.S.[15,25] The recognized geographic range of the tick *A. americanum* is expanding, thus suggesting that the area of risk for ehrlichial pathogens transmitted by this vector should be considered dynamic.[26] Most HGA cases have occurred in the north central and northeastern states, particularly New York, Connecticut, Minnesota, and Wisconsin.[15] The principal tick vector is the black-legged tick, *Ixodes scapularis*, the same tick that transmits *Borrelia burgdorferi*.[27] In the western U.S., *Ixodes pacificus* is the main vector of *A. phagocytophilum*.[28] In Europe, *Ixodes ricinus* has been incriminated in transmission of *A. phagocytophilum* to humans.[29]

Ticks in the genus *Ixodes* can transmit several other pathogens, including *Babesia* species, flaviviruses, and *Borrelia burgdorferi*; dual infection with *A. phagocytophilum* and *Borrelia burgdorferi* has been reported.[30] In some children, the concurrent presence of anaplasmosis and Lyme disease resulted in severe disease complicated by meningoencephalitis and disseminated intravascular coagulation.[31]

CLINICAL MANIFESTATIONS

As in adults, the most severe disease in children is associated with infection by *E. chaffeensis*. However, few detailed descriptions of *A. phagocytophilum* or *E. ewingii* infection in children have been published. Immunosuppressive conditions, including chemotherapy[32] and organ transplantation,[33] may predispose children to more severe disease by *E. chaffeensis*. Presumably, the same or similar conditions predispose children to infection by *E. ewingii*; the only report of disease attributable to *E. ewingii* was in an 11-year-old boy receiving immunosuppressive therapy after kidney transplantation.[25] Although numbers are few (3 cases), African American children have been reported with severe disease requiring hospitalization and, in one case, mechanical ventilation for a child with underlying sickle-cell β-thalassemia.[33,34]

The incubation period typically is 5 to 10 days after a recognized tick bite.[17,20] Most children (55% to 85%) recall a tick bite several days to weeks before the illness.[8,19,33] Common symptoms in children include fever, myalgia, and headache (Table 170-2). Among reported pediatric patients infected with *E. chaffeensis*, rash occurs in approximately two-thirds of cases, whereas only about 25% of adult patients experience rash.[17,19] The rash, which typically involves the trunk, with sparing of the hands and feet, may be macular, papular, maculopapular, or occasionally petechial. Less than 5% of patients infected by *A. phagocytophilum* exhibit a rash.[20,35] Gastrointestinal tract symptoms, including nausea, vomiting, anorexia, and diarrhea, are observed in approximately 60% of children with ehrlichiosis, a figure only slightly greater than that reported in adults with *E. chaffeensis* infection.[17] Adults with HGA have gastrointestinal tract symptoms less frequently (<40%).[35]

Moderate to severe headache is a common feature regardless of the etiologic agent (see Table 170-2). However, encephalitis or meningitis is reported most commonly with HME.[36] Long-term neurologic sequelae, including bilateral footdrop, speech impairment, and diminished reading and fine motor ability, have been described in children after severe disease.[19,32,33] Infections can

TABLE 170-2. Common Clinical Features of Ehrlichiosis and Anaplasmosis in Children

Symptom	No. (%)
Fever	40/40 (100)
Myalgia	20/30 (67)
Rash	23/35 (66)
Headache	17/27 (63)
Anorexia or nausea or vomiting	19/33 (58)
Hepatomegaly or splenomegaly	10/25 (40)

Data from references 18, 32, 34, and 38.

TABLE 170-3. Common Laboratory Features of Ehrlichiosis and Anaplasmosis in Children

Finding	No. (%)
Leukopenia	27/38 (71)
Lymphopenia	27/33 (82)
Thrombocytopenia	30/36 (83)
Elevated serum aspartate transaminase	28/31 (90)
Hyponatremia	15/23 (65)
Anemia	12/32 (38)

Data from references 18, 31, 34, and 38.

result in severe pulmonary disease, and acute respiratory distress syndrome in adults[37] as well as children.[33] Intubation and mechanical ventilation have been required for severe cases of *E. chaffeensis* ehrlichiosis.[19,33,38]

Opportunistic ehrlichiosis can occur in patients as a result of deficient neutrophil and CD4+ lymphocyte function.[7] Disseminated candidiasis, invasive pulmonary aspergillosis, *Cryptococcus neoformans* pneumonia, herpes simplex, and cytomegalovirus infections have been noted in these patients.[20,39,40] Reinfection with *A. phagocytophilum* also has been reported.[41]

LABORATORY FINDINGS

Irrespective of age, leukopenia (<4000/mm³), thrombocytopenia (<150,000/mm³), and elevations in serum hepatic levels (aspartate aminotransferase (AST) >55 U/L) characteristically develop in patients early in the course of illness (Table 170-3). These laboratory findings provide early presumptive clues to the diagnosis of ehrlichiosis or anaplasmosis regardless of the specific agent.[17,19,33,35] Leukopenia occurs with both *E. chaffeensis* and *A. phagocytophilum* infection, with the nadir typically between 1000 and 4000/mm³.[40] Lymphocytopenia is common in patients with HME and HGA (see Table 170-3), and neutropenia is reported in adults with HGA.[35] Thrombocytopenia is reported in >70% of patients, with platelet counts generally between 50,000 and 150,000/mm³.[19,40] Anemia is reported in about one-third of children with HME (see Table 170-3). The bone marrow of cytopenic patients frequently is normocellular or hypercellular, thus suggesting that the leukopenia and thrombocytopenia are due to peripheral sequestration or destruction of these elements.[42]

Mildly or moderately elevated serum levels of AST occur in most children infected by *E. chaffeensis* (see Table 170-3).[17,19,35] Alkaline phosphatase levels are less affected. Electrolyte abnormalities, particularly mild to moderate hyponatremia, are noted frequently in children and adults with severe disease.[18,19,43]

Cerebrospinal fluid (CSF) pleocytosis, elevated protein levels, or both are most often reported in patients with HME, as are episodes of confusion, disorientation, or delirium.[36] Morulae of *E. chaffeensis* have been identified in mononuclear cells in the CSF, and this organism has been isolated from the CSF of patients with ehrlichiosis.[44]

The differential diagnosis for ehrlichiosis and anaplasmosis is remarkably broad and encompasses various infectious and noninfectious diseases. Early in the illness, the nonspecific findings of fever, headache, myalgia, nausea, and malaise can be mistaken for various viral syndromes, upper respiratory tract illness, septicemia, urinary tract infection, or gastroenteritis. A history of a tick bite is helpful; however, infections can cause symptoms similar to those of other illnesses associated with pathogens transmitted by ticks, including Lyme disease, RMSF, tularemia (*Francisella tularensis*), Colorado tick fever (Coltivirus), and babesiosis (*Babesia* species).[45] Differences between ehrlichiosis and anaplasmosis compared with RMSF are that: (1) rash is present in 90% of patients with progressive RMSF, (2) leukopenia and absolute lymphopenia and neutropenia are uncommon in RMSF, (3) morulae are not observed in RMSF, and (4) histopathologic vasculitis is a hallmark of RMSF but not of ehrlichiosis and anaplasmosis.

DIAGNOSIS

The diagnosis of ehrlichiosis or anplasmosis can be established by several laboratory methods. In order of routine application, these methods are: serologic tests to measure specific antibody, detection of DNA by polymerase chain reaction (PCR) assays on blood or CSF, detection of morulae in leukocytes in peripheral blood (Figure 170-1) or CSF, direct detection of *Ehrlichia* in tissue samples by immunohistochemistry, and isolation of the bacteria (not yet accomplished for *E. ewingii*).

The serologic gold standard for diagnosing these diseases is the indirect immunofluorescence assay (IFA).[46] IFA can be used to detect immunoglobulin IgG or IgM antibodies in a patient's serum or plasma that are reactive with *E. chaffeensis* or *A. phagocytophilum* antigens. Antibodies cross-reactive with *E. chaffeensis* antigens have been useful in diagnosing some cases of *E. ewingii* infection.[25] However, because cross-reactivity among *Ehrlichia* and *Anaplasma* species occurs in sera from 10% to 30% of patients, sera should be tested against both antigens when ascribing a specific etiology in areas where the pathogens coexist.[46] Confirmation of the diagnosis can be made in a person with compatible illness who has a 4-fold change in IgG antibody titer between acute- and convalescent-phase serum samples. The acute sample should be obtained as early in the disease process as possible, and the convalescent sample should be obtained 2 to 4 weeks after the acute sample. Detection of IgG and IgM antibodies by IFA frequently is negative in the first week of illness, when most patients initially seek care, so a negative serologic result for the acute-phase sample does not exclude the diagnosis.[47,48] IgM titers can remain elevated

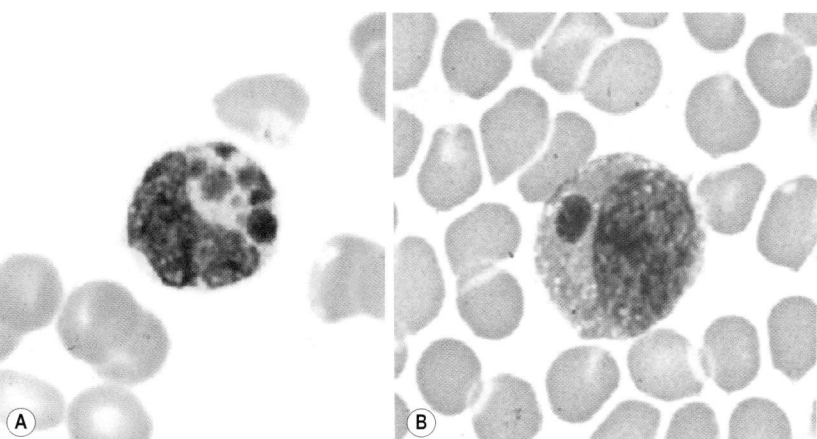

Figure 170-1. Morulae of *Ehrlichia chaffeensis* as seen on Wright stain of mononuclear cells in the peripheral blood of patients with human monocytic ehrlichiosis (**A**, multiple morulae; **B**, single).

for lengthy periods after treatment and resolution of disease (months to years), so presence of IgM is not always indicative of an acute infection.

PCR amplification assays to identify DNA from *Ehrlichia* and *Anaplasma* species are becoming more available at commercial and public health laboratories. Frequently, positive results can be obtained from acute-phase whole blood samples when serologic findings are negative.[47] PCR is most sensitive during early infection and detectability declines rapidly after the first 24 to 48 hours of antibiotic treatment. A variety of assays have been described for *E. chaffeensis* and *A. phagocytophilum*,[49] and specific gene targets for *E. ewingii* are now available.[50,51]

Identification of intraleukocytic morulae in blood smears, CSF sediment, or bone marrow aspirates has the advantages of being rapid and simple to perform, but does not differentiate genus and species. Artifacts, toxic granules, and overlying platelets sometimes can be misinterpreted as morulae. The peripheral blood smear should be stained with an eosin-azure type of stain (e.g., Wright, Diff-Quik, Giemsa). Morulae more often are identified in blood samples from patients with HGA (~25% to 75%) than HME (~25%), and therefore diagnostic sensitivity can be low.[47]

Isolation of *Ehrlichia* or *Anaplasma* by culture of blood, CSF, or other tissue samples requires a research laboratory, and primary isolation can take up to 7 weeks.[48,52] The sensitivity of other laboratory procedures compared with isolation has been investigated in only a few circumstances because isolation of these organisms is seldom undertaken.[47,53]

TREATMENT

When any rickettsial disease is suspected, treatment should be initiated before laboratory results are available. Doxycycline is the drug of choice for adults and children of all ages infected with all *Ehrlichia* and *Anaplasma* species.[20,33] For children, 4 mg/kg per day in 2 divided doses is recommended. For older children and adults, the dose is 100 mg twice daily. Most patients can be treated with oral therapy, but severely ill patients or patients unable to tolerate oral medications should receive doxycycline parenterally. Treatment length is variable, but typically is 7 to 10 days.

With appropriate therapy, most patients defervesce within 24 to 48 hours. Failure to respond to a tetracycline antibiotic within the first 3 days should suggest infection with another agent. Other symptoms generally subside over the next 2 weeks, although headaches, generalized weakness, and malaise can persist for several weeks after recovery from the acute febrile illness. Neurologic

sequelae and diminished performance in school have been reported in some children after severe *E. chaffeensis* disease.[19,33]

Chloramphenicol appears ineffective against *E. chaffeensis* when tested in cell culture systems,[54] and treatment failure has been reported with this drug in some patients.[17,55]

Antibiotics used frequently for empiric treatment of bacterial infections in febrile patients (e.g., β-lactam agents, macrolides, aminoglycosides, and fluoroquinolones) are ineffective in treating ehrlichiosis and anaplasmosis. Rifampin has been used successfully in the treatment of children with ehrlichiosis but is not the drug of choice.[56] Anecdotal evidence suggests that sulfa-containing antimicrobial agents may increase the severity of disease. Descriptions of pediatric patients with severe or fatal infections include reports of children in whom sulfonamides were administered for a week or longer before the disease was diagnosed correctly.[38,39,57] Whether use of sulfa drugs results in delayed diagnosis or exacerbation of infection remains unclear.

Special Considerations

Certain circumstances may warrant alternative treatment or prolonged treatment of infections. HGA has been treated successfully with rifampin during the third trimester of pregnancy.[58,59] In the two instances described, healthy uninfected infants were delivered after treatment of the pregnant mothers at 25 and 39 weeks' gestation.[59] Prolonged doxycycline therapy for over 2 weeks may be required in patients coinfected with *A. phagocytophilum* and *B. burgdorferi* (Lyme disease).[60]

PREVENTION

Avoidance of tick-infested habitats is the key to preventing ehrlichiosis, anaplasmosis, and other tickborne infections. However, because recreational activities of children in the spring and summer frequently occur in these environments, this measure may be impractical. In these circumstances, children exposed to tick-infested habitats should be subjected to prompt and careful inspection for crawling or attached ticks. Rapid discovery and removal of recently attached ticks lessen the risk of infection because ticks may require 24 to 48 hours of attachment before bacteria can be transmitted.[61] Application of approved skin and clothing repellents is a good protective measure. Prophylactic administration of doxycycline after a tick bite is not indicated because the overall risk of infection is low. No vaccine is available currently for humans.

Key Points. Diagnosis and Management of Anaplasmosis and Ehrlichiosis

MICROBIOLOGY AND VECTORS OF *ANAPLASMA* SPECIES IN THE U.S.

- Anaplasmosis is caused by the bacterium *Anaplasma phagocytophilum*
- The black-legged tick (*Ixodes scapularis*) is the vector to humans in New England and the north central U.S. and the western black-legged tick (*Ixodes pacificus*) is the vector in northern California

MICROBIOLOGY AND VECTORS OF *EHRLICHIA* SPECIES IN THE U.S.

- Ehrlichiosis is caused by at least two bacteria in the U.S., *Ehrlichia chaffeensis*, and less commonly, *E. ewingii*. A third species of *Ehrlichia*, most closely related to *E. muris* (*E. muris*-like), is a cause of human ehrlichiosis in the upper midwestern U.S.
- The lone star tick (*Amblyomma americanum*) is the primary vector of *E. chaffeensis*. The role of other tick species in transmission is unclear. *I. scapularis* is the suspected vector of the *E. muris*-like bacterium, but it has not been implicated clearly

DIAGNOSIS

- PCR of whole blood is available commercially, can be performed during the early acute phase of illness, and is highly specific; however, sensitivity decreases after 48 hours of appropriate treatment
- IFA serology for IgG antibodies to demonstrate a 4-fold increase in titers between acute and convalescent samples is the gold standard for serodiagnosis. IgM is less specific than IgG, and due to persistence, IgM may not indicate acute infection
- Visualization of morulae in leukocytes in peripheral blood during the first week of illness is possible in ≥20% of patients

TREATMENT

- Doxycycline is the treatment of choice for adults and children of all ages and is most effective if started within 5 days of symptom onset. Treatment should not be postponed while awaiting laboratory confirmation. Alternative antibiotics may not be as effective at preventing severe complications or death
- Recommended doxycycline dosage is 4 mg/kg/day orally/intravenously divided q12 hours, maximum dose 200 mg/day
- Treatment duration is at least 3 days after fever subsides and clinical improvement is documented (7 to 10 days total)

DESCRIPTION OF PATHOGEN AND EPIDEMIOLOGY

Francisella tularensis, the etiologic agent of tularemia, is a small, fastidious, nonspore-forming, aerobic gram-negative coccobacillus, which is nonmotile and nonpiliated and has a thin capsule composed mostly of lipid. Tularemia is a zoonotic disease; in addition to humans, who are accidental hosts, more than 100 animal species are affected, particularly ground squirrels, rabbits, hares, voles, and muskrat.[1] Organisms most frequently are transmitted by ticks and biting flies,[2] but infections can be transmitted by direct contact with rabbits (other than domesticated rabbits) or other infected animals or their aerosols, especially related to skinning, dressing, or eating infected animals.[3] Infections also can be transmitted through contaminated food or water[4] (possibly facilitated by the organism's survival within amebas), and by other biting vectors such as mosquitoes, fleas, and mites.[1,2,5]

Tularemia is the third most commonly reported tickborne disease in the United States. Domestic animals, especially cats[6] but also sheep, hamsters,[7] and prairie dogs,[8] occasionally have been implicated.[1,9] Fomites have been involved rarely, but person-to-person spread through contact with infected ulcers is not an important mode of transmission.[10] There is a potential use of *F. tularensis* as a biologic weapon by intentional aerosol release of organisms.

Although there are four subspecies, human disease is due primarily to two subspecies: *F. tularensis* subsp. *tularensis* (type A) and *F. tularensis* subsp. *holarctica* (formerly *palaearctica*; type B).[11] Type A strains are more virulent and are almost exclusively found in North America while type B strains are found primarily in Europe and Asia. Cottontail rabbits and three ticks, *Amblyomma americanum* (Lone Star tick), *Dermacentor andersoni* (wood tick), and *D. variabilis* (dog tick), are the main reservoir of the type A subspecies.[12] In the U.S. most cases occur from June through September, the season correlating with increased tick activity. Approximately 100 to 200 cases of tularemia have been reported annually. In 2007, 137 cases of tularemia were reported to the Centers for Disease Control and Prevention; the states with the highest numbers of cases were Missouri, Massachusetts, Arkansas, and South Dakota.[12] Approximately one-third of cases occurred in children and children 1 through 14 years of age had the highest attack rate.[12]

Subspecies B is less virulent and often results in subclinical infection, but can cause typhoidal infection in immunocompromised patients.[13] Subspecies B undergoes a waterborne cycle predominantly, with aquatic rodents such as muskrats, beavers, and ground voles as reservoirs. Transmission occurs via these rodents and mosquitoes. Subspecies B has a worldwide distribution in the northern hemisphere between latitudes 30°N and 71°N, which includes the continents of Europe, Asia, and North America.[11]

PATHOGENESIS AND IMMUNITY

The portal of entry most commonly is the skin via a tick bite, crushing of a tick found on an animal,[14] or a wound, but entry also can occur through the conjunctivae, oropharynx, respiratory tract, or rarely, the gastrointestinal tract. *F. tularensis* is highly contagious; an inoculum size as small as 10 organisms through the skin is sufficient to induce tularemia in experimental infection of humans.[15] Regardless of the route of inoculation, bacteria usually invade regional lymph nodes and are disseminated to other organs and lymph nodes via bacteremia. *F. tularensis* is a facultative intracellular pathogen that survives and multiplies within macrophages. Infection generally results in humoral and cellular immune responses and protection against reinfection.[16]

Protection is chiefly mediated by a cellular immune process in which bacteria are killed by macrophages activated by specifically committed T lymphocytes and producing nitric oxide,[17] but humoral immunity also has been demonstrated to contribute to immunity.[18] Protective immunity develops approximately 2 weeks after infection and is long-lasting.

CLINICAL MANIFESTATIONS

Important clues to the diagnosis of tularemia are a history of a tick bite, exposure to live or dead rabbits or squirrels (or other wild or domestic animals, including other rodents), or consumption of poorly cooked game meat. Clinical manifestations appear after an incubation period of 2 to 10 days (ranging up to 21 days). The most common clinical syndromes are ulceroglandular and glandular tularemia, which account for 80% of reported cases. Other manifestations include oropharyngeal (the second most common finding in children in some series[19]), oculoglandular, typhoidal, gastrointestinal, and pleuropulmonary syndromes (Table 171-1). Overall, the most common clinical sign is regional lymphadenopathy, which was present in 76% of 250 patients from Arkansas with tularemia.[5] Children with tularemia have constitutional symptoms, including fever, chills, malaise, and fatigue, and gastrointestinal symptoms more frequently than do adults.[9]

Ulceroglandular and Glandular Disease

Ulceroglandular disease is manifest as swollen tender lymph nodes in the inguinal, cervical, or axillary regions, usually from the bite of a bloodsucking arthropod. Lymphadenopathy can be accompanied by systemic symptoms and typically is preceded by a painful, swollen papule or at times a vesicle distal to the involved lymph nodes that can evolve into an ulcer with raised edges. Ulcers on the upper extremities usually result from exposure to infected mammals and occur in hunters and ranchers. Ulcerated lesions can persist for weeks if untreated. Lymphadenopathy in the inguinal region develops more frequently in patients with tick-associated infection than in those with rabbit-associated

TABLE 171-1. Clinical Forms of Tularemia

Clinical Form	Features
Glandular	Most common form; painful adenitis with or without a papule that becomes an ulcer distal to the adenitis; several lymph nodes or groups of lymph nodes can be involved; late suppuration common
Oculoglandular	Nodular conjunctivitis; painful preauricular lymphadenopathy
Oropharyngeal	Can simulate diphtheria; fever common; may have oral ulcers; associated with ingestion of contaminated meat or water
Typhoidal tularemia	Caused by ingestion of contaminated food; can have gastrointestinal tract ulceration; "sepsis" manifestation; high, prolonged fever usual
Gastrointestinal	Caused by ingestion of contaminated food; diarrhea and abdominal or back pain
Pneumonia	Rare in children; caused by aerosol exposure or hematogenous dissemination to lung; can be rapidly fatal

infection.[5] Frequently, multiple enlarged lymph nodes can be observed. In one pediatric series, most children had enlarged nodes in more than one cervical location or in a cervical chain and another regional location.[9,19] With mosquito-borne infection by type B strains in northern Finland, children had high fever and lymphadenopathy for 2 to 4 days, followed by low-grade fever and, commonly, a draining skin ulcer at the site of the mosquito bite.[11] Symptoms lasted a median of 26 days.

Oculoglandular Infection

Oculoglandular disease results from conjunctival infection, usually acquired from contaminated fingers. Multiple, small, well-demarcated nodules and ulcers can be seen on the conjunctiva in association with inflammation and edema. Pain is a major symptom, causing the patient to seek medical care early in the course of the infection, at times prior to the development of preauricular lymphadenopathy. The associated enlarged preauricular lymph node is painful, a feature unique to oculoglandular infection with this pathogen and with *Coccidioides*, which distinguishes it from the oculoglandular syndrome in cat-scratch disease, sporotrichosis, tuberculosis, and syphilis.[20]

Oropharyngeal Infection

In the oropharyngeal form of tularemia, organisms enter the oropharyngeal mucosa from ingestion of inadequately cooked infected meat or contaminated milk or water.[21] The clinical presentation is tonsillitis with throat pain out of proportion to the visible lesions and cervical lymphadenitis. Oral ulceration can develop and there may be an oropharyngeal pseudomembrane similar to infection with *Corynebacterium diphtheriae*. Fever and other systemic symptoms can occur and the lymphadenitis may suppurate. In the U.S., this form occurs most commonly in children.

Typhoidal Tularemia

The symptoms and signs of typhoidal tularemia are similar to those of acute septicemia of any etiology and include high fever, chills, malaise, headache, vomiting, myalgia, and on occasion, photophobia. Hepatosplenomegaly is seen frequently and diarrhea is seen occasionally, but lymphadenopathy is not a prominent feature. When typhoidal tularemia results from the ingestion of contaminated food, necrotic lesions can occur in the bowel.[5] Patients generally do not have cutaneous ulcers or adenopathy. Untreated cases can have a fatal outcome or resolve after persistent fever for 2 to 3 weeks or longer. Patients also can have persistent diarrhea and abdominal or low-back pain from gastrointestinal tract tularemia without septicemic symptoms.

Pneumonia

The pneumonic form of tularemia occurs almost exclusively in adults but has been reported in children exposed to an aerosol from an infected rabbit carcass run over by a lawn mower.[22] Intentional aerosol release as a biologic weapon would most commonly cause pneumonia (or typhoidal tularemia).[23] Pneumonia is the most common manifestation of tularemia acquired by laboratory workers. The usual abnormality is a unilateral lower-lobe infiltrate, at times with associated pleural effusion and/or hilar adenopathy. This form of infection can be severe or fatal. Pneumonia also can result from hematogenous dissemination to the lungs from typhoidal (30% to 80% of cases) or ulceroglandular (10% to 15% of cases) infections. A case of fever and a pulmonary nodule secondary to *F. tularensis* has been reported in a stem cell transplant recipient.

Occasional Sites

Rare manifestations of infection have included subcutaneous nodules resembling sporotrichosis, meningitis with a mononuclear cell predominance and hypoglycorrhachia,[24] encephalitis,

pericarditis, endocarditis, peritonitis, and osteomyelitis.[10] A variety of rashes, including maculopapular, pustular, and erythema nodosum, have been seen.

LABORATORY FINDINGS AND DIAGNOSIS

Gram-stain smears prepared from exudate or tissue sections rarely show weakly staining gram-negative coccobacilli in an extracellular or intracellular location. Organisms can be identified using an indirect immunofluorescent antibody test. The histopathology of affected lymph nodes shows follicular hyperplasia with conglomerates of macrophages, epithelioid cell granulomas, and caseating necrosis, findings similar to those seen in tuberculosis[16] or *Bartonella* infection. A polymerase chain reaction assay to detect bacterial DNA in clinical specimens such as swabs of ulcers showed good sensitivity and excellent specificity.[25-27]

Culture of *F. tularensis* is not routinely performed in clinical laboratories because of the potential for aerosol inhalation and infection of laboratory personnel. Additionally, specimens should be collected cautiously and the laboratory notified when specimens suspected of harboring *F. tularensis* are submitted. Biosafety level 2 is recommended for clinical laboratory work and transfer of cultures to biosafety level 3 as soon as *F. tularensis* is suspected.[28] An enriched medium such as cysteine heart blood agar supplemented with 9% chocolatized sheep blood, chocolate agar, or buffered charcoal yeast extract agar (used for culture of *Legionella*) incubated aerobically is required for isolation of *F. tularensis* from clinical specimens.[28] Colonies are 1 to 2 mm in diameter, blue-grey, round, smooth, and slightly mucoid. Direct isolation can be achieved from ulcer scrapings, lymph node biopsy specimens, gastric washings, sputum, and occasionally, culture of blood using a radiometric or nonradiometric technique.[29] Inoculation of laboratory animals such as mice or rabbits is a sensitive means of isolation of *F. tularensis* but is no longer used routinely for diagnosis.

The laboratory diagnosis of tularemia is most often confirmed by serologic testing using a tube agglutination or microagglutination assay. Antibodies generally are detectable at the end of the second or during the third week of illness. A fourfold increase or decrease in titer using a serum agglutination test is diagnostic; a single titer of >1 : 160 by tube agglutination or >1 : 128 by microagglutination is a presumptive positive result but can reflect past infection.[28] Infected patients can have convalescent titers >1 : 1000 and a prozone phenomenon can be observed. Nonspecific cross-reactions can occur in patients infected with bacteria from the genus *Brucella* and certain other gram-negative bacteria.[30] The microagglutination assay is more sensitive than the tube agglutination test.[31] An enzyme immunoassay using lipopolysaccharide antigens and immunoblot confirmation[32] or outer-membrane proteins[33] is highly sensitive. An immunochromatographic test (ICT) to rapidly detect *F. tularensis*-specific antibodies in sera has been developed and has similar sensitivity and specificity to the microagglutination assay.[34] Assay for immunoglobulin M (IgM) antibodies is not useful because IgM antibodies are not present earlier than IgG antibodies and can persist for years.[28,33] Empiric antimicrobial therapy must often be initiated before serologic confirmation of infection is possible.

TREATMENT

A 7-day course of streptomycin, gentamicin,[35] or amikacin is the treatment of choice for tularemia and is expected to produce defervescence within a few days and is associated with a low relapse rate.[5] Streptomycin is given intramuscularly twice daily at a dose of 30 to 40 mg/kg per day (which can be reduced by half after 3 days of therapy); gentamicin is given every 8 hours and can be administered intramuscularly or intravenously. A Jarisch–Herxheimer reaction has been described early during streptomycin treatment.[10] Ciprofloxacin given for 10 to 14 days (or possibly imipenem-cilastatin) is the best alternative to aminoglycosides or is used after relapse following aminoglycoside therapy.[36,37] Although ciprofloxacin is not approved for treatment of children with tularemia, courses of at least 10 days have been used successfully to treat infected children.[37,38] Treatment with tetracycline or chloramphenicol results in a prompt clinical response, but these agents are not bactericidal and relapse occurs in at least half of patients after cessation of therapy. A limited number of cases of pneumonia have been treated successfully with erythromycin.[10] In vitro susceptibility does not necessarily predict clinical efficacy. For example, *F. tularensis* is susceptible to third-generation cephalosporins in vitro, but all of 8 children treated with ceftriaxone failed to improve, indicating that this therapy is ineffective.[39] Suppurative lymph nodes may require surgical drainage. In one pediatric series, late suppuration after antibiotic therapy was noted in 33% of children. In these cases, the aspirated or excised material was sterile.[9] The mortality rate for tularemia currently is <3%.[9,10]

In Finnish patients infected with *F. tularensis* subsp. *holarctica* (type B) organisms, the impact of antibiotics on the clinical course was uncertain.[11] By in vitro susceptibility testing, strains are susceptible to tetracyclines, aminoglycosides, quinolones, chloramphenicol, and rifampin. Strains generally are resistant to β-lactam antibiotics, carbapenems, aztreonam, and macrolide antibiotics.[40,41]

PREVENTION

The key to preventing tularemia is interruption of transmission, which can be achieved by prevention or timely detection of tick bites, avoidance of handling sick or dead rabbits or rodents, use of rubber gloves to handle game meat, and thorough cooking of meat. An investigational live-attenuated vaccine given pre-exposure using a multiple puncture technique was used in the U.S. for research personnel with exposure to *F. tularensis* but is no longer available. This vaccine prevents respiratory tract infection in laboratory personnel but does not prevent ulceroglandular infection.[2,17,42] A 14-day course of doxycycline or ciprofloxacin has been recommended for prophylaxis of exposed persons following an intentional aerosol release of organisms or exposure in a laboratory.[23]

Key Points. Diagnosis and Management of Tularemia

MICROBIOLOGY
- Small, aerobic gram-negative coccobacillus
- Nutritionally fastidious, requires enriched medium

EPIDEMIOLOGY
- Zoonotic infection
- Transmitted primarily by ticks, biting flies, or by direct contact with rabbits or other infected animals or their aerosols
- Summer occurrence
- Potential for bioterrorism via intentional aerosol release of organisms

CLINICAL FEATURES
- Incubation period: 2 to 10 days (up to 21 days)
- Most common presentation is lymphadenitis ("glandular") with or without painful papule or ulcer at inoculation site; often lymphadenitis occurs at more than one site
- Other presentations: oropharyngeal, oculoglandular, typhoidal, gastrointestinal, pleuropulmonary
- Fever is common

DIAGNOSIS
- Fourfold rise in serum IgG antibody titer is confirmatory
- Organism can be isolated from ulcers using enriched medium but is a biohazard for laboratory personnel

TREATMENT
- Gentamicin, streptomycin, or amikacin for 7 days
- Alternative: ciprofloxacin for 10 or more days
- Ceftriaxone is ineffective; relapses occur after tetracycline

---

172 *Haemophilus influenzae*

Joseph W. St. Geme III

Haemophilus influenzae was first isolated by Pfeiffer during the 1889 influenza pandemic.[1] For a time, *H. influenzae* was believed to be the causative agent of influenza and originally was called the *influenza bacillus*. However, subsequent studies demonstrated the fallacy of this notion, and the organism ultimately was given the genus name *Haemophilus*, meaning *blood loving*. The species name was chosen to reflect the historical association with influenza.

In 1995, the nucleotide sequence of the entire genome of *H. influenzae* strain Rd KW20 was published, representing the first organism to be sequenced completely. The annotated sequence of this strain is available at http://www.ncbi.nlm.nih.gov/bioproject. More recently, a number of additional clinical isolates have been sequenced[2] (see http://www.ncbi.nlm.nih.gov/bioproject).

THE PATHOGEN

H. influenzae is a nonmotile, nonspore-forming, gram-negative bacterium and typically appears as small coccobacilli, roughly 1 × 0.3 μm in size, although some isolates grow as long filaments. *H. influenzae* can grow aerobically or anaerobically. Aerobic growth requires two supplements known as factors X and V, whereas anaerobic growth requires only factor X. Factor X can be supplied by heat-stable iron-containing pigments, including hemin and hemoglobin, both of which represent a source of protoporphyrin IX. Factor V can be supplied by nicotinamide adenine dinucleotide, nicotinamide adenine dinucleotide phosphate, or nicotinamide nucleoside. Factor V is present in erythrocytes but must be released to sustain growth; as a consequence, standard blood agar is an unsatisfactory medium for propagating *H. influenzae*. Optimal growth is achieved on media enriched with erythrocytes that have been disrupted by heating (e.g., chocolate agar) or by peptic digestion (e.g., Fildes medium). Incubation in the presence of 5% to 10% carbon dioxide has a beneficial effect on the growth of some strains and is thus recommended for primary isolation.

Isolates of *H. influenzae* are classified according to their polysaccharide capsule.[3] As detailed in Table 172-1, six structurally and antigenically distinct capsular types (serotypes) designated a through f exist. In addition, strains can be nonencapsulated; these strains are defined on the basis of their failure to react with typing antisera against capsular serotypes a through f and are referred to as nontypable. Worldwide, most clinical isolates are either type b or nontypable.[4,5]

Isolates also can be separated into subgroups called biotypes by using biochemical tests that determine the production of indole and the presence of ornithine decarboxylase and urease.[6] These

TABLE 172-1. Chemical Composition of the Capsule of *Haemophilus influenzae*

Type	Sugar	*N*-Acetyl	Phosphate
A	Glucose	–	+
B	Ribose, ribiol	–	+
C	Galactose	–	+
D	Hexose	–	+
E	Hexosamine	+	+
F	Galactosamine	+	+

TABLE 172-2. *Haemophilus influenzae* Biotypes

Biotype	Indole	Urease	Ornithine Decarboxylase
I	+	+	+
II	+	+	–
III	–	+	–
IV	–	+	+
V	+	–	+
VI	–	–	+
VII	+	–	–
VIII	–	–	–

reactions define eight biotypes designated I through VIII (Table 172-2). Data generated from biotyping studies indicate that type b isolates are predominantly biotype I.[7] Nontypable strains also can be biotype I but in most collections are more often biotype II or III.[8] Clinical isolates that are biotypes IV, V, VI, VII, or VIII are relatively uncommon and are almost always nontypable.

Multilocus enzyme electrophoresis and a variety of other molecular techniques have been used to examine relatedness of isolates of *H. influenzae*. Studies using multilocus enzyme electrophoresis demonstrate that the population structure of encapsulated *H. influenzae* is clonal, with most isolates falling into a few common clonal groups.[9] Nontypable strains are genetically distinct and more heterogeneous than encapsulated *H. influenzae* and appear to lack clonality.[10]

EPIDEMIOLOGY

In the past, *H. influenzae* type b (Hib) strains were found in the upper respiratory tract of 3% to 5% of children and a small percentage of adults. In general, colonization rates with type b strains are even lower now because of routine immunization of infants with conjugate Hib vaccines, although exceptions exist.[11] Non-type b encapsulated *H. influenzae* stains are present in the nasopharynx of <2% of individuals, whereas nontypable strains colonize the respiratory tract of 40% to 80% of children and adults.[12]

Until approximately 1990, Hib was the leading cause of bacterial meningitis in children younger than 5 years in the United States, accounting for 8000 to 10,000 cases per year.[13] Hib also was the predominant etiology of epiglottitis and a major cause of pyogenic arthritis, pneumonia, pericarditis, and facial cellulitis in young children. Approximately 1 in 200 children in the U.S. experienced invasive (bacteremic) disease with this organism before the age of 5 years, with a peak incidence at 6 to 7 months of age. Invasive disease was more frequent in boys, African Americans, Alaskan Eskimos, Apache and Navajo Indians, childcare center attendees, and children living in overcrowded conditions.[14–18] Medical conditions predisposing to invasive Hib disease included sickle-cell disease, asplenia, human immunodeficiency virus (HIV) infection, certain immunodeficiency syndromes, and

malignancies. Since 1990, the incidence of invasive Hib disease in the U.S. has fallen by over 95%, with a minority of cases now occurring in young children.[19–22] However, recent shortages of vaccine have resulted in small clusters of cases in underimmunized young children.[23] In addition, there has been a modest resurgence of cases in recent years in parts of the U.S. and other developed countries.[24,25] Some children fail to respond to Hib vaccination and develop invasive Hib diseases, in most cases reflecting underlying immunodeficiency.[25,26]

Despite the overall successful reduction in invasive Hib disease in the U.S. and other industrialized countries, Hib remains a common pathogen in many developing countries, where routine vaccines still are not available to most of the population. In these countries, Hib remains the leading cause of bacterial meningitis and the second leading cause of bacterial pneumonia.[5,27] Based on data from the World Health Organization, in 2009 vaccines against Hib were unavailable in 33 countries, most notably populous nations in Asia and parts of Africa (http://www.who.int/immunization/topics/hib/en/). Consistent with this information, as of 2009 only 38% of infants worldwide had received 3 doses of Hib vaccine by age 1 year (http://www.who.int/immunization/topics/hib/en/).

Nontypable strains of *H. influenzae* are a common cause of localized respiratory tract disease in both children and adults.[28,29] In children, these organisms are the most common cause of purulent conjunctivitis, the most common or second most common cause of otitis media, and a frequent etiology of sinusitis. In children in developing countries, nontypable strains are a frequent cause of pneumonia and an important source of mortality. In adults, nontypable *H. influenzae* is an especially common etiologic agent of community-associated pneumonia and exacerbations of underlying lung disease and also accounts for a substantial fraction of cases of otitis media and sinusitis. Beyond producing localized disease, nontypable *H. influenzae* is an occasional cause of serious systemic disease such as septicemia, meningitis, and pyogenic arthritis, especially in neonates and individuals with compromised immunity.[30,31]

Disease due to non-type b encapsulated strains occurs occasionally, in both developed and underdeveloped countries. For example, among children in Papua New Guinea, roughly one-quarter of *H. influenzae* isolates associated with acute lower respiratory tract infection and approximately 15% of isolates associated with meningitis are non-type b encapsulated strains.[32,33] Based on recent reports, in the U.S., Canada, and Europe, *H. influenzae* type a, *H. influenzae* type e, and *H. influenzae* type f invasive disease are increasing in frequency and are fatal in up to 20% of children and 30% of adults.[34–39]

PATHOGENESIS

Generally, *H. influenzae* is transmitted by airborne droplets or by direct contact with respiratory tract secretions. Colonization with a particular strain can persist for weeks to months, and most individuals remain asymptomatic throughout this period.[40] A variety of bacterial factors appear to influence the process of respiratory tract colonization. For example, the lipid A component of *H. influenzae* lipopolysaccharide (LPS), peptidoglycan fragments, and a surface-associated glycerophosphodiester phosphodiesterase called protein D or GlpQ (which allows choline to be transferred from the host to the bacterial surface) cause ciliostasis and thereby interfere with mucociliary clearance.[41–44] In addition, both pilus and nonpilus adherence factors exist and are known to mediate binding to mucus and to respiratory epithelium.[45–49] Like other mucosal pathogens, *H. influenzae* produces IgA1 protease, an enzyme that cleaves human IgA1 and presumably facilitates evasion of the local immune response.[50] Bacterial antigenic variation, entry into host cells, penetration between host cells (paracytosis), and biofilm formation may also promote evasion of local immunity and persistence on mucosal surfaces.[51–59]

In certain circumstances, colonization is followed by contiguous spread within the respiratory tract, resulting in local disease

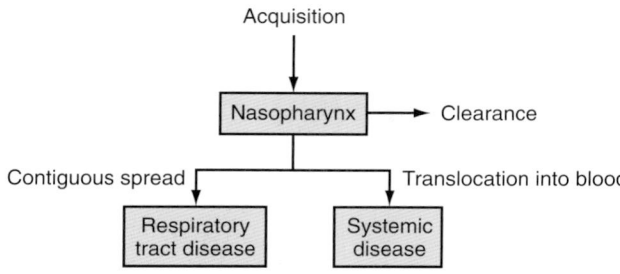

Figure 172-1. Pathogenic sequence for disease caused by *Haemophilus influenzae.*

in the middle ear, sinuses, conjunctiva, or lungs (Figure 172-1). Anatomic factors, deficiencies in local immune function, viral respiratory infection, exposure to cigarette smoke, and allergies predispose to localized respiratory tract disease.[28] On occasion, bacteria penetrate the nasopharyngeal epithelial barrier and enter the bloodstream (see Figure 172-1). The determinants of this event remain poorly defined but may include bacterial LPS.[60] Of note, penetration of the epithelial barrier appears to involve the separation of tight junctions, which allows bacteria to migrate between cells and into the subepithelial space.[61] In most cases, the bacteremia is probably transient. However, in nonimmune hosts, intravascular bacteria that express the type b capsule are sometimes able to survive, replicate, and disseminate to distant sites. In the absence of specific antibody, the type b polysaccharide capsule promotes resistance to serum bactericidal activity and to phagocytosis. A variety of other factors also have been implicated in resistance to serum killing.[62–64]

IMMUNITY

The age-associated susceptibility to Hib disease is inversely related to the presence of serum bactericidal antibody,[65] much of which is directed against the type b polysaccharide capsule.[66] Antibody against the type b capsule activates complement-mediated bactericidal killing and facilitates phagocytosis by opsonization.[67] Based on studies performed in the pre-Hib vaccine era, during the first 3 to 6 months of life, most infants have protective levels of maternally acquired anticapsular antibody. These levels gradually decline, reach a nadir by 6 to 12 months of age, and remain low for the next few years. By the age of 5 years, virtually all individuals have acquired anticapsular antibody,[68,69] in some cases as a result of colonization with Hib and in others probably from exposure to commensals (e.g., *Escherichia coli* K100) or ingested food possessing cross-reactive epitopes.[70] Antibodies to noncapsular antigens such as LPS and outer membrane proteins also contribute to serum bactericidal and opsonic activity.[71,72]

A number of investigators have examined the immune response to infection with Hib. At the time of infection, serum antibodies against the serotype b capsule are low or absent. In children younger than 2 years, levels remain low during convalescence[73] because of an age-related deficiency in the ability to respond to polysaccharide antigens (T-lymphocyte-independent antigens). In older children, infection stimulates a brisk increase in the level of anticapsular antibody. Natural infection also is associated with the formation of antibodies to LPS and surface-associated proteins, and these antibodies contribute to protection against recurrent Hib disease.

The complement system is critical in host defense against Hib disease, and patients with congenital deficiencies of certain complement components, including C2, C3, and C4, have increased susceptibility to Hib disease.[74] Type b organisms are capable of activating both the classic and the alternate complement pathways.[74,75] Early in the course of infection in nonimmune hosts, the alternate pathway probably is more important, whereas at later stages, the antibody-dependent classic pathway is more likely to predominate. Clearance of bacteremia with type b organisms also

requires an intact mononuclear phagocytic system, thus explaining the higher incidence of Hib septicemia in patients with splenic dysfunction.

Immunity to nontypable organisms involves both systemic and local antibody responses. Moreover, evidence suggests that systemic priming functions to enhance the local response. Based on studies of patients with otitis media and bronchitis, it appears that the immune response to nontypable *H. influenzae* often is strain specific. For example, Faden and colleagues observed a population of children prospectively for 2 years and identified 8 subjects who experienced 2 separate episodes of acute otitis media from nontypable *H. influenzae*.[76] In all 8 patients, the second episode was caused by a different strain. Serum was collected from 6 of these patients at the time of the second episode and was found uniformly to contain bactericidal antibody against the first strain. However, only 3 of these 6 samples possessed measurable bactericidal antibody against the second strain, thus indicating the absence of cross-reacting bactericidal activity. Consistent with these findings, Musher and associates found that adsorption of normal human serum with nontypable *H. influenzae* removed bactericidal activity against the adsorbing isolate but not necessarily against other nontypable strains.[77] Major targets of the antibody response to infection include the P2 major outer membrane protein, the HMW1/HMW2 and Hia adhesins, and LPS. Recent evidence indicates that the P6 outer membrane protein is a potent and selective inducer of macrophages and proinflammatory cytokines.[78]

CLINICAL MANIFESTATIONS

Haemophilus influenzae Type b Infection

Meningitis

Meningitis is the most common and most serious form of Hib disease. Symptoms typically include fever, irritability, lethargy, and vomiting. Antecedent symptoms of an upper respiratory tract infection are common. Occasionally, the course is fulminant, with rapid neurologic deterioration leading to respiratory arrest.[79] Shock is present in 20% of cases of meningitis and can be associated with coagulopathy and purpura.[80] An association of Hib meningitis and anemia is clear and appears to be related, at least partly, to adsorption of capsular antigen to the red cell surface with secondary immune-mediated hemolysis.[81] Complications of Hib meningitis include subdural effusion or empyema, ischemic or hemorrhagic cortical infarction, cerebritis, ventriculitis, intracerebral abscess, and hydrocephalus. The overall mortality rate is approximately 5%. Among survivors, between 5% and 10% have permanent sensorineural hearing loss, and about 30% have some other significant handicap. If subtle neurologic deficits are sought, up to one-half of survivors have sequelae.[82–84]

Epiglottitis

Epiglottitis is a life-threatening infection involving cellulitis of the epiglottis and the aryepiglottic folds. Complete obliteration of the vallecular and piriform sinuses is typical, and acute airway obstruction can occur. Most affected children are between 2 and 7 years of age. Symptoms often are sudden in onset, and classically include high fever, sore throat, stridor, and dyspnea progressing rapidly to dysphagia, pooling of secretions, and drooling. In children younger than 2 years, the fever can be low grade, a croup-like cough can be present, and dysphagia and drooling sometimes are lacking. Regardless of age, the patient usually is restless and anxious and adopts a sitting position with the neck extended and the chin protruding to reduce airway obstruction. Abrupt deterioration can occur within a few hours and result in death unless an artificial airway is established. Direct laryngoscopy at the time of controlled placement of an endotracheal tube reveals a red and swollen epiglottis and swollen aryepiglottic folds (Figure 172-2A, B). On a lateral neck radiograph, the swollen epiglottis produces the so-called *thumb sign* (see Figure 172-2C).

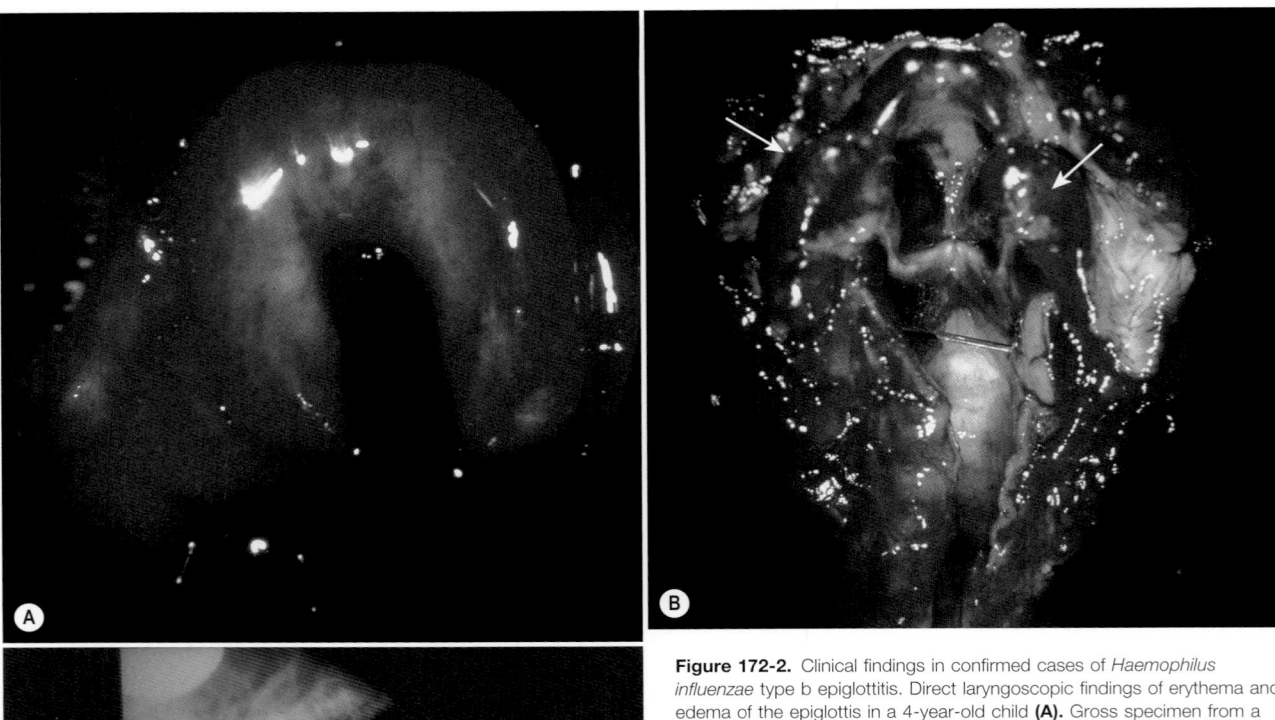

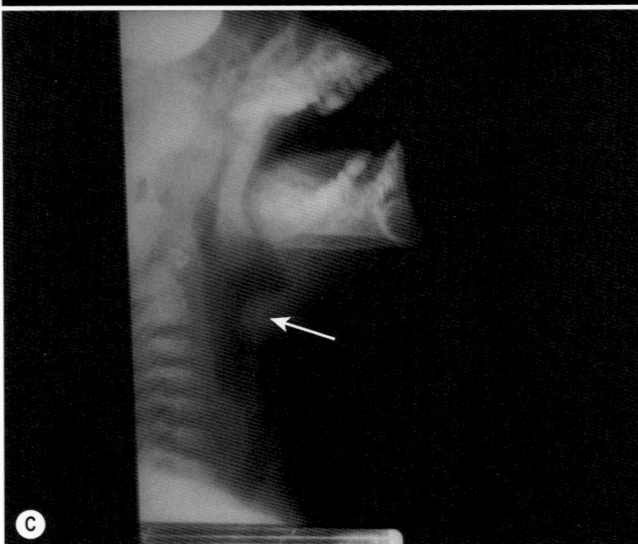

Figure 172-2. Clinical findings in confirmed cases of *Haemophilus influenzae* type b epiglottitis. Direct laryngoscopic findings of erythema and edema of the epiglottis in a 4-year-old child **(A).** Gross specimen from a fatal case shows erythema and edema predominantly of arytenoids structures (arrows) and aryepiglottic folds **(B).** Lateral neck radiograph in another case shows thumb-print appearance (arrow) of the swollen epiglottis **(C).** (Courtesy of S.S. Long.)

Pneumonia

Patients with Hib pneumonia typically have a consolidative pulmonary infiltrate. In 50% of cases, evidence of pleural involvement can be seen on the initial chest radiograph, and up to 90% of these patients have pleural fluid recoverable by thoracentesis. Generally, Hib pneumonia is more insidious in onset than is pneumonia from *Staphylococcus aureus* or *Streptococcus pneumoniae*. Nearly one-quarter of patients have concomitant meningitis or epiglottitis. An important complication is contiguous spread to the pericardium and subsequent purulent pericarditis, which is manifest as severe dyspnea (grunting in infants), tachycardia, and cardiac failure. Although patients with Hib pneumonia often have a persistent pleural reaction with secondary restrictive lung function at the time of hospital discharge, long-term abnormalities are rare.

Osteoarticular Infection

Historically, Hib was the most common cause of pyogenic arthritis in children younger than 2 years,[85] usually with a single large weight-bearing joint (hip, knee, or ankle) involved. In 10% to 20% of cases, contiguous osteomyelitis is present. Osteomyelitis alone is unusual. The response to systemic antibiotics combined with prompt drainage of the joint is dramatic, but long-term follow-up is important because residual joint dysfunction can occur. On occasion, culture-negative arthritis develops during treatment of *H. influenzae* meningitis, presumably as a result of immune complex deposition in the joint.[86] In 75% of patients with reactive arthritis, signs of joint inflammation begin 1 week or more after therapy is begun.

Bacteremic Cellulitis

Cellulitis is the result of a metastatic focus of bacteremia and is seen predominantly in young children. Typically, the patient is febrile and has a warm, tender area of erythema or violaceous discoloration on the cheek or in the periorbital area. Facial (buccal) cellulitis almost invariably occurs in children younger than 1 year. The age of the child, the location of the cellulitis, and the occasional distinctive violaceous color should suggest the etiology (Figure 172-3). Aspirate cultures, either from the center of

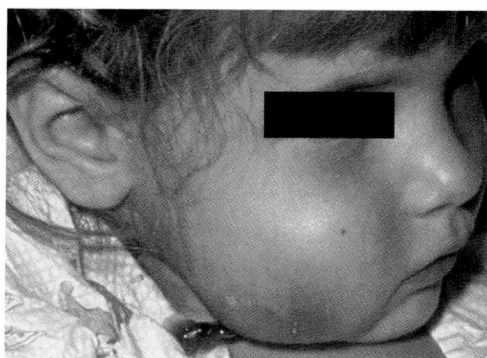

Figure 172-3. Buccal cellulitis in a 14-month-old girl whose blood culture yielded *Haemophilus influenzae* type b. Note distinctive site of cellulitis on the lower cheek and violaceous color. (Courtesy of S.S. Long.)

the lesion or the leading edge, usually yield the organism. Concomitant bacteremia is present in most patients, and another focus of infection such as meningitis develops in approximately 10% of cases.[87,88] Cellulitis that occurs as a complication of trauma to the skin is not caused by *H. influenzae*.

Other

Other manifestations of Hib disease include occult bacteremia (which is rarely self-limited), otitis media, orbital cellulitis, endophthalmitis, urinary tract infection, and peritonitis. In addition, purulent pericarditis can result from direct seeding from bacteremia.

Infection Due to Nontypable *Haemophilus influenzae*

Respiratory Tract Infection

Studies examining the bacteriology of acute otitis media (AOM) consistently demonstrate *H. influenzae* as the most common or second most common pathogen.[89–92] Among *H. influenzae* isolates, >90% are nontypable. According to studies reported from the U.S. and Scandinavia, the peak age-specific incidence of *H. influenzae* AOM occurs between the ages of 6 and 15 months.[93,94] Characteristic manifestations include ear pain, fever, irritability, sleep disturbance, and otorrhea. On examination, the tympanic membrane usually is red or yellow and bulging, with distorted landmarks. Pneumatic otoscopy reveals decreased mobility, indicative of middle ear fluid. In addition to producing AOM, nontypable *H. influenzae* is the pathogen implicated most commonly in otitis media with effusion and accounts for >40% of cases with positive tympanocentesis cultures.[95,96] Nontypable *H. influenzae* also has been associated with dual infection of the conjunctiva and the middle ear.[97] These infections occur primarily during the winter months and have been termed the *conjunctivitis-otitis syndrome*. Nontypable strains also are an important cause of isolated conjunctivitis (see Chapter 173, Other *Haemophilus* Species).

Among individuals with acute sinusitis, *S. pneumoniae* and *H. influenzae* account for nearly three-quarters of all bacterial isolates recovered,[98] with most *H. influenzae* strains being nontypable. The majority of patients with sinusitis have persistent nasal discharge or cough that lasts longer than 10 days without improvement. Others present acutely with high fever and purulent nasal discharge, and a third group have initial improvement of a respiratory tract illness with subsequent resurgence of fever and purulent discharge. Physical examination often reveals tenderness over the involved paranasal sinuses. Data on the microbiology of chronic sinusitis are limited but suggest that nontypable *H. influenzae* is a prominent pathogen.[99] Several studies have examined the predictive value of surface cultures of the nose, throat, or nasopharynx

in patients with acute or chronic sinusitis. Although the organisms isolated from direct aspiration of infected sinuses generally are recovered from surface cultures, they are not consistently the predominant organisms. As a result, surface cultures are of minimal value in establishing an etiologic agent.

Because sputum frequently is contaminated by pharyngeal bacterial flora, interpretation of the growth of *H. influenzae* from sputum culture is difficult. However, there is substantial evidence that nontypable *H. influenzae* causes bacterial pneumonia, especially in children in developing countries, elderly people, and patients with underlying lung disease or aspiration syndromes. Among children in developing countries with clinical evidence of pneumonia, lung aspiration studies demonstrate that bacteria can be recovered more than 60% of the time; up to half of these isolates are nontypable *H. influenzae*.[100]

Meningitis

Nontypable *H. influenzae* is an occasional cause of meningitis and usually spreads by direct extension from a contiguous focus of infection, thus contrasting with Hib. Most individuals with nontypable *H. influenzae* meningitis have a predisposing factor, such as sinusitis, otitis media, head trauma, or another anomaly resulting in cerebrospinal fluid (CSF) leak. In patients with recurrent bacterial meningitis, nontypable *H. influenzae* is the second most common cause (after *S. pneumoniae*) and generally enters the central nervous system via a communication between a parameningeal site and the subarachnoid space.[101]

Neonatal Infection

Nontypable *H. influenzae* is a well-recognized neonatal pathogen.[102–106] (Non-type b encapsulated strains occasionally also have been implicated in this setting.) In most cases, *H. influenzae* produces an early-onset neonatal syndrome similar to that caused by group B streptococci. Disease occurs primarily in premature neonates and is associated with a mortality rate of nearly 50%. Symptoms develop in most infants within the first few hours of life, with pneumonia and respiratory distress dominating the clinical picture. Meningitis occurs infrequently. *H. influenzae* usually can be isolated from the genitourinary tract of mothers of infected infants, often in association with maternal postpartum endometritis. Paired maternal–infant isolates have been confirmed to be the same strain by a variety of methods.[107,108] Studies have indicated that a large percentage of these isolates are biotype IV, a subgroup of nontypable *H. influenzae* found uncommonly at other sites of infection.[104] Analysis of these biotype IV strains by multilocus enzyme electrophoresis indicates divergence from other *H. influenzae*, and chromosomal DNA hybridization studies and 16S rRNA gene sequencing suggest that these strains represent a distinct *Haemophilus* species most similar to *H. haemolyticus*,[109,110] leading to the designation *Haemophilus* cryptic genospecies.

Other

Nontypable *H. influenzae* has been reported rarely as a cause of endocarditis, pericarditis, pyogenic arthritis, osteomyelitis, epiglottitis, cellulitis, urinary tract infection, intra-abdominal infection, and occult bacteremia.[28]

DIAGNOSIS

Consideration of the diagnosis of meningitis, epiglottitis, pneumonia, pyogenic arthritis, or cellulitis usually is prompted by the history and physical examination. In most cases of invasive Hib disease, blood cultures are positive. When meningitis is present, bacteria almost always can be recovered from CSF. In patients with epiglottitis, culture of the epiglottis usually is positive, but specimens should be obtained only after establishment of an artificial airway. *H. influenzae* often is cultivated from samples of pleural fluid, joint fluid, or pericardial fluid in affected patients. In roughly 70% of patients with *H. influenzae* meningitis, Gram stain of the

CSF is positive for gram-negative coccobacilli. The sensitivity of CSF Gram stain correlates with bacterial density and ranges from 0% in the presence of <10^3 colony-forming units per milliliter to nearly 100% when the density is ≥10^5 colony-forming units per milliliter.[111] (The sensitivity of Gram stain is higher when CSF is cytocentrifuged.)

Type b capsular polysaccharide is secreted during bacterial growth, and detection of capsular antigen can aid in diagnosis. Methods available for this purpose include latex particle agglutination, coagglutination, countercurrent immunoelectrophoresis, and enzyme immunoassay. Serum, CSF, urine, and other normally sterile body fluids are suitable for examination for capsular antigen. Antigen detection techniques can be useful in patients who have previously received antibiotic therapy and have sterile cultures. In cases of culture-proven meningitis, capsular antigen is detected roughly 90% of the time in CSF and even more frequently in concentrated urine. False-positive reactions occur occasionally as a result of cross-reactivity with E. coli, S. pneumoniae, staphylococci, or meningococci. Of note, Hib conjugate vaccines can produce positive reactions in urine and CSF for days to weeks after vaccination.[112–116]

Because H. influenzae is a common commensal organism in the upper respiratory tract, establishing H. influenzae as an etiology of localized respiratory tract disease is challenging. Procedures such as tympanocentesis, sinus aspiration, tracheal or lung aspiration, bronchoscopy, and bronchoalveolar lavage can provide a definitive diagnosis, but these procedures generally are reserved for circumstances in which a specific microbiologic diagnosis is required, as in patients with persistent or recurrent infection or underlying immunodeficiency.

TREATMENT

Historically, ampicillin was effective therapy for invasive H. influenzae disease. However, resistance to ampicillin now is common in isolates of H. influenzae, with the incidence in the range of 40% in some communities.[117,118] Ampicillin should never be used alone as empiric therapy of invasive disease. Ampicillin resistance usually is related to plasmid-mediated production of β-lactamase but occasionally is due to decreased affinity of certain penicillin binding proteins (in particular PBP3).[119] To detect both forms of resistance, a β-lactamase assay should be performed along with disk or broth-dilution susceptibility tests. The third-generation cephalosporins are the therapy of choice for H. influenzae meningitis. Both cefotaxime and ceftriaxone have potent activity against H. influenzae (including isolates that produce β-lactamase and isolates with an altered penicillin-binding protein) and achieve high levels in CSF. For infections outside the central nervous system, cefuroxime or ampicillin-sulbactam are effective as suitable alternatives.

In patients with invasive H. influenzae disease, antibiotic therapy represents only one component of management. For patients with meningitis, optimal ventilation and judicious administration of fluid are important (see Chapter 40, Acute Bacterial Meningitis Beyond the Neonatal Period). In addition, dexamethasone therapy

in a dose of 0.15 mg/kg every 6 hours for the first 2 or 4 days of treatment appears to decrease the likelihood of neurologic sequelae, including hearing deficit.[120–122] Dexamethasone should be initiated before the first dose of antibiotic whenever possible. Patients with epiglottitis require placement of an artificial airway, and children with pneumonia often need treatment with supplemental oxygen. When pleural empyema, purulent pericarditis, or pyogenic arthritis is present, prompt drainage is essential for optimal outcome.

Otitis media and sinusitis are treated effectively with oral agents to which the causative strain is susceptible. Table 172-3 shows comparative minimal concentrations inhibitory to 90% of isolates (MIC90) for selected oral antibiotics.

PREVENTION

Vaccination

First-generation vaccines against Hib were purified type b capsular material, polyribosylribitol phosphate (PRP). These vaccines were not effective in children younger than 24 months and had variable efficacy in children 24 months and older.[123,124] Second-generation vaccines contain PRP or a derivative of PRP conjugated to an immunogenic carrier protein, are effective in infants, and have replaced the earlier vaccines and are recommended universally in infancy. Currently, three conjugate vaccines are licensed, all differing to some extent in the size of the polysaccharide, chemical

TABLE 172-3. In Vitro Activity of Selected Oral Agents against Haemophilus influenzae

Antibiotic	MIC$_{90}$ (mg/mL)
Cephalexin	8
Cefaclor	8
Cefprozil	8
Cefdinir	1
Cefuroxime	0.5
Cefpodoxime	0.06
Cefixime	0.06
Cefditoren	0.03
Amoxicillin	16
Amoxicillin-clavulanate	1
Trimethoprim-sulfamethoxazole	0.5
Clarithromycin	8
Azithromycin	1

MIC, minimal inhibitory concentration.

TABLE 172-4. Haemophilus influenzae Type b Conjugate Vaccines

Vaccine	Trade Name	Polysaccharide	Linkage	Protein Carrier
PRP-OMP[a]	PedvaxHIB	Medium	Thioether	Neisseria meningitidis outer membrane protein
PRP-T[a]	ActHIB	Large	6-Carbon	Tetanus toxoid
HbOC	HibTITER	Small	None	CRM$_{197}$ mutant Corynebacterium diphtheriae toxin

PRP, polyribosylribitol phosphate; OMP, outer membrane protein; HbOC, oligosaccharide-CRM$_{197}$ conjugate Haemophilus influenzae type b vaccine.

[a]Additional combination vaccines have been licensed that include these conjugate vaccines. PRP-OMP-HepB (Comvax) contains PRP-OMP and hepatitis B vaccine; DTaP/PRP-T (TriHIBit) contains DTaP vaccine and PRP-T; DTaP-IPV/PRP-T (Pentacel) contains DTaP vaccine, inactivated poliovirus vaccine, and PRP-T.

linkage between the polysaccharide and the carrier, and the type of protein carrier[125] (Table 172-4). Among these three vaccines, PRP-T (PRP-tetanus toxoid) and PRP-OMP (PRP-*Neisseria meningitidis* outer membrane protein) are available in the U.S. As a result of differences in immunogenicity, the primary series in infancy consists of three doses (at 2, 4, and 6 months of age) for PRP-T and two doses (at 2 and 4 months) for PRP-OMP. Regardless of the particular vaccine used during the first year of life, a booster dose should be administered between 12 and 15 months of age. Two combination vaccines that contain a Hib conjugate formulation are licensed and available currently in the U.S., namely PRP-OMP/HepB (Comvax) and DTaP-IPV/PRP-T (Pentacel).

Children with sickle-cell disease, anatomic or functional asplenia, HIV infection, or IgG2 subclass deficiency, patients receiving chemotherapy for malignancies, and patients who have undergone bone marrow transplantation have an increased risk of invasive Hib disease. Conjugate vaccine should be considered for those who are unvaccinated. Two doses (at least 1 month apart) are recommended for children 12 to 59 months of age and one dose for those 60 months or older. (For further consideration, see the *2009 Red Book* by the American Academy of Pediatrics Committee on Infectious Diseases[125] and Chapter 6, Active Immunization.)

All Hib conjugate vaccines are well tolerated, with the most common adverse effect being short-lived redness and swelling at the site of injection. Postlicensing studies indicate that the existing conjugate vaccines are highly effective against Hib disease and reduce rates of nasopharyngeal colonization. These vaccines confer no protection against non-type b or nontypable strains.

A 10-valent pneumococcal vaccine using conjugation with nontypable *H. influenzae* protein D was examined recently in a randomized, double-blind efficacy trial and was found to be associated with an efficacy against nontypable *H. influenzae* otitis media of 35.3% (95% confidence interval, 1.8% and 57.4%).[126] This vaccine has been licensed in over 40 countries but is not currently licensed in the U.S. A variety of other nontypable *H. influenzae* surface proteins are under study as candidate vaccine antigens.[127]

Chemoprophylaxis

Chemoprophylaxis is an important intervention for preventing invasive Hib disease.[114] The intent is to eradicate nasopharyngeal colonization and thereby interrupt transmission. In households with one or more infants younger than 12 months who have not received the complete Hib primary vaccine series, all household contacts should receive rifampin prophylaxis. The same applies in households with children younger than 4 years who are incompletely vaccinated and in families with a fully vaccinated but immunocompromised child. In addition, when two or more cases of invasive disease occur within a 60-day period in attendees of a group childcare facility and incompletely vaccinated children attend the facility, rifampin is recommended for all attendees and supervisory personnel. Management after a single case at a childcare facility is controversial and depends on the age and immunization status of the attendees and the duration of daily contact between attendees and the index patient. In-home group childcare settings are managed like families.

Treatment of the index case with cefotaxime or ceftriaxone eradicates Hib colonization, eliminating the need for prophylaxis in this individual. However, index patients who are treated with other agents (e.g., ampicillin or meropenem) and who are younger than 2 years of age or have a susceptible household contact should receive rifampin prophylaxis at the end of systemic treatment for invasive disease.

Chemoprophylaxis also is a consideration in children who have recurrent otitis media from nontypable *H. influenzae* (or other typical pathogens). In this situation, chronic prophylaxis with either amoxicillin or sulfisoxazole may be effective in reducing infectious episodes.

Key Points. Diagnosis and Management of *Haemophilus influenzae* Infection

MICROBIOLOGY

- Nonmotile, nonspore-forming, gram-negative coccobacillus
- Grows aerobically and anaerobically; requires factor X and factor V for aerobic growth and factor X for anaerobic growth
- Optimal growth is achieved on media enriched with erythrocytes that have been disrupted by heating (e.g., chocolate agar) or by peptic digestion (e.g., Fildes medium)
- Isolates are classified according to polysaccharide capsule (encapsulated forms are designated serotypes a–f; nonencapsulated forms are designated nontypable)

EPIDEMIOLOGY

- Normal nasopharyngeal flora; type b and non-type b encapsulated stains generally colonize nasopharynx of <3% of individuals, whereas nontypable strains colonize the nasopharynx of 40% to 80% of children and adults
- Hib was leading cause of bacterial meningitis and other invasive diseases in children younger than 5 years in the United States until routine infant immunization in 1990; remains a common pathogen in young children in countries without routine immunization
- Type a, type e, and type f invasive disease appears to be increasing in frequency in the U.S., Canada, and Europe
- Nontypable strains are a common cause of localized respiratory tract disease in both children and adults

DIAGNOSIS

- Culture from a normally sterile site (blood, CSF, joint fluid, pleural fluid, pericardial fluid, epiglottis)
- Culture of fluid obtained by tympanocentesis, sinus aspiration, tracheal or lung aspiration, bronchoscopy, and bronchoalveolar lavage when specific microbiologic diagnosis is required

TREATMENT

- ~40% of isolates are ampicillin resistant, in most cases due to β-lactamase production
- Ampicillin should never be used alone as empiric therapy of invasive disease but can be used as definitive therapy for ampicillin-susceptible isolates
- A third-generation cephalosporin is the therapy of choice for meningitis
- A variety of β-lactam and other oral agents are suitable for otitis media, sinusitis, and most other respiratory tract infections

---

173 Other *Haemophilus* Species

Jennifer Vodzak

Of the *Haemophilus* species, *H. influenzae* causes by far the most human disease. Several other members of this genus, however, are capable of causing clinical illness. These include *H. aegyptius* (now termed *H. influenzae* biogroup *aegyptius*), *H. ducreyi*, *H. parainfluenzae*, *H. haemolyticus*, *H. parahaemolyticus*, and the ill-defined species *H. paraphrohaemolyticus*.[1] Three other *Haemophilus* species known to cause human disease have been reclassified into a new genus, *Aggregatibacter*, as follows: *H. aphrophilus*, and *H. paraphrophilus* are now the single species *A. aphrophilus* and *H. segnis* is now *A. segnis*.[2,3] Reclassification is based on phenotypic properties and molecular analyses (16S rRNA analysis and DNA-DNA hybridization studies). The genus name *Aggregatibacter* refers to "rod-shaped bacteria that aggregate with others," thus more aptly describing the tendency of these bacterial colonies to adhere to test tube walls.

The genus *Haemophilus* is classified in the family Pasteurellaceae. Members of this genus are small, pleomorphic, facultatively anaerobic, gram-negative coccobacilli. *Haemophilus* species can be distinguished from one another based on need for X factor (hemin) and/or V factor (nicotinamide) for in vitro growth, ability to lyse horse erythrocytes, and production of catalase (Table 173-1). With the sole exception of *H. ducreyi*, all *Haemophilus* species ferment glucose. *H. ducreyi* grows optimally at 33 °C, whereas other species do so between 35 °C and 37 °C. In general, haemophili grow best in a humid environment enriched with 5 to 10% carbon dioxide.[1] Both *A. aphrophilus* and *A. segnis* are small gram-negative rods that do not require X factor, have variable dependence on V factor, and ferment glucose.[2]

HAEMOPHILUS INFLUENZAE BIOGROUP AEGYPTIUS

The "Koch–Weeks bacillus" that was originally observed in Egyptian children with conjunctivitis by Koch in 1883 and further characterized by Weeks in 1886 was formally designated *Haemophilus aegyptius* in 1950.[4] Controversy over whether *H. aegyptius*

merits classification as a separate species from *H. influenzae*, already extant at that time, has persisted. Several reports have described phenotypic and pathogenetic differences between *H. aegyptius* and *H. influenzae*.[4-8] No single characteristic unequivocally distinguishes the two organisms; however, DNA hybridization studies indicate that they are highly related.[9,10] For these reasons, the Koch–Weeks bacillus is presently considered a distinct subgroup of *H. influenzae* biotype III and termed *H. influenzae* biogroup *aegyptius*.[8]

In the United States, *H. influenzae* biogroup *aegyptius* has been a cause of seasonal acute conjunctivitis in southern states during the warmer months of the year. Studies performed in Texas[11] and Georgia[12] found this organism to be the leading cause of acute purulent conjunctivitis among children in the 1930s to 1950s. Some studies have suggested that the eye gnat (*Hippelates pusio*) might serve as a transmission vector (hence the lay term, "gnat sore eyes"), though this role has not been proven.

H. influenzae biogroup *aegyptius* also can cause severe infection, Brazilian purpuric fever (BPF). The first known cases of BPF occurred in 1984 in rural Brazil, when 10 children died from a rapidly progressive illness characterized by fever, abdominal pain, vomiting, purpura, and vascular collapse.[13] Epidemiologic investigation found infection strongly associated with a recent history of purulent conjunctivitis. When another outbreak occurred in Brazil in 1986, the etiology of BPF was established.[14] *H. influenzae* biogroup *aegyptius* was isolated from 9 blood cultures and 1 hemorrhagic cerebrospinal fluid culture from 10 clinically affected children.

Reported patients with BPF have ranged in age from 3 months to 10 years of age, with the peak incidence between 1 and 4 years. About 90% of patients have a recent history of conjunctivitis, and about 70% of identified cases have been fatal.[15,16] In Brazil, epidemic and sporadic cases have been reported from the states of São Paulo, Paraná, and Mato Grosso.[13-16] Single cases of BPF with bloodstream infection due to *H. influenzae* biogroup *aegyptius* have been reported from Australia[17] and the U.S.[18] Molecular studies showed that isolates were unique clones.[18,19] Extensive analyses of the bacterial isolates, including examination of protein profiles, ribotyping, plasmid restriction patterns, seroagglutination and multilocus sequencing,[20] indicate that the isolates causing BPF in Brazil belong to a single clone that is distinct from other strains of *H. influenzae* biogroup *aegyptius* in Brazil and other countries.[10]

Interestingly, there have been no reports of BPF since the mid-1990s; speculation about the apparent "disappearance" of this illness includes natural history of a bacterial species, underrecognition and/or underreporting of the disease, and potential rapid acquisition of immunity in a previously nonimmune population.[21] No explanation completely accounts for the unusual disease pattern, and investigations into the pathogenesis of BPF are ongoing.

Potential virulence factors of BPF strains include lipooligosaccharides, capsular polysaccharides, pilus proteins, immunoglobulin (Ig) A proteases, membrane-associated proteins, and extracellular proteins.[22] BPF strains express both pilus and non-pilus adhesins that presumably facilitate mucosal colonization.[23] Compared with non-BPF strains, BPF strains resist lysis following incubation with normal adult human serum[24] and are cytotoxic for microvascular endothelial cells.[25] Additionally, BPF strains produce an extracellular hemagglutinating protein purported to be responsible for the hemorrhagic manifestations of BPF.[26]

TABLE 173-1. Some Differential Characteristics of *Haemophilus* Species

	Growth Factor Requirement		Hemolysis	Catalase	CO$_2$ Enhances Growth
	X	V			
***HAEMOPHILUS* SPP.**					
H. influenzae	+	+	−	+	−
H. aegyptius	+	+	−	+	−
H. parainfluenzae	−	+	−	D	−
H. ducreyi	+	−	−	−	+
H. haemolyticus	+	+	+	+	−
H. parahaemolyticus	−	+	+	+	−
***AGGREGATIBACTER* SPP.**					
A. aphrophilus[a]	−	D	−	−	+
A. segnis[b]	−	+	−	D	D

D, differences are encountered; V, nicotinamide; X, hemin.

[a]Previously *H. aphrophilus* and *H. paraphrophilus*.

[b]Previously *H. segnis*.

Early systemic antibiotic therapy can improve clinical outcome in patients with BPF. Appropriate therapeutic options include ampicillin, chloramphenicol, cefotaxime, or ceftriaxone; most isolates of the BPF clone are resistant to trimethoprim-sulfamethoxazole.[10] In a randomized trial of children with *H. influenzae* biogroup *aegyptius* conjunctivitis, systemic therapy with rifampin (20 mg/kg orally once daily for 4 days) eradicated the organism in 12 of 12 children, compared with only 7 of 16 children treated with topical chloramphenicol 0.5% (administered every 4 hours for 7 days).[27] This finding led to speculation that oral rifampin therapy for such children might prevent the development of BPF.

HAEMOPHILUS DUCREYI

H. ducreyi is the causative agent of chancroid, a sexually transmitted disease characterized by genital ulceration and inguinal adenitis.[28] This organism, which was first described by Ducrey in 1889, is a fastidious coccobacillary gram-negative bacterium that requires X factor for growth. Studies of DNA homology and ribosomal RNA gene sequences indicate that, although *H. ducreyi* is correctly assigned to the family Pasteurellaceae, classification in the genus *Haemophilus* should be reconsidered.[29,30]

Chancroid occurs sporadically in developed countries, but is a major cause of genital ulcer disease in developing countries.[28] In the U.S., chancroid usually occurs in discrete outbreaks, and reported cases increased markedly during the 1980s to a high of 5001 cases in 1988. Since then, reported cases have declined steadily, with only about 300 reported cases from 2000 to 2007 (less than 50 cases per year since 2004) and only 28 cases reported in 9 states in 2008.[31] Poverty, sex for money or drugs, and illicit drug use are well-recognized risk factors. Chancroid is an important cofactor in the transmission of human immunodeficiency virus (HIV). In addition, as many as 10% of patients with chancroid are coinfected with syphilis or herpes simplex virus (HSV).[32]

Transmission of *H. ducreyi* occurs through sexual contact, putatively gaining tissue inoculation via epithelial microabrasions. After an incubation period of 3 to 10 days, a papule develops. Papules typically surrounded by erythema, evolve over 2 to 3 days into pustules which ultimately rupture to form tender, friable, sharply circumscribed ulcers with grey or yellow purulent exudates. In the absence of effective antibiotic therapy, ulcers resolve only after several weeks or months. Chancroid occurs more frequently in men than women. Moreover, depending on the locations of ulcers, women can have subtle symptoms such as dysuria, dyspareunia, vaginal discharge, dyschezia, or rectal bleeding. Rarely, extragenital lesions occur. About 50% of patients develop painful, tender enlarged inguinal lymph nodes, which can become fluctuant and, if not aspirated or drained surgically, rupture spontaneously. Occasionally, ulcers can appear and resolve, with development of suppurative inguinal adenitis 1 to 3 weeks later.[28]

Although the pathogenesis of *H. ducreyi* infection is not completely understood, several potential virulence factors and host immune responses have been described.[33-35] These include lipooligosaccharide,[36-39] pili,[40] soluble cytolethal distending toxin,[41-43] hemoglobin-binding outer-membrane protein,[44,45] cytotoxic hemolysin,[46,47] copper-zinc superoxide dismutase,[48,49] filamentous hemagglutinin-like protein,[50] and zinc-binding periplasmic protein.[51] In addition, two proteins that likely facilitate *H. ducreyi* persistence within genital epithelium are HgbA, which mediates hemoglobin binding,[52] and Dsr, which mediates serum resistance.[53-55]

In the U.S., the most common causes of genital ulcer disease in sexually active patients are HSV infection, syphilis, and chancroid. In developing countries, the differential diagnosis also includes granuloma inguinale and lymphogranuloma venereum.[56] Definitive diagnosis of chancroid requires recovery of *H. ducreyi* on special culture media, which often is not available readily. Even under optimal conditions, culture is no more than 80% sensitive compared with polymerase chain reaction (PCR); however, no Food and Drug Administration-approved PCR test for *H. ducreyi* currently exists.[56] Direct examination of gram-stained clinical material can be misleading (owing to the polymicrobial flora of most genital ulcers) and is not recommended as a diagnostic test.[28,57] The diagnosis of chancroid, therefore, is based on clinical findings and the exclusion of other causes of genital ulcers.[32] Current guidelines from the Centers for Disease Control and Prevention indicate that a probable diagnosis of chancroid can be made in a patient with all of the following features: (1) one or more painful genital ulcers; (2) no evidence of syphilis (i.e., by darkfield examination of ulcer exudate *or* by a serologic test for syphilis performed at least 7 days after onset of ulcers); (3) clinical presentation, appearance of genital ulcers and, if present, regional lymphadenopathy; and (4) a negative test for HSV performed on the ulcer exudate.[56]

Effective antibiotic regimens in the treatment of chancroid include: ceftriaxone (250 mg) as a single dose intramuscularly, azithromycin (1 g) as a single dose orally, ciprofloxacin (500 mg) twice daily for 3 days orally, and erythromycin base (500 mg) thrice daily for 7 days orally.[56] Worldwide, there have been reports of isolates with intermediate resistance to either ciprofloxacin or erythromycin.[56] HIV-infected patients who receive single-dose ceftriaxone or azithromycin therapy should be monitored closely, as data are limited regarding the efficacy of these regimens in this population.[56] Patients should be re-examined 3 to 7 days after initiation of therapy. If therapy is successful, symptoms improve within 3 days and ulcers begin to resolve objectively after 7 days. Possible reasons for therapeutic failures include: incorrect diagnosis, coinfection with another sexually transmitted infection, coinfection with HIV, nonadherence to therapy, and infection with an *H. ducreyi* strain resistant to the prescribed antimicrobial. Large ulcers can take longer than 2 weeks to heal completely. Fluctuant lymphadenopathy may require needle aspiration or incision and drainage despite otherwise successful medical therapy. Uncircumcised men and patients with HIV infection do not respond as well to treatment as do those who are circumcised or HIV-negative.[56] Patients with chancroid should be evaluated for other sexually transmitted infections at the time of diagnosis and should be re-tested for syphilis and HIV infection 3 months later if the initial test results are negative. Sex partners (i.e., contact within the 10 days preceding symptom onset) of patients with chancroid should be examined and treated even if asymptomatic.[32,56]

ORAL AND PHARYNGEAL HAEMOPHILUS SPECIES

Haemophilus species (including those reclassified as *Aggregatibacter* spp.) account for about 10% of the cultivable flora normally colonizing the oral cavity and upper respiratory tract of healthy children. *H. parainfluenzae* comprises about three-fourths of pharyngeal *Haemophilus* isolates. In contrast, nonencapsulated *H. influenzae*, though present in 80% of healthy children, makes up less than 2% of the total pharyngeal flora.[58] *Aggregatibacter* spp. (formerly *H. aphrophilus*, *H. paraphrophilus*, and *H. segnis*) can be found in dental plaque specimens, particularly from adults, and *H. haemolyticus* has been encountered in gingival crevices.[1,58] Moreover, *H. parainfluenzae* and *H. influenzae* occasionally are isolated from urethral and vaginal specimens from adults and children.[59,60] On rare occasions, these haemophili depart from their role as harmless commensals and cause disease. The infections most consistently associated with *H. parainfluenzae* in children have been endocarditis (discussed below) and meningitis;[61,62] however, it is possible that *H. influenzae* isolates that were misidentified as *H. parainfluenzae* account for many of the reported meningitis cases.[1,62] Other pediatric infections reportedly caused by *H. parainfluenzae* include bacteremia, septic arthritis, urinary tract infection, peritonitis, and abscesses of the liver, brain, soft tissue, and head and neck spaces.[61-65] Historically, *A. aphrophilus* (formerly *H. aphrophilus*) was associated with a similar spectrum of diseases in children, along with rare cases of cervical lymphadenitis[66-70] Bacteremia and secondary brain abscesses have been associated with recent dental work, including one case associated with manipulation of dental braces in a pediatric patient.[71] *A. aphrophilus* (formerly *H. paraphrophilus*) has been reported to cause epiglottitis[72] and fatal pneumonia[73] in infants and septic arthritis in an adolescent.[74] *H. parahaemolyticus* was reported to cause periorbital cellulitis in a toddler.[75] *H. haemolyticus* and *A. segnis* (formerly *H. segnis*) have not been described as pediatric pathogens.

"*Haemophilus* species" (when *Aggregatibacter* were *Haemophilus* species) cause approximately 3% to 5% of cases of infective endocarditis in adults[76] and children.[77,78] A recent literature review[65] identified 17 pediatric cases of *Haemophilus* species endocarditis reported between 1965 and 2001; of these, etiologic agents were *H. parainfluenzae* in 13 cases and *A. aphrophilus* in 4 cases. *A. paraphrophilus*, which rarely causes endocarditis in adults, has not been reported to do so in a child. Of the 17 reported patients with "*Haemophilus* species" endocarditis, 10 had underlying cardiac abnormalities, 8 suffered embolic complications, 6 required cardiac surgery, and 2 died.

Ampicillin has historically been the drug of choice for infections caused by *Haemophilus* species, and remains so for susceptible isolates. Ampicillin resistance can occur among these organisms, however, resulting from either β-lactamase production or alterations in penicillin binding proteins.[1] In studies from southern Europe, 10% to 57% of respiratory *H. parainfluenzae* isolates produced β-lactamase; moreover, 40% were resistant to trimethoprimsulfamethoxazole and 40% were resistant to clarithromycin. More recently there have been reports that some *Haemophilus* spp. can produce extended-spectrum β-lactamases, although this is still uncommon.[79] Because antimicrobial susceptibility testing has not been well standardized for *A. aphrophilus*, resistance rates for these organisms remain unclear. For treatment of serious infections caused by *Haemophilus* species and *A. aphrophilus*, cefotaxime or ceftriaxone should be administered intravenously until antibiotic susceptibility test results are available. For uncomplicated native valve endocarditis, the minimum duration of antimicrobial therapy is 4 weeks.

174 *Helicobacter pylori*

Benjamin D. Gold

Helicobacter pylori demonstrates declining prevalence in developed countries and yet is one of the most common human infections worldwide. The primary period of acquisition is early childhood via fecal–oral, oral–oral and gastro–oral mechanisms. Although a number of zoonotic mechanisms for transmission have been postulated, nonhuman reservoirs have not been demonstrated definitively. *H. pylori* infection causes gastritis, duodenal and gastric ulcers, as well as gastric adenocarcinoma and mucosal-associated lymphoid type (MALT) lymphoma. *H. pylori* also has been associated with extragastric conditions including growth failure, iron-deficiency anemia, and chronic idiopathic thrombocytopenia purpura (ITP). El-Omar et al.[1,2] have demonstrated that outcome of *H. pylori*-associated diseases is not dictated merely by the bacterial virulence factors or by the host immune function, finding that bacterial virulence, host factors, and potentially environmental exposures play a role in the type of gastroduodenal inflammation and in *H. pylori* disease outcome. Evidence-based clinical practice guidelines now recommend eradication of *H. pylori* in infected children, especially if there are primary family members with gastric cancer. There is urgent need for more research due to the growing prevalence of antimicrobial resistance among *H. pylori* strains. Multicenter, multinational studies of *H. pylori* infection in children, which include specific, randomized controlled eradication trials, are essential to extend current knowledge and develop better predictors of disease outcome.

THE PATHOGEN

H. pylori is a gram-negative, motile, spiral-shaped bacillus that resides in a unique biological niche, the human gastric mucosa. Although studies indicate that *H. pylori* itself or bacterial components may translocate to other places in the gastrointestinal tract (contributing to Crohn disease),[3–5] or to the coronary arteries (facilitating plaque development and myocardial infarction[6]) and to carotids (leading to cerebral vascular incidents[7]), the stomach is *H. pylori*'s definitive home in its human host. Numerous studies also provide compelling evidence of colonization of the oral cavity; whether *H. pylori* colonization is transient or persistent remains unclear.[8–13] Meta-analysis demonstrates a close relation between *H. pylori* colonization in the oral cavity and stomach, and *H. pylori* in the oral cavity.[14] Further research is needed to further characterize the potential relevance of this "pre" gastric biologic niche.

The pattern of gastric mucosal colonization by *H. pylori* and resultant gastric inflammation appears to play a major role in influencing disease phenotype.[15–17] A Nobel Prize in Medicine was awarded in 2005 to Barry Marshall and Robert Warren for their 1982 discovery of *H. pylori* (then called *Campylobacter pyloridis*) and its association with duodenal and gastric ulcer disease.[18] *Helicobacter* constitutes group III of the rRNA superfamily VI, which also includes *Campylobacter* (group I) and *Arcobacter* (group II).[19–22] A number of *Helicobacter* species have been identified, with *H. pylori* being the most common and the primary pathogen associated with human disease.[23–25]

H. pylori is a microaerophilic bacterium that devotes over half of its energy to producing significant quantities of the urease enzyme to successfully maintain persistence in the human stomach. *H. pylori* urease is a potent stimulus for memory CD8+ T lymphocytes, showing a 15-fold greater response to urease in infected compared with uninfected subjects,[26] which may have important implications for development of more severe disease outcomes.[27] Much attention has been focused on *H. pylori* virulence, specifically on a portion of the bacterial genome called the cytotoxin-associated gene pathogenicity island.[21,28] Although *H. pylori* "typing" based on genotype–phenotype relationships is problematic due to the genetic heterogeneity of strains, a great number of the genes found responsible for disease outcomes in the infected host are contained within this pathogenicity island.[29–31] Genetic variability is the rule with *H. pylori* and these genetic modifications have led investigators to label variant strains a type of "quasi-species."[32–34]

H. pylori infection elicits a variety of phenotypic responses in cultured gastric epithelial cells, including the expression of proinflammatory genes and changes in the actin cytoskeleton. Both responses are mediated by the type IV secretion system (TFSS) encoded by the *cag* pathogenicity island (*cag* PAI) that contains over 31 genes.[20,27,35] TFSS is unique among bacteria and is postulated to be a key mechanism in *H. pylori*-associated carcinogenesis.[31] In addition, BabA-mediated binding of *H. pylori* to Le(b) on the epithelial surface augments TFSS-dependent *H. pylori* pathogenicity by triggering the production of proinflammatory cytokines and precancer-related factors.[36] *H. pylori* produces other enzymes, including catalase and oxidase (use in biochemical confirmation), mucinase, and a vacuolating cytotoxin (VacA) responsible for epithelial cell damage.[37] *H. pylori* adheres intimately to epithelial cells in the gastric mucosa and expresses several surface proteins, including a blood group antigen-binding adhesin, BabA.[38–40] Lewis (Le)-associated antigens, carbohydrates related biochemically to the ABO blood groups, also are thought to play a role in *H. pylori* adhesion to gastric mucosa. *H. pylori* is one of the few known microbes to be able to utilize its host glycoproteins (i.e., Lewis[x] and Lewis[y] antigens) within its outer membrane to facilitate immune evasion. Moreover, both as a mechanism to facilitate persistence in colonization and facilitate immune cell evasion, *H. pylori* contains a fucosyltransferase gene ($\alpha 1,3,4$-*FUT*) expressed in the bacterial outer membrane as lipopolysaccharide moieties strikingly similar to Lewis[x] and Lewis[y] epitopes.[36,38,41,42]

EPIDEMIOLOGY

H. pylori resides in the stomachs of >50% of the world's population. Prevalence varies widely by geographic area, age, race, and socioeconomic status. In developing countries or developing populations in developed countries, such as the Native Canadian and Native Alaskan population with poor water sanitation and socioeconomic conditions, up to 90% of the population is infected.[43,44] Prevalence of infection is determined substantially by socioeconomic status.[45] In poor populations, infection usually is acquired early in childhood; i.e., with most infections acquired before 10 years of age.[43–47] Conversely, although there are no population-based incidence studies published, large seroprevalence studies demonstrate that *H. pylori* infection has decreased substantially for the last 5 decades, with a <15% prevalence by 10 years of age[45,48–52] (Figure 174-1). Data suggest that acquisition is decreasing in age cohorts born more recently worldwide, and such decreases are more prevalent in developed countries.[45,48,52,53] It appears that over a century ago, nearly all humans carried *H. pylori* in their stomachs, demonstrated in a serosurvey of a large cohort of indigenous Amazon natives.[54] In this cohort, overall seroprevalence was 92%, with >80% of children positive by 3 years of age. Interestingly, *H. pylori* seroprevalence in this Amazon cohort did not correlate with the length of contact with the outside world, suggesting that *H. pylori* was indigenous.[54] The specific reason for declining prevalence is unknown, although better living conditions, less

crowding, smaller family size, clean, chlorinated water, and the widespread use of antibiotics may contribute.[55,56] More recently, numerous investigators have focused on the human microbiome as the model "system" by which answers to the development and prevention of many human diseases can be ascertained.[57–60] Provocative theories have included speculation that not all *H. pylori* strains are pathogenic, and that at some point during the microbe and/or human evolution *H. pylori* may have been a constituent of the human gastrointestinal microbiome.[5,61,62]

Despite overall decline in prevalence, childhood is the period in which most new *H. pylori* infections are acquired, especially in developing countries.[56,63–65] Studies have shown that Irish children are most at risk for acquiring infection prior to the age of 3 years.[66] Turkish children acquire *H. pylori* infection 2.5 times higher than they lose infection;[67] following eradication of infection, children, particularly adolescents, become reinfected more frequently than adults.[68] Authors of the last study concluded that close contact with children >5 years of age, especially siblings, could be a more important risk factor for recurrent infection than age at initiation of treatment.[68]

In the United States, ethnic differences are notable in the prevalence of *H. pylori* infection. African American and Hispanic populations, as well as immigrant populations, have a 2- to 6-fold increased risk of seropositivity compared with white people of higher socioeconomic status.[48,52,53] Overall, sex is not associated with prevalence of *H. pylori* infection but may play a role in the disease outcome.[69] Poor hygiene in the living environment, particularly during childhood, correlate with higher prevalence.[44,46,70,71] Socioeconomic status of the family in which the child is raised is inversely associated with *H. pylori* prevalence.[56,72,73] Relative role of mothers versus fathers in infection transmission is controversial, although most data infer the predominant role of mothers simply due to overall contact with infants and young children in whom acquisition primarily occurs.[44,74–76] Diet, such as increased consumption of fruits and vegetables and vitamin C supplements, reduces the probability of acquisition of *H. pylori* infection, but more importantly, the severity of disease outcomes.[77,78]

Most evidence for routes of *H. pylori* transmission include person-to-person, waterborne, and iatrogenic spread through contaminated medical equipment.[79–82] Person-to-person transmission is predominant and includes fecal–oral, gastro–oral and oral–oral routes, with much higher risks associated with neurologically impaired persons residing in an institutionalized setting where contact with feces and vomitus is frequent.[83–86] Multiple, large family studies, some multigenerational, show clearly increased risk of intrafamilial transmission, especially mother to offspring, younger to older sibling, and between spouses.[84,87–91] A number of studies demonstrated that *H. pylori* isolates from family members are homologous by DNA fingerprinting.[92–94,95] In a study of a binational family of four *H. pylori*-infected members, from El Paso, Texas and Juarez, Mexico, all four family members were infected with the same *H. pylori* genotype *vac*A s1a/m2.[96] Similarly, MacKay et al.[97] demonstrated further that the fecal–oral route is the predominant mode of acquisition and that DNA purification followed by *H. pylori* polymerase chain reaction (PCR) analysis is an effective tool for harvesting *H. pylori* DNA isolates from the feces of children.[97]

Oral–oral transmission also can occur in certain populations, and may not be associated solely with premastication of food by mothers.[44] Saliva, dental plaque, reflux of gastric contents, and vomiting are considered the primary sources of *H. pylori*.[86,98–103] *H. pylori* genetic material has been detected by a variety of molecular methods performed on the stool of infected individuals.[96,104] However, primary isolation of *H. pylori* from stool is difficult, although some research-based laboratories have been able to recover ~50% from infected persons.[63,86,105] Although transmission through contaminated, poorly sanitized water is debated, the evidence is compelling.[106–113] Two studies have demonstrated isolation of *H. pylori* from well water and from sewage contaminated water.[114–117] Iatrogenic spread also is important, even in the developed world.[79,118] The occupational risks of healthcare personnel (HCP) for acquisition of *H. pylori* were reviewed in a meta-analysis

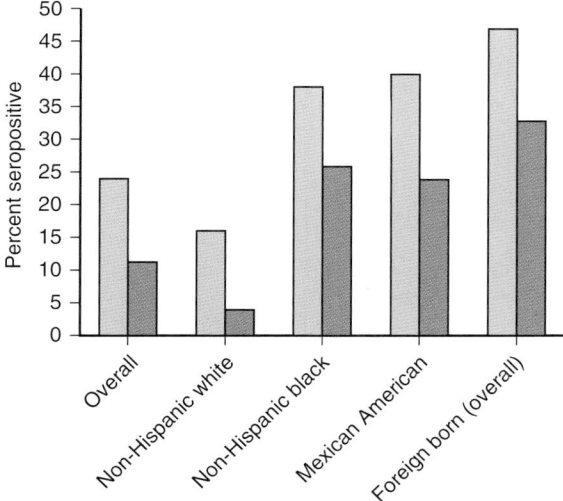

Figure 174-1. Declining seroprevalence of *H. pylori* in U.S. children, using sera from NHANES III (1988–1991) (pale blue bars, 2795 subjects) and NHANES (1999–2000) (purple bars, 2898 subjects). Change in seroprevalence over time periods has P < 0.001. (Redrawn from Gold BD, Kruszon-Moran D, Sobel J, et al. Decreasing seroprevalence of *Helicobacter pylori* infection in U.S. children ages 6–19 years. J Pediatric Gastroenterol Nutr 2003;37:360.)

spanning 10 years.[118] The risks are highest for gastroenterologists, some nurses, and employees caring for persons with mental disability; however, results for other groups are conflicting.[79] Moreover, the use of improperly disinfected endoscopes increases the risk of infection, whereas disinfection of endoscopes by soaking in glutaraldehyde cleaning agents and more importantly, cleansing of the channels by vigorous brushing, reduces the risk of *H. pylori* acquisition.[79,119]

PATHOGENESIS

H. pylori infection and its long-term effects, including peptic ulcer, MALToma, and gastric adenocarcinoma, result from a complex interaction between the strain's virulence properties, the host's susceptibility to infection and immune response, and environmental factors that might modulate susceptibility to infection or disease outcomes or both.[15,120–123]

Colonization of gastric mucosa by the motile *H. pylori* is initiated by a unique and specific tropism for gastric epithelial cells rich in Lewis[b] blood group antigen.[36,38,124–127] Avoidance of the gastric acidity is efficiently addressed by the *H. pylori* urease enzyme, which converts urea into ammonium and bicarbonate, thereby creating an alkaline microenvironment that permits survival despite gastric acidity.[128,129] Attachment to the gastric epithelial cell Lewis[b] receptor is mediated by the bacterial blood group antigen-binding adhesin BabA.[130] Although other bacterial adhesins may contribute to colonization, BabA has been

associated with duodenal ulcer and gastric adenocarcinoma.[38,127] The vacuolating cytotoxin VacA also is associated with an increased risk for gastroduodenal ulcers and, to a lesser extent, gastric cancer.[131–133] Polymorphisms, and the two main variable regions of the *vacA* gene, the signal sequence (*s*) and the mid region (*m*) properties, facilitate typing of isolated strains.[134] Expression of these regions reflects production of the vacuolating toxin; s1-m1, s1-m2, and s2-m1 genotypes correspond to high, medium, and low toxin-producing strains, respectively. However, the overall correlation between *vacA* and disease phenotype remains equivocal.

H. pylori is a potent inducer of gastric mucosal inflammation through various mechanisms, the most important of which is CagA.[135–137] TFSS are macromolecular assemblies, which are widespread in pathogenic bacteria, and often are used to deliver effectors into host cells. Encoded for in the *cag* pathogenicity island, *H. pylori* encodes Cag-TFSS that mediates the injection of the toxin CagA into gastric epithelial cells, where it undergoes tyrosine phosphorylation by host cell kinases.[36,138] CagA then activates nuclear factor κB (NF-κB), the intracellular signaling pathway that regulates induction of the proinflammatory cytokines interleukin-8 (IL-8) and IL-1β.[139,140] The relative ability of *H. pylori* strains to induce epithelial cell inflammation is dependent on the presence of an intact *cag* pathogenicity island (PAI) containing the *picB* gene.[141] Strains that possess the complete PAI induce pangastritis, which evolves to gastric ulceration, atrophy, intestinal metaplasia, and eventually, distal gastric cancer.[141] *CagA*[+] variant strains that have an incomplete *cag* PAI (because of deletions or mutations)

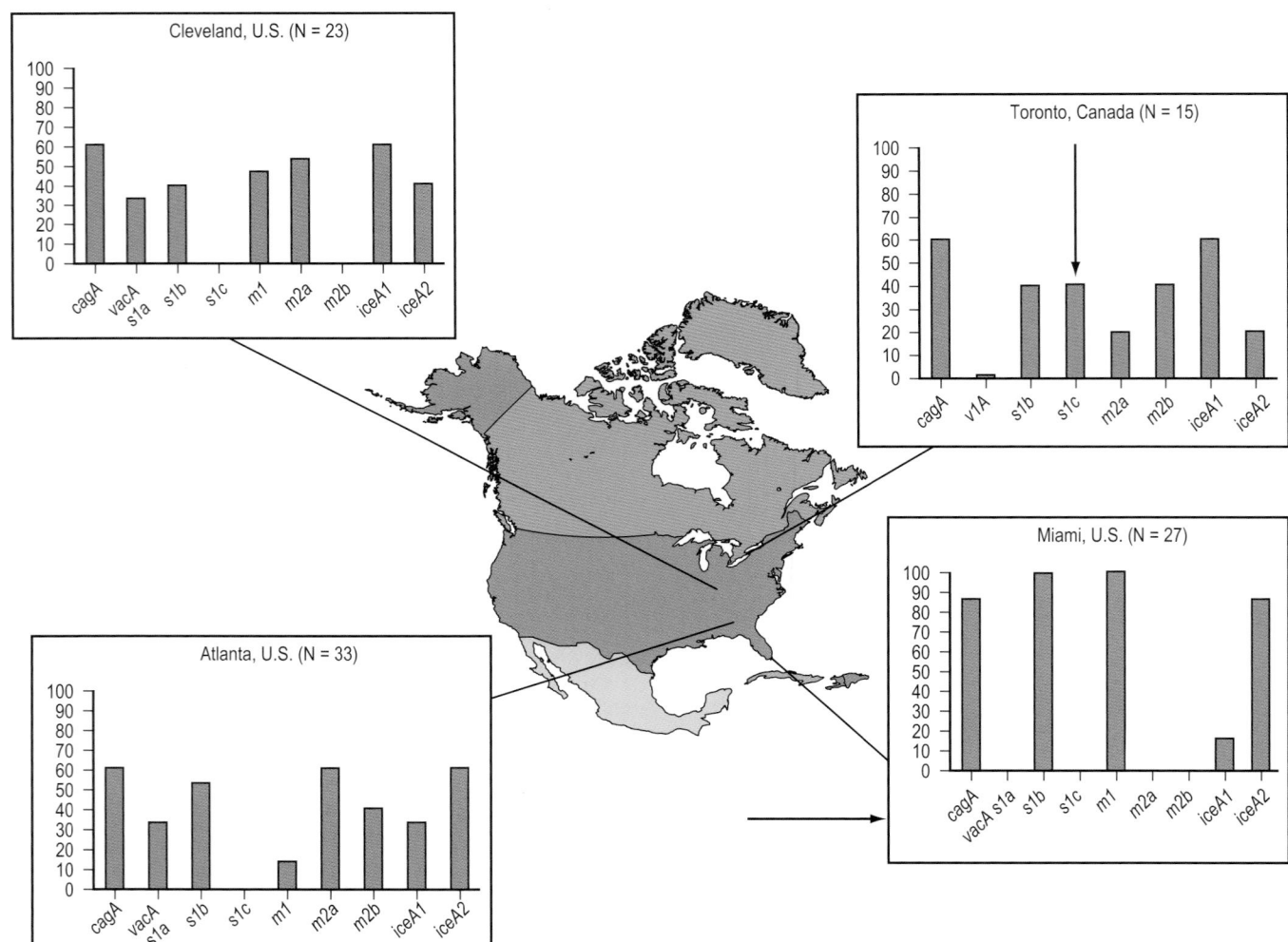

Figure 174-2. Genotyping of *H. pylori* strains isolated from children from 4 cities in North America, evaluating *vacA*, *cagA*, and *iceA*. (Redrawn from Gold BD, van Doorn LJ, Guarner J, et al. Genotypic, clinical, and demographic characteristics of children infected with *Helicobacter pylori*. J Clin Microbiol 2001;39:1348–1352.)

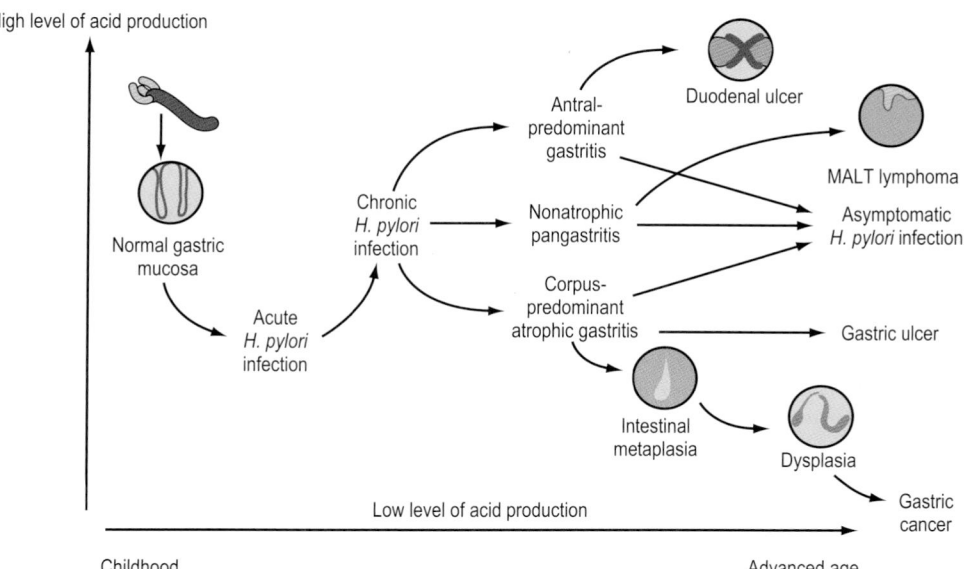

High level of acid production

Normal gastric mucosa

Acute *H. pylori* infection

Chronic *H. pylori* infection

Antral-predominant gastritis

Nonatrophic pangastritis

Corpus-predominant atrophic gastritis

Duodenal ulcer

MALT lymphoma

Asymptomatic *H. pylori* infection

Gastric ulcer

Intestinal metaplasia

Dysplasia

Gastric cancer

Low level of acid production

Childhood

Advanced age

Figure 174-3. Pathogenesis and natural history of *H. pylori*. Bacterial, host, and environmental determinants affect disease outcome. (Modified from Suerbaum S, Michetti P. *Helicobacter pylori* infection. N Engl J Med 2002;347: 1175–1186.)

Host/environmental factors	Bacterial factors
Oxygen free radicals	Antigen mimicry
Nitrosamines, nitrates	Cytotoxin
Ascorbic acid (vitamin C)	Signal transduction
Genetic co-factors (IL-1β polymorphisms)	Heat shock protein
•Increased gastrin	Urease
•Salt intake	Type IV secretion
•Smoking, alcohol abuse	CagA status

induce antral-predominant gastritis, more likely leading to duodenal ulcer than to distal gastric cancer.[31,141]

H. pylori displays remarkable genetic diversity. Strain presence of the toxigenic *vacA s1* allele, a complete *cag* PAI, *cagA* alleles containing multiple EPIYA phosphorylation sites, and expression of BabA adhesin correlates with development of gastroduodenal disease in adults. *H. pylori* strains infecting 47 North American children with a variety of gastroduodenal pathologies were assessed to identify genomic content and prevalence of mixed infection.[142] Random amplified polymorphic DNA analysis of multiple *H. pylori* clones from each patient and microarray-based comparative genomic hybridization were used. A range of EPIYA motif configurations were observed for the *cagA* gene, which was present in strains from 47% of patients, but only 41% contained a complete *cag* PAI. Sixty-four percent of children were infected with a strain having the *vacA s1* allele, and 60% had the *babA* gene. The presence of a functional *cag* PAI correlated with ulcer disease (P = 0.0095). At least 11% of patients had mixed infection. Pediatric strains differ in their spectrum of strain-variable genes and percentage of absent genes compared with adult strains. Moreover, in this novel study, most children were infected with *H. pylori* strains lacking the *cag* PAI, but the presence of a complete *cag* PAI (in contrast to other virulence markers) was associated with more severe gastroduodenal disease.[142] Although *H. pylori* strains that possess the *cag* PAI and secrete a functional cytotoxin induce more severe gastric injury and further augment the risk for developing distal gastric cancer, carcinogenesis also is influenced by host genetic diversity, particularly involving immune response genes such as *IL-1ss* and *TNF-α*.

H. pylori urease binds to major histocompatibility complex class II molecules expressed on the surface of gastric epithelial cells, which in turn induces apoptosis and thus modulates cell growth.[143-145] A second mechanism is the induction of Fas-Fas ligand-regulated apoptosis through two different proinflammatory cytokines: (1) production of interferon (IFN)-γ induced by a Th1 immune response triggered by *H. pylori* colonization and (2) induction of IL-1β by CagA.[146-148] CagA is one of the primary *H. pylori*-produced stimuli of production of the proinflammatory cytokine IL-1β, which also is a potent inhibitor of gastric

acid secretion.[123,149,150] Gastric acidity may be further reduced in *H. pylori*-infected individuals with particular polymorphisms of the IL-1β gene promoter, thereby increasing the risk of atrophic gastritis and gastric adenocarcinoma.[150,151] Another virulence marker of *H. pylori* is the *iceA* gene, so called because its expression is induced after contact with epithelial cells.[133] The gene has two distinct genotypes, *iceA1* and *iceA2*, but the overall relevance of genotypes to disease phenotype remains unclear.[152-155]

Although >50% of the world's population is infected, the majority of individuals remain clinically asymptomatic, suggesting that not all *H. pylori* strains are pathogenic. Why ~15% to 20% develop gastroduodenal ulcer disease and <1% develop gastric adenocarcinoma remains unclear.[15,156] Thus, optimal cost-effective public health strategies would be to characterize markers that predict more severe disease outcomes in order to target eradication treatment. In both children and adults, studies to determine associations between BabA, VacA, CagA, and PicB with peptic ulcer and gastric cancer continue to reveal conflicting results.[36,39,40,154,155] While *cag* PAI appears to be the one marker of inflammation and clinical disease found in clinical isolates of *H. pylori*, other virulence factors appear to be markers of geographic distribution (Figure 174-2) rather than predictors of disease outcome (Figure 174-3).[152,157,158]

CLINICAL MANIFESTATIONS

Intestinal Disease

H. pylori infection in children generally does not result in clinically apparent symptoms. However, once there is persistent colonization, mucosal inflammation is associated almost universally. Although there are a number of reports of spontaneous elimination of *H. pylori* infection in children, many of these studies are limited by the methodology used to determine infection presence/absence.[46,159-161] The rate of spontaneous clearance of infection in children is not known. Nodular gastritis appears to be observed more commonly in children; however, the time to development of these endoscopically visible nodules and their natural history remains uncharacterized.[162-165] Additionally, it is not clear which children with lymphofollicular gastritis will progress to develop MALToma, and over what time period.[166,167] Studies have demonstrated that eradication of *H. pylori* in children with MALT lymphoma results in resolution of the mucosal disease, both gastric and extragastric.[167,168]

Although only case reports describe development of gastric cancer in children, early childhood acquisition of *H. pylori* significantly increases the risk of gastric cancer.[169,170] Atrophic gastritis and intestinal metaplasia, precursor lesions for gastric cancer, occur in *H. pylori*-infected children.[171,172] In an endoscopic study of 173 children from countries with high incidence of gastric cancer (58 from Korea, median age of 14 years; 115 from Colombia, median age of 13 years), *H. pylori* was present in 85% of Colombian children and 17% of Korean children. Atrophic mucosa near the antrum–corpus border was present in 16% of children, primarily as pseudopyloric metaplasia (31%, intestinal metaplasia; 63%, pseudopyloric metaplasia; 6%, both). The median age of children with corpus atrophy was 15 years. Investigators also suggested that identification of this specific disease phenotype requires targeted biopsies to include the lesser and greater curve of the gastric corpus, in addition to biopsies targeting the antrum and cardia.[172]

Landmark studies by El Omar et al.[1] demonstrated that IL-1 gene cluster polymorphisms are associated with an increased risk of *H. pylori*-induced hypochlorhydria and gastric cancer. Compared with healthy controls, relatives of patients with gastric cancer had a higher prevalence of hypochlorhydria (27% vs. 3%) but a similar prevalence of *H. pylori* infection (63% vs. 64%).[151,173] Relatives of cancer patients matched for *H. pylori* prevalence also had a higher prevalence of atrophy (34%) than patients with non-ulcer dyspepsia (5%). Increased prevalence of precancerous gastric abnormalities in relatives is limited to those with *H. pylori* infection. Because of these findings, pediatric guidelines have been changed to target eradication or prevention strategy in selected patients.[174,175]

The natural history of *H. pylori* infection appears to occur in phases. In studies of adult volunteers, an initial phase of intense bacterial proliferation with gastric inflammation is observed and can be associated briefly with upper gastrointestinal symptoms and hypochlorhydria. Relationships of phases to *H. pylori* acquisition in either high- or low-endemic regions remain unclear. A chronic phase follows in which the inflammatory response is reduced to either a chronic diffuse superficial gastritis (with normal and or increased gastric pH), or antral predominant gastritis that results in increased gastric acid output and higher predilection for ulcer disease.

To date, a causal relationship between *H. pylori* infection and recurrent abdominal pain of childhood has not been established definitively. Additionally, although a relationship between ulcer disease and abdominal symptoms is apparent, it is unclear whether chronic gastritis causes symptoms in children. Results from studies around the world have been conflicting, precluding a definitive recommendation for treatment of *H. pylori* found in the child with gastrointestinal symptoms but no demonstrable disease. For example, a study from India reported association of *H. pylori* with recurrent abdominal pain (RAP) in 65 *H. pylori*-positive children (age: 3 to 12 years), 83% of whom had complete symptomatic relief after eradication therapy.[176] However, the study was not randomized or double-blinded, did not use a validated symptom assessment instrument, and did not include assessment of control of the socioeconomic status as a confounding variable.[176] In another study of this nature, Bode et al.[177] analyzed the relationship between social and familial factors, *H. pylori* infection, and RAP in children in a population-based cross-sectional study among 1221 preschool children aged 5 to 8 years. Results did not show an association between RAP (i.e., symptoms) and *H. pylori* infection, but a clear association between RAP and social and familial factors.[177]

Further, *H. pylori* infection in children does not appear to cause any specific symptoms. Epigastric pain, abdominal pain causing nocturnal wakening, hematemesis, recurrent vomiting, are not predictive of *H. pylori* infection because no difference has been found between colonized and noncolonized children.[178] In the only randomized placebo-controlled treatment trial to date (with strong methodology and long-term follow-up), 20 children with RAP and *H. pylori* infection all had evidence of gastritis; 8 of 10 in the treatment group and none in the placebo group had eradication of *H. pylori*. At 52 weeks, however, bacterial eradication and healing of gastric inflammation did not lead to symptomatic relief of chronic abdominal pain.[179]

The true incidence of gastric and duodenal ulcer disease in children is unknown. However, children with duodenal or gastric ulcers in general have symptoms similar to those of adults, including a sharp, "burning" type of pain, located primarily in the epigastrium that generally occurs with an empty stomach, between meals, and during the early morning hours. In addition, signs of occult (e.g., guaiac-positive stools) as well as frank bleeding can occur. In children, most, if not all primary ulcers (the majority of which are *H. pylori*-associated) occur in the duodenum and are seen in older children. Gastric ulcers are less common, and usually secondary, e.g., due to another disease process such as Crohn disease or produced by chemical irritation of the gastric mucosa as caused by aspirin or nonsteroidal anti-inflammatory drugs.[180]

A number of studies provide compelling evidence that *H. pylori*-infected children are more at risk for diarrhea due to enteric infections.[181,182] A study in Peru showed a high incidence of diarrhea in infected children, probably as a result of the transient achlorhydria that occurs during the acute phase of infection.[182] Increased rates of enteric infection in the face of early *H. pylori* infection likely are due to poor water sanitation and/or poor hygiene resulting in increased exposure to enteric pathogens. Conversely, an epidemiologic study from a developed country indicated that *H. pylori* colonization is associated with protection from childhood diarrhea.[183] These conflicting observations may be explained by the geographic region in which the child resides (hence the overall bacterial load, both *H. pylori* and the enteric pathogens) and/or the stage at which infection is detected, as protection against diarrhea occurs when the pH returns to acid. Furthermore, the presence of *H. pylori* augments the local and systemic immune response to enteropathogens, as has been demonstrated in *Vibrio cholerae*.[184,185]

The controversy surrounding whether *H. pylori* infection is protective, causative, or unrelated to gastroesophageal reflux disease (GERD) in adults and children has for the most part been settled. *H. pylori* at most is an innocent bystander and is not protective against GERD or its sequelae in both children and adults.[48,186,187] Although there is reverse prevalence of GERD in countries with a high and low prevalence of *H. pylori*, conclusion of causality is overly simplistic.[188] In a study of 95 children and adolescents who were recruited and completed an eradication trial with a mean follow-up of 11.2 months, the distribution of outcomes for each GER symptom (better, worse, unchanged) was similar before and after eradication and did not depend on prior *H. pylori* status.[189] These data and other case series allowed the Canadian, as well as the European Society for Paediatric Gastroenterology, Hepatology and Nutrition (ESPGHAN) and the North American Society for Pediatric Gastroenterology, Hepatology and Nutrition (NASPGHAN) guidelines committees to recommend the following: *H. pylori* eradication is recommended in children with GERD who are undergoing endoscopy.[174,175] However, when the diagnosis of GERD is made clinically or by pH monitoring, it is not necessary to screen for *H. pylori*.

Extraintestinal Disease

There are a number of extragastric diseases with sufficient evidence of association with *H. pylori* infection. In children, these are iron-deficiency anemia and short stature. There are a number of reports from around the world with sufficiently powered samples sizes that demonstrate a positive association between the infection and iron-deficiency anemia. Among 700 children in 10 villages in Alaska, a high prevalence of iron deficiency was demonstrated among school-aged children; active *H. pylori* infection was independently associated with iron deficiency and iron-deficiency anemia.[190] Additionally, a U.S. population-based study demonstrated a positive association between *H. pylori* infection and anemia.[191,192] In a Centers for Disease Control and Prevention's National Health and Nutrition Examination Survey (NHANES) (1999 to 2000), *H. pylori* infection was associated with iron deficiency and iron-deficiency anemia among 7462 survey participants ≥3 years of age, *H. pylori* infection was associated with decreased serum ferritin levels, but not with levels of free erythrocyte protoporphyrin, transferrin saturation, or hemoglobin. *H. pylori* infection was associated with the prevalence of iron-deficiency anemia and, to a lesser degree, other types of anemia. *H. pylori* infection was associated with a 40% increase in the prevalence of iron deficiency after controlling for relevant covariates. Although multicenter, sufficiently powered, randomized controlled treatment trials have not been performed, evidence suggests that anemia and iron deficiency may benefit from eradication.

The role of *H. pylori* in idiopathic thrombocytopenic purpura (ITP) in adults was supported by a number of publications.[193–196] In a recent review and in case series, eradication of *H. pylori* has been associated with platelet recovery in adults and children with ITP.[196,197] In a study of 17 children with ITP, *H. pylori* infection was not found.[198] In contrast, an investigation of 22 children with ITP using polyclonal *H. pylori* antigen stool testing found *H. pylori* infection in 9 of them; following eradication therapy, 5 of these 9 children had increased platelet counts that persisted throughout the 24-month follow-up period.[199] In addition, a case report of a 12-year-old boy with chronic ITP observed a complete platelet recovery after the eradication of *H. pylori*.[200] The eradication of *H. pylori* has been associated with remission of ITP in approximately one-half of eradicated patients. Further controlled studies in children are needed; data are limited to small case series. Of 244 screened patients <18 years of age with chronic ITP from 16 centers in Italy, 50 (20%) had *H. pylori* infection, 37 of whom received eradication therapy and completed follow-up. Eradication was successful in 89%; platelet recovery occurred in 39% of patients after eradication whereas spontaneous remission occurred in 10% of *H. pylori*-negative patients ($P < 0.005$).[201]

The first reports of *H. pylori* infection effects on growth retardation were published from Gambia and demonstrated convincingly that *H. pylori* could be a co-factor for growth disturbance in children infected early in life.[202] Longitudinal studies in children have demonstrated a link between short stature and *H. pylori* infection, especially in girls, although the association of infection with failure to thrive needs further study.[203,204] In a large Colombian cohort study, 105 children (30%) became infected with *H. pylori*. A significant decrease in growth velocity was observed during the first 4 months after infection, without height catch-up in infected children. At 8 months after acquisition, an infected child had a cumulative difference of 0.24 cm (growth velocity) compared with uninfected children.[205] In at-risk populations, potential interventions that target infected preschool children are likely to prevent growth retardation.

Other clinical conditions that have also been associated with *H. pylori* infection include: protein-losing gastropathy, periodontal disease, rosacea, food allergy, and in adults, coronary artery disease. However, studies were poorly designed and associations remain speculative.

DIAGNOSIS

There are no specific symptoms or constellation of signs and symptoms that predict the presence of gastritis or peptic ulcer in children. Furthermore, the majority of *H. pylori* infections and associated gastritis remain asymptomatic. However, children with warning symptoms or alarming signs such as severe chronic abdominal pain, anorexia and failure to thrive, or persistent vomiting require investigation. The presence of occult blood in feces, particularly in the face of iron deficiency and/or iron-deficiency anemia, should lead to investigation. The severity of symptoms determines the need for endoscopy; endoscopy and biopsy is performed to determine the cause of symptoms, not merely to investigate for *H. pylori* infection.[174,175]

Two groups have updated management guidelines recently based on best evidence. Updated Canadian *H. pylori* study group recommendations[175] are: (1) Population-based screening for *H. pylori* in asymptomatic children to prevent gastric cancer is not warranted. (2) Testing for *H. pylori* in children should be considered if there is a family history of gastric cancer. (3) The goal of diagnostic interventions should be to determine the cause of presenting gastrointestinal symptoms and not the presence of *H. pylori* infection. (4) Recurrent abdominal pain of childhood is not an indication to test for *H. pylori* infection. (5) *H. pylori* testing is not required in patients with newly diagnosed GERD. (6) However, *H. pylori* testing may be considered before the use of long-term proton pump inhibitor therapy. (7) Testing for *H. pylori* infection should be considered in children with refractory iron-deficiency anemia when no other cause has been found. (8) When investigation of pediatric patients with persistent or severe upper abdominal symptoms is indicated, upper endoscopy with biopsy is the investigation of choice. (9) The ^{13}C-urea breath test currently is the best noninvasive diagnostic test for *H. pylori* infection in children. (10) There currently is insufficient evidence to recommend stool antigen tests as acceptable diagnostic tools for *H. pylori* infection. (11) *H. pylori* serologic antibody tests are not recommended as diagnostic tools for infection in children.[174]

ESPGHAN-NASPGHAN guidelines, including grading of evidence, recommend: (1) The primary goal of clinical investigation of gastrointestinal symptoms is to determine the underlying cause of symptoms and not solely the presence of *H. pylori* infection. (2) Diagnostic testing for *H. pylori* infection is not recommended in children with functional abdominal pain. (3) In children with first-degree relatives with gastric cancer, testing for *H. pylori* may be considered. (4) In children with refractory iron-deficiency anemia, in which other causes have been ruled out, testing for *H. pylori* infection may be considered. (5) For the diagnosis of *H. pylori* infection during esophagogastroduodenoscopy (EGD) gastric biopsies (antrum and corpus) should be obtained for histopathology. (6) Initial diagnosis of *H. pylori* infection can be based on either positive histopathology plus positive rapid urease test or a positive culture. (7) The ^{13}C-urea breath test (UBT) is a reliable noninvasive test to determine eradication of *H. pylori*. (8) A validated enzyme immunoassay (EIA) test for *H. pylori* antigen in stool is a reliable noninvasive test to determine eradication of *H. pylori*. (9) Tests to detect antibodies (IgG, IgA) against *H. pylori* in serum, whole blood, urine, and saliva are not reliable for clinical use. (10) Clinicians need wait at least 2 weeks after stopping proton pump inhibitor (PPI) therapy and 4 weeks after stopping antibiotics to perform biopsy-based and noninvasive tests (UBT, stool test) for *H. pylori*.

The gold standard for the diagnosis of *H. pylori* infection is identification of the organism in culture and histologic examination of gastric biopsy samples. Compared with histologic changes in adults children have a higher density of *H. pylori* within the pits and on the surface of epithelial cells and a milder degree of infiltration with neutrophils, plasma cells, and eosinophils;[206] similar degree of infiltration with mononuclear cells and atrophy;[206,207] and less frequent ulcers and intestinal metaplasia.[207] In children, mucosal ulceration is located in the duodenum and is uncommon in the gastric corpus but can be seen in the gastric antrum.[208] Hematoxylin and eosin staining of gastric secretions is not as sensitive as other methods such as using Warthin–Starry silver stain, acridine orange, or Giemsa stain; the sensitivity of hematoxylin and eosin staining of gastric secretions is 77% versus 88% for biopsy specimens taken by endoscopy.[175,208] Because *H. pylori* is a fastidious organism, biopsy material can be transported in saline if it is to be processed within 3 hours, otherwise transport medium must be used, and the specimen should be kept on ice before inoculation. Gastric biopsy material can be tested using a rapid urease test that exploits the urease enzyme of *H. pylori* and can be performed in the endoscopy suite.[209] In the Entero-test, a noninvasive method to obtain a sample for culture for *H. pylori*, a capsule attached to a highly absorbent nylon string is swallowed. Amplification of several genes (urease, 16S RNA, 29-kd antigen, *cag*, and *vacA*) by PCR was demonstrated to be a successful alternative to culture and histology for diagnosis.[210] Although 16S RNA may be more sensitive for the detection of *H. pylori*, amplification of the *cag* or *vacA* genes gives more information on the infecting strain.[133,211,212] Biopsy specimens from the gastric antrum and corpus are inoculated onto enriched horse or sheep blood agar supplemented with antibiotics (vancomycin, amphotericin B, and cefoperazone) and incubated at 37°C in a microaerophilic atmosphere with 7% nitrogen. Few clinical microbiology laboratories have the capacity to perform culture for *H. pylori*.

The UBT using techniques such as a novel laser associated ratio analysis (LARA)-^{13}C, and the stool antigen tests (particularly new-generation monoclonal tests) have been studied extensively in both adults and children.[96,171,174,175,213–217] Investigations clearly demonstrated utility of these assays in children both for diagnosis and as a test for cure in a wider range of age groups.[213,218,219] Further validation of these assays is required for children <6 years of age. The polyclonal stool antigen test demonstrated variable performance and had less favorable accuracy compared with the UBT and newer-generation monoclonal stool antigen tests.[215,220]

Another method to diagnose *H. pylori* infection in children is detection of specific antibodies in serum, urine, or saliva.[221,222] Detection of serum immunoglobulin (Ig) G antibodies by EIA and Western blot (WB) is the most widely used.[223,224] The sensitivity of most commercially available EIAs, however, is much lower in children than in adults.[225] Recently developed EIAs that use recombinant CagA and VacA antigens require further evaluation in children. Moreover, three original pediatric *H. pylori* guidelines[226–228] as well as revised Canadian and ESPGHAN-NASGPHAN guidelines for children[175] clearly recommend against clinical use of serology.

The "string test" is a novel, relatively noninvasive method (requiring swallowing, 1-hour dwell time, and retrieval) that can provide both isolation of the organism for typing and antimicrobial susceptibility testing.[229–234] In a recent study, string test was compared with endoscopy and biopsy for detecting and analyzing *H. pylori* infection in 44 people with gastric complaints. In addition to culture and standard histologic evaluation, molecular assays (i.e., randomly amplified polymorphic DNA, RAPD, and PCR for urease B gene) were performed on both biopsies and string test samples.[230] *H. pylori* was cultured from 80% of strings and detected by PCR from 91% of strings from participants whose biopsies were culture-, PCR-, and histology-positive. Strains recovered from strings and biopsy specimens yielded identical or closely related RAPD profiles in each of 24 cases tested.[230] Genotypes of *H. pylori* from members of 62 shantytown households in Peru were compared using cultures and/or DNA assays by the string test.[233] The RAPD fingerprints of 70% of child–mother pairs did not match, nor did the diagnostic gene sequences (>1% DNA sequence difference), independent of the child's age (range, 1 to 39 years). Most strains from siblings or other paired family members also were unrelated. Data suggest that *H. pylori* infections in the society studied often are community acquired. This small but novel study infers that effective prevention of *H. pylori* infection and associated gastroduodenal disease will require anti-*H. pylori* measures applied community-wide. Although both studies are small in size, they provide evidence that the string test is useful clinically, especially in settings such as in rural communities or areas where pediatric gastroenterologists are not available.

TREATMENT

Treatment Guidelines

ESPGHAN-NASPGHAN clinical practice guidelines[174] make the following recommendation: (1) In the presence of *H. pylori*-positive peptic ulcer disease, eradication of *H. pylori* is recommended. (2) When *H. pylori* infection is detected by biopsy-based methods in the absence of peptic ulcer disease, treatment may be considered. (3) A "test and treat" strategy is not recommended in children. (4) In infected children whose first-degree relative has gastric cancer, treatment may be offered. (5) First-line eradication regimens are the following: triple therapy with a PPI plus amoxicillin plus clarithromycin or an imidazole or bismuth salts plus amoxicillin plus an

imidazole or sequential therapy. (6) The duration of triple therapy should be 7 to 14 days. Cost, compliance and adverse effects should be taken into account. (7) If treatment has failed, 3 options are recommended: (i) EGD with culture and susceptibility testing (including alternative antibiotics), if not performed before; (ii) fluorescence in situ hybridization (FISH) on previous paraffin-embedded biopsies if clarithromycin susceptibility testing was not performed previously; (iii) modification of therapy by adding an antibiotic, using different antibiotics, adding bismuth, and/or increasing the dose and/or duration of therapy.[174] Additionally, both the updated Canadian recommendations and the recent ESPGHAN-NASPGHAN guidelines make strong suggestions to screen asymptomatic people with a family history of gastric cancer, and to treat if infected.[174,175] ESPGHAN-NASPGHAN guidelines provide an algorithm for evaluation of a child with suspected *H. pylori* infection (Figure 174-4). The most effective anti-*Helicobacter* therapy currently accepted for children is a 2-week, triple therapy regimen that includes a PPI, such as omeprazole (1 mg/kg/day) or lansoprazole, plus clarithromycin and amoxicillin.[235] Box 174-1 lists accepted, evidence-based most effective eradication therapies for children. In a study of 63 French children with gastritis, 1 week of triple therapy resulted in *H. pylori* eradication in 74%.[236] According to updated Canadian and the combined ESPGHAN-NASPGHAN guidelines, *H. pylori* culture and antibiotic sensitivity testing should be made available to monitor population antibiotic resistance and to manage treatment failures. In studies in adults, quadruple therapy that also includes bismuth subsalicylate or citrate for 7 days has been demonstrated to be highly effective. Quadruple therapy in children as well as levofloxacin-based therapy requires additional studies for approval.[237,238] Ranitidine bismuth citrate plus two antibiotics also has been shown to have a high *H. pylori* eradication rate; however, in children further validation in the pediatric population is required.[239] In adults, triple therapy including levofloxacin now is recommended as an important component of salvage therapeutic regimens for treatment failures and is being used more widely as part of first-line therapy.[240,241] A recent meta-analysis showed that rescue therapy with levofloxacin is better tolerated and more effective than quadruple therapy (i.e., PPI plus two antibiotics with a bismuth base).[242]

Antibiotic Resistance and Follow-Up

Antibiotic resistance influences the efficacy of eradication treatment and clinical relapses are invariably associated with failure to eradicate the organism. Treatment should be guided by knowledge of specific geographic susceptibility patterns. Emerging resistance makes options for therapy less definitive. In a large multicenter, multinational European study of 1233 patients from northern (3%), western (70%), eastern (9%), and southern Europe (18%), primary resistance rate of *H. pylori* strains obtained from unselected children was high; use of antibiotics for other indications was deemed a major risk factor for primary resistance.[243] In this large pediatric study, overall resistance to clarithromycin was 24%, with higher rates in boys, in children <6 years compared with >12 years of age, and in patients living in southern compared with northern Europe. Overall resistance to metronidazole was 25%, and was higher in children born outside of Europe.

Recent reports in the U.S. and Europe show resistance rates of 21% to 41% for clarithromycin, 43% to 46% for metronidazole, and up to 5% for amoxicillin.[175,243,244] Metronidazole resistance in developing countries is even greater, up to 80%.[245,246] Follow-up to confirm cure and eradication should be performed using either UBT or *H. pylori* stool antigen test on weeks 4 to 6 after treatment. Reinfection rate appears to be <1% in developed countries, but is much higher in developing populations and if >1 family member is infected. Monitoring is justified only when the risk of reinfection is increased.

Novel Therapies

Novel therapies proposed for the treatment of *H. pylori* infection range from chewing gum to honey and green tea.[247] Emerging data

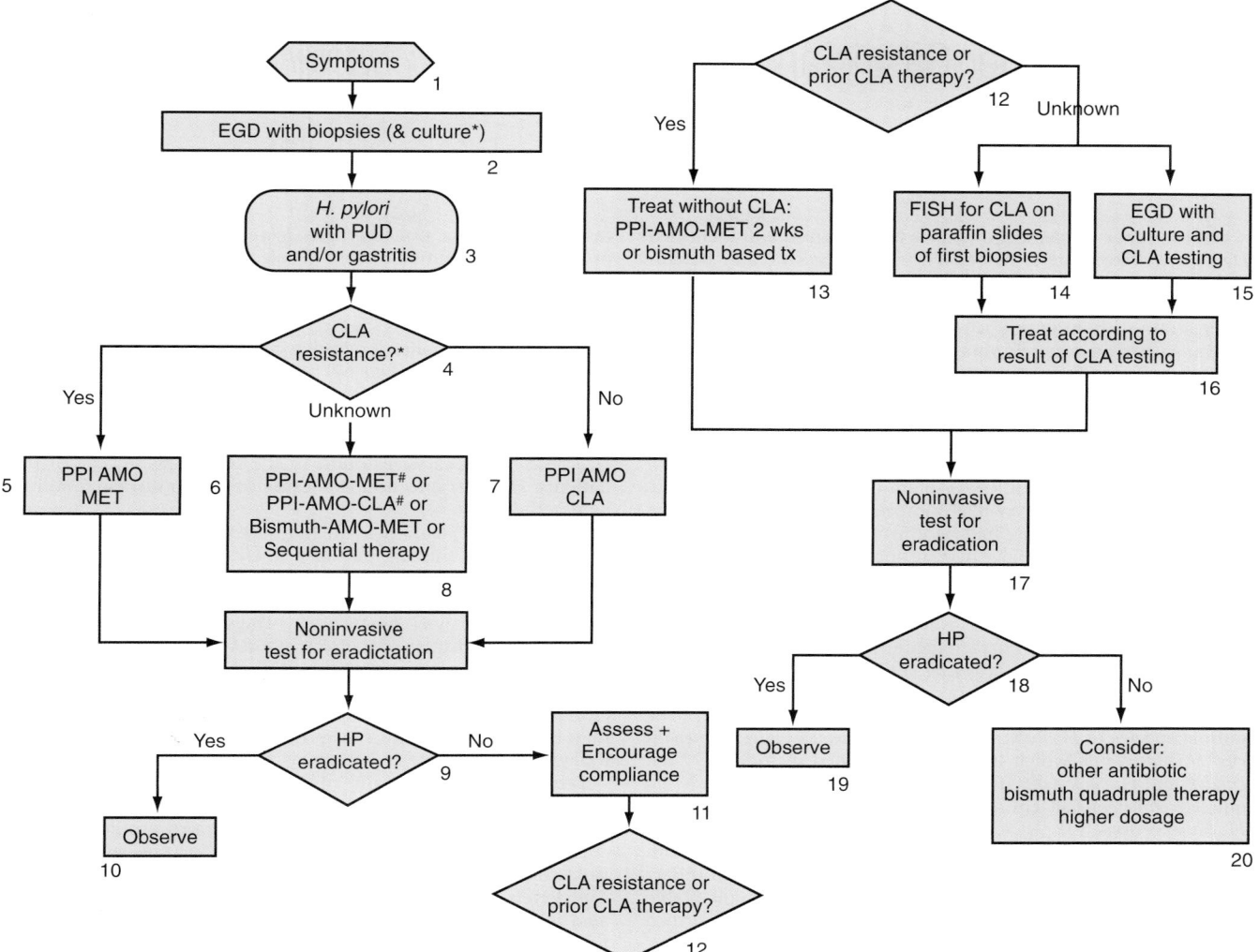

Figure 174-4. Algorithm for treatment of *H. pylori* infection in children. EGD, esophagogastroduodenoscopy; PUD, peptic ulcer disease; CLA, clarithromycin; AMO, amoxicillin; MET, metronidazole; PPI, proton pump inhibitor; FISH, fluorescence in situ hybridization; HP, *Helicobacter pylori;* tx, therapy. *In areas or populations with a primary clarithromycin resistance rate of >20% or unknown background antibiotic resistance rates, culture and susceptibility testing should be performed and the treatment should be chosen accordingly. #If susceptibility testing has not been performed or has failed, antibiotics should be chosen according to the background of the child.[1]

BOX 174-1. First-Line Treatment Recommendations for *H. pylori* Eradication in Children

- PPI + amoxicillin + metronidazole
- PPI + amoxicillin + clarithromycin
- Bismuth salts (bismuth subsalicylate or subcitrate) + amoxicillin + metronidazole
- PPI + amoxicillin for 5 days; then PPI + clarithromycin + metronidazole for 5 days

Doses are: PPI, 1–2 mg/kg/day; amoxicillin, 50 mg/kg/day; metronidazole, 20 mg/kg/day; clarithromycin, 20 mg/kg/day; bismuth salts, 8 mg/kg/day. Therapy is given in 2 divided doses daily for 10–14 days. Maximum daily doses are: amoxicillin, 2 g; metronidazole, 1 g; clarithromycin, 1 g.

PPI, proton pump inhibitor.

---

support the potential role for probiotics in treatment regimens for *H. pylori*. One randomized, blinded placebo-controlled found that *Lactobacillus casei* as a supplement to standard triple therapy was associated with higher eradication rates (84.6% vs. 57.5%, P = 0.0019).[248] Another study of probiotic administered alone versus standard triple therapy demonstrated superiority of standard treatment.[249,250] A Cochrane Database review of the role of probiotics in *H. pylori* infection concluded that probiotics do not eradicate *H. pylori* but likely suppress levels in the stomach, and in combination with antibiotics, may increase eradication rates and/or decrease adverse effects of the multidrug treatment regimens.[251]

Prebiotics also have been proposed as an adjuvant to traditional/standard eradication therapy. Reports suggest a modest bacteriostatic effect of foodstuffs such as berry juice and some milk proteins on *H. pylori*. Regular intake of these and other dietary products might constitute a low-cost, large-scale alternative solution applicable for populations at risk for *H. pylori* colonization.

175 Other Gastric and Enterohepatic *Helicobacter* Species

Benjamin D. Gold

A great number of investigators have characterized and identified *Helicobacter*-like bacteria associated with the gastric and enterohepatic disease of humans and other animals as a direct result of the discovery of *Helicobacter pylori* and demonstration of its causal association with human gastroduodenal disease (i.e., gastritis, ulcers, gastric adenocarcinoma).[1-4] There are now >20 formally named species in the genus *Helicobacter*.[3,5-7] In addition, there are a number of provisional species that have been named but not yet validated. Genomic advances in non-*H. pylori Helicobacter* include description of the complete genome of *H. canadensis*, delineation of two *H. bilis* genomospecies, and identification of a novel *cis*-regulatory RNA.[2] In addition, 3 gram-negative, microaerophilic bacteria with a corkscrew-like morphology isolated from the gastric mucosa of cats have had rigorous biochemical and molecular analyses applied and have been proposed as constituting a new taxon corresponding to "*Candidatus* H. heilmannii" or *H. heilmannii* sp. nov. previously demonstrated in the stomach of humans, wild Felidae, cats, and dogs.[2] New insights concerning growth conditions, biochemical characterization, and the effect of certain dietary compounds on *Helicobacter* spp. have also been reported. Other non-*pylori Helicobacter* spp. are found in a wide variety of animals, both in the stomach and lower intestinal tract.[8] The animal species of *Helicobacter* include *Helicobacter bilis*, *H. hepaticus*, *H. muridarum* which have been identified in rodents,[9-11] *H. cinaedi* and *H. cholecystus* in gerbils and hamsters,[12-16] *H. pullorum* and *H. pametensis* in chickens and birds,[17] *H. felis* in cats, and *H. canis* in dogs.[5,13,18,19]

In addition, there are *H.* non-*pylori* infections associated with gastritis, gastric ulcers, and MALT lymphomas; hepatobiliary disease; and enteritis, proctitis, and septicemia in humans (Table 175-1). Although there are no epidemiologic studies performed on a population-based level, approximately 20% to 40% of these are caused by *Helicobacter* spp. commonly found in dogs and cats, including *H. felis* and two "newer" identified *Helicobacter* species, *H. bizzozeronii* and *H. salomonis*.[13] Intestinal *Helicobacter* species: *H. cinaedi*, *H. fennelliae*, *H. pullorum*, *H. westmeadii*, *H. canadensis*, and "*H. rappini*" have been isolated from patients with enteritis and proctitis. *H. fennelliae*, *H. cinaedi*, *H. westmeadii*, and "*H. rappini*" have been isolated also from patients with septicemia.[15] Animal models for these bacteria have not been established, however, nor have other experimental studies validated Koch postulates for these organisms as human pathogens. Except for the

cases of septicemia, none of these *Helicobacter* species yet has been proven to cause human disease. A role for *Helicobacter*-like organisms in inflammatory bowel diseases has been postulated.[15,20] In one study,[21] mucosal fragments were obtained from the ileum, different colonic regions, and rectum of 43 patients with Crohn disease and of 74 patients without inflammatory bowel disease.[21] *H. pylori* strains, identified by 16S rRNA gene sequencing, were more frequently isolated and detected by polymerase chain reaction (PCR) in the intestinal mucosa of patients with ulcerative colitis-like Crohn disease than in the control group. No other *Helicobacter* species were found in the intestinal mucosa of the patients. *H. pylori* infection as a cause of Crohn disease is still to be determined.[21-23]

Hepatobiliary *Helicobacter* include several species isolated from bile and liver of animals, but only *H. bilis* has been isolated from the human gallbladder and *H. pylori* from the human liver.[6,24,25] A unique model of carcinogenesis, however, has been characterized in mice infected by *H. hepaticus*.[26-28] The study of this *Helicobacter* species and its disease sequelae may provide insight into hepatic carcinoma development as well as cholangiocarcinoma etiopathogenesis. *H. bilis* has been isolated from dogs, cats, mice, and rats. Non-*pylori Helicobacter* species usually are difficult to culture and may be more frequently causes of human disease than realized today.[29-30]

Taxonomic classification of *Helicobacter* is determined by sequences of bases in their 16S ribosomal DNA, DNA-DNA hybridization, protein profile, cellular fatty acid profile, and biochemical characterization.[2-3,5] Other *Helicobacter* species have been isolated from the stomachs of various mammals, including dogs, cats, ferrets, pigs, monkeys, and cheetahs, all of which are associated with various degrees of gastritis in their hosts.[31] The other formally named *Helicobacter* organisms have been assigned GenBank 16 ribosomal RNA accession numbers.[3,5]

H. pylori is the most frequently identified *Helicobacter* species in humans. However, other gastric and enterohepatic species have been identified from the human and animal stomachs[4,32-37] and from other locations in the intestinal tract or from hepatic sources.[6,38-52] The complete spectrum of disease syndromes associated with the "other" *Helicobacter* species has not been defined fully and could provide a model for understanding chronic diseases in both the gastrointestinal tract and extra-gastrointestinal locations. As more non-*pylori Helicobacter* species become identified, it is clear that all of the potential zoonotic infections in humans have not been characterized. This chapter provides an overview of gastric and enterohepatic infections in children by *Helicobacter* spp. other than *H. pylori*.

EPIDEMIOLOGY

The relationship between disease and infection with other *Helicobacter* spp. is generally believed to be host specific.[5,38,53] Zoonotic transmission of *H. pylori* from animals to humans has been examined in many studies, such as from sheep (i.e., shepherds, sheep milk, food supply),[54-57] as well as transmission of both *H. pylori* and *H. heilmannii* from cats[2,4-5,13,18,58] and dogs[4,18,59-62] and *H. pylori* from flies.[63,64] Although a number of models have compelling biologic plausibility, a definitive nonhuman host(s) that then transmits both *H. pylori* and non-*pylori Helicobacter* to humans remains to be validated.

In addition, there have been reports demonstrating one species of *Helicobacter* originally thought to infect one host type actually infecting other host species.[65-70] In an important study by Dubois

TABLE 175-1. Gastric and Enterohepatic *Helicobacter* Species Identified in Humans

Taxon	Location
H. heilmannii	Gastric
H. pylori	Gastric
H. bilis	Enterohepatic
H. canadensis	Enterohepatic
H. canis	Enterohepatic
H. cinaedi	Enterohepatic
H. fennelliae	Enterohepatic
H. flexispira taxon 5	Enterohepatic
H. mainz	Enterohepatic
H. pullorum	Enterohepatic
H. westmeadii	Enterohepatic

et al.,[70] four rhesus monkeys that had been cured of their natural *H. pylori* colonization were challenged with a mixture of 7 *H. pylori* strains of human origin. Bacteria recovered from the monkeys during periodic videogastroscopy were DNA fingerprinted. Interestingly, 3 animals carried mixtures of several strains for 4 months, after which strain J166 predominated.[70] In the fourth animal, only strain J238 was isolated from the earliest phase of colonization through 7 months, but strain J166 again became predominant by 10 months after the challenge. Gastritis scores, plasma gastrin, and immunoglobulin (Ig) G anti-*H. pylori* titers reached levels observed in naturally colonized animals by 4 months after the challenge; however, no plasma IgA response was observed up to 10 months. The authors concluded that: (1) natural colonization does not elicit protective immunity against subsequent *H. pylori* challenge; (2) individuals differ in susceptibility to different *H. pylori* strains during initial stages of colonization; and (3) certain strains are better suited than others for long-term survival in different hosts. In another study by Fernandez et al.,[68] *H. cinaedi* was isolated from captive rhesus monkeys. *H. cinaedi* can cause proctocolitis or bloodstream infection (BSI) in men who have sex with men infected with human immunodeficiency virus infection, or occasionally in other immunocompromised hosts. Microaerophilic cultures of feces from 5 of 16 asymptomatic rhesus monkeys (*Macaca mulatta*) (31%) were positive for *H. cinaedi*.[68] Hornsby et al.[65] utilized the rhesus macaque model to study the effects of the *cag* pathogenicity island (*cag* PAI) on the *H pylori* host–pathogen interaction. *H. pylori*-specific pathogen-free (SPF) monkeys were challenged experimentally with wild-type (WT) *H. pylori* strain J166 (J166WT, n = 4) or its *cag* PAI isogenic knockout (J166Δ*cag* PAI, n = 4). Animals underwent endoscopy before and 1, 4, 8, and 13 weeks after challenge. Gastric biopsies were collected for quantitative culture, histopathology, and host gene expression analysis. Microarray analysis showed that of the 119 upregulated genes in the J166WT-infected animals, several encode innate antimicrobial effector proteins, including elafin, siderocalin, DMBT1, DUOX2, and several novel paralogues of human beta-defensin-2. Quantitative reverse transcription (RT)-PCR confirmed that high-level induction of each of these genes depended on the presence of the *cag* PAI. The authors concluded that one function of the *cag* PAI is to induce an antimicrobial host response that may serve to increase the competitive advantage of *H. pylori* in the gastric niche and could even provide a protective benefit to the host.[65] Thus, there may be reservoirs other than man that could promote infection under the right circumstances and these reservoirs could serve as biologically relevant models for understanding *H. pylori*-associated pathogenesis and for the evaluation of novel eradication strategies for human infection.

Although early observations of *H.* non-*pylori* infections were made in cats and dogs. Organisms also have been identified in many animals, including macaques, ferrets, pigs, cattle, cheetahs, mice, rats, hamsters, chickens, sheep, and birds.[18,39,65,71–77] Other unlikely hosts include ocelots, mountain lions, dolphins, and whales.[35–36,78–82] Gastric ulcerations in dolphins have been reported for decades.[35,83,84] Other *Helicobacter* spp. and a novel species (proposed name *H. cetorum*) have been identified in gastric mucosa of affected Atlantic and Pacific dolphins and a beluga whale.[84–86] Infections associated with other *Helicobacter* spp. can for the most part, be associated with the presence of host disease.

Increasing evidence supports the causal relationship between infection with an organism originally called *Gastrospirillum hominis*, now designated *H. heilmannii*, and human gastroduodenal disease, specifically in children.[2,87–91] These organisms are found in the stomachs of mammals, including humans. The prevalence and overall epidemiology of *H. heilmannii*-like organisms in humans is not clearly defined but estimates are from <0.5% to 2% among patients undergoing upper gastrointestinal tract endoscopy.[3,92,93] In one of the larger clinical-pathologic correlation studies performed, 2 antral and 1 corpus full-thickness random endoscopic gastric mucosal samples (6077 biopsies) obtained from 946 patients with duodenal ulcers and 1794 biopsies from 281 patients with nonsteroidal anti-inflammatory drug (NSAID)-associated gastric ulcers were analyzed.[94] *H. heilmannii* was

detected in 6 (0.5%) of 1227 patients (14; 0.2% of 7871 biopsies). Of these, 4 (0.4%) of 946 were patients with duodenal ulcers (9; 0.2% of 6077 biopsies), and 2 (0.7%) of 281 were patients with NSAID-associated gastric ulcers (5; 0.28% of 1794 biopsies).[94] Thus, it appears that *H. heilmannii* has a "worldwide" epidemiology that is yet to be characterized completely. To date, reports of children with gastritis and ulcers and associated *H. heilmannii* infection have been published from Bulgaria, Brazil, southern England, the United States, Japan, and other parts of Asia.[2–3,53,92–93,95–99] Overall prevalence of *H. heilmannii* may be higher in people in countries other than the U.S., and in contrast to infection in humans, infection is common in other mammals, namely, cats, primates, pigs, and carnivorous mammals.[95,99–102]

The enterohepatic *Helicobacter* spp. differ from the gastric *Helicobacter* spp. in that the former normally do not colonize the gastric mucosa but have been identified in the intestinal tract, liver, or both of humans, other mammals, and birds.[1,5,7,25,38,53,103–108] These organisms have ultrastructural and physiologic features in common with gastric *Helicobacter* spp. In addition, enterohepatic species are considered a component of the normal intestinal tract flora of many animals. Two specific pathogens, *H. cinaedi* and *H. fennelliae*, are associated with lower gastrointestinal human disease particularly in immunocompromised hosts.[1,68,109–114] Both of these *Helicobacter* species also have been shown to produce disease in a primate model. Reports of the isolation of other gastric and enterohepatic *Helicobacter* strains from children have been published but are uncommon.[5,115–118] Although these organisms have been associated with gastroenteritis, hepatitis, and other diseases in humans and other animals, the underlying pathobiology as a cause of human disease has not been defined.

Because *H. heilmannii*, *H. pullorum*, and *H. bilis* are so common in animals, it is believed that infection with one of these organisms in humans may represent zoonotic transmission. This observation is supported by the findings of similar organisms in humans and their pet dogs[34,119–123] and cats[5,18,124,125] and of animal contact among infected humans.[1,113,126–131] In one study from 3 centers, gastric biopsy specimens of 108 human *Helicobacter*-like organism-infected patients (42 women and 66 men) were screened for the presence of *H. pylori* and animal gastric *Helicobacter* species by PCR, using assays targeting the 16S rDNA region of the three known canine and feline *Helicobacter* species (*H. bizzozeronii*, *H. salomonis*, and *H. felis*), "*Candidatus H. suis*," and "*Candidatus H. bovis*." Non-*pylori Helicobacter* species commonly colonizing the stomachs of cats and dogs were found in 48.5% (49/101) of the patients and *H. pylori* in 13 patients (12.9%); 11 stomachs (10.9%) were infected with at least two different *Helicobacter* species.[4]

The potential relationship between *Helicobacter* spp. and inflammatory bowel disease has been suggested. In particular, Helicobacteraceae DNA was investigated in intestinal biopsies collected from 179 children undergoing colonoscopy (Crohn disease 77, controls 102) using a Helicobacteraceae-specific PCR. Members of the Helicobacteraceae were detected in 32/77 children with Crohn disease (41.5%) compared with 23/102 controls (22.5%) (P = 0.0062). Non-*pylori Helicobacter* also were significantly higher in patients than in controls (P = 0.04). Phylogenetic analysis of *H. pylori* sequences showed that the *H. pylori* strains identified in Crohn disease patients did not group with gastric *H. pylori* included in the analysis, but rather clustered with other *H. pylori* strains detected in the intestine, gallbladder, and liver, indicating that different *H. pylori* strains may adapt to colonize extragastric niches.[129]

CLINICAL MANIFESTATIONS

Of the other *Helicobacter* organisms, the majority of the clinical literature describes *H. heilmannii*,[2,18,93,95–97,99] *H. cinaedi*,[1,15,41,68,110,125,132,133] and *H. fennelliae*[1,113,132,134] infections. *H. heilmannii* involves the stomach, whereas *H. cinaedi* and *H. fennelliae* predominantly colonize and are associated with enterohepatic manifestations of disease.

Gastritis and mucosal ulceration has been associated with *H. heilmannii* infection, although some studies suggest that the overall inflammation and mucosal response is less severe than that associated with *H. pylori*. In addition, *H. heilmannii* infection has been associated with acute and chronic gastritis and dyspepsia and also has been described in asymptomatic individuals.[96,99,102,128,135] In one published prospective, pediatric cohort study of 580 patients, 26.4% of all examined dyspeptic children were infected with spiral-shaped organisms, and 0.9% of patients were found to be infected with spiral *H. heilmannii*-like organisms.[93] Mucosal associated lymphoid type tissue (MALT) lymphomas also have been associated with *H. heilmannii*. In a Japanese study of both adults and children, gastric biopsy materials of 4074 consecutive Japanese patients undergoing esophagogastroduodenoscopy were reviewed.[95] From this cohort, 15 patients had *H. heilmannii* infection (11 chronic gastritis, 4 mucosa-associated lymphoid tissue (MALT) lymphoma). In chronic gastritis, the gastric mucosa was endoscopically normal (13.3%), had erythema (33.3%), or had erosions (53.3%). Histologic evaluation of biopsies showed no epithelial change, mild mononuclear cell infiltration, and slight and focal neutrophil infiltration.[95] Eradication of *H. heilmannii* in this study resulted in remission of MALT lymphoma.[95] MALT lymphoma has been replicated in animals. This histologic response increased in severity with the length of infection, with the development of overt lymphoma in some animals 18 months after infection. In a murine study (BALB/c mice), MALT lymphomas were detected in up to 25% of *H. heilmannii*-infected animals, and the prevalence of lymphoma was dependent on the length of infection and the origin of the infecting isolates.[37] An association with gastric lymphoma and particularly the remission of MALT lymphoma has been described in 5 patients after treatment of *H. heilmannii* infection.[90,95,98,102] In the Morgner et al.[90] study, patients received 40 mg omeprazole and 750 mg amoxicillin 3 times per day for 14 days. PCR was used to detect rearrangement of immunoglobulin heavy-chain genes before treatment and during follow-up. Treatment resulted in the cure of *H. heilmannii* infection in each of 5 cases and complete histologic and endoscopic remission of tumors.[90] Three of 5 patients showed monoclonal B cells before treatment, 2 of whom remained PCR positive. Within a median follow-up period of 24 months, no relapse of the lymphoma or reinfection with *H. heilmannii* occurred.

H. cinaedi and *H. fennelliae* (originally identified as *Campylobacter* spp.) cause invasive disease as well as gastroenteritis in humans, particularly persons with underlying immunosuppression.[3,72,111,136,137] Persons with acquired immunodeficiency syndrome (AIDS) are especially prone to these *Helicobacter* infections including recurrent infections that are difficult to eradicate.[136] *H. cinaedi* has been associated with proctocolitis, enterocolitis, and diarrhea in immunocompromised hosts.[15,110,113–114,132,138] However, BSI without gastroenteritis has been associated more commonly with *H. cinaedi* and *H. fennelliae* in immunocompromised people with AIDS or other underlying conditions.[136–137,139–141] These species also are described to cause cellulitis and pyogenic arthritis, BSI due to *H. cinaedi* in immunocompetent children and adults without diarrhea, and BSI and meningitis in a neonate.[5,137,141,142]

Other diarrheal enteropathogens in the *Helicobacter* genus also have been associated with human disease. In addition to *H. pylori*, the 5 species are: *H. pullorum*, *H. canis*, "*H. rappini*," *H. fennelliae*, and *H. cinaedi*. Fox and his colleagues[133] analyzed 11 *Helicobacter* isolates cultured from diarrhea patients in Canada. These isolates had been originally characterized biochemically and by restriction fragment length polymorphism (RFLP; AluI, HhaI) analysis as *H. pullorum*. However, 4 isolates differed biochemically from *H. pullorum*; when complete 16S rRNA analysis was used, the 4 strains clustered near *H. pullorum* but had a sequence difference of 2% and therefore represent a novel species, *H. canadensis*. This novel *Helicobacter* could also be distinguished from *H. pullorum* by RFLP analysis using ApaLI.[133] Thus, the number of novel *Helicobacter* spp. associated with gastrointestinal disease in humans and animals is increasing rapidly.

Enterohepatic disease also has been associated with other *Helicobacter* spp., but additional studies are needed to demonstrate causality. In one recent study, liver samples from 28 patients with hepatocellular carcinoma (HCC) diagnosed histopathologically were studied using multiple molecular and tissue techniques.[143] The culture-positive rate in HCC of 10.7% (3/28) provided circumstantial evidence that *H. non-pylori* species may be involved in carcinogenesis outside of the stomach.[143] In another pathology-based study,[144] *Helicobacter* species 16S rDNA (predominantly but not solely *H. pylori*) was found in 8 of 20 samples of primary liver carcinoma, whereas none of the controls harbored this rDNA.

A pediatric study was performed on 61 liver biopsies of patients with miscellaneous diseases and on autopsy liver tissue from 10 control subjects with no evidence of pre-existing liver disease. Multiple molecular methods and a semi-nested PCR assay for *H. ganmani* were used; 40/61 patient samples and 4/10 control samples were positive in the genus-specific *Helicobacter* PCR. The nucleotide sequences of 16S rDNA fragments were 99% to 100% similar to *Helicobacter* sp. "liver" and *H. ganmani*. PCR products similar to *H. canis* and *H. bilis* also were found. The 16S rDNA of control specimens showed similarity to *Helicobacter* sp. "liver"; in the *H. ganmani*-specific PCR analysis, 19 patients but no control sample was positive.[145] Possible causal link between *Helicobacter* species and liver diseases in adults and children requires further prospective studies.

H. canis, *H. flexispira*, *H. canadensis*, and *H. pullorum* have been isolated from children with diarrhea.[1,5,15,105,116,133,145,146] Several strains, including *H. mainz* and *H. westmeadii*, have been associated with invasive disease in people with AIDS and X-linked agammaglobulinemia.[141,147,148]

DIAGNOSIS

The majority of other *Helicobacter* spp. have been identified initially in tissue and by molecular techniques. Culture and primary isolation of *H. non-pylori* has been more difficult and taxonomy has been a slow process in humans and in animals.[149–153]

The urea breath test may have promise for screening for any urease producing *Helicobacter*-like organism, but may not be specific. This technology, however, has been applied to animals for diagnosis as well as a "test of cure." The urea breath test was successfully used for *H. heilmannii*-infected cats.[154]

Growth of other *Helicobacter* spp. is complex and requires special conditions, including a microaerobic environment; many strains grow better in an atmosphere of 5% to 10% hydrogen. The *Helicobacter* spp. grow slowly and can be overgrown easily by contaminating enteric or gastric flora. Organisms from stool usually have been identified through the use of methods for isolating *Campylobacter* spp. However, some *Helicobacter* spp. are susceptible to common antimicrobial agents added to commercial *Campylobacter* media. Susceptibility to nalidixic acid and cephalothin varies among strains.

All of the other *Helicobacter* spp. except *H. canis* product catalase, and most species identified in humans have bipolar flagella, except *H. pullorum* and *H. westmeadii*, which have monopolar flagella. *Helicobacter* spp. such as *H. cinaedi* and *H. fennelliae* can be recovered by an automated blood culture instrument, usually from the aerobic bottle. Most isolates are detected after 5 or more days of incubation as slightly elevated growth indices.[19,149,155–157]

H. heilmannii is well visualized and can be distinguished from *H. pylori* in gastric tissue on light-microscopic examination of paraffin sections stained with hematoxylin and eosin stains or Warthin–Starry silver stain. Transmission and electron microscopy has enabled various morphologic forms of the other *Helicobacter* spp. to be described. A phylogenetic tree for validated *Helicobacter* spp. and additional provisional species based on 16S rRNA sequence has been published.[2–3,38,72,107,158]

TREATMENT

Determining whether *H. heilmannii* infection causes gastrointestinal tract symptoms and gastric pathologic changes is difficult because of the low prevalence of infection, lack of susceptibility testing of organisms, and absence of clinical trials. This observation also can hold true for the variety of *Helicobacter* organisms listed in this chapter. Although randomized controlled clinical trials have not been performed for eradication of *H. non-pylori*, overwhelming evidence based on the literature reviewed is that the same guidelines for *H. pylori* eradication should be employed. When a *Helicobacter* sp. such as *H. fennelliae* or *H. cinaedi* is identified from a nongastric site, the significance of the organism should be assessed, and if treatment is warranted, antimicrobial susceptibility testing should be performed.

176 *Kingella* Species

Pablo Yagupsky and David Greenberg

The genus *Kingella* comprises four species: *Kingella denitrificans*, which is a rare cause of endocarditis,[1] pediatric vaginitis,[2] chorioamnionitis,[3] and septicemic granulomatosis in AIDS patients;[4] *Kingella oralis*, which has been found in association with periodontitis;[5,6] *Kingella potus*, which has been isolated from a wound caused by an animal bite;[7] and *Kingella kingae*, which is emerging as an invasive pathogen of young children and will be discussed in detail in this chapter.

MICROBIOLOGY

Kingella kingae is a facultative anaerobic β-hemolytic bacterium that appears as short chains of plump bacilli with tapered ends (Figure 176-1).[8] *Kingella kingae* grows on blood- and chocolate-agar producing marked impressions on the medium's surface, fails to grow on MacConkey or Krigler agar, and its growth is enhanced by a CO_2-enriched atmosphere.[8] *Kingella kingae* is nonmotile, exhibits oxidase positivity, and has no catalase, urease, or indole activity. The organism produces acid from glucose and maltose but not from other sugars, and can be readily identified by commercial systems such as API NH or VITEK 2 (bioMérieux, Marcy-l'Etoile, France).

VIRULENCE AND PATHOGENESIS

The pathogenesis of invasive *K. kingae* disease is believed to begin with colonization of the oropharynx. Organisms recovered from the blood of children with invasive infections are genotypically identical to those isolated from the tonsils.[9] Colonization involves adherence to epithelial cells, which is mediated by type IV pili that share homology with the major pilin of other gram-negative pathogens.[10-12] *K. kingae* disease frequently occurs in children who exhibit symptoms consistent with a viral infection, herpetic gingivostomatitis or buccal ulcers, suggesting that breach of the mucosal lining facilitates bloodstream invasion.[13-15] In addition, the organism produces a potent extracellular toxin that belongs to the RTX family, capable of lysing epithelial, synovial, and macrophage cells.[16] This toxin may disrupt the respiratory epithelium and contribute to pathogenesis by damaging skeletal tissues.[16] Preliminary studies suggest that *K. kingae* elaborates a polysaccharide capsule to promote survival in the bloodstream, explaining the tendency of the organism to infect young children who have not yet developed a mature T-lymphocyte independent immune response.

IMMUNITY

In a longitudinal study, titers of IgG antibodies against *K. kingae* outer membrane proteins were high at 2 months of age, reached a nadir at the age of 6–7 months, remained low until the age of 18 months, and increased at 24 months, whereas serum IgA levels were lowest at 2 months and also peaked in the second year.[17] The low attack rate of disease, absence of pharyngeal carriage, and high levels of IgG but no IgA antibodies in early infancy suggest that immunity to colonization and disease is conferred by maternal antibodies. The high pharyngeal prevalence of *K. kingae* and the increased incidence of invasive disease among children 6 to 24 months of age coincide with the age at which antibody levels are lowest. Increasing antibody levels in older children presumably reflect immunologic maturation and cumulative experience with *K. kingae* or with cross-reacting antigens, resulting in an efficient reduction of carriage and burden of disease.[17] Because of the relative rarity of invasive infections, asymptomatic pharyngeal colonization probably is the immunizing event. Exposed epitopes, however, are polymorphic and the immune response appears to be incomplete and strain-specific, and does not prevent colonization by an antigenically different organism.[18]

EPIDEMIOLOGY

Carriage

K. kingae is carried asymptomatically on the tonsillar surfaces and is almost never isolated from nasopharyngeal cultures.[19,20] Children usually acquire *K. kingae* after the age of 6 months and carriage is characterized by frequent turnover of strains.[19-21] The colonization rate increases to 9% to 12% at the ages of 12 through 24 months and gradually declines thereafter, paralleling the age-related incidence of invasive disease (Figure 176-2). *K. kingae*

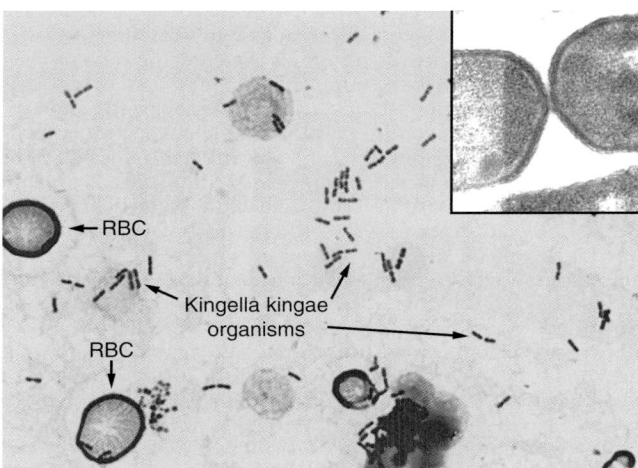

Figure 176-1. Gram stain of a positive Bactec 9240 blood culture vial showing pairs and short chains of gram-negative coccobacilli typical of *K. kingae* organisms. RBC, red blood cells. Right upper corner insert: electron microscopic picture showing the characteristic gram-negative cell wall structure (75,000×).

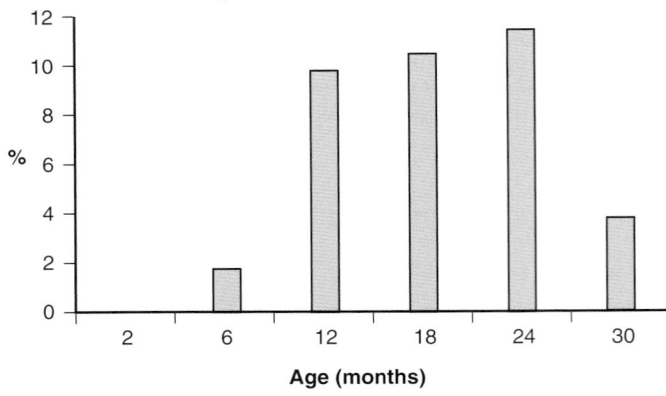

Figure 176-2. Point prevalence of pharyngeal carriage of *K. kingae* in a cohort of 716 children sampled sequentially between the ages of 2 and 30 months.

spreads from child to child by close contact between siblings and playmates, and daycare center attendance increases the risks for colonization and transmission.[19,20] A carriage rate of 28% has been found among children in daycare[19] and clusters of invasive infections have been detected in daycare facilities in the U.S.[22,23] and Israel.[24] When surveillance cultures were obtained from asymptomatic children attending classrooms where *K. kingae* outbreaks occurred, many were found to be colonized by organisms identical to those recovered from the index patients, indicating that the outbreak strains were highly transmissible and successful as respiratory tract colonizers.[22–24]

Invasive Infections

K. kingae infections are almost limited to children. Of a total of 128 patients identified over a 23-year period in southern Israel, only one was an adult; 126 of the 127 children were younger than 4 years, yielding an annual incidence of invasive disease of 9.4/100,000 in this age group.[25] The disease is rare in the first 6 months of life (Figure 176-3).

Most infected children younger than 4 years are otherwise healthy, whereas older children and adults often have immunosuppressing conditions, malignancy, or cardiac valve pathology.[15,25,26] In a multicenter Israeli study, none of 291 previously healthy children with an invasive *K. kingae* infection were older than 48 months, whereas 9 of 22 (41%) children with underlying diseases were >48 months of age.[25] The disease is more common among males, with a male-to-female ratio of 1.3.[25]

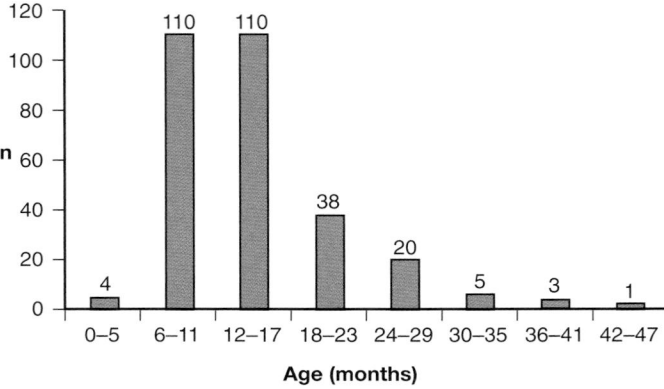

Figure 176-3. Age distribution of 291 previously healthy Israeli children with culture-proven invasive *K. kingae* infections.

Invasive *K. kingae* infections occur throughout the year and are most common during November and December and least common between February and April.[15,25,27]

CLINICAL MANIFESTATIONS

Pediatric patients with *K. kingae* infections other than endocarditis are usually considered to be only mildly or moderately ill.[15,26,28–33] Generally a single focus of infection is detected.[34] Most children have moderate fever, but 23% are afebrile, and acute-phase reactants frequently are normal or only slightly elevated.[25,31] In a series of children with culture-proven *K. kingae* disease, 172 of 301 (57%) had a white blood cell (WBC) count <15,000/mm³, and 18 of 82 (22%) had normal C-reactive protein values.[25] In the 321 children with invasive *K. kingae* infection enrolled in a nationwide collaborative study in Israel, involvement of the skeletal system was observed in 169 (53%), bacteremia with no focus in 140 (44%), endocarditis in 8 (2%), and pneumonia in 1 (1%).[25]

Skeletal System Infections

Pyogenic arthritis. Pyogenic arthritis is the single most common presentation of *K. kingae* infections. The disease usually affects the knee, ankle, or hip.[25] Less frequently, *K. kingae* invades the wrist, shoulder, elbow, and small articulations such as metacarpophalangeal, sternoclavicular, and tarsal joints, which are rarely infected by other bacteria.[15,25,35,36]

Lack of leukocytosis has been observed in 76 of 149 (51%) children with *K. kingae* arthritis, and 18 of 78 (23%) had <50,000 WBC/mm³ in synovial fluid.[25] The synovial fluid Gram stain usually is negative, probably due to the low bacterial concentration in the exudate.[15,25,37–39] Because of the mild symptomatology and benign laboratory findings, diagnosis of *K. kingae* arthritis requires a high index of suspicion. Blood culture drawing and use of nucleic acid amplification techniques, when available, are recommended in children younger than 4 years presenting with minimal orthopedic symptoms.[40]

Osteomyelitis. *K. kingae* osteomyelitis especially affects the long bones,[41] although involvement of the calcaneus, talus, sternum, or clavicle also can occur.[15,25,31,35] Patients with *K. kingae* osteomyelitis have a significantly more prolonged duration of symptoms before admission compared with children with pyogenic arthritis (9.2 ± 9.4 days vs. 3.2 ± 3.0 days, respectively), and have lower body temperature (37.7 ± 1.0°C *vs.* 38.4 ± 0.9°C, respectively).[25] Despite the diagnostic delay of *K. kingae* osteomyelitis, chronicity and orthopedic sequelae are exceptional.[15,42]

Spondylodiskitis. *K. kingae* is the most common etiology of hematogenous spondylodiskitis in the 6 to 48 months age group.[31,43–45] Circulating organisms appear to reach the intervertebral disks through a network of vessels that enter the annulus from the cartilaginous vertebral endplates.[45] *K. kingae* spondylodiskitis generally involves the lumbar disks, followed by the thoracolumbar, lumbosacral, and cervical intervertebral spaces. Patients present with limping, lumbar pain, back stiffness, refusal to sit or walk, neurologic symptoms, or abdominal complaints. Plain radiograph or MRI demonstrates narrowing of the intervertebral space. Because blood cultures are negative in the majority of patients and obtaining a tissue specimen for culture if difficult, nucleic-acid amplification techniques play an important role in establishing the etiology.[45,46] Children with *K. kingae* spondylodiskitis respond well to antibiotic therapy and recover without sequelae.[15]

Abortive skeletal system infections. Although bone and joint infections are not considered self-limited diseases, transient involvement of the skeletal system during a bacteremic *K. kingae* episode has been reported.[40,47,48] Children with this condition present with limping or refusal to walk or bear weight, but without objective signs of osteoarthritis and with normal peripheral blood WBC count and imaging studies and, by the time blood cultures become positive, symptoms and fever have resolved. As a matter of caution, however, adequate antimicrobial therapy should probably be administered to all patients from whom *K. kingae* is isolated from a normally sterile site.

Soft-Tissue Infections

Soft-tissue infections, including cellulitis,[49] tenosynovitis, dactylitis,[15,50] bursitis,[51] subcutaneous,[52] and presternal abscesses[35,53] also have been reported.

Bloodstream Infections

Bloodstream infection (BSI) without focus is the second most frequent presentation of pediatric *K. kingae* infections.[13,15,25,26,48] In a large study, only half of children with this condition had a body temperature ≥39°C, and one-third had a leukocyte count <15,000 WBC/mL; therefore the current guidelines for managing young febrile children with no apparent focus, which rely on the height of fever and WBC count for obtaining blood cultures, may be not sensitive to detect *K. kingae* BSI.[26,54] A maculopapular rash, resembling disseminated neisserial infection, has been described in a few patients.[37,55-57]

Endocarditis

K. kingae is included in the HACEK group of organisms that is collectively responsible for up to 5% of cases of bacterial endocarditis. In contrast to other *K. kingae* infections, endocarditis has been diagnosed also in older children and adults.[15] In approximately one-half of patients the infection affects a native valve. Predisposing cardiac malformations or rheumatic disease are observed commonly, but some patients have previously normal valves.[15,23,58-61] Typically the left side of the heart is involved, usually the mitral valve. Despite the remarkable susceptibility of *K. kingae* to antibiotics, and the benign clinical picture observed in other invasive *K. kingae* infections, the course of endocarditis is severe and characterized by life-threatening complications such as cardiac failure, septic shock, mycotic aneurysms, pulmonary infarctions, meningitis, and cerebrovascular accidents in half of the patients, and a case-fatality rate of 16%.[23,58-61] Because of the potential gravity of endocardial involvement, routine echocardiographic evaluation of all individuals from whom *K. kingae* is isolated from a normally sterile site has been recommended.[62]

Lower Respiratory Tract Infections

K. kingae has been isolated from the blood or respiratory secretions of previously healthy and immunocompromised adult and pediatric patients with epiglottitis, laryngotracheobronchitis, pneumonia, or pyothorax, suggesting that the organism can cause lower respiratory tract infections.[15,25]

Meningitis

K. kingae meningitis has been described as a primary infection,[63-67] or as a complication of endocarditis.[34,68,69] The age distribution of patients with *K. kingae* meningitis is noticeable in that half of the cases have occurred in adolescents and young adults.[15]

Ocular Infections

K. kingae has been isolated from patients with a variety of ocular infections such as orbital cellulitis,[70] eyelid abscess,[71] endophthalmitis,[37,72] and a corneal ulcer.[73]

DIAGNOSIS

Culture Detection

Attempts to isolate *K. kingae* on routine solid media frequently are unsuccessful, and recovery of the organism can be substantially improved by inoculating synovial fluid aspirates and bone exudates into blood culture vials of the BACTEC (Becton Dickinson, Cockeysville, MD),[74] BacT/Alert (Organon Teknika Corporation, Durham, NC),[75,76] Hemoline DUO (bioMérieux, Paris, France),[77]

and Isolator 1.5 Microbial Tube (Wampole Laboratories, Cranbury, NJ)[39] systems, suggesting that pus exerts an inhibitory effect upon the bacterium, and dilution of clinical specimens in a large broth volume decreases the concentration of detrimental factors enabling bacterial growth.[74] In two studies in which the blood culture vial method was used routinely for culturing joint fluid aspirates from young children with arthritis, *K. kingae* was isolated in half of the patients with culture-proven infections.[30,78]

Nucleic Acid Amplification

Because of the difficulties in recovering *K. kingae* in culture, the organism is a natural candidate for detection by nucleic acid amplification techniques. The entire procedure can be completed in a few hours compared with the 3 to 5 days required for the culture detection and biochemical identification of *K. kingae*.[79] Using home-made nucleic acid amplification assays, enhanced detection of *K. kingae* in bone and joint specimens demonstrates that *K. kingae* is responsible for a large proportion of culture-negative cases of pyogenic arthritis and osteomyelitis, and is the leading etiology of skeletal system infections in children 6 to 48 months of age.[31-33,80,81]

TREATMENT

K. kingae is almost always susceptible to penicillins, cephalosporins, aminoglycosides, macrolides, trimethoprim-sulfamethoxazole, and fluoroquinolones, and β-lactamase production is exceptional.[82-86] The organism exhibits decreased susceptibility to oxacillin and is fully resistant to trimethoprim and glycopeptide antibiotics.[15,83] Nearly 40% of isolates are resistant to clindamycin.[83]

Because of the lack of specific guidelines for the treatment of *K. kingae* infections, patients have been treated with different antibiotics and drug combinations or according to protocols developed for infections caused by more traditional pathogens.

Bone and Joint Infections

The empiric drug therapy for skeletal infections in children usually consists of intravenous administration of a second- or third-generation cephalosporin, pending culture results. Because vancomycin or clindamycin is used for empiric treatment for skeletal system infections in children younger than 4 years in areas where community-associated methicillin-resistant *Staphylococcus aureus* is prevalent and these drugs are not adequate for *K. kingae*, a β-lactam drug should be administered in addition.[84,87]

When *K. kingae* is detected, therapy frequently is changed to parenteral ampicillin (once β-lactamase production is excluded), cefuroxime, or a third-generation cephalosporin. Normalization of body temperature, improvement of local signs, and decreasing erythrocyte sedimentation rate and C-reactive protein levels are used to guide a change to oral antibiotics and to determine the duration of therapy.[88,89] Treatment has varied from 17 days to 3 months for *K. kingae* arthritis,[15] from 3 weeks to 6 months for osteomyelitis,[15,77] and from 3 to 12 weeks for spondylodiskitis.[43,44]

Bloodstream Infection

Children with *K. kingae* BSI and no focal infection generally are treated with an intravenous cephalosporin and subsequently are given oral β-lactam antibiotics. Patients respond favorably to a 1- to 2-week antibiotic course.[13,15]

Endocarditis

Patients with *K. kingae* endocarditis usually are treated with a β-lactam drug alone intravenously or in combination with an aminoglycoside for 4 to 7 weeks. Careful assessment and early surgical intervention is necessary for life-threatening complications unresponsive to medical therapy.[15,58-60]

177 *Legionella* Species

Lorry G. Rubin

Investigation of an outbreak of pneumonia among attendees at an American Legion Convention in Philadelphia in 1976 revealed a previously unrecognized causative pathogen, *Legionella pneumophila*.[1,2] The illness was called legionnaire disease, or legionellosis. *L. pneumophila* also was shown to have been the cause of Pontiac fever, a previously described outbreak in Michigan of a short-incubation, self-limited influenza-like illness primarily affecting adults and causing symptoms of fever, malaise, myalgia, chills, and headache.[3,4]

The genus *Legionella* in the family Legionellaceae currently consists of at least 50 species and at least 60 serogroups.[5–7] *L. pneumophila* serogroup 1 is responsible for 50% to 90% of human infections.[7–9] Other *L. pneumophila* serogroups, especially serogroup 6 and *L. longbeachae*, *L. bozemanii*, and *L. micdadei*, cause most of the remainder of human infections.[7,9] Patients with infections caused by *Legionella* species other than *L. pneumophila* are more likely to be immunocompromised.[7] *Legionella* are nutritionally fastidious, motile, nonspore-forming aerobic bacilli. In tissue, *Legionella* organisms appear as short bacilli or coccobacilli with nonparallel sides tapering to rounded ends. In vitro growth of *Legionella* from clinical specimens requires a source of amino acids, iron, and L-cysteine such as buffered charcoal-yeast extract (BCYE) agar enriched with α-ketoglutarate.[5] Following recovery on artificial media, *Legionella* stain as gram-negative organisms.

PATHOGENESIS AND EPIDEMIOLOGY

Legionella species are facultative intracellular pathogens capable of surviving and multiplying both in mammalian cells to cause human infection and in free-living amebas to survive in the environment. Virulent, avirulent, and variant strains of *L. pneumophila* have been isolated and some virulence factors have been identified.[5,10] A number of genes, e.g., *dot, icm*, are required for growth of *Legionella* in amebas,[11] and such growth enhances their virulence. *Legionella* species attach to and are internalized by monocytes and macrophages in the alveolar spaces. In human lung tissue, *L. pneumophila* serogroup 1 enters macrophages by phagocytosis in an antibody-independent process. Macrophages exhibit an oxidative burst, but phagosomal acidification and lysosomal fusion do not occur, and the organism survives and multiplies within the cytoplasm with eventual cell lysis.[5,10,11] Cell-mediated immunity (i.e., sensitization of lymphocytes that release cytokines, which in turn activate macrophages) probably is more important to recovery than antibody. The pathogenesis of Pontiac fever may involve a host response to endotoxin from lipopolysaccharide of *Legionella* or other bacteria without multiplication of *Legionella* in the host.[12]

Infection with *L. pneumophila* is not transmitted from human to human. Infection most commonly results from the inhalation of contaminated aerosol from environmental or aquatic sources.[13–18] *Legionella* species naturally occur in natural freshwater habitats such as lakes, rivers, and ground water. From these sources organisms gain entry into water systems of buildings, including hospitals. These bacteria thrive in warm water (temperatures between 30°C and 54°C) but are killed at temperatures above 60°C.[11] *Legionella* have been found in cooling towers and evaporative condensers, shower heads, respiratory therapy devices, air conditioners, whirlpool spas, and humidifiers.[14,15] Survival and persistence of these nutritionally fastidious organisms in the environment make it likely that protozoa, particularly amebas, act as

TABLE 177-1. *Legionella* Pneumonia in Children

Patient Population	Features
Neonates	Previously healthy or premature infants, can have bronchopulmonary dysplasia, corticosteroid therapy, or congenital heart disease; frequently nosocomial; typically healthcare-associated, frequently unsuspected and diagnosed at autopsy
Immunocompetent children hospitalized with pneumonia	Mild to moderate severity; recovery can occur without the use of effective antibiotics; most cases diagnosed by serology
Children with underlying pulmonary disease or receiving mechanical ventilation	Nosocomial source is common
Immunocompromised children receiving corticosteroid, anticancer, or antiorgan rejection therapies; children with severe combined immunodeficiency or chronic granulomatous disease	Nosocomial or community-acquired; onset often within weeks of transplantation or induction chemotherapy for malignancy

reservoirs in water sources. Legionnaire disease due to *L. longbeachae* has been associated with exposure to potting soil.[7]

Nosocomial infections and hospital outbreaks due to *L. pneumophila* or other *Legionella* spp. have occurred. The source generally is water, most commonly the hot water supply.[14–17] Strains associated with nosocomial infection can colonize water supplies over long periods.[17] Community-acquired outbreaks of legionnaire disease are almost always due to *L. pneumophila*[7] and such outbreaks have frequently been associated with a nearby cooling tower, as proven by isolation of the same strain as confirmed by DNA-based molecular typing techniques from infected patients, the cooling tower, and aerosols from the cooling tower.[13,14] In addition, outbreaks have been associated with whirlpool baths, including the use of a whirlpool bath on a cruise ship,[18] decorative fountains, and ultrasonic mist machines used to humidify fresh produce in a grocery store.[15] Sporadic cases of legionellosis have been linked to home water heaters, particularly electric water heaters. In 40% of 20 sporadic cases studied, isolates identical to the infecting isolates were found in the potable water at the patient's home or workplace, or at an ambulatory medical facility visited by the patient.[19]

Most cases of legionnaire disease occur in susceptible elderly or middle-aged adults. Based on the outbreak in Philadelphia, the incubation period is estimated to range from 2 to 10 days, with a mean of approximately 7 days.[1] Risk factors for infection in adults include cigarette smoking, alcoholism, chronic lung or heart disease, and treatment with high doses of corticosteroids or other immunosuppressive drugs, including those given to prevent rejection of transplanted organs and tumor necrosis factor-α antagonists.[1,15,20] Legionellosis is an occasional cause of pneumonia in adults with acquired immunodeficiency syndrome, in whom it accounts for 1% to 3% of pneumonia episodes.[21] *L. pneumophila* has caused pneumonia in patients infected with 2009 pandemic influenza A:H1N1.[22] In the United States during 2008, higher numbers of cases were reported during the summer months but no clustering of cases by state or geographic region was observed.[23]

Legionellosis is uncommon in children. Only 0.44% of cases of legionellosis reported to the Centers for Disease Control and Prevention in 2008 were patients younger than 15 years.[23] *Legionella* bacteria probably are responsible for 1% to 5% of episodes of pneumonia in immunocompetent children[24–27] and are being recognized increasingly in neonates.[28–30] In pediatric legionellosis, risk factors for serious infection are neonatal age group, immune compromise as a result of cancer or organ transplantation and their treatments, corticosteroid therapy, primary

immunodeficiency, or underlying lung disease[16,31,32] (Table 177-1). The majority of published cases of legionellosis in children are hospital-acquired but this may represent a reporting bias.[32] In a review of legionellosis in children the overall mortality rate was 33%, with the highest mortality rates in immunosuppressed children and children younger than 1 year of age.[32]

CLINICAL MANIFESTATIONS

Legionella infection can be classified into the following four categories: (1) pneumonia; (2) subclinical infection; (3) nonpneumonic disease, referred to as Pontiac fever; and (4) extrapulmonary inflammatory disease. The most important clinical infection in children and adults is pneumonia, which is manifest as an acute febrile illness with cough, and often with respiratory distress.[32] Initially, nonpulmonary symptoms can predominate and include chills, abdominal pain, myalgia, confusion, malaise, anorexia, and diarrhea. Extrapulmonary manifestations, particularly confusion and diarrhea, are common, but the combination of pulmonary and extrapulmonary clinical findings is not sufficiently specific to differentiate *Legionella* pneumonia from community-acquired or nosocomial pneumonia of other etiologies.[33] The nonproductive cough suggests atypical pneumonia, which needs to be differentiated from *Mycoplasma pneumoniae*, viral, and *Chlamydophila pneumoniae* infections in outpatients.

Chest radiographs show patchy alveolar rather than interstitial infiltrates. In the majority of cases pulmonary disease is unilateral. Pulmonary nodules with or without cavitation can develop, particularly in immunocompromised hosts.[31,32,34–37] Pleural effusion occurs, with an incidence similar to that of other bacterial pneumonias. Progressive respiratory distress and respiratory failure can develop over a period of several days. Copathogens have been recovered from respiratory tract specimens in only a few cases. The fatality rate in previously healthy, appropriately treated individuals is about 6%.[8] *Legionella* infection causing fever and pulmonary nodules is relatively common in adult renal or cardiac transplant recipients and occurs within several weeks of transplantation. Alternatively, these patients may have prodromal symptoms of malaise, myalgia, and headache followed by an abrupt onset of symptoms indicative of pneumonia: dyspnea, cough, and pleuritic chest pain.[38,39]

Serious or fatal *Legionella* pneumonia is increasingly being reported in neonates.[28,29,30,34] Many of the infants were born at term, presenting with septicemia, pneumonia, or both, but several were born prematurely or had congenital heart disease. An outbreak of 11 cases of *Legionella* pneumonia in term neonates from a single nursery included 3 fatal cases; evaluation implicated a *Legionella*-contaminated humidifier in the nursery.[29] *L. pneumophila* pneumonia was diagnosed in a 7-day-old infant following vaginal delivery in a hospital birthing pool.[40] Mortality rate of neonatal legionellosis is high and survival correlates with macrolide/azalide treatment.

Infections in immunocompromised hosts and neonates represent the most severe form of pediatric disease. At the other end of the clinical spectrum, *Legionella* species are probably responsible for 1% to 5% of cases of community-acquired pneumonia in healthy children;[24] infections usually resolve without treatment with effective antibiotic therapy. Subclinical infection also occurs, as evidenced by data that anti-*Legionella* antibody titers generally increase with age,[24,25,27] and by antibody rises in the absence of recognized episodes of pneumonia.

Epidemic, nonpneumonic disease, also known as Pontiac fever, is characterized by a high attack rate in exposed individuals. After a short incubation period of 12 to 48 hours, the infection is characterized by the abrupt onset of an influenza-like illness without pneumonia. Prominent signs and symptoms include fever, malaise, myalgia, and cough. The illness is self-limited, although a cluster of cases with respiratory compromise has been described.[41] The initial outbreak was caused by *L. pneumophila* serogroup 1, but other *Legionella* species have been associated with outbreaks.[12]

In adults, many extrapulmonary infections have been documented, including sinusitis, perirectal abscess, pyelonephritis, peritonitis, pancreatitis, pericarditis, and endocarditis.[33] In children, extrapulmonary sites of infection in the liver, spleen, and brain have been documented at autopsy.[28,42] Localized extrapulmonary infection, such as infection of postoperative wounds after wound irrigation with *Legionella*-contaminated tap water, also can occur.

LABORATORY DIAGNOSIS

Nonspecific laboratory abnormalities in legionellosis include leukocytosis with a left shift of neutrophils, hyponatremia, proteinuria, or elevated serum concentrations of hepatic enzymes. In adults, hyponatremia is significantly more frequent in the initial stage of legionellosis than in pneumonia of other etiologies.

A specific laboratory diagnosis can be established by: (1) isolation of the organism in culture; (2) direct detection of organisms, bacterial antigens, or nucleic acids in clinical specimens; or (3) documentation of a serologic response to the organism.[43] Although culture is the gold standard for diagnosis, urine antigen testing has almost equal sensitivity and specificity for *L. pneumophila* type 1 and may be more sensitive than culture in clinical laboratories inexperienced in isolation of *Legionella*. A useful clue to the diagnosis is the presence of inflammatory cells without bacteria on a Gram-stained preparation of lower respiratory tract secretions. This staining pattern is due to the fact that *Legionella* induces a neutrophilic inflammatory response but stains poorly with Gram stain. However, the absence of significant numbers of neutrophils does not exclude the diagnosis.[44] Microscopic screening protocols of sputa evaluating the presence of leukocytes, commonly used to determine the adequacy of the specimen for bacterial culture, are not useful for selecting samples to be cultured for *Legionella*. *Legionella* species, particularly *L. micdadei*, may stain with acid-fast stain;[45] modified acid-fast stain can be useful.

Culture

Legionella grow on enriched BCYE agar supplemented with dyes to aid identification of colonies and antimicrobial agents such as vancomycin, polymyxin B (but not cefamandole, which can inhibit the growth of *L. micdadei* and *L. bozemanii*), and anisomycin to inhibit the overgrowth of other bacteria and yeast.[5,46] Heating or washing sputum specimens with acid before inoculation reduces contamination and enhances recovery.[5,47] Although BCYE agar is available commercially, some lots exhibit poor clinical performance. Colonies take 3 or more days to appear and exhibit a ground-glass morphology. *L. pneumophila* has been isolated from both aerobic and anaerobic broth blood culture systems, but only after blind subculture. The laboratory should be apprised when legionellosis is suspected.

Bacterial Detection

Antigen detection tests are used most frequently to diagnose legionellosis. Detection of *L. pneumophila* serogroup 1 lipopolysaccharide antigens in urine by commercially available immunochromatographic membrane assays, enzyme immunoassay (EIA), or radioimmunoassay (RIA) is possible as early as a few days after the onset of infection (Binax).[48] These assays have high specificity and a sensitivity of 80% to 90%. The immunochromatographic assay is rapid and easy to perform and has a sensitivity and specificity comparable with that of RIA and EIA.[48] Another commercial EIA (Biotest *Legionella* UrineAntigen EIA) is designed to detect other *L. pneumophila* serogroups and other *Legionella* species in urine. The sensitivity of these tests is increased when urine is concentrated prior to testing and when incubation time was prolonged.[49] Both tests had similar sensitivity and specificity for detection of *L. pneumophila* serogroup 1 and both detected antigen from some patients infected with nonserogroup 1 *L. pneumophila* or other *Legionella* species.[50,51] The sensitivity of urine antigen testing is higher in patients with more severe pneumonia.[52] Antigenuria typically is prolonged beyond resolution of clinical infection and should not be used to judge the adequacy of therapy.[53] In one outbreak, urine antigen assay was useful in diagnosing Pontiac fever.[54]

Detection of organisms on smears of respiratory tract secretions by direct (or indirect) immunofluorescence assay (DFA) using polyclonal or monoclonal antibody is rapid; the mean sensitivity approximates 60%, and the specificity, 95% to 99%. Failure to detect bacilli on a Gram-stained smear increases the confidence that a positive DFA is a true positive. DFA testing (or culture) of pleural fluid from patients with pneumonia generally has not been useful in diagnosis.

Nucleic acid probes also have been developed to detect *Legionella* DNA in respiratory specimens, but false-positive results have been reported.[55] Polymerase chain reaction (PCR)-based assays to detect DNA from all *Legionella* species in respiratory specimens have been developed. These assays have a sensitivity comparable with or superior to that of culture or urinary antigen detection and have excellent specificity but are not available widely.[43,56–58]

Serology

Confirmation of infection using serology requires documentation of a fourfold rise in antibody titer to ≥1:128 in specimens, typically taken 3 to 6 weeks apart, using an indirect immunofluorescence assay (IFA); optimally both specimens should be assayed in the same run. Enzyme immunoassay kits are commercially available but are less specific than IFA assays and are best considered a screening assay.[43] Serology is useful to confirm infection due to *L. pneumophila* type 1; the utility of serology to confirm infection with other serotypes or species has not been established firmly. In the setting of sporadic disease neither a single elevated IFA titer nor measurement of IgM antibody is useful for diagnosis.[5,43] Although elevated serum antibody can be found during acute illness, seroconversion may take up to 9 weeks and may not occur in all patients. In one study of infected adults who demonstrated a serologic response, seropositivity occurred in only 35% after 2 weeks from the onset of infection and in only 60% after 4 weeks.[59] "Seroconversion" occasionally is due to cross-reaction after infection with another organism such as *Citrobacter freundii*,[60] *Bacteroides fragilis*, *Chlamydophila psittaci*, or *Coxiella burnetii*.[61] A false-positive serologic test is frequent in patients with cystic fibrosis and is related to cross-reaction with *Pseudomonas* species.[62] Although infected children <1 year of age have been thought not to undergo seroconversion,[63] seroconversion has been documented in several young children with legionellosis.[25,64,65] Almost all cases of Pontiac fever are diagnosed using serologic tests.

TREATMENT

Options for antibiotic treatment of legionellosis are summarized in Table 177-2. Based on clinical experience, intravenously administered azithromycin is the antibiotic of choice for the treatment of *Legionella* infection in healthy children while levofloxacin is the antibiotic of choice for the treatment of *Legionella* infection in immunocompromised children. In five observational studies in adults with *Legionella* pneumonia, patients treated with a fluoroquinolone, primarily levofloxacin, had a more rapid defervescence and a trend toward a shorter hospital stay than patients treated with a macrolide or azalide.[66,67] Azithromycin is preferred over intravenous erythromycin because of its ease of administration (one versus four daily doses, smaller fluid volume, and less vein injury), superior activity in vitro and in an animal model of infection, higher lung levels, and better intracellular penetration.[8,68] Oral azithromycin can be substituted after definite clinical response to complete a 5- to 10-day course of therapy. The longer duration of therapy is used for immunocompromised patients. The addition of rifampin has not been demonstrated to enhance the efficacy of azithromycin or levofloxacin and some treated patients have developed elevated bilirubin levels.[67] When treating recipients of transplanted solid organs, caution is required because erythromycin and azithromycin inhibit the metabolism of cyclosporine.[38]

Many antibiotics show activity against *Legionella* in vitro, but only antibiotics with intracellular penetration are effective. Testing of antibiotics in vitro against intracellular *Legionella* in a

TABLE 177-2. Antimicrobial Therapy for Legionellosis[a]

Antimicrobial Agent(s)	Intravenous Dose		Oral Dose	
	Pediatric	**Adult**	**Pediatric**	**Adult**
FIRST CHOICE				
Normal host: azithromycin	10 mg/kg per day	500 mg daily	10 mg/kg per day	500 mg daily
Immunocompromised host: levofloxacin[b]	Not approved <18 years for routine use. Age 6 mos–4 y: 10 mg/kg every 12 hours; 5–17 y: 10 mg/kg every 24 hours (maximum, 750 mg)	750 mg every 12–24 hours	Not approved <18 years for routine use. Age 6 mos–4 y: 10 mg/kg every 12 hours; 5–17 y: 10 mg/kg every 24 hours (maximum, 750 mg)	750 mg every 12–24 hours
SECOND CHOICES				
Erythromycin[c]	40 mg/kg per day	1 g every 6 hours	40 mg/kg per day	500 mg every 6 hours
Clarithromycin	Not available	Not available	15 mg/kg per day	500 mg every 12 hours
Ciprofloxacin[d]	Not approved <18 years for routine use; 10 mg/kg q 8 hours	400 mg every 12 hours	Not approved <18 years for routine use; 15 mg/kg q 12 hours	750 mg every 12 hours
POTENTIAL ALTERNATIVES				
Moxifloxacin	Not approved <18 years	400 mg every 24 hours	Not approved <18 years	400 mg every 24 hours
TMP-SMX	15 mg TMP/kg per day	160 mg TMP every 8 hours	15 mg TMP/kg per day	160 mg TMP every 12 hours
Doxycycline	2–4 mg/kg per day[e]	200 mg every 12 hours twice; then 100 mg every 12 hours	2–4 mg/kg per day[d]	100 mg every 12 hours

TMP-SMX, trimethoprim-sulfamethoxazole.

[a]*The duration of therapy is 2–3 weeks, except for therapy with azithromycin, which is 5–10 days.*

[b]*In severely ill patients, combination therapy with levofloxacin and azithromycin can be considered but clinical experience is very limited.*

[c]*Intravenous erythromycin doses up to 100 mg/kg per day have been administered to children without difficulty.*

[d]*Approved for children younger than 18 years with a complicated urinary tract infection; dose 30 mg/kg per day every 12 hours orally or 20–30 mg/kg per day every 8 hours intravenously; active against* Legionella *pneumonia but not against pneumococcal pneumonia.*

[e]*Generally not used in children younger than 9 years.*

Legionella-infected cell line or in vivo (e.g., with a guinea pig model of infection) may more accurately predict the effectiveness of an antibiotic against human infection.[8] For example, β-lactam antibiotics are active in vitro but are ineffective in treating *Legionella* pneumonia. Clindamycin and aminoglycosides also are ineffective.[7] Fluoroquinolone antibiotics, unlike erythromycin, are bactericidal for *Legionella* and may be superior to macrolide/azalide therapy.[8,66,68] Doxycycline or trimethoprim-sulfamethoxazole has been used successfully in some patients. In a few cases of infection with *L. micdadei*, patients who failed treatment with erythromycin responded to trimethoprim-sulfamethoxazole.[8]

PREVENTION

Attempts to prevent healthcare-associated *Legionella* infection in healthcare facilities where cases have occurred or in which *Legionella* has been detected in the water systems are directed toward treating water distribution systems to inactivate organisms.[69,70] An evidence-based review was published recently.[69] Methods include: (1) copper-silver ionization by electrolysis;[11,58] (2) chlorine dioxide, monochloramine, or hyperchlorination followed by continuous chlorination (to 1 to 2 mg of free residual chlorine per liter); (3) periodic superheating to temperatures greater than 60°C and flushing of distal sites (with or without maintenance of the water temperature above 50°C); (4) point-of-use filtration; or (5) UV light. Copper-silver ionization may be the method of choice,[71,72] although this requires relatively expensive equipment and its effectiveness may wane after several years because of the emergence of *Legionella* strains tolerant of silver ions.[73] Over time, continuous chlorination can cause corrosion of pipes and leakage and chlorination is associated with the production of carcinogenic trihalomethane by-products.[7,71] Superheating is advantageous in that it can be instituted rapidly to interrupt an outbreak. In one hospital with a high incidence of nosocomial *Legionella* pneumonia in renal transplant patients, prophylactic erythromycin therapy was successful.[74] A vaccine is not available.

Key Points. Epidemiology, Clinical Features, and Diagnosis of *Legionella* Infection

EPIDEMIOLOGY

- Risk groups
  - elderly
  - immunosuppressed adults and children particularly organ transplant recipients
  - adults and children treated with corticosteroids
  - adults and children with chronic lung disease
  - neonates
- Bacterial reservoir: freshwater habitats and potable water
- Mode of transmission: inhalation of *Legionella*-contaminated water
- Pediatric infections frequently are nosocomial

CLINICAL FEATURES

- Pneumonia most common manifestation
- Clinical manifestations: fever, nonproductive cough, respiratory distress
- Chest radiograph: patchy alveolar infiltrates, usually unilateral, at times nodular

DIAGNOSIS

- Urine antigen detection is most practical diagnostic test.
  - high specificity
  - sensitive for *Legionella pneumophila* serotype 1
  - occasionally detects other serotypes or species

178 *Rickettsia rickettsii* (Rocky Mountain Spotted Fever)

Jennifer H. McQuiston, Joanna J. Regan, and Christopher D. Paddock

DESCRIPTION OF THE PATHOGEN

Rickettsia rickettsii, the etiologic agent of Rocky Mountain spotted fever (RMSF), is a small (0.3 to 0.7 μm × 1.0 to 2.0 μm) coccobacillary intracellular bacterium. Although *R. rickettsii* can infect several different cell types, including macrophages and vascular smooth muscle, the primary targets of infection in mammalian hosts are the endothelial cells lining the small vessels of all major tissues and organ systems.[1,2] Damage to endothelium in the dermis, skeletal muscle, and vital organs such as brain, heart, lungs, kidneys, and gastrointestinal tract results in the moderate to severe systemic manifestations characteristically observed in people with RMSF.

R. rickettsii is a tickborne pathogen that is inoculated into the skin of humans or natural vertebrate hosts by a tick vector when the arthropod obtains a bloodmeal. *R. rickettsii* attaches to its host cell by using a major rickettsial outer membrane protein (rompA),[3] and subsequently is endocytosed by the host endothelial cell. Intracellular movement of *R. rickettsii* and spread to adjacent endothelium involves rickettsia-mediated polymerization of host-cell actin. Oxidative injury to host cells leads to diffuse microvascular injury and fluid leakage into extravascular spaces.[4-8]

In vitro, different strains of *R. rickettsii* produce varying levels of injury to cultured human endothelial cells;[6,9] however, these differences have not been characterized in vivo, and severe or fatal disease has resulted from infections with most genetically distinct strains of *R. rickettsii*.[10]

EPIDEMIOLOGY

RMSF occurs throughout much of the western hemisphere, and is maintained in nature in a complex cycle involving several species of ticks and mammals. Humans are incidental hosts and become infected with *R. rickettsii* from the bite of an infected tick. In North America, *Dermacentor variabilis* (the American dog tick) and D.

andersoni (the Rocky Mountain wood tick) are considered primary tick vectors.[11,12] *Rhipicephalus sanguineus* (the brown dog tick) is also a primary vector in some regions, particularly in Mexico and the southwestern U.S.[13-16]

The reported incidence of RMSF has increased dramatically in the last decade[17] (Figure 178-1). During 2000 through 2007, reported incidence increased from 1.7 to >7 cases per million persons. The incidence is highest in North Carolina, Oklahoma, Arkansas, Tennessee, and Missouri (Figure 178-2). Demographic risk factors include being male or of American Indian race.[17] The majority of U.S. cases are reported in April through September, corresponding with periods of increased host-seeking activity of ticks. Only 4% of reported U.S. cases have a winter onset;[17] such cases have a higher risk for failed diagnosis.[18]

Contemporary surveillance data suggest that RMSF infections occur more frequently in adults than in children (Figure 178-3).[17,19-21] However, pediatric patients experience severe outcomes disproportionately compared with adults. Over 35% of patients with RMSF ≤4 years of age are hospitalized, and the highest case-fatality rate (2.6%) was reported among patients aged 5 through 9 years of age (Figure 178-3).[17]

The prevalence of *R. rickettsii* antibodies appears to increase with age, likely as a function of increased risk of exposure to either *R. rickettsii* or other rickettsial organisms over time.[22,23] A survey of approximately 2000 children from the southeast and south central regions of the U.S. reported a 12% seroprevalence of *R. rickettsii* antibodies using standard serum diagnostic assays.[24] Seroprevalence may reflect, in part, infections caused by *Rickettsia* species other than *R. rickettsii* because serologic assays are not species specific.[25,26]

RMSF usually occurs sporadically, but family clusters have been reported associated with similar tick exposures.[27-30] Community clusters also may be related to focal infection with *R. rickettsii* in tick populations in neighborhoods or parks.[31] Recognition of this feature is important because multiple infections can occur simultaneously or sequentially in the same household after identification of an index case, leading providers to suspect a communicable infection.[27]

CLINICAL MANIFESTATIONS

RMSF can be difficult to diagnose in early stages, even by experienced physicians. While most patients seek care within the first 3 days after onset of fever, the prodromal signs and symptoms are nonspecific, and even in areas where awareness of the disease is high as many as 60% to 86% of patients with RMSF are not diagnosed correctly on their first visit for medical care.[32-34] A history of outdoor activity, contact with animals, or exposure to ticks may be helpful; however, many patients do not recall a tick bite during the days or weeks that preceded illness.[33-35]

Approximately 1 week (range, 3 to 12 days) after the bite of an infected tick, disease begins with the abrupt onset of fever often accompanied by severe frontal headache, nausea, vomiting, and generalized myalgia. The temperature generally is high (38.9°C to >40°C). Headache, which is noted less commonly in very young children, often is intractable to therapy.[29,36] Other findings recorded consistently in pediatric case series include irritability, severe abdominal pain, splenomegaly, conjunctivitis, and periorbital edema.[37,38]

A generalized maculopapular rash consisting of 1- to 5-mm blanching macules is considered a hallmark feature of RMSF. However, the rash can be absent until 2 to 5 days after fever onset,

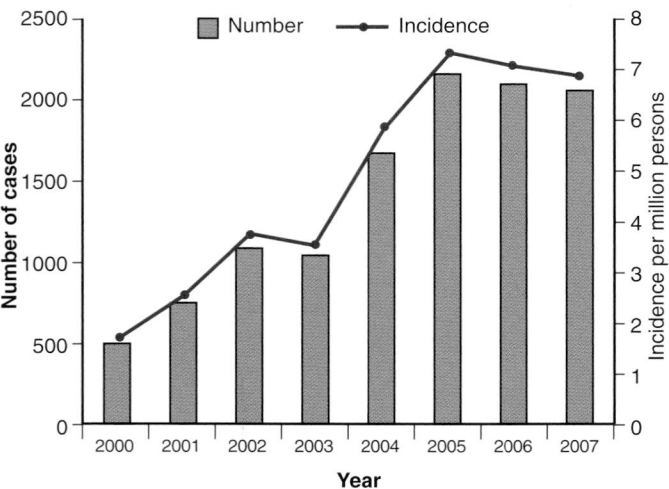

Figure 178-1. Number and incidence of reported cases of Rocky Mountain spotted fever (RMSF) in the United States, 2000–2007. (Data derived from the Centers for Disease Control and Prevention, National Electronic Telecommunications System for Surveillance for 2000–2007.)

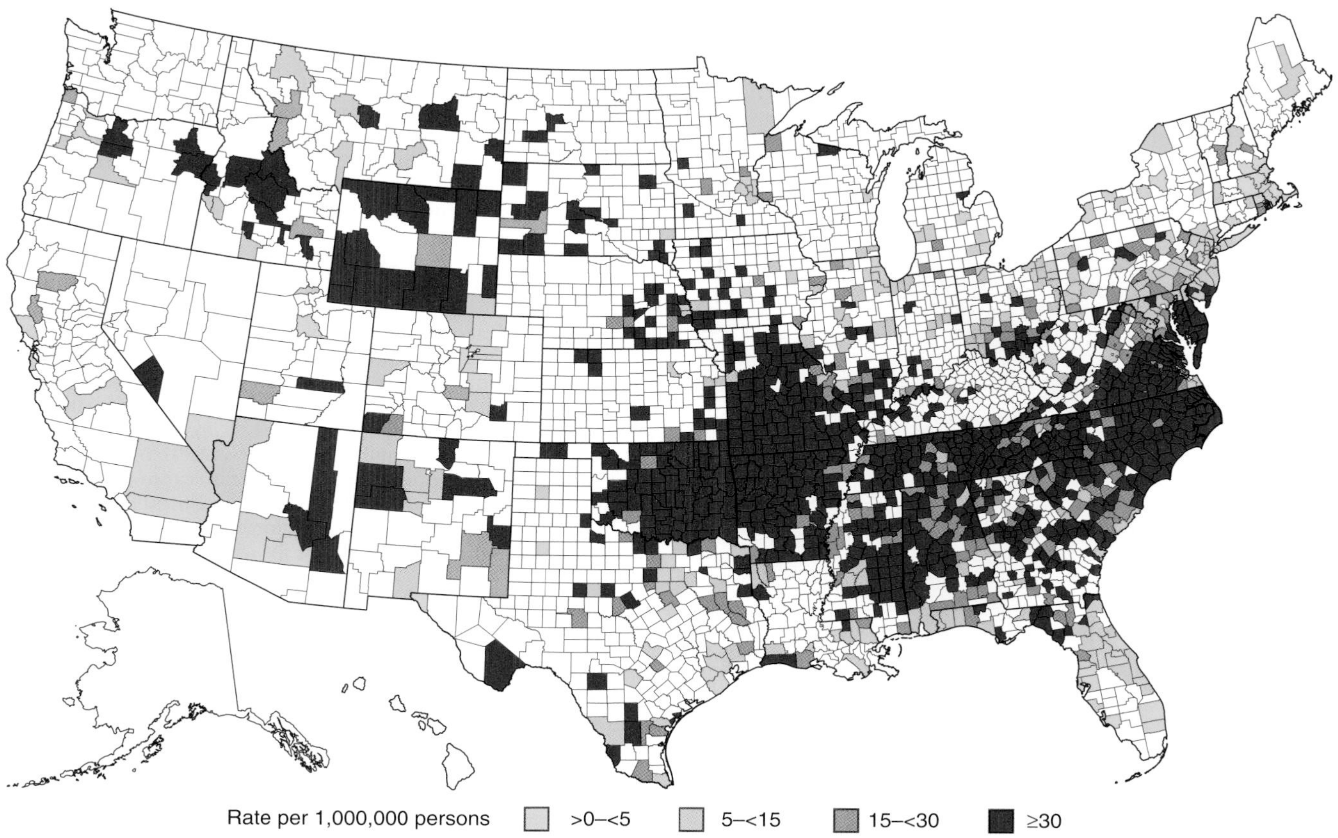

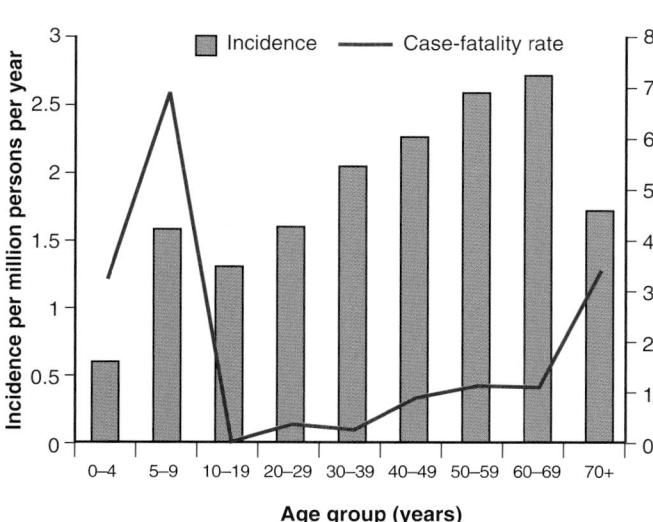

Figure 178-2. Annual reported incidence and geographic distribution of Rocky Mountain spotted fever by county, 2000–2007, United States. (Data from the Centers for Disease Control and Prevention, National Electronic Telecommunications System for Surveillance for 2000-2007.)

Rate per 1,000,000 persons   >0–<5   5–<15   15–<30   ≥30

Figure 178-3. Age-specific incidence of Rocky Mountain spotted fever per million U.S. population, and case-fatality rate by age group, 2000 to 2007. (Incidence data derived from the Centers for Disease Control and Prevention (CDC), National Electronic Telecommunications System for Surveillance. Case-fatality rates calculated from CDC RMSF Case Report Forms for 2000–2007.)

especially in older patients.[32-38] Therefore, clinicians must not await appearance of the distinctive rash to initiate therapy. In most cases, the rash begins on the wrists, ankles, and forearms then spreads centrally to involve the legs, buttocks, trunk, and face (Figure 178-4). The rash can appear on the palms and soles. The mucous membranes of the palate and pharynx also can be affected.[37,39] In later stages, the exanthema is petechial and can coalesce to form large ecchymoses. Unlike some other spotted fever rickettsiosis, an eschar is rarely present in RMSF. In approximately 10% of patients, the rash is fleeting, evanescent, atypical in distribution, or is absent entirely.[29,32,35,40]

RMSF can progress rapidly to catastrophic disease involving multiple organ systems. Severe manifestations include interstitial pneumonitis, acute respiratory distress syndrome, myocarditis, disseminated intravascular coagulopathy, meningoencephalitis, acute renal failure, and gangrene.[41-44] Before introduction of effective antirickettsial therapies in the 1940s, an estimated 20% to 80% of patients with RMSF died.[36,45] With advances in effective treatment and medical care, the currently reported case-fatality rate derived from national surveillance data is <1%.[17] However, among confirmed RMSF cases, the case-fatality rate during 2000–2007 was 3%,[17] and the case-fatality rate in some defined outbreaks approaches 10%.[14,15]

RMSF historically has been considered a disease with a high risk of fatal outcome, and several contemporary estimates of case-fatality rates range from 3% to 20% among pediatric series.[15,34,42,46] Most deaths are attributable to delayed diagnosis and failure to initiate specific antimicrobial therapy within the first several days of illness.[19,41,47-49] Timely administration of appropriate therapy is critical because at least one-half of all deaths occur within the first 8 days of illness.[47-49]

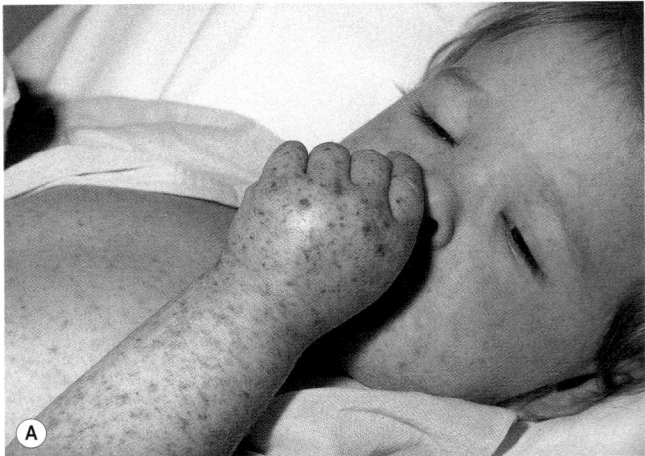

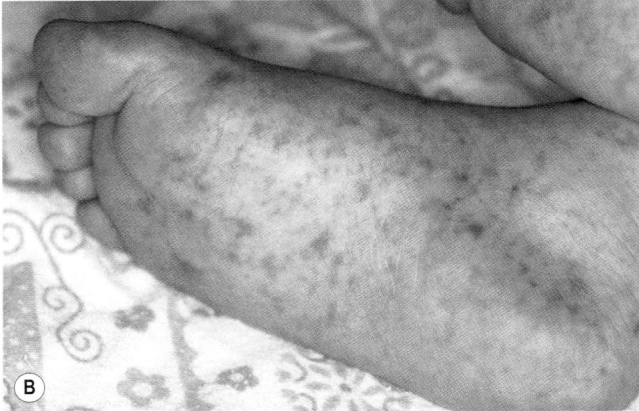

Figure 178-4. A 2-year-old girl with Rocky Mountain spotted fever admitted on day 8 of fever, and day 6 of rash that was maculopapular initially and then became petechial and purpuric. She had hyponatremia, thrombocytopenia, and meningitis. Note the typical character and distribution of rash, and edema. (Courtesy of M.C. Fisher and S.S. Long, St. Christopher's Hospital for Children, Philadelphia, PA.)

LABORATORY FINDINGS AND DIAGNOSIS

Decisions to treat are guided principally by epidemiologic clues garnered during a careful history and by clinical findings.[49,50]

Abnormalities in routine laboratory tests in RMSF can help direct a clinical diagnosis, and include hyponatremia, hypoalbuminemia, anemia, and thrombocytopenia; such findings reflect vascular injury and increasing vascular permeability.[43,50] Low serum sodium levels or diminished platelet counts occur in approximately 50% to 60% of all patients. The white blood cell count usually is normal, but leukocytosis can occur in up to 30% of patients.[29]

The diagnosis can be confirmed by serology, polymerase chain reaction (PCR) assays, immunohistochemical (IHC) staining of tissue specimens, or isolation of *R. rickettsii* in cell culture. Indirect immunofluorescence antibody assay (IFA) detecting antibodies to *R. rickettsii* in paired sera is the most widely available and frequently used method of confirmation, permitting a quantitative evaluation of antibody titers.[50] In approximately 50% of patients, diagnostic levels of antibody do not appear until the second week of disease, and a serum sample collected during the acute phase of illness can be negative. Evaluation of a second serum sample taken 2 to 4 weeks later with detection of a ≥4-fold change in IFA titer confirms a diagnosis of spotted fever rickettsiosis. A single IFA serum titer ≥1:64 suggests only a probable diagnosis.[50] Tests detecting IgG antibody titers are preferred over tests evaluating IgM antibody titers alone, as the latter is prone to false-positive results.

Enzyme immunoassay (EIA) has become available recently for serologic diagnosis of RMSF, but this qualitative assay is limited in ability to confirm active infection; furthermore, IgM EIA tests are prone to false-positive test results. In recent years, use of EIA to diagnose RMSF has risen dramatically and provided the primary form of laboratory assessment for some patients, accounting for 38% of all case reports during 2005–2007.[17] However, testing of paired sera by IFA is considered a superior technique for discriminating prior versus acute infection, and remains the recommended serologic test for RMSF.

Skin biopsy at a site of exanthem is an effective tool to aid in the diagnosis of acute RMSF; both PCR assay and IHC staining techniques can be used.[50] These assays also can be applied to tissues obtained at autopsy.[46] While offered by the Centers for Disease Control and Prevention and some specialty laboratories, these assays are not available widely. PCR assay of whole blood is not highly sensitive and is not recommended for most patients. In specialized laboratory settings, *R. rickettsii* can be isolated in cell culture, but this technique is restricted to research laboratories using biosafety level-3 precautions.[50] *R. rickettsii* cannot be isolated via standard blood cultures available through clinical laboratories. Tissue specimens for PCR, IHC, or culture should be obtained prior to or soon after initiation of antimicrobial therapy.

TREATMENT

RMSF is a life-threatening illness and appropriate antimicrobial therapy should be initiated immediately on the basis of clinical and epidemiologic findings when the disease is suspected. Empiric therapy is given while awaiting results of diagnostic tests, and should not be delayed or discontinued on the basis of an initial negative test result.

A tetracycline, most often doxycycline, is the treatment of choice. Patients treated with a tetracycline within the first 5 days of symptoms are significantly less likely to die than people treated later, or people treated with ineffective antibiotics.[41,48] The American Academy of Pediatrics Committee on Infectious Diseases considers doxycycline the drug of choice for treating RMSF in children of all ages,[51] with dosage of 4 mg/kg/day PO/IV, maximum dose 200 mg/day, divided every 12 hours.[50,52] Doxycycline generally is preferred over other tetracyclines because of its reduced phototoxicity, safety in patients with renal insufficiency, lower binding to calcium, and longer plasma half-life. Most patients with uncomplicated RMSF who receive doxycycline defervesce within 24 to 48 hours after initiation of therapy. Severely ill patients can have slower resolution, especially people with damage to multiple organ systems; however, absence of clinical improvement within 72 hours should suggest the need to consider a possible alternative diagnosis. Therapy should be continued for at least 3 days after unequivocal evidence of clinical improvement (usual duration, 7 to 10 days). While older tetracycline-class antibiotics were associated with cosmetic staining of permanent teeth, these effects have not been associated with the dose and duration of doxycycline that is recommended for therapy of RMSF. Clinical evaluation of children <8 years of age receiving doxycycline treatment has shown no detectable cosmetic staining of permanent teeth.[53–55] To minimize pediatric mortality, doxycycline should always be prescribed to children when a diagnosis of RMSF is suspected.

Chloramphenicol is the only other antimicrobial agent with recognized clinical efficacy against *R. rickettsii*, but it is no longer available in the oral form in the U.S.. In addition, epidemiologic data suggest that patients with RMSF treated with chloramphenicol have a higher risk for severe illness and death than children treated with a tetracycline.[19,48] In addition, treatment with chloramphenicol carries a risk for idiosyncratic aplastic anemia, and must be used with caution in the third trimester of pregnancy because of the risk of grey-baby syndrome. In vitro evidence suggests that chloramphenicol also may not be effective treatment of infections caused by *Ehrlichia* and *Anaplasma* spp., which commonly manifest with clinical syndromes similar to RMSF.[56,57] The pediatric parenteral dose of chloramphenicol is 50 to 100 mg/kg per day in 4 divided doses.[52] Reversible dose-related toxicities associated with this drug include bone marrow suppression and cardiomyopathy, and monitoring of serum levels is advisable when treating patients <2 years of age, patients with hepatic disease, or people receiving therapy for >5 days. Peak serum levels of chloramphenicol should be maintained within the range of 10 to 30 µg/mL.[52]

Prophylactic antibiotic therapy in asymptomatic people with a recent history of a tick bite is not warranted. Tetracyclines and chloramphenicol are bacteriostatic drugs; therefore, presumptive therapy before onset of symptoms is unlikely to prevent infection, and instead can result in a delayed onset of disease.[58]

SPECIAL CONSIDERATIONS

Penicillins, cephalosporins, macrolides, aminoglycosides, and sulfa-containing antimicrobial agents are ineffective in treating RMSF. Sulfonamides have no activity against *R. rickettsii* and may exacerbate the disease.[32,39,59] Some fluoroquinolones demonstrate strong bacteriostatic activity against *R. rickettsii* in vitro,[60] have been effective in treating dogs with RMSF,[61] and have been used in Europe as effective therapy for Mediterranean spotted fever caused by *R. conorii*.[62] However, efficacy data are not available for the treatment of RMSF in humans.

Tetracyclines generally are contraindicated in pregnant women because of the risks associated with malformation of teeth and bones in the fetus and hepatoxicity and pancreatitis in the mother. Chloramphenicol has been used successfully to treat women with RMSF in the third trimester of pregnancy[63,64] Because chloramphenicol crosses the placenta, low maternal dosages are given if the drug is administered during labor, to avoid grey-baby syndrome in the neonate. However, because of the increased risk of fatal outcome in patients treated with chloramphenicol compared with tetracyclines,[48] clinical judgment is warranted to manage RMSF during pregnancy. For pregnant patients experiencing severe or life-threatening complications due to RMSF, use of doxycycline still may be advised.[50]

Because early clinical findings of invasive *Neisseria meningitidis* infection can overlap findings of RMSF, empiric treatment for both diseases usually is necessary, using a third-generation cephalosporin in addition to doxycycline.[50]

Severely ill patients can have hypotension, oliguria or anuria, edema, and coma. Close hemodynamic and electrolyte monitoring coupled with pressor support and administration of intravenous fluids is warranted in these patients; however, because of increased capillary permeability, avoidance of pulmonary or cerebral edema is necessary.

Long-term sequelae, including hearing loss, peripheral neuropathy, bladder and bowel dysfunction, vestibular and motor disorders, and limb amputations, can occur in people who survive severe disease.[65] In a series of 93 children with RMSF, 3 died and 13 had neurologic deficits at hospital discharge.[34] In children, behavioral disturbances and learning disabilities are among the neurologic sequelae most frequently described and generally occur in patients in whom severe alterations in consciousness occurred during the acute illness.[34,66] These sequelae can result in permanent deficits.

PREVENTION AND CONTROL

No rickettsial vaccine is available commercially in the U.S. Limiting exposure to ticks is the most effective way of reducing the likelihood of acquiring RMSF and primarily depends on avoidance of tick-infested sites. Ticks can be controlled through habitat modification, such as removing dense underbrush and mowing grass frequently, or through application of appropriate pesticides. Because several important tick vectors of *R. rickettsii* (i.e., *D. variabilis* and *R. sanguineus*) live on dogs, tick prevention for family pets, including use of collars, sprays, or topical medications, is important. Although dogs do not pose a direct communicable disease risk to humans, they can carry questing ticks into the home environment where humans can be exposed; dogs also can be important sentinels for human risk.[67,68]

When engaging in outdoor activities, especially during spring and summer months, application of up to 30% *N,N*-diethyl-*m*-toluamide (DEET) can be recommended safely for use on children >2 months of age.[69,70] Additional personal protective measures that permit easy visualization of ticks include wearing light-colored clothing. Parents whose children are frequently exposed to tick habitats should employ a daily tick check, removing ticks as soon as possible to reduce the chance of disease transmission (which takes several hours).[71] Ticks can attach to concealed areas, including the scalp, axilla, and perineum, so careful searches for ticks are necessary. To remove an attached tick, blunt curved forceps or tweezers should be used to grasp the tick as close to the skin surface as possible; the tick is then removed by pulling upward with steady, even pressure. The person removing the tick should avoid crushing the body of the tick. Folk remedies (e.g., petroleum jelly, hot matches, isopropyl alcohol) are ineffective.[72]

Because RMSF can be difficult to diagnose clinically, and requires specialized laboratory assays to confirm a suspected diagnosis, many cases likely are missed, misdiagnosed, or underreported. RMSF is a nationally notifiable disease, and cases should be reported promptly to local or state public health authorities. Accurate and timely reporting is essential for assessing the magnitude and distribution of cases of RMSF in order to develop effective public health education programs and prevention strategies.

Key Points. Diagnosis and Management of Rocky Mountain Spotted Fever (RMSF)

MICROBIOLOGY AND VECTORS IN THE U.S.

- RMSF is caused by the bacterium *Rickettsia rickettsii*
- The American dog tick (*Dermacentor variabilis*) and the Rocky Mountain wood tick (*D. andersoni*) are common tick vectors throughout much of the U.S. In eastern Arizona and possibly other areas, the brown dog tick (*Rhipicephalus sanguineus*) is a vector

DIAGNOSIS

- Most patients present with a fever and headache, and may not always recall a tick bite
- A maculopapular to petechial rash commonly develops by day 3 to 5 of illness
- Thrombocytopenia, hyponatremia, and elevated serum hepatic transaminase levels are common
- Treatment must be initiated as soon as the disease is suspected, and never postponed while awaiting laboratory confirmation

- IFA serology for IgG antibodies to demonstrate a 4-fold increase in titers between acute and convalescent samples is the standard. IgM is less specific for RMSF than IgG, and is not specific for acute illness
- PCR testing of skin from the rash site or other tissue specimens for RMSF is highly sensitive and is recommended. PCR is specific; however, sensitivity decreases after 48 hours of appropriate antibiotic treatment. PCR of whole blood may not be useful to detect *R. rickettsii* during the acute phase of illness

TREATMENT

- Doxycycline is the treatment of choice for adults and children of all ages and is most effective if started within 5 days of symptom onset
- Recommended doxycycline dosage is 4 mg/kg/day (maximum dose 200 mg/day) divided q12h PO/IV
- Duration of therapy is at least 3 days after defervescence (usual, 7 to 10 days)

179 Other *Rickettsia* Species

Marina E. Eremeeva and Gregory A. Dasch

RICKETTSIA PROWAZEKII (CLASSIC LOUSE-BORNE EPIDEMIC TYPHUS; BRILL-ZINSSER DISEASE OR RECRUDESCENT TYPHUS; SYLVATIC OR FLYING SQUIRREL-ASSOCIATED TYPHUS)

Description of Pathogen

Rickettsia prowazekii is a small, gram-negative, obligately intracellular, rod-shaped bacterium. *R. prowazekii* possesses a regularly arrayed surface protein (OmpB) layer external to the cell envelope that has a peptidoglycan sacculus located between the inner cytoplasmic and outer membranes. It does not possess flagella. Both humoral and cellular immune responses are directed against the surface layer protein and result in protective immunity. *R. prowazekii* grows freely in the cytoplasm of infected host cells and preferentially infects endothelial cells in humans.[1,2] *R. prowazekii* is the prototype species of the typhus group (TG), which is differentiated from the more diverse and numerous rickettsial agents in the spotted fever group (SFG) by its lipopolysaccharide (LPS) group antigen and some biologic characteristics. Unlike SFG rickettsiae, which can survive and replicate for several days after death of their host cells, TG rickettsiae rapidly die after killing their host cells. However, *R. prowazekii* can retain high aerosol infectivity and viability in dried louse feces.[3] Similarly, it remains highly infectious following drying in media with high osmolarity and has been weaponized so it could be used as an agent of bioterrorism. Consequently, *R. prowazekii* is a "select agent," whose possession and distribution is tightly regulated in the United States and other countries.[4] Genetic variants of *R. prowazekii* with different geographic distributions are known.[5,6]

Epidemiology

Classic epidemic typhus is spread from infected to uninfected people by migration of the human body lice, *Pediculus humanus corporis*, away from febrile hosts.[7,8] Infected lice defecate during feeding and excrete copious amounts of rickettsiae in their feces. Transmission occurs to nonimmune humans when louse fecal material or crushed lice are inoculated into the bite site or skin abrasions or conjunctiva (more rarely), or when they are inhaled. The lice die from the rickettsial infection within 2 weeks but desiccated dead lice and fecal materials may remain infectious for much longer. Epidemic typhus is one of the classic plagues of humankind, having infected and killed millions of people in the preantibiotic era during epidemics until the middle of the 20th century. However, major outbreaks still occur infrequently in sub-Saharan Africa and sporadic cases continue to be reported from North Africa, Ethiopia, Peru, Russia, and the U.S.[9–12] Body lice live in clothing; classic epidemic typhus occurs typically in conditions where poverty, famine, and war, frequently accompanied by cold weather, lead to unhygienic conditions favoring louse infestation. Head and pubic lice have not been shown to be significant human vectors for epidemic typhus although head lice can be infected with *R. prowazekii* and are closely related to body lice.[13]

Humans are the primary reservoir for *R. prowazekii* where the organism persists despite strong humoral and cellular immune responses. Formerly infected people can suffer a relapse of typhus, known as Brill–Zinsser disease or recrudescent typhus.[14] The precise factors causing relapses are not well understood but recrudescence of disease is thought to constitute the source of *R.*

prowazekii that permits initiation of new outbreaks of louse-transmitted typhus. Because infestation with body lice is now uncommon in much of the world and fewer people who experienced primary epidemic typhus now exist in the population, both primary epidemic typhus and herd immunity have declined throughout the world in the last 40 years. Indigenous louse-borne epidemic typhus has not occurred in the U.S. since 1922 but Brill–Zinsser disease occasionally is seen among immigrants from historically endemic foci of epidemic typhus or people infected in concentration camps. Healthcare personnel and military personnel may be at particular risk of infection. The last major Burundi outbreak was first detected because of the fatal infection of an evacuated Swiss Red Cross worker.[15]

Bozeman and colleagues first reported a sylvatic cycle of *R. prowazekii* in flying squirrels and their ectoparasites from Florida and Virginia.[16] *R. prowazekii* can be transmitted experimentally between flying squirrels by squirrel lice (*Neohaematopinus sciuropteri*) and their fleas (*Orchopeas howardi*).[17] About 40 cases of human sylvatic typhus infections, including several cases in children, have been reported in the eastern U.S.[18,19] Onset usually is during the winter months when squirrels may enter houses; many such patients reported contact with the southern flying squirrel (*Glaucomys volans*) or their nests and associated ectoparasites. The mechanism by which disease is transmitted to humans is unclear but squirrel fleas occasionally bite humans. It also is possible that humans become infected by inhalation of contaminated feces from the squirrel ectoparasites. One patient previously diagnosed with sylvatic typhus may have experienced a recurrent episode of febrile rickettsial illness like Brill–Zinsser disease.[20]

R. prowazekii has been detected in *Hyalomma* ticks in Ethiopia[21] and in *Amblyomma* ticks from Mexico.[22] If confirmed, this unusual source may account for sporadic cases of epidemic typhus in the Americas that are not associated with human body lice, infected flying squirrels, or prior infections.[12]

Clinical Manifestations

Epidemic typhus is fatal in 10% to 50% of untreated patients and is more likely to be clinically severe or fatal in people with concurrent malnourishment or other disease.[6,8,23] Onset of epidemic typhus is abrupt and occurs 7 to 14 days post exposure while Brill–Zinsser disease can occur >40 years after primary infection. Patients manifest high prostrating fever with severe headache, limb pains, and vomiting. The patient often appears vacant and semi-mute, and can have epistaxis (or a nosebleed) and a dry cough. The classical macular or maculopapular, sometimes petechial, rash which can become purpuric appears 5 to 7 days after onset of symptoms. The exanthem, which may be difficult to see on dark skin, begins on the trunk and spreads to the arms and legs but rarely involves the palms, soles or face. Constipation is common and paralytic ileus can occur. Typhus infrequently induces diarrhea or splenomegaly, which helps in its differentiation from typhoid and malaria, respectively. A cough and pneumonia is observed in two-thirds of patients and nervous system involvement (drowsiness, disorientation, and delirium) is frequent. In severe cases, a meningoencephalitic syndrome occurs with meningismus, tinnitus, and hyperacusis, followed by deafness, dysphoria, agitation, and coma. Thrombocytopenia, jaundice, and abnormal liver function can occur in severe cases. Survivors can experience hemiparesis, acute transverse myelitis, or peripheral neuropathy. Complications include secondary bacterial infections, myocarditis, and peripheral gangrene or venous thromboembolism. Convalescence is rapid and uneventful if appropriate antibiotic therapy is initiated early after onset of disease. Classic epidemic typhus in pediatric patients often is a milder illness and has a lower fatality rate compared with adults and elderly people. Intoxication syndrome, cardiovascular and neurologic symptoms usually are less pronounced. Observations from the preantibiotic era indicate that epidemic typhus in pregnant women clinically resembles Brill–Zinsser disease (see below) with a good prognosis and low mortality; however, spontaneous abortion and premature birth can occur in 20% to 50% of pregnant patients.

In contrast to primary epidemic typhus, delirium is rarely noted in recrudescent typhus. Although Brill–Zinsser disease often is considered to be milder than primary disease, exceptions occur. Late in the second week of illness, fever and headache subside abruptly, and patients feel generally well. The clinical presentation of flying squirrel-associated typhus fever also appears to be milder than that observed in louse-borne epidemic typhus. Whether this difference in clinical presentation is related to the different strains associated with sylvatic *R. prowazekii* or to the relatively good nutrition, health, and supportive care in U.S. cases is unknown.[18]

Clinical diagnosis of epidemic typhus can be difficult because of resemblance to influenza, typhoid, meningococcal meningitis, hemorrhagic fevers, infectious mononucleosis, sepsis, measles, and malaria.

Laboratory Findings and Diagnosis

The white blood cell count frequently is reduced with a relative lymphocytosis during the first week of epidemic typhus, and can be elevated as disease progresses.[24] Eosinophils are decreased or absent during the entire febrile period. Anemia and increased erythrocyte sedimentation rate frequently are detected but return to normal following treatment. Nephritis, typified by azotemia and moderate amounts of albumin and granular casts in urine, is expected.

Diagnosis of epidemic typhus generally is suspected because of specific epidemiologic circumstances and clinical findings. Diagnosis of acute epidemic typhus can be made by polymerase chain reaction (PCR) assay for rickettsial DNA extracted from whole blood or the buffy coat fraction, or biopsies of the rash; PCR is sensitive and specific.[12,25] Detection of rickettsial DNA in squirrel tissues and ectoparasites provides alternative identification of the etiologic agent.[18,26] Immunohistochemical procedures also can be applied to biopsy and ectoparasite samples.[8,15,27] However, these procedures are available only in specialty laboratories, and prompt submission and correct handling of samples is essential for agent detection. Isolation is possible from acute-phase blood and biopsy samples collected before initiation of antimicrobial therapy, in laboratories with access to embryonated chicken eggs, susceptible animals, or antibiotic-free cell cultures.[2,28] Isolation can require up to several weeks. Isolates of *R. prowazekii* are differentiated readily from other species of *Rickettsia* by genetic, biologic, and antigenic criteria.[5,29]

The indirect immunofluorescence assay is the current gold standard for serologic diagnosis of epidemic typhus.[30] Diagnosis is based on a 4-fold rise in IgG antibody titers between acute and convalescent paired sera to *R. prowazekii* antigen or a high single titer of antibody with compatible clinical symptoms. Other serologic procedures for the specific detection of TG antibodies include enzyme immunoassay (EIA), complement fixation, latex agglutination, dip-sticks, and chromatographic flow assays. Commercial testing usually employs IFA or EIA methods. The nonspecific Weil–Felix febrile agglutination test, which detects IgM antibodies to a typhus cross-reactive LPS epitope found in *Proteus* OX19 antigen, is not used in the U.S., but may be available in less developed countries. Serologic cross-reactions can occur between TG and SFG of *Rickettsia*, and IgM antibodies can react with some species of *Legionella* and other strains of *Proteus*.[31] Cross-absorption of sera for IFA testing or Western blotting analysis differentiates epidemic and murine typhus and excludes other cross-reactions.[32]

Treatment

Treatment must be instituted before the diagnosis of epidemic typhus is confirmed by laboratory testing. Tetracyclines and chloramphenicol are effective against all forms of typhus infections while ciprofloxacin and azithromycin have failed in the treatment of primary disease and Brill–Zinsser disease, respectively.[15,33,34] Doxycycline is the preferred treatment for both adults and children since the risk of tooth staining is low compared with the threat of this disease.[35] Dosage is 4 mg/kg/day (maximum dose 200 mg/day), PO or IV divided into doses every 12 hours, for 7 to 10 days. A single dose of 200 mg of oral doxycycline for adults and 100 mg for children is efficient in the control of epidemics where continuous patient management can be difficult. Chloramphenicol (50 mg/kg/day divided into doses every 6 hours for children for 7 to 10 days) also is effective; however, the use of chloramphenicol has been associated with increased risk of fatal outcome and relapses in Rocky Mountain spotted fever and typhus.[36] Marked improvement with cessation of fever should be apparent within 48 hours after treatment with either antibiotic but other symptoms can persist for up to a week. Development of specific immune responses is important for full recovery because the antibiotics of choice are bacteriostatic, not bactericidal.

Prevention and Control

Sporadic cases of Brill–Zinsser disease can occur in the U.S. primarily among immigrants from areas endemic for epidemic typhus but they pose little risk for spread except from individuals infested with body lice. Head lice have never been associated with outbreaks of epidemic typhus but body lice continue to be present in many regions of the world and can serve as a source of infestation in areas that presently are free of lice. No licensed vaccine for epidemic typhus is available. Exclusion of flying squirrels and their nests from domiciles to prevent concomitant exposure to their ectoparasites, use of pyrethrin-containing insecticides, and decontamination of infested clothing by washing with detergent at high temperatures are recommended for prevention and control.

RICKETTSIA TYPHI (MURINE TYPHUS; ENDEMIC OR FLEA-BORNE TYPHUS)

Description of Pathogen

Rickettsia typhi is a member of the TG of rickettsiae and closely resembles the other member of that group, *R. prowazekii*, in its genetic, biologic, and immunologic properties.[1,2,37] *R. typhi* replicates to higher titers in the yolk sacs of embryonated chicken eggs and is more infectious for laboratory mice and guinea pigs than *R. prowazekii* but it is not regulated as a "select agent" in the U.S.

Epidemiology

Commensal rats of the genus *Rattus* are the primary zoonotic reservoirs for *R. typhi*.[38] The oriental rat flea, *Xenopsylla cheopis,* is the classic vector that transmits murine typhus to humans but six genera and seven species of flea, including the cat flea (*Ctenocephalides felis*), have been found to be naturally infected with *R. typhi*. Cats and peridomestic opossums infested with cat fleas have been implicated in the maintenance of *R. typhi* in the U.S.; however, murine typhus from this source is likely to be a rare event.[39,40] Fleas are infected for life after feeding upon *R. typhi* infected rodents. The fleas shed organisms in their feces, and humans become infected through contact between flea feces and abraded skin, or possibly through inhalation of fecal material. Besides rats, fleas may be an important reservoir of *R. typhi* since they can transmit the organism transovarially to their progeny.[41]

Murine typhus has been diagnosed throughout the world but is reported most frequently from warmer climates and coastal areas where *Rattus* and fleas flourish.[38,42-47] Typically, seaports, coastal areas, and the major commercial arteries are disease-endemic sites. While only 333 cases of murine typhus were described in 1931 and 2000 cases in 1933, by World War II, more than 5000 cases were documented annually in the U.S.[48,49] After World War II, flea and rodent control programs caused a precipitous drop in the number of reported cases. Since the 1980s, the prevalence and distribution of murine typhus in the U.S. are poorly known. In the U.S., infection has been reported most commonly from focal areas in California, Texas, and Hawaii.[40,50,51] Both sporadic cases and small outbreaks occur. Disease can be imported by travelers returning to the U.S. from southern Europe, Asia, and Africa.[52,53]

Clinical Manifestations

Murine typhus manifests with fever, chills, headache, and myalgia. Although the disease generally is mild clinically, up to 10% of adults require intensive care with mortality approaching 4% for untreated cases. Most cases of murine typhus in the U.S. occur in adults but children are infected frequently in many parts of the world. An extensive series of 96 serologically confirmed cases of murine typhus in children <1 to 16 years of age from Texas provides the most accurate clinical pediatric data available.[54] Fever occurred in all patients 8 to 16 days after exposure; headaches occurred in 76% with frontal distribution and dengue-like intensity. Rash occurred in 63% with a median onset at 6 days of illness, while the clinical triad of rash, fever, and headache was found in only 49% of patients. Rash generally was macular (50%) or maculopapular (25%) and less frequently erythematous, petechial, or papular. While flea bites were reported in only 34% of patients, potential patient contact with animal reservoirs that likely were flea-infested was found in 85% of the cases.

Nausea and vomiting occur during the early stage of illness in almost all infected adults. In contrast, children tolerate the early disease symptoms well, with gastrointestinal tract symptoms, (anorexia, vomiting, nausea, diarrhea, and abdominal pain), occurring in 27% to 46% of children, and pharyngitis, lymphadenopathy, and cough in 15% to 20%.[54] Pneumonitis, stupor, conjunctivitis, or photophobia occurred in only 5% to 12% of children. Splenomegaly and hepatomegaly were not common in this series but these symptoms have been described previously in populations in the tropics.[42,55] The difference may be ascribed to early treatment in the pediatric group from Texas or to coinfection with other common diseases in the tropics. Neurologic findings appear to be more common in adults (15% to 45% in different studies) than children.

Most patients with murine typhus are hospitalized and many patients have signs of shock and sepsis. Complications of murine typhus can include meningitis, meningoencephalitis, facial paralysis, hearing loss, ocular abnormalities, myocarditis, renal and respiratory failure.[56–58] Severe hemolysis has been associated with glucose-6-phosphate dehydrogenase deficiency.[59] Splenic rupture has been reported in a 10-year-old child.[60]

Laboratory Findings and Diagnosis

Laboratory findings are nonspecifically abnormal in murine typhus in children.[54] In the case series, 81% had high erythrocyte sedimentation rate, 77% had a left shift in differential leukocyte count, 68% had absolute neutropenia, 51% had absolute lymphopenia. Serum hepatic enzyme levels were measured infrequently but generally were abnormal. Serum electrolyte changes included hyponatremia (58%), hypokalemia (21%), and elevated serum creatinine (21%).

Although all patients in the pediatric case series were confirmed serologically by IFA, diagnostic titers were present in only 15% of patients at 7 days and 62% by 14 days after onset of illness. More than 28 days were required for all patients to exhibit diagnostic titers. Serologic tests for murine typhus use *R. typhi* antigen and detect cross-reactive antibodies that usually are elicited during both epidemic and murine typhus infections but less frequently in SFG infections.[30,32] With murine typhus, antibody titers to *R.*

typhi may be higher than to *R. prowazekii*; antibody cross-absorption studies often are necessary to clearly distinguish murine and epidemic typhus.[32] Since circulation of *R. felis* also has been demonstrated in states traditionally endemic for murine typhus,[39,40,43] and *R. typhi* and *R. felis* share a number of cross-reactive antigens, differential serology of these flea-borne agents also may be necessary. Genetic tests that readily discriminate *R. typhi*, *R. prowazekii*, and *R. felis* also are available. Because fleas have high-density infections with *R. typhi*, PCR and direct fluorescent antibody staining of the agent in fleas are effective assays.[61–63]

Treatment

Treatment regimens for suspected *R. typhi* infections are the same as those for *R. prowazekii* and other rickettsial infections. Relapses have been reported in patients treated with chloramphenicol but not those treated with tetracyclines, indicating that tetracycline or tetracycline analogs are preferable.[64] Ciprofloxacin also has been used successfully for treating adults with murine typhus. In a cohort of 87 adult patients from Greece, doxycycline treatment led to defervescence in 2.9 days (median), chloramphenicol in 4.0 days, and ciprofloxacin in 4.2 days.[65] Treatment regimens combining doxycycline with chloramphenicol or ciprofloxacin did not improve the clinical effectiveness of doxycycline. In children median time to defervescence was 2 days for tetracycline and 2.5 days for chloramphenicol.[54]

Prevention

No vaccine is available for preventing murine typhus. Avoidance or elimination of rodent-infested areas are the best methods for preventing infection.[38] Rodent and flea eradication programs are recommended for areas where harborages already exist. Essential measures include rat proofing of homes and buildings, elimination of crowded and unsanitary housing conditions, and elimination or reduction of agricultural food sources and rat harborages in the domestic environment. Workers trapping and removing rats or working in rat harborages can use aerosol sprays of pyrethroid insecticides and protective clothing and masks to reduce risk of infection from fleas seeking new hosts and from residual flea feces. Control of opossums and their fleas has not yet been shown to be a necessary or effective strategy for murine typhus.

RICKETTSIA FELIS (CAT FLEA RICKETTSIOSIS)

Description of Pathogen

Rickettsia felis was first discovered by electron microscopy in the midgut epithelium and ovaries of the cat flea, *Ctenocephalides felis*, where it is maintained by transovarial passage.[66] *R. felis* can be grown in South African clawed toad XTC-2, *Drosophila* S2, mosquito C6/36, or tick ISE6 cells at 28°C. By comparative genomic analysis *R. felis* appears to be related most closely to *R. akari* and *R. australis*.[67] As with *R. akari*, its LPS differs from that of prototypical SFG rickettsiae like *R. rickettsii* and *R. conorii*. Like other rickettsiae, *R. felis* has large surface layer protein antigens (Sca proteins) that are important targets in immune responses, but little is known about their biologic properties.[66,68,69]

Epidemiology

The epidemiology of cat flea rickettsiosis is ill-defined.[66,70,71] *Rickettsia felis* was discovered in 1990 in a commercial stock of fleas collected in 1969 from cats at a rodent-infested granary in the central valley area of California. The colony of fleas was shown to maintain *R. felis* transovarially. Cat fleas infected with *R. felis* have been collected in many states including California, Florida, Georgia, Louisiana, New York, North Carolina, Oklahoma, Tennessee, and Texas. *R. felis* also was found in *Pulex irritans* collected from a dog in Georgia and *X. cheopis* in Hawaii and California.[43,62] Fleas containing *R. felis* have been collected from opossums in Tennessee, Texas, California, and Georgia. The fleas are not affected by the presence of *R. felis* despite their location in midgut epithelial linings, tracheal matrix, muscle, ovaries, and epithelial sheath of the testes. *Rickettsia felis*-infected cat fleas can acquire *R. typhi* during a blood meal and maintain *R. typhi* for up to 9 days; however, effects of coinfection on the subsequent transovarial transmission of each agent were not determined.[63] *R. felis* also can coinfect fleas with *Bartonella quintana, B. henselae,* and *Wolbachia pipientis*.[72] *R. felis* has a worldwide distribution in association with many flea species and animal hosts.[66,70]

The ability of vertebrate hosts to be infected or to act as reservoirs for *R. felis* is not fully understood. *Rickettsia felis* DNA has been detected by PCR in opossums.[39,40] As many as 11% of cats surveyed are seropositive for *R. felis*.[73] About 30% of U.S. households have cats; if only 5% of these animals are infected with *R. felis,* potentially 285,000 cats may act as hosts of infected fleas, suggesting human exposure to this agent.

Given these findings, it is surprising that so few PCR confirmed cases of infection with *R. felis* have been identified worldwide.[70,74-77] Lack of communication between laboratories able to identify *R. felis,* lack of diagnostic tests in patients with relatively mild or influenza-like symptoms of infection, low human susceptibility or low pathogenicity of this agent, may account for low case numbers. Alternatively, *R. felis* may vary in pathogenicity for humans and other vertebrates. *R. felis* was detected by PCR followed by restriction enzyme analysis and hybridization in one patient from Corpus Christi, Texas with murine typhus-like symptoms; this is the only confirmed U.S. case.[71] Serologic evidence of *R. felis* infection has been reported for patients from several countries.[70,75] Six cases of *R. felis* infection were diagnosed by PCR in the Yucatan.[77] Low rate of sporadic cases does not account for relatively high seroprevalence (5.6%) of antibodies to SFG rickettsiae found in this area even though *R. felis* frequently was detected among 1800 ticks, fleas, and lice.[70] Probably, cross-reactivity of antibody among rickettsial species explains the discrepancy. In Texas patients, of 32 human serum samples positive for antirickettsial antibodies, only 3 were found positive for *R. felis* while the others reacted to *R. typhi* antigen,[78] although *R. felis* was more common than *R. typhi* in fleas and opossums.[39]

Clinical Manifestations

Few human cases of *R. felis* infection with reliable laboratory support have been described. Clinical presentations of *R. felis* illnesses diagnosed in different countries vary. The *R. felis* case from Texas initially was diagnosed as murine typhus as the patient presented with a fever and headache, and no apparent rash.[71] Two French cases were first diagnosed clinically as murine typhus or Mediterranean spotted fever.[70] Five patients treated in Mexico and Brazil had rash and systemic symptoms including fever, headache, and myalgia;[79] 4 patients had visceral involvement with abdominal pain, nausea, vomiting, and diarrhea; and 4 patients had involvement of the central nervous system (photophobia in 2 patients, hearing loss and signs of meningismus in 1 patient, and coma in 1 patient). One patient also had conjunctivitis. Some of the Mexican cases in the Yucatan had dengue-like illness, and others presented with pulmonary symptoms, a skin lesion consistent with an ulcer, or peripheral erythema.[77] Complications of *R. felis* infection in humans include hepatitis, polynephropathy, and splenic infarction.[74,77,80]

Laboratory Findings and Diagnosis

Patients with *R. felis* infection can have thrombocytopenia and increased levels of serum aspartate transaminase or anemia, leukocytosis, thrombocytosis, and prolonged prothrombin time, or leukopenia.[70]

Most cases of suspected *R. felis* infection lack detectable antibodies to rickettsiae in acute serum samples. Convalescent sera contain high antibody to *R. felis* (IFA IgG of ≥1 : 512 and IgM titers of ≥1 : 64). Because *R. felis* shares antigens with typhus and SFG rickettsiae, cross-absorption of sera is necessary for specific diagnosis.[75]

Definitive diagnosis requires detection of *R. felis* DNA by PCR amplification.[70,74,76,77,80] PCR amplification and sequencing of *R. felis* DNA from skin biopsy, whole blood, and serum samples is done with primers for the *Rickettsia* 17-kd protein gene, 120-kd protein gene (*sca*4), *omp*A, *omp*B, and *R. felis* plasmid genes.

No isolates have been obtained directly from patients. *R. felis* from different flea populations exhibits variable genetic features that suggests substantive diversity of biological and antigenic properties.[69,81]

Treatment and Prevention

R. felis infections are treated with doxycycline as for other rickettsial diseases. Chloramphenicol frequently is used as an alternative medication when doxycycline is not available.[77] In vitro quantitative PCR data indicate that *R. felis* is susceptible to doxycycline (minimum inhibitory concentration, MIC 0.06 to 0.125 µg/mL), rifampin (MIC 0.06 to 0.25 µg/mL), thiamphenicol (MIC 1 to 2 µg/mL), and fluoroquinolones (MIC 0.5 to 1.0 µg/mL); gentamicin, erythromycin, amoxicillin, or trimethoprim-sulfamethoxazole are not suitable for treatment.[82]

Rickettsia felis appears to be maintained primarily in cat fleas infesting opossums in central and south central Texas and Los Angeles and Orange counties in California. Rodents and other fleas may be involved in other parts of the world. Cat fleas are promiscuous feeders on free-ranging wild and domestic cats and dogs, and their owners. Opossums are opportunistic marsupials which have adapted well to destruction of their natural habitats by moving into hospitable urban and suburban areas. They are found in more than 40 states in the U.S. Elimination of open food sources like garbage, as well as trapping and removal of opossums and flea control of domestic animals are recommended for prevention of cat flea rickettsiosis.[83]

RICKETTSIA AKARI (RICKETTSIALPOX)

Description of Pathogen

Until the discoveries of *R. felis* and other rickettsiae associated with other arthropods, *Rickettsia akari* was considered the most unusual species of *Rickettsia* because it is transmitted by mites rather than ticks. The SFG LPS of *R. akari* is unusual because it does not elicit typical OX2 and OX19 Weil–Felix agglutinin responses in humans. Its surface protein antigens are important in protective immune responses and properties, separating it from other SFG species. Isolates of *R. akari* differ in resistance of inbred strains of mice to intraperitoneal challenge. Molecular differences between U.S. and Ukrainian isolates also have been detected. Antigenically, *R. akari* is distinguished readily from other species of SFG rickettsiae with immune mouse sera in indirect fluorescent antibody tests.[84]

Epidemiology

Although *R. akari* appears to be distributed widely in the world, its natural history is incompletely understood. In the U.S. *R. akari* is best known for causing focal urban outbreaks of rickettsialpox in areas following the bite of the house mouse mite, *Liponyssoides sanguineus*. Following its discovery in 1946 in Queens, New York, cases have been reported in Boston, Cleveland, Philadelphia, Pittsburgh, Salt Lake City, Tucson, Champaign, Indianapolis, Washington, DC, West Hartford, and Baltimore.[83,85] Although over 800 cases have been reported in the U.S., 500 were reported within the first 3 years after discovery of rickettsialpox, most of them in New York City. By the 1960s a sharp decline occurred in reported cases of rickettsialpox.[86] It is unclear whether the incidence of rickettsialpox has continued to decline or it is recognized rarely since only 13 cases were reported in a New York City hospital from 1980 to 1989.[87] Increasing alertness due to the anthrax investigation in New York City during 2001–2003 led to identification of recent cases of rickettsialpox in the U.S.[88,89] Human cases of rickettsialpox also have been reported from the former Yugoslavia, Turkey, and Mexico.[90-92] A major outbreak in Ukraine occurred during 1949–1952, but no subsequent cases were reported there following elimination of the endemic foci.[93] *Liponyssoides sanguineus* is the major reservoir of *R. akari* since it maintains the agent by both transtadial and transovarial passage. Isolates also have been obtained from infected house mice and other rodents and they can transmit *R. akari* to uninfected mites. *R. akari* has been isolated from commensal rats in the Ukraine and from voles in Korea.[94,95] However, the importance of rodents as reservoirs of *R. akari* in nature is unclear. *Liponyssoides sanguineus* is a parasite of house mice *(Mus musculus)* and rats *(Rattus norvegicus* and *Rattus rattus)* but voles and gerbils can be infected in the laboratory. Dogs in New York City have been shown to have antibodies to *R. akari*,[96] and *R. akari* was detected in *Rhipicephalus sanguineus* collected from a sick dog in Mexico.[97]

The mite abandons the host after feeding and can be found in mouse bedding and walls of infested rooms. Rickettsialpox appears to occur primarily when mice and rats are not available as the primary vertebrate hosts as can happen following lymphocytic choriomeningitis virus (LCMV) infections of rodents when the mites feed on humans as an available alternative host.[98] The decline in rickettsialpox in the inner city may be due to replacement of *L. sanguineus* with the tropical rat mite, *Ornithonyssus bacoti*, which can maintain *R. akari* by transovarial passage but is an inefficient vector of rickettsialpox.[85]

Clinical Manifestations

Rickettsialpox is a relatively mild illness and is rarely fatal, although more severe cases have been reported from Mexico.[92,93] Rickettsialpox affects males and females equally and has no age dependence. Three features are characteristic of the disease. First, following an incubation period of 7 to 14 days after the bite of the mite, the skin inoculation site has a firm red papule 1 to 1.5 cm in diameter. Shortly thereafter, the painless lesion vesiculates and becomes filled with cloudy fluid. As the lesion dries, it leaves a brown to black crust surrounded by a 0.5 to 3 cm area of induration. The initial lesion can be located anywhere on covered areas of the body; more than one lesion is rare. Regional draining lymph nodes often are swollen but lymphangitis has not been reported. In the second stage, an influenza-like syndrome begins abruptly about 1 week after exposure (up to 17 days later) with chills, fever, sweats, and myalgia. The peak temperature usually is 39°C to 40°C; without treatment, fever persists for about 7 to 11 days. Other common symptoms include profuse diaphoresis and headache (usually frontal) and photophobia; occasionally vertigo, rhinorrhea, cough, sore throat, nausea, vomiting, and constipation are present. Finally, usually within 1 to 3 days after the onset of constitutional symptoms, an exanthem appears as a single crop, with 5 to 100 discrete, firm erythematous papules on the face, trunk, and extremities; lesions are 2 to 10 mm in diameter and can develop a small vesicle or pustule in the center. Lesions can involve the palate, tongue, and pharynx but less frequently (<10%) the palms or soles. In about 1 week, vesicles dry and form scales that do not scar but can result in postinflammatory hyperpigmentation. Untreated rickettsialpox usually resolves uneventfully in 2 to 3 weeks. Rickettsialpox most often is confused with chickenpox but chickenpox lacks a primary eschar, and the vesicles rest on an erythematous base. The appearance of the eschar in rickettsialpox resembles the skin lesion developed in patients with cutaneous anthrax; rickettsialpox should be included in the differential diagnostic panel of urban diseases as was done in 2001 in New York City.[88,89]

Laboratory Findings and Diagnosis

Leukopenia (2400 to 4000 cells/mm³) with relative lymphocytosis usually is detected during the early febrile stage of rickettsialpox. Hematocrit, hemoglobin, erythrocyte sedimentation rate, and electrolyte and serum transaminase values are normal; urinalysis can show mild proteinuria.[86–88]

Specific diagnosis typically requires a combination of clinical and epidemiologic findings in conjunction with group-specific serologic tests. Patients with a compatible illness and known or possible mite exposure should be tested for antibodies to SFG rickettsiae. *R. rickettsii* typically is used as a surrogate antigen because it is antigenically related to *R. akari* and is more widely available. Seroconversion in a clinically compatible case provides good evidence of rickettsialpox but definitive evidence requires cross-absorption with SFG rickettsial antigens.[99] Direct fluorescent antibody tests or immunohistochemical staining of punch biopsies taken from skin lesions also have been used to confirm the diagnosis of rickettsialpox but use of a species-specific antibody is necessary to confirm *R. akari* infection.[88,89,100,101] PCR amplification of a rickettsial 17-kd protein gene fragment or OmpB gene fragment followed by DNA sequencing has good diagnostic efficiency.[92,100] *R. akari* can be isolated from skin biopsy samples.[100]

Treatment and Prevention

No fatalities have been reported for rickettsialpox. Uncontrolled studies show that treatment with tetracyclines hastens defervescence and abatement of systemic symptoms within 48 hours. Dosage is the same as for other rickettsial infections; duration generally is 3 days following defervescence. Chloramphenicol can be used as an alternative treatment when doxycycline is not available.[92]

No vaccine has been developed. Disease can be prevented by enforcing sanitary measures that preclude development of urban rodent harborages. Rodent eradication programs can eliminate infestation problems; insecticides and acaricides must be applied so that the ectoparasites do not seek alternative human hosts and initiate an outbreak.[83,93,98]

RICKETTSIA PARKERI (MACULATUM DISEASE)

Description of Pathogen

Rickettsia parkeri, also called "maculatum agent," is an SFG rickettsia that was first recovered from the tick *Amblyomma maculatum* in 1939.[102] Phylogenetically and microbiologically, *R. parkeri* clusters in a genetic lineage together with *R. africae*, *R. sibirica*, and the unnamed isolate "S" obtained from *Rh. sanguineus* ticks in Armenia.[103] Another new genetic type related to *R. parkeri* has been detected in skin biopsy of patients from Brazil.[104,105]

Epidemiology

The ecology and distribution of *R. parkeri* is not completely understood. In North America the Gulf Coast tick, *A. maculatum*, is the primary vector of *R. parkeri*.[106] *R. parkeri* is transmitted transovarially and transtadially in these ticks. While *A. maculatum* is found in southeastern states that border the Gulf of Mexico and along the southern Atlantic coast to Virginia, inland populations also exist in Kansas and Oklahoma. *R. parkeri* has been found in *A. maculatum* ticks collected in Alabama, Georgia, Mississippi, Texas, Florida, Kentucky, and South Carolina. *A. maculatum* also is found in some countries of Central and South America and some Caribbean islands. *R. parkeri* also can infect *A. cajennense*; its DNA has been detected in *A. triste*, *A. tigrinum*, and *A. nodosum* from South America.[22,107,108] Human cases due to *R. parkeri* infection have been diagnosed in at least 9 states in the U.S.[109–111]

Clinical Manifestations, Laboratory Findings and Diagnosis

Patients present with fever, headache, diffuse myalgia, and arthralgia. Single or multiple eschars are present in >90% of cases; the multiple eschars suggest that transmission by exposure to larval tick nests may be common. An erythematous maculopapular rash develops on the trunk and spreads to the extremities, including the palms and soles. Some patients have a diffuse nonpruritic maculopapular and vesicular rash.

A mild leukopenia, elevated levels of serum hepatic enzymes, lactate dehydrogenase, and total bilirubin were detected in the blood of acutely ill patients. Paired acute and convalescent serum specimens show rises of IgG antibodies reactive with SFG rickettsiae. Since significant cross-reactivity exists among SFG rickettsiae, cross-absorption and Western blotting analyses are necessary to obtain specific serologic diagnoses. Histopathologic evaluation of biopsy specimens obtained from the rash or eschar reveal the presence of rickettsiae and lymphohistiocytic perivascular infiltrates. PCR amplification and sequencing of DNA from skin biopsy samples and sequencing allows precise identification of the rickettsial etiologic agent.[109,110] Isolation in cell culture provides the best confirmation of the specific rickettsial etiology and permits further characterization of the properties of the organism.

Treatment, Prevention and Control

Patients are treated with doxycycline as for other rickettsial doses. Fever resolves within 24 to 48 hours, while malaise and rash has more gradual resolution. Laboratory test values return to normal within 1 month.

Prevention measures rely on reduction of exposure to ticks by avoiding tick habitat, reducing tick abundance in tick-infested areas, wearing protective clothing, and checking for and removing ticks after exposure. Wearing long pants, long sleeves, and long socks will reduce tick attachment, but tucking pant legs into socks or boots and tucking shirts into pants is more effective. Light-colored clothing also can aid in spotting ticks more easily. Using insect repellent with 20% to 30% DEET (*N,N*-diethyl-*m*-toluamide) on skin and clothing to prevent tick attachment is recommended. DEET is not recommended for use on children under 2 months of age. Permethrin is another repellent that also kills ticks on contact. One application to pants, socks, and shoes is effective through several washings. Permethrin should not be applied directly to skin.

Prophylactic antibiotic therapy is not recommended for people with attached ticks because it may only delay onset of disease and many ticks are not infected. People should remove attached ticks properly without crushing to avoid aerosolization and contamination of skin wounds.

RICKETTSIA SPECIES 364D

Description of Pathogen

Rickettsia sp. 364D is an SFG rickettsia that was first detected in the Pacific Coast tick, *Dermacentor occidentalis*, in the 1970s.[112] Its microbiologic characteristics are typical of other SFG rickettsiae; however, its in vitro cytopathic effect is significantly milder than that of *R. rickettsii*. *Rickettsia* sp. 364D is a close relative of *R. rickettsii*; however, it has a sufficient number of unique genetic characteristics to satisfy current molecular criteria to be classified as a new species, *Rickettsia philipii* sp. nov.

Epidemiology

The vector of *Rickettsia* sp. 364D is *D. occidentalis*,[113] a tick with a limited distribution spanning from Baja, Mexico to southern Oregon. Approximately 7% of *D. occidentalis* in southern and northern California are infected with *Rickettsia* sp. 364D, compared with <1% with *R. rickettsii*.[114] Among California ticks, *Rickettsia* sp. 364D has been identified only in *D. occidentalis*, a species that occasionally bites humans and is common throughout much of California except the very dry regions of the central valley and the southeastern desert. In northern California, adult *D. occidentalis* are most active March through May, whereas nymphal *D. occidentalis* are encountered more commonly during June through August, the peak occurrence of disease.

Clinical Manifestations

Rickettsia sp. 364D infection causes nonspecific clinical symptoms including fever, fatigue, headache, and lymphadenitis

or lymphadenopathy; no rash has been reported.[115] The presence of a single ulcerated eschar on the forearm, shoulder, or hip associated with a previous tick bite at that site is a significant diagnostic clue for clinical diagnosis. Severe manifestations or complications have not been observed and no patients required hospitalization.

Treatment, Prevention and Control

The treatment of 364D rickettsiosis is the same as for other rickettsial diseases and requires a full course of doxycycline. Prescription of sulfa drugs when other etiologies are suspected may worsen the course of rickettsial infection and prolong clinical symptoms and healing of skin lesions. For prevention, see *R. parkeri* above.

OTHER TRAVEL-ASSOCIATED RICKETTSIOSES (AFRICAN TICK BITE FEVER, MEDITERRANEAN SPOTTED FEVER OR BOUTONNEUSE FEVER, TIBOLA/DEBONEL, LYMPHANGITIS-ASSOCIATED RICKETTSIOSIS, OTHER SPOTTED FEVERS, SCRUB TYPHUS)

Epidemiology and Description of Pathogens

As international travel and ecotourism have become increasingly popular, physicians may need to treat patients that have become infected with other rickettsial agents that are transmitted by ticks and mites.[53,116,117] The SFG rickettsiae comprise a large number of pathogenic agents with varied geographic distributions that are dependent upon the presence of their different tick vectors (Table 179-1).[117,118] *Rickettsia africae*, the agent of African tick-bite fever, is the most common cause of rickettsial infections in travelers.[119,120] Boutonneuse fever (Mediterranean spotted fever) is caused by *R. conorii* subsp. *conorii*;[121,122] its distribution is throughout Africa to southern Europe and the Indian subcontinent. Whether *R. conorii* subsp. *caspia* and *R. conorii* subsp. *israelensis* are limited just to the Mediterranean–Caspian region is unknown.[117,122,123] *R. conorii conorii* and *israelensis* can cause severe disease. *Rickettsia massiliae* appears to cause rifampin-resistant cases of rickettsiosis in Catalonia, Spain.[117,124] *R. massiliae* infections have been identified in Sicily, France, and Argentina.[125] It has been isolated from a *Rh. sanguineus* tick in eastern Arizona and detected in California and South America.[22,126,127] *R. honei* is distributed widely in Southeast Asia.[118] *Rickettsia honei* strain "marmionii" occurs in Queensland, Tasmania, and South Australia.[128] *Rickettsia japonica* can cause a severe illness.[129] *Rickettsia heilongjiangensis* was detected in *Dermacentor silvarum* ticks in Heilongjiang Province of China in 1982[130] and later in patients. The range of *R. heilongjiangensis* extends to the Far East of Russia, where 13 patients infected with *R. heilongjiangensis* were identified,[131] and to Japan.[132] It has a different seasonal peak at the end of June and July from Siberian tick typhus (STT), which is caused by *Rickettsia sibirica* sensu stricto. *Demacentor* ticks transmit STT in a large area of Asia from Russia to India and southern China.[117,118] *Rickettsia sibirica* subsp. *mongolotimonae* causes infections in southern Europe, Africa, and Asia.[133] *Rickettsia aeschlimannii* is implicated in human cases reported from Africa and southern Europe,[134] and similar rickettsiae are found in ticks from southern Europe and the Middle East to Kazakhstan.[117,134] *R. slovaca* and *R. raoultii* cause sporadic and atypical rickettsioses in Eurasia.[135,136] *Rickettsia helvetica* is found throughout the wide distribution of *Ixodes ricinus*. It is implicated as a cause of febrile illness.[137,138] The closely related etiologic agent of scrub typhus, *Orientia tsutsugamushi*, was removed from the genus *Rickettsia* because it lacks peptidoglycan and LPS, and because it does not share any major surface antigens with *Rickettsia*, and it differs in its cell wall structure, staining properties, and morphology.[139] This antigenically diverse agent is transmitted by numerous species of trombiculid mites (chiggers) in the Asia-Pacific region from Australia to Russia and from New Guinea to Afghanistan.[140] Recently

TABLE 179-1. Differential Characteristics of Spotted-Fever Rickettsioses Acquired Outside the United States

Rickettsia sp.	Disease	Arthropod Vector	Location	Season	Outbreaks	Eschar	Rash	Lymphadenopathy	Fatality
			Epidemiologic Features				**Clinical Features**		
R. africae	African tick bite fever[a]	Amblyomma hebraeum, Amblyomma variegatum	Sub-Saharan Africa, West Indies	Year-round	Common	Yes (95–99%), often multiple	Maculopapular (49%) or vesicular (50%)	Enlarged lymph nodes (43%)	None reported
R. aeschlimannii	Unnamed spotted fever rickettsiosis[a]	Hyalomma marginatum marginatum, Hyalomma marginatum rufipes, Rhipicephalus appendiculatus	Southern Europe, northern Africa, South Africa	Year-around	Not reported	Yes[c]	Maculopapular[c]	Not reported	None reported
R. akari	Rickettsialpox	Liponyssoides sanguineus	Europe, Africa, Asia, Mexico	Year-round	Originally discovered as outbreaks, sporadic cases now	Yes (100%)	Papulovesicular (100%)	Lymphadenopathy of regional nodes (100%)	None reported
R. australis	Queensland tick typhus	Ixodes holocyclus, Ixodes tasmanii	Eastern Australia	June to November	None reported	Yes (65%)	Vesicular (94–100%)	71–84%	2%
R. conorii subsp. conorii	Mediterranean spotted fever	Rhipicephalus sanguineus	Southern Europe, Africa	Summer months	Sporadic cases	Yes (94–100%)	Maculopapular (93%)	Enlarged lymph nodes (1%)	2.3–2.5%
R. conorii subsp. caspia	Astrakhan spotted fever	Rhipicephalus sanguineus, Rhipicephalus pumilio	Volga delta of Russia, Kosovo, Chad	May through September	Sporadic cases	Yes (23%)	Maculopapular (94–100%)	Regional lymphadenitis (15.6%)	None reported
R. conorii subsp. israelensis	Israeli spotted fever[a]	Rhipicephalus sanguineus	Southern Europe from Portugal to Italy and Israel	Summer months	Sporadic cases	Yes (10–44%)	Maculopapular (87–100%)	Lymphadenitis (23–26.9%)	23%
R. felis	Cat flea rickettsiosis	Ctenocephalides felis	Worldwide	Year-round	Sporadic cases	Yes (25%)	Maculopapular (75%)	Not reported	None reported
R. heilongjiangensis	Far Eastern spotted fever	Dermacentor silvarum	Far east of Russia, Northern China	Summer months	Sporadic cases	Yes (92%)	Macular or maculopapular (92%)	Lymphadenopathy (15%), enlarged lymph nodes (77%)	None reported
R. honei	Flinders Island spotted fever	Aponoma hydrosauri, Ixodes granulatus	Southeastern Australia, Thailand	December to January	Sporadic cases	Yes (25%)	Maculopapular (85%)	Lymphadenopathy (55%)	None reported
R. honei strain marmionii	Flinders Island spotted fever	Haemaphysalis novaeguineae	Eastern seaboard of Australia	February to June	Sporadic cases	Yes[c]	Maculopapular or vesicular (43%)	Lymphadenopathy (29%)	Yes
R. japonica	Oriental (Japanese) spotted fever	Ixodes ovatus, Dermacentor taiwanensis, Haemaphysalis longicornis, Haemaphysalis flava	Japan, Korea, Taiwan	April to October	Sporadic cases	Yes (90–91%)	Macular progressing into petechial (100%)	Not reported	Yes
R. massiliae	Unnamed rickettsiosis	Rhipicephalus sanguineus Rhipicephalus turanicus	Mediterranean countries, Africa, South America	Spring and summer months	Sporadic cases	Yes (100%)	Maculopapular to purpuric (100%)	Not reported	None reported
R. parkeri	Maculatum infection	Amblyomma maculatum, Amblyomma cajennense, Amblyomma triste Amblyomma tigrinum Amblyomma nodosum	Argentina, Bolivia, Brazil, Uruguay	Spring to summer months	Sporadic cases	Yes (100%)	Maculopapular to vesicular[c]	Not reported	None reported

TABLE 179-1. Differential Characteristics of Spotted-Fever Rickettsioses Acquired Outside the United States—cont'd

Rickettsia sp.	Disease	Arthropod Vector	Location	Season	Outbreaks	Eschar	Rash	Lymphadenopathy	Fatality
			Epidemiologic Features			Clinical Features			
R. raoultii	Tick-borne lymphadenopathy (TIBOLA), *Dermacentor*-borne necrosis and lymphadenopathy (DEBONEL)	*Dermacentor marginatus Dermacentor reticulatus*	Europe to Asia	March–May to September–November	Sporadic cases	Yes (20%)	Yes (100%)	Yes	None reported
R. rickettsii	Rocky Mountain spotted fever, São Paulo exanthematic typhus, Minas Gerais exanthematic typhus, Brazilian spotted fever[a]	*Amblyomma cajennense Rhipicephalus sanguineus Amblyomma imitator*	Mexico, Costa Rica, Panama, Brazil, Argentina	Spring to fall months	Sporadic cases, also outbreaks and family cluster cases can occur	Most cases present without eschar	Macular progressing into papular or petechial (90%)	Enlarged lymph nodes (27%)	10–30%[d]
R. sibirica	Siberian tick typhus[a]	*Dermacentor nuttalli, Dermacentor marginatus, Dermacentor silvarum, Haemaphysalis concinna*	Europe, Asia	Spring to summer months	Sporadic cases	Yes (77%)	Maculopapular (100%)	Regional lymphadenopathy (100%)	None reported
R. sibirica subsp. *mongolotimonae*	Lymphangitis-associated rickettsiosis	*Hyalomma asiaticum, Hyalomma reticulatus*	Southern France, Asia, Africa[b]	Late spring to early summer	Sporadic cases	Yes (75–89%), multiple eschars	Maculopapular (63–78%)	Lymphangitis (25–44%), enlarged lymph nodes (55%)	None reported
R. slovaca	Tickborne lymphadenopathy (TIBOLA), *Dermacentor*-borne necrosis and lymphadenopathy (DEBONEL)	*Dermacentor marginatus, Dermacentor reticulatus*	Europe, Asia	October through May	Sporadic cases	Yes (64–100%)	Maculopapular (10 to 23%)	Cervical lymphadenopathy and enlarged lymph nodes (100%)	None reported

[a]*Indicates diseases reported for international travelers from endemic areas.*

[b]*Original isolation of a reference strain of* R. sibirica *subsp.* mongolotimonae *was made from* Hyalomma asiaticum *ticks from Northern China.*[130]

[c]*Prevalence has not been reported if numbers in parentheses are not shown.*

[d]*The case fatality rate due to* R. rickettsii *infection depends on patient's age and time of initiation of antibiotic therapy.*

a related agent, *Orientia chuto*, was identified from Dubai.[141] Chiggers are found in areas infested by rodents, particularly in areas of vegetation that have been disturbed but also in urban and suburban areas.

Clinical Manifestations

Differential clinical features of these rickettsioses are described in Table 179-1. A characteristic of many but not all of these infections is the development of an eschar (also called a tache noire) at the site of tick or mite bite in many patients, either immediately prior to or coincident with the onset of constitutional symptoms.[100,109,115,123,129,131,133,142,143] Depending on ectoparasite abundance, their likelihood for biting humans, and the prevalence of each rickettsial agent in its host arthropods, different rickettsioses can be associated with either single or multiple eschars; multiple eschars are common in African tick bite fever and *R. parkeri* rickettsiosis. Illness typically occurs one week following a tick bite, and is characterized by the abrupt onset of fever, headache, lymphadenopathy, and malaise. For *R. conorii* and *R. australis*, a maculopapular rash usually first appears between days 3 and 5, and typically affects the extremities first before spreading to include the trunk. *R. africae* infections may be less likely to cause a rash;

this infection also is characterized by a delayed antibody response compared with Mediterranean spotted fever and is the most common travel-associated rickettsiosis.[117,119,120] Other symptoms include hepatomegaly, splenomegaly, conjunctivitis, and gastrointestinal tract manifestations. These agents cause mild to moderate disease, with occasional severe complications reported including neuropathy and skin necrosis. Case fatalities up to 2.5% have been reported for *R. conorii* subsp. *conorii*, with similar case fatalities for *R. australis*, *R. japonica*, and *R. honeii* subsp. *marmionii*. Tickborne lymphadenopathy (TIBOLA) also is called *Dermacentor*-borne necrosis and lymphadenopathy in Spain (DEBONEL).[135,136] It is caused by *R. slovaca* and *R. raoultii* and often is diagnosed in children and women. Patients have a large eschar on the scalp and enlargement of the cervical lymph nodes, but only one third of patients develop mild fever. Peak incidence is March through May and September through November, when *Dermacentor* ticks are most active. Patients infected with *R. helvetica* develop acute illness with rash, meningitis, or persistent myasthenia.[137,138] Most cases of scrub typhus have a heralding eschar. Scrub typhus can cause multiorgan involvement, pulmonary complications, meningoencephalitis, renal failure, jaundice, hepatitis, gastrointestinal tract dysfunction, and sepsis complicated by secondary bacterial, viral, fungal, or parasitic infections.[142,144–146]

Diagnosis

Serologic diagnosis of these rickettsioses is most commonly made retrospectively by IFA.[117] Because specific tests are available only in specialty laboratories in the U.S., assays employing *R. rickettsii* are used as a surrogate cross-reactive antigen. Antigen-specific serologic tests for most of the SFG rickettsioses and scrub typhus are available upon request from the Centers for Disease Control and Prevention. Confirmed infections exhibit a 4-fold change in antibody titer between acute and convalescent serum specimens. A single high titer with a clinically compatible illness may be considered as a probable case. Acute-phase samples, particularly whole blood and skin biopsy samples collected prior to antibiotic treatment, can be used for the direct identification of rickettsial DNA by PCR amplicon sequencing. Rickettsial etiology also can be confirmed by immunohistochemistry tests performed on formalin-fixed paraffin-embedded tissues or direct cell culture isolation of rickettsiae from appropriately collected specimens and identification of the specific agent by subsequent molecular methods.

Treatment

Therapy is given empirically using drugs and dosage as for other rickettsioses. Doxycycline is the drug of choice for children and adults. For patients in whom life-threatening reactions to doxycycline have been documented, intravenous chloramphenicol is an alternate antibiotic. Rifampin should be excluded as an antibiotic of choice if infection with *R. massiliae* and *R. aeschlimannii* is suspected since these rickettsiae are resistant to this drug.[147] Cases of scrub typhus from northern Thailand which responded poorly to doxycycline and chloramphenicol have been described but 900 mg of daily rifampicin was effective.[148] Azithromycin can be used for treatment of scrub typhus in patients for whom tetracyclines and chloramphenicol are not recommended. One clinical trial indicated that a single 500 mg dose of azithromycin was as effective as a 1-week course of daily 200 mg doses of doxycycline

for treatment of mild scrub typhus in Korea.[149] Effectiveness of the azithromycin course in a 19-week pregnant woman (1.0 g on the first day followed by 500 mg on the second and third days) and a 26-week pregnant woman (500 mg on the first day followed by 250 mg for the next 4 days) has been demonstrated.[150,151] In both cases defervescence occurred 24 to 36 hours following drug administration with no recurrence of symptoms after the treatment was completed. Azithromycin in a single dose of 1000 mg (14-year-old) or 250 mg for 3 days (9-year-old) was used to treat cases of scrub typhus that developed after visiting Papua New Guinea.[152] However, response to treatment with azithromycin should be followed closely and therapy extended if necessary due to the risk of relapse or therapeutic failure.[143]

Prevention

Vaccines are not available for any rickettsial agent. Prevention depends upon avoiding arthropod bites and rodent- and ectoparasite-infested habitats. When traveling in these environments, people should wear long sleeves and pants, with the ends tucked into socks or sealed with tape. Use of permethrin-treated clothing may help repel ticks and mites. Repellents containing DEET can be applied to the skin, but should be used with caution on children due to the risk of adverse reactions. Adults should perform a body check on themselves and children daily following exposure to wild habitats and carefully and immediately remove any ticks and mites that are found in order to reduce the likelihood of transmission of rickettsiae.

Acknowledgments

The findings and conclusions in this report are those of the authors and do not necessarily represent the views of the Centers for Disease Control and Prevention or the Department of Health and Human Services of the United States.

180 *Streptobacillus moniliformis* (Rat-Bite Fever)

Lorry G. Rubin

Streptobacillus moniliformis is the only species in the genus *Streptobacillus*. The organism is a fastidious, nonmotile, gram-negative, pleomorphic and often filamentous, beaded, facultative anaerobic bacillus. The organism can exist in two phases, the bacillary phase and the cell wall-deficient L-phase.[1,2] In addition to being the main etiologic agent of a systemic illness called rat-bite fever, *S. moniliformis* causes two other syndromes, Haverhill fever and an arthritis known as erythema arthriticum epidemicum. Sodoku (spirillary rat-bite fever), an extremely rare disease in the United States, is the name given to rat-bite fever caused by *Spirillum minus*, which manifests 1 to 4 weeks after a bite with relapsing fever and ulceration at the site of the bite with associated regional lymphadenopathy. *S. minus* is a spiral gram-negative coiled bacillus with two or more helical turns and is motile. *S. minus* has not been isolated on solid media and diagnosis relies on visualization by darkfield microscopic examination of an ulcer or blood smear or using a Giemsa- or Wright-stained smear. This infection responds rapidly to therapy with penicillin.[2]

EPIDEMIOLOGY

The natural habitat of *S. moniliformis* is the upper respiratory tract of rodents where carriage is common and causes no symptoms.

The organism can be excreted in rat urine. Humans are infected by the bite of a rat (or mouse, squirrel, cat, or weasel) or, less commonly, from a scratch by a rat, from rat contact with a break in the skin, from handling a dead animal, or from contact with rat-eating carnivores such as a dog.[1,2] In some cases a pet rat had died recently of an unknown illness.[3] In some persons with no history of rodent contact, infection may have been acquired through ingestion of milk or water contaminated with rat excreta, as occurred in epidemic form in 1916 in Haverhill, Massachusetts, and in the 1980s in England.[4] Approximately 50% of cases of rat-bite fever are reported in children.

CLINICAL FINDINGS

Two to 10 days (or up to 3 weeks) after a rat bite, there is an abrupt onset of fever accompanied by chills, headache, vomiting, myalgia, and a rash that is maculopapular in appearance and frequently includes petechiae and at times pustules.[3] The rash is most prominent on the extremities and frequently involves the palms and soles. The bite wound usually has healed and exhibits no or minimal inflammation. Generalized or regional lymphadenopathy occurs commonly. Fifty percent of patients experience a migratory polyarthritis or polyarthralgia (erythema arthriticum epidemicum) typically involving the knees and ankles. Young children may have diarrhea and weight loss. Clinical features can be similar to Rocky Mountain spotted fever, rheumatoid arthritis, or septicemia due to *Neisseria meningitidis* or another bacterial species.

Untreated, *S. moniliformis* infection usually follows a relapsing course for a mean of 3 weeks, but a mortality rate of up to 10%,[5] or arthritis persisting for several months can occur.[2] Cases of a disseminated, rapidly fatal infection have been reported in adults and in infants.[1,6] Other reported manifestations are fever without a focus, bacterial endocarditis, myocarditis, meningitis, focal abscesses including brain and skin,[7] pyogenic arthritis typically with polyarticular involvement but without rash, fever, or bacteremia,[8] pneumonia, hepatitis, nephritis, and amnionitis.[2,6]

When the infection is acquired through ingestion of the organism from water, milk, or food contaminated with rat excrements, it is known as Haverhill fever. Fever, chills, headache, pharyngitis, and vomiting are prominent and are often followed by rash and polyarthralgia/polyarthritis.

DIAGNOSIS

The diagnosis is established by recovery of the organism from cultures of blood, joint fluid, or abscess specimens in broth or on solid media. Media enriched with horse serum, sheep or rabbit blood, or ascites fluid and yeast extract and incubation in a 5% to 10% CO_2 atmosphere are required to recover *S. moniliformis*.[2,9] On solid media, small round grey colonies are noted within 3 days; in addition, mycoplasma-like colonies with a fried-egg appearance can develop. Isolation of the more fastidious L-phase variants requires an enrichment medium such as heart infusion supplemented with horse serum and yeast extract. Sodium polyanethol sulfonate (SPS) can inhibit *S. moniliformis*.[9,10] Although Bactec blood culture medium contains SPS, *S. moniliformis* has been recovered using Bactec Peds-Plus and Bactec Plus media,[7] perhaps

because they contain resin. Growth in broth appears as "puffball" colonies at the bottom of the vial after 2 to 6 days. Occasionally, gram-negative pleomorphic bacilli are visualized in a smear of a clinical specimen such as a skin lesion or bacilli are visualized on a blood smear.[6]

Diagnosis can be established by polymerase chain reaction amplification of a segment of the 16S rRNA gene using broad-range primers followed by sequencing from a clinical specimen or incubated blood culture media.[9,11] At least 25% of patients infected with *S. moniliformis* have a false-positive reaction to the Venereal Disease Research Laboratories (VDRL) test for syphilis.[2]

TREATMENT

Penicillin is the drug of choice for treatment of persons with rat-bite fever, although penicillin-resistant strains have been reported rarely.[2] Strains are resistant to trimethoprim-sulfamethoxazole, nalidixic acid, and colistin.[9] Sulfonamides are ineffective.[2] Organisms are susceptible in vitro to penicillin, ampicillin, cefuroxime, cefotaxime, clindamycin, tetracycline (doxycycline), streptomycin, and vancomycin.[2] Doxycycline is an acceptable alternative agent to penicillin.[12] Failure of erythromycin treatment and successful treatment with clarithromycin have been described.[7,13] The L-phase of *S. moniliformis* is resistant to penicillin but responds to tetracycline.[1] For therapy of endocarditis caused by *S. moniliformis*, the addition of streptomycin to high dosages of penicillin should be considered.[2]

PREVENTION

Avoiding contact with rodents and their excreta is the best means of prevention. The rate of rat-bite fever after a rat bite is approximately 10%. Individuals who sustain rat-bite wounds should be observed closely; penicillin prophylaxis seems reasonable.

---

181 Other Gram-Negative Coccobacilli

Lorry G. Rubin

A large number of gram-negative coccobacilli have been reported to cause infections in humans. This chapter describes four coccobacilli not discussed in other chapters. These organisms are important in specific epidemiologic and clinical situations and present special problems of diagnosis and therapy.

AGGREGATIBACTER SPECIES

Aggregatibacter (formerly *Actinobacillus*) *actinomycetemcomitans*,[1] a small, fastidious gram-negative coccobacillus, is a cause of endocarditis, of periodontal infection, and, in conjunction with *Actinomyces israelii*, of pneumonia and soft-tissue abscesses (see Chapter 187, Anaerobic Bacteria: Classification, Normal Flora, and Clinical Concepts; Chapter 195, Anaerobic Gram-Positive Nonsporulating Bacilli (Including Actinomycosis)). The other species of this newly formed genus are *Aggregatibacter* (formerly *Haemophilus*) *aphrophilus* and *Aggregatibacter* (formerly *Haemophilus*) *segnis*. The other *Actinobacillus* species – *A. equuli* subspecies *equuli*, *A. equuli* subspecies *haemolyticus*, *A. lignieresii*, *A. ureae*, and *A. hominis* – occasionally are associated with human disease; the first three primarily infect animals.

A. actinomycetemcomitans commonly is part of the normal flora of the mouth of humans, especially the gingival and supragingival

crevices, and also can be found in various animal species.[2] The incidence of carriage is markedly higher in individuals with refractory periodontitis and in people with juvenile periodontal disease.[2] The organism may be transmitted among household members.[2]

A. actinomycetemcomitans contributes to the AACEK (formerly HACEK) acronym for a group of fastidious gram-negative coccobacilli that also include *Aggregatibacter* (formerly *Haemophilus*) *aphrophilus*, *Cardiobacterium hominis*, *Eikenella corrodens*, and *Kingella kingae* that cause endocarditis. Poor dentition or recent dental manipulation is a risk factor for *A. actinomycetemcomitans* endocarditis and most patients are adults with underlying valvular heart disease. Infection manifests subacutely with a mean interval from onset of symptoms to diagnosis of 3 months. Symptoms include fever, chills, malaise, anorexia, and weight loss.[3] Hepatosplenomegaly and peripheral stigmata, including petechiae, are common clinical findings. The incidence of embolic phenomena is similar to that in persons with endocarditis from other causes. Anemia and an elevated erythrocyte sedimentation rate are common laboratory findings.

The most common illness associated with *A. actinomycetemcomitans* is juvenile periodontal disease. *A. actinomycetemcomitans* also causes soft-tissue abscesses, particularly of the chest wall or mandibular area, often as a coinfection with *A. israelii*. Chest wall lesions often are associated with pulmonary or pleural lesions and lesions of the mandibular area typically are associated with dental caries or periodontal disease. Cases of pneumonia, empyema, osteomyelitis, septic arthritis, brain abscess, cervical lymphadenitis, intra-abdominal abscess, and urinary tract infection have been reported with *A. actinomycetemcomitans* as a sole pathogen or copathogen.

Isolation of the organism is hampered by slow and fastidious growth; a carbon dioxide-enriched environment improves growth. Growth in nutrient broth, such as trypticase soy or Schaedler, can occur without turbidity in blood culture bottles including radiometric blood culture bottles or can appear as tiny puffballs growing in the blood cell layer or as granules that adhere to the sides or bottom of the bottle. *A. actinomycetemcomitans* grows on blood or chocolate agar forming small colonies after up to 7 days of incubation but grows poorly on MacConkey agar.[4]

Although penicillin or ampicillin has been used commonly to treat infections caused by *A. actinomycetemcomitans*, resistance can occur and response to ampicillin may be unsatisfactory. Strains are uniformly susceptible to the third-generation cephalosporin antibiotics cefotaxime and ceftriaxone and either of these agents can be considered the drug of choice. Isolates usually are susceptible to aminoglycosides, rifampin, tetracycline, trimethoprim-sulfamethoxazole, fluoroquinolones, azithromycin, imipenem, and chloramphenicol and generally are resistant to antistaphylococcal penicillins, clindamycin, vancomycin, and erythromycin.[2,3,5]

Clinical experience suggests that treatment of endocarditis with penicillin and gentamicin usually is successful. Cefotaxime or ceftriaxone with or without an aminoglycoside or rifampin may be optimal therapy for endocarditis.[3] Oral ciprofloxacin also has been used successfully. Severe periodontal disease usually is treated with mechanical debridement in combination with oral tetracycline or the combination of metronidazole and amoxicillin.[6]

BARTONELLA SPECIES

Bartonella bacilliformis is a member of the family Bartonellaceae and the genus *Bartonella*.[7] In addition to *B. bacilliformis*, human pathogens and their main clinical syndromes in this genus include: *B. clarridgeiae* (cat-scratch disease), *B. elizabethae* (neurologic, bacteremia, neuroretinitis, endocarditis), *B. henselae* (cat-scratch disease, bacillary angiomatosis, endocarditis), *B. koehlerae* (endocarditis), *B. quintana* (trench fever, bacillary angiomatosis, endocarditis), and *B. vinsonii* subsp. *berkhoffi* and subsp. *arupensis* (endocarditis).[7] *B. bacilliformis* is the etiologic agent of bartonellosis or Carrión disease. The organism is motile by means of flagella and is transmitted to humans through the bite of the nocturnal sandfly (*Lutzomyia verrucarum*), which is endemic solely in the Andes regions of Peru, Ecuador, and Colombia at elevations between 2000 and 8000 feet (600 and 2400 meters). The incubation period is approximately 2 to 3 weeks and one-half of cases occur in children and adolescents.[8–10] The organism adheres to and invades erythrocytes and endothelial cells.

Carrión disease manifests in two distinct stages.[9,11,12] Bacteremic illness (Oroya fever) is the first stage of infection, in which erythrocytes are parasitized, generally resulting in an acute onset of illness associated with severe hemolytic anemia. The most common findings are sustained fever, pallor, malaise, hepatomegaly, and lymphadenopathy.[10] There also is transient immune suppression that can result in disseminated opportunistic infections such as septicemia due to *Salmonella* or other gram-negative bacteria or reactivation and dissemination of latent toxoplasmosis, tuberculosis, or histoplasmosis.[9] Without antibiotic therapy, this stage of infection is fatal in up to 40% of cases, with death due to complications of profound anemia or opportunistic coinfection during the immune deficiency state or both. Some infected individuals experience fever, headache, and musculoskeletal pain but do not have anemia. Subclinical infection, documented by asymptomatic bacteremia or seroconversion, occurs commonly.[13]

There is a 1- to 2-month or longer interval before the onset of the secondary or eruptive stage of infection.[9] Cutaneous lesions occur after bacterial invasion of capillary endothelial cells with stimulation of cellular proliferation; lesions may contain bacteria.[9] In this stage, one of three types of lesions known as verruca peruana are observed: miliary lesions that are the most common and consist of multiple 1 to 4 mm papular, erythematous, round lesions that frequently are on the lower extremities and are pruritic; nodular raised lesions with normal overlying skin; and mular lesions that are >5 mm in diameter, erythematous, and bleed easily.[10] Patients can manifest verruca peruana without a preceding fever.[13]

Diagnosis of Oroya fever can be made through examination of a blood smear, which reveals bacteria adherent to the majority of erythrocytes. The organism can be isolated by inoculation of blood or material from cutaneous lesions onto supplemented brain-heart infusion agar and incubation for 1 to 2 weeks at 25°C to 30°C in 5% carbon dioxide. During an outbreak of acute bartonellosis, detection of the organism on a blood smear had a sensitivity of only 36% compared with bacterial isolation.[14] A serum titer of ≥1:256 on an indirect fluorescence antibody assay has been shown to have a sensitivity of 86% for diagnosis of infection in a highly endemic area.[11] Diagnosis of verruca peruana is confirmed by biopsy of a cutaneous lesion that characteristically demonstrates hyperplasia of endothelial cells with swollen nuclei, abundant mitosis, and proliferation of capillaries.

Chloramphenicol, penicillin, tetracycline, or erythromycin is effective treatment for Oroya fever, although spontaneous resolution of erythrocyte parasitism occurs in milder cases after a few days.[8,9] Verruca peruana lesions can be self-limited[11] or may respond to treatment with rifampin or streptomycin; ciprofloxacin can be used but some isolates exhibit in vitro resistance to fluoroquinolones.[15] Large lesions may require surgical excision.

CARDIOBACTERIUM HOMINIS

Cardiobacterium hominis, a microaerophilic, pleomorphic gram-negative bacillus, is one of the AACEK organisms. *C. hominis* is a component of the normal flora colonizing the nose and throat. The principal clinical disease caused by *C. hominis* is endocarditis,[16] but focal soft-tissue infection and peritoneal dialysis-related infection has occurred.[17] Endocarditis occurs almost exclusively in adults with pre-existing valvular disease; it has an insidious, subacute onset, often occurring after an oral infection, a dental procedure, or upper gastrointestinal endoscopy. Prosthetic valve endocarditis has been reported.[18] Common signs and laboratory findings are moderate fever, splenomegaly, cutaneous signs such as petechiae, an elevated erythrocyte sedimentation rate, and mild anemia. Large vegetations and large vessel emboli are characteristic. At least 6 cases of aortic valve endocarditis in adults have been reported due to the recently described *Cardiobacterium valvarum*, a *Cardiobacterium* species also found in the oral cavity.[19,20]

Diagnosis is made through recovery of *C. hominis* in blood culture, which takes an average of 5 days of incubation. In broth culture, growth can occur adjacent to the red cell layer in the absence of turbidity and can remain undetected if blind subculture is not performed. The organism grows on sheep blood, chocolate, Mueller–Hinton, and trypticase soy agars, provided that incubation conditions include high humidity and ≥3% CO_2 concentration. In cases of culture-negative endocarditis, the diagnosis has been made using broad-range PCR assay performed on heart valve tissue.[20,21]

Isolates generally are susceptible to penicillin, ampicillin, cephalosporins, fluoroquinolones (including ciprofloxacin and levofloxacin), chloramphenicol, and tetracycline.[5] However, penicillin-resistant, β-lactamase-producing strains have been described rarely.[22] Susceptibility to vancomycin, aminoglycosides, erythromycin, and clindamycin is variable. Penicillin with or without an aminoglycoside is the therapy of choice for susceptible isolates and achieves a high cure rate; a third-generation cephalosporin with an aminoglycoside is recommended until the results of antibiotic susceptibility testing are available.

PSYCHROBACTER IMMOBILIS

Psychrobacter immobilis is a psychrotropic (cold-loving), gram-negative coccobacillus and a member of the family Neisseriaceae that grows best at 20°C. Previously called *Moraxella*-like, *P. immobilis* is related to *Moraxella* and *Acinetobacter*. *P. immobilis* is associated with fish, processed meat, and poultry and has been isolated from various clinical sites.[23] Clinically significant isolates have been recovered from the blood of a hospitalized adult with AIDS,[24] cerebrospinal fluid of a 2-day-old infant in Micronesia with low-grade meningitis, and a conjunctival swab of a 12-day-old infant in Guatemala who experienced bilateral purulent conjunctivitis while receiving penicillin.[25,26] The isolate recovered from the 2-day-old infant was initially thought to be *Neisseria gonorrhoeae*. The isolates were recovered on sheep blood agar incubated at 35°C, although growth is best at 20°C. Isolates were resistant to penicillin and/or ampicillin, 2 of 3 were susceptible to gentamicin, and the isolate causing septicemia in the man with AIDS was susceptible to cefotaxime, ceftazidime, piperacillin, amikacin, and ciprofloxacin.

182 *Treponema pallidum* (Syphilis)

Sarah A. Rawstron and Sarah J. Hawkes

Four diseases are associated with pathogenic treponemes: (1) venereal syphilis, caused by *Treponema pallidum* subsp. *pallidum*; (2) yaws, caused by *T. pallidum* subsp. *pertenue*; (3) endemic syphilis, or bejel, caused by *T. pallidum* subsp. *endemicum*; and (4) pinta, caused by *Treponema carateum*. These diseases are thought to have diverged from a single disease 10,000 to 100,000 years ago under the influence of population migration and environmental factors.[1] The pathogenic treponemes cannot be distinguished serologically or morphologically,[2] but new molecular techniques can distinguish *T. pallidum* from the other treponemes.[3] Serologic tests (nontreponemal and treponemal) are reactive in any treponemal infection and cannot be used to distinguish between them. Treponemal diseases share other similarities. They evolve over many years in three symptomatic stages: a primary stage, marked by a single highly contagious cutaneous or mucous membrane lesion; a secondary stage, the consequence of disseminated organisms, which results in highly infectious cutaneous and mucous membrane lesions, with other organs also affected; an asymptomatic latent stage; and a tertiary symptomatic stage, marked by destructive lesions. These diseases also share an early immune response that modifies the course but does not prevent the disease from progressing. In all cases, a cure is achievable by relatively small doses of penicillin, and humans are the only host.

Treponemal diseases can be differentiated by epidemiology and mode of transmission (sexual contact and congenital infection for syphilis, skin contact for yaws and pinta, and oral mucosa for bejel). Syphilis occurs globally; yaws in tropical South and Central America and Africa; bejel in North Africa, the Middle East, and southwest Asia; and pinta in South and Central America. *T. pallidum* subsp. *pallidum* is the subject of this chapter.

MICROBIOLOGY AND PATHOGENESIS

Between 1905 and 1910, Schaudinn and Hoffman identified *T. pallidum* as the cause of syphilis, Wasserman described a diagnostic serologic test, and Ehrlich discovered that salvarsan (an arsenic-based compound) could be used for treatment. The inability to sustain the growth of treponemes in vitro has hampered research, but application of modern molecular techniques is providing an increased understanding of the interaction between treponemes and the host.[4-6] *T. pallidum* cultivation in the laboratory still requires propagation in rabbit testes.[7] The *T. pallidum* Nichols strain DNA sequence was published in 1998[8] and this has led to other advances in understanding the structure and function of the organism.[9-11] Molecular techniques have been described to subtype *T. pallidum*[12] and this technique has been used to investigate the epidemiology and spread of syphilis in local areas,[13-15] with newer modifications creating a more discriminating typing system.[16]

Treponemes are tapered, thin spiral bacilli (5 to 15 μm in length, 0.15 μm in width) that exhibit corkscrew locomotion. Infection starts with penetration through minor abrasions in the skin or intact mucous membrane. Only spirochetes that adhere to cells replicate, and cell division occurs every 30 to 33 hours. At least 50 *T. pallidum* organisms are necessary to initiate infection; larger inocula decrease the incubation period. *T. pallidum* structure consists of outer and cytoplasmic membranes, a thin peptidoglycan layer, and three endoflagella that lie in the periplasmic space at each end and are responsible for motility.[17] The outer membrane contains a small number of poorly immunogenic transmembrane proteins (*T. pallidum* rare outer membrane proteins, or TROMP), but does not contain lipopolysaccharide.[18] Highly antigenic lipoproteins (47, 34, 17, and 15 kd) are localized to the subsurface cytoplasmic membrane and are not exposed on the cell surface.[18,19] Host reaction to infection includes cellular and humoral immune responses with more than 60 specific antibodies identified by SDS–polyacrylamide gel electrophoresis. Antibodies directed to the prominent 47 kd treponemal antigen are the earliest detected by Western blot. Macrophages activated in the presence of specific antibody ingest and destroy large numbers of organisms.[20] However, it is unclear why this and other immune reactivity hasten healing of the primary lesion but do not halt infection. Various hypotheses suggest that: (1) a lack of antigenic reactivity in the outer membrane acts as an immunologic barrier; (2) a change in membrane-bound immunoproteins after dissemination allows organisms to evade antibody-mediated immunity; or (3) treponemes surround themselves with host material, thus delaying host cell response.

Spirochetes preferentially adhere to endothelial cells. Vasculitis with a predominance of mononuclear and plasma cells surrounding the involved vessels is typical of syphilitic lesions. In primary and secondary disease, infectious treponemes are demonstrated easily in lesions. These lesions heal completely, whereas tertiary lesions result in irreversible tissue destruction and fibrosis. Tertiary lesions consist of gummas and cardiovascular and central nervous system disease. Gummas are large granulatomous lesions with a central necrotic mass surrounded by plasma cells, lymphocytes, and monocytes; multinucleated giant cells are not present. Organisms usually are not found in these lesions, which are thought to represent a hypersensitivity phenomenon. Gummas occur in both acquired and congenital disease. Cardiovascular syphilis, another tertiary manifestation, is associated with pathologic changes in the proximal aorta, consisting of inflammation-induced obliterative endarteritis of the vasa vasorum, leading to medial necrosis. Although inflammatory changes begin in the early stages of infection, clinical manifestations appear 10 to 40 years later. Tertiary neurosyphilis is the result of chronic meningeal inflammation, which affects primarily the meninges but also can include the brain and spinal cord.[21] Meningeal, meningovascular, parenchymatous, and gummatous neurosyphilis also occur after untreated congenital infection.

EPIDEMIOLOGY

Syphilis is acquired by sexual contact (including oral sex)[22] and, extremely rarely, by other forms of close contact. Congenital syphilis is a consequence of undiagnosed, untreated, or inadequately treated maternal syphilis. Syphilis occurs worldwide, with the highest incidence in young people. An understanding of transmission, the development of serologic tests to detect asymptomatic infections, and an effective treatment (penicillin) led to a steady decline in the number of cases in western Europe and the United States after a peak during World War II. Reported cases of syphilis in the U.S. remained at low levels until 1986, when the number of cases increased sharply, with the epidemic peaking in 1990.[23] This epidemic started in large cities but spread nationwide to smaller cities and rural areas. The epidemic was associated mostly with heterosexual transmission, poverty, use of crack cocaine, human immunodeficiency virus (HIV) infection, and minority (predominantly black) ethnic background. Primary and secondary syphilis rates declined from 1990 to 2000, but have risen again.[24] Much of the recent increase is in men who have sex with men (MSM). However, recent outbreaks in Alabama[25] and Arizona[26] have been predominantly through heterosexual contact. The highest incidence in the U.S. currently is in urban areas in the southeast (largely heterosexual transmission), with rising rates among MSM in large cities.[27] Rates of primary, secondary, and congenital syphilis continue to be higher among black than white populations in the U.S. – in 2005, the rate of congenital syphilis was almost 20 times higher among African Americans than whites.[28]

The prevalence of seroreactivity in pregnant women in some areas of the world approaches 5% or higher; in the U.S., it is below 1%, although rates between 2% and 3% have been recorded in high-risk locales.[29] The syphilis epidemic of the early 1990s was associated with an increase in congenital syphilis in the U.S.[30] Although there was an increase in symptomatic congenital disease, the Centers for Disease Control and Prevention expanded the criteria for case surveillance in 1989 to include asymptomatic infants born to mothers with untreated or inadequately treated infection, and this also contributed to the increase in reported cases.[31] The number of cases of congenital syphilis had declined since 1991;[32] however, from 2005 to 2008, a 23% increase in congenital syphilis was noted, primarily in the south.[28] Risk factors associated with vertical transmission of syphilis include (in addition to those described for acquired syphilis) lack of prenatal care, first prenatal visit late in pregnancy, and lack of maternal screening and treatment. Because the most important risk is birth to a mother who received no prenatal care, tests for syphilis always should be performed when pregnant women at risk seek healthcare, even if care is sought for matters unrelated to pregnancy.[33]

CLINICAL MANIFESTATIONS

Acquired Syphilis

Primary Syphilis

Untreated syphilis becomes a chronic disease evolving in three symptomatic stages. Primary syphilis occurs in about 30% of sexual exposures. The incubation period of 1 to 4 weeks is influenced by the number of organisms in the original inoculum. The typical primary chancre is a single painless papule that erodes to form an ulcer with a reddened base and rolled edges. A small inoculum may produce only a papule. Primary lesions can occur in both the genital and oral areas.[22] Women may not notice primary disease because a chancre in the vagina or on the cervix is not visible. Both men and women may ignore a visible lesion, because it is painless (unless it becomes secondarily infected) and

heals completely in 3 to 6 weeks. Painless nonsuppurative enlargement of local lymph nodes accompanies the chancre and can persist for months. Primary lesions contain infectious treponemes, and hematogenous dissemination of treponemes begins within hours after superficial organism invasion and continues throughout primary and secondary disease.

Secondary and Latent Syphilis

Secondary syphilis is a systemic, multiorgan disease that begins 6 to 12 weeks after infection. In 15% of patients, the primary chancre is still present when symptoms of secondary disease begin. Mucocutaneous lesions are common, usually beginning on the trunk and eventually involving most of the body, including palms and soles. Salmon-pink macules, 5 to 10 mm in size, evolve to copper-colored papules that occasionally develop a follicular or pustular appearance. In untreated patients, regressing skin lesions often appear as hypopigmented or hyperpigmented papules that persist for months. Painless generalized lymphadenopathy is found in 85% of patients. In 10% of patients, raised, enlarged, broad, flat papules (condyloma lata) develop in warm moist areas (vulva, anus, scrotum, and axilla). White-to-grey patches on mucous membranes also are detected in 10% of patients. Fewer than 10% of patients develop transient patchy alopecia and loss of other body hair, including eyebrows and beard, due to spirochetal invasion of hair follicles. Arthritis, osteitis, gastritis, hepatitis, splenomegaly, and nephrotic syndrome occur in some patients. Central nervous system involvement is common in secondary syphilis and, although usually asymptomatic, 1% to 2% of patients have acute meningitis. Lukehart, using the rabbit infectivity test, demonstrated that 40% of patients with early syphilis had either treponemes in the cerebrospinal fluid (CSF) or a reactive CSF Venereal Disease Research Laboratory (VDRL) test result.[34] The most common constitutional symptoms, fever, malaise, aches, pains, and sore throat, are nonspecific; if there is no history of exposure or characteristic lesion, the diagnosis may not be suspected.

Even without treatment, complete resolution of secondary syphilis occurs after 3 to 12 weeks, and the disease enters the latent phase. Early latent syphilis is defined as the first year after infection and late latent syphilis as more than a year after infection. Relapses of secondary syphilis occur in about 25% of untreated patients during early latent syphilis, but late latent syphilis is asymptomatic. Although patients in the latent stage of syphilis are asymptomatic, CSF examination is included in their evaluation because CSF abnormalities have been correlated with subsequent symptomatic tertiary neurosyphilis.[35] A history of previous syphilitic lesions or reactive serology is necessary for categorizing these asymptomatic patients. A study evaluating CSF findings in adults with syphilis (the majority who had late latent syphilis and also were infected with HIV) showed that a serum RPR titer ≥1:32 was predictive of neurosyphilis in all individuals, and a CD4+ T-lymphocyte count of ≤350 cells/mm³ was a second risk factor in adults with HIV.[36] Patients' immunity during late latency seems to protect against relapse, but it does not prevent progression to the tertiary stage.

Tertiary Syphilis

Tertiary disease occurs in about 30% of untreated patients; manifestations are divided into three main subgroups: neurosyphilis, cardiovascular syphilis, and late benign syphilis (gummas).

Tertiary neurosyphilis includes several clinical syndromes: meningeal, meningovascular, and parenchymatous syphilis (including general paresis and tabes dorsalis). Manifestations appear within a few months of primary infection (meningeal syphilis) or 20 to 30 years later. Meningeal syphilis manifests as cranial nerve palsies, sensorineural deafness, and hydrocephalus. Meningovascular syphilis causes a stroke syndrome caused by infarction secondary to syphilitic endarteritis, with the middle cerebral artery the most common site. The findings of general paresis can be summarized by the mnemonic PARESIS: Personality, Affect,

Reflexes (hyperactive), Eye (Argyll Robertson pupils, which react to accommodation but not to light), and abnormalities of Sensorium (illusions, delusions, hallucinations), Intellect (decreased recent memory, orientation, judgment, insight), and Speech.[37] Tabes dorsalis describes the symptoms and signs of demyelination of the posterior column and roots of the spinal cord. Patients can have more than one form of neurologic disease. Treatment can arrest the disease; however, the extent of underlying pathology determines whether signs and symptoms resolve.

Cardiovascular syphilis, which occurs from 10 to 40 years after infection, is seen in 10% of patients with tertiary disease. An aneurysm in the ascending portion of the aorta, aortic insufficiency due to aortic root dilation, and coronary artery disease are commonly recognized signs.

The "benign tertiary" form of disease refers to gummatous lesions found in skin, bones, and, rarely, in other organs. The lesions vary in size from microscopic to clearly visible. Gummas are considered benign because they rarely involve vital body structures, but gummas can be destructive. Cutaneous gummas can ulcerate, and bone lesions are painful. Failure to treat or delay in treatment is associated with disfiguring scars.

Syphilis Associated with HIV Infection

Syphilis and HIV exhibit "epidemiologic synergy"[38] and coinfection is common.[39-41] The presence of HIV infection is thought to alter the clinical expression of syphilis, response to therapy, and the results of serologic tests.[38] Antibody titers can higher than expected, but occasionally false-negative results or delayed seroreactivity can occur.[41] In addition, people with HIV and early syphilis may be at higher risk for both neurologic complications and treatment failure with currently recommended regimens.[42] Adults with neurosyphilis and HIV are less likely to revert from a reactive CSF VDRL than adults without HIV.[43] Persons with syphilis should be offered testing for HIV infection – and vice versa. Those with coinfection require careful and more frequent follow-up.

Congenital Syphilis

Congenital syphilis has been divided into early disease (detected before the patient is 2 years of age) and late disease (detected after 2 years of age); most with early disease are <3 months of age.

Early-Onset Disease

Early-onset disease is the result of transplacental transmission of spirochetes. Transmission is higher (60% to 90%) in untreated maternal primary or secondary syphilis, decreasing to 40% in early latent syphilis, and to <10% in late latent syphilis; overall it is estimated that approximately 70% of women with untreated syphilis in pregnancy will experience an adverse outcome (stillbirth, neonatal death, low birthweight, infected infant).[44-47] Placental and umbilical cord abnormalities are common; the placenta can appear larger and more pale, and immature villi and focal villitis with endovascular and perivascular proliferation are seen microscopically. Changes are not pathognomonic, although necrotizing funisitis within the matrix of the umbilical cord is considered highly indicative of syphilis. *T. pallidum* usually can be identified by silver or immunofluorescent stains in the tissue specimens. Fetal infection can occur at any time during pregnancy, but the risk of infection increases as pregnancy progresses. Approximately 60% of infants with congenital syphilis are asymptomatic at birth.

Congenital syphilis lacks a primary stage, because it is a consequence of hematogenously disseminated *T. pallidum* and is similar to secondary syphilis. The typical stillborn or highly symptomatic newborn is born prematurely, has an enlarged liver and spleen, skeletal involvement, and often has pneumonia (pneumonia alba) and skin lesions. Less affected infants have a variety of signs. Hepatomegaly is reported in almost 100%, and biochemical evidence of liver dysfunction usually is observed; serum alkaline phosphatase levels are elevated but elevation of hepatic transaminase levels may occur only after treatment is initiated and an

immune response has occurred.[48] Approximately 40% to 60% of infected infants have one or more of the following: hepatosplenomegaly, rash, generalized lymphadenopathy, skeletal abnormality, or nasal discharge. The rash usually is maculopapular, and initially erythematous, changing to a papular desquamating rash of coppery color and often involving the palms and soles. Petechial lesions, secondary to thrombocytopenia, can also be seen. Pemphigus syphiliticus is a rash unique to the infected newborn and consists of vesiculobullous lesions that contain many organisms. These lesions rupture easily, leaving a macerated appearance.

Radiographic abnormalities are common in early syphilis; 95% of symptomatic infants and up to 20% with asymptomatic disease have bony abnormalities.[49] Lesions include metaphysitis, periostitis, and osteitis. Findings are symmetric and involve multiple long bones; the lower extremities are almost always affected. Metaphyseal lesions (osteochondritis) (Figure 181), which vary from punctate lucencies to more destructive changes, are seen earlier than periostitis. Wimberger sign ("cat bite") describes osteitis and destruction of the proximal medial tibial metaphysis (see Figure 182-1B) and, although occasionally seen in other conditions, it is highly suggestive of congenital syphilis. Occasionally, the lesions are painful, resulting in pseudoparalysis of the affected limb (pseudoparalysis of Parrot). Periostitis appears radiographically as multiple layers of periosteal new bone formation.

The CSF is abnormal in 50% of infected infants with symptoms and in up to 10% of those who are asymptomatic. The diagnosis of

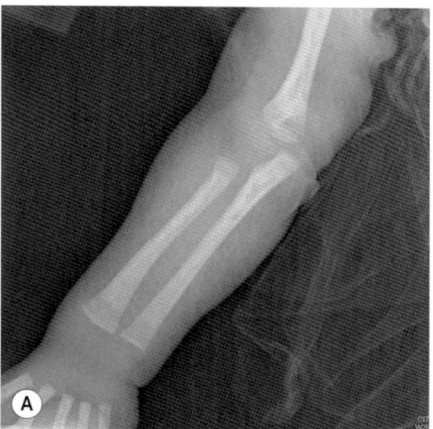
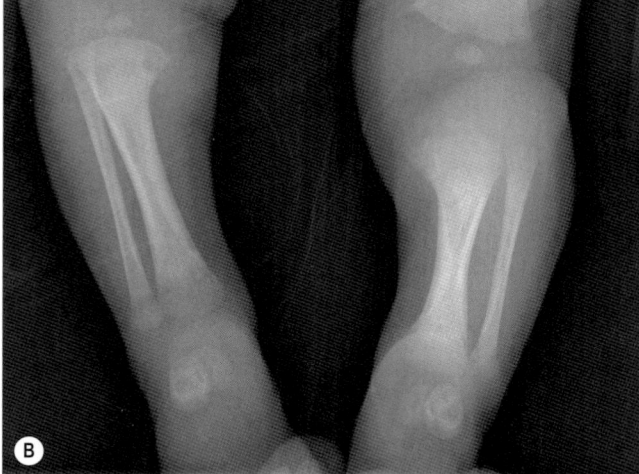

Figure 182-1. Plain radiographs of an infant with congenital syphilis. Note decreased mineralization of the metaphyses of long bones of the upper **(A)** and lower extremities **(B),** as well as bilateral lytic lesions of the talus, calcaneus, and proximal tibia (Wimberger sign) medially **(B).** (Courtesy of J.H. Brien©.)

neurosyphilis is made with a reactive CSF VDRL test, or abnormal elevation of CSF white blood cell (WBC) count or protein levels (although the definition of "abnormal" varies).[38] However, this standard for diagnosing neurosyphilis is insensitive in comparison with rabbit infectivity testing (RIT) in infants with congenital syphilis.[50] Although no single laboratory test identifies all those with neurosyphilis as confirmed by RIT, most infants with neurosyphilis are identified by conventional testing (physical examination, complete blood count, bone radiography, and lumbar puncture), and the addition of IgM immunoblotting and PCR tests identifies almost all others. Even when CSF is abnormal, neurologic symptoms or signs usually are absent. Rhinitis, or "snuffles," occurs rarely now and it consists of a clear nasal discharge (containing many spirochetes) that becomes chronic and turns bloody as a result of mucosal erosion. Nephrotic syndrome, which occurs less commonly than other manifestations, is caused by immune complex disease rather than direct invasion by treponemes.[51] Hematologic disturbances are seen in symptomatic infection; more than 75% of infants have anemia, and 50% of them have an elevated WBC count with a significant monocytosis.

The appearance of symptomatic congenital syphilis after discharge from the nursery most often is caused by a failure to perform maternal serologic testing at delivery or to obtain results of serologic tests before discharge. Infants born to recently infected mothers whose serology is negative at delivery may continue to escape detection until symptomatic. In such cases, onset of symptoms before 3 months of age is expected, with a spectrum of disease similar to that seen in symptomatic newborn infants, except that fever can be a prominent initial complaint.[29]

Late-Onset Disease

Late-onset disease is seen in patients >2 years of age and is not considered contagious. Malformations in bones (frontal bossing, saddle nose (a result of osteochondritis), and saber shins), teeth (Hutchinson peg-shaped, notched central incisors, mulberry multicusped first molars), and skin (rhagades, or linear scars, fanning out from the corner of the mouth) result from growth disturbances in these organs. Other manifestations, such as interstitial keratitis and eighth nerve deafness, result from long-standing chronic inflammation. Symmetric, chronic painless swelling of the knees (Clutton joints) has been described in a few affected patients. Asymptomatic neurosyphilis is more common in these children than is symptomatic disease. Pathologic changes in the nervous system and mental, motor, and sensory deficits are similar to those of acquired tertiary disease. During the 19th century, Hutchinson noted that the triad of defects in the incisors, interstitial keratitis, and eighth nerve deafness was unique to congenital syphilis. A more recent review, encompassing 271 cases of congenital syphilis, reconfirmed the pathognomonic constellation.[52]

Other Adverse Outcomes of Pregnancy

The classic symptoms and signs of an infected infant (as noted above) are estimated to occur in approximately 20% of cases in which the mother is undiagnosed or untreated in pregnancy.[44–46] In addition, historical records and surveys conducted among women who have not received any prenatal care suggest that untreated syphilis in pregnancy can cause late abortion or stillbirth in 25% of women, prematurity or low birthweight in 13%, and neonatal death in 11%.[44–47]

DIAGNOSIS

Antibody Tests

Serology is the most commonly used method to identify asymptomatic infection and confirm clinical diagnosis. Seroreactivity is present in all stages of disease but cannot be used to distinguish among stages. Serologic tests include nontreponemal and treponemal tests.

Nontreponemal Tests

Nontreponemal tests are performed easily and detect IgM and IgG antibodies to cellular lipids and lecithin. The two commonly used nontreponemal tests are the rapid plasma reagin (RPR) test and the VDRL test. Reactive sera produce flocculation of the antigenic material. Nontreponemal antibodies appear from 4 to 8 weeks after infection; seroreactivity is present in 70% of patients within 2 weeks of the eruption of a chancre and in 100% who have secondary and latent disease. No nontreponemal serologic test is reactive in the first weeks of infection. Nontreponemal tests can be quantified by serial serum dilution; a two-tube (fourfold) change or more in reactivity is significant. A fourfold to eightfold decrease in titer 6 to 12 months after successful treatment is expected for all patients with early disease (primary and secondary) with a slower decline in treated later stages.[53] A titer that does not fall or that rises after initial significant decline indicates inadequate therapy or new infection. Seroreversion to negative occurs after treatment in some patients and depends on the original titer and the stage of disease during therapy.[53] For others, titers fall significantly but persist at low levels; such individuals are considered to be serofast. Untreated individuals remain seroreactive for life, although titers fall with time even without treatment. The VDRL is used less frequently for screening but remains the only test approved for testing CSF. A false-positive nontreponemal serum test result usually has a titer ≤1:4 and can occur with connective tissue disorders, viral diseases (such as hepatitis, chickenpox, and infectious mononucleosis) and in about 10% of injecting drug users and, occasionally, from pregnancy. A false-negative reaction can result from excess antibody concentration (the prozone effect) that inhibits formation of the antigen–antibody lattice needed for flocculation; prozone effect is overcome by serial serum dilutions. The prozone effect must be considered when a neonate shows signs of congenital syphilis and the mother is seronegative. Nontreponemal tests are useful for screening and monitoring therapy. Treponemal tests are required for confirmation that the nontreponemal reactivity is caused by syphilis or another treponemal infection.

Treponemal Tests

Treponemal tests include the fluorescent treponemal antibody-absorbed test (FTA-ABS), microhemagglutination test for *T. pallidum* (MHA-TP), and the *T. pallidum* particle agglutination test (TP-PA). Characteristics of treponemal tests are: positivity slightly earlier than nontreponemal tests, positivity for life. They are more expensive and more difficult to perform, and do not reflect activity of infection. Treponemal tests are not recommended for screening in the U.S. False-positive treponemal tests can be seen in various conditions, especially spirochetal infections, including Lyme disease (in which the nontreponemal test shows negative results).[54] New treponemal assays, including enzyme immunoassays (EIAs),[55,56] chemiluminescence immunoassays (CIAs), and recombinant *T. pallidum* antigen tests,[57] are automated and easily adapted for population level screening. These tests have been used for initial screening in Europe and in some states in the U.S., with additional confirmation testing in reactive specimens using a second different treponemal test and a quantitative RPR or VDRL.[58,59] This practice, called reverse sequence testing (*Treponema* EIA/CIA first), is not recommended.[38,60] The U.S. Centers for Disease Control and |Prevention (CDC) analyzed data from five laboratories during 2006 to 2010. Of persons with positive treponemal EIA/CIA, 57% had a nonreactive RPR test; among these, 32% did not have a confirmatory TP-PA test.[60] In many developing countries, a new generation of point-of-care treponemal tests, which use whole blood, have been evaluated and are being promoted as a useful adjunct to existing testing algorithms – for example as initial screening tests.[61,62] The impact of using these point-of-care tests is enhanced when combined with health systems strengthening approaches to improve the overall functioning of the antenatal care system for pregnant women.[62a]

Tests for Organisms

The most sensitive diagnostic method for identifying viable treponemes in CSF and exudate is the RIT,[63] which involves serial passage of infected material in the testes of rabbits. Although not clinically useful, this is the gold standard for measuring infectivity and for determining the sensitivity of other *T. pallidum* detection methods, including those under development, such as PCR.[50] Darkfield microscopy can be used to examine exudates; motile organisms too thin to be seen by light microscopy can be visible. Drawbacks include the need for specialized equipment, personnel skilled in its use, and urgency of examination before drying immobilizes treponemes.

The direct fluorescent antibody-*T. pallidum* test (DFA-TP), uses a fluorescein-labeled rabbit or monoclonal *T. pallidum* antibody for identifying organisms in body fluids and exudate. The DFA-TP test also has been modified for use on biopsy and autopsy material.[64] A negative test does not exclude the diagnosis because the number of organisms present in the sample affects sensitivity. Treponemes in tissue specimens can be visualized with silver stain, but this is less specific than the fluorescent antibody technique.

LABORATORY EVALUATION AND DIAGNOSIS OF CONGENITAL SYPHILIS

A screening test for syphilis should be performed at the first antenatal visit and repeated at delivery. In high-risk individuals, an additional serologic test at the beginning of the third trimester also is suggested.[65] In one report, 13% of women found to be seroreactive at delivery were seronegative earlier in the pregnancy.[29] When syphilis treatment is offered to a pregnant woman, treatment also should be offered to her sexual partner(s).

A number of problems confound diagnosis of congenital syphilis, particularly in an asymptomatic infant. Any nontreponemal or treponemal test performed on the infant may reflect maternal antibody titers and does not prove congenital infection.[66,67] Passively acquired nontreponemal antibody usually reverts to negative by 6 months, whereas treponemal antibody can persist for 1 year or longer. An infant treated for congenital syphilis could have similar test results. Children who retain reactive nontreponemal and treponemal antibody at 18 months of age or older should be re-evaluated (see Acquired Syphilis section).[68] Treponemal IgM tests can be useful to identify infants who are producing their own treponemal antibodies (i.e., congenital infection) because IgM antibodies do not cross the placenta. However, not every infant with congenital syphilis produces IgM antibodies.[69] Identification of treponemes in lesions, or in the placenta or umbilical cord, can identify infected infants but are not seen in every infected infant, and the tests are not available readily. Additional tests, such as CSF VDRL and skeletal radiographs, can identify infected asymptomatic babies, but the sensitivity of these tests is not known.

To optimize testing and to maximize treatment of potentially infected infants, the CDC has developed a broad definition of congenital syphilis. A *confirmed* case is one in which spirochetes are demonstrated by darkfield microscopy, fluorescent antibody, or other specific stains, or the neonate's nontreponemal serologic titer is fourfold greater than that of the mother. A *presumed* case (symptomatic or asymptomatic) is an infant born to a mother with reactive serology (1) whose mother was not treated, was inadequately treated, or was treated less than 1 month before delivery; (2) or an infant who has physical signs, CSF abnormalities, or evidence of congenital disease on skeletal radiographs.[31] The definition of a presumed case of congenital syphilis ensures that all possible cases are treated, although all may not be infected.

Evaluation for Congenital Syphilis

The evaluation of each newborn infant whose mother has a positive serologic test for syphilis requires careful and individualized

attention (Figure 182-2). The CDC recommends that all infants born to seroreactive mothers should have a quantitative nontreponemal serum test performed (because umbilical cord blood can be falsely positive or negative).[38,67] In addition to obtaining the maternal history, all infants born to seroreactive mothers should be examined for physical evidence of congenital syphilis (e.g., hepatosplenomegaly, rash). Examination of the placenta and umbilical cord by a pathologist using DFA is suggested. Additional tests to evaluate congenital syphilis (CSF analysis by VDRL, WBC count, protein level, long bone x-rays, complete blood cell count, and serum hepatic enzyme levels) should be performed if the infant is suspected of having congenital syphilis or has any abnormal physical findings.

Unfortunately, confirming a diagnosis of congenital syphilis has not improved in the U.S. as validated serologic tests for *T. pallidum* IgM antibodies, and tests for treponemal antigens or DNA, have not become available widely. Despite carefully designed screening programs, some neonatal infections are missed because recently acquired maternal infection can be associated with seronegativity at birth in mother and neonate.[29]

Evaluation of Syphilis with Other Adverse Outcomes of Pregnancy

Given the strong association between maternal syphilis infection and adverse outcomes of pregnancy (including late fetal loss, stillbirth and low birthweight), the World Health Organization recommends screening, and treating as appropriate, all women (and their partners) who present with one of these pregnancy outcomes.[70]

Acquired Syphilis in Children

Children can acquire syphilis after the neonatal period, predominantly from sexual abuse, but syphilis is rare in sexually abused children.[71] Adolescents can acquire syphilis through sexual activity, and they should be evaluated and managed as appropriate for the stage of syphilis. In younger children, determining whether syphilis is congenital or acquired can be difficult in the absence of physical findings or a clear history.[72,73] Similarly, children immigrating from areas of the world endemic for other treponematoses who have reactive serologic tests pose a diagnostic problem. An algorithm to help in evaluating and treating refugee and other immigrant children is available (http://www.cdc.gov/std/syphilis/treponemalalgorithm.pdf).[74] Important information includes maternal history of syphilis, titer results and treatment during pregnancy, maternal and infant titers, and evaluation and treatment for congenital syphilis at birth. If there are no physical findings, a reactive nontreponemal test result (confirmed by treponemal test) can be the result of either congenital or acquired disease. In these cases, the child should be fully evaluated for congenital syphilis including a lumbar puncture to evaluate for possible neurosyphilis, skeletal radiographs, an eye examination, and complete blood cell count. Positive results on an FTA-ABS test can be retained in an infant who has been appropriately treated for congenital syphilis at birth.[68] If the nontreponemal test is negative, further workup is not recommended; however, if the nontreponemal test is positive at ≥18 months, the infant should be re-evaluated fully and treated for congenital syphilis.

TREATMENT

Syphilis has been treated successfully for more than 50 years using penicillin. Treatment regimens are updated regularly by the CDC (http://www.cdc.gov/std/treatment), and the AAP[65] (Table 182-1).[38,75] Treatment failures are uncommon; more than 95% of otherwise healthy individuals with primary disease and approximately 90% of patients with secondary and early latent disease are cured with one injection of benzathine penicillin G. Failure to

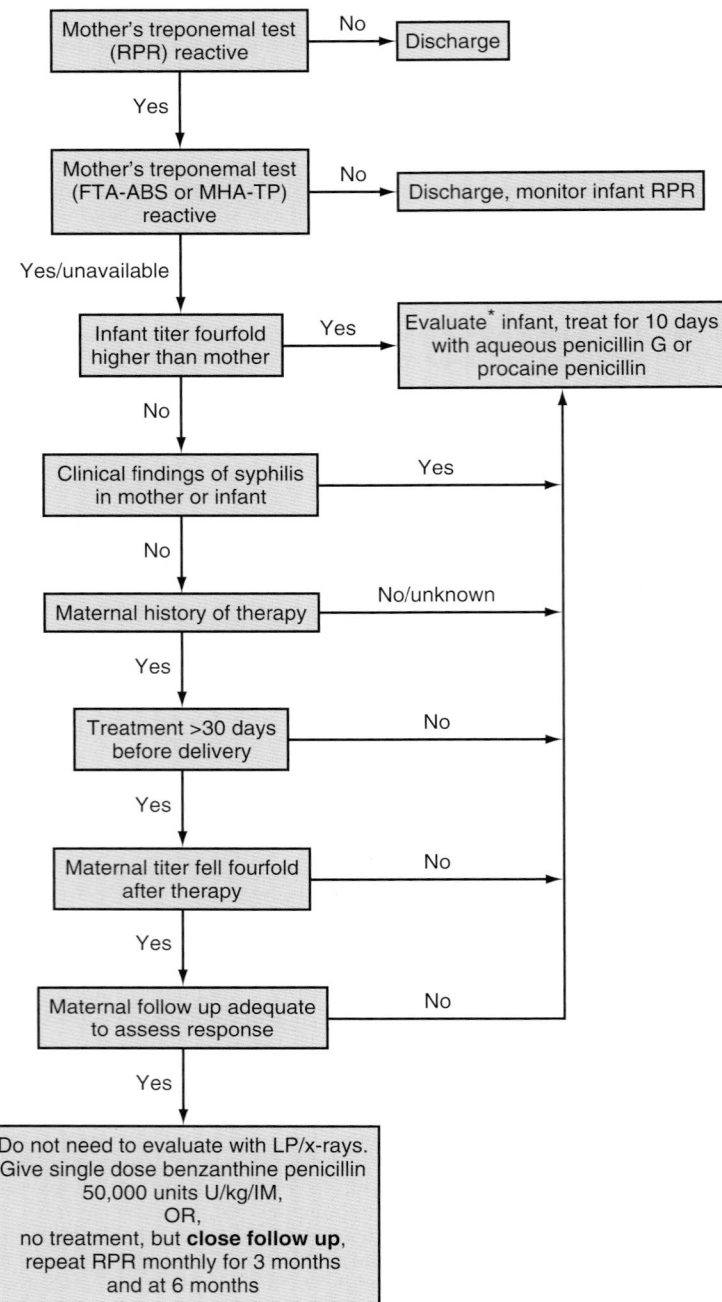

Figure 182-2. Assessment and management of congenital syphilis. *Evaluation includes physical examination, pathologic study of placenta (with direct fluorescent antibody (DFA) test, if possible) and cerebrospinal fluid (CSF) (including VDRL, white blood cell (WBC) count, protein levels); complete blood cell (CBC) count; and other tests as clinically indicated, such as long bone and chest radiographs, liver function tests, cranial ultrasonography ophthalmologic examination, and auditory brainstem response. (Based on Centers for Disease Control and Prevention. Sexually transmitted diseases treatment guidelines, 2010. MMWR Recomm Rep 2010;59(RR-12):26–39 and American Academy of Pediatrics. Syphilis. Data from Pickering LK, Baker CJ, Kimberlin DW, Long SS, eds. Red Book: 2009 Report of the Committee on Infectious Diseases 28th ed. Elk Grove Village, IL: American Academy of Pediatrics;2009:638–651.)

cure acquired disease may be more common in patients with symptomatic secondary disease and in those infected with HIV. Some practitioners treat patients with symptomatic secondary disease with a second injection of benzathine penicillin 1 week after the initial dose. HIV-infected patients with primary disease and *T. pallidum* in CSF are not always cured with the recommended single injection of benzathine penicillin G.[34] Musher has suggested that HIV-infected individuals should be treated with higher doses of penicillin,[76] which also are not always sufficient to cure CNS disease.[42]

Prenatal treatment that has effectively cured maternal disease has sometimes failed to prevent congenital disease.[77,78] In one report, 60 (14%) of 437 infants with congenital disease were born to mothers who were treated during pregnancy.[78] Failures were highest with treatment in the third trimester, especially in the month before delivery. Failure of maternal treatment also is

associated with preterm delivery.[79] Pregnant patients should be treated only with penicillin regimens, appropriate for their stage of syphilis.

Congenital infection, either proved or presumed, is treated with a 10-day course of aqueous penicillin G or procaine penicillin G. Azimi et al.[80] noted that, in some neonates, the level of penicillin in CSF 18 to 24 hours after a dose of procaine penicillin G was below that considered to be treponemidical and suggested that, for infants with severe or proven CNS disease, aqueous penicillin G might be superior therapy. The CDC guidelines suggest that benzathine penicillin G might be used when risk of congenital syphilis is low, i.e., an infant born to a mother treated in the month before delivery when the baby has no symptoms and has normal results on evaluation. However, the development of congenital syphilis in some infants whose mothers were treated toward the end of pregnancy and the failure of benzathine

TABLE 182-1. Syphilis Therapy

Condition	Treatment[a]	Comments
ACQUIRED DISEASE		
Primary, secondary, early latent disease (normal host)	Adults: 2.4 million U BPG × 1 Children: 50,000 U/kg BPG × 1	Penicillin-allergic adult may be treated with tetracycline 500 mg orally q6h or doxycycline 100 mg bid for 2 weeks; penicillin-allergic child (<age 8) should be desensitized and treated with penicillin
Late latent disease, disease of unknown duration, gumma, aortitis	Adults: 2.4 million U BPG weekly × 3 Children: 50,000 U/kg BPG weekly × 3	Perform lumbar puncture if neurologic or ophthalmologic signs or symptoms, active tertiary syphilis or treatment failure; if CSF is abnormal, treat for neurosyphilis
Neurosyphilis	Adults: 18–24 million U/day APG, divided into q4h doses (3–4 million U/dose) or continuous IV infusion for 10–14 days; or APPG 2.4 million U once daily IM and probenecid 500 mg 4 times daily for 10–14 days Children: 200,000–300,000 U/kg/day APG divided into q4–6h doses for 10 days	Penicillin-allergic patients should be densensitized and treated with penicillin
Pregnancy	Treat as for acquired disease; see text	Penicillin is the only drug used in pregnancy; penicillin-allergic individual should be densensitized and treated with 10-day course of APG
HIV infection	Treat as for acquired disease; see text	Perform lumbar puncture for same indications as late latent disease; strongly consider lumbar puncture if serum nontreponemal antibody titer does not fall fourfold 6–12 months after therapy. If CSF is abnormal, treat for neurosyphilis; if penicillin-allergic, desensitize and treat with APG penicillin
CONGENITAL DISEASE	≤4 weeks of age: 100,000 U/kg/day APG IV divided into q12h doses during first 7 days of life and 150,000 U/kg/day APG divided into q8h doses thereafter for total of 10 days *or* 50,000 U/kg once/day APPG IM × 10 days >4 weeks of age: 200,000–300,000 U/kg/day APG divided into q4–6h doses × 10 days	See text

APG, aqueous penicillin G; APPG, aqueous procaine penicillin G; BPG, benzathine penicillin G; CSF, cerebrospinal fluid.

[a]Children who weigh >50 kg are treated with adult dosing schedule.

From Larsen SA, Steiner BM, Rudolph AH. Laboratory diagnosis and interpretation of tests for syphilis. Clin Microbiol Rev 1995;8:1–21.

penicillin G to cure early congenital syphilis suggest that such infants might optimally be treated with a 10-day regimen of aqueous or procaine penicillin G.[77,78,81] In the future, tests currently under investigation to detect the presence of spirochetes or spirochetal DNA in CSF should better determine CNS infection and provide a more precise basis for therapy.[82]

Patients who are allergic to penicillin and who are not pregnant can be given tetracycline or doxycycline for early, latent, and tertiary disease that has not affected the CNS. Because oral tetracycline or doxycycline must be given daily for 2 weeks, it should be used only for patients in whom adherence and follow-up are assured. Children with acquired syphilis who are aged 8 years or younger, pregnant women, HIV-infected patients, and adults with later stages of syphilis or tertiary disease who are allergic to penicillin should be desensitized and treated with penicillin.[38] Although single-dose azithromycin in the treatment of early syphilis showed equivalent treatment efficacy in comparison with the recommended penicillin regimen,[83] recent reports of macrolide resistance in *T. pallidum* in several geographic areas has decreased enthusiasm for this new therapy.[84–86] In addition, treatment failures resulting in congenital syphilis have been reported with the use of azithromycin in pregnant women.[87] Erythromycin is not considered an acceptable alternative therapy for the penicillin-allergic pregnant woman.

The Jarisch–Herxheimer reaction, the major complication of therapy, occurs most commonly among those with early syphilis, both children and adults. Fever is the major symptom and can be accompanied by headache and myalgia. Hypotension, tachycardia, and an increase in respiratory rate occur in some patients. During pregnancy, the Jarisch–Herxheimer reaction can cause uterine contractions, decreased fetal activity, and occasionally can result in premature delivery or fetal death.[88]

Follow-up

Persons with primary, secondary, or early latent syphilis should be re-examined clinically and serologically at 6 and 12 months after therapy. Late latent syphilis requires a further re-examination at 24 months after therapy. Persons with HIV infection and syphilis require careful clinical and serologic follow-up at 3, 6, 9, 12, and 24 months after therapy for early syphilis; and at 6, 12, 18, and 24 months for those with latent syphilis. Infants with congenital syphilis and all seroreactive infants, regardless of infection status, should be examined and have repeated quantitative nontreponemal tests every 2 to 3 months until nonreactivity is documented.

PREVENTION

Prevention of congenital syphilis requires a multifaceted approach,[89,90] including the following: (1) information, education and counseling regarding syphilis transmission and prevention (including promotion of safer sexual activity); (2) adequate and equitable healthcare for all, including access to comprehensive and integrated reproductive and sexual healthcare for those at highest risk of infection; (3) comprehensive partner management (notification and treatment) for all sexual partners of primary patients; (4) access to early and comprehensive prenatal care for all pregnant women, including syphilis testing at the first visit and at time of delivery, and adequate treatment; (5) detection and treatment of congenital infection before appearance of symptoms; and (6) primary recognition and treatment of symptomatic infection when it occurs after the neonatal period. A systematic review and meta-analysis of these types of interventions showed that the syphilis-attributable incidence of stillbirth and perinatal death could be reduced by 50% if these measures were implemented.[62a]

Key Points. Epidemiology, Clinical Features, Diagnosis, and Treatment of Syphilis

EPIDEMIOLOGY

- Worldwide, but more common in low-income settings
- Epidemiology varies by region; more common in U.S. males who have sex with males and among minority populations
- Acquired transplacentally (congenital syphilis), or by sexual contact

CLINICAL FEATURES

- Primary stage: painless genital chancre with regional lymphadenopathy
- Secondary stage: disseminated disease with rash (especially palms and soles), constitutional symptoms, condylomatous lesions
- Tertiary stage: cardiovascular, neurologic, gummas
- Mother-to-child transmission results in: stillbirth, late fetal loss, low birthweight baby, neonatal death, infant with congenital syphilis

- Congenital syphilis: early (<2 years), symptomatic (hepatosplenomegaly, small for gestational age, rash, bone, CSF findings), or asymptomatic
- Congenital syphilis: late (>2 years), bone or dental findings, hearing loss

DIAGNOSIS

- Serology:
  (a) nontreponemal test (RPR, VDRL) for screening and to follow adequacy of treatment
  (b) treponemal test (FTA-ABS, TP-PA) for confirmation of nontreponemal test as due to syphilis

TREATMENT

- Penicillin
- Alternative: doxycycline (>8 years and not pregnant)
- Follow nontreponemal titers to monitor for success (i.e., fourfold decrease in titer)

---

183 Other *Treponema* Species

Sarah A. Rawstron

YAWS

Yaws (*Treponema pallidum* subsp. *pertenue*) is an infectious disease of childhood. It is seen in warm, humid tropical regions in rural, often inaccessible areas, in association with poverty, overcrowding, poor hygiene, and lack of access to health services. "Yaws begins where the road ends."[1] Endemic areas include Africa, Southeast Asia, the Western Pacific, and South and Central America. Yaws is also known as framboesia, pian, parangi, paru, bouba, and buba.

Mass treatment campaigns of approximately 50 million people in the 1950s and 1960s helped eradicate yaws from most areas. However, there was resurgence of the disease in the 1980s, particularly in parts of West and Central Africa and Southeast Asia.[2,3] Resurgence has been ascribed to the persistence of severely impoverished living conditions and a lack of follow-up surveillance and treatment programs. Control of yaws depends on treatment of all patients with active disease and their contacts. The recent successful yaws eradication campaign in India[4] has renewed energy and efforts for elimination of yaws worldwide.[1]

Clinical Manifestations

Yaws is passed from child to child through nonsexual contact with primary or secondary skin lesions. The primary lesion, the mother yaw, generally occurs on the lower half of the body at sites of minor trauma. The lesion begins as a painless erythematous papule that enlarges, ulcerates, and becomes covered by a honey-colored crust 9 to 90 days after inoculation. Painless, regional lymphadenopathy occurs. The primary lesion heals after several weeks to months.

Organisms disseminated during the primary stage form the basis of secondary disease. This stage manifests as multiple cutaneous lesions (daughter yaws), which resemble the mother yaw both clinically and histologically but are smaller, and painful periostitis involving bones of the extremities, especially the hands and feet. Secondary lesions heal spontaneously and without scarring.

The pathology of primary and secondary lesions resembles that seen in sexually acquired syphilis. Latent yaws is characterized by intermittent relapses of skin lesions at intervals for up to 5 years, but congenital infection is not seen. Experimental infections of guinea-pigs have confirmed the lack of congenital infection in yaws.[5]

Tertiary yaws, which develops in about 10% of untreated patients after several years, consists of destructive lesions of bone, cartilage, soft tissue, and skin. Characteristic findings are: palmar-plantar hyperkeratosis; goundou, a rare lesion in which symmetric involvement of the nasal processes of the maxilla leads to excessive bone formation and obstruction of the airway; gangosa (destructive ulcerative rhinopharyngitis); and chronic osteitis leading to saber tibia.

Diagnosis

In endemic areas, the diagnosis is made clinically. In addition, treponemes are identified easily with darkfield microscopy of exudate from primary and secondary lesions and serologic tests for syphilis show reactions. Vorst[6] has called attention to an "attenuated" form of the disease, seen in areas of low prevalence, in which one or just a few small, dry, flat lesions, confined mainly to moist skin folds, are seen. The Centers for Disease Control and Prevention (CDC) has recommended screening children who come from areas of the world with endemic treponematoses using nontreponemal serologic tests.[7] This recommendation includes an algorithm to aid in the evaluation and treatment of children with reactive nontreponemal and treponemal tests as serologic tests do not distinguish yaws from congenital and acquired syphilis (www.cdc.gov/std/syphilis/treponemalalgorithm.pdf).

ENDEMIC SYPHILIS (BEJEL)

Endemic syphilis (bejel), caused by *Treponema pallidum* subsp. *endemicum*, is found in areas with a hot, dry climate in North

Africa, Southwest Asia, and the eastern Mediterranean. Until 1960, disease also was present in Bulgaria and Yugoslavia; a treatment and prevention program eliminated these foci. Imported cases have been recognized in some European cities.

Infection occurs in childhood and is acquired from contaminated fomites, such as communal drinking vessels, or through oral-oral contact. The primary lesion, a small, painless papule or ulcer in the mouth, usually is not detected. The secondary stage, resulting from treponemal dissemination, is characterized by numerous highly infectious mucous membrane patches, often accompanied by hoarseness from syphilitic laryngitis, and regional lymphadenopathy. Axillary and anogenital condylomata can be seen, and osteoperiostitis of the long bones can cause nocturnal leg pain.

After a latent period, untreated bejel progresses to tertiary symptoms in most patients, and sometimes is characterized by destructive lesions (gummas) involving the nasopharynx, skin, and bones, but involvement of other organs, including the eye, can occur. As living conditions improve in endemic areas, a form of the disease has been observed in which the number of lesions as well as the signs and symptoms are less severe.

The disease has some similarities to sexually acquired syphilis. However, the method of acquisition, the site of the primary lesion, the lack of congenital disease, and the absence of cardiovascular and neurologic symptoms in endemic syphilis differentiate the two diseases. When symptoms consistent with either endemic syphilis or venereal syphilis occur in an area where both diseases exist, epidemiologic features of an outbreak can be useful for differentiation.

PINTA

Pinta (*Treponema carateum*), which occurs only in the Western hemisphere, has been described in Central and South America, Cuba, and the Caribbean islands. Control with penicillin has made this a rare disease. Pinta begins during childhood and adolescence, and the clinical stages are confined to the skin, with lymphadenopathy the only systemic manifestation. The word

pinta is taken from the Spanish verb to paint and is indicative of the various colors seen as the skin lesions mature – red, white, violet, blue, brown, or black.

Pinta is transmitted through contact with broken skin, and the primary lesion occurs mainly on the lower leg, dorsum of the foot, forearm, or back of the hands. One to 8 weeks after inoculation, a tiny erythematous papule or cluster of papules appears, which enlarges and coalesces. An irregular and heaped border surrounds the erythematous, scaly central lesion. Dissemination from the primary site results in secondary skin lesions known as *pintids*, which develop 3 to 9 months after the initial inoculation and before the primary lesion has healed completely. Secondary lesions are indistinguishable clinically and histologically from the primary lesion.

Primary and secondary lesions are highly contagious and heal slowly. Three months to many years later, tertiary disease, manifesting as achromic, atrophic lesions, appears. These lesions are not considered infectious.

TREATMENT

Treatment of all nonvenereal treponematoses is the same. One dose of benzathine penicillin (1.2 million units for adults and 0.6 million units for children younger than 10 years) is curative. Family members, contacts, and patients with latent infection should receive the same dose as those with active disease.[8] Later treatment results in slower healing, and serologic reactivity can persist.

In an outbreak of yaws in New Guinea in 1998, a substantial rate (28%) of treatment failures following penicillin was noted (although patients responded to additional penicillin treatment).[9] Investigators suggested that failures were due to reduced susceptibility of the organism to penicillin, although reinfection could not be ruled out, and susceptibility tests were not performed.

A study of the efficacy of a targeted yaws control program in Guyana using oral penicillin V therapy for 7 to 10 days appears promising,[10] but parenteral benzathine penicillin remains the recommended therapy.[11,12]

184 *Leptospira* Species (Leptospirosis)

Eugene D. Shapiro

PATHOGENESIS

The *Leptospira* genus is comprised of a group of motile, finely coiled, catalase-producing spirochetal bacteria that are obligate aerobes. *Leptospira* are classified into two species based on phenotypic differences: *Leptospira biflexa*, a free-living saprophytic organism that is found in water and soil and does not cause human disease, and *Leptospira interrogans*, the many different serotypes (also known as serovars, for example, *L. interrogans* serovar *icterohaemorrhagiae*) of which are responsible for leptospirosis in humans. Stimson, who first saw the organism under the microscope in 1907, named it *interrogans* because it was shaped like a question mark.

L. interrogans infects humans through intact mucous membranes or disrupted skin, invades the bloodstream, and disseminates rapidly to multiple organs. Although the precise mechanism by which *L. interrogans* causes disease has not been defined, tissue injury is apparently mediated by direct toxic effects of the bacterium.

L. interrogans has a predilection for infecting the liver and kidney, although any tissue can be infected. The organism causes hepatocellular dysfunction, which can lead to jaundice, in most instances without producing necrosis. *L. interrogans* also can cause renal tubular dysfunction resulting in renal failure, and hemorrhagic vasculitis. The signs and symptoms of leptospirosis during the initial "septicemic" phase of the illness are due to a direct effect of the organism; inflammation during the second or "immune" phase of the illness is related to antigen–antibody complexes.

EPIDEMIOLOGY

Leptospirosis is a zoonosis,[1] and infection with *L. interrogans* is widespread in both wild and domestic animals throughout the world.[2] Humans, who are incidental hosts, rarely transmit the organism to other humans or to animals, and are unimportant in the maintenance of *L interrogans* in nature. By contrast, *L. interrogans* can be shed in the urine of wild animals such as rodents (particularly mice and rats) and by domestic animals such as dogs, cows, and pigs, for long periods. Such animals serve as reservoirs for the organism and, because of their close association with people, are the sources of most human infections.

The epidemiology of human leptospirosis largely is determined by the nature of the contact between humans and infected animals and the level of sanitation in the community. In the United States, most cases are reported from the southern states, which may reflect high year-round potential for exposure.[3] In developing countries, rats are the primary reservoir for leptospirosis. In the U.S., dogs and farm animals are important reservoirs in addition to rats.[3] However, *L. interrogans* also has been identified in many wild mammals such as raccoons, foxes, skunks, opossums, and wolves.[3] Although any animal can be infected with any serovar of *L. interrogans,* certain serovars seem to infect certain species preferentially. For example, *L interrogans* serovar *pomona* is isolated most frequently from cows and pigs, serovar *canicola* from dogs, and serovar *icterohaemorrhagiae* from rats and mice. The prevalence of infection in certain animal species is high. Up to 90% of Norway rats have been found to be infected with *L interrogans*; once infection is established in rats, *L interrogans* is shed for life. Many other animals, such as dogs (even those immunized), cattle, and pigs, can shed high concentrations of *L interrogans* in urine for months after the initial infection, but shedding diminishes substantially or halts within 6 to 12 months. Organisms survive for 3 months or more in neutral or slightly alkaline water but not in acidic environments.

Infection in humans often occurs through contact with the urine of infected animals, either directly or via contaminated water or soil; human infection also can occur through contact with organs of infected animals. People with occupational, recreational, or accidental contact have an increased risk of leptospirosis. A case-control study conducted in France found that skin lesions, canoeing, contact with wild rodents, and residing in the country were independently associated with leptospirosis, showing that leisure activity is an important risk factor for this illness.[4] In recent years, dogs have been implicated as the major source of cases in the U.S.[3] People who live or work on dairy, cattle, or pig farms, as well as abattoir (slaughterhouse) workers and veterinarians, are at increased risk. Up to 15% of abattoir workers have serologic evidence of past infection. Field workers, even in developed countries, also may have increased risk of leptospirosis.[5]

The incidence of leptospirosis is unknown because most cases either are asymptomatic or diagnosed incorrectly. The diagnosis is made most often in teenage boys and young men, presumably because their activities expose them more frequently to the urine of infected animals. However, infection can occur regardless of age or sex.[3-6] Children usually become infected via exposure to stagnant, urine-contaminated water. Common-source outbreaks have occurred after swimming in contaminated ponds.[7] Outbreaks have occurred in athletes who participated in triathlons.[8]

CLINICAL MANIFESTATIONS

The incubation period is approximately 10 days (usual range, 7 to 14 days), although incubation can be as short as 2 days and as long as 25 days. Clinical manifestations are divided into the initial "septicemic" phase and the subsequent "immune" phase.[9-12] The severity of illness ranges from the classic, icteric Weil syndrome (which affects about 10% of patients) to the more common, less severe anicteric form of leptospirosis.[9-12] The correlation between fever, other clinical findings, and the presence of organisms in body fluids in the different stages of disease is shown in Figure 184-1.

Anicteric Leptospirosis

Symptoms of leptospirosis begin abruptly, with viral-like illness marked by fever, headache, and myalgia. Abdominal pain, vomiting, diarrhea, anorexia, and conjunctival suffusion can be present. Rarely, circulatory collapse ensues. During this phase of illness, organisms are present in the bloodstream and cerebrospinal fluid. The severity of illness varies substantially during this phase; symptoms usually last 4 to 7 days and resolve spontaneously.

Some patients have a second, immunologic phase of the illness that begins 1 to 3 days later with low-grade or no fever. During this phase, headache, myalgia, rash, conjunctival suffusion, and hepatomegaly are typical. Nausea, vomiting, and abdominal pain also are common. Typically, the headache is severe and may be associated with nuchal rigidity. These manifestations of aseptic meningitis usually last for several days, although they can persist occasionally for 2 to 3 weeks. Other much less frequent manifestations of immune-mediated nervous system disease include encephalitis, Guillain–Barré syndrome, radiculomyelitis, and mononeuropathy or polyneuropathy of the cranial or peripheral nerves.

Interstitial nephritis also is common; manifestations range from incidental pyuria, hematuria, and proteinuria to renal failure.

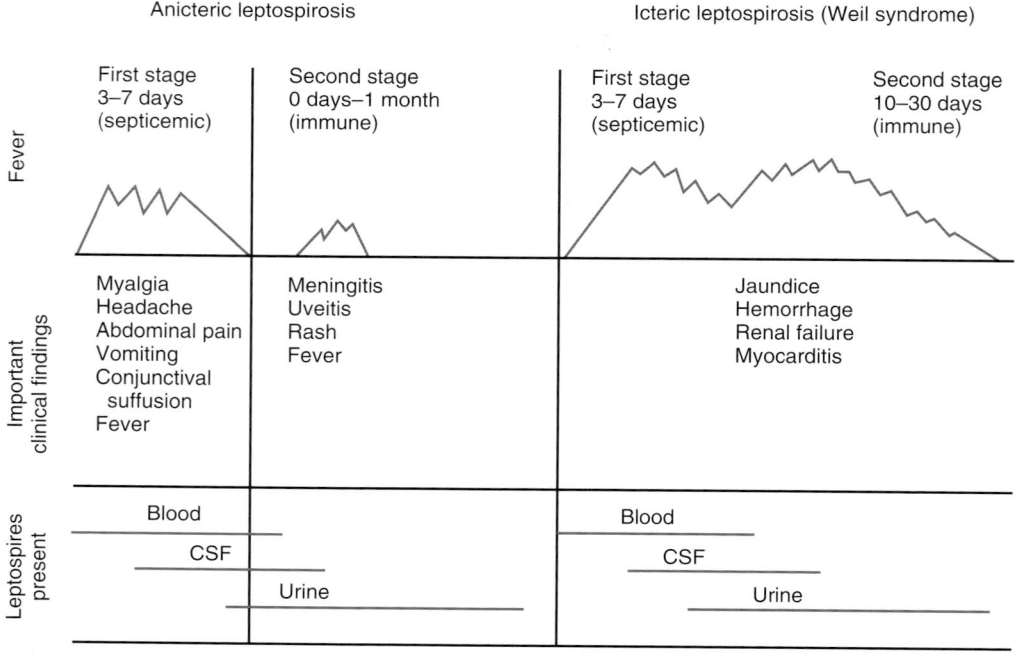

Figure 184-1. Stages of anicteric and icteric leptospirosis. Correlation between clinical findings and the presence of leptospires in body fluids. (Redrawn from Feigin RD, Anderson DC. Human leptospirosis. CRC Crit Rev Clin Lab Sci 1975;5:413–467.)

Patients can have right upper quadrant abdominal pain and a mass from acalculous cholecystitis with hydrops of the gallbladder. Pulmonary involvement also can occur. The rash of leptospirosis is immune-mediated and nonspecific and can be macular, maculopapular, urticarial, petechial, or purpuric. The infectious and immune phases of anicteric leptospirosis usually resolve within 2 weeks of the onset of symptoms.

Icteric Leptospirosis (Weil Syndrome)

The severe, icteric form of leptospirosis, also called Weil syndrome, can be caused by any serovar of *L. interrogans*, is indistinguishable in the early phase from the benign, anicteric form of leptospirosis, but has a mortality rate of 5% to 10%. The hallmarks of Weil syndrome – jaundice, azotemia, and hemorrhage – become apparent 4 to 6 days after the onset of symptoms and can progress through the second week of the illness. Persistent fever (lasting up to 2 to 3 weeks) and the severity of the illness obscure the biphasic characteristics of the symptomatology.

Although hepatomegaly, hepatocellular injury, and jaundice are prominent features of Weil syndrome, necrosis and frank hepatic failure do not occur, and there is no residual hepatic damage in survivors. By contrast, renal impairment, which occurs to a varying degree in both forms of leptospirosis, can be profound in patients with Weil syndrome.[10-13] Bacterial-mediated toxicity to the renal tubules can be aggravated by shock and, rarely, by hemoglobinemia from hemolysis and leads to acute tubular necrosis and renal failure. Because of advances in supportive care, the survival rate has improved substantially in recent years. Renal dysfunction is reversible in most but not all cases.

Significant cardiac dysfunction is rare, although many patients have nonspecific electrocardiographic abnormalities (such as first-degree heart block) during the first week of the illness. Rarely, congestive heart failure and cardiovascular collapse develop in patients with Weil syndrome.

LABORATORY FINDINGS AND DIAGNOSIS

A wide variety of laboratory abnormalities are present in patients with leptospirosis, depending on the severity and phase of the illness and the organ systems involved. None is specific. Weil syndrome is associated with leukocytosis and neutrophilia, especially during the early phase of the illness. Anemia is unusual in anicteric leptospirosis but can be severe in Weil syndrome. Serum concentrations of hepatic enzymes, creatinine, and blood urea nitrogen usually are elevated modestly (if present at all) in patients with anicteric leptospirosis but can be extremely elevated in Weil syndrome. Approximately half of patients with leptospirosis have clinical signs of meningitis during the immune phase of the illness, and three-quarters have cerebrospinal fluid (CSF) pleocytosis; neutrophils predominate very early in the illness, but a change to mononuclear cells occurs rapidly; protein concentration is normal or elevated; glucose usually is normal. In the early phase of the illness, the urine usually contains protein, red and white blood cells, and cellular casts.

The number of conditions that could be included in the differential diagnosis of leptospirosis is myriad. Most often, leptospirosis must be differentiated from viral illness and other causes of aseptic meningitis or meningoencephalitis. Leptospirosis can mimic Kawasaki disease and other causes of hepatitis, acute tubular necrosis, interstitial nephritis, and hepatorenal syndrome.

The diagnosis is confirmed by recovery of *L. interrogans* from fluid or tissue or by 4-fold or greater rise in antileptospiral antibodies by the microscopic agglutination test in acute and convalescent sera in a patient with a compatible clinical illness. A presumptive diagnosis of leptospirosis can be made in a patient who has a clinically compatible illness and either a titer of antileptospiral antibodies of ≥1 : 100 by the microscopic agglutination test or a positive macroscopic agglutination test. *L. interrogans* cannot be visualized with routine light microscopy; organisms can be seen by the use of modified silver stains on tissue or fluorescent

antibody techniques on urine or tissue specimens. Rarely, *L. interrogans* can be visualized by darkfield microscopy when the density of organisms is high.

Culture

L. interrogans can be isolated from blood or CSF during the septicemic phase, and from urine during the immune phase of leptospirosis. Special media are required and include Tween 80-albumin, Fletcher, and Ellinghausen–McCullough–Johnson–Harris semisolid media; Tween 80-albumin is available commercially and may be superior. Solid media are less reliable for primary isolation of organisms but are useful for secondary isolation of *L. interrogans* from semisolid media contaminated with other organisms. Because of difficulty isolating *L. interrogans* and inexperience in clinical microbiology laboratories, specimens for culture from suspected cases should be sent to the National Leptospirosis Laboratory at the Centers for Disease Control and Prevention. Polymerase chain reaction assays for *L. interrogans* are under development.[14,15]

Serology

The macroscopic slide agglutination test is the most useful test for rapid screening.[16,17] Twelve serotypes of killed *L. interrogans* (representing strains responsible for most infections in the U.S.) are included in this test. The microscopic agglutination test uses live organisms and is the "gold standard" for detecting antibodies to *L. interrogans*.

Generally, agglutination tests are not positive until after the first week of infection; antibody levels peak 3 to 4 weeks after the onset of symptoms and can persist for years, although concentrations may decline over time. Demonstration of a 4-fold or greater rise in antibodies between acute and convalescent serum samples tested together is most definitive. Newer serologic tests may become useful in making the diagnosis of leptospirosis and include indirect hemagglutination tests, a passive microcapsule agglutination test, and enzyme immunoassays.[18-22]

TREATMENT

Because leptospirosis occurs only sporadically, is generally self-limited, and cannot be confirmed early in the course of infection, clinical trials of efficacy of treatment are difficult to perform. Treatment, even if begun late in the course of a relatively severe infection, potentially is beneficial. This positive effect of treatment is based on limited data from clinical trials,[23,24] in vitro susceptibility of *L. interrogans*, the efficacy of antimicrobial treatment of experimental leptospirosis in animal models (when treatment is begun early), and numerous case reports.[25] An open-label randomized clinical trial conducted in Thailand found that for treatment of patients with severe leptospirosis, penicillin G, cefotaxime, and doxycycline all were highly efficacious.[26] Frequent occurrence of a Jarisch–Herxheimer reaction also supports an effect of treatment.[27]

Treatment should begin as early in the course of the illness as possible. Aqueous penicillin G (200,000 to 250,000 U/kg/day in divided doses administered every 4 to 6 hours; maximal dose, 12 million U/day) is recommended for serious infection. Less seriously ill patients can be treated with doxycycline orally (2 mg/kg/day divided into 2 doses with maximum of 100 mg twice a day, only for children 8 years or older) or amoxicillin (50 mg/kg/day in divided doses three times a day; maximum of 500 mg per dose). Therapy is continued for 7 to 14 days.

SPECIAL CONSIDERATIONS

Congenital Leptospirosis

Although leptospirosis commonly causes abortion in pregnant animals, little information is available on the effect of leptospirosis on the human fetus. The limited information is primarily derived from pregnant women with relatively severe disease. A review of 16 reported cases of leptospirosis during pregnancy revealed that 5 of 8 women (63%) who aborted had leptospirosis during the first or second trimester.[28] Four of the 16 infants were born with evidence of congenital infection (hepatosplenomegaly), 3 were treated successfully, and 1 who died on the second day of life had leptospires seen on stained tissue specimens from the liver and kidneys. Three women with untreated anicteric leptospirosis late in the third trimester gave birth to children who were not infected. No congenital malformations were observed.

Pregnant women in whom leptospirosis develops should be treated promptly with penicillin or ampicillin administered intravenously. At the time of delivery, infants should be examined carefully, and if signs of congenital leptospirosis (jaundice, hepatomegaly) are present, they should be treated promptly with parenterally administered penicillin.

PREVENTION

Widespread infection with *L. interrogans* in animals precludes elimination of leptospirosis. Good sanitation reduces the population of the rodent reservoir. Immunization of domestic animals reduces the risk of disease and decreases but does not eliminate leptospiruria.[29] People with occupational exposure to *L. interrogans* should take precautions (such as wearing gloves), especially when in direct contact with potentially infected fluid, water, or soil. Children should not swim in potentially contaminated ponds; pools should be chlorinated adequately. Doxycycline (200 mg, once weekly) administered to soldiers in Panama reduced the risk of leptospirosis; prophylaxis might be considered in extraordinary circumstances for travelers who are expected to be at risk for a limited time.[30]

---

185 *Borrelia burgdorferi* (Lyme Disease)

Eugene D. Shapiro

PATHOGENESIS AND IMMUNITY

Lyme disease is caused by the spirochete *Borrelia burgdorferi*,[1-3] a cylindrical, fastidious, microaerophilic bacterium that replicates very slowly and requires special medium for in vitro growth. Its cell membrane is covered by flagella and a loosely associated outer membrane. The three major outer-surface proteins, OspA, OspB, and OspC (which are highly charged basic proteins with molecular weights of about 31, 34, and 23 kd, respectively), as well as the 41-kd flagellar protein, are important targets for the immune response of humans. Biologic differences in strains of *B. burgdorferi* sensu lato presumably are responsible for differences in the clinical manifestations of Lyme borreliosis in Europe and in the United States. *B. burgdorferi* sensu stricto is the only genomospecies that causes disease in the U.S., while there is considerable variation in the genomospecies, which also include *B. garinii*, *B. afzelii*, and a number of others, that cause disease in Europe.[4] The greater frequency of radiculoneuritis in Europe and of arthritis in the U.S. likely are related to these differences.

Lyme disease is a zoonosis with complex pathogenesis.[3] *B. burgdorferi* is inoculated by the tick into the skin and begins to spread locally. Local inflammation results in erythema migrans in most patients with symptomatic infection (~90%). Days to weeks later, the spirochete can disseminate, via the bloodstream, to many other sites, including eye, muscle, bone, synovial tissue, central nervous system, and heart. Despite the low density of organisms and the fastidious nature of growth in vitro, *B. burgdorferi* has been isolated from blood or from affected tissues at all stages of illness. Relatively few organisms invade. Host mediators amplify the inflammatory response and cause much of the tissue damage. Preferring cell surfaces, the spirochete can adhere to a wide variety of cell types, which may explain clinical manifestations of involvement in a broad array of organ systems. Because the organism can persist in tissues for prolonged periods when untreated, symptoms can appear months after infection. The host's immune response is an important element in the pathogenesis of Lyme disease.[4] Symptoms of early localized disease, early disseminated disease, and late disease (see discussion of clinical manifestations) usually are due to inflammation as a direct result of the spirochete's presence. However, in rare patients with refractory symptoms of late Lyme disease (chronic recurrent Lyme arthritis), symptoms may have an immunogenic basis.[5] Some people with Lyme disease who

are treated early in the course of infection do not develop antibodies and remain susceptible to subsequent infections. People with late Lyme disease rarely develop erythema migrans again, even with repeated exposure to ixodid ticks in endemic areas, suggesting they have developed immunity.

EPIDEMIOLOGY

Disease in Humans

Although Lyme disease occurs throughout the world, endemicity varies widely. In the U.S., from 1993 to 2006, 93% of reported cases came from 10 states (Figure 185-1).[6] Most cases occur in southern New England and in the eastern Mid-Atlantic states. Fewer cases occur in Minnesota, Wisconsin, and parts of Michigan. Rarely, cases occur along the northern Pacific coast. In Europe, most cases occur in the Scandinavian countries and in central Europe, although the disease has been reported throughout the region.

Although frequency has increased and the geographic distribution of Lyme disease in the U.S. has expanded, the incidence of Lyme disease varies substantially from region to region and within local areas.[1-2,6] The annual number of reported cases in the U.S. increased from 9908 cases in 1992 to 19,931 cases in 2006. This is likely due both to an increased incidence and to improved recognition and reporting of disease. Estimates of the incidence of disease are complicated by reliance, in most instances, on passive reporting of cases as well as by the high frequency of misdiagnosis of disease. Furthermore, seroepidemiologic studies indicate that some patients in whom there is evidence of recent infection with *B. burgdorferi* are asymptomatic.[7,8] The reported annual incidence in the most highly endemic areas, such as Connecticut, is about 75 cases per 100,000 persons, although in certain localized areas in which the disease is hyperendemic (e.g., Lyme, CT), the annual incidence may be as high as 1000 or more per 100,000 persons. The reported incidence is highest among children 5 to 14 years old. Most cases occur during the summer months.

Ecology

Lyme disease is a zoonosis.[3,9] *B. burgdorferi* is transmitted by ticks of the *Ixodes* genus. In the U.S., vectors are *I. scapularis* (the deer

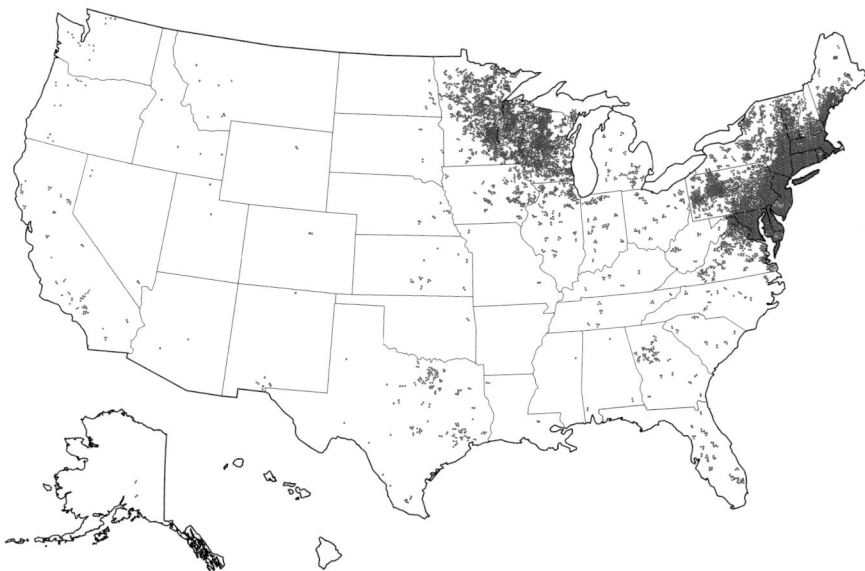

Figure 185-1. Average incidence of Lyme disease (per 100,000 persons) by county of residence – United States, 1992 to 2006. (From: Centers for Disease Control and Prevention. Surveillance for Lyme Disease – United States, 1992–2006. MMWR 2008;57(SS-10):5.)

1 dot placed randomly within county of residence for each confirmed case

tick) in both the Northeast and Midwest and *I. pacificus* (the Western black-legged tick) in the Pacific states. The life cycle of these ticks consists of three stages – larva, nymph, and adult – that develop during a 2-year period. Larvae are usually not infected with *B. burgdorferi*, because transovarial transmission rarely occurs. Ticks become infected as they feed on infected small mammals, such as *Peromyscus leucopus* (the white-footed mouse), which are natural reservoirs for the bacteria. Deer are important in the life cycle of the tick but are not a competent reservoir for the bacterium.

Multiple factors affect the risk of transmission of *B. burgdorferi* from ticks to humans. The first is the likelihood that a tick is infected. The proportion of infected ticks varies tremendously by geography as well as by species and stage of life cycle. Most cases of Lyme disease are transmitted by nymphal deer ticks, because they outnumber adult ticks, are active during times of the year when many more people are outdoors, and are very small and therefore less likely to be detected and removed before transmitting infection. *I. pacificus* often feeds on lizards, which are not a competent reservoir for *B. burgdorferi* and their blood contains factors that kill the bacteria. Consequently, fewer than 10% of these ticks are infected with *B. burgdorferi*. By contrast, *I. scapularis* feeds on small mammals that constitute the natural reservoir for *B. burgdorferi*. In southeastern Connecticut and in Westchester County, New York, which have very high incidences of Lyme disease, rates of infection for *I. scapularis* are approximately 2% for larvae, 15% to 25% for nymphs, and 30% to 50% for adults.

CLINICAL MANIFESTATIONS

Lyme disease generally is divided into three clinical stages: early localized disease, early disseminated disease, and late disease.[1,2] Box 185-1 shows the major clinical features of these stages. The tick bite that transmits the infection often is not recognized.

Early Localized Disease

The first clinical manifestation of Lyme disease is a typical annular rash, erythema migrans (Figure 185-2). Approximately two-thirds of children with symptomatic infection have a single erythema migrans lesion, which occurs at the site of tick bite (though typically the bite was not recognized).[10] Onset of rash is usually 7 to 14 days after the bite (range, 3 to 32 days). The rash most often is uniformly erythematous, but it can appear as a target lesion with

central clearing, or occasionally it can have a vesicular or a necrotic center. The rash can be pruritic, painful, or asymptomatic. Associated systemic symptoms, such as fever, myalgia, headache, and malaise, are variably present. Untreated, the rash gradually expands (hence the name *migrans*) to an average diameter of

---

BOX 185-1. Clinical Manifestations of Lyme Disease in Children According to Stage of the Disease

EARLY LOCALIZED DISEASE (3–32 DAYS AFTER TICK BITE)

- Erythema migrans (single) sometimes accompanied by any of the following nonspecific symptoms or signs:
  - Myalgia
  - Headache
  - Fatigue
  - Fever
  - Lymphadenopathy (regional or generalized)

EARLY DISSEMINATED DISEASE (3–10 WEEKS AFTER TICK BITE)

- Erythema migrans (multiple)
- Cranial neuritis (especially facial palsy)
- Meningitis
- Carditis (especially heart block)
- Radiculoneuritis

All of the above may be accompanied by any of the following nonspecific symptoms or signs:
- Myalgia
- Headache
- Fatigue
- Fever
- Lymphadenopathy (regional or generalized)
- Conjunctivitis
- Neck pain and stiffness

LATE DISSEMINATED DISEASE (2–12 MONTHS AFTER TICK BITE)

- Arthritis (usually monoarticular or pauciarticular with involvement of the knee)

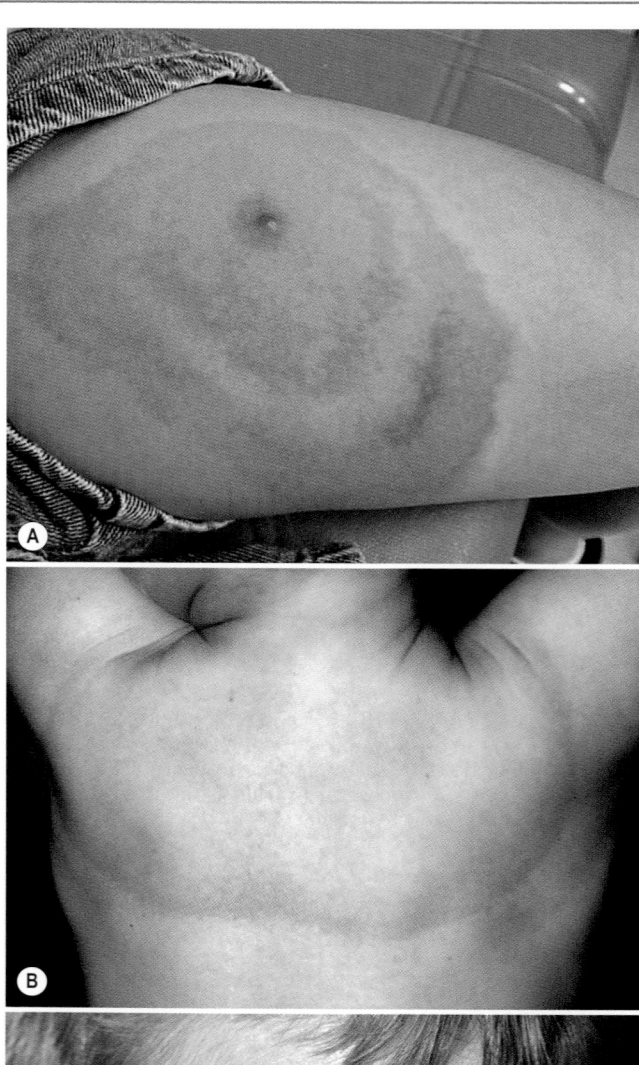

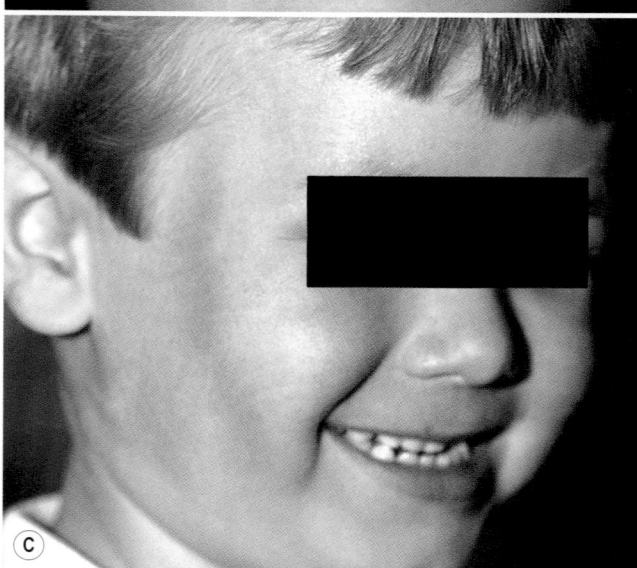

Figure 185-2. (A) Typical expanding annular lesion of erythema migrans at the site of a tick bite. The central area underwent minor necrosis. (Case courtesy of J. Capra, Abilene, Texas.) **(B, C)** A 5-year-old boy had a giant expanding lesion of erythema migrans with central clearing on his back and another on his face probably from bacteremic dissemination. (Courtesy of M. Weir, Temple, Texas.)

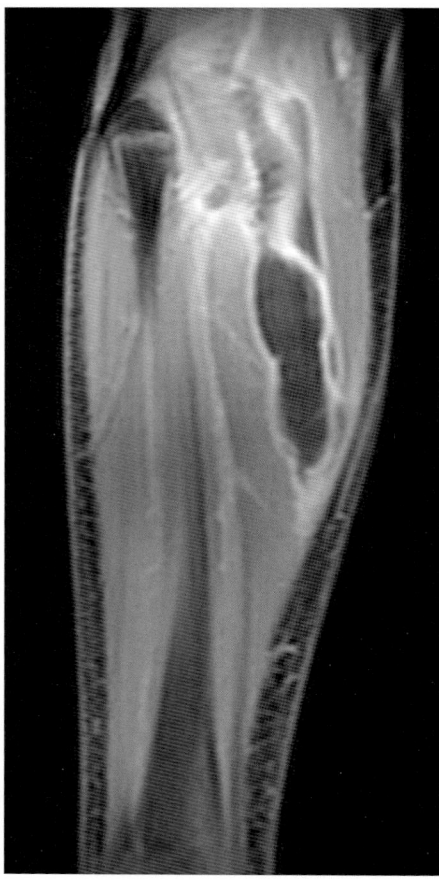

Figure 185-3. A 12-year-old boy came to attention after 2 weeks of pain and swelling in his knee and then in his calf, which was warm, swollen and tender. Fat-suppressed T_1-weighted coronal MRI with contrast shows enhancing multilobulated fluid-filled mass (Baker cyst) with atypical inferior extension. Fluid had 140,000 white blood cells per mm^3 and was sterile. Serum Lyme antibody was 13 EU/mL.

15 cm (although lesions larger than 30 cm can occur) and persists for at least 1 to 2 weeks. Lesions can occur anywhere on the body, although they are more common in the head and neck area in children than in adults.

Early Disseminated Disease

Approximately one-quarter of children with Lyme disease are initially diagnosed with early disseminated infection when, as a consequence of bacteremic dissemination to multiple sites, they develop secondary erythema migrans lesions days or weeks after initial infection.[10] Secondary lesions usually are smaller than the primary lesion and often are accompanied by fever, myalgia, headache, and fatigue; conjunctivitis and lymphadenopathy also can develop. Aseptic meningitis with clinical evidence of meningeal irritation, such as nuchal rigidity accompanied by a headache, is the presentation in about 1% of patients. Carditis, usually marked by varying degrees of heart block, can occur at this stage, but complete heart block is rare (<1% of patients).

Focal neurologic involvement, in particular cranioneuropathy, is a manifestation of early disseminated infection. The most common sign, paralysis of the facial (7th cranial) nerve, is relatively common in children (3% to 5% of cases) and may be the only manifestation of Lyme disease. Paralysis usually lasts from 2 to 8 weeks and resolves completely. Rarely, palsy resolves partially or not at all. There is no evidence that the clinical course of facial palsy is affected by antimicrobial therapy. Radiculoneuritis, manifested as radicular pain with motor and sensory abnormalities of peripheral nerves, has been reported in children in the U.S., although it is more common among adults and in Europe.

Late Disease

Arthritis, the usual manifestation of late Lyme disease, is the presenting complaint in approximately 7% of children with Lyme disease. Large joints are affected primarily, the knee being involved in more than 90% of cases. Characteristically, the affected joint is swollen, tender, and has an effusion, although pain and limitation of motion usually are modest and are less marked than in other bacterial arthritides. With treatment, the primary episode of arthritis usually abates over 4 to 7 days, with complete resolution over 2 to 6 weeks. Arthritis recurs in approximately 5% to 10% of treated patients and usually resolves with retreatment. In virtually all untreated patients, arthritis recurs, often in other joints, but symptoms and signs eventually resolve even without treatment.[11] Baker cyst is a well-described complication of Lyme arthritis and can occur unilaterally or bilaterally; with or without frank arthritis; and before, during, or after therapy (Figure 185-3).[12–14] An immune-mediated chronic arthritis associated with Lyme disease is rare in adults and is extremely rare in children. Likewise, late manifestations of Lyme disease of the central nervous system have been reported only rarely in children.

LABORATORY FINDINGS AND DIAGNOSIS

Except for erythema migrans, the clinical manifestations of Lyme disease are nonspecific. Erythema migrans can be confused with a number of other skin lesions (ringworm, nummular eczema, cellulitis, granuloma annulare, and insect bites), but its rapid and continuing expansion is distinctive. Lyme meningitis tends to be more prolonged than typical aseptic meningitis due to enteroviruses and papilledema often occurs.[15] Lyme arthritis usually is subacute in onset, with effusion out of proportion to pain or disability, but sometimes it can mimic acute pyogenic arthritis.

Routine laboratory tests rarely aid diagnosis of Lyme disease, because most laboratory abnormalities also are nonspecific. Not uncommonly, mild cerebrospinal fluid pleocytosis can be found in patients with facial nerve palsy despite the absence of clinical manifestations of meningitis.[16]

Isolation of *B. burgdorferi* in a specimen from a symptomatic patient is diagnostic of Lyme disease; however, appropriate medium is expensive, time to isolation can be 4 weeks, and sensitivity of culture is poor. In addition, an invasive procedure is required to obtain appropriate material for culture. Diagnostic tests based on the identification of either antigens or DNA of *B. burgdorferi*, including the polymerase chain reaction, suffer from similar problems in addition to the substantial risk of a false-positive result because of contamination. Consequently, laboratory diagnosis of Lyme disease usually rests on detection of antibodies to *B. burgdorferi*.[17]

Typical antibody responses to acute infection with *B. burgdorferi* are well described. Specific immunoglobulin (Ig) M antibody appears 3 to 4 weeks after infection begins, peaks by 6 to 8 weeks, and subsequently declines. However, prolonged (years) elevation of IgM antibodies despite clinical cure is not unusual.[18] Specific IgG antibody usually appears 4 to 8 weeks after onset of infection, peaks 3 to 6 months later, and can remain elevated indefinitely after cure of infection.[18,19] Effective antimicrobial therapy may or may not be associated with a decline in specific IgG or IgM antibody level.[18,19]

Enzyme immunoassay (EIA) is the most widely used procedure for the detection of antibodies against *B. burgdorferi*. The procedure is associated with false-positive results because of cross-reactive antibodies in patients with other spirochetal infections (e.g., syphilis, leptospirosis, or relapsing fever), certain viral infections (e.g., varicella), certain autoimmune diseases (e.g., systemic lupus erythematosus), or from antibodies that cross-react with spirochetes of normal oral flora. The immunoblot test (Western blot) is used to detect serum antibodies against specific proteins of *B. burgdorferi*. Because many uninfected patients have

antibodies against certain proteins of *B. burgdorferi* (especially against the 41-kd flagellar protein), guidelines have been established for diagnosing Lyme disease with the immunoblot test.[1,17] Currently, a two-tier approach to diagnose Lyme disease is recommended, beginning with a sensitive EIA and, if that result is either positive or equivocal, then a Western blot to validate the result.[17,20] Western blot tests generally should not be ordered alone. A one-step EIA assay (VIsE C6) for IgG antibody to the variable major protein-like sequence-expressed (VlsE) sixth invariant region (C6) has good sensitivity but is somewhat less specific than the two-step approach for determining the presence of specific antibody.[21] Additional studies are needed before it can be used routinely to replace two-step testing.

Antibody test results often are negative in patients with early infection, such as those with a single erythema migrans lesion, since the lesion often precedes detectability of specific antibody. Persons with disseminated or late Lyme disease virtually always have a strong IgG response to *B. burgdorferi*. Antibody response against erythema migrans can be abrogated if invading organisms are killed when patients are treated early in the course of infection.

There are multiple pitfalls in performance and interpretation of serologic test results for Lyme disease. The commercially produced kits in wide use have poor specificity, standardization, and reproducibility.[22] In addition, some commercial laboratories are performing tests for Lyme disease by using assays the accuracy and clinical usefulness of which have not been established.[23] Serologic tests performed in several reference laboratories throughout the U.S. are relatively accurate, with good sensitivity and specificity. However, the predictive value of a positive result, even of a Western blot, depends primarily on the pretest likelihood (on the basis of the clinical and epidemiologic history and the results of the physical examination) that the patient's problem is due to Lyme disease. Although nonspecific, subjective symptoms such as fatigue, arthralgia, or headache can accompany Lyme disease, such widely prevalent symptoms alone, in the absence of a specific objective sign of infection such as erythema migrans, facial nerve palsy, or arthritis, almost never signify Lyme disease. Positive antibody test results in such patients are almost always false-positive results.[24,25] Such nonspecific symptoms may be due to a variety of causes, including fibromyalgia or medically unexplained symptoms.[26,27]

Serologic tests for Lyme disease, even those performed by reference laboratories, should be performed selectively to confirm specific clinical findings suggestive of Lyme disease. A positive serologic test result for Lyme antibody does not necessarily denote active infection. It may reflect previous asymptomatic infection or previously cured clinical infection.[17–19] Test results generally cannot be used to assess either activity of or relapse of past infection.

TREATMENT AND OUTCOMES

Antimicrobial treatment of Lyme disease is highly effective; expert guidelines for management are published.[28] Box 185-2 lists the recommended therapy for children with Lyme disease. Children younger than 8 years are not treated with doxycycline because it may permanently discolor teeth. Patients who are treated with doxycycline should be alerted to the risk of drug-related, sun-induced dermatitis.

Some patients experience a Jarisch–Herxheimer reaction within 48 hours after treatment, which occurs as a result of bacteriolysis and release of cellular products. Symptoms of fever, sweating, and myalgia resolve spontaneously within 1 to 3 days. Treatment with nonsteroidal anti-inflammatory agents may be useful in treating Jarisch–Herxheimer reaction as well as myalgia, arthralgia, headache, and other symptoms of Lyme disease; duration of anti-inflammatory therapy is determined empirically.

Cefuroxime is preferable to a macrolide as an alternative for patients for whom both doxycycline and amoxicillin are contraindicated. There is little need for new agents because the results of treatment with standard therapy (e.g., amoxicillin or doxycycline)

BOX 185-2. Antimicrobial Treatment of Lyme Borreliosis[25]

EARLY DISEASE

- **Erythema migrans and early disseminated disease**

  Doxycycline, 4 mg/kg/day divided bid (maximum 100 mg/dose) for 14 days (range: 10–21 days; do not use in children <8 years) or amoxicillin, 50 mg/kg/day divided tid (maximum 500 mg/dose) for 14 days (range: 10–21 days)

  Alternative agent for those who cannot take either amoxicillin or doxycycline: cefuroxime axetil (preferred), 30–50 mg/kg/day divided bid (maximum 500 mg/dose) or erythromycin, 50 mg/kg/day divided qid (maximum 250 mg/dose) or clarithromycin, 15 mg/kg/day divided bid (maximum 500 mg/dose) all for same duration as above or azithromycin, 10 mg/kg/day (maximum 500 mg/dose) in a single daily dose for 7–10 days

- **Seventh nerve palsy or palsy of other cranial nerves**

  Treat as for erythema migrans for 14–21 days (doxycycline preferred if possible); do not use corticosteroids

- **Carditis**

  First- or second-degree heart block: same treatment as above

  Third-degree heart block: treat as for meningitis

- **Meningitis**[a]

  Ceftriaxone, 75–100 mg/kg/day in a single daily dose (maximum 2 g) for 14 days (range: 14–28 days administered IV or IM) or cefotaxime, 150–200 mg/kg/day (maximum 6 g/day) divided q8h administered IV for 14 days (range: 14–28 days) or penicillin G, 200,000–400,000 units/kg/day (maximum 20 million units/day) divided q4h administered IV for 14–28 days

LATE DISEASE

- **Neurologic (central or peripheral nervous system)**[b]

  Same as for meningitis

- **Arthritis**

  Initial treatment is the same as for erythema migrans, except treatment should be given for 28 days; if swelling fails to resolve after 2 months or there is a recurrence, consider a second course of oral therapy, or use parenteral therapy and treat as for meningitis

[a]There is evidence that oral doxycycline is as effective as IV ceftriaxone to treat Lyme meningitis.[52]

[b]For isolated palsy of the facial nerve or other cranial nerves (see above).

have been excellent.[10,28] Reinfection after treatment of localized erythema migrans can occur, but is rare after either early disseminated or late Lyme disease. Clinicians should also keep in mind the possibility of coinfection with pathogens (*Babesia microti* and *Anaplasma phagocytophilum*) that are also transmitted by *Ixodes* ticks.

A growing body of literature indicates that the outcomes for persons with Lyme disease who receive conventional antimicrobial treatment is excellent.[10,28–34] The most common reason for "failure" of treatment of Lyme disease is that the diagnosis was erroneous.[22,24,25,35–38] Although patients with Lyme disease who are successfully treated may have fatigue, arthralgia, or myalgia that resolves over weeks to months after completion of therapy, there is little evidence that such symptoms are related to persistence of the organism. Repeated courses of antimicrobial agents do not speed the resolution of persistent musculoskeletal pain, neurocognitive symptoms, dysesthesia, or fatigue.[28,38–41] Misinterpretation of the cause of persistent symptoms or of antibody test results, augmented by inaccurate information on the internet and in the lay press,[42] has led to unfounded anxiety about the long-term consequences of Lyme disease among both the public and physicians.

SPECIAL CONSIDERATION: CONGENITAL LYME DISEASE

Because another spirochete, *Treponema pallidum*, is transmissible transplacentally, there is concern that *B. burgdorferi* could be transmitted from an infected pregnant woman to her fetus. Case reports have documented isolation of *B. burgdorferi* from abortuses and infection in a few liveborn infants with congenital anomalies, but placentas, abortuses, and tissue in which the spirochete was identified did not show histologic evidence of inflammation. In addition, no consistent pattern of congenital malformation has been observed, unlike with other diseases due to intrauterine infections.

Two serosurveys conducted in endemic areas found no difference in the prevalence of congenital malformations among women who tested seropositive versus seronegative for *B. burgdorferi*. In the largest study of Lyme disease in pregnancy, investigators prospectively observed 2000 pregnant women in Westchester County, New York, 79 of whom had Lyme disease according to history or serologic test results. Although the number of infected women was relatively small (15 had Lyme disease during the pregnancy), no association was found between maternal exposure to *B. burgdorferi* before conception or during pregnancy and fetal death, prematurity, or congenital malformations.[43] An extensive survey of 162 pediatric neurologists in endemic areas revealed that none had observed a clinically significant neurologic disorder either attributable to congenital Lyme disease or after Lyme disease during pregnancy.[44]

There is no definite evidence that *B. burgdorferi* causes congenital disease. If congenital Lyme disease exists, it is extremely rare. Pregnant women with Lyme disease should be treated as stage and severity of illness dictate (although doxycycline is contraindicated). Transmission of *B. burgdorferi* through breastfeeding has not been documented.

PREVENTION

In areas where deer ticks are prevalent, children are commonly bitten. The overall risk of acquiring Lyme disease is approximately 1% to 3% in areas where the disease is highly endemic.[45–47] The risk of becoming infected is greater if the tick is in the nymphal stage and is engorged when discovered (indicating substantial feeding time, which is necessary for transmission of the organism to occur). Treatment of infection, if it develops, is highly effective. Consequently, routine administration of antimicrobial prophylaxis after a deer tick bite is not recommended.[28,48] On the other hand, in endemic areas of the Northeast or the Upper Midwest in the U.S., if the tick is reliably identified as either a nymphal or an adult deer tick that is engorged and the child is ≥8 years of age, treatment with a single dose (4 mg/kg up to 200 mg maximum) of doxycycline (administered with food to minimize nausea) may be indicated.[46–48] The routine testing of ticks that have been removed from humans for infection with *B. burgdorferi* also is not recommended, because the sensitivity, specificity and predictive values of the results of such tests on ticks for predicting infection of the human who was bitten are unknown. Hypersensitivity reactions to tick products frequently result in erythematous or nodular lesions <2 cm in diameter that do not expand and should not be misinterpreted as erythema migrans. Topical antimicrobial treatment of a tick bite has successfully prevented dissemination of infection in an animal model but has not been tested in humans.[49]

A reasonable approach to avoiding Lyme disease consists of: (1) wearing appropriate protective clothing (such as lightweight long pants tucked into socks) when entering tick-infested areas; (2) checking for ticks after spending time in such areas; and (3) removing them promptly.[50,51] Insect repellents also may provide temporary protection.

Antibodies against the OspA protein protect against Lyme disease in animal models. A recombinant OspA vaccine was licensed for persons 15 to 70 years of age,[8] but it was removed from the market in 2002 by the manufacturer because of poor sales.

186 Other *Borrelia* Species and *Spirillum minus*
Eugene D. Shapiro

BORRELIA SPECIES (RELAPSING FEVER)

Microbiology

Members of the genus *Borrelia* are microaerophilic spirochetal bacteria characterized morphologically by coarse and irregularly shaped coils, with a cell wall and an inner cytoplasmic membrane, between which are multiple flagella that provide a corkscrew-like motility. Substantially thicker than the *Treponema* spp., *Borrelia* spp. stain easily with aniline or acid dyes and can be visualized on light microscopy in Wright- or Giemsa-stained blood smears. Isolation of the organism is difficult, requiring special media, and growth is slow.[1]

Borrelia spp. can change the antigenic structure of their surface proteins by transposition of structural genes on a linear plasmid.[2] This ability allows them temporarily to elude host defenses, resulting in "relapsing fever" in infected humans.[3,4] The resolution of symptomatic stages of the illness correlates with peak concentrations of antibodies against specific antigens.[5] Borreliae cause vasculitis, with a predilection for capillaries and small arterioles of any organs, especially the reticuloendothelial system, bone marrow, and central nervous system.

Epidemiology

Ticks and lice are vectors that transmit the bacterium to humans. Epidemiology of the disease is determined by environmental conditions conducive to vectors and, in the case of the ticks, to contact with humans.[6] Risk factors, organisms, and vectors associated with each form of disease are shown in Table 186-1.

Louse-borne relapsing fever, caused by *Borrelia recurrentis*, is transmitted by the body louse, *Pediculus humanas*. Crab lice (*Phthirus pubis*) cannot transmit this organism. There is no animal reservoir for *B. recurrentis*; its existence depends on human-to-human transmission by lice. Bacteria multiply in the hemolymph of the louse, but infected fluid is not inoculated into humans. Human infection occurs when the louse is crushed (usually inadvertently) and the organisms come in contact with skin or mucous membranes. Infection with *B. recurrentis* is associated with crowding and poor hygiene; epidemics are associated with war, famine, and natural disasters such as earthquakes. A major epidemic of

louseborne recurrent fever occurred in Europe during World War II. The disease is endemic in Ethiopia and Sudan. Infection with *B. recurrentis* is virtually unknown in the United States.

Tickborne relapsing fever, caused by a number of species of *Borrelia*, is transmitted by soft ticks of the genus *Ornithodoros*. Many small animals (chipmunks, rats, mice, squirrels, and others) serve as reservoirs for *Borrelia* spp. and as hosts for *Ornithodoros* ticks. There is variable transovarial transmission of bacteria to larval ticks, and an enzootic cycle is well established in certain areas of the U.S. Ticks thrive in warm, humid environments and at altitudes from 1500 to 6500 feet (450 to 2000 meters).

Unlike hard ixodid ticks that transmit *B. burgdorferi* only after feeding for days, soft ticks feed for less than an hour yet are able to transmit *Borrelia* during this relatively brief period. Transmission occurs via inoculation of saliva from an infected tick. Ticks often feed at night and the human host rarely is aware of the bite, which may be associated with up to a 50% risk of disease if the tick is infected. Unlike with louseborne recurrent fever, humans are incidental hosts for bacteria that cause tickborne relapsing fever. Humans become infected when they enter environments in which the ticks thrive, such as old cabins and caves. Tickborne recurrent fever has a worldwide distribution. The disease is endemic in parts of East Africa, Asia, and South America. Most cases in the U.S. occur in rural areas in the Western states. Outbreaks have occurred among tourists staying in log cabins at Western parks and among spelunkers.[7–9]

Clinical Manifestations

Tickborne and louseborne relapsing fevers are indistinguishable from each other clinically, although louseborne disease tends to have fewer (though more severe) recurrences.[10–15] Exact time of exposure usually is unknown, because lice typically cause chronic infestations and the bites of ticks often are unrecognized. Symptoms begin 5 to 10 days after exposure, with sudden onset of fever and chills usually accompanied by headache, myalgia, arthralgia, photophobia, and cough. Common physical findings include petechiae or frank purpura, conjunctivitis, and abdominal tenderness (often with an enlarged and tender liver or spleen). Nuchal rigidity often occurs,[16] and some patients have jaundice, epistaxis, or gastrointestinal hemorrhage. This phase of the illness is associated with bacteremia, usually lasts for 3 to 7 days, and resolves spontaneously.

During the next (crisis) phase, patients are afebrile or have low-grade fever and may have a diffuse maculopapular rash. Diaphoresis, extreme fatigue, and, occasionally, hypotension characterize this phase. Borreliae are not found in the blood but presumably are present in organs such as the spleen and liver, where antigenically variant strains propagate.

The relapse phase of illness, which typically occurs 5 to 7 days after primary spirochetemia resolves, is marked by rapid onset of high fever and chills as well as the other signs and symptoms of the initial spirochetemic phase. In untreated patients, three to five relapses are typical (though many more are possible) in tickborne infections, and up to two or three relapses occur in louseborne infections. Relapsing fever usually resolves even in untreated patients, although deaths have occurred. During some epidemics, mortality rates as high as 20% to 30% have been reported; poor general health and poor nutrition may be responsible. Severe hepatitis, lobar pneumonia, myocarditis,

TABLE 186-1. Causes of *Borrelia* Relapsing Fever

Vector	Bacteria	Risk Factors
LOUSE		
Pediculus humanus	*B. recurrentis*	Crowding, poverty, war, famine
TICK		
Ornithodoros ticks[a]	*B. duttoni*[b]	Exposure to environments in which rodents thrive: old cabins, caves, primitive huts
O. hermsi	*B. hermsii*	
O. parkeri	*B. parkeri*	
O. tholozani	*B. persica*	
O. talaje	*B. mazzottii*	

[a]These are only some of the many species that are vectors for relapsing fever.

[b]These are only some of the many species that cause relapsing fever.

ruptured spleen, and cerebral hemorrhage are rare causes of death. Pregnant women who become infected often have spontaneous abortion, in most instances because of thrombocytopenia and retroplacental hemorrhage. Long-term sequelae are uncommon among survivors, although iridocyclitis can result in scars and impairment of vision.

Laboratory Findings and Diagnosis

Laboratory abnormalities are nonspecific. Leukocytosis (with a left shift) and a markedly elevated erythrocyte sedimentation rate are typical. Cerebrospinal fluid often is abnormal, usually with 10 to 2000 predominantly mononuclear white blood cells per mm^3, elevated protein, and normal glucose concentrations.

Awareness of epidemiology is crucial to making the diagnosis. Louseborne relapsing fever usually occurs in epidemics at times of unstable social conditions; in those circumstances, the symptoms are rarely confused with those of any other condition except epidemic typhus, which also is transmitted by the body louse. By contrast, except in certain developing countries, tickborne relapsing fever is uncommon and occurs sporadically. For patients with compatible symptoms, history of recent exposure to old cabins, caves, or other environments in which rodents reside should lead to consideration of relapsing fever.

Culture is an insensitive method for confirming diagnosis, which is best made by examination of peripheral blood during febrile episodes by using darkfield microscopy, Wright or Giemsa staining.[17] Diagnostic yield may be enhanced by staining of a smear with acridine orange and use of fluorescence microscopy. Polymerase chain reaction assay is a promising diagnostic test but is not available generally.[18]

Treatment

Tetracycline (500 mg/dose administered four times a day) or doxycycline (2 mg/kg/day divided into 2 doses with maximum dose of 100 mg twice a day) are the drugs of choice for relapsing fever.[10,15] Treatment is administered for 7 to 10 days; however, for louseborne relapsing fever, 100 mg of doxycycline or 500 mg of either tetracycline or erythromycin given once orally has been effective.[19–21] In children younger than 8 years, erythromycin (30 to 50 mg/kg/day divided into 4 doses) is preferred, although penicillin also is effective.

If vomiting is severe, the initial dose of the antimicrobial agent can be administered intravenously, although a severe Jarisch–Herxheimer reaction can occur. This reaction, marked by rigors, increased fever, and, in severe cases, hypotension, typically occurs within a few hours after initiation of antimicrobial therapy and cannot be prevented by prior administration of corticosteroid. Nonsteroidal anti-inflammatory medications and, in severe instances, intravenously administered fluids have been used for treatment of this reaction.

Prevention

The primary means of preventing relapsing fever consists of control and avoidance of vectors that transmit the disease. Ticks that transmit relapsing fever are dispersed widely throughout the world. The use of insecticides around the inner walls of primitive buildings and huts (where ticks often are found) in developing countries has reduced the frequency of disease.[22] Postexposure chemoprophylaxis with 5 days of doxycycline was highly effective in persons thought to be at high risk after a tick bite.[23] The risk of louseborne disease can be controlled through good personal hygiene and prompt treatment if an infestation occurs.

SPIRILLUM MINUS (RAT-BITE FEVER)

Spirillum minus, a short spiral bacterium, is one cause of rat-bite fever.[24–28] *S. minus* is more common in Asia than in the U.S. and elsewhere in North America, where most cases of rat-bite fever are caused by *Streptobacillus moniliformis*. In Japan, the disease is known as *sodoku* (so, "rat"; *doku*, "poison").

S. minus is a tightly coiled, gram-negative spiral bacillus. Infection is due to inoculation during the bite of a rat. Up to one-fourth of rats are colonized with *S. minus* in sputum, conjunctiva, blood, or nasopharynx. Unlike streptobacillary rat-bite fever, *S. minus* infection has not followed ingestion of the organism. Transmission of infection between humans does not occur.

One to 4 weeks after the bite, patients have abrupt onset of fever, chills, and headache, usually in association with an inflamed, tender, ulcerated wound at the site of the rat bite. Typically, the wound, which had healed previously, ulcerates concurrently with onset of systemic symptoms. Musculoskeletal symptoms (arthralgia or myalgia) are less common in infections due to *S. minus* than in streptobacillary rat-bite fever. Most patients have a generalized red or purple macular rash that can be urticarial. The rash, usually prominent during the first week of illness and during febrile periods, may fade with resolution of symptoms. In untreated patients, high fever and systemic symptoms last for 3 to 7 days, remit, and recur 3 to 10 days later, followed by recurring cycles for 3 to 8 weeks. In severe cases, pneumonia, meningitis, myocarditis, or (especially in patients with pre-existing valvular disease) endocarditis can develop.

S. minus has not been cultivated on artificial media but can be identified on darkfield microscopy and, occasionally, in Wright- or Giemsa-stained smears of peripheral blood. There is no serologic test. Organisms can be identified in the blood of a guinea pig 2 to 3 weeks after intraperitoneal inoculation of infected blood.

S. minus is exquisitely susceptible to penicillin. Excellent response is expected with the use of procaine penicillin given intramuscularly (20,000 to 50,000 units/kg once daily), penicillin G given intravenously, or penicillin V given orally (1 to 2 g/day divided into 3 doses).[24–26] Streptomycin and tetracycline are effective altrnative agents. Therapy is given for 10 to 14 days.

187 Anaerobic Bacteria: Classification, Normal Flora, and Clinical Concepts

Itzhak Brook and Sarah S. Long

CLASSIFICATION

Anaerobic bacteria predominate in normal skin and the bacterial flora of mucous membranes.[1,2] Infections caused by anaerobic bacteria are common, arise from the sites where they are normal flora (endogenous) and can be serious or life-threatening. Anaerobic bacteria are fastidious, difficult to isolate, and often overlooked. Their recovery requires proper methods of collection, transportation, and cultivation.[3–6] Their ubiquity on mucocutaneous surfaces often interferes with obtaining meaningful cultures.

TABLE 187-1. Classification of Microorganisms by Conditions of Replication

Class	Requirement for Replication	Examples
Strict anaerobe	Requires reduced oxygen tension; does not replicate on agar surface in air or 10% CO_2	*Bacteroides, Prevotella, Peptostreptococcus,* and *Fusobacterium* spp.
Microaerophilic organism	Replicates poorly on agar surface in presence of oxygen but distinctly grows better under 10% CO_2 in air or anaerobically	Most streptococci of normal oropharyngeal flora
Facultative anaerobe	Replicates in presence or absence of oxygen	Groups A, B, and C streptococci, *Streptococcus pneumoniae, Staphylococcus* spp., *Escherichia coli*
Strict aerobe	Replicates only in presence of oxygen	Most *Pseudomonas* and *Mycobacterium* spp.

TABLE 187-2. Genera of Clinically Significant Anaerobic Bacteria

GRAM-NEGATIVE BACILLI	NONSPORE-FORMING GRAM-POSITIVE BACILLI
Bacteroides (*B. fragilis* group and others)	*Actinomyces*
Fusobacterium	*Arcanobacterium*
Porphyromonas	*Bifidobacterium*
Prevotella	*Eubacterium*
Other Bacteroidaceae (Bilophila, Centipeda, Leptotrichia, Mobiluncus, Seleonomonas, Sutterella)	*Lactobacillus*
	Propionibacterium
Campylobacter	**ENDOSPORE-FORMING GRAM-POSITIVE BACILLI**
	Clostridium
GRAM-NEGATIVE COCCI	**GRAM-POSITIVE COCCI**
Veillonella	*Gemella*
	Parvimonas
	Peptococcus
	Peptostreptococcus
	Ruminococcus
	Staphylococcus (*S. saccharolyticus*)
	Streptococcus[a] (*S. anginosus, S. constellatus, S. intermedius*)

[a]*Microaerophilic streptococci.*

Although there is no universally accepted or simple and accurate way to classify microorganisms according to conditions required for their replication, Table 187-1 presents a useful framework for the clinician. Nevertheless, differences between strains exist within the same species.

Anaerobic bacteria do not replicate in the presence of oxygen; however, they exhibit substantial differences in lethal effect of oxygen. In general, anaerobic organisms found exclusively as normal flora are strict anaerobes (i.e., die within minutes in <0.5% oxygen), whereas those of clinical significance are somewhat aerotolerant (i.e., tolerate 2% to 8% oxygen). Strict anaerobes do not grow in 10% CO_2 in air; microaerophilic bacteria can grow in 10% CO_2 in air or under aerobic or anaerobic conditions, and facultative organisms can grow in the presence or absence of air. The physiologic basis for oxygen sensitivity is not well understood. Common teaching is that negative oxidation-reduction potential (Eh) of the environment is the critical factor. However, studies with *Bacteroides fragilis* reveal that oxygen has a direct toxic effect; chemical manipulation of oxidation-reduction potential has no effect if oxygen is not introduced. Furthermore, aerotolerance, and possibly virulence, of anaerobic bacteria correlates with ability to induce the protective enzyme superoxide dismutase on exposure to oxygen.[4]

Although Louis Pasteur is credited with discovery of the first true anaerobe, *Clostridium butyricum* in 1861,[4] and Altemeier[7] made landmark observations of their importance in intra-abdominal infections in the 1930s, major advances occurred in the 1960s with the increased ability to isolate and classify these bacteria and the potential to treat related infections.

The clinically important anaerobic genera are shown in Table 187-2. The taxonomy of anaerobic bacteria has changed because of improved characterization through the use of genetic studies.[3,5] The ability to differentiate between similar strains enables better characterization of the type of infection and prediction of antimicrobial susceptibility. The genera/groups most frequently isolated from clinical infections, in descending order of frequency, are: *Bacteroides* spp., *Peptostreptococcus* spp., *Clostridium* spp., *Fusobacterium* spp., gram-positive bacilli, and gram-negative cocci.[2,3]

The use of DNA technology (e.g., determination of DNA G+C mol%, ribosomal RNA homology, gel electrophoresis sequencing) and chemotaxonomic analyses (e.g., analysis of peptidoglycans, gas–liquid chromatography of whole-cell fatty acids) has enlightened taxonomic relationships among anaerobic bacteria. Wide-ranging taxonomic changes have affected the family Bacteroidaceae and anaerobic gram-positive cocci. *Bacteroides melaninogenicus*, a single species until 1977, now encompasses two genera (*Prevotella*

and *Porphyromonas*) and >15 species.[8] Minor changes have been made in the classification of gram-positive bacilli, and the genus *Eubacterium* remains heterogeneous and inadequately examined.

INDIGENOUS FLORA

Establishment and Composition of Normal Flora

Frequency of recovery of anaerobic bacteria as normal flora varies by body site and age and so also does their importance in site-related infections. Table 187-3 shows sites of colonization of clinically important anaerobic bacteria. Mucocutaneous surfaces in humans have a complex indigenous flora composed of anaerobic, microaerophilic, facultative, and aerobic bacteria. Flora is remarkably predictable within days after birth, depending on type of delivery, feeding, and receipt of antibiotics.[9] Successive colonization of the gut simulates that in germ-free laboratory animals after exposure to peers.[10] Facultative organisms, such as oral streptococci, intestinal *Escherichia coli*, and skin staphylococci, precede anaerobic species, but by the end of the first few weeks of life, flora is complex and predictable. Infants fed human milk exclusively have a relatively simple, fermentative gut flora with predominance of *Bifidobacterium*, fewer *Bacteroides* and facultative gram-negative bacilli, and *Enterococcus* spp., whereas infants fed cow's milk have putrefactive flora similar to that of adults, with gram-negative anaerobic and facultative bacilli predominating.[11,12] Early colonization at <3 weeks with *B. fragilis* has been associated with risk of asthma at a later age.[11a] There is remarkable perturbation of gut flora at weaning from human milk,[13] and disruption of flora occurs with use of antibiotics, especially in infancy.

Colonization of the mouth similarly is rapid and predictable. Viridans streptococci and *Streptococcus salivarius* are present and predominate, usually within 12 hours after birth, with successive representation by facultatively anaerobic *Neisseria* and *Staphylococcus* spp. and then anaerobic streptococci, *Veillonella*, and *Bifidobacterium* spp. on the second day.[14–16] Nasopharyngeal and oropharyngeal *Streptococcus pneumoniae*, nontypable *Haemophilus influenzae*, and *Moraxella catarrhalis* follow and remain as facultative flora throughout childhood. *Prevotella melaninogenica* becomes predominant at gingival crevices, seemingly under hormonal influences, at puberty.[14,15] Predominant oral flora are *Prevotella, Porphyromonas, Fusobacterium*, and non-*fragilis Bacteroides* species.

Colonization of skin varies by site and age.[16,17] Coagulase-negative staphylococci (or *Staphylococcus aureus* in nurseries where it is prevalent) appear, followed by Enterobacteriaceae at diapered sites. *Propionibacterium acnes* becomes the dominant anaerobe, quantitatively accounting for almost one-half of cultivable flora at

TABLE 187-3. Selected Anaerobic Bacteria of Normal Flora

Bacteria	Body Site (Ratio of Total Anaerobic:Aerobic Flora)[a]					
	Mouth (1000:1)	Upper Respiratory Tract (4:1)	Upper Intestine (1:1)	Lower Intestine (1000:1)	Lower Genitourinary Tract (5:1)	Skin (2:1)
GRAM-POSITIVE BACILLI						
Actinomyces spp.	+	+	±	+	±	
Bifidobacterium spp.	+	+	±	++	+	
Eubacterium spp.	+	±		+	+	±
Lactobacillus spp.	+			++	++	
Propionibacterium spp.	+	+	±	+	+	++
Clostridium perfringens, C. ramosum			±	++	+	
GRAM-POSITIVE COCCI						
Gemella spp.	++	+		+	+	
Peptostreptococcus spp.	++	++	+	++	++	+
Streptococcus anginosus, S. constellatus, S. intermedius	++	+				
GRAM-NEGATIVE BACILLI						
Bacteroides fragilis	±	±	±	++	±	
Bacteroides spp. (other)	+	+	±	++	++	
Fusobacterium spp.	++	+	±	+	+	
Porphyromonas spp.	++	+		+	++	
Prevotella melaninogenica	++	++		+	++	
Prevotella spp. (other)	++	+		+	++	
Wolinella spp.	+	+		+		±
GRAM-NEGATIVE COCCI						
Veillonella spp.	++	+	±	+	++	

±, irregularly present; +, usually present; ++, usually present in large numbers.

[a]Mouth includes gingiva, teeth, saliva, anterior mucosa; upper respiratory tract includes nasal passages, nasopharynx, oropharynx, and tonsils; upper intestine includes duodenum, jejunum, mid-ileum; lower intestine includes lower ileum, colon, rectum; lower genitourinary tract includes vagina, urethra, genital skin in adults.

Data from Shah,[8] Hentges,[16] and Finegold SM. Anaerobic bacteria: their role in infection and their management. Postgrad Med 1987;81:141–148.

most anatomic sites; anaerobic cocci also are important. Anaerobic bacteria predominate in vaginal flora, even prepubertally, with gram-positive bacilli and cocci and *Prevotella* highly represented.[18]

Clostridium ramosum and *C. perfringens* are dominant clostridial species in intestinal flora. *Clostridium difficile* is found in only 1% to 4% of healthy adults and children >6 months of age. Finding of asymptomatic colonization in up to 60% of infants in neonatal intensive care units in occasional studies probably reflects unusual nosocomial phenomena.[19]

The qualitative and quantitative complexity of flora and the difficulty of its study cannot be overestimated. Within the mouth, for example, the gingival crevice has an oxidation-reduction potential of −300 mV (similar to that in the colon); the ratio of anaerobes to aerobes is 1000:1, yet saliva and teeth have ratios closer to 1:1. The normal flora of the colon contain more than 500 obligate anaerobic species in a total concentration of 10^{11} to 10^{12} colony-forming units (CFU) per gram of feces and most are unculturable.[20] The predominant gram-negative anaerobes are *Bacteroides* and *Fusobacterium* spp. Although <0.1% of normal flora consists of facultative or aerobic organisms (e.g., 10^8 CFU/g of feces), ease of recovery from endogenous infections has led to overestimation of their importance in the microbial ecology of the gut. Similarly, there is an erroneous tendency to focus on the clinically most significant anaerobic bacteria as critical in ecology. *B. fragilis*, for example, is quantitatively among the least important species of the *Bacteroides* group in normal flora. Animal models and continuous-flow in vitro culture models have been established to study microbial ecology, mechanisms of microbial interaction, and the importance of microbes in health; studies are painstaking, and conclusions are difficult to establish.[21]

Anaerobes reach a concentration of 10^6 organism/mL in vaginal secretions, with predominance of *Prevotella*, *Bacteroides*,

Fusobacterium, and *Clostridium* spp. Anaerobes isolated most commonly from clinical specimens are *Prevotella bivia* and *P. disiens*.[16]

Role of Indigenous Flora

Multiple observations support the theory that indigenous, especially anaerobic, flora provide resistance to colonization and invasion by nonindigenous microorganisms. Anaerobic bacteria that make up most of the endogenous gastrointestinal, vaginal, and oral flora possess interference capabilities. Ability to interfere with potential pathogens has been observed in *B. fragilis*, *Prevotella oralis*, *Peptostreptococcus anaerobius*, *Veillonella* spp., and *Bifidobacterium* spp. A few such observations follow:

1. Infants in an intensive care nursery are at higher risk of pharyngeal colonization with potentially pathogenic organisms if they are not colonized initially with viridans streptococci.[15]
2. Children who are colonized with group A streptococcus (GAS), have recurrent GAS tonsillitis, or have recurrent otitis media or sinusitis are less likely to have inhibitory facultative (α-hemolytic streptococci) and anaerobic (*Prevotella* and *Peptostreptococcus* spp.) oropharyngeal flora.[22]
3. *Propionibacterium* spp. hydrolyze triglycerides, thus producing free fatty acids that are inhibitory to GAS and *S. aureus*.[16]
4. Primary metabolic byproducts of anaerobes, volatile fatty acids, inhibit the multiplication of nonindigenous organisms in the intestine.[16]
5. *Lactobacillus* spp. produce hydrogen peroxide, which is bactericidal for *P. bivia* and *Gardnerella vaginalis* (agents of bacterial vaginosis); presence in vaginal flora is inversely related.[23]
6. Susceptibility of germ-free mice to colonization and outgrowth of *Clostridium botulinum* can be manipulated

dramatically by selective colonization, especially with anaerobic flora.[24]

7. Infant botulism occurs exclusively in the first year of life, especially at the time of perturbation of anaerobic gut flora at weaning.[13]

8. *C. difficile* pseudomembranous colitis is highly associated with the use of antibiotics. Protection from colonization or cure of disease can be afforded animals and humans by intestinal administration of fecal organisms or *Lactobacillus*.[25–27]

9. Experimental infectivity of *Salmonella* or *Shigella* spp. is enhanced by pretreatment of animals with antibiotics; infectivity is reduced when germ-free animals are fed mixed cultures of pathogens with anaerobic bacteria.[28]

10. Susceptibility of children <2 years of age to all enteric pathogens correlates with the relative ease of disruption of indigenous flora.

11. In a double-blind, placebo-controlled trial, infants 5 to 24 months old who were admitted to a chronic care facility and whose formula was supplemented with *Bifidobacterium bifidum* and *Streptococcus thermophilus* had significantly less diarrhea and shedding of rotavirus.[29]

12. Prophylactic administration of a probiotic mixture of *Lactobacillus acidophilus* and *Bifidobacterium infantis* given to very-low-birthweight infants reduced the incidence of all cases of necrotizing enterocolitis (NEC) as well as severe stage III NEC.[30]

Mechanisms by which normal flora provide resistance to colonization have been reviewed.[22,31,32] They include: (1) production of bacteriocins and other metabolic products, such as volatile fatty acids, that inhibit multiplication of nonindigenous flora at local conditions of pH and oxidation-reduction potential; (2) competition for limited nutrients; and (3) competition for available attachment sites. Host factors undoubtedly provide exquisitely specific microbial niches by means of their unique properties of epithelial surfaces, enzymes, secretory immunoglobulins (Igs), pH, nutrients, exfoliation of skin and mucous membranes, motility of gastrointestinal tract, and mucociliary movement in the respiratory tract. Coliforms are present in oropharyngeal or nasopharyngeal flora of only about 3% of healthy adults[33] and children.[34,35] Severe noninfectious illness, viral infection, malignancy, diabetes, chemotherapy, antibiotic therapy, and antacid therapy affect changes in colonization. Changes in attachment properties of epithelial cells for bacteria in vitro correlate with changes in flora.[36] Relative or absolute increase in nasopharyngeal *S. pneumoniae, H. influenzae,* or *M. catarrhalis* occurs in association with viral illness and acute otitis media, predicting concordant middle ear pathogens in the latter disease.[34,35]

Besides resistance to colonization, normal anaerobic intestinal flora have broadly ranging metabolic effects, mainly through provision of catabolic enzymes for organic compounds that cannot be digested by enzymes of eukaryotic origin. The enzymes are necessary to: (1) process diverse dietary and host polysaccharides thus aiding human digestion;[32a] (2) catabolize cholesterol, bile acids, and steroid hormones; (3) hydrolyze a number of flavonoid glycosides of plant origin to anticarcinogens; and (4) detoxify certain carcinogens and drugs.[37] Erythromycin or tetracycline treatment raises the serum digoxin level 50%, almost certainly by reducing gut *Eubacterium lentum*, which inactivates digoxin through hydrogenation of the double bond of its lactone ring.[38]

Normal flora provide stimulation to the host's immune system from birth onwards. Germ-free animals (and probably heavily antibiotic-exposed infants) have immune defects, such as in production of complement and immunoglobulins, and in reticuloendothelial and lymphoid tissues.[34a] *B. fragilis* zwitterionic polysaccharide A regulates an immunologic equilibrium in the intestine by balancing colonic Th1 and Th2 T lymphocytes and promotes anti-inflammatory IL-10 production.

Effect of Antimicrobial Agents

The effect of antibiotics on normal flora is extremely complex and varies with dose and route of administration, spectrum of antimicrobial activity (breadth, potency, and specificity for anaerobes), and chemical and pharmacokinetic properties. Clinical impact depends on duration of antibiotic use, presence and severity of underlying conditions, exposure to nonindigenous pathogens (*Pseudomonas, C. difficile*), and host susceptibility to indigenous and nonindigenous microbes (underlying valvular heart disease, malignancy, surgery, inserted devices, and age). In general, agents that have a major impact on anaerobic flora cause the greatest disruption of homeostasis.

The main determinant of effect on oropharyngeal flora is secretion of the agent in saliva or from mucous membranes, which correlates with lipophilicity. Clindamycin, erythromycin, and rifampin are present in high concentrations; penicillins and ampicillin, despite relatively low concentrations, have potent activity against oral facultative and anaerobic bacteria. Use of β-lactam antibiotics (even penicillin) may not supplant a species from its microbial niche but can select for organisms with reduced antimicrobial susceptibility (*S. pneumoniae,*[39] viridans streptococci)[40] or β-lactamase production (*Moraxella, Prevotella* spp.).[41]

Administration of antimicrobial agents can influence the composition of nasopharyngeal flora.[41,42] The oral flora are depleted of organisms with interference protective potential more with amoxicillin-clavulanate therapy than with a narrower-spectrum agent.[42]

The most profound effects on gut flora occur with administration of agents that have exquisite activity against anaerobic bacteria, which are present in high concentration at the ileal-colonic mucosa. The pharmacodynamics of specific agents is important. Exquisite activity against anaerobes (clindamycin, amoxicillin-clavulanate), high biliary excretion (ceftriaxone, cefoperazone), or use of oral nonabsorbable agents (neomycin, gentamicin) ensures an effect on flora, but high absorption of oral agents does not necessarily predict low colonic concentrations, because antibiotic is delivered to the mucosal site by blood (amoxicillin).[43] Outgrowth of *Enterococcus* and *Candida* spp. occurs rapidly when potent agents have selective nonactivity (aztreonam, ceftriaxone, cefoxitin)[44–47] or poor activity (imipenem) for enterococci.[48] The β-lactamases of certain facultative organisms (the SPACEY group: *Serratia, Pseudomonas, Acinetobacter, Citrobacter, Enterobacter,* and *Yersinia* spp.) can be induced by cefoxitin and several third-generation cephalosporins;[49] β-lactamase production by anaerobes can increase;[50] or resistant nosocomial pathogens can be acquired. Use of broad-spectrum, exquisitely active cephalosporins and other agents with profound effect on normal flora undeniably has changed the incidence, microbiology, and susceptibility of superinfecting microbes in children.[49,51,52] Attempts to reconstitute flora, as with lactobacilli, have an overall positive but uncertain impact.[22,53]

PATHOGENESIS

Anaerobic infections are predictable, because organisms are not intrinsically highly pathogenic. Most anaerobic infections are caused by the host endogenous flora and occur at sites contiguous or related to sites of their normal residence, under permissive or instigating circumstances. Such circumstances include: (1) access to deep tissue through surgery, trauma, tuberculous lesions, endoscopic procedure, right-to-left cardiac shunt, perforation of viscus, or massive aspiration of oropharyngeal flora; (2) impairment of normal clearance of a hollow viscus (obstruction by a foreign body, stricture, tumor, lymph node), decreased patency of a respiratory passage (chronic otitis media and sinusitis), or dysfunctional mucociliary movement, cough, or alveolar macrophage function; and (3) lowering of oxygen-reduction potential through tissue necrosis (surgery, trauma), impairment of blood supply, the presence of infection due to aerobic bacteria or foreign material (aspirated foreign body, sutures, catheter, intrauterine device).

Traditionally defined host susceptibility factors (such as disorders of complement, hypofunction of spleen, human immunodeficiency virus infection, and cellular immune deficiencies) increase risk of infection due to facultative and aerobic pathogens but generally not to anaerobic infections. Severe debilitation, malnutrition, diabetes, corticosteroid use, collagen vascular disease, cytotoxic drugs, neutropenia or neutrophil dysfunction, malignancies, and lymphopenia are associated with anaerobic necrotizing soft-tissue infections and other invasive disease. Certain specific associations have been observed between some underlying diseases and infections involving anaerobic bacteria. They include acatalasemia with oral gangrene, trisomy 21 or human immunodeficiency virus infection with severe periodontal disease, colon cancer and neutropenia with clostridial infection and colitis, and diabetes mellitus with cholecystitis and osteomyelitis.[2,3] In an animal model, T-lymphocyte-mediated responses govern protection from B. fragilis.[54] B. fragilis bacteremia was reported in several children who underwent elective appendectomy at the time of renal transplantation and corticosteroid therapy; infection was correlated with severity of lymphopenia.[55,56]

A few anaerobic infections are of exogenous origin. These include gas gangrene after trauma, C. difficile-associated disease, C. perfringens food poisoning or diarrhea, botulism (including wound botulism), and tetanus and C. botulinum and C. tetani wound infections.

Anaerobes responsible for infection do not always correlate with their quantitative presence in normal flora. B. fragilis, F. necrophorum, F. nucleatum, P. melaninogenica, and Actinomyces israelii are highly overrepresented, implying specific virulence. Bilophila wadsworthia is associated specifically with acute appendicitis,[57] C. septicum with typhlitis and septicemia in hematologic malignancy,[58] Eubacterium and Actinomyces spp. with intrauterine devices,[59] and Peptostreptococcus and Propionibacterium spp. with prosthetic devices,[60] implying specific microbial niches. Additionally, spore-forming anaerobes, C. botulinum, C. difficile, and C. tetani, each produce potent exotoxins that are responsible primarily for disease manifestations.

Virulence factors of anaerobic bacteria have been reviewed;[61] they include the following:

- Promotion of adhesion by capsular polysaccharide and fimbriae (B. fragilis) and lectin (F. nucleatum).
- Invasion by phospholipase C (C. perfringens), lipopolysaccharides (Porphyromonas gingivalis, F. nucleatum, F. necrophorum, Prevotella spp.), and protease (B. fragilis, F. nucleatum, F. necrophorum, Prevotella spp.).
- Tissue infection and damage by multiple exoenzymes, such as fibrinolysin, neuraminidase, heparinase, N-acetylglucosaminidase (B. fragilis, Porphyromonas, and others), and collagenase (C. perfringens).
- Capsular resistance to phagocytosis, macrophage migration, and lysis by IgA protease (B. fragilis, Porphyromonas, Prevotella spp.).[62] The capsule of B. fragilis activates the host CD4+, T lymphocytes, the release of interleukin (IL)-17 and chemokines,[63] and tumor necrotic factor-α and IL-1β from peritoneal macrophages. These cytokines lead to an increase in neutrophil adherence to the mesothelial cells and abscess formation.[64]
- Production of other toxins and enzymes (elastase, hydrolytic enzymes, fibrinolysin, chondroitin sulfatase, lipase, lecithinase, gelatinase, immunoglobulin protease, botulism toxin, tetanolysin, tetanus toxin, neuraminidase, leukocidin), various other leukotoxins (volatile fatty acids, hemolysins, hemagglutinins, lysophospholipase, proteases), endotoxins, deoxyribonuclease (DNase), ribonuclease (RNase), phosphatase, heparinase, other proteases, and other sulfatases.
- Production of metabolites that are harmful to other bacteria, such as volatile fatty acids, sulfur compounds, and amines (most anaerobes).
- Production of lipopolysaccharide (F. necrophorum) that stimulates host-mediated damage.
- Production of superoxide dismutase and catalase that permits aerotolerance.

Certain clinical findings that typify anaerobic infection – such as abscess production (B. fragilis), burrowing through tissue planes (A. israelii), phlebitis, thrombosis, and persistent bacteremia (Bacteroides, Fusobacterium spp.), and putrid purulence – are due to specific components of organisms or their metabolic byproducts.[65] Although Fusobacterium spp. produce biologically active endotoxin, the endotoxins of B. fragilis and P. melaninogenica are chemically different and biologically inactive compared with those of coliforms.

An experimental animal model of intra-abdominal infection and septicemia has been studied extensively, and corollaries in the pathophysiology of human infection have been observed.[66] In summary, intraperitoneal inoculation of cecal contents, with an adjuvant such as barium sulfate or hog mucin, led to death in almost half of animals in the first 4 days after challenge, always from E. coli septicemia (although the inoculum was polymicrobic). All surviving animals later demonstrated abscesses, with predominant isolation of B. fragilis. "Antibiotic probes" confirmed relative bacterial roles; after microbial challenge, administration of clindamycin (which activity excludes E. coli) did not reduce mortality rate compared with untreated animals, but only 5% of the surviving animals had abscess, whereas administration of gentamicin (which activity excludes B. fragilis) reduced the mortality rate to 4%, and 98% of the surviving animals had abscesses. Administration of both antibiotics showed salutary advantages of each. Although these experiments of biphasic intra-abdominal infection suggest separate roles of microorganisms, a synergistic role of anaerobe with anaerobe, and with facultative anaerobe and aerobe is more likely. Synergistic pathogenesis is supported by the observation of complexity of anaerobic infections (average of 3 to 6 microbial species) as well as by unsuccessful attempts to induce singular anaerobic infections in experimental models. The "synergy" provided could be creation of a favourable milieu or pH, provision of an obligatory vitamin, or an enzyme to enhance tissue spread.

Anaerobic bacteria can produce certain growth factors that confer themselves selective advantage or can facilitate synergistic capabilities with other bacteria. These factors include hemin, succinate, menadione, peptides, amino acids, and steroids. Critical study remains elusive; simple therapeutic elimination of the facultative partner or partners does not reliably eradicate existent infection.[61]

CLINICAL CLUES AND APPROACH

Although anaerobic infections overall are not common in children, accounting for <2% of bloodstream infections (BSI) in childhood, certain clinical settings or characteristics of infection are so typical as to make diagnosis of anaerobic infection almost certain (Table 187-4). Equally important, confirmation of an anaerobic infection mandates explanation or investigation for a predisposing event or circumstance. For example, bronchoscopy is indicated for unexplained anaerobic lung abscess or empyema in children (if congenital pulmonary sequestration or cyst is not likely) or to remove a foreign body (despite forgotten or negative history) or obstructing granulation tissue. Repeated pneumonia, bronchiectasis, or hemorrhage otherwise will result.

Intra-abdominal polymicrobic abscess in children is almost always due to subacute ruptured appendix.[67] Table 187-5 lists infections that commonly (chronic sinusitis, aspiration pneumonia) or virtually always (brain, bite, or periappendicular abscess) involve anaerobic bacteria. Characteristic syndromes occur, such as that of Lemierre,[68] (see Chapter 193, Fusobacterium Species). The triad of parenchymal lung infection, osteomyelitis of a contiguous rib, and soft tissue abscess is typical of actinomycosis[69] (see Chapter 195, Anaerobic Gram-Positive Nonsporulating Bacilli). Putrid odor of breath can be the clue to the presence of a nasal foreign body or anaerobic lung abscess.[70]

MICROBIOLOGIC METHODS

Specimen Collection

Appropriate documentation of anaerobic infection requires collection of appropriate specimens followed by their expeditious transportation and careful laboratory processing. The use of inadequate techniques or media can lead to the assumption

TABLE 187-4. Clinical Clues to Infection Due to Anaerobic Bacteria

Predisposition/Characteristics	Examples/Comments
PREDISPOSITION	
Infection contiguous to site of mucosal colonization	Sinuses, periodontal, oropharyngeal-orofacial (noma) pulmonary, periappendiceal, intra-abdominal, perirectal sites
Obstruction or perforation of hollow viscus	Nasal or pulmonary foreign body or anatomic abnormality, bronchiectasis, perforated appendix, chronic cervicitis/salpingitis, surgical breach of mucosa
Disruption of normal clearance mechanism	Impaired cough, gag, laryngopharyngeal function, mucociliary movement, alveolar macrophage function; unconsciousness
Excessive bacterial inoculation	Periodontal disease, massive aspiration, bite wound, right-to-left cardiac-pulmonary shunt, surgical peritoneal soilage
CHARACTERISTICS	
Marked tendency to tissue necrosis and abscess formation	Necrotizing pneumonia or lung abscess, tubo-ovarian or intra-abdominal abscess
Necrotizing cellulitis or myositis, sometimes with gas or gangrene and abscess formation	Meleney synergistic gangrene, noma[97] and omphalitis (severe underlying malnutrition, crush injury, or ischemic tissue expected); *Clostridium, Peptostreptococcus, Bacteroides* spp. produce gas, but so do coliforms and *Pseudomonas*
Putrid exudate, putrid breath	Pathognomonic but present in less than half of anaerobic abscesses, related to volatile fatty acid byproducts; severe hallitosis can be the initial or predominant complaint in nasal foreign body or lung abscess
Marked tendency to septic thrombophlebitis	Pelvic thrombophlebitis with appendiceal or genital tract infection; jugular vein thrombosis with oropharyngeal infection; clues are persistently positive blood culture and/or pulmonary septic emboli
Polymicrobial Gram stain of exudate	Pathognomonic; irregular uptake of Gram stain and pleomorphic, gracile, beaded, or branched morphologies also a clue
Failure to isolate pathogens in aerobic cultures or isolation of facultative normal flora	"Sterile pus," despite positive Gram stain, especially if processing inadequate; isolation of microaerophilic streptococci or *Aggregatibacter* (formerly *Actinobacillus*) *actinomycetemcomitans*
Failure to respond to antibiotic(s) without activity against anaerobes	Failure of monotherapy aminoglycoside for *Escherichia coli* intra-abdominal abscess, penicillin for lung abscess, cephalosporin for brain abscess

TABLE 187-5. Infections Commonly Involving Anaerobic Bacteria in Children and Adolescents

Oropharyngeal Flora	Intestinal/Genital Flora
Chronic sinusitis	Wound abscess after intestinal,
Chronic otitis media	genitourinary surgery
Subacute/chronic, tonsillar/	Perirectal, pilonidal abscess
parapharyngeal/peritonsillar/	Infection related to enterocutaneous
parotid abscess	or genitourinary fistula (acquired
Gingivitis, odontofacial cellulitis/	or congenital)
abscess, noma	Peritonitis and abdominal abscess
Ludwig angina (sublingual and	secondary to intestinal
submandibular infection)	perforation (spontaneous or
Lemierre infection (posterior and	surgical)
lateral pharyngeal infection)	Periappendiceal, subphrenic,
Bite or clenched fist, fight injury	guttural abscess
abscess	Hepatic, pancreatic, splenic,
Paronychia	nephric abscess
Septicemia or metastatic infection	Obstructive cholangitis
related to lymphoreticular	Septicemia or metastatic abscess
malignancy	related to intestinal tumor or
Infection of congenital cyst	abdominal infection
(pulmonary, cervical,	Meningitis, brain abscess
thryroglossal)	associated with anterior
Aspiration pneumonia	meningomyelocele; after
Necrotizing pneumonia	instrumentation, dilation, surgery,
Pneumonia with empyema	or trauma to colon or rectum;
Lung abscess	metastatic from *Bacteroides*
Pneumonia–rib osteomyelitis–soft-	*fragilis* bacteremia in neonate
tissue abscess triad	Bartholin abscess
Superinfected bronchiectasis	Infection related to vaginal or
Subdural/epidural emypema	endometrial foreign body,
Brain abscess (after sinopulmonary	surgery, or instrumentation
infection or surgery, tracheal or	Pelvic inflammatory disease
esophageal instrumentation for	Tubo-ovarian abscess
dilatation, congenital heart	Suppurative pelvic thrombophlebitis
disease)	Puerperal septicemia

that only aerobic organisms are present in a mixed infection (Table 187-6).[3] Specimens must be obtained with techniques that bypass the normal flora. Direct needle aspiration or surgical exposure is the best method of obtaining a specimen for culture (Table 187-6).

Transport

Transportation of specimens should be prompt unless transport devices are used. These devices generally contain an oxygen-free environment, provided by a mixture of carbon dioxide, hydrogen, and nitrogen, plus an aerobic condition indicator. Specimens should be placed into an anaerobic transporter immediately. Liquid or tissue specimens always are preferred to swabs. A liquid specimen is inoculated into an anaerobic transport vial. A syringe also could be used after all air bubbles are expelled. Because air gradually diffuses through the plastic syringe wall, however, specimens should be processed in <30 minutes. Swabs are placed in sterilized tubes containing carbon dioxide or pre-reduced, anaerobically sterile Carey and Blair semisolid media. A tissue specimen can be transported in an anaerobic jar or in a sealed plastic bag that has been rendered anaerobic.

A number of transport systems have been developed and are useful in certain settings, such as for smaller specimens, with delayed processing, or unavoidable use of a swab specimen (Table 187-7). Compared with the Vacutainer anaerobic specimen collector, Port-a-Cul was found to be superior for isolation of anaerobic bacteria from abscesses in one study, especially when transit time was >24 hours.[71]

Direct Examination

The general appearance (necrosis, purulence) and putrid odor of the specimen can suggest the presence of anaerobes. Inspection of clinical specimens might reveal sulfur granules, which are pathognomonic for *Actinomyces* infection. Gram stain can provide

TABLE 187-6. Methods for Collection of Specimen for Anaerobic Bacteria

Infection Site	Methods
Abscess or body cavity	Aspiration by syringe and needle
	Incised abscesses – syringe or swab (less desirable); specimen obtained during surgery after skin is cleansed
Tissue or bone	Surgical specimen using tissue biopsy or curette
Sinuses or mucus surface abscesses	Aspiration after decontamination or surgical specimen
Ear	Aspiration after decontamination of ear canal and membrane; in perforation, cleanse ear canal and aspirate through perforation
Pulmonary	Transtracheal aspiration, lung puncture, bronchoscopic aspirate[a]
Pleural	Thoracentesis
Urinary tract	Suprapubic bladder aspiration
Female genital tract	Culdocentesis after decontamination, surgical specimen
	Transabdominal needle aspirate of uterus
	Intrauterine brush[a]

[a]Using double-lumen catheter and quantitative culture.

TABLE 187-8. Media Used for Recovery of Anaerobic Bacteria

Media	Purpose
NONSELECTIVE MEDIA	
Anaerobic blood agar: *Brucella*, brain-heart infusion with yeast extract, Columbia, CDC, Schaedler	Supports growth of anaerobic and facultatively anaerobic bacteria; requires vitamin K supplementation; CDC agar best for cocci, *Brucella*; Schaedler best for gram-negative bacilli
SELECTIVE MEDIA	
Bacteroides bile esculin (BBE) agar	Selects growth of *Bacteroides fragilis* group, and most hydrolyze esculin to brown-black colonies; contains bile and gentamicin, which inhibit most other organisms
Kanamycin-vancomycin laked blood (KVLB) agar	Selects growth of *Bacteroides* and *Prevotella* spp.; enhances pigment production of *Prevotella melaninogenica*
Phenylethyl alcohol (PEA) sheep blood agar	Supports growth of anaerobic bacteria; inhibits coliforms
Colistin-nalidixic acid blood agar	Selects growth of gram-positive bacteria; inhibits gram-negative bacteria
Cycloserine-cefoxitin-fructosec agar (CCFA)	Selects growth of *Clostridium difficile*
ENRICHMENT BROTHS	
Enriched thioglycolate (BBL-135C), chopped meat broth	Used in addition to agar(s), as holding, enrichment media for slow-growing organisms and for heat shock treatment for selection of spore-forming bacteria; requires vitamin K and hemin

important clues, as follows:[4] (1) presence of multiple species typifies anaerobic infection; (2) certain morphologies are discernible (pale-staining pleomorphic *Bacteroides*, gracile fusiform *Fusobacterium*, tiny gram-negative coccal *Veillonella*, branching *Actinomyces*, boxcar *Clostridium*); and (3) findings aid interpretation of the relative importance of subsequent isolates or a sterile culture result. Immunofluorescence staining of specimens can be helpful in detection of special organisms, such as *Propionibacterium propionicum* and *Actinomyces* spp. However, this method is not yet sufficiently refined to be used for the detection of gram-negative anaerobic rods. Direct analysis for characteristic short-chain fatty acids by gas–liquid chromatography has been applied to blood cultures and exudate specimens, as have detection methods for *C. difficile* to stool specimens (see Chapter 190, *Clostridium difficile*). Each examination method has limitations of practicality, sensitivity, or cost. Nucleic acid probes have been developed for detection and identification of anaerobic organisms (especially for *Bacteroides* spp. and potential periodontal pathogens) and polymerase chain reaction (PCR) for detection of oral anaerobes, *C. difficile*, and toxins.[3] Also 16S rRNA gene sequencing can be used for strains that cannot be identified phenotypically.

TABLE 187-7. Specimen Transport System for Anaerobic Bacteria

Type of System	Examples
HOLDING SYSTEM	
Enclosed tube or vial, anaerobic atmosphere, isotonic agar, moist environment	Port-A-Cul system (BBL Microbiology Systems)
	Anaerobic transport medium (Anaerobe Systems)
	Agar gel transport swab[a] (Copan Diagnaostics)
PREREDUCED MEDIA SYSTEM	
Tube with anaerobic atmosphere and prereduced, anaerobically sterilized (PRAS) medium	Anaerobic transport system (Starplex Scientific Inc)
	Anaerobic Transport Medium (Anaerobe Systems)

[a]Care should be taken to flick off excess gel when preparing Gram stain as gel itself can contain non-viable but Gram-stainable organisms.

Primary Isolation

Table 187-8 lists media used for primary isolation of anaerobic bacteria. Because the majority of infections are polymicrobial, optimal recovery requires use of nonselective and selective aerobic and anaerobic media. A minimum for isolation of anaerobic bacteria is inoculation onto supplemented blood agar and a medium selective for growth of *B. fragilis* and *Prevotella* groups (see Chapter 286, Laboratory Diagnosis of Infection Due to Bacteria, Fungi, Parasites, and Rickettsiae).

Susceptibility Testing

Antimicrobial susceptibility patterns of anaerobes have become less predictable. Resistance to several antimicrobial agents, especially by gram-negative bacilli, has increased.[72,73] Screening of anaerobic gram-negative bacilli isolates for β-lactamase activity may be helpful. However, occasional strains can be resistant through other mechanisms. Susceptibility testing of anaerobes should be performed primarily to determine activity of new agents and to monitor local, national, or international susceptibility patterns periodically. Testing of an individual patient's isolates may be required for serious or chronic infection, such as endocarditis, bacteremia, osteomyelitis, brain abscess, or device-related infection, or when serious infection is due to an organism with unpredictable antibiotic susceptibility.[74]

Problems in antimicrobial susceptibility testing of anaerobic bacteria include lack of standardization of techniques, idiosyncrasies and fastidiousness of bacterial growth, appropriate choice of antimicrobial susceptibility breakpoints, clustering of isolates at breakpoints, lengthy testing period, and limited clinical correlation of in vitro observations. Treatment usually is based on statistical knowledge of suspected or proven pathogens and antimicrobial susceptibility patterns as tested in batches in reference laboratories. Problems with the latter include sources of test strains (clinical isolates versus laboratory strains versus normal flora), currency, number and relevance of representative species, and accuracy of identification.

There is no standard testing method, because of the lack of reproducibility and inability to grow all clinically significant anaerobes on a standard medium. Agar dilution and broth macrodilution and microdilution currently are acceptable; agar disk diffusion and broth disk elution are inappropriate. The E-test compares favorably with broth microdilution and may be cost-effective, because only a few agents need to be tested.[75] Nitrocefin (chromogenic cephalosporin) testing is useful for the detection of β-lactamase production and attendant resistance of *Bacteroides* spp. and *P. melaninogenica* to β-lactam agents; however, resistance of some *Bacteroides* (especially *B. gracilis* and *B. distasonis*) can occur by other mechanisms, and hydrolysis of imipenem and cefoxitin may not be predicted accurately.[76,77]

MECHANISMS OF RESISTANCE

Mechanisms of the antibiotic resistance of anaerobic bacteria are at least as broad as those for facultative and aerobic organisms; they include β-lactamase inactivation, hydrolysis, blocking of drug target site, alteration in affinity of penicillin-binding proteins, ribosomal protection or alteration, active efflux, RNA methyltransferase, and production of adenyltransferase and acetyltransferase.[77] Determinants of resistance are transferable by multiple mechanisms, such as a conjugation-like process, transposons, plasmid self-transfer, and mobilization. At the genetic level, some resistance determinants are highly specific for one or several anaerobes or can exhibit homology with genes from facultative bacteria.[76,78]

TREATMENT

Principles of Management

Managing principles for anaerobic infections are: (1) neutralization of toxins; (2) prevention of local proliferation of bacteria by changing the environment; and (3) deterrence of bacterial spread.[79] Toxin neutralization by specific antitoxins is essential in infections caused by certain clostridia (tetanus and botulism). Control of the environment is achieved by debriding necrotic tissue, draining pus, improving circulation, alleviating the obstruction, and increasing the tissue oxygenation. Debridement and removal of foreign bodies are essential for successful therapy of anaerobic infection. Drainage of abscess also is important, although certain small or multifocal tubo-ovarian, brain, and intra-abdominal abscesses can respond to antimicrobial therapy alone or in combination with percutaneous aspiration or catheter

drainage.[80-83] Lung abscess commonly drains spontaneously, or bronchoscopy is performed for diagnostic and therapeutic reasons; empyema must be drained. Lobectomy or decortication should not be performed, because resolution, even of necrotizing infection, is surprisingly complete.

The use of clostridial antitoxin for gas gangrene is still controversial, because: (1) necessity is less clear with aggressive surgical debridement; and (2) immediate anaphylaxis and delayed serum sickness are attendant risks.[84] Use of specific antitoxins for management of botulism, tetanus, and diphtheria is addressed in subsequent chapters.

Certain types of adjunctive therapy, such as hyperbaric oxygen therapy (HBO) for infection due to spore-forming gram-positive anaerobic rods is controversial, but may be useful. Uncontrolled reports demonstrate efficacy in individual cases.[85] Use of HBO is contraindicated when it could delay other essential procedures. The topical application of oxygen-releasing compounds may be useful.

Surgical therapy is the most important, and sometimes the only, form of treatment required. This includes drainage, debridement, resection, restoration of airspaces, or maintenance of blood supply. Some of these procedures can be performed percutaneously when assisted by computed tomography (CT), magnetic resonance imaging (MRI), or ultrasonography.

There are few controlled, comparative efficacy studies of treatments of anaerobic infections and no clinical data at all for many microbes and antimicrobial agents. Additionally, most studies involve adults or are case reports involving children. Investigations in the 1970s showed lower mortality rates in patients with anaerobic BSI who were treated with appropriate antimicrobial agents. Later case reports and series of BSIs related to devices or malignancy collectively suggest clinical failure of therapy with agents that have no activity in vitro.[86,87] The notion that treatment of facultative or aerobic copathogens is sufficient for cure may be correct early in the course of certain infections, such as aspiration pneumonia and paranasal sinusitis, especially when drainage can be promoted. Established, necrotizing infections, abscesses, or BSI, however, require specific use of effective agents. Randomized clinical studies have shown superiority of clindamycin over penicillin[88,89] and of clindamycin over metronidazole[90] for treatment of anaerobic lung abscess or necrotizing anaerobic pneumonia.

Antimicrobial Agents

Susceptibility of anaerobic bacteria to antimicrobial agents is shown in Table 187-9, and drugs of choice are listed in Table 187-10. Certain agents have activity against virtually all anaerobes:

TABLE 187-9. Susceptibility of Anaerobic Bacteria to Antimicrobial Agents[a]

Bacteria	Penicillin	A Penicillin and a β-Lactamase Inhibitor	Ureido-Carboxy-penicillin	Cefoxitin	Chloram-phenicol	Clindamycin	Macrolides	Metronidazole	Carba-penems	Tigecycline
Peptostreptococcus spp.	4	4	3	3	3	3	2–3	2	3	3
Fusobacterium spp.	3–4	3–4	3	3	3	2–3	1	3	3	3
Bacteroides fragilis group	1	4	2–3	3	3	3–4	1–2	4	4	2–3
Prevotella and *Porphyromonas* spp.	1–3	4	2–3	3	3	3–4	2–3	4	4	3
Clostridium perfringens	4	4	3	3	3	3	3	3	3	3
Clostridium spp.	3	3	3	2–3	3	2	2	3	3	3
Actinomyces spp.	4	4	3	3	3	3	3	1	3	3

[a]Degrees of activity: 1, minimal; 2, moderate; 3, good; 4, excellent.

TABLE 187-10. Drugs of Choice for Infections Caused by Anaerobic Bacteria

Bacteria	First Choice	Alternative
Peptostreptococcus spp.	Penicillin	Clindamycin, chloramphenicol, cephalosporins
Clostridium spp.	Penicillin	Metronidazole, chloramphenicol, cefoxitin, clindamycin
Clostridium difficile	Metronidazole, vancomycin	Bacitracin
Gram-negative bacilli (BL⁻)[a]	Penicillin	Metronidazole, clindamycin, chloramphenicol
Gram-negative bacilli (BL⁺)[a]	Metronidazole, imipenem, a penicillin and β-lactamase inhibitor, clindamycin	Cefoxitin, chloramphenicol, piperacillin

BL, β-lactamase.

[a]*Bacteroides fragilis* group; *Prevotella* spp., *Porphyromonas* spp., *Fusobacterium* spp.

carbapenems (imipenem, meropenem, doripenem), chloramphenicol, and β-lactam agents combined with β-lactamase inhibitor.[91,92] Metronidazole is the most bactericidal agent against *Bacteroides* spp. and other gram-negative anaerobes but has variable or minimal activity against important gram-positive cocci and bacilli, including *Actinomyces* and *Lactobacillus* spp., and some *Propionibacterium* spp. Clindamycin has excellent activity against most *B. fragilis*, *Prevotella melaninogenica*, *Porphyromonas*, and most gram-positive anaerobes. Resistance of *B. fragilis* can vary geographically, and within *Bacteroides fragilis* group, non-*fragilis* members such as *Bacteroides thetaiotaomicron*, *B. distasonis*, and other bile-resistant *Bacteroides* spp. have higher rates of resistance, as do *Bacteroides* species outside the *B. fragilis* group (*B. gracilis*).

Penicillin and ampicillin, first-, second- and third-generation cephalosporins, and vancomycin are active against most gram-positive anaerobes but have unpredictable or little activity against most anaerobic gram-negative bacilli.[91,92] Penicillin derivatives, isoxazoyl penicillins, and nafcillin are considerably less active than penicillin G against most anaerobes. The extended spectrum of ticarcillin or piperacillin compared with penicillin is somewhat artificial, related primarily to use of larger doses of agents and higher in vitro breakpoints; the β-lactamases of anaerobes inhibit activity of these agents. Cefoxitin is the most active cephalosporin, exhibiting a similar pattern, but is more affected by changing in vitro conditions; additionally, some *Clostridium* and *Fusobacterium* spp. are resistant. Cefotetan and ceftizoxime have fairly good activity against anaerobes, but ceftriaxone, cefoperazone, and cefotaxime are not reliable enough against gram-negative anaerobes to be useful, and ceftazidime and cefepime have poor activity against

both gram-positive and gram-negative anaerobes. Vancomycin has good activity against many gram-positive anaerobes, including *Clostridium* and *Actinomyces* spp., but has not been studied clinically.

The activity of clarithromycin is superior generally compared with erythromycin and azithromycin against anaerobes but is reliable only for some *Prevotella*, *Porphyromonas*, *Propionibacterium*, and *Eubacterium* spp.[93] For penicillins, extended-spectrum penicillins, cephalosporins (not carbapenems), and chloramphenicol (for *B. fragilis*), minimal inhibitory concentrations effective against susceptible anaerobic bacteria are high (requiring use of maximal doses of agents), vary by inoculum size and other in vitro conditions, and cluster around breakpoints – all features leading to interassay, interlaboratory, and interstudy variability in reports of percentage of resistant organisms. Tetracyclines and older fluoroquinolones have unreliable activity against anaerobes, and aminoglycosides and monobactams have none. Doxycycline and minocycline are more active than the parent compound. Some broad-spectrum fluoroquinolones (gatifloxacin and moxifloxacin) and tigecycline have significant anti-anaerobic activity. Meropenem has excellent activity in vitro against most clinically relevant gram-positive and gram-negative anaerobes (including *Bacteroides* and *Prevotella* species) except *C. difficile*.

Antimicrobial resistance of anaerobes has increased in recent years for clindamycin, cefoxitin, cefotetan, cefotaxime, and piperacillin. Resistant isolates have been recovered infrequently for the carbapenems, metronidazole, and the combinations of β-lactam/β-lactamase inhibitors.[74,94,95] The production of β-lactamase is the resistance mechanism of the *B. fragilis* group, as well as increasing numbers of other *Bacteroides*, *Prevotella*, *Porphyromonas*, and *Fusobacterium* spp.

Choice of antibiotics for presumed anaerobic infection is empiric, based on knowledge of likely organisms, expected in vitro susceptibility, and pharmacodynamics of agents. Fortunately, the types of anaerobes involved in many infections and their antimicrobial susceptibility patterns tend to be predictable. Some excellent anaerobe-antimicrobial agents, such as metronidazole, have limited range of activity and cannot be administered as a single agent in mixed infections. Others (i.e., carbapenems and tigecycline) have a wide spectrum of activity against Enterobacteriaceae and anaerobes. Treatment of mixed infection should cover most of the aerobic and anaerobic pathogens.[67] Combination therapy is always required for intracranial abscess (such as with penicillin or vancomycin plus metronidazole plus a third-generation cephalosporin) and is time honored for intra-abdominal infection (such as with ampicillin plus clindamycin and gentamicin), although cefoxitin or ceftizoxime (which are not active against *Enterococcus* spp.) or piperacillin-tazobactam is as good as combination therapy for most polymicrobial gastrointestinal or pelvic infections studied.[67] A retrospective cohort study of monotherapy (piperacillin-tazobactam, meropenem, cefoxitin, or ceftriaxone) versus aminoglycoside-based triple antibiotic therapy for children with ruptured appendicitis showed at least equal efficacy of monotherapy.[96] Nosocomial acquisition affects antibiotic choice, especially to include agents with activity against expected or proven facultative or aerobic organisms.

188 *Clostridium tetani* (Tetanus)

Itzhak Brook

Tetanus is caused by a neurotoxin produced by *Clostridium tetani*. It is common in warmer climates. The worldwide incidence of tetanus is about one million cases annually. Although a major cause of morbidity and mortality in developing countries, tetanus

is rare in the United States, with about 35 to 70 cases reported annually to the Centers for Disease Control and Prevention (CDC).[1] It is estimated that reported cases represent 60% of actual cases. Tetanus remains a likely diagnosis in certain clinical situations even in developed countries, and individual patients suffer severe morbidity. Most cases of tetanus occur in unvaccinated individuals and in adults; persons older than 60 years account for 60% of the cases and for 75% of deaths from tetanus in the U.S.

In the U.S., the current average annual incidence is less than 0.1 per 100,000 population compared with 0.39 per 100,000 in 1947.[2] The decline reflects the efficacy of the effective immunization program. About 70% of cases of tetanus in the U.S. follow acute injuries, less than half of which occur outdoors. Chronic wounds and abscesses, wounds associated with a foreign body (e.g., splinters, thorns), surgical wounds, major trauma, parenteral drug abuse, and animal-related injuries are responsible for 25% of the tetanus-associated injuries; approximately 20% of wounds are from unknown circumstances, and in 5% of cases of tetanus, no wound source can be identified. Rare causes of tetanus are burns and otitis media.

MICROBIOLOGY AND PATHOGENESIS

C. tetani is a slender, gram-positive, nonencapsulated, motile, obligatively anaerobic bacillus. It exists in vegetative and sporulated forms. The genome of the organism has been sequenced.[3] The sporulated form has a characteristic drumstick microscopic appearance because of the terminal position of spores. Spores are highly resistant to disinfection by chemicals or heat, but vegetative forms are susceptible to the bactericidal effect of heat (autoclaving at 121°C and 103 kPa (15 psi) for 15 minutes), chemical disinfectants (iodine, glutaraldehyde, hydrogen peroxide), and a number of antibiotics.

Spores are ubiquitous in soil; they are dormant and nonpathogenic in soil or contaminated tissue until conditions are favorable for transformation to the vegetative, pathogenic form. Such conditions are those of locally decreased oxygen reduction potential as created in devitalized tissue by foreign body, trauma (especially crush injury), or suppurative infection.

The organism is noninvasive and does not cause inflammatory response or tissue destruction. Disease is initiated by exotoxins. Two toxins are produced, tetanolysin (of uncertain importance) and tetanospasmin (a potent neurotoxin responsible for clinical tetanus). Tetanospasmin, often referred to as "tetanus toxin," is encoded on a plasmid present in all toxigenic strains,[4] and is released with growth of *C. tetani* at the site of infection. Tetanospasmin affects the neuromuscular endplates and the motor nuclei of the central nervous system, causing skeletal muscle spasm and convulsions. Mechanisms of absorption and transport of tetanospasmin are not understood completely, but two mechanisms are speculated. If a large amount of tetanospasmin is produced, spread to neurons via the bloodstream and lymphatic system occurs, causing spasm at sites distant from the site of infection, first affecting muscles with the shortest neural pathway. Lockjaw and risus sardonicus, often seen in generalized tetanus, reflect this pathophysiology and are associated with rapidly progressive, severe disease. From the site of production, small amounts of neurotoxin also can ascend the neural axis (and sometimes the spinal axis cranially), causing localized tetanus. Timing of onset of muscle involvement is proportional to the neural distance from the site of injury.

Tetanospasmin primarily gains access to the nervous system via the neuromuscular junction, where it migrates retrograde trans-synaptically, protected from neutralizing antitoxin, predominantly thought to affect inhibitory synapses where it prevents release of acetylcholine.[5] Uninhibited lower motor neurons increase tone of agonist and antagonist muscles, thereby causing characteristic localized spasms and rigidity.

Tetanospasmin also can prevent transmission at neuromuscular junctions, causing paralysis. The effect of the toxin on the brain is controversial; direct inoculation can cause seizures, but spasms of tetanus probably result from spinal rather than supraspinal action of tetanospasmin. Affected patients are fully conscious. Some clinical manifestations of tetanus suggest involvement of the sympathetic nervous system. The effect of tetanospasmin is permanent; recovery depends on ultrasprouting of neurons.

CLINICAL MANIFESTATIONS

Tetanus is divided into clinical patterns that reflect host factors and site of inoculation: generalized, localized, cephalic, and neonatal. In most cases, the site of injury, which often is minor, can be determined. Inability to identify a portal of entry does not exclude the diagnosis, especially in unimmunized individuals. Appearance of a wound is not helpful in diagnosis, but circumstances of occurrence are (e.g., severity of crush injury and soil contamination). In the U.S., most cases of tetanus occur after puncture wounds, farming or gardening activities,[2] or the use of illicit drugs.

The interval between the time of injury and appearance of symptoms has important prognostic significance; the shorter the interval (<7 days), the worse the prognosis. The portal of entry also is an important prognostic factor. Certain injuries (e.g., compound fracture, puncture wound in drug user) or infections (e.g., that following abortion, infection of neonate's umbilical stump, burn wound) have poor prognoses. Involvement of the autonomic nervous system portends a poor prognosis. Such data have been used to develop scoring systems to predict severity and prognosis.[4]

Generalized Tetanus

Generalized tetanus, which is a neurologic disease manifesting as trismus and severe muscular spasms, is the most common manifestation of tetanus, usually occurring as a complication of localized tetanus that is recognized only in retrospect. The onset can be insidious over a period of 1 to 7 days. Trismus (lockjaw), the most common presenting symptom, commonly is mistaken as a manifestation of parapharyngeal infection or temporomandibular joint problems. History of stiffness of the back or rigidity of the neck or abdomen frequently is recognized in retrospect. Subtle "sarcastic smile" (risus sardonicus) may be noticed, and rigidity of abdominal muscles is detectable on examination.

As the disease progresses, additional muscle groups become involved, the most striking involvement being of the paraspinal musculature. The most dramatic feature of generalized tetanus is the very painful, generalized tetanic, opisthotonic spasm manifest as arching of the back (sometimes with just head and feet touching the bed) to resemble decorticate posture (Figure 188-1). The force can produce fractures of vertebrae or other bones and hemorrhage into muscles. The periodicity of tetanic spells can cause confusion with seizures; however, patients with tetanus, unlike those with seizures, do not lose consciousness. The spasms often are triggered by sensory stimuli. Respiratory compromise during

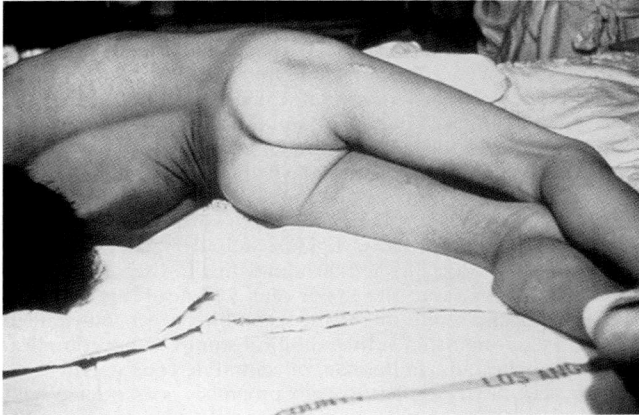

Figure 188-1. The patient is displaying opisthotonic posturing due to *Clostridium tetani* exotoxin. (Courtesy of U.S. Centers for Disease Control and Prevention.)

the tetanic spells can be life-threatening; upper airway obstruction is common, and with additional involvement of abdominal and diaphragmatic muscle, apnea can occur.

Symptoms of autonomic overactivity generally are manifest in early phases as irritability, restlessness, sweating and tachycardia. In later phases, profuse sweating, cardiac arrhythmias, labile hypertension or hypotension, and fever commonly are present.[5] Episodes of bradycardia and hypotension can lead to cardiac arrest. Cardiac arrest also has been attributed to myocardial damage caused by the high catecholamine level[6] and toxic damage to the brainstem.[7] Fever can be due to the sympathetic overactivity or superinfections, such as pneumonia.[8] Spasms and cardiovascular complications occur most commonly during the first week and resolve slowly during the ensuing 2 to 4 weeks.

Even with available treatment, generalized tetanus usually worsens in the first 2 weeks after diagnosis, with recovery occurring over the subsequent 3 to 5 weeks. If antitoxin is not given, disease persists for weeks to months, until cessation of production and binding of tetanospasmin and the formation of new neuromuscular junctions.

Localized Tetanus

Localized tetanus is an unusual presentation. Muscles near the entry wound become painful and weak within 2 to 3 days after the injury and then become rigid; deep tendon reflexes are hyperactive. Rigidity usually persists for weeks to months and resolves spontaneously without progressing, although disease can progress to generalized tetanus. Localized tetanus has a mortality <1%. In partially immune individuals, neutralization of local toxin and heightened production of antitoxin can prevent generalized tetanus.

Cephalic Tetanus

Cephalic tetanus is a rare presentation, the result of decreased neuromuscular transmission of the lower cranial nerves affected because of wounds on the head and neck. Clinical manifestations usually occur 1 to 2 days after injury and can include facial palsy, dysphagia, paresis of extraocular muscles (ophthalmoplegic tetanus),[9] and supranuclear oculomotor palsies.[10] The mechanism of the last clinical manifestation is not clear. Usually, cephalic tetanus has a poor prognosis, although some patients have good outcome. Cephalic tetanus has been reported in individuals after complete immunization. Cephalic tetanus can precede generalized tetanus.

Neonatal Tetanus

Neonatal tetanus is a generalized form of the disease that occurs only in infants born to inadequately immunized mothers. Tetanus usually follows infection of the umbilical stump, which can result from poor obstetric procedure, delivery outside of a healthcare environment, inadequate postnatal care, or cultural practices such as application of cow dung or soil to the umbilical stump. Immunization of adolescent girls and women of childbearing age, appropriate training of midwives, and topical application of antibiotics can reduce the risk of neonatal tetanus. Neonatal tetanus remains a significant problem in developing countries.[11]

Weakness and inability to suck are the most common manifestations, often appearing between 7 and 14 days of age. Later, generalized tetanic spasms, rigidity and opisthotonus occur (Figure 188-2). Mortality is >90% and may be secondary to a hypersympathetic state. The major causes of death are apnea in the first week and septicemia in the second week, generally due to infection that originated at the umbilical stump. Other complications are pneumonia, pulmonary or central nervous system hemorrhage, and laryngeal spasm. Poor prognosis is associated with risus sardonicus, fever, age <10 days, and delayed presentation for medical care.

Improvement is heralded by defervescence (usually within 3 to 7 days), decrease in the number of episodes of spasm, and slow

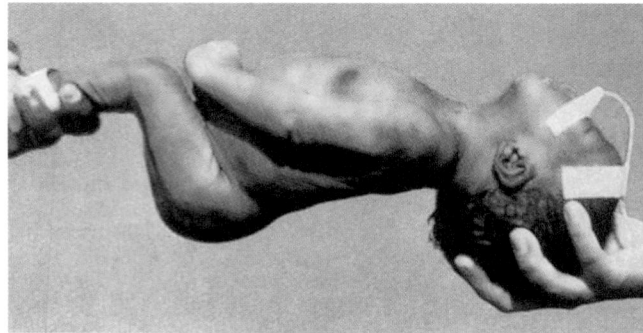

Figure 188-2. This infant with neonatal tetanus is displaying body rigidity produced by *Clostridium tetani* exotoxin. (Courtesy of U.S. Centers for Disease Control and Prevention.)

resolution of rigidity. Complete resolution may take up to 6 weeks. Developmental disability often occurs in survivors.

DIAGNOSIS AND DIFFERENTIAL DIAGNOSIS

The diagnosis of tetanus is made from clinical findings in a setting of risk and by excluding other causes of tetanic spasms. Recovery of *C. tetani* from wounds is not helpful because presence does not necessarily indicate toxin production. Laboratory tests are useful only to exclude other diseases; management cannot be delayed until test results are available. Although generalized tetanus and cephalic tetanus are recognized easily, diagnosis can be unsuspected if no portal of entry is identified. Given the clinical suspicion, history should be elicited regarding chronic otitis media, otitis externa, recent intramuscular injection, a minor surgical procedure, intravenous drug abuse, and rectal or vaginal instrumentation. Neonatal tetanus becomes apparent shortly after initial manifestations. Localized tetanus can be unrecognized until generalized manifestations occur. Trismus must be differentiated from manifestations of parapharyngeal and retropharyngeal infections.

The differential diagnosis of generalized tetanus includes stiff-man syndrome,[12] pseudotetanus,[13] meningitis, encephalitis, hypocalcemic tetany, seizures, rabies, dystonic reactions to neuroleptic drugs or other central dopamine antagonists (for which treatment with an anticholinergic agent is rapidly effective), hysterical conversion reaction, and strychnine poisoning. Although strychnine poisoning is the most commonly confused intoxication, patients with such poisoning lack trismus and abdominal rigidity between spasms. Biochemical analysis of blood and urine for strychnine is performed in cases of suspected generalized tetanus. Conversely, tetanus always should be considered when strychnine poisoning is suspected.

TREATMENT AND OUTCOME

The goals of management of tetanus are: eradication of *C. tetani*, neutralization of toxin, and provision of specific supportive care.

Providing aggressive yet restrained, supportive care with a minimum of stimulation is challenging. Transfer to an optimal setting should be accomplished early in the disease, before the severity of spasms precludes moving the patient. Survival depends on minimizing morbid or fatal spasms over a prolonged period. The patient is protected from stimuli by isolation in a noise-free, darkened room, with a nurse in the room at all times, monitors silenced, and a sentry nurse positioned outside the door to limit entry and to reinforce minimal examination and manipulation of the patient.

The child with tetanus should be sedated and human tetanus immune globulin (TIG) administered immediately. TIG neutralizes circulating tetanospasmin. Recommended dosage and administration of TIG is shown in Table 188-1.[14,15] Local infiltration of part of the dose around the wound is recommended. However, the efficacy of this has not been proven. In countries where TIG

TABLE 188-1. Treatment of Tetanus

Agent	Dosage/Administration
Tetanus immune globulin, human (TIG)	Single dose, 3000–6000 units IM[a]
Tetanus antitoxin (TAT)[b]	Single dose, 50,000–100,000 units after appropriate testing is performed for sensitivity and desensitization if necessary; part of dose (20,000 units) is given IV, and the remainder IM
Immune globulin intravenous (IGIV)	Single dose of 200 to 400 mg/kg IV can be considered if TIG is not available; not approved for this indication
Metronidazole	30 mg/kg/day (maximum, 4 g/day) divided into q6h doses PO or IV for 10–14 days
Penicillin G	100,000 units/kg/day (maximum, 12 million units/day) divided into q6h doses IV for 10–14 days
Tetracycline	25–50 mg/kg/day; an alternative; not approved for children < 8 years old

IM, (given) intramuscularly; IV, (given) intravenously; PO, (given) orally.

[a]*Some experts recommend a single dose of 500 units IM, which appears to be as effective and causes less discomfort.*[14,15]

[b]*TAT is not available in the United States; it should be used elsewhere only if TIG is not available.*

TABLE 188-2. Complications of Tetanus

Complication	Comment
Cardiomyopathy	Direct toxic effect
Phrenic nerve palsy	Direct toxic effect
Laryngeal nerve palsy	Direct toxic effect
Respiratory compromise	Secondary to spasms
Rhabdomyolysis	Secondary to spasms
Myositis ossificans circumscripta	Secondary to spasms
Vertebral compression fracture	Secondary to spasms
Hypoxic cerebral injury	Secondary to respiratory compromise
Acute renal failure	Secondary to rhabdomyolysis
Psychologic	Most prominent after recovery

is not available, equine tetanus antitoxin (TAT) is an alternative. It is administered after adequate testing for sensitivity and desensitization if needed. Immune globulin intravenous (IGIV) may be given if TIG is not available.

Local wound care is essential. Foreign bodies, if present, are removed; the wound is irrigated vigorously and debrided to remove devitalized tissue. Extensive debridement of puncture wounds is not needed. Excision of necrotic tissue may be required, but excision of the umbilical stump is no longer recommended in cases of neonatal tetanus.

C. tetani is susceptible to penicillins, cephalosporins, metronidazole, macrolides, tetracyclines, and imipenem. Although the utility of antimicrobial therapy in tetanus is controversial, specific therapy should be given (Table 188-1). Oral or intravenous metronidazole or parenteral penicillin G is appropriate. Oral tetracycline and intravenous vancomycin are effective against *C. tetani*, but the cephalosporins are not reliably active.

A single, nonblinded clinical study performed in Indonesia compared oral metronidazole with intramuscular penicillin for treatment of tetanus.[16] Patients treated with metronidazole had less progression of disease (i.e., severity and frequency of spasms), shorter hospital stay, and better overall survival. The validity of these findings may have been compromised by an inadequate dose of penicillin given intramuscularly, the administration of which can increase the severity and frequency of tetanic spasms. Although theoretically, penicillin could act synergistically with tetanospasmin to worsen neuromuscular effects,[17] extensive experience has been accrued for penicillin treatment of tetanus.

Sedation and muscle relaxation in mild cases should be accomplished, generally with diazepam, 0.1 to 0.2 mg/kg given intravenously every 4 to 6 hours. Ventilatory assistance is imperative at higher doses. Other benzodiazepines (lorazepan or midazolam) are equally effective. Additional sedation with a phenothiazine drug is appropriate; use of phenothiazine alone is less effective than sedation with diazepam. If spasms are not controlled effectively, therapeutic paralysis is necessary. Neuromuscular blockade can be achieved with curariform drugs. The agents used most often are pancuronium and vecuronium.

Suppression of excessive catecholamine release (which induces the autonomic dysfunction) can control the dysautonomia. Labetalol (0.25 to 1.0 mg/min) frequently has been administered because

of its dual alpha and beta blocking potential. Beta blockade alone (i.e., with propranolol), should be avoided because of the danger of sudden death.[18] Morphine sulfate (0.5 to 1.0 mg/kg per hour by continuous intravenous infusion) is used commonly to induce sedation and to control autonomic dysfunction by reducing sympathetic tone in the heart and the vascular system, thus controlling cardiac instability without causing cardiac compromise.[19] Other agents available for the treatment of various autonomic events are atropine, clonidine, and epidural bupivacaine.

Of the above drugs only magnesium sulfate was evaluated in a randomized clinical trial,[20] and in clinical series for controlling spasms.[21-24] The results of these studies brought about the use of magnesium titrated to clinical endpoints as a first-line agent in the management of tetanus. Magnesium is a vasodilator, and reduces catecholamine release from the adrenal medulla[25] and adrenergic nerve endings.[26]

In a randomized, double-blind study of 256 patients, magnesium sulfate infusion (loading dose 40 mg/kg over 30 minutes, followed by continuous infusion of 2 g per hour for patients >45 kg or 1.5 g per hour for patients ≤45 kg) was compared with placebo.[20] Magnesium sulfate significantly reduced the need for other drugs to control muscle spasms and patients were 4.7 times (95% CI, 1.4 to 15.9) less likely to require verapamil to treat cardiovascular instability than those in the placebo group.

Hypotension if present is treated initially with saline; unresolved, a pulmonary catheter is placed for monitoring and fluid, dopamine, or norepinephrine are administered as indicated.

Nutritional support should be initiated as soon as possible to sustain the patient's high caloric and protein needs. Enteral feeding is preferred; percutaneous endoscopic gastrostomy tube is used commonly to limit gastroesophageal reflux compared with nasogastric tube. Prophylactic administration of sucralfate or acid blocking agent can prevent gastroesophageal hemorrhage from stress ulcers. Prevention of thromboembolism can be attained with heparin, low molecular weight heparin or other anticoagulants, and should be begun early. Because patients often become disabled because of the drug-induced paralysis and immobilization, physical therapy should be initiated as soon as spasms have abated.

Complications of tetanus are shown in Table 188-2.

PREVENTION

There is no reliable natural immunity to tetanus. Prevention consists of providing neutralizing antibody to tetanospasmin in case *C. tetani* contaminates and multiplies in a wound.

Primary Prevention

Primary prevention is pre-exposure immunization, consisting of primary immunization followed by booster doses of tetanus toxoid-containing vaccines (TT) throughout life.[27] Schedules are

TABLE 188-3. Prevention of Tetanus

PRIMARY IMMUNIZATION[a]

Age	Vaccine
2 months	DTaP
4 months	DTaP
6 months	DTaP
12–18 months	DTaP
4–6 years	DTaP
11–12 years	Tdap

SECONDARY IMMUNIZATION[b]

History/Dose of Tetanus Toxoid Administration	Clean Minor Wound		All Other Wounds[f]	
	TIG	Td[d]	TIG	Td[d]
<3 doses or unknown	No	Yes	Yes	Yes
≥3 doses[c]	No	No[e]	No	No[g]

DTaP, diphtheria and tetanus toxoids, and acellular pertussis vaccine; Td, tetanus and diphtheria; Tdap, tetanus and diphtheria toxoid and reduced acellular pertussis antigens; TIG, tetanus immune globulin.

[a]If an infant has contraindications to pertussis vaccine, diphtheria/tetanus toxoid (DT) is given on the same schedule; if primary immunization is begun at 7 years, Td/Tdap is used. (see Chapter 162: Bordetella pertussis (Pertussis) and Other Bordetella Species).

[b]See text for important details.

[c]If the patient has received only three doses of fluid toxoid, a fourth dose of toxoid, preferably an adsorbed toxoid, should be given.

[d]For children <7 years old, DTaP (DT if pertussis vaccine is contraindicated) is preferred to tetanus toxoid alone; for persons >7 years old, Td is preferred to tetanus toxoid alone. For children and adolescents, Tdap should be used when Td is indicated if the individual has not already received Tdap.

[e]Yes, if >10 years since last dose.

[f]Such as, but not limited to, wounds contaminated with dirt, feces, soil, or saliva; puncture wounds; avulsions; and wounds resulting from missiles, crushing, burns, and frostbite.

[g]Yes, if >5 years since last dose (more frequent boosters are not needed and can accentuate side effects).

shown in Table 188-3.[28] The goal of immunization is to provide a continuous serum concentration of 0.01 IU/mL of neutralizing antitoxin.[29,30] Protection between levels of 0.01 and 1.0 IU/mL is not absolute; some authorities consider an antibody level of 0.15 IU/mL or greater as protective.[31]

A number of long-term follow-up studies indicate that protective antitoxin levels persist in 91% to 96% of individuals 10 years after receipt of the initial 3-dose series of TT as infants.[32-34] In one study, 70% of the individuals >6 years of age living in the U.S. had antibody levels ≥0.15 IU/mL.[35] Presence of protective antibody dropped with age, from >90% in children 6 to 9 years of age to 80% in those 10 to 16 years, to <28% in individuals ≥70 years of age. Rates reflect the time since immunization or the lack of immunization (especially in older women). There was no effect of race, but poverty, lower educational status, and birth outside the U.S. were associated with lower antibody levels.

Immunodeficient individuals may not acquire adequate response to TT and require passive immunization. Stem cell or bone marrow transplant recipients need to be revaccinated with at least two doses.[36] Even though only 38% of HIV-infected children and adolescents had protective tetanus antibody levels the majority developed and maintained levels after booster.[37] Severe anaphylactic reactions, brachial neuritis, and Guillain–Barré syndrome following TT administration have been rarely reported.

Secondary Prevention

Secondary prevention consists of administration of vaccine and antitoxin (TIG) after a tetanus-prone injury (see Table 188-3), the need determined by the type of injury and the patient's immunization history. Although wounds with major tissue injury are most tetanus prone, any type of wound, if contaminated, can lead to tetanus. Immunization is given immediately if the patient's tetanus immunization history is not available or is uncertain, or if 60 months or more have elapsed since the last TT booster dose. When indicated by immunization history, TIG is given intramuscularly in a dose of 250 U (regardless of age or weight). IGIV or equine tetanus antitoxin is recommended if TIG is unavailable. Decisions on the need for TIG for infants <6 months of age who have not received a full 3-dose primary vaccine series should be based on the mother's TT immunization status at the time of delivery. Additional circumstances warrant the use of TIG in immunized individuals, including anticipated impairment of response to vaccine such as infection with HIV, and certain wounds, such as major burns, frostbite, crush injury, or injury by avulsion, puncture, or missile.

Hyperimmunization (multiple booster doses of toxoid over a short time) can cause severe local reactions at the injection site, such as swelling of the entire arm. Individuals with such reactions have high antitoxin levels. Preformed antitoxin forms complexes with administered toxoid and induces an Arthus type II hypersensitivity response. Use of tetanus toxoid in situations where it is not indicated is inappropriate.

Tertiary Prevention

Tertiary prevention consists of antitoxin and immunization given after clinical tetanus is manifest. Tetanus does not provide protective immunity, probably because the minute amount of toxin produced is insufficient to elicit an immune response. All patients should complete a series of immunizations with tetanus toxoid, beginning at presentation.

189 *Clostridium botulinum* (Botulism)

Sarah S. Long

Botulism is a neuroparalytic disease caused by the action of a heat-labile neurotoxin produced almost exclusively by *Clostridium botulinum*. Potential modes of acquisition are: (1) foodborne botulism, which results from the ingestion of preformed toxin, elaborated in food naturally contaminated with spores and improperly preserved; (2) wound botulism, which results from outgrowth and toxin production in wounds contaminated with spores; (3) infant botulism, which was first recognized in 1976 and results from intestinal colonization and in vivo toxin elaboration after incidental exposure to spores; (4) adult intestinal toxemia botulism, which can occur rarely as a result of intestinal colonization and in vivo toxin production, usually in the context of abdominal surgery, gastrointestinal tract abnormalities, or recent antibiotic treatment; (5) inhalational botulism, which could occur by deliberate dissemination of toxin by aerosol; and anecdotally (6) iatrogenic botulism, which has been reported following high-dose injection of toxin for treatment of muscular movement disorders or after injection of an unlicensed product for cosmetic purposes.[1-5]

More than 1500 cases of infant botulism have been confirmed in the United States since it became a nationally notifiable disease in 1985, and more than 2900 cases worldwide.[4,6,7] Infant botulism is the most common form of botulism, accounting for approximately 63% of all cases annually, with a mean of 87 cases annually from 2001 through 2009.[6] Infant botulism is the primary focus of this chapter as children have only rarely accounted for cases of all other forms.

ETIOLOGY AND PATHOGENESIS

Organisms and Toxins

C. botulinum represents a heterogeneous group of gram-positive, anaerobic, spore-forming bacilli, individual strains of which can produce one of seven serologically distinct neurotoxins (types A to G). More than 95% of cases of infant botulism in the United States are due to type A or B; rare cases due to types C,[8] E,[7,9,10] F,[11,12] and G[13] are reported in the U.S. or elsewhere. *Clostridium butyricum*[8,9] is responsible for rare cases due to botulinal neurotoxin type E, and *Clostridium baratii* is responsible for type F cases of infant botulism, especially in neonates.[11,12] Molecular techniques demonstrate that unexpressed botulinum toxin genes can be found in a variety of clostridial species, and more than one toxin type in a single *C. botulinum* strain.[14]

Botulinum toxins are large, single polypeptides of similar structure. After systemic absorption, toxin is concentrated at the plasma membrane of the neuron, and is taken into the synaptic vesicle where it binds irreversibly to receptors on presynaptic cholinergic and adrenergic nerve endings; a portion is internalized, cleaving protein components of the neuroexocytosis apparatus within the cell to shut down the synaptic vesicle cycle.[15] Release of acetylcholine is blocked. Neutralizing antitoxin is effective only before internalization of the toxin molecule. Recovery depends on ultrasprouting of nerve endings. With intoxication at 70% or more junctions, impairment of voluntary muscular and autonomic function ensues; diaphragmatic function is preserved until 90% involvement occurs.

Botulinum toxins are the most potent toxins known; 10^{11} molecules (0.3 ng) reaching neuromuscular junctions are enough to cause clinical botulism. Type A is the most avidly binding, most potent toxin, and is associated with the most severe clinical disease. Spores of *C. botulinum* are heat-resistant, withstanding 100°C for hours. For destruction of spores, food must be heated under pressure to temperatures of 116°C. Toxin is acid- and enzyme-resistant but can be destroyed by heating of food to boiling point (100°C) for 10 minutes. Certain environmental conditions promote outgrowth of vegetative forms and production of toxin in food, such as anaerobic conditions, pH >4.6, warm temperature (>39°C), and high moisture content.

Pathophysiology

Infant botulism results from unrecognizable ingestion of botulinal spores in most cases in the U.S. following the recommendation to avoid feeding honey to infants.[2,4,5] Honey may still be a significant source of spores for cases in other countries.[16] The gastrointestinal tract of children and adults is resistant to outgrowth of *C. botulinum* spores, but in infants younger than 12 months occasionally is permissive of such outgrowth. Age-related vulnerability is related at least partially to lack of competitive flora and possibly to pH and motility. Multiple observations and experimentations in a mouse model provide compelling evidence for importance of competitive flora in protection,[17,18] such as: (1) age-limited (7 to 13 days)

natural susceptibility to intestinal colonization by *C. botulinum* spores; (2) ongoing susceptibility in germ-free adults; (3) acquisition of resistance in germ-free adults after replacement of normal cohort colony for 3 days; (4) resistance after establishment of selective, limited intestinal flora; and (5) loss of resistance after antibiotic suppression of intestinal flora.

The necessary components of resistance are undoubtedly complex, but *Bacteroides*, *Lactobacillus*, and other *Clostridium* spp. are inhibitory to *C. botulinum*. Stool flora of seven infants delineated at first manifestations of botulism showed relative paucity of *Bacteroides* and *Lactobacillus* spp.[19] The putrefactive intestinal flora of the infant fed formula and the fermentative flora of the infant fed human milk would be expected to be inhibitory. Epidemiologic data support the theory that the period of permissiveness of the gut of the infant fed formula is brief (i.e., competing flora is established rapidly[20]), and that of the infant fed human milk is extended and especially heightened during perturbation of flora during weaning.[21] Natural occurrence of infant botulism in horses (shaker foal syndrome) and ducks (limberneck) suggests similar age-related vulnerability to colonization in animals. The rare cases of intestinal toxemia botulism in older persons have been associated with underlying gut anomaly[3] or presumed alteration of gut flora, pH, or motility by surgery and drugs.[22]

EPIDEMIOLOGY

Environmental Exposure

Potential sources of *C. botulinum* spores are the environment and naturally contaminated foodstuffs (e.g., honey and corn syrup). Soil-dwelling *Clostridium* species other than *C. botulinum* have been isolated from U.S. manufactured powdered infant formulas suggesting their potential as a source of neurotoxigenic clostridia.[23] *C. botulinum* spores are ubiquitous worldwide, found in cultivated and virgin soil, in aquatic sediment and marine life, and in the intestinal content of birds. *C. botulinum* producing types A, B, and F toxins generally are found in areas of low rainfall and moderate temperature, whereas those producing types D and E are associated with water.[7,24] In the most recent soil survey in the U.S., types A, B, C, D, and E strains were found; 23% of soil samples contained botulinal spores.[25]

The geographic distribution of *C. baratii*-producing toxin F is less certain as the organism would not be detected by microbiologic screening for *C. botulinum*; source in cases of infant botulism from California and Iowa was apparently the environment, and contaminated food in an adult.[12,26,27] Soil sampling in Argentina showed that 23% of samples were positive for a variety of *C. botulinum* types; distribution was uneven, with higher prevalence in cultivated soil.[28]

In the U.S., almost all type A spores are found west of the Mississippi River, where the Rocky Mountain cordillera rise out of the Middle and Great Plains (Figure 189-1). Type B spores have a more general east–west distribution but are confined almost totally to areas between 35 and 55 degrees north latitude and occur in soil with high organic content. Type E-producing bacteria are found in marine life and sediment around fresh water from the Pacific northwest and the Great Lakes region of the U.S.[7,24] Type F strains have been isolated from marine sediment from the Pacific coast and from crabs in the Chesapeake Bay. Reasons for this geographic distribution of spores producing different neurotoxins largely are unknown.

Botulism and botulinum toxin types in humans (and animals) mirror the geography and density of *C. botulinum* spores in the environment. Infant botulism undoubtedly is underrecognized but cases have been reported from 5 continents and in 46 states in the U.S.[29] The highest reported incidence of disease in the U.S. is the Delaware–Pennsylvania–New Jersey region arching Philadelphia, followed by California and Utah.[6] Argentina, Australia, Canada, Italy, and Japan, respectively, have reported the next largest number of cases.[29]

Among cases of infant botulism, approximately half are caused by toxin type A and half by toxin type B. Other types are associated

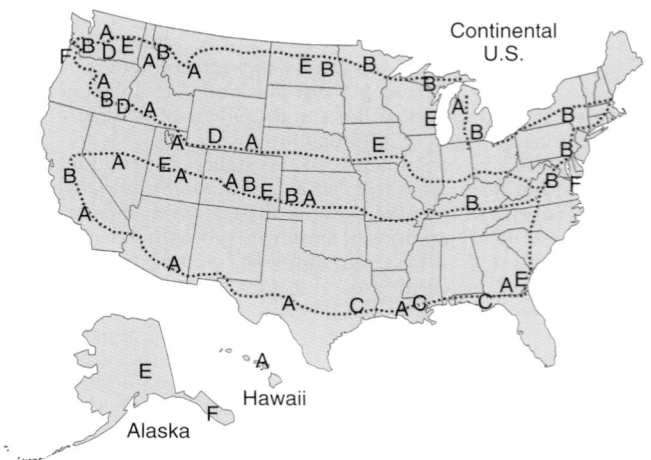

Figure 189-1. Natural occurrence of *Clostridium botulinum* spores by toxin type. Data primarily represent four east–west crossings of the United States (dotted lines) during which soil samples were collected every 50 miles. Multiple samplings were positive in some states (not shown). (Data from Smith LDS. The occurrence of *Clostridium botulinum* and *Clostridium tetani* in the soil of the United States. Health Lab Science 1978;15:74–80.)

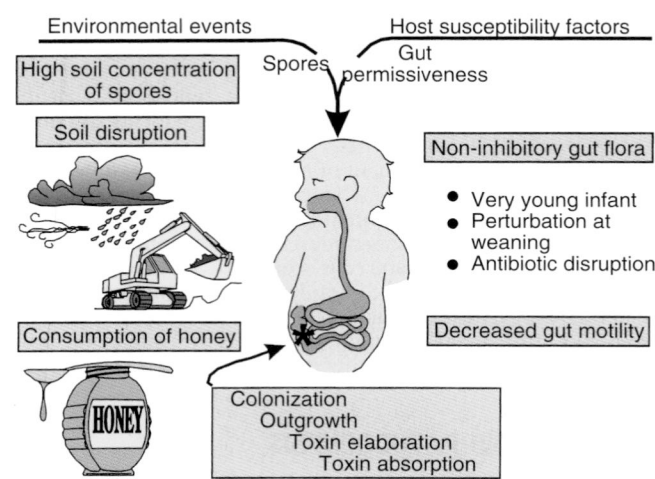

Figure 189-2. Schematic representation of pathophysiologic events in infant-type botulism.

rarely. Cases in California are divided between types A and B,[30] but type B organisms account for >90% of cases in Pennsylvania.[19] One or more samples from an affected infant's environment, such as yard soil, vacuum cleaner dust, crib, father's shoes, or consumed honey, usually yield growth of *C. botulinum*, always of matching toxin type.[19,30] Samples do not contain preformed toxin.

Unusual epidemiologic findings suggest uneven distribution of spores within limited geographic areas. In one Pennsylvania study, for example, residences of 83% of the 53 patients with botulism formed an arc around Philadelphia, with remarkable sparing of the city itself, of counties surrounding the arc, and of the western parts of the state.[21] In Colorado, 3 of only 6 cases reported between 1977 and 1985 were from the same town of 800 people; 2 of 3 infants shared a crib (years apart), and all samples from their environments (including the crib) yielded *C. botulinum* producing type A toxin.[31] Nearly all of 39 infants with botulism in Utah over a 20-year period resided within a 70-mile metropolitan corridor including Salt Lake City, Ogden, and Provo.[32] A cluster of 12 cases occurring over 2 years in Utah suggested association with wind and rain;[33] such a correlation was not found in Pennsylvania.[19]

Many parents of infants with botulism report nearby soil disruption (such as home or commercial construction or road work) or a dusty "event" before onset of the infant's illness.[19,33] Nearby construction was common but was not significantly associated with botulism in a prospective case-control study performed by the U.S. Centers for Disease Control and Prevention (CDC).[34] In Pennsylvania, 50% of infants' fathers had occupations that required daily contact with soil; spores were found on work shoes or at a work site in most cases for which such samples were taken.[19] Organisms of matching toxin type were found in yard soil and drinking water in cases in Australia,[35] and also in vacuum cleaner dust in a case in Finland.[36]

Honey and light and dark corn syrups have been found to harbor *C. botulinum* spores, testing positive in from 0.5% to 20% of samples.[37,38] Following changes in corn syrup production, the Food and Drug Administration (FDA) laboratory found that samples tested negative for *C. botulinum*.[39] Consumption of honey is a clear risk factor for infant botulism (odds ratio (OR) = 9.8 in one study)[30,34] but accounts for <15% of cases currently in the U.S. Corn syrup has not been a proven vehicle for spores in any case of infant botulism. A single case of infant botulism in the U.K. was linked to isolation of *C. botulinum* spores from powdered infant formula; non-botulinal clostridial spores have been found in commercial powdered formula in the U.S.[23,39a]

Host Susceptibility

Infant botulism has a striking age group for susceptibility and association with feeding. The youngest reported patient had onset of disease at 38 hours of age,[26] and the oldest at 11.7 months.[34] Most cases occur between 6 weeks and 6 months of age. Median age at onset of infant botulism is significantly earlier in infants fed formula (7.6 weeks) than in infants fed human milk (13.7 weeks).[19,33] Median age at onset was 7.6 days for 5 type F cases (due to *C. baratii*) in the U.S. and 9 days for a single case due to *C. botulinum*-producing type E toxin; these are significantly younger than the median 84 days for types A and B.[27] Breastfeeding is a risk factor for infant botulism, present in 66% to 100% of cases in published series.[19,33,34] It was not a risk factor for infants with disease before 2 months of age in one study.[34] Long and associates[19] found that 66% of breastfed infants with botulism who had received human milk exclusively had been introduced to the first nonhuman food substances (cereal, formula, fruit) within 2 to 4 weeks before onset of symptoms.

Other socioeconomic and racial factors associated with infant botulism probably are markers for breastfeeding. In one study, human milk appeared to be protective against rapidly fatal infant botulism. Additional age-specific risk factors are: (1) living in a rural or farming area for infants younger than 2 months (OR = 6.4); (2) having less than one bowel movement per day for at least 2 months (OR = 2.9); and (3) ingestion of corn syrup (OR = 5.2) for infants 2 months of age or older.[34] A schematic summary of environmental and host factors and pathophysiologic events in infant-type botulism is shown in Figure 189-2.

Immunity

C. botulinum is not part of normal intestinal flora. There is no apparent natural acquisition of immunity to the organism or its toxin. Infants recovering from botulism have demonstrable specific antibody to toxin,[40] despite continued presence of toxin in stool. The extent and duration of protective effect are not known. There are no cases of distant recurrences; occurrence after 12 months of age is rare in all individuals.

CLINICAL MANIFESTATIONS

The clinical manifestations of botulism are similar regardless of mode of acquisition. The spectrum of infant botulism is broad, with sudden infant death syndrome (SIDS) an occasional presentation at one extreme and transient mild weakness and hypotonia, slow feeding, or constipation alone at the other. Clinical manifestations have not changed over 3 decades.[5,33]

TABLE 189-1. Symptoms and Signs at the Time of Hospitalization in 251 Infants with Botulism

Finding	Percent Occurrence Across Studies	
	Average	Range
HISTORY		
Decreased bowel movements	83	65–100
Poor feeding, weak suck	92	79–100
Floppiness, weakness	93	88–100
Weak cry	65	18–100
PHYSICAL EXAMINATION		
Temperature ≥38.3°C	14	–
Decreased spontaneous movement	82	–
Decreased phonation	80	–
Poor head control	97	96–98
Ptosis	84	75–97
Sluggish pupils	55	50–79
Ophthalmoplegia	55	18–61
Facial weakness	75	69–84
Decreased gag reflex	89	75–100
Difficulty swallowing	90	75–92
Hyporeflexia	54	52–57
Absence of reflexes	6	0–7
Flushed robust appearance	18	–
Decreased tears or saliva	18	18–79

Data from references 19, 32, 33, 41, 42. Not all findings were reported in all studies.

Classic Manifestations

History

After an unknown incubation period, symptoms of descending symmetrical paralysis progress over 6 hours to 20 days (median 4.2 days)[19] before medical recognition or hospitalization. Function of cranial nerves is affected before that of others that control muscles of trunk, extremities, and diaphragm. Subtly flat facial expression, quiet voice, and less avid suck are noted first, usually only by parents. The relative frequency of symptoms and signs is shown in Table 189-1.[19,32,33,41,42] Decreased frequency of bowel movements is common. Floppiness, poor feeding, gurgling, and drooling are noted almost universally by the time of hospitalization.

Physical Examination at Hospitalization

The most notable immediate impression is the infant's quiet, still demeanor. Poor head control and hypotonia (inability of sustained postural control and movement against gravity) are universal. Although frequently misinterpreted as "lethargic" and "septic," the infant is alert (but paralyzed and thus unable to smile, regard, vocalize, or move), and skin color is normal or robust. Diagnosis should not be made in the absence of cranial nerve palsies as first neurologic manifestations. Swallowing function is most affected and corneal reflexes most preserved (Figure 189-3). Disconjugate gaze precedes ophthalmoplegia. Pupils are dilated or sluggishly reactive. Hyporeflexia is unimpressive early in the course relative to profound hypotonia, but can progress over time. Respiratory difficulty at the time of hospitalization is present in <20% of patients, but is variable by case, age, and promptness of diagnosis.

Autonomic dysfunction is underrecognized. Decreased tearing and salivation can be misinterpreted as dehydration. Erythema of

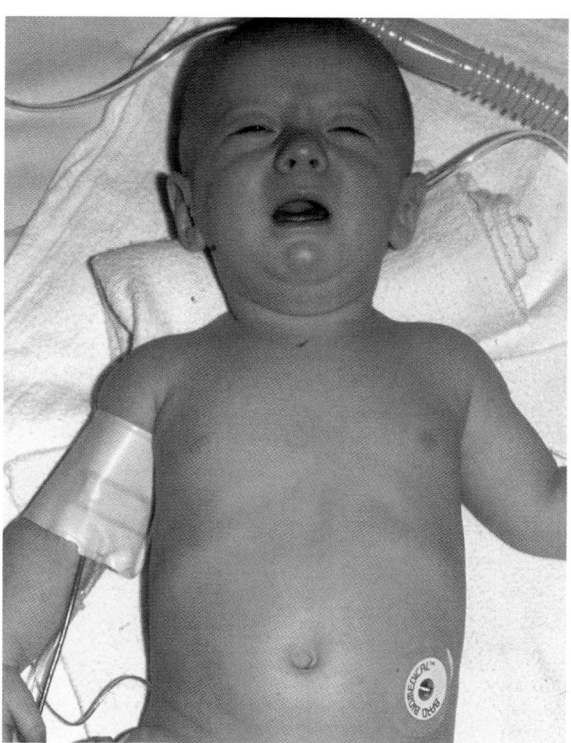

Figure 189-3. Three-month-old infant with botulism just prior to intubation. Note bilateral ptosis and facial palsy, and absence of tears.

oral mucosa can be misinterpreted as pharyngitis. Blood pressure, heart rate, and skin tone fluctuate frequently. Harlequin flushing can occur. Decreased intestinal motility, poor anal sphincter tone, and bladder atony are present commonly.

Infants Younger than 2 Months

Progression of disease and functional effects are more severe in infants younger than 2 months.[34,43] Hypotonia leads rapidly to inability to protect the airway and collapse of hypopharyngeal support. Obstructive apnea can manifest within hours of the appearance of subtle clues of poor feeding or muscle weakness or can be the sentinel event. Very young infants with *C. baratii* type F have not had heralding constipation.[27]

Sudden Infant Death Syndrome

Sudden apnea, fulminant paralysis, apparent life-threatening event, or SIDS[43] can occur in young infants with botulism. Arnon and colleagues[44] proposed a significant association by the age of epidemic curves of botulism and SIDS and further associated SIDS presentation of botulism with formula feeding (and, possibly, iron fortification). Spika and associates[34] showed botulism to be extremely severe in infants younger than 2 months regardless of type of feeding. In two studies, *C. botulinum* was isolated from intestinal contents in 4%[44] and 15%[13] of SIDS cases; in the latter study performed in Switzerland, unusual toxin types, such as C, F, and G, were identified.[13] A prospective study in Australia failed to confirm the presence of *C. botulinum* in 248 victims of SIDS.[45]

DIFFERENTIAL DIAGNOSIS

Several disorders with weakness or hypotonia can mimic infant botulism superficially,[46,47] but the constellation of findings in the setting of age, feeding history, and exposures usually is classic, and the possibility of another diagnosis is remote. Table 189-2 shows differentiating features of conditions frequently considered. Tick paralysis (rare in infants) causes symmetrical ascending flaccidity,

TABLE 189-2. Differentiating Features of Conditions Considered or Misdiagnosed in Infants with Botulism Condition

Condition	Expected Findings
Septicemia	Fever, lethargy, mottling
Meningitis/encephalitis	Fever, irritability, nuchal rigidity; specific/predominant CNS abnormalities; abnormal CSF
Cerebrovascular event	Focal neurologic deficits; abnormal CT/MRI
Genetic metabolic disorder	Onset with vomiting, irritability, or intellectual or neurologic abnormality; no weakness
Hypothyroidism	Hypotonia, lethargy, poor development; onset over weeks–months
Myasthenia gravis	Neonatal, or older age at onset; ptosis usually sole finding early
Spinal muscular atrophy	Inherited, progressive hypotonia and weakness; involvement tongue, face, jaw sparing extraocular muscles and sphincters; areflexia
Anticholinergic poisoning	Agitation, coma, extrapyramidal movements
Poliomyelitis	Asymmetric, spotty paralysis; aseptic meningitis; spasms
Guillain–Barré syndrome	Rare before 2 years of age; progressive symmetrical ascending paralysis; areflexia; CSF proteinosis

CNS, central nervous system; CSF, cerebrospinal fluid; CT, computed tomography; MRI, magnetic resonance imaging.

with gait abnormality the usual first manifestation. In the Miller Fisher variant of Guillain–Barré syndrome (rare in infants), ataxia and areflexia occur early in the course of ophthalmoplegia. In a case of a 9-week-old infant, biopsy for possible Hirschsprung disease because of constipation was performed before neurologic abnormalities were noted.[48]

DIAGNOSIS

Routine laboratory tests are not useful in diagnosis. Complete blood count, erythrocyte sedimentation rate, and cerebrospinal fluid values are normal. Definitive diagnosis requires isolation of the organism or detection of the toxin in stool. Mouse bioassay for toxin is the preferred method for diagnosis and results are positive in all likely cases of infant botulism. *C. botulinum* organisms and toxin have been identified in stool of affected infants as late as 5 months and 4 months, respectively, after onset of symptoms. Fluorescent antibody or enzyme immunosorbent assays for detection of toxin or organism are inferior. Polymerase chain reaction testing is promising as a rapid and less cumbersome test, but is not standardized.[14,49]

Isolation of Organisms

Specimens for culture should be refrigerated if inoculation is not to be prompt. *C. botulinum* can be isolated from stool, intestinal contents from autopsy specimens, food specimens, or dust or dirt with the use of enrichment in chopped meat broth and then anaerobic incubation on selective egg yolk agar. Density of organism in stool can be as high as 10^8 colony-forming units per gram. *C. botulinum*-producing toxins types A through F produce lipase, which is detected as an iridescent film surrounding colonies. Vegetative cells are straight or slightly curved, motile, gram-positive bacilli with oval subterminal spores. Identity is confirmed by carbohydrate fermentation, biochemical reactions, and gas chromatography; typing is assigned according to toxin production utilizing mouse toxin neutralization assay.

C. botulinum type G, neurotoxigenic *C. butyricum* type E,[10] and *C. baratii* type F[4,47] are lipase-negative and thus may not be detected by usual screening and isolation techniques. *C. botulinum* type G also is asaccharolytic. Isolation of *C. botulinum* type E from the stool of an affected infant was successful only after enrichment following identification of the toxin gene by PCR testing of culture supernatant.[7]

Identification of Toxin

Mouse inoculation toxin neutralization assay on stool filtrate is the only reliable confirmatory test for infant botulism. Serum assay results are positive in <10% of infants with botulism, and implicated honey does not have preformed toxin. In cases of foodborne, wound, or unclassified botulism, appropriate specimens include stool, gastric aspirate or vomitus, serum, wound, and foodstuff. Serum has the highest yield of positive results in foodborne botulism, but the positive yield from stool is almost equal in such cases.

Passed stool is the preferred specimen, but effluent obtained after a small-volume enema using sterile, nonbacteriostatic water is acceptable. In the latter instance, subsequent specimens are collected if the initial test result is negative and diagnosis is likely. Specimens for toxin assay should be refrigerated but not frozen pending shipping directions from public health officials.

Neurologic Tests

Electromyographic (EMG) findings characteristic of botulism are: (1) motor unit action potentials of brief duration and small amplitude (BSAP; brief small action potential) that are overly abundant for the amount of stimulus (so-called BSAP pattern); (2) enhancement of compound action potential in response to rapidly repetitive nerve stimulation at 30 Hz; (3) normal velocity of nerve conduction; and (4) no significant clinical response to injection of edrophonium chloride or neostigmine. Findings of electromyography depend on stage of disease and the timing and amount of nerve stimulation.[48,49] Post-tetanic facilitation of compound muscle action potential, thought to be sensitive and pathognomonic for botulism,[49] requires 10-second stimulation at 50 Hz. Because the age and clinical findings are unique and the diagnosis can always be proved by toxin assay, painful EMG is usually not justified; it provides no additional prognostic information. Tensilon test to exclude myasthenia gravis rarely is performed in infants as safe doses for infants are not established and borderline positive tests have been reported in adults with botulism. Electroencephalogram and neuroimaging studies usually are normal, barring an hypoxic event. Cerebrospinal fluid values are normal. Abnormal auditory and visual evoked potentials reflect involvement of respective cranial nerves. Seizures, which occur in 2% to 5% of cases, are rarely unexplained. Raised intraocular pressure has been reported.[50]

HOSPITAL COURSE

Disease Progression

Respiratory Compromise

The natural course of a typical case is progressive weakness over 2 to 10 days in hospital, remaining at a nadir for 1 to 2 weeks, followed by regaining of abilities slowly.[3,19,33,51,52] Mean duration of hospitalization in California was 3.8 weeks for type B botulism and 5.4 weeks for type A.[51] Manifestations of disease progression are shown in Table 189-3.[19,41,51] Most infants have progressive inability to swallow or protect the airway, leading to discontinuation of oral feeding, and 75% require intubation. Some patients require protection of the airway without the need for mechanical ventilation. Acute respiratory distress syndrome, reported in 5% of patients with botulism in one study,[19] was associated with the artificial ventilation but otherwise was unexplained.

TABLE 189-3. Associated Events and Complicating Conditions in 111 Hospitalized Infants with Botulism

Associated Events	Average	Range
Percent Occurrence Across Studies		
Intubation required	77	20–89
Seizures	4	2–5
Acute respiratory distress syndrome	5	–
Failure of oral feeding	89	77–93
Excessive production of antidiuretic hormone	17	16–18
Autonomic instability	11	11
Complications		
Acute otitis media	30	–
Pneumonia	15	7–25
Urinary tract infection	6	0–11
Septicemia	3	0–5

Data from references 19, 41, 51. Not all findings were reported in all studies.

Fluid and Electrolyte Disorders

Seizures are uncommon but are difficult to note clinically in the paralyzed infant; sudden tachycardia is a clue. Seizures are related almost invariably to hypoxia or hyponatremia. The syndrome of excessive secretion of antidiuretic hormone (ADH), reported anecdotally[33] and in 17% in two series,[19,41] is almost certainly due to venous pooling in the paralyzed infant, decreased left atrial filling, and subsequent stimulus to ADH production. Hyponatremia and hypo-osmolality can be profound. Hyponatremic seizure occurred in one patient in Philadelphia as a result of extreme hyponatremia of the mother's milk (a recognized consequence of stress).

Complications

Except for complications directly related to muscular dysfunction, secondary infections are most common in botulism (see Table 189-3), predominantly acute otitis media, aspiration pneumonia, and urinary tract infection. Schechter and associates[53] reported five cases of *Clostridium difficile* colitis in infants during or after hospitalization for botulism; toxic megacolon and necrotizing enterocolitis distinguished two cases.

MANAGEMENT

The challenge of management is to recognize the diagnosis promptly and before catastrophic events, to administer antitoxin urgently, and to prevent complications until neuromuscular function recovers. Successful treatment depends on meticulous attention to protection of the airway and prevention of sudden catastrophic hypoxia, provision of adequate ventilation and nutrition, and prevention of nosocomial complications. It must be remembered that the sensory system is unaffected and intellectual function is preserved throughout (as documented in adults paralyzed from foodborne botulism).

Antitoxin Therapy

All infants with the clinical diagnosis of botulism should be treated urgently with human botulism immune globulin intravenous (BIG-IV), which neutralizes botulinum toxins. Treatment halts progression of neuromuscular blockade and should not be delayed for confirmatory testing. This pentavalent antitoxin product is derived from plasmapheresis of donors who have received at least 5 doses of A, B, C, D, E toxoid vaccine (usually for at-risk laboratory work). BIG-IV does not cover the rare occurrence of type F disease.

A 5-year, placebo-controlled (with immune globulin intravenous), randomized clinical trial of the efficacy of BIG-IV was performed in 129 California infants under the sponsorship of the Orphan Drug Program of the FDA and the California Department of Health Services (CDHS).[5] Infants treated with BIG-IV had duration of hospitalization reduced by 3.1 weeks (from 7.7 weeks to 2.6 weeks), mechanical ventilation by 2.6 weeks, tube or intravenous feedings by 6.4 weeks, and mean hospital charges by $88,600 (in 2004 U.S. dollars).[5] No serious adverse events were attributable to BIG-IV. In open-label use of BIG-IV in 366 infants with laboratory-confirmed botulism who were treated within 7 days of hospitalization, duration of hospitalization was significantly shorter for those treated before 4 days (2.0 weeks) compared with those treated on days 4 to 7 (2.9 weeks). In 2003, BIG-IV was licensed by the FDA to the CDHS as BabyBIG. Drug is obtained through the CDHS Botulism Treatment and Prevention Program (510-231-7600; http://www.infantbotulism.org). The product is administered as a single dose intravenously. The January 2012 price was $45,300. The mean serum half-life of BabyBIG is 27.7 days, which is reassuring in light of prolonged intraluminal toxin production in infants. Equine antitoxin should not be given to infants with botulism and BabyBIG is not licensed, appropriate, or available for use in other forms of botulism.

Antimicrobial Therapy

Antibiotic therapy is indicated only for the treatment of secondary bacterial infection. Antibiotics with bactericidal activity against *C. botulinum* (e.g., β-lactam agents) do not have an apparent beneficial or detrimental effect on the course of paralysis. Aminoglycosidic agents are avoided because they contribute to neuromuscular blockade and have been associated temporally with rapid deterioration. Fever and an abnormal white blood cell count suggest a complicating infection. Ampicillin or amoxicillin is appropriate for treatment of pneumonia, acute otitis media, or sinusitis.

Respiratory Management

Respiratory arrest is the primary cause of mortality and sequelae and either can follow days of progressive paresis or occur suddenly, sometimes before or as the diagnosis is suspected. In infants older than 2 months, the tempo of progression is apparent over 24 hours; respiratory failure usually is predictable and is due to weakness of intercostal muscles and then the diaphragm. In younger infants, obstruction, aspiration, and weakness are concurrent problems, requiring pre-emptive intubation.

The patient is observed in an intensive care unit with continuous monitoring to determine progression of disease. In general, rapid onset of impairment (over 24 hours rather than days) portends total paralysis and a certain requirement for ventilation. Nasotracheal or endotracheal intubation is performed when the patient's ability to cough, gag, swallow, or move against gravity is substantially impaired. Waiting for the appearance of fatigue, apnea, tachypnea, hypercarbia, or hypoxemia is inappropriate, because a life-threatening hypoxic event can occur suddenly.

Positioning with elevation of the planar mattress to 30 degrees at the head allows flow of saliva by gravity to the posterior hypopharynx, where it is swallowed most easily. Placement of a small blanket roll behind the neck minimizes neck flexion, which can compromise the airway. Optimal positioning with frequent suctioning and the use of nasogastric feeding can avert endotracheal intubation in more mildly affected patients. A cloth "bumper" placed below the buttocks prevents sliding and elevates the legs slightly to minimize venous pooling.

Tracheostomy was performed because of prolonged intubation or for fear of subglottic stenosis postextubation in approximately 50% of infants with botulism in one institution in Philadelphia before 1981,[41] but not in another institution in the same city,[19] and in <1% of infants reported from California. With careful selection of endotracheal tube size and proper care, tracheostomy is rarely needed and should not be performed prophylactically.

Immediate or late sequelae of airway trauma is unusual, even when intubation was required for >1 month in the pre-antitoxin era.

Atelectasis and pneumonia can be minimized by careful physiotherapy, suctioning, and positioning and by provision of periodic sighing respirations (even for intubated patients who do not require continuous ventilation). Plugging of the tube and accidental extubation largely are avoidable; experienced personnel must be vigilant and capable of immediate intervention when necessary.

Criteria for extubation are return of gag, cough, and sustained motion against gravity. Mean duration of intubation calculated for all studies before the use of antitoxin was approximately 21 days, with relatively longer duration for type A disease.

Nutrition

Enteral feeding is well absorbed and well tolerated because of an apparent relative sparing of paralytic effect on the small bowel. Additionally, enteral feeding stimulates gut motility (which may help purge organisms and toxin), protects integrity of the enteric mucosa and obviates the need for an indwelling intravenous catheter. Continuous small-volume nasoenteric (usually nasojejunal) feeding is begun within 48 hours of hospitalization. Caloric needs of the immobile, ventilated infant are approximately two-thirds of predicted. A small enema is used judiciously to obtain a stool sample for diagnosis; a therapeutic benefit is not apparent, and vigorous enema or use of cathartic is contraindicated. Human milk or formula is appropriate for feeding.

Oral feedings are not resumed until strong swallow, gag, and suck reflexes return, the infant has sustained strength against gravity, and bolus nasogastric feedings have been tolerated.

Weight and fluids and electrolytes are monitored carefully through the nadir of muscular function, to correct initial dehydration and observe for hyponatremia. Intravenous catheters and an indwelling urinary bladder catheter are unnecessary, and their use carries risks of mechanical and infectious complications.

Infection Control

No case of person-to-person transmission of botulism in the home or hospital has been reported. No special isolation of hospitalized infants is recommended. Infants' stools are likely to contain *C. botulinum* organisms and toxin for the duration of hospitalization and beyond. Careful handwashing practices and disposal of diapers as contaminated waste are important. After the patient's discharge, circumstances for potential fecal–oral transmission to other infants (such as the sharing of cribs) should be avoided for 3 to 4 months.

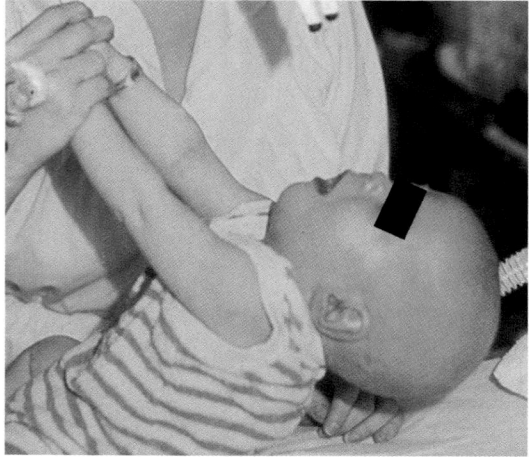

Figure 189-4. Severe head lag in a 4-month-old infant 2 months after infant botulism (1 month after extubation).

OUTCOME AND PREVENTION

Patients in whom supportive care is begun before an hypoxic episode have an excellent prognosis, with <1% mortality rate even before the availability of human BIG. Full recovery without neurologic or neuromuscular sequelae depends on maintaining vigilance and meticulous supportive care while minimizing interventions that increase complications. Peripheral muscular strength and muscles of cranial nerve intervention recover quickly, while strength to control the head and trunk recovers slowly (Figure 189-4).

Botulism is uncommon despite unavoidable, frequent environmental exposure to spores. Honey is an avoidable source of spores. The American Academy of Pediatrics and CDC recommend avoidance of honey for children younger than 12 months.[54]

FOODBORNE BOTULISM

Foodborne botulism in the U.S. rarely occurs in children. The 20 to 30 cases occurring annually in adults over the past several decades have been related to improper preparation, preservation, or storage of food in the home, in restaurants and in traditional ethnic foods. Most cases are sporadic and most outbreaks are small, involving 2 or 3 persons. Larger outbreaks, however, occur from commercial and restaurant sources.[55] Toxin types other than A and B (which were responsible for more than 90% of cases before 1980) have emerged, especially *C. botulinum* type E in Arctic regions globally[24] and foodborne cases due to *C. baratii* toxin type F.[12,47]

Of 160 foodborne botulism events occurring in the U.S. from 1990 to 2000, 39% of cases and 58% of events occurred in Alaska. Toxin type E caused 90% of cases in Alaska, reflecting its marine habitat and the Eskimo diet.[4,56] Multiple restaurant-associated outbreaks have occurred, however, most recently ascribed to prepared chopped garlic (type B),[57] sautéed onions (type A),[58] roasted eggplant (type B),[59] foil-wrapped baked potatoes (type A) held at ambient temperature,[60] and improperly stored chili sold at a salvage store.[61] Foods kept in oil, which probably promotes anaerobic conditions, were notably responsible. Outbreaks have occurred related to commercially prepared cheese sauce (type A),[62] chili sauce (type A),[63] and carrot juice (type A).[64]

Symptoms of descending symmetrical paralysis begin 12 to 36 hours (range 6 hours to 8 days) after ingestion of the contaminated food (which usually does not taste tainted). Classic symptoms, including dysphagia, diplopia, dilated and fixed pupils, and dry mouth and throat, occur in an alert patient and are followed by musculoskeletal weakness, postural hypotension, and respiratory paralysis. Ocular symptoms can be heralding manifestations, including blurred near or distant vision (i.e., impairment of accommodation) and diplopia.[65] Type E intoxication has the shortest but variable incubation period (1 to 8 days) and commonly is heralded by nausea and vomiting. Type A disease is most severe; the rates of required intubation for types A, B, and E intoxications are 67%, 52%, and 39%, respectively.[66] Atypical features, such as asymmetrical weakness, paresthesia, and sensory abnormalities, have been documented.

Diagnostic methods for foodborne botulism are similar to those for infants, except that toxin assays on serum and potential food source are always performed and expected to be positive; culture and toxin assays on stool also are positive in approximately one-third of cases. Antitoxin and supportive care are mainstays of therapy. A suspect case should be reported to the state health department and equine antitoxin administered urgently. Antitoxin reduces the mortality rate from type A intoxication from 46% to 26% and shortens hospital stay as well.[2,67,68] In March, 2010 a heptavalent equine botulinum antitoxin (HBAT, containing antitoxin to types A, B, C, D, E, F, and G; made through contract by the Department of Human Services to Cangene Corporation in Canada) replaced previous A, B, and E products as the only product available in the U.S. for naturally occurring non-infant botulism.[68] HBAT is available only through a CDC-sponsored Food and Drug Administration Investigational New Drug (FDA

IND) protocol (770-488-7100; information at http://www.bt.cdc.gov/agent/botulism). Hypersensitivity reaction or serum sickness illness following administration of modern antitoxin is infrequent.[24,68]

WOUND BOTULISM

Wound botulism was rare in the U.S. in the last half century until the early 1990s when a dramatic and continuing increase in cases occurred, especially in the western U.S. and almost exclusively in injection drug users.[4] "Black tar heroin" and "skin popping" are especially associated. The same phenomenon has been seen in the U.K.[69] Recent incidence of wound botulism in the U.S. is between 20 and 40 cases annually.[6] Wound botulism results from infection and toxin production by *C. botulinum* in a wound that typically is traumatic and contaminated with soil. When neuroparalytic symptoms and signs begin the wound itself is clinically unimpressive, with minimal erythema, induration, and serosanguineous discharge, and no crepitus or warmth. Gastrointestinal symptoms are less common than in foodborne botulism. Toxin types mirror the soil distribution of *C. botulinum*. Children are affected usually after accidental crush injury, with direct major soil contamination.[70]

Diagnostic methods include serum toxin assay and unroofing of lesions to obtain specimens for culture and toxin assay. Although toxin is detectable in serum less commonly than with foodborne disease, equine antitoxin is used, and the wound is debrided and irrigated vigorously. An anticlostridial agent, such as penicillin or vancomycin, usually is given parenterally, although this therapy has no known beneficial effect on the course of disease. Wound botulism has occurred despite use of antibiotic prophylaxis at the time of accidental injury. Debridement of devitalized tissue and vigorous irrigation of wounds are the most effective means of prevention.

VACCINES

The only vaccine available in the U.S. currently is a pentavalent (types A–E) botulinum toxoid (PBT) produced by the Michigan Department of Public Health and used under an IND held by the CDC (for at-risk workers) and the U.S. Army Office of the Surgeon General (for military personnel at risk during deployment). Vaccination requires 5 doses and annual boosters. Recombinant subunit vaccines are in development and a papain-fragmented (H_C) bivalent vaccine (rBVAB) is being evaluated in a phase II clinical trial.[71] Immunity to botulism would preclude potential benefits of therapeutic botulinum toxin.

Key Points. Infant Botulism

- Age of onset is 2 days through 11 months (median age onset formula fed, 7.6 weeks; human milk fed, 13.7 weeks)
- Beginning of weaning is a period of heightened risk for infants fed human milk exclusively
- Exposures to *C. botulinum* spores usually are incidental and unavoidable
- Nearby soil disruption (e.g., construction, dust) or bringing soil into the home (e.g., shoes of construction worker) is common in history
- Constipation is a heralding feature
- Descending symmetric paralysis over hours to days with primary cranial nerve and bulbar involvement is universal
- All infants in whom diagnosis is considered should be monitored in an intensive care unit
- All infants should be treated urgently with BabyBIG
- Administration of BabyBIG is associated with an average reduction of hospital stay by 3.1 weeks, of mechanical ventilation by 2.6 weeks, and tube feedings by 6.4 weeks

---

190 *Clostridium difficile*

Nalini Singh and David Y. Hyun

DESCRIPTION OF PATHOGEN

Clostridium difficile is an anaerobic spore-forming gram-positive bacillus that was first described as part of a study of the intestinal flora of newborn infants. Recovery of *C. difficile* requires selective agar containing cycloserine, cefoxitin, and fructose (CCFA). Isolation can be enhanced further by addition of taurocholate or lysozyme.[1,2] *C. difficile* can exist in vegetative or spore forms. Once spores reach the colon, they convert to the functional vegetative form in which the organism becomes susceptible to antimicrobial agents and begins producing toxins A and B.

Pathogenesis of *C. difficile* infections begins with disruption of the colonic microflora, usually as a result of antimicrobial therapy. Alteration of the intestinal ecosystem decreases resistance to *C. difficile* colonization.[3] Subsequent ingestion and colonization of *C. difficile* leads to production of toxins A and B, which cause intestinal mucosal injury, inflammation, and diarrhea. In vitro and animal model studies have demonstrated that these toxins disrupt the cytoskeleton and tight junctions of epithelial cells and cause apoptosis.[4,5] Toxin B has been shown to be 10 times more potent than toxin A in causing human colonic mucosal damage, and certain *C. difficile* strains that produce only toxin B have been described to cause significant and severe disease in the absence of toxin A.[6,7] Molecular diagnostic tools such as pulsed field gel electrophoresis

have been utilized for epidemiologic investigations. *C. difficile* outbreaks in health care facilities in the United States and Canada were linked to a strain identified as NAP1 (North American pulsed field type 1) by pulsed field gel electrophoresis and by restriction-endonuclease analysis.[8] The epidemic strain NAP1 has an upregulated production of toxin A and B compared with other strains, likely secondary to genetic differences in regulatory genes.[8,9] NAP1 strains also produce an additional binary toxin, but its pathogenic role is not well delineated.[10]

EPIDEMIOLOGY

The epidemiology of *C. difficile* in children has been evolving from healthcare-associated to community-acquired in the past decade.[11,12] *C. difficile* spores are present in asymptomatic neonates, healthy young infants, soil, and healthcare and daycare environments. *C. difficile* spores are resistant to heat, acidic environment, antibiotics, and most antiseptics, which allow the organisms to survive in the environment for prolonged periods.[13] *C. difficile* can be acquired from infected or colonized individuals and from contaminated environment or equipment. Neonates can become colonized without developing symptomatic illness. In 2001, the Centers for Disease Control and Prevention reported a 26% increase in reported hospital discharge diagnoses of *C.*

difficile-associated diarrhea (CDAD).[14] Among children evaluated for diarrhea in a hospital emergency department in Seattle, *C. difficile* was found to be the third most common cause, after viral and other bacterial causes.[15] A similar trend, peaking in 2004–2005, occurred when an increased number of CA-CDAD episodes were documented in children with fewer prior antibiotic exposures.[11] In a study utilizing administrative data, CDAD increased from 7.24 to 12.80 cases per 10,000 from 1997 through 2006 in the U.S. Incidence was lowest for newborns and young children.[16] CDAD in adults is associated with significant economic burden.[17,18] The hypervirulent NAP1 strain of *C. difficile* has emerged in a small number (20%) of affected children.[19]

Selected states in the U.S. and Canada currently require hospitals to report incidence rates of CDAD.[20,21] Newer molecular diagnostic tests and public reporting should help define further the incidence of CDAD. Modifiable risk factors associated with CDAD include exposure to antimicrobial therapy. Other risk factors include use of antineoplastic agents, repeated enemas or use of gastrointestinal stimulants, underlying bowel disease such as inflammatory bowel disease or Hirschsprung disease, gastrointestinal surgery, and renal insufficiency.[22–27] CDAD has been associated with almost every antibiotic but is associated more frequently with penicillins, macrolides, clindamycin, cephalosporins, and fluoroquinolones.[28]

CLINICAL MANIFESTATIONS

The spectrum of clinical manifestations associated with *C. difficile* infection ranges from asymptomatic colonization with toxigenic strains to pseudomembranous colitis. Asymptomatic colonization and toxin production are common in infants, with up to 50% of children under one year of age being carriers. The most common clinical presentation of CDAD is mild to moderate diarrhea, with some patients having mucus or blood in stool. Children with pseudomembranous colitis can have diarrhea, fever, abdominal distention, cramps, pain, and systemic toxicity such as malaise, anorexia, and dehydration. Occasionally, some children develop severe disease associated with complications such as toxic megacolon. Other complications such as sepsis, ascites, intestinal perforation, intussusception, pneumatosis, and rectal prolapse have been reported rarely.[29,30] Severe cases of CDAD occur most frequently in neutropenic children with leukemia and with inflammatory bowel disease. Extraintestinal manifestations of *C. difficile* are extremely rare, but cases of bacteremia, osteomyelitis, reactive arthritis, and splenic abscesses have been reported.[31–34] Disease characteristically begins while the child is hospitalized and receiving antimicrobial therapy, but can occur weeks after hospital discharge. Coinfection with enteric virus, such as rotavirus and calicivirus, has been reported in severe cases of CDAD requiring intensive therapy.[35]

LABORATORY FINDINGS AND DIAGNOSIS

Detection of *C. difficile* toxins in stool specimens provides the most practical and clinically relevant method of diagnosis for *C. difficile*-associated diseases. *C. difficile* testing should be performed on diarrheal stool samples from children who have received antibiotics within the previous 2 months or whose diarrhea began 72 hours after hospitalization, especially in patients with other risk factors. Testing also is appropriate for children with community-associated colitis whose cultures do not reveal other bacterial pathogens. Cell culture cytotoxicity assay is considered the gold standard for toxin detection. The sensitivity of this assay ranges from 67% to 100%,[36,37] and is influenced by the type of cell lines used, as well as storage and handling of samples (i.e., immediate assay or freezing of stool sample) with the potential for rapid inactivation of toxin B. Due to the cost, slow turnaround time, and need for special expertise in performing cytotoxicity assays, commercially available enzyme immunoassay (EIA) kits for toxins A and B have become the preferred method of toxin detection in most laboratories in the U.S. EIA kits are more rapid but less sensitive compared with cytotoxin assays. The sensitivity and specificity for EIA kits are reported to be 63% to 94% and 75% to 100%, respectively.[28,38]

C. difficile can be isolated by using selective culture medium (CCFA), which remains the most sensitive testing method. However, culture cannot distinguish between toxigenic and nonpathogenic colonization without adjunctive toxin detection. Culture is used primarily for epidemiologic and outbreak investigations. Another highly sensitive test method for *C. difficile* is enzyme-linked immunoassay (EIA) detection of *C. difficile* glutamate dehydrogenase (GDH) antigen, an enzyme constitutively produced by all isolates.[39] As in culture isolation, this method cannot distinguish between toxigenic and non-toxigenic strains. Several 2-step algorithms have been developed and investigated in studies of adults using GDH detection as an initial rapid screening step, followed by toxin detection.[40,41] This 2-step method may be preferred for rapidity of reporting negative result if step 1 is negative, and in decreasing a false-positive result when toxin assay is used alone. Real-time polymerase chain reaction (rPCR) testing for toxin A and B genes is available commercially, and initial studies have demonstrated high sensitivity and specificity for this method.[42] Further data and experience are needed to determine whether rPCR is appropriate for routine clinical use.

Direct visualization of mucosal plaques or pseudomembranes on colonic mucosa by sigmoidoscopy or colonoscopy can help establish the diagnosis of pseudomembranous colitis. Due to the cost and risk associated with the procedure, endoscopy should be reserved for patients in whom other disease processes are being considered or for severely ill patients with strong clinical suspicion for *C. difficile* infection despite negative noninvasive results such as an EIA toxin assay.[43]

DIFFERENTIAL DIAGNOSIS

Viral gastroenteritis due to agents such as rotavirus, adenovirus, and enterovirus can have similar presentations to mild *C. difficile* infections. For moderate to severe presentations, bacterial causes such as *Salmonella*, *Shigella*, *Yersinia*, *Campylobacter*, or toxigenic *E. coli* should be considered, as these infections can cause local and systemic inflammation. Parasitic infections such as *Giardia* or *Cryptosporidium* also should be considered, especially if the course of diarrhea is protracted and stools are not bloody. Noninfectious causes such as inflammatory bowel disease also can mimic *C. difficile* infections. Appendicitis, intussusception, necrotizing enterocolitis, or other acute intra-abdominal diseases should be considered in extremely ill patients.

TREATMENT

Treatment for initial episodes of *C. difficile* infection consists of discontinuation of precipitating antimicrobial agent and initiation of metronidazole (oral or intravenous) or vancomycin (oral only) therapy.[28] The efficacy of these antimicrobial regimens for *C. difficile* infection has been demonstrated in randomized studies, mostly involving adult patients.[44,45] Oral metronidazole (30 mg/kg/day in 4 divided doses, maximum 2 g/day) is the drug of choice for initial treatment of mild to moderate *C. difficile* infections. Oral vancomycin (40 mg/kg/day in 4 divided doses, maximum of 125 mg/dose) is indicated in patients with severe disease who are critically ill and hospitalized in the intensive care unit, patients with underlying intestinal disease, or patients who are unresponsive to metronidazole therapy; efficacy is modestly superior to metronidazole.[46,47] Vancomycin is not effective if given intravenously. For patients with severe disease and complications such as shock, ileus, or megacolon, addition of intravenous metronidazole to oral vancomycin therapy is recommended. The duration of therapy for any regimen should be a minimum of 10 days, with most patients demonstrating clinical improvement within 24 to 48 hours of initiation of therapy, and resolution of diarrhea within 4 to 5 days. Toxin testing as a routine follow-up study is not recommended.

In addition to antimicrobial therapy, supportive care with fluid, electrolyte, and nutrition replacement should be provided.

Anti-motility drugs should not be administered to patients with *C. difficile* infections due to the associated risk of developing ileus or toxic megacolon.[48] Surgical intervention, such as colectomy, can be life-saving in selected patients with complications such as intestinal perforation or toxic megacolon.[49]

Relapses of *C. difficile* infection are observed in up to 25% of patients after initial therapy is discontinued. First relapse episodes are treated with the same regimen as the initial episode. For second or later relapses, oral vancomycin regimen in the form of tapered (e.g., over weeks) or pulse therapy (e.g., repeatedly interspersed week of therapy followed by week without therapy) is preferred based on studies involving adults.[50] Use of metronidazole beyond the first relapse episode should be avoided due to the potential for cumulative neurotoxicity.[47] Investigational therapies, including nitazoxanide, rifaximin, immune globulin, and instillation of stool from a healthy donor, have been reported as effective in single cases or small studies.[51–54] Cholestyramine and other anion-exchange resins also have been investigated, but a paucity of efficacy data limits their recommendation for routine use.[55] In addition, these resins bind vancomycin and therefore these agents should not be used concurrently. Studies evaluating the efficacy of the probiotic *Saccharomyces boulardii* in preventing relapses have been inconclusive;[56] caution must be taken as *S. boulardii* has been associated with fungemia in immunocompromised patients and patients with a central venous catheter.[57]

PREVENTION

Meticulous hand hygiene with soap and water should be performed before and after donning gloves when any contact is expected with patients infected with *C. difficile*. All healthcare personnel (HCP) should use glove and gown precautions when in contact with the patient *and* the surrounding environment.[58,59] Waterless gel is ineffective in killing spores of *C. difficile*. Cases of HA-CDAD in HCP have occurred. Children with CDAD should not attend out-of-home childcare facilities while symptomatic with diarrhea.

Environmental contamination plays an important role in the transmission of *C. difficile*.[28] *C. difficile* has been transmitted via electronic thermometers.[60] Endoscopes have not been implicated in *C. difficile* transmission. The degree to which the environment becomes contaminated is proportionate to the severity of disease in the patient. Diluted sodium hypochlorite successfully eradicates spores whereas routine hospital cleaning agents such as quaternary ammonium compounds are ineffective. Vaporized hydrogen peroxide delivered via a special apparatus is successful in reducing environmental contamination of *C. difficile*.[61] This procedure can be carried out in vacant hospital rooms and requires that the room be sealed off to ensure efficacy and avoid inadvertent exposure to patients. The effectiveness of this new technology needs further evaluation. Antimicrobial stewardship programs promoting judicious use of antimicrobial agents can also reduce the risk of CDAD.[62]

Key Points. Diagnosis and Management of *Clostridium difficile* Infection

EPIDEMIOLOGY
- Acquired from infected individuals or contaminated environments, especially healthcare environments
- Evolving from healthcare-associated to community-acquired disease
- Exposure to antibiotic therapy is a risk factor for developing disease
- Neonates can be colonized without symptomatic illness

CLINICAL FEATURES
- Most commonly manifests as mild to moderate diarrhea with or without mucous or blood in stool
- Pseudomembranous colitis
- Complications include toxic megacolon, intestinal perforation, sepsis, ascites, intussusception, and pneumatosis

DIAGNOSIS
- Detection of *C. difficile* toxins
  - Enzyme immunoassay (EIA) kits for toxins A and B
  - Cell culture cytotoxicity assay is gold standard but associated with high cost and slow turnaround time

- Culture isolation of *C. difficile* cannot distinguish between toxigenic and nonpathogenic colonizing strains
- Two-step identification of organism's glutamate-dehydrogenase (GDH) antigen, followed by EIA toxin assay if GDH positive, holds promise because of rapidity and high predictive values

TREATMENT
- Discontinuation of precipitating antibiotic
- Initial infection:
  - Mild to moderate disease: oral metronidazole (30 mg/kg/day in 4 divided doses, max. 2 g/day)
  - Severe disease in patients who have underlying intestinal disease, or are unresponsive to metronidazole therapy, or are critically ill: oral vancomycin (40 mg/kg/day in 4 divided doses, max. 125 mg/dose)
  - Severe disease with shock, ileus, or megacolon: oral vancomycin and intravenous metronidazole
  - Duration of therapy is minimum of 10 days
- Relapse infection:
  - First relapse: same regimen as the initial episode
  - Second or later relapse: oral vancomycin in therapeutic and then tapered or pulsed therapy

---

191 Other *Clostridium* Species

Itzhak Brook

Clostridia are gram-positive spore-forming bacilli that cause up to 10% of anaerobic infections[1–5] and occur at diverse clinical sites. Of the more than 200 recognized species of *Clostridium*, <20 are associated with invasive and toxigenic human diseases. Clostridial species vary in oxygen tolerance, nutritional needs, motility, and optimal temperature for growth. They can cause distinct clostridial histotoxic syndromes due to specific clostridial toxins (e.g., gas gangrene,

food poisoning) and other, nonsyndromic clostridial infections (e.g., bloodstream infection, BSI). Clostridia also are recovered from various sites as part of polymicrobial infection,[4,5] including intra-abdominal, biliary tract, female genital tract, pleuropulmonary, central nervous system, and skin and soft-tissue infections.[3]

Clostridia are members of normal human flora, present primarily in the intestinal tract and vagina,[4] and colonize the gut of other vertebrates, and insects, and are ubiquitous in soil. Clostridia are part of the phylum Firmicutes and based on 16S rDNA sequence analysis can be divided into 11 homology groups. The majority of the clinically significant species are part of group 1.[6] Most clostridial infections in children are polymicrobial and arise from the site of endogenous colonization, the organisms gaining access when normal mucocutaneous barriers are disrupted as from surgery, trauma, a perforated viscus, necrotizing enterocolitis, or chemotherapy-related mucositis.[3] Devitalized tissue and low oxidation-reduction potential enhance the growth of clostridia. Contamination of existing wounds or surgical sites with organisms from soil, unsanitary water, contaminated objects, and human and animal feces can lead to infection.

Clostridial species that cause gas gangrene produce a number of extracellular toxins or possess virulence factors such as enzymes or lysis factors. Clostridia that cause gastrointestinal disease produce enterotoxins.[7]

Clostridium perfringens is the most common clinical isolate of the genus. It is a ubiquitous bacterium associated with several exotoxin-mediated clinical diseases. *C. perfringens* has 12 recognized toxins, and the species is divided into types A through E on the basis of toxins produced.[7] *C. perfringens* causes food poisoning, necrotizing enteritis, and gas gangrene.

CLINICAL MANIFESTATIONS

Histotoxic Infections

Table 191-1 shows characteristics of histotoxic infections and the likely responsible *Clostridium* spp. *C. perfringens* is the most common pathogen associated with gas gangrene.[8] Other responsible organisms that can also produce exotoxins are *C. bifermentans, C. sordellii, C. septicum, C. novyi*, and *C. histolyticum*. The spectrum of infection includes cellulitis, necrotizing fasciitis, and severe myonecrosis (gas gangrene).[9] The last often is a polymicrobial infection that occurs after bacteremic spread from an intestinal site of colonization to traumatized soft tissue.

In adults, the predisposing factor for BSI often is colorectal or hematologic malignancy, inflammatory bowl disease, or hemodialysis[10,11] Trauma to the colon or female genital tract or injection

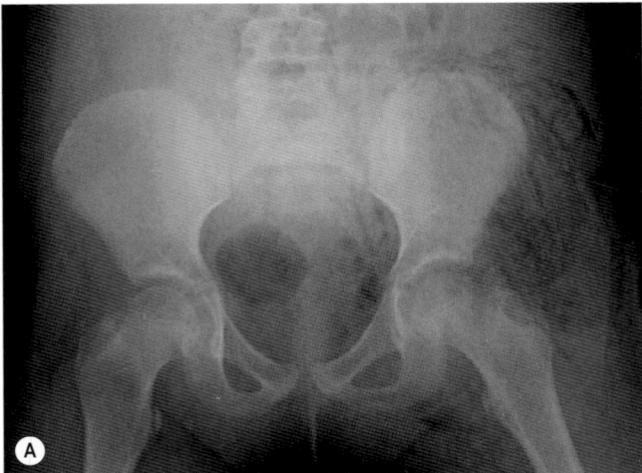
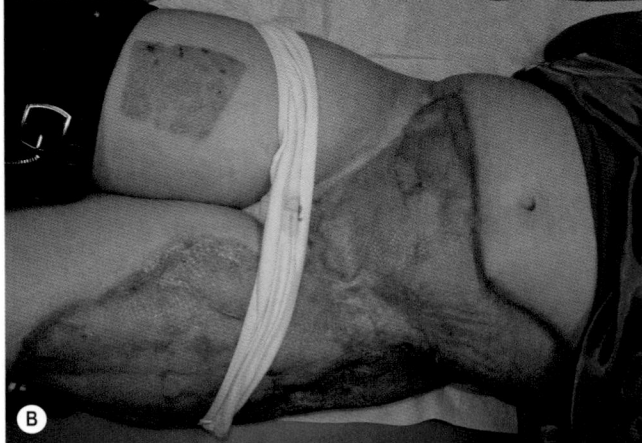

Figure 191-1. A 9-year-old girl with MyD88 deficiency (due to myeloid differentiation primary response gene) had a 5-day history of abdominal pain and acute onset of left thigh and buttock pain. Frontal radiograph **(A)** shows diffuse left-sided linear radiolucencies indicative of gas in muscle planes and soft tissues. Urgent, widely-extensive and frequent operative debridement procedures were performed and then muscle flap and grafting **(B)**. *Clostridium septicum* was isolated from tissue. (Courtesy of D. Conway, W. Davis, and S.S. Long, St. Christopher's Hospital for Children, Philadelphia, PA.)

drug abuse is present in most BSIs. *C. sordellii* and *C. septicum* deserve special note because of generally rapidly fatal course. *C. septicum* septicemia in children usually is associated with profound neutropenia (as a primary genetic disorder or related to malignancy or chemotherapy). Typhlitis, mucositis, or necrotizing enterocolitis frequently is present but some cases occur spontaneously.[12] In such cases, BSI and generalized soft-tissue infection progress rapidly and gas production is evident clinically at widely distributed body sites (Figure 191-1), Survival is unusual. *C. septicum* septicemia can complicate hemolytic uremic syndrome caused by *Escherichia coli* O157:H7,[13] bowel ischemia or trauma, and often is fatal.[14] *C. sordellii* infections occur in previously healthy individuals following induced or spontaneous abortion, childbirth, genital tract surgery, skin or soft-tissue trauma, or injection drug abuse.[15] Lethal and hemorrhage toxins are thought to be responsible for typical leukemoid reaction and high fatality.[15] Clostridial endocarditis is rare. Clostridial bacteremia can be transient, without clinical consequence, or represent a contamination.[16] In infants, BSI can be associated with necrotizing enterocolitis.[16]

Gas gangrene affects muscle tissue that has been compromised by surgery, trauma, or vascular insufficiency and is contaminated with *C. perfringens* spores, usually from foreign material, such as clothing, dirt, or a medical device.[17] The ubiquitous nature of *C. perfringens* spores in dirt, soil, and clothing and on skin,

TABLE 191-1. Clinical Manifestations of Histotoxic Clostridia

Disease	Comment
Localized skin/ soft-tissue infection	Polymicrobic; related to trauma or ischemia; frequently remains localized but with extensive necrosis; perirectal abscess, decubitus ulcers
Spreading cellulitis/ fasciitis	*Clostridium ramosum, Clostridium perfringens, Clostridium septicum* usual pathogens; compartment syndromes; 50% mortality rate
Myonecrosis (gas gangrene)	*C. perfringens, C. sordellii* responsible for >75%; related to trauma or ischemia; extremities or abdominal wall; aggressive surgical débridement required; usually fatal
Disseminated myonecrosis	*C. septicum, C. sordellii*, or *C. perfringens* usually responsible; no predisposing trauma; highly associated with profound neutropenia, colorectal or hematologic malignancy, intestinal insult; spreading cellulitis and crepitation; survival rare
Suppurative visceral infection	Polymicrobic, with *C. perfringens, C. ramosum* especially; associated with cholangitis, pancreatic disease, pelvic infections, intra-abdominal abscess, pulmonary aspiration
Bacteremia/septicemia	*C. perfringens* associated sometimes with relatively benign course; *C. septicum* and *C. sordellii* rapidly progressive, causing disseminated gas gangrene

especially of the lower trunk, provides multiple opportunities for inoculation of wounds. The metabolic requirements of *C. perfringens* for growth are the major factors in the establishment of clostridial myonecrosis.

After inoculation and outgrowth of *C. perfringens* in the muscle, the severe, rapidly progressive myonecrosis results from toxins elaborated, principally the α-toxin.[7] The α-toxin is a lecithinase that rapidly lyses cell membranes and causes hemolysis, myofibrillar injury, and vascular permeability. Severe systemic manifestations accompany local infection and may be toxin related. The patient has fever, tachycardia, and diaphoresis and is alert, anxious, and apprehensive or apathetic. Shock and attendant multiorgan failure ensue in most cases.

Gas gangrene characteristically begins 1 to 4 days (range 6 hours to 21 days) after an injury.[18] Onset is heralded by sudden and persistent pain at the site of injury and an accompanying limb "heaviness." Overlying skin appears normal at the onset but quickly becomes cool, pale, and waxy due to ischemia. Local tense swelling, tenderness, pallor, and a thin hemorrhagic exudate are noted first; pallor gives way to a bronze or magenta discoloration, and hemorrhagic (purplish) bullae appear. Pain remains the most prominent symptom. Soft-tissue crepitation can be present, but if the amount of gas is small, this may be noted first on a plain radiograph or other imaging study. As the condition worsens, a peculiar offensive odor (sometimes described as sweet) is noted, and brown serosanguineous discharge is present. Gram stain of discharge shows large numbers of gram-positive bacilli with few or no white blood cells. Involved muscle can be edematous and pale initially, advancing to a mottled appearance and greenish black gangrene. Consistency of the muscle changes from pasty and mucoid to friable and liquefied.

Tachycardia, widespread myalgia, anxiety, and diaphoresis despite low-grade fever appear early and progress rapidly to hypotension, poor perfusion, disseminated intravascular coagulation, and mental status changes. Without definitive therapy, the disease progresses inexorably, with high fever (often with rigors), shock, renal failure, metabolic acidosis, and coma, to death. Clostridial septicemia can occur terminally.

Food Poisoning

Acute self-limiting gastroenteritis due to contaminated food products (mostly meat products) often is associated with *C. perfringens* and its toxins. *C. perfringens* has been documented as the third most common cause of outbreaks of foodborne disease (after *Salmonella* and *Staphylococcus aureus*). Food poisoning occurs as a result of ingestion of vegetative forms of *C. perfringens* that develop in foods standing at a temperature between 30°C and 50°C.[19] Primary contamination of meat with *C. perfringens* spores is common. The temperature of cooking meat must exceed 120°C to ensure that spores are killed. With cooking at lower temperatures, spores can be converted to vegetative forms during cooling of food, risking the growth of *C. perfringens* in the gastrointestinal tract.

Although the symptoms of *C. perfringens* food poisoning are attributable largely to the action of enterotoxins, these usually are formed in the gut after ingestion of organisms. Ingestion of preformed toxin results only in diarrhea if gastric acidity has been neutralized. The enterotoxin formed in vivo is a 35-kd polypeptide that is heat and acid labile and is inactivated by some proteolytic enzymes.[7] The enterotoxin gene *cpe* can be used to detect illness-causing strains. The toxin inhibits absorption of glucose and secretion of water, sodium, and chloride, and it strips the epithelium of villous tips. The in vitro cytotoxic effect is similar to that of *Shigella* toxin but differs from that of cholera or *E. coli* enterotoxins. Adenyl cyclase appears not to be involved in the mediation of *C. perfringens* toxin activity. The resultant gastroenteritis demonstrates components of secretory and inflammatory diarrhea.

C. perfringens food poisoning is an acute, self-limiting diarrheal illness with an onset 6 to 24 hours after consumption of contaminated food.[19] Crampy abdominal pain commonly accompanies watery diarrhea, which does not contain blood or mucus. Fever, nausea, and vomiting occur rarely. The duration of disease is commonly <24 hours, and medical intervention usually is not warranted or sought, except in the case of outbreaks. It is difficult to differentiate food poisoning due to *C. perfringens* from that due to *Bacillus cereus*.

Differentiating this acute diarrheal disease from the numerous other viral, bacterial, and toxic causes of diarrhea on clinical grounds can be difficult unless an outbreak has occurred. The absence of fever, nausea, vomiting, and blood or mucus in stools in a patient with *C. perfringens* diarrhea makes *Salmonella*, *Shigella*, *Campylobacter*, *Yersinia*, and rotavirus unlikely. The duration of infection caused by these pathogens usually is more prolonged than *C. perfringens* food poisoning. Diagnosis can be confirmed only by isolation of large quantities of *C. perfringens* from the suspect food (above 10^6 colony-forming units per gram) and the patient's fecal samples. The enterotoxin can be detected using a cytopathic toxin neutralization assay, latex agglutination, or enzyme immune assays. However, this is not useful in clinical diagnosis.

Miscellaneous Infections

Clostridia can participate in various polymicrobial infections in children, including arthritis, osteomyelitis, skin and soft tissue (often after trauma or foreign body penetration), intra-abdominal, pulmonary, intracranial, and pelvic infections and abscesses.[5] Clostridial septicemia is rare in children without malignancy, aplastic anemia, or immunodeficiency and usually follows an ischemic gastrointestinal insult, such as with neonatal necrotizing enterocolitis or toxic megacolon.[5] Pneumatosis cystoides intestinalis is present and extensive. Highly lethal enteritis necroticans, uncommon in the United States, is associated with consumption of undercooked pork (pigbel); *C. perfringens* with type C enterotoxin is usually the cause.[20] Neutropenic enterocolitis (typhlitis) is seen with congenital neutropenia, leukemia, or neutropenia resulting from cytotoxic chemotherapy and usually is associated with *C. septicum* but other clostridia have been implicated.[21] *Clostridium* spp. of normal flora (especially *C. perfringens* and *C. ramosum*) also are associated with septic abortion and puerperal septicemia, for which mortality is high. *C. perfringens* has been reported to cause panophthalmitis in children.[22]

DIAGNOSIS

Gas gangrene is a clinical diagnosis. Myonecrosis and crepitation are classic findings but are not pathognomonic, because a number of facultative and anaerobic bacteria produce gas. Synergistic non-clostridial anaerobic myonecrosis can have local clinical manifestations similar to those of gas gangrene but usually with less severe systemic symptoms. Localized anaerobic cellulitis is more likely to have gradual onset, less pain, or systemic toxicity and is difficult to distinguish locally from group A streptococcal infection associated with exotoxin A-producing strains. A pre-existing wound in streptococcal disease, however, usually is minor, whereas in anaerobic cellulitis and myonecrosis, severe crush injury is the expected predisposing injury.[23]

Gram stain of local lesions reveals gram-positive bacilli, usually in the absence of neutrophils. Isolation of *C. perfringens* from a wound is not diagnostic of gas gangrene, and inability to isolate *C. perfringens* does not exclude the diagnosis.[23,24] Isolation from a deep tissue site should be attempted (see Chapter 187, Anaerobic Bacteria: Classification, Normal Flora, and Clinical Concepts).

TREATMENT AND PREVENTION

Histotoxic Infections

Early and aggressive surgical debridement of affected tissues is critical to successful outcome. Urgent intervention may require radical debridement to decompress fascial compartments and prevent further tissue anoxia and to provide drainage. Amputation of extremities may be required. Commonly, several surgical procedures must be performed to remove all necrotic tissue and any compromised tissue as it becomes necrotic.

Specific antimicrobial therapy directed at *Clostridium* spp. should be administered, recognizing that the anoxic and acidic environment of dead muscle is not conducive to antimicrobial efficacy. Penicillin G has excellent activity against most *Clostridium* spp. and always should be included in regimens for treatment of rapidly spreading clostridial cellulitis, myonecrosis, or septicemia. However, increasing resistance of *Clostridium* spp. to penicillin has been noted. Clindamycin, cefoxitin, and metronidazole are clinically inferior, and some *Clostridium* spp. (especially *C. ramosum, C. tertium, C. sporogenes*) are resistant. The drug of choice is penicillin G in a dose of 200,000 to 400,000 U/kg/day given intravenously in divided doses every 4 hours. Clindamycin has an advantage over penicillin because it suppresses the bacterial toxin synthesis. The combination of penicillin and clindamycin was found to be more effective than penicillin alone in a mouse model.[25] Other effective antimicrobial agents are chloramphenicol, later-generation cephalosporins, the carbapenems, and vancomycin. Treatment should be continued until BSI has cleared and symptoms have resolved.

Aggressive supportive care is essential and, predictably, is complex. Although no controlled data are available and pediatric studies are lacking, hyperbaric oxygen (HBO) appears to be useful in treating gas gangrene.[26] However, if fasciotomy is indicated, it should not be delayed for HBO therapy nor should aggressive support be forfeited. The major advantage of HBO may be in minimizing tissue loss and diminishing the extent of debridement required. Complications, including oxygen toxicity, mental status changes, and tympanic membrane perforation, are significant; survival may not exceed that obtained by an aggressive surgical approach. The use of polyvalent antitoxin (of equine origin) has been advocated, but substantive supportive data are not available. Other adjuvant therapies include G-CSF, granulocyte transfusions, and immunoglobulin intravenous.[14]

The prognosis for survival depends on the location and extent of disease and promptness of appropriate debridement. Death is virtually certain if surgical treatment is delayed (e.g., in a wartime situation). The overall survival rate, however, approaches 75% to 90% with early, modern, aggressive treatment.

Food Poisoning

Because of the self-limiting nature of *C perfringens* food poisoning, medical intervention rarely is warranted. Oral rehydration with hypotonic fluids generally suffices, although in unusual circumstances, particularly in infants, intravenous hydration may be required. Antibiotics serve no useful purpose in this disease and should not be used; no antitoxin is available.

PREVENTION

Histotoxic Infections

The key to prevention of histotoxic infections is adequate cleaning and debridement of contaminated wounds. Antimicrobial treatment, best considered therapeutic rather than prophylactic in this setting, should be administered to patients with heavily contaminated wounds, and care should be taken to avoid the anaerobic environments created by closing the wounds. Meticulous attention to the principles of surgical wound management prevents most cases of surgical wound gas gangrene.

Food Poisoning

The best means of preventing food poisoning due to *C perfringens* is appropriate handling of cooked foods (especially meats). Meats should reach at least 120°C during cooking and, if not consumed while hot, should be stored at <5°C. Meat allowed to stand at room temperature is permissive to growth of *C. perfringens*. Preformed toxin is destroyed with reheating to serving temperature, although this temperature does not affect spores. Inhomogeneous heating, as can occur in microwave ovens, can leave some toxin undestroyed and should be avoided.

192 *Bacteroides* and *Prevotella* Species and Other Anaerobic Gram-Negative Bacilli

Itzhak Brook

Clinically important anaerobic gram-negative bacilli (AGNB) include *Bacteroides, Prevotella, Porphyromonas,* and *Fusobacterium. Fusobacterium* is discussed in Chapter 193, *Fusobacterium* Species. Infection due to *Porphyromonas* and *Prevotella* (previously mainly *Bacteroides* species) is not common in children, except for *Prevotella melaninogenica* and *Prevotella intermedia*.[1,2] Changing taxonomy has caused considerable clinical confusion in recategorization of *Bacteroides* species (see Chapter 187, Anaerobic Bacteria: Classification, Normal Flora, and Clinical Concepts).

Bacteroides and *Prevotella* are gram-negative, obligate anaerobic bacteria that constitute a major part of the normal flora of the mouth, gastrointestinal tract, and female genital tract.[3] The *Bacteroides fragilis* group comprises the species of Bacteroidaceae that occur with greatest frequency in clinical infections. They are resistant to penicillins mostly through the production of β-lactamase.[4] The group includes *B. fragilis* (the most commonly recovered member), *B. ovatus, B. thetaiotaomicron,* and *B. vulgatus*.[5] *B. distasonis* is classified now as *Parabacteroides distasonis*.[6]

Bacteroides reside primarily in the large intestine and predominate in infections and infections that originate from gut flora (e.g., perirectal abscesses following perforation or surgery, intra-abdominal abscesses, decubitus ulcers). A heterogeneous group of *Bacteroides* species (*B. ureolyticus, B. gracilis, B. forsythus*) have a less clear taxonomic relationship and may be more closely related genetically to *Campylobacter*. Pigmented *Prevotella*, previously called the *Bacteroides melaninogenicus* group (*P. melaninogenica* and *P. intermedia*), and *Porphyromonas* (*Porphyromonas asaccharolytica*) and nonpigmented *Prevotella* (*P. oralis, P. oris*) are part of the normal oral and vaginal flora and are the predominant gram-negative anaerobic species isolated from contiguous oral respiratory tract infections, such as aspiration pneumonia, lung abscess, chronic otitis media, chronic sinusitis, abscesses around the oral cavity, human bites, paronychia, brain abscesses, and osteomyelitis. *Prevotella bivia* and *P. disiens* (previously also called *Bacteroides*) are important in obstetric and gynecologic infections.

Bacteroides species possess virulence factors or special characteristics to compete successfully for microbial niches, including pili and fimbriae (which enhance adherence),[1,7] hemagglutination, enzymes (collagenase, phospholipase A, hemolysin, peroxidase, protease, fibrolysin, heparinase, neuraminase, superoxide dismutase),[8-10] and lipopolysaccharide and capsular polysaccharide (which enhance invasion and evasion from host phagocytosis). *B. fragilis* and *P. melaninogenica* are associated more frequently with infection than their relative density in normal flora would predict, and are especially associated with abscess formation (see Chapter 187, Anaerobic Bacteria: Classification, Normal Flora, and Clinical Concepts).

PATHOPHYSIOLOGY

Most infections with AGNB originate from the endogenous mucosal flora. This knowledge allows for logical selection of antimicrobial agents for the treatment of infections predictably due to anaerobic bacteria AGNB infections generally are polymicrobial, and the number of unique isolates can reach 5 to 10. The type of other copathogens depends on the site and circumstances of the infection. AGNB promote infection through synergy with their aerobic and anaerobic counterparts. An indirect pathogenic role of AGNB is conferred by their ability to produce a β-lactamase enzyme. Such organisms may protect not only themselves but also other penicillin-susceptible organisms from the activity of penicillins.

CLINICAL MANIFESTATION AND PREDICTION OF PATHOGENS

Central Nervous System Infections

Anaerobic bacteria, including AGNB, can cause a variety of intracranial infections: brain abscess, subdural empyema, epidural abscess, and meningitis.[11,12] Infection generally is polymicrobial, mixed with microaerophilic streptococci. The main source of brain abscess is an adjacent, generally chronic infection in the middle ear, mastoid, sinus, oropharynx, teeth, or lungs. Middle ear or mastoid infections tend to spread to the temporal lobe or cerebellum, whereas sinusitis often causes abscess of the frontal lobe. Hematogenous spread often occurs after dental, oropharyngeal, or pulmonary infection.[13,14] Rarely, bloodstream infection (BSI) has another origin or endocarditis can lead to CNS infection. Meningitis is rare and can follow respiratory tract infection or occur as a complication of a cerebrospinal fluid shunt. Ventriculoperitoneal shunt infection with the *B. fragilis* group can have enteric origin after perforation of the gut.[15]

At the stage of encephalitis, antimicrobial therapy can prevent the formation of abscesses. Once an abscess has formed, excision or drainage generally is needed, combined with 4 to 8 weeks of antibiotics. Administration of antibiotics for an extended period is an alternative approach that may replace surgical drainage in selected patients. Depending on the organism(s) isolated and β-lactamase production, metronidazole, penicillins, and chloramphenicol frequently are chosen because of their spectrum and favorable pharmacodynamic profile.

Head and Neck Infections

Anaerobic bacteria are recovered from a variety of head and neck infections, especially in their chronic form.[16]

Odontogenic infections. Most dental infections involve anaerobic bacteria, including *Prevotella* and *Porphyromonas* of oral flora origin.[17] These include pulpitis and periodontal and endodontal (gingivitis and periodontitis) infections, periapical and dental abscesses, and perimandibular space infections. Vincent angina (trench mouth or acute necrotizing ulcerative gingivitis) is an acute destructive ulcerative gingivitis that causes severe pain and putrid breath odor. Oral fusospirochetes and other oral flora are causative.[18]

Peritonsillar, lateral pharyngeal, and retropharyngeal abscesses. The predominant anaerobes isolated are *Prevotella, Porphyromonas, Fusobacterium,* and *Peptostreptococcus* spp. *Streptococcus pyogenes* is isolated in about one-third of cases.[19] More than two-thirds of abscesses contain β-lactamase-producing organisms.[19] Systemic antimicrobial therapy should be given in large doses; when pus is formed, adequate surgical drainage is needed. Untreated abscesses can rupture spontaneously into the pharynx, causing aspiration. Other complications are lateral extension or dissection into the posterior mediastinum and the prevertebral space.

Deep neck infections. These infections generally follow oral, dental, and pharyngeal infections, usually are polymicrobial, and involve the organisms that caused the primary infection. Mediastinitis after esophageal perforation or extension of a retropharyngeal abscess or cellulitis often involves anaerobic bacteria, including AGNB.[20]

Chronic otitis media[21] and chronic mastoiditis.[22] AGNB can be recovered from patients with chronic suppurative otitis media, chronic mastoiditis, or infected cholesteatoma and lead to complicating intracranial abscesses.

Sinusitis. AGNB become involved when the sinusitis is chronic and oxygen levels decline.[23] Anaerobic bacteria are isolated from 10% of patients with acute maxillary sinusitis (most often in disease secondary to periodontal infection)[24] and in up to 67% of chronic infections (average of 3 species per aspirate).[25] Infection can spread via anastomosing veins or contiguously, causing orbital cellulitis, meningitis, cavernous sinus thrombosis, and epidural, subdural, and brain abscesses.[14]

Cervical lymphadenitis and cysts. AGNB can be isolated in cervical lymphadenitis,[26] especially in association with dental, periodontal, or tonsillar infection. Thyroglossal duct cysts, cystic hygromas, branchial cleft cysts, laryngoceles, and dermoid cysts can become infected.[27]

Infection after head and neck surgery. These infections follow exposure of the surgical site to the oropharyngeal flora. Infections generally are polymicrobial, which warrants the use of proper prophylaxis.[28]

Chronic tonsillitis. AGNB can be involved in acute and chronic tonsillitis and their complications, including internal jugular vein thrombophlebitis. Evidence of pathophysiology of anaerobes in nonstreptococcal tonsillitis includes reduction of fever and clinical symptoms in patients treated with metronidazole compared with untreated children;[29] detectable immune response against AGNB in patients with tonsillitis, peritonsillar cellulitis or abscess, and infectious mononucleosis;[30] isolation of AGNB from the cores of tonsils of children with recurrent tonsillitis[23] and peritonsillar and retropharyngeal abscesses;[31] and isolation of aerobic and anaerobic β-lactamase-producing organisms from the tonsils of more than 75% of children with recurrent streptococcal tonsillitis.[32] The ability to measure β-lactamase activity in the core of tonsils and patients' responses to agents effective against β-lactamase-producing bacteria (i.e., clindamycin or amoxicillin plus clavulanic acid) support the role of AGNB in children in whom penicillin has failed to eradicate streptococcal tonsillitis.[32]

Pleuropulmonary Infections

Aspiration of oropharyngeal or gastric secretions and periodontal or gingival disease are risk factors for the development of anaerobic (including AGNB) pleuropulmonary infection. Infection can progress from pneumonitis to necrotizing pneumonia and abscess, with or without empyema. AGNB can be recovered from patients with community and nosocomially acquired aspiration pneumonia[33] and pneumonia associated with tracheostomy[34] with and without mechanical ventilation, in which case AGNB generally are recovered along with Enterobacteriaceae, *Pseudomonas,* and *Staphylococcus aureus.* Anaerobes can be recovered in empyema associated with aspiration pneumonia, lung abscess, subdiaphragmatic abscess, and abscesses of dental or oropharyngeal origin.[35]

Management of these infections includes drainage of the pleural space when indicated and antimicrobial therapy.

Intra-Abdominal Infections

Intra-abdominal infections characteristically are biphasic; initial peritonitis is associated with *Escherichia coli* sepsis and later intra-abdominal abscesses are caused by *B. fragilis*.[36]

Perforated appendicitis, inflammatory bowel disease with perforation, gastrointestinal surgery, obstruction, infarction or trauma often are predisposing factors to secondary peritonitis and intra-abdominal abscesses, which invariably are polymicrobial (average of 12 isolates).[37] The predominant isolates are AGNB (including *Biophila wadsworthia*).[38] Similar aerobic and anaerobic bacteria are found in pyogenic liver,[39] splenic,[40] pancreatic,[41] and retoperitoneal abscesses.[42] In neonates, peritonitis and abscesses often occur as a result of necrotizing enterocolitis.[43] Management of intra-abdominal infections requires the use of agents effective against aerobic and anaerobic pathogens, as well as surgical correction and drainage. Single and easily accessible abscesses can be drained percutaneously.

Therapy directed at Enterobacteriaceae and AGNB can be achieved with combinations or single agents in certain circumstances.[44] Potential single agents could be a carbapenem (imipenem, meropenem) or a penicillin plus a β-lactamase inhibitor (e.g., piperacillin-tazobactam, ticarcillin-clavulanate). Combination therapy includes an anti-Enterobacteriaceae agent (e.g., aminoglycoside, fluoroquinolone, third-generation cephalosporin) plus an anti-anaerobic agent. The need to add amoxicillin or vancomycin routinely for *Enterococcus* therapy is controversial.

Antimicrobial prophylaxis before colonic surgery could be an oral preparation such as erythromycin plus neomycin or a parenteral agent such as cefoxitin. The use of prophylaxis has reduced the rate of postsurgical wound infection.

Enterotoxigenic *B. fragilis* (ETBF) has been associated with acute diarrhea, colitis, and colonic inflammatory bowl disease.[45] Abdominal pain and nonfebrile inflammatory diarrhea are usual manifestations.[46]

Female Genital Tract Infections

These infections are polymicrobial and include bacterial vaginosis, soft-tissue perineal, vulvar and Bartholin gland abscesses, endometritis, pyometra, salpingitis, tubo-ovarian abscesses, adnexal abscess, and pelvic inflammatory disease. The last includes pelvic cellulitis and abscess, amnionitis, septic pelvic thrombophlebitis, intrauterine device-associated infection, septic abortion, and postsurgical obstetric and gynecologic infections.[1,2]

AGNB play a role in prostatitic and scrotal infections including Fournier gangrene.[47] Therapy should include agents effective against all potential aerobic and anaerobic pathogens. Additionally, coverage against sexually transmissible pathogens should be provided.

Skin and Soft-Tissue Infections

AGNB can cause superficial infections such as infected cutaneous ulcers, cellulitis, secondary diaper rash, gastrostomy or tracheostomy site wounds, infected subcutaneous sebaceous or inclusion cysts, eczema, scabies or kerion infections, paronychia, hidradenitis suppurativa, and pyoderma.[48] Subcutaneous tissue infections and postsurgical wound infection also can include skin flora and AGNB.[28,37] Such infections include cutaneous and subcutaneous abscesses, decubitus ulcers,[49] infected diabetic (vascular or trophic) ulcers, breast abscesses, bite wounds,[50] anaerobic cellulitis and gas gangrene, bacterial synergistic gangrene, infected pilonidal cyst or sinus, Meleney ulcers, and burn wound infection. Deeper anaerobic soft-tissue infections are necrotizing fasciitis, necrotizing synergistic cellulitis, gas gangrene, and crepitus cellulitis.[51] These infections can involve only the fascia, the muscle surrounded by the fascia (inducing myositis and myonecrosis), or both the fascia and the muscle.

The organisms recovered from soft-tissue infections vary according to the type and location of the infection and the circumstances leading to the infection. Wound and subcutaneous tissue infections and abscesses of the rectal area (decubitus ulcer, perirectal abscess) or those originating from gut flora (e.g., diabetic foot infection) tend to yield colonic flora. Sites in and around the oropharynx (e.g., paronychia, bites) generally contain oral flora. Skin flora organisms such as *S. aureus* and *Streptococcus* or nosocomially acquired organisms (gram-negative aerobic bacilli) can be isolated at all body sites. In addition to oral flora, human bite infections often contain *Eikenella* species, and animal bite infections can include *Pasteurella multocida*. Anaerobic infections (e.g., decubitus ulcers, diabetic foot ulcer) generally are polymicrobial and often are complicated by osteomyelitis or BSI. Deep tissue infections such as necrotizing cellulitis, fasciitis, and myositis often involve clostridia or *Streptococcus pyogenes* or are polymicrobial; they contain gas and grey, thin, putrid-like pus and are associated with BSI and substantial mortality.

Management of deep-seated soft-tissue infection includes surgical debridement and drainage, improvement in the blood supply when indicated, and administration of hyperbaric oxygen, especially in clostridial infection.

Osteomyelitis and Pyogenic Arthritis

Osteomyelitis is associated with AGNB in patients with peripheral vascular disease and decubitus ulcers and when infection occurs in long bones and in cranial and facial bones.[52] Cranial and facial bone osteomyelitis generally is due to spread from a contiguous soft-tissue source or from sinus, ear, or dental infections. Osteomyelitis of long bones generally is due to hematogenous spread, trauma, or the presence of a prosthetic device.

Recovery of AGNB is associated with certain settings: *Prevotella*, *Porphyromonas*, and *Fusobacterium* with skull osteomyelitis and bites; *B. fragilis* with vascular disease or neuropathy; and clostridia with long bone osteomyelitis, especially in wounds contaminated after trauma.[53]

Most cases of pyogenic arthritis due to anaerobic bacteria are monomicrobial and occur after hematogenous and contiguous spread, trauma, and arthritis associated with prosthetic joints. The predominant isolates are peptostreptococci and *Propionibacterium acnes* (often in prosthetic joint infection), *B. fragilis* and fusobacteria (often in infections of hematogenic origin), and clostridia (associated with trauma).

Bloodstream Infection

AGNB are responsible for up to 5% to 15% of BSIs. Common isolates are the *B. fragilis* group (60% to 75% of isolates). The *B. fragilis* group and clostridia are associated with a gastrointestinal source, pigmented *Prevotella* and *Porphyromonas* and *Fusobacterium* with oropharyngeal and pulmonary sites, *P. bivia* and *P. disiens* with the female genital tract, *P. acnes* with foreign bodies, and peptostreptococci with all sources, but especially with oropharyngeal, pulmonary, and female genital tract sources.[54]

Predisposing factors include neoplasms, hematologic disorders, organ transplantation, recent gastrointestinal, obstetric or gynecologic surgery, intestinal obstruction, decubitus ulcers, dental extraction, diabetes mellitus, the postsplenectomy state, and the use of cytotoxic agents or corticosteroid therapy. Features typical of BSI with AGNB include metastatic lesions, hyperbilirubinemia, and suppurative thrombophlebitis. Shock and disseminated intravascular coagulation are less common compared with aerobic gram-negative BSI. Mortality is 15% to 30% but improves with early appropriate antimicrobial therapy and aggressive management of the root cause.

Anaerobic bacteremia in newborns is caused by AGNB, *Clostridium* and *Peptostreptococcus* spp., and is associated with perinatal maternal complications (primarily premature rupture of membranes and chorioamnionitis), prematurity, and necrotizing enterocolitis.[55]

TREATMENT

In most cases, surgical therapy is of critical importance. Surgical treatment includes draining abscesses, debriding necrotic tissues, identifying the primary source of infection, removing devitalized tissue, decompressing closed-space infections, and relieving obstructions. In selected cases, an abscess can be drained with the use of imaging modalities to guide catheter placement without surgery or laparoscopy. When surgical drainage is not performed, the infection can persist and serious complications can develop. The duration of antimicrobial therapy for anaerobic infections generally is longer than that for infections with aerobic and facultative organisms.

Resistance to antimicrobial agents has a broad basis, but β-lactamase production has the most clinical significance. All *B. fragilis* group strains produce β-lactamase, as do many clinical isolates of *Prevotella, Porphyromonas, Fusobacterium, B. wadsworthia,* and *Bacteroides splanchnicus* which renders them resistant to penicillins. Agents active in vitro against β-lactamase-producing AGNB include metronidazole, clindamycin, chloramphenicol, cefoxitin, carbapenems, and combinations of a penicillin and a β-lactamase inhibitor (e.g., ampicillin-sulbactam, ampicillin-clavulanate, ticarcillin-clavulanate, and piperacillin-tazobactam) (see Chapter 187, Anaerobic Bacteria: Classification, Normal Flora, and Clinical Concepts). Large databases in the latest decade show the following resistance rates of the *B. fragilis* group in the United States and Europe, respectively: clindamycin 26% and 32%, moxifloxacin 34% and 14%, cefoxitin 10% and 17%, tigecycline 4% and, 2%, ampicillin-sulbactam/amoxicillin-clavulanate 3% and 10%, piperacillin-tazobactam <1% and 3%, meropenem/imipenem <1% and 1%, and metronidazole <1%.[56,57] *Prevotella, Fusobacterium,* and *Porphyromonas* species isolates are more likely than *B. fragilis* group to be susceptible to clindamycin. Although antibiotic susceptibility of *Prevotella melaninogenica* and *P. intermedia* can vary geographically, the majority are β-lactamase producing (penicillin resistant), 10% are resistant to clindamycin, and none is metronidazole resistant.[58] *B. gracilis* group, found primarily in gingival crevices, is more likely than *B. ureolyticus* (now *Campylobacter ureolyticus*) to be recovered from serious, deep infections and is more resistant to antibiotics (e.g., clindamycin and metronidazole), but it is sensitive to gentamicin;[59] *Sutterella wadsworthensis* is predominantly responsible for resistant organisms in the former *B. gracilis* group, with clindamycin resistance of 15% to 30%[60] in some areas. Despite difficulties in breakpoint determinations and exact clinical correlation with in vitro results, agents active in vitro are more likely to be associated with a good clinical outcome and vice versa.[61] The choice of agents depends on the site and stage of infection and the probable coinfecting pathogens. Although early infection such as aspiration pneumonia can be treated effectively with agents active primarily against facultative and some anaerobic organisms (not necessarily *Bacteroides* or *Prevotella*), necrotizing infection or abscess is best treated with specifically directed therapy.

The role of hyperbaric oxygen in the treatment of anaerobic infections remains unclear, with some suggestion of benefit as adjunctive therapy to surgical debridement and antibiotics.[62,63]

PREVENTION

Elimination of acute infection can prevent chronic infections in which AGNB and other anaerobes predominate. When anaerobic infections are anticipated complications of surgery at heavily colonized mucosal sites, proper antimicrobial prophylaxis reduces their rate. Early treatment of conditions that may lead to anaerobic infection also can reduce their rate. Preventing aspiration of oral flora by improving the patient's neurologic status, suctioning, improving oral hygiene, and maintaining lower stomach pH can reduce the risk of aspiration pneumonia and its complications.

Skin and soft-tissue infections can be prevented by irrigation and debridement of wounds and necrotic tissue, drainage of pus, and improvement of perfusion. Prophylaxis generally is instituted before surgery when contamination by normal flora is expected at the operative site.[64] Cefazolin is effective prophylaxis at sites distant from the oral or rectal areas. Cefoxitin is the drug of choice in procedures that involve the oral, rectal, or vulvovaginal surfaces.

193 *Fusobacterium* Species

Robert W. Tolan, Jr

Fusobacteria are nonspore-forming, nonmotile, pleomorphic, gram-negative (Figure 193-1), obligate anaerobic bacilli increasingly recognized to cause human disease, most notoriously (but not most frequently) septic thrombophlebitis of the internal jugular vein (known as or Lemierre syndrome, post-anginal sepsis, or necrobacillosis).[1-15] *F. nucleatum* and *F. necrophorum* subspecies *funduliforme* are the most common fusobacteria identified in human disease.[1,6,16,17]

DESCRIPTION OF THE PATHOGEN

The genus *Fusobacterium* includes 9 disease-causing species that are part of the normal flora of the human oral cavity and gastrointestinal and/or genitourinary tracts: *F. nucleatum* (subspecies *nucleatum, polymorphum, vincentii, animalis, fusiforme,* and *canifelium*[6]), *F. necrophorum* (subspecies *necrophorum* and *funduliforme*), *F. ulcerans, F. gonidiaformans, F. mortiferum, F. naviforme, F. necrogenes, F. russii,* and *F. varium*.[6,7,17-25] Because molecular techniques are redefining the taxonomy and role of fusobacteria as commensals and pathogens, this compilation is evolving.[6,24]

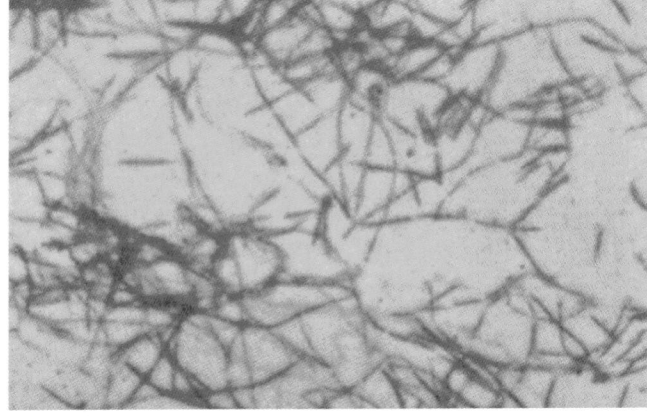

Figure 193-1. Gram stain of *Fusobacterium nucleatum*, magnification 1000×. (From Baron EJ, Finegold SM. Bailey and Scott's Diagnostic Microbiology. St. Louis: Mosby, 1990, with permission.)

Unlike other anaerobes, *F. necrophorum* produces lipopolysaccharide, which contributes to its intrinsic virulence.[4,5] Overall, one-third of fusobacterial infections are polymicrobial[26] and animal studies demonstrate increased virulence of *F. necrophorum* in the presence of fecal organisms.[27] Additional, but less well-characterized, virulence factors include production of leukocidins, hemolysins, lipases, DNAases, hemagglutinins, β-lactamases (by *F. nucleatum*), and the ability to aggregate platelets (*F. necrophorum*).[4,5,14,17] Recently, molecular thrombophilic predisposition has been identified in children with invasive fusobacteriosis,[28-31] as has a single nucleotide polymorphism in the toll-like receptor 5 gene in an affected child,[28] suggesting that underlying host factors also may predispose to infection.

EPIDEMIOLOGY

Well recognized in the pre-antibiotic era, invasive fusobacteriosis was rarely reported after the advent of antibiotic therapy for pharyngitis[32] and it became known as the forgotten disease.[5] During the past 2 to 3 decades, incidence (and reporting of the infection) clearly is increasing.[4,33-35] In addition to burgeoning literature, actual increase in incidence likely results from decreased empiric use of antibiotics for sore throat, fewer tonsillectomies, increased use of corticosteroid therapy for mononucleosis or sore throat, superior blood culture methods, improved techniques for diagnosis of anaerobic infections, and use of nonculture-based molecular diagnostic tools.[1,4,5,14] Estimates of incidence range from 0.8 to 3.6 cases per million people.[26,33,36] A prospective study in Denmark demonstrated an incidence of Lemierre disease of 14.4 cases per million persons aged 15 to 24 years.[36] There may be a peak in late winter.[32] Males are more commonly afflicted.[1-4,32]

Three age-related disease patterns are observed for both localized and disseminated fusobacteriosis (Table 193-1).[1,4,36,37] Localized head and neck disease tends to arise from the middle ear (and, occasionally, cervical lymph nodes) in children, the throat and tonsil in adolescents, and the sinuses and carious teeth and gums in adults.[37] Older adults also can have localized infection arising from the gastrointestinal or genitourinary tract. Similarly, invasive or disseminated fusobacterial infection tends to vary with age. Children tend to develop infection, often associated with otitis media,[37] that can disseminate systemically but more often results in intracranial complications.[1,38] Otogenic Lemierre disease was reported in persons aged 2 months to 51 years, with a median age of 5 years, while pharyngitis-associated Lemierre disease occurred in those aged 8 months to 63 years, with a median age of 19 years.[1] Others note a peak age of Lemierre disease at 16 to 23 years of age,[34] with a median age for reported cases ranging from 17 to 21.5 years.[26,39,40] Another series noted an age range of 2 months to 78 years; median age 22 years; and distribution of 51%, 20%, and 8% of cases in the second, third, and first decades of life, respectively.[2] Finally, disseminated fusobacteriosis is seen less frequently arising from the gastrointestinal or genitourinary tract in elderly people (median age 62 years[26]), most (72%) of whom have underlying medical conditions,[26] and in whom the infection has a higher fatality rate.[1,36,37] In a prospectively collected series of 391 isolates of *F. necrophorum* from localized and disseminated infection, 342 (87%) were found to be *F. necrophorum* subspecies *funduliforme*, 1 (0.003%) was *F. necrophorum* subspecies *necrophorum*, and 48 (12%) were not subspeciated.[36,37]

CLINICAL MANIFESTATIONS

Fusobacterial infection can be divided into invasive disease and localized disease (exemplified by peritonsillar abscess), the latter occurring more frequently though it is reported rarely. Lemierre disease can be diagnosed by clinical manifestations.[41] The most common symptoms and findings include sore throat, fever, rigors, neck mass, neck pain, trismus, tenderness along the neck vasculature, anorexia, malaise, cough, chest pain, shortness of breath, and prostration.[1-5] Typically, a previously healthy adolescent male develops sore throat, followed by fevers and rigors (a distinctive feature of this disease) on the fourth or fifth day, and painful swelling in the neck (often mistakenly attributed to lymphadenopathy, which is tender but rarely is painful).[1-5] Metastatic foci of infection appear in the lungs, but also can arise in joints, muscles, bones, the liver, the skin, the spleen, and endocardium.[1]

Otogenic disseminated fusobacteriosis more often results in intracranial complications, including meningitis[38,42-48] and vascular thrombosis,[47,48] but rarely results in internal jugular involvement.[48] Meningitis also can complicate fusobacterial sinusitis in older children and adults,[49-51] as can brain abscesses, but the latter occur more often secondary to periodontal disease with bloodstream infection (BSI).[52-54]

BSI in adults usually is associated with predisposing conditions;[36,55] BSI has been reported in healthy[56] and neutropenic[3] children.

The most common clinical manifestations of fusobacterial infection are pharyngitis (particularly recurring and persisting pharyngitis that is poorly responsive to typically-prescribed antibiotic therapy – the persistent sore throat syndrome[57]),[20,57-59] tonsillitis,[23] and peritonsillar abscess.[37,60-62] Using appropriate culture and PCR-based techniques, *F. necrophorum* subspecies *funduliforme*

TABLE 193-1. Prospectively Collected Series of 388 Cases of *F. necrophorum* Infection[36,37]

Classification	Source of Infection	Number of Cases	Age Range (Years)	Median Age (Years)
Localized disease (*n* = 288)	Otogenic	7	0–26	4
	Cervical lymphadenitis	9	0–46	3
	Tonsillitis	26	13–57	20
	Peritonsillar abscess	215	4–72	19
	Sinus- or teeth-associated	10	29–73	44
	Localized disease caudal to the head and neck	21	9–83	38
Disseminated disease (*n* = 100)	Otogenic Lemierre disease	5	0–16	2
	Oropharyngeal-associated Lemierre disease	37	6–66	20
	Disseminated disease originating from sinus or teeth	16	7–89	24–55[a]
	Disseminated disease originating from the gastrointestinal tract	30	5–89	61
	Disseminated disease originating from the genitourinary tract	6	25–96	78
	Disseminated disease originating from an unknown focus	6	66–87	76

[a]Group subdivided with two medians reported in Hagelskjær Kristensen L, Prag J. Lemierre's syndrome and other disseminated *Fusobacterium necrophorum* infections in Denmark: a prospective epidemiological and clinical survey. Eur J Clin Microbiol Infect Dis 2008;27:779–789.

can be isolated in 10% to 21% of cases of persistent sore throat or tonsillitis.[20,23,57,58] In a Finnish study, *F. nucleatum* and *F. necrophorum* were isolated from 26% and 38% of peritonsillar abscesses, respectively (compared with 45% for *Streptococcus pyogenes*).[60] In Denmark, a prospective study identified *F. necrophorum* in 21% of 1001 peritonsillar abscesses.[37] Another Danish series of 847 patients with peritonsillar abscess noted that *F. necrophorum*

was the most frequent cause (23%, compared with 17% for *S. pyogenes*).[62]

Less common manifestations of fusobacteriosis include pyogenic arthritis, which most frequently involves the knee, hip, ankle, shoulder, elbow, sacroiliac, or sternoclavicular joint[38,63,64] and osteomyelitis, affecting the facial bones more often than the vertebrae, pubic bone, or extremities.[65] Wound and zoonotic

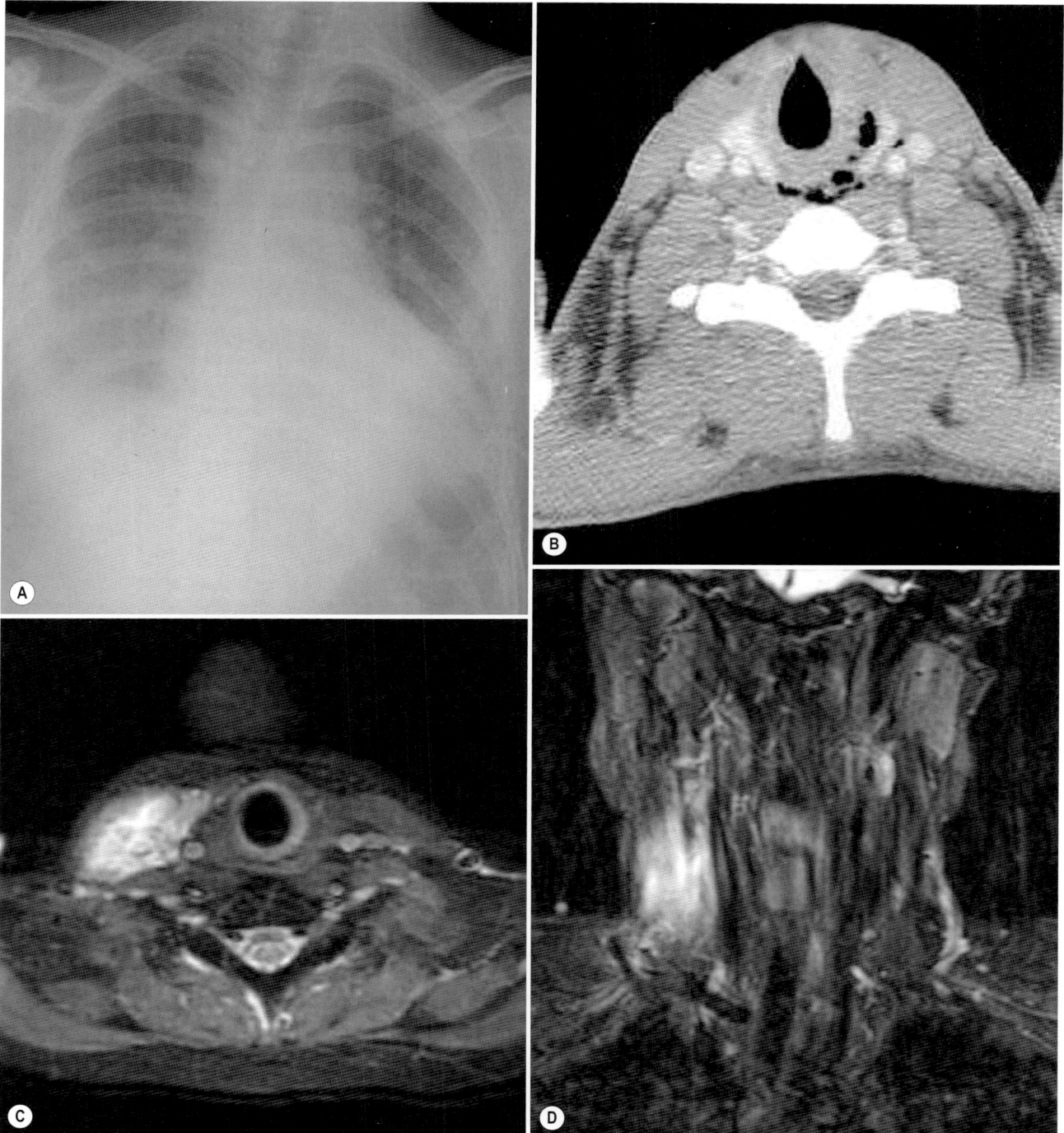

Figure 193-2. Images of two adolescents with Lemierre disease. **(A)** Chest radiograph shows left lower lobe consolidation, bilateral pleural effusions, and widened mediastinum. **(B)** Axial computed tomography of the neck shows left-sided soft-tissue swelling and perivascular gas, which extended into the mediastinum. **(C, D)** Axial and coronal magnetic resonance imaging of the neck in another patient shows right-sided soft-tissue swelling, perivascular edema, and filling defects in the internal jugular vein. (Courtesy of S. Underberg-Davis and S. Schonfeld, the Children's Hospital at St. Peter's University Hospital, New Brunswick, NJ.)

infections occur rarely.[4,6,17] Multiple cranial nerve involvement[64] and sensorineural hearing loss[38] each has been reported in one patient. Finally, *F. necrophorum* has been implicated in orofacial gangrene (cancrum oris or noma)[66-68] and tropical ulcer.[19]

LABORATORY FINDINGS AND DIAGNOSIS

Laboratory findings are nonspecific;[1-3] leukocytosis with increased band forms is common, as is elevated C-reactive protein.[2,3,36,37,62] Abnormal results of hepatic biochemical tests, particularly hyperbilirubinemia, are found in 11% to 49% of cases of Lemierre disease.[26,36,40] Less commonly, thrombocytopenia and/or evidence of disseminated intravascular coagulopathy are present in Lemierre disease.[36,64] Culture confirmation of *Fusobacterium* infection requires adequate/protected specimen collection, and optimized transport, culture medium, and identification. Increasingly, PCR-based methods are applied to diagnose fusobacterial infections.[16,20,23,69]

Imaging studies generally are helpful to confirm clinical suspicion and evaluate the intravascular, local, and metastatic complications of infection (Figure 193-2).[70] Multiple imaging modalities may be employed, as patients often are quite ill and the extent of the disease may not be established on clinical grounds alone.

TREATMENT

F. nucleatum isolated from children often produces β-lactamase.[71] In one series, 15% of isolates of *F. necrophorum* were resistant to erythromycin, 2% to penicillin, and 1% to tetracycline.[34] In the absence of comparative studies, most experts recommend antibacterial therapy with metronidazole (in combination with a penicillin for severe or invasive disease), since metronidazole resistance has not been reported among isolates of *Fusobacterium* and clinical outcomes (particularly with central nervous system disease) seem to be improved when metronidazole is included.[1,4,72] Combination therapy is preferable to monotherapy for serious infection because cultures may not be properly obtained, infections occasionally are polymicrobial, and infection with other organisms

can mimic fusobacteriosis.[1,4,72] Median duration of fever after initiation of appropriate antibiotic therapy for Lemierre disease is 8 to 12 days.[4] Duration of reported therapy ranges from 9 to 84 days, with a median of 42 days,[13] but some recommend a 2- to 3-week course of antibiotics parenterally followed by oral therapy to complete 6 weeks if the clinical course is reassuring.[1] Important adjunctive therapy includes operative intervention as necessary to drain abscesses.[4] Ligation of the thrombosed internal jugular vein rarely is necessary in the antibiotic era, unless the thrombus progresses or repeated embolism occurs despite medical therapy.[73] The role of anticoagulation remains controversial, with inadequate data to make recommendations.[29-31,73]

SPECIAL CONSIDERATIONS

F. nucleatum infections have been implicated in preterm delivery and chorioamnionitis.[3,74,75] In one series, 36% of women with preterm delivery (compared with 0% who delivered at term) had *F. nucleatum* isolated from the vagina.[74] *F. nucleatum* is the organism most frequently isolated from the amniotic fluid of women with preterm labor and intact membranes.[75] The subspecies identified, *F. nucleatum* subspecies *nucleatum* and *vincentii*, are found in the oral cavity rather than the lower genital tract, suggesting that hematogenous infection of the amniotic fluid and resultant preterm labor was the result of periodontal disease.[75]

PREVENTION

Most fusobacterial infection cannot be prevented. However, optimized oral hygiene can be recommended. Furthermore, a thoughtful approach to the patient with throat infection seems prudent. Withholding empiric antibiotic therapy for simple pharyngitis in the absence of evidence of streptococcal disease is appropriate. However, patients (particularly adolescents and young adults) without coryza, who have high fever >3 days (especially with rigors) with neck pain/swelling/tenderness, and/or who have severe sore throat >3 days deserve special attention.[5,59]

194 Anaerobic Cocci

Debrah Meislich and Anat R. Feingold

The anaerobic cocci are major components of the normal flora of the mouth, upper respiratory tract, gastrointestinal tract, vagina, and skin.[1] Gram-positive cocci and gram-negative cocci (*Veillonella* spp.) and microaerophilic *Streptococcus* spp. are the anaerobic bacteria most commonly isolated from clinical specimens.[2,3] They occur in pure cultures, however, in only 8% to 10% of cases.[4,5] Of the anaerobic cocci, *Finegoldia magna* is most likely isolated in pure culture.[6] While anaerobic bloodstream infection (BSI) is rare in children, anaerobic cocci have been isolated, especially in cases of polymicrobial BSI.[7] The classification of anaerobic gram-positive cocci is changing continually; new species are added and old species renamed. Currently, the six genera of anaerobic gram-positive cocci that can be isolated from human specimens include: *Peptostreptococcus, Peptoniphilus, Parvimonas, Finegoldia,* and *Anaerococcus*; the genus of the sixth group has not yet been determined.[8] *Peptostreptococcus, Peptoniphilus,* and *Anaerococcus* are the most common human isolates. Of the three genera of anaerobic gram-negative cocci, only one, *Veillonella*, is found in clinical isolates.

There are seven species of *Veillonella*; *V. parvula* is the species most commonly isolated from human specimens.[8]

PATHOPHYSIOLOGY AND PREDISPOSING CONDITIONS

Infection by anaerobic cocci occurs at sites contiguous to their commensal habitats. Anaerobic coccal infections can occur in all body sites, including the central nervous system, head, neck, chest, abdomen, pelvis, skin, and soft tissues.[3,5] These organisms can be sole pathogens in osteoarticular infections, occasionally in soft-tissue infections, and in BSI. Soft-tissue and visceral infections generally are polymicrobial (virtually always involving aerobic, facultative, and other anaerobic organisms).[3,5]

Synergy has been found between anaerobic gram-positive cocci and their aerobic and anaerobic counterparts.[9-11] Synergy is indicated by mutual enhancement of the induction of sepsis, higher mortality, greater ability to induce abscesses, and enhancement of the growth of the bacterial components in mixed infection. The ability of anaerobic gram-positive cocci and microaerophilic streptococci to produce capsular material is one of probably several important virulence mechanisms.[9,12]

Veillonella parvula, the most significant anaerobic gram-negative coccus, is an uncommon significant clinical isolate but occasionally causes serious infection in association with malignancy, corticosteroid use, previous surgery, indwelling devices, or intravenous drug use or rarely in otherwise healthy individuals.[13,14] *V. parvula* usually is recovered as part of a polymicrobial infection, but has been isolated in pure culture from various sites and is a recognized pathogen.

CLINICAL MANIFESTATIONS

Central Nervous System Infections

Anaerobic gram-positive cocci and microaerophilic streptococci can be isolated from subdural empyema and brain abscesses that develop as sequelae of chronic infections of the ear, mastoid, sinuses, teeth, and pleuropulmonary infections.[15] Anatomic abnormality leading to communication with a mucosal site should be sought if a predisposing infection is not found. Anaerobic gram-positive cocci and microaerophilic streptococci have been isolated from 46% of brain abscesses.

Upper Respiratory Tract and Dental Infections

Anaerobic gram-positive cocci and microaerophilic streptococci often are recovered from acute and chronic upper respiratory tract infections. They have been reported to be recovered in 15% of cases of chronic mastoiditis,[16] in 30% of cases of chronic otitis media[17] and chronic sinusitis,[18] in 33% of cases of peritonsillar[19] and retropharyngeal[20] abscesses, and in 50% of purulent parotitis.[21] These organisms accounted for two-thirds of isolates from periodontal abscesses in one study.[22] In >90% of cases, other organisms of oral flora are found with anaerobic gram-positive cocci and microaerophilic streptococci.

Anaerobic Pleuropulmonary Infections

Anaerobic gram-positive cocci and microaerophilic streptococci account for 10% to 20% of anaerobic isolates recovered from properly obtained specimens of pulmonary infections,[23] most commonly aspiration pneumonia, lung abscess, and empyema associated with aspiration pneumonia. Sampling by transtracheal aspiration, aspiration through double-lumen catheter, or direct lung puncture is required to obtain meaningful specimens.

Intra-Abdominal Infections

Anaerobic gram-positive cocci are recovered from about 20% of specimens of intra-abdominal infections, such as peritonitis and abscesses of the liver, spleen, and abdomen.[24] Generally, these organisms are recovered with other organisms of intestinal origin, including *Escherichia coli*, the *Bacteroides fragilis* group, and *Clostridium* spp.

Female Pelvic Infections

Anaerobic gram-positive cocci and microaerophilic streptococci can be isolated from 25% to 50% of cases of endometritis, pyoderma, pelvic abscess, Bartholin glands abscess, postsurgical infections of the pelvis, and pelvic inflammatory disease. The origin of these organisms is most probably the vaginal and cervical flora. BSI with anaerobic gram-positive cocci and microaerophilic streptococci often is associated with septic abortion. Anaerobic gram-positive cocci generally are found along with *Prevotella* species.

Osteomyelitis and Arthritis

Anaerobic gram-positive cocci account for 40% of anaerobic isolates of osteomyelitis caused by anaerobic bacteria, and 20% of anaerobic isolates of arthritis caused by anaerobic bacteria.[25] Most patients with infections involving these organisms have previously undergone orthopedic surgery and placement of prosthetic material. Management of these infections requires a prolonged course of antimicrobial therapy, and outcome is enhanced by removal of foreign material.

Skin and Soft-Tissue Infections

Anaerobic gram-positive cocci and microaerophilic streptococci often are recovered in polymicrobial skin and soft-tissue infections, where they are found with other organisms specific to the site or injury. Such infections include necrotizing synergistic gangrene, necrotizing fasciitis,[26] decubitus ulcers,[27] paronychia,[28] burns,[29] human or animal bite infections,[30] infected cysts,[31] and abscesses of the breast,[32] rectum, and anus.[33] Gastrointestinal flora is associated with decubitus ulcers of the buttocks, rectal abscesses, and diabetic foot infections. Vaginal and cervical flora can cause scalp wound infection in neonates after fetal monitoring. Because anaerobic gram-positive cocci and microaerophilic streptococci are part of the normal skin flora, care must be used in obtaining specimens to avoid contamination by normal flora.

Bloodstream Infection

Anaerobic gram-positive cocci and microaerophilic streptococci can be responsible for 4% to 15% of isolates from blood cultures of patients with clinically significant anaerobic BSI.[34] The most common associated sources are oropharyngeal, pulmonary, female genital tract, abdominal, and skin and soft-tissue infections. The most frequent predisposing conditions are malignancy, recent surgery (gastrointestinal, obstetric, or gynecological), immunosuppression, and following dental procedures. Microaerophilic streptococci account for 5% to 10% of cases of endocarditis.

TREATMENT

It is rare for the anaerobic gram-positive cocci to be the only pathogens isolated from clinical specimens.[4,5] Most often, infection is polymicrobial, and treatment is empiric, without laboratory confirmation and susceptibility testing. Knowledge of trends of antimicrobial resistance of anaerobes comes from multicenter surveys.[6,35] Most infections due to anaerobic gram-positive cocci and microaerophilic streptococci can still be treated with penicillin G. A large multicentered European study reported that 7% of the gram-positive anaerobic cocci isolated from clinical specimens were resistant to penicillin and/or clindamycin.[36] The majority of resistant strains were *F. magna*. All clinical isolates were susceptible to metronidazole, vancomycin, imipenem, and linezolid.[36] However, in other studies, strains of anaerobic gram-positive cocci and aerotolerant strains were resistant to metronidazole.[6] Another European survey that included fewer gram-positive anaerobic isolates, found no β-lactam resistance. However, 22% of the anaerobic gram-positive cocci were resistant to clindamycin.[37] These large surveys also have determined trends in fluoroquinolone resistance of anaerobic gram-positive cocci in clinical isolates. One study found that moxifloxacin was more potent than ofloxacin and ciprofloxacin; no isolate was resistant to moxifloxacin.[37] Another Belgian multicenter survey found that only 68% of anaerobic cocci isolates were susceptible to moxifloxacin.[38] In the laboratory, linezolid has shown excellent activity against these organisms, however, clinical experience is more limited.[38]

In mixed infection with bacteria that produce β-lactamase, anaerobic gram-positive cocci and microaerophilic streptococci can survive penicillin or cephalosporin therapy because of the protection provided by the free enzyme. In such instances, agents with wider spectrum of activity may be more effective. An agent with activity against gram-negative enteric bacteria generally is added to cover Enterobacteriaceae for treatment of intra-abdominal infections.

In most cases, surgical drainage of abscesses, debridement of necrotic tissues, decompression of closed-space infections, and

relief of obstruction is critical. When surgical drainage is not used, the infection can persist, and serious complications develop.

Duration of therapy for anaerobic infections generally is prolonged but must be individualized. In some cases, the treatment course may be 6 to 8 weeks; therapy may be shortened in association with proper surgical drainage.

195 Anaerobic Gram-Positive, Nonsporulating Bacilli (including Actinomycosis)

Anat R. Feingold and Debrah Meislich

Anaerobic gram-positive, nonsporulating bacilli of clinical significance include *Actinomyces, Bifidobacterium, Eubacterium, Lactobacillus, Mobiluncus,* and *Propionibacterium. Actinomyces* and *Propionibacterium* are the most common clinical pathogens and can be differentiated by biochemical reactions and metabolic products. Both *Actinomyces* and *Propionibacterium* show indole-positive reactions in the laboratory. Typically, *Propionibacterium* produces copious amounts of propionic acid and acetic acid, whereas *Actinomyces* produces acetic acid plus succinic and lactic acid. *Actinomyces* and *Propionibacterium* do not have mitochondria or a nuclear membrane. *Actinomyces* has diaminopimelic and muramic acid in the cell wall, whereas *Propionibacterium* has lysine. The genus *Mobiluncus* consists of gram-variable or gram-negative, curved rods with tapered ends, sometimes occurring in pairs with a gullwing appearance. Previously aligned with Bacteroidaceae, *Mobiluncus* is more closely related to *Actinomyces*.

PROPIONIBACTERIUM SPECIES

Propionibacterium species are pleomorphic, occasionally branching bacilli that are normal flora of the skin, conjunctiva, external ear canal,[1] and exposed mucous membranes. On the skin, this organism colonizes hair follicles and sebaceous glands. *P. acnes* infections are most common in children with altered host defenses. Predisposing conditions include: history of surgical manipulation, presence of a foreign body/medical device, trauma, malignancy, and primary or acquired immune deficiency.[2] *Propionibacterium* spp.[3] (especially *P. acnes*) can cause bloodstream infection (BSI) in immunocompromised individuals. *P. acnes* is catalase-positive and has caused pneumonia in children with chronic granulomatous disease[4] as well as endocarditis in individuals with prosthetic or damaged heart valves;[5] conjunctivitis in contact lens wearers; and infections related to ventriculoperitoneal (VP) shunts, prosthetic joints, peritoneal dialysis, or intravascular catheters.[3] *P. acnes* osteomyelitis most often follows orthopedic surgical procedures or instrumentation and placement of hardware as following spinal fusion[6] *P. acnes* causes inflammation of acne lesions.[7] In otherwise healthy adolescents with moderate to severe acne, even in the absence of orthopedic surgery or instrumentation, *P. acnes* can be a rare cause of osteomyelitis.[8] *P. acnes* also is a rare cause of delayed VP shunt infections, identified only when cerebrospinal fluid (CSF) and shunt catheters routinely are cultured anaerobically. *P. acnes* VP shunt infections more often follow valve puncture or distal catheter revision due to distal obstruction. Compared with other causes of infection, children with *P. acnes* VP shunt infections tend to be less systemically ill, have only mild CSF pleocytosis, and minor changes in CSF glucose and protein. Because of its slower rate of growth CSF and catheter tips must be incubated for 5 to 7 days anaerobically when *P. acnes* is suspected.[9-11] Uncommonly, *P. acnes* is isolated alone, or more

commonly is mixed with other aerobic or anaerobic bacteria in brain abscesses, subdural empyema, parotid, pulmonary or dental infections, peritonitis, and osteomyelitis.[2] Isolation, however, most frequently represents skin contamination of cultures. Repeated isolation or visualization of *Propionibacterium* on Gram stain is required to distinguish true infection.

Surgical debridement, incision and drainage, and removal of foreign material are important in the management of *Propionibacterium* infections. Topical and oral antibiotics play a role in the treatment of moderate to severe acne. A recent study of children and adults with moderate to severe acne found that antibiotic-experienced patients were more likely to be colonized with *P. acnes* resistant to clindamycin, erythromycin, and tetracycline than were those individuals who had not taken antibiotics in the preceding 2 to 6 months.[12] When non-skin clinical isolates of *P. acnes* were examined for antimicrobial susceptibility, 2.6% were resistant to tetracycline, 15.1% were resistant to clindamycin, and 17.7% were resistant to erythromycin. None of the isolates were resistant to linezolid, penicillin, or vancomycin.[13] Metronidazole does not have predictable activity against *Propionibacterium* and cannot be used for therapy.[14]

ACTINOMYCES SPECIES

Actinomyces species are filamentous, branching, gram-positive, pleomorphic nonspore forming, catalase-negative anaerobic or microaerophilic bacilli. On Gram stain, *Actinomyces* cannot be distinguished from *Nocardia*.[15] However, *Nocardia* species grow aerobically and stain with acid-fast technique and *Actinomyces* species do not. With the use of 16S rRNA sequencing, at least 21 species of *Actinomyces* have been identified in humans.[16] *Actinomyces israelii* is the predominant species causing disease; however, other *Actinomyces* species, including *A. naeslundii, A. meyeri, A. odontolyticus, A. gerencseriae,* and *A. viscosus,* as well as *Propionibacterium propionica,* also have been implicated.[17,18] Most actinomycotic infections are polymicrobial, involving other aerobic and anaerobic bacteria. Co-isolates depend on the source/site of infection and include *Aggregatibacter* (formerly *Actinobacillus*) *actinomycetemcomitans, Eikenella corrodens, Bacteroides, Fusobacterium, Capnocytophaga,* aerobic and anaerobic streptococci, *Staphylococcus,* and Enterobacteriaceae.

Pathogenesis

Actinomyces species, generally have low virulence and are part of the normal flora of the mouth and gastrointestinal tract, and female genital tract. *Actinomyces* species colonize the oral cavity in early childhood with prevalence rate increasing from 31% to 97% within the first 2 years of life; organisms reside in periodontal pockets, carious teeth, dental plaque, and tonsillar crypts.[19]

Infections are infrequent in children[20,21] but are underrecognized,[22–25] probably because of fastidious growth requirements. *Actinomyces* take advantage of infection, trauma, or surgical injury to penetrate mucosal barriers. Having attained access to tissues by a breach in the mucous membranes or by aspiration, they can become pathogenic.[26] Cervicofacial and oral disease often are associated with trauma, dental procedures, eruption of a molar tooth, oral surgery, or dental infection. Pulmonary infections usually follow aspiration of oropharyngeal or gastrointestinal secretions. Other less common routes of infection are extension from cervicofacial disease or spread from the abdomen and, rarely, dissemination through blood from other sites of infection (e.g., pelvic or orofacial). Gastrointestinal infection frequently follows loss of mucosal integrity, as can occur with appendicitis, trauma, or foreign bodies. The use of an intrauterine contraceptive device is linked to the development of actinomycosis of the female genital tract.

Actinomyces infections are uncommon, indolent, and invasive. Infection generally is polymicrobial and can involve any body organ,[27] including the heart. Other copathogens with *Actinomyces* act synergistically by enhancing the spread of infection through inhibition of host defenses and reduction of local oxygen tension. Diagnosis often is delayed because of nonspecific and prolonged symptoms.[28] Patients with chronic granulomatous disease have an unusual susceptibility to *Actinomyces* infection.[29]

Clinical Manifestations

Unique characteristics of actinomycosis are indolent inflammation with spreading ("burrowing") through soft and bony tissue planes to contiguous or remarkably distant sites. The hallmark of actinomycosis is spread that fails to respect tissue or fascial planes. Classically, small abscesses form at the site of origin, with extension to form multiple sinus tracts that can drain yellow, gritty, purulent material (sulfur granules) composed of spheroid colonies of radiating club-shaped filaments, neutrophils, debris, and granulomatous reaction. *Actinomyces* grows in tissues in microscopic or macroscopic clusters of tangled filaments surrounded by neutrophils. The differential diagnosis includes other chronic infections at these sites, including tuberculosis, nocardiosis, and complications of foreign bodies. The most common sites of infection are cervicofacial, abdominopelvic, thoracic, and in the central nervous system.

Cervicofacial Actinomycosis

Most infections in immunocompetent individuals are cervicofacial. Depending on the composition of the concomitant synergistic flora, the onset can be acute, subacute, or chronic. The most commonly recognized manifestations are: "lumpy jaw," which is a slowly enlarging, fluctuant painless swelling over the lower border of the mandible, or a widely spread infection that involves the submandibular area; or osteomyelitis of the mandible or maxilla. Infection spreads slowly without regard to tissue planes, and draining fistulas can occur (usually to the mucosal side) and can be accompanied by trismus.[20,21] Fever or systemic illness usually is absent. Chronic tonsillitis, dental decay, mastoiditis, and otitis media are risk factors, but some patients have no recognizable disorder or preceding event. Periostitis or osteomyelitis can develop if the infection extends to the facial and maxillary bones (or rarely can complicate primary disorder of bone such as fibrous dysplasia) (see Figure 78-6). Primary infection can develop in the palate, scalp, salivary glands, maxilla, paranasal sinuses, tongue, larynx, hypopharynx, and trachea.[30] Meningitis also can occur if the process extends into the cranial bones through sinus tracts.[31] The prognosis is excellent with extremely prolonged antimicrobial therapy (sometimes more than 1 year), frequently without surgical intervention. In a review of 19 cases of actinomycosis presenting as osteomyelitis in children, the mandible was most commonly affected, age was predominantly young school age, half had one predisposing factor, and mandibular cases required >1 debridement procedures for cure.[32]

Abdominal and Pelvic Actinomycosis

The appendix is the most frequent gastrointestinal site. Appendicitis with perforation is the most common predisposing event; unrecognized foreign body perforation (e.g., needle, pin) also has occurred. The inciting event can precede the diagnosis by months to years. Chronic nonspecific symptomatology consisting of fever, chills, weight loss, diarrhea or constipation, abdominal pain, and night sweats, with few abdominal symptoms, is typical and can mimic tuberculosis or lymphoreticular malignancy. Infection can spread to other intra-abdominal (e.g., hepatic) and pelvic viscera. Primary pelvic infection can complicate abortions, retained surgical sutures, intrauterine devices, endometritis, tubo-ovarian abscess, or pelvic inflammatory disease.[33] Patients can have an indolent vaginal discharge, abdominal or pelvic pain, menorrhagia, fever, and weight loss.

Thoracic Actinomycosis (Figure 195-1)

Thoracic actinomycosis usually starts as undetected aspiration pneumonia in a predisposed host. Neurologically impaired children who are at increased risk of aspirating and often have poor dentition account for some cases. In review of thoracic actinomycosis in 55 children only 5 (9%) children had this risk factor.[28] The most common clinical finding is a chronic indolent and slowly progressing pneumonia with or without pleural involvement. Tachypnea, chest pain, and productive cough are not prominent. Fever and weight loss may be the only manifestations. A high index of suspicion is required. Infection typically burrows through ribs (causing an osteolytic lesion) and then can manifest as a subcutaneous mass on the thorax with or without a draining sinus.[17,18,23] Infection can mimic malignancy, tuberculosis, and lung abscess. Thoracic infection can traverse tissue planes to the soft tissues of distal extremities or through the diaphragm into the abdomen.[34]

Diagnosis and Treatment

Histologic identification of sulfur granules is pathognomonic but is not a universal finding in actinomycosis. Gram and acid-fast stains are helpful in differentiating probable *Actinomyces* from other genera causing similar clinical manifestations. Isolation of organisms is extremely important to confirm the diagnosis. Frequently, a less fastidious copathogen, *A. actinomycetemcomitans*, is the sole isolate and predicts the presence of *Actinomyces*.[20,21,34] A singular role of *Aggregatibacter* is possible, and some patients have responded poorly to therapy when clindamycin, erythromycin, or vancomycin was used (to which *Aggregatibacter* but not *Actinomyces* is resistant).[27,34] Prolonged antimicrobial therapy is the cornerstone of treatment. Usually, cervicofacial infection responds to antibiotics alone. Drainage of large thoracic, abdominal, or soft-tissue abscesses, extensive resection of affected tissues, and excision of sinus tracts generally are required. *Actinomyces* and *Aggregatibacter* are exquisitely susceptible to penicillin and extended-spectrum penicillins;. *Actinomyces* are susceptible in vitro to a wide range of β-lactam agents and these, when combined with a β-lactamase inhibiting agent, are regarded as agents of first choice when polymicrobial infection is likely.[35] The duration of therapy is more important than the route of administration. Initially, aqueous penicillin G (250,000 U/kg/day in 4 divided doses) can be used intravenously (depending on the patient's clinical status), followed by 6 to 12 months of oral penicillin or amoxicillin, with or without probenecid.

OTHER GRAM-POSITIVE BACILLI

Other gram-positive anaerobic bacilli include *Lactobacillus*, *Bifidobacterium*, and *Eubacterium* species. These genera are part of the normal flora of the female genital tract, oral cavity, and gastrointestinal tract.[36] Polymicrobial infection usually occurs contiguous to body sites where organisms are normal inhabitants, e.g., periodontal disease and infections of the female genital tract and abdominal viscera. Rarely, BSI also can occur. Most *Bifidobacterium*

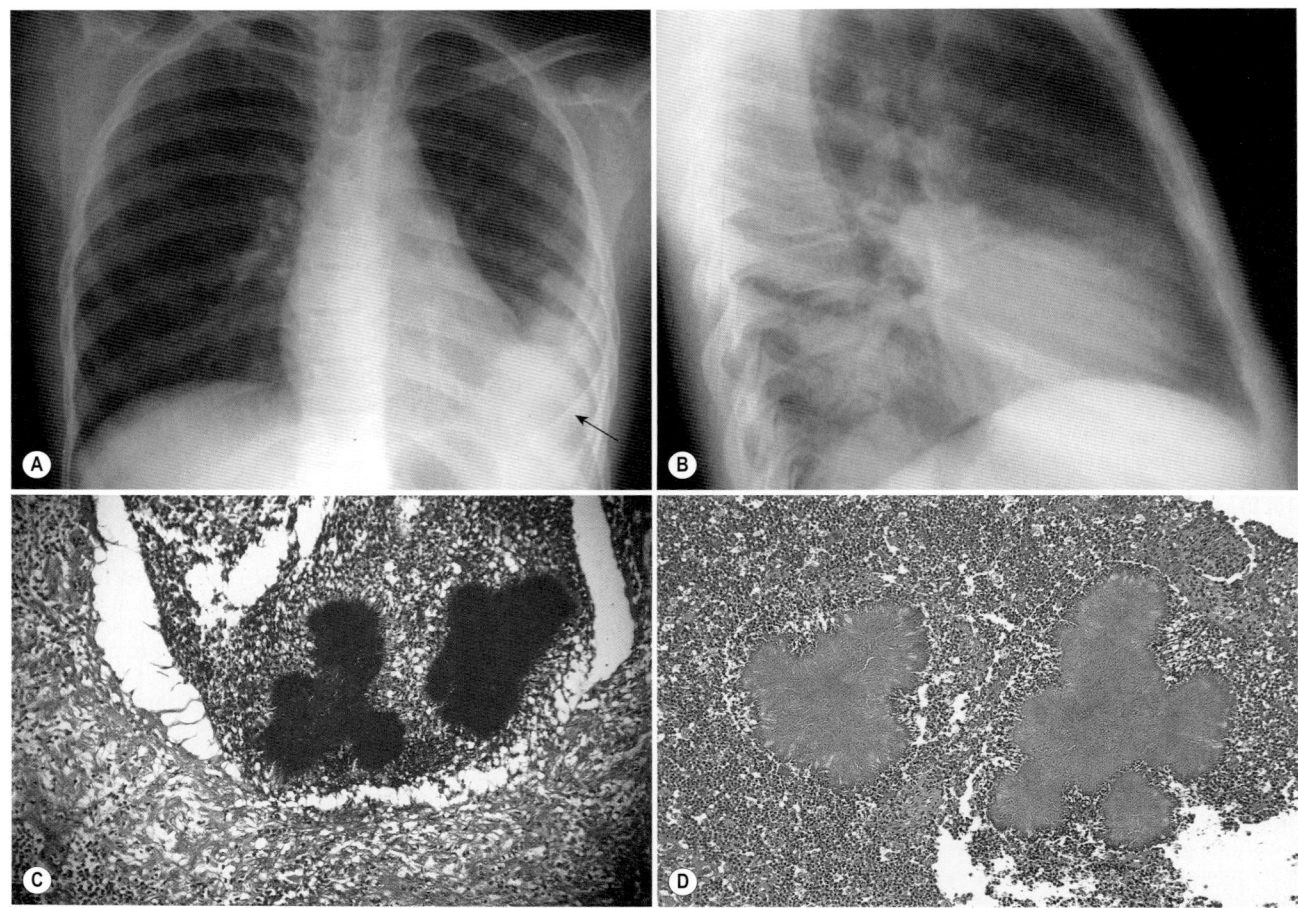

Figure 195-1. Thoracic actinomycosis. A 9-year-old girl had a lump noted on her chest wall. She was afebrile and had no respiratory tract complaints or physical finding except a nodular lesion on the tenth rib anteriorly. She had a history 8 months prior to admission of left lower lobe pneumonia and atelectasis. Chest radiograph shows left lower lobe pneumonia, loculated pleural collection, and a lytic lesion of the rib (arrow) **(A, B).** Biopsy of the rib lesion stained by periodic acid–Schiff **(C)** and hematoxylin-eosin stain **(D)** show histologic findings of chronic osteomyelitis and sulfur granules. Culture of specimens from lung, pleura, and rib yielded growth of *Actinobacillus actinomycetemcomitans* and *Actinomyces israelii.* (Case courtesy of D.V. Schidlow and E.N. Faerber, St. Christopher's Hospital for Children, Philadelphia, PA.)

isolates are recovered from chronic otitis media, abscesses, peritonitis, aspiration pneumonia, and paronychia. Most *Eubacterium* isolates are associated with abscesses, peritonitis, decubitus ulcers, and bite wound infections. *Lactobacillus* is recovered mainly from abscesses, aspiration pneumonia, BSI, and conjunctivitis.[36] Predisposing conditions associated with these anaerobic bacilli are previous surgery, malignancy, corticosteroid therapy, and immunodeficiency. These genera usually are susceptible to penicillins, carbapenems, and clindamycin. However, *Lactobacillus*, some *Eubacterium*, and other facultative anaerobes, are resistant to nitroimidazoles. Cephalosporins, erythromycin, and tetracycline have variable activity.

Key Points. *Actinomyces* Species

DESCRIPTION

- Filamentous branching gram-positive catalase-negative bacillus
- Anaerobic or microaerophilic
- *Actinomyces israelii* is predominant species causing disease

EPIDEMIOLOGY

- Colonizes human oral cavity early in childhood
- Normal flora of mouth, gastrointestinal, and female genital tracts
- Attains access to tissue via breach in mucous membranes, i.e., following trauma, or by aspiration
- Infections usually are polymicrobial
- Special hosts at risk: patients with chronic granulomatous disease

CLINICAL FEATURES

- Infections are indolent
- Diagnosis often is delayed

- Hallmark is spread that fails to respect tissue or fascial planes
- Development of sinus tracts also is characteristic
- Most common sites of infection:
  - Cervicofacial (normal hosts)
  - Abdominopelvic
  - Thoracic
  - Central nervous system

DIAGNOSIS AND TREATMENT

- "Sulfur granules" (clumps of microorganisms in vivo) can be seen
- Bacteriologic identification confirms diagnosis
- Prolonged antimicrobial therapy is key to successful treatment
- Penicillins, clindamycin, cephalosporins all are active

196 *Mycoplasma pneumoniae*
Samir S. Shah

THE PATHOGEN

Mycoplasma pneumoniae is a member of the class Mollicutes, which includes bacterial pathogens and commensals found in many animals and plants. These pathogens comprise the smallest self-replicating prokaryotes known to cause infection in humans.[1] *M. pneumoniae* is approximately 120 to 150 nm, about the size of myxoviruses, and passes easily through membrane filters intended to prevent bacterial contamination. Humans are the only known natural host for *M. pneumoniae*.

The absence of a cell wall distinguishes *Mycoplasma* from other pathogenic bacteria and results in the following additional characteristics: (1) growth on cell-free media only if sterols and other nutrients are provided by yeast extract and animal serum; (2) pleomorphism, preventing classification as either cocci or bacilli in the manner of conventional eubacteria, and variable ability to take up bacteriologic dyes such as Gram stain; (3) resistance to penicillins and cephalosporins, which act by inhibiting cell wall synthesis; and (4) susceptibility to desiccation, a factor that mandates proper handling of clinical specimens for culture as well as close contact for transmission of infection from person to person.

PATHOGENESIS

The organism gains access to the respiratory tract through aerosolized droplets spread among close contacts. Specific attachment to the respiratory epithelial tissue occurs primarily through interaction between a host epithelial cell receptor and the organism's P1 attachment protein, a 169-kd surface antigen.[2-4] Other structures that participate in cytadherence also have been identified.[5] Following attachment, hydrogen peroxide and superoxide radicals synthesized by *M. pneumoniae* act in concert with endogenous toxic oxygen molecules generated by host cells to induce oxidative stress in the respiratory epithelium.[6] Once *M. pneumoniae* reaches the lower respiratory tract, the organism may be opsonized by complement or antibodies. Activated macrophages begin phagocytosis, and undergo chemotactic migration to the site of infection. CD4+ T lymphocytes, B lymphocytes, and plasma cells infiltrate the lung. Further amplification of the immune response occurs in association with lymphocyte proliferation, production of immunoglobulins, and release of tumor necrosis factor-α, interferon-γ, and various interleukins.[7] Lymphocyte activation and cytokine production either can minimize disease by controlling infection or exacerbate disease by stimulating immune-mediated lung injury.

Extrapulmonary complications of *M. pneumoniae* infection can occur as a consequence of immune-mediated injury or direct invasion. *M. pneumoniae* has been identified by polymerase chain reaction (PCR) in cerebrospinal fluid (CSF)[8] and serum,[9] indicating that dissemination occurs in some cases. Effects of cross-reactive antibody with host tissues remain the proposed mechanism for hemolysis and cutaneous manifestations.[10]

EPIDEMIOLOGY

The age at which *M. pneumoniae* should be considered among causes of lower respiratory tract infection is uncertain. Although primarily a disease in adolescents and young adults,[11-13] *M. pneumoniae* has been recognized as a cause of lower respiratory tract infection in young children.[14-22] In Finland, *M. pneumoniae* was the cause of community-acquired pneumonia (CAP) in 9% of children 0 to 4 years of age and in 40% of children 5 to 9 years

of age.[18] *M. pneumoniae* accounts for approximately 20% to 40% of cases of CAP in junior high and high school students and for up to 50% of cases among college students and military recruits.[23-27] Incidence of endemic *M. pneumoniae* CAP ranges from 1 to 2 per 1000 children <5 years of age, 3 to 4 per 1000 children 5 to 15 years of age, and <1 per 1000 adults <70 years of age.[13,26,28]

Epidemic *M. pneumoniae* occurs at 3- to 7-year intervals in the United States, superimposed on low-level endemic disease.[26,29] Community epidemics can be unrecognized until clusters of extrapulmonary complications occur because testing is not performed routinely in the office setting and *M. pneumoniae* is not a publicly reportable disease.[30] Factors that facilitate the occurrence and persistence of outbreaks of *M. pneumoniae* infection in institutional and military settings include the difficulty of making a rapid diagnosis, the long incubation period (2 to 3 weeks), and prolonged respiratory tract shedding (weeks to months following infection).[31,32] Persistence of the organism in many cases despite antibiotic therapy contributes to protracted outbreaks.[33]

Epidemics of *M. pneumoniae* commonly begin in the fall and can persist for months. Young children often serve as the index case within a family; they commonly have symptoms of upper respiratory tract infection or few overt symptoms.[12] Sequential transmission to family members frequently occurs with 2- to 4-week lapses between cases; approximately 40% of family members develop infection.[11,31,33] The attack rate is approximately 25% in other closed populations, including nursing homes.[27,34] Smoking appears to modify the relationship between pre-existing specific antibodies and risk of infection. During an epidemic among military trainees, pre-existing IgG anti-*M. pneumoniae* was protective in nonsmokers, with an attack rate of 30%, while the attack rates in antibody-positive smokers and antibody-negative nonsmokers ranged from 77% to 86%.[35]

Longitudinal community surveillance and studies of military recruits demonstrate that *M. pneumoniae* infection provides at least short-term protection from subsequent infection and that immunity after pneumonia lasts longer than that after asymptomatic infection or upper respiratory tract disease alone.[36-38] The relatively mild course of infection in very young children has led to speculation that infection in early childhood results in a sensitizing immunologic response necessary for the development of lower respiratory tract involvement later in life.

CLINICAL MANIFESTATIONS

Respiratory Tract Disease

M. pneumoniae was first isolated during efforts to determine the cause of the clinical syndrome referred to as "primary atypical pneumonia."[39] Failure of patients with this infection to respond to penicillin or sulfonamide therapy – the standard therapy for pneumococcal pneumonia – was considered "atypical."

In young children, *M. pneumoniae* can be indistinguishable from viral causes of respiratory tract infection; concomitant *Mycoplasma* and viral infection also occurs.[40-42] *M. pneumoniae* infection in young children can be asymptomatic or can cause rhinorrhea, pharyngitis, otitis media, croup, bronchiolitis, or pneumonia.[11,19,29,43,44] *M. pneumoniae* infection in older children and adolescents can cause upper or lower respiratory tract infection. Initial symptoms typically are general malaise, myalgia, sore throat, retrobulbar headache, and fever.[29,45] Sinus pain or fullness and ear pain often are described. These symptoms are indistinguishable from those due to influenza and other respiratory viruses. Physical

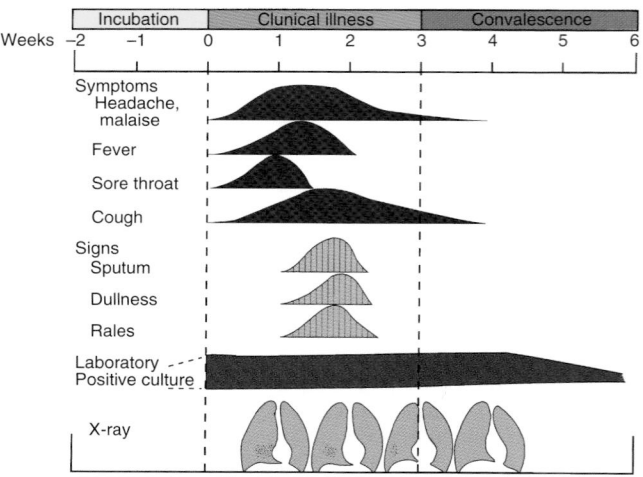

Figure 196-1. Characteristic clinical course of pneumonia due to *Mycoplasma pneumoniae*. (Redrawn from Denny FW, Clyde WA Jr, Glezen WP. *Mycoplasma pneumoniae* disease: clinical spectrum, pathophysiology, epidemiology, and control. J Infect Dis 1971;123:74, © 1971, the University of Chicago Press.)

findings reflect the sites of respiratory tract involvement. The patient can have sinus tenderness, nonexudative posterior pharyngeal erythema, and otitis media. Bullous myringitis was thought to be pathognomonic for *M. pneumoniae* infection following the observation of bullous myringitis in inoculated, nonimmune adults.[46] However, numerous other causes of bullous myringitis have been identified.[47,48] Additionally, *M. pneumoniae* was isolated by culture of middle ear fluid in only 1 of 771 children with otitis media.[49] *M. pneumoniae* was not detected by PCR in any of 37 children with either bullous or hemorrhagic myringitis.[50]

Patients with *M. pneumoniae* pneumonia can have chills, chest pain, nausea, vomiting, and diarrhea. The characteristic course of pneumonia is depicted in Figure 196-1. Dry, nonproductive cough, which develops 3 to 5 days after the initial symptoms, can become productive of mucopurulent or blood-streaked sputum. Cough usually brings the patient to medical attention 5 to 7 days after onset of symptoms; cough can be paroxysmal and worse at night. Coughing from either tracheobronchitis or pneumonia can persist for ≥2 weeks after resolution of fever and other constitutional signs and symptoms, resulting in a 4-week illness that can resemble pertussis.[51] Palpation of the neck can produce paroxysms of coughing. Physical findings of lower respiratory tract disease can be absent during the first week of the illness, but in the second week of illness, as fever, myalgia, and other constitutional symptoms resolve, sputum production begins and auscultation of the chest frequently reveals crackles or wheezes or both – thus the appellation "walking pneumonia". *M. pneumoniae* has been documented to cause parapneumonic effusions and necrotizing pneumonitis in children.[52-54] Severe and sometimes fatal *M. pneumoniae* pneumonia is reported in both adults and children.[55-61]

M. pneumoniae infections frequently are associated with exacerbations of asthma. In a prospective study, *M. pneumoniae* was detected by either PCR or serology in 20% of children hospitalized for exacerbation of asthma and in 50% of children hospitalized for first-episode wheezing; in contrast, *M. pneumoniae* infection was diagnosed in only 5% of control children with either stable asthma or allergic rhinitis.[62] *M. pneumoniae* also may have a role in chronic lung disease. Mice experimentally inoculated with *M. pneumoniae* into the respiratory tract were more likely than control mice to have chronic pulmonary disease characterized by airway hyperreactivity, airway obstruction, and histologic inflammation.[63] In children, lung abnormalities, including reduced pulmonary clearance and airway hyperresponsiveness, can persist for months to years following *M. pneumoniae* infection.[64,65]

Numerous case reports describe severe respiratory illness caused by *M. pneumoniae* in immunodeficient children. *M. pneumoniae* was detected in 2% of bronchoalveolar lavage specimens from human immunodeficiency virus-infected patients with pneumonia.[66] Serologic evidence of *M. pneumoniae* infection was demonstrated in 9% of 538 children with sickle-cell disease and acute chest syndrome.[67] Patients with sickle-cell disease or sickle-related hemoglobinopathies often develop severe respiratory illness as a consequence of *M. pneumoniae* infection.[68-71]

Extrapulmonary Disease

Extrapulmonary complications of *M. pneumoniae* infection occur (Table 196-1).[72-98] Certainty about a causative role has been increased with PCR detection at extrapulmonary sites, but many reports remain anecdotal, with diagnosis resting on elevation of cold agglutinin or complement-fixing (CF) antibody values. Because CF antibodies can cross-react with human tissue,

TABLE 196-1. Extrapulmonary Disease Associated with *Mycoplasma pneumoniae*[a]

Organ System	Manifestation
Dermatologic	Discrete maculopapules
	Erythema multiforme
	Stevens–Johnson syndrome
	Gianotti–Crosti syndrome
	Urticaria
	Morbilliform exanthem
	Vesicles/bullae
	Ulcerative stomatitis
	Erythema marginatum
Hematologic	Complement-dependent, Coombs-positive, anti-I antigen, immunoglobulin M antibody
	Thrombosis (transient antiphospholipid antibody response)
	Thrombotic thrombocytopenic purpura
Central nervous system disease	Encephalitis/meningoencephalitis
	Transverse myelitis
	Guillain–Barré syndrome
	Focal encephalitis
	Polyradiculitis
	Bell palsy
	Asymmetrical paralysis
	Cerebellar ataxia
	Psychosis
	Cerebral infarction
Arthritis	Acute/chronic course
	Monoarticular/migratory/polyarticular arthritis
Cardiac disease	Pericarditis
	Myocarditis
	Heart block
	Myocardial infarction
	Congestive heart failure
Hepatic dysfunction	Mild hepatic enzyme elevation[b]
Pancreatitis	Acute inflammation
Ocular disease	Conjunctivitis
	Glomerulonephritis
	Iritis
	Optic disk edema
Other	Rhabdomyolysis

[a]Organ system/finding occurs in <10% of cases except where noted.
[b]Occurs in approximately 30% with pneumonia.

particularly brain and pancreas, elevation can occur during inflammation or destruction of tissue due to other causes. In the context of family and community outbreaks of *M. pneumoniae* infection, however, and in individuals with concomitant pulmonary involvement, reports of extrapulmonary involvement are more credible.[99-102] Additionally, occasional isolation of *M. pneumoniae* from blood, cerebrospinal fluid, synovial fluid, and skin lesions (primarily in immunocompromised patients) indicates that dissemination rather than an immune-mediated mechanism occurs in some cases. PCR testing has confirmed the role of *M. pneumoniae* in cases of encephalitis and transverse myelitis,[8,103-105] pleural effusion,[53] and bacteremia.[9]

The central nervous system (CNS) appears to be the most common extrapulmonary site of *M. pneumoniae* infection. Of 1988 patients enrolled in the California Encephalitis Project, 111 (5.6%) had evidence of recent or current *M. pneumoniae* infection.[106] In some series, CNS involvement is reported in 1% to 7% of patients requiring hospitalization for *M. pneumoniae*.[79,107,108] Neurologic symptoms of children with *M. pneumoniae* in the California Encephalitis Project included altered consciousness (58%), seizures (40%), focal neurologic signs (37%), and hallucinations (18%).[106] Respiratory tract symptoms, reported in >80% of children with CNS involvement, precede neurologic symptoms by 7 to 10 days.[79,108] In patients with *M. pneumoniae* encephalitis or meningitis, CSF findings often are normal, but a mild, predominantly mononuclear pleocytosis (up to 200 cells/mm³) and protein elevation up to 70 to 80 mg/dL can occur; higher CSF white blood cell counts (WBC) (>900 cells/mm³) and protein concentrations (>170 mg/dL), although uncommon, have been described.[80-82,106]

Joint involvement in children appears to be less common than in adults. Monoarthritis, polyarthritis, and migratory arthritis mimicking acute rheumatic fever have been described.[86,87,109-114] Limited information is available regarding synovial fluid analysis in patients with *M. pneumoniae*-associated arthritis; synovial pleocytosis has ranged from 1000 WBCs/mm³ in a child with hypogammaglobulinemia to approximately 50,000/mm³ in an otherwise healthy child.[87,112] *M. pneumoniae*-associated glomerulonephritis has been described.[115-120] Glomerulonephritis appeared concomitantly with other symptoms in some cases and 5 to 10 days later in other cases. Serum C3 complement level is decreased initially in some cases. Hematologic complications include the development of hemolytic anemia attributable to cross-reacting cold agglutinins,[76,105,121] thrombotic thrombocytopenic purpura,[122] and transient antiphospholipid antibodies.[123,124]

LABORATORY FINDINGS AND DIAGNOSIS

Pathogen-specific Identification

Culture

Many *Mycoplasma* species grow best in 5% to 10% carbon dioxide, but *M. pneumoniae* also grows well under aerobic conditions. The fermentation of simple carbohydrates, such as glucose, xylose, mannose, and maltose, provides a method for recognizing the growth of *Mycoplasma* in the laboratory. The complex nutritional requirements and slow growth on artificial media make identification by culture impractical for most laboratories and of limited value clinically. Because *M. pneumoniae* can persist in the respiratory tract for weeks to months after symptomatic or asymptomatic infection, recovery of the organism from the throat or sputum does not necessarily confirm causation of current disease.[25,44]

Cold-agglutinins

Cold-reacting antibodies against red blood cells can be detected in the serum of patients with primary atypical pneumonia.[39] Cold-agglutinating antibodies are immunoglobulin M (IgM) autoantibodies directed against the I antigen on human erythrocytes, which appear within 7 to 10 days of initial symptoms and drop sharply after 2 to 3 weeks.[29,45,125,126] In the laboratory, the highest

dilution of serum causing hemagglutination or "clumping" of type O erythrocytes at 4°C is reported as the cold agglutinin titer. Titers >1:64 are present at the time of acute illness in approximately 75% of adults with pneumonia due to *M. pneumoniae*. The test is less well studied in children. Specificity of a titer <1:64 is low because a variety of other respiratory tract pathogens provoke modest increases in cold agglutinins. For example, 18% of military recruits with adenoviral pneumonia had a cold agglutinin titer of ≥1:32.[127] Cold agglutinin antibodies should not be used for the diagnosis of *M. pneumoniae* infections if other methods are available. Bedside cold agglutinin testing lacks rigorous standards for performance and interpretation and is not recommended.

Serology

Methods to measure serum antibody include complement fixation (CF), indirect fluorescence (IFA), enzyme-immunoassays (EIA), and rapid EIA cards. Although CF testing has been the most widely available assay for detection of antibody to *M. pneumoniae*,[128] CF measures mainly IgM antibody, limiting its diagnostic value to initial rather than repeated infections.[96] An elevated CF antibody titer should also be interpreted with caution in patients with nonrespiratory disease since the antigens used in the CF test can cross-react with human tissue.[94-96]

CF tests have largely been replaced by less time-consuming and labor-intensive immunoglobulin assays, including EIA and immunofluorescence assay, and an indirect hemagglutination assay. These assays can be performed on a single serum specimen obtained during the acute infection; they all appear to be as sensitive as the CF test in children with pneumonia.[96,129-131] In adults, *M. pneumoniae* frequently represents a second infection and IgM response does not occur reliably.[132,133]

EIA IgM assays are reported to be sensitive in children with pneumonia.[130] The Immunocard rapid IgM test (Meredian Bioscience, Cincinnati, OH) compared with other serologic tests (but not with PCR), using IFA as the gold standard, had sensitivities ranging from 74% compared with EIA to 96% compared with CF; specificities ranged from 85% compared with the IgM-specific EIA to 98% compared with the IgM-specific IFA.[134] Results were similar in a subsequent study of 145 children tested for *M. pneumoniae*.[135] False-positive IgM tests can occur, however, and predictive values of test results depend on prevalence/likelihood of *M. pneumoniae* infection. The specificity of IgM detection during a university and community outbreak of *M. pneumoniae* pneumonia was only 43% for children 10 to 18 years of age and 82% for those ≥19 years of age compared with a case-definition gold standard for diagnosis.[136] A combined IgG/IgM assay (Remel, Themo Fisher Scientific, Lenexa, KS) assessed during this outbreak had a higher specificity in children 10 to 18 years of age (74%) but a lower sensitivity (52%) compared with IgM detection (89%).[136] Other immunoglobulin M assays appear to be as sensitive as PCR for detection of *M. pneumoniae* in CAP in children.[130]

IgG anti-*M. pneumoniae* can persist for months to years following infection. Testing for both IgM and IgG in paired specimens collected 2 to 3 weeks apart may provide the most accurate serologic diagnosis.[137] A ≥4-fold rise in antibody indicates a recent or current *M. pneumoniae* infection. Therefore, accurate diagnosis often is made only retrospectively.

Molecular Methods

Molecular assays to detect *M. pneumoniae* are available.[130,131,138-143] PCR testing has detected *M. pneumoniae* in a variety of syndromes. Use of primers against two different targets maximizes the ability to detect the organism; potential targets include the ATPase operon gene, P1 gene, conserved regions of 16S RNA, and the *tuf* gene.[144-148] Direct comparison of studies utilizing PCR is difficult since specimens were obtained from different sites (e.g., nasal wash, nasopharyngeal swab, throat, sputum) and different primer sets and amplification techniques were used. Compared with seroconversion, sensitivity of some PCR-based tests has ranged from 79% for pharyngeal specimens to 90% for nasopharyngeal

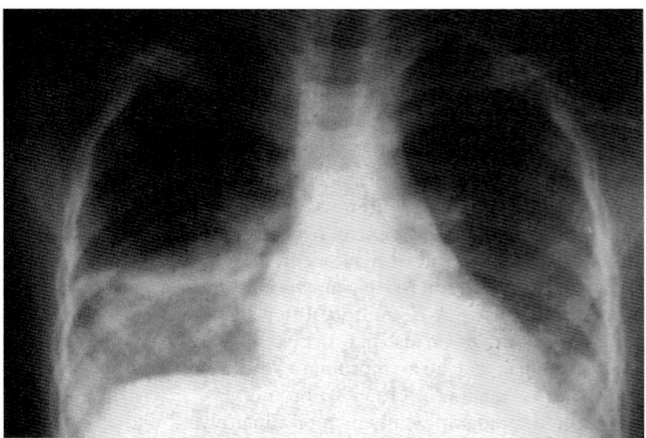

Figure 196-2. Chest radiograph of a 10-year-old girl with *Mycoplasma pneumoniae* pneumonia.

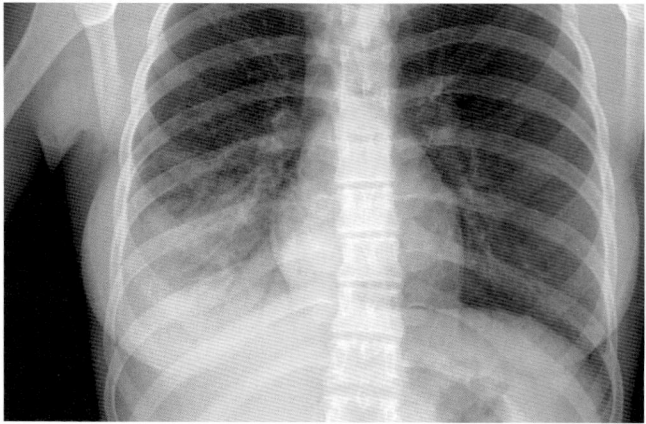

Figure 196-3. Chest radiograph in a 14-year-old boy with lobar pneumonia. Air bronchograms can be seen in the right lower lobe. *Mycoplasma pneumoniae* genome was detected in his nasopharynx and throat by PCR testing.

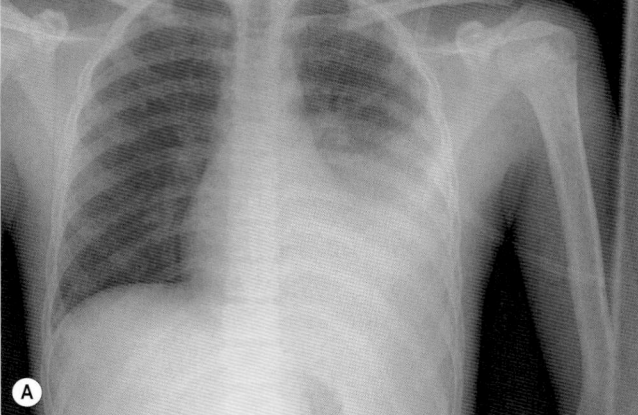

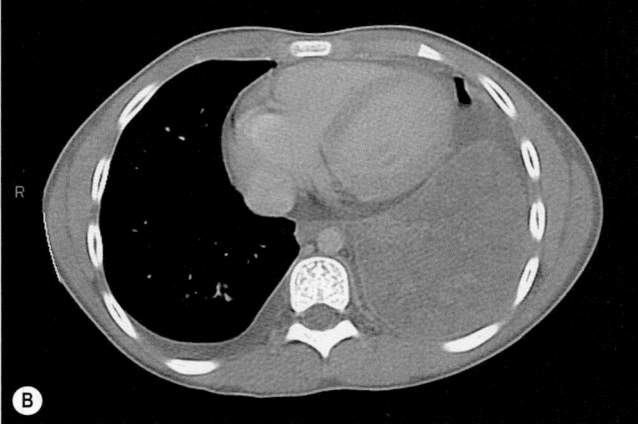

Figure 196-4. (A) Radiograph and **(B)** computed tomography (CT) of the chest of a 13-year-old girl with *Mycoplasma pneumoniae* pneumonia complicated by parapneumonic effusion. The radiograph demonstrates opacification of the left lung base with a moderate pleural effusion. CT of the same patient also demonstrates a small right-sided pleural effusion and a trivial pericardial effusion.

specimens; specificity was 98% when using these specimens.[148] Compared with culture, PCR has the advantage of ability to detect *M. pneumoniae* genome in clinical settings when the organism may no longer be viable, such as in contaminated specimens or from tissue that has already been processed for histologic examination. Additionally, PCR test can be positive earlier in the course of infection than serologic tests.

Testing of Extrapulmonary Specimens

Verification of extrapulmonary complications attributable to *M. pneumoniae* is challenging. Among children with encephalitis attributable to *M. pneumoniae* (defined by the presence of IgM anti-*M. pneumoniae* in acute or convalescent serum), intrathecal *M. pneumoniae* antibodies were detected rarely; IgM was found in 1 (3%) of 32 and IgG in 2 (12%) of 17 CSF samples.[106] CSF PCR was positive in 1 of 62 children with *M. pneumoniae* encephalitis; the subject with a positive CSF PCR also had positive CSF IgM anti-*M. pneumoniae*.[106] Smaller case series have yielded similar findings.[149,150]

Additional Tests

Routine laboratory studies are not likely to distinguish between respiratory tract infections caused by *M. pneumoniae*, viruses, or other bacteria. The peripheral blood WBC count is normal or

slightly elevated, with neutrophilia. Reported erythrocyte sedimentation rates range from 20 to >100 mm/h with higher rates reflecting more severe pulmonary disease.[40,151-153]

Chest radiograph documents lower respiratory involvement, but few features differentiate *M. pneumoniae* from viral or other bacterial pathogens. Chest radiograph in *M. pneumoniae* infection can show significant abnormality despite insignificant clinical symptoms. Bilateral interstitial infiltrates as well as patchy, unilateral, segmental, or subsegmental consolidation are described (Figures 196-2 and 196-3).[154-156] Pleural effusions, reported in 20% of patients in one study when lateral decubitus views were obtained, usually are small and bilateral,[153-157] although large pleural effusions occur occasionally (Figure 196-4).[52-54] Hilar lymphadenopathy, observed in 34% of children in one study, is seen more commonly in *M. pneumoniae* pneumonia than in pneumonia from most other causes.[154]

THERAPY

Antimicrobial Therapy

M. pneumoniae is inhibited in vitro by tetracyclines, macrolides, ketolides, and fluoroquinolones.[158-160] Fluoroquinolones appear bactericidal for *M. pneumoniae* whereas macrolides, ketolides, and tetracyclines primarily are bacteriostatic;[158] significance in patient outcomes is not known. The minimum inhibitory concentration (MIC_{90}) for levofloxacin ranges from 0.25 to 2 µg/mL;[158,161-164] the minimum bactericidal concentration (MBC) is 2-fold higher.

Moxifloxacin and gatifloxacin have somewhat greater activity in vitro compared with levofloxacin and ofloxacin; $MICs_{90}$ for all fluoroquinolones generally are several-fold higher than those of macrolides.[159,160] For azithromycin, clarithromycin, and telithromycin, the MIC_{90} values range from 0.001 to 0.015 µg/mL; MBC values often are 8- to 16-fold higher.[158,159,161] Linezolid has minimal activity against *M. pneumoniae* (MIC_{90} >64 µg/mL).[163] Several other agents, including streptogramins, clindamycin, chloramphenicol, and aminoglycosides demonstrate activity in vitro but are not effective clinically. β-Lactam and glycopeptide antibiotics have no activity against mycoplasmas.

The efficacy of antibiotic treatment of *M. pneumoniae* respiratory tract infections is uncertain. Azithromycin improves microbiologic, histologic, and immunologic markers of disease in experimental *M. pneumoniae* pneumonia in mice.[165] Studies comparing β-lactam and macrolide agents in the treatment of CAP in children included too few patients with *M. pneumoniae* to draw meaningful conclusions.[166] However, several lines of evidence suggest a possible therapeutic benefit. First, prophylactic oxytetracycline administered to family members of patients with *M. pneumoniae* infection prevented symptomatic infection (but not seroconversion).[167] Second, during epidemic *M. pneumoniae* infections in institutional settings, subjects receiving azithromycin prophylaxis had significantly lower secondary attack rates than those not receiving prophylaxis.[34,168] Third, small retrospective studies have shown that among children with atypical CAP (including *M. pneumoniae*), those treated with macrolides had a shorter duration of fever[169] and were less likely to have persistence or progression of signs and symptoms after 3 days of therapy.[170,171] In adults, Shames et al.[172] found a shorter duration of fever and hospitalization among erythromycin recipients compared with controls. No data suggest benefit of therapy for respiratory tract infections other than pneumonia.

Macrolide-class antibiotics also have been explored as potential treatments for *M. pneumoniae* due to their anti-inflammatory properties.[173-177] The importance of anti-inflammatory properties is supported by studies showing clinical cure in patients treated with macrolides despite persistence of *M. pneumoniae* organisms,[11,29,178,179] clinical improvement despite the administration of doses that provide tissue levels below the MIC of the organism,[180-182] and clinical cure in patients with macrolide-resistant *M. pneumoniae*.[183,184] The relative importance of the antimicrobial and anti-inflammatory effects of macrolide antibiotics in the treatment of *M. pneumoniae* is not known.

Therapy, if prescribed, may be more effective when started within 3 to 4 days of illness onset.[28,178,185] Therapeutic options for children include erythromycin (30 to 40 mg/kg/day divided into 4 doses for 7 to 14 days), clarithromycin (15 mg/kg/day divided into 2 doses for 7 to 14 days), or azithromycin (10 mg/kg once on the first day, followed by 5 mg/kg/day once daily for the next 4 days). Studies comparing erythromycin with clarithromycin[14,186] or azithromycin[187,188] for treatment of pneumonia did not identify a difference in frequency of therapeutic failure between the two

groups; however, patients receiving erythromycin were twice as likely to have a drug-related adverse event, usually related to the gastrointestinal system. For adolescents, doxycycline (100 mg twice daily for 7 to 14 days), clarithromycin (500 mg twice daily for 7 to 14 days), azithromycin (500 mg on day 1, and 250 mg on days 2 to 5) or levofloxacin (500 mg once daily for 7 to 14 days) can be used. As few as 2% of patients with *M. pneumoniae* pneumonia require hospitalization, even in the presence of radiographic pneumonia.[28] Antibiotic therapy of *M. pneumoniae* infections has important limitations. The organism persists in many patients despite the antibiotic therapy; thus, contagiousness extends through and after treatment. Because of pathogen persistence, relapsing infection should be considered in patients whose symptoms recur. Increasing resistance of *S. pneumoniae* to macrolides should prompt caution against using these agents alone for treatment of CAP.

The prevalence of clinically significant antibiotic resistance among *M. pneumoniae* isolates is not known; organisms from acute infection rarely are isolated in culture or tested in vitro for susceptibility to antibiotics. Macrolide resistance was reported in 12 (6.2%) of 195 clinical isolates in Japan.[189] The median MIC values were >32 µg/mL for azithromycin, clarithromycin, and telithromycin and 8 µg/mL for josamycin; however, the MIC values for minocycline and levofloxacin were similar between macrolide-susceptible and macrolide-resistant *M. pneumoniae* isolates.[189] Mutations in the peptidyl transferase loop of domain V of the 23S rRNA gene reduces the affinity of macrolides for ribosomes in both experimental models and clinical isolates.[183,190]

No controlled studies of antibiotic or immunologic therapies for the nonrespiratory manifestations of *M. pneumoniae* infection have been conducted; no consistent benefit has been noted with antibiotic or corticosteroid therapy in individual patients. Because of the possibility of severe disseminated infection in immunocompromised individuals, it is reasonable to administer an antibiotic with antimycoplasmal activity to patients with arthritis, CNS disease, hemolysis, or cardiac disease when *M. pneumoniae* infection is suspected.

Adjunctive Therapy

The effect of systemic or inhaled corticosteroids on infection-induced airway inflammation is poorly understood. Inhaled corticosteroids do not increase the infectious load of *M. pneumoniae*.[191] However, there is currently no compelling evidence for their efficacy. In experimentally infected mice, dexamethasone alone did not reduce *M. pneumoniae*-induced lung inflammation substantively compared with either placebo or clarithromycin monotherapy; however, combination therapy with clarithromycin and dexamethosone showed a significant reduction in lung inflammation compared with the other treatment regimens.[192] Anecdotal reports in children with *M. pneumoniae* pneumonia reveal temporal improvement of fever and radiologic abnormalities in association with corticosteroid therapy.[193]

Key Points. Diagnosis and Management of *Mycoplasma pneumoniae* Infection

MICROBIOLOGY

- Pleomorphic bacteria without a cell wall, making it resistant to β-lactam antibiotics

EPIDEMIOLOGY

- Primarily a cause of upper and lower respiratory tract infection, although extrapulmonary complications occur
- Highest prevalence in school-aged children and adolescents, although younger children have less overt symptoms
- Attack rate among close contacts is 25% to 40%
- Clusters of infection occur in closed populations such as in institutionalized children and the military

DIAGNOSIS

- Clinical findings are suggestive
- Serology (IgM anti-*M. pneumoniae* detection in children or ≥4-fold rise in IgM or IgG) or PCR testing of nasopharyngeal washing or throat swab specimen

TREATMENT

- Role of antibiotic treatment for pneumonia uncertain
- Generally susceptible in vitro to macrolides, fluoroquinolones, and tetracyclines

197 Other *Mycoplasma* Species

Samir S. Shah

Many Mollicutes colonize the mucosal surfaces of humans (Table 197-1). Of these, only *Mycoplasma genitalium, M. hominis, M. pneumoniae* (see Chapter 196, *Mycoplasma pneumoniae*), and *Ureaplasma urealyticum* (see Chapter 198, *Ureaplasma urealyticum*) are known to be pathogenic for healthy humans. Other *Mycoplasma* species have been isolated in pure culture from nonmucosal sites in immunocompromised individuals, indicating that commensal species can cause disease in some circumstances. In addition, animal *Mycoplasma* spp. occasionally cause local wound infection in humans.[1]

MYCOPLASMA HOMINIS

M. hominis commonly colonizes the lower genitourinary tract of healthy adult men and women. In general, women are more likely to be colonized than men and the likelihood of colonization increases with the number of sexual partners.[2-4] *M. hominis* is found in <5% of asymptomatic men and in as many as 20% of men attending sexually transmitted disease clinics.[5] The rate of colonization in asymptomatic women ranges from 10% to 30%;[6,7] the rate of isolation may be higher in women with bacterial vaginosis,[8,9] urethritis, or cervicitis.[10] Adolescent girls and boys are colonized infrequently, with reported rates of approximately 5% and 2%, respectively.[11] *M. hominis* seldom colonizes the upper respiratory tract; it has been recovered from the oral or respiratory tracts of 1% to 3% of healthy adults and in a greater proportion of those who engage in oral-genital sexual practices.[12]

The respiratory and genitourinary tracts of neonates also can be colonized (incidence 2% to 7%), particularly after birth complicated by prolonged rupture of amniotic membranes or amnionitis.[7]

Isolation of the organism from normally sterile sites and documentation of immunologic response to infection have implicated *M. hominis* as a cause of the conditions listed in Table 197-2. Numerous case reports implicate *M. hominis* as a cause of amnionitis, postpartum fever,[13-20] and other postpartum infections.[21] However, the clinical importance of neonatal *M. hominis* infection is less clear.[22] Neonatal central nervous system infections attributed to *M. hominis* include ventriculitis,[23] meningitis,[24-31] meningoencephalitis,[32,33] and subdural empyema.[34] Several studies have identified *M. hominis* in cerebrospinal fluid (CSF). *M. hominis* was isolated from the CSF of 5 (5%) of 100 preterm infants 1 to 6 days of age;[27] the single infant with CSF pleocytosis had 71 white blood cells/mm[3] and a mononuclear cell predominance.[27] In another study, *M. hominis* was isolated from 9 (13%) of 69 neonates undergoing lumbar puncture; the CSF white blood cell count ranged from 0 to 28 white blood cells/mm[3].[25] *M. hominis* also was isolated from the CSF in 9 (2.8%) of 318 infants evaluated by lumbar puncture in the peripartum period at 4 community hospitals;[26] the single infant who died had concomitant *Haemophilus influenzae*

TABLE 197-1. Sites of Colonization or Infection of Mollicutes in Humans

Species	Primary Site
Acholeplasma laidlawii	Oropharynx
Acholeplasma oculi	?
Mycoplasma amphoriforme	Oropharynx
Mycoplasma buccale	Oropharynx
Mycoplasma faucium	Oropharynx
Mycoplasma fermentans	Lower genital tract, respiratory tract
Mycoplasma genitalium	Oropharynx, genital tract
Mycoplasma hominis	Lower genital tract, oropharynx
Mycoplasma lipophilum	Oropharynx
Mycoplasma orale	Oropharynx
Mycoplasma penetrans	Genital tract
Mycoplasma pirum	?
Mycoplasma pneumoniae	Oropharynx, trachea, bronchial tree, lung, pleural fluid
Mycoplasma primatum	Genital tract
Mycoplasma salivarium	Oropharynx
Mycoplasma spermatophilum	Cervix, sperm
Ureaplasma parvum	Genital tract
Ureaplasma urealyticum	Genital tract

Adapted from Tully G. Current status of the mollicute flora of humans. Clin Infect Dis 1993;17(Suppl 1):S2.

TABLE 197-2. Infection Associated with *Mycoplasma hominis*[a]

Age Group	Type of Infection
Neonate	Septicemia
	Meningitis
	Ventriculitis
	Brain abscess/subdural empyema
	Pneumonia
	Pericarditis
	Wound infection
	Submandibular adenitis
	Subcutaneous abscess
Infants and children	Septicemia
	Ventriculitis
	Pleural effusion
Adolescents and adults	Amnionitis
	Postpartum fever
	Pyelonephritis/perinephric abscess
	Septicemia
	Wound infection
	Intravascular infection
	Arthritis
	Ventriculitis
	Upper respiratory tract infection (parapharyngeal abscess)
	Pneumonia/pleural infection

[a]Nongenitourinary infections almost always occur in patients with immune compromise because of severe burns, collagen-vascular disease, severe trauma, malignancy, organ transplantation, or congenital immunodeficiency, particularly hypogammaglobulinemia.

sepsis. Neonates who did not receive specific therapy for *M. hominis* in these studies did not appear to have any apparent clinical consequence of infection.[25-27] On the other hand, a term infant with early-onset meningoencephalitis attributed to *M. hominis* identified by both culture and polymerase chain reaction (PCR) of the CSF had improvement in CSF findings that coincided with the administration of ciprofloxacin.[32]

Recovery of *M. hominis* from the respiratory or urinary tract of neonates generally has not been associated with clinical illness.[35,36] However, neonates with *M. hominis* isolated from sterile sites appear to have worse clinical outcomes. In a study of 351 preterm infants (23 to 32 weeks of gestational age), *M. hominis* was isolated from cord blood cultures alone (n = 21, 6.0%) or in combination with *Ureaplasma urealyticum* (n = 18, 5.1%).[37] Earlier gestational age correlated with a higher rate of positive umbilical cord blood cultures.[37] Furthermore, infants with positive cord blood cultures were more likely to have systemic inflammatory response syndrome compared with infants with negative cord blood cultures.[37]

There have been numerous anecdotal reports of *M. hominis* infection occurring outside the genitourinary system in other populations, including immunocompromised patients[38-46] and those undergoing intracranial surgery.[47] In a series of 36 adult patients with extragenital *M. hominis* infection, patients most commonly had abdominal wound infections following genitourinary tract surgery.[48]

M. hominis infection should be considered when specimens from localized purulent infection, especially following genitourinary tract exposure (e.g., neonate) or manipulation, fail to yield a pathogen by conventional laboratory methods. Isolation and identification of *M. hominis* require inoculation and initial incubation in beef heart infusion broth containing horse serum and yeast extract, available commercially as pleuropneumonia-like-organism (PPLO) broth. Arginine, which is metabolized by *M. hominis*, is added to the broth, along with phenol red. Metabolism of arginine increases the pH, so that growth can be detected by a change in the color of the broth, usually within 24 to 48 hours. Subculture onto solid agar and incubation in 95% nitrogen and 5% carbon dioxide yields, within 7 days, colonies of 200 to 300 μm, which develop a characteristic "fried egg" appearance. *M. hominis* (but not *M. pneumoniae* or *U. urealyticum*) also grows on conventional blood agar and in most broth media used for blood culture. Laboratory personnel should be alerted to look for pinpoint, translucent colonies that develop within 2 to 3 days on blood agar that should be subcultured as described. Recognition of *M. hominis* growth in blood culture broth depends on blind subculture, even if Gram stain of broth is negative. Growth causes little turbidity in broth, but radiometric assays show a positive growth index within 5 to 7 days.[20] Automated, continuous-monitoring blood culture systems do not permit recovery of *M. hominis* reliably.[49] Multiplex PCR[50] and PCR-based microtiter plate hybridization assays[51] have been described; their accuracy and usefulness in the clinical setting remains to be determined.

Generally, *M. hominis* is susceptible to tetracyclines, fluoroquinolones, and clindamycin.[52-55] The minimum inhibitory concentration (MIC$_{90}$) values are lower for levofloxacin (0.19 to 0.5 μg/mL), gatifloxacin (0.063 μg/mL), and moxifloxacin (0.063 μg/mL) than for ciprofloxacin (0.5 to 1 μg/mL).[52,54,56] Chloramphenicol, rifampin, and linezolid (MIC$_{90}$, 8.0 μg/mL) demonstrate modest in vitro activity.[57] Up to 20% of *M. hominis* clinical isolates are resistant to tetracycline and doxycycline.[52,58] Fluoroquinolone resistance occurs occasionally.[38,59] Unlike the other pathogenic mycoplasmas, *M. hominis* is almost always resistant to macrolides, azalides and ketolides, including erythromycin, azithromycin, clarithromycin, and telithromycin.[57,60,61] The benefit of immune globulin intravenous (IGIV) therapy in patients with hypogammaglobulinemia and *M. hominis* infection is not known.

MYCOPLASMA GENITALIUM

M. genitalium was first isolated in 1980 from urethral specimens of two homosexual men with symptoms of nongonococcal urethritis.[62] Clarifying the subsequent role of *M. genitalium* in human disease has been hampered by its slow growth, fastidious cultivation requirements, and serologic cross-reactivity of surface antigens with *M. pneumoniae*.[63] The high rate of detection of *M. genitalium* in sexual partners (38% to 63%) of affected index cases compared with uninfected control patients (6%) suggests that the infection is sexually transmitted.[64,65] Numerous studies using PCR confirm the association of *M. genitalium* with nongonococcal urethritis in men.[65-69] Fewer studies of *M. genitalium* have been carried out in women. The prevalence of *M. genitalium* of 6% among asymptomatic women attending a sexual-health clinic was comparable to that of *Neisseria gonorrhoeae* and *Chlamydia trachomatis*.[70] *M. genitalium* has been detected using PCR techniques in women with acute and chronic urethritis and pelvic inflammatory disease.[71-73] Women with pelvic inflammatory disease attributed to *M. genitalium* have a milder spectrum of symptoms compared with women with gonococcal pelvic inflammatory disease.[74]

Re-examination of presumed *M. pneumoniae* isolates from respiratory specimens obtained in the 1970s and from synovial fluid of a patient with hypogammaglobulinemia and polyarthritis has shown that some of these isolates were actually mixed strains of *M. pneumoniae* and *M. genitalium*.[75,76] Although *M. genitalium* is associated with nongonococcal urethritis in men, its association with other human diseases of the genitourinary or respiratory tract remains uncertain. The twofold higher prevalence of *M. genitalium* among HIV-infected persons also warrants investigation into potential clinical associations.[77]

The organism typically is detected by PCR of urethral or cervical swabs or urine specimens.[78-80] *M. genitalium* is susceptible to tetracyclines, fluoroquinolones, and macrolides.[81,82] However, doxycycline does not consistently eradicate *M. genitalium* from the genitourinary tract.[83-85] Among 398 men with urethritis enrolled in a randomized clinical trial, 13% of azithromycin-treated men remained *M. genitalium* positive compared with 55% of doxycycline-treated men.[85] In another study, colonization persisted in 20 (67%) of 30 patients treated with doxycycline but in 0 of 36 patients treated with azithromycin.[84]

OTHER *MYCOPLASMA* INFECTIONS

Mycoplasma spp., including *M. fermentans*, *M. penetrans*, and other "nonpathogenic" species, have been isolated from patients, including children, with human immunodeficiency virus (HIV) infection and acquired immunodeficiency syndrome (AIDS).[86-88] In most instances, infection has appeared to be asymptomatic, but serious and fatal disease has been reported.[89,90] There is speculation that *Mycoplasma* spp. may enhance the pathogenicity of HIV by a variety of mechanisms, but evidence is insufficient to prove that *Mycoplasma* spp. are more than opportunistic pathogens.

Human infections with *Mycoplasma* spp. that infect animals have been reported predominantly in immunocompromised patients[91] and in individuals in whom trauma and wound contamination have occurred.[1] Because these infections appear to be uncommon, routine attempts to recover *Mycoplasma* spp. are not warranted. However, in unusual circumstances, such as an immunocompromised patient with negative results on routine bacterial cultures or a patient with an infected wound after a seal bite, culture for *Mycoplasma* spp. should be considered. "Seal finger," an infection known to occur in seal hunters and wildlife workers, results from seal bites or from skinning or handling seals.[1,92,93] Several different species of marine mycoplasma found in mouths and respiratory tracts of seals are the presumed cause. Tetracyclines are considered first-line therapy for seal finger.

A number of illnesses including chronic fatigue syndrome, Gulf War syndrome, and fibromyalgia have been associated with positive results for one or more *Mycoplasma* spp. by PCR testing.[94,95] These associations should be considered speculative, at best. Additional studies in subjects with Gulf War syndrome have shown no such association.[96] Although such reports warrant further well-designed studies, PCR testing for *Mycoplasma* spp. should not be considered part of the clinical investigation for such patients.

198 Ureaplasma urealyticum

Samir S. Shah

MICROBIOLOGY

Members of the family Mycoplasmataceae are small pleomorphic bacteria, which characteristically lack a cell wall. Shapes range from filamentous to spherical, with diameters up to 0.8 μm. The genus *Ureaplasma* is biochemically unique in that all members possess urease and therefore hydrolyze urea to produce adenosine triphosphate. Ammonia also is produced, which increases the pH and limits growth in culture. *Ureaplasma urealyticum* was first described by Shepard in 1950; he noted minute colonies growing amid larger *Mycoplasma* colonies in specimens taken from the urethra and urine of men with nongonococcal urethritis.[1] These bacteria were initially called "T-strain" *Mycoplasma* because of their tiny colony size. The knowledge that urease was produced allowed their placement in a separate genus within the family Mycoplasmataceae and formed the basis of the name *Ureaplasma urealyticum*.

U. urealyticum, a human pathogen, historically has been divided into 14 serotypes. The serotypes are divided into two distinct biovars on the basis of biochemical and genetic features. Genetic study suggests that the two biovars may represent two separate species; *U. urealyticum* biovar 1 (*parvum* biovar or the proposed *Ureaplasma parvum*) includes serovars 1, 3, 6, and 14, and *U. urealyticum* biovar 2 is further divided into three subtypes. Subtype 1 includes serovars 2, 5, 8, and 9. Subtype 2 includes serovars 4, 10, 12, and 13, and subtype 3 includes serovars 7 and 11.[2] The entire genome of *U. urealyticum* has been sequenced.[3] It is the smallest sequenced prokaryotic genome, except for *Mycoplasma genitalium*, and consists of only 75 DNA kilobase pairs. At least 50% of the 652 identified genes have, as yet, unknown function. The description of the genome should lead to an improved understanding of the mechanism of disease caused by these elusive organisms.

EPIDEMIOLOGY

Ureaplasma spp. colonize the urogenital tract of healthy adults and adolescents. *Ureaplasma* spp. can be found on the mucosal surfaces of the cervix or vagina of 40% to 80% of asymptomatic women. Reported rates of asymptomatic urethral carriage of *U. urealyticum* among adult males typically range from 20% to 50%; however, most studies have assessed only sexually active men in the context of medical visits for urologic evaluation or sexually transmitted infection.[4-7] Urethral carriage was detected in only 8 (7%) of 114 asymptomatic male volunteers recruited from the hospital staff and from primary care practices.[8] Though colonization occurs less frequently among adolescents and young children, its presence is related to both sex and sexual activity. Foy et al. isolated *Ureaplasma* spp. from the urine of 1% of adolescent boys and 15% of adolescent girls;[9] girls who reported dating members of the opposite sex were more likely to be colonized. The organism was not recovered from any of 101 children younger than 13 years of age.[9] Approximately 50% of colonized mothers transmit the organisms to their infants.[10-12] Peripartum colonization occurs most often in infants born >1 hour following rupture of membranes[10] and in those weighing <1000 g.[11] Sites of infant colonization, in order of decreasing frequency, include the vagina, nasopharynx and throat, rectum, and conjunctiva.[10-12] Colonization persisted at 3 months of age in 37%, 68%, and 33% of infants with initial vaginal, throat, or conjunctival colonization, respectively, in one study.[12] Other studies have noted disappearance of peripartum colonization by 2 years of age.[13]

CLINICAL MANIFESTATIONS

A causal relationship between *U. urealyticum* and various clinical syndromes has been difficult to confirm. Studying these organisms poses a challenge given the relatively high frequency of asymptomatic carriage and the difficulty in collecting samples from normally sterile sites. Furthermore, many published studies have failed to adjust for potentially important confounding variables or were underpowered to detect significant associations. Nevertheless, *U. urealyticum* has been shown to cause urethritis. In pregnant women, it has been implicated as a cause of chorioamnionitis, spontaneous abortion, stillbirth, preterm delivery, and postpartum endometritis. *U. urealyticum* also has been associated with long-term sequelae such as chronic lung disease in preterm infants. Invasive infections also have been reported, predominantly in neonates and immunocompromised individuals. The reported association with infertility in adults is controversial.

Urethritis

Nongonococcal urethritis in men appears to be associated with biovar 2 but not biovar 1 (*U. parvum*).[14] Clinical symptoms do not distinguish *Ureaplasma* spp. infection from other causes of nongonococcal urethritis. Among men, biovar 2 has been isolated 2 to 3 times more frequently from men with nongonococcal urethritis than from asymptomatic men.[5,6,15] Among men with *U. urealyticum* detected in urine by 16S rRNA polymerase chain reaction (PCR), quantitative loads were significantly higher in men with urethritis compared with those without symptoms.[14] Coinfection with *U. urealyticum* also conferred a 3.6-fold greater odds of postgonococcal urethritis (urethritis that persists after successful eradication of laboratory-confirmed gonococcal infection).[16] Although young boys usually are not colonized, recurrent urethritis was attributed to *U. urealyticum* in a 7-year-old boy.[17]

Intrauterine and Neonatal Infection

Ureaplasma spp. infection is associated with fetal demise, chorioamnionitis, and postnatal complications. *Ureaplasma* spp. have been isolated from the placenta and fetus after spontaneous abortions in individual case reports.[18,19] *U. urealyticum* was isolated from the placenta more often in cases of spontaneous abortion, stillbirth, or neonatal death (31%) than in control liveborn infants (9%) in one study.[20] Several studies support the association between *U. urealyticum* and chorioamnionitis. In a case-control study, Abele-Horn et al. demonstrated a dose–response relationship between the density of vaginal colonization with *U. urealyticum* and clinical chorioamnionitis risk; chorioamnionitis was more likely in women with moderate (odds ratio (OR), 2.5; 95% confidence interval (CI), 1.0 to 5.9) or heavy (OR, 7.2; 95% CI, 3.3 to 15.5) vaginal colonization than in noncolonized women.[21] Histologic evidence of chorioamnionitis is present more frequently when *U. urealyticum* is isolated from either the amniotic fluid[22] or the newborn infant.[23] Colonization was detected in 18 (38%) of 48 infants whose placentas exhibited histologic evidence of chorioamnionitis and in 22 (19%) of 116 infants with normal placentas (P = 0.02).[23] While smaller studies have not shown a difference in the frequency of *U. urealyticum* isolation from the amniotic fluid of patients with or without chorioamnionitis,[24] a nonrandomized study of women colonized with *U. urealyticum* revealed significantly fewer midtrimester losses in the 35 women who received oral erythromycin (11%) compared with the 9 who were not treated (44%; P = 0.04).[25]

Isolation of *U. urealyticum* from the amniotic fluid but not from the lower vaginal tract appears to be associated with preterm delivery. *U. urealyticum* has been detected in the amniotic fluid of approximately 9% of patients in preterm labor and is associated with a higher risk of preterm delivery and adverse neonatal outcomes in this setting.[26-28] Cytokines elaborated in the amniotic fluid in response to the presence of microorganisms, including *U. urealyticum*, trigger prostaglandin synthesis, which may lead to uterine contractions and cervical dilation.[29] In contrast, Carey et al. prospectively evaluated 4934 women from five medical centers for vaginal colonization with *U. urealyticum* between 23 and 26 weeks' gestation and followed them to delivery.[30] Preterm delivery was not associated with *U. urealyticum* vaginal colonization after adjustment for medical and sociodemographic factors (OR, 1.0; 95% CI, 0.8 to 1.2).[30]

U. urealyticum also appears to have a causal role in chronic lung disease of prematurity, perhaps by stimulating the production of proinflammatory mediators, including neutrophils, tumor necrosis factor-α, and interleukin-8.[31,32] Animal models support this assertion. Rodent macrophage cell lines release nitric oxide in the presence of *U. urealyticum*.[33] Premature baboons artificially colonized with *U. urealyticum* develop classic hyaline membrane disease and necrotizing bronchiolitis.[34,35] In a meta-analysis conducted in 1995, the relative risk for the development of chronic lung disease in colonized neonates was 1.72 (95% CI, 1.50 to 1.96) compared with noncolonized neonates.[36] Many subsequent studies have addressed this issue[37-45] but comparison is complicated by differences in study design, study population, and method of identification of *Ureaplasma*. Waites et al. analyzed prospective studies that used requirement for supplemental oxygen at 28 days postnatal age (23 studies that included 2216 infants) or 36 weeks postmenstrual age (8 studies that included 751 infants) as outcome measures.[46] There was a significant association between *U. urealyticum* colonization of the lower respiratory tract and development of chronic lung disease in both groups. More recently, *U. parvum* was detected in tracheal secretions more than twice as often as *U. urealyticum*; there was no difference between infants harboring *U. parvum* versus *U. urealyticum* in development of chronic lung disease.[41] However, detection of both species simultaneously occurred more often in infants with than without chronic lung disease (17 versus 7 infants, respectively) (OR, 3.0; 95% CI, 1.2 to 7.7; P = 0.01).

U. urealyticum can cause invasive disease in the neonate. Individual cases of congenital pneumonia have been associated with *Ureaplasma* spp.[47] Cassell et al. demonstrated concomitant *U. urealyticum* bacteremia in 26% of preterm neonates with *U. urealyticum* isolated from endotracheal aspirates.[48] The clinical manifestations of infants with *U. urealyticum* isolated from cerebrospinal fluid (CSF) specimens range from subclinical infections with complete recovery to suppurative infections associated with long-term sequelae. In one study, *U. urealyticum* was isolated from the CSF of 8 (8%) of 100 infants undergoing lumbar puncture either for suspected meningitis or treatment of hydrocephalus;[49] some infants had the organisms isolated from multiple separate CSF specimens. The CSF white blood cell counts ranged from 0 to 5240 cells/mm[3].[49] Rao et al. reported a 3-week-old infant with brain abscess attributed to mixed infection with *U. urealyticum* and *Mycoplasma hominis*.[50] However, Valencia et al. describe a neonate with *Ureaplasma* isolated from CSF who remained well, even though specific therapy was not administered.[51] *U. urealyticum* was isolated from the CSF of a premature infant with intraventricular hemorrhage; CSF findings included an elevated protein concentration and low glucose concentration but no pleocytosis.[52] The prognosis and long-term neurodevelopmental outcomes of infants with CSF *Ureaplasma* spp. infections have not been studied.

OTHER INFECTIONS

Several reports suggest an etiologic role for *U. urealyticum* in several focal infections, including pneumonia,[53-58] arthritis,[59-61]

meningitis,[62] renal abscesses,[63,64] and postoperative mediastinitis.[65] Focal infections typically, though not exclusively, have been reported in immunocompromised patients. *U. urealyticum* has been recovered in cultures of respiratory tract secretions (usually in combination with other respiratory pathogens) obtained from both immunocompetent and immunocompromised infants with lower respiratory tract infections.[53,55-58] *U. urealyticum* was isolated from culture of bronchoalveolar lavage fluid in 3 children with cancer during a period of acute respiratory deterioration.[54] Pyogenic arthritis has occurred in patients with agammaglobulinemia with identification of *U. urealyticum* in blood[60] or joint fluid.[59] The organism was detected in the joint fluid by PCR in a patient with reactive polyarthritis.[61] Meningitis[62] and renal abscesses[63,64] have been described in adults following renal transplantation.

LABORATORY FINDINGS AND DIAGNOSIS

Ureaplasma spp. are fastidious. Body fluid specimens or material collected on calcium alginate or Dacron-tipped swabs should be inoculated at the bedside into special transport/growth medium, such as Shepard 10B broth, and then inoculated onto solid media as soon as possible. Freezing decreases viability, but if the sample must be held, freezing at −70°C is recommended. Inoculation onto A8 or a commercial solid medium that contains urea allows rapid growth, generally within 2 to 5 days. An indicator dye added to the medium to detect hydrolysis of urea permits early identification of *Ureaplasma* spp.

In culture, the organisms are ovoid in shape. On solid media, the organism shares the upside-down "fried egg" appearance typical of Mycoplasmataceae. They vary in size but are approximately 350 nm in diameter, too small to be seen with a light microscope. Growth can be detected in broth or on agar when specialized culture medium is used. Distinct small colony morphology (on appropriate media) and passage in selective broth allow culture identification, although serovar classification is more difficult and generally is not performed in clinical laboratories.

PCR offers a more practical approach to identifying *Ureaplasma* spp. Gene targets include the urease,[66] 16S rTNA,[67] and the multiple-banded antigen[68,69] genes. Amplification of the multiple-banded antigen gene allows biovar and, possibly, serovar identification.[2,68-70] PCR testing also has the advantage of not requiring specific growth media and time for culture. In addition, biovar and serovar information can be obtained easily. The disadvantage of PCR testing is that minute contamination can lead to false-positive results. A multiplex PCR for simultaneous detection of *U. urealyticum*, *Trichomonas vaginalis*, and *Mycoplasma hominis* has been described.[71] The sensitivity of multiplex PCR for detection of *U. urealyticum* was 96% compared with a gold standards of culture or one of several PCR assays.[71]

TREATMENT

There are no well-established breakpoints for determining susceptibility of *U. urealyticum* to any antibiotics. However, most *Ureaplasma* spp. have minimal inhibitory concentrations (MICs) for erythromycin in the range of 0.125 to 4 µg/mL, which suggests susceptibility. Resistant strains (MIC, 8 µg/mL) have been reported.[72] The MICs of azithromycin (range, 0.125 to 2 µg/mL) and clarithromycin (range, 0.06 to 2 µg/mL) are slightly lower compared with erythromycin.[73-76] MICs of doxycycline range from 0.016 to 1 µg/mL,[72,73] although acquisition of the *tet*M determinant mediates tetracycline resistance.[77,78] More than 90% of clinical isolates are susceptible to levofloxacin, moxifloxacin, ofloxacin, and chloramphenicol, whereas fewer than 50% are susceptible to ciprofloxacin or clindamycin.[73,74,76,79,80] Quinupristin/dalfopristin and telithromycin also appear to have adequate activity against *U. urealyticum* (MIC$_{90}$ < 0.25 µg/mL).[76] Although some *Ureaplasma* spp. isolates appear to be susceptible to aminoglycosides in vitro these agents do not have clinical efficacy. Since *Ureaplasma* spp. lack peptidoglycan, they are not affected by β-lactam agents or vancomycin.

Urethritis can be treated with azithromycin, doxycycline, or newer generation fluoroquinolones such as ofloxacin. In a randomized, double-blind multicenter trial, microbiological cure rates of *U. urealyticum* urethritis among men were 45% for those receiving azithromycin (1 g, single dose) and 47% for those receiving doxycycline (100 mg, twice daily for 7 days).[81] A subsequent randomized trial reported microbiologic eradication at 2 weeks post-diagnosis in 8 of 10 men treated with a single 1 g dose of azithromycin.[82] Women with >3 weeks of symptoms had higher rates of clinical cure and eradication after the administration of azithromycin at a dose of 500 mg daily for 6 days than after a single dose of 1 g.[83] Macrolides may be less effective than doxycycline in the acidic environment of the female genital tract.[76,84]

Making specific recommendations for treating invasive *Ureaplasma* spp. infections in neonates is difficult since the spectrum of disease in this population has not been elucidated fully. Furthermore, drug options are limited in this population, clinical studies of antibiotic efficacy are not available, conditions under which treatment should be offered are controversial, and the optimal duration of therapy, when prescribed, is not known. The proven ability of *U. urealyticum* to induce inflammation in the lung and CSF and their isolation from normally sterile sites including the blood and CSF justify specific therapy when the organisms are isolated from an affected site and when no other organisms are detected. Erythromycin (25 to 40 mg/kg/day in 4 divided doses) is the drug of choice for treating infections that do not involve the central nervous system. In older children, azithromycin is associated with less gastrointestinal discomfort and better compliance. Therapy generally is continued for 5

(azithromycin) or 10 days (erythromycin or clarithromycin). If therapy for central nervous system infection is considered, an agent with better penetration of the blood–brain barrier than erythromycin should be selected. In such cases, it may be prudent to document recovery of the organism from multiple CSF samples before initiating therapy with either macrolides or doxycycline. Rao et al. treated a neonate with a brain abscess attributed to *U. urealyticum* and *M. hominis* with a combination of doxycycline and erythromycin for 6 weeks; a doxycycline concentration of 1.0 μg/mL in ventricular fluid was documented using a dose of 4 mg/kg/day.[50]

Treatment of colonized neonates does not improve their outcome.[85] Chronic lung disease developed in 13 (38%) of 34 ventilated preterm infants receiving erythromycin intravenously for prophylaxis and in 11 (27%) of 41 untreated control infants (relative risk (RR), 1.4; 95% CI, 0.7 to 2.7).[86] Only 3 infants in the treatment group and 6 infants in the control group had *U. urealyticum* isolated from respiratory specimens; 1 colonized infant in each group developed chronic lung disease. Chronic lung disease developed in 9 (64%) of 14 colonized infants receiving erythromycin and in 10 (71%) of 14 colonized but untreated controls in one study (RR, 0.9; 95% CI, 0.5 to 1.5).[87] In another study no difference in respiratory status between *U. urealyticum* colonized and noncolonized extremely-low-birthweight infants was found; however, all infants with positive results of culture received erythromycin intravenously, precluding assessment of treatment efficacy.[88] There is also insufficient evidence to know whether giving antibiotics to women with *Ureaplasma* vaginal colonization will prevent preterm birth;[89] thus, such treatment is not recommended.

199 Kawasaki Disease

Anne H. Rowley

Kawasaki disease (KD) is the most common cause of acquired heart disease in children in the developed world.[1] The epidemiology and clinical features of the illness point to an infectious etiology, but the cause remains unknown. KD is a unique disorder, an acute vasculitis that occurs in previously healthy young children that can result in serious long-term coronary artery disease or death.[2] Approximately 25% of children with KD who are not treated with intravenously administered immune globulin (IGIV) develop coronary artery abnormalities.[3]

KD is named after Dr Tomisaku Kawasaki, who first recognized the clinical features of the illness in Japanese children in the 1960s.[4] By 1970, the coronary artery sequelae became apparent when some children who were recovering from KD suddenly died from coronary artery aneurysms with thrombosis and myocardial infarction. Before Dr Kawasaki's description of the clinical features of the illness, the disease was recognized only at autopsy and was termed *infantile periarteritis nodosa* by pathologists.[5] The illness is now recognized worldwide and affects children of all ethnic groups. Careful epidemiologic records developed by the Japanese Kawasaki Disease Research Committee indicate that over 240,000 cases were diagnosed in Japan by the year 2008.[6] The total number of cases diagnosed to date in the United States and other countries is uncertain. Symptomatic or fatal ischemic coronary artery disease in adolescents and young adults with angiographic characteristics highly suggestive of KD sequelae has been increasingly recognized by cardiologists.[7,8]

ETIOLOGY AND EPIDEMIOLOGY

KD is an illness of infants and young children. Approximately 80% of patients are under the age of 5 years.[6,9] Children older than 8 years account for only a small percentage of KD patients, and the diagnosis may be delayed in this age group.[10] Males are more commonly affected than females (3:2). Epidemics of KD have been observed in Japan and other countries, with a geographic wavelike spread of cases as the epidemic progresses.[11,12] The illness recurs in about 3% of Japanese children; the recurrence rate in the U.S. likely is lower.[6]

The annual incidence of KD in Japanese children is about 215 cases per 100,000 children <5 years of age.[6] Thus, approximately 1% of Japanese children develop KD by age 5 years. Asian children who live in non-Asian countries continue to experience high rates of KD. The attack rate of the illness in white children is 10-fold lower than in Asians, and African Americans appear to have an intermediate incidence. Attack rates can increase substantially during epidemics in all ethnic groups; a calculated annual attack rate during an outbreak of KD in the Rochester, NY area increased from about 10 to 180 cases per 100,000 children <5 years of age.[13]

Epidemiologic features strongly suggest a ubiquitous microbe as the causative agent. The rarity of KD in infants <3 months is compatible with protection from passive maternal antibody, and the virtual lack of KD in adults suggests widespread immunity. The presence of a winter-to-spring predominance of cases in temperate climates, epidemics of illness, and the wavelike spread of illness during outbreaks are all consistent with an infectious cause. Little evidence of person-to-person spread of KD exists. However, because most ubiquitous microbes result in asymptomatic infection in the majority of the population, person-to-person spread may be difficult to document without knowledge of the causative agent. In a study of Japanese children with KD, the risk of developing a second case in a family within 1 year after onset of the first case was significantly higher than the risk of KD for the general population of age-matched children. Moreover, more than half of the second cases in families developed within 10 days after the first case.[14] These findings suggest common exposure to an infectious agent in genetically predisposed individuals. Children with KD generally are healthy before the onset of illness and are not more likely than unaffected children to develop subsequent autoimmune disease or recurrent infections.

A variety of known infectious agents have been proposed to be causative agents of KD, but none has been associated consistently with the illness. This has led some investigators to propose multiple causes for KD. However, recent data in acute KD patients indicate that a single monoclonal antibody identifies cytoplasmic inclusion bodies in ciliated bronchial epithelium and other tissues, that the structures resemble protein/RNA aggregate inclusion bodies formed by viruses, and that viral-like particles are observed in close proximity to the inclusion bodies.[15-17] These findings increase the probability that KD results from infection with a single, unidentified respiratory viral agent.

PATHOLOGY

In acute KD, inflammatory cells including macrophages, monocytes, and CD8+ T lymphocytes as well as immunoglobulin IgA plasma cells infiltrate the vascular wall, particularly the coronary artery,[18-20] and selective nonvascular tissues.[21] This remarkable IgA immune response suggests a mucosal portal of entry of the etiologic agent.

The stimulus for inflammatory cell infiltration in tissues in acute KD patients is unclear. Possibilities include direct infection of tissues by the etiologic agent or an immune response to self, perhaps triggered by a mechanism of molecular mimicry. The former seems more likely because the inflammatory process resolves spontaneously within a few months after onset. The end result of inflammation in the coronary artery wall can be catastrophic for the patient. Elastin and collagen fibers in the vessel can be disrupted, and the wall loses its structural integrity. The weakened wall can balloon and form an aneurysm. Sluggish blood flow in these abnormal vessels encourages coronary thrombosis with resultant myocardial infarction. If the wall is severely weakened, it can rupture, causing sudden death. Myocarditis can be marked and can result in arrhythmia. Pericarditis resulting in pericardial effusion commonly occurs.

Marked immune activation in acute KD is manifest by upregulation of cytokines in the peripheral blood.[22,23] Although some investigators have proposed that cytokine activation in acute KD is the result of an etiologic agent that produces a superantigen, conventional antigens can give rise to cytokine activation.[24] More importantly, the hallmark of superantigen-mediated disease, paralysis of the adaptive immune response,[25] is not observed in acute KD. The detection of robust oligoclonal, antigen-driven immune responses in T lymphocytes[26] and IgM and IgA B lymphocytes[27,28] attest to intact adaptive immune responses in acute KD. Other immunologic findings include a decrease in CD8+ T lymphocytes in the peripheral blood[29,30] and elevation of all serum immunoglobulins in the subacute phase of illness.[31]

Although the inflammatory process gradually subsides within 2 to 3 months after onset in most cases, pathologic changes of severely affected arteries can persist over time.[32] In large aneurysms, myofibroblasts can proliferate at the site of damaged endothelium and lead to stenosis of the vessel, with the potential for myocardial ischemia and infarction.

CLINICAL MANIFESTATIONS

The clinical course of KD can be divided into three phases. The acute phase usually lasts 7 to 14 days and manifests as: fever; conjunctival injection without exudate; oral and pharyngeal redness, "strawberry tongue," and red, cracked, bleeding lips without oral ulcerations; swelling and erythema of the hands and feet; polymorphous rash; and cervical lymphadenopathy. These findings form the basis for the classic diagnostic criteria (Box 199-1), which require fever plus four of five of the above clinical features of illness. Young children are very irritable and often refuse to walk or bear weight during the acute phase. Marked tachycardia, resulting from myocarditis, is common. Although cervical lymphadenopathy is the least common of the five clinical features of KD, it can be the predominant symptom. Enlarged cervical lymph nodes in KD usually are tender to palpation, occasionally erythematous, and usually unilateral, with a diameter of >2 cm. In such cases, patients often are treated for bacterial adenitis, without success, and referred with that diagnosis.[33] Careful examinations, sometimes over days, reveal other clinical features supporting the diagnosis of KD. The rash in KD can be maculopapular, scarlatiniform, or erythema multiforme-like (Figure 199-1). Vesicles and bullae do not occur. Perineal accentuation of the rash occurs in two-thirds of patients.[34] Perineal involvement commonly is misdiagnosed as candidal diaper dermatitis; it also occurs in toilet-trained children. Associated features of the illness are described in Table 199-1.[3,35-50]

On rare occasion, patients with KD can present in shock, often resulting in a delay in diagnosis; these patients are more likely to have refractory KD and thus could be at higher risk of developing coronary artery abnormalities.[51,52]

In the subacute phase, fever, rash, and lymphadenopathy resolve, but conjunctival injection and irritability often persist. Periungual desquamation of the fingers and toes, arthritis, and thrombocytosis are characteristic of the subacute phase, which occurs from about day 10 to day 25 after the onset of fever. Beau lines (transverse grooves in the nails) can be observed in the late subacute stage. Temporary hair loss can occur. The convalescent phase begins when all clinical signs of illness have resolved and continues until the erythrocyte sedimentation rate (ESR) becomes normal, usually 6 to 8 weeks after the onset of illness. Prolonged fever and recurrence of fever after apparent resolution are associated with an increased risk of coronary artery sequelae.[53]

Incomplete KD is a particular challenge. Incomplete KD (preferred to "atypical" KD) refers to the *lack* of full diagnostic criteria for KD, *not* atypical or extra clinical findings. Worldwide, young children, often infants, with KD can have fever and fewer than four of the other five clinical features of the illness. Unfortunately, infants are at higher risk than older children for developing coronary artery abnormalities.[54] Patients with incomplete KD appear to have laboratory features similar to patients with classic presentations. The Committee on Rheumatic Fever, Endocarditis, and

---

BOX 199-1. Diagnostic Criteria for Kawasaki Disease

Fever persisting for at least 5 days[a]
Four of the following clinical findings:
- Bilateral conjunctival injection
- Erythema of the oropharynx, with fissuring of the lips and "strawberry tongue"
- Erythema and swelling of the hands and feet, with subsequent periungual desquamation
- Erythematous rash
- Cervical lymph node enlargement to >1.5 cm in diameter

Illness not explained by other known disease process

[a]The diagnosis of Kawasaki disease may be made by experienced physicians before the fifth day of fever.

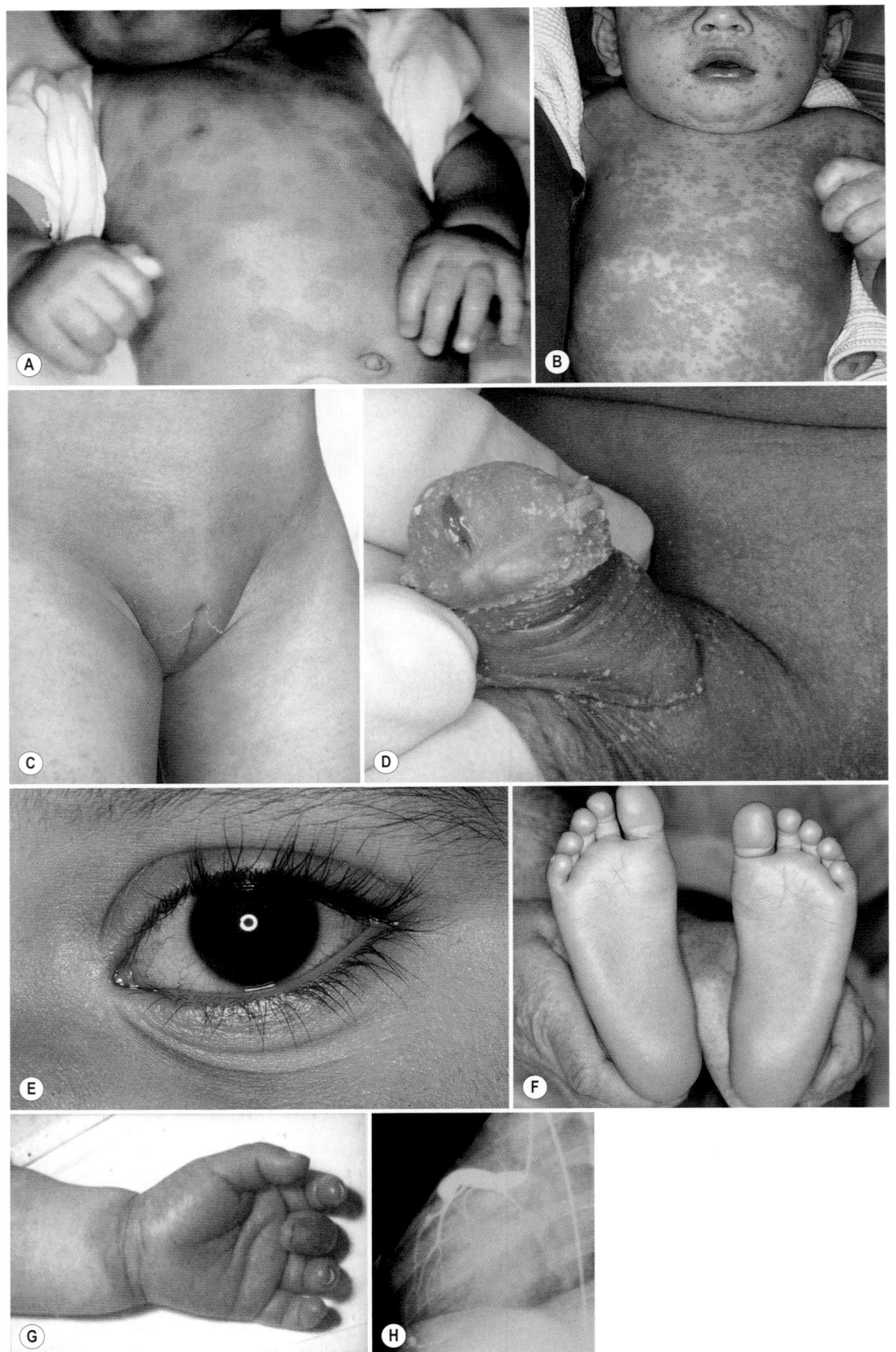

Figure 199-1. Clinical manifestations of Kawasaki disease. **(A)** Erythema multiforme-like rash and swollen hands. **(B)** Morbilliform rash. **(C)** Erythematous desquamating perineal rash. **(D)** Desquamating periurethral rash. **(E)** Bulbar conjunctival erythema. **(F)** Erythema and edema of feet (loss of plantar creases). **(G)** Glove-like distribution of erythema of hand with dusky finger. **(H)** Saccular aneurysm of the right coronary artery on day 8 of fever in 6-month-old-boy. (Courtesy of A.H. Rowley **(A)**, J.H. Brien© **(B–F)**, S.S. Long **(G, H)**.)

TABLE 199-1. Features of Kawasaki Disease

Feature	Incidence	References
CARDIOVASCULAR		
Coronary artery aneurysms	25% untreated; 4% IGIV treated	3, 35
Other systemic artery aneurysms	2%	36
Myocarditis	>50%	37
Pericarditis	25%	36
Valvular disease	1%	36
NEUROLOGIC		
Extreme irritability	>90% in infants; less common in older children	38
Aseptic meningitis	40%	39
Facial palsy	<1%	40
GASTROINTESTINAL		
Hepatitis	50%	41
Jaundice	<10%	41
Pancreatitis	Unknown; probably common but usually mild	42, 43
Gallbladder hydrops	10%	38
Diarrhea	25–50%	38
GENITOURINARY		
Urethritis	50–90%	44
Hydrocele	25–50%	45
MUSCULOSKELETAL		
Arthralgia and arthritis	33% untreated; 8% IGIV treated	46
RESPIRATORY		
Preceding respiratory illness	50–90%	13
Pneumonitis, radiologic but not clinical evidence	15%	47
OTHER FINDINGS		
Anterior uveitis	25–50%	48
Erythema and induration at BCG inoculation site	50%	49
Peripheral gangrene	<1%	50

BCG, bacille Calmette–Guérin; IGIV, immune globulin intravenous.

Kawasaki Disease of the American Heart Association published an algorithm incorporating clinical features, laboratory data, and echocardiographic findings to assist the clinician in decision-making regarding diagnosis and treatment for suspected incomplete KD.[55]

LABORATORY FINDINGS AND DIAGNOSIS

Certain laboratory findings in KD are characteristic, although none is diagnostic (Table 199-2).[35,38,39,41,44,46,54–56] Thrombocytosis occurs at a mean time of 2 weeks after onset and is therefore not useful in making a diagnosis in the acute stage, during which therapy should be instituted. IGIV therapy does not appear to prevent thrombocytosis.[55] The ESR usually is elevated markedly; values of ≥35 mm/hour, by the Wintrobe method, and ≥80 mm/hour, by the Westergren method, are common. The ESR can be artifactually low in the acute phase in a subset of KD patients; the C-reactive protein level in these children is very high.[57] A persistently elevated ESR for 4 to 6 weeks after fever onset is characteristic of KD in IGIV-treated and untreated patients; a transient increase in ESR can occur in IGIV-treated patients due to the effect of immune globulins on red blood cell sedimentation. Therefore, after administering IGIV, the C-reactive protein may be a more useful assay for monitoring inflammation in a persistently febrile child.

A baseline echocardiographic study should be obtained at diagnosis, 1 to 2 weeks later, and 6 to 8 weeks after fever onset. Additional studies may be unnecessary if all three of the studies are normal. If a patient demonstrates abnormalities on any of the three echocardiograms, additional studies are necessary.

KD can be difficult to differentiate from other febrile illnesses of childhood (Box 199-2). Measles and group A streptococcal or staphylococcal infections most closely resemble KD. In uncomplicated measles, the white blood cell count and sedimentation rate usually are low; a measles IgM antibody test can confirm the diagnosis. Occasionally, it is difficult to differentiate acute infection due to group A streptococcus from KD in a group A streptococcal carrier. Treatment with penicillin for 24 to 48 hours followed by clinical reassessment usually clarifies the diagnosis, because patients with KD do not respond to antibiotic therapy.

Although some of the clinical findings in KD are present in a variety of infectious and inflammatory diseases of childhood, certain clinical features strongly suggest KD as the diagnosis.[58] Conjunctival injection in KD is primarily bulbar and usually without exudate. Lip redness and swelling can be severe enough

TABLE 199-2. Characteristic Laboratory Findings in Kawasaki Disease

Finding	Incidence	Comment	References
Leukocytosis	All	≥15,000/mm³, or left shift	3, 35
Anemia[a]	50–90%	Normochromic, normocytic	53, 55, 56
Hypoalbuminemia[a]	10–50%		56
Elevated acute-phase reactants	>90%	ESR usually >35 mm/hour (Wintrobe), >80 mm/hour (Westergren)	3, 35
Sterile pyuria	50–90%	Can be intermittent	44
Proteinuria	<10%		38
Serum transaminase elevation	37%	Mean serum ALT of 100 U/L	40
Serum bilirubin elevation	13%		40
Arthritis	33% untreated	Cell count >25,000/mm³, predominantly neutrophils, in 80% of patients	46
	8% IGIV treated		
CSF pleocytosis	40%	Median cell count 20 cells/mm³ with 90% neutrophils, 10% mononuclear cells; glucose and protein levels usually normal	39
Thrombocytosis	>90%	In subacute phase, 500,000 to 2,000,000/mm³	35, 54

ALT, alanine aminotransferase; CSF, cerebrospinal fluid; ESR, erythrocyte sedimentation rate; IGIV, immune globulin intravenous.

[a]Severity correlates with risk of coronary artery disease.

BOX 199-2. Conditions That Share Clinical Features with Kawasaki Disease

- Measles
- Group A streptococcal infection (including scarlet fever)
- Toxic shock syndrome
- Stevens–Johnson syndrome
- Drug reactions
- Juvenile rheumatoid arthritis
- Adenovirus infection
- Leptospirosis
- Rocky Mountain spotted fever

to cause cracking and bleeding, and "strawberry tongue" is characteristic. Oral ulcerations and exudative pharyngitis are not features. Firm induration of the hands and feet with or without palmar and/or plantar erythema is distinctive and is rarely seen in other childhood febrile illnesses. Perineal accentuation of the rash without accentuation at other skin folds is common in KD but not in other disorders. Vesicles, bullae, petechiae, and purpura are not seen.

TREATMENT

Current therapy for KD during the acute phase of illness is aimed at reducing clinical symptoms, reducing inflammation in the myocardium and in the coronary artery wall (thus preventing coronary aneurysm formation), and preventing thrombosis by inhibiting platelet aggregation. Discovery of the cause of KD will allow more specific treatment.

IGIV was first used in Japan to successfully treat KD.[59] The mechanism of action of IGIV in KD is unknown. Subsequent multicenter studies in the U.S. confirmed the efficacy of IGIV with aspirin for KD; IGIV given within the first 10 days of illness hastens resolution of fever and a decrease in levels of acute-phase reactants and reduces the prevalence of coronary artery abnormalities from about 20% in aspirin-treated patients to about 5% in those treated with IGIV and aspirin.[3,35] Patients should be treated as early as possible after diagnosis; it is not necessary to wait until the fifth day of fever in patients who clearly have the disease. Data regarding treatment after the 10th day of illness are lacking; however, patients who remain febrile are likely to benefit from IGIV even after the 10th day. In patients who receive IGIV but nonetheless develop coronary aneurysms, there is a higher rate of resolution of aneurysms than in untreated patients.

The recommended dosage of IGIV is 2 g/kg, given as a single infusion over 10 to 12 hours.[35] Patients should also receive anti-inflammatory doses of aspirin, 80 to 100 mg/kg daily, given orally in divided doses every 6 hours; high doses are needed because of poor aspirin absorption and increased clearance in acute KD. The aspirin dose generally is reduced to 3 to 5 mg/kg daily, for antithrombotic effects, at the 14th day of illness, and when the patient has been afebrile for at least 48 hours. Low-dose aspirin therapy is discontinued 6 to 8 weeks after onset of disease if coronary artery disease is absent by echocardiography and if the ESR is normal. Aspirin therapy can be interrupted if the patient develops an illness suspected to be varicella or influenza to reduce the risk of Reye syndrome. In patients at particularly high risk for myocardial infarction, the use of an alternative antiplatelet agent should be considered.

The majority of KD patients have a dramatic response to IGIV; however, about 10% continue to be febrile 48 hours after completing the IGIV infusion. A second 2 g/kg dose of IGIV appears to be effective in most of these patients,[60–62] although a controlled study of retreatment has not been performed. Cases of apparent response to corticosteroid therapy after two doses of IGIV have been reported.[63,64] Pulse methylprednisolone therapy at 30 mg/kg daily for 1 to 3 days has been administered to such patients.[62,64]

Recently, IGIV-nonresponders have been treated with infliximab, a monoclonal antibody to tumor necrosis factor α, with apparent response.[65,66] Such reports are difficult to interpret, since the clinical features of acute KD are self-limited. Optimal treatment for IGIV nonresponders remains uncertain.

Corticosteroid therapy was commonly used as primary therapy to treat KD in Japan in the 1960s and 1970s; patients treated with this therapy appeared to have rates of coronary disease similar to those treated with aspirin alone.[67] An early Japanese study that demonstrated worsening of coronary artery disease in corticosteroid-treated patients has been criticized.[64,68] Potential complications of corticosteroid use in KD include prothrombotic effect and the possibility of interference with the host immune response to the causative agent of KD. A multicenter, randomized, double-blind, placebo-controlled clinical trial to determine whether addition of IV methylprednisolone to conventional therapy (IGIV and aspirin) improves outcomes for primary therapy of acute KD showed no benefit in coronary outcomes or fever days;[69] thus, corticosteroids are not indicated for primary therapy of acute KD.

In patients who develop persistent coronary artery abnormalities, long-term low-dose aspirin therapy at 3 to 5 mg/kg daily is indicated. Such therapy often is recommended for patients with coronary artery abnormalities that have resolved, as determined by echocardiography, because studies show that regressed aneurysms have impaired endothelial function and a thickened neointima.[70–73] KD patients with large aneurysms may benefit from warfarin therapy. Occasionally, acute thrombolytic therapy is needed in patients with thrombosis of large aneurysms; such decisions should be made in consultation with a pediatric cardiologist. Long-term management of coronary artery sequelae of KD has been summarized by the AHA Committee.[55] Rarely, patients with KD require intervention such as transluminal coronary angioplasty, transluminal coronary rotational ablation, coronary atherectomy or stent implantation,[74] coronary artery bypass surgery,[75] or heart transplantation.[76] Long-term prognosis depends on the severity of coronary artery disease; patients with giant aneurysms are most likely to require multiple catheter interventions or bypass procedures; long-term survival is likely to be shortened. Patients with less severe or no coronary artery disease may be at increased risk of atherosclerosis as adults, but data regarding the risk are lacking.

The routine administration of live-attenuated viral vaccines, such as measles, mumps, rubella and varicella vaccines, should be delayed 11 months after IGIV treatment for KD. Schedules for administration of other routine childhood vaccinations need not be interrupted.

SPECIAL CONSIDERATIONS

Coronary artery aneurysms form in the second to third week after the onset of illness, ranging from the 10th to the 25th day after fever begins. The development of aneurysms after the sixth week of illness is rare. Identifiable risk factors for the development of coronary disease have formed the basis for several clinical scoring systems; these risk factors include age <1 year, duration of fever longer than 16 days, recurrence of fever after an afebrile period of at least 48 hours, anemia, thrombocytopenia, and hypoalbuminemia.[53,55,56] However, such scoring systems do not predict with certainty which patients will develop coronary aneurysms, and selective treatment with IGIV on the basis of risk factors cannot be recommended. At 1 year after onset of KD, echocardiographic resolution of coronary aneurysms occurs in 50% of patients. However, intracoronary ultrasonography demonstrates that these vessels have persistent abnormalities, such as intimal thickening.[72,73] Patients with giant coronary artery aneurysms, which historically were defined by an internal diameter of at least 8 mm, but are more accurately defined as coronary artery diameter z-scores of ≥10, are at greatest risk of developing coronary thrombosis, stenosis, and myocardial infarction.[2,77]

Prevention of KD is not possible until the cause of the disorder is identified.

Key Points. Diagnosis and Management of Kawasaki Disease

EPIDEMIOLOGY

- Most patients 6 months to 5 years of age, but can occur in younger and older children
- Highest attack rate in Asian children, 1% of Japanese children develop KD by age 5
- Epidemics with a geographic wavelike spread
- Probably due to a ubiquitous infectious etiologic agent that results in KD in a small subset of genetically predisposed children

CLINICAL FEATURES

- Classic KD: fever for ≥5 days with four of the five other findings (see Box 199-1)
- Incomplete KD: prolonged fever with fewer than 4 of the 5 clinical findings, with compatible laboratory and echocardiographic findings and no other explanation for illness
- Most serious complication is coronary artery dilatation and aneurysm formation
- KD is a multisystem inflammatory disorder (see Table 199-1)

DIAGNOSIS

- Diagnosis is based on clinical criteria in classic KD
- Diagnosis of incomplete KD is based on clinical, laboratory, and echocardiographic findings

TREATMENT

- IGIV (2 g/kg) given over 10–12 hours with aspirin, 80–100 mg/kg/day divided every 6 hours
- Aspirin is reduced to 3–5 mg/kg/day as a single daily dose when the patient has been afebrile for at least 3 days, to be continued until acute-phase reactants and echocardiogram are normal at 6–8 weeks after onset of fever, or indefinitely if coronary artery abnormalities develop/persist

200 Chronic Fatigue Syndrome

Gary S. Marshall and Bryan D. Carter

Chronic fatigue syndrome (CFS) consists of profound, debilitating fatigue associated with subjective complaints and resulting in impaired daily functioning. Symptoms usually are abrupt in onset and persist for years. Interest in CFS increased in the 1980s with the description of patients with persistent fatigue and evidence of Epstein–Barr virus (EBV) infection,[1-4] as well a cluster of cases in Incline Village, Nevada.[5] The proposed connection with EBV led to the use of terms like "chronic mononucleosis" and "chronic EBV infection", terms that now are disfavored because a specific, universal causal relationship with EBV has not been established. Use of the term "myalgic encephalomyelitis" has persisted in Europe.

Skepticism about CFS as a distinct diagnosis has yielded to acceptance.[6] Clinicians usually have little difficulty suspecting the syndrome but may have great difficulty diagnosing by exclusion, sorting out comorbidities, and guiding patients through recovery.

CASE DEFINITION AND SUBGROUPS

A case definition that was formulated in 1994,[7] modified in 2003,[8] and validated in 2005[9] is still widely used in research. The key feature of CFS by this definition is unexplained, persistent or relapsing fatigue for ≥6 months that results in substantial reduction in previous activities (those with fatigue for 1 to 5 months are considered to have "chronic fatigue," not CFS). Certain medical and psychiatric conditions are considered permanent exclusions, and the concurrent occurrence of at least 4 symptoms is required. In practice, few adults who present with fatigue meet this case definition,[10-15] and making a diagnosis of CFS is complicated by overlap with other unexplained syndromes and comorbid conditions.[7,8,16-20] CFS in adults is a heterogeneous disorder.[9,21-23] A recent international study identified 5 distinct symptom domains: musculoskeletal pain/fatigue, neurocognitive difficulties, inflammation, sleep disturbance/fatigue, and mood disturbance.[24]

Genetically defined subgroups appear to correlate with particular symptom complexes (see below).

Published definitions of CFS are difficult to apply to children,[25-29] and none has been adopted universally. Most experts agree that ≥3 months of fatigue warrants investigation.[16,25-27,30] Profound fatigue in children also is heterogeneous, and only a subset of children have adult-like CFS. Factor analysis has identified distinct phenotypes in children, including sore throat, musculoskeletal, and migraine subtypes.[31]

EPIDEMIOLOGY

Separate studies in Wichita, Kansas and Chicago, Illinois estimated the prevalence of CFS among adults to be around 200 to 400 per 100,000.[32,33] In the most comprehensive study to date, random-digit dialing was used to identify cases (and controls) in Georgia.[34] A total of 19,381 respondents were screened for "unwellness," which is arguably more sensitive than screening for fatigue, and validated and standardized instruments were used to identify cases. Overall, the prevalence of CFS was a remarkable 2.5% and did not differ by geographic region. CFS was less prevalent among men in metropolitan areas (0.4%) than in rural areas (2.9%), such that in metropolitan areas the prevalence among women was 11 times higher than among men. Overall, there was no relationship with race, level of education, or income. Similar overall prevalence rates have been found in England[35] and Australia.[36]

Other studies have suggested higher rates of CFS among women than men.[32,33,37] Some have shown high rates in minority and lower socioeconomic groups;[32,33,37] overrepresentation of upper middle class individuals is suggested in other studies.[2-5,13,38-40] Although clusters of CFS have been reported,[41,42] there is no evidence of person-to-person transmission.

Fatigue is extremely common among adolescents,[43-45] and persistent fatigue is a common reason for referral to pediatric infectious diseases specialists (see also Chapter 15, Prolonged,

Recurrent, and Periodic Fever Syndromes).[46,47] Few children, however, meet case definitions for CFS.[43] The prevalence of CFS in Australian children was estimated at 48 per 100,000.[48] Studies in both the United States and United Kingdom suggest that CFS-like illness is very rare in children under 12 years of age.[49–51] Whereas the Wichita study identified no adolescents who met the 1994 case definition, CFS-like illness was seen in 338 per 100,000.[52] Gender was not correlated with CFS-like illness, although other population-based studies show a predominance of girls,[28,50,51] and girls are overrepresented in clinic populations.[46,47,53–57]

POTENTIAL ETIOLOGIC FACTORS

Infectious Agents

Onset after a distinct infectious mononucleosis (IM)- or flu-like illness, as well as reports of disease clusters, immunologic aberrations, and activation of antiviral pathways, suggest that CFS may be an infectious disease. However, no single infectious agent has been found to cause CFS. Table 200-1 lists some of the agents that have been investigated.[46,58–127] Organisms have come under suspicion because of their association with similar clinical syndromes, known biologic properties, or popularization in the lay press. Invariably, initial excitement has yielded to skepticism as more rigorous studies have been done.

A good example of this was the 2009 report suggesting that 67% of CFS patients were carriers of xenotropic murine leukemia virus-related virus (XMRV),[108] a rodent retrovirus associated with human prostate cancer. Three studies in Europe[109–111] and one in the U.S.[112] were unable to replicate the original findings. It is possible that XMRV infections are geographically circumspect (it is notable that the original study used specimens from the outbreak of CFS in Incline Village).[128] As of 2010, the issue remains unresolved.[129]

The complex relationship between infectious agents and CFS is illustrated by EBV. First, EBV-induced IM can result in fatigue for >6 months in over 20% of patients.[130,131] Second, all EBV infections are "chronic" in that the virus establishes lifelong latency. Initial serologic findings suggested that CFS patients had continued active EBV infection, but subsequent studies showed inconsistencies in serologic results, nonspecifically elevated antibodies to several viruses, and failure of virus detection to identify cases (see Table 200-1). Patients with true chronic active EBV infection have end-organ involvement and low levels of antibody to EBV nuclear antigen,[132] findings that are absent in CFS.

Third, a distinct, disabling persistent fatigue syndrome can follow a variety of acute infections.[133] In the case of EBV, postinfectious fatigue syndrome (PIFS) is not associated with increased viral load or lytic replication.[66] In addition, whether associated with EBV or other infectious agents, PIFS is not associated with increased cytokine production, a surprising finding given overlap between the physiologic effects of cytokines and symptoms of CFS.[134,135] Thus, some CFS patients may have PIFS "triggered" by EBV, but the condition is not specifically "driven" by the virus. The most consistent predictor of prolonged fatigue following IM is poor physical functioning at onset and during recovery, suggesting that the acute illness leads to deconditioning which leads to perpetuation of symptoms.[136]

Immunology

Patients with CFS do not manifest immunodeficiency in the classic sense, with recurrent or opportunistic infections. However, symptoms of the illness suggest viral infection, and reactivation of latent viruses suggests relaxation of immunologic surveillance; allergy symptoms are common and autoantibodies have been reported.[137,138]

As summarized in Table 200-2, no consensus has emerged from controlled immunologic studies.[13,39,114,135,139–178] Any proposed connection between laboratory abnormalities and clinical manifestations is complicated by interactions among psychological wellbeing, the neuroendocrine system, and immune function.

Cardiovascular Physiology

Some studies suggest an etiologic role for orthostatic intolerance in CFS,[179–182] whereas others provide less convincing evidence for altered autonomic function.[183,184] Many children and adolescents with CFS have orthostatic tachycardia associated with hypotension, acrocyanosis, and peripheral edema.[185,186] In a matched case-control study, 50% of 26 children and adolescents with CFS and 20% of controls had orthostatic intolerance demonstrated on tilt-table test.[187] Additional evidence of autonomic dysfunction comes from the demonstration of abnormal catecholaminergic-dependent thermoregulatory responses.[188]

In the Wichita surveillance study, tilt-table testing caused orthostatic instability in 30% of adult CFS subjects and 48% of non-fatigued controls.[189] These results were particularly powerful because subjects were drawn from the general population rather than tertiary center clinics. It seems unlikely that pre-existing orthostatic intolerance causes CFS; rather, the inciting event and ensuing decrease in activity may lead to deconditioning and orthostatic intolerance that is detectable in the laboratory.[187]

Connective Tissue Disease

Joint hypermobility was reported more frequently in children with CFS than in controls,[190] and Ehlers–Danlos syndrome has been diagnosed in adolescents with CFS.[191] However, a study of 32 adolescents with CFS and 167 controls failed to demonstrate evidence of constitutional laxity or differences in collagen metabolism.[192]

Hypothalamic-Pituitary-Adrenal (HPA) Axis

Some studies in adults with CFS suggest mild central adrenal insufficiency.[193–195] Whereas modest improvements have been seen

TABLE 200-1. Infectious Agents Investigated as a Chronic Fatigue Syndrome

Agent or Disease	Reason for Suspicion	Evidence Against Causation
HERPESVIRUSES		
Epstein–Barr virus	Causes mononucleosis	Serologic results inconsistent[5]
	Serologic pattern[1–4,58]	Serology does not distinguish cases[5,41,60–63]
	Lymphocyte transformation[59]	Virus detection does not distinguish cases[13,63,64]
		Genome detection in blood does not distinguish cases[65]
		Cellular viral load does not distinguish cases[66]
Cytomegalovirus	Causes mononucleosis	Serology does not distinguish cases[13,62]
	Elevated antibodies[5,67]	Genome detection in blood does not distinguish cases[63,65]
	IgM antibodies to nonstructural proteins[68]	
Herpes simplex virus	Viral persistence and reactivation	Serology does not distinguish cases[62]
		Genome detection in blood does not distinguish cases[65]

Continued

TABLE 200-1. Infectious Agents Investigated as a Chronic Fatigue Syndrome—cont'd

Agent or Disease	Reason for Suspicion	Evidence Against Causation
Human herpesvirus 6	Isolated from cases[40,69] Elevated antibodies[65,70] Genome detected in blood[71] Coinfection with human herpesvirus 7 detected[72]	Infection is almost universal[73,74] Serology does not distinguish cases[13,41,46,62,63,74] Genome detection in blood does not distinguish cases[63,65,74,75]
Human herpesvirus 7	Viral persistence and reactivation Coinfection with human herpesvirus 6 detected[72]	Genome detection in blood does not distinguish cases[63,65,71,74]
Human herpesvirus 8	Viral persistence and reactivation	Genome detection in blood does not distinguish cases[65,75]
Varicella-zoster virus	Viral persistence and reactivation	Serology does not distinguish cases[7,65]
OTHER VIRUSES		
Arboviruses	Central nervous system dysfunction	No serologic evidence[7]
BK virus	Nonspecific	Genome detection in blood does not distinguish cases[65]
Borna disease virus	Central nervous system dysfunction Genome detected in blood[76]	No serologic evidence[77,78] Gene transcripts not detected in blood[78]
Enteroviruses	Elevated antibodies[79,80] Circulating VP1 antigen[81] Genome in muscle or serum[82-85] Possible defective virus[86] VP1 and genome detected in gastric mucosa[87,88]	Serology does not distinguish cases[62,89,90] Circulating VP1 antigen does not distinguish cases[90,91] Genome detection in muscle does not distinguish cases[90] Genome detection in stool does not distinguish cases[90]
GB virus-C	Persistent viremia	Serology does not distinguish cases[93] Genome detection in blood does not distinguish cases[93]
Hepatitis B virus or vaccine	Canadian press reports	No epidemiologic or serologic evidence[62,94]
Hepatitis C virus	Chronic infection	No serologic evidence[62,95]
Inoue–Melnick virus	Central nervous system dysfunction	Serology does not distinguish cases[96]
JC virus	Nonspecific	Genome detection in blood does not distinguish cases[65]
Measles virus	Subacute sclerosing panencephalitis	Serology does not distinguish cases[62]
Parvovirus	Persistent fatigue and arthralgia after acute infection[97] Genome detected in gastrointestinal biopsies[98] Antibody to nonstructural protein[99]	Serology does not distinguish cases[62] Genome detection in blood does not distinguish cases[65,100]
Respiratory viruses	Flu-like illness precedes CFS	Serology does not distinguish cases[62]
Retroviruses	HTLV-II *gag* sequences[101] Electron microscopy[102]	Genome not detected[103-105] Epidemiologically implausible[103] No serologic evidence[41,62,103-106]
Rubella	Low-grade fever and arthralgia	Serology does not distinguish cases[62]
"Stealth" virus	Tissue culture isolation[107]	Findings not replicated
Xenotropic murine leukemia virus-related virus	Genome and virus detected in peripheral blood mononuclear cells[108]	Findings not replicated[109-112]
BACTERIA, FUNGI, AND PARASITES		
Bartonella henselae	Adenopathy	No serologic evidence[62]
Borrelia burgdorferi	Nonspecific symptoms	No serologic evidence[113,114]
Candida	The "yeast connection"[115]	No connection[62,117] Antifungal therapy ineffective[118]
Chlamydia	Persistent intracellular infection	No serologic evidence[62,119]
Ehrlichia	Intracellular infection	No serologic evidence[62]
Gram-negative enteric bacteria	Increased serum IgA against lipopolysaccharide[120]	
Gram-positive enteric bacteria	Increased D-lactic acid producing organisms[121]	
Mycoplasma	Genome detected in blood[122-124]	No serologic evidence[125] Genome not detected in blood[126]
Rickettsia	Intracellular infection	No serologic evidence[62]
Toxoplasma	Causes mononucleosis	Serology does not distinguish cases[13]
16S rDNA sequences	Broad-range amplification of bacterial sequences in plasma	No unique or predominant bacterial sequences in CFS patients[127]

CFS, chronic fatigue syndrome; HTLV-II, human T-lymphocyte leukemia/lymphoma type II virus.

TABLE 200-2. Findings of Controlled Studies of Immune Function in Chronic Fatigue Syndrome

Immune System Component	Study Findings[a]			Immune System Component	Study Findings[a]		
	Normal	Increased	Decreased		Normal	Increased	Decreased
T LYMPHOCYTES				**NATURAL KILLER CELLS**			
Number	139–146		147	Number	139, 140, 143, 145	148, 151, 163	141, 164
Helpers (CD4)	139, 141–144, 146, 148	13	140, 147	Activated cells (e.g., CD25, HLA-DR, CD69)	139	163	146
Activated helpers (e.g., CD25, HLA-DR)	139, 140	141	146	Function	149	13	148, 164
Suppressors (CD8)	13, 139–141, 143, 144, 146	148	142, 147	Intracellular perforin			165
Activated suppressors (e.g, 12, ICAM-1, HLA-DR)	140, 141, 144	139, 148, 149	146	L-Arginine enhancement of function			166
Naive T lymphocytes (CD4/CD45RA)	143		140, 148	**NEUTROPHILS**			
				Apoptosis		167	
Memory T lymphocytes (CD45RO)	143	140		**IMMUNOGLOBULINS**			
				IgG	141, 147, 149		168
Delayed-type hypersensitivity			142, 147, 150	IgA, IgM	141, 147, 149		
Mitogen response	13, 141, 145, 149, 151, 152		140, 142, 147, 148	IgG subclasses	110		147, 168
Antigen response	149, 152		141	**CIRCULATING CYTOKINES, CYTOKINE PRODUCTION, SOLUBLE RECEPTORS, AND OTHER INFLAMMATORY OR ANTIVIRAL MARKERS**			
Th2 responsiveness		153		IL-1α	144	39	
B LYMPHOCYTES				IL-1β	39, 114, 144, 151, 156, 169		
Number	139–141, 143–146, 148			IL-2	170	171	
In vitro antibody synthesis	151			IL-4	156, 172		
MONONUCLEAR CELLS				IL-6	39, 114, 151, 156	149, 169, 173	
IL-1 production	154, 155	151		IL-10	156		174
IL-1β production	156			TNF-α	114, 144, 151, 156, 170, 175	174, 176	
IL-2 production	151		13	TGF-β	114, 144	149, 151	
IL-4 production	156			IL-2R, soluble CD8	39		149
INF-γ production			148	IFN-α	170, 175	174	
IL-6 production	155,156	151	145, 157	IFN-γ	39, 149, 170, 175		172
IL-8 production	156			Neopterin	39, 175	173	
IL-10 production	155, 156			Cerebrospinal fluid IFN-α		175	
TGF-β production			151, 158	35 different cytokines, chemokines, and growth factors	135		
TNF-α production	155, 156	151	145, 157	CRP		177, 178	
Activation markers (e.g., HLA-DR, CD25, IL-2R)	139, 151	147					
Adhesion markers (e.g., LFA-1, ICAM-1)	139	141					
RNAse-L production	159	160–162					
PKR production	159						

ICAM, intercellular adhesion molecule; Ig, immunoglobulin; IFN, interferon; IL, interleukin; LFA, leukocyte function-associated antigen; PKR, RNA-regulated protein kinase; RNase L, ribonuclease latent; TGF, transforming growth factor; TNF, tumor necrosis factor.

[a]*Numbers refer to references. Studies were done with varying degrees of methodological rigor.*

with the use of low-dose hydrocortisone,[196,197] significant adrenal suppression probably outweighs the potential benefits.[196]

One can easily postulate connections between HPA axis abnormalities and both orthostatic intolerance and immune dysfunction. It is possible that HPA axis disturbance evolves over time and is related to factors like inactivity, sleep disturbance, psychiatric comorbidity, and stress.[198] One study, however, showed decreased salivary cortisol awakening responses in a population-based sample of CFS subjects who had experienced childhood trauma, suggesting that HPA axis disturbance in CFS may have its origins before symptoms are manifest.[199]

Neurobiology and Sleep

Parallels have been drawn between CFS and postpolio syndrome.[200,201] Of particular interest are reports of patients with CFS in whom punctate subcortical white matter hyperintensities were visualized on magnetic resonance imaging (MRI).[40,202,203] Some functional studies demonstrate alterations in regional cerebral blood flow and metabolic activity,[204–207] but others do not.[208] Whereas the significance of these findings is unclear, there is evidence of neuropsychological impairment in patients with CFS.[209,210] Other evidence for neurobiologic alterations includes sleep disturbance[211–214] and the possibility of a central mechanism for muscle fatiguability.[215,216] Metabolic defects in skeletal muscle also have been proposed.[217,218]

Genomics

Early studies in CFS patients suggested differential expression of genes involved in immunologic, neuronal, and mitochondrial function,[219,220] as well as dramatic differences in exercise-responsive genes.[221] The most extensive study published to date used a micro-array and subsequent quantitative polymerase chain reaction to examine gene expression in a total of 55 CFS patients and 75 controls.[222] Overall, 39,174 genes were probed; 85 were found to be upregulated and 3 downregulated. Seven distinct subtypes were seen based on the pattern of gene expression, and those subtypes were associated with different clinical phenotypes.[223] In a follow-up study that included 62 new CFS patients, there was evidence of subtype-specific relationships for EBV and enterovirus infection, consistent with the idea that these viruses can "trigger" CFS.[224]

Psychology

In a recent population-based study, 89% of adults with CFS had at least one lifetime psychiatric diagnosis.[225] Some studies suggest that psychiatric illness is more likely to precede the onset of CFS than to follow it.[226] Other studies show that the premorbid incidence of psychological disturbance in adults with CFS is similar to that in general medical populations,[227] and that the development of prolonged fatigue is not related to initial levels of psychological stress.[228] In addition, premorbid psychiatric disorders and psychological distress do not seem to predict prolonged fatigue following IM,[229–231] and gene expression patterns in CFS patients differ markedly from those with endogenous depression.[224]

Adolescents with CFS, however, report high levels of premorbid physical, psychological, and family problems,[232] and longitudinal studies suggest that depression and anxiety are risk factors for the development of chronic fatigue.[43–45] The psychological distress found in youth with CFS is not attributable solely to the stress of having a chronic illness.[233] Compared with peers who have routine medical problems[53] or are healthy,[47,234] youth with chronic fatigue demonstrate higher levels of depressive symptomatology. As many as three-fourths of pediatric patients with chronic fatigue meet diagnostic criteria for affective disorder.[47] Structured diagnostic interviews, however, can lead to overdiagnosis of psychiatric syndromes in these patients. Therefore, a multi-method assessment,

TABLE 200-3. Psychological Studies of Pediatric Chronic Fatigue Syndrome

Study	Subjects	Significant Findings in Cases
Smith et al. (1991)[53]	15 adolescents 205 adolescent controls 50 depressed controls	Depression criteria met in 5 but magnitude less than depressed controls; endorsed more secondary than primary depressive symptoms
Walford et al. (1993)[234]	12 children/adolescents 12 cystic fibrosis controls 12 healthy controls	Depression criteria met in 5; higher levels of fatigue, somatic symptoms, and depression than either control group
Carter et al. (1995)[47]	20 children/adolescents 20 healthy controls 20 depressed controls	One or more psychiatric diagnosis in 15; level of depression higher than healthy controls but lower than depressed controls; somatization higher than in both control groups
Carter et al. (1999)[233]	19 children/adolescents 19 healthy controls 19 juvenile rheumatoid arthritis controls	Physical and social impairment similar to juvenile rheumatoid arthritis controls but psychological distress higher
Garralda et al. (1999)[244]	25 children/adolescents 15 healthy controls	Reduced self-esteem and social competence; half of cases had clinical levels of anxiety and depression
Rangel et al. (2000)[245]	25 children/adolescents 15 healthy controls	Higher levels of conscientiousness, vulnerability, emotional lability, feelings of worthlessness, and symptoms associated with decreased social competence
van Middendorp et al. (2000)[232]	36 adolescent girls	High incidence of premorbid physical, psychological, and family problems; internalizing distress, internal locus of control, palliative coping strategies; normal self-esteem and social abilities
Smith et al. (2003)[238]	97 adolescents 179 migraine controls 32 healthy controls	High rates of school absenteeism, anxiety, and depression
Garralda et al. (2004)[239]	28 adolescents 30 juvenile rheumatoid arthritis controls 27 emotional disturbance controls	High rates of school impairment, illness worry; decreased problem-solving and coping strategies; resignation to nonattendance in academic and social situations
Richards et al. (2005)[246]	30 adolescents 30 inflammatory bowel disease (IBD) controls	50% scored in clinical range on emotional symptoms index, compared with 30% with IBD; subjects had more functional disability, school absences and favored rest over exercise in service of recovery
Richards et al. (2006)[236]	21 adolescents and their parents	Majority of subjects and parents endorsed belief in a unitary infectious cause of illness; many endorsed belief that recovery involves refraining from activity
van de Putte et al. (2007)[241]	40 adolescents 36 healthy controls	Higher scores on Identifing Feelings subscale of alexithymia measure, which correlated with scores on measures of depression and anxiety; only 30% fulfilled criteria for alexithymia

with data obtained from the child, parents, siblings, and teachers, is advisable for both research and clinical practice.

Compared with children who have primary affective disorders, children with chronic fatigue are much less likely to report primary symptoms of depression, including suicidal ideation and severe dysphoria. Symptoms are typified by multiple somatic complaints,[235] reduced physical and social activity,[234] and difficulty experiencing pleasure in activities formerly enjoyed.[47] Although adjustment appears to be normal for social abilities and self-esteem, adolescents with CFS experience diminished competence in such domains as athletics, recreational activities, and romantic involvement.[232] Unlike adults with CFS, adolescents seem to employ palliative coping strategies, such as distraction, escape, and optimism, as well as adoption of a more internal locus of control. In one investigation, the majority of adolescents attributed the cause of CFS to an infectious process and endorsed activity reduction and resting as their primary approach to symptom management.[236] In contrast, there are indications that children and adolescents with CFS who experience a more favorable outcome are those who see a relationship between psychological factors and illness manifestation and recovery, and those whose parents encourage participation in activities and have higher expectations about performance of responsibilities.[237]

School absenteeism and identification of school issues as illness disability-related are disproportionately higher among pediatric chronic fatigue patients than among children who have migraine[238] or juvenile rheumatoid arthritis.[239] CFS patients tend to be anxious, to worry more about illness, to internalize symptoms, and to exhibit particular coping strategies. One study found that parents' estimations of their child's IQ were higher for children with CFS than healthy controls, suggesting that stress associated with unrealistic expectations may play a role.[240]

Some adolescent CFS patients have difficulty identifying, labeling, and expressing affective states (something known as alexithymia), and this is associated with higher levels of affective disturbance.[241] Interestingly, mothers of adolescents with CFS exhibit fatigue and psychological symptoms similar to their children, suggesting the influence of both environmental and genetic variables.[242] Adolescent offspring of mothers with CFS manifest fatigue slightly more often than peers with unaffected mothers.[243]

Table 200-3 lists psychological studies of pediatric CFS.[47,53,232–234,236,238,239,241,244–246] Healthcare professionals should resist the temptation to align themselves with either the organic or the psychological "camp." Although frustration experienced by providers makes it inviting to ascribe CFS symptoms to psychological causes, transcendence of this mind–body dualism is crucial to effective treatment.

PATHOGENIC MODELS

It is unlikely that CFS is caused by a specific, persistent infectious agent. Rather, CFS may be the final common pathway of a variety of insults, including infection and stress, which cause activation and dysregulation of the immune system in genetically and/or psychologically susceptible hosts. Dysregulation may result in cytokine release, inflammation, and epiphenomena such as reactivation of latent viruses, all of which contribute to fatigue and associated symptoms;[247] deconditioning sustains and magnifies the problem. The PIFS model suggests that symptoms are triggered by an acute infection and are perpetuated in the absence of a sustained systemic inflammatory response.[133,134] Support for this model comes from the finding of gene expression pattern subtypes that are associated with infection.[223,224] The severity of the acute illness is predictive of PIFS; accordingly, the syndrome follows relatively severe infectious syndromes like IM,[133] Lyme disease,[248] dengue,[249] viral meningitis,[250] Ross River virus infection,[133] and Q fever,[133] but not minor upper respiratory infections.[251] Demographic or premorbid psychological factors do not seem to play a role.

CFS is not simply a psychological disorder. Rather, patients may enter a cycle of attribution and avoidant behaviors after an acute infectious or immunologic event associated with fatigue.[252] They attribute their symptoms to an external agent ("my virus") and retreat from an active lifestyle into a state of learned helplessness; self-esteem is preserved because the cause is perceived to be external and beyond control. Vulnerability genes, early life experiences, and comorbid conditions may play a role in magnifying stress responses and symptoms.[178] Of interest in this regard, early childhood trauma is associated with a 6-fold increased risk for CFS with neuroendocrine dysfunction, suggesting that in some patients CFS is a disorder of adaptation promoted by early environmental insults.[199] Avoidant behavior further reduces tolerance for physical activity, and re-exposure to activity elicits further symptomatic behavior. Repeated common viral illnesses perpetuate the cycle of symptoms, attribution, avoidance, fatigue, and withdrawal; immunologic and neuroendocrine abnormalities, which are epiphenomenal rather than primary, contribute to the symptom complex. In support of this model, both children and adults with CFS maintain strong convictions that the fatigue is physiologic, rejecting psychological explanations.[234,252] In addition, medical illness beliefs correlate with functional impairment.[253–256]

CLINICAL MANIFESTATIONS AND EVALUATION

The sentinel complaint is profound, debilitating, pervasive fatigue that dramatically interferes with normal activity. Fatigue begins suddenly and stands in marked contrast to the patient's previous wellbeing. Patients may complain that they simply "never recovered" from "that virus." Children often experience disruption in school attendance and extracurricular activities.[210,257,258] Accompanying complaints in adults[38,39,139,148,259–261] and children[47,53–55] are summarized in Table 200-4. Many are subjective and nonspecific, and sometimes they are odd (see Box 17-4). Symptoms are manifested to a pathologic degree and are continuous; objective confirmation is difficult.

TABLE 200-4. Symptoms Frequently Associated with Chronic Fatigue Syndrome[a]

Symptom	Percentage of Adults (*N*)	Percentage of Children and Adolescents (*N*)
Myalgia	89 (272)	31 (141)
Arthralgia	82 (272)	23 (141)
Prolonged post-exertional fatigue	76 (357)	(Infrequently reported)
Neuropsychiatric disturbance	74 (419)	29 (141)
Sleep disturbance	71 (419)	72 (83)
Fever	70 (272)	37 (141)
Headache	69 (419)	60 (141)
Muscle weakness	68 (392)	(Infrequently reported)
Sore throat	56 (419)	54 (141)
Abdominal pain	52 (147)	43 (141)
Lymphadenopathy/lymphodynia	52 (419)	32 (141)
Dizziness	44 (177)	28 (141)
Depressed mood	40 (177)	24 (93)
Nausea/vomiting	32 (177)	28 (141)

[a]*Data collated from the following references: Adults meeting criteria of U.S. Centers for Disease Control and Prevention (CDC) for chronic fatigue syndrome: Lane et al[38] (n = 60); Linde et al[39] (n = 35); Landay et al[139] (n = 147); Klimas et al[148] (n = 30); Straus et al[259] (n = 27); Peterson et al[260] (n = 28); Strayer et al[261] (n = 92). Pediatric studies (many patients did not meet CDC criteria): Carter et al[47] (n = 20); Smith et al[53] (n = 15); Feder et al[54] (n = 48); Krilov et al[55] (n = 58).*

TABLE 200-5. Case Series of Pediatric Chronic Fatigue[a]

Feature	Marshall[46]	Smith[53]	Feder[54]	Carter[47]	Krilov[55]	Bell[56]	Gill[57]
					Study		
Location	Philadelphia, PA	Seattle, WA	Farmington, CT	Louisville, KY	Long Island, NY	Lyndonville, NY	Sydney, Australia
Years of study	1986–1988	1991	1986–1990	1990–1992	1989–1994	1984–2000	1993–2001
Number	23 (14 girls)	15 (9 girls)	48 (35 girls)	20 (13 girls)	58 (41 girls)	35 (24 girls)	49 (33 girls)
Age (years)	4–17	13–17	7–21	8–19	7–21	5–18	14 (mean)
School absences	70% ≥2 weeks	4 weeks per 6 months	42% ≥9 weeks	55% ≥20 days	81% >20 days	37% ≥6 months[b]	23 days (median)[b]
Follow-up (years)[c]	1.4–3.3	1.1–2.7	2–6	1.5	1–4	13[b]	4.1 (mean)[b]
Improved (%)[c]	76	53	94	100	95	80[b]	56[b]

[a]Not all patients in each study met the 1994 U.S. Centers for Disease Control and Prevention (CDC) case definition of chronic fatigue syndrome.

[b]Patients meeting CDC case definition.

[c]Follow-up data were not available for every subject in each study.

The typical teenage patient referred for chronic fatigue is previously energetic, athletic, high achieving, and female. She is from an upper middle class suburban family and has been affected for many months, with exacerbations and remissions. Significant social, family, or interpersonal changes often predate the onset of illness. There may be a close relative with CFS. Some patients participate in usual activities but complain of exhaustion afterward, while others virtually are bedridden. Some patients are overcome by worry, distress, and frustration, while others are seemingly indifferent.

OUTCOME

The overall prognosis for adult patients is guarded.[253,262] In adolescents, fatigue per se is a relatively stable complaint;[43,44] most case series document a favorable prognosis (Table 200-5),[263] with rates of improvement ranging from 53% to 100% over a period of several years.[46,47,53–57] Relentless deterioration and the discovery of alternative diagnoses are rare.

MANAGEMENT

The following set of principles directs the approach to the patient with CFS (see also Box 17-5).

Acknowledgment

The patient's conviction that "something is wrong" should not be dismissed, even in the face of normal physical findings and laboratory test results. While a willingness to listen is crucial, the physician must be careful not to endorse unfounded pathogenic theories, because further psychological investment in such theories can increase the patient's helplessness, frustration, and isolation.

Medical Evaluation

A clinically useful guideline for diagnosis is summarized in Box 200-1.[30] The approach is similar for those who do and do not meet these criteria. The initial history, physical examination, and laboratory evaluation focus on discovering other causes for the patient's symptoms; clues to alternative diagnoses that can present with persistent fatigue are listed in Box 200-2.[30] The suggested laboratory workup listed in Box 200-3[7,30] should suffice to rule out most major underlying causes of persistent fatigue. While EBV serology has no diagnostic value in CFS per se, some children referred for fatigue are simply convalescing from recent EBV infection.[47] Other tests are considered only if specifically indicated; these might include antinuclear antibody, creatine kinase, immunoglobulins, lead level, serum cortisol, drug screening, skin tests for anergy, a tilt-table test, and serologic analysis for specific pathogens. Routine use of commercial testing packages that include, for example,

BOX 200-1. When to Suspect Chronic Fatigue Syndrome

FATIGUE WITH ALL OF THE FOLLOWING FEATURES
- New or of specific onset (i.e., not lifelong)
- Persistent and/or recurrent
- Not explained by other conditions
- Resulting in substantial reduction in activity level

AND AT LEAST ONE OF THE FOLLOWING SYMPTOMS
- Exacerbation of symptoms with physical or mental exertion[a]
- Cognitive dysfunction (e.g., difficulty thinking, inability to concentrate, impairment of short-term memory, difficulty with word-finding, planning or organizing thoughts, and information processing)[a]
- Difficulty sleeping (e.g., insomnia, hypersomnia, unrefreshing sleep, disturbed sleep–wake cycle)[a]
- Multifocal muscle and/or joint pain without evidence of inflammation[a]
- Headaches
- Painful lymph nodes without pathological enlargement
- Sore throat
- General malaise or "flu-like" symptoms
- Dizziness and/or nausea
- Palpitations without cardiac pathology

Adapted from reference 30.
[a]Absence of at least one of these symptoms calls the diagnosis into question.

immunophenotyping, is unwarranted.[7] The possibility of psychiatric morbidity should be addressed formally, but clinicians should anticipate resistance.

Quantification of symptoms (e.g., duration of illness, hours spent sleeping per day, changes in grades, weeks of school missed,

BOX 200-2. When to Suspect an Alternative Diagnosis Causing Fatigue

- Focal neurologic signs
- Signs and symptoms of inflammatory arthritis or connective tissue disease
- Signs and symptoms of cardiorespiratory disease
- Significant weight loss
- Sleep apnea
- Clinically significant lymphadenopathy

Adapted from reference 30.

BOX 200-3. Medical Laboratory Evaluation for Children with Chronic Fatigue

ROUTINELY PERFORMED TESTS

Test	Representative alternative diagnoses screened for
Complete blood count	Anemia, hematologic malignancy
Comprehensive metabolic panel	Electrolyte disturbance, diabetes, occult hepatopathy, renal insufficiency, eating disorder, adrenal insufficiency
Urinalysis	Chronic urinary tract infection, nephritis, nephrosis, diabetes
Thyroid-stimulating hormone and free thyroxine	Hypothyroidism
Erythrocyte sedimentation rate and C-reactive protein	Chronic infection, malignancy, auto-inflammatory or rheumatologic disorder
IgA anti-endomysial antibody or IgA anti-tissue transglutaminase antibody	Gluten-sensitive enteropathy
Creatine kinase	Myopathy, myositis
Serum ferritin	Iron deficiency anemia
Epstein–Barr virus serology panel	Infectious mononucleosis[a]

OTHER DIAGNOSES AND TESTS TO CONSIDER

Diagnosis	Representative test (indication)
Vitamin B_{12} or folic acid deficiency	Serum cobalamin and folate concentration (macrocytosis)
Chronic bacterial infection	*Brucella* serology (exposure history)
Human immunodeficiency virus infection	Human immunodeficiency virus serology (risk factors, lymphadenopathy, etc.)
Chronic viral hepatitis	Hepatitis B virus and hepatitis C virus serology (risk factors, transaminase elevation, etc.)
Latent viral infection	Epstein–Barr virus, cytomegalovirus, and *Toxoplasma gondii* serology (signs of reactivation disease)
Rheumatologic disease	Antinuclear antibody and rheumatoid factor (prominent joint complaints, acute-phase reaction, etc.)

TESTS THAT SHOULD NOT BE PERFORMED ROUTINELY

Head-up tilt-table test
Auditory brainstem responses
Electrodermal conductivity
Immunophenotyping

[a]Prolonged symptoms after acute Epstein–Barr virus-induced infectious mononucleosis are common among adolescents. Testing for IgG and IgM antibodies to the viral capsid antigen as well as IgG antibodies to the nuclear antigen can help to understand the time of onset and immunologic resolution of infection. Adapted from references 7 and 30, with modifications by the authors.

and time spent in social, sporting, or recreational activities) provides useful objective measurements for baseline assessment and follow-up. Documentation of illnesses or exposures preceding the onset of fatigue, provocative and palliative factors, occurrence of CFS in family members, and recent major psychosocial changes is sought. The patient's experience with healthcare providers and beliefs about diagnosis are elicited. The evaluation process helps solidify the doctor–patient relationship, assures the patient that the illness is being taken seriously, and protects the patient from unnecessary procedures.

For some patients, labeling the illness as CFS provides a sense of relief from diagnostic confusion. For others, adopting the CFS label leads to further withdrawal by focusing on illness rather than on rehabilitation.

Psychological Evaluation

A comprehensive psychological evaluation, including measures of cognitive function, depression, somatiform disorder, family dynamics, and neuropsychological functioning is warranted. Physicians can aid the family's acceptance of such intervention by pointing out that any chronic condition has psychological concomitants that play a role in coping and recovery. Psychological services should be an integrated part of assessment and treatment programs so as to minimize patient and family resistance to referral.

Medical Intervention

Controlled trials demonstrate benefit from graded exercise programs and cognitive behavior therapy (CBT).[264] Therapies with antiviral agents, immunoglobulin, psychoactive drugs, corticosteroids, dietary supplements, and complementary/alternative measures all have shown inconsistent results, although many studies show strong placebo effects. Therapies targeted at specific comorbidities may be useful, such as antidepressants for patients with concomitant depressive illness and sleep aids for patients with profound sleep disturbance. A host of unconventional therapies have been advocated in CFS, almost all of which have no theoretical basis for utility. Medical therapies should be undertaken or recommended only in the context of controlled clinical trials, and the physician has a responsibility to protect the patient from unproven therapies.

Psychological Intervention

Psychotherapeutic interventions are likely to be rejected by parents and patients unless they are integrated with medical care and physical therapies. The most success has come from CBT, which attempts to modify maladaptive thinking and attributional patterns in order to enhance feelings of self-efficacy and decrease activity avoidance. Improvement in adult CFS patients has been demonstrated.[252,265–267]

Supportive counseling combined with behavioral techniques and increased physical activity can benefit some children.[268] Success has been reported using a program focused on breaking the association between experiencing symptoms and stopping activity.[269] In a randomized trial, CBT was effective in reducing the severity of fatigue, improving physical functioning, and increasing school attendance.[270] Decreases in fatigue associated with CBT are associated with decreases in reported pain.[271] CBT was found to reduce self-reported cognitive impairment but did not improve performance on specific neuropsychological tests;[272] this suggests that distorted perception of cognitive processes may be more central to CFS than actual cognitive performance.

Multidimensional cognitive behavioral approaches show promise. In one such program,[273] patients and parents are educated in a holistic understanding of CFS that discourages adopting exclusively physical or psychological models of illness. Vicious cycles that exacerbate illness are explained, including nutrition, sleep patterns, physical deconditioning, social isolation, and loss of self-esteem; tailored gradual return to school and social activity are planned, and adaptive coping strategies are emphasized. Improvement in several areas of physical and emotional functioning have been seen.[274]

Some centers have adopted the multidisciplinary inpatient rehabilitation model employed by many pediatric chronic pain programs.[275] A 4-week inpatient program produced modest gains in volitional time to fatigue and peak oxygen uptake, moderate improvements in mood, and more substantial improvements in upper body strength and function,[276] although only 13% of patients reported improvement in fatigue severity. In a randomized controlled study of adolescents with CFS, family-focused CBT resulted in more rapid return to school, but at 6- and 12-month follow-up was no more effective than psycho-education alone.[277]

Reassurance

Patients should be reassured that the natural history of chronic fatigue in children is favorable, but they also should be prepared for lifestyle adjustments and periodic exacerbations.

Activity

Return to physical activity and schoolwork is an essential part of treatment. Excused absences from school must be time-limited and linked to gradual increases in activity and integration. There is no scientific evidence that such activity prolongs the course of the illness or leads to complications. Committing to gradual increases in activity and keeping formal records may engender feelings of self-efficacy and hopefulness. Clinical trials of graded exercise programs in adults have shown benefits.[278-281] A rehabilitative program for children and adolescents with CFS demonstrated improvements in wellness scores and school attendance compared with patients receiving supportive care alone.[282] However, a controlled study showed no benefits of hospitalization for physical therapy, graded exercise, and psychiatric evaluation.[57]

General Health Maintenance

Adequate nutrition and avoidance of harmful activities such as cigarette smoking and alcohol abuse are important. Immunizations are given on the standard schedule.

Follow-Up

Regular medical and psychological follow-up visits are an important part of treatment. A multidisciplinary team approach may be beneficial. Serial evaluations enable the physician to monitor for alternative, potentially treatable diagnoses and to repeat some laboratory tests as indicated. Follow-up visits allay the patient's fear of abandonment and provide reassurance through exacerbations until improvement occurs.

SECTION B: Viruses

201 Classification of Human Viruses

Robert David Siegel

The "viral family" concept is fundamentally important in understanding the biologic classification of viruses.[1] By specifying the family to which a virus belongs, a great deal may be inferred about the physical, chemical, and biological properties of that virus as well as its evolutionary relationships and modes of gene expression.[2] Viral families are designated with the suffix *-viridae*.[3] Families are distinguished largely on the basis of physiochemical properties, genome structure, size, morphology, and molecular processes.[4] Table 201-1 lists some criteria that are used to differentiate human virus families.

Twenty-four virus families have been implicated in human disease;[5] they are listed in Table 201-2. In some cases, humans serve as a reservoir for the viruses and the link to human disease is clear cut. In other cases, humans may be incidental hosts or the link to disease may be more tenuous. Table 201-3 lists specific viruses within each family that are linked to human disease.

Facilitated by advances in molecular methods, the discovery of new viruses and more careful characterization of known viruses[6,7] have resulted in frequent changes in family taxonomy. Some examples of such changes include: (1) de novo creation of a virus family (e.g., Anelloviridae);[8] (2) splitting a new family off of an existing one (e.g., Hepeviridae from Caliciviridae);[9] (3) dividing a family into two new families (e.g., Papovaviridae into Papillomaviridae and Polyomaviridae);[10] and (4) uniting formerly separate families (e.g., the incorporation of Toroviridae into Coronaviridae).[11,12] Working groups[13] within the International Committee on Taxonomy of Viruses (ICTV)[14] have the responsibility of approving new names and making changes in classification. Figures 201-1, 201-2, and 201-3 illustrate the relationships between human virus families in terms of key biologic criteria listed in Table 201-1.

Families hierarchically are subdivided in a variety of ways including into subfamilies (suffix *-virinae*), genera (suffix *-virus*), and species (suffix *-virus*).[15] In the past, the conventions for naming species were somewhat arbitrary and varied from family to family. The ICTV has instituted a more uniform system. A virus species, as defined by van Regenmortel, is "a polythetic class of viruses that constitutes a replicating lineage and occupies a particular ecologic niche."[16] *Polythetic* refers to the fact that viruses grouped within a species share many but not all properties in common. Species criteria may include genetic structure, sequence homology, host range, tissue tropism, biological reservoir, route of transmission, immunologic cross-reactivity, epidemiology, and pathogenicity.[17] With the advent of rapid nucleic acid sequencing, sequence homology has taken precedence over other species classification criteria.[18]

The current system of species classification does not always correspond to common usage or historical concepts of viral species. For example, the three immunologically distinct viruses targeted by the trivalent poliovirus vaccine are now considered to be the

TABLE 201-1. Major Criteria for Classifying Human Viral Families

Criterion	Basis of Classification
Type of genomic nucleic acid	DNA or RNA
Nucleic acid strandedness	ds, ss, partially ds
"Sense" of ss nucleic acid	+, −, − with ambisense
Capsid morphology	Icosahedral, helical, or complex
Envelope	Present or absent
Genome segmentation	Number of segments
Genomic structure	For example, type of RNA cap, location of structural genes or repeat sequences
Electron micrographic (EM) appearance	For example, bullet-shaped rhabdoviruses or star-shaped astroviruses
Size of virion and/or genome	For example, large genome DNA viruses like pox or herpesviruses versus small genome viruses like picornaviruses, parvoviruses, or hepadnaviruses
Nature of gene expression: (including nature and number of mRNA transcripts)	For example, use of genomic polyproteins (picornaviruses, flaviviruses); use of reverse transcriptase (retroviruses, hepadnaviruses); use of multiple 3′ nested genes (coronaviruses); use of RNA ambisense coding (arenaviruses, bunyaviruses)

ds, double stranded; ss, single stranded.

TABLE 201-2. Families of Viruses that Infect Humans[2]

Name	Derivation of Family Name	Genome	Segmentation	Capsid Morphology	Envelope
Adenoviridae	"Gland"	dsDNA	1	Icosahedral	Naked
Anelloviridae	"Ring-shaped"	ssDNA(−)[f]	1	Icosahedral	Naked
Arenaviridae	"Sand"	ssRNA(−)[g,h]	2	Helical	Enveloped
Astroviridae	"Star"	ssRNA(+)[i]	1	Icosahedral	Naked
Bornaviridae[a]	Location in Germany	ssRNA(−)[g]	1	Helical	Enveloped
Bunyaviridae	Location in Uganda	ssRNA(−)[g,h]	3	Helical	Enveloped
Caliciviridae	"Cup" or "chalice"	ssRNA(+)[i]	1	Icosahedral	Naked
Coronaviridae[b]	"Crown"	ssRNA(+)[i]	1	Helical	Enveloped
Filoviridae[a]	"Thread"	ssRNA(−)[g]	1	Helical	Enveloped
Flaviviridae	"Yellow"	ssRNA(+)[i]	1	Icosahedral	Enveloped
Hepadnaviridae	"Liver", DNA	Partially ssDNA	1	Icosahedral	Enveloped
Hepeviridae	"HEPatitis E"	ssRNA(+)[i]	1	Icosahedral	Naked
Herpesviridae[c]	"Creeping"	dsDNA	1	Icosahedral	Enveloped
Orthomyxoviridae	"True"; "slime or mucus"	ssRNA(−)[g]	6–8	Helical	Enveloped
Papillomaviridae	"Bumpy"; "tumor"	dsDNA	1	Icosahedral	Naked
Paramyxoviridae[a]	"Alongside"; "slime or mucus"	ssRNA(−)[g]	1	Helical	Enveloped
Parvoviridae	"Little"	ssDNA	1	Icosahedral	Naked
Picornaviridae[d]	"Little"; RNA	ssRNA(+)[i]	1	Icosahedral	Naked
Polyomaviridae	"Many"; "tumor"	dsDNA	1	Icosahedral	Naked
Poxviridae	"Pustule"	dsDNA	1	Complex	Variable
Reoviridae	Respiratory-enteric-orphan	dsRNA	10–12	Icosahedral	Naked
Retroviridae	"Backwards"	ssRNA(+)[i]	1 but diploid	Complex	Enveloped
Rhabdoviridae[a]	"Rod"	ssRNA(−)[g]	1	Helical	Enveloped
Togaviridae	"Cloak"	ssRNA(+)[i]	1	Icosahedral	Enveloped
(delta)[e]	"Fourth" hepatitis group	ssRNA(−)[g]	1	Icosahedral	Enveloped

[a]*Mononegavirales.*

[b]*Nidovirales.*

[c]*Herpesvirales.*

[d]*Picornavirales.*

[e]*"Floating genus" – This genus is not currently assigned to a viral family. It bears some similarities to viroid pathogens of plants.*

[f]*ssDNA(+) indicates the mRNA coding strand.*

[g]*ssRNA(−) indicates the complement of message sense strand.*

[h]*Some segments are ambisense.*

[i]*ssRNA(+) indicates message sense strand.*

TABLE 201-3. Human Viral Infections Listed by Family[a]

Name	Representative Viruses[b]
Adenoviridae	Human adenovirus types 1 to 57 in seven species (human adenovirus species A to G)[22a]
Anelloviridae[8]	TT (transfusion-transmitted or Torque-Teno) virus[c]
Arenaviridae	Lassa virus, lymphocytic choriomeningitis virus, Junin virus, Machupo virus, Guanarito virus, Sabiá virus, Whitewater Arroyo virus,[23] Chapare virus[24]
Astroviridae	Human astroviruses – eight serotypes
Bornaviridae	Borna disease virus (BDV)
Bunyaviridae	California encephalitis virus, Sin Nombre virus, La Crosse virus, Hantaan virus, Muerto Canyon virus, Crimean–Congo hemorrhagic fever virus, Sandfly fever viruses, Rift Valley fever virus, and many others
Caliciviridae	Norwalk and Norwalk-like viruses, Sapporo and Sapporo-like viruses
Coronaviridae	SARS coronavirus, Human coronaviruses OC43,[24a] 229E, NL63,[25] and HKU1;[26] human torovirus and other human enteric coronaviruses
Filoviridae	Ebola viruses (e.g. Ebola Zaire), Marburg virus
Flaviviridae	Genus Alphavirus: dengue virus, yellow fever virus, Japanese encephalitis virus, West Nile virus, Murray Valley encephalitis virus, Kyasanur encephalitis virus, tick-borne encephalitis virus, Zika virus, and others Genus Hepacivirus: hepatitis C virus (HCV) Genus Pegivirus:[d] GB virus-C[c] (GBV-C, formerly hepatitis G virus or HGV)[26a]
Hepadnaviridae	Hepatitis B virus (HBV)
Hepeviridae[9]	Hepatitis E virus (HEV)
Herpesviridae	Herpes simplex virus type 1, herpes simplex virus type 2, varicella-zoster virus, cytomegalovirus, Epstein–Barr virus, human herpesvirus 6, human herpesvirus 7, human herpesvirus 8 (Kaposi sarcoma-associated herpesvirus), herpes simian B virus
Orthomyxoviridae	Influenza A virus (e.g. subtype H1N1), influenza B virus, influenza C virus, Thogoto virus, Dhori virus[26b]
Papillomaviridae	Human papilloma virus – more than 150 types of varying oncogenicity[26c]
Paramyxoviridae	Measles (rubeola) virus, mumps virus, respiratory syncytial virus, parainfluenza viruses, human metapneumoviruses, Hendra virus, Nipah virus, Menangle virus[27]
Parvoviridae	Human parvovirus B-19, human bocavirus,[28] adeno-associated viruses[c,e]
Picornaviridae[28a]	Genus Enterovirus: human rhinoviruses (more than 100 serotypes), enteroviruses (including poliovirus 1–3, coxsackie A and B viruses, echoviruses, other human enteroviruses) Genus Hepatovirus: hepatitis A virus (HAV) Genus Parechovirus: human parechoviruses Genus Kobuvirus: Aichi virus Genus Cosavirus: human cosaviruses[29] Genus Cardiovirus: Vilyuisk humanencephalomyelitis virus, Saffold viruses[30] Genus Salivirus: human klassevirus,[31] salivirus A Genus Senecavirus: Seneca Valley virus[f] Unassigned: Syr-Darya Valley fever virus
Polyomaviridae	JC virus, BK virus, KI virus, WU virus, Merkel cell polyomavirus, lymphotropic polyomavirus, human polyomavirus 6, human polyomavirus 7, trichodysplasia spinulosa-associated polyomavirus, human polyomavirus 9[32,32a]
Poxviridae	Molluscum contagiosum virus, variola (smallpox) virus, monkeypox virus, vaccinia virus, orf virus, pseudocowpox virus, Tanapox virus, Yaba monkey tumor virus[32b]
Reoviridae	Human rotavirus, Colorado tick fever virus, human reovirus,[c] Kemerovo virus
Retroviridae	Human immunodeficiency viruses 1 and 2, human T-lymphocyte lymphotropic viruses,[33] xenotropic murine leukemia virus-related virus,[g] human endogenous retroviruses (HERVs), simian foamy virus
Rhabdoviridae	Rabies virus, vesicular stomatitis virus
Togaviridae	Rubella virus; eastern equine, western equine, and Venezuelan equine encephalitis viruses; Ross River, Sindbis, and Semliki Forest viruses
(Delta)[h]	Hepatitis delta virus[e] (HDV)

[a]Examples listed correspond to common usage and do not necessarily comply with the official ICTV designations of virus species.

[b]Some zoonoses are included.

[c]Orphan virus for which a link to human disease has not been determined.

[d]Proposed genus name.

[e]Satellite virus requiring coinfection with heterologous virus for replication.

[f]Porcine virus being used clinically in humans as an oncolytic agent.[34]

[g]Possible laboratory contaminant.

[h]"Floating genus", See Table 201-2.

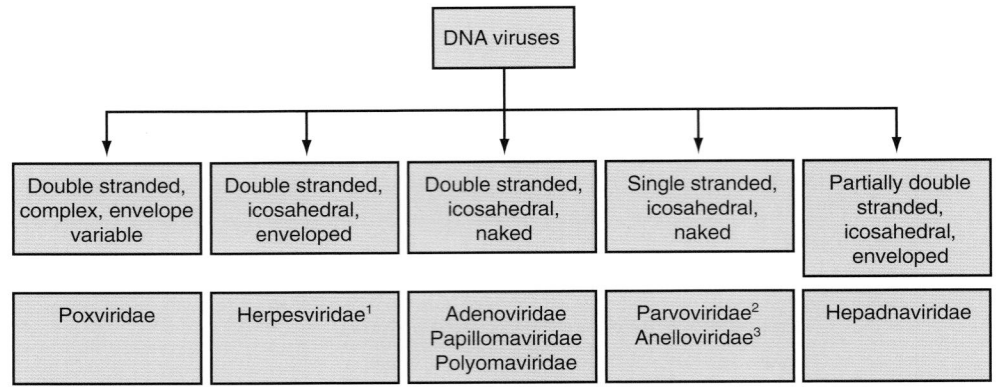

Figure 201-1. Organizational chart of the eight human virus families with DNA genomes. The chart groups virus families using the strandedness of the viral genome, the structure of the capsid, and the presence or absence of an envelope. All of these viruses are nonsegmented. Like retroviruses, hepadnaviruses contain reverse transcriptase.

[1]This family of viruses has been assigned to the Herpesvirales order of viruses.

[2]Parvoviruses vary in the percentage of positive and negative sense ssDNA genomes that are packaged, depending on the genus.

[3]Anelloviruses package negative sense ssDNA genomes. This is the strand that will be transcribed into mRNA.

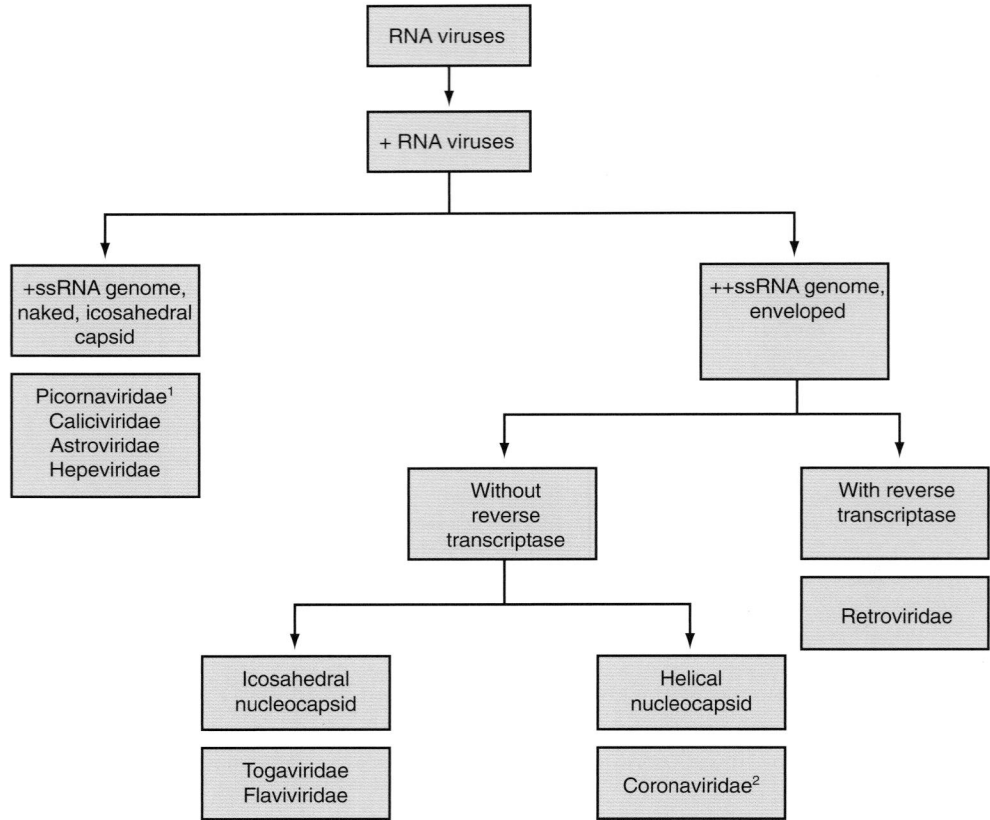

Figure 201-2. Organizational chart of the eight human virus families with positive-sense RNA (mRNA-like) genomes. The chart groups virus families using the presence or absence of an envelope, the presence of reverse transcriptase, and the structure of the capsid. All of these viruses have a single-stranded, nonsegmented viral genome.

[1]This family of viruses has been assigned to the Picornavirales order of viruses.

[2]This family of viruses has been assigned to the Nidovirales order of viruses.

same species: human enterovirus C.[19,20] This species includes at least 18 additional serotypes with diverse clinical presentations.[20a] The practicality of distinguishing such serotypes is emphasized by the eradication of wild poliovirus type 2 in 2000.[21]

Species can be subdivided further into groups, clades, types, subtypes, serotypes, variants, and isolates – depending on the family involved and the degree of similarity. Selected representatives called "type viruses" may be used to illustrate the properties of a particular taxon.

A number of virus families now are assigned to higher level "orders" designated with the suffix *-virales*. Examples are Herpesvirales, Mononegavirales, Picornavirales, and Nidovirales.[22] These are indicated by footnotes in Table 201-2. Most families currently are unassigned to orders.

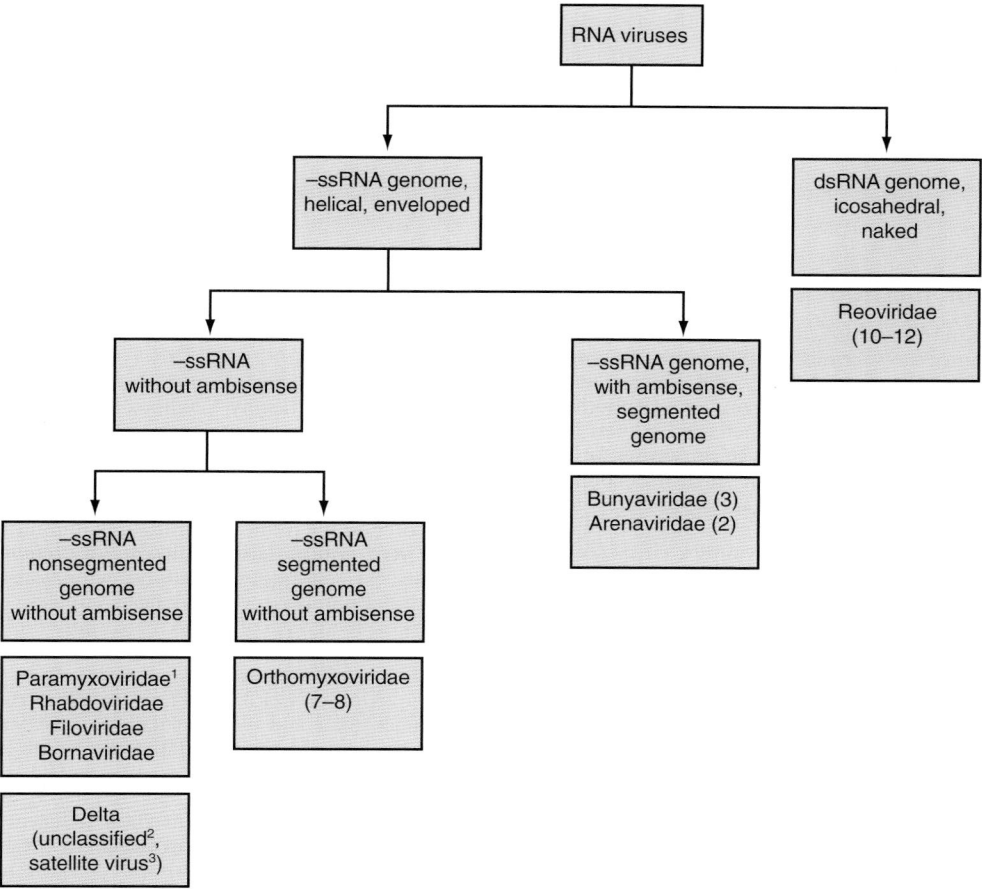

Figure 201-3. Organizational chart of the remaining eight human RNA virus families including the negative singled-stranded (complementary to message sense) and double-stranded RNA viruses. The chart groups the families using the structure of the genome, presence or absence of an envelope, and the presence or absence of ambisense gene expression. For segmented viruses, the number of genome segments is listed in parentheses.
[1]This group of virus families is assigned to the Mononegavirales (for monosegmented, negative stranded, order of viruses) order of viruses.
[2]"Floating genus" – This genus is not currently assigned to a viral family. It bears some similarities to viroid pathogens of plants.
[3]Satellite virus refers to the fact that hepatitis D virus (HDV) is dependent upon HBV, a genomically unrelated virus for its successful replication.

BOX 201-1. Common Routes of Viral Transmission to Humans

- Respiratory (droplet, aerosol, respiratory secretions on the hands and elsewhere, oral exchange): e.g., influenza virus, varicella-zoster virus, human rhinovirus, human adenovirus, respiratory syncytial virus, parainfluenza virus, metapneumovirus
- Fecal–oral: e.g., polioviruses, Coxsackie viruses, hepatitis A virus, rotavirus, astrovirus, Norwalk virus
- Direct contact: e.g., human papillomavirus (HPV), molluscum contagiosum, HSV-1
- Sexual: e.g., HIV-1, HTLV-1, HBV, HPV 16 &18, HSV-2
- Urine-associated: e.g., CMV
- Parenteral (blood and blood products, transplantation, tattooing, and scarification): e.g., HIV-1, HBV, HCV
- Animal bite: e.g., rabies virus
- Vertical (germline, intrauterine, perinatal, human milk): e.g. HIV-1, HTLV-1, germline transmission of endogenous retroviruses

- Arthropod-borne (mosquitos, ticks, sandflies): e.g., Japanese encephalitis virus, West Nile virus, dengue virus, yellow fever virus, and many others
- Rodent-associated: e.g., lassa fever virus, sin nombre and other hanta viruses
- Bat-associated transmission: e.g., rabies virus, Nipah virus, Ebola virus, SARS CoV
- Monkey associated: e.g., herpes B virus, monkeypox virus, orf virus
- Other zoonotic associations (cows, sheep, etc.): e.g., orf virus, cowpox virus

---

In addition to biologic classification, viruses often are categorized according to their clinical presentation (syndromic classification), epidemiology, or mode of transmission. Box 201-1 lists the major routes of transmission in humans, with representative examples of viruses transmitted by each route.

Understanding viral classification can lead to important generalizations regarding the prevention and treatment of viral infection as well as insights into the distribution and evolution of viruses.

Acknowledgments

I wish to acknowledge the invaluable contributions of David Mitchell and Charles Prober.

202 Poxviridae

Zack S. Moore

DESCRIPTION OF PATHOGEN

Since the eradication of smallpox, the only remaining poxviruses of clinical significance are vaccinia (the virus used for smallpox vaccination), molluscum contagiosum, and several relatively uncommon zoonotic viruses. In recent years, concern about smallpox as a bioterrorist weapon has led to renewed interest in poxvirus research. At the same time, interest in poxviruses as vaccine vectors and potential immunotherapeutic agents has contributed to a rapid expansion of knowledge regarding poxvirus genetics and pathogenesis.

Poxviruses are the largest and most complex viruses infecting humans. Virions range from 220 to 450 nm in length and have a characteristic brick-shaped appearance on electron microscopy (except the ovoid parapoxviruses).[1] The genome consists of linear double-stranded DNA ranging from 130 to 300 kbp. Four genera within subfamily Chordopoxvirinae contain recognized human pathogens (Table 202-1).

Poxviruses share several features. All poxviruses replicate in the cytoplasm, and therefore encode for the proteins necessary for replication.[2] In addition, poxviruses are notable for their ability to evade or subvert the host immune system. Several poxviruses encode for proteins that either mimic or inhibit mediators of the host inflammatory response.[3–5] Poxviruses exhibit varying degrees of tropism for host species and cell types through mechanisms that are not understood fully.[6,7]

VARIOLA AND VACCINIA

Epidemiology

Variola, the virus causing smallpox, was among the most feared viruses in human history. Smallpox has had a tremendous impact on human civilizations throughout history. Significant milestones are listed in Box 202-1. Currently, smallpox is primarily of concern as a potential weapon of bioterrorism.

Smallpox is a strictly human disease. The lack of an animal reservoir and the induction of lifelong immunity following infection were critical factors allowing for eradication. Smallpox spreads via respiratory secretions, with transmission generally resulting from close or prolonged contact. In pre-eradication studies, 37% to 88% of unvaccinated household members developed smallpox after contact with a known case, compared with 90% for measles or pertussis.[1,8–10]

Acquisition of variola infection usually occurs via the respiratory tract. Skin and eye inoculation and transplacental spread also have been documented.[1] The incubation period averages 10 to 14 days with a range of 7 to 19 days.[1,11,12] During incubation the virus replicates in the upper respiratory tract, then reaches the reticuloendothelial system via a transient primary viremia. Respiratory viral shedding and infectivity are highest during the febrile prodrome, which corresponds to a massive secondary viremia.

TABLE 202-1. Poxvirus Diseases of Humans

Genus and Species	Clinical Syndrome	Lesion Type	Frequency	Geography	Animal Hosts
ORTHOPOXVIRUS					
Variola virus	Febrile rash illness (smallpox)	Vesicopustular	Eradicated	Laboratory only	None
Monkeypox virus	Febrile rash illness (monkeypox)	Vesicopustular	Rare	West-central Africa, United States[a]	Rodent, monkey
Vaccinia virus	Localized skin lesions	Vesicopustular	Rare	Worldwide	Indian milking buffalo, cattle
Cowpox virus	Localized skin lesions (cowpox)	Vesicopustular	Rare	Eurasia	Rodent, cat, cow, others
MOLLUSCIPOXVIRUS					
Molluscum contagiosum	Multiple skin lesions	Epidermal hyperplasia	Common	Worldwide	None
PARAPOXVIRUS					
Orf virus	Localized skin lesions (orf, ecthyma contagiosum)	Proliferative	Rare	Worldwide	Sheep, goat
Paravaccinia virus	Localized skin lesions (milker's nodules, pseudocowpox)	Proliferative	Rare	Worldwide	Dairy cow
Bovine papular stomatitis virus	Localized skin lesions	Proliferative	Rare	Worldwide	Calves, beef cattle
Deerpox, sealpox viruses	Localized skin lesions	Proliferative	Rare	Variable	Various
YATAPOXVIRUS					
Tanapox virus	Localized skin lesions	Skin thickening	Rare	East-central Africa	Monkey
Yaba-like disease virus of monkeys, Yaba monkey tumor virus	Localized skin lesions	Skin thickening	Rare	West Africa	Monkey

[a]*Single outbreak in Midwestern United States, 2003.*

Vaccinia is the virus used for smallpox vaccination. Its origins are unclear; phylogenetic analysis indicates that it was not recently derived from either variola or cowpox.[2] Eradication of smallpox using the smallpox vaccine is among the greatest achievements in public health; significant milestones are listed in Box 202-2.

Vaccinia has a broader host range than most poxviruses, which has allowed it to be used as a model for smallpox infection in laboratory animals. Certain strains have become endemic in domesticated animals, resulting in occasional zoonotic transmission.[13-16] These infections are generally localized and self-limited.

Clinical Manifestations

Smallpox begins abruptly with a prostrating febrile prodrome characterized by high fever, chills, headache, backache, vomiting, and severe abdominal pain. In "ordinary type" smallpox, the first lesions appear in the oropharynx 1 to 4 days after the onset of fever. Skin lesions develop first on the face or forearms, and then spread to the rest of the body. The highest concentration of lesions is on the face and distal extremities. The palms and soles are commonly involved. Lesions develop slowly from macules to papules to vesicles to pustules, with each stage lasting approximately 2 days. Lesions on any one part of the body are characteristically in the same stage of development at any given time. Crusting of lesions is usually complete within 2 to 3 weeks following onset of rash.[1]

Variola major produced several distinct clinical syndromes and had an overall mortality rate of ~30%,[11,17] although mortality was higher in very young children.[1] Approximately 90% of cases in the largest series were "ordinary type" smallpox, characterized by round, firm, well-circumscribed pustules 7 to 10 mm in diameter.[17] The mortality rate was approximately 10% for patients with discrete lesions and 60% for patients with confluent lesions.[17] Less common clinical presentations were characterized by flat or hemorrhagic lesions, and were associated with case-fatality rates greater than 90%. Modified smallpox (2% of unvaccinated and 25% of vaccinated cases) was similar to "ordinary type" smallpox, but had a more mild and accelerated course. Fever and other constitutional symptoms without rash (variola sine eruptione) was known to occur in rare instances.[1,17] Variola minor (alastrim) generally produced milder disease and was rarely fatal.

Laboratory Findings and Diagnosis

To aid those evaluating patients with rash illnesses suspicious for smallpox, the Centers for Disease Control and Prevention (CDC) and collaborating organizations created an algorithm based on the clinical features of "ordinary type" smallpox. Three major criteria and five minor criteria are combined to assess the risk of smallpox (low, medium, or high risk) (Table 202-2). Specific

TABLE 202-2. Major and Minor Smallpox Criteria and Risk of Smallpox

MAJOR SMALLPOX CRITERIA	RISK OF SMALLPOX
Febrile prodrome: occurring 1–4 days before rash onset; fever ≥101°F (38°C) and at least one of the following: prostration, headache, backache, chills, vomiting, or severe abdominal pain	**High risk of smallpox (report immediately)**
	Febrile prodrome AND
	Classic smallpox lesion AND
Classic smallpox lesions: deep-seated, firm/hard, round, well-circumscribed vesicles or pustules; as they evolve, lesions may become umbilicated or confluent	Lesions in same stage of development
Lesions in same stage of development: on any one part of the body (e.g., the face or arm) all the lesions are in the same stage of development (i.e., all are vesicles, or all are pustules)	**Moderate risk of smallpox (urgent evaluation)**
	Febrile prodrome AND
	One other MAJOR smallpox criterion
MINOR SMALLPOX CRITERIA	OR
Centrifugal distribution: greatest concentration of lesions on face and distal extremities	Febrile prodrome AND ≥4 MINOR smallpox criteria
First lesions on the oral mucosa/palate, face, or forearms	**Low risk of smallpox (manage as clinically indicated)**
Patient appears toxic or moribund	No febrile prodrome
Slow evolution: lesions evolve from macules to papules to pustules over days (each stage lasts 1–2 days)	OR
	Febrile prodrome AND
Lesions on the palms and soles	<4 MINOR smallpox criteria

Source: Centers for Disease Control and Prevention (http://www.bt.cdc.gov/agent/smallpox/diagnosis/evalposter.asp).

diagnostic measures are recommended based on the risk level (Figure 202-1). Laboratory testing for variola is not recommended for low or moderate risk cases in the absence of known circulating smallpox.[18] The positive predictive value of such tests is extremely low, and the public health implications of false-positive results could be considerable.[19,20] If undertaken, variola testing should be performed at a biosafety level (BSL)-4 laboratory designated by national authorities. Polymerase chain reaction (PCR) testing is the preferred method for laboratory confirmation, although electron microscopy, serologies, and other methods also may be useful for diagnosis.[21] CDC guidelines for laboratory testing of suspected smallpox cases are available at http://www.bt.cdc.gov/agent/smallpox.

Some illnesses that could be confused with smallpox are listed in Box 202-3. Chickenpox is the illness most commonly confused with smallpox. Important features useful in distinguishing these two diseases are listed in Table 202-3. Monkeypox also can be difficult to distinguish from smallpox in the absence of epidemiologic clues, although lymphadenopathy is more prominent with monkeypox.[1]

Treatment

Prior to eradication, treatment of smallpox largely was supportive. Vaccination of contacts within the immediate postexposure period may prevent or modify disease.[8–10,22] Cidofovir inhibits the poxvirus DNA polymerase and has proven effective against other poxvirus infections in humans[23] and against lethal orthopox virus infections in animal models.[24,25] A newer lipid ester derivative of cidofovir with improved oral bioavailability and decreased renal toxicity has proven effective against orthopoxvirus infections in

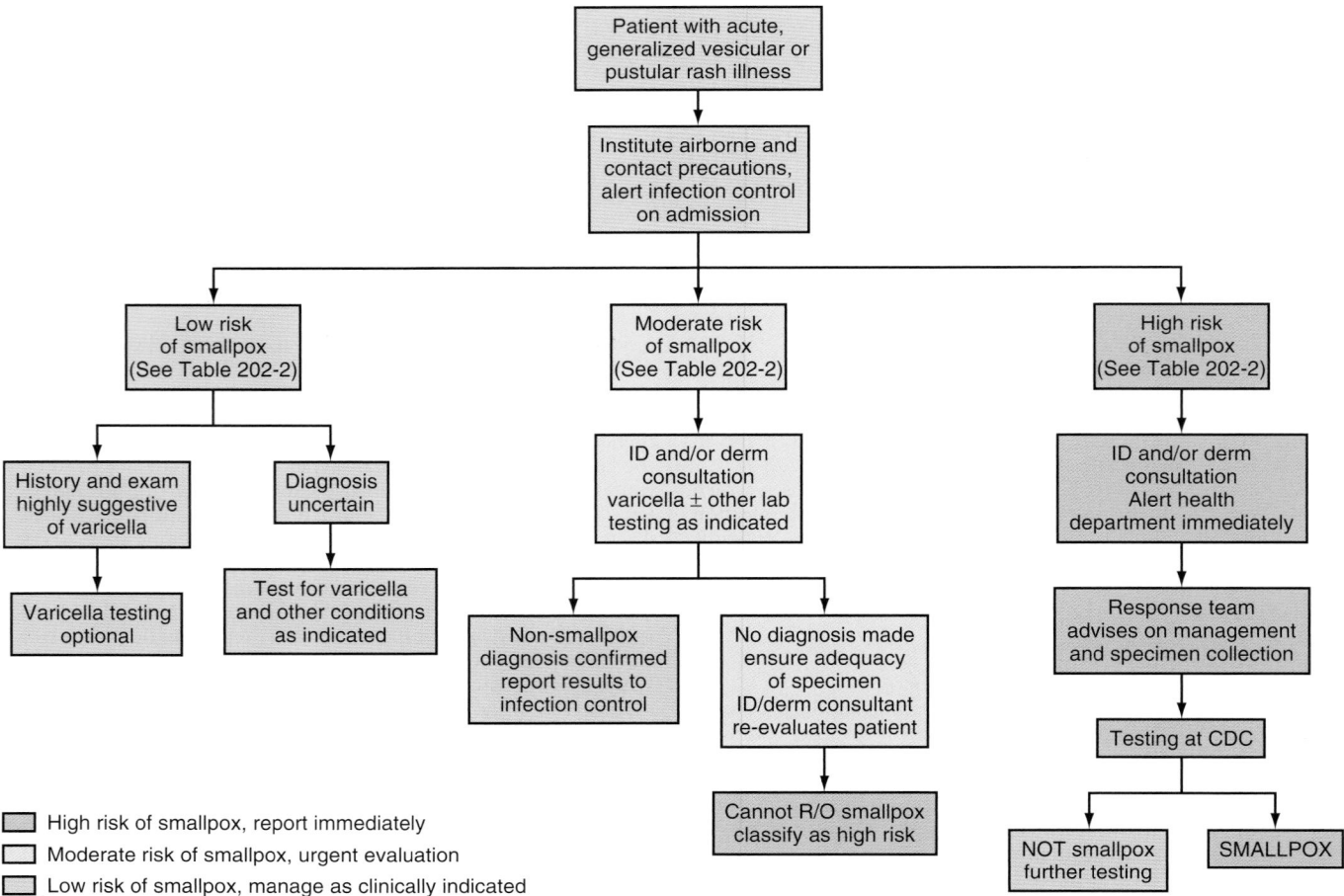

Figure 202-1. Algorithm for evaluating patients for smallpox. ID, infectious diseases; R/O, rule out. (Redrawn from Centers for Disease Control and Prevention. http://www.bt.cdc.gov/agent/smallpox/diagnosis/evalposter.asp.)

BOX 202-3. Conditions That Might be Confused with Smallpox by Stage

MACULAR/PAPULAR	VESICULAR/PUSTULAR
Measles	Chickenpox
Rubella	Disseminated herpes zoster
Drug eruptions	Disseminated herpes simplex virus
Secondary syphilis	Drug eruptions
Erythema multiforme	Contact dermatitis
Scabies/insect bites	Erythema multiforme (including
Acne	Stevens–Johnson syndrome)
Scarlet fever	Enteroviral infections
	Secondary syphilis
	Acne
	Generalized vaccinia
	Monkeypox
	Impetigo
	Scabies/insect bites
	Disseminated molluscum
	contagiosum

animal models.[26–29] Another orally bioavailable compound (ST-246) that prevents release of virus from infected cells also has proven effective against orthopoxvirus infections – including variola – in vitro and in animal models.[30–33] Evidence from animal studies suggests that these compounds could function synergistically for treatment or prevention of orthopoxvirus infections.[34,35]

Prevention

Several types of smallpox vaccine have been developed. First-generation vaccines contain live vaccinia grown in animals then purified and treated to ensure stability.[1] Second-generation vaccines are single clones that have been isolated and grown in cell culture. These vaccines are generally similar to first-generation vaccines with regard to safety and immunogenicity.[36] Third-generation vaccines are single clones further attenuated by serial passage or genetic manipulation. These vaccines appear to be safer than earlier vaccines.[37–40] Third-generation vaccines protect against orthopoxvirus infection in animal models[38,41–43] and attenuate response to first-generation vaccines in humans,[44,45] but their ability to protect against smallpox has not been documented. Moreover, evidence suggests that third-generation vaccines might be less immunogenic than first-generation vaccines.[38,46] Subunit

and DNA-based vaccines have shown promise in animal models.[47–51]

The first-generation vaccine that was used in the United States until recently (Dryvax, Wyeth) was derived from the New York City Board of Health (NYCBOH) strain, one of the strains recommended by the World Health Organization (WHO) during the eradication campaign.[1] A second-generation vaccine derived from NYCBOH virus (ACAM2000, Acambis), was licensed in 2007[36,52] and has replaced Dryvax in the U.S. for ongoing vaccination and use in the strategic national stockpile.[53] No third-generation vaccines are available currently.

Smallpox vaccine is delivered by multiple punctures with a bifurcated needle. Normally, a papule appears 3 to 4 days after inoculation and progresses to a vesicle and then a pustule, which crusts and separates by approximately 12 days post vaccination. Virus can be recovered from vaccination sites for up to 3 weeks. Therefore, covering the site with a porous bandage (e.g., gauze) is recommended.[54] Fever, local swelling, headache, and nonspecific rashes are all common following vaccination. Images of a normal vaccination "take" and selected adverse reactions are available at http://www.bt.cdc.gov/agent/smallpox/vaccineimages.asp.

Severe adverse events include postvaccinial encephalitis, progressive vaccinia, eczema vaccinatum, and fetal vaccinia.[55] Generalized vaccinia occurs more commonly and is usually self-limited. Accidental inoculation of self or others (Figure 202-2) (including ocular inoculation) also occurs.[55,56] Myocarditis and pericarditis

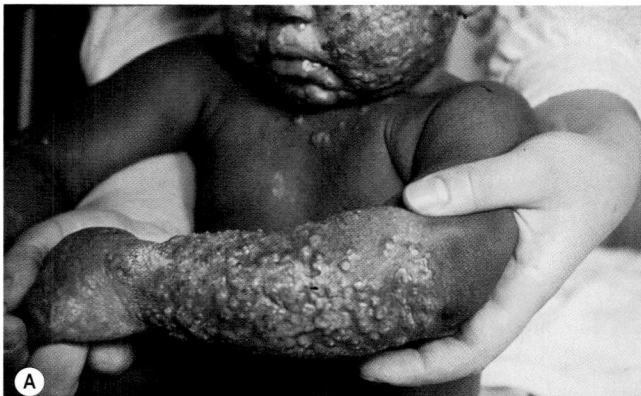

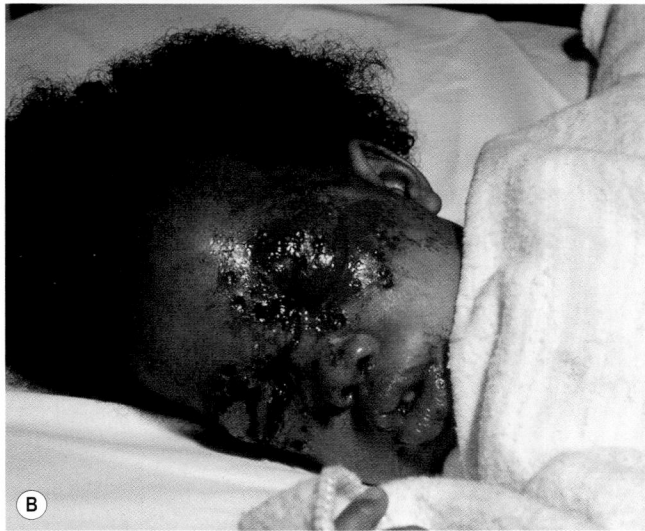

Figure 202-2. (A) A 6-month-old infant developed eczema vaccinatum after exposure to his vaccinated sibling. **(B)** An 18-month-old toddler had accidental self-inoculation of his eye and face. (Cases from Philadelphia in the 1960s. Courtesy of S.S. Long.)

TABLE 202-3. Features Distinguishing Smallpox from Chickenpox

Feature	Smallpox	Chickenpox
Prodromal symptoms	Frequent, severe	Infrequent, usually mild
Mature lesion morphology	Firm, well-circumscribed pustules	Superficial vesicles
Lesion development	Same stage on any one part of body	Different stages on any one part of body
Lesion distribution	Centrifugal	Centripetal
Location of first lesions	Mouth, face, forearms	Face, trunk
Patient appearance	Often toxic or moribund	Rarely toxic or moribund
Lesion evolution	Slow; 1–2 days per stage	Rapid; <24 hours per stage
Palmar/plantar lesions	Frequent	Rare

both occurred at a higher than expected rate among persons vaccinated in the U.S. since 2002.[57,58] The reasons for this are not clear. Vaccinia immune globulin (VIG) is indicated for certain adverse reactions, and is available from the CDC.[59] Orally bioavailable antiviral agents hold promise for treatment of certain vaccine complications.[60]

In the absence of known circulating smallpox, vaccination is contraindicated for several groups, including those with atopic dermatitis or other exfoliative skin conditions, those with diseases or treatments causing immunosuppression, pregnant women, and those with household members in any of these groups. Vaccination also is contraindicated for breastfeeding women, children less than 12 months old, persons with previous allergy to the vaccine, and those with moderate or severe illness or cardiac disease. Nonemergent vaccination of children less than 18 years old is not recommended by the Advisory Committee on Immunization Practices (ACIP).[61]

ZOONOTIC POXVIRUSES

Epidemiology

Three orthopoxviruses are capable of causing zoonotic infection: Vaccinia, monkeypox, and cowpox. Vaccinia has become endemic in a variety of animal species. Both monkeypox and cowpox have been reported increasingly during recent years, possibly reflecting a decline in population-level immunity to orthopoxviruses following the end of the smallpox eradication campaign.[62]

Because of its similarity to smallpox, monkeypox was not recognized as a cause of human illness until 1970, 3 years after the start of the WHO's intensified smallpox eradication program.[63] Prior to 2003, monkeypox was limited to parts of central and western Africa, where it is endemic in several species of small mammals.[64] In 2003, an outbreak of human monkeypox in the U.S. resulted in 47 confirmed and probable cases.[65] The outbreak was linked to prairie dogs that had been housed with exotic animals shipped from Ghana.[66]

Genomic analysis has confirmed the existence of two monkeypox clades, Congo Basin and West African. Morbidity, mortality, and transmissibility are all higher among persons infected with the Congo Basin clade.[67] Overall, studies of African outbreaks indicate that 8% to 15% of unvaccinated household contacts develop infection.[63,68]

Cowpox is an emerging infection that currently is limited to Europe and Central Asia, where it is endemic in several species of rodents.[69–71] Despite the name, infection is most commonly contracted from domestic cats. Transmission from rats and other animals also has been reported.[71–73]

Several parapoxviruses also cause zoonotic infections. The most frequently reported is orf, also known as ecthyma contagiosum or contagious pustular dermatitis. Orf is contracted by exposure to saliva of infected sheep or goats.[74,75] Bovine papular stomatitis (caused by the bovine papular stomatitis virus) and milker's nodules/pseudocowpox (caused by the paravaccinia virus) are clinically identical to orf, but occur following exposure to cattle.[1,76] Other parapoxviruses reported to cause human disease include reindeerpox and sealpox.[16,77]

Tanapox is a mild zoonotic illness endemic to equatorial Africa. Only five cases have been reported in the U.S., and all had recent travel to endemic areas or exposure to laboratory animals.[78] Epidemiologic evidence suggests transmission from nonhuman primate hosts via an arthropod vector or, rarely, by direct contact.[79,80] Two other yatapoxviruses have caused localized skin lesions in animal handlers.[21]

Clinical Manifestations

Clinically, monkeypox begins with a smallpox-like prodrome following a 10- to 14-day incubation period. The rash is similar to smallpox, but may be less extensive. Lymphadenopathy is prominent and may be useful in distinguishing monkeypox from smallpox.[1] Monkeypox is more common and more severe among

children. Of 247 cases in Zaire between 1970 and 1984, 98% of severe cases and 100% of fatalities occurred among children.[1] Overall case-fatality rates range from 0% to 11%.[1,63,66,68]

Cowpox infection presents with lesions similar to those following smallpox vaccination. Lesions develop at sites of inoculation approximately 7 days after exposure, usually in association with localized lymphadenopathy, fever, and malaise. Eschars form after the lesions crust and residual scarring is common. Cowpox has been mistaken for cutaneous anthrax, although anthrax lesions evolve more rapidly and generally are not painful.[69] Cowpox is usually mild and self-limited, although disseminated disease and fatalities have been reported in patients with atopic dermatitis.[81,82]

The lesions of orf, bovine papular stomatitis, and milker's nodules/pseudocowpox develop at the site of exposure (usually hands or arms) following a 3- to 7-day incubation period and classically progress over 14 to 72 days.[76,83] Fever, regional lymphadenopathy, and erythema multiforme can occur. Severe or widespread lesions have been reported in immunocompromised patients.[84,85]

Yatapox infections present with fever and other systemic symptoms which usually precede skin lesions by 1 to 4 days. Lesions are solitary in >75% of cases. They are characterized by slow evolution from macule to papule to nodule (with frequent ulceration), and often are accompanied by regional lymphadenopathy.[78,79]

Laboratory Findings and Diagnosis

Monkeypox can be difficult to distinguish from chickenpox.[86] Options for laboratory diagnosis include PCR, electron microscopy, and serology.[87] Lesion characteristics and animal exposure history are critical factors in diagnosing and differentiating localized zoonotic poxvirus infections. Diagnostic options include histopathology, serologic testing, and performance of electron microscopy or PCR.[74,75,78]

Treatment

Treatment for monkeypox primarily is supportive, although vaccinia immune globulin or cidofovir can be considered.[88] Cidofovir and poxvirus egress inhibitors have proven effective against monkeypox and cowpox in animal models, but human data are lacking.[23–25,27,31,32] Parapoxvirus and yatapoxvirus infections are self-limited in most cases. Treatment of orf with topical cidofovir or topical imiquimod has been reported to be effective.[84,89] However, excision and even amputation have been required in severe cases among immunocompromised patients.[85]

Prevention

The likelihood of acquiring a zoonotic poxvirus infection can be decreased by observing appropriate hygiene measures around animal contact and by limiting exposure to ill or exotic animals. Smallpox vaccination is effective in preventing monkeypox transmission, and vaccination following exposure may prevent or ameliorate disease.[63,88] Antiviral prophylaxis also has proven effective in animal models.[27,34]

MOLLUSCUM CONTAGIOSUM

Epidemiology

Molluscum contagiosum is a common infection worldwide. Incidence is highest among children younger than 5 years and those with atopic dermatitis.[90] Transmission results from direct contact or through fomites such as towels. Molluscum contagiosum can be spread by sexual contact, with resulting lesions on the genitalia, inner thighs, and abdomen. Autoinoculation is common, particularly in individuals with conditions that compromise the epidermal barrier. Autoinoculation is believed to be the most common cause of lesions on the genitalia of infants and young children. However, the possibility of sexual abuse should be considered.[91] Vertical transmission also has been reported.[92] The incubation period varies from 2 weeks to 6 months. Molluscum contagiosum has been associated with outbreaks,[93] but usually occurs sporadically.

Clinical Manifestations

Infection results in multiple, small (1 to 5 mm), umbilicated papules that are pearly white or flesh-colored. In approximately 10% of cases, localized eczematous dermatitis ("molluscum dermatitis") develops around a molluscum papule.[94] Four clinically indistinguishable subtypes have been identified, with MCV1 predominating.[90] Molluscum contagiosum is a common opportunistic infection in patients with the acquired immunodeficiency syndrome (AIDS), cancer, or neutropenia, and can be problematic in primary immunodeficiency syndromes, especially hyperimmunoglobulinemia E syndromes.[95-98] The extensive and unusual molluscum lesions observed in these patients include multiple papules and giant hyperkeratotic lesions. Keratoconjunctivitis can develop secondary to eyelid lesions.[97]

Laboratory Findings and Diagnosis

The diagnosis of molluscum usually is clinical, but can be confirmed by examination of smears of lesions for the presence of intracytoplasmic inclusion bodies.[90] Biopsy generally is not required. Molecular diagnostic assays have been developed,[99] but are not used widely. Molluscum contagiosum cannot be isolated in tissue culture. The presence of genital lesions in sexually active adolescents should prompt evaluation for other sexually transmitted infections.[91]

Treatment

Molluscum lesions usually resolve spontaneously within 6 to 18 months, and recurrences are rare. Intervention often is warranted for patients with underlying skin conditions or immunodeficiency. Several topical treatments are available, including imiquimod, tretinoin, and cantharidin.[90,100,101] Therapeutic options are listed in Box 202-4. Molluscum lesions in patients with AIDS often spread despite aggressive therapy.[95] Topical cidofovir and other investigational treatments have been used in refractory

cases.[90,102] Surgery may be required for removal of large solitary lesions.

Prevention

Isolation or exclusion of infected children from school or child-care settings is not warranted. The likelihood of transmission can be decreased by restricting sharing of towels and other potential fomites with infected persons. Genital lesions in adolescents should be treated to prevent sexual transmission.[103]

BOX 202-4. Treatment Options for Molluscum Contagiosum

PHYSICAL DISRUPTION
- Curettage
- Cryotherapy
- Laser
- Electrosurgery

CHEMICAL DISRUPTION
- Cantharidin (topical)
- Podophyllin (topical)
- Trichloroacetic acid (topical)
- Silver nitrate (topical)
- Potassium hydroxide (topical)

IMMUNE MODULATION
- Imiquimod (topical)
- Tretinoin cream (topical)
- Cimetidine (systemic)
- Interferon-α (intralesional)[a]
- OK-432 (intralesional)[a]

ANTIVIRAL
- Cidofovir (topical or systemic)[a]

UNKNOWN
- Taping/Occlusion

[a]Investigational therapies reserved for severe cases.

---

203 Introduction to Herpesviridae

Charles G. Prober

The family Herpesviridae contains three subfamilies, Alphaherpesvirinae (herpes simplex-like viruses), Betaherpesvirinae (cytomegaloviruses and cytomegalo-like viruses), and Gammaherpesvirinae (lymphocyte-associated viruses).[1] Eight herpesviruses that are human pathogens are represented in six different genera. Genus and typical characteristics of subfamilies of the eight human herpesviruses are shown in Table 203-1.

Herpesviridae share several features (summarized in Box 203-1). The architecture of the virion best defines family membership. The typical herpes virion is roughly spherical and 150 to 200 nm in diameter. The virion consists of a core of linear, double-stranded DNA wrapped around a fibrillar core spool, an icosadeltahedral capsid containing 162 capsomeres, a layer of amorphous, asymmetrically distributed material surrounding the capsid called the tegument, and a surrounding, lipid-containing envelope containing multiple embedded glycoprotein protrusions.

The most important biologic property of members of the Herpesviridae family is their ability to establish a latent state with lifetime persistence in infected hosts after primary infection. The different sites of latency, as noted in Table 203-1, are a distinguishing feature of the three Herpesviridae subfamilies. The viral genome takes the form of closed circular molecules within latently infected cells, but with reactivation, the genome again becomes linear, and each replication cycle results in local cellular destruction. Clinical correlation of this biologic cycle is virus-specific and is observed through a lifelong risk of viral reactivation, with or without recrudescence of symptoms. Primary infection generally results in more severe symptoms than reactivated infection. However, mild or subclinical primary infection can be followed by more severe reactivated infection.

TABLE 203-1. Members of Herpesviridae Family

Subfamily	Characteristics	Genus	Member
Alphaherpesvirinae	Short reproductive cycle Efficient destruction of infected cells with release of viral progeny Rapid spread in culture Latency in sensory ganglia	Simplexvirus Varicellovirus	Herpes simplex virus type 1 Herpes simplex virus type 2 Varicella-zoster virus
Betaherpesvirinae	Long reproductive cycle Slow cell-to-cell spread in culture Enlargement of infected cells Multiple nonganglionic sites of latency	Cytomegalovirus Roseolovirus	Cytomegalovirus Human herpesvirus 6 Human herpesvirus 7
Gammaherpesvirinae	Replication in lymphoblastoid cells Latency in lymphoid tissue Monocytes and B lymphocytes	Lymphocryptovirus Rhadinovirus	Epstein–Barr virus Human herpesvirus 8

BOX 203-1. Common Features of Members of Herpesviridae Family

GENERAL FEATURES

Viral particle size, 150–200 nm
More than 30 structural proteins
Icosahedral nucleocapsid with 162 capsomers, 100 nm in diameter
Surrounded by an envelope, acquired via budding through inner lamella of nuclear envelope
Multiple surface projections embedded in envelope

DNA

Linear double-stranded genome wrapped around a fibrillar spool core
Contains terminal and internal reiterated sequences; variability in number of reiterations between members

Genomic size, 120–230 kb; size variation related to number of sequence reiterations
Specifies a large number of enzymes involved in nucleic acid metabolism

FEATURES OF REPLICATION AND PERSISTENCE

Complex replication occurs in nucleus
Destruction of infected cell accompanies production of progeny
Latency follows primary infection with lifetime persistence in infected hosts
Potential for reactivation exists

---

204 Herpes Simplex Virus

Charles G. Prober

Herpes simplex virus types 1 and 2 (HSV-1 and HSV-2) belong to the Alphaherpesvirinae subfamily of herpesviruses.[1] Characteristics of these large DNA viruses include: a short reproductive cycle, rapidly productive of lytic infection in tissue culture and the propensity for latency in sensory neural ganglia. After infection of the oral mucosa by HSV-1, the site of latency of the virus is the trigeminal ganglia; after genital infection by HSV-2, the site of latency is the sacral ganglia. In common with other herpesviruses, the HSV core of linear, double-stranded DNA is contained within an icosahedral capsid that consists of 162 capsomeres. The capsid is surrounded by a tightly adherent membrane of tegument protein and a phospholipid-rich envelope. The complete virion has an approximate diameter of 110 to 120 nm. Complete DNA sequencing demonstrates a greater than 90% homology between HSV-1 and HSV-2.

The HSV genome encodes at least 84 different polypeptides. They include: (1) glycoproteins embedded in the viral envelope; (2) capsid proteins; (3) DNA polymerase, protein kinase, and other viral enzymes; (4) DNA-binding proteins involved in viral replication; and (5) multiple other proteins with poorly understood biologic functions.[2] Attachment of HSV to cell-surface receptors initiates infection. After attachment, the HSV envelope fuses to the plasma membrane, allowing the viral capsid to be transported to the nucleus where DNA is released. Transcription, DNA synthesis, capsid assembly, DNA packaging, envelopment, and release of new viral progeny ensue in susceptible cells.[2]

Several viral surface glycoproteins (g) appear to be important determinants of virulence. For example, gB and gC mediate cellular attachment, whereas gD is required for viral entry into cells. gE is required for efficient expression of late genes and, with glycoprotein I (gI), forms a potent Fc receptor.[2]

The first set of viral gene products to be synthesized is the 6 immediate early proteins; 5 regulate the reproductive cycle of the virus, and 1 protein blocks the presentation of antigenic peptides on the cell surface. The second set of proteins produced is the early proteins. These proteins, which include thymidine kinase and DNA polymerase, primarily are responsible for viral nucleic acid metabolism and are the main targets of antiviral therapy. The third set of proteins, known as late proteins, assembles to form the capsid and tegument. These proteins ultimately facilitate viral envelopment.

PATHOPHYSIOLOGY

Infection of the susceptible host occurs when virus penetrates through abraded skin or mucosal surfaces. It is hypothesized that HSV enters cutaneous neurons after minimal replication at the site of inoculation and then migrates along innervating axons to the sensory ganglia, where infectious virus is synthesized.[3] Visible lesions result when virus subsequently travels back to the inoculation site via peripheral sensory nerves, replicates, and destroys epithelial cells.[4] Histology of skin lesions shows sequential changes of balloon degeneration of infected cells, with condensation of nuclear chromatin, degeneration of cell nuclei and plasma membranes, and formation of multinucleated giant cells. Initially, vesicular lesions appear between epidermal and dermal layers and contain large amounts of virus, cell debris, and inflammatory cells. As additional inflammatory cells are recruited, pustular lesions replace vesicles, and healing ensues. Mucosal membrane lesions are more ulcerative than skin lesions, because the thin layer of epithelium in mucosal lesions ruptures readily. Histologic changes observed in primary infection usually are more severe than those of recurrent episodes.

Occasionally, spread occurs beyond the dorsal root ganglia or the localized mucocutaneous eruption, leading to generalized infection. When the host is unable to limit viral replication, viremia can result in multiorgan involvement. Disseminated clinical infection occurs most often in neonates and patients with compromised immune systems but also occurs rarely in immunocompetent hosts.

Establishment of lifelong latency, interrupted by bouts of recrudescence, is an important feature of HSV infections. Maintenance of the latent state probably depends on several factors, including the number of neurons infected during the primary episode, the number involved with each reactivation, and the possible incremental involvement of additional neurons with each recurrent episode.[5] During latency, the HSV genome is maintained in a repressed, noninfectious, static state. Transcriptional latency patterns of HSV-1 and HSV-2 are similar.[6] The molecular basis of latency and reactivation involves the active expression of only a single diploid gene encoding latency-associated transcripts.[7] Maintenance of the virus in this nonreplicating state is compatible with the survival and normal function of host ganglion cells.

Periodic reactivation of HSV and centrifugal spread down the neuraxis are associated with the development of recurrent lesions or asymptomatic viral excretion. A number of stimuli can precipitate recurrent infections, including manipulation of nerve roots, direct trauma to ganglia or skin/mucosa innervated by peripheral nerve, exposure to ultraviolet light, stress, hormonal changes such as those accompanying menses, administration of immunosuppressive agents, and intercurrent infections. Likelihood of reactivation is related to virus type and interaction between the virus and the host's immunologic systems. Recurrences are common after primary orolabial infection with HSV-1 and genital infection with HSV-2. By contrast, when primary orolabial infection is caused by HSV-2 or primary genital infection is caused by HSV-1, recurrences are less common. For example, <25% of people have recurrences after first-episode infections of the genital tract caused by HSV-1, whereas >60% have recurrences after genital HSV-2 infections.[8,9] The likelihood that recurrences are associated with symptoms depends on the quantity of reactivated virus, virus–cell interactions, and host immune factors.

IMMUNITY

The immune response to HSV appears to be initiated as a "containment" strategy and continues as a "curative" strategy.[10] The usual result in normal hosts is the localization of virus to a limited anatomic area with neutralization of infectivity, followed by establishment of latency. Despite extensive investigation, specific immunologic factors that modulate the clinical course and outcome of HSV infections are not understood completely. Although HSV infections tend to be more severe in patients with cellular rather than humoral immunodeficiencies, both antibody- and cell-mediated responses are important in influencing the acquisition of disease, the severity of infection, and the frequency of recurrences.[11] The important role of antibody in HSV infections is evident from investigations of neonates exposed to HSV at the time of delivery. Those exposed to HSV-2 in the presence of transplacentally acquired neutralizing antibody are significantly less likely to contract infection[12] and, if infected, usually have localized disease manifesting later in the neonatal period.[13] Additionally, titers of antibodies that mediate antibody-dependent cellular cytotoxicity (ADCC) correlate inversely with severity of neonatal infection.[14]

Humoral immunity also seems to be relevant to the pathogenesis of HSV infections beyond the neonatal period. For example, HSV-1 seropositive stem-cell transplant recipients who have HSV-1 seropositive donors have less frequent and shorter episodes of HSV-1 infection than those who have HSV-1 seronegative donors.[15] Also, low levels of mononuclear cell ADCC activity in patients with leukemia correlate with greater susceptibility to HSV infections.[16] Furthermore, antibodies against HSV-1 provide partial protection against HSV-2 infection. Prior HSV-1 infection reduces the risk of contracting HSV-2 infection by about 50%,[17] and a first episode of genital infection caused by HSV-2 is less severe if people have pre-existing HSV-1 antibodies.[18] Investigations focused on local defense mechanisms have identified the protein targets of antibodies to HSV and their appearance in mucosal secretions.[19] These studies underscore the role of humoral immune response in HSV infections.

It is well established that the cellular immune response is critical for the control of HSV infections, but which HSV antigens are the most important inducers of protective responses remains unknown. Substantially diminished HSV antigen-stimulated lymphocyte proliferation and reduced interferon production are observed in infected neonates and postpartum women compared with responses in nonparturient adults.[20]

EPIDEMIOLOGY

Most infections caused by HSV are asymptomatic or nonspecific. Therefore, defining the epidemiology of HSV has depended on seroepidemiologic studies, which have been confounded by extensive antigenic similarities between HSV-1 and HSV-2. The development of type-specific assays for antibodies unique to HSV-1 and HSV-2 now provides a means of reliably determining prior infection with each virus.[21]

Beyond the neonatal period, primary infection with HSV-1 usually occurs in infancy or childhood, whereas primary infection with HSV-2 occurs after the onset of sexual activity. HSV infections occur throughout the world, with humans serving as the only reservoir. Acquisition of virus follows intimate mucocutaneous contact between a susceptible host and a host who is shedding virus during primary infection or reactivation. Because HSV infection results in lifelong latency, the prevalence in any population is cumulative. Transmission and acquisition of virus usually occur in the absence of symptoms, so the spread of infection throughout a population can be silent. These factors account for worldwide endemic HSV infection.

Infections caused by HSV have no seasonal predilection; however, geographic location, socioeconomic status, age, and race influence the prevalence of infection in most studies.[3] Approximately one-third of children from lower socioeconomic populations have serologic evidence of HSV infection by 5 years of age, with prevalence rising to more than three-fourths by adolescence. In contrast, only about 20% of middle-class individuals have HSV infection by 5 years of age, and there is no substantial increase in frequency until the second or third decade of life. Presumably, greater direct person-to-person contact occurring in crowded living conditions partially accounts for these differences.

Beginning in the mid-1960s, population-based studies of genital herpes revealed a rising incidence of clinically evident genital disease, with most first infections occurring in those 18 to 36 years of age.[22] Estimating the prevalence of HSV-2 infection on the basis of clinically apparent genital disease has two major limitations. First, an increasing proportion of genital herpes infections are caused by HSV-1; especially among young adults.[23] Second, most HSV-2 infections either are inapparent or are not recognized as genital herpes.[24]

Population-based serosurvey studies, which have utilized type-specific assays that reliably detect antibodies to HSV-2, demonstrated an increase of >30% in the prevalence of HSV-2 infections between 1976 and 1980 and between 1988 and 1994.[25] Subsequently HSV-2 seroprevalence in the United States has decreased and the current seroprevalence of HSV-2 among young adults is 15% to 20%.[26] Age, race, gender, and past history of other sexually transmitted infections (STIs) affect seroprevalence rates. In general, HSV-2 infection rates are comparatively higher among black persons, among women, and among persons attending STI clinics.[25] Seroprevalence of HSV-2 in pregnant women has ranged consistently from 15% to 30%.[27]

Transmission of HSV-2 typically results from contact with an asymptomatic sexual partner. In one study evaluating contacts of 66 individuals who had recently experienced genital herpes, only one-third of source partners reported recent genital herpetic lesions, one-third described genital symptoms that were atypical of genital herpes, and one-third had no prior symptoms.[28] In another prospective study evaluating 144 heterosexual partners in whom one partner was seronegative and the other had symptomatic, recurrent genital HSV, 70% of all transmissions resulted from contact during periods of asymptomatic viral shedding.[29] The reported risk of acquisition of infection in such cohorts is approximately 10% per year.[29,30]

CLINICAL SYNDROMES

Orolabial Infection

Primary Infection

Most HSV infections occurring above the waist are caused by HSV-1 and are localized to the mouth and oropharynx (Figure 204-1). Limited data suggest that only about 10% to 30% of cases

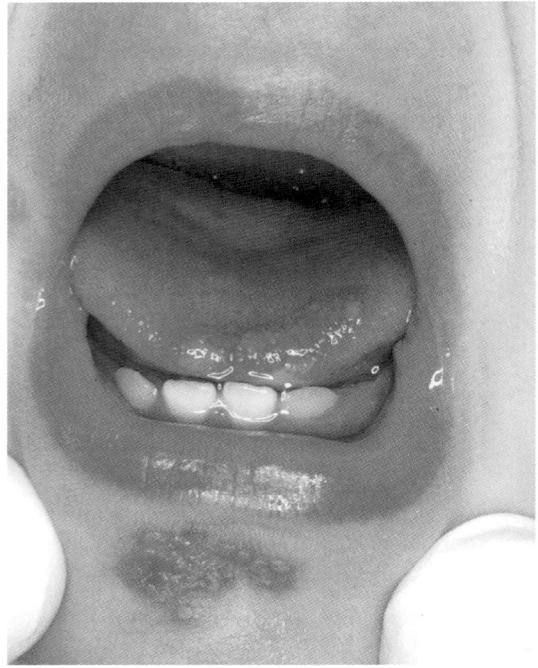

Figure 204-1. Toddler with 3 days of high fever and poor intake has typical HSV vesico-ulcerative lesions on tongue and cluster of vesiculo-bullous lesions below the lip. (Courtesy of J.H. Brien©.)

of perioral HSV infections in children are associated with signs and symptoms of illness.[31,32] Thus, the classic clinical presentation of extensive orolabial HSV lesions with primary HSV infection in the young child is an extreme manifestation. When such symptomatic disease occurs, high fever, irritability, tender submandibular lymphadenopathy, and mucocutaneous eruption evolves after a mean incubation period of 3 to 4 days. Viremia, demonstrated by polymerase chain reaction (PCR), has been demonstrated in about one-third of these symptomatic children.[33] Vesiculo-ulcerative lesions can involve the palate, gingiva, tongue, lip, and facial area.[34,35] Intraoral edema and pain are associated with lesions that evolve from vesicles to shallow ulcers on an erythematous base. The most common reason for hospital admission is dehydration resulting from impaired eating and drinking. Symptomatic primary infection is lengthy, ranging from 2 to 3 weeks.

Pharyngitis is a common manifestation of primary HSV infection in older children and adults; HSV has been isolated from the posterior pharynx of 5% to 24% of college students with pharyngeal symptoms.[36,37] HSV pharyngitis cannot be distinguished clinically from other viral and bacterial infections; common manifestations of illness are pharyngeal erythema, exudative or ulcerative lesions on the posterior pharynx and tonsils, enlarged cervical lymph nodes, and fever.[36,37]

Reactivation

Reactivation of HSV from the trigeminal ganglia usually is not associated with clinical findings. It is estimated that silent excretion of virus in healthy, previously infected individuals occurs on about 1% of days for children and 5% to 10% of days for adults.[38] Reactivation of infection commonly follows manipulation of the trigeminal nerve route[39] or dental manipulation,[40] or can occur in response to certain patient-specific stimuli. Some of these stimuli are fever, exposure to ultraviolet radiation or wind, and nonspecific stresses. The frequency of recurrences is highly variable but, on average, approximately one-third of people with prior infection experience clinically evident recurrences.[41] Signs and symptoms associated with clinical recurrences usually are mild.[42] Unilateral clusters of lesions on skin along trigeminal nerve distribution, with or without conjunctivitis, are not unknown (see Figure 83-1). Many patients have prodromal symptoms of pain, burning, or tingling that precede the eruption by 1 to 2 days. The most common site of recurrent orolabial lesions is the outer edge of the vermilion border. On average, 3 to 5 lesions are present. Lesions begin as vesicles, evolve into pustules or ulcers in 1 to 2 days, and heal completely within 8 to 10 days. Pain is greatest at the onset of eruption and resolves within 4 to 5 days. Viral excretion and, thus, infectivity last only 2 to 3 days; titer of virus varies from <10 plaque-forming units (PFU)/mL in the prodromal phase to almost 10^5 PFU/mL in the vesicular phase.

Genital Infection

Familiarity with the serologic classification of genital herpes infection is important to the understanding of the biologic and clinical features of the disease.[43] Primary infection occurs in the absence of pre-existing antibodies to HSV, either HSV-1 or HSV-2. First-episode nonprimary infections occur in the absence of any previous signs or symptoms of genital herpes, but in the presence of pre-existing heterologous antibodies. Most first-episode nonprimary infections are caused by HSV-2 in persons with pre-existing antibodies against HSV-1. More rarely first-episode nonprimary infections are caused by HSV-1 in persons with pre-existing antibodies to HSV-2. Recurrent genital herpes occurs in persons who have had prior outbreaks and therefore also pre-existing homologous antibodies to the reactivating HSV.

Historically, most first-episode genital herpes infections were caused by HSV-2. However, an increasing proportion, especially among young adults, are caused by HSV-1. Whereas only 5% to 10% of adults in the U.S. have a history suggestive of prior genital herpes infection, seroepidemiologic studies show that approximately 1 in 4 persons >30 years of age have been infected with HSV-2.[44] Seroprevalence rates exceed 40% among attendees of STI clinics in the U.S., with comparatively higher rates in women and in blacks.[45]

Primary Infection

About 40% of men and 70% of women seeking medical care for primary genital herpes have constitutional symptoms. Headache, fever, myalgia, and backache develop after a mean incubation period of 7 days; symptoms peak within 4 days of onset of lesions and gradually abate over 7 to 10 days. Local symptoms such as itching and pain usually precede visible lesions by 1 to 2 days. New lesions appear over 7 to 8 days. Lesions evolve from vesicles and pustules to wet ulcers over approximately 10 days and then crust and heal during the ensuing 10 days. Lesions are distributed over the labia majora, labia minora, mons pubis, vaginal mucosa, and cervix in women. In men, lesions typically occur over the shaft of the penis. About 85% of women have vaginal discharge, and 25% of men have urethral discharge; >80% of women and >40% of men have dysuria for 7 to 10 days. Tender inguinal lymphadenopathy typically appears during the second or third week of illness in about 80% of both sexes and generally is the last sign to resolve. Mean duration of viral shedding is 11 days. Extragenital complications of primary HSV infections include aseptic meningitis, mucocutaneous lesions beyond the genital area, pharyngitis, and visceral dissemination. These complications are more common in women than in men.[18]

Nonprimary First Episode Infection

Almost one-half of people with their first clinical outbreak of genital herpes have pre-existing antibodies to the heterologous herpes virus. Presumably as a result of the pre-existing immunity to shared HSV antigens, such people have lower frequencies of systemic symptoms and extragenital complications, fewer lesions, shorter duration of pain, and more rapid healing than patients with primary infections.[18]

Reactivation

Most recurrences of genital herpes are asymptomatic. About 1% of individuals previously infected with HSV-2 have active viral shedding without symptoms on any given day.[46] Shedding of HSV from the genital tract occurs in individuals seropositive for HSV-2, even if they have no prior history of genital herpes.[47] Average duration of episodes of asymptomatic viral shedding is 1.5 days. Recurrent clinical genital herpes usually is mild, with constitutional symptoms present in only 5% of men and 10% of women. Of those who have symptoms, >40% of women and >50% of men have local prodromal symptoms for several hours to 3 days.[18] Genital lesions, which are few and confined, typically increase in size over the first 3 days, reach a plateau at 6 days, and resolve rapidly. Mean time to complete healing is 9 to 10 days, and duration of viral shedding is 4 days. Tender lymphadenopathy, dysuria, vaginal discharge, and systemic complications occur less commonly. Factors implicated in precipitating recurrences include emotional stress, menses, and sexual intercourse. Genital shedding of HSV-2 in women, as determined by PCR, also is increased in the presence of hormonal use, bacterial vaginosis, and high-density vaginal colonization with group B streptococcus.[48]

Keratoconjunctivitis

HSV-1 is the usual cause of ocular herpes infection beyond the neonatal period. Approximately 300,000 cases of HSV infection of the eyes are diagnosed each year in the U.S.[3] Infection involves one or both eyes with a typical course of follicular conjunctivitis associated with pain, photophobia, and tearing, followed by chemosis, periorbital edema, and preauricular lymphadenopathy.[49] Periocular skin involvement can occur. As infection progresses, diffuse punctate lesions occur on the cornea, followed within days by the appearance of serpiginous ulcers. Pathognomonic branching dendritic lesions (see Figures 84-1, 84-2, and 84-3) of the cornea appear and are associated with blurred vision. Deeper stromal structures can be injured, especially after injudicious use of topical corticosteroids. Healing can require >1 month. After primary ocular HSV infection, recurrences are observed in about one-third of individuals during the ensuing 5 years. Recurrences can include reappearance of dendritic ulcerations or deep stromal injury that can threaten sight.

Cutaneous Infections

HSV can infect skin outside the perioral and genital areas. Infection of the pulp or nail bed of the finger is a typical site and is referred to as *herpetic whitlow.* Whitlow is most common in medical and dental professionals, in whom it results from digital contamination with genital and oral secretions, respectively.[50] Young children experience herpetic whitlow as a result of autoinoculation of HSV-1 during primary oral herpes infection or when an infected adult inoculates virus while trimming the child's nails by biting them[51] (Figure 204-2). In adolescents and adults herpetic whitlow usually follows autoinoculation of HSV-2 from genital secretions.[52] Discrete vesicular or pustular lesions, which coalesce over several days, appear over the distal phalanx. These lesions often are confused clinically with bacterial cellulitis. Surgical intervention is contraindicated. Crusting of the lesions occurs after about 10 days and is followed by healing and reappearance of normal skin. Infection is associated with local tingling, burning pain, erythema, and edema and is accompanied by fever, lymphangitis, and tender swelling of related lymph nodes. The affected area often appears purple and dusky. Lesions recur but at rates lower than those observed with oral or genital disease.

HSV-1 causes cutaneous infection among athletes participating in contact sports, such as wrestling and rugby, referred to as *herpes gladiatorum* and *scrum-pox,* respectively.[53,54] Viral inoculation results from close contact between abraded skin and oral secretions.[55] Surveys of athletic trainers suggest that this infection is endemic among young competitive wrestlers.[56] In the largest outbreak of herpes gladiatorum reported, infection was diagnosed in 60 high school wrestlers;[57] 73% of infected wrestlers had lesions on the head, 42% on the extremities, and 28% on the trunk. About 25% of all the infected boys had fever, chills, and headache, and 40% had sore throat.

Herpes infections of skin damaged by diaper dermatitis, thermal burns, or atopic dermatitis/eczema (eczema herpeticum) can be

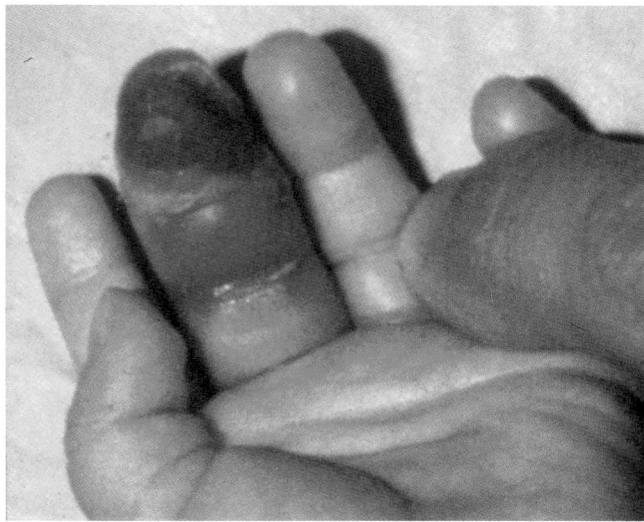

Figure 204-2. Herpetic whitlow due to HSV-1 in an infant whose mother trimmed his nails with her teeth. (Courtesy of S.S. Long.)

particularly severe.[58-60] Rapidly spreading eruptions and visceral dissemination can occur.

HSV is the most commonly recognized precipitating factor for recurrent erythema multiforme, being identified as the precipitant in about one-quarter of these patients.[61] In one study, HSV type-common glycoprotein antigen was found in 12 of 16 skin biopsy specimens of lesions from patients with erythema multiforme.[62]

Central Nervous System Infections

HSV causes a variety of peripheral and central nervous system (CNS) illnesses, both infectious and postinfectious. HSV is the

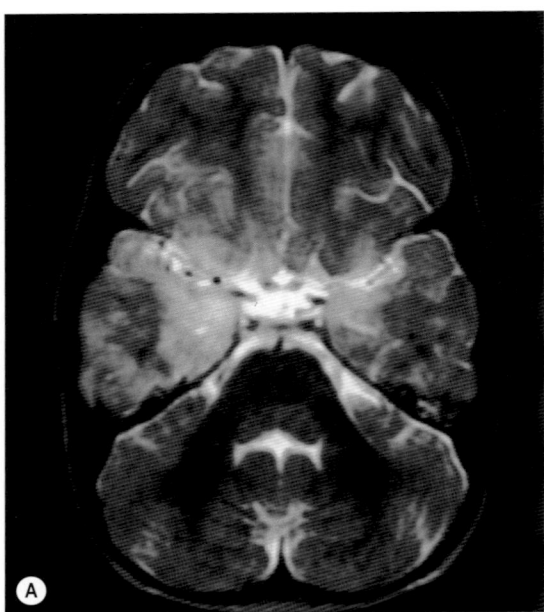

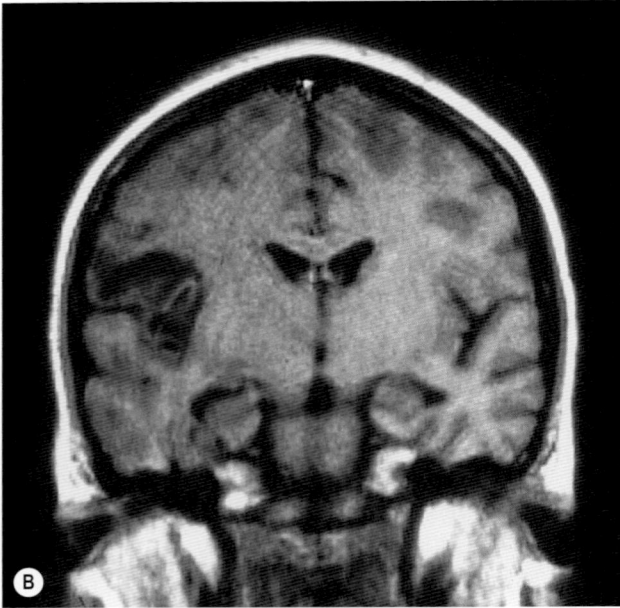

Figure 204-3. (A) Axial T₂-weighted MR image of a 27-day-old infant with HSV-2 encephalitis. Image shows edema with necrosis of the temporal lobes bilaterally, with lesser involvement of parietal lobes. Mother had only a distant history of genital HSV >15 years prior to this pregnancy with no clinical recurrence within several recent years. **(B)** Coronal T₁-weighted MR image of a 13-year-old adolescent with acute onset of left-sided seizures due to HSV-1 encephalitis. Note right-sided temporal lobe necrosis and edema. (**A,** Courtesy of S.S. Long, **B,** Courtesy of J.H. Brien©.)

most common cause of severe sporadic fatal encephalitis, accounting for approximately 10% to 20% of cases of all viral encephalitis in developed countries.[63,64] Beyond the neonatal period, HSV encephalitis virtually is always caused by HSV-1. Encephalitis has a biphasic age predilection, occurring in people 5 to 30 years of age and in those >50 years of age. Encephalitis can occur as a result of primary infection or, more commonly, reactivation. Typically, patients have fever, altered consciousness, unusual behavior, and focal neurologic abnormalities, with signs and symptoms consistent with temporal lobe involvement. Although antiviral therapy has resulted in a dramatic decrease in mortality, a substantial number of survivors are left with varying degrees of neurologic impairment, including cognitive deficits, behavioral disorders, and recurrent seizures.

Approximately one-half of patients with HSV encephalitis have an increased number of red blood cells in CSF; counts >1000/mm³ are not uncommon, and counts >25,000/mm³ have been observed.[60] Typically, CSF has a few hundred white blood cells (WBCs)/mm³ with a predominance of lymphoid cells (75% to 100%). However, pleocytosis varies from a few to >1000 WBCs/mm³ and, occasionally, neutrophils predominate; 10% to 20% of CSF specimens may be acellular, especially if obtained early in the disease.[65] Protein concentration is normal in about one-half of CSF specimens obtained during the first week of illness, but thereafter, concentrations as high as 500 to 1200 mg/dL are observed.[65] Production of HSV-specific antibody in the CNS occurs by the second week of illness, resulting in an increased ratio of CSF-to-serum concentration of HSV antibody.[65] Virus rarely is isolated from CSF. The presence of HSV DNA in CSF, identified by PCR testing, has proven to be sensitive and specific for the diagnosis of HSV encephalitis.[66] However, CSF obtained before the third day of disease can be falsely negative by PCR.[67,68] Therefore, if index of suspicion remains high, a repeat CSF analysis with testing by PCR is performed.

Electroencephalography typically reveals focal spike and slow-wave abnormalities early in the course of HSV encephalitis. A characteristic finding of paroxysmal lateralizing epileptiform discharges (PLEDs) has been described. Neurodiagnostic images can be normal at the onset of infection but, within days, edema associated with focal infection or hemorrhagic necrosis is evident; magnetic resonance imaging is a more sensitive early test than computed tomography (Figure 204-3).[69]

A number of unusual CNS manifestations attributed to HSV have been described. These include recurrent aseptic meningitis (Mollaret meningitis), brainstem encephalitis, ascending myelitis, and parainfectious encephalomyelitis (acute disseminated encephalomyelitis) and encephalomyeloradiculitis.[70] In addition, HSV has been implicated in the pathogenesis of several other neurologic syndromes, including Bell palsy, atypical pain syndromes, trigeminal neuralgia, vestibular neuritis, and temporal lobe epilepsy.

Other Infections

A number of unusual clinical manifestations of HSV have been described in immunocompetent hosts. They include visceral dissemination, esophagitis, tracheobronchitis, pneumonitis, and hepatitis. Viremia with visceral dissemination can result in infection of any organ. Beyond the neonatal period, disseminated infection is more common in adults, especially pregnant women, than in children.

Isolated esophageal involvement has been described in about 60 patients, with a mean age of 35 years.[71] Almost all infections were caused by HSV-1, and most were primary. Symptoms suggestive of esophageal HSV include retrosternal chest pain and odynophagia.

Necrotizing and exudative tracheobronchitis precipitates bronchospasm, often necessitating mechanical ventilation. Almost all reported cases have involved elderly adults or immunocompromised hosts.[72] Pneumonitis can result from spread down the tracheobronchial tree, extension from esophageal involvement, or hematogenous dissemination.

TABLE 204-1. Characteristics of Neonatal Herpes Simplex Virus Infections

Feature	Skin/Eye/Mucous Membrane Infection	CNS Infection	Disseminated Infection
Usual age at onset (days)	7–14	14–21	5–10
Clinical findings	Vesicles on a red base at sites of trauma; conjunctivitis	Lethargy, irritability, fever, seizures	Shock, hepatomegaly, jaundice, bleeding, respiratory distress
Diagnostic testing	DFA and culture of skin lesions	DFA and culture of skin lesions if present; analysis, culture, and PCR of CSF; EEG; neuroimaging studies, brain biopsy	DFA and cultures of skin lesions; culture of nasopharynx, rectum, buffy coat, CSF
Mortality if treated (%)	0	15	54
Sequelae if treated (%)	5	54	38

CNS, central nervous system; DFA, direct fluorescent antibody test; EEG, electroencephalogram; PCR, polymerase chain reaction.

Hepatic infection caused by HSV rarely occurs in normal hosts but, rather, affects neonates, pregnant women, and persons with underlying conditions.[73] Infection usually is fulminant in nature, with death commonly ensuing as a result of severe hepatic necrosis and consequent uncontrolled liver failure and coagulopathy.

Acute retinal necrosis can occur as a reactivation-immunologic event, reported as long as 9 years after perinatally acquired infection.[74]

Intrauterine and Perinatal Infections

Congenital (in utero) infection due to intrauterine exposure to HSV is uncommon; 63 cases were published between 1963 and 2009.[75] Manifestations of congenital infection usually include skin lesions and scars, chorioretinitis, microcephaly, hydranencephaly, and microphthalmia. Hydrops fetalis has been reported as a rare manifestation of intrauterine HSV infection.[76]

In contrast to in utero infection, most neonatal HSV infections result from exposure to infectious maternal genital secretions at delivery.[77] The risk of neonatal infection largely is influenced by the HSV antibody status of the mother. About one-half of neonates exposed to maternal primary infection acquire HSV infection, whereas infection occurs in <5% of those exposed to recurrent infection at delivery.[12]

Neonates infected with HSV manifest infection in three ways, with considerable clinical overlap (Table 204-1). Signs of neonatal infection are invariably evident by 4 to 5 weeks of age; illness with onset after this time is unlikely to be caused by perinatally acquired HSV. Approximately one-third of neonatal HSV infections are localized to the skin, eyes, and mouth (SEM), one-third are limited to the CNS, and one-third are disseminated.[78] SEM disease (Figure 204-4) typically manifests during the first 2 weeks of life, occasionally with skin lesions evident in the delivery room. Skin lesions tend to appear at sites of trauma, such as the site of attachment of fetal scalp electrodes, the bulb syringe trauma site on palatal mucosa, the margin of the eyes, or at a circumcision site, or over the presenting body part; they evolve rapidly from macules to vesicles on a red base. HSV infection should be considered whenever any vesicle appears on a neonate. Outcome of SEM disease is excellent if diagnosis is made quickly and antiviral therapy is administered. When the disease is not treated, about 75% of cases progress to disseminated or CNS disease.[78,79]

HSV infection of the CNS manifests later in the neonatal period than other forms of HSV infection. Typically, fever and lethargy appear between 2 and 3 weeks of age, followed by the sudden onset of seizures, which may be focal and difficult to control; skin lesions are present in about 45% at the time of presentation. CSF examination usually reveals <100 WBCs/mm³ (predominantly mononuclear), a slightly reduced glucose level, and a modestly to markedly elevated protein concentration (as high as 500 to 1000 mg/dL). The electroencephalogram typically is abnormal diffusely. Computed tomography can be normal early in the course; magnetic resonance imaging is a more sensitive study. Temporal lobe involvement is typical, but diffuse infection can occur. Without therapy, most neonates with herpes infection of the CNS die, and survivors sustain severe neurologic impairment.

Disseminated infection often mimics severe bacterial infection, with onset during the first several days of life. Common clinical findings include cardiovascular instability, hepatomegaly, jaundice, bleeding, and respiratory dysfunction. Nearly 70% of patients demonstrate skin lesions some time during their illness, but lesions often are absent at the onset of symptoms. Progression of infection is rapid, with death caused by unremitting shock, progressive liver failure, bleeding, respiratory failure, or neurologic deterioration.[79]

Infection in Compromised Hosts

HSV infection in immunocompromised hosts is a frequent source of morbidity but is uncommonly fatal. Risk of severe HSV parallels the extent of compromise of cellular immune responses. The most frequent complication of HSV infections among these patients is severe ulcerations that develop on both keratinized and nonkeratinized mucosal surfaces.[80] Oral and genital lesions progress slowly, with accompanying tissue damage and necrosis. Healing takes an average of 6 weeks. Local cutaneous dissemination can occur. Contiguous mucosal spread of infection can result in esophageal, tracheal, or pulmonary involvement or visceral dissemination.[81]

LABORATORY FINDINGS AND DIAGNOSTIC TECHNIQUES

Identification of Virus

Culture is the most specific method for diagnosing an active HSV infection. Samples from skin lesions should be obtained by: (1) aspiration of the contents of intact skin lesions; (2) swabbing of the bases of denuded skin lesions; or (3) swabbing of the mucosal sites of prior outbreaks. Premoistened cotton swabs are preferred for collection of specimens for culture, because calcium alginate-impregnated swabs inhibit virus isolation.[82] If direct inoculation onto culture media at the time of collection is not feasible, specimens should be placed into 1 to 2 mL of medium for viral transport. Specimens transported to reference laboratories at room temperature within 3 days yield adequate recovery of HSV.[83] For prolonged storage, specimens should be maintained at −70°C. Both freezing at −20°C before processing and multiple cycles of freezing and thawing reduce the viability of HSV.

The typical cytopathic effect of HSV in vitro is foci of enlarged, refractile cells in the monolayer of a variety of cell culture lines. Time required to observe cytopathic effect after incubation depends on the concentration of virus in the sample; cytopathic effect is evident within 24 hours if the sample contains high concentrations of virus, and within 4 to 5 days if there is a low concentration. Timing of specimen collection is critical; HSV can be recovered from >90% of genital herpes lesions sampled during the vesicular stage but only from about 25% sampled during the crusted stage.[84] The availability of HSV-specific monoclonal antibody has facilitated the confirmation of virus isolated and the

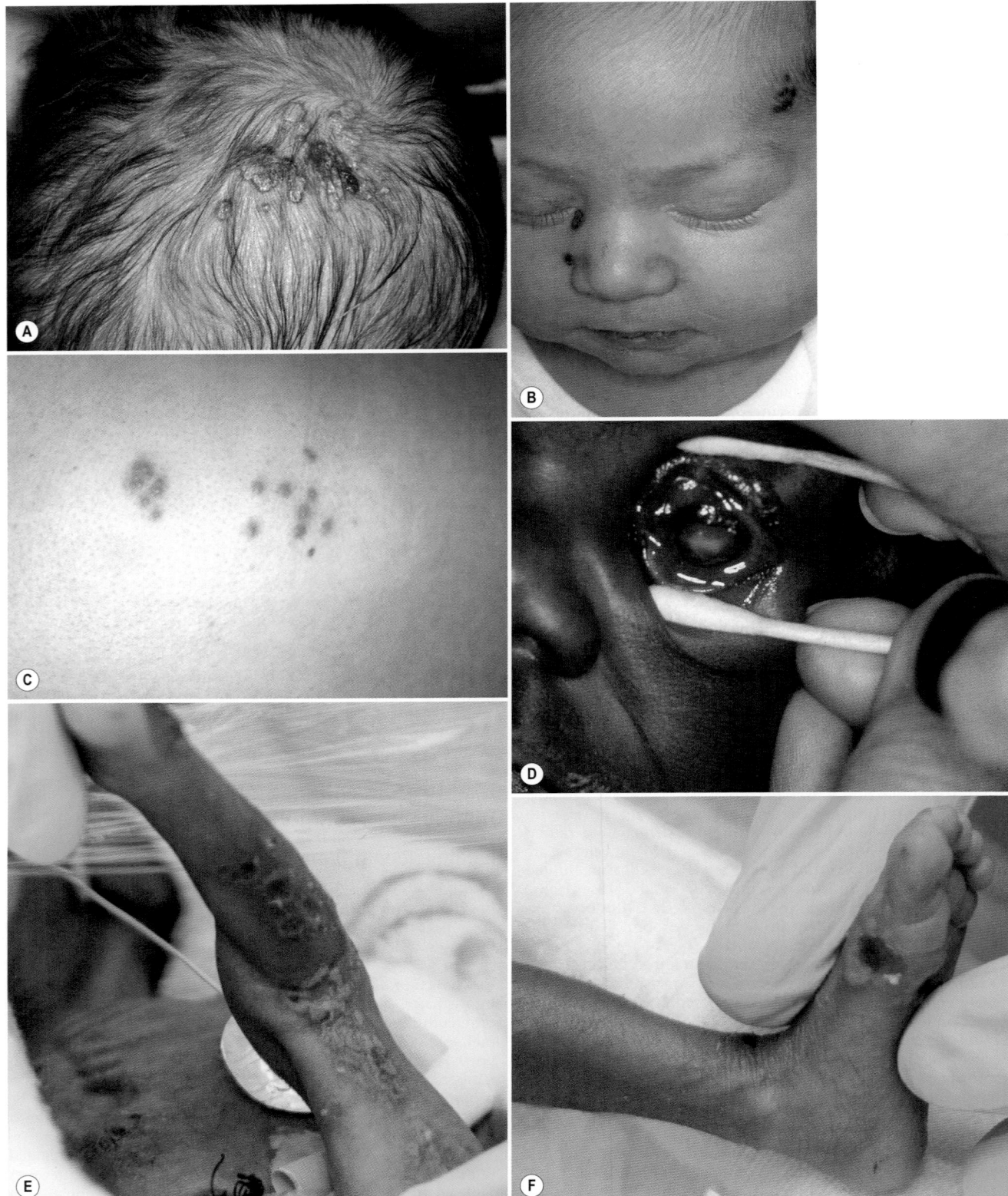

Figure 204-4. Mucocutaneous manifestations of HSV in the neonate. Clusters of vesicular lesions at the scalp electrode site **(A)** and on the face **(B)** of one infant and early skin vesicles in another infant **(C)**. This infant was discharged from the nursery at 2 days of age with the diagnosis of "chemical" conjunctivitis. He returned at 8 days of age with keratoconjunctivitis **(D).** HSV-2 was isolated from the conjunctiva. Infant born at 25 weeks of gestation 72 hours after rupture of membranes (footling presentation) had onset of raised vesicular-bullous lesions on day-of-life 4 with rapid spread down the leg and ulceration **(E, F).** HSV-2 was recovered from mucocutaneous sites, and PCR was positive on blood and CSF. (**A, B, C,** Courtesy of J.H. Brien©. **D,** Courtesy of S.S. Long. **E, F,** Courtesy of Pinniti SG, Feja KN, Hiatt M, Tolan RW, Jr; The Children's Hospital at Saint Peter's University Hospital, New Brunswick, NJ.)

specification of type.[85] Specificity of these reagents corresponds well with typing of isolates by restriction enzyme analysis.[86]

Rapid, reliable direct methods have been developed to detect HSV in specimens obtained from mucocutaneous lesions; the most commonly used method is direct immunofluorescent staining.[86] The best method for specimen collection consists of unroofing a lesion to expose its base, removing cells with the blunt end of a cotton applicator stick, and streaking the sample onto a glass slide. With the use of fluorescein-conjugated monoclonal HSV antibody, direct staining of samples from lesion scrapings is 80% to 90% as sensitive as tissue culture isolation, with few false-positive reactions.[85,87] The Papanicolaou stain or Tzanck test can be used to demonstrate cytologic changes in specimens obtained from suspected HSV lesions, but these methods are less sensitive and are not specific for HSV.[79]

PCR amplification of HSV DNA has been developed as a sensitive and specific diagnostic technique for infections caused by HSV. The most important application of HSV PCR testing is in the diagnosis of HSV encephalitis. The utility of PCR testing for the evaluation of patients with encephalitis was first reported in 1990.[88] Subsequently, a number of studies from several laboratories confirmed utility of PCR for the diagnosis of HSV encephalitis, sensitivity and specificity consistently exceeding 90%.[66,89–93] PCR testing is now considered the gold standard for the laboratory diagnosis of HSV CNS disease.[66]

Serology

A number of sensitive serologic assays detect the presence of HSV immunoglobulin (Ig) G antibody. The most popular assays are kits using enzyme immunoassay or latex agglutination procedures.[94] Unfortunately, these assays did not reliably differentiate HSV-1 from HSV-2 infections because of extensive cross-reactivity; reports based on these assays that list HSV-1 and HSV-2 antibody titers separately are likely to be misleading. Newer serologic methods have overcome the problem of HSV-1 and -2 cross-reactions. Monoclonal antibodies to the unique glycoprotein G of HSV-2 are used to capture protein from an HSV-infected cell sonicate in a solid-phase enzyme immunoassay or to prepare immunoaffinity-purified antigen for use in a dot blot assay.[95]

Serologic tests that detect immunoglobulin G antibodies cannot be used to diagnose recurrent HSV infection, because a rise in antibody titer does not always occur. Primary infections can be confirmed by documenting seroconversion between samples of acute and convalescent sera. Presence of IgM anti-HSV does not distinguish primary infection, because reactivation can cause production of IgM antibody.

TREATMENT

Acyclovir (or a derivative) is the drug of choice for most HSV infections (Table 204-2).[96] Available formulations include topical ointment, oral tablets and liquid, and a preparation for intravenous delivery. The mechanisms of action, pharmacokinetics, dosages, and toxicities are detailed in Chapter 295, Antiviral Agents.

Orolabial Infection

The effect of oral acyclovir on the course of primary herpetic gingivostomatitis has been reported in a study of 72 children. Children with documented HSV disease who received acyclovir had a shorter duration of oral lesions (4 versus 10 days) as well as earlier disappearance of fever, extraoral lesions, and drinking and eating difficulties than children who received placebo. Duration of viral shedding also was significantly shorter in the group treated with acyclovir (1 versus 5 days).[97]

Both topical and oral acyclovir regimens have been evaluated in the treatment of recurrent herpes labialis. Topical acyclovir is not effective, and oral acyclovir, even when administered immediately at the onset of symptoms, affords marginal benefit in immunocompetent hosts.[98,99] Prophylactic administration of oral

TABLE 204-2. Role of Systemic Acyclovir Therapy in the Management of Herpes Simplex Virus Infections

Type of Infection	Comments on Potential Usefulness
Orolabial	Possibly effective in severe, primary gingivostomatitis
	Marginally effective in recurrent infections
	Useful prophylactically in limited circumstances
Genital	Effective in treatment of first episode and, to a limited extent, recurrent infections
	Effective in suppressing frequently recurrent attacks
Keratoconjunctivitis	Topical therapy beneficial (vidarabine, trifluridine, or acyclovir)
Cutaneous	Possibly effective in severe eruptions in those with compromised integument (e.g., burns and eczema)
	Possibly effective in whitlow infections
	Possibly effective prophylactically in limited circumstances
Central nervous system	Effective in reducing mortality and morbidity of encephalitis
Neonates	Effective in reducing mortality and morbidity
Compromised hosts	Effective for therapy of localized and disseminated infections
	Effective prophylactically against recurrent infection
	Resistance can emerge during long-term therapy

acyclovir may be useful in persons with frequently recurrent herpes labialis. In one randomized, double-blind, placebo-controlled study, 56 adults who previously experienced >6 recurrent episodes of herpes labialis a year experienced a 53% reduction in clinical recurrences while receiving suppressive therapy with oral acyclovir.[100] Oral acyclovir also has been shown to have some benefit in reducing the extent of herpes labialis outbreaks in individuals who are prone to recurrences as a result of certain precipitants, such as ultraviolet light exposure[101] and alpine skiing.[102]

Genital Infection

Acyclovir is useful in the management of patients with genital herpes, affording greatest benefit in first-episode primary infections and least benefit in recurrent genital herpes.[103,104] Valacyclovir and famciclovir, two antiviral agents with superior bioavailability for oral dosing, are safe and effective in the therapy of genital herpes.

Intravenous and oral administrations of acyclovir are more effective than topical therapy for primary and nonprimary first clinical episodes of genital HSV infections.[105] Oral administration is preferred for ambulatory patients because it is almost equal in efficacy to intravenous therapy. For primary infection, treatment reduces the duration of viral shedding and the time to complete healing by >1 week. In some studies, acyclovir therapy also shortens the duration of new lesion formation, pain, dysuria, and other symptoms. Treatment does not prevent the establishment of latency or reduce the frequency of subsequent recurrences. Acyclovir has a beneficial although less pronounced effect on the course of recurrent genital herpes, resulting in a reduction of viral shedding and time-to-healing by 1 to 2 days; the effect on pain and itching is less.[105,106] Patients who tend to have more severe recurrent attacks, with multiple lesions persisting for >1 week, may benefit most from treatment. To ensure maximum benefit of therapy, patients who typically experience severe recurrent attacks of genital herpes could be given a prescription for acyclovir tablets with instructions to begin the drug at the first indication of reactivation.

Long-term suppressive therapy with acyclovir has substantial value for frequently recurrent genital herpes. Recurrences are reduced by >75%, and when lesions occur, they are more likely to be mild. Although the frequency of asymptomatic shedding of HSV is substantially reduced during long-term suppressive therapy, it is not eliminated, and therefore sexual transmission of the virus still can occur.[107]

Keratoconjunctivitis

Ocular infections caused by HSV usually are treated topically (in conjunction with parenteral therapy in the neonate). Either trifluridine or vidarabine ophthalmic drops are used commonly (see Chapter 84, Infective Keratitis). Oral acyclovir as prophylaxis against recurrent stromal keratitis appears to be effective at reducing long-term scarring from herpes infection.[108]

Cutaneous Infections

Sparse data exist regarding treatment of cutaneous HSV infections in the normal host beyond the neonatal period. One study of 9 evaluable subjects with recurrent lesions on the hand caused by HSV-2 concluded that oral acyclovir therapy had a beneficial effect on the duration of symptoms, signs, and culture positivity.[109] Treatment of cutaneous infections should be considered for burned patients or patients with eczema, because infections in these hosts are potentially serious.

Central Nervous System Infection

In a study published >3 decades ago, vidarabine was shown to significantly improve the outcome of patients with HSV encephalitis.[110] Mortality was reduced from 70% in placebo recipients to 44% in drug recipients. A subsequent controlled intervention trial determined acyclovir to be superior to vidarabine.[111] Mortality was reduced from 54% in vidarabine recipients to 28% in acyclovir recipients. Survival was significantly affected by the age of the patient and the Glasgow Coma Scale score and duration of disease at onset of therapy. Age and Glasgow score also significantly influenced morbidity observed 6 months after diagnosis. Outcome was best for those <30 years of age with a Glasgow score >10 at the onset of therapy.[111] A subsequent uncontrolled evaluation of acyclovir in the management of HSV encephalitis in adults observed poorer long-term prognosis in subjects with a poor physiology score upon admission to hospital and in those for whom therapy was delayed >2 days following hospital admission.[112] A low Glasgow score and age <3 years appear to be predictors of poor outcome of HSV encephalitis in children treated with acyclovir.[92] The presence of seizures at the time of onset of therapy among young infants with HSV CNS disease is almost invariably a predictor of long-term neurologic morbidity.[113]

Other Infections

There are no controlled data regarding the effectiveness of antiviral therapy in patients with unusual manifestations of HSV infection. It is prudent to administer parenteral acyclovir to those with severe, life-threatening infections.

Intrauterine and Perinatal Infections

Antiviral therapy is beneficial for neonates with HSV infections. Vidarabine was the first agent demonstrated to benefit neonates with HSV infection, reducing mortality for infants with disseminated or CNS infection from 70% in placebo recipients to 40% in vidarabine recipients. Acyclovir is now the drug of choice.[113] An open-label evaluation of increasing dosages of intravenous acyclovir support the use of a 21-day course of 60 mg/kg/day to treat neonatal CNS and disseminated infection.[114] Best therapeutic results are obtained with localized SEM infection; with

commencement of treatment before progression, all infants survive, and >90% appear to be developmentally normal, although almost one-half have recurrent skin lesions within 6 months of completion of therapy.[113] By contrast, >50% of infants with disseminated infection die.[113] There have been anecdotal reports of recovery/survival from fulminant hepatic failure following liver transplantation (and while receiving plasmapheresis/hemofiltration awaiting transplantation). About 15% of infants with CNS disease die despite therapy, and <50% of survivors are normal at 1 year of age.[113] Recurrence of CNS symptoms with abnormal CSF findings occurs in about 8% of survivors of disseminated or CNS disease.[113] Six months of suppressive oral acyclovir, begun immediately after initial therapy of CNS infection, appears to improve neurodevelopment outcome assessed at 12 months of age.[115] Dose used in the National Institute of Allergy and Infectious Diseases-sponsored trial was 300 mg/m^2 per dose, 3 times a day.

Neonates with proven HSV infections should receive acyclovir; the role of empiric acyclovir therapy is not clear. Clinical settings in which empiric therapy should be considered include: (1) the appearance of skin lesions typical of HSV while awaiting results of diagnostic tests; (2) fever or other unexplained signs of infection in a neonate known to have been exposed to HSV at delivery; (3) progressive clinical deterioration in an infant initially suspected to have bacterial sepsis for whom bacterial culture results are negative; and (4) unexplained encephalitis in a neonate with unremitting seizures. Whether or not antiviral therapy is initiated under these circumstances, specimens obtained from the nose, eyes, mouth, pharynx, rectum, CSF, and buffy coat should be submitted for viral culture. Specimens of CSF and peripheral blood mononuclear cells also should be tested for HSV DNA by PCR.

Compromised Hosts

Acyclovir is the drug of choice for management of progressive mucocutaneous HSV in patients with compromised immune function. Therapy speeds healing of localized lesions and reduces morbidity and mortality caused by visceral dissemination.[116] Emergence of HSV strains resistant to acyclovir is more common in the management of HSV infections in immunocompromised hosts than in normal hosts.[117] The prevalence of acyclovir-resistant strains in immunocompromised hosts varies according to the type and degree of immunosuppression, but generally ranges between 5% and 10%.[118] HSV strains resistant to both acyclovir and foscarnet, isolated from patients in whom sequential therapy with the two drugs failed, have been reported.[119]

PREVENTION

A number of candidate HSV vaccines have been developed from extracts of infected cells or recombinant virus glycoproteins; newer vaccine approaches include DNA-based vaccines and replication-impaired viruses.[120–122] To date, no tested vaccine effectively prevents infection or establishment of latency; thus, prevention of HSV infection depends on reducing transmission and reactivation. Prevention of transmission of genital HSV infection would require sexual abstinence, because most infections are subclinical; consistent condom use provides some protection.

Reduction in the vertical transmission of HSV could be accomplished by reducing maternal infections or the likelihood of transmission to the neonate. Although prophylactic acyclovir reduces clinical HSV reactivation, it does not eliminate asymptomatic viral shedding.[107] Furthermore, most women infected with HSV-2 have no history of genital herpes. Therefore, it is unlikely that this method will be a practical approach to reducing the risk of infection of neonates born to previously infected mothers. Preventing the acquisition of new infections during pregnancy is complicated by the high proportion of genital infections transmitted from partners not known to be infected with HSV-2.

Strategies to identify women who are shedding virus at parturition and thereby prevent transmission by cesarean delivery have been confounded by the need to recognize clinical lesions before progression of labor. Such strategies are further frustrated by the occurrence of asymptomatic viral shedding, even in primary episodes. Use of prenatal cultures fails to predict shedding of virus at delivery and is not recommended.[123]

Long-term suppressive therapy with acyclovir reduces reactivation of latent genital and orolabial HSV infections.[100,107] Once-daily suppressive valacyclovir therapy, administered to the infected partner of immunocompetent, heterosexual, monogamous couples, discordant for HSV-2 infection, has been shown to reduce transmission of HSV to the uninfected partner.[124] Prophylactic acyclovir also has been used successfully in immunocompromised hosts, including bone marrow and renal transplant recipients, patients with cancer, and other immunodeficient patients. In these immunocompromised hosts, the frequency of

HSV reactivation typically is reduced from 60% to 80% among placebo recipients to 0% to 10% among acyclovir recipients.[125] Prophylactic antiviral therapy is not recommended at this time for neonates inadvertently exposed to HSV at delivery.[27] Availability of rapid virus identification and specific serologic tests could inform a graded approach in the future. The American Academy of Pediatrics has given guidance for management of the neonate in specific circumstances of maternal HSV status and delivery.[126] The neonate with HSV infection should be hospitalized and managed with contact precautions. Relapse of HSV at sites in skin, eyes, mouth, and CNS can occur after cessation of treatment in the neonate; the rate of recurrence of skin vesicles is 60% to 80%, with 1 to 12 recurrences in the first year. Orally administered acyclovir for 6 months after the initial infection appears to reduce the likelihood of cutaneous recurrences.[115]

Key Points. Diagnosis and Management of Perinatal HSV Infections

EPIDEMIOLOGY
- Rate of neonatal infection ranges from 8 to 60 per 100,000 live births in the U.S.
- Infections acquired in utero (congenital) are uncommon, representing less that 5% of all cases
- Most infections result from exposure at delivery to mothers shedding virus in the absence of symptoms
- Maternal primary infections are associated with a higher neonatal attack rate than maternal reactivated infections

CLINICAL FEATURES
- Three classic presentations, each occurring with similar frequency:
  - skin/eye/mucous membrane infection characterized by skin vesicles at sites of trauma, mucosal lesions, and conjunctivitis
  - disseminated infection resembling bacterial sepsis with shock, liver failure, bleeding, and respiratory failure
  - central nervous system infection with irritability, lethargy; typified by seizures

- Usual age of onset, 5 to 21 days; disseminated infection typically is earlier; CNS infection typically is later
- High (>70%) untreated mortality rate
- With antiviral therapy: reduced mortality rate but substantial morbidity, except for SEM infection

DIAGNOSIS
- DFA and culture of skin lesions
- Viral cultures of specimens obtained from skin, mucosal surfaces, buffy coat, and CSF
- CSF analysis, including HSV PCR
- EEG and brain MRI

TREATMENT
- Intravenously administered acyclovir, 60 mg/kg/day in 3 divided doses for 14 (SEM infection) to 21 (disseminated and CNS infection) days

---

205 Varicella-Zoster Virus
Ann M. Arvin

Varicella-zoster virus (VZV) is an alphaherpesvirus that is related most closely to herpes simplex virus (HSV). Primary infection with VZV causes varicella, commonly called *chickenpox*. VZV establishes latent infection in dorsal root ganglia and can reactivate to cause herpes zoster, often referred to as *shingles*. The double-stranded DNA genome of the virus encodes more than 70 proteins, including regulatory and virion structural proteins as well as envelope glycoproteins.[1,2] VZV replication usually involves synthesis of a viral thymidine kinase, making the virus susceptible to inhibition by acyclovir and related antiviral agents.

PATHOGENESIS

The pathogenesis of primary VZV infection, shown in Figure 205-1, begins with mucosal inoculation by virus transferred via the respiratory route or by direct contact with skin lesions of patients with varicella or herpes zoster. T lymphocytes from tonsils are highly susceptible to VZV infection. Since tonsillar crypts are lined with

epithelial cells, VZV is presumed to gain access to lymphocytes in lymphoid tissues of the oropharynx, initiating a cell-associated viremia. Studies in the SCID-hu mouse model of VZV pathogenesis show that the virus is transported by infected human T lymphocytes to skin xenografts within 24 hours. These experiments indicate that VZV reaches skin early but viral replication is countered by an innate antiviral response, characterized by interferon-α/β production.[3] The 10- to 21-day incubation period appears to be the interval required for VZV to overcome this vigorous innate epidermal cell response (see Figure 205-1). VZV viremia then is enhanced as uninfected T lymphocytes traffic through infected skin; replication in reticuloendothelial tissues also may contribute to amplification.[4] VZV is carried back to respiratory mucosal sites during the late incubation period, as is evident from transmission to susceptible contacts exposed 24 to 48 hours before the appearance of cutaneous lesions in the index case.[5] The release of infectious virus into respiratory droplets is a pathogenic characteristic that differentiates VZV from other human herpesviruses. Latent

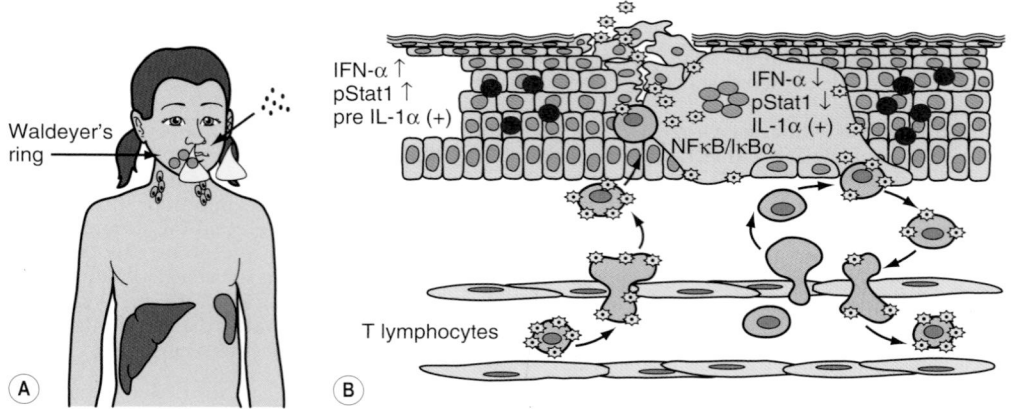

Figure 205-1. Modeling the pathogenesis of varicella. **(A)** Primary infection with VZV is initiated by inoculation of respiratory epithelial cells from which the virus gains access to highly permissive T lymphocytes in the tonsillar lymphoid tissues that comprise Waldeyer's ring. During the incubation period, which lasts from 10 to 21 days, the virus is transferred to skin sites of replication and may also replicate in reticuloendothelial organs, e.g., liver and spleen. Replication in epidermal cells causes the characteristic rash of varicella often referred to as *chickenpox.* The virus reaches neurons in sensory ganglia during primary infection, either by the hematogenous route or by anterograde transport along neurons from skin lesions, where it establishes latency. **(B)** The formation of skin lesions that penetrate the skin surfaces requires 10 to 21 days, because cell–cell spread of the virus after T lymphocyte transfer is countered by potent innate antiviral responses of epidermal cells. Uninfected T lymphocytes that traffic through sites of VZV lesion formation may amplify VZV viremia. This well-regulated virus–host interaction in skin enhances opportunities for VZV transmission. IFN-α, interferon-alpha; pStat1, phosphorylated Stat-1; pre IL-1α, pre-interleukin-1α; NF-κB, nuclear factor-κB. (Modified from Cohen J, Straus S, Arvin A. Varicella-zoster virus. In: Fields BN, Knipe DH, Chanock R, et al (eds) Virology, 5th ed. Philadelphia, Lippincott-Raven, 2007, pp 2774–2808.)

infection of cells in dorsal root ganglia appears to be an invariable consequence of primary VZV infection; VZV persists predominantly or exclusively in neurons.[1]

VZV reactivation causes a localized vesicular rash that usually involves the dermatomal distribution of a single sensory nerve. Infectious VZV is present in herpes zoster lesions, but the virus does not appear to be released into respiratory secretions during reactivation. Although subclinical reactivation has been difficult to document, it is likely to occur (unless maintenance of VZV latency is unusually effective compared with that of other herpesviruses).[1] Reinfection with VZV is rare; apparent second episodes of varicella are encountered in clinical practice, but laboratory diagnosis of the first episode usually is lacking, and vesicular rashes in childhood have many possible causes. Immunocompromised patients who have had varicella can have scattered cutaneous lesions suggesting reinfection, but most of these cases probably represent generalized atypical reactivation of latent virus without limitation to a dermatomal distribution.

Primary VZV infection elicits immunoglobulin (Ig) G, IgM, and IgA antibodies directed against viral proteins.[6,7] Antibodies to VZV proteins have neutralizing activity and mediate destruction of infected cells by antibody-mediated cellular cytotoxicity. However, intact cellular immunity appears to be critical for the host to terminate viremia and virus replication at localized cutaneous sites.[8] Children with untreated agammaglobulinemia generally have uncomplicated varicella, whereas those with primary cell-mediated immunodeficiency diseases often die. Among children with malignancy, failure to acquire T lymphocytes that recognize VZV antigens correlates with persistent viremia and a high risk of visceral dissemination.[1] Early nonspecific immunity, such as natural killer cell cytotoxicity and the induction of interferon-α production, also may be beneficial; exogenous interferon-α has been shown to modify the severity of varicella in immunocompromised children.[9]

Primary VZV infection elicits memory T lymphocytes that exhibit helper and cytotoxic activity as well as continued production of specific antibodies. Immune subjects also have delayed-type hypersensitivity responses to VZV skin test antigens. Persistent VZV immunity may be maintained by periodic re-exposure to the virus during annual epidemics or by repeated antigenic stimulation from subclinical reactivation. Diminished T-lymphocyte recognition of VZV antigens probably accounts for the increased risk of herpes zoster in immunocompromised children.[6] The short interval between primary and recurrent VZV infections in children

with human immunodeficiency virus (HIV) infection and herpes zoster in young children after intrauterine or early postnatal varicella probably reflects poor induction of cell-mediated immunity.[10–13]

EPIDEMIOLOGY

VZV is restricted to the human host and is found worldwide. Before the licensure of varicella vaccine, an estimated 4 million cases of varicella occurred annually in the United States, which is equivalent to the annual birth cohort. In temperate climates, 90% to 95% of individuals acquire VZV in childhood as a result of annual varicella epidemics that occur during the late winter and spring. Adults with herpes zoster provide a continuing source for potential exposures to VZV, causing varicella in susceptible contacts; these sporadic cases of varicella lead to the infection of many more susceptible children because of the relative efficiency of VZV transmission by the respiratory route and high titers of cell-free infectious virus in skin lesions.[1,2] The attack rate for previously uninfected household contacts exposed to varicella is approximately 90%, whereas the transmission rate from less sustained exposures, such as in school classrooms or hospitals, is much less predictable and may be as low as 12% to 33%. For unexplained reasons, the attack rates for varicella are much lower in tropical areas, so more adults remain susceptible. Molecular analyses of viral isolates from various geographic areas do not point to major alterations in the pathogen that could account for variations in geographic prevalence.[14]

Herpes zoster shows no seasonal variation in incidence because it is due to the reactivation of endogenous, latent virus. Herpes zoster is uncommon in children younger than 10 years, occurring in this group at a rate of 0.74 cases, compared with 3.4 cases in 1000 persons per year among the general population.[15] The incidence of herpes zoster is higher among children with prior VZV infection who are immunocompromised.[10] Primary VZV infection acquired in utero or during the first year of life also is associated with an increased risk of herpes zoster in early childhood.[11–13]

Wild-type strains of VZV that cause annual epidemics of varicella do not exhibit changes in virulence, as judged from the clinical severity of primary VZV infections from year to year. The risk of severe or life-threatening primary or recurrent VZV infections appears to depend on host factors rather than alterations of the virus.

VARICELLA

Clinical Manifestations

The incubation period of primary VZV infection is 10 to 21 days; symptoms most commonly begin between 14 and 16 days.[1,2] Varicella often is mild enough to escape diagnosis, but subclinical varicella is rare when exposed, susceptible children are examined prospectively during the period of risk.[16] About half of children have prodromal symptoms, including fever, malaise, anorexia, headache, and, occasionally, mild abdominal pain, for 24 to 48 hours before the appearance of rash. Constitutional symptoms are prominent during the 24 to 72 hours after the first cutaneous lesions develop, but significant respiratory or gastrointestinal symptoms are unusual. Temperature elevation usually is moderate, ranging from 37.8°C to 38.8°C, but can be as high as 41.1°C.

Varicella lesions appear first on the scalp, face, or trunk. The initial exanthem consists of erythematous macules that evolve to form clear, fluid-filled vesicles; vesicles with surrounding irregular margin of erythema are often described as resembling "dewdrop on a rose petal" (Figure 205-2). Varicella lesions in their early stages usually are pruritic. After 24 to 48 hours, fluid becomes cloudy, and some lesions exhibit characteristic umbilication as crusting begins. As initial lesions begin to resolve, new crops form on the trunk and then the extremities. Late lesions may disappear without progressing to vesicle formation. Crusts are sloughed during the final phase as new epithelium is generated beneath the lesion site. Vesicles or small ulcers on mucous membranes of the oropharynx, conjunctivae, and vagina are common.

In otherwise healthy children, new lesions appear for 1 to 7 days. In a prospective study of 521 children, more than half demonstrated new lesions for 3 to 6 days, whereas only 1 child had new lesions for 7 days.[16] The total number of varicella lesions ranged from 12 to 1968 per child, with most children having <300 lesions. The duration of fever and new lesion formation is likely to be longer among children who have varicella after household exposure.[16,17] The severity of the illness also increases with increasing age. Pre-existing skin trauma, such as eczema or trauma acquired during the incubation period (e.g., sunburn or surgery), exacerbates the exanthem at those sites. Extensive scarring is unusual, but hypopigmentation often persists for several weeks, especially in older children or children with darker skin. A single, shallow scar on the forehead is a common consequence of varicella because the initial lesions, which often occur along the hairline or eyebrow, involve deeper layers of the skin.

Varicella eruption must be distinguished from vesicular rashes associated with infections caused by other common pathogens, such as enterovirus or *Staphylococcus aureus*, or from rashes due to drug reactions, contact dermatitis, or insect bites. Early skin lesions may be particularly difficult to recognize clinically.

Complications in Healthy Children

Bacterial Infections

Secondary bacterial infections constitute the most common cause of morbidity in otherwise healthy children.[18-26] *S. aureus* and *Streptococcus pyogenes* are usual pathogens (see Figure 118-3). "Impetigo" often is diagnosed but is difficult to differentiate from larger lesions caused by the virus alone. Bullous varicella can represent an unusual presentation of cutaneous lesions caused directly by VZV or can be due to bacterial superinfection. Cellulitis is the most common diagnosis, but lymphadenitis and subcutaneous abscesses also occur. Cellulitis of the soft tissues of the neck can result in severe edema that compromises the airway. Life-threatening varicella gangrenosa, rare in the last quarter-century, increased with the resurgence of exotoxin A-producing *S. pyogenes*. Typically, the skin around a single varicella lesion, usually on the trunk or an extremity, becomes erythematous, warm, and painful. The erythematous area enlarges rapidly over a few hours, often turning a dusky, dark-red color, and extensive edema develops in the soft tissue around the lesion, producing necrotizing fasciitis (Figure 205-3). Varicella lesions provide a portal of entry occasionally resulting in transient bacteremia or septicemia associated with high fever, cardiovascular collapse, and disseminated intravascular coagulopathy. Varicella can be complicated by methicillin-resistant *S. aureus*.[27] Hematogenous spread of the bacteria can result in focal infection, including pneumonia, arthritis, and osteomyelitis.

Neurologic Complications

Neurologic complications are the second most common indication for hospitalization of immunocompetent children with varicella.[19-29] Varicella accounted for 13% of reported encephalitis cases of known etiology in the U.S. between 1972 and 1977.[24] The incidence of central nervous system morbidity is highest among patients younger than 5 and older than 20 years.[20,26] Neurologic manifestations include cerebellar disease as well as encephalitis, with some overlap of signs occurring in individual patients. Meningoencephalitis manifests as sudden onset of seizures,

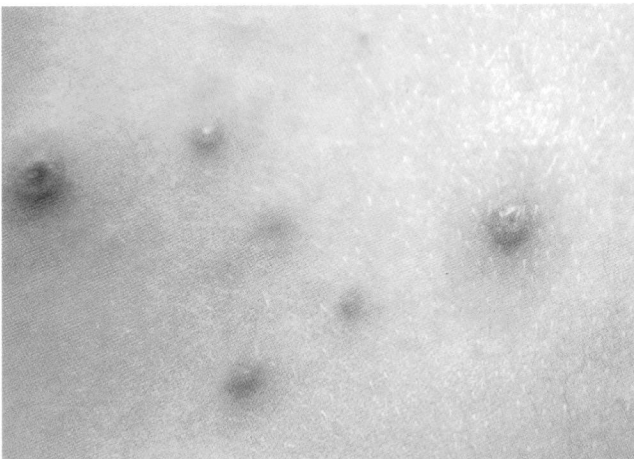

Figure 205-2. Early varicella lesions in various stages, including "dewdrop on a rose petal".

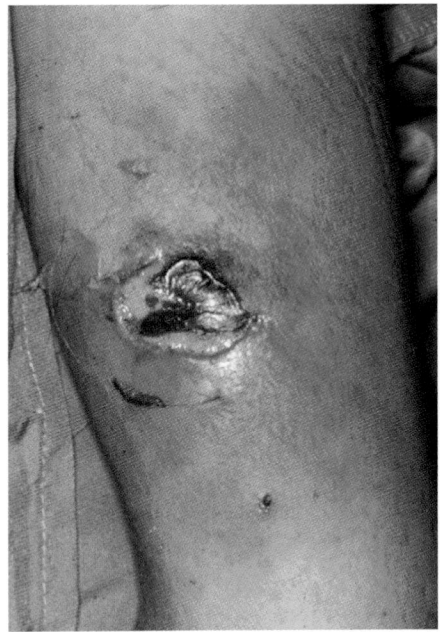

Figure 205-3. Group A streptococcal necrotizing fasciitis complicating otherwise mild varicella. (Courtesy of J.H. Brien©.)

diminished level of consciousness, nuchal rigidity, and extensor plantar reflexes. Some patients have meningitis only, without seizures or altered consciousness. Cerebellar ataxia is characterized by a more gradual evolution of gait disturbance, nystagmus, and slurred speech. Signs of varicella encephalitis and of cerebellar ataxia have been described during the incubation period and after resolution of cutaneous disease, but in most cases the neurologic symptoms occur between 2 and 6 days after the onset of the rash.[7,28,29] These neurologic syndromes may have a vasculitic or immune-mediated pathogenesis. Although fatal cases are reported, the recovery from VZV-related encephalitic symptoms often is rapid, occurring within 24 to 72 hours; chronic neurologic sequelae are rare, although seizures recur and neurologic deficits persist in some cases. Symptoms of cerebellar ataxia last for several days and sometimes weeks, but resolution is almost always complete.

Reye syndrome can accompany varicella, but is rare now that salicylates are known to be contraindicated in children with varicella.[30] Transverse myelitis has been described as a complication of varicella; Guillain–Barré syndrome is reported rarely.

Other Complications

In a prospective study of healthy children with varicella, 49% had mild elevations of aspartate aminotransferase (AST) (32 to 50 IU/L) and 28% had AST concentrations >50 IU/L. Varicella hepatitis usually is subclinical, although some children with the highest elevations of AST (range, 200 to 800 IU/L) have severe vomiting.[31] These cases can be differentiated from stage I Reye syndrome only by liver biopsy.

Acute thrombocytopenia, associated with petechiae and purpuric skin lesions, hemorrhage into the varicella vesicles, epistaxis, hematuria, and gastrointestinal bleeding, is a reported complication of varicella.[1] Clinical manifestations usually are brief, but platelet counts can remain low for days to weeks. Some patients have postinfectious thrombocytopenia beginning more than 1 or 2 weeks after varicella; bleeding complications persist for an average of 5 weeks. Purpura fulminans, due to arterial thrombosis, is a rare but life-threatening complication of varicella.

Renal complications of primary VZV infection are rare.[1] Nephritis with hematuria, diffuse edema, and hypertension is described within 3 weeks after varicella exanthem; many of these cases represent poststreptococcal glomerulonephritis. Nephrotic syndrome and hemolytic uremic syndrome have been reported in a few children with varicella. Viral arthritis is an infrequent complication of varicella, but VZV has been isolated from joint fluid; arthritis resolves spontaneously within 3 to 5 days and is not associated with residual joint disease. Other rare complications of varicella are myocarditis, pericarditis, pancreatitis, and orchitis. Many children have vesicular lesions on the eyelids and conjunctivae, but serious ocular complications of varicella are unusual.

Complications in High-Risk Populations

Progressive disease caused by primary VZV infection occurs in older adolescents and adults, immunocompromised children, pregnant women, and neonates.

Adolescents and Adults

Clinically significant varicella pneumonia is rare in children, but otherwise healthy adults are more susceptible, a factor that accounts for most of the increased morbidity and mortality caused by primary VZV infection in this age group.[26,32,33] VZV pneumonia is associated with cough and dyspnea usually beginning within 1 to 6 days (average 3 days) after the onset of the rash.[34,35] Patients have cough, with or without cyanosis, pleuritic chest pain, and hemoptysis. Hypoxemia often is more severe than is suggested by the physical findings. The chest radiograph may be normal or may show diffuse bilateral infiltrates with small nodular densities, especially in the perihilar area. Varicella pneumonia often is transient, resolving completely within 24 to 72 hours, but in severe cases, interstitial pneumonia can progress rapidly to respiratory failure.

Pregnancy

Varicella acquired during pregnancy can have severe consequences for both the mother and the fetus. Because most adults born in the U.S. are immune, the incidence of maternal varicella is low, affecting 0.7 in 1000 women in a study of 30,000 pregnancies in the 1960s.[36] Varicella pneumonia is the major cause of maternal morbidity and mortality.[37-39] Spontaneous abortion, fetal demise, and premature delivery can occur, although the frequency of these complications is low.[37-40]

In rare instances, maternal varicella results in congenital varicella syndrome (Box 205-1).[2] The highest risk of severe embryopathy accompanies varicella acquired during the first 20 weeks of gestation and is estimated to occur in fewer than 2% of cases of maternal varicella.[2,36-41] Infants affected after maternal varicella contracted later in pregnancy are described, but defects are limited to cutaneous scarring, diminished limb growth, or unilateral ocular defects.[41] The most striking anomalies of the congenital varicella syndrome are unusual cutaneous defects with cicatricial skin scars, atrophy of an extremity, and evidence of damage to the autonomic nervous system. Many affected infants have microcephaly and cortical atrophy secondary to probable intrauterine VZV encephalitis; seizures and mental retardation are common sequelae. Chorioretinitis, microphthalmia, and cataracts also occur. Dysfunction of the autonomic nervous system produces neurogenic bladder, hydroureter, hydronephrosis, and severe gastroesophageal reflux with recurrent aspiration pneumonia.[42] Limb anomalies and other sequelae of intrauterine varicella can be detectable with fetal ultrasonography.[43] Some infants who are asymptomatic at birth have been infected in utero, as shown by VZV-specific immunity or the occurrence of herpes zoster in infancy, without any intervening episode of varicella. Although a few cases of fetal abnormalities have been reported after maternal herpes zoster, clinical evidence indicates that recurrent VZV infection does not cause the congenital varicella syndrome or neonatal varicella.

When maternal varicella occurs during the last few days of gestation, the infant is at risk for neonatal varicella, with an attack rate

---

BOX 205-1. Clinical Manifestations of the Congenital Varicella Syndrome

SKIN

Cutaneous defects
Cicatricial scars
Hypopigmentation
Bullous lesions

EXTREMITIES

Hypoplastic limb
Muscular atrophy and denervation
Joint abnormalities
Absent or malformed digits

EYE

Chorioretinitis
Microphthalmia
Anisocoria

CENTRAL NERVOUS SYSTEM

Intrauterine encephalitis with cortical atrophy
Seizures
Mental retardation

URINARY TRACT

Hydronephrosis/hydroureter

GASTROINTESTINAL TRACT

Esophageal dilation/reflux

of approximately 20%.[43,44] Infants who are born at least 5 days after the onset of varicella in the mother are not at high risk; these infants have lesions at birth or within the first 5 days of life but are protected from severe disease because the interval between maternal infection and delivery permits transplacental transfer of maternal IgG antibodies to VZV. Those who are born within 4 days after or 2 days before the onset of maternal varicella can exhibit progressive varicella, with an untreated mortality rate of 30%. Exposure of an infant to nonmaternal contacts with varicella rarely causes varicella in the infant because most infants are born to seropositive mothers. Rare cases of postnatally acquired varicella that have occurred in infants younger than 2 months who were born to seronegative mothers do not suggest a severe course, but careful observation of such infants is warranted. Occasionally, infants born to immune mothers who have close household exposure to varicella have mild varicella or subclinical infection that manifests as herpes zoster later in childhood.[11-13]

Malignancy

Without effective antiviral drugs, 32% to 50% of children with lymphoproliferative malignancies or solid tumors experience visceral dissemination; varicella pneumonia occurs in 20% of cases of varicella, and the mortality rates range from 7% to 17%.[45-48] Progressive disease is characterized by a prolonged period of new lesion formation, pneumonia, hepatitis, encephalitis, and disseminated intravascular coagulopathy.[1,2] The risk of progressive varicella is highest if chemotherapy is given during the incubation period, especially within 5 days before the appearance of the rash, and when the absolute lymphocyte count is <500 cells/mm³ at the onset of the rash. Pneumonia is the most common life-threatening complication; in one large series, all varicella-related deaths occurred within 3 days after the diagnosis of varicella pneumonia.[48] Hemorrhage into cutaneous lesions, or severe abdominal or back pain is associated with potentially life-threatening varicella. Some patients experience progressive encephalitis with coma, but varicella encephalitis is rarely the immediate cause of death among immunocompromised patients. The syndrome of inappropriate secretion of antidiuretic hormone can accompany disseminated varicella with or without clinical encephalitis. Disseminated VZV infection in children with cancer also can be associated with pancreatitis, necrotizing splenitis, esophagitis, and enterocolitis.

Other Immunodeficiency States

Children who acquire varicella after organ transplantation are at risk of progressive VZV infection unless they receive antiviral therapy.[48-52] Thrombocytopenia and hepatitis are the major clinical complications in renal transplant recipients. Children receiving long-term, low-dose corticosteroid therapy for asthma usually are not at risk of serious varicella. However, fatal varicella is described in patients who receive higher doses of prednisone, especially during the incubation period.[53] Untreated varicella is severe or fatal in children with defects of T-lymphocyte function, including severe combined immunodeficiency, cartilage hair hypoplasia–short-limbed dwarfism, Wiskott–Aldrich syndrome, and ataxia telangiectasia.[6] Unusual clinical findings in varicella, including lesions that develop a unique hyperkeratotic appearance and formation of new lesions for weeks or months, have been described in children with HIV infection, but varicella does not appear to accelerate the progression of HIV disease.[54-57]

HERPES ZOSTER

Clinical Manifestations

Herpes zoster is unusual in children. When it occurs, the cutaneous eruption is mild, and symptoms of acute neuritis are minimal or absent. Herpes zoster is characterized by vesicular lesions clustered unilaterally in the dermatomal distribution of one or more adjacent sensory nerves (Figure 205-4). Discrete vesicles resembling varicella lesions appear first and then enlarge and coalesce

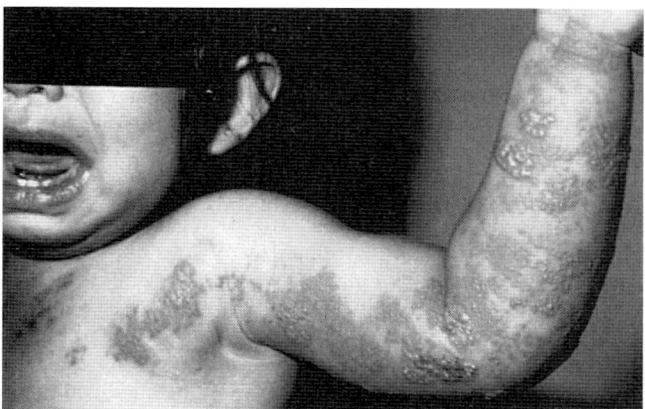

Figure 205-4. Characteristic unilateral dermatomal distribution of discrete and coalescent vesicles in a 10-month-old child with herpes zoster.

as the exanthem evolves. The rash is preceded or accompanied by localized pain, hyperesthesias, and pruritus. In healthy individuals, formation of new lesions in the primary dermatome stops within 3 to 7 days, and crusting occurs within 2 weeks. VZV reactivation without skin lesions (zoster sine herpete) has been diagnosed in adults with idiopathic facial palsy or other pain syndromes, but this entity rarely occurs in children.

Complications

Healthy children are not at risk for the complication of postherpetic neuralgia, which causes debilitating chronic pain in adults.[1] Complications of herpes zoster involving cranial nerves include conjunctivitis, dendritic keratitis (Figure 205-5), anterior uveitis, iridocyclitis, retinitis, and facial palsies.[58] Neurogenic bladder dysfunction or ileus with intestinal obstruction can accompany lumbosacral herpes zoster. Transverse myelitis is a rare, severe complication that produces transient or persistent paralysis and sensory deficits.

Herpes zoster in immunocompromised children can result in severe local dermatomal infection and visceral dissemination.[48] Cutaneous lesions outside the primary dermatome or an adjacent dermatome indicate that the patient has VZV viremia and provide evidence of risk for visceral dissemination. Hematogenous spread of reactivated VZV can cause pneumonia, hepatitis, encephalitis, and disseminated intravascular coagulopathy. Atypical nonlocalized herpes zoster occurs in severely immunocompromised patients, especially bone marrow transplant recipients; the widely scattered vesicular lesions cannot be distinguished from varicella.

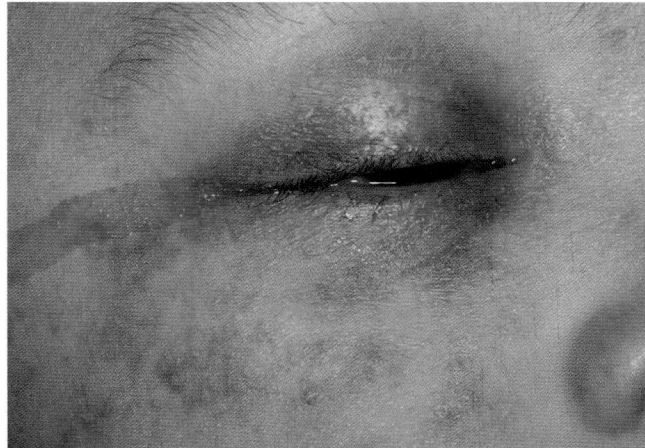

Figure 205-5. Zoster with keratitis in an otherwise healthy child. (Courtesy of J.H. Brien©.)

Severely immunocompromised children, particularly those with HIV infection, can have unusual chronic or relapsing cutaneous disease, retinitis, and central nervous system infections that occur without associated cutaneous disease or that progress after resolution of signs of herpes zoster.[54–57] Unusual neurologic complications, such as multifocal leukoencephalopathy, are described in patients with prolonged, severe immunosuppression.

LABORATORY FINDINGS AND DIAGNOSIS

Laboratory evaluation is not necessary for management of previously healthy children with varicella. Abnormal laboratory values are common. The total white blood cell count often is decreased during the first 72 hours of rash, followed by lymphocytosis; lymphoblasts, and prolymphocytes can be noted in peripheral blood.[6] Slight to moderate abnormalities of serum hepatic enzyme values are common. The cerebrospinal fluid (CSF) in patients with neurologic complications of varicella usually shows a mild lymphocytic pleocytosis with fewer than 100 cells/mm³ and a slight to moderate elevation of protein (<200 mg/dL); glucose concentration is usually normal. CSF pleocytosis and protein concentrations are higher in patients with encephalitis than in those with cerebellar disease.[28] Patients with uncomplicated herpes zoster can have CSF pleocytosis consisting predominantly of mononuclear cells as well as elevated protein concentration.

In contrast to the disease in healthy children, specific diagnosis of VZV often is important to guide decisions about antiviral therapy when varicella or herpes zoster is suspected in immunocompromised children. The definitive diagnosis of VZV infection requires the recovery of infectious virus with the use of tissue culture methods.[7] However, VZV is difficult to isolate in tissue culture, and the time to viral identification is 3 to 7 days; therefore, viral cultures primarily serve to confirm diagnoses made with rapid antigen detection methods. Rapid diagnosis of cutaneous VZV infection is accomplished by obtaining epithelial cells from the base of a newly formed vesicle and staining the specimen with immunohistochemical reagents that detect viral proteins in infected cells.[7] Cytologic methods can be used to detect multinucleated giant cells in lesion specimens or tissue sections, but false-negative results are common, and these methods do not differentiate VZV from HSV. Enzyme immunoassay methods can be used to detect VZV antigens in solubilized preparations of cells and vesicle fluid from cutaneous VZV lesions.

VZV can be detected in clinical specimens through in situ hybridization or polymerase chain reaction (PCR) testing, but must be done by a laboratory with experience using these methods.[59,60] The use of PCR to diagnose unusual manifestations of VZV unassociated with cutaneous lesions, or for assessing fetal risk after maternal varicella during pregnancy, is particularly problematic for quality control reasons. In the case of fetal exposures, interpretation of results is difficult because infection can occur without damaging the fetus.[37,38,40]

Antibodies are not present in serum during most of the incubation period, but can be measured in low concentrations at the time of onset of the varicella exanthem. IgG anti-VZV is detectable in almost all patients within 3 days and exhibits a marked increase during convalescence. IgG anti-VZV persists for life after primary infection. Many laboratory methods can be used to detect IgG anti-VZV, but serologic diagnosis is rarely useful because it is retrospective and available methods have limitations in sensitivity. Testing for IgM anti-VZV should not be used for clinical diagnosis because false-positive and false-negative results are unavoidable with all commercially available methods. Assays for IgG antibodies to VZV are valuable: to determine the immune status of individuals whose clinical history of varicella is unknown or equivocal; to evaluate the risk of primary VZV infection in exposed individuals or the risk of reactivation in patients who are receiving immunosuppressive therapy; and to guide decisions about the need for varicella immunization.[61,62]

Immunofluorescence testing performed with unfixed, VZV-infected cells is a highly sensitive method for detecting IgG anti-VZV, but involves complex methodology; immunofluorescence

testing using fixed cells is subject to false-positive interpretation. Commercial enzyme immunoassay methods to assess VZV antibodies usually have a high degree of specificity, generating few false-positive results, but they are not as sensitive as research methods; from 10% to 15% of individuals who are immune to VZV may be identified as susceptible. Latex agglutination methods are somewhat more sensitive and specific than enzyme immunoassay, providing a simple and rapid alternative for detecting IgG anti-VZV.[63,64] A positive history of varicella predicts immunity in >95% of individuals; likelihood of immunity in an adult with a negative history also is high, unless the patient's childhood was spent in an area such as the tropics, where varicella is less common. Serologic testing after varicella vaccination has limited value because false-negative results may be even more common with commercially available serologic methods than is observed in naturally immune individuals.

TREATMENT

Acyclovir is used most commonly to treat varicella and herpes zoster (Box 205-2).[17,45,46,65] Famciclovir and valacyclovir, nucleoside analogues that are structurally similar to acyclovir, are

---

BOX 205-2. Use of Acyclovir for the Treatment of Varicella

ACYCLOVIR INDICATED

Patients

Malignancy, bone marrow or organ transplantation, high-dose steroid therapy
Congenital T-lymphocyte immunodeficiencies
Human immunodeficiency virus infection
Neonatal varicella after maternal varicella beginning within 5 days before or 2 days after delivery
Associated pneumonia or encephalitis

Administration

Initiate as soon as possible after initial lesions appear
Intravenous route[a]

Dosage

<1 year old: 30 mg/kg/day divided into 8-hourly doses given as 1-hour infusion
>1 year old: 1.5 g/m²/day divided into 8-hourly doses given as 1-hour infusion
Duration: 7 days or until no new lesions have appeared for 48 hours

ACYCLOVIR OPTIONAL

Patients

Chronic cutaneous disorders
Chronic diseases that may be exacerbated by acute VZV infection, such as cystic fibrosis or other pulmonary disorders, diabetes mellitus, or disorders requiring chronic salicylate therapy or intermittent corticosteroid therapy
Otherwise healthy children, especially those >12 years old or secondary household contacts

Administration

Initiate within 24 hours after the initial lesions appear
Oral route

Dosage

80 mg/kg/day divided into 4 doses (maximum 800 mg/dose)
Duration: 5 days

[a]Selected patients who are considered at relatively low risk for varicella-zoster virus (VZV) dissemination can be treated with oral acyclovir and carefully monitored for progression.

absorbed more efficiently after oral administration. These drugs have been licensed for treatment of herpes zoster in adults, but experience in children is limited.[65]

Acyclovir is metabolized to the triphosphate form within VZV-infected cells; the phosphorylated compound functions as a competitive inhibitor and chain terminator of viral DNA polymerase. The antiviral activity of acyclovir is lower against VZV than against HSV. The relatively lower sensitivity of VZV to acyclovir has clinical significance, because ensuring that plasma concentrations are several-fold higher than in vitro inhibitory concentrations for most VZV isolates requires the use of high doses. Prolonged exposure of VZV isolates to acyclovir in vitro selects for thymidine kinase-negative mutants. Resistant strains of VZV have been recovered from severely immunocompromised patients who have been treated with acyclovir for repeated or chronic episodes of VZV infection.[65]

Varicella

Healthy Children and Adolescents

Placebo-controlled clinical studies show that orally administered acyclovir diminishes the clinical symptoms of varicella in otherwise healthy children, adolescents, and adults when administered within 24 hours after the appearance of the initial cutaneous lesions.[17,66-68] In a study in which healthy children 2 to 12 years old were treated with 80 mg/kg per day (20 mg/kg per dose 4 times a day; maximum 800 mg/dose) of acyclovir administered orally for 5 days, reductions in fever, pruritus, number of days of new lesion formation, and total number of cutaneous lesions were observed.[17] Acyclovir recipients also had fewer lesions that progressed from the maculopapular to the vesicular stage. Among younger children, immediate acyclovir therapy converted all cases of varicella to the mildest form of illness that might be observed without treatment, in which fever and new lesion formation continue for 3 days or less and the total number of cutaneous lesions is fewer than 300.[17] No effect on the risk of secondary bacterial infection or other serious sequelae of varicella was documented; the overall frequency of these complications was low.

The impact of orally administered acyclovir on varicella in adolescents (age 13 to 18 years) and in young adults was similar to that observed in young children. However, the effects have more clinical relevance because varicella is more severe among untreated patients in these older age groups.[67] Adolescents in the treated group were significantly less likely to have residual hypopigmented skin lesions at 4 weeks, suggesting that drug therapy minimized the spread of virus to cells deeper in the dermis. Although study groups were not large enough to document it, the evidence of diminished viremia and cutaneous viral replication supports the assumption that oral acyclovir would reduce the risk of varicella pneumonia in otherwise healthy adults. In adults, as in young children, acyclovir must be given within 24 hours after initial lesions to have demonstrable clinical efficacy.[32] All patients with varicella pneumonia should receive acyclovir intravenously.

Oral acyclovir is licensed for the treatment of varicella in healthy children and adults. Acyclovir therapy does not have a detrimental effect on the host response to VZV.[17,68] The American Academy of Pediatrics recommends that acyclovir be considered for patients with varicella who are 12 years or older, who have chronic cutaneous or pulmonary diseases requiring long-term salicylate therapy, or who are being treated with short or intermittent courses of corticosteroids or aerosolized corticosteroids.[69]

Immunocompromised Patients

Acyclovir therapy diminishes the clinical severity of varicella in immunocompromised children by terminating cell-associated viremia in spite of impaired host response.[70,71] Early antiviral therapy prevents progressive varicella and visceral dissemination; mortality is decreased particularly because the risk of varicella pneumonia is reduced. When acyclovir was given intravenously to children with malignancy in a placebo-controlled trial, the incidence of varicella pneumonia was decreased from 45% to 0.[72] The dosage of acyclovir for varicella in high-risk patients is 1.5 g/m² per day, administered intravenously in 3 divided doses for 7 days.

The optimal use of acyclovir in immunocompromised children with varicella requires initiation of treatment within the first 24 to 72 hours after the onset of rash. Intravenous administration should be started immediately if the patient has signs of pneumonia, hepatitis, thrombocytopenia, or encephalitis. Waiting to initiate treatment until prolonged new lesion formation has been documented is inappropriate, because visceral dissemination occurs during the same period. In addition to preventing life-threatening dissemination, early acyclovir therapy can be expected to minimize cutaneous disease, possibly reducing the risk of secondary bacterial infections. Oral administration of acyclovir, famciclovir, or valacyclovir has not been evaluated in clinical trials among high-risk children. The use of these agents should be considered only in selected patients with minimal immunosuppression and requires careful follow-up during the illness.

Herpes Zoster

Acyclovir has been shown to be effective for the treatment of herpes zoster in healthy and immunocompromised patients participating in placebo-controlled trials.[65,70] For patients who are at high risk for disseminated disease, the dose of acyclovir is 1.5 g/m² per day or 30 mg/kg per day divided into doses every 8 hours and given intravenously. Acyclovir is given for a total of 7 days or for 2 days after the cessation of new lesion formation, whichever is longer. Acyclovir therapy initiated within 72 hours after the onset of VZV reactivation reduces the duration of new lesion formation to only about 3 days rather than 1 week or longer. Antiviral treatment is associated with earlier cessation of acute pain and crusting as well as complete healing by 2 to 3 weeks. Although early acyclovir treatment is likely to produce the best results, clinical benefit is observed even when therapy is delayed for more than 3 days in immunocompromised patients. Relapse of herpes zoster is a clinical problem in some immunocompromised patients, but most patients show response to treatment with a second course of acyclovir. Oral acyclovir administration for herpes zoster in high-risk patients is reserved for patients who are considered to be at low risk for visceral dissemination. Famciclovir and valacyclovir are effective oral agents for herpes zoster.[71,73] Ganciclovir has in vitro activity against VZV that is equivalent to acyclovir but is more toxic. Foscarnet is the drug of choice for the treatment of infections due to acyclovir-resistant VZV.[74]

PREVENTION

Preventing the transmission of VZV to susceptible individuals is difficult because infected individuals are contagious for 24 to 48 hours before the onset of clinical signs of varicella. For example, restrictions on attendance do not alter the course of varicella epidemics in schools.[75] Infection control practices, including caring for infected patients in isolation rooms with filtered air systems, are essential in hospitals that care for immunocompromised children. Filtration is necessary because VZV has been transmitted to hospitalized patients via airflow systems and VZV can be detected in air samples by PCR testing.[76-78] Susceptible healthcare personnel (HCP) who have had a close exposure to varicella should not care for high-risk patients during the incubation period, because secondary cases have occurred in this clinical setting. Similar precautions should be taken in vaccinated HCP who have had close exposures; breakthrough varicella is not uncommon in adults although the infection is much less severe. Serologic testing is not helpful in these individuals because breakthrough infection can occur in those with or without detectable IgG anti-VZV.

Passive Antibody Prophylaxis

Varicella-zoster immune globulin (VZIG), which was prepared from high-titer immune human serum, reduced the attack rate for varicella when given just after exposure.[79–82] Breakthrough infections occurred, but the extent of exanthem and risk of varicella pneumonia were diminished. VZIG given after the appearance of varicella rash did not alter the disease process. However, VZIG is no longer available in the U.S.; the alternative preparation, VariZIG, which is an investigational high-titer VZV immune globulin, is available through a new drug expanded access program (FFF Enterprises, Temecula, CA; 24-hour telephone 800-843-7477).[83] Immune globulin intravenous (IGIV, 400 mg/kg) may be given to high-risk patients exposed to varicella as an alternative to VariZIG.[69,83,84]

The decision to administer VariZIG (or IGIV) depends on three factors: (1) the likelihood that the exposed person is susceptible to VZV; (2) the probability that the exposure will result in infection; and (3) the likelihood that VZV infection would be severe or complicated[69] (Box 205-3). VariZIG (or IGIV) should be given to susceptible high-risk patients within 96 hours, and if possible within 48 hours, after a close exposure to an individual with varicella or herpes zoster. Passive antibody prophylaxis is recommended for immunocompromised children, pregnant women, and neonates exposed to mothers with onset of varicella 5 days or less before delivery or within 48 hours after delivery.[42,82] VariZIG (or IGIV) is not indicated for healthy, full-term infants exposed postnatally, including those whose mothers' rash developed more than 48 hours after delivery. If possible, pregnant women should be tested for IgG anti-VZV before passive antibody administration, because many adults with no clinical history of varicella are immune.

The administration of passive antibody prophylaxis does not eliminate the possibility of disease in high-risk patients.[44,82] The incidence of varicella despite VZIG prophylaxis was significantly higher after household exposures. In one study, passive administration of antibody preparations to immunocompromised children lowered the risk of severe varicella significantly, but 11% of the children still experienced pneumonitis.[45] Immunocompromised patients who have received high-dose IGIV (100 to 400 mg/kg) for other indications within 2 to 3 weeks before the exposure can be expected to have serum antibodies to VZV.[84] Because passive antibody titers decline by 2 weeks in some patients and by 4 weeks in most, a second dose should be given if a new exposure occurs more than 2 weeks later. Although the risk of VZV transmission from an individual with herpes zoster is low, close contact between a susceptible high-risk patient and a patient with herpes zoster justifies administration of VariZIG or IGIV. Administration of VZIG can prolong the incubation period to 28 days; whether other passive antibody preparations will have this effect is not known. Passive antibody prophylaxis does not reduce the risk of VZV reactivation in high-risk populations or alter the clinical course of herpes zoster when given after the onset of symptoms.

BOX 205-3. Use of Varicella-Zoster Antibody Post Exposure

PATIENTS AT RISK

- Immunocompromised child with no history of varicella or varicella immunization
- Pregnant woman with no history of varicella and no antibody to VZV[a]
- Newborn infant whose mother had onset of chickenpox within 5 days before or 48 hours after delivery
- Hospitalized preterm infant <28 weeks' gestation or birthweight <1000 g regardless of maternal history of chickenpox or VZV serostatus
- Hospitalized preterm infant ≥28 weeks' gestation whose mother lacks a reliable history of chickenpox, or lacks antibody to VZV

CRITERIA FOR CLOSE EXPOSURE

- Household: residing in the same household
- Playmate/schoolmate/other: face-to-face indoor contact[b]
- Hospital:
  Varicella
  – In the same 2- to 4-bed room, or in an adjacent bed in an open ward
  – Face-to-face contact with a contagious staff member, visitor, or other individual[b]
  Herpes zoster
  – Intimate contact (e.g., touching or hugging) with a person deemed contagious
  – Newborn infant
  – Onset of chickenpox in the mother within 5 days before or 48 hours after delivery (VariZIG is not indicated if mother has herpes zoster)

ADMINISTRATION OF VariZIG

- VariZIG should be administered as soon as possible and at least within 96 hours after exposure
- Dose: 1 vial (125 U)/10 kg body weight (maximum 5 vials) by intramuscular injection. VariZIG cannot be given intravenously. The minimum dose is 125 U.

[a]Serologic testing is recommended if results can be obtained immediately because most adult women with no history of varicella are immune.
[b]Experts differ in estimate of minimum duration of contact to be considered significant, from 5 minutes to >1 hour.
Data from American Academy of Pediatrics. Varicella-zoster infections. In: Pickering LK (ed) 2009 Red Book: Report of the Committee on Infectious Diseases, 28th ed. Elk Grove Village, IL, American Academy of Pediatrics, 2006, p. 717; see also: Centers for Disease Control and Prevention (CDC) A new product (VariZIG) for postexposure prophylaxis of varicella available under an investigational new drug application expanded access protocol. Morb Mortal Wkly Rep 2006;55:209–210. Availability of VariZIG: FFF Enterprises (Temecula, CA); 24 hour telephone: 800-843-7477.

Antiviral Prophylaxis

Although the use of acyclovir as prophylaxis against varicella has been described, it is not recommended because data are limited. In one study, the attack rate after household exposure was reduced to 16% when oral acyclovir (40 or 80 mg/kg/day in 4 divided doses for 7 days) was given to 25 healthy children beginning 7 to 9 days after the onset of varicella in the index case; seroconversion was observed in 84% of the patients.[85] Additional data about acyclovir prophylaxis is needed because of the potential for interference with the host response, which may predispose to early recurrent infection or incomplete protection from subsequent exposures, and enhanced selection of resistant VZV. In most circumstances, the objective of modifying the severity of varicella can be achieved by following the patient closely and giving the drug immediately after the onset of symptoms. However, if follow-up cannot be assured, chemoprophylaxis with acyclovir (80 mg/kg/day divided into 4 doses of 20 mg/kg, for 7 days) may be considered.

Acyclovir prophylaxis reduces the risk of recurrent VZV infection in bone marrow transplant recipients, but VZV reactivation occurs when acyclovir is discontinued. Acyclovir prophylaxis for herpes zoster is not essential because the prompt initiation of acyclovir for the treatment of recurrent VZV infections is effective in reducing morbidity and mortality among immunocompromised patients.[65] In some centers, acyclovir prophylaxis is used in the early months post transplant, and sometimes is continued for 12 months. However prolonged low-dose administration of acyclovir has the potential to result in the emergence of drug-resistant VZV.

Varicella Vaccine

The development and initial clinical evaluation of a live-attenuated varicella vaccine were first reported by Takahashi[86] in 1974. Live-attenuated varicella vaccine, made from the Oka strain, was the first human herpesvirus vaccine licensed for clinical use in several countries. The varicella vaccine was licensed in the U.S. in 1995 and 2 doses are now recommended for universal administration

BOX 205-4. Indications for and Contraindications to the Administration of Live-Attenuated Varicella Vaccine

INDICATIONS

- Age 12 months to 13 years; 2 doses at minimum 3-month interval in patients susceptible according to history[a]
- Age 13 years to young adult; 2 doses, at 4–8-week interval; consider serologic testing to evaluate susceptibility
- Postexposure prophylaxis for unvaccinated people without other evidence of immunity

CONTRAINDICATIONS

- Congenital or acquired immunodeficiency, or systemic immunosuppression therapy, blood dyscrasia
- Leukemia, lymphoma, other malignancy until chemotherapy has been terminated for at least 3 months[b]
- Symptomatic human immunodeficiency virus infection
- High-dose systemic corticosteroids (≥2 mg/kg/day of prednisone for ≥1 month, or 20 mg daily)
- Pregnancy
- Anaphylaxis to neomycin or other vaccine component

PRECAUTIONS

- Intercurrent illness (if more than minor)
- Immunoglobulin or other blood products within 3 to 11 months depending on the product (similar to measles vaccine)
- Salicylates should be avoided for 6 weeks after vaccination[c]
- Thrombocytopenia

[a]One dose is 0.5 mL SC. Simultaneous administration with measles, mumps, rubella (MMR) vaccine is acceptable but requires the use of separate syringes and injection sites. Quadrivalent MMRV is associated with a higher risk of febrile seizures after the first dose.
[b]Vaccination of children with acute lymphocytic leukemia who are in remission and who do not have evidence of immunity to varicella should be undertaken only with expert guidance and with availability of antiviral therapy should complications ensue.
[c]Unless the risk of natural varicella is considered to outweigh the theoretical risk of Reye syndrome.
Committee on Infectious Diseases, American Academy of Pediatrics. Prevention of varicella: recommendations for use of varicella vaccine in children, including a recommendation for a routine 2-dose varicella immunization schedule. Pediatrics 2007;120:221–231.
Marin M, Güris D Chaves SS, et al. Prevention of varicella: recommendations of the Advisory Committee on Immunization Practices (ACIP). MMWR 2007;56(RR-04):1–40.

in early childhood.[87,88] The recommendations and contraindications for its use are outlined in Box 205-4.

Before its licensure, the investigational live-attenuated varicella vaccine (Oka-Merck strain) was administered to more than 7000 children and more than 1600 healthy susceptible adults in the U.S.[89] The vaccine, given as a high titer preparation, induced protection against household exposure, with an efficacy rate of more than 95% in an initial placebo-controlled study.[90–93] Subsequent evaluations of children immunized in the clinical trials demonstrated high seroconversion rates by the glycoprotein enzyme immunoassay (gpEIA) method. Mild breakthrough infections were observed in some children, but disease was modified to <50 cutaneous lesions without associated fever in most cases.[94,95] In 2163 vaccinees evaluated at one center, varicella developed in 114 children at a median of 44 months after immunization; the median number of skin lesions was 18, and the incidence of transmission to other vaccinated children in the household from these cases was 12%.[94] Persistence of VZV immunity over an interval of 1 to 6 years was documented in 94% to 100% of children by means of assays for IgG antibodies and T-lymphocyte proliferation to VZV.[95–97] Sustained protective efficacy of 95% was shown among vaccine recipients from the original placebo-controlled trial, who were monitored for 7 years.[90]

Based on the prelicensure studies, the varicella vaccine was introduced for routine use as a single-dose regimen in children from 12 months to 12 years old. As anticipated, routine varicella immunization in childhood has had a substantial impact on varicella morbidity and mortality in the U.S.[98–101] However, active and passive surveillance studies demonstrate that many vaccinated children develop breakthrough varicella following close exposure and may transmit the virus.[102–105] This postlicensure experience, along with evidence of enhanced immunogenicity and better long-term efficacy, led to the recommendation of a two-dose varicella vaccine schedule, with dose 1 given at 12 to 15 months of age and dose 2 at 4 to 6 years of age. The second dose is given to ensure that infants and children who have a primary vaccine failure or a limited initial immune response have more complete and persisting protection.[106] The second dose can be administered at an earlier age, with a minimum interval of 3 months. Catch-up immunization is recommended for children, adolescents, and young adults who previously received only one dose. Children and adults who do not have evidence of VZV immunity should be vaccinated. The criteria for immunity are documentation of two doses of vaccine; birth in the U.S. before 1980; verification of a history of varicella, diagnosed by HCP; or laboratory evidence of immunity or disease.[69]

Varicella vaccine elicits VZV immunity when administered concurrently with measles, mumps, and rubella vaccines and as a quadrivalent MMRV formulation.[107–110] A single dose of the quadrivalent vaccine (MMRV) elicited VZV antibody responses in young children that were comparable with those in children who were given a single dose of varicella vaccine; seroconversion rates were approximately 90%.[109,110] A two-dose regimen of MMRV was substantially more immunogenic.[109,110] Postlicensure surveillance showed that young children given MMRV were more likely to have fever than those who received MMR and varicella vaccine as separate inoculations (21.5% vs. 14.9%) at the time of their first immunization.[111,112] MMRV recipients aged 12 to 23 months had a 2.3 times higher relative risk for febrile seizures than those given separate inoculations. These risks of fever and febrile seizures were not observed with the second MMRV dose. MMRV can be given for initial vaccination if after informing parent, the combination is preferred; otherwise MMR, with varicella vaccine given at separate sites, is given. MMRV is preferred for the second dose.[113]

Two doses of varicella vaccine must be given to susceptible adolescents and adults.[60] Adults are more likely than children to have transient local reactions and rash and to have less persistent VZV antibodies. However, immunization of susceptible adults has important clinical benefit because of their tendency to develop serious varicella and because protection or modified severity of illness is documented despite lower antibody titers.

When it causes skin lesions in healthy recipients, the vaccine virus can be transmitted to susceptible close contacts. In one case, a pregnant woman had generalized cutaneous lesions due to vaccine virus after exposure to a vaccine-related rash in her child; no spread to the fetus was detected.[103]

The Oka-Merck varicella vaccine has been given to children with acute leukemia in remission, reducing the attack rate after household exposure to 13%.[61] Seroconversion in these patients is associated with a high level of protection, but most children required two doses of the vaccine to elicit immunity. There no longer is a protocol held by the manufacturer for immunizing children with leukemia. The varicella vaccine virus has caused disseminated and chronic infection in children with immunodeficiencies that were not recognized before vaccination and that would be expected to be associated with severe natural varicella.[113,114] Susceptible healthy household contacts should be immunized with varicella vaccine to reduce the risk of household exposure of the high-risk child.[115]

VZV reactivation has been described in a few healthy vaccine recipients,[116] but changes in herpes zoster epidemiology have not been detected as varicella incidence has declined.[117] When the incidence of herpes zoster was assessed in children with leukemia who had vaccine-induced immunity or past natural infection, vaccine virus reactivation was less common than wild-type VZV.[118] Vaccine virus is inhibited by acyclovir, so episodes of vaccine-related herpes zoster can be treated with antiviral therapy if necessary. Generalized rashes that occur late after immunization have been shown to be breakthrough infections caused by wild-type VZV.[119] Herpes zoster due to natural VZV can occur after subclinical infection in vaccinated individuals.[120]

An analysis of medical and other costs related to the annual epidemics of varicella indicates that universal immunization programs directed at healthy children and susceptible adults are cost effective as well as safe.[121] Use of varicella vaccine has been documented to reduce the incidence of varicella in the U.S. and has been associated with reduction of invasive group A streptococcal infections; further benefits are expected with the change to a two-dose regimen for early childhood vaccination.[122,123]

206 Cytomegalovirus

Robert F. Pass

Cytomegalovirus (CMV) is the most common cause of congenital infection in the United States. Approximately 10% to 20% of affected infants suffer sensorineural hearing loss, ocular damage, or impairment of cognitive or motor function. In addition, CMV is an important opportunistic pathogen in patients with impaired T-lymphocyte function, especially organ transplant recipients and patients with acquired immunodeficiency syndrome (AIDS), in whom it can cause a variety of clinical problems.

THE VIRUS

Human CMV is a member of the β-herpesvirus group which also includes HHV-6A, HHV-6B, HHV-7, and a large number of related viruses that infect other mammals. Human CMV is a large, complex virus with characteristic morphology and a distinctive focal cytopathic effect in tissue culture. The virus is approximately 200 to 300 nm in diameter; the complete virion is composed of a linear, double-stranded DNA genome within an icosahedral capsid of 162 capsomeres. The capsid is contained within the amorphous tegument comprised mostly of numerous virus-encoded proteins; the tegument is surrounded by a lipid bilayer envelope derived from host cell endoplasmic reticulum–Golgi complex intermediate compartment and containing more than 20 virus-encoded glycoproteins.[1] The genome of human CMV is composed of approximately 235,000 base pairs with 166 protein coding genes.[1] Reiterated terminal and internal base pair sequences divide the genome into unique long (U_L) and unique short (U_S) regions.

Many different cell types are infected by CMV. The virus is able to enter the cell by fusion of specific envelope glycoproteins (gB, gH, gM/gN) with cell surface proteins including heparan sulfate, cellular integrins, and platelet derived growth factor-α receptor.[1-3] Cytomegalovirus is also capable of employing an endocytic pathway dependent on proteins from the UL128, UL130, UL131 gene complex.[4,5] Viral proteins involved in attachment and entry are important targets for neutralizing antibody. As with other herpesviruses, synthesis of CMV proteins is directed by sequential transcription of genes. Viral DNA replication, protein synthesis, and assembly of nonenveloped particles take place within the nucleus, where the accumulation of nucleocapsids accounts for the typical "owl's eye" appearance of the intranuclear inclusion. Envelopment of the virus appears to be a multistep process initiated by budding through the nuclear membrane and continued with acquisition of endosomal membranes in the cytoplasm. Virus is transported via the Golgi apparatus to the cell surface for release through exocytosis. The typical cytoplasmic inclusion seen in CMV-infected cells represents the accumulation of nucleocapsids and dense bodies (enveloped tegument without nucleocapsid or DNA) in the Golgi complex.

PATHOGENESIS

Cytomegalovirus infection in humans involves a complex balance between virus and host, the usual outcome of which is clinically inapparent, persistent infection with establishment of latency. Human CMV encodes numerous genes for proteins that could influence host cell activation, leukocyte movement, inflammatory response, and both innate and adaptive immunity in ways that favor persistence of CMV in the human host.[6]

Dissemination, Tissue Tropism, and Persistence

The usual site of inoculation of CMV in the healthy host is a mucosal surface in the upper respiratory or genital tract. Viremia is the likely mechanism for dissemination of CMV to tissues in many different organs, with infection of leukocytes and vascular endothelial cells playing a role. CMV-encoded chemokines, chemokine receptors, and cytokines have the potential to influence the level of viremia by modulating cell trafficking, intracellular signaling, and host cell activation.[1,7]

Cytopathology due to CMV is often found in many organs (salivary glands, lung, kidney, liver, pancreas, adrenals, intestinal mucosa), even in persons (healthy hosts, as well as immunocompromised patients) with no premortem evidence of CMV disease.[1] After initial infection, virus is readily isolated from urine, saliva, tears, semen, cervical secretions, and human milk. On the basis of experience with perinatal, transfusion, and organ transplant transmission of CMV, viral shedding begins around 4 to 6 weeks after acquisition of CMV. Viremia is often detectable at this time and can persist for months even in the healthy host with asymptomatic infection.[8] Shedding of virus in saliva, urine, and genital secretions typically continues for months to years. Active CMV replication persists in the face of antibody response and more slowly developing cell-mediated immune response. Viral mechanisms for evading the host immune response may account for this remarkable persistence. Human CMVs carry multiple genes with the ability to interfere with host immune response at different times in the virus replication cycle and via multiple mechanisms.[9,10] Specific functions that appear to trap or destroy major histocompatibility complex (MHC) class I molecules, interfere with antigen processing and presentation, degrade MHC class II proteins, and inhibit natural killer (NK) cell killing have been identified.[1,9,10] Cytomegalovirus employs multiple mechanisms for evading host interferon response to infection.[11] Persistence of CMV in humans is thought to be due to maintenance of the viral genome in stem cells in bone marrow, though persistent replication in epithelial cells of kidney and salivary glands could play a role.[1]

Immune Response

The frequency and severity of disease due to CMV parallels the extent of impairment of host immunity. Patients who are immunocompromised because of chemotherapy, organ transplantation, or AIDS shed CMV from multiple sites, often have persistent viremia, and frequently develop CMV-related disease. Antibody plays an important role in modifying infection or preventing infection. Infections in transplant recipients who are CMV antibody negative are more likely to be associated with morbidity than infections in patients who are CMV antibody positive prior to transplant. Disease from transfusion-acquired CMV infection in small, premature neonates almost always occurs in those who lack maternal antibody. Passive and active immunization of seronegative recipients of kidney transplants from seropositive donors reduces the severity of primary CMV infection.[12,13] In addition, immunization with a CMV glycoprotein B (gB) vaccine that stimulates robust antibody responses is able to prevent infection in seronegative young women and reduce the impact of infection in solid-organ transplant patients.[14,15] The critical role of cell-mediated immunity in controlling CMV infections is supported by the observation that most severe infections occur in patients with profound impairment of cell-mediated immunity: solid-organ transplant recipients treated with antithymocyte globulins, bone marrow transplant recipients, and patients with AIDS who have very low numbers of CD4 T lymphocytes. The success of adoptive transfer of CMV-specific cytotoxic T lymphocytes as a prophylactic intervention in bone marrow transplant patients supports the critical role of cell-mediated immunity.[16–18]

Pathogenesis of Congenital Infection

Autopsy studies of fetuses or newborns with congenital infection show that CMV infects numerous cell types and damages multiple organs. A study of 34 fetuses with congenital CMV infection diagnosed in utero reported immunohistochemical detection of CMV in placenta and pancreas from all subjects; lung and kidney were each positive in 87%, liver in 71%, brain in 55%, and heart in 44%.[19] Inflammatory infiltrates were present in CMV-positive organs and correlated with organ damage. Brain cells of many different types (nervosa, glia, ependyma, choroid plexus, meninges, vascular endothelium) have cytopathologic lesions and inclusions, but involvement is typically patchy with focal areas of necrosis. Inclusion-bearing epithelial cells are found in the semicircular canals, vestibular membrane, cochleae, and other structures of the ear.[20,21] Temporal bone anomalies with cochlear, vestibular, and auditory canal defects (Mondini dysplasia) have been associated with deafness in infants with congenital CMV infection. Cytomegalic cells and focal necrosis can be seen in the retina. Examination of liver specimens reveals periportal lymphoid infiltration, bile stasis, inclusion-bearing cells in bile ducts, giant cell transformation, and necrosis of parenchymal cells.[22] Inclusion-bearing cells, without necrosis or inflammatory cell infiltrate, usually are found in abundance in glandular epithelial cells (salivary, pancreas, endocrine) as well as in lung and kidney. Results with an animal model suggest that CMV damages the developing brain through a number of mechanisms, including lytic infection of cells, interference with neuronal migration, loss of neuronal stem cells, and vascular compromise.[23]

In addition to direct effects on the fetus, CMV impairs fetal development through placental infection as evidenced by villitis, villous necrosis, and vascular lesions.[24] The predominant placental cell type infected is a fixed connective tissue or stromal cell, but CMV also is found in placental macrophages, endothelial cells, and syncytiotrophoblast cells.[25,26] In an in vitro model, CMV infection impaired the ability of cytotrophoblasts to differentiate and invade, suggesting that CMV infection could impair placental function.[27]

Newborns with congenital CMV infection and infants who acquire CMV perinatally do not control the infection as well as adults, shedding virus for much longer, sometimes up to years. Developmental immaturity of the immune response to CMV probably contributes to the severity of fetal infection and the inability of infants to control ongoing virus replication. Fetuses have cellular immune responses to CMV as early as 22 weeks of gestation.[28] A study of mothers with primary CMV infection and their fetuses with congenital infection showed that they had similar levels of activated and memory CD8+ T lymphocytes, but fetuses had lower numbers of pp65 (CMV tegument protein) specific cytotoxic T cells.[29] Newborns with congenital CMV infection have virus specific, functional CD8+ T cells that are present in numbers similar to those measured in healthy adults with CMV infection.[30] After in vitro CMV infection, myeloid dendritic cells from cord blood produced lower levels of immunomodulatory cytokines than did dendritic cells from adult peripheral blood, deficiencies that could impact T-cell responses to infection.[31] Impaired lymphocyte proliferative responses to CMV and lower numbers of interferon-γ-producing CD4+ T cells are found in infants with both congenital and acquired CMV infection.[32–34]

Cytomegalovirus can be transmitted from mother to fetus even if the mother was infected years before conception.[35] Transmission of CMV to the fetus of a mother with established immunity could be due to reactivation of latent virus or, more commonly, reinfection with new strains.[36,37] There is strong evidence that preconception maternal immunity reduces the risk of congenital CMV infection by 3- to 4-fold.[38] Long-term follow-up of children with congenital CMV infection suggests that sequelae, such as deafness and impaired cognitive function, are more common and more severe when congenital CMV infection is due to primary gestational infection (Table 206-1).[39–42]

Overall around 35% to 40% of maternal primary infections are transmitted to the fetus. The transmission rate is higher in late gestation compared to early gestation infection.[43] However, first trimester maternal infections are more likely to cause congenital infections that are manifest at birth and to be associated with sequelae (retinitis, deafness, mental retardation) than are late gestation infections. Abnormalities (by prenatal ultrasound, fetal autopsy, or neonatal examination) were found in 26% of cases when primary maternal infection occurred prior to 20 weeks of

TABLE 206-1. Sequelae in Children with Congenital Cytomegalovirus Infection, According to Type of Maternal Infection

Sequela	Primary (% with Sequela)[a]	Recurrent (% with Sequela)[b]
Sensorineural hearing loss	15	5[c]
Bilateral hearing loss	8	0[c]
Speech threshold ≥60 dB[d]	8	0[c]
IQ ≤70	13[e]	0[c,f]
Chorioretinitis	6	2
Other neurologic sequelae[g]	6	2
Microcephaly	5	2
Seizures	5	0
Paresis or paralysis	1	0
Any sequela	25	8[c]

[a]Number evaluated equals 112–125 except where noted otherwise.

[b]Number evaluated equals 54–65 except where noted otherwise.

[c]P ≤0.05 for difference between maternal primary and recurrent infection.

[d]For the ear with better hearing.

[e]Number evaluated equals 68.

[f]Number evaluated equals 32.

[g]Four of eight affected children (50%) had more than one abnormality.

Adapted from Fowler KB, Stagno S, Pass RF, et al. The outcome of congenital cytomegalovirus infection in relation to maternal antibody status. N Engl J Med 1992;326:663.

gestation compared with 6.2% when maternal infection was later in gestation.[44] A study of newborns with congenital CMV infection reported that central nervous system (CNS) sequelae occurred in 32% when primary maternal infection occurred in the first trimester, compared with 15% with later infection.[45] A similar study reported hearing loss in 4 of 5 affected infants following first trimester infections, one of 12 following second trimester infections, and none of 11 following third trimester CMV infections.[46]

EPIDEMIOLOGY

Age-Related Prevalence and Modes of Transmission

Age-related prevalence of CMV infection varies widely, depending on living circumstances and social customs. Where rate of maternal seropositivity is high and breastfeeding is common, more than half of all infants acquire CMV during the first year of life.[47] Group care of children facilitates spread of CMV (especially in toddlers) and leads to higher prevalence of infection in children attending daycare centers and their caregivers.[48] A seroepidemiologic survey of CMV prevalence based on sera collected from 1988 to 1994 from a random sample of the U.S. population found that the overall prevalence for the U.S. was 58.9%.[49] Prevalence was higher in females than males, 63.5% versus 54.1%, and notably higher in non-Hispanic blacks (75.8%) and Mexican-Americans (81.7%) than among non-Hispanic whites (51.2%). A follow-up report based on sera collected a decade later observed similar rates and reported that CMV seropositivity was independently associated with older age, female sex, foreign birthplace, low household income, household crowding, and low household education.[50] In Africa, Asia, and Latin America, the majority of children are infected by CMV prior to adolescence. Breastfeeding, child-rearing practices, crowding, sanitation, and sexual behavior probably all influence age-related variations in CMV prevalence.

Exposure to young children and sexual contacts are important sources of CMV infection for young women. Young children readily transmit CMV to peers and caregivers, including parents and childcare workers.[48] Oral shedding is common and persists for months or longer; the high frequency of mouthing behaviors in toddlers facilitates transmission of CMV through saliva directly, on toys or surfaces or hands of children and workers. Sexual transmission of CMV is important among adolescents and adults. Early sexual debut, greater number of partners, nonwhite race, and presence of other sexually transmitted diseases are associated with higher prevalence of CMV infection among attendees of clinics for sexually transmitted diseases and among adolescents.[51-53] Restriction enzyme studies of viral DNA provides evidence for transmission of CMV among toddlers and their caregivers in daycare centers, between sex partners, and from child to mother to fetus.[54-56] A population-based study of CMV seropositivity and sexual activity in the U.S. concluded that sexual activity significantly influences rates of CMV infection and that prevention efforts should address this risk.[57]

Cytomegalovirus can be transmitted from mother to offspring transplacentally, at delivery by exposure to virus in the maternal genital tract, and by breast milk.[58,59] Approximately 10% of seropositive mothers shed CMV in the genital tract at delivery, and about 50% of neonates exposed to CMV during birth are infected. Cytomegalovirus can be detected in the breast milk of 30% to 70% of CMV-seropositive mothers by culture[60] and up to 95% by PCR.[61,62] Around 50% of infants nursed by mothers with virolactia acquire infection.[60] Infants who are infected early in life shed virus for years; they are an important source of CMV for other children and caregivers.

Epidemiology of Congenital Infection

Congenital CMV infection is worldwide in distribution; rates range from about 0.2% to 3.9% of live births.[58,59,63] Rates are higher in developing countries and in low-income groups in developed countries. Rates of congenital CMV infection tend to parallel those of maternal seropositivity; populations with a high prevalence of maternal CMV infection also have higher rates of congenital CMV infection. Young maternal age, single marital status, and nonwhite race are associated with higher rates of congenital CMV infection in the U.K. and U.S.[64,65]

Nosocomial Infection

Most hospital-acquired CMV infections result from transfusions or transplantation. Banked human milk could be a source of infection for newborns, though use of donor milk banks is an uncommon practice. Transfusion-acquired CMV infections in healthy hosts are usually asymptomatic. Among bone marrow transplant recipients, blood products, especially leukocytes, can be an important source of CMV infection and disease.[66] Risk of acquiring CMV from blood products is greatest if CMV-seronegative recipients are given multiple transfusions from CMV-seropositive donors. In one study, 9.7% of 93 CMV-seronegative children undergoing open heart surgery demonstrated seroconversion; risk of post-transfusion CMV infection was estimated to be 2.7% per unit.[67] Infection rates of 13.5% and 9.2% were reported in transfused offspring of seronegative mothers in two other studies.[68,69] Risks of infection and disease acquired through transfusion or human milk are increased in neonates with birthweight <1250 g compared with larger infants.[70]

Occupational Risk of Infection

Nurses, other patient care personnel in hospitals, daycare workers, school teachers, and mothers have frequent close contact with young children; women of childbearing age constitute the majority of individuals in each of these areas. Among hospital workers, risk of CMV infection does not appear to be increased, suggesting that handwashing and other routine precautions in hospitals reduce CMV transmission.[71-73] In contrast, studies of daycare workers in the U.S. and Canada consistently have shown higher incidence of CMV infection, with rates from 8% to 20% per year, compared with an expected rate of approximately 2% per year.[48] The risk of acquisition of CMV is higher for daycare workers who have contact with younger children.

CLINICAL MANIFESTATIONS

Acquired Infection in Healthy Hosts

CMV infection among immunologically normal children and adults is usually asymptomatic, although it is a common cause of heterophil antibody-negative mononucleosis. Mononucleosis syndrome due to CMV is clinically indistinguishable from that due to Epstein–Barr virus (EBV). Malaise, headache, fever, and fatigue are common among patients with mononucleosis due to either virus. Fever is present in >90% of adults with mononucleosis caused by CMV.[74] High temperatures (39°C to 40°C) are common; the mean duration of fever is >2 weeks. Other clinical findings include: pharyngitis, tonsillitis, lymphadenopathy, hepatomegaly, and splenomegaly. Splenomegaly and exudative pharyngitis are less common with CMV than with EBV infection. A review of clinical findings in 116 immunocompetent adults hospitalized with symptomatic CMV infection reported chills in 39% of patients, sweats in 35%, abdominal pain in 17%, and weight loss in 10%.[75] Rash associated with ampicillin therapy is common with both CMV and EBV mononucleosis.

Elevated serum hepatic transaminase levels occur in >90% of patients with mononucleosis caused by CMV; peak alanine transferase levels are rarely >300 mIU/mL.[74] Elevation of bilirubin level above 2 mg/dL occurs in <5% of patients. Lymphocytosis with atypical lymphocytes (usually 10% to 35%) occurs consistently. Children with CMV mononucleosis are less likely than adults to have fever (43% versus 94%) but more likely to have hepatomegaly (100% versus 53%) and splenomegaly (86% versus 53%).[76]

The expected outcome of CMV mononucleosis in healthy hosts, including those with transfusion-acquired infection, is recovery without sequelae. However, symptoms can persist for 4 weeks or longer. A laboratory-based study that identified 124 immuno-competent, symptomatic adults with serologic evidence of recent CMV infection reported that symptoms persisted for an average of 7.8 weeks.[77]

Severe illness due to CMV infection in normal hosts has been described in a small number of patients.[78,79] Complications infrequently associated with CMV infection in the healthy host include: venous thromboembolism, uveitis with iris atrophy, persistent thrombocytopenia, hemolytic anemia, myocarditis, gastrointestinal ulceration, transverse myelitis, Guillain–Barré syndrome, and encephalitis.[1,80] A review of 21 normal hosts with encephalitis attributed to CMV infection found that patients presented with confusion, coma, seizures, aphasia, dysphasia, and cranial nerve abnormalities; recovery was slow and some patients had persistent abnormalities.[81] Severe CMV infection in the normal host is sufficiently uncommon that when it is suspected, a careful evaluation of host immunocompetence is warranted.

Congenital Infection

The clinical manifestations of congenital CMV infection can be divided into findings in the neonate and signs of CNS damage that are usually not fully apparent until later in childhood. More than 90% of neonates with congenital CMV infection appear healthy at birth. A study of 267 cases of congenital CMV infection, identified by virologic screening of >27,000 neonates, found that 7% of infected subjects had petechiae, hepatosplenomegaly, microcephaly, thrombocytopenia, or jaundice with conjugated hyperbilirubinemia and the remainder had no signs of congenital infection at birth.[65]

Clinical and laboratory findings for 106 neonates with symptomatic congenital CMV infection are summarized in Tables 206-2 and 206-3. Symptomatic congenital CMV infection portends

TABLE 206-3. Laboratory Abnormalities in Infants with Congenital Cytomegalovirus Infection Who Were Symptomatic at Birth

Test	Abnormal/Total Examined (%)
Elevated ALT (>80 units/L)	46/58 (83)
Thrombocytopenia	
<100 x 10³/mm³	62/81 (77)
<50 x 10³/mm³	43/81 (53)
Conjugated hyperbilirubinemia	
Direct serum bilirubin >2 mg/dL	55/68 (81)
Direct serum bilirubin >4 mg/dL	47/68 (69)
Hemolysis	37/72 (51)
Increased cerebrospinal fluid protein (>120 mg/dL)[a]	24/52 (46)

[a]Determinations made in the first week of life.

From Boppana SB, Pass RF, Britt WJ, et al. Symptomatic congenital cytomegalovirus infection: neonatal morbidity and mortality. Pediatr Infect Dis J 1992;11:93.

significant morbidity; 13 of 106 (12%) of the affected infants died by 6 weeks of age, and the mean duration of hospitalization was 16 days.[82] Evidence of CNS involvement (microcephaly, lethargy–hypotonia, poor suck, seizures, optic atrophy, decreased hearing sensitivity, or intracranial calcifications) is present in around two-thirds of symptomatic neonates.[82,83]

Infants with symptomatic congenital CMV infection at birth are likely to have CNS and sensory impairments including mental retardation, cerebral palsy, sensorineural hearing loss, and vision loss. A review of 15 studies that screened infants for congenital CMV infection reported that 40% to 58% of symptomatic newborns and 13.5% of those without symptoms at birth had permanent sequelae with the caveat that these are likely to be underestimates.[84] Neonates with symptomatic congenital CMV infection should be considered at high risk for sequelae, even if clinical findings are mild. Chorioretinitis, microcephaly, and neurologic abnormalities are associated with increased risk of mental retardation.[85,86] Computed tomography, ultrasound, and magnetic resonance techniques can provide evidence of CNS involvement in newborns with congenital CMV infection, and abnormal imaging results are predictive of CNS sequelae.[86–89] Abnormalities noted in patients with symptomatic congenital CMV infection include periventricular calcifications, lenticulostriate vasculopathy, periventricular cysts, ventricular dilatation, cortical atrophy, cerebellar hypoplasia, polymicrogyria, and lisencephaly. Although CNS imaging usually is performed only in newborns with signs of congenital infection, CNS abnormalities have been found in a small number of newborns who were detected by virologic screening but had no signs of congenital infection. Ultrasound has been recommended as the initial neuroimaging study.[89] It does not require sedation nor does it involve exposure to radiation, and ultrasound findings have correlated with outcome. In contrast with the high rate of CNS impairments among infants with symptomatic congenital CMV infection, over 90% of infected newborns, detected in large studies that employed virologic screening of those with no clinical abnormalities at birth, remained free of sequelae. However, infants with asymptomatic congenital CMV infection have higher than expected rates of sensorineural hearing loss that is similar in severity and clinical course to hearing loss in symptomatic patients. Congenital CMV infection is a leading cause of sensorineural deafness and of mental retardation in children.

Hearing loss due to congenital CMV infection is often progressive during childhood. Children with normal hearing at birth can develop hearing loss later, and a high proportion of infants with hearing loss experience further decline in hearing sensitivity.[90–92] Late-onset or progressive hearing loss usually occurs during the

TABLE 206-2. Clinical Findings in 106 Infants with Congenital Cytomegalovirus Infection Who Were Symptomatic at Birth

Abnormality	%[a]
Prematurity[b]	34
Small for gestational age[c]	50
Reticuloendothelial abnormality	
Petechiae	76
Jaundice	67
Hepatosplenomegaly	60
Purpura	13
Neurologic abnormality; one or more of the following:	68
Microcephaly[d]	53
Lethargy/hypotonia	27
Poor suck	19
Seizures	7

[a]Number evaluated equals 102–106.

[b]Gestational age <38 weeks.

[c]Weight <10th percentile for gestational age.

[d]Head circumference <10th percentile based on Colorado Intrauterine Growth Charts for premature newborns.

From Boppana SB, Pass RF, Britt WJ, et al. Symptomatic congenital cytomegalovirus infection: neonatal morbidity and mortality. Pediatr Infect Dis J 1992;11:93.

first 2 years of life, but decline in hearing sensitivity has been observed in school age children with congenital CMV infection. Retinitis also can reactivate, leading to further impairment of vision.[93] There is little evidence for postnatal progression of brain lesions, but this is a difficult area to study in young infants. A case of congenital CMV infection with computed tomography evidence of progressive brain destruction during the first months of postnatal life has been reported.[94]

Premature Newborns

Studies of transfusion-acquired CMV infection in newborns described a clinical syndrome of hepatosplenomegaly, atypical lymphocytosis, thrombocytopenia, worsening of respiratory status, and a septic appearance that occurred at the time of onset of CMV infection in a small percentage of premature newborns.[95,96] The risk for CMV infection and disease was related to very low birthweight (<1250 g), exposure to multiple units of blood, and birth to a seronegative mother.[68,69] Fortunately, transfusion-acquired CMV infection in newborns is now prevented by limiting them to blood products from seronegative donors or blood that has been filtered through cotton wool to remove leukocytes.[68,97,98] However, some small premature newborns acquire CMV from a maternal source and develop clinical syndromes similar to those observed with transfusion-acquired infection.[99] Postnatal CMV infection was found in 59% of newborns of less than 32 weeks' gestation and less than 1500 g birthweight who were fed mother's milk which was positive for CMV.[61] The onset of CMV infection was accompanied by symptoms in approximately half of patients. A sepsis-like syndrome (apnea, bradycardia, gray pallor, bowel distention), with onset of infection during the first 2 months after birth, occurred in some of the more premature newborns. Laboratory abnormalities including leucopenia, thrombocytopenia, abnormal liver function, and elevated C-reactive protein also were observed.[61,100] Compared with term infants, premature newborns have lower levels of transplacentally acquired maternal CMV IgG, especially those born prior to the third trimester, and their levels of antibody decline rapidly after birth due to repeated blood sampling. Whether CMV infection in small premature newborns is an independent cause of CNS sequelae is controversial.[62] At this time there is no consensus as to what steps, if any, should be taken to prevent or treat CMV infections acquired from a maternal source in very low birthweight premature newborns.

CMV Infection in Transplant Recipients

Solid-Organ Transplantation

When either the donor or the recipient of an organ is seropositive, CMV infection occurs in 50% to 100% of patients after immunosuppression and transplantation. The principal sources of infection are reactivation of endogenous latent virus, the transplanted organ or tissue, and use of untreated blood from seropositive donors. Disease attributed to CMV is most common among seronegative recipients of solid organs or tissue from seropositive donors, though immunosuppression can lead to severe disease in transplant recipients who are CMV seropositive before transplantation. Prior to the widespread use of antivirals for prevention of CMV disease, CMV infection occurred in the majority of CMV-seronegative solid-organ transplant recipients who received organs from CMV-seropositive donors (D+/R−) and in approximately 5% to 25% of CMV-seropositive recipients. Studies from more than a decade ago reported that CMV disease increased the duration of hospitalization by 10 to 18 days and costs by approximately $22,000 to $42,000 per solid-organ transplant recipient.[101,102]

The onset of viremia, viral shedding, and CMV disease is usually between 4 and 12 weeks after transplantation. The hallmarks of CMV disease in solid-organ transplant recipients are fever, malaise, arthralgia, leukopenia or pancytopenia, and laboratory evidence of hepatitis. More serious consequences of CMV infection include pneumonitis, retinitis, and gastrointestinal ulceration. Indirect

effects attributed to CMV infection include coinfection with opportunistic pathogens (e.g., *Pneumocystis carinii*, *Aspergillus*), and deterioration of graft function. Primary CMV infection in renal transplant recipients is associated with graft rejection or acute glomerular injury. Persistent hepatitis and hepatic failure are associated with CMV infection in liver transplant recipients. Pneumonitis is more common in CMV infection in recipients of lung or heart–lung transplants than in other solid-organ transplant recipients. Accelerated development of coronary artery atherosclerosis has been associated with CMV infection in cardiac transplant recipients. Whether CMV is a primary cause of damage in transplanted organs or of graft failure or simply a marker for host–graft incompatibility and more intense immunosuppression is controversial. Rates of CMV disease vary widely among transplant centers. Risk factors for greater severity of CMV infection in transplant recipients include primary infection, intensive T-lymphocyte suppressive regimens, and high levels of viremia. Recent reviews provide detailed discussions of the clinical manifestations, diagnosis, and management of CMV infection in solid-organ transplantation.[103–105]

Hematopoietic Stem Cell Transplantation

Sources of CMV among hematopoietic stem cell transplant (HSCT) recipients are similar to those among solid-organ recipients. Clinical abnormalities similar to the CMV syndrome (fever, malaise, leukopenia, hepatitis) that sometimes accompanies onset of CMV infection in solid-organ transplant patients also occur in HSCT patients. The two most troublesome manifestations of CMV disease in HSCT patients are pneumonitis and gastrointestinal disease. Prior to the routine use of antivirals to prevent CMV disease in HSCT patients, interstitial pneumonia occurred in around 20% to 40%; CMV was responsible for approximately 50% of cases and mortality as high as 90% was observed.[106] In a review of CMV disease among patients receiving allogeneic HSCT over a 20-year period, 8.6% of transplants in which either donor or recipient were CMV positive pretransplant developed CMV disease.[107] Among patients with CMV disease, 63.6% had pneumonitis alone, 18.2% gastrointestinal disease alone, and 9.1% pneumonitis plus gastrointestinal disease; there was one case each of retinitis, hepatitis, and encephalitis. Indirect effects of CMV disease in HSCT patients include greater frequency of opportunistic bacterial and fungal infections and possibly greater mortality, though the latter is controversial. Factors associated with increased risk of CMV disease among HSCT patients include D+/R− transplants, donor–recipient histoincompatibility, myeloablative conditioning regimens, graft-versus-host disease, and immunosuppressive regimens that induce lymphopenia or profound impairment of T lymphocytes (high-dose steroids, mycophenolate mofetil, T-cell depletion, anti-CD52 or antithymocyte globulin).[108]

Prevention of CMV disease in D+ or R+ HSCT patients during the first 90 to 120 days post transplant, largely by the use of antivirals, has reduced the rate of CMV disease during this period to less than 5%.[107,109] However, late-onset CMV disease has become a problem. Among HSCT patients who received either prophylactic or pre-emptive antiviral therapy to prevent CMV disease in the first 100 days post transplant, 17.8% experienced late-onset CMV disease at an average of 5.5 months after transplant.[110]

CMV Infection in Acquired Immunodeficiency Syndrome

Treatment with combination, highly active antiretroviral therapy (HAART) has dramatically reduced the occurrence of CMV disease among adults and children with HIV or AIDS. Most CMV disease in adult patients with AIDS occurs in those with extremely low CD4 counts, usually less than $50/mm^3$. The most common manifestations of CMV disease in adults with AIDS are retinitis which accounts for about 85% of cases, esophagitis, colitis, or some combination of these.[111] Encephalitis, peripheral neuropathy, polyradiculoneuritis, pneumonitis, gastritis, hepatitis, adrenalitis, skin lesions, oral mucosal ulceration, and sialoadenitis are less common.[112] Cytomegalovirus disease has similar manifestations in children. In HIV-infected infants, CMV disease is not as strongly associated with profoundly low CD4 counts as it is in adults.[113] Prior to the control of HIV infection with antiretroviral drugs, coinfection with CMV was associated with more rapid progression to AIDS.[113,114] Data from the Perinatal AIDS Collaborative Transmission Study showed a more than 10-fold reduction in non-ocular CMV disease and a similar dramatic reduction in retinitis in the era of HAART compared with pre-HAART.[113] Cytomegalovirus disease is now rarely encountered in children with HIV infection in the U.S. The rate of congenital CMV infection in HIV-uninfected infants born to HIV-infected mothers has also decreased from 3.5% to 1.2% in the post-HAART era according to data from the French Perinatal Cohort.[115]

LABORATORY DIAGNOSIS

Serologic Tests

Although serologic methods are of limited value for diagnosis of CMV infection in immunocompromised patients, they are widely used for screening and they provide the basis for distinguishing primary infection from past infection in the healthy host (Box 206-1). Enzyme immunoassays are commonly used for detection of both IgG and IgM antibodies to CMV.

Serum IgG antibody to CMV is used to screen for past CMV infection in order to determine risk of transmitting virus (blood and organ donors), risk of reactivation disease in immunocompromised patients, and risk of acquiring virus for those likely to be exposed. Although CMV IgM antibody assays are widely used to detect primary infection, they vary in accuracy for this purpose. Demonstration of low-avidity CMV IgG antibody testing improves the specificity of a positive CMV IgM result.[116,117]

Diagnosis of Congenital Infection

The diagnosis of congenital CMV infection is proven by detection of virus in body fluids within the first 3 weeks of life. Urine and saliva are the preferred specimens for testing. CMV is detected by characteristic cytopathic effect in tissue culture, by PCR, or by rapid, centrifugation-enhanced culture (shell vial) using monoclonal antibody to early antigens to identify infected cells after 24 hours of incubation. Prenatal diagnosis of fetal infection is made by detection of CMV in amniotic fluid by culture or PCR. After 3 weeks of age, laboratory detection of virus does not prove congenital infection; excretion of CMV may be due to acquisition during birth or through breast milk. Serologic methods should not be used for diagnosis of congenital CMV infection. High levels of CMV in blood, measured by quantitative competitive or real-time PCR, have been associated with increased risk of hearing loss and other sequelae.[87,118,119] However, quantitative PCR results vary considerably from one laboratory to another and a threshold of CMV in blood or urine that can be used as a basis for management decisions has not been demonstrated.

Diagnosis of CMV Disease in Immunocompromised Patients

The isolation of CMV from immunocompromised hosts does not prove that clinical findings are related to CMV. However, because primary CMV infection commonly causes disease, the development of antibodies to CMV or documentation of viremia or viral excretion in a previously seronegative patient provides strong support for a causal role. In transplant recipients with primary CMV infection, viremia, virus excretion, seroconversion, and clinical abnormalities usually occur between 4 and 12 weeks after transplantation. In immunocompromised patients with reactivated CMV infection, neither antibody response nor excretion of virus in urine, saliva, or respiratory tract secretions is a reliable indicator of CMV disease.

In both solid-organ transplantation and HSCT, all donors and recipients should be tested for CMV IgG antibody prior to immunosuppression and transplantation. Following transplant the laboratory tests that are most widely used to identify patients with or at risk for CMV disease are assays that estimate the quantity of virus in blood. The quantity of CMV DNA in blood that is predictive of disease varies with the method of measurement, the type of sample (whole blood, plasma, leukocytes), and the clinical setting. The antigenemia assay identifies white blood cells (WBC) that contain the abundant CMV tegument protein pp65, using immunofluorescent staining with a monoclonal antibody. Results are expressed as the number of positive WBCs per 2×10^5 WBCs visualized and usually range from 0 to 200. In allogeneic HSCT patients any positive WBC in an antigenemia assay is considered significant and should prompt the initiation of antiviral therapy. In renal transplant patients, the threshold for initiation of intervention usually is 20 to 50 positive WBCs per 2×10^5. Real-time PCR is gaining in popularity due to its sensitivity, ability to accurately quantitate viral DNA in clinical specimens over a wide range of concentrations, and its adaptability to automation. The lack of standardization in laboratory assays and the fact that the level of CMV in blood that predicts disease varies with the clinical setting make it difficult to make recommendations regarding significant levels. For example, a study in solid-organ transplant patients reported that a real-time PCR result of 130 genome equivalents was approximately equivalent to an antigenemia assay result of one pp65-positive cell per 2×10^5 WBCs.[120] A similar study by a different group reported that a real-time PCR result of 125,000 genome equivalents was equivalent to an antigenemia result of 10 pp65 positive cells per 2×10^5 WBCs.[121] Comparison of real-time PCR to the pp65 antigenemia assay shows that PCR detects CMV in more patients and earlier after transplant than detection of antigen.[122,123] Because of the lack of standardization in assays for quantitation of CMV, it is important to consult with the laboratory performing the assays in order to develop local data on clinical correlations.

TREATMENT

Treatment of CMV mononucleosis in the immunologically normal host is not indicated. Resolution of illness without sequelae is the expected outcome. Severe or life-threatening CMV disease in immunologically normal hosts has been reported, and treatment of these patients is recommended.[78]

BOX 206-1. Clinical Use of CMV Serology

CMV IgG
- Screening to determine if subject has ever been infected
  - Blood and organ donors
  - Organ transplant candidates
  - Immunocompromised patients
  - Pregnant women
- Detect seroconversion from CMV IgG-negative to -positive, proving primary infection

CMV IgM
- Test for recent CMV infection in immunocompetent patient with compatible illness
- Test pregnant women for primary CMV infection, using CMV IgG avidity for confirmation
- Not useful in immunocompromised patients
- Not recommended for diagnosis of congenital infection

Congenital Infection

Studies of ganciclovir and valganciclovir indicate that antiviral treatment of newborns with symptomatic congenital CMV infection may be beneficial in some cases. A randomized trial that included neonates with severe, symptomatic congenital CMV found that subjects treated with intravenous ganciclovir had improved hearing and developmental outcome compared with untreated subjects.[124,125] Eligibility for this trial required the presence of signs of CNS disease and was thus limited to patients at high risk for serious CNS sequelae. Treatment was associated with neutropenia, which was reversible with dosage adjustment or discontinuation of ganciclovir, in about half of treated patients. Animal studies indicate the potential for reproductive toxicity and carcinogenicity at levels similar to those achieved in treating humans but similar toxicity has not been reported in humans. Although treatment of newborns with symptomatic congenital CMV infection with ganciclovir appears to be beneficial, an expert panel has cautioned against ganciclovir treatment of patients with milder disease than those included in the clinical trial.[126] Valganciclovir is the mono-valyl ester of ganciclovir; it has improved oral bioavailability compared with the parent drug. In infants with congenital CMV infection, a 16 mg/kg dose of oral valganciclovir achieved pharmacokinetic and pharmacodynamic results similar to a 6 mg/kg intravenous dose of ganciclovir. The safety and efficacy of prolonged oral treatment of infants with symptomatic congenital CMV infection is being studied.[127]

Infection in Immunocompromised Patients

HIV/AIDS Patients

Detailed guidelines for preventing and treating CMV disease in HIV/AIDS patients are available from www.cdc.gov/mmwr/mmwr_rr/rr_pvol.html and from www.aidsinfo.nih.gov.[113,128] Ganciclovir prophylaxis is recommended for HIV-infected adults, adolescents and children who are CMV-seropositive and have CD4+ T-lymphocyte counts of <50 cells/μL. In addition, education of patients regarding the importance of visual symptoms and the performance of regular eye examinations are recommended in order to allow prompt recognition and treatment of CMV retinitis. Prophylaxis with intravenous ganciclovir is recommended for all HIV/AIDS patients with previous CMV end-organ disease. Discontinuing prophylaxis for CMV should be considered for patients who have sustained (≤6 months) increases in CD4+ T-lymphocyte counts in response to antiretroviral therapy. When CMV disease is recognized in patients with HIV/AIDS, an induction treatment of 14 to 21 days (or until symptomatic improvement) is usually followed by chronic maintenance therapy. Maintenance therapy is not recommended for patients with disease limited to the lungs or gastrointestinal system. Treatment recommendations for children are similar to those for adults, though there is little experience with alternative antivirals (cidofovir and foscarnet) in children. Treatment of symptomatic congenital CMV infection in HIV-exposed or infected infants with intravenous ganciclovir, 6 mg/kg of body weight every 12 hours for 6 weeks, is recommended.[113]

Prevention and Treatment of CMV Infection in Transplant Patients

Antivirals are used more commonly to prevent than to treat CMV disease in transplant patients and success with preventive strategies has substantially decreased the occurrence of CMV disease. However, CMV disease still occurs in patients who were judged to be at low risk and not placed on any preventive program, in those with late-onset disease after the preventive regimen has been completed, or as breakthrough disease in patients on prophylaxis or pre-emptive regimens.

Intravenous ganciclovir (5 mg/kg/dose every 12 hours) is the preferred antiviral agent for treatment of CMV disease in transplant recipients. Ganciclovir is given until clinical and laboratory abnormalities related to CMV infection show substantial improvement and viral load declines. This usually is accomplished after 2 weeks of therapy. If viral load is used to assess the effectiveness of treatment, antiviral therapy usually is continued until the quantity of virus in blood drops below the threshold that would trigger initiation of treatment. Failure to clear viremia has been associated with recurrence of CMV disease. After initial control of CMV infection is achieved, maintenance therapy with either 5 days per week of intravenously administered ganciclovir once per day or daily oral ganciclovir or valganciclovir usually is recommended.[66] Maintenance therapy often is continued through the first 100 days after transplant in HSCT patients. Foscarnet may be used as an alternate agent if CMV is resistant to ganciclovir, the patient fails to respond to treatment, ganciclovir is not tolerated, or marrow suppression is a concern.

Antiviral agents commonly are used to prevent CMV disease in transplant patients either as a prophylactic regimen given from transplantation through the time of greatest risk for CMV disease or in a pre-emptive approach in which laboratory surveillance for CMV in blood is used to identify patients for antiviral therapy. The prophylactic approach is chosen more often for patients at great risk of CMV disease, such as D+/R− transplants. The use of prophylactic therapy avoids the need for frequent laboratory surveillance and it is very effective. Antiviral prophylaxis has the disadvantage of exposing many patients to antivirals who would not develop CMV disease and it could increase the prevalence of drug-resistant virus. The pre-emptive strategy has the advantage of substantially reducing antiviral use, but it has the disadvantage of requiring a laboratory capable of generating viral load results rapidly. Transplants in which donor and recipient are CMV-seronegative have little or no risk of CMV disease. Assuming steps are taken to prevent infection through blood products; D−/R− transplants should not receive a preventive antiviral regimen. Either prophylactic or pre-emptive regimens should be considered for both R+ and D+/R− transplants, though other factors can influence the approach to prevention, such as type of organ transplanted, donor–recipient histocompatibility, immunosuppressive regimen, and underlying disease.

Guidelines from consensus panel and literature reviews of published studies of prophylactic and pre-emptive approaches to prevention of CMV disease in solid-organ transplant patients provide recommendations.[129–134] Most recommendations endorse universal prophylaxis for D+/R− solid-organ transplant patients and consideration of prophylaxis for R+ patients at greater risk of severe disease because of immunosuppressive regimen or type of transplant (heart–lung). Although ganciclovir is the most widely recommended antiviral, valganciclovir also is recommended and valacyclovir has been found to be similar in efficacy for prophylaxis in renal transplant patients. Prophylaxis is usually continued for at least 90 days after transplant. Pre-emptive therapy is considered an acceptable approach among R+ kidney, liver, pancreas, and heart transplant recipients. Some centers choose to observe low-risk R+ patients and not use a preventive strategy.

Cytomegalovirus immune globulin (CMVIG) is used commonly in solid-organ transplantation as part of a prophylactic regimen for prevention of CMV disease.[135] A multicenter, randomized, placebo-controlled clinical trial of CMVIG in D+/R− renal transplant patients showed a statistically significant reduction in CMV disease and opportunistic fungal and parasitic infections among treated patients compared with placebo controls, though the rate of CMV infection was not reduced.[12] Randomized, placebo-controlled clinical trials in seronegative recipients of allogeneic stem cells have failed to show efficacy of CMVIG for prevention of CMV disease.[136,137] A panel of experts did not list CMVIG in any regimens recommended for prophylaxis of CMV infection in HSCT patients.[66]

A consensus panel of experts from the Centers for Disease Control and Prevention (CDC), the Infectious Diseases Society of America, and the American Society of Blood and Marrow Transplantation issued guidelines for prevention of opportunistic infections including CMV infection in HSCT patients.[66] Use of a CMV disease prevention program for all R⁺ and all D⁺/R⁻ HSCT patients from the time of engraftment until 100 days after transplant is recommended. Either prophylactic or pre-emptive treatment with intravenous ganciclovir was recommended for recipients of allogeneic hematopoietic cells; foscarnet was listed as an alternative antiviral for prophylaxis. Although autologous HSCTs are considered low risk for CMV disease, weekly monitoring for viral load for 60 days after transplant was recommended for CMV-seropositive HSCT recipients who have underlying hematologic malignancies or receive intense immunosuppressive regimens.

CMV Antiviral Drug Resistance

Resistance of CMV to antiviral treatment is encountered in situations in which prolonged treatment is required and ongoing viral replication cannot be effectively suppressed. Relatively high rates of CMV resistance to ganciclovir were common in adult patients with AIDS in the pre-HAART era. Transplant patients often require prolonged use of antivirals for treatment of CMV infection and rates of antiviral drug resistance of 5% to 10% have been reported with higher rates associated with more severe CMV disease.[138] Antiviral drug resistance should be suspected in patients with CMV disease who are not improving clinically on treatment and in whom a decrease in viral load in blood or plasma is not achieved. The three currently licensed CMV antivirals (ganciclovir/valganciclovir, foscarnet, and cidofovir) all act on the viral DNA polymerase. Ganciclovir requires phosphorylation by a viral kinase before it can complete phosphorylation by cellular kinases. Mutations in the CMV gene, *UL97*, that encodes the viral kinase as well as mutations in the viral DNA polymerase gene, *UL54*, can lead to ganciclovir resistance. Resistance to foscarnet and cidofovir is mediated by mutations in the DNA polymerase gene. Genotypic testing for resistance mutations is available from specialty laboratories. Management of patients in whom antiviral resistance is suspected or proven is challenging as these are usually patients who are severely immunocompromised, have high levels of CMV in blood despite treatment, and have uncontrolled CMV disease. Their management should include consideration of modification of immunosuppressive regimens as well as changing the antiviral regimen. Depending on the results of genotypic resistance testing, it might be advantageous to increase the dose of ganciclovir to overcome *UL97* mutations that confer low level resistance, to change to foscarnet, or use combination therapy. If ganciclovir resistance is due to *UL54* mutations, resistance to cidofovir also is likely. For a more detailed discussion of this topic, a review of the biology and clinical significance CMV antiviral resistance is recommended.[138]

PREVENTION

Transmission of CMV appears to require direct contact with infected body fluids. The two leading sources of community-acquired CMV infection are contact with young children and intimate contact. Prevention of these exposures is challenging because they are a normal part of family and social life and child-rearing. Because CMV infection in the normal host is almost always clinically silent, it is best to assume that contact with saliva, urine or other body fluids from anyone is a potential source of CMV.

Prevention of Maternal and Congenital Infection

Handwashing and careful attention to hygiene are recommended to prevent CMV infection in pregnant women. The CDC has listed specific steps for pregnant women to take to avoid exposure to body fluids that might contain CMV (Box 206-2).[139] Similar steps are recommended for prevention of CMV infection in persons who care for infants and children.[140]

BOX 206-2. Steps Recommended by the Centers for Disease Control and Prevention for Reducing CMV Exposure in Pregnant Women and Thus Reducing the Risk of Fetal Infection

- Wash your hands often with soap and water for 15 to 20 seconds, especially after
  - changing diapers
  - feeding a young child
  - wiping a young child's nose or drool
  - handling children's toys
- Do not share food, drinks, or eating utensils used by young children
- Do not put a child's pacifier in your mouth
- Do not share a toothbrush with a young child
- Avoid contact with saliva when kissing a child
- Clean toys, countertops, and other surfaces that come into contact with children's urine or saliva

---

Studies in pregnant women suggest that providing them with information on CMV risk and clear steps for prevention will result in reduced rates of infection during pregnancy.[141,142] Cytomegalovirus immune globulin treatment of pregnant women with primary CMV infection has been reported to prevent transmission to the fetus and to improve the condition at birth of infected fetuses.[143] The study was not randomized and did not include an appropriate control group. Although no conclusions regarding efficacy of CMVIG for preventing transplacental transmission of CMV infection can be drawn, the results should lead to further evaluation of this approach to prevention of congenital CMV infection. Most primary CMV infections in pregnant women are not recognized because they are asymptomatic. Prenatal screening for CMV infection is not recommended in the U.S., Canada, or the United Kingdom.[144-146]

Prevention of Hospital-Acquired CMV Infection

Nosocomial CMV infections occurring through transmission between patients and healthcare workers are rare – probably because of the handwashing and body fluid precautions that are part of routine hospital care. Transfusion-acquired CMV infections can be prevented by either filtration of blood to remove WBCs or screening donors so that only seronegative blood products are provided to seronegative high-risk patients. These two strategies are not equally effective for high-risk HSCT patients; some unexpected CMV infections still occur in patients receiving filtered blood products.[147] There is the potential for transmission of CMV through assisted reproductive technology. The American Society for Reproductive Medicine has published guidelines for screening sperm and oocyte donors and for prevention of CMV infection in recipients.[148,149]

CMV Vaccine

No vaccine for prevention of CMV infection and disease is approved for use. The Towne strain live-attenuated virus vaccine showed limited efficacy for prevention of severe disease in renal transplant recipients.[13] The Towne vaccine was unable to prevent infection in either transplant recipients or healthy adults exposed to young children shedding CMV.[13,150] Results of phase II, randomized, placebo-controlled clinical trials of a recombinant, subunit CMV vaccine based on the envelope glycoprotein gB are encouraging. This vaccine is the first to prevent CMV infection in humans; it achieved 50% efficacy for prevention of maternal infection in high-risk young women.[14] In addition pretransplant immunization with CMV gB vaccine improved control of CMV infection in solid-organ transplant patients.[15] A number of other CMV vaccines are in development.[151]

Key Points. Cytomegalovirus Infections

VIROLOGY

- Large, complex virus, member of herpesvirus family
- Double-stranded DNA with ~160 open reading frames
- Much of genome is devoted to immune evasion or interaction with host immune functions
- Persists in latent form indefinitely

EPIDEMIOLOGY

- Endemic in all human populations
- Prevalence increases with age but varies depending on child-rearing and other practices
- Perinatal transmission is an important epidemiologic feature
- Transmission of CMV is primarily by direct contact with body fluids
- CMV is shed in body fluids for months to years after primary infection
- Transplacental transmission infects about 0.7% of fetuses worldwide

CLINICAL FEATURES

- Almost all infections in normal hosts are clinically silent
- CMV rarely causes a mononucleosis syndrome
- Approximately 10% of fetal infections have typical signs of congenital infection at birth
- Congenital infection is leading cause of hearing loss and CNS impairments

- CMV is a major cause of morbidity in immunocompromised patients

DIAGNOSIS

- Serum IgG antibody identifies subjects who have ever been infected
- Congenital infection is diagnosed by detection of virus in body fluids
- Quantity of virus in body fluids is used to identify immunocompromised at risk for disease

PREVENTION

- Specific measures are used to prevent disease in immunocompromised patients
- Specific measures are recommended for avoiding exposure during pregnancy

TREATMENT AND CHEMOPROPHYLAXIS

- Newborns with symptomatic congenital CMV infection may benefit from ganciclovir treatment
- Antiviral chemoprophylaxis is used to prevent CMV disease in immunocompromised patients
- CMV disease in immunocompromised patients is treated with antiviral agents
- Immunocompromised patients who develop CMV disease may require maintenance antiviral treatment to prevent recurrent disease

---

207 Human Herpesviruses 6 and 7 (Roseola, Exanthem Subitum)

Caroline Breese Hall and Mary T. Caserta

HUMAN HERPESVIRUS 6

Human herpesvirus 6 (HHV-6) was first isolated from the peripheral blood lymphocytes of adults with lymphoproliferative diseases and human immunodeficiency virus (HIV) infection and was named human B-lymphotropic virus.[1] When additional isolates were found in CD4[+] lymphocytes, further characterization indicated the virus was a herpesvirus. Since it was the sixth member of the herpesvirus family, it was renamed human herpesvirus 6 (HHV-6). Two years after its initial isolation, HHV-6 was discovered in the lymphocytes of four infants with roseola.[2] Subsequently, HHV-6 was established as the prime cause of this common illness of the young, which for many decades was prophetically known as "the sixth exanthematous disease of childhood." HHV-6 is an important pathogen in young children globally and, as characteristic of most herpesviruses, HHV-6 subsequently establishes persistent, latent, and lifelong infection.

Description of the Pathogen

HHV-6 and HHV-7 comprise the *Roseolovirus* genus of the β-herpesviruses. They have the characteristic human herpesvirus family's morphology and structure: an electron-dense nucleic acid core encased in an icosahedral capsid surrounded by proteins

collectively known as the tegument, and an outer envelope containing proteins and glycoproteins in a lipid bilayer. The linear, double-stranded DNA genome of 160 to 170 kilobases (kb) has a unique central region (U), which contains open reading frames (ORFs) U1–U100 bounded on each end by terminal direct repeats (tDR). HHV-6 is most closely related to HHV-7. Both share limited homology to human cytomegalovirus (CMV), the only other human β-herpesvirus.[3–5] Two subgroups of HHV-6, variants A and B, are distinguishable by their genetic, biologic, and epidemiologic characteristics.[4,5] Indeed, some have proposed the two variants be classified as separate viruses.[6] Their overall nucleotide sequence identity is approximately 90%, but less in the direct repeats (85%) and U86–U100 (72%).[7–9] HHV-6A and HHV-6B are colinear with minimal (<1%) intragroup strain variation.[4,5]

HHV-6B causes almost all primary infections in infants and is the predominant variant associated with reactivated infection in older immunocompetent and immunocompromised individuals.[4,10,11] However, in some African populations, most of the infant infections are associated with variant A.[12] Elsewhere, HHV-6A strains primarily have been isolated from immunocompromised patients with reactivated disease. HHV-6A has not been clearly associated with a distinct disease.

HHV-6 infects mature T lymphocytes, especially activated CD4[+] cells. In contrast to in vitro studies, HHV-6 replicates more efficiently in monocytes/macrophages during acute infection than CD4+ cells. HHV-6 can also infect multiple other cell types, including B lymphocytes, fibroblasts, natural killer cells, neuronal, epithelial, and endothelial cells.[13-15] Growth is characterized by cellular ballooning, lysis, and cell death.

HHV-6 uses CD46 as a cellular receptor, a glycoprotein expressed on the surface of all human nucleated cells, which may partly explain HHV-6's wide cellular tropism and tissue distribution.[3,4,9] Viral binding occurs primarily via the interaction of glycoprotein H (gH) with CD46, which requires active replication.[16] However, gH does not appear to be the only ligand for CD46. Different receptors may be used by HHV-6A versus HHV-6B strains, and even by strains of the same variant.[9] Fusion between cells expressing CD46 has been produced by some non-replicating HHV-6A strains and by HHV-6B strains using novel multiglycoprotein complexes as ligands.[9]

After primary infection both HHV-6A and HHV-6B establish latency in monocytes and macrophages, and possibly in other sites, such as the central nervous system (CNS).[4,11] Persistent infection can occur in saliva.[11,17] The structure of the HHV-6 genome during latency appears to be maintained by chromosomal integration and/or by closed circular molecules, similar to episomes of other herpesviruses, and only a few viral genes are expressed.[9,18]

Reactivation occurs with multiple, but poorly defined, stimuli and may be asymptomatic or result in organ-specific diseases.[19-21] Usually reactivation in the normal host is clinically occult. Occasionally primary infection with a closely related virus, such as HHV-7, may result in HHV-6 reactivation associated with viremia and febrile illness.[22]

Immunity

Neutralizing antibodies to multiple HHV-6 proteins, especially to linear and conformational epitopes of the glycoproteins, develop with primary HHV-6 infection. IgM antibody usually appears in the first week of illness and disappears within 1 to 2 months. IgG antibody appears during the second week after the onset of illness, and concentrations and avidity peak within 1 to 2 months.[4,5,11,23] The antibody response to primary infection occurs despite the presence of maternal antibody, but may be dampened by high levels of passive antibody. Humoral antibody appears protective as illness is uncommon during the first few months of life when maternal antibody is present in high concentration (Figure 207-1).[20] As transplacental antibody concentrations decline, infants rapidly acquire HHV-6 infection.[20] HHV-6 IgG antibody titers subsequently fluctuate and can be boosted by infection with other closely related herpesviruses. However, the immunologic response after primary infection usually protects against repeated viremia and subsequent clinical illness. HHV-6 antibody is detectable throughout life as evidenced by its almost universal presence in the cord blood of neonates.[24]

Clinical observations suggest that cellular immunity is critical in the control, persistence, and reactivation of HHV-6 infection. Patients with compromised cellular immunity, especially bone marrow and solid-organ transplant recipients, are most prone to developing disseminated infection with HHV-6 reactivation.[21] HHV-6's effects on the innate and adaptive cellular responses are incompletely defined, but appear complex. Multiple observations indicate that HHV-6 has the capability to modulate and circumvent the host immune response which enhances the pathogenesis of primary infection and favors the persistence and lifetime survival of the virus.[4,5,25]

HHV-6 may evade host immune defenses by depleting CD4+ T lymphocytes, which may partly explain the lymphopenia observed in children with primary illness.[13] In vitro and during acute infection HHV-6 induces an array of cellular immune modulating mediators, including interleukin-1β, interferon-α, interferon-γ, TNF-α, and natural killer cell cytotoxicity.[4,26-29] HHV-6 targets monocytes and monocyte-derived dendritic cells which are involved in the transport of HHV-6 to CD4+ T-cells, a function integral to the virus's pathogenesis and immunosuppressive effects during acute infection.[5,14,30] HHV-6 further evades the immune

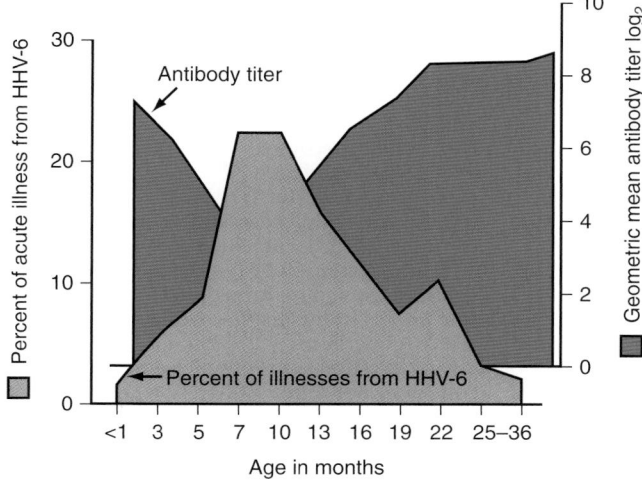

Figure 207-1. The proportion of visits to an emergency department in Rochester, NY, for acute febrile illnesses caused by HHV-6 primary infection for children from birth to 36 months of age is shown in relation to the average titer (log₂) of antibody to HHV-6 present in children ≤36 months of age. (Data from Hall C, Long C, Schnabel K, et al. Human herpesvirus-6 infection in children: a prospective study of complications and reactivation. N Engl J Med 1994;331:432–438.)

response by impairing expression of intracellular signaling of toll-like receptors in dendritic cells.[31] In addition, the virus can inhibit spontaneous apoptosis of naïve T lymphocytes, monocytes, and memory CD4+ and CD8+ T-lymphocyte subsets, which favors viral persistence.[30,32] HHV-6 encoded proteins also have been identified that suppress immune mediator responses and interfere with immune recognition of T-cell receptors essential to T-cell activation and adaptive immunity.[5,33,34]

Epidemiology

HHV-6 infection is worldwide in distribution and has no seasonal or gender predilection.[11,20,35,36] Primary infection usually occurs between 6 months and 3 years of age,[17,20] which matches the typical age distribution of roseola.[37,38] Studies of HHV-6 primary illness in Japan and the United States show similar age distributions, with relatively few cases before 6 months or after 2 to 3 years of age.[35,39] The peak period of acquisition occurs between 6 and 12 months, with a median of about 8 months of age.[11,17,20,40]

HHV-6 is a major cause of acute febrile illness in infants 6 to 18 months of age and is responsible for about 20% of visits to emergency departments for acute illness in infants 6 to 12 months of age (see Figure 207-1).[20] Infection is ubiquitous and in most areas where studied essentially all adults are seropositive.[11,20,35] Some geographic differences may exist and in some countries the age of acquisition of initial infection and seropositivity is later than in the United States.[41-43]

Mode of Transmission

Postnatal Infection

The major mode of transmission of HHV-6 to young children appears to be via respiratory secretions containing HHV-6 DNA that is asymptomatically shed by close contacts. In a prospective study of the epidemiology of roseola in 1941, Breese[37] observed that infants with roseola lacked a history of contact with children with similar disease and, thus, suggested that roseola was acquired from the asymptomatic shedding of a viral agent in secretions by family members. Kempe and colleagues[38] in 1950 demonstrated that the serum, as well as the respiratory secretions, of an infant with clinical roseola could transmit the disease after an incubation period of 10 days in humans and after about 5 days in monkeys.

Subsequent molecular and epidemiologic studies confirmed that HHV-6 DNA can be detected after primary infection in the peripheral blood mononuclear cells and in the saliva and salivary glands.[8,11,17,44,45] Although HHV-6 persists in the salivary glands, isolation of HHV-6 from oropharyngeal secretions is rare.[39,46,47] Genomic analysis of HHV-6 detected in the saliva of a few mothers, when compared with isolates recovered from their infants, has confirmed mother-to-child transmission.[45,48]

Although the incubation period for HHV-6 infection has not been established, the Kempe study[38] suggests it is about 10 days, and primary infection has been documented in the first several weeks of life.[17,20,49,50] The detection of HHV-6 DNA in the genital secretions of pregnant women and in the peripheral blood mononuclear cells of some infants in the first few weeks of life further indicate perinatal HHV-6 infection.[20,49,51–54] Human milk is not a likely source of perinatal infection as the prevalence among breast- and bottle-fed infants does not differ, and HHV-6 DNA has not been identified from human milk.[55,56]

HHV-6 is latent in bone marrow progenitor cells and, thus, may be transmitted to recipients of bone marrow transplants or to those receiving solid-organ transplants.[57–61] HHV-6 infection with chromosomally integrated virus (CI-HHV-6), characterized by high viral loads, may also be established in bone marrow recipients after transplantation from a donor with CI-HHV-6.[62–65]

Congenital Infections

Congenitally acquired infections determined by detection of HHV-6 DNA in cord blood occur in about 1% of newborns.[24,48,66] Intrauterine HHV-6 infections may result from transplacentally passed maternal infection or from CI-HHV-6 passed through the germline.[51,67] The latter appears to account for most (86%) congenital infections. HHV-6 has the unique ability among human β-herpesviruses to integrate as a whole, partial, or rearranged genome into chromosomes of some normal and immunocompromised individuals.[65,68–76] CI-HHV-6 is estimated to occur in 0.2% to 1% of Japanese, United Kingdom, and American populations.[67,68,75,77] Among the small number of individuals with CI-HHV-6 reported, integration has occurred invariably in the telomeric region of one chromosome's short arm or long arm.[18,67,68,78,79] At least 8 different chromosomes thus far have been identified.[75]

When CI-HHV-6 is passed through the germline the HHV-6 genome is present in every nucleated cell,[62,63,65,67] resulting in these individuals having high viral loads in all blood and other specimens.[62,63,65,67] These distinctive biologic characteristics allow the diagnosis of congenital infections from CI-HHV-6 by detection of HHV-6 DNA in all cells of two different lineages, such as cord or peripheral blood mononuclear cells and hair follicles, or by demonstrating constantly and persistently high viral loads in peripheral blood mononuclear cells.[62,63,65,67] A sizeable proportion of these congenital infections are HHV-6A, in contrast to HHV-6B which is detected in essentially all postnatally acquired infections.[80] Children with CI-HHV-6 congenital infection have no distinctive clinical findings at birth.[67] However, it is not yet known if neurodevelopmental or other abnormalities may develop in subsequent years. The recent evidence suggesting that CI-HHV-6 can reactivate and replicate supports this as a possibility.[18,81]

Children with transplacentally acquired congenital infection also usually appear normal at birth. The initial diagnosis requires detection of HHV-6 DNA in cord blood mononuclear cells.[51,67] HHV-6 DNA subsequently can be detected in peripheral blood mononuclear cells and saliva, but not consistently or in the high viral loads observed with CI-HHV-6 congenital infections. A recent study suggests that some, possibly all, transplacental congenital infections may result from maternal reactivated CI-HHV-6.[81]

Clinical Manifestations

Yamanishi and associates[2] first isolated HHV-6 from four Japanese infants with roseola (exanthem subitum), the major clinical expression of primary HHV-6 infection in Japan.[82–84] In the U.S. a

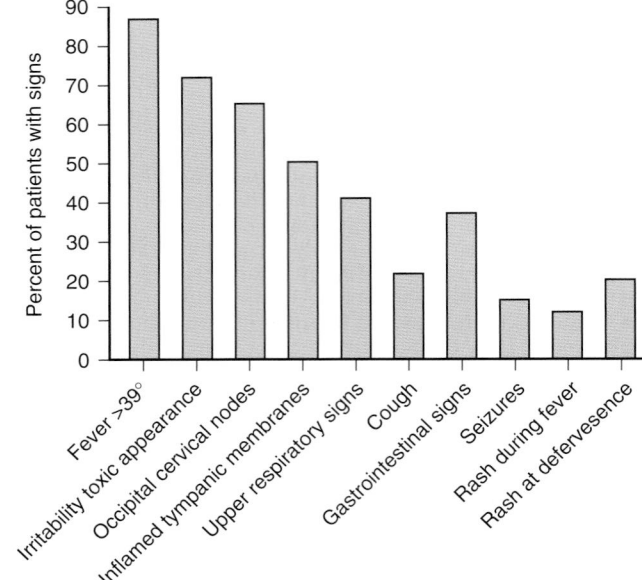

Figure 207-2. Clinical signs associated with primary HHV-6 infection and the proportion of children with primary HHV-6 infection manifesting each sign as documented by both viremia and seroconversion in 335 children studied in Rochester, NY. (Data from Hall C, Long C, Schnabel K, et al. Human herpesvirus-6 infection in children: a prospective study of complications and reactivation. N Engl J Med 1994;331:432–438 and Hall CB. Human herpesvirus 6, 7, and 8. In: Gershon A, Katz S, Hotez P (eds) Krugman's Infectious Diseases in Children, 11th ed. Philadelphia, PA, Mosby, 2003, pp 277–291.)

wide spectrum of febrile illnesses occur in infants with primary infection (Figure 207-2), with roseola being the clinical diagnosis in 10% to 30% (Figure 207-3).[17,20,40,85] Initial HHV-6 infection mimics a myriad of common, often nonspecific, illnesses of young children, thus making clinical differentiation difficult. Some features, however, provide clues to the diagnosis of HHV-6 infection, especially if the child is 6 to 24 months old. The abrupt onset of high fever (average, 40°C) is characteristic (Figures 207-2 and 207-4). Children with HHV-6 infection have substantially higher average temperatures and appear more acutely ill and irritable than age-matched children with acute febrile illnesses attributable to other etiologies.[20,40]

Among children ill with primary HHV-6 infection, about one-third have fever with no localizing signs, half manifest nasal congestion and other upper respiratory tract signs, and in about one-third diarrhea and vomiting are prominent. Diffuse pharyngeal erythema, a mild maculopapular enanthem on the soft palate and uvula (Nagayama spots), and inflamed tympanic membranes are common. The eyelids may appear puffy and the palpebral conjunctivae erythematous. A maculopapular rash occasionally may be present during the early febrile phase rather than appearing later at defervescence as is classic for roseola. Although mild cervical and postoccipital lymphadenopathy can be present at the initial evaluation, the distinctive prominent nodes in the posterior occipital region usually appear around days 3 to 4.[37,40]

The course of acute illness in most infants is 3 to 7 days. Fever usually remains high for 3 to 5 days (see Figure 207-4). Recovery generally is rapid and complete after defervescence. Ten percent to 15% of infants with HHV-6 infection are hospitalized. The usual indications for admission include a toxic appearance and CNS manifestations, including seizures, a bulging fontanel, and encephalopathy.

Central Nervous System Manifestations

CNS manifestations are common among infants with primary HHV-6 infection.[20,86,87] Case reports have noted the association

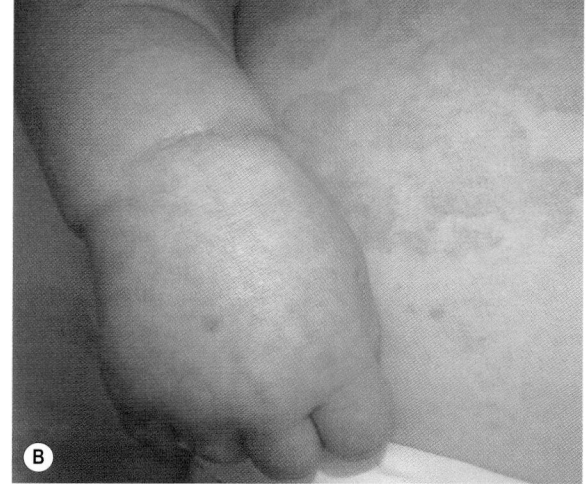

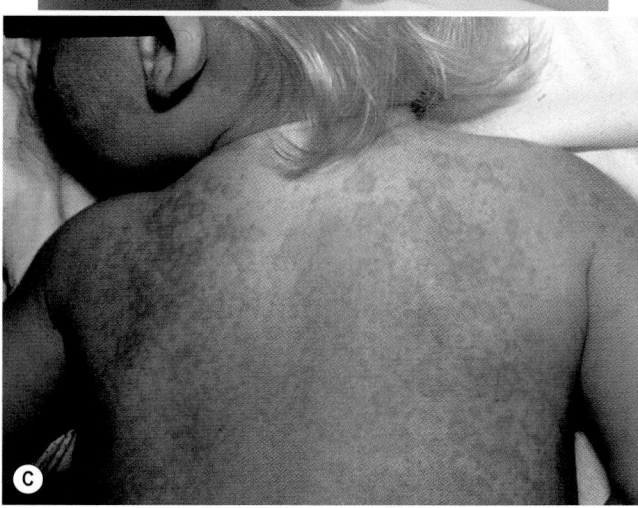

Figure 207-3. Exanthems associated with roseola. The rash observed with roseola was historically described as the "rash of roses" and denoted the sudden blooming of a pink to red exanthem. The lesions tend to appear first on the trunk, with spread to the face and extremities, and they can be morbilliform or rubella-like, with 1 to 3 mm macular, blanching lesions that sometimes coalesce into patches. As shown in **A to C,** the rash can be variable in its appearance and extent.

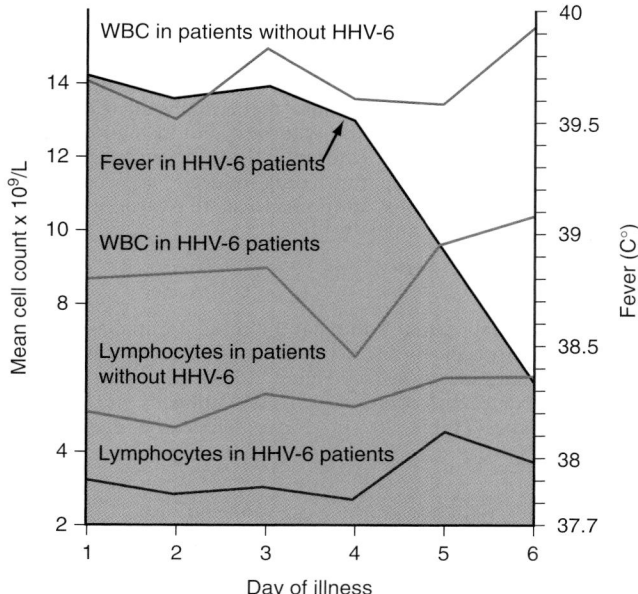

Figure 207-4. In patients with primary HHV-6 infection, the mean total white blood cell (WBC) and lymphocyte counts are shown by day of illness in relation to the average course of fever. In comparison, the mean WBC and lymphocyte counts are shown for children matched for age and season with similar acute febrile illnesses not caused by HHV-6. (From Pruksananonda P, Hall C, Insel R, et al. Primary human herpesvirus 6 infection in young children. N Engl J Med 1992;326:1445–1450.)

between roseola and CNS signs, particularly a bulging anterior fontanel which occurs in up to one-fourth of patients with roseola.

Seizures are the most common manifestation of CNS involvement among infants with primary infection.[20,40,87,88] HHV-6 has been identified as the cause of 10% to 20% of febrile seizures.[20,89] Among approximately 200 children <24 months of age with primary HHV-6 infection, presenting with acute illness to the emergency department, 13% developed febrile seizures, which sometimes were recurrent or prolonged.[20] Only about half of the seizures developed on the initial day of fever. In a prospective study of children with febrile status epilepticus, one-third had primary HHV-6 infection.[90] An association also appears to exist between the development of mesial temporal lobe epilepsy and HHV-6 persistent or reactivated infection of the hippocampus and of temporal lobe years after primary infection.[86] These observation are consistent with the recognized link between complicated febrile seizures and damage to the hippocampus with subsequent mesial temporal sclerosis. HHV-6 infection of astrocytes with aberrant glutamate transport is one proposed mechanism linking viral infection with epilepsy.[91]

Reported cases of encephalitis and encephalopathy associated with HHV-6 have been variable in spectrum, severity, and outcome, but neurologic sequelae are frequent.[87,92–95] However, the incidence of HHV-6 encephalitis/encephalopathy and the associated clinical findings are unclear as mild cases in children likely are underreported. A national survey in Japan estimated that 62 cases of exanthem subitum-associated encephalitis/encephalopathy occurred yearly.[96] Neurologic sequelae were reported in 47% of cases, and 25% died.

Clinical and laboratory findings associated with HHV-6 CNS disease generally are not distinctive from other infectious causes of encephalitis/encephalopathy. Cerebrospinal fluid (CSF) abnormalities are infrequent.[96] Magnetic resonance imaging may be negative, show transient involvement of cerebral white matter, or involvement of multiple areas of the brain, including the temporal lobe, hippocampus, and amygdala.[97–99] The presence of insomnia, hallucinations, or short-term memory loss with imaging abnormalities in the hippocampus, amygdaloid complex, or entorhinal cortex have been suggested to be compatible with a distinct entity of limbic encephalitis, observed among transplant recipients and associated with HHV-6.[99,100]

The diagnosis of HHV-6 as a cause of CNS disease often is made by detection of HHV-6 DNA in the CSF and sometimes in CNS tissue. However, the diagnosis is confounded by the ability of HHV-6 to become latent in the CNS, and thus is detected in the

CNS of normal and diseased individuals.[101–104] HHV-6 DNA is commonly detected in the CSF of children during primary HHV-6 infection and subsequently in asymptomatic children.[95,103,105–109]

Many uncommon findings have been associated with primary HHV-6 infection, but HHV-6's causal role remains unclear. Among these are a severe febrile course with recurrent rash and arthritis, hepatitis, hemophagocytic syndrome, thrombocytopenia, granulocytopenia, cardiomyopathy, drug-induced hypersensitivity syndrome, an infectious mononucleosis-like syndrome, and Gianotti–Crosti syndrome.[23,110–114]

Diagnosis

No clinical or laboratory finding at the time of initial assessment is sufficiently specific or distinctive to assure accurate diagnosis of HHV-6 primary infection (see Figure 207-4). Multiple assays are available to detect infectious virus, HHV-6 antigens, nucleic acids, and antibodies (Table 207-1). Nevertheless, the diagnosis of HHV-6 infection is confounded by the ubiquity of infection and subsequent latency, making differentiation of acute from past latent infection difficult. HHV-6 primary infection can be ascertained by the isolation of HHV-6 from peripheral blood mononuclear cells (limited to research laboratories) and seroconversion, or serologic confirmation of new infection. Diagnosis based solely on rise in antibody titers, seroconversion, or even viral isolation can be misleading (Table 207-1). Viremia occurring in healthy children is rare except during primary infection. However, viremia has been described during reactivation in immunocompromised hosts and occasionally in immunocompetent children experiencing primary infection with other β-herpesviruses.[22,115] Marked fluctuations in antibody titer may result from changes in the replicative state of latent virus and from cross-reactive antibodies. Absence of detectable seroconversion in infants may result from presence of passive maternal antibody. However, some currently available assays for viral antigen and HHV-6 DNA and RNA allow differentiation of active, productive versus latent infection (Table 207-1).

TABLE 207-1. Diagnosis of HHV-6 and HHV-7 Infections

Assay[a]	Specimen	Acute Primary	Recent Active	Past/ Latent	Reactivated	Comments
SEROLOGY[b]						
Antibody titers:	Serum/Plasma					
IgG titers		+	+	+	±	Sensitive. Seroconversion indicates primary infection HHV-6 variants are not differentiated HHV-6 and HHV-7 cross-reactivity is limited depending on assay used Results are not available during acute illness as requires testing of 2 or more serial specimens Single specimen, if antibody negative, DNA positive, suggests early, primary infection Maternal antibody can be present <6 months of age and confounds results
IgM titers		+	+			Not detected in all primary infections May be detected in small percentage of normal individuals and in some reactivated infections
Avidity titers		+	+	+		Single specimen testing indicates acute infection within 6 weeks (low avidity) or >6 weeks (high avidity)
DNA/RNA DETECTION						
DNA PCR	Mononuclear cells in blood and other specimens	+	+	+	+	DNA detection can indicate acute and/or past infection; requires serology and/or RT-PCR for clarification Differentiates HHV-6 variants
	Serum/Plasma or whole blood	+			+	Lysis of peripheral blood mononuclear cells can produce appreciable proportion of false-positive results[7,214]
Real-time DNA PCR	Serum/Plasma or whole blood	+			+	Quantitative, very sensitive, costly Lysis of peripheral blood mononuclear cells can produce appreciable proportion of false-positive results[7,214]
RNA PCR						
RT-PCR	Mononuclear cells	+			+	Very sensitive, semi-quantitative Differentiates HHV-6 variants, costly
Real-time RT-PCR	Mononuclear cells	+			+	Very sensitive, quantitative, costly
VIRAL GROWTH	Mononuclear cells of blood and other specimens	+			+	Available only in research laboratories HHV-6 variants can be differentiated Results usually not available during acute illness
VIRAL ANTIGEN DETECTION	Blood, secretions	+			+	Suggests active replication, semi-quantitative Differentiates HHV-6 variants Sensitivity and specificity variable

[a]Congenital infection with HHV-6 can confound interpretation of diagnostic tests; see text on Congenital Infections.

[b]Multiple serologic tests are available including immunofluorescent assays (IFA), neutralizing antibody assays, enzyme immunoassays (EIA), immunoblots, anti-complement assays.[2,11,76,212,213]

Management and Therapy

Since primary HHV-6 infection is generally benign and self-limited, management consists mainly of supportive treatment, control of fever, and adequate fluid intake.

Antiviral therapy has been used primarily in patients who are immunocompromised or who have severe disease, such as encephalitis. No antiviral agent, however, has been approved for the treatment or prophylaxis of HHV-6 infections. Currently available antiviral agents that have been used for HHV-6 infections are ganciclovir, foscarnet, valganciclovir, and cidofovir.[4,76,116] All these agents inhibit replication in vitro, whereas acyclovir shows relatively little antiviral activity. Most commonly used are ganciclovir and foscarnet, or the combination. Results of treatment have been mixed, but no controlled trials exist. Resistant HHV-6 strains have been reported.[76,117] Among the many new antiviral compounds being developed which appear promising are both nucleoside/nucleotide analogues and non-nucleoside analogues, including the antimalaria drug artesunate.[4,76,118]

Complications in Special Populations

The role of HHV-6 in the genesis of cancer is unclear and complicated by viral latency in diverse body sites.[21] Reactivation of HHV-6 occurs in 20% to 50% of immunocompromised patients. The highest rates are observed in bone marrow and solid-organ transplant recipients.[4,17,21,23,57,119,120] HHV-6 reactivation usually occurs early, in the first 2–4 weeks after transplantation, and can be accompanied by viremia. Whether disease is associated with the reactivation of endogenous HHV-6 infection or reactivation associated with transplantation is less clear and complicated by the presence of other opportunistic infections.[121,122] Most HHV-6 reactivations are asymptomatic, but a variety of associated findings and symptoms have been reported. Most frequent are fever and rash, sometimes with leukopenia. Myelosuppression, delayed engraftment, graft-versus-host disease, interstitial pneumonitis, and hepatitis also have been associated with HHV-6 reactivation.[4,17,21,23] Encephalitis and other CNS manifestations noted with HHV-6 reactivation have been reported to occur in 1% to 8% of stem cell and cord blood recipients, and may be severe.[21,123–126] The risk of HHV-6 reactivation has been correlated with the degree of immunosuppression, unrelated solid-organ and cord blood transplantation, low anti-HHV-6 antibody titers before transplantation, younger age, and the concurrence of other herpesvirus infections.[21]

HHV-6 has been shown in vitro to act as a cofactor in augmenting HIV infection and simian immunodeficiency disease (SIV) in a macaque animal model.[127–129] However, the adverse consequences of HHV-6 infection in patients with HIV/acquired immunodeficiency syndrome (AIDS) are less clear. Poorer prognosis and development of malignancies have been associated with HHV-6 detection and reactivation, and patients with increased HIV loads have been reported as more likely to develop viremic HHV-6 reactivation and clinical complications, such as encephalitis and pneumonitis.[130–133] However, progression of HIV disease from HHV-6 reactivation has not been proven.[21,134]

Interest in HHV-6's contribution to the development of demyelinating disease, primarily multiple sclerosis (MS), has been sparked by the identification of HHV-6 DNA in the oligodendrocytes of MS plaques and the greater frequency of detection of HHV-6 DNA and proteins in MS than in control specimens.[135–138] Furthermore, active HHV-6 replication in blood, CSF, and CNS specimens has been observed in some patients, such as those with relapsing and remitting MS.[135,139–141] However, findings associating HHV-6 with MS are inconsistent and require further clarification.[142]

HUMAN HERPESVIRUS 7

The discovery of HHV-7 in the peripheral blood lymphocytes of a healthy adult was reported 4 years after the initial isolation of HHV-6.[143] HHV-7 and HHV-6 are closely related biologically.[5,23]

As with HHV-6, primary infection with HHV-7 occurs in most individuals during childhood and establishes a persistent infection in the salivary glands. In contrast to HHV-6, however, HHV-7 may be easily isolated from saliva of previously infected individuals.[5,46] Furthermore, clinical expression of HHV-7 infection appears to be substantially less common, and its virologic characteristics and cellular tropism differ from those of HHV-6.

Description of the Pathogen

HHV-7 belongs to the *Roseolovirus* genus of the Betaherpesvirinae subfamily. Among human herpesviruses, HHV-7 is most closely related to HHV-6 and CMV.[5] The genomic structure and properties of HHV-7 and HHV-6 are similar. They have genetically colinear genomes with analogous gene arrangements. The HHV-7 genome, however, is more compact, and the length is about 10% less. The amino acid sequence identity between HHV-6 and HHV-7 ranges from 22% to 75%. The antigenic relatedness between the two viruses is sufficient to result in serologic cross-reactivity. No variant groups have been identified for HHV-7 as little variation among strains exists (about 0.1%). The HHV-7 genome encodes at least 84 different proteins, some of which appear to be unique to the Betaherpesvirinae.[5,46,144]

HHV-7's growth properties and cytopathic effects in cell culture resemble those of HHV-6.[46,145] HHV-7 is tropic for CD4+ T lymphocytes and, in contrast to HHV-6, utilizes the CD4+ molecule for at least part of its essential receptor for entry into target cells.[146] Isolation of HHV-7 requires growth in primary phytohemagglutinin-stimulated CD4+ T lymphocytes from peripheral blood mononuclear cells or cord blood, or in a continuous CD4+ lymphoblastic cell line, SupT1. The cytopathic effect, characteristic of both HHV-6 and HHV-7, is ballooning, refractile, multinucleated giant cells.[46] HHV-7, however, usually grows more slowly and is less cytopathic than HHV-6.

HHV-7 establishes both active and latent infection in CD4+ T lymphocytes and readily produces ongoing persistent infection in salivary glands.[46] HHV-7 latent or persistent infection also has been detected in a wide range of tissues, including skin, lungs, mammary glands, tonsils, liver, and kidney. In vitro, HHV-7 infects, but does not replicate, in monocytes and macrophages. HHV-7 also infects CD34+ hematopoietic progenitor cells and CD68+ monocytes/macrophages in lesions of Kaposi sarcoma.[147–149]

Epidemiology

The epidemiology of HHV-7 has been determined mostly from seroepidemiologic studies.[11,46,150,151] HHV-7 is a ubiquitous infection of childhood, which is acquired more slowly and later than HHV-6 infection.[22,152] The median age of acquisition is generally about 2 years. In Rochester, New York, about 20% of healthy children have acquired HHV-7 by 1 year, 50% by 2 years of age, and 75% by 5 years of age.[22,152] The prevalence of HHV-7 antibody gradually rises thereafter to reach 80% to 98% in adults, and passive antibody is present in almost all newborns.[22,153] HHV-7 and HHV-6 infection appear to be acquired independently, but cross-reacting antibodies from the initial infection of one possibly may exert some protective effect against the acquisition or clinical expression of the other.[11,22,46,154]

Transmission of HHV-7 likely occurs most frequently from contact with the saliva of previously infected individuals. Infectious virus is shed in the saliva of >90% of adults.[11,46] The detection of HHV-7 DNA in 3 of 29 human milk samples suggests another possible means of transmission to infants.[155] Antibody to HHV-7 also has been detected in human milk, and breastfeeding has been associated with a lower risk of early acquisition of HHV-7 infection.[152,155] Although HHV-7 infection occurring during the first months of life is uncommon, perinatal transmission may result from contact with infected maternal cervical secretions at birth.[22,51,156,157] HHV-7 DNA has been detected in the cervical swabs of 2.7% to 9.6% of pregnant women, and in 0% to 3% of non-pregnant control women.[51,54,157] Despite this, and in contrast to HHV-6, intrauterine transmission of HHV-7 does not appear to occur.[24,51]

Clinical Manifestations

The clinical presentation of primary HHV-7 infection in the relatively small number of reported cases resembles that of HHV-6.[22,154,158–162] Acute HHV-7 infection has been identified in a few children with febrile illnesses which may explain the occasional second or recurrent cases of roseola. However, clinical disease with confirmed primary infection has been reported infrequently, thus suggesting that most primary HHV-7 infections are asymptomatic or mild.

Among the few reported cases of primary HHV-7 infections, the most common presentation is a nonspecific, highly febrile illness.[22,154,158–162] However, CNS manifestations, especially febrile seizures, have occurred in a high proportion.[87] Of eight children with primary HHV-7 infection, demonstrated by isolation of the virus from the blood and seroconversion, six had seizures accompanying their febrile illness (Table 207-2).[154] HHV-7 also has been associated with more serious neurologic manifestations, including encephalitis and hemiplegia.[23,103,163–165] HHV-7 DNA has been detected in the CSF from a few patients with and without neurologic disease, and in about 5% of brain tissue samples from normal adults.[11,23,103,164,166–170]

Much interest currently exists in the potential immunomodulatory effects of HHV-7 infection. As with HHV-6, HHV-7 encodes genes that can alter, inhibit, and evade the immune response elicited to HHV-7 infection, which results in cytokine and chemokine release from cells of myeloid lineage, enhanced natural killer cell activity, and apoptosis.[5] HHV-7 can downregulate the expression of CD4[+] on T lymphocytes and encode functional β-chemokine receptors via open reading frames N12 and N51, which are in the same location as the HHV-6 homologues.[38,146,171–175]

The downregulation of CD4[+] expression on T lymphocytes potentially can exert a beneficial effect in patients with HIV infection. Both HHV-7 and HIV-1 use CD4[+] cells as a receptor for infection of T lymphocytes, and HHV-7 infection has been shown to produce an antagonistic effect on HIV infection of CD4[+] T

lymphocytes. This appears not to be dependent on viral replication but more likely represents competition for the CD4[+] receptor.[176–179] HHV-7 DNA has been found more frequently among HIV-seropositive than HIV-seronegative patients, and among HIV patients who were long-term, non-progressors, than among those with progressive disease.[176] However, no relationship between viral loads of HHV-7 and HIV or CD4[+] T lymphocytes were observed. The clinical correlates of these findings of HHV-7 infection on HIV infection and disease require further study.[176]

HHV-7's role in causing disease among immunosuppressed patients appears similar to that of HHV-6, and often both are reactivated simultaneously.[120,180,181] HHV-7 infection in these patients is most likely reactivation of latent endogenous infection, considering the high prevalence of HHV-7 infection at an early age. However, primary infection can occur, especially among seronegative young children, via secretions of close contacts or from donor-positive transplants. Information on the frequency of active HHV-7 infection occurring in immunodeficient populations is limited. Among solid-organ transplant recipients, active HHV-7 infection has been estimated as occurring in 0% to 46%, and, like HHV-6, occurring early, about 2 to 4 weeks, after transplantation.[120,182]

HHV-7 has been suggested to be less pathogenic than HHV-6 in this population, possibly in part because of HHV-7's more limited cellular tropism.[180,183] Nevertheless, HHV-7's pathogenicity and role in causing disease are difficult to assess in immunocompromised hosts because HHV-7 infection is ubiquitous and multiple other infections simultaneously occur in these patients.[121]

Although symptomatic disease due to HHV-7 has not been clearly demonstrated in transplant recipients, fever and CNS disease have been reported with reactivated HHV-7 infection.[120,184,185] Diminished survival time and acute graft-versus-host disease also have been associated with HHV-7 infection, but, unlike that observed with HHV-6, the circulating load of HHV-7 does not correlate with disease.[120,180,186,187] Reactivated HHV-7 infection also has been suggested to be a cofactor in CMV reactivation and the development of disease in solid-organ transplant recipients, but the evidence is conflicting.[188–191]

Multiple studies have explored the association between HHV-7 infection and varied skin diseases, especially pityriasis rosea, but HHV-7's role has been unclear and confounded by HHV-7's detection in normal skin.[192–198] HHV-7 has been detected more frequently in biopsy specimens from patients with pityriasis rosea than in controls, and HHV-7 has been isolated from peripheral blood mononuclear cells of pityriasis rosea patients during acute illness. Other studies, however, have not confirmed HHV-7 as a cause of pityriasis rosea.[199–201] HHV-7 has been associated anecdotally with a variety of other syndromes, including connective tissue and autoimmune diseases, chronic fatigue syndrome, hepatitis, a mononucleosis-like syndrome, and Kawasaki disease, but these associations remain unproven.[46,202–211]

Diagnosis

Many diagnostic tests can detect the presence of HHV-7 infection, but do not determine the correlation with acute clinical manifestations because they do not differentiate primary, past, latent, and reactivated HHV-7 infection (Table 207-1). Furthermore, those that can show active infection, like viral isolation, are primarily performed by research laboratories. HHV-7 infection is most commonly identified by HHV-7 DNA detection. Active or acute infection can be identified by the detection of HHV-7 RNA or suggested by detection of HHV-7 at multiple times in some specimens, such as plasma, or combined with determination of viral loads or serology (Table 207-1).[11,76,212–214]

Treatment

Specific antiviral therapy for HHV-7 is rarely needed since most primary and reactivated HHV-7 infections are asymptomatic or mild, and transient in normal children and even among

TABLE 207-2. Clinical and Laboratory Findings in Patients with Primary HHV-7 and HHV-6 Infection

	HHV-7	HHV-6	P
Median age (months)[215]	26	9	0.001
Range	3–34	1–28	
Mean temperature (°C)	39.8	39.8	NS
Range (°C)	38.9–40.4	37.8–40.6	
Seizures (%)	6 (75)	5 (17)	0.004
Irritability (%)	7 (88)	20 (69)	NS
Vomiting or diarrhea (%)	3 (38)	10 (34)	NS
Rash (%)	1 (13)	14 (48)	0.11
Hospitalized (%)	1 (13)	5 (17)	NS
Mean days of fever	3	4	NS
Mean WBC count (× 10³/mm³)	7.44	6.31	NS
Range (× 10³/mm³)	4.2–13.3	3.6–13.9	
Mean absolute lymphocyte count (× 10³/mm³)	1.85	2.63	NS
Mean absolute neutrophil count (× 10³/mm³)	4.93	2.86	0.018

From Caserta T, Hall CB, Schnabel KC, et al. Primary human herpesvirus 7 infection: a comparison of human herpesvirus 7 and human herpesvirus 6 infections in children. J Pediatr 1998;133:386–389.

immunocompromised children.[120,154] Although compounds similar to those that inhibit HHV-6 have suppressed the growth of HHV-7 in vitro, the clinical benefit of antiviral agents for HHV-7 infection has not been adequately determined, and no controlled trials currently exist.[215] Antiviral drugs, therefore, are not usually recommended therapeutically or prophylactically. More effective may be measures that reduce the immunosuppression that augments both the reactivation of HHV-7 and, more importantly, the manifestations associated with other commonly concurrent opportunistic viruses, such as CMV.

208 Epstein–Barr Virus (Mononucleosis and Lymphoproliferative Disorders)

Ben Z. Katz

Epstein–Barr virus (EBV), a ubiquitous herpesvirus of humans, was discovered in 1964. The causal relationship between EBV and infectious mononucleosis (IM) was first observed in 1968.[1] The spectrum of infections associated with EBV ranges from self-limited mononucleosis in normal hosts to progressive infections in patients with acquired or inherited disorders of immunity.[2]

DESCRIPTION OF PATHOGEN

EBV is a gammaherpesvirus. Mature, infectious particles, which are composed of a 172-kb, double-stranded DNA genome, capsid, protein tegument, and lipid-containing outer envelope, are 150 to 200 nm in diameter. The viral capsid has icosahedral symmetry and is composed of 162 capsomeres.[3] The entire nucleotide sequence of three strains is known.[4] EBV, like other herpesviruses, is easily degraded, and has a latent and a lytic life cycle.

Latent and Lytic Life Cycles

Cells that are latently infected with EBV grow continuously, the viral genome is maintained as a circle (plasmid), a limited number of regions of the EBV genome are transcribed, and a relatively small number of viral proteins are synthesized. One of these latent proteins, Epstein–Barr nuclear antigen-1 (EBNA-1), is necessary for plasmid maintenance. Cells that are permissive for the lytic life cycle of EBV linearize the EBV genome, transcribe a larger portion of the genome than latently infected cells, synthesize more proteins, release infectious EBV, and perish.

In vitro, the virus has a narrow host range and infects B lymphocytes of humans and other primates. In vivo, the virus can also be found in epithelial cells, T or natural killer (NK) cells.[5-7]

B-Lymphocyte Immortalization and Activation

EBV generally infects B lymphocytes, and confers upon them the ability to grow continuously in cell culture, a process termed *immortalization*. B-lymphocyte immortalization is the hallmark of EBV infection. EBV latent membrane protein (LMP)-1 mimics B-lymphocyte activation antigen CD40,[8] promoting B-lymphocyte activation and immortalization, by preventing programmed cell death (apoptosis). The role played by EBV latent proteins in the immortalization process has been reviewed.[9]

EBV Antigens

Up to 11 mRNAs and 9 EBV antigens are expressed during latency. EBNA, the classic EBV-induced latent neoantigen defined by immunofluorescence microscopy, is composed of 6 proteins (including EBNA-1). About 60 mRNAs are produced when the virus replicates lytically. Early antigens (EAs) are lytic proteins

produced by the virus before viral DNA replication; these antigens consist mainly of viral enzymes necessary for genome replication. The classic EA complex consists of diffuse (EA-D) and restricted (EA-R) components. The viral capsid antigen (VCA) is the classic EBV late antigen and is synthesized after EBV DNA replication. Genes encoding some of the classic EBV lytic antigens (e.g., EA-D, EA-R, and VCA) have been identified.[3]

EPIDEMIOLOGY

In developing countries and in lower socioeconomic populations in industrialized nations, up to 90% of children contract EBV infection by 8 years of age. In contrast, in higher socioeconomic groups, anywhere from 30% to 75% of adolescents are EBV sero-negative[10] (Figure 208-1).

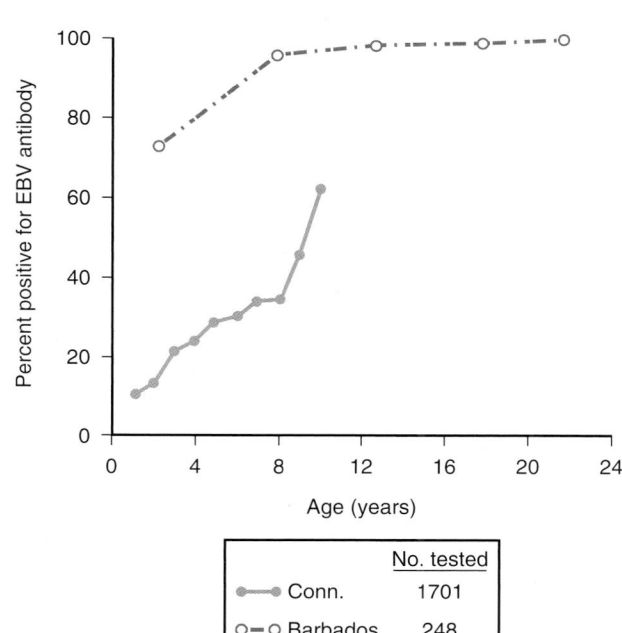

	No. tested
●—● Conn.	1701
○−○ Barbados	248

Figure 208-1. Differences in rates of acquisition of Epstein–Barr virus (EBV) by socioeconomic status. In Connecticut, by 8 years of age, only 30% of children are EBV-seropositive, whereas in Barbados, by the age of 8 years, 90% have been infected with the virus. (Modified from Evans AS, Niederman JC. Epstein–Barr virus. In: Evans AS (ed) Viral Infections of Humans: Epidemiology and Control, 3rd ed. New York, Plenum, 1991, p 265.)

Young children who acquire primary EBV infection usually do so asymptomatically, or with only mild, nonspecific symptoms. Infectious mononucleosis (IM) occurs mainly in adolescents and adults of higher socioeconomic groups. Approximately 1% to 5% of susceptible adolescents and adults contract EBV infection annually, about half of whom develop symptomatic IM.[11] Many of the symptoms of IM are secondary to the immune response to EBV. The annual incidence of IM in the United States is about 500 per 100,000; peak ages affected are 15 to 24 years.[10]

EBV is shed in oropharyngeal secretions during acute infection and intermittently thereafter; these secretions are the major source of infectious virus. It is not clear how EBV transitions between B lymphocytes and oral epithelium; however, because patients with X-linked agammaglobulinemia do not contract EBV infection, B lymphocytes must play a critical role in this process.[8,12]

Infection usually is transmitted through close personal contact. EBV can also be contracted sexually.[11,13,14] Infection is only modestly communicable and secondary attack rates are low. Rarely, transmission of IM has been documented after blood transfusion.

PATHOGENESIS AND DISEASE IN PREVIOUSLY HEALTHY CHILDREN

Infection in a susceptible person probably begins in the epithelial cells of the buccal mucosa or salivary glands. Subsequently, virus gains access to B lymphocytes (probably resting memory B lymphocytes,[15] the primary site of EBV persistence), in the lymphoid tissue of the pharynx, and disseminates to the entire lymphoid system (Figure 208-2). CD21, the major B-lymphocyte receptor for EBV, binds to the viral glycoprotein gp350. Various HLA molecules can act as coreceptors, and other viral glycoproteins allow the virus to penetrate the cell.[16,17]

Early in the course of primary EBV infection, up to 20% of circulating B lymphocytes are infected and immortalized, and EBV DNA is present within the nucleus. Most of the characteristic lymphocytes of IM are activated, EBV-specific cytotoxic/suppressor T lymphocytes, which account for up to 30% of the CD8+ T cells in blood; they can kill EBV-infected B lymphocytes, and are themselves subject to enhanced apoptosis.[18,19] NK lymphocytes that lyse EBV-infected B lymphocytes also are produced. Probably due to this CD8+ T- and NK-cell activity, a transient general depression

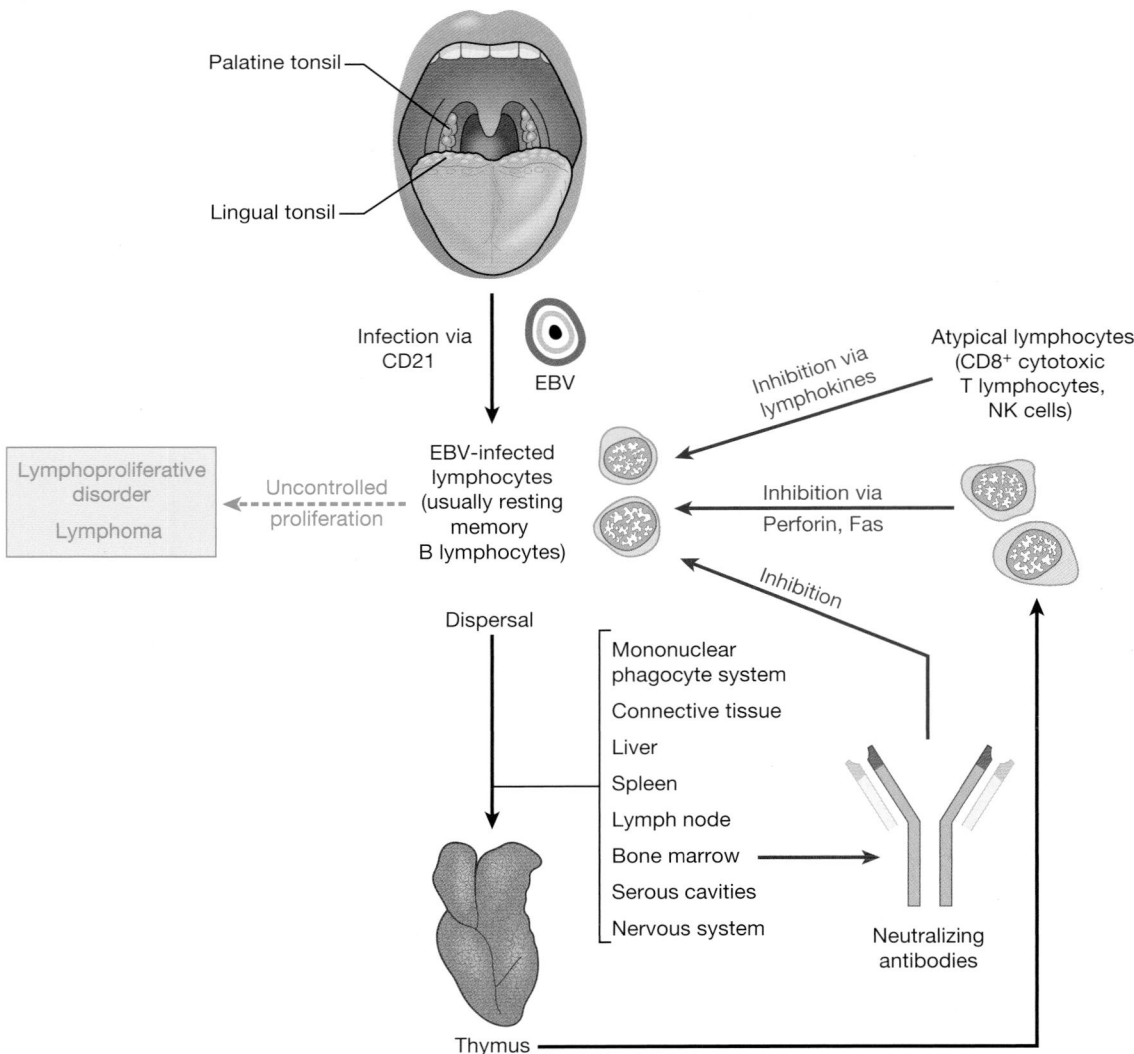

Figure 208-2. Pathogenesis and control (or lack therefore) of primary Epstein–Barr virus (EBV) infection. (Figure not drawn to scale.) EA, early antigen; EBNA, Epstein–Barr nuclear antigen-1; HLA, human leukocyte antigen; NK, natural killer; VCA, viral capsid antigen.

in cellular immunity can occur, with anergy to skin test antigens and decreased lymphocyte responses to plant mitogens, soluble antigens, and mixed leukocyte culture.[1,20]

INFECTIOUS MONONUCLEOSIS

Clinical Manifestations

EBV causes almost all cases of heterophil-positive and most cases of heterophil-negative IM. Other causes of heterophil-negative mononucleosis include cytomegalovirus, toxoplasmosis, human immunodeficiency virus (HIV), rubella, hepatitis A and B virus, human herpesvirus 6, 7, and 8, and adenovirus. Pharyngitis, lymphadenopathy, and hepatitis tend to be more severe in EBV-induced cases.[21-25]

The incubation period for IM is approximately 4 to 6 weeks.[26-28] Infection often is heralded by 3 to 5 days of mild headache, malaise, and fatigue. Major clinical manifestations include fever, sore throat/pharyngitis, and lymphadenopathy; hepatosplenomegaly, jaundice, and rash also are seen.[29] Recurrences are rare.[30]

Body temperature usually rises to 39.4°C and gradually falls over about 6 days. In severe cases, temperature may remain greater than 40°C for 2 weeks or longer.[31,32]

Generalized lymphadenopathy is a hallmark of IM. Involvement of anterior and posterior cervical nodes is most common. Enlarged nodes usually are single, firm, tender, 2 to 4 cm in diameter, and not matted. Massive mediastinal and hilar lymph node enlargement leading to respiratory embarrassment can occur. Mesenteric lymphadenopathy can be confused with acute appendicitis. Lymphadenopathy gradually subsides over days to weeks.[31,32]

Pharyngitis caused by EBV can be indistinguishable from that caused by group A streptococci. The tonsils are enlarged, reddened, and covered with exudate in more than 50% of patients. Petechiae appear on the palate between days 5 and 17 of illness in up to 25% of patients, characteristically at the junction of the hard and soft palate.[31-33]

Moderate enlargement of the spleen occurs in about 20% of cases between the second and third weeks of illness, and usually is asymptomatic.[34] Once splenomegaly is detected, repeated splenic examination should be avoided because of the rare possibility of precipitating splenic rupture,[35] which can follow trauma or, less commonly, can occur spontaneously, leading to hemorrhage, shock, and death. Splenic rupture should be suspected in any patient with acute infectious mononucleosis and abdominal pain, especially if there are signs of peritoneal irritation, hemorrhage, shock, tachycardia, or shoulder pain.[36] Spontaneous, atraumatic splenic rupture occurs in 1/500 to 1/1600 cases of IM.[37,38] Most cases of splenic rupture occur within 3 weeks of the diagnosis of IM,[39] although rupture can occur as late as 7 weeks.[10,40] Splenic infarction also has been reported.[41]

Whereas hepatomegaly is present in 10% to 35%[34] and hyperbilirubinemia in up to 25%, moderately elevated serum concentrations of hepatic transaminases are found in more than 65% of patients.[34,42] Jaundice develops in less than 5% and usually is mild; direct hyperbilirubinemia is typical. Hepatitis can be associated with anorexia, nausea, and vomiting.

An exanthem occurs in 3% to 19% of cases of IM.[31-33,43-45] The rash usually is located on the trunk and arms; rarely, palmar dermatitis occurs.[46] Rash appears during the first few days of illness, lasts 1 to 6 days, and can be erythematous, macular, papular, or morbilliform. Sometimes, an urticarial or scarlatiniform eruption or acrocyanosis is observed.[47-50] Rarely, the rash can be petechial, vesicular, umbilicated, or hemorrhagic.[51] Rashes can resemble those of Gianotti–Crosti syndrome and secondary syphilis.[52,53] Eyelid edema occurs in up to 50% of patients early in the disease.[33]

In 1967, Pullen and colleagues[54] and Patel[55] observed an increased incidence of rash in patients with IM who received ampicillin. The copper-colored exanthem is mainly over the trunk, but can progress into an extensive, confluent, maculopapular pruritic eruption that includes the palms and soles, and can persist for up to 1 week, with desquamation occurring over several more days. The rash also has been reported with the administration of amoxicillin,[56] methicillin,[57] cefprozil,[58] and azithromycin.[59] A rash can develop in 40% to 95% of patients with IM treated with one of these agents.[10] Exanthems do not represent hypersensitivity to the antibiotic, which can be used safely when the infection subsides.[60-63]

Paroxysmal cough and radiographic findings of patchy alveolar and interstitial pneumonia develop in a small percentage of patients. Pleural effusion also can occur.[64]

Neurologic complications occur in 1% to 5% of cases of IM,[10] and include aseptic meningitis, encephalitis, Guillain–Barré syndrome, optic neuritis, cranial nerve palsy, transverse myelitis, acute cerebellar ataxia, dysautonomia, subacute sclerosing panencephalitis, peripheral neuritis, optic neuritis, psychosis, Parkinson-like syndrome, acute disseminated encephalomyelitis, and central nervous system (CNS) lymphoma.[65-69] These can occur as the singular manifestation of EBV or in association with typical IM.[70]

Hematologic complications generally are mild and can occur in about 25% of cases.[10] Transient thrombocytopenic purpura and hemolytic anemia are most common.[71] Rare hematologic complications include aplastic anemia, agranulocytosis, agammaglobulinemia, hemolytic uremic syndrome, and disseminated intravascular coagulation.[10]

Unilateral or bilateral orchitis lasting 2 to 4 weeks can occur. Renal complications include interstitial nephritis, acute renal failure, and glomerulonephritis.[72,73] Electrocardiographic abnormalities, as well as pericarditis and myocarditis, have been reported.[74] Endocrinopathies include thyroiditis and polyglandular syndrome.[75,76] Arthritis, pancreatitis, proctitis, ocular involvement, genital ulcerations, necrotizing epiglottitis, cholecystitis, extrahepatic biliary obstruction, and hydrops of the gallbladder also have been observed.[77-85]

Deaths from infectious mononucleosis in previously healthy individuals are rare. In a review of the literature from 1932 to 1970, only 20 well-documented deaths were attributable to IM. Causes of death, in decreasing frequency, include neurologic complications, secondary infections, splenic rupture, hepatic failure, and myocarditis. Mortality rate was estimated to be less than 1 per 3000 cases.[86]

Laboratory Findings and Diagnosis

IM usually is diagnosed on the basis of typical clinical features, hematologic abnormalities, and a positive heterophil agglutination antibody test. Antibodies to specific EBV antigens can be used to confirm the diagnosis. Younger children often experience primary EBV infection in the absence of characteristic symptoms, hematologic abnormalities, and heterophil antibody response; a specific antibody response to EBV antigens is present, however.[87,88] Pathology can resemble that of a lymphoma.[89]

During the first week of illness, leukopenia or leukocytosis can be so prominent that leukemia is suspected. An absolute increase in the number of atypical lymphocytes is characteristic during the second week of illness. Downey cells are a hallmark of IM. These cells vary markedly in size and shape. After Wright staining, the cytoplasm of these cells is dark blue and vacuolated, with a foamy appearance. Their nuclei are round, bean-shaped, or lobulated and contain no nucleoli.

Greater than 10% atypical lymphocytes is characteristic, although not specific, for infectious mononucleosis.

Serologic Response

The heterophil antibody is principally immunoglobulin (Ig) M that appears during the first or second week of illness, and gradually disappears over 6 to 8 months. Differential absorption increases specificity for the diagnosis of EBV infection. Typically, serum from patients with IM causes agglutination of sheep red blood cells after absorption with guinea pig kidney antigens, but not after absorption with beef red blood cells. Rapid heterophil slide tests show a high correlation with standard Paul–Bunnell

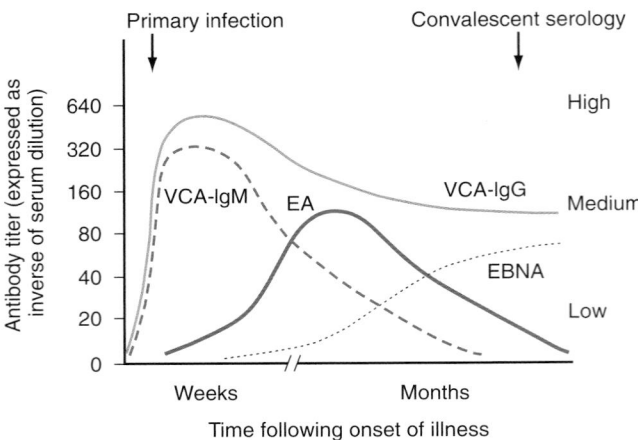

Figure 208-3. Idealized time course for the development of antibody to different Epstein–Barr virus antigens after primary infection with the virus. EA, early antigen; IgM, immunoglobulin M; VCA, viral capsid antigen.

heterophil test results,[90] and the specificity of the test for EBV infection is high (90% in most studies). False-positive heterophil test results may occur with rubella, cytomegalovirus, adenovirus, hepatitis C, HIV, malaria, systemic lupus erythematosus, leukemia, and lymphoma.[90–94]

The first antibodies produced during the course of primary EBV infection are directed against VCA (Figure 208-3). IgM antibodies against VCA are transient, usually disappearing in 4 to 8 weeks,[10] whereas IgG antibodies to VCA persist for life. Antibodies against the EA complex appear later in the course of acute infection and usually disappear after 6 months; however, low levels of antibody (mainly to the R component) of the EA complex can be detected in up to 20% of healthy individuals for years after infectious mononucleosis.[95]

Antibodies against the EBNA complex usually take 1 to 6 months to become detectable, and unlike antibodies to VCA and EA, they rise during convalescence. Therefore, all late convalescent sera from healthy, previously infected individuals contain (high titers of) antibodies against EBNA. Thus, the presence of IgG antibody against VCA and the absence of antibody to EBNA is diagnostic of primary EBV infection. IgM antibody to VCA also denotes acute infection; however, this assay is technically difficult and may yield false-positive reactions in the presence of rheumatoid factor. Extremely elevated antibody to VCA or EA in the presence of antibody to EBNA is compatible with secondary or reactivated EBV infection (Table 208-1).[96]

Autoantibodies, including antinuclear antibody, rheumatoid factor, a false-positive reagin test for syphilis, and false-positive mumps and rubella IgM tests occur occasionally during IM.[97,98] Some EBV-induced antibodies can have clinical importance. For example, IgM and IgG antiplatelet antibodies can be associated with thrombocytopenia,[99] and anti-I,[100] anti-i, and anti-HLA class I antibodies can cause severe hemolytic disease.[100,101] Hypogammaglobulinemia or isolated IgA deficiency also can occur.[102,103]

TABLE 208-1. Typical Serologic Findings Related to the Stage of Epstein-Barr Virus Infection

Stage of Infection	Presence of Antibody
Primary	VCA IgM or IgG (usually high) ± EA (usually high), no (or low) EBNA
Convalescent/past	VCA IgG ± EA (low), EBNA (high)
Reactivation	VCA IgG (high) ± EA (high), EBNA

EA, early antigen; EBNA, Epstein–Barr nuclear antigen; IgG, immunoglobulin G; VCA, viral capsid antigen.

Detection of EBV

The immortalization assay assesses the ability of patient's specimen (saliva, peripheral blood, lymph node tissue) to cause lymphoblastic transformation of laboratory cultured lymphocytes (usually umbilical cord cells). The test is time-consuming (6 to 8 weeks), and requires specialized tissue culture facilities.

Immunofluorescence or immunoperoxidase staining, or Western or immunoblotting of proteins. can be used to demonstrate latent viral antigens (e.g., EBNA) in tissue. The most specific method for demonstrating EBV in pathologic material, however, is nucleic acid hybridization. Two techniques are currently used: (1) in situ hybridization, which identifies the cells that contain EBV nucleic acid; and (2) polymerase chain reaction (PCR), which amplifies a segment of DNA. PCR generally is more sensitive than immortalization assays.[104]

In many cases of acute infection, EBV DNA can be detected in blood by PCR. EBV DNA load in the blood correlates with severity of disease; median amounts of EBV DNA in the blood during acute IM are 10^3 to 10^4 genome copies/mL.[105,106] In situ hybridization for the abundant EBV-encoded small RNAs (EBERs, which are expressed in latency[107] and can play multiple roles in the growth transformation of B lymphocytes[108]) is a specific and sensitive technique for detecting EBV-infected cells in pathologic specimens; often, the number and type of infected cells can be determined.[109]

Treatment

IM is a self-limited disease; treatment chiefly is supportive. Bedrest is indicated in the acute stage of disease. Most patients resume normal activities in 2 to 3 months.[10] Acetaminophen and saline gargles can be used to control the discomfort caused by enlarged lymph nodes and pharyngitis; in severe cases, codeine or meperidine (Demerol) may be required.

A Cochrane review concluded that there was insufficient evidence to recommend corticosteroid therapy for symptomatic relief of uncomplicated IM.[110] Although often prescribed,[111] caution is warranted because of reports of neurologic complications and secondary bacterial infections following corticosteroid use.[112,113] Corticosteroid therapy should optimally only be considered for the treatment of severe complications such as obstruction of the airway or thrombocytopenic purpura.

Sports should be avoided until patients are fully recovered and the spleen is not palpable, which usually is 3 to 4 weeks after onset of illness.[40]

Acyclovir and ganciclovir act only on the lytic phase of EBV replication. Ganciclovir can also inhibit EBV-induced B-lymphocyte immortalization[114] and its antiviral effect after drug withdrawal is more prolonged than that of acyclovir.[115] Valacyclovir is a prodrug of acyclovir with better bioavailability.[116]

Parenteral administration of acyclovir to patients with acute infectious mononucleosis reduces the replication of oropharyngeal EBV; however, there is little effect on clinical course.[117,118] Acyclovir is therefore not recommended for the treatment of IM. A randomized, double-blind, placebo-controlled treatment trial of oral acyclovir plus prednisolone in 94 adolescents and young adults also showed no significant effect of treatment.[119] One small, unblinded, non-placebo-controlled trial using a nonvalidated symptom questionnaire showed a trend towards clinical improvement with valacyclovir use.[116] In cases of severe EBV-related complications (e.g., encephalitis) or in the immunocompromised host, treatment often is considered based on anecdotal data.[120]

PATHOGENESIS AND DISEASE IN IMMUNOSUPPRESSED CHILDREN

After primary infection, EBV persists in a small population of immortalized, latently infected B lymphocytes. These infected cells periodically undergo lytic replication to produce cell-free virus. Neutralizing antibodies (to viral envelope glycoprotein, gp$_{350/220}$[121]) and cytotoxic lymphocytes (which include NK lymphocytes and CD8$^+$ cytotoxic T lymphocytes directed mainly against EBNA-3[121,122]), limit primary infection and keep the immortalized, EBV-infected B-lymphocyte pool in check. Cytotoxic T cells and NK lymphocytes exert their effect at least partly via the secretion of a protein termed *perforin*, which causes their target cells (in this case, EBV-infected B lymphocytes) to undergo programmed cell death.[123] CD4$^+$ T lymphocytes also may play a role inhibiting B lymphocytes recently infected by EBV.[124] If the immune response is dysfunctional, however, the normally small pool of EBV-infected cells can expand, perhaps allowing an EBV-activated B lymphocytes to transform into a lymphoma cell (Figure 208-2).

Posttransplant Lymphoproliferative Disorder (PTLD)

Recipients of solid organ or bone marrow/stem cell transplants (HSCT) can develop PTLD as a result of immunosuppression. In solid organ transplant recipients, the immunosuppression is due to ongoing medications given to prevent rejection. In HSCT recipients immunosuppression is due to the conditioning regimen. The greater the immunosuppression, the greater the risk for developing PTLD. In organ transplant recipients, immunosuppressive therapies that produce greater immunosuppression and risk are agents such as calcineurin inhibitors (cyclosporine and tacrolimus (FK-506)). For HSCT recipients, risk factors include the use of antibodies against T lymphocytes (especially antithymocyte globulin or anti-CD3 antibody) or use of an HLA-mismatched donor.

EBV-naiveté prior to transplant (especially when receiving an organ from an EBV-seropositive donor) is a major risk factor for PTLD in solid organ recipients;[125] such individuals have a 5- to 10-fold higher risk of developing PTLD. Unfortunately, due to their scarcity, it is not feasible to use only EBV-naive donors for EBV-naive recipients.

The risk of developing PTLD is greatest (50% to 90%) in the first year after transplant. Because HSCT recipients usually have immune reconstitution within 1 year of transplantation; PTLD rarely occurs >1 year following transplantation. In solid organ recipients, PTLD can occur many years after transplantation.

Most PTLD lesions are B lymphocyte in origin, and most are EBV-positive; however, only 15% to 40% of lesions occurring >1 year following solid organ transplant are EBV-positive, and some can have T-lymphocyte origin.[126] PTLD can range from a self-limited IM-like illness to a fatal illness characterized by solid tumors that usually resemble large-cell non-Hodgkin lymphoma (NHL). A substantial number of PTLD tumors developing in solid organ recipients involve the CNS, gastrointestinal tract, or grafted organ.[121]

The histology of PTLD ranges from plasmacytic, hyperplastic or polymorphic lesions to lesions that can be monomorphic or lymphomatous. Plasma cell hyperplasias usually are polyclonal and often regress with decreased immunosuppression. Polymorphic PTLD lesions can contain subpopulations of genetically monoclonal cells, however, which are less likely to regress with tapering immunosuppression. However, even frank lymphomas occasionally regress when immunosuppression is reduced.[127] Recurrences, which develop about 5% of the time, are more likely to be clonal and more aggressive than the original lesion.[128]

The diagnosis of PTLD can be difficult. Serologic evidence of disease includes a primary or reactivated EBV response and/or decreasing EBNA titers.[129,130] Virologic evidence of disease includes demonstrating the presence of EBV within the lesion by PCR or in situ hybridization. A definitive diagnosis of PTLD can only be made histologically.[131]

Increasing levels of EBV DNA in the peripheral blood, as measured by PCR, correlate with the development of PTLD in both solid organ and stem cell recipients.[132] Wide variability in reported EB viral load, depending upon the units and the laboratory used, precludes cutpoints that are generalizable.[133] Knowledge of the ranges of EB viral load that correlate with disease for each laboratory is crucial.

There is no proven method to prevent PTLD, and not everyone with high EB viral loads in the blood develops PTLD.[134,135] Most transplant physicians follow trends in EB viral loads to determine which patients are at highest risk for PTLD, so that diagnostic testing can be done and therapy initiated as early as possible.[136] There are some retrospective data suggesting that ganciclovir or acyclovir can reduce the risk of PTLD. This effect may be due to the antiviral agents' direct activity against lytic EBV or due to the prevention of cytomegalovirus infection, which is a possible risk factor for PTLD.[137] Pre-emptive therapy in HSCT recipients with increased EBV loads using rituximab or cytotoxic T-cell infusions (see below) has been evaluated.[138]

Treatment of PTLD is not optimal; recent estimates of mortality range from 10% to 35%, and may be higher in adolescence.[125] While there are no controlled trials to guide therapy, there have been attempts to standardize management.

Reduction of immunosuppression[127] is the first line of treatment for PTLD in solid organ recipients, despite the risk of rejection.[121] Usually, azathioprine or mycophenolate mofetil are discontinued and doses of cyclosporine, tacrolimus, and/or prednisone are halved. Reducing immunosuppression in asymptomatic solid organ transplant recipients with rising EBV loads is practiced increasingly,[139] but is controversial due to lack of controlled data and because of the possibility of precipitating rejection.

Several groups have systematically examined the use of four weekly infusions of the anti-CD20 monoclonal antibody, rituximab, following failure of reduction of immunosuppression.[136,140] Normal B lymphocytes and most B-cell malignancies express CD20. By eliminating all CD20$^+$ lymphocytes within days, rituximab eliminates most PTLD lesions. The complication rate following rituximab therapy is low (about 5% have profound neutropenia and/or serious infection), while the PTLD remission rate is as high as 60%.[141,142] Rituximab does not penetrate the CNS well; thus, CNS lesions are unlikely to respond.[143] The recurrence rate following rituximab therapy is about 20%, usually occurring after the biologic effect of rituximab wanes, i.e., after about 6 months, or due to the development of PTLD lesions that are CD20 negative.[144,145]

In patients who fail rituximab therapy, chemotherapy yields about a 75% response rate, but with a rate of toxicity of approximately 25%.[146–148] Low-dose chemotherapy (with or without rituximab) also has been used.[149] Antiviral agents generally are not recommended for treatment of PTLD.[136] For treating focal PTLD tumors, local radiation and/or surgery may be useful.[150]

Disease Associated with Acquired Immunodeficiency Syndrome (AIDS)

Four major EBV-associated conditions can develop in patients with HIV infection: (1) lymphocytic interstitial pneumonitis (LIP); (2) non-Hodgkin lymphoma (NHL); (3) oral "hairy" leukoplakia; and (4) leiomyosarcoma. These conditions have become uncommon since the advent of combination antiretroviral therapy.[151]

Lymphocytic Interstitial Pneumonitis

Before the AIDS epidemic, LIP usually was observed only in adults with immunologic abnormalities.[152] LIP in children with AIDS is associated with generalized lymphadenopathy and parotitis, and may be part of a more diffuse, predominantly CD8$^+$ lymphoproliferative process, whose dominant manifestations are bilateral, diffuse reticulonodular densities on chest radiography.[153–155] Diagnosis is confirmed by lung biopsy.

EBV DNA has been detected in the lungs of approximately 80% of children with LIP.[156–158] In a case-control study, all children with LIP had evidence of primary or reactivated EBV infection compared with significantly fewer of matched, HIV-infected control subjects.[159] In a prospective study, LIP developed in 1 of 18 HIV-infected children 7 months after primary EBV infection.[160] LIP is uncommon in adults with AIDS because LIP is a manifestation of primary EBV infection. LIP has been reported to regress with acyclovir, although corticosteroids may be more effective;[161] resolution following combination antiretroviral therapy also has been reported.[155,162] LIP is not a lymphoma, and has a better outcome than other opportunistic infections seen in HIV-infected children.

Non-Hodgkin Lymphoma

In the general population, Hodgkin disease is more prevalent than NHL. In immunocompromised individuals, however, NHL is more common. The NHL seen in patients with AIDS is more aggressive, more likely to be manifest at extranodal sites, and more likely to be composed mainly of oligoclonal B lymphocytes.[163-170]

EBV has been detected in at least half of the NHL lesions examined from patients with AIDS. EBV load has correlated with cancer risk in pediatric HIV-infected patients with CD4 counts >200/mm³. More than 90% of CNS lymphomas are EBV-associated.[171,172] PCR of cerebrospinal fluid has been used to distinguish AIDS-associated CNS NHL from other CNS mass lesions; this test is sensitive but not specific.[173]

Oral "Hairy" Leukoplakia

A new form of oral leukoplakia was recognized in HIV-seropositive men who had sex with men, beginning in 1984. This entity has been reported rarely in children.[174] Oral hairy leukoplakia principally is found on the lateral surface of the tongue. Lesions resemble flat warts.[175] Evidence supporting the etiologic role of EBV includes the presence of EBV DNA and antigens in biopsy material, documented lytic EBV DNA replication in the epithelial cells of lesions,[176] and regression of lesions with acyclovir.[176,177] EBV DNA also has been identified in esophageal ulcers in HIV-infected patients, the pathology of which resembles oral hairy leukoplakia.[178]

Leiomyosarcoma

Leiomyosarcomas are malignant cancers of smooth muscle, and are rare in childhood. Paradoxically, cases associated with EBV have been seen mainly in children and young adults with AIDS, and in transplant recipients. The tumors are monoclonal, biclonal, or oligoclonal. Serologic data revealed a reactivated EBV infection in 1 of 3 patients with AIDS.[179,180] Surgery is the mainstay of therapy, although reduction of immunosuppression and radiation therapy also have been used.[181,182] Prognosis is poor.

X-Linked Lymphoproliferative Syndrome/Infection-Associated Hemophagocytic Syndrome/Chronic Active EBV Infection

X-linked lymphoproliferative syndrome (XLPS), infection-associated hemophagocytic syndrome (IAHS), and chronic active EBV infection (CAEBVI) are three clinically overlapping syndromes associated with EBV infection. All three likely are related to the inability of NK and/or cytotoxic T lymphocytes to regulate EBV proliferation, and all three are usually classified under the rubric of hemophagocytic lymphohistiocytoses (HLH), which are disorders of NK cells, cytotoxic T lymphocytes, and macrophages and characterized by hypercytokinemia.[183]

HLH was first described in 1939, recognized as possibly being familial in 1952, and first associated with viral infections in 1979.[184] The cardinal symptoms of HLH include fever, hepatosplenomegaly, and CNS involvement. Lymphadenopathy and rash also can be present. Laboratory abnormalities include cytopenias, coagulopathy, hypertriglyceridemia, elevated serum ferritin level, and hemophagocytosis.

Some forms of HLH are genetic. Other forms are triggered by infection, malignancy, or rheumatologic conditions, although it is suspected that there are as yet unknown genetic predisposing

factors in the acquired forms as well. Both forms can be associated with EBV.[183] In some of these conditions, EBV infects T or NK cells, rather than B cells.

X-Linked Lymphoproliferative Syndrome (XLPS)

Rare individuals, because of an X-linked genetic predisposition, are incapable of mounting a normal immune response to primary infection with EBV. Thus this disorder has *both* a known genetic mutation and a known extrinsic trigger (EBV infection). Up to 90% of patients with X-linked lymphoproliferative disorder have evidence of hemophagocytosis.[183,185,186]

A progressive *proliferative* response develops in approximately 60% of individuals affected by XLPS (Box 208-1). The cause of death in these individuals is usually liver necrosis secondary to infiltration of lymphoid cells. Pathologic examination reveals widespread mononucleosis-like changes in two-thirds of patients and malignant B-cell lymphoma, usually of the Burkitt type, in one-third of patients. Approximately one-third of patients with XLPS survive the initial EBV infection, and an *aproliferative* disease develops. Findings in these patients include hypogammaglobulinemia, aplastic anemia, agranulocytosis, increased susceptibility to bacterial infection, and the development of malignancies.[185,186]

Most patients with XLPS have normal responses to viral and bacterial infections of childhood, and have normal cell-mediated immune responses and T- and B-lymphocyte numbers.[187] Immunologic evaluation of patients with XLPS during the course of their acute EBV infection reveals exaggerated CD8+ T-lymphocyte activity against EBV-infected B lymphocytes. In survivors, a global deficiency in immunoglobulin production, T-lymphocyte and NK-cell function is observed. In addition, almost all survivors fail to produce or lose antibody to EBNA and have abnormalities in VCA antibody production, suggesting an inability to regulate primary EBV infection.[185]

The (SAP) genetic defect found in about 80% of patients with XLPS is a defect in an inhibitory T-lymphocyte signaling pathway important for T-cell development and function.[185,186] SAP normally is upregulated in response to EBV infection and is important for the control of T-cell activation, NK-cell activation and cytotoxicity, and memory B-cell development.[186,188] Untreated, about 75% of boys with the SAP defect die within a month of primary EBV infection.[189] It has been postulated that a pro-apoptotic defect of cytotoxic T lymphocytes might lead to the fatal IM phenotype due to an inability to downregulate the cytotoxic T-cell response against EBV, while a pro-apoptotic defect of B-lymphocyte subpopulations might lead to B-cell lymphomas.[186] A second genetic defect (XIAP) has been observed in most of the remaining patients with XLPS;[190] to date, lymphomas have not been reported in these patients, perhaps explaining some of the phenotypic heterogeneity of XLPS, although exact genotype–phenotype correlation remains incomplete. Flow cytometry may prove useful for diagnosis in the future.[191]

Therapeutic options for XLPS are limited. Patients with proliferative responses often are treated with regimens similar to those

---

BOX 208-1. Major Manifestations of X-Linked Lymphoproliferative Syndrome

PROLIFERATIVE

Fatal infectious mononucleosis
Malignant lymphoma
Associated with hemophagocytic syndrome

APROLIFERATIVE

Hypogammaglobulinemia
Aplastic anemia
Agranulocytosis
Associated with bacterial infections, late malignancies

used for IAHS (described below).[192] The only definitive therapy is stem cell transplantion.[183,185] Boys who are discovered prior to acquiring infection with EBV have been treated with monthly immune globulin intravenous (IGIV) therapy to prevent acquisition of EBV, and occasionally have been pre-emptively treated with rituximab, corticosteroids, immunoglobulin, and ganciclovir after acquiring primary EBV infection.[193,194]

Infection-Associated Hemophagocytic Syndrome

Familial HLH is a genetic syndrome associated with defect(s) in the pro-apoptotic perforin (or related) gene pathway(s) in cytotoxic T lymphocytes and NK cells, resulting in excessive and persistent activation of macrophages and hypercytokinemia; untreated, the 3-year survival is about 10%.[123,195,196] IAHS is a secondary, acquired form of HLH; the most common infectious trigger is primary EBV infection. A similar syndrome can be triggered by malignancies or rheumatologic disorders, when HLH is called macrophage activation syndrome (MAS).[183] Patients diagnosed with IAHS, by definition, do not have any of the known gene mutation characteristic of familial HLH or XLPS.[197] Children diagnosed with familial HLH often are younger (<1 year of age) than those diagnosed with IAHS (or other acquired forms of HLH). (See Box 208-2.)[183]

The signs and symptoms of IAHS are the same as those of HLH. IAHS appears to be due to macrophages reacting against EBV-infected CD8+ T lymphocytes.[198] Etoposide, which reduces macrophage activation, and dexamethasone, with or without cyclosporine, are used to treat HLH. The 3-year survival for presumed nonfamilial cases (those with no affected sibling) is 55%; for those >1 year old at onset the overall survival is 70%. Definitive therapy and potential cure requires stem cell transplantation; 7-year survival following stem cell transplantation is 50% to 70%.[185] (See Chapter 12, Hemophagocytic Lymphohistiocytosis and Macrophage Activation Syndrome.)

Chronic Active EBV Infection (CAEBVI)

CAEBVI has been reported mainly in Asians, and appears to have two subtypes: a T-lymphocyte form and an NK-cell form, depending upon which cells are infected with EBV.[199] Clinically, patients with CAEBVI have chronic or recurrent mononucleosis-like symptoms including fever, lymphadenopathy, and hepatosplenomegaly for at least 3 months. Hepatitis, pancytopenia, uveitis, interstitial pneumonitis, skin manifestations (e.g., photosensitivity), sicca syndrome, neuropathy, cardiomyopathy/carditis, neutropenia, eosinophilia, thrombocytopenia, and hyper- or hypogammaglobulinemia also can occur; a similar "cytokine storm" as is seen with HLH can be present.[200] Occasionally, the disease can mimic leukemia. Rarely, coronary artery ectasia or aneurysms (as can occur in Kawasaki disease) are observed.[201] Patients have prolonged, severe, relapsing, and often fatal courses. Death can be associated with respiratory failure secondary to interstitial pneumonia, or with diffuse T-lymphocyte infiltrate, lymphoma or hemophagocytic syndrome.[202,203] Distinguishing clinically between CAEBVI and IAHS is difficult.

Patients with CAEBVI have abnormal EBV serologic responses, such as extremely high levels of antibody to the EA and VCA complexes and low or absent antibody to EBNA. Some patients have selective absence of antibody to EBNA-1.[204] Impaired cytotoxic T-lymphocyte responses against EBV-infected NK cells have been reported.[205] EBV loads typically are extremely high, especially in patients with complications. Elevated EBV load in cerebrospinal fluid in patients with CNS involvement is reported.[206-209] There is no evidence of a prior immunologic abnormality. These patients do not have the gene defect associated with XLPS,[210] although there is a case report of a patient with CAEBVI and a perforin gene defect.[211]

The NK-cell form of CAEBVI is characterized by high EBV DNA loads, high serum IgE, NK-cell lymphocytosis, and hypersensitivity to mosquito bites. The T-lymphocyte form of the disease is associated with anemia, and a worse prognosis. Other poor prognostic signs of CAEBVI are age >8 years and platelet counts <12,000/mm^3.[212]

Several families have been described in which this syndrome has occurred in multiple members.[213] Stem cell transplantation[214] or autologous cytotoxic T-lymphocyte infusions are the most effective therapies;[215] chemotherapy also has been used.[216]

Chronic active EBV infection must not be confused with *chronic fatigue syndrome* (CFS).[217] In CFS, few, if any, objective signs of illness exist. EBV does not play an etiologic role in most cases of CFS,[218] despite the finding that a few patients have elevated antibody titers to EA complex[219] and may lack antibody to EBNA-1,[204] and in some adolescents, the disease follows an episode of infectious mononucleosis.[220]

Congenital Infection

Rare infants with birth defects attributed to congenital infection following maternal primary EBV infection have been reported. One infant had bilateral congenital cataracts, cryptorchidism, hypotonia, and mild micrognathia. A "celery stalk" appearance of long bones was noted radiographically, similar to that seen with congenital rubella.[221] However, a prospective study of more than 4000 pregnant women failed to document intrauterine EBV infection.[222] Another report described nearly 700 pregnant women with serologic evidence of EBV infection during pregnancy. Pregnancies were several times more likely to result in early fetal death, premature labor, or delivery of an infant who became ill soon after birth;[223] however. the association of these conditions with EBV infection is unknown. A comprehensive review of this topic recently has been published.[224]

209 Human Herpesvirus 8 (Kaposi Sarcoma-Associated Herpesvirus)

Caroline Breese Hall and Mary T. Caserta

In 1872, Moritz Kaposi, a Hungarian dermatologist, first described in five men an aggressive, pigmented, multicentric sarcoma of the skin which disseminated to multiple body sites.[1] It was rare, and received little attention until a century later when similar lesions were observed in African children and adults and subsequently found in association with human immunodeficiency virus (HIV) infection in the 1980s. Although the cause of Kaposi sarcoma (KS) was suspected from these epidemiologic associations to be infectious, it was not confirmed until 1994 when Chang et al.[2] isolated two novel DNA fragments with homologies to two oncogenic gammaherpesviruses from a sarcoma in an HIV-infected patient. This led to classification of HHV-8 as a lymphotropic gammaherpesvirus. Except for an endemic form observed primarily in Africa, HHV-8 disease rarely occurs in children.

CHARACTERIZATION OF THE VIRUS

HHV-8 is the only human gamma-2 herpesvirus, a rhadinovirus. Epstein–Barr virus (EBV), a gamma-1 herpesvirus, is the most closely related human virus. HHV-8 is a large, double-stranded, enveloped DNA virus. Its genome has a central unique region of about 140 kb, which encodes all the known open reading frames and is flanked by terminal repeat sequences that contain important signals for packaging and cleavage.[3,4] The HHV-8 genome contains cellular homologs that are related to human oncogenes, which inhibit tumor suppressor pathways by affecting control of cellular growth and inhibition of apoptosis.[4,5]

HHV-8 infects multiple cell types, suggesting that one or more ubiquitous host cell surface molecules are involved in viral attachment and cell entry. Proposed candidates are four structural HHV-8 glycoproteins.[3,5,6] After initial infection, the HHV-8 genome persists as covalently closed episomal circles, establishing lifelong latent infection. Monocytes and B lymphocytes are the major reservoir.[3,6] Latent virus can be activated to a lytic phase from multiple stimuli, including inflammatory mediators and coinfections, as with HIV.

HHV-8 can be propagated in cell cultures, but most are latently infected and lytic infection must be induced.[7] Most frequently used are continuous, chronically infected cell lines derived from HHV-8 primary effusion lymphomas that produce relatively low titers of cell-free virus.

EPIDEMIOLOGY

In contrast to other herpesviruses, HHV-8 does not cause ubiquitous worldwide infection. Its prevalence predominantly mirrors the incidence of KS.[3,7,8] Seropositivity rates show wide geographic variation, with the highest rates in sub-Saharan Africa, ranging from 20% to 80%.[9–12] In Cameroon, Ghana, Uganda, and Tanzania, 40% to 60% of children <10 years of age are seropositive.[8] Seroprevalence is 6% to 20% in most Mediterranean countries, and lowest, 0% to 5%, in northern Europe, United States, Latin America, and Asia. However, seropositivity and HHV-8 disease can vary widely among countries within the same region. Furthermore, high-risk groups exist even in countries with low HHV-8 seroprevalence. In the U.S., 15% to 40% of men who have sex with men (MSM) are seropositive, with the highest rates occurring among HIV-infected MSM.[9,12,13] Seroprevalence is not as high among other HIV-infected populations, especially children.[14]

The putative modes of acquisition of HHV-8 include nonsexual and sexual horizontal transmission, vertical transmission, blood transfusions, and organ transplantation.[10,15–18] In areas with low HHV-8 prevalence, as in the U.S., transmission is mainly sexual and predominantly among teenage and adult MSM. In areas with high HHV-8 seroprevalence, transmission appears to be nonsexual horizontal, occurring among families and close contacts, with high seropositivity present among children prior to adolescence and little increase thereafter.[9,11,18,19] Secretions, primarily saliva, are likely the major source of infection.[12]

Viral DNA has been detected most frequently and in highest levels in saliva, but also is in semen and peripheral blood mononuclear cells.[12,18,20] Blood transfusions have been correlated with HHV-8 seropositivity among children from endemic countries, but appear to have no appreciable role in transmission in the U.S.[12,15] No evidence exists for transmission via breastmilk.[12,20] Vertical transmission has been suggested by detection of HHV-8 DNA in the blood of a few neonates.[21]

CLINICAL MANIFESTATIONS

HHV-8 has a clear causal role only in KS, primary effusion lymphomas, and multicentric Castleman disease.[7,22] Many diseases have been associated with HHV-8 infection, but not confirmed casually, including multiple myeloma, sarcoidosis, and basal and squamous cell carcinomas in transplant recipients.

Clinical manifestations of HHV-8 infection primarily are associated with KS, a multifocal neoplasm of vascular endothelium.[3,7] KS lesions are vascular, purplish nodules that range from isolated cutaneous lesions to widespread disease involving the lung, biliary tract, and other viscera (Figure 209-1).

HHV-8 infection is a major, but not the only, factor contributing to the development of KS.[15,23] Four KS variants have been described:

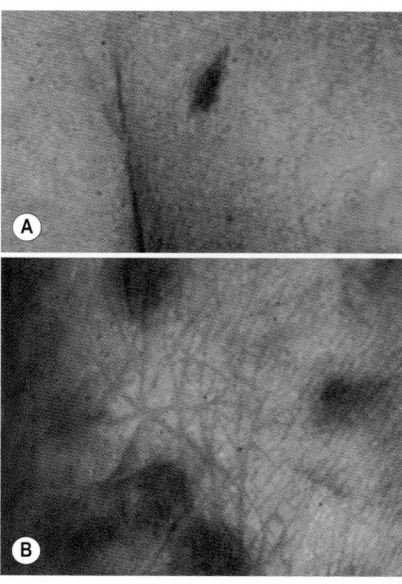

Figure 209-1. Kaposi sarcoma lesions of the chest **(A)** and foot **(B)**. (Courtesy of Susan Cohn, MD, Northwestern University, Evanston, IL.)

(1) classic; (2) endemic/sub-Saharan African; (3) epidemic (AIDS-associated); and (4) immunosuppression-associated forms. The classic type, primarily affecting older men from Mediterranean and eastern European countries, is indolent, involves mainly the skin, and is associated with long survival. The endemic form occurs predominantly in parts of sub-Saharan Africa and affects both adults and children.[3,24] In some areas of Central Africa, KS is among the most common tumors, causing up to 10% of all childhood malignancies.[7,24–26] Endemic HIV-negative KS in African children is distinct from the adult endemic form and characteristically is a more aggressive, often fatal, lymphadenopathic disease and usually has no cutaneous manifestations.[24,27] Endemic KS has been reported in children born to consanguineous parents, suggesting inherited immunodeficiency as one mechanism of KS disease development in children in areas of high HHV-8 prevalence.[28]

Epidemic KS associated with AIDS usually is aggressive with widespread cutaneous and visceral involvement, and is associated with a poor prognosis in adults.[3,7,23,24,29] Epidemic KS in children more closely resembles the endemic form, with lymphadenopathy a prominent feature and a variable prognosis.[23] KS associated with immunosuppression not related to HIV most frequently occurs in endemic areas in solid-organ transplant recipients with previous HHV-8 infection.[14]

Descriptions of primary infection are limited, especially among children, but indicate that most are likely asymptomatic. Clinical expression varies geographically and according to comorbidities.[3,8,24] Among young immunocompetent children residing in endemic areas, primary infection was identified in 7% of those presenting with acute febrile illnesses.[19] Clinical manifestations included fever, upper respiratory tract signs, and a nonspecific maculopapular rash. All children recovered before seroconversion occurred 3 to 12 months later. A mononucleosis-like illness also has been described in several children.[30]

Among immunocompromised patients, primary infection often also is asymptomatic, but sometimes manifests as a febrile illness of varying severity, with lymphadenopathy, splenomegaly, arthralgia, pancytopenia, and occasionally with acute onset of KS.[3,8,26]

DIAGNOSIS

Laboratory methods for diagnosing HHV-8 infection are evolving rapidly. Many polymerase chain reaction (PCR) and serologic assays are available, but their sensitivity, specificity, and clinical usefulness vary widely.[3,14,24,27,31] These tests combined with histopathology and immunocytochemistry, however, allow accurate diagnosis of KS and other HHV-8 associated lymphoproliferative disorders.

Serologic tests include indirect immunofluorescence assays (IFAs) to detect latency-associated nuclear antigen (LANA) and lytic antigens, enzyme immunoassays (EIAs), and immunoblot assays.[3] Their usefulness for diagnosing and differentiating HHV-8-associated diseases is highly dependent on which antigens are detected, as gene expression varies among different HHV-8-related entities.[31] Combining several serologic assays generally increases the sensitivity and specificity of detecting HHV-8 infection.[14]

Qualitative and quantitative PCR assays can detect HHV-8 infection in peripheral blood and tissue biopsy specimens. However, clinical diagnostic accuracy of PCR assays is confounded by the variable and often low number of HHV-8 genomic copies present in infected tissue and peripheral blood, and by the occurrence of asymptomatic viremia.[24,27,32] PCR assays have been used to support the diagnosis of HHV-8-associated disorders, detect exacerbations, and help determine prognosis.[33]

THERAPY

No antiviral therapy is currently approved in the U.S. for HHV-8 infection. HHV-8 shows variable susceptibility to several antiviral agents in vitro, including foscarnet, ganciclovir, and cidofovir, but clinical therapeutic evaluation is limited.[34] Also, whether any observed clinical benefit is directly related to the inhibition of HHV-8 replication or to an effect on concurrent infections is unclear.[7,26,34] Valganciclovir administered for 8 weeks to a small group of HHV-8-infected men has been associated with decreased frequency and quantity of HHV-8 shedding.[34]

Treatment of KS has included excision of small singular lesions, and combinations of radiation, cryotherapy, cryo- and laser surgery, and chemotherapy for more severe disease.[24] Augmenting immunity in immunosuppressed patients is important. For HIV-associated KS, highly active antiretroviral therapy has been combined with chemotherapy. Antiviral therapy is not recommended for asymptomatic HHV-8 infection, even among immunosuppressed patients.[24,35]

210 Adenoviruses

Upton D. Allen and Gail J. Demmler

Adenoviruses are relatively small, nonenveloped double-stranded DNA viruses belonging to the family Adenoviridae (from *adenos*, the Greek word meaning "gland," because they were first isolated from adenoid tissue). There are at least 54 human adenovirus serotypes defined by biological characteristics, including immunochemical methods, such as serum neutralization and hemagglutination.[1–5] Additional novel candidates "serotypes" have been proposed based on characterization using genomics and bioinformatics.[6] The serotypes are classified according to their biochemical, structural, biologic, and immunologic characteristics into seven subgroups A to G.[1–5] Adenoviruses in subgroup B and C (notably C) have the ability to cause latent infections in lymphoid cells.

EPIDEMIOLOGY

Transmission mainly is by direct spread from person to person through contact with infected respiratory tract secretions, fomites and aerosols; enteric strains are transmitted by the fecal–oral route. Transmission also can occur through organ transplantation. Among transplant recipients, reactivation of latent or persistent virus from the host may occur after the start of immunosuppressive therapy.[7,8] Reinfections (which are often asymptomatic) with the same serotype may occur.[9]

While not having the definite seasonality seen with other respiratory viruses, adenoviruses can produce sporadic outbreaks, most commonly in winter, spring, and early summer. No differences in incidence are apparent between males and females or among races or ethnic groups. However, the incidence of infection with adenoviruses appears greatest in lower socioeconomic groups and in situations of crowding. Epidemic adenoviral disease also occurs commonly in military recruits. Outbreaks, especially of pharyngoconjunctival fever, have occurred following exposure at swimming pools, summer camps, childcare centers, and in health-care settings.

Adenovirus infection occurs in all age groups; however, the incidence peaks between the ages of 6 months and 5 years and adenoviruses are a leading cause of febrile illnesses in children seeking urgent care. The use of molecular detection techniques in recent years has indicated a greater burden of adenoviral infections among children in group childcare than had been previously determined.[10] The most common serotypes associated with respiratory tract disease are serotypes 1 through 7, and 21: military recruits are most commonly infected with serotypes 4 and 7; types 8 and 37 are associated most commonly with epidemic kerato-conjunctivitis; and serotypes 3, 7, 32, 40, and 41 have been associated with diarrhea. Disseminated adenovirus disease is associated most often with infection with serotypes 3, 7, and 23, causing serious or fatal disease in both normal and immunocompromised children (Table 210-1).[1,7,11,12] In 30 children hospitalized in Buffalo, NY with adenovirus infection, serotypes 1, 2, 3, 5, and 41 were most common; specific serotypes were associated with symptoms and season.[13]

Nosocomial adenovirus infections also occur. The virus can spread rapidly and cause serious morbidity and substantial mortality, especially if outbreaks occur in neonatal intensive care or hematopoietic stem cell transplant (HSCT) units.[14–21] Factors contributing to the spread of adenoviruses include transmission of virus from the contaminated hands of healthcare workers,[16] infected ophthalmologic specula, retractors and solutions,[14] and equipment such as pneumotonometers,[19,22] endotracheal tubes, and suction catheters.[16] Disinfection of hands or equipment is not accomplished by alcohol, detergents, or chlorhexidine, because adenoviruses are nonenveloped viruses and therefore resistant to these agents. Instruments contaminated with adenoviruses can be disinfected, by immersion in a 1% solution of sodium hypochlor-ite for 10 minutes[23] or by steam autoclaving.[24] Adenoviruses can persist on hands despite handwashing for 10 seconds; therefore, disposable gloves that are changed between contacts with patients should be used to help control institutional outbreaks.[19,22] The use of gowns and masks is recommended for tracheostomy care.[17] Other measures to control adenovirus nosocomial infections are isolation and cohorting of ill patients.[14,15,19] Healthcare workers with epidemic keratoconjunctivitis should not have direct contact with patients until 14 days after the onset of disease in the second eye.[19] The incubation period of respiratory tract infection usually is 2 to 14 days, while for gastrointestinal infection, it is 3 to 10 days.[24]

CLINICAL DISEASE

Adenoviruses cause a variety of syndromes, due to one or more different serotypes (see Table 210-1). The specific symptoms are

TABLE 210-1. Clinical Illnesses and Serotypes Associated with Adenoviral Infections

Syndrome	Signs and Symptoms	Serotypes Involved	
		Frequently	**Infrequently**
Upper respiratory illness	Coryza, pharyngitis, fever, tonsillitis, with diarrhea	1–3, 5, 7	4, 6, 11, 18, 21, 29, 31
Lower respiratory illness	Bronchitis, laryngotracheobronchitis, bronchiolitis, pneumonia, fever, coryza, cough	3, 4, 7, 21	1, 2, 5, 6, 14, 35
Pertussis-like cough illness	Paroxysmal cough, vomiting, fever, with upper respiratory tract symptoms	5	1–3, 12, 19
Infectious mononucleosis-like or Kawasaki-like illness	Fever, malaise, irritability, cervical lymphadenopathy, pharyngitis, rash, conjunctivitis	ND	ND
Pharyngoconjunctival fever	Pharyngitis, conjunctivitis, fever, coryza, headache, rash, adenopathy, with diarrhea	2, 3, 4, 7, 14	1, 5, 6, 8, 11, 16, 19, 37
Epidemic keratoconjunctivitis	Keratitis, headache, preauricular adenopathy, with pharyngitis, diarrhea	3, 8, 19, 37	2, 4, 7, 10, 11, 13, 17, 20, 21, 23
Acute hemorrhagic (follicular) conjunctivitis	Chemosis, subconjunctival hemorrhage, preauricular adenopathy, fever	11	1, 2–8, 9, 10, 14, 15–17, 19, 20, 22, 34, 37
Genitourinary tract disease	Cystitis (usually hemorrhagic), nephritis, orchitis, urethritis, cervicitis, ulcerative genital lesions, with pharyngitis and fever	2, 11, 37	1, 5, 7, 18, 19, 21, 31, 34, 35
Gastrointestinal disease	Gastroenteritis with diarrhea and vomiting; abdominal pain with intussusception, pseudoappendicitis syndrome, or mesenteric lymphadenitis	3, 5, 7, 31, 40, 41	1, 2, 8, 12–17, 21, 25, 26, 29
Central nervous system disease	Meningitis, encephalitis, Reye syndrome	7	3, 26, 32
Cardiac disease	Myocarditis, pericarditis	7, 21	ND
Infection in immunocompromised hosts	Diarrhea, rash, upper respiratory tract illness, pneumonia, hepatitis, hemorrhagic enterocolitis, cystitis, disseminated disease	1, 2, 3, 5, 7,11, 34, 35	21, 29–31, 37–39, 43, 45
Fetus and newborn	Hydrops fetalis, myocarditis, pneumonia, hepatitis, disseminated disease	3	35

ND, not determined.

Modified from Hierholzer JC. Adenoviruses. In: Balows A (ed) Manual of Clinical Microbiology, 6th ed. Washington, DC, American Society for Microbiology, 1994, pp 947–955.

affected by host age and immune status, as well as the site of infection. Many of the endemic adenoviruses, such as subgenus C, types 1, 2, 5, and 6, can cause infection throughout the year and are commonly associated with prolonged but asymptomatic fecal excretion of virus.[25] Other adenoviruses are associated with epidemic disease, common environmental exposure, or novel virus types to which most hosts are susceptible. Among asymptomatic individuals, virus can be present in peripheral blood lymphocytes, lung tissue, and normal duodenal epithelium.[26-29]

Respiratory Infections

Adenoviruses cause 2% to 5% of respiratory tract infections, including upper respiratory tract infections (URIs), such as otitis media, pharyngitis, exudative tonsillitis, cervical adenopathy, and the common cold, as well as mid and lower respiratory tract infections (LRIs), such as bronchitis, laryngotracheobronchitis, pertussis-like syndrome, bronchiolitis, pneumonia, pleural effusions, and hyperlucent lung syndrome.[29]

Tonsillitis is a common feature of adenoviral infections. This tends to occur in younger children (less than 3 years of age) compared with group A streptococcal tonsillitis, which occurs in an older age group (5 to 17 years of age).[30,31] Adenoviruses have been reported to account for approximately 10% to 20% of childhood pneumonias.[32,33] The most severe respiratory tract infections are due to adenovirus types 3 and 7, serotypes that also can cause necrotizing diseases.[16,34-36] The adenovirus serotype 7 has a virulent variant, genome type 7h, which was isolated from children in Argentina, and was associated with all 6 fatalities among 73 children with adenovirus LRI.[35] Retrospective evaluations of lower respiratory tract infections due to adenovirus 7h noted that 10 of 29 children died in Argentina[35] and 2 of 66 in Chile.[36] Death has been recently reported among individuals (predominantly adults) infected with serotype 14 in the United States.[37-39] Obliterative bronchiolitis can develop in children with severe respiratory compromise associated with adenovirus LRI.[40,41] This complication is most common in those who require intensive care, mechanical ventilation, oxygen supplementation, corticosteroid therapy, or β-agonist agents for recovery.[24,40] Hyperlucent lung syndrome, bronchiectasis, and bronchopulmonary dysplasia in premature infants also have been attributed to prior adenovirus infections.[14,18] Pertussis and pertussis-like cough illness can be caused by adenovirus alone or associated with a mixed infection with *Bordetella pertussis*.[42]

Pharyngoconjunctival Fever and Keratoconjunctivitis

Adenoviral pharyngoconjunctival fever is a constellation of conjunctivitis, fever, pharyngitis, and cervical or preauricular lymphadenopathy. Eye involvement consists of acute follicular conjunctivitis; sequelae are rare.

Epidemic keratoconjunctivitis, caused mainly by types 3, 8, 19, and 37, is a severe eye disease that usually occurs in adults.[43] Novel serotypes recently have been shown to be associated with this condition.[5,6] The clinical course is characterized by slow progression from foreign body sensation and photophobia to impaired vision, swelling of conjunctiva and eyelids, and subconjunctival hemorrhage.[19] Acute symptoms can last for 4 to 6 weeks and can be associated with pharyngitis. Diffuse epithelial engorgement can progress to punctate epithelial lesions followed by subepithelial keratitis, which may persist. Preauricular lymphadenopathy often is present. Epidemic keratoconjunctivitis can progress to pseudomembranous conjunctivitis and eyelid erythema and edema mimicking periorbital bacterial cellulitis.[18,41]

Gastrointestinal Infections

Adenovirus types 40 and 41 of subgroup F[44,45] and serotypes 3, 5, 7, and 31[46] are associated most commonly with a gastroenteritis

syndrome, especially in children younger than 2 years of age. Other serotypes, including serotypes 2 and 8, also have been implicated.[35] Enteric adenoviruses are a common cause of infantile diarrhea.[46-49] Illness associated with enteric adenovirus infection, notably the rate of fever and dehydration, is comparable to that associated with group A rotavirus infection.[49-52] However, enteric adenovirus diarrhea usually has no seasonality, lasts longer than most other infectious diarrhea syndromes, and is associated with more vomiting than that caused by rotavirus infection.[50,53]

Adenoviruses also have been associated with mesenteric lymphadenitis, appendicitis, and intussusception. Fulminant hepatic necrosis has been described in patients with disseminated adenoviral disease and in immunosuppressed patients.

Genitourinary Infections

Genitourinary tract infection can result in acute hemorrhagic cystitis in both healthy and immunocompromised patients. Infection has been associated with nephritis, orchitis, and hemolytic uremic syndrome. In bone marrow transplant recipients, adenovirus-associated hemorrhagic cystitis can be prolonged and associated with substantial morbidity, including severe pain and the need for blood transfusions. If infection occurs during the first 100 days after transplantation, disseminated disease can develop and mortality may be high.[12,54,55] Coinfection with other DNA viruses, such as BK virus (a polyomavirus), also can occur.[54]

Cardiac Infections

Adenoviruses have been detected in specimens of pericardial fluid and myocardial tissue obtained from patients with acute myocarditis and pericarditis.[56-58] Intrauterine adenoviral myocarditis with cardiac failure rarely causes nonimmune fetal hydrops.[59,60]

Neurologic Infections

Neurologic disease, including aseptic meningitis, encephalitis, and transverse myelitis, associated with adenovirus infection is rare. Adenoviruses have been detected in cerebrospinal fluid by cell culture and by polymerase chain reaction (PCR), and in brain tissue by histopathology using immunohistochemical staining.[61,62] Central nervous system involvement can occur as part of severe, disseminated disease, especially in immunocompromised patients. Adenoviruses also have been associated with febrile convulsions.[63]

Other Illnesses

Adenoviruses can cause prolonged fever without a focus.[64,65] Other clinical entities include an infectious mononucleosis (IM)-like syndrome as well as a Kawasaki-like syndrome.[66,67]

Immunocompromised and Special Hosts

Adenoviruses are important pathogens in immunocompromised hosts, especially hematopoietic stem cell transplant (HSCT) and solid-organ transplant recipients.[1,2,68-72] In HSCT recipients, the rates of adenovirus infections are 4% to 18%, with reported fatality rates of up to 75%.[73] Most infections occur during the first months after transplantation, before engraftment. Fever, pneumonia, hepatitis, hemorrhagic cystitis, gastroenteritis, and colitis are the most common clinical presentations, and widespread virus dissemination also occurs, often with fatal outcome.[73-78] Risk factors for adenoviral infection and death in HSCT recipients include graft-versus-host disease, total-body irradiation, type of marrow graft, pulmonary disease, isolation of the virus from more than one site and the type of immunosuppressive regimen.[72,75]

Adenovirus infections occur in approximately 10% of liver transplant recipients, often causing hepatitis in the transplanted organ or disseminated disease, with an overall fatality rate of

53%.[1,79-82] Adenovirus infection in lung transplant recipients can be severe and can cause pneumonia, obliterative bronchiolitis, and disseminated disease.

Adenovirus infections occur in approximately 10% of renal transplant recipients. Acute hemorrhagic cystitis, with hematuria, frequency, dysuria, and fever, and rarely renal impairment can result.[83]

Children with malignancy and patients with acquired immuno-deficiency syndrome (AIDS) can be infected with a wide variety of adenovirus serotypes, and serious, even fatal disease, involving liver and lungs, has been reported.[84,85]

Adenovirus infections in the fetus and newborn are rare but typically are severe.[86-93] Fetal death can result from nonimmune hydrops.[59,60,87,88] In addition, most infections in the first month of life are fatal, and can be acquired nosocomially during outbreaks in neonatal special care units, perinatally from the mother, or postnatally from family members or other close contacts.[14-16,90,91,93] Risk factors for perinatal adenovirus disease include premature labor, prolonged rupture of membranes, and maternal fever with upper respiratory tract illness at the time of delivery.[90] The illness usually manifests with lethargy, fever, and hepatosplenomegaly, with onset within 10 days of birth. After a brief period of apparent stabilization, virus disseminates and hepatitis, pneumonia, disseminated intravascular coagulation, and death ensue.

DIAGNOSIS

The method used to detect adenovirus infection varies according to the nature of the disease that is being investigated. Conventional methods include electron microscopy to detect adenovirus particles in feces or respiratory tract secretions, histopathology with immunohistochemical staining of tissue, virus isolation by culture, direct antigen detection, and PCR.[67,94,95]

Adenoviruses can be isolated in a variety of cell culture systems.[95] Isolation of adenovirus from the nasopharynx, throat, urine, and stool support the diagnosis of acute infection, although isolation of virus from these sites can occur in the absence of disease. Isolation of virus from blood, pleural, pericardial, or cerebrospinal fluid, or tissue provides strong evidence of invasive disease. Adenovirus produces a characteristic rounded "cluster of grapes" cytopathic effect in cell culture, usually within 3 to 5 days of incubation; virus-specific immunofluorescence assays can be used for definitive identification. Identification of adenovirus serotype requires neutralization or hemagglutination-inhibition tests. Some serotypes of adenovirus, such as types 40 and 41, are fastidious, and culture is not a sensitive or reliable method for their detection. Some serotypes may be excreted for prolonged periods, thereby making the association between diseases and virus isolation challenging.

Adenovirus antigens can be detected in respiratory tract secretions by direct fluorescence assay using commercially available reagents. Results can be available within 24 hours, which is rapid enough to impact clinical decisions.[67] Other rapid antigen detection methods include immunochromatography and latex agglutination, which are particularly useful for stool samples. A commercially available rapid immunochromatographic test detects most adenovirus serotypes, in a wide variety of specimens, including feces, nasopharyngeal and respiratory tract secretions, eye and conjunctival swabs, and urine. The test is simple to perform and results are available in less than 30 minutes.[96] Studies suggest that the test is sensitive and specific compared with reference standards such as viral culture and DNA detection by PCR. False-positive reactions have been documented with the local eye anesthetic oxybuprocaine.[97] Caution with interpretation of antigen-detection test results in neonatal stools is warranted; 50% of Sure-Vue adenovirus tests (SA Scientific, San Antonio, TX) in 56 infants in a neonatal intensive care unit were falsely positive (i.e., negative by isolation, PCR and RT-PCR) for undetermined reasons.[98]

Molecular methods of detection are favored by many laboratories. These methods can detect and/or quantify adenovirus DNA in respiratory tract secretions, feces, blood, and urine. Gene amplification techniques, such as PCR, are sensitive and can detect any adenovirus or specific adenovirus serotypes using unique genomic regions of primers, probes, or both.[99-101] In addition, serial quantitative PCR assays can be used to monitor transplant recipients prospectively.[102] If high or rising viral DNA levels are detected by serial quantitative PCR assays, intervention with antiviral and immunomodulating therapies, as well as adjustment of immunosuppression regimens, are indicated to prevent serious or fatal disease.[103] Assays that amplify and detect partial or unique regions of the hexon genomic region also have been used to study the molecular epidemiology of adenoviruses.[45,104] Other test modalities (e.g., DNA microarray technology) are the subject of research and are not available for routine clinical application.[105-107]

Serologic methods can detect significant rises in levels of antibodies between serum specimens collected during acute illness and convalescence 2 to 4 weeks later. Serologic methods include testing for group-reactive antibody (complement fixation test, enzyme immunoassay) or type-specific antibody (neutralization or hemagglutination-inhibition assay). However, sensitivity may be 50% or less in acute infections in normal hosts. Serologic methods are even more unreliable in the immunocompromised host and are not recommended for routine clinical diagnosis of infection.

TREATMENT AND PREVENTION

While most adenovirus infections in otherwise healthy individuals are self-limited, symptomatic infection of immunocompromised hosts should be treated with antiviral agents and reduction of immunosuppression, if possible. While early antiviral treatment is desirable, no consensus exists regarding the optimal management of asymptomatic patients with detectable adenovirus viremia.

Trifluridine, ribavirin, and cidofovir are active in vitro against adenoviruses.[108-110] However, there are only anecdotal case reports or uncontrolled case series of treatment for serious adenovirus disease with antiviral agents. Ribavirin has been administered with variable success, depending on the location and extent of the infection and immune function of the host.[11,109-111] Cidofovir has emerged as the preferred antiviral agent for treatment of adenoviral disease.[7] Cidofovir at a dosage of 5 mg/kg administered intravenously once weekly or at a reduced dosage of 1 to 1.5 mg/kg administered intravenously 3 times weekly has demonstrated clinical and virologic benefit in some patients.[112-115] The drug should be administered with intravenous hydration and oral probenicid to reduce renal toxicity. Lipid esters of cidofovir are being evaluated to overcome the toxicity of conventional cidofovir.[116,117] Ganciclovir has activity against adenoviruses; however, studies are needed to clarify its effectiveness and role in the management of adenoviral disease.[118,119]

Treatment of hypoxemia or respiratory failure may require oxygen supplementation, mechanical ventilation, inhaled nitric oxide, or extracorporeal membrane oxygenation.[120]

Immunoglobulin for intravenous use has been used to treat patients with acute myocarditis, as well as immunodeficient patients with pneumonia and disseminated disease due to adenovirus.[121,122] Novel immunoadoptive therapies that transfer virus-specific T-lymphocyte immunity to hosts with no specific adenovirus T-lymphocyte immunity are being explored as therapeutic options in HSCT recipients.[71,123,124]

Prevention of adenovirus infections by active immunization is not available outside of the military setting. Passive immunization with immunoglobulin has not been proven to be effective for immunoprophylaxis or outbreak control. Careful hand hygiene by caregivers, and adequate disinfection of instruments and objects in the environment remain primary tools for preventing the spread of adenovirus in home, group childcare and healthcare settings.

211 Human Papillomaviruses

Loris Y. Hwang and Anna-Barbara Moscicki

Papillomaviruses are species-specific and widely distributed among mammals and non-mammalian animal species. Human papillomaviruses (HPVs) are strictly epitheliotropic and cause infections and cancer of the skin and mucous membranes. Clinical conditions include anogenital infections and cancers, oral infections and cancers, and recurrent respiratory papillomatosis.

THE VIRUS AND PATHOGENESIS

HPVs are nonenveloped, double-stranded DNA viruses with a small circular genome of approximately 8000 basepairs. HPV genes are classified by their expression being either early or late in the viral replication cycle. The early gene E6 disrupts the anti-oncogene p53. E7 disrupts the E2F/pRb complex, leading to activation of E2F, an important cellular transcription factor.[1] Both events lead to abnormal cellular proliferation. E6 and E7 also activate telomerase to lengthen telomeres, leading to the prolonged life of epithelial cells and blockade of apoptosis. E6 and E7 transcription is regulated by E2. Interestingly, viral integration, which occurs in over 80% of HPV-related cancers, results in E2 loss and the enhanced transcription of E6 and E7.

HPV infection begins with viral invasion of the epithelial basal cells particularly in the setting of epithelial disruption due to minor abrasions or inflammation. In the basal and parabasal layers, only the early viral genes are expressed, and viral DNA is replicated in low copy numbers, which likely contributes to evasion of the host immune system. In the more differentiated upper layers of the epithelium, expression of the late genes, L1 and L2, produces capsid antigens that allow the release of fully infectious viral particles with physiologic epithelial desquama-

tion. Inflammatory signals are absent as initial HPV infection does not induce cell death.

Extensive study of HPV as a cause of invasive cervical cancer has formed the basis of our understanding of HPV pathogenesis. Cervical cancer originates in the cervical transformation zone where the proximal single-layered columnar epithelium transitions to the distal stratified squamous epithelium. At this juncture, the physiologic process of squamous metaplasia transforms the columnar cells into squamous cells. Squamous metaplastic activity is thought to be triggered by pubertal hormonal changes, and thus is most common during adolescence and young adulthood, when initial HPV infection also commonly occurs.[2,3] However, the time between initial HPV infection and the development of invasive cancer is several decades in most healthy women. Active viral replication results in the benign changes of mild basal cell proliferation and perinuclear halos. These changes are described using different nomenclature when evaluated by cytology and by histology. Cytology results are reported according to the Bethesda system; benign changes are referred to as atypical squamous cells of undetermined significance (ASC-US) and low-grade squamous intraepithelial lesion (LSIL) (Table 211-1).[4] Based on histology, these benign lesions are reported according to the World Health Organization terminology and referred to as cervical intraepithelial neoplasia (CIN) 1. The cytologic term high-grade squamous intraepithelial lesion (HSIL) and the histologic term CIN 2 and 3 refer to precancerous lesions. The histologic changes of aneuploidy, altered chromatin texture, and increased nuclear volume are thought to be related to E6 and E7 expression in the epithelial stem cells. These cells have lost the ability to differentiate and demonstrate mutagenic consequences including damage of

TABLE 211-1. Terminology Used to Describe the Cervical Epithelium

Bethesda Terminology for Cytology	Equivalent WHO Terminology for Histology
SQUAMOUS CELL ABNORMALITIES	
Atypical squamous cells of undetermined significance (ASC-US)[a]	Squamous atypia
Atypical squamous cells, cannot exclude HSIL (ASC-H)[b]	
Low-grade squamous intraepithelial lesion (LSIL)[a]	Mild dysplasia, condylomatous atypia, HPV-related changes, koilocytic atypia, cervical epithelial neoplasia 1 (CIN 1)
High-grade squamous intraepithelial lesion (HSIL)[b]	Moderate dysplasia (CIN 2), severe dysplasia (CIN 3), carcinoma in situ
GLANDULAR CELL ABNORMALITIES	
Atypical glandular cells (AGC)[c]	
Endocervical adenocarcinoma in situ (AIS)[c]	
Adenocarcinoma[d]	

[a]*Repeat cytology in 12 months.*

[b]*Refer to a gynecology specialist for colposcopy.*

[c]*Refer to a gynecology specialist for colposcopy including endocervical sampling; consider endometrial sampling depending on clinical history.*

[d]*Refer to gynecology specialist.*

chromosomal integrity, recombination of diverse DNA, and viral integration. The final mechanisms leading to invasive cancer remain unexplained.

IMMUNITY

Cell-mediated immunity is critical for HPV control, as evidenced by the increased risk of HPV-related anogenital cancer in individuals with depressed cell-mediated immunity.[5] Likely both genetic and epigenetic factors influence the host immune response. The primary mechanism for HPV persistence is thought to be evasion of both innate and adaptive immune responses. The antibody response to natural HPV infections is relatively low in titer compared to other systemic viral infections and is not universally detected.[6] Antibodies associated with natural infection may not be protective since women with HPV-associated invasive cervical cancer are more likely to have antibodies than women without cancer. In contrast, antibody levels induced by HPV vaccines are 60 to 100 times higher than those found in natural infections.[7]

EPIDEMIOLOGY AND CLINICAL FEATURES

The more than 100 HPV types are catalogued into the genera alpha, beta, gamma, mu, and nu.[8] Alpha types are further divided according to their natural tropism for cutaneous or mucosal sites. The types associated with cutaneous warts include HPV types 1, 2, 3, and 10. Of the 40 mucosal alpha types found in the anogenital or oral tracts, several are termed "high-risk" (types 16, 18, 31, 33, 35, 39, 45, 51, 52, 56, 58, 59, 66, 68, 73, 82) based on their association with cancers of these regions.[9] Notably, HPV-16 and -18 are responsible for approximately 70% of cervical cancers; HPV-16 is associated with over 70% of anal cancers and 20% to 30% of head and neck squamous cell carcinomas; and HPV-18 is associated with adenocarcinoma of the cervix. High-risk types are also associated with 50% of vulvar, vaginal, and penile cancers, although this association is highly dependent on histologic type.

The more common low-risk anogenital types (types 6, 11, 40, 42, 43, 44, 54, 61, 72, 73, 83) cause benign or low-grade cervical cellular changes and anogenital warts. Anogenital warts are caused most commonly by HPV-6 and -11. HPVs associated with cutaneous warts are likely transmitted via nonsexual skin-to-skin contact. However, fomite reservoirs exist since risk factors for plantar warts include bare feet in communal bathrooms and showers. Anogenital HPV transmission occurs predominantly through sexual contact. Perinatal transmission can occur at birth from an infected mother to her newborn. Although consequent clinical disease in infants is rare, HPV-6 and -11 can cause juvenile-onset recurrent respiratory papillomatosis or anogenital warts.

Anogenital Tract Infections

Initial HPV infection in the female anogenital tract typically occurs within 3 years of sexual debut. Lifetime risk reaches 80% in sexually active individuals. In developed countries, women aged 15 to 25 years exhibit the highest prevalence rates of 25% to 40%. Prevalence rates decline to approximately 15% in women 30 years and older, and plateau at 10% around age 40 years. The strongest risk factors for infection are new sexual partners and lack of condom use in women of any age. Ninety percent of infections detected by DNA testing resolve spontaneously within 6 to 9 months.[10] Thus, infection by high-risk HPVs is common in the female anogenital tract and by itself is not concerning. Most young women with HPV demonstrate either no detectable lesion by cytology or only LSIL. LSIL is a benign manifestation of HPV, and studies show that the vast majority of CIN1 lesions regress spontaneously.

Recurrent infections with both new HPV types and the same types are common in young women.[11] Whether recurrence of the same type represents repeated new infections or reactivation of latent infection remains controversial. However, the rare persistent infection with a high-risk type is known as the necessary step for progression to cervical cancer. HPV infection detected in an older woman likely represents a persistent infection originally acquired years before. Hence HPV DNA testing is proposed as a primary screening tool in women over 30 years of age.[12]

HPV prevalence in the male anogenital tract is estimated at 50%, but varies widely from 1% to 73% according to sampling techniques, and the number of HPV types and genital areas tested.[13] In contrast to women, prevalence does not vary with age,[14] prompting the hypotheses that male infections are primarily transient without inducing a protective immune response. Supporting this hypothesis is the finding that within 6 months, most men experience clearance of the initial HPV type detected.[15] Antibody titers are lower in men than women at all ages despite the prevalence of DNA detection being higher in men than women at all ages.[16] As with cervical infection, HPV persistence is essential to the development of penile cancer. Information about anal infection has been derived predominantly from studies of men who have sex with men (MSM). Prevalence of anal infection is approximately 60% in HIV-negative persons and approaches 100% in HIV-positive persons.[17-19] Anal HPV also is common in women including adolescents.[20] The cumulative 1-year incidence of anal HPV in women was 70% in one study.[21] Clearance of anal HPV is slightly faster than cervical HPV infection. Persistent anal intraepithelial neoplasia (AIN) 2 and AIN3 are precancerous and can progress to anal cancer.

Anogenital Cancers

Cervical cancer is the second most common female malignancy worldwide, following breast cancer. About 500,000 new cases of cervical cancer are diagnosed annually worldwide, with 12,200 new cases projected for the United States during 2010.[22] The age-adjusted incidence is 8.1 per 100,000 women. U.S. rates have decreased significantly due to the availability of routine cervical screening and management of precancerous lesions. However, barriers to healthcare remain a contributing factor for new cases.

The rates for cancers of the vulva, vagina, anus, and penis are considerably lower than the rates for cervical cancer. In the U.S., the projected number of newly diagnosed cases during 2010 was 3900 for vulvar cancer; 2300 for vaginal cancer; 5260 for anal cancer; and 1250 for penile cancer.[22] Age-adjusted incidence rates for anal cancer are 1.4 per 100,000 women and 1.0 per 100,000 men. Rates are increased in MSM (non-HIV-infected) to 37 per 100,000.[23,24] Risk factors for anal cancer in women include a history of cancers of the cervix, vulva, or vagina, and CIN 3.[25-27]

Oral Infections and Cancers

The prevalence of oral HPV infection has been reported at 4% to 5%;[28] however, sampling techniques likely are inadequate in detecting HPV from the areas around the tonsils and base of the tongue. Most cases of oral cancers are associated with alcohol and tobacco use. However, approximately 25% of head and neck cancers are HPV-associated.[29] This association is increased in cancers at the tonsils and base of the tongue.

HPV Infection in Immunocompromised Individuals

Individuals who are HIV-infected or otherwise immunocompromised experience increased HPV prevalence, persistence, and progression to cancer. In HIV-infected MSM, the incidence of anal cancer is approximately 78 per 100,000 person-years.[17-19,24] Prevalence of cervical HPV infection reaches 80% in HIV-infected women, who also experience increased rates of cervical, vulvar, and anal cancers.[30] Invasive cervical cancer is an AIDS-defining condition.

Anogenital Warts

Warts (condylomas) are the most common clinical manifestations of anogenital HPV. U.S. physicians see more than 1 million individuals yearly for anogenital warts, and 6% of sexually active 18- to 59-year-olds report a history of anogenital wart diagnosis.[31] Approximately 90% of warts are caused by infections with HPV-6 and -11 which almost never are associated with invasive cancers.

Anogenital warts are found in the external genitalia, upper thighs, inguinal folds, vagina, uterine cervix, and periurethral, intraurethral, perianal and intra-anal areas. Anogenital warts can be papular, cauliflower-shaped, keratotic, flat, or pedunculated; and single or multiple. Individuals with a history of receptive anal sex are at higher risk of intra-anal warts. Infants can acquire anogenital warts perinatally from an infected mother. Congenital infection is rare. Anogenital warts in children of any age may indicate sexual abuse, with a particularly higher association with abuse in those older than 3 years.

Cutaneous Warts

Cutaneous warts commonly are papular, cauliflower-shaped, and keratotic. Plantar and palmar warts typically are flat. Cutaneous warts can occur in the perineal skin, but these HPVs rarely infect mucosal surfaces. Skin warts are most prevalent in school-aged children and young adults. Malignant transformation of skin warts is almost never seen in immunocompetent individuals. In contrast, immunocompromised patients can experience extensive skin warts with the potential for malignant transformation.

Recurrent Respiratory Papillomatosis

Juvenile-onset recurrent respiratory papillomatosis (JORRP) is a rare but serious disease usually caused by HPV-6 or -11 acquired at birth. Incidence is estimated at 1 to 4 cases per 100,000 births annually.[32] Risk factors for JORRP are first-order birth, young

maternal age, and maternal condylomas at delivery. Most cases are diagnosed by 5 years of age. Although most cases are isolated to the larynx, mucosal papillomas can affect the nasopharynx, oropharynx, trachea, and esophagus. Infants can exhibit a hoarse or weak cry, stridor, feeding difficulties, and failure to thrive. Older children can manifest hoarseness, stridor, and dysphonia. Rare cases of bronchopulmonary involvement with malignant degeneration have been reported. Papillomas are not precancerous, but airway obstruction is a serious consequence. Diagnosis is by direct laryngoscopic visualization and histologic analysis. Management can require extensive surgical excisions and chemotherapy. Many patients experience frequent recurrences necessitating multiple surgeries.

Epidermodysplasia Verruciformis

Epidermodysplasia verruciformis (EV) is a rare genetic disorder characterized by susceptibility to persistent and extensive cutaneous HPV warts with malignant transformation in up to one-half of cases.

LABORATORY SCREENING AND DIAGNOSIS

Cutaneous and anogenital warts are diagnosed reliably by history and examination by experienced clinicians. However, if therapy is ineffective, biopsy may be warranted to verify the diagnosis.

The primary mode of screening for cervical precancers and cancers is by cytology (Papanicolaou smear or liquid-based cytology). Sampling should include both ectocervical scrapings and brush sampling within the cervical os to assure sampling of the squamocolumnar junction. Screening guidelines, updated in 2009 by both the American Society for Colposcopy and Cervical Pathology (ASCCP) and the American College of Obstetricians and Gynecologists (ACOG), are found at www.asccp.org.[33,34] Routine cervical cytology is now recommended to begin at 21 years of age. Subsequent scheduling of ongoing screening varies somewhat, but new guidelines are expected in 2012 from the U.S. Preventive Services Task Force, American Cancer Society, the American Society for Colposcopy and Cervircal Pathology and American Society for Clinical Pathology (www.uspreventiveservicestaskforce.org/recommendations, www.asccp.org). Preliminary draft guidelines indicate that nonimmunocompromised women ages 21–29 years will be advised to receive screening every 3 years. HIV-infected or immunocompromised women of any age should have cytology screening twice during the first year after diagnosis of HIV and annually thereafter.

Direct cervical visualization is warranted in patients with bleeding, dyspareunia, or other symptoms. Overt cancer may be visualized without the assistance of magnification.

Abnormal cytology (see management section below) may warrant further diagnostic verification by colposcopy and histology sampling. Colposcopy at 10–16× magnifications with application of 3% to 5% acetic acid enhances vascular and tissue abnormalities and guides the clinician to appropriate biopsy sites.

Screening for anal precancers and cancers remains controversial. However, since HIV-infected MSM have the highest incidence, many clinicians perform anal cytologic screening.[35] Anal screening practices must be conducted by skilled clinicians and supported by appropriate referrals. Some advocate for screening in women with a history of cervical or vulvar cancer or CIN 3. At a minimum these women should have routine digital rectal examinations. There are no screening recommendations for vulvar, vaginal, penile, or oropharyngeal cancers.

MANAGEMENT

Current treatments for cutaneous and anogenital warts are directed toward destruction or excision of visible lesions. Treatment of cutaneous warts usually is for cosmetic reasons since the risk of malignant transformation is exceedingly low and

---

BOX 211-1. Recommended Therapy for Genital Warts

PATIENT-APPLIED

Podofilox 0.5% solution or gel. Apply with swab or finger to visible warts twice daily for 3 days, followed by 4 days without treatment. Repeat this cycle for up to 4 cycles, using a maximum of 0.5 mL per day.

or

Imiquimod 5% cream. Apply once daily 3 times per week, for up to 16 weeks. Wash the treatment area with soap and water 6–10 hours after the application.

or

Sinecatechins (Veregen® ointment 15%). Apply 3 times daily for up to 16 weeks.

PROVIDER-ADMINISTERED

Cryotherapy with liquid nitrogen or cryoprobe. Repeat every 1–2 weeks.

or

Trichloroacetic acid (TCA) or bichloroacetic acid (BCA) 80–90%. Apply small amounts to each wart weekly, followed by air drying. Take care to avoid applying to normal skin.

or

Surgical removal by scissor excision, shave excision, curettage, or electrosurgery.

ALTERNATIVE

Intralesional interferon

or

Photodynamic therapy

Adapted from Centers for Disease Control and Prevention. Sexually transmitted diseases treatment guidelines, 2006. MMWR 2010;59(RR-12):70–74.

---

immune-mediated regression of lesions over a period of months to a few years is expected. Noteworthy exceptions are warts that cause bleeding, pruritus, or pain, especially plantar and subungual warts. Warts typically require costly repeated treatments associated with significant discomfort and high failure rates.

Cutaneous warts are treated with provider-applied cryotherapy, electrocautery, laser therapy, surgical excision, or patient-applied combinations of acetic acid–salicylic acid. External anogenital warts are treated with cryotherapy, surgical excision, or application of caustic agents. The 2010 Centers for Disease Control and Prevention (CDC) guidelines for patient-applied and provider-administered treatment of external anogenital warts are summarized in Box 211-1.[36] Recently, the provider-administered podophyllin resin 10–25% has lost favor due to unreliable potency. Sinecatechins (Veregen ointment 15%) has been approved by the Food and Drug Administration (FDA) for topical application to anogenital warts 3 times daily for up to 16 weeks.

The 2006 ASCCP guidelines for the management of abnormal cervical cytology in females of all ages are found at www.asccp.org. Although routine cervical cytology screening is not recommended until age 21 years, implementation of these guidelines may take several years. A key point for women under 21 years of age is that ASC-US or LSIL should be observed with repeat cytology every 12 months for 24 months since many cases self-resolve.[33,37] Women with persistent ASC-US or LSIL at 24 months of follow-up or HSIL at any visit should be referred for further evaluation by colposcopy. Immediate treatment using excisional therapy without histologic confirmation of HSIL is unwarranted in adolescents. Adolescents with CIN 2 or 3 on histology should be referred for further management by a gynecology specialist. CIN 1 on histology can be followed similarly to ASC-US or LSIL. In HIV-infected

or immunocompromised women, referral to colposcopy should be made if ASC-US is found at two consecutive visits, or if LSIL or HSIL are found at any time.

Currently, HPV DNA testing serves as a triage test for risk stratification of women 21 years and older who have a cytologic diagnosis of ASC-US. Adults with ASC-US and a positive high-risk HPV DNA test result require colposcopy. Those with ASC-US but a negative HPV result can resume routine screening. The current FDA-approved assays detect the presence of one or more of 13 to 14 of the high-risk HPVs. Women 20 years and younger should not receive HPV DNA testing under any circumstances because infection is highly prevalent and the vast majority resolve.

PREVENTION

Genital HPV infection is avoided by sexual abstinence, and decreased by delayed sexual debut, monogamy, and fewer sexual partners. Condom use reduces the risk of infection and hastens LSIL resolution.[38,39] Cesarean delivery to prevent perinatal transmission is not recommended.

Two HPV vaccines are licensed by the FDA. The recombinant quadrivalent vaccine Gardasil, containing the L1 protein of HPV-6, -11, -16, and -18, is licensed for females (2006) and males (2009) aged 9 to 26 years.[40,41] The bivalent vaccine Cervarix, containing only the L1 of HPV-16 and -18, is licensed for females (2009) aged 9 to 26 years.[42] Both vaccines demonstrate >90% efficacy in preventing cervical cancer precursor lesions caused by their respective HPV vaccine types, among females who have not already been infected with those types.[43–48] Additionally, Gardasil is efficacious in preventing vaginal and vulvar precancer lesions and anogenital warts in males and females caused by the HPV vaccine types.[49,50] Preliminary studies of MSM suggest high vaccine efficacy in reducing anal precancer lesions. There is no evidence of protection against any HPV disease in patients already infected with the vaccine types before vaccination.

The target group for HPV vaccination is adolescents who have not initiated any sexual activity. The Centers for Disease Control and Prevention and American Academy of Pediatrics recommend either vaccine for routine universal vaccination of females aged 11 to 12 years, with "catch-up" vaccination up to age 26 years (Box 211-2). Gardasil has a permissive recommendation for males aged 11 to 12 years, with "catch-up" up to age 26 years. Immunization can begin as young as age 9 years. Either vaccine requires 3 doses (0.5 mL each) intramuscularly at 0, 1–2, and 6 months. The absolute minimum intervals are 4 weeks between the first and second dose, and 12 weeks between the second and third dose. An Australian study has already demonstrated the public health impact of marked drops in genital wart diagnoses after vaccine introduction.[51] Other potential benefits may include prevention of penile, anal, and oropharyngeal cancers. Clinicians should remain alert for future vaccine updates and evolving information on the long-term duration of immunity.

BOX 211-2. Recommendations for Quadrivalent and Bivalent HPV Vaccine[a]; Advisory Committee on Immunization Practices, Centers for Disease Control

- Quadrivalent or bivalent vaccine for girls, quadrivalent vaccine for boys
- Routine vaccination of girls and boys 11–12 years of age
- Vaccination series can be started as young as 9 years of age at discretion of provider and parent
- Catch-up vaccination for adolescent and young women and men 13–26 years of age who have not been vaccinated previously

[a]Vaccination is a series of 3 doses of quadrivalent HPV vaccine.

---

212 BK, JC, and Other Human Polyomaviruses

Veronique Erard and Michael Boeckh

VIRUSES, PATHOGENESIS, AND EPIDEMIOLOGY

The Polyomaviridae constitute a family of small DNA viruses infecting a variety of hosts. In humans, polyomaviruses can cause central nervous system (CNS), urinary tract, and skin infection exclusively in immunosuppressed individuals.

Six human polyomaviruses have been identified. BK virus (BKV) and JC virus (JCV) in 1971,[1,2] WU polyomavirus (WUPyV) and KI polyomavirus (KIPyV) in 2007, Merkel cell polyomavirus (MCV) in 2008,[3] and trichodysplasia spinulosa virus (TSV) in 2010.[4]

Polyomaviruses belong to the Papovaviridae family. They are small (diameter 40 nm) nonenveloped viruses with a double-stranded DNA genome, and an icosahedral capsid composed of three structural proteins, VP1, VP2, and VP3. The viral DNA is a supercoiled, circular, double-stranded DNA of around 5000 base pairs. The genome is organized in three regions (early, late, and regulatory), each of which has specific functions.[5,6]

The outcome of polyomavirus infection is species specific. In a permissive host, a lytic infection generally occurs, while in non-permissive hosts a block to viral replication leads to abortive infection or oncogenesis. Infection of the human cells by the human-specific viruses generally is limited to epithelial cells, fibroblasts, lymphocytes, or cells derived from the CNS.

Seroprevalence rates for the human polyomaviruses are: 82% for BKV, 39% for JCV, 55% for KIPyV, 69% for WUPyV, 25% for MCV strain 350, 42% for MCV strain 339, and 2% for SV40.[7] Age-specific prevalence studies have been performed for BKV and JCV. BKV seroconversion peaks during childhood. JCV seroprevalence increases steadily from childhood to the sixth or seventh decade of life.[8,9]

Fecal–oral, oral, and respiratory routes of transmission have been suggested for different human polyomaviruses. Studies in urban sewage samples suggest the possibility of JC and BK virus acquisition through fecally contaminated water, food, and fomites.[10,11] The detection of salivary shedding of BKV implicates oral transmission as another route of infection.[12] KIPyV and WUPyV have been isolated from respiratory secretions of children,[13,14] and exceptionally in immunosuppressed adults.[15–17] MCV DNA can be detected in respiratory tract specimens of symptomatic individuals (mainly adults).[18,19]

BK VIRUS

BK virus was first reported to be a human pathogen in 1971, when a renal transplant recipient, with the initials BK, presented with ureteric stenosis.[1] In the last decade, BK virus has become an emerging pathogen in the setting of kidney transplantation with a propensity to cause severe nephritis in the allograft resulting in graft loss in up to 80% of cases.[20,21] In the hematopoietic stem cell transplant (HSCT) population, the association of BK virus infection and hemorrhagic cystitis was reported first in the mid-1980s.[22,23]

Primary infection during childhood generally is asymptomatic or is associated with fever and mild upper respiratory tract symptoms,[24] or occasionally self-limited hemorrhagic cystitis.[25] Primary infection is followed by virus dissemination to the sites of persistent infection, principally the urinary tract.[26]

Intermittent replication occurs as evidenced by periodic excretion of BK virus in the urine of immunocompetent individuals and pregnant women.[27] The control of persistent infection by the host innate, humoral and cellular immunity is incompletely understood.[28]

Hematopoietic Stem Cell Transplant Recipients

Hemorrhagic cystitis. Hemorrhagic cystitis (HC) is characterized by hemorrhagic inflammation of the bladder mucosa leading to painful micturition and urinary frequency and urgency with hematuria. HC ranges from a mild and brief (grade I) to a severe and life-threatening (grade IV) illness.[29,30] In HSCT recipients, HC occurs in the early (before engraftment) or late (after engraftment) transplantation period. Early-onset HC usually is caused by drug toxicity and is commonly associated with conditioning regimens containing high-dose cyclophosphamide and busulfan.[31-34] Late-onset HC usually is attributed to BK virus, adenovirus, and, rarely, cytomegalovirus (CMV) infection.[35,36] There is a direct relationship between BK viruria, late-onset HC, and the quantity of BK virus in the urine. Several studies have reported an association between presence and level of BK virus in urine and late onset HC.[37-40] An association between HC and high levels of BK viremia detected by polymerase chain reaction (PCR), also has been observed in some,[34,41,42] but not all,[43-45] studies.

Viral loads of 10^9 to 10^{10} copies/mL in urine, BK viruria increasing by more than 3 $\log_{10}$ from baseline, or BK viremia, $>10^4$ copies/mL of plasma has been associated with an increased risk of late HC.[34,41-43,46,47]

BK nephritis. Cases of BK nephritis have been reported sporadically in HSCT recipients and patients with leukemia.[48-53] This complication is severe, invariably leading to permanent renal failure. Therefore, patients with any unexplained significantly deteriorating kidney function should be evaluated for BK virus infection. Testing of urine and blood for BK virus, by PCR followed by renal biopsy for immunostaining, usually is indicated.

Other organ manifestations. BK virus infection also has been reported to cause disseminated disease – meningitis, encephalitis, and pneumonitis – in patients with cancer.[52,54-57]

Kidney Allograft Recipients

The kidney is the most commonly reported site of BK virus reactivation.[58,59] BK viruria is present in up to 50% of renal transplant recipients and is asymptomatic in the majority of cases.[1,60] In some patients BK virus infection can cause ureteral stenosis, transient allograft dysfunction, and irreversible graft failure due a tubulo-interstitial nephritis.[61] BK virus nephritis occurs in up to 8% of adult renal allograft recipients.[21,61-66] Reported risk factors for BK virus nephritis include prior tubular injury from rejection, or drugs, surgical injury, warm ischemia and reperfusion injury during implantation of the graft, higher HLA mismatches, and transplant into a seronegative recipient.[67-69] The use of potent immunosuppressive agents such as mycophenolate mofetil and tacrolimus has been associated with an increased incidence of infection.[70] However, the current consensus is that the degree of immunosuppression, rather than the specific type of immunosuppression predisposes to BK virus nephritis.[71] The majority of cases of BK nephritis occur within the first year after transplantation.[20] BK virus nephritis typically manifests as an elevation in serum creatinine level and mimics rejection or drug toxicity. Graft loss occurs in a median of 44% of cases (range 0–100) and appears to depend on renal functional status at the time of diagnosis.[68]

The definitive diagnosis of BK virus disease requires renal biopsy. Because of the focal nature of polyomavirus nephritis two core biopsy samples, including the medulla, should be obtained.[72] The histologic hallmark is intranuclear viral inclusion bodies, seen in epithelial cells and focal necrosis of tubular cells.[69] In situ hybridization, or in situ PCR is used to identify BK virus in tissue.[64,73] Plasma BK virus DNA detection is a useful diagnostic tool, having a reported sensitivity of 100%, a positive predictive value of 85%, a specificity of 90% and negative predictive value of 100%.[74] Detection of plasma BK virus DNA can occur months before the histologic diagnosis or clinical manifestations of BK virus nephritis.[61,67,74,75]

The incidence of BK virus nephritis following a second transplantation for patients in whom a first graft failed due to BK virus

nephritis has not been established. However, re-transplantation is not considered to be contraindicated.[68,76]

Limited information has been published regarding BK virus-associated nephritis in pediatric kidney transplant recipients.[77-79] The largest retrospective cohort, which included 173 children transplanted between 1984 and 2002, observed that biopsy-proven BK virus nephritis caused late graft dysfunction in 3.5% of children.[80]

Treatment

The optimal treatment of BK virus-associated disease in HSCT and kidney allograft recipients is unknown. In HSCT recipients, the treatment of HC mainly is supportive, including analgesia, hyperhydration with forced diuresis, and continuous bladder irrigation.[31,81,82] Cystectomy may be necessary in the extreme circumstance of intractable bleeding.[33,83]

First-line treatment of BK virus-associated disease is reduction of immunosuppression.[68,72] Low-dose cidofovir (0.25 to 1 mg/kg up to twice a week) without probenecid, and leflunomide, are available for treatment; however, neither of these agents has been systematically evaluated or approved for treatment.[50,84-92] Hypogammaglobulinemia, if present, usually is corrected; benefit for BK in the management of BK virus-associated disease is not known.

JC VIRUS

JC virus is associated with progressive multifocal leukoencephalopathy (PML). The infectious nature of the disease was suggested by electron microscopy studies in the mid-1960s, when polyoma-like virions were found within intranuclear inclusion bodies of oligodendrocytes.[93] A few years later the virus was cultured from human brain tissue obtained from patients with PML.[2] PML gained attention in the late 1980s because of association with acquired immunodeficiency syndrome (AIDS). The disease rarely has been reported in patients with hematologic malignancies or in transplant recipients.[94-98] Recently, PML has emerged among patients treated with immunomodulatory drugs used for hematologic malignancy or autoimmune disease. These drugs include natalizumab, rituximab, and efalizumab.[99-101] Other neurologic disorders attributed to JCV infection include JCV granule cell neuropathy, JCV encephalopathy, and possibly meningitis.[102]

After asymptomatic primary infection,[9,103] the virus remains latent in tonsillar tissues, kidney tubular epithelial cells, bone marrow, and brain.[104,105]

Progressive Multifocal Leukoencephalopathy

PML is a demyelinating disease of the CNS occurring as a consequence of active JC virus replication in oligodendrocytes and astrocytes in immunocompromised individuals. Predominant symptoms include cognitive dysfunction, gait imbalance, difficulty with coordination, limb paresis, and rarely seizures.[106] PML usually is fatal.

Brain biopsy is the gold standard for the diagnosis of PML, with sensitivity of 64% to 96% and specificity of 100%. A more conservative approach is the demonstration of virus DNA in cerebrospinal fluid (CSF) by PCR; CSF usually shows mild pleocytosis and slight protein elevation. Detection of virus by PCR in the CSF has sensitivity of 72% to 92% and specificity of 92% to 100%.[98,107]

Typical neuroimaging findings are multiple white matter lesions, sparing the cortex and not corresponding to particular vascular territories. These lesions are classically located in the subcortical white matter or in the cerebellar peduncles, occasionally in thalamus and basal ganglia. Magnetic resonance imaging is the preferred diagnostic modality.

There is no specific treatment for PML. For HIV-infected persons, antiretroviral therapy should be implemented or optimized.[108] In uninfected persons, if immunosuppressive therapy is being administered, it should be discontinued.[109] Cidofovir has activity in vitro; however, little is known about its in vivo efficacy.[110]

Interleukin-2, cytarabine, chlorpromazine, the serotonin 5-HT2A receptor blocking agents (e.g., ziprasidone, risperidone, olanzapine, and mefloquine) have been prescribed for individual patients.[98,111]

KI POLYOMAVIRUS (KIPyV) AND WU POLYOMAVIRUS (WUPyV)

In 2007, KI polyomavirus (KIPyV) and WU polyomavirus (WUPyV) were isolated in respiratory secretions from children with acute respiratory tract infection.[13,14] KIPyV and WUPyV are named for the institutions in which they were discovered, Karolinska University Hospital (Stockholm, Sweden) and Washington University School of Medicine (St. Louis, Missouri, USA).

Seroprevalence studies show that KIPyV is detected in 55% and WUPyV in 69% of healthy blood donors.[7]

The association between KIPyV and WUPyV and respiratory tract infection remains inconclusive, even in immunocompromised patients.[112]

TRICHODYSPLASIA SPINULOSA-ASSOCIATED POLYOMAVIRUS (TSV)

Trichodysplasia spinulosa (TS) is a rare skin disease characterized by development of papules and alopecia on the face and is observed exclusively in immunocompromised patients.[113-115] In 2010, the trichodysplasia spinulosa-associated polyomavirus (TSV) was discovered and identified from the skin lesion from a child who developed trichodysplasia spinulosa following cardiac transplantation.[4,116] A confirmed second case has been reported in a 7-year-old girl with leukemia.[116] The presence of the virus in clinically unaffected individuals suggests that the virus can cause subclinical or latent infection.[4]

HUMAN POLYOMAVIRUS AND CANCER

The oncogenic potential of natural and experimental polyomavirus infections in animals has been reported.[117] The exact causative and oncologic potential of polyomaviruses in humans is controversial except for Merkel cell tumor.

Merkel cell carcinoma (MCC) is an uncommon aggressive skin cancer with an overall age-adjusted incidence of 0.24 per 100,000 person-years.[118] The tumor typically affects elderly and immunosuppressed individuals.[119,120] There is a strong correlation between genome detection and MCC.[3,121-124] The pathogenesis of the virus is unknown. There is no specific antiviral therapy.

Given the increasing use of immunosuppressive treatment it is probable that the incidence of polyomavirus-associated diseases will increase over the years. Thus, a significant need for more effective and specific antiviral treatment is expected.[125,126]

213 Hepatitis B and Hepatitis D Viruses

Kathy K. Byrd, Trudy V. Murphy, and Dale J. Hu

HEPATITIS B VIRUS

DESCRIPTION OF THE PATHOGEN

Hepatitis B virus (HBV), a member of the Hepadnaviridae family, is a major global infectious pathogen. HBV is a spherical particle that is 42 to 47 nm in diameter and is known as a Dane particle. It contains partially double-stranded DNA, DNA polymerase with reverse transcriptase activity, and hepatitis B core antigen (HBcAg), all surrounded by hepatitis B surface antigen (HBsAg, or Australia antigen). HBsAg is also found in serum as filamentous and spherical particles that are 20 nm in diameter. These particles do not contain viral DNA and are not infectious.

The 3200-basepair, partially double-stranded genome consists of 4 open-reading frames that code for several key proteins (Figure 213-1). Unlike replication of most other DNA viruses, DNA replication of HBV occurs via an RNA intermediate. HBcAg and hepatitis B e antigen (HBeAg) are translated from a common gene but display different antigenic properties. HBcAg, the nucleocapsid protein, is found in liver tissue in patients with acute or chronic HBV infection. HBeAg is a soluble protein that is detectable in blood of patients with high viral loads; it might function as a modulator of the host immune response.[1]

HBV has been subclassified by two separate classification systems: serologic subtype and genotype. Nine serologic subtypes of HBV (adrq+, adrq-, ayr, ayw1, ayw2, ayw3, ayw4, adw2, and adw4) initially were described on the basis of the serologic heterogeneity of HBsAg.[2] At least eight HBV genotypes have been described, designated A through H, on the basis of an approximately 8%

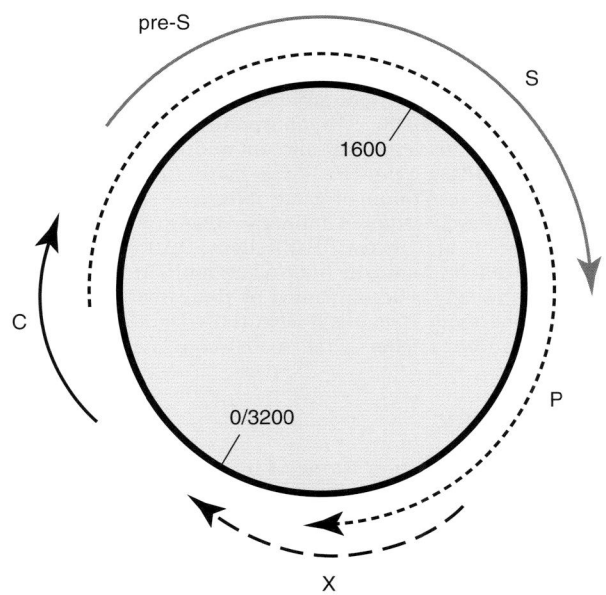

Figure 213-1. Structure and organization of the hepatitis B virus genome. Four overlapping reading frames: 1, P (DNA polymerase/reverse transcriptase, primase, RNAse); 2, S (surface glycoproteins HBsAg, preS1, preS2); 3, X (X protein); 4, C (HBcAg, HBeAg).

TABLE 213-1. Geographic Distribution of Hepatitis B Virus Genotypes and Serotypes

Genotype	Serotype	Geographic Location
A	*adw2, ayw1*	Northwest Europe, North America, Central America
B	*adw2, layw1*	Indonesia, China, Vietnam
C	*adw2, adr⁻, adrq⁺, ayr*	East Asia
D	*adw2, ayw3*	Mediterranean, Turkey, Middle East, India
E	*ayw4*	Sub-Saharan Africa
F	*adw4q⁻*	American Natives, Polynesia
G	*adw2*	United States, France
H	–	Central and South America

difference in nucleotide sequence. HBV serotypes and genotypes vary geographically (Table 213-1).[3,4]

PATHOGENESIS

HBV-associated liver damage is not a direct cytopathic effect of the virus but rather the consequence of the host immune response to infection (e.g., cytotoxic T-lymphocyte-mediated lysis of infected hepatocytes).[5,6] Viral clearance and resolution of infection or development of chronic infection appears to depend on the effectiveness and specificity of the initial cytotoxic T-lymphocyte response. For patients in whom acute HBV infection resolves, the response is vigorous, with cytokine-mediated control of viral replication and relative sparing of infected cells.[7] For patients in whom chronic infection develops, the initial T-lymphocyte response might be suboptimal and more narrowly focused, with enough cytokines produced to suppress some viral gene expression but insufficient to clear the virus. Persistent infection develops because of "immune tolerance."[8,9] HBV integrates into human DNA, potentially resulting in oncogene activation and carcinogenesis by insertional mutagenesis. Some studies suggest that regenerative hyperplasia resulting from chronic inflammation eventually might lead to carcinogenesis.[10]

Hepatitis B antigens and markers of infection. Hepatitis B surface antigen (HBsAg) indicates either acute or chronic HBV infection. People with positive HBsAg are infectious and can transmit the virus to others. The IgM subclass of antibody to the hepatitis B core antigen (IgM anti-HBc) indicates acute infection while total IgG anti-HBc is a nonspecific marker of infection which can indicate acute, chronic, or resolved acute infection. Antibody to HBsAg (anti-HBs) is a marker of immunity and is present after resolution of acute infection, after vaccination, or through passively acquired antibody. HBeAg indicates ongoing viral replication and increased infectivity. Antibody to HBeAg (anti-HBe) can be found in both acute and chronic infection; its presence usually is accompanied by decreased viral load and decreased infectivity. Hepatitis B DNA (HBV DNA) is a marker of viral replication. Higher viral loads correlate with greater infectivity.

EPIDEMIOLOGY

Worldwide, HBV infection is one of the leading causes of infectious disease-related morbidity and mortality. An estimated 2 billion people – one-third of the world's population – have serologic evidence of past or present HBV infection, and 350 million people are infected chronically. Each year, an estimated 620,000 people die from HBV-related liver disease, including cirrhosis and hepatocellular carcinoma (HCC).[11] In the United States, HBV infection is responsible for an estimated 2000–3000 deaths annually (Centers for Disease Control and Prevention (CDC), unpublished data).

Transmission

The principal modes of HBV transmission are: (1) percutaneous, (2) sexual, and (3) perinatal.[12] HBV is present in high titers in blood and exudates (e.g., skin lesions) of acutely and chronically infected people. Moderate viral titers are found in semen, vaginal secretions, and saliva. Other body fluids that do not contain blood or serous fluid, such as feces or urine, are not a source of HBV. Although HBV is found in human milk, breastfeeding has not been shown to increase HBV transmission.[13–15] Transmission between household contacts, especially in developing countries, can occur through contact with skin lesions such as eczema or impetigo; sharing of potentially blood-contaminated objects such as toothbrushes and razor blades; and in rare instances, in association with human bites.[16–18] All people who are HBsAg-positive are potentially infectious and can transmit the virus to others.

The virus is stable in the environment for at least 7 days and can be found in high titers on environmental surfaces even in the absence of visible blood.[19] Inoculation can occur from contact with environmental surfaces or equipment contaminated with HBV. The virus is inactivated by household bleach solution.[20]

Percutaneous and permucosal transmission of HBV results from transfusion of unscreened blood, injection-drug use, occupational exposure (e.g., needlestick injuries), and other nosocomial exposures (e.g., unsafe injections, breach in aseptic technique). In the U.S., blood transfusion is no longer a significant mode of transmission because all donor blood is screened for HBV markers. However, blood transfusion remains an important source of infection in many developing countries. Globally, unsafe injection practices are thought to account for 32% of new HBV infections annually;[21] the burden of disease from other unsafe medical practices is unknown. Nosocomial transmission is not limited to developing countries; in the U.S. and other developed countries, nosocomial transmission is associated with improper infection control and continues to occur despite long-standing infection control recommendations and guidelines.[22–25] Over the past decade, nosocomial HBV outbreaks have involved reuse of fingerstick devices (meant for individual use) for multiple persons, during assisted blood glucose monitoring, and reuse of single-use vials or devices for multiple patients.[26]

Horizontal transmission (or intrafamilial or household transmission) refers to percutaneous transmission from infected family members within the household (most often mothers and older siblings to young children).[27–37] Although this mode of transmission is most important in countries of high HBV endemicity, its occurrence in the U.S. has been well documented.[38–41]

Sexual transmission of HBV results from sexual contact (heterosexual or homosexual) with an infected person and has been associated with: ≥1 sexual partners in a 6-month period; history of another sexually transmitted infection; and sexual practices that facilitate HBV transmission, such as anal intercourse.[42] Among men who have sex with men (MSM), the prevalence of past or current HBV infection has been reported to be as high as 60%.[42,43]

Perinatal HBV transmission occurs during delivery and is highly efficient. In utero transmission is relatively rare, accounting for <3% of vertical infections.[44–48] Risk of perinatal transmission is related to the HBeAg status of the mother; presence of HBeAg indicates increased viral load and infectivity. The risk of perinatal transmission is 70% to 90% for infants born to mothers who are both HBsAg- and HBeAg-positive, and 5% to ≥20%, for infants born to mothers who are HBsAg-positive but HBeAg-negative.[49–57]

Reported Risk Factors for Acute Infection

The most commonly reported risk factors for acute hepatitis B in the U.S. are high-risk heterosexual activity (e.g. multiple sex partners), MSM, and injection-drug use, which accounts for approximately half of all reported cases.[58] Acquisition of HBV infection from transfused blood is rare in the U.S.[59] The most commonly reported risk factors for acute infection among persons 12 to 21 years of age are high-risk sexual behaviors and injection-drug use.

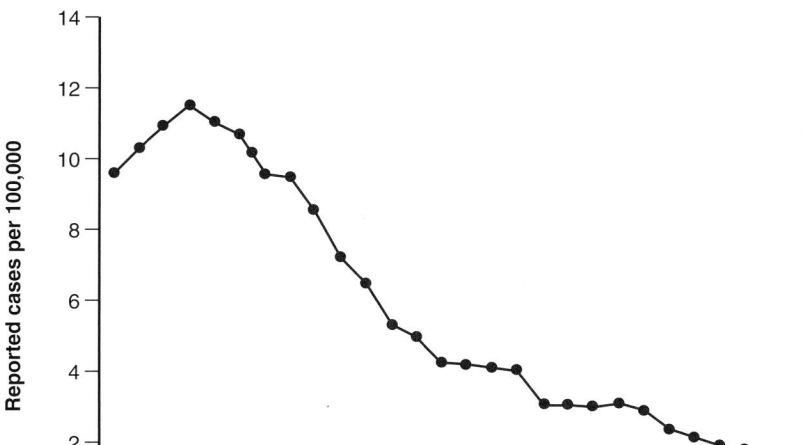

Figure 213-2. Reported incidence of acute hepatitis B in the U.S.

Other characteristics found in HBV-infected adolescents are homelessness and having run away.[60,61]

Prevalence of Infection in the United States

Data from the Third National Health and Nutrition Examination Survey (1999–2006), indicated that the prevalence of lifetime HBV infection in the U.S. population was 5% while chronic HBV infection was present in 0.3% of the population, corresponding to 1.5 million chronically infected people.[62] The prevalence of past or current HBV infection was higher among non-Hispanic blacks and persons of "other" race than among non-Hispanic whites and Mexican-Americans, and prevalence was significantly higher among foreign-born people. The U.S. prevalence of past or current HBV infection was 0.6% among those 6 to 19 years of age and 5% among those 20 to 49 years of age.[62] Mortality data for 2000 to 2003 suggest that HBV infection is responsible for 2000 to 3000 deaths annually in the U.S., the majority from cirrhosis and HCC (CDC, unpublished data).

Incidence of Infection in the United States

During the past two decades, incidence of acute hepatitis B in the U.S. has declined significantly. National surveillance data indicate that incidence decreased from 11.5 per 100,000 population in 1985 to 1.3 per 100,000 in 2008 (Figure 213-2). Incidence is estimated to be about 10 times the reported number of cases after adjustment for underreporting of cases and asymptomatic infections. In 2008, an estimated 38,000 people were newly infected (http://www.cdc.gov//hepatitis/PDFs/disease_burden.pdf).

The impact of hepatitis B vaccination is reflected in the dramatic decline in incident cases among the cohort of children for whom recommendations for routine infant and adolescent catch-up vaccination have applied.[58] From 1990 through 2007, hepatitis B incidence declined 93% (from 1.2/100,000 to 0.02/100,000) among children <15 years of age. From 1990 through 2002, the majority of new cases, in children <15 years of age, was among international adoptees and other non-U.S. born children who were not vaccinated appropriately.[63]

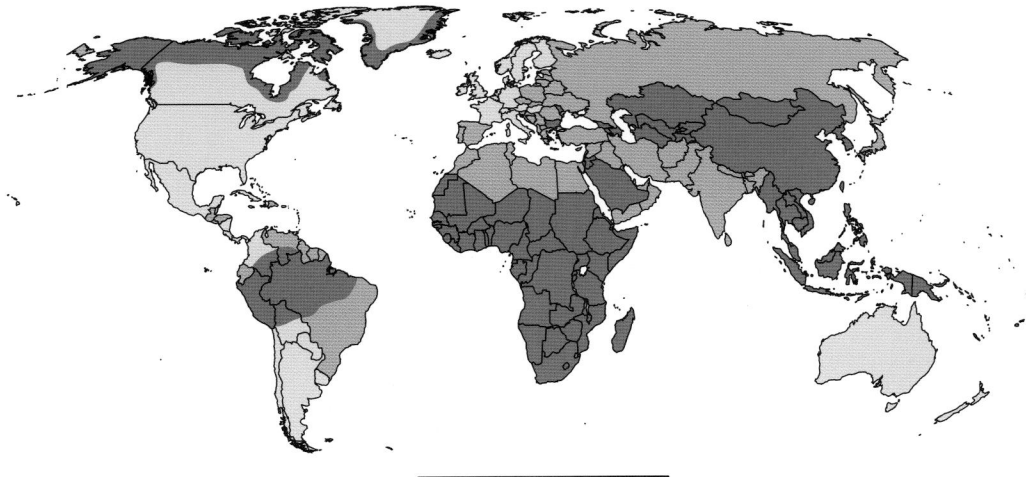

Figure 213-3. Geographic distribution of chronic hepatitis B virus infection. Note: For multiple countries, estimates of prevalence of hepatitis B surface antigen (HBsAg), a marker of chronic HBV infection, are based on limited data and might not reflect current prevalence in countries that have implemented routine childhood hepatitis B vaccination. In addition, HBsAg prevalence rates might vary within countries by subpopulation and locality.

HBsAg prevalence
≥8% = high
2–7% = intermediate
<2% = low

Global Prevalence of Infection and Patterns of Transmission

Countries and regions can be divided into areas of low, intermediate, and high HBV endemicity based on the prevalence of chronic HBV infection in the general population (Figure 213-3). Approximately 45% of the world's population lives in high-endemic countries where the prevalence of chronic HBV infection is ≥8% and the lifetime rate of infection is >60%. Most high-endemic countries are in Asia and Africa. In high-endemic countries, most new infections occur among infants and young children. Perinatal and horizontal transmission, as well as unsafe injections and other unsafe medical practices, account for most infections. Because most perinatal and early childhood HBV infections are asymptomatic, acute infection is rarely recognized in high-endemic countries.

Intermediate-endemic countries (HBsAg prevalence of 2% to 7%) constitute 43% of the world's population; in these countries, 20% to 60% of the population have serologic evidence of chronic or resolved infection. All modes of transmission contribute to HBV disease burden in these countries.

In low-endemic countries (HBsAg prevalence of <2%), most new infections occur among adolescents and adults and result from sexual exposures and injection-drug use. However, even in low-endemic areas, perinatal and early childhood infections account for a significant proportion of chronic infections and HBV-related deaths.

CLINICAL MANIFESTATIONS

Acute Infection

The usual incubation period for HBV infection is about 3 months but can vary from 6 weeks to 6 months. Clinical manifestations range from asymptomatic infection to fulminant hepatitis. The likelihood that symptoms will develop is age dependent. Perinatal HBV infections usually are subclinical, whereas symptomatic illness is noted in 5% to 15% of children 1 to 5 years of age and in 33% to 50% of older children, adolescents, and adults.[64] However, fulminant infection and death can occur at any age, including among infants with perinatal HBV infection.

Clinical signs and symptoms of acute HBV infection can include nausea, abdominal pain, vomiting, fever, jaundice, dark urine, changes in stool color, hepatomegaly, or splenomegaly. Malaise and anorexia might precede jaundice by 1 to 2 weeks. Fulminant hepatitis B is uncommon (<1%) but frequently leads to death or liver failure necessitating liver transplantation.

Chronic Infection

Chronic infection is associated with progressive liver disease including cirrhosis, liver failure, and hepatocellular carcinoma (HCC). Chronic infection is defined as persistence of HBsAg in serum for at least 6 months after acute infection.

The majority of chronically infected people remain asymptomatic until development of cirrhosis or end-stage liver disease.[65] Cirrhosis can lead to development of liver failure manifest by coagulopathy, ascites, encephalopathy and increased risk for HCC. Among people with chronic infection, the overall annual incidence of cirrhosis is 2% to 3%.[66,67] The survival rate of people with compensated and uncompensated cirrhosis is 84% and 14% at 5 years, respectively.[68] Risk factors for HBV-related cirrhosis and HCC include earlier age at infection, prolonged immune active phase of chronic infection, HBeAg positivity, and prolonged elevation of HBV DNA.[69] Although severe HBV-related liver disease is uncommon in childhood, chronic infection during infancy and childhood can lead to development of cirrhosis and HCC as early as the first decade of life.[70] Up to 25% of infants and older children with chronic infection eventually develop HBV-related cirrhosis or HCC.[71,72]

Extrahepatic Manifestations

Both acute and chronic HBV infection can be associated with extrahepatic clinical entities including: polyarteritis nodosa, membranous and membranoproliferative glomerulonephritis, polyradiculoneuritis, essential mixed cryoglobulinaemia, porphyria cutanea tarda, polyneuritis, papular acrodermatitis and thyroid dysfunction.[73-78] Urticarial rashes, arthralgia, and arthritis commonly are associated with acute HBV infection; thrombocytopenia preceding jaundice also has been reported.[79]

NATURAL HISTORY OF CHRONIC INFECTION

There are 4 phases of chronic HBV infection: (1) immune tolerant, (2) immune active, (3) immune inactive, (4) and reactivation (or HBeAg-negative immune active).[68,80]

People in the *immune tolerant phase* are HBsAg-positive, HBeAg-positive, have high HBV DNA levels (>20,000 IU/mL), normal serum alanine aminotransferase (ALT) levels and no to minimal hepatic inflammation or fibrosis.[68] Most chronically infected children will remain in the immune tolerant phase until late childhood or adolescence.[81]

The *immune active phase* is characterized by an active immune response resulting in inflammation (with or without fibrosis), hepatocyte damage and a resultant rise in serum ALT levels. People in the immune active phase are HBsAg-positive, have HBV DNA levels >2000 IU/mL, and can be either HBeAg-positive or HBeAg-negative and anti-HBe-positive.[68] People who remain in the immune active phase for prolonged periods are at high risk of developing cirrhosis and HCC.[69]

People in the immune *inactive phase* are HBsAg-positive, have HBV DNA <2000 IU/mL, are HBeAg-negative, anti-HBe-positive, and have improvement of hepatic inflammation and fibrosis.[68] Risk of progression to HCC is lower among persons in the inactive phase than among persons in the active phase.[82]

People in the *reactivation phase* (or *HBeAg-negative immune active phase*) are HBsAg-positive, HBeAg-negative, and anti-HBe-positive with HBV DNA levels >2000 IU/mL. There is active liver inflammation (with or without fibrosis) and serum ALT levels can be elevated or normal.[68] HBeAg-negative immune active disease often is caused by a mutant hepatitis B virus, which can be more virulent than nonmutant forms.[83]

Chronically infected people do not necessarily pass through the phases of chronic infection in a linear fashion. Chronically infected people may spend little to no time in the immune tolerant phase. Twenty percent of HBeAg-negative people will revert back to HBeAg positivity;[84] 10% to 30% of HBeAg-negative/anti-HBe-positive persons will remain in the immune active phase with elevated serum ALT and HBV DNA levels; and 10% to 30% of HBeAg-negative/anti-HBe-positive people will revert from the inactive phase to an anti-HBe-positive hepatitis with elevated serum ALT and HBV DNA levels.[85-87] As such, the current practice guidelines of the American Association for the Study of Liver Diseases recommend lifelong follow-up with repeated testing to monitor changes in the phase of chronic infection.[82]

Influence of Age and HBeAg

Age at time of acute infection is the primary determinant of progression to chronic infection. More than 90% of perinatally infected infants develop chronic infection. Between 25% and 50% of children infected between 1 and 5 years of age become chronically infected, whereas only 6% to 10% of acutely infected older children and adults develop chronic infection (Figure 213-4).[64,88] Elderly adults have higher rates of developing chronic infection,[89,90] as do patients who have acute HBV infection while immunosuppressed or concurrently with an underlying chronic illness.[71]

Perinatally infected children usually remain in the immune tolerant phase for extended periods whereas chronic infection acquired during later childhood or adolescence usually is accompanied by more active liver disease and elevated serum ALT

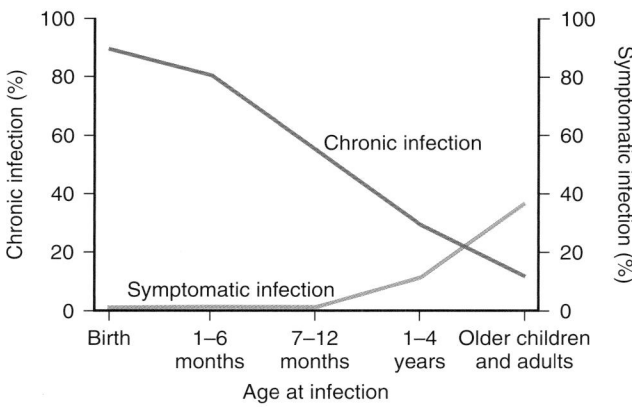

Figure 213-4. Outcome of hepatitis B virus infection by age of infection.

values.[91] Children infected perinatally have lower annual rates of HBeAg loss than children infected later in childhood or in adolescence. Of Taiwanese children infected perinatally, HBeAg seroconversion occurred in <2% annually during the first 3 years of life, and only in one-third by 10 years of age.[92,93] Children infected horizontally clear HBeAg more rapidly; in one study, 35% of older Asian children cleared HBeAg >5 years after infection,[93] and 83% of European children cleared HBeAg during an average of 13 years of follow-up.[94]

Presence of HBeAg indicates ongoing viral replication. HBeAg-positive patients usually have high serum levels of HBV DNA and HBsAg. Clearance of HBeAg and development of anti-HBe (HBeAg seroconversion) is accompanied by reductions in serum HBV DNA and ALT levels and might be preceded by a temporary exacerbation of liver disease. HBeAg seroconversion occurs at a rate of 5% to 10% per year.[84] Most patients who seroconvert have little to no progression of liver disease (immune inactive phase). In these patients, the risk of HCC is reduced but remains higher than in patients without chronic infection.[95] Serologic reversion (reappearance of HBeAg) is common in the absence of anti-HBe. However, reversion to HBeAg positivity also can occur with loss of anti-HBe.[85]

HBeAg positivity during pregnancy greatly increases the risk of perinatal transmission. In the absence of appropriate post-exposure prophylaxis, nearly all neonates born to mothers who are both HBsAg- and HBeAg-positive become infected and 90% develop chronic infection. Clearance of HBeAg and development of anti-HBe is associated with decreased risk of perinatal transmission; approximately 25% of newborns to HBsAg- and anti-HBe-positive mothers become infected and 10% to 15% develop chronic infection.[96]

Influence of Genotype

The clinical significance of HBV genotypes remains unclear. Existing studies suggest that genotype influences the time to HBeAg seroconversion and response to treatment. Among Alaska Natives, the median time to seroconversion is approximately 18 years among people with genotype C, 8 years among people with genotype F, and less than 6 years among people with genotypes A, B, and D.[97] Reversion to HBeAg positivity is more common among Alaska Natives infected with genotypes C and F.[97] Since genotype influences the rate of HBeAg seroconversion during childbearing years, genotype might play a role in the risk of perinatal transmission.

An improved response to treatment with interferon alfa-2b has been observed in adults with genotype A compared with adults with genotype D[98] and among adults with genotype B compared with genotype C.[99] Studies in children have shown mixed results. In one study, Chinese children with genotype B had an improved response to interferon-alfa compared with children with genotype

C.[100] In another study, Taiwanese children showed no difference in treatment response by genotype.[101]

Resolved Acute Infection and the "Recovery Phase" of Chronic Infection

Resolved acute infection is defined as the clearance of HBsAg, loss of detectable HBV DNA, and normalization of serum ALT levels; development of anti-HBs might occur. Resolved acute infection is not a risk factor for subsequent chronic liver disease or HCC.[102] However, viral clearance still might be incomplete; patients with a history of acute hepatitis B and apparent resolution (anti-HBs positivity and HBsAg negativity) can experience reactivation of hepatitis B if they become immunosuppressed,[103] and HBV DNA has been detected in blood of patients 20 years after resolution of acute infection.[104]

People with chronic infection who clear HBsAg enter what is often called the *recovery phase*. During childhood, the annual clearance rate of HBsAg is <1%.[82,105] People who clear HBsAg generally have a better prognosis with improvements in hepatic inflammation and fibrosis over time.[106,107] However, HCC still can develop in HBsAg-negative people,[106,107] and HBV DNA can be found in serum of a significant minority of HBsAg-negative people. Practice guidelines recommend continued follow-up for previously chronically infected, HBsAg-negative people, to monitor for HCC.[108]

SCREENING

Serum HBsAg and anti-HBs are the most useful screening tests for chronic HBV infection or immunity to HBV. HBsAg is present in most chronically infected persons, even when HBV DNA levels are undetectable. Lack of anti-HBs in an HBsAg-negative person indicates susceptibility to HBV infection.

Routine HBsAg screening is recommended for the following people: (1) all pregnant women; (2) all neonates born to HBsAg-positive women after completing the vaccination series; (3) immigrants from regions of high or intermediate HBV endemicity (e.g., most areas of Asia, Africa, the Middle East, and Pacific Islands); (4) U.S. born people, who were not vaccinated as infants, whose parents were born in regions with HBsAg prevalence ≥8%; (5) people with elevated serum ALT/AST levels of unknown etiology; (6) people with behavioral risks including MSM and injection drug users; and (7) and hemodialysis patients.[69]

Screening for HBsAg is recommended at the first prenatal visit for all pregnant women.[109] Women in labor without HBsAg test information should have HBsAg serology upon arrival. In addition, pretested women who have a history of high-risk behaviors (e.g., HBsAg-positive sexual partner, injection-drug use) should be retested at the onset of labor. A copy of the original HBsAg test result should be placed in the infant's medical chart (in addition to the mother's chart) to avoid errors in communication or interpretation of the laboratory report.[110]

All HBsAg-positive tests should be reported to the state or local health department, including HBsAg-positive tests from pregnant women for referral to the Perinatal Hepatitis B Prevention Program.

SEROLOGIC DIAGNOSIS

Acute Infection

Following infection, the first serologic markers to become detectable are HBsAg and IgM anti-HBc, which appear within 1 to 2 months and are present when initial symptoms appear (Figure 213-5; Table 213-2). IgM anti-HBc is diagnostic of recent HBV infection. The presence of HBeAg, also detectable in acute infection, reflects viral replication and increased infectivity.

Resolution of Acute Infection

During resolution of acute infection, IgM anti-HBc is replaced by antibody of the IgG subclass (IgG anti-HBc) and anti-HBs

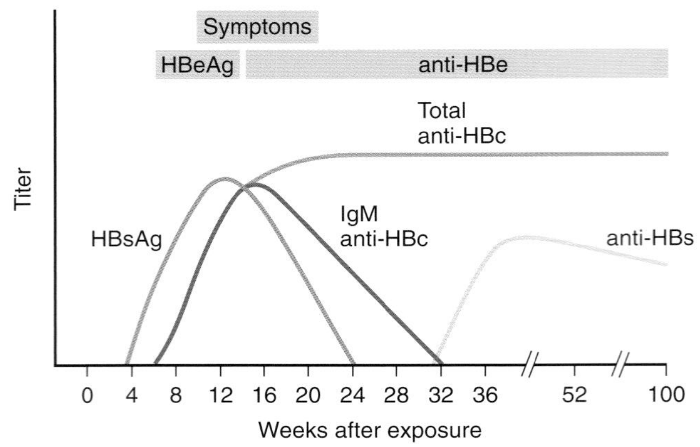

Figure 213-5. Serologic response to hepatitis B virus infection with recovery. Anti-HBc, antibody to hepatitis B core antigen; anti-HBe, antibody to hepatitis B e antigen; anti-HBs, antibody to hepatitis B surface antigen; HBeAg, hepatitis B e antigen; HBsAg, hepatitis B surface antigen; IgM anti-HBc, antibody of the immunoglobulin M subclass to hepatitis B core antigen.

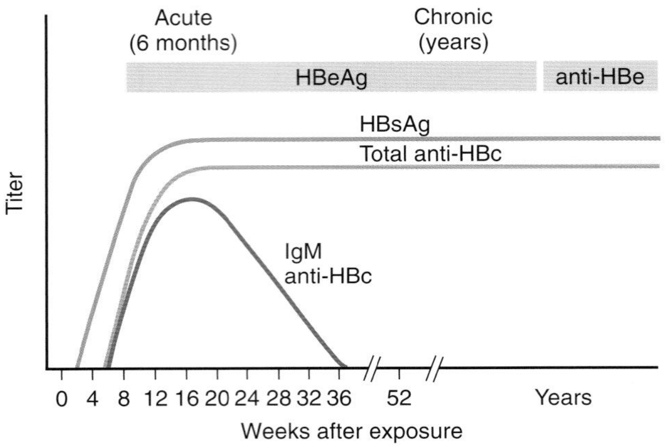

Figure 213-6. Serologic response to hepatitis B virus (HBV) infection with progression to chronic HBV. Anti-HBc, antibody to hepatitis B core antigen; anti-HBe, antibody to hepatitis B e antigen; HBeAg, hepatitis B e antigen; HBsAg, hepatitis B surface antigen; IgM anti-HBc, antibody of the immunoglobulin M subclass to hepatitis B core antigen.

develops (Figure 213-5; Table 213-2). Anti-HBs is a protective, neutralizing antibody and its presence indicates recovery from acute infection and immunity to reinfection. The period when all HBsAg has been neutralized by anti-HBs, and neither HBsAg nor anti-HBs is detectable is referred to as the window period. During the window period, the only serologic marker of infection is IgM anti-HBc. During resolution, anti-HBe replaces HBeAg. In people with past HBV infection, IgG anti-HBc usually remains detectable for life, but anti-HBs might become undetectable in remote infection.

Chronic Infection

In chronic infection, HBsAg persists for >6 months and anti-HBs does not develop. (Figure 213-6; Table 213-2). People initially identified as HBsAg-positive should be retested 6 months later to document clearance or chronic infection. Similar to acute infection with resolution, in chronic infection, IgM anti-HBc disappears and is replaced by IgG anti-HBc. HBeAg is variably present in chronic infection. When HBeAg is not present, anti-HBe usually is detectable.

TABLE 213-2. Interpretation of Serologic Markers for HBV Infection

Serologic Marker[a]				
HBsAg	**Anti-HBs**	**IgM Anti-HBc**	**Total Anti-HBc**	**Interpretation**
–	–	–	–	Susceptible; never infected
+	–	–	–	Acute infection, early incubation; transient, up to 3 weeks after vaccination
+	–	+	+	Acute infection
–	–	+	+	Acute infection, resolving
–	+	–	+	Past infection, recovered and immune
+	–	–	+	Chronic infection
–	–	–	+	False positive (i.e., susceptible) past infection, or "low level" chronic infection
–	+	–	–	Immune from vaccination

[a]HBsAg = hepatitis B surface antigen; anti-HBs = antibody to hepatitis B surface antigen; IgM anti-HBc = IgM antibody to hepatitis B core antigen; Total anti-HBc = Total antibody to hepatitis B core antigen.

Perinatal Infection

Because maternal HBsAg generally does not cross the placenta, HBsAg found in serum of an infant shortly after birth usually indicates infection, but can result from specimen contamination.[111] IgG anti-HBc and anti-HBs are transferred from mother to fetus through the placenta, and neither is a useful diagnostic marker of infection in infants. Passively acquired maternal anti-HBs and anti-HBc usually disappear within the first 1 to 2 years of life.[112,113]

Special Serologic Considerations

Anti-HBs, with no other serologic marker of infection, is present after hepatitis B vaccination. HBsAg alone, with no other markers of infection, might be present very early in infection, before development of IgM anti-HBc, or immediately after hepatitis B vaccination (Figure 213-5; Table 213-2). Transient HBsAg positivity from vaccine antigen, within the first 3 weeks after vaccination, has been documented in infants, adolescents, and adults.[114–116]

Anti-HBc without other markers of infection might be detected in three situations: (1) false-positive result; (2) remote, past infection with the loss of detectable anti-HBs levels; or (3) chronic infection in which the HBsAg level is below the level of detection for commercial assays. In the latter situation, person-to-person transmission is unlikely to occur.[117]

ASSESSMENT, MONITORING, AND REFERRAL

While chronic HBV infection in childhood usually is asymptomatic, sequelae can become manifest in adolescence or adulthood. Chronically infected children are at increased risk of developing cirrhosis and HCC; as such, they require lifelong monitoring for disease progression.

HBsAg-positive people should be retested 6 months later to determine if they have developed chronic infection. Initial evaluation of chronically infected children includes laboratory testing for serum ALT, white blood cell (WBC) count, platelet count, HBeAg, anti-HBe, HBV DNA, and α-fetoprotein (AFP) level. Hepatitis B serology and serum ALT level are used to determine the phase of chronic infection. Decreased WBC and platelet counts can indicate liver fibrosis; AFP is a nonspecific marker for HCC. Family history of liver cancer and liver disease should be elicited and a baseline hepatic ultrasound performed.[83]

An expert panel commissioned by the Hepatitis B Foundation recommends that children in the immune tolerant and immune inactive phases of chronic infection have serum ALT and AFP levels tested every 6 to 12 months and HBeAg and anti-HBe tested annually. To determine if children in the immune inactive phase have entered the reactivation phase, annual HBV DNA testing also may be useful. Children with elevated ALT, elevated AFP (≥10 ng/mL), a family history of liver cancer or liver disease, and children in the reactivation phase should be referred to a pediatric liver specialist for further evaluation.[83]

TREATMENT

No specific treatment is available for people with acute HBV infection. Neither hepatitis B immune globulin (HBIG) nor corticosteroids are effective.[118,119]

An expert panel commissioned by the Hepatitis B Foundation recommends treatment for children with chronic infection based on ALT levels, age, liver biopsy findings, comorbidities, and family history of liver disease and liver cancer.[120] Children with normal serum ALT levels should be monitored regularly. Children with persistently elevated serum ALT levels (>1.5 times the laboratory upper limit of normal or >60 IU/mL on at least two occasions over 6 months in HBeAg-positive children or on at least 3 occasions over 12 months in HBeAg-negative children) are divided into two categories: children in the immune active phase and those in the reactivation phase. Treatment is indicated for children in the reactivation phase with persistently elevated serum ALT levels and moderate to severe hepatic inflammation and/or fibrosis. Benefit from treatment is unclear among children in the immune active phase with elevated serum ALT levels and minimal or mild hepatitis inflammation and/or fibrosis.[120]

Treatment response is not assessed until at least 6 months after completion of therapy. A response usually is defined as clearance of HBeAg. Other measurable markers of response are: (1) development of anti-HBe, (2) clearance of HBsAg, (3) normalization of serum ALT levels, (4) reductions in serum levels of HBV DNA, and (5) improvement in histologic features of the liver.[105] The natural history of chronic HBV infection is an important consideration in the evaluation of results from clinical trials because spontaneous improvement occurs in many untreated patients.[121]

U.S. Food and Drug Administration (FDA)-approved therapies for chronic hepatitis B in the U.S. are interferon alfa-2b (IFN-α), pegylated interferon alfa-2a (peg-IFN), lamivudine, adefovir, entecavir, tenofovir, and telbivudine. Only IFN-α, lamivudine, adefovir, and entecavir are approved for use in children. The youngest age of approved use is 12 months for IFN-α, 3 years for lamivudine, 12 years for adefovir, and 16 years for entecavir. Emtricitabine has activity against HBV but currently is approved only for treatment of human immunodeficiency virus (HIV) infection.

Interferon-Based Therapies

Few data are available for children treated with IFN-α. Available studies in western countries report success (defined as HBeAg seroconversion) from 20% to 58% among treated children and 8% to 17% among untreated, control subjects.[122-125] Treatment success is less prevalent for children from Asian countries with normal serum ALT levels.[126] In the largest randomized, controlled trial reported to date, chronically infected children with consistently elevated serum ALT levels treated with IFN-α for 6 months were more likely than untreated controls to lose HBeAg (35% versus 11%) and HBsAg (10% versus 1%). No difference in treatment success was reported between children born in Asian or western countries. For children who responded to treatment, serum ALT levels normalized and liver histologic features improved.[125] A meta-analysis of six other studies concluded that children treated with IFN-α had significantly increased clearance of HBV DNA and HBeAg compared with untreated controls.[127] In

addition, other studies have shown that children <5 years of age have improved response to treatment.[123,128] IFN-α might accelerate the rate of HBeAg clearance in children who would eventually clear HBeAg without treatment; the long-term benefits of accelerated clearance are not known.[129]

Generally, the pediatric treatment regimen for IFN-α is 5 to 10 million units/m² injected intramuscularly three times a week for 4 to 6 months. Adverse effects of IFN-α can be moderate to severe including fever, headache, myalgia, neutropenia, worsening hepatitis, and depression or irritability limiting a patient's ability to tolerate full doses or to complete a course of treatment.[91] Interferon therapy is contraindicated in patients with cirrhosis; therapy has been associated with exacerbation of hepatitis and hepatic decompensation. A European working group concluded that interferon therapy is most appropriate for children without cirrhosis who have intermediate to low HBV DNA levels, have abnormal serum ALT levels, and are ≥2 years of age.[91]

Antiviral Agents

Nucleoside and nucleotide analogues have emerged as alternative treatments for chronic hepatitis B. These agents have fewer adverse events than interferon-based therapies. In one study, adults treated with lamivudine for 1 year were more likely than untreated patients to have a histologic response and to undergo HBeAg seroconversion.[130] Long-term treatment (up to 5 years) with lamivudine also has been shown to delay progression of clinical disease and decrease development of HCC in patients with hepatitis B-related advanced fibrosis or cirrhosis.[131] However, lamivudine treatment selects for mutations in the HBV polymerase (YMDD mutants), which limits its usefulness as monotherapy.[132] Adefovir and entecavir, provide similar or more effective response rates than lamivudine and induce resistance mutations at a slower rate.[133-137] Both are effective in treatment of patients infected with YMDD mutants. Combining lamivudine with interferon has not proven more effective than interferon monotherapy.[138,139] Recent data suggest that combining adefovir with lamivudine for patients with lamivudine resistance provides better response rates and decreases the risk for developing further antiviral resistance compared with sequential monotherapy.[140] Treatment with antiviral agents does not eradicate HBV (<2% become negative for HBsAg), and relapse occurs in the majority of patients when the drug is stopped. Relapse can result in severe exacerbation of liver disease, with hepatic decompensation and death.[141]

A randomized clinical trial indicated that chronically infected children with elevated serum ALT levels who received oral lamivudine at a dose of 3 mg/kg per day (maximum, 100 mg) once daily for 52 weeks were significantly more likely to have a virologic response (loss of HBV DNA and HBeAg) compared with children receiving placebo (23% versus 13%). This response was maintained in 89% of participants at 24 months after discontinuing therapy. Patients from this study who did not respond to 1 year of treatment were continued for 24 additional months. Further clinical response was observed at 3 years, with an additional 21% achieving a virologic response. However, lamivudine resistance developed in 19%, 49%, and 64% of participants at 1, 2, and 3 years, respectively.[142,143] Children (151) were followed for an additional 2 years (5 years total); 75% of controls maintained HBeAg seroconversion compared with 82% who received 1 year of treatment and 90% who received at least 2 years of treatment. Elevated serum ALT levels, prior to treatment, were associated with treatment success.[144] Lamivudine treatment was well tolerated.[142,143]

In a randomized controlled study of adefovir, 173 HBeAg-positive children with elevated serum ALT levels were treated for 48 weeks. Children 12 through 17 years of age in the treatment group reached the treatment endpoint (HBV DNA <1000 copies/mL and normal serum ALT levels) more often than the untreated controls (23% versus 0%). Treated children 2 through 11 years of age did not have a significantly different outcome from untreated counterparts. No viral mutations were noted among any of the treated children and treatment generally was well tolerated.[145]

There are no published studies on entecavir in children although clinical trials are ongoing.

Management of Patients with Chronic HBV Infection and Their Contacts

Chronically infected patients should be counseled to limit alcohol consumption to avoid acceleration and progression of disease and should be immunized against hepatitis A.[146] Household, sexual, and needle-sharing contacts of chronically infected people should be identified. Unvaccinated contacts should be screened and receive the first dose of hepatitis B vaccine; contacts who are susceptible should complete the vaccination series. Sex partners of HBsAg-positive people should be counseled to use methods to protect themselves from sexual exposure until they are proven to be nonsusceptible.

PREVENTION AND CONTROL

The primary goals of hepatitis B prevention programs are to prevent acute hepatitis B, and to reduce chronic infection and HBV-related chronic liver disease. During the past two decades, a comprehensive immunization strategy was developed to eliminate HBV transmission in the U.S. The strategy has four components: (1) prevention of perinatal infection through HBsAg screening of all pregnant women, and postexposure immunoprophylaxis and vaccination of infants born to HBsAg-positive women; (2) routine vaccination of newborns prior to hospital discharge; (3) routine vaccination of adolescents and all previously unvaccinated children; and (4) vaccination of adults at high risk for HBV infection (Box 213-1).[109] This strategy addresses the need to prevent perinatal and early childhood HBV infection and to vaccinate adolescents before they engage in high-risk behaviors.

Hepatitis B vaccination has resulted in a significant decrease in incident hepatitis B cases in the U.S. (Figure 213-2). Incidence has decreased most notably among children and adolescents since the 1991 Advisory Committee on Immunization Practices recommendation for universal infant hepatitis B vaccination, and later recommendations for vaccinating older unvaccinated children and adolescents.[147] Further declines in HBV infection are expected with continued routine vaccination and aging of the vaccinated cohort. Worldwide, >170 countries have initiated routine infant hepatitis B vaccination as recommended by the World Health Organization. Over the next 30 to 50 years, routine infant immunization programs worldwide with implementation of a birth dose of vaccine are expected to result in significant reductions in the incidence of death from cirrhosis and HCC.

Vaccines and Schedules

Hepatitis B vaccines (HepB) are composed of HBsAg adsorbed to an adjuvant of aluminum hydroxide or aluminum hydroxyphosphate sulfate.[148,149] HBsAg elicits development of the neutralizing antibody, anti-HBs, which confers protection from infection. Plasma-derived vaccines were manufactured from HBsAg purified from the plasma of people with chronic HBV infection and were available worldwide. Recombinant vaccines have replaced plasma-derived vaccines and are produced through the insertion of the gene for HBsAg into yeast cells (*Saccharomyces cerevisiae*, or baker's yeast) and, less commonly, mammalian cells (Chinese hamster ovary cells). Recombinant vaccines are considered equivalent to plasma-derived vaccines in their immunogenicity and effectiveness. HepB vaccines are formulated to contain 5 to 40 μg of HBsAg protein per dose of vaccine, and in the U.S., do not contain the preservative thimerosal.

In the U.S., Hib-HepB and DTaP-HepB-IPV are the only combination vaccines currently licensed for use in pediatric populations (infants and children through 10 years of age).[150–152] Combination vaccines should not be administered to infants aged <6 weeks of age; monovalent HepB should be used for the birth dose.[109]

BOX 213-1. Immunization Strategy to Eliminate Hepatitis B Virus Transmission in the United States

- Prevention of perinatal HBV infection through:
  - Routine screening of all pregnant women for hepatitis B surface antigen (HBsAg), and
  - Immunoprophylaxis of infants born to HBsAg-positive women and infants born to women with unknown HBsAg status
- Universal routine vaccination of infants, beginning at birth
- Routine vaccination of previously unvaccinated children and adolescents <19 years of age
- Vaccination of previously unvaccinated adults at increased risk for HBV infection:
  - Adults at risk by sexual exposure (e.g., sex partners of HBsAg-positive people, people with >1 sex partner in the previous 6 months, people seeking treatment for sexually transmitted infection, men who have sex with men)
  - Adults at risk by percutaneous or mucosal exposure to blood (e.g., household contacts of HBsAg-positive people, current or recent injection-drug users, healthcare and public safety workers, people with end-stage renal disease)
  - Other adults (international travelers to areas with high or intermediate levels of endemic HBV infection (HBsAg prevalence ≥2%), people with chronic liver disease)
- Vaccination of adults in settings in which a high proportion of people have risk factors for hepatitis B virus (HBV) infection:
  - Sexually transmitted infection treatment facilities
  - Human immunodeficiency virus testing and treatment facilities
  - Facilities providing drug-abuse treatment and prevention services
  - Healthcare settings targeting services to injection-drug users
  - Correctional facilities
  - Healthcare settings targeting services to men who have sex with men
  - Chronic hemodialysis facilities and end-stage renal disease programs
  - Institutions and nonresidential daycare facilities for developmentally disabled people

HepB typically is administered as a three-dose series on a variety of vaccination schedules. In the U.S., the recommended schedule is administration of a first dose, followed by a second dose in 1 to 2 months and a third dose 6 to 12 months after the first dose (i.e., 0, 1–2, and 6–12 months).[109] For routine infant immunization, the first dose of vaccine should be administered at birth before hospital discharge, and the third dose should not be given before age 6 months (24 weeks).[109] A two-dose series for adolescents 11 through 15 years of age,[153] and a four-dose series also are approved for use in the U.S.[109]

Prevention of Perinatal Hepatitis B Infection

Infants born to HBsAg-positive women have a 90% risk of developing chronic infection if infected at birth. Infants not infected at birth remain at risk from transmission within the household. HepB combined with HBIG is highly effective in preventing perinatal and household HBV transmission when administered within 12 hours of birth followed by completion of the vaccination series. Women whose HBsAg status is unknown at delivery should receive immediate testing for HBsAg and their term infants administered HepB within 12 hours of birth. HBIG should be administered as soon as possible but within 7 days when the mother's HBsAg-test result is positive or remains unknown.

Infants born to HBsAg-positive pregnant women should receive postvaccination serologic testing (anti-HBs and HBsAg) 1 to 2 months after completion of the vaccination series to determine their response to vaccination and their chronic HBV infection status. Infants who fail to respond to an initial HepB series, and are not infected, should be revaccinated with 3 additional doses and retested. Infants who fail postexposure prophylaxis (develop chronic HBV infection) should be referred for appropriate follow-up and care.

A high HBV viral load (HBV DNA $\geq 10^8$ copies/mL) during pregnancy is associated with an increased risk of perinatal transmission despite appropriate infant postexposure prophylaxis. Some evidence suggests that antiviral treatment of these HBsAg-positive women during the third trimester of pregnancy might lower perinatal transmission risk.[154] However, no current recommendation exists for routine determination of viral load among HBsAg-positive pregnant women.

Immunization of Infants with Birthweight <2000 Grams

Routine HepB immunization of preterm infants weighing <2000 grams at birth should be delayed until the infant is 1 month of age or is discharged from the hospital, whichever is first, and the 3-dose series completed at intervals of 1 to 2 months and 6 months from the first dose. If the infant's mother is HBsAg-positive or her HBsAg status is unknown,[109] the infant should receive HepB and HBIG within 12 hours of birth and complete three additional doses on a 0, 1, 6 months schedule (i.e., the birth dose does not count as part of the vaccine series for infants weighing <2000 grams).[109]

Vaccine Dosage and Administration

The vaccine dosage varies by manufacturer and age of recipient. The typical dosage for infants, children, and adolescents ranges from 5 to 10 µg, and for adults from 10 to 20 µg.[109] A dosage of 40 µg is recommended for people with certain immunocompromising conditions such as dialysis dependence.[155] Vaccines from different manufacturers can be used interchangeably, provided that each vaccine is given at the dosage recommended by the manufacturer. If a low dosage of vaccine is administered, the dose should be repeated with the appropriate dosage.[109]

HepB should be administered intramuscularly, in the anterior thigh of children <2 years of age and in the deltoid muscle in older children and adolescents. HepB should not be administered in the buttock or intradermally as this has been associated with decreased immunogenicity. Administration with a standard 1-inch needle has been associated with decreased immunogenicity among obese adolescents; improved immunogenicity is achieved when vaccine is administered with a 1.5-inch needle.[109,156] If a dose of vaccine is missed, the vaccine series does not need to be restarted. The missed dose should be given as soon as possible and the vaccine series completed. HepB can be administered concurrently with other indicated vaccines. A total of 4 doses can be given when a monovalent HepB dose is administered at birth, followed by 3 doses in combination vaccines.

Vaccine Immunogenicity and Efficacy

A seroprotective immune response to HepB is defined as development of anti-HBs ≥ 10 mIU/mL at 1 to 2 months after completion of the vaccine series. HepB are highly immunogenic, with seroconversion rates of $\geq 95\%$ in healthy infants, children, and adolescents after completion of the 3-dose series.[157] Seroconversion rates, however, vary depending on the numbered dose in the vaccine series with much lower seroconversion after one dose compared with after series completion. Concurrent administration of HBIG does not reduce seroconversion rates. Lower rates of seroconversion are associated with administration at older age (>40 years) and in people with immunocompromising conditions.[158,159] In studies among infants and children infected with HIV, 20% to 78% attained seroprotective levels of anti-HBs after series completion.[160–165]

HepB starting at birth is 70% to 90% effective in preventing perinatal HBV infection; and HBIG administered within 12 hours of birth with completion of the vaccine series is 85% to 95% effective.[166,167]

Prevaccination and Postvaccination Testing

Prevaccination testing for immunity is not indicated before routine vaccination of infants, children, and adolescents. However, children born in high- or intermediate-endemic countries should be tested before or at the same time the first dose of vaccine is given.

Because HepB is highly immunogenic, postvaccination serologic testing is not indicated after routine vaccination, except for the following groups: (1) infants born to HBsAg-positive mothers; (2) healthcare providers; (3) people with immunosuppressive conditions, including those undergoing long-term hemodialysis; and (4) sex partners of HBsAg-positive people.[109,155,168] Postvaccination serology should be performed 1 to 2 months after administration of the last dose of vaccine. In people who do not respond to the primary series (i.e., anti-HBs concentration <10 mIU/mL), revaccination is recommended. Revaccination (usually 3 doses) is not associated with an increase in adverse events and substantially increases the rates of seroprotection in low- or non-responders. People who do not respond to a second series should be tested for HBsAg to determine if they are chronically infected.[109] Persons who are not chronically infected and do not respond to two vaccine series are unlikely to respond to further vaccination.

Vaccine Safety

The safety of HepB has been demonstrated in a large, prospective clinical trial[169] and in postlicensure safety analyses.[170] Pain at the injection site (3–29%) and increased temperature >37.7°C (1–6%) are the most frequently reported adverse events.[169] The incidence of anaphylaxis to HepB is estimated to be 1 case per 1.1 million doses of vaccine distributed.[171] Several case reports of demyelinating or other neurologic diseases temporally associated with HepB have been reported, but no association has been observed in large, controlled studies.[172–175] Expert reviewers have found no supportive evidence for an association between HepB and neurologic disease.[176–178]

HepB is contraindicated for people with a history of hypersensitivity to yeast or to any vaccine component.[109] Pregnancy is not a contraindication to vaccination. People with a history of a serious adverse event (e.g., anaphylaxis) after receipt of HepB should not receive additional doses.

Hepatitis B Immune Globulin (HBIG) and Postexposure Prophylaxis

HBIG is prepared from plasma containing high concentrations of anti-HBs. HBIG provides short-term protection (i.e., 3 to 6 months) from infection. Currently, HBIG administered in conjunction with HepB is recommended for: (1) infants born to HBsAg-positive mothers; (2) unvaccinated sexual contacts of a person known to be or at high risk of being HBsAg-positive; and (3) unvaccinated persons with a percutaneous exposure (e.g., needlestick injury, sharing of injection-drug equipment) from someone who is known to be or at high risk of being HBsAg-positive. Administration of HBIG alone is the primary means of protection after exposure to HBV in known non-responders to vaccination.[109] HBIG also is used in patients with HBV-related chronic liver disease who have undergone liver transplantation to reduce the incidence of recurrent HBV infection.[179] HepB at birth, with or without HBIG, eliminates any theoretical risk of virus transmission through breastfeeding.[180–182]

Long-term Protection

HepB provides long-term protection against HBV infection. Despite the loss of detectable levels of anti-HBs, people who

TABLE 213-3. Long-term Protection from Hepatitis B Vaccines

Study Location, by Age Group of Vaccinees	n	Years of Follow-up	Anti-HBs Positive (%)	HBsAg Positive (%)	Anti-HBc Positive (%)	Reference
INFANTS[a]						
Taiwan[b]	78	15	70	1.2	33	187
England[b]	64	14	50	0	1.5	188
Alaska[b]	16	12	24	0	0	189
Alaska[c]	17	12	24	0	0	189
Taiwan[b]	805	10	85	0.4	14	190
Taiwan[b]	118	10	67	0	12	195
Italy[b]	53	10	68	0	0	196
Alaska[b,c]	350	2–10	8–45	2	2	191
Micronesia[c]	105	15	40	0	0	197
OLDER INFANTS AND CHILDREN						
Hong Kong	88	18	61	0	3	192
China	52	15	50	2	6	194
United States	18	13	83	0	0	193
Gambia	429	15	34	0.4	18	199
ADULTS						
United States[d,e]	783	15	41–77	0.2	2	200
Italy	310	10	85	0	0	201
United States[d]	493	22	60	0	1	198

anti-HBc, antibody to hepatitis B core antigen; anti-HBs, antibody to hepatitis B surface antigen; HBsAg, hepatitis B surface antigen; P, plasma-derived vaccine; R, recombinant vaccine.
[a]Vaccinated beginning at birth.
[b]Born to HBsAg-positive mothers.
[c]Born to HBsAg-negative mothers.
[d]Includes children and adolescents.
[e]Includes persons who did not respond to the initial vaccine series (i.e., nonresponders).

responded to vaccination remain protected, and a booster dose of vaccine is not recommended currently.[109,155,168,183–186] In most studies among infants and children who responded to the primary vaccine series, 40% to 85% had detectable levels of anti-HBs 10 to 22 years after vaccination (Table 213-3).[187–199] Although breakthrough infections have been observed in a small proportion of children and adolescents as evidenced by development of anti-HBc, chronic infection (i.e., development of HBsAg) occurred rarely and there were no reports of clinically apparent acute hepatitis B. Long-term studies among vaccinated adults have shown similar findings (Table 213-3).[198,200,201]

Long-term protection from HepB is thought to be related to sensitization of B lymphocytes to HBsAg in the vaccine and development of an anamnestic antibody response upon HBV challenge.[184,186] Booster dose studies have been used to simulate natural infection with HBV. In studies of children and adolescents who were vaccinated in infancy and childhood and who had a documented response to the primary vaccine series and lost detectable levels of anti-HBs, most (>90% in most studies) responded to a booster dose of vaccine 10 to 15 years after the initial vaccine series.[183,187–189,195,196] In people with immunosuppressive conditions, vaccine-induced protection might persist only as long as antibody levels remain >10 mIU/mL. In hemodialysis patients, anti-HBs levels should be tested annually and booster doses given when antibody levels are <10 mIU/mL; for other immunocompromised people (e.g., HIV-infected persons, hematopoietic stem cell transplant recipients) repeat testing may be considered.[109]

HEPATITIS DELTA VIRUS

PATHOGENESIS

Hepatitis delta virus (HDV) is an RNA virus which was first detected in hepatocytes of patients infected with HBV. HDV is a

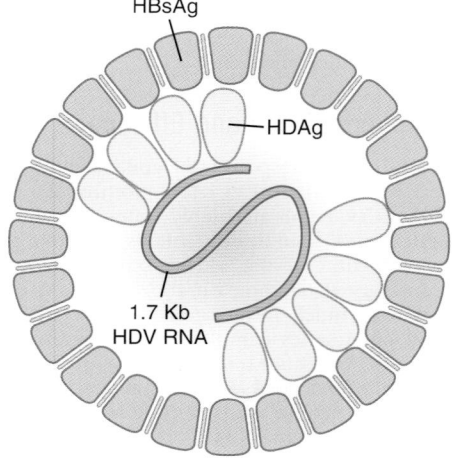

Figure 213-7. Schematic diagram of hepatitis D (delta) virus.

unique pathogen which is distinct molecularly from other hepatitis viruses in that it can only infect cells and cause disease in the presence of HBV. As such, HDV is classified as a satellite virus or subviral agent because of its inability to encode its own envelope protein. HDV encodes a single protein, the delta antigen (HDAg), which is encapsulated with HBsAg encoded by HBV (Figure 213-7). Because of the unique requirement for HBV, infections with HDV occur in two forms: HBV-HDV coinfection and HDV superinfection. In HBV-HDV coinfection, HBV and HDV are transmitted simultaneously to a person who is susceptible to HBV infection. People who are immune to HBV infection, through either prior infection or vaccination, cannot be infected with HDV. In HDV superinfection, HDV is transmitted to a person with pre-existing chronic HBV infection which provides the HBsAg needed to establish the HDV infection.

EPIDEMIOLOGY

The epidemiology of HDV infection is similar to that of HBV infection. Percutaneous transmission of HDV is very efficient, as evidenced by the high prevalence of HDV among people who have frequent percutaneous exposures such as injection-drug users. Worldwide, approximately 15 million people are infected with HDV with areas of high endemicity limited primarily to parts of the Mediterranean basin, several countries in Africa, and the Amazon basin in South America.[202-204] In the U.S., the prevalence of serologic markers of past or present HDV among HBsAg carriers ranges from 4% in the general population to as high as 73% among some populations of HBsAg-positive injection-drug users.[205,206] In low-endemic area, such as the U.S., transmission usually results from coinfection in well-defined high-risk groups with frequent percutaneous exposures, such as injection-drug users and people with hemophilia. Although most HDV infections in low-endemic areas occur sporadically, outbreaks of HBV-HDV coinfection and HDV superinfection among injection-drug users and their sexual contacts have been described.[207] In high-endemic areas, transmission of HDV occurs primarily through person-to-person contact, especially in households, and usually results from HDV superinfection.

CLINICAL MANIFESTATIONS

The incubation period for HBV-HDV coinfection ranges from 6 to 24 weeks. One feature that might distinguish HBV-HDV coinfection from other viral hepatitides is a biphasic course of illness, with two peaks of liver cell damage; the first is related to the appearance of HBV antigens in the liver, and the second to the appearance of HDV antigens. Approximately 2% of coinfected people become chronically infected.[208] In people who are HBV-HDV coinfected, fulminant hepatitis develops more often than in people with HBV monoinfection.[209]

The incubation period for HDV superinfection ranges from 2 to 8 weeks. Fulminant hepatitis occurs more often with HDV superinfection than with acute HBV infection alone.[210] In contrast to HBV-HDV coinfection, HDV superinfection results in chronic HDV infection in up to 90% of patients, and the majority of patients progress to cirrhosis.[211,212]

LABORATORY FINDINGS AND DIAGNOSIS

HDV-infected people produce both IgM and IgG antibodies to the hepatitis delta antigen (anti-HDV). During acute HBV-HDV coinfection, antibodies are produced to both HBV and HDV antigens, but the anti-HDV response often is weak and might be delayed by several months. Because anti-HDV might not be present until several weeks after onset of illness, diagnosis of HDV infection might require testing of acute and convalescent sera; HDV infection also can be diagnosed using PCR assays.[213] Often, anti-HDV does not persist, making diagnosis of past coinfection difficult. In contrast, HDV superinfection produces a brisk anti-HDV response that persists throughout chronic infection.[214] Acute HBV-HDV coinfection usually can be distinguished from HDV superinfection by the presence of IgM anti-HBc. The IgM anti-HDV response is not useful for distinguishing acute from chronic HDV infection, as IgM anti-HDV production persists throughout chronic infection.[215]

TREATMENT

Interferon alfa-2a (IFN-α) is the only therapy approved by the FDA for chronic hepatitis D. Data are limited on the effectiveness of IFN-α in children. In a study using 3 to 5 MU/m^2 of IFN-α, clearance of HDV viremia occurred in 2 of 13 (15%) children treated for 24 months; however, no significant improvement in liver histology was noted.[216]

Liver transplantation for end-stage chronic hepatitis D has a 5-year survival rate as high as 88%. The success of liver transplantation for chronic hepatitis D is attributed to the suppressive effect of HDV on HBV replication, which greatly reduces the posttransplant HBV reinfection rate in the grafted liver. When HBIG is used for prophylaxis before liver transplantation for end-stage chronic hepatitis D, the HBV-HDV reinfection rate is approximately 10%, compared with close to 100% HBV reinfection rate due to HBV alone.[217]

PREVENTION

Hepatitis B vaccine is the single most important tool to prevent HBV-HDV coinfection. Administration of HepB, and HBIG if indicated, at birth provides protection against HBV infection and HBV-HDV coinfection.[109] No vaccine exists to prevent HDV superinfection in HBV-infected persons; prevention depends on modification of behaviors, such as safer sexual and drug-injection practices.

214 Human Parvoviruses

Eileen Schneider

Parvoviruses, small (20 to 25 nm), nonenveloped, icosahedral, single-stranded DNA viruses with a linear genome of between 4500 and 5500 nucleotides, are common infectious agents of animals, including birds and insects, as well as humans.[1] At least four different types of parvovirus have been detected in humans, adeno-associated viruses, parvovirus B19, Parv4/5 viruses, and human bocavirus. Parvovirus B19 is the best characterized and definitively linked to human disease. Human bocavirus (HBoV) has been identified in respiratory secretions of young children with acute wheezing and lower respiratory tract infections.[2-7] However, the contribution of HBoV as an etiologic pathogen for respiratory disease is currently unclear, since HBoV is often found in the presence of other pathogens.

PARVOVIRUS B19

Parvovirus B19 replication occurs only in human erythrocyte precursors, and is classified as a member of the *Erythrovirus* genus. The viral genome encodes one nonstructural protein, which mediates cytotoxicity,[8] and two capsid proteins, VP1 and VP2, which self-assemble to form virus-like particles in vitro.[9] Based on viral sequence, parvovirus B19 can be divided into three distinct genotypes (genotypes 1, 2, and 3),[10] but only a single parvovirus B19 antigenic type has been described.[11]

Pathogenesis

Parvovirus B19 replication and production of infectious virus occur preferentially in late erythroid progenitor cells in bone marrow. Virus-induced cytotoxicity results in reticulocytopenia and arrest of red cell production. Therefore, parvovirus B19 infection causes transient aplastic crisis in patients who have increased erythropoiesis, such as those with sickle-cell anemia. Parvovirus B19 also causes chronic anemia in patients who are immunosuppressed and unable to control the infection. Erythroid specificity is in part due to the tissue distribution of the receptor for parvovirus B19, the blood group P antigen.[12] This antigen, also known as *globoside*, is found in the erythrocyte precursors in bone marrow as well as in a variety of other tissues, including megakaryocytes, endothelial cells, placenta, fetal myocardium, and fetal liver. Rare individuals who lack the blood group P antigen are naturally resistant to parvovirus B19 infection.[13] Some of the clinical consequences of parvovirus infection, including fifth disease, are immune mediated.

After infection there is a brisk viremia, which peaks at $>10^{12}$ virus particles (international units) per mL of blood (Figure 214-1). Viremia often is accompanied by a nonspecific febrile illness. In immunocompetent individuals, as viremia resolves an immunoglobulin (Ig)M and IgG antibody response is mounted. The second, immune-mediated phase of illness begins 2 to 3 weeks after infection, as the IgM response peaks. Typical manifestations of this phase of the illness are the rash of fifth disease, arthralgia, and arthritis. In normal hosts, there usually is no clinical evidence of residual infection, although parvovirus B19 DNA can be detected by polymerase chain reaction (PCR) in blood and tissues for months to years after acute infection.[14] Chronic, high-titer viremia can occur in immunocompromised individuals, who do not make neutralizing antibody.[15]

Epidemiology

Parvovirus B19 infection is a common illness of childhood; by 15 years of age, approximately 50% of children have detectable IgG.[16,17]

In temperate climates, most infections occur in the spring, with mini-epidemics occurring at regular intervals several years apart. Secondary infection rates approach 50% in households,[18] but are lower for adults in schools or other institutions.[19] Transmission is

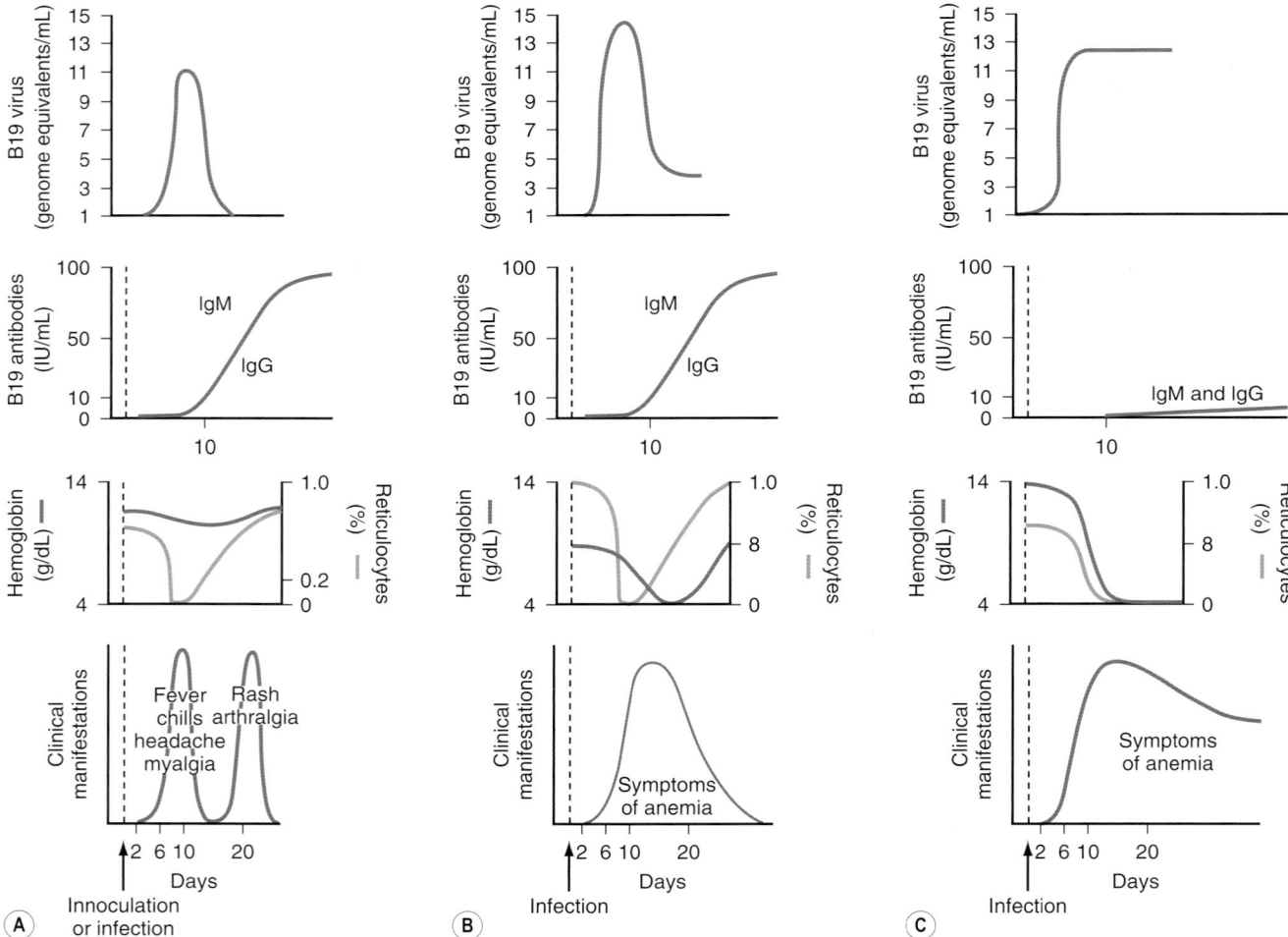

Figure 214-1. Schematic of the time course of parvovirus B19 infection, showing the associations of viremia, antibody production, and clinical symptoms in three groups of individuals: **(A)** fifth disease; **(B)** transient aplastic crisis; and **(C)** chronic bone marrow failure. (Redrawn from Young NS, Brown KE. Parvovirus B19. N Engl J Med 2004;350:586–597.)

predominantly via the respiratory route, probably by droplet spread, and is highest at the time of viremia, before the onset of rash or arthralgia.

Persons who have hemolytic anemias or decreased red cell production are at increased risk of severe anemia or transient aplastic crisis when infected with parvovirus B19. Globally, many children have severe anemia due to malaria, chronic parasitic infections (e.g., hookworm), and nutritional deficiencies (e.g., iron, vitamin A, vitamin B$_{12}$). Recently, several studies have investigated the relationship between parvovirus B19 and these conditions.[20-22] Although study results have been mixed, some studies have indicated that parvovirus B19 infection may be an important contributor to severe anemia, especially in malaria endemic regions.

Parvovirus B19 infections also can occur as a result of transfusion of blood or blood products.[23] Most reported cases of transfusion-related infection are due to pooled components, especially factor VIII and IX concentrate, rather than individual units. Parvovirus B19 is resistant to both heat and to solvent-detergent inactivation.[24] In July 2009, the United States Food and Drug Administration (FDA) issued a guidance for nucleic acid testing of blood to reduce the risk of transmission parvovirus B19 by plasma-derived products.[25]

Clinical Manifestations

Most infections caused by human parvovirus are asymptomatic or mild. When infection is associated with symptoms, a variety of disease manifestations, depending on the immune status of the host, can be observed (Table 214-1).

Erythema Infectiosum

The most common manifestation of parvovirus B19 infection is erythema infectiosum, a mild febrile illness with rash.[26] Erythema infectiosum also is known as "fifth disease" or "slapped cheek disease." Studies in adult volunteers demonstrated a minor febrile illness that began approximately 8 days after nasal inoculation of virus and was associated with mild hematologic abnormalities during the second week and facial rash at 17 to 18 days (see Figure 214-1A).[27]

In naturally infected children, medical care often is sought when the classic "slapped cheek" rash appears (Figure 214-2). The rash subsequently can spread to the extremities in a lacy reticular pattern (see Figure 214-2B). The rash can be exacerbated by exercise, emotion, hot baths, or sunlight. The intensity and distribution of the rash varies. Among adults, the "slapped cheek" may not be apparent. The rash can be difficult to appreciate in dark-skinned individuals and to distinguish from other viral exanthems, such as rubella (see Figure 214-2D).

Polyarthropathy Syndrome

Although uncommon in children, arthropathy occurs in ~50% of adults and is more common in women than men.[28] The joint distribution often is symmetrical, with arthralgia and even frank arthritis affecting the small joints of the hands and occasionally

the ankles, knees, and wrists. Resolution usually occurs within a few weeks, but persistent or recurring symptoms can continue for years.

Transient Aplastic Crisis

Transient reticulocytopenia followed by rebound reticulocytosis occurs in most subjects infected with parvovirus B19.[29] This transient marrow suppression is not associated with symptoms in most individuals. However, among those who depend on continual rapid production of red blood cells, parvovirus B19 infection often causes transient aplastic crisis (see Figure 214-1B).[18] Affected individuals include those with hemolytic disorders (e.g., hereditary spherocytosis), hemoglobinopathies (e.g., sickle-cell disease, thalassemia), red cell enzymopathies (e.g., glucose-6'-phosphate dehydrogenase deficiency, pyruvate kinase deficiency, pyrimidine-5' nucleotidase deficiency) and autoimmune hemolytic anemias.[30] Aplastic crises precipitated by parvovirus B19 infection often necessitate treatment with blood transfusions, and can be associated with a high rate of severe complications. In one retrospective study, there was a significantly increased risk of cerebrovascular complications within 5 weeks after parvovirus B19-associated aplastic crises in patients with homozygous sickle-cell disease.[31] Patients with aplastic crisis are viremic and therefore infectious at the time of clinical presentation.

Chronic Bone Marrow Failure and Pure Red Cell Aplasia

Persistent parvovirus B19 infection resulting in pure red cell aplasia has been reported in a wide range of immunosuppressed patients, including those with congenital immunodeficiency (e.g., Nezelof syndrome), acquired immunodeficiency syndrome, and lymphoproliferative disorders (especially acute lymphoblastic leukemia) as well as transplant recipients.[32] Patients manifest persistent anemia associated with reticulocytopenia, absence or low levels of parvovirus B19-specific antibody, and high levels of parvovirus B19 DNA in serum (see Figure 214-1C). Bone marrow examination often reveals the presence of scattered giant pronormoblasts. Temporary reduction of chemotherapy may result in an immune response to parvovirus B19 and resolution of infection. Alternatively, administration of immunoglobulin can lead to a prompt drop in viral DNA titers in the blood and resolution of infection.

Other Hematologic Complications

Although parvovirus B19 primarily targets the red cell precursor, other hematologic lineages can be affected. Transient neutropenia, lymphopenia, and thrombocytopenia have been observed during acute parvovirus B19 infection.[27] Parvovirus infection occasionally is associated with a hemophagocytic syndrome.[33]

Rare cases of idiopathic thrombocytopenia (ITP) and Henoch–Schönlein purpura have been reported to follow parvovirus B19 infection.[34] Transient erythroblastopenia of childhood and aplastic anemia do not appear to be caused by the virus.

Unusual Manifestations

A large number of unusual clinical presentations associated with detection of parvovirus DNA in serum and tissue have been reported[35,36] (Box 214-1). However, the observation that parvovirus B19 DNA can be detected by PCR for years in normal tissue in healthy individuals[36,37] confounds the interpretation of parvovirus B19 association with disease. Papular-purpuric gloves and socks syndrome has been associated with parvovirus B19 infection for decades, and also has been described in infections due to herpesviruses, measles and enteroviruses.[38]

Infection and the Fetus

Maternal infection with parvovirus B19 during pregnancy can lead to miscarriage or the development of hydrops fetalis.[39,40] The risk

TABLE 214-1. Diseases Associated with Human Parvovirus B19 Infection

Disease	Host(s)
Fifth disease (erythema infectiosum)	Healthy children
Polyarthropathy syndrome	Healthy adults (especially women)
Transient aplastic crisis	Patients with increased erythropoiesis
Persistent anemia/pure red cell aplasia	Immunodeficient or immunocompetent patients
Hydrops fetalis/congenital anemia	Fetus (<20 weeks)

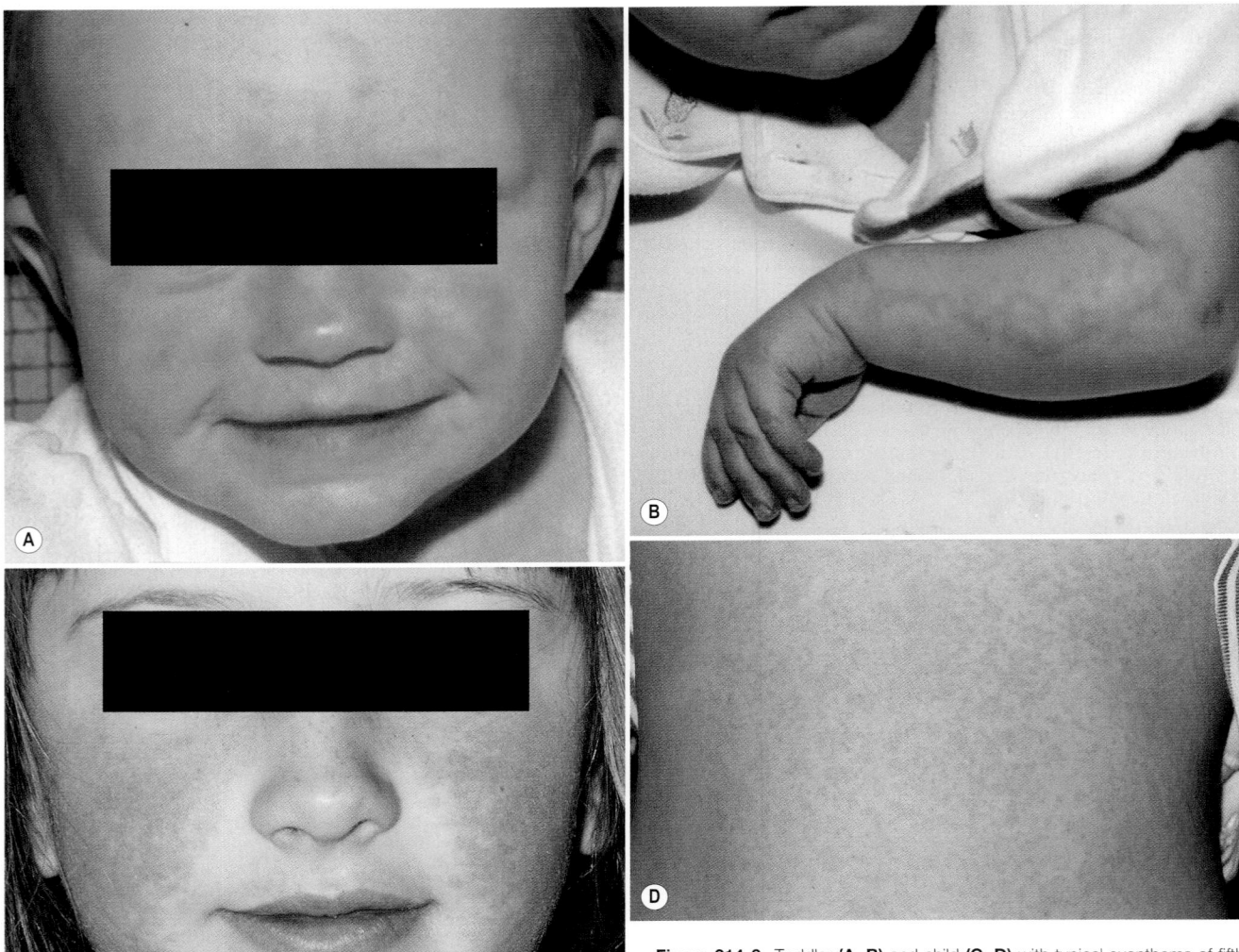

Figure 214-2. Toddler **(A, B)** and child **(C, D)** with typical exanthems of fifth disease. (Courtesy of J.H. Brien© and M. Prober.)

BOX 214-1. Unusual Manifestations of Parvovirus B19 Infection

Hepatitis
Myocarditis
Vasculitis
Glomerulosclerosis
Neurologic disease
Encephalitis
Brachial neuropathy

of adverse outcome appears to be limited to maternal infection occurring during the first half of gestation. In a British study of 427 pregnant women who contracted parvovirus B19 infection during gestation, excess fetal loss was observed only among those infected during the first 20 weeks of pregnancy. The observed risk of fetal hydrops was 2.9% (95% CI, 1.2 to 5.9).[41] In another study, conducted in Japan, the outcomes of 13 pregnancies for which the

timing of gestational parvovirus B19 infection could be established were reported. All 5 infants with adverse consequences (3 with nonimmune hydrops, 1 spontaneous abortion, and 1 liveborn infant who was small for gestational age) resulted from exposure to maternal infection contracted between 3 and 19 weeks' gestation. Eight fetuses appeared to have had no adverse clinical outcomes following maternal infection between 6 and 33 weeks' gestation, but parvovirus B19 DNA was detected in serum at birth from all 8 infants.[42] Although parvovirus B19 does not appear to be teratogenic, anecdotal cases of possible eye damage and central nervous system abnormalities in infants whose mothers were infected with parvovirus B19 during pregnancy have been reported.[43] In addition, several cases of congenital anemia following maternal gestational infection have been described.[44]

Parvovirus B19 probably causes 10% to 20% of all cases of nonimmune hydrops.[45] The pathogenesis is a combination of cardiac decompensation due to severe anemia and parvovirus B19-induced fetal myocarditis. Intrauterine blood transfusion can prevent fetal loss in some cases.[46,47]

Attempts have been made to estimate the risk of fetal loss when erythema infectiosum is recognized in the community.[48,49] Because approximately 50% of pregnant women are susceptible to parvovirus infection and about 30% of susceptible hosts exposed to a community outbreak become infected, the likelihood that a susceptible woman will contract infection is approximately 15%. Considering that no more than 10% of fetuses exposed to maternal infection during the second trimester die, the overall risk of fetal death would be <2%. This estimate is consistent with the findings of a prospective study of gestational parvovirus B19 infections conducted in Spain.[39] Household exposure increases risk of transmission of infection to susceptible individuals to approximately 50%.[18]

Diagnosis

Parvovirus B19 is difficult to isolate in culture. Detection of virus in serum, tissues, or cells depends on DNA hybridization or PCR techniques.

Because viremia is transient (2 to 4 days) in immunocompetent individuals, the diagnosis of acute parvovirus B19 infection usually is based on detection of IgM antibodies.[17] Original assays utilized virus derived from serum as a source of antigen, limiting the availability of assays to research laboratories. However, commercially available, reliable assays based on recombinant virus-like particles expressed in insect cells are now available. IgM antibodies can be detected at the time of rash in fifth disease and by the third day of aplastic crisis in patients with hematologic disorders. IgM antibodies remain detectable for 2 to 3 months after primary infection.

IgG antibodies are detectable several days after the appearance of IgM antibodies and remain detectable thereafter for life. Because >50% of the population has parvovirus B19 IgG antibodies, the test is not as useful for diagnosis of acute infection, but can be helpful in determining prior infection.

PCR assays are highly sensitive and specific tests that can be used to identify acute and chronic B19 infection. These tests can also be used for parvovirus B19 screening of blood products. PCR is particularly valuable in identifying patients with acute aplastic crisis before the development of an antibody response and patients with chronic infection who may have a weak or absent antibody response, and also in diagnosis of fetal infection based on detection of virus in amniotic fluid and placental tissue.

Parvovirus B19 DNA can be detected by PCR for many months after acute infection, although levels fall rapidly after acute infection.[50] In acute infection, viremia peaks at $>10^{12}$ parvovirus B19 DNA genome copies/mL of serum and falls rapidly within days. Patients with aplastic crisis or pure red cell aplasia due to parvovirus B19 generally have $>10^5$ parvovirus B19 DNA genome copies/mL of serum at the time of the crisis. Results from parvovirus B19 PCR assays must be carefully interpreted in the context of clinical history and findings because of potential for false-positive results from amplicon contamination and because low viral loads may not be indicative of acute parvovirus B19 infection.

Treatment and Prevention

No antiviral drug is available for treatment of parvovirus B19 infection. However, because the humoral immune response plays a prominent role in controlling parvovirus B19 infection, commercial immune globulin preparations from healthy blood donors can clear or ameliorate persistent parvovirus B19 infection in immunosuppressed patients.[51,52] Treatment of patients with polyarthropathy is symptomatic only; administration of immunoglobulin is not beneficial. There are no definitive guidelines for clinical management of pregnancies complicated by intrauterine parvovirus B19 infection and fetal hydrops; however, the American College of Obstetrics and Gynecology has published guidelines that recommend serologic testing and serial ultrasound examinations.[53]

Once classic symptoms (e.g., rash) appear in persons with erythema infectiosum, the risk of transmission is low. In contrast, persons with transient aplastic crisis or chronic parvovirus B19 infection generally are viremic, and thus are contagious for longer periods. Therefore, consistently maintaining good personal hygiene (e.g., proper handwashing) is one of the mainstays of prevention.[54] For hospitalized persons, Droplet Precautions, in addition to Standard Precautions, are recommended for a duration of time that depends upon the presentation of parvovirus B19 infection and the patients' clinical status and immunologic competency.[54,55]

No vaccine is approved for parvovirus B19, although research of candidate vaccines is ongoing. A vaccine would be advantageous in specific populations where parvovirus B19 potentially can cause substantial morbidity, such as those who are pregnant, immunocompromised, and those with underlying hemolytic disorders or increased red cell production.

Key Points. Erythema Infectiosum (Fifth Disease)

EPIDEMIOLOGY

- Erythema infectiosum is the most common manifestation of parvovirus B19 infection
- In temperate climates, most infections occur in the spring, with epidemics occurring every several years
- ~50% of persons aged ≥15 years have evidence of past infection
- Transmission is predominantly via the respiratory route. Once the rash appears, the risk of transmission is very low

PATHOGENESIS

- Parvovirus B19 replication occurs in late erythroid progenitor cells in bone marrow

CLINICAL FEATURES

- Initially, a nonspecific febrile illness appears ~1 week after infection. This is followed by an immune-mediated phase which typically begins with a "slapped cheek" rash which may spread to the extremities in a lacy reticular pattern. Adults often will present with arthralgias instead of rash. A transient anemia may also appear

DIAGNOSIS

- Primarily based on epidemiologic and clinical presentation
- Laboratory diagnostic tests include:
  - Detection of IgM antibodies – appear at the time of rash and remain detectable for 2 to 3 months
  - Detection of IgG antibodies – appear several days after IgM antibodies and remain detectable thereafter for life. Helpful in determining past infection, especially among pregnant women
  - Polymerase chain reaction (PCR) assays – highly sensitive and specific tests that can be used to detect acute and chronic B19 infection, as well as screening of blood products

TREATMENT

- No antiviral drug or vaccine is available for treatment of parvovirus B19 infection

---

215 Coltivirus (Colorado Tick Fever)

Marc Fischer and J. Erin Staples

BOX 215-1. Colorado Tick Fever: Agent and Epidemiology

AGENT

Colorado tick fever virus, *Coltivirus* genus, Reoviridae family

VECTOR

Dermacentor andersoni, Rocky Mountain wood tick

NATURAL RESERVOIR

Rodent, small mammal–tick cycle

DISTRIBUTION

Western United States and southwestern Canada at elevations from 4000 to 10,000 feet

SEASONALITY

March–September with an April–July peak

RISK FACTORS

Outdoor exposure in an endemic area
One transfusion-acquired case and 16 laboratory-associated cases reported

Colorado tick fever (CTF) is an acute febrile illness caused by the Colorado tick fever virus (CTFV). CTFV is a double-stranded RNA virus assigned to the *Coltivirus* genus of the family Reoviridae (Box 215-1).[1,2] The virus is transmitted to humans through the bite of an infected Rocky Mountain wood tick, *Dermacentor andersoni* (Figure 215-1).

TICK VECTOR AND VERTEBRATE HOSTS

CTFV is maintained in an epizootic cycle between *D. andersoni* and small mammals, principally rodents.[3–11] The virus-amplifying mammal hosts develop apparently silent infections but remain viremic for weeks to months. Larval ticks become infected as a

result of feeding on viremic mammals. Infection then passes from larval ticks to the nymphal and adult stages. Humans usually are infected by bites of adult ticks.[5,7,10]

EPIDEMIOLOGY

D. andersoni is found in the western United States and southwestern Canada at elevations from 4000 to 10,000 feet, typically in areas with pine–juniper–sagebrush vegetation (Figure 215-2).[3,8–10] Approximately 90% of CTFV-infected persons report a recent history of tick bite or outdoor exposure in *D. andersoni*-endemic areas.[12–14] Most human cases occur between April and July.[12–14] Although infection is thought to be more common among people aged 10 to 49 years, one recent study found a higher incidence of CTF among older adults.[12–14]

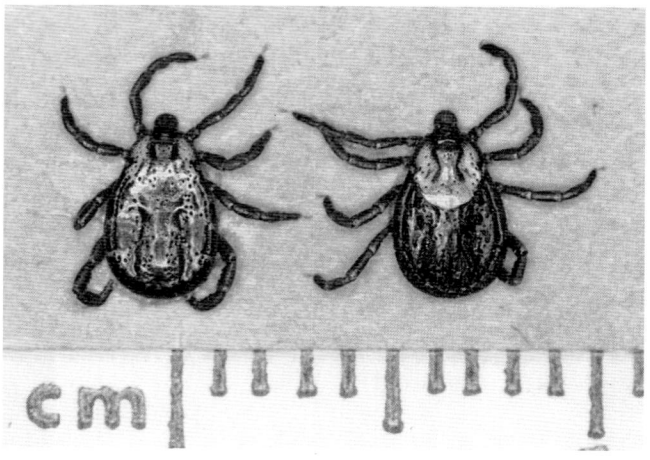

Figure 215-1. Both adult male (left) and female (right) *Dermacentor andersoni* ticks can transmit Colorado tick fever virus.

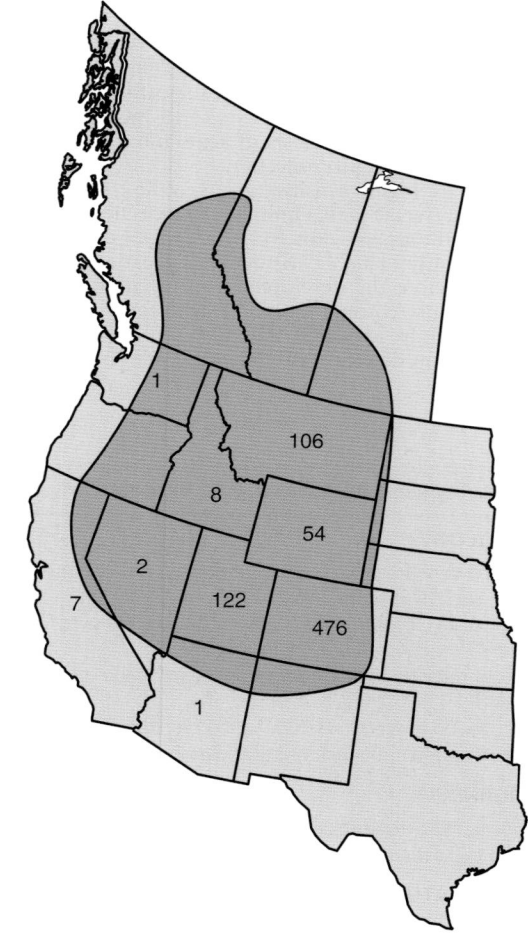

Figure 215-2. Approximate geographic distribution of *Dermacentor andersoni* (Rocky Mountain wood tick) and numbers of CTF cases reported to state health departments, United States, 1987 to 2001. (Redrawn from Marfin AA, Campbell GL. Colorado tick fever and related *Coltivirus* infections. In Goodman JL, et al. (eds) Tick-Borne Diseases of Humans, 1st ed. Washington, DC, American Society for Microbiology 2005, pp. 143–149.)

CTF is not a nationally notifiable disease but it is reportable in some states where the disease is endemic. Between 1987 and 2001, CTF cases were reported from nine U.S. state health departments, with Colorado, Utah, Montana, and Wyoming accounting for the vast majority (Figure 215-2).[8] From 1995 through 2003, the average reported annual incidence of CTF in Utah, Montana, and Wyoming was 2.7 cases per 1,000,000 population (range, 1.4 to 7.2).[14] The average annual incidence in these three states decreased over time from 3.9 per 1,000,000 in 1995–1997, to 2.7 in 1998–2000, to 1.7 in 2001–2003.[14] This decreased incidence likely reflects changes in testing and reporting practices. However, changes in the environment or human exposure also may have played a role. A survey in one endemic area suggested that only 10% of CTF cases were reported.[3] One transfusion-acquired and 16 laboratory-associated cases of CTF have been reported.[15-20]

CLINICAL AND LABORATORY FINDINGS

The incubation period for CTF is usually 3 to 4 days (range, 1 to 14 days).[3,12,13] Symptoms include fever, chills, headache, myalgias, and lethargy (Box 215-2).[12,13,21] Sore throat, vomiting, abdominal pain, and stiff neck are less common manifestations. Physical examination may reveal conjunctival injection, pharyngeal erythema, lymphadenopathy, or hepatosplenomegaly. A maculopapular or petechial rash has been reported in 5% to 16% of patients.[12-14,21]

Leukopenia is the most characteristic laboratory finding in CTF (Box 215-3).[12,21-23] There usually is a relative lymphocytosis with atypical lymphocytes. Moderate thrombocytopenia can occur.[11,24] CTFV infects erythrocytic precursors in the bone marrow. Although red blood cells remain infected for their lifespan, anemia is rare.[12,18,23,25] Patients with central nervous system involvement typically have lymphocytic pleocytosis and elevated protein in their cerebrospinal fluid.[13]

About half of all patients experience a biphasic illness. In these cases, symptoms remit after 2 to 4 days, but then recur 1 to 3 days later.[12,13,21] Patients often are bedridden and approximately 1 in 8 require hospitalization.[13,14] A prolonged convalescence characterized by weakness and fatigue is common but age-dependent, with symptoms often continuing for >3 weeks in persons >30 years of age.[12]

Life-threatening complications and deaths due to CTF are rare; all reported fatalities have been children and most have been

---

BOX 215-3. Colorado Tick Fever: Complications, Laboratory Findings, and Diagnosis

COMPLICATIONS

Life-threatening complications and deaths rare
Meningoencephalitis or disseminated intravascular coagulation
Hepatitis, pericarditis, myocarditis, pneumonitis, epididymo-orchitis also have been reported

LABORATORY FINDINGS

Leukopenia (2000–4000/mm^3) is the most characteristic laboratory finding
Relative lymphocytosis with atypical lymphocytes
Moderate thrombocytopenia (20,000–60,000/mm^3) common

DIAGNOSIS

Viral isolation from whole blood or red blood cells
Immunofluorescent staining of peripheral blood smear
Polymerase chain reaction (PCR) assay on serum or whole blood
Serologic assays (e.g., indirect fluorescent antibody and plaque-reduction neutralization)

---

associated with disseminated intravascular coagulation or meningoencephalitis.[3,11,13,21,26] Other reported complications include hepatitis, pericarditis, myocarditis, pneumonia, and epididymo-orchitis.[12,17,26-29] Teratogenic effects and fetal loss have been found in mice experimentally infected with CTFV, but this association has not been clearly established in humans.[3,30,31]

DIAGNOSIS

A history of exposure to an enzootic location is the most helpful clue to the diagnosis. The differential diagnosis includes other vector-borne infectious diseases (e.g., tularemia, Rocky Mountain spotted fever, tickborne relapsing fever, and mosquito-borne arboviral fevers), and non-arthropod-borne infections such as enteroviruses and leptospirosis.[1,8] Distinguishing CTF from Rocky Mountain spotted fever can be difficult. However, a biphasic fever pattern, prominent leukopenia, and absence of a hemorrhagic rash, all favor a diagnosis of CTF. The geographic distributions of other tickborne diseases such as human anaplasmosis (i.e., human granulocytic ehrlichiosis), human monocytic ehrlichiosis, and babesiosis have minimal overlap with that of CTF; therefore, residence and travel history may help in the differentiation of these diseases.

CTFV can be isolated from whole blood or red blood cells in suckling mice or cell culture.[3,8,18,32] CTFV antigens also can be detected in peripheral blood smears by immunofluorescent staining.[33] Although culture and immunofluorescent staining are most sensitive during the acute illness, CTFV has been isolated from nearly 50% of patients 4 weeks after onset, and viral antigen can be detected in red blood cells in peripheral blood smears for 20 weeks.[12,18,32] Real-time reverse transcriptase-polymerase chain reaction (rRT-PCR) assays can detect CTFV RNA in serum or whole blood reliably during the first 2 weeks of illness and for up to 6 weeks after onset.[34-36]

The most commonly used serologic assays for CTF are indirect fluorescent antibody (IFA) and plaque-reduction neutralization testing.[1,34,37-39] Antibodies to CTFV are slow to develop with <50% of patients having detectable antibodies by 2 weeks after illness onset.[37,38] However, by 30 days, >90% of patients have neutralizing antibodies, with titers peaking around 20 weeks after onset.[12] Other tests that have been used to detect CTFV antibodies include enzyme immunoassay (EIA), complement fixation, and Western blot. IgM antibodies measured by EIA usually do not appear until 14 to 21 days after illness onset and decline abruptly after 6 weeks.[1,37] Complement-fixing antibodies develop late after CTFV infection, and are not detected in 25% of patients.[1,38]

BOX 215-2. Colorado Tick Fever: Clinical Features

HISTORY

Recent tick bite or outdoor exposure in endemic areas within 2 weeks of illness onset

INCUBATION PERIOD

Usually 3–4 days; range 1–14 days

SYMPTOMS

Fever, chills, headache, myalgias, lethargy
Sore throat, vomiting, abdominal pain, and stiff neck are less common
Absence of respiratory symptoms

SIGNS

Elevated temperature, conjunctival injection, pharyngeal erythema, lymphadenopathy, or mild hepatosplenomegaly
Maculopapular or petechial rash (5–12% of cases)

CLINICAL COURSE

Fever and symptoms remit in 2–4 days
Recurrence of symptoms after 1–3 days (50% of cases)
Prolonged convalescence especially among persons >30 years old

---

Testing for CTFV and CTFV-specific antibodies are available only at a few reference laboratories. Many laboratory tests for CTF have not been adequately standardized or evaluated.

TREATMENT AND PREVENTION

Patients with CTF should be given supportive care under standard infection control precautions. No specific therapy is available. Ribavirin variably inhibits CTFV growth in vitro,[40] but safety and efficacy data in humans are lacking. Patients with CTF should defer blood and bone marrow donation for at least 6 months after recovery.[8,18,41]

Persons with outdoor exposures in endemic areas should wear protective clothing, spray clothing with permethrin, apply repellent to exposed skin, and periodically check for and remove

ticks.[3,8] CTFV should be handled under Biosafety Level 2 conditions to minimize risk of laboratory-acquired infection.[20]

OTHER RELATED TICKBORNE COLTIVIRUSES

Historically, coltiviruses have been divided into subgroup A (North American and European species) and subgroup B (Asian species). However, the subgroup B mosquito-borne viruses were recently reassigned to a new genus designated *Seadornavirus* (Southeast Asian dodeca RNA virus).[1,42] Two other tickborne coltiviruses rarely have been associated with human disease. Salmon River virus was isolated from a patient with CTF-like illness in Idaho, and Eyach virus may cause neurologic disease in Europe.[1,8,11,43,44]

216 Rotaviruses

Catherine Yen and Margaret M. Cortese

Rotaviruses are the most common cause of severe infant and childhood gastroenteritis worldwide and are responsible for over half a million deaths and approximately 40% of all diarrheal hospitalizations among children under 5 years of age annually.[1] To mitigate this substantial burden of disease, rotavirus vaccines have been developed and now are licensed in many countries.

DESCRIPTION OF THE PATHOGEN

Rotaviruses were first discovered in humans in 1973 by Bishop and colleagues when they observed wheel-shaped particles in the duodenal mucosa from biopsies from infants with severe gastroenteritis in Australia using immune electron microscopy (Figure 216-1).[2,3] Rotaviruses are 100 nm, nonenveloped RNA viruses belonging to the family Reoviridae.[4,5] Viral particles contain a

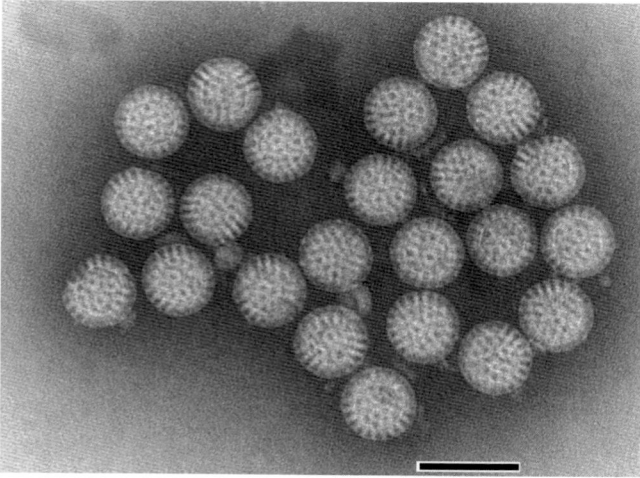

Figure 216-1. Electron micrograph of rotavirus particles in stool specimens, visualized by negative staining. Note typical double-shelled appearance of intact virions. Spikes formed by VP4 and protruding from the outer shell are not apparent in this image. (Courtesy of Charles D. Humphrey, PhD, CDC, Atlanta, GA).

triple-layered capsid surrounding a viral genome of 11 segments of double-stranded RNA.[5] These RNA segments code for 6 structural proteins (VP1–VP4, VP6, and VP7) and 6 nonstructural proteins (NSP1–NSP6). The VP7 protein (a glycoprotein, or G-type protein) and VP4 protein (a protease-activated protein, or P-type protein) comprise the outer layer of the capsid. These proteins are the principal targets of neutralizing antibodies, and therefore are critical to vaccine development. The VP6 protein comprises the middle layer of the capsid and is the protein to which common immune diagnostics are directed. The other three structural proteins comprise the inner core of the capsid (VP2) or are associated with viral RNA (VP1 and VP3). The NSP4 protein is an enterotoxin that mediates some of the early symptoms and signs of disease and may be a protein to which antibodies are developed in the immune response to infection.[4]

Rotaviruses most commonly are classified according to group and serotype. Seven groups of rotavirus have been described (A–G), and are based on genetic and antigenic differences in the VP6 protein.[5] Only those viruses in groups A, B, and C are known to cause disease in humans. Group A rotaviruses are the principal cause of human disease and the main subject of this chapter. Group B rotaviruses have been associated with epidemic gastroenteritis in Asia,[6–8] and group C rotaviruses have been associated with sporadic mild gastroenteritis.[9–11] Of note, several animal species are susceptible to rotavirus infection (e.g., primates and cows). However, the rotavirus strains that infect these animals differ from those that infect humans, and animal-to-human transmission appears to be uncommon.[12,13]

Group A rotaviruses are further classified by serotype based on their VP7 (G type) and VP4 (P type) proteins. G types commonly are determined by either enzyme immunoassays (EIA) using type-specific monoclonal antibodies for predominant serotypes or by reverse transcription-polymerase chain reaction (RT-PCR).[12,14] P types usually are determined using molecular methods, such as RT-PCR or sequencing, since characterization by more traditional methods is difficult. To date, 14 G serotypes and 32 P genotypes have been described.[15] Globally, five G types (G1–4 and G9) and three P types (P[4], P[6], and P[8]) predominate.[12,14–16] Although the genes that code for VP7 and VP4 segregate independently, five combinations of these common types generally account for more than 90% of circulating viruses: P[8]G1, P[4]G2, P[8]G3, P[8]G4, and P[8]G9.[16]

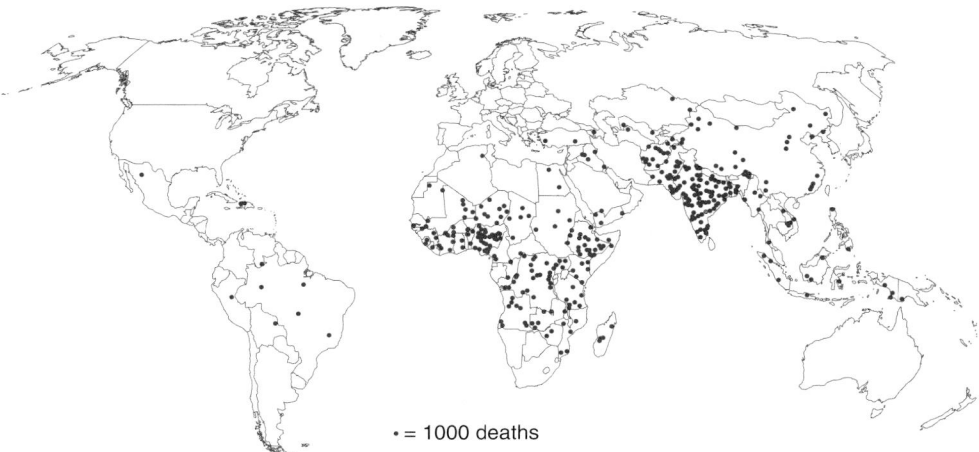

Figure 216-2. Estimated distribution of rotavirus deaths among children <5 years of age, by country. Each dot represents 1000 deaths. (Adapted from Parashar UD, Burton A, Lanata C, et al. Global mortality associated with rotavirus disease among children in 2004. J Infect Dis 2009;200:S9–S15.)

• = 1000 deaths

EPIDEMIOLOGY

Rotaviruses are the most common cause of severe, dehydrating gastroenteritis among children worldwide.[1,17] However, the epidemiology of infection in different settings can be distinct. Worldwide, an estimated 527,000 children under 5 years of age die each year from rotavirus disease, translating to approximately 1440 deaths due to rotavirus per day. More than 85% of these deaths occur in low-income countries (Figure 216-2).[1] Overall, among children under 5 years of age, rotavirus has been estimated to account for about 29% of all diarrheal deaths and 5% of all deaths. Although deaths due to rotavirus are rare in economically developed countries,[18,19] hospitalizations due to rotavirus are common in both developed and economically developing countries.[20,21] In the United States, prior to implementation of the rotavirus vaccination program in 2006, rotavirus gastroenteritis accounted for approximately 55,000 to 70,000 hospitalizations, 205,000 to 272,000 emergency department (ED) visits, and 410,000 physician visits annually, with total annual direct and indirect costs of approximately $1 billion.[22–26] Studies in countries in Asia estimate that approximately 24% to 44% of gastroenteritis hospitalizations are attributable to rotavirus.[27–29] These estimates are similar to those from Africa and Latin America.[30,31]

In temperate climates, rotavirus disease occurs in distinct winter seasonal peaks.[21,32–36] Prior to introduction of vaccine in the U.S., rotavirus activity usually began in early winter in the southwest and moved across the country, ending in northeastern states in the spring.[34] In tropical settings, rotavirus can circulate year-round, but often has seasonal peaks during the cool or dry months.[20,31,37,38] Rotaviruses are spread through fecal–oral contamination, predominantly by close person-to-person contact.[5] Spread also likely occurs through contaminated fomites, especially in out-of-home-care settings and hospitals.[39–41] Very few infectious virions are needed to cause disease in susceptible hosts.[42] While probable waterborne transmission has been described,[43] spread through food and water is likely to be rare. Transmission through airborne droplets has been hypothesized because of rapid seasonal transmission through populations, but is not proven.[5,44]

Almost all children are infected at least once with rotavirus by the age of 5 years.[45,46] The highest rates of rotavirus gastroenteritis occur among children 4 to 23 months of age, who also are more likely to experience severe, dehydrating rotavirus gastroenteritis.[45,47–49] Infants younger than 3 months of age have lower rates of infection and full-term neonates are more likely to be asymptomatic when infected, possibly due to protection from passively transferred maternal antibody.[50,51] After a single natural infection, 38% of children are protected against subsequent rotavirus infection, 77% are protected against subsequent rotavirus gastroenteritis, and 87% are protected against severe rotavirus gastroenteritis; second and third infections confer progressively greater protection

against rotavirus gastroenteritis.[46] Because natural infection confers protection against subsequent infection and disease, symptomatic illness is less common among those older than 5 years of age.[46,50] Even so, rotavirus can cause gastroenteritis among older children and adults, often in households with young children, or among adults who care for young children with rotavirus.[52,53]

CLINICAL MANIFESTATIONS

Rotavirus infects the villus enterocytes of the proximal small intestine, leading to destruction of the absorptive enterocytes, downregulation of the expression of absorptive enzymes, functional changes in tight junctions between enterocytes, and production of an enterotoxin.[4] This leads to symptoms of gastroenteritis, following a mean incubation period of 1 to 3 days.[5] The initial manifestations of illness are often fever and abrupt onset of vomiting.[54–59] Most children have profuse, frequent diarrhea that can occur 8 to 20 times per day. Vomiting often resolves in 1 to 3 days, while diarrhea can persist for 5 to 8 days.[17,60] Some children can have fever without gastrointestinal tract symptoms at the first medical visit, presumably early in the illness.[60] Complications and fatalities are related almost exclusively to the adverse effects of dehydration, electrolyte imbalance, and acidosis. Symptoms and asymptomatic viral shedding can be prolonged in immunocompromised patients, such as those with primary immunodeficiencies and those who have undergone bone marrow or solid-organ transplantation.[61–64] Rotavirus infection does not appear to cause more severe disease in children infected with human immunodeficiency virus (HIV).[65] An important feature of rotavirus is that it is associated with more severe gastroenteritis than other enteric pathogens and is more likely to result in dehydration.[57]

Rare cases of meningoencephalitis possibly due to rotavirus have been reported.[66] Other extraintestinal rotavirus manifestations have been described including acute myositis, hepatitis, hemophagocytic lymphohistiocytosis, and polio-like paralysis, but their relationship to rotavirus infection remains unclear.[67] Rotavirus antigenemia and viremia have been identified in children with rotavirus disease,[68–70] but the clinical significance of these findings is unclear. Rotavirus has been detected in some surveys of children with intussusception, although the studies usually are uncontrolled, and the results variable.[71] A large case-control study did not find an association between rotavirus infection and intussusception.[73] Rotavirus is not thought to be a principal cause of intussusception.[72,73]

LABORATORY FINDINGS AND DIAGNOSIS

Stool examination from patients infected with rotavirus reveals watery or soft stools, which rarely have gross blood and usually are guaiac-test negative. Fecal leukocytes generally are not observed.

Patients can demonstrate electrolyte abnormalities associated with accompanying dehydration.[55] Additionally, rotavirus causes a transient rise in serum hepatic enzyme levels (i.e., alanine aminotransferase levels elevated to twice normal) in about two-thirds of children hospitalized for rotavirus gastroenteritis.[74]

The diagnosis of rotavirus primarily is made by testing of fresh, whole stool samples using a variety of commercial kits that detect group A rotavirus antigen by enzyme immunoassay (EIA), immunochromatography, and latex agglutination.[75] EIA assays are the most widely used because of their high sensitivity and specificity.[75,76] Rotavirus can be detected in stool using EIA tests during the symptomatic period, and immediately prior to onset and for days following resolution of symptoms.[77,78] Virus also can be identified in stool by electron microscopy, electrophoresis and silver staining, and RT-PCR assay for detection of viral genomic RNA. RT-PCR is more sensitive than antigen detection for rotavirus infection, but remains primarily a research tool.

TREATMENT

No specific therapies exist for rotavirus infection. Care requires assessment of hydration status, appropriate correction of fluid loss and electrolyte disturbances, and maintenance of adequate hydration and nutrition. Oral rehydration using appropriate solutions is sufficient for most patients. Intravenous rehydration is required for some patients. Continuation or early reintroduction of oral feeding according to management guidelines should be a priority.[79] Breastfed infants should continue to nurse on demand. Infants fed with formula should continue their usual formula immediately upon rehydration. Children receiving semisolid or solid foods should continue to receive their usual diet during episodes of diarrhea, although it may be useful to avoid substantial amounts of foods high in simple sugars (e.g., carbonated soft drinks, juice, gelatin desserts) because the osmotic content might worsen diarrhea. Human or bovine colostrums and human serum immunoglobulin contain antibodies to rotavirus and may be beneficial in decreasing or preventing rotavirus diarrhea, but are not used in routine practice.[63,80–82]

PREVENTION

Rotavirus Vaccines

Live, orally administered rotavirus vaccines are the current best strategy for prevention of rotavirus morbidity and mortality. All rotavirus vaccines are attenuated strains given in multiple doses, and are designed to replace a child's first exposure to wild-type rotavirus with exposure to strains that will not cause disease but will generate a protective immune response.[83] Even so, distinct approaches to rotavirus immunization have been taken with respect to strain type (including the use of attenuated, human strains, nonhuman strains, and human–animal reassortants), the number of strains in a vaccine (monovalent versus polyvalent), and the number of doses.[83,84] Two rotavirus vaccines are used in immunization programs globally: RotaTeq (RV5) (Merck and Company, Whitehouse Station, New Jersey) and Rotarix (RV1) (GlaxoSmithKline Biologicals, Rixensart, Belgium). Both are licensed for use in the U.S.

RV5 is a live, pentavalent human-bovine reassortant vaccine that contains 5 separate reassortant viruses, 4 expressing a unique human G-type protein (G1–G4) and 1 expressing a human P-type protein (P[8]).[85] The vaccine is given to infants in the U.S. in three orally administered doses, at ages 2, 4, and 6 months.[86] Prior to licensure, a large efficacy trial performed predominantly in the U.S. and Finland demonstrated a vaccine efficacy of 74% against G1–G4 rotavirus gastroenteritis of any severity through the first full rotavirus season following vaccination. Efficacy was 98% against severe G1–G4 rotavirus gastroenteritis.[85] Vaccine trials performed in Africa and Asia where disease burden is higher demonstrated lower efficacy; vaccine efficacy against severe rotavirus gastroenteritis was 64% in a trial conducted in Ghana, Kenya, and Mali and 51% in a trial conducted in Bangladesh and Vietnam.[87,88] This lower efficacy

is consistent with the performance of oral vaccines in developing country settings.[89] In these settings, the immune response to oral vaccines may be reduced because of higher levels of transplacental maternal antibody, interference by immune and nonimmune components of human milk, micronutrient malnutrition (e.g., vitamin A and zinc), interfering gut flora, and the disease state of the infant (e.g., HIV infection or concomitant diarrhea).[89,90] (See Chapter 6, Active Immunization, for recommendations.)

RV1 is a live, monovalent vaccine that contains an attenuated, human P[8]G1 strain. The vaccine is given to infants in the U.S. in two orally administered doses, at 2 and 4 months of age.[86] RV1 vaccine trials performed in Latin America and Europe demonstrated a vaccine efficacy of 85% and 96% against severe rotavirus gastroenteritis through the first year of life following completion of a 2-dose series, respectively, and efficacy in Europe against rotavirus disease of any severity of 87%.[91,92] In both Latin America and Europe, efficacy against non-G1 strains was observed. Clinical trials conducted in Africa demonstrated lower vaccine efficacy against severe rotavirus gastroenteritis, ranging from 49% in Malawi to 77% in South Africa.[93] Despite lower vaccine efficacy, the number of rotavirus cases prevented per 100 infants vaccinated was substantial – 7 cases per 100 vaccinated in Malawi and 4 cases per 100 vaccinated in South Africa.[93] (See Chapter 6, Active Immunization, for recommendations.)

Vaccine Impact

Many countries have documented substantial declines in the burden of rotavirus disease shortly after rotavirus vaccine introduction.

In the U.S., RV5 was licensed in February 2006, and RV1 was licensed in April 2008. Data from a national laboratory surveillance network have demonstrated delayed, shorter rotavirus seasons and a sustained reduction in the number of rotavirus antigen-positive tests through the 2009–2010 rotavirus season compared with pre-vaccine years (Figure 216-3).[94] Additionally, several studies have observed substantial declines in diarrhea-related and rotavirus-specific healthcare visits (i.e., hospitalizations, emergency department and outpatient visits) among children under 5 years of age following rotavirus vaccine introduction.[95–98] An estimated 40,000 to 60,000 fewer gastroenteritis-related hospitalizations occurred in the 2008 season compared with pre-vaccine seasons among children under 5 years of age.[97] Declines in disease also were noted among those children under 5 years of age who were age-ineligible to receive vaccine, suggesting possible indirect benefits of vaccination.

In Latin America, where rotavirus vaccines have been integrated into the national immunization programs of many countries since 2006–2007, reductions in both mortality and morbidity have been observed. In Mexico, diarrhea-related mortality rates decreased by 41% among infants 0 to 11 months of age in 2008 compared with pre-vaccine years, at a time when RV1 coverage was greater than 70% for this age group.[99] Additionally, the number of diarrhea-related hospitalizations among infants in this age group decreased by 52% by 2009.[100] In Brazil, a 48% reduction in the number of diarrhea-related hospitalizations occurred among infants under 1 year of age in 2007 following introduction of RV1;[101] and in El Salvador, a sustained decrease of >65% in the rate of rotavirus hospitalizations among children under 5 years of age was observed in 2008 and 2009, following introduction of RV1.[102]

In Australia, where both RV5 and RV1 were introduced in 2006, a 43%–45% decrease in the proportion of rotavirus tests with a positive result among children under 2 years of age residing in Queensland in 2007 and 2008 and a 53% to 68% decline in the number of rotavirus hospitalizations among children from Victoria in 2007 to 2009 have been observed following vaccine introduction.[103,104]

Vaccine Safety

Neither RV1 nor RV5 was found to be associated with intussusception in prelicensure trials.[85,91] Concerns that these vaccines might

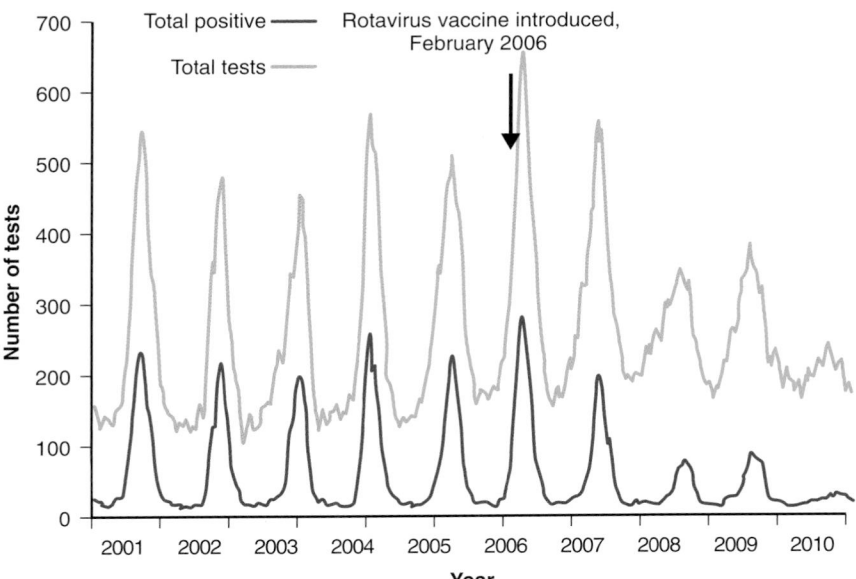

Figure 216-3. Number of total rotavirus EIA tests performed and number of positive rotavirus EIA tests from 25 continuously reporting laboratories in the U.S. National Respiratory and Enteric Viruses Surveillance System (NREVSS), by week of year, June 2000–July 2010, 3-week moving average. (Adapted from Tate JE, Mutuc JD, Payne DC, et al. Sustained decline in rotavirus detections in the United States following introduction of rotavirus vaccine in 2006. Pediatr Infect Dis J, 2011;30:S30–S34.)

be associated with an increased risk for intussusception following vaccination are based on the demonstrated association between a previous quadrivalent, human-rhesus reassortant rotavirus vaccine (Rotashield, Wyeth Laboratories) and intussusception.[105,106] This vaccine was estimated to cause one excess case of intussusception per 10,000 infants vaccinated[73] and was withdrawn from use in 1999, less than a year after being licensed and introduced in the U.S.[107] Post-marketing surveillance for intussusception associated with the current rotavirus vaccines is ongoing in many countries, and data from Mexico and Australia suggest a low level risk of intussusception, primarily in the first week after the first vaccine dose.[108,109] The estimated risk is substantially lower than that observed with Rotashield. On September 22, 2010, the U.S. Food and Drug Administration approved a label change for RV1 to advise practitioners of new data regarding intussusception from an evaluation in Mexico by GSK.[110]

While a risk has not been documented with RV1 or RV5 in the U.S.,[111] available U.S. data are not able to exclude a risk of the magnitude seen in other settings. Considering currently available data that suggest only a small possible risk of intussusception caused by rotavirus vaccine and considering that the benefits of rotavirus vaccination are great, the Centers for Disease Control and Prevention continues to recommend both RV1 and RV5 to prevent severe rotavirus disease in U.S. infants and children.[110]

Future Vaccines

Additional rotavirus vaccines are in various stages of development.[84] While most vaccines in clinical development are live, orally administered vaccines, parenterally administered vaccines also are being investigated.[83]

Other Preventive Measures

Nonvaccine approaches to prevention include breastfeeding and hand hygiene. Breastfeeding may protect young infants against rotavirus infection through anti-rotavirus antibodies and other nonimmunologic factors in human milk.[112] Appropriate hand hygiene practices should be encouraged, particularly in institutional settings such as childcare centers and hospitals.

Acknowledgment

This chapter was updated from the previous version written by Joseph Bresee.

---

217 Togaviridae: Alphaviruses

Edward B. Hayes and J. Erin Staples

Alphaviruses are arthropod-borne members of the family Togaviridae. They are small, enveloped viruses containing a single strand of positive-sense RNA that comprise serologically differentiated complexes.[1,2] Members of the western equine encephalitis virus (WEEV), eastern equine encephalitis virus (EEEV), and Venezuelan equine encephalitis virus (VEEV) complexes cause encephalitis in horses and humans, whereas members of the Semliki Forest virus (SFV) complex, such as chikungunya (CHIKV), o'nyong nyong (ONNV), and Ross River virus (RRV), cause epidemic fever, arthralgia, arthritis, and rarely neurologic disease.[3]

VIRUSES

Chikungunya Virus

CHIKV is transmitted from one human to another primarily by infected *Aedes aegypti* and *Ae. albopictus* mosquitoes in tropical areas of Africa and Asia. Enzootic transmission cycles between forest-dwelling mosquitoes and wild mammals occur in Africa.[4,5] From 2004 through 2007, CHIKV swept out of Kenya across islands in the Indian Ocean and into India causing epidemics of chikungunya and acquiring an adaptive mutation which enhanced transmission by *Ae. albopictus* mosquitoes.[4,6] Previously unrecognized clinical manifestations and transmission dynamics were described following the large epidemics on Reunion Island and in Asia. In 2007, an infected traveler brought the virus from India to northeastern Italy, sparking an outbreak transmitted by local infestations of *Ae. albopictus* mosquitoes.[7]

After an incubation period of typically 3 to 7 days (range 2 to 12 days), chikungunya manifests with fever and severe symmetric polyarthralgia that most commonly affects ankles, knees and fingers, but can affect other joints as well.[4] Headache, arthritis, myalgias, lymphadenopathy, rash, diarrhea, vomiting, abdominal pain, photophobia, conjunctivitis, myocarditis, uveitis, and retinitis occur with varying frequency.[4,7–10] Neurologic manifestations, recognized increasingly, include encephalitis, meningitis, flaccid paralysis, and Guillain–Barré syndrome.[4,11,12] Hemorrhagic manifestations occasionally are reported.[4,11,13,14] During the recent outbreaks, vesiculobullous skin blistering was noted in infants and aphthous-like skin ulcers were reported in adults.[15,16] Chikungunya can be confused with dengue, but arthralgia and arthritis are more common with chikungunya, while thrombocytopenia and hemorrhage are more common with dengue.[4,9] In some patients with CHIKV infection joint pain can last for months or years.[17,18] There is no specific treatment for acute illness but nonsteroidal anti-inflammatory drugs (NSAIDs) may be beneficial for persisting arthritis.[17,18] While increased overall mortality and fatal cases of chikungunya have been described during recent outbreaks, fatalities among people with no underlying illness are rare.[11,19–22]

Congenital CHIKV infection was first described during the epidemic on Reunion Island in 2005 and 2006.[23] Infected neonates most commonly had pain, rash, fever, and edema, but intracerebral and gastrointestinal hemorrhage as well as severe encephalopathy with seizures also were reported.[13,14] The frequency of intrauterine transmission was low for mothers infected early in pregnancy but nearly 50% for mothers infected just prior to delivery.[13,24]

O'nyong Nyong Virus

ONNV is unusual among arboviruses in that it is transmitted between humans in Africa by infected anopheline mosquitoes, primarily *Anopheles funestus* and *An. gambiae*, which also are vectors of malaria.[25,26] After an incubation period of about 8 days, ONNV causes epidemic febrile polyarthralgia often accompanied by headache, pruritic rash, prominent lymphadenopathy (frequently in the cervical area), and conjunctivitis.[27] There is no specific treatment; virtually all patients recover completely, but many are incapacitated for up to 2 weeks during the illness.[27]

Ross River Virus

RRV is transmitted to humans in Australia and the Western Pacific Islands by a broad range of mosquito vectors, primarily *Ae. vigilax*, *Ae. camptorhyncus*, *Culex annulorostris*, and *Ae. polynesiensis*.[28–31] The virus is transmitted enzootically between mosquitoes and kangaroos, horses, and other vertebrates; human–mosquito–human transmission also occurs.[29,32] After an incubation period of 3 to 21 days, RRV causes sudden onset of arthralgia, arthritis, rash, myalgias, and fatigue; many patients do not have fever.[28,31,32] Glomerulonephritis and suspected encephalitis have been reported rarely.[28,31] Disease affects primarily those between 20 and 60 years of age; symptomatic illness is rare in children.[31,33,34] Infection generally is not life-threatening and symptoms usually resolve within 6 months.[28] Joint pain and inflammation can be treated with NSAIDs.[28,31]

Venezuelan Equine Encephalitis Virus

VEEV is transmitted in tropical areas of the western hemisphere by a variety of arthropod vectors including the mosquitoes *Psorophora confinnis*, *Ps. columbiae*, *Ae. sollicitans*, and *Ae. taeniorhynchus*, which transmit epizootic VEEV strains, and *Cx. (Melanoconion)* species, which transmit enzootic VEEV strains.[35] Enzootic VEEV strains are transmitted in sylvatic cycles between mosquitoes and rodents, whereas equines are the primary amplifying hosts for epizootic VEEV strains. The potential for human–mosquito–human transmission varies depending on local ecology.[35–38] Direct human-to-human transmission appears to be rare, but the virus has been isolated from the oropharynx of ill humans, aerosol transmission has occurred in laboratories, and VEEV has been considered a possible bioterrorism threat.[35–37,39] Following an incubation period of about 2 to 5 days, VEEV causes the abrupt onset of fever, headache, malaise, tremor, and myalgia, often accompanied by nausea and vomiting.[35,40] A high proportion of fatal cases in one epidemic had pneumonia.[41] During an outbreak in Colombia, less than 5% of all symptomatic infections were estimated to result in neurologic disease, but among hospitalized cases neurologic disease was seen most frequently in children, as was also noted in a review of 42 people infected with enzootic strains of VEEV in Panama.[37,40]

Eastern Equine Encephalitis Virus

EEEV is transmitted in enzootic cycles between mosquitoes and birds in wetland habitats of tropical and temperate areas of the western hemisphere. In eastern regions of North America, EEEV is maintained by *Culiseta melanura* mosquitoes in an avian cycle but these mosquitoes do not tend to bite mammals. Instead, the virus is sporadically transmitted to horses and humans, which are dead-end hosts, by bridging mosquito vectors such as *Coquillettidia perturbans* and *Ae. vexans*.[42,43] South American strains of EEEV have been found in *Culex* spp. (*Cx. pedroi* and *Cx. taeniopus*) and have been associated with equine but not human disease typically.[44] EEEV has also been experimentally transmitted to animals via aerosols.[45] Following a typical incubation period of about 5 to 7 days, EEEV causes the abrupt onset of fever, headache, and often abdominal symptoms, then rapid deterioration into lethargy, weakness, paralysis, seizures, and coma.[42,43,46,47] Mortality is about 30%, and survivors often have permanent neurologic damage.[43,46]

Other Alphaviruses of Medical Importance

A variety of other alphaviruses have been reported to cause either epidemic or sporadic illness in humans. WEEV is transmitted between mosquitoes and birds in rural farm and range lands in the western hemisphere.[43] In recent years WEEV disease in humans has not been documented despite continued enzootic transmission.[48,49] Aerosol transmission of WEEV in laboratories has been reported.[50] The risk of symptomatic infection, with manifestations ranging from mild febrile illness to meningitis or encephalitis, is highest in young children, particularly among infants.[42] Overall mortality is less than 5%; most adults recover completely but young infants may have lasting neurologic sequelae.[3,42,43] Sindbis virus has been reported from Europe, Africa, Asia, and Australia, causing fever, rash and arthritis.[1,51] Closely related Ockelbo, Pogosta, and Karelian fever viruses cause fever and arthralgia in Scandinavia and Russia.[1,51,52] Mayaro virus causes dengue-like febrile illness with rash and arthralgia in South America.[51,53] Barmah Forest virus disease appears to be similar to Ross River in its epidemiology and clinical manifestations, resulting in epidemic fever, arthralgia, arthritis, and rash in Australia.[51,54]

LABORATORY DIAGNOSIS

Routine clinical laboratory tests will not distinguish alphavirus infections from many other viral infections. Initial peripheral leukopenia with thrombocytopenia and eventual lymphocytosis occur.[55] Peripheral leukocytosis with a left shift is common with EEEV infection.[43] In patients with alphaviral encephalitis, cerebrospinal fluid (CSF) examination can show an initial neutrophilic and then lymphocytic pleocytosis; CSF protein is normal or elevated and CSF glucose usually is normal.[42,43,56] Hyponatremia can develop in some cases due to inappropriate secretion of antidiuretic hormone.[43] A variety of abnormalities on brain imaging have been reported.[12,14,46,57]

A specific diagnosis can be determined by finding virus, viral antigen, or viral RNA in serum, CSF, or tissues; however, most cases are diagnosed by detecting virus-specific immunoglobulin M (IgM) antibody in CSF or serum using enzyme immunoassays (EIA).[42,43] The IgM EIA distinguishes between alphaviruses of different serogroups but can be cross-reactive for viruses of the same serogroup.[58] A fourfold rise in specific neutralizing antibody titers between two serum samples obtained several weeks apart can confirm the infecting virus. CHIKV and ONNV can be isolated from serum obtained early after illness onset, or can be detected in serum by reverse transcriptase-polymerase chain reaction (RT-PCR).[4,59] Isolation of the encephalitis viruses from CSF is variably successful; tests for viral RNA in CSF are more sensitive.[60] Diagnostic assays are available through many state health departments and the U.S. Centers for Disease Control and Prevention (tel. 970-221-6400), http://www.cdc.gov/ncidod/dvbid/index.htm.

PREVENTION

Alphavirus infection can be prevented by avoiding exposure to mosquitoes that transmit these viruses. Personal protective strategies include wearing repellent, staying in screened or air-conditioned dwellings, and avoiding outdoor activities during times when the vectors are most avidly seeking blood meals. Vaccines against VEEV, EEEV, WEEV, and CHIKV have been used to protect laboratory workers and others with occupational exposure to these viruses, but are not available for public use.

Acknowledgment

The authors gratefully acknowledge the contributions of Dr. Ted Tsai to previous editions of this chapter. The findings and conclusions in this chapter are those of the author(s) and do not necessarily represent the views of the Centers for Disease Control and Prevention.

218 Flaviviruses

Edward B. Hayes and Marc Fischer

The flaviviruses are single-stranded, enveloped RNA viruses that are transmitted to humans primarily through the bites of arthropods.[1] While over 40 arthropod-borne flaviviruses have been described, this chapter will discuss those that are most important in causing human illness: yellow fever virus (YFV), dengue viruses, Japanese encephalitis virus (JEV), West Nile virus (WNV), and tickborne encephalitis virus (TBEV). Yellow fever and dengue viruses tend to cause systemic febrile syndromes and severe hemorrhagic fever. The encephalitic flaviviruses are neurotropic and cause encephalitis and focal neurologic manifestations in addition to nonspecific febrile illness. Other flaviviruses not discussed in this chapter can cause sporadic or epidemic human illness and elicit cross-reactive antibody.

SPECIFIC AGENTS

Yellow Fever Virus

YFV, the prototype flavivirus, is transmitted to humans primarily by infected *Aedes* and *Haemogogus* mosquitoes in tropical areas of Africa and South America. Sporadic human infections occur following exposure to the enzootic mosquito vectors (*Haemogogus* species in South America and *Aedes africanus*, *Ae. furcifer*, *Ae. vittatus*, *Ae. luteocephalus*, and *Ae. simpsoni* in Africa).[2] These mosquitoes acquire YFV from infected monkeys and transmit the virus to humans who enter or live in the forest or savannah. Large urban outbreaks occur when viremic humans infect peridomestic *Ae. aegypti* mosquitoes, which can then transmit the virus to other humans after an "extrinsic" incubation period in the mosquito of about 8 days. Direct person-to-person transmission of YFV has not been reported. However, the live-attenuated vaccine strain of the virus can be transmitted transplacentally, through breastfeeding, and through blood transfusion.[3-5]

Most YFV infections are asymptomatic. In symptomatic infection, following an incubation period in humans of 3 to 6 days, yellow fever begins with the acute onset of headache, fever, chills, and myalgia, often accompanied by photophobia, back pain, anorexia, vomiting, and restlessness.[2] During this phase patients are viremic. Viremia usually clears about 4 days after illness onset, as fever and other symptoms subside ("period of remission"). Most patients remain anicteric and then fully recover. About 15% of all infected people develop moderate or severe yellow fever with jaundice. These patients enter a "period of intoxication," characterized by return or persistence of fever, development of jaundice, nausea, vomiting, epigastric tenderness, oliguria, and hemorrhage.[2] Some patients develop myocardial dysfunction. Viral invasion of the central nervous system is rare, but neurologic manifestations can include delirium, convulsions, and coma. The case-fatality rate of severe disease ranges from 20% to 50%. Laboratory abnormalities include elevated aspartate and alanine aminotransferases, proteinuria, thrombocytopenia, leukopenia, and prolonged blood coagulation.

Patients with severe disease require intensive supportive care with careful attention to optimizing fluid and metabolic balance.[2] Secondary bacterial infections should be treated with appropriate antibiotics. Antibiotics may be indicated for patients with persistent neutropenia.[6] Commercially available preparations of immunoglobulin in the United States may contain measurable neutralizing antibody against YFV due to prior vaccination among donors. Passive immunization has a protective effect against yellow fever when given to monkeys during the incubation period; however, it is not known whether administration of immunoglobulin to humans with yellow fever would be of any benefit.[2,7] Interferon protects monkeys from YFV infection, if they are treated before or shortly after inoculation ; it is not protective if given 24 hours after experimental infection.[2,8] In the event of a known YFV exposure such as a laboratory accident in an unimmunized person, prophylactic immunoglobulin or interferon could be considered.[2]

An effective live-attenuated vaccine against yellow fever has been available since 1937, and is recommended for persons who reside in or travel to endemic areas beginning at 9 months of age.[9] The vaccine is contraindicated in infants less than 6 months of age, and should only be given to infants aged 6 through 8 months of age when the risk of yellow fever outweighs the risk of adverse events in this age group.[9] In children 9 months of age and older, serious adverse events are rare but have been described, including cases of neurotropic and viscerotropic disease. The vaccine virus can be transmitted across the placenta and through breastfeeding.[9] While limited data suggest that vaccination during pregnancy does not increase the risk of congenital malformations or other adverse pregnancy outcomes, at least one infant developed encephalitis after acquiring yellow fever vaccine virus through breastfeeding.[4,9] Thus, yellow fever vaccine should not be given to pregnant or breastfeeding women unless they have a clear risk of acquiring yellow fever.[9]

Dengue Viruses

There are four serotypes of dengue viruses, designated as DENV-1, DENV-2, DENV-3, and DENV-4; all are transmitted from human to human through the bite of certain species of *Aedes* mosquitoes, primarily *Ae. aegypti* and *Ae. albopictus*.[10] Each serotype of dengue virus produces long-term immunity only to that specific serotype. Dengue occurs in tropical areas on all continents.[11] Major outbreaks of dengue have occurred in many countries of Latin America and the Caribbean from the 1980s through the present. In recent years, indigenous transmission of dengue in the U.S. has recurred in Texas, Hawaii, and Florida.[12–14]

The incubation period of dengue is usually from 4 to 10 days.[11] Most infections with dengue viruses are asymptomatic or cause a relatively mild systemic illness. Previously, three somewhat overlapping syndromes of dengue were described: classic dengue fever, dengue hemorrhagic fever, and dengue shock syndrome. However, recent World Health Organization (WHO) guidelines have simplified the clinical classification of dengue into two categories: nonsevere dengue and severe dengue.[11] Nonsevere dengue can be incapacitating acutely but is self-limited and usually resolves without sequelae. Severe dengue, which is reported in less than 1% of all cases, is manifest by one or more of the following: increased vascular permeability with plasma leakage and extravascular fluid accumulation, severe hemorrhage, or severe organ dysfunction. If not appropriately treated, severe dengue has a high case-fatality rate.[11,15] Severe dengue can occur following a primary dengue virus infection, but more commonly occurs following a secondary infection.[11] Rarer manifestations of DENV infection include hepatitis, myocarditis, and neurologic symptoms.[11]

Current WHO guidelines divide the clinical course of dengue into three phases: acute, critical, and recovery.[11] The acute phase typically begins with abrupt onset of fever and headache (often retro-orbital) that frequently is accompanied by body pain, joint pain, and a maculopapular rash.[11,16] Other manifestations that occur with varying frequency include anorexia, vomiting, conjunctival injection, leukopenia, and thrombocytopenia.[11,16] Many patients with dengue have a positive tourniquet test (appearance of greater than 20 petechiae in a 2.5-cm square patch of skin following inflation of a blood pressure cuff), and some patients have mild hemorrhagic manifestations such as epistaxis or gum bleeding. Differentiating acute-phase dengue from other acute febrile illnesses is difficult, and the discriminating manifestations may vary with age. In a report from one endemic area, the presence of retro-orbital pain was predictive of laboratory confirmation of dengue in patients of all ages, while rash was predictive of dengue only in patients older than 9 years of age.[16] Leukopenia was predictive of dengue in patients older than 20 years, while thrombocytopenia was predictive for those younger than 10 years.

The critical phase of dengue begins from 2 to 7 days after the onset of illness, often corresponding with defervescence. At this point, most patients improve and their illness resolves, sometimes after a recurrence of fever. Some patients develop increased capillary permeability associated with progressive leukopenia, thrombocytopenia and a rising hematocrit, harbingers of severe dengue.[11] The clinical warning signs for development of severe dengue include abdominal pain, persistent vomiting, extravascular fluid accumulation, severe mucosal bleeding, lethargy, restlessness, hepatomegaly, and increasing hematocrit with decreasing platelet count.[11] A chest radiograph or abdominal ultrasound may reveal pleural effusion or ascites. Plasma leakage can progress to shock, often associated with narrowed pulse pressure and disseminated intravascular coagulation.[11] In rare cases severe hemorrhage or critical organ dysfunction occurs without evidence of plasma leakage or shock.[11] Detailed WHO guidelines for treatment and

management of severe dengue with carefully monitored intravenous fluid administration are available at http://www.who.int/csr/disease/dengue/en/. The high fatality rate of severe dengue is reduced to <1% with early detection and appropriate fluid management.[11,17]

With good management the critical phase of dengue usually resolves within 48 hours and patients enter the recovery phase, characterized by reabsorption of extravascular fluid over the ensuing 2 to 3 days.[11] Some patients develop a confluent erythematous rash with "isles of white," pruritus, bradycardia, or electrocardiographic abnormalities during this phase.[11] Pulmonary edema or congestive heart failure can occur, particularly with excessive fluid administration.[11]

Patients with nonsevere dengue who do not have warning signs or other indications for hospitalization can be managed as outpatients with rest, vigilant monitoring of clinical parameters, attention to hydration, and pain management with acetaminophen (paracetamol).[11] Aspirin and ibuprofen should be avoided.[11] WHO provides more detailed guidelines for management of nonsevere dengue as well as criteria for hospitalization (http://www.who.int/csr/disease/dengue/en/).[11]

Congenital DENV infection has been described but accurate estimates of the risk of materno-fetal transmission are not available.[18] Some studies have suggested that maternal dengue infection during pregnancy might increase the risk of preterm birth and low birthweight.[18] Neonates with congenital dengue have had clinical manifestations ranging from fever with thrombocytopenia to pleural effusions, severe hemorrhage, and shock.[18]

Several dengue vaccines are under development and some are entering phase III trials, but none is available commercially at this writing.[19]

Japanese Encephalitis Virus

JEV is the leading vaccine-preventable cause of encephalitis in Asia. Japanese encephalitis (JE) occurs throughout most of Asia and parts of the western Pacific.[20,21] JEV is maintained in an enzootic cycle between mosquitoes and amplifying vertebrate hosts, primarily pigs and wading birds.[22,23] The virus is transmitted to humans through the bites of infected mosquitoes. Humans usually do not develop a level or duration of viremia sufficient to infect mosquitoes and, therefore, are dead-end hosts.[24] Direct person-to-person spread of JEV does not occur except rarely through intrauterine transmission.[25,26] *Culex* mosquitoes, especially *Cx. tritaeniorhynchus*, are the principal JEV vectors.[22,27] The risk of JE is increased in rural areas with irrigated fields and where pigs are raised close to human dwellings.[28] In temperate areas of Asia, transmission is seasonal and human disease usually peaks in summer and fall.[22,23,29] In the subtropics and tropics, seasonal transmission varies with monsoon rains and irrigation practices, and may be extended or even occur year-round. Most JE cases occur among children, but in areas of recent viral introduction or where population immunity has waned, adults also develop the disease.[22,23,29]

The majority of human JEV infections are asymptomatic; <1% of infected people develop clinical disease.[23,29] Acute encephalitis is the most commonly identified clinical syndrome; aseptic meningitis or undifferentiated febrile illness also can occur but have been reported more commonly among adults.[23,30,31] Among patients who develop clinical symptoms, illness usually begins with acute onset of fever, headache, and vomiting, following an incubation period of 5–15 days. Mental status changes, seizures, focal neurologic deficits, generalized weakness, parkinsonism, and other movement disorders often develop over the next few days. Acute flaccid paralysis, with clinical and pathological features similar to poliomyelitis, also has been associated with JEV infection.[32] Laboratory findings can include a moderate leukocytosis, mild anemia, and hyponatremia.[30,31] Cerebrospinal fluid (CSF) typically shows a mild to moderate pleocytosis with a lymphocytic predominance, slightly elevated protein, and normal glucose concentration. The case-fatality rate is approximately 20% to 30%.[30] Among survivors, 30% to 50% have significant neurologic, cognitive, or psychiatric sequelae.[20] There is no specific treatment.[33] Supportive care includes maintenance of adequate cerebral perfusion and management of increased intracerebral pressure, aspiration, seizures, hypoglycemia, hyponatremia, and secondary infections.

Two JE vaccines are licensed in the U.S., an inactivated mouse brain-derived vaccine (JE-Vax) and an inactivated Vero cell culture-derived vaccine (Ixiaro).[20] JE-Vax has been licensed in the U.S. since 1992 for use in travelers ≥1 year of age. In 2006, production of JE-Vax was discontinued, and remaining supplies are limited. Ixiaro was approved in March 2009 for use in persons ≥17 years of age. Thus as of January, 2011, JE-Vax is the only JE vaccine approved for use in young children in the U.S. and the limited remaining JE-Vax inventory is reserved for use in children 1 to 16 years of age. Other inactivated and live-attenuated JE vaccines are manufactured and used in Asia but are not licensed for use in the U.S.

West Nile Virus

WNV is transmitted primarily through the bite of several species of *Culex* mosquitoes.[34,35] WNV is found in most of Africa, much of Asia, Australia, Europe, North America, and in some focal areas of Latin America and the Caribbean. Following the first detection of WNV in the western hemisphere in New York City in 1999, the virus spread over the entire continental U.S., with most intense transmission occurring in the central and western plains states.[36] From 1999 through 2007, there were 1478 pediatric cases of WNV disease reported in the U.S.; 443 (30%) were West Nile neuroinvasive disease (WNND), 1009 (68%) were West Nile fever (WNF), and 26 (2%) had unknown clinical presentation.[37] For up-to-date WNV surveillance data see http://www.cdc.gov/ncidod/dvbid/westnile/index.htm.

Mosquitoes that acquire WNV from birds incidentally infect humans. In immunocompetent people, viremia usually lasts <7 days and viral concentrations in blood are too low to effectively infect mosquitoes.[34,35] However, WNV can be transmitted through transfusion of infected blood and organ transplantation.[35] Screening of blood donations for WNV began in 2003 and has substantially reduced the risk of transmission through transfusion, but rare instances of "breakthrough" transmission can occur.[38] Occupationally acquired WNV infection has raised the possibility of aerosol transmission.[39,40]

Transplacental transmission of WNV and possible transmission through breastfeeding have been described but appear to occur infrequently.[41-43] Most women known to have been infected with WNV during pregnancy have delivered infants without evidence of infection or clinical abnormalities.[43] In the most well-documented case of confirmed congenital WNV infection, the mother developed neuroinvasive WNV disease during the 27th week of gestation, and the infant was born with cystic destruction of cerebral tissue and chorioretinitis.[44] One infant who apparently acquired WNV infection through breastfeeding remained healthy.[45]

The majority of WNV infections are asymptomatic. Following an incubation period of 2 to 14 days, about 20% of infected people develop self-limited WNF. Less than 1% develop WNND.[35] The risk of WNND is highest in the elderly and in solid-organ transplant recipients; children accounted for only 4% of reported WNND in the U.S. from 1999 through 2007.[37] While encephalitis, tremor, and flaccid paralysis have all been described in children, meningitis is the most commonly reported manifestation of WNND in children and young adults.[37,46,47]

Patients with WNF typically have an abrupt onset of fever, headache, myalgia, and weakness, variably accompanied by abdominal pain, nausea, vomiting, diarrhea, and a maculopapular rash.[35,46,47] The acute phase of illness usually resolves within several days, but fatigue, malaise, and weakness can linger for weeks. Patients with WNND can present with neck stiffness and headache, mental status changes, movement disorders such as tremor or parkinsonism, seizures, or acute flaccid paralysis with or without meningitis or encephalitis.[35,46,47] Routine clinical laboratory results are variably and nonspecifically abnormal. CSF reveals

neutrophilic pleocytosis early in the infection evolving over several days to lymphocytosis. Isolated limb paralysis can occur without fever or apparent viral prodrome.[48,49] Flaccid paralysis caused by WNV infection is similar clinically and pathologically to poliomyelitis caused by poliovirus, with damage of anterior horn cells. Progression can occur to respiratory muscle paralysis requiring mechanical ventilation. Guillain–Barré syndrome can follow WNV infection and can be distinguished from anterior horn cell damage by CSF findings of elevated protein with few white cells and electrophysiologic findings indicating damage to peripheral myelin. Chorioretinitis, cardiac dysrhythmias, myocarditis, rhabdomyolysis, optic neuritis, uveitis, orchitis, pancreatitis, and hepatitis have been reported.[35] Mortality following WNND in adults is over 10%; the case-fatality rate for WNND in children in the U.S. is <1%.[35,37]

Treatment of WNV disease is supportive.[50] Ribavirin, and interferon have been given to patients with WNND with inconclusive results; there are anecdotal reports of improvement of WNND following administration of high-titer anti-WNV immunoglobulin, but evidence from clinical trials is lacking.[51] Several vaccines against WNV disease are under development but none is available currently.[52,53]

Tickborne Encephalitis Virus

Tickborne encephalitis (TBE) is endemic in focal areas of Europe and northern Asia, with approximately 10,000 cases reported annually.[54,55] Over the past 30 years, the geographic range of TBEV has expanded and the number of reported TBE cases has increased. TBEV infections are usually acquired in forested areas during outdoor occupational or recreational activities. Most cases occur from April through November, with peaks in early and late summer. The incidence and severity of disease are highest in persons >50 years of age.

There are three subtypes of TBEV: European, Siberian, and Far Eastern.[54] Each is transmitted to humans through the bite of an infected *Ixodes* tick, primarily *I. ricinus* (European subtype) or *I. persulcatus* (Siberian and Far Eastern subtypes). TBEV transmission can also occur through ingestion of unpasteurized dairy products, slaughtering viremic animals, and laboratory exposure.[54] Direct person-to-person spread of TBEV does not occur except rarely through blood transfusion or breastfeeding.[54]

Approximately two-thirds of TBEV infections are asymptomatic.[56,57] In people who develop clinical illness, the median incubation time is about 8 days but ranges from 2 days to several weeks.[54,58,59] Typically, patients infected with the European subtype have a biphasic illness. The first (viremic) phase consists of a nonspecific febrile illness, often followed by a remission of symptoms. Approximately one-third of these patients then develop the second, more severe (neuroinvasive) phase of illness, resulting in meningitis (approximately 50%), encephalitis (approximately 40%), or myelitis (approximately 10%). Laboratory abnormalities include leukopenia and thrombocytopenia in the first stage followed by leukocytosis in the second stage, and pleocytosis that can be polymorphonuclear progressing to monocytic, with elevated CSF protein.[54] The case-fatality rate associated with the European and Siberian subtypes is approximately 1% to 3%. The Far Eastern subtype typically causes a more severe monophasic illness with a case-fatality rate of approximately 20% and neurologic sequelae in up to 80% of survivors. Most children with TBE recover without sequelae, although some residual neurologic and cognitive deficits have been reported and there is a need for better data regarding long-term outcomes.[54]

There is no specific antiviral treatment; therapy consists of supportive care and management of complications.[54] No TBE vaccines are licensed in the U.S.[60] Two safe, effective inactivated TBE vaccines are available in Europe, in adult and pediatric formulations: FSME-IMMUN (Baxter, Austria) and Encepur (Novartis, Germany).[61] The adult formulation of FSME-IMMUN is also licensed in Canada.[62] Although no formal efficacy trials of these vaccines have been conducted, indirect evidence suggests that their efficacy is above 95%. For both vaccines, the primary vaccination series consists of three doses administered over 6 to 15 months. However, an accelerated schedule with three doses administered on days 0, 7, and 21 has been shown to result in similar seroconversion rates.[60]

Other Flaviviruses of Medical Importance

Many other flaviviruses can cause sporadic or epidemic illness in humans and may cross-react in serologic tests for the viruses discussed above.[1] St. Louis encephalitis virus and Murray Valley encephalitis virus are mosquito-borne viruses in the same antigenic complex with JEV and WNV. Kyasanur Forest disease virus, louping ill virus, Omsk hemorrhagic fever virus, and Powassan virus (which causes encephalitis in the U.S., Canada, and Russia) are tickborne and genetically related to TBEV. Other flaviviruses reported to cause human illness are Apoi, Bagaza, Banzi, Bussuquara, Dakar bat, Ilheus, Koutango, Kunjin (a subtype of WNV), Langat, Modoc, Ntaya, Rocio, Sepik, Spondweni, Usutu, Wesselsbron, and Zika viruses.[1]

DIAGNOSIS

Flavivirus infections are confirmed most frequently by measurement of virus-specific antibody in serum or CSF. Acute-phase serum specimens should be tested for virus-specific immunoglobulin (Ig) M antibody using an enzyme immunoassay (EIA) or microsphere immunoassay (MIA). With clinical and epidemiologic correlation, a positive IgM test has good diagnostic predictive value, but cross-reaction with related arboviruses from the same family can occur. For most flavivirus infections, IgM is detectable 3 to 8 days after onset of illness and persists for 30 to 90 days, but longer persistence has been documented. Therefore, a positive IgM test result occasionally can reflect a past infection. Serum collected within 10 days of illness onset may not have detectable IgM, and the test should be repeated on a convalescent sample. IgG antibody generally is detectable shortly after IgM and persists for years. Plaque-reduction neutralization tests (PRNTs) can be performed to measure virus-specific neutralizing antibodies. A 4-fold or greater rise in virus-specific neutralizing antibodies between acute- and convalescent-phase serum specimens collected 2 to 3 weeks apart may be used to confirm recent infection or discriminate between cross-reacting antibodies in primary flavivirus infections. In patients who have been immunized or infected with another arbovirus from the same virus family in the past (i.e., who have secondary flavivirus infections), cross-reactive antibodies in both the EIA and neutralization assays may make it difficult to identify which flavivirus is causing the patient's illness.

Viral culture and nucleic acid amplification (NAA) tests for RNA can be performed on acute-phase serum, CSF, or tissue specimens. YFV and dengue viruses are more likely to be detected using culture or NAA tests than are the neurotropic flaviviruses. Immunohistochemical staining (IHC) can detect specific viral antigen in fixed tissue.

Antibody testing for common flavivirus diseases is performed in most state public health and many commercial laboratories. Confirmatory PRNT, viral culture, NAA testing, IHC, and testing for less common flaviviruses are performed only at the Centers for Disease Control and Prevention (CDC) and selected other reference laboratories.

PREVENTION

Flaviviral infection can be prevented by avoiding exposure to the arthropods that transmit these viruses. Personal protective strategies including wearing repellent, staying in screened or air-conditioned dwellings, and avoiding outdoor activities during times when the vectors are most avidly seeking blood meals. The times of peak feeding vary between vectors; for example, *Ae. aegypti*, the principal vector of urban yellow fever and dengue, feeds primarily at dawn and dusk but not usually at night. The *Culex* vectors of WNV disease and JE typically feed from dusk to dawn. Thus, sleeping under insecticide-impregnated bednets may help reduce the risk of JE but not the risk of dengue.[20,63] Wearing light-colored clothing and checking one's body for ticks and removing them promptly may decrease the risk of TBEV infection. Programs to decrease abundance of vector mosquitoes are important to reduce risk of yellow fever, dengue, WNV disease, and JE, but may be difficult to implement and maintain. Effective vaccines are available for prevention of yellow fever, JE, and TBE; vaccines against dengue and WNV disease are under development.

219 Bunyaviruses

Adam MacNeil and Pierre E. Rollin

DESCRIPTION OF PATHOGEN

The family Bunyaviridae contains five genera of viruses, including four which have important human pathogens: *Hantavirus, Nairovirus, Phlebovirus,* and *Orthobunyavirus*.[1] A wide range of clinical syndromes in humans exist among the pathogenic bunyaviruses, with severity of human infections ranging from mild febrile illnesses to illnesses with high case fatalities. Important clinical diseases include hantavirus pulmonary syndrome (HPS; *Hantavirus* genus), hemorrhagic fever with renal syndrome (HFRS; *Hantavirus* genus), Crimean-Congo hemorrhagic fever (CCHF; *Nairovirus* genus), Rift Valley fever (RVF; *Phlebovirus* genus), and encephalitis caused by California serogroup viruses (*Orthobunyavirus* genus). Owing to pathogenic potential and human-to-human transmission, CCHF virus is considered a biosafety level 4 agent (BSL-4) and hantaviruses and RVF virus are biosafety level 3 agents.[2]

The biology, including reservoirs and transmission modalities is diverse. Humans are incidental hosts for all pathogenic bunyaviruses and all have a zoonotic component. In addition, viruses of the *Nairovirus, Phlebovirus,* and *Orthobunyavirus* genus involve an arthropod vector as part of the long-term ecologic maintenance of the virus, with vector-borne transmission commonly involved in human infection. In contrast, hantaviruses are directly maintained in rodent reservoirs without a vector-borne component to the transmission cycle.

EPIDEMIOLOGY (Table 219-1)

Hantaviruses

Hantavirus pulmonary syndrome (HPS) is caused by a wide variety of New World hantaviruses. All have rodent reservoirs, and pathogenic viruses are known to exist in the United States, Canada,

TABLE 219-1. Taxonomy and Epidemiologic Characteristics of Select Bunyaviruses

Genus	Species	Geographic Location	Reservoirs	Infection Route
Hantavirus	Important HPS-associated viruses include Sin Nombre virus and Andes virus; many other species exist	Large portions of North and South America	Rodents	Inhalation of rodent excreta, rodent bite
	Important HFRS-associated viruses include Hantaan virus, Dobrava virus, Saaremaa virus, Seoul virus, Puumala virus; other species exist	Large portions of Europe and Asia	Rodents	Inhalation of rodent excreta, rodent bite
Phlebovirus	Rift Valley fever virus	Central and South Africa, Egypt, Saudi Arabia, Yemen	Mosquitoes, ruminants serve as amplifying hosts	Blood or tissue of infected animals, mosquito bite
Nairovirus	Crimean-Congo hemorrhagic fever virus	Africa, eastern Europe, Middle East, central Asia	Maintained between ticks and small mammals, farm animals can be infected	Tick bite, blood or tissue of infected animals; nosocomial and person-to-person transmission
Orthobunyavirus	La Crosse virus	Eastern United States	Mosquitoes, rodents are amplifying hosts	Mosquito

HPS, hantavirus pulmonary syndrome; HFRS, hemorrhagic fever with renal syndrome.

Panama, and across a large portion of South America.[3] Within the U.S., most cases are due to Sin Nombre virus infection and occur in the western portion of the country.[4,5] A number of species of hantavirus are associated with HPS across South America.[6,7] The route of infection is typically through inhalation of rodent urine or feces or by bite from an infected rodent. Infections are often associated with cleaning or other activities that result in the aerosolization of infectious material from buildings or structures with rodent contamination.[8-10]

Multiple species of Old World hantavirus cause hemorrhagic fever with renal syndrome (HFRS). Pathogenic Old World hantaviruses are found across Europe and Asia, with Hantaan and Seoul viruses associated primarily with China, Korea, and far east Russia, and Dobrava and Puumala viruses found in western Russia and Europe. Puumala virus infections are also a common occurrence in Scandinavia.[11-15] In addition, cases of HFRS due to Seoul virus have been documented in North America (Woods et al.,[16] and CDC unpublished observations) and serologic evidence suggests the presence of the virus in rodent populations in a number of cities in North and South America.[17] As with HPS, hantavirus infections resulting in HFRS occur through inhalation of rodent excreta or by rodent bite.

Rift Valley Fever (RVF)

RVF is known for explosive outbreak potential. The causative virus is maintained though transovarian transmission in mosquitoes (most commonly *Aedes* species) and infected eggs can exist dormantly for long periods of time in dried waterbeds and flood plains, with no evidence of activity. Outbreaks typically occur following flooding periods, in which increased mosquito breeding results in large numbers of infected mosquitoes from reservoir pools. Domestic ruminants (cattle, sheep, goats) serve as amplifying hosts. RVF is a severe disease, with high death and abortion rates in many ruminants, and evidence of RVF activity in animals often precedes evidence of human infections during outbreaks.[18,19]

Human RVF infections occur through direct contact with blood or bodily fluids of infected animals, often through slaughtering or handling meat, and infections often occur in farmers, abattoir workers, and among other persons with occupational exposures to animals.[20,21] Though less common, humans also can be infected by bite from a mosquito carrying the virus. There is no evidence of person-to-person or nosocomial transmission. RVF is endemic across a large portion of Africa,[19,22] and in recent decades, outbreaks also have occurred in the Middle East (Saudi Arabia and Yemen).[23,24] Major outbreaks have recently occurred in Kenya, Tanzania, Sudan (2006–2007),[25-27] Madagascar (2008–2009),[28] and South Africa (2010).[29]

Crimean-Congo Hemorrhagic Fever (CCHF)

CCHF virus is a tickborne virus that has been documented across a large portion of central Africa, South Africa, the Middle East, central Asia, and southeastern Europe.[30-32] Although not apparent prior to 2002, numbers of cases in Turkey have rapidly increased and in recent years have accounted for more cases of CCHF than any country in the world.[33] CCHF virus is maintained through a tick–vertebrate–tick transmission cycle. The typical zoonotic hosts are believed to be small mammals, although livestock can serve as secondary hosts. Overt symptomatic disease is known to occur only in humans. Human infection occurs through transmission from the bite of ticks from the *Hyalomma* genus, or by contact with tissues, blood, or milk from infected animals.[34-36] Due to asymptomatic infection in farm animals, infection commonly occurs among farmers and abattoir workers.

California Serogroup Viruses

The California serogroup viruses include a number of viruses endemic to the U.S.; however, the majority of human disease is associated with La Crosse virus.[37] La Crosse virus is the most common severe mosquito-borne cause of encephalitis reported in the U.S.[38,39] It is maintained in *Aedes triseriatus* through transovarial transmission and small rodents serve as amplifying hosts.[40,41] The virus is endemic in the eastern half of the U.S., with highest numbers of pediatric cases in West Virginia, North Carolina, and Tennessee.[42,43] Infections peak in the summer months of July–September.[42]

CLINICAL MANIFESTATIONS (Table 219-2)

Hantavirus Pulmonary Syndrome

The incubation of HPS is from 1 to 5 weeks.[44] Cases begin with a prodromal syndrome, with symptoms including fever, myalgia, nausea, vomiting, and diarrhea, followed by the rapid onset of bilateral noncardiogenic pulmonary edema, which may radiographically resemble acute respiratory distress syndrome.[4,45-47] Myocardial depression occurs in severe cases of HPS, with death often due to shock[48] and case fatality as high as 40%. Clinically, HPS is similar in children and adults.[49,50]

Hemorrhagic Fever with Renal Syndrome

HFRS typically progresses through five clinical stages: febrile, hypotensive, oliguric, polyuric, and convalescent.[51] Severe manifestations of HFRS include renal insufficiency, shock, and

TABLE 219-2. Clinical Characteristics of Bunyavirus Diseases

Disease	Viruses	Common Symptoms	Treatment
Hantavirus pulmonary syndrome	Important viruses include Sin Nombre virus and Andes virus; many other species exist	Febrile prodrome followed by acute respiratory distress	Supportive; extracorporeal membrane oxygenation as possible salvage therapy
Hemorrhagic fever with renal syndrome	Hantaan virus, Dobrava virus, Saaremaa virus, Seoul virus, Puumala virus; other species exist	Febrile prodrome, possible renal failure, hemorrhage, and shock	Supportive; ribavirin if administered early in disease (patients usually seen late)
Rift Valley fever	Rift Valley fever virus	Febrile illness, possible hemorrhage, hepatitis, meningitis, retinitis	Supportive
Crimean-Congo hemorrhagic fever	Crimean-Congo hemorrhagic fever virus	Febrile prodrome, myalgia, nausea/vomiting, diarrhea, hemorrhage; high case fatality	Supportive: ribavirin if administered early in disease
La Crosse encephalitis	La Crosse virus	Commonly asymptomatic or nonspecific febrile illness; possible encephalitis or meningitis	Supportive

hemorrhage.[11,52,53] Prognosis of HFRS varies, depending on the viral species. The most severe disease is associated with Hantaan and Dobrova/Saaremaa viruses (with case-fatality rates as high as 15%). Case fatality is around 1% for Seoul virus.[11,51,52] A generally less severe form of disease, neuropathica epidemica (NE), is caused by Puumala virus, endemic to central and northern Europe. While clinical symptoms of NE may be similar to HFRS, overall case fatality is less than 0.1%.[54]

Rift Valley Fever

Most human cases of RVF result in mild febrile illness, with myalgias, nausea, and vomiting. Only a small proportion of cases result in severe disease.[20] Severe RVF may result in the acute onset of hemorrhagic symptoms, hepatitis, or encephalitis. Hepatitis or retinitis also may develop at later stages (1 to 4 weeks), following onset of illness.[20,55,56] Overall case fatality due to RVF is 1% to 2%.

Crimean-Congo Hemorrhagic Fever

CCHF has an estimated incubation period of 3 to 7 days.[57] Disease is heralded by the onset of the prehemorrhagic stage of the disease, characterized by fever, headaches, dizziness, myalgias, nausea, vomiting, abdominal pain, and diarrhea.[34,35] Of the bunyaviruses, CCHF has the highest propensity for hemorrhagic manifestations that can include petechiae, epitaxis, hematemesis, melena, gingival bleeding, hematuria, and vaginal bleeding.[30,34,58] Case-fatality rates range from 1% to over 50%.

La Crosse Encephalitis

Most infections tend to be mild or inapparent.[59-61] Severe infections are most common in children, and manifest as meningitis or encephalitis, with a clinical presentation similar to other viral causes of meningitis or encephalitis. Focal or generalized seizures occur in severe cases.[37,62,63] Clinical management is supportive. While recovery occurs without specific interventions, long-term neurologic sequelae have been reported.[64]

LABORATORY FINDINGS AND DIAGNOSIS

Bunyaviruses result in acute infections in humans, with a short period of viremia and no long-term or latent maintenance of the virus. In most instances, symptoms are directly associated with the presence of the virus, whereas for some syndromes (for instance, California serogroup viruses, and neurologic and ocular manifestations of RVF), presenting symptoms occur after the virus has largely been cleared from the organism. Serologic assays (immunofluorescent assay, electroimmunoassay (EIA), and neutralization assay) are useful particularly in the diagnosis of bunyavirus infections. For some diseases (CCHF, RVF), direct detection of the virus can be performed (PCR, antigen detection EIA, viral culture) during acute stages of disease.

TREATMENT

Hantavirus pulmonary syndrome. Ribavirin is not efficacious in the treatment of HPS and no specific antiviral therapies are available.[65,66] Some studies suggest the utility of extracardiopulmonary oxygenation (ECMO) as a salvage therapy in the management of HPS.[67,68]

Hemorrhagic fever with renal syndrome. Data suggest efficacy of ribavirin in improving the course of HFRS (due to Hantaan virus), when administered early in clinical disease.[69]

Rift Valley fever. Treatment is supportive.

Crimean-Congo hemorrhagic fever. The efficacy of ribavirin remains controversial. Some data suggest efficacy if administered as postexposure prophylaxis, as well as possible improved disease prognosis if administered early in the disease.[70]

La Cross encephalitis. Treatment is supportive.

PREVENTION

While veterinary vaccines are available for RVF, no commercially licensed human vaccines are available for any of the bunyaviruses, with the exception of hantavirus vaccines available in Korea and China.[71,72] In North America, there is no evidence of person-to-person or nosocomial transmission of hantaviruses, whereas person-to-person transmission of Andes virus in Argentina and Chile has been documented,[73-75] and thus contact precautions are advised when handling suspected cases in endemic areas. Person-to-person, particularly nosocomial, transmission of CCHF has been documented.[76,77] Transmission is most probable following contact with blood or body fluids of infected individuals; standard contact precautions are recommended for handling confirmed or suspected CCHF cases.

220 Hepatitis C Virus

Rania A. Tohme, Deborah Holtzman, and Scott D. Holmberg

In the 1970s, after development of routine diagnostic testing for hepatitis A and hepatitis B viruses, a small proportion of acute viral hepatitis could not be attributed to these or other known pathogens. The search for the major etiologic agent of "non-A, non-B hepatitis" (NANBH)[1] culminated in 1989 with discovery of hepatitis C virus (HCV).[1] Although substantially more prevalent among the adult population, HCV infection does occur among the pediatric age group and should be considered as a potential source of infection when relevant clinical or epidemiologic factors are present.

PATHOGEN

HCV is an enveloped single-stranded RNA virus, of approximately 9500 nucleotides, belonging to the Hepacivirus genus in the Flaviviridae family. There are at least six genotypes of HCV, numbered 1 through 6, the nucleic acid sequences of which differ by 30% to 40%.[2] More than 50 subtypes that differ by 20% to 25% also have been described. The most common subtypes are 1a, 1b, 2a, and 2b.[3] The prevalence of the six genotypes varies by continent and region of the world. For example, genotype 1 accounts for 75% of infections in the United States and 64% of infections in Europe; genotype 3 is prevalent primarily in Australia and the Indian subcontinent; genotype 4 in Africa and the Middle East, especially Egypt; genotype 5 in southern Africa; and genotype 6 in Southeast Asia and Australia.[3]

Data on environmental survival, disinfection, sterilization, and decontamination procedures for HCV are limited. Techniques to culture HCV have been developed,[4] are difficult to perform, and are not always reliable. The inability to culture HCV easily has limited many research efforts including development of vaccines. One study suggests that HCV in dried plasma can cause infection in experimental animals when left at room temperature for at least 16 hours but not after 4 days.[5] Use of chemical germicides that are capable of producing at least an intermediate level of disinfection activity (e.g., 0.1% glutaraldehyde or 500 ppm free chlorine from sodium hypochlorite – 2 tablespoons of household bleach in one gallon of water) or conventional sterilization processing such as steam autoclaving is thought to be suitable for inactivating HCV.[6]

PATHOGENESIS AND IMMUNITY

The primary site of hepatitis C viral replication is the hepatocyte. In the acute phase, histopathologic findings in the liver are typical of acute viral hepatitis and include ballooning degeneration, focal necrosis, and hepatocellular apoptosis.[7,8] These findings are believed to be due to the immune response to virus-infected cells rather than to a direct cytopathic effect of the virus.

The high rate of chronicity with HCV infection in adults is partly attributable to failure of the virus to elicit effective neutralizing antibody. High rates of mutation in the single-stranded RNA genome of HCV are believed to play a role in the pathogen's ability to evade the immune system. In an infected person, several closely related but genetically distinct strains of HCV, termed *quasispecies*, generally occur.[9] Typically, one dominant variant accounts for the majority of circulating virus at any given time. Over time, this variant often loses dominance and is replaced by a new dominant variant.[10,11] Presumably, evolution of quasispecies is a result of the immune response to the dominant variant, resulting in sequential selection of resistant mutants. In addition, sequential infection

with different genotypes has been observed in humans.[12,13] Mechanisms associated with persistence and clearance of HCV are not well understood and likely involve both host and viral factors. The heterogeneity of HCV prevents development of conventional vaccines, allows the virus to escape eradication by the host's immune system, and affects the completeness of the response to antiviral therapies.[14]

EPIDEMIOLOGY

Prevalence and Incidence

In the U.S., the National Health and Nutrition Examination Survey (NHANES) conducted during 1999 to 2002 found that 1.6% of the population had been infected with HCV.[15] Fewer than 5% of all HCV infections in the U.S. are among persons <20 years of age. Among persons aged 6 through 11 years and 12 through 19 years, the prevalence of anti-HCV is 0.2% and 0.4%, respectively.[16] The prevalence of HCV infection among adolescents with risk factors for HCV infection, such as injection drug use, has been shown to be higher than in the general pediatric population. In a survey of newly incarcerated adolescent detainees, 2% had evidence of HCV infection, 95% of whom reported injection drug use.[17] In a survey of homeless adolescents, of whom one-third were injection drug users (IDUs), the prevalence of HCV infection was 4.4%.[18]

The incidence of HCV infection in the U.S. reached a peak in the 1980s with approximately 250,000 infections per year, but fell rapidly during the early 1990s. In 2008, an estimated 18,000 new infections occurred.[19] If the incidence remains relatively low, the prevalence of HCV infection among women of childbearing age will continue to decline and the prevalence among children and adolescents should decline as well.

Transmission

HCV is transmitted most efficiently through direct percutaneous exposure to blood. Mucous membrane exposures to blood also can result in HCV transmission but this route is less efficient. Although HCV can be detected in saliva, semen, human milk, and other body fluids of some infected persons, these body fluids are not believed to be efficient vehicles of transmission.[20] HCV does not penetrate intact skin spontaneously and airborne transmission does not occur.[21]

In pediatric practice, perinatal infection currently accounts for most cases of HCV infection, although older children and adolescents can be at risk for HCV infection from injection drug use, sexual transmission, or from blood, blood products, and solid-organ transplants received before 1992.

Perinatal Transmission

Among HCV-infected infants and young children in developed countries, perinatal exposure is the most common source of infection. The rate of vertical transmission of HCV is estimated to be 5% with rates varying between 0% and 25%.[22-25] Most infected infants do not have a positive RNA test during the first month after birth, suggesting that infection occurs at the time of delivery rather than in utero. By 3 months of age, 90% of infected infants test positive for HCV RNA, and by 6 months of age, almost all test positive.[23,26-29] Because maternal antibody can remain detectable in uninfected infants for more than a year, anti-HCV testing is not recommended before 18 months of age.[30]

Risk Factors for Perinatal Transmission

HCV viremia. Perinatal transmission is almost always limited to women with detectable HCV RNA,[24,28,29,31–33] although a few transmissions have been reported from women without HCV RNA.[31–33] The level of viremia has been shown to be a determinant of perinatal transmission in some studies. For example, women with viral loads below 10^5 copies per mL were less likely to transmit HCV[34–36] even if they were coinfected with HIV.[37] However, other studies have failed to demonstrate this association.[23,28,38]

Maternal HIV coinfection. The risk for transmission of HCV is 2- to 7-fold higher in infants born to mothers coinfected with HCV and HIV compared with children born to mothers infected with HCV alone.[23,39–41] Higher HCV RNA levels among HIV coinfected women may explain in part the increased risk of vertical transmission. HIV infection also was shown to facilitate entry and replication of HCV in blood cells which might increase the risk of perinatal transmission.[42,43] In addition, compared with infants who do not become infected with HIV, infants of coinfected mothers who develop HIV infection have a higher risk of developing HCV infection.[37]

Prolonged rupture of membranes. Rupture of membranes ≥6 hours before delivery has been associated with higher rates of transmission in several studies.[23,26,32,44]

Obstetric procedures. Data remain limited on the role of obstetric procedures in promoting HCV transmission. Internal fetal monitoring was shown to be associated with transmission of infection.[23,45] One study linked amniocentesis to HCV transmission in infants;[46] however, another study showed that only 6% of women who underwent amniocentesis during the fourth month of pregnancy had HCV in their amniotic fluid.[47]

Sex of the infant. A few studies have indicated that the rate of perinatal transmission of HCV infection is two times higher in female compared with male newborns,[32,48] suggesting that hormonal or genetic factors may influence susceptibility or response to infection.

Factors Not Associated with Perinatal Transmission

Mode of delivery. Based on well-controlled cohort studies, the mode of delivery (vaginal versus cesarean) does not appear to affect risk of transmission.[24,28,38,44,49,50]

Breastfeeding. More than 20 prospective cohort studies have not shown any increased risk for HCV infection among breastfed infants compared with formula-fed infants despite 2 years of follow-up after delivery.[22,24,27,28,32,38,44,45,49,50–61] Only one prospective study showed potential perinatal transmission of HCV through breastfeeding. In this study, all three women who transmitted the infection to their babies developed symptomatic liver disease during the transmission period and had high HCV RNA titers in serum.[62]

Transmission through Injection Drug Use

HCV is spread efficiently through sharing of equipment used to inject drugs. Several studies have demonstrated that, in addition to sharing of needles/syringes, sharing of paraphernalia used to inject drugs (e.g., water for rinsing needles/syringes or dissolving drugs, "spoons" or "cookers" used for preparing drugs, and "cottons" used to filter the drug solution as it is drawn into the syringe) also plays an important role in transmitting HCV.[63–65] In the U.S., injection drug use accounts for about 60% of infections. Historically, approximately 80% of IDUs became infected within the first 2 years of beginning to inject, with >90% infected within 5 years.[65] The incidence of HCV infection among IDUs in the past

---

BOX 220-1. Recommendations for Hepatitis C Virus (HCV) Testing

PERSONS WHO SHOULD BE TESTED ROUTINELY FOR HCV INFECTION ON THE BASIS OF THEIR RISK FOR INFECTION

- Persons who ever injected illegal drugs, including those who injected once or only a few times many years ago
- Persons with selected medical conditions, including:
  - Persons who received clotting factor concentrates produced before 1987
  - Persons who ever received long-term hemodialysis
  - Persons with persistently abnormal serum alanine aminotransferase levels
- Prior recipients of transfusions or organ transplants, including:
  - Persons who were notified that they received blood from a donor who later tested positive for HCV infection
  - Persons who received a transfusion of blood or blood components before July, 1992
  - Persons who received an organ transplant before July, 1992

PERSONS WHO SHOULD BE TESTED ROUTINELY FOR HCV INFECTION ON THE BASIS OF A RECOGNIZED EXPOSURE

- Healthcare, emergency medical, and public safety personnel after needlesticks, sharps, or mucosal exposures to HCV-positive blood
- Children born to HCV-positive women:
  - Testing of infants for anti-HCV should be performed no sooner than 18 months of age
  - If earlier diagnosis of HCV infection is desired, reverse transcriptase-polymerase chain reaction testing for HCV RNA can be performed at 1–2 months of age and repeat at 6 months of age

PERSONS FOR WHOM ROUTINE HCV TESTING IS NOT RECOMMENDED (UNLESS THEY HAVE RISK FACTORS FOR INFECTION)

- Healthcare, emergency medical, and public safety workers
- Pregnant women
- Household (nonsexual) contacts of HCV-positive persons
- The general population

PERSONS FOR WHOM ROUTINE HCV TESTING IS OF UNCERTAIN NEED

- Settings not confirmed as risk factor or in which prevalence of infection unknown:
  - Recipients of transplanted tissue (e.g., corneal, musculoskeletal, skin, ova, sperm)
  - Users of intranasal cocaine and other noninjecting illegal drugs
  - Persons with a history of tattooing or body piercing
- Settings confirmed as risk factor but in which prevalence of infection low:
  - Persons with a history of multiple sex partners or sexually transmitted infections
  - Long-term steady sex partners of HCV-positive persons

ANY PERSON

- Anyone who wishes to know or is concerned regarding their HCV infection status should be provided the opportunity for counseling, testing, and appropriate follow-up

Adapted from Centers for Disease Control and Prevention. Recommendations for prevention and control of hepatitis C virus (HCV) infection and HCV-related chronic disease. MMWR 1998;47(RR-19):1–39.

decade may be lower, but is still in the range of 15% to 20% per year.[66] As a consequence, people who have ever injected drugs, even if only briefly, may have been infected with HCV and should be screened for evidence of infection (Box 220-1).

Sexual Transmission

Sexual contact is not an efficient mode for transmission of HCV infection.[67] Based on available data, there is no increased risk of transmission of HCV among heterosexual couples in monogamous relationships. However, the risk is almost double among people having multiple sexual partners (although this association may be confounded by increased likelihood of injection drug use with increased number of partners) or among those already having a sexually transmitted infection. In addition, the risk of HCV infection through sexual contact increases 4-fold among HIV-infected men and women.[67]

Transmission among Household Contacts

Although rare, transmission among nonsexual household contacts also can occur. The presumed mechanism of transmission is direct or inapparent percutaneous or permucosal exposure to infectious blood or body fluids containing blood.[68] In one documented episode, an HCV-infected mother transmitted HCV to her hemophiliac child during performance of home infusion therapy, presumably when she sustained an unintentional needlestick injury and subsequently used the contaminated needle in the child.[69]

Transmission in Healthcare Settings

HCV can be spread through exposures in the healthcare setting. Some body fluids, including cerebrospinal fluid, synovial fluid, pleural fluid, peritoneal fluid, and amniotic fluid, are considered potentially infectious. Feces, nasal secretions, saliva, sputum, sweat, tears, urine, and vomitus are not considered potentially infectious unless they contain blood. Transmission between patients in the healthcare setting generally is associated with inadequate infection control practices, such as reuse of needles and syringes and other failures of aseptic technique, contamination of multidose vials,[70] or inadequate cleaning of equipment.[71,72]

There are no formal screening recommendations for people who may have undergone injections or medical procedures in settings with inadequate infection control practices. Nonetheless, clinicians should be aware that infection control procedures in many parts of the world are poor and patients may have been exposed to HCV via unsafe injection practices and failure to follow appropriate aseptic techniques during provision of medical care.

Transmission from Transfusion of Blood and Blood Products

Transfusion-acquired HCV infection probably accounted for most HCV infections in children in the 1970s and 1980s, particularly among children undergoing cancer chemotherapy[73,74] or open-heart surgery.[75] A preliminary survey of cancer survivors who received blood transfusions at St. Jude Children's Research Hospital, in Memphis, Tennessee, from 1961 to March 1992 found 6.6% to be infected with HCV.[73] Prevalence was highest (10.7%) in children who received transfusions before 1986. Since 1992, when second-generation HCV enzyme immunoassay (EIA) screening was implemented, the risk of HCV infection from a single transfusion was considered to be <1 per 100,000 units.[76] Nucleic acid testing (NAT) of all donors for HCV RNA, implemented in 1999, has reduced this risk even further to 1 per ≥2 million blood units.[77]

Plasma-derived products such as clotting factor concentrates frequently were contaminated with HCV until 1987,[78] when manufacturers incorporated effective viral inactivation steps into their purification processes. Consequently, people with hemophilia who were treated with factors XIII and IX manufactured before 1987 have a high prevalence of HCV infection.[79] Since December 1994, all immunoglobulin products (intravenous and intramuscular) commercially available in the U.S. must undergo an inactivation procedure or be confirmed as not containing HCV RNA before release.

CLINICAL MANIFESTATIONS AND NATURAL HISTORY

Infants with vertically acquired HCV infection do not usually become icteric or symptomatic, and a substantial proportion have normal or only mildly elevated serum alanine aminotransferase (ALT) levels.[33,48,80] In the 20% to 30% of acutely infected older children and adults who are symptomatic, symptoms usually are mild and indistinguishable from symptoms of other acute viral hepatitides, including jaundice, nausea, anorexia, and right upper-quadrant abdominal pain.[81] Fulminant hepatitis C has been reported, including cases in an infant and a child,[82] but is rare.

The natural history of HCV infection in children differs slightly between perinatally acquired and transfusion-acquired infections (Figure 220-1). Although the long-term progression of liver disease in HCV infection acquired in infancy and childhood is

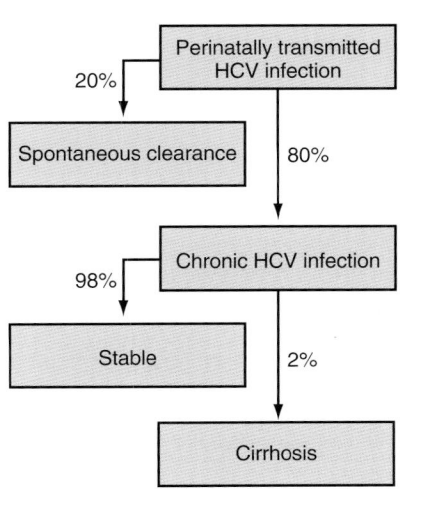

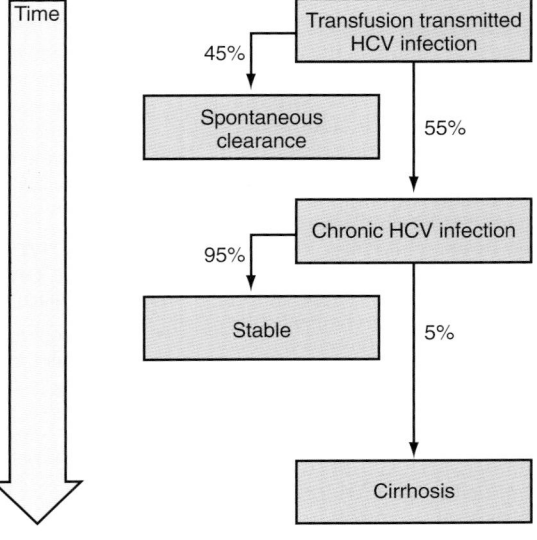

Figure 220-1. Natural history of HCV infection in children.

not yet well understood, longitudinal studies conducted to date indicate a milder progression of HCV infection in children compared with adults. Infections acquired in infancy are more likely to resolve spontaneously than infections acquired during adulthood. Around 20% of perinatally infected children clear the virus during the first two years of life and up to 55% of children with post-transfusion acquired HCV have been shown to clear the virus.[48,75,83,84] Most children with chronic infection are asymptomatic and hepatomegaly is observed in only 10%. However, fatigue, particularly in teens and young adults, is associated commonly with persistent HCV infection.

During chronic infection, about 23% of children have normal serum ALT levels while 25% have consistently high serum ALT levels.[83,85,86] Progression to fibrosis increases with age and development of advanced liver disease in children is uncommon until >20 years have elapsed since infection. Patients with anorexia, weight loss, abdominal pain, hepatomegaly, and splenomegaly are likely to have advanced liver disease. A study in a quaternary referral center showed that 7 of 91 (8%) children developed cirrhosis at a mean age of 11.7 years. Four of the 7 required transplantation, all of whom had recurrent HCV infection after transplantation and two of whom died.[87] The authors recommended treatment to clear the infection before transplantation in order to achieve better prognosis. In another study, 5 of 121 infected children had bridging fibrosis, and two had cirrhosis. Children with fibrosis were older and more likely to have higher serum ALT levels and inflammation (on biopsy), suggesting that likelihood of fibrosis increases with time.[88] In another series of 332 HCV-infected children with persistent viremia, 6 children (2%) progressed to decompensated cirrhosis with a mean duration of 9.9 ± 5.9 years between HCV exposure and diagnosis of cirrhosis.[48] Children with genotype 1 are more likely to progress to advanced disease compared with those with genotype 3. Vertically infected children develop cirrhosis earlier than transfused children with no underlying systemic disease. In a study of 67 adolescents and young adults (mean age, 19.8 years) who tested positive for anti-HCV and had received blood transfusions as infants or young children, 45% of participants cleared the infection and only 3 had histologic evidence of progressive liver damage, 2 of whom also had congestive heart failure.[75] The median time to develop end-stage liver disease among 392 patients with post-transfusion HCV infection was 33 years for those infected between the ages of 21 and 30 years and only 4% of patients infected below the age of 20 years had cirrhosis.[89]

Progression of HCV infection and development of severe liver disease is accelerated in the presence of comorbid conditions such as thalassemia, iron overload, childhood cancer, and HIV coinfection. Children who received blood transfusions for thalassemia are at risk for liver injury from hemochromatosis[90] and following HCV infection have higher risk of progression to cirrhosis.[91,92] A nationwide survey of complications of thalassemia major in North America revealed cirrhosis rates to be 4.3%, 9.7%, and 15% for people 0–15, 16–24, and 25 years of age or older, respectively.[93] In addition iron overload also may diminish the response to treatment for HCV infection.[94] Children with hemophilia have higher risk for morbidity and mortality due to HCV infection, although end-stage liver disease is uncommon before adulthood.[95] Among children with leukemia, advanced liver disease did not develop during 13 to 27 years of follow-up.[96] In a study of the natural history of HCV among children with inherited bleeding disorders, cirrhosis developed in 75% of children with HIV coinfection and death was reported in one child also coinfected with HIV.[84]

Hepatocellular carcinoma has been reported rarely among HCV-infected children. A retrospective survey of survivors of childhood cancer from a single medical center who had received blood transfusions prior to donor screening identified 2 HCV-infected patients who developed cirrhosis and died of hepatocellular carcinoma approximately 25 years after they were likely to have been infected.[97]

A number of extrahepatic conditions associated with HCV infection in adults, including cryoglobulinemia, glomerulonephritis, and porphyria cutanea tarda, are not common in children.

Data from people infected with HCV at a young age indicate that one-third or more apparently resolve their infections. Among the other two-thirds, chronic liver disease appears to progress slowly, and serious sequelae are rare during the first two decades after infection. The slower progression of HCV in childhood probably is related to the reduced frequency of comorbid factors such as alcohol consumption, hemochromatosis, and non-alcoholic fatty liver disease compared with adults.

SCREENING AND DIAGNOSIS

Screening

Healthcare professionals should ascertain the risk of HCV infection in all patients including pregnant women and adolescents. In addition, any person with persistent, unexplained elevations in serum ALT level, regardless of history of risk factors, should be tested for HCV. Furthermore, because people with HCV infection

---

BOX 220-2. Key Counseling Messages for Persons Who Test Positive for Hepatitis C Virus (HCV) Infection

TO PROTECT THE LIVER FROM FURTHER HARM, HCV-POSITIVE PERSONS SHOULD:

- Not start any new medicines, including over-the-counter and herbal medicines, without checking with their physician
- Be vaccinated against hepatitis A and B
- Avoid drinking alcohol

HCV-POSITIVE PERSONS SHOULD BE ADVISED:

- HCV is **not** spread by sneezing, hugging, coughing, food or water, sharing eating utensils or drinking glasses, or casual contact
- HCV-positive persons should **not** be excluded from work, school, play, childcare, or other settings on the basis of their HCV infection status
- To cover cuts and sores on the skin to keep from spreading infectious blood or secretions
- Not to share toothbrushes, dental appliances, razors, or other personal-care articles that might have blood on them with other people
- To discuss the risk of transmitting HCV with their sexual partners. Although risk of transmission is low, they may decide to use barrier precautions (e.g., latex condoms)

FOR HCV-POSITIVE WOMEN CONSIDERING PREGNANCY OR WHO HAVE HAD CHILDREN:

- No evidence exists that mode of delivery (vaginal versus cesarean) is related to transmission; therefore, determining the need for cesarean delivery versus vaginal delivery should not be made on the basis of maternal HCV infection status
- Data indicate that breastfeeding does not transmit HCV, although HCV-positive mothers should not breastfeed if their nipples are cracked or bleeding

HCV-POSITIVE PERSONS SHOULD BE EVALUATED FOR PRESENCE OR DEVELOPMENT OF CHRONIC LIVER DISEASE, INCLUDING:

- Assessment for biochemical evidence of chronic liver disease
- Assessment for severity of disease and possible treatment according to current practice guidelines in consultation with, or by referral to, a specialist knowledgeable in this area

Adapted from Centers for Disease Control and Prevention. Recommendations for prevention and control of hepatitis C virus (HCV) infection and HCV-related chronic disease. MMWR 1998;47(RR-19):1–39.

might be reluctant to disclose certain risk factors, any person concerned about his or her infection status should be given appropriate counseling and testing.[30]

Infants of women known to be HCV infected should be screened for HCV RNA on two occasions between the ages of 2 and 6 months and/or be tested for anti-HCV after 18 months of age. HCV testing should be offered routinely to people most likely to be infected with the virus (see Box 220-1). Routine HCV testing is not recommended for household contacts of HCV-positive persons unless a history exists of a direct (percutaneous or mucosal) exposure to blood. Identification of people at risk for HCV infection provides an opportunity for testing to determine their infection status, medical evaluation to determine their disease status if infected, and antiviral therapy if appropriate. It also provides the infected person an opportunity to obtain information about how to prevent further liver damage and prevent transmitting infection to others (Box 220-2).

The incubation period for HCV infection averages 6 to 7 weeks, with a range of 2 weeks to 6 months. The time from exposure to development of viremia is usually 1 to 2 weeks. Because HCV infection is asymptomatic in the majority of cases, diagnostic testing in the pediatric age group is recommended in the following circumstances:[30]

- Infants born to HCV-infected women and infants born to mothers with risk factors for HCV infection such as history of injection drug use.

- People who have received blood products or have a history of care in a neonatal intensive care unit prior to 1992.
- Adolescents with risk factors for HCV infection including history of drug use and multiple sexual partners. Although HCV is not efficiently transmitted through sexual contact, adolescents with multiple sexual partners are more likely to engage in other high-risk behaviors, notably drug use.[98]

Demonstration of HCV infection is based on detection of antibody or RNA in serum or plasma. In humans, HCV RNA can be detected in peripheral blood beginning 1 to 3 weeks after infection.[99] Among patients with chronic infection, serum concentrations of HCV RNA generally range from 10^5 to 10^8 genome equivalents per mL and are relatively stable within individual patients.[100] Box 220-1 summarizes the recommendations for HCV testing. A suggested testing algorithm for people with suspected HCV infection is provided in Figure 220-2.

Serologic Assays

The primary method for diagnosis of previous HCV infection is serologic testing for anti-HCV. Initial anti-HCV testing is performed using one of the approved enzyme immunoassays (EIAs). The current EIAs for anti-HCV are 97% sensitive and more than 99% specific but antibody testing cannot distinguish among acute, chronic, and resolved infections. A high signal-to-cutoff ratio on the EIA confirms HCV infection. The recombinant immunoblot

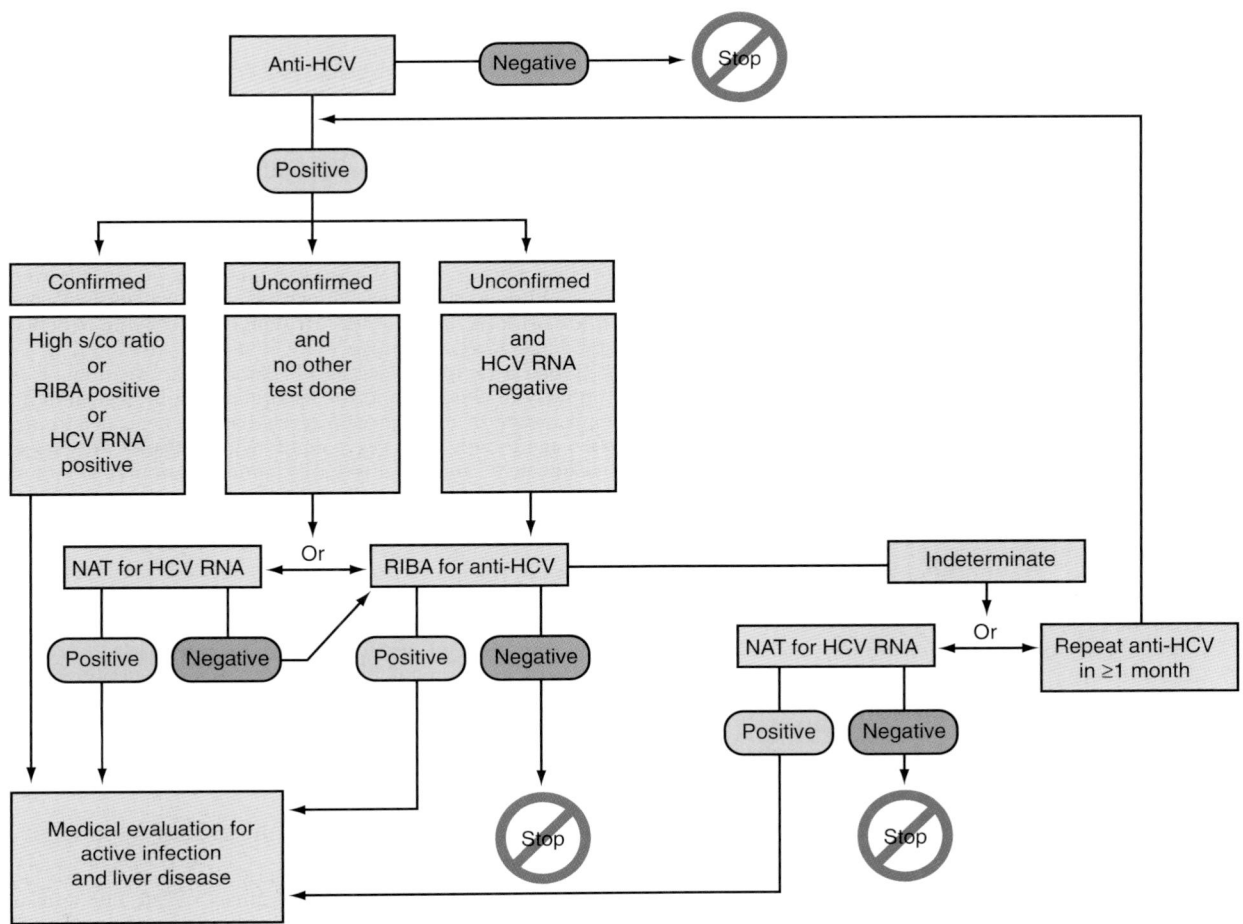

Figure 220-2. Testing algorithm for persons with suspected hepatitis C virus (HCV) infection. Anti-HCV, antibody to HCV; NAT, nucleic acid testing; RIBA, recombinant immunoblot assay; RNA, ribonucleic acid; s/co, signal-to-cutoff. HCV RNA levels can fluctuate. A single negative HCV RNA nucleic acid test does not rule out the possibility of chronic HCV infection. (Adapted from: Centers for Disease Control & Prevention. Guidelines for laboratory testing and result reporting of antibody to hepatitis C virus. MMWR 2003,52(RR-3):1–16.)

assay (RIBA) is a supplemental anti-HCV test with high specificity that is used to confirm infection in specimens with a low signal-to-cutoff ratio on EIA tests.[101] Infants who are infected perinatally should not be tested for anti-HCV before 18 months of age because passively acquired maternal antibodies might be detected up until 18 months.

There are important limitations of antibody testing for HCV in the setting of acute hepatitis. Because seroconversion occurs on average 8 to 9 weeks after infection[102] and can be delayed up to 6 months after exposure, a small percentage of people with acute hepatitis C have negative antibody test results at the onset of symptoms. Thus, serologic testing too early in the course of the infection may not detect and cannot rule out HCV as the cause of acute hepatitis.

Currently, there is no FDA-approved serologic test that indicates higher virus levels or active HCV replication, but a hepatitis C core-antigen test, well correlated with detectable HCV viral levels, and used in Europe, may be approved in the near future for use in the U.S.

Nucleic Acid Testing (NAT)

Reverse transcriptase polymerase chain reaction (RT-PCR) is the most widely used method for demonstrating the presence of HCV RNA. The qualitative RT-PCR assay can detect viral RNA in concentrations as low as 10 copies/mL, although the actual sensitivity of the assay can vary markedly from sample to sample. Quantitative assays also are available commercially to determine HCV viral load and are used primarily to monitor response to antiviral therapies. Compared with qualitative assays, quantitative assays are less sensitive and should not be used as primary tests to confirm or exclude the diagnosis of HCV infection or to monitor the end-point of treatment.

Most clinicians now use HCV RNA detection to confirm positive results of anti-HCV EIA testing. NAT indicates whether a patient has active HCV infection and thus is at risk for progression to chronic liver disease. However, a single negative HCV RNA test result cannot rule out chronic hepatitis C, because some patients are viremic only intermittently. People with a negative NAT result and a positive EIA test for anti-HCV require additional testing with RIBA to verify the anti-HCV result and determine the need for further medical evaluation (Figure 220-2). The presence of HCV RNA in the mother and infant is the most reliable means of detecting perinatal transmission of HCV. Infants born to HCV-positive mothers can be tested for HCV RNA on two occasions between the ages of 2 and 6 months to detect perinatal transmission.

Viral Genotyping

Among people infected with HCV, genotyping is recommended for guiding the duration of therapy and predicting the response to treatment regimens. Treatment of HCV genotypes 1 and 4 requires twice as long as treatment of genotypes 2 and 3 – currently 48 versus 24 weeks. These latter genotypes also are much more likely to be treated "successfully."

MANAGEMENT OF HCV INFECTION

There are no specific recommendations for management of HCV infection in children and adolescents and most management strategies are derived from adult studies. However, in view of the long duration of infection among children and adolescents compared with adults, regular follow-up for chronic HCV infection is necessary.

Serum Aminotransferase Levels

Normal serum ALT levels are not reliable indicators for lack of hepatic inflammation; however, elevated serum ALT levels are suggestive of hepatic inflammation. Therefore, serial measurement of serum ALT can be used to monitor disease activity. HCV-infected children can be followed regularly by physical examination and measurement of serum ALT level every 6 to 12 months.[103] More frequent follow-up is needed in children suffering from comorbidities such as HIV coinfection, thalassemia, or malignancy.

Evaluation of Liver Damage

Liver biopsy is the best method to assess the severity of liver damage in patients with hepatitis C. Neither viral load nor liver enzyme levels correlate well with severity of disease. Liver biopsy specimens are evaluated for the grade and stage of disease, which, respectively, are measures of the severity of ongoing disease and the extent of damage already incurred. Most pathologists now use a standard system to describe liver fibrosis, such as the Knodell fibrosis score, as modified by Ishak, the METAVIR score, or the histologic activity index.[104] Although liver biopsy often is viewed as a "gold standard," the accuracy of liver biopsy is affected by sampling and interpretation errors. Obtaining an adequate number of biopsy samples of appropriate size and using standard grading and staging criteria improve diagnostic accuracy.

For clinicians, the most important use of liver biopsy is in determining whether to proceed with therapy. For children and young adults with HCV infection, decisions regarding liver biopsy can be based on genotype and age of infection:[105,106]

- Children and young adults with genotype 2 or 3 do not need a liver biopsy to guide treatment decisions as they are highly likely to respond to combination therapy and treatment is indicated at any stage of disease.
- Because infection with genotype 1 is less responsive to treatment than genotype 2 or 3, liver biopsy can be offered to help guide treatment decisions. However, for people who acquired HCV infection recently through horizontal transmission (e.g., IDU), liver biopsy is not necessary as advanced liver disease is unlikely if infection is of short duration.

Because liver biopsy has several limitations, including patient acceptability, there is great interest in identifying indirect markers of liver fibrosis. Several serologic assays are under development, and although some have shown promise in identifying patients with cirrhosis, they are less accurate in identifying patients with moderate levels of fibrosis.

Progression to cirrhosis and hepatocellular carcinoma is highly unlikely in children and the usefulness of ultrasonography (US) and testing of α-fetoprotein levels has not been determined for this age group. However, patients with cirrhosis or a coexisting malignancy can be followed by annual measurement of serum α-fetoprotein level and a liver US.[106]

TREATMENT

Treatment aims to prevent complications and death from HCV infection. Several virologic measures are used to document response to treatment. The most important is sustained virologic response (SVR) defined as the absence of HCV RNA 24 weeks after discontinuation of therapy. The majority of patients who achieve an SVR show definitive absence of viremia and normal liver function.[105]

Treatment of Acute Infection

Several studies of adult patients have examined the effectiveness of antiviral agents during the early phase of infection and suggest higher SVR rates among people acutely infected compared with response rates observed among people with chronic HCV infection.[107–109] Currently, there is no consensus on the type or duration of therapy required or the timing of initiation of therapy.

Only one study reported treatment of acute HCV infection (genotype 4) in a pediatric patient with pegylated interferon α-2b and the child achieved SVR.[110] Treatment of acute HCV infection is a rapidly evolving area of research and more specific guidelines for treatment of acute HCV infection in children are likely to be forthcoming.

Treatment of Chronic Infection

HCV is the only chronic viral infection that can be "cured" – i.e., achievement of SVR for 24 or more weeks, usually permanently, after cessation of treatment. However, treatment is difficult for the patient, who frequently is debilitated with fatigue, depression, and malaise during the treatment course; and treatment with injected interferon and ribavirin is expensive, currently with estimated costs of $15,000 for a 48-week course. The decision to treat chronic HCV infection varies depending on the age, severity of the disease, efficacy of the chosen therapy and its adverse events, as well as assessed adherence with treatment and willingness to complete the regimen.

Because of the possibility of spontaneous clearance of the virus among children <3 years of age, and the adverse effects of current medications, which include spastic diplegia, treatment of children in this age group has not been approved.[105,111] In 2008, the FDA approved the use of peginterferon alfa-2b (PEG-INF α-2b) in combination with ribavirin for treatment of children ≥3 years of age. Recently, in 2011, the FDA approved the use of PEG-INF α-2a with ribavirin in children ≥5 years of age. The key points box depicts the currently approved FDA treatment regimens for chronic hepatitis C in children and adolescents. Prior to treatment initiation, it is necessary to know the viral genotype since this will affect the response to therapy. Higher SVR rates are achieved for infections due to genotypes 2 and 3 compared with genotypes 1 (the most common genotype in the U.S. and Europe) and 4.[103,105,106,112] The duration of therapy is 24 weeks for genotypes 2 and 3 and 48 weeks for genotypes 1 and 4.

Combination treatment with PEG-INF α-2b and ribavirin achieved the best SVR rates in all genotypes in the pediatric age group.[112] Large trials that included more than 100 children ≥3 years of age showed SVR rates ranging from 44% to 53% for genotype 1 and 80% to 100% for genotypes 2 and 3.[113–115] PEG-INF α-2b should be discontinued temporarily if the neutrophil count falls below 750 to 1000 cells/mm^3 and is resumed once the count increases.[112] Compared with regular interferon-α-2b, PEG-INF α-2b is more convenient because of the once weekly administration and limited duration of influenza-like symptoms.[113–117] Ribavirin in combination with PEG-INF α-2b enhances the second and third phases of viral decay, which reduces the probability of relapse.[118]

The most common adverse events associated with interferon are influenza-like symptoms, particularly fever, headache, fatigue, and irritability, which are almost universal after the first few doses but usually resolve in children by the second or third week of therapy.[114,116,119] Weight loss also is common but a compensatory catch-up weight gain occurs after completion of treatment.[114–116] In addition, a temporary decrease in height growth also is noted as a result of therapy, which also resolves after discontinuation of therapy.[114–116] Bone marrow suppression is the most severe adverse event which can lead to neutropenia or thrombocytopenia, but can be managed by reduction of the interferon dosage.[114–116,119,120] With therapy, mood disturbances and suicidal ideation are common and more so among adolescents and those with pre-existing mood disorders.[112] Depression occurred in 13% of participants in one study.[119] Abnormalities of thyroid function also can occur but normalize after completion of treatment.[113,114,119] Hemolysis is a common adverse effect of ribavirin and can require discontinuation of the drug. Teratogenicity is a major concern for men as well as women, who should avoid conception during therapy and for 6 months thereafter. Treatment with interferon is contraindicated in patients with certain comorbid conditions such as depression, psychiatric conditions, seizures, renal insufficiency, and autoimmune hepatitis.[112]

Special attention is needed for children with anemia and thalassemia. Erythropoietin and darbapoietin might be used to decrease the hemolytic effect of ribavirin therapy in patients with pre-existing anemia. However, the effect of erythropoietin on SVR is unknown.[121] Children with thalassemia may require more transfusions and chelation therapy as a result of hemolysis due to ribavirin therapy and iron overload.[121,122]

In summary, the efficacy of combined therapy in children reflected by SVR rates of 50% and 90% in genotype 1 and genotypes 2 and 3, respectively, warrants its use. However, longitudinal studies are needed to investigate adverse events after completion of therapy such as thyroid function abnormalities and growth alterations.

Future Treatments

Therapy for hepatitis C is a rapidly evolving field with numerous drugs under development. A recombinant protein of INF-α-2b genetically infused with albumin is being evaluated as a monthly rather than weekly injection.[123] Viramidine and taribavirin, ribavirin analogues with less risk for hemolytic anemia, are under study and show promising results.[124,125]

Because treatment success rates are poorer for patients with genotype 1, and for those who have failed therapy previously, there has been special interest in oral agents, such as protease and polymerase inhibitors, as additions to or replacements for pegylated interferon-ribavirin "backbone" therapy. There are at least 10 such agents currently under development and in stages of clinical trial. In particular, two – telaprevir and boceprevir – have emerged in the last two years as valuable therapeutic agents. The addition of 12 weeks of telaprevir therapy to pegylated interferon–ribavirin treatment has resulted in substantial improvements in rates of achievement of SVR in initial[126] or previously unsuccessfully treated[127] adults with chronic HCV genotype 1 infections. Duration of therapy also may be reduced when telaprevir is added to "backbone" therapy. Likewise, the addition of boceprevir to standard therapy after a 4-week lead-in doubled the rates of achievement of SVR in treatment-naive HCV genotype 1 patients in North America and Europe.[128] However, telaprevir use may be associated with rash that, with other adverse events, can increase treatment discontinuation rates.[126] Boceprevir use is limited substantially because of concerns with its frequent resultant anemia (55% of treated patients).[128] Nonetheless, these and other agents mark major improvements in chronic HCV therapy and may offer a route to oral, non-injection (interferon) therapy as well as better adherence.

PREVENTION

Comprehensive recommendations for prevention and control of HCV infection have been published.[30] For example, immunoglobulin has not been shown to be effective for postexposure prophylaxis of hepatitis C and its use is not recommended.[30,129] There is no recommendation to screen women for HCV infection either before or during pregnancy, unless they have risk factors for HCV infection. Currently, both the American Academy of Pediatrics and the American College of Obstetricians and Gynecologists support breastfeeding in HCV-infected women. However, HCV-infected women should abstain from breastfeeding if their nipples are cracked or bleeding. Box 220-2 provides key counseling messages for persons with HCV infection. Regardless of risk factors, all children should be immunized against hepatitis A and B.[130,131] Development of a vaccine for hepatitis C has been challenging given the genetic heterogeneity of HCV, the high mutation rate, and the lack of a cell culture system. However, novel vaccine candidates based on molecular technology are being explored.[132,133]

221 Rubella Virus

Yvonne A. Maldonado

Rubella is a benign, self-limited viral illness. Acquired rubella is characterized by an exanthem and lymphadenopathy, although infants and children with rubella frequently are asymptomatic. Much of the morbidity attributed to rubella virus results from infection in utero. Sequelae of congenital rubella syndrome (CRS) include growth retardation, deafness, congenital heart disease, and mental retardation. Routine vaccination in childhood has resulted in elimination of rubella and CRS in the United States, and more recently concerted efforts in the western hemisphere have virtually eliminated CRS in this region of the world,[1] but this syndrome still occurs in areas of the world that lack routine rubella vaccination programs.

DESCRIPTION OF THE PATHOGEN

Rubella virus is the only member of the *Rubivirus* genus within the Togavirus family. It is a spherical virus, 50 to 70 nm in diameter, that has a single-stranded positive-sense RNA genome. The nucleoprotein core is surrounded by a glycolipid envelope; the lipid component is host cell-derived. There is only one antigenic type of rubella virus. Although humans are the only natural hosts of rubella virus, experimental infection can occur in a wide range of vertebrate species.

Rubella virus contains three major structural proteins, E1, E2, and C. E1 and E2 are glycosylated envelope proteins that make up the spiked 5- to 6-nm surface projections of the viral surface. Monoclonal antibodies directed against epitopes of both E1 and E2 have neutralizing activity. E1 is the viral hemagglutinin that binds both hemagglutination- and hemolysis-inhibiting antibodies. C protein is the nucleoprotein.

Rubella virus is readily inactivated by chemical agents such as chlorine, deoxycholate, formalin, β-propiolactone, and ethylene glycol, and by lipid solvents such as ether, chloroform, and acetone. The virus is also inactivated by heat (>56°C), cold (−10°C to −20°C), ultraviolet light, and extremes in pH (<6.8 and >8.1). Infectious virus can be maintained for long periods at −60°C, and

in the presence of protein, infectivity can be maintained for weeks at 4°C.

Rubella virus grows well in a variety of primary and continuous cell lines. In most primary cell lines, rubella produces persistent infection without evidence of cytopathic effect (CPE). The virus does produce CPE in some continuous cell lines, such as Vero, RK13, and SIRC cells. Rubella virus also can be detected in cell culture on the basis of its ability to interfere with growth of enteroviruses in vervet monkey kidney cell lines.

Pathogenesis of Acquired Rubella Infection

Rubella is most likely transmitted by aerosolized particles from the respiratory tract secretions of infected individuals. Infectivity, which correlates with virus shedding from the nasopharynx, begins between 3 and 8 days after exposure and lasts for approximately 11 to 14 days. Individuals who experience the rash illness are infectious from 5 days before until 6 days after the onset of rash.

After exposure, the virus first attaches to and invades respiratory epithelium and then spreads hematogenously to regional lymphatics. Virus replicates in both local and distant reticuloendothelial sites, followed by secondary viremia that occurs between 6 and 20 days after infection. Cell-associated virus can be recovered from peripheral blood lymphocytes and monocytes for up to 4 weeks after infection.[2] Within 8 to 14 days after exposure, active viral replication occurs throughout the body and can be recovered from numerous sites, including the respiratory tract, skin, lymph nodes, urine, cerebrospinal fluid, and breast milk.[3-5] This also is the period of maximal nasopharyngeal shedding. Clinical manifestations of infection appear during this period, coincident with development of a humoral immune response.

Immune Response in Acquired Rubella Infection

Humoral immunity to both natural and vaccine rubella virus is characterized by development of a variety of antibody types

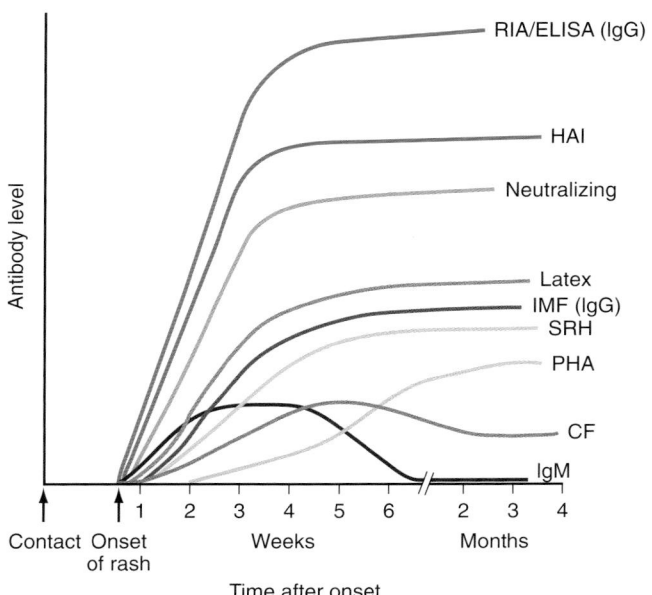

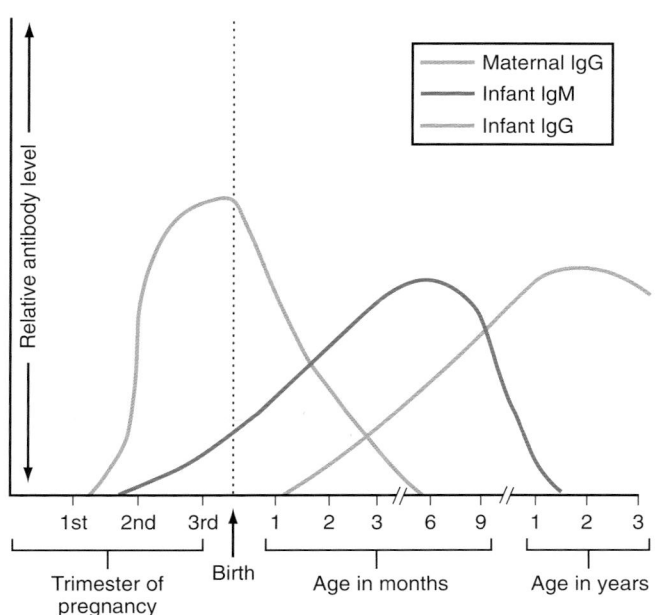

Figure 221-1. Antibody responses in acute rubella infection. CF, complement fixing; EIA, enzyme immunosorbent assay; HAI, hemagglutination inhibition; IgG, immunoglobulin G; IMF, immunofluorescence; PHA, passive hemagglutination; RIA, radioimmunoassay; SRH, single radial hemolysis. (Redrawn from Best JM, O'Shea S. Rubella virus. In: Lennette EH, Schmidt NJ (eds) Diagnostic Procedures for Viral, Rickettsial, and Chlamydial Infections, 6th ed. Washington, DC, American Public Health Association, 1989, pp 731–795.)

Figure 221-2. Immune responses in congenitally acquired rubella after maternal infection in the first trimester of pregnancy. IgG, immunoglobulin G; IgM, immunoglobulin M. (Redrawn from Best JM, O'Shea S. Rubella virus. In: Lennette EH, Schmidt NJ (eds) Diagnostic Procedures for Viral, Rickettsial, and Chlamydial Infections, 6th ed. Washington, DC, American Public Health Association, 1989, pp 731–795.)

reactive to distinct viral antigens, including viral hemagglutinins, complement-fixing (CF) antigens, and precipitating antigens (Figure 221-1).[6] Development of hemagglutination inhibition (HAI) and neutralizing antibodies occurs with the onset of the rash illness, and CF antibodies are detected 1 week later. Peak titers of HAI and neutralizing antibodies occur approximately 2 weeks after onset of rash; CF antibodies peak about 2 weeks later. HAI and neutralizing antibodies persist for life. Although the antibody titers induced by the RA 27/3 vaccine virus currently used in the U.S. are lower than those induced by natural infection, the nature of the antibody response is similar to the response to natural infection.

Cell-mediated immunity to rubella virus develops at least 1 week before the development of humoral immunity. Transient suppression of cellular immunity and a decrease in numbers of leukocytes (neutrophils and lymphocytes) can occur after natural infection or vaccination.[7] Clinically significant immunosuppression has not been described in immunocompetent individuals after acquired rubella infection.

Pathogenesis of Congenital Rubella

In contrast to acquired rubella infection, congenital infection results in a persistent, progressive infection. Placental and fetal infection with rubella virus occurs most consistently after maternal infection during the first trimester of pregnancy, and early fetal infection, especially during organogenesis, is associated with increasing risk of fetal death or teratogenicity.[8,9] Maternal rubella infection in the first trimester of pregnancy results in fetal infection rates of 80% to 100%. By 16 weeks of gestation, the fetal infection rate drops to 10% to 20%, but it rises again to 60% or higher after 30 weeks of gestation.[10,11]

Factors associated with the greater susceptibility of the placenta and fetus to rubella virus during the first trimester are unknown. Pathologic effects of congenital infection primarily are the result of a generalized virus-induced, progressive necrotizing vasculitis. The resulting parenchymal hypoplasia produces characteristic clinical findings associated with CRS. Other pathologic effects are

focal inflammation, edema, and granulomatous changes. Evidence of mitotic arrest and chromosomal defects has been identified in congenitally infected fetuses and in chronically infected human embryonic cells and may represent other pathologic mechanisms leading to reduced cell numbers and hypoplasia. The spectrum of fetal infection varies from extensive involvement of multiple organs when infection occurs early in the first trimester, to focal involvement of few organs, especially of the eye and auditory system, which occurs in fetal infections after 11 to 12 weeks of gestation.

Immune Response in Congenital Rubella Infection

Both humoral and cell-mediated immune responses in congenital rubella infection are distinct from those observed after acquired infection (Figure 221-2). With congenital infection, fetal immunoglobulin (Ig) M antibodies to rubella virus can be detected as early as 20 weeks of gestation, and fetal IgG can be detected by the middle of the second trimester. Levels of both IgM and IgG continue to rise throughout the first few months of life; IgM levels decline by about 6 months of age, and IgG levels persist for many years.[12] However, maternal antibody titers persist longer, and the geometric mean titers in mothers are higher than those in their congenitally infected infants 5 years after birth. Cell-mediated responses to congenital rubella, such as delayed-type hypersensitivity reactions, lymphocyte-mediated cytotoxicity, phytohemagglutinin-induced lymphocyte transformation, and interferon production, are decreased compared with responses after acquired infection. The most depressed cell-mediated immunity responses are observed in infants infected earliest in gestation.[13,14]

EPIDEMIOLOGY

Rubella infection occurs most often in late winter and throughout spring. In unvaccinated populations, epidemics occur in 2- to 4-year cycles; larger epidemics occur at 6- to 9-year intervals. Although rubella is endemic worldwide, the natural history of

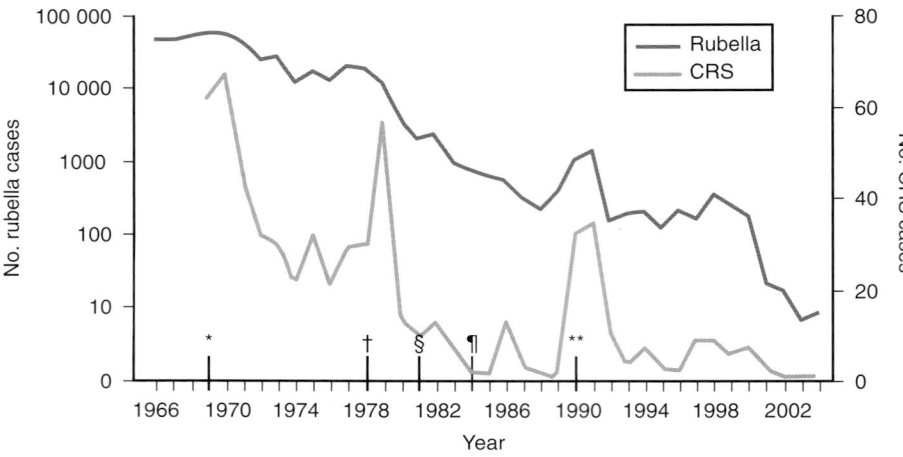

Figure 221-3. Number of reported cases of rubella and congenital rubella syndrome (CRS), by year, and chronology of rubella vaccination recommendations by the Advisory Committee on Immunization Practices – United States, 1966–2004. (Adapted from Centers for Disease Control and Prevention. Achievements in Public Health: Elimination of Rubella and Congenital Rubella Syndrome – United States, 1969–2004. MMWR 2005;54:279–282.)

* 1969 – First official recommendations are published for the use of rubella vaccine. Vaccination is recommended for children aged 1 year to puberty.

† 1978 – Recommendations for vaccination are expanded to include adolescents and certain adults, particularly females. Vaccination is recommended for adolescent or adult females and males in populations in colleges, certain places of employment (e.g., hospitals), and military bases.

§ 1981 – Recommendations place increased emphasis on vaccination of susceptible persons in training and educational settings (e.g., universities or colleges) and military settings, and vaccination of workers in health-care-settings.

¶ 1984 – Recommendations are published for vaccination of workers in daycare centers, schools, colleges, companies, government offices, and industrial sites. Providers are encouraged to conduct prenatal testing and postpartum vaccination of susceptible women. Recommendations for vaccination are expanded to include susceptible persons who travel abroad.

** 1990 – Recommendations include implementation of a new 2-dose schedule for measles-mumps-rubella vaccine.

acquired rubella is not well described because clinical manifestations are nonspecific and produce few important sequelae. The association between maternal rubella and congenital defects was described in 1941. Detailed clinical and epidemiologic information about rubella was only available after the rubella pandemics that occurred in 1941 and 1963.[15] In the U.S., rubella was not a reportable disease until 1966. Since the licensure of rubella vaccines in the U.S. in 1969, dramatic decreases in epidemic and endemic rubella occurred until 2004, when it was concluded that rubella was no longer endemic in the U.S. (Figure 221-3).[16]

Rubella attack rates among susceptible individuals in closed communities, such as college dormitories and military facilities, range from 75% to 90%; however, attack rates can approach 100% among household contacts. The rubella attack rate in an open population is unknown.

Between 1966 and 1968, the estimated incidence of acquired rubella was 24 cases in 100,000 individuals, compared with rates of 0.06 to 0.09 in 100,000 between 1992 and 1994.[17-19] In the prevaccine era, infants and young children were most susceptible to rubella infection, the highest attack rate for rubella being among 3- to 9-year-old children. Most individuals therefore experienced rubella in childhood, and most adults were not susceptible during cyclic epidemics. Because most infants now receive rubella vaccine, older unvaccinated individuals are most susceptible to infection. For example, 88% of cases reported in 1994 occurred in individuals 5 years of age and older. In 2004 only 9 rubella cases were reported and from 2001 to 2004 only 4 congenital rubella cases were reported in the U.S.[16] About half of the acquired cases and 3 of the 4 congenital cases occurred among persons born outside the U.S., most of whom were born outside the western hemisphere. Rubella now is most likely to occur in small outbreaks of illness among susceptible populations in the U.S., such as religious groups who traditionally refuse vaccination, unvaccinated recent immigrants, and communities with large numbers of unvaccinated adolescents and young adults.[20] Unfortunately, in the developing world, the burden of congenital rubella remains substantial.[21]

Rubella immunization programs in the U.S. include two strategies: universal immunization of all infants and targeted vaccination of susceptible prepubertal girls and women of child-bearing age. Success has been achieved primarily with the universal immunization of infants. By 1998, more than 90% of 2-year-old children in the U.S. had received at least one dose of a measles-containing vaccine, usually measles, mumps, rubella vaccine.[22] The current epidemiology of rubella seropositivity in the U.S. reflects the interaction between the immunization program and the natural history of rubella. Based upon serum specimens from the third National Health and Nutrition Examination Survey (1988 to 1994), rubella seropositivity rates were 92% in persons aged 6 to 11 years, 33% in persons aged 12 to 19 years, 85% in persons aged 20 to 29 years, 89% in persons aged 30 to 39 years, and >93% in those >40 years of age.[23]

CLINICAL MANIFESTATIONS

Acquired Rubella

The incubation period from exposure to onset of exanthem is 14 to 21 days (mean, 18 days). Nonspecific prodromal symptoms, which can occur 1 to 5 days before onset of exanthem, consist of fever, eye pain, sore throat, arthralgia, and gastrointestinal complaints. Prodromal symptoms are less common among infants and young children than among adolescents and adults.

The characteristic clinical findings are rash and suboccipital adenopathy. The course of the exanthem can be quite variable. Rash usually begins on the face, spreads in a cephalocaudal direction to involve the entire body over the next 24 hours, and fades during the ensuing 2 or 3 days, also in a cephalocaudal direction. Duration ranges from <1 day to >5 days. Usually erythematous and maculopapular, the rash can also be scarlatiniform, morbilliform, or macular; in adolescents, the rash can be confused with acne. In adults, the rash may be pruritic. Other symptoms of the exanthemous phase are low-grade fever and lymphadenopathy. Lymphadenopathy almost always occurs with rubella infection and can be noted for up to 1 week before onset of the exanthem. Usually, the posterior auricular and suboccipital lymph nodes are involved, but generalized involvement can occur.

Reinfection is uncommon. Reinfection that occurs during pregnancy and produces fetal infection has been documented but is extremely rare.[24-29] Reinfection is usually subclinical and

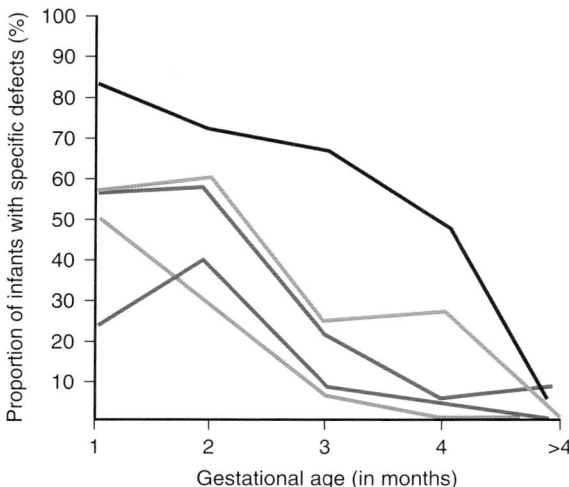

Figure 221-4. Clinical manifestations of congenital rubella and time of maternal infection. ━━, deafness; ━━, central nervous system deficit; ━━, heart disease; ━━, cataract/glaucoma; ━━, neonatal purpura. (Redrawn from Best JM, O'Shea S. Rubella virus. In: Lennette EH, Schmidt NJ (eds) Diagnostic Procedures for Viral, Rickettsial, and Chlamydial Infections, 6th ed. Washington, DC, American Public Health Association, 1989, pp 731–795.)

nonspecific and therefore must be diagnosed by means of serologic methods.

Congenital Rubella

Clinical manifestations of congenital rubella reflect the chronic, progressive nature of the infection.[30-32] Fetal infection can lead to early miscarriage, spontaneous abortion, or stillbirth. Up to 20% of maternal infections occurring in the first 8 weeks of gestation result in miscarriage. Among live births, the risk of congenital rubella infection and subsequent congenital defects is inversely related to gestational age at the time of maternal infection. Congenital defects occur in >80% of infants infected in the first trimester, and virtually no defects are identified in infants infected after the first 16 weeks of gestation (Figure 221-4). The gestational age at the time of infection also affects the distribution of congenital defects among infected infants. Infants infected in the first trimester are more likely to have multiple congenital defects, whereas those infants infected after 11 to 12 weeks of gestation are more likely to have only deafness or retinopathy as a clinical manifestation. Clinical manifestations of congenital rubella can be evident at birth or, more commonly, can result in normal-appearing infants with late-onset sequelae. In addition, early clinical manifestations can be transient or progressive (Table 221-1).

Transient, early clinical manifestations of congenital rubella reflect acute nonspecific immunologic responses to congenital viral infection. Signs and symptoms include generalized lymphadenopathy, hepatosplenomegaly, intrauterine growth retardation, hepatitis, jaundice, hemolytic anemia, pneumonitis, meningoencephalitis, cloudy corneas, bony radiolucencies, and diarrhea.[33-38] Thrombocytopenic purpura with petechiae and "blueberry muffin" lesions, which usually represent focal areas of dermal erythropoiesis, are associated with rubella more than with other congenital viral infections. Transient manifestations typically resolve within days to weeks, usually without long-term sequelae. More than 50% of newborns with clinically apparent congenital rubella have low birthweight, and persistent postnatal growth retardation or failure to thrive occurs in many.

Permanent or progressive manifestations of congenital rubella can occur in any organ. The organ systems most commonly involved are the heart, eye, brain, and auditory system. Deafness is the most common manifestation of congenital rubella. Deafness is usually bilateral and can be peripheral or central in origin. Cardiac anomalies are present in >50% of infants born with

TABLE 221-1. Clinical Features Associated with Congenital Rubella Syndrome

Category	Common	Uncommon
PRESENT AT BIRTH		
Transient	Low birthweight	Cloudy corneas
	Thrombocytopenic purpura	Hepatitis
	Hepatomegaly	Generalized lymphadenopathy
	Splenomegaly	Hemolytic anemia
	Bone lesions	Pneumonitis
Permanent	Sensorineural deafness	Severe myopia
	Peripheral pulmonary stenosis	Thyroid disorders
	Pulmonary valvular stenosis	Dermatoglyphic abnormalities
	Patent ductus arteriosus	Glaucoma
	Ventricular septal defect	Myocardial abnormalities
	Retinopathy	Sensorineural deafness
	Cataract	
	Microphthalmia	
	Psychomotor retardation	
	Cryptorchidism	
	Inguinal hernia	
	Diabetes mellitus	
DELAYED		
	Peripheral pulmonary artery stenosis	Severe myopia
	Mental retardation	Thyroiditis
	Central language defects	Hypothyroidism
	Diabetes mellitus	Growth hormone deficiency
	Immune complex disease	Chronic rash
	Hypogammaglobulinemia	Pneumonitis
		Progressive panencephalitis

Modified from Banatvala JE, Best JM. Rubella. In: Brown F, Wilson R (eds) Topley and Wilson's Principles of Bacteriology, Virology, and Immunity, vol. 4, 7th ed. London, Edward Arnold, 1984, pp 271–302.

symptomatic congenital rubella. The most common lesions are patent ductus arteriosus, pulmonary arterial stenosis, and pulmonary valvular stenosis. The most common ocular manifestations are "salt-and-pepper" retinopathy and cataracts.[39] Retinopathy occurs in 20% to 50% of infants with symptomatic infection and is usually unilateral. Cataracts occur in up to a third of infants with retinopathy; they are bilateral in about 50% of affected infants and are associated with microphthalmia in about 60%.

Late-onset manifestations of congenital rubella may not be identified until 2 years or longer after birth.[40,41] Findings include endocrinopathies, chronic immunologic defects, auditory and ocular dysfunction, and vascular and central nervous system disease. The most common endocrinopathy is insulin-dependent diabetes mellitus,[42-44] occurring at four times or greater the rate in unaffected children. The highest rate was reported in a series from Australia, in which 20% of young adults with symptomatic CRS had diabetes mellitus.[45] Thyroid disorders, such as hyperthyroidism, hypothyroidism, and thyroiditis, occur in up to 5% of infections.[46-50] Glaucoma as well as abnormalities of the cornea and lens also can have late onset. Retinal neovascularization secondary to congenital retinal vascular atrophy can result in visual disturbances, and renal vascular stenosis can lead to hypertension.

Central nervous system defects associated with congenital rubella may be present at birth. In some cases, these are transient manifestations with no permanent sequelae; in others, the symptoms are progressive. Additionally, some infants demonstrate new central nervous system manifestations later in life.[51,52] Permanent neurologic defects include developmental delay, microcephaly, behavioral disorders, and chronic encephalitis. Developmental delay can be the result of intrauterine damage of the central nervous system, acute and chronic encephalitis in the immediate postnatal period, or progressive effects of generalized failure to thrive. Microcephaly may not be associated with developmental delay if the decrease in head circumference is a result of generalized growth retardation without failure to thrive.[53] Psychiatric manifestations, such as reactive or neurotic behavior disorders and autism, occur in up to a third of preschool and school-aged children.[34,52] Late-onset progressive panencephalitis is a rare complication that usually becomes manifest in the second decade of life.[54]

Permanent manifestations of congenital rubella are common, resulting in long-term sequelae in 80% or more of infected infants. The most common complications are hearing deficits that can progress or can develop even after years of normal hearing. The overall incidence of hearing deficits in children with congenital rubella infection is about 50%, but may be identified only after 4 to 6 years of age in up to 20% of children. Ophthalmologic defects, which occur in up to 50% of infants with clinically apparent infection at birth, can result in progressive visual disturbances, especially in children with retinopathy in whom progressive macular scarring develops. Cardiac defects may require surgical intervention. Developmental delay and behavioral disorders are usually progressive; the overall prevalence of permanent central nervous system involvement is about 10% in infants with symptomatic infection at birth. It is important to evaluate auditory and visual acuity in such children because of the possibility that hearing or vision disturbances are the primary cause of learning disorders.[55]

LABORATORY FINDINGS AND DIAGNOSIS

Acquired Rubella

Laboratory abnormalities during acquired rubella infection include leukopenia and relative neutropenia. Because the rubella exanthem is nonspecific, infection can rarely be diagnosed on the basis of clinical presentation alone; serologic tests are usually necessary to confirm the diagnosis. Testing acute and convalescent sera for rubella HAI antibodies is the standard serologic technique used, but enzyme immunoassays that detect rubella-specific IgA, IgG, and IgM antibodies are most available.[56-60] Detection of rubella neutralizing antibodies is a more sensitive marker of past infection, but is labor-intensive; HAI, CF, and enzyme immunoassay tests are suitable for the diagnosis of acute infection. Rubella virus can be cultured from nasopharyngeal secretions and urine, but this is impractical compared with serologic assays.

A fourfold or greater rise in antibody titer between paired sera collected 2 weeks apart, or a single elevated IgM titer, indicates recent infection (see Figure 221-1). Interpretation of serologic results must be based on the timing of the serum samples relative to the onset of the rash, because IgM antibodies may only be detectable from 1 to 2 weeks until 3 weeks after onset of rash.[61] Visualization of rubella virus antigen by immunofluorescent methods and detection of rubella virus genome by polymerase chain reaction methods also have been described.[62]

The differential diagnosis of rubella infection includes other benign rash illnesses of childhood, such as enteroviral infections, exanthem subitum, adenovirus and Epstein–Barr virus infections, and streptococcal infections. Infection due to *Mycoplasma pneumoniae* and drug rashes can also mimic rubella infection.

Congenital Rubella

A maternal history of rubella during pregnancy or neonatal manifestations suggestive of congenital infection, such as microcephaly, hepatosplenomegaly, generalized lymphadenopathy, thrombocytopenia, or ocular abnormalities, should prompt evaluation for multiple causes. The diagnosis of congenital rubella requires virologic or serologic confirmation. Rubella virus can be isolated for up to a year or more from nasopharynx, buffy coat of the blood,

TABLE 221-2. Frequency of Virus Excretion with Age of Infants with Congenitally Acquired Rubella

Age	Number with Positive Culture (%)
0 through 1 month	71/85 (84)
1 through 4 months	50/81 (62)
5 through 8 months	26/80 (33)
9 through 12 months	11/98 (11)
13 through 20 months	4/115 (3)
3 through 15 years	0/20 (0)

Data from Cooper LZ, Krugman S. Clinical manifestations of postnatal and congenital rubella. Arch Ophthalmol 1967;77:434–439, copyrighted 1967, American Medical Association.

cerebrospinal fluid, and urine of infants with congenital infection (Table 221-2).[63,64]

The serologic confirmation of congenital rubella is difficult. Rubella-specific IgM can be measured in cord blood or neonatal serum but is associated with false-positive reactions in the presence of rheumatoid factor or maternal IgG and with false-negative reactions if maternal infection occurred late in pregnancy.[65-67] Serial measurement of IgG may therefore be necessary; specimens drawn at 3 and 6 months of age should be tested in parallel; persistence of rubella-specific HAI or enzyme immunoassay antibodies is considered diagnostic of congenital infection.

TREATMENT

No specific therapy is available for congenital or acquired rubella infection. The infant with presumed or proven congenital rubella infection should undergo complete evaluation for associated congenital defects, including ophthalmologic, auditory, cardiac, and neurodevelopmental assessments.

COMPLICATIONS OF ACQUIRED RUBELLA

Arthropathy is the most common complication of acquired rubella, occurring in up to 20% of children and in almost three-fourths of adults older than 30 years of age. Women are more often affected than men. Clinical manifestations can include arthritis and arthralgia of multiple joints; fingers, knees, and wrists are involved most often. Onset is usually 1 to 6 days after onset of rash, and symptoms persist for a mean of 9 days. An association between acquired rubella infection and rheumatoid arthritis has been reported.[68] Higher prevalence of rubella HAI antibodies has been demonstrated in individuals with rheumatoid arthritis than in matched controls, and rubella virus and antigens have been detected in the synovial fluid of a few patients with juvenile rheumatoid arthritis. A cohort study of >3000 women failed to demonstrate an association between rubella vaccination and new-onset chronic arthropathy.[69]

Acute encephalitis occurs in approximately 0.02% of cases and usually manifests within 4 days of the onset of rash.[70-72] Cerebrospinal fluid analysis demonstrates a mild pleocytosis, usually <300/mm^3 (>50% lymphocytes), a normal or slightly elevated protein concentration, and a normal glucose concentration. Rubella encephalitis has a variable course. In most individuals, illness is mild and self-limited, but deaths have occasionally occurred. Symptoms of peripheral neuritis are commonly reported. Rarely, subacute sclerosing panencephalitis can occur in patients after acquired rubella.[73] The clinical course is similar to that seen with subacute sclerosing panencephalitis caused by rubeola virus.

Thrombocytopenia with purpura occurs in 0.03% of individuals.[74] The prevalence is higher in children than in adults and occurs more often in girls than in boys. Thrombocytopenia usually is self-limited but can last days to months. Rare complications of rubella are myocarditis, pericarditis, follicular conjunctivitis, hemolytic anemia, and hepatitis.

PREVENTION

Active Immunity

Rubella vaccination programs in the U.S. targeted universal immunization of infants to eliminate the CRS in subsequent generations.[75–78] Selective vaccination of prepubertal women or women of reproductive age also has been recommended. The Centers for Disease Control and Prevention (CDC) and the American Academy of Pediatrics (AAP) recommend universal rubella vaccination at 12 to 15 months of age, with a second dose prior to school entry (4 to 6 years) or at entry to junior high or middle school (11 to 12 years), as part of the two-dose measles vaccine recommendation. The second dose of vaccine is intended to provide immunity to those children who do not seroconvert after the first dose.

The RA 27/3 strain of live-attenuated rubella virus is the rubella vaccine currently licensed for use in the U.S. The vaccine is prepared in WI38 human embryonic lung tissue culture, and it produces a mild, noncommunicable infection. It is immunogenic in 98% of recipients and confers lifelong immunity to >90% of vaccinees.[79,80] Vaccine is available in a monovalent formulation as well as in combination with mumps and measles. A quadrivalent vaccine, including measles, mumps, rubella, and varicella, was licensed in the U.S. in 2005. In two postlicensure studies, the quadrivalent vaccine was found to be associated with one additional febrile seizure 5 to 12 days after vaccination per 2300 to 2600 children immunized at ages 12 through 23 months, who had received the first dose of MMRV vaccine compared with children who had received the first dose of MMR vaccine and varicella vaccine administered as separate injections at the same visit. These data did not suggest that children aged 4–6 years who received the second dose of MMRV vaccine had an increased risk for febrile seizures after vaccination compared with children the same age who received MMR vaccine and varicella vaccine administered as separate injections at the same visit. CDC and AAP currently recommend that at age 12 through 47 months children receive either separate MMR and varicella vaccines or the combined MMRV vaccine. However, unless the parent or caregiver expresses a preference for MMRV vaccine, MMR vaccine and V vaccine should be administered separately for the first dose in toddlers. For the second doses at any age (15 months to 12 years) and for the first dose at age ≥48 months, use of MMRV vaccine generally is preferred over separate injections of MMR vaccine and varicella V).[81]

Adverse reactions to rubella vaccine include rash, fever, and lymphadenopathy in up to 15% of vaccine recipients. Joint pains occur in <1% of children, but arthritis and arthralgia occur in up to 25% of postpubertal women after vaccination;[82,83] arthropathy begins 1 to 3 weeks after vaccination and is transient. Persistent arthropathy has been reported but is uncommon. Rarely, transient peripheral neuropathy, thrombocytopenia, and central nervous system manifestations have been described.

Rubella vaccine should not be given to pregnant women or to women who are considering pregnancy within 3 months of vaccine administration.[84–88] The risk of congenital rubella infection after vaccination is based on accumulated data from 226 seronegative women who received rubella vaccine inadvertently during the first trimester of pregnancy and demonstrated seroconversion. Two percent of infants of these women had serologically confirmed rubella infection with no clinical manifestations; no infant had congenital defects.

Although administration of live-virus vaccine is contraindicated in immunosuppressed children, the one exception is administration of MMR vaccine to children infected with the human immunodeficiency virus (HIV), because of the higher risk of morbidity and mortality associated with measles in this population. HIV-infected children without severe immunosuppression should receive MMR vaccine at the generally recommended ages, although primary vaccine failure among HIV-infected individuals may be substantial. Persons who have received immune globulin, blood or blood products, or immunosuppressive therapy should not be vaccinated for at least 3 months, and longer if a high dose of immune globulin was given intravenously (see Chapter 6, Active Immunization).

Passive Immunity

Immune globulin (IG) can modify or prevent clinical manifestations of acquired rubella infection among exposed susceptible individuals. However, absence of clinical infection may not indicate absence of viremia and infants with congenital rubella have been born to women who received IG soon after exposure to rubella during pregnancy. IG therefore is not recommended routinely for postexposure prophylaxis of susceptible pregnant women and should only be considered if termination of the pregnancy cannot be considered. IG can be given intramuscularly at a dose of 0.55 mL/kg; the maximum dose is 15 mL.

Public Health Measures

Children with acquired rubella should be excluded from school or group childcare until 7 days after the onset of rash. Infants with congenital rubella should be considered contagious until 1 year of age unless results of multiple urine and nasopharyngeal cultures for rubella virus performed after 3 months of age are negative.

Healthcare, childcare, and military personnel as well as college students should be screened for rubella immunity, and susceptible individuals should be immunized to prevent infection with and transmission of the virus.[89–92] Routine serologic screening of postpubertal women is not recommended.

Isolation Procedures

Contact isolation of persons with postnatal rubella is indicated for 7 days after onset of rash. Contact isolation is also required for neonates with suspected congenital rubella.

---

222 Human Coronaviruses

Susan M. Poutanen

Coronaviridae are enveloped nonsegmented, single-stranded, positive-sense RNA viruses named after their corona- or crown-like surface projections seen on electron microscopy that correspond to large surface spike proteins (Figures 222-1 and 222-2). Coronaviruses are host-specific and can infect humans as well as a variety of different animals, causing diverse clinical syndromes.[1] Three serologically and genetically distinct groups of coronaviruses have been described. Human coronaviruses (HCoVs) are part of groups 1 and 2 and primarily cause a variety of respiratory tract infections[1] (Table 222-1).

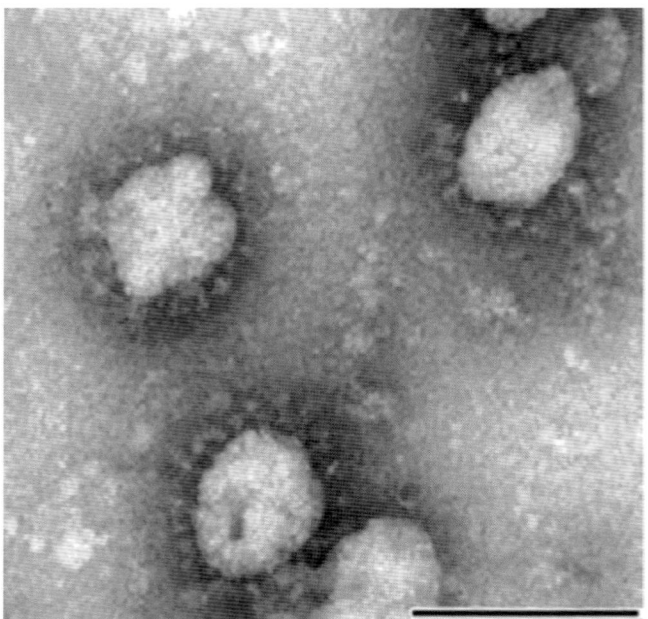

Figure 222-1. Electron micrograph of a typical coronavirus. Negative-contrast electron micrograph of severe acute respiratory syndrome coronaviruses (SARS-CoV). The typical crown-like spike proteins on the surface of the coronavirus particles are shown. Bar = 100 nm. (From Kuiken T, Fouchier RA, Schutten M, et al. Newly discovered coronavirus as the primary cause of severe acute respiratory syndrome. Lancet 2003;362:263–270.)

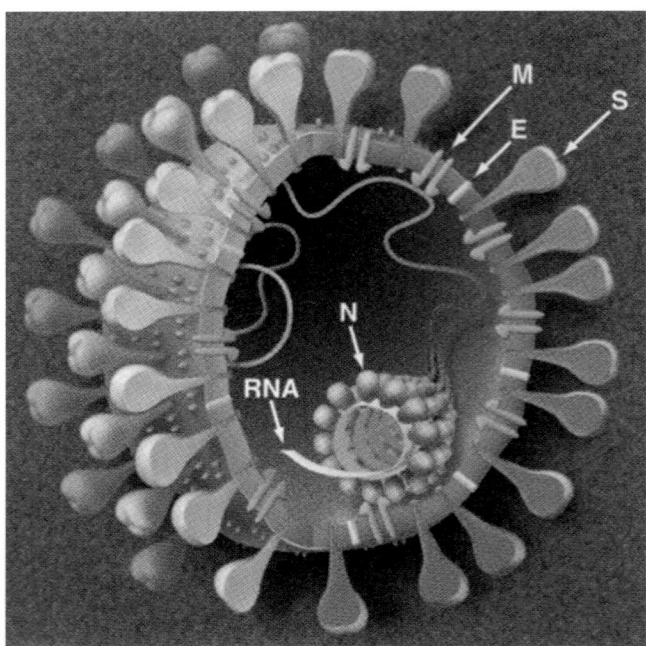

Figure 222-2. Pictorial illustration of a typical coronavirus. The organization of the spike (S), membrane (M), and envelope (E) glycoproteins is shown. The RNA is protected by the nucleocapsid proteins (N). (From Holmes KV, Enjuanes L. The SARS coronavirus: a postgenomic era. Science 2003;300:1377–1378.)

TABLE 222-1. Human and Representative Animal Coronaviruses (CoV)

Group	Common Name of Virus	Acronym	Host	Associated Diseases
1	Human CoV-229E	HCoV-229E	Human	Respiratory tract infection
	Human CoV-NL63	HCoV-NL63	Human	Respiratory tract infection
	Feline infectious peritonitis virus	FIPV	Cat	Hepatitis, respiratory tract, enteric, and neurologic infection
2	Human CoV-OC43	HCoV-OC43	Human	Respiratory tract infection
	Human CoV-HKU1	HCoV-HKU1	Human	Respiratory tract infection and possibly gastroenteritis
	Severe acute respiratory syndrome-CoV[a]	SARS-CoV[a]	Human	Severe acute respiratory syndrome (SARS)
	Mouse hepatitis virus	MHV	Mouse	Hepatitis, encephalitis, and enteric infection
3	Infectious bronchitis virus	IBV	Chicken	Respiratory tract and enteric infection

[a]*SARS-CoV appears to be an outlier of group 2 but some phylogenetic analyses suggest it is the first member of a fourth group of coronaviruses.*[131]

EPIDEMIOLOGY

In the 1930s, coronaviruses were recognized as disease agents in animals.[2] Thirty years later, coronaviruses were identified as agents of respiratory tract infections in humans. The first recognized HCoVs included 229E and OC43. Less well recognized strains, such as B814, OC16, OC37, and OC48, also were described but were not investigated further and to date little is known regarding their prevalence and associated clinical illnesses.[3–5] Coronavirus-like particles also have been detected in stool as possible enteric pathogens, primarily in infants with gastroenteritis and necrotizing enterocolitis, but further characterization has been possible because viruses have not been culturable from these specimens.[6–8] Dramatically, in 2003, severe acute respiratory syndrome (SARS)-CoV was identified as a novel respiratory pathogen responsible for a global outbreak of SARS. This outbreak lasted 9 months and ultimately resulted in 8098 people infected and 774 deaths.[9–13] Most experts believe SARS-CoV evolved from a natural reservoir of SARS-CoV-like viruses in horseshoe bats, with civet cats serving

as intermediate hosts.[14–18] Finding a novel HCoV initiated a renewed interest in CoV research and 2 years later, NL63 (referred to in various publications as NL and NH) and HKU1 were identified as newly recognized HCoVs.[19–21] HCoV-NL63 has since been shown to have been present in human respiratory samples as early as 1981.[22] How HCoV-NL63 and HCoV-HKU1 relate to HCoVs originally described in the 1960s, such as B814, OC16, OC37, and OC48, or the enteric coronavirus-like particles detected in stool, is unclear.[23]

HCoVs other than SARS-CoV are found worldwide and cause disease predominantly in winter and spring months in temperate climates.[22,24] Seroprevalence data suggest that exposure is common in early childhood.[25] Approximately 90% of adults are seropositive for HCoV-229E, HCoV-OC43, and HCoV-NL63 and 60% for HCoV-HKU1.[26] SARS-CoV, on the other hand, has not been identified since December 2003/January 2004 when 4 sporadic cases of SARS with no associated transmission were identified in China[27], community-acquired and 13 cases of laboratory-acquired SARS (2 isolated cases and a cluster of 11 cases with 1 death) were identified in Southeast Asia related to breaches in biosafety practices in different laboratories cultivating SARS-CoV.[28–30] Modes of transmission for HCoV other than SARS-CoV have not been well studied. However, based on studies of other respiratory viruses, it is likely that transmission occurs primarily via a combination of droplet and direct and indirect contact spread.[31] Which mode is most important remains to be determined, and the possible role of aerosol spread needs further study. Droplet and direct contact spread are likely the most common modes of transmission for SARS-CoV, although evidence for indirect contact spread and aerosol spread also exists.[32–39] There is no evidence of vertical transmission of SARS-CoV.[40,41]

Based on data for HCoV-229E and HCoV-OC43, HCoVs other than SARS-CoV are most likely to be transmitted during the first few days of illness when symptoms and viral load in the respiratory tract is highest.[42,43] Further study is needed to confirm if this also is the case for the more recently identified HCoV-NL63 and HCoV-HKU1. SARS-CoV, on the other hand, is most likely to be transmitted during the second week of illness when both symptoms and viral load in the respiratory tract peak.[44–46]

The incubation period for HCoV-229E is 2 to 5 days (median 3 days).[43,47] Further study is needed to confirm the incubation periods for the other non-SARS-HCoVs. The incubation period for SARS-CoV is 2 to 10 days (median 4 days).[44]

PATHOGENESIS AND IMMUNITY

The pathogenesis of HCoV has been best described for 229E and SARS-CoV. For SARS-CoV, most evidence is from infections in adults given that few children were affected by the 2002–2003 outbreak.[48] More study is needed to further understand the pathogenesis of other HCoVs.

HCoV-229E infections are initiated through inoculation of mucosal surfaces of the respiratory tract. HCoV-229E infection is associated with nasal mucosal plasma exudation and increased levels of interferon-γ (IFN-γ) in nasal lavage specimens, which correlate with symptom severity.[49,50] Viral load in respiratory tract specimens peaks within the first 3 days after infection and drops off dramatically at 1 week, correlating with development and subsequent improvement in symptoms.[42,51] Antibodies can be detected starting at 1 week, correlating with the drop in viral load, and reach a maximum levels approximately 1 week later.[52] Thereafter, antibody titers decline slowly. Immunity is not complete and reinfection is common.[52,53] Higher circulating antibody levels and especially levels of specific IgA anti-HCoV correlate with reduced virus shedding and reduced symptoms upon re-exposure.[52,54]

SARS-CoV infection most likely is initiated through inoculation of the respiratory tract mucosa. Subsequent viremia is followed by predominant replication in the lung and gastrointestinal tract.[55,56] Replication at other sites also likely occurs given the wide distribution of SARS-CoV in tissues examined at autopsy.[57,58] Peak viral loads in nasopharyngeal specimens are noted during the second week of symptoms.[45,56] A rise in SARS-CoV specific antibodies typically is seen starting at week 2 after infection. Increasing antibody titers and symptomatic improvement during the second and third week are associated with a fall in the quantity of SARS-CoV, as measured by reverse transcriptase polymerase chain reaction (RT-PCR).[45,59] Paradoxically, despite a fall in SARS-CoV viral load and a rise in SARS-specific antibodies, clinical deterioration is observed in some patients. This suggests that host immune responses likely are responsible for clinical deterioration.[45] Indeed, SARS is associated with an elevation of IFN-γ, inflammatory cytokines interleukin (IL)-1, IL-6, and IL-12 as well as elevations in neutrophil chemokine IL-8, monocyte chemoattractant protein 1, and IFN-γ-inducible protein-10. Levels of IL-6 correlate with severity of disease.[60,61]

CLINICAL MANIFESTATIONS

HCoVs 229E, OC43, NL63, and HKU1, are commonly associated with the common cold, typically characterized by rhinorrhea, nasal congestion, sore throat, sneezing, and cough that may be associated with fever.[20,22,51,62–65] Together, they are the next most common cause of the common cold after rhinoviruses.[66,67] Based on data for HCoV-229E, symptoms typically peak on day 3 or 4 of illness and are self-limiting.[51,68] These HCoVs also may be associated with acute otitis media or exacerbations of asthma.[22,63,65,69,70] Less frequently, these viruses are associated with lower respiratory tract infections including bronchiolitis and pneumonia, primarily in infants and immunocompromised children and adults.[21,21,63,65,71–79] Compared with other HCoVs, HCoV-NL63 more frequently is associated with croup, being the next most common isolate after parainfluenza virus type 1.[80,81] A possible association of HCoV-NL63 with Kawasaki disease was not substantiated.[82,83] HCoV-HKU1 has been associated with symptoms of gastroenteritis, including vomiting and diarrhea, that typically occur along with respiratory symptoms.[65,70,84] HCoV-HKU1 also appears to be more frequently associated with febrile seizures compared with other HCoVs.[65,70]

Compared with other HCoVs, SARS-CoV is associated with more severe symptoms.[85–87] SARS-CoV disproportionately affects adults, who typically manifest fever, myalgia, headache, malaise, and chills followed by a nonproductive cough and dyspnea 3 to 5 days later. Approximately 25% develop watery diarrhea. Respiratory distress progresses to require intubation and ventilation in 25% of cases. The overall associated mortality rate is approximately 10%, most deaths occurring in the third week of illness.[86] The case-fatality rate in persons over the age of 60 approaches 50%.[88] Typical laboratory abnormalities include lymphopenia and increased serum lactate dehydrogenase and creatine kinase levels.[89,90] The majority have progressive unilateral or bilateral ill-defined air-space infiltrates on chest imaging.[89,91–93] Pneumothoraces and other signs of barotrauma are common in critically ill patients receiving mechanical ventilation.[86]

Infants and children appear to be protected against SARS-CoV infection, and clinical manifestations in infected children are less severe. Notably no infants or children died due to SARS-CoV infection in the 2002–2003 outbreak.[48,94–97] Infants and children <12 years of age who develop SARS typically manifest fever, cough, and rhinorrhea. Associated lymphopenia is less severe and radiographic changes are milder and generally resolve more quickly than in adolescents and adults. Adolescents who developed SARS had clinical courses more closely resembling that of adults, manifesting fever, myalgia, headache, and chills. Adolescents are more likely to develop dyspnea, hypoxemia, and worsening chest radiographic findings. Laboratory abnormalities are comparable with those in adults.

Women infected with SARS-CoV during pregnancy who survive have an increased risk of spontaneous miscarriage, preterm delivery, and intrauterine growth restriction.[40,41,98] Two neonates born to mothers with SARS in the 2002–2003 outbreak developed gastrointestinal complications (jejunal perforation, necrotizing enterocolitis with ileal perforation) shortly after birth but neither had clinical evidence of SARS-CoV infection.[41] It is unclear whether these findings were related to complications of maternal SARS-CoV infection or treatments used during pregnancy, such as ribavirin and corticosteroids.

DIAGNOSIS

In the past, the diagnosis of infections due to HCoVs typically was not attempted in clinical settings outside of outbreak situations or epidemiologic surveys. However, the 2002–2003 SARS outbreak renewed interest in identifying the etiology of respiratory tract infections and some specialized laboratories now offer comprehensive diagnostic testing for respiratory tract specimens primarily based on RT-PCR; some panels include detection of HCoV.[65,99] Antibody tests also are available for SARS-CoV.[100]

Upper and lower respiratory tract specimens are the most appropriate samples for viral detection when testing is available.[42,56,63,65,101] Stool samples frequently are positive in patients with SARS and have been positive in some children with HCoV-HKU1 infection.[56,70,84,101] Serum samples may be positive in patients with SARS-CoV. For HCoV-299E and HCoV-OC43, specimens are most likely to be positive during the first few days of illness;[42] whether this also is true for HCoV-NL63 and HCoV-HKU1 needs further study. For SARS-CoV, serum samples for RT-PCR testing are most likely to be positive in the first week of illness,[55,102] but respiratory and stool specimens may not be positive until the second week of illness when symptoms and viral loads peak.[45,56] Compared with adults, infants and children with SARS-CoV infections are less likely to have positive specimens. This is consistent with the milder symptoms and presumed correspondingly lower viral loads in children.[94,95]

Laboratory guidance for SARS-CoV diagnostic testing is available on the Centers for Disease Control and Prevention website.[103] Given the potential for false-positive results and the associated public health implications, testing for SARS-CoV in the absence of known person-to-person transmission of SARS-CoV only should be done with caution, preferably in consultation with regional public health departments, and when there is a high degree of clinical suspicion with no alternative diagnosis.

TREATMENT

Because of mild symptoms and the self-limited nature of HCoV infections other than SARS-CoV, few treatment studies have been performed. Generally, care is supportive. SARS-CoV infections are more serious. Corticosteroids, type 1 IFN agents, convalescent plasma, ribavirin, and lopinavir/ritonavir all have been used to treat SARS.[89,104–107] For most of these treatments, anecdotal reports suggest benefit, and in vitro assays and animal models are supportive.[89,104–116] Despite some reports of anecdotal clinical improvement with ribavirin, however, in vitro studies do not support likely efficacy.[113,117,118] Since the SARS outbreak, other agents have been tested in vitro and appear promising. These include viral entry and protease inhibiting agents, RNA interfering agents, and glycyrrhizin.[119] However, no definitive conclusions can be drawn regarding efficacy of these treatments. This is noteworthy because controlled studies have not been performed for any of these agents, and there are reports of uneventful recovery for patients given supportive care alone. In the event that SARS-CoV re-emerges, clarification of the effectiveness of these treatments through controlled clinical trials will be needed.

PREVENTION

Meticulous hand and respiratory hygiene is the most useful and easily implemented control measure to curb the spread of all respiratory viruses including HCoVs.[120,121] Other preventive measures have been assessed. Prophylactic intranasal IFN-α has been shown to reduce the duration and severity of 229E infection in research settings but has not been used clinically.[122,123] IFN-α has not been studied for prevention of other HCoVs. A proprietary extract of the roots of North American ginseng (*Panax quinquefolium*) has been shown to reduce the number of colds as well as the severity and duration of cold symptoms in adults when taken daily, presumably due to immune stimulation.[124–127] Efficacy for decrease in colds specifically due to HCoVs has not been studied.

Healthcare personnel should wear a mask when evaluating persons with a cough illness and should use a gown, gloves, mask, and eye protection for the duration of illness when caring for children hospitalized with signs and symptoms of a respiratory tract infection.[128] The same precautions, with the replacement of the mask with a respirator, if available, plus negative-pressure isolation are recommended for patients with SARS-CoV infection for the duration of illness or 10 days after resolution of fever, provided respiratory symptoms are absent or improving.[128] Cleaning and disinfection of environmental surfaces that are frequently touched by infected persons, using standard disinfectants, should decrease the potential for indirect transmission of HCoVs via fomites.[129]

The control of the 2002–2003 SARS outbreak is credited to the rapid identification of cases and early implementation of infection control and public health measures including contact tracing and quarantine. If SARS-CoV re-emerges, all measures should be implemented quickly in an attempt to prevent a recurrent worldwide outbreak.[130,131]

Key Points. Epidemiology, Clinical Manifestations, Diagnosis, and Treatment of Human Coronavirus (HCoV) Infections

EPIDEMIOLOGY

- HCoVs 229E, OC43, NL63, and HKU1 – found worldwide; exposure common in early childhood; in temperate climates, primarily causes infections in winter and spring months
- SARS-CoV – not identified in the world since January 2004 (soon after the 2002–2003 global outbreak of SARS); possibility/probability of a large-scale re-emergence of SARS is unknown
- Most common modes of transmission are through droplet and direct and indirect contact

CLINICAL MANIFESTATIONS

- HCoVs 229E, OC43, NL63, and HKU1 – associated with the common cold, acute otitis media, asthma exacerbations, and less frequently, bronchiolitis and pneumonia; HCoV-NL63 – also associated with croup; HCoV-HKU1 – also associated with vomiting and diarrhea frequently with respiratory tract symptoms; appears to be associated more frequently with febrile seizures compared with other HCoVs
- SARS-CoV – associated with SARS with an attendant mortality rate of 10% which primarily affects adults and adolescents; children <12 years of age who develop SARS typically have less severe manifestations (fever, cough, and rhinorrhea)

DIAGNOSIS

- Upper and lower respiratory tract specimens can be tested by HCoV RT-PCR
- Stool samples frequently are positive in patients with SARS-CoV and have been positive in some children with HCoV-HKU1 infection; antibody tests also are available for SARS-CoV

TREATMENT

- HCoVs 229E, OC43, NL63, and HKU1 – supportive care
- SARS-CoV – no definitive treatment can be recommended because of lack of controlled trials

223 Parainfluenza Viruses

Asunción Mejías and Octavio Ramilo

Human parainfluenza viruses (HPIVs) were first identified in humans in the late 1950s.[1] Initially described in children with croup, the role of HPIVs as an important cause of acute respiratory tract infections in patients who are immunocompromised, have chronic conditions, or are elderly, has been recognized increasingly.[2–5] In otherwise healthy children, HPIVs commonly cause upper respiratory tract infections (URIs), pneumonia, and exacerbations of reactive airway disease.[3,6] Studies have shown that HPIVs are responsible from 6% to 11% of total hospitalizations in children less than 5 years of age, highlighting the need for effective vaccines.[3,7]

DESCRIPTION OF THE PATHOGEN

Microbiology

HPIVs are pleomorphic enveloped RNA viruses that belong to the Paramyxoviridae family. There are four antigenically distinct types, types 1, 2, 3, and 4, with two antigenic subtypes, 4A and 4B.[8–10] The five parainfluenza viruses are divided into two different genera based upon complement fixation and hemagglutinating antigens. Parainfluenza types 1 and 3 belong to the *Paramyxovirus* genus, and parainfluenza types 2, 4A, and 4B belong to the *Rubulavirus* genus.

Other viruses in this family include mumps, measles, Hendra and Nipah viruses, respiratory syncytial virus (RSV), and human metapneumovirus (HMPV).[11,12] The HPIV serotypes and subtypes display substantial serologic cross-reactivity. The single-stranded negative-sense nonsegmented RNA genome (-ssRNA) of HPIV contains 15,000 to 16,000 nucleotides that encode at least six common structural proteins. The viral envelope is derived from the host cell and it is covered with glycoprotein spikes. There are two mayor glycoproteins that play a major role in pathogenesis, the hemaglutinin-neuraminidase (HN) and fusion (F) proteins. HN is coupled with the activated F protein to allow the virion entry into the cell. Activation of the F protein is mediated by cellular proteases. The specific localization of these proteases may influence specific member-HPIV cellular tropism.

Pathogenesis and Immunity

HPIVs replicate exclusively in cells of the respiratory epithelium.[13] Clinically, HPIVs most commonly affect the large airways of the lower respiratory tract causing croup.[14] Viral tropism for this anatomic location seems to be related to the ciliated epithelial cells that are abundant in the respiratory tract.[15] In more severe cases, infection spreads to the lower respiratory tract with the development of bronchiolitis or pneumonia.[16] The mechanism of airway and parenchymal injury and resulting symptoms probably are a combination of direct viral cytopathic effect and indirect effects of the host immune response.[17]

HPIVs induce the production of different cytokines and chemokines in animal models, in in vitro systems, and in children with acute infection.[18–20] The magnitude of the cytokine response probably is related to the clinical syndrome and viral type. Local production of interferon (IFN)-γ was detected in 30% of children with HPIV-lower respiratory tract disease and local concentrations of interleukin (IL)-8 were significantly higher in children infected with HPIV-3 compared with other HPIV types.[20,21] In addition, significant concentrations of MIP-1α (macrophage inflammatory protein-1α) and RANTES (regulated upon activation, normal T lymphocyte expressed and secreted), chemokines with potent effects on the recruitment and degranulation of eosinophils and

basophils, were found in nasopharyngeal (NP) samples of children with acute HPIV URI.[22] A disruption in the mechanism that regulates metalloproteinases has been associated with increased disease severity in infants with bronchiolitis caused by both HPIV and RSV.[23] Peripheral blood mononuclear cells (PBMCs) exposed to HPIV-3 produced large amounts of IL-10. This immunoregulatory cytokine has been shown to contribute to viral inhibition, decreased T-lymphocyte proliferation and to protect T lymphocytes from HPIV-3 mediated apoptosis.[24]

Necrosis and occasionally proliferation of the bronchiolar epithelium accompany the destruction of ciliated epithelial cells in children with pneumonia and bronchiolitis.[25] A peribronchiolar infiltrate of lymphocytes, plasma cells, and macrophages appears along with edema and excessive mucus production. Interalveolar walls thicken with mononuclear cell infiltrates, and if pneumonia is prominent, the alveoli fill with fluid.[17,26]

Host defense against HPIVs is mediated largely by humoral immunity towards epitopes on the surface glycoproteins of the virus – HN and F.[13] Mucosal immunity appears to play a key role in controlling the disease. Studies in adults, after experimental challenge with HPIV-1 and HPIV-2, indicate that local neutralizing antibody in secretions correlates better with protection than does serum antibody.[27,28] In children, secretory antibodies appear 7 to 10 days after the onset of symptoms and peak at about 2 weeks after disease onset.[29] Parainfluenza-specific mucosal IgE antibody responses at the time of illness were greater in infants with HPIVs bronchiolitis than in those with only upper respiratory tract infections.[30]

Most children are born with neutralizing antibodies to all four HPIV types. Titers fall sharply during the first 6 months of life. Most antibody responses involve serum immunoglobulin G1 (IgG1), but levels of serum IgG3, IgG4, IgA, and IgM rise significantly in 30% of adults.[31] HPIVs are monotypic antigenically and although antigenic variations have been described they are related to the heterogeneity within HPIV viruses rather than antigenic viral drifts.[32] Thus reinfections, which occur many times throughout life, most likely reflect waning immunity. After several infections, antibodies may develop that cross-neutralize different parainfluenza strains. This cross-reactivity is most noted within Paramyxoviridae subfamilies (e.g., HPIV-1 and -3, or HPIV-2 and -4).

In immunocompetent individuals, reinfections are more likely to cause only upper respiratory tract symptoms.[33] In epidemiologic studies, HPIV-3 was isolated in 143 children (50% of all HPIV isolates) <5 years of age. Of those, 9% had subsequent reinfections with isolation of the same virus type >1 month after the initial infection. Although reinfections are thought to induce increased resistance to lower respiratory tract infections (LRIs) by the infecting serotype, protection does not seem to be entirely based on increased humoral immunity.[31,33] In these studies, the clinical manifestations of the reinfection episodes did not differ from those of the initial episode. No reinfections were seen with HPIV-1 or HPIV-2.[6,34]

Results of studies conducted in animal models of acute HPIV infection suggest that CD8+ T-lymphocyte-mediated immune responses are critical for viral clearance.[35,36] Infants with HPIV-induced croup have defective regulation of cell-mediated immune responses compared with children with simple URI, suggesting that abnormal cellular immunity contributes to the pathogenesis of the disease.[37] Moreover, the prolonged viral shedding and severe disease manifestations observed in individuals with defective cell-mediated immunity indicate the important role of T lymphocytes in controlling infection.[38–40]

TABLE 223-1. Clinical and Epidemiologic Characteristics of Human Parainfluenza Virus Infections

	HPIV-1	HPIV-2	HPIV-3	HPIV-4
Age	1–5 years	2–6 years	<6 months	Unknown
Seasonality	Fall, odd-numbered years	Fall, follows HPIV-1	Endemic; spring/summer	Not defined
Most common clinical manifestation	Croup	Croup	LRI	URI[10]
Viral shedding	1 week	1 week	3 weeks	Unknown
Hospitalization rates[7]	0.32–1.59/1000	0.1–0.86/1000	0.48–2.6/1000	Unknown

LRI, lower respiratory tract infection; URI, upper respiratory tract infection.

EPIDEMIOLOGY

The different serotypes of HPIV have distinct epidemiologic patterns that can vary depending on the geographic location, but overall HPIV seasonal patterns are predictable, and cyclic. HPIVs are transmitted from close person-to-person direct contact and exposure to contaminated nasopharyngeal secretions through respiratory tract droplets and fomites.

HPIV-3 is the most frequently recovered HPIV, is endemic, with more prominent isolation during spring and summer but often continuing into autumn, especially when other HPIV outbreaks are absent.[6,33] HPIV-1 causes the largest, most defined outbreaks of croup, in the fall of odd-numbered years. Outbreaks of HPIV-2, although more erratic, usually follow HPIV-1 outbreaks.[26] A major increase in the number of cases of croup in the autumn usually indicates a parainfluenza type 1 or 2 outbreak. HPIV-4A and -B are isolated rarely and seasonality is not well described (Table 223-1).[41,42] The age of primary infection varies by serotype. By 12 months of age, 50% of infants have serologic evidence of infection by HPIV-3 and by 5 years of age, almost all children have been infected with all HPIVs.[43,44] A prospective surveillance study conducted in Houston, Texas, showed that rates of primary infection in the first and second year of life were 62 and 81 per 100 child-years, respectively. The risk of LRI associated with primary infection was approximately 10% in the first, and 20% in the second year of life (Figure 223-1).[33]

Infection with HPIV-3, the HPIV type that most closely resembles RSV, frequently occurs in infants <6 months of age and is a prominent cause of LRI. Infections with HPIV-1 and HPIV-2 viruses are seen most commonly in children between 1 and 5 years of age. Age at acquisition of HPIV-4 infection is not well established (Table 223-1). Traditionally, HPIVs have been considered the second most common cause of hospitalization for respiratory disease in children.[1] Reports on the annual rates of HPIV hospitalization in children <5 years of age have varied from 1.0 to 5.1 per 1000 children.[6,7] Based on a 4-year longitudinal study, rates of hospitalization for children <5 years of age in the United States are similar for HPIVs, HMPV, and influenza virus; 1.02/1000, 1.2/1000, and 0.9/1000 children, respectively. In comparison, rates of hospitalization for RSV in the same population are three-fold higher (3.0/1000).[3,45] HPIVs are responsible for 18,000 to 35,000 pediatric hospitalizations for croup each year.[46,47] The costs associated with a typical annual HPIV-1 or -2 fall outbreak have been estimated to be ~ $190 million.[48] In addition, these viruses are associated with acute respiratory illness with substantial morbidity in immunocompromised patients, those with underlying chronic cardiopulmonary conditions, and elderly people.[49–51]

Transmission

HPIVs, particularly HPIV-3, are highly transmittable. In closed settings, HPIV-3 infection occurs in virtually all exposed children. Secondary attack rates for HPIV-1 and HPIV-2 are 65% to 79%.[2] The usual incubation period for HPIV infection is 2 to 4 days.[16] Depending on the serotype, children with primary HPIV infection can shed virus from 1 week before the onset of symptomatology to more than 3 weeks after symptoms resolve. Children with primary HPIV-1 infection shed virus for an average of 4 to 7 days.

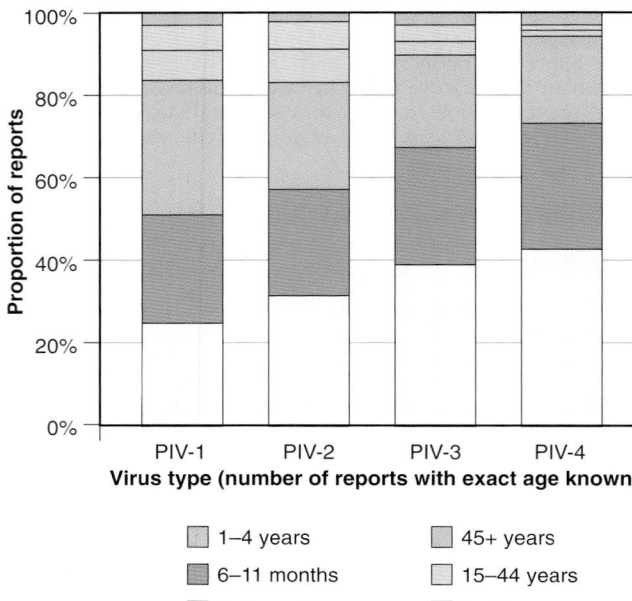

Figure 223-1. Proportion of reports of different parainfluenza virus (PIV) serotypes by age from laboratories in England and Wales from 1985 to 1997. (Redrawn from Laurichesse H, Dedman D, Watson JM, et al. Epidemiologic features of parainfluenza virus infections: laboratory surveillance in England and Wales, 1975–1997. Eur J Epidemiol 1999;15:475–484.)

In the Houston Family Study, ~17% of children infected with HPIV-3 shed virus for as long as 3 to 4 weeks.[52]

Climatologic factors may impact the shedding of HPIVs; in vitro studies have shown that aerosol particles of HPIV-3 survive longer when the relative humidity is 20% rather than 50% or 80%.[53] If kept from drying, all HPIVs survive on porous surfaces for up to 4 hours and on nonporous surfaces for as long as 10 hours.[54] Infection most likely is transmitted by contamination of hands with secretions containing virus, followed by autoinoculation. A study in adult volunteers testing this mode of transmission showed that, after 20 minutes on contaminated hands, HPIV was not transferable readily to the fingers of volunteers.[55] Outbreaks of HPIV-3 infection are associated with high attack rates and variable morbidity and have been reported in neonatal nurseries, pediatric wards, and bone marrow transplant units.[38,39,56–59]

CLINICAL MANIFESTATIONS

HPIVs cause a variety of respiratory tract illnesses (Figure 223-2), dependent upon age, virus serotype, and season. In healthy children, most illnesses involve the upper respiratory tract and up to 50% are associated with otitis media.[60] In general, HPIV-1 and HPIV-2 are associated with croup whereas HPIV-3 causes bronchiolitis and pneumonia. Croup is the most common HPIV-associated diagnosis.[3,61] Lack of specific epidemiologic data on HPIV-4 limits understanding of the clinical significance of this serotype.[6,48,62,63]

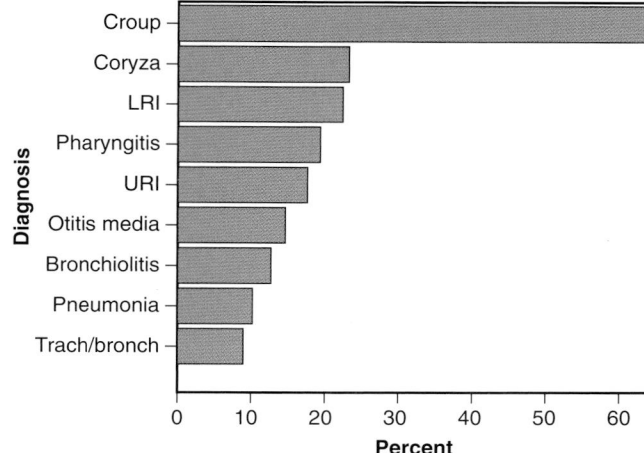

Figure 223-2. Clinical illnesses caused by parainfluenza viruses. LRI, lower respiratory tract infection; trach/bronch, tracheobronchitis; URI, upper respiratory tract infection. (Redrawn from Reed G, Jewett PH, Thompson J, et al. Epidemiology and clinical impact of parainfluenza virus infections in otherwise healthy infants and young children <5 years old. J Infect Dis 1997;175:807–813.)

Upper Respiratory Tract Disease

In children, HPIVs account for 18% to 45% of all URIs.[6,64] Infection typically starts with coryza, rhinorrhea, pharyngitis without cervical lymphadenopathy, and low-grade fever. All four serotypes have been recovered from children and adults with the common cold. Upper respiratory tract illness (URI) is the typical manifestation of HPIV infection in immunocompetent adults.

Laryngotracheichitis (Croup)

Croup (laryngotracheitis) is a term used to encompasses a heterogeneous group of illnesses that affect the larynx, the trachea, and the bronchi. Croup affects about 3% of children in a given year, with a peak incidence between ages 6 months and 3 years.[65,66] HPIVs are the most frequent cause of croup, accounting for almost 75% of all cases. HPIV-1 is the most common and is estimated to cause 18% of all cases of croup.[6,64] Croup is characterized by fever, hoarse barking cough, laryngeal obstruction, dyspnea, and inspiratory stridor. Typically, in mild to moderate disease symptoms last 3 to 5 days; progression is unpredictable, and sudden respiratory failure can occur.[28] In cases presenting with severe stridor, differentiation from epiglottitis can be facilitated by lateral neck radiography. The typical finding in those with croup is subglottic narrowing or the "steeple sign".[67] In some children, repeated episodes of spasmodic croup may occur. Whether these episodes are separate illnesses is not clear. Old studies in infants with a history of croup (particularly recurrent croup) identified abnormalities in lung function that can persist for several years.[68,69] Whether these abnormalities were present as a result of laryngotracheitis or whether they preceded and contributed to the laryngotracheitis is unknown.

Bronchiolitis

Historically, HPIVs have been considered the second in frequency to RSV as a cause of bronchiolitis.[70] However, the introduction of more sensitive molecular diagnostic tools has identified other respiratory viruses more frequently than HPIV as etiologic agents of bronchiolitis.[71–73] All four types of HPIV can cause bronchiolitis, but HPIV-3 typically has been reported most commonly.[3,7] Over 80% of cases of bronchiolitis occur during the first year of life, the majority in infants under 6 months of age. HPIV-1 and HPIV-3 cause 5% to 15% of bronchiolitis cases in children, and 2.8 of every 1000 children with such infections require hospitalization.[6,26,74] Most hospitalizations for bronchiolitis occur from November through April. A study conducted in the U.S. using National Hospital Discharge survey data over 18 years showed that among children <1 year of age, bronchiolitis hospitalizations related to HPIVs peaked earlier during odd-numbered years than even-numbered years, resulting in a longer season.[7] Bronchiolitis caused by RSV, HMPV, or HPIVs are clinically indistinguishable. Predominant symptoms include fever, tachypnea, retractions, expiratory wheezing, rales, and air trapping.

Asthma

Virus-induced asthma and asthma exacerbations are more commonly associated with respiratory viruses other than HPIVs.[75,76] Nevertheless, asthma is diagnosed commonly in children >2 years of age with any type of HPIV infection.[3] In adults, HPIVs have not been associated strongly with asthma exacerbations.[77]

Pneumonia

Pneumonia has been associated with all HPIV types. HPIV-1, HPIV-2, and HPIV-3 are responsible for ~10% of outpatient pneumonia cases and for 8% to 15% of inpatient pneumonia cases in children of all ages.[78–82] The percentage of hospitalized children diagnosed with HPIV pneumonia, including those requiring admission to a pediatric intensive care unit, is higher in the first year of life and, as with bronchiolitis, mostly associated with HPIV-3 infection.[3,26,63,70,80–84] HPIV pneumonia occurs more frequently and is more severe in chronically ill or immunocompromised children.[63,85] In hematopoietic stem cell transplant (HSCT) recipients, HPIV infection can result in refractory pneumonia with prolonged viral shedding, viral dissemination, and a high (~40%) mortality rate.[86–89]

Otitis Media

Acute otitis media can follow HPIV URI in 30% to 50%[6,60,64,90] of children 3 to 4 days after the onset of URI, and frequently is a mixed viral-bacterial infection.[91,92] In a study conducted over 20 years in previously healthy children <5 years old, the rate of acute otitis media was higher for HPIV-3 than for HPIV-1 and HPIV-2.[6,93–95]

Other Manifestations

Neonates, particularly premature infants infected with HPIV, can manifest apnea.[3] An association between sudden infant death syndrome and infection caused by any of the HPIV types has been described.[96,97] Fever and febrile seizures have been reported in young infants with HPIV infections. A recent study conducted over 4 years in 2798 children <5 years of age showed that HPIVs accounted for 6.8% of all hospitalizations for fever, acute respiratory illness, or both.[3] High fever is observed in <10% of HPIV illnesses.[6] Conjunctivitis occurs in >35% of children with no specific association with viral type.[6] Rarely, HPIVs have been isolated in patients with parotitis, myopericarditis, aseptic meningitis, encephalitis, or Guillain–Barré syndrome.[3,6,93–95,98–100] This, coupled with the close family homology of HIPV with neuroinvasive paramyxoviruses, including measles, Hendra, and Nipah viruses, suggests that some strains of HPIV may be neurotropic. Disseminated infection can occur in immunosuppressed people.[87]

LABORATORY FINDINGS AND DIAGNOSIS

Specific diagnosis requires isolation of the virus or detection of viral antigens or viral RNA in respiratory secretions. HPIVs rarely are isolated in otherwise healthy asymptomatic children, thus detection of the virus in the context of an acute respiratory illness strongly suggests causality.[101] Respiratory specimens for viral diagnosis should be collected early in the course of illness. Nasopharyngeal (NP) aspirates or swabs are the preferred method for sample collection. Studies suggest that the rates of HPIV detection may be similar with either NP swabs or NP aspirates.[102] In immunocompromised hosts or HSCT recipients with involvement of the lower respiratory tract, direct sampling via bronchoalveolar lavage or lung biopsy may be necessary to recover the virus. Adequate specimen collection and handling is critical for the success of isolating the virus. After collection, samples should be placed immediately on ice (or refrigerated at 4 °C) and transported promptly to the laboratory. Isolating the virus by tissue culture remains the gold standard. Primary monkey kidney (LCC-MK2) or human embryonic kidney cell cultures are optimal for viral recovery, usually in 5 days, except for HPIV-4, which requires up to 3 weeks of incubation.[103] Rapid antigen diagnostic tests using indirect immunofluorescence (IF) are available, and although specific, are less sensitive than culture.[103,104] Reverse transcriptase-polymerase chain reaction (RT-PCR) has been shown to be highly sensitive and specific, it has replaced tissue culture and IF techniques, and is becoming the preferred diagnostic assay in many laboratories.[105] It is the preferred method for the diagnosis of HPIV-4 and has proved to be especially useful for the diagnosis of HPIV infections in adults and immunocompromised patients in whom viral shedding is low.[106,107] Serologic assays based on hemagglutination inhibition or enzyme immunoassays can be used to detect serum IgM or IgG antibodies against HPIV but have limited value in patient management.

TREATMENT

No specific antiviral therapy is available for HPIV. In general, most HPIV infections are self-limited in immunocompetent hosts and do not require treatment. Ribavirin has demonstrable in vitro activity against HPIVs. The use of ribavirin, mostly inhaled, has been reported in immunocompromised children and adults with severe HPIV pneumonia with or without concomitant administration of immune globulin intravenous (IGIV); however, controlled studies are lacking.[108–110] Treatment of bronchiolitis and croup is supportive. During the acute infection, efforts should be aimed at decreasing healthcare-associated infections. In addition to standard precautions, contact precautions are recommended for hospitalized infants and young children for the duration of illness. Prevention of environmental contamination by respiratory tract secretions and careful hand hygiene should control healthcare-associated spread.

SPECIAL CONSIDERATIONS

Immunocompromised Hosts

Parainfluenza infections are associated with substantial morbidity and mortality in children and adults with congenital or acquired immunodeficiencies. Most cases of HPIV pneumonia in immunocompromised hosts undergoing HSCT have been associated with

HPIV-3.[59,86,109] Solid organ transplant recipients also have increased HPIV-associated mortality and substantial morbidity, including chronic rejection. HPIV infection has been associated with the development of bronchiolitis obliterans in lung transplant recipients.[86,111–113] Airflow decline has been linked not only to parainfluenza pneumonia, but also to HPIV upper respiratory infections in HSCT recipients.[114] The most severe illnesses and 90% of the deaths related to HPIV pneumonia occur in the first 100 days after transplantation, when lymphopenia is most pronounced. Use of unrelated donors and systemic corticosteroids have been identified as risk factors for progression to pneumonia.[108,109] HPIV-3 pneumonia has been associated with other pulmonary copathogens, including *Aspergillus* spp., in approximately half of HSCT cases.[115]

Patients with primary immunodeficiencies can have prolonged shedding of HPIVs, particularly parainfluenza type 3.[116] For example, fatal pneumonia has been described in children with severe combined immunodeficiency and interferon-γ receptor deficiency syndrome.[87,117,118] In children infected with the human immunodeficiency virus (HIV)-1, HPIV infections have been associated with increased morbidity and mortality in developing countries.[85,119] Although prolonged shedding occurs in HIV-infected children, HPIV infections do not appear to be more severe in developed countries.[118]

PREVENTION

The lack of durable immunity and full understanding of the mechanisms responsible for immune protection has hampered the development of HPIV vaccines.[120] The first attempts to develop an HPIV vaccine were conducted in the late 1960s. The formalin-inactivated vaccine preparations used in infants were immunogenic and did not cause enhanced disease, but they did not confer protection.[121] Currently, viral protein subunit vaccines consisting of HN or F protein have shown some efficacy in animals, but have not been entered into clinical trials.[122] Two strategies have been used for the development of live-attenuated HPIV-3 vaccines: the use of an antigenically related strain (bovine-PIV-3), and the use of a cold-adapted HPIV-3 strain. Both candidate vaccines have shown to be safe, well tolerated, and immunogenic when administered intranasally to seropositive and seronegative children.[123–125] Other approaches to develop an HPIV-1 vaccine and live-attenuated HPIV-2 vaccines using reverse genetic manipulations of the L-protein gene have been reported.[126,127]

Key Points. Diagnosis and Management of Human Parainfluenza Virus (HPIV) Infections

MICROBIOLOGY
- Enveloped negative-sense single-stranded RNA paramyxovirus
- Five HPIV types: HPIV-1, -2, -3, -4A, and -4B

EPIDEMIOLOGY
- Different HPIVs have distinct epidemiologic patterns:
  - HPIV-3 is endemic
  - HPIV-1 and HPIV-2 cause outbreaks of croup
- Age of primary infection varies for each serotype
- By age 5 years, almost all children have been infected with all HPIVs
- HPIV does not confer protective immunity and reinfections are common throughout life
- HPIVs are transmitted from person-to-person by direct contact and exposure to contaminated droplets and fomites

CLINICAL FEATURES
- HPIVs account for 18% to 45% of all upper respiratory tract illnesses in children
- Acute otititis media occurs in 30% to 50% of children after HPIV upper respiratory tract infection
- HPIV-3 is associated predominantly with bronchiolitis and pneumonia (children <1 year)

- HPIV-1 and -2 are the most frequent causes of croup in children 1 to 5 years of age
- Full spectrum of HPIV-4 is not well understood
- In hematopoietic stem cell transplant patients, HPIV infection can result in refractory pneumonia with ~40% of mortality rates

DIAGNOSIS
- Direct fluorescent antibody, PCR, or viral culture from respiratory secretions (nasopharyngeal swab or aspirate)
- PCR is preferred method for HPIV-4 confirmation and in immunocompromised/elderly persons
- Respiratory samples should be collected early on the course of disease and transported on ice to the laboratory
- Bronchoalveolar lavage or lung biopsy in immunocompromised or HSCT

TREATMENT
- Symptomatic
- Ribavirin (inhaled) with or without IGIV has been used in immunocompromised persons with severe pneumonia
- No vaccine is available

224 Mumps Virus

Kathleen Gutierrez

Mumps is an acute viral infection of childhood that typically involves swelling of one or both parotid glands, although many different organs can be infected. Childhood mumps is uncommon in the United States since the implementation of widespread immunization. Recent mumps outbreaks involving highly vaccinated populations have prompted re-evaluation of current strategies for mumps prevention.[1-3,3a]

DESCRIPTION OF THE PATHOGEN

Mumps virus is a member of the Rubulavirus genus in the Paramyxoviridae family. Mumps is an enveloped negative-stranded RNA virus with an irregular spherical shape ranging in size from 100 to 600 nm. The viral genome is contained in a helical nucleocapsid enclosed in a trilayered envelope studded with glycoproteins possessing hemagglutinin and neuraminidase (HN protein) and cell fusion (F-protein) activities. The virus contains seven structural proteins, including nucleocapsid-associated protein (NP), a (V and I)/phosphoprotein (P), membrane or matrix protein (M), a high-molecular-weight protein (L), SH protein, HN protein, and F protein. There is one serotype of virus. The gene for the SH protein is the most variable part of the mumps virus genome and amplification of a sequence of the SH gene region by polymerase chain reaction (PCR) is used to classify the virus into 12 genotypes.[4,5]

Mumps virus grows well in a number of cell lines, including primary rhesus monkey kidney cells, green monkey kidney cells, Vero cells, and HeLa cells. The typical cytopathic effect in tissue culture includes rounding and fusion of cells into giant multinucleated syncytia and the presence of intracytoplasmic inclusions.[5]

EPIDEMIOLOGY

In the U.S., the reported incidence of mumps declined following introduction of mumps vaccine in 1967 and recommendation for its routine use in 1977. After expanded recommendations for a 2-dose measles, mumps, and rubella (MMR) vaccine schedule for measles control in 1989, mumps cases declined further.[6] During 2001 to 2003, fewer than 300 mumps cases were reported each year – a 99% decline from the 185,691 cases reported in 1968. However, an increase in cases occurred late in 2005 (Figure 224-1).[7] Following a first case of mumps on a college campus in eastern Iowa in December 2005, outbreaks in 8 midwestern states resulted in 6584 cases (Figure 224-2). The virus strain isolated was

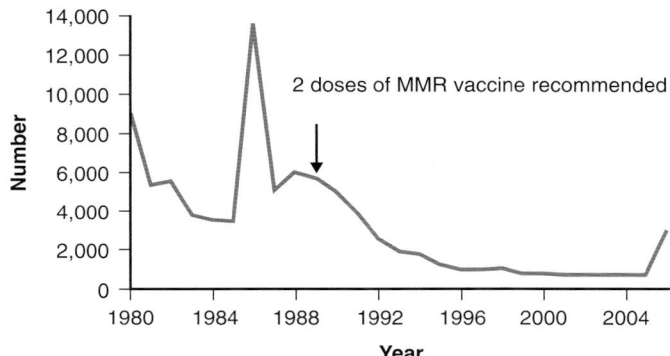

Figure 224-1. Number of reported cases of mumps by year – United States, 1980 to 2006. MMR, measles, mumps, and rubella.

Figure 224-2. Outbreak-related mumps by state, January 1 to May 2, 2006.

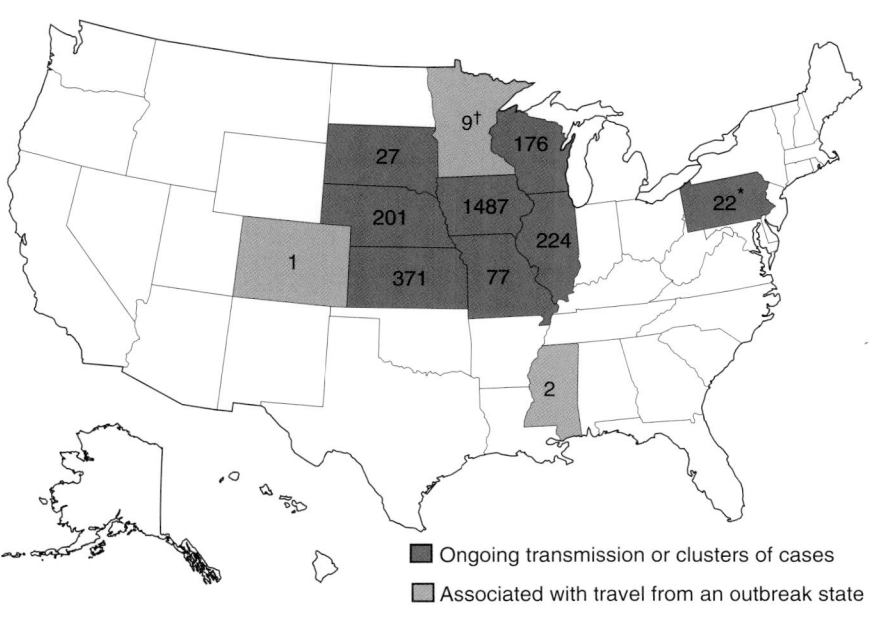

■ Ongoing transmission or clusters of cases

□ Associated with travel from an outbreak state

[†]Three cases related to outbreak
[*] Twelve cases related

of genotype (G) lineage. Almost 40% of cases were 18 to 24 years of age.[8] Parotitis was reported in the majority of individuals; complications of orchitis, meningitis, encephalitis, deafness, oophoritis, mastitis, and pancreatitis also occurred. A smaller outbreak in 2006 involved students at the University of Virginia. Genetic analysis suggested that the virus was not linked to the strain associated with the outbreak in the midwest.[9] In June of 2009, an 11-year-old boy traveled to the United Kingdom during a time when several thousand cases of mumps were reported in that country.[10] Shortly after his return, he attended a summer camp for tradition-observant Jewish boys and developed mumps at camp. Subsequently, as of January 2010, more than 1500 mumps cases were reported in the New York–New Jersey area. The outbreak generally was confined to members of the tradition-observant Jewish community and most cases occurred in vaccinated persons. Current outbreaks have occurred in settings where prolonged close contact may facilitate transmission of virus, even in immunized individuals.[3] Transmission of mumps within a hospital setting has been reported.[11]

Endemic mumps infections are most common in winter and early spring. Although rates of infection are similar in males and females, males are more likely to have complications.

The incubation period ranges from 12 to 25 days. An estimated 80% to 90% of nonimmune household contacts become infected.[12] Attack rates for development of clinically apparent disease are substantially lower in recent outbreaks, especially for those who received 2 doses of MMR vaccine.[13] Patients are most contagious 1 to 2 days before the onset of symptoms and for 5 days thereafter; virus has been isolated from saliva 7 days before symptoms and up to 9 days after the appearance of parotid swelling. Both clinical and subclinical infections provide lifelong immunity; reinfection occurs rarely. Children with subclinical disease are infectious.[14]

PATHOGENESIS

Mumps infection is acquired after contact with infected respiratory tract secretions. Viral replication in the nasopharyngeal mucosa and regional lymph nodes is followed by primary viremia, which results in spread of infection to multiple organs, including the central nervous system (CNS) and glandular epithelium.[15] Pathologic changes in the salivary gland include diffuse interstitial edema and serofibrinous exudate with infiltration of lymphocytes and macrophages. The ductal epithelium undergoes degenerative changes with intraluminal accumulation of lymphocytes and debris.[16]

Mumps orchitis results from direct viral infection of the testes; virus has been isolated from testicular biopsy specimens of the affected gland within the first few days of symptoms.[17] Histologic changes within the testes include interstitial edema and lymphocytic infiltration.[18] Focal destruction of the germinal epithelium can occur.

Mumps infection of the CNS is common. The virus probably enters the CNS through the choroid plexus and infects the choroidal epithelium and ependymal cells lining the ventricles.[19] Mumps encephalitis occurs when infection spreads to the brain parenchyma along neuronal pathways.

IMMUNE RESPONSE

Specific immunoglobulin (Ig) M, IgA, and IgG antibodies are produced in response to mumps infection.[20-23] Virus-specific secretory IgA appears concurrently with the cessation of viral shedding in saliva. Intrathecal synthesis of mumps IgG and IgM antibodies has been demonstrated, as well as production of interferon-γ by activated cytotoxic T lymphocytes in the cerebrospinal fluid (CSF).[24-27]

CLINICAL MANIFESTATIONS

One-third of patients with mumps infection have subclinical or mild respiratory tract illness.[28-31] The most common manifestation is parotid swelling, which usually is unilateral at the onset of

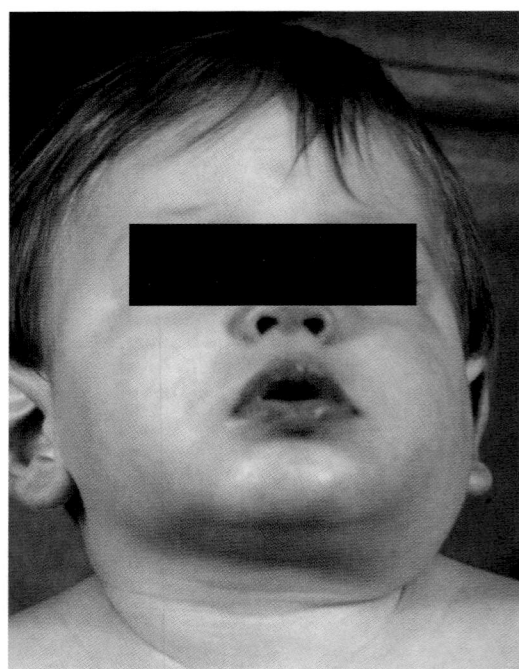

Figure 224-3. Toddler with mumps parotitis. (Courtesy of A. Margileth.)

illness, later becoming bilateral in 70% of cases. Prodromal symptoms, including headache, vague abdominal discomfort, and loss of appetite, typically precede the parotid swelling by 12 to 24 hours. Earache on the side of parotid involvement and discomfort with eating or drinking acidic food are common.

The swollen parotid gland lifts the earlobe upward and outward, and the angle of the mandible is obscured (Figure 224-3); the opening of the Stensen duct on the buccal mucosa is edematous and erythematous. Trismus (spasm of the masticatory muscles) can occur. Other salivary glands such as the submandibular and

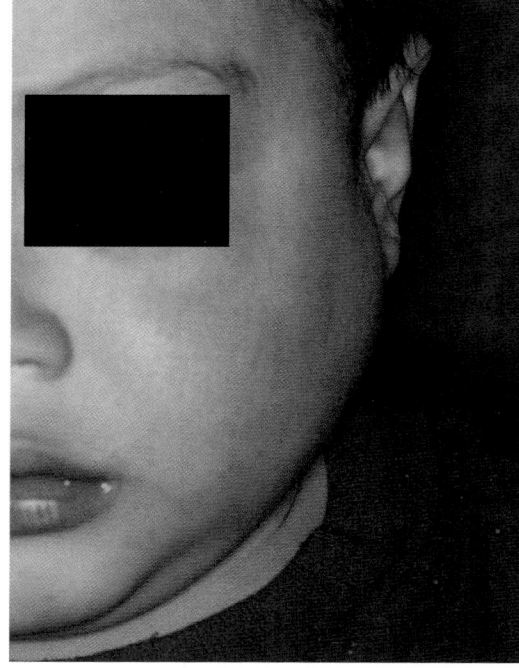

Figure 224-4. Boy with parotitis not due to mumps virus. (Courtesy of J.H. Brien©.)

sublingual glands can also be involved. Presternal edema can be notable. Morbilliform rash has been reported.[32]

Systemic symptoms, including fever, usually resolve within 3 to 5 days, and parotid swelling subsides within 7 to 10 days. Adolescents and adults have more severe disease than young children.

For purposes of surveillance, the Council of State and Territorial Epidemiologists (CSTE) has established a case definition of mumps infection based on clinical and laboratory criteria (link at http://www.cdc.gov/ncphi/disss/nndss/casedef/mumps_current).[33] Studies have shown that failure to use a strict case definition or confirmatory laboratory testing can lead to an overestimation of the number of cases of mumps in a population.[34]

The differential diagnosis of parotitis is broad and includes bacterial (suppurative) parotitis, parotid duct stone, drug reactions, recurrent parotitis of childhood, parotid tumor, and Sjögren syndrome. Other viruses, such as Epstein–Barr virus, influenza, coxsackievirus A, echovirus, and parainfluenza viruses 1 and 3, can cause parotitis and are usually responsible for "recurrent mumps" (Figure 224-4). Children with human immunodeficiency virus (HIV) can have chronic bilateral parotid swelling that is not due to mumps virus infection.

COMPLICATIONS

Central Nervous System Infection

Mumps virus is neurotropic and the degree of neuropathogenicity may depend on the genotype of the virus.[35] CSF pleocytosis occurs in >50% of individuals with mumps parotitis, but only 1% to 10% of patients have clinical evidence of meningitis or encephalitis.[36,37] Parotitis does not develop in about 50% of patients with mumps meningitis.[38] Virus can be isolated from CSF in approximately 40% to 50% of individuals with mumps meningitis.[39]

Mumps infection of the CNS is diagnosed three times more often in males than in females, with meningitis more common than encephalitis.[37,40] Symptomatic CNS disease typically occurs 3 to 10 days after the onset of parotitis, but it can precede or occur without parotitis. Symptoms of meningitis include headache, fever, lethargy, nuchal rigidity, delirium, and vomiting. Seizures occur in 20% of patients.[38]

The CSF white blood cell count is usually less than 1000 cells/mm^3, with lymphocytes predominating. CSF protein is normal or mildly elevated, and CSF glucose is decreased in 30% of cases (rarely <20 mg/dL).[41] CSF pleocytosis can persist for prolonged periods, suggesting persistent infection.[42]

In general, infection of the CNS is self-limited, with no sequelae. However, some children develop ataxia, behavioral problems,[43] aqueductal stenosis with hydrocephalus,[44-46] and sensorineural hearing impairment.[47,48] In Japan, where mumps remains endemic because measles-rubella vaccine is used instead of MMR vaccine, the incidence of hearing loss in children with mumps is 1/1000 cases.[49] Other complications of mumps include paralysis[50] and neuroretinitis.[51] Death occurs in approximately 1.4% of cases of encephalitis.[52]

Orchitis

Orchitis develops in 14% to 35% of males with mumps virus infection.[53,54] The highest risk is in those 15 to 29 years of age. Orchitis is uncommon in prepubertal males.[12,29] Symptoms usually begin 4 to 8 days after the onset of parotid swelling, but orchitis can occur before or in the absence of parotitis. Testicular involvement usually is unilateral, and epididymitis is associated with orchitis in most cases.[55] Clinical findings include fever, malaise, vomiting, lower abdominal pain, and testicular pain. The testicle typically is swollen and tender for 3 to 7 days. Mumps virus has been cultured from seminal fluid and mumps virus RNA has been detected in semen several weeks after infection.[56] Elevated C-reactive protein is frequently seen with mumps orchitis.[57]

Treatment of mumps orchitis is symptomatic, with bedrest and the use of scrotal support, ice packs, and anti-inflammatory agents.[54] Approximately 50% of males with mumps orchitis recover completely, and 50% have some testicular atrophy. Infertility rarely occurs, although a decrease in sperm count and sperm motility has been described.[55,58]

Other Sites of Infection

Hematuria and proteinuria can occur in children with mumps, and transient alterations in creatinine clearance are reported.[59-61] Glomerulonephritis usually is self-limited, but rare reports of death from renal failure have appeared.[62]

Arthralgia, polyarticular migratory arthritis with effusion, and monoarticular arthritis are described.[63-65] Signs usually appear 1 to 3 weeks after the onset of parotitis, but can occur before or in the absence of parotitis. Joint complaints are three to four times more common in males; the average age at occurrence is 24 years.[63,66] Large joints are affected most frequently and include the knee, hip, wrist, ankle, and shoulder. Although the duration of joint symptoms ranges from 2 days to 6 months, recovery with no evidence of persistent or recurrent symptoms is usual.

Electrocardiographic abnormalities consistent with myocarditis have been noted in 4% to 15% of patients with mumps, most commonly in adults.[67-69] Abnormalities generally resolve within 2 to 4 weeks, although sequelae are reported.[70]

The incidence of pancreatitis with mumps infection is poorly defined; involvement usually is associated with mild epigastric pain, but severe hemorrhagic pancreatitis has been reported.[71,72] The role of mumps virus in the development of insulin-dependent diabetes mellitus is controversial. Cases have been noted to follow outbreaks of mumps, but no causal relationship has been established.[73,74]

Oophoritis, mastitis,[12] thyroiditis,[75,76] thrombocytopenic purpura,[77] and hepatitis with acute cholecystitis[78] have been associated with mumps virus infection.

PREGNANCY

Compared with uninfected women, women with mumps during pregnancy have no increase in the risk of delivering an infant with congenital malformations.[79] The rate of spontaneous abortion in women who acquire mumps during the first trimester of pregnancy is increased.[80] Gestational mumps infection has been implicated in the development of endocardial fibroelastosis (EFE) in offspring. Although many infants with EFE have had positive skin test responses to mumps antigen[81,82] (which is not a highly specific test), mumps virus has not been isolated from affected infants.[83,84] Analysis using PCR has found the mumps viral genome in >70% of samples from 29 patients with autopsy-proven EFE.[85]

Perinatal mumps infection with parotid swelling, pneumonia, and pulmonary hypertension has been reported.[86-88a]

DIAGNOSIS

The diagnosis of mumps is suspected in patients with parotitis for 2 days or longer and no other apparent cause. Laboratory findings include increased serum amylase level during the first week of illness. The white blood cell count usually is low or normal with a relative lymphocytosis. Mumps infection can be confirmed by the presence of a positive serum mumps IgM, demonstration of a rise in IgG antibody titers to mumps virus antigens in acute and convalescent serum, positive mumps virus culture, or detection of the viral genome by reverse transcriptase PCR (RT-PCR).[33,89]

Practitioners should consult their local health department for recommendations for optimal specimen testing and submission.[90] If a patient has clinical features compatible with mumps a buccal and oral swab should be obtained and blood should be drawn for serologic testing. Suitable specimens for mumps virus isolation include a swab of the pharynx or area around the duct of Stensen obtained after massaging the affected parotid gland for 30 seconds, CSF, and urine. Virus can be isolated from the oropharynx 1 week before the onset of symptoms and up to 9 days after symptoms appear.[91] Virus is found in urine for up to 2 weeks and in CSF for

8 to 9 days after the appearance of symptoms.[92] Samples for virus detection should be collected as soon as mumps is suspected. This is particularly important in patients with a history of vaccination, since quantity and duration of virus shedding may be decreased.[93] Cell culture shows typical cytopathic effect of cellular degeneration and syncytium formation.[94] The presence of virus should be confirmed by the use of hemagglutination inhibition (HAI) assays or immunofluorescent antigen detection.[95]

Mumps infection is confirmed by a positive mumps IgM antibody test or by demonstrating a ≥4-fold rise in mumps-specific IgG antibody between acute and convalescent titers. Mumps antibodies can be measured by enzyme immunoassay (EIA),[96] immunofluorescence (IF) or HAI assay,[89] complement fixation,[97] or neutralization assays.[98] The Centers for Disease Control and Prevention (CDC) currently test for mumps using a nonquantitative capture IgM EIA. The antigen utilized is a recombinant mumps nucleocapsid protein. IFA assays also perform well for diagnosis of acute infection. A positive IgM test indicates current or recent mumps infection. Mumps IgM is less likely to be positive if the mumps patient has previously received either 1 (50% positive)[99] or 2 doses of mumps vaccine (13–15%).[9,93]

IgG is detected utilizing a commercial indirect EIA. A positive IgG response indicates either recent or past exposure to wild-type virus or vaccine. A second sample of serum should be obtained 2 to 3 weeks after onset of symptoms. It may be difficult to demonstrate seroconversion in previously vaccinated individuals since mumps IgG can be quite elevated already in the acute phase sample.

PCR is now used to detect viral RNA in clinical specimens and in CSF samples from children with aseptic meningitis.[100,101] RT-PCR also is useful to detect mumps virus RNA in previously vaccinated individuals who developed clinical symptoms of mumps in recent outbreaks.[9,93]

A commercially available mumps skin test antigen is no longer available because of its poor specificity and sensitivity in predicting immunity.[14,102,103]

TREATMENT AND PREVENTION

No specific antiviral therapy is available for mumps infection. Treatment is supportive.

Mumps Vaccine

The live-attenuated Jeryl Lynn strain (genotype A) of mumps virus vaccine currently used in the U.S. was licensed in 1967.[104,105] Neutralizing antibodies develop in more than 90% of vaccine recipients after a single dose.[106] Levels of neutralizing antibody are considerably lower after vaccination than after natural infection,[104] but vaccine-induced immunity is relatively long-lasting.[107,108] Although the vaccine was licensed for use in 1967, universal immunization was not recommended until 1977. Between 1985 and 1988, an increase in the number of mumps cases was observed (see Figure 224-1), primarily in older school-aged children, college students, young adults, and children too young to be vaccinated.[109–113] One explanation for the resurgence in mumps during that time was failure to vaccinate all susceptible individuals during the 10 years after licensure of the mumps vaccine; this failure to vaccinate resulted in a cohort of nonimmune older individuals.[114]

Numbers of cases of mumps increased dramatically in England and Wales beginning in 2003 to 2004. The highest attack rate was in adolescents and young adults born between 1983 and 1986. These individuals would not routinely have been offered MMR vaccination when it was introduced in 1988, and many in this age group may have received no vaccine or only one dose.[115] Declining rates of immunization in the U.K. may account for an increase in recent cases in younger children.[116]

Outbreaks of mumps have been reported in highly vaccinated populations in the U.S. Infection is due to primary vaccine failure or, less commonly, to waning immunity.[114,117,118] The protective

efficacy of 1 dose of vaccine based on information from outbreaks between 1973 and 1989 ranges from 75% to 91%.[111,112,114,119] In the midwestern U.S. outbreak of 2006, receipt of 2 doses of mumps vaccine was associated with substantially higher individual protection and a lower attack rate (2%) in one college with higher 2-dose vaccination coverage compared with an attack rate of 3.8% in another college with lower coverage.[7]

Analyses of outbreaks suggest that adolescents or young adults who receive 2 doses of vaccine, but who reside in low population communities where opportunities for natural boosting by exposure to endemic disease is low, may be at higher risk for mumps infection when they move to more crowded living situations.[3] One hypothesis is that current population immunity of approximately 90%[120] is lower than that needed to achieve herd immunity. Higher rates of vaccination or more effective mumps vaccine strategies may be required.[3a,121]

Vaccine Recommendations

Two doses of mumps vaccine administered subcutaneously to children at 12 months of age or older and at 4 to 6 years of age are recommended.[122,123] Key changes in recommendations for mumps vaccine are shown in Box 224-1. Mumps vaccine is given in combination with measles and rubella immunization (MMR) or with measles, rubella and varicella immunization (MMRV). Mumps immunization is of particular importance for children approaching puberty. Children who have not received a second dose of vaccine should do so at a routine provider visit by 11 to 12 years of age. Routine use of mumps vaccine is not recommended for individuals born before 1957. Immunization is not contraindicated in immune individuals.

BOX 224-1. Key Changes in Recommendations for Mumps Vaccine

ACCEPTABLE PRESUMPTIVE EVIDENCE OF IMMUNITY

- Documentation of adequate vaccination is now 2 doses of a live mumps virus vaccine instead of 1 dose for:
  - school-aged children (i.e., grades K–12)
  - adults at high risk (i.e., persons who work in healthcare facilities, international travelers, and students at posthigh-school educational facilities)

ROUTINE VACCINATION FOR HEALTHCARE WORKERS

- Persons born during or after 1957 without other evidence of immunity; 2 doses of a live mumps virus vaccine
- For unvaccinated personnel born before 1957 who lack laboratory evidence of mumps immunity or laboratory confirmation of disease, healthcare facilities should consider vaccinating personnel with 2 doses of MMR vaccine at the appropriate interval

FOR OUTBREAK SETTINGS

- Children aged 1–4 years and adults at low risk; if affected by the outbreak, consider a second dose[a] of live mumps virus vaccine
- Healthcare workers born before 1957 without other evidence of immunity: healthcare facilities should recommend 2 doses of MMR vaccine during an outbreak of mumps

[a]Minimum interval between doses = 28 days.
From Centers for Disease Control and Prevention. Updated recommendations of the Advisory Committee on Immunization Practices (ACIP) for the Control and Elimination of Mumps. MMWR 2006;55:1–2; Centers for Disease Control and Prevention. Immunization of health care personnel: recommendations of the Advisory Committee on Immunization Practices (ACIP). MMWR 2012;60:14–16.
Note: MMRV not licensed for use in individuals >12 years old.

Vaccine Adverse Reactions

Allergic reactions, possibly secondary to the gelatin or neomycin component of the vaccine, are uncommon. Severe allergic reactions, including anaphylaxis, are rare. Reported adverse events with a temporal association to vaccination, including fever, febrile seizures, meningitis, encephalitis, orchitis, and parotitis, are extremely rare. Reported rates of all CNS reactions with the Jeryl Lynn strain of vaccine range from 1 in 50,000 to 1,000,000 doses of vaccine, a frequency lower than the background incidence observed in the normal population.[124]

An increase in the expected number of mumps vaccine-associated cases of meningitis occurred in several countries, including Canada, Japan, and the U.K., during a period when the Urabe Am 9 strain of mumps virus was used in combination with measles and rubella vaccine.[125-128] Virus isolated from CSF in many cases was identified as the mumps vaccine strain by determination of the nucleotide sequences of the P gene.[126,127]

Vaccine Contraindications

Vaccine virus has been isolated from the placenta of nonimmune women immunized 7 to 10 days before therapeutic abortion.[129] Virus has not been isolated from fetal tissue of immunized women, and no cases of mumps vaccine-associated embryopathy have been reported. However, because of theoretical risks to the fetus, pregnant women should not be immunized, and conception should be avoided for 28 days after vaccination. Mumps vaccine is not transmitted from vaccinees to contacts and can be given to children whose mothers are pregnant.

Persons who are allergic to neomycin or gelatin should receive vaccine in a setting where they can be monitored and after consultation with an allergist or immunologist. Most children with egg hypersensitivity can be immunized with MMR. Skin testing of children allergic to eggs is not recommended because it is not predictive of reactions to MMR vaccine.[130] Children with a significant hypersensitivity reaction after the first dose of MMR should be tested for immunity and, if immune, should not receive a second dose or, alternatively, could receive evaluation and possible skin testing before receiving a second dose. Children with anaphylactic reactions to vaccine should not be reimmunized.

Immune globulin preparations interfere with the serologic response to live-attenuated virus vaccines. Mumps vaccine should be given at least 2 weeks before or 3 months after standard administration of immunoglobulin preparations or blood transfusions and for longer periods after high-dose intravenous immune globulin. Children with compromised immunity should not be given mumps vaccine. The American Academy of Pediatrics (AAP) does not recommend MMR vaccine for children with most immunodeficiency diseases including those: receiving immunosuppressive therapy, such as with corticosteroids, alkylating agents, antimetabolites, or radiation; with malignancies who are receiving immunosuppressive therapy; who have undergone bone marrow transplantation.[130] Children can be immunized with mumps vaccine if they have not received immunosuppressive therapy for at least 3 months and their underlying disease is in remission. Patients with HIV should receive mumps vaccine as part of the MMR vaccine unless they are severely compromised.[131] The second dose of vaccine can be administered as early as 4 weeks after the first to induce seroconversion as early as possible.

Nonimmune contacts of immunosuppressed individuals should be immunized because vaccinated persons do not transmit attenuated mumps virus.

Control Measures

The CDC and AAP now recommend a 5-day isolation period after onset of parotitis for isolation of persons with mumps, with use of standard and droplet precautions.[132] Immune globulin does not offer effective postexposure prophylaxis, and mumps vaccine is not effective in preventing illness after exposure. Vaccination programs conducted during outbreaks are effective in preventing disease after subsequent exposure.

Key Points. Diagnosis and Management of Mumps Infection

MICROBIOLOGY
- Negative stranded RNA virus
- Member of Rubulavirus genus in the Paramyxoviridae family
- One serotype but at least 12 genotypes based on variability in SH gene

EPIDEMIOLOGY
- Humans are the only known host
- Virus is spread by respiratory secretions
- In pre-vaccine era mumps infections were most common during winter–spring in children <10 years
- Incubation period is 12 to 25 days
- Patients are most contagious 1 to 2 days prior to onset of symptoms and for 5 days after symptoms appear

CLINICAL FINDINGS
- One or more salivary glands can be swollen
- In 30% of cases, patient has only upper respiratory infection symptoms
- Other manifestations of infection include:
  - Meningitis/Encephalitis
  - Orchitis
  - Thyroiditis
  - Myocarditis
  - Sensorineural hearing loss
  - Hepatitis
  - Arthritis
  - Oophoritis
  - Glomerulonephritis
  - Pancreatitis
  - Transverse myelitis
  - Thrombocytopenic purpura

DIAGNOSIS
- Virus can be identified from buccal swabs, other respiratory secretions or CSF
- PCR may detect mumps virus RNA
- Positive serum mumps IgM antibody confirms acute infection. IgM test can be negative in previously immunized individuals
- Mumps IgG also can be used to diagnose infection if acute and convalescent titers are obtained and significant rise in titer is noted

ISOLATION
- Hospitalized patients: standard and droplet precautions for 5 days after onset of symptoms
- School and daycare: children should be excluded from attending for 5 days after onset of symptoms

225 Respiratory Syncytial Virus

H. Cody Meissner

Respiratory syncytial virus (RSV) is among the great threats to child health, causing illness and death by inflammatory disease of the lower respiratory tract. Since its discovery in 1956,[1,2] investigators have worked to understand the pathogenesis and immunity of this virus, which is one of the most infectious human viruses. Nearly all humans are infected with RSV in the first years of life but that immunity is not complete or sustained. The importance of immunity in recovery and protection is underscored by the enhanced severity of RSV disease in immunodeficient patients. Successes in preventing severe RSV disease with RSV-specific antibody preparations provide optimism that continuing scientific work will provide the means to protect children effectively from yearly RSV epidemics. Those who care for children will manage RSV disease often. Attention to current knowledge about RSV disease will equip clinicians to balance risk and benefit in treating RSV infection, and to prevent its spread to the most vulnerable children. Recent knowledge of RSV disease in healthy, elderly adults living in the community as well as adults with chronic heart or lung disease and adult patients hospitalized with acute cardiopulmonary conditions emphasizes the importance of this virus as a cause of morbidity and mortality at both ends of the age spectrum.[3]

DESCRIPTION OF THE PATHOGEN

RSV is a member of the virus subfamily Pneumovirinae, which also includes the pediatric respiratory pathogen human metapneumovirus (hMPV). RSV is a member of the Paramyxoviridae virus family, along with other viruses that frequently cause morbidity and mortality in children, including measles, mumps, and parainfluenza viruses, and the recently discovered Nipah and Hendra viruses. The pleomorphic RSV virion contains a nucleocapsid surrounded by a viral envelope derived from the plasma membrane of the host cell. The viral nucleocapsid is composed of viral proteins in complex with the RSV genome, which is a single strand of negative-sense RNA encoding 11 proteins. These proteins include components of the nucleocapsid and RNA-dependent RNA polymerase complex (nucleoprotein (N), phosphoprotein (P), large, polymerase protein (L), and two regulatory proteins (M2-1, and M2-2)), the matrix (M) protein important for viral structure, the three surface glycoproteins fusion protein (F), glycosylated attachment protein (G), and short hydrophobic protein (SH), and the nonstructural proteins NS-1 and NS-2 that modulate host response to infection.[4]

The viral surface glycoproteins F and G are integral membrane proteins that are primary targets for host neutralizing antibodies, and are important determinants of viral infectivity and pathogenesis. The G protein mediates viral attachment to target cells and is the most genetically and antigenically diverse RSV protein. The F protein mediates penetration of the virus into the target cell cytoplasm by fusion of the virus and host cell plasma membranes. RSV F protein also mediates the formation of characteristic syncytia, or multinucleated aggregates of cells sharing fused plasma membrane, seen following inoculation of RSV onto susceptible cell lines, such as HEp-2 or HeLa cells. However, the characteristic syncytial cytopathic effect for which RSV was named and which is useful for virus detection in vitro is rarely observed in patient specimens or experimental infection of primary respiratory epithelial cell cultures.

All RSV strains belong to a single serotype. However, sufficient antigenic dimorphism exists to allow assignment of strains to one of two antigenic subgroups, designated A and B, based on reciprocal cross-neutralization studies using polyclonal immune sera or anti-RSV monoclonal antibodies.[5] These subgroups are quite divergent and show antigenic relatedness of about 25%. G-protein antigenic relatedness between subgroups is just 1% to 7%, while the more highly conserved F protein exhibits 50% antigenic relatedness between subgroups.[4-12] There is considerable antigenic variation within viruses of each RSV subgroup, and a number of smaller virus groupings have been identified by genotyping studies. Molecular epidemiology studies show that viruses of RSV subgroup A and B can circulate simultaneously in the population, and that temporally and geographically distinct RSV epidemics are caused by viruses of multiple subgroups and subtypes. These divergent, co-circulating RSV lineages distribute broadly from a geographic standpoint.[13-15]

Some studies have demonstrated considerable genetic diversity among circulating RSV strains; however, studies of RSV F-protein genetic and antigenic features suggest a high level of stability over time. Over a 30-year period it was found that antibody epitopes on the RSV F protein of circulating RSV strains remained remarkably stable, and that mutations that confer escape from host immunity directed at major neutralizing antibody determinants did not occur. These data suggest that there was little antigenic drift in the RSV F protein over this period,[15] in stark contrast to the continual antigenic drift of influenza antigens. Thus, RSV shows remarkable strain diversity but a slow accumulation of new mutations that result in antigenic escape. The role of subgroup diversity in RSV epidemics and disease severity is not well understood, although some studies suggest that infection with a virus of the heterologous subgroup may be more common after primary infection.

EPIDEMIOLOGY

RSV infection occurs worldwide, in yearly epidemics that vary in severity and occur in the winter and spring in temperate climates[16-19] (Figure 225-1). Efforts to relate RSV activity (including onset and end of yearly outbreaks) to climate conditions suggest a complex interaction with latitude, temperature, humidity, and ultraviolet radiation.[17,18] Virtually all children are infected within the first few years of life, and RSV causes a tremendous disease burden in this population. Approximately 2% to 3% of all otherwise healthy infants require hospitalization for bronchiolitis during the first 12 months of life, and about 2% to 5% of hospitalized children require mechanical ventilation.[20] One prospective longitudinal study showed that about one-half of infants were infected during their first RSV epidemic, and nearly all were infected at least once after two epidemics.[21] By 6 months of life, maternally acquired serum antibodies to RSV wane, and studies consistently show that more than 20% of infants experience lower respiratory tract disease with their first RSV infection.[22-25]

RSV is the leading viral pathogen associated with childhood acute respiratory tract illness requiring hospitalization.[26] In one study, RSV accounted for 17 hospitalizations per 1000 United States children <6 months of age and 3 per 1000 children <5 years of age.[27] The risk of hospitalization attributable to RSV is 3 to 5 times higher in high-risk infants and young children compared with other children.

An estimated 55,000 to 120,000 children are hospitalized with RSV in the U.S. each year. During peaks of RSV epidemics approximately 75% of children hospitalized for acute lower respiratory

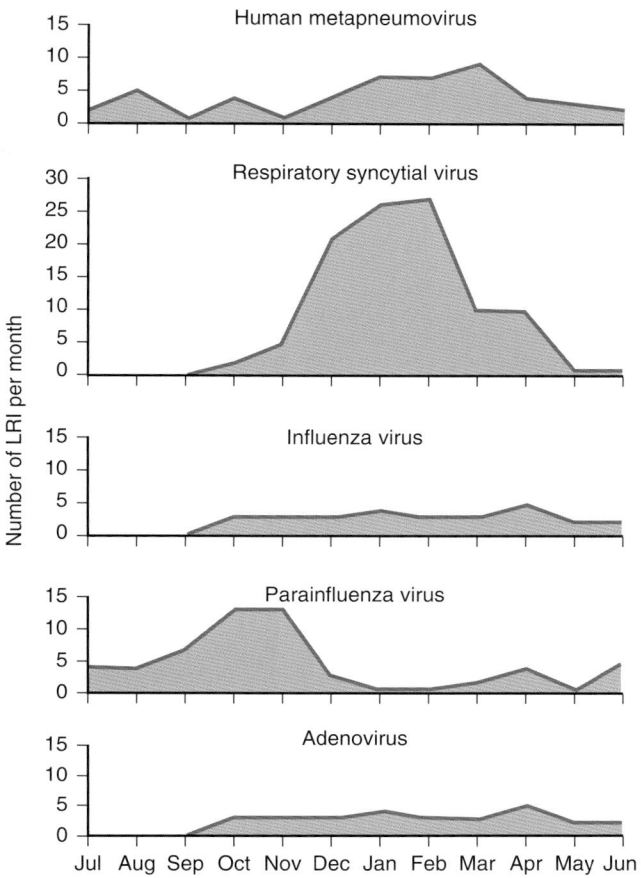

Figure 225-1. Epidemiologic pattern of lower respiratory illness with respiratory syncytial virus and other viruses. Data are combined from 25 years of surveillance in the Vanderbilt Vaccine Evaluation Clinic. Used with permission.

BOX 225-1. Medical Conditions Associated with Increased Risk for Severe Respiratory Syncytial Virus Infection

HOST FACTORS

Congenital heart disease
Bronchopulmonary dysplasia
Chronic pulmonary disorders (e.g., cystic fibrosis, asthma)
Immunosuppression
- Congenital: HIV/AIDS, immunodeficiency
- Acquired: HIV/AIDS, chemotherapy, high-dose corticosteroid therapy
Malnutrition
Prematurity
Advanced (elderly) age

DEMOGRAPHIC FACTORS[a]

>1 sibling and a crowded household
Maternal smoking
Male sex
White race
Maternal education <12 years

AIDS, acquired immunodeficiency syndrome; HIV, human immunodeficiency virus.
[a]Most exert only a minor effect; based on reference 28. Group childcare increases the risk of acquisition of respiratory syncytial virus.

tract illness (LRTI) have RSV infection.[27-29] Comparative analysis of virus-attributable deaths in the United Kingdom over 11 winters revealed that influenza and RSV accounted for similar numbers of deaths in children.[30] RSV is increasingly recognized as an important cause of mortality in adults[31] and was found to be associated with approximately 17,000 all-cause deaths per year among persons of all ages in the U.S.[32]

RSV reinfection is common in persons of all ages.[23,32,33] Most reinfections are symptomatic and are limited to the upper respiratory tract and occur despite the presence of RSV-specific neutralizing antibodies.[34-36] RSV subgroup diversity may contribute to the prevalence of reinfection, but strain diversity is not required for reinfection.[37,38] Healthy adults manifest upper respiratory tract signs and symptoms in about one-half of cases of natural or experimental infections, despite numerous previous infections. Reports addressing whether RSV subgroup A strains cause more severe disease than RSV subgroup B viruses have been conflicting.[39-42]

Persons at increased risk for severe RSV disease include premature infants, infants with chronic lung disease or congenital heart disease, patients with immunodeficiency, including human immunodeficiency virus (HIV) disease, and the elderly[43-51] (Box 225-1). Numerous factors have been associated with an increased risk of RSV hospitalization. Boys have a higher incidence of RSV LRTI than girls.[52-54] Other factors reported to increase the risk of RSV hospitalization include poverty, malnutrition, exposure to environmental pollutants such as second-hand tobacco smoke, household crowding, daycare attendance, lower level of maternal education, altitude, and lack of breastfeeding. However, many of these risk factors are inconsistent from study to study and in most

instances the impact on increased hospitalization is small[55-59] (see Box 225-1).

Transmission of RSV occurs through respiratory tract secretions, and RSV can survive on nonporous surfaces for >24 hours.[60-65] Transmission occurs through close contact and by large respiratory droplets (but not by small-particle aerosols) or fomites;[61] nasal and conjunctival mucous membrane inoculation are efficient means of transmission. The incubation period is about 5 days, and viral shedding can occur in healthy infants for up to 3 weeks.[64,65] Hospital infection control practices that can limit RSV spread include careful hand hygiene, contact/droplet precautions for patient isolation, use of gowns and gloves, cohorting of infected patients, and use of facemasks and goggles.[66-69] RSV rapid diagnostic testing enhances hospital infection control by identifying RSV-infected patients.[70] Importantly, the sensitivity of rapid antigen tests is not sufficient to detect the low amount of virus present early or late in infection or during asymptomatic infection. Low amounts of virus are sufficient for nosocomial transmission; therefore a negative rapid RSV antigen test should not be the only basis for discontinuing isolation of hospitalized patients recovering from RSV.

Healthcare-associated (HA) transmission of RSV is an important, preventable cause of RSV disease in hospitalized patients,[68-75] including severe disease in immunocompromised patients.[71-83] Failure to adhere strictly to hospital infection control procedures during RSV epidemics and hospital outbreaks can result in fatal HA-RSV infections. RSV epidemiology and copathogenicity contribute to the epidemiology of bacterial diseases. RSV upper respiratory tract infection frequently is complicated by bacterial otitis media. Antibiotic therapy does not alter the course of uncomplicated RSV bronchiolitis or pneumonia. Annual RSV and influenza virus epidemics correlate directly with the period of peak incidence of invasive pneumococcal disease (IPD) in epidemiologic studies.[84] Provocative evidence for RSV and pneumococcal copathogenicity in severe pneumonia has emerged from a double-blind, randomized, placebo-controlled trial of pneumococcal conjugate vaccine that shows vaccine-attributable reduction in rates of childhood viral pneumonia requiring hospitalization, caused by any of seven respiratory viruses, including RSV.[85] The impact of RSV infection on IPD is unknown and the subject of ongoing investigation.

PATHOGENESIS AND IMMUNE RESPONSE

RSV replicates to high titer in cells of the nasopharynx and can spread to the lower respiratory tract via aspiration of secretions or by cell-to-cell spread to cause bronchiolitis or pneumonia.[86] Infection of monocytes and macrophages also can contribute to RSV respiratory tract spread,[87-89] and infection of these circulating cells could contribute to disseminated RSV disease in immunocompromised patients.[90,91] However, RSV is restricted to the respiratory tract in most cases. Early pathologic findings in RSV bronchiolitis include lymphocytic peribronchiolar infiltration with edema, progressing to proliferation and necrosis of bronchiolar epithelium.[92] Mucus and sloughed respiratory tract epithelium block the small bronchiolar lumens of infants, and the resulting resistance to pulmonary airflow is greatest during expiration when thoracic pressures are normally highest. Air trapping and hyperinflation result from partial airway obstruction and increased expiratory resistance.[93] RSV causes extensive damage to the bronchiolar ciliary apparatus,[94] resulting in impaired clearance of debris. During the acute stage of disease, large numbers of RSV-infected respiratory epithelial cells are present. Late in the disease course, after the acute stage has passed, tissue samples from lungs of patients with bronchiolitis can show few epithelial cells that are RSV-positive by antigen testing using immunofluorescence techniques.[92] While the immune response is felt to contribute to the pathogenesis of RSV disease, several studies demonstrate a direct correlation between the quantity of RSV in respiratory tract secretions of infants, disease severity, and prolonged hospitalization.[95] In tissues or samples from immunocompetent patients, it is unusual to find syncytia that are so commonly seen in vitro in cell line cultures, and for which the virus was named. It is not clear in humans that cell–cell fusion leading to syncytium formation contributes to RSV pathogenesis.

RSV pneumonia can be severe, especially among immunocompromised patients. Pathologic examination shows fluid-filled alveoli and interalveolar wall thickening with mononuclear cell infiltration.[86] Patients with RSV pneumonia can show extensive RSV immunofluorescence staining of respiratory tract epithelial cells.[92]

The importance of the immune system in RSV pathogenesis is dramatically underscored by the formalin-inactivated, randomized RSV vaccine (Lot 100) clinical trial, conducted in 1966 to 1967 in children aged 2 months to 9 years. Following natural exposure to RSV, RSV vaccine recipients were not protected from infection compared with children receiving the control parainfluenza virus vaccine. In fact, 80% of RSV vaccinees needed hospitalization compared with 5% of children receiving the control vaccine, and 2 vaccinated children subsequently died of severe RSV respiratory disease.[96,97] Postmortem examination of respiratory tissues revealed an intense inflammatory infiltrate suggesting immunopathologic disease. A number of immune mechanisms have been proposed to account for enhanced RSV disease seen in this vaccine trial.[98] In general, the formalin inactivation appears to have preserved the immunogenicity of antigens leading to induction of harmful T-lymphocyte inflammation, but altered the antigen to eliminate its ability to induce protective neutralizing antibodies. Thus the children appear to have been primed for an enhanced inflammatory state on re-exposure that did not reduce the magnitude of the virus infection. This tragedy markedly impeded subsequent RSV vaccine development.[99]

RSV infection induces both cellular and humoral immune responses, and although immune protection is incomplete, the adaptive immune system is critical for recovery from RSV disease and for protection against reinfection. Intact cell-mediated immunity is required for control of established infection and termination of viral shedding.[100,101] Immunocompromised persons deficient in cell-mediated immunity suffer prolonged and severe RSV disease, and may shed virus for prolonged periods of time (e.g., months).[102-104] Cell-mediated immunity may also contribute to short-term protection against RSV reinfection; however, robust activation of antigen-specific T lymphocytes generally is short-lived.

Although young infants are susceptible to severe primary RSV bronchiolitis at an age when maternally acquired RSV-specific antibodies are present, transplacentally derived RSV antibodies do appear to have an ameliorating effect. For example, among prematurely born infants, some studies correlate milder RSV illness with higher levels of maternal RSV-specific immunoglobulin (Ig) G.[105] Long-term protection from RSV reinfection is incomplete; however, resistance to severe disease appears to correlate with the level of RSV-specific serum antibodies and local secretory IgA antibodies. Additionally, secretory IgA antibodies[106] and B lymphocytes[107] are important in termination of RSV shedding and resistance to RSV reinfection.

Stated broadly, humoral immunity primarily mediates protection from RSV reinfection, and cell-mediated immunity is required for control of established infection and termination of viral shedding. The roles of innate immunity and toll-like receptors, interferons, surfactants, the inflammatory response, and viral immune evasion in RSV disease are all under study and underscore the complexity of RSV immunity and immunopathogenesis.

CLINICAL MANIFESTATIONS

RSV infection usually causes upper respiratory tract symptoms[108-111] and can cause LRTI, including clinically distinct but often overlapping syndromes of bronchiolitis and pneumonia. Older children can develop laryngotracheobronchitis or croup (Box 225-2). After an incubation period of 3 to 5 days, RSV-infected infants develop upper respiratory tract illness, including rhinorrhea and congestion, sometimes with fever. Fewer than 40% of infants progress to LRTI with cough and wheezing, varying in severity from mild disease to life-threatening respiratory failure and cyanosis. Infants with bronchiolitis have dyspnea with nasal flaring, intercostal retractions, and prolonged expiration; chest auscultation reveals crackles and wheezing. Chest radiograph typically shows hyperinflation, peribronchiolar thickening, and atelectasis.[112-114] Infants with RSV bronchiolitis also can have pneumonia with radiographic signs of airway consolidation.[115] Infants with severe RSV LRTI can deteriorate rapidly, and close monitoring of arterial oxygen saturation is recommended;[116,117] severe disease can lead to hypercarbia and respiratory failure. In a previously healthy infant, supplemental oxygen is indicated if oxyhemoglobin saturation falls persistently below 90%. Duration of uncomplicated RSV illness in most infants is 1 to 3 weeks.[118] RSV infection is associated with about 5% to 10% of cases of croup.[119]

During the first few weeks of life, particularly among preterm infants, infection with RSV may produce minimal respiratory tract signs. Lethargy, irritability, and poor feeding, sometimes accompanied by apneic episodes, may be the presenting manifestations in these infants.[119-121] Although RSV is not an established cause of sudden infant death syndrome, evidence of RSV infection has been found in some infants with this syndrome.[122-128] Neurologic

---

BOX 225-2. Common Clinical Manifestations of Respiratory Syncytial Virus Infection at Various Ages

INFANCY

Bronchiolitis
Pneumonia
Croup
Apnea
Upper respiratory tract infection
Otitis media

OLDER CHILDREN/ADULTS

Upper respiratory tract infection
Bronchitis
Pneumonia (elderly)
Exacerbation of asthma

complications associated with RSV bronchiolitis include seizures and acute encephalopathy.[129,130] Acute neurologic abnormalities occur in patients with non-RSV respiratory infections as frequently as in those with RSV respiratory infections.[131] Rarely, RSV has been associated with meningitis, encephalitis, and myelitis.[132-134] There are rare reports of RSV associated with myocarditis and arrhythmias,[135-137] and exanthems.[138] However, most RSV infections in otherwise healthy children do not cause systemic disease.

Upper respiratory tract symptoms are the most common manifestations of RSV infection in older children and adults. Symptoms include nasal congestion, cough, and low grade fever.[35] Otitis media frequently is associated with RSV infection in infants and young children.[139-145] Apart from otitis media, the risk of bacterial infection in infants and children with RSV lower respiratory tract disease probably is low.[146-155] RSV and other respiratory viruses can precipitate wheezing in people with asthma.[156] Most studies have observed that infants hospitalized with wheezing associated with viral lower respiratory tract infection have high rates of asthma and pulmonary function abnormalities during the first decade of life.[157-165] The hypothesized role of RSV infection in the future development of asthma and associated atopy has been studied intensely. Recent studies generally fail to show a causative role for RSV in asthma and atopy,[156-160] with exceptions. Some studies support a more important role for rhinovirus infection in persistent wheezing.[166-168] The impact of improved respiratory virus control and disease prevention on the epidemiology of asthma may provide new insights regarding the causative role of viruses in chronic pulmonary disease.

RSV is an important pathogen in the elderly and in adults with chronic heart or lung disease.[3,169] In one study, RSV infection accounted for >10% of hospitalizations for pneumonia and chronic obstructive pulmonary disease, and >5% of hospitalizations for asthma and congestive heart failure in these patients.[3] Other studies confirm that RSV causes a high percentage of cases of pneumonia requiring hospitalization in adults.[170,171] Outbreaks of RSV occur in long-term care facilities among elderly[172,173] and institutionalized young adults.[110]

Children with underlying conditions have a high risk for severe RSV disease.[26] These include children with chronic lung disease or prematurity, and congenital heart disease.[173-179] Additionally, Native American and Alaska Native children have increased risk for severe RSV LRTI.[180-182]

RSV is an important cause of severe pulmonary disease in immunocompromised people.[183] Patients with defects in cell-mediated immunity that are congenital (severe combined immunodeficiency) or acquired (immunosuppression from malignancy or transplantation) have a high incidence of severe RSV disease, with mortality rates that can approximate 50%.[183-188] Patients with defects in phagocytic function, including chronic granulomatous disease and interferon-γ receptor deficiency, also can develop severe RSV LRTI.[188] Although RSV is not a prominent opportunistic pathogen in HIV-infected children, studies in these patients show increased susceptibility to RSV pneumonia and prolonged RSV shedding.[189,190] RSV infection causes severe pulmonary disease in lung transplant recipients and may contribute to the pathogenesis of obliterative bronchiolitis in these patients.[191-193]

LABORATORY DIAGNOSIS

Specific diagnosis is made by RSV detection in respiratory tract secretions by viral culture or by rapid diagnostic tests, including enzyme immunoassays, direct immunofluorescence assays, and reverse transcriptase-polymerase chain reaction (RT-PCR) assays. Proper specimen collection and handling impact each test's performance. Sampling is performed routinely by collection of a nasopharyngeal aspirate or nasal swab. Studies show increased rates of RSV detection by nasal aspiration compared with swab collection.[194-197] RSV is labile, and specimens for viral culture should be kept cold and inoculated into tissue culture as quickly as possible. Characteristic syncytial cytopathic effect can be seen in RSV-infected cells within 3 to 7 days; time to RSV detection in culture can be reduced by the use of shell vial cultures and immunostaining.[197] Rapid RSV diagnostic tests for antigen or nucleic acid detection generally perform well compared with RSV culture techniques, with reported test sensitivities exceeding 90%. Rapid RSV tests enhance hospital infection control efforts and in many cases can be performed with little technical expertise. Microscopy using direct fluorescent antibody staining is labor-intensive but permits assessment of adequacy of the specimen. Viral culture and RT-PCR techniques have several orders of magnitude higher sensitivity than rapid antigen tests. Serologic studies have limited usefulness in patient management.

TREATMENT

Treatment of RSV lower respiratory tract disease is supportive, including supplemental oxygen for hypoxemia, management of respiratory secretions, and mechanical ventilation for respiratory failure. Advances in pediatric critical care are primarily responsible for decreases in morbidity and mortality from RSV. Infants hospitalized for RSV disease should be monitored for apnea.[198,199] The role of nitric oxide[200,201] and mixtures of helium and oxygen (heliox),[202,203] as well as surfactant in the support of infants with severe RSV disease is controversial and under study.

Nebulized α- and β-adrenergic receptor agonists cause bronchodilation and are widely used in the treatment of RSV bronchiolitis despite the absence of convincing data demonstrating efficacy. Clinical Practice Guidelines from the American Academy of Pediatrics state that "bronchodilators should not be used routinely in the management of bronchiolitis."[198] Some physicians may use bronchodilator therapy out of concern that reactive airway disease may be misdiagnosed as RSV bronchiolitis, but repeat doses of a bronchodilator should only be continued in patients who demonstrate a well-documented improvement in respiratory status after the dose. Studies of corticosteroid therapy for RSV bronchiolitis do not show clinically significant benefit and use is not indicated.[204] In fact, corticosteroid treatment may prolong RSV shedding. A placebo-controlled trial of montelukast (an anti-inflammatory agent and cysteinyl leukotriene antagonist) in the treatment of RSV bronchiolitis found no benefit.[205]

Ribavirin is a synthetic guanosine nucleoside analogue that inhibits RSV replication and is the only Food and Drug Administration-approved specific treatment for RSV LRTI. Aerosolized ribavirin therapy has been shown in small clinical trials of RSV-infected immunocompetent patients to improve oxygenation and provide short-term clinical benefit, but decreases in mechanical ventilation and duration of hospitalization have not been proved.[206] Considering conflicting results of clinical trials, high drug cost, cumbersome administration apparatus, and concern regarding toxicity to healthcare providers, ribavirin generally is not indicated for treatment of RSV bronchiolitis in immunocompetent patients.[207] Ribavirin therapy may be more effective in treating RSV disease in some severely immunocompromised patients such as those who have undergone bone marrow or solid-organ transplantation. There are no controlled prospective studies to demonstrate efficacy, however.

PREVENTION

Careful infection control is critical in the protection of vulnerable, immunocompromised patients from severe RSV disease in the hospital setting. Successes in passive RSV immunoprophylaxis began with studies showing significant reductions in RSV-associated hospitalizations and severity of disease following monthly administration of intravenous human immunoglobulin with high RSV neutralizing activity (RSV-IGIV or RespiGam).[208-210] In 1996 this product was licensed for use in children at high risk of severe RSV disease. Inconvenience due to need for intravenous cannulation, high infusion volumes, concern for adventitious agents, supply problems, and potential for interference with childhood vaccinations due to broad antibody content stimulated the development of RSV-specific monoclonal antibodies for RSV immunoprophylaxis. In 1998 a humanized mouse monoclonal antibody palivizumab (Synagis) was licensed for RSV prophylaxis following studies demonstrating its safety and efficacy.[211-216] Palivizumab is recommended for administration by intramuscular injection monthly through the RSV season (not to exceed 5 doses) and has been widely used in high-risk patients with premature birth at <32 weeks' (i.e., through 31 weeks and 6 days) gestation; chronic lung disease; hemodynamically significant heart disease; or premature birth at 29 to <32 weeks' gestation if <6 months of age during the RSV season; or premature birth at 32 to <35 weeks' (i.e., through 34 weeks and 6 days) gestation with other additional, uncontrollable epidemiologic risk factors for severe RSV disease.[217] Indications for this effective but costly prophylactic medication remain a topic of study and debate.[215]

Ultimate control of RSV disease will require development of a safe and effective vaccine for infants. Nonreplicating RSV protein vaccines are problematic for use in infants given their potential for disease enhancement, as well as overall poor immunogenicity in this population. However, an RSV protein vaccine might be useful in boosting immunity in RSV-experienced older children and adults who are at increased risk of severe RSV disease due to underlying disease or advanced age and in pregnant women. The current best hope for a safe and immunogenic RSV vaccine for widespread use in infants is in the development of a live-attenuated intranasal RSV vaccine. A live-attenuated vaccine would not be expected to cause disease enhancement, and intranasal administration circumvents interference in immunogenicity of maternal anti-RSV antibodies. Clinical trials of a safe, live-attenuated RSV vaccine for intranasal administration have shown restriction of viral replication in infants following administration of a second dose.[217] Additional attenuated vaccine candidates are being developed.[218]

226 Human Metapneumovirus

John V. Williams and James E. Crowe, Jr

PERSPECTIVE

Human metapneumovirus (HMPV) is a paramyxovirus that is a leading cause of respiratory disease in humans worldwide. All humans appear to contract primary HMPV infection during infancy and early childhood, and reinfections are common. Clinical manifestations of HMPV infection generally are similar to those caused by other respiratory viruses and include bronchiolitis, croup, pneumonia, and asthma exacerbation. HMPV is associated with a substantial number of upper respiratory infections (URIs) and episodes of acute otitis media (AOM). Hospitalizations occur in otherwise healthy children, but are more common in patients with underlying conditions such as prematurity, asthma, immune compromise, or cardiopulmonary disease. Numerous studies have defined much of the epidemiology of this emerging virus, but less is known regarding pathogenesis and immunity. Despite the recent discovery of HMPV, candidate vaccines are already in development.

DESCRIPTION OF PATHOGEN

HMPV was first described in 2001 by Dutch investigators who collected a number of unidentified virus isolates over a 20-year period.[1] The virus grew slowly in cell culture with minimal cytopathic effects. Electron micrograph and biochemical studies of the virus showed that it was pleomorphic with a lipid bilayer envelope (Figure 226-1). Reverse transcriptase-polymerase chain reaction (RT-PCR) and nucleotide sequence analysis of the virus genome identified it as a member of the Pneumovirus subfamily of the Paramyxoviridae family that includes respiratory syncytial virus (RSV). HMPV is most closely related by sequence homology to avian pneumovirus type C, the sole previous member of the metapneumovirus genus. Avian pneumovirus, discovered in 1979, is a major pathogen of poultry, causing severe respiratory disease in chickens and turkeys with ensuing economic losses.[2] Evolutionary genetic analysis suggests that HMPV diverged from avian pneumovirus C several hundred years ago.[3,4]

HMPV has a negative-sense, single-stranded RNA genome which encodes 9 proteins (Table 226-1 and Figure 226-2). The fusion (F) protein has domains analogous to those of other paramyxovirus fusion proteins and mediates fusion of the virus and cell membranes.[5-8] Studies using animal models show that F is the major target for neutralizing antibodies.[9-12] The other major HMPV membrane protein is G, a heavily glycosylated protein that may serve as an attachment protein for interaction with host cells. In contrast to all other paramyxovirus accessory glycoproteins, HMPV G does not appear to be a protective antigen.[11,13,14] Analysis of the predicted amino acid sequences of the remaining HMPV proteins suggests that they are similar in function to analogous proteins of other paramyxoviruses, although there is little directly conserved sequence.

Complete and partial sequences for many HMPV strains worldwide now are available, and phylogenetic analysis of these sequences defines two major genetic subgroups of HMPV, designated A and B, each with two minor subgroups.[3,4,15] These subgroups of viruses are presently defined as genogroups. The F protein is highly conserved, with 93% to 95% amino acid identity between major subgroups and ~97% amino acid identity within subgroups. In contrast, the G protein is only 30% to 35% conserved between major subgroups of HMPV, and 70% within subgroups. Reinfection with either homologous or heterologous strains of HMPV occurs readily, even during early childhood.[16-18] It is not clear whether the ability of HMPV to reinfect humans is

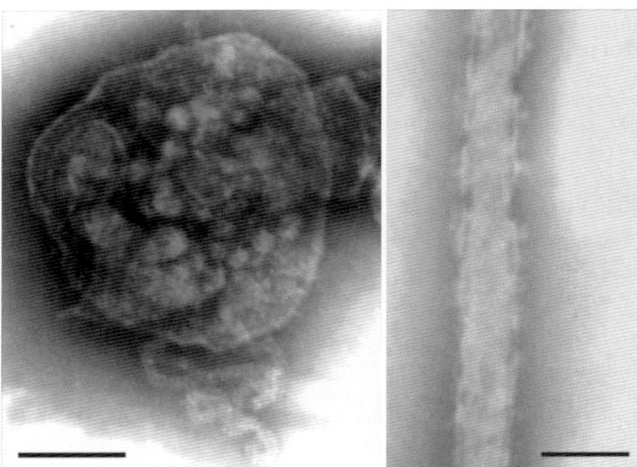

Figure 226-1. Electron micrographs of human metapneumovirus. Left panel shows whole virion. Glycoprotein spikes are visible in viral membrane and extruded nucleocapsid is visible below. Right panel shows a filamentous viral particle; a herringbone pattern of coiled nucleocapsid is visible within the virion. Bar in each image represents 100 nm.

TABLE 226-1. Genes and Proteins of Human Metapneumovirus

Designation	Nucleotides (mRNA)	Molecular Weight (kd)	Function
N	1200	44	Nucleoprotein; structural protein, replication
P	885	33	Phosphoprotein; structural protein, replication
M	765	28	Matrix; structural protein
F	1620	59	Attachment and fusion of virus with the host cell membrane; target of neutralizing antibodies
M2-1	564	21	Unknown; likely regulates RNA transcription/replication
M2-2	204	8	Unknown; likely regulates RNA transcription/replication
SH	552	21	Short hydrophobic; function unknown
G	657–714	~75	Glycosylated protein; attachment to host cells
L	6018	231	Large protein; the RNA polymerase

and organizing lung injury, with diffuse alveolar damage and hyaline membrane formation; cytoplasmic inclusion bodies were noted.[23] Another study of bronchoalveolar lavage fluid from six HMPV-infected patients described the presence of sloughed, degenerated epithelial cells with eosinophilic cytoplasmic inclusions, multinucleated giant cells, and histiocytes.[24] A major limitation of these reports is that all of the patients had underlying diseases, and thus these findings may not reflect what occurs during HMPV infection in otherwise healthy humans.

Detailed analysis of the pathologic features of HMPV infection has been described in mice, cotton rats, and cynomolgus macaques.[25-28] Histopathologic changes included disruption of respiratory epithelial architecture, sloughing of epithelial cells, loss of ciliation, and inflammatory infiltrates in the lungs. Histopathologic changes or evidence of infection were not detected in other organs or tissues. Immunohistochemical staining for HMPV in the macaques and cotton rats revealed localization of viral antigen almost exclusively at the apical surface of ciliated respiratory epithelial cells.[26,27]

Preliminary studies in humans and animals show that HMPV infection stimulates the production of varied cytokines and chemokines and invokes T-lymphocyte responses.[25,29-33] The genome of HMPV contains open reading frames analogous to all those of RSV, except that HMPV lacks the equivalent of the immunomodulatory RSV nonstructural (NS) genes NS1 and NS2. This fact provides a unique opportunity to compare pathogenesis and host immune responses between these two important viruses that cause clinically similar diseases, but that vary in their capacity to stimulate host responses.

EPIDEMIOLOGY

HMPV infections occur in annual epidemics during the late winter and early spring months in temperate locations. The HMPV season overlaps with those of RSV and influenza viruses, but the peak incidence of HMPV usually occurs 1 to 2 months later than the peak of RSV. Prospective surveillance studies conducted over a 25-year period showed that HMPV was present in every season, although the prevalence varied from year to year.[16,34] Different lineages of HMPV frequently circulate in a community during the same winter season, although one subgroup may predominate in a given year.[34] Viruses from each subgroup appear capable of causing severe lower respiratory tract disease; different subgroups have not been associated convincingly with differing severity of disease. In most studies of patients with acute respiratory tract infection, the percentage of HMPV detection varies from 6% to 15%. HMPV infection usually causes symptoms; HMPV is rarely detected in nasal specimens from asymptomatic children.[16,35-38]

Studies of hospitalized and outpatient children in many countries have found HMPV to be associated with between 6% and 40% of acute respiratory illnesses in a given season[16,34,37,39-69] The average prevalence of infection is 5% to 10%, although it may be much higher during the peak months of HMPV circulation. HMPV generally ranks after RSV in most studies and has prevalence comparable with that of influenza or parainfluenza viruses.[47]

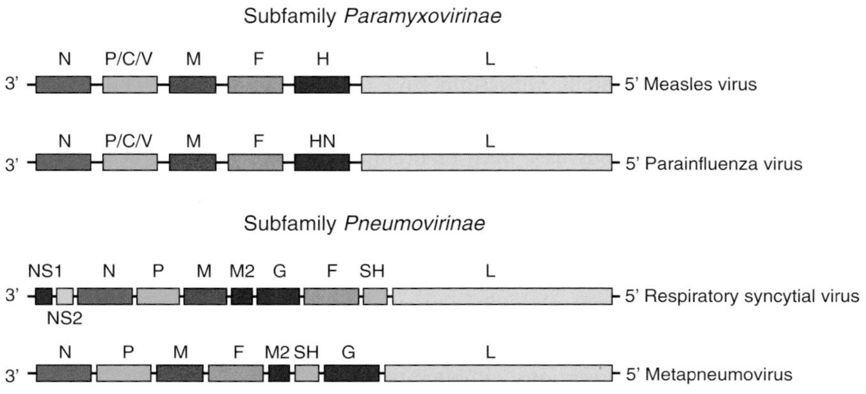

due to infections with different subgroup viruses that are antigenically distinct, incomplete induction of immunity, or waning immunity. Serum neutralizing titers in adults appear to correlate with risk for reinfection.[19] There are no definitive human data determining the degree of cross-protection between different HMPV subgroups. However, animal studies of the antigenic diversity between HMPV subgroups suggest that there is cross-protective immunity in hamsters and primates that protects the lungs against reinfection.[11,15,20-22] These findings have important implications for the development of candidate vaccines or passive antibody interventions for prophylaxis.

There are few data describing the pathogenesis or histologic findings of HMPV infections in humans. HMPV has been detected only in respiratory tract specimens, suggesting that replication is limited to the respiratory tract epithelium. One study of lung transplant recipients infected with HMPV described both acute

Figure 226-2. Schematic of the genomic organization of human metapneumovirus in comparison to other paramyxoviruses. Gene segments drawn roughly to scale.

BOX 226-1. Clinical Manifestations of Human Metapneumovirus Infection at Various Ages

INFANCY

Bronchiolitis
Pneumonia
Croup
Asthma exacerbation
Upper respiratory tract infection
Acute otitis media

OLDER CHILDREN/ADULTS

Upper respiratory tract infection
Croup
Laryngitis
Bronchitis
Asthma exacerbation
Pneumonia
Exacerbation of chronic obstructive pulmonary disease

TABLE 226-2. Percentage of Children with Presenting Signs/Symptoms and Clinical Diagnoses Associated with Human Metapneumovirus (HMPV) Infection in Eight Clinical Studies

Reference	4	43	37	41	16	34	47	56
Number of HMPV-Infected Patients	**12**	**32**	**25**	**53**	**49**	**118**	**29**	**50**
Fever	67	100	61	77	52	54	76	44
Rhinorrhea	92	38	80	64	88	82	72	90
Cough	100	90	72	68	90	66	86	90
Wheezing	83	28	24	51	52	NA	38	56
Vomiting	25	—a	—a	—a	10	20	—a	36
Diarrhea	8	6	—a	—a	17	14	—a	14
Rash	0	12	—a	—a	4	3	—a	—a
Abnormal chest radiograph	—a	68	62	56	50	NA	—a	
Bronchiolitis	67	9	—a	—a	59	NA	38	48
Pneumonia	17	38	—a	—a	8	NA	24	34
Croup	0	—a	—a	—a	18	NA	10	
Asthma	—a	19	—a	—a	14	NA	24	
Acute otitis media	50	12	—a	—a	37	50	—a	

NA, not applicable.

aNot reported.

References 37, 40, 41, 43, and 56 include only hospitalized children.
Reference 16 includes only children with lower respiratory illness.
Reference 34 includes only children with upper respiratory illness.

Multiple studies have reported that the peak age of hospitalization for HMPV occurs between 6 and 12 months of age, substantially later than the 2-month peak age of hospitalization for RSV.[37,40-43,51,56,60,61,64,66,70] The biological reasons for peak susceptibility to HMPV at this age are not known. Males appear to be at greater risk of lower respiratory tract infection due to HMPV compared with females, similar to sex difference in severity observed for other respiratory viruses. HMPV infections appear to be more severe in patients with underlying medical conditions; 30% to 85% of children hospitalized with HMPV have chronic conditions, such as asthma, prematurity, cardiac disease, or cancer.[37,40,41,56,60,61,70]

HMPV infection has been associated with acute respiratory illness in adults as well. In several studies, HMPV accounted for 5% to 15% of all hospitalizations for acute respiratory illnesses in older patients; most of the hospitalized adults had chronic heart or lung disease.[71-73] Other reports in adults have noted that hospitalizations attributed to HMPV occur most frequently in patients with chronic underlying conditions, such as asthma, chronic obstructive pulmonary disease, or cancer.[72-82] The clinical manifestations of HMPV infection differ slightly between younger and older patients (Box 226-1).

CLINICAL MANIFESTATIONS

HMPV has been associated with a variety of respiratory symptoms and diagnoses (Table 226-2). Children with HMPV infection typically present with upper respiratory tract symptoms, including rhinorrhea, cough, and fever. Conjunctivitis, vomiting, diarrhea, and rash are occasionally reported but are not prominent in most studies. Only one study found evidence by RT-PCR of HMPV in patient serum,[42] suggesting that HMPV infection is limited to the respiratory tract. Lower respiratory tract syndromes most frequently associated with HMPV infection are bronchiolitis, croup, pneumonia, and asthma exacerbation. These illnesses are neither clinically nor radiographically distinct from the same clinical syndromes caused by other common respiratory viruses. HMPV can cause severe and fatal disease. Limited human and animal data suggest that pneumococcal superinfection occurs in some cases.[83,84] Reinfection with HMPV occurs, although repeat infections are more likely to be limited to the upper respiratory tract in otherwise healthy children.[16,17,34] A substantial proportion of children infected with HMPV develop AOM and viral RNA has been detected in middle-ear fluid from patients with AOM.[85-87]

Transmission of HMPV probably occurs via respiratory droplets and secretions, similar to RSV. Infectious HMPV particles can persist in the environment for hours[88] and numerous nosocomial outbreaks have been reported.[74,78,89-91] Preliminary data suggest that the duration of virus shedding in the nasopharynx is 1 to 2 weeks in otherwise healthy children, but can last for weeks to months in immunocompromised patients.[16,34,37,57,92,93]

LABORATORY FINDINGS AND DIAGNOSIS

Traditional viral culture techniques are insensitive for detection of HMPV. The virus grows slowly in a limited number of cell types and requires trypsin for replication in culture.[1,88,94-96] These stringent requirements for virus culture procedures are presumed to be the reasons why HMPV was not detected previously. There is no commercial rapid antigen test for HMPV, although immunofluorescent detection has been reported and HMPV-specific monoclonal antibodies, direct fluorescent antibody reagents, and RT-PCR-based assays are available commercially. In general, rapid and reliable diagnosis of HMPV currently depends on molecular techniques based on standard or real-time RT-PCR. Several RT-PCR methods have been reported in research settings that are sensitive and specific, although they are labor-intensive.[97-103]

TREATMENT

The majority of children infected with HMPV can be managed at home with supportive care. For infants and children who require hospitalization, the primary therapies are supplementary oxygen and intravenous hydration. Bronchodilators and corticosteroids have been used empirically, but there are no controlled trials of these medications for HMPV. Studies conducted in cotton rats have suggested potential benefit of bronchodilator and corticosteroid treatment.[104] Aerosolized ribavirin is the only currently licensed antiviral agent for treatment of the related virus, RSV. In one study, ribavirin and polyclonal human immunoglobulin possessed in vitro virus-inhibiting activity against HMPV equivalent to activity against RSV.[105] There are no published animal or human data studying the effects of these interventions, although they may be worthy of consideration in immunocompromised hosts with severe infection due to HMPV. Anecdotal reports of ribavirin, administered to profoundly immunocompromised HMPV-infected patients, often in conjunction with immune globulin intravenous (IGIV), have been published but there are no controlled studies; this therapy should be considered experimental.[106–109]

SPECIAL CONSIDERATIONS

HMPV infection has been associated with exacerbations of underlying asthma in adults and children.[16,38,110–112] Two reports suggest that HMPV infection during infancy is associated with asthma or impaired lung function later in life;[113,114] however, all such studies are complicated by the difficulty of assigning the diagnosis of asthma during infancy, when acute wheezing is frequently associated with viral infections.

HMPV can cause severe and fatal infections in immunocompromised hosts. Several studies suggest that HMPV is a relatively common cause of acute respiratory tract infection in children and adults with malignancy or hematopoietic stem cell transplant, HIV, and lung transplant.[82,107,115–119] Further long-term prospective

studies are needed to characterize fully the extent and severity of disease due to HMPV in immunocompromised hosts.

PREVENTION

The molecular biology cloning technique termed *reverse genetics* to generate recombinant live paramyxoviruses from DNA copies of virus genomes allows the incorporation of specific mutations or entire genes into recombinant viruses. These techniques have now been developed for HMPV. A recombinant chimeric bovine/human parainfluenza virus type 3 vaccine that expressed HMPV F was immunogenic and protective against challenge with HMPV in hamsters.[12] Investigators have generated recombinant HMPV strains that lack various genes, including the small hydrophobic (SH), G, M2-1, or M2-2 genes, or that possess avian metapneumovirus gene insertions.[120–124] Many of these recombinant viruses caused attenuated infection in rodents or nonhuman primates but were highly immunogenic, inducing neutralizing antibodies and protection against challenge with wild-type HMPV. HMPV-specific monoclonal antibodies similar to palivizumab have shown preventive and therapeutic efficacy in rodent models.[125,126]

Key Points. Epidemiology, Clinical Features, Diagnosis, and Treatment of Human Metapneumovirus

EPIDEMIOLOGY

- Distributed worldwide
- Affects all age groups, but most serious disease is in young children or persons with underlying chronic respiratory diseases or immunosuppression
- Transmission: direct person-to-person contact, droplets, and contact with contaminated environmental surfaces

CLINICAL FEATURES

- Acute upper and lower respiratory infections
- Disease characterized most frequently by
  - Rhinorrhea, cough, wheezing
  - Associated acute otitis media common

- Bronchiolitis, pneumonia, croup, and asthma exacerbation common lower respiratory syndromes
- Hypoxemia most common complication in young and elderly
- Duration of viral shedding: 1 to 2 weeks

DIAGNOSIS

- Detection of metapneumovirus by reverse transcriptase polymerase chain reaction testing of respiratory specimens
- Detection of metapneumovirus by fluorescent antibody testing of respiratory specimens

TREATMENT

- Supplemental oxygen, trial of bronchodilators
- No highly effective antiviral drugs or vaccine available

---

227 Rubeola Virus (Measles and Subacute Sclerosing Panencephalitis)

Yvonne A. Maldonado

Before the use of effective measles vaccines in the United States, rubeola infection was an almost universal occurrence during childhood; infection frequently occurred in large, cyclic epidemics reflecting the changing pool of susceptible individuals in the community. Measles continues to be a major cause of morbidity and mortality in unvaccinated infants and children, especially those living in developing countries where measles vaccines are not universally available.

DESCRIPTION OF THE PATHOGEN

Rubeola (measles) virus is a member of the Morbillivirus genus of the Paramyxoviridae family, which also includes mumps, parainfluenza viruses, human metapneumovirus, and respiratory

syncytial virus. Rubeola virus contains a single-stranded, negative-sense linear RNA genome. The virus is pleomorphic, ranges in diameter from 100 to 250 nm, and consists of a helical RNA protein core surrounded by a lipid envelope derived from the host cell. Although only one antigenic type is known, minor antigenic shifts occur in some measles strains.[1–3] These antigenic shifts have not compromised long-lasting immunity. Measles virus infects only humans and primates.

Measles virus contains six major structural proteins: two of these, the hemagglutinin (H) protein and the fusion (F) protein, as well as surface envelope glycoproteins, are important in the development of neutralizing antibodies. The H protein, which mediates viral attachment to host cells, is essential for primary infection. The F protein enhances cell-to-cell spread of the virus.

Matrix (M) protein, which is located on the inner surface of the virus envelope, is important in viral assembly. Neutralizing antibodies confer lifelong immunity to measles and are primarily directed against the H protein. The nucleoprotein (NP), polymerase phosphoprotein (P), and large protein (L) are internal to the virus. L and P proteins are important in RNA polymerase activity, and NP is a structural nucleocapsid protein.

Because measles virus has a lipid envelope, it is inactivated by lipid solvents such as ether and chloroform; the virus is also inactivated by heat (>37°C), cold (<20°C), ultraviolet light, and extremes in pH (<5 and >10). Infectious virus can be maintained for long periods at −70°C.

PATHOGENESIS

Measles is transmitted by aerosolized particles from the respiratory secretions of infected individuals directly to susceptible hosts. The particles also can persist in the environment for more than 1 hour and be acquired by inhalation.[4] Individuals with measles are most contagious during the prodromal stage (which occurs 7 to 10 days after exposure) through the fourth day after the onset of rash. Measles is highly contagious, and symptomatic infection develops in most susceptible exposed individuals.

After exposure, measles virus enters the nasopharynx, attaches to and invades the respiratory epithelium, and spreads to the regional lymphatics; cell-associated viremia follows on the second or third day after exposure. Virus continues to replicate in both local and distant reticuloendothelial sites, and secondary viremia occurs between 5 and 7 days after infection. Cell-associated viremia primarily involves leukocytes,[5] especially monocytes.[6] Within 7 to 14 days after exposure, active replication of measles virus occurs throughout the body, including the respiratory tract, skin, and other organs. Active replication is manifest clinically as upper respiratory tract symptoms, fever, and rash.[7] The development of both humoral and cellular immunity by 15 to 17 days after exposure aborts further viral replication, and in normal hosts, clinical illness resolves.[8,9]

Pathologic changes associated with viremia include lymphoid hyperplasia of the adenoids, tonsils, lymph nodes, spleen, and intestinal tract. Multinucleated giant cells are found most commonly during the early stage of measles in the respiratory tract, especially in the nasopharynx and bronchial mucosa. Syncytial epithelial cells also can be observed. Mononuclear infiltration with peribronchial inflammation occurs in the respiratory tract.

IMMUNE RESPONSE

Both humoral and cellular responses are important in developing and maintaining normal immunity to rubeola. Neutralizing antibodies confer lifelong immunity to measles.[10,11] However, it appears that neutralizing antibodies to both H and F proteins are necessary for protection. Individuals vaccinated with killed virus in whom atypical measles developed after exposure to measles virus had neutralizing antibodies to H protein but lacked neutralizing antibody to F protein.[12] By contrast, recipients of live-attenuated vaccine demonstrate neutralizing antibody to both H and F proteins and are immune to infection. Whereas humoral immunity is important in preventing measles infection, the cellular immune response appears to be important in aborting clinical symptoms during acute infection.[13,14] Among children with congenital hypogammaglobulinemia, for example, measles infection follows a normal clinical course in the absence of a specific antibody response, whereas a congenital or acquired deficiency in cellular immunity predisposes children and adults to severe or fatal infection.[15]

A striking feature of the immune response to measles virus is the induction of transient cellular immunosuppression after infection or vaccination. Delayed-type hypersensitivity responses, such as reactivity to purified protein derivative, are transiently suppressed, and defects in lymphocyte proliferation in response to various mitogens are observed in vitro. Anergy can persist for as long as 2 to 6 weeks after infection. This response is characteristic of cytokine-mediated immune suppression.[16,17]

EPIDEMIOLOGY

Measles is endemic worldwide, with the exception of a few isolated, closed populations. Before the advent of measles vaccination in the U.S., virtually all children contracted infection. Epidemics of measles occurred with regular frequency in 2- to 3-year cycles. In the U.S., measles epidemics occurred most often in late winter through early spring, most frequently in crowded, urban areas. Until the late 1990s, measles accounted for almost 1 million deaths a year in developing countries.[18-20] However, measles deaths worldwide have decreased by 78%, from

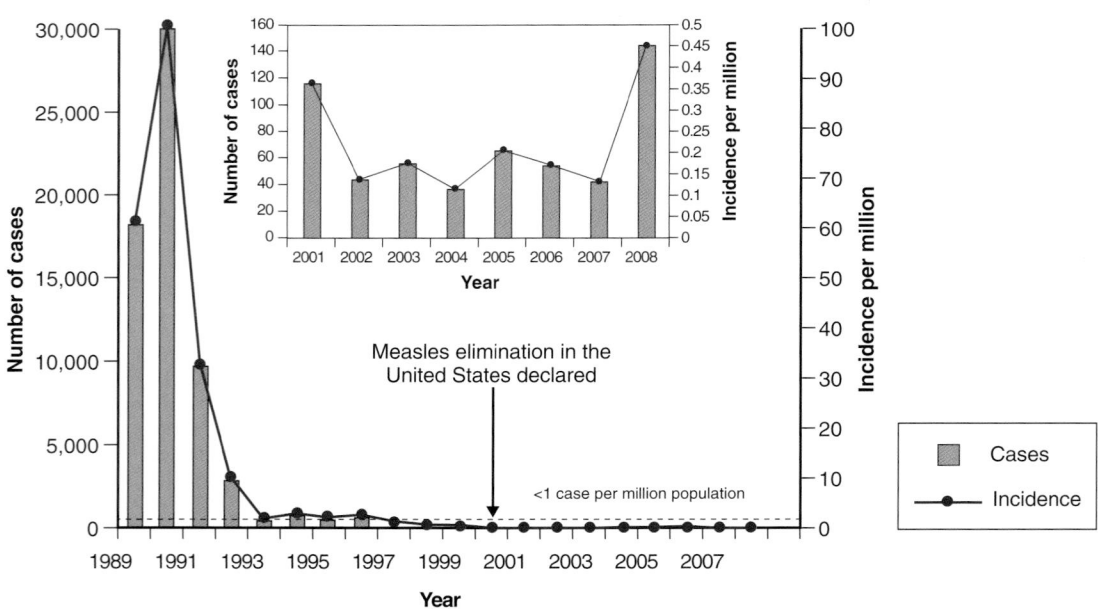

Figure 227-1. Incidence of measles cases, by year – United States, 1989 to 2008. (From Fiebelkorn AP, Redd SB, Gallagher K, et al. Measles in the United States during the postelimination era. J Infect Dis 2010;202:1520–1528.)

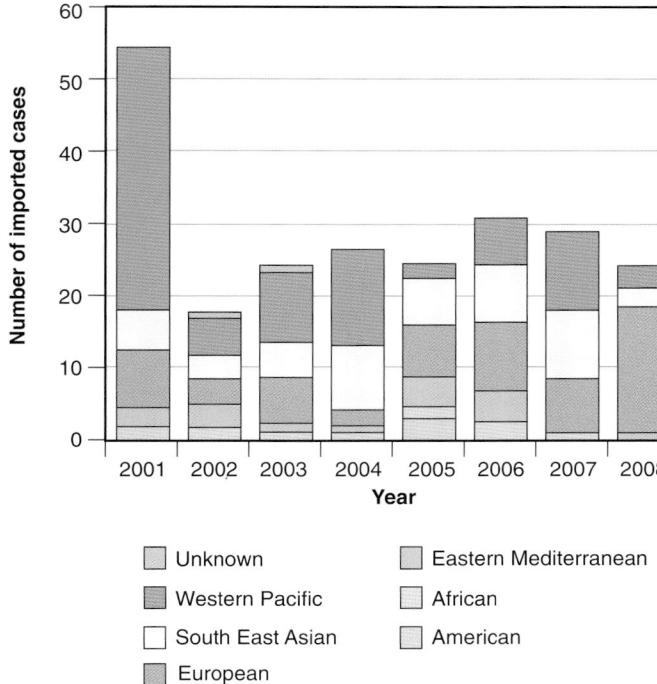

Figure 227-2. Importations of measles cases to the United States by WHO region, 2001 to 2008. (From Fiebelkorn AP, Redd SB, Gallagher K, et al. Measles in the United States during the postelimination era. J Infect Dis 2010;202:1520–1528.)

approximately 733,000 in 2000 to 164,000 in 2008 because of increased global immunization efforts.[21]

Measles vaccines initially were licensed in the U.S. in 1963. The first vaccines used included both killed (inactivated) and live-attenuated vaccines. Inactivated vaccines were found to provide only partial immunity on subsequent exposure to measles, and their use was discontinued after 1968.[22,23] Since licensure of measles vaccine, a 99% reduction in cases had been observed until 1984, when reported numbers of measles cases increased from a low of 1497 in 1983 to 6282 in 1986.[24,25] Reported cases have

fluctuated since that time, with a peak of 27,786 indigenous cases of measles in 1990,[26,27] followed by a record low of 37 cases reported in 2004.[28] The 1990 resurgence of measles was mainly due to two factors: decreased measles vaccination rates in infants and children younger than 2 years, particularly in crowded, urban areas,[29,30] and an increase in susceptible adolescents because of primary vaccine failure in childhood.[31,32]

Approximately 26% of 16,819 cases occurring from 1985 to 1988 were nonpreventable, defined as measles cases in infants younger than 16 months, in individuals born before 1957, in those with a previous physician diagnosis of measles, or in patients with medical contraindications to vaccination. An additional 42% of cases occurred in appropriately vaccinated individuals, and the remaining 32% occurred in unvaccinated individuals for whom vaccine was indicated. Based on this resurgence of measles, an intensified effort to provide two-dose measles vaccine coverage in the U.S. was undertaken. As a result of these efforts, more recent data on the incidence and prevalence of measles in the U.S. strongly suggest that measles is no longer endemic in this country[28,33,34] (Figures 227-1 and 227-2). Similar data from the entire region of the Americas suggest that intensive measles vaccination programs have reduced measles rates substantially throughout the Americas[35] (Figure 227-3). Measles, however, is endemic in the WHO European region, which was the source of 39% of U.S. measles imports during 2005–2008. In the first two months of 2011, 13 imported cases of measles occurred in U.S. residents, the majority of whom (7) were 6 to 23 months of age and none of whom received MMR vaccine prior to travel.[36] Limited cyclic epidemics of measles probably will continue to occur, even in highly vaccinated populations, until global eradication of measles is achieved.[37] If a vaccine with 95% efficacy is used, mathematical estimates indicate that eradication of measles in a closed population requires that virtually all susceptible individuals be immunized.[38] This model is validated by observations in which transmission of measles occurred in populations with up to 99% vaccination rates.[39-41] The currently available vaccine is approximately 95% effective, but 100% vaccination rates have not been achieved in the U.S. and small outbreaks continue to occur.[41]

Infants and young children are most susceptible to measles. In local measles outbreaks, up to 40% of cases occur in children younger than 16 months.[42,43] In the prevaccine era, most individuals contracted measles in childhood (highest attack rate, 5 to 9 years of age), and therefore most adults were not susceptible during cyclic epidemics. In the vaccine era, infants and younger

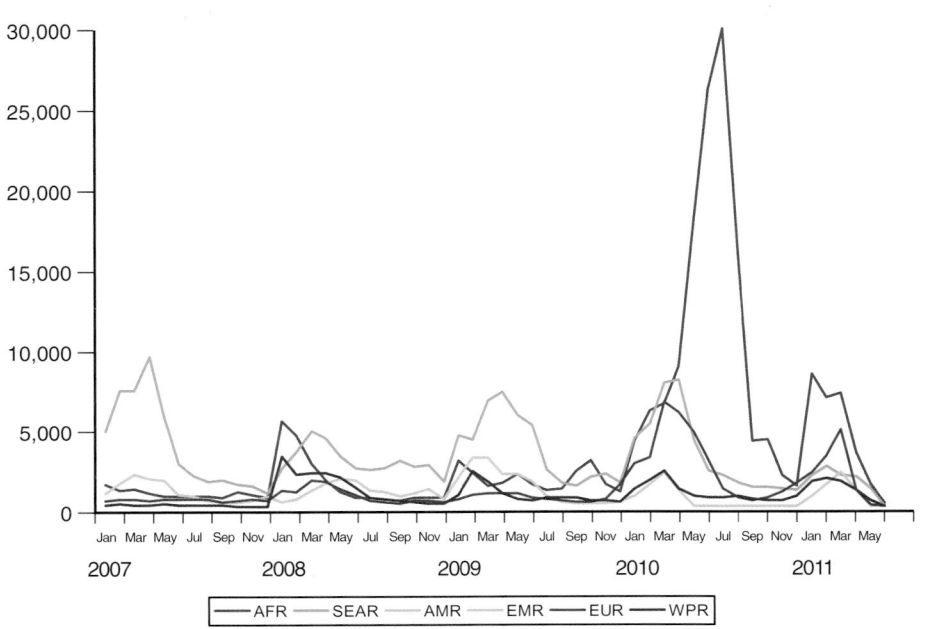

Figure 227-3. Measles case distribution by month and WHO regions, 2006 to 2010. World Health Organization Measles Surveillance Data at http://www.who.int/immunization_monitoring/diseases/measles_monthlydata/en/index.html (last accessed January 16, 2012.)

children are most susceptible to measles infection. In 1991, 9643 cases of indigenous measles were reported in the U.S., with the highest attack rate of 46.9 per 100,000 population occurring in children younger than 12 months.[44] The morbidity and mortality attributable to measles likewise are highest in the youngest age groups.[42,43,45] The severity of measles may also be higher in secondary household cases, when compared with community-acquired cases.[46-50]

Protective transplacental immunity to measles is conferred to infants whose mothers have either had measles infection or received measles vaccine. However, measles antibody titers are higher after natural infection;[51-54] infants whose mothers had measles infection have maternally derived passive measles antibody for longer periods than do infants whose mothers received measles vaccine. Over time, therefore, more infants will be susceptible to measles infection at younger ages because women born after universal immunization in 1963 will constitute a larger proportion of those giving birth.[55,56]

CLINICAL MANIFESTATIONS OF MEASLES

Typical Measles

After an 8- to 12-day incubation period, fever, a hacking or brassy cough, nonpurulent conjunctivitis, photophobia, and coryza develop. Within 2 to 3 days, white macular 1-mm lesions appear on the buccal mucosa. These lesions, called Koplik spots, initially are discrete and appear anywhere on the buccal mucosa, including the hard and soft palate, but characteristically are located opposite the lower premolars. Lesions eventually coalesce and spread rapidly throughout the buccal mucosa. Enanthem is present for 12 to 72 hours.

The rash typically begins at the peak of the respiratory symptoms, generally about 14 days after exposure and 2 to 3 days after the appearance of Koplik spots. Rash is erythematous and initially maculopapular, starts on the forehead or posterior occipital area, and spreads within 3 days to the trunk and extremities (Figure 227-4). The rash is more likely to be confluent over the head and upper extremities than over the trunk and lower extremities (Figure 227-5). After 2 to 3 days, the rash fades from red to copper to brown, also in a cephalocaudal direction; fine desquamation follows. The rash can become mildly hemorrhagic and petechiae are noted occasionally. In general, the severity of illness is proportional to the extent and degree of confluence of the rash. Symptoms during the exanthematous phase include high fever (up to 40°C) that peaks 2 to 3 days after the development of rash,

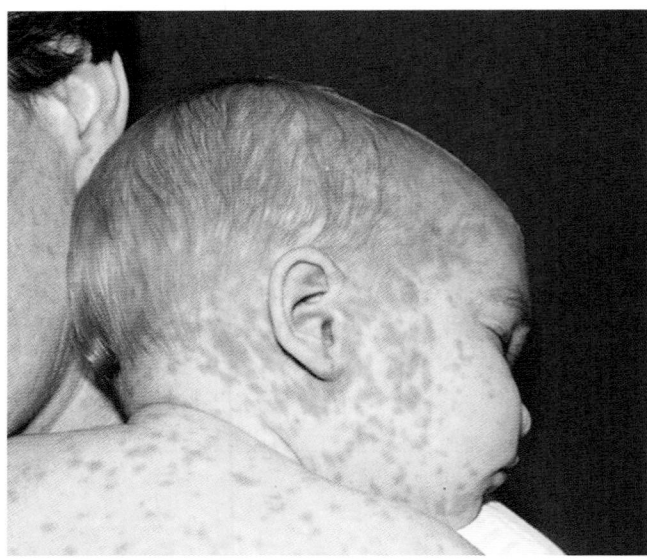

Figure 227-5. Rash on day 5 of measles showing typical confluence and density on head with scattered lesions on the trunk. (Courtesy of J.H. Brien©.)

continued respiratory symptoms, nonpurulent conjunctivitis, pharyngitis, and cervical adenopathy. Once the fever peaks, it usually resolves rapidly; persistent fever is a possible indication of secondary bacterial infection. Occasionally, gastrointestinal symptoms occur, including diarrhea, vomiting, and abdominal pain. In developing countries, diarrheal illness is a major complication of measles.

Severe hemorrhagic measles, or black measles, is most common in infants in developing countries and is characterized by a sudden onset of high fever accompanied by seizures or altered mental status. Pneumonia, a hemorrhagic exanthem and enanthem, bleeding from the mouth, nose, and gastrointestinal tract, and disseminated intravascular coagulation follow.

Transient anicteric hepatitis has been documented in young adults with measles.[57-59] An abnormal chest radiograph in the absence of clinical pulmonary signs and an abnormal electroencephalograph (EEG) in the absence of central nervous system symptoms are common.[60]

Atypical Measles

Atypical measles occurs in individuals infected with natural virus who had previously received killed measles vaccines between 1963 and 1968.[61-63] These persons have a sudden onset of high fever accompanied by abdominal pain, cough, vomiting, and pleuritic chest pain. Koplik spots rarely are present, and rash begins distally and progresses in a cephalad direction, with little involvement of the face and upper part of the trunk. The rash is not as generalized and confluent as in typical measles, and although it is erythematous and maculopapular, it often has a vesicular component. Cough and conjunctivitis are not prominent features of atypical measles. Pulmonary symptoms accompanied by radiographic evidence of pneumonia, hilar adenopathy, and pleural effusions are common. Recovery from atypical measles may take 2 weeks or longer.

Modified Measles

Modified measles is an attenuated form of infection that may occur in individuals who have received immune globulin after exposure to measles. The clinical manifestations of modified measles are milder than those of typical infection, and the incubation period is prolonged from 14 to 20 days. Complications are rarely observed after modified measles.

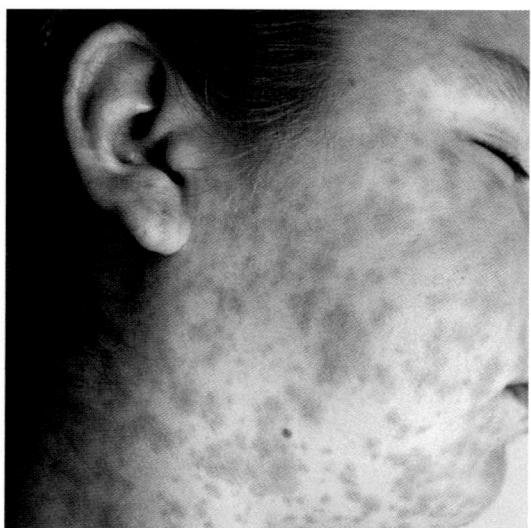

Figure 227-4. Typical rash on day 2–3 of measles. (Courtesy of J.H. Brien©.)

LABORATORY FINDINGS AND DIAGNOSIS

Laboratory abnormalities during measles infection include leukopenia and marked lymphopenia. Serologic tests that can be used to establish the diagnosis include complement fixation, hemagglutination inhibition, and enzyme immunoassays. Although neutralizing antibody assays are more sensitive than the other tests in diagnosing previous infection, performance is expensive and time-consuming. Antibody levels begin to rise 1 to 3 days after the onset of rash and peak 2 to 4 weeks later. A 4-fold or greater rise in antibody titer from paired sera or a single elevated immunoglobulin (Ig) M level is indicative of recent infection. IgM antibody usually is detectable 1 to 2 days after the onset of rash and persists for 30 to 60 days.[64-66] Measles virus can sometimes be isolated from blood, urine, and nasopharyngeal secretions, but isolation is difficult, and serology is the preferred diagnostic method. Detection of measles virus antigen in respiratory epithelial cells or tissue by immunofluorescent methods and detection of viral genome by PCR also have been reported.[67,68]

The differential diagnosis of measles includes rubella, enteroviral infection, exanthem subitum, and adenovirus, Epstein–Barr virus, *Mycoplasma pneumoniae,* and streptococcal or staphylococcal infections. Hypersensitivity to drugs, leptospirosis, and Kawasaki disease also can be confused with measles.

TREATMENT

No specific therapy is indicated for measles. Ribavirin is active against measles virus in vitro and has been used to treat immunocompromised patients with measles pneumonia and encephalitis. Ribavirin has not been evaluated in controlled clinical trials and is not licensed for the treatment of measles.[69-71]

In developing countries where the morbidity and mortality associated with measles are high, administration of vitamin A to children with active measles decreases measles complications such as diarrhea and pneumonia.[72-74] Vitamin A can function as an immunomodulator by boosting antibody responses to measles.[75-77] Studies conducted in the U.S. have demonstrated low levels of vitamin A in selected pediatric populations with measles.[78-80] Some studies have demonstrated increased measles morbidity in children with low vitamin A levels.

The World Health Organization and the United Nations International Children's Emergency Fund recommend that vitamin A be administered to children with measles who live in areas with high measles mortality rates and known vitamin A deficiency. In the absence of well-controlled studies of the effect of vitamin A on measles infection in the U.S., the Centers for Disease Control and Infection (CDC) recommends consideration of supplementation during measles in selected populations at increased risk for complications, such as children hospitalized 6 months to 2 years of age, older than 6 months with immunodeficiency, evidence of vitamin A deficiency, impaired intestinal absorption, moderate to severe malnutrition, or recent immigration from areas with high rates of mortality from measles.[81] Limited data are available regarding the safety and efficacy of vitamin A in infants younger than 6 months. The recommended dose of vitamin A is 100,000 IU orally for infants 6 through 11 months of age and 200,000 IU orally for children 12 months of age and older.

SPECIAL CONSIDERATIONS AND COMPLICATIONS

Respiratory Tract and Other Complications

Even in developed countries, death from measles occurs in 1 of every 1000 cases, usually from pneumonia or encephalitis. Complications of measles are due to the intense inflammatory response to viral replication, particularly in the respiratory tract, possibly compounded by downregulation of immune function. The most common complication of measles in children is acute otitis media (AOM), which occurs in 7% to 9% of cases. Extension of measles infection or secondary bacterial superinfection of the lower respiratory tract, or both, occurs in 1% to 6% of children with measles and accounts for up to 60% of mortality.

Clinical manifestations of measles infection include bronchopneumonia, bronchiolitis, laryngotracheobronchitis, and interstitial or lobar pneumonia.[42,43,59,82,83] Other uncommon complications include thrombocytopenia, hepatitis, appendicitis, ileocolitis, pericarditis, myocarditis, glomerulonephritis, hypocalcemia, Stevens–Johnson syndrome, and toxic shock syndrome.

In developing countries, mastoiditis, pneumonia, and diarrhea are the most common life-threatening complications of measles, especially in malnourished children. In developed countries, most complications, with the exception of encephalitis, resolve without sequelae.

Acute Encephalitis

Central nervous system (CNS) complications of measles include acute encephalitis, subacute sclerosing panencephalitis (SSPE), and subacute encephalitis in immunocompromised hosts.[84-86] Acute encephalitis occurs in approximately 0.01% to 0.1% of measles cases. Fever, headache, lethargy, and other changes in mental status usually occur 2 to 6 days after the appearance of rash. Lumbar puncture demonstrates mild to moderate lymphocytic pleocytosis (40 to 400 cells/mm^3), elevated protein levels (50 to 250 mg/dL), and normal glucose levels.[87-90] The pathophysiology of measles encephalitis is ill defined, but probably results from an immune response to infection, although virus has been isolated from the central nervous system of some patients. Measles encephalitis is mild and self-limited in most children, but about 15% of patients have rapidly progressive fatal disease within 24 hours of diagnosis; about one-fourth of survivors have long-term sequelae such as seizures, hearing loss, developmental delay, and paralysis.

Subacute Sclerosing Panencephalitis

SSPE is a rare complication of measles infection that is characterized by progressive, ultimately fatal neurologic deterioration as a result of persistent CNS infection.[91-98] It is classified as a slow virus disease because of the long latency period and slowly progressive clinical course. The incidence of SSPE in the U.S. in the prevaccine era was 1 in 100,000 measles cases. Despite concern that SSPE could develop after the administration of live measles vaccines, the disease has become uncommon in the U.S. since universal vaccination, rarely occurs in vaccinated children, and even in those can be proved to be caused by wild measles virus.[99]

SSPE is associated with the acquisition of measles before 2 years of age. Travel of infants to countries where measles is prevalent, before receipt of vaccine, can be a clue to SSPE. A review of 453 cases of SSPE reported to the CDC between 1960 and 1976 revealed a mean annual incidence of 3.5 in 10 million persons younger than 20 years. SSPE was 2.3 times more likely to develop in males, and the median age at onset was 9 years. Between 1976 and 1983, 84 cases of SSPE were reported in the U.S.; the mean time from measles infection to the onset of SSPE was 10.8 years. In more recent cases confirmed in brain tissue by the CDC using molecular techniques, wild measles virus was identified with genotype identical to the epidemic strain causing >55,000 cases of measles in the U.S. in 1989 to 1991. Risk of SSPE following measles was estimated to be 10-fold greater than recorded previously.[99]

Microscopic examination of the brain in SSPE demonstrates panencephalitis with lymphocytic and plasma cell perivascular infiltrate, as well as type A and type B intranuclear Cowdry inclusion bodies. Electron microscopic examination of the inclusion bodies reveals paramyxovirus-like structures. Both an abnormal immune response to measles virus and the presence of defective or mutant measles virus strains may be important in the pathogenesis of SSPE. Although patients with SSPE have high antibody levels to measles virus in serum and cerebrospinal fluid (CSF), cellular immune responses are limited. Strains of defective measles virus can produce incomplete infection in the CNS and remain latent in host cells. Phenotypic and genotypic differences in strains of measles virus isolated from patients with SSPE and typical measles have been demonstrated, but the relevance is not clear.

SSPE causes progressive deterioration in behavioral and intellectual function. Early symptoms can include subtle mood disturbances, hyperactivity, and decrease in mental capacity. As the disease progresses, myoclonic seizures and motor disturbances, increasing mental and neurologic deterioration (leading to stupor), dementia, and coma supervene. Death usually occurs within 6 to 9 months after the onset of symptoms. The characteristic EEG finding is a "burst-suppression" pattern with paroxysmal high-amplitude bursts and background suppression. Typical CSF

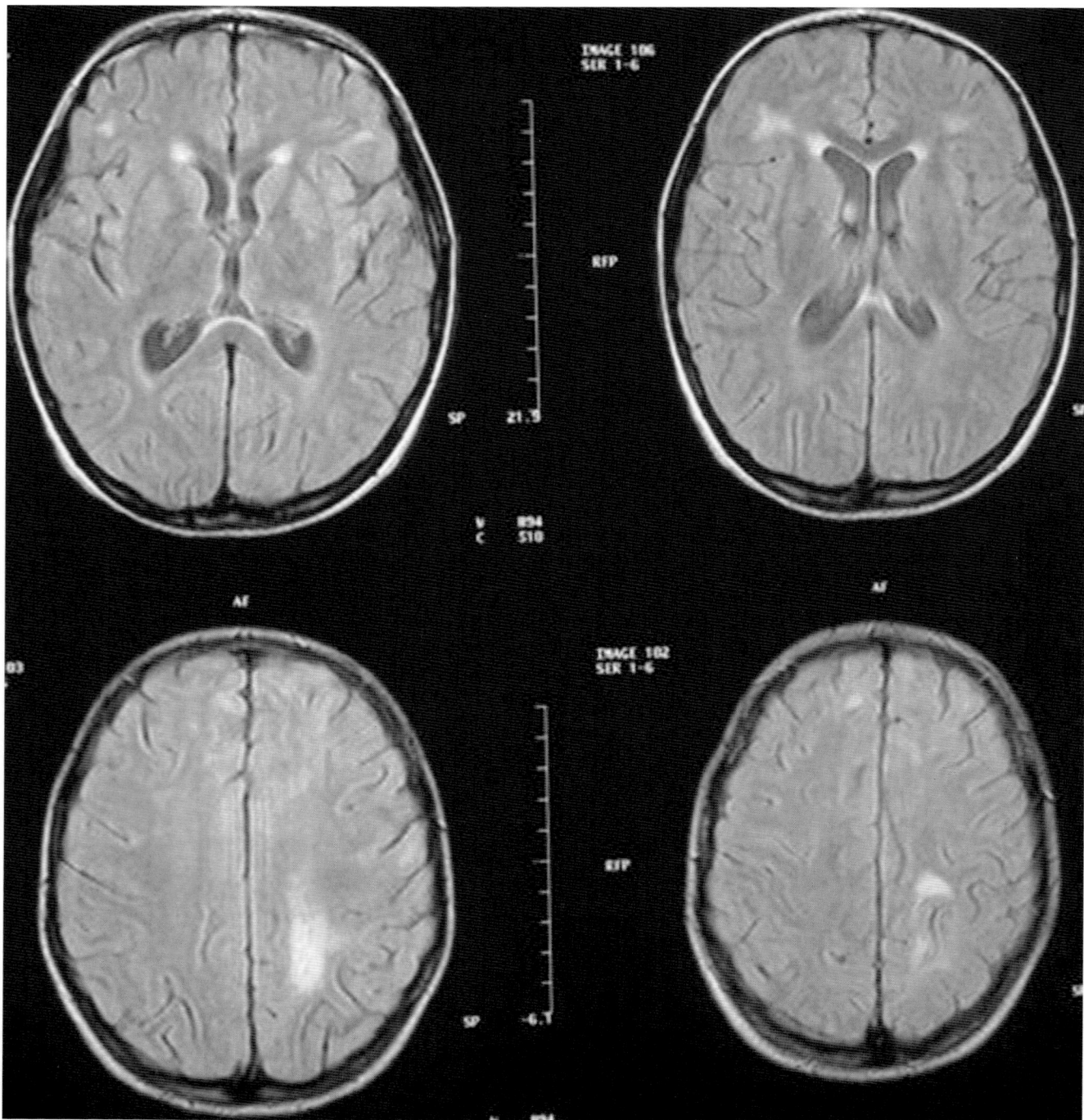

Figure 227-6. In 2006 an 8-year-old girl had clumsiness and decrease in school performance that progressed over 13 weeks to weakness of the right face and extremities, hyperreflexia, jerking movements, decreased intellectual capacity and alertness, seizures, and death. Initially diagnosed and treated as acute disseminated encephalomyelitis, evaluation of the clinical course and electroencephalogram to show slowing with burst suppression led to consideration of subacute sclerosing panencephalitis. Serum measles indirect fluorescent antibody titer was 1:8192 and cerebrospinal fluid 1:512. The patient visited Turkey from age 7 to 10 months and had a 1-day febrile exanthematous illness. Axial magnetic resonance imaging fluid attenuation inversion recovery (FLAIR) images show brain atrophy and white-matter lesions in the frontal (bilateral) parietal and temporal lobes. (Courtesy of E.N. Faerber, J.J. Melvin, and S.S. Long, St. Christopher's Hospital for Children, Philadelphia, PA.)

findings include marked elevations in γ-globulin and measles antibody titers. Frequently, measles antibody in the CSF is oligoclonal. Serum measles hemagglutination inhibition (HI) and complement fixation (CF) antibody levels also are markedly elevated (>1 : 1280), and CSF levels range from 1 : 8 to 1 : 64 or higher. Computed tomography demonstrates cortical brain atrophy. Magnetic resonance imaging findings in one patient are shown in Figure 227-6. Brain biopsy is diagnostic, although the triad of clinical symptoms, characteristic EEG burst-suppression pattern, and elevated measles oligoclonal bands in the CSF is sufficient to make the diagnosis. Therapeutic interventions have included treatment with corticosteroids, immunomodulating agents, plasmapheresis, ribavirin, amantadine, inosiplex, and immunomodulating therapy such as intrathecal interferon-α and -β. None has been successful. Patients with SSPE are not contagious.

MEASLES IN IMMUNOCOMPROMISED HOSTS

Primary viral pneumonia (giant cell pneumonia) and encephalitis are common in malnourished or immunosuppressed children,[100,101] especially those with absent or defective T-lymphocyte function because of congenital defects, receipt of chemotherapy for cancer, or human immunodeficiency virus (HIV) infection.[102–105] Rash can be absent. Measles virus can be isolated persistently from blood and nasopharyngeal tissue for up to 1 month after onset of the rash. Antibody response may be limited. Death usually results from progressive pneumonia. In one study, the case-fatality rate in immunosuppressed patients with measles was 70% for patients with cancer and 30% for HIV-infected patients. HIV-infected patients who had received measles vaccine had lower mortality rates than unvaccinated patients.[106]

Subacute measles encephalitis in an immunocompromised host develops 1 to 7 months after acute infection. Symptoms include seizures, altered level of consciousness, hemiparesis, hemiplegia, ataxia, aphasia, slurred speech, and visual effects. Fever usually is absent, and CSF findings generally are normal. The EEG shows nonspecific abnormalities, and computed tomography of the brain is normal. Brain biopsy is the only reliable method of diagnosing subacute measles encephalitis. Mortality in immunocompromised hosts is high, especially those with T-lymphocyte deficiencies.

Data on the effect of measles on the outcome of pregnancy are limited, and reports of congenital measles are sporadic. Infants born to mothers who acquire measles late in pregnancy can be born with a congenital measles exanthem or an exanthem can develop within the first 10 days of life. No distinct congenital measles syndrome has been described, but the severity of the systemic illness in pregnant women with measles infection can cause spontaneous abortion, premature onset of labor, and low birth in offspring.[107–109]

PREVENTION

Immunization

Interference by passive measles antibody is the most important obstacle to successful immunization of young infants with live-attenuated measles vaccine. Measles vaccines were given at 9 months of age until 1965, at 12 months until 1976, and at 15 months of age thereafter. The increasing age at vaccination was based on documented reduced seroconversion rates in infants vaccinated with the live-attenuated vaccine when younger than 12 months. Increasing vaccine failure rates of up to 95% with decreasing age at vaccination below 12 months of age have been observed, and several studies have confirmed a correlation between vaccine failure with young age and high maternal measles antibody titer.[110,111] Measles vaccine efficacy rates of 95% are reported in populations that received vaccine at ages older than 12 months.[112]

Most women currently of reproductive age have vaccine-induced immunity to measles, which is associated with lower titers of transplacentally acquired antibody (than following natural infection) and is present in offspring for shorter periods of time after birth.[38,51–54,81,113] An earlier loss of protective antibody results in a longer interval of susceptibility to infection before immunization is initiated. Prospective studies conducted in North America in the 1980s suggested that most infants lose maternal antibody by 9 months of age.[55,61] Because of low risk of exposure to measles, The CDC and the American Academy of Pediatrics (AAP) currently recommend routine measles vaccination at 12 to 15 months of age, with a second dose at 4 to 6 years or 11 to 12 years of age.[114] The second dose of vaccine is intended to provide immunity to children who have primary vaccine failure after the first dose.[115,116] A third dose of measles vaccine only is recommended for children who received their initial dose of measles vaccine before their first birthday. Further studies may prompt further changes in the age at routine administration of measles vaccine.[117–119] It is extremely important that infants 6 months through 11 months of age be given measles vaccine (as MMR) prior to travel to countries where measles is endemic; two doses should be given on return after the first birthday.

The Moraten strain of live-attenuated measles is the exclusive measles vaccine currently licensed for use in the U.S. The vaccine is prepared in chick embryo cell culture and produces a mild, noncommunicable infection. The vaccine is available in the U.S. only in combination with mumps and rubella (MMR). A quadrivalent vaccine (MMRV), including measles, mumps, rubella, and varicella, was licensed in the U.S. in 2005. In two postlicensure studies, one additional febrile seizure per ~25,000 children aged 12 to 23 months, was observed in those who had received MMRV compared with those who received MMR vaccine and V vaccine administered as separate injections at the same visit. There was no increased risk of febrile seizures after the second dose of MMRV at 4 to 6 years of age. Based on these data, the CDC and AAP recommend the administration of MMR and V vaccine as two injections at a single visit at age 12 to 47 months, unless the parent or caregiver expresses a preference for the MMRV vaccine. For the second dose of measles, mumps, rubella, and varicella vaccines at any age (15 months to 12 years) and for the first dose at age ≥48 months, use of MMRV vaccine generally is preferred over separate injections.[120]

Despite the lack of evidence that measles vaccine given during pregnancy causes fetal infection, it is not recommended for pregnant women or for those considering pregnancy within 3 months of vaccination. Measles vaccine is contraindicated in immunosuppressed children, except for those selected children infected with HIV, who have a high risk of morbidity and mortality from natural measles. HIV-infected children without severe immunodeficiency and their susceptible household contacts who themselves are not severely immunocompromised should receive MMR, but the primary vaccine failure rate among HIV-infected children may be substantial.[100,101]

Adverse reactions to measles vaccine include fever with temperatures ≥39.4°C in up to 15% and transient rash in up to 5% of recipients. Febrile reactions generally occur 7 to 12 days after vaccination and persist for 1 to 2 days. Allergic reactions related to allergies to egg or egg products or neomycin are uncommon. Patients with a history of nonanaphylactic egg allergies or contact dermatitis from neomycin may receive measles vaccine; those with a history of anaphylactic reactions may require skin testing and desensitization before receiving measles vaccine.[121,122] Hypothesized associations between measles vaccination and the development of Crohn disease, other inflammatory bowel disease, and autism have not been supported by several rigorous prospective and retrospective studies.[123–126]

Recommendations for measles vaccination in developing areas of the world have undergone modification during the 1990s.[20,127,128] In areas in which endemic measles is an important cause of infant morbidity and mortality, vaccination of infants as early as 3 months of age is encouraged. However, this strategy is associated with substantial vaccine failure because of interference by persistent passive antibody. The introduction of high-titer measles vaccines as opposed to standard-titer measles vaccines in these areas of the world resulted in improved immunogenicity in young infants. Longitudinal follow-up, however, revealed that recipients (especially females) of high-titer vaccine had an increased mortality rate compared with recipients of standard-titer vaccines.[129-131] An immunosuppressive effect of vaccine virus infection has been postulated to be causative, and high-titer measles vaccines have been abandoned. Barring new strategies, the WHO recommends that the two-dose vaccine program for infants and children should be adopted in all areas of the world as the only avenue for global elimination of measles.[128,132]

Passive Immunity

Serum immune globulin (IG) can be used to prevent or modify measles in susceptible contacts, particularly household contacts of measles cases, infants younger than 12 months, and pregnant women. To be effective, IG must be given within 6 days of exposure.[133] Infants younger than 6 months generally have protective passive maternal antibody and may not need prophylaxis; however, IG should be given to infants or other unimmunized children if measles has been diagnosed in the mother. IG can be given intramuscularly at a dose of 0.25 mL/kg; for immunocompromised individuals the dose is 0.5 mL/kg (maximum dose, 15 mL).

To assure immunogenicity, measles vaccine must be deferred after immune globulin administration. The period of deferment depends on the dose and type of immune globulin therapy.[114] Measles vaccination should be postponed for 3 to 6 months after the administration of immune globulin intramuscularly for prophylaxis against tetanus, hepatitis A and B, rabies, measles, and varicella. When immune globulin intravenous (IGIV) is used as replacement therapy or for the treatment of idiopathic thrombocytopenic purpura or Kawasaki disease (400 mg to 2 g/kg), vaccination should be deferred for 8 to 11 months, and when blood or blood products are given, vaccination should be deferred for 3 to 7 months. No delay in vaccination is necessary after the administration of packed washed red blood cells. Children with

symptomatic HIV infection or unknown HIV infection status born to HIV-infected women should receive IG prophylaxis after exposure to measles regardless of their measles immunization status. Children who receive monthly IGIV do not routinely require additional IG postexposure prophylaxis if the IGIV was given within 3 weeks.

Public Health Measures and Outbreak Control

Measles vaccine may provide protection against measles if given within 72 hours of exposure.[134-136] In institution-associated measles outbreaks (e.g., childcare centers, primary and secondary schools, colleges, and other institutions), all students and their siblings should be vaccinated unless they have documentation of immunity or have received two doses of measles vaccine at or after 12 months of age. School personnel born after 1956 who have not had documented measles or vaccination also should be vaccinated. For measles outbreaks in preschool-aged populations, vaccination effort is directed at the youngest susceptible populations, including infants ≥6 months of age, and at ensuring immunization of children ≥12 months of age. Infants <12 months who are vaccinated during an outbreak must be revaccinated at 12 to 15 months of age and again before school entry.

Healthcare personnel should be screened for measles immunity and susceptible individuals vaccinated to prevent nosocomial transmission of measles.[137-140]

Isolation Procedures

Isolation of household or school contacts alone is not effective in preventing transmission because excretion of virus occurs before the onset of symptoms. Hospitalized patients exposed to measles should be cared for in respiratory airborne from days 5 to 21 after exposure. Immunocompetent patients with measles should be isolated until 5 days after the onset of rash; immunocompromised individuals should be isolated for the duration of their illness.[140]

Key Points. Epidemiology, Clinical Features, Diagnosis, and Prevention of Measles

EPIDEMIOLOGY

- Distributed globally
- Affects all susceptible age groups but most are infected in infancy and early childhood
- Airborne (aerosol) transmission; highly contagious
- Natural infection results in lifelong immunity

CLINICAL FEATURES

- All infections are symptomatic
- Incubation period 8–12 days; patient contagious day 7 after exposure (before rash illness occurs) until 4 days after rash appears
- Disease characterized most frequently by:
  - Classic triad: "Cough, coryza, conjunctivitis" with fever
  - An erythematous maculopapular rash, which spreads in a cephalocaudal direction
  - Evanescent enanthem (Koplik spots) that appears on the lower buccal mucosa adjacent to the molars
  - Common complications include otitis media, pneumonia, croup, and diarrhea; encephalitis in 1 of 1000 cases; rare deaths from pneumonia and neurologic complications
- Case fatality highest among infants

DIAGNOSIS

- Clinical diagnosis based on symptoms described above in conjunction with serologic tests for measles IgM (IgM can be negative in 72 hours after rash onset)

TREATMENT

- Vitamin A treatment results in reduced risk of mortality in deficient children
- No antiviral drugs available
- Treat secondary bacterial complications (otitis media, pneumonia)

PREVENTION

- Measles immunization at 12–15 months of age with a second dose at 4–6 years of age

228 Rabies Virus

Rodney E. Willoughby, Jr

THE VIRUS

Rabies virus and related viruses, including Lagos, Mokola, and Duvenhage viruses, are members of the Rhabdoviridae family, genus Lyssavirus (which is derived from the Greek word *lyssa*, meaning "madness." *Rabies* derives from the Sanskrit word *rabhas*, which means "to do violence"). Rabies virus causes human encephalitis through zoonotic infection, predominantly of bats in the Americas.[1]

The lyssaviruses differ antigenically but are morphologically similar and neurotropic.[2] Rabies virus is an enveloped bullet-shaped virus, 180 nm long and 75 nm wide, composed of five structural proteins (Figure 228-1). Rabies virus contains one copy of a single-stranded, nonsegmented, negative (noncoding) RNA of approximately 12,000 nucleotides. The virus envelope contains glycosylated G-protein spikes that bind to cells. The matrix (M) protein is located on the inner virus envelope, inside which the virus nucleoprotein (N) tightly binds the viral RNA to form the nucleocapsid core. This core, along with a large transcriptase protein (L) and a phosphorylated protein (P), is the rabies virus nucleocapsid (RNP).[3]

PATHOGENESIS

The incubation period after rabies virus inoculation begins with an ill-defined local latent phase prior to neuronal entry that can involve replication in muscle or skin for canine or bat rabies variants, respectively. This step in pathogenesis is the basis of the rationale for recommendations of local wound care and instillation of neutralizing antibody (i.e., to reduce the rabies infectious inoculum). Neutralizing antibodies actually can penetrate the infected cells.[4] Response to the rabies vaccine then generates further neutralizing antibody.

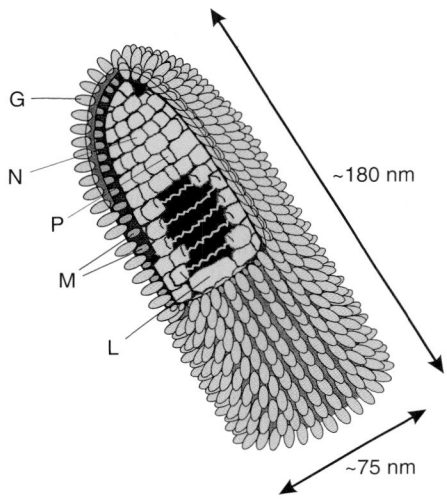

Figure 228-1. Hypothetical model of the rabies virion. The surface is covered by G glycoprotein (G) embedded in lipid membrane derived from the host cell. Matrix proteins (M) associate with the lipid membrane. Within this envelope is a ribonucleoprotein core composed of RNA closely associated with protective nucleoprotein (N), virion transcriptase (L), and phosphoprotein (P).

After local tissue replication over weeks to months, the virus attaches to nicotinic acetylcholine receptors that provide access to the peripheral nervous system through neuromuscular spindles or muscle motor endplates.[5] Sensory and autonomic nerves also are infected. Other host receptors for rabies virus include specific carbohydrates, the neuronal cell adhesion molecule (NCAM), and the p75 neurotrophin receptor (p75NTR).[6] Direct virus entry into neuroepithelial cells of the olfactory end organ has been implicated in acquisition of rabies by aerosol exposure.

Rabies virus moves centripetally along peripheral nerves, without virus replication, at rates of 100 mm/day or higher. Once in the spinal cord, virus spreads rapidly to brain tracing neurons in retrograde fashion across synapses, one synapse per day.[7] Centrifugal spread then occurs along motor, sensory, and autonomic axons into host body tissues (usually restricted to nerves innervating organs, including hair follicles) and particularly into the salivary and lacrimal glands.[8-10] Pathologic features are minimal. *Negri bodies* are rabies-specific eosinophilic inclusions in the cytoplasm of neurons that contain virus antigens, but vary by brain region and may not be found in 30% of cases.[11] Histologic damage results from limited perivascular leukocytosis, neuronal degeneration, and neuronophagia. Inflammation of the dorsal root ganglia correlates with focal neurologic prodromes.[12] In the less common paralytic form of rabies, axonal loss mimics acute motor axonal neuropathy and other polio-like diseases.[13] Minimal histologic damage is in stark contrast to the severity of clinical rabies. Rabies viremia has not been observed as a mechanism of virus spread.

VIRULENCE AND IMMUNITY

Host factors that reduce the incubation period are: (1) young age; (2) immunocompromised state, including corticosteroid use; (3) greater severity of the wound; (4) closeness of the wound to the central nervous system; and (5) large inoculum. Neuroinvasiveness itself is determined by the virus G protein. In animal models, a single-point mutation at position 333 of the G protein renders strains avirulent as a result of alteration in the ability of the virus to spread from cell to cell.[14]

The G protein and the RNP are the major targets of the protective host response. The G glycoprotein is the major target of virus-neutralizing antibody and also of cellular immunity.[15] Antigenicity of the G protein of rabies virus is broad enough to induce protective immunity to all rabies virus strains, but may not protect against other lyssaviruses.[16] A combination of two monoclonal antibodies is sufficient to neutralize most clinical rabies virus isolates.[14]

EPIDEMIOLOGY

Rabies primarily is an animal infection. Humans become infected through exposure to infected animals. The control of rabies requires both knowledge of the endemic animal source of rabies and the geography of infection and an understanding of virus transmission in nature.[17] Any warm-blooded animal can become infected, but some animal species are more susceptible, and some rabies strains are more infectious, than others.[18,19] The duration of virus shedding in saliva and the rapidity of death vary among animal species. Skunks shed virus for up to 18 days before death, whereas foxes succumb rapidly. A single animal species harbors the majority of rabies infections in each geographic area. In North America, the source of rabies has shifted from domestic animals

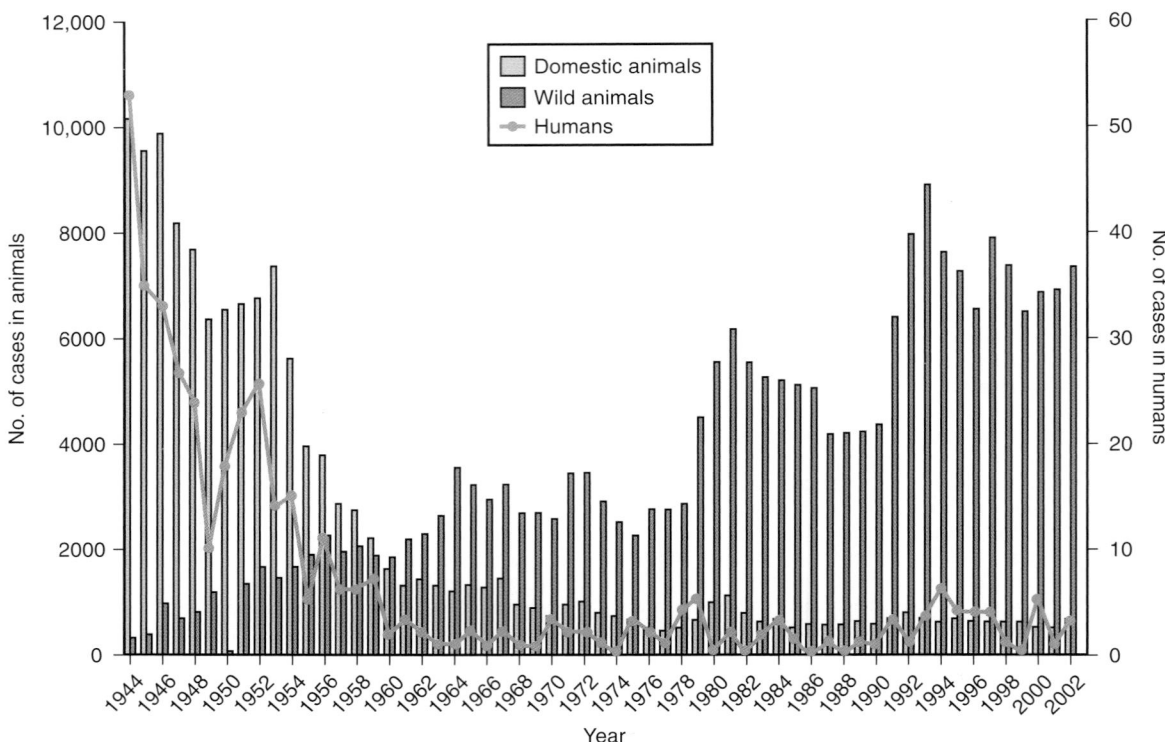

Figure 228-2. Temporal trends in animal and human rabies in the United States. (Redrawn from Rupprecht CE, Gibbons RV. Clinical practice. Prophylaxis against rabies. N Engl J Med 2004;351:2626–2635.)

to wildlife (Figure 228-2). Six separate rabies enzootics exist. Outside North America, wildlife rabies enzootics involve other animals (Table 228-1). Other bat lyssaviruses have been isolated in Europe, Africa, and Australia and can cause sporadic human encephalitis with fatal outcome.[16] Genetic sequencing and typing by monoclonal antibody panels may distinguish rabies enzootics and whether humans are infected with local or imported rabies virus strains.[20,21]

The dog remains the principal vector for transmission of rabies virus to humans in most parts of the world (outside the United States and Europe). Cats usually are second in importance in these areas. The incubation period for rabies in dogs usually is 1 to 3 months but can be >1 year. The first manifestations of rabies in

dogs are a change in disposition, restlessness, and fear. After 3 to 5 days, the dog demonstrates the "furious" phase (snapping, increased restlessness, drooling) or the "dumb" phase (lethargy, paralysis) of illness followed by death, which usually occurs within 10 days after the onset of illness. There are rare reports of dogs who survive up to 1 month after spreading rabies to humans.[20] Rabies in wild animals is characterized mainly by loss of nocturnal habits or fear of humans. Other signs are similar to those described in dogs.

The vehicle of virus transmission is infected animal saliva, which can be inoculated by a bite or scratch. Contact of infected animal saliva with human mucous membranes also can transmit infection.[22] In addition to animal transmission of rabies virus, 14 human-to-human transmissions have occurred after transplantation of infected tissue.[23] Human rabies cases also have been observed secondary to aerosol transmission of virus, as has occurred after exposure in caves containing bats and from laboratory accidents. Nine of 13 human cases of rabies reported in the U.S. between 1980 and 1990 resulted from exposure to animals outside the country.[20] The majority of human rabies contracted within the U.S. in recent years have been determined by molecular techniques to have been acquired from bats.[24] Because a history of bat exposure often is absent, it is assumed that certain insectivorous bats inflict unperceived bites on sleeping persons.[22]

Endemic rabies infection occurs on every continent except Antarctica and Australia and on selected islands such as Hawaii and the United Kingdom. Worldwide data on human rabies epidemiology are incomplete because of the hopelessness, stigma, and extreme poverty associated with rabies. It is estimated that 50,000 to 60,000 people die annually from rabies. Most cases of rabies occur in males and children.[17]

CLINICAL MANIFESTATIONS

Clinical stages of human rabies correspond to steps in pathophysiology.[25,26] The asymptomatic first phase is the virus incubation period, which generally lasts from 10 to 90 days but ranges from

TABLE 228-1. Endemic Rabies in Wildlife

Geographic Region	Principal Species with Endemic Rabies[a]
United States and Canada	
Central United States and Canada	Striped skunk
Mid-Atlantic, southeast United States	Raccoon
New York, Quebec, Ontario	Red fox
Northwest territories	Arctic fox
Arizona	Grey fox
Texas	Grey fox
Caribbean	Mongoose
Europe	Red fox
Iran	Wolf
Africa	Jackal

[a]The bat is always considered endemically rabid. The dog is the principal vector for transmission of rabies around the world, except for North America and Europe.

4 days to 7 years.[25,26] The long incubation period lowers the yield of obtaining a history of an antecedent animal exposure. A retaking of the history, focused on travel and animal exposures, is critical.[27]

The second, or prodromal, period lasts for 2 to 10 days and correlates with viral invasion of the central nervous system. Early symptoms in up to half of patients are a nonspecific febrile illness, frequently accompanied by behavioral, sleep, and emotional changes. Local pruritus, pain, paresthesia, weakness, or myoclonic jerks occur at the site of inoculation in approximately 50% of cases and are most helpful at bringing rabies into consideration. This stage correlates with virus infection of the dorsal root ganglia, spinal cord, brainstem, and limbic system.[25,26]

The third stage is the development of neurologic signs of disease and correlates with widespread infection of brain. The "furious" form of rabies comprises aggressiveness (biting, hitting, yelling), excitement, hyperactivity, and hallucinations that last for brief periods and alternate with normal behavior progressing to confusion or delirium. Fever can be intermittent but is present universally. More than 50% of patients experience hydrophobia (with attempts to drink liquids) or aerophobia (when air is blown on the face). These reactions result from violent diaphragmatic contractions as an exaggerated respiratory protective reflex, and are sufficient to cause pneumothorax. Hypersalivation, lacrimation, and difficulty swallowing increase the risk of aspiration. Status epilepticus, marked dystonia, parkinsonian signs, or opisthotonus are uncommon and should suggest other diagnoses. Clinical presentation at this stage can mimic that of intoxication, meningitis, encephalitis, myoclonic epilepsy, tetanus, polio, or Guillain–Barré syndrome.

The "paralytic" form of rabies occurs in approximately 20% of patients and is slower to evolve. Flaccid paralysis progresses to quadriparesis, bulbar abnormalities, and respiratory insufficiency. Hypersalivation and hydrophobic spasms can occur. Guillain–Barré syndrome often is considered but findings of fever, pain, sensory or sphincter disturbance, and more prominent involvement of proximal musculature are more suggestive of rabies.[12] In developing countries, where tissue-derived rabies vaccines are produced, vaccine-associated autoimmune encephalitis is a consideration. Other diagnostic possibilities include hysteria, botulism, and elapid snake bite.

The fourth stage of rabies is coma. Examinations consistent with brainstem death are distinctively discordant with electroencephalogram (EEG) or magnetic resonance imaging (MRI) findings.[28–30] Hypoxic-ischemic insults or progressive decline in EEG activity are terminal events. Death usually occurs within 7 days in furious rabies and 21 days in paralytic rabies; critical care can prolong survival considerably. Early deaths can result from respiratory arrest or cardiac dysrhythmias, including asystole. Coma is correlated with generalized spasm of the basilar arteries measured by transcranial doppler ultrasonography.[31] Complications associated with the immune response include complete heart block in dog rabies, and cerebral edema in bat rabies. Nine survivors of rabies are known, and seven received rabies vaccine prior to the onset of clinical illness.

LABORATORY DIAGNOSIS

Rabies often is misdiagnosed clinically.[32] Cerebrospinal fluid (CSF) findings are typical of viral meningoencephalitis. CSF is normal in approximately one-third of cases during the first week of illness. EEG, computed tomography, and MRI of the brain also can be normal.[33]

Specific laboratory tests that are not widely available are required for diagnosis. Aside from studies performed on brain tissue, virus-specific studies require tissue from sites reflecting the centrifugal movement of virus. Detection of rabies virus antigen by immunofluorescence testing or culture of specimens obtained by skin-punch biopsies of the hair follicles at the nape of the neck has 50% to 94% sensitivity and almost 100% specificity. The earliest to yield a positive result, but technically challenging due to virus heterogeneity, is a reverse transcriptase-polymerase chain reaction

(RT-PCR) test for rabies nucleic acid performed on the patient's saliva or skin.[34–36] Virus can also be isolated or its genome amplified from skin, CSF, urine, and respiratory secretions. Fluorescent immunohistology is a more sensitive method than both histologic examination of brain tissue for Negri bodies and virus culture of brain. Consideration should be given for brain biopsy at the time of placement of intracranial pressure-monitoring devices in patients with idiopathic encephalitis.

Rabies-specific antibodies in serum or CSF can be measured by enzyme immunoassay and neutralizing antibody by the rapid fluorescent focus inhibition test (RFFIT). Antibodies can be detected in serum as early as 6 days (and in CSF within 13 days) after the onset of symptoms.[24] Only clinical rabies (and not rabies immunization) produces detectable rabies antibodies in the CSF.[24]

TREATMENT

Patients are intermittently alert until coma supervenes. Care should emphasize minimization of environmental stimuli that precipitate spasms, meticulous respiratory care, and control of pain and anxiety. Since the 1970s, intensive medical care often came close to producing survivors. Two case series report an upper limit of 5% survival.[32,37] A recent case report suggests a continuum of disease.[38] Limited animal experiments and human case reports suggest that inflammation is accentuated, paralytic disease precipitated, or death accelerated when persons with rabies are "treated" with rabies vaccine or rabies-specific immune globulin.[39,40] Use of broad-spectrum antiviral agents (vidarabine, ribavirin, interferon) is unsuccessful and associated with massive brain necrosis.[41,42] A teenage girl recently survived rabies without prior receipt of post-exposure prophylaxis (PEP). Her therapy included deep sedation to minimize dysautonomia. Administration of rabies vaccine and immune globulin were avoided.[43] Three more survivors have been registered, all with bat-associated rabies. An updated protocol and case-registry of similarly treated patients are available at www.mcw.edu/rabies.

PREVENTION

Vaccines Available

Schedule and indications for administration of rabies vaccine and human-derived rabies immune globulin (HRIG) are shown in Tables 228-2 and 228-3. Three rabies vaccines are licensed in the U.S.: human diploid cell vaccine (HDCV), primary chick embryo

TABLE 228-2. Rabies Immunization Schedules

	Dose	Route of Administration	Days
PRE-EXPOSURE PROPHYLAXIS			
Vaccine	1.0 mL	IM	0, 7, and 21–28
	0.1 mL	ID[a]	
POSTEXPOSURE PROPHYLAXIS			
Vaccine	1.0 mL	IM	No previous immunization: 0, 3, 7, 14 Previously immunized: 0, 3
Human rabies immune globulin (HRIG)	20 IU/kg	Infiltrated at site of exposure	Immediately (if not immunized previously)

ID, intradermal; IM, intramuscular.

[a]Not an approved route in all countries.

TABLE 228-3. Schedule of Postexposure Prophylaxis for Rabies in the United States, 2009

Vaccination Status, Treatment	Regimen[a]
NOT PREVIOUSLY VACCINATED	
Wound cleansing	All postexposure treatment should begin with immediate, thorough cleansing of all wounds with soap and water. If available, a virucidal agent such as a povidone-iodine solution should be used to irrigate the wounds
Human RIG	Administer at a dose of 20 IU/kg of body weight. If anatomically feasible, *full dose* should be infiltrated around the wound(s), and any remaining volume should be administered IM at an anatomic site distant from vaccine administration. RIG should not be administered in the same syringe as the vaccine. Because human RIG can partially suppress the active production of antibody, no more than the recommended dose should be given
Vaccine (HDCV or PCECV)	One 1-mL dose IM (deltoid area[c]) on days 0,[c] 3, 7, 14
PREVIOUSLY VACCINATED[d]	
Wound cleansing	All postexposure treatment should begin with immediate thorough cleansing of all wounds with soap and water. If available, a virucidal agent such as a povidone-iodine solution should be used to irrigate the wounds
Human RIG	RIG should *not* be administered
Vaccine (HDCV or PCECV)	One 1-mL dose IM (deltoid area[b]) on days 0,[c] 3

HDCV, human diploid cell culture vaccine; IM, intramuscularly; PCECV, purified chick embryo cell culture vaccine; RIG, rabies immune globulin.

[a]*These regimens are applicable for all age groups, including children.*

[b]*Deltoid area is the only acceptable site of vaccination for adults and older children. For younger children, the outer aspect of the thigh can be used. Vaccine should never be administered in the gluteal area.*

[c]*Day 0 is the day on which the first dose of vaccine is administered.*

[d]*Any person with a history of pre-exposure vaccination with HDCV, RVA, or PCVEC; prior postexposure prophylaxis with HDCV, RVA, or PCECV; or previous vaccination with any other type of rabies vaccine and a documented history of antibody response to the prior vaccination.*

From Use of a reduced (4-dose) vaccine schedule for postexposure prophylaxis to prevent human rabies recommendations of the advisory committee on immunization practices. MMWR Recomm Rep 2009;59(RR-2):1–9.

cell vaccine (PCECV), and rhesus lung cell vaccine (RVA), although RVA is no longer being produced. Outside the U.S., additional vaccines include purified Vero cell vaccine (PVRV) and purified duck embryo vaccine (PDEV). All of these vaccines can be used interchangeably, although it is preferable to use the same vaccine for the entire course of immunizations. In the U.S., intramuscular administration is recommended.[44] In other countries, many of the cell culture vaccines are administered intradermally to reduce dose volume/expense. Nerve tissue vaccines and suckling mouse brain vaccines are in declining use and should never be used where there is access to cell-culture-derived vaccines.[45]

Pre-exposure Prophylaxis

Pre-exposure prophylaxis with vaccine should be offered to individuals in veterinary medicine, wildlife management, and rabies laboratory work, spelunkers, and selected persons who travel to areas where canine rabies is endemic. It is not necessary to measure

the antibody response, except in immunosuppressed persons or if risk is ongoing.[22,44] Aside from local and systemic reactions, which are generally mild, side effects include immune complex-mediated reactions (hives, angioedema, arthritis), most often after booster doses. Cell culture-derived vaccine-associated neurologic diseases are unproven.[46] Pregnancy is not a contraindication to rabies vaccine.[46] Chloroquine interferes with antibody production following HDCV.[22]

Postexposure Prophylaxis (PEP)

Postexposure management of a patient wounded by an animal begins with aggressive care of animal-induced wounds, including tetanus prophylaxis. Steps are: (1) complete and thorough washing and repeated flushing (especially of larger wounds) with soap or detergent and water or water alone; (2) avoiding suturing; and (3) avoiding occlusive dressings. Failure of PEP often is ascribed to wound closure for cosmetic indications or lack of administration of rabies immune globulin.

A decision must then be made whether a rabies exposure has been likely.[47] Close communication with public health officials is recommended to gain information regarding locally infected animal species and to ensure proper examination of animals. Two-thirds of PEP courses can be avoided by submission of the suspect animal for examination of the brain.[46] Prophylaxis generally is not required for contact with a vaccinated animal or when contact with a rabid animal has not violated the individual's skin barrier or involved a mucous membrane. Because few cases of human rabies have occurred from rodent bites, vaccination generally is not recommended after these exposures.[22] In developed countries, bites from dogs and cats who remain healthy after 10 days of observation do not warrant prophylaxis. However, in developing countries where the risk of animal rabies is higher, vaccination should be given immediately, and should only be discontinued if the observed animal remains healthy.

Immediate administration of rabies immune globulin and commencement of immunization are required for persons who are bitten by wild carnivores and bats, as well as by dogs or cats known or suspected to be rabid. Because bats have infected people in the absence of a recognized bite, rabies prophylaxis is recommended for children and other individuals who were asleep or unattended in a room with a bat, and others for whom it is impossible to exclude direct contact with a bat.

Passive immunization should be administered as early as possible to exposed individuals not previously immunized. Human rabies immune globulin (HRIG) should be given at a dose of 20 IU/kg, with the entire dose infiltrated into the wound if feasible. The volume can be diluted if insufficient to infiltrate the entire wound. Unused immune globulin can be injected intramuscularly into the gluteal or anterolateral thigh muscle with a different syringe and injection site from those used for the vaccine. HRIG is safe and free from serious side effects. It should be given at the time of the first vaccine dose, but HRIG is not beneficial if given later than 7 days after the first vaccination. Equine rabies immune globulin often is used outside North America, in a dose of 40 IU/kg. As the product is purified, it is well tolerated and equally as effective as HRIG.

Postexposure immunization for previously unimmunized individuals requires 4 doses given into the deltoid muscle (never in the gluteal region) over 14 days.[44] It is not necessary to measure the antibody response, except in immunosuppressed persons. Children produce an immune response equivalent to that of adults. The immunization series can be stopped if the brain of the suspected rabid animal tests negative for rabies virus on direct fluorescent antibody testing or if the domestic dog or cat remains healthy during 10 days of observation.[47] Regimens for immunization are summarized in Table 228-3.

Theoretically, human-to-human transmission can occur but transmission to healthcare workers has not been documented.[46,48] The patient should be placed in an isolation room, and gowns, gloves, masks, and goggles are worn by anyone who has direct contact with the patient. Healthcare workers who experience mucous membrane or parenteral exposure to potentially infected tissues or saliva should be considered for PEP. When rabies is not considered ante mortem, an average of 80 to 150 healthcare workers receive prophylaxis.[27] There are no data to support chemoprophylaxis with oral ribavirin or amantadine.

Ultimately, improved rabies prevention depends on immunization of domestic animals and wildlife vectors of rabies. Wildlife exposures are increasing (see Figure 228-2).[46] Rabies is increasing internationally where deforestation displaces bat colonies, affluence increases pet ownership, or there is an increase in feral dog packs. Wildlife can be efficiently immunized against rabies by the oral route through the use of baits containing live-attenuated strains or recombinant poxviruses that produce G glycoprotein.[49] There is a need for more inexpensive rabies vaccine and immune globulin, especially in countries with a high incidence of human rabies.[45]

Key Points. Characteristics of Rabies Virus and Infection

VIROLOGY
- Single negative-stranded RNA viruses of the family Lyssaviridae
- Marked tropism for the nervous system

EPIDEMIOLOGY
- Emerging, major zoonosis causing encephalitis, with 55,000 deaths annually in Africa and Asia alone
- Dogs are the major vectors worldwide, with bats predominant in the Americas. Wild animal reservoirs vary geographically
- Predilection for children and males
- Prolonged and variable incubation period

CLINICAL
- Major "furious" form characterized by febrile encephalitis with focal myoclonus and paresthesias, and characteristic hydrophobia and aerophobia (when present); intermittent consciousness until late in the disease
- Minor "paralytic" form often confused with Guillain–Barré syndrome, but rabies shows sphincter disturbances and more sensory phenomena
- Prominent vascular and metabolic dysfunction contribute to rabies encephalitis

DIAGNOSIS
- Requires sending skin biopsy, saliva, serum, and CSF specimens to a WHO rabies reference laboratory

TREATMENT
- Conventional therapy is palliative
- Milwaukee protocol (www.mcw.edu/rabies) consists of sedation to minimize dysautonomia and prophylaxis against generalized vasospasm of the basilar arteries
- Immunization and human rabies immune globulin (HRIG) are avoided once symptomatic

PREVENTION
- Pre-exposure prophylaxis (3 doses over 21–28 days) indicated for travel to rabies-endemic areas and for high-risk occupations. Boosters (2 doses) are then required after an exposure
- Postexposure prophylaxis (aggressive washing of wound, then 4 doses of vaccine over 14 days, plus HRIG). Immunocompromised patients receive 5 doses and require serologic confirmation

---

229 Influenza Viruses

Fatimah S. Dawood, Kanta Subbarao, and Anthony E. Fiore

Influenza viruses cause annual winter epidemics of respiratory illness in temperate climates and have resulted in four influenza pandemics since 1900. Although most data on influenza burden come from temperate countries, the burden of influenza in other countries, including tropical countries with varied seasonal transmission patterns, increasingly is appreciated.[1] In the United States, influenza is estimated to result in 3000 to 49,000 deaths[2] and 55,000 to 431,000 hospitalizations annually.[3] Among children, influenza virus infections are common, and influenza-associated hospitalization rates among children are highest in those <2 years of age[4–9] and those with underlying medical conditions.[6,10,11] Although >90% of seasonal influenza-associated mortality occurs among persons ≥65 years of age, patients with cardiopulmonary disease, and those with compromised immunity,[12] 40 to >200 influenza-associated deaths are estimated to have occurred annually in children in the U.S. during 1977 through 2007.[13] During the 2009 influenza A (H1N1) pandemic, children were disproportionately affected by 2009 H1N1 influenza and experienced the highest pandemic influenza attack rates and hospitalization rates.[14] Influenza vaccination is the best method of influenza prevention and influenza vaccines are currently approved for use in children 6 months of age and older.[15]

MICROBIOLOGY

Three antigenic types of influenza virus (A, B, and C) are recognized, with influenza A viruses being further subdivided into multiple subtypes. Influenza A and B viruses contain eight segments of negative-sense, single-stranded RNA that code for 10 and 11 proteins, respectively.[16] Influenza viruses are irregular spherical (80 to 120 nm) or filamentous structures; their surfaces are studded with rod-shaped hemagglutinin (HA) and neuraminidase (NA) spikes (Figure 229-1).[17] These surface glycoproteins are the major targets of the protective host immune response.[18–20] Influenza C virus lacks NA.[21]

HA is the attachment protein and is synthesized as a single polypeptide chain that undergoes proteolytic cleavage to yield HA1 and HA2.[16,22] Cleavage of HA is required for infectivity, and increased cleavability is associated with excess virulence.[23,24] HA is expressed on the surface as a trimer and binds to sialic acid, which

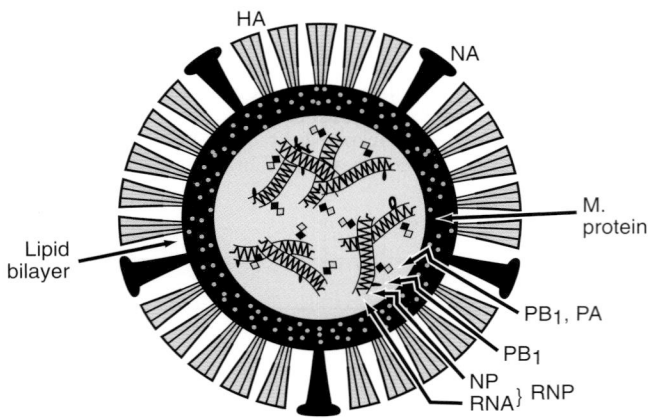

Figure 229-1. The influenza virus virion. (Modified from Betts RF. Influenza virus. In: Mandell GL, Bennett JE, Dolin R (eds) Principles and Practice of Infectious Disease, 4th ed. New York, Churchill Livingstone, 1995, p 1546.)

is the receptor for influenza viruses. Avian and human influenza A viruses preferentially bind to sialic acids with different oligosaccharide side chains.[25,26] NA is synthesized as a single polypeptide chain and is expressed on the surface as a tetramer.[27] This protein destroys sialic acid, the receptor recognized by HA, thereby facilitating the release of progeny virions from the infected cell.

Aquatic birds are the natural hosts of influenza A viruses, and viruses bearing all subtypes of HA and NA have been isolated from birds.[28] Influenza A viruses of a few distinct subtypes have been isolated from pigs, horses, seals, whales, and humans. Influenza B and C viruses have been shown to infect only humans. The standard convention for nomenclature of influenza viruses takes into account the variability in influenza surface proteins. Virus designations specify type, host (for strains of animal origin), geographic source, strain number, and year of isolation, followed by the HA and NA subtypes in the case of influenza A viruses (Box 229-1).[29]

Antigenic Drift and Antigenic Shift

Changes in viral HA, and to a lesser extent, in NA are responsible for the ability of influenza viruses to cause annual worldwide epidemics. Minor changes in antigenicity of the HA and NA of both influenza A and B viruses, called *antigenic drift*, result from an accumulation of point mutations in the genes encoding these proteins. Antigenic variants responsible for annual epidemics arise continually when point mutations allow viruses to escape neutralization by antibodies directed against previously circulating strains.[30]

Antigenic shift is a major antigenic change that occurs when an influenza A virus that bears a novel HA (or novel HA and NA) emerges in the human population. Antigenic shift is a rare event that is responsible for worldwide epidemics or pandemics, and occurs solely in influenza A viruses. Antigenic shift occurs either when a nonhuman influenza virus directly infects human hosts or when a new virus is generated by genetic reassortment between nonhuman and human influenza viruses.[30] The segmented genome of influenza viruses facilitates such reassortment events. Swine are thought of as "mixing vessels" for the emergence of novel recombinant viruses derived from human and avian viruses because swine possess both sialic acid alpha 2,3-galactose linked receptors to which avian influenza viruses preferentially bind and sialic acid alpha 2,6-galactose linked receptors to which human influenza viruses preferentially bind.[31] However, reassortant viruses can be generated in any host that is coinfected with two influenza A viruses.

Influenza Pandemics of the 20th and 21st Centuries

Since 1900, four pandemics have occurred with the emergence of novel influenza A viruses: the 1918 H1N1 "Spanish flu" pandemic, the 1957 H2N2 "Asian flu" pandemic, the 1968 H3N2 "Hong

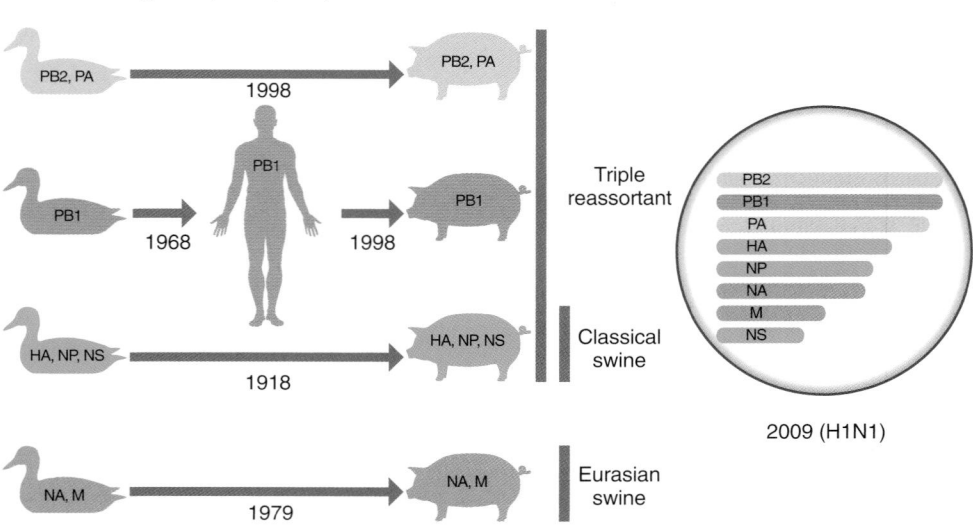

Gene segments, hosts, and years of introduction

Figure 229-2. Host and lineage origins for the gene segments of the 2009 influenza A (H1N1) virus. (Modified from Garten RJ, Davis CT, Russell CA, et al. Antigenic and genetic characteristics of swine-origin 2009 A(H1N1) influenza viruses circulating in humans. Science 2009;325:197–201.)

PB2: polymerase basic; PB1: Polymerase basic1; PA: polymerase acidic; HA: hemagglutinin; NP: nucleoprotein; NA: neuraminidase; M: matrix gene; NS: nostructural gene

Kong flu" pandemic, and the 2009 H1N1 pandemic. During the 1918, 1957, and 1968 pandemics, the strains that emerged were novel influenza A subtypes that subsequently replaced the previously circulating subtype and became established as the predominant circulating influenza A subtype. In 1977, H1N1 viruses reappeared after a 20-year absence (since the 1957 H2N2 pandemic) and caused disease in children and young adults who lacked previous exposure to H1N1 viruses. H1N1 viruses subsequently began circulating in the human population but did not replace the H3N2 viruses; instead, influenza A H1N1 and H3N2 viruses continued to cocirculate. In April 2009, cases of human infection with a novel influenza A (H1N1) virus were identified; this novel virus possessed a unique combination of gene segments including genes that originated from swine, avian, and human influenza viruses that were established in pigs in North America and Europe (Figure 229-2). By June 2009, this virus (now referred to as 2009 pandemic influenza A (H1N1)) was causing widespread illness throughout the world.[32,33]

Sequence analysis of 1918 pandemic influenza A (H1N1) viruses suggests that the 1918 pandemic virus resulted from adaptation of avian H1N1 influenza A viruses to the human population.[34] In general, the HA of avian influenza viruses exhibits receptor-binding specificity for sialic acid residues with alpha 2-3 linkages expressed in the gastrointestinal tract of waterfowl and the lower respiratory tract of humans, whereas the HA of human influenza viruses exhibits receptor-binding specificity for sialic acid residues with alpha 2-6 linkages expressed in the upper respiratory tract of humans. Some 1918 pandemic viruses possess dual binding specificity for both sialic acid alpha 2,3 and alpha 2,6-galactose linked receptors,[35] but it is unclear whether this dual specificity accounts for the increased virulence attributed to these viruses.[36]

PATHOGENESIS

Influenza virus transmission is believed to occur primarily through large-particle respiratory droplets. Transmission by contact with contaminated surfaces also occurs.[37-39] Airborne transmission over long distances (via small-particle residue (≤5 μm) of evaporated droplets that might remain suspended in the air for long periods of time) has not been observed with influenza; however, short-distance small-particle droplet nuclei transmission is thought to be possible based on limited data.[38,40-42]

Influenza viruses infect the columnar epithelial cells of the respiratory tract. Peak virus replication occurs 1 to 3 days after inoculation; virus shedding continues for 6 to 8 days in adults and can persist for more than 13 days in young children or immunocompromised persons.[43,44] Necrosis of epithelial cells, edema, and inflammation occur rapidly.[45] Most infections are largely confined to the upper airways, but infection can spread to involve smaller airways such as the bronchioles and alveoli. In the absence of bacterial superinfection, epithelial cell recovery begins within 3 to 5 days, but complete restoration of ciliary function and mucus production takes about 2 weeks.

In experimental human influenza A virus infection in healthy adults, interleukin (IL)-6 and interferon-alpha (IFN-α) concentrations in nasal lavage fluid peak on day 2 and correlate directly with viral titers, temperature, mucus production, and symptom scores.[46] Tumor necrosis factor-α (TNF-α) responses peak later as viral shedding and symptoms are subsiding, and IL-8 responses peak late in the course of illness (days 4 to 6) and only correlate with lower respiratory symptoms. A study that enrolled patients with community-acquired influenza found that plasma and nasal lavage levels of IL-6 correlated best with symptoms,[47] whereas TNF-α correlated with fever but not with other symptoms and peaked only after fever and other symptoms had already declined.

IMMUNITY

During influenza infection, death of virus-infected cells is mediated by antibody-dependent cellular cytotoxicity, antibody plus complement, cytotoxic T lymphocytes (CTLs), or apoptosis.[48,49] The development of influenza-specific CTLs is important for clearance of virus and recovery from illness; clearance of virus is delayed in individuals with T-lymphocyte immunodeficiency states.[50] CD8+ class I histocompatibility antigen-restricted CTL subsets recognize CTL epitopes in surface glycoproteins and internal proteins and confer both subtype-specific and cross-reactive species immunity.[51] Subsets of lymphocytes with a CD4+ class II histocompatibility antigen phenotype augment B-lymphocyte-mediated antibody production and CD8+ cell proliferation.[51] Intracellular targeting of processed antigen or interaction with the major histocompatibility complex may lead to differential recognition by class I- and class II-restricted CTLs.

Influenza virus infection induces the production of local and humoral antibodies to HA and NA. Antibodies to HA are critical for virus neutralization, and those to NA reduce virus replication.[16,19] Although antibodies to nucleocapsid and matrix protein are detectable, they do not appear to provide protection.[19] Protection afforded by either CTL or cross-reactive antibody is limited; subtype-specific antibody-mediated protective immunity to influenza is durable over many years, but antigenic variation in HA and NA may compromise such immunity.[52]

EPIDEMIOLOGY

In temperate climates, influenza epidemics occur annually, typically during the winter months, whereas in some tropical climates, influenza viruses circulate year-round or circulate more during rainy seasons.[53-55] Influenza A and B viruses can circulate at the same or different times, and the severity of influenza epidemics varies substantially from year to year depending upon the predominant circulating strains. In temperate climates, epidemics of influenza and respiratory syncytial virus (RSV) or other respiratory viruses often occur at about the same time during the winter.[56,57]

Influenza A H3N2 viruses appear to cause the most severe influenza epidemics (as measured by overall mortality), while influenza A H1N1 and influenza B viruses result in relatively milder epidemics.[58] Mortality and hospitalization rates might not reflect the full impact of influenza in some seasons. For example, during the 2009 H1N1 pandemic, which had a disproportionate impact on children and younger adults, overall severe morbidity and mortality was lower than in some influenza A (H3N2) predominant seasons in which the majority of severe infections occur among older persons with comorbidities.[59]

The Impact of Seasonal Influenza in Children

Influenza virus infection and illness occur most commonly among school-age children.[60,61] Children play an important role in sustaining community epidemics of influenza A and B both due to the high attack rate of influenza among young children and because they shed infectious virus for longer periods and at higher titers than adults. Adults in homes with young children have a significantly higher risk of influenza illness than do adults without child contact.[60,62] Peaks of influenza in children generally precede peaks of influenza in adults,[63] and early in an epidemic, school absenteeism precedes work absenteeism. In a prospective survey of 313 schoolchildren, influenza accounted for an excess of 28 illness episodes, 63 missed school days, 22 secondary illnesses in families, and 20 days of missed parental work per 100 children.[64]

Influenza results in a substantial number of both outpatient and inpatient visits among children. In the U.S., an estimated 500 to 950 clinic visits and 60 to 270 emergency department visits per 10,000 children occur due to influenza annually,[8] and influenza-associated hospitalization rates are high among children <5 years of age (Table 229-1). Among infants <6 months of age, an estimated 9 to 104 hospitalizations occur per 10,000 children,[4,7,8,11,65] and hospitalization rates exceed hospitalization rates seen in healthy adults ≥65 years of age during some seasons.[66] Influenza-associated hospitalization rates are higher among children with cardiac and pulmonary conditions than among healthy

TABLE 229-1. Influenza-Associated Hospitalization Rates Among Children

Study Years	Population	Age Group	Hospitalizations/ 100,000 persons
1973–1993	Tennessee Medicaid[a]	<6 months	1038
		6–11 months	496
		1–2 years	186
		3–4 years	86
		5–14 years	41
1973–1993	Tennessee Medicaid[b]	0–11 months	1900
		1–2 years	800
		3–4 years	320
		5–14 years	92
1992–1997	Two health maintenance organizations[c]	<2 years	86–112
		2–4 years	0–15
		5–17 years	5–7
2000–2001	Two counties[d]	<1 year	170
		1 year	50
		2–4 years	20
2001–2004	Large children's hospital[d]	<6 months	253
		6–11 months	113
		1 year	96
		2 years	36
2000–2004	Three counties[d,f]	<6 months	230–720
		6–23 months	40–150
		2–4 years	4–60
1994–2000	Health maintenance organization[e,g]	6–23 months	51–213
		2–4 years	32–142
2000–2004	Large children's hospital[d,h]	0–23 months	416
		2–4 years	70
		5–11 years	19
		12–17 years	18
2003–2008	10 states[d,f]	<6 months	90–300
		6–23 months	30–110
		2–4 years	10–40
		5–17 years	3–8

[a]Outcomes were for acute cardiac or pulmonary conditions among healthy children. Rates are the average annual rate during the study period. Study included only healthy children.

[b]Outcomes were for acute cardiac or pulmonary conditions among children with asthma and other chronic medical conditions. Rates are the average annual rate during the study period.

[c]Outcomes were for acute pulmonary conditions among healthy children. Rate range reflects rates in the two health maintenance organizations.

[d]Laboratory-confirmed influenza.

[e]Rate is per 100,000 person months of observation.

[f]Rate range includes seasonal rates for influenza seasons included in the study period.

[g]Low estimate is for healthy children and high estimate is for children with one or more medical conditions.

[h]Rate is per 100,000 person years of observation.

Modified from Fiore AE, Shay DK, Haber P, et al. Prevention and control of influenza. Recommendations of the Advisory Committee on Immunization Practices (ACIP), 2007. MMWR Recomm Rep 2007;56:1–54.

children.[66,67] In addition, children with neurologic and neuromuscular conditions are at increased risk for respiratory failure associated with influenza.[68]

During the 2003–2004 influenza season, a substantial number of influenza-associated deaths occurred among children in the U.S. Mortality rates were highest in children <6 months of age and

next highest in 6- through 23-month-old children. Two-thirds of the deaths occurred in children who had underlying conditions, and of those, half occurred in children with chronic neurologic and neuromuscular disorders.[69] The 2003–2004 experience prompted new interest in the contribution of influenza to severe respiratory illness among children, and deaths among children attributed to laboratory-confirmed influenza became a nationally reportable disease in 2004. The surveillance data collected during the following three influenza seasons (2004–2007), documented an increase in the proportion of pediatric influenza-related deaths associated with bacterial coinfections, from 6% during the 2004–2005 season to 34% during the 2006–2007 influenza season.[70] *Staphylococcus aureus* was the most frequently identified bacterial pathogen among patients with influenza and bacterial coinfection; 64% of *S. aureus* isolates were methicillin resistant.[70]

The 2009 Influenza A (H1N1) Pandemic

During the spring of 2009, a novel influenza A (H1N1) virus that resulted in a pandemic was identified.[32] An estimated 61 million illnesses, 274,000 hospitalizations, and 12,400 deaths associated with the 2009 H1N1 virus occurred in the U.S. during the first year.[71] The highest estimated attack rates occurred in children and young adults, the highest estimated hospitalization rates occurred in children <5 years of age, and about 90% of deaths occurred in persons <65 years of age.[14] In one estimate, the mean age among persons whose deaths were attributed to the 2009 H1N1 influenza pandemic was 37 years, compared with a mean age of 76 years among deaths attributed to seasonal influenza A (H3N2).[72] During the 2009 pandemic, adults ≥60 years of age experienced lower attack rates compared with typical influenza seasons. This was attributed to cross-protective antibodies from prior exposure to antigenically similar influenza A H1N1 viruses that circulated prior to 1957.[73]

Severe illnesses and deaths among pregnant women, an epidemiologic trend that had been observed in previous influenza pandemics, also were observed during the 2009 pandemic;[74-76] in addition, severe infections among postpartum women were documented.[75] Persons with severe and morbid obesity were overrepresented among persons with fatal infection. It is unclear whether obesity was an independent risk factor for severe illness with 2009 H1N1 virus infection or simply a marker for comorbid high-risk medical conditions.[77,78]

CLINICAL MANIFESTATIONS

Some of the manifestations of illness caused by influenza virus vary according to the age of the host (Table 229-2). Infants with influenza virus infection can manifest irritability, difficulty feeding, or fever alone and can have clinical presentations that are difficult to distinguish from that of bacterial sepsis. In neonates, influenza virus infection can result in apnea.[79]

Among preschool and school-age children, fever and signs of respiratory tract involvement including laryngotracheobronchitis are common. Gastrointestinal symptoms including nausea, vomiting, and diarrhea also can occur and are more common in preschool-aged children than in older age groups.[80,81] Older children and adults are more likely to have an abrupt onset of fever and chills accompanied by headache, sore throat, myalgia, malaise, anorexia, and a dry cough.[30]

The younger the child, the greater the overlap between influenza illness and syndromes caused by other viruses, particularly infections caused by RSV, adenovirus, and parainfluenza virus.[82,83] In a study of hospitalized children <6 years of age, fever and cough together had a sensitivity of 54% to detect influenza virus infection but a positive predictive value of only 16%, which increased to 25% when the analysis was limited to periods when at least one influenza virus infection was detected per week among study participants.[57] In another study that included children up through 17 years of age, the triad of cough, headache, and pharyngitis as a predictor of laboratory-confirmed influenza in children during influenza season had a sensitivity of 80% and specificity of 78%.[84]

TABLE 229-2. Common Manifestations of Influenza Illness in Children

Age	Manifestation	Frequency
Infant, toddler <5 years old	Afebrile URI	+
	Febrile URI	+++
	Acute otitis media	++
	Pneumonia	+
	Laryngotracheobronchitis	+
	Bronchiolitis	+
	"Sepsis syndrome"	+
Child ≥5 years old	Afebrile URI	+
	Flu-like syndrome[a]	+++
	Acute otitis media	++
	Pneumonia	+
	Myositis	+
	Myocarditis	Rare
	Encephalopathy	Rare

URI, upper respiratory tract infection.

+++, most common manifestation; ++, common manifestation; +, infrequent manifestation.

[a]*Fever, cough, headache, myalgia, malaise.*

Upper respiratory tract illness caused by influenza is characterized by a dry, hacking cough that peaks after 3 to 4 days and persists for more than 1 week after other symptoms resolve. Sore throat occurs frequently but is not associated with exudative pharyngitis. Patients may complain of rhinorrhea and eye discomfort (tearing, photophobia, or burning). Croup syndrome associated with influenza tends to be more severe than that associated with parainfluenza virus; secretions are tenacious, and fever is typically higher. Airway compromise is often more severe and is sometimes complicated by bacterial superinfection.[85]

Most episodes of bronchopneumonia are mild and associated with complete recovery. A history of high fever (often above 39°C), epidemic influenza in the community, and recent "flu-like" symptoms in other family members may help differentiate influenza pneumonia from infections caused by other respiratory viruses. Rarely, pneumonia secondary to influenza can be fatal in previously healthy individuals.[86-88]

COMPLICATIONS

Complications involving the upper and lower respiratory tract of influenza include acute otitis media (AOM), sinusitis, bronchiolitis, croup, and pneumonia. AOM was diagnosed in 35% of children 6 months through 3 years of age presenting with influenza-associated upper respiratory tract infections (URI) in one prospective study.[89] In other studies, influenza virus was isolated from middle ear fluid in 3% of all children with AOM and accounted for 5% to 28% of all cases of viral otitis media.[90,91] AOM associated with viral URI typically manifests 3 to 4 days after the onset of the URI.[92]

Radiographically confirmed pneumonia has been reported in 8% to 16% of children hospitalized with influenza,[93-95] which can be primary viral pneumonia or secondary bacterial pneumonia. When present, bacterial pneumonia usually is caused by *Streptococcus pneumoniae* or *Staphylococcus aureus*.[96,97] Secondary bacterial pneumonia is characterized by the appearance of fever and a productive cough during convalescence, along with radiologic evidence of lobar consolidation.[30] In addition to severe, progressive pneumonia, *S. aureus* superinfection also has been associated with bacterial tracheitis and toxic shock syndrome.[85,98] Infection with *S. aureus* is thought to enhance cleavage of viral HA, thus increasing the virulence of influenza viruses.[99]

Myocarditis and evidence of cardiac muscle damage associated with electrocardiographic changes, disturbances in cardiac rhythm,

and elevated levels of cardiac enzymes are rare complications after influenza A and B infection.[30] Febrile convulsions are associated with influenza infection in infants and young children and have been reported in up to 20% of children aged 6 months through 5 years hospitalized with influenza.[100,101] Encephalitis and encephalopathy are unusual complications of influenza infection. Sporadic cases of influenza-associated encephalitis or encephalopathy have been reported from several countries including the U.S.,[102,103] but the majority of reported cases have occurred in Japan. In two large case series of patients with influenza-associated encephalitis or encephalopathy in Japan, the majority of reported cases occurred in children <5 years of age. Patients presented with a range of neuropsychiatric symptoms including seizures, altered consciousness, and psychotic behavior; up to 28% of patients had persistent neurologic sequelae, and 27% to 32% of patients died.[104,105] Other neurologic complications associated with influenza include transverse myelitis, Guillain–Barré syndrome, and Reye syndrome.[30] Reye syndrome (encephalopathy and fatty degeneration of the liver) has become uncommon since the recognition of the association between Reye syndrome and concomitant aspirin use and influenza in children.[106,107] Myositis, characterized by acute pain and tenderness in the gastrocnemius and soleus muscles that is severe enough to limit walking, can occur within 1 to 3 days of influenza symptom onset. Myositis has been observed more often following influenza B compared with influenza A virus infection.[108] Serum creatine kinase concentrations often are transiently elevated. Complete recovery usually occurs in 3 to 4 days. Associated rhabdomyolysis and renal failure occur rarely.

Influenza virus infection can cause exacerbations of underlying illness, particularly in children with pre-existing pulmonary disease such as asthma and cystic fibrosis. Patients with cystic fibrosis with influenza virus infection have lower expiratory flow rates than those with other nonbacterial infections.[109,110]

Although most cases of 2009 H1N1 virus infection were self-limited, associated complications such as encephalitis and encephalopathy, myocarditis, and hemorrhagic pneumonia occurred in children.[111-113] One study that compared symptoms among persons with 2009 H1N1 influenza to those of persons with seasonal influenza concluded that the risk of pneumonia, hospital admission, and intensive care unit admission was not elevated in adults or children with 2009 H1N1 influenza.[114] Thus, the increase in the number of deaths and hospitalizations among children and young adults observed during the 2009 H1N1 pandemic may be attributable primarily to the increased attack rates observed during the pandemic compared with typical influenza seasons.

LABORATORY FINDINGS

The peripheral white blood cell count usually is normal. Relative lymphopenia is typical in older children, and neutrophilia with a left shift occasionally is observed in infants. The radiographic appearance of influenza lower respiratory tract infection is not distinguishable from that of infection caused by other respiratory viruses.[115] Peribronchial infiltrates, hyperexpansion, and segmental or lobar atelectasis are common; interstitial infiltrates and pleural effusions are uncommon. Influenza pneumonia can evolve from peribronchial infiltrates to a more diffuse alveolar process in fatal disease.[87]

DIAGNOSIS

Because of overlap with the clinical presentation of other respiratory tract infections influenza cannot be diagnosed definitively on the basis of clinical signs and symptoms or epidemiologic patterns.[56] In one study, the diagnosis of influenza in children, based on clinical signs and symptoms during the influenza season, was 38% sensitive and 91% specific compared with laboratory confirmation of influenza virus infection.[116] Establishing the diagnosis of influenza through laboratory testing, especially in hospitalized patients and those at high risk for severe influenza, can limit

TABLE 229-3. Influenza Diagnostic Testing Options

Diagnostic Test	Advantages	Disadvantages
Rapid antigen test	Provides results in 30–60 minutes May differentiate influenza types High specificity (63–100%)	Variable sensitivity
DFA and IFA stain	Provides results in 2–4 hours High specificity (>90%)	Sensitivity depends on technical skill of operator
RT-PCR	Can provide results in 6–8 hours High sensitivity and specificity	Not as widely available
Viral culture	Considered gold standard diagnostic test High sensitivity and specificity	May take 2–7 days to obtain results
Influenza serology	Useful during outbreak investigations and epidemiologic studies	Requires acute and convalescent sera. Results usually not available to inform clinical decision making in acute setting

inappropriate antibiotic use, guide antiviral therapy, and provide data for influenza surveillance purposes.

Currently available influenza diagnostic tests based upon examination of nasopharyngeal aspirates or nasal swabs include: tissue or cell culture, real-time reverse transcriptase-polymerase chain reaction (rtRT-PCR), rapid antigen detection tests, and immunofluorescence assays (Table 229-3).[117] Sensitivity of these diagnostic tests is affected by the quality of the respiratory specimen and the timing of specimen collection. Nasopharyngeal specimens generally are preferred to throat swab specimens. Diagnostic yield is highest when specimens are collected within the first few days of illness when influenza virus shedding is at its peak.[118]

Virus culture is considered the "gold standard" for identification of influenza viruses and yields isolates that can be typed, subtyped, and characterized antigenically and genetically. With conventional culture, results are not available for ≥3 days. The shell vial culture technique provides results sooner than conventional techniques with results within 18 to 48 hours.[117] Real-time RT-PCR may be more sensitive than viral culture,[119] provides results within 6 to 8 hours, can be combined with detection of other respiratory viruses in a multiplex format,[120–122] and allows for typing, subtyping, and strain identification by sequence analysis of influenza viruses.

Rapid diagnostic tests have sensitivity ranging from 39% to 100% and specificity ranging from 62% to 100% for detecting influenza in specimens from children compared with virus culture.[123] Rapid tests can provide results within 30 to 60 minutes, and some can differentiate between influenza A and B viruses. There are currently no licensed rapid tests that can differentiate influenza A virus subtypes. Given the potentially low sensitivity of influenza rapid tests, results must be interpreted in the context of local influenza surveillance data. If the influenza rapid test is negative, but the patient has symptoms consistent with influenza, the patient may still have influenza and clinicians should use clinical judgment when deciding whether to obtain additional influenza testing (e.g., rtRT-PCR or culture) or initiate antiviral therapy. Interpretation of a positive rapid influenza test result also

is problematic when the prevalence of influenza among persons with respiratory illness is low.[124]

Direct and indirect fluorescent antibody tests have a specificity >80%, but highly variable sensitivity compared with virus culture.[123] Serologic testing of acute and convalescent specimens for the presence of antibodies to influenza viruses can be useful for clinical studies and outbreak investigations, but do not provide timely data.

TREATMENT

Two classes of antiviral drugs are available for the treatment of influenza: the adamantanes, which are ion channel inhibitors and are active against influenza A viruses but not against influenza B viruses, and the NA inhibitors, which are effective against both influenza A and influenza B viruses. The adamantanes have not been recommended for treatment of influenza during most recent influenza seasons because of widespread resistance among circulating influenza viruses.[125,126]

Adamantanes

The adamantanes include the oral medications amantadine and rimantadine. These drugs block the M2 ion channel on influenza A viruses that maintains the acidity of the Golgi microenvironment and permits virus uncoating.[127] Amantadine and rimantadine are approved by the Food and Drug Administration (FDA) for prophylaxis of influenza in children 1 year of age and older, but only amantadine is approved for treatment in children.

In studies of the use of adamantanes for the treatment of influenza in adult patients, amantadine or rimantadine therapy begun within 48 hours of the onset of symptoms was associated with a rapid reduction in fever, systemic complaints, and virus shedding.[128–130] Data on the effectiveness of adamantane treatment in children are limited. Treatment with rimantadine appears to reduce viral shedding rapidly in most patients, but shedding of resistant virus late in therapy has been observed.[131,132] The clinical significance of this finding for the individual patient is unclear, but transmission of rimantidine-resistant influenza A viruses among family members has been documented.[133]

Amantadine is excreted renally and dosage adjustments must be made for patients in renal failure.[134] Rimantadine is also renally excreted and requires substantial hepatic metabolism prior to clearance necessitating dosage adjustments for patients with hepatic dysfunction or renal failure.[134]

Neuraminidase Inhibitors

The NA inhibitors licensed for treatment of influenza include zanamivir, which is available as an inhalational agent, and oseltamivir, which is available as a liquid suspension or tablet. The NA inhibitors bind to the influenza neuraminidase enzyme active site thereby inhibiting the release of virions from the infected cells.[127] Inhaled zanamivir is approved by the FDA for treatment in children ≥7 years of age and for chemoprophylaxis in children ≥5 years of age. Oseltamivir currently is approved for treatment or chemoprophylaxis of influenza in children ≥1 year of age. In addition, two NA inhibitors, intravenous peramivir and intravenous zanamivir, currently are under investigation for use in the treatment of influenza.[15]

Both zanamivir and oseltamivir reduce the duration of illness due to influenza when treatment is initiated early in the course of illness. In one randomized, placebo-controlled trial involving children 4 to 12 years of age and three trials involving adults and children 12 years of age and older, zanamivir shortened the duration and severity of influenza symptoms when initiated within 48 hours of illness onset.[135–139] In a randomized, placebo-controlled trial of children 1 through 12 years of age, treatment with oseltamivir within 48 hours of illness onset reduced the length of illness by a median of one and half days, the overall illness severity, and the incidence of AOM.[140] Oseltamivir reduced the incidence of asthma exacerbations and improved pulmonary function during the illness period in a study of children with asthma and influenza. Oseltamivir also reduced the incidence of pneumonia[141] and sinusitis[142] in adults with influenza. In a retrospective study of medical and pharmacy benefit data, treatment with oseltamivir within 1 day of influenza diagnosis was associated with a reduction in risk for non-pneumonia respiratory illness, AOM, and hospitalization during the 2 weeks after influenza diagnosis.[143]

Zanamivir is concentrated in the respiratory tract; 10% to 20% of the active compound reaches the lungs, and the rest is deposited in the oropharynx. Only 5% to 15% of the total dose is absorbed and excreted in the urine. Therefore, zanamivir dosage adjustment is not required for patients with renal failure. The concentration of the drug in the respiratory tract has been estimated to be >1000 times the 50% inhibitory concentration (IC_{50}) for NA and the inhibitory effect begins within 10 seconds. Postlicensure reports indicate that zanamivir can cause cough, bronchospasm, and reversible decrease in pulmonary function. Therefore, if patients with pulmonary dysfunction receive zanamivir, they should have a fast-acting bronchodilator available and discontinue zanamivir if respiratory difficulty develops.[127] Oseltamivir is readily absorbed from the gastrointestinal tract and is converted by hepatic esterases to the active form of the compound that is widely distributed in the body. The half-life of oseltamivir is 6 to 10 hours. Oseltamivir is excreted primarily through the kidneys, and the dosage must be modified in patients with renal insufficiency. The most commonly reported side effects are nausea, vomiting, and diarrhea.

Antiviral Treatment in Infants

None of the currently licensed influenza antiviral medications are approved by the FDA for use in children less than 1 year of age. However, during the 2009 H1N1 pandemic, the FDA issued an Emergency Use Authorization (EUA) approving the use of oseltamivir in children less than 1 year of age for treatment or chemoprophylaxis of 2009 H1N1 influenza. The EUA subsequently was removed in June 2010. Observational studies conducted while the EUA was in effect provide limited data about the use of neuraminidase inhibitors in children <1 year of age. In a study of 36 premature infants given oseltamivir prophylaxis after exposure to a healthcare worker with 2009 H1N1 influenza, a 1 mg/kg dose of oseltamivir given twice daily produced oseltamivir carboxylate (the active metabolite of oseltamivir) levels similar to a 3 mg/kg dose given twice daily in older children.[144] A retrospective cohort study of 115 children less than 1 year of age treated with oseltamivir or an adamantane found no difference in the incidence of neurologic adverse events in the two treatment groups.[145] A retrospective cohort study of antepartum exposure to antiviral therapy also found no association with adverse pregnancy and fetal outcomes among women who received antiviral treatment during pregnancy.[146]

Indications for Antiviral Treatment

Treatment of children with influenza virus infection should be based on the severity of disease, presence of underlying medical conditions, and the time since symptoms started. Empiric treatment is recommended for all persons with suspected or confirmed influenza requiring hospitalization and for persons with progressive or complicated illness regardless of previous health or vaccination status.[14,147,148] Empiric antiviral therapy also is recommended for persons who are at a higher risk for influenza complications (Box 229-2), such as children with underlying medical conditions, pregnant women, and children <5 years of age.[147]

Antiviral treatment should be started as soon as possible after illness onset. Early initiation of treatment for severely ill patients has been associated with reduced morbidity and mortality.[14,77,149] Empiric treatment often is necessary, and initiation should not be delayed while waiting for confirmatory diagnostic test results. Patients should continue to receive antiviral treatment regardless of the initial test results until an alternative diagnosis can be established.[14,147] Treatment of severely ill patients, such as those

---

BOX 229-2. Persons at Higher Risk for Influenza Complications

- Children <5 years of age, particularly children <2 years of age
- Adults 50 years of age and older
- Persons with the following underlying medical conditions: chronic pulmonary (including asthma), cardiovascular (except hypertension), renal, hepatic, hematologic (including sickle-cell disease), neurologic, neuromuscular, or metabolic (including diabetes mellitus) disorders
- Persons with immunosuppression caused by medications or underlying medical conditions (including HIV infection)
- Women who are pregnant or postpartum (within 2 weeks after delivery)
- Persons <19 years of age who are receiving long-term aspirin therapy
- American Indians and Alaskan Natives
- Adults who are morbidly obese (body-mass index ≥40)
- Residents of nursing homes and other chronic-care facilities

---

who require hospitalization, is recommended regardless of illness duration. Several studies conducted among adults have shown that hospitalized patients benefit from treatment even when initiated more than 48 hours after illness onset.[150,151]

Antiviral Resistance

Resistance to the adamantane compounds occurs as a result of mutations in the gene encoding the M2 protein and resistance to the NA inhibitors occurs as a result of mutations in the HA or NA genes. Starting with the 2005–2006 influenza season, widespread adamantane resistance was observed among circulating influenza A (H3N2) viruses.[125] During the 2007–2008 influenza season, widespread resistance to the NA inhibitor oseltamivir was observed among circulating seasonal influenza A (H1N1) viruses that shared a single point mutation at amino acid residue 275 on the viral neuraminidase gene, but viruses with oseltamivir resistance remained susceptible to the NA inhibitor zanamivir.[126] Since the emergence of the 2009 H1N1 virus in April 2009 up through November 2011, the majority of influenza A and B viruses tested were resistant to the admantanes but were sensitive to both oseltamivir and zanamivir.[151a] Oseltamivir-resistant 2009 H1N1 viruses have been detected sporadically and have been associated with subtherapeutic treatment with oseltamivir in some instances.[152] The emergence and rapid evolution of antiviral resistance among circulating influenza strains necessitates careful monitoring of local influenza surveillance data to determine which influenza strains are circulating and the prevalence of antiviral resistance among circulating strains and frequent reassessment of influenza antiviral treatment strategies.

SPECIAL CONSIDERATIONS

Immunocompromised Hosts

Immunocompromised hosts frequently acquire infection through nosocomial transmission, and they can shed virus for extended periods, especially if T-lymphocyte function is compromised.[50,153-157] Influenza A and B cause substantial morbidity and mortality in recipients of solid-organ and hematopoietic stem-cell transplants;[156,158,159] fatal pulmonary and neurologic syndromes have been reported.[155,159] Pneumonia occurs in about 75% of adults with leukemia and bone marrow transplant recipients who are infected with influenza virus. The attendant mortality rate is up to 40%.[160] Guidelines for the prevention of influenza in hematopoietic stem-cell transplant recipients have been published.[161] There have been reports of the development of influenza viruses resistant to antiviral medications in immunocompromised patients exposed to antiviral medications.[162,163] Influenza immunization is recommended by the American Society of

Transplantation for recipients of solid-organ transplants before transplantation and starting again 6 months after transplantation.[164]

HIV-Infected Individuals

Some studies suggest that HIV-infected persons have an increased susceptibility to influenza virus infection compared with the general population.[165,166] Some HIV-infected children with influenza have prolonged viral shedding.[167] Influenza vaccination with trivalent inactivated vaccine (TIV) has been documented to produced adequate antibody responses in HIV-infected children receiving highly active antiretroviral therapy and to have a similar safety profile in HIV-infected children compared to HIV-uninfected children.[168-170] Annual influenza vaccination is recommended for all HIV-infected persons in the U.S.[171]

Pregnancy

Although no evidence supports influenza as a teratogen or cause of abortion, influenza pneumonia is associated with high morbidity and mortality in pregnant women. Risk of hospitalization with influenza among pregnant women increases with gestational age[172,173] and women in the third trimester of pregnancy were hospitalized at a rate comparable to that of nonpregnant women who had high-risk medical conditions.[173] Concerns about the risk for influenza complications among pregnant and early postpartum women have led to a much greater emphasis on empiric treatment of any pregnant woman with suspected influenza. Influenza vaccination remains the primary strategy for reducing influenza complications among pregnant women.[147]

PREVENTION

Vaccine

Two types of influenza vaccines are available in the U.S.: an injectable inactivated virus vaccine and a live, attenuated inhaled vaccine. Both vaccine types are trivalent preparations containing three vaccine strains selected to match the strains considered most likely to circulate in the upcoming influenza season: an influenza A (H1N1), an influenza A (H3N2), and an influenza B strain.

The U.S. Advisory Committee on Immunization Practices (ACIP) of the CDC recommends influenza immunization annually for all persons 6 months of age or older with a continued emphasis on immunization of persons at increased risk for severe influenza including: children <5 years of age; persons 50 years of age and older; persons with chronic underlying medical conditions or immunosuppressive conditions; children receiving chronic aspirin therapy; women who are or will be pregnant during the influenza season; residents of long-term care facilities; American Indians and Alaska Natives; and persons who are morbidly obese.[15] In addition, household contacts and caregivers (including healthcare personnel, homecare providers, and employees of assisted-living and long-term care facilities) of persons at increased risk for severe influenza should be vaccinated.[15] Immunization of all healthcare personnel is recommended by the ACIP, and mandatory immunization of healthcare personnel is recommended by the Infectious Diseases Society of America[174] and the American Academy of Pediatrics.[175] Immunization of close contacts of children <6 months of age is particularly important because these children cannot be immunized with currently licensed vaccines. Coverage in all groups, including healthcare personnel and young children, remains below levels that are likely to reduce substantially the impact of annual influenza epidemics.[15] Influenza vaccine is contraindicated in persons with known anaphylactic hypersensitivity reactions to eggs or other components of the influenza vaccine who have not been desensitized.[15] Most children with presumed egg allergy, however, stratified by history, can receive influenza vaccine in the provider's office without consultation with an allergist.[175a]

School-aged children often have the highest attack rates of influenza, and play a key role in the introduction and transmission of influenza viruses in communities.[176-178] Observational studies and several randomized trials[179-182] in which immunization of children was associated with reductions in influenza or respiratory illness among their household contacts or persons living in the same community provide support for a universal recommendation for immunization of children. Reductions in community-wide rates of influenza also have been predicted by modeling studies.[183]

The efficacy of influenza vaccines depends on the age of the vaccine recipient, closeness of antigenic match between the vaccine strains and epidemic strains, and the endpoints used for the measurement of efficacy. Clinical efficacy studies that use laboratory-confirmed influenza as an endpoint have higher estimates of protection than effectiveness studies that use clinical illness endpoints. Currently available influenza vaccines are challenging to manufacture quickly and do not provide reliable protection against strains that are antigenically different from the vaccine strain. In addition, the continuous antigenic changes that occur among influenza viruses result in the need for annual revaccination. Efforts to improve influenza vaccines are an active area of research, and urgency in creating more immunogenic vaccines in shorter timeframes was underscored by the challenges posed by the 2009 H1N1 pandemic.[184]

Inactivated Influenza Vaccine

Trivalent inactivated seasonal influenza vaccines (TIV) available in the U.S. are split virus or virus subunit vaccines, and generally are considered interchangeable when given in the standard doses. The immunogenicity of TIV is inconsistent but is generally poor in infants <6 months of age. TIV is licensed for use in persons ≥6 months of age. Seroresponse rates increase with increasing age, reaching 70% to 100% in adolescents. However, immunologic priming is important for response to TIV, and a single dose of vaccine is ineffective in inducing immunity in children lacking previous experience with the matching influenza type or subtype.[185] Young children require several years of exposure to influenza epidemics or two doses of vaccine to ensure a reliable response to all three vaccine antigens after the administration of inactivated vaccine.[186] Therefore, two doses of TIV administered ≥4 weeks apart are recommended for children <9 years during their first season of influenza immunization.[187]

In a large, randomized placebo-controlled trial that evaluated TIV in children 1 to 15 years of age, vaccine efficacy ranged from 77% to 91%.[188] Other studies conducted during seasons with a suboptimal match between vaccine strains and circulating influenza strains have estimated vaccine effectiveness ranging from no significant effectiveness to up to 57% effectiveness among fully vaccinated children.[189-191] Studies on the effectiveness of TIV against AOM have produced conflicting results. The incidence of AOM in two childcare center studies was lower among TIV recipients than among unimmunized children.[192,193] However, a randomized placebo-controlled study of children 6 to 24 months of age failed to show decreases in the incidence of AOM or duration of middle-ear effusion in vaccine compared with placebo recipients.[194]

Fewer data are available on vaccine efficacy and effectiveness in children with underlying chronic medical conditions. However, the immunologic response to TIV in children with asthma has been documented to be the same as in healthy children,[195] and TIV is safe for administration to adults and children with asthma.[151] Some studies suggest that TIV also protects against acute asthma exacerbations.[196,197] Data on influenza vaccine efficacy among persons with HIV infection are largely from studies of adults with HIV. Several studies, including one conducted among children with HIV, have documented that vaccination with TIV produces protective antibody titers in persons with HIV without AIDS defining symptoms,[169,198,199] but protective antibody titers may not be achieved in persons with advanced HIV and lower CD4 lymphocyte counts.[199] Results of a non-randomized study conducted during an influenza outbreak at a residential care facility, determined that vaccination with TIV was 65% effective among persons with HIV infection and CD4+ T-lymphocyte cell counts >100/mm³.[166]

Vaccination of pregnant women with TIV provides protection to their infants, presumably through passive transfer of antibodies against influenza.[200,201] Influenza vaccination of pregnant women was 63% effective in preventing laboratory-confirmed influenza among infants of vaccinated women through 6 months of age in a randomized controlled trial[202] and resulted in a 41% reduction in laboratory-confirmed influenza among infants through 6 months of age in a prospective cohort study.[203]

In 2009, a higher-dose vaccine (4-fold increase in vaccine antigen) was licensed in the U.S. for persons ≥65 years of age, and has demonstrated superior immunogenicity in several studies.[15] In 2011, the U.S. FDA licensed a reduced-dose (9 μg hemagglutinin per strain) intradermal, inactivated vaccine for use in persons 18 through 64 years of age.[203a] The newly licensed intradermal vaccine uses a 1.5 mm microneedle to deliver vaccine consistently into the dermis. Administration of influenza vaccine intradermally might better induce cell-mediated immunity through vaccine delivery into the skin, which is heavily populated by dendritic cells important for antigen presentation.[203b] Studies currently underway will determine whether intradermal vaccines are more effective in preventing influenza compared with intramuscular vaccines. New formulations of inactivated vaccines that might improve immunogenicity and effectiveness are likely to be available in the future, such as adjuvanted vaccines.

Live-Attenuated Influenza Vaccines

Live-attenuated influenza vaccines (LAIV), in which 6 internal protein genes of a temperature-sensitive, attenuated, cold-adapted parent influenza virus are combined with wild-type HA and NA genes, are recommended for use in healthy nonpregnant persons from 2 through 49 years of age.[15] Multiple studies have shown that LAIV is safe for healthy school-age children[204] and adolescents. In the largest randomized controlled trial conducted in children <6 years of age, those with medically diagnosed or treated wheezing within 42 days before enrollment or with a history of severe asthma were excluded. Among children aged 24 through 59 months who received LAIV, the rate of medically significant wheezing, using a prespecified definition, was not greater compared with those who received TIV.[205] Wheezing was observed more frequently only among younger LAIV recipients aged 6 through 23 months in this study. However, a significantly increased risk of wheezing was observed in children 18 through 35 months of age in another study.[206] In a pooled analysis of 20 studies evaluating LAIV compared to either placebo or TIV in children 2 through 17 years, children 24 through 35 months of age who received LAIV did not have higher rates of wheezing than those who did not.[206a] Based on these observations, LAIV is not approved for use among children <24 months old, and the ACIP recommends that children 2 through 4 years of age with a history of wheezing or children of any age with asthma should not receive LAIV.[15]

In studies of children who have received LAIV, shedding of virus has been documented;[207,208] when genotype analysis was performed, shed virus retained the attenuated phenotype.[209] The frequency of transmission of LAIV from immunized young children to unimmunized contacts has been estimated to be <2% and is likely lower among older children and adults who shed less virus.[207,208] Transmission of vaccine virus from an immunized person to an unimmunized contact has not been shown to cause significant illness.[15,208] LAIV virus is shed for a shorter duration and at lower titer than wild-type influenza virus.[210] LAIV should not be given while the recipient is receiving influenza antiviral medication since antivirals decrease influenza viral replication and may interfere with the immune response to LAIV; persons who receive influenza antiviral medications during the 2 days before to 14 days after LAIV receipt should be reimmunized after cessation of antiviral therapy.[15]

Persons who receive LAIV develop mucosal immunity, which is challenging to measure. Clinical studies demonstrate that LAIV has excellent efficacy against influenza, particularly among children. In one randomized controlled trial comparing LAIV with placebo, LAIV was 94% effective against culture-confirmed influenza in children who received two doses of LAIV and 89% effective in children who received one dose during a season when the vaccine strains were well matched against circulating strains and 86% effective during a season when the predominant circulating strain was drifted from the vaccine strain.[211,212] The efficacy of LAIV against laboratory-confirmed seasonal influenza in young children in other studies has ranged from 64% to 89%.[204,213] A case-control study evaluating the 2009 H1N1 monovalent LAIV found that a single dose was 82% effective in preventing influenza in children 2 through 9 years of age but did not demonstrate effectiveness in persons 10 through 49 years of age.[213a]

The safety, immunogenicity, and efficacy of LAIV and TIV have been compared in several studies.[205,214–217] Both vaccines are well tolerated and effective but elicit significantly different immune responses.[216,217] In randomized controlled comparative trials in young children, vaccination with LAIV was more effective against laboratory-confirmed influenza regardless of match between circulating strains and vaccine strain and provided greater cross-protection during seasons when vaccine strains were not well matched against circulating influenza virus strains.[214,218] In a study comparing immune responses to a 2-dose sequence of TIV, LAIV, or a combination of the 2 vaccines in children 6 through 35 months of age, both vaccines induced similar humoral antibody responses but only LAIV induced cell-mediated responses thought to be important for heterosubtypic immunity.[218a] In contrast, in a series of randomized controlled studies comparing placebo, LAIV, and TIV in healthy young adults, TIV was more effective.[219–221] In a single study conducted among adults, LAIV was more effective in those who had never received influenza vaccine in the past.[222]

CHEMOPROPHYLAXIS

If given before or shortly after influenza virus exposure, chemoprophylaxis with an influenza antiviral agent can effectively prevent symptomatic influenza virus infection. Oseltamivir postexposure chemoprophylaxis (PEP) in household contacts of persons with influenza has been shown to be 68% to 89% effective in preventing laboratory-confirmed influenza when given soon after exposure.[223,224] Several studies have documented similar efficacy for zanamivir when it is given as PEP.[225,226]

PEP is considered for persons who are at high risk for developing severe influenza and have not been vaccinated or have received vaccine <14 days prior to exposure.[66,147] In general, chemoprophylaxis should be given for 10 days and within 48 hours after the time of exposure.[148] Occasionally, extended periods of prophylaxis are indicated for patients who cannot be immunized.[227] The choice of antiviral agent used for chemoprophylaxis should be guided by local surveillance data on antiviral resistance when available. Influenza virus infection can occur in persons receiving antiviral chemoprophylaxis,[152] and sporadic cases of antiviral-resistant influenza virus infection have been identified in persons taking chemoprophylaxis.[224] Therefore, clinicians should advise patients taking chemoprophylaxis to seek care at the first signs of respiratory illness and providers should consider antiviral-resistant influenza virus as a potential etiology in such instances. In most situations, counseling patients about signs and symptoms of influenza and encouraging early treatment if signs or symptoms develop is a preferable alternative to chemoprophylaxis for persons with a suspected exposure to influenza virus. Clinical judgment based on consideration of the patient's age, severity of underlying illness, ability to comply with a chemoprophylactic regimen, and access to medical care should be used when considering postexposure chemoprophylaxis.

ZOONOTIC INFLUENZA

Influenza viruses are known to infect many animal species in addition to humans. Interspecies transmission has been documented including human infections with avian and swine influenza viruses. Human infection with novel or nonhuman influenza A virus strains, including influenza A viruses of animal origin, is a notifiable disease in the U.S.[228]

Sporadic cases and clusters of human infection with avian H5N1, H7N2, H7N3, H7N7, and H9N2 viruses prove that avian influenza A viruses can be transmitted directly to humans without passage through an intermediate host and without acquiring human influenza gene segments by genetic reassortment.[229,230] The first case of human infection with an avian influenza A H5N1 virus was identified in a child in Hong Kong in 1997 who died as a result of the infection.[231] A few months later, 17 additional cases occurred with five additional deaths.[232] The 1997 outbreak ended, but progenitors of the Hong Kong H5N1 viruses continued to circulate in avian species in the region. In late 2002, outbreaks of highly pathogenic H5N1 avian influenza were reported in 10 countries in Asia and human cases were reported in Vietnam and Thailand.[233,234] Since then, H5N1 viruses have spread to other countries in Asia, Europe, and Africa, and more than 500 cases of human infection and more than 300 deaths have been reported (http://www.who.int/csr/disease/avian_influenza/en).

The incubation period in human cases of H5N1 virus infections ranges from 2 to 5 days, but longer incubation periods have been reported.[235] The majority of patients with H5N1 virus infection have a history of contact with sick poultry, but there are instances of probable person-to-person transmission among family clusters with close contact.[236,237] Although most cases have febrile respiratory illnesses (sometimes with dyspnea),[238] there have been reports of atypical infections,[239] including infections in two children who had diarrhea and coma without respiratory tract symptoms.[240] Laboratory findings include lymphopenia, thrombocytopenia, and, in some cases, abnormal hepatic transaminases.[241,242] Reported complications include progression to acute respiratory distress syndrome, shock and renal failure.[242-245] The diagnosis of H5N1 virus infections is based on molecular methods.[246] In a review of 308 persons infected with H5N1, oseltamivir treatment initiated up through 6 to 8 days after symptom onset reduced mortality by 49%.[247] Although treatment with oseltamivir provides a survival benefit, the case-fatality rate in treated patients remains high, and H5N1 viruses resistant to oseltamivir or amantadine have been reported.[248,249]

Highly pathogenic H5N1 virus has not been identified in wild or domestic birds or in humans in the U.S. Guidance for testing suspected cases of H5N1 virus infection among persons in the U.S. and follow-up of contacts is available.[250,251] Human H5N1 cases have continued to occur from 2009 through 2011, including in the Middle East and Southeast Asia.

Sporadic cases and clusters of human infection with swine influenza viruses have been reported in the U.S. and elsewhere since 1958 and include infection with classical swine influenza viruses and triple reassortant swine influenza viruses containing genes from human, avian, and swine influenza viruses.[252] In 2011, sporadic cases of human infection with a newly identified swine-origin triple reassortant influenza A (H3N2) virus containing genes from a swine-origin A (H3N2) virus known to be circulating in North American pigs and the matrix gene from the 2009 H1N1 virus were identified, including a case cluster in which limited human-to-human transmission might have occurred.[255a,255b] The majority of patients with swine influenza virus infection have had mild, self-limited illnesses that are clinically indistinguishable from seasonal influenza,[253] although severe and fatal cases also have been reported.[252] The incidence of human infection with swine influenza viruses is unknown since testing for influenza viruses is not always conducted in patients presenting with influenza-like illness, but serologic studies suggest that these infections might occur more frequently among persons with occupational exposure to swine and close contacts of such persons.[254,255] Swine influenza virus infections should be considered in the differential diagnosis of persons with febrile respiratory illness and recent swine exposure. If swine influenza virus infection is suspected, clinicians should obtain a nasopharyngeal swab from the patient and contact their local health department to facilitate testing.

PANDEMIC INFLUENZA

The introduction and global spread in humans of a novel influenza A virus is referred to as antigenic shift. The prerequisites for a pandemic are: (1) isolation from humans of a novel influenza virus to which the general population has little or no immunity; (2) ability of the virus to replicate and cause disease in humans; and (3) sustained and efficient transmissibility of the virus from person to person.[256] Novel influenza viruses with pandemic potential can arise through reassortment of gene segments between avian, swine, or human influenza viruses in humans or an intermediate host or can be wholly avian or swine influenza A viruses that cross the species barrier and directly infect humans.[257] As demonstrated in 2009, a pandemic can result if a virus emerges with antigenic characteristics that are novel to most humans; an entirely new hemagglutinin gene is not necessarily required.[33]

History and the biology of influenza viruses indicate that future influenza pandemics are inevitable; however, the timing of a pandemic, the subtype that will cause it, and the impact of the pandemic cannot be predicted. Specific measures for the control of influenza pandemics include vaccines and antiviral drugs. Candidate vaccines, including vaccines with adjuvants that elicit broad cross-clade immune responses, have been developed for different subtypes of avian influenza but are still under evaluation in clinical trials.[258-261] The U.S. Department of Health and Human Services maintains a stockpile of the two currently licensed classes of antiviral drugs, the adamantanes and the neuraminidase inhibitors.[262] The U.S. government pandemic preparedness plan is available at www.pandemicflu.gov.

Acknowledgments

This work was supported in part by the Intramural Research Program of the National Institutes of Health, NIAID.

Key Points. Influenza Virus Infections

MICROBIOLOGY

- Three antigenic types of influenza viruses are recognized: A, B, and C
- The surface proteins hemagglutinin (HA) and neuraminidase (NA) are the major targets of the protective immune response; minor changes in these surface glycoproteins are responsible for the ability of influenza viruses to evade immunity acquired from infection in previous seasons and cause annual epidemics of respiratory illness
- The emergence of influenza A viruses with novel HAs that are antigenically distinct from previously circulating influenza A

viruses have resulted in 4 influenza pandemics during the 20th and 21st centuries in 1918, 1957, 1964, and 2009

EPIDEMIOLOGY

- Among children, influenza-associated hospitalization rates are highest among infants <6 months of age
- Persons at increased risk for severe seasonal or 2009 pandemic H1N1 influenza include children <5 years of age, persons ≥50, persons with chronic medical conditions, pregnant women, residents of long-term care facilities, American Indians and Alaska Natives, and persons who are morbidly obese

- Annual influenza immunization is recommended in the U.S. for all persons 6 months of age and older

DIAGNOSIS

- Clinical signs and symptoms often are not distinctive; laboratory testing is the only reliable way to distinguish influenza from other respiratory infections
- Virus culture is the "gold standard" for diagnosis; rRT-PCR may be more sensitive and provide results more quickly
- Rapid diagnostic tests have variable sensitivity and specificity; during periods when influenza viruses are known to be circulating in the community, a patient with a negative rapid test still can have influenza and clinicians should use clinical judgment to decide whether to initiate antiviral therapy or obtain additional diagnostic testing

TREATMENT

- Immediate empiric treatment is recommended for persons with suspected influenza requiring hospitalization or with progressive or complicated illness
- Treatment is recommended for persons with chronic medical conditions, pregnant women, and children <5 years old
- Two classes of antiviral drugs are available: the adamantanes (rimantidine and amantadine) and the neuraminidase inhibitors (oseltamivir and zanamivir)
- In recent years, neuraminidase inhibitors have been the mainstay of treatment
- Local surveillance and prevalence of antiviral resistance should be used to guide antiviral treatment strategies

230 Filoviruses and Arenaviruses

Margot Anderson and Daniel G. Bausch

THE VIRUSES

Viruses of the families Filoviridae and Arenaviridae comprise single-stranded RNA in lipid envelopes.[1,2] The Filoviridae comprise five species of Ebola virus and one Marburg virus (Table 230-1). Arenaviruses are taxonomically divided into Old World (i.e., Africa) and New World (i.e., the Americas) viruses. Along with viruses from the Flaviviridae and Bunyaviridae families (see Chapter 218, Flaviviruses, and Chapter 219, Bunyaviruses), filoviruses and arenaviruses are the principal causative agents of viral hemorrhagic fever (HF), an acute and sometimes severe systemic illness classically involving fever, a constellation of initially nonspecific signs and symptoms, and a propensity for bleeding and shock.[3,4] The exception is lymphocytic choriomeningitis virus (LCMV), an Old World arenavirus that has now been disseminated worldwide, which is associated with febrile illness and central nervous system (CNS) disease.[2] Many of these viruses are considered potential bioweapons.[5]

EPIDEMIOLOGY

Maintenance in Nature and Transmission to Humans

Filoviruses and arenaviruses are zoonotic, and therefore the endemic area for each virus is restricted by the distribution of its animal reservoir. With the exception of Lassa virus, human infection is relatively rare and plays no role in virus maintenance in nature. Recent findings suggest that fruit bats are the filovirus reservoir,[6,7] while pathogenic arenaviruses are maintained in rodents,[2,8] with strict pairing between the specific virus and animal reservoir (Table 230-1). Miners, spelunkers, forestry workers, and others with exposure to environments where bats typically roost are at risk of filovirus infection.[9–11] The rodents that transmit Lassa and Machupo viruses and LCMV commonly invade domestic environments, whereas the reservoirs for Junin, Machupo, and Guanarito viruses typically inhabit agricultural fields, wood lots, or other rural habitats.[2,8]

Transmission to humans likely usually occurs via inadvertent exposure to animal excreta or saliva or, in some cases, blood when the animals are hunted and consumed.[1,2,12] Nonhuman primates, especially gorillas and chimpanzees, and other wild animals often serve as intermediate hosts for filoviruses.[13–15] These animals presumably are infected by exposure to bats and develop severe and usually fatal disease similar to human HF. Since the HF viruses are rapidly inactivated by heating, infection likely occurs through exposure during preparation, rather than via consumption of cooked meat. LCMV also has been transmitted to humans via contact with infected laboratory mice and cell lines, as well as pet rodents, especially hamsters.[2,16]

Human-to-Human Transmission

Secondary human-to-human transmission can occur but attack rates generally are low (15% to 20% even for Ebola Zaire virus, which is probably the most transmissible) (Table 230-1).[17,18] Transmission is through direct contact with blood or body fluids and probably usually occurs through exposure to oral or mucous membranes, most often in the context of providing care to a sick family member (community) or patient (nosocomial transmission).[19] Large outbreaks almost always have fuelled by nosocomial transmission in resource-poor regions where basic infection control practices cannot be maintained.[20] The role of aerosols is controversial; infectious aerosols have been produced artificially in the laboratory, a finding of concern with regard to potential biowarfare. But epidemiologic and limited laboratory-based data generally do not suggest aerosol transmission between humans in natural settings.[17,19,21–24]

Infectivity parallels the clinical state; persons are most infectious late in the course of severe disease.[25] Transmission during the incubation period or from asymptomatic persons is negligible. Funeral rituals that entail the touching of the corpse have played significant roles in transmission, especially for Ebola virus.[26,27] Transmission through breast milk and congenital transmission have been documented.[28] Infection through fomites cannot be excluded but probably is not common unless the object is obviously contaminated with blood or body fluids.[28,29] Sexual transmission months after recovery from acute disease has been reported.[30]

TABLE 230-1. Filoviruses and Arenaviruses Known to Cause Human Disease

Virus	Disease	Principal Reservoir/Vector	Geographic Distribution of Disease	Annual Cases	Disease-to-Infection Ratio	Human-to-Human Transmissibility	Case Fatality
FILOVIRIDAE							
Ebola	Ebola HF	Fruit bat ("Egyptian fruit bat" or *Rousettus aegyptiacus,* perhaps others)	Sub-Saharan Africa, Philippines[b]	–[a]	1:1	High	25–85% depending upon species[b]
Marburg	Marburg HF	Fruit bat ("Egyptian fruit bat" or *Rousettus aegyptiacus,* perhaps others)	Sub-Saharan Africa	–[a]	1:1	High	25–85%
ARENAVIRIDAE[c]							
Old world							
Lassa	Lassa fever	Rodent ("multimammate rat" or *Mastomys natalensis)*	West Africa	30,000–50,000	1:10	Moderate	5–50%
Lujo[d]	Lujo HF	Unknown. Presumed rodent	Zambia	Unknown	Unknown	Moderate-to-high	80%
Lymphocytic choriomeningitis	Lymphocytic choriomeningitis	Rodent ("house mouse" or *Mus musculus).* Transmission from pet rodents also documented	Worldwide	Unknown. Infection probably frequent but under-recognized	3:10	None	<1%
New world							
Junin	Argentine HF	Rodent ("corn mouse" or *Calomys musculinus)*	Argentine pampas	<50	1:1.5	Low	15–30%
Machupo	Bolivian HF	Rodent ("large vesper mouse" or *Calomys callosus)*	Beni department, Bolivia	<50	1:1.5	Moderate	15–30%
Guanarito	Venezuelan HF	Rodent ("cane mouse" or *Zygodontomys brevicauda)*	Portuguesa state, Venezuela	<50	1:1.5	Low	30–40%
Sabiá[e]	Brazilian HF	Unknown. Presumed rodent	Rural area near Sao Paulo, Brazil?	–[e]	1:1.5	Low?	33%
Chapare[f]	Chapare HF	Unknown. Presumed rodent	Cochabamba, Bolivia	Unknown	Unknown	Unknown	Unknown

HF, hemorrhagic fever.

[a]Although some endemic transmission of the filoviruses (Ebola > Marburg) occurs, these viruses have most often been associated with outbreaks. Filovirus outbreaks are typically less than 100 cases and have never been greater than 500.

[b]Five species of Ebola virus are known with varying associated case-fatality ratios: Ebola Zaire, 85%, Ebola Sudan, 55%, Ebola Bundibugyo, 25%, Ebola Cote d'Ivoire, zero (only one recognized case), Ebola Reston, zero (not pathogenic to humans). All are endemic to sub-Saharan Africa, with the exception of Ebola Reston virus which is found in the Philippines.

[c]In addition to the arenaviruses listed in the table, Flexal and Tacaribe viruses have caused human disease as a result of laboratory accidents. Another arenavirus, Whitewater Arroyo, has been noted in sick persons in California but its role as a pathogen has not been clearly established.

[d]Discovered in 2008 in an outbreak of 5 cases (4 of them fatal) in South Africa. The index case to South Africa from Zambia.

[e]Discovered in 1990. Only 3 cases (1 fatal) of Sabiá virus infection have been noted, 2 of them from laboratory accidents.

[f]Discovered in 2003 from a small outbreak in Cochabamba, Bolivia. Chapare virus was isolated from a fatal case but few other details from the outbreak have been reported.

PATHOBIOLOGY

After inoculation into mucous membranes or deposition in the lungs and initial replication in local tissues, virus migrates to regional lymph nodes and ultimately through the blood to a broad range of tissues.[31] The liver, endothelium, and adrenal glands appear to be particularly important targets. The CNS is particularly affected in LCMV and New World arenavirus infections.[2]

Microvascular instability and impaired hemostasis are the hallmarks of viral HFs.[3,4] Impaired hemostasis can entail endothelial cell, platelet, and/or coagulation factor dysfunction. Disseminated intravascular coagulopathy (DIC) is common, with the exception of Lassa fever.[32] Contrary to common belief, bleeding is not always seen and exsanguination usually is not a key factor in death. Rather, severe disease results from immune cell activation precipitating an inflammatory and vasoactive process consistent with the systemic inflammatory response syndrome (see Chapter 11, The Systemic Inflammatory Response Syndrome (SIRS), Sepsis, and Septic Shock), with insufficient effective circulating intravascular volume, cellular dysfunction, and multiorgan system failure.[31,33] Cardiac inotropy can be inhibited, especially in Lassa fever. In severe disease viremia remains unchecked and there is little or no antibody response.[25] Inflammatory cell infiltrates likewise are mild.[34]

Immune cell activation also is the fundamental process in the pathogenesis of LCMV, although without the same effects on endothelial cell function and hemostasis as in HF.[2] CNS involvement typically occurs a week or two after disease onset, after virus has cleared from the blood, and is thought to be immune mediated, although virus can still be recovered from the cerebrospinal fluid.

CLINICAL MANIFESTATIONS

Viral Hemorrhagic Fever

Filovirus and arenavirus infections occur in both sexes and all age groups, with a spectrum from asymptomatic infection (especially for arenaviruses) to rapidly fatal disease.[9,35-39] Generally it is not possible to distinguish disease produced by a specific virus on clinical grounds, especially at disease onset. The syndrome produced by the New World arenaviruses usually is collectively referred to as "South American HF".

After an incubation period of 8 to 10 days (range 3 to 21 days), patients typically manifest nonspecific signs and symptoms, including fever, general malaise, anorexia, headache, chest or retrosternal pain, sore throat, myalgia, arthralgia, lumbosacral pain, and dizziness. The onset of illness typically is abrupt with filovirus infection and more gradual with the arenaviruses. The pharynx can be erythematous or even exudative in Lassa fever, incorrectly leading to a diagnosis of streptococcal pharyngitis. Gastrointestinal signs and symptoms readily ensue, including nausea, vomiting, epigastric and abdominal pain, abdominal tenderness (especially over the liver in filovirus infection), and diarrhea. Misdiagnosis as acute appendicitis or another abdominal emergency sometimes occurs. A dry cough with a few scattered rales is common, but prominent pulmonary symptoms are uncommon early in the course of the disease. Jaundice is not typical and should suggest a different diagnosis.

A subset of patients, especially with filovirus infections, progress to vascular instability. Clinical manifestations include conjunctival injection (not accompanied by itching, discharge, or rhinitis), facial flushing, edema, bleeding, hypotension, shock, and proteinuria. The likelihood of clinically discernible hemorrhage is highest for filovirus infections and the South American HFs. Hematemesis, melena, hematochezia, metrorrhagia, petechiae, purpura, epistaxis, and bleeding from the gums and venepuncture sites may develop, but hemoptysis and hematuria are infrequent (Figure 230-1). Bleeding is almost never seen in the first few days of illness. Swelling in the face and neck is sometimes seen in Lassa fever and is relatively specific to this disease (see Figure 230-1).[39] Anasarca (the "swollen baby syndrome") also has been described in Lassa fever but may have been related to aggressive rehydration.[40]

Morbilliform, maculopapular, petechial, and ecchymotic skin rashes can occur. Maculopapular rash on the torso or face may be one early and relatively specific, although not sensitive, indicator of filovirus infection. Rash almost always occurs in eight-skinned people but, for unclear reasons, is rare in dark-skinned people.

CNS manifestations, including disorientation, tremor, gait anomalies, convulsions, and hiccups, can be noted in end-stage disease, especially in South American HF, particularly Argentine HF.[2] Renal insufficiency or failure is common. Pregnant women often present with spontaneous abortion and vaginal bleeding. Maternal and fetal mortality approaches 100% in the third trimester.[41,42]

Common clinical laboratory findings in are summarized in Table 230-2. Radiographic and electrocardiographic findings generally are nonspecific and usually correlate with the physical examination.[43,44]

Death occurs in fatal cases around 8 to 10 days after onset for the filoviruses and 10 to 14 days for arenaviruses. Shock, bleeding, neurologic manifestations, high levels of viremia, elevated levels of aspartate aminotransferase (>150 IU/L), and pregnancy (especially during the third trimester) are indicators of a poor prognosis.[39,45] Viremia clears rapidly in survivors, who can be discharged without concern of subsequent transmission at home once acute symptoms resolve.[25,46] However, clearance of virus may be delayed for weeks to months from a few immunologically protected sites, such as the kidney, chambers of the eye, and gonads.[47]

Survivors usually suffer no obvious long-term sequelae, with the notable exception of sensorineural deafness in up to 30% of patients after Lassa fever and sometimes after Venezuelan HF.[48] Convalescence can be prolonged, with the potential for persistent myalgia, arthralgia, anorexia, weight loss, alopecia, pancreatitis,

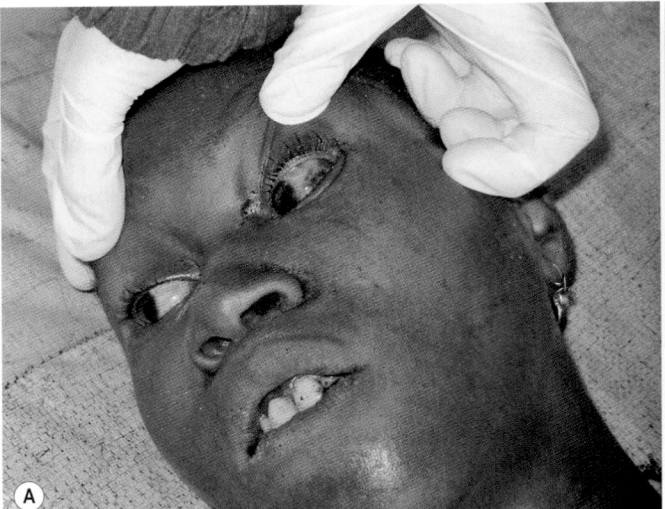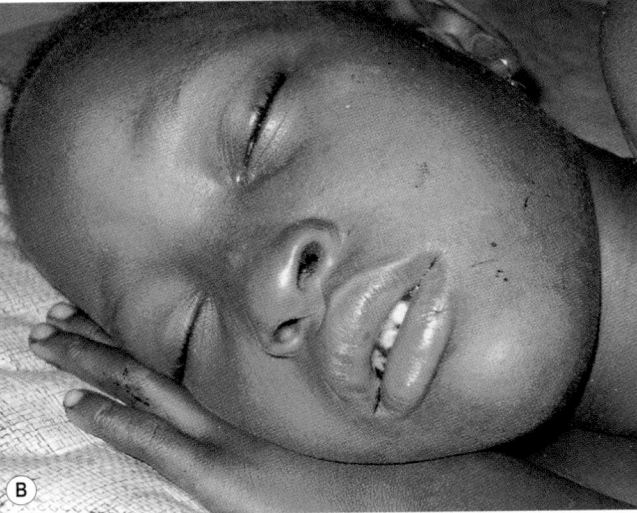

Figure 230-1. (A and B) Subconjunctival hemorrhage, oral bleeding, and facial swelling in patients with Lassa fever (Courtesy of Victor Lungay.)

TABLE 230-2. Clinical Laboratory Tests Indicated and Characteristic Findings in Filovirus and Arenavirus Infections

Test	Characteristic Findings and Comments
Leukocyte count	Early: moderate leukopenia, sometimes with atypical lymphocytes. Later: leukocytosis with left shift
Hemoglobin and hematocrit	Hemoconcentration
Platelet count	Mild-to-moderate thrombocytopenia
Electrolytes	Sodium, potassium, and acid–base perturbations, depending upon fluid balance and stage of disease
Lactate	Level >4 mmol/L (36 mg/dL) may indicate persistent hypoperfusion and sepsis
BUN/creatinine	Renal failure can occur late in disease
AST, ALT, amylase	Increased, usually AST > ALT level
Coagulation studies (PT, PTT, fibrinogen, fibrin split products, platelets, D-dimer)	DIC common except for Lassa fever
Urinalysis	Proteinuria common
Blood culture	Useful early to exclude VHF and later to evaluate for secondary bacterial infection
Stool culture	Useful to exclude VHF (in favor of hemorrhagic bacillary dysentery)
Thick and thin smears or other assay for malaria	Negative in VHF unless coinfection with malaria
Febrile agglutinins or other assay for *Salmonella* Typhi	Negative in VHF unless coinfection with *Salmonella* Typhi
Cerebrospinal fluid analysis	Lymphocytic choriomeningitis: moderately increased protein (50–150 mg/dL), normal or decreased glucose, mononuclear pleocytosis up to 5000 cells/mm³ (although neutrophils can comprise as much as 25%). Usually normal in VHF

ALT, Alanine aminotransferase; AST, aspartate aminotransferase; BUN, blood urea nitrogen; DIC, disseminated intravascular coagulation; PT, prothrombin time; PTT, partial prothrombin time; VHF, viral hemorrhagic fever.

uveitis, and orchitis up to a year after infection. The psychological effects also can be significant, with some patients experiencing depression or posttraumatic stress.

Lymphocytic Choriomeningitis

Many LCMV infections are asymptomatic or result in a nonspecific febrile illness, sometimes accompanied by photophobia.[49] After 7 to 14 days of illness, and often a brief period of defervescence, CNS manifestations ensue in a minority of patients, running a spectrum from aseptic meningitis (the most common) to fulminant encephalitis with cranial nerve palsies, abnormal reflexes, focal seizures, polyneuritis, flaccid paralysis, and papilledema. CNS symptoms also can occur without recognized febrile illness. Rarer manifestations and complications of LCMV infection include hydrocephalus, transverse myelitis, Guillain–Barré syndrome, hearing loss, arthritis, parotitis, orchitis, myocarditis, mucosal bleeding, and pneumonia. Congenital infection has been associated with spontaneous abortion in early pregnancy and, when occurring later in pregnancy, a variety of neurologic deficits can result, including psychomotor retardation, microcephaly and macrocephaly, hydrocephalus, chorioretinitis with visual loss, and seizures (Figure 230-2). LCMV infection in organ transplant recipients resulted in a highly fatal syndrome resembling viral HF.[50]

DIAGNOSIS

The nonspecific presentation of filovirus and arenavirus infections results in a broad differential diagnosis that varies by geographic region, but usually includes malaria, typhoid fever, leptospirosis, and many other systemic febrile illnesses.[51] Clinicians should focus on making the general diagnosis of viral HF and then seek laboratory support to confirm the syndrome and specific infecting virus. For LCMV, the arboviral causes of meningitis and herpes encephalitis must be excluded.

A diagnosis of viral HF should be considered in patients with a clinically compatible syndrome who, within 3 weeks prior to disease onset, (1) traveled in areas where an HF virus is known or suspected to be endemic, (2) had potential direct contact with blood or body fluids of a person with viral HF during their acute illness (this group most often comprises healthcare workers), (3) had contact with live or recently killed wild animals (especially rodents and nonhuman primates) in or recently arriving from an area where an HF virus is endemic, (4) worked in a laboratory or animal facility where HF viruses are handled, or (5) had sex with someone recovering from a viral HF in the previous 3 months. However, viral HF is rare even in persons possessing one of the above risk factors, so alternative diagnoses should always be

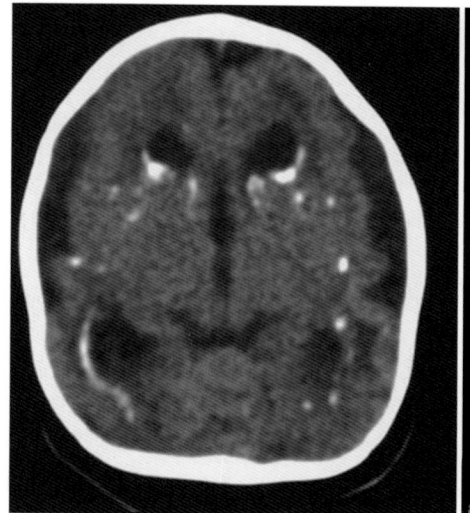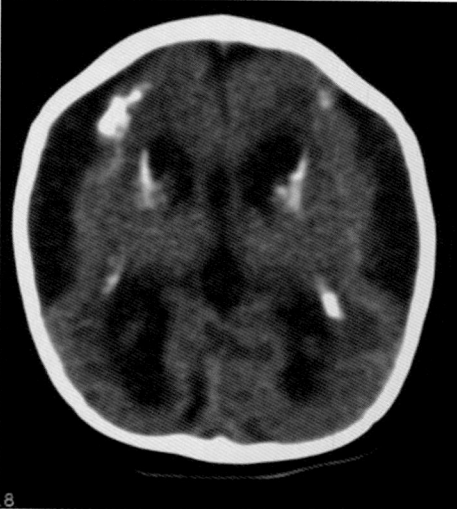

Figure 230-2. Computed tomography at 5 months of age of an infant with profound developmental delay and chorioretinitis due to intrauterine lymphocytic choriomeningitis virus infection. Scan shows microencephaly, lissencephaly, and calcifications that are periventricular, intracerebral, and over the convexities of the brain. Serum immunofluorescent antibody titer was >1:1024. Mother had no known illness or exposure to rodents during pregnancy. (Courtesy of G.L. Rodgers and S.S. Long, St. Christopher's Hospital for Children, Philadelphia, PA.)

sought aggressively, especially malaria and typhoid fever. Acts of bioterrorism must be considered if viral HF is seen in a patient without any of the above criteria, especially if there are clusters of cases.[5] All confirmed cases should be reported immediately to local, state, and federal health authorities.

Laboratory Testing

Prompt laboratory diagnosis is imperative. Enzyme immunoassay (EIA) and reverse transcription polymerase chain reaction (RT-PCR) are the mainstays of diagnosis, with sensitivities and specificities usually >90%.[52-57] No commercial assays are available but testing can be arranged through a few specialized laboratories, such as the U.S. Centers for Disease Control and Prevention (001-404-639-1115).

TREATMENT

The overall management of patients with viral HF is as for septic shock (Chapter 11, The Systemic Inflammatory Response Syndrome (SIRS), Sepsis, and Septic Shock).[26,32,58-63] Impaired gas exchange is not typically a prominent feature and mechanical ventilation should be avoided because of the risk of barotrauma and pleural-pulmonary hemorrhage. When required, low tidal volumes (i.e., lung-protective ventilation) are optimal. The possibility of DIC should be assessed and treatment with appropriate blood products implemented. Because of the risk of bleeding and hematomas at insertion sites, intravascular catheters (with the exception of peripheral intravenous lines), intramuscular and subcutaneous injections, arterial puncture, and use of procoagulants (such as nonsteroidal anti-inflammatory drugs) should be avoided. To the extent possible, hemodynamic and respiratory status should be monitored by blood pressure cuff and pulse oximetry, respectively.

Broad-spectrum antibacterial and/or antiparasitic therapy, with specific consideration of antimalarial agents and doxycycline for tickborne rickettsial diseases, should be given until a diagnosis can be confirmed. If fever persists or begins anew after about 2 weeks of illness, secondary bacterial infection should be suspected.

Treatment with ribavirin (30 mg/kg, maximum 2 g, loading dose; followed by 15 mg/kg, maximum 1 g every 6 hours for 4 days; followed by 7.5 mg/kg, maximum 500 mg, every 8 hours for another 6 days) administered intravenously for 10 days decreases mortality in severe Lassa fever, although the drug is not approved by the U.S. Food and Drug Administration for this indication.[64] Ribavirin should be diluted in 0.9% saline and infused slowly, with the dose diminished in persons with a creatinine clearance <50 mL/min. Based on limited data, the drug appears to be efficacious for the South American HFs as well.[65,66] No specific antiviral treatment is available for filovirus infection.

The main side effect of ribavirin is a dose-dependent, mild-to-moderate hemolytic anemia that infrequently necessitates transfusion and disappears with cessation of treatment. Rigors can occur when ribavirin is infused too rapidly.[64] Relative contraindications in children include severe anemia or hemoglobinopathy, renal insufficiency, decompensated liver disease, and known hypersensitivity. Hemoglobin, hematocrit, and bilirubin levels should be monitored.

Transfusion of appropriately titered convalescent plasma within the first 8 days of illness reduces mortality in Argentine HF.[65] However, this therapy has been associated with a convalescent-phase neurologic syndrome characterized by fever, cerebellar signs, and cranial nerve palsies in 10% of those treated. Direct comparison of the efficacy of convalescent plasma and ribavirin for Argentine HF has not been conducted. Animal studies show convalescent plasma to be efficacious in Lassa fever as well, but only if it contains a high titer of neutralizing antibody (which cannot be assumed uniformly) and there is a close antigenic match between the infecting viruses of the donor and recipient.[67] Furthermore, in most countries, no stockpile of immune serum is available for patients with viral HF. Convalescent plasma does not appear to be efficacious in filovirus infections.[68]

Recognition that disturbances in the procoagulant–anticoagulant balance as well as overactive immune responses play important roles in septic shock have prompted trials of various immune and coagulation modulators. Two anticoagulant therapies, activated protein C and rNAPc2, diminished mortality in Ebola virus-infected monkeys.[69,70] However, efficacy of these drugs for shock or viral HF in children has not been established and their use should be considered experimental. Another experimental approach under investigation is the use of anti-sense oligomers.[71] Statins, which have anti-inflammatory properties and other stabilizing effects on the vasculature, were included in the treatment of a surviving case of Lujo virus infection, along with the antioxidant and free radical scavenger N-acetylcysteine.

The treatment of LCMV infection is supportive. Anti-inflammatory drugs, such as corticosteroids, can be considered with severe CNS disease. The single surviving patient in a cluster of LCMV cases related to transplanted organs received ribavirin, as well as a reduction of immunosuppressive therapy.[50]

Management of Convalescence

Clinical management during convalescence includes the use of warm packs, acetaminophen, nonsteroidal anti-inflammatory drugs, cosmetics, anxiolytics, antidepressants, nutritional supplements, and nutritional and psychological counseling.[32,59,61] Transmission through toilet facilities or eye secretions has not been noted, but simple precautions to avoid contact with these potentially infected body fluids are prudent, including separate toilet facilities and regular handwashing.

PREVENTION

All patients with a syndrome compatible with viral HF should be presumed infectious and kept isolated under standard HF precautions until a specific diagnosis is made. Placement in a negative airflow room is prudent, but hermetically sealed isolation chambers are not required.[72] Access to the patient should be limited to designated staff and family members with specific training on infection control guidelines and the use of personal protective equipment.

Personal Protection and Precautions for Healthcare Workers

Although specific viral HF isolation precautions (surgical mask, double gloves, gown, protective apron, face shield, and shoe covers) are recommended for added security, routine strict barrier nursing is protective in most cases.[26,59,72] Positive-airway pressure masks and other small-particle aerosol precautions should be used when performing procedures that may generate aerosols, such as endotracheal intubation. Items that were in direct contact with a patient with viral HF can be decontaminated using ordinary 5% chlorine bleach, a 1 : 100 (1%) solution for reusable items and 1 : 10 (10%) solution for disinfecting excreta, corpses, and items to be discarded, or one of various commercially available lysis buffers.

Contact Tracing

Persons with unprotected direct contact with a patient during the symptomatic phase of illness should be monitored daily for evidence of disease for 3 weeks after their last contact. Contacts should check their temperature daily and record the results in a log. Confinement of asymptomatic persons is not warranted, but those who develop signs and symptoms suggestive of viral HF should be isolated immediately until the diagnosis can be excluded. Fortunately, the low secondary attack rates of filoviruses and arenaviruses afford a measure of reassurance, even when cases go unrecognized, as long as proper barrier nursing is maintained. Furthermore, since mild cases, which may be more difficult to recognize, are usually not very infectious, missed or delayed diagnosis of these patients is unlikely to pose a problem from an infection control standpoint.

Vaccines

The live attenuated vaccine Candid #1 decreases morbidity and mortality of Argentine HF and may also protect against Bolivian HF, although it does not appear to cross-protect against other arenaviruses.[73] However, the vaccine is not approved in the U.S. and supplies are insufficient even in Argentina where it is produced. A number of experimental vaccine candidates show promise for both filoviruses and arenaviruses.[2,74,75]

Postexposure Prophylaxis

Postexposure prophylaxis with oral ribavirin (35 mg/kg loading dose, maximum 2.5 g, followed by 15 mg/kg, maximum 1 g, 3 times daily for 10 days) may be considered for persons with direct unprotected contact with blood or body fluids (such as a needle-stick injury or splash of blood to mucous membranes) from an infected person.[76,77] Prophylaxis never should be given if the only exposure was during the incubation period.

Convalescent plasma is efficacious as postexposure prophylaxis for Argentine HF.[65] No postexposure prophylaxis is available for filovirus infection, although an experimental vaccine for Ebola HF was administered on a compassionate use basis to a laboratory worker after a needle-stick injury with no apparent detrimental effect.[78] Efficacy could not be assessed. Small interfering RNAs also show promise for prophylaxis.[79]

Reservoir and Vector Control

Effective and sustainable control measures usually entail avoidance of known reservoir habitats or, when this is not feasible, implementation of measures to prevent direct contact with virus vectors and reservoirs and their excreta. Most successful prevention programs integrate biological and chemical control measures with education and/or regulation to change human behaviors that put them at risk. Trapping of rodents occasionally may be useful in outbreaks and perhaps, more routinely, for control of house mice and LCMV inside homes.

231 Introduction to Retroviridae

Katherine Luzuriaga

The Retroviridae are a large family of viruses (seven genera) that primarily infect vertebrates.[1] Retroviruses are RNA viruses that require the generation of a DNA genome and integration within host DNA for the production of viral progeny. Retroviral integration can modify the host genome to produce transforming genes, or oncogenes. Research into this process has provided insights into the molecular bases of carcinogenesis. Retroviruses also have medical importance as potential vectors for gene transfer and gene therapy.[2]

Human endogenous retroviruses (HERV) consist of proviral DNA or partial genomes that have been integrated into host genomes.[3] HERV constitute up to 8% of human genomic DNA. HERV proviral DNA in germline cells can be passed from parents to their offspring. Transcription of HERV elements does not result in the generation of infectious viruses, but may produce functional proteins, which have been shown to play a role in normal physiologic processes. HERV have also been implicated in several diseases, although the precise role of HERV as etiologic or contributing agents of disease remains to be elucidated.[3,4]

Retroviruses that are passed horizontally through blood, sexual secretions, or breast milk are known as *exogenous* retroviruses. Human pathogens include human T-cell lymphotropic virus types 1 and 2 (HTLV-1 and HTLV-2; associated with T-lymphocyte lymphomas and neurologic disease) and human immunodeficiency virus types 1 and 2 (HIV-1 and HIV-2; causative agents of acquired immune deficiency syndrome).

Retroviruses are composed of lipid-enveloped particles roughly 80 to 100 nm in diameter, with a protein core that contains two linear, positive-sense, 7 to 11 kb single-stranded RNA genomes. Viral enzymes important in viral replication (protease, reverse transcriptase, and integrase) are also included in the core. Glycoprotein spikes in the lipid membrane envelope determine the host range of retroviruses through their interaction with target cell surface receptors and coreceptors. After virus entry into the cell, linear double-stranded DNA (provirus) is made from the single-stranded viral RNA by the viral reverse transcriptase enzyme. Integration of the provirus into the host genome is mediated by the viral enzyme integrase and is necessary for the production of viral particles. The stability of the integrated provirus and its transmission to the cell's progeny provide the basis for persistence of the retrovirus over the lifetime of the host.

Regulatory sequences (long terminal repeats) on either end of the proviral genome flank the coding regions for viral structural (gag) proteins, envelope (env) proteins, and enzymes (reverse transcriptase and integrase; pol). Some retroviral genomes (including those of human immunodeficiency viruses) contain at least two additional genes, *tat* and *rev*, that are essential for viral replication. Retroviral genomes can also contain variable sets of accessory genes, which may modify the replication kinetics and pathogenicity of these viruses.

Recombination and errors in reverse transcription provide the basis for the generation of genomic diversity of retroviruses. Various selective pressures (e.g., virus cell tropism and growth fitness, host immune responses, antiretroviral therapies) can then drive the evolution of a genetically diverse group of viral variants (or *quasispecies*) over the course of infection. The evolution of the quasispecies provides a mechanism by which retroviruses can evade potential mechanisms of control such as host immune responses and antiretroviral therapies.

The virus uses host cell machinery to synthesize and process viral genomes, messenger RNA, and proteins necessary for the generation of progeny viral particles. Virion assembly requires encapsidation of viral RNA and takes place primarily at the cell plasma membrane. As the virion buds through cellular membranes, it picks up a lipid bilayer along with the viral envelope glycoproteins and several host cell membrane proteins.

232 Human T-Cell Lymphotropic Viruses

Katherine Luzuriaga

EPIDEMIOLOGY

Human T-cell lymphotropic (or lymphoma) viruses (HTLVs) are delta-retroviruses. The two most clinically important HTLVs are HTLV type 1 (HTLV-1) and HTLV type 2 (HTLV-2).[1,2] Infections with two additional HTLVs (HTLV-3 and HTLV-4) have been identified in central African populations but their clinical significance is unclear.[3,4]

HTLV-1 and HTLV-2 are most prevalent in southwestern Japan, the Caribbean, Melanesia, and parts of Africa. Around the world, approximately 10 to 20 million people are infected with HTLV-1.[5] In the United States, only about 1 in 6250 volunteer blood donors has antibodies to HTLV-1 or HTLV-2. However, foci of HTLV-1 infection have been reported from the Gulf Coast states and from New York City among people who were either born in the Caribbean or had sexual contact with such individuals. Endemic foci of HTLV-2 infection now exist among the Guayani Indians of Panama and certain North American Indians living in Florida and New Mexico. In the U.S., Europe, South America, and Asia, HTLV-2 infection is four times more common than infection with HTLV-1 among injection drug users.

Genomic similarities between HTLV and simian T-lymphotropic viruses (STLVs) suggest that the human viruses are derived from viruses transmitted to humans from nonhuman primates. Human populations that are exposed to nonhuman primates through hunting, butchering, or keeping primates as pets appear to have particular risk for acquiring HTLV infections. STLVs do not appear to be transmitted to humans through occupational exposure to nonhuman primates (e.g., through employment in primate centers or laboratories). HTLVs are spread by three modes: sexual contact, infusion of blood or blood products, and breastfeeding. Heterosexual transmission from infected men probably is the most efficient route of infection; about 60% of the susceptible female sexual partners of infected men become infected in this way. However, female-to-male sexual transmission is rare; fewer than 1% of susceptible men contract infection from a seropositive female partner. About 50% of those exposed to HTLV-1-contaminated blood become infected.

Since 1988, all U.S. blood donors have been screened for HTLV-1 and HTLV-2 antibodies and excluded if seropositive. HTLV-3 and HTLV-4 appear to be serologically indistinguishable from HTLV-1 and HTLV-2.[4] Because the viruses are only infectious when present in lymphocytes, there is no risk of infection from serum or clotting factors, and individuals with hemophilia do not have high rates of seropositivity. HTLV-1 and HTLV-2 infection occurs in childhood and appears to be associated principally with transmission through breast milk.[6] The risk of transplacental or perinatal transmission of viruses from an infected mother is about 5% for an infant who is not breastfed, whereas the risk of infection is about 25% for the breastfed child. Therefore, infected women should not breastfeed their infants. HTLV-1 is not transmitted by casual contact, and medical workers are not at risk of contracting infection if they observe universal precautions.[7]

CLINICAL MANIFESTATIONS

HTLV-1

Infection with HTLV-1 causes two devastating human diseases: adult T-cell leukemia/lymphoma (ATLL) and HTLV-1-associated myelopathy/tropical spastic paraparesis (HAM/TSP).[8] The cumulative lifetime risk of developing either of these diseases is approximately 5% in infected individuals.[5]

ATLL is a clonal malignancy of well-differentiated CD4$^+$ T lymphocytes, occurring in about 2% to 4% of HTLV-1 infected individuals.[9] Whereas both CD4$^+$ and CD8$^+$ T lymphocytes are infected, the leukemic cells are exclusively CD4$^+$.[10,11] The HTLV-1 DNA provirus is integrated into the genome of malignant cells. Infection appears to have a long latency period, generally manifesting clinically in persons 40 to 60 years of age, after many years of asymptomatic infection. The disease typically is aggressive and rapidly fatal. It is associated with hypercalcemia and characteristic lytic lesions of bone, which have been ascribed to the ability of virus-encoded *trans*-activating factor *tax* to activate genes for parathyroid hormone production.

HAM/TSP is a slowly progressive neurologic disease associated with permanent weakness in the legs, paresthesias, long tract neurologic abnormalities, and urinary incontinence.[12] Although these manifestations of infection are evident in fewer than 1% of all persons infected with HTLV-1, they occur in about 20% of those infected by contaminated blood. Antibodies to HTLV-1 are present in the cerebrospinal fluid of patients with this disorder. Treatment with corticosteroid or other immunosuppressive agents is only modestly beneficial. HAM/TSP affects patients of all ethnic groups, but it is most prevalent in geographic regions where HTLV-1 has been endemic for a long time.[13]

HTLV-1 also has been associated with isolated cases of uveitis, arthritis, polymyositis, and panbronchiolitis. HTLV-1-infected individuals commonly come to medical attention with skin lesions. Skin manifestations are observed in 43% to 72% of ATLL cases.[14] Children can manifest infective dermatitis associated with HTLV-1 (IDH), a severe form of chronic eczema associated with *Streptococcus pyogenes* and *Staphylococcus aureus* infections.[15]

HTLV-2

HTLV-2 appears to have originated in Africa several thousand years ago.[16] DNA provirus has been detected in breast milk,[17] and maternal–child transmission, probably due to breastfeeding, is documented.[18] Rare cases of mycosis fungoides and large granular lymphocytic leukemia have been detected in HTLV-2-infected individuals, but causality has not been proven. HTLV-2 does appear to be associated with an HAM/TSP-like neurodegenerative disease and other neurologic disorders.[19] Bacterial skin infections have been described in persons coinfected with HTLV-2 and HIV-1.

233 Human Immunodeficiency Viruses

Katherine Luzuriaga

Human immunodeficiency virus types 1 and 2 (HIV-1 and HIV-2) are members of the primate lentivirus group of the Lentivirus genus of the Retroviridae family.[1] HIV-1 and HIV-2 appear to have entered humans as a result of cross-species transmission of simian immunodeficiency viruses (SIV). HIV-1 is similar to an SIV that infects chimpanzees (SIV_cpz; Table 233-1), and HIV-2 is similar to SIV strains that infect sooty mangabeys (SIV_sm). Interestingly, the simian viruses do not cause disease in their natural hosts. Comparative genomic analyses of SIV_cpz and HIV-1 have documented at least three independent transmissions of SIV_cpz strains to humans. The current HIV-1 pandemic likely resulted from one of these transmission events in the first half of the 20th century.[2,3] Similar analyses also suggest that HIV-2 resulted from the transmission of SIV_sm to humans in West Africa in the first half of the 20th century.[4]

HUMAN IMMUNODEFICIENCY VIRUS TYPE 1

Life Cycle

The mature HIV-1 virion is approximately 110 nm in diameter and is composed of a core surrounded by a lipid bilayer envelope. The virion core consists of a structural shell composed of a protein (p24) processed from the gag precursor polypeptide. Within this shell are two copies of single-stranded RNA, two transfer RNA primers of host cell origin, and multiple copies each of the virus-encoded reverse transcriptase (RT), integrase, and RNAse H enzymes. Matrix protein (p17), another product of the gag polypeptide precursor, surrounds the virion core and is associated with the transmembrane glycoprotein of the viral envelope (gp41). At least three more virus-encoded proteins (vpr, vif, and nef) are packaged within the virion. These proteins are active early in the intracellular life cycle of HIV-1 and contribute to the efficiency of infection. Trimers of an external glycoprotein (gp120), anchored by gp41, protrude from the lipid bilayer envelope. The gp120 glycoproteins contain binding sites for the cell surface HIV-1 receptor (CD4 molecule) and coreceptors (chemokine receptors)

and therefore are functionally important in viral attachment and entry.

Virus–cell membrane fusion begins with the interaction of gp120 with the first immunoglobulin-like domain of the CD4+ molecule expressed on the cell surface. This interaction causes conformational changes in gp120 that allow binding of gp120 to the coreceptor. The binding results in the exposure of a hydrophobic domain in gp41, which, in turn, leads to the insertion of this domain into the cell membrane and the initiation of viral envelope–cell membrane fusion.

The 9-kb HIV-1 genome is similar in organization to that of other retroviruses, but has at least six other genes (*tat, rev, vpr, vpu, vif,* and *nef*) that are not found in nonprimate retroviruses. Each of these genes encodes a protein that has been implicated in viral replication and pathogenicity.[5]

After internalization and uncoating of the viral core, a new viral life cycle begins with the generation of a DNA transcript of viral RNA through the activity of the viral reverse transcriptase. As the linear, double-stranded DNA provirus is generated, it remains associated with RNA, matrix proteins, and the viral integrase enzyme as a preintegration complex. For completion of the viral replication cycle, the preintegration complex must be transported from the cytoplasm to the nucleus and integrated into host genomic DNA. The extent to which integration and subsequent virion synthesis occur appears to depend on the cell cycle stage and activation state of the infected cell.[6] Cells with integrated provirus represent long-lived reservoirs for viral persistence and barriers to eradication of the virus from infected individuals.

Virion assembly takes place primarily at the cell plasma membrane. Structural (*gag*, envelope) and viral enzyme genes encode precursor proteins that are processed and cleaved to produce multiple gene products. Cleavage of the gag structural proteins by the viral protease enzyme occurs during viral assembly and is essential for the proper assembly of infectious virions. Antiretroviral agents that inhibit the protease enzyme thus prevent the production of infectious virions. As the virus buds through cellular membranes, it acquires a lipid bilayer along with viral envelope glycoproteins.

Early Infection

The CD4 molecule is the primary cellular receptor for HIV-1; cells that express this molecule on their cell surfaces (CD4+ T lymphocytes and cells of monocyte or macrophage lineage) are major targets for HIV-1 infection. Members of the chemokine receptor family are coreceptors for HIV.[7] Cell surface chemokine receptors are 7-transmembrane, G-protein-coupled receptors that transduce chemokine binding into intracellular signals, which in turn lead to the activation and migration of leukocytes. The configuration of cysteine motifs in chemokines is the basis for structural groupings (C-C-C or CC-chemokines; C-X-C or CXC-chemokines) that determine differences in biologic activities. Most HIV-1 strains use the CCR5 or CXCR4 (also known as LESTR or fusin) coreceptors.

CCR5 appears to be important especially in the initial establishment of infection. HIV-1 infection is uncommon in individuals with a homozygous 32-basepair deletion in CCR5; their lymphocytes do not express this chemokine receptor on cell surfaces and are relatively resistant to infection with primary HIV-1 isolates in vitro. Nonetheless, several HIV-1-infected individuals, homozygous for this defect, have been identified, suggesting that under some circumstances, other coreceptors might be utilized in

TABLE 233-1. Comparison of Human Immunodeficiency Viruses Types 1 (HIV-1) and 2 (HIV-2)

	HIV-1	HIV-2
Source virus	Chimpanzee simian immunodeficiency virus	Sooty mangabey simian immunodeficiency virus
Geographic distribution	Worldwide	West Africa; India
Transmission	Sexual; contaminated needles; blood transfusion; mother-to-child	Sexual; mother-to-child; blood transfusion; lower overall transmissibility than that of HIV-1
Mother-to-child transmission	25–35%[a]	≤4%[a]
Clinical manifestations	Lymphadenopathy; wasting syndrome; central nervous system disease; CD4+ lymphocyte depletion and immunodeficiency	Same as those of HIV-1 but generally less rapid disease progression

[a]*Transmission rates without antiretroviral therapy.*

the establishment of infection. Although heterozygosity for the CCR5 deletion mutant does not appear to protect from the acquisition of infection, studies in both adults and children indicate that it might protect against disease progression.

Following virus entry, HIV-1 proteins can interact with multiple cellular proteins to enhance viral replication.[8] For example, HIV-1 Tat interacts with the cellular protein cyclin-T1 to increase the efficiency of proviral transcription; the interaction of HIV-1 Gag with tumor suppressor gene 101 (TSG-101) enhances viral budding from the plasma membrane. Several cellular proteins have also been identified that restrict the replication of primate lentiviruses. CEM-15 is a member of the APOBEC 3 family of proteins. These proteins are cytidine deaminases that are packaged into retroviruses; during reverse transcription, they introduce G to A hypermutations that alter the integrity of the proviral DNA. HIV-1 Vif restores HIV-1 infectivity by complexing with CEM-15 and targeting it for proteosomal degradation, thus preventing its incorporation into virions. TRIM-5α is a cellular restriction factor that appears to interfere with uncoating of the viral RNA following entry.

The vertical transmission of HIV-1 can occur during gestation (in utero), during delivery (intrapartum), or postpartum through breastfeeding. Although admixture of maternal–fetal blood is a potential mechanism for in utero and intrapartum transmission, the majority of infections are thought to occur after mucosal (ocular or gastrointestinal) exposure to maternal blood and cervicovaginal fluids during delivery or to breastmilk after birth. Dendritic cells initially are infected and facilitate infection of CD4+ T lymphocytes, which then become the major source of viral production and dissemination throughout the body. Regardless of the route of infection, the gastrointestinal tract appears to be a major site of viral replication, persistence, and CD4+ T-cell depletion throughout infection.[9,10]

HIV-1 DNA can be detected by means of polymerase chain reaction (PCR) assay in peripheral blood mononuclear cells of infected infants at birth, suggesting in utero infection. In nonbreastfed populations, results of PCR assay are negative in the majority of infected infants (up to 75%) at birth, but become positive in those 2 to 4 weeks of age, suggesting the intrapartum transmission of HIV-1. In breastfeeding cohorts, up to 40% of infants can acquire HIV-1 through breastmilk transmission. The administration of antiretroviral therapies can markedly reduce the risk of mother-to-child HIV-1 transmission.[11]

Rapid increases in the plasma HIV-1 RNA copy number to 10^5 to 10^7 copies/mL have been documented in vertically infected infants during the first weeks of life. By contrast, plasma HIV-1 RNA levels gradually decrease in infants over the first 1 to 2 years of life, but mean plasma HIV-1 RNA levels do not drop below 10^5 copies/mL until at least the third year of life. A continued reduction in plasma HIV-1 RNA (mean −0.2 to −0.3 log decline per year) has been observed in vertically infected children through 5 to 6 years of age. Plasma HIV-1 RNA levels during infancy do not

appear to distinguish those with rapid and slow disease progression. However, after 3 to 4 years of age, plasma HIV-1 RNA levels are predictive of disease progression. Reductions in plasma HIV-1 RNA after antiretroviral therapy have been associated with clinical benefit. Several studies have demonstrated significant benefit to the initiation of antiretroviral therapy in early infancy;[12–14] early diagnosis and treatment of infants is now recommended, irrespective of symptoms or CD4 counts.[11,15]

HUMAN IMMUNODEFICIENCY VIRUS TYPE 2

HIV-2 was first isolated in the mid-1980s from individuals with acquired immunodeficiency syndrome (AIDS) in West Africa. Since then, most cases of HIV-2 infection have been reported from West Africa, although cases have also been reported from Zimbabwe and India.[16] The distribution of HIV-2 infections in West Africa coincides with the natural habitat of the sooty mangabey. HIV-2 is thought to be a zoonosis resulting from cross-species transmission of SIV_{sm}. HIV-2 and SIV_{sm} are genomically similar and share an accessory gene, vpx, not found in other primate lentiviruses.

To a lesser extent, HIV-2 also shares structural and genomic similarities with HIV-1. The HIV-2 gag and pol genes share approximately 60% homology with corresponding HIV-1 genes, whereas the env genes share only 30% to 40% homology. Viral genomic differences form the basis for molecular assays that distinguish between HIV-1 and HIV-2. Corresponding differences in viral proteins form the basis for antibody tests that distinguish between infections with these viruses.

Heterosexual and mother-to-child transmission of HIV-2 has been documented. Transmission through blood transfusion also occurs. Transmission through contaminated needles is postulated but not well documented. Overall, heterosexual and mother-to-child transmissions of HIV-2 appear to occur less readily than transmission of HIV-1. Antiretroviral therapy also can reduce the risk of mother-to-child transmission of HIV-2.

The clinical manifestations of HIV-2 infection are similar to those of HIV-1. Lymphadenopathy, wasting syndrome, central nervous system disease, and CD4+ depletion are common findings. Opportunistic infections and malignancies are common complications. The rate of CD4+ depletion after HIV-2 infection is much slower, and the median time from infection to the development of AIDS is longer, after HIV-2 infection than after HIV-1 infection. HIV-1 and HIV-2 coinfection occurs and follows a clinical course similar to that in individuals infected with HIV-1 alone.

The bases for the reduced transmissibility and pathogenicity of HIV-2 are unclear. Peripheral blood proviral load in HIV-2 infection is similar to that in HIV-1 infection, but plasma RNA levels are much lower in HIV-2-infected individuals than in HIV-1-infected individuals. Improvements in molecular techniques to detect, quantify, and characterize HIV-2 should allow improved understanding of the pathogenesis of HIV-2 infections in humans.

---

234 Introduction to Picornaviridae

John F. Modlin

The family Picornaviridae represent a large group of small (pico), positive-strand RNA viruses that infect a wide variety of hosts throughout the animal kingdom and are now classified by RNA sequence alignment (Table 234-1).[1] Included in the Picornavirus family are three genera commonly associated with human infection: Enterovirus, Parechovirus, and Hepatovirus.

Seven enterovirus species (human enterovirus A through D and human rhinovirus A through C), the human parechovirus species and hepatitis A virus, the only member of the Hepatovirus genus (see Chapter 237, Hepatitis A Virus), cause human infection. The enteroviruses, rhinoviruses, and parechoviruses each contain multiple serotypes, which are differentiated from one another by both

TABLE 234-1. Classification of the Human Picornaviruses

Genus	Species
Enterovirus	Human enterovirus A
	Human enterovirus B
	Human enterovirus C
	Human enterovirus D
	Human rhinovirus A
	Human rhinovirus B
	Human rhinovirus C
Parechovirus	Parechovirus
Hepatovirus	Hepatitis A virus

BOX 234-1. Major Physical Characteristics of the Picornaviridae

Size: 24–30 nm
Symmetry: Icosahedral
Envelope: None
Genome: Single-stranded RNA, 2.3–2.8×10^6 daltons (7.5 kb)

BIOLOGY

The major physical characteristics of picornaviruses are shown in Box 234-1. Picornavirus infection at the cellular level requires the presence of specific host cell membrane proteins that serve as receptors for viral attachment.[2] The receptors for many of the human picornaviruses have been identified and characterized.

Penetration, uncoating, and release of the positive-strand RNA genome into the cytoplasm occurs within minutes at 37°C. The RNA functions as a monocistronic messenger, the product of which is a large polyprotein that is cleaved in a series of steps into both structural and nonstructural regulatory proteins. Four capsid proteins (VP1, VP2, VP3, and VP4) are assembled in equimolar amounts into the capsid. Progeny RNA are copied from the genome via a negative-strand RNA intermediary and encapsidated to complete the replication cycle. In vitro infection produces about 10^4 to 10^5 particles per cell but the number of infectious particles is 10- to 1000-fold lower. Host protein and RNA synthesis are compromised within 3 hours of cell infection, and cell lysis occurs within 8 hours, with release of the progeny virions.

Picornaviruses are resistant to ether, chloroform, and alcohol but are inactivated by formaldehyde, phenol, and irradiation. They are rapidly inactivated at temperatures in excess of 50°C.

RNA sequence and by neutralization with immune serum. Important clinical and epidemiologic characteristics are associated with viral serotype and some biologic and genetic diversity also exists within each serotype.

Enteroviruses, rhinoviruses, and hepatitis A virus can be distinguished from one another on the basis of certain biophysical, clinical, and epidemiologic properties. Rhinoviruses replicate optimally at 33°C, reflecting their adaptation to the nasal mucosa. They are unstable at a pH <6 and can be recovered only from the respiratory tract. The enteroviruses and hepatitis A virus, which remain stable over a wide pH range, survive the acid environment of the stomach and are shed in the feces. Enteroviruses replicate in diverse tissues and cause many different diseases. Hepatitis A virus replication is limited to liver cells, and extrahepatic clinical manifestations of hepatitis A infection are rarely reported. The physical, clinical, and epidemiologic properties of the parechoviruses are indistinguishable from the enteroviruses.

235 Polioviruses

Stephanie B. Troy and Yvonne A. Maldonado

PATHOGEN AND PATHOPHYSIOLOGY

Polioviruses are single-stranded RNA viruses belonging to the family Picornaviridae. They have a naked protein capsid with a dense central core. The capsid consists of four structural proteins, VP1, VP2, VP3, and VP4. The genomic RNA is approximately 7440 to 7500 nucleotides in length. Three serotypes of poliovirus are antigenically distinct, but all three have 70% nucleotide identity.[1] Polioviruses are stable and can be stored indefinitely at −20°C and are inactivated by formaldehyde, chlorination, and ultraviolet light.

Humans are the only known natural host; however, poliovirus can replicate in other primates. The virus is exclusively propagated in cultured cells of primate origin because other cell lines lack a functional receptor molecule. Since identification and molecular cloning of the viral receptor, transgenic mice have been developed that are susceptible to all three serotypes of poliovirus.[2]

Poliovirus is transmitted primarily by the fecal–oral route and replicates in the pharynx and lower intestinal tract (Table 235-1). Only small amounts of infectious virus are needed to cause infection. Virus is shed in the pharynx for 1 to 3 weeks and in the gut for 4 to 8 weeks after primary infection. During reinfection, pharyngeal shedding is rare and fecal shedding is reduced to less than 3 weeks. The incubation period generally is 7 to 14 days but can be as short as 3 days and as long as 35 days. The virus spreads quickly

from the alimentary tract to regional lymph nodes. After several days, a minor viremia ensues, and a number of sites, such as muscle, fat, liver, spleen, and bone marrow, become infected. If virus is contained at this point, subclinical infection occurs. Further replication of virus in these tissues leads to major viremia and the onset of clinical symptoms. The central nervous system (CNS) is seeded during the viremic phase in approximately 1% of infections. The virus can also infect the CNS via axonal transport from skeletal muscle;[3] such infection may correlate with the intense myalgia seen at the onset of paralysis in affected individuals.

Poliovirus replicates within neurons; the anterior horn cells of the spinal cord are involved most often. Neurons in nuclei of

TABLE 235-1. Pathogenesis of Poliovirus Infection

Site of Virus Replication	Time (Days)	Clinical Illness
Pharynx and intestine	0–1	Asymptomatic
Regional lymph nodes	1–3	Asymptomatic
Blood (minor viremia), muscle, fat, liver, spleen, bone marrow	3–7	Minor illness
Blood (major viremia), central nervous system	7–21	Major illness

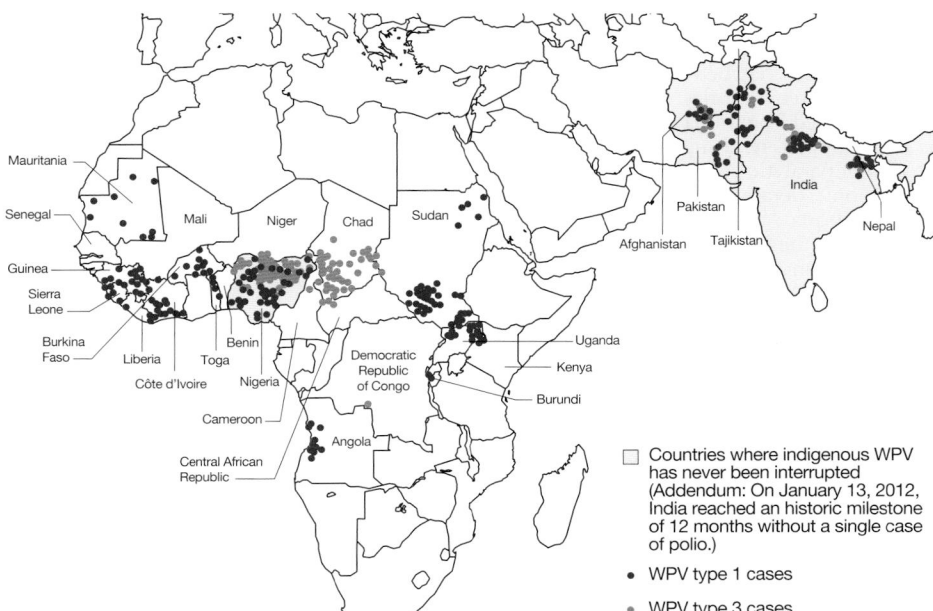

Figure 235-1. Countries with active transmission of wild poliovirus in 2009. (Data as of May 5, 2010. Figure taken from Centers for Disease Control and Prevention. Progress toward interruption of wild poliovirus transmission – worldwide, 2009. MMWR 2010;59(18):545–550.)

☐ Countries where indigenous WPV has never been interrupted (Addendum: On January 13, 2012, India reached an historic milestone of 12 months without a single case of polio.)

• WPV type 1 cases

• WPV type 3 cases

the medulla, vermis of the cerebellum, midbrain, thalamus and hypothalamus, palladium, and motor cortex of the cerebrum also can be involved. Rarely, the posterior horn cells and dorsal root ganglia are infected. Although poliovirus infection usually destroys neurons, injury occasionally is reversible.

Serum neutralizing antibody develops after about 1 week and protects against paralysis but not reinfection. Immunity to poliovirus infection is type specific, without any cross-protection, and persists for life. Local antibody appears 1 to 3 weeks after infection and limits virus replication at the mucosal level. Reinfection occurs; however, the duration of shedding is reduced and viremia does not occur. Immunodeficient individuals are at considerable risk of disseminated infection.

EPIDEMIOLOGY

Poliovirus infection occurs primarily in summer and fall in temperate climates and year round in tropical areas. Warm weather favors the spread of virus. Before the industrial revolution, poliomyelitis occurred predominantly in an endemic form, infecting most infants early in life before the disappearance of passively acquired maternal antibody. Most infections with poliovirus were inapparent; paralytic disease developed in a small proportion of infections.

As hygiene and sanitation improved, especially in the more temperate countries, epidemics appeared. Change occurred because of lack of contact with the virus by the youngest population, and a large group of older children and adults became susceptible. The first large epidemic of paralytic poliomyelitis in the United States occurred in Vermont in 1894 and involved approximately 130 people. Epidemics increased in size and frequency and peaked in 1952, when 57,879 cases were reported in the U.S. Introduction of the inactivated vaccine in 1955 led to a sharp decline in the number of cases.

In 1988, the World Health Assembly developed the goal of global eradication of poliomyelitis by the year 2000.[4] This objective was determined to be feasible because poliovirus has no animal reservoir, does not survive for long periods in the environment, and induces lifelong immunity after disease or vaccination. Global eradication strategies were developed and implemented, and annual polio cases dropped over 99%, from 350,000 in 1988 to 1,606 in 2009 (for further information, refer to www.polioeradication.org).[5] Wild poliovirus type 2 has been eradicated globally. The Americas, Australia, and Europe have

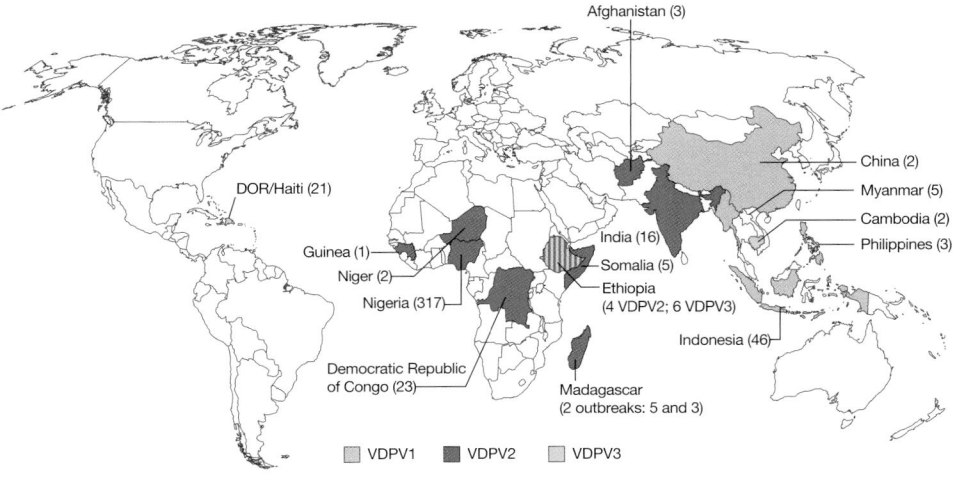

Figure 235-2. Outbreaks of circulating vaccine-derived poliovirus (VDPV), 2000–2010. The numbers indicate the number of cases of acute flaccid paralysis. Outbreaks are defined as those associated with at least two cases of acute flaccid paralysis. The Niger and Chad cases are linked to the Nigeria outbreak. Madagascar had two different outbreaks in 2001/2 and 2005. Ethiopia had two different outbreaks in 2008/9 and 2009/10. (Data from www.polioeradication.org. Site last accessed December 9, 2011.)

☐ VDPV1 ☐ VDPV2 ☐ VDPV3

been declared polio-free, and only four countries remain with uninterrupted wild poliovirus transmission (Afghanistan, India, Nigeria, and Pakistan). Unfortunately, wild poliovirus has been exported from Nigeria and India to previously polio-free countries in Africa. Further, in 2010, wild poliovirus was exported from India to Tajikistan, where vaccination coverage had dropped, resulting in an epidemic that has caused over 450 cases of paralytic poliomyelitis (Figure 235-1). Sustaining immunization coverage, even in polio-free countries, is critical to eradication efforts.

One complicating factor in global eradication was the discovery in 2000 that vaccine-derived polioviruses (VDPV) can cause outbreaks of poliomyelitis. While oral polio vaccine (OPV) has long been known to rarely cause vaccine-associated paralytic poliomyelitis (VAPP) in vaccinees or their close contacts, at a rate of about one case per million births, it was discovered only recently that with prolonged replication, OPV can mutate to form VDPV capable of causing poliomyelitis outbreaks in undervaccinated communities.[6] From 2000 to 2010, outbreaks in 15 countries have been identified (Figure 235-2). The attack rates and severity of disease associated with VDPV are similar to those seen with wild poliovirus.[7]

CLINICAL MANIFESTATIONS

Infection with poliovirus most often is inapparent. From 90% to 95% of infections produce no symptoms or nonspecific minimal symptoms, such as fever, malaise, anorexia, and sore throat. Aseptic meningitis develops in 4% to 8% of children, but patients usually recover completely in 5 to 10 days; <2% of infections lead to paralytic disease.

Paralytic illness in children often is biphasic, with an initial self-resolving, minor illness. The child then experiences high fever and intense muscle pain accompanied by a decrease or loss of reflexes. The appearance of paralysis is sudden and progresses to complete loss of motor function in one or more extremities over a period of several hours. Maximal loss of function develops within 5 days of onset. The hallmark of poliomyelitis is asymmetric paresis or paralysis, with proximal limb muscles involved more frequently than distal, and lower limbs more often affected than upper limbs. Bladder paralysis and bowel atony commonly occur but improve over a period of 1 to 3 days. Pain, spasticity, nuchal and spinal rigidity, and hypertonia occur early and are due to lesions in the brainstem, spinal ganglia, and posterior columns. In general, the paralysis tends to subside over time, with maximal improvement by 6 months. Cranial nerve dysfunction occurs in 5% to 35% of patients with paralysis. Sensory abnormalities are rare except in the most severe cases.

Hypoxia is a common complication of poliomyelitis and can result from weakness in the respiratory muscles, involvement of the respiratory center in the brainstem, or infection of the 9th, 10th, and 12th cranial nerves. Cranial nerve involvement results in paralysis of the pharynx, soft palate, and vocal cords, with subsequent respiratory compromise. Respiratory failure is responsible for most deaths attributable to paralytic poliomyelitis.

Most patients with limb paralysis improve; however, 60% of affected individuals exhibit some degree of residual deficit. Currently, <7% of individuals with spinal poliomyelitis die, usually of respiratory failure. In contrast, as many as 60% of individuals with bulbar paralysis died before modern methods of assisted ventilation became available.

Other diseases can mimic poliomyelitis. Nonpoliomyelitis enteroviruses, especially coxsackievirus A7 and enterovirus 71, cause sporadic cases, as well as small outbreaks of paralytic disease. Guillain–Barré syndrome causes ascending symmetric paralysis and infant botulism causes descending symmetric paralysis. West Nile encephalitis can cause flaccid paralysis and Lyme disease can cause neuropathy.

DIAGNOSIS

Routine laboratory studies are not distinctively abnormal. The complete blood cell count and differential cell count usually are

unremarkable. Examination of cerebrospinal fluid demonstrates changes consistent with aseptic meningitis. Poliovirus can be recovered readily from the throat and stool and rarely from the cerebrospinal fluid of infected individuals. Virus is shed from the throat for 1 to 3 weeks and from stool for 4 to 8 weeks. The virus produces cytopathogenic effects in monkey kidney cell and human cell monolayers within 1 week. Vaccine- and wild-type polioviruses, as well as other enteroviruses, cannot be distinguished without further specific studies such as PCR. Neutralizing antibody to specific poliovirus serotypes can be detected in serum as early as 1 week after infection.

TREATMENT

Supportive care is the mainstay of treatment. Analgesics and bedrest are indicated. Manual decompression of the bladder, medication to relieve severe muscle spasms, intermittent catheterization, or the short-term use of a parasympathetic stimulant may be necessary if bladder paralysis exists. Ventilator support may be necessary for individuals with respiratory compromise.

SPECIAL CONSIDERATIONS

Pregnant women have an increased risk of paralytic disease. Rarely, poliovirus causes an intrauterine infection resulting in abortion or premature delivery; malformations are not a consequence. Infection acquired from a mother incubating the virus at the time of delivery often results in paralytic disease in the newborn. Immunocompromised individuals are prone to the development of progressive, often fatal disease. Persons with B-lymphocyte immunodeficiency are susceptible to chronic or disseminated infection from wild and attenuated vaccine virus.

New neurologic symptoms develop in approximately 25% to 35% of individuals with paralytic disease 25 to 35 years after infection.[8] This "postpolio syndrome" is characterized by muscle weakness, pain, atrophy, and fatigue. The muscles involved are the same as those involved in the original illness. The causes of these changes remain unclear, with postulations of neuronal "fallout," slow infection, or immunopathologic mechanisms.

PREVENTION

Use and Efficacy of Salk and Sabin Vaccines

Poliomyelitis reached pandemic proportions in the U.S. in the first half of the 20th century. During the early 1950s, paralytic disease developed in 10,000 to 20,000 people annually during the summer and fall. Although paralytic illness represented approximately 1% of the total infections, millions of infected individuals participated in the spread of virus throughout communities.

The first inactivated poliovirus vaccine (IPV, Salk) was introduced in 1955, just 6 years after the virus had been successfully propagated in tissue culture of nonneurogenic origin.[9] It was followed by an immediate decline in paralytic poliomyelitis from 37 to 0.8 cases per 100,000 population in 1961.[10,11] In 1961 to 1962, live OPV (Sabin) was introduced and quickly supplanted the use of IPV because it was easy to administer, induced lifelong immunity, provided local immunity, and secondarily immunized contacts through fecal shedding of virus. Paralytic cases of poliomyelitis continued to decline substantially with the widespread administration of Sabin vaccine.[12]

The initial use of OPV in the U.S. and elsewhere has resulted in a dramatic reduction in the global incidence of poliomyelitis. In most developing nations, OPV is still used for routine and mass immunization programs and has resulted in a dramatic decline in paralytic disease in these regions. However, seroconversion rates have been suboptimal in developing countries, especially tropical countries, and outbreaks of poliomyelitis have occurred in countries with relatively high rates of vaccine coverage. Possible explanations for the failure of OPV in the tropics include vaccine instability, the vaccine formulation, concurrent enteric infections, malnutrition, and the presence of inhibitory substances in the intestine.[13,14] In the U.S., concurrent viral infections have been reported to impair the immune response to poliovirus vaccines; however, the effects are minimal and are insignificant clinically.[15]

VACCINE-ASSOCIATED PARALYTIC POLIOMYELITIS

After the dramatic reduction in cases of poliomyelitis in the U.S., concern about VAPP increased. From 1980 through 1995, 132 cases of VAPP were reported in the U.S.[12] Of these cases, approximately 40% occurred in previously healthy vaccine recipients, 31% in healthy contacts of vaccine recipients, and 24% in immunodeficient individuals. Individuals with congenital immunodeficiency have a risk of VAPP that is approximately 2000-fold higher than that in normal children. Most immunologic abnormalities in affected individuals are congenital isolated B-lymphocyte deficiency or combined immunodeficiencies. The incidence of VAPP remained steady at about 4 cases annually, until the transition to the exclusive use of IPV in the U.S., beginning in 2000. A high rate of vaccine-strain associated paralytic disease in Romania was associated with intramuscular injections within 30 days of immunization with OPV. This "provocation paralysis" was previously only associated with wild-type poliovirus infection.[16]

Type 3 poliovirus is the most common isolate from patients with VAPP in the U.S. and type 1 poliovirus is the least common. In an analysis of 62 virologically confirmed cases of VAPP reported in the U.S. between 1980 and 1989, 60% of isolates were type 3 and 15% were type 1 polio.[10] The attenuated type 3 poliovirus in OPV probably is excessively associated with VAPP because it is genetically more unstable than the other two viruses.[17]

ROLE OF IPV VERSUS OPV IN ROUTINE IMMUNIZATION

The role of IPV for routine immunization in the U.S. has been reassessed continually. Inactivated vaccines had previously required the administration of booster doses because of a decline in antibody titer. However, one long-term follow-up study of standard IPV immunization in Sweden demonstrated persistent immunity to each of the three polioviruses for as long as 25 years in this population, where the immunization rate was 99%.[18]

Despite a good record of clinical efficacy, several countries using IPV as the predominant vaccine have had outbreaks of poliomyelitis in the past several decades. In 1984, Finland experienced a unique epidemic that involved 9 cases of paralytic disease caused by type 3 virus. Investigation demonstrated an unexpectedly low rate of seropositivity (i.e., 60%) to type 3 poliovirus in the population. The decline in the seropositivity rate from earlier years was attributed to a decline in the type 3 poliovirus content of vaccine and a slight change in the immunologic and molecular characteristics of the epidemic virus compared with the vaccine virus.[19] Extensive spread of virus in the community was documented during this outbreak, with at least 100,000 individuals estimated to be infected, thus suggesting that IPV vaccine failed to induce sufficient mucosal immunity to halt person-to-person transmission.

Newer, enhanced-potency IPV (eIPV) offers distinct advantages over older preparations. It contains 40, 8, and 32 D antigen units per dose of poliovirus types 1, 2, and 3, respectively, compared with 20, 2, and 4 D antigen units per dose in the original Salk vaccine. The increased antigenic content is associated with a higher seroconversion rate after the administration of fewer doses. The schedule for administration is the same as for OPV, with seroconversion rates of 99% after as few as two doses of eIPV, in contrast to earlier preparations of IPV, which required three or four doses to achieve the same rate of seroconversion.[20–22]

One dose of OPV or IPV is not associated with a significant rise in neutralizing antibody in 2-month-old infants, whereas 95% or more of children exhibit antibody after two doses of either vaccine.[21,22] Each vaccine produces high neutralizing antibody titers after three doses.[22] Type 2 vaccine virus elicits the highest

antibody response after OPV. Detectable serum antibody to all three types persists in more than 90% of vaccinees 4 years after primary immunization with either OPV or eIPV.[23]

Before 1996, the use of a combined schedule, eIPV followed by OPV, had been proposed to avoid some cases of VAPP and to boost the response to OPV. Studies performed in the U.S. have shown that sequential dosing of IPV and OPV results in excellent systemic and local immune responses.[21,22] Four years after the third dose of vaccine, the combined schedule yields higher antibody titers than does exclusive immunization with OPV or IPV.[23]

Poliovirus-specific immunoglobulin A (IgA) is detected in 100% of individuals after three doses of OPV or eIPV.[22] OPV-immunized children tend to have higher IgA-specific antibody levels than do children who receive IPV exclusively.[22,23] When challenged with OPV, children immunized with IPV shed lower concentrations of virus for a shorter period than do nonimmune individuals. Virus shedding is less in recipients of eIPV than in recipients of the previously available IPV.[24] Children immunized with OPV shed virus in a manner similar to rechallenged, naturally immune subjects.[25]

Significant differences in poliovirus-specific local antibody are observed between OPV- and IPV-immunized children when trypsin-treated poliovirus is used as the antigen for antibody determination. The local neutralizing antibody titer against enzyme-cleaved virus is significantly higher than that against whole virus in the OPV vaccines.[26] This observation suggests that the secretory antibody response is directed against distinct epitopes or antigenic sites of the poliovirus that are not expressed in IPV, thus providing further explanation for the superior production of mucosal immunity induced by OPV.

Recently, monovalent OPV (mOPV) against type 1 or type 3 polio has been reintroduced for use in mass immunization campaigns in countries where wild poliovirus is endemic or has been imported. mOPV leads to approximately three times more type-specific antibody concentrations than trivalent OPV,[7,27,28] although mOPV1 and mOPV3 use in place of the trivalent vaccine may have contributed to an outbreak of type 2 circulating VDPV in Nigeria.[7] Efforts have been made to make IPV more affordable for developing countries. IPV has been combined with other injectable vaccines into pentavalent and even hexavalent vaccines without decreasing its immunogenicity.[29] Another strategy is to use one-fifth the standard dose of IPV intradermally. Two studies comparing fractional dose intradermal IPV to full dose intramuscular IPV have been conducted. In one study, seroconversion rates were the same but in the second study, the seroconversion rate was reduced in those receiving the fractional dose intradermally. Both studies demonstrated that the fractional dose given by the intradermal route resulted in lower titers of antibody.[30,31]

Current Poliovirus Immunization Schedule in the United States

Because of the absence of indigenous transmission of wild-type poliovirus in the U.S. and the rare but continued occurrence of VAPP, the U.S. Public Health Service recommended a sequential IPV–OPV vaccination schedule from 1997 through 1999, with two doses of IPV at ages 2 and 4 months, followed by two doses of OPV at 12 to 18 months and 4 to 6 years of age.[12] The subsequent schedule, begun in January 2000, consists of a 4-dose series of IPV exclusively – at 2, 4, and 6 to 18 months and 4 to 6 years (see Chapter 6, Active Immunization). The change from OPV to IPV does not appear to have had a negative impact on vaccine coverage and has resulted in the elimination of VAPP in the U.S.[32] Canada and most of Europe also use IPV, with schedules recommending between 3 and 7 doses depending on the country. Preterm infants mount systemic and local antibody responses similar to term infants.[33]

In the U.S., OPV has not been used since 2000, and currently is recommended only for use as the vaccine of choice for mass vaccination in the event of a polio outbreak. OPV should not be used in individuals with immune deficiency, in unvaccinated adults, and in children who live in households with immune-deficient individuals. Although in general live vaccines are contraindicated during pregnancy, OPV has been administered to pregnant women during mass immunization programs without adverse effect and is advised if protection is required.[34] Travelers to countries where OPV is used, who are previously unimmunized or who have not received a booster dose of IPV, should be aware of the risk of VAPP in these settings, and should consider immunization. Those who have received an incomplete series should complete the series, not repeat it. For previously immunized adult travelers to polio-endemic areas, vaccination with one dose of IPV should be considered; for adult travelers who have not previously been immunized, three doses of IPV should be given with intervals of at least 4 weeks between doses. Available information suggests that only one lifetime booster dose of IPV is necessary. Current information regarding polio-endemic areas can be obtained at www.polioeradication.org and updated polio immunization information can be obtained at www.cdc.gov.

236 Enteroviruses and Parechoviruses

John F. Modlin

The human enteroviruses and parechoviruses are members of the Picornavirus family that are commonly transmitted by enteric and respiratory routes and cause a wide spectrum of illnesses in persons of all ages.

The enteroviruses are divided among four species within the genus Enterovirus, human enterovirus A, B, C, and D, based on RNA sequence relatedness. Enterovirus species C polioviruses and 3 additional genus Enterovirus species, human rhinovirus A, B, and C, are discussed in separate chapters. Before the availability of viral genome sequencing, the human enteroviruses were distinguished from the rhinoviruses by their relative acid stability and were subdivided into several classes based on differences in host range and into individually numbered serotypes within each class on the basis of differential neutralization by immune sera (Table 236-1). The three poliovirus serotypes are the prototypic enteroviruses which can be transmitted to nonhuman primates and replicate in primate cell culture. The coxsackieviruses were originally distinguished from polioviruses by their ability to cause paralysis and death in suckling mice. They are divided into group A and group B according to the type of disease produced in these animals (see Table 236-1). Group B coxsackieviruses are readily isolated in primate cell culture, whereas most group A coxsackieviruses grow poorly in cell culture. Echoviruses (enteric cytopathic human orphan viruses) are not pathogenic for mice and monkeys, but are recovered readily in primate cell culture. All enterovirus serotypes identified since 1970 are designated simply as enterovirus. More than 100 poliovirus, group A coxsackievirus, group B coxsackievirus, echovirus, and enterovirus serotypes are now distributed among the 4 human enterovirus species A to D (Table 236-2).

Parechoviruses share many of the same biological, clinical, and epidemiologic characteristics with enteroviruses, but differ sufficiently in genomic sequence to be classified in a separate genus.[1] The prototypic parechovirus serotypes 1 and 2 originally were designated echovirus 22 and 23, respectively; 14 parechovirus serotypes are recognized currently.

PATHOGENESIS

The pathogenesis of enterovirus infections has been investigated most extensively with poliovirus infection in monkeys and humans. Although comparable data are not available for the non-polio enteroviruses, it is assumed that the pathogenic events are similar although tissue and organ tropism is highly variable.

Human enteroviruses are acquired directly or indirectly by the ingestion of virus that is shed in the feces or upper respiratory tract of infected contacts. Initial viral replication occurs in the upper

TABLE 236-1. Traditional Biologic Classification of the Human Enteroviruses

| Subgroup | Serotypes | Experimental Host Range | | Cell Culture |
		Primates	Newborn Mice	
Polioviruses	1–3	++	–[a]	++
Coxsackievirus A	1–24[b]	–[c]	+++	±[d]
Coxsackievirus B	1–6	–	+++	++
Echoviruses	1–34[e]	–	–[f]	++
Enteroviruses	68–72[g]	Variable	Variable	+

[a]Rare strains (e.g., Lansing strain of poliovirus 2) have been adapted to mice.

[b]Coxsackievirus A23 has been reclassified as echovirus 9, which leaves 23 coxsackieviruses in group A. Antigenic interrelationships exist between coxsackievirus types A3 and A8, A11 and A15, and A13 and A18.

[c]Coxsackievirus A7 is pathogenic for the central nervous system of primates.

[d]Most coxsackievirus serotypes of group A are not readily isolated in cell cultures, but exceptions exist (e.g., types A9 and A16), and additional serotypes have been adapted to cell cultures.

[e]Echovirus 10 has been reclassified as reovirus 1 and echovirus 28 as rhinovirus 1A. Echovirus 34 is a variant of coxsackievirus A24; a total of 31 serotypes of echovirus therefore remain from the original 34. Antigenic interrelationships exist between echovirus types 1 and 8, 12 and 29, and 6 and 30. Echoviruses 22 and 23 are now reclassified in the novel genus Parechovirus.

[f]Except echovirus 21.

[g]Hepatitis A virus was designated as enterovirus 72, but now is classified as a separate Picornavirus genus.

TABLE 236-2. Classification of Human Enteroviruses by RNA Sequence

Enterovirus Species	Enterovirus Serotypes
A	Coxsackievirus A serotypes 2–8, 10, 12, 14, 16
	Enterovirus serotypes 71, 76, 89–92
B	Coxsackievirus A serotype 9
	Coxsackievirus B serotypes 1–6
	Echovirus serotypes 1–7, 9, 11–21, 24–27, 29–33
	Enterovirus serotypes 69, 73–75, 77–88, 93, 97, 98, 100, 101, 106, 107
C	Coxsackievirus A serotypes 1, 11, 13, 17, 19–22, 24
	Poliovirus serotypes 1–3
	Enterovirus serotypes 95, 96, 99, 102, 104, 105, 109
D	Enterovirus serotypes 68, 70, 94

Adapted from reference 100.

respiratory tract and distal small bowel. Infectious virus is detectable in ileal lymphoid tissue 1 to 3 days after the ingestion of virus, and fecal shedding can be detectable for ≥6 weeks. Generally, enteroviruses are recovered from the gastrointestinal tract in greater density and for longer periods than from the upper respiratory tract.

Viral replication in submucosal lymphoid tissue gives rise to a transient "minor" viremia that distributes virus to reticuloendothelial tissue in distant lymph nodes, liver, spleen, and bone marrow. Further replication in these organs leads to sustained "major" viremia and dissemination of virus to target organs such as the central nervous system (CNS), heart, and skin.

Many infected persons control infection before the major viremia and experience only transient symptoms or asymptomatic infection. The onset of symptomatic disease including fever and other systemic manifestations coincides with the major viremia, and organ-specific disease (i.e., poliomyelitis, myocarditis) results from virus-induced cell necrosis and the accompanying inflammatory response. Early viral replication does not cause histopathologic changes in the gastrointestinal tract or lymphoreticular tissue.

Both experimental and clinical data suggest that certain host factors enhance the severity of enterovirus infection, including exercise during the incubation period, cold stress, malnutrition, and B-lymphocyte immunodeficiency.

IMMUNITY

Protective immunity to enterovirus infection is serotype specific. Infection leads to production of neutralizing humoral antibodies that protect against recurrent disease but not against asymptomatic reinfection. Passive antibody provided by immune globulin[2] or transplacental maternal antibody[3] effectively prevents enterovirus disease. Secretory IgA antibodies appear in nasal and duodenal secretions 2 to 4 weeks after primary infection and persist for at least 15 years.[4] Secretion of IgA antibodies at each mucosal site is dependent on local virus replication.[5] Upon enterovirus re-exposure, secretory IgA antibodies prevent or substantially reduce subsequent replication. Secretory IgA antibodies also are found in colostrum and milk of immune women. Antibodies in human milk may interfere with the replication of attenuated polioviruses given to breastfed infants during the first month of life.[6]

Persons with isolated B-lymphocyte immunodeficiency syndromes develop persistent enterovirus infections, suggesting that humoral antibodies are necessary for viral clearance.[7] Administration of intramuscular immune serum globulin does not affect the course of acute poliomyelitis,[8] but controlled trials of immune globulin administered intravenously (IGIV) in both CNS and non-CNS enterovirus infections have not been performed. Studies in a well-characterized murine model show that inhibition of T-lymphocyte function has little effect on the course of enterovirus infection, although T lymphocytes participate in immunopathologic events contributing to the cytotoxicity that accompanies infection.[9] These data may explain the observation that patients with T-lymphocyte immunodeficiency or immunosuppression do not appear to be at risk for severe or prolonged enterovirus infection. In contrast, experimental studies suggest that macrophage function is critical to the clearance of virus and recovery from infection.[10]

EPIDEMIOLOGY

Infections occur in all human populations, although rates of infection vary markedly by geography, season, age, and other host factors. Transmission occurs throughout the year in most locations, although much higher rates occur in temperate climates in summer and fall.[11] Seasonal periodicity is more pronounced (i.e., higher density of infection during short seasons) with increasing latitudes in both hemispheres. Conversely, seasonal fluctuations diminish in tropical latitudes.

Although enterovirus infections and disease occur in all age groups, infants and young children have the highest rates. Infants <1 year of age are infected at several-fold higher rates than children and adults; and within the first year of life, enterovirus infections are recognized most often clinically in infants <3 months of age.[12-14] Males' risk of disease exceeds that of females by as much as 50%. Infants of low socioeconomic status have a higher risk of infection that is attributable to crowding and poor hygiene.

The contribution of different enterovirus serotypes to human infection and disease varies markedly. From 30% to 80% of adults have antibody to the more common enterovirus serotypes (e.g., group B coxsackieviruses 1 to 5 and some echoviruses). A small number of serotypes cause endemic disease with annual regional variation in the United States. Other serotypes (e.g., echoviruses 9, 11, and 30) are responsible for widespread outbreaks in which the epidemic strain accounts for >30% of all isolated enteroviruses, followed by several years of relative quiescence.[15] The reasons for appearance and disappearance of particular serotypes are unknown, although accumulation of a "critical mass" of susceptible young children may be necessary to sustain epidemic transmission.[16] Periodic reappearance of the same serotype is marked by strain variation as measured by oligonucleotide fingerprinting or genomic sequencing.[14,17] Between 1970 and 2005, 10 serotypes (all species B enteroviruses) represented 71% of all enterovirus isolates submitted from state and local public health laboratories to the National Enterovirus Surveillance System of the Centers for Disease Control and Prevention (Table 236-3).[18] In

TABLE 236-3. Most Common Enterovirus Serotypes Submitted by State and Local Public Health Laboratories to Centers for Disease Control and Prevention, 1970 to 2005[18]

Enterovirus Serotype	Percentage
Echovirus 9	11.8
Echovirus 11	11.4
Echovirus 30	10.1
Coxsackievirus B5	8.7
Echovirus 6	6.1
Coxsackievirus B2	5.2
Coxsackievirus A9	4.8
Echovirus 4	4.6
Coxsackievirus B4	4.2
Echovirus 7	4.0
Total	70.9

contrast, some enterovirus serotypes (e.g., echovirus 1, coxsackie-virus B6, and enteroviruses 68 and 69) rarely are recognized clinically and appear to have little epidemic potential. These data may underestimate infections by group A coxsackieviruses because only some serotypes (e.g., types 9 and 16) are readily isolated in cell culture.

TRANSMISSION

Enteroviruses are shed in the upper respiratory tract for 1 to 3 weeks and in the feces for 2 to 8 weeks after primary infection, suggesting both respiratory and fecal–oral routes of transmission. Studies of naturally occurring and attenuated polioviruses demonstrate that fecal (but not oropharyngeal) shedding also occurs during reinfection, albeit at lower titer and for a shorter duration. A notable exception to this pattern is enterovirus 70, the agent of acute hemorrhagic conjunctivitis, which is shed in tears and spread via fingers and fomites.[19] Both direct fecal–oral and indirect mechanisms of person-to-person transmission are postulated. Secondary infection rates exceed 50% in household contacts.[20] Infants, particularly those in diapers, appear to be the most efficient transmitters of infection. Indirect transmission is abetted by poor sanitary conditions and can occur via numerous routes, including contaminated water, food, and fomites. The relative role of virus shedding by symptomatic and asymptomatic persons is not known, but it is likely that both are important.

The incubation period for enteroviral infection is difficult to determine precisely and may vary according to the clinical syndrome. Brief febrile illnesses occur after an average incubation period of 3 to 5 days. Detailed studies of poliovirus infection have indicated that CNS manifestations (i.e., aseptic meningitis, poliomyelitis) usually are not observed until 9 to 12 days after exposure.[21]

CLINICAL MANIFESTATIONS

Most enterovirus infections in children are asymptomatic. The proportion of infections that result in illness varies widely within a serotype and is affected by a variety of host factors. Table 236-4 shows clinical syndromes commonly associated with nonpolio enterovirus infections in children. Some enteroviral diseases (e.g., nonspecific febrile illness, pharyngitis, and aseptic meningitis) are

associated with multiple serotypes of group B coxsackievirus and echovirus,[20,22] whereas others are associated with specific subgroups (e.g., myopericarditis with group B coxsackieviruses and herpangina with group A coxsackieviruses) or a limited number of serotypes (e.g., acute hemorrhagic conjunctivitis with coxsackievirus A24 or enterovirus 70).

Nonspecific Acute Febrile Illnesses

Nonpolio enteroviruses are the most commonly identified cause of fever without an apparent focus in infants <3 months of age.[23,24] During the summer and fall, enteroviruses account for at least one-half of cases.[13,14,25] Fever often occurs alone or in association with irritability, lethargy, poor feeding, vomiting, diarrhea, exanthems, or signs of upper respiratory tract infection.[26] Approximately one-half of infants infected with an enterovirus have aseptic meningitis,[24,26] often in the absence of meningeal signs.[26] Most infants with fever or aseptic meningitis recover within 2 to 10 days without complications.

Exanthems and Enanthems

Enteroviruses are common causes of a broad array of acute cutaneous eruptions and mucous membrane lesions (Figure 236-1). Exanthems can resemble those of measles, rubella, or roseola, or can be vesicular, petechial, purpuric, or urticarial. Exanthems are reported more commonly with infections due to echoviruses than other enteroviruses.

Herpangina is a distinctive enanthem characterized by painful vesicular lesions on the soft palate, uvula, tonsils, and posterior of the oropharynx, often accompanied by fever, headache, and sore throat. Mucosal lesions begin as punctate macules and evolve over a 24-hour period to 2- to 4-mm vesicular lesions that ultimately ulcerate centrally. Fever subsides in 2 to 4 days, but lesions can persist for a week.

Coxsackievirus A16 (and less commonly other group A and group B coxsackieviruses) and enterovirus 71 cause *hand-foot-and-mouth (HFM) disease*, a syndrome characterized by vesicular stomatitis and cutaneous lesions of the distal extremities) (Figure 236-2). Children <10 years of age are affected most commonly. Fever, sore throat, and refusal to eat are common complaints. Oral lesions occur chiefly on the buccal mucosa and tongue and can coalesce

TABLE 236-4. Spectrum of Illness Caused by the Enteroviruses

	Group A Coxsackieviruses	Group B Coxsackieviruses	Echoviruses	Newer Enteroviruses
EXANTHEMS/ENANTHEMS				
Herpangina	+++	+	+	−
Hand-foot-and-mouth disease	+++	+	−	+++
Nonspecific rash	++	+	+++	++
CENTRAL NERVOUS SYSTEM INFECTIONS				
Aseptic meningitis	+	+++	+++	++
Encephalitis	+++	++	++	++
Motor paralysis	++	+	+	+++
DISEASES OF MUSCLE				
Pleurodynia	+	+++	+	−
Myositis	++	++	++	−
Myopericarditis	+	+++	+	−
OPHTHALMIC INFECTIONS				
Acute hemorrhagic conjunctivitis	+++	−	−	+++
SYSTEMIC INFECTIONS				
Neonates	+	+++	+++	−
B-lymphocyte immunodeficiency	+	+	+++	−

+++, characteristic; ++, occasionally reported; +, rarely reported; −, no known association.

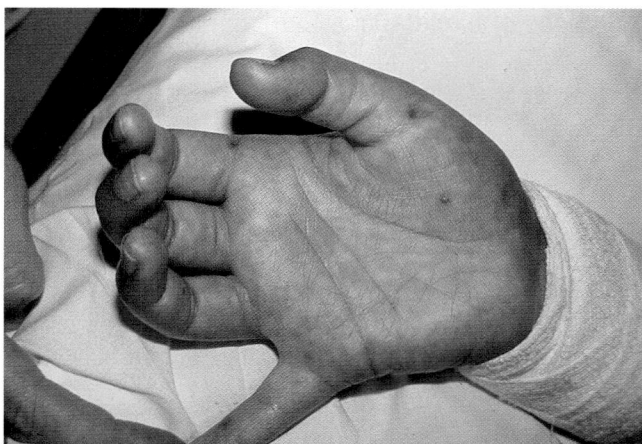

Figure 236-1. Typical hand lesions of coxsackie A virus in an infant with a febrile illness. No other exanthem was present. (Courtesy of M.C. Fisher and S.S. Long, St. Christopher's Hospital for Children, Philadelphia, PA.)

and ulcerate by the time of the initial examination. Cutaneous lesions occur in approximately 75% of cases and are found mainly on the hands, feet, wrists, ankles, and buttocks or genitalia. Lesions are tender papules or vesicles with a surrounding zone of erythema and resemble the lesions of herpes simplex virus (HSV) infections. HFM disease generally is self-limited, with average 7-day duration.[25] When caused by enterovirus 71 (EV-71), however, HFM disease can herald the onset of more serious CNS disease, including acute motor neuron disease and brainstem encephalitis.[27–29]

Central Nervous System Infections

Meningitis

Most cases of community-associated aseptic meningitis are caused by viruses, 90% of which are group B coxsackieviruses and echoviruses.[22] Although many serotypes cause meningitis, coxsackievirus serotypes B2 and B5 and echovirus serotypes 4, 6, 9, 11, 16, and 30 are most commonly reported. Not all enteroviruses that infect young infants are equally likely to cause meningitis. In one study, febrile infants infected with certain serotypes (e.g., the group B coxsackieviruses and echovirus serotypes 11 and 30) were more likely to have meningitis; group A coxsackieviruses caused <5% of cases.[26]

Infants <3 months of age appear to have the highest rate of aseptic meningitis, perhaps in part because lumbar puncture commonly is performed for evaluation of fever in this age group.[13] A minority of infants have clinical manifestations suggestive of neurologic disease.[13,25,26] The severity of meningeal symptoms and other signs of neurologic involvement in older children and adults with aseptic meningitis varies widely. Onset can be gradual or abrupt. Typically, the patient has a brief prodrome of fever, chills, and headache. Meningismus, when present, varies from mild to severe. Kernig and Brudzinski signs are present in only one-third of older children and adults.

The diagnosis of enterovirus meningitis usually is made by detection of enterovirus RNA in cerebrospinal fluid (CSF) by PCR, which is more sensitive than cell culture and produces a faster result, thus enabling a shorter length of hospital stay.[30,31]

Most cases of enteroviral meningitis are uncomplicated. Fever and signs of meningeal irritation resolve in 2 to 7 days, but CSF pleocytosis can persist. Adults compared with children appear to

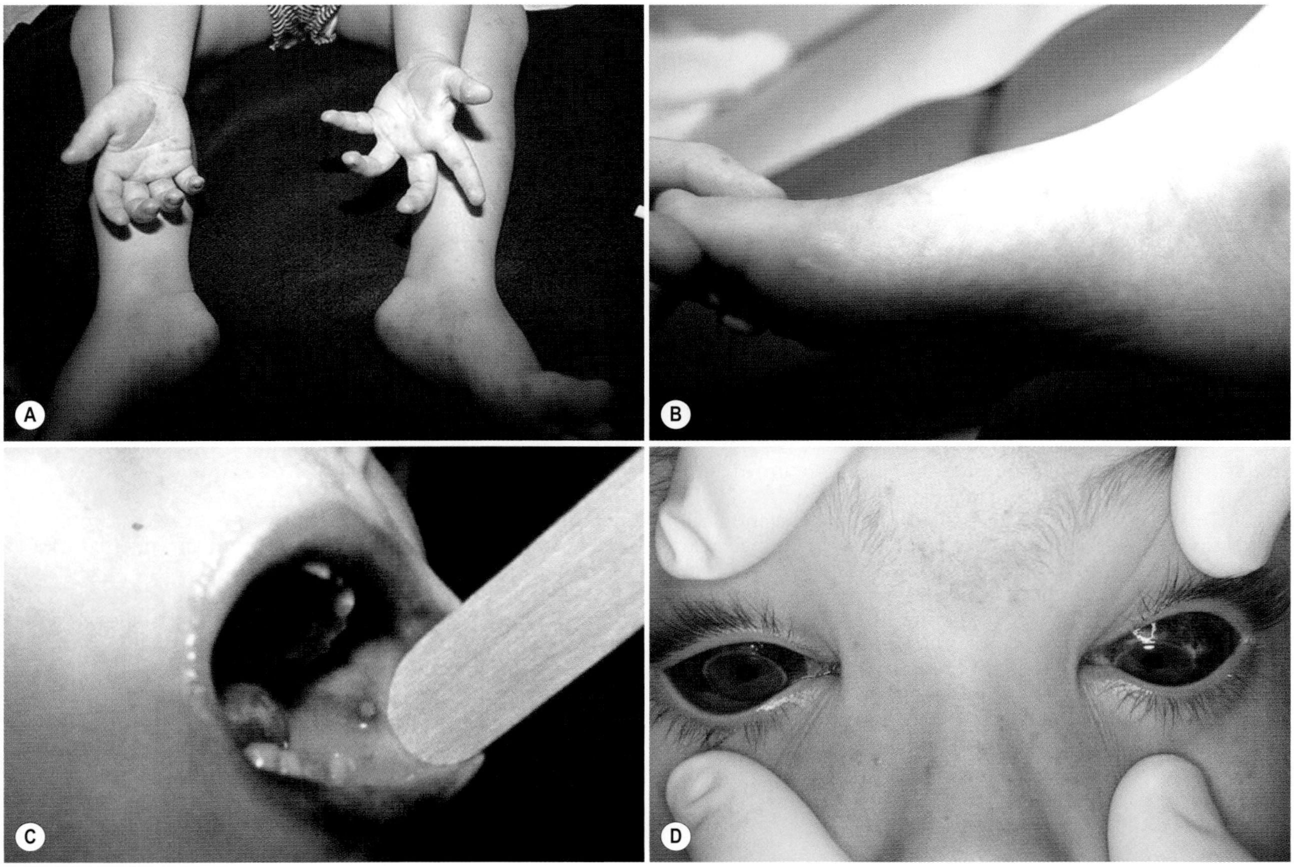

Figure 236-2. Characteristic findings of hand, foot and mouth disease include petechial, maculopapular or vesicular lesions on hands and feet **(A, B)** and ulcerative lesions with erythema on the oral mucosa **(C).** Acute hemorrhagic conjunctivitis with hemorrhage and edema of the conjunctivae **(D).** (Courtesy of J.H. Brien©.)

have more severe and prolonged symptoms.[32] Approximately 10% of infants hospitalized with aseptic meningitis experience acute CNS complications such as seizures, obtundation, or increased intracranial pressure.[13,33] Although some early reports suggested that infants with viral meningitis at an early age had a moderate risk of long-term neurologic and cognitive sequelae,[34] prospective studies indicate no measurable effect,[35,36] (including infants with neurologic findings during the acute illness).[13]

Encephalitis

Enteroviruses account for about 5% of all cases of acute encephalitis when comprehensive diagnostic testing is performed.[37] Many nonpolio enterovirus serotypes have been identified in patients with encephalitis. Group A coxsackieviruses have been isolated from infants and children with focal enteroviral encephalitis.[38]

Clinical manifestations of enterovirus encephalitis range from mild, reversible changes in mental status to coma, decerebration, and death. Patients with focal encephalitis can manifest partial motor seizures, hemichorea, or acute cerebellar ataxia. Initial findings in some cases suggest a diagnosis of HSV encephalitis.[38,39] Because CSF findings in enteroviral encephalitis are similar to those of aseptic meningitis, the term *meningoencephalitis* commonly is used interchangeably with *encephalitis*. Brain imaging and the electroencephalogram usually reflect the extent and severity of disease. Encephalitis occurring as a manifestation of generalized neonatal infection (see Special Considerations, later) often is fatal or results in permanent neurologic sequelae. The prognosis for older infants and children is better; although static neurologic sequelae and rare deaths occur, most patients recover fully.

Poliomyelitis-Like Illness

Nonpolio enteroviruses rarely can cause a syndrome of acute motor weakness and acute flaccid paralysis (AFP) that is clinically and pathologically indistinguishable from poliomyelitis. Outbreaks of acute paralysis caused by EV-71 have involved hundreds of people, mostly children, in eastern Europe and Southeast Asia, as well as smaller numbers of patients in Southeast Asia and parts of the U.S.[29,40–42] Coxsackievirus A7 has caused small outbreaks of AFP in Scotland and Russia. Sporadic cases of AFP can be caused by numerous enteroviruses, most commonly EV-71, group A coxsackievirus types 7 and 9, group B coxsackievirus types 1 to 5, and echovirus types 6 and 9. The myelitis caused by nonpolio enteroviruses tends to be less severe than that caused by polioviruses (i.e., less persistent muscle weakness and less common bulbar involvement).

Brainstem Encephalitis

A distinctive, life-threatening brainstem encephalitis occurred during epidemics of EV-71 infection in Malaysia and Taiwan.[28,29,42,43] Most cases occur in children <5 years of age and in association with HFM disease. Affected children have myoclonus, vomiting, ataxia, nystagmus, and oculomotor palsies. The most severely affected patients die rapidly from noncardiac pulmonary edema, which is postulated to be caused by dysregulation of sympathetic outflow and overload of the pulmonary vascular bed.[29,44] Neuronal degeneration and mononuclear cell infiltration in the grey matter of the pons and medulla are found at postmortem examination; EV-71 has been isolated from brainstem tissue, but virtually never from CSF.[42,43] A small number of similar cases have occurred sporadically in the U.S.[45,46]

Other Neurologic Syndromes

Guillain–Barré syndrome is reported in a limited number of patients infected with group A coxsackievirus types 2, 5, and 9 and echovirus types 6 and 22. Acute transverse myelitis has been attributed to coxsackievirus A9, coxsackievirus B4, and echovirus 5.

Infections of Skeletal and Cardiac Muscle

The myotropic nature of the group A and group B coxsackieviruses has been recognized since their discovery. Group B coxsackievirus types 1 to 5 are the principal causes of the myotropic diseases, although pleurodynia and myopericarditis rarely have been associated with some group A coxsackieviruses and echovirus types.

Pleurodynia (Epidemic Pleurodynia, Bornholm Disease)

Pleurodynia, an acute, communicable disease involving the intercostal and abdominal muscles, is characterized by fever and sharp, spasmodic pain in the chest wall or abdomen. Local outbreaks of pleurodynia with high attack rates within affected households have occurred, and major epidemics can take place every 10 to 20 years. Many reported outbreaks have occurred in sparsely populated areas. The diagnosis of pleurodynia is more common in older children and adults. Involvement of the abdominal muscles is more common in younger children than in older children and adults, who most often manifest thoracic pain. Paroxysmal nature of the pain is a hallmark. Involvement of the intercostal and other muscles of respiration results in enhanced pain with deep breathing and a sensation of "pleuritic" pain that can result in splinting of the chest and rapid, shallow breathing. Muscle inflammation can be detected by finding tenderness on direct palpation or, less commonly, by observing localized swelling. Fewer than 10% of patients have a pleural friction rub or pleural fluid evident on chest radiograph. Pain is most severe initially and typically diminishes over 4 to 6 days, although pain can persist up to 3 weeks. Analgesic medications and limitation of physical activity are helpful in reducing pain.

Myositis

Involvement of other muscles is less common; sporadic cases are caused by coxsackieviruses A9, B2, and B6 and by echoviruses 9 and 11. Both focal and generalized myositis can occur. Focal myositis often involves the thigh muscles. Generalized myositis frequently is manifest as polymyositis syndrome with an abrupt onset of fever, chills, and weakness, tenderness, and edema of the involved muscle groups. Myoglobinemia, myoglobinuria, and elevated serum levels of skeletal muscle enzymes are characteristic. Most cases occur in adults, who recover rapidly. An unusual case of systemic echovirus 11 infection with extensive myositis was reported in a 3-month-old infant; virus was recovered from muscle tissue at postmortem examination.[47]

Myopericarditis

Enteroviruses are a major cause of acute infection of cardiac muscle and pericardium. Although most patients have symptoms and signs of either pericarditis or myocarditis, the term *myopericarditis* is preferred because pathologic studies reveal that both the pericardium and myocardium usually are involved. Group B coxsackievirus types 2 to 5 are the predominant enteroviruses and account for one-third to one-half of sporadic cases[48,49] and almost all epidemic cases of myopericarditis.[50] Many other enterovirus serotypes have been reported to cause acute heart disease. Enteroviral myopericarditis is indistinguishable clinically from disease caused by other cardiotropic viruses.

The pathophysiology of group B coxsackievirus myopericarditis has been studied extensively in animals, principally in the mouse model, in which initial viral replication in myocytes results in scattered necrosis and focal infiltration, with inflammatory cells persisting for weeks to months after disappearance of virus. Some investigators consider the late phase of the inflammatory response to be due to virus-induced, cytotoxic T-lymphocyte destruction of myocytes, whereas others postulate development of a myocardial neoantigen[51] or cross-reactivity between viral and myocardial cell antigens.[52] Healing is accompanied by interstitial fibrosis and loss of myocytes.

Enteroviruses cause myopericarditis in all age groups. Physically active adolescents and young adults may have the highest risk, and males have at least twice the risk of females.[53] Approximately two-thirds of patients have a febrile upper respiratory tract illness preceding the symptoms of substernal chest pain, exercise intolerance, and dyspnea.[54] Auscultation reveals a pericardial friction rub in 35% to 80% of cases and a gallop rhythm or other signs of ventricular failure in ~20%. Electrocardiographic (ECG) abnormalities invariably are present. Echocardiography (ECHO) may confirm the presence of acute ventricular dilation or a diminished cardiac ejection fraction. Serum levels of myocardial enzymes frequently are elevated.

Although the acute course of myopericarditis often is complicated by congestive heart failure or cardiac arrhythmia, most children recover uneventfully. Fatality during the acute illness is <5%. However, ECG or ECHO abnormalities persist in 10% to 30%, and a similar proportion have persistent or recurrent congestive heart failure.

IGIV may have beneficial immunomodulatory effects.[55] In one study using historical controls, improved cardiac function and a trend toward increased survival was found in children with acute myopericarditis treated with IGIV.[56] However, randomized, controlled trials have not been reported. Although corticosteroid and other immunosuppressive therapies have been used,[57,58] experimental evidence suggested adverse rather than beneficial effects,[59] and a large prospective randomized trial of prednisone combined with either cyclosporine or azathioprine versus supportive treatment showed no differences in outcome.[60]

Chronic dilated cardiomyopathy is the final result of multiple infectious and noninfectious cardiac insults,[61] including up to one-third of cases of acute myopericarditis and, in some instances, unrecognized past enterovirus infection.[49,62,63] A case-control study of idiopathic dilated cardiomyopathy in adults in the United Kingdom and Italy suggested a possible association with group B coxsackieviruses.[64] Enteroviral RNA has been detected in cardiac tissue months to years after the onset of dilated cardiomyopathy in some studies,[65,66] but not in others using similar methods.[67-70]

Ophthalmic Infections

Acute hemorrhagic conjunctivitis is a highly contagious infection characterized by eye pain, eyelid swelling, and subconjunctival hemorrhage (Figure 236-2D). Widespread epidemics of acute hemorrhagic conjunctivitis have occurred in many parts of the world, particularly in the tropics. Two enterovirus serotypes have been responsible for almost all cases. EV-70 was the cause of the original pandemic in 1969 that spread globally during the early 1970s.[71] Since 1970, the epidemiology of disease caused by a variant of coxsackievirus A24 has intertwined with that of EV-70.[72] Both viruses have caused epidemics throughout Southeast Asia and the Indian subcontinent. Disease in the West has been confined to seasonal outbreaks in the Caribbean, Central America, and south Florida.[73]

Acute hemorrhagic conjunctivitis is transmitted directly from person to person via fingers and fomites. Both EV-70 and coxsackievirus A24 are readily isolated from tears, but only infrequently from other sites. Contagion is favored by crowding and poor sanitation; reuse of water for bathing and sharing of towels contribute to the spread of infection. After an incubation period of 1 to 2 days, symptoms of ocular pain, photophobia, watery discharge, and swelling of the eyelids appear abruptly. Fever and headache occur in 20% of cases. The distinctive physical finding is subconjunctival hemorrhage, found in 70% to 90% of EV-70 cases but in fewer coxsackievirus A24 cases. Conjunctival edema and follicle formation, punctate epithelial keratitis, and pre-auricular lymphadenopathy are present commonly. Symptoms and signs peak on the first day of illness and resolve within a few days without residual eye complications. Unusual cases of concomitant motor paralysis have been reported during some EV-70 outbreaks.

Other Infections

The role of enteroviruses in gastrointestinal disease is unsettled. Conflicting data comparing rates of enterovirus isolation from children with acute diarrheal illness and matched healthy control children are reported. Some echoviruses, particularly types 11, 14, and 18, have been implicated in outbreaks of diarrhea in young infants. The role of enteroviruses in nonbacterial gastroenteritis probably is minor. Enteroviral hepatitis beyond the neonatal period appears to be rare.[74,75] Pancreatitis is reported in patients infected with group B coxsackievirus types 1 to 5 and echovirus types 6, 11, 22, and 30. Prospective studies of acute pancreatitis have demonstrated concurrent enterovirus infection in 2% to 20% of cases.[76,77]

Acute parotitis occasionally is reported in association with herpangina caused by group A coxsackieviruses and also during group B coxsackieviruses and EV-70 infections. Orchitis can occur in adolescents during coxsackievirus A9, group B coxsackieviruses 2, 4, and 5, and echovirus 6 infections.

Enterovirus 71 Infections

Enterovirus 71 (EV-71) is a species A enterovirus closely related to coxsackievirus A16 that has caused large outbreaks of HFM disease, aseptic meningitis, and serious CNS disease in young children.[45,78-87] Paralytic disease similar to poliomyelitis has occurred in localized outbreaks involving small numbers of patients over several years[79,88-90] and regional epidemics affecting thousands of persons within a single season.[28,84,91-93] Although EV-71 infections occur globally, in the past two decades several genetic lineages of EV-71, most recently genotype C4, have caused widespread disease in infants and young children throughout Southeast Asia.[28,43,94-96] Affected patients can develop acute flaccid paralysis and/or a rapidly progressive brainstem encephalitis characterized by cardiovascular collapse, pulmonary edema, and high mortality.[42,43,87] Other less common manifestations include generalized maculopapular rash,[79] interstitial pneumonia,[87] and myocarditis.[87,92]

The diagnosis depends on isolation of virus in cell culture or by polymerase chain reaction (PCR) in respiratory secretions or feces as the virus is not readily detected in CSF by either method.[97] Treatment is symptomatic and supportive. There is interest in development of an EV-71 vaccine.[27,98]

Parechovirus Infections

With the introduction of viral RNA sequencing, it was discovered that the previously designated echovirus serotypes 22 and 23 diverged sufficiently from other enteroviruses to be re-assigned to a new Picornavirus genus as parechovirus serotypes 1 and 2, respectively.[99] Twelve parechovirus serotypes now are recognized;[100] serotypes 1 and 3 are mostly commonly associated with disease.[101] The spectrum of attributable disease is similar to echoviruses, including fever, respiratory tract infections, exanthems, viral meningitis, encephalitis, myocarditis, and serious neonatal infections.[1,101-106]

Enteroviruses and Diabetes Mellitus

Although genetic susceptibility is established clearly, enterovirus infection may initiate and possibly maintain an inflammatory insult to pancreatic islet cells and thereby contribute to the development of type 1 diabetes mellitus.[107] Evidence for the involvement of group B coxsackieviruses is most abundant, but other species B and C enteroviruses also are implicated.[108-111] Cases of new-onset diabetes occur in seasonal patterns[112,113] and sometimes in clusters or small outbreaks, often peaking 1 to 2 months after peak enterovirus activity.[114,115]

Two major theories on the pathophysiology of enterovirus-induced diabetes exist. The "direct hit" hypothesis, which posits destruction of pancreatic islets by direct viral infection, derives support from murine studies showing specific destruction of beta cells in the islets of Langerhans, from in vitro demonstration of enterovirus tropism for human beta cells, from detection of enteroviral RNA in serum and intestinal mucosa at the onset of type 1 diabetes, and from postmortem isolation of coxsackievirus serotypes B4 and B5 from the pancreatic tissue of children dying of new-onset ketoacidosis.[116-119] Demonstration of IgM serum antibody to group B coxsackievirus in children with recent-onset diabetes supports the direct-infection hypothesis,[108,109,120] although this finding has been inconsistent in different studies.[121,122]

A second theory focuses on acute viral infection as a trigger for an autoimmune response to pancreatic islet cells because of similarity between the antigens of the virus and islet cells.[123] This concept is supported by the induction of chronic islet cell inflammation by enteroviral infection in genetically susceptible mice,[124] observation that most children with diabetes have humoral anti-islet cell antibodies at diagnosis, and demonstration of a temporal association between the development of islet cell antibodies and seroconversion to group B coxsackievirus.[125,126] Some investigations suggest that molecular mimicry between a nonstructural coxsackievirus protein and a beta-cell enzyme may permit autoimmune destruction of pancreatic islet cell tissue.[127]

Although persistent enterovirus infection also is considered a possible mechanism of islet cell damage, no widely accepted evidence has been presented that enteroviruses are capable of persisting in an immunocompetent human host. Reviews of the role of enteroviruses in type 1 diabetes have been published.[107,115,128,129]

INFECTION IN SPECIAL HOSTS

Infections in Pregnancy

Nonpolio enterovirus infections do not appear to be more serious in pregnant women although a distinctive syndrome of fever and severe abdominal pain (probably secondary to mesenteric lymphadenitis) is described in late pregnancy in association with perinatal transmission to neonates.[130,131] While enterovirus infection during pregnancy undoubtedly is common, documented intrauterine infection is rare, perhaps because of an effective placental barrier.[3,132] Rare cases of fetal hydrops and stillbirth are reported,[133] but there is no convincing evidence that fetal infection is associated with congenital malformation.

Neonatal Infections

Neonates are at risk of serious, often fatal disease resulting from enterovirus infections acquired during the perinatal period. The echoviruses and group B coxsackieviruses are responsible for most neonatal infections, especially echovirus serotypes 6, 9, and 11 and group B coxsackievirus serotypes 1 to 5.[134] Serious neonatal group B coxsackievirus serotype 1 disease was widely reported during 2007 and 2008 when this serotype circulated prominently in the U.S.[135] Parechoviruses, especially parechovirus serotype 3, are reported to cause neonatal encephalitis, severe hepatitis, rash with fever, and other syndromes identical to those caused by enteroviruses.[103]

Neonates who acquire enterovirus infections perinatally as a result of vertical transmission from infected mothers develop illness within the first week of life. Onset of serious infection beyond 10 days of age is rare. During seasonal outbreaks, approximately 3% of pregnant women excrete enteroviruses at term.[3] The outcome of neonatal infection is strongly influenced by the presence or absence of passively acquired maternal antibody specific for the infecting enterovirus serotype.[3,136,137] Thus, the timing of maternal infection in relation to delivery is probably the most critical factor in the outcome of neonatal enterovirus infection.

Nosocomial postnatal infection occurs less frequently.[131,138,139] Infant-to-infant spread within nurseries occurs via the hands of healthcare personnel engaged in mouth care, gavage feeding, and other activities affording close direct contact.[140]

Although a wide range of clinical disease has been reported in neonates, including nonspecific febrile illnesses, exanthems, and aseptic meningitis, the most severe manifestations include myocarditis with or without encephalitis, hepatitis, and pneumonia.

Myocarditis

Neonatal myocarditis is most frequently caused by group B coxsackievirus serotypes 2 to 5. The onset often is abrupt, with respiratory distress, tachycardia, cyanosis, jaundice, and diarrhea. Initial examination frequently reveals temperature instability, tachycardia, arrhythmia, hepatomegaly, and signs of poor peripheral circulation. The ECG can show low-voltage and other electrophysiologic abnormalities, and ECHO often indicates poor left ventricular or biventricular function. Approximately one-third of illnesses are biphasic, with lethargy, poor feeding, or mild respiratory distress preceding the onset of cardiac manifestations by 2 to 5 days.

Infants with group B coxsackievirus myocarditis often have concomitant meningoencephalitis, pneumonia, hepatitis, pancreatitis, or adrenalitis. Although a limited number of organs can be involved pathologically, the degree of involvement often is severe, which has given rise to the use of terms such as *disseminated, systemic,* or *overwhelming* group B coxsackievirus disease in the neonatal period. Mortality in infants with myocarditis alone is generally reported to be 30% to 50%, but it is higher when other organs are involved.

Hepatitis

Neonatal hepatitis can occur as the sole manifestation of infection or can accompany myocarditis and other sequelae of neonatal group B coxsackievirus disease. Echovirus 11 has been implicated most frequently,[131] but cases caused by echovirus serotypes 6, 7, 9, 14, 17, 19, and 21 and parechovirus serotype 3 are described.

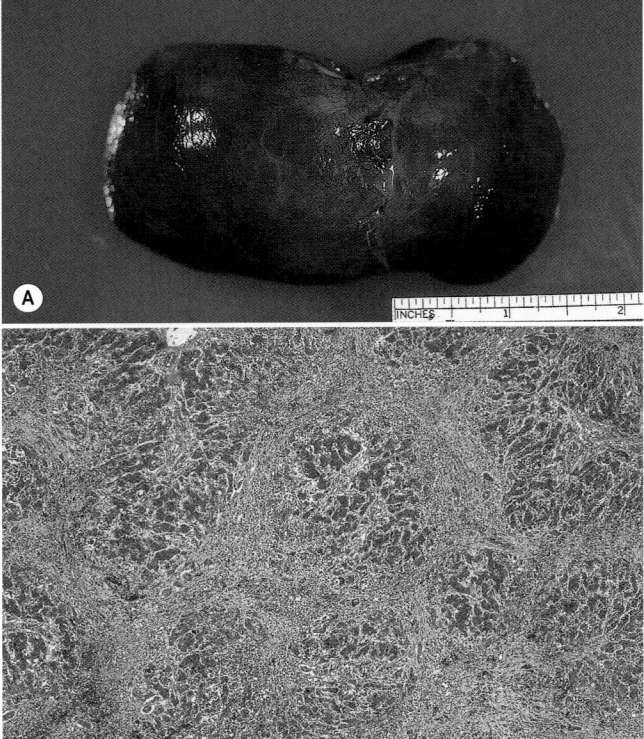

Figure 236-3. A term infant whose mother had a respiratory illness at delivery had onset of "overwhelming sepsis" at 3 days of age, which was fatal. Cultures of multiple organs and stool yielded enterovirus. No bacteria was isolated. Autopsy findings included a small hemorrhagic liver **(A)**, which on microscopic examination (×400) reveals extensive hepatocellular necrosis **(B)**. (Courtesy of S.S. Long.)

The degree of hepatic involvement varies, but a severe form of hepatitis unique to this age group is characterized by extensive necrosis of the liver and fulminant hepatic failure. Initial signs and symptoms of severe hepatitis resemble those of septicemia, with lethargy, poor feeding, apnea, and jaundice. Within 2 to 3 days, evidence of hypocoagulability appears, along with ecchymoses and prolonged bleeding at puncture sites. Anemia, marked prolongation of the prothrombin time and partial thromboplastin time, and extreme elevations of serum transaminase levels occur.[130,131] Marked hypocoagulability, more attributable to hepatic failure than to disseminated intravascular coagulation, causes spontaneous hemorrhage into the skin, lungs, gastrointestinal tract, kidneys, and brain. The mortality rate is high. Infants dying of hepatitis have massive hepatic necrosis (Figure 236-3) and extensive hemorrhage into the cerebral ventricles, pericardial sac, renal medulla, and interstitial spaces of many solid organs. Necrosis commonly is limited to the liver and adrenal glands, sparing the heart, brain, meninges, and other organs. Cirrhosis and chronic hepatic insufficiency can develop in survivors.

Central Nervous System Infection

Extreme lethargy, seizures, hemiparesis, flaccid paralysis, and coma herald the more serious form of meningoencephalitis that occurs in the neonate as isolated CNS disease or accompanying myocarditis or hepatitis. Inflammation of the brain or spinal cord is found in approximately two-thirds of infants dying of myocarditis.[141] Distinctive periventricular white matter lesions have been observed by MRI in many neonates with enterovirus and parechovirus encephalitis and postmortem microscopy demonstrates diffuse or scattered perivascular inflammation with lesions in the cerebrum, cerebellum, pons, medulla, and spinal cord.[142,143]

Pneumonia

Echovirus serotypes 6, 9, and 11 have been associated with a small number of reported cases of perinatal pneumonitis.[144] Some cases characterized by the onset of symptoms within hours of birth suggest prenatal exposure, and have a high mortality rate. Less severe neonatal pneumonitis has been described with echovirus serotypes 7 and 22.[145] Pathologic evidence of pneumonitis can be seen with group B coxsackievirus myocarditis in newborns, but generally is limited to focal areas of interstitial inflammation.[141]

Chronic Infections in Patients with Immunodeficiency

Enteroviruses cause persistent, sometimes fatal infections of the CNS, gastrointestinal tract, and skeletal muscle in patients with hereditary or acquired defects in B-lymphocyte function. Most reported patients are children with X-linked agammaglobulinemia or severe combined immunodeficiency syndrome[7] or adults with common variable immunodeficiency. Cases of chronic meningoencephalitis as a complication of X-linked hyper-IgM syndrome have been reported.[146] Chronic infections also occur in bone marrow transplant recipients.[147] Echoviruses are responsible for most of these infections; individual cases caused by group A coxsackievirus types 4, 11, and 15 and by group B coxsackievirus types 2 and 3 have been reported.[7]

Chronic meningoencephalitis, the most common clinical syndrome, typically begins insidiously with headache, lethargy, mild meningismus, motor dysfunction, or seizures; abnormalities fluctuate in severity, disappear, or slowly progress. Persistent CSF pleocytosis and a high CSF protein concentration are characteristic. Virus is recovered persistently in high titer from the CSF of many patients.[7] Subtle abnormalities such as developmental arrest or regression are not uncommon, especially in IGIV-treated individuals, and PCR rather than culture may be necessary to confirm the presence of virus in CSF.[146,148]

Chronic myositis in a subset of patients produces an illness similar to dermatomyositis. Recovery of virus from muscle tissue

in at least one case suggests ongoing viral replication.[149] Isolation of enteroviruses from other tissues such as the brain, lung, liver, spleen, kidney, and bone marrow suggests that infection is widely disseminated in at least some cases.

The prognosis for immunodeficient children who are persistently infected is poor. The efficacy of IGIV in the treatment of chronic enterovirus meningitis has been inconsistent. Some patients have experienced clinical improvement when IGIV was injected directly into the ventricles,[149] but relapse of infection occurs even after long-term intraventricular IGIV therapy. Pleconaril therapy has been used under compassionate release.[150,151]

LABORATORY DIAGNOSIS

Polymerase Chain Reaction

PCR using primers that identify conserved sequences in the 5′ non-coding region of the enterovirus genome is more sensitive than culture for identification of enteroviruses in CSF, respiratory tract secretions, and urine.[14,152,153] PCR also has been used to detect enteroviral RNA in cardiac tissue from patients with myocarditis,[66] although the relative sensitivity and specificity of the technique in these patients are not defined. PCR testing of fecal specimens has been less successful because of the presence of substances that inhibit the polymerization step.

Virus Isolation

Isolation of viruses in cell culture remains an important method laboratory diagnosis. Success of isolation varies widely between enterovirus classes and among serotypes within a class. Generally, three or four primate cell lines must be used to support isolation of most enteroviruses. Cytopathic effect usually is evident between 2 and 5 days after the inoculation of cell monolayers. Once isolated, the virus serotype can be identified for most of the common enteroviruses with use of the Lim Benyesh–Melnick intersecting equine antiserum pools or by RNA sequencing. The optimal method for isolation of group A coxsackieviruses is newborn mouse inoculation.

An etiologic diagnosis is confirmed by the isolation of virus from CSF, pericardial fluid, tissue, or blood. The opportunity to recover a virus in cell culture is optimized by sampling multiple sites. Isolation of virus from stool is less definitive because unrelated intercurrent asymptomatic infections can occur. However, because background rate of shedding from the gastrointestinal tract is low, isolation of enterovirus from any site is strong presumptive evidence of causation.

Serology

The microneutralization test is the method used most widely for determining enterovirus antibodies. This serotype-specific assay has limited usefulness in the routine diagnosis of nonpolio enterovirus infections because it is not feasible to incorporate all relevant live viral antigens into the assay and methods based on neutralization are relatively insensitive, poorly standardized, and labor intensive. Type-specific immunoassays now are available commercially for measuring antibodies against the more common enterovirus serotypes, but they often are not well standardized. Serum IgM antibody has been detected early in the course of infection with group B coxsackieviruses, echovirus 30, and enterovirus 70. However, enteroviral IgM assays are not serotype specific[154,155] and appear to lack sensitivity.[156]

TREATMENT

Immune serum immunoglobulin and IGIV are reported to suppress or eradicate persistent enterovirus infections in some, but not all patients with immunoglobulin deficiency,[7] and one uncontrolled trial of IGIV, 2 g/kg, suggested benefit in children with acute myopericarditis.[56] However, little or no evidence of the efficacy of immunoglobulin has been observed in the treatment of other serious or acute enterovirus infections. A prospective, randomized trial of IGIV (750 mg/kg) for treatment of enterovirus infections in newborn infants did not reduce the daily incidence of viremia or viruria overall, although there may have been benefit when the IGIV lot contained a neutralization titer of ≥1:800 to virus isolated from the patient.[157]

The antiviral compounds in clinical development are more promising than immune-based therapy. The oxazoline class of antiviral agents exhibit potent in vitro activity against many human enteroviruses by binding avidly to a pocket in the viral capsid, thereby preventing virus attachment and uncoating.[158] One compound, pleconaril, an orally administered drug with a favorable pharmacokinetic and toxicity profile has been studied in clinical trials and shown to have a modest benefit in adults and children with enterovirus meningitis.[159–162] Uncontrolled experience in immunocompromised patients with persistent enterovirus infections and patients with serious, potentially fatal infections also suggests substantial clinical benefit.[32,150,163] The National Institute of Allergy and Infectious Diseases is conducting a randomized placebo-controlled, phase II trial of pleconaril for treatment of neonates with enteroviral sepsis syndrome (http://clinicaltrials.gov/ct/show/NCT00031512).

PREVENTION

Because pre-exposure administration of immune serum globulin reduces the risk of paralytic poliomyelitis, it is possible that nonpolio enterovirus infections could be prevented in the same manner. Although commercial preparations of IGIV contain variable concentrations of antibody against some enterovirus serotypes, no data are available regarding the protective efficacy of these preparations. Active immunization against the nonpolio enteroviruses is not practical because of the large number of serotypes, although several candidate vaccines for enterovirus 71 infection are under development.

Simple hygienic measures such as handwashing and careful disposal of soiled diapers should reduce transmission. It is prudent to advise pregnant women and children who are immunocompromised to avoid contact, whenever possible, with persons suspected of having enterovirus infection.

237 Hepatitis A Virus

Roxanne E. Williams and Umid M. Sharapov

Hepatitis A virus (HAV) is a nonenveloped RNA virus and a member of the Picornaviridae family.[1] The single-stranded RNA genome is approximately 7500 nucleotides long, and contains a single long open reading frame. The encoded polyprotein includes structural proteins for the 27- to 28-nm diameter capsid, nonstructural proteins with protease or polymerase activities, and other proteins which functions have not been fully determined.[2,3]

Among infected people, HAV replicates in the liver, is excreted in bile, and found in high concentrations in stool. The incubation period averages 28 days (range, 15 to 50 days). Peak viral concentrations in stool and greatest infectivity are during the 2 weeks before onset of symptoms. Virus concentrations in stool diminish markedly within 1 week after onset of symptoms. However, polymerase chain reaction (PCR) assays have been used to demonstrate low levels of viral RNA in stools of infected neonates for up to 6 months after infection.[4] In older children, HAV RNA can be detected in stools for as long as 10 weeks after symptoms begin, but the clinical significance of these findings is uncertain.[5] Viremia occurs soon after infection and persists at least through the period of elevation of hepatic enzymes in serum.[6,7]

The pathogenesis of HAV infection is not completely understood. However, absence of cytopathic changes in cell culture and demonstration of HAV-directed natural killer and lymphokine-activated killer cells in vitro suggest that cell-mediated immunity is responsible for hepatocellular damage.[8]

HAV is a single serotype.[9] Immunity resulting from HAV infection is lifelong. In contrast to infection with hepatitis B virus (HBV) and hepatitis C virus (HCV), HAV infection does not result in chronic infection or chronic liver disease.

EPIDEMIOLOGY

The principal mode of HAV transmission is person to person, by the fecal–oral route. Transmission occurs most commonly among close contacts, including household and sexual contacts of people infected with HAV. Hepatitis A also is transmitted by contaminated food, most often from an infected food handler but also in association with food contaminated before retail distribution, such as produce contaminated during growing or processing.[10–12] Transmission by contaminated water is rare. Because transient viremia occurs in HAV infection, bloodborne HAV transmission can occur, such as among injection drug users.[13] On rare occasions, HAV infection has been transmitted by transfusion of blood or blood products collected from donors during the viremic phase of infection.[14] In addition, outbreaks have been reported in Europe and the United States among patients who received factor VIII and factor IX concentrates prepared with use of solvent detergent treatment.[15] However, changes in viral inactivation procedures, high hepatitis A vaccine coverage, and improved donor screening have nearly eliminated the risk for HAV transmission from clotting factors.[16] Vertical transmission to offspring from pregnant women who develop hepatitis A during the third trimester of pregnancy has been reported, but the risk appears to be low. In approximately 50% of people with sporadic, community-acquired hepatitis A, no source of infection is identified.[17]

Because most young children have asymptomatic or unrecognized infections, they play an important role in the epidemiology of hepatitis A, often serving as sources of infection for others. In several studies in which serologic testing of household contacts was performed, 25% to 40% of contacts <6 years of age had serologic evidence of acute HAV infection.[18,19] In one study in the U.S., 52% of households of adults without an identified source of infection included a child <6 years of age, and the presence of a young child was associated with HAV transmission in the household. In this study, transmission chains were identified that involved as many as 6 generations and >20 cases.[18]

The relationship between risk of infection and likelihood of asymptomatic infection during childhood is key to understanding HAV transmission patterns worldwide and to developing prevention strategies. Level of economic development, as indicated by hygienic and sanitary conditions for example, also are correlated with global HAV transmission patterns (Figure 237-1).

In areas where seroprevalence of anti-HAV is high even among young children (e.g., parts of Asia, Africa, Central and South America), the lifetime risk of infection is greater than 90% and occurs primarily in early childhood.[20] Asymptomatic infection

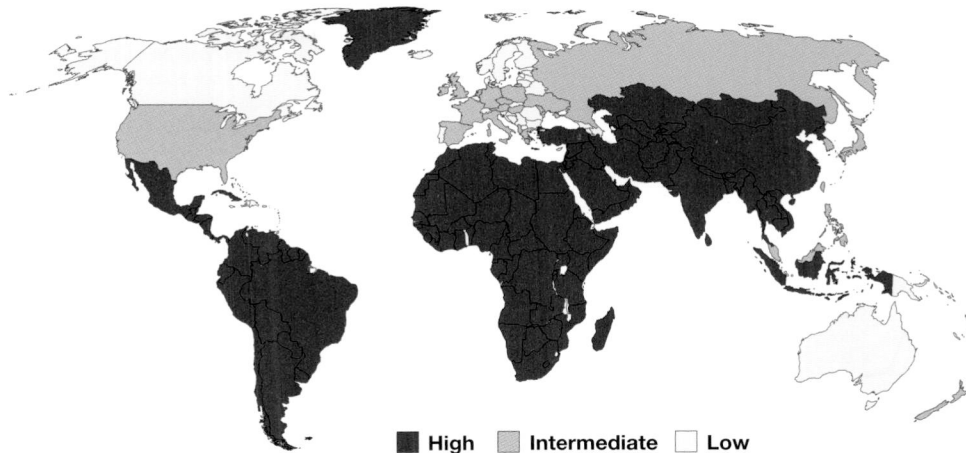

Figure 237-1. Prevalence of antibody to hepatitis A virus, 2006. Geographic distribution of hepatitis A virus (HAV) infection endemicity. For multiple countries, estimates of prevalence of antibody to hepatitis A virus (anti-HAV), a marker of previous HAV infection, are based on limited data and might not reflect actual prevalence. In addition, anti-HAV prevalence rates might vary within countries by subpopulation and locality. As used on this map, "high," "medium," and "low" reflect available evidence of how widespread infections are within each country rather than precise quantitative assessments. (From Centers for Disease Control and Prevention. Prevention of hepatitis A through active or passive immunization: recommendations of the Advisory Committee on Immunization Practices. MMWR 2006;55(RR-7):1–23.)

■ High   ■ Intermediate   □ Low

predominates, and nearly the entire population is infected before reaching adolescence. The high rates of HAV transmission during childhood might not be recognized because typical clinical manifestations of hepatitis A are uncommon in children. The incidence of clinical hepatitis A generally is low, and outbreaks are rare because most adults are immune. However, adults who remain susceptible to infection in these areas are at high risk for HAV infection. Travelers to high endemic areas from the developed world also are at high risk.

In areas of moderate endemicity (e.g., eastern Europe), HAV is not transmitted as readily because of better sanitation and living conditions, and the average age of infection is older than in areas of high endemicity. However, transmission among young children remains relatively common. Paradoxically, the potential for large outbreaks can be increased (compared with highly endemic areas) because of the relatively larger pool of susceptible older children and adults who are at high risk for infection and who, when infected with HAV, are likely to develop symptomatic illness.[21] Unimmunized travelers from the developed world to these areas also are at risk.[22]

In some instances, countries undergoing rapid development accompanied by improvement in sanitation standards and clean water supplies have experienced changes in the epidemiologic pattern of HAV. In these countries, HAV is likely to become a more serious problem.[23] The resultant decline in childhood and adolescent HAV seroprevalence leads to susceptibility at a later age at which there is greater associated morbidity and mortality.[20]

In most developed countries, the incidence of both HAV infection and hepatitis A clinical disease is low. The prevalence of anti-HAV increases gradually with age, primarily reflecting declining incidence, changing endemicity, and resulting lower childhood infection rates over time.[24] Most cases occur in the context of cyclic, community-wide outbreaks that feature transmission among preschool and school-aged children and their adult contacts.[25] As endemicity continues to decline in some parts of the developed world (e.g., Scandinavia), most cases are identified in defined risk groups, such as travelers returning from endemic areas and injection drug users.[21]

In the U.S., before hepatitis A vaccine was widely available, hepatitis A occurred in large nationwide epidemics approximately every decade, with the last increase in 1995 (Figure 237-2). In 2004, 5683 cases were reported to the Centers for Disease Control and Prevention (CDC), although the disease is believed to be substantially underreported.[22] One model of HAV incidence estimated an average of 271,000 infections per year during 1980 to 1999, 10.4 times the average reported number of clinical cases

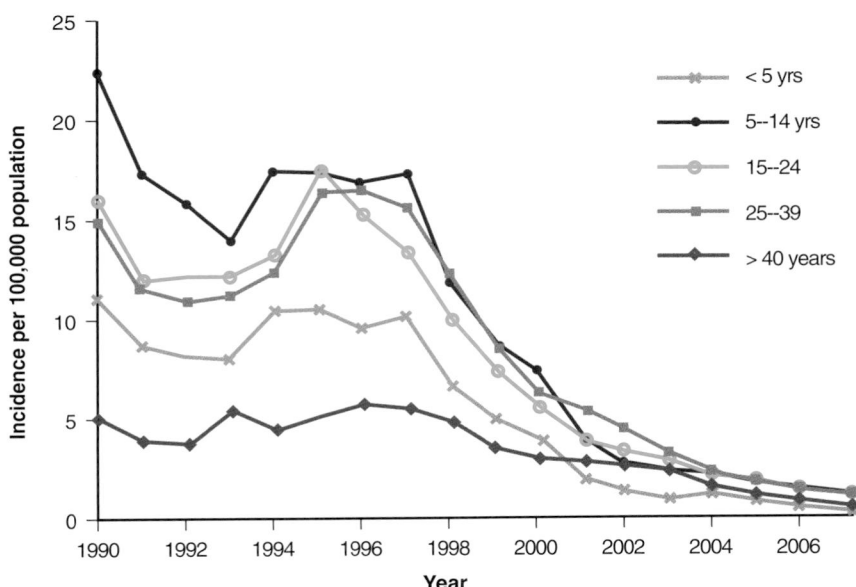

Figure 237-2. Incidence rates of reported hepatitis A, by age group and year, United States, 1990–2007. Incidence rates are per 100,000 population. National Notifiable Diseases Surveillance System, 2007. (From Centers for Disease Control and Prevention. Surveillance for acute viral hepatitis, United States 2007. MMWR 2009;58:1–27.)

Legend:
─✕─ < 5 yrs
─●─ 5--14 yrs
─○─ 15--24
─■─ 25--39
─◆─ > 40 years

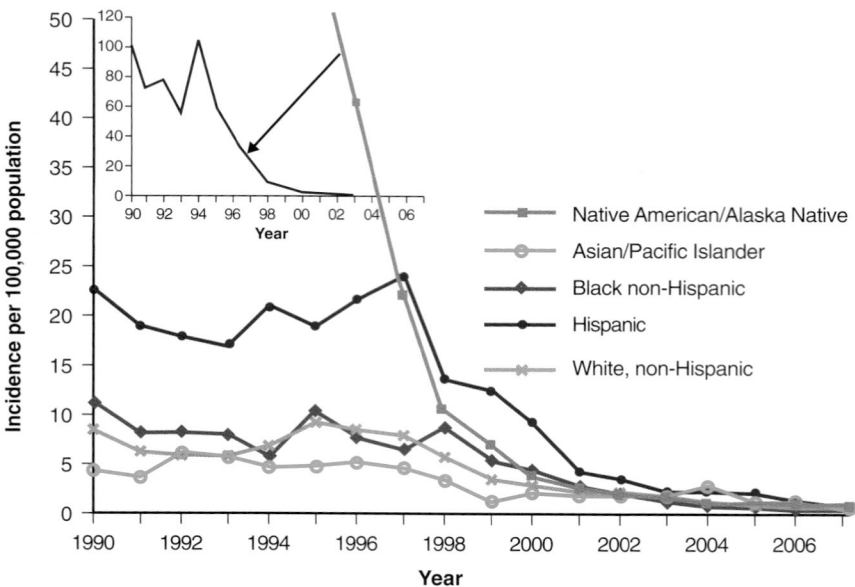

Figure 237-3. Rate of reported hepatitis A, by race/ethnicity and year, United States, 1990–2007. Incidence rates per 100,000 population. National Notifiable Diseases Surveillance System, 2007. (From Centers for Disease Control and Prevention. Surveillance for acute viral hepatitis, United States 2007. MMWR 2009;58:1–27.)

during that period. More than one-half of these infections were estimated to have occurred among children <10 years of age and the majority among children 0 to 4 years of age.[26]

Until 2001, the highest rates of HAV infection in the U.S. were observed among children 5 to 14 years of age, with approximately one-third of reported cases involving children <15 years of age (see Figure 237-2).[29–29] The highest rates and the majority of cases occurred in the western and southwestern states.[27,28] Most cases occurred in the context of periodic community-wide outbreaks that persisted for a year or longer and were difficult to control. Cases were identified across all age groups and involved extended person-to-person transmission.[18,25] Disease surveillance systems indicated that the most commonly recognized source of infection was personal contact (household or sexual) with a case of hepatitis A (12% to 26% of reported cases). Approximately 10% to 15% of reported cases occurred among childcare center attendees, employees, or their contacts, but whether contact with childcare centers is associated with a higher risk of hepatitis A has not been evaluated in studies using an adequate comparison group.[27] The proportion of cases associated with men who have sex with men or with users of illicit drugs varied widely from year to year, accounting for up to 15% of reported cases nationwide, as a result of periodic outbreaks occurring in these groups in some communities.[28,30,31] Other potential sources of infection (e.g., recognized foodborne or waterborne outbreaks and international travel) were reported by 3% to 6% of cases. In >50% of cases of hepatitis A, the source of infection is never identified.[22]

Since licensure of the first hepatitis A vaccines in 1995, incidence rates have declined sharply (Figures 237-2 and 237-3).[29] Declines have been especially prominent since implementation of recommendations made in 1999 for routine statewide vaccination during childhood in the western and southwestern states with consistently elevated hepatitis A rates with respect to the average during the prevaccine era.[27,32] Historic lows in incidence have been recorded in each year since 2000, with rates declining >75% compared with rates during the early to mid-1990s. Declines among children have exceeded 85%, reaching or declining below rates among adults in recent years (see Figure 237-2). In the past decade, age, regional, ethnic, and racial differences in incidence rates of hepatitis A virtually have been eliminated, indicating fundamental shifts in hepatitis A epidemiology; see Figure 237-3).[17,33,34]

In the U.S., international travel is the most frequently reported risk factor among patients contracting HAV, although nearly 70% of cases have no specific risk factor identified.[35] Cases recognized

in the context of childcare centers have declined. In addition, the large community-wide outbreaks that once accounted for the majority of cases have become unusual events. International adoption has been a recently recognized risk for acquiring HAV and has resulted in an update of recommendations for use of hepatitis A vaccination by the American Academy of Pediatrics (AAP) and the Advisory Committee on Immunization Practices (ACIP).[35]

Although outbreaks of HAV related to childcare centers and hospitals have declined markedly, these settings retain challenges for prevention efforts.[36,37] Once HAV is introduced into a childcare center, high rates of spread are associated with larger numbers of children in diapers.[38] Because infection often is asymptomatic among young children, outbreaks usually are recognized only when staff members or family contacts of attendees become ill. Nosocomial hepatitis A outbreaks have been reported most often in neonatal intensive care units, in which transmission has occurred to other infants and staff from an infant infected by transfusion of blood donated by a person incubating HAV infection.[37] HAV transmission between students at elementary and secondary schools is uncommon, and cases in schools usually reflect disease acquired in the community.[39]

Methods to isolate and sequence HAV from sera of infected people and to define the genetic variation of HAV are advancing understanding of the epidemiology. The resulting database of HAV genome sequences[40] has been useful in investigations of foodborne outbreaks by demonstrating links among apparently sporadic cases and suggesting possible sources of contamination.[10,41]

CLINICAL MANIFESTATIONS

HAV infection can be *inapparent* (patient is asymptomatic with no elevation in serum hepatic enzymes), *subclinical* (asymptomatic with elevation of hepatic enzymes), *anicteric* (symptomatic without jaundice), or *icteric* (symptomatic with jaundice). The likelihood of having symptoms with HAV infection is related directly to age. Most children <6 years of age have asymptomatic infection or mild nonspecific symptoms with hepatitis A; <10% of children in this age group have jaundice.[42] Among older children and adults, 76% to 97% have symptoms when infected with HAV, and 40% to 70% of patients with symptoms are icteric.[43]

When symptoms occur, the majority of patients have onset of low-grade fever, myalgia, anorexia, malaise, nausea, and vomiting. These symptoms are followed several days later by specific symptoms and signs of hepatic dysfunction, including dark urine, light-colored stools, jaundice, and scleral icterus.[43] Many children

(60%) and some adults (20%) have diarrhea. Some children (<20%) have upper respiratory tract symptoms (cough, coryza, sore throat). Urticaria can occur at onset of illness.[44] Physical findings are variable and can include jaundice, scleral icterus, hepatomegaly, right upper-quadrant tenderness, and splenomegaly. Abdominal ultrasonography showed edema of the gallbladder wall in about 50% of children with uncomplicated hepatitis A who were studied prospectively; transient ascites occurred in a few patients.[45]

The symptoms of hepatitis A last for several weeks on average and usually not longer than 2 months, although some people can have prolonged or relapsing signs and symptoms for up to 6 months (see Special Considerations, below).

LABORATORY FINDINGS AND DIAGNOSIS

During HAV infection, inflammation of the liver is accompanied by abnormalities in serum hepatic enzymes, with increases in serum levels of alanine aminotransferase (ALT), aspartate aminotransferase (AST), alkaline phosphatase (AP), and γ-glutamyltranspeptidase (GGTP). Usually in acute hepatitis A, ALT and AST values are between 200 and 5000 IU/L; the ALT value is higher than the AST value; and AP levels are only mildly elevated. Elevations in ALT and AST can precede symptoms by a week or more and generally peak 3 to 10 days after onset of symptoms (Figure 237-4).

The pattern and magnitude of abnormalities of hepatic enzymes are not distinct for hepatitis A. The specific diagnosis of hepatitis A relies on serologic testing. Virtually all people with acute hepatitis A have detectable immunoglobulin (Ig) M antibodies to HAV (IgM anti-HAV) during the acute or early convalescent phase of infection (see Figure 237-4).[46] IgM anti-HAV generally disappears within 6 months after onset of symptoms, although people who test positive for IgM anti-HAV >1 year after infection or with no known history of infection have been reported.[47,48] IgG anti-HAV, which appears in the convalescent phase of infection, remains detectable in serum for the lifetime of the individual and confers protection against disease. Commercial enzyme immunoassays are available for detection of IgM and total anti-HAV in serum. Because total anti-HAV frequently is performed first in laboratories, care must be taken to order and see a positive stand-alone IgM anti-HAV test result before making the diagnosis of HAV hepatitis.

PCR assays can be used to detect HAV RNA in stool specimens and sera of people with HAV infection, although these tests only are available in a few research laboratories.[3,6] To date, PCR assays cannot determine whether a person is infectious because incomplete virus particles can be detected. On the basis of epidemiologic studies, peak infectivity occurs during the 2 weeks before onset of

symptoms. For practical purposes, people with hepatitis A can be assumed to be noninfectious 1 week after onset of jaundice.

Light microscopy of liver specimens in acute hepatitis A reveals pathologic features common to all forms of viral hepatitis, including hepatocellular necrosis, inflammatory infiltration of lymphocytes and other mononuclear cells, and regeneration of hepatocytes. The extent of involvement varies with the stage and severity of hepatitis and age of the patient. Liver biopsy typically is not indicated for diagnosis or management of hepatitis A.

TREATMENT

Treatment generally is supportive. Hospitalization may be necessary for patients who are dehydrated from nausea and vomiting or who have fulminant hepatitis A. No specific diet or restriction of activity is necessary. Medications that might cause hepatic damage or that are metabolized by the liver should be used with caution. For the infrequent presentations of cholestatic or relapsing hepatitis A (see Special Considerations, below), a short course of corticosteroid therapy has been reported as effective in limiting symptoms and hastening recovery, but no controlled trials have evaluated this approach.[49,50]

Liver transplantation is successful in some people with acute liver failure. Criteria for choosing patients for liver transplantation are difficult to establish because survival without transplantation is high (50% to 70%), even for patients who have coma, and no single factor is predictive of a poor outcome.[51]

SPECIAL CONSIDERATIONS

HAV infection occasionally results in fulminant hepatitis and death. In addition, hepatitis A has several atypical manifestations, including relapsing hepatitis A, cholestatic hepatitis, "triggering" of autoimmune hepatitis, and extrahepatic symptoms.

Fulminant hepatitis A is an infrequent occurrence.[52] The case-fatality rate from fulminant hepatitis among reported cases of hepatitis A in all age groups is approximately 0.4%.[22] Host factors associated with a higher risk for fulminant hepatitis A include older age (>50 years old) and underlying chronic liver disease.[53] Molecular studies have not shown an association between fulminant hepatitis A and any type of viral variant. Of 348 children with acute liver failure from the U.S., Canada, and the United Kingdom entered into a registry, only 3 had acute hepatitis A.[54] Spontaneous recovery occurs in 30% to 60% of people with fulminant HAV infection, with survivors generally regaining full liver function. Prognosis is influenced by age, clotting-factor level, stage of course and presence of renal disease.[17] In approximately 10% to 15% of patients with hepatitis A, relapsing hepatitis occurs and approximately 20% of these patients have multiple relapses.[17,50] These patients typically have another episode of hepatitis 1 to 4 months after initial acute hepatitis. The relapse is accompanied by elevation of serum hepatic enzymes and persistence of IgM anti-HAV. Molecular studies have demonstrated the presence of HAV in stool specimens during relapse. Most patients recover completely within several weeks.

Cholestatic hepatitis occurs rarely following infection with HAV.[49] Patients with this disorder have substantially elevated concentrations (>10 mg/dL) of bilirubin in serum and jaundice persisting for an extended period (in some cases >3 months). This syndrome can be distinguished from obstructive jaundice by normal abdominal ultrasonographic findings. A short course of corticosteroids can reduce symptoms and hasten disease resolution.[17]

Several case series have been described in which HAV infection is followed by autoimmune chronic active hepatitis, in some instances requiring long-term corticosteroid therapy.[55] Laboratory studies have demonstrated a T-lymphocyte defect in affected patients, suggesting a genetic predisposition to development of autoimmune hepatitis that is "triggered" by HAV infection.

Extrahepatic manifestations of hepatitis A include pruritus, arthralgia, cutaneous vasculitis, cryoglobulinemia, and hemophagocytic syndrome (anemia and thrombocytopenia, with

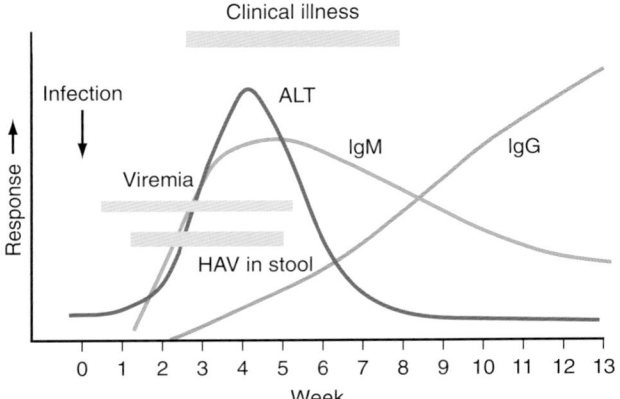

Figure 237-4. Typical serologic profile of hepatitis A virus (HAV) infection. ALT, serum alanine aminotransferase level; Ig, immunoglobulin.

hemophagocytosis apparent on biopsy of bone marrow). These manifestations are rare and resolve with resolution of hepatitis.

PREVENTION

The methods of prevention of hepatitis A include: (1) general measures of good personal hygiene (with an emphasis on hand hygiene), provision of safe drinking water, and adequate disposal of sanitary waste; (2) pre-exposure or postexposure prophylaxis with immune globulin (IG) or hepatitis A vaccine.

Immune Globulin

IG is a solution of antibodies prepared from human plasma by serial ethanol precipitation for intramuscular administration. In the U.S., IG is produced only from plasma that has tested negative for hepatitis B virus (HBV), antibody to human immunodeficiency virus (HIV), and antibody to hepatitis C virus (HCV). In addition, the manufacturing process must include a virus inactivation step or the final product must test negative for HCV RNA. The efficacy of IG in preventing hepatitis A is >85% when administered before exposure to HAV or within 2 weeks after exposure.[56,57]

IG is indicated for postexposure prophylaxis of household and sexual contacts of people with hepatitis A and for use in institutions (e.g., hospitals and residences for the developmentally disabled) when an outbreak is recognized.[27] Aggressive use of IG is recommended for control of HAV transmission in childcare centers when a child or employee is diagnosed with hepatitis A.[27,36] In selected situations, IG is recommended for patrons at food establishments when a food handler is identified as acutely infected with HAV.[58,59]

The dose for postexposure prophylaxis is 0.02 mL/kg body weight. Because hepatitis A vaccine is only licensed for people 12 months of age or older, IG also is recommended for children younger than 12 months of age who are traveling internationally.[27] Although hepatitis A is often asymptomatic in this age group, prophylaxis is indicated because rare severe cases do occur and because infants and young children can transmit HAV to others after returning from travel abroad. The dose for pre-exposure prophylaxis is 0.02 mL/kg for travel of <3 months and 0.06 mL/kg for travel of ≥3 months duration. For extended trips, IG must be readministered every 5 months.

Vaccine

Hepatitis A vaccines available in the U.S. are licensed for people 12 months of age or older. Inactivated hepatitis A vaccines are prepared by methods similar to methods used for inactivated poliovirus vaccines, including growth in cell culture; purification by ultrafiltration or other methods; inactivation with formalin; and adsorption to an aluminum hydroxide adjuvant.[60,61] Two single-antigen hepatitis A vaccines are available in pediatric and adult formulations and are licensed in a two-dose series, with the second dose given 6 to 18 months after the first. The route of administration is intramuscular. A formulation that combines hepatitis A and hepatitis B vaccines is available for persons ≥18 years of age, and is licensed in a three-dose series.[62]

Inactivated hepatitis A vaccines have been studied extensively in children and adults. In general, after one dose of vaccine, 95% to 100% of children and adults respond with levels of antibody considered to be protective; a second dose is necessary 6 to 18 months later to boost antibody levels for long-term protection.[63,64] Delayed administration of the second dose beyond 18 months does not appear to reduce immunogenicity, and the series can be completed rather than restarted.[65] Available data indicate that the vaccines are safe and immunogenic in children <12 months of age who do not have passively acquired maternal antibody.[66] However, final antibody concentrations in infants with passively acquired maternal antibody are one-third to one-tenth of those of anti-HAV-negative infants who are vaccinated according to the same schedule, and fewer have detectable anti-HAV 6 years after vaccina-

tion compared with children vaccinated as infants who did not have passively acquired maternal antibody.[66,67]

Inactivated hepatitis A vaccine is highly efficacious in preventing clinical hepatitis A. In a large study conducted in Thailand among children 1 to 16 years of age, efficacy of vaccine was 94% after two doses of vaccine administered 1 month apart.[68] In another study conducted in New York among children 2 to 16 years of age and with a different inactivated vaccine, efficacy was 100% starting 17 days after administration of one dose.[69]

The duration of protection after vaccination is unknown.[70] Anti-HAV has been shown to persist in vaccine recipients for at least 12 years.[71] A review by an expert panel concluded that estimates of antibody persistence derived from kinetic models of antibody decline indicate that protective levels of anti-HAV could be present for at least 25 years in adults and at least 14 to 20 years in children.[72]

Surveillance data and population-based studies are being used to monitor long-term protective efficacy of hepatitis A vaccine and to determine the possible need for a booster dose.[73] In the longest such follow-up study reported to date, no cases of hepatitis A were reported among children followed for 10 years after vaccination.[70]

Hepatitis A vaccination has shown efficacy compared with placebo when given up to 14 days after exposure to a person with HAV infection.[74,75] A controlled study that compared the efficacy of hepatitis A vaccine with that of IG when given after exposure showed performance of vaccine to be similar to that of IG in healthy children and adults 12 months through 40 years of age.[75,76] The CDC recommends that for healthy people 12 months through 40 years of age who have been exposed to HAV recently and who have not received hepatitis A vaccine in the past, single antigen hepatitis A vaccine at the age-appropriate dose is preferred to IG. For persons older than 40 years of age and people with underlying medical conditions, IG is preferred because of lack of data in this age group and among people with underlying medical conditions.[75–77]

In prelicensure clinical trials among children, the most frequently reported local reaction following hepatitis A vaccination was soreness at the injection site (15% to 19%).[64,65] Since licensure of the vaccines, >188 million doses of hepatitis A vaccine have been administered worldwide. No serious adverse events among children or adults that could be attributed definitively to the vaccine, and no increases in serious adverse events among vaccinated people compared with baseline rates, have been identified.[78,79]

Recommendations for use of hepatitis A vaccine were first issued in 1996 by the Advisory Committee on Immunization Practices (ACIP) of the CDC, the American Academy of Pediatrics (AAP), and other groups.[80] ACIP guidelines were updated in 1999 to include recommendations for routine vaccination of children living in the 17 states with persistently elevated incidence rates during the prevaccine era.[27] By 2004, first-dose coverage rates among children 24 through 35 months of age living in these states had reached 25% to 50%.[81] The impact of even limited routine vaccination of children on hepatitis A incidence was evidenced by historic reductions in incidence rates.[32] In 2006, ACIP extended recommendations to routine vaccination of children, beginning at or after 1 year of age, throughout the U.S. in order to achieve a sustained reduction in the national incidence of hepatitis A. (Table 237-1).[82] The estimated hepatitis A vaccination rate among children 19 through 35 months of age for receiving ≥2 doses of vaccine was 40% in 2008, with a slight increase to 47% in 2009.[83]

In 2007, the ACIP began considering reports of HAV infection among people in close contact with new adoptees from countries of high or intermediate hepatitis A endemicity. In 2009, ACIP updated guidance by further recommending hepatitis A vaccination for all previously unvaccinated persons who anticipate close personal contact with an international adoptee from a country of high or intermediate endemicity during the first 60 days following arrival of the adoptee in the U.S.[84] Vaccination of people at

TABLE 237-1. Advisory Committee on Immunization Practices (ACIP) Recommendations for Routine Pre-Exposure Use of Hepatitis A Vaccine

Group	Comments
All children at 12 through 23 months of age[a]	Integrate into routine childhood immunization schedule; children who are not vaccinated by 2 years of age can be vaccinated at subsequent visits
Children 12 through 18 years of age	Maintain existing programs.[b] Can be considered in areas without existing programs
International travelers	Except people traveling to Canada, western Europe, Japan, Australia, or New Zealand, who are at no greater risk than in the United States
Men who have sex with men	Includes adolescents
Illicit drug users	Includes adolescents
People with chronic liver disease	Increased risk of fulminant hepatitis A
People receiving clotting factor concentrates	
People who work with HAV in research settings	
Anyone wishing to obtain immunity	

HAV, hepatitis A virus.

[a]Hepatitis A vaccine is not licensed for children <12 months of age.

[b]Areas covered by 1999 ACIP recommendations (AR, AK, AZ, CA, CO, ID, MT, MO, NV, NM, OK, OR, SD, TX, UT, WA, WY, and selected areas in other states).[25]

From Centers for Disease Control and Prevention. Prevention of hepatitis A through active or passive immunization. Recommendations of the Advisory Committee on Immunization Practices. MMWR 2006;55(RR-7):1–23.

increased risk for hepatitis A also is recommended (Table 237-1 and Figure 237-1).[74] In 2008, CDC published the first study providing estimates of self-reported hepatitis A vaccination coverage among persons 18 through 49 years of age in the U.S. Among this age group, 12% had received ≥2 doses of hepatitis A vaccine in 2007. Since hepatitis A vaccination is only recommended for adults at risk, which is estimated to be 15% to 25% of the U.S. adult population, coverage among this population is expected to be low.[85] The effectiveness of using vaccination to control community-wide epidemics has been variable, depending on the type of community. In small, relatively well-defined communities with the highest hepatitis A rates in the U.S. historically, rapid achievement of high first-dose vaccination coverage (65% to 80%) of preschool and school-aged children has effectively interrupted ongoing outbreaks.[86,87] In larger, more heterogeneous communities in which vaccination programs targeting children were implemented, first-dose coverage generally has been low (20% to 45%) and the impact of vaccination often has been limited to reducing disease rates in the targeted age groups, which might not represent the majority of cases.[88] Because of logistic difficulties, accelerated vaccination as an additional measure to control outbreaks should be undertaken with caution. Efforts probably are better directed towards sustained routine vaccination of children, as is now recommended in the U.S. and several other countries, to maintain high levels of immunity and prevent future epidemics.

Vaccination of successive cohorts of young children should lower significantly the incidence of hepatitis A in the U.S. over time and eventually provide the opportunity to eliminate HAV transmission. To achieve this goal, high vaccination coverage among children throughout the U.S. must be achieved. This effort would be facilitated by the availability of combination vaccines that include hepatitis A vaccine.

Key Points. Diagnosis and Management of Hepatitis A Virus Infection

MICROBIOLOGY

- Nonenveloped RNA virus and member of the Picornaviridae family
- Replicates in the liver, is excreted in bile and found in high concentrations in stool
- Average incubation period of 28 days, range 15 to 50 days
- Greatest infectivity is 2 weeks before onset of symptoms

EPIDEMIOLOGY

- Primarily fecal–oral transmission by person-to-person contact or consumption of contaminated food or water
- Endemic in many developing countries; infection occurs mainly in childhood
- Low prevalence in developed countries; infection occurs typically among adolescents and adults
- In U.S., international travel is the most frequently reported risk factor
- International adoption is a risk factor

CLINICAL FEATURES

- Symptoms range from none to acute debilitating disease
- Symptomatic infection generally is characterized by acute onset and:

  - early symptoms, including low-grade fever, myalgia, anorexia, malaise and vomiting
  - later symptoms/signs, including hepatic dysfunction, dark urine, light-colored stools, jaundice and scleral icterus
- Likelihood of developing symptoms increases with patient's age
- Average duration is 2 months; overall case-fatality rate is 0.3% to 0.6%

DIAGNOSIS

- Presence of serum antibodies to HAV: IgM detectable 5 to 10 days before onset of symptoms; IgG appears in convalescent phase and is lifelong
- PCR assay can be used to detect viral RNA in blood and/or stool, but is not widely available and is used typically only in outbreak investigations

TREATMENT

- Supportive care

PREVENTION

- General measures of good personal hygiene, provision of safe drinking water, and adequate waste disposal
- Pre-exposure or postexposure prophylaxis with hepatitis vaccine or immune globulin

238 Rhinoviruses

Diane E. Pappas and J. Owen Hendley

Rhinoviruses (*rhino*, nose) are the most common cause of the common cold, accounting for at least 50% of upper respiratory tract infections in children and adults. Rhinoviruses are difficult to detect, but the development of sensitive PCR-based assays has led to the identification of three distinct groups of rhinovirus (HRV-A, HRV-B, and HRV-C).[1] Although infection results in serotype-specific lasting immunity, rhinovirus infections are common because there are >100 different serotypes.

DESCRIPTION OF PATHOGEN

Rhinovirus belongs to the picornavirus family. The virus is composed of single-stranded RNA within a capsid with icosahedral symmetry. Canyons on the surface of the virus provide an attachment site for receptors on the surface of susceptible target cells. The attachment site for most rhinoviruses is the intercellular adhesion molecule-1 (ICAM-1) on human respiratory tract epithelium. Viral infectivity is neutralized when host immunoglobulin (Ig) G binds to the surface of the virus, thereby blocking interaction between the host cell receptor and the receptor binding site located at the base of the canyon.[2]

EPIDEMIOLOGY

Rhinovirus is found worldwide and causes infection throughout the year. In temperate climates, there is a sharp increase in the number of rhinovirus infections in September after the return of children to school.[3] Schoolchildren frequently transfer rhinovirus to family members; in one study, 73% of infections in the home could be traced via serotype to infection in a child.[4] There is a smaller peak of rhinovirus infections in the spring.

Rhinovirus infection of humans is restricted to respiratory tract epithelium, primarily the nose and nasopharynx. It does not appear to infect the submucosa. The temperature of normal nasal mucosa is 33°C to 35°C, the optimal temperature for growth of rhinovirus in vitro. Rhinovirus also can infect the lower respiratory tract.[5-7] Rhinovirus RNA has been detected in blood, but rhinoviremia has not been demonstrated by culture.[8] It has not been detected in stool. It has not been recovered from domestic animals (dogs and cats); the only animal model of infection is in primates.

Transmission of rhinovirus occurs via small-particle aerosol, large-particle aerosol, or direct contact.[9] To cause infection, virus must be deposited on the nasal mucosa or conjunctiva; oral inoculation is not sufficient.[10,11] In studies of experimental[12,13] and naturally acquired[10,14] rhinovirus infections, virus often can be recovered from the hands of infected individuals. Virus also can be recovered from objects touched by infected persons, including toys in a physician's waiting room.[12,14,15] Studies of young adults showed efficient transfer during brief hand contact and inoculation by finger onto conjunctival or nasal epithelium.[12] Sneezing and coughing were inefficient methods of transfer.[14] In a different experimental model, it appeared that infection also could be transmitted by aerosol.[16,17] Transmission routes under natural conditions have not been definitely established, but in one study, interruption of hand transmission alone reduced secondary attack rates in mothers after introduction of virus by a family member.[9]

CLINICAL MANIFESTATIONS

The symptoms of a rhinovirus cold largely are subjective; nasal congestion or discharge, sore or scratchy throat, and cough are typical complaints. In adults, physical findings may be limited to mild erythema of the nasal mucosa and pharynx. In addition, children also can have fever during the first 2 to 3 days and moderate enlargement of the anterior cervical nodes. Illness generally lasts 5 to 7 days in adults, but can persist for 10 to 14 days in children.

Both in vivo and in vitro studies have demonstrated that the respiratory tract epithelium remains intact during infection. Nasal biopsy specimens taken during and after illness showed no histologic change in the nasal mucosa other than an influx of neutrophils early in the course of infection.[18,19] Similarly, rhinovirus replication in vitro produced no apparent damage to a monolayer of nasal epithelial cells.[20]

Infection with rhinovirus begins with inoculation of the nasal mucosa. Studies using in situ hybridization techniques show that viral replication occurs in only a small number of epithelial cells at any point in time.[21,22] Infected epithelial cells initiate an inflammatory cascade by release of cytokines and chemokines, including interleukin 8 (IL-8), a potent chemoattractant for neutrophils. Vascular leakage allows plasma containing albumin and other serum proteins to flood the nasal mucosa. Evaluation of nasal washings has shown that viral titers and concentrations of serum albumin, neutrophils, IL-8, and kinins all peak about 48 hours after inoculation and then decline, paralleling the course and severity of symptoms (Figure 238-1).[23] Localized inflammatory response limits viral replication, and symptoms improve. Between 2 and 3 weeks, sufficient neutralizing antibody is produced to block viral replication, and the infection ends.

LABORATORY FINDINGS AND DIAGNOSIS

Laboratory confirmation is not useful in clinical practice. If desired, diagnosis can be confirmed with detection of rhinovirus in cell culture; nasal wash samples are superior to nasal swab specimens.[24,25] Optimally, two sensitive cell lines (WI-38 human embryonic lung fibroblasts and susceptible HeLa cells) are inoculated. Using either cell line alone misses 20% to 35% of culture-positive samples;[24] use of both cell lines increases sensitivity

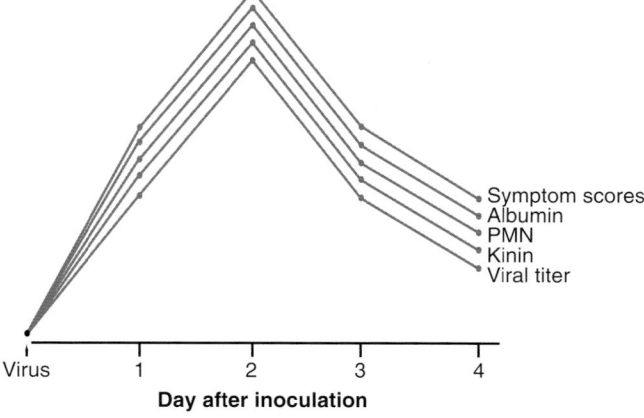

Figure 238-1. Schematic composite of kinetics of average symptom scores compared with concentrations of markers of inflammation and virus in nasal washes after inoculation of rhinovirus. (Redrawn from Hendley JO. Clinical virology of rhinoviruses. Ad Virus Res 1999;54:463.)

from 76% to 82%.[26,27] Using detection by cell culture, rhinovirus was associated with about 30% of symptomatic colds. Reverse transcriptase-polymerase chain reaction (RT-PCR) technology detects rhinovirus with a sensitivity of 98% to 100%. Studies utilizing both cell culture and RT-PCR for detection of rhinovirus from nasopharyngeal secretions of adults and children with naturally acquired colds have shown that rhinovirus is associated with 50% of all colds during year-round surveillance[26,28] and 80% of colds occurring in the fall.[27] The group C rhinoviruses detected with RT-PCR have not been grown in available cell lines.

TREATMENT

There is no effective treatment for rhinovirus colds, although the capsid-binding agent pleconaril had activity (but is no longer being investigated),[29] and interferon-α[30] is under investigation. Antihistamines, decongestants, and antitussives have not been shown to be effective in children with colds. Echinacea preparations are commonly believed to be effective, but a placebo-controlled, double-blind study showed no significant effect on the rate of rhinovirus infection or its symptoms.[31]

SPECIAL CONSIDERATIONS

Although rhinovirus infections are considered benign, self-limited infections, certain populations may experience more serious consequences. In one study, preterm infants with rhinovirus infection were severely compromised and all required respiratory support.[32] In another study, rhinovirus (predominantly HRV-C) was identified in young infants admitted with a diagnosis of apparently life-threatening event (ALTE).[33] Children with underlying medical conditions such as chronic pulmonary or neurologic disease also can experience more severe disease manifestations.[34,35]

PREVENTION

Vaccination for prevention of rhinovirus infection is impractical because of the large number of serotypes and the serotype specificity of immunity. Transmission can be interrupted, at least in part, by the simple physical removal of virus on fingers by handwashing prior to self-inoculation of nasal or conjunctival mucosa.

239 Caliciviruses

Aron J. Hall and Marc-Alain Widdowson

DESCRIPTION OF PATHOGENS

Caliciviruses were discovered in 1972 by electron microscopy of stool samples from children affected by an outbreak of gastroenteritis in a school in Norwalk, Ohio, several years previously.[1] This discovery of the subsequently named Norwalk virus marked the first identification of a virus as a cause of gastroenteritis. Named for the marked cup-like depressions in the capsid (*calyx* = cup in Latin) (Figure 239-1), the family Caliciviridae are small, non-enveloped single-stranded RNA viruses divided into five genera: Norovirus, Sapovirus, Lagovirus, Vesivirus, and the recently added Nebovirus.[2,3] Noroviruses and sapoviruses include human pathogens, with main characteristics shown in Table 239-1. Lagoviruses, vesiviruses, and neboviruses are animal pathogens and have not been detected in naturally occurring human illnesses.

Noroviruses are classified into five genogroups: viruses of genogroups I, II, and IV cause human disease, whereas genogroups III and V contain viruses only found in animals. These five genogroups are further subdivided into at least 31 genotypes,[4,5] among which genogroup II type 4 (GII.4) viruses have emerged as the leading cause of norovirus outbreaks worldwide.[6] Animal noroviruses have not been found in humans, but strains infecting pigs and dogs have been identified within genogroups II and IV, respectively.[5,7] Additionally, serologic evidence of human infection with bovine noroviruses suggests the potential for zoonotic transmission.[8] Sapoviruses similarly are divided into five genogroups, four of which (genogroups I, II, IV, and V) contain viruses affecting humans.[9]

Noroviruses and sapoviruses infect villi of the small intestine, and likely cause diarrhea by a variety of mechanisms, including both disruption of the epithelial barrier and active anion secretion.[10] Mechanisms of immunity to norovirus infection remain unclear. Immunity to one infecting strain does not appear to confer cross-protection and may only be temporary, with people becoming susceptible to reinfection with the same strain after 6 months or less.[11,12] High levels of antibody seem to be a marker for susceptibility, rather than protection, whereas some people may be entirely refractory to infection with a particular strain.[12] This apparent paradox has been explained in part by studies demonstrating genetic factors related to susceptibility and resistance to norovirus infection. Innate resistance has been associated with mutations in the genes for the secretor enzyme 1,2-fucosyltransferase (FUT2), leading to lack of expression of histo-blood group antigens (HBGAs).[13-16] These antigens are expressed on the surface of intestinal cells and serve as receptors for norovirus; thus, people who express HBGAs ("secretors") are associated with strain-specific susceptibility and typically have higher antibody levels.[13,14,16-19]

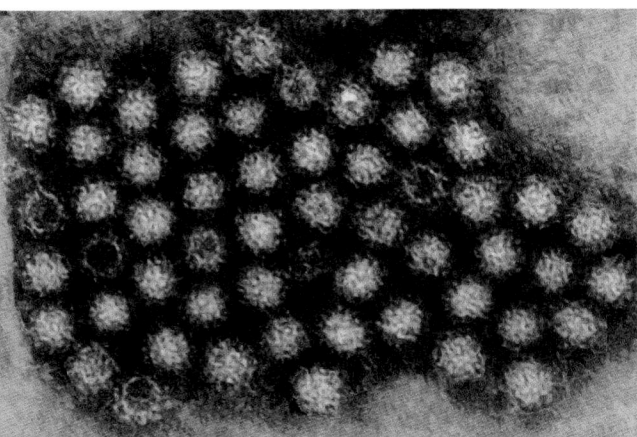

Figure 239-1. Transmission electron micrograph of norovirus virions revealing typical structural morphology. (Courtesy of Charles D. Humphrey, Centers for Disease Control and Prevention.)

TABLE 239-1. Comparison of Main Characteristics of Noroviruses and Sapoviruses

	Noroviruses	Sapoviruses
Appearance by electron microscopy	27–35 nm virus with appearance of cup-like indentations in capsid (Figure 239-1)	27–35 nm virus with striking cup-like depressions with hollow in middle leading to "star of David" configuration
Other names	Small round structured viruses, "Norwalk-like" viruses	"Classical" caliciviruses, "Sapporo-like" viruses
Name of prototype virus	Norwalk virus	Sapporo virus
Genogroups (G)	I–V (GIII exclusively bovine viruses, GV exclusively lion, canine, and murine viruses)	I–V (GIII exclusively porcine viruses)
Immunity	Short-term (<6 months) homologous acquired immunity, genetic resistance/susceptibility factors	Largely unknown
Affected age groups	All ages	Mainly children
Clinical symptoms	Primarily vomiting and/or diarrhea	Mild gastroenteritis with less vomiting
Asymptomatic infections	30% in volunteer studies	Common: possibly up to 75% of infections among children in childcare outbreaks
Percent of diarrheal hospitalizations among children <5 years of age	10–15%	<5%
Outbreak potential	High	Moderate
Modes of transmission	Fecal–oral: direct person-to-person; contaminated food, water or fomites; droplet spread from vomitus	Fecal–oral: person-to-person spread likely the predominant modes; occasionally contaminated food

EPIDEMIOLOGY

Caliciviruses, specifically noroviruses, are the most common infectious cause of gastroenteritis in people of all ages, and second only to rotavirus among children <5 years of age.[20,21] In a systematic review, noroviruses accounted for 12% of severe gastroenteritis in children <5 years of age and 12% of mild to moderate gastroenteritis across all ages.[20] Noroviruses are estimated to cause 21 million cases of diarrhea annually in the United States, including 71,000 hospitalizations.[20,22,22a,23] Although rotavirus remains the leading cause of severe gastroenteritis among young children, caliciviruses also play a substantial role. A prospective study of Finnish children <2 years of age reported rotavirus in 29% of sporadic gastrointestinal tract illness, norovirus in 20%, and sapoviruses in 9%.[23] Among young children hospitalized for gastroenteritis in a German hospital, rotavirus was detected in 47% and noroviruses in 21%.[24] With introduction of universal rotavirus immunization of infants in many countries and consequent reduction of the burden of rotavirus disease, the relative importance of noroviruses in severe pediatric gastroenteritis is expected to increase in these settings.

Noroviruses are highly infectious, transmitted through the fecal–oral route, either directly from person to person or indirectly via contaminated food and water[25] (Figure 239-2). Droplet spread from vomitus also can infect people in the vicinity,[26] as well as contaminate environmental surfaces, where norovirus can persist and remain infectious for several days.[27,28] These characteristics help make noroviruses the leading cause of gastroenteritis outbreaks in the U.S. and Europe, responsible for approximately 50% of all reported gastroenteritis outbreaks.[29] Although outbreaks occur year round, they are more common in the winter months.[30] Periodic increases in norovirus outbreaks also have occurred in association with emergence of new viral strains, particularly those within GII.4, resulting in seasons with increased norovirus activity.[31,32]

Figure 239-3 shows the setting of 773 confirmed norovirus outbreaks with specimens submitted to the Centers for Disease

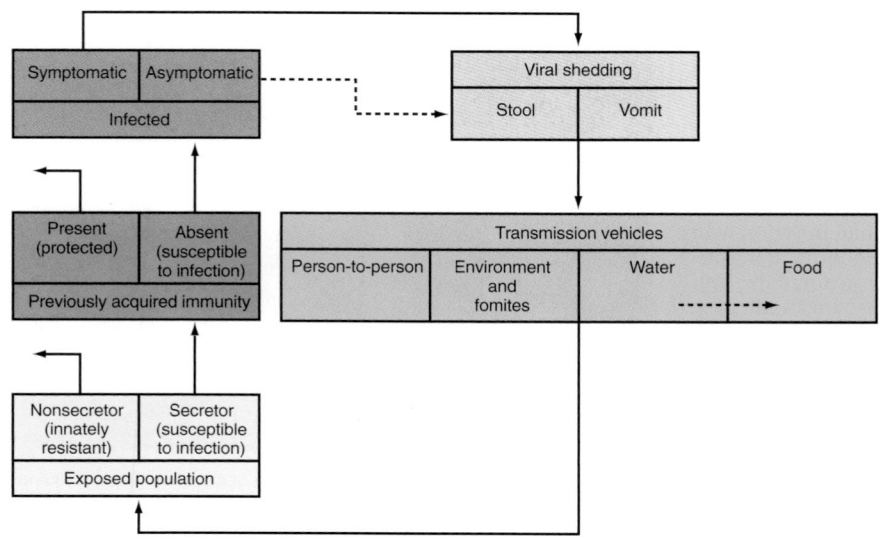

Figure 239-2. Transmission cycle of norovirus, beginning with infected individuals (red box), including both symptomatic and asymptomatic infections. Virus is shed in stool and vomit of symptomatic individuals (blue box), as well as stool of asymptomatic individuals (dashed arrow). Subsequent transmission vehicles may include raw or ready-to-eat foods, drinking or recreational water, contaminated fomites or environments, and direct person-to-person contact (green box). Cross-contamination may occur among these vehicles, such as contamination of fresh produce with irrigation water or shellfish with wastewater. Individuals exposed to contaminated vehicles include both innately susceptible and resistant individuals, as conferred in part by secretor status (yellow box). Among exposed individuals without innate resistance, a proportion previously will have acquired immunity and therefore be protected from infection (orange box). Those without innate or acquired immunity then become infected and the cycle begins again.

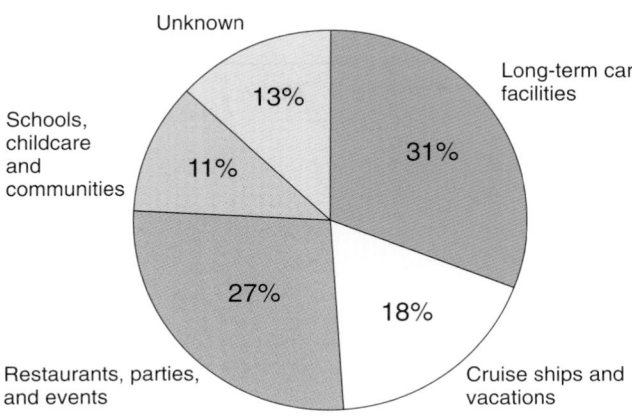

Unknown 13%
Long-term care facilities 31%
Schools, childcare and communities 11%
Restaurants, parties, and events 27%
Cruise ships and vacations 18%

Figure 239-3. Setting of 773 outbreaks with stool specimens submitted to the Centers for Disease Control and Prevention for viral testing and confirmed due to norovirus, 1994–2006. (Derived from Zheng DP, Widdowson MA, Glass RI, Vinje J. Molecular epidemiology of genogroup II-genotype 4 noroviruses in the United States between 1994 and 2006. J Clin Microbiol 2010;48:168–177.)

Control and Prevention (CDC) for diagnostics during 1994–2006.[31] The most common setting of reported U.S. norovirus outbreaks is long-term care facilities, in which the predominant transmission route is person-to-person.[32a,33] Outbreaks also frequently occur in schools and childcare facilities.

Noroviruses also are the leading cause of foodborne disease outbreaks in the U.S. During 2006–2007, noroviruses accounted for 35% of foodborne disease outbreaks reported to the CDC, more than all other known causes combined.[33,34] Outbreaks have been associated with consumption of oysters that concentrate viruses from contaminated waters,[35,36] raspberries presumed contaminated in fields,[37] and delicatessen meat contaminated during processing;[38] however, outbreaks usually are linked to ready-to-eat foods (e.g., salads, sandwiches) contaminated at the point of service.[39]

The epidemiology of sapoviruses is less well studied. Although sapoviruses are a common infection of infants with seroprevalence similar to that of genogroup II noroviruses,[40,41] infections often are mild or asymptomatic.[42] Outbreaks of sapovirus illness are much less common than outbreaks of norovirus, but have been reported in schools,[43] childcare facilities,[44] adult long-term care facilities,[45] and hospitals,[46] as well as in occasional foodborne outbreaks.[47] The broad age range of people affected in these outbreaks suggests that sapovirus infection may not be restricted to young children. Furthermore, an emergent genotype of sapovirus (genogroup I type 4) has been associated with an increased number of outbreaks in Europe, which primarily affected older adults.[48]

CLINICAL MANIFESTATIONS

Norovirus infection usually manifests as acute-onset vomiting with watery, nonbloody diarrhea, after an incubation period of 12 to 48 hours. Other symptoms include abdominal cramps, nausea, and occasionally low-grade fever; thus the term "stomach flu" is commonly used to describe the illness, although it is not related to influenza. Although illness generally is self-limiting and full recovery can be expected in 1 to 4 days, symptoms can be debilitating and lead to dehydration and its sequelae requiring medical attention, especially in people who are very young or elderly, or who are hospitalized.[17,49] Deaths associated with norovirus also have been reported among elderly people and during outbreaks in nursing homes.[50,51] Calicivirus infections do not appear to result in long-term sequelae, although secondary features that have been reported include necrotizing enterocolitis in neonates,[52] chronic diarrhea in immunosuppressed patients,[53] postinfectious irritable bowel syndrome,[54] and neurologic manifestations such as infantile seizures

and encephalopathy.[55,56] More data are needed to confirm these observations and determine their relative frequency.

Generally, norovirus illness is less severe than rotavirus disease although hospitalized children infected with either virus have similar severity scores.[57] Clinical sapovirus infection manifests with similar but milder symptoms than norovirus infection and with less vomiting.[42,58] Volunteer studies suggest that 30% of norovirus infections may be asymptomatic.[59] Importantly, norovirus can be shed in stools for an average of 4 weeks after infection, although peak shedding occurs 2 to 5 days after infection.[60] Children and those with suppressed immune systems have been reported as shedding for longer periods.[17] It is unclear at what point an infected person ceases to represent a significant risk of contagion.

LABORATORY FINDINGS AND DIAGNOSIS

Human caliciviruses cannot be grown in vitro, a feature that has hampered development of diagnostic tests. Reverse transcriptase-polymerase chain reaction (RT-PCR) is the state-of-the-art tool for diagnosing calicivirus infection,[61,62] replacing electron microscopy and serology that were insensitive, nonspecific, and generally difficult to perform. Real-time platforms using Taqman probes that allow for simultaneous detection and quantification generally have replaced conventional RT-PCR platforms for the purposes of diagnosis.[63,64] However, these assays are not approved for clinical laboratory use and are limited to public health laboratories and research settings, predominantly for detecting caliciviruses in gastroenteritis outbreaks or for etiologic studies. Enzyme immunoassays for antigen detection also have been developed and some have been approved for use in specific settings and circumstances, but exhibit poor sensitivity and generally are not recommended for clinical diagnosis of sporadic gastroenteritis cases, although they may have utility in rapid diagnosis of multiple outbreak specimens.[65,66,67]

TREATMENT

No specific treatment exists for calicivirus illness. Similar to therapy for other causes of viral gastroenteritis, recommended supportive treatment includes therapy for dehydration and electrolyte imbalances. First-line therapy for uncomplicated viral gastroenteritis should be oral rehydration, while severe dehydration or shock may warrant intravenous fluid therapy.[68] Antiemetics, and antimotility agents generally are not recommended.[69,70] Antimicrobial agents are of no benefit. Research and development of potential antiviral agents against noroviruses is ongoing, although no clinical trials have been conducted.[71]

PREVENTION

Prevention of infection should focus on standard hygienic precautions, including frequent hand hygiene, environmental disinfection, proper disposal of fecal or vomit-soiled materials, and limited contact with ill persons.[67] Washing with soap and water for a minimum of 20 seconds is the preferred method of hand hygiene to prevent calicivirus transmission, with alcohol-based hand sanitizers used only as an adjunct in between proper handwashing and when hands are not visibly soiled.[67,72] Whenever possible, contact with ill people should be limited during the period of peak infectiousness (acute illness through 72 hours postrecovery). Ill staff members in healthcare facilities, food handlers, and childcare workers should be excluded from work until 48 to 72 hours after symptom resolution. Potentially contaminated environmental surfaces should be disinfected using a chlorine bleach solution with a concentration of 1000 to 5000 ppm (1:50 to 1:10 dilution of household bleach (5.25%)) or another approved disinfectant.[67,72-74] City and state health departments should be notified of outbreaks so that stool can be collected for diagnosis and the outbreak reported to the CDC via the National Outbreak Reporting System.[67] Current vaccine development efforts utilizing virus-like particles have shown promise, although to date, no vaccines against human caliciviruses are available.[75,76]

240 Astroviruses

Jacqueline E. Tate and Joseph S. Bresee

Astroviruses were first described in 1975 when detected by electron microscopy in stool specimens of infants with gastroenteritis.[1,2] Since 1990, with development of sensitive and specific diagnostic methods, including enzyme immunoassays (EIAs) and reverse transcriptase-polymerase chain reaction (RT-PCR),[3–6] astroviruses have been appreciated to be relatively common causes of community-acquired and hospital-acquired gastroenteritis. Astroviruses are one of the most common viral causes of gastroenteritis among children after rotaviruses and noroviruses.[7]

DESCRIPTION OF PATHOGEN

Astroviruses are nonenveloped, positive-sense single-stranded RNA viruses in the family Astroviridae.[8,9] By electron microscopy, astroviruses are 28 to 30 nm in diameter with a smooth edge, and sometimes have a characteristic star-like appearance in the center (Greek, *astron* meaning "star")[10,11] (Figure 240-1). There are at least 8 distinct serotypes (HastV 1–8) of human astrovirus, defined both antigenically and by genetic sequence differences, with several novel species described since 2008.[12–14] Serotype 1 viruses are detected most commonly, but more than one serotype may circulate in communities during each season.[12,15] Nonserotype 1 viruses can predominate in a season, and greater serotype diversity may be found in developing countries.[12,16–20]

EPIDEMIOLOGY

Like rotaviruses and caliciviruses, astroviruses have a worldwide distribution and have been detected in all countries where sufficiently sensitive detection methods have been used, both as a cause of sporadic gastroenteritis and of outbreaks.[21–25] In both economically developed and developing countries, astroviruses generally have been detected in 5% to 14% of young children treated for gastroenteritis in outpatient clinics or in hospitals. The lower proportions reported from some studies (<1% to 3%)

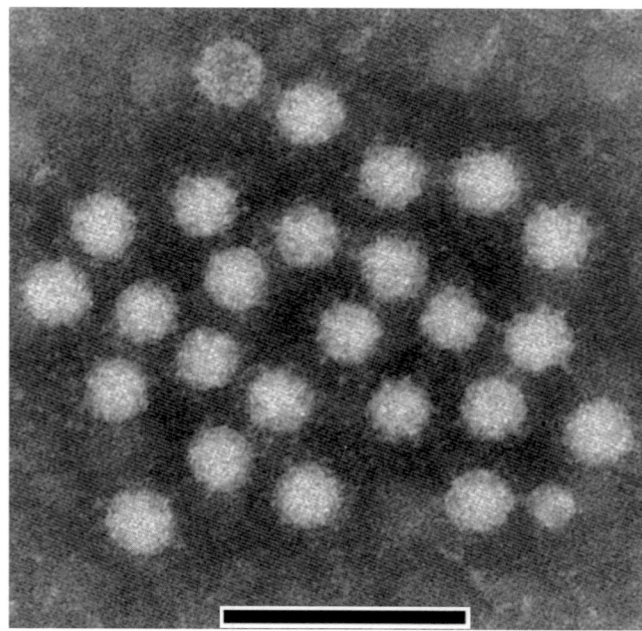

Figure 240-1. Astroviruses are 28 to 30 nm, have a smooth edge, and a distinctive 5- or 6-pointed star on some particles when fecal suspension derived virus is viewed. The smooth surface is not always present on astroviruses grown in culture and can resemble miniature versions of noroviruses. Scale bar = 100 nm. (Courtesy of Charles D. Humphrey, PhD, CDC, Atlanta, GA.)

may reflect insensitive detection methods rather than true prevalence.[7,23,26-32]

Outbreaks of astrovirus gastroenteritis have been reported in closed settings such as schools,[33,34] childcare centers,[22,35] hospitals,[21,36,37] nursing homes,[38,39] and households.[34,40] Outbreaks can be associated with high attack rates, particularly in closed populations such as group childcare settings. Astroviruses have been reported to be responsible for 5% to 16% of cases of nosocomial gastroenteritis in children's hospitals.[36,41,42]

Although astroviruses have been detected in all age groups, most infections occur in children <2 years of age.[21,25,30,43] Most adults have serum antibodies against astroviruses that are acquired early in life.[44] Disease in adults is uncommon. In volunteer studies, most adults challenged with virus did not become infected or develop diarrhea.[45] However, illness among teachers during school outbreaks have been described, perhaps as a result of a large dose of virus in this type of setting or a different mechanism of spread.[33,34] Outbreaks among elderly people may be due to waning immunity associated with increasing age.[37-39] Astroviruses also have been associated with disease in immunocompromised adults.[46]

Transmission is by the fecal–oral route, generally through person-to-person contact, but transmission occasionally can occur via contaminated food and water.[33,34] The infectious dose has not been established. In temperate climates, astrovirus shows a similar seasonal distribution to rotavirus with a peak in winter,[16,23,28] but seasonality is less clear in tropical settings.[31,43,47]

CLINICAL MANIFESTATIONS

The incubation period for astrovirus infections is 1 to 4 days.[45] Symptomatic illness occurs more commonly and with increased symptoms in infants and young children, although asymptomatic infections can occur in all ages.[22,24] Clinical symptoms generally are milder but similar to symptoms caused by rotavirus, with 2 to 5 days of watery diarrhea, often accompanied by vomiting and less often by high fever and abdominal pain.[30,36,43,48] Illness generally is mild and self limited,[30] but malabsorption and lactose intolerance have been reported following infection.[43,49] Stools do not contain blood or mucus. Children can shed virus 1 to 2 days prior to illness and for a median of 5 days after onset of symptoms.[22,35,36] Prolonged diarrhea has been reported among children with malnutrition and in immunocompromised patients. Asymptomatic excretion among healthy children has been reported

for 3 weeks when more sensitive detection methods have been used.[22] Persistent excretion occurs in immunocompromised patients.[50] Because illness is largely confined to young children and elderly people, infection probably confers protection which is relatively durable.

LABORATORY FINDINGS AND DIAGNOSIS

Since 1990, there have been many improvements in diagnostic methods for astroviruses, including adaptation to grow in continuous cell lines, sequencing and elucidation of the structure of the genome, and development of improved methods of detection, including EIAs and RT-PCR.[7] Commercial EIA assays to detect viral antigen in stool are available in many countries and offer a sensitive and specific method to diagnose infections; none is yet available in the United States.[3,6,7] Other diagnostic methods include RT-PCR,[35] serum EIA for astrovirus antibodies, and electron microscopy; these are used primarily in research settings.[7]

TREATMENT

No specific therapies exist for any of the viruses that cause acute gastroenteritis. The mainstay of management is rapid assessment, correction of fluid loss and electrolyte disturbances, and maintenance of adequate hydration. Oral rehydration therapy with appropriate glucose-electrolyte solutions is sufficient for most patients. Intravenous rehydration is required for children with severe dehydration with shock or intractable vomiting. Children should maintain caloric intake as best as possible, with maintenance of diet.[51] Breastfed infants should continue to nurse on demand, and formula-fed infants should continue formula immediately upon rehydration. Children receiving semisolid or solid foods should continue to receive their usual diet during episodes of diarrhea, although substantial amounts of foods high in simple sugars (carbonated soft drinks, juice, gelatin desserts) should be avoided because the osmotic load might worsen diarrhea.

PREVENTION

No vaccine is available to prevent astrovirus infections, and none is in clinical trials. Prevention of astrovirus infections is best accomplished through good hygiene and attention to appropriate hand hygiene practices.

241 Hepatitis E Virus

Eyasu H. Teshale and Saleem Kamili

HEPATITIS E VIRUS

Hepatitis E virus (HEV), the major etiologic agent of enterically transmitted non-A hepatitis worldwide, is a spherical, non-enveloped, single-stranded, positive sense RNA virus that is approximately 32 to 34 nm in diameter.[1] HEV is the sole member of the family Hepeviridae, genus *Hepevirus*.[2] The HEV genome, which is approximately 7.2 kilobases, consists of three open reading frames (ORF 1, ORF 2, and ORF3). HEV is classified into four major genotypes, which represent a single serotype.[3] Genotype 1 includes Asian and African strains; genotype 2 includes a single Mexican strain and some African strains. Both genotypes 1 and 2 are associated with large epidemics. Genotype 3 includes strains from sporadic human cases from industrialized countries including the United States, and Japan, and countries in

Europe, and animal strains from swine; genotype 4 includes strains from sporadic human cases in Asia and animal strains from swine.

Following HEV infection, both immunoglobulin (Ig) M and IgG antibodies to HEV (anti-HEV) are elicited (Figure 241-1). IgM anti-HEV generally is detectable at the time of symptom onset or liver enzyme elevations; levels decline during early convalescence.[4] IgG anti-HEV persists and appears to provide at least short-term protection against disease,[5] but duration of immunity after infection has not been determined. One study demonstrated persistence of IgG anti-HEV in approximately 50% of people studied at least 14 years after infection.[6]

Histopathologic features of HEV infection include both classic acute viral hepatitis with focal hepatocellular necrosis, ballooned hepatocytes, acidophilic degeneration of hepatocytes, and chole-

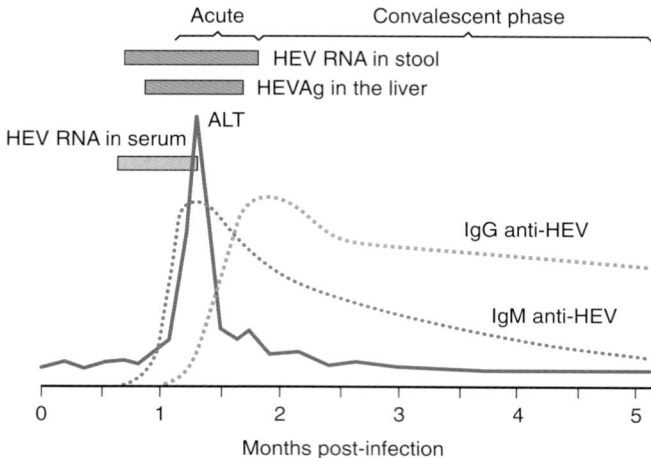

Figure 241-1. Typical serologic and biochemical response to hepatitis E virus infection. (Courtesy of Dr. K. Krawczynski.)

static hepatitis with bile stasis in canaliculi and glandlike transformation of hepatocytes.[7,8]

EPIDEMIOLOGY

HEV infection manifests two distinct clinicoepidemiologic patterns mainly related to viral genotype.[9] In hepatitis E epidemics, HEV (genotype 1 or 2) is transmitted primarily by the fecal–oral route. Fecally contaminated drinking water is the most commonly documented vehicle of transmission, and outbreaks usually occur during the rainy season sometimes affecting thousands of people.[5,7,10] HEV infection also accounts for the majority of acute sporadic hepatitis cases in both children and adults in endemic countries.[11–13] Risk factors for sporadic hepatitis E have not been well defined.

Most cases of HEV infection from the U.S. and western Europe have been reported among travelers returning from HEV genotype 1 endemic areas.[14–16] Although outbreaks of HEV do not occur in the U.S. and western Europe, autochthonous cases unrelated to travel are being reported increasingly.[17,18] The HEV strains isolated from these patients belong to HEV genotype 3 and have close

genetic resemblance to the swine HEV strains isolated from local farms, suggesting that swine might serve as zoonotic source for human disease. However, the mechanism of transmission from swine to humans in these autochthonous cases is unknown.

The worldwide distribution of hepatitis E has not been determined fully, in part due to lack of well-standardized serodiagnostic tests.[19,20] However, given the high prevalence of anti-HEV in different populations,[21] high seroprevalence in animals,[22] frequent occurrence of outbreaks, and that a significant proportion of sporadic acute viral hepatitis are caused by HEV,[23,24] the infection is endemic globally. Large outbreaks of HEV have been documented over a wide geographic area, primarily in developing countries with inadequate environmental sanitation (Figure 241-2).[10,25–30]

Identification of anti-HEV IgG in animal species in many regions of the world provides credence to speculation that HEV is a zoonotic agent.[31,32] HEV can be transmitted by food, as evidenced by disease following consumption of uncooked offal meat from wild boar and sika deer in Germany and Japan, and consumption of raw figatellu, a traditional pig liver sausage in France.[33–35] Vertical transmission of HEV from infected mother to the fetus is common.[36] In epidemic settings person-to-person transmission may contribute to significant transmissions.[37] Nosocomial transmission, presumably by person-to-person contact and by transmission through blood transfusion, has been reported.[38,39]

CLINICAL MANIFESTATIONS

HEV infection can be asymptomatic, clinically inapparent, or can result in clinically evident disease. The incubation period after exposure to HEV ranges from 15 to 60 days (mean, 40 days). Typical acute clinical signs and symptoms are indistinguishable from those of other types of viral hepatitis, consisting of jaundice, malaise, anorexia, nausea, vomiting, abdominal pain, dark urine, fever, and hepatomegaly.[10,12,13,40,41] Other less common signs and symptoms are diarrhea, arthralgia, pruritus, and urticarial rash. The period of infectivity after acute infection has not been determined, but virus excretion in stool has been demonstrated beginning approximately 2 weeks before elevation of serum hepatic enzyme levels and ending by the time levels return to normal.[42,43] In most outbreaks of HEV infection, the highest rates of clinically evident disease have occurred in young to middle-aged adults; lower disease rates in younger age groups might be the result of anicteric or subclinical infections.[5,19,25,28] In contrast, most autochthonous HEV infections occur among older (usually >40 years of

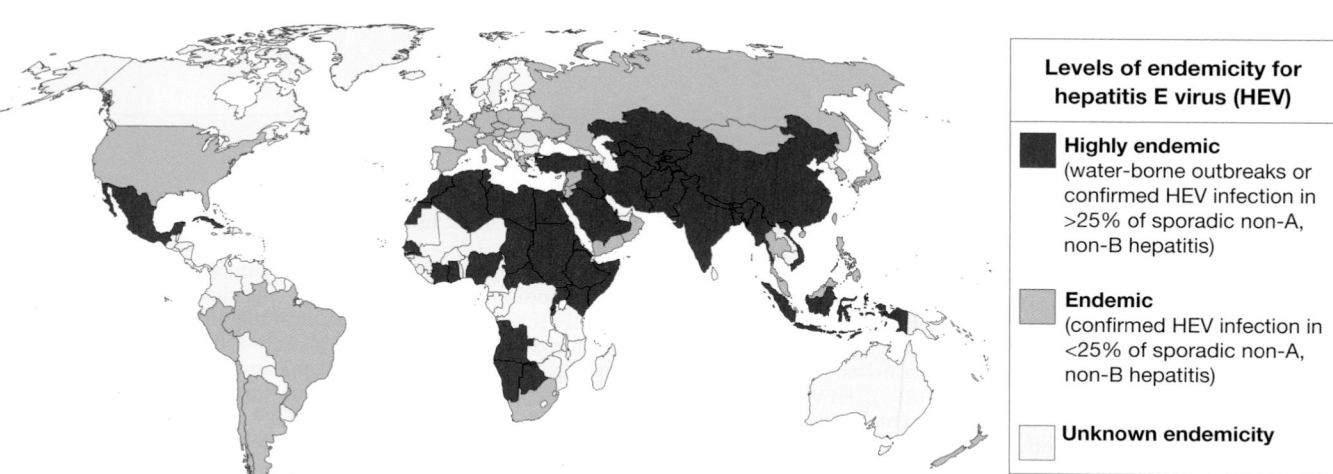

Figure 241-2. The global pattern of HEV infection. (Courtesy of Dr. Chong Gee Teo.)

TABLE 241-1. Interpretation of Hepatitis E Test Results in People with Clinical Hepatitis

Specimen	Assay	Result	
		Positive	**Negative**
Serum	IgM anti-HEV	Consistent with current or recent HEV infection; in most cases, IgG anti-HEV also is detected	Consider other causes of hepatitis; if acute hepatitis E is suspected, test for IgG anti-HEV, HEV RNA
	IgG anti-HEV	Consistent with past or current HEV infection; test for IgM anti-HEV or HEV RNA to confirm current or recent infection	If acute hepatitis E is suspected, test for IgM anti-HEV or HEV RNA
Serum or stool	HEV RNA	Current infection	Cannot exclude current infection

HEV, hepatitis E virus; Ig, immunoglobulin.

Modified from Ticehurst JR. Hepatitis E virus. In: Murray PR, Baron EJ, Pfaller MA, et al. (eds) Manual of Microbiology, 7th ed. Washington, DC, American Society for Microbiology, 1999.

age) men.[44] No evidence of chronic HEV infection has been detected in long-term follow-up of otherwise healthy people.[45] However, there are reports of chronic infection among solid organ transplant recepients,[46] people with AIDS,[47] and people with hematologic malignancies.[48] Association of autochthonous hepatitis E with neurologic signs and symptoms including Guillain–Barré syndrome[49,50] is recognized increasingly, as is cirrhosis in immunosuppressed populations.[51] Whether a proportion of cases of presumed drug-induced liver injury are actually cases of HEV infection[52] needs further elucidation. HEV also causes severe hepatic decompensation in patients with chronic liver disease.[53,54]

The mortality rate observed during epidemics of hepatitis E is approximately 0.5% to 4%. However, fulminant hepatitis occurs more frequently among pregnant women, particularly in the third trimester, and case-fatality rates can reach 25%.[55–57] Investigations have revealed that mortality in young children could be high.[55,58] Serious outcomes of HEV infection also have been observed in countries of low endemicity among pregnant women who acquired infection by travel to regions of high endemicity.[59] The reason for the high mortality among pregnant women is unknown;[60] causes of death include hepatic encephalopathy and disseminated intravascular coagulation.[61] In a prospective study of 26 pregnant women with HEV infection, 15 patients had fulminant hepatic failure (FHF) and 11 patients had non-fulminant disease. Five mothers died undelivered, two aborted, four had premature delivery, and 15 delivered full-term infants. Fifteen (79%) of the 19 liveborn infants had evidence of HEV infection at birth (12 IgM anti-HEV positive and 10 HEV RNA positive). Neonates had icteric hepatitis (7), anicteric hepatitis (5), and jaundice with normal hepatic enzymes (3). In the first week of life 7 infants died from prematurity (1) and HEV infection (6); 5 of 6 mothers of infants who died had FHF. Vertical transmission of HEV to the fetus with poor perinatal outcome has occurred in 30% to 100% of mothers with HEV infection.[62]

LABORATORY FINDINGS AND DIAGNOSIS

Laboratory findings are similar to other viral hepatitides and include elevated serum levels of bilirubin, alanine aminotransferase, aspartate aminotransferase, alkaline phosphatase, and γ-glutamyltransferase.[8,9,41] Resolution of hyperbilirubinemia and serum aminotransferase elevations generally occurs within 1 to 6 weeks after onset of illness.

Enzyme immunoassays to detect IgM and IgG anti-HEV in serum are available commercially but none is FDA approved for clinical use in the U.S. The sensitivity and specificity of these tests vary significantly.[20] Reverse-transcriptase polymerase chain reaction can be used to detect HEV RNA in serum and stool but is not available routinely in diagnostic laboratories. Other tests initially used to detect HEV infection are immunohistochemistry to identify HEV antigen in liver tissue and fluorescent antibody-blocking assay to identify anti-HEV reacting to HEV antigen in serum. However, both these assays have limited sensitivity and are available only in a few research laboratories. Western blot assays can detect IgM and IgG anti-HEV in serum but are less sensitive. Interpretation of test results can be difficult, and in low endemic regions a definitive diagnosis generally requires use of multiple tests, consideration of risk factors, and exclusion of other causes of acute hepatitis (Table 241-1).

Treatment

Treatment is supportive. Data are not available to evaluate efficacy of antiviral agents or other specific therapies. In solid organ recipients with chronic hepatitis E, discontinuation of immune suppressor drugs is associated with sustained virologic response.[63] In a few instances, pegylated interferon and ribavirin were used successfully to treat chronic HEV infection.[64,65]

Prevention

Prevention of HEV infection relies primarily on provision of clean drinking water. Prudent hygienic practices when traveling to developing countries consist of avoiding drinking water (and beverages with ice) of unknown purity, and eating uncooked fruits and vegetables that are not peeled and prepared by the traveler.

Studies conducted during outbreaks of HEV infection have demonstrated that anti-HEV from prior exposure protects against clinical disease.[5] Passive immunoprophylaxis with convalescent serum in nonhuman primates has been shown to prevent disease but not infection.[66] However, immune globulin (IG) prepared from plasma collected in low endemic areas is not effective in preventing clinical disease in humans.[39] The efficacy of IG prepared from plasma collected in high endemic areas is unclear.[39,67,68] In studies of prototype recombinant vaccines, animals were protected against disease but not against infection, as indicated by detectable viremia and viral excretion.[69,70] A recombinant protein vaccine based on the capsid protein was found to be safe and efficacious in a phase II/III clinical trial among human volunteers in Nepal.[71] In a large phase III trial, another recombinant protein vaccine (truncated ORF-2 protein) was found to be safe and effective in preventing hepatitis E.[72]

NEWLY IDENTIFIED VIRUSES

Patients with acute hepatitis in whom recognized viral and nonviral causes have been excluded are considered to have non-A-through-E (non-A–E) hepatitis.[73] Within the past two decades, new viruses, which include GBV agents (previously known as hepatitis G virus),[74] transfusion transmitted virus, and Sendai virus, have been identified as possible causes of non-A–E hepatitis.[75-77] However, their role in the etiology of non-A–E hepatitis has not been established and their pathogenic role is not clear.

Studies have shown that GBV does not replicate in the liver of people coinfected with HCV and GBV, suggesting that GBV is not a hepatotropic virus.[78,79] While it is possible that a viral etiology for non-A–E hepatitis exists, efforts to find the potential etiologic agent have not yet succeeded.

SECTION C: Fungi

242 Classification of Fungi

Martin B. Kleiman

Although only a few hundred of the estimated quarter-million fungal species have been considered primary pathogens of humans, newly recognized opportunistic pathogens in immunocompromised patients have increased this number.[1-4] The medically important fungi are relatively avirulent, opportunistic environmental saprophytes. Human infection plays a dead-end role in their life cycles. The only property that most agents of human infections appear to share is the ability to grow at body temperature. Although efforts to characterize and classify these diverse agents and the illnesses that they cause can be confusing due to taxonomic changes, alterations in disease terminology, and subjective pathologic categorizations about which experts may disagree, some basic generalizations benefit understanding.

THE AGENTS

Fungi are eukaryotic; that is, they have a nucleus surrounded by a nuclear membrane, multiple chromosomes, and a mitotic apparatus. Their rigid cell walls contain chitin, cellulose, or both. Cytoplasmic membranes contain sterols. The principal action of amphotericin B and the azole antifungal drugs is disruption of sterol-containing cytoplasmic cell membranes.

With some exceptions, fungi can be divided into two morphologic forms termed yeasts and molds. Yeasts are unicellular structures that generally are round or oval. Most yeasts reproduce by budding, but a few important pathogens do so by internal segmentation of their cytoplasm (e.g., *Coccidioides immitis*). On solid media, yeast colonies are discrete and circular and appear pasty or mucoid. Distinguishing microscopic features that are used to assign yeasts to taxa include size and shape, method of budding (conidiogenesis), the presence of true hyphae or pseudohyphae, and the presence of sexual spores. The term "yeast", however, is not a taxon, and some microbiologists use it to refer to a group of ascomycetes that produce ascospores in a free ascus. The term "yeastlike" is used for fungi that have budding morphology but do not have ascospores; examples include the dimorphic fungi. Although morphologic criteria are used primarily to distinguish yeasts at the genus level, the ability to use specific carbohydrates and nitrogen-containing compounds for growth also is considered in the assignment of species.

Molds usually are multicellular and are composed of tubular structures, or hyphae, that grow by longitudinal extension and branching. Hyphae interweave to form mycelia. Mold colonies appear "wispy" on solid agar. Some fungi can grow as either yeast or mold forms and are termed dimorphic fungi. Among dimorphic fungi that are important human pathogens are the agents of histoplasmosis, blastomycosis, sporotrichosis, coccidioidomycosis, paracoccidioidomycosis, and penicilliosis. The spore-bearing mold forms in the environment usually are the source of exposure to these pathogens. Mold forms of these agents grown in the laboratory also can be a hazard to personnel. Molds generally are differentiated by morphologic characteristics, including size, presence or absence of cross-walls (septa) within the tubular

structures, and the way in which spores (conidia) are formed within specialized reproductive hyphae (conidiophores). In some cases, molecular methods have differentiated species that are indistinguishable using standard morphologic and biochemical techniques. A detailed taxonomic classification of medically important fungi is available elsewhere.[5-8]

In addition to growth by budding, branching, and apical extension, fungal growth also occurs through spore formation. Spores can result from asexual (mitotic) or sexual (meiotic) reproduction. The taxonomy of some important pathogens has been reclassified as a result of induction of some fungi first recognized in the asexual (imperfect) state to the sexual (perfect) state. For example, *Histoplasma capsulatum* and *Blastomyces dermatitidis* are names given to the asexual forms of these fungi; the term *anamorph* is synonymous with asexual forms. The teleomorphic, or sexual, stage of these agents is classified in the ascomycetous forms as *Ajellomyces capsulatus* and *A. dermatitidis*, respectively. Because clinical laboratories isolate these fungi as anamorphs, the terms *H. capsulatum* and *B. dermatitidis* are used. However, nonmicrobiologists should recognize this distinction in texts and journals.

Although the pathogenic fungi are a diverse group of organisms, familiarity with a few general principles can help clinicians understand the role played by the laboratory in evaluation of a suspected mycosis. Aside from superficial dermatophyte and candidal infections, fungal infections are uncommon, and many clinical laboratories may perform only microscopic examination and preliminary isolation procedures and then refer isolates to reference laboratories for further testing.

Laboratory personnel should be informed of suspected diagnoses so that methods of specimen collection and processing and duration of incubation can be optimized.[5] Specimens should be fresh, kept from drying, and transported and processed promptly. Although microscopic examination of a wet mount prepared with a 10% potassium hydroxide solution is simple and rapid, considerable skill is required to differentiate fungal elements from background artifact. A wet mount using calcofluor white stains cell walls and clearly differentiates fungal elements, but reading requires a fluorescence microscope. Some yeast cells can stain with the Gram stain (gram-positive) but Gram stain might not stain hyphal elements reliably. Common Gram-stained artifacts can resemble yeasts. Tissue specimens should be examined for fungus with specialized stains because the standard hematoxylin and eosin preparation, although useful, is less reliable. Gomori methenamine silver (GMS) stain renders cell walls strikingly brownish black against a faint background and facilitates recognition of low numbers of organisms. The periodic acid–Schiff (PAS) procedure stains the cell walls of viable organisms and, in contrast with GMS, retains details of cellular architecture. The Giemsa stain also is useful. Standard fungal culture media include Sabouraud dextrose agar and brain–heart infusion (BHI) agar supplemented with 5% sheep blood. Duplicate plates are incubated at 25°C and 35°C. Cultures should be maintained for 4 to 6 weeks. Blood culture is made more sensitive by using a large inoculum. The time to

TABLE 242-1. Association of the Etiologic Agents of Systemic Fungal Infections with Specific Predisposing Factors

Predisposing Factor	Etiologic Agent(s)
Traumatized skin	*Candida* spp.
	Candida (*Torulopsis*) *glabrata*
	Malassezia furfur[a]
Ketoacidosis	Agents of mucormycosis
Therapy with deferoxamine	Agents of mucormycosis
Intravenous drug abuse	*Candida* spp.
	Agents of mucormycosis
Malnutrition	*Candida* spp.
	Agents of mucormycosis
Neutropenia	*Candida* spp.
	Aspergillus spp.
	Agents of mucormycosis
	Scedosporium apiospermum
	(*Pseudallescheria boydii*)
	Trichosporon spp.
	Fusarium spp.
Chronic granulomatous disease	*Aspergillus* spp.
	Candida albicans
	Candida (*Torulopsis*) *glabrata*
Impaired cell-mediated immunity	*Candida* spp.[b]
	Cryptococcus neoformans
	Histoplasma capsulatum
	Coccidioides immitis
	Paracoccidioides brasiliensis
	Blastomyces dermatitidis
	Pneumocystis jirovecii

[a]*In patients who are receiving lipid emulsions intravenously.*

[b]*Infections tend to be limited to mucocutaneous areas without dissemination.*

Modified from Levitz SM. Overview of host defenses in fungal infections. Clin Infect Dis 1992;14(Suppl.):37–42.

detection of a positive culture is shortened by venting bottles to facilitate an aerobic environment (especially helpful for *Candida*), using lysis centrifugation methods, and culturing on biphasic media that combine an appropriate broth (BHI) with solid agar.

FUNGAL–HOST INTERACTION

The outcome of chance human exposure to environmental fungi is determined by the interplay of many factors, among which are species-specific fungal virulence factors,[8] inoculum size, breach of integumental barriers, and adequacy of host immune mechanisms critical to control of infection by the particular offending organism[1,9] (Table 242-1). Most systemic mycoses are acquired through inhalation of spores. Subcutaneous mycoses also can follow accidental inoculation of contaminated soil or vegetable matter.[10] Dermatophytes[10] and *Candida albicans* have adapted to humans and can be spread from person to person; however, most fungal infections cannot be transmitted in this manner.

CLINICAL MANIFESTATIONS

Only a few fungal species cause a distinct clinical illness. Even in these instances the spectrum and severity of infections, such as histoplasmosis and coccidioidomycosis, are broad and the functional integrity of the host's immune system is a major determinant of expression. A wide variety of agents, such as the dematiaceous fungi and the agents of mucormycosis, cause clinical and pathologic entities that can be indistinguishable. Mycetoma, a chronic, destructive localized infection of skin, soft tissue, fascia, and bone, can be caused by a variety of true fungi (eumycotic mycetoma), as well as several aerobic actinomycetes (actinomycotic mycetoma). Invasive candidiasis and cryptococcosis are frequent infections in immunocompromised hosts. However, superficial candidal infections occur in healthy infants, and cryptococcal infections can occur in otherwise healthy persons. Thus, it is impossible to develop a comprehensive method to precisely classify infections caused by this diverse group of microorganisms. Nonetheless, a useful preliminary approach divides the medically important fungi into three broad categories

TABLE 242-2. Classification of Human Infections Caused by the Medically Important Fungi

Clinical Category	Principal/Representative Causes
PRIMARY SYSTEMIC MYCOSES	
Histoplasmosis	*Histoplasma capsulatum*
Coccidioidomycosis	*Coccidioides immitis*
Blastomycosis	*Blastomyces dermatitidis*
Paracoccidioidomycosis[a,b]	*Paracoccidioides brasiliensis*
OPPORTUNISTIC MYCOSES[c]	
Invasive candidiasis	*Candida* spp., *Torulopsis* spp.
Invasive aspergillosis	*Aspergillus* spp.
Cryptococcosis	*Cryptococcus neoformans*
Agents of mucormycosis[a,d]	*Absidia* spp., *Mucor* spp., *Rhizomucor* spp., *Rhizopus* spp., *Mortierella* spp., *Cunninghamella* spp., etc.[e]
Hyalohyphomycosis[f]	*Penicillium* spp., *Acremonium* spp., *Fusarium* spp.
INOCULATION/CONTAMINATION MYCOSES	
Superficial mycoses (dermatophytosis)[a,g]	*Microsporum* spp., *Trichophyton* spp., *Epidermophyton* spp.
Pityriasis (tinea) versicolor	*Malassezia furfur*
Sporotrichosis	*Sporothrix schenckii*
Chromoblastomycosis[a,h]	
Phaeohyphomycosis[a,i]	Dematiaceous fungi[j]
Mycetoma[a,k]	
Pseudallescheriasis[a,l]	*Scedosporium apiospermum* (*Pseudallescheria boydii*)[l]

[a]*Synonymous, obsolete, overlapping, or incomplete terminology for the clinical entities.*

[b]*South American blastomycosis.*

[c]*A complete list of agents is encyclopedic (see text).*

[d]*Phycomycosis, zygomycosis.*

[e]*Saksenaea* spp., *Cokeromyces* spp., *Syncephalostrum* spp., *Conidiobolus* spp., *Basidiobolus* spp.

[f]*Many nondematiaceous molds; colorless cell walls in hematoxylin & eosin-stained sections.*

[g]*Ringworm (tinea).*

[h]*Chromomycosis.*

[i]*Cerebral chromomycosis, chromoblastomycosis, chromomycosis, cladosporiosis, phaeomycotic cyst, pheosporotrichosis, subcutaneous mycotic cyst.*

[j]*Group of fungi with a pale brown to black color in the cell walls of vegetative cells, conidia, or both; ubiquitous saprophytes of soil and plants. Examples include* Alternaria *spp.,* Bipolaris *spp.,* Cladosporium *spp.,* Curvularia *spp.,* Fonsecaea *spp.,* Phialophora *spp.,* Rhinocladiella *spp., and* Wangiella *spp.*

[k]*Madura foot, maduromycosis.*

[l]*Allescheriasis, allescheriosis, petriellidosis, pseudallescheriosis; Pseudallescheria boydii renamed Scedosporium apiospermum.*

(Table 242-2). The first, the primary systemic mycoses, includes a group of infections virulent enough to infect an immunocompetent host. Examples include histoplasmosis, coccidioidomycosis, blastomycosis, and paracoccidioidomycosis. The second, termed the opportunistic mycoses, are caused by less virulent agents that almost never cause primary invasive disease in immunocompetent hosts and almost always occur in immunocompromised persons or people with indwelling foreign bodies. Examples include invasive candidiasis, aspergillosis, cryptococcosis, and mucormycosis.

The third category of infections, the inoculation/contamination mycoses, usually affects immunocompetent people. Infections can be superficial or deep and result from skin contamination or inoculation through compromised integumental barriers. An example of the former is dermatophytosis; examples of the latter include mycetoma and the cutaneous manifestations of mucormycosis. Immunocompromised patients are at high risk for acquiring almost all fungal infections and often experience aggressive, life-threatening clinical illnesses.

243 *Candida* Species

P. Brian Smith and William J. Steinbach

Advances in medical therapy have allowed for the improved survival of increasingly immunocompromised and critically ill patients. These improvements have augmented the frequency as well as the morbidity and mortality associated with *Candida* infection. In this chapter, epidemiology, risk factors, clinical manifestations, diagnosis, and treatment options available for *Candida* infections, will be discussed, focusing on invasive disease in infants and children.

EPIDEMIOLOGY

Although there are over 200 identified species of *Candida*, only 12 appear to cause disease in children. These species are *C. albicans, C. parapsilosis, C. tropicalis, C. glabrata, C. krusei, C. lusitaniae, C. stellatoidea, C. kefyr, C. pseudotropicalis, C. dubliniensis, C. intermedia,* and *C. guilliermondi.*[1–4]

C. albicans is the most commonly isolated species in children.[4–6] In a prospective (1994 to 2000) study of neonatal candidiasis, *C. albicans* was isolated as the causative organism in 66% (38/58) of cases.[4] Similarly, *C. albicans* was isolated in 54% (31/57) of pediatric patients with candidiasis in the first year following hematopoietic stem cell transplantation (HSCT).[7] However, the epidemiology of candidiasis is changing, and the percentage of cases caused by *C. albicans* has declined from over 80% to as low as 29% in some centers.[6,8] Despite these trends, *C. albicans* continues to be associated with higher rates of end-organ damage and higher attributable mortality relative to other *Candida* species.[9,10]

C. parapsilosis is increasing in importance as a cause of candidiasis in both neonatal and pediatric patients.[4,11] A study of neonatal candidiasis found that 5% (1/22) of cases from 1981 through 1990 were due to *C. parapsilosis.*[2] However, the percentage of cases due to *C. parapsilosis* increased to 60% (53/89) from 1991 to 1995. In a cohort of infants <1000 g birthweight with invasive *Candida* infections, 43% (132/307) of cases were caused by *C. parapsilosis.*[12] *C. parapsilosis* also is the most common species found colonizing the hands of healthcare workers,[13] suggesting a possible vehicle of transmission. *C. parapsilosis* is less virulent than other *Candida* species in animal models and has been associated with overall lower mortality.[4,10,14]

C. glabrata and *C. krusei* are less commonly isolated species but are important because they often are resistant to fluconazole.[15] In adult patients, where use of fluconazole for prophylaxis is more widespread, *C. glabrata* is increasing in incidence and is the second or third most common cause of candidiasis.[16,17] *C. tropicalis* is considered to be the second most virulent species behind *C. albicans* and has been isolated increasingly in recent years.[8] *C. lusitaniae,* which is resistant to amphotericin B, is isolated less

frequently but is important given its unique resistance pattern. *C. dubliniensis,* once thought to be an atypical *C. albicans* isolate, is a separate species often found in human immunodeficiency (HIV)-infected patients.[18] *C. guilliermondii* has been reported as a cause of bloodstream infections (BSIs) in patients with cancer and *C. kefyr* as a cause of esophagitis.[19,20]

Candida species are the third most common pathogen in nosocomial BSIs among premature infants.[21–23] A prospective study of 2847 infants admitted to 6 neonatal intensive care units (NICUs) revealed a cumulative incidence of 0.3% (3/1139) in infants weighing more than 2500 g, 3% among very low birthweight (VLBW, <1500 g birthweight) infants, and 7% among extremely low birthweight (ELBW, <1000 g birthweight) infants.[24,25] The mean age at diagnosis was 15 to 33 days of life.[5,26] Mortality from all *Candida* species in premature infants has been reported consistently at 20% from large multicenter studies.[10,14,21,23,24] In addition to a high mortality rate, candidiasis in infants is associated with significant morbidities in survivors, including poor neurodevelopmental outcome, periventricular leukomalacia, chronic lung disease, and severe retinopathy of prematurity (ROP).[27–30]

Candida also is isolated commonly in hospitalized older pediatric patients. In an examination of over 3400 BSIs in patients ≤16 years of age, *Candida* was the third most commonly isolated organism.[31] A study of over 500 patients in 35 pediatric intensive care units (PICUs) revealed *Candida* to be the second most common cause of nosocomial infections.[32] Mortality also is substantial in pediatric patients. Candidemia was associated with a mortality rate of 16% in 1108 pediatric cases diagnosed outside the neonatal period,[33] and the mortality rate in another cohort of 64 PICU patients with candidemia (70% of which were non-*albicans* species) was 28%.[34]

CLINICAL MANIFESTATIONS

Superficial and Mucosal Infections

Oropharyngeal Candidiasis (Thrush)

Thrush, commonly found in infants and immunocompromised children, is characterized by pearly, white, curdish, material visible on the buccal and gingival mucosa.[35] The underlying mucosa can appear erythematous or normal in color. Often painful, thrush can lead to inadequate nutritional intake and subsequent dehydration. Thrush occasionally progresses to esophagitis, laryngitis (Figure 243-1), or invasive disease in severely immunocompromised patients. Newborn infants often are colonized from the mother's genital tract. In hospitalized infants, the median age of

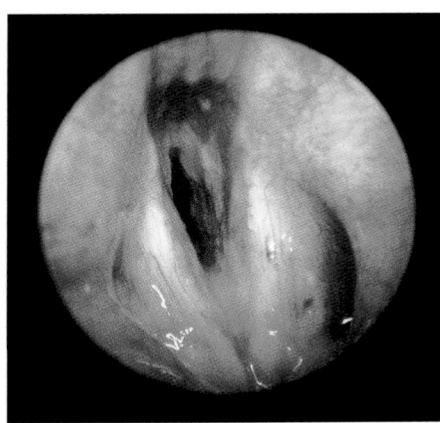

Figure 243-1. Endoscopic view of *Candida albicans* laryngitis in a 12-year-old girl with systemic lupus erythematous receiving high-dose glucocorticoid therapy and antibiotics. She did not have oral candidiasis. (Courtesy of S.S. Long.)

onset is 9 to 10 days. *C. albicans* consistently is the most commonly isolated species.[36]

Diaper Dermatitis

Candida diaper dermatitis is characterized by a confluent erythematous rash with satellite pustules.[37] In term infants, diaper dermatitis is most common from 7 to 9 months of age but manifests earlier in premature infants. As with thrush, diaper dermatitis in term infants rarely is associated with systemic disease. However, in a prospective study of VLBW infants, 32% of infants with mucocutaneous involvement (largely diaper dermatitis) developed invasive candidiasis.[38]

Esophagitis

Candida esophagitis occurs most often in severely immunocompromised individuals such as HIV-infected patients. Esophagitis can occur in the absence of thrush.[39] Patients commonly present with dysphagia or odynophagia. Definitive diagnosis requires endoscopy for biopsy, but often the diagnosis can be suspected by clinical presentation or observation of mucosal irregularities on barium esophagram. In immunocompromised patients, including people with acquired immunodeficiency syndrome (AIDS), *Candida* esophagitis can occur simultaneously with cytomegalovirus and herpes simplex infection.

Chronic Mucocutaneous Candidiasis

Persistent or recurrent infections of the skin, mucous membranes, and nails with *Candida* is termed chronic mucocutaneous candidiasis.[40] This is a group of disorders in which patients have heterogeneous defects in T-lymphocyte-mediated immunity and a poor proliferation response specifically to *Candida* species. Although often phenotypically similar, the diverse group of underlying disorders and conditions predisposing patients to chronic mucocutaneous candidiasis includes HIV, inhaled corticosteroid use, autoimmune polyendocrinopathy–candidiasis–ectodermal dystrophy, and Job syndrome.[41,42]

Vulvovaginitis

Although vulvovaginitis occurs in 75% of healthy women over the course of their lifetimes, certain conditions are associated with increased risk, including HIV infection, pregnancy, diabetes mellitus, and exposure to broad-spectrum antibiotic agents.[43] Over 80% of cases of vulvovaginitis are caused by *C. albicans*.[44] Symptoms of infection are nonspecific but include pruritus, vaginal discharge, and dysuria.

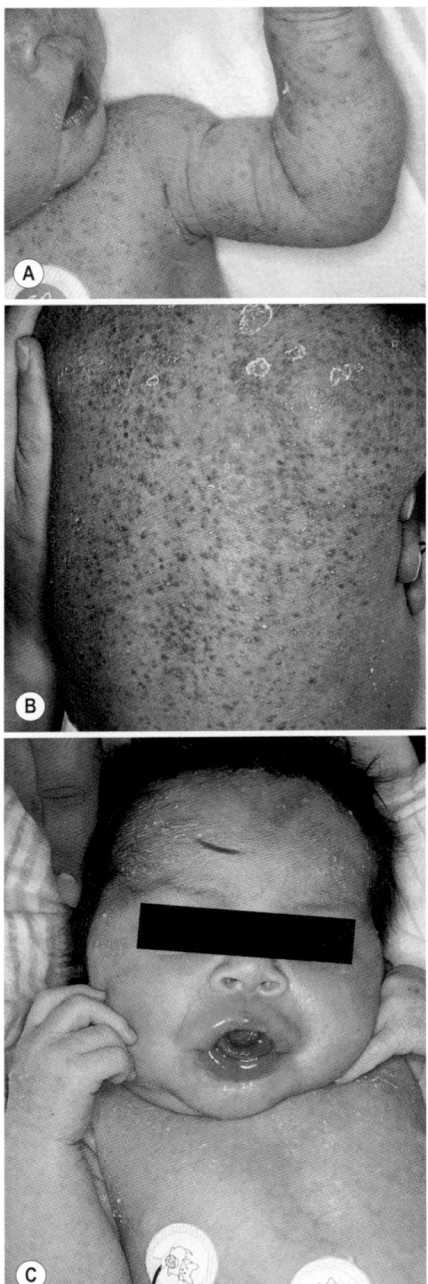

Figure 243-2. Term neonate with the typical exanthem of congenital cutaneous candidiasis on the first day of life **(A, B).** Note superficial papulopustules with erythema. Clearing within a few days is expected **(C).** This infant was treated with amphotericin B. (Courtesy of J.H. Brien©.)

Unique Neonatal Presentations

Congenital cutaneous candidiasis is caused by an ascending infection into the uterus prior to birth. An uncommon clinical condition, the infant at birth has a diffusely erythematous papular rash (Figure 243-2).[45] The papular rash becomes pustular followed by the development of vesicles and bullae. The rash also can develop as a bright red "burn-like" dermatitis usually associated with positive cerebrospinal fluid (CSF), blood, and urine cultures. Infants >1500 g most often experience a benign clinical course. Systemic involvement is more likely in preterm infants and is frequently associated with a markedly elevated white blood cell counts

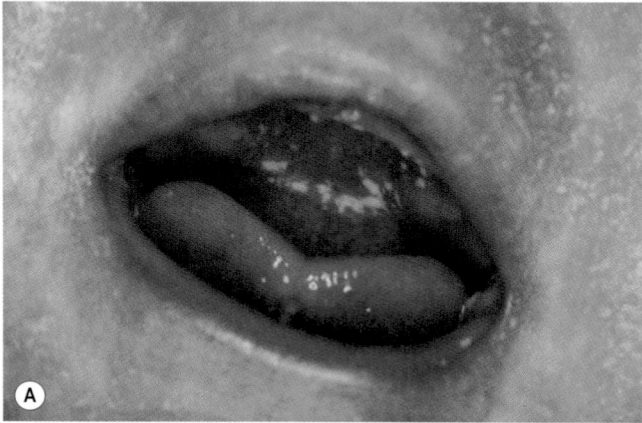

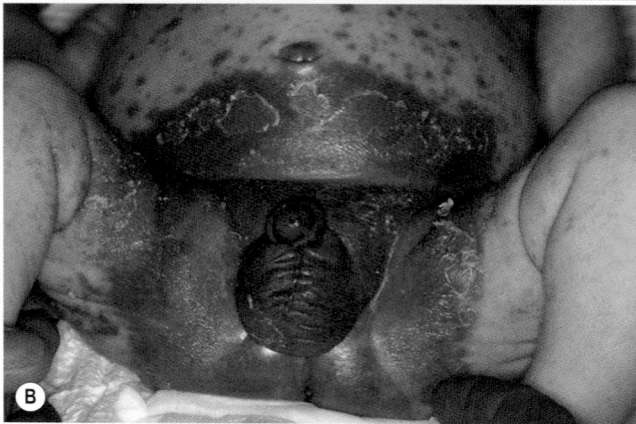

Figure 243-3. One-week-old infant with cutaneous dissemination of *Candida albicans* infection associated with oral thrush **(A)** and extensive diaper dermatitis **(B)**. (Courtesy of J.H. Brien©.)

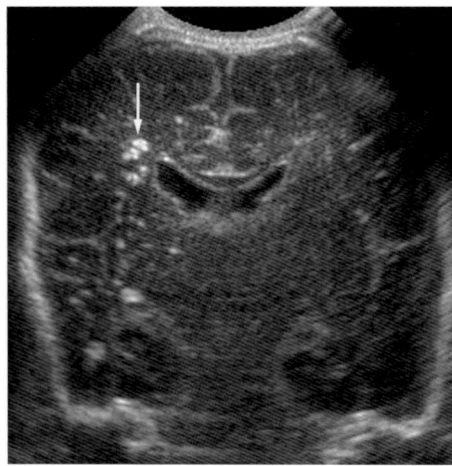

Figure 243-4. Cranial ultrasound showing fungal abscesses seen as hyperechoic regions in a 22-day-old ex-25-week neonate with *Candida albicans* candidemia.

(WBC: >100,000/mm^3). Risk factors for congenital cutaneous candidiasis include the presence of maternal intrauterine device and cerclage placement.[46]

A second dermatologic manifestation in infants is invasive fungal dermatitis. Unlike congenital cutaneous candidiasis, lesions develop after birth but within the first 2 weeks of life (Figure 243-3).[46] The skin is the point of entry and risk factors for development include extreme prematurity, vaginal birth, hyperglycemia, and postnatal corticosteroid administration. The rash of invasive fungal dermatitis is erosive and crusting and is associated with a high incidence of BSI. Definitive diagnosis is made by biopsy.

Invasive *Candida* Infections

Candidemia is defined as isolation of *Candida* from blood cultures. Candidiasis describes all deep-seated *Candida* infections, including candidemia, as well as infections of deep organ(s) (liver, spleen, bone, brain, etc). Candidiasis is rare in immunocompetent children. Infants with candidiasis typically are extremely premature, and children with candidiasis are often immunocompromised due to hematologic malignancy, transplantation, or other primary or secondary immunodeficiency conditions. In addition to poor immunologic status, these patients commonly are exposed to a host of other risk factors, discussed below.

Signs and symptoms of candidemia often are nonspecific and subtle, especially in infants, and can include temperature instability, lethargy, apnea, hypotension, respiratory distress, abdominal distention, hyperglycemia, and feeding intolerance.[11,47] The presentation of candidemia cannot be distinguished readily from bacteremia. In immunocompromised pediatric patients, candidemia often manifests as persistent fever despite antibiotic therapy. Presenting signs and symptoms can result from end-organ (central

nervous system (CNS), renal, hepatic) dissemination following periods of candidemia. Although longer periods of candidemia are associated with increased risk of dissemination, dissemination can occur in the setting of only a single positive blood culture.[11,48]

Meningoencephalitis

Among infants, meningitis is found in approximately 15% of cases of candidemia – a decrease over the past 30 years, but still substantially higher than the incidence of meningitis observed in adults with candidemia.[9] This decrease may be due to more aggressive use of empiric antifungal therapy. The incidence of meningitis in children with cancer and candidemia also is higher than in adult counterparts (11% vs. 1%).[49] This fact has important implications for diagnostic evaluation and therapeutic approaches, as clinicians cannot assume that the CNS is not involved in otherwise seemingly straightforward candidemia.

CNS candidiasis is described most accurately as meningoencephalitis because infection often results in granulomas, parenchymal abscesses, and vasculitis (Figure 243-4). As a result, unremarkable CSF findings in the presence of CNS infection are common.[5,27] Only 25% of infants with *Candida* meningitis had abnormalities noted on CSF examination in one study.[29] Complications of CNS infection include obstructive hydrocephalus, calcifications, and thrombosis.[50] Once involvement of the CNS is suspected or confirmed, imaging (head ultrasound or computed tomography) should be considered.

Renal and Urinary Tract Infections (UTIs)

Candida infections of the renal system include isolated candiduria, fungal debris within the renal collecting system, and renal parenchymal involvement (Figure 243-5).[51] Renal disease can manifest as pyelonephritis, rising creatinine, hypertension, flank mass, or acute urinary obstruction from fungal mycetoma.[52,53] In addition to severely immunocompromised patients at risk for *Candida* infections, children with anatomic obstructions, congenital malformations of the urinary tract, or neurogenic bladder causing urinary stasis are at increased risk for *Candida* urinary tract infection.[51]

Patients with candiduria should have a renal ultrasound performed to evaluate for the two types of renal involvement: nonshadowing echogenic foci and parenchymal infiltration.[52] Often, imaging findings persist despite proper therapy, negative cultures, and clinical recovery.[54] However, caution must be employed in interpreting ultrasound results as blood clots and renal stones can also have a similar appearance to collections of infected

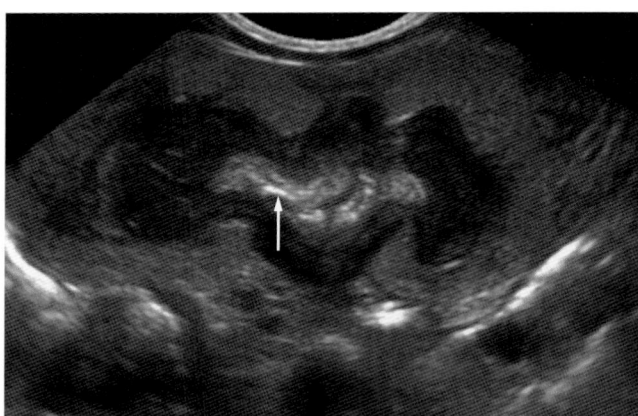

Figure 243-5. Renal ultrasound showing fungal abscess seen as echogenic material within the renal collecting system of a 7-year-old child with acute myelogenous leukemia undergoing induction chemotherapy.

material.[51,52] Fortunately, systemic antifungal therapy is usually sufficient treatment for renal involvement. Surgical intervention usually is indicated only in instances of complete urinary obstruction.[52] Non-neutropenic pediatric patients with uncomplicated candiduria with a Foley catheter in place should have the catheter removed, or replaced, if removal is not possible and do not need systemic antifungal therapy.[55]

Optic Complications

Optic infections can result in chorioretinal infections or, more rarely, lens abscesses.[56,57] As with meningitis, the incidence of chorioretinal lesions complicating candidemia is decreasing.[58,59] Although chorioretinal lesions were found in 28% of adults with candidemia in one series,[60] a review of 123 VLBW infants with candidemia found only 1 patient with optic involvement.[59] Similarly, no ocular findings were discovered in a cohort of 30 pediatric patients with candidemia.[61]

Infants with candidemia in the absence of direct optic infections are at increased risk for the development of severe ROP.[27,28,30,56,62] Although the reason for this association is unclear, cytokines produced in reaction to the infection may play a role.[56] Because of the risk of endophthalmitis and the increased risk of severe ROP among infants, ophthalmologic examination should be considered in all cases of candidemia. These examinations are especially important for the term and near-term infant with candidemia because these infants are not routinely followed for ROP. Systemic antifungal therapy usually is sufficient therapy for chorioretinal infections, but infections of the lens, an avascular structure, may require surgery.[56,63]

Hepatosplenic Candidiasis

Hepatosplenic candidiasis (chronic disseminated candidiasis) (Figures 243-6 and 243-7) occurs predominantly in leukemic patients but can occur in any patient at risk for candidemia. Children can manifest nausea and vomiting, right upper quadrant pain, hepatomegaly, or splenomegaly.[64] Often patients present after recovery of immune function. Blood cultures are positive in as few as 20% of patients with chronic disseminated candidiasis, and biopsy is considered the gold standard for diagnosis.[65]

Other Affected Organs

Endocarditis is documented in 5% or fewer cases of candidemia. Central vascular catheters can cause localized damage to the endocardium and increase the risk for endocarditis, especially in infants.[66,67] Other risk factors for *Candida* endocarditis in children include immunosuppression, congenital heart disease, and corrective surgery for congenital heart disease.[67]

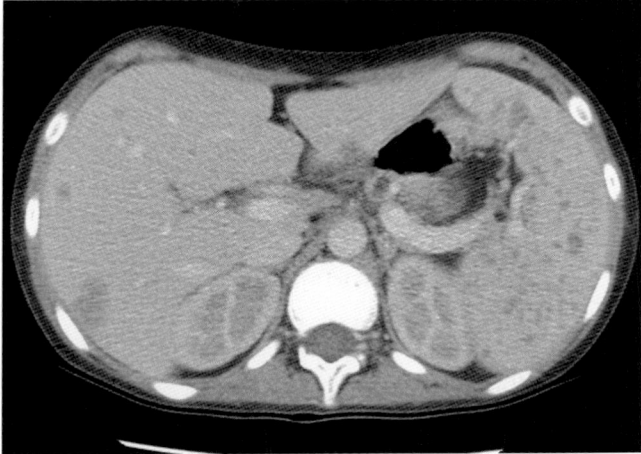

Figure 243-6. Abdominal computed tomography without contrast showing multiple hypodense areas in the spleen and liver due to disseminated *Candida albicans* infection in a 12-year-old child who underwent an unrelated cord blood transplant for acute lymphoblastic leukemia.

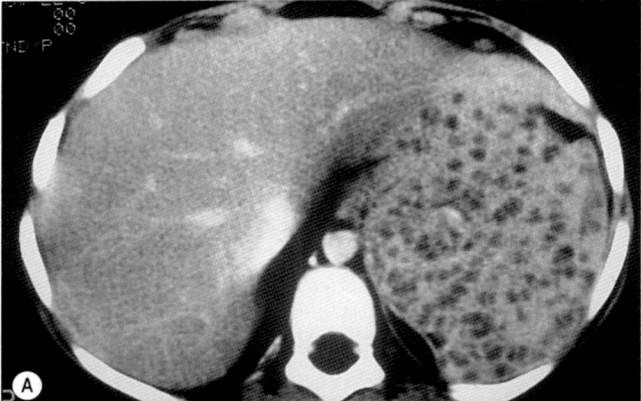

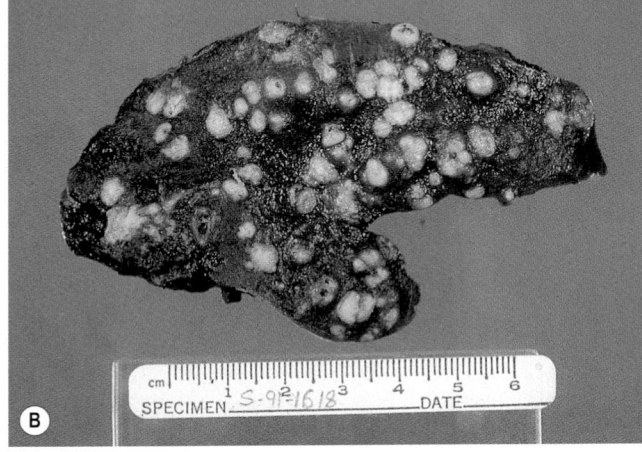

Figure 243-7. Computed tomography **(A)** and gross specimen **(B)** showing multiple granulomatous lesions of *Candida albicans* in a 5-year-old boy with acute lymphoblastic leukemia and prolonged granulocytopenia, and fever despite amphotericin B therapy. (Courtesy of S.S. Long.)

Candidemia also can result in infections of bones and joints, which can become evident days to weeks after control of BSI. Assessment for end-organ damage in the presence of neonatal candidemia should include an ultrasound of the head and abdomen, lumbar puncture, ophthalmologic examination, and an echocardiogram. Candidemia in a pediatric patient should prompt a careful CNS examination, echocardiogram, and ophthalmologic examination.

LABORATORY FINDINGS AND DIAGNOSIS

Routine Tests

Although WBC counts often are used as markers for systemic infections, only 60% of infants with candidiasis have abnormal WBC count.[6] Thrombocytopenia is a more sensitive marker and was found in 84% of VLBW infants with candidemia.[68] However, the specificity of thrombocytopenia is low.[68] Unexpected hyperglycemia can be associated with candidemia in neonates receiving parenteral alimentation.

Blood Culture

The sensitivity of a standard bacterial culture typically is equivalent to using specific fungal culture media. However, the sensitivity of either type of culture is lower for fungi compared with bacteria.[69–71] *Candida* species exhibit a tissue tropism that often leads to deep organ involvement in the absence of prolonged candidemia. Blood culture sensitivity increases with an increasing number of infected deep organs. In an adult study using autopsy reports, sensitivity of blood culture was found to be <30% with a single infected site but increased to 80% when four or more organs were involved.[69] Sensitivity of blood culture in pediatric patients is further compromised by the small volume of blood collected (as little as 0.5 mL in preterm infants vs. >10 mL in adult patients). Although sensitivity is poor, blood culture specificity approaches 100%. Isolation of *Candida* from a blood culture should never be considered a contaminant.

Serology

Serology to detect *Candida* antibodies is seldom used for diagnosis of *Candida* infections.[72] Sensitivity is compromised in the profoundly immunocompromised child with limited antibody production. Specificity also is low as colonized patients often produce antibodies.

Antigen Detection

Limitations to antigen assays include rapid antigen removal by the immune system, use of polyclonal antibodies causing variability in results between assays, variability of cutpoints, and poor assay sensitivity.[72] Also, several assays require the antigen to undergo processing by the immune system, which may not occur reliably in immunocompromised patients. The two antigens used to detect *Candida* are (1,3)-β-D-glucan and mannan.

(1,3)-β-D-glucan is a cell wall component found in most species of *Candida* (and *Aspergillus*) and can be detected in elevated amounts in serum of patients with invasive disease. Using a cutoff value of 60 pg/mL, the assay demonstrated a sensitivity and specificity of 70% and 87%, respectively, in a series of 333 adults with invasive disease.[73] A second study in adults receiving antifungal prophylaxis found the assay to be 90% specific with a 100% negative predictive value.[74] Finally, a study of healthy blood donors and non-neutropenic adults with candidemia found a sensitivity of 93% and specificity of 100%.[75] However, the assay can produce many false-positive results.[76] False-positive tests can be due to a variety of causes, including hemodialysis with a cellulose membranes and exposure of sample to gauze.[77,75]

Two antigen test kits are currently commercially available (Fungitec® G-test, Seikagaku Corporation, Tokyo, Japan; Fungitell®, Associates of Cape Cod, Inc.). There are increasingly more patients evaluated with these newer molecular diagnostic tools, but to date no large pediatric or neonatal series have been conducted.[72,74] A second fungal antigen, mannan, has been found to correlate with invasive disease but assays have limitations of low sensitivity and specificity. Assay sensitivity can be improved by testing at multiple time points.

Fungal Metabolites

D-arabinitol, a sugar alcohol, is produced by *C. albicans*, *C. parapsilosis*, and *C. tropicalis*. D and L-arabinitol are present in normal human urine and serum.[78] Serum D-arabinitol/creatinine ratios were shown to correlate with antifungal treatment response in adults with cancer.[79] In children with invasive candidiasis, the urinary D-arabinitol/L-arabinitol ratio (DA/LA ratio) was noted to be elevated, including all 10 of the children with confirmed invasive candidiasis.[80] In a separate study, the urine DA/LA ratio was found to be elevated in 6 infants infected with *C. albicans* compared with the ratio determined in 40 healthy control infants.[78] Limitations to D-arabinitol as a diagnostic test include low specificity, as colonized patients are known to have elevated D-arabinitol/creatinine levels, the need for GC-mass spectrophotometer equipment, and little or no D-arabinitol production by several pathogenic species of *Candida*.[81] At present this test is not commercially available.

DNA Polymerase Chain Reaction (PCR)

In preliminary studies in adults, PCR is both sensitive and specific for *Candida* as a qualitative diagnostic test,[82] detecting 1 colony-forming unit (CFU)/mL of specimen.[83,84] Sensitivity of PCR as a diagnostic test is optimized by targeting ribosomal DNA genes that contain highly conserved areas (18S, 5.8S, and 28S) which are separated by internal transcribed sequences (ITS1 and ITS2) containing variable, species-specific regions. These genes are present in multiple copies within the *Candida* genome and are an attractive target for amplification as the number of copies of the gene may improves PCR assay sensitivity.[83] Real-time PCR offers several advantages over conventional PCR techniques, including faster detection of amplicon (as detection occurs during cycling) and minimization of contamination (as the reaction vials do not have to be opened). Additionally, real-time PCR allows for the quantification of the amount of starting DNA in the clinical sample, which could aid assessment of response to antifungal therapy.[85]

TREATMENT

Superficial Infections

Thrush typically is treated with oral nystatin suspension. Azole antifungal agents (fluconazole, voriconazole) also are alternatives in recalcitrant disease. *Candida* dermatitis is treated with topical nystatin or miconazole. *Candida* vulvovaginitis is treated with topical antifungal formulations or oral azole agents.

Invasive Infections

If a diagnosis of candidemia is confirmed in a patient with a central venous catheter (CVC) (tunneled, non-tunneled, subcutaneously implanted, or peripherally inserted), the catheter should be removed within 24 hours.[86] Delayed removal of CVC is associated consistently with increased mortality as well as other morbidities, including poor neurodevelopmental outcome in infants.[12] This is a critical tenet of management. Due to the extremely rapid development of *Candida* biofilms on catheters, the notion of treating invasive candidiasis with a contaminated catheter still in place is incorrect.

There are few well-powered randomized controlled trials for treatment of candidiasis in children. A comparison of micafungin (2 mg/kg/day) versus liposomal amphotericin B (3 mg/kg/day) found no difference in treatment success, 73% (35/48) and 76% (38/50) for the micafungin and liposomal amphotericin B groups, respectively.[87] The incidence of adverse events was lower in the micafungin group (4%) compared with the liposomal amphotericin B group (17%). Length of therapy generally should be 3 weeks for infants as CNS involvement should be assumed. In older children, therapy should continue for 2 weeks following documentation of clearance of *Candida* from the bloodstream.

Most clinically important species of *Candida* are susceptible to amphotericin B deoxycholate with the exception of *C. lusitaniae* and occasionally *C. glabrata* and *C. krusei*.[88] Amphotericin B deoxycholate generally is better tolerated in infants compared to older children and adults.[89] Because immediate hypersensitivity reactions are less common in infants, test doses of the drug are not indicated in this population.[90] Lipid preparation of amphotericin B often are used because of renal insufficiency or in patients unable to tolerate amphotericin B deoxycholate. Relatively increased doses of the parent drug can be administered with less associated toxicity. In the one randomized controlled trial of amphotericin B products in infants for the treatment of candidemia, 56 infants (including 36 ELBW infants) were given amphotericin B deoxycholate if their serum creatinine was <1.2 mg/dL ($n = 34$) or either of two liposomal formulations ($n= 22$).[91] No statistical difference in mortality was noted among the three cohorts.

Flucytosine (5-FC) is not an option as monotherapy for candidiasis because resistance develops rapidly. Use of 5-FC for candidiasis is further limited by lack of a parenteral formulation in the United States and adverse effects (predominantly intestinal mucosal damage and neutropenia). The use of flucytosine in preterm neonates is not recommended because of the immaturity of the preterm infant's renal system and need for monitoring of serum levels.[92] However, 5-FC occasionally is administered in combination with other antifungal agents for *Candida* meningoencephalitis because of good CNS penetration.[93] In a cohort of 17 cases of *Candida* meningitis (including 11 infants), improvement was noted in 15 patients receiving combination therapy of amphotericin B deoxycholate and 5-FC.[94]

Fluconazole is used commonly to treat candidiasis in infants and children.[95] The two most common species of *Candida* found in infants and children, *C. albicans* and *C. parapsilosis*, almost always are susceptible to fluconazole. However, 50% of *C. glabrata* and 100% of *C. krusei* isolates are resistant to fluconazole.[96] Children >3 months of age require 6–12 mg/kg per day to achieve comparable adult exposures. In premature infants, 12 mg/kg per day is necessary to achieve exposures similar to older children and adults,[97] and a loading dose of 25 mg/kg may be needed to achieve steady-state concentrations sooner than the traditional dosing scheme.[98] Voriconazole has a wider spectrum of activity against *Candida* than fluconazole and is active in vitro against some isolates of *C. glabrata* and *C. krusei* that are resistant to fluconazole. The pharmacokinetics of voriconazole have been described in children as young as 2 years of age (Table 243-1).[99-101]

Echinocandins (micafungin, anidulafungin, and caspofungin) are fungicidal for all clinically significant species of *Candida*. Side effects are minimal in older patients, and the tolerability to echinocandins is superior to amphotericin B deoxycholate.[102] Recent studies have examined the pharmacokinetics of the echinocandins in pediatric subjects (Table 243-1).[103-108] Although micafungin levels are undetectable in the CSF,[109] the drug penetrates and cures invasive fungal infections in CNS tissue in animal models.[109] Higher systemic exposures in the premature infant are thought to be important to drive the antifungal agent into the CNS.[110]

SPECIAL CONSIDERATIONS

Development of invasive disease is the result of an interaction between the virulence factors of the *Candida* species, colonization burden, and host immunologic function. Specific risk factors for invasive disease tend to fall in one of two categories: those that increase colonization of mucosal surfaces or those that disrupt or impair immune function.[111]

Risk Factors Increasing Colonization

Infants are initially colonized by vertical transmission during birth or horizontally by parents or caregivers.[112,113] On admission to the NICU, 5% to 10% of all infants were found to be colonized with *Candida* when cultures were taken from the oropharynx, skin, endotracheal tube aspirate, and rectum.[114] VLBW infants were found to be colonized at slightly higher rates. By 7 days of life colonization rates increased to 50%, and later rose to 64% by 1 month of age.[112,115,116]

Risk Factors Increasing Invasion

After *Candida* colonization of the gastrointestinal (GI) tract and skin, any penetration of the epithelial barrier through immature neonatal skin or iatrogenic delivery of medical care allows for hematogenous dissemination.[112,115,117] A study of VLBW infants found that invasive disease developed in 8% (3/39) of those with *Candida* colonization and in none of the non-colonized infants.[114] Endotracheal colonization has been associated with a sixfold increased risk of candidiasis.[116] In a trial of fluconazole prophylaxis, there was a threefold increase in risk for the development of invasive disease with each additional skin site of *Candida* colonization.[118] A study of pediatric liver transplant recipients also identified colonization as a risk factor for candidiasis.[119]

Use of broad-spectrum antibiotics enhances *Candida* colonization and density by destroying competing bacterial flora.[5] In a cohort of over 6000 infants, expanded-spectrum cephalosporin or carbapenem use in the previous 7 days was associated with candidiasis.[120]

High serum glucose levels provide substrate for fungal growth and have been reported in a higher percentage of infants with candidiasis.[121] Hyperglycemia also can lead to decreased neutrophil mobility, upregulation of genes for adhesion proteins and proteins impairing the ability of complement to opsonize fungus.[122] Gastric acidity is considered to be protective against *Candida* infection by suppressing fungal growth in the upper GI tract. Acid-reducing drugs such as histamine-2 (H_2)-blocking and proton pump-inhibiting agents have been shown to increase *Candida* overgrowth in the GI tract of adults.[123] The use of H_2-blockers has been linked to an increase risk of candidemia in infants.[25] H_2-blocking agents also can increase the risk of infection by inhibiting neutrophil function.[124]

In almost every instance, candidiasis affects patients in whom the immune function is compromised. Prematurity is the strongest risk factor for invasive disease in infants. The immune system of the preterm infant has defects in chemotaxis, cytokine and antibody production, and phagocytosis.[48,125] In addition to defects in both cellular and humoral immune response, the need for invasive medical devices such as CVCs and endotracheal tubes compromises an already underdeveloped layer of skin and places the preterm infant at an especially high risk for candidiasis.

TABLE 243-1. Dosing of Pediatric Antifungal Agents for Candidiasis

Drug	Formulation	Pediatric Dose	Infant Dose
POLYENES			
Amphotericin B deoxycholate	IV	0.5–1 mg/kg/day	1 mg/kg/day
TRIAZOLES			
Fluconazole	IV, PO	6–12 mg/kg/day	12 mg/kg/day
Voriconazole	IV, PO	16 mg/kg/day divided q12h	N/A
ECHINOCANDINS			
Caspofungin	IV	50 mg/m²/day (70 mg/m²/day loading dose)	25 mg/m²/day
Micafungin	IV	4–8 mg/kg/day	10 mg/kg/day
Anidulafungin	IV	1.5 mg/kg/day (3 mg/kg loading dose)	1.5 mg/kg/day (3 mg/kg loading dose)[a]

IV, intravenous; PO, oral; N/A, not available.

[a]*Does not include neonates.*

A defect in neutrophil function or number is an important risk factor for the development of candidiasis.[126,127] These defects in neutrophil number or function can be the result of primary immune defects (chronic granulomatous disease) or secondary defects (cytotoxic chemotherapy). The role of neutrophils includes phagocytosis of yeast and hyphal elements, as well as the elaboration of cytokines stimulating other components of the immune system.[128]

The presence of a CVC, commonly used in immunocompromised patients, also allows formation of a thrombin sheath to which *Candida* can adhere and grow. The thrombin sheath protects the growing organisms from host immune defenses. Presence of a CVC has been associated with the development of candidemia in both infants and children.[6,129] In addition, some *Candida* isolates are able to produce a biofilm, providing additional protection from immunologic attack and antifungal drug activity. The ability to produce a biofilm occurs more often in non-*albicans* species such as *C. parapsilosis* and *C. tropicalis*.[130] Persistence of candidemia may be related to biofilm development, as reported in one study in which 100% (22/22) of *C. parapsilosis* isolates from adults with multiple positive blood cultures produced biofilms, compared with only 62% (8/13) of isolates from patients with only one positive culture.[130]

The use of corticosteroids such as hydrocortisone and dexamethasone is associated with increased risk of candidiasis in infants and children.[49,131–133] Corticosteroids, in addition to immune system suppression, can upregulate *Candida* virulence genes,[134] and corticosteroid-induced hyperglycemia also can predispose to infection.[22]

Among adult ICU patients, patients in surgical ICUs have the greatest risk of candidiasis.[135] Abdominal surgeries that compromise the barrier of the intestinal lumen may allow translocation of *Candida* into the bloodstream.[25,47,136] Surgical patients are also at heightened risk because of frequent exposure to broad-spectrum antibiotics and CVCs.[136]

PREVENTION

Non-Absorbable Oral Agents

Use of non-absorbable oral agents for prevention of neonatal candidemia is controversial. A randomized controlled trial of 65 infants given nystatin or placebo demonstrated a significant decrease in both colonization rates and invasive *Candida* infections (6% in the nystatin group versus 32% in the placebo group).[137] However, no difference in mortality or duration of stay

was noted, and the significance of this decrease is difficult to interpret as the infection rate for the control group is substantially higher than the rate predicted from other multicenter trials.[14,24] No decrease in candidiasis was observed in a placebo-controlled trial of 600 infants <1750 g birthweight given oral miconazole gel.[138] A small randomized study of 50 pediatric patients comparing oral nystatin (50,000 units/kg per day divided into doses every 6 hours) to oral fluconazole (3 mg/kg per day) demonstrated no difference in the cumulative incidence of candidiasis (8% in the nystatin group versus 4% in the fluconazole group).[139] Large multicenter randomized trials of oral agents for prophylaxis are needed before recommendations can be made regarding their efficacy.[140]

Fluconazole

The pharmacokinetics of fluconazole make it an attractive drug for prophylaxis. Fluconazole has good enteral absorption, excellent CSF penetration, and a long half-life allowing for long dosing intervals.[98] The drug is metabolized by the kidney and is excreted 80% unchanged in the urine.[141]

Several placebo-controlled trials have evaluated fluconazole prophylaxis in preterm infants. The first study enrolled 103 VLBW infants and demonstrated decreased rates of colonization but no difference in invasive disease.[115] The second study of 100 ELBW infants found a significant decrease in the incidence of candidiasis.[118] The placebo arm in this study had one of the highest rates (20%) of invasive candidiasis reported in ELBW infants, making the results of the study difficult to interpret. Neither study demonstrated a statistical difference in mortality between cohorts. A randomized multicenter study of 322 VLBW infants showed significant reductions in invasive candidiasis in fluconazole versus placebo recipients but no difference in all-cause mortality.[142] Again, the rate of candidiasis (13%) in the control group was much higher than generally is reported.

Experience with fluconazole as an agent for prophylaxis in older children has also been mixed. A randomized study in pediatric patients compared oral fluconazole with oral nystatin in 50 children undergoing cancer chemotherapy.[139] One patient in the fluconazole group developed *Candida* colitis. An additional patient in the fluconazole group and two patients in the nystatin group required empiric antifungal therapy. A second, nonrandomized study of fluconazole prophylaxis in afebrile neutropenic pediatric patients demonstrated three breakthrough fungal infections among the 24 treated patients,[143] including two fluconazole-resistant *Candida* species and one *Aspergillus* infection.

Key Points. Diagnosis and Management of *Candida* Infection	
EPIDEMIOLOGY • *Candida albicans* is the most common species • Non-*albicans Candida* species are increasing in many centers **CLINICAL FEATURES** • Certain patient populations are at highest risk (surgical intensive care, neutropenic) • *Candida* meningitis is underdiagnosed in the neonatal population • Known neonatal risk factors include cephalosporin or carbapenem use **DIAGNOSIS** • Blood cultures still are the standard, yet often are not sensitive (especially in neonates due to blood volume issues) • Newer PCR and molecular testing are in research stages currently • Negative culture results do not rule out disease definitively	**TREATMENT** • Echinocandin therapy is preferred for more severe disease/ill-appearing patients • Azole therapy is adequate for less severe disease/stable patients • Antifungal resistance is increasing, especially in non-*albicans Candida* species • Optimal antifungal dosing for pediatric patients is crucial • *Candida*-contaminated central venous catheters should be removed as soon as possible; biofilm formation begins rapidly **DURATION OF THERAPY** • Treatment for candidemia is at least 14 days after first negative culture • Evaluation for dissemination is recommended (see text)

244 *Aspergillus* Species

William J. Steinbach

Although yeasts such as *Candida* species remain the most common invasive fungal infections in children, the incidence of *Aspergillus* infections is increasing and carries a dismal mortality.[1-3] Invasive aspergillosis is likely gaining prominence due to more intensive chemotherapies for certain malignancies, immunosuppressive therapies for graft-versus-host disease (GvHD), increased use of mismatched or unrelated donor transplantations, newer preparative regimens to avoid rejection or relapse, and increase in early posttransplantation survival rate due to better control of bacterial and cytomegalovirus (CMV) infections.[1,4]

MICROBIOLOGY

The genus *Aspergillus* contains nearly 200 separate species, only approximately two dozen of which are known to cause human disease. Human disease is primarily caused by *A. fumigatus, A. flavus, A. niger, A. terreus,* and *A. nidulans,* with each species at times generating unique clinical entities. *A. fumigatus* is responsible for the vast majority of clinical disease with invasive and chronic aspergillosis,[5] specifically pulmonary, sinus, and central nervous system infection. Isolated sinus disease can also be caused by *A. niger* and *A. flavus,*[6] and ear disease in immunocompetent children can often be due to *A. niger.* A review of *Aspergillus* cultures found that amphotericin B-resistant *A. terreus* accounted for only 3% of isolates in cases of invasive aspergillosis, but was found exclusively in cases of invasive disease and not in patients with colonization.[6]

The ecological niche of *Aspergillus* species is the soil, especially thriving in compost, where they function as saprophytic fungi growing on organic debris and recycle carbon and nitrogen throughout the environment.[7] No defined sexual stage has been identified for *A. fumigatus,* although it possesses the genetic machinery, and this fact has long hampered molecular investigation of this most pathogenic *Aspergillus* species. *A. nidulans* is the more distantly related model organism that also can cause human disease. *A. nidulans* is easily trackable genetically and more often is studied in the laboratory, yet it is unclear how general pathogenesis findings translate from the model organism to *A. fumigatus.* Asexual reproduction in all *Aspergillus* species is abundant and is characterized by the production of green pigmented asexual conidia (spores). The conidia are produced in long chains radiating from phialides, and this reproductive structure is where the genus name *Aspergillus* is derived – from the aspergillum used to spread holy water during the Catholic Mass.

Aspergillus aerosolize conidia, which immunocompetent people asymptomatically breathe everyday; it has been estimated that most people inhale several hundred *A. fumigatus* conidia per day. Invasive infection in severely immunocompromised patients, or allergic or chronic infection in immunocompetent and less immunocompromised patients, usually is acquired through inhalation of airborne conidia. Two lines of host defense against *Aspergillus* exist, macrophages and neutrophils, and it appears that both are required for resistance to invasive disease. The first defense is formed by alveolar macrophages and in vitro murine studies have suggested that resident pulmonary macrophages are responsible for eliminating inhaled *Aspergillus* conidia from the lung.[8,9] If inhaled conidia escape, conidia germinate into the invasive *Aspergillus* hyphae and become susceptible to neutrophil killing through the release of toxic reactive oxygen species.[10] The host can develop disease through neutropenia, high challenge doses of conidia overcoming macrophages, or corticosteroid suppression of macrophage conidiacidal activity.[11]

A. fumigatus, in particular, is highly successful in colonizing and causing invasive disease in immunocompromised patients. *A. fumigatus* has several characteristics that allow it to be a successful saprophyte and opportunistic pathogen. The ability to grow at 37 °C is crucial for the development of human disease and *A. fumigatus* is thermotolerant and thrives at human body temperature. Conidia are small (2.5 to 3 µm in diameter) and this size allows them to remain buoyant in the air for prolonged periods of time and be inhaled deep into the lung alveoli. When inhaled by an immunocompetent person, conidia rarely have deleterious effects as they are cleared by the phagocytic cells of the innate immune system. However, severe allergic disease can occur with repeated exposure to large doses of conidia.

Whole genome sequencing of several *Aspergillus* species has spurred molecular advances, coupled with newer proteomic techniques. Various suspected putative *Aspergillus* virulence factors have been exhaustively reviewed[12] and gene disruption studies have examined proteases, toxins, hemolysins, melanin pigmentation, and other gene products with little insight into true pathogenesis. Species of *Aspergillus* are also well known for their production of secondary metabolites, including the carcinogen aflatoxin produced by some strains of *A. flavus,* which plays an unclear role in human invasive fungal disease. The true virulence of *A. fumigatus* is likely multifactorial, and likely also weighs heavily on the host condition.

CLINICAL PRESENTATION

Aspergillus species produce a spectrum of disease, including allergic bronchopulmonary aspergillosis (ABPA), aspergilloma, chronic necrotizing aspergillosis, and various forms of invasive aspergillosis.[12] The most common forms of invasive aspergillosis are acute pulmonary aspergillosis, acute invasive rhinosinusitis, cerebral aspergillosis, and disseminated disease. As with most invasive mold infections, the clinical signs and symptoms are nonspecific. Unfortunately, the most immunocompromised patients are those least likely to have symptoms and progress most rapidly, whereas less immunocompromised patients (e.g., patients with diabetes mellitus or chronic corticosteroid use) usually have more indolent symptomatic presentations.[5]

Pulmonary Infection

Separate clinical manifestations in different patient populations have been reviewed,[5] but disease in most immunocompromised patients often is bilateral diffuse pulmonary infection (Figure 244-1). The most common presentation is unremitting fever in a high-risk patient,[3] but high fever can be absent in patients receiving corticosteroid therapy.[13] Other early symptoms of pulmonary disease include a dry cough, and possibly chest pain. Dyspnea is more common is patients with diffuse disease, and the presentation in some patients is similar to that of a pulmonary embolism. Hemoptysis can occur and can be fatal with the first presenting episode,[14] while in neutropenic patients, pneumothorax also is an occasional presenting feature.[5]

Invasive pulmonary aspergillosis is the leading cause of mortality in patients with chronic granulomatous disease (CGD), and can be the first manifestation of CGD. Invasive aspergillosis in patients with CGD usually manifests within the first 20 years of life; invasive aspergillosis in a child or adult without a known predisposing risk factor should prompt an evaluation for CGD. Patients with CGD can lack typical clinical symptoms (including

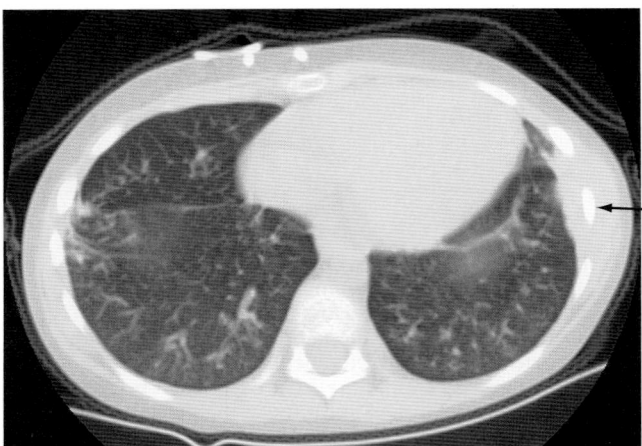

Figure 244-1. Axial CT of the chest (lung window) in a 12-year-old child with history of acute myelobastic leukemia and cord blood transplant showing diffuse interstitial disease, with pleural thickening and soft-tissue involvement on the left (arrow). Bronchoalveolar lavage culture grew *Aspergillus terreus*.

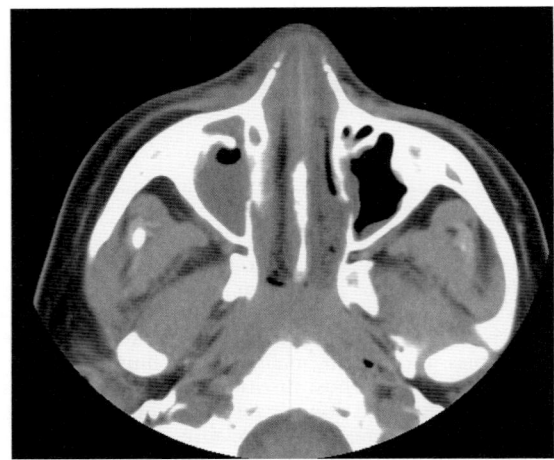

Figure 244-3. Axial CT of the sinuses in a 17-year-old with combined variable immunodeficiency showing opacification of the right maxillary sinus and minor thickening of the left maxillary sinus. Sinus aspirate culture grew *Aspergillus fumigatus*.

being completely asymptomatic), or can be afebrile and have only an elevated erythrocyte sedimentation rate (ESR). In a review of clinical findings at diagnosis of invasive aspergillosis in 23 patients with CGD, only one-third were symptomatic, only one-fifth were febrile; one-half had white blood count <10,000 cells/mm³, and almost one-half had ESR <40 mm/hour.[15]

In early disease in a patient with CGD there is an acute neutrophilic response, and neutrophils surround hyphae. However, hyphae remain intact due to impaired neutrophil-mediated killing. In this setting, pulmonary aspergillosis is a chronic progressive infection that can spread locally to involve pleura, vertebrae, and the chest wall (Figure 244-2). In contrast to patients with neutropenia, hyphal angioinvasion is not a feature of disease in patients with CGD. The halo sign (angioinvasion with surrounding tissue ischemia), cavitated lesions, and pulmonary infarcts seen in neutropenic patients are not seen typically in CGD. Areas of tissue destruction are secondary to reactive acute and granulomatous inflammatory process rather than due directly to growth of the hyphae.[16] Infection with *A. nidulans* is more common in patients with CGD, with pulmonary disease more likely to involve adjacent bone, more likely to cause disseminated disease, generally refractory to intensive antifungal therapy, and more likely to require surgery in CGD than in non-CGD patients.[17]

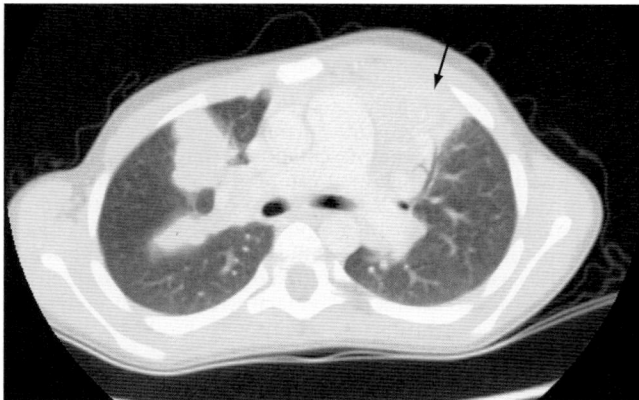

Figure 244-2. Axial CT of the chest (lung window) postcontrast in an 11-year-old child with chronic granulomatous disease and cord blood transplant, showing chest mass extending to soft tissues (arrow), bilateral consolidations, and lymphadenopathy. Chest mass biopsy culture grew *Aspergillus fumigatus*.

Invasive Sinusitis

Invasive *Aspergillus* sinusitis likely is underdiagnosed due to lack of detailed examination, but patients can come to medical attention with ear pain or discharge, facial pain or swelling, localized pallor of the nasal septum or turbinate mucosa, epistaxis, orbital swelling, or headache.[5,13] The maxillary sinus is involved most commonly (Figure 244-3), followed by the ethmoid, sphenoid, and frontal sinuses.[18] A careful rhinoscopic examination is needed to look for insensitive areas with decreased blood flow, frank crusting or ulceration, or blackened necrotic foci. One study reviewed 11 patients with invasive fungal sinusitis after bone marrow transplantation, including 8 patients with *Aspergillus*. The mean interval from bone marrow transplantation to diagnosis of fungal sinusitis was 22 days and all patients had maxillary sinus involvement, one-half also had ethmoid sinusitis, and the majority of patients showed extension into the orbits, bone, or brain.[18] One major difficulty is the critically important diagnostic distinction between zygomycosis and aspergillosis, due to the divergent therapeutic approaches. In one study evaluating pulmonary aspergillosis and pulmonary zygomycosis, concomitant sinusitis was significantly associated with zygomycosis and not aspergillosis in patients with radiographic pulmonary disease.[19]

Cerebral Infection

Cerebral involvement occurs in up to 40% of patients with invasive aspergillosis.[3,20] The pathogenesis is thought to be hematogenous dissemination from an extracranial focus, most commonly the lung, or direct extension through the sinuses. *Aspergillus* hyphae are angioinvasive and thrombose arteries to create hemorrhagic infarcts, which then become abscesses (Figure 244-4). Cerebral aspergillosis is the most common brain abscess in hematopoietic stem cell transplant (HSCT) recipients; in one study 58% of brain abscesses were caused by *Aspergillus* and 87% of these patients had concomitant pulmonary infection.[21] In another report of 18 patients with invasive aspergillosis, 10 patients had cerebral involvement, including 3 patients who presented with neurologic signs and no pulmonary symptoms.[22] The classic features of abscesses such as headache, nausea, and vomiting can be present in <10% of cases, with more prevalent features including altered mental status, confusion, hemiparesis, and cranial nerve palsies. Multiple lesions in the corticomedullary junction are consistent with infarct due to *Aspergillus* vasculopathy, with dilated cortical vessels located in the central portion of the lesions in the corticomedullary junction often a distinctive sign of cerebral aspergillosis.[23] Definitive diagnosis requires a brain biopsy, but

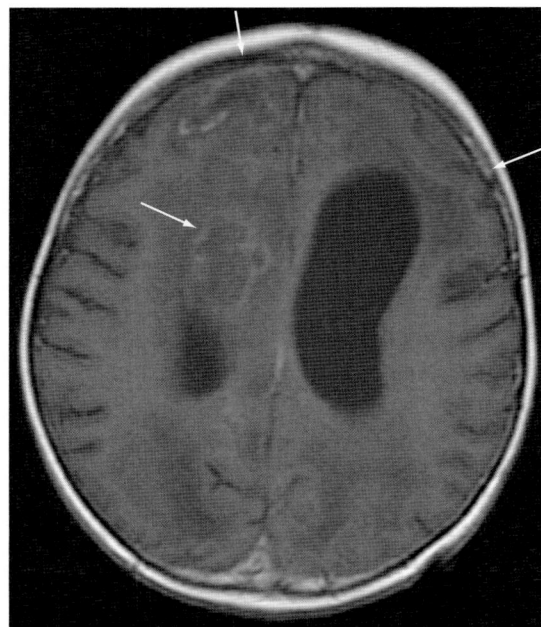

Figure 244-4. Axial contrast-enhanced MRI in a 3-year-old child with history of medulloblastoma showing ventricular dilatation and multifocal abscesses (arrows). Brain biopsy culture grew *Aspergillus fumigatus*.

these patients often are too coagulopathic for the diagnostic operation.

Cutaneous Infection

Cutaneous aspergillosis can be either primary, usually from skin injury or traumatic inoculation, or secondary from contiguous extension of hematogenous dissemination. In general, burn victims, neonates, and solid-organ transplant recipients develop cutaneous inoculation after prolonged local skin injury. HSCT recipients often develop secondary disease from contiguous extension of infected structures under the skin or from hematogenously disseminated embolic lesions.[24] In a review of >4000 patients with malignancy, 15 had documented *Aspergillus* cutaneous infection,[25] while in another review, embolic skin lesions were present in approximately 11% of patients with disseminated aspergillosis.[26]

Cutaneous aspergillosis often begins as an area of raised erythema that progresses to include pain; skin involvement can be the first presenting sign of invasive infection.[27] The center of the lesion changes from red to purple, and then to black, and can ulcerate.[5] Infections arising at the site of an intravenous catheter puncture typically begin with erythema and induration and progress to necrosis that extends radially.[28] Compared with wound mucormycosis, patients with primary cutaneous aspergillosis appear to present with significantly less necrosis and systemic toxicity.[24]

Chronic Pulmonary Aspergillosis

Acute invasive aspergillosis almost uniformly occurs in patients with profound immunosuppression and displays rapid progression with poor outcome. However, some patients clearly have a more chronic *Aspergillus* infection. Chronic aspergillosis previously has been known by several different terms, most notably semi-invasive aspergillosis, chronic invasive pulmonary aspergillosis, and symptomatic pulmonary aspergillosis. The blurred entity of chronic aspergillosis has been reclassified[29] to include chronic cavitary pulmonary aspergillosis, in which imaging findings are formation and expansion of multiple cavities with some containing fungus balls; chronic fibrosing pulmonary aspergillosis, which denotes progress to marked and extensive pulmonary fibrosis; and chronic necrotizing pulmonary aspergillosis, or

subacute invasive pulmonary aspergillosis. These patients have a mild or moderate defect in immune function, and their course is unlike that of the other two chronic classifications in which there is a slow and progressive enlargement of an *Aspergillus*-containing cavity. Surgery appears to play a smaller role in managing chronic aspergillosis, and the mainstay of treatment is long-term antifungal therapy to halt the progression of disease. While there have been no randomized clinical trials demonstrating the benefit of antifungal therapy in chronic aspergillosis, anecdotal evidence suggests slow improvement.[29]

Pulmonary Aspergilloma

Aspergilloma is considered a "saprophytic", or noninvasive, form of infection in which *Aspergillus* colonizes pre-existing pulmonary cavities due to tuberculosis, sarcoidosis, bullous emphysema, bronchiectasis, or other etiologies. Aspergilloma develops in approximately 15% to 25% of patients with cavitating lung disease due to tuberculosis.[30] Disease can be divided into simple and complex aspergillomas based on radiographic criteria. The simple aspergilloma can be differentiated from the complex aspergilloma by the absence of constitutional symptoms, paracystic lung opacities, cyst expansion, or progressive pleural thickening.[31] In one study of 62 cases of pulmonary aspergilloma, chest radiograph showed a "fungus ball" in the cavities of 42 (67%) and thickening of the cavity wall in 16 (26%) cases.[32] Patients with aspergilloma can be asymptomatic, but many have persistent and productive cough, hemoptysis, and weight loss. Surgical management to completely eradicate the aspergilloma is the preferred treatment. Although the postoperative morbidity rate is higher in complex aspergilloma, in one series of 88 patients, surgical management led to nearly equivalent (80%) survival rates in both patients with simple or complex aspergilloma.[33] Systemic antifungal therapy often is unsuccessful as penetrance of the antifungal agent into the cavity is poor. Percutaneous intracavitary instillation of antifungal therapy designed to fill the cavity and create an anaerobic environment for the *Aspergillus* has led to some success,[34] but should be reserved for inoperable patients.[35]

Allergic Bronchopulmonary Aspergillosis

Allergic bronchopulmonary aspergillosis (ABPA) is a hypersensitivity lung disease resulting from sensitization to environmental exposure to allergens of *A. fumigatus*. In this condition, *A. fumigatus* grows saprophytically to colonize the bronchial lumen and results in persistent bronchial inflammation. Conidia trigger an IgE-mediated allergic inflammatory response in the bronchial airways, leading to bronchial obstruction. ABPA is primarily a disease of patients with asthma (1% to 2%) or cystic fibrosis (1% to 15%). The disease manifestations are due to the immunologic responses to the *A. fumigatus* antigens and include wheezing, pulmonary infiltrates, bronchiectasis, and fibrosis. Immunologic manifestations include peripheral blood eosinophilia, immediate cutaneous reactivity to *A. fumigatus* antigen, elevated total levels of serum IgE, presence of precipitating antibody to *A. fumigatus*, and elevated specific serum IgE and IgG antibodies to *A. fumigatus*.[36]

The mainstay of therapy for ABPA is corticosteroid therapy for attenuation of the inflammation and immunologic activity, while antifungal therapy is used to decrease the fungal burden and therefore the antigen load. In a randomized, double-blind study, itraconazole was found to be superior to placebo for treatment of ABPA.[37] While data are questionably sufficient to recommend itraconazole for initial therapy for ABPA exacerbation, itraconazole should be added to therapy if there is a slow or poor response to corticosteroids[36] as part of a two-armed approach to optimize therapy.

EPIDEMIOLOGY AND RISK FACTORS

Epidemiology

In a review of over 5500 patients who underwent HSCT during a 15-year period, >7% had mold infections, including 342 patients with proven or probable *Aspergillus*, 31 patients with *Fusarium*, 29 with Zygomycetes, and 10 with *Scedosporium* infections.[1] Aspergillosis is the leading cause of infectious death in HSCT recipients and one study showed that 36% of all confirmed nosocomial pneumonia in these patients was caused by *Aspergillus*, with an attendant crude mortality of 95%.[38] The incidence of *Aspergillus* infection in HSCT recipients has ranged from 3% to 7%,[14,20] but the true incidence is likely dependent on the follow up duration of individual studies. In a retrospective review of 409 patients, 13% had invasive aspergillosis, which accounted for 17% of all isolated pathogens in allogeneic transplant recipients and nearly 4% in autologous transplant recipients.[39] A review of patients from 1990 through 1998 found an increasing incidence of invasive aspergillosis in both allogeneic transplants (5% increasing to 12%) and autologous transplants (1% increasing to 5%). Importantly, the incidence of non-*A. fumigatus* species as the cause of invasive pulmonary disease also increased dramatically after 1995 (18% increasing to 34%).[1] In another study of HSCT patients with invasive aspergillosis, the risk of developing the disease was 12.8 times higher among recipients of allogeneic than autologous HSCT.[40] The incidence of invasive aspergillosis is possibly higher in unrelated donors due to more complicated immunobiology and more immunosuppressive treatment regimens required.

There is a well-characterized bimodal distribution of aspergillosis in HSCT recipients, which correlates with pre-engraftment neutropenia with a median of 16 days, and the peak of GvHD with a median of 96 days.[41] This likely relates to the two major mechanisms of protection against invasive aspergillosis, alveolar macrophages and neutrophils. Most patients with autologous transplants were diagnosed with invasive aspergillosis while neutropenic, while patients with allogeneic transplants were at greatest risk after engraftment or during impairment of cell-mediated immunity due to CMV or GvHD.[41] As early posttransplant management and survival improves, the peak of invasive aspergillosis appears to be shifting to the outpatient setting. In large reviews of patients undergoing allogeneic HSCT, invasive aspergillosis was diagnosed at a mean of 88 to 115 days post transplantation,[3,22,40,42] with mortality exceeding 80%. In some studies most cases were diagnosed after posttransplant day 30,[40,42] and in another study no cases of invasive aspergillosis were diagnosed during the neutropenic period following transplantation.[43]

Risk Factors

The risk of invasive aspergillosis is calculated to increase from 1% per day after the first 3 weeks of neutropenia to 4% to 5% per day after 5 weeks,[44] with a 70% incidence after neutropenia exceeds 34 days.[45] Prolonged or marked macrophage dysfunctions that occur as a result of underlying disease and its treatment also can predispose patients to invasive aspergillosis. Therefore, risk of infection is higher with advanced underlying disease, transplantation during relapse of malignancy or chemotherapeutic rescue therapy, GvHD, or concurrent infection such as CMV.[44] In a survey of 24 medical centers of 148 invasive aspergillosis patients, 30% also had a bacterial infection, 20% also had a viral infection, and 19% also had another fungal infection.[6]

Numerous studies repeatedly have shown risk factors for invasive aspergillosis to be: older age, receipt of an HSCT from an HLA-mismatched or unrelated donor, and underlying disease.[1,41] Corticosteroids are a well-known major risk factor for the development of invasive aspergillosis and can suppress the ability of monocytes/macrophages to kill conidia through inhibition of nonoxidative processes and impairment of lysosomal activity. Corticosteroids also inhibit polymorphonuclear neutrophils in their chemotaxis, oxidative bursts, and activity against hyphae.[46] Generally, corticosteroids suppress macrophages while cytotoxic chemotherapies decreased neutrophil number and function. Corticosteroids also greatly accelerate the growth of *A. fumigatus*, in one study decreasing the doubling time to only 48 minutes.[47]

In several HSCT patient risk factor studies only moderate-severe GvHD and corticosteroid prophylaxis for GvHD[3,42,48,49] or total body irradiation[48] were significant variables in the multivariate analyses. In one study several factors in the period from HSCT to diagnosis of fungal infection influenced survival, all of which were related to cumulative dose of prednisolone. In multivariate analysis, relative risk of death from invasive aspergillosis was 8.8 in patients with acute active GvHD (grade 2 or more) or extensive chronic GvHD combined with a cumulative total prednisolone dose of >7 mg/kg dose in the week prior to diagnosis.[3]

There have been few pediatric studies performed to examine risk factors for invasive aspergillosis. One study found that the highest incidence of invasive aspergillosis was seen in children who had undergone allogeneic bone marrow transplantation (4.5%) and those with acute myelogenous leukemia (4%). Specifically, the incidence of invasive aspergillosis in patients with acute myelogenous leukemia was significantly greater than the incidence in patients with acute lymphoblastic leukemia (relative risk, 5.6; 95% confidence interval, 4.6 to 7.0).[50]

DIAGNOSIS

Cultures

A definitive diagnosis of aspergillosis requires isolation of the mold from culture and histologic demonstration.[51] The "gold standard" of tissue biopsy often is considered too invasive and can be complicated by bleeding or secondary infection in HSCT patients. In a prospective study of 3857 clinical specimens from 230 patients, a mold was isolated from 86 patients, 95% of which was an *Aspergillus* species.[48] A one-year retrospective study found that 12% of patients with positive cultures for *Aspergillus* met criteria for invasive aspergillosis. Among high-risk patients a positive culture was associated with invasive aspergillosis in 50% to 65% of cases, among intermediate risk patients in 8% to 28%, while patients with low risk rarely had invasive aspergillosis.[6]

In one study the predictive value of respiratory tract cultures was 40% to 100% for patients with invasive pulmonary aspergillosis.[52] Even in patients with established diagnosis, sputum specimens commonly are negative,[13,53] which likely is because invasive pulmonary aspergillosis is predominantly infiltrative and does not have aerial growth in the bronchial tree.[13] Colonization with *Aspergillus* species has been a marker for reduced short-term survival, as 12% of colonized patients died within 3 months. Invasive pulmonary aspergillosis was diagnosed in 12% of patients with a positive culture, but this is likely an underestimate because diagnosis often was made by radiographic imaging and culture specimens were not always obtained.[6]

Aspergillosis rarely is diagnosed by blood culture. There has been speculation that only 32 cases of true *Aspergillus* fungemia have been correctly documented in patients with hematologic disease.[54] In a study of 1477 separate positive *Aspergillus* cultures there were more than a dozen positive blood cultures, but most were associated with pseudofungemia or terminal events noted at autopsy.[6] In general, the *Aspergillus* hyphal mass that develops in the lumen during angioinvasion remains in place until the force of blood flow causes hyphal breakage, which then allows the mass to circulate. The likelihood is small that a blood culture would capture these irregularly and infrequently discharged units. This difficulty in detection of *A. fumigatus* in blood culture stands in contrast to other angioinvasive filamentous fungi (e.g., *Fusarium* species, *Paecilomyces lilacinus*, *Scedosporium prolificans*, *Acremonium* species) that have the ability to discharge a steady series of unicellular spores into the bloodstream, which are more likely to be captured in a blood sample. This ability to sporulate in tissue and blood has been termed adventitious sporulation.[55] As *A. terreus* also displays adventitious sporulation, histopathology and potassium hydroxide examination of these spores also can allow rapid, presumptive identification of *A. terreus*. Therefore, a positive blood culture with *A. terreus* or another fungi that demonstrate adventitious sporulation should not be ignored.

Radiology

A review of 27 pediatric patients showed that radiographic changes that developed after HSCT but before diagnosis of pulmonary fungal infection included unilateral infiltrates (52%) slightly more often than bilateral infiltrates. At the onset, infiltrates were interstitial (41%), alveolar (41%), and mixed (18%). Hilar or mediastinal lymphadenopathy or pleural effusion/thickening was rare. By the time of diagnosis of pulmonary fungal infection the infiltrates usually were bilateral (66%) and alveolar or nodular (74%), including 22% of patients having cavitary lesions.[56] Invasive pulmonary aspergillosis characteristically manifests on radiographs as multiple, ill-defined, 1 to 3 cm peripheral nodules that gradually coalesce into larger masses or areas of subsegmental and segmental consolidation. Lobar or diffuse pulmonary consolidation are common findings.[57] Although chest radiographs usually are abnormal, in one series radiographs were normal in approximately 30% of patients in the week preceding death.[58]

There are two classic radiologic signs of invasive pulmonary aspergillosis. The "halo sign" occurs in neutropenic patients with a hemorrhagic nodule due to angioinvasion. An early computed tomography (CT) finding of the halo sign is a rim of ground-glass opacity surrounding the nodule. In one study, the halo sign was seen in all patients with biopsy-proven invasive pulmonary aspergillosis, but it is nonspecific and also is seen in patients with mucormycosis or entomophthoramycosis (formerly zygomycosis), organizing pneumonia, or pulmonary hemorrhage.[59] These early lesions subsequently change into a cavitary lesion or lesion with an "air crescent sign" 2 to 3 weeks later when neutrophils recover.[57,60] In one study, the air crescent sign was seen in 48% of patients 3 to 10 days after recovery from neutropenia.[22] The appearance of the air crescent sign had no relationship to duration of neutropenia, and showed a tendency to appear in large lesions such as a consolidation or a mass rather than in small lesions like nodules.[61] Cavitation of the nodules or masses occurs in about 40% of patients and is characterized by an intracavitary mass composed of sloughed lung and a surrounding rim of air. The use of CT has increased the sensitivity of radiologic diagnosis. In one study of 37 cases with invasive pulmonary aspergillosis the mean time to diagnosis in HSCT recipients was reduced from 7 days to 1.9 days using chest CT.[62]

There may be radiologic differences for invasive aspergillosis between adult and pediatric patients. In adult series of pulmonary aspergillosis, approximately 50% of cases show cavitation and 40% show air crescent formation.[63] In one 10-year review of pediatric patients (mean age 5 years), there was central cavitation of small nodules in only 25% of children and no evidence of air crescent formation within any area of consolidation.[64] In another pediatric report there was a 22% (6/27) rate of cavitation on chest radiography[65] and in another there was a 43% (6/14) rate of cavitation by CT.[66] In these last two pediatric series, mean ages were older than in the other report of lower rates of cavitation and no air crescent formation. This suggests there is a spectrum of radiologic disease presentation related to age, with cavitation and air crescent formation more likely in the older child and adult than in the younger child.

Findings by thoracic magnetic resonance imaging (MRI) are not as characteristic as CT findings, and the typical MRI sign is the "target sign", a nodular lesion with a lower signal in the center compared with higher, contrast-enhancing signal intensity in the rim on T_1-weighted images. This sign is highly suggestive of late stage disease.[67] MRI is the modality of choice for diagnosing cerebral aspergillosis, and is more sensitive than CT. Findings often show multiple lesions located in the basal ganglia that include an intermediate signal intensity, lack of contrast enhancement, and absence of mass effect.[68] CT of the head often reveals one or multiple hypodense, well-demarcated lesions. Hemorrhage and mass effect are unusual, but for patients with adequate neutrophil counts a ring enhancement and surrounding edema are more frequent.[5] In evaluating sinus disease, T_2-weighted MRI images show markedly decreased signal intensity compared with that of bacterial sinusitis, which show increased signal intensity.[5]

Bronchoalveolar Lavage (BAL)

The BAL was analyzed in 23 consecutive patients with histologically proven invasive aspergillosis, and only 7 patients (30%) had BAL specimens diagnostic for invasive aspergillosis. In the BAL-positive group, 71% had multiple changes on thoracic CT compared with 25% of patients with a negative BAL. The diagnostic yield of BAL was not associated with clinical symptoms or duration of neutropenia. A thorough review of the diagnostic yield of BAL specimens in histologically proven invasive aspergillosis yielded sensitivities of approximately 40% (range 0 to 67%),[69] but in one study BAL had a sensitivity of only 50% even in patients with focal invasive aspergillosis.[70] The sensitivity of respiratory tract culture specimens in general has ranged from 15% to 69%,[6] and in one study it increased to 50% to 70% in high-risk invasive aspergillosis groups. Therefore, a negative BAL in a high-risk patient does not exclude the possibility of invasive aspergillosis.

Serologic Testing

Serologic testing for antibodies to *Aspergillus* antigens is helpful to diagnosis aspergilloma or allergic bronchopulmonary aspergillosis in immunocompetent individuals, but unfortunately serology plays little role in the immunocompromised patient since *Aspergillus* growth does not correlate with an increase in anti-*Aspergillus* antibody titers.[12] Serologic examination of 18 patients with invasive aspergillosis showed anti-*Aspergillus* antibody detection was negative in all cases, likely due to profound immunosuppression.[22]

Galactomannan Antigen Testing

Galactomannan (GM) is a major cell wall component of *Aspergillus* and it is known that the highest concentrations of GM are released in the terminal phases of the disease.[12] An enzyme-immunosorbent assay (EIA) was introduced using a rat anti-GM monoclonal antibody, EB-A2, which recognizes the 1→5-β-D-galactofuranoside side chains of the GM molecule.[71] A sandwich EIA was introduced in 1995[72] and by using the same antibody as both a capture and detector antibody in the sandwich EIA (Platelia® Aspergillus, Bio-Rad, France) the threshold for detection can be lowered to 1 ng/mL. This sandwich EIA is the current commercially-available assay.

Positive findings are suggestive of invasive disease, but false-positive results can be high during the neutropenic period following HSCT. A 3-year prospective trial showed that sensitivity of serial monitoring was 90%, specificity 98%, and negative predictive value was 98%. All 30 patients with proven invasive aspergillosis tested positive, with no false-negative results. GM detection preceded the development of infiltrates on chest radiograph in 68% of patients. The false-positive rate was 14%, and therefore the improved sensitivity over latex agglutination is counterbalanced by the loss of specificity and greater false-positive rate.[73] Other studies have reported false-positive rates of 5% to 8% and suggested they were due to cytotoxic agents, increased resorption of GM, or cross-reacting factors from the intestines.[74]

Serial testing at least twice a week has been recommended.[75] In one study an increase in value during the first week of observation was predictive of progressive disease in allogeneic HSCT patients.[76] In a large prospective study of hematology and HSCT patients with confirmed or probable invasive aspergillosis, GM was detected in 65% of patients an average of 8.4 days before positive CT or culture, and GM was detected in 40% of patients before the onset of clinical symptoms by a mean of 6.9 days. The sensitivity of GM detection in bone marrow transplant patients was 89%, with a specificity of 98%.[77] Unfortunately the GM assay has decreased sensitivity in the setting of a patient receiving *Aspergillus* antifungal therapy, while the specificity for detection does not change.[78]

Diagnosis of pediatric invasive aspergillosis with the GM assay was once deemed impossible as earlier studies repeatedly showed a higher rate of false-positive results in children.[79,80] Theories to explain increased false-positivity in children ranged from presence of *Bifidobacterium bifidum* in the gut microflora that could mimic the epitope recognized by the EB-A2 in the EIA test[81] to GM-positive infant formula used in children.[82] However, more recent studies have shown that the GM assay is very effective in children and carries a low (1% to 2%) false-positivity rate.[83,84] Caution should be used with concurrent use of certain antibiotics, most notably piperacillin-tazobactam and ampicillin-sulbactam, that cause false-positive reactions in the GM assay. The test has lower sensitivity in solid-organ transplant recipients than in patients with hematologic malignancies, HSCT and neutropenia.[85] False-negative GM results occur in specific pediatric patients such as those with CGD. One report details a 4-year-old child with CGD and invasive aspergillosis diagnosed by lung biopsy who had persistent false-negative serum GM testing.[86] Another study evaluated 10 patients with CGD and 6 with Job syndrome who had invasive aspergillosis; GM antigenemia was detected in only 4 cases compared with 24 of 30 cases in patients with all other immunocompromising conditions (P = 0.0004).[87]

(1,3)-β-D-Glucan

(1,3)-β-D-glucan is an integral cell wall component and, in contrast to GM, normally is not released from the fungal cell.[12] Factor G, a coagulation factor of the horseshoe crab, is a highly sensitive natural detector of (1,3)-β-D-glucan.[88] The "G-test" detects (1,3)-β-D-glucan via a modified limulus endotoxin assay and detects *Aspergillus, Candida,* and other fungi, but does not identify the genus of the fungi detected.[88] The G-test is widely used in Japan; however, these tests may yield positive results only at advanced stages of infection in some patients.[89] A 1-year prospective study of patients with hematologic malignancy and controls found sensitivities of 79% for real-time PCR, 58% for GM, and 67% for G-test, with specificities of 92%, 97%, and 84%, respectively.[90]

In a study comparing (1,3)-β-D-glucan with galactomannan, the sensitivity, specificity, and positive and negative predictive values for GM and β-glucan were identical. False-positive reactions occurred at a rate of 10.3% in both tests, but the patients showing false-positive results were different in each test. Both tests anticipated the clinical diagnosis and CT abnormalities, but the G-test tended to become positive earlier than GM. A combination of the two tests improved the specificity (to 100%) and positive predictive value (to 100%) of each individual test without affecting the sensitivity and negative predictive values.[91]

Another study compared galactomannan, PCR, and (1,3)-β-D-glucan in patients with hematologic disorders; the receiver-operating characteristic (ROC) analysis showed that area under the curve was greatest for the galactomannan assay, using two consecutive positive results. This study suggest that the galactomannan was the most sensitive at predicting the diagnosis of invasive aspergillosis in high-risk patients with hematologic disorders.[92] A recent meta-analysis of 23 studies describes infections and usefulness in the proper setting and with considerations of interpretation.[93]

Polymerase Chain Reaction (PCR)

Although GM assays created a noninvasive test with improved sensitivity and specificity, recent efforts have focused on defining an optimal primer sequence for a PCR detection method. At present this diagnostic method is not available commercially, and reports can be difficult to interpret due to the lack of standardization between centers. Due to the ubiquitous nature of the mold, the value of this test likely will be its high negative predictive value. Issues remaining unresolved in the use of PCR are the best source of material (e.g., whole blood, serum, plasma, BAL specimens), the amplification protocol (e.g., real-time, sample volume, extraction methods), and primer selection (e.g., "panfungal", 18S rRNA, 28S rRNA, mitochondrial DNA).[94] Using PCR for BAL specimens compared with blood samples seems less promising due to the higher number of false-positive results. Real-time PCR assays seem to decrease the risk of false-positive results and have better reliability than conventional PCR.[95]

In numerous retrospective reports of PCR, reported sensitivities are 55% to 100%, with negative predictive value (NPV) generally around 100%.[96] The high NPV is consistent with PCR as a sensitive marker for any colonizing or infected *Aspergillus;* negative PCR in a patient with suspected invasive aspergillosis suggests that the patient does not have aspergillosis.[97] PCR has been used to detect *Aspergillus* in BAL specimens, but does not distinguish colonization from invasive disease. A prospective evaluation of 197 BAL samples in febrile, neutropenic patients with lung infiltrates showed that all immunocompromised patients with a negative PCR had no evidence of fungal disease, and only a few immunocompetent patients with a positive result had no evidence of disease. Further dividing the tested population into a high-risk group (patients with acute leukemia undergoing chemotherapy), the negative predictive value of PCR was 100%.[98] A two-step PCR was shown to detect as few as 10 fg *Aspergillus* DNA (approximately 5 colony-forming units per mL) and was tested in 100 BAL specimens from consecutive patients and 278 consecutive blood samples. BAL PCR was positive in 17 immunocompromised patients, with a specificity of 93%, and negative predictive value of 100%. Comparatively, in the blood samples sensitivity was only 20%, but negative predictive value was 100%.[99]

TREATMENT

For years the response rate for invasive aspergillosis was only approximately 30% using either amphotericin B or itraconazole treatment.[100] Amphotericin B was previously the "gold standard" since its approval in 1958, but currently voriconazole is the clear choice for primary therapy of invasive aspergillosis. In the pivotal study comparing voriconazole to amphotericin B deoxycholate,[101] voriconazole showed a statistically superior response rate (53%) versus amphotericin B (32%). This response rate also translated into improved patient survival (71% vs. 58%) for initial therapy with voriconazole. While some criticized this study for the use of other licensed antifungal agents after initial randomization to voriconazole or amphotericin B deoxycholate, a subsequent analysis revealed the strategy of initial therapy with voriconazole also was superior to subsequent use of liposomal amphotericin B.[102] An additional open-label study confirmed the benefit of voriconazole as primary therapy versus salvage therapy,[103] highlighting the importance of using the best available antifungal therapy first.

Voriconazole is now the guideline-recommended primary therapy for all forms of invasive aspergillosis.[104] However, there is no defined optimal alternative in the case of recalcitrant disease or in the event of voriconazole side effects. If "salvage" therapy is required after the first agent fails clinically or unacceptable toxicities develop, options include therapeutic drug monitoring of voriconazole levels to document adequate exposure to the guideline-approved first agent, switching antifungal therapy to likely include a different class of agent, or the addition of another antifungal agent to utilize combination antifungal therapy.

Voriconazole trough levels do not correlate exactly with clinical outcome, and there are no accepted minimum standards. While most experts would agree that a serum level should exceed the expected minimum inhibitory concentration for voriconazole of the infecting *Aspergillus* isolate (generally 0.5 μg/mL), different studies report the need for levels of at last 1.0 μg/mL or 2.0 μg/mL. It is clear that voriconazole pharmacokinetics show great interpatient variability, so dosing and levels cannot be extrapolated easily between patients. In the largest pediatric report of voriconazole use in 58 children in open-label, compassionate use evaluation, voriconazole was administered as a loading dose of 6 mg/kg every 12 hours on day 1 followed by 4 mg/kg every 12 hours thereafter (see Chapter 293, Antifungal Agents). Posaconazole is another triazole with excellent activity against *Aspergillus* and a study has demonstrated excellent activity as salvage therapy.[105]

One option for failed voriconazole therapy is to switch antifungal classes; amphotericin B products or an echinocandin are excellent options. A study comparing two doses of liposomal amphotericin B (3 mg/kg/day vs. 10 mg/kg/day) found no difference in clinical outcome, yet greater toxicity associated with the higher amphotericin B dose.[106] The echinocandin antifungal agents appear to act primarily on the growing hyphal tip of the *Aspergillus*.[107] In the large open trial examining caspofungin as salvage therapy for invasive aspergillosis, there was a 45% (37/83) favorable response rate,[108] suggesting an option for salvage therapy if initial antifungal therapy should fail. Micafungin also has been studied as primary therapy for invasive aspergillosis with similar results.[109]

In the past, combination antifungal therapy for invasive aspergillosis was of little consequence since there were only a handful of possible permutations available, including the use of other agents such as rifampin and flucytosine, which are no longer recommended. However, the recent surge of newer antifungal drugs has created numerous potential combinations.[110] Although there have been concerns of antagonism, especially with polyene–azole interaction, these concerns generally have not been clinically relevant.[100,110] While there are reports of success with combination antifungal therapy for invasive aspergillosis,[111] laboratory data suggest a myriad of effects ranging from antagonism to synergy. Future clinical combination trials will be crucial to determine optimal therapy for patients failing monotherapy.

Surgery has value for treatment of local pulmonary aspergillosis, patients with significant hemoptysis, and for lesions impinging on great vessels or major airways.[5,112,113] Marrow recovery induces cavitation, which creates a major risk of massive hemorrhage when the *Aspergillus* lesion is located near a main pulmonary artery or branch.[114] When marrow recovery occurs, the granulocyte count increases and proteolytic enzymes are released from leukocytes at the site of infection, potentially damaging lung tissue. Radical debridement also is a crucial adjunct in sinusitis, and may help contribute to the improved survival.

PROGNOSIS

The outcome of invasive aspergillosis absent immune reconstitution generally is poor, highlighting the paramount importance of recovery of immune function in order to survive. The mortality associated with untreated invasive aspergillosis is nearly 100% in most patient groups, and the overall survival among patients treated with amphotericin B consistently had been approximately 34%[115,116] but now is generally improved to approximately 50%.[101] Cerebral disease is rapidly and near uniformly fatal irrespective of treatment.[21] Prognosis for focal pulmonary aspergillosis is more favorable than for diffuse bilateral disease, as focal disease tends to progress more slowly. However, focal disease carries an increased risk of hemoptysis, which often is life-threatening.[5] In one series, the median duration of survival of patients diagnosed with invasive aspergillosis was 29 days.[1] In another series median survival after invasive aspergillosis diagnosis was 36 days, with a one-year survival rate estimated to be 22%, while mean survival for 11 patients with central nervous system disease was only 19 days.[3]

Key Points. Diagnosis and Management of *Aspergillus* Infection

EPIDEMIOLOGY
- *Aspergillus fumigatus* is the most common species
- Ubiquitous mold in the soil

CLINICAL FEATURES
- Bimodal peak incidence of disease in stem cell transplant recipients – during periods of neutropenia and periods of graft-versus-host disease
- Increasing number of cases of invasive aspergillosis in non-classically immunocompromised patients (e.g., chronic obstructive pulmonary disease, patients in intensive care)
- Pulmonary disease is the most common clinical presentation
- Disease is more indolent in patients with chronic granulomatous disease (CGD)

DIAGNOSIS
- High-resolution computed tomography is the imaging standard
- Serum galactomannan assay is the ideal noninvasive method; performance is best when patients are screened twice weekly during periods of greatest risk
- Negative culture result on bronchoalveolar lavage specimen does not exclude disease

TREATMENT
- Voriconazole is the preferred antifungal agent for primary therapy
- For salvage therapy (when primary therapy fails), options are switching antifungal classes or considering adding another antifungal agent
- Azole resistance is developing slowly
- Optimal antifungal dosing is crucial in pediatric patients; physicians should strongly consider measuring voriconazole levels

DURATION OF THERAPY
- No defined recommendations, but at least 6 to 12 weeks
- Continue therapy during periods of immunosuppression

---

245 Agents of Hyalohyphomycosis and Phaeohyphomycosis

Thomas F. Patterson and Deanna A. Sutton

Agents of hyalohyphomycosis and phaeohyphomycosis are ubiquitous filamentous molds. (Moulds is the preferred spelling by many mycologists.) These molds are soil saprophytes and plant pathogens that have gained notoriety as emerging pathogens in immunocompromised hosts, including children. The pathogenesis of infections due to these organisms is not clearly established as many are minimally pathogenic in humans. However, these fungal conidia can cause infection in severely immunocompromised children, frequently in the paranasal sinuses or lungs, due to inhalation of aerosolized conidia.[1,2] Some of these organisms, like *Fusarium* spp., also can gain entry through the gastrointestinal tract, central venous catheters, or skin.[3,4] Direct inoculation of these organisms into tissues following trauma can lead to infection in both immunocompromised as well as immunocompetent children.[5–7]

AGENTS OF HYALOHYPHOMYCOSIS (*FUSARIUM, PSEUDALLESCHERIA BOYDII* COMPLEX, *PAECILOMYCES, TRICHODERMA,* AND *PENICILLIUM* SPECIES)

Agents of hyalohyphomycosis are a diverse group of molds whose tissue form is hyaline. Colonies may be of various colors or lightly pigmented. The most important of these organisms is *Aspergillus* (discussed in Chapter 244, *Aspergillus* Species), but other molds, such as *Fusarium* species, the *Pseudallescheria boydii* species complex, *Chrysosporium* species, *Penicillium* species, *Paecilomyces,* and others, also cause infection in severely immunosuppressed children. These organisms appear similar to each other and to *Aspergillus* in tissue, so that cultures are needed to confirm the specific agent causing the disease.[8,9] As with other fungi, recent molecular and phenotypic studies have resulted in taxonomic changes in these molds so that many are reported clinically as a species complex (such as *Pseudallescheria boydii* species complex and *Fusarium solani* species complex, which may contain a large number of distinct species).[10,11] The risk factors for these infections include significant immunosuppression such as immunosuppression associated with hematopoietic stem cell (HSCT) or marrow transplantation, profound neutropenia, malignancy, and inherited immunodeficiencies.[12,13]

Epidemiology

An increasing number of agents of hyalohyphomycosis have been reported to cause invasive mycoses in severely immunosuppressed children.[14,15] The epidemiology and risk factors for infection with these agents are similar to those associated with *Aspergillus*, and the clinical presentations of these infections are similar to manifestations of invasive aspergillosis.[1,13] Clinical presentations include sinusitis, pulmonary infection, localized abscesses, cutaneous infection, and disseminated infection. Some of these infections have characteristic epidemiology, including *Fusarium* species, which has been associated with inhalation of contaminated aerosols from hospital water as well as infection following a primary paronychial or skin infection.[1,3] In 2006, 164 confirmed cases of *Fusarium* keratitis were reported in soft contact lens-wearers, leading to corneal transplantation in 34%.[16,17] In a case-control study, cases were associated with use of a single solution, although *Fusarium* was not found in unopened bottles.[16] *S. apiospermum* infection has been reported in patients after an episode of near-drowning.[10,18–20]

Clinical Manifestations

Fusarium infections are among the most common of these agents and cause a spectrum of disease: toxin-mediated (mycotoxin syndrome), locally invasive, catheter-related, allergic bronchopulmonary, and disseminated infection. Toxin-mediated disease results from ingestion of contaminated grains. Symptoms range from mild gastroenteritis to bone marrow suppression resulting in aplasia and eventual death. Locally invasive diseases include mycotic keratitis, endophthalmitis, sinusitis, brain abscess, cystitis, cutaneous and subcutaneous infections, and paronychial and ungual infections.[12,13,21–23] Penetrating trauma has been associated with osteomyelitis and pyogenic arthritis. Locally invasive infections can occur in immunocompetent and immunocompromised hosts.[24–26]

Disseminated fusariosis, which is limited to immunocompromised hosts, especially hosts with a hematologic malignancy or HSCT, is characterized by fungemia, skin lesions, and multiple organ involvement. Fungemia is detected in 50% to 60% of patients diagnosed with disseminated infection and is the only mold commonly associated with fungemia.[12] Skin lesions are macular or papular, often with a necrotic center, and occur predominantly on extremities and are characteristic for this infection (Figure 245-1).[3,23] Disseminated fusarial infection often is fatal;

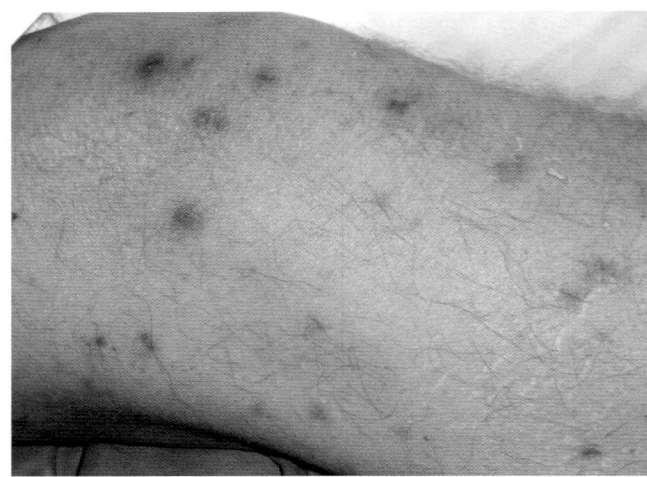

Figure 245-1. Typical necrotic-appearing skin lesions of *Fusarium* infection on the arm of a patient with disseminated disease.

mortality rates between 60% and 100% are reported despite antifungal therapy.[13,27,28]

Scedosporium apiospermum is the lightly pigmented asexual form of the heterothallic teleomorph (sexual form) previously thought to be *Pseudallescheria boydii* but now recognized as *Pseudallescheria apiosperma. Scedosporium boydii* is now recognized as the anamorph of the homothallic teleomorph, *Pseudallescheria boydii,* an ascomycete that produces dark, round sexual structures in culture. *Scedosporium boydii* is now recognized as the anamorph of the homothallic teleomorph *Pseudallescheria boydii.*[11] A large number of other distinct species also can be identified by molecular studies in the *P. boydii* species complex.[10,11] In tissue, hyaline, septate hyphae of *P. boydii* species complex resemble *Aspergillus* species.[29] In immunocompetent hosts, *S. apiospermum* is a major cause of fungal mycetoma, but in immunosuppressed hosts, widely disseminated infection occurs, including involvement of brain.[10,19,30] This organism can be resistant to amphotericin B, with activity of extended-spectrum azoles, voriconazole and posaconazole, shown in adults and children.[14,31–33]

Clinical manifestations of other hyalohyphomycoses are not distinctive and mimic invasive aspergillosis, including pulmonary infection, sinus infection, central nervous system (CNS) disease, osteomyelitis, and locally invasive infections like keratitis, and skin and soft-tissue infection.

Laboratory Evaluation and Diagnosis

In tissue, all of these organisms appear as branched, septated hyphae that are indistinguishable from hyphae of *Aspergillus* and other hyaline molds. Specific diagnosis requires isolation of the organism from culture of tissue (Figure 245-2A). Some of these organisms are resistant to amphotericin B clinically and in vitro, including *Fusarium* and *S. apiospermum,* with better susceptibility reported to the newer azoles, voriconazole and posaconazole.[32,33] Blood cultures can be useful in *Fusarium* but are rarely positive with infection due to other agents of hyalohyphomycosis. Serologic testing and nonculture-based methods like polymerase chain reaction for these agents are not available commercially.

Therapy and Prevention

Because some of these organisms, including *Fusarium* and *S. apiospermum,* are resistant to amphotericin B, responses to amphotericin B are poor, although successful outcomes with the use of lipid formulations of amphotericin B have been reported.[34,35] Posaconazole and voriconazole have been used with success in the treatment of both *S. apiospermum* and *Fusarium* infections and are likely the drugs of choice for agents of hyalohyphomycosis.[31,32,36–38] Voriconazole appears effective against *S. apiospermum,*

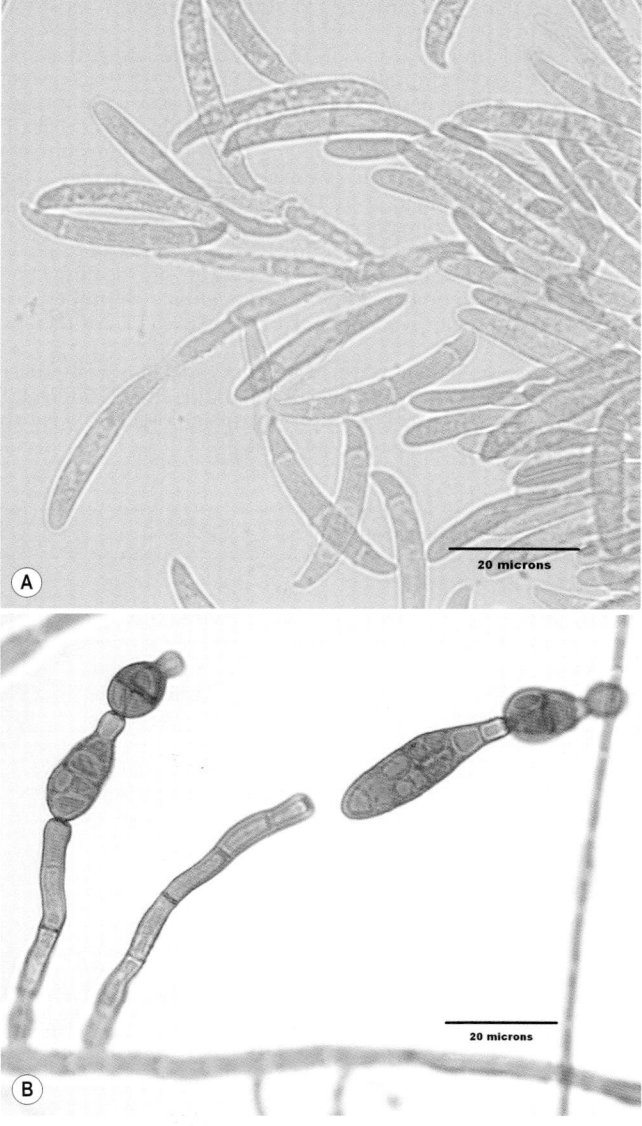

Figure 245-2. (A) Crescent-shaped macroconidia of *Fusarium* spp. **(B)** Club-shaped conidia of *Alternaria* spp.

with 63% of 27 patients responding in one study.[14,32] Similar responses have been reported with salvage use of posaconazole. Itraconazole also has activity against many of these organisms but, because of variable bioavailability, the role of itraconazole is limited to children with less severe infection. Antifungal agents to prevent these mycoses are not specifically indicated because infection is rare, although prophylaxis with posaconazole has been shown to reduce *Aspergillus* infections and would presumably prevent emergence of infections with these mycoses as well.[39,40]

AGENTS OF PHAEOHYPHOMYCOSIS (*BIPOLARIS, ALTERNARIA, EXOPHIALA, CLADOPHIALOPHORA* SPECIES, AND *SCEDOSPORIUM PROLIFICANS*)

Agents of phaeohyphomycosis comprise a group of opportunistic molds that are dematiaceous, i.e., lightly or darkly pigmented in both tissue and culture.[7,9] Although phenotypic characteristics traditionally have been used to identify these organisms, molecular techniques have resulted in reclassification of many of these

organisms as well as the recognition of species complexes of distinct separate species. Examples of genera include *Bipolaris, Alternaria, Scedosporium prolificans, Exophiala, Exserohilum, Cladosporium, Curvularia, Cladophialophora, Scopulariopsis,* and many others.[2,5,7,41–52] These emerging molds rarely are reported to cause infection in children.

Epidemiology

Over 150 and 70 genera of dematiaceous fungi have been implicated in human and animal disease, respectively, some of which have been considered relatively nonpathogenic but can cause serious – even fatal – infection in severely immunocompromised children.[7] Some infections are associated with specific characteristics, such as *Cladophialophora bantiana* with predilection for causing CNS infection, but generally these fungi do not cause syndromes specific to children.[2,7,53]

As with other molds, infection usually occurs by inhalation of conidia and generally starts in the sinuses or the lungs. Alternatively, infection can follow percutaneous inoculation.[2,6,54] Fungemia also can occur, although is less common compared with fusariosis.[55]

The organisms are found in decaying vegetation and are abundant in nature but of sufficiently low virulence that only scattered infections occur. These fungi thrive best in an acidic, glucose-rich environment and are killed by neutrophils. Neutropenia and uncontrolled diabetes are risk factors for infection. Traumatic inoculation from soil or plants is a major mode of infection.

Clinical Manifestations

The pathogenicity of agents of phaeohyphomycosis and resulting clinical manifestations are quite variable. In immunocompetent children or children with minimal host defense abnormalities, phaeohyphomycosis can be associated with the development of sinusitis or pneumonia that can follow a subacute course developing over months to years, and there can be direct invasion of brain from the sinuses.[2,7,53] There also can be a significant component of hypersensitivity, with eosinophils and Charcot–Leyden crystals in sinus aspirates.

Locally invasive diseases include mycotic keratitis, paranasal sinusitis, osteomyelitis, and cutaneous infections. The paranasal sinuses are the most commonly infected sites, particularly in immunocompromised hosts with malignancy. Characteristic lesions associated with sinonasal infections appear as superficial ulcers of the nasal septum, plaque-like necrotic lesions, and hemorrhagic crusts that are indistinguishable from lesions of aspergillosis or other fungi. Cutaneous lesions appear as nonhealing ulcerative or papular lesions with dry crusts. Subcutaneous lesions can enlarge gradually over months. Some, such as *Cladophialophora, Ochroconis gallopava, Rhinocladiella,* and others are neurotropic and cause brain abscesses.[7,56] Disseminated disease, including infection of the CNS, has been reported in severely compromised hosts, including children undergoing HSCT.

Laboratory Findings and Diagnosis

Agents of phaeohyphomycosis are characterized by the production of black melanin pigment, which can be seen histopathologically and in gross lesions. They are a diverse group of organisms characterized by septate, dematiaceous, branched or unbranched fungal elements in tissue that may appear moniliform, bead-like, or swollen.[8,9] Species identification is made by examining conidia in culture (Figure 245-2B). Unfortunately, these mycoses can manifest in culture as "mycelia sterilia", a mold culture that does not readily sporulate and thus does not allow identification. Masson–Fontana staining of tissue specimens is useful for staining the melanin in the hyphae, and allows a specific diagnosis of an agent of phaeohyphomycosis. Culture specimens are best obtained from normally sterile sites (e.g., biopsy of a subcutaneous lesion or sinus aspirate). These organisms can be found as commensals colonizing the respiratory tract from sputum samples, so a tissue biopsy may be needed to establish a diagnosis of invasive infection. Although blood cultures are not positive as frequently as with infections due to *Fusarium*, fungemia can occur.[57]

Treatment and Prevention

Therapy commonly has been amphotericin B. However, in vitro and in vivo activity of itraconazole and extended-spectrum azoles, posaconazole and voriconazole, has been demonstrated against many of the agents of phaeohyphomycosis, so these drugs are possible alternatives, especially for long-term suppressive therapy.[58–60]

Although many of the black molds are susceptible to the extended-spectrum azoles, *S. prolificans* is one resistant pathogen.[2,31] The darkly pigmented *S. prolificans* (previously known as *S. inflatum*) is distinguished from the usually lightly pigmented *S. apiospermum* by the lack of sexual structures and the characteristic inflated conidiophore in the former. *S. prolificans* causes bone and soft-tissue infections, as well as disseminated disease.[2] Outcomes

are poor, even with treatment with the new antifungal agents, often prompting attempts at combination therapy or local debridement.[61]

Voriconazole and posaconazole (usually used as salvage therapy) have been effective clinically in a few patients.[53,56,62] Itraconazole usually is reserved for patients with less severe infection.[63] Although pediatric doses of voriconazole or posaconazole are not established, voriconazole doses of 7 to 8 mg/kg every 12 hours intravenously have been suggested to give exposures similar to that of the usual adult dose (4 mg/kg every 12 hours). Posaconazole typically has been started at 12 mg/kg per day in 2 to 4 divided doses. Therapeutic drug monitoring of both drugs should be useful to guide therapy. The echinocandins also have activity in vitro against some agents of phaeohyphomycosis, but there is limited clinical experience and they are not recommended as single agents for therapy for these infections.[64,65]

There are no known ways to prevent infection with these unusual mycoses, although infection control efforts similar to those used to reduce risk of invasive aspergillosis are likely to reduce nosocomial airborne acquisition.

Key Points. Diagnosis and Management of Agents of Hyalohyphomycosis and Phaeohyphomycosis

MICROBIOLOGY

- Agents of hyalohyphomycosis: molds that are hyaline in tissue; variously colored or light pigmented in culture, associated with soil, water, decomposing vegetation. Species include *Aspergillus* and other genera including *Fusarium,* the *Pseudallescheria boydii* species complex, *Paecilomyces, Chrysosporium, Penicillium,* and others
- Agents of phaeohyphomycosis: melanized or dematiaceous (darkly pigmented) molds or yeastlike fungi, associated with soil, water, decomposing vegetation. Over 150 species and 70 genera including *Bipolaris, Alternaria, Scedosporium prolificans, Exophiala, Exserohilum, Cladosporium, Curvularia, Cladophialophora, Scopulariopsis,* and others
- Many now referred to as a species-complex due to phylogenetic, phenotypic, and physiologic differences in strains

EPIDEMIOLOGY

- Occur worldwide, most commonly in severely immunocompromised children usually following inhalation of conidia
- Can follow direct inoculation from trauma or localized infection (keratitis, sinusitis, otitis)
- Specific exposures associated with some organisms (water aerosols for *Fusarium;* or near-drowning for *Pseudallescheria boydii* species complex; outbreaks due to contaminated solutions – *Fusarium* keratitis)

CLINICAL FEATURES

- Cutaneous infection: follows trauma in immunocompetent or compromised children; slowly increasing nodular or ulcerative lesions; also can reflect disseminated infection (fusariosis)
- Pulmonary: follows inhalation; including productive cough, fever, weight loss, shortness of breath, hemoptysis; nonspecific radiographic infiltrates
- Disseminated: severely immunocompromised children; neurotropism with brain abscess common for some organisms (agents of phaeohyphomycosis such as *Cladophialophora bantiana*)

DIAGNOSIS

- Recovery of organism from body fluids or tissue
- Microscopic examination of pathologic material – nonspecific histopathology for agents of hyalohyphomycosis; beaded irregular appearance of pigmented hyphae for agents of phaeohyphomycosis
- Melanin staining by Masson–Fontana method useful for agents of phaeohyphomycosis

TREATMENT

- Traditionally amphotericin B (or lipid formulation) but many species resistant to polyenes. Activity and clinical use of voriconazole or posaconazole reported in case series; itraconazole reserved for less seriously ill

---

246 Agents of Mucormycosis (Zygomycosis)

Thomas F. Patterson and Deanna A. Sutton

Mucormycosis (formerly zygomycosis) is an uncommon but emerging infection that occurs in immunocompromised patients, including children and neonates.[1–6] Previously, the term zygomycosis was used to refer to syndromes of mucormycosis and entomophthoramycosis, but updates in taxonomy have determined

that the class name Zygomycota is invalid.[7] Since the class Zygomycota no longer exists, the term zygomycosis has become obsolete.[1,7] Molds causing these infections are now in the subphyla Mucoromycotina and Entomophthoromycotina, respectively.[1,7] Infectious syndromes produced by agents in the order

Entomophthorales, such as *Conidiobolus* and *Basidiobolus*, produce distinct cutaneous and subcutaneous disease syndromes that are discussed here.[8-11] As clinically significant genera are in the subphylum Mucoromycotina, order Mucorales, the term mucormycosis is a useful clinical and valid mycologic reference.[1,7] Organisms in this order are characterized by the formation of broad, aseptate or rarely septate hyphae and by sexual reproduction with formation of zygospores. The Mucorales are divided into 6 families of significance in human or animal disease, although most cases of human infection are caused by members of the family Mucoraceae. These families have undergone taxonomic revisions based on molecular, physiologic, and phylogenetic studies, including the reclassification of the family Absidiaceae to Lichtheimiaceae for pathogenic species that are able to survive at temperatures of ≥37°C.[7,12] The family Mucoraceae produces *sporangiospores* (asexual spores) in a closed sac-like structure called a *sporangium*, which are released when the wall ruptures. The sporangium is attached to the hyphal substratum with a stalk-like structure called a *sporangiophore*. Different species are distinguished by microscopic appearance of the sporangiophores, sporangia, and sporangiospores, as well as by the presence or absence of rhizoids (root-like structures) that anchor sporangiophores to the substratum.[13] In the family Mucoraceae, members of the genera *Rhizopus, Mucor, Actinomucor, Rhizomucor,* and *Apophysomyces* all have been implicated in human disease. Less frequently reported species in human disease in other families include *Cunninghamella, Saksenaea, Syncephalastrum, Cokermyces,* and *Lichtheimia.*[1]

The species isolated from cases of human infection are ubiquitous in decomposing organic matter such as spoiled bread, fruit, and other food items, as well as in soil. The most commonly encountered human pathogen is *Rhizopus oryzae*, but many other species have been implicated.[3,6] All of these organisms cause similar syndromes in children and neonates.[3-5]

Mucormycosis generally is acquired through inhalation of spores; the lungs and sinuses are the most common initial sites of infection. Less commonly, disease can arise after ingestion of contaminated foods or by direct inoculation following trauma or vascular catheters, which is an important route of nosocomial transmission in neonates.[3,14] In an immunocompetent host, pulmonary macrophages ingest and kill inhaled sporangiospores.[15,16] In diabetic hosts and other immunosuppressed patients, macrophages fail to suppress spore germination.[17] Once infection is established, neutrophils have a pivotal role in killing hyphae. Severe neutropenia increases the risk of invasive infection as does ketoacidosis in diabetic patients because of abnormal neutrophil function.[18]

EPIDEMIOLOGY

The spores of Mucorales are ubiquitous in the environment, but only rarely cause infection without predisposing host factors.[6] Certain predisposing conditions are associated with specific clinical manifestations of disease. For example, patients who have diabetic ketoacidosis typically experience rhinocerebral mucormycosis. Patients with leukemia and other causes of neutropenia receiving cytotoxic chemotherapy can develop rhinocerebral, pulmonary, or disseminated disease. Infants and children with severe malnutrition can have gastrointestinal tract mucormycosis.[5,19] Patients receiving deferoxamine for iron overload states also are at increased risk for mucormycosis.[6,15]

Prolonged neutropenia is well recognized as an important risk factor for mucormycosis among patients with leukemia and recipients of bone marrow or hematopoietic stem cell transplant (HSCT).[20] Other contributing factors in these patients are the use of corticosteroids and broad-spectrum antibacterial agents.[3,5,21,22] Prolonged use of antifungal agents without activity against Mucorales (especially voriconazole, but also the echinocandins and fluconazole) in severely immunosuppressed patients has been reported as a risk factor for mucormycosis.[23-26]

In children, mucormycosis often develops in settings similar to those seen in adults, including neutropenia, solid-organ transplantation, HSCT or bone marrow transplantation, burns, and deferoxamine treatment for management of iron overload.[3,6] Infection occurs in distinct settings in children and neonates as well. These conditions include diabetes mellitus in children, particularly with uncontrolled diabetic ketoacidosis, and cutaneous infection in neonates.[3,14]

Nosocomial outbreaks of mucormycosis have been linked to construction work as well as to contaminated air-conditioning systems.[27,28] Nosocomial clusters of cutaneous infections, especially in neonates, have been traced to use of contaminated biomedical devices, such as wooden tongue depressors, or have been associated with use of various adhesive bandages used in the hospital setting, such as elastic bandages or tape.[29,30] However, most cases of mucormycosis in hospitalized patients are sporadic, so that it is difficult to determine the site of inoculation or source of infection.[3,6]

CLINICAL MANIFESTATIONS

There are several clinical presentations of mucormycosis. Rhinocerebral and pulmonary infections are by far the most common. Other common clinical manifestations are gastrointestinal, cutaneous, and disseminated infection, which can include central nervous system (CNS) involvement. Like other angioinvasive molds, a characteristic feature of mucormycosis is vascular invasion, which results in thrombosis, infarction, and necrosis of surrounding tissue. Mucormycosis often is characterized by a rapid onset of a necrotic lesion, followed by a fulminant course that requires rapid and aggressive medical and surgical therapy.

Rhinocerebral Infection

Rhinocerebral mucormycosis often begins with a necrotic lesion in the paranasal sinuses that then spreads to involve the orbit, face, palate, and brain. The disease classically occurs in patients with diabetic ketoacidosis, but also can occur in patients with neutropenia and other immunocompromising conditions. Most commonly, rhinocerebral mucormycosis progresses rapidly and requires extensive surgical debridement combined with antifungal therapy.

Initial symptoms can include nasal or sinus congestion or pain, and epistaxis, along with fever. Black necrotic lesions on the nasal or palatine mucosa are a characteristic diagnostic sign but the diagnosis often is not established early in infection. Infection can spread into the orbits, periorbital or perinasal tissues and is associated with induration, necrosis, and edema. Ptosis, proptosis, dilatation and fixation of the pupil, and loss of vision can occur. Infection can spread into the cavernous sinus and brain, resulting in abscess formation and necrosis of the frontal lobes.

Studies using computed tomography (CT) or magnetic resonance imaging (MRI) are needed to assess the anatomic extent of suspected infection. The results of cerebrospinal fluid examination are nonspecific and do not assist in diagnosis.

Pulmonary Infection

Pulmonary mucormycosis is most common in severely neutropenic and other severely immunocompromised children, including children undergoing marrow or HSCT, particularly in the setting of graft-versus-host disease.[3,6,20,31] The clinical presentation usually is nonspecific and is similar to pneumonia due to other angioinvasive molds (*Aspergillus*), and can include pleuritic chest pain, cough, fever, and hemoptysis. The radiologic signs also can be nonspecific but can include nodular lesions, cavitation, and a "halo" sign, which can mimic invasive pulmonary aspergillosis. Mortality is high due to unsuspected diagnosis in many patients as well as persistence of the underlying severe immunosuppression that predisposed to infection.

Gastrointestinal Tract Infection

Mucormycosis of the gastrointestinal tract is rare but occurs in malnourished infants and children. In one review, 19 of 34 children with this condition were <1 year of age.[3,32] All segments of the gastrointestinal tract can be involved, but the most commonly affected sites are the stomach, large and small intestine, and esophagus.

Symptoms reflect the site affected but are not specific and include abdominal pain and hematemesis or gastrointestinal tract bleeding. Gastrointestinal mucormycosis can be complicated by perforation, perirenal abscess, and renal infarction. The course of the disease can be rapid, and survival is rare due to severe immunocompromise in the host and difficulty in making the diagnosis.

Cutaneous Infection

Traumatic implantation of spores from soil can lead to extensive necrotic cutaneous infections.[33–36] Cutaneous mucormycosis has developed at the sites of surgical incisions and infected burn wounds.[3,37] *Rhizopus* spp. and other Mucorales have caused necrotizing cellulitis in premature infants and children with leukemia in whom contaminated biomedical devices or adhesive products have been applied to the skin near sites of catheter insertion or wounds.[29,30,35,38–40] Cutaneous infection due to the emerging mold *Apophysomyces elegans* has been reported increasingly following traumatic inoculation in otherwise immunocompetent people, including children.[36] These infections can be difficult to diagnose and identify because of the lack of growth from homogenized tissues and poor sporulation on routine media.[41–44] Children with leukemia also can manifest cutaneous lesions that result from hematogenous dissemination from another site.

Cutaneous lesions typically begin with erythema and edema and progress to raised indurated lesions with a black, necrotic center. Lesions are painful and are indistinguishable from those caused by *Aspergillus* or other molds, and can resemble ecthyma gangrenosum. Cutaneous mucormycosis can progress rapidly, requiring extensive surgical debridement as well as optimal antifungal therapy.[45]

Disseminated Infection

Dissemination can follow any primary site of mucormycosis but usually is seen in severely neutropenic children following pulmonary infection.[3] The most frequent and feared site of dissemination is to the brain, but metastatic necrotic lesions can occur in any organ. Cutaneous lesions may be an initial site of diagnosis that actually reflects disseminated infection.

Focal cerebral infection usually occurs in children as a result of disseminated infection but in adults also can occur as an isolated event in association with injecting drug abuse. The diagnosis of CNS mucormycosis is difficult but should be considered in a severely immunocompromised child with systemic mucormycosis who becomes lethargic, confused, or obtunded and is found to have a focal brain lesion by an imaging study.

DIAGNOSIS

Early diagnosis of mucormycosis is essential for successful treatment. Unfortunately, diagnosis of these infections is difficult because infection often is not suspected early in the course, blood cultures rarely are positive and cultures of infected tissues are undertaken reluctantly. Nonculture-based methods are not available commercially. Agents of mucormycosis usually can be distinguished from other molds, such as *Aspergillus*, by their characteristic broad, rarely septate or aseptate hyphae with right-angled branching. However, in histopathologic samples with only hyphal fragments identified, specific distinction can be difficult. It also is notable that homogenization of tissue samples can render culture for Mucorales negative. In patients suspected of having mucormycosis, communication between the clinician and microbiologist to inoculate a nonhomogenized sample may increase the yield.

TREATMENT

If treatment of mucormycosis is to be successful, the underlying immunologic or metabolic defects that precipitated the infection must be corrected, infected necrotic tissue must be debrided, and aggressive antifungal therapy must be administered.[3] Amphotericin B has consistent activity against Mucorales, but toxicity limits usefulness. Lipid formulations of amphotericin B and introduction of posaconazole, the first extended-spectrum azole with activity against these fungi, may reduce toxicity and improve outcomes of mucormycoses. Adjunctive measures should include surgical excision of infected tissues and discontinuation or reduction in immunosuppressive therapies or iron chelation treatment if possible. Hyperbaric oxygen therapy has been advocated by some investigators but its efficacy remains unproven.[46–48]

Amphotericin B is the recommended therapy with high doses (1.0 to 1.5 mg/kg per day) often recommended. Unfortunately, this dose frequently is not tolerated and outcomes have been extremely poor. Lipid formulations of amphotericin B (in doses ≥5 mg/kg per day) are less toxic, are as active as amphotericin B deoxycholate, and should be considered as primary therapy for most patients with this disease.[1,3,49–53] Posaconazole has been shown to have activity in salvage therapy of mucormycosis and offers the advantage of long-term oral therapy.[54,55] The pediatric dose of posaconazole is not established, although 12 mg/kg per day in 2 to 4 divided doses has been the initial dose in a limited number of pediatric patients given salvage therapy.

The duration of therapy is dependent on clinical response, extent of surgical excision, and persistence of the underlying immunosuppression. Long-term oral therapy with posaconazole has been associated with good response.[54,55]

The mortality rate of mucormycosis among patients with cancer remains high, despite more rapid diagnosis and aggressive surgical and antifungal treatment.[1,3,31,56,57] Although rates of successful salvage therapy with either posaconazole or liposomal amphotericin B are as high as 80%, selection of patients to receive these agents likely influences reported favorable response rates.[52,54,55] Better responses also occur with infection that is surgically excised or debrided, such as isolated renal, cerebral, or cutaneous infection.

PREVENTION

Preventive measures should focus on reducing underlying risk factors that lead to the development of mucormycosis. These preventive measures include control of diabetes mellitus, use of iron chelating agents other than deferoxamine, and limiting use of aluminum-containing buffers in dialysis.[6,15,58] Limiting exposure of severely immunosuppressed patients to soil and plants as well as use of laminar air filtration and limitation of exposure to hospital construction have been recommended to reduce the occurrence of aerosolization of molds, which include Mucorales.[59] Use of nonsterile items (which often become contaminated with environmental molds) on skin and mucous membranes in low-birthweight infants and other immunocompromised patients should be avoided or initiated with caution.[30,39,60] In addition, reports of mucormycosis in patients receiving long-term prophylactic therapy with voriconazole raise concerns about its extended use in high-risk patients.[61] Although prophylaxis studies with posaconazole were not powered to show reduction in mucormycosis, it may be reasonable to consider posaconazole prophylaxis as a means of reducing mucormycosis and other mold infections in high-risk patients.[62,63]

Key Points. Diagnosis and Management of Mucormycosis (Zygomycosis)

MICROBIOLOGY

- Agents of mucormycosis: broad, aseptate, or rarely septate ribbon-like hyphae with right-angle branching
- Organisms now classified in the subphylum Mucoromycotina (which has replaced Zygomycota); predominately in order Mucorales so that mucormycosis is useful clinically and mycologically
- Order Mucorales with 6 families contains most agents of human disease. Taxonomic revisions due to phylogenetic, phenotypic, and physiologic differences in strains including the reclassification of the family Absidiaceae to Lichtheimiaceae for pathogenic species which are able to survive ≥37°C
- Family Mucoraceae members (*Rhizopus, Mucor, Actinomucor, Rhizomucor,* and *Apophysomyces*) all implicated in human disease. Species in other families (*Cunninghamella, Saksenaea, Syncephalastrum, Cokermyces,* and *Lichtheimia*) less frequently reported in human disease

EPIDEMIOLOGY

- Spores of Mucorales are ubiquitous in the environment but usually cause infection only with predisposing host risk factors
- Risk factors for infection include: neutropenia, diabetes mellitus, ketoacidosis, iron overload, iron chelation, severe malnutrition, transplantation, corticosteroids, antifungals without activity against agents of mucormycosis, burns, contaminated wounds, and intravenous catheters

CLINICAL FEATURES

- Cutaneous infection: associated with intravenous catheters and wound dressings; burns; traumatic implantation into normal children especially with *Apophysomyces elegans*

- Pulmonary: usually in severely neutropenic children; nonspecific presentation following inhalation of organism including productive cough, fever, shortness of breath, hemoptysis; nonspecific infiltrates with "halo"
- Gastrointestinal: rare but occurs in malnourished infants and children; can affect any area of gastrointestinal tract with symptoms including perforation and abscess
- Rhinocerebral: classically associated with diabetic ketoacidosis; but occurs with prolonged neutropenia and immunocompromise; requires aggressive medical/surgical treatment
- Disseminated: severely immunosuppressed children with prolonged neutropenia and in solid-organ or stem cell transplantation; high mortality rates especially with CNS involvement

DIAGNOSIS

- Recovery of organism from body fluids, tissue; no commercial nonculture-based methods
- Microscopic examination of pathologic material – broad, ribbon like hyphae with few or no septations
- Cultures of nonhomogenized tissue may increase yield

TREATMENT

- Polyenes (amphotericin B deoxycholate or lipid formulation) drugs of choice; activity of posaconazole demonstrated in salvage trials and for long-term therapy
- Adjunctive therapy: echinocandins (may increase host responses, especially in combination), hyperbaric oxygen, deferasirox, immune modulation, white blood cell infusion (all anecdotal)
- Preventive therapy: posaconazole presumed to have activity but not completely protective

247 Malassezia Species

Deanna A. Sutton and Thomas F. Patterson

MICROBIOLOGY

Malassezia (obsolete name *Pityrosporum*)[1] is a genus of lipophilic, basidiomycetous yeasts lacking ballistospores and classified in the order Malasseziales. Its phylogenetic placement within the Ustilaginomycotina (Basidiomycota) appears to be highly supported;[2-5] however, Hibbert's recent taxonomic treatment placing the order in the Ustilaginomycotina *incertae sedis* highlights its still somewhat unresolved phylogenetic placement.[6] *Malassezia* increasingly is recognized as an opportunist affecting both humans and animals.[7,8] Newer identification methods have made the characterization of several new species possible, and also have enhanced our understanding of the ecology and clinical associations of the genus.[9] The genus is responsible for various superficial skin infections of humans, including pityriasis (tinea) versicolor (PV),[10,11] and *Malassezia* folliculitis (MF).[11] The association of *Malassezia* with seborrheic eczema/dermatitis also has been reconfirmed although the implication of the immune system in this disease is critical.[12,13] Less commonly, members of the genus cause invasive disease in premature infants and other immunocompromised and debilitated individuals.[1] *Malassezia* species also have been implicated in atopic dermatitis, confluent and reticulate papillomatosis,[11] and neonatal cephalic pustulosis.[14,15] Various species of *Malassezia* form part of the normal microbial flora of the skin of humans and other warm-blooded animals, and most infections are endogenous in origin.

Until the 1990s, only 3 *Malassezia* species were recognized; these were 2 lipid-dependent species, *Malassezia furfur* and *M. sympodialis,* and 1 nonobligate lipophile, *M. pachydermatis.* After genomic and ribosomal sequence comparisons of a large number of human and animal isolates, the genus *Malassezia* was enlarged into 7 species, consisting of the 3 former taxa, *M. furfur, M. pachydermatis,* and *M. sympodialis,* and 4 new taxa named *M. globosa, M. obtusa, M. restricta,* and *M. slooffiae.*[16] More recently, 6 new species have been described and reported; *M. dermatis,*[17] *M. japonica,*[18] *M. nana,*[19] *M. yamatoensis,*[20] *M. caprae,*[21] and *M. equina*[21] (also published under the invalid name *M. equi*).[22] With the exception of *M. pachydermatis,* 12 of the 13 *Malassezia* species are lipid-dependent. Their isolation in culture requires the use of a lipid-enriched culture medium. If a conventional medium, such as Sabouraud dextrose agar, is used, the surface must be covered with a thin layer of sterile olive oil; however, this method only yields recovery of *M. furfur, M. pachydermatis,* and *M. yamatoensis.* Other selective media useful for a wider range of species include Dixon, modified Dixon, and Leeming and Notman agars.[23] The mostly non-lipid-dependent species *M. pachydermatis* usually can be isolated on Sabouraud dextrose agar. Incubation temperature also is an important consideration as many cutaneous species have optimum growth temperature between 32°C and 34°C rather than 37°C. Methods have been developed to separate the species of *Malassezia* on the basis of morphologic and physiologic differences; however, these are somewhat cumbersome and species identification can be difficult. Commonly used physiologic tests include urease, catalase, and β-glucosidase activities, growth at 37°C and 40°C and evaluation of growth in four water-soluble lipid supplements (Tweens 20, 40, 60, 80) and in Cremophor EL (castor oil) using a diffusion method in Sabouraud glucose agar.[24–27] The dependence on lipid precludes the use of conventional assimilation tests.

Molecular methods utilized in the detection and characterization of *Malassezia* species in humans and animals include biotyping using enzymatic methods, pulsed-field gel electrophoresis (PFGE), random amplification of polymorphic DNA (RAPD), DNA sequence analysis, restriction analysis of PCR amplicon of ribosomal sequences, amplified fragment length polymorphism (AFLP), denaturing gradient gel electrophoresis (DGGE), and terminal fragment length polymorphism (tFLP). These methods have confirmed the robustness of the new classification of *Malassezia* species, all species having their own characteristic karyotype.[28–31] Although PCR–restriction endonuclease analysis has been found to be a rapid and reliable method for the molecular differentiation of *Malassezia* species, AFLP currently appears to be the method of choice for strain identification, epidemiology, phylogeny, and characterization of new species.[9,31] DNA-based culture-independent methods such as quantitative real-time PCR methods using TaqMan probes that can detect as few as 10 copies of *Malassezia* DNA currently are the most reliable methods for detecting *Malassezia*.[31]

Although 13 species of *Malassezia* have thus far been recovered from humans and animals,[5] they appear not to be of equal clinical importance. While many clinicians have previously considered all clinical isolates to be *M. furfur*, this assumption is no longer valid as the host, sources of infections, and routes of transmission vary by species.

EPIDEMIOLOGY

Malassezia species form part of the normal cutaneous flora of humans and other warm-blooded animals. The prevalence of skin colonization depends on age, anatomic site, and, to a lesser extent, race. Cutaneous *Malassezia* is found immediately after birth. In a British study of skin swabs from 245 neonates, 31% were positive for *Malassezia*[32] and in 195 neonates from Iran, 68% were positive with a distribution of *M. furfur* and *M. globosa* of 60% and 7%, respectively.[33] A recent study from Korea demonstrated 19 healthy individuals between the ages of 17 and 55 years who were colonized with *M. dermatis*.[34]

The incidence of skin colonization with *Malassezia* species increases with age, rising from about 25% in children[35] to almost 100% in adolescents and adults. The density of colonization in postpubertal individuals is greater in anatomic sites that contain pilosebaceous glands; *Malassezia* spp. have been isolated from 100% of samples taken from the back of adults, but from only 75% taken from the face and scalp. Studies have shown that the degree of colonization with *Malassezia* species is closely aligned with age-related changes in sebaceous gland activity,[36,37] with increased fatty acid concentration occurring primarily at puberty. Pityriasis versicolor is worldwide in distribution but is most prevalent in hot, humid tropical and subtropical climates, where 30% to 40% of the adult population can be affected.[8] In temperate climates, the disease affects 1% to 4% of the adults and is most common during the hot summer months. *Malassezia* folliculitis also is more prevalent in tropical countries, and is more common during the summer months in temperate regions.[8]

The precise conditions that lead to the development of pityriasis versicolor and other forms of superficial *Malassezia* infection have not been defined, but host-specific adaptations are important factors, since the transition from commensal to pathogenic states appears to be a continuum rather than a discrete entity.[38] The lesions of pityriasis versicolor and seborrheic dermatitis have a predilection for anatomic sites that are well supplied with sebaceous glands, and patients with the latter condition have been shown to have higher concentrations of lipids on their skin than other individuals.[8] Instances in which noncohabiting members of the same family have demonstrated pityriasis versicolor suggest a genetic predisposition. The higher incidence of *Malassezia* folliculitis and seborrheic dermatitis in persons with immunosuppressive disorders, including acquired immunodeficiency syndrome (AIDS), and in persons undergoing corticosteroid or other immunosuppressive treatment suggests that the relationship between *Malassezia* species and the immune system is important.

Exposure to lipid-rich intravenous infusions through a central venous catheter is the single most important risk factor for systemic *Malassezia* infection in both adults and infants.[39–46] Among neonates, other risk factors include low birthweight (LBW), early gestational age, and length of hospitalization. An investigation of one outbreak of *M. furfur* infection among LBW infants, most of whom received intravenous lipids, identified long duration of antimicrobial treatment as an additional risk factor for disease.[42]

Human-to-human transmission of *Malassezia* species is possible, either through direct contact or via contaminated clothing or bedding. In practice, however, cutaneous infection is endogenous in most cases, and spread between persons is uncommon. No cases of occupational infection among healthcare personnel (HCP) have been reported.

Although most infections appear to be sporadic, healthcare-associated (HA) outbreaks of systemic *Malassezia* infection have been reported since the late 1980s in LBW infants and debilitated adults and children who were receiving parenteral lipid nutrition through indwelling vascular catheters.[40–44] An investigation of one outbreak of *M. furfur* infection among low-birthweight infants provided evidence that the organism can be transmitted from an infected or colonized infant to other infants via the hands of HCP.[42] HA outbreaks of *M. pachydermatis* infection also have been reported.[22–24] In one outbreak, patient-to-patient transmission of the organism was documented in a neonatal intensive care unit (NICU), but the source of the outbreak was not identified.[45] In another outbreak that involved 15 infants in a NICU, *M. pachydermatis* was introduced into the unit on the hands of HCP after being colonized from pet dogs at home.[46] The organism persisted in the unit through patient-to-patient transmission.

CLINICAL MANIFESTATIONS

Superficial Skin Disorders

Pityriasis Versicolor

A disfiguring but otherwise harmless condition, pityriasis versicolor (PV) most commonly affects the trunk, neck, and upper portions of the arms. While commonly ascribed to *M. furfur* under the old taxonomic classification, molecular studies have shown that most cases in northern countries are attributed to *M. globosa*, which is present in the yeast state on healthy adult skin but produces clinical lesions of PV after developing into the pseudohyphal state.[11] In tropical and subtropical climates, lesions more often are localized on the face and attributed to *M. furfur*. The characteristic lesions consist of patches of fine brown scaling that may become confluent and progress to cover large areas of the skin of the trunk and proximal extremities. Pruritus, which occurs in less than one-third of adolescents and adults with PV, can be a prominent feature in young children. The disease is exacerbated by sunlight and sweating. Occasionally, there is an inflammatory component to the rash, manifesting as erythema and fine vesicles. In light-skinned persons, lesions are hyperpigmented and range in color from red to brown. In dark-skinned or tanned individuals, the lesions are hypopigmented and white. In contrast to adults who seldom have facial involvement, prepubescent children with

PV often have hypopigmented nummular lesions with fine scaling on the face.

In most cases, the diagnosis of PV is made clinically. Hyperpigmented lesions must be distinguished from a number of conditions, including erythrasma, nevi, seborrheic dermatitis, and tinea corporis. Hypopigmented lesions can be confused with pityriasis alba and vitiligo. Wood light examination can be useful if the diagnosis is uncertain. On exposure to ultraviolet light, infected skin, particularly the scaly borders of the most recent lesions, emit a pale yellow fluorescence. If the diagnosis is in question, material for direct microscopic examination can be obtained by taking scrapings from the affected skin or by gently pressing a transparent tape to the skin and then removing and examining the tape.

Malassezia Folliculitis

Malassezia folliculitis (MF) is a chronic disorder primarily affecting adults with chronic debilitating disease and persons who are immunosuppressed.[11,47] A minor outbreak of 11 cases of MF over a 4-month period was reported in an ICU in cardiac transplant recipients.[48] MF also is seen quite often in persons with AIDS. Little information exists about MF in infants and children. The typical lesions are small, erythematous, follicular papules that slowly enlarge and often become pustular. The condition often is associated with troublesome pruritus. Lesions occur on the back, chest, upper arms, and sometimes the neck, but seldom on the face. Pruritus and lack of comedones differentiate the condition from acne vulgaris. However, the two diseases often coexist with nonitching acne lesions on the face and itching lesions of MF on the trunk and upper arms. It is sometimes necessary to perform a skin biopsy to make a definitive diagnosis. As with PV, M. globosa appears to be the predominant causative agent.[11]

Seborrheic Eczema/Dermatitis

The role of Malassezia species in seborrheic eczema (SE) or seborrheic dermatitis (SD) has previously been questioned; however, recent studies have reaffirmed its association.[12,49,50]

The clinical forms of seborrheic dermatitis include infantile seborrheic eczema (ISE) on the scalp and trunk, and adult seborrheic eczema (ASE) with an erythematous rash with scaling found on the scalp, face, ears, chest, and the upper part of the back. Dandruff is the mildest manifestation of the disease. Scaling of the eyelid margins and around the nasolabial folds is a common presentation. Itching is common on the scalp. The course of the disease is chronic, with regular flare-ups. In temperate climates, the disease often improves during the summer months. The most common species associated with SE/SD include M. globosa and M. restricta, followed by M. sympodialis, M. furfur, and M. slooffiae.[26,51]

Systemic Infections

Systemic Malassezia infection has become a well-recognized complication of lipid-supplemented parenteral alimentation, with most cases occurring in low-birthweight infants younger than 1 month. Life-threatening systemic Malassezia infections have also been reported in older children and adults, all of whom received lipid emulsions through indwelling central venous catheters for periods ranging from a few days to many months. Predisposing diseases in this setting include Crohn disease, continuous ambulatory peritoneal dialysis, other chronic illnesses, invasive procedures, intensive care, and long-term antibiotic administration. Reported systemic infections range from localized organ infections to fulminant fungemia and death.

In infants, Malassezia fungemia can manifest with fever, apnea, or both and bradycardia; interstitial pneumonia and thrombocytopenia are common. The most common symptoms of systemic infection are fever and respiratory distress with or without apnea. Less common symptoms and signs are poor feeding and hepatosplenomegaly. No signs of infection have been noted at catheter insertion sites, nor has rash been seen in infants with systemic Malassezia infection.

Predominant pathologic changes in patients with systemic Malassezia infection involve the heart and lungs and include mycotic thrombi around the tips of indwelling catheters, vegetations on the endocardium, vasculitis, and inflammation of alveoli, bronchi, and bronchioles. Predominant organisms in invasive disease include M. furfur and M. pachydermatis.

DIAGNOSIS

Superficial Infections

Direct microscopic examination of scrapings from lesions usually is sufficient to permit the diagnosis of PV if clusters of round to oval budding yeast cells and short, seldom-branching pseudohyphae are seen. Because Malassezia species are part of the normal cutaneous flora, their isolation in culture must be correlated with clinical findings. Additionally, with the exception of most strains of M. pachydermatis, these organisms cannot be isolated on routine mycologic media unless lipid is added. In Malassezia folliculitis, microscopic examination of biopsy specimens reveal inflammatory cell infiltration of the pilosebaceous apparatus, keratin plugging, and round budding yeast cells in the dilated hair follicles.

DNA-based culture-independent molecular methods such as quantitative real-time PCR methods using TaqMan probes currently are the most reliable methods for detecting Malassezia in skin samples.[31] Isolates from nosocomial outbreaks can be analyzed by PCR fingerprinting, PFGE, and AFLP analysis.[39]

Systemic Infections

The diagnosis of Malassezia septicemia should be considered in any febrile patient (particularly if there is clinical and radiologic evidence of pneumonia) who is receiving lipid-containing alimentation through a central venous catheter, especially if results of routine blood cultures are sterile. If the catheter can be removed, the tip of the catheter should be inoculated onto Sabouraud dextrose agar overlaid with olive oil or another medium supplemented with long-chain lipids. When catheter removal is not feasible, blood for culture is obtained through it. The lipid concentration of conventional broth and agar media usually is insufficient to support the growth of Malassezia species (with the exception of M. pachydermatis), but it would appear that the blood of patients receiving parenteral alimentation often contains sufficient lipids to support initial growth of these organisms in culture. Although yield is low, microscopic examination of Giemsa-stained smears of blood obtained through the catheter may be helpful.

TREATMENT

Skin Infections

Most patients with pityriasis versicolor show response to topical treatment, but more than 50% experience relapse within 12 months. Selenium sulfide lotion (2.5%) should be applied to the lesions for 15 to 30 minutes nightly for 1 to 2 weeks and then once monthly to avoid recurrences. Ketoconazole shampoo is applied for 3 to 5 minutes once daily for 5 days. For extensive involvement in adolescents, or in infections unresponsive to topical therapy, both itraconazole (200 mg once daily for 1 week) and ketoconazole (200 mg once daily for 1 week) are effective oral treatments.

Treatment with a topical imidazole or selenium sulfide often is effective in Malassezia folliculitis, but oral treatment with ketoconazole (in doses of 200 mg/day for 1 to 2 weeks) may be required in patients with extensive or recalcitrant lesions. To prevent recurrence, maintenance treatment should be given once or twice per week. Ketoconazole shampoo, used twice per week for 2 to 4 weeks, is an effective treatment for seborrheic dermatitis and dandruff of the scalp. Thereafter, it should be used at 1- or 2-week intervals to prevent recurrence. Oral ketoconazole (in doses of

200 mg/day for 1 to 2 weeks) should be reserved for cases not responding to topical treatment. Ciclopirox olamine 1% shampoo also appears to be a safe agent for treatment of scalp SD.[52]

Systemic Infections

The most important factor in successful management of *Malassezia* fungemia in preterm infants is prompt removal of the colonized vascular catheter, whether or not antifungal treatment is given. Lipid supplements should be discontinued in almost all patients, and an antifungal imidazole agent, such as parenteral fluconazole (in doses of 5 mg/kg/day), should be administered to those with more serious infection. The extended-spectrum azoles, voriconazole and posaconazole, have in vitro activity but clinical data

regarding efficacy are extremely limited. No data support the activity of echinocandins against these basidiomycetous yeasts. Oral fluconazole or itraconazole may be adequate therapy for less ill patients. The duration of therapy depends on persistence of fungemia, presence of metastatic foci of infection, and removal of the catheter. While in vitro antifungal susceptibility testing of *Malassezia* species is currently unstandardized, several methods are published.[53-55] These methods testing a variety of species (*M. furfur, M. dermatis, M. globosa, M. obtuse, M. restricta, M. sloofiae, M. sympodialis, M. pachydermatis*) against several antifungal agents (amphotericin B, itraconazole, ketoconazole, fluconazole, voriconazole, posaconazole, terbinafine) demonstrated species-dependent in vitro data. The reader is referred to these papers for species-specific susceptibility.

Key Points. Diagnosis and Management of *Malassezia* Infections

MICROBIOLOGY

- Lipophilic, basidiomycetous yeasts in the order Malasseziales
- Genus includes 13 species, 12 of which require lipid-enriched culture medium for growth
- *M. pachydermatis* is non-lipid-dependent

EPIDEMIOLOGY

- *Malassezia* is part of normal flora of humans and warm-blooded animals
- Skin colonization begins at birth, increases to 25% in children, and almost to 100% in adults
- Degree of colonization is related to sebaceous gland activity at puberty
- Lipid-rich intravenous infusions are important risk factor for systemic disease
- Most infections are sporadic although nosocomial systemic outbreaks have been reported

CLINICAL FEATURES

- Superficial skin disorders
  - Pityriasis versicolor – commonly affects trunk, neck, upper arms; lesions are hyperpigmented in light-skinned individuals, and hypopigmented in dark-skinned persons
  - *Malassezia* folliculitis – primarily affects adults with debilitating disease – lesions are small, erythematous, follicular papules that often enlarge and become pustular

  - Seborrheic eczema/dermatitis – clinical forms include infantile and adult seborrheic eczema with dandruff being the mildest manifestation
- Systemic infections – severity ranges from localized organ infections to fulminant fungemia

DIAGNOSIS

- Superficial infections – direct microscopic examination of lesions, culture, molecular methods
- Systemic infections – cultures of central venous catheter and blood

TREATMENT

- Skin infections
  - Pityriasis versicolor – topical selenium sulfide lotion 2.5% or oral imidazoles
  - *Malassezia* folliculitis – topical imidazole or selenium sulfide; oral ketoconazole may be required; maintenance treatment may be required to prevent recurrence
  - Seborrheic dermatitis – ketoconazole shampoo or ciclopirox olamine 1% shampoo usually is effective; oral ketoconazole for recalcitrant infections
- Systemic infections
  - Remove vascular catheter promptly in preterm infants with fungemia; discontinue lipid supplements; give parenteral fluconazole in doses of 5 mg/kg/day
  - In vitro activity of various antifungal agents is species-dependent

---

248

Sporothrix schenckii (Sporotrichosis)

Thomas F. Patterson and Deanna A. Sutton

Sporotrichosis is a chronic subcutaneous fungal infection caused by a thermally dimorphic fungus, *Sporothrix schenckii*. This organism is found worldwide in soil, on decomposing vegetation, and on plant materials, such as sphagnum moss, hay bales, rose bushes, and wood. In nature, *S. schenckii* grows as a filamentous mold, but in tissue, it forms small budding yeast cells. Sporotrichosis has worldwide distribution but is most common in warm, temperate, or tropical regions where the temperature ranges between 16°C and 22°C. Phylogenetic, phenotypic, and physiologic differences have been identified among strains

previously referred to as *Sporothrix schenckii*, so that isolates are now reported as being members of the *Sporothrix schenckii* complex. In addition to *S. schenckii*, other distinct species in the complex include *S. mexicana, S. globosa, S. luriei, S. albicans, S. inflata,* and *S. brasiliensis*.[1,2] The typical rosettes produced by these species are mostly indistinguishable; however, the sessile conidia display varying morphologies. *S. luriei* lacks sessile conidia and has a thick-walled budding yeast form.[3] Calmodulin gene sequences are the most informative for species identification. Varied in vitro susceptibility may be responsible for varying clinical responses.[4]

EPIDEMIOLOGY

Cutaneous infection, which is the most common presentation in children and adults, usually follows traumatic implantation of *S. schenckii*.[5] Minor trauma from thorns or wood splinters is a typical route of exposure. Lesions usually appear 1 to 4 weeks after inoculation. Pulmonary disease is less common but is acquired by inhalation. Animal-to-human transmission, usually from cats with lesions, can occur but is not common, although large outbreaks associated with cats have occurred and transmission from other animals including armadillos has been reported.[6-8]

Infection with *S. schenckii* occurs in all age groups and is independent of race and gender, although some studies report male predominance, possibly due to increased exposures. Infections often are sporadic, occurring following outdoor exposures, although common source outbreaks are described and can be traced to activities that result in contact with contaminated moss, hay, or wood.[9-12] Ongoing zoonotic transmission from cats has been associated with a large epidemic of sporotrichosis in Brazil.[7,8,13-15] Investigation of outbreaks has led to insights into the epidemiology of sporotrichosis in the epidemic setting, but there is less information about disease in areas where sporotrichosis is hyperendemic.[16] Pappas et al. described 238 cases occurring in a remote region of the central highlands of Peru.[16] The incidence of disease ranged from 48 to 60 cases per 100,000 population and was highest among children 7 to 14 years of age, approaching 1 case per 1000. This report indicates that sporotrichosis in children is more common than is recognized, particularly in economically developing countries. Risk factors for sporotrichosis among children living in Peru included increased skin trauma, such as living in homes with dirt floors and contact with cats.[17]

CLINICAL MANIFESTATIONS

Most cases of sporotrichosis are localized to skin and lymphatic tissues. In contrast to sporotrichosis in adults, which can occur at any anatomic site, in children the disease most commonly affects the face and limbs, particularly hands and fingers.[16,18] Pulmonary and extrapulmonary infection, including joints, bones, central nervous system, and other tissues, occurs but is less common. Systemic infection is more likely to occur in patients with altered host defenses, including people with diabetes, alcoholism, injecting drug use, and other immunocompromised people, including people with AIDS. Systemic forms of sporotrichosis are rare in children.[16]

After inoculation, the fungus replicates at the site of infection and then invades the regional lymphatics. In 25% of cases, the infection remains confined to the initial site of inoculation, which is common in facial lesions. Such "fixed" infections are more common in children than in adults.[5,19] Cutaneous sporotrichosis develops as a small, firm painless papule or vesicle that initially is mobile but later becomes fixed. The lesion slowly enlarges over several weeks, and the skin and subcutaneous tissues surrounding the lesion become indurated and red. Within 10 days to 2 weeks after appearance of the lesion, skin necrosis occurs, leaving a minimally painful superficial ulcer with irregular borders. In most cases, infection spreads to the regional lymph nodes that drain the site of the primary infection. The resulting ascending chain of nontender, mobile, subcutaneous nodules with overlying erythematous skin is the classic manifestation of sporotrichosis. Untreated, the nodules slowly enlarge, soften, and can evolve into draining ulcers, even though involved skin may not be painful (see Figure 20-2).

In disseminated cutaneous sporotrichosis (which occurs in <1% of patients), numerous small papules or vesicles progress to necrotic, ulcerated nodules over the trunk and limbs. This form generally follows lymphatic or hematogenous spread from an initial cutaneous or pulmonary site of infection, but also can be due to multiple cutaneous inoculations. The diagnosis of cutaneous or lymphocutaneous sporotrichosis should be suspected in any patient with papulovesicular or ulcerative lesions of the skin that are unresponsive to antibacterial treatment. Sporotrichosis should be suspected with the following triad: painless skin ulcer, nodules along ascending lymphatics, and unresponsiveness to antibacterial treatment. Other infectious etiologies that should be considered include blastomycosis, chromoblastomycosis, paracoccidioidomycosis, and leishmaniasis, in the appropriate epidemiologic setting. "Fixed" cutaneous infections without lymphangitic spread are difficult to differentiate clinically from actinomycosis, nocardiosis, and nontuberculous mycobacterial disease.

Pulmonary sporotrichosis usually manifests as subacute or chronic pneumonia, which can be indistinguishable clinically from other chronic pulmonary infections. Symptoms are nonspecific, including productive cough, fever, weight loss, anorexia, shortness of breath, and hemoptysis, which can be massive. The radiographic findings are nonspecific and can mimic tuberculosis, usually involving the upper lobes, which can cavitate. Hilar adenopathy and pleural involvement can occur. Disseminated sporotrichosis, which is uncommon in children, generally develops after lymphatic or hematogenous spread from an initial cutaneous infection or after pulmonary infection.[5] Skeletal involvement has been reported in up to 80% of patients with extracutaneous disease. A chronic destructive arthritis of the knee and other large weight-bearing joints is the most typical presentation, although the small joints of the hand and wrist can be involved. Meningitis is a rare but severe manifestation of disseminated sporotrichosis.

DIAGNOSIS

The laboratory diagnosis of sporotrichosis can be difficult and depends on direct microscopy and culture of pathologic material. Direct microscopic examination can be negative due to the paucity of organisms in clinical samples, such as skin scrapings or exudates. Detection of typical oval or cigar-shaped cells or asteroid bodies of *S. schenckii* in stained histologic sections confirms the diagnosis. Immunofluorescence is a sensitive and specific method but is not widely available for clinical use.[20]

The diagnosis of sporotrichosis depends on isolation of the organism from a soft-tissue exudate or a tissue biopsy specimen. With visceral organ or osteoarticular infection, cultures of tissue rather than sputum, synovial, or other body fluids, increases the yield. Culture incubated at room temperature usually is positive within a week.

Serology has not proved to be useful for diagnosis of sporotrichosis, and nonculture-based tests are not available.

TREATMENT

Guidelines for therapy for treatment of sporotrichosis have been published.[21] Lymphocutaneous sporotrichosis uncommonly resolves without treatment.[13] Permanent scarring and disfigurement are common, as is bacterial superinfection. Oral itraconazole (in doses of 6 to 10 mg/kg/day up to a maximum of 400 mg/day) is recommended for children with cutaneous or lymphocutaneous sporotrichosis, although lower doses (100 mg/day) also have been effective.[21,22] Therapy should be continued for 2 to 4 weeks after lesions have resolved; for most patients therapy is required for 3 to 6 months and is successful in >90% of patients.[21,23] Fluconazole is less effective and should be regarded as a second-line agent for children who cannot tolerate other therapies or who do not absorb itraconazole.[21,24] Ketoconazole has less efficacy and should not be used. Data for use of posaconazole or voriconazole for sporotrichosis are very limited but *Sporothrix* species frequently are resistant in vitro to voriconazole, which should not be used.[4,25] Oral terbinafine (at doses up to 500 mg twice daily) is effective for lymphocutaneous disease in small clinical studies in adults but with very limited data in children.[26,27] Saturated potassium iodide solution (SSKI) is the least costly option for lymphocutaneous infection and can be administered to children, but SSKI is associated with many side effects and thus is poorly tolerated by children and adults. Dose-limiting side effects include a strong metallic taste, gastrointestinal tract intolerance, salivary gland swelling, rash, and fever.[28] In children, a dose of 50 mg or 1 drop 3 times daily in water or juice is given initially and increased as tolerated by 1 drop per dose per day (up to a maximum of 1 drop/kg or 40 to 50 drops 3 times daily, whichever is lower).[21,29] Local application of heat, by a variety of warming devices or baths, has been reported as an effective alternative treatment for fixed cutaneous lesions, but should be reserved for patients in whom antifungal drugs are contraindicated or not tolerated.[30]

For patients with life-threatening systemic or pulmonary sporotrichosis, amphotericin B (0.7 to 1 mg/kg/day) or liposomal amphotericin B (3 to 5 mg/kg/day) is recommended.[21] Itraconazole can be used for less seriously ill patients and as oral sequential therapy after an initial response to therapy with amphotericin B. Surgical resection, when possible, combined with antifungal therapy may improve outcome. Osteoarticular sporotrichosis

usually is treated with itraconazole, which should be continued for 1 to 2 years.[21] Unfortunately, joint function uncommonly returns to normal. SSKI or terbafine should not be used for osteoarticular sporotrichosis.[21]

PREVENTION

Sporotrichosis can be prevented by reducing skin trauma in high-risk settings (from hay bales, moss, plants, rose bushes, and trees) by wearing protective clothing, such as long sleeves and gloves, by limiting animal exposures in specific epidemiologic settings such as epidemic transmission from cats, or by avoiding exposure completely.[7,10,16]

Key Points. Diagnosis and Management of Sporotrichosis

MICROBIOLOGY
- Thermally dimorphic fungus – grows as a mold in nature, with small budding yeast cells in tissue; grows within a week on routine microbiologic media
- Isolated in soil, decomposing vegetation – sphagnum moss, hay, rose bushes, wood
- Now referred to as *Sporothrix schenckii* complex due to phylogenetic, phenotypic, and physiologic differences in strains; additional distinct species include *S. mexicana*, *S. globosa*, *S. luriei*, and *S. brasiliensis*

EPIDEMIOLOGY
- Occurs worldwide, most commonly as cutaneous or lymphocutaneous infection
- Typically associated with minor trauma from thorns or wood splinters
- Zoonotic transmission – uncommon, usually from cats (which has led to current epidemic in Brazil); other animals such as armadillos also implicated

CLINICAL FEATURES
- Cutaneous or lymphocutaneous infection: especially common in children including face perhaps due to autoinfection
  - Fixed lesion – painless papule with erythema and induration

- Lymphocutaneous – more common; superficial ulcer with ascending lymphangitic chain of nontender, mobile, subcutaneous nodules or ulcers over erythematous skin
- Pulmonary: subacute or chronic pneumonia following inhalation of organism; nonspecific presentation including productive cough, fever, weight loss, shortness of breath, hemoptysis; nonspecific infiltrates
- Disseminated: uncommon, especially in children; can involve bone and central nervous system

DIAGNOSIS
- Recovery of organism from body fluids, tissue
- Microscopic examination of pathologic material – oval or cigar-shaped cells or asteroid bodies
- Immunofluorescent tissue stain is sensitive and specific but not available widely

TREATMENT
- Lymphocutaneous or cutaneous: itraconazole is preferred therapy, usually for 3 to 6 months
- Life-threatening disseminated or pulmonary: amphotericin B or liposomal amphotericin B followed by itraconazole
- Osteoarticular or extrapulmonary: extended course of itraconazole

---

249 *Cryptococcus* Species

George R. Thompson III and Thomas F. Patterson

Cryptococcus species are encapsulated, basidiomycetous yeasts. Although >30 species are included in the genus *Cryptococcus*, the pathogenic yeasts of cryptococcosis are currently classified in 2 species: *C. neoformans* and *C. gattii*.[1,2] These species were previously separated into 3 varieties: *C. neoformans* var. *neoformans*, *C. neoformans* var. *grubii*, and *C. neoformans* var. *gattii*, which were classified into 8 molecular genotypes and 5 serotypes based on capsular polysaccharide antigens. Serotypes A and D and the hybrid diploid AD strains belong to *C. neoformans* and serotype B and C strains are classified as *C. gattii* (Table 249-1). Serotype A strains are designated as *C. neoformans* var. *grubii* and serotype D strains are designated *C. neoformans* var. *neoformans*.[3–5] *C. neoformans* var. *grubii* has a worldwide distribution and is the most common causative agent of cryptococcosis in people with acquired

immunodeficiency syndrome (AIDS) and other immunocompromised people, accounting for >95% of cryptococcal cases.[4,6] In contrast, *C. gattii* usually affects immunocompetent people living in the tropics and subtropics and has been associated with eucalyptus trees, which were considered its major environmental niche. As reported in 2004, *C. gattii* has caused a substantial outbreak of cryptococcal infections on Vancouver Island, further expanding its geographic boundaries and demonstrating its association with other trees.[7]

Several factors contribute to the virulence of *C. neoformans*, including the ability to grow in the environment as well as at 37°C, production of a polysaccharide capsule, and the ability to produce melanin. Acapsular strains of *Cryptococcus* exhibit a marked decrease in virulence. Genetic knockout studies in mice

TABLE 249-1. Characteristics of the Genus *Cryptococcus*

	Cryptococcus Species		
Characteristic	***Cryptococcus neoformans***		***Cryptococcus gattii***
Varieties	*grubii*	*Neoformans*	–
Serotype	A	D	B, C
Sexual state	*Filobasidiella neoformans*	*Filobasidiella neoformans*	*Filobasidiella bacillispora*
Geographic distribution	Worldwide (95% of cryptococcal cases)	Northern Europe	Tropics and subtropics; recent outbreak on Vancouver Island
Natural sources	Avian guano	Avian guano	Eucalyptus trees; other trees
Isolation from AIDS patients	Common	Common	Uncommon

using an acapsular mutant strain with deletion of the capsular *CAP59* gene demonstrated a marked reduction in virulence.[8] The ability to produce melanin is thought to play a role in both the virulence and the neurotropism of *C. neoformans*, as melanin-deficient mutants are less virulent in mice and the central nervous system (CNS) is rich in precursors for production of melanin.[9] Primary infection with cryptococcosis usually follows inhalation into the lungs. The organism is controlled principally by cell-mediated immunity in conjunction with phagocytosis.[10] Initially, neutrophils play a role in containing the yeast in lungs, followed by activity of monocytes. CD4+ T lymphocytes have been shown to be essential in containing CNS infection, which may account for the much higher incidence of cryptococcosis in people with AIDS. Although antibody and complement cannot kill cryptococci directly, both enhance opsonization.[6]

EPIDEMIOLOGY

C. neoformans and *C. gattii* differ in their natural habitat and geographic distribution. *C. gattii* causes infection in tropical and subtropical regions of the world and is associated with several species of eucalyptus trees as its ecologic niche, although the outbreak of *C. gattii* infections on Vancouver Island has demonstrated association with other trees, including firs and oaks, and an expanded geographic zone.[7] For *C. neoformans*, both *C. neoformans* var. *grubii* (serotype A) and *C. neoformans* var. *neoformans* (serotype D) are isolated most frequently from soil contaminated with pigeon or other bird guano.[11] The two varieties differ in their geographic distribution: serotype A has been isolated throughout the world, usually infecting people with AIDS or other immunocompromising conditions, whereas infections with serotype D are more prevalent in certain geographic areas, such as northern Europe.[6]

Although *Cryptococcus* species can be isolated from pigeon droppings, documentation of infection following this type of exposure is limited.[12] Molecular strain typing has not yet linked a specific environmental source with cryptococcosis but has demonstrated that some clinical and environmental isolates are indistinguishable.[13] Host factors are important in determining the risk of developing cryptococcosis. HIV infection is now the most common immunocompromising illness in patients with cryptococcosis, although the incidence of cryptococcosis has decreased with the institution of active antiretroviral therapy (ART). However, in areas worldwide where ART is not available, cryptococcosis remains the most common life-threatening fungal infection.[6] In people with HIV infection, cryptococcosis usually occurs in patients with CD4+ lymphocyte counts of <100 cells/mm³.[14] Other immunocompromised hosts with cell-mediated immunologic defects, such as patients with lymphoma and sarcoidosis, and people receiving corticosteroid treatment, also have increased risk for both *C. neoformans* and *C. gattii* infections.[14a] No association between cryptococcosis and race has been detected.[14]

Until the AIDS epidemic began, cryptococcosis was rare. Population-based active surveillance conducted in four areas of the United States during 1992 to 1994 showed that cryptococcosis developed in 2% to 5% of people with AIDS per year.[14] The rate of cryptococcal infection in HIV-infected people decreased dramatically after the introduction of ART, decreasing by 46% in one study and from an incidence as high as 66 per 1000 to 2–7 per 1000 in another study.[15,16] Also notable is the fact that, of the 1083 cases of cryptococcosis detected during a population-based surveillance before ART, only 4 occurred in people <18 years of age, 2 of whom were HIV-infected.[14] These data were confirmed by other studies that showed cryptococcal infection was less common in HIV-infected children than adults, with occurrence rates of 1% and 1.4%.[17,18] Most of the cases of cryptococcosis occurred in children 6 to 12 years of age; 9 of 13 cases diagnosed after 1990 occurred in children with vertical HIV infection. Similarly, *C. gattii* infection is uncommon in children, with only 3 confirmed cases (all pulmonary and in HIV-negative patients) reported.[19]

Occasional cases of cryptococcosis occur in children without HIV infection, the most common underlying conditions being lymphoproliferative disorders and immunosuppressive treatment.[20] Rare cases occur in apparently healthy children. The reasons for the lower incidence reported in children is unknown but may relate to differences in environmental exposures or immunologic factors.

CLINICAL MANIFESTATIONS

Cryptococcosis is acquired by inhalation of infectious airborne particles. The incubation period is unknown and could be weeks, months, or even longer. Whether the infectious particles are desiccated acapsular yeast cells or basidiospores of the sexual state of the fungus is unclear, but the encapsulated yeast cells are thought to be too large to penetrate the defenses of the upper respiratory tract. After inhalation, organisms then disseminate in immunocompromised patients from lungs to other sites, with or without evident pulmonary infection. Any organ can be affected, including bone and soft tissue, but the most serious form of the disease is meningitis or meningoencephalitis, which is fatal if untreated.[6]

The clinical manifestations of cryptococcosis in children with AIDS are similar to those in adults.[17,18,20] The presentation of cryptococcosis in patients with AIDS more commonly involves extrapulmonary disease, including cryptococcemia, and extensive CNS infection with a high burden of organisms, as manifest by positive India ink examinations and antigen titers, as well as a limited cerebrospinal fluid (CSF) inflammatory response.[21]

Pulmonary Manifestations

Primary cryptococcosis is asymptomatic in up to one-third of immunocompetent people after inhalation of *C. neoformans*.[22] Even in immunocompromised patients, including people with AIDS, primary pulmonary infection may not be diagnosed until extrapulmonary dissemination, particularly meningitis, occurs.[23] More persistent pulmonary cryptococcosis often develops in people with HIV infection. Most patients come to medical attention with headache, fever, cough, dyspnea, and weight loss, and some have pleuritic chest pain and hemoptysis. The most frequent radiographic findings are focal or diffuse interstitial infiltrates and hilar lymphadenopathy. Unlike in patients with filamentous fungal infections, nodular and alveolar infiltrates are rare, as are large mass lesions and pleural effusions.[22,24]

Neurologic Manifestations

Infection of the CNS is the most common clinical presentation of cryptococcosis and the complication most frequently associated with mortality. Although cryptococcal meningitis can be acute, it most often follows an indolent course with asymptomatic periods. In people with AIDS, the most common symptoms are headache, fever, and altered mental status; meningeal signs are uncommon. Focal neurologic signs are initially uncommon and occur in about 10% of patients. If focal lesions are detected, especially in patients with AIDS, another diagnosis, such as brain abscess due to another infectious cause (toxoplasmosis, tuberculosis, bacterial abscess, or other causes) or malignancy (primary CNS lymphoma) should be considered as CNS mass lesions (cryptococcomas) have not been reported in HIV-infected children.[25] Increased intracranial pressure is common in patients with CNS cryptococcosis, especially those with AIDS, and represents a life-threatening complication. These patients present with severe headache, abnormal mental status, visual disturbance, and frequently with hearing loss.[26,27] The underlying mechanism is unclear, but it is thought to be due in part to interference with CSF reabsorption in the arachnoid villi as a result of the accumulation of fungal polysaccharide. Aggressive management of elevated intracranial pressure by means of repeated lumbar CSF drainage is perhaps the most important factor in reducing mortality and minimizing the morbidity of acute cryptococcal meningitis.[26]

About 90% of patients with cryptococcal meningitis who are not HIV-infected have abnormal CSF findings, including increased opening pressure (65%), elevated protein concentration (90%), lowered glucose concentration (75%), and a lymphocytic pleocytosis. In people with AIDS, the CSF can appear normal, with normal protein and glucose concentrations and minimal or absent pleocytosis[28]

Skin Manifestations

Cryptococcal skin lesions occur in 10% to 15% of patients with disseminated disease as a result of hematogenous spread. Direct extension from a bone lesion can also occur. Single or multiple pustules or papules are most common and sometimes progress to ulcers or abscesses. These lesions typically are described as molluscum contagiosum-like but cannot be distinguished without a biopsy and culture from other infections such as those due to *Histoplasma capsulatum, Coccidioides immitis,* or *Penicillium marneffei.*[29] Infiltrated plaques resembling cellulitis also have been reported. Although the most common site for skin lesions is the face and scalp, the trunk or limbs also can be involved.

Other Sites

Bone infection occurs in about 5% to 10% of patients with disseminated cryptococcosis. Pain and swelling can be present, but bone lesions often are found incidentally. Radiographs reveal well-defined osteolytic lesions without marginal sclerosis or periosteal change. Joint involvement is rare. Eye involvement with cryptococcal meningitis can occur and manifests as retinitis. Cryptococcosis can involve any organ system, including adrenal glands, heart, liver, spleen, and prostate.

DIAGNOSIS

Diagnosis is not usually difficult and requires isolation of *Cryptococcus* in culture or detection of cryptococcal capsular antigen in blood, CSF, or urine.

Encapsulated *C. neoformans* often can be seen on direct microscopic examination of CSF or other body fluids and secretions mounted in India ink, mucicarmine, or other stains, such as nigrosin. In people with AIDS, *C. neoformans* cells usually are plentiful in the CSF, although care must be taken not to confuse organisms with lymphocytes in CSF. Budding of the organism can be useful for that distinction.

C. neoformans can be isolated from CSF in 75% to 90% of cases of cryptococcal meningitis and is even more likely to be positive in

patients with AIDS due to the high burden of organisms.[28] In patients with negative cultures, periodic high-volume CSF samples (>10 mL) may increase the yield. The organism grows well on standard microbiologic media and fungal media such as Sabouraud glucose agar, but it is inhibited in media containing cyclohexamide. *C. gattii* grows as deep blue colonies on canavanine–glycine–bromothymol culture (CGB) media while *C. neoformans* is unable to grow on this media. Growth is enhanced at 30°C to 35°C; incubation should be extended for up to 2 weeks in suspected cases. Blood and urine cultures also can be positive. Isolation of *Cryptococcus* from respiratory tract samples, including sputum, bronchoalveolar lavage fluid, or lung tissue, may be useful in pulmonary infection. Immunocompromised patients with pulmonary cryptococcosis should be evaluated for CNS disease.

Testing for cryptococcal capsular antigen in serum, CSF, urine, or bronchoalveolar lavage specimens is one of the most reliable nonculture-based methods of fungal diagnosis. The antigen test is positive in >90% of patients with untreated cryptococcal meningitis, but it is somewhat less sensitive in patients without CNS disease. The test is highly specific, and false-positive results are seen primarily in other basidiomycetous yeast infections such as those caused by *Trichosporon* spp. False-negative test results can occur if the organism load is low or if organisms are not well encapsulated. Tests to detect serum antibodies to *C. neoformans* have been less helpful because such antibodies are seldom found in patients with untreated meningeal or disseminated infection, although their presence may indicate a favorable prognosis.[30]

Antigen tests should be performed on all CSF specimens at the time of initial diagnosis and can be measured on subsequent CSF specimens to evaluate response to treatment, although serial CSF antigen titers have a limited role in management.[31] Serum antigen levels are even less useful in monitoring response to treatment, likely due to persistence of polysaccharide capsule. Various commercial tests are available for detection of cryptococcal antigen, which now are performed by enzyme immunoassay rather than the original latex agglutination assay.

TREATMENT

Without treatment, cryptococcal meningitis is fatal.[32] Treatment for cryptococcal disease has not been studied in a controlled manner in pediatric patients, so that data from adult trials have been used in recommendations for treating cryptococcal infection in children.[25,33] Combination therapy with amphotericin B and flucytosine for 2 weeks followed by another 8 weeks of therapy with fluconazole is recommended for most patients with severe cryptococcosis and cryptococcal meningitis.[25,34] This approach is associated with a mortality of <10% and a mycologic response >70%.[33,35]

Amphotericin B deoxycholate remains the standard agent for treating serious cryptococcal infection, despite the fact that it must be administered parenterally and is associated with dose-limiting toxicities.[34] Amphotericin B usually is given at a dose of 0.7 to 1.0 mg/kg per day in combination with flucytosine at 100 mg/kg per day in 4 divided doses for 2 weeks followed by therapy with fluconazole or itraconazole for 8 weeks or until cultures are sterile.[25,34] Lipid-based formulations of amphotericin B reduce toxicities of amphotericin B.[36,37] Although the optimal doses of these agents have not been established, a dose of 4 mg/kg per day has been effective.[36,37] Cost remains a serious obstacle to their routine use.

Flucytosine is an orally bioavailable antifungal agent with potent activity against *C. neoformans,* but resistance develops rapidly when the drug is used as a single agent. When flucytosine is given in combination with amphotericin B, relapses are reduced and cultures become negative more quickly.[35] Studies of combination therapy in animals and randomized clinical studies support their use, although data documenting superior outcomes are limited.[38] Flucytosine has the potential for considerable toxicities, including bone marrow suppression, nausea and vomiting, skin and kidney toxicities, especially in patients with abnormal renal function.

The triazole antifungal agents, including fluconazole and itraconazole, as well as the extended-spectrum triazoles, voriconazole and posaconazole, have excellent activity against *C. neoformans.*[39] Fluconazole crosses the blood–brain barrier, achieves good CSF concentrations, and is well tolerated, so it has become the primary azole used in cryptococcal meningitis. For children with mild-to-moderate cryptococcosis that does not involve the CNS or is confined to the lungs, fluconazole alone can be considered for primary therapy. However, higher failure rates and increased mortality are associated with fluconazole as primary therapy of cryptococcal meningitis, so that use as a single agent is not recommended in most patients with more severe infection or meningitis.[34] For children with cryptococcal meningitis completing a 2-week induction course of amphotericin B combined with flucytosine, fluconazole (at a dosage of 10 to 12 mg/kg per day divided into 2 doses daily, either intravenously or orally) then is recommended for a minimum of 8 weeks.[25] Itraconazole is an alternative, but it does not penetrate well into the CSF and is associated with significant drug interactions and gastrointestinal tract intolerance.[25]

Refractory infection occurs and usually is related more to the severe immunocompromised condition of the host rather than to antifungal resistance, which is uncommon.[39] Susceptibility testing of *Cryptococcus* is of limited clinical value. More important clinically is confirming the diagnosis, establishing drug compliance and lack of interactions that limit drug exposure. Alternative agents are available, including voriconazole and posaconazole, which have both been shown in anecdotal series to have activity, although overall responses are not favorable due to their use almost exclusively as late salvage therapy in very immunosuppressed hosts.[40,41] The echinocandins do not have activity against *Cryptococcus* species due to a difference in fungal cell wall and should not be used.[42]

Prevention of relapse after successful treatment requires long-term suppressive treatment.[25] After 10 weeks the fluconazole therapy dosage can be reduced to an adolescent or adult dose of 200 mg/day, depending on the patient's clinical status. The safety of discontinuing secondary prophylaxis in HIV-infected children following immune reconstitution with ART has not been studied extensively, but it appears from cases in adults and adolescents that risk of relapse is low after the CD4+ lymphocyte count has risen to >200 cells/mm³.[25] Suppressive therapy should be reinitiated if the CD4+ lymphocyte count decreases to <200 cells/mm³ at a later time.

SPECIAL MANAGEMENT CONSIDERATIONS

In all cases of cryptococcal meningitis, careful attention to management of intracranial pressure is essential to ensure an optimal clinical outcome.[26,27] The principal intervention for reducing elevated intracranial pressure is percutaneous lumbar drainage of CSF. Radiographic imaging of the brain is recommended before performance of the initial lumbar puncture to rule out a space-occupying lesion.[34] Lumbar drainage should remove enough CSF to reduce the opening pressure by 50%. In cases in which repeated lumbar punctures or use of a lumbar drain fail to control elevated pressure symptoms or when persistent or progressive neurologic deficits are present, a ventriculoperitoneal shunt is indicated.[34] Adjunctive treatment with corticosteroid therapy is not recommended in HIV-infected patients.[34] Use of acetazolamide therapy was associated with increased toxicity, including severe acidosis in one trial in adults, and is not recommended.[43]

The use of ART has significantly improved the long-term outcomes associated with cryptococcal infection in HIV-infected patients and has decreased the incidence of disease. However, an immune reconstitution inflammatory syndrome (IRIS) has been reported in the last decade following initiation of ART in the acute treatment phase of opportunistic diseases in both adults and children.[44,45] Only positive baseline serum cryptococcal antigen titers have been found to correlate with cryptococcal IRIS.[46] Symptoms include elevated intracranial pressure, CSF pleocytosis, fever, headache, and meningismus, which can make it difficult to distinguish IRIS from relapse or progression of disease.[47,48] IRIS (which also can occur in non-HIV-infected patients with a rapidly recovering immune system) generally occurs within the first 1 to 2 months

after starting ART, so that delaying ART until completion of 8 to 10 weeks of antifungal therapy for cryptococcal infection should be considered.[47,48]

PREVENTION

Guidelines have been published for prevention of opportunistic infections, including cryptococcosis, in people with HIV infection.[49] Several studies have demonstrated that prophylactic administration of fluconazole to HIV-infected people at high risk for cryptococcosis can significantly reduce the risk of development of the disease.[50,51] However, use of fluconazole to prevent cryptococcal infection is not recommended because of the relative lack of frequency of infection and the unfavorable cost-to-benefit ratio in that setting.[49] No vaccine is available.

Key Points. Diagnosis and Management of Cryptococcal Infections

MICROBIOLOGY

- Encapsulated, basidiomycetous yeasts; grow well on routine microbiologic media
- Two species (*C. neoformans* and *C. gattii*) account for the majority of invasive infections
- *C. gattii* grows as deep blue colonies on canavanine–glycine–bromothymol blue media while *C. neoformans* is unable to grow in the presence of canavanine

EPIDEMIOLOGY

- Occurs worldwide, but only rarely causes disseminated infection in immunocompetent people
- Estimated one million cases in adults and children worldwide per year with 700,000 deaths
- Major risk factors: AIDS, prolonged glucocorticoid treatment, organ transplantation, hematologic malignancy, sarcoidosis, or use of other immunosuppressive medications
- Cryptococcosis is uncommon in children (even those with AIDS) compared with adults – reasons are unknown

CLINICAL FEATURES

- Central nervous system: often indolent with headache, fever, and altered mental status most common; focal neurologic deficits present in 10%; increased intracranial pressure very common
- Pulmonary: cough, pleuritic chest pain, hemotypsis, and focal or diffuse interstitial infiltrates with hilar lymphadenopathy
- Cutaneous: typically in those with disseminated disease; can mimic molluscum contagiosum
- Other: any organ system can be affected including adrenals, heart, liver, spleen, and prostate

DIAGNOSIS

- Recovery of organism from body fluids or tissue
- Microscopic examination of CSF on India ink-stained wet mounts
- Detection of cryptococcal capsular antigen in blood, CSF, or urine

TREATMENT

- CNS: combination amphotericin B and flucytosine for 2 weeks followed by fluconazole for 8 weeks. Fluconazole should be continued until immune reconstitution is observed (CD4+ lymphocyte count >200 cells/mm³ for at least 6 months)
- CNS: attention to intracranial pressure and attempt to reduce urgently if elevated
- Immune reconstitution inflammatory syndrome (IRIS): can occur following recovery of immunologic responsiveness; complicates management

250 *Histoplasma capsulatum* (Histoplasmosis)

Martin B. Kleiman

Histoplasmosis, the most common primary systemic mycosis in the United States, affects millions of people in urban and rural areas of the East and Midwest,[1,2] mostly in the Ohio and Mississippi river valleys. The fungus is also endemic to Central and South America,[3] parts of Australia, Africa, and eastern Asia.[4]

THE PATHOGEN

Microbiology

Histoplasmosis is caused by the dimorphic fungus *Histoplasma capsulatum* var. *capsulatum*. A common soil saprophyte, *H. capsulatum* grows as a spore-bearing mold below 35°C and as a yeast-like organism at 37°C. In its mold form, tuberculate macro conidia 8 to 14 μm in diameter are an identifying morphologic feature (Figure 250-1A). Co-culture of opposite mating types can produce altered sporulating structures in which genetic recombination occurs. This perfect state (teleomorph) is termed *Ajellomyces capsulatus*. Morphologic methods for identification of *H. capsulatum* isolates are slow, laborious, and hazardous; DNA probe technology shortens the time required for identification.[5] The infectious particles are the microconidia, spores 2 to 5 μm in diameter that are produced by the mold form. Yeastlike forms are 2 to 3 μm by 3 to 4 μm in diameter and typically are found in infected tissues (Figure 250-1B and C).

Pathogenesis

After inhalation, microconidia germinate within distal bronchioles and pulmonary alveoli where they undergo transition to yeastlike forms. Acute inflammatory changes then ensue. Lympho-hematogenous fungal dissemination occurs early in infection, even in self-limited disease.[6] The successful pathogenesis[7,8] of *H. capsulatum* results from its transition to the yeast phase, entry into and proliferation within macrophages,[9] and its ability to survive[10,11] and retain its ability to reactivate. In the normal host, after 1 month, specific T-lymphocyte immunity develops and interleukin (IL)-12 and interferon (IFN)-γ stimulate macrophages to kill the fungus, thereby controlling disease. Tumor necrosis factor-α (TNF-α) is also critical for effective host immunity.[12] Histopathologic changes include granulomas with Langerhans giant cells, typical yeastlike forms, and caseous necrosis.[13] Lesions heal by fibrous encapsulation and can calcify. In some patients, albeit rarely in children, an exuberant fibrous reaction destroys or obstructs major vessels, bronchi, or lung parenchyma, and/or critical mediastinal structures. In immunocompromised hosts or those with progressive disseminated infection, granulomas can be poorly formed and the large fungal burden can overwhelm the reticuloendothelial system.[14,15] Findings compatible with macrophage activation syndrome can occur in this setting.[16]

Immunity

Humoral immunity is measurable about 1 month after infection, but antibodies do not play a major role in controlling infection. In normal hosts, the cell-mediated immune response[17] significantly alters lymphocyte subpopulations,[14,18] aborts fungal growth, and provides a degree of protection against reinfection.[19] Reinfection usually results from re-exposure; recurrences have shorter incubation periods and are generally milder than primary infections. Although recrudescence of latent infection has been well

documented in HIV-infected people,[20] in recipients of transplanted organs from infected donors,[21] and in people receiving corticosteroids[22] or TNF-α inhibitors,[12,23–27] debate exists about the frequency of reactivation versus re-exposure-induced infection.[28] Progressive disseminated infections that occur in otherwise immunocompetent hosts, especially infants, can cause a transient T-lymphocyte deficiency that resolves after eradication of the organism.[14,15]

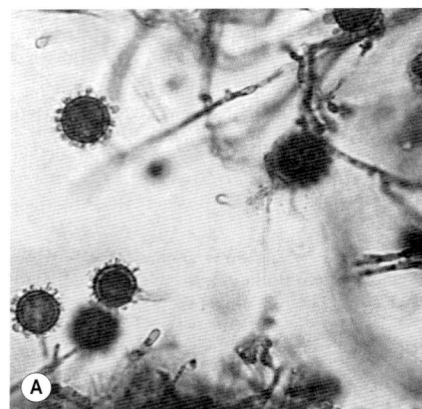

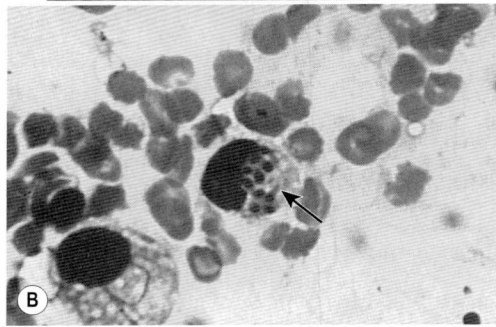

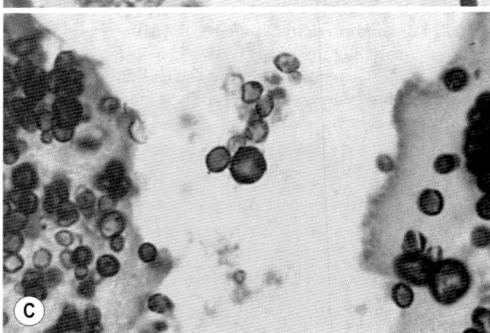

Figure 250-1. (A) Characteristic appearance of the tuberculate macroconidia of the mold form of *Histoplasma capsulatum* (lactophenol cotton blue stain, ×400). **(B)** Yeastlike forms of *H. capsulatum* in tissue. Yeastlike forms are typically found phagocytosed by histiocytes (see arrow) and are 2 to 3 μm in diameter (Giemsa stain, ×400). **(C)** Yeastlike forms of *H. capsulatum* in tissue stained with Gomori methenamine silver nitrate stain. Although cellular detail is lost with this stain, the characteristic yeastlike forms are easily identified (×1250).

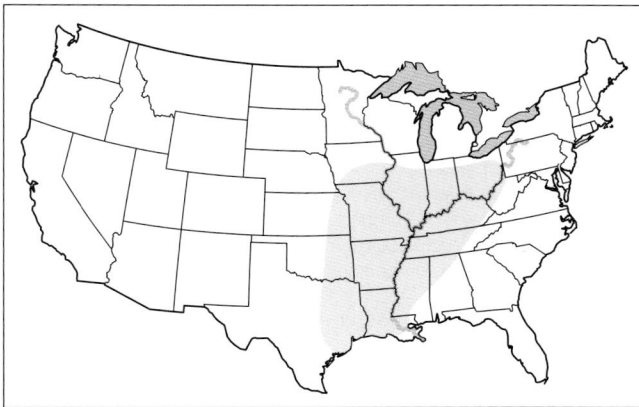

Figure 250-2. United States map showing the most highly endemic region for *Histoplasma capsulatum* – the Ohio and Mississippi river valleys.

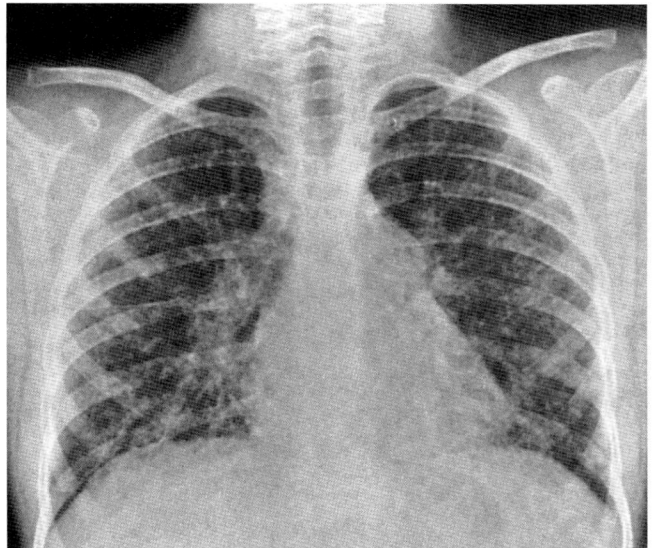

Figure 250-3. Chest radiograph of a severely ill 4-year-old child exposed to a large inoculum of *Histoplasma capsulatum* spores when her parents cleaned the fireplace of an abandoned house. Note the diffuse reticulonodular infiltrate and hilar lymph node enlargement.

EPIDEMIOLOGY

Skin test reactivity is common in residents of endemic regions. Areas of high incidence include the Mississippi and Ohio river valleys (Figure 250-2), where skin test reactivity in hyperendemic areas can develop in as many as 80% of people by 18 years of age.[2,29] Infections can occur sporadically or in clusters.[30,31] A single epidemic of over 100,000 cases of infection has been described in Indianapolis.[1] Bird and bat excrement promote fungal growth in the environment. Inhalation of aerosols generated when contaminated sites are disturbed are risk factors for infection. Box 250-1 shows a summary of the microfoci[31,32] and activities that most often predispose to infections in children. Contaminated air in closed spaces can cause intense exposure and serious illness (Figure 250-3). Large outbreaks have been reported to occur in industrial settings and in a school.[33-35] Increasingly, infections have been reported among travelers returning from endemic areas.[36-42] Vertically acquired disseminated histoplasmosis and HIV infection have been reported in a 5-week-old infant.[43]

CLINICAL MANIFESTATIONS

In non-outbreak settings, symptomatic infection occurs in fewer than 5% of infected individuals, and clinical manifestations vary widely. The outcome of exposure to *H. capsulatum* is influenced by: (1) inoculum size; (2) the functional integrity of host's cellular immunity;[14,17,18] (3) strain-specific virulence factors; and (4) pre-existing immunity.

Immunocompetent Host

The spectrum of principal clinical manifestations of histoplasmosis in childhood is summarized in Box 250-2. In a single source, high inoculum outbreak[35] at a high school, 523 persons developed serologic evidence of recent infection, 77% of whom

---

BOX 250-1. Point Sources/Activities Associated with Sporadic Childhood Histoplasmosis

Cleaning/renovating basements, attics, wall insulation of older homes
Cutting firewood/tree stumps
Cleaning abandoned building
Digging at sites of former bird roosts
Gardening
Playing in a barn
Playing in hollow trees
Exploring caves
Being downwind of excavation/demolition of contaminated sites

---

BOX 250-2. Principal Clinical Manifestations of Histoplasmosis in Children

RESPIRATORY TRACT

Pulmonary infarction
Cavitary pneumonia
Asthma
Pleural effusion
Anterior mediastinal lymphadenopathy
Acute/chronic bronchial obstruction
Isolated cervical/supraclavicular lymphadenopathy
Superior vena cava syndrome
Mediastinal granuloma/fibrosis
Vocal cord granuloma
Vocal cord paralysis
Hemoptysis
Broncholithiasis with lithoptysis
Chylothorax
Diaphragmatic weakness/paralysis

OTHER

Meningitis/focal cerebritis
Arthritis
Parotitis
Interstitial nephritis
Nephrocalcinosis
Hypercalcemia
Gastrointestinal tract ulceration/hemorrhage
Gastrointestinal tract pseudomalignancy
Biliary obstruction
Cutaneous or conjunctival inoculation and regional adenitis
Choroiditis
Endocarditis
Esophageal diverticulum/fistula
Adrenal mass

---

developed symptoms. Most began from 2 to 3 weeks following exposure. Principal complaints were headache (90%), fatigue (79%), fever (79%), cough (73%), myalgias (71%), non-pleuritic chest pain (66%), and arthralgias (52%). Symptoms usually last 2 or 3 days. In about 5% of children, symptoms are subacute, persist longer than 2 weeks, and include lethargy, poor appetite, and weight loss. Rhematologic manifestations including erythema nodosum and/or arthralgia[44] can occur, often in adolescents. In about 10% of symptomatic children, pericardial effusion develops and, albeit infrequently, can become large enough to impair diastolic filling.[45,46] Pericardial fluid is almost always sterile and usually results from inflammation caused by infected contiguous lymph nodes. Hypercalcemia, occasionally seen with other granulomatous infections, can occur in histoplasmosis.[47] Many mediastinal and abdominal manifestations result from irritation, compression, or destruction of structures adjacent to infected lymph nodes.[48,49] Other manifestations include chylothorax,[50] pleural effusion,[51] multifocal choroiditis,[52] and cystic duct obstruction.[53] Except in cases of massive exposure (see Figure 250-3), fatality is rare in otherwise healthy, older children.

Fungal dissemination that occurs early in infection almost always is self-limited in normal individuals. The term *progressive disseminated histoplasmosis* is applied to instances of continued and overwhelming reticuloendothelial infection; and is fatal if untreated.[15,48] This manifestation often suppresses cellular immune function[14,15] in previously immunocompetent hosts, and is a common opportunistic infection in individuals with acquired or congenital cellular immune dysfunction. An infrequent manifestation of progressive dissemination occurs in otherwise healthy infants. Termed *progressive disseminated histoplasmosis of infancy*, its initial symptoms are subacute, sometimes lasting several weeks, although progressive. Complaints and signs include fever, weight loss,[15] and progressive hepatosplenomegaly (Figure 250-4). Meningitis occurs in about 60% of affected infants.[15] Pancytopenia and disseminated intravascular coagulopathy (DIC) are ominous signs; infection is fatal if untreated.

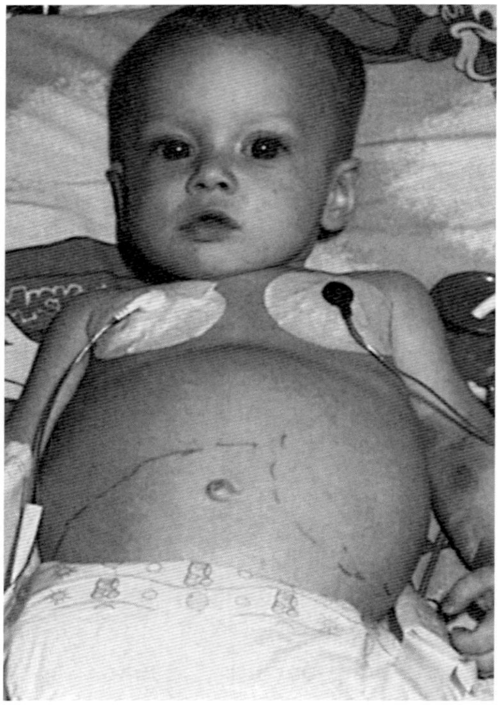

Figure 250-4. Six-month-old boy with disseminated histoplasmosis. He had a 1-month history of failing to thrive and a "swollen abdomen". Note the characteristic appearance with massive hepatosplenomegaly, early signs of cachexia, and yet a bright, responsive facial appearance.

BOX 250-3. Risk Factors for Severe Histoplasmosis in Human Immunodeficiency Virus Infection

Risk factors

Black race
Partial thromboplastin time >45 seconds
Alkaline phosphatase >2.5 times the upper limit of normal
Bilirubin serum level >1.5 mg/dL
Serum creatinine level >2.1 mg/dL
Aspartate aminotransferase serum level >2.5 times the upper limit of normal
Albumin serum level <3.5 mg/dL

Independent risk factors for death within 30 days of treatment

Dyspnea
Platelet count <100,000/mm³
Lactic dehydrogenase serum level >2 times the upper limit of normal

Immunocompromised Host

Impaired cellular immunity markedly increases the risk of progressive dissemination and life-threatening infection.[18,54–56] In addition to patients undergoing immunosuppressive therapy for malignancies or transplantation,[57,58] increased risk has also been associated with use of TNF antagonists that are used to treat inflammatory conditions.[23,59–61] Illness usually begins with fever, followed by cough, diffuse pulmonary infiltrates, and ultimately hypoxia. Patients with HIV infection may have only prolonged fever and weight loss and no pulmonary findings.[48,54,56] Large necrotic masses of infected lymph nodes can develop occasionally. Although data for children are lacking, Box 250-3 identifies risk factors that, when present in adults with HIV infections complicated by histoplasmosis, are predictive of shock, respiratory failure, or death.[62,63] Patients who are receiving highly active antiretroviral therapy (HAART) may, as a result of immune reconstitution, develop recurrence of symptoms caused by histoplasmosis.[64,65]

LABORATORY FINDINGS AND DIAGNOSIS

Nonspecific Tests

In self-limited histoplasmosis in an immunocompetent host, hemograms may show only mild anemia. The erythrocyte sedimentation rate almost always is elevated. Pancytopenia and DIC often are seen in untreated, progressive disseminated histoplasmosis. Hemophagocytosis can occur in disseminated infections in immunocompromised hosts.[66] Histopathologic features of histoplasmosis in the immunocompetent host show well-formed necrotizing granulomatous inflammation. In immunocompromised patients histology shows poorly formed granulomas with sheets of histiocytes containing typical yeasts.[67]

Chest radiographic findings in persons with acute infections can be normal or show middle mediastinal adenopathy[68] and/or localized pulmonary infiltrates (Figure 250-5). Computed tomography of the chest is more sensitive than plain radiography. In high inoculum exposure, a diffuse reticulonodular infiltrate can be observed (see Figure 250-3). Radiographs of asymptomatic residents of endemic regions often reveal single or multiple calcified nodules in the lungs and hilar lymph nodes and, occasionally, calcifications in the spleen or liver. These findings usually are the result of previous, often unrecognized infections.

Specific Laboratory Tests

Serologic tests, culture, tissue and body fluid examination, and quantitative enzyme immunoassay (EIA) for *Histoplasma* antigen in the urine, serum, cerebrospinal fluid, and bronchoalveolar

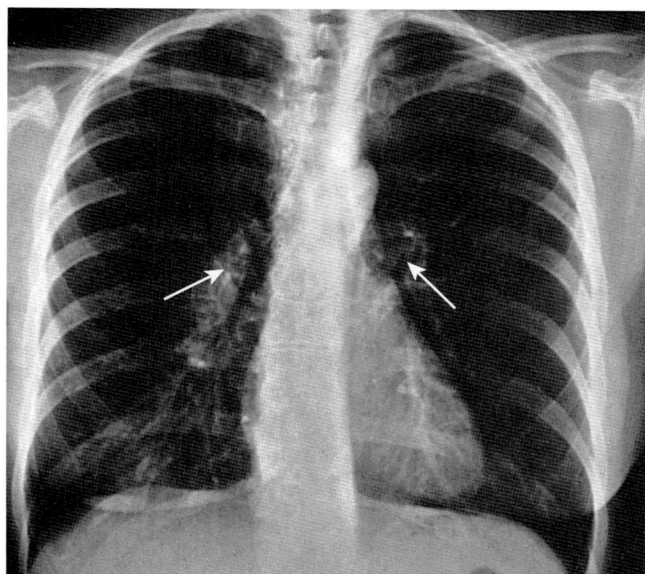

Figure 250-5. Chest radiograph of an adolescent with acute histoplasmosis and erythema nodosum. Radiographic findings are typical of mild histoplasmosis and show a minor pulmonary infiltrate (right lower lobe) and hilar lymph node enlargement (arrows).

lavage fluid[69-73] are the principal laboratory tests used for diagnosis. Table 250-1 is an interpretive guide. Multiple positive tests, especially in children with clinically compatible illnesses, increase the positive predictive value of marginal serologic results.

Immunodiffusion and complement fixation assays that detect *Histoplasma*-specific antibody are positive in about 90% of infections in immunocompetent patients.[69] The titer of antibody by the

complement fixation test is directly proportional to severity of illness and degree of exposure.[35,74] In acute self-limited infections, measurable antibody appears 4 to 6 weeks after infection and can revert to negative after 12 to 18 months. Although more sensitive than the immunodiffusion test, the complement fixation test is less specific, showing 18% cross-reactivity with antigens of *Blastomyces*, *Paracoccidioides*, and *Coccidioides* as well as other fungi.[31] Clinical features, exposure and travel histories, and results of other diagnostic data aid in differentiating these entities. In the immunodiffusion precipitin test, H bands are found in only 23% of patients with acute pulmonary infection but are more highly suggestive of active infection compared with M bands; M bands are found in 76%. The immunodiffusion assay is quite specific, showing cross-reactions in only 5%.

A positive culture is confirmatory, but growth may take up to 6 weeks. The sensitivity of culture is low in all but severe, progressive dissemination and chronic pulmonary infection. Lysis centrifugation methods should be used. In the presence of a compatible illness and the probability of exposure, the observation, by an experienced examiner, of yeastlike forms compatible with *H. capsulatum* in tissue, bone marrow, bronchoalveolar lavage fluid, or peripheral blood often is diagnostic (see Figure 250-1). Exceptions can include instances in which typical, though nonviable, organisms are observed within granulomas in patients with past infections.[75] Although progress has been made in molecular methodology that can detect *H. capsulatum* in tissue samples,[76-79] techniques are not available commercially.

A rapid EIA[4,73,80] that quantifies *Histoplasma* antigen in urine, serum, bronchoalveolar lavage,[81] and cerebrospinal fluid is available for diagnosis. The EIA demonstrates high sensitivity in serious manifestations of infection including early primary pulmonary infection and serious and life-threatening histoplasmosis. EIA is especially useful for immunocompromised patients in whom serologic tests can be falsely negative. In a highly endemic region, antigenuria was detected in 100% of children with progressive, disseminated histoplasmosis. Since the assay also reflects fungal burden, it is also used both to monitor the effectiveness

TABLE 250-1. Interpretive Guidelines for Laboratory Tests in Children with Acute Histoplasmosis

Test	Result	Immunocompetent	Immunocompromised
Serum complement fixation antibody assay[a]	≤1:8	−	[−]
	1:16	+	+
	≥1:32	++	++
Serum immunodiffusion antibody assay[a]	M and H negative	−	[−]
	M present only	+	+
	H present only	++	++
	M and H present	++	++
Urine antigen	None detected	[−][b]	[−][b]
	Positive	++[c]	++[c]
Histologic findings			
Node/mass	Negative	−	−
Infected organ	Granulomas, no yeast form	++	++
	Granulomas, yeast forms	+++	+++
Bone marrow/blood	No yeast forms	[−]	[−]
	Yeast forms seen	+++[c]	+++[c]
Culture any site	Negative	[−]	[−]
Culture any site	Positive	+++	+++
Culture bone marrow/blood	Positive	+++[c]	+++[c]

[−], does not exclude infection; −, recent infection unlikely (≤5% probability); +, recent infection possible; ++, strongly suggestive of acute or recent infection; +++, confirms current infections; M, M bands; H, H bands.

[a]Seroconversion confirms acute/recent infection.

[b]Progressive disseminated infection unlikely.

[c]Strongly suggestive of progressive disseminated infection.

of treatment and thereafter, to detect relapse. The EIA is highly sensitive with its calibration curve linear only up to concentrations of 39 ng/mL. Therefore, serum specimens (in which simultaneously measured concentrations are substantially lower than those of urine) should be used to monitor effectiveness of treatment in individuals whose urine concentrations exceed this value. When antigen becomes undetectable in the serum, urine specimens can be used for follow-up thereafter. Following completion of therapy, the EIA on urine samples can be used to detect early relapse in individuals at high risk for recurrence.[71,72] Although reasonably specific, the *Histoplasma* antigen assay can cross-react with *Paracoccidioides brasiliensis, Blastomyces dermatitidis, Coccidioides immitis* and *C. posadasii,* and *Penicillium marneffei.*[82] However, differentiation of these endemic mycoses usually is straightforward when clinical manifestations, serologic tests, and geographic considerations are evaluated. False-positive results have been observed in patients who receive rabbit anti-thymocyte globulin;[83] however, modifications in the current assay have eliminated this problem.[84]

Differential Diagnosis

The differential diagnosis of symptomatic pulmonary histoplasmosis usually includes tuberculosis, with which the clinical and radiographic findings often overlap. Other subacute infections that cause similar findings include blastomycosis and coccidioidomycosis. When middle mediastinal/hilar lymphadenopathy disproportionate to the degree of pulmonary infiltrates is present, histoplasmosis can mimic lymphoma, particularly in patients with fever and weight loss. In a series of patients residing in an endemic area, all children with middle mediastinal adenopathy and complement fixation titers ≥1:32 were diagnosed accurately with histoplasmosis.[68] Progressive disseminated forms of histoplasmosis can mimic septicemia or reticuloendothelial or primary gastrointestinal tract neoplasm[85] when the initial signs include hepatosplenomegaly, anemia, thrombocytopenia, leukopenia,

coagulopathy, hemorrhage from gastrointestinal ulceration, or any combination of these conditions.[55]

Since severe, disseminated, or recurrent histoplasmosis can represent opportunistic infection, evaluation should include screening for a previously unrecognized acquired or congenital immunodeficiency disorder.[64,65,86]

TREATMENT

Key factors used to determine whether antifungal therapy for histoplasmosis is needed are clinical manifestations, severity of symptoms, and functional integrity of the immune system. Recommendations for treatment are reviewed in Table 250-2. Inasmuch as controlled trials have not been performed in children, most recommendations for treatment are derived from results of trials conducted in adults[87] and opinions of experts.

Healthy children whose chest radiographs show findings compatible with previous histoplasmosis require no therapy. Symptomatic histoplasmosis in immunocompetent children usually is self-limited, and few children benefit from antifungal treatment. The only disease manifestations that uniformly require therapy in otherwise immunocompetent children are progressive disseminated infection and serious respiratory infections resulting from high inoculum exposure. Other infections for which antifungal therapy often is used are pulmonary infection with clinical symptoms that last >4 weeks and granulomatous adenitis that obstructs or occludes blood vessels, bronchi, the esophagus, or other critical structures. The lymphocytolytic effect of corticosteroids also can provide prompt relief of obstruction;[49] in these instances, concomitant antifungal treatment is needed to prevent progressive dissemination. Neither antifungal nor corticosteroid therapy is of benefit if inflammation has progressed to fibrosis. Presumed ocular disease, rheumatologic syndromes, and isolated pericarditis do not require antifungal therapy. Patients with histoplasma pericarditis usually improve, sometimes dramatically, with indomethacin.[45,46]

TABLE 250-2. Summary of Treatment Recommendations for Children with Histoplasmosis

Manifestation	Severe Illness	Moderate or Mild Illness
Acute pulmonary	AmB,[a] then Itr for 12 weeks	Symptoms <4 weeks: none; persistent symptoms >4 weeks: Itr for 6–12 weeks
Disseminated (without HIV)	AmB[b] or AmB followed by Itr for 6 months[c]	Itr for 6–18 months or the same as for severe illness
Disseminated (with HIV)[d]	AmB[e] or AmB followed by Itr for life[f]	Itr treatment, then Itr suppression for life[e]
Meningitis	AmB for 3 months, then Flu or Itra for 12 months	Same as for severe illness because of poor outcome
Granulomatous mediastinitis	AmB, then Itr for 6 months	Itr for 6–12 months
Fibrosing mediastinitis	Itr for 3 months[g]	Same as for severe illness
Pericarditis	Pericardial drainage for severe tamponade + an NSAID, for 2–12 weeks	NSAID 2–12 weeks (indomethacin preferred)
Rheumatologic	NSAID for 2–12 weeks	Same as for severe illness
Compression of contiguous structures by granulomatous lymphadenopathy		Corticosteroid, concurrent Itr (see text)

AmB, amphotericin B; Flu, fluconazole; HIV, human immunodeficiency virus; Itr, itraconazole; NSAID, nonsteroidal anti-inflammatory agent.

[a]*The effectiveness of concomitant corticosteroids is controversial.*

[b]*If amphotericin B is used for the entire course of treatment, a total of 30 mg/kg should be given over a 4-week period.*

[c]*Therapy should continue until the Histoplasma antigen concentration in serum is undetectable and the Histoplasma urine antigen concentration is less than 2 µg/mL and stable. (Low urine concentrations can be present for extended periods following successful therapy.)*

[d]*Liposomal amphotericin B should be used (see text).*

[e]*Therapy may be continued for 4–6 weeks.*

[f]*See text regarding discontinuation of secondary prophylaxis after highly active antiretroviral therapy with regimen outlined in reference 94.*

[g]*Probably ineffective if fibrotic; when granulomatous mediastinitis could be present, it may be considered.*

Modified from Rychly DJ, DiPiro JT. Infections associated with tumor necrosis factor-alpha antagonists. Pharmacotherapy 2005;25(9):1181–1192.

Immunocompromised hosts with any manifestation of active histoplasmosis should be treated with an antifungal agent because the risk for progressive dissemination is high. Patients who are asymptomatic and in whom a biopsied pulmonary nodule reveals granulomatous inflammation, sometimes containing typical yeast like organisms,[75] do not benefit from treatment.

Amphotericin B is the preferred agent for initial treatment of severely ill patients because it induces a faster clinical response than the azole agents. However, the effectiveness, convenience of administration, and lesser toxicity of the azoles have established important therapeutic roles for these agents, as well.[88] Azoles can be used either as consolidation therapy following induction with amphotericin B, or as monotherapy in mildly or moderately ill patients.[87] In patients with progressive, disseminated infections, antigenuria should be monitored at monthly intervals to ensure that the urine antigen level decreases. Low-level antigenuria <2 ng/mL can persist in asymptomatic infants for several weeks after adequate treatment with disseminated histoplasmosis.[51] In these instances, antifungal therapy can be stopped safely provided that the infant is clinically well and the recommended duration of treatment has been completed. Patients should be followed to ensure that antigenuria resolves.

Liposomal amphotericin B has been shown to decrease the duration of fungemia and antigenemia more quickly than itraconazole.[89-92] A controlled clinical trial in adults with AIDS complicated by disseminated histoplasmosis found that liposomal amphotericin B was associated with improved survival compared with amphotericin B deoxycholate.[90] Prior to the availability of HAART, microbiologic cure could not be achieved reliably in persons with HIV infection. Since cessation of treatment was often followed by relapse, long-term antifungal suppressive therapy[91] with itraconazole is recommended (see Table 250-2). Ketoconazole is not effective. Fluconazole, although not recommended for treatment of acute infections, can be used for suppression if itraconazole is not tolerated.[91] Itraconazole results in more rapid sterilization of blood cultures than fluconazole, despite no demonstrable difference in urine antigen clearance.[92] Fluconazole resistance has been reported to develop during therapy.[93] With availability of HAART therapy, a controlled trial in adults[94] found that discontinuation of secondary prophylaxis is safe provided that HAART was given for at least 6 months, CD4+ T-lymphocyte count was >150 cells/mm³, antifungal therapy had been given for 1 year, fungal blood cultures were negative, and serum and urine antigen levels were <4.1 units.[5] Infected patients with non-HIV-induced cellular immune disorders in whom antigenuria persists or relapse occurs after adequate therapy should be considered candidates for long-term antifungal suppression. Voriconazole has been used successfully as salvage therapy in a small number of patients.

Large necrotic masses that do not diminish with medical treatment should be drained only if they obstruct critical structures.[95] Excision of densely fibrotic lesions involving the lung parenchyma, blood vessels, and/or bronchi is rarely helpful, and is associated with a high risk of uncontrolled hemorrhage.[96]

SPECIAL CONSIDERATIONS

Adrenal insufficiency, nephrocalcinosis,[47] and hypercalcemia (perhaps caused by hypersensitivity to vitamin D) have been associated with disseminated infections. Gastrointestinal tract ulcerations[85] can cause bleeding, mimic neoplastic disorders, or obstruct the gastrointestinal or biliary tracts.[49,85,97] Transplacental infection has been reported in an infant born to a mother with HIV infection and disseminated histoplasmosis during pregnancy.[98] Presumed ocular histoplasmosis is a destructive retinal lesion; evidence that this entity is caused by histoplasmosis is weak.[99,100] This entity, as well as mediastinal fibrosis,[101] chronic histoplasmosis, central nervous system infections,[102-104] and endocarditis,[105] are manifestations that occur almost exclusively in adults.

PREVENTION

In endemic regions, patients with cellular immunodeficiencies or HIV infection or people who receive immunosuppressive drugs should be counseled concerning high-risk activities (see Box 250-1). If such activities are unavoidable, protective masks should be used. Advances in vaccine development have been reviewed.[106,107]

Key Points. Microbiology, Epidemiology, and Clinical Aspects of Histoplasmosis

MICROBIOLOGY AND ACQUISITION

- The spore-bearing, mycelial form of *H. capsulatum* grows in the environment; bird and bat excreta stimulate growth. Inhaled spores convert to the yeastlike (parasitic) form that replicates at 37°C and is recovered from sites of infection
- Infection results from inhalation of microconidia (spores) produced by the mycelial form of the endemic, dimorphic fungus *Histoplasma capsulatum* var. *capsulatum*

EPIDEMIOLOGY

- Distributed worldwide; highly endemic in Ohio and Mississippi River valleys of the U.S., in which as many as 80% of individuals demonstrate skin test reactivity by 18 years of age
- Infections occur both sporadically and when contaminated sites are disturbed

CLINICAL FEATURES

- Severity is proportionate to inoculum size and the degree of functional impairment of cellular immune function; 90% of infections in healthy hosts are subclinical
- Common symptoms include low-grade fever, chest pain, weight loss, headache, myalgias, and erythema nodosum (in adolescents)

- Life-threatening, progressive disseminated infection can occur during infancy, or in children with acquired or congenital cellular immune dysfunction

DIAGNOSIS

- In patients within, or having visited endemic regions, focal pulmonary infiltrates with middle mediastinal lymphadenopathy is compatible
- Strongly compatible laboratory findings:
  - Complement fixation antibody titer ≥1:32 to yeast or mycelial phase
  - Detection of antigen in urine and/or serum
  - Histopathologic demonstration of granulomatous inflammation associated with yeastlike forms characteristic of *H. capsulatum*

TREATMENT

- Most mild infections in healthy children resolve without antifungal treatment
- Non-disseminated infections associated with persistent symptoms can be treated with itraconazole
- Seriously ill patients, including those with signs of progressive dissemination, require induction therapy with amphotericin B followed by itraconazole

251 *Pneumocystis jirovecii*

Francis Gigliotti and Terry W. Wright

DESCRIPTION OF PATHOGEN

Pneumocystis jirovecii (formerly *P. carinii*) is an opportunistic parasite possessing some common features of protozoa, but molecular studies have shown greater genetic homology to fungi.[1] *Pneumocystis* organisms exhibit a high degree of host species specificity, with organisms infecting humans designated as *P. jirovecii*.[2] Alternative acceptable nomenclature retains the use of *P. carinii* but uses the annotation *forma specialis* or *f. sp.* to identify the host of origin, such that *P. carinii* infecting humans, rats, or mice would carry the *f. sp.* designation *hominis, ratti,* or *muris,* respectively. Clinicians should be aware that any of these variations may appear in the medical literature.

To date, reliable axenic culture of *Pneumocystis* from any mammalian host has not been achieved. However, specific developmental life forms of *Pneumocystis* have been identified in infected tissue. The 5- to 7 µm cyst contains up to eight pleomorphic intracystic bodies (sporozoites). Once excysted, sporozoites are believed to become trophic forms (trophozoites). All these forms reside in the alveoli of the lung. Most immunocompetent children have acquired asymptomatic infection by the age of 4 years. *Pneumocystis* pneumonia (PCP) occurs almost exclusively in severely compromised hosts, and the infection remains localized to the lungs with rare exception. Although pneumonia in immunocompromised patients was presumed to represent reactivation of latent infection, animal studies have called into question the capacity of *Pneumocystis* to persist as a latent infection.[3]

EPIDEMIOLOGY

Animal-to-animal transmission of *Pneumocystis* by the airborne route has been demonstrated, and DNA sequences identical to those of *Pneumocystis* have been detected in samples of ambient air. Human-to-human transmission has not been proved, but clusters of cases of pneumonia have been reported in immunocompromised patients. Animal-to-human transmission is unlikely because of the well-established genetic and antigenic diversity of the organism related to the host of origin. A natural habitat has not been found but the infection has a global distribution. Serologic studies demonstrate that a high proportion of the population has evidence of infection and that seroconversion occurred during childhood. A prospective longitudinal study demonstrated that seroconversion begins in the first few months of life and by 20 months of age 85% of the infants had seroconverted.[4] Animal studies have demonstrated that *Pneumocystis* can be transmitted from normal host to normal host, producing very mild disease in the process.[5] This finding, along with the observation of early seroconversion in children, provides a potential explanation of how *Pneumocystis* is maintained in the human population.

Overt disease in the form of pneumonia develops only in immunocompromised hosts. The occurrence of PCP is related to the extent of immunosuppression, especially impairment in cell-mediated immunity.[6] For example, PCP occurs in about 40% to 50% of infants and children with acquired immunodeficiency syndrome (AIDS) or severe combined immunodeficiency syndrome (SCIDS), in 12% of children with acute lymphocytic leukemia, and in 6% of recipients of an organ transplant if no prophylaxis is given.

CLINICAL MANIFESTATIONS

The signs and symptoms of PCP are directly related to the organisms and the inflammatory response in the alveolar lumen, septum, or both. Two somewhat different clinical patterns have been observed that differ only in intensity of expression.

The endemic infantile form of PCP, originally described in outbreaks in European nursing homes for infants, is an interstitial plasma cell pneumonitis.[7] Its onset is subtle in debilitated infants at 4 to 6 months of age. A bronchiolitis-like illness can occur, with prominent tachypnea and dyspnea in the absence of fever. Intercostal retractions are marked, and as the course progresses, flaring of the nasal alae and cyanosis can be observed, and crackles are heard bilaterally. The untreated course is prolonged over many days to a few weeks, and at least half of these patients die.

PCP in older children and adults with an underlying, non-AIDS immunodeficiency disorder such as cancer or organ transplantation begins abruptly with fever, tachypnea, and cough. Intercostal retractions and flaring of the nasal alae may occur, but breath sounds are normal and rales are not heard. The untreated course is progressive, and all untreated patients die within a month.

The spectrum of clinical manifestations in patients with AIDS can vary from the subtle variety seen in the infantile type to the acute fulminating type. Without treatment, the course ends in fatality in almost all patients.

Clinical observations in humans suggest that a poor prognosis in PCP correlates with evidence of inflammation. For example, elevated levels of neutrophils or interleukin-8 in bronchoalveolar lavage fluid, but not increased numbers of organisms, correlate with poorer oxygenation and decreased survival. Some insight into these observations comes from animal models. Physiologic studies of mice with SCIDS demonstrate that lung injury (decreased compliance, hypoxia, and surfactant dysfunction) is directly related to the *Pneumocystis*-specific inflammatory response rather than to the organism burden per se.[8] It also appears that $CD8^+$ T lymphocytes are critical in producing injury in the absence of effective $CD4^+$ T-lymphocyte-mediated immunity. Thus, in the future, developing better means of controlling the inflammatory response could result in an improved outcome in patients with PCP.

LABORATORY FINDINGS AND DIAGNOSIS

In all clinical types of PCP, the arterial oxygen tension (PaO_2) is decreased and reflects the severity of the disease. In moderately severe cases, the PaO_2 is less than 70 mmHg and the alveolar-arterial oxygen gradient exceeds 35 mmHg. The white blood cell count is unaffected by the infection. In patients with AIDS-related PCP, the $CD4^+$ T-lymphocyte count is usually below the normal range and often less than 200 cells/mm³ in patients above 6 years of age. Determining the risk of PCP based on $CD4^+$ T-lymphocyte counts in patients on immunosuppressive medicines is complicated by the fact that those $CD4^+$ cells present may not be fully functional.

The role of antibody in the control of *Pneumocystis* has been underappreciated. Early descriptions of patients with PCP included patients with primary antibody deficiencies.[9] More recently, patients with hyper-IgM syndrome have been observed to be at high risk for PCP.[10,11] These patients lack CD40 ligand on their T lymphocytes and as a result these cells are unable to interact properly with B lymphocytes for the production of specific IgG.

Mouse models have confirmed the importance of antibody. For example, blocking CD40 ligand in mice prevents resolution of PCP, consistent with observations in patients with the hyper-IgM syndrome.[12] B-lymphocyte-deficient mice (MuMT), which are incapable of normal antibody production but largely have preserved T-lymphocyte function, are naturally susceptible to *Pneumocystis*.[13] Finally, passive administration of *Pneumocystis*-specific antibody to immunosuppressed mice limits the extent of infection with *Pneumocystis*.[14]

The chest radiograph typically shows bilateral alveolar disease, first appearing in the perihilar area and then progressing peripherally, often with the apical areas spared (Figure 251-1). In some cases, no radiographic abnormality is detectable at the onset of symptoms. In such cases, a gallium scan may reveal the pulmonary disease, but the finding is not unique to PCP. Definitive diagnosis requires the demonstration of *Pneumocystis* in the pulmonary parenchyma or in fluid from the lower respiratory tract.[15] The least invasive method for obtaining diagnostic specimens is inducement of sputum. This procedure requires the cooperation of the

TABLE 251-1. Specimens for Identification of *Pneumocystis*

Method	Sensitivity (%)[a]	Comments
Induced sputum	20–40	5 years of age and older
Tracheal aspirate	50–60	First step in intubated patients
Fiberoptic bronchoscopy bronchoalveolar lavage	75–95	Procedure of first choice in most patients; both bronchoalveolar lavage and biopsy are preferred
Transbronchial biopsy	75–95	
Open-lung biopsy	90–100	Most sensitive and informative specimen

[a]*Estimates of the percentage of specimens expected to be positive in cases of* Pneumocystis *pneumonia.*

patient and is usually limited to children 5 years of age and older. Typically, 20 to 30 minutes of inhaling a nebulized mist of 3% saline from an ultrasonic nebulizer is required to stimulate adequate expectoration. The sputum specimen is diluted 1:1 in sterile saline, treated with dithiothreitol, and processed for cytologic examination and culture. About 20% to 40% of specimens reveal organisms in patients with PCP (Table 251-1). The organism is more likely to be found in the sputum of PCP patients with AIDS than in patients without AIDS because of the greater infectious burden in the former condition.

Bronchoalveolar lavage usually is the method of first choice for most patients because it can be performed through a flexible fiberoptic bronchoscope with 1% lidocaine anesthesia topically. A transbronchial lung biopsy can also be performed at the time of bronchoscopy. A successful biopsy should provide at least 20 alveoli for study. With these combined procedures, PCP can be identified in nearly 100% of cases.

Open-lung biopsy provides a larger specimen for evaluation of the histopathology of the disease process and for culture of viruses, bacteria, and fungi. Open biopsy, however, has the disadvantage of requiring general anesthesia and can be complicated by pneumothorax and bleeding.

Specimens should be stained with Giemsa, Grocott–Gomori, or fluorescein-labeled antibody stains (Figure 251-2). Other useful

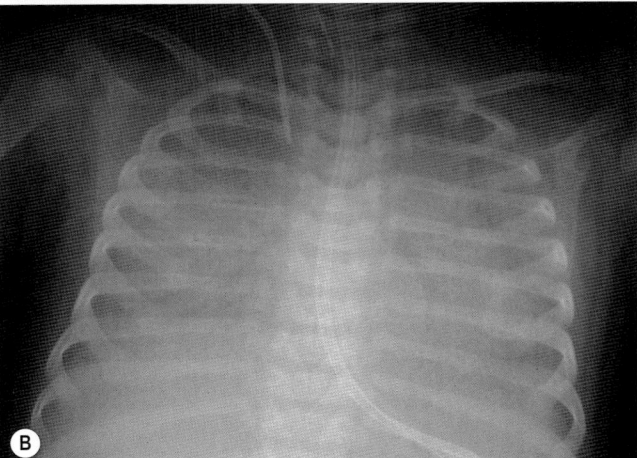

Figure 251-1. Typical *Pneumocystis* pneumonia as the presenting manifestation of human immunodeficiency virus (HIV) infection in a 6-month-old infant in foster care who had a 5-day history of fever and congestion. Physical examination revealed tachypnea, retractions, flaring, and hypoxia, but no rales. Plain radiograph shows bilateral diffuse air-space lung disease **(A)**, which progressed peripherally over 2 days **(B)**. Note apical sparing. (Courtesy of E.N. Faerber, J. Chen, and J. Foster, St. Christopher's Hospital for Children, Philadelphia, PA.)

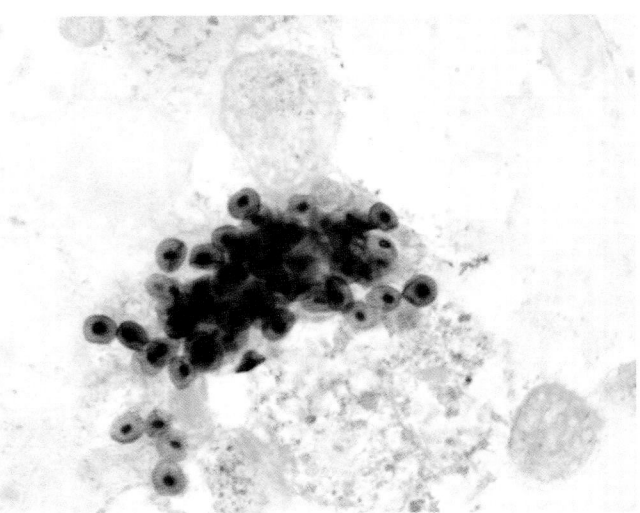

Figure 251-2. A bronchoalveolar lavage specimen stained by the Grocott–Gomori method shows the dark staining (brown to black) of *Pneumocystis* cysts. These cysts measure 5 to 6 μm in diameter. The method stains background tissue light green.

stains include toluidine blue O and Gram–Weigert stains. Specimens also should be inoculated onto culture media for bacteria, fungi, and viruses (especially cytomegalovirus). Polymerase chain reaction test to identify *Pneumocystis* in a sputum or lavage sample is being performed in many research laboratories. These investigations may lead to diagnostic assays that can be adapted to clinical laboratories.

SPECIAL CONSIDERATIONS

Under certain circumstances, forgoing an invasive diagnostic procedure and treating the patient on the basis of a presumptive diagnosis of PCP may be prudent. Examples include children with terminal stages of untreatable cancer and patients with uncontrollable bleeding disorders. When planning an invasive diagnostic procedure, knowing that *Pneumocystis* persists in the lungs for many days after the onset of specific therapy is useful. For example, if conditions for performance of a diagnostic procedure or monitoring are not optimal, therapy can be initiated immediately and the procedure performed a few hours later.

TREATMENT

The drugs and dosage schedules used for the treatment of PCP are shown in Table 251-2. Trimethoprim-sulfamethoxazole (TMP-SMX) is the drug of choice and is available for oral as well as intravenous therapy. The oral route of administration can be used in mild cases if patients can take and retain oral medication dependably. However, most patients require treatment by the intravenous route. The course of treatment is 2 to 3 weeks for most children. Because posttreatment prophylaxis is necessary for all immunocompromised patients, the dose of TMP-SMX is reduced to the prophylaxis dose after recovery, and continued indefinitely or until the immunodeficiency has resolved.

Adverse reactions to TMP-SMX occur infrequently in non-AIDS patients (around 5%) but are frequent in children with AIDS (around 40%). An erythematous maculopapular rash is the most common adverse effect. The rash often is transient and may clear without withdrawal of the drug, but progressive intensive rashes, especially urticaria, require discontinuation of therapy with the drug. Rarely, Stevens–Johnson syndrome can occur secondary to the sulfonamide and can have serious consequences. Other adverse effects include neutropenia, megaloblastic or aplastic anemia, renal dysfunction, nausea, vomiting, and diarrhea.

Patients who cannot tolerate or who fail to respond to TMP-SMX should be treated with intravenous pentamidine isothionate. If intravenous access is not available, the drug can be given by deep intramuscular injection, but serious reactions at the injection site, such as soft-tissue necrosis and abscess, are common. Other adverse reactions occur in up to 70% of cases and include renal and hepatic dysfunction, thrombocytopenia, anemia, hypotension, abnormally high or low blood glucose concentrations, and rash.

TABLE 251-2. Recommended Treatment of Infants, Children, and Adolescents with *Pneumocystis* Pneumonia[a]

Drug	Infant and Child Dosage	Adolescent and Adult Dosage
Trimethoprim-sulfamethoxazole (TMP-SMX) (drug of first choice)	**TMP** 15–20 mg/kg per day, PO or IV, divided into 4 doses **SMX** 75–100 mg/kg per day, PO or IV, divided into 4 doses	**TMP** 15–20 mg/kg per day, PO or IV, divided into 4 doses **SMX** 75–100 mg/kg per day, PO or IV, divided into 4 doses
Pentamidine (alternate of first choice)	4 mg/kg per day, as single dose by aerosol	4 mg/kg per day, as single dose by aerosol
Atovaquone	3–24 months of age: 45 mg/kg per day, PO, divided into 2 doses 1–3 months and over 24 months: 30 mg/kg per day, PO, divided into 2 doses (maximum daily dose 1500 mg)	1500 mg/day, PO, divided into 2 doses, with food
Dapsone plus trimethoprim	**Dapsone** 2 mg/kg per day (maximum 100 mg), PO, once daily **Trimethoprim** 15 mg/kg per day, PO, divided into 3 doses	**Dapsone** 100 mg per day, PO, once daily **Trimethoprim** 15 mg/kg per day, PO, divided into 3 doses
Primaquine plus clindamycin	**Primaquine** 0.3 mg/kg per day (maximum 30 mg), PO, once daily **Clindamycin** 40 mg/kg per day, IV, divided into 4 doses (no pediatric data for this regimen)	**Primaquine** 15–30 mg, PO, once daily **Clindamycin** 800 mg per day, IV, divided into doses every 8 hours
Trimetrexate plus leucovorin	**Trimetrexate** 45 mg/m² per day, IV or PO, once daily **Leucovorin** 20 mg/m² per day, IV or PO, divided into doses every 6 hours (continue 3 days beyond trimetrexate)	**Trimetrexate** 45 mg/m² per day, once daily, or <50 kg: 1.5 mg/kg per day, IV, once daily 50–80 kg: 1.2 mg/kg per day, IV, once daily >80 kg: 1.0 mg/kg per day, IV, once daily **Leucovorin** <50 kg: 0.8 mg/kg per day, IV or PO, divided into doses every 6 hours >50 kg: 0.5 mg/kg per day, IV or PO, divided into doses every 6 hours (continue 3 days beyond trimetrexate)

AIDS, acquired immunodeficiency syndrome; IV, intravenous; PO, orally; TMP-SMX, trimethoprim-sulfamethoxazole.

[a]*General duration of therapy is 3 weeks in patients with AIDS and 2 weeks in other immunosuppressed patients. Prednisone is recommended as adjunctive therapy to any antimicrobial therapy for moderate or severe PCP pneumonia (room air PaO₂ of ≤70 mmHg or an alveolar–arterial gradient of ≤35 mmHg).*

Several other drugs have been shown to have activity against *Pneumocystis* but have not been studied extensively in children. These drugs include atovaquone, an oral hydroxynaphthoquinone; trimetrexate, a drug for intravenous use that must be given concomitantly with leucovorin; TMP-dapsone orally; pyrimethamine-sulfadoxine (Fansidar) orally; clindamycin plus primaquine orally; and aerosolized pentamidine.

Supportive measures are important in the management of PCP. The PaO_2 should be maintained above 70 mmHg, and, if possible, the inspired oxygen fraction (FiO_2) should be kept below 50 vol%. If the PaO_2 cannot be maintained at 60 mmHg or greater, assisted ventilation is usually indicated. Anemia should be corrected with packed red blood cell transfusion.

Several studies in adults suggest that administration of a corticosteroid in severe and moderately severe cases of PCP improves survival. Limited data in children indicate similar effects.[16] It is reasonable to consider corticosteroid administration at the onset of treatment in patients with a PaO_2 less than 70 mmHg or an alveolar-arterial gradient of 35 mmHg and greater. Methylprednisolone, 2 mg/kg per day, has been used in children. The dose should be tapered and the corticosteroid discontinued in the recovery stage of pneumonia. The effect of corticosteroid in this setting probably is modulation of the inflammatory response.

The animal data[8] linking pulmonary morbidity with the *Pneumocystis*-induced inflammatory response suggest that better means of controlling this inflammatory response could result in improved outcomes in patients with PCP.

PREVENTION

Four drugs are available for prevention of PCP (Table 251-3). TMP-SMX or aerosolized pentamidine are used most frequently, but only TMP-SMX has been studied in children. Comparative studies in adults show that TMP-SMX is superior to aerosolized pentamidine in the prevention of PCP in patients with AIDS, although the frequency of adverse reactions is greater with the former drug. The prophylactic dose is 5 mg TMP and 25 mg SMX/kg per day in 2 divided doses. The drug can be given daily or only 3 days per week. The 3-day-a-week schedule should be on consecutive days, such as Monday, Tuesday, and Wednesday.[17] Some evidence suggests that TMP-SMX also may prevent certain bacterial infections in addition to *Pneumocystis*. When this effect is sought, it is advisable to use the daily dosage schedule.

For patients who cannot tolerate TMP-SMX, aerosolized pentamidine can be tried in children who are old enough and cooperate with administration.[18] Most children 5 years and older can tolerate treatment with aerosolized pentamidine. A dosage has not been established, but 300 mg delivered in a Respirgard II nebulizer once monthly is reasonable and well tolerated. The main adverse effects are cough and bronchospasm. For patients younger than 5 years of age and those who cannot tolerate aerosolized pentamidine or TMP-SMX, dapsone orally at a dose of 2 mg/kg per day or 4 mg/kg once weekly can be used. Dapsone is effective in the prevention of PCP, but adverse reactions similar to those caused by sulfonamides can occur. The total dose should not exceed 100 mg per day or 200 mg per dose weekly. Atovaquone at a dose of 1500 mg orally once daily appears to be equal to pentamidine or dapsone for the prevention of PCP in adults. Atovaquone has not been studied well in children, but a dose of 30 mg/kg once daily has been suggested for children 1 to 3 months old or those older than 24 months of age and 45 mg/kg once daily for children between 4 and 24 months of age.[19]

Several risk factors have been recognized as guides to the selection of candidates for PCP prophylaxis, including immunosuppressed patients who have had one episode of PCP; children with severe cell-mediated immunodeficiency such as SCIDS, organ transplant recipients, and those with AIDS; and children with lymphoproliferative malignancies and other types of malignancy that require intensive chemotherapy.

Infants and children with AIDS can be selected for primary prophylaxis by the $CD4^+$ T-lymphocyte count or percentage.[19] Approximately one-half of the cases of PCP in infants with AIDS, however, occur as the initial manifestation of AIDS, with high mortality. All human immunodeficiency virus (HIV)-exposed or -infected infants should receive PCP prophylaxis between 1 month and 1 year of age or until HIV infection has been ruled out, because of the high risk of pneumonia in this age group. After 1 year of age, the $CD4^+$ lymphocyte count and percentage serve as the guide (Table 251-4).

Administration of chemoprophylaxis does not ensure complete protection from PCP. Breakthrough infections occur in at least 6% of those receiving TMP-SMX and about 12% of those receiving aerosolized pentamidine or oral dapsone. For children who have adverse reactions to TMP-SMX, desensitization can be attempted by escalating from extremely small doses to full doses.[20] This scheme has been successfully applied in patients with AIDS. Prophylaxis is effective only during times when drugs are being administered, so effort must be made to ensure adherence in high-risk patients and to continue prophylaxis when patients are hospitalized.

In HIV-infected adults receiving highly active antiretroviral therapy, primary and secondary prophylaxis against PCP can be discontinued safely after the $CD4^+$ lymphocyte count has increased to $200/mm^3$ for more than 3 months.[21] A similar approach is recommended for children who have received at least 6 months of highly active antiretroviral therapy and whose $CD4^+$ lymphocyte counts have returned to normal levels for age.[19]

TABLE 251-3. Recommended Prophylaxis for Recurrence of *Pneumocystis* Pneumonia after Treatment in HIV-Infected Infants, Children, and Adolescents

Age Category	First Choice	Alternatives
Infants and children	TMP-SMX orally	Dapsone orally *or* Aerosolized pentamidine *or* Pentamidine intravenously
Adolescents	TMP-SMX orally	Dapsone orally *or* Dapsone + pyrimethamine + folinic acid orally *or* Aerosolized pentamidine *or* Atovaquone orally

HIV, human immunodeficiency virus; TMP-SMX, trimethoprim-sulfamethoxazole.

TABLE 251-4. Recommended Primary Prophylaxis for Pneumocystis in HIV-Infected Infants and Children by Age and $CD4^+$ Count or $CD4^+$ Percentage

Age	$CD4^+$ Count	$CD4^+$ %
1–12 months[a]	All infants	All infants
12–23 months	$<750/mm^3$	<15
24 months to 5 years	$<500/mm^3$	<15
6 years and older	$<200/mm^3$	<15

[a]Includes all infants 1 to 4 months old born to women infected with human immunodeficiency virus (HIV).

252 *Blastomyces dermatitidis* (Blastomycosis)

Martin B. Kleiman

Blastomycosis is an endemic primary systemic mycosis that occurs sporadically or in isolated clusters. An infrequent infection, blastomycosis affects children less often than adults. The spectrum of clinical manifestations is similar to that seen in adults[1] ranging from an asymptomatic or accidentally discovered self-limited illness to a rapidly progressive, multisystem, fatal infection.[2-5]

MICROBIOLOGY

Blastomycosis is caused by *Blastomyces dermatitidis*, a thermal dimorphic fungus that exists in an asexual (imperfect, anamorphic) or sexual (perfect, teleomorphic) state. The term *B. dermatitidis* refers to the asexual state, which exists either as a mold form, if grown at temperatures below 37°C, or as a multinucleate yeast form, if grown at 37°C. The mold form grows in the environment and bears spores, which measure 2 to 10 μm in diameter and, when inhaled, are the infectious form of the fungus. Spores convert to yeast forms in infected tissue where they appear as broad-based, round, thick-walled, "double-contoured" budding forms, 8 to 15 μm in diameter, and are easily identified (Figure 252-1).

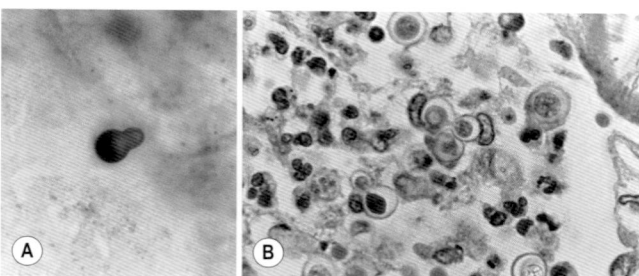

Figure 252-1. (A) Cutaneous blastomycosis. Touch preparation of a skin biopsy showing single *Blastomyces dermatitidis* yeastlike cell with a broad-based bud. (Gomori methenamine silver nitrate stain, ×1000.) **(B)** Acute pulmonary blastomycosis. Single yeastlike cells with doubly contoured walls and two prominent, budding, yeastlike cells of *B. dermatitidis* are present within a suppurative exudate. In histopathologic sections of involved tissues, the finding of yeasts of 8 to 15 μm in diameter with single broad-based buds is considered diagnostic. The inflammatory reaction can be acute, suppurative, or granulomatous. (Hematoxylin and eosin, ×1000.)

The teleomorph of *B. dermatitidis* is termed *Ajellomyces dermatitidis*. In this state, two compatible mating types are required for spore formation. Methodologies based on polymerase chain reaction (PCR) have identified considerable genetic diversity, especially among strains from different geographic regions.[6,7]

The yeast forms of *B. dermatitidis*[8,9] have antiphagocytic properties attributed to structural and chemical surface components. In vitro studies comparing cell surface components of strains of differing virulence for mice have identified alterations of expression of a unique protein (WI-1, now termed BAD1)[10] and a cell surface carbohydrate,[11-13] which participate in complement activation, macrophage recognition, binding, tumor necrosis factor-α suppression, and fungal cell killing.[14-17] The presence of a 25-amino-acid tandem repeat of the adhesin domain of the WI-1 protein has been shown to be indispensable for pathogenicity.[18] Yeast forms of *B. dermatitidis* produce melanin, which has been found to be a virulence factor in other pathogenic fungi.[19]

PATHOGENESIS AND IMMUNITY

Inhaled spores convert to yeast forms in the lung and are phagocytosed by pulmonary macrophages and acute suppurative inflammation follows (see Figure 252-1B). Lymphohematogenous dissemination is a uniform feature of early infection. After development of cell-mediated immunity, acute and granulomatous changes can be present concurrently. Caseous necrosis and calcification do not occur. Extrapulmonary infection can result from early dissemination, progression of pulmonary disease or, rarely, reactivation of endogenous disease (Figure 252-2). Extrapulmonary infection in children most commonly affects the lungs, skin, and bones.[1] In contrast to extrapulmonary manifestations in adults, genitourinary and central nervous system (CNS) infections are unusual in children. Skin lesions caused by direct inoculation have been reported,[15-17,20-22] but the majority result from hematogenous dissemination.

The humoral immune response plays a minor role in blastomycosis, as evidenced both by satisfactory control of fungal infection by patients with hypogammaglobulinemia and in experiments in which antibody to WI-1 did not improve outcome in murine models.[12,23]

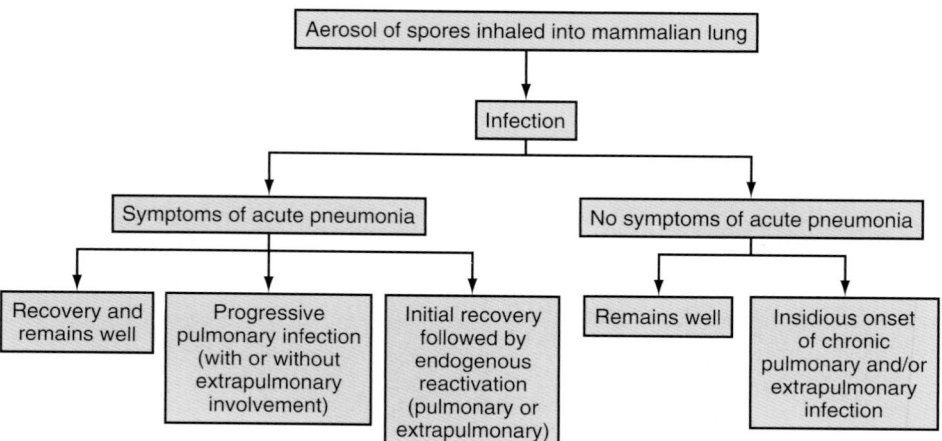

Figure 252-2. Spectrum of clinical illness in blastomycosis. (Redrawn from Sarosi GA, Davies SF. Blastomycosis. Am Rev Respir Dis 1979;120:911–938.)

Yeast forms contain chemotactic factors that attract neutrophils and monocytes. Neutrophils have some fungicidal capabilities. However, the cellular immune response, mediated by antigen-specific T-lymphocyte and lymphokine-activated macrophages, appears to play the principal role in aborting fungal growth and providing some degree of protection following re-exposure. Severe manifestations of blastomycosis have been recognized in patients with AIDS.[24] Specific lymphocyte reactivity to purified antigens has been demonstrated in children 21 months after infection[25] but wanes with time.[26]

EPIDEMIOLOGY

The lack of reliable skin and serologic tests, and difficulty in isolating *B. dermatitidis* from the environment, have hampered epidemiologic study.[4] On the basis of reports of human and canine disease in the United States, endemic areas include the Mississippi and Ohio River basins, to some extent the Missouri River basin, and western New York, eastern Ontario, and areas along the St. Lawrence River[27] (Figure 252-3). Proximity to water is a risk factor for canine infection.[28] These areas partially overlap regions in which histoplasmosis is endemic (see Chapter 250, *Histoplasma capsulatum* (Histoplasmosis)). Sporadic cases[3] of blastomycosis occur in a much wider area of the midwestern and southeastern U.S.,[29] and in Africa. Infections that occur in nonendemic areas often result in delayed diagnosis.[30,31] Although blastomycosis has been studied most systematically in outbreak investigations, the majority of cases are sporadic.

In endemic regions, *B. dermatitidis* has been found in soil, especially in microfoci of moist, acidic, organically rich soil in proximity to waterways.[32-34] Molecular analyses of clinical and soil isolates recovered during a large outbreak showed dissimilarity; more than one strain was present in the environment and among clinical isolates.[6] Acquisition through a dog bite, perinatal exposure, and through conjugal contact have been reported, but person-to-person or zoonotic transmission is rare.[35] Infections in children constitute a minority of sporadic cases but comprise 15% to 25% of outbreak-related cases. A 4:1 to 15:1 reported male preponderance in sporadic adult infections has been attributed to occupational and recreational activities. Sex distribution is equal among affected children. In 73 cases occurring over 11 years in a hyperendemic region, most occurred between December and April and in immunocompetent individuals who lived or visited within 500 meters of rivers or associated waterways.[36] In an endemic area, patterns of disease suggested that summer environment exposure led to localized pneumonia within 1 to 6 months. This was followed 4 to 9 months thereafter by slow progression of asymptomatic infection resulting in isolated extrapulmonary or disseminated hematogenous disease in the minority.[37]

CLINICAL MANIFESTATIONS

Nonspecific Symptoms

Among 46 children and 2 adults who acquired infections following exposure to a beaver pond, 54% experienced symptoms[32] within 21 to 106 days (median, 45 days). Cough, headache, chest pain, weight loss, fever, abdominal pain, and/or night sweats occurred in >50% of patients. Symptoms are not distinctive, and this may contribute to delayed diagnostic consideration. Canine susceptibility makes inquiry regarding symptoms in pet dogs a useful clue to diagnosis in patients with pulmonary symptoms.[38]

The full clinical spectrum of extrapulmonary blastomycosis is summarized in Figure 252-2.[39] Progressive pulmonary infection and disseminated infection are life-threatening conditions that occur in 10% of reported cases.

Pulmonary Manifestations

Acute Pulmonary Infection

Acute pulmonary infection is the most common manifestation of blastomycosis in children.[1,40-43] As in adults,[44] the spectrum of severity of related symptoms ranges from absent or mild illness (Figure 252-4) to respiratory failure.[45] Associated symptoms include fever, chills, and cough productive of purulent sputum. Infection can resolve spontaneously (usually within 2 to 4 weeks) before the diagnosis is established. In endemic regions, persistence of symptoms despite treatment for bacterial infection should prompt consideration of blastomycosis.[46] Erythema nodosum[47] sometimes occurs in association with respiratory tract symptoms.

Chronic Pulmonary Infection

Symptoms of chronic pneumonia include weight loss, night sweats, fever, cough, and chest pain; complaints can persist for 2 to 6 months. Additional diagnostic considerations include tuberculosis, other mycoses, and neoplasms.

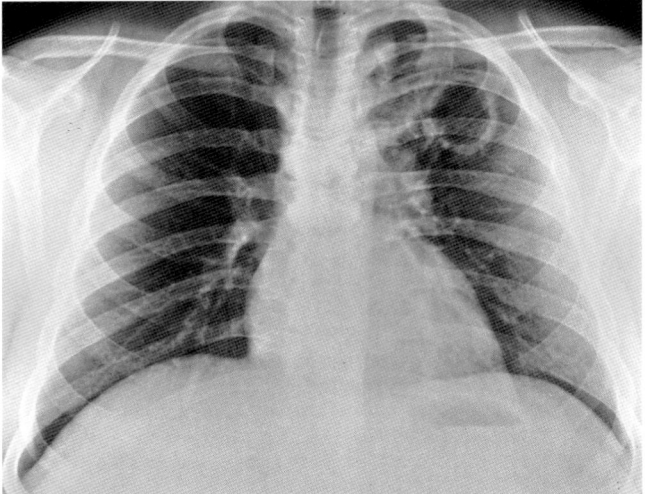

Figure 252-4. Chest radiograph of an 18-year-old insulin-dependent diabetic man with hemoptysis of 2 days' duration who described no fever or any antecedent respiratory symptoms. The radiograph showed a large cavitary lesion in the left upper lobe and enlargement of a left hilar lymph node. *Blastomyces dermatitidis* was isolated from bronchoscopy specimens, although the results of direct examination were negative. No additional focus of infection was identified with extensive evaluation; a 6-month course of ketoconazole was given, the patient remained well, and radiographic findings showed improvement.

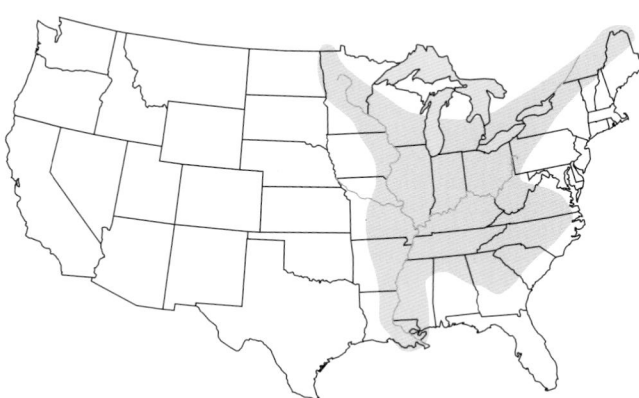

Figure 252-3. United States map showing the most highly endemic region for *Blastomyces dermatitidis*.

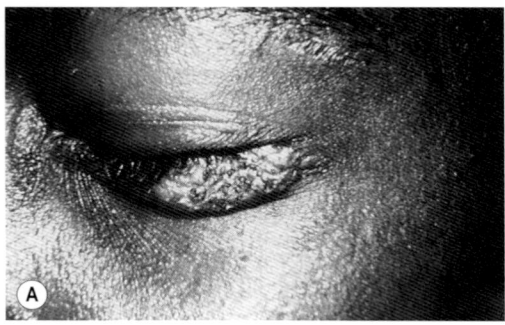 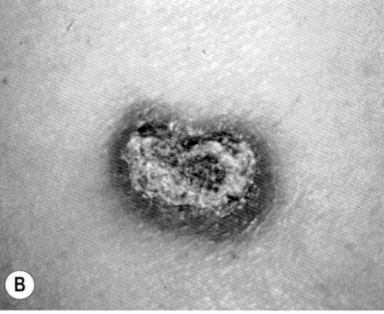

Figure 252-5. Cutaneous lesion of blastomycosis. Lesions are generally painless and most commonly appear on the face and extremities; lymphangitis and regional lymphadenopathy are usually absent.
(A) Verrucous lesion characterized by crusting and induration; areas of healing with scarring and pigmentary changes are common.
(B) Ulcerated lesions, which usually follow the stage of papulopustular nodules.

Extrapulmonary Manifestations

Although primary blastomycosis almost always results from a pulmonary focus, extrapulmonary manifestations can affect many structures and organ systems (see Figure 252-2). In these instances, pulmonary symptoms may be absent and chest radiographs often show abnormalities but may also be normal.

Cutaneous Manifestations

Skin lesions are common in disseminated infections, observed most often in sporadic cases and infrequently in epidemic settings.[48] They begin as minimally tender papules and can evolve into verrucous or ulcerative lesions; both types can be present simultaneously. Verrucous lesions have raised irregular borders, crusting, and purulent drainage (Figure 252-5A). In ulcerative forms, borders are sharp and heaped up, and granulation tissue and exudate are seen centrally (Figure 252-5B). Chronic disseminated cutaneous blastomycosis has been reported rarely.[49]

Osseous Manifestations

Symptoms typical of acute or subacute suppurative osteomyelitis occur in 25% to 50% of children with blastomycosis.[1] Long bones, vertebrae, ribs, skull, sacrum, or pelvis can be affected (Figure

TABLE 252-1. Prevalence of Extrapulmonary Blastomycosis by Site in Adults

Site	Prevalence (%)
Skin	69
Bone and joints	19
Genitourinary tract	15
Reticuloendothelial system (liver, spleen, lymph nodes, bone marrow)	9
Subcutaneous nodules	5
Larynx, oropharynx, nose	4
Thyroid	2

From Deepe GS, Gomez AM. Blastomyces and paracoccidioides. In: Gorbach S (ed) Infectious Diseases. Philadelphia: WB Saunders, 1992, p 2367.

252-6). Abscesses and sinus tracts in adjacent soft tissue are common. Lesions sometimes are asymptomatic and identified using bone imaging methodologies.

Unusual Manifestations

Metastatic foci of infection in adults can result in a variety of presentations of low frequency, most of which also can occur in children (Table 252-1).[8,40-43] Meningitis and focal parameningeal and parenchymal intracranial abscesses can occur, frequently in association with immunosuppression.[8,24,40,43] Infections of the prostate gland or epididymis, although common in adults, are not reported in prepubescent children.[40]

LABORATORY FINDINGS AND DIAGNOSIS

Nonspecific Abnormalities

Hematologic findings in blastomycosis are not distinctive; mild anemia, leukocytosis (with mild increase in band forms), and elevated erythrocyte sedimentation rate occur commonly. Chest radiographic findings include consolidation, mass lesions, nodules, miliary disease, cavities, pleural effusion, fibrosis, and/or interstitial disease.[50] The most commonly reported finding in children was consolidation in one or several lobes.[51] Osseous lesions usually are lytic, often are multiple (see Figure 252-6), can affect long and/or flat bones, and can mimic findings caused by other pathogens or some neoplasms.[52] Lytic lesions of vertebrae, ribs, pelvis, or skull should raise suspicion of blastomycosis.[53]

Specific Laboratory Diagnosis

Direct Examination and Culture

A rapid diagnosis can be established through identification of pyogranulomatous inflammation and observation of typical

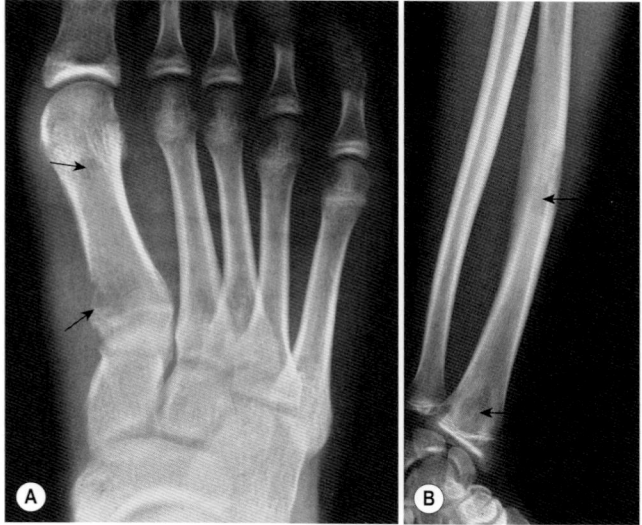

Figure 252-6. Radiographs of a 16-year-old boy with complaints of pain of 2 months' duration in his right foot and right forearm. He had no fever but had lost 5.9 kg (13 lb). Radiographs show **(A)** radiolucent areas in the proximal and distal first metatarsal (arrows) and **(B)** lucent areas of the distal metaphysis and midshaft of the radius (arrows). The chest radiograph was normal. A large abscess of the radius and surrounding soft tissue was drained; fluid showed yeast forms of *Blastomyces dermatitidis*, and culture results were positive. The patient recovered fully after receiving amphotericin B for 8 weeks.

organisms in tissue or in sputum, bronchial washings, or other body fluids.[54] *B. dermatitidis* is never a commensal. Typical yeast-like fungi can be seen in wet mounts and in tissue stained with hematoxylin and eosin or Gomori methenamine silver nitrate (see Figure 252-1). The periodic acid–Schiff stain also is useful for tissue because it stains the fungal cell wall and preserves histologic detail. In endemic regions, if observers are experienced and clinical features are compatible with blastomycosis, a morphologic diagnosis can be secure. In patients with subacute meningitis, examination of cerebrospinal fluid rarely is definitive; ventricular fluid is more likely to be diagnostic.[55,56] Histologic findings in skin lesions include papillomatosis, downward proliferation of epidermis, intraepidermal abscesses, and multinucleated giant cells.

B. dermatitidis can be isolated from cultures of infected tissue or body fluids; cultures have been found to be positive in 10% of instances in which organisms were not observed in surgical/cytopathologic specimens.[57] The organism grows on Sabouraud dextrose agar, brain–heart infusion, and other enriched media; media that inhibit bacteria and other fungi should be used for specimens from nonsterile sites. Laboratory confirmation of an isolate requires conversion (at 37°C) of the mold to the yeast form, and a positive result of a confirmatory test using a nucleic acid probe[58] or detection of exoantigen.[59] Growth in culture takes 2 to 4 weeks and may not be required if typical organisms are observed in primary specimens. PCR methods for identification of *B. dermatitidis* in clinical samples are not available.[60]

Serologic Tests

Serologic tests used to establish the diagnosis of blastomycosis are suboptimal.[8,61] This was demonstrated in a large outbreak investigation in which the complement fixation (CFA), immunodiffusion (ID), and enzyme immunoassay (EIA) were found to be positive in 9%, 28%, and 77%, respectively.[32,62] Thus, even in immunocompetent hosts, negative antibody assays do not exclude infection and should be interpreted in tandem with clinical, microbiologic, and histopathologic findings.

The CFA using yeast antigens suffers from both cross-reactivity, especially with antigens of *Histoplasma capsulatum*, and poor sensitivity.[59] The use of purified antigen A and WI-1 has improved serodiagnosis.[59,62-65] Commercially available macro-ID tests use purified antigen A and positive control sera. Serum specimens that produce lines of identity with the A band are considered positive. A positive ID test result is compatible with recent or active blastomycosis, although bands can persist for several months after infection. Although quite specific, the ID test has a sensitivity range of 52% to 79%; sensitivity is lower in patients with localized disease or people with symptoms of <50 days' duration. EIA[66] using protein A antigen and a radioimmunoassay method that uses WI-1[59] have been developed but neither is available commercially.

Cross-reactions of *H. capsulatum* antigens with antigens of *B. dermatitidis* and other endemic mycoses make the *Histoplasma* urine antigen test useful for evaluation.[61,67,68] In this setting, distinguishing between these infections should take into consideration clinical, epidemiologic, and other diagnostic laboratory data. An immunoassay for *B. dermatitidis* antigenuria also has been reported;[69] sensitivity was 93% and included 89% of disseminated and 100% of pulmonary infections; specificity was 79%. Cross-reactions were common with *Histoplasma* (96%), *Paracoccidioides* (100%), and *Penicillium marneffei* (70%). Rare cross-reactions occur with *Aspergillus* and *Cryptococcus* (1.8%). A more sensitive and specific assay is available commercially (MiraVista Diagnostics/Mirabella Technologies, Indianapolis) and may be useful for monitoring response to therapy and for detecting relapse.[70] Antigen concentration is highest in urine, but antigen may be detected in cerebrospinal,[71] bronchoalveolar lavage,[72] and other sterile body fluids.

TREATMENT

Although mortality rates of 60% were reported before availability of effective therapy, not all immunocompetent persons with mild pulmonary infection require treatment.[66,67,73,74] Observation for 1 or 2 weeks without antifungal treatment may be appropriate for mildly ill patients who are improving or in individuals with acute pneumonia whose symptoms resolve before a definitive diagnosis is established. In these latter settings, experts recommend that consideration be given to treatment in order to prevent extrapulmonary dissemination.[8,35,73,74] In all such instances, a search performed for extrapulmonary infection should be negative, and long-term follow-up should be ensured.

Systemic antifungal treatment is required for blastomycosis causing moderate to severe pneumonia, disseminated infection, or infection in immunocompromised patients.[73,75] Amphotericin B (a lipid preparation or deoxycholate)[73] and the azole drugs (itraconazole, fluconazole, and ketoconazole) have been used to treat blastomycosis. Itraconazole has emerged as the preferred oral therapy for both adults and children.[5,73] Choice of agents is based upon considerations that include: immune status, severity of illness, anatomic site of infection, drug tolerance, expected adherence to the therapeutic regimen, and cost.

In a trial of itraconazole, 90% of 48 adults with nonmeningeal, nonlife-threatening infection who received doses of 200 to 400 mg/day for 6 months were cured.[76] Itraconazole is more effective and better tolerated than ketoconazole.[5,76,77] Fluconazole has been used successfully in adult trials[78] and has the advantage of reaching effective concentrations in cerebrospinal fluid. Drug interactions, absorption, distribution, and toxicity of the azoles are complex; knowledge of these issues is essential (see Chapter 293, Antifungal Agents).

Experience with newer antifungal agents is limited. Voriconazole and posaconazole show good in vitro activity against *B. dermatitidis*. Voriconazole, owing to its excellent penetration into the CNS, has been used successfully[79,80] in cerebral blastomycosis in patients who either failed to respond, had a recurrence following treatment, or were intolerant of recommended regimens.[73]

Recommendations

Recommendations for treating blastomycosis are derived from clinical trials in adults and the clinical experience of experts. Current clinical practice guidelines for the management of blastomycosis,[73] are summarized in Table 252-2 and include recommendations for the treatment of children. In all instances, long-term follow-up is required to identify late dissemination or relapse. Adherence to therapy should be assessed prior to the start of treatment with any oral antifungal agent and should be reassessed if a patient fails to improve.

Moderately severe to severe pulmonary disease and/or dissemination in children[73] is treated with full dosage of either amphotericin B deoxycholate or a lipid amphotericin B preparation for 1 to 2 weeks or until improvement occurs. Thereafter, itraconazole is used for 12 months. For these manifestations, and any manifestation of blastomycosis for which itraconazole is used, the maximum dose is 400 mg/day; serum concentrations should be determined after 2 weeks of treatment and dosage adjusted to ensure adequate drug exposure. Children with mild to moderate pulmonary infection can be treated with oral itraconazole for 6 to 12 months. When blastomycosis is diagnosed and treated during pregnancy, the newborn should receive therapy if there is evidence of infection. Although data are few, amphotericin B should be used for treatment. Consultation with experts may be needed for unusual or severe cases.

Liposomal amphotericin B is preferred for treating CNS infections since it has been determined in animal models that it attains higher concentrations within the CNS than does amphotericin B deoxycholate. Treatment should be at full dosage for 4 to 6 weeks, and followed thereafter by an azole (fluconazole, itraconazole, or voriconazole) for at least one year.[73] Dosage of itraconazole should be at the upper range of that recommended. Ketoconazole or fluconazole can be used if itraconazole is not tolerated. Suboptimal response or relapse may require retreatment with amphotericin B or a higher dose of itraconazole. A recent multicenter

TABLE 252-2. Summary of Recommendations for Treatment of Blastomycosis

Manifestation/Patient Population	Preferred Treatment	Comments
Moderately severe to severe pulmonary	Lipid AmB, 3–5 mg/kg per day, or deoxycholate AmB, 0.7–1.0 mg/kg per day, for 1–2 weeks; followed by itraconazole,[a] 200 mg bid for 6–12 months	The entire course can be given with deoxycholate AmB to a total of 2 g; most clinicians prefer to use step-down therapy after the patient's condition improves. Lipid formulations of AmB have fewer side effects
Mild to moderate pulmonary disease	Itraconazole,[a] 200 mg once or twice per day for 6–12 months	
Moderately severe to severe disseminated disease	Lipid AmB, 3–5 mg/kg per day, or deoxycholate AmB, 0.7–1.0 mg/kg per day, for 1–2 weeks; followed by itraconazole,[a] 200 mg bid for 6–12 months	The entire course can be given with deoxycholate AmB to a total of 2 g; most clinicians prefer to use step down therapy after the patient's condition improves. Lipid formulations of AmB have fewer side effects. Treat osteoarticular disease for 12 months
Mild to moderate disseminated disease	Itraconazole,[a] 200 mg once or twice per day for 6–12 months	Treat osteoarticular disease for 12 months
Central nervous system disease	Lipid Amb, 5 mg/kg per day for 4–6 weeks is preferred;[b] followed by an oral azole for at least one year	Step-down therapy can be with fluconazole, 800 mg per day; itraconazole,[a] 200 mg 2–3 times per day; or voriconazole, 200–400 mg 2 times per day. Longer treatment may be required for immunosuppressed patients
Disease in Immunosuppressed patients	Lipid AmB, 3–5 mg/kg per day, or deoxycholate Amb, 0.7–1 mg/kg per day, for 1–2 weeks; followed by itraconazole,[a] 200 mg bid for 12 months	Lifelong suppressive treatment may be required if immunosuppression cannot be reversed
Disease in pregnant women	Lipid Amb, 3–5 mg/kg per day	Azoles should not be used during pregnancy
Moderately severe to severe disease in children	Deoxycholate AmB, 0.7–1.0 mg/kg per day, or lipid Amb, 3–5 mg/kg per day, for 1–2 weeks; followed by itraconazole,[a] 10 mg/kg per day for 12 months	Children tolerate deoxycholate AmB better than adults; maximum dose of itraconazole should be 400 mg per day
Mild to moderate disease in children	Itraconazole, 10 mg/kg per day for 6–12 months	Maximum dose, 400 mg per day

AmB, amphotericin B; bid, twice per day.

[a]*In any regimen for which itraconazole is used, serum concentrations should be determined after 2 weeks of treatment and, if needed, dosage adjusted to ensure adequate drug exposure.*

[b]*In animal models of fungal meningitis, liposomal AmB achieves higher CNS levels than other lipid formulations. Hence, many infectious diseases experts recommend liposomal AmB as the preferred lipid formulation for the treatment of CNS fungal infections.*

review[71] of 22 adults concluded that initial treatment with a lipid formulation of amphotericin B followed by a prolonged course of an azole orally, preferably voriconazole, appeared to be effective.[81] In the latter review, 55% were immunocompromised and 18% died during follow-up. Although amphotericin B is the drug of first choice, fluconazole can be considered for use after a 6-week course of amphotericin B; fluconazole should be used at the upper dose range and continued for 6 months. For patients unable to tolerate amphotericin B, fluconazole is considered for primary therapy. Voriconazole has been used successfully.[3,71,79,82] Azoles used to treat bone infection, either after amphotericin B induction or as monotherapy, should be continued for 1 year.

SPECIAL CONSIDERATIONS

Blastomycosis has been reported to occur in pregnant women whose offspring have been uninfected, but fatal perinatal infections also have occurred.[83-86] Blastomycosis should therefore be treated if it is identified during pregnancy. Since azole agents potentially are teratogenic, amphotericin B is the drug of choice.[87]

In conjunction with antifungal therapy, surgical drainage of large abscesses, excision of devitalized bone and purulent material, drainage of purulent empyema or pericardial effusion, or excision of an established fistula often hasten recovery and lessen the likelihood of relapse. Surgical resection without concomitant antifungal therapy is not curative.

Blastomycosis, although not a common opportunistic infection in patients with human immunodeficiency virus (HIV) infection,[24,88,89] can cause severe, diffuse pulmonary involvement and extrapulmonary dissemination that sometimes is associated with CNS infection. Mortality is 30% to 40%. Transplant recipients and patients receiving immunosuppressive agents, including tumor necrosis factor-α inhibitors,[90-92] also are at risk for severe blastomycosis. Complications are similar to complications in patients with HIV infection, although CNS infection is less frequent.[89] Treatment of immunosuppressed hosts should be initiated with amphotericin B. Since relapses have been reported after completing therapy, chronic suppressive treatment with itraconazole should be considered; fluconazole suppression can be used following treatment for CNS infection.[73]

PREVENTION

Avoidance of exposure to the microfoci associated with outbreaks of blastomycosis should be discussed when immunodeficient patients are counseled about decreasing the risk of acquiring opportunistic infections.

Progress in vaccine development[93-96] has included the development of a live recombinant strain of *B. dermatitidis* that is deficient in the WI-1 surface antigen and is immunogenic in animals. At present, there is no human vaccine available to prevent blastomycosis.

253 *Coccidioides immitis* and *Coccidioides posadasii* (Coccidioidomycosis)

Martin B. Kleiman

Coccidioides immitis and *C. posadasii* cause coccidioidomycosis (San Joaquin Valley fever), an endemic primary systemic mycosis that is asymptomatic or mild in 95% of cases but that also causes life-threatening infections in immunocompetent and immuno-compromised hosts.[1,2]

THE PATHOGEN

Microbiology

Coccidioides spp. are dimorphic fungi that exist as spore-forming saprophytic molds in soil and as endosporulating spherules in their parasitic form (Figure 253-1).[3] Two species have been identified using molecular and biogeographic characteristics. The two species show little or no phenotypic, antigenic, virulence, or morphologic differences. *C. immitis* is found in California whereas *C. posadasii* is found in Mexico and areas of Central and South America.[4-7] Isolates demonstrate extensive genetic diversity.[1,8]

The infectious forms of this unique fungus are the multinucleate spores (arthroconidia), which are barrel-shaped structures with thick hydrophobic walls that are released from the mold when the thin-walled intervening cells lyse. Arthroconidia propagate the mold in soil; inhalation of only a few spores can cause infection in humans. Following inhalation, the spores germinate in the lung, and become spherules 10 to 200 μm in diameter in about 3 to 4 days. Spherules undergo internal cleavage and septation and eventually release large numbers (sometimes 500 to 800) of uninucleate endospores 2 to 5 μm in diameter (Figure 253-2). Endospores then propagate in the host, thereby amplifying the number of fungal elements and completing the life cycle of the parasitic phase. Growth of endospores and their release are stimulated by progesterone, 17β-estradiol, and testosterone.[9] The mold form is rarely found in human tissue.[10]

Pathogenesis

Primary infection occurs in the lungs. Factors that govern transition from the saprobic to the invasive form of the fungus are not understood fully. Neutrophils, lymphocytes, and monocytes influence fungal dimorphism toward the spherule phase.[3] A fungal enzyme with elastase activity may facilitate spread of infection and increase inflammation.[11] *C. posadasii* perturbs pulmonary surfactant proteins, potentially enabling disease progression.[12,13] Molecular techniques have been used to examine specific genes that affect virulence.[14,15] Virulence has been attributed to a gene coding for a cell surface glycoprotein that is produced early in spherule development and which acts as an adhesin.[16] An initial neutrophilic inflammatory response does not control infection, and granulomatous inflammation eventually predominates. A characteristic histologic finding is pyogranulomatous inflammation containing spherules and endospores (see Figure 253-2).

Primary pulmonary infection, whether clinically apparent or asymptomatic, often is accompanied by lymphohematogenous dissemination of the fungus. Whereas symptoms resulting from extrapulmonary infection occur in only 1% of infected patients, chorioretinal lesions can be found in as many as 40%.[17]

Immunity

Despite complement-dependent chemoattraction induced by fungal elements, neutrophils and macrophages have little capacity to damage or kill arthrospores, endospores, and, in particular, spherules.[18] Phagocytosis is made difficult physically by the size of fungal elements, especially the spherules. A metalloproteinase produced during endosporulation interferes with host recognition, thereby impairing phagocytosis when these fungal elements are most susceptible.[19] Fibrillar surface matrices also can both prevent effective leukocyte contact with spherules and isolate endospores from phagocytic fungicidal mechanisms.[20]

Natural infection results in lifelong immunity.[21] Polyclonal B-lymphocyte activation and increased complement fixation antibody (CFA) titers develop in disseminated infection, especially when coupled with loss of skin test reactivity, but humoral immunity is not protective. Protection has been firmly related to induction of Th1-associated immune responses. Coccidioidal antigens are processed and presented to T lymphocytes by macrophages and dendritic cells. This induces the production of interferon (IFN)-γ and other Th1 cytokines which act by recruiting and activating immune effector cells.[21,22] Stimulated coccidioidal-immune

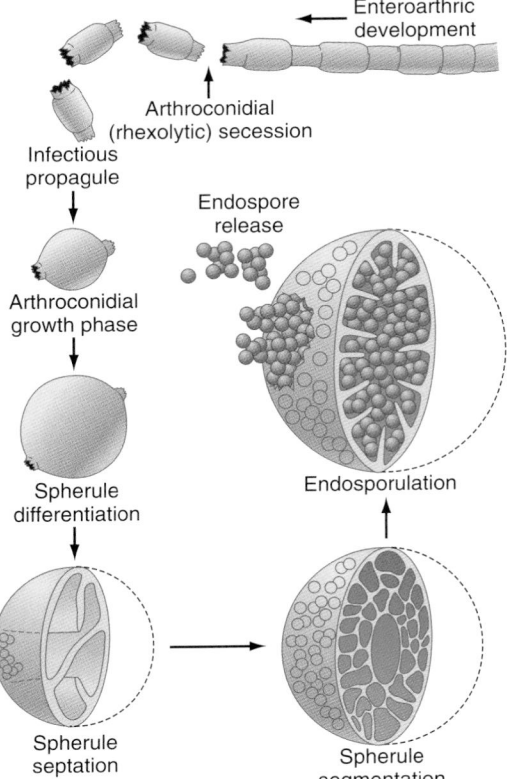

Figure 253-1. Life cycle of *Coccidioides immitis*. (Redrawn from Cole GT, Sun SH. Arthroconidium–spherule–endospore transformation in *Coccidioides immitis*. In: Fungal Dimorphism: With Emphasis on Fungi Pathogenic for Humans. New York, Plenum Press, 1985, p 281.)

Enteroarthric development

Arthroconidial (rhexolytic) secession

Infectious propagule

Endospore release

Arthroconidial growth phase

Spherule differentiation

Endosporulation

Spherule septation

Spherule segmentation

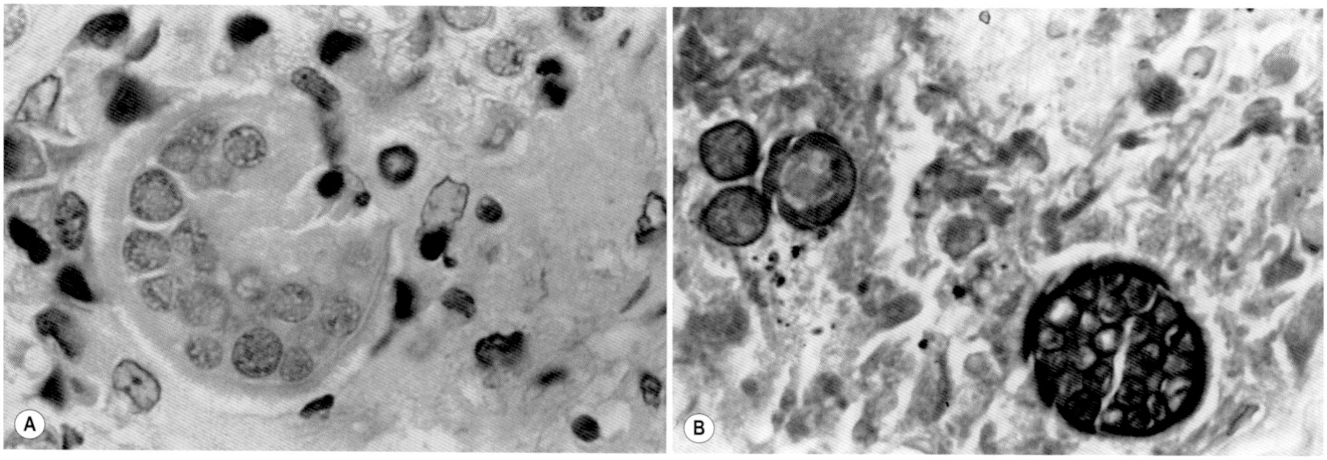

Figure 253-2. Specimens from a patient with acquired immunodeficiency syndrome and pneumonia caused by *Coccidioides immitis*. **(A)** Ruptured endosporulating spherule containing endospores 2 to 5 μm in diameter (hematoxylin and eosin stain, ×1250). **(B)** Typical intact, large endosporulating spherule and three immature spherules (Gomori methanamine silver nitrate stain, ×1000).

T lymphocytes interact with and activate macrophages and enhance phagosome–lysosome fusion and killing. A diminished Th1 response to *C. immitis* antigens has been demonstrated in patients with disseminated infections when compared with Th1 responses in otherwise healthy subjects.[23] A variety of contributing factors may include high concentrations of fungal antigen, circulating immune complexes, and direct suppression of immunity by fungal products or suppressor cells.[24] Congenital or acquired impairment of cellular immunity is a major risk factor for serious primary infection or relapse of past infection.

EPIDEMIOLOGY

Coccidioidomycosis occurs in hot, arid regions of the southwestern United States and is endemic to southern California, Arizona, western and southern Texas, and New Mexico (Figure 253-3). Infection also occurs in regions of Mexico and Central and South America where biogeographic distribution probably resulted from

a co-dispersal of the human host population and its pathogen.[5] Environments with hot summers, infrequent freezes, alkaline soil, and alternating periods of rain and drought support fungal growth and aerosolization of arthroconidia. Analyses of epidemic strains have shown that outbreaks result from environmental occurrences and population changes rather than the emergence of pathogenic fungal clones.[8,25,26]

Infection usually is acquired during recreational[27] or occupational activities that expose susceptible people to aerosolized arthroconidia. Examples include archeologic digs, recreational events, construction projects, and military training.[27-32] A large outbreak in Ventura County, California, followed exposure to dust clouds generated by an earthquake in January, 1994.[33] The incidence of infections has increased in California from 2000 to 2007.[34] Infections can be overlooked or undiagnosed when they occur in people who travel to high-risk regions but who reside and seek care in nonendemic areas.[22,35-41] Outbreaks of coccidioidomycosis also have been recognized after visits to areas not previously

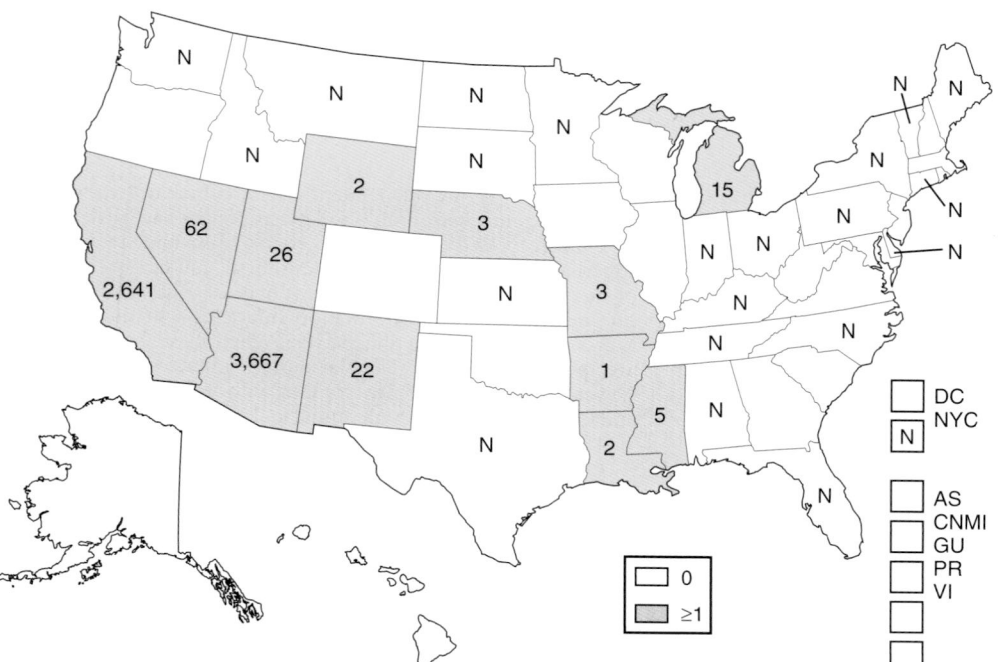

Figure 253-3.
Coccidioidomycosis reported cases – United States and United States territories, 2004. N, Not notifiable. (Data from Centers for Disease Control and Prevention. Summary of notifiable diseases – United States, 2003. Morbid Mortal Wkly Rep MMWR 2006;53:45.)

recognized as endemic.[30,42,43] Fomites, such as dusty clothing or agricultural products, also have been implicated as sources of infection; such cases are sometimes reported from nonendemic areas.[44,45] Growth of mold forms in dressings contaminated by purulent drainage rarely have been implicated.[45]

An estimated 25,000 to 150,000 new infections occur annually in the U.S.[15,21,46] Rates are highest in summer and early fall. Coccidioidomycosis has become increasingly important as migration to sunbelt states and the numbers of elderly[47] and immunosuppressed[14,48] populations grow. Conversely, significant reduction in coccidioidin skin test reactivity in Kern County, California, observed over a period of 58 years, has been attributed to decreased amounts of *C. immitis* in the soil resulting from increasing cultivation, irrigation, and urbanization.[21,49] Skin test positivity has been found in 17% of children living in a highly endemic area for up to 1 year and in 77% of children living in an endemic area for ≥10 years.

CLINICAL MANIFESTATIONS

Infection is subclinical in about 60% of infected people, and most others have self-limited, primary pulmonary infections. Pulmonary complications occur in <5% and disseminated infections in <1% of infected people. Pulmonary complications and extrapulmonary infections can occur without recognized antecedent illness. Illnesses in children requiring hospitalization mirrored the increased incidence of disease in 2005–2006 and were more common among patients with comorbid conditions and those requiring surgical drainage.[50]

Primary Pulmonary Infection

The incubation period is 10 to 16 days (range, 1 to 4 weeks). Malaise, chest pain, and fever are common symptoms.[51] Cough is variable, and hemoptysis is unusual in children. Acute, diffuse, erythematous rash and erythema multiforme are common in children. Erythema nodosum and fever can follow onset of symptoms by 3 to 18 days. Such progression occurs most often in girls and is termed *valley fever*. Erythema nodosum and transient arthritic complaints (*desert rheumatism*) are mediated by the cellular immune response. Occasionally, pulmonary symptoms are absent, and only hypersensitivity manifestations occur.

Symptoms usually improve without treatment in a few days to 1 month. Granulomas eventually can calcify. In adults, 5% to 10% of infections result in residual pulmonary nodules or thin-walled cavities.[46] Rarely, primary pulmonary infections that result from exposure to large inocula are severe and progress to involve multiple areas of the lungs, and can cause symptoms of adult respiratory distress syndrome.

Chronic Pulmonary Complications

Chronic pulmonary complications are uncommon in children and usually occur in adults with diabetes mellitus or an immunocompromising condition. Chronic progressive pneumonia, lung cavities, and pulmonary nodules are the most common manifestations (Figure 253-4). Peripheral thin-walled cavities sometimes rupture into the pleural space and cause pyopneumothorax.

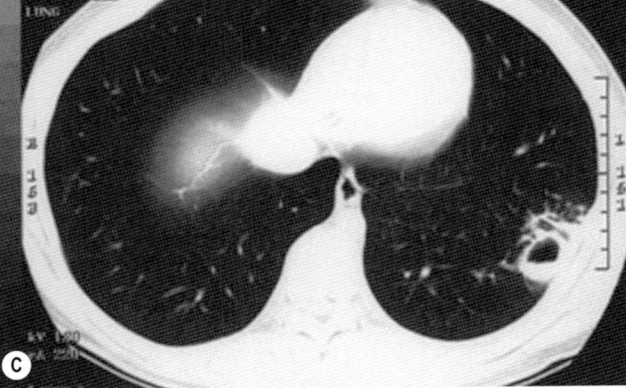

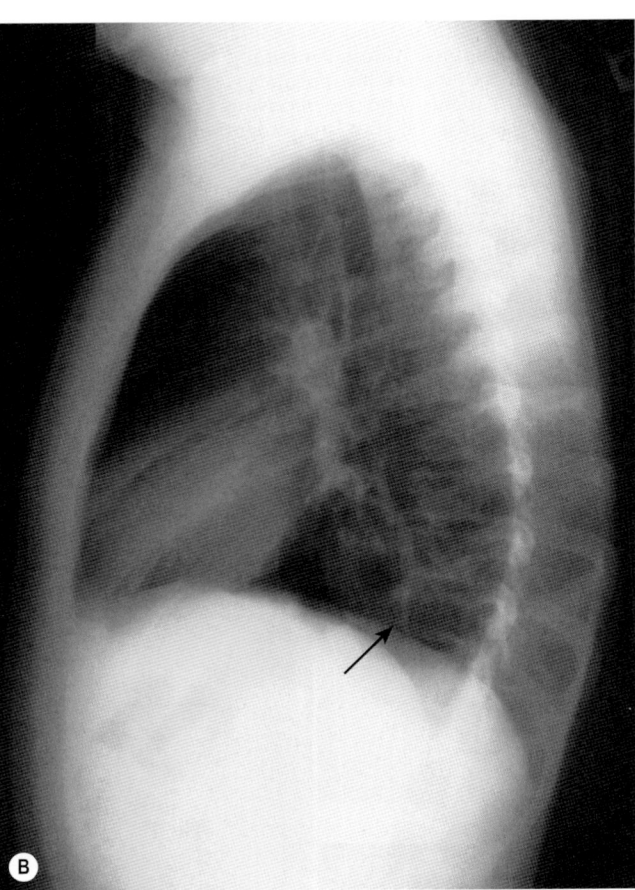

Figure 253-4. A 14-year-old boy with type 2 diabetes mellitus had a 6-month history of occasional chest pain and 13.6 kg (30 lb) weight loss. Chest radiographs **(A, B)** show peripheral left lower-lobe lung abscess (arrows); computed tomography (lung window) shows air–fluid level **(C)**. Aspirate yielded growth of *Coccidioides immitis*. (Courtesy of J.H. Brien©.)

Extrapulmonary Manifestations (Dissemination)

Clinical manifestations of dissemination[52] to extrapulmonary sites occur in about 0.5% of patients, usually within several months of the primary pulmonary infection and rarely after 1 year. Dissemination is less frequent in children than in adults.[46] Persistent fever is common and frequently affected sites include the lungs, skin, bones, joints, and central nervous system (CNS). Those at highest risk are neonates and young infants, immunosuppressed patients,[53–56] Filipinos, African Americans, Native Americans, Hispanics,[57,58] and women in late pregnancy[59] and the early postpartum period. Patients who are receiving tumor necrosis factor (TNF)-α antagonists[60,61] also are recognized to be at risk (Box 253-1).

Osteomyelitis and Arthritis

Osteomyelitis is subacute or chronic, often multifocal, and occasionally is associated with decompression into adjacent soft tissues.[62] Common sites are the hands and feet, ribs, skull, and vertebrae. Vertebral involvement can result in collapse, articular instability, paraspinal abscess,[63] or in some instances, meningitis. Monoarticular arthritis, often of the knee or ankle, occurs in 20% of adults with disseminated infection and can be chronic. Isolated osseous lesions can resemble neoplasms.[64]

Cutaneous Disease

Most skin infections represent extrapulmonary manifestations arising by bloodstream spread from a primary pulmonary focus.[65]

Lesions begin as papules or pustules that enlarge and can ulcerate. Verrucous plaques, subcutaneous cold abscesses, and wart-like lesions also occur (Figure 253-5). Lesions can occur anywhere but are common on the face, along the nasolabial folds. Cutaneous lesions, accompanied by regional adenitis, rarely occur after accidental inoculation.[66,67]

Meningitis

Meningitis[68–70] can occur acutely but often is subacute with transient periods of remission. Symptoms often include headache; altered sensorium, ataxia, vomiting, and focal neurologic deficits also occur. Fever is variable and meningismus occurs in only 50% of patients. Meningeal vasculitis, often associated with cerebral infarction, is recognized increasingly; a retrospective review[71] reported a mortality rate of 70% with this complication. Basilar meningeal reaction can interfere with cerebrospinal fluid (CSF) resorption and cause obstructive or communicating hydrocephalus. If untreated, meningitis is fatal within 1 to 2 years.[57] Long-term, often lifelong, treatment is required to prevent relapse.

DIAGNOSIS

Symptoms of coccidioidomycosis are not distinctive. A careful history of travel to endemic areas and inquiry about high-risk activities often prompts consideration of the diagnosis, particularly for patients residing in nonendemic regions.[15,35,36]

Nonspecific Tests

The erythrocyte sedimentation rate usually is increased, and mild peripheral eosinophilia occurs in 5% to 10% of patients with primary infection; extreme eosinophilia can occur with dissemination.[72] In patients with meningitis, CSF shows moderate hypoglycorrhachia, elevated protein concentration, and pleocytosis with a predominance of mononuclear cells although neutrophils can predominate; eosinophilia is reported in 15% of cases.[69] Specific antibody is present in the CSF of patients with meningitis. CSF can be normal in some CNS infections. The chest radiograph can be normal or show parenchymal infiltrates, hilar lymphadenopathy, thin-walled cavities, or parapneumonic effusion.[72] Osseous lesions usually are lytic, but scintigraphy of bone is more sensitive than plain radiography. Magnetic resonance imaging is useful for demonstrating bone marrow signal abnormalities and sites of decompression into soft tissue or joints.[73,74]

Direct Examination and Culture

The observation of spherules containing endospores 2 to 5 μm in diameter is diagnostic. Spherules do not take up Gram stain but can be identified in infected body fluids with potassium hydroxide preparations or the Calcofluor white stain. Stains of infected CSF usually are negative. In tissue samples, pyogranulomatous

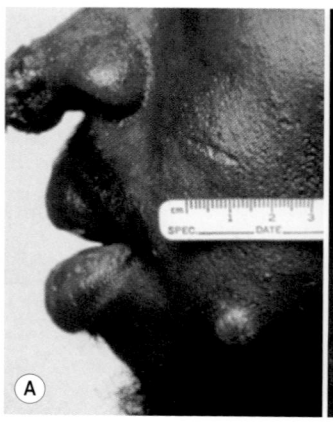
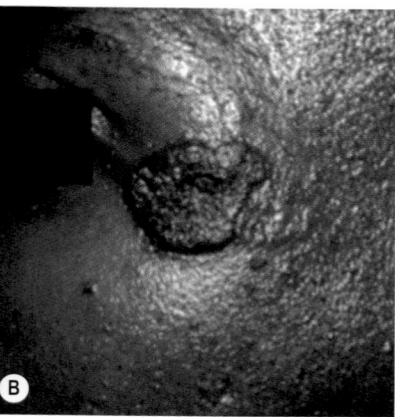

Figure 253-5. Cutaneous manifestations of disseminated coccidioidomycosis. **(A)** Raised nodules on the nose and cheek. **(B)** Hyperpigmented verrucoid plaque lateral to outer canthus. (From Sanders CV, Nesbitt LT Jr. The Skin and Infection. Philadelphia, Williams & Wilkins, 1995.)

inflammation with endosporulating spherules is seen readily with hematoxylin and eosin stain (see Figure 253-2) or periodic acid–Schiff stain. Spherules also stain well with Gomori methenamine silver nitrate. (see Figure 253-2). Mold forms are rarely seen in body fluid or tissue specimens.[75]

If organisms are not visualized in body fluid specimens or tissue, the diagnosis can be confirmed by culture. The mold is a hazard to laboratory personnel;[76] therefore, the clinical laboratory should be informed if coccidioidomycosis is suspected. Slants rather than agar plates are inoculated; growth of *Coccidioides* spp. is supported by many conventional laboratory media at 30°C to 37°C. Yield from respiratory tract secretions can be enhanced by chemical digestion of purulent specimens. Cultures of blood infrequently are positive.[77] Culture of purulent material from other infected sites usually is positive, although urine, peritoneal fluid, and CSF cultures can be negative despite infection at these sites. In situ methods have been developed that identify *C. immitis* in infected tissue.[78] The fungus is isolated in culture in its mycelial phase and can be confirmed as *Coccidioides* spp. using exoantigens or nucleic acid probes.[79] Formaldehyde pretreatment of isolates can cause a false-negative result in the nucleic acid probe and therefore should be avoided.[80] Progress in development of molecular diagnostic techniques that can identify *Coccidioides* spp. in clinical specimens has been reviewed.[81] Polymerase chain reaction testing in a clinical setting has been shown to identify negative results accurately while showing sensitivity similar to that of fungal culture.[82]

Skin Test

Four weeks after exposure, almost all infected people have positive intradermal skin tests (induration ≥5 mm) to coccidioidal antigen prepared from spherule forms (Spherulin).[15] Although recent conversion of skin test reactivity is diagnostic, reactivity persists after infection, thereby relegating the skin test to use as an epidemiologic tool. Cutaneous anergy in infected, symptomatic patients suggests the presence of disseminated infection. Conversely, conversion to skin test positivity correlates with improvement. The coccidioidal skin test is not available in the U.S.[55,83]

Serologic Tests

Assays for coccidioidal antibody are valuable diagnostic and prognostic tools,[84,85] but false-negative results can occur early in infection and in immunocompromised patients. Cross-reactions with *H. capsulatum, B. dermatitidis,* and *Penicillium marneffei* may occur.[86,87] Current antigen detection methodology[88] utilizes a more specific *Coccidioides* antigen enzyme immunoassay (EIA) which is positive in 71% of patients with coccidioidomycosis, and negative in 99% of uninfected individuals. Cross-reactions with other endemic mycoses occur in only 11% of cases. Dissociation of immune complexes improves the sensitivity for detecting antigenemia.[89]

Specific-immunoglobulin (Ig) M anti-*Coccidioides* is detectable in 75% of patients 1 to 3 weeks after onset of symptoms and is usually absent after 6 months. Presence indicates recent infection. IgM is detected by the tube precipitin test but more often by the sensitive immunodiffusion tube precipitin (IDTP) technique. Sensitive latex particle and EIA methods are available as screening tests for IgM anti-*Coccidioides* but positive results must be confirmed using more specific methods.[90]

Complement fixation assay (CFA) detects IgG-specific antibody and is positive in about 50% of patients at 4 weeks and in 83% at 3 months after infection. CFA titers become undetectable in several months if infection resolves. Standardized CFA titers >1:16 directly correlate with the presence and severity of extrapulmonary disease. A qualitative immunodiffusion complement fixation (IDCF) test for detecting IgG antibody also is available and should not be confused with the IDTP test. The IDTP and IDCF techniques are useful qualitative screening tests. The CFA usually is performed if the latter is positive.[57] The IDCF method is useful for sera that are anti-complementary. The EIA for coccidioidal IgG and

IgM antibodies correlates well with the titer of IDCF.[91] An experienced laboratory should confirm positive tests and compare results with a database of localized primary versus disseminated disease.[15]

CFA antibody is present in the CSF of 95% of patients with coccidioidal meningitis, although serial samples may be required. Titers decline during effective therapy. A parameningeal focus of coccidioidal infection can cause a positive CSF CFA.

TREATMENT

Fewer than 5% of people with coccidioidomycosis require antifungal treatment. Decision to treat is based on specific features and severity of the initial illness and the presence of risk factors for progressive dissemination, a poor outcome, or both[21,24,46] (see Box 253-1). Treatment is required for patients with primary or acquired immunodeficiency including those receiving TNF-inhibiting agents, fulminant infections, extrapulmonary manifestations, or prolonged symptoms. In a review of experience with outcomes in adults with primary pulmonary coccidioidomycosis with clinical severity for which therapy with azoles was elected, complications were observed only among those who received treatment but in whom treatment was discontinued.[92]

Published reports of the results of amphotericin B treatment (the first antifungal agent used), are limited to nonrandomized open-label studies of chronic pulmonary infections and extrapulmonary disease. Accumulated experience with intrathecal and intracisternal[91] instillation of amphotericin B for the treatment of meningitis also has been reported.[93,94] The toxicity and inconvenience of amphotericin B have made use of alternative agents desirable and the effectiveness and relative safety and convenience of the oral azoles very attractive. Amphotericin B generally is reserved for use in the initial management of respiratory failure or rapidly progressive disease. Amphotericin B also is used for women during pregnancy since the azole agents have the potential for teratogenicity.[59,95] Some experts reserve amphotericin for use as salvage therapy.[91] No clinical evidence supports greater efficacy of lipid formulations of amphotericin B.

Fluconazole and itraconazole are the principal agents used for treatment. Ketoconazole has the advantage of being less costly. Selection of an azole agent is based on proven efficacy for the disease manifestation, tolerability, and cost. The availability of a generic preparation of fluconazole has decreased cost. Although better tolerated than amphotericin B, these agents have adverse effects, pharmacokinetic properties, and drug interactions that must be considered (see Chapter 293, Antifungal Agents). Most trials with the triazole agents have been conducted in open-label, nonrandomized, multicenter studies in adults and have differed in design and follow-up;[46] a comparative study is reported.[96] Recommendations for children are derived from published experience in adults. However, generalization of these results to children disregards differences in host factors that predict outcome, including children's improved response and tolerance of therapy. Physicians who treat children with coccidioidomycosis should consider seeking consultation from experts.

RECOMMENDATIONS

Primary Infection

Immunocompetent patients without risk factors for poor outcome (see Box 253-1) and who have mild primary respiratory tract infections usually do not require treatment. However, they should be assessed at 3 to 6 month intervals for up to 2 years to ensure that both symptoms and radiographic abnormalities have resolved.[46] Severe, prolonged, or progressive primary respiratory tract infections require antifungal therapy. Firm criteria for severity are not established in children, but useful indicators in adults include: weight loss >10% of body weight, symptoms for ≥3 weeks, pulmonary infiltrates involving more than one-half of one lung or occurring bilaterally, prominent hilar lymphadenopathy, chest pain, and standardized CFA titers ≥1:16.[46] Although the azole agents have

supplanted amphotericin B as a primary drug, the use of amphotericin B results in a more rapid clinical response and is recommended for initial management of severe or rapidly progressing
infections that do not involve the CNS. In adults, amphotericin B
is given until substantial improvement is observed, and then for up
to several weeks with cumulative doses of 1 g. An oral azole agent
is then used for the remainder of treatment. A similar approach is
used for children, in whom the total dose of amphotericin B deoxycholate can vary based upon severity of symptoms and the rapidity
of response. Duration of treatment can be several months to a year.
Important determinants of improvement include resolution of
respiratory tract and constitutional symptoms, and decrease of CFA
titers. In mild to moderately severe primary pulmonary infections
for which treatment is elected, azole agents may be used as monotherapy. The duration of treatment is individualized but probably
should be at least 3 months beyond the resolution of symptoms.
Itraconazole or fluconazole can be used. Periodic reassessment is
needed for at least 1 to 2 years thereafter.

Nonmeningeal Extrapulmonary Infection

Treatment is indicated for all extrapulmonary manifestations of
coccidioidomycosis and in all immunocompromised patients
including people with human immunodeficiency virus (HIV)
infection and pregnant women.[46] In patients with severe illness or
rapid progression of disease, amphotericin B is used initially. The
dose and duration of amphotericin B depend on the severity of
symptoms, rapidity of response, and host-related risk factors. The
remainder of the course of treatment can be completed with an
oral azole agent, except during pregnancy when amphotericin
should be continued. Total duration of therapy should be at least
1 year and extend for 3 months beyond complete resolution of
symptoms. Because late relapse can occur, usually within 2 years of
apparently successful treatment, long-term follow-up is required.

The azole agents have been evaluated in treatment of extrapulmonary manifestations of coccidioidomycosis in adults. Although
ketoconazole is effective,[97] fluconazole[98–102] (400 mg/day) and
itraconazole[103–105] (200 mg twice daily) are effective, better tolerated, and have been associated with lower rates of relapse. The
primary endpoint of a comparative trial[96] of these agents in adults
with prolonged (>3 months) pulmonary or nonmeningeal
extrapulmonary infection showed neither fluconazole nor itraconazole to have superior efficacy despite a trend toward slightly
greater efficacy with itraconazole at the doses studied. Subanalyses
showed itraconazole to be more effective for treatment of skeletal
lesions and superior when analyzed 12 months after commencement.[46] Relapse rates after cessation of a 12-month course of
therapy were 18% for itraconazole and 28% for fluconazole (difference not statistically significant). Apparent inferiority of fluconazole versus itraconazole for treatment of skeletal infections in
this trial contrasts with previous reports.[102] Based on these data,
itraconazole[106] is a reasonable first choice for treating children
with nonmeningeal dissemination. The dose range for itraconazole in children is 5 to 10 mg/kg per day; the suspension is better
absorbed and is preferred (adult dose, 100 to 200 mg twice daily).
The dose range for fluconazole is 3 to 6 mg/kg per day (adult dose,
400 to 800 mg/day).

Meningeal Infection

Amphotericin B, given both systemically and either intrathecally
or directly instilled into the cerebral ventricles or cisterna
magna,[15,93,107] was the mainstay of therapy for coccidioidal meningitis before availability of the azole agents.[68] The inconvenience
and toxic effects of amphotericin, as well as the irritative arachnoiditis resulting from intrathecal instillation, have relegated
amphotericin to second-line therapy if response to an azole agent
is suboptimal. Although ketoconazole[108] and itraconazole[105] have
been shown to be effective in treating meningitis in adults, the
relative safety, acceptability, and comparatively superior ability of
fluconazole[46,98–100] to penetrate the blood brain barrier have made
fluconazole the treatment of choice for coccidioidal meningitis.

Doses effective in adults are 400 mg/day, but some experts begin
therapy with 800 to 1000 mg/day.[46,68] Response rates to fluconazole range from 67% to 80%. Children should be treated with
fluconazole at doses in the upper end of the recommended range
(12 mg/kg/day).[100,101] Indicators of improvement are a reduction
in CSF cell count and a decrease in CSF CFA titer.

Despite excellent response rates to azole agents, cure is infrequent; relapse of infection after cessation of therapy was reported
in 14 of 18 patients treated with an azole agent.[24,109] Relapses
occurred 2 weeks to 30 months after treatment cessation with
courses of 8 to 101 months. Because clinical or laboratory factors
predictive of relapse are not identified, fluconazole therapy should
be continued indefinitely and the CSF assessed every 3 months for
life.[68,109]

Patients who fail to respond to treatment with an azole agent
may improve with systemic therapy and direct instillation[93] of
amphotericin B into the intrathecal, ventricular, or intracisternal
spaces, with or without continuation of azole treatment.[46] Pleocytosis and elevated CFA titers in the CSF can indicate relapse before
clinical symptoms occur. Periodic examination of the CSF at
6-week intervals should continue for up to 2 years after cessation
of therapy.[93] An increased incidence of chronic arachnoiditis has
been observed in patients treated exclusively with fluconazole; in
these circumstances improvement has been seen following change
to intrathecal amphotericin B.[68] The optimal management of CNS
vasculitis is unclear.[68]

The persistent basilar inflammation resulting from meningitis
caused by *Coccidioides* spp. commonly results in obstructive hydrocephalus necessitating placement of a CSF shunting device.
Whereas the abnormal dynamics of CSF flow interferes with distribution of intrathecally administered amphotericin B, the use of
fluconazole, which crosses the blood–brain barrier more easily,
simplifies management in these instances. Development of hydrocephalus is not necessarily indicative of treatment failure and does
not itself require any alteration in antifungal management unless
accompanied by other findings suggestive of treatment failure.
However, treatment failure resulting from biofilm on a ventricular
shunt device has been reported.[75]

SPECIAL CONSIDERATIONS

Acquired or inherited cellular immune dysfunction is a risk factor
for aggressive and disseminated coccidioidomycosis. Although
highly active antiretroviral therapy (HAART) has decreased
incidence of coccidioidomycosis, it remains an important opportunistic infection in patients with HIV.[110,111] In this setting diagnosis often rests on clinical suspicion, histopathologic findings, and
culture. Skin test anergy and seronegativity do not exclude the
diagnosis.[112] Although the incidence of coccidioidomycosis is
highest in residents of endemic areas, infections can occur in residents of nonendemic areas,[113] resulting from exposure during
travel or from recrudescence of past infection. Patients are at high
risk for active coccidioidomycosis if the CD4+ lymphocyte count
is <250/mm3.[110] People with no apparent symptoms of active
infection but who have elevated coccidioidal antibody titers also
are at risk for having active coccidioidomycosis.[114] Symptoms
include fever and dyspnea, often in association with diffuse reticulonodular pulmonary infiltrates. Treatment strategies are similar
to those for HIV-uninfected people and include amphotericin B
for severe or diffuse pulmonary disease, followed by fluconazole
or itraconazole.[111,112,115–117] For mild disease, monotherapy with fluconazole or itraconazole is recommended. Following treatment,
lifelong antifungal suppression with fluconazole or itraconazole
is needed to prevent relapse.[112] Immune reconstitution inflammatory syndrome presenting as superior vena cava syndrome secondary to *Coccidioides* lymphadenopathy has been reported in an
HIV-infected patient.[118]

Recrudescence of coccidioidomycosis is common in patients
who receive organ or hematopoietic stem cell transplants.[116] Seropositive transplant recipients and/or people with previous clinical
coccidioidomycosis should receive prophylactic antifungal
therapy; fluconazole has been used successfully.[116,117] Severe

coccidioidomycosis has been reported in recipients of organs from donors with unrecognized infections.[48,119] In these instances, diagnosis can be delayed if transplants are done in nonendemic regions using organs procured from patients from endemic areas.

Limited clinical information is available for newer therapeutic agents. Posaconazole,[63,120] an extended-spectrum triazole with activity against *Coccidioides* spp., was shown to be effective in 6 patients with lung infections, 3 of whom also had nonmeningeal dissemination; all were refractory to treatment with azole agents (6) and amphotericin B (5). An open-label study of oral posaconazole given to 15 adults with refractory pulmonary (7) and disseminated (8) infections found a 73% response rate.[121] Voriconazole, another extended-spectrum triazole, was effective in treating coccidioidal meningitis that failed to respond to fluconazole.[122] Voriconazole also has been used successfully in combination with caspofungin in 3 children with refractory extrapulmonary infection, 1 of whom also had meningeal infection. Voriconazole was effective in an adult with disseminated, nonmeningeal coccidioidomycosis that was refractory to an extended course of amphotericin B, fluconazole and caspofungin.[123] Voriconazole also was used successfully as salvage therapy in 4 of 7 patients who had failed or did not tolerate standard therapy.[124] Caspofungin alone was successful in treating disseminated coccidioidomycosis in a renal transplant patient who was intolerant of fluconazole.[125] Adjunctive IFN-γ was effective in a critically ill patient with respiratory failure who failed to improve after extensive treatment with amphotericin B preparations and fluconazole.[126] The roles of these new agents for treating coccidioidomycosis await results of clinical trials.

Coccidioidomycosis that occurs during late pregnancy[127,128] or during the postpartum period can disseminate and require antifungal therapy; however, most women have favorable outcomes without treatment and with close observation.[59] Infection of the newborn is rare, even in gestational infections, but infected neonates and infants are at high risk for dissemination and require treatment.

Among two series of children hospitalized with coccidioidomycosis, 45% had operative procedures involving the CNS, as well as drainage of focal chest, joint, bones, or soft-tissue sites.[50,129] Although unusual in children, removal of cavitary lung lesions is necessitated by bleeding, enlargement, or intrapleural drainage. In bone infections, drainage of soft-tissue abscesses and resection of sequestra (sometimes performed with direct instillation or irrigation of antifungal agents) are helpful in concert with systemic antifungal therapy. Synovectomy for chronic joint infection is sometimes helpful in association with medical management. Management of vertebral disease can require drainage of paraspinal abscess and, if the spine is unstable, operative repair to stabilize affected joints.[91]

PREVENTION

Substantial evidence supports the feasibility and usefulness of an effective vaccine.[22,130] Attempts to immunize with a killed spherule vaccine were unsuccessful. Candidate immunizing agents and approaches are under development and have been reviewed.[22,131–134] Primary prophylaxis with an azole is not recommended for patients with HIV infection.[135] In endemic areas, exposure to activities that may aerosolize spores in heavily contaminated sites should be avoided, especially for immunosuppressed persons. If unavoidable, respiratory filtration devices should be used.

Key Points. *Coccidioides immitis* and *Coccidioides posadasii*

MICROBIOLOGY
- *Coccidioides* spp. are endemic, dimorphic fungi that exist as saprophytic molds in the environment and as endosporulating spherules in parasitic forms
- Multinucleate spores (arthroconidia) released from the mold result in a primary respiratory tract infection following inhalation
- Conversion to spherules within the host releases large numbers of endospores that amplify infection.

EPIDEMIOLOGY
- *C. immitis* is found in California; *C. posadasii* primarily in Mexico and regions of Central and South America
- Hot summers, alkaline soil, infrequent freezes, and alternating rain and drought favor growth
- Isolated and epidemic outbreaks can result from activities and environmental conditions that favor fungal growth and aerosolization of spores

DIAGNOSIS
- Diagnosis is confirmed by culture or observation of endosporulating spherules in tissue specimens
- Antigen detection in urine is sensitive and, if negative, makes the diagnosis unlikely; cross-reactions with other endemic fungi can occur

- In immunocompetent individuals, IgM-specific antibody is found in 75% within 1 to 3 weeks of symptoms; IgG-specific antibody is present in 50% by 4 weeks and 83% by 3 months
- Standardized complement fixation (CF) titers >1 : 16 correlate with the presence and severity of extrapulmonary disease
- CF antibody is present in CSF of 95% of patients with meningitis

TREATMENT
- Fewer than 5% of infections require antifungal therapy; follow-up of all patients is required for 2 years to ensure resolution
- Antifungal therapy is required for severe, prolonged (>6 weeks) primary infections, all extrapulmonary infections and in patients with risk factors for poor outcome (Box 253-1)
- Fluconazole and itraconazole are effective; itraconazole is preferred for bone infections; fluconazole achieves effective levels in CSF and is preferred for CNS infections
- Amphotericin B is preferred for severe, rapidly progressive, nonmeningeal infections; following induction, azole agents are used to complete therapy
- Management of meningeal infections is complex and consultation with experts is recommended

254 Dermatophytes and Other Superficial Fungi

Caroline Diane Sarah Piggott and Sheila Fallon Friedlander

Dermatophytes are aerobic fungi that can invade and infect the keratinized layers of skin, hair, and nails. Three genera of fungi, *Trichophyton, Microsporum,* and *Epidermophyton,* account for most dermatophytic infections. These fungi are found worldwide and infection is acquired by contact with infected humans or animals, or from exposure to contaminated soil or fomites (e.g., combs, brushes). Dermatophytes often are classified by their host preferences – anthropophilic and zoophilic species primarily infect human and animal species, respectively; geophilic species reside in soil. Direct contact can result in transmission of zoophilic or geophilic dermatophytes to humans. Dermatophytes do not cause invasive disease except in immunocompromised hosts. The clinical disease attributable to dermatophytes varies by organism, site of infection, and host immunologic responses.

Infection is often termed *tinea,* from the Latin word for worm, because infections originally were thought to derive from parasitic worms transmitted from cats or dogs. The modifying term (e.g., capitis) refers to the body site infected.

TINEA CAPITIS

Microbiology and Epidemiology

Tinea capitis is likely the most common pediatric dermatophyte infection worldwide and a common cause of hair loss in prepubertal children.[1] Precise incidence is unknown; infection is most common in elementary school-aged children and occasionally affects postpubertal individuals.[2,3] Prepubertal age prevalence may relate to lack of fungistatic properties of sebum fatty acids, which are more abundant post puberty.[4]

Prevalence and pathogens vary widely; *Trichophyton tonsurans* is most common in the United States, while *Microsporum canis* is most common in the Mediterranean area; *T. soudanense* is the major cause of disease in many parts of Africa.[5] *T. soudanense* infections have been noted in immigrant populations in Scandinavia and other European countries.[5]

T. tonsurans is the predominant cause of tinea capitis in North and Central America, responsible for >90% of cases.[6] In a recent survey of elementary school-aged children in Alabama, the incidence of *T. tonsurans*-positive scalp cultures was ~11%, with symptomatic disease in 3%. In another study of >10,000 U.S. children, ~6% were culture positive.[7,8] A retrospective study utilizing International Classification of Diseases (ICD)-9 codes for symptomatic tinea capitis, identified a much lower rate (0.1%) of infection.[9] *M. canis, M. audouinii, Trichophyton mentagrophytes,* and *T. violaceum* are less common causes of infection in North America. *T. tonsurans* is transmitted human to human; animals are the usual vectors for *M. canis.* Infection can be insidious, and asymptomatic scalp colonization is common in endemic regions. *T. tonsurans* often is isolated from asymptomatic family members of infected individuals;[10,11] this may be an important mode of spread. Family contacts of cases have a high risk of infection (46% of siblings in one small study).[12] In this same study, reservoirs of infection (e.g., combs) were documented in 4 of 10 families. There is no evidence that hair care practices (e.g., use of pomades, braiding) facilitates infection.

Clinical Manifestations

Tinea capitis has protean manifestations, including patchy areas of dandruff-like scaling, focal or diffuse hair loss, pustules, large crusts, scalp erythema, and boggy edema (Figure 254-1). Involved areas can show scattered broken hairs of various lengths or discrete

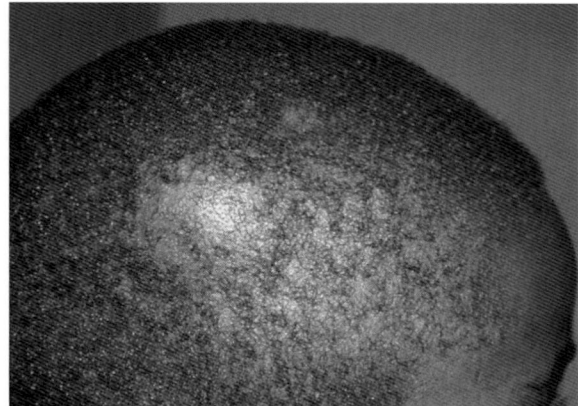

Figure 254-1. Tinea capitis. Note the focal alopecia and scaling.

areas of hair loss containing broken stubs of hair (black dot ringworm). Occipital or posterior cervical lymphadenopathy is a clue to diagnosis.[13]

Kerion is an inflammatory form of tinea characterized by a boggy, indurated mass, often with superimposed vesicles and pustules (Figure 254-2). Fever, lymphadenopathy, leukocytosis, and purulent drainage can lead to misdiagnosis as cellulitis or bacterial abscess. Kerion represents an extreme local immunologic response to infection.[14] Pruritic, papulovesicular, or eczematous eruptions involving the face, trunk, or extremities (*dermatophytid* or *id*) can accompany tinea capitis. This eruption is a hypersensitivity response to the infecting fungus and does not represent infection at the sites of the rash.

Tinea capitis should be suspected in any prepubescent child with unexplained hair loss, particularly if the hair loss is focal, patchy, and accompanied by scaling or lymphadenopathy. Although a presumptive diagnosis can be made clinically, confirmation should be attempted when possible. Wood light examination of the area of hair loss can establish *M. canis* or *M. audouinii* infection. These dermatophytes invade the outer hair shaft (ectothrix) and fluoresce yellowish-green when exposed to ultraviolet light. By contrast, the

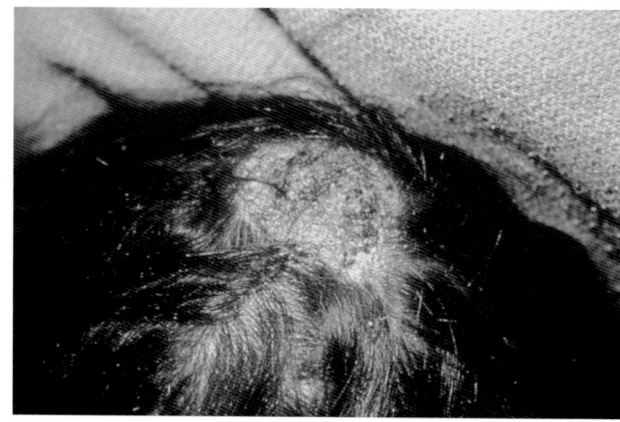

Figure 254-2. Kerion associated with tinea capitis from *Trichophyton tonsurans.*

more common *T. tonsurans* invades the inner core (endothrix) of the hair shaft and cannot be detected using ultraviolet light. Potassium hydroxide (KOH) preparation of affected hairs/scale and culture are standard evaluations. Samples are obtained by scraping or plucking hair. KOH examination reveals arthroconidia or spores within and/or around the hair shaft. Hyphae can be noted from scales within the area. A less distressful method to obtain a culture consists of rubbing a moistened cotton-tipped applicator or toothbrush over involved scalp and then placing the sample in a culturette transport system (such as bacterial specimens).[15] Family members should be queried regarding symptoms, and many experts recommend treatment of all family members empirically with twice weekly topical antifungal shampoo.

The differential diagnosis includes seborrheic dermatitis, atopic dermatitis, psoriasis, alopecia areata,[16] traction alopecia, trichotillomania, folliculitis, impetigo, and lupus erythematosus. Alopecia areata usually manifests as focal hair loss without inflammation or scaling. Fractured hairs of different length and unusual patterns and excoriations of the scalp are hallmarks of trichotillomania; patchy hair loss of eyebrows and eyelashes also is typical. Seborrheic dermatitis, atopic dermatitis, and psoriasis typically are not associated with alopecia, although scratching can cause secondary scalp and hair changes mimicking tinea capitis.

Treatment

Daily griseofulvin, 20 mg/kg daily (maximum, 1 g) in micronized form (available in suspension), or 10 to 15 mg/kg daily (maximum, 750 mg) in ultramicronized form, is standard treatment. In recent years, higher doses of micronized griseofulvin (up to 25 mg/kg daily) and longer durations sometimes are required for cure.[17] Administration of griseofulvin with a fatty meal (e.g., milk, ice cream, peanut butter) enhances drug absorption. Duration of treatment generally is 6 to 8 weeks. Monitoring laboratory tests are not required unless therapy exceeds 8 weeks. A prospective trial utilizing micronized griseofulvin (20 mg/kg/day) with twice weekly selenium sulfide shampoo topically for 6 weeks showed mycologic, clinical, and complete cure rates of 89%, 66% and 49%, respectively.[18] Side effects of griseofulvin include nausea, headache, and photosensitivity reactions.

Many experts consider terbinafine another option for *T. tonsurans* therapy. Terbinafine is approved by the Food and Drug Administration (FDA) for children and because a 2- to 4-week course usually results in cure, adherence is more likely.[19] A large, multinational randomized controlled trial of >1500 children compared oral griseofulvin (10 to 20 mg/kg/day) with terbinafine oral granules (5 to 8 mg/kg/day) utilizing weight-based dosing for both products; complete clinical and mycologic cure were significantly higher for terbinafine, particularly in *T. tonsurans* infections.[20] Other studies have shown high cure rates with 2-week courses of terbinafine using a weight-based sliding scale dosage utilizing standard 250 mg terbinafine tablets: $\frac{1}{4}$ tablet (62.5 mg) for <20 kg, $\frac{1}{2}$ tablet (125 mg) for 20 to 40 kg, and adult tablet (250 mg) for >40 kg patient.[21] Treatments with oral fluconazole or itraconazole utilizing daily or pulse regimens also are effective for tinea capitis, perhaps with shorter duration of therapy, but limited data are available in children.[17,19,22] All newer agents rarely cause hepatic inflammation. Patients treated with terbinafine should have baseline measurement of serum hepatic enzymes, with repeat testing if clinical abnormalities suggest hepatotoxicity.

M. canis disease often is more difficult to treat than *T. tonsurans*, requiring longer duration of therapy and higher doses of griseofulvin to achieve resolution.[23,24] In conjunction with oral therapy, selenium sulfide shampoo (1% or 2.5%), ciclopirox shampoo 1%, or other topical antifungal agents such as ketoconazole shampoo may reduce numbers of surface fungi, and thus infectivity. Topical therapies alone are not sufficient for treatment.[25–27] A comparison of selenium sulfide shampoo 1% and ciclopirox shampoo 1% as adjunctive agents showed equivalency.[27] Systemic corticosteroids have not been shown to accelerate healing significantly or reduce the incidence of postinflammatory scarring.[28–30] Antibiotic therapy or surgical intervention is not indicated.[31]

Key Points. Diagnosis and Management of Tinea Capitis

MICROBIOLOGY
- Most common cause in North America is anthropophilic dermatophyte *Trichophyton tonsurans*
- Other causes: *Microsporum canis, M. audouinii, T. mentagrophytes, T. violaceum*

EPIDEMIOLOGY
- Highest prevalence in children 3 to 10 years of age; family members at risk
- More common in urban settings
- Can be transmitted (particularly *T. tonsurans*) from human to human
- *M. canis* can be transmitted from pets (dogs, cats)

DIAGNOSIS
- Direct microscopy with KOH examination
- Fungal culture
- Wood light for *M. canis* and *M. audouinii*: fluoresce bright yellow color

TREATMENT
- Oral griseofulvin (20 to 25 mg/kg/day of micronized) is the treatment of choice; must be taken with a fatty meal
- Terbinafine is an FDA-approved alternative that often requires shorter duration of therapy but may be more expensive
- Second-line therapies: itraconazole or fluconazole
- Adjunctive antifungal shampoo (selenium sulfide 2%, ketoconazole, or ciclopirox) twice a week decreases infectivity

DURATION OF THERAPY
- For griseofulvin, 6 to 8 weeks of therapy is recommended. Some recommend treatment 2 weeks beyond clinical resolution of disease
- For other agents, shorter courses can be used (e.g., terbinafine 4 to 6 mg/kg/day for 2 to 4 weeks)

TINEA PEDIS (ATHLETE'S FOOT)

Microbiology and Clinical Manifestations

Tinea pedis is a superficial fungal infection of the epidermis commonly caused by *T. mentagrophytes, T. rubrum,* or *Epidermophyton floccosum.*[32] Tinea pedis is less common prepubertally, but has been reported in 2% to 4% of school-aged children in some studies.[33] Data from human volunteer study suggests that the fungi responsible for tinea pedis do not invade normal skin.[34] A moist environment and maceration of the skin appear to be important predisposing factors. The role of bacteria in tinea pedis is poorly defined; however, some evidence indicates that subclinical bacterial infection may permit pathogenic fungi to invade the cornified epithelium.

There are three clinical forms of tinea pedis. The most common form, caused by a variety of dermatophytes, manifests as *maceration, peeling, and fissuring* of the intertriginous areas of the toes. Pruritus is the most prominent symptom. A second form, caused by *T. mentagrophytes,* manifests as *vesicles, small bullae, and occasionally erosions* on the instep of the plantar surface of the foot. As the lesions heal, plaques and scales form. This inflammatory condition is subacute, and can be associated with an eczematous rash or vesicles on the hands (*dermatophytid* or *id*). The least common form shows *chronic, diffuse scaling and hyperkeratosis* of the plantar surface of the feet and heels (moccasin foot) and usually is caused by *T. rubrum.*

Common conditions mimicking tinea pedis in children are irritant, allergic contact, or atopic dermatitis. Occasionally pitted keratolysis can be confused, but is associated with a strong foul odor, and usually manifests as small crateriform depressions of the sole and heel. In adolescents and adults, tinea pedis must be differentiated from erythrasma, bacterial infection, plaque or pustular psoriasis, and primary irritant dermatitis. Erythrasma can be diagnosed by utilizing a Wood lamp which will reveal coral-red fluorescence; axillae are affected typically. Dermatitis generally spares the intertriginous areas of the toes. The vesiculobullous form of tinea pedis can be confused with scabies or dyshidrosis. Although some providers treat patients empirically, KOH and/or cultures should be obtained from children who have resistant or atypical disease.

Treatment

Topical antifungal agents (e.g., imidazoles or allylamines) are effective for most forms of tinea pedis. Systemic therapy with griseofulvin or terbinafine may be necessary for treatment of diffuse moccasin-foot type of infection; alternatively, 40% urea cream plus a topical antifungal, which is thought to help loosen the thick plantar scale and allow increased absorption of the antifungal agent, can be used.[35]

TINEA CORPORIS (RINGWORM)

Microbiology and Clinical Manifestations

Tinea corporis is a superficial skin infection that occurs worldwide in all age groups. It has a predilection for males and almost 50% of cases in the U.S. occur in children <15 years of age.[36] Any dermatophyte can cause disease, but the predominant pathogen varies geographically. *T. rubrum, T. tonsurans, T. mentagrophytes, M. canis,* and *E. floccosum* are the most common causes of tinea corporis in the U.S. Acquisition is through direct contact with infected humans or animals (primarily dogs and cats) and, less commonly, contaminated fomites. Infectivity and inflammatory potential vary by species. Outbreaks among wrestlers are common and have been termed *tinea gladiatorum* (tinea capitis also can be present in affected individuals).[37] *T. tonsurans* is the most common cause of tinea gladiatorum in the U.S.[38]

Three forms of clinical disease can occur. *Papulosquamous* disease, the most common, manifests as an erythematous papule or plaque that transforms rapidly into an annular ring lesion with well-defined margins – the classic *ringworm*. Infection spreads similarly to involve the surrounding normal skin, often with central skin clearing. *Inflammatory* tinea corporis, such as occurs especially with *M. canis*, manifests with fine vesicular lesions at the plaque's advancing edge. Generally, lesions remain discrete; however, coalescence can occur. *Granulomatous* tinea corporis, the least common, occurs predominantly in children whose initial infection was misdiagnosed and treated with topical corticosteroid agents, in immunocompromised hosts, or in females who have re-inoculated the fungus while shaving their legs.[39] The granulomas occur when dermatophytes in hair follicles subsequently rupture into the dermis, causing an inflammatory response. The infection is subacute or chronic and manifests as firm, nontender skin nodules with an overlying crust or plaque; lesions associated with leg shaving are follicular or perifollicular and often have a circumferential scale on an erythematous base.

Isolated lesions of nummular eczema can mimic tinea corporis, as can the herald patch of pityriasis rosea. If tinea corporis is erroneously treated with topical corticosteroids, the classic features of ringworm may not be evident. In such cases, the term *tinea incognito* has been coined; KOH examination will help identify the dermatophyte. Granuloma annulare can be mistaken for tinea corporis and often is the cause of "resistant tinea corporis". Granuloma annulare is distinguished by the absence of scale; a KOH preparation or biopsy is useful in equivocal cases.

Treatment

Most forms of tinea corporis can be treated with once- or twice-daily topical antifungal therapy for 14 to 21 days. Optimal duration of therapy and comparative efficacy of topical agents have not been evaluated extensively. Patients with widespread cutaneous lesions or a granulomatous reaction sometimes are given systemic therapy with griseofulvin, terbinafine or alternative antifungal agents.

Key Points. Diagnosis and Management of Tinea Corporis

EPIDEMIOLOGY
- 50% of cases in the U.S. occur in children <15 years of age
- More commonly affects males than females
- Most infections result from human-to-human transmission
- Outbreaks among wrestlers relatively common, termed tinea gladiatorum

CLINICAL FEATURES
- Papulosquamous (most common): annular plaque with ring of scale and central clearing, classically termed "ringworm"
- Inflammatory or vesicular: plaques with vesicles at the advancing edge
- Granulomatous (Majocchi granuloma): nontender skin nodules with overlying crust or plaque, follicular based
- Manifestations can be atypical ("tinea incognito") if erroneously treated with topical corticosteroids

DIAGNOSIS
- Direct microscopy with KOH examination reveals hyphae

TREATMENT
- Topical triazoles: ketoconazole, clotrimazole or econazole once or twice a day
- Topical allylamines: e.g., terbinafine
- Rare resistant cases, especially Majocchi granuloma, may require adjunctive oral antifungal agent; e.g., fluconazole

DURATION OF THERAPY
- 14 to 21 days for topical therapy
- Duration for oral antifungal therapy depends on agent chosen, e.g., ~2 weeks for fluconazole

---

TINEA CRURIS (JOCK ITCH)

Tinea cruris is an acute or subacute superficial fungal infection of the perineum and inner aspect of the thighs that occurs primarily in males. There is an increased incidence in postpubertal females who wear close-fitting exercise garments or panty hose. Increasing incidence of tinea cruris in adolescents may be related to increases in diabetes mellitus and obesity.[40] Infection is more common in warm, humid climates.

T. rubrum, T. mentagrophytes, and *Epidermophyton floccosum* are the most common pathogens. The incidence of *T. rubrum* is increasing in the U.S.[6]

Red to reddish brown, usually symmetrical scaly lesions with well-demarcated borders and/or fine, oozing vesicles are typical. Local pruritus is common. Chronically involved skin can manifest as brownish discoloration with well-defined borders.

Differential diagnosis includes primary irritant or allergic contact dermatitis, erythrasma (*Corynebacterium minutissimum* infection), seborrheic dermatitis, psoriasis, and candidal intertrigo. Often, secondary infection with *Candida albicans* develops in obese individuals with chronic tinea cruris. KOH examination of specimen from the advancing edge of the lesion can show hyphae. Erythrasma can be identified by its coral red-colored fluorescence when exposed to ultraviolet light.

Treatment consists of drying the weeping areas with Burow solution compresses and application of topical antifungal agents. For those with *Candida* superinfection, the addition of nystatin powder is helpful due to its anti-infective and drying properties. Nystatin powder should not be mixed with the antifungal cream as this can form a gritty irritating mixture. When tinea cruris occurs with a concurrent dermatophyte infection of the fingernails or toenails (onychomycosis), treatment of both disorders may be required for cure.

TINEA FAVOSA

Tinea favosa (favus) is a chronic fungal infection of the scalp most commonly caused by *T. schoenleinii*. Tinea favosa does not occur in the U.S., except in new immigrants or residents of a few well-localized, endemic geographic areas. Friable yellowish brown crusts that have a peculiar cup-shaped configuration (*scutulum*) are typical. The scalp beneath the crusts is erythematous, boggy, and oozing with focal ulceration. Permanent scarring alopecia can occur in untreated cases. The differential diagnosis and treatment of tinea favosa are similar to those of tinea capitis.

TINEA UNGUIUM (ONYCHOMYCOSIS)

Tinea unguium, a dermatophytic infection of the nails, is commonly associated with tinea pedis. Prevalence increases with age and is uncommon in prepubertal children. *T. rubrum, T. mentagrophytes,* and *E. floccosum* are the primary pathogens.[41,42] The clinical findings vary. The most common clinical form is invasion of keratin along the distal and lateral aspect of the nail, which slowly spreads proximally along the nail.[33] The nail becomes "soft" and disfigured with subungual debris and nail discoloration. A less common superficial form has focal, irregular opaque lesions on the nail.

Onychomycosis must be differentiated from congenital and acquired conditions causing nail dystrophy including *Candida* infection, psoriasis, alopecia areata, and atopic dermatitis. *Candida* infection often has an associated paronychia and rarely causes subungual deposits. Nail and subungual debris should be obtained for direct microscopy and culture. Fungal elements can be visualized by direct microscopy of KOH-treated scrapings or by microscopic evaluation of paraffin-embedded nail clippings stained with periodic acid–Schiff. Chronic mucocutaneous candidiasis should be considered in the differential diagnosis of any child with candida onychomycosis.

Griseofulvin often is used for the treatment of tinea unguium in children. Alternatives include terbinafine, itraconazole, and fluconazole. The duration of therapy for griseofulvin is prolonged (6 to 12 months), and recurrences are common. Terbinafine and the triazoles can be administered for shorter durations or administered as pulse regimens. They are not FDA-approved for the treatment of pediatric onychomycosis.[43,44] Topical antifungal agents generally are ineffective because of inability to penetrate to the lowest portions of the nail bed. Children with onychomycosis often have affected family members.[43]

TINEA VERSICOLOR (PITYRIASIS VERSICOLOR)

Tinea versicolor is a common superficial dermatophyte infection caused by *Pityrosporum orbiculare* (also known as *Malassezia furfur*). *Pityrosporum* spp. generally are considered to be normal skin flora, but in patients affected by tinea versicolor, there is overgrowth of both filamentous and yeast forms likely due to genetic and environmental factors.[45] Most commonly, asymptomatic dark or light skin patches are noted on the neck and upper trunk. Facial involvement, particularly on the temple, can be seen in children. Pink, hyper- or hypopigmented discrete and coalescent macules are noted, often with a fine white scale (Figure 254-3). KOH examination of scrapings reveals a "spaghetti and meatball" appearance of blastoconidia and pseudomycelium, confirming the diagnosis. Wood lamp examination reveals yellow fluorescence.

First-line treatment generally consists of topical antifungal cream, selenium sulfide shampoo, or other antifungal shampoos. Patients should be advised that it may take months for the skin to become repigmented, and that recurrence is common. For resistant or extensive cases, oral fluconazole or ketoconazole, given once and repeated in one week, is effective.[46,47] Vigorous physical activity (causing sweating) within a few hours after taking

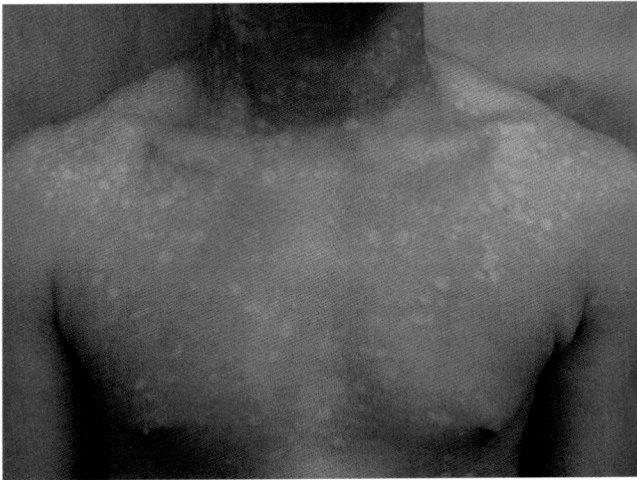

Figure 254-3. Tinea versicolor. Hypopigmented patches with fine scale.

the medicine increases penetration into the skin.[47] *Pityrosporum* species also can cause folliculitis which is most concentrated in the sebum-bearing areas (face, chest, back) and resembles acne, but lacks comedones. It occurs most often in adolescents, particularly those who have been treated with long-term oral antibiotics, and in immunosuppressed patients. Oral antifungal therapy with fluconazole often is required, although immunocompetent patients may respond to topical antifungal therapies.

Key Points. Epidemiology, Clinical Features, Diagnosis, and Treatment of Tinea Versicolor

EPIDEMIOLOGY

- Distributed throughout the U.S.
- Commonly affects adolescents and young adults
- *Pityrosporum orbiculare (Malassezia furfur)* is causative organism, but also considered normal skin flora

CLINICAL FEATURES

- Often comes to medical attention during summer months with complaint of skin not "tanning" normally
- Hypo- or hyperpigmented patches and plaques with fine white scale
- Commonly distributed on neck, trunk, proximal upper extremities
- Pruritus is minimal or absent

DIAGNOSIS

- Direct microscopy of KOH preparation shows "spaghetti and meatballs" appearance of blastoconidia and pseudomycelium
- Special medium required for culture

TREATMENT AND DURATION OF THERAPY

- Topical antifungal cream and shampoo generally is sufficient therapy
- Discoloration can persist for months despite clearance of infection
- Oral antifungal agent (e.g., ketoconazole or fluconazole, taken once and repeated in one week) for resistant cases

---

TINEA NIGRA

Rare in the U.S., tinea nigra is a superficial dermatophyte infection of the stratum corneum that manifests as black, dark brown or grey patches on the palms and soles. Scale can be present, but typically is minimal. Patients with hyperhidrosis or those living in moist climates are more commonly affected. Occasionally confused with a melanocytic neoplasm due to its dark color, entities can be differentiated visually using dermoscopy.[48] Tinea nigra is caused by *Hortae werneckii (Exophiala werneckii)*, and can be visualized using KOH preparation and direct microscopy. Topical antifungal therapy and drying solutions (e.g., aluminum chloride 20% solution) generally are sufficient for treatment.[49] Treatment of hyperhidrosis alone sometimes leads to cure. Topical keratolytics (e.g., 3% topical salicylic acid) also are helpful in some cases.[49]

PIEDRA

White and black piedra are superficial fungal infections of the hair caused by the *T. beigelii* and *Piedraia hortae*, respectively. More

commonly occurring in tropical climates, they manifest as is soft concretions attached to scalp hair (sometimes in the axilla, pubis, and beard area). Concretions can be confused easily with nits, hair casts, and other hair disorders; upon KOH examination, masses of septate hyphae (pigmented in the case of black piedra) are visualized within the concretion.[49] Treatment for both piedras includes clipping or shaving the affected area and topical antifungal therapy.[50] Ketoconazole 2% shampoo also is effective.[49,51]

Acknowledgment

The authors acknowledge substantial use of the work of John Browning and Moise Levy from previous editions.

255 Agents of Eumycotic Mycetoma: *Pseudallescheria boydii* (Anamorph *Scedosporium apiospermum*)

Martin B. Kleiman and Elaine Cox

A mycetoma (maduromycosis, Madura foot) is a noncontagious, localized chronic infection that affects skin, subcutaneous tissue, fascia, muscle, and bone. Characteristic clinical features of mycetomas include localized swelling, fistulous tracts, and suppurative drainage that contains dense colonies (called granules, sclerotia) of the offending pathogen. Mycetomas can be divided into two general categories based on the causative agent. Mycetomas caused by one of the filamentous fungi are termed *eumycotic mycetomas*, and those caused by Actinomycetes are termed *actinomycotic mycetomas*. Striking geographical differences occur in the proportion of mycetomas caused by true fungi and mycetomas caused by Actinomycetes.[1] Agents of eumycotic mycetoma are considered in this chapter and agents of actinomycotic mycetoma are considered in Chapter 195, Anaerobic Gram-Positive Nonsporulating Bacilli (Including Actinomycosis).

MICROBIOLOGY

At least 32 species of filamentous fungi (Eumycetes) are recognized as causes of eumycotic mycetoma[2,3] (Box 255-1). All are common saprophytes of soil and vegetable matter. *Madurella mycetomatis*, the most common cause worldwide, accounts for 70% of eumycotic mycetoma infections, and *Pseudallescheria boydii* (anamorph *Scedosporium apiospermum*) and *Leptosphaeria senegalensis* each account for 10% of infections.[2] *P. boydii, Fusarium falciforme, M. mycetomatis, Madurella grisea*, and *Exophilia jeanselmei*, in decreasing order of frequency, are the most common causes of eumycotic mycetoma in the United States. Within these groups, additional species have been recognized that are separate phylogenetically and have distinct clinical spectra and antifungal susceptibilities.[4] *Scedosporium aurantiacum, Pseudallescheria minutispora*, and *Madurella pseudomycetomatis* are among those recognized most recently.[5]

The agents of eumycotic mycetoma grow on Sabouraud dextrose agar, with optimal growth occurring between 25°C and 37°C. Isolation is facilitated if the agar contains chloramphenicol to inhibit growth of bacteria and cycloheximide to inhibit growth of extraneous molds, although cycloheximide also can inhibit growth of *P. boydii*. Incubation may be required for up to 6 weeks for growth. Identification of isolates is based on morphology and pigmentation of colonies, mechanisms of conidia production, and morphology of conidiophores and conidia. *Madurella*

BOX 255-1. Etiologic Agents of Eumycotic Mycetoma

ASCOMYCOTA

Emericella nidulans (anamorph *Aspergillus nidulans*)
Leptosphaeria senegalensis[a]
Leptosphaeria tompkinsii
Neotestudina rosatii[a]
Pseudallescheria boydii (anamorph *Scedosporium apiospermum*)[a]

MITOSPORIC FUNGI (FUNGI IMPERFECTI)

Acremonium kiliense
Acremonium recifei
Aspergillus flavus
Aspergillus nidulans
Curvularia geniculata[a]
Curvularia lunata[a]
Corynespora cassicola
Cylindrocarpon cyanescens
Cylindrocarpon destructans
Exophilia jeanselmei[a]
Fusarium falciforme[a]
Fusarium solani var. *coeruleum*
Fusarium solani var. *minus*
Fusarium verticillioides
Madurella grisea[a]
Madurella mycetomatis[a]
Phaeoacremonium species
Phialophora verrucosa
Plendomas avramii
Polycytella hominis
Pseudochaetosphaeronema larense
Pyrenochaeta mackinnonii[a]
Pyrenochaeta romeroi[a]
Rhinocladiella atrovirens

---

[a]Among the causative agents described most commonly.
Adapted from De Hoog GS, Ahmed AOA, McGinnis MR, Padhye AA. Fungi causing eumycotic mycetoma. In: Murray PR, Baron EJ, Pfaller MA (eds) Manual of Clinical Microbiology, 9th ed. Washington, DC, American Society of Microbiology, 2007, p 1919.

species, *Neotestudina rosatii*, and *Pyrenochaeta* species do not sporulate readily, so special sporulation media and physiologic tests for carbohydrate and nitrate utilization may be needed to identify these agents. Detailed information on isolation and identification of the fungi that cause eumycotic mycetoma is available.[2]

VIRULENCE AND IMMUNITY

The agents of eumycotic mycetoma are relatively avirulent, opportunistic pathogens that do not invade intact skin. Infection results from direct fungal inoculation or contamination of wounds. Factors that predispose an exposed person to mycetoma have not been determined. Impaired cellular immunity may be important but has not been observed consistently in patients with mycetoma. Fungal agents act as chemoattractants that stimulate the complement system to induce chemotaxis. This leads to the accumulation of neutrophils around granules, and in the centers of abscesses and sinus tracts. However, this immune response appears to be an ineffective mechanism for inhibiting fungal replication.[6]

Antibodies to some antigens of the offending agent are produced after established infections and can be measured by counter-immunoelectrophoresis, immunodiffusion, and immunoblot methods.[7,8] Specific IgG and IgM antibody directed against the causative organism also can be measured by enzyme immunoassay (EIA).[7,8] In endemic regions, antibodies to fungi that cause mycetoma can be detected by EIA in infected patients, as well as in uninfected people.[7] The effect of specific antibody on the course of infection has not been established. Antibody titers decrease in some patients after appropriate treatment. In some endemic regions, resolution of precipitation arcs identified with counter-immunoelectrophoresis techniques are used to guide therapy.[6]

PATHOGENESIS

Infection usually begins with a skin wound caused by a thorn contaminated with the causative fungus. Organisms proliferate, with development of localized skin and subcutaneous infection appearing as a papular lesion. Often unrecognized, the lesion enlarges slowly and painlessly over a period of weeks to months. Inflammation also can advance along fascial planes; hematogenous dissemination does not occur, although lymphatic spread has been described and is estimated to occur in approximately 2% of cases.[9]

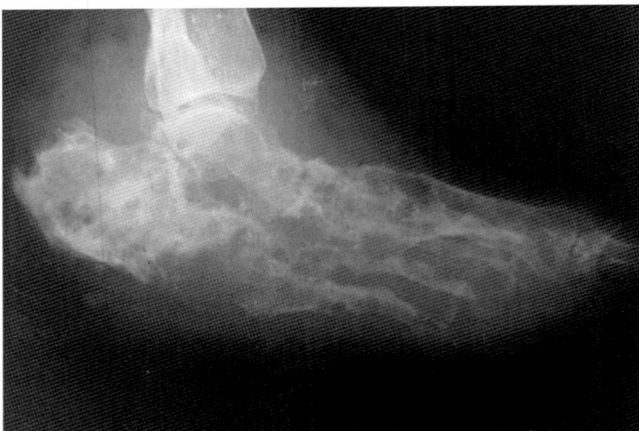

Figure 255-1. Radiograph of the foot of a 43-year-old farm worker with an 8-year history of foot swelling and fistulous drainage of suppurative material. *Madurella mycetomatis* was isolated from exuded granules. The radiograph shows extensive destruction of all bones of the foot with characteristic multiple lytic cavities and almost complete loss of normal bony architecture.

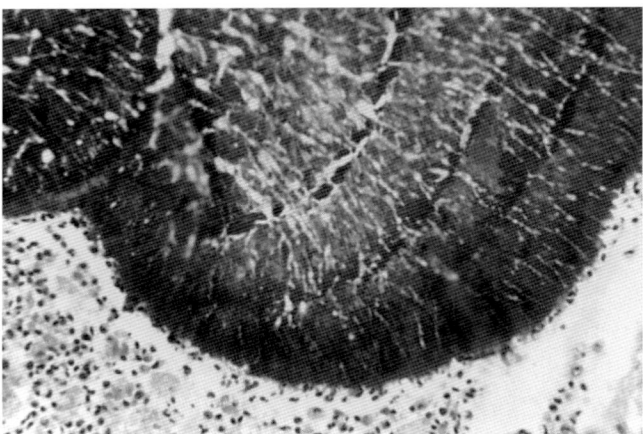

Figure 255-2. Hematoxylin and eosin-stained section of a brownish granule of *Madurella mycetomatis* containing radially oriented hyphae within a matrix of cement-like material. The granule is located within an abscess and is surrounded by acute inflammatory cells (×200).

The process slowly destroys contiguous soft tissues and has a predilection for infecting and permanently damaging bone (Figure 255-1). Multiple sinus tracts are common and exuded drainage contains granules consisting largely of densely packed fungal colonies. Some matrix substances found in granules in vivo are not found in cultures grown in vitro and may represent antigenic material derived from the fungus or the host. The size, shape, and color of fungal filaments and presence or absence of matrix material within granules are features that vary with the offending agent.

Except for the granules, histopathologic findings in mycetoma are nonspecific. Localized abscesses containing neutrophils and necrotic material surround single or multiple granules. A subacute and chronic inflammatory response consisting of plasma cells, lymphocytes, multinucleated giant cells, and epithelioid cells surrounds the abscess (Figure 255-2). An eosinophilic deposit (referred to as Splenore–Hoeppli reaction) surrounds the granule and is thought to represent an immunologic response. Fibrosis eventually ensues and contributes to the gross anatomic deformities.

EPIDEMIOLOGY

Most mycetomas occur in tropical or subtropical regions, mainly in areas where rainy seasons alternate with lengthy dry periods. Mexico, India, large regions of Africa, and Central and South America have the highest incidence of reported infections. Eumycotic mycetomas are rare in the most temperate regions of the world and are extremely rare in the U.S. Clinical diagnosis is becoming more common in individuals who travel to endemic regions.[8]

In endemic areas, the agents of eumycotic mycetoma commonly occur in soil and on plants. Thorn injuries, abrasions caused by solid objects, and occupational activities that predispose to skin trauma and soil contamination lead to infection. Infection occurs most frequently in men 30 to 50 years of age and is rare in children. Mycetoma is more common in men than women with a ratio of 4:1.[10,11] Poor nutrition or concomitant infections, often seen in people in underdeveloped rural areas, are thought to increase the likelihood that exposure will lead to infection.

CLINICAL MANIFESTATIONS

The initial lesion usually is a small subcutaneous nodule attached to the overlying skin. Fistulous tracts and sinus formation begin early, usually within several months to 1 year following infection. The purulent drainage contains granules. Subcutaneous

TABLE 255-1. Anatomic Alterations Attributable to Mycetoma

Tissue	Abnormality
Skin and subcutaneous fatty tissue	Fistulas, granulomas, change in color, zones of fibrosis
Muscle	Degenerative myositis
Tendon	Few alterations because of resistance
Nerve sheath	Hypertrophy
Lymphatics	Inflammatory reaction; embolization of granules possible
Lymphatic ganglia	Hypertrophy; dissemination rare
Bone	Periostitis, osteolysis, osteofibrosis
Peripheral nerve	Altered by sclerosis

From Magana M. Mycetoma. Int J Dermatol 1984;24:221–236.

nodules slowly enlarge, additional nodules appear, and new sinuses form as old sinus tracts heal. The progress of infection is slow, and medical attention frequently is not sought for many months or years. Extension contiguously and along fascial planes can lead to chronic bone infection. Systemic symptoms are absent unless secondary bacterial infection intervenes. Pain is not a characteristic feature and presence of pain often is associated with secondary bacterial infection of bone, or progression of fistulous tracts.

Although infection can begin at any superficial anatomic site, mycetomas usually occur on extremities. About 70% affect feet and 12% to 15% involve hands; other sites on extremities and on the head and neck account for most of the remaining cases. Chronic changes and destruction eventually affect most underlying structures[12] (Table 255-1). The eventual result is a disfigured, scarred, swollen site with draining sinuses and functional impairment.

LABORATORY FINDINGS AND DIAGNOSIS

In the presence of a lesion with tumefaction (indurated swelling), fistulous sinus tracts, and drainage that contains granules, the clinical diagnosis of mycetoma is straightforward. However, because treatment and prognosis differ for mycetomas caused by *Actinomyces* species or filamentous fungi, a specific diagnosis is necessary and biopsy is required. Histopathologic findings in mycetoma are nonspecific and consist of acute and chronic inflammation, granulomatous changes, and fibrosis. On biopsy specimen, "grains" may or may not be observed because they are scattered along sinus tracts and vulnerable to sampling error. When present, they are large and surrounded by neutrophils. Careful examination of granules in tissue (see Figure 255-2) or purulent material suggests the causative agent. Accurate confirmation requires fungal culture. Granules range in size from 0.2 to 5.0 μm and are often visible to the unaided eye. The color, texture, size, and shape of the granules provide important clues to the etiologic agent. Eumycotic mycetomas have granules that are black or white and soft or hard, with a cement-like matrix. Gomori methenamine silver nitrate staining of eumycotic granules shows wide, interwoven septate hyphae 2 to 5 μm in diameter; large swollen cells up to 15 μm in diameter also may be present at the periphery of granules. Actinomycotic infections have gram-positive, interlaced, thin filaments 0.5 to 1.0 μm in diameter, with coccoid and bacillary forms.

To facilitate recovery of fungus, granules obtained from purulent material or tissue should be washed in normal saline that contains antimicrobial agents added to inhibit growth of contaminating bacteria. Sabouraud dextrose agar is inoculated and incubated at 25°C and 37°C and examined for growth at 2-day

intervals for 6 weeks. A secure etiologic diagnosis is established when a single agent is isolated from several granules.

Other modalities, including radiographic findings, have been used to aid in diagnosis. Radiographic abnormalities can be seen in soft tissue and bone and include areas of increased soft-tissue density (caused by granulomas) adjacent to normal soft tissue. Osseous lesions have a variable appearance (see Figure 255-1); most are lytic cavities in bone that may contain large numbers of granules. Cortical bone also can be eroded by extrinsic irritation from contiguous soft-tissue inflammation. Periosteal new bone formation can be seen as spicules oriented perpendicular to the long axes of long bones. Osteopenia results from disuse or impairment of perfusion. Some radiographic improvement can occur in response to successful treatment. Although serologic tests have been investigated for use in diagnosis and to monitor therapy, standardized reagents are not available commercially.

TREATMENT AND SPECIAL CONSIDERATIONS

Eumycotic mycetomas respond less favorably to treatment than do mycetomas caused by *Actinomyces* species with low cure rates overall. Optimal management includes medical and surgical interventions. Initial surgical debulking generally is necessary, although medical therapy is a beneficial adjunct to attempt to avoid amputation.[13] In general, the response of mycetoma to antifungal agents is poor, perhaps because of changes within fungal cell walls that enable them to act as barriers to penetration of drug. These alterations also serve both to make the cell wall less penetrable to the respiratory burst products of inflammatory cells and to impair leukocyte adhesion to the fungal cell wall.[3]

Most clinical experience with antifungal therapy has been with mycetomas caused by *M. mycetomatis*. Antifungal susceptibility testing might be helpful since there is considerable strain-to-strain variation in susceptibility. However, testing is not available widely and standard cutoff values have not been well established.[6] Treatment with amphotericin B often is ineffective due to inherent resistance. Limited efficacy has been observed in a few patients treated with liposomal amphotericin formulations.[14] Ketoconazole (200 mg per dose given twice daily in adults) historically was the most frequently used agent and was successful in approximately 70% of cases.[15] However, ketoconazole was not successful in treating eumycetomas caused by *M. grisea*,[16] *P. boydii* (*S. apiospermum*), and *Acremonium* species.[17] For patients who did not respond to ketoconazole, griseofulvin (500 mg per dose given three times daily in adults) was used but improvement has been infrequent. Itraconazole has shown only marginal benefit with 40% of patients showing a favorable response,[15,18–20] none of whom were cured. Fluconazole is ineffective.[9] Of the newer azoles, voriconazole has been used successfully for treatment of subcutaneous infections with *S. apiospermum* when used intravenously and then followed by oral administration as an adjunct to debridement in localized infections.[13,21] Serum concentrations should be monitored. Posaconazole has been evaluated in clinical studies and has been shown to be more effective than voriconazole in treating *P. boydii* in certain clinical scenarios.[9,22,23] The echinocandin class appears to have little to no therapeutic potential in early clinical studies although there is some evidence of in vitro activity of caspofungin for *P. boydii*.[9,24] Although there are no controlled studies regarding duration of treatment, antifungal therapy should be continued for at least 10 months or at least 3 months after resolution of inflammation.[6] Decreasing antibody titer may be a marker of effective therapy;[6] however, standardized serologic tests are not available.

Surgical management is an important adjunctive therapy. Incision and drainage of abscesses, debulking of large masses, and excision of sinus tracts facilitate healing, reduce pain, and may avoid amputation. Length of therapy often can be reduced with adequate debulking procedures. Excision can be curative if performed when lesions are small and have not involved bone; a wide margin of uninfected tissue should be removed in such cases.[15] Without antifungal therapy, relapse after resection occurs in more than one-half of cases. Other treatment modalities, such as topical negative pressure, have been reported with minimal success.[25]

PREVENTION

In endemic areas, prevention requires protection from injuries that are prone to contamination by soil or vegetable matter. Improvements in hygienic standards, reduction of occupational injuries, and use of adequate footwear and protective clothing should reduce the frequency of mycetoma. Education of people at risk to seek medical intervention early, when cure is more likely and loss of limb can be avoided, is essential.

PSEUDALLESCHERIA BOYDII (SCEDOSPORIUM APIOSPERMUM)

P. boydii (*S. apiospermum*) is a saprophytic fungus with worldwide distribution in soil, water, and feces of domesticated animals. *P. boydii* is an opportunistic pathogen that rarely causes infection in healthy, immunocompetent hosts. *P. boydii* causes approximately 10% of eumycotic mycetoma and also is responsible for a variety of other localized and systemic infections, especially in immunocompromised people.[2,26] Nonmycetomatous infections caused by *P. boydii* are termed pseudallescheriasis.

Microbiology

P. boydii is a member of the class Ascomycetae and, in contrast to most pathogenic fungi, exists in tissue in its teleomorphic (sexual) form. The anamorph (asexual form) is termed *Scedosporium apiospermum* and can cause infection that is clinically indistinguishable from infection caused by the teleomorph. The mold grows on Sabouraud and most standard media, and matures in 7 days. Growth can be inhibited by cycloheximide contained in some selective agars used for primary isolation. On oatmeal agar, white colonies grow rapidly at 25°C and later turn to grey. Hyphae are yellow-brown and 2 to 3 µm in diameter. Asci are 12 to 18 µm × 9 to 13 µm in diameter and contain 8 ascospores. Two morphologic types of asexual conidia are produced, the most common being *Scedosporium* type and a smaller *Graphium* type. In tissue sections, the hyphae of *P. boydii* are branched, septate, hyaline, and hematoxylin stain positive. Morphologic distinction of *P. boydii* hyphae from hyphae of *Aspergillus* and other hyaline molds is not possible, and direct immunofluorescent testing is needed.[27] *P. boydii* likely does not represent a single entity but rather is a complex with at least 6 known species.[28,29]

Epidemiology

P. boydii is a common contaminant of water, soil, and manure, and usually gains entry to a host through accidental trauma or contamination of aspirated material. Although worldwide in distribution, considerable regional differences occur in the frequency of isolation of *P. boydii* from people with clinical illnesses. This discrepancy may be attributable to differences in strain virulence.[30]

Clinical Manifestations

Almost 99% of infections caused by *P. boydii* are mycetomas. The presence of granules (sclerotia) is a distinguishing feature of true mycetomas. Infections caused by traumatic implantation of *P. boydii*, but which do not contain granules, are termed pseudallescheriasis. The nomenclature previously has referred to these nonmycetomatous infections as allescheriasis, petriellidiosis, and monosporiosis.[31]

P. boydii occasionally is found as a commensal in pre-existing lung cavities and in paranasal sinuses. Respiratory tract illnesses attributed to *P. boydii* have included pneumonitis caused by inhalation of contaminated material (similar to the process that occurs with allergic aspergillosis) and fungus balls in lung cavities and paranasal sinuses. Infections that occur in immunocompetent children often are localized and result from contaminated puncture injuries. Sites most commonly affected are an eye and periorbital structures, skin and subcutaneous tissue, and osteoarticular structures.

Infections in an immunocompromised host can be localized but are increasingly reported to result in invasive and disseminated disease. These life-threatening manifestations occur most often in patients with solid-organ transplants,[32] hematologic stem cell transplants,[33] hematologic malignancies,[34] HIV infection, chronic granulomatous disease, and people receiving immunosuppressive therapy.[35] In these groups of patients, systemic infection, meningitis, brain abscess, keratitis and endophthalmitis, otomycosis, endocarditis, indwelling device-related infection, central nervous system infections, and other invasive infections are common.[36] Mortality rates as high as 75% are reported in patients with central nervous system and progressive disseminated infections.[26,37-39] Clinical findings in these settings often mimic findings caused by *Aspergillus* or *Fusarium* infections.

Diagnosis

Diagnosis is confirmed by isolating the offending agent from a normally sterile site. Culture has been the gold standard but identification by polymerase chain reaction is increasingly important and used more widely.[40,41] Illnesses caused by *P. boydii* can mimic illness caused by *Aspergillus*. Since antifungal susceptibility patterns differ for these organisms, laboratory confirmation is needed.[42] Rare instances of coinfections have been identified.

Treatment

P. boydii often is resistant to amphotericin B[43] and its therapeutic use in these infections has been associated with poor clinical response and recurrence following seemingly effective therapy.

Development of the first triazoles provided new, but limited therapeutic options. Fluconazole has no activity against *P. boydii*.[35] Itraconazole[44-46] and ketoconazole[47] have been used clinically, although with mixed results. Voriconazole and posaconazole have each been shown to have activity in vitro.[23,43,48-55] Voriconazole has been used successfully in cutaneous infections,[13,21] disseminated disease,[37-39] and pulmonary infections.[56] Voriconazole appears to have good penetration into the cerebrospinal fluid and has been used in treating central nervous system disease.[37,39,55,57-61] Due to the wide spectrum of disease manifestations that appear to respond favorably, voriconazole is considered by most experts to be the drug of choice.[9] Posaconazole also has been shown to have good activity in vitro against *Scedosporium apiospermum*[38] but also has adequate penetration into the central nervous system. Posaconazole has been used successfully to treat brain abscesses in immunocompromised hosts who were refractory to treatment with other agents.[55,62,63] An isolated report suggests a potential role for potassium iodide.[64] Drainage or excision of infected tissue, when possible, is an important adjunct to therapy.[39] Mortality in invasive infections is high if operative management is not feasible.

The optimal duration of antifungal therapy has not been established and must be individualized. In immunocompetent hosts in whom lesions can be excised, antifungal treatment may be discontinued after 3 to 6 months. Patients with underlying conditions that make clearance of the fungus unlikely (e.g., chronic pulmonary disease, immunocompromised states) may require treatment for years, or indefinitely. Consultation with experts is recommended in managing such patients.

Key Points. Eumycotic Mycetoma (Maduramycosis, Madura Foot)

DEFINITION

- Noncontagious, chronic infection of skin, subcutaneous tissue, fascia, muscle, and bone caused by a variety of filamentous fungi

MICROBIOLOGY

- *Madurella mycetomatis* (70%); *Pseudallescheria boydii* (anamorph *Scedosporium apiospermum*) (10%); *Leptosphaeria senegalensis* (10%)
- At least 32 species of filamentous fungi (Box 255-1)

EPIDEMIOLOGY

- Tropical, subtropical areas with rainy seasons and dry seasons. Mexico, India, large regions of Africa, Central and South America. Rare in temperate regions; rare in children
- Skin injury predisposes to inoculation of contaminated wounds

CLINICAL FEATURES

- Lesions often affect feet (70%), hands (15%)
- Subcutaneous nodule(s) early; fistulous tracts in weeks to months

- Purulent drainage contains granules
- Lesions usually are painless and systemic symptoms are absent unless secondarily infected with bacteria
- Slow progression along fascial planes often leads to bone infection

DIAGNOSIS

- Tumefaction, fistulous sinus tracts, and drainage containing granules often are present
- Clinical, radiographic, and histopathologic findings are similar in actinomycotic mycetoma. Examination/culture helps distinguish between entities and informs appropriate antimicrobial therapy

TREATMENT

- Eumycotic mycetomas respond less favorably than infection caused by *Actinomyces*
- Surgical debulking and drainage of abscesses is needed in association with antifungal therapy

---

SECTION D: Human Parasites and Vectors

256 Classification of Parasites

Peter J. Hotez

Although all infectious agents of humans are parasites, by convention, parasitic diseases often are defined as diseases caused by protozoa or helminths. Parasitic protozoa and helminths sometimes are referred to as animal parasites to distinguish them from bacteria, fungi, and viruses. This distinction has an historical basis. Parasitology (the study of animal parasites) emerged as a separate discipline from microbiology as a result of 19th century scientific investigations conducted outside the mainstream of science in Europe. Animal parasites were considered "exotic" because many initially were described by European investigators working in the tropics. The life cycle of filariasis was elucidated by Manson (British) in China, malaria by Ross (British) in India, ancylostomiasis by Looss (German) in Egypt, and schistosomiasis by Bilharz (German) in Egypt. Within the last decade, the study of microbiology has begun to encompass eukaryotic microorganisms.

The animal parasites of humans and their vectors constitute a diverse array of eukaryotic organisms that span many phyla (Box 256-1).[1] The major endoparasitic helminths of humans belong to the phyla Platyhelminthes (flatworms) and Nematoda (roundworms). The endoparasitic protozoa are a diverse group of several thousand eukaryotic unicellular animals.[2] Together, the parasites exert an enormous toll on human life and health. The malaria parasite, *Plasmodium falciparum*, causes almost one million deaths annually,[2] while the other human parasites combine to cause an estimated 500,000 annual deaths.[3,4] Using the disability-adjusted life year (DALY) as a metric, human parasites also cause an enormous disease burden with more than 100 million DALYs annually by some estimates.[3,4] This value exceeds the global disease burden from HIV-AIDS. Despite their public health importance, most of the human parasitic diseases have been neglected by the scientific, medical, and public health communities.[3,4] Their neglect stems from the observations that parasitic diseases generally occur

among the poor, and more often than not occur in remote and rural areas where they are hidden from view. Moreover, parasitic diseases not only occur predominantly in the setting of poverty, but often because they result in chronic disability they are themselves poverty-promoting. In some cases parasitic diseases have stigmas attached. Hence, the major chronic parasitic infections of humans often are referred to as *neglected tropical diseases*.[3-5] Since 2006, global efforts have been implemented to provide low-cost or drug company-donated treatments for seven of the most common neglected tropical diseases, i.e., the three major soil-transmitted helminth infections plus schistosomiasis, lymphatic

---

BOX 256-1. Major Kingdoms and Phyla of Animal Parasites with Representative Genera

KINGDOM ARCHEOZOA

Phylum Metamonada (*Giardia*)
Phylum Microspora (*Enterocytozoon*)

KINGDOM PROTOZOA

Phylum Parabasala (*Trichomonas*)
Phylum Euglenozoa (*Leishmania*)
Phylum Ciliophora (*Balantidium*)
Phylum Apicomplexa (*Toxoplasma*)
Phylum Rhizopoda (*Entamoeba*)

KINGDOM ANIMALIA

Phylum Platyhelminthes (*Schistosoma*)
Phylum Nematoda (*Ascaris*)

filariasis, onchocerciasis, and trachoma, in programs of mass drug administration.[3-5] However, the commercial markets for new drugs, vaccines, and diagnostics are extremely small and there have been few incentives for pharmaceutical companies to undertake drug discovery and development programs for parasitic and neglected tropical diseases. As a result, many of the drugs still in use today for parasitic infections were first discovered in the middle of the 20th century.[4] There is some optimism that the recent creation of new nonprofit product development will accelerate development and clinical testing of new drugs and vaccines for neglected tropical disease.[4]

PARASITIC ARCHEOZOA AND PROTOZOA

Some investigators are of the opinion that the old classification, in which a single phylum of protozoa encompassed all unicellular eukaryotic microorganisms, is not validated by the wealth of new ultrastructural and molecular taxonomic data. Armed with newly developed molecular probes, tools, and approaches to cladistic analysis, biologists are re-examining the classification of these organisms. For instance, the parasite *Giardia lamblia* has been shown to lack mitochondria and to contain ribosomal RNA sequences that more closely resemble those of bacteria.[6,7] It has been proposed that this organism represents an evolutionary transition between prokaryotic and eukaryotic microorganisms.[8] Similarly, the obligate intracellular microsporidia have ultrastructural features, such as ribosomes and a unique complex extrusion apparatus, that are distinctly different from those found ordinarily in protozoa. Some experts think that these parasites are different

---

TABLE 256-1. Classification of Representative Archeozoa and Protozoa According to Modes of Transmission

Mode of Transmission	Representative Genera
Enteric	*Balantidium*
	Cryptosporidium
	Cyclospora
	Dientamoeba
	Entamoeba
	Giardia
	Sexual *Trichomonas*
Arthropod	*Babesia*
	Leishmania
	Plasmodium
	Trypanosoma

---

enough to justify exclusion from Protozoa. Corliss[1] reclassifies them as Archeozoa, a term that reflects their evolutionary transitional nature. Typically, members of Archeozoa primitively lack certain organelles such as mitochondria, peroxisomes, and typical Golgi bodies. In contrast, one or more of these organelles is present characteristically in Protozoa.

In response to these observations some microbiologists have elevated both the Archeozoa and Protozoa to the status of a taxonomic kingdom to more accurately describe the diversity of these two groups (Box 256-2). In this classification, the former subphyla of protozoa, specifically, Apicomplexa, Ciliophora, and Rhizopoda, are raised to independent phyla within the kingdom of Protozoa. Clinicians prefer to identify unicellular eukaryotic microorganisms on the basis of their mode of transmission (e.g., enteric, arthropod-borne; Table 256-1) or site of parasitism within humans (e.g., blood, gastrointestinal tract). However, a sound taxonomic understanding of these microorganisms fosters an understanding of their pathophysiology and predicts the activity of antiparasitic agents. For instance, albendazole might be useful for treatment of Microspora but not for more conventional protozoa.

Almost certainly our knowledge about classification and biology of the Archeozoa and Protozoa will increase substantially in the coming decade. The new knowledge will be derived from the dozen or more protozoan genome projects completed within the last five years. The projects include completion of genomes for some of the most important protozoan pathogens including the kinetoplastid parasites *Trypanosoma cruzi*, *T. brucei*, and *Leishmania major*, which reveal a conserved core proteome of about 6200 genes in large syntenic polycistronic gene clusters, as well as many species-specific genes that include large surface antigen families,[9] the complete genome of the malaria parasite *Plasmodium falciparum* and its mosquito vector,[10,11] as well as *Entamoeba histolytica*,[12] and *Cryptosporidium parvum*,[13] with others in progress. In every case, these genome projects are revealing promising drug targets and new insights into evolution of parasitic protists.

PARASITIC ANIMALIA

The endoparasitic worms of humans belong to the phyla Nematoda and Platyhelminthes.

Nematodes are nonsegmented cylindroid roundworms that predominantly are free-living forms inhabiting the soil and water. Many species of nematodes also are plant parasites of enormous agricultural and economic importance. Almost every vertebrate can harbor one or more species of endoparasitic nematodes. Humans are no exception, and nearly one-fourth of the world's population is infected with at least one species of nematode. For instance, an estimated 600 to 800 million people are infected with the intestinal nematodes *Ascaris lumbricoides*, *Trichuris trichiura*, and the major human hookworm, *Necator americanus*.[14]

BOX 256-2. Representative Human Parasite Genera of the Kingdoms Protozoa and Archeozoa

KINGDOM ARCHEOZOA

Phylum Archamoebae
Phylum Metamonada
 Giardia
 Chilomastix
Phylum Microspora
 Enterocytozoon
 Nosema

KINGDOM PROTOZOA

Phylum Percolozoa
Phylum Parabasala
 Dientamoeba
 Trichomonas
Phylum Euglenozoa
 Leishmania
 Trypanosoma
Phylum Opalozoa
Phylum Mycetozoa
Phylum Choanozoa
Phylum Dinozoa
Phylum Ciliophora
 Balantidium
Phylum Apicomplexa
 Babesia
 Cryptosporidium
 Cyclospora
 Plasmodium
 Toxoplasma
Phylum Rizopoda
 Acanthamoeba
 Entamoeba
Phylum Heliozoa
Phylum Radiozoa

TABLE 256-2. Major Human Parasitic Nematodes Classified by Mode of Transmission

Mode of Transmission	Common Mode of Acquisition
SOIL TRANSMITTED	
Ancylostoma duodenale (hookworm)	Skin penetration by or ingestion of larvae
Ascaris lumbricoides (human roundworm)	Ingestion of embryonated egg
Necator americanus (hookworm)	Skin penetration of larvae
Strongyloides stercoralis (threadworm)	Skin penetration of larvae
Toxocara canis (dog roundworm)	Ingestion of embryonated egg
Trichuris trichiura (whipworm)	Ingestion of embryonated egg
PARATENIC	
Anisakis spp.	Ingestion of fish
Trichinella spiralis	Ingestion of pork
ARTHROPOD-BORNE	
Brugia malayi	Bite of mosquito
Dracunculus medinensis	Ingestion of cyclops (crustacean)
Loa loa	Bite of mango fly (Chrysops spp.)
Onchocerca volvulus	Bite of blackfly
Wuchereria bancrofti	Bite of mosquito

TABLE 256-3. Major Human Parasitic Platyhelminths Classified by Mode of Transmission

Parasite	Common Mode of Acquisition
DIGENETIC TREMATODES (FLUKES)	
Clonorchis sinensis	Ingestion of EMc in fish
Fasciola hepatica	Ingestion of EMc in vegetation
Fasciolopsis buski	Ingestion of EMc in vegetation
Paragonimus spp.	Ingestion of EMc in crustaceans
Schistosoma spp.	Skin penetration of cercaria
CESTODES (TAPEWORMS)	
Diphyllobothrium latum	Ingestion of pleurocercoids in fish
Dipylidium caninum	Ingestion of cysticercoids in fleas
Hymenolepis diminuta	Ingestion of cysticercoids in insects
Hymenolepis nana	Ingestion of embryonated eggs
Taenia saginata	Ingestion of cysticerci in beef
Taenia solium	Ingestion of cysticerci in pork
INFECTIONS BY LARVAL CESTODES	
Cysticercosis	Ingestion of Taenia solium eggs
Hydatid disease	Ingestion of Echinococcus granulosus eggs

EMc, encysted metacercariae.

Human parasitic nematodes vary enormously in length from just over 200 μm (microfilariae) to more than 120 cm (Dracunculus). Their size, however, does not correlate with pathogenicity. One of the smallest nematodes, Strongyloides stercoralis, is among the most virulent of human pathogens. Nematodes are surrounded by a resistant cuticle and move by means of a complex muscular system; their digestive system is divided into an oral (buccal) cavity, esophagus, midgut, hindgut, and anus. Frequently, these structures are modified in the parasitic forms. For instance, the oral cavity of hookworms is enlarged and armed with teeth or cutting plates to ingest intestinal mucosa, and the esophagus is equipped with large exocrine glands that may contain hydrolytic enzymes for exodigestion.[14] The reproductive organs are highly developed in parasitic nematodes, particularly in females, and reflect their capacity to give rise to progeny. An adult female ascarid can release 200,000 eggs per day. Most nematodes have one or more life cycle stages, such as an egg or larva, that develop outside the host. It is convenient to categorize nematodes on the basis of their site of external development and the mechanism of entry into their definitive human host. Therefore, we frequently group endoparasitic nematodes according to whether they are transmitted through contact with soil (Ascaris); have an invertebrate intermediate host such as an insect (Wuchereria), crustacean (Dracunculus), or mollusk (Angiostrongylus); or have another vertebrate host with acquisition by the ingestion of undercooked meat (Trichinella) (Table 256-2). Several new genome projects for human nematode parasites are underway (http://www.nematodes.net and http://www.nematodes.org), which should add considerably to our fundamental knowledge.

Two endoparasitic classes of the phylum Platyhelminthes are important medically: trematodes and cestodes (Table 256-3). Human trematodes include blood flukes (schistosomes), intestinal flukes, and tissue flukes. Each species of human trematode also has external life cycle stages in one or more intermediate hosts. At least one intermediate host is always a mollusk. The adult fluke is either monoecious, having both sexes (hermaphroditic), or diecious, having separate sexes. Monoecious flukes reproduce by self- or cross-fertilization, whereas diecious trematodes live in copula as separate sexes. Except for the schistosomes, all human trematodes are monoecious. Eggs released by adult flukes typically hatch in water and give rise to free-living ciliated miracidia that seek their molluscan intermediate host. Miracidia are pluripotent and, once inside the snail, ultimately generate large numbers of cercariae. Cercariae exit the snail and enter their definitive human host by direct skin penetration (schistosomes) or encyst as metacercariae in a second intermediate host such as fish (Clonorchis) or vegetation (Fasciola) before ingestion. In terms of prevalence and chronic disease burden, the two most important trematodes are Schistosoma haematobium and S. mansoni. Almost 200 million people are infected with either of these two parasites, most in Africa,[15] although some estimates suggest that this number could be two or more times higher.[16] Two schistosome genome projects have been completed.[17]

In their definitive vertebrate host, cestodes are parasitic tapeworms with a gastrointestinal tract attachment apparatus (scolex) and a series of proglottid segments (strobila). Each proglottid segment contains both male and female reproductive organs and typically fills with eggs before detachment in feces. Ingestion of eggs by an intermediate host results in the liberation of larvae that frequently migrate to muscle as a final destination. Humans acquire tapeworms when they ingest the larval stage contained within arthropods or uncooked meat. Much more severe disease results when humans serve as the "accidental" intermediate host for cestodes by ingesting tapeworm eggs. Such intake can result in cysticercosis after ingestion of the eggs of Taenia solium or in hydatid disease after ingestion of the eggs of Echinococcus granulosus. Cysticercosis is emerging as an important cause of epilepsy in children, including children living in North America.

257 Ectoparasites (Lice and Scabies)

Dirk M. Elston

PEDICULOSIS

The Parasites, Virulence, and Pathogenesis

Pediculosis is an infestation by one of several species of sucking lice of the phylum Arthropoda, class Insecta, order Phthiraptera, suborder Anoplura, family Pediculidae or family Pthiridae. The three types of lice that infest humans are *Pediculus humanus capitis* (the head louse), *Pediculus humanus humanus* (the body louse), and *Phthirus pubis* (the crab louse).

Louse infestation spreads readily and the host response offers little protection against reinfestation. Resistance to chemical pediculicides is widespread, especially knockdown resistance to permethrin related to a double gene mutation (*T929I* and *L932F*). Glutathione-S-transferase-based resistance also has been implicated in pyrethroid resistance. Monooxygenase-based resistance is common, but can be overcome by synergistic agents such as piperonyl butoxide.

Transfer of lice is optimal when hairs are parallel and slow-moving, as when two individuals are sleeping or napping. Except in very humid climates, head lice lay nits very close to the scalp (within 1 to 2 mm). The nymphs hatch within 1 week and mature over a period of 1 week. In most climates, head lice can survive for about 24 hours off of the scalp.

Epidemiology

Head louse infestation affects about 6 to 12 million people per year in the United States alone, with highest prevalence among children between the ages of 3 and 12 years. Transmission occurs by means of direct contact or through fomites such as hats and scarves. Crab lice usually are spread sexually. Adolescents with pubic lice are roughly twice as likely as uninfested adolescents to have chlamydial or gonococcal infection. Among the homeless, body lice serve as vectors for *Bartonella quintana* endocarditis, epidemic typhus, louseborne relapsing fever, and trench fever.

Clinical Manifestations and Diagnosis

Head louse infestation manifests with pruritus of the scalp and posterior cervical lymphadenopathy. Body louse infestation produces a widespread dermatitis that can mimic a viral exanthem. The finding of characteristic bluish hued to copper-colored skin discoloration, *maculae cerulea* (caused by bite of a louse or flea), should prompt a search for body lice or nits in the seams of clothing. Crab louse infestation involves pubic hairs as well as hair on the chest, abdomen, and legs. Patients can present with generalized pruritus. Maculae cerulea (Figure 257-1) identical to those seen in body louse infestation can be present in crab louse infestation, and underwear commonly is stained with bloody louse excrement.

The diagnosis is made by finding lice or nits in the hair or seams of clothing (Figures 257-2 to 257-5).

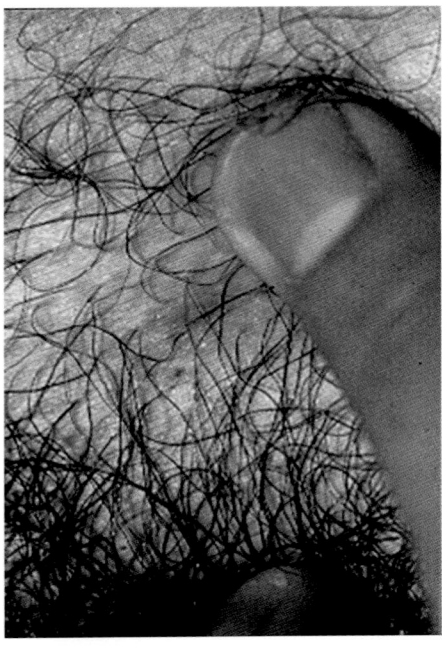

Figure 257-1. Maculae cerulae caused by bite of the body louse.

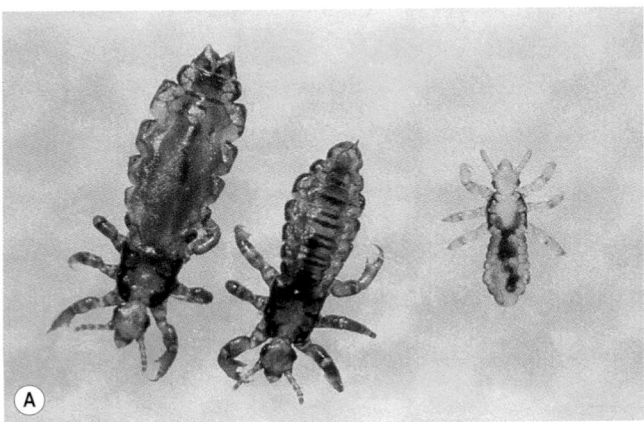
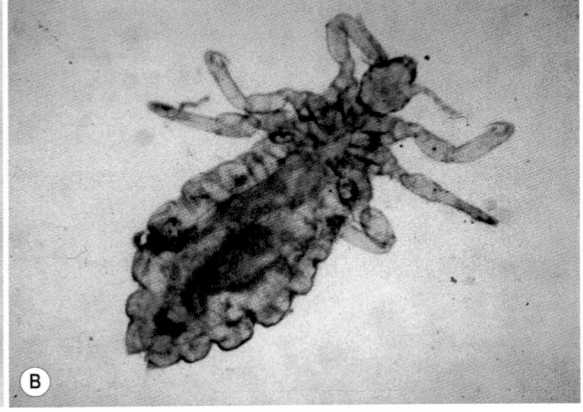

Figure 257-2. (A and B) *Pediculus humanus* (head and body louse).

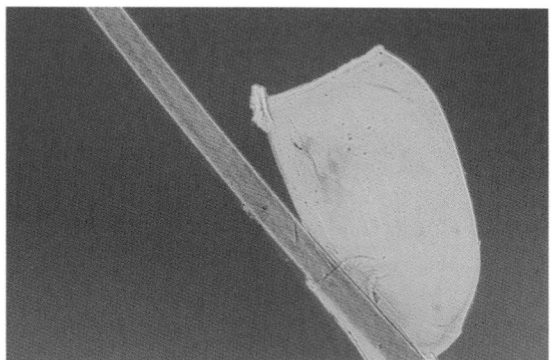

Figure 257-3. Empty egg case on shaft of hair.

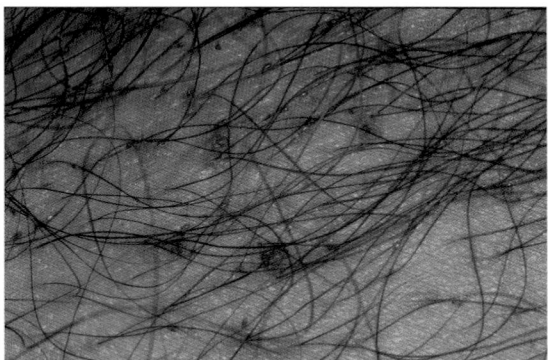

Figure 257-5. Crab lice in pubic hair.

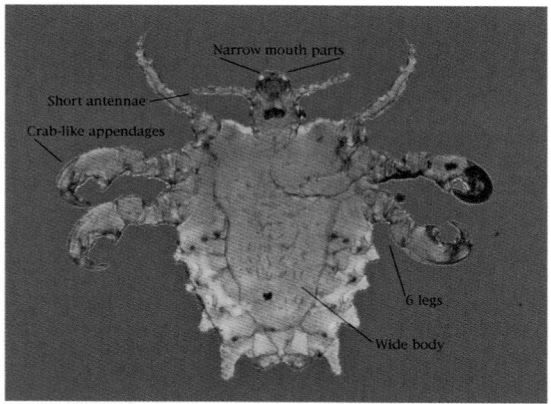

Figure 257-4. *Phthirus pubis* (crab louse).

Labels on figure: Narrow mouth parts; Short antennae; Crab-like appendages; 6 legs; Wide body

Treatment

Shaving of all parasitized hair will eradicate head and pubic lice, but is not cosmetically acceptable in most societies. Mechanical removal via wet-combing is labor-intensive and compliance is poor. Dilute solutions of vinegar or formic acid are not capable of dissolving nit cement, but can facilitate combing by flattening the hair cuticle.

Topical products (Table 257-1) are recommended treatment for louse infestations, and with the exception of lindane, should be applied twice with a 10-day interval between treatments.

Treatment of Choice

Benzyl alcohol (Ulesfia 5% lotion). Benzyl alcohol lotion 5% (Ulesfia) is the first FDA-approved non-neurotoxic louse treatment available in the U.S., approved for children ≥6 months of age. Benzyl alcohol occludes the respiratory spiracles of the louse, and the quantity applied must be sufficient to saturate the hair completely. Treatment achieved 100% efficacy after both 10- and 30-minute applications in a phase II trial. Phase III trials

TABLE 257-1. Treatments for Pediculosis and Scabies

Name	Evidence[a]	Instructions for Use	Precautions
TOPICAL TREATMENTS LABELED FOR THE TREATMENT OF PEDICULOSIS			
First line			
Benzyl alcohol	IB	Apply topically to dry scalp for 10 minutes, then rinse off; repeat in one week	Allergic/irritant dermatitis
Second line			
Permethrin 1%	IA	Apply topically to body or dry scalp for 5–10 minutes, then rinse off; repeat in one week	Allergic/irritant dermatitis
Pyrethrins	IIB	Apply topically to body or dry scalp for 5–10 minutes then rinse off; repeat in one week	Allergic/irritant dermatitis
Malathion	IB	Apply topically to body or dry scalp for 8–12 hours then rinse off; repeat in one week	Respiratory depression
Third line			
Lindane	IA	Apply topically to body or dry scalp for 5–10 minutes, then rinse off	Risk of seizures
TREATMENTS FOR SCABIES			
First line			
Permethrin 5%	IA	Apply topically[b]	Risk of leukemia
Precipitated sulfur	IIB	Apply topically[b]	Offensive odor
Benzyl benzoate	IB	Apply topically[b]	Neurotoxicity
Ivermectin	IB	200 µg/kg orally	Neurotoxicity
Second line			
Lindane	IA	Apply topically[b]	Neurotoxicity
Crotamiton	IIA	Apply topically[b]	Marginal efficacy

[a]Levels of evidence: IA, meta-analysis of randomized controlled trials; IB, at least one randomized controlled trial; IIA, at least one controlled study without randomization; IIB, at least one other type of quasi-experimental study.

[b]The cream should be applied to the entire body, including the head in infants. Care should be taken to apply a thick coat under the nails, in the umbilicus, axillae, web spaces, wrists, ankles, and genitalia. Close contacts should be treated concurrently.

comparing the product to vehicle placebo for two 10-minute applications showed it to be safe and effective (P<0.001).[1] Benzyl alcohol can induce histamine release and produce scalp itching, but overall is very well tolerated.

Second-Line Treatments

Pyrethrin/piperonyl butoxide (RID, A200). Pyrethrins are botanically derived pediculicides that act as neurotoxins. Piperonyl butoxide typically is added to potentiate the insecticidal effect. Allergic contact dermatitis can occur in people who are sensitive to Compositae plants and ragweed.

Permethrin (Nix). Permethrin is a synthetic pyrethroid neurotoxin available over the counter as a 1% cream rinse. Permethrin acts on sodium-gated channels resulting in paralysis (knockdown) and subsequent death of the louse. Knockdown resistance is now widespread and identified readily via gene mutation or lack of initial immobilization. Resistance to permethrin commonly crosses over to pyrethrins as well as to the other pyrethroids.[2]

Malathion (Ovide). Malathion is a weak organophosphate cholinesterase inhibitor that acts as a neurotoxin. Currently, malathion resistance is rare in the U.S., but is more common in the United Kingdom.[3] Although malathion is labeled for patients ≥6 years of age, recent studies showed no cholinesterase inhibition in patients 2 to 6 years of age. Flammability of malathion compounded in isopropyl alcohol has resulted in human injury about once in >1 million prescriptions filled. Efficacy for eradication of louse infestation in the U.S. is 97% to 98%.[4]

Carbaryl. Carbaryl is a carbamate insecticide once used commonly in the U.K., where over-the-counter sales have been restricted because of concerns about carcinogenicity. Acetylcholinesterase-based resistance is emerging.

Lindane. Lindane (gamma benzene hexachloride) is an organochloride neurotoxin with a long half-life in adipose tissue. If used, a single application is prescribed. Lindane is banned in California and should be avoided in patients with a history of seizure disorder or an impaired cutaneous barrier. California's ban on use of lindane does not appear to have had an adverse effect on outcomes of treatment of head lice and scabies (using other agents).[5] With effective and safer treatments available, lindane need not be used for treatment of louse infestation.

Alternative Agents

Ivermectin. Ivermectin may have some potential for neurotoxicity, and safety and efficacy in the setting of pediculosis remains to be established. A study comparing oral ivermectin (at a dose of 400 μg/kg of body weight) with 0.5% malathion lotion, each given on days 1 and 8, found ivermectin to be more effective. It should be noted that the dose of ivermectin used was twice that typically prescribed for this indication.[6]

Others. Dimeticones kill head lice by physical means and appear promising as an alternative to neurotoxins.[7] Crotamiton (Eurax) is better known as a second-line anti-scabetic agent but also has some activity as a pediculicide. A combination product containing 50% isopropyl myristate and 50% cyclomethicone was approved in Canada in 2006 and marketed under the name Resultz. Trimethoprim-sulfamethoxazole once was thought to act on lice by killing bacterial flora necessary for the synthesis of B vitamins in the louse's gut, but recent evidence suggests limited efficacy.[8] A wide variety of botanical oils are marketed through the internet for the treatment of pediculosis. Some of the ingredients have demonstrated pediculocidal activity, but many also are common contact allergens. Lice in clothing can be killed by ironing or machine laundering at 50°C and machine drying on a hot cycle.[9]

Special Considerations

Variations in cerebral p-glycoprotein, cytochrome P450 monooxygenases, esterases, and alcohol and aldehyde dehydrogenases make some individuals more susceptible to toxic effects of pesticides.[10] Reports suggesting a possible association between

pesticides and childhood leukemia have raised concern about the use of pediculicides in children, particularly pyrethroids.[11] Congenital leukemia with a *11q23/MLL* rearrangement has been reported in a child whose mother had heavily abused aerosolized permethrin during pregnancy. Laboratory evidence that incubation of a BV173 cell line with permethrin can induce MLL cleavage suggests a possible causal association.[12]

Prevention

"No-nit" policies have not been shown to reduce the incidence of louse infestation, but exclude many children from school. A better approach is through community education and louse inspections during outbreaks. Piperonal is a pediculicide that also exhibits repellent effects.

Key Points. Diagnosis and Management of Louse Infestation

MICROBIOLOGY
- Bloodsucking lice of the phylum Arthropoda, class Insecta, order Phthiraptera, suborder Anoplura, family Pediculidae or family Pthiridae

EPIDEMIOLOGY
- Transmission occurs by direct contact or through fomites such as hats and scarves
- Crab lice usually are spread sexually

TREATMENT
- Benzyl alcohol lotion 5% (Ulesfia) is the first FDA-approved non-neurotoxic louse treatment available in the United States
- Second-line treatments include a number of neurotoxic agents including pyrethrins with piperonyl butoxide, permethrin, malathion, and carbaryl
- Alternative agents include ivermectin, dimeticones, crotamiton, and isopropyl myristate/cyclomethicone

DURATION OF THERAPY
- Most topical products should be applied twice, with a 10-day interval between treatments

---

SCABIES

The Parasites, Virulence, and Pathogenesis

Human scabies usually is caused by the mite *Sarcoptes scabiei* var. *hominis*, an obligate human parasite and member of the class Arachnida, subclass Acari, order Astigmata, and family Sarcoptidae. Animal mange mites occasionally can produce symptoms in humans.

Sarcoptes scabiei elicits a mixed type I/type IV hypersensitivity reaction. Cross-reactivity occurs between the scabies mite and the house dust mite. During infestation, there is marked increase in the secretion of interleukin-6 (IL-6) and vascular endothelial growth factor (VEGF). IL-6 activates Th1 CD4+ lymphocytes to secrete IL-2, promoting lymphocyte proliferation and differentiation.

Direct skin-to-skin contact for 15 to 20 minutes is required for transfer of mites.

The average person harbors only between 5 to 12 mites, but those with crusted scabies can shed mites by the thousands.

Epidemiology

Roughly 300 million cases of scabies occur in the world each year. Risk factors include overcrowding, immigration, poor hygiene, poor nutritional status, homelessness, dementia, and sexual contact. In developing countries, scabies infestation and associated impetigo appear to be important risk factors for chronic kidney disease. Spread from healthcare personnel is documented, most recently to infants in a newborn nursery over a period of months.[13]

Clinical Manifestations and Diagnosis

The diagnosis should be suspected in anyone with intense, intractable, generalized pruritus. Often, multiple family members are affected, and the itch typically is worse at night. The eruption has a predilection for anterior axillary folds, periumbilical skin, the nipple area in females, volar surface of the wrists, interdigital web spaces, the belt line, penis, scrotum, and ankles (Figures 257-6 to 257-8). Mite burrows are serpiginous 1- to 4-mm keratotic lines, often punctuated by a small vesicle at one end, which houses the mite. In infants and young children, scalp, face, and neck can be heavily involved. Pustules on the palms and soles are typical in infantile scabies. After puberty, genital nodules are common. In endemic areas, widespread impetigo generally is presumed to indicate scabies infestation. Crusted scabies in children with Down syndrome appears with whitish flaky crusts with striking involvement of the hands and ears. In infants and young children, a dense Langerhans cell infiltrate can result in misdiagnosis as Langerhans cell histiocytosis.

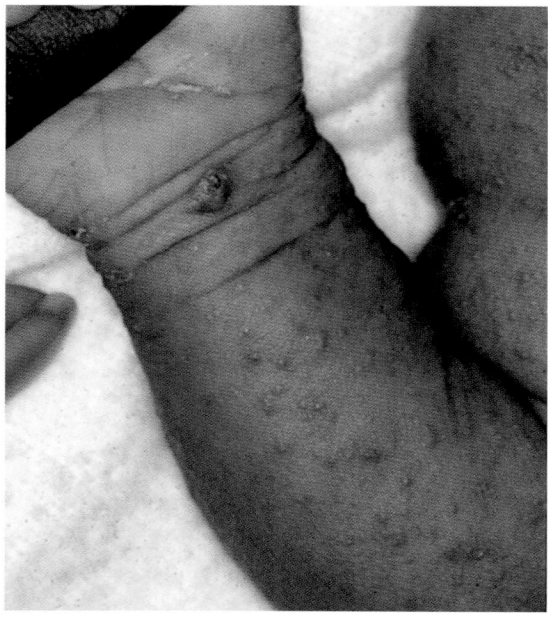

Figure 257-6. Scabies in infant.

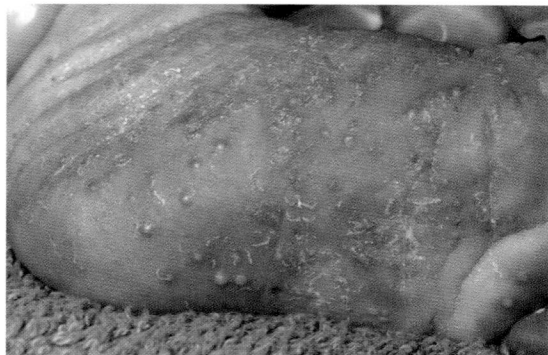

Figure 257-7. Acral pustules of scabies.

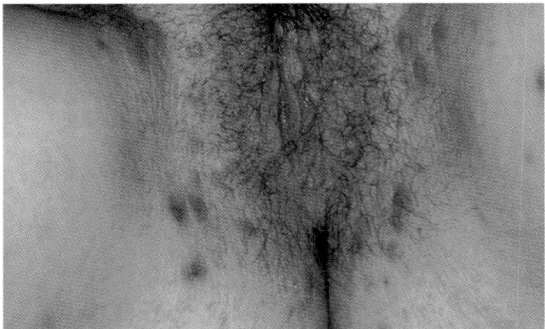

Figure 257-8. Scabies nodules.

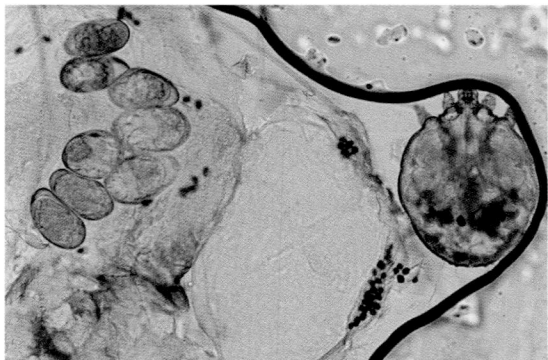

Figure 257-9. Microscopic appearance of mites, ova and feces of scabies.

The diagnosis is confirmed by identification of the mites, eggs, or fecal pellets in scrapings from burrows (Figure 257-9). Fluorescent microscopy can be used to highlight fecal debris and fragments of ova. *S. scabiei* DNA polymerase chain reaction assays exist, but are rarely used in clinical practice.

Treatment (Table 257-1)

First-Line Treatments

Permethrin 5%. Permethrin cream 5% should be applied to the entire body, including the head in infants, left on for at least 8 hours and repeated in 7 to 10 days. A Cochrane group review of interventions for scabies concluded the following: topical permethrin remains the most effective treatment for scabies, ivermectin appears to be an effective oral alternative; more research is needed on the effectiveness of malathion.[14] Direct comparisons of permethrin with oral ivermectin have shown mixed results.[15-17]

Precipitated sulfur 6% to 10% in petrolatum. Sulfur is the oldest recorded treatment modality for scabies, and remains in common use worldwide. Despite a lack of controlled clinical trials, it is generally acknowledged to have a high degree of efficacy, even in the setting of crusted scabies.

Benzyl benzoate 10% to 25%. Benzyl benzoate remains one of the most commonly prescribed agents for scabies in many parts of the world and compares favorably with other topical agents and oral ivermectin.[17,18] Benzyl benzoate is not available in the U.S. or Canada. The 25% emulsion is applied below the neck, with 3 applications during a 24-hour period. In young adults or children, the concentration can be reduced to 12.5%. Use can be complicated by allergic contact dermatitis, and benzyl benzoate should not be used during pregnancy, or in lactating women, infants, or children <2 years of age because of the risk of neurotoxicity.

Oral ivermectin. For the off-label treatment of scabies, ivermectin is given orally as a single dose of 200 µg/kg repeated in 7 to

10 days. High doses can cause embryotoxicity in animals, and some have suggested it should not be used during pregnancy, although ivermectin often has been used in this setting in the treatment of onchocerciasis. Comparisons with permethrin, benzyl benzoate, and lindane have shown mixed results. In scabies-endemic areas, ivermectin has been shown to reduce the incidence of streptococcal disease and renal damage in children.[19]

Second-Line Treatments

Lindane (gamma benzene hexachloride 1%). Lindane is applied overnight for 6 to 8 hours. Levels in breast milk are 60 times higher than in blood and lindane should be avoided during breastfeeding. Convulsions and death have been reported in children or infants with intentional misuse of the product or overexposure related to an altered skin barrier. Other effective and safe treatments should replace the use of lindane for treatment of scabies.
Crotamiton 10%. Crotamiton 10% is applied twice daily for 2 to 5 consecutive days. Although efficacy is low, crotamiton sometimes is used as an adjunctive agent because of its inherent antipruritic effect.

Special Considerations

Crusted scabies may require treatment with both oral ivermectin and a topical agent. The author has found 10% precipitated sulfur to be most effective. Keratolytics should be used to improve penetration of treatment agents. The nails should be trimmed and

brushed with a scabicidal agent. Patients with scabies are highly infectious and require isolation.

Prevention

In some countries, soaps containing monosulfiram have been used for prophylaxis in communities with high infestation.

Key Points. Diagnosis and Management of Scabies Infestation

MICROBIOLOGY
- *Sarcoptes scabiei* var. *hominis* is a member of the class Arachnida, subclass Acari, order Astigmata, and family Sarcoptidae

EPIDEMIOLOGY
- Transmission occurs through close physical contact
- Fomites such as bed sheets are an important means of spread in the setting of crusted scabies

TREATMENT
- First-line treatments include permethrin, precipitated sulfur, benzyl benzoate, and oral ivermectin
- Second-line treatments include crotamiton

DURATION OF THERAPY
- Most topical products should be applied twice, with a 7- to 10-day interval between treatments

---

258 *Babesia* Species (Babesiosis)
Robert W. Tolan, Jr

Babesiosis is a malaria-like tickborne parasitic zoonosis resulting from infection by *Babesia* species.[1-10] Symptomatic infection is more frequently diagnosed and reported in asplenic adults,[11] those older than 50 years of age,[8] and compromised hosts;[12] but neonates,[13] infants,[14] and children[15] also are infected in endemic areas following a tick bite, blood product transfusion,[14] and via congenital or perinatal transmission.[13,14] Although as many as 7 species of *Babesia* have been implicated in human babesiosis,[3] *B. microti* is most common in the northeastern and upper midwestern United States,[1] *B. duncani* in the western U.S.,[16] and *B. divergens* in Europe.[2] Fever, malaise, and hemolytic anemia typify clinical disease,[17] which tends to be milder in *B. microti* infection[5] and more severe in *B. divergens* infection.[7] Clinical diagnosis is confirmed by identification of the parasite in a blood smear or detection of *Babesi* DNA in serum by polymerase chain reaction (PCR).[18] Atovaquone and azithromycin are considered the treatment of choice for most symptomatic cases.[19] Avoidance of exposure to the tick vector is the best measure to prevent babesiosis.[1]

DESCRIPTION OF THE PATHOGEN

The *Babesia* species belong to phylum Apicomplexa (with *Cryptosporidium*, *Plasmodium*, and *Toxoplasma*) due to the presence of apical organelles, class Aconoidasida, order Piroplasmidora (with Theileriidae) based upon their pear-shaped morphology, and family Babesiidae.[5] *Babesia* organisms directly infect erythrocytes (without the pre-erythrocytic–hepatic stage that some plasmodia exhibit) where they divide by sporogony (budding).[3] Since

sporogony is asynchronous in the human host, massive hemolysis usually does not occur (e.g., in contrast to malaria).[15,20]

Recent analyses of 18S rRNA sequence data[21] suggest that the human *Babesia* species can be divided into four clinically relevant clades[3,6,21,22]: clade 1 contains *B. microti* and *B. microti*-like parasites, the most common cause of human babesiosis to date (primarily the northeastern and upper midwestern U.S.); clade 2 includes *B. duncani*[16] (initially isolates were named WA1, WA2, CA5, and CA6; for Washington State 1 and 2 and California 5 and 6) and *B. duncani*-like (CA1, CA3, CA4) organisms causing infection in the western U.S.; clade 3 comprises species causing human disease in Europe,[2,23] including *B. divergens*, *B. divergens*-like (similar disease, but clearly different organisms), and *B. venatorum* (previously designated EU1, for Europe 1),[24] and single *B. divergens*-like[4] cases in Missouri (MO1),[25] Kentucky (KY),[26] and Washington State;[27] clade 4 organisms are rarely transmitted to humans but include the human isolate from Korea (KO1).[28] Morphologically, trophozoites from clades 1 and 2 are typically small, measuring 1 to 2.5 μm, while those from clades 3 and 4 are large, measuring 2.5 to 5 μm.[6,8] Clinically, human infection by the organisms in clades 3 and 4 tends to occur in older or asplenic individuals, many of whom describe significant cattle exposure, and disease tends to be much more severe than that seen in infection caused by organisms of clades 1 and 2.[3] All clinical human babesiosis is more frequent, and potentially more severe, in immunocompromised individuals.[8]

Indigenous human babesiosis occurs only in regions where ixodid ticks (the only recognized vectors) are found. Since these ticks also transmit *Borrelia burgdorferi* and *Anaplasma phagocytophilum*, the causative agents of Lyme disease and human granulocytic anaplasmosis, respectively, coinfection with *Babesia* can occur.[29,30] The primary hosts for the ticks carrying *B. microti* are the rodent (the white-footed mouse in the northeast U.S.) for the larvae and nymphs and deer and other large mammals for the adult ticks.[15] Proximity to white-tailed deer perpetuates the population of ixodid ticks, which transmit the organism to humans as incidental hosts.[31] Human babesiosis results from the confluence of parasite, vector, primary hosts (e.g., mice and deer) and accidental hosts (humans).

EPIDEMIOLOGY

First described as pathogens of cattle in 1888 and humans beginning in 1956 in Europe and the 1960s in the U.S. (Nantucket fever), babesial parasites have caused sporadic human infection throughout Europe and endemic babesiosis along the coast of

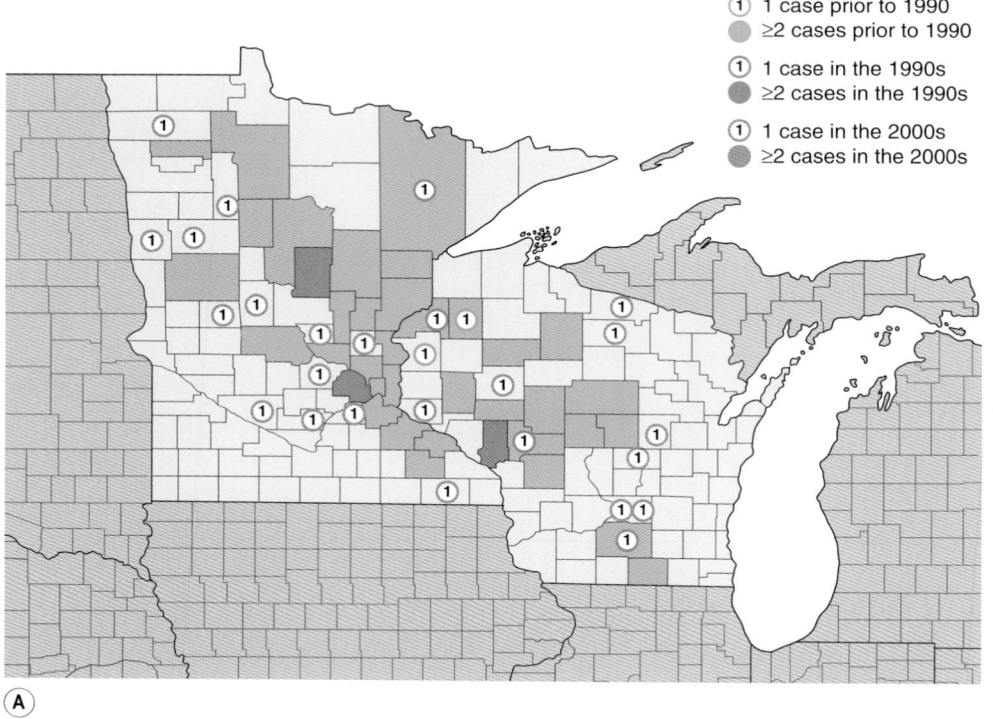

- ① 1 case prior to 1990
- ◯ ≥2 cases prior to 1990

- ① 1 case in the 1990s
- ● ≥2 cases in the 1990s

- ① 1 case in the 2000s
- ● ≥2 cases in the 2000s

Ⓐ

Figure 258-1. Expanding endemicity of indigenous babesiosis in the upper midwest and northeast U.S. by county of residence (or acquisition if available) and decade. Blue denotes cases reported prior to 1990; orange denotes cases reported during the 1990s; green denotes cases reported during the 2000s. Data assembled from internet sources, the medical literature, and courtesy of personnel at the state health departments of the states depicted, including Erica Berl, DVM, MPH (VT); Elizabeth R. Daly, MPH (NH); Paula Eggers, RN, BS (DE); Katherine Feldman, DVM, MPH (MD); Jennifer L. Hallisey, MPH (NY); Dawn Heisey-Grove, MPH (MA); James Kazmierczak, DVM, MS (WI); Melissa M. Kemperman, MPH (MN); Sara Robinson, MPH (ME); and Kirsten Waller, MD, MPH (PA). Babesiosis became a reportable disease in many states only recently; data included may reflect less rigorous case definitions and less than optimal case investigations. (Figure created by Jeremy Bechtel, Jeremy@JeremyBechtel.co.uk.)

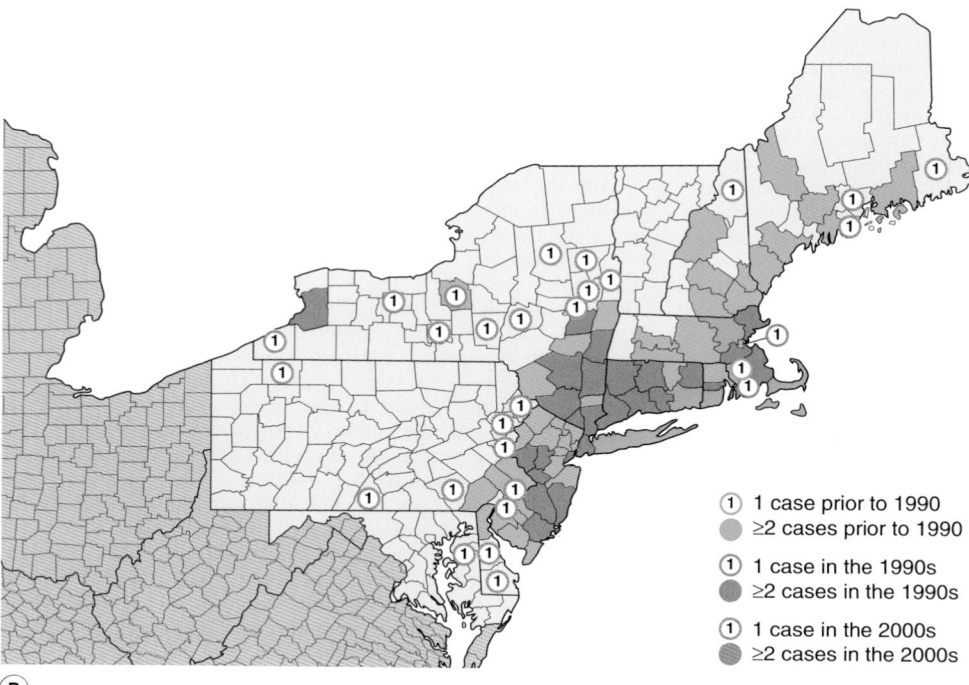

- ① 1 case prior to 1990
- ◯ ≥2 cases prior to 1990

- ① 1 case in the 1990s
- ● ≥2 cases in the 1990s

- ① 1 case in the 2000s
- ● ≥2 cases in the 2000s

Ⓑ

New England and the upper midwest in the U.S.[3] Initially, *B. microti* was found to be endemic in Massachusetts (Nantucket Island, Martha's Vineyard, Elizabeth Islands, and Cape Cod), Rhode Island (Block Island), southeastern Connecticut, and New York (Shelter Island, Fire Island, and eastern Long Island).[32] In Europe, much less common, but more severe disease in splenectomized adults has been recognized due to *B. divergens*.[7,33] In the past decade, however, this understanding of the epidemiology of babesiosis has been found to be too simplistic.[3] New species have been identified;[16,34] biologic and morphologic taxonomy have yielded to molecular analysis;[21] recognition of cases in more varied populations (including transfusion-associated[35-37] and congenital/perinatal[13,14] cases) has ensued; and an appreciation that the regions of endemicity have expanded dramatically (in the U.S., in particular) (Figure 258-1). At the end of 2010, human babesiosis was reportable in the U.S. states of California, Connecticut, Delaware, Indiana, Maine, Maryland, Massachusetts, Minnesota, Nebraska, New Hampshire, New Jersey, New York, Rhode Island, Vermont, Washington, and Wisconsin. As of January 2011, babesiosis became a reportable disease in all of the U.S. (with reporting in each state to follow if such regulations are enacted).

Currently, human babesiosis due to indigenous *B. microti* infection is endemic in the northeastern,[32,38-43] and upper midwestern (Wisconsin[44] and Minnesota) U.S. (see Figure 258-1), with thousands of cases having been reported to date (more than 1800 in New York State alone as of 2009). Seroprevalence among Long Island blood donors in 1984 was 15.8%.[45] Only one seroprevalence study (on Block Island, Rhode Island[46]) has been published in the past 20 years.[47] The seroprevalence of babesiosis in children aged 0 to 19 years on Block Island between 1991 and 2000 was 1632/100,000 (compared with 1287/100,000 for Lyme disease) while that in adults aged 20 to 89 years was 1618/100,000 (compared with 2183/100,000 for Lyme disease).[47] In that study, children aged 0 to 19 years had significantly fewer symptoms, significantly shorter duration of illness, and were rarely hospitalized, particularly compared with people >50 years of age.[47] Cases also have been reported in Vermont, Maryland, Indiana, California, Washington, and elsewhere. Rarely, *B. duncani* infection has been described in Washington and California.[16,34] Finally, *B. divergens*-like infections have occurred in Washington, Missouri, and Kentucky.[4,27]

In Europe, human babesiosis results from *B. divergens* infection in asplenic individuals,[2,7,22,33,48] although it is much less common than in the U.S., with reported cases numbering <100.[2] Babesiosis has been reported in Croatia (initially); France, the United Kingdom, Ireland (most frequently); and Spain, Sweden,[49] Switzerland,[50] elsewhere in the former Yugoslavia, the former Soviet Union, Austria,[24] Germany,[51,52] Italy,[24,53] Portugal,[54] and Finland[55] (sporadically). Three cases of disease due to *B. venatorum* (EU1) have been described.[24,52] Autochthonous (indigenous) *B. microti* was first reported in Germany,[56] but the disease likely is under-recognized and under-reported due to its less fulminant course and lack of cross-reactivity with serologic tests for *B. divergens*.[22,23] Human babesiosis also has been reported in Canada,[57] Korea,[28] Japan, China, Egypt, Mexico, South Africa, Taiwan, and Australia.[10,33]

CLINICAL MANIFESTATIONS

Most babesial infection, particularly in the pediatric population, is asymptomatic.[46] When clinical disease occurs, it is most often a nonspecific, influenza-like illness and the diagnosis is rarely made.[46] More severe manifestations of infection are a malaria-like illness with fever, fatigue, malaise, and manifestations of hemolytic anemia.[1,8] The case-fatality rate for *B. microti* infection is approximately 5%.[3] Typically, *B. divergens* infection is more fulminant,[33] often including disseminated intravascular coagulopathy, acute renal failure, and cardiorespiratory complications – resulting in a case-fatality rate of 42%.[3]

The incubation period following a tick bite is up to 33 days[3] (although the tick bite often goes unnoticed since the unengorged nymph measures <2 mm) and 1 to 9 weeks following transfusion.[19] Most infections occur between May and September, when

TABLE 258-1. Common Symptoms of *B. microti* Infection

Symptom	Percentage of All Patients (*n* = 299)
Fever	87
Fatigue	82
Chills	68
Sweats	57
Headache	50
Myalgia	46
Anorexia	38
Cough	29
Arthralgia	26
Nausea	24

Modified from Vannier E, Krause PJ. Update on babesiosis. Interdiscip Perspect Infect Dis 2009;2009:984568; Krause PJ, McKay K, Thompson CA, et al. Disease-specific diagnosis of coinfecting tickborne zoonoses: babesiosis, human granulocytic ehrlichiosis, and Lyme disease. Clin Infect Dis 2002;34:1184–1191; Krause PJ, Lepore T, Sikand VK, et al. Atovaquone and azithromycin for the treatment of babesiosis. N Engl J Med 2000;343:1454–1458.

the nymphal ticks are most actively feeding.[3] The most common symptoms seen in *B. microti* infection are summarized in Table 258-1. Others reported in two series of 84 total patients[58,59] include emotional lability in 50%, neck stiffness in 48%, sore throat in 31%, vomiting in 20%, joint swelling in 11%, and conjunctivitis in 11%. Individuals noted 9 separate symptoms lasting 10 weeks, on average.[58]

Physical findings often are limited to fever in mild cases, although icterus, pallor, mild hepatosplenomegaly, and/or dark urine may be present.[17] Noncardiac pulmonary edema has been described in adults.[59] Ocular manifestations, such as retinal lesions, appear to be rare.[60]

B. divergens infection results in a more fulminant illness,[7] with evidence of cardiorespiratory compromise, bleeding diathesis, poor perfusion, hypotension, and other complications possible. Risk factors for severe babesiosis, in addition to infection with *B. divergens*, include age >50 years; male gender; functional, anatomic, or operative asplenia;[11] other immune compromising conditions,[61] including acquired immunodeficiency syndrome (AIDS);[62] and coinfection with *Borrelia* or *Anaplasma* or both.[12,29,30,58,63] Manifestations of severe disease can include acute respiratory distress syndrome, disseminated intravascular coagulopathy, congestive heart failure, acute renal failure, myocardial infarction,[12,17] splenic infarction,[64] splenic rupture,[65] septic shock,[66] and death.[54,55] Furthermore, patients found to have anemia (hemoglobin concentration <10 g/dL) or parasitemia >10% are more likely to have complications.[17]

LABORATORY FINDINGS AND DIAGNOSIS

Laboratory findings can be unremarkable or nonspecifically abnormal in asymptomatic or mild cases. Among hospitalized patients with *B. microti* infection, thrombocytopenia and elevated serum hepatic transaminases were more commonly present than in febrile adults with other infections.[17] Low haptoglobin, anemia, and evidence of hemolysis can be present.[12] Occasionally, parasites may be identified during performance of a manual differential of peripheral white blood cells.

Laboratory confirmation of human babesiosis primarily employs thin blood smear, PCR,[67] and species-specific serology.[18,47,68] Characteristic findings on thin smear are shown in Figure 258-2. The tetrad ("Maltese cross") is pathognomonic for the small babesial parasites. Findings on thin smear for *Babesia* and *Plasmodium* are contrasted in Table 258-2. PCR, although generally only available at reference laboratories, is necessary for

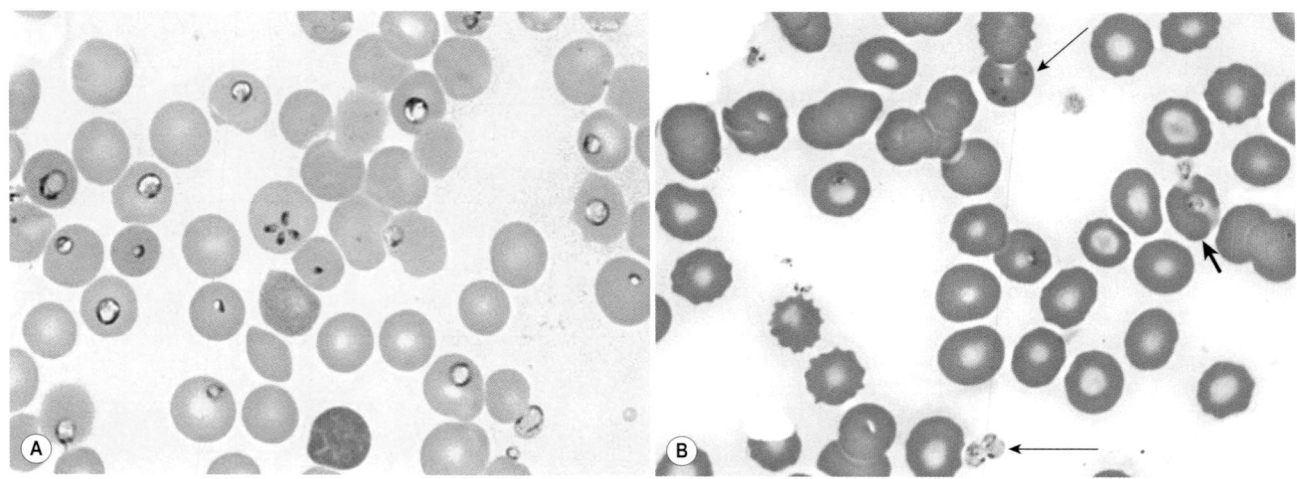

Figure 258-2. Wright- **(A)** and Giemsa-stained **(B)** peripheral blood smear from a 26-day-old infant with transplacentally acquired babesiosis and ~15% parasitemia.[13] The smear demonstrates typical features, including thrombocytopenia, parasites of variable size and morphology, and absence of hemozoin pigment. A pathognomonic tetrad (open arrowhead) and typical basket cells (arrowheads and throughout) are seen in image **A,** while image **B** demonstrates an extracellular syncytium (long arrow) and multiple parasites per erythrocyte (short arrows). Magnification ×1000.

TABLE 258-2. Comparison of Findings on Thin Blood Smear Between *Babesia* and Plasmodium Infections

Finding	*Babesia* Species (Figure 258-2)	*Plasmodium* Species
Ring appearance	Pleomorphic more common (Figure 258-2A)	Monomorphic more common
Morphology present	Only ring forms (Figure 258-2A)	Ring forms and/or schizonts and gametocytes
Intracellular parasites	Polyparasitism common (may have ≥4) (Figure 258-2B, short arrows)	Rarely >4 intracellular parasites per erythrocyte
Food vacuole	Refractory white vacuole often present (Figure 258-2A)	Rare (in early trophozoite stages)
Chromatin dots	1–3 present (Figure 258-2A)	1–2 present in ring forms
Tetrads (Maltese Cross)	Present (*B. microti*) (Figure 258-2A, open arrowhead)	Absent
Red blood cell morphology	Normal (Figure 258-2A and B)	Can be normal, unchanged, small, enlarged, or fimbriated
Erythrocyte stippling	Absent (Figure 258-2A and B)	Maurer,[a] Schüffner,[b] or Ziemann[c] stippling
Hemozoin (partially digested hemoglobin)	Absent (Figure 258-2A and B)	Present
Extracellular parasites	Common (Figure 258-2B, long arrow)	Uncommon

[a]*Irregular mauve/red dots in* P. falciparum-*infected erythrocytes.*

[b]*Pink- or red-staining dots in* P. ovale- *or* vivax-*infected erythrocytes.*

[c]*Eosinophilic dots in* P. malariae-*infected erythrocytes.*

Modified from Pantanowitz L, Ballesteros E, De Girolami P. Laboratory diagnosis of babesiosis. Lab Med 2001;32:184–187.

TABLE 258-3. Overview of Diagnostic Approaches for Human Babesiosis

Diagnostic Method	Advantages	Disadvantages
Blood smear	Inexpensive, rapid; reliable with high parasitemia	Can be confused with malaria, especially with inexperienced reader; can be negative with low-lowel parasitemia
Immunofluorescent antibody assay (serology)	The only commercially available serology	Expensive; requires reference laboratory confirmation; cross-reactivity; species-specific
Enzyme immunoassay (serology)	Less cross-reactivity	Not commercially available (investigational)
Hamster inoculation	Effective for low-parasitemia disease	Slow, labor-intensive; can be negative with fastidious organisms
Microaerophilous stationary phase in vitro culture	Effective for low-parasitemia disease	Impractical for human disease diagnosis
PCR assay	Reliable; accurate if assay is standardized and performed well	Expensive; requires reference laboratory

Modified from Schuster FL. Cultivation of Babesia *and* Babesia-*like blood parasites: agents of an emerging zoonotic disease. Clin Microbiol Rev 2002;15:365–373.*

accurate speciation. Commercially-available serology employs immunofluorescent antibody testing and is species-specific. An enzyme-immunosorbent assay[69] and immunoblot testing[70] also have been described. Examination of formalin-fixed tissues via an immunohistochemical approach also has been proposed.[71] Available diagnostic techniques for clinical and research purposes are compared in Table 258-3.[72]

Decision to treat depends upon the presence of symptoms and positive thin blood smear or PCR assay, rather than serologic results. However, serology is useful to confirm suspected infection, as it often is positive at the time parasitemia becomes detectable.[47]

TREATMENT

Initially, human babesiosis was treated with quinine and clindamycin,[19,47,73] during which prolonged parasitemia and adverse events were common (~75%) and therapeutic failure occurred occasionally.[74] A randomized trial comparing quinine plus clindamycin therapy with a combination of atovaquone[75] plus azithromycin,[74] demonstrated equivalent cure rates with significantly fewer toxicities (~15%); therefore, the latter has become the treatment of choice in most situations. Atovaquone and azithromycin therapy generally is well tolerated and has been successful in the treatment of neonates.[13,76] Duration of therapy typically is 7 to 10 days in the otherwise healthy individual.[19,47] Severe illness may necessitate the use of quinine and clindamycin, however, if the newer treatment regimen fails. In addition to supportive care, exchange transfusion is beneficial, particularly with severe infection, significant hemolysis, renal/hepatic/pulmonary compromise, poor response to initial antiparasitic therapy, and/or high parasitemia.[1] This intervention seems to be less frequently necessary in the infected pediatric patient,[13,14] for reasons which remain unclear. While routine screening of healthy individuals for post-treatment relapse is not recommended, those found to have positive thin blood smears or PCR >3 months after completing therapy should be retreated, irrespective of symptoms.[1]

Even with no therapy, almost all healthy individuals become asymptomatic and eventually clear their parasitemia. Those with underlying immune compromising conditions, however, can develop persistent or relapsing disease; such patients should be monitored for recurrence of symptoms and have thin blood smears or PCR or both checked only if symptoms arise. Treatment of these persons may include a variety of agents (often in combination), including atovaquone, azithromycin, clindamycin (intravenous route is preferred[1]), doxycycline, proguanil, pentamidine, quinine, and trimethoprim-sulfamethoxazole, for multiple and prolonged courses.[61] While a particular combination of agents is not recognized as superior, it is clear that continuation of treatment for ≥2 weeks beyond clearance of parasitemia by thin blood smear, and, generally ≥6 weeks in total, is associated with more frequent cure.[61] No adjunctive immunomodulating therapies have yet been identified. Recently, parasites resistant to atovaquone and azithromycin have been identified in immunocompromised people with babesiosis in Connecticut and New York State.[77]

SPECIAL CONSIDERATIONS

Babesiosis is a particular problem for the immunocompromised host.[61] Almost all cases of *B. divergens* infection in Europe have occurred in asplenic individuals,[7] in whom the case-fatality rate is high (42%).[3] Similarly, widespread *B. microti* infection was first recognized among asplenic hosts,[11] although the disease is less severe than that caused by *B. divergens*. In those with AIDS, babesiosis can manifest as fever of unknown origin,[62] as well as persistent or relapsing disease. Transfusion-associated babesiosis is an emerging problem,[35-37] particularly in transplant patients[63] and among neonates.[14,35,45,73,78,79] Although two cases of tick-transmitted babesiosis in neonates were reported from Long Island,[80] most of the cases in neonates have been transfusion-associated.[14] To date, four cases of congenital/perinatal babesiosis have been reported.[13,81-83]

PREVENTION

The best way to prevent babesiosis is to avoid exposure to the tick vector.[1] Similarly, screening of the blood supply for evidence of contamination should decrease the incidence of transfusion-associated infection.[18] Measures to decrease infection of pregnant women would likely impact congenital/perinatal transmission. If exposure to the vector is unavoidable, several measures are appropriate to decrease the likelihood of being bitten or having infection transmitted during a bite. These include wearing protective clothing (long pants, tucked into socks or boots, and long sleeves), use of tick repellants, daily careful examination of the entire body for ticks, and prompt removal of any ticks identified. Prevention of unrecognized infection is supported by education of healthcare personnel about babesiosis and careful observation for development of any associated symptoms for a month or so after tick removal. There is no role for antibiotic prophylaxis, examination of removed ticks for parasites, or laboratory testing of asymptomatic individuals following tick removal.[1]

Although animal vaccines exist, there is no role for passive or active immunoprophylaxis for human babesiosis. Aside from transfusion- (and, potentially, organ-)[63] associated transmission, no human-to-human transmission has been documented and no particular infection prevention measures are necessary.

Key Points. Diagnosis and Management of *Babesia* species (Babesiosis) Infection

MICROBIOLOGY
- Apicomplexan parasite transmitted to humans by ixodid tick bites
- The same vector transmits *Borrelia burgdorferi* and *Anaplasma phagocytophilum*
- *B. microti* most common in U.S.; *B. divergens* in Europe; other species much less common

EPIDEMIOLOGY
- Endemic in CT, DE, MA, ME, MN, NH, NJ, NY, PA, RI, WI in the U.S.
- Sporadic cases in CA, IN, KY, MD, MO, VT, WA in the U.S.; Europe and elsewhere worldwide
- Range of endemicity is expanding rapidly
- Chief risk factors are age >50 years, asplenia, male gender, and immunocompromising conditions
- Transfusion-transmitted infection is recognized increasingly
- Congenital/perinatal transmission is rare, but is well documented

DIAGNOSIS
- Thin blood smear is rapid, inexpensive, and diagnostic with appropriate expertise
- Speciation requires polymerase chain reaction (PCR)
- Serology can confirm clinical suspicion, but should not drive therapy

TREATMENT
- Atovaquone plus azithromycin is the combination treatment of choice
- Severe cases may require therapy with quinine and intravenous clindamycin
- Exchange transfusion is beneficial in severe cases

DURATION OF THERAPY
- Prolonged parasitemia (>7 days) can occur despite clinical improvement
- Duration of therapy typically is 7 to 10 days for the immunocompetent host
- In the compromised host, therapy should continue for 2 weeks after negative thin blood smears and PCR, or for 6 weeks (whichever is longer)

---

259 *Balantidium coli*

Frank E. Berkowitz

Balantidium coli is the largest protozoan, and the only ciliated one, known to infect human and nonhuman primates. The parasite thrives in the large intestine of a wide range of animals,[1,2] but domestic pigs are considered the most important reservoir host.[1,3,4] Water is the vehicle for most cases of balantidiasis, but human-to-human transmission also can occur. No intermediate host is needed. Infected people can be asymptomatic, or can develop diarrhea or dysentery accompanied by abdominal colic, tenesmus, and emesis.

THE PATHOGEN

B. coli exists in two forms, the trophozoite form, which causes disease, and the cyst form, which is the infectious ingested form.[1] Cysts excyst in the intestine, and the trophozoites that emerges infect the colon (Figure 259-1). Cysts are resistant to environmental stresses such as drying. The trophozoite form is somewhat pear-shaped, measuring 30 to 150 µm in length and 25 to 120 µm in width (Figure 259-2). The size depends on the amount of material ingested. The cyst form is round, measuring 40 to 60 µm in diameter (Figure 259-3).[5] The trophozoite has an oral end (narrow end), a cytopyge ("anus") at the rounded posterior end, a macronucleus and a micronucleus, and contains mitochondria-like organelles that might serve as hydrogenosomes. *B. coli* can survive in both anaerobic and aerobic conditions, uses carbohydrates for energy production, and reproduces asexually by fission, but sexual reproduction by conjugation has been reported. The surface is covered by longitudinal rows of cilia that function as the organs of locomotion and give the trophozoite its characteristic morphology.[5]

Several species of *Balantidium* can infect many different animals, both vertebrate and invertebrate. The species infecting humans is *B. coli*.

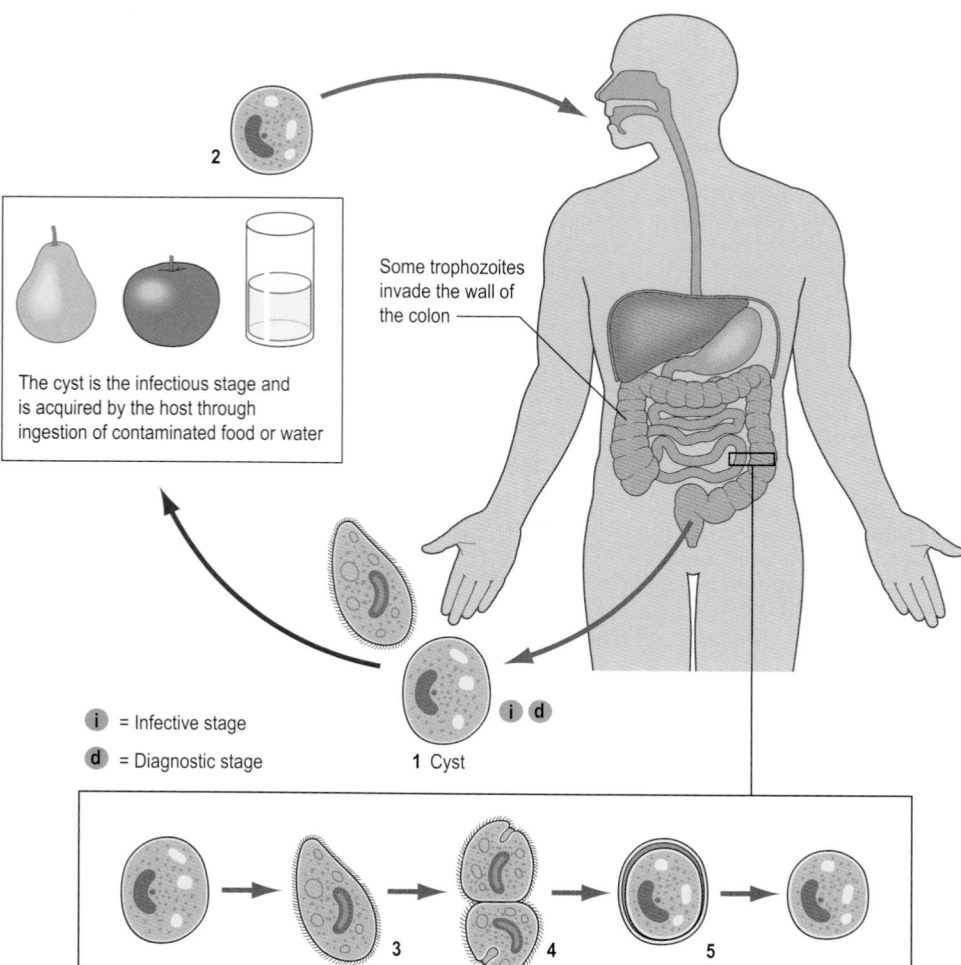

Figure 259-1. Life cycle of *Balantidium coli* and pathogenesis of balantidiasis. (Courtesy of the Centers for Disease Control and Prevention.)

Some trophozoites invade the wall of the colon

The cyst is the infectious stage and is acquired by the host through ingestion of contaminated food or water

i = Infective stage

d = Diagnostic stage

1 Cyst

i **d**

Cyst   Trophozoite

2   3   4   5

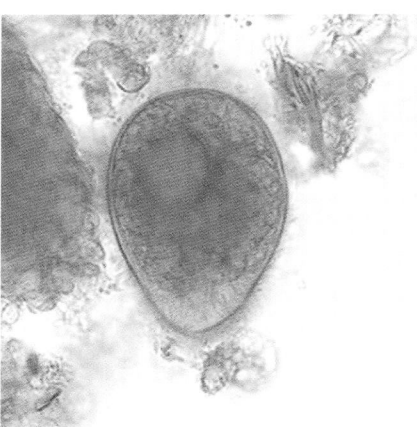

Figure 259-2. Pear-shaped trophozoite form of *B. coli* in stool specimen (Courtesy of DPDx image library, CDC.)

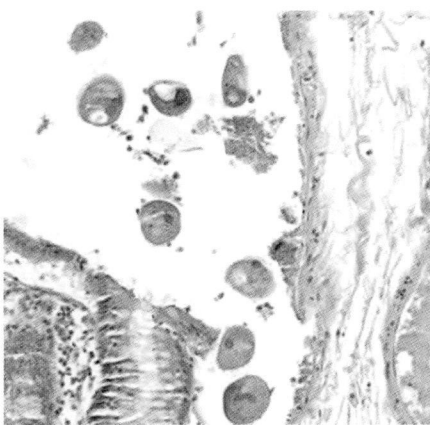

Figure 259-4. Biopsy of colon shows excystation of *B. coli* with emergence of trophozoites. (Courtesy of DPDx image library, CDC.)

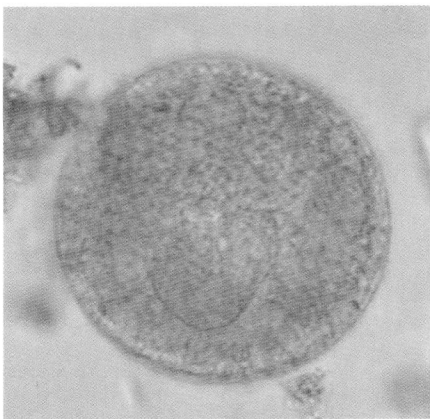

Figure 259-3. Round cyst form of *B. coli* in stool specimen. (Courtesy of DPDx image library, CDC.)

EPIDEMIOLOGY

B. coli is zoonotic, occurs worldwide and is found in pigs, rodents, cattle, reptiles, birds, fish, annelids, arthropods, and many simian hosts. The pig is the most common and heavily parasitized animal, usually is asymptomatic, and is the main source of infection for humans.[6] Humans are relatively refractory to infection with *B. coli* of porcine origin, but once the parasite has become established in humans, rarely it can spread from person to person by the fecal–oral route.[7] Achlorhydria, a heavy inoculum, and immunosuppression are likely to increase the risk for infection in humans. Efforts to infect human volunteers fed gelatin capsules containing *B. coli* cysts were not successful.[8]

Although infections have been reported from most parts of the world, a relatively high prevalence has been found in some tropical and subtropical areas, including New Guinea, southern Iran, South and Central America, central Asia, the Philippines, and some Pacific islands.[1,9] In Papua New Guinea, where pigs are a common domestic animal, the prevalence of infection is high (28%).[10,11] In Peru, 6% of a studied population was found to be infected with *B. coli*,[12] and in 11 of 22 Bolivian Altiplano communities surveyed, the prevalence of infection with *B. coli* was 1% to 5%.[13] An epidemic of balantidiasis was associated with contamination of the water supply by pig feces during a typhoon in the Pacific island of Truk.[14] In countries like Iran, wild boars probably are another source of *B. coli*.[9] In the United States and other economically developed countries, sporadic infections have been reported in facilities for the handicapped where poor conditions of personal hygiene prevailed.[15] Human infection is rare in indus-

trialized countries, but infection can occur in susceptible immunocompromised people.[16,17]

CLINICAL MANIFESTATIONS

Most infected humans are asymptomatic. However, the organism can invade mucosa of the cecum and colon causing clinical illness (Figure 259-4), which takes two main forms, diarrhea, which can become chronic, and dysentery. Colonic perforation, appendicitis, and spread to the genitourinary tract has been reported.[18] In most people, recovery occurs without treatment in mild balantidiasis, but in a few cases, especially in malnourished or immunosuppressed hosts, the course can be fulminating and fatal.[19] The course usually is chronic, with intermittent episodes of diarrhea of varying severity and constipation associated with abdominal pain, anorexia, weight loss, and weakness. Sometimes, symptoms in the cecal region mimic appendicitis. The differential diagnosis includes amebic and bacillary dysentery as well as noninfectious causes including inflammatory bowel disease. Rarely, parasites perforate the intestinal wall by penetrating through the muscular layers into the peritoneal cavity. Extraintestinal infections affecting the liver, lungs, and genitourinary tract have been reported.[16,20,21] *B. coli* should be considered in immunocompromised people with diarrhea.[16,19–21] Factors predisposing to clinical illness are malnutrition, alcoholism, hypochlorhydria and other causes of immunosuppression, such as malignancies.

DIAGNOSIS

The diagnosis is made by visualizing organisms in a fecal specimen or in scrapings taken from the periphery of ulcers or by endoscopic biopsy of an ulcer. The large size and spiraling motility make the protozoa easy to recognize. *B. coli* is shed irregularly, and repeated examination of feces may be necessary. Motile trophozoites are present when stools are watery or dysenteric; cysts are found in semiformed or formed stools. Because trophozoites disintegrate rapidly in fecal specimens, samples must be examined immediately after collection or be placed in preservative solutions. *B. coli* do not stain well on permanent stained smears, so direct preparations of fresh or concentrated material should be used for identification.[1,5] A phase contrast microscope can be used to help identify *B. coli* features such as the oral apparatus, somatic ciliation, and the macronucleus.[1]

TREATMENT AND PREVENTION

Tetracycline, which should not be given to pregnant women and children younger than 8 years of age, is the drug of choice.[22,23] Tetracycline (40 mg/kg/day orally in 4 divided doses; maximum, 2 g/day) for a course of 10 days is effective. Alternative therapies are metronidazole (35 to 50 mg/kg/day orally in 3 divided doses;

maximum 750 mg 3 times a day) for 5 days, or iodoquinol (30 to 40 mg/kg/day orally in 3 divided doses; maximum 650 mg 3 times a day) for 20 days.[22,23]

Prevention of contamination of the environment with pig feces is important. Reducing human contact with infected pigs and with

contaminated food and water as well as improvement in conditions of personal hygiene and nutrition are additional methods of control. Control of cockroaches, which are an important reservoir for cysts of *B. coli*, is important especially in areas where people use pit latrines.[24]

260 *Blastocystis* Species

Frank E. Berkowitz

Blastocystis is a protozoan organism that infects the lower intestine of humans and many animals. Although *B. hominis* has been implicated as a cause of various gastrointestinal tract symptoms, its role as a pathogen, mechanism of transmission, and life cycle have been the subject of debate.[1–4] A clinical syndrome of self-limited abdominal pain, diarrhea, nausea, anorexia, and flatulence has been described in several series of predominantly adult patients.[5–7] When no other cause of disease has been identified in a patient, *B. hominis* should be considered as a possible agent of intestinal disease. Because the actual species of organism cannot be determined by routine diagnostic tests, it should be reported as *Blastocystis* sp., not as *B. hominis*.

PATHOGEN

Blastocystis is a protist organism placed within the kingdom Chromista. It is diverse genetically, which might explain the controversies around whether it is a pathogen.[1,2] *Blastocystis* spp. infect a wide variety of animals, and have been reported in humans from around the world. There are 9 main subtypes, with humans infected most commonly with subtype 3. Several distinct morphologic stages have been characterized: vacuolar, granular, ameboid, and cystic. The vacuolar form is observed most frequently in clinical samples; it usually divides by binary fission, generally is spherical, and usually ranges from 5 to 14 μm in diameter but can vary from 3 to 120 μm.[1] The granular form is found primarily in older cultures and rarely in fecal specimens. The ameboid form is observed in culture and occasionally in diarrheal stools where it can resemble leukocytes. The cystic form ranges from 2 to 5 μm, is the transmissible form, and is able to survive at room temperature for up to 19 days but is fragile at extremes of heat and cold and when exposed to commonly used disinfectants. Following ingestion of an infectious cyst, the organism lives in the lumen of the cecum and proximal colon where excystation occurs. Cysts then develop into vacuolar forms and undergo encystations before being excreted as the cyst form, which, if eaten, completes the cycle.[1–3]

EPIDEMIOLOGY

B. hominis is distributed throughout the world. Surveys of intestinal parasites in population groups in developing countries documented prevalence rates of 54% in Papua New Guinea and 33% among travelers and foreign residents with diarrhea in Nepal.[8,9] In the United States, surveillance data from clinical microbiology laboratories report prevalence rates in the range of 10% to 18% of stool samples examined.[1,2] In a 2000 study of fecal specimens from 48 states and the District of Columbia, *B. hominis* was identified in 23% of 5792 stool specimens.[10]

There are few reports of *Blastocystis* infection in children.[1,11–15] A laboratory-based report described *Blastocystis* in 5% of samples from children through 18 years of age in the U.S. A community-based survey northeast of Mexico City reported a frequency of 7%

in children <14 years of age.[11] A study of the prevalence of enteroparasites in a facility for orphaned and homeless children in Argentina found 44% of stool samples had *B. hominis*.[16] A similar study of children living in residential institutions and street communities in metropolitan Manila, Philippines found *B. hominis* in 41% of children examined.[15] A community-based study in Papua New Guinea found that >65% of children <18 years of age had *Blastocystis*.[8]

Little is known about the mode of transmission among humans, although by analogy with other intestinal protozoa, fecal–oral spread is the suspected mechanism. Infections have been associated with recent travel to the tropics and consumption of untreated water.[1,17,18] *Blastocystis* spp. have been documented in nosocomial diarrhea and in children attending childcare centers.[13,19] Sexually active homosexual men have *Blastocystis* spp. infection rates as high as 52%,[10] a finding consistent with person-to-person transmission. Limited data suggest that illness due to *Blastocystis* may be more severe in patients with acquired immunodeficiency syndrome (AIDS) and other immunocompromising disorders.[20,21] Isolation of *Blastocystis* spp. has been reported from a variety of animals, birds, reptiles, and insects.[22] Working closely with animals increases the risk of becoming infected with *Blastocystis* spp.[23]

CLINICAL MANIFESTATIONS

Whether *Blastocystis* causes disease is controversial, and the possible mechanism of pathogenicity is unclear.[1,4,5] Symptoms associated with infection are abdominal pain, diarrhea, nausea, anorexia, bloating, and flatulence. The apparent differences in pathogenicity might be due to the genetic variability of the organism. Nevertheless, presence of this organism in stool suggests that the individual is exposed to fecally contaminated food or water. Symptoms last for 3 to 10 days but can persist for weeks to months.

The mechanism by which *Blastocystis* mediates intestinal disease is unclear. Attempts to infect germ-free guinea pigs did not provide convincing evidence of pathogenicity, except when large numbers of organisms were inoculated with normal enteric flora.[1–3] Gross pathologic effects were limited to mild intestinal hyperemia. Microscopic examination revealed a slight increase in cellularity and intraepithelial penetration by *Blastocystis*. A case-control study examining the association between acquisition of *Blastocystis* and presence of mucosal lesions by upper gastrointestinal endoscopy and sigmoidoscopy failed to demonstrate intestinal pathology.[24]

DIAGNOSIS

Diagnosis is made by detection of the organism by staining of a fixed fecal specimen with iron hematoxylin or trichrome stain[1] (Figure 260-1). This method is superior to iodine staining of a wet mount. When detected, quantification should be reported. The presence of >5 organisms per high power field (×400) or per oil-immersion field (×1000) has been used for quantification in different studies. Recognition of the organism can be difficult because of large variation in size and form. *Blastocystis* organisms can be grown in culture in Jones medium. Polymerase chain reaction (PCR) has been shown to be highly sensitive, and specific, but PCR is not standardized or available widely.[25,26] Serology is not helpful in diagnosing *Blastocystis* infection.

TREATMENT AND PREVENTION

Detection of the organism in feces should not automatically lead to administration of antimicrobial therapy since the clinical significance of these organisms is controversial. Most children in whom *Blastocystis* is found should not be treated. Therapy should be considered when there is persistent, significant diarrhea and when no other cause is found. Drugs that should be considered are metronidazole, iodoquinol, and trimethoprim-sulfamethoxazole (TMP-SMX).[27] Egyptian patients[11,28] with diarrhea and *Blastocystis* as the sole identified cause treated with nitazoxanide, Mexican and Italian patients[29] treated with metronidazole, and patients in Turkey[30] treated with TMP-SMX resolved their symptoms and had eradication of organisms.

Prevention of *Blastocystis* infection involves adequate sanitation, careful handwashing, avoidance of untreated water, and use of enteric precautions to interrupt person-to-person spread.

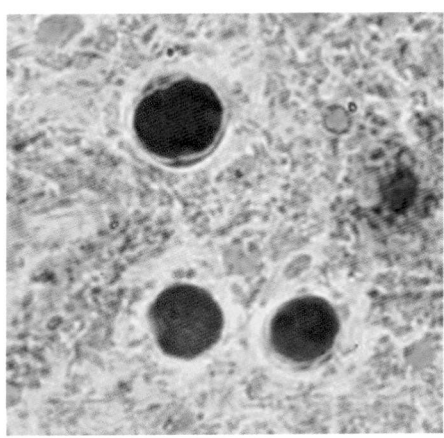

Figure 260-1. Cyst-like forms of *Blastocystis* stained with trichrome stain. (Courtesy of DPDx image library, CDC.)

261 *Cryptosporidium* Species

Patricia M. Flynn

Human disease caused by *Cryptosporidium* sp. was first described in 1976 and became recognized increasingly during the acquired immunodeficiency syndrome (AIDS) epidemic. Improved detection of oocysts in feces has shown *Cryptosporidium* to be a common cause of diarrhea in both immunocompetent and immunocompromised hosts.[1] *Cryptosporidium* is one of 10 enteric organisms in the Centers for Disease Control and Prevention's Foodborne Disease Active Surveillance Network (FoodNet).[2]

THE PATHOGEN

Organisms of the genus *Cryptosporidium* are 2- to 6-μm coccidian parasites that infect epithelial cells lining the digestive and respiratory tracts of vertebrates, including fish, birds, reptiles, and mammals as well as humans. The organism lacks host specificity; however, most human infections are caused by *Cryptosporidium hominis* or *C. parvum*.[3–5] The life cycle of *Cryptosporidium* is similar to that of other true coccidia that infect mammals. Infectious oocysts excyst within the lumen of the intestine and release sporozoites. The released sporozoites penetrate host cells, where they develop into trophozoites. Trophozoites can undergo asexual division resulting in autoinfection in adjacent cells or undergo sexual reproduction resulting in formation of oocysts. After fertilization of gametes, a thick-walled oocyst is formed. The oocysts of *Cryptosporidium* undergo sporogony within the host cells and are infectious when released in feces.[3]

EPIDEMIOLOGY

Oocysts of *Cryptosporidium* withstand adverse environmental conditions and can survive for long periods if stored moist and cold.[6] Oocysts are resistant to common disinfectants, including disinfectants recommended for hospital use. One study reported that ammonia concentrations >50% and formalin concentrations ≥10% were necessary to kill the organism.[7]

Infection occurs following ingestion or, possibly, inhalation of infectious spores.[8] In healthy adult volunteers with no serologic evidence of past infection with *C. parvum*, the median infective dose was 132 oocysts.[9] Spread to humans occurs via person-to-person transmission[10,11] and from ingestion of environmentally contaminated water[3] or contaminated food.[12] An increase in cases reported in 2007–2008 is attributable partially to multiple large recreational water-associated outbreaks.[13] Transmission also has been linked with close association with infected animals.[14,15] Person-to-person transmission is responsible for cryptosporidiosis outbreaks in childcare centers and hospitals and is most often caused by *C. hominis*.[16] *Cryptosporidium* also causes traveler's diarrhea.[3] In the United States, reported cases of cryptosporidiosis peak in the summer and early fall (June through October), especially in young children.[17]

Zoonotic transmission from calves has been well documented, and other animals such as rodents, puppies, and kittens probably also serve as reservoir hosts.[3,18] Zoonotic transmission occurs in people living and working in close association with animals and is most often caused by *C. parvum*. Outbreaks of cryptosporidial infection have been associated with contaminated community water supplies in several states in the U.S. and in the United Kingdom.[18,19] In 1993, a waterborne outbreak in Milwaukee, Wisconsin caused approximately 400,000 cases of diarrhea.[20] Consumption of untreated surface water or inadequate water filtration has occurred in some, but not all, waterborne outbreaks. Swimming pool water and water from decorative fountains have been linked to outbreaks.[18] An accidental fecal spillage into a community swimming pool resulted in 44 persons contracting diarrhea in one outbreak. Attack rates in different groups of swimmers ranged from 47% to 100% of exposed group members, with the highest rate in people with prolonged water exposure.[21] Waste water in the form of raw sewage and runoff from dairies and grazing lands can contaminate drinking and recreational water.[3,18] Molecular techniques allow specific linkages of outbreaks of

Cryptosporidium disease to human versus animal contamination of water.[4]

Cryptosporidiosis is associated with diarrheal illness worldwide, but is more prevalent in underdeveloped countries and in children <2 years of age.[3,22-24] Surveys of selected populations have shown that infection rates in developed countries range from 0.6% to 20% compared with rates as high as 32% in less developed countries.[25] Seroprevalence studies confirm that cryptosporidiosis is more common in developing countries. In Europe and North America, approximately 25% to 35% of people have antibodies against *Cryptosporidium*, compared with 64% in Peru and Venezuela.[3] Increased infection rate probably is due to poor sanitation, lack of clean water, crowded living conditions, and close association with animals.[3]

CLINICAL MANIFESTATIONS

Cryptosporidiosis is characterized by profuse watery diarrhea that can contains mucus but rarely contains white or red blood cells. Fifty percent of affected people have crampy abdominal pain, nausea, and vomiting. Nonspecific symptoms such as myalgia, fatigue, weakness, headache, anorexia, weight loss, and low-grade fever also may occur as well as asymptomatic infection.[3,6,17,25-27] Severity of symptoms correlates with density of oocyst shedding, which can be intermittent. Symptomatology may vary based on the species of infecting *Cryptosporidium*.[28] Malabsorption, lactose intolerance, dehydration, and malnutrition often occur in severe cases. Radiographic findings are nonspecific and include prominent mucosal folds and thickening of intestinal walls.[6]

The incubation period is 2 to 14 days. Infection can be asymptomatic, self-limited, or protracted with severity linked to immunosuppression. Most immunocompetent hosts have a self-limited diarrheal illness that usually resolves within 10 to 14 days, although diarrhea can persist for as long as 5 weeks.[29] Oocyst shedding can continue for up to 2 weeks after clinical improvement.[21] Prolonged, debilitating disease can occur in immunocompromised hosts, including people with HIV infection, malignancy, CD40 ligand deficiency, severe combined immunodeficiency syndrome, other T-lymphocyte abnormalities, selective IgA deficiency, solid-organ or stem cell transplant, or in people who are undernourished.[5]

Biliary tract disease is well documented in immunocompromised hosts and is characterized by fever, right upper quadrant pain, nausea, vomiting, and diarrhea. Jaundice and elevated serum levels of alkaline phosphatase, γ-glutamyltranspeptidase, and bilirubin can occur. The gallbladder can appear dilated and thick-walled on radiography and ultrasonography. If stenosis of the common bile duct occurs, the extrahepatic ducts usually are dilated.[30] Approximately 15% of patients with AIDS who have cryptosporidiosis have biliary tract involvement. *Cryptosporidium* also has been detected in the pancreatic duct of a child with AIDS and has been associated with pancreatitis and sclerosing cholangitis in an immunocompetent host.[3,6,25,31]

Cryptosporidium has been detected in people with respiratory tract symptoms including cough, shortness of breath, wheezing, croup, and hoarseness. These symptoms can occur with and without diarrhea. Oocysts have been identified in sputum and bronchoalveolar lavage specimens. Not all respiratory tract symptoms can be attributed to cryptosporidiosis because other pathogens often are present, especially in HIV-infected patients. Further study of respiratory tract disease, including the potential for airborne spread of the organism, is warranted.[3,8,32]

LABORATORY DIAGNOSIS

Most clinical laboratories use enzyme immunoassays (EIA) or immunofluorescence assays (IFA) to diagnose infection. These tests use antibodies against *Cryptosporidium* antigens to detect organisms in stool specimens. Polymerase chain reaction (PCR) analysis also has been reported to have increased sensitivity over light microscopy.[33] In addition, PCR may be beneficial as an epidemiologic tool.

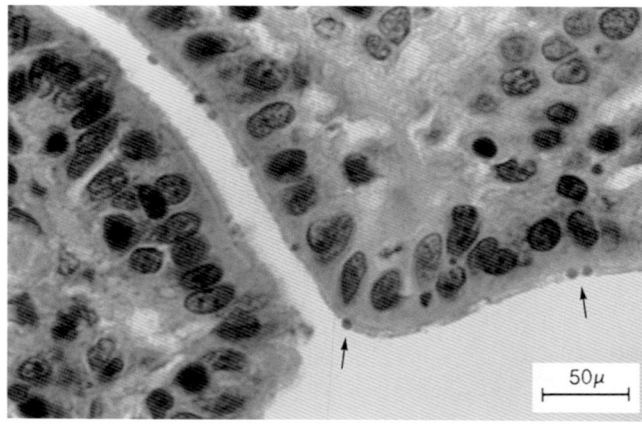

Figure 261-1. Cryptosporidia can be seen along the luminal border of the small bowel in a patient with AIDS.

The definitive diagnosis of cryptosporidial infection relies on identifying oocysts in feces or body fluids, or along the epithelial surface of biopsy tissue (Figure 261-1). On hematoxylin–eosin-stained sections, oocysts appear as small, spherical, basophilic bodies located along the microvilli of the epithelium lining of the gastrointestinal tract. Because not all areas of the intestinal tract may be affected, sampling errors can occur. An indirect IFA can be used to detect oocysts in embedded tissue.[3] Histologic sections reveal villous atrophy and blunting, epithelial flattening, and inflammation of the lamina propria.

Fresh stool specimens should be placed in a fixative before submission to the laboratory, to prevent infection of laboratory workers. At least 3 specimens should be examined in immunocompetent hosts and 2 specimens in immunocompromised hosts.[34] Serodiagnostic assays are available for epidemiologic study; however, the role of serodiagnosis in acute diarrheal disease is undefined.[3]

TREATMENT

In most immunocompetent hosts, cryptosporidiosis is self-limited and requires no therapy except maintenance of adequate hydration. In severe cases, including immunocompromised hosts, a variety of antimicrobial agents have been used with no consistent success. Nitazoxanide is the only approved therapy for cryptosporidiosis and is approved for this condition in children. Clinical trials have demonstrated reductions in duration of diarrhea and oocyst shedding following treatment.[35-38] However, in studies of HIV-infected children in Zambia, nitazoxanide, including prolonged high-dose therapy, did not appear to be beneficial.[37,39] The recommended dose is 200 mg twice a day for 3 days for children 4 through 11 years of age, and 100 mg twice a day for children 12 through 47 months of age. The dose of nitazoxanide in people ≥12 years of age is 500 mg twice a day for 3 days.

Clarithromycin, azithromycin, roxithromycin, and paromomycin, a nonabsorbable aminoglycoside, have been reported to be successful in managing cryptosporidial diarrhea in immunocompromised patients.[40-48] However, randomized trials show conflicting results.[44,47,48] Combination therapy with paromomycin and azithromycin has been proposed but limited clinical experiences preclude recommendations.[49]

Immunologic therapy may be beneficial in patients with cryptosporidiosis. Breastfeeding may be protective.[50] Oral administration of hyperimmune bovine colostrum, dialyzable leukocyte extract (a cell-free supernatant from the lymph nodes of immunized cows), and human serum immune globulin have all been reported to attenuate diarrhea and other symptoms associated with cryptosporidiosis.[25,51,52]

In addition to specific antiparasitic agents, use of nonspecific antidiarrheal agents such as kaolin plus pectin, loperamide, diphenoxylate, bismuth subsalicylate, or opiates have been helpful in management of symptoms, as well as the long-acting parenteral somatostatin analogue octreotide acetate.[25]

SPECIAL CONSIDERATIONS

HIV-infected people have high rates of cryptosporidial infection. Prior to the availability of highly active retroviral therapy (HAART), approximately 10% to 15% of AIDS patients in the U.S. had reported cryptosporidiosis, whereas the prevalence in developing countries, such as in Haiti and countries in central Africa, is as high as 50%. Infections in HIV-positive people can be self-limited or chronic; rarely, asymptomatic infection can occur. A retrospective review indicated that patients with CD4+ T-lymphocyte counts >180 cells/mm³ often have spontaneous resolution of infection. In patients with more severe immunosuppression, chronic disease is likely to develop.[53] Improvements in symptoms and clearance of shedding of oocysts can occur following treatment with HAART.[32] This may be due to improvement in the immune system as well as some effect of protease inhibitors on the parasite's life cycle.[54]

Outbreaks of *Cryptosporidium* infection in childcare centers are reported with increasing frequency[55–57] (see Chapter 3, Infections Associated with Group Childcare). Childcare centers with toddlers most often are involved, and the attack rate can be as high as 67%.[56] In addition, family members have been infected by attendees[58] Transmission of infection within closed pediatric hospital units also has been documented.[59]

PREVENTION

Because the organism most commonly is spread by person-to-person transfer, handwashing helps prevent infection. Alcohol-based hand cleaners are not effective against *Cryptosporidium* spp.[17] Universal precautions should be used for hospitalized patients >6 years of age; diapered or incontinent children <6 years of age should be managed with contact precautions. Infected people in hospitals can be cohorted to limit the spread of disease. Children with diarrhea should not attend childcare. Immunocompromised people should take special precautions around animals. People should avoid swallowing recreational water; avoid drinking water from shallow wells, lakes, rivers, streams, ponds, and springs; and avoid drinking untreated water during community-wide outbreaks caused by contaminated drinking water.[15]

Key Points. Diagnosis, Clinical Features, and Treatment of Cryptosporidiosis

MICROBIOLOGY
- Most infections are caused by *Cryptosporidium hominis* or *C. parvum*, 2- to 6-μm coccidian parasites that infect epithelial cells lining the intestinal and respiratory tracts
- Oocysts are infectious when released from the infected host

EPIDEMIOLOGY
- Infection occurs through person-to-person transmission, from ingestion of environmentally contaminated water or contaminated food, and through zoonotic transmission
- Outbreaks have been associated with contaminated community water supplies, swimming pool and recreational water exposure, and childcare center attendance

CLINICAL FEATURES
- Profuse watery diarrhea without white or red blood cells is most common

- Infection also can be associated with myalgia, fatigue, weakness, headache, anorexia, weight loss, and low-grade fever; asymptomatic infection can occur
- Symptoms are more severe in immunocompromised hosts

DIAGNOSIS
- Enzyme immunoassays or immunofluorescence assays on stool specimens, or identification of oocysts in feces
- Multiple samples improve sensitivity of testing

TREATMENT
- Self-limiting in immunocompetent hosts
- Nitazoxanide is the only approved therapy
- In HIV-infected patients, treatment with combination antiretroviral therapy may improve clinical symptoms

---

262 *Endolimax nana*

Frank E. Berkowitz

Parasites of the genus *Endolimax* consist of nonpathogenic amebas that inhabit the alimentary tracts of their hosts. The clinical significance of *Endolimax nana* is differentiating it from pathogenic amebas (*Entamoeba histolytica*). *E. nana* is an indicator of fecal contamination of food and water.

THE PATHOGEN

Other amebas within this group are *Entamoeba coli*, *Entamoeba hartmanni*, *Entamoeba polecki*, and *Iodamoeba buetschlii*. These organisms have the same life cycle (Figure 262-1), characterized by a trophozoite stage, which lives in the colon, and a cyst stage, which is infectious. These organisms are differentiated from one another by their morphology.[1,2] *E. nana* trophozoites (Figure 262-2) measure 5 to 12 μm in diameter. The cytoplasm is granular with multiple vacuoles that contain ingested bacteria and debris. The nucleus is small and when stained, the nuclear chromatin characteristically is distributed against the nuclear membrane. The mature cysts (Figure 262-3) are ovoid to round in shape (similar in size to trophozoites), contain 4 nuclei, and also can have small, slightly curved chromatoid rods and glycogen vacuoles. Immature cysts containing 2 nuclei rarely are seen in stool specimens.

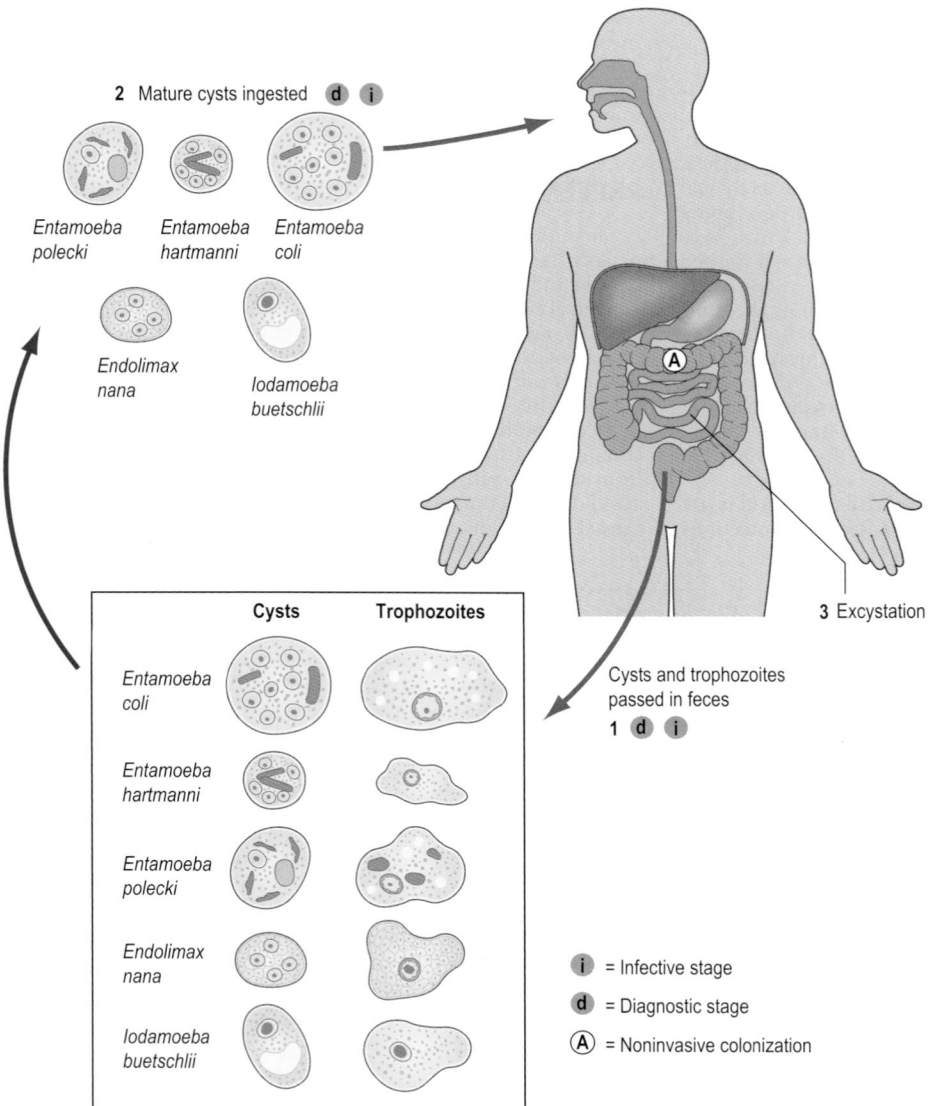

Figure 262-1. Life cycle of *Endolimax nana, Entamoeba coli, Entamoeba hartmanni, Entamoeba polecki,* and *Iodamoeba buetschlii.* (Courtesy of DPDx image library, CDC.)

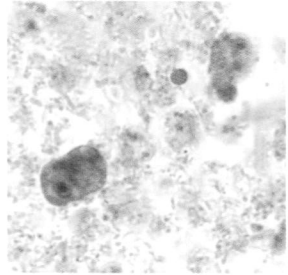

Figure 262-2. Trophozoites of *E. nana* in stool specimen. (Courtesy of DPDx image library, CDC.)

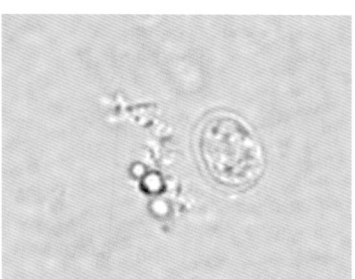

Figure 262-3. Mature cyst of *E. nana* in stool specimen. (Courtesy of DPDx image library, CDC.)

EPIDEMIOLOGY AND CLINICAL MANIFESTATIONS

E. nana has a worldwide distribution, is more prevalent in warmer climates, and has been found in stools of varying proportions of people in different studies, ranging from 4% to 83% of people living in rural areas of tropical regions.[3,4] Human infection results from ingestion of infectious cysts in contaminated food or water and indicates the potential presence of multiple other species of intestinal protozoa.

DIAGNOSIS AND TREATMENT

Confirmation of parasitosis is by microscopic identification of the characteristic cysts or trophozoites in stool specimens. However, cysts and live trophozoites are difficult to differentiate from other amebas, such as *E. histolytica, Dientamoeba fragilis,* and *E. hartmanni.* Cysts can be identified in direct wet mount preparations after concentration sediment or flotation surface film techniques.[5,6] Typical ovoid cysts are identified easily in iodine- and hematoxylin-stained fecal samples. Because *E. nana* is a commensal, treatment is not indicated.

263 *Entamoeba histolytica* (Amebiasis)

Candice McNeil and Upinder Singh

In 1993, two morphologically identical but genetically distinct species were reclassified: the pathogenic *Entamoeba histolytica* (Schaudinn, 1903), an invasive disease-causing parasite; and the commensal *Entamoeba dispar* (Brumpt, 1925), a noninvasive parasite.[1]

DESCRIPTION OF THE PATHOGEN

E. histolytica is a pseudopod-forming, nonflagellated protozoan parasite. It is the only invasive species of parasites in the *Entamoeba* genus infecting humans (including *E. histolytica, E. dispar, E.*

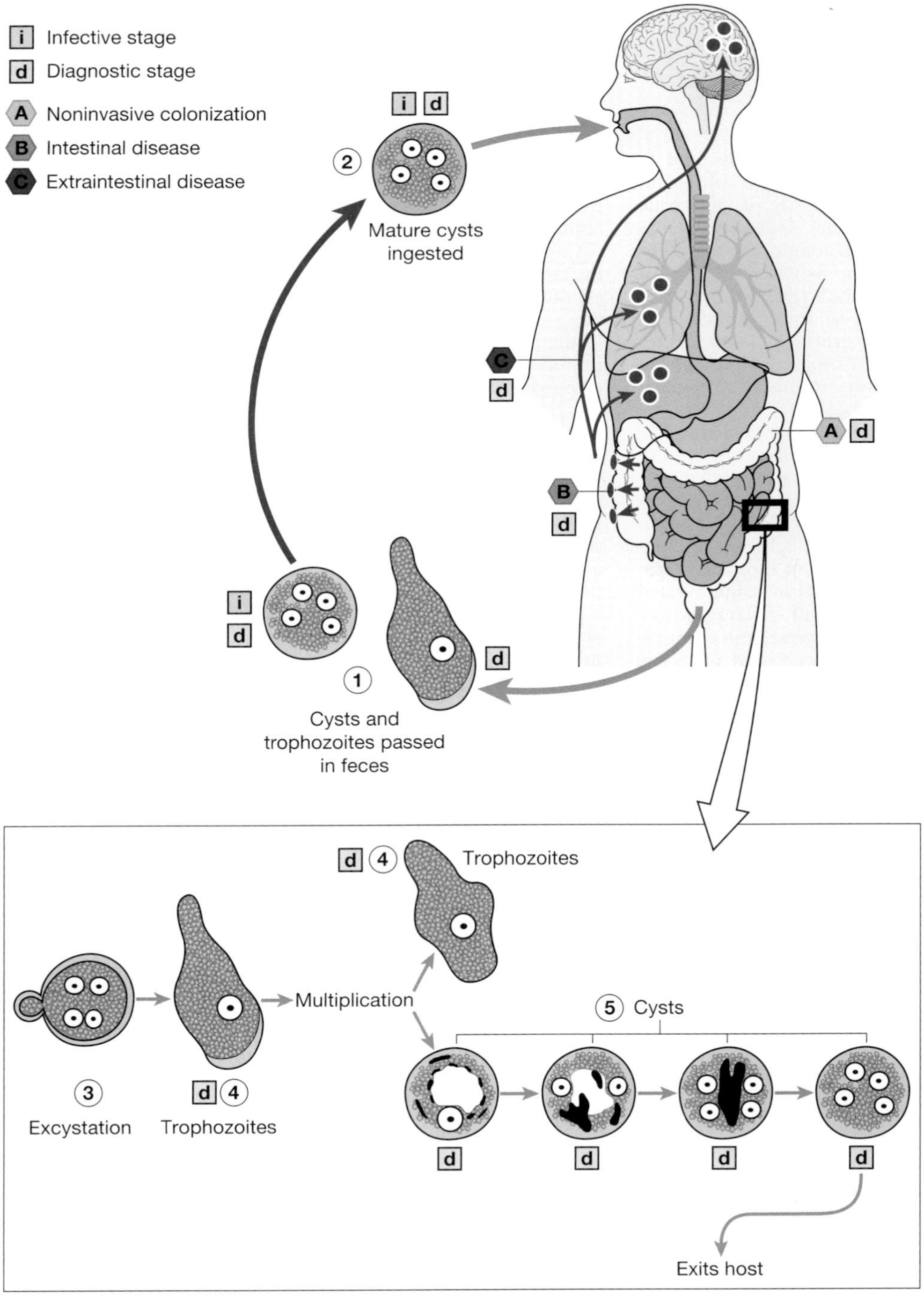
i Infective stage
d Diagnostic stage
A Noninvasive colonization
B Intestinal disease
C Extraintestinal disease
i d
2
Mature cysts ingested
C
d
A d
B
d
i
d
d
1
Cysts and trophozoites passed in feces
d 4 Trophozoites
Multiplication
5 Cysts
3
Excystation
d 4
Trophozoites
d
d
d
d
Exits host

Figure 263-1. Life cycle of *Entamoeba histolytica*. Cysts and trophozoites are passed in feces (1). Cysts are typically found in formed stool, whereas trophozoites are typically found in diarrheal stool. Infection by *Entamoeba histolytica* occurs by ingestion of mature cysts (2) in fecally contaminated food, water, or hands. Excystation (3) occurs in the small intestine and trophozoites (4) are released, which migrate to the large intestine. The trophozoites multiply by binary fission and produce cysts (5), and both stages are passed in the feces. Because of the protection conferred by their walls, the cysts can survive days to weeks in the external environment and are responsible for transmission. Trophozoites passed in the stool are rapidly destroyed once outside the body, and if ingested would not survive exposure to the gastric environment. In many cases, the trophozoites remain confined to the intestinal lumen (A: noninvasive infection) of individuals who are asymptomatic carriers, passing cysts in their stool. In some patients the trophozoites invade the intestinal mucosa (B: intestinal disease), or, through the bloodstream, extraintestinal sites such as the liver, brain, and lungs (C: extraintestinal disease), with resultant pathologic manifestations. It has been established that the invasive and noninvasive forms represent two separate species, respectively *E. histolytica* and *E. dispar*. These two species are morphologically indistinguishable unless *E. histolytica* is observed with ingested red blood cells (erythrophagocystosis). Transmission can also occur through exposure to fecal matter during sexual contact (in which case not only cysts, but also trophozoites could prove infective). (Courtesy of the CDC DPDx.)

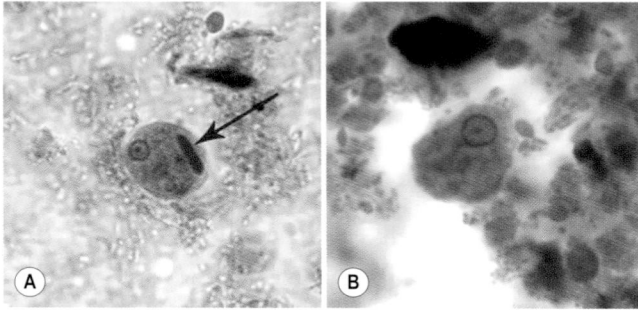

Figure 263-2. Light microscopy of *Entamoeba histolytica* in stool. **(A)** Cyst of *E. histolytica/E. dispar* stained with trichrome. Notice the chromatoid body with blunt, rounded ends (arrow). **(B)** Trophozoite of *E. histolytica*. The specimen was preserved in polyvinyl alcohol (PVA) and stained in trichrome. PCR was performed on this specimen to differentiate between *E. histolytica* and *E. dispar* (Courtesy of CDC DPDx.)

moshkovski, E. hartmanni, E. polecki, E. coli, E. gingivalis, and *E. chattoni*) and the only member of the group to cause colitis and amebic liver abscess (ALA). Molecular phylogeny of eukaryotic organisms based on small subunit ribosomal RNA places *Entamoeba* on the lowermost branches of the eukaryotic tree, closest to the social ameba *Dictyostelium discoideum*,[2] whereas analysis of elongation factor 1 α shows that *E. histolytica* is likely an outgroup of *Euglena* and higher eukaryotes.[3,4] However, the organism most closely resembles lower eukaryotes in structure. Trophozoites contain a single nucleus, which divides by binary fission without formation of condensed metaphase chromosomes. No sexual forms of the parasite have been identified.

The life cycle of *E. histolytica* (Figure 263-1) consists of an infectious cyst and an invasive trophozoite. The infectious cyst is 10 to 16 μm in diameter, contains four nuclei, and is surrounded by a refractile wall (Figure 263-2A). Trophozoites are 10-60 μm in diameter, and have one nucleus with a central karyosome or endosome (Figure 263-2B). The quadrinucleate cyst is highly resilient and can survive in the environment for weeks to months. *E. histolytica* infection occurs when cysts are ingested in contaminated food or water. Excystation occurs in the small or large bowel, giving rise to 8 daughter trophozoites. Trophozoites can colonize or invade the large bowel, but cysts are never found in tissue. Approximately 10% of colonized individuals develop invasive disease characterized by flask-shaped colonic ulcers due to disruption of the intestinal mucosal barrier by the trophozoite. Hematogenous spread of trophozoites to and from other organs is thought to occur via the portal vein. Interaction of the amebic strain with bacterial flora as well as host factors (malnutrition, diet, sex, age, immune status) may influence whether infection results in colonization or invasive disease.

PATHOGENESIS

A well-defined sequence of events occurs during amebic invasion of the colonic mucosa.[5–7] First, trophozoites adhere to colonic mucins and epithelial cells via interaction of an amebic galactose/N-acetyl-D-galactosamine (Gal/GalNAc) inhibitable adherence lectin to host glycoconjugates.[8,9] Then, secreted proteolytic enzymes disrupt the intestinal barrier and facilitate tissue penetration by trophozoites.[10,11] Trophozoites kill host epithelial and immune cells, resulting in tissue destruction. This process was demonstrated as a three-part process in vitro including adherence, cytolysis, and phagocytosis. In vitro, *E. histolytica* trophozoites can destroy a variety of tissue culture cell lines as well as neutrophils, T lymphocytes, erythrocytes, macrophages, and bacteria. Target cell killing is contact dependent and mediated by the amebic Gal/GalNAc inhibitable lectin.[12,13] The heavy subunit of lectin is encoded by a multigene family, is highly expressed in trophozoites,[14] and highly conserved in *E. histolytica* isolates worldwide,

thus having important implications for vaccine development.[15] Contact-dependent target cell lysis is reduced in the presence of galactose and a monoclonal antibody against the heavy subunit, which is able to inhibit cytolysis in part without blocking adherence. Lectin also mediates serum resistance by inhibiting assembly of the membrane attack complex of human complement on the surface of the ameba.[16]

The mechanism of cytolysis has been the subject of intense investigation. In lymphocytes killed in vitro by *E. histolytica*, compaction of nuclear chromatin, cytoplasmic condensation, and membrane blebbing occur, suggesting an apoptotic mechanism of cell killing.[17] The importance of apoptotic cell killing has been studied in intestinal invasion in a mouse model of colitis. Furthermore, activation of host cell caspases occurs within minutes of contact by trophozoites, and caspase 3 inhibitors significantly block cell killing.[18] A 5-kd polypeptide with pore-forming activity in liposomes, *amebapore*, has been identified that may be a major effector molecule mediating the cytolytic activity.[19] Purified amebapore possesses cytolytic activity against bacteria and eukaryotic cells, but cells killed by purified amebapore do not die by apoptosis.[20] Amebapore may co-act with other virulence factors, perhaps by facilitating entry of amebic proteases into host cells analogous to perforin/granzyme-mediated cell killing by cytotoxic T lymphocytes. Finally, within seconds of contact by an amebic trophozoite, the target cell's cytoplasmic calcium level rises approximately 20-fold, and cell death occurs in 5 to 15 minutes.[21]

Chelation of extracellular calcium with EDTA or treatment of the target cells with slow sodium-calcium channel-blocking agents significantly reduces amebic killing.[22] Upon incubation of Chinese hamster ovary (CHO) cells with purified amebic Gal/GalNAc lectin, a nonlethal, reversible rise in intracellular calcium concentration occurs, suggesting that amebic adherence lectin may be cytotoxic directly.[21,23]

EPIDEMIOLOGY

The greatest morbidity and mortality due to *E. histolytica* occurs in developing nations. Disease is more severe in elderly, young, malnourished individuals, and pregnant individuals. Reports have documented the bidirectional relationship between malnutrition and morbidity associated with diarrhea.[24–30] A fulminating form of amebiasis can occur in pregnancy.[31] Intestinal amebiasis occurs equally in males and females; however, 90% of amebic liver abscesses in adults (but not children) occur in males.[32–34] *E. histolytica/E. dispar* infect approximately 500 million people worldwide. Fortunately, the majority of people previously believed to be infected with *E. histolytica* carry *E. dispar*, which does not cause human disease.[1] The best estimate is that approximately 40 to 50 million symptomatic *E. histolytica* infections occur worldwide annually.[35] In Hue City, Vietnam, the annual incidence of amebic liver abscess was 21 cases per 100,000.[36] Seroprevalence studies in Mexico demonstrated 8.4% seroprevalence. Similarly, in an urban slum (Fortaleza, Brazil), high rates of *E. histolytica* antibodies were detected. In Bangladesh, seroprevalence is approximately 50% by age of 5 years.[37] Worldwide, approximately 100,000 deaths occur from amebiasis annually.[38]

Groups at increased risk in developed nations include immigrants from endemic areas, long-term visitors to endemic areas, people in group homes and institutions for mentally disabled, men who have sex with men (MSM), and people with acquired immunodeficiency syndrome (AIDS).[39–41] In the United States, amebiasis is the third most common cause of parasitic infections,[42] with combined prevalence of *E. histolytica/E. dispar* estimated at 4%.[41] High prevalence (40% to 50%) was described in MSM in New York City and San Francisco during the late 1970s,[43] although invasive disease seemed uncommon (likely due to predominant species *E. dispar*). Approximately 2900 cases of amebiasis were reported to the U.S. Centers for Disease Control and Prevention (CDC) in 1993 and 1994. In 1993, 33% of patients reported were Hispanic, and 17% were either Asians or Pacific Islanders.[44] Since 1994, amebiasis is no longer a U.S. nationally notifiable disease.

IMMUNITY

Innate immunity. Amebas encounter natural "barriers" in the intestine and systemic circulation after extraintestinal invasion. In the gut, innate barriers prevent potential pathogens and antigens from gaining access to the underlying epithelium, a process called nonimmune exclusion. Gastrointestinal tract mucins are the first line of host defense against enteric pathogens, including *E. histolytica*. Binding sites of mucins have been shown to compete with binding sites of underlying epithelium, preventing attachment of pathogens to the intestinal wall.[45]

The human complement system is an important early host defense against bloodstream dissemination of *E. histolytica*. The major *E. histolytica* extracellular proteinase, a 56-kd neutral cysteine proteinase, activates complement in the fluid phase.[46]

Acquired immunity. Tissue invasion results in rapid development of acquired immune responses. In a prospective cohort study conducted in Bangladesh, children with IgA anti-Gal/Gal NAc lectin in stool on enrollment developed 64% fewer *E. histolytica* infections during the first 5 months of follow-up compared with antibody-negative children.[47] Apart from serum and secretory IgA, the dominant class of antibodies produced against *E. histolytica* appears to be IgG.[48]

In one study, higher median interferon-γ (IFN-γ) levels in children were associated with >50% reduction in risk of *E. histolytica* diarrhea and longer survival without *E. histolytica* diarrhea.[49] IFN-γ production was lower in malnourished children, which has been associated with *E. histolytica* infections. Innate and acquired IFN-γ responses were not distinguished.[49]

CLINICAL MANIFESTATIONS

Noninvasive Intestinal Infection

Noninvasive intestinal infection with an ameba identified morphologically as *E. histolytica* most likely is due to nonpathogenic *E. dispar*. Examination of stool samples typically reveals no occult blood or amebic trophozoites containing ingested red blood cells. Colonization with *E. dispar* does not require treatment.[50] In some parts of the world, i.e., in rural Mexico, a high frequency of *E. histolytica* asymptomatic infection, higher than *E. dispar* infection (13.8% versus 9.6%), was detected by polymerase chain reaction (PCR), suggesting a predominant distribution of *E. histolytica* strains of low invasive potential in this community.[51]

Amebic Colitis (Intestinal Amebiasis)

Patients with *E. histolytica* colitis typically have a 1- to 3-week history of worsening diarrhea progressing to grossly bloody dysenteric stools with abdominal pain and discomfort. Children can have rectal bleeding without diarrhea.[52] Illness lasts >4 weeks in ~20% of patients. Constitutional symptoms frequently are mild. Whereas fever is present in one-third of patients, weight loss is common. Fecal leukocytes may not be present, but virtually all patients have heme-positive stools (Table 263-1; Figure 263-3).[53-55] Patients with chronic, nondysenteric intestinal amebiasis may complain for months to years of abdominal pain, flatulence, intermittent diarrhea, mucus in stools, and weight loss. One-third of patients with amebic colitis in central Virginia reported symptoms for >1 year. Chronic nondysenteric intestinal amebiasis has been misdiagnosed mistakenly as ulcerative colitis, with significant adverse consequences after administration of corticosteroid therapy.

Amebic colitis can be confused with inflammatory bowel disease (IBD) in children, leading to delayed treatment with corticosteroid if IBD or to a fulminant course if amebic colitis. Amebic colitis also can exacerbate IBD. A high index of suspicion should be maintained in children from endemic regions, travelers, and those with compromised immune systems.[56] The differential diagnosis in patients with bloody diarrhea include causes that are infectious (*Entamoeba*, *Shigella*, *Salmonella*, and *Campylobacter* species, *Clostridium difficile*, enteroinvasive and enterohemorrhagic

TABLE 263-1. Signs and Symptoms of Amebic Colitis

Sign or Symptom	Percentage of Patients Affected
Symptoms >1 week	80
Diarrhea	94–100
Dysentery	94–100
Abdominal pain	12–80
Weight loss	44
Fever >38°C	10
Heme (+) stools	100
Immigrant from or traveler to endemic area	>50
Prevalence (male/female)	50/50

Escherichia coli, and *Balantidium coli*) and noninfectious diseases (IBD and gastrointestinal tract bleeding due to diverticulitis). Often, the diagnosis of amebic colitis is difficult, as manifestations can be insidious or chronic, bleeding can occur without diarrhea, fever is an unusual finding, a single stool examination for parasites is insensitive, histopathologic confirmation of infection in biopsy specimens can be difficult, and serologic tests have limited utility in the acute setting.

Acute Fulminant or Necrotizing Colitis

Fulminant or necrotizing amebic colitis (Figure 263-3) is an unusual (about 0.5% of cases) and severe complication of amebic colitis occurring more frequently in patients inappropriately treated with corticosteroid therapy; surgical intervention usually is required, and mortality exceeds 40%.[57,58] With full colonic involvement, mortality rates may be >90% in children and adults.[59] Abdominal pain, distention, and rebound tenderness are present in most patients with fulminant colitis, although frank guarding is uncommon. Indications for surgery include failure to respond to antiamebic therapy instituted after intestinal perforation and localized abscess formation, persistence of abdominal distention and tenderness after institution of antiamebic therapy, and toxic megacolon. Early diagnosis and surgical intervention is associated with improved prognosis. Poor prognostic indicators include prolonged duration of symptoms, invasion of trophozoites into the bowel wall, and a low peripheral white blood

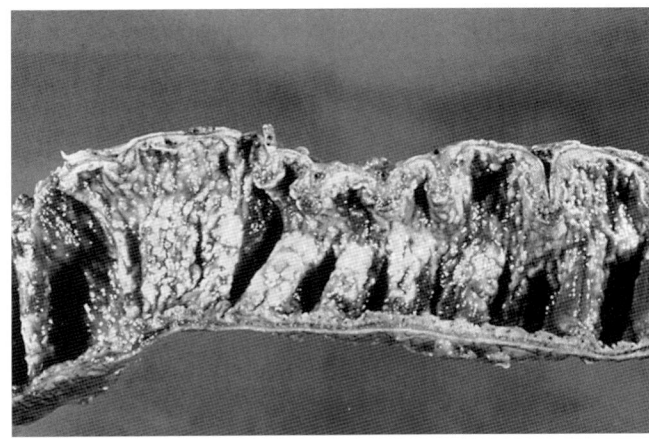

Figure 263-3. Fulminant amebic colitis. Amebic ulcers in the colon varying from superficial to transmural. The intervening normal mucosa shows prominent lymphoid nodules and areas that are obscured by a pseudomembrane.

cell count.[59] Partial colectomy with colostomies is recommended over primary anastomosis for localized colonic disease as the friable bowel wall predisposes to incompetent anastomoses. For extensive disease, total colectomy has achieved better results.[57,58]

Ameboma

Ameboma, a segmented mass of granulation tissue in the cecum or ascending colon, represents the hyperplastic granuloma related to amebic abscess in the bowel wall. Ameboma occurs in 0.5% to 1.5% of adults and children with intestinal amebiasis. Presentation usually is with a tender, palpable, abdominal mass. At diagnosis amebic dysentery is present concurrently in two-thirds of patients. An ameboma typically appears as single or multiple "apple-core" lesions on a barium enema study, with irregular margins and distortion of the folds; the diagnosis is established with colonoscopy and biopsy. Lesions usually resolve with antiamebic therapy and do not require surgery.[53–55] In a case report of surgery performed for intussusception with a lead mass expected to be a lymphoma, an ameboma, was found.[56]

Intestinal stricture occurs in the colon in <1% of patients with amebic dysentery; *E. histolytica* can be identified in the granulation tissue. Strictures usually respond to antiamebic therapy without surgical intervention.

Liver Abscess

ALAs are considered one of the most common extraintestinal manifestations of amebiasis; 5% occur in children. Even in endemic regions, ALA in infants <1 year of age and neonates is exceptionally rare. Adults and young children typically have fever, abdominal pain, and tender hepatomegaly; neonates tend to have fulminant onset of symptoms that mimic sepsis.[34,60] Infants with ALA are more likely than adults to have colitis concurrently despite negative stool examinations for ova and parasites.[34] In adults (but not in children) ALA occurs predominantly in males and can manifest as an acute or chronic illness. In one study, 85% of patients who had symptoms for <10 days had fever and abdominal pain. Chronic illness (2 to 12 weeks of symptoms) is more common and manifests with hepatomegaly and weight loss. Hepatic tenderness is common, but peritoneal signs and jaundice are unusual. Atelectasis, elevation of the right hemidiaphragm, and serous pleural effusion occurs in 75% of patients with ALA, and in itself does not represent primary thoracic disease (Table 263-2).[32–34,54,61–65]

Uncommon extraintestinal manifestations include: pleuropulmonary amebiasis, which is the most common complication of an amebic liver abscess, occurring in up to 35% of patients; empyema and pericardial effusions resulting from direct extension from a hepatic abscess; amebic abscess of the brain, which usually is detected at autopsy; cutaneous amebiasis, which occurs perianally from an enterocutaneous fistula or as an amebic ulceration of the penis or cervix; and genitourinary amebiasis.[54,61]

Growth and Cognitive Complications

Diarrheal illness significantly impacts morbidity of children in developing nations. Among 298 Bangladeshi children aged 2 to 5 years enrolled in a prospective observational study, *E. histolytica* infection occurred at least once in 90% and repeat infection in 68% of children observed over 8.2 years. *E. histolytica* infection had a significant impact on growth, and stunting was more frequent with *E. histolytica* infection compared with *Cryptosporidia*, enterotoxigenic *E. coli* (ETEC), and *Giardia* associated diarrheal illness. Moreover, the relative risk of diarrheal illness also was higher in malnourished children.[66,67] Children with *E. histolytica* dysentery, compared with other etiologies, had lower Wechsler Abbreviated Scale of Intelligence scores after adjusting for environmental factors.[68]

LABORATORY FINDINGS AND DIAGNOSIS

Ultrasonography, computed tomography, and magnetic resonance imaging studies of the liver are equally sensitive for detecting ALA (see Figure 263-4). However, none differentiates amebic from pyogenic abscess.[69–72] Six months after therapy, resolution of liver lesions by ultrasonography occurs only in one-third to two-thirds of cases, thus follow-up studies are not helpful in evaluating response to treatment.

Microscopy-based methods are not capable of differentiating pathogenic *E. histolytica* from *E. dispar* and *E. moshkovskii*, thus microscopy should not be used to make the diagnosis of amebiasis. The possible exception is visualization of trophozoites containing ingested red blood cells, which does favor *E. histolytica* infection over *E. dispar* colonization.[73–75]

Among several antigen detection assays for diagnosis of human amebiasis, a commercially available enzyme immunoassay (EIA) (TechLab *E. histolytica* II test, TechLab, Blacksburg, VA) is the best available test for specific diagnosis in clinical settings. The sensitivity and specificity of this assay on stool in dysentery disease is >96%.

TABLE 263-2. Signs and Symptoms of Amebic Liver Abscess

Sign or Symptom	Percentage of Patients Affected
Symptoms >4 weeks	21–51
Fever	85–90
Weight loss	33–50
Diarrhea	20–33
Cough	10–30
Jaundice	6–10
Abdominal tenderness	84–90
Hepatomegaly	30–50
Immigrant from or traveler to endemic area	>50
Prevalence (male/female)	50/50 in children; 90/10 in adults

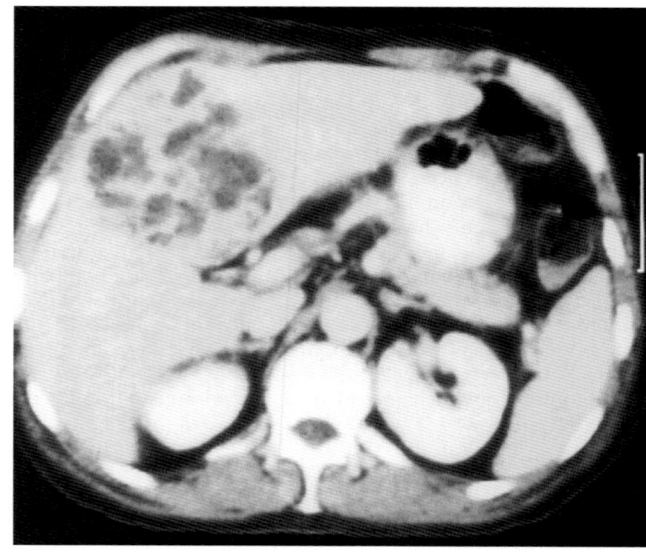

Figure 263-4. Computed tomographic image of hepatic amebic abscess. (From Ravdin JI, Petri WAJ. *Entamoeba histolytica*. In: Mandell GL, Bennett JE, Dolin R (eds) Principles and Practice of Infectious Disease, 4th ed. New York, Churchill Livingstone, 1995, pp 2798–2807.)

Colonoscopy remains important to evaluate other potential causes of disease. Cathartic or enema preparation of the patient can interfere with visualization of trophozoites. The colonic mucosa appears hemorrhagic in patients with amebic colitis, with discrete, shallow ulcers with raised edges. Wet preparations aspirated or scraped from the ulcer base should be examined for trophozoites. Biopsy should be confined to the ulcer margins; special stains, such as periodic acid–Schiff, facilitate identification of *E. histolytica*.[76-78]

Serologic tests for antiamebic antibodies are an important adjunct to diagnosis; >90% of patients develop antibodies to *E. histolytica*, which can be detected by indirect hemagglutination (IHA), EIA, counter-immunoelectrophoresis, or agar gel diffusion. IHA is positive in 88% of patients with amebic dysentery, in 70% to 80% of patients with ALA, and in only 5% of the general population in developed nations. Antibody persists for years after infection; presence cannot be used to distinguish current from prior infection. In endemic areas, 5% to 30% of the population may have antibodies by IHA.[79] An EIA for *E. histolytica* galactose-inhibitable lectin antigen and salivary immunoglobulin (IgG) antibodies to a recombinant cysteine-rich lectin-derived protein (LC3) is more sensitive and specific for acute amebic colitis compared with EIA for serum anti-LC3 IgG antibodies.[80] Other serologic methods, including dot-EIA and rapid dipstick assay, have been used for diagnosis of different forms of human disease, and also can be used for the diagnosis of amebiasis.[81]

Molecular methods have been used to diagnose human amebiasis and to differentiate pathogenic *E. histolytica* from nonpathogenic *E. dispar*. In stool samples, PCR is more sensitive than the best currently available EIA kit for detection of *E. histolytica* antigens.[82] PCR testing for short tandem of tRNA-linked gene repeats also can separate genotypes, and has been used for virulence and epidemiologic studies.[83] Real-time (rt) PCR assay has been used to diagnose intestinal infection and liver abscess in Bangladeshi patients.[84] The sensitivity of rt-PCR was higher than both traditional PCR and the antigen detection test.

Diagnosis of ALA is made by serologic testing as stool tests and abscess aspirate frequently are unrevealing.[85] *E. histolytica* antibody can be detected in serum with IHA assay in 70% to 80% of cases, and, prior to treatment, the TechLab *E. histolytica* II EIA can detect amebic antigen in serum of approximately 96% of patients with ALA.[86]

TREATMENT

Asymptomatic infection with *E. histolytica* should be treated with an intestinal luminal agent alone (Box 263-1). Drugs effective against luminal infection are: diloxanide furoate (Furamide) available (in the U.S. through the CDC), paromomycin (Humatin) (25 to 35 mg/kg/day by mouth in 3 divided doses), and iodoquinol (30 to 40 mg/kg/day (maximum dose, 2 g) in 3 divided doses). A 10-day course of diloxanide furonate has an 85% eradication rate. All three agents are relatively well tolerated; the recommended duration of treatment is 7 days for paromomycin, 10 days for

---

> **BOX 263-1.** Treatment of *Entamoeba histolytica* Infections
>
> **Asymptomatic amebiasis:**
> Due to *Entamoeba dispar* infection: No treatment required
> Due to *E. histolytica* infection: A luminal agent (paromomycin, diloxanide furoate, or iodoquinol)
> **Amebic colitis:** Metronidazole and a luminal agent
> **Amebic liver abscess:** Metronidazole and a luminal agent

---

diloxanide furoate, and 20 days for iodoquinol.[87-89] Metronidazole should not be used as sole therapy to treat asymptomatic people, since this drug often fails to eradicate organisms from the lumen.

Invasive amebiasis should be treated with metronidazole plus a luminal agent. Fever from amebic liver abscess is expected to defervesce after 3 to 4 days of treatment with metronidazole (35 to 50 mg/kg/day (maximum dose 750 mg)) in 3 divided doses for 10 days followed by iodoquinol (30 to 40 mg/kg/day (maximum dose, 2 g) by mouth) in 3 divided doses for 20 days, or paromomycin (25 to 35 mg/kg/day by mouth) in 3 divided doses for 7 days. Alternative regimens include tinidazole for patients ≥3 years of age (50 mg/kg/day (maximum dose, 2 g) by mouth) in 1 dose daily for 3 days followed by iodoquinol or paromomycin as above.[89] Chloroquine, dehydroemetine, and percutaneous drainage of the liver abscess each has been used successfully in addition to metronidazole for the unusual case not responding to metronidazole alone.[89-92] Percutaneous drainage is not required for most ALAs and does not speed recovery.[92] In one study, almost 50% of patients with ALA failed to respond to metronidazole alone and required aspiration.[93] Metronidazole does not eliminate intestinal colonization in up to 50% of patients with invasive amebiasis unless therapy is given for a minimum of 10 days (which is difficult for some patients to complete due to nausea and abdominal discomfort). Shorter courses of metronidazole therapy are associated with relapse of invasive infection months later.[90,91] Repeated stool EIA studies should be performed to document eradication. Systemic tetracycline or erythromycin followed by a luminally active agent are effective alternatives for patients with mild amebic colitis who are not able to tolerate metronidazole. However, these regimens do not eradicate parasites in the liver and care must be taken to assess the patient for hepatic involvement.

PREVENTION

Prevention of *E. histolytica* requires disruption of the fecal–oral spread of amebic cysts. People should be advised of the risk of traveling to endemic areas, safeguards to prevent ingesting colonic organisms, and the risk involved in sexual practices that include oral–anal contact. Because humans and primates are the only known reservoirs of *E. histolytica*, a successful vaccine potentially could eliminate amebiasis.[1,94]

> **Key Points. Epidemiology, Clinical Features, and Diagnosis of *Entamoeba histolytica* Infection**
>
> **MICROBIOLOGY AND HISTOPATHOLOGY**
> - Pseudopod-forming, nonflagellated protozoan parasite
> - Life cycle involves a quadrinucleate cyst and invasive trophozoite
> - Flask-shaped colonic ulcers can be found in invasive disease
>
> **EPIDEMIOLOGY**
> - Approximately 40 to 50 million symptomatic infections occur annually worldwide
> - Up to 100,000 deaths occur annually worldwide
> - Amebiasis is the third most common cause of parasitic death worldwide
>
> - Increased risk of severity in the elderly, young, malnourished individuals, and pregnant women
>
> **CLINICAL FEATURES**
> - Asymptomatic colonization
> - Intestinal amebiasis and associated complications
>   - Amebic colitis
>   - Acute fulminant or necrotizing colitis
>   - Ameboma
>   - Liver abscess
> - Growth and cognitive complications

Key Points. Epidemiology, Clinical Features, and Diagnosis of *Entamoeba histolytica* Infection—cont'd

- Other uncommon manifestations include pleuropulmonary disease, empyema and pericardial effusions, amebic brain abscess, and cutaneous amebiasis

DIAGNOSIS

- Microscopic identification of the parasite in stool, liver abscess, or biopsy is not sensitive
- Stool antigen detection is highly sensitive and specific (>96%)
- Real-time PCR is a highly sensitive, research-based test for the diagnosis of intestinal and liver infections

- Serum antibody testing can detect infection in 70% to 80% of acute cases and 96% of patients prior to the institution of treatment
- Colonoscopy is an important tool to evaluate for other diseases. Wet preparation of material from the ulcer base and special stains such as periodic acid–Schiff should be performed for diagnosis
- Imaging with ultrasound, CT, and MRI cannot differentiate pyogenic from amebic abscesses and are equally sensitive for detecting amebic liver abscess

---

264 Other *Entamoeba*, Amebas, and Intestinal Flagellates

Candice McNeil and Upinder Singh

Pseudopod-forming nonflagellated protozoan parasites that infect the human intestinal tract in addition to *Entamoeba histolytica* include *E. dispar, E. hartmanni, E. polecki, E. chattoni, E. coli,* and *E. gingivalis. E. invadens* does not infect humans but is of great value as a laboratory model in human research of amebiasis. The highly virulent species *E. histolytica* is distinguished from the other, mostly nonpathogenic, intestinal pseudopod-forming protozoa by morphologic appearances of the cyst and trophozoite forms or, in the case of *E. dispar*, by differences in antigens or DNA sequences (see Chapter 263, *Entamoeba histolytica* (Amebiasis)).

ENTAMOEBA DISPAR

E. dispar is a nonpathogenic intestinal commensal protozoan that is indistinguishable morphologically from *E. histolytica* on light microscopy (see Chapter 263, *Entamoeba histolytica* (Amebiasis)). Approximately 90% of the asymptomatic intestinal infections previously attributed to infection with *E. histolytica* actually were due to *E. dispar*. Although *E. dispar* has been shown to cause intestinal ulcerations in animal models, symptomatic *E. dispar* infection has not been demonstrated in humans.[1] The prevalence of amebic intestinal colonization in some male homosexual populations is as high as 33%, and *E. dispar* commonly is found in stool specimens from patients with acquired immunodeficiency syndrome. However, invasive *E. dispar* infection has not been reported in this population.[2] A stool antigen detection test that differentiates nonpathogenic *E. dispar* from the morphologically identical and pathogenic *E. histolytica* is available commercially (TechLab E. histolytica II test, TechLab, Blacksburg, VA).[3]

ENTAMOEBA MOSHKOVSKII

E. moshkovskii is morphologically identical to *E. histolytica* and *E. dispar*; however, improved diagnostic techniques have allowed for its identification in human specimens worldwide.[4] Though earlier studies of *E. moshkovskii* failed to show an association with clinical illness, studies from Bangladesh and India suggest a potential role in symptomatic gastrointestinal tract illness.[5,6] Future studies will be important in defining the pathogenic potential of this *Entamoeba* species.

ENTAMOEBA POLECKI

E. polecki is a common parasite of pigs, wild boars, and monkeys in the tropics and subtropics.[7] Humans acquire infections accidentally, and whether this organism can produce disease in humans

is unknown. In Papua New Guinea, where pigs are the main domestic animals, up to 30% of people can be colonized.[8] The trophozoite stage of *E. polecki* has a frothy cytoplasm and resembles that of *E. histolytica, E. dispar,* and *E. coli,* although the *E. polecki* cyst contains a single nucleus and may contain inclusion bodies and abundant fragmented chromatoidal bars with angular, pointed, or thread-like ends. *E. polecki* has been treated successfully with one of three antiparasitic drugs, i.e., metronidazole, ornidazole, and furamide, with metronidazole given in a regimen similar to that used for *E. histolytica* infection.[9]

ENTAMOEBA CHATTONI

E. chattoni is a parasite of nonhuman primates, although accidental human infections have been reported on rare occasions, mainly from people who had contact with monkeys.[10] *E. chattoni* produces uninucleated cysts. There is no evidence that this species produces clinical disease in humans; however, its uninucleated cysts have been confused with cysts of *E. histolytica*.[11]

ENTAMOEBA INVADENS

E. invadens is a pathogenic species in snakes, producing symptoms similar to human amebiasis. Others reptilian creatures such as turtles act as asymptomatic reservoir hosts.[12] *E. invadens* is not important medically, but has been used extensively as a laboratory model in the study of *E. histolytica* encystation.[13]

ENTAMOEBA GINGIVALIS

E. gingivalis is found only in the mouth and is associated with poor dental hygiene. *E. gingivalis* has no cyst form and can be confused with *E. histolytica* when sputum is examined in patients with pyogenic lung abscess or suspected pulmonary amebic abscess.[14] In patients infected with human immunodeficiency virus type 1, *E. gingivalis* infection is associated with periodontal disease, although a causal relationship has not been established.[15] On rare occasions, *E. gingivalis* has been recovered from other sites, including neck nodules[16] and the uterus.[17] Treatment with metronidazole has been reported to be effective.[15]

ENTAMOEBA HARTMANNI

Previously known as the small race of *E. histolytica*, *E. hartmanni* is a nonpathogenic organism also found in the colon. This organism is identical morphologically to *E. histolytica*, except for its smaller size. Trophozoites of *E. hartmanni* are <12 μm, and cysts are <10 μm in diameter on a wet preparation of stool.[14]

ENTAMOEBA COLI

E. coli is a nonpathogenic protozoan and the most prevalent human ameba. *E. coli* has a wide geographic distribution. This organism can be distinguished from *E. histolytica* because of the larger cyst (>15 μm in diameter), the presence of 5 to 8 (and rarely up to 18) nuclei, and an eccentric karyosome. The presence of this organism in stool is not an indication for treatment but is a useful indicator of fecal–oral exposure.[14]

DIENTAMOEBA FRAGILIS

D. fragilis is a protozoan, most commonly with a binucleated trophozoite. Trophozoites are variable in size but typically range from 5 to 12 μm in diameter. The prevalence of *D. fragilis* is been reported to be 0.4% to 42% worldwide,[18] and up to 50% in groups at high risk for fecal–oral transmission, including children, people in institutional settings, and settings with inadequate hygiene.[19]

D. fragilis has no known cyst form and is unable to survive the gastric environment. The mode of transmission for *D. fragilis* remains unclear. Several studies have shown an association of concurrent pinworm *Enterobius vermicularis* with *D. fragilis* parasitosis; others have not.[19-22] Symptomatology has been observed in 20% to 58% of people infected with *D. fragilis*.[19] Common complaints include abdominal pain and loose stools. Additional presenting symptoms include nausea, anorexia, vomiting, bloating, flatulence, weight loss, and fever.[18,19,22] Chronic symptoms have been reported, with up to 32% of patients having persistent diarrhea.[21] There also have been reports of associations of *D. fragilis* with irritable bowel syndrome[23] and appendicitis.[24]

The diagnosis of *D. fragilis* is based on microscopic examination of stool. Multiple fresh samples should be examined with a permanent stain such as hematoxylin, trichrome, or celestine blue B. Molecular methods also have been used to identify the parasite directly in stool.[4,25] Treatment is recommended when significant symptoms occur. Iodoquinol, metronidazole, tetracycline, paromomycin, and secnidazole each has been effective in eradicating the parasite in the limited number of patients studied.[22,26,27]

CHILOMASTIX MESNILI

The most prevalent nonpathogenic flagellate, *C. mesnili* can be distinguished from *Giardia intestinalis* on the basis of its lemon-shaped cyst and a single nucleus. Some identical forms have been found in other animals but it is not clear that these animals have any role in the epidemiology of human infections.[7]

IODAMOEBA BUTSCHLII

I. butschlii, a nonpathogenic commensal of the colon, can be distinguished from *E. histolytica* in trophozoite form because of its smaller size and sluggish motility, and in the cyst form because of its characteristic large glycogen vacuole, which stains with iodine on a wet preparation.[14]

265 *Giardia intestinalis* (Giardiasis)

Larry K. Pickering and Andreas Konstantopoulos

Giardia intestinalis is a flagellated protozoan that infects the duodenum and upper small intestine. *Giardia* is the most commonly identified enteric parasite in the United States and Canada. Infection can be asymptomatic or associated with a variety of intestinal manifestations. Factors contributing to this variation include genotype of the *Giardia* strain, the number of cysts ingested, the age of the host, and the status of the host's immune system. Diagnosis is made by detection of cysts or trophozoites in stool specimens, duodenal fluid, or small bowel biopsy or by detection of *Giardia* antigens in stool specimens. Several drugs are effective in treating people infected with *Giardia*. Prevention occurs by use of appropriate hand hygiene and prevention of ingestion of contaminated food and water, including contaminated recreational water.

PATHOGEN AND PATHOGENESIS

Giardia, an intestinal flagellate in the division Protozoa, is distributed globally and has been detected in nearly all classes of vertebrates, including domestic animals and wildlife. Molecular typing of *Giardia* strains reveals that human strains are placed in two of seven specialized genetic groups referred to as assemblages,[1-4] which are species specific. Assemblages A and B of *G. intestinalis* infect primarily humans and primates although other mammalian hosts can be infected. Assemblages C through G do not appear to infect humans. These findings suggest that *G. intestinalis* does not have as high a level of potential transmission as a zoonotic disease as thought previously.[3-5]

After ingestion, excystation of *Giardia* cysts occur in the proximal small intestine releasing trophozoites[6] that undergo repeated mitotic division and form environmentally resistant cysts in response to bile salts and other conditions. Attachment to intestinal epithelium by the adhesive disk located on the flat ventral surface of the trophozoite results in colonization.[7] Trophozoites are 10 to 20 μm in length and 5 to 15 μm in width, with a convex dorsal surface, two nuclei, four symmetrically placed flagella originating at the anterior pole of the nucleus, and the ventrally located adhesive disk (Figure 265-1). The disk is composed of microtubules, microribbons, and cross-bridges consisting of proteins referred to as giardins. *G. intestinalis* trophozoites divide by longitudinal binary-fission in vitro, with a doubling time in culture of 6 to 12 hours. *Giardia* undergoes frequent antigenic variations during infection of humans and animals during encystations and during culture in vitro.[8-10]

As detached trophozoites pass through the intestinal tract, they encyst to form smooth, oval-shaped, thin-walled cysts that measure 8 to 12 μm in length and 8 to 10 μm in width. Cysts are passed in feces, and are the infective form. In patients with watery diarrhea and rapid transit time, trophozoites may be found in stool specimens, but are not stable once passed. After ingestion of *G. intestinalis* cysts, an incubation period of 3 to 25 days (median, 7 to 10 days) ensues before onset of symptoms.

After colonization, morphologic damage to intestinal epithelial cells and their brush borders can occur.[10] Varying degrees of villous atrophy ranging from normal microvilli to subtotal atrophy have been observed in intestinal biopsy specimens from people with giardiasis.[11,12] Most people have normal or relatively mild villus shortening. The degree of mucosal abnormality correlates with severity of diarrhea.[13]

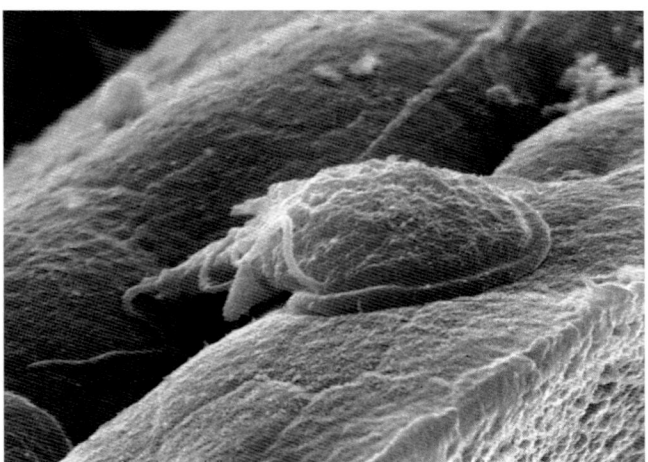

Figure 265-1. Scanning electron micrograph of a *Giardia* intestinalis trophozoite attached to the microvillous border of the small intestine (×1680). (Courtesy of Stanley Erlandsen, MD.)

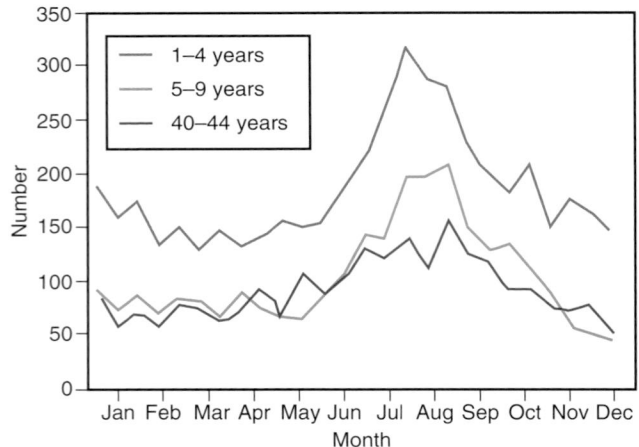

Figure 265-2. Number of giardiasis case reports, by selected age group and date of illness onset, National Notifiable Disease Surveillance System, United States, 2006 to 2008.[39]

Disaccharidase deficiencies, usually of lactase, in the microvillous membrane have been documented in humans and in the mouse model of *G. muris* infection.[14,15] Malabsorption associated with *Giardia* infection in humans affects protein, fat-soluble vitamins, and D-xylose.[16,17] Decreased intestinal absorption of oral antimicrobial agents also occurs and leads to treatment failure of other infections.[18] Simultaneous colonization of the small intestine with *Giardia* and Enterobacteriaceae may contribute to malabsorption by deconjugation of bile salts in some patients.[19] Production of enterotoxin has not been demonstrated.

The pathogenesis of diarrhea in giardiasis is thought to be related to several factors, including: (1) the number of organisms ingested, (2) the specific infecting strain, (3) nonantibody protective factors in the gastrointestinal tract, and (4) the immune response of the host.[20]

Studies in adults show that ingestion of as few as 10 to 100 fecally derived cysts is sufficient to initiate infection[21] and studies in children document person-to-person transmission in childcare centers (see Chapter 3, Infections Associated with Group Childcare). *Giardia* cysts are infectious immediately upon being excreted in feces and remain viable for 3 months in water at 4°C.[4,22] Freezing does not eliminate infectivity completely,[23] whereas heating, drying, and seawater are likely to do so.[22,24]

Relatively little is known about protective responses in human giardiasis. Both B and T lymphocytes appear to play a role in protective immunity,[6,25] as shown by the predisposition to giardiasis in patients with common variable immunodeficiency and in children with X-linked agammaglobulinenia.[6,26–28] Anti-*Giardia* IgG can be found in >80% of patients during symptomatic infection.[20,29,30] IgG antibody tends to persist, thus limiting usefulness in distinguishing current from past infection in individual patients.[30] An association between the presence of anti-*Giardia* IgG and protective immunity is not clear. Serum IgM antibodies increase early in infection and decrease rapidly after 2 to 3 weeks.[30,31] Serum IgA antibodies can be absent in symptomatic people; measurement has limited diagnostic value. Secretory IgA (sIgA) is presumed to be important in host protection.[20] Human milk is protective against giardiasis in infants;[32–34] this protection correlates with the amount of specific anti-*Giardia* sIgA.[32,35] Human milk is lethal to *Giardia* trophozoites through action of free fatty acids, which are liberated from milk triglycerides by bile salt-stimulated lipase.[36–38]

EPIDEMIOLOGY

Giardiasis occurs worldwide and is the most commonly identified human intestinal parasite in the U.S. and Canada.[39,40] Giardiasis

has been a nationally notifiable gastrointestinal tract illness in the U.S. since 2002. Reporting of giardiasis occurs in 45 states (exclusions are Indiana, Kentucky, Mississippi, North Carolina, and Texas).[39] Age-specific prevalence rates are highest in children 1 through 9 years of age (Figure 265-2), followed by people 40 through 44 years of age.[39] In the 45 reporting states, the total number of reported giardiasis cases from 2006 through 2009 ranged from 19,140 to 19,794.[40] The mean number of cases per 100,000 population varied by state with a range of 2.2 to 33.8 cases per 100,000 population. Most cases were reported between June and October, and were associated with the summer recreational water season and with camping.[39] Males accounted for approximately 56% of reported cases from 2006 through 2009. Although reporting of giardiasis is required by 45 states, because diarrheal diseases often are underreported, these rates underestimate the disease burden attributable to *Giardia*.

Transmission of *G. lamblia* is common in certain high-risk groups, including (1) children and employees in childcare centers, (2) travelers to disease-endemic areas of the world, (3) close contact with infected people, (4) people who swallow contaminated drinking water or recreational water, (5) people exposed to infected domestic and wild animals (dogs, cats, cattle, deer, and beaver), (6) people who take part in outdoor activities (e.g. camping or backpacking) who consume unfiltered or untreated water, and (7) men who have sex with men.[39] The relative contribution of person-to-person, animal-to-person, and foodborne and waterborne transmission to sporadic human giardiasis is not well understood.[41–52] Ingestion of surface water treated by faulty or inadequate purification systems has been a commonality of waterborne outbreaks. In addition, drinking untreated mountain stream water is a major risk for hikers. During 1997 to 2006, *Giardia* was identified as a causal agent of 6 of 162 (4%) reported recreational water associated outbreaks and in 15 of 141 (11%) reported drinking water associated outbreaks of gastroenteritis in the U.S.[43,50–52] *Giardia* is one of the most frequently identified parasites associated with waterborne disease outbreaks in the U.S.,[43,50,53] while foodborne outbreaks of giardiasis are reported rarely.[46,54] During 1998 to 2007, of 7650 foodborne outbreaks with an identified etiology, 15 (0.2%) were associated with *Giardia*.[39,54] Because the infectious dose in adults is only 10 to 100 cysts,[21] person-to-person spread also occurs, particularly in areas of low hygienic standards, crowding, and frequent fecal–oral contact. Person-to-person spread occurs frequently in childcare centers and in families of children with diarrhea.[55–57] As with other enteropathogens, individual susceptibility, lack of toilet training, crowding, and fecal contamination of the environment all contribute to transmission of *Giardia* in childcare centers.[57]

CLINICAL MANIFESTATIONS

After excystation and colonization, a broad spectrum of clinical manifestations can occur (Table 265-1): (1) asymptomatic excretion of organisms, (2) acute infectious diarrhea, or (3) chronic diarrhea with failure to thrive or persistent gastrointestinal tract symptoms. Symptoms vary by age,[58,59] with symptomatic infections more frequent in children than in adults. Short-lasting, acute diarrheal disease with or without low-grade fever, nausea, and anorexia is usual; an intermittent or more protracted course occurs occasionally and is characterized by diarrhea, abdominal cramps, bloating, malaise, flatulence, nausea, anorexia, and weight loss[37,41,58,59] (Table 265-2). Stools can be profuse and watery initially and later become greasy, foul smelling, and buoyant. Blood, mucus, and fecal leukocytes are absent. Varying degrees of malabsorption can occur, and abnormal stool patterns can alternate with periods of constipation and normal bowel movements. Giardiasis should be considered in any patient with a history of contact with an index case or a young child who attends a childcare center, has traveled recently to an endemic area, or has gastrointestinal tract symptoms, including persistent or intermittent diarrhea and constipation, malabsorption, crampy abdominal pain, abdominal bloating, unexplained gastrointestinal tract symptoms, failure to thrive, or weight loss. Extraintestinal involvement is unusual, but trophozoites occasionally migrate into bile or pancreatic ducts. Infrequently associated conditions with giardiasis include reactive arthritis,[60] urticaria,[61,62] and retinal changes.[63]

The asymptomatic carrier rate of *G. intestinalis* is estimated to be 3% to 7% in the U.S. and as high as 20% in southern regions. In prevalence studies of children younger than 36 months of age enrolled in childcare centers, *Giardia* cysts have been found in 21% and 26% of asymptomatic children.[64,65] Longitudinal studies have shown that asymptomatic infections are well tolerated.[64,66] Thus, neither testing of case contacts nor treatment of asymptomatically infected people is indicated routinely.

Humoral immunodeficiencies, including common variable hypogammaglobulinemia and X-linked agammaglobulinemia, predispose humans to chronic symptomatic giardiasis.[6,26–28] People with sIgA deficiency appear to have an increased risk for *Giardia* infection.[67,68] Children with severe T-lymphocyte deficiencies from thymic dysplasia (DiGeorge syndrome) and patients with acquired immunodeficiency syndrome with a low CD4+ T-lymphocyte count do not have persistent or severe diarrheal episodes from *Giardia*.[20] People with cystic fibrosis have a higher incidence of *Giardia* infection,[69] probably as a result of local factors such as an increased amount of mucus, which may protect the organism in the duodenum.

DIAGNOSIS

A definitive diagnosis is established by detection of *Giardia* trophozoites or cysts in stool specimens, duodenal fluid or small-bowel tissue by microscopic examination using staining methods such as trichrome or direct fluorescent antibody (DFA) assays; by detecting soluble stool antigens using enzyme immunoassays (EIA); or by using molecular techniques including polymerase chain reaction (PCR).[70–73] The traditional method used was identification of trophozoites and cysts on direct smears or concentrated specimens of stool. Trophozoites are fragile and more likely to be present in unformed stools as a result of rapid intestinal transit time. Stools should be examined fresh, or placed in a preservative fluid. Laboratories can reduce reagent and personnel costs by pooling specimens submitted for detection of *Giardia* from different patients before evaluation by EIA.[74,75] Because variability in concentration of *Giardia* organisms in stool can make infection difficult to diagnosis,[76] fecal immunoassays that do not require microscopy (EIA) and rapid immunochromatogenic cartridge assays, which are rapid and more sensitive and specific, are preferred by many laboratories.[77] These rapid diagnostic tests can be positive both before [78] and after[31] detection of organisms by

TABLE 265-1. Clinical Symptoms of Giardiasis

Symptom	Percent Range
Diarrhea	64–100
Malaise, weakness	72–97
Abdominal distention	42–97
Flatulence	35–97
Abdominal cramps	44–81
Nausea	14–79
Foul-smelling, greasy stools	15–79
Anorexia	41–73
Weight loss	53–73
Vomiting	14–35
Fever	0–28
Constipation	0–17

Data from references 41, 58, 59.

TABLE 265-2. Oral Antimicrobial Therapy for Giardiasis

Antimicrobial Agent[a]	Pediatric Dose	Adult Dose
Albendazole (Albenza)	15 mg/kg/day for 5 days (max, 400 mg/day)	400 mg/day for 5 days
Furazolidone (Furoxone)	6 mg/kg/day divided into 3–4 doses for 7 to 10 days	100 mg qid for 7 to 10 days
Metronidazole (Flagyl)	15 mg/kg/day divided into 3 doses for 5 days	250 mg tid for 5–7 days
Nitazoxanide (Alinia)	12 through 47 months: 200 mg/day divided into 2 doses with food for 3 days 4 through 11 years: 400 mg/day divided into 2 doses with food for 3 days	500 mg bid with food for 3 days
Paromomycin[b]	Not recommended	500 mg tid for 7 days
Quinacrine[c] (Atabrine)	6 mg/kg/day divided into 3 doses for 5 days (max, 300 mg/day)	100 mg tid for 5 days
Tinidazole (Tindamax)	≥3 years of age, 50 mg/kg as a single dose (max, 2 g) with food	2 g as a single dose with food

bid, twice a day; tid, three times a day; qid, four times a day.

[a]*For refractory cases, metronidazole and quinacrine for 14 days.*

[b]*Not absorbed; may be useful for treatment of giardiasis in pregnancy.*

[c]*Not available commercially but can be compounded (contact Professional Compounding Centers of America 800-331-2498 or www.pccarx.com).*

microscopic examination. Antigens shared by trophozoites and cysts excreted in stool specimens include the 65-kd antigen used in commercial diagnostic assays.[70,71,79,80] Direct fluorescent antibody (DFA) testing is a sensitive and specific method and is considered the "gold standard" by many laboratories.[77,81-88] Only molecular testing (e.g., PCR) can be used to subtype *Giardia*.

When giardiasis is suspected and stool specimens are negative, the string test,[82] duodenal aspiration, or biopsy can be performed. In a fresh specimen, trophozoites usually can be visualized on direct wet mount. Duodenal biopsy is the optimal method for diagnosis. The biopsy sample can be used to make touch preparations for identifying *Giardia* in tissue sections and for histologic examination, and to identify abnormalities not associated with *Giardia*. Small intestinal biopsy should be considered in patients with characteristic clinical symptoms, negative stool and duodenal fluid specimens, and one of the following: abnormal radiographic findings (such as edema and segmentation in the small intestine), abnormal lactose tolerance test, absent sIgA, hypogammaglobulinemia, or achlorhydria.

Identification of *Giardia* can be difficult because of intermittent excretion of cysts. Additionally, medications, including antimicrobial agents, antacids and antidiarrheal compounds, and certain enema and laxative preparations, can interfere with identification of the organism by altering morphology or by causing a temporary disappearance of parasites from stool specimens. Such compounds should be withheld for 48 to 72 hours before collection of stool for identification of *Giardia*. Because contrast material, such as barium used for imaging studies, also masks the presence of parasites, stools should be examined before performing tests with these materials.

Specific antibodies to *Giardia* have been detected and quantified by immunodiffusion, hemagglutination, immunofluorescence, and EIA, but a diagnostic serologic test is not available commercially. Radiographic studies of the small intestine can show nonspecific findings such as irregular thickening of mucosal folds. The peripheral blood leukocyte count usually is normal; giardiasis is not associated with eosinophilia.

TREATMENT

Children with acute or chronic diarrhea with failure to thrive, malabsorption, or other gastrointestinal tract symptoms should be treated with an antiprotozoal agent if *Giardia* is identified in stool or a duodenal specimen. Several drugs are available in the U.S. for treatment of giardiasis[89-98] (see Table 265-2). Tinidazole, nitazoxanide, and metronidazole are the drugs of choice.[90] Tinidazole and metronidazole are members of the nitroimidazole family. Tinidazole, which is used as single-dose therapy,[91-95] was approved by the Food and Drug Administration (FDA) in 2004 for children 3 years of age and older and for adults for treatment of giardiasis. Nitazoxanide was approved by the FDA in 2003 for use in children with giardiasis and cryptosporidiosis, and more recently for giardiasis treatment in adults.[89-91,97,98] Quinacrine and furazolidone are not available from any U.S. manufacturer, although the drugs can be obtained from several U.S. compounding pharmacies. Furazolidone, a nitrofuran derivative and a monoamine oxidase inhibitor, is approved by the FDA for treatment of giardiasis. Paromomycin, a luminally active aminoglycoside that is not absorbed, is less effective than other agents but can be used for treatment of pregnant women.[99] Albendazole is effective against many helminths, making it useful for treatment when multiple intestinal parasites are identified or suspected.[89,90]

A review of comparative trials on treatment of giardiasis[100] reported that cure rates for patients treated with metronidazole (92% of 219) were higher than for patients treated with furazolidone (84% of 150) (P<0.001). Approximately 7% of metronidazole-treated patients and 10% of furazolidone-treated patients had side effects that were adverse enough to report. A

meta-analysis of 31 publications on treatment of giardiasis also showed that metronidazole administered for >3 days appears to achieve a better parasitologic cure than do other long-term treatment regimens.[92] Single-dose tinidazole was as effective as longer-term treatments.[92] The clinical response rate of tinidazole was 85% compared with 80% for metronidazole (tinidazole package insert). In one study furazolidone, which is available in a pediatric liquid formulation, had a cure rate of 92% after a 10-day course.[101] Metronidazole can be formulated into liquid preparations by special request. Asymptomatic excreters generally are not treated except in specific instances, such as repeated antibiotic treatment failures (possibly related to decreased antibiotic absorption),[19] outbreak control, and prevention of household transmission by toddlers to pregnant women, or people with hypogammaglobulinemia or cystic fibrosis.[102]

Symptomatic giardiasis recurs in some immunologically normal people despite appropriate therapy and in cases in which reinfection cannot be documented. The ability to isolate trophozoites axenically in culture[103] permits in vitro susceptibility testing of *Giardia* strains, although testing is not standardized,[103-106] and study of mechanisms of resistance.[107] Variable strain susceptibility, as well as resistance, has been demonstrated. Switch to a drug of a different class or combined therapy may be considered for patients whose infection persists after single-drug therapy[104,105,108-110] (assuming that the medication was taken as prescribed and that reinfection is unlikely). Combination therapy with standard doses of metronidazole and quinacrine given for 3 weeks has been effective when studied in a small number of refractory infections.[109]

PREVENTION

Prevention of giardiasis involves good hygiene, and avoidance of water and food that might be contaminated.[39] Infected people and people at risk especially should adhere to strict hand-hygiene techniques after contact with feces, notably caregivers of diapered infants in childcare centers where diarrhea is common and carrier rates are high. People with diarrhea, especially children in diapers, should avoid all swimming venues until diarrhea subsides. Information about recreational water illnesses and control measures is available at www.cdc.gov/healthyswimming/ and www.cdc.gov/healthywater/hygiene/.

Methods adequate to purify public water supplies include chlorination, sedimentation, and filtration. Inactivation of *Giardia* cysts by chlorine requires attention to multiple variables such as the chlorine concentration, water pH, turbidity, temperature, and contact time. These variables cannot be controlled appropriately in all municipalities and are almost impossible to control in swimming pools and other water venues.[111-114] People should avoid swallowing recreational water; drinking water from shallow wells, lakes, rivers, streams, ponds, and springs; and drinking untreated water during community-wide outbreaks caused by contaminated drinking water. Travelers to endemic areas are advised to avoid drinking untreated water and uncooked foods that might have been grown, washed, or prepared with water that potentially was contaminated.

Purification of drinking water can be achieved by heating the water to a brisk boil for at least 1 minute or by using a filter that has been tested and rated by the National Safety Foundation (NSF) standard 53 or NSF standard 58 for cyst removal. Filtered water will need additional treatment to kill or inactivate bacteria or virus. Treatment with halazone (5 tablets/L) for at least 30 min, saturated crystalline iodine, or similar chlorine and iodine preparations may be less effective against *Giardia* than boiling or filtering because they are affected by temperature, pH, and cloudiness of the water.[111,114] Additional information about water purification including use of water filters can be found at www.cdc.gov/travel/foodwater.htm/ or at www.cdc.gov/crypto/gen_info/filters.html/.

266 *Cystoisospora (Isospora)* and *Cyclospora* Species

Patricia M. Flynn

Cystoisospora belli (formerly *Isospora belli*) has been renamed and included in the *Cystoisospora* genus. Both *C. belli* and *Cyclospora* spp. infect the small intestine and have been implicated in diarrheal disease. *C. belli*, which first was linked with disease in 1915, is believed to infect only humans.[1] Prior reports of diarrhea associated with "Cyanobacteria-like" or "coccidian-like" bodies in stools are now thought to have been caused by *Cyclospora* spp.[2,3] Interest in *C. belli* and *Cyclospora* has increased because of association with the acquired immunodeficiency syndrome (AIDS) epidemic and identification in water and foodborne outbreaks, respectively.

PATHOGENS

Both *C. belli* and *C. cayetanensis* are intestinal coccidia of the phylum Apicomplexa. Noninfectious, unsporulated oocysts are passed in stools. Sporulation outside the host usually occurs within 7 to 15 days under ideal conditions (23 °C to 27 °C). When sporulation occurs, oocysts presumably become infectious to a susceptible host. *C. belli* can be distinguished from *Cyclospora* spp. by their size and the number of sporozoites in each sporocyst; *C. belli* have four sporozoites per sporocyst, compared with two sporozoites per sporocyst in *Cyclospora* spp.[1,2]

EPIDEMIOLOGY

C. belli infection is endemic in developing countries, especially in South America and Africa, because of poor sanitation, and in tropical and subtropical climates.[1] The organism has been reported as an etiologic agent of traveler's diarrhea in visitors to endemic areas[4-6] and has been implicated in outbreaks in facilities for handicapped people.[1,7,8] Cystisosporiasis has been documented in 15% of patients with AIDS in Haiti but in <0.2% of patients with AIDS in the United States.[1] The presence of the organism almost always is associated with symptoms, and in the U.S., reports of *C. belli* usually involve persons with AIDS.

Cyclospora cayetanensis infections have been documented in both immunocompetent and immunocompromised hosts worldwide.[9-12] Epidemiologic studies in Peru and Nepal have demonstrated seasonal variation in the number of infections. In Peru, infections peaked between April and June,[2] and in Nepal, no infections were diagnosed in the cooler, dry months between December and April.[9] Asymptomatic carriage of the organism has been noted in Peruvian natives.[2] However, in studies of tourists and foreign residents in Nepal, identification of the organism was always associated with diarrhea.[9]

Infection with *C. belli* and *Cyclospora* follows ingestion of mature oocysts.[6] Because sporulation occurs outside of the host, direct person-to-person transmission does not occur. Both *Cystisospora* and *Cyclospora* have been linked to contaminated food and water, although *Cyclospora* is a more frequent food- and waterborne pathogen. The first reported outbreaks of diarrheal illness associated with *Cyclospora* in the U.S. occurred among employees and physicians in a Chicago hospital in 1990; stagnant water supplied to the physicians' dormitory was implicated.[13] Multiple outbreaks associated with contaminated foods, including berries, lettuce, snow peas, and basil, and water have been reported.[14-23] *Cyclospora* is one of the enteric pathogens monitored by the Foodborne Diseases Active Surveillance Network (FoodNet) of CDC's Emerging Infections Program.[18]

CLINICAL MANIFESTATIONS

Clinical signs and symptoms associated with either organism usually are evident within 1 week (range, 3 to 14 days) of infection. Diarrhea is the hallmark of infection for both organisms but may not be the presenting or predominant symptom for patients with *Cyclospora* infection.[1–3,6,16,24] Described as profuse, foul-smelling, and watery, diarrhea can result in dehydration or weight loss. Affected people can have intermittent, crampy abdominal pain, flatulence, nausea, vomiting, and anorexia. Biliary tract disease also has been reported.[25–27] Diarrhea can alternate with constipation in cyclosporiasis.[3] Fever is more common in cystisosporiasis. In immunocompetent hosts, both organisms produce a self-limited infection, although diarrhea can persist for several weeks. Chronic diarrhea is common in patients infected with human immunodeficiency virus (HIV), and onset of diarrhea can be more insidious than in immunocompetent hosts.[1,24] In patients with AIDS, symptoms and shedding of oocysts can continue indefinitely. In immunocompetent hosts with self-limited disease, shedding can persist for several weeks after resolution of symptoms. Bouts of acute and relapsing diarrhea are described as well.[13]

LABORATORY FINDINGS AND DIAGNOSIS

Infection with either organism is best diagnosed through identification of oocysts in stained smears of stool. Although staining frequently is variable, both organisms can be identified with use of a modified acid-fast stain.[12] *Cyclospora* also are detectable with phenosafranin stain and through autofluorescence.[2] Oocysts are round and resemble *Cryptosporidium*, but their size, 8 to 10 μm, is twice that of *Cryptosporidium* (Figure 266-1). *Cyclospora* do not stain with the monoclonal antibody specific for *Cryptosporidium* sp.[2,15] *C. belli* oocysts are oval, measuring 23 to 33 μm long by 10 to 19 μm wide (Figure 266-2).[1] Polymerase chain reaction and flow cytometry have been used to detect *Cyclospora* in clinical and environmental samples but these tests are not available commercially.[28–30] Serologic assays are not available for detection of antibody to either organism.

Small bowel biopsy reveals pathologic changes, including blunting and atrophy of villi, acute and chronic inflammation, and hyperplasia of crypts.[6,7] The extent of histopathologic changes correlates with severity of clinical symptoms, including malabsorption.[2]

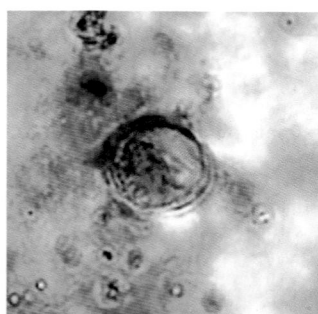

Figure 266-1. Oocyst of *Cyclospora cayetanensis* stained with safranin.

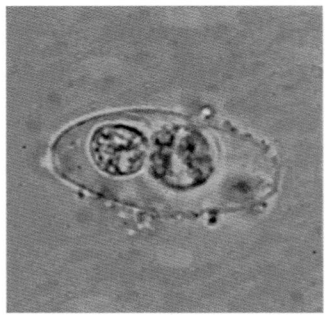

Figure 266-2. Wet mount demonstrating *Cystoisospora belli* oocyst in stool.

TREATMENT

C. belli is effectively treated with trimethoprim-sulfamethoxazole (TMP-SMX).[31] In a study of administration of oral TMP (160 mg) and SMX (800 mg) four times daily for 10 days and then twice daily for 3 weeks to adults who were infected with human immunodeficiency virus, diarrhea ceased within 2 days in all patients; however, relapse occurred in 47%.[24] In another study, initial therapy with TMP (160 mg) and SMX (800 mg) four times daily for 10 days, followed by prophylaxis with either TMP (160 mg) and SMX (800 mg) three times a week or sulfadoxine (500 mg) and pyrimethamine (25 mg) given weekly was equally effective in eliminating diarrhea and preventing relapse in patients infected with HIV.[32] Daily pyrimethamine (75 mg), alone or with folinic acid, followed by daily pyrimethamine at the reduced dose of 25 mg is effective in patients with adverse reactions to sulfonamide drugs.[33] Nitazoxanide and ciprofloxacin also have been reported to be effective.[34,35]

Similar success with TMP-SMX treatment has been reported in *Cyclospora* infections.[16,31,36–38] Patients with HIV were treated successfully with a regimen of 160 mg TMP and 800 mg SMX, given four times a day for 10 days; diarrhea resolved in all patients within 2.5 days. Recurrence was prevented with secondary prophylaxis consisting of TMP-SMX administered thrice weekly.[38] Treatment with 160 mg TMP and 800 mg SMX, administered twice daily for 7 days, successfully eradicated the organism from immunocompetent hosts in Nepal.[37] Ciprofloxacin is acceptable therapy for patients who cannot tolerate TMP-SMX.[26,34] Nitazoxanide also has been proposed as effective therapy in patients with sulfa intolerance.[26,39]

As with all causes of diarrhea, supportive care, including replenishment of fluids and electrolytes, is essential.

PREVENTION

To date, nosocomial spread has not been reported. Nonetheless, careful handwashing by both the caregiver and the patient is recommended. Travelers to endemic areas should avoid untreated water as well as consumption of unpeeled fruits and vegetables, all of which can be contaminated.

267 *Leishmania* Species (Leishmaniasis)

Frank E. Berkowitz

Leishmaniasis consists of a group of infections caused by members of the genus *Leishmania,* which targets tissue macrophages. The obligate, intracellular, flagellated parasite *Leishmania* is transmitted to mammals by the bite of female sandflies of the genera *Phlebotomus* (Old World) and *Lutzomyia* (New World).[1,2] Leishmanial infections are caused by nearly two dozen distinct *Leishmania* species,[3-5] each of which can produce more than one clinical syndrome. Organisms occur in nature in a wide range of vertebrate hosts but are particularly common in canids, rodents, and primates, including humans.[2] Organisms invade the host mononuclear-phagocytic system and can cause inapparent infection or result in one of three distinct clinical syndromes: *cutaneous, mucosal,* and *visceral leishmaniasis,* often with a fatal outcome. Symptomatic disease is subacute or chronic, diverse in presentation, and outcome and intracellular infection most likely is lifelong. Diagnosis depends on visualizing parasites in tissue, by use of serology, or by polymerase chain reaction (PCR) if available. Leishmaniasis occurs in widely scattered foci over 5 continents with an estimated annual case incidence exceeding 1.5 million in children and adults (1–1.5 million cutaneous and 0.5 million visceral cases).[3,5]

PATHOGEN

The genus *Leishmania* has been divided into two subgenera: *Viannia* and *Leishmania.*[6,7] All forms of *Leishmania* infection have three pathogenic features in common: (1) resident tissue macrophages are targeted and support intracellular parasite replication; (2) the immunoinflammatory response of the host regulates expression and outcome of disease; and (3) persistent infection in tissue is characteristic. The parasite exists in two forms: in the sandfly as promastigotes, which are flagellated, and measure 2–3 × 15–30 μm; and in the mammalian host as amastigotes, which measure 3–4 × 4–5 μm. (Figure 267-1). The amastigotes are obligate intracellular parasites of macrophages (Figure 267-2) and the stage that causes clinical manifestations of disease.

EPIDEMIOLOGY

Leishmania species traditionally have been classified based on biologic, clinical, geographic, and epidemiologic criteria as belonging to three major clinical disease groups, with examples of causative *Leishmania* species: (1) local *cutaneous* form, typically self-healing

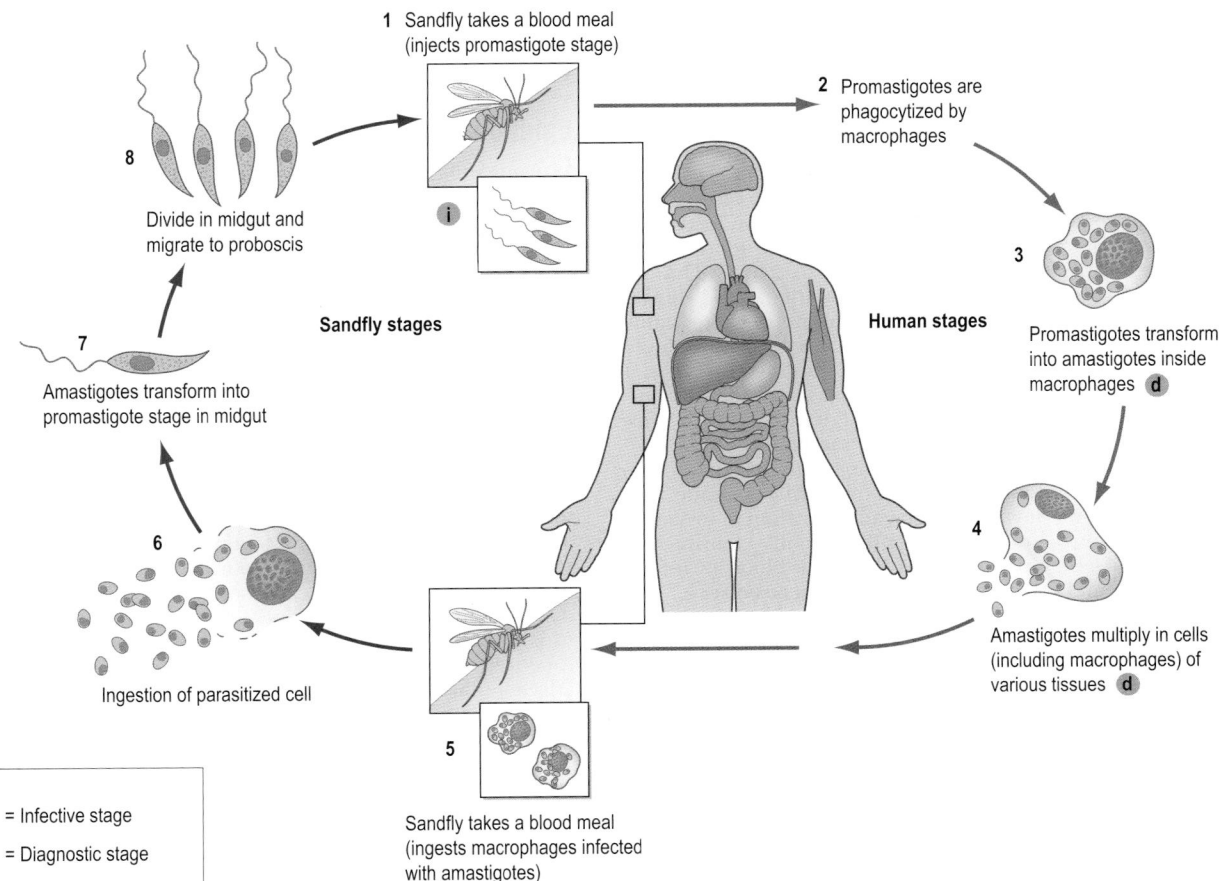

1 Sandfly takes a blood meal (injects promastigote stage)

2 Promastigotes are phagocytized by macrophages

3 Promastigotes transform into amastigotes inside macrophages **d**

4 Amastigotes multiply in cells (including macrophages) of various tissues **d**

5 Sandfly takes a blood meal (ingests macrophages infected with amastigotes)

6 Ingestion of parasitized cell

7 Amastigotes transform into promastigote stage in midgut

8 Divide in midgut and migrate to proboscis

Sandfly stages

Human stages

i = Infective stage

d = Diagnostic stage

Figure 267-1. Life cycle of *Leishmania* species showing the sandfly stage and the human stage. (Courtesy of the CDC.)

All references are available online at www.expertconsult.com

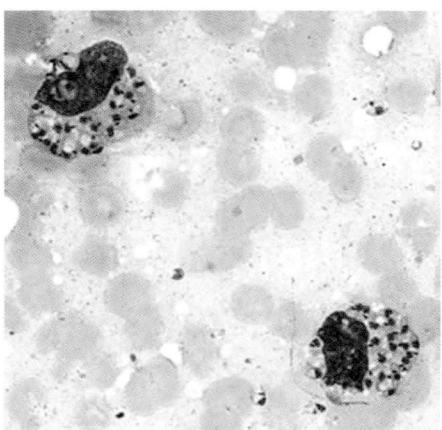

Figure 267-2. Bone marrow smear showing *Leishmania* amastigotes inside macrophages. The kinetoplasts are the small rod-shaped structures adjacent to the nucleus. (Courtesy of DPDx image library, CDC.)

and caused by *L. tropica, L. major, L. amazonesis,* and *L. mexicana;* (2) *mucocutaneous* disease with progressive destruction of the nasal, oral, or pharyngeal mucous membranes, caused by *L. braziliensis* and *L. aethiopica;* and (3) *visceral* form, in which the parasite spreads systemically, caused by *L. donovani, L. infantum, L. tropica,* and *L. amazonensis.*[1,6,7]

Leishmaniasis affects about 12 million people worldwide, most cases being cutaneous disease. About 1 to 1.5 million cases of cutaneous leishmaniasis (CL), 500,000 cases of visceral leishmaniasis (VL), and 70,000 deaths from disease occur annually.[3-5] There are three main geographic zones in which 90% of VL occur: (a) India (primarily Bihar State), Sudan, and Brazil.[1,2] Approximately 90% of CL occur in the Middle East, including Saudi Arabia, Iran, Syria; in Brazil and Peru; and in Afghanistan in central Asia.[3,5]

Most leishmaniasis is zoonotic (transmitted to humans from animals), and humans become infected only when accidentally exposed to the natural transmission cycle of *Leishmania* of infected wild animals, transmitted by phlebotomine sandfly vectors. Sandflies have a short flight range, generally are inactive in daylight, and breed in dark and moist places. Sandflies live approximately 2 weeks, are capable of disease transmission 3 to 7 days after acquiring the parasite, and remain infective until they die. Females, which require a blood meal for each generation of eggs to mature, feed on a variety of warm- and cold-blooded hosts, including humans, cats, dogs, rodents, cattle, bats, birds, and lizards. In endemic areas, there is seasonal variation in the incidence of new cases, with peak incidence approximately 3 months after the onset of the rains, which hasten emergence of sandflies.

In some areas there is a reservoir mammalian host, particularly rodents, hyraxes, and canines (zoonotic), while in some areas, especially India, the infection is spread from human-to-sandfly-to-human (anthroponotic). In anthroponotic transmission, female sandflies become infected if they suck blood of infected human beings and can cause visceral or cutaneous disease.[1] Most mammalian hosts have adapted well to *Leishmania* infection and are asymptomatic, but dogs can develop severe disease. Although leishmaniasis is primarily a vector-borne disease, infection can be transmitted by blood and tissues, through blood transfusion, sharing of needles, and organ transplantation, and transplacentally to the fetus.[1,3,4]

CLINICAL MANIFESTATIONS

Parasitic characteristics (infectivity, pathogenicity, virulence) as well as host factors and host responses, regulate the various expressions of disease and clinical manifestations, which also are affected by parasitic species and endemic region.[1,8,9] Factors for susceptibility and disease expression include age, nutritional status, and efficacy of the innate and timely acquired T-lymphocyte-dependent immune responses.[10-14] Although most clinical infections remain localized in skin or adjacent lymph notes, dissemination indicates differing parasite properties including temperature sensitivity, tissue tropism, and immunoevasive and persistence abilities.[15-18] Host responses include T-lymphocyte activation and cytokine-induced macrophage activation.[8,13,19-24] Regional variations include local parasite properties, population characteristics, mode of transmission (zoonotic and anthroponotic), risk of recurrence, and treatment and prevention approaches.[1,3] The main forms of leishmaniasis (cutaneous, mucocutaneous, and visceral) result from infections occurring in many different geographic areas. Although many different *Leishmania* species can cause any disease, most cases of specific diseases in specific areas are caused by a few species.

Although a clear humoral antibody response is induced during leishmanial infection in humans and experimental hosts, the protective immune response appears primarily to be cell-mediated. Acting in coordination, innate and acquired immune responses dictate overall outcome of infection, including spontaneous healing, prevention of reactivation, and responses to therapy.[1]

VISCERAL LEISHMANIASIS

Visceral leishmaniasis is a strongly immunosuppressive, generalized infection of the reticuloendothelial system resulting in a spectrum of symptoms and findings including chronic progressive disease that often is fatal without treatment. In the Indian subcontinent, late stage VL is referred to as kala-azar (black sickness) because of the associated hyperpigmentation. Most cases of VL are caused by *L. donovani* complex parasites that occur in widely scattered areas throughout the world, and cause classic VL in Asia. *L. infantum* causes VL in the Mediterranean region (referred to as infantile splenomegaly) and Middle East. *L. tropica* and *L. amazonensis* have been isolated sporadically from patients with typical VL, although they are associated most frequently with CL.[1,3,6,7]

Epidemiology

Transmission depends on presence of the sandfly vector, susceptible human hosts and a suitable reservoir. In India, northwestern China, and Kenya, human beings appear to be the only reservoir; elsewhere, all forms of the disease are zoonoses. In India, the domestic sandfly vector *Phlebotomus argentipes* feeds solely on humans. Around the Mediterranean, domestic dogs are the main reservoir, and the disease is urban. Dogs also are important reservoirs in China and in Latin America. In southern France and central Italy, foxes are the reservoir, and the disease primarily is rural. Foxes and domestic cats also are reservoirs in Brazil, and rodents and dogs are responsible for sporadic, rural cases in the Middle East and central Asia. In East Africa, suggested reservoirs include rodents and small carnivores. Humans also can serve as a reservoir during epidemics. Other reported mechanisms of transmission are congenital exposure, blood transfusion, sexual contact, accidental inoculation in the laboratory, and contamination of mucosa and wounds with infectious material.[1,3-5] Animals can be infected by eating infected carcasses.

In countries bordering the Mediterranean littoral, infection usually occurs in children from 1 to 4 years of age. In South America, China, and southwest Asia, young children also are affected most frequently, but in Africa and India, VL usually is a disease of adolescents and young adults.[25] Men are infected twice as frequently as women, due probably to greater occupational exposure. Sporadic leishmaniasis can affect people of all ages and can occur when susceptible people (i.e., tourists, migrants) enter an endemic area. Outbreaks have been associated with movement of large numbers of susceptible people (i.e., agricultural or refugee settlements, military personnel) into endemic areas or may be related to population upsurges of reservoir hosts.[26] Lowered resistance due to malnutrition or other immunosuppressive disease probably predisposes to clinical disease. Mortality of untreated persons with established disease ranges from 75% to 95%. The incubation period usually is 2 to 6 months but can vary between 2 weeks and 24 months.

Pathology and Pathogenesis

Skin lesions where promastigotes are inoculated by the sandfly usually are not apparent in people with VL. Organisms enter skin macrophages, become amastigotes, multiply locally, spread to local lymph nodes and then hematogenously within macrophages to the liver, spleen, and bone marrow, where they are ingested by fixed macrophages (see Figure 267-1). Bone marrow infiltration compromises both erythropoietic and granulocytic cells, resulting in leukopenia with granulocytopenia, anemia, and relative monocytosis.

The spleen is greatly enlarged and congested, with marked hyperplasia of reticuloendothelial cells, atrophy of paracortical zones and areas of infarcts, and fibrosis. The liver shows hyperplasia and infection of Kupffer cells, fatty acid degeneration, focal granulomas, and fibrosis, leading to hypoalbuminemia and hypoprothrombinemia. The lymph nodes usually are enlarged, and parasitized cells can be found in lymph spaces. The intestinal submucosa is infiltrated, especially around Peyer patches. Characteristically, there is polyclonal B-lymphocyte activation that results in hypergammaglobulinemia and reversal of the albumin–globulin ratio. Interstitial nephritis or mild proliferative glomerulonephritis can occur secondary to deposition of immune complexes.[1] Parasites also can be found in the skin, heart muscle, adrenal glands, lungs, meninges, and parotid glands.

Clinical Manifestations

In all endemic areas, fully developed clinical manifestations are similar and include prolonged fever, weight loss, hepatosplenomegaly, pancytopenia, and hypergammaglobulinemia. The incubation period may be years but generally is from 2 to 6 months. The onset in subacute or chronic cases generally is insidious, with intermittent low-grade fever, sweating, weakness, weight loss, and progressive enlargement of the liver and spleen.[27,28] Fever can be continuous, intermittent, or remittent, often reaching 40°C. In the acute presentation in people without immunity, the course of disease is more rapid (e.g., high fever, chills, malaise), and death can occur within a few weeks.

The primary lesion at the site of inoculation appears as a small papule or a cutaneous ulcer, but the lesion usually has resolved by the time the patient seeks medical attention. The patient often is weak and emaciated, with marked abdominal distention secondary to enlargement of the spleen and liver. Femoral and inguinal lymph nodes are moderately enlarged, but generalized lymphadenopathy is uncommon. Darkening of the skin, especially on hands, feet, abdomen, and forehead, commonly occurs in light-skinned patients, giving rise to the name kala-azar (black fever) in India. In dark-skinned people, warty eruptions can develop. Jaundice, petechiae, ecchymoses, and purpura also can occur. Oral and nasopharyngeal mucosal lesions occasionally occur in patients in India, East Africa, and Sudan, appearing as nodules or ulcers of the gum, palate, tongue, or lip. Lesions of the nasal mucosa can cause perforation of the septum. Renal involvement in VL is common.[29]

Anemia, which invariably is present and often is severe, is secondary to multiple factors, including hypersplenism, autoimmune mechanisms, bone marrow infiltration, and coexistent iron deficiency. The Coombs test result usually is positive, with both C3 and immunoglobulin (Ig) G deposits on red blood cells. The differential blood cell count reveals neutropenia, relative lymphocytosis, and absence of eosinophils, and thrombocytopenia. Serum hepatic enzyme concentrations are mildly elevated, and the prothrombin time is prolonged.

Death usually occurs within 2 years as a complication of intercurrent bacterial infection, hemorrhage, or progressive emaciation. Bacterial pneumonia can develop as a consequence of severe neutropenia. Pulmonary tuberculosis is a common complication. Patients with HIV infection can have a shorter duration of symptoms, a poor response to treatment, a higher rate of relapse after therapy, and higher mortality.[30] VL also can occur as an opportunistic infection in other immunosuppressed people, including people with renal transplants and hematologic malignancies.[30,31]

Dermal leishmaniasis occurs following treatment of VL (kala-azar). This form of disease appears to indicate reversal of the agent from viscerotropic to dermatotropic, most likely representing a modification of the host immune status. Dermal leishmaniasis occurs in up to 10% of people following treatment for VL in India and 50% in Sudan.[23,32] Dermal leishmaniasis is rare following treatment in Latin America or the Mediterranean region. The lesions are polymorphic, consisting of nodules and hypopigmented macules that can coalesce to form irregular patches. These lesions occur predominantly on the face and, to a lesser extent, on forearms, arms, upper trunk, and legs; otherwise, the patient has no evidence of systemic illness. Parasites can be isolated readily from papular and nodular lesions and may represent an important source of infection for the sandfly.

Diagnosis

Diagnostic consideration should be undertaken in patients in or from endemic areas with prolonged fever, progressive weight loss, weakness, significant enlargement of liver and spleen, cytopenias and hypergammaglobulinemia. There are several methods for diagnosing leishmaniasis including visualization of the organism, on smears, scrapings, aspirates and imprints (cytologic examination), or of biopsy material (histologic examination) after staining with Giemsa stain or immunoperoxidase stain.[51] Direct visualization of amastigotes within macrophages is the diagnostic gold standard (see Figure 267-2). The main differential diagnosis of this pathologic finding is histoplasmosis. The presence of a kinetoplast in the organism confirms the identification of *Leishmania*. Material for diagnosis includes the base or the inflammatory edge of ulcers, biopsy of other lesions, bone marrow aspirate, liver biopsy, or splenic puncture aspirate. Splenic puncture has the highest sensitivity, but can be hazardous. Amplifying *Leishmania*-specific DNA from biopsy tissue or blood by PCR can be performed if available.[52] This improves the sensitivity, and allows for DNA analysis for species identification; which has relevance for chemotherapy. In addition *L. braziliensis* is difficult to grow and isolate in culture, making PCR especially useful.[37] Several different tests measure antibodies to *Leishmania*, including IFA and EIA. They are of limited value, because of cross-reactions with other parasitic infections and inability to distinguish current from past infection; the direct agglutination test and the rk39 immunochromatographic test have been developed for field use.[1,3]

Parasitologic diagnosis of VL can be confirmed by visualization of amastigotes in tissue, isolating promastigotes from culture, or by PCR.[23-37] Direct visualization of amastigotes in macrophages in clinical specimens is the diagnostic gold standard. Diagnostic sensitivity for smears of aspirates varies for spleen (>95%), bone marrow (55% to 90%) and lymph nodes (60%).[35] Parasites can be found 7 days after inoculation of appropriate culture media; incubation should be maintained for 21 days, however.[36] Finding serum anti-leishmanial IgG in high titer is diagnostic, using standard serologic assays.[1,34,35] In symptomatic patients, anti-K39 strip test sensitivity is >90%[36,38,39] but specificity can vary by region.[35,36] Urine can be tested by latex agglutination.[40,41] Leishmanial DNA can be detected by PCR testing, using peripheral blood or serum.[34-37,42,43]

CUTANEOUS LEISHMANIASIS OF THE OLD WORLD

Cutaneous leishmaniasis (CL) of the Old World is characterized by chronic nodular or ulcerative skin lesions, the classic form of which was referred to as "oriental sore." CL is caused by three distinct species, all transmitted by sandflies: *L. tropica*, a natural infection of dogs and humans that occurs in urban areas; *L. major*, a parasite of desert rodents that occasionally infects humans as a rural zoonosis; and *L. aethiopica*, a parasite of the hyrax that infects people who explore mountain slopes. The spectrum of disease of Old World CL includes single or multiple, localized cutaneous ulcers; diffuse CL; post-kala-azar dermal leishmaniasis; and leishmaniasis recidivans.

Epidemiology

CL of the Old World usually is sporadic in endemic areas but epidemics occur when susceptible people gather in large numbers as during refugee movement. The vectors are *Phlebotomus papatasi* and other *Phlebotomus* species. Both sexes and all ages are susceptible. However, most children in endemic areas are infected between 2 and 3 years of age, and men are infected more frequently than women, probably as a result of occupational exposure.

L. major infects desert rodents (primarily great gerbils) and humans in arid and rural regions of the Middle East, Africa and central Asia, and has been a problem for troops located in endemic areas of the Middle East.[26,44] *L. tropica* infects dogs and humans in urban areas of the Middle East and cities in the Mediterranean littoral, India, and Pakistan. *L. aethiopica* is endemic in the highlands of Kenya, Ethiopia, and southwest Africa. Primary vectors are the tree and rock hyraxes and rodents.

Pathogenesis

In the skin, an intense granulomatous inflammatory response to parasites develops, composed of infected and uninfected mononuclear phagocytes, variable lymphocyte and plasma cell infiltration, and tissue necrosis. This response is followed by progressive thinning of the epidermis, ulceration, and hyperplasia at the margins of the lesion. Amastigotes are eliminated after macrophage activation by sensitized lymphocytes; epithelioid and giant cells appear, fibroblasts invade the lesion, and thin epithelium grows to cover the fibrous tissue. If the epidermis remains intact, initial lesions are dry and nodular. Granulomas can be seen in local lymph nodes. In leishmaniasis recidivans, there is a granulomatous reaction without caseation, with numerous lymphocytes, some epithelioid and giant cells, but few amastigotes. By contrast, in diffuse cutaneous leishmaniasis, massive infiltration with parasite-filled macrophages, and few surrounding lymphocytes, occurs.

Independent of the etiologic agent, Old World CL is self-limited and confers lifelong protective immunity to the homologous *Leishmania* species. Immunity depends on a cell-mediated response. Delayed-type hypersensitivity appears early in cases of simple CL and leishmaniasis recidivans, but is absent in diffuse CL.

Clinical Manifestations

The lesion, which begins as a firm, small papule at the site of the sandfly bite, either grows over several months into a nodular lesion covered by fine, dry, papery scales and an infiltrate border, or progresses to a large, nonpainful ulcer with a depressed granulating center and well-defined, raised, indurated borders (Figure 267-3). Satellite lesions are common and may fuse with the original ulcer. Lesions tend to be multiple, painless, rapidly ulcerating, and covered with a serous discharge. Lesions appear most commonly on exposed areas of the body (i.e., face, ears, neck, arms, hands, legs, and feet), rarely on the trunk, and never on the palms, soles, or hairy scalp. Local lymph nodes may be involved. Healing is complete in 6 to 12 months.

L. tropica lesions typically are dry, single, crusted, slowly enlarging, and may not ulcerate. The incubation period is about 2 months, and the total course of the lesion from onset to healing is 1 to 2 years. *L. major* lesions are moist with an exudate, are larger, mature more rapidly, and typically heal after many months. *L. aethiopica* infections resemble the dry form but produce more

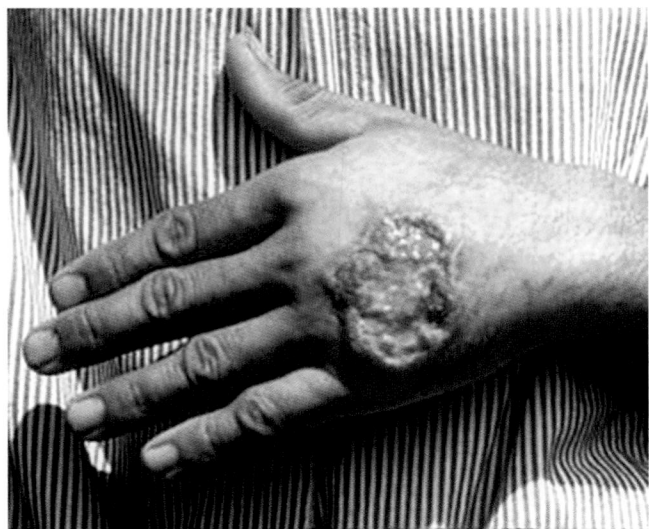

Figure 267-3. Cutaneous leishmaniasis. (Courtesy of the CDC.)

chronic lesions lasting several years. Viscerotropic *L. tropica* infection was reported in military personnel in Saudi Arabia during Operation Desert Storm and also from Kenya and Israel.[44,45] The most common complication is bacterial superinfection of the open lesions. The differential diagnosis includes pyogenic nodules, insect bites, tertiary syphilis, yaws, tuberculosis of the skin, lupus vulgaris, and leprosy.

Leishmaniasis recidivans is a relapsing form of cutaneous disease that usually has been associated with *L. tropica* infections. The lesions often begin on the face and may persist for 20 years or more. Satellite lesions appear at the margins of healing primary lesions, forming small, painless, hard papules. Parasites are rare, the delayed skin test reaction is positive, and the condition is considered to be a hypersensitive reaction with an intense cell-mediated immune response.

Diffuse cutaneous leishmaniasis is a disseminated chronic form associated with *L. aethiopica* infection and anergy to leishmanial antigens with negative *Leishmania* skin test reaction. Diffuse cutaneous leishmaniasis is characterized by thickening of the skin in plaques, papules, or multiple nodules, particularly on the face and limbs, that resemble lesions of lepromatous leprosy. Macrophages containing amastigotes are abundant, with scanty lymphocytic infiltrate.

Diagnosis

Definitive diagnosis of Old World CL depends on one or more chronic skin lesions, history of exposure in an endemic area, and identification of amastigotes in appropriate tissue specimens, isolation of promastigotes in culture or by amplifying *Leishmania*-specific DNA by PCR.[1,35,37] The margin of the most recent or an active lesion is scraped; the material is used to prepare smears and is stained with Giemsa. Alternatively, a slit incision or biopsy specimen from the edge of the lesion can be used for tissue impression smears, histologic study, and culture. In addition, serous tissue fluid from the lesion can be inoculated into NNN or Schneider culture medium and inspected regularly for up to 4 weeks. Inoculation of material into either a susceptible BALB/c mouse or the footpad or nose of a golden hamster can improve diagnostic yield, but it may take 2 to 3 months for the animal to show clinical lesions.

Speciation of isolated parasites with specific monoclonal antibodies, isoenzyme analysis, or use of DNA probes is desirable.[37] The *Leishmania* skin test reaction is negative in diffuse cutaneous leishmaniasis but is positive in patients with simple CL and leishmaniasis recidivans, and remains positive for life. Serologic assays generally are not helpful in diagnosis of CL.

NEW WORLD CUTANEOUS LEISHMANIASIS

New World CL is a rural zoonosis caused by members of the *L. mexicana* and *Leishmania (Viannia)* complexes, which are transmitted by ground-dwelling or arboreal sandflies of the genus *Lutzomyia* spp. The disease, which is found in the Americas, is characterized predominantly by skin ulcers and severe diffuse or destructive mucocutaneous lesions.

Epidemiology

New World CL is endemic in the Americas, from southern Texas to most of Central and South America as well as the Caribbean.[46] The disease usually is restricted to tropical and subtropical regions and to altitudes <2500 feet (760 m), although in Peru, infection occurs at elevations >3600 feet (1100 m). Human infections are sporadic and occur in people residing in rural areas, travelers to forested areas (explorers, tourists, scientists, missionaries, hunters, and military personnel), and temporary workers in forested regions.[47]

At least 13 distinct *Leishmania* species are recognized as causing cutaneous disease in the Americas.[6,47] In general, *L. mexicana* subspecies and *Leishmania (Viannia)* species are the agents of cutaneous disease, and *Leishmania (Viannia) braziliensis* is responsible for mucocutaneous lesions. *L. infantum/L. chagasi*, the agent of American VL, also has been associated with cutaneous lesions, apparently without visceral involvement.

L. mexicana has been isolated mainly in Mexico, Guatemala, and Belize, but is responsible for American CL from Argentina to Texas where a small number of autochthonous cases have been reported.[48,49] It is transmitted among forest rodents by *Lutzomyia olmeca*. An unidentified subspecies of *L. mexicana* probably is responsible for cases acquired in the United States.[48,49]

L. amazonensis is distributed mainly in the Amazon region. The vector *Lutzomyia flaviscutellata* primarily infects forest rodents and rarely causes infection in humans. Marsupials and foxes can be secondary hosts. *L. braziliensis* causes cutaneous and mucocutaneous leishmaniasis (espundia) in Brazil, neighboring countries, and Central America and has occurred in American tourists returning from Belize and other areas of Latin America. The main vector, *Lutzomyia wellcomei*, infects forest rodents and humans living in newly cleared forest areas. It is the species most commonly associated with human disease, which includes cutaneous and mucosal leishmaniasis, and the most widely distributed species in the Americas. *L. peruviana* is the agent of uta in the Andean villages of Peru.

Pian bois or bush yaws is caused by *L. guyanensis* in the northern Amazon basin. The incubation period of localized cutaneous leishmaniasis ranges from 3 weeks to 6 months, although latent periods of several years have been reported.

Pathology and Pathogenesis

The initial lesion is characterized by a large number of parasitized macrophages as well as mild infiltration with granulocytes, mononuclear cells, and eosinophils in association with hyperplasia of the epidermis and necrosis of the dermis. Subsequently, there is heavy infiltration with lymphocytes and plasma cells, and a granulomatous reaction with epithelioid, multinucleated giant cells and few parasites. Mucous membranes are infected by direct extension or lymphatic or hematogenous dissemination. Mucosal lesions show massive necrotizing inflammation with a variable number of lymphocytes, small histiocytes, plasma cells, and few amastigotes. There is an exaggerated, antigen-specific, cell-mediated immune reaction, and levels of serum antibodies are high.

In diffuse cutaneous leishmaniasis, large numbers of infected mononuclear cells are seen, but lymphocytic infiltration is negligible. Both in vivo and in vitro, antigen-specific cell-mediated immune reactions are absent. The antibody response, however, is conserved and often is increased.

Clinical Manifestations

The primary lesion developing at the site of the bite of the sandfly in New World CL consists of an erythematous, painless papule. Over 2 to 3 weeks, the lesion evolves to nodules and eventually to ulcers with raised, indurated margins and granular bases covered by a serous discharge. *L. mexicana* lesions occur on the face and ears (40% to 60% of the cases) and usually are single papules, nodules, or ulcers that heal spontaneously in about 6 months; however, ear lesions (chiclero ulcer) with destruction of the pinna are more persistent. *L. braziliensis* produces large single or multiple lesions that require 6 to 18 months to heal. Regional adenopathy may precede development of CL by 1 to 12 weeks.[50] As the skin ulcer develops, systemic symptoms and lymphadenopathy subside. Both *L. guyanensis* and *L. panamensis* produce multiple skin ulcers and involvement of lymphatic nodules, but nasopharyngeal lesions are rare. In *L. guyanensis* infection, a chain of nodules (which mimic sporotrichosis) may occur along lymphatic proximal to the lesion, especially on the extremity.

Mucocutaneous lesions occur in <5% of people with *L. braziliensis* infection several months to many years (within 2 years of infection in 50% of cases) after the initial cutaneous lesion has healed. Patients have symptoms of nasal blockage, stuffiness, discharge, or epistaxis. Inflammation of the nasal, pharyngeal, and oral mucosa is followed by progressive ulceration and destruction of the nasal septum, nasal turbinate tissue, palate, lips, pharynx, and larynx. The uvula is swollen and subsequently can be destroyed. Rarely, trachea, bronchi, and esophagus can be involved. Death occurs from compromise of the respiratory system, aspiration pneumonia, starvation, or secondary bacterial infection.

Diagnosis

Generally, in clinical syndromes characterized by a robust cell-mediated immune response, such as leishmaniasis recidivans and mucocutaneous leishmaniasis, there are few parasites and a poor antibody response, while in syndromes associated with a poor cell-mediated immune response, such as visceral leishmaniasis and diffuse cutaneous leishmaniasis, there are many parasites and a good antibody response.

TREATMENT OF LEISHMANIASIS

Because infection is heterogeneous regarding the species and strains associated with different clinical syndromes in different geographic areas, firm generalizable recommendations for therapy cannot be made. Several different drugs can be used for treatment, but several drug-related factors should be considered: the balance between the adverse effects (which are significant) and the benefits of therapy, the ease of administration, the capacity of the patient and the healthcare system for several-week hospitalization, and cost.

Treatment of Visceral Leishmaniasis (Table 267-1)

VL is a life-threatening disease, and affected patients always should be treated. Pentavalent antimonial agents are the drugs of choice except in Bihar State, India, where drug resistance is present in up to 60% of cases,[1,53-69] and North America and other settings where cost is not a limiting factor. In the U.S., liposomal amphotericin B is the drug of choice and is the only drug licensed by the Food and Drug Administration for treatment of visceral leishmaniasis.[57,58] For consultation, including obtaining antiparasitic drugs in the U.S., contact the Division of Parasitic Disease at the Centers for Disease Control and Prevention (CDC) at 770-488-7778; for after-hours emergencies, call 770-488-7100.

In the future, combination therapy might be used more, having the advantages of reduced duration of therapy and reduced

TABLE 267-1. Evaluation of Drugs for Treatment of Visceral Leishmaniasis[a]

Drug	Disadvantages	Advantages	Category
Sodium stibogluconate or meglumine antimonate	Cardiotoxic, arrhythmias, pancreatitis; administered IV or IM	Inexpensive, effective except in India	Drug of choice
Amphotericin B liposomal	Nephrotoxic, hypokalemia, expensive; administered IV	Effective, safe	Drug of choice
Miltefosine	Teratogenic, GI effects, epididymitis, oculotoxicity	Administered orally; effective	Drug of choice
Amphotericin B deoxycholate	Nephrotoxic, hypokalemia, IV	Inexpensive, effective	Alternate
Paromomycin	Nephrotoxic, ototoxic, elevated transaminases; administered IM	Inexpensive, effective	Alternate

IV, intravenous; IM, intramuscular.

[a]See Chapter 296, Antiparasitic Agents, for dosing regimens.

probability of the development of drug resistance.[62-64] The following drugs are used for treatment.[65]

Pentavalent antimonial compounds. Two pentavalent antimonial compounds are available (sodium stibogluconate and meglumine antimonate), are effective, have been used for decades, and are the drugs of choice. In the U.S., the pentavalent antimonial compounds are not licensed for use but sodium stibogluconate is available from the Drug Service of the CDC. They must be given by intravenous or intramuscular injection and can cause cardiotoxicity, pain at the injection site, chemical evidence of pancreatitis, elevation of transaminase levels, bone marrow suppression, rashes, and myalgia and arthralgia.

Amphotericin B. Liposomal amphotericin B, a lipid formulation of amphotericin B, has been used as an antifungal agent for decades.[57,58] The drug must be given by intravenous infusion. Amphotericin B deoxycholate, the parent compound, is associated with infusion fever and chills during infusion, some degree of nephrotoxicity, and renal loss of potassium. Although these adverse effects occur with liposomal amphotericin B, they occur much less commonly and larger doses of the drug can be used. Clinical improvement can be noted after one or two doses, and short courses are effective.[58]

Miltefosine. Miltefosine is an alkylphosphocholine analogue with an unknown mode of action, is well absorbed from the intestinal tract after oral administration, and is distributed widely in tissues. It causes vomiting and diarrhea frequently, and can cause serum elevation of transaminases and creatinine, decreased sexual function, and ocular toxicity. It is teratogenic, and therefore is contraindicated in pregnancy. Miltefosine has been used successfully in India with a final cure rate of 82%.[59,60]

Paromomycin. Paromomycin is an aminoglycoside that is given by intramuscular injection. It carries the same ototoxicity and nephrotoxicity as other aminoglycosides.[61]

Treatment of Cutaneous Leishmaniasis

Since cutaneous leishmaniasis usually resolves spontaneously over a period of several months, treatment usually is not indicated. Under normal circumstances CL is not fatal, is self-limited, and confers lasting protection. Specific treatment is recommended for cases with large or multiple lesions, involvement of lymphatics, invasive mucous membrane lesions for leishmaniasis recidivans, in diffuse CL, or when there is a risk (as in cases of infection with *L. braziliensis* or *L. panamensis*) of later development of mucocutaneous leishmaniasis, and in *L. amazonensis* infections to avoid late disseminated cutaneous leishmaniasis.[70-72] Treatment should be continued until lesions are free of parasites; however, in leishmaniasis recidivans and diffuse CL, total cure is difficult to achieve, and relapses occur frequently when the drug is stopped. In patients with extensive tissue destruction, plastic surgery may be necessary after parasitologic cure has been achieved. *L. guyanensis* infection responds slowly to therapy and frequently relapses; treatment is the same as for espundia. Disseminated cutaneous disease usually responds to initial therapy with antimonial agents, but relapses are the rule and do not respond to additional antimonial therapy.

Many forms of treatment have been used with varying degrees of success, but optimal therapy requires individualization based on the geographic area of disease acquisition.[70,71,73,63-65] Pentavalent antimonial agents have been used successfully for many years, but are associated with significant adverse effects. Cochrane reviews have been published for both Old World and New World CL.[15,72] The authors reviewed 38 trials involving 2728 subjects with American cutaneous leishmaniasis or mucocutaneous leishmaniasis. For *L. braziliensis* infections, they concluded that parenteral antimonials plus oral allopurinol seemed better than other forms of therapy, while for infections caused by *L. panamensis*, parenteral meglumine antimonate, oral ketoconazole, intramuscular paromomycin, oral allopurinol, oral miltefosine, and topical paromomycin plus methylbenzethonium each had some effect. Authors emphasize the need for better randomized control trials for treatment of CL. A review of the wide variety of treatments for CL has been published.[74] Geographic location determines which species and strains cause the infection, which likely affect drug efficacy.[74] See Chapter 296, Antiparasitic Agents, for specifics of therapy.[65]

Treatment of Mucocutaneous Leishmaniasis

The main drugs used for treatment of mucocutaneous leishmaniasis are amphotericin B, pentavalent antimonial agents, or miltefosine.[65] Reviews of the variety of treatments used for patients with this condition have been published.[75,76] Specifics of therapy can be found in Chapter 296, Antiparasitic Agents.

PREVENTION AND CONTROL

Prevention can be approached on an individual and community basis. Individually there is no vaccine available to prevent any form of leishmaniasis and no form of chemoprophylaxis for travelers is available. Prevention depends on reducing transmission from reservoirs to the vector sandflies, and from the flies to human beings. Use of insecticide-treated dog collars can reduce transmission to children. Measures of control include treatment of infected people, reduction of reservoir hosts, and spraying to eliminate vector insects. Where humans are the sole reservoir, as in India, case detection and treatment help contain the spread of disease. Where canines are important reservoirs, identification and destruction of infected dogs is effective, but when rodents or sylvatic mammals are involved, reservoir control is difficult. Vector control using bednets impregnated with pyrethroids or DDT and other residual insecticides has had a significant effect in reducing visceral leishmaniasis in many parts of the world. Insect repellents containing DEET, protective clothing, and fine mesh netting can provide temporary protection.[77] In addition, it is desirable to have sleeping quarters on the roof or upper floor, because sandflies do not fly high above ground level.

268 Microsporidia

Patricia M. Flynn

Before 1985, few human microsporidial infections had been reported. Since then, the number of cases has increased dramatically because of recognition of this pathogen in patients infected with human immunodeficiency virus (HIV). Although most reported infections have occurred in HIV-infected people, the organism is being recognized increasingly as pathogenic in immunocompetent hosts.[1,2]

PATHOGEN

Microsporidia are obligate, intracellular, spore-forming parasites that have been reclassified from protozoa to fungi[3] (Figure 268-1). They are ubiquitous and infect most animal groups, including humans (Table 268-1). At least 14 species of microsporidia have been reported to be pathogens in humans.[4,5] Microsporidia are characterized by spore size, nuclear configuration, and relationship between the organism and its host cell. Replication occurs within the cytoplasm of the host cell via both binary fission (merogony) and multiple fission (schizogony) and culminates in spore production (sporogony). Maturing spores accumulate within a vacuole that eventually ruptures and releases the spores.[6] All microsporidial spores contain a complex tubular extrusion mechanism that injects the infectious substance (sporoplasm) from an infected cell into an uninfected host cell.[6]

EPIDEMIOLOGY

The epidemiology of microsporidial disease is not defined clearly. Antibodies against *Encephalitozoon cuniculi* are relatively common in selected human populations, thus suggesting that latent human infection may occur.[7]

Transmission is thought to occur from person to person and through ingestion of contaminated water and food.[3] Following ingestion, infectious spores travel to the intestine, where their contents are injected into cytoplasm of host cells. Intracellular division produces new spores that can spread to nearby cells, disseminate to other host tissues, or be passed into the environment via feces. Spores also have been detected in urine and respiratory tract epithelium, thus suggesting that related body fluids also can be infectious and that transmission also can be airborne.[3,8] Once in the environment, microsporidial spores remain infectious for up to 4 months.[8] Zoonotic transmission has been proposed as has vectorborne transmission.[3,9] The potential for vertical transmission of infection from an infected mother has not been documented in humans but occurs in other mammals.[3]

CLINICAL MANIFESTATIONS

Microsporidial infection has been implicated in a number of disorders (see Table 268-1), including corneal infections, diarrhea associated with HIV infection, cholecystitis, cholangitis, encephalitis, sinusitis, myositis, pneumonitis, hepatitis, nephritis, peritonitis, and disseminated disease.[1-13] Corneal infections in HIV-infected patients are characterized by conjunctival irritation, photophobia, foreign body sensation, and decreased visual acuity. Slit-lamp examination reveals conjunctival hyperemia, mixed follicular-papillary tarsal conjunctival reaction, and punctate epithelial keratopathy.[8] In immunocompetent hosts, keratopathy is reported to extend deeper into the cornea than in HIV-infected patients.

Microsporidia-associated diarrhea is intermittent; stools are copious, watery, and nonbloody and contain no fecal leukocytes.

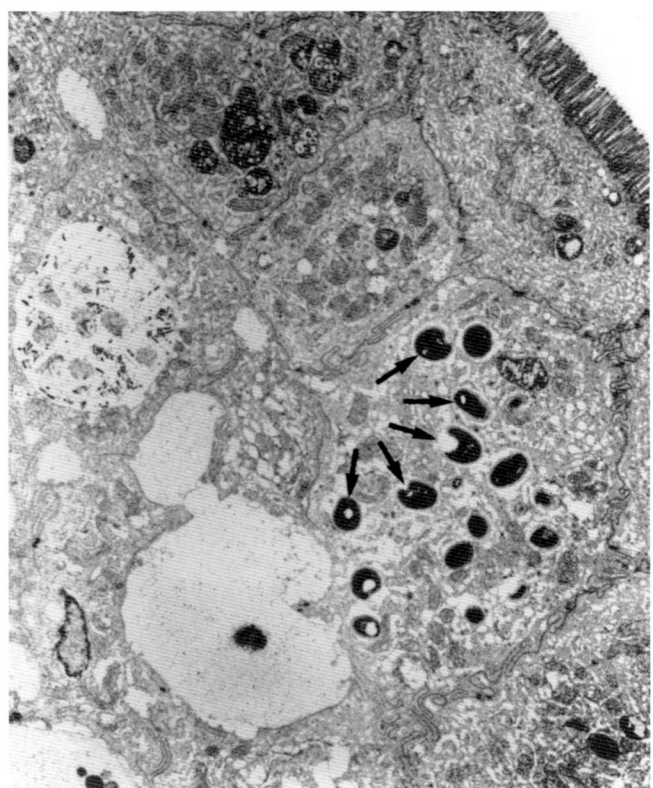

Figure 268-1. Electron micrograph of mature spores (arrows) of *Enterocytozoon bieneusi* in a duodenal biopsy specimen (original magnification, ×10,000). (Reproduced with permission from Gyorkey F, Genta RM, et al. The role of Microsporidia in the pathogenesis of HIV-related chronic diarrhea. Ann Intern Med 1993;119:895.)

TABLE 268-1. Clinical Diseases Associated with Microsporidia

Organism	Disease
ANNCALIIA SPP.	
A. algerae	Myositis, disseminated disease, keratopathy, skin infection
A. connora	Disseminated disease, keratopathy
A. vesicularum	Myositis
ENCEPHALITOZOON SPP.	
E. cuniculi	Encephalitis, hepatitis, peritonitis, keratopathy, sinusitis, osteomyelitis, pulmonary disease, disseminated disease
E. hellem	Keratopathy, disseminated disease, sinusitis, pneumonitis, nephritis, urethritis, cystitis
E. intestinalis	Diarrhea, cholangitis, disseminated disease, nodular skin lesions
Enterocytozoon bieneusi	Diarrhea, cholangitis, pulmonary disease
MICROSPORIDIUM SPP.	
M. africanum	Keratopathy
M. ceylonensis	Keratopathy
Nosema ocularum	Keratopathy
Pleistophora ronneafiei	Myositis, disseminated disease, sinusitis
TRACHIPLEISTOPHORA SPP.	
T. hominis	Myositis, cardiac disease, disseminated disease
T. anthropophthera	Disseminated disease, encephalitis, keratopathy
Vittaforma corneae	Keratopathy, urinary tract infection, diarrhea

Clinical symptoms include crampy abdominal pain and weight loss; fever is not present usually. Whether chronic diarrhea in HIV-infected patients is due to microsporidia remains controversial. Some studies have implicated microsporidia as causal,[14–16] whereas others have shown the presence of diarrhea and this organism to be independent of one another.[17] Because microsporidia have been found in the bile, ductal biliary cells, and gallbladder tissue of several HIV-infected patients with cholangitis, these organisms have been suggested to have a causal role in cholangitis.[10,12] Disseminated disease has been shown to involve liver, kidneys, brain, bladder, lung, bone, and sinuses.

LABORATORY FINDINGS AND DIAGNOSIS

Microsporidial infection is diagnosed by microscopic demonstration of the organism in tissue or body fluids. All microsporidia range in size from 1.5 to 5 μm in width and 2 to 7 μm in length.[6] The organism can be detected with hematoxylin–eosin, Giemsa, acid-fast, fluorescent brighteners (e.g., Calcofluor, Fungifluor), Gram, modified trichrome stain, periodic acid–Schiff staining, and immunofluorescence assay.[3,18,19] Nonetheless, the organism can be overlooked because of its small size, variable staining, and lack of an inflammatory response. Polymerase chain reaction (PCR) has been reported to be a sensitive and specific diagnostic tool but is not available commercially.[20–22] Identification of species can be made by electron microscopy, immunofluorescence, or PCR.[2,3,20] Current serologic tests are not helpful in diagnosis.

TREATMENT

There is no proven therapy for microsporidial infections. Early cases of encephalitis in immunocompetent hosts appeared to respond to sulfa drugs. Metronidazole, albendazole, atovaquone, nitazoxanide, fluoroquinolones, and fumagillin are reported to decrease diarrhea and other symptoms but not to eradicate the organism.[23–31] Encephalitozoon intestinalis infections of the gastrointestinal tract usually respond to albendazole, but infections due to Enterocytozoon bieneusi are more difficult to treat. Improvement in symptoms and less frequent detection of the organism have been reported with the use of protease inhibitor therapy in HIV-infected patients.[32] In a small, placebo-controlled trial of fumagillin (60 mg per day for 2 weeks), therapy was effective in AIDS patients with E. bieneusi; neutropenia and thrombocytopenia were frequent adverse events.[33]

PREVENTION

Because transmission probably occurs by passage of infectious spores in feces, isolation precautions should be considered for hospitalized patients. Patients and caregivers should perform careful handwashing. Immunocompromised individuals should avoid untreated water as well as unpeeled fruits and vegetables, all of which can be contaminated.[3]

269 *Naegleria fowleri*

Candice McNeil and Upinder Singh

Naegleria fowleri is a free-living ameba from the vahlkampfiid family, and is the only known pathogenic species of the genus *Naegleria* that causes primary amebic meningoencephalitis (PAM) in humans and animals.[1,2] Some 30 other species have been identified according to sequencing data, some of which, like *N. australiensis* and *N. italica,* are known to cause death of experimental animals.[3,4] The organism is a facultative pathogen that occurs worldwide in soil and warm freshwater ponds, hot springs, streams, rivers, pools, thermally polluted streams, and tap waters. The parasite is thermophilic and thermotolerant, proliferates in naturally and artificially warmed waters, and has an optimum activity at 37 °C. The majority of human PAM cases are caused by *N. fowleri,* which can grow at temperatures as high as 45 °C.

The life cycle includes (Figure 269-1) vegetative trophozoite (the infective stage) and resistant cyst phases. The trophozoite measures 10 to 30 μm has a distinctive limacine (slug-like) pattern of locomotion, and has ≥1 ectoplasmic pseudopods (Figure 269-2). Distinctive characteristics of *Naegleria* include a transient, nonfeeding and nondividing flagellated stage, an unusual mitosis that retains the nuclear membrane, cysts that are double-walled and of approximately 9 μm with pores through which the trophozoites excyst, and transformation into a nonreproductive flagellate form in response to unfavorable environmental conditions.[5] The most remarkable thing about the molecular biology of *Naegleria* species is that the rRNA genes are carried on a 14-kb plasmid that is present as a multicopy (4000) episome.[6] The

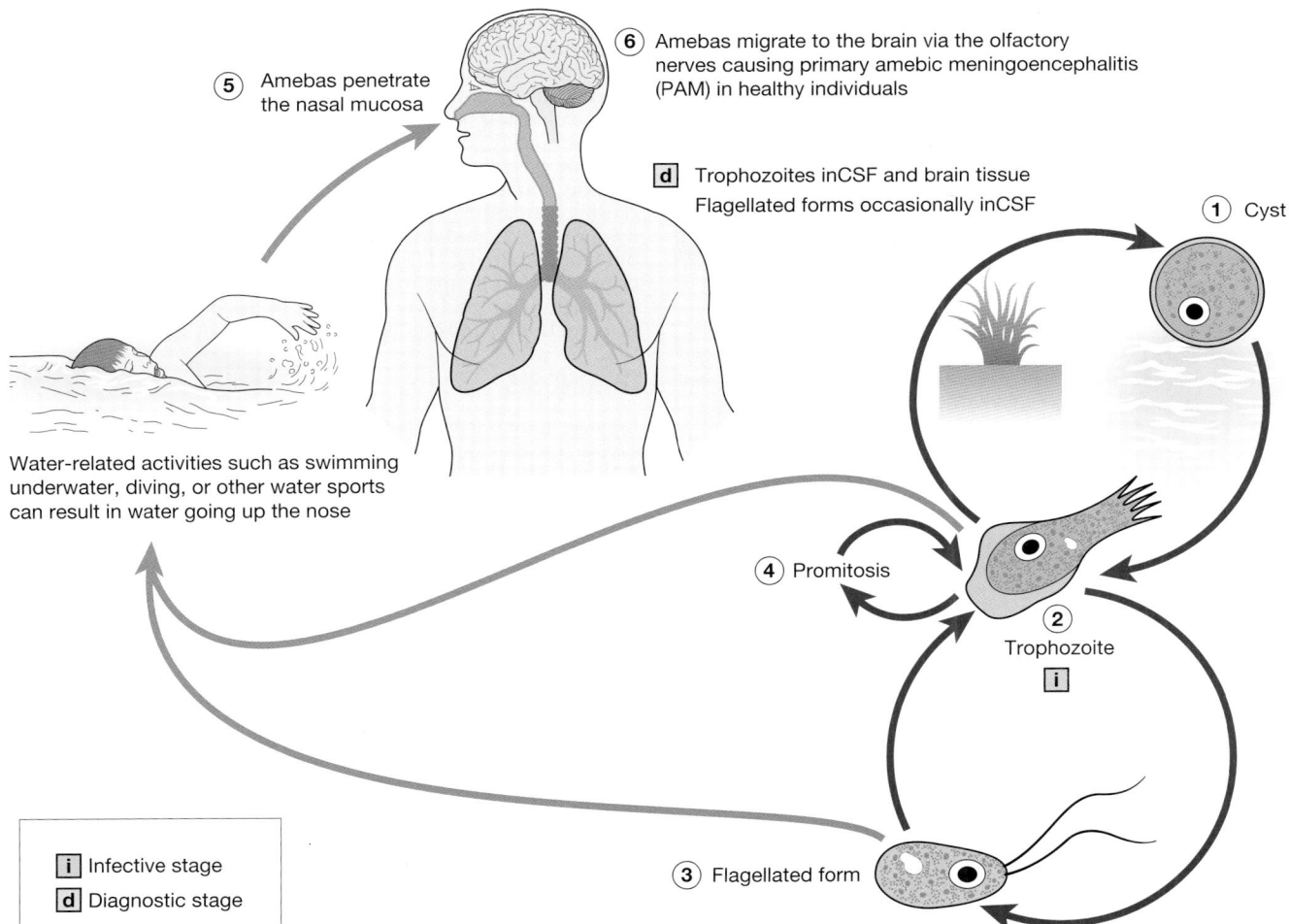

5 Amebas penetrate the nasal mucosa

6 Amebas migrate to the brain via the olfactory nerves causing primary amebic meningoencephalitis (PAM) in healthy individuals

d Trophozoites inCSF and brain tissue
Flagellated forms occasionally inCSF

1 Cyst

Water-related activities such as swimming underwater, diving, or other water sports can result in water going up the nose

4 Promitosis

2 Trophozoite i

3 Flagellated form

i Infective stage
d Diagnostic stage

Figure 269-1. Life cycle of *Naegleria fowleri*. *Naegleria fowleri* has 3 stages in its life cycle: cysts (1), trophozoites (2), and flagellated forms (3). The trophozoites replicate by promitosis (nuclear membrane remains intact) (4). *N. fowleri* is found in fresh water, soil, thermal discharges of power plants, heated swimming pools, hydrotherapy and medicinal pools, aquariums, and sewage. Trophozoites can turn into temporary nonfeeding flagellated forms, which usually revert back to the trophozoite stage. Trophozoites infect humans or animals by penetrating the nasal mucosa (5) and migrating to the brain (6) via the olfactory nerves, causing primary amebic meningoencephalitis (PAM). *N. fowleri* trophozoites are found in cerebrospinal fluid (CSF) and tissue, while flagellated forms occasionally are found in CSF. Cysts are not seen in brain tissue. (Courtesy of the CDC DPDx.)

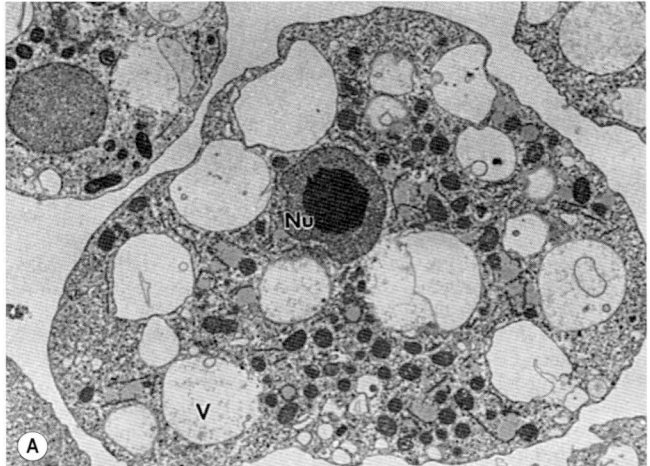

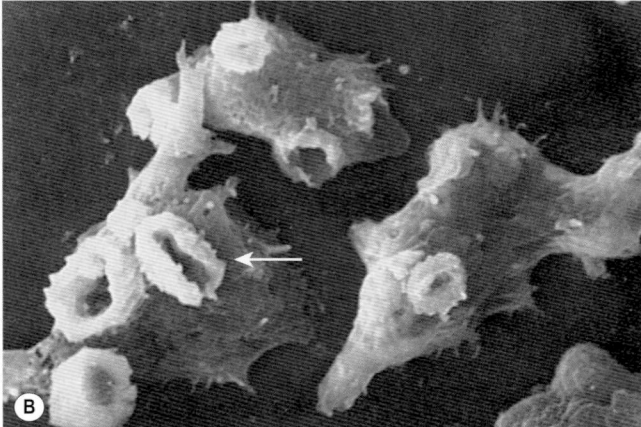

Figure 269-2. Transmission **(A)** and scanning **(B)** electron micrographs of *Naegleria fowleri*. Trophozoites of pathogenic *N. fowleri* (LEE strain) ameba, isolated from a human case of primary amebic meningoencephalitis in 1968, were grown axenically in Cline medium at 37°C. Food-cup surface structures (arrow) are abundant on the surface of the amebas. These structures are used to ingest bacteria, yeast, or mammalian cells. Nu, nucleus; V, vacuole. (Courtesy of Francine Marciano-Cabral, MD.)

free-living *Naegleria* feed on bacteria, and unlike other pathogenic protozoa, they have no known intermediate hosts.[7]

EPIDEMIOLOGY

In 1965, Fowler and Carter demonstrated that free-living amebas can invade the human brain causing a rapidly fatal meningitis. In the United States from 1937 to 2007, a total of 121 cases were reported. The majority of cases occurred in the summer months in the setting of warm freshwater exposure. In all, 15 southern states, Arizona, Arkansas, California, Florida, Georgia, Louisiana, Mississippi, Missouri, Nevada, New Mexico, North Carolina, Oklahoma, South Carolina, Texas, and Virginia, have reported cases of PAM.[8] Over 50% of PAM cases have occurred in the states of Florida and Texas.[9] Worldwide prevalence cannot be estimated reliably; however, over 16 countries have reported cases of PAM in the past 40 years.[9]

PAM is a fulminant disease, in contrast to the more indolent course with granulomatous amebic encephalitis (caused by *Acanthamoeba* and *Balamuthia* spp.). In the U.S. the age of patients has ranged from 8 months to 66 years with a median age of 12 years. Among the cases where sex of the patients was documented, 78% were male.[8,9] In general, the predilection for young people may reflect behavior (e.g., more likely to remain in the water for longer periods of time, more activity in the water, and more diving and

underwater swimming) that stirs bottom sediment that may contain amebas. Primarily young healthy individuals are affected, and they have a history of swimming, especially diving, in warm, fresh water or of other exposure to water within a week before the onset of symptoms. The organism has been isolated from swimming pools, but this feature has not been reported as the mechanism of exposure in the U.S. Clustering of cases from a common environmental exposure has been observed. A few cases have not followed exposure to water, being attributed to inhalation of cysts.

Amebas enter the nasal cavity, are phagocytosed by sustentacular cells of the olfactory neuroepithelium, and migrate along the unmyelinated axonal fibers of the olfactory nerve, through the cribriform plate, and into the subarachnoid space. The incubation period varies from 2 to 7 days but can be as long as 15 days after exposure. The olfactory bulbs, the base of the frontal and temporal lobes, and the cerebellum primarily are involved in a hemorrhagic, necrotizing process.[10–12]

CLINICAL MANIFESTATIONS

Due to the rapid progression and significant mortality associated with PAM, a high degree of clinical suspicion should be maintained in the setting of children and young adults presenting with acute neurologic symptoms and history of recent freshwater exposure. The initial presentation of patients with PAM can be indistinguishable from acute bacterial or pyogenic meningoencephalitis.[13] In 94% to 100% of patients, initial symptoms of PAM consist of severe bifrontal headaches not responsive to analgesics, fever ranging from 38°C to 41°C, pharyngitis, nasal congestion or discharge, nausea, vomiting, and altered mental status.[1,14] Some people initially notice an altered sense of smell and taste. Somnolence, confusion, signs of meningeal irritation, and convulsions are followed by coma in approximately two-thirds of patients, often progressing so rapidly that focal neurologic signs do not develop. Intracranial pressure is increased terminally, commonly causing herniation of the uncus and cerebellar tonsils. The mortality rate is >95%, and death usually occurs within 3 to 10 days after onset of symptoms.[1,15] Diffuse or focal subclinical myocarditis has been identified in approximately one-half of patients at autopsy. Although neutrophils are identified in the myocardium, amebas have not been found outside the central nervous system in humans.

DIAGNOSIS

Because human naegleriasis is an acute disease, early diagnosis is essential so that appropriate antimicrobial therapy can be initiated to limit extensive amebic damage. Primary amebic meningoencephalitis should be suspected in previously healthy adolescents who have purulent meningitis without identifiable bacteria and who recently have been exposed to warm water. Computed tomography or magnetic resonance imaging demonstrates cerebral edema and obliteration of the subarachnoid space. Images obtained after intravenous infusion of contrast material can show marked meningeal enhancement, particularly in the basilar areas.[12,14,16]

The cerebrospinal fluid (CSF) pressure can be increased, and the fluid is cloudy and slightly hemorrhagic. Pleocytosis can be modest initially, but increases to 400 to 26,000 cells/mm³, with predominance of neutrophils. CSF glucose concentration is normal or decreased (mean, 43 mg/dL; low, 2 mg/dL), and the protein concentration usually is increased (mean, 413 mg/dL; high, 1170 mg/dL). Rapid diagnosis is made by microscopic examination, preferably using phase-contrast, of freshly drawn CSF, to visualize motile amebas. Amebas can be seen on Wright- or Giemsa-stained CSF preparations. Trophozoites have a clear nucleus with a prominent, dark-staining central nucleolus that aids in distinguishing them from macrophages. The amebic cytoplasm usually contains phagocytosed material, including erythrocytes and myelin fragments. Some trophozoites can be binucleate. Fresh CSF preparations collected within 30 minutes of evaluation and centrifuged at slow speeds (250 × gravity) also should be examined for motile trophozoites.[1,17,18] *Naegleria* are destroyed by

TABLE 269-1. Characteristics of *Naegleria* and *Acanthamoeba*

	Naegleria	**Acanthamoeba**
Disease	Primary amebic meningoencephalitis	Granulomatous amebic encephalitis (also causes *Acanthamoeba* keratitis)
Agent	*N. fowleri*	More than 20 implicated *Acanthamoeba* species
Protozoology	Trophozoite 10–15 µm in diameter	Trophozoite 14–40 µm in diameter
	Round cyst with pores	Double-walled cyst
	Transient flagellate form	
Epidemiology	History of recreational water sports	History of poor health Immunocompromised (AIDS)
	Previous good health	
Incubation period	2–7 days, up to 15 days	Uncertain, >10 days
Clinical course	Acute, fulminant	Chronic
Portal of entry	Olfactory neuroepithelium	Lung, skin, eyes
CSF findings	Active trophozoites present	Organism rarely isolated from CSF
	Neutrophils predominant	Lymphocytes predominant, neutrophils increased
Pathology	Acute purulent leptomeningitis	Chronic granulomatous encephalitis
	Only trophozoites in brain tissue	Cysts and trophozoites in brain tissue

AIDS, acquired immunodeficiency syndrome; CSF, cerebrospinal fluid.

refrigeration. Suspending amebas in 1 mL of distilled water can further confirm the identity of the amebas as *Naegleria*, by watching for development of actively swimming flagellates forms in 1 to 2 hours.[1,19] Brain biopsy of grey matter can reveal trophozoites localized around blood vessels. Indirect immunofluorescence or immunoperoxidase staining can be used to speciate amebas in formalin-fixed, paraffin-embedded tissue sections. *Naegleria* cysts rarely are present in tissue, and identification of cysts should raise suspicion of another infective ameba, such as *Acanthamoeba* (Table 269-1).[20] The peripheral white blood cell count can be elevated with neutrophilia.

CSF polymerase chain reaction (PCR) testing has been proposed as a means of rapid diagnosis of PAM; however, PCR is not available widely.[21] Serologic tests generally are not helpful, because the acutely infected patient usually succumbs before mounting a significant antibody response. In addition, antibody can be present in the healthy population, suggesting the possibility of subclinical infection. Further corroboration can be obtained by isolation of the amebas from CSF or macerated brain tissue on a non-nutrient agar plate that has been spread with a lawn of *E. coli*, and incubated overnight at 37°C. The amebas grow in large numbers, feeding on the bacteria. Tissue culture, especially on monkey kidney cells, also has been used to cultivate *Naegleria*.[22]

TREATMENT

Survival from PAM is rare with only a few well-documented cases in the literature. In the absence of clear guidelines, amphotericin B is the most widely accepted drug for the treatment of PAM.[23] Amphotericin B intrathecal therapy also has been used as an adjunct to intravenous amphotericin with reported success.[24,25] Amphotericin targets the parasite's plasma membrane by binding to ergosterol in the membrane, producing pores and causing loss of small molecules. From in vivo and in vitro evaluations, *N. fowleri* appears to be highly sensitive to amphotericin B, but delay in diagnosis and the fulminant nature of the disease result in few survivors,[26] and even with appropriate treatment selection, relapses have occurred.[27]

Numerous anecdotal cases have reported success in treating *Naegleria* infections with combination therapy. These regimens have included amphotericin B in combination with rifampin, or amphotericin B in combination chloramphenicol, fluconazole, or ketoconazole.[26,28–30] Regimens including amphotericin and azithromycin also have been suggested as possible synergistic agents in vitro and in mouse models of PAM.[31] The optimal duration of therapy is not known, but at least 10 days of treatment has been used in survivors.[24,25]

PREVENTION

Avoidance of the free-living amebas is virtually impossible since they are ubiquitous in the environment, as evidenced by the presence of antibodies in screened human populations.[32] *N. fowleri* is so common in the environment that surveillance is not indicated unless several people are infected after a common exposure.[22,33,34] The incidence of PAM is low despite populations of amebas >1 organism/25 mL of water (as found in water tested in late summer in Florida) and despite millions of exposures to recreational waters. Protective factors are unknown. *Naegleria fowleri* is susceptible to ≤1 mg/L chlorine.[1] Proper chlorine disinfection of water in swimming pools and whirlpools and avoidance of diving and of introduction of water into the nostrils appear to be reasonable measures in order to avoid development of amebic encephalitis.[1] Recommendations include use of chlorine in swimming pools at 1 mg/L if the water temperature is <26°C, at least 2 mg/L if the temperature is >26°C, and 3 mg/L for temperatures >28°C.[1] Cysts are destroyed after 1 hour of exposure to pool or tap water at these concentrations.

270 *Acanthamoeba* Species

Candice McNeil and Upinder Singh

PATHOGEN

Castellani first described the presence of an ameba in *Cryptococcus pararoseus* cultures in 1930.[1] Since then nearly 25 named species and 15 genotypes of *Acanthamoeba* have been identified worldwide. Previously these groups were distinguished based on morphology and cyst size into three groups (I, II, III); however, newly available molecular techniques have led to species identification based on genetic similarities.[2] Like *Naegleria fowleri*, *Balamuthia mandrillaris*, and *Sappinia diploidea*, *Acanthamoeba* are classified as free-living amebas due to their lack of dependence on animals to complete their life cycle. The organism has two phases in its life cycle: a motile trophozoite and a resilient infective cyst stage. Both forms tend to have a wide distribution in nature. As such, this ubiquitous organism has been isolated from soil, water, and numerous anatomic sites.[1,3] *Acanthamoeba* is the causative agent of granulomatous amebic encephalitis (GAE), amebic keratitis (AK), and cutaneous and sinus disease in human immunodeficiency virus (HIV)-infected and other immunocompromised people.

Several species of *Acanthamoeba* are known pathogens in humans. *A. castellanii, A. culbertsoni, A. polyphagia, A. astronyxis, A. palestinensis, A. healyi,* and *A. divionensis* usually cause a fatal, subacute disseminated disease with GAE in immunocompromised hosts.[1,3] Additionally, *A. polyphagia, A. castellanii, A. culbertsoni, A. hatchetti, A. rhysodes, A. quina, A. lugdunensis,* and *A. griffini* can cause AK, a vision-threatening disorder predominantly seen in contact lens wearers.[1]

EPIDEMIOLOGY

Acanthamoeba species have been isolated readily from water (including treated water, brackish water, seawater, swimming pools, sewage, domestic tap water, bottled mineral water, cooling, heating, and humidifying units, hot tubs, hospitals and dialysis units, dental irrigation units, eyewash stations, contact lenses and associated paraphernalia), soil, dust, air, sediments, and as contaminants in cell cultures.[3] Limited seroprevalence surveys of healthy humans have demonstrated antibodies from IgM and IgG classes to *Acanthamoeba* species, indicating that asymptomatic infections likely occur.[4,5] Persons with a compromised immune system such as individuals with diabetes mellitus, chronic liver disease, renal failure, systemic lupus erythematosus, transplant patients, persons receiving corticosteroids chronically, pregnant women, and HIV/AIDS-infected people are at risk for severe manifestations of *Acanthamoeba* infections such as disseminated disease and GAE.[6,7] Difficulties in diagnosing GAE limits ability to capture the true incidence of disease; for the most part, cases have been reported in adults. There have, however, been several reports of disseminated disease including GAE in HIV-infected children 8 months to 8 years of age.[8-10] Although central nervous system (CNS) disease with *Acanthamoeba* occurs predominantly in immunocompromised individuals, cases in both the adult and pediatric literature have been reported in individuals with an intact immune system.[11-17]

First described in 1974, AK cases parallel the use of homemade contact lens solutions.[18] Estimated annual incidence ranges from 1.65 to 2.01 cases per 1,000,000 contact lens wearers[19] to as high as 1 per 10,000 contact lens wearers.[20] Unfortunately, the incidence has not declined with the advent of disposable contact lenses and cases. Rarer ocular infections include uveitis, endophthalmitis, and optic neuritis. Water contamination is a critical factor in acquisition of *Acanthamoeba* keratitis. *Acanthamoeba* has been isolated from a wide variety of water sources.[1,21] Over 90% of soft contact lens users admit to risk factors such as unsterile contact lens solutions and swimming while wearing contact lenses.[21,22] There are reported cases of AK occurring in patients without predisposing contact lens use. In such cases ocular trauma and exposure to unclean water appeared to be the requisite exposures. However, there are reported adult and pediatric cases in which no predisposing factor was identified.[22,23]

CLINICAL MANIFESTATIONS

Acanthamebic encephalitis usually is termed *granulomatous amebic encephalitis* (GAE) because of its pathologic appearance. The disease generally occurs after infection at other sites, thus implying that trophozoites reach the CNS by hematogenous dissemination.[7] The route of infection is thought to be inhalation of amebae through the nasal passages and lungs or introduction through skin lesions. Although the incubation period for *Acanthamoeba*

infections is unknown, it can be several weeks or months. The neurologic symptoms of GAE have an insidious onset and include focal deficits such as hemiparesis, diplopia, cranial nerve palsies (especially of cranial nerves III and VI), and cerebellar ataxia. Nonfocal neurologic manifestations include personality changes, seizures, headache, meningismus, nausea, stiff neck, lethargy, altered mental status, signs of increased intracranial pressure and coma. Low-grade intermittent fever, nausea, and vomiting also can occur. The disease usually is fatal after an average of 39 days of illness (range, 7 to 120 days).

The symptoms of *Acanthamoeba* keratitis often begin with the sensation of a foreign body in the eye, followed by severe (usually unilateral) ocular pain, redness, photophobia, tearing, blurred vision, and lid edema. Physical signs include corneal ulceration (initially a dendritic pattern and then a stromal one), a characteristic corneal ring infiltrate, cataracts, and iritis. Waxing and waning of symptoms and physical signs are common and often result in delayed diagnosis. In rare circumstances, *Acanthamoeba* can spread from the cornea to the retina, causing chorioretinitis. On these occasions, the spread of the *Acanthamoeba* has been postulated to have been facilitated by a combined keratoplasty, extracapsular cataract extraction, and intraocular lens insertion.[24]

Cutaneous infections often are a reflection of disseminated disease caused by *Acanthamoeba* and are most common in patients with AIDS.[25-27] The cutaneous form of the disease is characterized by the presence of hard erythematous nodules or skin ulcers.[28] Early manifestations include the presence of firm papulonodules that become abscesses, drain purulent material and then develop into nonhealing indurated ulcerations.[1,29] The mortality rate from cutaneous infection in individuals without CNS involvement is approximately 73%, while the mortality rate from cutaneous infection accompanied by CNS disease is 100%.[25] Other manifestations of *Acanthamoeba* infections in HIV-infected patients include sinus infection which manifests with the typical symptoms of sinusitis.[30]

DIAGNOSIS

The diagnosis of GAE depends on isolation or histologic demonstration of *Acanthamoeba* from a brain biopsy specimen (Figure 270-1). A variety of stains (e.g., hematoxylin and eosin, Wright, Giemsa, periodic acid–Schiff, and Calcofluor white) highlight the trophozoites or cysts in tissue, which in the brain often localize to the perivascular spaces. Indirect immunofluorescent and immunoperoxidase staining methods can be used to confirm the diagnosis. Cerebrospinal fluid (CSF) and radiologic findings are nonspecific. Computed tomography of the head has shown mass lesions that resemble abscesses, tumors, or hemorrhage.[1,31] These

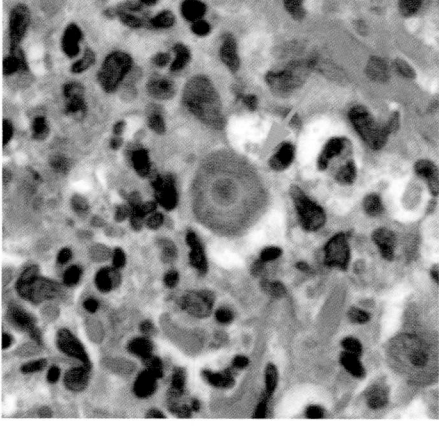

Figure 270-1. *Acanthamoeba* trophozoite (arrow) in a biopsy tissue (hematoxylin and eosin stain; ×1000). (Courtesy of CDC, DPDx.)

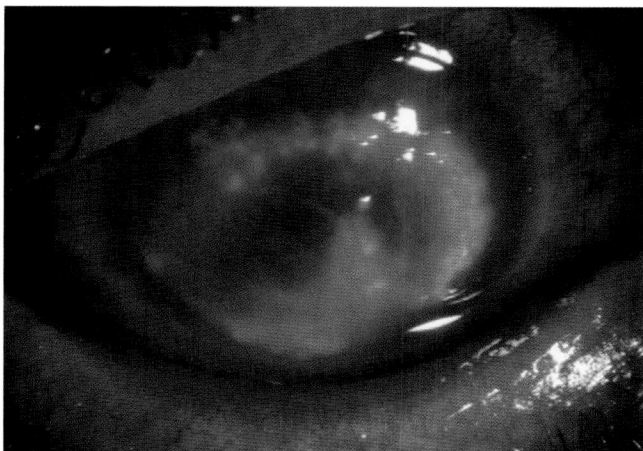

Figure 270-2. Ring infiltrate and severe scleritis in advanced *Acanthamoeba* keratitis. (From Dart JKG, Saw V, Kilvington S. *Acanthamoeba* keratitis: diagnosis and treatment update 2009. Am J Ophthalmol 2009;148:487–499.e2.)

lesions often are multifocal and occasionally nonenhancing and occur throughout the cortex, brainstem, and spinal cord. Lumbar puncture may be contraindicated because of these space-occupying lesions, but, when performed, the CSF has elevated opening pressure, lymphocytic pleocytosis, and moderately elevated protein, and low glucose concentrations. Although the CSF traditionally has been considered sterile, there have been reports of motile trophozoites and positive cultures from the CSF samples from children.[11,32] Culture requires that tissue be inoculated onto non-nutrient agar overlaid with *Escherichia coli* or *Enterobacter aerogenes,* which serve as food sources for the ameba.[33,34] The organism also can be isolated from culture of skin lesion swabs, and in suspected cases biopsy should be performed on skin lesions.

The diagnosis of AK depends on isolation or demonstration of *Acanthamoeba* in corneal scrapings or corneal biopsy specimens (1- to 2-mm biopsy). Scrapings should be examined for motile trophozoites or cysts as a wet mount before drying or fixation. Newer alcohol-based fixatives and centrifugation protocols are being investigated.[35] Staphylococci, streptococci, or other bacteria have been isolated concurrently in a number of cases and can confound the diagnosis. *Acanthamoeba* has been isolated from contact lenses, lens cases, lens-cleaning solutions, and corneal tissues.[34] Early ophthalmologic findings include a dendriform epithelial pattern in the cornea with patchy stromal infiltrates. Treatment at this early stage can save vision. The characteristic ring infiltrate of the cornea is a late sign[36] (Figure 270-2).

TREATMENT

CNS Infections

Treatment of GAE is rarely successful probably because of a combination of late diagnosis and antimicrobial failure. There is no standard regimen; however, anecdotally successful regimens have involved combination therapy including pentamidine, sulfadiazine, flucytosine, and either fluconazole or itraconazole.[3] Treatment of GAE in immunocompromised hosts such as HIV-infected individuals can be particularly challenging; however, treatment success has been reported with combination therapy using fluconazole, pyrimethamine, and sulfadiazine along with surgical resection of the CNS lesion.[37] Oral regimens including a combination of trimethoprim-sulfamethoxazole, rifampin, and ketoconazole have been used successfully to treat children with chronic *Acanthamoeba* meningitis.[11]

Cutaneous Disease

Patients with cutaneous acanthamebiasis have been treated with various drugs. Successful treatment of a patient with AIDS with cutaneous and sinus lesions using 40 mg/kg of 5-fluorocytosine orally for 2 weeks has been reported.[38] Topical therapy with miltefosine[39] also is a consideration in the immunocompromised host. Of note, some treatment regimens that may be successful in one patient may yield a poor outcome in another. For instance, intravenous pentamidine plus topical chlorhexidine and 2% ketoconazole cream, followed by itraconazole orally has been used successfully;[40] however, failure of a similar regimen was reported in another patient.[41] *Acanthamoeba* isolates have shown varied susceptibility patterns between species and among strains of the same species; thus susceptibility testing is recommended to guide therapy.[42]

Keratitis

Treatment of AK can be effective, particularly when initiated during the early dendriform epithelial pattern stage of infection. Treatment entails use of topical antiamebic agents and, in more severe cases, surgical debridement. There are no clear guidelines for treatment of this disease; however, combination therapy with topical chlorhexidine, or propamidine isethionate (PHMB) and dibromopropamidine (Brolene), are commonly used successfully.[1,34] Adjunctive oral and topical therapies such as ketoconazole and itraconazole can be considered.[43] The use of adjunctive topical corticosteroids is controversial. Although there are some reports of corticosteroid therapy controlling inflammation, pain, and ulceration,[44] use has been complicated by crystalline keratopathy due to viridans streptococci (including *Streptococcus oralis*) and *Staphylococcus aureus.*[45] In cases where medical therapy with debridement has failed, penetrating keratoplasty, corneal transplantation, and even enucleation have been required.[34]

PREVENTION

The ubiquitous nature of *Acanthamoeba* argues against complete prevention of GAE in highly immunocompromised people untenable. *Acanthamoeba* keratitis, however, is largely a preventable disease if proper contact lens care techniques are followed and swimming with contact lenses is avoided. Additional appropriate prevention measures include thermal disinfection of contact lenses, use of hydrogen peroxide-containing solutions (two-step processes are better than one-step), good lens case care, and the use of an amebicidal storage solution (a combination of PHMB and chlorhexidine appears to be ideal).[46,47] Sterile saline containing benzalkonium preservatives (chlorine-based solutions are not effective against *Acanthamoeba*) should be used for lens storage. Homemade saline solutions should never be used for cleaning or storing lenses.[21] No vaccine is available, but, in animal models of *Acanthamoeba* keratitis, an ocular IgA antibody response appears to protect against infection.[48,49]

271 *Plasmodium* Species (Malaria)

Aarti Agarwal, Meredith McMorrow and Paul M. Arguin

Clinicians in the United States encounter cases infrequently, yet up to two-thirds of the world's population is exposed to malaria annually. In the U.S., most cases occur in people who have traveled to or emigrated from endemic areas.[1] Rarely, malaria is acquired from blood transfusion, through congenital transmission, or through transmission from an imported case. It is important to have a high index of suspicion for malaria in people who have traveled to malarious areas because infection can be rapidly fatal. This chapter focuses on malaria as it is likely to be encountered in the U.S.

DESCRIPTION OF THE PATHOGEN

Four species of malarial parasites commonly infect humans: *Plasmodium falciparum, P. vivax, P. ovale,* and *P. malariae. P. falciparum* is the most lethal and the most drug-resistant. Of the human species, *P. vivax* was the most widely distributed geographically and best adapted to survive in temperate climates. However, successful mosquito eradication programs in the U.S. and Europe essentially eliminated *P. vivax* from these regions. *P. falciparum* is the most prevalent in sub-Saharan Africa. *P. ovale* mainly occurs in the western areas of sub-Saharan Africa.

Recently, *P. knowlesi,* a species that normally infects macaques in Southeast Asia, has been found to be the cause of significant numbers of malaria cases in humans. Different stages of *P. knowlesi* closely resemble *P. malariae,* making it difficult to diagnose by microscopy. In contrast to the usually benign infections with *P. malariae,* infection with *P. knowlesi* can be rapidly fatal, so it is important to consider this possibility when treating patients from this region, or who have traveled to this region, to minimize morbidity and mortality.[2]

The life cycles of all human malarial parasites are illustrated in Figure 271-1. Sporozoites are inoculated into humans by the bite of an *Anopheles* mosquito and invade hepatic parenchymal cells within minutes. The parasites undergo asexual multiplication, or schizogony, in this tissue phase of their life cycle, also called exo-erythrocytic schizogony. After a period of development and amplification (7 to 10 days for *P. falciparum, P. ovale,* and *P. vivax,* and 10 to 14 days for *P. malariae* and *P. knowlesi*), merozoites emerge to invade erythrocytes and begin what will become the symptomatic phase of the illness. Parasites of the two relapsing species of *Plasmodium, P. ovale* and *P. vivax,* also can differentiate into a quiescent stage, the hypnozoite, which later can enter into schizogony and reemerge to invade erythrocytes. *P. malariae* has the potential to persist at very low levels in the circulation for decades if not recognized and treated.

Each species has developed an efficient strategy for erythrocyte invasion that relies on a specific, complex interaction of certain surface proteins or glycoproteins on the erythrocyte and a specific ligand of the parasite. For example, *P. vivax* preferentially invades erythrocytes bearing the Duffy blood group antigen,[3] an antigen that is rarely found on erythrocytes in persons from West and central Africa. *Plasmodium falciparum* most efficiently invades erythrocytes with intact glycosylated forms of the glycophorin family of proteins.[4] Parasitic ligands that facilitate interactions with these erythrocyte molecules have been identified in *P. falciparum* and *P. vivax.*[5] *P. ovale* and *P. falciparum* invade erythrocytes of all ages while *P. vivax* preferentially invade reticulocytes, and *P. malariae* and *P. knowlesi* preferentially invade mature erythrocytes. Once inside the erythrocyte, parasites can undergo either asexual schizogony or sexual differentiation to produce gametocytes.

During asexual schizogony, the parasites are known as trophozoites once they are established inside the erythrocyte; the early trophozoite forms often are called rings because of their apparent lack of central cytoplasmic staining. Parasites in this stage ferment homolactate and actively digest the host cell hemoglobin, which they use as a source of amino acids and energy.[6] This activity is

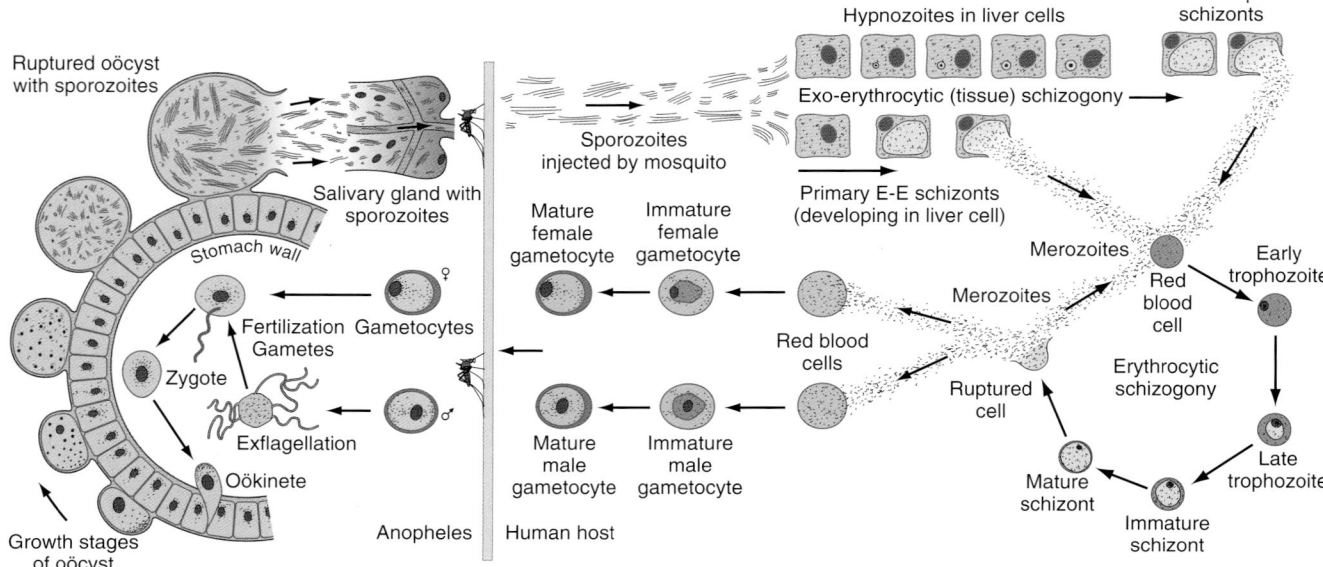

Figure 271-1. Generalized life cycle of malarial parasites in the anopheline mosquito vector and in humans. (Redrawn from Bruce-Chwatt LJ. Essential Malariology, 2nd ed. New York, John Wiley & Sons, copyright ©1985. Reprinted by permission of John Wiley & Sons, Inc.)

accomplished through a set of highly adapted proteinases in a singularly adapted organelle, the food vacuole.[7] The residue of hemoglobin degradation is an intact tetrapyrrole ring, ferriprotoporphyrin IX, which the parasites detoxify through polymerization and which can be seen microscopically as malarial pigment.[8] This polymerization step is thought to be the site of action of quinoline-containing antimalarial compounds, including chloroquine.[9,10]

The last few hours of the erythrocytic stage of the parasite's life cycle, when the parasite is called a schizont, comprise the actual replicative phase in which the parasite undergoes mitosis and subdivides and differentiates into merozoites. It is the subsequent rupture and release of merozoites that lead to fever and other malarial symptoms. If infections are synchronized, the periodicity of symptoms is 48 hours in *P. ovale* and *P. vivax* malaria, whereas it is 72 hours in *P. malariae* infections, and just 24 hours in *P. knowlesi* infections.[11] While periodicity may be every 48 hours in *P. falciparum* infections, it often is irregular. Indeed, the parasite's reproductive cycles often are not synchronized with any of the species and the absence of periodicity does not exclude malaria being the cause of fevers.

Parasites in the erythrocytic stages also can undergo sexual differentiation, a step that is necessary for transmission. Male and female gametes, which are produced by each *Plasmodium* species, remain inside the erythrocyte until they are ingested by the mosquito. At this point, they undergo further differentiation and join to form a zygote, which differentiates into an ookinete and invades the mosquito midgut to form the reproductive oocyst. Sporozoites emerge from the oocyst and migrate to the salivary gland, where they can reinfect a human during a subsequent blood meal.

In general, all of the erythrocytic asexual and sexual developmental stages of *P. ovale, P. vivax, P. malariae,* and *P. knowlesi* occur in circulating blood and can be visualized in the peripheral blood smear. The late trophozoite stages of *P. falciparum* rarely are seen in the peripheral circulation because of the development of "knobs" on infected erythrocytes that lead to adherence of the parasitized erythrocytes to the capillary endothelium.[12] Sequestration of parasites in various organs is believed to be responsible for the clinical manifestations that occur with *P. falciparum* infections, such as central nervous system (CNS) and pulmonary complications.

No strict immunity per se develops to malaria, but rather an acquired ability to tolerate *Plasmodium* infections occurs, which is a selective process related to the degree of exposure to a variety of strains.[13] Most deaths from malaria occur in children younger <5 years of age in areas of high transmission of *P. falciparum.* Although *P. falciparum* can cause lethal infection in young children or nonimmune individuals, asymptomatic parasitemia is common in older age groups in highly endemic areas. In the U.S., most malaria cases occur among first- and second-generation immigrants returning to their countries of origin to visit friends and relatives and who do not feel it is necessary or are unaware of the need to take prophylaxis while traveling, despite their loss of immunity.[1]

EPIDEMIOLOGY

The epidemiology of malarial infections is intricately linked to the distribution and habits of the anopheline vectors in any particular region. In highly endemic areas, mosquito breeding can take place nearly year round, and reproductive capacity in the mosquito is maximized by a tropical climate.[14] In areas of seasonal transmission, prevalence is particularly related to rainfall or other ecologic events that affect the mosquito population. Malaria also can be related to occupation when only certain segments of the population are exposed to the vectors.

The estimated worldwide incidence of malaria is 243 million (5th to 95th centiles, 190 to 311 million) clinical malaria episodes per year, with an estimated 863,000 deaths (5th to 95th centiles, 708,000 to 1,003,000) in 2008, most of which occur in children younger than 5 years.[15] Almost all deaths are due to *P. falciparum,* with more than 80% occurring in sub-Saharan Africa. Prior to the 1950s, malaria was endemic throughout the southeastern U.S. During the late 1940s, a combination of improved housing and socioeconomic conditions, water management, vector-control efforts, and case management was successful in interrupting malaria transmission. In the U.S. today, almost all cases occur in persons who have traveled to or are emigrating from malarious areas,[1] although transmission occasionally occurs congenitally or through transfusion or transplantation. Anopheline vectors still are present in most areas of the U.S., and, infrequently, localized outbreaks of malaria occur because of transmission from imported human cases.[16]

CLINICAL MANIFESTATIONS

The clinical features of malaria are dependent on the malaria-specific immune status of the host and the infecting species of *Plasmodium.* Nonimmune people, such as those who have not resided in an endemic area or have moved away from an endemic area, generally have symptomatic infection. Infections with *P. falciparum* are more likely to become severe than infections with the other four species that infect humans, though *P. vivax* and *P. knowlesi* also can cause severe disease.

The febrile paroxysm is the hallmark of malaria and typically lasts from 10 to 12 hours and consists of a period of severe rigors or chills, followed by high fever that can induce a febrile seizure; profuse sweating occurs with defervescence. Other nonspecific complaints at the time of fever include headache, malaise, myalgia, and arthralgia. Gastrointestinal tract symptoms, including abdominal pain, vomiting, and diarrhea, can occur. Although prostrated during febrile episodes, people otherwise can be remarkably asymptomatic between episodes.

Given the variable and nonspecific clinical findings and the potential for rapidly fatal disease, a high index of suspicion for malaria is necessary in ill travelers who have returned from an endemic area. Another complicating factor is that nonimmune individuals can have clinical symptoms despite low levels of parasitemia. Thus, 3 thick and thin blood smears separated by 12 to 24 hours are recommended to exclude malaria.

Significant morbidity and mortality from *P. falciparum* infections is due to cerebral effects.[17] Delirium and confusion can occur with the high fever of malaria, but actual declining mental status is more ominous and indicates the need for urgent treatment. Symptoms can progress rapidly to coma. Whereas meningismus, generalized seizures, and symmetrical upper motor neuron dysfunction can be seen, focal seizures or localizing neurologic signs are uncommon in malaria. The rapid recovery of CNS function with treatment and the general lack of sequelae suggest metabolic encephalopathy as the probable mechanism of dysfunction. The highest risk for neurologic sequelae is in patients with multiple seizures, prolonged coma, hypoglycemia, and clinical features of intracranial hypertension.[18,19]

The combination of respiratory compromise and renal dysfunction with *P. falciparum* infection also is associated with increased mortality.[20] Respiratory distress syndrome can occur and can be exacerbated by vigorous fluid resuscitation. Renal dysfunction most commonly is acute tubular necrosis, probably secondary to hypoperfusion from hypotension or hypovolemia. Although reported in children, this complication is observed more frequently in nonimmune adults. Nephrotic syndrome and glomerulonephritis have been associated with chronic infections with *P. malariae* in children, but are not common.

Hyperparasitemia (≥5% red blood cells (RBCs) infected) with *P. falciparum* in nonimmune individuals frequently is associated with hypotension, metabolic acidosis, and hypoglycemia.[17,20] These signs all can be attributed to parasitemia and associated cytokine disturbances, although concomitant gram-negative bacillary septicemia has been reported, particularly in association with severe gastrointestinal tract symptoms.[20] Hypoglycemia must be managed aggressively and monitored carefully, particularly when using quinine or quinidine therapy.

Anemia is an expected consequence of malaria, especially with hyperparasitemia. Hemolysis from erythrocytic parasitosis, sequestration and RBC destruction resulting in hypersplenism, and dyserythropoiesis have been identified as mechanisms contributing to anemia.[21] Thrombocytopenia is common in malaria but rarely leads to a bleeding diathesis. Evidence of a consumptive coagulopathy is rare but can occur with *P. falciparum* infection in nonimmune individuals and usually develops in the setting of "algid" malaria, a septic shock-like syndrome. Brisk hemolysis with hemoglobinuria, called blackwater fever, can occur with hyperparasitemia in nonimmune individuals, but it is more common as an epiphenomenon in individuals residing in endemic areas and is associated with prolonged quinine intake (which is no longer recommended) or in glucose-6-phosphate dehydrogenase (G6PD)-deficient people using oxidant antimalarial drugs.

LABORATORY FINDINGS AND DIAGNOSIS

The most important step in making the diagnosis of malaria is including it in the differential. Many of the deaths from malaria in the U.S. are related to a delay in diagnosis.[22] Malaria should be considered the primary diagnosis until proven otherwise in any febrile patient who has traveled to or emigrated from an endemic area. Malaria also should be considered in patients who develop fever within days to a few months after blood transfusion.

The diagnosis of malaria is made by identifying parasites in thick or thin blood films stained with common hematologic stains, most typically Giemsa-based stains. The thick-film preparation is the more sensitive technique, but it is more difficult to interpret by inexperienced examiners. Speciation usually is performed with a thin smear. For initial clinical management, it is most important to identify the presence or absence of malaria parasites. If present, determining the percent parasitemia is essential for managing the patient as patients with ≥5% infected RBCs have greater incidence of complications and require immediate therapy intravenously. *P. falciparum* is strongly suggested by RBC parasitemia >2%, RBCs containing multiple parasites, the exclusive presence of ring forms, and lack of schizonts. *P. falciparum* is identified pathognomonically by the banana-shaped gametocyte form; its presence is helpful, but its absence does not rule out the diagnosis. Late trophozoite stages of *P. falciparum* rarely are seen except in the setting of high parasitemia. A quantitative assessment of the initial parasitemia also is useful in assessing response to therapy.

Various test kits are available to detect antigens derived from malaria parasites. Such tests most often use a dipstick or cassette format, and provide results in 15 to 20 minutes. These rapid diagnostic tests (RDTs) offer a useful alternative to microscopy in situations where reliable microscopic diagnosis is not available. One malaria RDT, Binax NOW® Malaria, was approved for use in the U.S. by the Food and Drug Administration (FDA) in 2007. This RDT uses histidine-rich protein 2 (HRP2) to detect *P. falciparum* malaria, as well as a panmalarial aldolase to detect the presence of other species. The sensitivity of this test to detect *P. falciparum* malaria is reported to be 95%, while sensitivity for *P. vivax* is only about 69%.[23] It is important to note that the sensitivity is considerably lower in patients with low parasitemia (<200 parasites/µL). In a recent World Health Organization RDT product testing, Binax NOW® detected 91% of *P. falciparum* isolates at 200 parasites/µL but only 10% of *P. vivax* isolates at 200 parasites/µL.[24] While RDTs can be useful in making a rapid diagnosis, all Binax NOW® tests, negative or positive, must be followed by microscopic evaluation of a blood smear.

Parasite nucleic acids are detected by polymerase chain reaction (PCR), which may be a useful complement to microscopy, for example when species determination cannot be made by blood smear. However, PCR requires a specialized laboratory and is not available widely.

Serology (immunofluorescence assay) detects antibodies against malaria parasites, but because of the time required for development of antibody and also the persistence of antibodies, serologic testing is not useful for routine diagnosis of acute malaria. Commercially available enzyme immunoassays for malaria antibodies should not be used as none have been FDA-approved for the diagnosis of malaria.

While no other laboratory findings are diagnostic for malaria, a number of laboratory findings support the diagnosis and can be useful to assess the severity of infection. Generally, patients have a normocytic, hemolytic anemia with a variable white blood cell count and differential count. Thrombocytopenia often is present. In the setting of cerebral malaria when meningitis also must be excluded, lumbar puncture can reveal raised opening pressure, and cerebrospinal fluid (CSF) analysis can show mildly elevated protein levels and mild lymphocytic pleocytosis. Electrolyte disturbances are common in severe malaria and usually are multifactorial in origin, including dehydration, vomiting, renal failure, and tissue hypoxia. Hypoglycemia can occur. Urinalysis generally is normal except for proteinuria during high fever. Urinalysis also can reveal hemoglobinuria in the setting of brisk hemolysis, proteinuria associated with nephrotic syndrome, or RBCs with glomerulonephritis. Mildly elevated serum hepatic transaminase levels and indirect hyperbilirubinemia can be present; hepatic failure is uncommon.

TREATMENT

Once the diagnosis of malaria is made, multiple factors must be assessed to establish an appropriate strategy for treatment. The first factor to consider is whether the patient has uncomplicated or severe malaria (Box 271-1). Other factors that affect therapy are the geographic region in which malaria was acquired and the use of antimalarial chemoprophylaxis.[25,26] See Chapter 296, Antiparasitic Agents, for a discussion of specific properties of antiparasitic agents.

Patients with *P. falciparum* malaria and those in whom *P. falciparum* cannot be excluded because the species has not been determined at the time of diagnosis should be hospitalized for therapy and monitored because of the rapid clinical deterioration that can occur even if the patient initially appears stable (Box 271-2). Therapy should be started immediately and supportive care given as necessary. If the patient has severe malaria or is unable to tolerate oral therapy, intravenous quinidine in combination with doxycycline, tetracycline, or clindamycin should be used in a setting in which cardiovascular status and hypoglycemia can be monitored closely and managed urgently[27,28] (Table 271-1). As newer

---

BOX 271-1. Manifestations of Severe Malaria

- Cerebral malaria, defined as unarousable coma not attributable to any other cause in a patient with *P. falciparum* malaria
- Seizures
- Severe normocytic anemia with hematocrit <15%
- Hypoglycemia
- Metabolic acidosis with respiratory distress
- Fluid and electrolyte disturbances
- Acute renal failure
- Acute respiratory distress syndrome
- Hypotension, shock, septicemia ("algid malaria")
- Abnormal coagulation
- Hemoglobinuria
- Hyperparasitemia (>5% of red blood cells infected)

BOX 271-2. Management of Individuals with Severe Malaria

- Hospitalize
- Initiate intravenous antimalarial therapy immediately
- Correct fluid balance and electrolyte abnormalities cautiously
- Monitor, prevent, and correct hypoglycemia
- Correct anemia as needed
- Provide antipyretic therapy
- Protect the airway in patients with altered mental status
- Consider exchange transfusion for parasitemia >10% or end organ complications
- Avoid harmful adjuvant therapies

TABLE 271-1. Guidelines for the Treatment of Malaria in the United States

Clinical Diagnosis/ *Plasmodium* Species	Region Infection Acquired	Recommended Drug and Adult Dose	Recommended Drug and Pediatric Dose *Pediatric dose should NEVER exceed adult dose*
Severe malaria	All regions	**A. Quinidine gluconate plus one of the following: Doxycycline, Tetracycline, or Clindamycin** **Quinidine gluconate:** 6.25 mg base/kg (= 10 mg salt/kg) loading dose IV over 1–2 hours, then 0.0125 mg base/kg/min (= 0.02 mg salt/kg/min) continuous infusion for at least 24 hours. An alternative regimen is 15 mg base/kg (= 24 mg salt/kg) loading dose IV infused over 4 hours, followed by 7.5 mg base/kg (= 12 mg salt/kg) infused over 4 hours every 8 hours, starting 8 hours after the loading dose. Once parasite density is <1% and patient can take oral medication, complete treatment with oral quinine, dosed as below. Quinidine/quinine course = 7-day course for Southeast Asia; = 3-day course for all other regions **Doxycycline:** 100 mg PO bid × 7 days. If patient is not able to take oral medication, give 100 mg IV every 12 hours and then give oral doxycycline as soon as patient can tolerate oral medication. Treatment course = 7 days **Tetracycline:** 250 mg PO qid × 7 days **Clindamycin:** 20 mg kg/day PO divided tid × 7 days. If patient is not able to take oral medication, give 10 mg base/kg loading dose IV followed by 5 mg base/kg IV every 8 hours. Give oral clindamycin (oral dose as above) as soon as patient can tolerate oral medication. Treatment course = 7 days	**A. Quinidine gluconate plus one of the following: Doxycycline, Tetracycline,[a] or Clindamycin** **Quinidine gluconate:** Same mg/kg dosing and recommendations as for adults **Doxycycline:[a]** 4 mg/kg/day PO divided bid × 7 days. Can be used in children ≥8 years old. If patient is not able to take oral medication, may give IV. For children <45 kg, give 2.2 mg/kg IV every 12 hours and then give oral doxycycline (dose as above) as soon as patient can take oral medication. For children ≥45 kg, use same dosing as for adults **Tetracycline:[a]** 25 mg/kg/day PO divided qid × 7 days **Clindamycin:** 20 mg base/kg/day PO divided tid × 7 days. If patient is not able to take oral medication, give 10 mg/kg loading dose IV followed by 5 mg/kg IV every 8 hours. Switch to oral clindamycin (oral dose as above) a soon as patient can take ora medication
		B. Investigational new drug: Contact CDC for more information **Artesunate** followed by one of the following: **Atovaquone-proguanil (Malarone™), Doxycycline (Clindamycin** in pregnant women), or **Mefloquine**	**B. Investigational new drug: Contact CDC for more information** **Artesunate** followed by one of the following: **Atovaquone-proguanil (Malarone™), Doxycycline (Clindamycin** in pregnant women), or **Mefloquine**
Uncomplicated malaria/ *P. falciparum* or species not identified If "species not identified" is subsequently diagnosed as *P. vivax* or *P. ovale*: see *P. vivax* and *P. ovale* (below) re. treatment with primaquine	Chloroquine sensitive (Central America west of Panama Canal; Haiti; the Dominican Republic; and most of the Middle East)	**A. Chloroquine phosphate (Aralen™ and generic formulations)** 600 mg base (= 1000 mg salt) PO immediately, followed by 300 mg base (= 500 mg salt) PO at 6, 24, and 48 hours Total dose: 1500 mg base (= 2500 mg salt)	**A. Chloroquine phosphate (Aralen™ and generic formulations)** 10 mg base/kg PO immediately, followed by 5 mg base/kg PO at 6, 24, and 48 hours Total dose: 25 mg base/kg
		B. Hydroxychloroquine 620 mg base (= 800 mg salt) PO immediately, followed by 310 mg base (= 400 mg salt) PO at 6, 24, and 48 hours Total dose: 1550 mg base (= 2000 mg salt)	**B. Hydroxychloroquine** 10 mg base/kg PO immediately, followed by 5 mg base/kg PO at 6, 24, and 48 hours Total dose: 25 mg base/kg

Continued

TABLE 271-1. Guidelines for the Treatment of Malaria in the United States—cont'd

Clinical Diagnosis/ *Plasmodium* Species	Region Infection Acquired	Recommended Drug and Adult Dose	Recommended Drug and Pediatric Dose *Pediatric dose should NEVER exceed adult dose*
	Chloroquine resistant or unknown resistance[b] (All malarious regions except those specified as chloroquine sensitive listed in the box above. Middle Eastern countries with chloroquine-resistant *P. falciparum* include Iran, Oman, Saudi Arabia, and Yemen	**A. Quinine sulfate[c] plus one of the following: Doxycycline, Tetracycline, or Clindamycin** **Quinine sulfate:** 542 mg base (= 650 mg salt) PO tid × 3 to 7 days **Doxycycline:** Treatment as above **Tetracycline:** Treatment as above **Clindamycin:** Treatment as above	**A. Quinine sulfate[c] plus one of the following: Doxycycline,[a] Tetracycline[a] or Clindamycin** **Quinine sulfate:[c]** 8.3 mg base/kg (= 10 mg salt/kg) PO tid × 3 to 7 days **Doxycycline:[a]** Treatment as above **Tetracycline:[a]** Treatment as above **Clindamycin:** Treatment as above
		B. Atovaquone-proguanil (Malarone™) **Adult tablet = 250 mg atovaquone/ 100 mg proguanil** 4 adult tablets PO qd × 3 days	**B. Atovaquone-proguanil (Malarone™)** **Adult tablet = 250 mg atovaquone/ 100 mg proguanil** **Pediatric tablet = 62.5 mg atovaquone/ 25 mg proguanil** 5–8 kg: 2 pediatric tablets PO qd × 3 days 9–10 kg: 3 pediatric tablets PO qd × 3 days 11–20 kg: 1 adult tablet PO qd × 3 days 21–30 kg: 2 adult tablets PO qd × 3 days 31–40 kg: 3 adult tablets PO qd × 3 days >40 kg: 4 adult tablets PO qd × 3 days
		C. Mefloquine (Lariam™ and generic formulations) 684 mg base (= 750 mg salt) PO as initial dose, followed by 456 mg base (= 500 mg salt) PO given 6–12 hours after initial dose Total dose = 1250 mg salt	**C. Mefloquine (Lariam™ and generics)** 13.7 mg base/kg (= 15 mg salt/kg) PO as initial dose, followed by 9.1 mg base/kg (= 10 mg salt/kg) PO given 6–12 hours after initial dose Total dose = 25 mg salt/kg
		D. Arthemeter-lumefantrine 1 tablet = 20 mg arthemeter and 120 mg lumefantrine 3 day weight-based treatment course: 1 tablet initially followed by one tablet after 8 hours. Then 1 tablet PO bid × 2 days. 5–<15 kg = 1 tablet per dose 15–<25 kg = 2 tablets per dose 25–<35 kg = 3 tablets per dose >35 kg = 4 tablets per dose	**D. Arthemeter-lumefantrine** 1 tablet = 20 mg arthemeter and 120 mg lumefantrine 3 day weight-based treatment course: 1 tablet initially followed by one tablet after 8 hours. Then 1 tablet PO bid × 2 days. 5–<15 kg = 1 tablet per dose 15–<25 kg = 2 tablets per dose 25–<35 kg = 3 tablets per dose >35 kg = 4 tablets per dose
Uncomplicated malaria *P. malariae* or *P. knowlesi*	All regions	**Chloroquine phosphate:** Treatment as above *OR* **Hydroxychloroquine:** Treatment as above	**Chloroquine phosphate:** Treatment as above *OR* **Hydroxychloroquine:** Treatment as above
Uncomplicated malaria *P. vivax* or *P. ovale*	All regions[d] Note: for suspected chloroquine resistant *P. vivax*, see below	**Chloroquine phosphate *or* Hydroxychloroquine plus Primaquine phosphate** **Chloroquine phosphate OR Hydroxychloroquine:** Treatment as above **Primaquine phosphate:** 30 mg base PO qd × 14 days	**Chloroquine phosphate *or* Hydroxychloroquine plus Primaquine phosphate** **Chloroquine phosphate OR Hydroxychloroquine:** Treatment as above **Primaquine phosphate:** 0.5 mg base/kg PO qd × 14 days
Uncomplicated malaria *P. vivax*	**Chloroquine-resistant[d]** (Papua New Guinea and Indonesia)	**A. Quinine sulfate[c] plus either Doxycycline or Tetracycline, plus Primaquine phosphate** **Quinine sulfate:** Treatment as above **Doxycycline or Tetracycline:** Treatment as above **Primaquine phosphate:** Treatment as above	**A. Quinine sulfate[c] plus either Doxycycline[a] or Tetracycline,[a] plus Primaquine phosphate** **Quinine sulfate:[c]** Treatment as above **Doxycycline[a] or Tetracycline:[a]** Treatment as above **Primaquine phosphate:** Treatment as above

Continued

TABLE 271-1. Guidelines for the Treatment of Malaria in the United States—cont'd

Clinical Diagnosis/ *Plasmodium* Species	Region Infection Acquired	Recommended Drug and Adult Dose	Recommended Drug and Pediatric Dose *Pediatric dose should NEVER exceed adult dose*
		B. Mefloquine plus Primaquine phosphate	**B. Mefloquine plus Primaquine phosphate**
		Mefloquine: Treatment as above	**Mefloquine:** Treatment as above
		Primaquine phosphate: Treatment as above	**Primaquine phosphate:** Treatment as above
		C. Atovaquone-proguanil plus Primaquine phosphate	**C. Atovaquone-proguanil plus Primaquine phosphate**
		Atovaquone-proguanil: Treatment as above	**Atovaquone-proguanil:** Treatment as above
		Primaquine phosphate: Treatment as above	**Primaquine phosphate:** Treatment as above

[a]*Doxycycline and tetracycline are not indicated for use in children less than 8 years old. For children less than 8 years old with chloroquine-resistant P. falciparum, quinine (given alone for 7 days or given in combination with clindamycin) and atovaquone-proguanil are recommended treatment options; mefloquine can be considered if no other options are available. For children less than 8 years old with chloroquine-resistant P. vivax, quinine (given alone for 7 days) or mefloquine are recommended treatment options. If none of these treatment options are available or are not being tolerated and if the treatment benefits outweigh the risks, doxycycline or tetracycline may be given to children less than 8 years old.*

[b]*There are three options (A, B, or C) available for treatment of uncomplicated malaria caused by chloroquine-resistant P. falciparum. Options A and B are equally recommended. Because of a higher rate of severe neuropsychiatric reactions seen at treatment doses, we do not recommend option C (mefloquine) unless options A and B cannot be used. For option A, because there are more data on the efficacy of quinine in combination with doxycycline or tetracycline, these treatment combinations generally are preferred to quinine in combination with clindamycin.*

[c]*For infections acquired in Southeast Asia, quinine treatment should continue for 7 days. For infections acquired in Africa and South America, quinine treatment should continue for 3 days.*

[d]*For treatment of chloroquine-resistant P. vivax infections, options A and B are equally recommended.*

anti-arrhythmic drugs have replaced quinidine for many cardiac indications, some hospitals and other healthcare facilities have dropped quinidine gluconate from their formularies. Clinicians providing care for patients with malaria should be aware of the inpatient availability of quinidine to avoid delays in treatment.

Patients with severe malaria should be given an intravenous loading dose of quinidine unless they have received >40 mg/kg of quinine in the preceding 48 hours or if they have received mefloquine within the preceding 12 hours. Consultation with a cardiologist and a physician with experience treating malaria is advised when treating patients with malaria using quinidine. Electrocardiogram should be performed prior to initiation of quinidine therapy to determine baseline QTc interval. During administration of quinidine, monitoring of blood pressure (for hypotension) and continuous cardiac monitoring (for widening of the QRS complex and/or lengthening of the QTc interval) are required, and blood glucose should be evaluated (for hypoglycemia) periodically.[29] Cardiac complications, if severe, may warrant temporary discontinuation of the drug or slowing of the intravenous infusion. Exchange transfusion should be considered strongly if the initial parasitemia is >10% or if altered mental status, acute respiratory distress syndrome (ARDS), or renal complications are present.[28-30] The percentage of infected RBCs should be monitored to assess response to therapy. Exchange transfusion should be continued until the parasitemia is <1% (usually requires replacement of 1 to 2 blood volumes). Intravenous quinidine administration should not be delayed for an exchange transfusion and can be given concurrently throughout the exchange transfusion.

Clinical deterioration can occur in the first 24 hours of therapy, particularly in patients with high-level parasitemia. Supportive care during this period is critical and should include careful monitoring for hypoglycemia and anemia, careful management of fluid and electrolyte disturbances, monitoring for respiratory and renal compromise, and protection of the patient's airway if declining mental status is evident. Adjunctive therapies such as corticosteroids, heparin, epinephrine, desferrioxamine, cyclosporine, prostacyclin, or osmotic agents for cerebral edema have not proven effective for severe malaria, and considerable evidence suggests potential harm from some of these treatments.

When intravenous quinidine is not available, contraindicated, or not tolerated, intravenous artesunate, an investigational drug available through the Centers for Disease Control and Prevention (CDC), may be provided. Artesunate is not FDA-approved, but has been accepted widely for the treatment of malaria in other countries.[31-33] The CDC should be contacted through the Malaria Hotline (770-488-7788 during working hours, 770-488-7100 after hours and weekends) for any cases for which use of this investigational drug may be indicated.

Complications of malaria generally are limited to the acute illness; prolonged convalescence is common. In general, full recovery from any pulmonary, renal, or CNS compromise is the rule. The exception occurs in children with cerebral malaria in whom up to 10% may have residual neurologic deficits.[19]

Parasitemia should decrease substantially after the first 48 hours of therapy. Parasites generally clear by 72 hours and their persistence should prompt evaluation of possible causes, including inadequate dosage or possible drug resistance. Gametocytes of *P. falciparum* are not killed by most therapies used and can be seen for weeks after the initiation of therapy; this finding should not be considered a sign of drug failure and no additional antimalarial therapy is required.

Oral chloroquine can be used in individuals with uncomplicated malaria due to *P. falciparum* if infection was acquired in parts of the world free of widespread chloroquine resistance (see CDC website for most up-to-date listings, http://www.cdc.gov/malaria/travelers/country_table/a.html) and if the patient is able to take oral medication (Table 271-1). Individuals with *P. falciparum* malaria acquired in all other geographic areas should be treated with artemether-lumefantrine, atovaquone-proguanil, or with oral quinine sulfate plus either tetracycline, doxycycline, or clindamycin, depending on the age of the patient, because of the high risk of chloroquine resistance. Artemether-lumefantrine is a newer antimalarial agent that is highly malariacidal and results in rapid parasite clearance. For patients with malaria acquired in Southeast

Asia, treatment with quinine should be continued for 7 days (instead of 3 to 7 days) because of evidence of declining efficacy. Doxycycline, tetracycline, or clindamycin should not be used alone for malaria therapy because of the delayed onset (48 hours) of action of these drugs.

Mefloquine is an alternative treatment for *P. falciparum* infections acquired in areas with chloroquine resistance if the other regimens cannot be used. Its use is limited by the higher rate of neuropsychiatric reactions seen at treatment doses and thus is considered second-line therapy. Mefloquine should not be given at the same time as quinine or quinidine due to concern for cardiotoxicity. Additionally, mefloquine should not be used in patients who have acquired infection in Southeast Asia due to high levels of resistance.

Patients who do not have *P. falciparum* infection and who have no signs of severe disease can be treated with chloroquine or hydroxychloroquine (Plaquenil) as outpatients, depending on their overall clinical status, and if they are monitored for symptomatic improvement (Table 271-1). Chloroquine treatment failure rates are high among *P. vivax* infections acquired in Papua New Guinea and Indonesia, and thus *P. vivax* infections acquired in these areas should be treated with mefloquine or a combination of quinine plus doxycycline.[34] If the patient cannot take oral medication, intravenous quinidine is the drug of choice. If the patient does not respond to treatment with chloroquine, the treatment should be changed to a regimen effective against chloroquine-resistant *P. vivax*.

If the infecting species is identified as *P. vivax* or *P. ovale*, treatment with primaquine also is necessary to prevent relapse from latent hypnozoite forms in the liver (Table 271-1). G6PD deficiency must be excluded prior to giving primaquine. Ideally, primaquine therapy should be initiated concomitantly with the blood schizonticide as there is evidence that this results in greater efficacy in eradicating hypnozoites. However, if there is a delay in determining the species, or in obtaining G6PD testing results, primaquine still should be given even if the person has already completed their acute treatment. Individuals with G6PD deficiency who are not able to take primaquine should be retreated with chloroquine if relapses occur, or given weekly chloroquine prophylaxis for 1 to 2 years. The recommended course of primaquine is 0.5 mg/kg daily for 14 days with a target total dose of >6 mg/kg. Patients weighing >70 kg may require treatment for >14 days to achieve the target total dose. Failure of primaquine to eradicate hypnozoites is very unusual if this total dose is attained. However, in many cases adherence cannot be assured. If relapse occurs, the patient should be retreated with chloroquine and primaquine. Primaquine should not be used during pregnancy.

Physicians desiring consultation regarding the management of patients with malaria can call the Malaria Branch of the CDC at (770) 488-7788 during working hours or at (770) 488-7100 during nights and weekends. Up-to-date treatment recommendations also are available on CDC website at http://www.cdc.gov/malaria/diagnosis treatment/treatment.htm.

PREVENTION

Travelers to endemic areas can prevent malaria through the use of chemoprophylaxis and personal protective measures such as insect repellents. The risk of acquiring malaria is highest in sub-Saharan Africa and Oceania and is more variable for other regions. The evolving picture of drug resistance complicates recommendations for chemoprophylaxis. Malaria prophylaxis recommendations are available in the bi-annual publication "Health Information for International Travel" and the CDC malaria website at www.cdc.gov/malaria. Breastfed infants should receive appropriate malaria prophylaxis since they will not receive enough drug in the breast milk to protect them.

Chloroquine (or hydroxychloroquine) can be used for prophylaxis in areas where chloroquine resistance has not been reported. Primaquine is the drug of choice for areas where *P. vivax* is the predominant malaria species (Table 271-2). Chloroquine is available only in tablet form in the U.S., and the taste is bitter when crushed. Reported side effects include gastrointestinal disturbance, headache, dizziness, blurred vision, insomnia, and pruritus, but often these effects do not require that the drug be discontinued. Chloroquine has been reported to exacerbate psoriasis.

In areas where drug resistance (other than chloroquine resistance) is not a concern, atovaquone-proguanil, doxycycline, and mefloquine are equally recommended prophylactic options for persons traveling to areas where malaria transmission occurs (Table 271-2). The most common adverse effects reported in persons using atovaquone-proguanil for prophylaxis include abdominal pain, nausea, vomiting, and headache. Atovaquone-proguanil should not be used in children weighing <5 kg, pregnant women, women breastfeeding infants weighing <5 kg, or patients with severe renal impairment (creatinine clearance <30 mL/min). Atovaquone-proguanil should be given with food. Because atovaquone-proguanil is considered a *causal prophylactic agent* (i.e., kills the initial hepatic stage of malaria parasites), it needs to be given for only 7 days after leaving a malarious area.

Daily doxycycline is another option for travelers who are ≥8 years old. Gastrointestinal complaints, photosensitivity, and candidal vaginitis are reported adverse effects. Doxycycline should be taken with an ample amount of fluid and should not be taken prior to sleep to minimize the risk of esophagitis. Photosensitivity associated with the use of doxycycline can be lessened with sunscreen use. Doxycycline is contraindicated during pregnancy.

Mefloquine can be used in children of any weight (Table 271-2). Nausea and vomiting have been problematic in children. Other reported side effects include headache, insomnia, abnormal dreams, visual disturbances, depression, anxiety disorder, and dizziness. Rare serious adverse reactions include acute reversible severe neuropsychiatric reaction, seizures, and cardiac conduction abnormalities. Mefloquine is safe to use in pregnancy although data on use in the first trimester is limited. Mefloquine is contraindicated in persons with active depression, a recent history of depression, generalized anxiety disorder, psychosis, schizophrenia, other major psychiatric disorders, or seizures (but not including typical febrile seizures). Mefloquine should be used with caution in persons with prior psychiatric disturbances or a previous history of depression. It is not recommended for persons with cardiac conduction abnormalities. Resistance to mefloquine has been reported in Southeast Asia, where doxycycline or atovaquone-proguanil should be used for prophylaxis.[35]

Travelers who reject the advice to take prophylaxis, who choose a suboptimal drug regimen (e.g., chloroquine in an area with chloroquine-resistant *P. falciparum*), or who require a less-than-optimal drug regimen for medical reasons are at greater risk for acquiring malaria. In addition, some travelers who are taking effective prophylaxis but who will be in very remote areas may decide, in consultation with their healthcare provider, to carry a reliable supply of a full course of an approved malaria treatment regimen. In the event that they are diagnosed with malaria, they will have immediate access to this appropriate treatment regimen, which if acquired in a developed country is unlikely to be counterfeit and will not deplete local resources. In rare instances when access to medical care is not available and the traveler develops a febrile illness consistent with malaria, the reliable supply medication can be self-administered empirically. Travelers should be advised that this self-treatment of a possible malarial infection is only a temporary measure and that prompt medical evaluation is imperative.

There are two malaria treatment regimens that can be prescribed as a reliable supply – atovaquone-proguanil or artemether-lumefantrine. The use of the same or related drugs that have been taken for prophylaxis are not recommended to treat malaria. For example, atovaquone-proguanil can be used for treatment by travelers not taking atovaquone-proguanil for prophylaxis.

Avoidance of mosquitoes and barrier protection are critical aspects of malaria prophylaxis given that no chemoprophylaxis guarantees complete protection. Anopheline mosquitoes feed from dusk to dawn. Avoiding nighttime exposure by staying in

TABLE 271-2. Drugs Used in the Prophylaxis of Malaria

Drug	Usage	Adult Dose	Pediatric Dose	Comments
Atovaquone-proguanil (Malarone®)	Prophylaxis in areas with chloroquine-resistant or mefloquine-resistant *P. falciparum*	Adult tablets contain 250 mg atovaquone and 100 mg proguanil hydrochloride. 1 adult tablet orally, daily	Pediatric tablets contain 62.5 mg atovaquone and 25 mg proguanil hydrochloride. 5–7 kg: ½ pediatric tablet daily 8–10 kg: ¾ pediatric tablet daily 11–20 kg: 1 pediatric tablet daily 21–30 kg: 2 pediatric tablets daily 31–40 kg: 3 pediatric tablets daily 41 kg or more: 1 adult tablet daily	Begin 1–2 days before travel to malarious areas. Take daily at the same time each day while in the malarious area and for 7 days after leaving such areas. Atovaquone/proguanil is contraindicated in persons with severe renal impairment (creatinine clearance <30 mL/min). Atovaquone/proguanil should be taken with food or a milky drink. Atovaquone/proguanil is recommended for children 5 kg, pregnant women, and women breastfeeding infants weighing <5 kg
Chloroquine phosphate (Aralen® and generic)	Prophylaxis only in areas with chloroquine-sensitive *P. falciparum*	300 mg base (500 mg salt) orally, once/week	5 mg/kg base (8.3 mg/kg salt) orally, once/week, up to maximum adult dose of 300 mg base	Begin 1–2 weeks before travel to malarious areas. Take weekly on the same day of the week while in the malarious area and for 4 weeks after leaving such areas. Chloroquine can exacerbate psoriasis
Hydroxychloroquine sulfate (Plaquenil)	An alternative to chloroquine for prophylaxis only in areas with chloroquine-sensitive malaria	310 mg base (400 mg salt) orally, once weekly	5 mg/kg base (6.5 mg/kg salt) orally, once a week. Max. dose = adult 310 mg base	Begin 2 weeks before travel to malarious region. Take weekly on the same day of the week while in malarious area and for 4 weeks after leaving malaria endemic area
Doxycycline (Many brand names and generic formulations)	Prophylaxis in areas with chloroquine-resistant or mefloquine-resistant *P. falciparum*	100 mg orally, daily	8 years of age or older: 2 mg/kg up to adult dose of 100 mg/day	Begin 1–2 days before travel to malarious areas. Take daily at the same time each day while in the malarious area and for 4 weeks after leaving such areas. Doxycycline is contraindicated in children <8 years of age and in pregnant women
Mefloquine (Lariam and generic formulations)	Prophylaxis in areas with chloroquine-resistant *P. falciparum*	228 mg base (250 mg salt) orally, once/week	9 kg and under: 4.6 mg/kg base (5 mg/kg salt) orally, once/week 10–19 kg: ¼ tablet once/week 20–30 kg: ½ tablet once/week 31–45 kg: ¾ tablet once/week 46 kg and over: 1 tablet once/week	Begin at least 2 weeks before travel to malarious areas. Take weekly on the same day of the week while in the malarious area and for 4 weeks after leaving such areas. Mefloquine is contraindicated in persons allergic to mefloquine or related compounds (e.g., quinine and quinidine) and in persons with active depression, recent history of depression, generalized anxiety disorder, psychosis, schizophrenia, other major psychiatric disorders, or seizures. Use with caution in persons with psychiatric disturbances, or a previous history of depression. Use is not recommended for persons with cardiac conduction abnormalities
Primaquine		30 mg base (52.6 mg salt) orally, daily	0.5 mg/kg base (0.8 mg/kg salt) up to adult dose orally, daily	Begin 1–2 days before travel to malarious areas. Take daily at the same time each day while in the malarious area and for 7 days after leaving such areas. Contraindicated in persons with G6PD deficiency. Also contraindicated during pregnancy and lactation unless the infant being breastfed has a documented normal G6PD level

G6PD, glucose-6-phosphate dehydrogenase.

screened-in or air-conditioned areas, using protective clothing, sleeping under insecticide-treated bed nets, and using repellents all are helpful. Topical mosquito repellents that contain *N-N*-diethyl-*m*-toluamide (DEET) or picaridin are the most effective in preventing malaria.[36] Permethrin-impregnated bed nets are effective, and permethrin sprays are available for use on clothing.

None of these measures is 100% effective, and therefore the diagnosis of malaria should be considered in anyone with a fever who has been in an endemic area. Most travelers in whom malaria is diagnosed manifest symptoms within a few weeks to months after return from the malaria endemic area, particularly with *P. falciparum* infection. Infections with the other species of malaria can appear months later. For persons emigrating from malaria-endemic areas, manifestations of *P. falciparum* infection would rarely occur after 1 year, whereas those with the other species of *Plasmodium* could occur years later.

Pregnancy increases the risk of complications from malaria in both nonimmune and partially immune women. Their clinical course can be more severe, and malaria during pregnancy carries an increased risk of premature birth or pregnancy loss. Pregnant women should avoid travel to malaria-endemic areas. If they must travel, chloroquine or mefloquine prophylaxis can be used during pregnancy. Doxycycline and atovaquone-proguanil are not recommended for use during pregnancy.

Traveling with children requires special preparation. In the U.S., antimalarial drugs are available only in tablet form and most taste bitter. Compounding pharmacies can pulverize tablets, weigh out the precise dose, and place the dose in a gelatin capsule; sufficient time will be needed before travel to allow preparation of appropriate dosages. The capsule can be opened at the time of administration and the medication mixed with sweet food items, such as applesauce, chocolate syrup, or jelly, to disguise the taste.[36]

Key Points. Epidemiology, Clinical Features, Diagnosis and Treatment of Malaria

EPIDEMIOLOGY

- Parasitic disease transmitted by anopheline mosquitoes
- Predominately in tropical climates
- 243 million cases per year
- 863,000 deaths per year, mostly in children <5 years of age
- Most deaths are due to *P. falciparum* and 80% occur in sub-Saharan Africa
- In the U.S., most cases occur in persons who have traveled to or emigrated from endemic areas.

CLINICAL FEATURES

- Cyclical fevers with chills, rigors
- Nonspecific symptoms such as myalgia, headache, arthralgia, fatigue
- Abdominal pain, diarrhea, vomiting
- Declining mental status can be a sign of cerebral malaria

DIAGNOSIS

- Malaria should be suspected in anyone with fever who recently was in an endemic area

- Microscopic examination of thick or thin blood films detect parasites
- Rapid diagnostic tests should be available if microscopy is not available on site
- PCR can be used to aid in speciation
- Thrombocytopenia is very common

TREATMENT

- Severe malaria (acquired in any region)
  - Quinidine IV followed by tetracycline, clindamycin, or doxycycline; *or*
  - Artesunate IV (investigational drug available via consultation with CDC), followed by atovaquone-proguanil, mefloquine, or doxycycline
  - See Table 271-1 for doses, duration, and age specifications
- Uncomplicated malaria
  - Consider prophylaxis regimen taken
  - Consider area of travel and resistance patterns
  - Consider species of *Plasmodium* identified
  - Consider age of patient and pregnancy status
  - See Table 271-1 to tailor therapy to above specifications

---

272 *Sarcocystis* Species

Frank E. Berkowitz

Sarcocystis was first observed in 1843 in mice, and since then more than 120 species have been reported from a range of wild and domestic animals.[1] The name *Sarcocystis* is due to the observation that the organism forms cysts in muscle. *Sarcocystis* is a zoonotic protozoan parasite, with an obligatory two-host cycle. Few of the >120 species infect human beings, which are incidental hosts, but they are an important cause of infection in wild and domestic animals.[1] The two main species infecting humans are *S. hominis* (from cattle) and *S. suihominis* (from pigs), acquired from ingestion of raw beef or poorly cooked pork containing tissue cysts.[1]

PATHOGEN

The life cycle of *Sarcocystis* is shown in Figure 272-1. *Sarcocystis* has an obligatory two-host cycle that mainly involves herbivorous

animals as intermediate hosts and carnivorous animals as definitive hosts. Definitive and intermediate hosts generally are species specific, but have not been identified for all *Sarcocystis* species. Thin-walled oocysts (containing two sporocysts) (Figure 272-2) or individual sporocysts (each containing four sporozoites) that have emerged from the oocyst are excreted in the feces of the definitive (carnivore) host. Sporocysts are ingested by cows and pigs and eventually form merozoites that penetrate muscle cells and develop into cysts containing crescent-shaped bradyzoites, which are the infective stage for the definitive host (Figure 272-3).

Humans can serve as incidental, intermediate hosts when food contaminated with sporocysts is ingested accidentally or serve as definitive hosts when raw or undercooked beef or pork is consumed.[1,2]

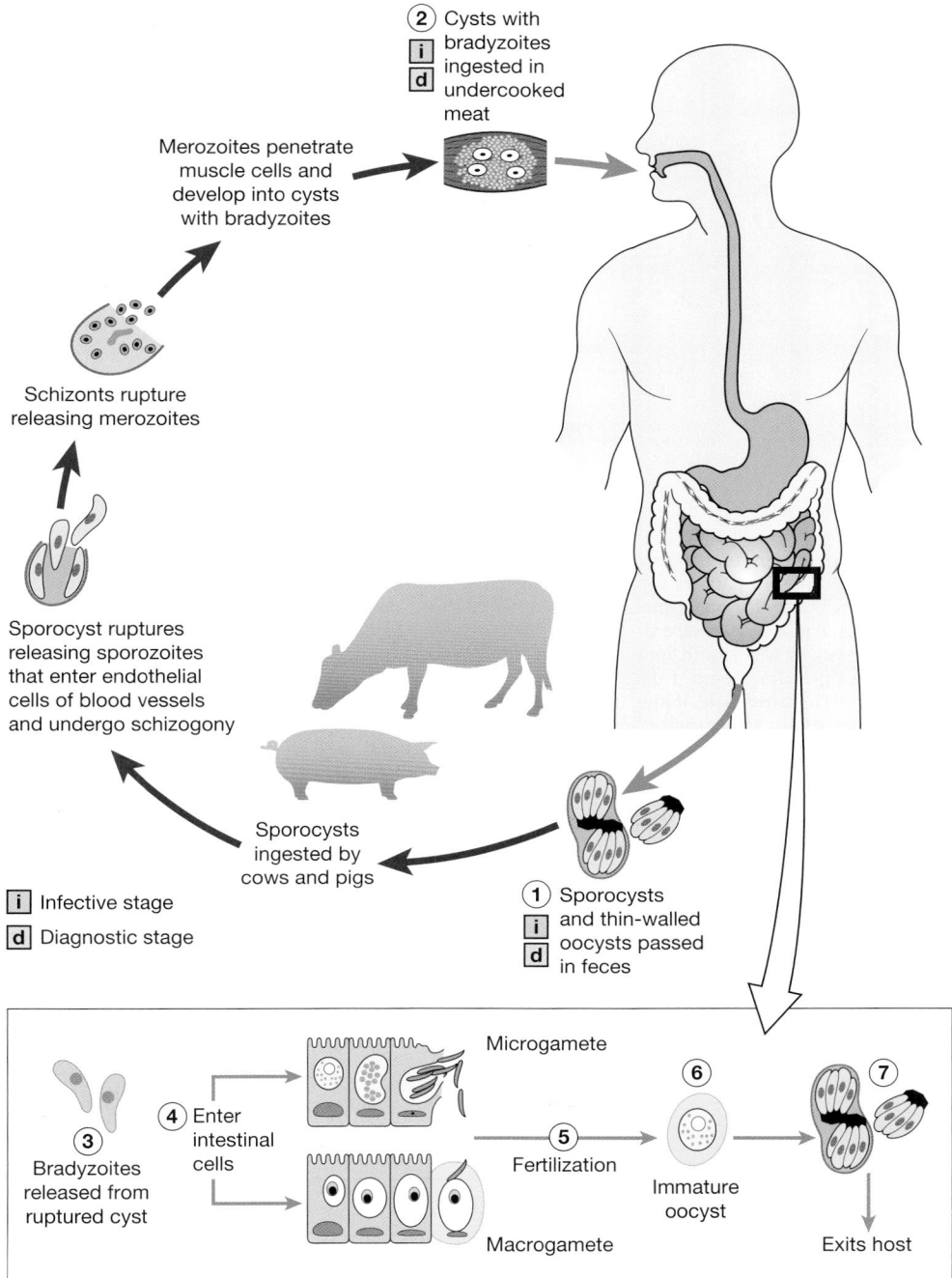

Figure 272-1. Life cycle of *Sarcocystis*. (Courtesy of DPDx image library, CDC.)

EPIDEMIOLOGY

Sarcocystis infection is a worldwide zoonosis with most cases reported from tropical and subtropical climates, mainly from Southeast Asia.[3–5] Identification of *Sarcocystis* in stool or muscle or antibodies in serum is most often an incidental finding.[6] High prevalence is explained by several conditions, including that a host can harbor any of several species of *Sarcocystis,* and many definitive hosts are involved in transmission, thereby facilitating spread of the parasite. Sporocysts are passed in feces in the infective form and are not dependent on weather conditions for maturation. In addition, large numbers of sporocysts are shed over a period of weeks or months and remain viable for several months in the environment. Oocysts and sporocysts are resistant to freezing, but can be killed by drying or exposure to 56°C for 10 minutes.

CLINICAL MANIFESTATIONS

Most people with *Sarcocystis* infection are asymptomatic. When humans consume infected meat, symptoms occur within 48 hours and include gastrointestinal tract disturbance, characterized by nausea, abdominal pain, and diarrhea, all of which are self-limited. These findings also were reported in human volunteers 3 to 6 hours after eating infected beef.[1,7]

Sarcocystis infection in muscle rarely is observed in humans and usually is an incidental discovery. Clinical findings reported in

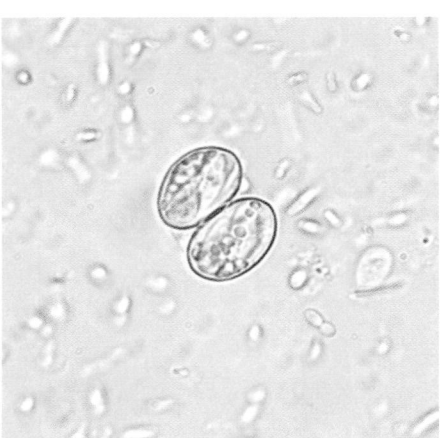

Figure 272-2. Sporulated oocyst of *Sarcocystis*. Wet mount. Magnification ×400. (Courtesy of DDx image library, CDC.)

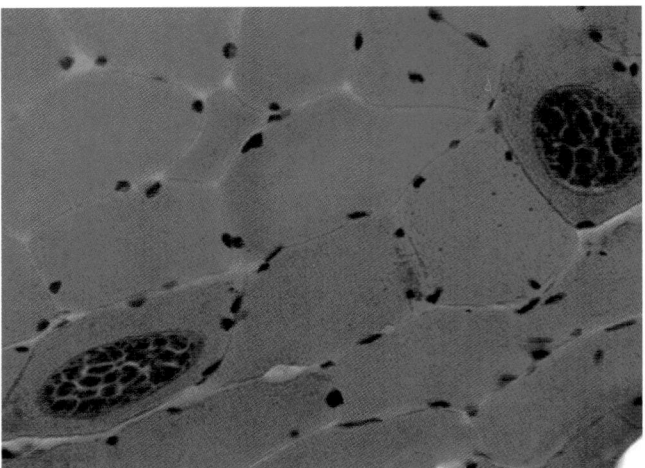

Figure 272-3. *Sarcocystis* in muscle tissue. Stained with hematoxylin and eosin. (Courtesy of DPDx image library, CDC.)

muscle infection include episodic muscular soreness or weakness and subcutaneous swelling in different parts of the body lasting 2 to 14 days, occasionally associated with fever, malaise, rash, and bronchospasm. Eosinophilia has been observed. Patients have been reported in whom *Sarcocystis* was found incidentally in the heart at autopsy following noncardiac death. Intact sarcocysts in human skeletal or cardiac muscle cause little, if any, inflammatory response. Muscle cysts vary greatly in size, ranging from 50 μm to 5 cm and persist in muscle for many years.[1,6] *Sarcocystis* was incriminated in an outbreak of acute eosinophilic myositis affecting military personnel in Malaysia. Illnesses were characterized by fever, myalgias, bronchospasm, rash, lymphadenopathy, subcutaneous nodules, and eosinophilia. *Sarcocystis* was found in a muscle biopsy of one of the cases.[8] A case of sarcocystosis affecting the intestine, liver, and muscle of a man with AIDS has been reported.[9]

DIAGNOSIS

Intestinal or intramuscular sarcocystosis should be suspected based on compatible symptoms in conjunction with a history of eating raw or undercooked beef or pork. The intestinal stage in humans can be diagnosed by examination of stool preparations made by high density-gradient centrifugation, in which sporocysts or occasionally oocysts can be seen as early as 2 weeks after ingestion.[1] Sarcocysts can be seen in muscle biopsies, or autopsy specimens stained with hematoxylin and eosin (see Figure 272-3). Such cysts must be differentiated from those of *Toxoplasma gondii* and *Trypanosoma cruzi*. The cyst wall of a *Sarcocystis* cyst has radial striations, which are not seen in *Toxoplasma*.[10] Molecular methods have been used in research studies in animals.[11] Serologic assays are not available commercially.

TREATMENT AND PREVENTION

Intestinal infection is self-limited and no specific treatment is available for this form of disease. Treatment of muscles disease is unsatisfactory once sarcocysts have formed. Albendazole has been reported to be efficacious for relief of symptoms.[7]

Prevention depends on avoiding exposure, namely by avoiding ingestion of raw beef or pork, or drinking water contaminated with feces of flesh-eating animals. Meat can be rendered noninfectious by heating and by freezing.

273 *Toxoplasma gondii* (Toxoplasmosis)

Despina Contopoulos-Ioannidis and Jose G. Montoya

Approximately one billion people worldwide are infected with *Toxoplasma gondii*. It is assumed that the parasite does not cause symptoms in most people during the acute or chronic stages of infection. However, *primary* infection can result in severe ocular disease in immunocompetent people, in significant neurologic and ocular sequelae in congenitally infected fetuses and children and, in certain tropical areas, in community-acquired pneumonia, disseminated disease, and even death among otherwise healthy individuals.[1,2] In addition, *reactivation* of chronic infection can occur in severely immunosuppressed individuals and cause life-threatening disease. Patients with profound T-lymphocyte-mediated immune compromise are at higher risk including those with the acquired immunodeficiency syndrome (AIDS),[3] hematopoietic stem cell transplants (HSCTs),[4] seronegative heart transplant recipients in whom a seropositive allograft is implanted,[5] those receiving high doses of corticosteroids and, likely, monoclonal antibodies such as alemtuzumab.[6] It is postulated currently that chronic infection may have more long-term consequences than thought previously; several investigators are addressing the possible impact of latent infection on psychiatric disorders and abnormal behaviors.

For definition, it is best to use the term *T. gondii infection* when referring to asymptomatic primary or chronic infection, and *toxoplasmosis* when primary infection or reactivation of chronic infection causes symptoms or signs or both.

THE PATHOGEN AND LIFE CYCLE

T. gondii is an obligate intracellular parasite with the capacity to infect almost any warm-blooded animal. The parasite has three infectious stages: *tachyzoites,* which are responsible for rapid spread of the parasite between cells and tissues, and the clinical manifestations of toxoplasmosis; *bradyzoites,* which are contained within tissue cysts, maintain chronic infection, and stay dormant for the life of the host unless the immune system is severely compromised; *sporozoites,* which are contained within oocysts, are shed by members of the felid family, and widely disseminate the agent in the environment.[7] Tachyzoites and bradyzoites are haploid, dividing asexually, while sporozoites are the product of meiosis. A sexual cycle only takes place in the small intestine of felids, allowing for the exchange of genetic material between strains and potentially generating variant strains in geographic areas where wild and large cats can travel long distances.[8,9]

The genome of *T. gondii* is available at http://toxodb.org. Genotyping studies have allowed the identification of several clonal lineages in Europe, North America, and South America. Types I, II, and III appear to be the most common strains observed in these areas; type II lineage is in Europe, whereas types I and III are reported predominantly from South America.[10] In addition, atypical strains are observed more commonly in North and South America. A type IV clonal ancestry has been reported recently from North America. Strains belonging to type I, atypical, and probably type IV groups have been associated with unusual and more aggressive clinical manifestations in humans. Children with congenital toxoplasmosis born in Brazil have a more aggressive ocular disease than those born in Europe.[11] Primary infections in adults have resulted in community-acquired pneumonia, acute hepatitis, fever of unknown origin, and death in HIV-negative and immunocompetent individuals in South America.[1]

Cats, domestic and wild, are the definitive host and are responsible for widespread existence of the parasite throughout the world. Although occasionally cats can become ill, most are asymptomatic during *T. gondii* infection and while shedding oocysts in their feces. Cats shed oocysts following the ingestion of any of the infectious stages of the parasite, tissue cysts and oocysts. As many as 10 million oocysts can be shed in a single day in the feces of the infected cat, for periods varying from 7 to 20 days. Oocysts can remain viable in moist soil for as long as 18 months; it is from this environmental source that other felids and intermediate hosts including humans can acquire infection. Eating meat of infected rodents, birds or other animals also can infect cats, and the consumption of infected meat can infect humans.[12]

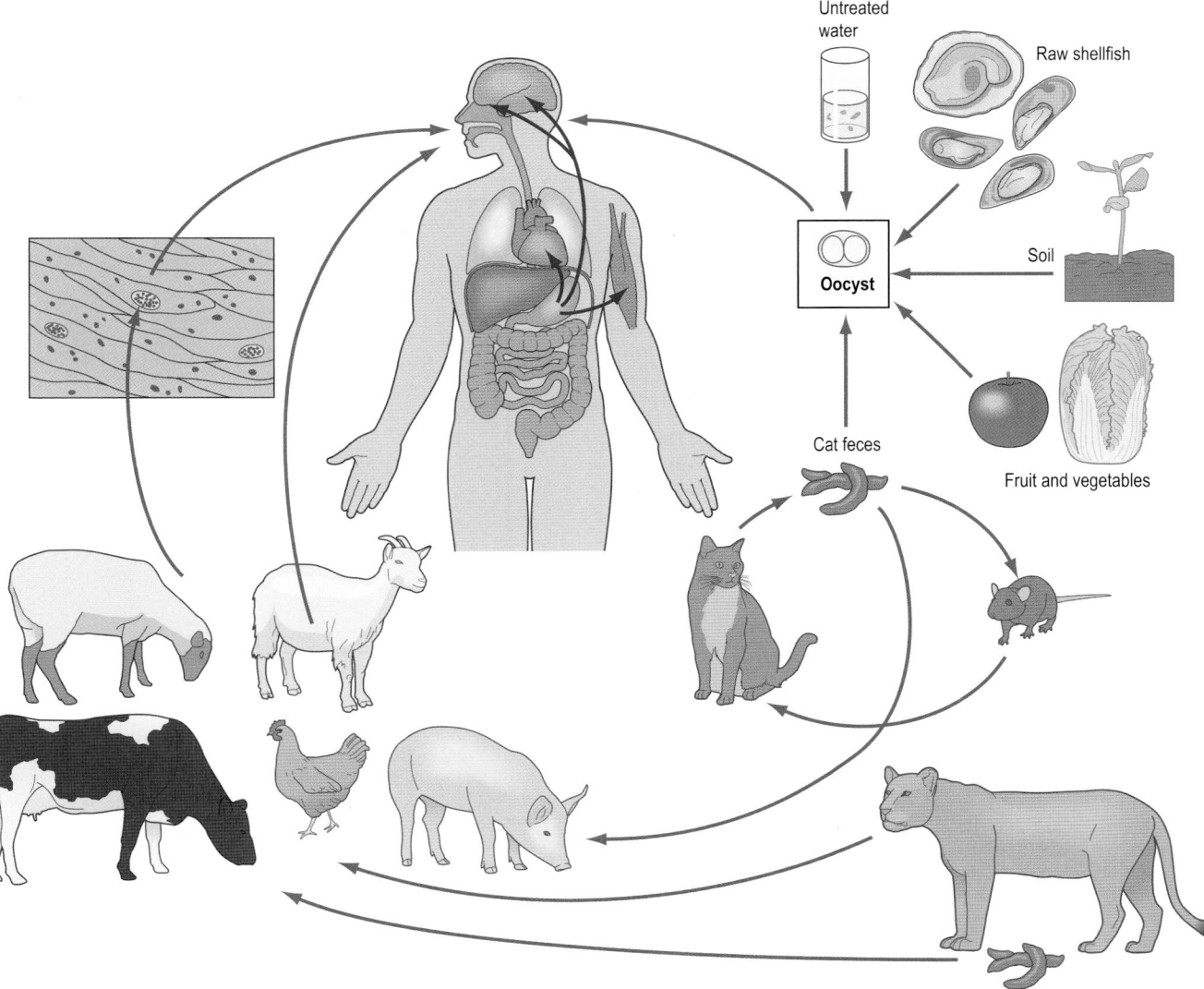

Figure 273-1. Life cycle of *Toxoplasma gondii.*

EPIDEMIOLOGY

Seroprevalence of *T. gondii* varies by geographic locale and by the socioeconomic strata of the population studied. Seroprevalence reflects the likelihood of a population or subgroup having been exposed to oocysts in soil, untreated water, vegetables, raw selfish, and other food items and to tissue cysts in uncooked or raw meat.[13–15] Seroprevalence can be as low as 7% (in England) and as high as 80% (in the Central African Republic).[2] The seroprevalence of *T. gondii* infection in the United States was reported recently as 11%; however, it may be as high as 30 to 40% in certain regions such as the northeast and within certain socioeconomic groups.[16] In most countries, including the U.S., prevalence is declining, whereas in certain areas of the world it appears stable or increasing. In all areas, seroprevalence increases with age (reflecting additive exposure) and usually is associated inversely with socioeconomic status, reflecting a strong influence of hygienic and alimentary habits in the transmission.

Humans and other vertebrates are incidental hosts and become infected primarily by the oral route, namely ingestion of contaminated food, water, or soil containing oocysts or infected meat containing tissue cysts (Figure 273-1). Vertical transmission from an infected mother to her offspring occurs during gestation. Humans also can acquire infection through receipt of an organ transplant from an infected donor and, more rarely, during a laboratory accident. Currently, main risk factors for acute *T. gondii* infection reported in the U.S. are: eating raw ground beef, rare lamb, locally produced cured, dried or smoked meat; working with meat; drinking unpasteurized goat milk or having ≥3 kittens.[14] An additional novel risk factor identified in this study was eating raw oysters, clams, or mussels. Drinking untreated water also showed increased risk but was not statistically significant.[14] Of note, untreated water has been reported to be the source of major outbreaks of acute toxoplasmosis in Canada and Brazil. In up to 50% of individuals with confirmed acute *T. gondii* infection, no known risk factor is found. Toxoplasmosis should not be excluded from the differential diagnosis of an ill patient based on a negative history for conventional risk factors for infection.

T. gondii is one of several microbes capable of crossing the placenta and infecting the developing fetus during pregnancy.[2] Congenital infection can occur when a woman acquires primary infection during gestation or within 3 months of conception. Women chronically infected with *T. gondii* prior to gestation can reactivate infection during gestation if significantly immunocompromised (e.g., by AIDS) and transmit the parasite to their offspring. Rare but well-documented cases are reported of chronically infected women who acquired a more virulent strain of *T. gondii* during gestation and gave birth to an infected infant.

The incidence of seroconversion during gestation for pregnant women in the U.S. has been estimated at 0.27%. Most countries report rates of seroconversion during pregnancy between 0.3 and 1.5%. The overall rate of transmission of the parasite from the infected mother to the fetus in women who seroconvert during gestation has been reported to be between 50% and 60% before the introduction of spiramycin and 25% to 30% thereafter.[2] Spiramycin was introduced in France in the 1970s in an attempt to prevent fetal transmission. Rate of vertical transmission increases whereas severity of disease decreases with advancing gestational age at the time of maternal infection (Figure 273-2A and B).[17] In treated women, vertical transmission rates can be as low as 6% at 13 weeks of gestation, 40% at 26 weeks, and 72% at 36 weeks (Figure 273-2A). In treated women, the risk of clinical signs in their infected fetus has been estimated at 61% if infection is acquired at 13 weeks of gestation, 25% if acquired at 26 weeks, and 9% if acquired at 36 weeks (Figure 273-2B). Because congenital infection is rare if the mother is infected in early pregnancy, estimates before 16 weeks of gestation should be interpreted with caution. After a diagnosis of acute maternal infection, when the infection status of the fetus is not known, the risk of clinical signs in the fetus or infant can be estimated by multiplying the risk of congenital infection (transmission) by the risk of signs among

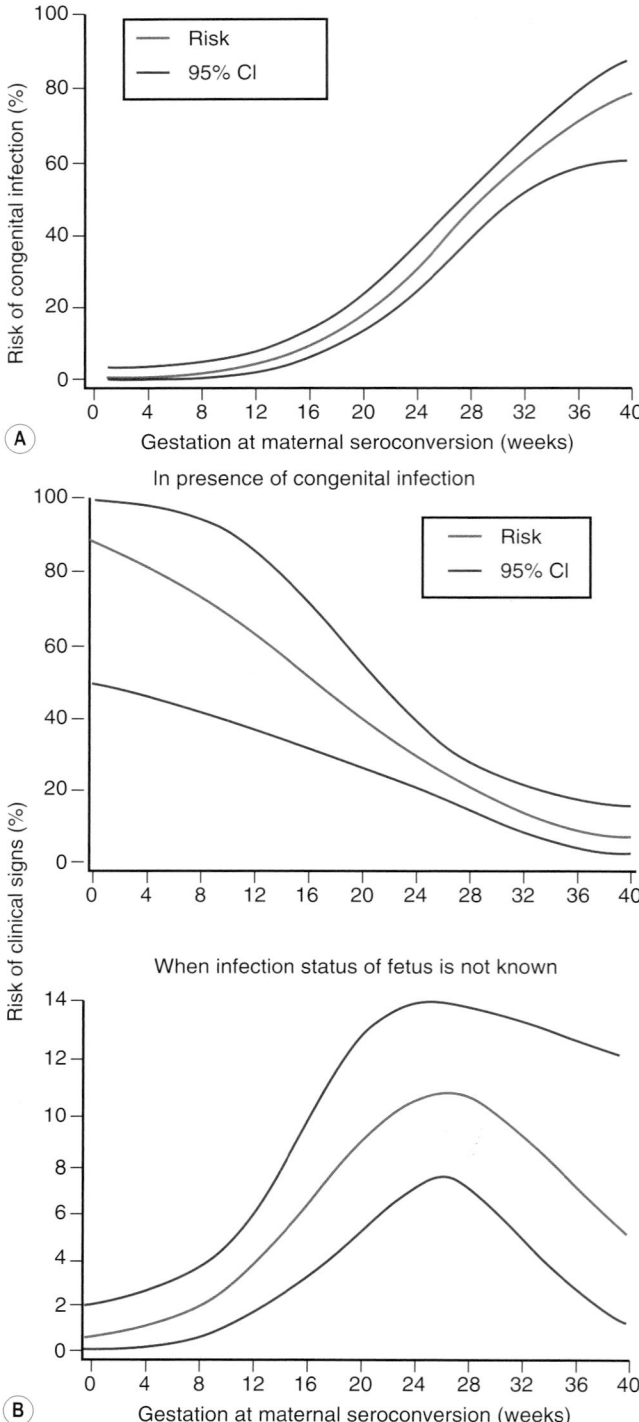

Figure 273-2. (A) Risk of congenital infection by age at gestational maternal seroconversion. (From Dunn et al. Lancet 1999;353(9167):1829–1833, with permission.) **(B)** Risk of developing clinical signs (not necessarily symptomatic) before the age of 3 years, according to gestational age at maternal seroconversion. (From Dunn et al. Mother-to-child transmission of toxoplasmosis: risk estimates for clinical counselling, Lancet 1999;353(9167):1829–1833, with permission.)

congenitally infected children. For instance, given a 40% risk of maternal–child transmission for maternal infection acquired at 26 weeks of gestation, and a 25% risk of clinical signs if transmission does occur, the overall risk of clinical signs is 10% (0.40 × 0.25) (Figure 273-2B). The maximum risk of giving birth to a symptomatic child is considered to be 10% (8% to 14%), which occurs around 24 to 30 weeks of gestation.[17]

The incidence of congenital toxoplasmosis in the U.S. is estimated to be 1 case per 10,000 live births.[18] These numbers are extrapolated from the New England Neonatal Screening program that includes universal neonatal screening for toxoplasmosis among 8 other diseases.[19] This incidence translates to 400 U.S. cases annually (extrapolating from approximately 4 million live births). Surveillance data in France have been determined on the basis of a national laboratory-based surveillance system.[20] The incidence rate for congenital toxoplasmosis is 2.9 cases per 10,000 live births and for symptomatic congenital toxoplasmosis is 0.34 cases per 10,000 live births.

PATHOGENESIS AND IMMUNE RESPONSE

Following oral ingestion of tissue cysts (e.g., in infected meat) or oocysts (e.g., in contaminated soil, water, or food), gastric juices disrupt cyst walls and release bradyzoites (from tissue cysts) and sporozoites (from oocysts), which are converted to tachyzoites. Because of their capacity to move by gliding, flexing, undulating and rotating, tachyzoites easily infect contiguous cells. Tachyzoites also can infect distant tissues by hematogenous or lymphatic spread. Tachyzoites likely infect Peyer patches and spleen first, followed by the lungs and liver. Bloodstream parasitemia can be detected for several days during the early stages of acute infection and probably lasts for approximately 14 days before IgG antibodies are detected. Tachyzoites ultimately arrive at sites such as the brain, eye, heart, and skeletal muscle where under the pressure of the immune system and other factors, they are converted into bradyzoites.

In immunocompetent hosts, an effective immune response controls the proliferation of the rapidly replicating tachyzoite and induces conversion to the metabolically slower bradyzoite, thereby facilitating the formation of tissue cysts (latent or chronic infection). Tissue cysts persist for the life of the host, most commonly in the brain, retina, and cardiac and skeletal muscles. Innate, humoral, and cellular immune responses are required to prevent the uncontrolled proliferation of tachyzoites including the activation of the monocyte-macrophage system, dentritic cells, natural killer cells, *T. gondii*-specific and cytotoxic CD4+ and CD8+ T lymphocytes; and interferon (IFN)-γ, interleukin (IL)-12, tumor necrosis factor (TNF)-α, IL-10 and other cytokines, transforming growth factor-β, costimulatory molecules (e.g., CD28, CD40 ligand), and, to a lesser degree, immunoglobulins.[21]

In immunocompromised patients previously infected with *T. gondii*, significant depletion of T-lymphocyte-mediated immune responses can facilitate the reactivation of infection (i.e., conversion of bradyzoites in tissue cysts into rapidly proliferating tachyzoites). Toxoplasmosis in this setting is generally fatal if untreated. Hydrocephalus in infants with congenital toxoplasmosis and toxoplasmic encephalitis in patients with AIDS appear to be associated with the HLA-DQ3 allele.

CLINICAL MANIFESTATIONS

Toxoplasmosis should be considered in the differential diagnosis of several clinical syndromes in immunocompetent children, congenitally infected infants, and immunocompromised children.[2] Symptoms and signs result from primary infection or reactivation of the parasite. In both forms, the rapid proliferation of the tachyzoite and its corresponding inflammatory immune response are responsible for clinical manifestations. Reactivation of chronic infection usually requires a profound depletion in T-lymphocyte-mediated control mechanisms. Primary infection can be asymptomatic in many infants and children, and conventional risk factors for the acute infection may not be present in a particular patient. If the goal is to detect each case of primary *T. gondii* infection in a given population of patients (e.g., pregnant women), or to diagnose toxoplasmosis in an ill patient, strategic laboratory testing is necessary. Testing of only symptomatic patients or those with conventional epidemiologic risk factors will miss a substantial portion of acute cases (probably ≥50%).[22]

Severity of toxoplasmosis during primary infection or reactivation can be influenced by the genetics of the infecting strain (e.g., type I or atypical strains appear to be associated with more severe disease),[23] inoculum size, infectious form (e.g., oocyst vs. cyst), immune competence and genetics of the host (e.g., presence of HLA-DQ3). Patients infected in certain geographic locales (e.g., South America) have more aggressive clinical presentations (both primary infection and reactivation) than those infected in Europe. Differences should be considered when evaluating ill travelers returning from endemic areas or patients emigrating from these areas.

Primary Infection in Immunocompetent Children, Adults, and Pregnant Women

Although most children and adults are asymptomatic at the time of primary infection, in ~10% of patients, the following symptoms or syndromes, alone or in various combinations, have been reported: fever (as high as 104°F/40°C), lymphadenopathy, headache, myalgia, arthralgia, sore throat, stiff neck, nausea, abdominal pain, anorexia, confusion, eye symptoms including eye pain, general malaise, fatigue; occasionally, skin rash and earache can occur. In outbreak settings or in certain tropical areas, the percentage of acutely infected individuals who are symptomatic is usually ~20% or greater.[24]

Lymphadenopathy can be localized or generalized. A solitary, occipital, and painlessly enlarged lymph node can be the sole manifestation of toxoplasmosis in a child, pregnant woman, or adult. However, more generalized cervical, axillary, and abdominal lymphadenopathy also occurs. Lymph nodes usually are 1 to 3 cm in size, and are nonsuppurative and nontender. Nodes usually regress within 3 months, but mild relapse of lymphadenopathy can occur between 3 and 6 months. Recurrence of lymphadenopathy beyond then is rare and should suggest an alternate diagnosis.

Chorioretinitis resulting in blurred vision, eye pain, decreased visual acuity, "floaters," scotoma, photophobia, or epiphora have been documented in postnatally acquired acute infection. Ocular toxoplasmosis as a manifestation of primary, postnatally acquired infection is more common in Europe and the U.S. than thought previously. Approximately 17% of acutely infected patients in South America (e.g., Brazil)[25] and in outbreaks (e.g., in Canada) have ocular manifestations.[24] People with postnatally acquired *T. gondii* also can develop chorioretinitis as a result of reactivation of chronic infection. The morphology of *T. gondii* retinal lesions on fundoscopic examination often is characteristic. An active whitish infiltrate usually is attached to the darkly pigmented border of an older scar. However, retinal lesions tend to be less typical in older or immunocompromised patients.

Other syndromes such as hepatitis, myositis, and myocarditis have also been described. Disseminated disease, pneumonia, and even death can occur in immunocompetent individuals infected with unusual strains of *T. gondii* in Latin America.

Disseminated or localized toxoplasmosis can occur in seronegative recipients of seropositive solid-organ transplants. Clinical presentations include fever of unknown origin, myocarditis, pneumonia, and encephalitis.

Congenital Toxoplasmosis

In countries where serologic screening and prenatal treatment is systematically offered to pregnant women, most fetuses and newborns infected with *T. gondii* do not exhibit any clinical signs of disease on initial evaluation. However, clinical manifestations of toxoplasmosis can be discovered years later. For instance, eye examination can reveal active or inactive toxoplasmic chorioretinitis and new lesions have been reported to occur in 31% of congenitally infected children observed through 12 years of age[26,27] (Figure 273-3). In contrast, among congenitally infected children whose mothers did not receive treatment during pregnancy and who were not treated during their first year of life, more than 70%

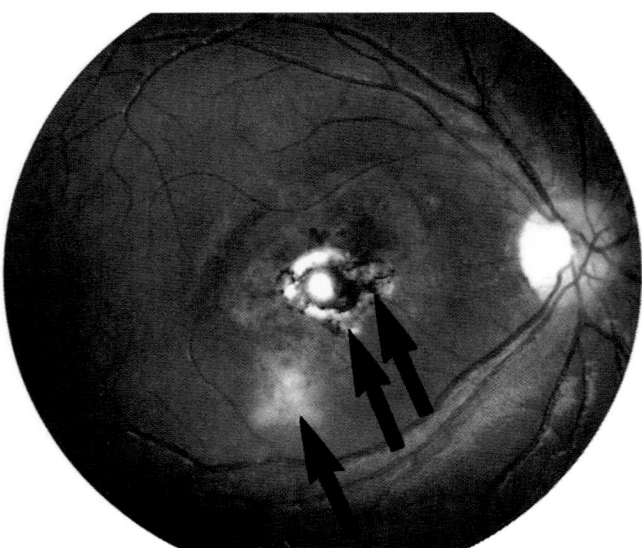

Figure 273-3. Toxoplasmic chorioretinitis in a congenitally infected child. The sharply demarcated quiescent scar is pigmented. Contiguous to this older lesion is a fluffy, active new lesion. (From Mets MB, Toxoplasmic Collaborative Study Group. Ophthalmologic findings in congenital toxoplasmosis. Invest Ophthalmol Vis Sci 1992;33:1094.)

developed new chorioretinal lesions; new lesions commonly were diagnosed after the first decade of life.[28]

Congenital infection can also result in fetal death, hydrocephalus, brain or hepatic calcifications, splenomegaly, ascites, pericarditis, and intrauterine growth retardation. Newborns can have a nonspecific illness or any of the following clinical manifestations, alone or in combination: chorioretinitis, strabismus, blindness, seizures, encephalitis, abnormal cephalic perimeter (microcephaly, macrocephaly, hydrocephalus), psychomotor or mental retardation, hepatosplenomegaly, pneumonitis, diarrhea, hypothermia, jaundice, petechiae, skin rash, and hearing loss.[29] Intracranial calcifications can be present in brain imaging studies. Many children suffer from chronic sequelae of congenital disease. The classic triad of chorioretinitis, hydrocephalus, and brain calcifications is highly suggestive of toxoplasmosis and primarily is seen in neonates whose mothers were not treated during pregnancy.

In a study of 281 congenitally infected children from the European multicenter EMSCOT study and 30 infected children from Brazil, *T. gondii* caused more severe ocular disease in Brazil compared with Europe. Observed differences in the frequency of chorioretinitis and in the size and number of ocular lesions might be attributed to more virulent strains implicated in South America[11] or lack of universal screening and treatment of pregnant women in the South American cohorts.

Chronic Infection in Immunocompetent Children

It appears that during the chronic stage of infection, *T. gondii* does not cause symptoms in the majority of immunocompetent individuals. However, toxoplasmic chorioretinitis can develop in chronically infected, immunocompetent individuals, most likely due to reactivation of the parasite and subsequent host immune response. Reactivation can occur in congenitally or postnatally infected people. Reactivation of congenital infection appears to occur more commonly between 10 and 30 years of age, and is more likely to involve the macula bilaterally. In contrast, ocular disease due to reactivation of a postnatally acquired and latent infection appears to occur in individuals >50 years of age, and it is more likely to cause peripheral and unilateral retinal lesions. Symptomatic ocular disease consists primarily of retinochoroiditis that manifests as blurred vision, eye pain, decreased visual acuity, "floaters," scotoma, photophobia, or epiphora. The morphology

of retinal lesions is thought to be characteristic, with an active whitish infiltrate usually attached to darkly pigmented border of an older scar. However, retinal lesions tend to be less typical in older or immunocompromised patients.

Reactivation of Chronic Infections in Immunocompromised Patients

Reactivation of chronic infection in immunocompromised individuals can be manifest as multiple brain abscesses, diffuse encephalitis, chorioretinitis, fever of unknown origin, pneumonia, myocarditis, hepatosplenomegaly, lymphadenopathy, and skin rash. Fever or pneumonia or both can occur as the only manifestations. Significant T-lymphocyte deficiency needs to be present for children to reactivate infection due to immunosuppression, and occurs in patients with AIDS or allogeneic HSCT. However, HIV-infected children (unlike adults) dually infected with *T. gondii* rarely develop toxoplasmic encephalitis.

DIAGNOSIS

Laboratory tools for the diagnosis of *T. gondii* infection and toxoplasmosis include serologic tests, the polymerase chain reaction (PCR), histologic and cytologic examination of tissue and body fluids, and attempts to isolate the parasite. Regardless of the presence or absence of symptoms, serologic tests can establish whether a patient is infected or not, and if infected, whether acutely or chronically. Available serologic tools include methods to detect *T. gondii*-specific IgG, IgM, IgA, IgE, and IgG-based avidity and differential agglutination (AC/HS).[30]

Acute and Chronic Infection

With the use of commercial kits for the detection of IgG and IgM, most laboratories can reliably diagnose the absence of *T. gondii* infection (negative IgG/negative IgM) and chronic infection (positive IgG/negative IgM). However, the diagnosis of acute infection cannot rest solely on a positive IgM test result. IgM antibody is observed during acute infection, but can remain positive for months to years without apparent clinical relevance. In addition, commercial IgM kits are not highly specific. Of patients with positive IgM results at non-reference laboratories, 60% are found to be chronically infected when their serum is tested at the national reference laboratory for the study and diagnosis of toxoplasmosis in the U.S. (Palo Alto Medical Foundation Toxoplasma Serology Laboratory (PAMF-TSL), Palo Alto, California; www.pamf.org/serology/; 650-853-4828; toxolab@pamf.org). At PAMF-TSL, a panel of confirmatory tests (avidity, differential agglutination, IgA, IgE) are available in addition to the "gold standard" dye test for IgG and the "double" sandwich capture enzyme-linked immunosorbent assay (ELISA) for IgM. These tests are used in various combinations, depending on the clinical scenario and the specific clinical question. For example, low positive IgG and positive IgM test results with a high IgG-avidity test result in a pregnant woman tested within the first 16 weeks of gestation will be interpreted as an infection acquired >16 weeks before the date of serum sampling and thus there is no risk of congenital toxoplasmosis; however, the same test results in an AIDS patient with multiple ring-enhancing brain lesions will be interpreted as supportive of the diagnosis of toxoplasmic encephalitis due to reactivation of chronic infection. At PAMF-TSL, three interpretations of *T. gondii* infection can be assessed by laboratory serologic test results: (1) *acute*, when results are consistent with a recently acquired infection; (2) *chronic*, when consistent with an infection acquired in the distant past; and (3) *equivocal*, when results cannot exclude a recently acquired infection (in which case an earlier or subsequent sample is required to attempt to establish whether the infection is acute or chronic). For serologic test results consistent with an acute infection, an attempt should be made to establish the approximate date of infection to help determine whether a patient's clinical symptoms can be attributed to toxoplasmosis.

Toxoplasmosis

The diagnosis of toxoplasmosis (due to primary infection or reactivation of chronic infection) requires the identification of tachyzoites in tissues or body fluids, the amplification of parasite DNA in any body fluid, or the visualization of tissue cysts surrounded by a strong inflammatory response. Tachyzoites can be visualized in histologic sections stained with hematoxylin and eosin or in cytologic preparations without any special staining, but are best visualized with Wright–Giemsa and *T. gondii*-specific immunoperoxidase stains. Real-time PCR has become a useful method for the diagnosis of toxoplasmosis; a positive test result in amniotic fluid during gestation is diagnostic of fetal infection, in cerebrospinal fluid of toxoplasmic encephalitis, in bronchoalveolar fluid of toxoplasmic pneumonia, in vitreous fluid of toxoplasmic chorioretinitis, and in peripheral blood and urine of disseminated toxoplasmosis. Isolation of the parasite in any body fluid is diagnostic of toxoplasmosis. In certain clinical settings the diagnosis of toxoplasmosis can be made presumptively by positive results in *T. gondii*-specific serologic test results along with characteristic histologic findings in a lymph node biopsy or retinal findings suggestive of ocular toxoplasmosis. PCR and isolation test results can be falsely negative in patients receiving anti-*Toxoplasma* treatment.

Pregnancy

The diagnosis of toxoplasmosis during pregnancy is primarily accomplished by the use of serologic tests, amniotic fluid PCR, and fetal ultrasound. For appropriate interpretation of results the consultant requires clinical information on the pregnant woman (including reason for testing, presence of clinical signs and symptoms of toxoplasmosis during gestation or shortly before conception, presence of immunosuppression including HIV infection, and gestational time at testing).

Maternal Serologic Tests

In countries where routine prenatal screening for evidence of seroconversion is applied, women are screened monthly (e.g., France) or every 3 months (e.g., Austria, Germany, Italy) until delivery. Seroconversion is defined as a change from undetectable to detectable IgG anti-*Toxoplasma*. In patients who seroconvert the IgM test becomes positive first, usually at high titers. Seroconversion during gestation is diagnostic of infection acquired during pregnancy.[2] However, in countries where no routine prenatal screening is used, prenatal diagnosis of *T. gondii* infection or toxoplasmosis is based on a single serum sample tested during gestation. If suspicion of toxoplasmosis during pregnancy is only raised when the patient has been identified as having conventional risk factors for the infection or has developed symptoms, approximately 50% of the infected women will be missed.

In non-reference laboratories, IgG-positive or -negative results, and IgM-negative results are reliable. If a pregnant woman has the ability to produce Ig and has negative IgG and IgM test results, there is no serologic evidence of prior *T. gondii* infection; it is recommended that she be tested for toxoplasma IgG and IgM every 4 to 8 weeks for the duration of gestation. If the IgG test is positive but at a low titer (e.g., near the cutoff of positivity for the IgG test or a dye test at PAMF-TSL ≤1:512) and the IgM test result is negative, the patient most likely has been infected for at least 6 months. IgG positive test results at high titers (e.g., ≥1:1024 at PAMF-TSL) even with negative IgM test results should be interpreted with caution and with the assistance of medical consultants at reference laboratories.

In pregnant women with positive toxoplasma IgG and IgM test results, the positive IgM test result alone cannot be used to confirm acute *T. gondii* infection or toxoplasmosis; additional confirmatory testing is performed. The battery of tests used varies with the gestational age at which the serum sample was obtained. For women screened at <16 weeks' gestation, the more cost-effective panel contains the IgG dye test, IgM ELISA, and IgG-avidity test. For women screened at >16 weeks' gestation, the differential agglutination test (AC/HS) is used in the panel instead for the IgG-avidity test. In most cases, results in these tests yield either of two interpretations: infection acquired during or shortly before gestation, or infection acquired in the distant past (i.e., prior to conception). However, when timing of infection is indefinite by these tests, additional or follow-up testing is recommended (which might include IgG-avidity, differential agglutination test AC/HS, IgA and/or IgE). If the results are consistent with an infection acquired in the distant past and prior to pregnancy, the incidence of congenital toxoplasmosis is extremely rare unless the woman is severely immunocompromised (i.e., HIV-positive, receiving corticosteroids or immunosuppressive drugs, etc.).[31] Cases of *T. gondii* reinfection during gestation of chronically infected women with different *T. gondii* strains are reported rarely.[32]

When maternal serology results are suggestive of a recently acquired infection (or cannot exclude the possibility), spiramycin therapy is recommended (unless contraindicated) to attempt to prevent congenital transmission. The request for spiramycin is made to the Food and Drug Administration.[31] Moreover, amniotic fluid sampling for PCR testing is recommended; positivity indicates fetal infection. Amniotic fluid examination should be performed, if feasible and safe, at 18 weeks' gestation. If the patient is >18 weeks' gestation, PCR results on amniotic fluid still can be helpful to determine whether treatment of the fetus is indicated. Amniotic fluid testing for *T. gondii* PCR generally should be avoided <18 weeks' gestation, as sensitivity and specificity has not been studied.

If a pregnant woman has a negative IgG dye test but a positive IgM test result, she may have been infected recently or have a false-positive IgM result. Sera should be submitted to a reference laboratory for confirmatory testing; follow-up testing 2 to 4 weeks later might be required. Follow-up IgG dye test positivity would be diagnostic of seroconversion and of a very recently acquired infection. In contrast, persistent IgG-dye negativity (even if the IgM remains positive) suggests infection acquired in the distant past, prior to gestation.

Interpretation of serologic test results performed late (>20 weeks) in gestation can be difficult to interpret unless serologic test results are clearly suggestive of an infection acquired in the distant past (e.g., >12 months before testing). In most cases, testing of a serum sample that might have been obtained and saved during the first 16 weeks of gestation would be required to determine the time of infection in such patients.

PCR Testing on Amniotic Fluid

Once the diagnosis of acute *Toxoplasma* infection or toxoplasmosis during pregnancy has been confirmed or is highly suspected, the next step is to determine whether the fetus has been infected. Amniotic fluid (AF) PCR is the laboratory method of choice. The diagnostic accuracy of AF-PCR varies according to the trimester of pregnancy during which maternal infection occurred. For pregnant women whose maternal infection was estimated to have been acquired during the first trimester, sensitivity of the AF-PCR test is reportedly 33% to 75%; during the second trimester, 80% to 97%, and during the third trimester, 68% to 88%.[33-35] In contrast, the specificity approaches 100%, as reported by several investigators and regardless of the trimester of maternal infection. Variation in sensitivity of PCR most likely reflects the lack of standardization of laboratory technique across centers (e.g., target gene, primers, amount of the sample required for testing, method used for extraction, amplification and probes). The negative predictive value (NPV) of PCR is 96% to 100% for infection acquired during the first trimester; 93% to 100% for the second trimester, and 48% to 98% for the third trimester.[35] The explanation for high NPV for infections acquired in the first trimester is that rates of transmission during this period are very low.

Fetal Ultrasound

Fetal ultrasonography also can help to determine whether the fetus has been affected. Ultrasound can reveal fetal death, or hydrocephalus, brain or hepatic calcifications, splenomegaly, ascites, or pericarditis.

Neonate

In the newborn, congenital toxoplasmosis can be diagnosed by having IgA or IgM anti-*T. gondii*, positive PCR, or isolation test results. The preferred method for the detection of IgM antibodies in the newborn is the immunosorbent agglutination assay (ISAGA) and for IgA the ELISA technique. Serum sample for serologic testing should be obtained from peripheral blood and not from cord blood (because of the high rate of maternal blood contamination). Of note, there still can be maternal blood contamination in the newborn's peripheral blood during the first 5 days of life with maternal IgM antibodies, and during the first 10 days of life with maternal IgA antibodies, but not thereafter. Thus, a positive IgM ISAGA (after 5 days of life) or IgA ELISA (after 10 days) is diagnostic of congenital disease. Congenitally infected babies can be positive for both; positive for either; or negative for both (occasionally). False-positive IgM ISAGA test results, particularly at low titers, can be seen in infants who have received transfusion of blood products.

A positive IgM anti-*T. gondii* in fluid (CSF) is diagnostic of congenital disease, but testing of the CSF by PCR rather than for IgM is strongly recommended because of the higher sensitivity of PCR testing. The diagnosis also can be made by a positive PCR in peripheral blood, CSF, or urine. The CSF of infected infants can exhibit high levels of protein (e.g., 1000 mg/dL) and eosinophilia in addition to mild to moderate lymphocytosis. Brain imaging studies of the newborn can reveal calcifications or hydrocephalus; CT scan is superior to ultrasound examination in the detection of central nervous system abnormalities. Calcifications also can be detected in the liver of infected infants.

Persistence of IgG anti-*T. gondii* in a child ≥12 months of age is diagnostic of congenital toxoplasmosis and is considered the "gold standard" for ultimate and definitive laboratory diagnosis. Maternal transplacental IgG antibodies usually disappear after 6 to 12 months of life. Initially, the titer of the IgG antibody in the infant should be similar to that of the mother. Then, the non-infected infant's IgG titers are anticipated to decrease according to the half-life of the IgG (4 weeks); *Toxoplasma* IgG titer should decrease by at least 50% every month. In performing serial testing, the infant's specimens should be tested simultaneously and expert consultation should be sought at reference laboratories. The kinetics of the child's IgG might be negatively affected by treatment for toxoplasmosis.

Immunocompetent Children

Systemic disease. In the vast majority of cases, immunocompetent children are tested because their symptoms and/or signs suggest the possibility of toxoplasmosis. If the patient has negative IgG and IgM test results, symptoms or signs should not be attributed to toxoplasmosis (assuming they are capable of producing immunoglobulins). If the serologic test results are consistent with a chronic infection, use of a reference laboratory can help to determine a minimum window of timing of infection in order to establish relevancy to clinical manifestations. Most immunocompetent children do not have clinically apparent reactivation of chronic infection. The only exception is ocular disease, which can reactivate in immunocompetent children. In addition, several investigators have hypothesized that chronic *T. gondii* infection may play a role in mental illness and behavior in infected animals and humans. Further investigation is required.

Lymphadenopathy due to toxoplasmosis, can result in histologic patterns that often are diagnostic: reactive follicular hyperplasia, irregular clusters of epithelioid histiocytes encroaching on and blurring the margins of the germinal centers, and focal distention of sinuses with monocytoid cells.[36]

Ocular disease. In patients with ocular disease, serologic tests for *T. gondii* always should be performed. Diagnosis of acute postnatally acquired infection can be made if IgM anti-*T. gondii* is present

(and results are confirmed at a reference laboratory) and symptoms started approximately at the same time as the infection was acquired. If serologic test results are consistent with distantly acquired infection, ocular symptoms can be ascribed presumptively to reactivation of *T. gondii* (likely acquired congenitally) if morphology of the retinal lesions are characteristic (see Figure 273-3) and there is adequate response to therapy for toxoplasmosis. In certain cases the possibility of an infection postnatally acquired cannot be excluded. In patients whose lesions are not typical for toxoplasmosis or in whom there is suboptimal response to therapy, sampling of ocular fluids for diagnosis should be considered.

Sampling of the aqueous humor, rather than vitreous fluid, has a lower risk of adverse events. The immune load (Goldmann–Witmer coefficient analysis of aqueous humor) is calculated as (IgG anti-*Toxoplasma* in aqueous humor/total IgG in aqueous humor)/(IgG anti-*Toxoplasma* in serum/total IgG in serum). A value of ≥2 is considered by some investigators as evidence of intraocular antibody synthesis in response to replicating tachyzoites. Vitreous fluid sampling, despite the greater risk of damage to the eye and retina, may be indicated when significant vitreal inflammation is observed, retinal lesions are difficult to visualize, or the patient is not responding to *Toxoplasma* therapy. For vitreal samples, detection of the parasite by DNA amplification (PCR) is preferred.

Immunocompromised Pediatric Patients

Clinicians should establish whether immunocompromised patients, or those about to become so, are at risk of reactivating latent *T. gondii* infection or acquiring primary infection through the oral route or a transplanted organ. All immunocompromised patients in whom cell-mediated immunity will be significantly compromised should be tested for anti-IgG *T. gondii*. Serologic testing following transplantation is unreliable; in the posttransplant period, serologic tests may be or become negative, not change or rise, without clinical relevance.

Establishing that the immunocompromised patient is chronically infected with *T. gondii* (IgG positive, IgM negative) also will facilitate anti-*Toxoplasma* prophylaxis. *T. gondii*-seropositive patients with AIDS, those who undergo allogeneic HSCT, or who receive drugs that target T-lymphocyte-mediated immunity should be closely followed and offered anti-*Toxoplasma* prophylaxis or preemptive therapy (if they become *Toxoplasma* PCR positive). Recipients of solid-organ transplants, and their donors, should be tested prior to transplant; donor-positive, recipient-negative individuals are at high risk of developing life-threatening toxoplasmosis.

Although pretransplant serologic tests can determine *T. gondii* infection and risk for toxoplasmosis, tests are of little value for diagnosis of disease. Methods of choice to establish toxoplasmosis in immunocompromised patients (due to reactivation of latent infection or acutely acquired primary infection) are testing of body fluids by PCR, examination of biopsy tissue by hematoxylin and eosin stain and *T. gondii*-specific immunoperoxidase, and isolation of the parasite. Real-time PCR possibly is the diagnostic test of choice for *Toxoplasma* encephalitis (performed on CSF), pneumonia (bronchoalvaolar lavage), disseminated disease (peripheral blood or urine), and chorioretinitis (vitreous fluid). Visualization of tachyzoites in any body fluid or tissue, or isolation from any body fluid (reference laboratories) also are diagnostic of toxoplasmosis.

TREATMENT

Effective treatment requires the combination of two drugs known to be effective against *T. gondii*; pyrimethamine is the most effective drug, and always should be prescribed in conjunction with folinic acid in order to prevent bone marrow toxicity. Other effective drugs include sulfadiazine, clindamycin, atovaquone, and trimethoprim-sulfamethoxazole. Drugs used clinically but with less efficacy include clarithromycin, azithromycin, and dapsone. Monotherapy is indicated only during pregnancy when attempting to prevent mother-to-child transmission; spiramycin alone is prescribed for women who acquired primary infection during gestation whose fetus has not been infected.

Pregnancy

Treatment of toxoplasmosis during gestation usually is aimed at preventing fetal infection or treating the infected fetus. If serologic testing suggests acquisition of the infection during the first 18 weeks of gestation or shortly before conception, maternal treatment with daily spiramycin orally (to attempt to prevent vertical transmission) is recommended by many clinicians in the U.S. and Europe[31] (Table 273-1). Spiramycin is not available commercially in the U.S. but can be obtained at no cost (drug compassionately provided by Sanofi-Aventis) and after consultation (with PAMF-TSL, telephone number (650) 853-4828, or the U.S. (Chicago, IL) National Collaborative Treatment Trial Study (NCCTS), telephone number (773) 834-4152) through the U.S. Food and Drug Administration (FDA), telephone number (301) 796-1600. Spiramycin should be continued throughout pregnancy even if amniotic fluid

PCR obtained at ≥18 weeks of gestation is negative (due to theoretical concerns of placental infection/transmission) later in gestation. If fetal infection is confirmed (i.e., PCR on amniotic fluid positive at ≥18 weeks), treatment with pyrimethamine, sulfadiazine, and folinic acid is recommended. (If the patient already is receiving spiramycin, combination therapy should replace spiramycin.) In some centers in Europe, change to combination therapy takes place as early as weeks 14 to 16. If serologic test results are consistent with acquisition of infection after 18 weeks of gestation, treatment with pyrimethamine, sulfadiazine, and folinic acid is recommended in an attempt to prevent or treat fetal infection, because of the high transmission rates after 18 weeks of gestation. In addition, pyrimethamine should be avoided earlier in gestation because it is potentially teratogenic. Combination therapy also is recommended when amniotic fluid PCR for *T. gondii* DNA is positive or when fetal ultrasound changes are highly suspicious for congenital toxoplasmosis.

There is no large, randomized controlled clinical trial that proves efficacy of spiramycin to prevent congenital toxoplasmosis. Thus, use has been questioned by some members of the European

TABLE 273-1. Antimicrobial Treatment for Pregnant Women Likely to Have Acquired *T. gondii* Infection During Gestation and Infants Suspected or Confirmed to Have Congenital Toxoplasmosis

	During Pregnancy	For Congenital Disease
Spiramycin	Recommended for pregnant women suspected or confirmed as having acquired their infection at <18 weeks of gestation. Spiramycin should be administered until delivery in those with negative amniotic fluid PCR tests and negative follow-up ultrasonography or low suspicion of fetal infection. Spiramycin is not teratogenic and is available in the U.S. only through the Investigational New Drug (IND) process at the U.S. Food and Drug Administration (FDA, (301) 796-1600). Consultation with experts in diagnosing/treating toxoplasmosis is strongly recommended[a] **Dose:** 1 g (3 million units) every 8 hours orally; total 3 g (9 million units) daily	Not recommended during pregnancy if the fetus is documented/suspected to be infected. In the setting of fetal infection, pyrimethamine/sulfadiazine/folinic acid should be instituted (see below)
Pyrimethamine *plus* Sulfadiazine *plus* Folinic acid[b]	Recommended for women ≥18 weeks of gestation suspected/confirmed to have acquired acute infection at or after 18 weeks of gestation or who have a positive amniotic fluid PCR test or abnormal ultrasonography suggestive of congenital toxoplasmosis. Pyrimethamine is teratogenic and should not be used during pregnancy before week 18 (or week 14 in some centers in Europe). Sulfadiazine should not be used alone **Doses:** Pyrimethamine: 50 mg every 12 hours orally for 2 days; followed by 50 mg once daily Sulfadiazine: 75 mg/kg (first dose); followed by 50 mg/kg every 12 hours orally (maximum dose 4 g/day) Folinic acid (leucovorin):[b] 10–20 mg daily (during and for 1 week after pyrimethamine therapy)	**Infant** (treatment regimen usually is recommended for one year): **Doses:** Pyrimethamine: 1 mg/kg every 12 hours orally for 2 days; followed by 1 mg/kg once per day orally for 2 or 6 months; followed by 1 mg/kg once per day every Monday, Wednesday, Friday Sulfadiazine: 50 mg/kg every 12 hours orally Folinic acid (leucovorin):[b] 10 mg three times weekly orally Prednisone (if CSF protein ≥1 g/dL or severe chorioretinitis): 0.5 mg/kg every 12 hours orally (until CFS protein <1 g/dL or resolution of severe chorioretinitis) **Older children with active disease** (treatment regimen usually is given for 1 to 2 weeks beyond resolution of clinical manifestations) **Doses:** Pyrimethamine: 1 mg/kg once every 12 hours orally (maximum 50 mg) for 2 days; followed by 1 mg/kg once per day orally (maximum 25 mg/day) Sulfadiazine: 75 mg/kg (first dose); followed by 50 mg/kg every 12 hours orally Folinic acid (leucovorin):[b] 10–20 mg three times weekly orally Prednisone (severe chorioretinitis): 0.5 mg/kg every 12 hours orally (maximum 40 mg/day); rapid taper

[a]*Palo Alto Medical Foundation Toxoplasma Serology Laboratory, PAMF-TSL; Palo Alto, CA; www.pamf.org/serology/; +1-650-853-4828; toxolab@pamf.org or U.S. (Chicago) National Collaborative Treatment Trial Study (NCCTS), telephone number (773) 834-4152.*

[b]*Folic acid should not be used as a substitute for folinic acid.*

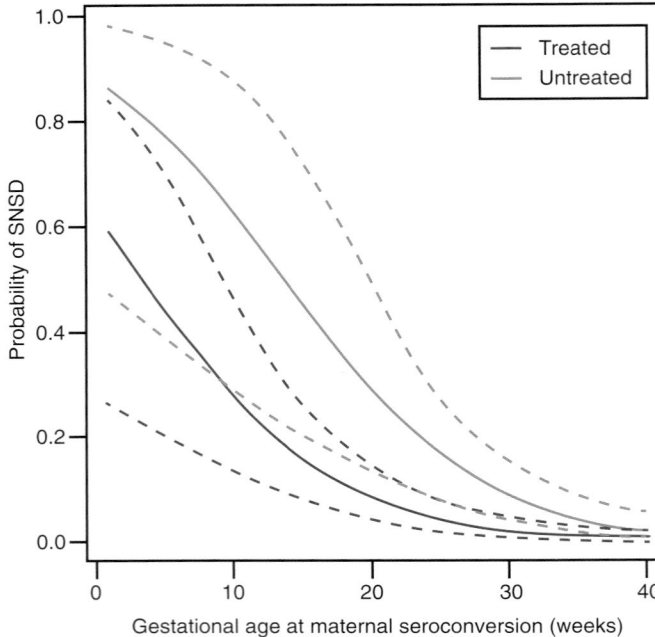

Figure 273-4. Probability of severe neurologic sequelae or death (SNSD) according to maternal treatment status (imputed gestational age at seroconversion, solid lines, and 95% Bayesian credible limits, hatched lines). (Cortina-Borja M, et al. (2010) Prenatal Treatment for Serious Neurological Sequelae of Congenital Toxoplasmosis PLoS Med 7(10) doi: 10.1371/journal. pmed.l000351 © 2010 Cortina-Borja et al. Made available through CCAL.)

Multicentre Study on Congenital Toxoplasmosis (EMSCOT).[37] Some data from Europe suggest that spiramycin might be more efficacious when administered early after seroconversion.[38] In a prospective observational EMSCOT study published in 2010, prenatal treatment with spiramycin and/or pyrimethamine, sulfadiazine, and folinic acid reduced the risk of composite severe neurologic sequelae or death by 76% (odds ratio, 0.24; 95% CI, 0.07 to 0.71) (Figure 273-4).[39] Until further data become available, it is our practice to recommend spiramycin treatment for women with suspected or confirmed acute *T. gondii* infection acquired during the first 18 weeks of gestation.

Neonate

Pyrimethamine/sulfadiazine/folinic acid therapy is recommended in infants <1 year of age when congenital toxoplasmosis is highly suspected or confirmed.[2] It is not known whether the infected but asymptomatic infant should be treated. Until appropriate data become available, treatment is recommended by several investigators for asymptomatic infants in an attempt to prevent late sequelae (see Table 273-1). No randomized trials on the effect of postnatal treatment for the development of eye disease have been performed; studies have been deemed unethical. Outcomes of treated patients often are compared with untreated historical controls. In these studies, infants who receive treatment develop significantly fewer new eye lesions; however, the role of selection bias in either group cannot be excluded.[40,41]

Among treated children (2 months pyrimethamine daily vs. 6 months pyrimethamine daily followed by pyrimethamine 3 times per week, in additional to sulfadiazine daily), 36% of infants who had moderate or severe neurologic disease at enrollment developed new eye lesions, whereas 8% of those with no substantial neurologic disease developed new eye lesions.

There are insufficient data on the effectiveness of other regimens such as trimethoprim-sulfamethoxazole (TMP-SMX) or pyrimethamine plus clindamycin plus folinic acid. However, if the pyrimethamine, sulfadiazine, and folinic acid regimen is in short supply or cannot be administered to the patient, these alternative regimens theoretically could be used.

Immunocompetent and Immunocompromised Children

Treatment is indicated for toxoplasmosis in immunocompetent children with acute *Toxoplasma* infection who have clinically significant myocarditis, myositis, hepatitis, pneumonia, brain lesions, or skin lesions (Table 273-2).[42] Treatment also is indicated in patients with *Toxoplasma* lymphadenitis accompanied by severe or persisting symptoms and in those with active ocular disease due to primary infection or reactivation of latent infection. In immunocompetent patients, treatment is prescribed for 3 to 4 weeks or until symptoms have subsided, whichever is longer. The drug regimen of choice is pyrimethamine plus sulfadiazine plus folinic acid. The use of alternative regimens such as TMP-SMX or pyrimethamine/clindamycin/folinic acid (Table 273-2) in these patients is supported by adult trials; unfortunately such data are not available in children.

TABLE 273-2. Antimicrobial Treatment Regimens[a] for Children with Primary Toxoplasmosis[b] and Immunocompromised Children with Toxoplasmosis Due to Reactivation

Pyrimethamine (PO)	1 mg/kg every 12 hours (maximum 50 mg/day) for 2 days; followed by 1 mg/kg once per day (maximum 25 mg/day)
plus	
Folinic acid[c]	10–20 mg three times weekly
plus	
Sulfadiazine (PO);	75 mg/kg (first dose); followed by 50 mg/kg every 12 hours (maximum 4 g/day)
or	
Clindamycin[d] (PO or IV)	
or	
Atovaquone[d] (PO)	
Trimethoprim-Sulfamethoxazole[d] (PO or IV) or Pyrimethamine *plus* folinic acid	Same doses as above
plus	
Clarithromycin[d] (PO)	
or	
Dapsone[d] (PO)	
or	
Azithromycin[d] (PO)	

PO, orally; IV, intravenously.

[a]Preferred regimens: pyrimethamine/sulfadiazine/folinic acid or trimethoprim-sulfamethoxazole. Assistance is available for the diagnosis and management of patients with toxoplasmosis at the US (Chicago, IL) National Collaborative Treatment Trial Study [NCCTS], telephone number (773) 834-4152) and the Palo Alto Medical Foundation Toxoplasma Serology Laboratory, PAMF-TSL; Palo Alto, CA; www.pamf.org/serology/; +1-650-853-4828; toxolab@pamf.org.

[b]Includes immunocompetent children with the acute infection particularly in the setting of myocarditis, myositis, hepatitis, pneumonia, brain, or skin lesions and lymphadenopathy accompanied by severe or persisting symptoms. Also indicated for those with active ocular disease due to primary infection or reactivation.

[c]Folinic acid = leucovorin; folic acid must not be used as a substitute for folinic acid.

[d]See text. Pediatric doses for these drugs have not been studied in the context of toxoplasmosis. Highest possible doses probably are needed in disseminated or severe cases.

PREVENTION

Primary Infection

Seronegative pregnant women and immunocompromised children should be educated on the known risks factors for acquisition of *T. gondii* and avoidance strategies (Table 273-3). All pregnant women and immunocompromised patients should be screened for IgG and IgM anti-*T. gondii* regardless of clinical or epidemiologic history. Seronegative pregnant women should be tested serially during gestation to diagnose seroconversion at the earliest time possible. In some countries, such as France,

TABLE 273-3. Recommendations for the Primary Prevention of *T. gondii* Infection in Seronegative Individuals[a]

Vehicle of Transmission	Recommendation
Meat and other edibles	Meat should not be "pink" in the center. Cook meat thoroughly to 67°C or to "well done"
	Freezing and thawing can kill *T. gondii* tissue cysts; freeze meat to −20°C for at least 24 hours
	Infected meat that has been smoked, cured in brine, or dried still can be infectious
	Wash hands carefully after contact with raw meat
	Avoid mucous membrane contact when handling raw meat
	Wash, wearing gloves, kitchen surfaces and utensils that have come in contact with raw meat
	Abstain from skinning or butchering animals without gloves
	Avoid drinking unpasteurized goat milk
	Avoid eating raw oysters, clams, or mussels
	Carefully wash fruits, vegetables, or any organic edibles
Untreated water	Refrain from drinking untreated water including that from wells or reservoirs that have not been secured from potential contamination by feces from wild or domestic cats
Cat feces and soil exposure	Avoid contact with materials potentially contaminated with cat feces, especially handling of cat litter or gardening
	Wearing gloves is recommended when these activities cannot be avoided

[a]Note that up to 50% of individuals can get infected with T. gondii *even without behaviors associated with the acute infection.*

seronegative pregnant women are mandated by law to be tested for IgG and IgM anti-*T. gondii* monthly.

Case-control studies from Europe, North America, and Latin America have identified ingestion of undercooked or raw meat as a significant risk factor associated with acute infection. Tissue cysts in contaminated meat can be rendered nonviable by γ-irradiation (0.4 kGy), heating throughout to 67°C, or freezing to −20°C for 24 hours and then thawing (Table 273-3). Cured, dried, or smoked meat has been associated with the acute infection and should not be considered *Toxoplasma* free. Potentially avoidable risks such as soil exposure, soil-related activities, and ingestion of untreated water are important in certain geographic areas (Latin America). Consumption of shellfish such as oysters, clams, and mussels is an avoidable risk factor.[14] Vegetarians can be infected with *T. gondii* by the ingestion of vegetables or other edibles contaminated with oocysts; thorough washing of fresh foodstuffs is recommended.

Seronegative solid-organ transplant recipients who receive an allograft from a seropositive donor should receive TMP-SMX prophylaxis for at least 6 months or pyrimethamine for at least 6 weeks. These regimens have been reported to be effective in the prevention of primary infection in the newly immunosuppressed patient.

Reactivation of Latent Infection

TMP-SMX and atovaquone have been used to prevent reactivation of latent infection in immunosuppressed adults. Dapsone plus pyrimethamine, and sulfadoxine plus pyrimethamine also have been reported to be effective, but use is limited by potential hematologic toxicity. Although likely effective in children, regimens should be tested in clinical trials. Prophylaxis against reactivation of latent infection has been successful in patients with AIDS dually infected with *T. gondii* (IgG seropositive) and whose CD4+ T lymphocyte counts are <200 cells/mm³. *Toxoplasma*-seropositive recipients of an allogeneic HSCT who develop graft-versus-host disease (GvHD) represent a unique challenge. Reactivation of *T. gondii* can be manifest as nonspecific illness (e.g., fever or pneumonia) yet be life-threatening; disease often is not recognized. Atovaquone prophylaxis has been proposed as an alternative regimen in these patients given the potential toxicity of TMP-SMX. Some investigators have proposed a pre-emptive strategy in which *Toxoplasma*-seropositive patients who receive an allogeneic HSCT and develop GvHD are monitored routinely (e.g., weekly for the first 100 days) with PCR tests. Those with positive PCR are given TMP-SMX or atovaquone pre-emptively. Discontinuation of prophylaxis against *Toxoplasma* encephalitis has proved safe in patients with AIDS receiving highly active antiretroviral therapy who demonstrate CD4+ T-lymphocyte counts ≥200 cells/mm³ and whose viral load has been undetectable for at least 6 months.

In patients with *Toxoplasma* chorioretinitis who experience frequent recurrences (e.g., >2 episodes per year), oral TMP-SMX for at least 12 months has been reported to be effective in the prevention of relapses.

274 *Trichomonas vaginalis*

Kimberly A. Workowski

Trichomonas vaginalis, a flagellated protozoan, was first described by Donné who in 1836 observed the organism in a preparation of fresh, vaginal discharge.[1] Although originally thought to be a harmless commensal, *T. vaginalis* now is recognized as a common sexually transmitted pathogen.

DESCRIPTION OF THE PATHOGEN

T. vaginalis is oval or fusiform, 10 to 20 μm wide, and is recognized readily in fresh specimens on microscopy by its characteristic, twitching motility (Figure 274-1). Organisms vary in size and

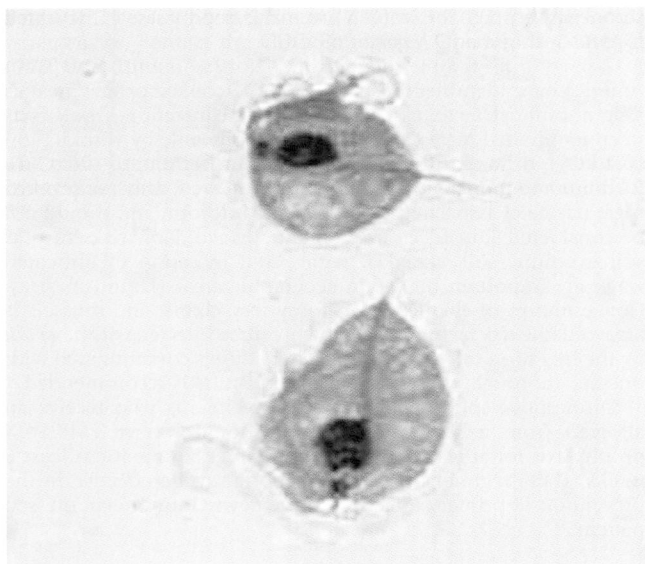

Figure 274-1. Two trophozoites of *Trichomonas vaginalis* obtained from in vitro culture (Giemsa stain). (Courtesy of the Centers for Disease Control and Prevention.)

shape, but each has four anterior flagella that appear to arise from a single stalk, a central axostyle, and an undulating membrane that extends across the organism. The microbe contains a large anterior nucleus and well-developed Golgi bodies. The organism generates metabolic energy in membrane-bound chromatic granules called hydrogenosomes.[1] All areas of the cell surface are capable of phagocytosis and can ingest bacteria, leukocytes, and erythrocytes. *T. vaginalis* readily attaches to mucous membranes via adhesion proteins[2] and appears to damage epithelial cells by direct contact.[3] Epithelial damage also can be caused by contact-independent mechanisms, including soluble and membrane-associated enzymes associated with phospholipase A activity, which can lyse nucleated cells in vitro and contribute to tissue damage and inflammation.[4–6] The organism reproduces by binary fission every 8 to 12 hours. *T. vaginalis* exists only in trophozoite form; cysts and other forms have not been described.[1]

T. vaginalis is facultatively anaerobic; utilizes a variety of carbohydrate sources; has limited biosynthetic capabilities; requires preformed purines, pyrimidines, fatty acids, and sterols; and grows in a variety of liquid and semisolid media or in cell culture.[1,7] Strains vary with respect to serotype, size, surface carbohydrates, protein profiles, hemolytic activity, and virulence properties.[1]

T. vaginalis induces both humoral and cell-mediated immune responses that are not fully protective, because persistent and repeated infections can occur. Neutrophils are the predominant cell type responding to natural infection and can kill the protozoa. Macrophages also can phagocytose and kill trichomonads in vitro. *T. vaginalis* activates serum complement via the alternate pathway, and the organism is susceptible to complement lysis.[1]

EPIDEMIOLOGY

Trichomoniasis is a common sexually transmitted infection (STI) that causes an estimated 7.4 million infections annually in the United States, and >180 million infections annually worldwide.[8] Most prevalence estimates have been limited to defined clinical situations and special populations. Among women, the prevalence of trichomoniasis has ranged from 3% in adolescent and student health clinics to over 45% in incarcerated women.[9–12] Among women, the rates of infection are highest among women with other STIs, older age, pregnancy, and drug use.[13,14] Among men, prevalence rates range from 10% to 21% in STI clinics and 45% in men who have had sexual contact with infected women.[15–17] A population-based prevalence study of

trichomoniasis demonstrated a 2.3% prevalence among young adults in the U.S.[18] The prevalence was slightly higher in women (2.8% versus 1.7% in men), increased with age, was higher in black women (10.5% versus 1.1% in white women), and Native American men (4.1% versus 3.3% in black and 1.3% in white men).

Nonsexual transmission of *T. vaginalis* is rare. Trichomoniasis can be transmitted to neonates during vaginal delivery.[1,19] Infection can be symptomatic during the first 3 to 4 weeks of life. However, the lack of estrogen and a shift in vaginal fluid pH to a more neutral level results in epithelial resistance to the organism and its usual disappearance. In older prepubertal girls, the diagnosis of vaginal trichomoniasis can indicate sexual abuse.[20,21] Infectivity is site-specific, and infection can occur only following intravaginal or intraurethral inoculation. The organism is sensitive to desiccation but can survive for a short time on moist objects.

CLINICAL MANIFESTATIONS

Trichomoniasis involves the urogenital tract almost exclusively.

Vaginitis

The incubation period for trichomonal vaginitis ranges from 5 to 28 days. Asymptomatic infection is common. When infection is evident clinically, symptoms and signs include vaginal discharge, vulvovaginal soreness or irritation, dysuria, and dyspareunia.[22] Discharge typically is homogeneous, yellow-green, frothy, and malodorous. Associated vulvar and vaginal erythema with copious frothy discharge that pools in the posterior vaginal fornix can be present. The external surface of the cervix usually is involved and can have a strawberry appearance, owing to punctate hemorrhages with ulcerations. Symptoms may begin or increase during menses. The differential diagnosis of vaginal discharge includes bacterial vaginosis, candidal vulvovaginitis, or cervicitis due to other organisms such as *Neisseria gonorrhoeae* or *Chlamydia trachomatis*. Trichomonal vaginitis has been associated with pelvic inflammatory disease and an increased risk of acquisition of human immunodeficiency virus.[23,24] Pregnant women who contract trichomoniasis can have an increased frequency of low-birthweight infants, preterm delivery, premature rupture of membranes, endometritis, and postcesarean infection.[25–27]

Urethritis in Males

Although many men infected with *T. vaginalis* are asymptomatic, some men can have urethral discharge. Additionally, *T. vaginalis* is responsible for approximately 1% to 15% of cases of nongonococcal urethritis.[15–18] Urethral discharge is common and dysuria and pruritus can occur. *T. vaginalis* urethritis cannot be distinguished clinically from nongonococcal urethritis due to other pathogens, such as *Chlamydia trachomatis* or *Mycoplasma genitalium*. *T. vaginalis* infection also has been associated with prolonged asymptomatic carriage and spontaneous resolution.

Neonatal Trichomoniasis

Neonates infected during vaginal delivery can manifest a self-limited vaginal discharge, urinary tract infection, or respiratory tract symptoms.[1,28,29]

LABORATORY DIAGNOSIS

Trichomonads can be identified in vaginal secretions using various diagnostic methods. Microscopic examination of a wet mount sample of vaginal secretions is the most frequently used diagnostic test, but has a sensitivity of only 60% to 70% and requires immediate evaluation by an expert examiner.[30] The wet-mount technique is performed by swabbing the anterior and posterior fornices, agitating the swab in 1 mL of saline in a test tube, and then placing a drop of the fluid on a microscope slide. The characteristic jerky movements of trichomonads are visualized readily with low (×100) or medium (×400) magnification. Neutrophils can be seen in wet mounts and epithelial cells appear normal. The vaginal fluid pH usually is >4.5. Culture is a sensitive and specific method of diagnosis. A commercially available culture system, In Pouch TV, permits easier transport and storage and appears to be comparable with traditional Diamond media. In women in whom trichomoniasis is suspected but not confirmed by microscopy, vaginal secretions should be cultured for *T. vaginalis*. Endocervical specimens for wet-mount examination or culture are not recommended because of their lower yield compared with vaginal fluid. Papanicolaou-stained smears of vaginal or cervical secretions also can suggest the diagnosis, but there is a high false-positive rate.[30] Point-of-care tests for vaginal trichomoniasis are more sensitive than vaginal wet prep; these tests include the OSOM Trichomonas Rapid Test (Genzyme Diagnostics), which uses an immunochromatographic capillary flow dipstick, and the Affirm VP III (Becton Dickinson), a nucleic acid probe test that can detect *Trichomonas vaginalis, Gardnerella vaginalis,* and *Candida albicans*. These tests are performed on vaginal secretions and have sensitivity >83% and a specificity >97%.[31-32] An FDA-cleared polymerase chain reaction (PCR) assay (Amplicor, manufactured by Roche Diagnostic Corp) has been modified for *T. vaginalis* detection in vaginal or endocervical swabs and in urine from women and men; sensitivity ranges from 88% to 97% and specificity ≥98%.[33]

Diagnosis of trichomoniasis is more difficult in men; both the type of specimen and the testing method influence test performance. Sensitivity of wet-mount microscopy or culture ranges from 60% to 80%.[34] Specimens from multiple sites and cultures of urethral swab, urine, and semen are required for optimal sensitivity. Nucleic acid amplification tests (PCR or transcription-mediated amplification) have superior sensitivity for diagnosis of *T. vaginalis* infection in men.[35]

TREATMENT

Nitroimidazoles, metronidazole and tinidazole, comprise the only class of drugs used for the treatment of trichomoniasis. Randomized controlled trials comparing a 2 g single dose of metronidazole or tinidazole suggest that tinidazole is equivalent to, or superior to, metronidazole in achieving parasitologic cure and resolution of symptoms.[36] Topical therapy with metronidazole is not recommended because therapeutic drug levels are not achieved in the urethra and periurethral glands.[37]

Most strains of *T. vaginalis* are susceptible to metronidazole. Low-level metronidazole resistance has been identified in 2% to 5% of cases of vaginal trichomoniasis.[38,39] If treatment failure occurs following a 2 g single dose of metronidazole and reinfection is excluded, metronidazole 500 mg orally twice daily for 7 days or tinidazole 2 g single dose is recommended.[37] Patients who fail either of these regimens should be given tinidazole or metronidazole, 2 g orally for 5 days. Failure of these therapies should be managed following in vitro susceptibility testing of *T. vaginalis* to metronidazole and tinidazole.[37]

Vaginal trichomoniasis has been associated with adverse pregnancy outcomes, particularly premature rupture of membranes, preterm delivery, and low birthweight of the infant.[25,26] However, data do not suggest that metronidazole treatment results in a reduction in perinatal morbidity. Some trials suggest the possibility of increased prematurity or low birthweight after metronidazole treatment. However, limitations of the studies prevent definitive conclusions about risks of treatment.[26,37,40] Treatment of *T. vaginalis* can relieve symptoms of vaginal discharge in pregnant women and can prevent respiratory or genital infection of the newborn and further sexual transmission. Clinicians should counsel patients regarding the potential risks and benefits of treatment. In lactating women, single-dose metronidazole therapy, with suspension of breastfeeding for 12 to 24 hours, is recommended.[37]

PREVENTION

Screening for *T. vaginalis* can be considered in people at high risk for infection (new or multiple partners, history of STIs, exchange of sex for payment, injection drug use).[37] Treatment and appropriate management of partner(s) results in relief of symptoms, microbiologic cure, and reduction of transmission. Male condoms, when used consistently and correctly, reduce the risk of many STIs that are transmitted in genital fluids, including trichomoniasis.[41]

275 *Trypanosoma* Species (Trypanosomiasis)
Frank E. Berkowitz

Organisms of the genus *Trypanosoma* are flagellated protozoan parasites that inhabit the blood and tissue of a wide variety of vertebrate hosts, including birds, reptiles, and mammals. The name is derived from the Greek, trypano (meaning auger) and soma (meaning body). The life cycle involves two hosts, and transmission to humans from insect vectors involves two different mechanisms. Trypanosomes have been classified into two groups according to the site of development in the invertebrate host. The *Salivaria* complete their development in the salivary glands of the vector and are transmitted by inoculation during the act of feeding. This group contains the subgenus *Trypanozoon*, which includes the species infecting humans, *Trypanosoma (Trypanozoon) brucei*. The *Stercoraria* are transmitted through infected feces of an arthropod vector. This group include the subgenus *Schizotrypanum* and contains one pathogen, *Trypanosoma (Schizotrypanum) cruzi*. The trypanosomes that infect humans in Africa (*T. brucei*) are transmitted by the bite of *Glossina* flies, whereas human trypanosomiasis in the Americas (*T. cruzi*) is transmitted by feces of triatomid insects.[1-3]

AFRICAN TRYPANOSOMIASIS

African trypanosomiasis (sleeping sickness) is one of the major health problems facing populations in sub-Saharan Africa. This disease is caused by two subspecies of the extracellular flagellate *Trypanosoma brucei*, namely *T. brucei gambiense*, which occurs in West and Central Africa, and which accounts for about 95% of all cases of African trypanosomiasis, and *T. brucei rhodesiense*, which occurs in East and south-central Africa.[1-8] Until recently, distribution of the two species did not overlap. However, there now is an overlap area in Uganda. This is of clinical significance because the laboratory differentiation between the two species is difficult and treatment varies by species.[1] African trypanosomes are transmitted by both sexes of flies of the genus *Glossina* ("tsetse flies"). These are aggressive flies that cause a painful bite. About 0.1% of tsetse flies are able to transmit mature trypanosomes in their saliva, from one mammalian host to another. Approximately 7 to 10 million km² of Africa are infested with the tsetse fly, and some 60 million people are at risk.[1] The principal clinical manifestations of the

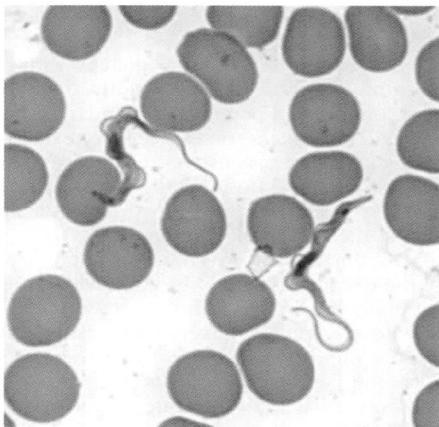

Figure 275-1. *Trypanosoma brucei* in a thin blood smear stained with Giemsa. (Courtesy of DPDx image library, CDC.)

disease are intermittent fever in the early stage, signs of reticuloendothelial hyperplasia, and in the advanced stage, neurologic manifestations. The disease is invariably fatal when untreated. WHO estimates that 300,000 to 500,000 people are infected, but accurate figures are not available.[1,9]

Description of the Pathogen

The African trypanosomes are members of the family Trypanosomatidae, genus *Trypanosoma*, and subgenus *Trypanozoon*.[1] All members of the two subspecies of *T. brucei* complex share a common morphology, biochemistry, and life cycle. After inoculation of infective metacyclic trypomastigotes into subcutaneous tissue by an infected tsetse fly, trypanosomes are converted to the pleomorphic bloodstream trypomastigotes (Figure 275-1), which are infective for the tsetse fly.

In the vertebrate host, African *Trypanosoma* always occurs in the trypomastigote form where it lives and multiples in blood, cerebrospinal fluid (CSF), interstitial space of the lymph nodes, spleen, and brain. The tsetse fly ingests bloodstream forms when taking a blood meal from an infected animal. Procyclic trypomastigotes eventually migrate through the esophagus toward the hypopharynx in the proboscis and into the salivary glands. In the salivary glands, they change into epimastigotes, attach to the epithelium, and finally become infective metacyclic trypomastigotes that are inoculated into the vertebrate host during a new blood meal.[1,7]

Epidemiology

Humans acquire *T. brucei* through the bite of infected male or female tsetse flies. Rarely, humans can acquire the infection transplacentally or by blood transfusion. The disease attacks all age groups and is equally frequent in females and males. Children are infected rarely, mainly because of a decreased risk of exposure, but in children the disease often is fulminant, with early central nervous system (CNS) involvement.

The insect vector is found in temperature conditions between 20°C and 30°C, high humidity, and an altitude below 1800 m. The development period in the tsetse fly takes about 3 weeks; infection is lifelong (up to 11 months) but it is not passed to the fly's progeny. *Glossina palpalis* and *G. tachinoides*, which inhabit dense vegetation along river banks, are the most common vectors of *T. b. gambiense*, whereas *T. b. rhodesiense* is transmitted to humans by *G. morsitans* and less frequently by *G. swynnertoni* and *G. pallidipes*, which inhabit the savannas and lake shores. By definition, *T. b. gambiense* is the trypanosome adapted to humans, and *T. b. rhodesiense* infects both animals and humans. Animal reservoirs play an important role in human transmission of *T. b. rhodesiense*, and natural infections occur in domestic animals, including cattle, sheep, and goats, and in various wild animals, including lions, hyenas, and several species of antelope. For *T. b. gambiense*, the period of incubation ranges from 2 to 23 days.

Pathogenesis and Pathology

After organisms are injected into the mammalian host with the saliva of the tsetse fly, they enter lymphatics and then the bloodstream (Figure 275-2). In about 20% of cases of *T. b. rhodesiense* infection, a chancre develops at the bite site 1 to 2 weeks after the bite. All organs can be affected. After a variable period, depending on the species, the organism enters the CNS where it causes meningoencephalitis. The severity of symptoms is related directly to the number of organisms. The lymph nodes are enlarged and show an increased number of lymphocytes and mononuclear cells. Histopathologic examination of the CNS reveals infiltration of plasma cells, macrophages and lymphocytes, with perivascular proliferation of endothelial and neuroglia cells, severe cerebral edema, and punctate hemorrhage. Demyelination and neuronal damage have been observed and can extend deeply into white matter. Chronic meningoencephalitis also can occur. Vasculitis associated with increased permeability of the capillary vessels is considered to be the essential factor in pathogenesis, and is suspected to be of immunopathogenic origin.[1,7,10]

Clinical Course

The disease appears in two stages, the first is the hemolymphatic stage and the second is the meningoencephalitis stage, which is characterized by CNS invasion. The specific clinical forms of African trypanosomiasis depend on the infecting trypanosome. Infection caused by *T. b. rhodesiense* causes acute and severe disease with few CNS symptoms and death within weeks or months. *T. b. gambiense* is characterized by a milder, chronic, progressive course with involvement of the lymph nodes, CNS invasion, and a fatal outcome after several years' duration. When the parasite crosses the blood–brain barrier, the disease progresses to the second stage, characterized by neurologic symptoms and, without treatment, evolves to body wasting, somnolence, coma, and death.[7,10] Disease caused by either of the two parasites leads to coma and death if left untreated.

Within a few days after infection, an indurated, erythematous, painful, warm, circumscribed, rubbery lesion (trypanosomal chancre) can develop at the site of the tsetse fly bite, more frequently in patients infected with *T. b. rhodesiense*. The lesion usually resolves within 3 weeks, but with residual scarring and depigmentation. The early parasitemic phase is accompanied by high fever, headache, and general malaise interspersed with relatively asymptomatic periods. As infection progresses, fever is intermittent and a papular rash and generalized enlargement of lymph nodes occurs, especially in the posterior cervical triangle *(Winterbottom sign)* and the submaxillary, inguinal, and femoral regions. The nodes are discrete, soft, and nontender and contain abundant parasites. The spleen and liver can be enlarged mildly. Dyspnea, chest pain, anemia, and loss of strength develop, and the patient becomes extremely emaciated. Endocrine abnormalities include increased or decreased thyroid function, decreased sexual function, and in women, amenorrhea is common. Arthralgia, weakness, and painful local edema of the hands, feet, and joints can be present. Deep hyperesthesia *(Kerandel sign)* often is reported in non-Africans; delayed, intense pain occurs when soft tissue is compressed.

The most common laboratory abnormalities include hemolytic anemia, elevation of serum hepatic enzymes, coagulation abnormalities, thrombocytopenia, and hypocomplementemia. The sedimentation rate is markedly elevated. Serum immunoglobulin levels (IgM), circulating immune complexes, heterophil antibodies, and rheumatoid factor are increased.

In the second stage, sleep disturbance and neuropsychiatric disorders dominate the clinical presentation. The neurologic disease is a meningoencephalitis, which can involve the spinal cord as well as the brain. There is leptomeningeal and perivascular infiltration of plasma cells, lymphocytes, and macrophages. The white

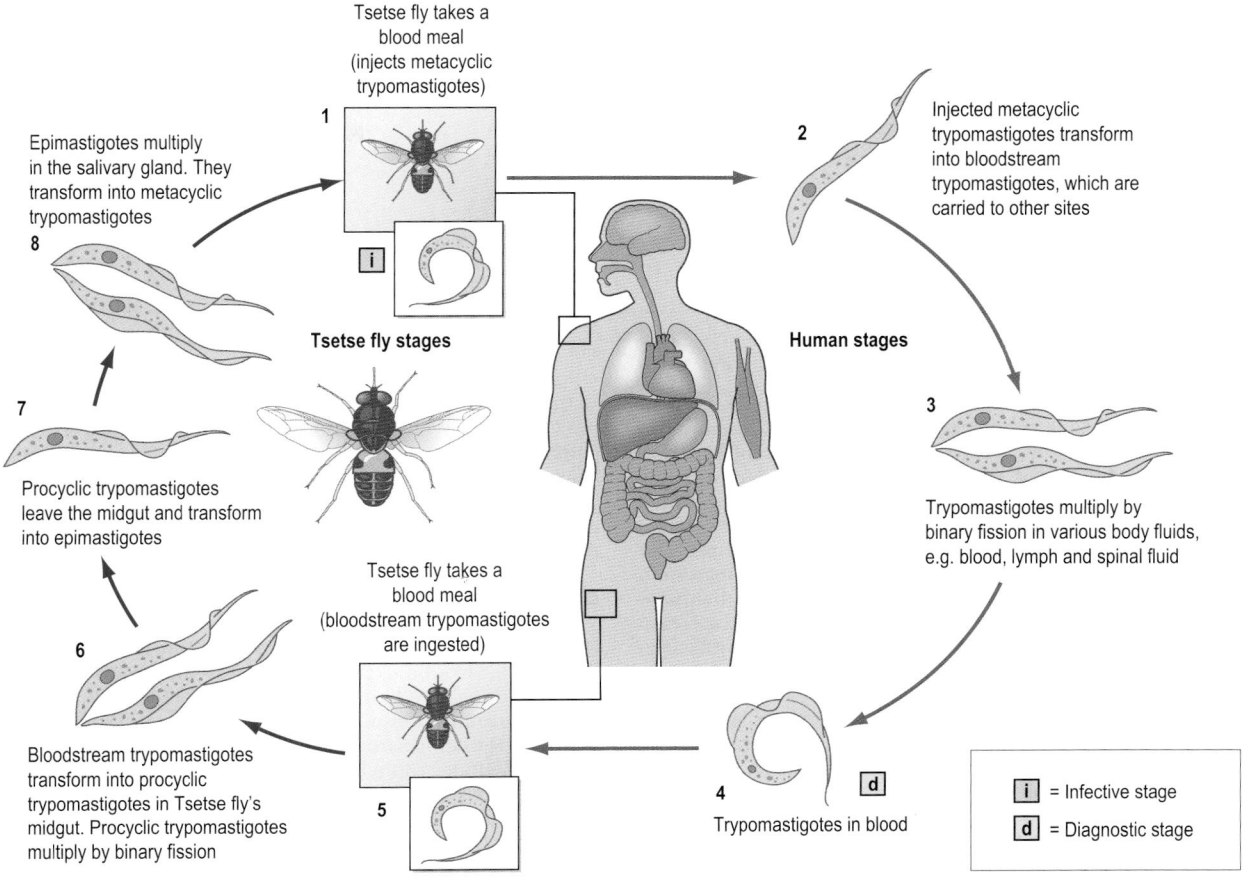

Figure 275-2. Life cycle of *Trypanosoma brucei* (African trypanosomiasis, African sleeping sickness). (Courtesy of the CDC.)

matter of the brain shows pathognomonic cells called morula or Mott cells, which are plasma cells containing large concentrations of IgM. With invasion of the CNS, the chronic or sleeping sickness stage of infection is initiated. The range of neurologic abnormalities is broad. Headache is severe, and irritability, personality and behavior changes, and gradual loss of cognitive function are common. Papilledema and headache reflect cerebral edema. Muscle spasms, ataxia, incoordination, tremor, alteration of reflexes, stiffness in the neck, and flaccid paralysis occur. Psychiatric manifestations include hallucinations, delusional states, and overt psychoses. Choreiform or oscillatory movements of the arms, head, neck, and trunk are frequent.[6–8,11]

Sleep disorders with diurnal somnolence, inappropriate episodes of sleeping, and nocturnal insomnia are a leading symptom of the second stage.[7,10] Progressive somnolence and convulsions develop and lead to deep coma and death. The CSF contains abnormal concentrations of white cells and IgM. At times, the heart is enlarged, and congestive heart failure, pericardial effusion, and electrocardiographic changes occur.[12] Death results from meningitis, heart failure, or complications such as bacterial pneumonia.

Congenital African trypanosomiasis due to *T. b. gambiense* has been reported rarely.[13,14]

The differential diagnosis of stage 1 includes other causes of febrile illness occurring in the area, namely malaria, typhoid fever, tuberculosis, brucellosis, syphilis, leptospirosis, hepatitis, borrelial relapsing fever, viral hemorrhagic fevers, and acute HIV infection. The differential diagnosis of causes of a chancre include cutaneous anthrax, in which there is marked swelling around the eschar, syphilis, and African tick bite fever, caused by *Rickettsia africae* and

R. conori. The differential diagnosis of stage 2 disease includes other causes of chronic meningoencephalitis, especially tuberculosis, cryptococcal infection, and syphilis.

Diagnosis

Diagnosis occurs at three levels: screening, diagnostic testing, and staging.

Screening. Screening can be performed for *T. b. gambiense* infection by use of a card agglutination test for trypanosomiasis (CATT), which utilizes a finger-prick drop of blood mixed on the card with a drop of reagent containing a freeze-dried trypanosomal antigen. Agglutination occurs within 5 minutes. This test can be performed in the field and has a sensitivity of 87% to 98%, and a specificity of 93% to 95%. False-negative results can occur in areas where the parasite does not express the specific antigen used in the test, and as a result of a prozone phenomenon. Other serologic tests include an immunofluorescent (FA) and an enzyme immunoassay (EIA) test, which cannot be performed readily in the field.[15,16]

Diagnostic testing. Diagnostic testing in a suspected case depends on visualizing the organism in blood, lymph node aspirate, bone marrow, or CSF in late stages of disease,[10,16] by microscopy. Examination of wet preparations of lymph node aspirates have a sensitivity of 40% to 80%. Because of periodicity of parasitemia, daily examination of blood films for 10 consecutive days is recommended. The diagnostic sensitivity of thick and thin blood smears, as are done for the diagnosis of malaria, is low for *T. b. gambiense* infection but high for *T. b. rhodesiense* infection, in which the degree of parasitemia is higher. The best method of testing blood for trypanosomes is thick and thin Giemsa-stained

TABLE 275-1. Antimicrobial Therapy for Patients with African Trypanosomiasis

Stage	Category of Recommendation	T. b. gambiense	T. b. rhodesiense
Hemolymphatic	Drug of choice	Pentamidine	Suramin
	Alternative	Suramin	None
Late-stage disease with CNS involvement	Drug of choice	Eflornithine *or* Eflornithine plus nifurtimox *or* Melarsoprol	Melarsoprol
	Alternative	None	None

For doses, see Chapter 296, Antiparasitic Agents.

smears of buffy coat preparations, which have a lower limit of detection of ~5000 parasites per mL of blood. Concentration methods can increase the sensitivity. The microhematocrit centrifugation technique (Woo test), in which 6 to 8 sealed microhematocrit tubes are centrifuged and the buffy coat is examined using a long-distance objective lens for motile parasites, has a lower limit of detection of ~500 parasites per mL. Quantitative buffy coat test, in which blood, EDTA and acridine orange stain are mixed and centrifuged, shows motile parasites with the use of fluorescence microscopy, and a miniature anion-exchange centrifugation technique has a lower limit of detection of ~100 parasites per mL. The last two tests cannot be performed readily in the field.

Staging. Staging determines whether or not there is nervous system involvement. Staging has important implications for therapy,[17] and depends on examination of CSF. WHO criteria for evidence of nervous system infection are: >5 leukocytes/mm³, visualization of trypanosomes, or protein concentration of >37 mg/dL. The presence of IgM in the CSF is an early and specific marker of CNS invasion.[18]

Intraperitoneal inoculation of 0.5 mL of heparinized blood or CSF into two mice is positive in 89% of cases of *T. b. rhodesiense*, with parasitemia developing within 2 weeks. Lymph node aspiration and CSF examination help define the extension and severity of the infection. Several highly sensitive and specific, conventional and real-time polymerase chain reaction (PCR) tests for rapid detection of trypanosomes in human blood samples have been developed.[19,20]

In *T. b. gambiense* infection, examination of lymph node aspirates is as sensitive as examination of blood. Trypanosomes also can be found in aspirates of bone marrow and serous effusions. Specific serum antibodies can be detected after the second week of infection by the indirect FA (IFA) test, latex agglutination, or EIA. The card agglutination test for trypanosomiasis is a fast and practical serologic test of value as a screening test for antibodies to *T. b. gambiense*.[17,21] The presence of elevated IgM in the CSF also is diagnostic. A monoclonal antibody-based EIA for detection of *Trypanosoma* antigens in serum and CSF has high specificity (>99%) and sensitivity (*T. b. gambiense*, 95%; *T. b. rhodesiense*, 92%).[9]

The diagnostic approach to *T. b. rhodesiense* infection differs from *T. b. gambiense* in the following ways: there is no serologic screening test for *T. b. rhodesiense*, parasitologic confirmation is easier for *T. b. rhodesiense*, and nonspecific biologic indices (hemoglobin and platelet counts) are abnormal more frequently in *T. b. rhodesiense* infection.[1]

Treatment

Few drugs are available to treat African trypanosomiasis, with selection based mainly on stage of disease and specific pathogen. Early treatment is essential because prognosis is poor once CNS involvement has occurred. In the absence of CNS disease, pentamidine and suramin are the drugs of choice.[22-25] Suramin sodium is useful only in treatment of early *T. b. gambiense* and *T. b. rhodesiense* infections because it does not cross the blood–brain barrier.[23]

Therapy is summarized in Table 275-1. Doses and side effects can be found in Chapter 296, Antiparasitic Agents. Treatment for patients with infection caused by *T. b. gambiense* and *T. b. rhodesiense* is different. When the implicated species can be suspected based on the geographic area of acquisition, appropriate therapy can be given. In areas where there is an overlap in distribution of the two subspecies this is more difficult.[26-30]

Prevention

Routine preventive measures include avoiding known foci of tsetse infestation, avoiding endemic areas, wearing wrist- and ankle-length dark-colored clothing, use of insect repellents, and routine use of mosquito nets. Clearing of vegetation around human settlements, limited destruction of game animals and potential wild reservoirs, and prophylactic treatment of cattle and domestic animals, as well as spraying of insecticides, have resulted in local eradication of the insect vector and a reduced incidence of human infection.[31,32] Chemoprophylaxis is no longer in use because of the poor risk–benefit ratio caused by adverse effects of the drugs.

AMERICAN TRYPANOSOMIASIS

Trypanosoma cruzi is the etiologic agent of Chagas disease, a chronic multisystemic disease that affects millions of people throughout the Americas. Approximately 25% of the Latin American population is living in an endemic area and is at risk of acquiring infection. Infection is a zoonosis transmitted to humans by bloodsucking insects of the family Reduviidae. Three clinical stages are recognized in Chagas disease: a short *acute stage*, a long, clinically asymptomatic *indeterminate stage*, and a long-lasting *chronic stage*.[2,3,33] Large-scale vector control programs and screening of blood donors have reduced disease incidence and prevalence.[34]

Description of the Pathogen

T. cruzi belongs to the genus *Trypanosoma*, subgenus *Schizotrypanum*. Members of this group develop in the lower gut and rectum of the triatomid vector (reduviid or kissing bug Figure 275-3), and transmission is through contamination. The developmental cycle of *T. cruzi* includes three morphologic forms: amastigotes, epimastigotes, and trypomastigotes. The trypomastigote (Figure 275-4), is found in the tissue and bloodstream (only stage found in blood) of infected mammals and is responsible for spread of infection from cell to cell and for transmission of the infection to the insect vector. The reduviid bug vector feeds on the vertebrate host, excretes the infectious forms in feces, which are rubbed or scratched into the bite wounds. The organisms also can enter the host through mucous membranes.

Epidemiology

T. cruzi infects humans and animals in temperate, subtropical, and tropical regions of the Americas and West Indies. Chagas disease originally was confined to rural areas of South and Central America, but in the past 25 years improved vector control blood donations and the number of cases of transfusion transmission has decreased substantially in all Latin American countries.[2,3]

Routine screening of blood in the U.S. began in 2007.[34] In a study conducted by the Red Cross in 2006–2007, 148,969 blood samples from the U.S. revealed that 32 donations (1 in 4655) were positive for *T. cruzi* antibodies.[34]

The increase in the number of immigrants from countries endemic for disease has resulted in Chagas disease becoming an important health issue in the U.S., Canada, and parts of Europe.[2,3,35] The most common destination for migrants from Latin America is the U.S., where an estimated 300,167 people with *T. cruzi* infection live, with most arriving from Mexico.[35] In addition 6 autochthonous insect-borne human cases of Chagas disease have been reported in the U.S.,[36] and cases of acute Chagas disease acquired through laboratory accidents and cases of imported infection have been reported to the Centers for Disease Control and Prevention (CDC).[37]

More than 100 species of Triatominae are recognized, and although more than 50 are known to transmit *T. cruzi*, relatively few of them feed on humans. Certain species show a considerable degree of adaptation to human habitation and are important vectors in transmission of Chagas disease. The domesticated species are large (2 to 3 cm or more in length), obligate hematophagous insects that hide in crevices in walls, dark corners, windows, and door frames or in the thatch of roofs and take their blood meals at night. They require a blood meal at each stage of development to grow and mature. Infection lasts for the life of the vector, which can be up to 2 years. Species of *Triatoma* vary from one geographic area to another. In the U.S., several southern states have host vectors and reservoirs for *T. cruzi*.[36–38]

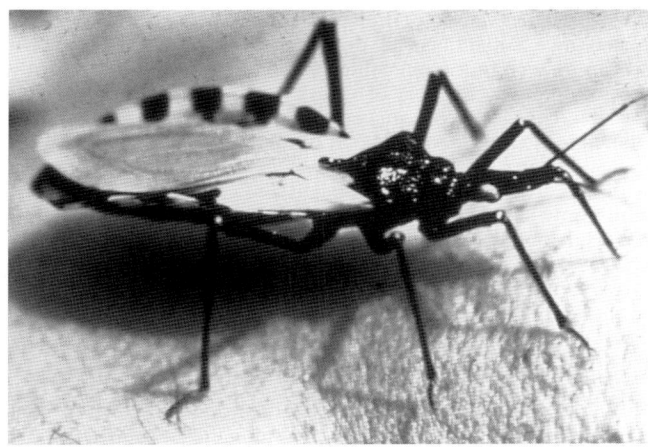

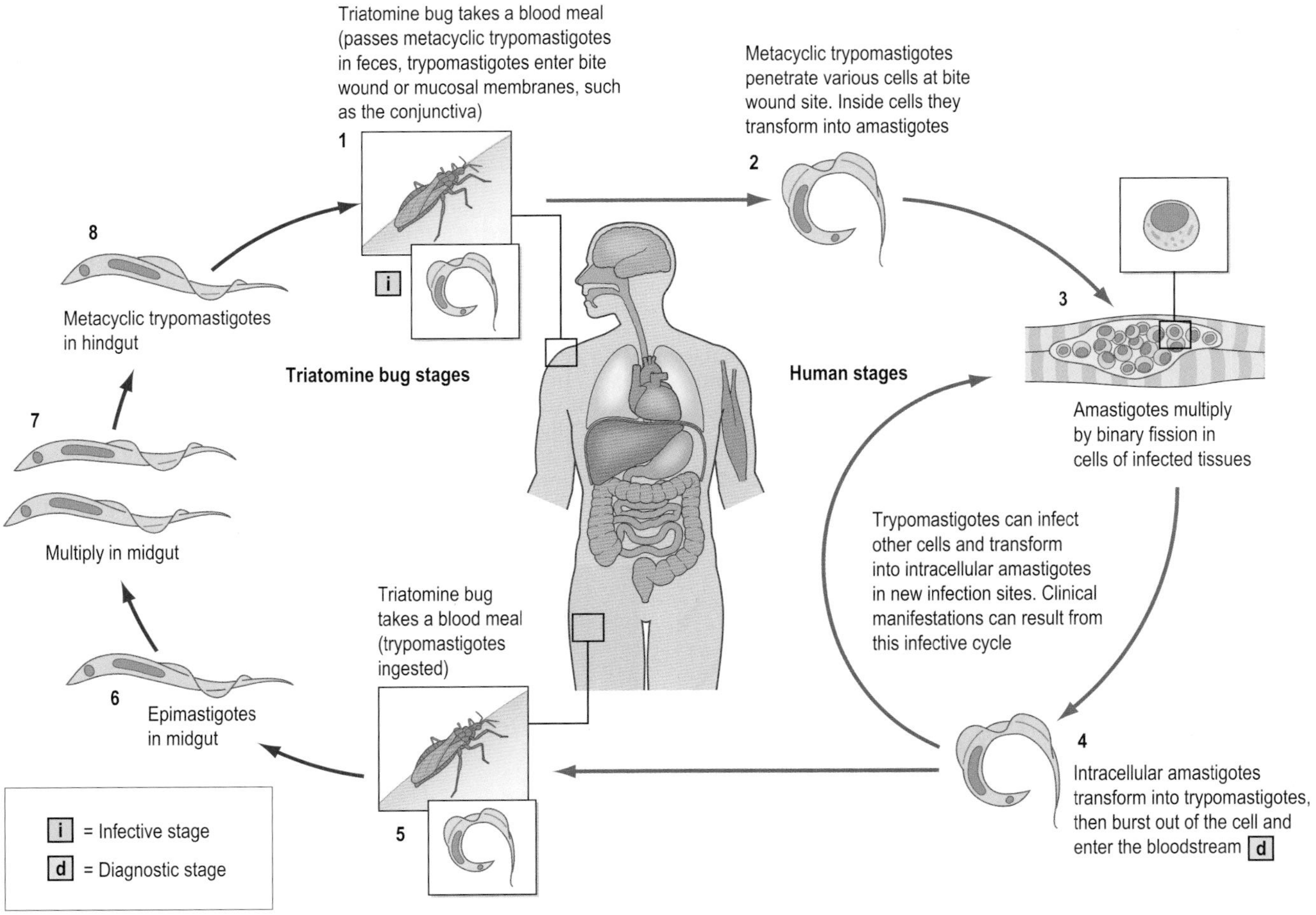

Figure 275-3. A triatomine bug *(Dipetalogaster maximus)* feeding on human skin. (Courtesy of World Health Organisation/Tropical Disease Research Library.)

programs and compulsory blood bank screening have reduced substantially new cases of infection.[2,3] In endemic areas the incidence of Chagas has decreased from 700,000 new cases per year to 40,000 and the annual number of deaths has fallen from more than 45,000 to 12,500.[2,3] Transmission of *T. cruzi* by the main domiciliary vector species, *Triatoma infestans*, was halted in Uruguay in 1997, Chile in 1999, and Brazil in 2006. Several endemic countries are now screening for *T. cruzi* in virtually all

Triatomine bug takes a blood meal (passes metacyclic trypomastigotes in feces, trypomastigotes enter bite wound or mucosal membranes, such as the conjunctiva)

Metacyclic trypomastigotes penetrate various cells at bite wound site. Inside cells they transform into amastigotes

Triatomine bug stages

Human stages

Metacyclic trypomastigotes in hindgut

Multiply in midgut

Epimastigotes in midgut

Triatomine bug takes a blood meal (trypomastigotes ingested)

Amastigotes multiply by binary fission in cells of infected tissues

Trypomastigotes can infect other cells and transform into intracellular amastigotes in new infection sites. Clinical manifestations can result from this infective cycle

Intracellular amastigotes transform into trypomastigotes, then burst out of the cell and enter the bloodstream **d**

i = Infective stage

d = Diagnostic stage

Figure 275-4. Life cycle of *Trypanosoma cruzi* (American trypanosomiasis, Chagas disease). (Courtesy of the CDC.)

A wide variety of animals are reservoirs, including opossums, armadillos, and canines. In sylvatic transmission, triatome bugs that live primarily in trees and tree holes transmit the infection among wild animals, and humans are accidental victims. In domestic transmission, bugs living in the cracks in walls of houses transmit the infection to humans; this explains predominant transmission in poor areas. Because the organism can be present in blood and in various tissues, infection can be transmitted by blood transfusion, sharing of syringes used for intravenous drug abuse, transplacentally,[39-46] and through transplantation of organs from infected donors.[47,48] Organisms also can be ingested in food and drink, such as sugarcane juice and palm juice contaminated by triatome feces. The epidemiology of Chagas disease has changed dramatically over the past 20 to 30 years due to the interventions of insecticide spraying and screening of blood for donation, which has been remarkably successful.[34,39-42]

Pathogenesis and Pathology

Pathologically, Chagas disease occurs in two phases: an acute phase (4 to 8 weeks), which is usually asymptomatic and is characterized by focal or diffuse inflammation mainly affecting the myocardium, and a chronic phase (lifetime) characterized by an inflammatory fibrotic reaction that damages the cardiac muscle and conduction system and the enteric nervous system. Two main hypotheses have been proposed to explain the mechanism of organ damage. One is that direct destruction of cells by the parasite prevails during the acute phase of the disease, when many parasites are present. The cardiac and digestive alterations characteristic of the chronic phase probably are caused by loss of ganglionic neurons and nerve fibers. Alternatively, pathology may be due to the inflammatory reaction resulting from an allergic response to parasitic antigens absorbed by host cells or due to autoimmune reactions resulting from the existence of antigens shared by the host and the parasite.[49-51]

The lesion at the portal of entry shows a local inflammatory response with infiltration of lymphocytes, monocytes, and giant cells. During the acute phase, parasites are distributed widely throughout tissues, but they show a preference for cells in cardiac, skeletal, and smooth muscle, for neural cells, and for cells of the reticuloendothelial system (Figure 275-5). The heart is enlarged and shows interstitial inflammation of the endocardium and myocardium, edema, and focal necrosis in the contractile and conducting system. The cellular infiltrates consist of lymphocytes, monocytes, and plasma cells, as well as parasitized muscle cells.

During the chronic phase, ganglion cells are progressively destroyed, with the affected organs showing variable tolerance to denervation. The heart becomes markedly enlarged with a characteristic thinning of the muscle wall, particularly the right atrium. Mural endocardial thrombosis and aneurysm can occur at the apex of the left ventricle. The myocardium is edematous and congested, myocardial fibers are degenerated, and dense foci of fibrosis can be seen in the interstitial space, but parasites infrequently are found (15% to 30% of cases). Inflammatory, fibrotic, and vascular changes occur in conductive tissue. The right bundle branch is the most damaged part of the system, and alterations in the atrioventricular conduction system are frequent. In people with digestive disease, the esophagus and colon are affected most commonly. Fibrosis is present in the myenteric plexus, as well as a considerable reduction in the number of neurons. Dysfunction is related directly to peristaltic abnormalities, which can lead to arrest in transit, extreme dilation of the organ, and hypertrophy of the muscle.

Clinical Course

Children often suffer early morbidity and mortality (which are relatively infrequent events), while adults suffer the late morbidity and mortality (which are frequent). Shortly after penetration into subcutaneous tissue, parasites elicit a local inflammatory reaction at the site of entry that gives origin to a *chagoma* (nodular skin lesion), which often is on the face and contains organisms; parasites and inflammation spread to regional lymph nodes within a few days causing the *Romaña* sign (unilateral periorbital edema, conjunctivitis, and preauricular lymphadenitis) if the initial inoculation was in the eye (Figure 275-6).[52] The *acute phase* of illness begins with headaches, irritability, tiredness, and fever that rarely exceeds 40°C but usually persists for several weeks when signs of systemic illness develop. Infection is not often recognized at this stage and is diagnosed in only 1% or 2% of all patients. Extensive lymphadenopathy and hepatosplenomegaly are observed frequently, and meningoencephalitis occurs occasionally. The most common (30% of cases) and severe manifestations are cardiovascular disturbances, including cardiac enlargement, functional murmurs, conduction blocks, and occasionally, heart failure. Mortality from acute myocarditis occurs in 2% to 3% of cases, but in people with meningoencephalitis, the mortality can be as high as 50%.[12]

People who survive enter the *indeterminate*, asymptomatic *phase* of the disease.[52] However, a low level of parasitemia persists and can be recognized by xenodiagnosis in 20% to 60% of cases. This phase can persist for years, even for the life of the patient, or the *chronic phase* of the disease can ensue. Up to 30% of people with the indeterminate form suffer from cardiac, digestive, or neurologic damage 10 to 20 years after having contracted the infection. The cardiac manifestations include palpitations, dizziness, syncope, dyspnea, and chest pain.[53] The most important complications are systemic and pulmonary embolism and sudden death. Ventricular fibrillation is the most frequent mechanism of sudden death. In many cases, a typical aneurysm develops at the apex of the left ventricle.

The digestive form of the disease occurs in 10% to 15% of patients and varies from minor changes in motility of the esophagus or intestine to two main syndromes of megaesophagus and megacolon. Patients have difficulty swallowing and regurgitation,

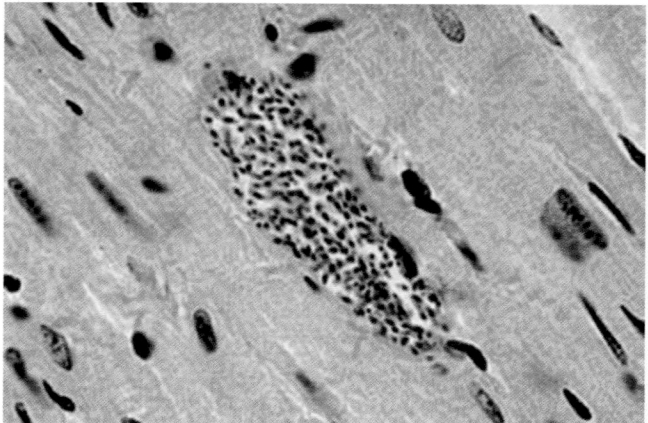

Figure 275-5. Cardiac muscle with a pseudocyst containing amastigotes of *T. cruzi*. (Courtesy of WHO/TDR/Stammers.)

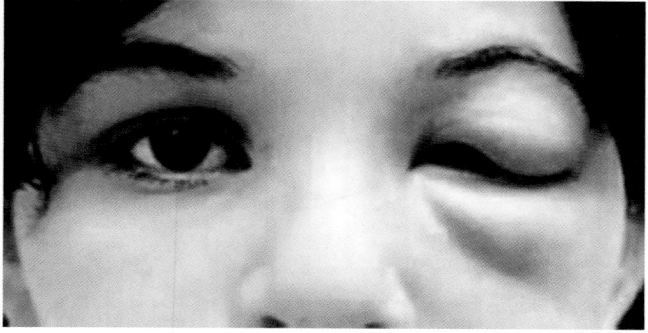

Figure 275-6. Child with acute Chagas disease demonstrating Romaña sign. (Courtesy of WHO/TDR.)

severe constipation, and abdominal pain. Esophagitis and cancer of the esophagus are the most common complications of megaesophagus, whereas fecaloma and volvulus can complicate megacolon.

Factors that account for differing clinical manifestations in different geographic areas might include different strains of parasite (there are two main zymodemes, namely I and II), and genetic differences in hosts. The gastrointestinal disease is common in central Brazil and southern South America, where zymodeme II is prevalent, but rare in northern South America and Central America, where zymodeme I is prevalent.

The prognosis depends on the clinical stage and complications that develop. The acute phase is most serious in children <2 years of age and is almost always fatal if heart failure or meningoencephalitis develops. In patients with chronic disease and pronounced cardiac manifestations, prognosis is poor and death usually occurs within 5 years of heart failure or pulmonary embolism. The prognosis in patients with the digestive form usually is good. Immunosuppression after organ transplantation or secondary to human immunodeficiency virus (HIV) can lead to reactivation of infection. Neurologic disease with brain lesions and meningoencephalitis caused by *T. cruzi* has been a major finding in HIV-infected patients.[52]

Acute Chagas disease should be considered in any child who has been in an endemic area and in whom myocarditis and an acute febrile illness with lymphadenopathy develop. The acute phase must be differentiated from typhoid fever, visceral leishmaniasis, brucellosis, tuberculosis, toxoplasmosis, malaria, schistosomiasis, cytomegalovirus infection, infectious mononucleosis, and brucellosis. Chronic disease must be distinguished from endomyocardial fibrosis, viral myocarditis, rheumatic heart disease, and carcinoma of the esophagus or colon.

Immunosuppression can result in severe systemic disease, which may have different manifestations from those in otherwise normal hosts. Posttransplant patients often have subcutaneous nodules, panniculitis, and myocarditis, while patients with AIDS may manifest with meningoencephalitis or focal brain lesions resembling those caused by toxoplasmosis.

Congenital Infection

Intrauterine infection can occur at any time during pregnancy and usually is asymptomatic.[42–46] In most reported cases, the mother was in the chronic or indeterminate stage. Patent parasitemia in the mother seems to have little relation to development of congenital infection. As the rates of infection caused by triatome bug transmission and by blood transfusion have decreased in many endemic areas as a result of insecticide use and screening of blood for donation, congenital transmission has assumed a greater role in the epidemiology. Although the highest risk for transmission is in infants born to mothers who have acute infection (when parasitemia is overt), most cases are born to women with chronic infection. It is estimated that in the year 2000 there were about 130,000 infected women between the ages of 15 and 44 years living in the U.S., and that there were between 170 and 640 cases of congenital infection.[38] Clinical illness may be present at birth or develop within the first few weeks of life. In a study of 530 mothers in Santa Cruz, Bolivia, 154 had serologic evidence of chronic *T. cruzi* infection, and the infants of 10 of these mothers were infected (6.5%).[46] Studies of infection during two periods in Cochabamba, Bolivia found a congenital rate of 5%.[42]

The most common findings of congenital infection are low birthweight, hepatosplenomegaly, fever, neurologic abnormalities (convulsions, hypotonia, hyporeflexia, and tremors), anasarca and petechiae.[42–46] Some patients manifest metastatic hemorrhagic chagomas in the skin or mucosa. Occasionally, intracranial calcifications and ocular lesions can occur. Cardiac involvement is rare and can manifest as heart failure. Megaesophagus and pneumonitis are reported. Laboratory findings can include anemia, thrombocytopenia, lymphocytosis, jaundice, and hyperglobulinemia. The CSF can show pleocytosis with predominance of lymphocytes and elevated protein concentration. A minority of patients survive,

and death frequently occurs during the first week of life. Severe neurologic sequelae consisting of mental deficiency or behavioral and learning disabilities develop in most survivors. Infants of seropositive mothers should be tested as soon as possible for the presence of circulating parasites and specific immunoglobulin (Ig) M antibody and should be monitored for a year after birth. A positive serologic test for specific IgG at 6 and 12 months of age is an indication for treatment.

The differential diagnosis includes all other congenital infections and enteroviral myocarditis, disseminated histoplasmosis, and HIV infection as well as noninfectious diseases, such as erythroblastosis fetalis and hemophagocytic syndrome. In addition to methods used to diagnose postnatally acquired Chagas disease, examination of the umbilical cord can show parasites. Infection of the placenta does not necessarily indicate infection of the baby.

Diagnosis

Visualization of the organism in blood smears is the optimal method of diagnosis during the acute phase (including early congenital infection) but is not sensitive in the chronic stage due to low-density parasitemia. Besides examination of stained thick and thin blood smears, examination of fresh blood for motile trypomastigotes can be performed. Concentration methods increase sensitivity. When smears are made, the angle of the "smearing" glass slide should be high, so as not to damage the trypanosomes, which are delicate. The parasite can be isolated in special culture media. Xenodiagnosis entails allowing laboratory-raised triatome bugs, previously fed on birds (which are not susceptible to the infection) to feed on the suspected case, with examination of the feces performed 20 to 25 days afterwards. PCR, where available, might become the optimal method for testing for acute infection, including chronic and congenital infections.[54] However, PCR is not standardized currently, and it is not sensitive in the chronic stage of the infection.

Several different serology methods, including EIA, IFA and indirect hemagglutination methods, are used for screening and diagnosing chronic infection. Diagnosis requires positivity with two different tests. If there is no exposure to vector-borne or blood-transmitted infection, seropositivity after the age of 9 months, by which age maternal antibodies would have disappeared, indicates congenital infection.

Treatment

The goals of treatment are to eradicate the parasite and to mitigate signs and symptoms of disease. Antitrypanosomal treatment is recommended for all cases of acute and congenital Chagas disease, reactivated infection, and for chronic *T. cruzi* infection in children younger than 18 years of age.[55] Drug therapy should be offered to adults 19 through 50 years of age without advanced Chagas heart disease. Drug therapy should not be given during pregnancy and to patients with severe renal or hepatic disease.

Two antimicrobial agents are available for treatment of Chagas disease, namely benznidazole and nifurtimox, neither of which is licensed for use in the U.S.[56–65] Treatment is prolonged (60 to 90 days). Therapeutic success is 60% to 85% in the acute stage of infection, >90% in congenital infection, and 60% (as measured by seroreversion) in early chronic disease in children. As the disease becomes chronic, therapeutic success decreases. Both drugs are well absorbed from the gastrointestinal tract, and are active against both trypomastigotes and amastigotes. They are both mutagenic, and should not be used during pregnancy. Before initiation of therapy, patients should have a blood count and serum chemistry performed and the blood count should be monitored every 2 to 3 weeks during therapy. The patient should be monitored for dermatologic side effects and peripheral neuropathy. Benznidazole must be compounded in a liquid form for children.[56] Congenital cases have been treated with nifurtimox.[55]

For assistance in diagnosis, management, and obtaining drugs for trypanosomiasis in the U.S., contact the CDC, Division of

Parasitic Diseases: normal hours: (770) 488-7775; for after-hours emergencies, contact the CDC Emergency Operations Center at (770) 488-7100.

Prevention

The main preventive method is spraying homes with pyrethroid insecticides that leave a residue, and by screening of blood for transfusion. There has been a concerted effort in southern South American countries to reduce the incidence of infection, by attacking the transmission by these two methods. In the U.S., blood donors are screened by an EIA and a radio-immunoprecipitation assay. For the future, better diagnostic tests and improved, safer drugs are needed.

Key Points. Comparison of African and American Trypanosomiases		
	AFRICAN TRYPANOSOMIASIS	**AMERICAN TRYPANOSOMIASIS**
Alternative name	African sleeping sickness	Chagas disease
Etiology	*Trypanosoma brucei*	*Trypanosoma cruzi*
Geography	*T. b. gambiense* – West Africa *T. b. rhodesiense*-East Africa	*T. cruzi* – Mexico, Central and South America
Vector	Tsetse fly (*Glossina* spp.)	Triatome ("kissing") bug
Infectious vector fluid	Saliva	Feces
Location in host	Extracellular	Intracellular (pseudocyst), extracellular
Target organs:		
Early	Systemic	Systemic
Late	Brain	Heart, esophagus, colon
Diagnosis	Visualization of parasite, serology, PCR	Visualization (early), serology, PCR
Outcome (untreated)	Fatal	Chronic heart or intestinal disease in 30% to 40%
	T. b. gambiense: months to years	
	T. b. rhodesiense: weeks to months	

276 Intestinal Nematodes

Michael Cappello and Peter J. Hotez

Intestinal nematode infections, sometimes referred to as soil-transmitted nematode (STN), soil-transmitted helminth (STH), or geohelminth infections, are among the most common parasitic infections in humans, affecting more than one-quarter of the world's population.[1] Studies have affirmed the negative health impact of intestinal nematodes, particularly *Ascaris lumbricoides*, *Trichuris trichiura*, and the hookworms *Necator americanus* and *Ancylostoma duodenale*, on child health and development. Intestinal nematode infection remains a major cause of physical growth delay, cognitive delay, and malnutrition throughout much of the developing world.[2–4] Chronic intestinal nematode infections during childhood adversely impact school performance and attendance, as well as future economic productivity.[5,6] Infection with these helminths also may impact susceptibility to or the clinical progression of other infectious diseases, including HIV-AIDS, tuberculosis, and malaria.[7–9] In most endemic populations, children are affected disproportionately by intestinal nematodes, often acquiring infections of high intensity relative to their adult counterparts living under similar conditions,[1,2] although the reasons for this difference are unknown. Furthermore, accurate interpretation of clinical studies of nematode infections is complicated by simultaneous infection with several different intestinal parasites in children.[1,10]

Intestinal nematode infections are encountered increasingly by pediatricians in the developed world.[11] In addition to travelers, children at particular risk include recent immigrants, refugees, and international adoptees.[12–14] Because *A. lumbricoides*, *Enterobius vermicularis*, and *Strongyloides stercoralis* are endemic to selected regions of the United States, including the American south and Appalachia, infection may be acquired in the absence of foreign exposure.[15]

Infection with intestinal nematodes generally occurs by one of two routes. For *A. lumbricoides*, *T. trichiura*, and *E. vermicularis*, infection results from ingestion of eggs, sometimes contained in food inadvertently contaminated with human feces. For *Strongyloides* (*S. stercoralis*, *Strongyloides fuelleborni*) and hookworms (*Ancylostoma duodenale*, *Ancylostoma ceylanicum*, *Ancylostoma caninum*, and *Necator americanus*), infective third-stage larvae, usually found in soil, penetrate host skin to begin the infective process. Infection with the larvae of *Ancylostoma* and *S. fuelleborni* also can be acquired orally. The clinical findings associated with intestinal nematode infections in children are summarized in Box 276-1. Recognized syndromes caused by perinatal infection with *A. lumbricoides*, *A. duodenale*, and *Strongyloides* are listed in Table 276-1.

The diagnosis of *Ascaris*, hookworm, and *Trichuris* infection is established most frequently by identification of characteristic eggs in feces (Figure 276-1). Pinworm eggs are found deposited on the perianal skin. In contrast, *Strongyloides* first-stage larvae, not eggs, are excreted routinely in feces. Serologic testing also can be useful in the diagnosis of strongyloidiasis, especially in lightly infected or asymptomatic people.

Benzimidazole anthelmintics remain the cornerstone of therapy for most intestinal nematode infections, including infections caused by *Ascaris*, hookworm, *Trichuris*, and pinworm.[16] Nitazoxanide is effective, with cure rates for most intestinal nematode infections that are comparable with albendazole.[17–19] Reductions in morbidity can be achieved even in the absence of complete eradication of parasites. This observation has catalyzed global efforts to reduce the morbidity from intestinal helminths through widespread use of these agents, which included a resolution passed at the 2001 World Health Assembly to deworm 75% of all

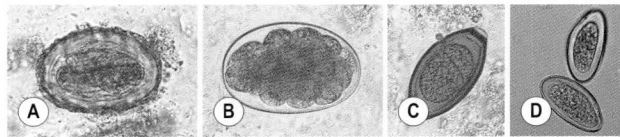

Figure 276-1. Photomicrographs showing the morphology of intestinal nematode eggs. *Ascaris lumbricoides* **(A),** hookworm **(B),** and *Trichuris trichiura* **(C)** infections routinely are diagnosed by fecal egg examination using light microscopy. *Enterobius vermicularis* **(D)** eggs are deposited on the perianal skin, and can be removed with adhesive tape and viewed under light microscopy. (From U.S. Centers for Disease Control http://dpd.cdc.gov/dpdx/HTML/Image_Library.htm)

BOX 276-1. Major Clinical Features of Intestinal Nematode Infections in Children

Ascaris lumbricoides

Löeffler pneumonia
Intestinal obstruction
Extraintestinal migration
Malabsorption
Eosinophilia

Trichuris trichiura

Chronic colitis
Dysentery
Intussusception
Rectal prolapse
Anemia

Ancylostoma duodenale and Necator americanus

Iron-deficiency anemia
Hypoproteinemia
Chlorosis
Eosinophilia
Developmental delays

Ancylostoma caninum

Eosinophilic enteritis
Aphthous ileitis

Ancylostoma ceylanicum

Enteritis
Eosinophilia

Strongyloides stercoralis

Eosinophilia
Epigastric pain
Autoinfection
Hyperinfection and disseminated disease

Enterobius vermicularis

Pruritus ani
Vaginitis
Extraintestinal migration

---

at-risk children by the year 2010.[20,21] Unfortunately, reinfection is common in children in endemic areas, thus necessitating repeated courses of therapy.[22] In addition, high treatment failure rates with mebendazole for human hookworm infection, decreasing efficacy with frequent and periodic use, and the possible emergence of drug resistance in human nematode infections raises important concerns about the widespread use of these agents.[21,23,24] However, in the absence of effective human vaccines, targeted chemotherapeutic interventions represent the best current option for control of the major health-related morbidity and mortality associated with intestinal nematode infections.[2]

TABLE 276-1. Neonatal Syndromes Caused by Intestinal Nematodes

Syndrome	Nematode Species	Speculated Routes of Transmission
Neonatal ascariasis	*Ascaris lumbricoides*	Transplacental
Infantile ancylostomiasis	*Ancylostoma duodenale*	Transmammary, perinatal
Infantile strongyloidiasis (swollen belly syndrome)	*Strongyloides fuelleborni* and *Strongyloides stercoralis*	Transmammary, perinatal

ASCARIS LUMBRICOIDES

Epidemiology

Ascariasis is the most common helminthic infection in humans, with more than 800 million people infected worldwide.[3] An estimated 51 million children suffer severe morbidity resulting from heavy infections with *A. lumbricoides*,[25] although the actual pediatric prevalence may be as high as 400 million. Ideally suited to warmer climates, *A. lumbricoides* eggs are resistant to a wide array of environmental stresses. For that reason, ascariasis frequently has both an urban and rural distribution and commonly affects children living in economically disadvantaged communities. Ascariasis still occurs in the U.S. as an imported infection, usually in recent immigrants from Latin America and Asia and in internationally adopted children.[13,14,26] Ascariasis also occurs as an autochthonous infection in the southeastern U.S., where the rate of infection in children ranges from 0.8% to 67%.[11,12,27]

Young children are affected more severely than adults, as evidenced by a larger worm burden and excessive vulnerability to parasite-induced malnutrition.[2] Chronic ascariasis in childhood is associated with impaired physical growth and intellectual development.[25,28,29] Young children also are more susceptible to life-threatening complications such as intestinal obstruction, perforation, and peritonitis. Globally, intestinal and biliary tract obstruction caused by *Ascaris* accounts for 10,000 to 100,000 deaths a year, mostly in children.[30,31] At one time in the U.S., children <6 years of age experienced intestinal obstruction caused by *A. lumbricoides* at a rate of 2 obstructions per 1000 infected children per year.[32] However, in the developing world, the rate of complications secondary to ascariasis ranges from 11% to 67%, with intestinal or biliary tract obstruction the most common serious sequela.[31] Transplacentally acquired neonatal ascariasis also has been described, and its global incidence may be underestimated.[33,34]

The life cycle of *A. lumbricoides* in humans begins with ingestion of embryonated eggs that have been deposited in moist soil. Bile salts and the alkaline pH of the small intestine cause the eggs to hatch, and emerging second-stage larvae penetrate the bowel wall, ultimately invading the microcirculation of the lamina propria. Once in the circulatory system, larvae are carried to the liver via the portal veins, and eventually are swept into the pulmonary vasculature where they lodge in capillaries and rupture into the alveolar space. After ascending the bronchi to the trachea, larvae are swallowed and again migrate to the small intestine. *Ascaris* larvae mature into sexually differentiated adults in the lumen of the small bowel, mate, and begin laying eggs. If egg laying precedes mating, infertile eggs are produced.

Clinical Manifestations

Illness associated with ascariasis can be attributed to the migration of both larvae and adult worms. As larvae migrate through the lung parenchyma, they cause both mechanical and immune-mediated damage. Pulmonary microhemorrhages from ruptured alveolar capillaries result in inflammation and exudation of fluid.

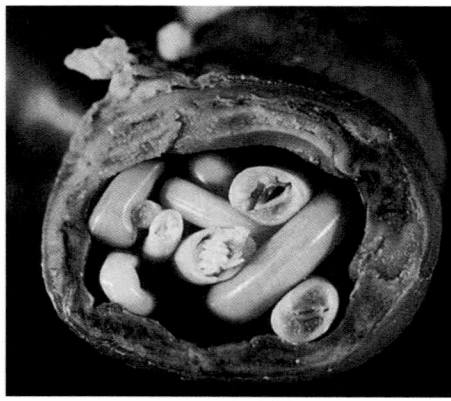

Figure 276-2. Surgical specimen showing adult *Ascaris lumbricoides* obstructing the small intestine. (From Meyers WM, Neafie RC, Marty AM, et al. Pathology of Infectious Diseases, Volume I (Helminthiases). Washington DC, American Registry of Pathology, 2000.)

Neutrophils and eosinophils are recruited to the lung, perhaps in response to secretory products released by the migrating larvae. Pulmonary infiltrates in association with cough, dyspnea, wheezing, and mild hemoptysis (Löeffler pneumonia) can occur and last up to 2 weeks. In some regions of the world this so-called "verminous pneumonia" is seasonal, occurring among cohorts of children following spring rains.[35] The intensity of illness caused by migrating larvae is proportional to their number, with lightly infected people often experiencing few, if any pulmonary symptoms. In rare instances, migrating adult worms can obstruct the airway and cause respiratory distress.[36]

Symptoms associated with the presence of adult *Ascaris* worms in the small bowel include epigastric pain and diffuse abdominal discomfort. Because adult worms can grow to 40 cm in length, heavy infestations can result in acute intestinal obstruction and perforation, especially in the region of the ileum, requiring emergency medical or surgical intervention (Figure 276-2). Migration of adult worms into the biliary tree and then to the liver or pancreas, sometimes elicited by ingestion of certain irritants, can precipitate acute cholecystitis, hepatitis, or pancreatitis. Hepatic abscess can occur if the intrahepatic ducts are obstructed.[31,37]

Chronic *Ascaris* infection has been associated with malnutrition, which is due partly to malabsorption of dietary protein, fat, and vitamin A. The pathogenesis of malabsorption probably is multifactorial.[25,28,38] It has been postulated that adult worms successfully compete for nutrients by secreting a variety of enzymes and protease inhibitors into the environment of the proximal part of the small intestine. Whether the physical and mental growth retardation syndromes associated with chronic ascariasis in childhood have a purely nutritional basis remains unknown. Furthermore, *Ascaris* infection frequently occurs in the setting of infection with other intestinal nematodes, especially *Trichuris* and hookworm, thus making it difficult to ascribe long-term sequelae to an individual parasitic species.

Laboratory Findings and Diagnosis

The diagnosis of *Ascaris* infection is best established by examination of stool for characteristic ova (Figure 276-1). Each adult female produces so many eggs that a single stool specimen usually is adequate. The presence of unfertilized eggs still mandates treatment because even a single adult worm represents a risk for serious illness associated with migration.

When migration of *Ascaris* larvae through the lungs is associated with peripheral blood eosinophilia and pulmonary infiltrates on a chest radiograph, examination of sputum can reveal eosinophils and Charcot–Leyden crystals. The differential diagnosis includes other causes of verminous pneumonia, including strongyloidiasis, toxocariasis (visceral larva migrans), and hookworm infection.

In areas endemic for *A. lumbricoides*, any child manifesting acute abdominal symptoms consistent with intestinal obstruction or perforation should be evaluated for ascariasis. Occasionally, an adult worm is present in vomitus. Abdominal radiographs after barium administration may reveal the nature of the intestinal obstruction caused by *A. lumbricoides*, whereas computed tomography with oral contrast may demonstrate cylindric filling defects.[39] Endoscopic retrograde cholangiopancreatography and ultrasonography can be helpful in identifying adult *Ascaris* worms in the intestinal tract or hepatobiliary tree.[40–43] Occasionally, however, the diagnosis of intestinal ascariasis is made at laparotomy.

Treatment

Benzimidazoles such as mebendazole (100 mg twice a day for 3 days or 500 mg once) and albendazole (400 mg in a single dose) are effective for treatment of intestinal ascariasis, with cure rates of greater than 90%.[2,44] Because of their teratogenic and tumorigenic potential, benzimidazoles generally are not given to children <2 years of age. However, wide experience with the use of these agents in children suggests that at a reduced dose (200 mg), administration of albendazole to children 12 to 24 months of age, or even children <12 months of age is not problematic. For this reason, benzimidazoles increasingly are being distributed in low- and middle-income countries with heavy disease burdens.[45–47] Nitazoxanide is comparable with albendazole for treatment of *Ascaris* infections, and is approved for use in children ≥12 months of age.[17,18,48,49] The recommended dose is 100 mg (5 mL) twice a day for children 12 through 47 months of age, 200 mg (10 mL) twice a day for children 4 through 11 years of age, and 500 mg twice a day for older children and adults, to complete a 3-day course. Pyrantel pamoate (11 mg/kg up to maximum 1 g per day for 3 days) is a suitable alternative.[7] In some heavily infected children, malnutrition, steatorrhea, and growth retardation are reversible with treatment; these children appear to demonstrate less dramatic catch-up growth after chemotherapy.[50]

In cases of partial small bowel obstruction caused by *Ascaris*, some physicians recommend alternative therapy with piperazine citrate, which paralyzes the worms and may abrogate the need for surgical intervention. However, this drug is no longer available in the U.S. It is important to note that piperazine and pyrantel pamoate are antagonistic and should not be given concurrently. Mineral oil or Gastrografin given orally or by nasogastric tube also can cause relaxation of the obstructing bolus of worms.

Standard supportive measures for treatment of small bowel obstruction also should be administered, including intravenous hydration, nasogastric suctioning, and monitoring of electrolyte status. Laparotomy to remove the adult worm bolus should be undertaken in people who do not respond to therapy with anthelmintic drugs.

Prevention

Prevention of ascariasis requires elimination of contact with soil contaminated by egg-containing feces. In tropical climates, poor sanitation is responsible for infection rates that approach 100% in endemic areas. Although *Ascaris* eggs are killed by prolonged exposure to sunlight or temperatures >40°C, they can survive extremely cold temperatures for many months and are resistant to many chemical disinfectants. *Ascaris* eggs survive in temperate climates and urban environments.

Diagnosis and effective treatment with improved sanitation practices are the most reliable means of preventing the spread of *Ascaris*. In endemic areas, where the prevalence of infection with *A. lumbricoides* is >50%, anthelmintic agents are recommended to be administered to school-aged children as part of a targeted deworming program,[38] or as a part of integrated preventive chemotherapy of ascariasis together with other soil-transmitted helminth infections, e.g., schistosomiasis, lymphatic filariasis, onchocerciasis, and trachoma.[47,51] However, the effects of a single intervention are likely to be short-term because of the inevitability of reinfection. Because ascariasis is an infection that is associated with poverty and malnutrition, sustained economic growth is the most effective means of long-term parasite control.

HOOKWORM (ANCYLOSTOMA DUODENALE, ANCYLOSTOMA CANINUM, ANCYLOSTOMA CEYLANICUM, AND NECATOR AMERICANUS)

Epidemiology

Approximately 600 million people harbor hookworms in their gastrointestinal tracts,[3] and hookworm infection remains a leading cause of iron deficiency, iron-deficiency anemia, and protein malnutrition in the developing world.[52] Children and women of reproductive age (especially pregnant women) are particularly vulnerable to the morbid effects of hookworm infection, often because dietary intake fails to compensate for intestinal losses of iron and serum proteins.[53] Although once highly endemic in the southeastern U.S., hookworm infection was essentially eradicated in the U.S. by the 1920s, in part because of the efforts of the Rockefeller Sanitary Commission.[54] Pockets of autochthonous hookworm infection still may be present in parts of the rural south, although hookworm is no longer a public health problem in the U.S.[15]

The two most common species of hookworm that infect humans are *A. duodenale* and *N. americanus*, with estimates from the 1940s suggesting that *N. americanus* is responsible for more than 80% of human infections worldwide.[55] *N. americanus* is significantly more common in the western hemisphere, Southeast Asia and Africa, although *A. duodenale* and mixed infections occur commonly. Other species that cause intestinal disease in humans include *A. ceylanicum* (Southeast Asia and India)[56] and *A. caninum* (the dog hookworm), which has been implicated as a zoonotic cause of eosinophilic enteritis in Australia and the U.S.[57,58]

The external life cycle of the hookworm begins when eggs are deposited in moist soil. Eggs develop optimally at ambient temperatures of 20°C to 30°C in the absence of direct sunlight. These conditions generally are achieved in association with cultivation of certain crops, such as mulberry leaves and sweet potatoes in China, tea in India, and coffee in Latin America. Thus, unlike ascariasis and trichuriasis, which can occur in urban slums, hookworm infection occurs primarily in rural areas. On hatching, the emerging larvae molt twice to nonfeeding, infective third-stage larvae, which can migrate vertically in the soil in response to changing conditions of moisture. Infection occurs by one of two routes, depending on the species of hookworm. Whereas both *Ancylostoma* and *Necator* can penetrate the skin, *Ancylostoma* larvae also are infective orally, and in some areas the oral route of infection predominates. Once in the host, third-stage larvae resume

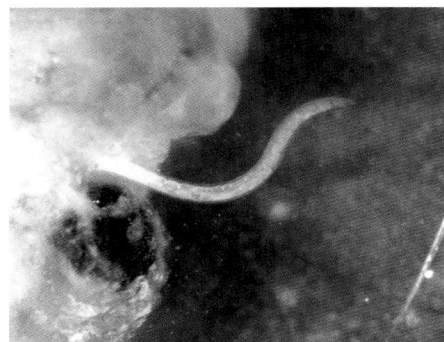

Figure 276-4. Photograph of an adult hookworm attached to the intestine of an experimentally infected animal. Note area of hemorrhage adjacent to site of attachment. (Courtesy of R. Bungiro.)

development while migrating via lymphatics and venules to the pulmonary circulation. After traversing the alveolar capillaries into the alveoli, larvae ascend the airways, are swallowed, and travel to the small intestine. Epidemiologic evidence indicates that some hookworm larvae of *A. duodenale* undergo developmental arrest within the host, where they await environmental or hormonal cues before resuming migration to the gut. This phenomenon may explain seasonal variations in fecal egg concentrations, as well as possible transmammary hookworm infection in newborn infants.[59,60]

Once in the small bowel, adults attach by their mouths to the intestinal mucosa and begin to feed (Figure 276-3). Equipped with teeth, cutting plates, or both, as well as powerful esophageal muscles and hydrolytic enzymes,[61,62] the hookworm digests the plug of tissue within its buccal capsule. At the same time, potent anticoagulants and inhibitors of platelet function are released and cause profound bleeding from lacerated capillaries in the lamina propria (Figure 276-4).[63-65] The ingested blood is acted upon by hemoglobin-digesting proteases lining the parasite gut.[66,67] Adult worms mate in the small intestine, and the females deposit fertilized eggs in the lumen. Approximately 5 to 9 weeks are required after acquisition for eggs to appear in the feces or longer in the case of developmentally arrested larvae.

Clinical Manifestations

Skin penetration by third-stage larvae can be associated with an intensely pruritic dermatitis called *ground itch*, which usually is localized to the site of hookworm entry.[68] Ground itch is followed within a week by cough, which occurs when hookworm larvae enter the lungs. Hookworm pneumonitis usually is less severe than the verminous pneumonitis resulting from ascariasis (Löeffler pneumonia), although it can last for several weeks. Wakana disease, a severe immediate hypersensitivity-like syndrome characterized by nausea, vomiting, dyspnea, and eosinophilia, can occur after oral ingestion of a large number of infective *A. duodenale* larvae.[69]

The presence of adult hookworms in the small intestine can cause nonspecific gastrointestinal tract symptoms including abdominal pain, even before onset of anemia. Blood loss secondary to hookworm infection generally is proportional to the worm burden and develops approximately 10 to 20 weeks after infection. *A. duodenale* infection usually is associated with greater blood loss than occurs with *N. americanus*.[70] Hookworm disease and anemia results when blood loss exceeds the host's iron reserves and dietary intake. Long-standing moderate or heavy hookworm infection causes serious iron-deficiency anemia associated with pallor, chlorosis (a greenish yellow skin discoloration), dyspnea on exertion, and fatigue. Occasionally, severe hookworm anemia can lead to congestive heart failure.

Children in the developing world are particularly vulnerable to the effects of hookworm anemia because of increased iron requirements and underlying nutritional deficiencies.[71] Growth and

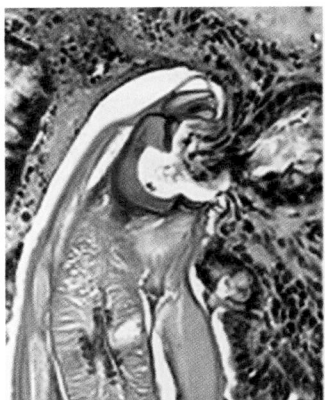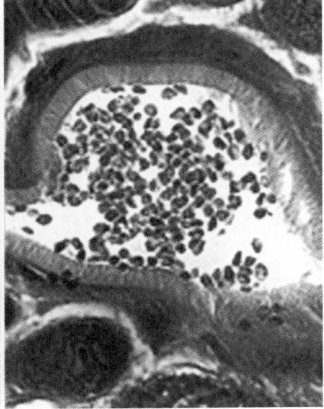

Figure 276-3. Left panel: Photomicrograph showing a sagittal section of an adult *Ancylostoma* hookworm attached to the intestinal mucosa. Right panel: Cross-section of an adult worm showing ingested host red blood cells within the parasite's intestine. (Courtesy of R. Bungiro.)

developmental delay, as well as learning disabilities, are common in chronically infected children.[72] Many of these effects can be attributed to iron deficiency, but hookworm-associated plasma protein loss and malabsorption also contribute to the clinical manifestations.[73,74] At least some of the malabsorption associated with hookworm infection may be due to the secretion of a potent inhibitor of digestive enzymes secreted by the adult parasite.[75,76] Hookworm disease also is an important problem in pregnant women in the developing world, and can result in severe maternal anemia as well as low birthweight and reduced infant survival.[52,77]

A fulminant form of gastrointestinal tract hemorrhage related to acute hookworm infection has been described in newborn infants. These children, often younger than 2 months of age, have melena, abdominal distention, and hypotension, with hematocrit values as low as 2% to 3%.[60,78] Seen primarily in children infected with hookworms of the genus *Ancylostoma*, it is speculated that larvae can be transmitted through the milk of chronically infected mothers. A similar route of vertical transmission has been shown to occur in Papua New Guinean infants infected with *S. fuelleborni*.

Infection of humans with the dog hookworm *A. caninum* has been implicated as a cause of eosinophilic enteritis, particularly in northeastern Australia.[57,58] This condition, characterized by intense abdominal pain and peripheral blood eosinophilia, can mimic appendicitis or intestinal perforation. Laparotomy often reveals only a single adult canine hookworm attached to the intestinal mucosa. In addition, asymptomatic aphthous ileitis with eosinophilia has been reported in association with zoonotic infection with *A. caninum*.[79]

Laboratory Findings and Diagnosis

Acute infection, characterized by symptoms associated with migration of infective hookworm larvae, is diagnosed on the basis of clinical findings. The characteristic rash of ground itch occurs on any skin surface and can be erythematous, papular, or vesicular.[68] Intense pruritus can lead to scratching, excoriation, and secondary bacterial infection. In contrast to *Ascaris*, the pulmonary symptoms of hookworm pneumonia usually are not severe.

Eosinophilia, which generally is mild, coincides with development of adult hookworms in the intestine.[80] Intestinal hookworm infection is detected by identifying the characteristic eggs in feces (Figure 276-1). Because most symptomatic people excrete large numbers of eggs, stool-concentrating techniques usually are not necessary to detect clinically relevant infections. Although hookworm secretory antigens can be detected in feces of infected laboratory animals,[81] fecal antigen tests are not available for diagnosing human infections. The eggs of *Ancylostoma* and *N. americanus* are similar under light microscopy and cannot be distinguished easily on the basis of morphology.

Treatment

Single doses of mebendazole are inadequate for treatment of human hookworm infection,[21] although higher cure rates have been reported after multiple doses of mebendazole (100 mg twice a day for 3 days) or albendazole (400 mg once). The safety of benzimidazoles in children has not been established definitively, although these compounds are the drugs of choice for children with intestinal helminth infections. Nitazoxanide may be effective in treatment of hookworm infections, although comparative data with albendazole are lacking. The recommended dose is 100 mg (5 mL) twice a day for children 12 through 47 months of age, 200 mg (10 mL) twice a day for children 4 through 11 years of age, and 500 mg twice a day for older children and adults, to complete a 3-day course. An alternative treatment is pyrantel pamoate (11 mg/kg/day, not to exceed 1 g/day, for 3 days), which has been reported to be effective in treatment of infantile ancylostomiasis. Unfortunately, reports suggest the possibility of emerging anthelmintic drug resistance among human hookworm isolates, based either on drug failure, or the observation of diminishing efficacy with increasing use.[23,24]

Mebendazole is absorbed poorly and thus may not eradicate developmentally arrested *Ancylostoma* larvae residing in extraintestinal tissues. Therefore, periodic follow-up stool examinations may be necessary to detect latent infection. Moreover, reinfection in endemic areas occurs so commonly that the effect of a single course of an anthelmintic drug is of questionable benefit. Iron supplementation reverses mild to moderate hookworm anemia and can lead to improvement in growth and intellectual development.[43] Severe and acute gastrointestinal tract hemorrhage caused by hookworm rarely can lead to hemodynamic compromise necessitating blood transfusion.

Prevention

At least short-term benefit in iron status has been demonstrated in heavily infected children treated with albendazole or mebendazole.[2,82,83] However, no evidence of naturally acquired resistance to hookworm infection has been reported, and children in endemic areas constantly are exposed to infective third-stage larvae. In addition, arrested larvae within the host may be resistant to currently available anthelmintic agents. For these two reasons, mass or targeted chemotherapy programs alone may not control hookworm infection in many parts of the developing world. As a result, renewed interest has been shown in development of vaccines.[84] To date, the most promising vaccine candidates are recombinant forms of two enzymes involved in parasite blood feeding, with a series of clinical trials planned in coming years.[85-88]

TRICHURIS TRICHIURA

Epidemiology

Approximately 600 million people worldwide are infected with the whipworm *T. trichiura*, which is distributed throughout the tropics and subtropics.[1,89] Named for its characteristic shape (Figure 276-5), the adult stage of *T. trichiura* is an important cause of inflammatory bowel disease in children from the developing world. Children with trichuriasis usually have greater numbers of whipworms than their adult counterparts and suffer disproportionately from clinical trichuriasis.

Fertilized *Trichuris* eggs require 3 to 4 weeks in a warm, moist environment to embryonate and become infectious. After ingestion, second-stage larvae hatch and penetrate mucosal epithelial cells of the cecum or colon. The worm expands intracellularly, ultimately creating tunnels within the epithelium to accommodate growth (Figure 276-6). The thickened posterior portion of the worm eventually ruptures the cell membrane and protrudes into the lumen of the large intestine. In this manner, *Trichuris* can disrupt the normal colonic architecture. However, a large component of the pathogenesis of trichuriasis results from the host inflammatory response mediated by cytokines produced by T lymphocytes[90] and macrophages.[91]

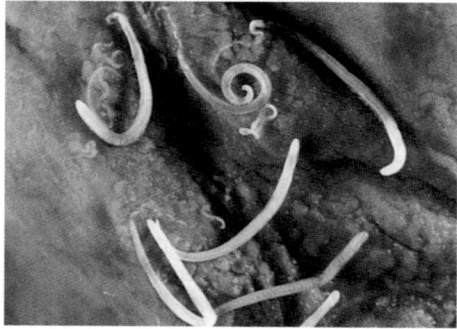

Figure 276-5. Photograph of adult *Trichuris trichiura* attached to the colonic mucosa. (From Meyers WM, Neafie RC, Marty AM, et al. Pathology of Infectious Diseases, Volume I (Helminthiases). Washington DC, American Registry of Pathology, 2000.)

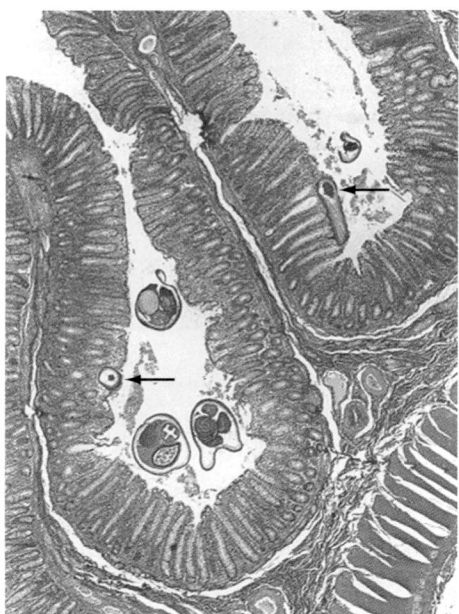

Figure 276-6. Photomicrograph of an intestinal biopsy specimen showing sections of *T. trichiura* in the colon. Note anterior portion of adult worm within the mucosa (arrows) and thicker posterior portion in the lumen. (From Meyers WM, Neafie RC, Marty AM, et al. Pathology of Infectious Diseases, Volume I (Helminthiases). Washington DC, American Registry of Pathology, 2000.)

Adult whipworms mate and females lay eggs in the colon, with approximately 5000 eggs deposited per day. About 90 days is required to complete the life cycle in humans from ingestion of eggs to development of mature egg-laying adults.

Clinical Manifestations

Although most whipworm infections are asymptomatic, two well-defined clinical entities are associated with heavy infection. The first, *Trichuris* dysentery, is an acute diarrheal disease associated with the passage of blood and mucus in stool.[89] Bleeding probably is due to the mucosal damage and inflammation caused by the attachment of adult worms to the colonic epithelium. No evidence shows that *T. trichiura* feeds on blood. The profound mucosal edema associated with *Trichuris* dysentery leads to tenesmus and, in protracted cases, can cause rectal prolapse or even colonic obstruction.[92]

Whipworm infection also can result in a chronic colitis that shares many clinical features with other inflammatory bowel diseases such as Crohn disease and ulcerative colitis. In particular, the factors that mediate delay of growth appear to be similar to those found in children with other causes of inflammatory bowel disease.[93] In heavy infections, worms also can spread proximally and cause ileitis. In some cases trichuriasis works in synergy with infection caused by *Campylobacter jejuni* to produce more severe disease.[94]

Diagnosis

Unlike *Ascaris* and hookworm, *Trichuris* commonly is associated with diarrhea. *Trichuris* dysentery can resemble dysentery caused by other pathogens, including enteric bacteria and *Entamoeba histolytica*. Examination of stool for characteristic *T. trichiura* eggs (Figure 276-1) is the most reliable means of diagnosis. Stool concentration techniques usually are not necessary to detect most symptomatic cases. If stool examination reveals the presence of Charcot–Leyden crystals, *Trichuris* infection is likely.

Important histologic findings distinguish *Trichuris* colitis from other types of inflammatory bowel disease. First, the pathologic changes in the colon resulting from whipworm infection are confined primarily to mucosal epithelium, with little involvement of the submucosa and muscularis layers. In addition, the dramatic symptomatology of *Trichuris* colitis characteristically is out of proportion to the modest inflammatory response seen histologically.

Laboratory tests rarely are helpful in making the diagnosis of trichuriasis. Iron deficiency is a common finding and can be acute (caused by gastrointestinal hemorrhage) or chronic, as occurs in long-standing cases of colitis. The erythrocyte sedimentation rate, which often is elevated in inflammatory bowel diseases, usually is normal in children with whipworm infection.[89]

Treatment

Trichuriasis is considered less responsive to anthelmintic therapy than are other intestinal nematode infections.[21] Albendazole and mebendazole are recommended routinely for the treatment.[44] A 3-day regimen with either may be necessary in heavy infections. A single-dose regimen of mebendazole (500 mg) has been shown to be more effective than single-dose albendazole (400 mg) in reducing fecal egg excretion in children with moderate *Trichuris* infection.[95] Nitazoxanide is effective for the treatment of *Trichuris* infections, and is approved for use in children ≥12 months of age.[18,19,49,96] The recommended dose is 100 mg (5 mL) twice a day for children 12 through 47 months of age, 200 mg (10 mL) twice a day for children 4 through 11 years of age, and 500 mg twice a day for older children and adults, to complete a 3-day course. An alternative regimen for the treatment of trichuriasis is a combination of albendazole (400 mg) and ivermectin (200 µg/kg), both given in a single dose orally.[47] A study of 155 children in Sri Lanka showed a cure rate of 79% after combination therapy, thus making the combination almost twice as effective as albendazole alone.[97] Although the benzimidazoles generally are considered safe in children, one recent study in asymptomatic children with trichuriasis opened the possibility that they could be associated with growth delay.[98] Other studies, however, have not supported this observation. Oxantel is an alternative drug for trichuriasis and frequently is formulated in a liquid suspension with pyrantel pamoate, which is suitable for young children. This preparation generally is not available in the U.S. Retreatment with anthelmintics may be necessary, especially in children who remain in endemic areas. Iron supplementation may help resolve the anemia of trichuriasis, as well as speed the rate of catch-up growth. Although treatment speeds physical "catch-up" growth dramatically, recovery of cognitive skills may be much less pronounced in heavily infected children.[99]

Prevention

Sanitary measures necessary to reduce the spread of other geohelminthic infections also have an impact on trichuriasis. However, some anthelmintic agents used in chemotherapy control programs may have less activity (especially in a single dose) against *Trichuris* than against other intestinal nematodes. In addition, raw fruits and vegetables grown in endemic areas where irrigation water is contaminated can harbor and transmit infective eggs.

ENTEROBIUS VERMICULARIS

Epidemiology

Along with toxocariasis, infection with the human pinworm *E. vermicularis* may be the most common helminthiasis in the U.S. and other developed countries.[15] Most infections occur in children, with high rates of transmission documented in group childcare facilities, nursery schools, and elementary schools.[12,100] Although enterobiasis is seldom if ever a cause of serious morbidity in children, it often is distressing for parents and guardians. Reassurance by healthcare providers is an important component in management of pinworm infection.

Infection with *E. vermicularis* occurs after ingestion of embryonated eggs that have been deposited by the adult female worm. Eggs frequently are identified on the perianal skin, thus implicating fecal–oral contamination as the most common route of infection in young children. However, infection by airborne eggs or contaminated fomites also has been described, as well as retroinfection, in which eggs deposited on the perianal skin hatch and give rise to motile larvae that migrate back into the rectum and develop into adults.

After ingestion, pinworm eggs hatch intraluminally, and the emerging larvae descend the small intestine and develop into mature adults on reaching the cecum. Adult female worms live primarily in the colon and migrate out onto the perianal skin, where they lay eggs. Worm migration frequently occurs at night. A female adult pinworm releases up to 10,000 fertilized eggs every 24 hours that embryonate and become infective within 6 hours. Although most eggs remain at the site of deposition, some can be dispersed into the air and contaminate environmental surfaces, or scratching can lead to transmission from contaminated fingers. Eggs can survive several days under conditions of high temperature and humidity. The complete life cycle of *E. vermicularis* can be completed in 4 to 6 weeks.

Clinical Manifestations

The most common symptom of people infected with pinworms is localized pruritus, probably caused by an allergic response elicited against the migrating adult pinworm as it lays its eggs on the perianal skin. Intense itching can result in scratching and excoriation of the area, occasionally leading to secondary bacterial cellulitis. In young girls and women, migrating pinworms can enter the vagina and cause a mild vaginitis or even enter the urethra and introduce bacteria that can lead to lower urinary tract infection. In one study, young girls with urinary tract infection were almost twice as likely to have pinworm (36% versus 16%) as those with no previous history of such infection.[101] Rarely, other sites of aberrant pinworm migration have been described, including the fallopian tubes,[102] ovaries,[103] and peritoneum.[104] Pinworms also have been associated with perianal cellulitis and granuloma or abscess formation.[105,106] It is controversial whether pinworm migration into the appendix is a common cause of acute appendicitis (Figure 276-7), but the incidence of pinworm-associated disease appears to be low even in highly endemic areas.[100,107,108]

The host-mediated inflammatory response to the intestinal stages of *E. vermicularis* is minimal, although eosinophilic ileocolitis has been reported.[109] However, the lack of prominent gastrointestinal tract complaints in the setting of this infection suggests that significant intestinal pathology is rare.

Laboratory Findings and Diagnosis

The most reliable means of diagnosing pinworm infection is examination of transparent adhesive tape that has been applied to the perianal skin. After removing the tape, it is placed on a

microscope slide and viewed for the presence of eggs (Figure 276-1). This procedure is best performed on arising in the morning, before bathing, and may have to be repeated on subsequent days to detect infection. *E. vermicularis* eggs are not excreted in the stool, so examination of feces is not helpful.

Serologic tests are not available to detect pinworm infection. Eosinophilia, which has been reported occasionally, is an unusual finding and therefore is not useful in the diagnosis. Adult pinworms, which are sometimes found in tissue specimens, are identified readily by the presence of bilateral cuticular ridges known as alae, which distinguish *E. vermicularis* from other intestinal nematodes of humans.

Treatment

Single-dose therapy with either mebendazole (100 mg), pyrantel pamoate (11 mg/kg, not to exceed 1 g), or albendazole (400 mg) is adequate treatment for pinworm infection.[44] Because none of these drugs is completely effective against eggs or developing larvae, a second treatment 2 weeks after the first is recommended. To date, resistance of *Enterobius* to benzimidazoles has not been reported.

Prevention

Because pinworm eggs can survive for days outside the host, all clothes and bed linens should be washed at the time of treatment. All family members should be treated as a group in situations in which multiple or repeated symptomatic infections occur. Within one institutional setting, a substantial reduction in the prevalence of pinworm was achieved through targeted chemotherapy of infected people and all potential contacts.[110] In this study, treating all infected people and their contacts with two doses of mebendazole 14 days apart reduced the prevalence of *E. vermicularis* infection from 24% to 1% over a 3-year period.

STRONGYLOIDES STERCORALIS AND *STRONGYLOIDES FUELLEBORNI*

Epidemiology

S. stercoralis can be found throughout both tropical and temperate climates, including parts of the U.S., particularly eastern Tennessee, Kentucky, and West Virginia.[15,111–114] The prevalence of strongyloidiasis probably is underestimated because of the relative difficulty in detecting subclinical infection. However, groups known to be at particularly high risk of harboring *Strongyloides* include veterans of World War II and Vietnam,[111] refugees from Southeast Asia,[115] and other immigrants to the U.S.[14] Epidemiologic studies have demonstrated an increased prevalence of strongyloidiasis in people who also are seropositive for human T-lymphocyte lymphotropic virus (HTLV) type I.[116–118] Dogs and other mammals also can harbor *S. stercoralis* and may serve as reservoir hosts inasmuch as zoonotic infections in animal handlers have occurred. A distinct and fulminant form of neonatal strongyloidiasis caused by *S. fuelleborni*, called *swollen belly syndrome*, has been described in neonates from Papua New Guinea.[119]

The life cycle of *Strongyloides* is complex and consists of both a parasitic (homogonic) cycle and a free-living (heterogonic) cycle. Human parasitism occurs initially when soil-borne third-stage filariform larvae penetrate the skin. Some, if not most of the infective larvae migrate via lymphatics and venules to the pulmonary circulation, penetrate the alveolar space, and migrate up the pulmonary tree, where they are swallowed and make their way to the small intestine. All parasitic adults found in the small bowel probably are female, and therefore reproduction within the host is likely to occur by parthenogenesis. Eggs deposited into the intestinal lumen release first-stage rhabditiform larvae (Figure 276-8) that are passed in the feces.

Under certain conditions, larvae do not exit the host in feces but instead molt intraluminally to the filariform stage during

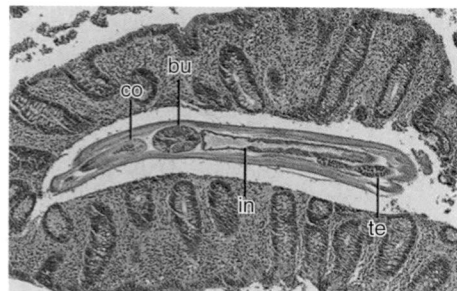

Figure 276-7. Photomicrograph of an intestinal biopsy specimen showing the anterior region of an adult pinworm (*Enterobius vermicularis*) lodged in the lumen of the appendix. Note the parasite's corpus (co), esophageal bulb (bu), intestine (in), and testis (te) visible by H & E stain. (From Meyers WM, Neafie RC, Marty AM, et al. Pathology of Infectious Diseases, Volume I (Helminthiases). Washington DC, American Registry of Pathology, 2000.)

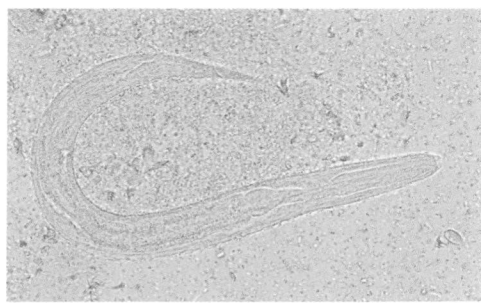

Figure 276-8. Photomicrograph of a *Strongyloides stercoralis* first stage (rhabditiform) larva excreted in feces. Unlike most intestinal nematodes, *S. stercoralis* eggs typically are not detected in fecal samples. (From U.S. Centers for Disease Control http://dpd.cdc.gov/dpdx/HTML/Image_Library.htm)

transit in the gut. These third-stage larvae can penetrate the intestinal mucosa or possibly the perianal skin and begin the infective cycle anew. This phenomenon, called *internal autoinfection*, allows *Strongyloides* to be maintained within the host for years after the initial infection. An important point is that the autoinfective cycle can be accelerated in an immunocompromised host and result in an often fatal condition known as *hyperinfection*.[118]

When first-stage larvae are deposited with feces, they develop in the soil to male or female adults, which mate and lay eggs. Eggs hatch, and larvae either can continue this free-living cycle for one or more generations or develop into parasitic filariform larvae and infect a suitable host.

Clinical Manifestations

Acute infection with *Strongyloides* larvae can elicit a cutaneous eruption at the site of skin penetration. This serpiginous urticarial rash, known as *larva currens* (racing larva), is thought to represent an allergic response to migrating filariform larvae.[120–122] In chronic infections, such an eruption can be caused by autoinfective larvae penetrating the perianal skin or buttocks.

In immunocompetent patients, strongyloidiasis is an important cause of irritable-bowel-like syndrome with intermittent abdominal cramping, and diarrhea alternating with constipation.[123] In children, strongyloidiasis is associated with chronic diarrhea, fever, cachexia, and failure to thrive.[112,124] Malabsorption of both fat and protein can lead to a celiac-like syndrome characterized by steatorrhea, hypoalbuminemia, and peripheral edema. Deficiencies of vitamin B_{12} and folate also are common in heavy infections.

A syndrome of infantile strongyloidiasis caused by *S. fuelleborni* has been described in Papua New Guinea.[119,125] Beginning in the first months of life, infected children often have diarrhea that becomes protracted, develop failure to thrive, protein malnutrition, and a kwashiorkor-like appearance attributable to hypoalbuminemia. Similar syndromes of infantile strongyloidiasis have been reported from parts of Africa. *Strongyloides* larvae have been detected in the milk of mothers with chronic infection, thus suggesting vertical transmission as a possible mode of neonatal disease.[126] Whether *S. stercoralis* also can be transmitted via human milk is not known, although this species has likewise been isolated from very young children.

The most serious complications of strongyloidiasis, hyperinfection and disseminated disease, occur during amplification of the autoinfective life cycle. A number of well-defined risk factors for the development of hyperinfection syndrome have been recognized.[123] Most commonly, severe disease develops in patients who are chronically infected with *S. stercoralis* after the initiation of immunosuppressive agents for a variety of underlying conditions. Severe strongyloidiasis has been reported most commonly in patients being treated for hematologic malignancies or after solid-organ transplantation.[127] Most of these patients were receiving corticosteroids as part of their antineoplastic or immunosuppressive regimens, which raises the possibility that glucocorticoid therapy, even in the absence of malignancy, may be the primary risk factor for hyperinfection syndrome.[128,129] *Strongyloides* hyperinfection also can occur in patients with generalized inanition and malnutrition, as well as in patients infected with HTLV-1.[117,118] In children with *Strongyloides* hyperinfection, the massive numbers of larvae migrating through the lungs can cause pulmonary infiltrates, dyspnea, and even respiratory collapse. These larvae often migrate aberrantly to distant organs, including the skin, brain, liver, heart, skeletal muscle, and lymph nodes, where they can elicit a vigorous immune response. Disseminated strongyloidiasis can be complicated by pyogenic abscess or meningitis caused by enteric bacteria transported from the colon by migrating worms.[130,131] Eosinophilia, found routinely in people with chronic strongyloidiasis, usually is absent in hyperinfection and disseminated disease. Untreated, *Strongyloides* hyperinfection has high mortality.

Laboratory Findings and Diagnosis

Definitive diagnosis of *Strongyloides* infection relies on identification of first-stage rhabditiform larvae in the feces of an infected person (see Figure 276-8). However, because female *S. stercoralis* nematodes release as few as 50 eggs a day, multiple stool specimens concentrated with the use of various techniques may be required to detect light or chronic infections. As a result, in most cases of uncomplicated strongyloidiasis a single fecal examination misses up to 70% of the cases.[132] Several techniques have been developed to increase the sensitivity of larval detection in the stools including an agar culture method.[132–134] Alternatively, the number of larvae recovered from feces can be amplified by allowing them to undergo the heterogonic life cycle in Baermann cultures.[129] In hyperinfective and disseminated strongyloidiasis, larvae can be recovered from extraintestinal sites, including sputum, bronchoalveolar lavage fluid, and in some cases, cerebrospinal fluid (Figure 276-9).[130]

Peripheral blood eosinophilia often is the only laboratory abnormality in chronic strongyloidiasis and probably represents an immune response to larvae migrating through host tissues. Eosinophilia frequently is absent in people experiencing hyperinfection. Serologic assays have been designed to detect subclinical *S. stercoralis* infection.[135] These assays can aid in diagnosis in people from endemic areas with unexplained eosinophilia.

Treatment

Because of the risk of hyperinfection, all people found to harbor *Strongyloides* should be treated, even in the absence of symptoms. The agent of choice is orally administered ivermectin (200 μg/kg/day for 2 days).[123] Cure rates are up to 97%.[136–140] Ivermectin has not been studied extensively in children. As an alternative drug, thiabendazole is administered at a dose of 25 mg/kg twice a day

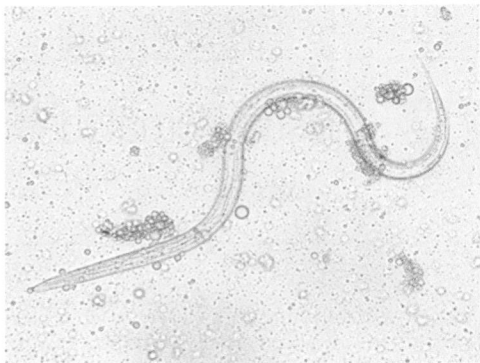

Figure 276-9. Photomicrograph of a *S. stercoralis* third stage (filariform) larvae. (From U.S. Centers for Disease Control http://dpd.cdc.gov/dpdx/HTML/Image_Library.htm)

(maximum, 3 g/day) for 2 days. Cure rates >80% have been reported, even in immunocompromised people with intestinal disease.[141] Unlike mebendazole, thiabendazole is well absorbed and has been associated with various side effects, including dizziness, nausea, and anorexia. Albendazole also has been used for treatment of strongyloidiasis, as have combinations of ivermectin together with albendazole.

The mortality rate from disseminated strongyloidiasis approaches 60%, even with aggressive treatment and supportive care. Therapy with ivermectin or ivermectin with albendazole should be continued for at least 7 days, preferably until the parasite can no longer be identified in clinical specimens. In some cases prolonged or repeated therapies with ivermectin may be required, and veterinary parenteral or enema formulations have been used in severely ill patients.[142] Concomitant bacterial infections should be treated aggressively with appropriate antibiotics,

and exogenous corticosteroid and other immunosuppressive therapy should be tapered quickly. Documenting cure may be difficult because the production of eggs usually is low before treatment. Monitoring the serologic response to treatment, as well as peripheral blood eosinophil counts, may be useful.[143]

Prevention

As with other helminths transmitted in soil, proper sanitation practices can help reduce the spread of *Strongyloides* infection in endemic areas. Prompt diagnosis and treatment of mild or asymptomatic infections should reduce the incidence of disseminated disease. People with unexplained eosinophilia, especially if they have lived in endemic areas, should be evaluated for strongyloidiasis before treatment with immunosuppressive therapy, especially glucocorticoids.

Key Points. Diagnosis and Management of Intestinal Nematode Infections

MICROBIOLOGY

- Intestinal nematodes (roundworms) are multicellular parasites with complex life cycles
- Infection is acquired by ingesting eggs or through skin contact by larvae
- Adult worms reside in the small intestine (*Ascaris,* hookworm, *Strongyloides*) or large bowel (*Trichuris, Enterobius*)

EPIDEMIOLOGY

- More than 2 billion people living in tropical and subtropical regions are infected with ≥1 intestinal nematode
- In the developed world, groups at significant risk for infection include immigrants, refugees, and children adopted from endemic regions
- Most infections acquired in the U.S. are caused by *Strongyloides stercoralis* or *Ascaris lumbricoides,* which are endemic in the southeast, or *Enterobius vermicularis* (pinworm), which is widespread and occurs in daycare and preschool settings

DIAGNOSIS

- Fecal microscopy is the diagnostic test of choice for most intestinal nematodes. In the case of *Strongyloides,* first-stage larvae, not eggs, are excreted in the feces

- Pinworm *(Enterobius vermicularis)* is diagnosed most commonly by visual inspection of the perianal area for evidence of adult worms, or by applying adhesive tape to the skin in order to recover eggs

TREATMENT

- Screening and treatment for intestinal nematode infections in immigrants and international adoptees is recommended, even in the absence of symptoms
- Benzimidazole anthelmintics (albendazole, mebendazole) remain the drugs of choice for treating *Ascaris,* hookworm, *Enterobius,* and *Trichuris* infections
- Ivermectin is the most effective treatment for *Strongyloides* infection, but only oral preparations are available routinely
- Nitazoxanide is a broad-spectrum agent for treatment of parasitic infections, and is effective against a number of intestinal nematodes

DURATION OF THERAPY

- Most infections are cured with 1 to 3 days of treatment
- Follow-up stool evaluations are recommended to establish cure or the need for additional treatment
- Despite therapy, disseminated strongyloidiasis in the compromised host is associated with significant mortality

---

277 Tissue Nematodes

Dickson D. Despommier and Peter J. Hotez

Parasitic nematodes are found in a variety of ecological settings that include human habitation. Many are transmitted to children due to pica, since the long-lived infectious eggs are contained in feces that contaminate most outdoor environments. Some nematode infections have zoonotic importance as disease-producing agents resulting in potentially serious childhood

infections. A few of these can permanently affect a child's ability to learn. This chapter covers clinical information relevant to nematodes that take up residence in the deep tissues: *Toxocara canis* and *T. cati, Baylisascaris procyonis, Anasakis* spp., *Angiostrongylus* spp., *Ancylostoma braziliense, Gnathostoma spinigerum,* and *Trichinella* spp.

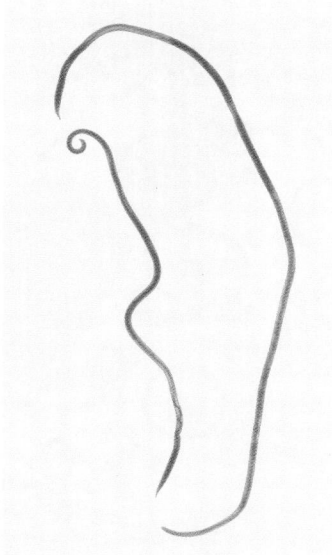

Figure 277-1. Adults of *Toxocara canis*. The male measures 6 cm and the female measures 9 cm in length.

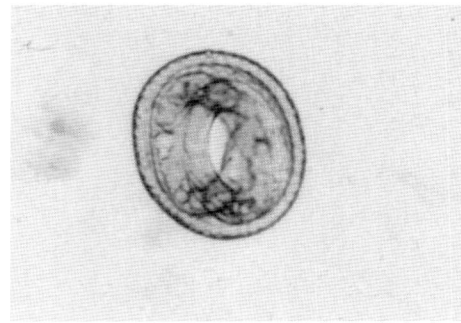

Figure 277-2. Embryonated egg of *Toxocara* species (65 μm).

VISCERAL AND OCULAR LARVA MIGRANS (VLM AND OLM) CAUSED BY *TOXOCARA CANIS*, *TOXOCARA CATI*, AND *BAYLISASCARIS PROCYONIS*

Visceral larva migrans (VLM) and ocular larva migrans (OLM) are two distinct clinical manifestations of a zoonotic infection commonly caused by the larval stages of *Toxocara canis* and *T. cati*, and, to a lesser extent, by the larva of *Baylisascaris procyonis*. Aberrant migration of these larvae through the viscera results in a series of serious conditions, most of which have a neurologic manifestation. The term *covert toxocariasis* also has been used to refer to *Toxocara* infection that is composed of some but not all of the signs and symptoms of VLM, including wheezing and eosinophilia.[1] On this basis some investigators have suggested toxocariasis is an important environmental cause of asthma, especially among underrepresented minority populations living in impoverished areas of the United States.[1] Today, toxocariasis may represent the most common helminth infection in the U.S.[1]

In the early 1950s, Beaver[2] published a series of articles describing children who had a high level of circulating eosinophils and severe multisystem disease caused by the larval stage of *T. canis* and *T. cati*. Both of these species are found commonly in dogs and cats, respectively, where their life cycle is similar to that of *Ascaris lumbricoides* in humans. The adults of *Toxocara* (Figure 277-1) are shorter than *Ascaris*, but all three species are similar regarding their biochemical and physiologic needs.

Clinical Features and Life Cycle

The major clinical features of VLM, OLM, and covert toxocariasis have been reviewed.[3] Infection in the human (abnormal host) begins when embryonated infectious eggs are ingested (Figures 277-2 and 277-3). This is a frequent event in those ecological settings throughout the world where children have unrestricted access to fecally contaminated soil. Urban parks and playgrounds are important settings for encountering the eggs of *Toxocara*. In the U.S., overall seroprevalence for toxocariasis (indicative of exposure to the parasite) is 14%, but exceeds 20% in non-Hispanic black populations, with the major risk factors being poverty, low head-of-household level of education, elevated blood lead levels, and dog ownership.[4] Coinfections with toxoplasmosis also are

*Toxocara canis and
Toxocara cati*

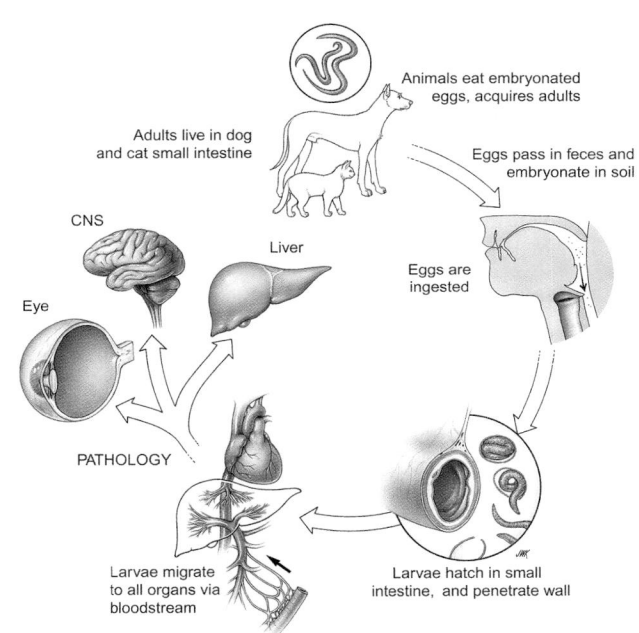

Figure 277-3. Life cycle of *Toxocara canis* and *T. cati*. (Redrawn from Despommier DD, et al. (eds) Parasitic Diseases, 5th ed. New York, Apple Trees Productions, 2005.)

common.[5] Pathology results when larvae hatch in the small intestine and migrate throughout the body, invading all organs. There still is controversy as to whether these are second- or third-stage larvae. The degree of host damage varies according to the number of eggs ingested and the kinds of tissues invaded: the liver, lungs, and central nervous system (Figure 277-4), especially the eyes, being the organ systems most seriously affected. After several months of wandering in the tissues, the larvae die. This event is followed by marked delayed-type and immediate-type hypersensitivity responses, with inflammatory responses manifesting primarily as eosinophilic granuloma. Immediate hypersensitivity reactions to dead and dying larvae in the viscera, including the lungs, liver, and brain, result in VLM. Larvae in the eye cause OLM and can affect the retina severely, where the granuloma can be misdiagnosed as retinoblastoma (Figure 277-5). Ocular disease frequently is diagnosed in the absence of systemic involvement, and vice versa. Unique strains of *T. canis* may have specific tropisms, or possibly VLM may reflect the consequences of a host inflammatory response to repeated insults of migrating larvae

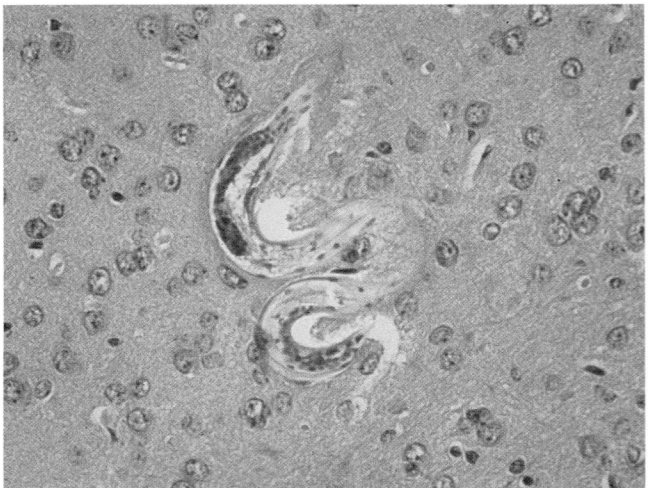

Figure 277-4. The third-stage larva of *Toxocara canis* in the brain of an experimentally infected mouse.

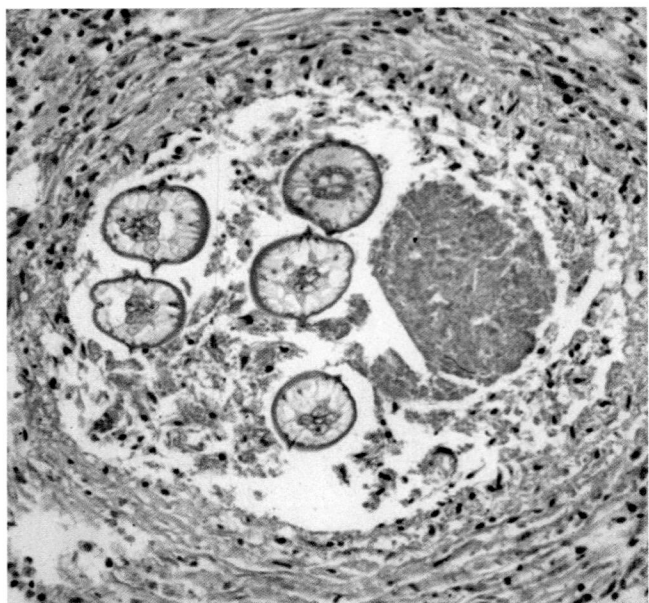

Figure 277-6. Larvae of *Baylisascaris procyonis* in brain of a child who died from the infection.

through the deep tissues, whereas OLM occurs in individuals who have not been exposed previously.[3,6]

VLM is a frequent condition of young children (<5 years of age).[7] Clinical disease includes fever, hepatosplenomegaly, lower respiratory tract symptoms (bronchospasm resembling asthma), circulating eosinophilia occasionally rising to over 70%, and IgM and IgG hypergammaglobulinemia. Myocarditis, nephritis, and central nervous system (CNS) involvement have been described, and can produce seizures, neuropsychiatric symptoms, eosinophilic meningomyelitis[3] and/or encephalopathy. Subclinical manifestations also can be induced by the migrating larvae that later emerge clinically. "Covert toxocariasis" ranges from asymptomatic infection to symptoms due to infection in specific organs.[8–10]

VLM can result in an asthma-like condition, indistinguishable from asthma due to other causes.[11,12] *T. canis* has been suspected as an environmental risk factor for asthma among some inner city populations.[1,10] *T. canis* larvae migrating throughout the brain have been implicated as one of the causes of "idiopathic" seizure disorders.[13] It also may cause functional intestinal disorders.[14] The full clinical spectrum of covert toxocariasis has not been defined completely.

OLM occurs mostly in adolescents as unilateral vision impairment, occasionally with strabismus.[15] Invasion of the retina,

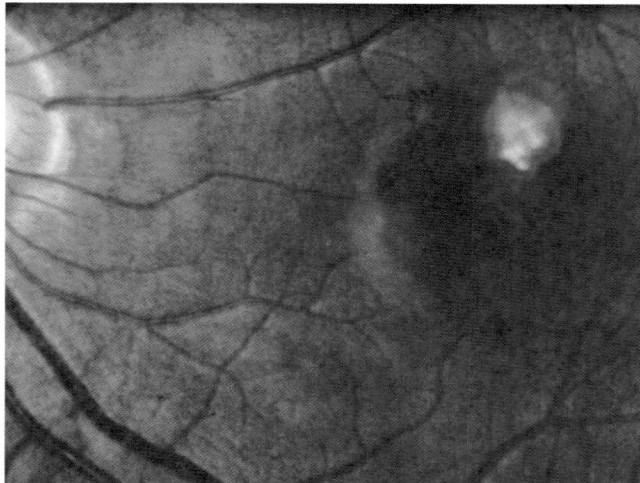

Figure 277-5. Larva of *Toxocara* in retina manifesting as granuloma.

leading to granuloma formation is the most serious manifestation of OLM. These granulomas tend to drag the retina, creating distortion, heteropia, or detachment of the macula.[16] The degree of impairment is correlated with the specific area of involvement, and blindness is common. OLM also can result in diffuse endophthalmitis or papillitis; secondary glaucoma often is a consequence.

Bayliascaris procyonis is a common infection of raccoons, but more recently patent infections also have been identified in dogs and in kinkajous.[17,18] An excellent review of all aspects of the infection has been published.[19] Infection in children is less common compared with *T. canis* and *T. cati*, but occurs in a similar fashion. Humans accidentally ingest the embryonated eggs. This can occur in woodland settings, as well as around suburban and urban dwellings. Raccoons routinely invade such human habitation areas as attics and the gutters of houses.[19,20]

Infection with the large larvae (up to 2 mm) of *B. procyonis* is more serious than that caused by the smaller larvae of *T. canis*. Damage is thought to occur by mechanical trauma produced during its migration through tissues (Figure 277-6).[19] Larvae migrating through brain tissue result in eosinophilic meningitis, which is associated with high mortality. This probably occurs because the larvae continue to grow during infection, as compared with larvae of *T. canis* and *T. cati*, which do not.[19,20]

OLM caused by *B. procyonis* has been described in nonhuman primates, and should be considered a possible etiologic agent in human ocular disease.[19,20] Antibodies to *B. procyonis* antigens do not cross-react with *T. canis*, so the excretory and secretory products of *B. procyonis* have been tested as a possible species-specific immunodiagnostic reagent.[21] An enzyme immunoassay (EIA) test has been developed with high specificity and sensitivity, but has limited availability.[19] Many human cases are diagnosed at autopsy, and since there are limited cases diagnosed to date, there is little experience with anthelmintic therapy for baylisascariasis.

Diagnosis

VLM should be suspected in any child with unexplained febrile illness and peripheral blood eosinophilia. Hepatosplenomegaly, evidence of multisystem disease, and history of pica suggest the diagnosis. Laboratory tests for VLM are based on serology.[22] The EIA, which uses secreted antigens of the larva, is the most reliable indirect measure of infection with *T. canis* and *T. cati;* EIA for VLM is highly sensitive (approximately 78%) and specific (approximately 92%) at a titer >1 : 32.

Other indicators include hypergammaglobulinemia and an elevated isohemoagglutin titer. Constellation of clinical disease, a history of pica, peripheral blood eosinophilia, and positive serology strongly support the diagnosis. Liver biopsy can reveal a granuloma surrounding a larva, but a successful diagnosis using this approach is fortuitous and is not recommended. Whether or not covert toxocariasis should be suspected in any child with wheezing and eosinophilia, or in children with asthma, is still not known. However, given its association in African American children and other groups considered high risk for asthma, the role of underlying toxocariasis is under investigation.[1]

Any child with unilateral vision loss and strabismus should be tested for OLM, and is diagnosed solely on the basis of clinical criteria during an ophthalmologic examination. Serological tests available for VLM are not reliable for OLM. In one study, only 45% of patients with proven OLM had serum titers >1 : 32.[22]

Treatment and Prevention

Albendazole is the drug of choice for all species of nematodes that cause toxocariasis.[23] Patients receiving a 5-day treatment course of albendazole (10 mg/kg/day in two divided doses) improved, compared with those receiving thiabendazole. The Medical Letter lists a dose of 400 mg of albendazole twice daily for 5 days (see Chapter 296, Antiparasitic Agents). The other commonly used benzimidazole, mebendazole, is poorly absorbed from the gastrointestinal tract. Therefore, this drug is second-line treatment, although some success has been reported in patients treated with >1 g for 21 days.[24]

Treatment of symptoms, including administration of corticosteroids, suppresses the intense manifestations of the infection. OLM is treated either by surgery (vitrectomy), anthelmintic chemotherapy, corticosteroids, or combinations of therapies.[15,16]

Toxocara spp. infection commonly occurs in young pets. Newborn puppies often harbor these worms, since the infection can be acquired transplacentally. Having a litter of puppies in the home is a significant risk factor.[25] Children with pica are at risk for ingesting the environmentally resistant, embryonated eggs from soil. Adults cared for in facilities for mentally handicapped people also are at risk.[26] Treatment of dogs and control of their feces are major control measures for this disease.

Medical Ecology

The physical environment plays a crucial role in maintaining and distributing the infective eggs of *T. canis* and *T. cati.* Developing effective control programs requires attention to the environment. Infective ascarid eggs of all species are viable for months to years outside the host under optimal conditions, due solely to a resistant outer shell composed of ascarosides. This acellular layer enables eggs to withstand various harsh chemicals (e.g., high concentrations of formalin, various inorganic acids), extreme temperature changes, and varying degrees of moisture. Novel strategies to reduce infectious eggs in soil must breach the egg shell barrier.

Earthworms and small mammals play a role in dispersing eggs from a point source. As Darwin pointed out in his essay, *On the Formation Of Vegetable Mould Through The Action of Worms With Observations On Their Habits,*[27] earthworms dump huge quantities of processed (i.e., partially digested) soil onto the surface of the ground, bringing it from depths as great 2 feet. Viable eggs become incorporated into their fecal pellets, and are then subject to random distribution throughout the local area by rain events and wind. Peridomestic mammals, such as dogs, cats, squirrels, and chipmunks, play a similar, albeit less efficient role, compared with earthworms, in dispersal of embryonated eggs.[28] Birds that feed primarily on the ground (e.g., pigeons, starlings, sparrows) can serve as paratenic hosts, carrying eggs on their feet and beaks from place to place, sometimes distant from the original source.

Drinking water is another mechanism for egg dispersal. In one study, public beaches adjacent to municipal drinking water supplies just outside the city limits of Moscow, Russia were implicated as a source of contamination.[29] The authors speculated that allowing dogs and cats free access to these recreational areas increased the likelihood that eggs of *Toxocara* would enter the water column of the lake. Bathers frequently and inadvertently drink water while wading and swimming, allowing for the possibility of ingesting infective eggs. In addition, this scenario also could lead to eggs contaminating tap water.

Some elements of soil, saprophytic fungi for example (*Paecilomyces lilacinus* and *P. marquandii*), have been shown under controlled conditions to have larvicidal activity against the juvenile worm within its eggshell.[30] Application of this finding to the control of *Toxocara* eggs in soil may prove intractably difficult, due to the high degree of unpredictability regarding the behavior of species of any kind that are introduced into new environments.[31]

VISCERAL LARVA MIGRANS (VLM) CAUSED BY *ANGIOSTRONGYLUS* SPP. AND *GNATHOSTOMA SPINIGERUM*

Angiostrongylus cantonensis is a major cause of VLM throughout Southeast Asia, Micronesia, Hawaii, Philippines, China, and Taiwan. Rats are the definitive hosts, and infected rodents can be found in all countries bordering on the Indian and South Pacific oceans.[32] A series of cases have been reported from Hawaii, and rats in Louisiana are infected.[33]

A. costaricensis infection has been reported throughout Central and South America, with more than 300 infections in humans reported annually from Costa Rica alone.[34] A case also has been reported from the U.S.[35]

The female adult *A. cantonensis* measures 400 mm in length and 28 mm in diameter, while the male measures 350 mm by 22 mm. The worms live and lay eggs in the pulmonary arteries of a number of species of wild rats, including the common wharf rat, *Rattus norvegicus*. Eggs spread to the capillaries of the lungs by the hematogenous route where they dissolve their way into the alveolar spaces and hatch. Larvae then migrate up the respiratory tree and across the epiglottis, and are swallowed.

The larvae pass out with the feces, incubate in the soil, and are eaten by mollusks and crustaceans. Humans are infected with *A. cantonensis* when they accidentally ingest the larval stages in uncooked land snails and slugs, or in raw vegetables contaminated by infected invertebrate secretions.[33] Adults of *A. costaricensis* live in the mesenteric arteries of wild rats and are infective only for one type of invertebrate, the slug. In Costa Rica, where most of the cases have been reported, the slug *Vaginulus plebius* serves as the intermediate host.

The pattern of clinical infection varies with each species of nematode. For *A. cantonensis*, the third-stage larvae migrate to the capillaries of the meninges, and induce eosinophilic inflammation, resulting in meningoencephalitis. Vascular thromboses and aneurysms also have been described.[36] Infection in the human host rarely has led to development of adult worms. Usually, larvae fail to complete their life cycle and die eventually, surrounded by an eosinophilic infiltrate. Pulmonary infiltrates have been observed in infants and young children with *A. cantonensis* infection.[37] Little is known regarding the pathogenesis of lesions. *A. costaricensis* larvae migrate to the mesenteric arterioles, inducing arteritis, thrombosis, and small infarcts. Necrotic ulcers form, leading to peritonitis and fistula formation.

Patients infected with *A. cantonensis* larvae complain of fever, headaches (which are typically bitemporal or frontal), and meningismus.[33] Vomiting also is a common sign.[33] In addition, patients may show focal findings of CNS involvement, such as parasthesias (about one-half of cases) and cranial nerve palsies (about one-fourth of cases).[38] Infection is accompanied by cerebrospinal fluid and peripheral blood eosinophilia. Most affected adults recover within 3 weeks with no apparent residual abnormalities; children frequently have more serious disease.

Patients infected with *A. costaricensis* can exhibit right iliac fossa pain and fever, and always peripheral blood eosinophilia. With advanced disease, abdominal masses representing eosinophilic granulomas are detectable upon palpation. Children with abdominal angiostrongyliasis sometimes are misdiagnosed as having acute appendicitis or Meckel diverticulum.[33]

Neither species of nematode parasite can be diagnosed serologically, but one study shows promise.[39] The disease must be suspected on the basis of clinical presentation, history of exposure or residence in endemic areas, and presence of peripheral blood eosinophilia. In the case of infection with *A. cantonensis*, cerebrospinal fluid eosinophilia suggests the diagnosis. Focal lesions on neuroradiographic imaging usually is not seen.[33] Symptomatic treatment with serial lumbar punctures to reduce elevated intracranial pressure is sometimes helpful and one prospective study showed improvement with a 2-week course of prednisone.[40] Albendazole combined with the use of corticosteroids may be the treatment of choice.[41] Widespread education about the proper cooking of food and vegetable washing, as well as the control of mollusks and planarians in vegetable gardens, can reduce the incidence of infections.[36]

There is no well-established treatment for abdominal angiostrongyliasis, although anthelmintics such as mebendazole and albendazole may shorten duration of symptoms. High doses of mebendazole were used with modest success in one case of abdominal angiostrongyliasis.[33] Because many patients have surgery for suspected appendicitis, definitive surgical resection of the eosinophilic granuloma frequently is performed.[36] Ivermectin kills migrating *A. cantonensis* larvae in experimental animal models, but there are no reports of its use in humans. Because of its superior absorption, albendazole may be a superior anthelmintic. In cases of severe discomfort and an intense inflammatory reaction, corticosteroid therapy is recommended.

Gnathostoma spinigerum is parasitic in various mammals, including cats, dogs, and the mongoose; the intermediate hosts include copepods in the genus *Cyclops*, and snakes, frogs, fish, and birds. Gnathostomiasis in humans is prevalent throughout Thailand, Asia, and Mexico, where infections are acquired commonly in and around Acapulco,[42] as well as elsewhere in Central and South America.[33]

Female adults are 25 to 54 mm in length, while males measure 11 to 25 mm. Adults live coiled in the wall of the small intestine in their definitive hosts. Eggs pass in feces and hatch in water, releasing larvae that are ingested by macroinvertebrate crustaceans of the genus *Cyclops*.[33] Fish, snakes, and birds eat infected crustaceans and develop the infective stage for humans. Humans eat these infected vertebrates and the larvae invade and migrate into deep tissues. Cutaneous, visceral, and CNS manifestations have been described.[33]

Skin manifestations include subcutaneous swellings, creeping eruption, and a panniculitis associated with pain, erythema, and pruritus.[33] Alternatively, ocular larva migrans, or even eosinophilic meningitis, can develop. CNS gnathostomiasis is associated with radicular pain and paresthesias, which result from larval migration along the cranial nerves or peripheral nerves into the spinal cord.[33] A diagnosis of gnathostomiasis is made on the basis of the presence of increased eosinophils in blood or cerebrospinal fluid and appropriate travel history and clinical manifestations. The disease can be self-limited. Surgical removal or a 21-day course of oral albendazole (400 mg once daily) is an effective regimen for treatment of gnathostomiasis.[41] Corticosteroids sometimes are helpful for CNS manifestations.

CUTANEOUS LARVA MIGRANS (CLM) CAUSED BY *ANCYLOSTOMA BRAZILIENSE*

CLM has a worldwide distribution. It is a zoonosis caused by larvae of one of the dog and cat hookworm *Ancylostoma braziliense* (Figure 277-7), but other hookworm species also have been implicated.[43] Zoonotic transmission from the dog hookworm

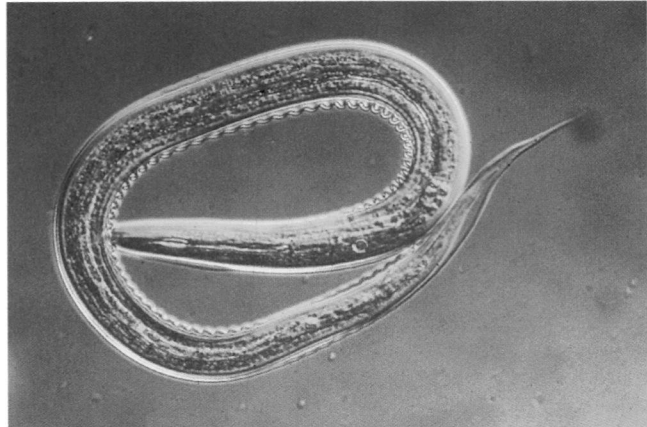

Figure 277-7. Third-stage larva of *Ancylostoma caninum*. (Courtesy of E. Gravé.)

Ancylostoma caninum also occurs in humans, but disease from this parasite usually causes eosinophilic enteritis rather than CLM. Other less common nematodes also can be responsible for CLM, including raccoon-transmitted *Strongyloides procyonis* that results in "duck hunter's itch."

The filariform larvae of *A. braziliense* survive in sandy, moist soils for several days. These larvae are especially common on beaches in India and Southeast Asia, Brazil, the Caribbean, and Puerto Rico, where dogs and cats are permitted to defecate.[44] In the U.S. a significant number of feral cats in Florida are infected with *A. braziliense*.[44] In the human host, infection begins when the filariform larvae penetrate unbroken skin but fail to receive the proper

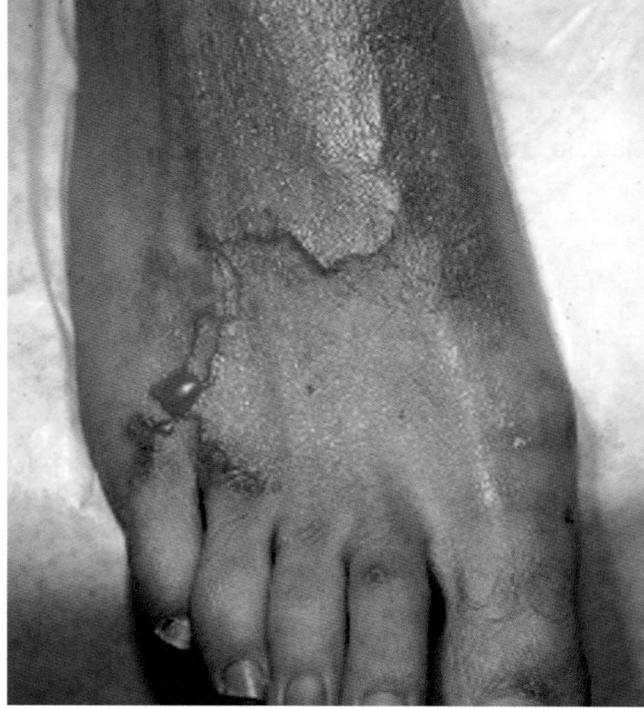

Figure 277-8. "Creeping eruption" caused by a larva of *A. caninum*. (Courtesy of G. Zalar.)

environmental cues. Instead of going further in the life cycle, larvae migrate laterally in the deeper layers of the epidermis and can survive there for about 10 days. An intense inflammatory reaction, associated with itching in the affected areas, develops within days after larvae enter the dermis, and is provoked by hydrolytic enzymes secreted by larvae.

The serpiginous lesions known as "creeping eruption" are evident (Figure 277-8) after an incubation period of 1 week. Secondary bacterial infection caused by scratching is common. In a review of 98 patients with CLM seen at a travelers' clinic in Munich, 73% of the lesions were found on the lower extremities, with the buttocks and anogenital region (13%) and trunk and upper extremities (7% each) affected less frequently. Some patients with CLM manifest peripheral blood eosinophilia, or elevated serum IgE level, but laboratory findings generally play little or no role in establishing a diagnosis of CLM.

The treatment of choice for CLM is either oral therapy with one of two anthelmintics. A single dose of ivermectin (200 µg/kg once, sometimes repeated) is considered more effective than a single dose of albendazole, but repeated treatments of albendazole (400 mg daily for 5–7 days) are comparable.[44] Some investigators recommend a 3-day course of albendazole (400 mg daily). Topical thiabendazole in a concentration of 10% to 15% 3 times daily for 5–7 days is an alternative treatment, but patient compliance sometimes is an issue. Cryotherapy with liquid nitrogen can cause blistering and ulceration of the skin and should not be performed.

VISCERAL LARVA MIGRANS (VLM) DUE TO ASCARIDS OF MARINE MAMMALS

Anisakiasis in humans is caused by a number of species of nematodes belonging to the genera *Anisakis, Phocanema, Terranova,* and *Contracoecum.* The adults of these parasites infect sea mammals, particularly dolphins, whales, sea lions, and seals,[45] and live in the lumen of the intestinal tract. Anasakid first-stage larvae infect a number of crustacean species. Second-, third-, or fourth-stage larvae infect a wide variety of teleosts (bony fishes).

Raw or undercooked saltwater fish, often in the form of sushi or sashimi, has become a popular style of cuisine throughout the world.[46,47] When an infected piece of raw fish is eaten, parasites in the muscle tissue are released by enzymes in the stomach, or more rarely, into the small intestine. Tissue invasion is facilitated by release of parasite hydrolytic enzymes.[48] All species of anasakid worms die within a few days in humans.

Dead parasites provoke an eosinophilic granulomatous infiltration. Initially, infection can be asymptomatic, but soon thereafter vague upper abdominal pain can develop. Symptoms can mimic gastric ulcer.[49] Radiographic evidence of infection resembles that of a tumor, which can lead to misdiagnosis as carcinoma of the stomach.

Definitive diagnosis and treatment is made by endoscopic removal of the parasite. Serologic tests using an *Anisakis*-specific monoclonal antibody is available in some countries.[50] Thorough cooking or freezing of seafood prior to ingestion can prevent infection by anisakid nematodes. Most sushi restaurants in the U.S. and elsewhere now inspect pieces of raw fish carefully prior to serving them. In recent years, the incidence of anisakid VLM in Europe and North America due to the consumption of raw fish has been reduced to a few sporadic cases annually.

TRICHINELLA SPIRALIS (TRICHINELLOSIS)

The genus *Trichinella* has undergone revision, due to the advent of reliable DNA probes.[51,52] There are 9 distinct genotypes and 7 recognized species (2 are provisional).[53] Members of the genus *Trichinella* are able to infect a broad spectrum of mammalian hosts, making them one of the world's most widely distributed nematode infections. *Trichinella* spp. are related genetically to *Trichuris trichiura* and *Capillaria* spp.; all belong to the family Trichurata. These roundworms constitute an unusual group of organisms

in the phylum Nematoda, in that they all live their lives as intracellular parasites.

Diseases due to *Trichinella* spp. are referred to collectively as trichinellosis. Currently, prevalence of trichinellosis is low in the U.S., occurring mostly as scattered outbreaks.[52] The majority of human cases are due to *Trichinella spiralis*, and the information that follows concentrates on this species. The domestic pig is the main reservoir host for *T. spiralis*. This species is significantly higher in prevalence in parts of Europe, Asia, and Southeast Asia than in the U.S. In Europe, and especially in eastern Europe, the rise of trichinellosis has been associated with a number of political and socioeconomic changes that resulted in a breakdown of the veterinary public health infrastructure.[53] Meat from horses and wild boar now account for a significant amount of European trichinellosis.[53] Trichinellosis is considered endemic in Japan and China, and a large outbreak occurred in Lebanon in 1997, infecting over 200 people.[54] *Trichinella spiralis* infection in humans also has been reported from Korea.[55] In contrast, *Trichinella* infections in wildlife in the U.S. are now thought largely to be due to the T5 strain, tentatively designated *T. murrelli.*[56]

An outbreak of *T. pseudospiralis* in Thailand has been reported.[57] This species also can infect birds of prey. Foci also have been described in Sweden,[58] Slovakia,[59] and Tasmania. *Trichinella paupae* (provisional), apparently similar in biology to *T. pseudospiralis*, has been described in wild and domestic pigs in Papua New Guinea.[60]

Humans also can be infected with *T. nativa*, and *T. britovi.*[61] Reservoir hosts for *T. nativa* include sled dogs, walruses, and polar bears. *T. britovi* is the sylvatic form of trichinellosis throughout most of Asia and Europe, with numerous reports of infections in foxes, raccoons, opossums, wild boars (as well as domestic pigs), domestic and wild dogs, and cats.[53]

T. nelsoni is restricted to mammals in equatorial Africa, such as hyenas, and the large predatory cats.[62] Occasionally people acquire infection from *T. nelsoni*. Most animals in the wild, regardless of their geographic location, acquire trichinella by scavenging. Puerto Rico and mainland Australia remain free of *Trichinella*. *T. pseudospiralis* has been isolated from the Tasmanian devil, but not from humans living in that part of Australia.[63]

Life Cycle

Infection is initiated by ingesting raw or undercooked meats harboring the nurse cell–larva complex (Figures 277-9 and 277-10). Larvae are released from muscle tissue by digestive enzymes in the stomach, and then locate to the upper two-thirds of the small intestine. The outermost cuticular layer (epicuticle) becomes partially digested,[64,65] enabling the parasite to receive environmental cues,[66] and to select an infection site within the small intestine. Immature parasites penetrate the columnar epithelium at the base of the villus where they live in a row, and are considered intramulticellular organisms.[67]

Larvae molt four times in rapid succession over a 30-hour period, developing into adults. The female measures 3 mm in length by 36 µm in diameter, while the male measures 1.5 mm in length by 36 µm in diameter.

Patency occurs within 5 days after mating. Adult females produce live offspring-newborn larvae (Figure 277-11), which measure 0.08 mm in length by 7 µm in diameter. The female produces offspring as long as host immunity does not develop. Eventually, acquired, protective responses interfere with the overall process of embryogenesis and create physiologic conditions in the local area of infection that force the adult parasites to egress and relocate further down the intestinal tract. Expulsion of worms from the host is the final expression of immunity, and may take several weeks.

The newborn larva is the only stage of the parasite that possesses a sword-like stylet located in the oral cavity, which is used to create an entry hole in potential host cells. Larvae enter the lamina propria in this fashion, and penetrate into the mesenteric lymphatics or the bloodstream. Most newborn larvae enter the general circulation, and become distributed throughout the body.

Trichinella spiralis

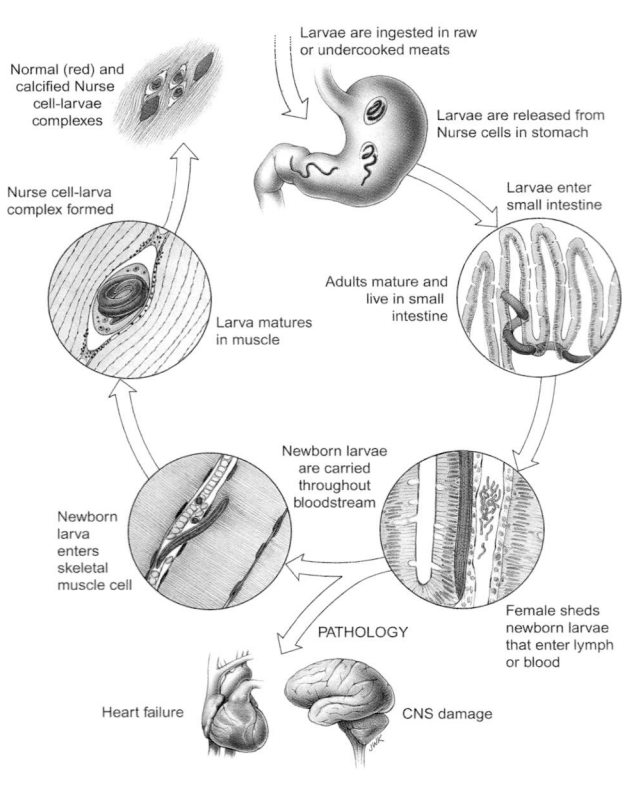

Larvae are ingested in raw or undercooked meats

Larvae are released from Nurse cells in stomach

Larvae enter small intestine

Adults mature and live in small intestine

Normal (red) and calcified Nurse cell-larvae complexes

Nurse cell-larva complex formed

Larva matures in muscle

Newborn larvae are carried throughout bloodstream

Newborn larva enters skeletal muscle cell

Female sheds newborn larvae that enter lymph or blood

PATHOLOGY

Heart failure   CNS damage

"Parasitic Diseases" 5ᵗʰ Ed. © Apple Trees Productions, LLC., Pub. P.O. Box 280, New York, NY 10032

Figure 277-9. Life cycle of *Trichinella spiralis*. (Redrawn from Despommier DD, et al. (eds) Parasitic Diseases, 5th ed. New York, Apple Trees Productions, 2005.)

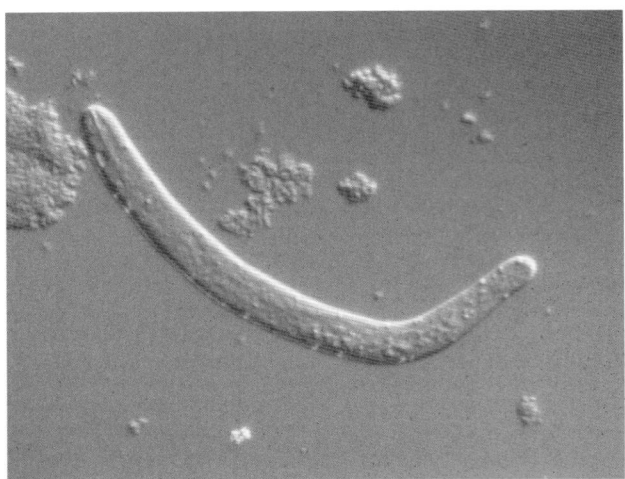

Figure 277-11. Newborn larva of *Trichinella spiralis* (80 μm × 7 μm).

Migrating newborns leave capillaries and enter cells (Figure 277-12). There appears to be no tropism for any particular cell type. Once inside, larvae either can remain or leave, depending upon environmental cues (yet to be determined) received by the parasite. Most cell types die as the result of invasion. Skeletal muscle cells are the only exception. Not only do the parasites remain inside them after invasion, they induce a remarkable series of changes, causing the fully differentiated muscle cell to

transform into one that supports the growth and development of the larva. This process is termed nurse-cell formation.[68] Parasite and host cell develop in a coordinated fashion. *T. spiralis* is infective by the 14th day of infection, but the worm continues to grow in size through day 20.[69] The significance of this precocious behavior has yet to be appreciated.

Parasites inside cells other than striated muscle cells fail to induce nurse cells, and either re-enter the general circulation or die. Nurse-cell formation results in an intimate and permanent association between the worm and its intracellular niche (Figure 277-10). At the cellular level, myofilaments and other related muscle cell components are replaced over a 14- to 16-day period by whorls of smooth membranes and clusters of dysfunctional mitochondria. The net result is that the host cell switches from an aerobic to an anaerobic metabolism. Nuclei enlarge and divide,[70] amplifying the host's genome within the nurse-cell cytoplasm. The nurse cell–parasite complex can live for as long as the host remains alive. Most do not, and are calcified within several months after forming. In order for the life cycle to continue, an infected host must die and be eaten by another mammal. Scavenging is a common behavior among most wild mammals, and this helps to ensure the maintenance of *T. spiralis* and its relatives in their respective host species.

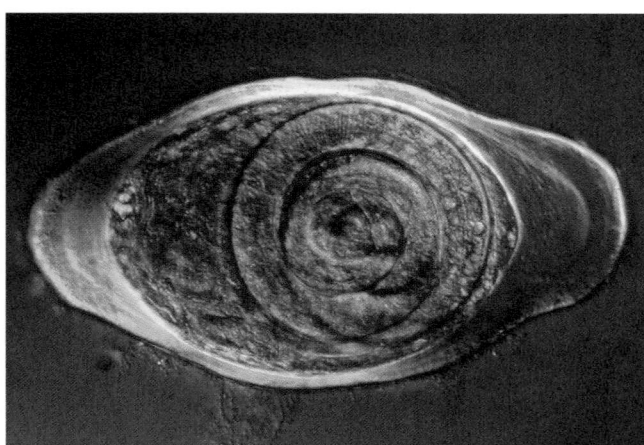

Figure 277-10. Nurse cell–larva complex of *Trichinella spiralis*.

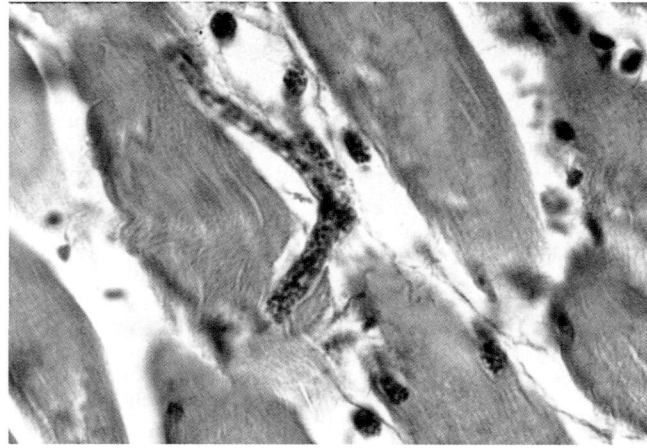

Figure 277-12. Migrating larva of *Trichinella spiralis* penetrating outward from a capillary.

Clinical Manifestations

The clinical features of mild, moderate, and severe trichinellosis have been reviewed.[71,72] The nature of the disease state varies over time, and as a result, resembles a wide variety of clinical conditions. Trichinellosis often is misdiagnosed for that reason. The severity of clinical trichinellosis is dose dependent; diagnosis based solely on symptoms is difficult. However, there are clues, even in the early stages of the disease, that should alert the physician to include trichinellosis in the differential diagnosis.

The first few days of the infection are characterized by gastroenteritis associated with diarrhea, abdominal pain, and vomiting. Enteritis ensues, and is secretory in nature.[73] This phase is transitory, and abates within 10 days after ingestion of infected tissue. A history of eating raw or undercooked meats, and of similar illness in others who ate the same meats is suspicious for trichinellosis.

The parenteral phase begins approximately 1 week after infection and can last several weeks. Typically, the patient has fever and myalgia, bilateral periorbital edema, and petechial hemorrhages, which are seen most clearly in the subungual skin, but also are observed in the conjunctivae and on other mucous membranes. Muscle tenderness is detected readily. Laboratory studies reveal a moderately elevated white blood cell count (12,000–15,000 cells/mm³), with eosinophilia ranging from 5% to 50%.

Larvae penetrating tissues other than muscle give rise to more serious sequelae. In many cases of moderate to severe infection, cardiovascular involvement leads to myocarditis.[74] Electrocardiographic (ECG) changes frequently are noted during this phase. Parasite invasion of the diaphragm and the accessory muscles of respiration results in dyspnea. Neurotrichinellosis also occurs in association with CNS invasion. Convalescent phase follows the acute phase, during which time many nurse cell–parasite complexes are destroyed.

Two clinical presentations have been described for *T. nativa* infections resulting from ingestion of infected polar bear or walrus meat: a classic myopathic form, and a persistent diarrheal illness. The second form is thought to represent a second infection in previously sensitized people.[75]

Diagnosis

Diagnosis is established on the basis of appropriate clinical and laboratory findings (including eosinophilia and increases in serum muscle enzyme levels, antibody detection, and/or detection of larvae in muscle), as well as epidemiologic investigations that identify a source and origin of infection.[53] Definitive diagnosis depends on finding the nurse cell–parasite complex in muscle biopsy by microscopic examination, or detection of *Trichinella*-specific DNA by PCR.[76] PCR is sensitive and specific for detecting small numbers of larvae in muscle tissue, but testing is expensive and usually is not available.

Muscle biopsy can be negative, even in high-density infections, due to sampling error. In addition, the larvae may be at an early stage of development, making them inconspicuous, even to the experienced pathologist. A rising, plateauing, and falling level of circulating eosinophils throughout the infection period is not confirmatory, but in the appropriate clinical context could warrant empiric therapy. Bilateral periorbital edema, petechiae under the fingernails, and high fever, coupled with a history of eating raw or undercooked meats, further solidifies a presumptive infection.

Wild mammals also can be sources of infection.[77] Outbreaks of trichinellosis have been traced to hunters and the recipients of their kills.

Muscle enzymes, such as creatine kinase and lactic dehydrogenase, are released causing an increase in serum levels. Serologic tests may be positive within 2 weeks; EIA can be positive as early as 12 days after infection.[72]

Treatment

An anthelmintic should be administered, with the recommended dose of albendazole (400 mg twice daily for 8–14 days).[53] Albendazole is preferred over mebendazole because of higher tissue levels of an active metabolite former that can be achieved following oral administration.[53] Use of the drug in pregnancy and in children <2 years of age requires consideration of potential risks versus benefits. In addition, it is thought that anthelmintics work best in the early stages of the infection; once muscle larvae are established, the clinical effectiveness of anthelmintics is reduced and larvae can survive for years to cause chronic myalgias.[53] Rapidly destroying larvae with anthelmintics can exacerbate host inflammatory responses and worsen disease (e.g., Jarisch–Herxheimer reaction). Corticosteroid therapy, particularly prednisone (30–60 mg/day) for 10 to 15 days is recommended if the diagnosis is secure and the symptoms are severe. Antipyretics and analgesics (aspirin, acetaminophen) are used in the myopathic phase and should be continued until fever and allergic signs recede.

Prevention

Within the last 10 years, outbreaks of trichinellosis in the U.S. have been rare and sporadic in nature. Generally, most cases have been associated with ingestion of raw or undercooked meats obtained from commercial sources.[52] However, pigs raised on family farms, as compared with commercial factory farm operations (such as exist in North Carolina), are more likely to be fed uncooked garbage, and thus acquire the infection. U.S. Department of Agriculture law, which bans feeding unprocessed garbage, is enforced only in large production facilities.

Hunters and those sharing in their kills of carnivorous mammals, including bear, fox, and cougar, have sometimes become infected. Herbivores can harbor the infection, since most plant eaters occasionally ingest meat when the opportunity arises. Epidemics due to eating raw horsemeat have been reported from France, Italy, and Poland.[78]

The scope of meat inspection in the U.S. does not include *Trichinella* species. In Europe, the countries in the European Union employ several strategies for examining meat for muscle larvae. Most serve to identify pools of meat sampled from given regions. If they are consistently negative, then a *Trichinella*-free designation is applied to that supply of meat. Nonetheless, rare outbreaks occur, despite this rigorous system of inspection.

Trichinellosis due to *Trichinella spiralis* can be prevented by either cooking meat thoroughly at 58.5°C for 10 minutes or by freezing it at −20°C for 3 days. Freezing is not effective with other species of *Trichinella* found mostly in wild animals. For example, bears and raccoons have substances in their muscles that prevent ice crystals from forming during their hibernation, inadvertently permitting survival of the larvae at temperatures below freezing. Hence, thorough cooking is the only way to render these meats safe.

In the U.S., most (90% to 95%) infections with *T. spiralis* can be traced back to a single episode of eating undercooked or raw pork purchased from commercial sources (e.g., sausage).[52] In addition, some outbreaks have been traced to ground beef adulterated with pork scraps.

In the U.S., tracing a sample of contaminated pork that was sold commercially back to its farm source often is futile because the origin of individual pigs is not identifiable after the animals are sold at auctions. Sporadic cases or outbreaks from pigs raised on small farms will continue to occur.

278 Blood and Tissue Nematodes (Filarial Worms)

LeAnne M. Fox

Human filariasis, a public health problem of global importance, is caused by infection with threadlike worms that have complex life cycles involving a human host, insect vectors, and, in some cases, other mammalian reservoirs. When an infected vector bites or takes a blood meal from a human host, filarial larvae penetrate the skin and migrate to specific tissues, where they develop into sexually mature adult worms. Months after infection, microfilariae are released by the fertile female worm and migrate to the skin or peripheral blood, where they are ingested by an insect vector when it bites or takes a blood meal. The development of the infective third-stage larvae in the insect completes the life cycle. Signs and symptoms of filarial infections are determined, in part, by the preferred locations of the adult worms and microfilariae (Table 278-1).

The chronic sequelae of filarial infections may not become evident for several years after infection. Thus, infected children living in areas where filariasis is endemic often are asymptomatic. People with no previous exposure who travel to endemic areas tend to have more vigorous immunologic responses to filarial infection, are less likely to have detectable microfilariae, and are more likely to have acute manifestations. For children with an appropriate travel history and signs or symptoms of filariasis or unexplained eosinophilia, the diagnosis can be confirmed by the finding of microfilariae in blood, in skin snips, or upon slit-lamp examination of the eye. For *Wuchereria bancrofti*, the most prevalent cause of lymphatic filariasis, a rapid test for circulating filarial antigen is available. Determination of serum antifilarial immunoglobulin (Ig)G may be helpful as an initial diagnostic test, particularly in expatriate visitors to endemic areas. This assay is available at the Parasitic Diseases Laboratory at the National Institutes of Health (telephone: 301-496-5398). If antifilarial antibodies are not detectable, filarial infection is unlikely. In the patient with antifilarial IgG, a careful clinical and travel history should guide selection of more specific serologic and parasitologic tests for filarial infection.

Many filarial nematodes contain rickettsia-like endosymbiotic bacteria of the genus *Wolbachia* that are important for normal development, viability, and fertility of the adult worm. These bacteria have been investigated as potentially important chemotherapeutic targets as well as disease-causing organisms, particularly for lymphatic filariasis and onchocerciasis.

LYMPHATIC FILARIASIS

Epidemiology

Lymphatic filariasis is caused by three species, *W. bancrofti, Brugia malayi*, and *Brugia timori*, which together infect an estimated 120 million persons in Africa, southern Asia, the western Pacific Islands, the Atlantic coast of South and Central America, and the Caribbean, particularly Haiti and the Dominican Republic (see Table 278-1).[1] More than 90% of these infections are caused by *W. bancrofti*. The three species cause similar signs and symptoms, although genital involvement occurs primarily with *W. bancrofti* infection.

The adult worms live in the lymphatic vessels for 5 to 10 years. Initial infection, detected as the presence of circulating filarial antigen, commonly occurs between the ages of 2 and 4 years.[2,3] In areas of intense transmission, prevalence of microfilaremia increases rapidly between the ages of 5 and 10 years. Chronic manifestations, such as hydrocele and lymphedema, occur infrequently in people younger than 20 years and generally increase in frequency with age.[3]

Clinical Manifestations

The clinical expression of lymphatic filariasis varies considerably. Most infected persons are asymptomatic. Filarial lymphadenopathy is seen commonly in infected children;[3-5] before puberty, adult worms can be detected by ultrasonography of the inguinal, crural, and axillary lymph nodes and vessels.[6,7] In boys after puberty, the adult worms tend to live in the intrascrotal lymphatic vessels.[6,7] Ultrasonography of lymphatic vessels can reveal motile adult

TABLE 278-1. Characteristics of Filarial Parasites of Humans

Species	Most Common Tissue Location		Geographic Distribution	Estimated No. Infected	Vector	Periodicity
	Adult	Microfilaria				
Wuchereria bancrofti	Lymphatics	Blood	Tropics worldwide	115 million	Mosquitoes	Nocturnal or subperiodic
Brugia malayi	Lymphatics	Blood	Southeast Asia	13 million	Mosquitoes	Nocturnal or subperiodic
Brugia timori	Lymphatics	Blood	Indonesia	Thousands	Mosquitoes	Nocturnal
Onchocerca volvulus	Connective tissue	Skin, eyes	Africa; South and Central America	37 million	Blackfly (*Simulium*)	None
Loa loa	Connective tissue	Blood	West and Central Africa	13 million	Deerfly (*Chrysops*)	Diurnal
Mansonella streptocerca	Skin	Skin	West and Central Africa	?	Midge (*Culicoides*)	None
Mansonella perstans	Serous cavities	Blood	Africa; South and Central America	?	Midge	None
Mansonella ozzardi	Serous cavities	Blood, skin	South and Central America, Caribbean	?	Blackfly, midge	None
Dirofilaria immitis	Lungs	—	Worldwide	?	Mosquitoes	—
Dirofilaria tenuis, Dirofilaria repens	Subcutaneous tissue	—	Worldwide	?	Mosquitoes	—

worms, termed the "filarial dance sign," examples of which may be viewed on the internet.[8] Even in asymptomatic people, the presence of living adult worms leads to lymphatic dilatation and abnormal lymph flow, which can be demonstrated by lymphoscintigraphy. These changes predispose the person to lymphedema.[9] Lymphatic vessel dilatation and lymph node enlargement and fibrosis also can be visualized when lymph nodes are examined histopathologically (Figure 278-1). Microscopic hematuria and proteinuria also are found.[10]

Acute filarial lymphangitis has been well documented in travelers to endemic areas. Two to 6 months after exposure, acute inflammation develops in a lymphatic vessel and its associated lymph nodes, most frequently in the leg, scrotal area, or arm. Characteristically, inflammation progresses distally along the lymphatic vessel, which becomes indurated, tender and erythematous, and resolves spontaneously within 3 to 7 days. Because biopsies reveal intense inflammation and nonliving adult worms, acute filarial lymphangitis is thought to be caused by the death of the adult worm.[11]

A separate and clinically distinct syndrome, which for years was confused with filarial lymphangitis, is acute dermatolymphangioadenitis, caused by bacterial infection of the small collecting lymphatic vessels in areas of lymphatic dysfunction.[11,12] Unlike true filarial lymphangitis, this syndrome develops in a reticular rather than a linear pattern and is more commonly associated with severe pain, fever, and chills.

Lymphedema occurs in the legs, scrotum, penis, and arms. In the legs and arms, it usually is unilateral. The most important factor involved in progression of filarial lymphedema to elephantiasis is repeated episodes of acute dermatolymphangioadenitis, originating from breaks in the epidermis, which contribute to further lymph stasis, secondary bacterial infection, and fibrosis.[9]

The pathogenesis of filarial hydrocele is unclear but is thought to be a consequence of lymphatic damage caused by living adult *W. bancrofti*.[9] In filariasis-endemic areas, clinically apparent hydrocele actually may be a chylocele, resulting from rupture of dilated intrascrotal lymphatic vessels and leakage of lymph into the cavity of the testicular tunica vaginalis.[9] Chyluria results from rupture of dilated retroperitoneal lymphatic structures into the renal pelvis.

Tropical pulmonary eosinophilia (TPE) is characterized by peripheral blood eosinophilia (>3000 cells/mm³), elevated serum IgE (>10,000 ng/mL), low-grade fever, lymphadenopathy, and a nonproductive cough that is more severe at night. Peripheral microfilaremia is absent in patients with TPE. Most cases of TPE have been reported in long-term residents from Asia. Men 20 to 40 years old most commonly are affected, but TPE has been reported in children.

Laboratory Findings and Diagnosis

The standard for diagnosis is microscopic detection of microfilariae on a thick blood film (Figure 278-2), but filtration of 1 to 5 mL blood through a 0.3- to 0.5-µm nucleopore filter is a more sensitive method.[13] In most endemic areas, the circulation of microfilariae in peripheral blood is periodic, with highest concentrations occurring at night; therefore, blood specimens should be collected between 10 pm and 2 am. Microfilariae of the three species are distinguished morphologically. Because infected children are frequently microfilaria negative, other tests may be helpful in making the diagnosis. Assays that detect circulating *W. bancrofti* antigen, primarily from the adult worm, are available (Table 278-2).[14] Elevated antifilarial IgG4 levels indicate active infection. Ultrasonography can be used to visualize the adult worms in children.[6,7] In postpubertal boys and men, the living adult worms are detected readily on ultrasonography of the scrotal area.[6,7,15] Polymerase chain reaction (PCR) to detect *W. bancrofti* in blood may be available in research laboratories.[16]

Treatment

Diethylcarbamazine (DEC) is the drug of choice for lymphatic filarial infection. DEC is both microfilaricidal and active against the adult worm. A single 6 mg/kg dose is as effective as the previously recommended dose of 6 mg/kg/day for 12 days, for killing the adult worm and long-term suppression of microfilariae.[17] The severity of systemic adverse reactions, including fever, myalgia, headache, and malaise, is related directly to microfilarial density before treatment. These symptoms develop within the first 2 days and usually are self-limited. Local adverse reactions, including the formation of tender nodules, can occur at the site of the adult worm, especially in the scrotal area. In the United States, DEC is available only through the Drug Service of the Centers for Disease Control and Prevention (during business hours: 404-718-4745; on evenings, weekends, and holidays: 770-488-7100). DEC is not recommended for treatment during pregnancy, although no teratogenic effects of the drug have been reported.

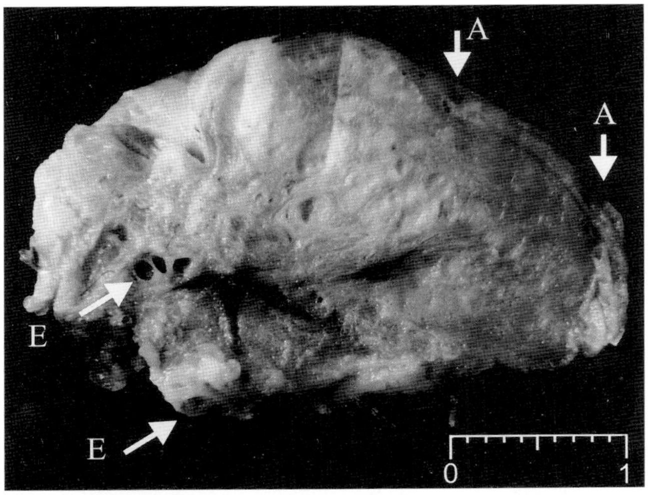

Figure 278-1. Gross appearance of a lymph node from a child infected with *W. bancrofti*. The capsule is thickened and the hilum distended. Afferent (A) and efferent (E) lymphatic vessels are dilated and tortuous. (From Figueredo-Silva J, Dreyer G. Bancroftian filariasis in children and adolescents: clinical-pathological observations in 22 cases from an endemic area. Ann Trop Med Parasitol 2005;99:759–769.)

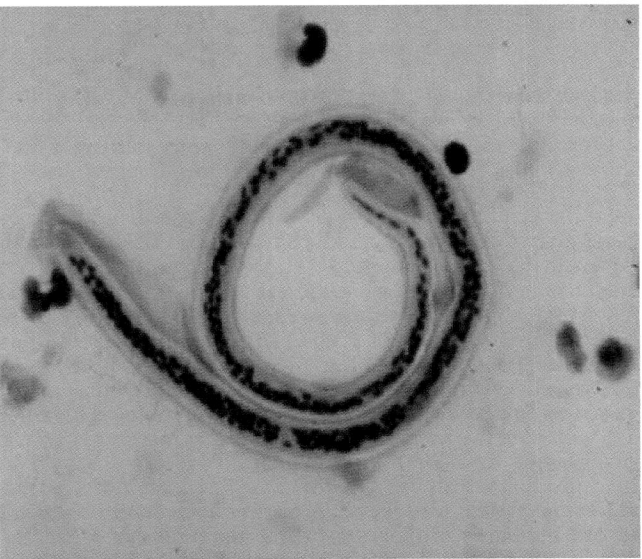

Figure 278-2. Microfilaria of *W. bancrofti* on a thick blood film stained with hematoxylin. (Courtesy of Mark L. Eberhard, PhD, Division of Parasitic Diseases and Malaria, Centers for Disease Control and Prevention, Atlanta, GA.)

TABLE 278-2. Diagnostic Test Results and Treatment for the Major Clinical Manifestations of Lymphatic Filariasis

Clinical Manifestation	Microfilaremia Detectable	Circulating Filarial Antigen	Filaria-Specific IgG4	Visualization of Worms on Ultrasound of Scrotal Area	Recommended Treatment
ACUTE					
Asymptomatic, infected	+	+	+	+	Diethylcarbamazine
Filarial lymphangitis	+/−	+/−	+	+/−	Supportive care[b,c]
Dermatolymphangioadenitis	−/+	−/+	−/+[a]	−/+	Supportive care; antibiotics[b]
CHRONIC					
Hydrocele	+/−	+/−	+/−[a]	+/−	Surgical repair[b]
Lymphedema and elephantiasis	−/+	−/+	−/+[a]	−/+	Hygiene, skin care, lymphedema care[b]
Chyluria	+/−	+/−	+/−[a]	−/+	Low-fat, high-protein diet[b]
Tropical pulmonary eosinophilia	−	+/−	+	+/−	Diethylcarbamazine

Ig, immunoglobulin; +, positive or detectable; −, negative or nondetectable; +/− likely positive; −/+, likely negative.

[a]Elevated if blood is positive for microfilaria or circulating filarial antigen.

[b]Treatment with diethylcarbamazine is given if patient has specific evidence of filarial infection (microfilaria or circulating filarial antigen detected, or living worms detected on ultrasonography).

[c]Treatment with diethylcarbamazine should be delayed until after the acute episode resolves.

Ivermectin is a potent microfilaricidal drug but does not kill the adult worm. Therefore, ivermectin is not recommended for treatment of the individual affected child, although it has an important role in community-based control programs in Africa. Albendazole appears to enhance the microfilarial suppression of DEC and ivermectin.[18] Initial trials of 4 to 8 weeks of antibiotic therapy directed against *Wolbachia* have suggested activity against *W. bancrofti* adult worms and microfilaria, but more research is needed.[19,20]

Most authorities recommend DEC treatment for infected people regardless of whether they have signs and symptoms of lymphatic filariasis. The goal of treatment is to clear the infection. There is little evidence that DEC alters the course of acute adenolymphangitis, or results in clinical improvement of long-standing lymphedema, elephantiasis, or hydrocele. There is, at present, one report that suggests that DEC and albendazole can reverse lymphatic pathology in children infected with *Brugia malayi*.[21] Children with TPE should be treated with DEC to prevent progression to chronic interstitial lung disease. Multiple courses (6 to 8 mg/kg/day for 21 days) may be required; if a clinical response and a decline in eosinophilia are not observed, alternative diagnoses should be considered.

There is growing evidence that lymphedema of the leg can be arrested and potentially reversed by measures such as proper hygiene, skin care, and treatment of skin lesions (e.g., with topical antifungal and antibacterial agents), elevation of the leg, exercise, and, in advanced cases, prophylactic antibiotics to prevent secondary infection.[22] Surgical repair is effective for hydrocele, but often is unsatisfactory for elephantiasis.

Special Considerations

Microfilariae have been observed infrequently in umbilical cord blood of infants born to infected mothers. Children born to infected mothers are more likely to have microfilaremia during childhood than children born to uninfected mothers.[23] It is unknown whether this apparent "tolerance" to infection is associated with higher or lower risk of disease.

Prevention

Recommendations for personal protection for travelers or visitors to endemic areas include use of insect repellent and bednets, wearing of clothing that covers the arms and legs, and avoidance of outdoor exposure between dusk and dawn. Prophylactic use of DEC has not been evaluated adequately. In 1997, the World Health Organization launched a global effort to eliminate lymphatic filariasis as a public health problem (website: http://

www.filariasis.org).[24] Recommended interventions include periodic mass treatment with DEC or ivermectin (in combination with albendazole), fortification of household salt with DEC, and vector control. Success in some areas has stressed the need to improve protocols and serologic tests to determine when annual mass drug administration can be interrupted and how surveillance should be performed subsequently.[25]

ONCHOCERCIASIS

Onchocerciasis, a leading cause of blindness worldwide, results from infection with *Onchocerca volvulus*. The infection is transmitted by blackflies of the genus *Simulium*, which breed near flowing water; hence the name "river blindness." An estimated 37 million people worldwide are infected; the disease is most prevalent in sub-Saharan Africa, but is also found in Yemen and in Central and South America.

In humans, the infective larvae mature in the subcutaneous and deeper connective tissues. Several adult worms of both sexes coil

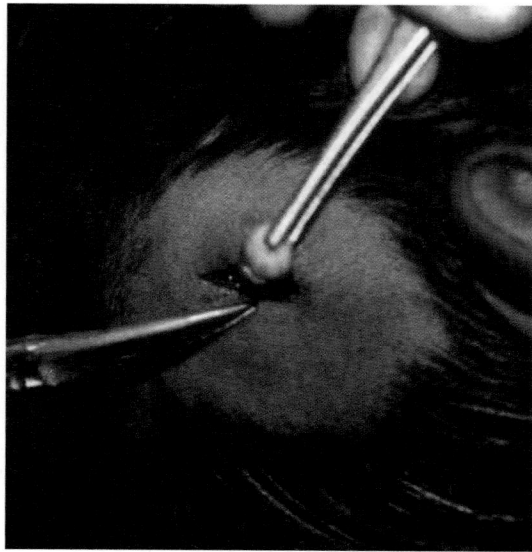

Figure 278-3. Onchocercal nodule being removed from the head of a Guatemalan child. (Courtesy of Frank O. Richards MD, The Carter Center, Atlanta, GA.)

together and form fibrous nodules 1 to 2 cm in diameter, which are most noticeable over bony prominences, including the skull (Figure 278-3). Adult females can live for 12 to 15 years and produce millions of microfilariae. These microfilariae, which are responsible for the signs and symptoms of onchocerciasis, migrate from the nodule to skin and connective tissues.

Epidemiology

The prevalence of infection increases dramatically during childhood. In hyperendemic areas of West Africa, for example, microfilariae can be detected in the skin of 1% to 2% of children 5 years or younger and in approximately 90% of children 15 years of age.[26] Transplacental infection of microfilariae has been documented. Blindness is rare in young children, but impaired vision secondary to onchocerciasis begins to occur by the second decade of life.

Clinical Manifestations

In addition to subcutaneous nodules, termed onchocercomas, the major clinical manifestations of onchocerciasis are dermatitis, lymphadenitis, and ocular disease. Inflammation surrounding dead microfilariae in the skin gives rise to pruritus, a common early symptom of onchocerciasis in children. Pruritic dermatitis, characterized by epidermal atrophy and loss of pigment, can develop in older children with high microfilarial density.

Ocular disease is the most serious complication of *O. volvulus* infection, yet is less common in people with brief exposures or light infections. Inflammation associated with death of microfilariae in the cornea causes punctate keratitis, an early ocular lesion commonly found in infected children. This lesion seems to resolve without intervention. Usually after years of exposure, vision loss and blindness can result from sclerotic keratitis, anterior uveitis, chorioretinopathy, or optic nerve atrophy.

Laboratory Findings and Diagnosis

Demonstration of microfilariae in the skin is the standard for diagnosis, although microfilariae often are not detectable in infected North American travelers returning from endemic areas. Skin snips are obtained with a sclerocorneal biopsy punch or by elevating a small cone (3 mm in diameter) of skin with a needle or straight pin and shaving it off bloodlessly with a scalpel or razor blade. The skin snip is then incubated in saline at room temperature for 30 minutes to 24 hours to allow the microfilariae to emerge, which can be visualized microscopically.[13] The diagnosis of onchocerciasis also can be made through excision of subcutaneous nodules and identification of the adult worms. Ultrasonography may be helpful in detecting impalpable nodules.[27] When present, microfilariae are detected readily in the anterior chamber of the eye on slit-lamp examination. The chances of detection are increased if patients are asked to sit with their head between their legs for up to 10 minutes prior to the examination. Microfilariae also can be observed in the cornea, vitreous, and retrolental space.

If results of all other tests are negative, including skin snips and ocular examination, and the diagnosis still is considered likely, a single 0.5 to 1.0 mg/kg dose of DEC can be administered diagnostically to provoke a so-called *Mazzotti reaction*. This reaction, which is associated with the death of microfilariae, occurs within a few hours and is characterized by pruritus, a maculopapular rash, fever, edema, and headache. Because these adverse reactions can be severe, this DEC provocative test is not recommended for routine diagnosis. As in lymphatic filariasis, measurement of total antifilarial IgG and IgG subclasses can be useful diagnostically. In addition, assays to detect specific antibodies to *Onchocerca* and PCR assays to detect onchocercal DNA in skin snips are available in specialized laboratories.[28,29]

Treatment

Ivermectin is the drug of choice for treatment of onchocerciasis. Ivermectin is available commercially in the U.S., but is not approved for use in children weighing <15 kg, pregnant women, and mothers nursing infants during the first week of life. Ivermectin is given in a single dose of 150 µg/kg on an empty stomach. Microfilarial densities in the skin are reduced by 85% to 95% 2 months after a single dose; ocular microfilarial densities decline more slowly. Unlike DEC, which formerly was used to treat onchocerciasis, ivermectin causes few adverse ocular reactions. A mild Mazzotti reaction after treatment can occur in 10% to 20% of patients. Patients coinfected with onchocerciasis and loiasis can develop encephalopathy when treated with ivermectin and it is recommended that coinfection with *Loa loa* be excluded prior to onchocerciasis treatment with ivermectin.[30] Ivermectin improves the pruritus and rash associated with onchocercal dermatitis and seems to reverse early disease in the anterior segment of the eye. However, it appears to be less effective in reversing chronic skin depigmentation or posterior ocular disease.

Although ivermectin interferes with release of microfilariae from the uterus of the adult female, the drug does not kill the adult worm. Therefore, repeated single doses of ivermectin are required, usually at 6- to 12-month intervals, particularly for people with ocular disease. All people with a diagnosis of onchocerciasis should undergo slit-lamp examination to assess the extent of ocular involvement. Expert ophthalmologic advice should be sought before treating eye lesions.

Antibiotic trials, with doxycycline, directed against *Wolbachia*, an endosymbiotic bacteria present in *O. volvulus*, have demonstrated decrease in onchocercal microfilaridermia with 6 weeks of therapy and macrofilaricidal activity when given with a single standard dose of ivermectin, but further trials, including those with shorter lengths of therapy, are needed.[31,32]

Prevention

The manufacturer, Merck & Co., has made ivermectin available free of charge for onchocerciasis control programs throughout Africa and Latin America. The following websites contain additional information about onchocerciasis control in Africa and Latin America: the African Programme for Onchocerciasis Control (APOC), http://www.who.int/apoc/en and the Onchocerciasis Elimination Program of the Americas (OEPA), http://www.cartercenter.org/health/river_blindness/oepa.html. To reduce exposure to blackflies, travelers should use insect repellent or wear protective clothing, particularly during the morning and evening, when the insects' biting activity is greatest. Individual prophylactic use of ivermectin has not been evaluated.

LOIASIS

Loa loa infection occurs in West and Central Africa and is transmitted by the bite of the deerfly *Chrysops*. The adult worms, which have a lifespan of up to 17 years, wander through the subcutaneous tissues and sometimes beneath the conjunctiva. Microfilariae circulate in the peripheral blood with a diurnal periodicity; peak microfilarial density occurs around noon.

Epidemiology

Microfilarial prevalence and density increase throughout childhood. Microfilaremia has been reported in a few neonates, but most studies have found no evidence for transplacental transfer of either microfilariae or microfilarial antigen. In areas of intense transmission, the prevalence of microfilaremia can reach 35% in adults, but the prevalence of infection probably is higher because 14% to 67% of persons with documented *L. loa* infection have no detectable microfilaremia.

Clinical Manifestations

The clinical manifestations of loiasis vary from asymptomatic infection to life-threatening complications, including encephalopathy, cardiomyopathy, and renal disease. Clinical signs and symptoms differ between visitors or temporary residents to loiasis-endemic areas and children born and raised in these areas, based on the immune response to the parasite.[33] Temporary residents often have no detectable microfilaremia; they are more likely to experience *Calabar swellings*, which are transient (up to several days' duration) pruritic areas of nontender erythematous angioedema that are several centimeters in diameter. These lesions typically occur on the extremities, such as the wrist or knee, and are thought to be associated with migration of the adult worm. By contrast, infected residents of endemic areas frequently have microfilariae in blood and commonly report subconjunctival migration of the worm across the eye, which can be accompanied by intense conjunctivitis and swelling of the eyelid.

Laboratory Findings and Diagnosis

The diagnosis can be confirmed through detection of microfilariae in peripheral blood obtained during the day or by identification of an adult *L. loa* worm removed either from subcutaneous tissue or from the conjunctiva of the eye. In expatriates, hypereosinophilia (>3000 cells/mm^3) is common, and serum IgE and antifilarial antibody titers are elevated.[34] A PCR test has been described, but is only available in research settings.[35]

Treatment

Because DEC is active against both microfilariae and the adult worm, it is the drug of choice for loiasis (8 to 10 mg/kg/day in 3 divided doses for 21 days), although several courses may be required for successful treatment.[36] Severe adverse reactions, including encephalopathy, are related to microfilarial density before treatment, but reactions can occur in people with moderate microfilaria levels (>2000 microfilariae/mL of blood) as well. Neither a gradual increase in DEC dose nor pretreatment with corticosteroids is completely effective in preventing encephalitis in such patients. Patients should be monitored closely during initiation of treatment and may require hospitalization. Plasmapheresis has been used to reduce the microfilarial load prior to treatment in persons with high numbers of circulating microfilariae prior to initiation of DEC and corticosteroid therapy. DEC should not be used in patients with concomitant onchocerciasis because of the risk of severe Mazzotti reactions, characterized by an intense pruritic rash, fever, hypotension, and possibly ocular damage (in those with microfilariae in the eyes). Ivermectin reduces microfilarial density but does not appear to kill the adult worm. Ivermectin has been associated with encephalopathy in persons with high *L. loa* microfilarial counts (>30,000 mf/mL) who are coinfected with *L. loa* and *O. volvulus* and is not recommended for the treatment of loiasis.[30] Preliminary observations indicate that albendazole may kill the adult stage of the parasite.[37] At present, there is no evidence for *Wolbachia* endosymbiosis with *L. loa*.[38]

Prevention

Personal protection measures from deerfly bites are recommended. A study of Peace Corps volunteers in West Africa suggested that DEC (300 mg once weekly) can be taken prophylactically to reduce the risk of infection.[39]

OTHER CAUSES OF FILARIASIS

Mansonella streptocerca

Mansonella streptocerca is transmitted by midges and is found in West and Central Africa. Adult worms live in the dermis and subcutaneous tissues. Microfilariae are found in the skin and can be diagnosed from skin snips or biopsies. Signs and symptoms include hypopigmented macular lesions over the thorax, pruritic dermatitis, and lymphadenopathy; asymptomatic infection is common. Treatment with DEC (6 mg/kg/day for 21 days) kills both adult worms and microfilariae. Ivermectin is effective against the microfilariae.[40] Both drugs can produce Mazzotti reactions.

Mansonella perstans

Mansonella perstans is transmitted by midges in sub-Saharan Africa, in Central and South America, and in focal areas of Algeria and Tunisia. The adult worms, which rarely are recovered, live in the peritoneal, pericardial, and pleural cavities and in associated connective tissue; microfilariae appear in the blood. The prevalence of microfilaremia rises with age. Infection has been reported in children as young as 2 years. Most people with microfilaremia are asymptomatic, but a variety of symptoms have been associated with infection, including arthralgias, pruritus, conjunctival granulomas, periorbital edema, angioedema similar to Calabar swellings, and, rarely, pericarditis.

Diagnosis is made through detection of microfilariae in the blood. Eosinophilia and coinfection with *L. loa, W. bancrofti*, or *O. volvulus* are common findings. Although chronic sequelae are poorly defined, treatment is recommended. Mebendazole (adult dose, 100 mg twice daily for 14 to 21 days), alone or in combination with DEC, appears to be more effective than DEC alone in clearing *M. perstans* microfilaremia.[41] Albendazole may be of value when given at a dose of 400 mg twice daily for at least 1 month. Repeated courses of DEC (6 mg/kg/day for 14 to 21 days) may not be effective and ivermectin has not proven effective. A recent trial has demonstrated that doxycycline (200 mg daily for 6 weeks) is effective.[42] Adverse reactions are similar to those associated with treatment of other filarial infections and are related to microfilarial levels. There is evidence for *Wolbachia* endosymbiosis in at least some isolates of *M. perstans*.[43]

Mansonella ozzardi

Mansonella ozzardi is transmitted by midges and blackflies in the Caribbean and Central and South America. Adult *M. ozzardi* live in serous cavities, particularly the thoracic and peritoneal cavities, and connective and subcutaneous tissues. Most infected persons are asymptomatic, although infection has been associated with arthralgia, pruritus, adenopathy, keratitis, and vague constitutional symptoms. Eosinophilia is a common finding. Little is known about the epidemiology of *M. ozzardi* infection in children. Diagnosis is made through detection of microfilariae in blood or skin snips. Treatment with DEC or albendazole is ineffective. A single 150 μg/kg dose of ivermectin reduces microfilaremia.[44]

DIROFILARIASIS

Pulmonary dirofilariasis in humans, a disease of adults, is caused by infection with *Dirofilaria immitis*, the agent of canine heartworm disease. The parasite is transmitted by mosquitoes. In humans, the worms migrate to the right ventricle of the heart, enter the pulmonary arteries, are carried to the periphery of the lung, and degenerate or calcify, causing solitary pulmonary nodules that classically appear as "coin lesions" on chest radiographs. They are unable to complete maturation in the human host. Although most affected people are asymptomatic, some experience cough, hemoptysis, or chest pain. Eosinophilia occurs in <15% of cases. Microfilaremia has not been observed in humans. Diagnosis is made by biopsy of the lung lesion and histologic examination. Although serologic tests are available, their sensitivity and specificity are not adequate for the diagnosis of human dirofilariasis. Antifilarial treatment is not necessary.

Subcutaneous dirofilariasis is caused by infection with *Dirofilaria tenuis*, which lives in the subcutaneous tissues of the raccoon, and *Dirofilaria repens*, which lives in the subcutaneous tissues of dogs and cats. In humans, the adult worms cause subcutaneous granulomas in the conjunctiva, eyelid, oral mucosa, extremities, scrotum, breast, and other tissues. These nodules can be tender, painful, and erythematous. Microfilaremia does not occur. The lesions can be excised surgically to confirm the diagnosis.

279 *Diphyllobothrium, Dipylidium,* and *Hymenolepis* Species

Frank O. Richards, Jr and Susan P. Montgomery

DIPHYLLOBOTHRIUM SPECIES

Description of the Pathogen

Pseudophyllidean cestodes of the genus *Diphyllobothrium* can cause intestinal tapeworm infections in humans. Adult tapeworms develop in mammals, and infection usually is contracted by eating raw or undercooked fish. First-stage larvae are found in crustaceans, and second-stage larvae develop in fish; for some *Diphyllobothrium* species, the second host is unknown. Although *Diphyllobothrium latum* (often called the *fish* or the *broad* tapeworm) is the best-known species infecting humans, about 14 other primarily zoonotic tapeworms (including *D. nihonkaiense, D. cordatum, D. dalliae, D. dendriticum, D. lanceolatum, D. pacificum,* and *D. ursi*) can cause human infection.[1,2] However, only *D. latum* has the ability to compete with its host for vitamin B_{12} and thus place the patient at risk for megaloblastic anemia.

The *Diphyllobothrium* adult-stage tapeworm attaches to the small intestinal mucosa with two sucking grooves (bothria) located on the ventral and dorsal surfaces of the scolex (head). The body of the tapeworm, or the strobila, can reach up to an amazing length of 12 m and is composed of thousands of proglottid segments. The proglottids break off the distal end of the worm and are passed, singly or in chains, during defecation. Each proglottid contains thousands of eggs, some of which can be released into feces during passage through the intestinal tract. Feces must be deposited promptly into fresh or salt water for an egg to hatch and release a free-swimming embryo (the coracidium). The coracidium is ingested by copepods (including *Cyclops* or *Diaptomus* species), enters the body cavity and develops into the first-stage larva, the procercoid. If the copepod is ingested by plankton-eating fish, the second-stage plerocercoid larva develops in the muscles. The size and shape of this larva may help identify the infecting species of *Diphyllobothrium.* Depending on the parasite species, freshwater, anadromous, or marine fish are second intermediate hosts. The second intermediate hosts for *D. latum* are freshwater fish such as trout, pike, turbot, and perch; *D. nihonkaiense* is found in salmon species in the northern Pacific Ocean; and larvae of *D. dendriticum* have been reported in Atlantic salmon and whitefish. The plerocercoid develops into the adult intestinal tapeworm after the infected fish is ingested by an appropriate mammalian or avian host, which for *D. latum* includes humans, dogs, cats, foxes, bears, and pigs; *D. nihonkaiense* is found in brown bear and humans; and another species commonly infecting humans, *D. dendriticum,* can use seagulls and mammals as its definitive host.[1,2]

Epidemiology

Diphyllobothriasis occurs worldwide and is primarily an infection of older children and adults, although infection of a 2-year old child with *D. nihonkaiense* has been reported.[3] Infection is most prevalent in populations whose culinary habits result in consumption of raw or undercooked fish flesh, liver, or roe. The recent development of molecular tools to identify the species of *Diphyllobothrium* causing human infections by polymerase chain reaction has provided new insight into the epidemiology of this disease. In the past, most infections have been attributed to *D. latum* but more recent information suggests other species may be implicated, based on species-specific second host preferences and geographic distribution as defined by molecular studies.[1,2,4,5] *D. latum* infections are most prevalent in the temperate and subarctic zones of Eurasia (particularly Finland, Sweden, and Lithuania). *D.*

latum and other *Diphyllobothrium* species occur in other populations of Europe (especially northern Italy, Romania, the lower Volga, and the Baltic nations), in Eskimos in Alaska and Canada, and Latin America (Peru, Chile, and Argentina). *D. dendriticum* is found in regions farther north than *D. latum*; most infections in polar regions are likely due to this species. The majority of human infections in Asia (Japan, Siberia, and Manchuria) are caused by *D. nihonkaiense.*[1] In the United States, infected salmon was implicated in 82% of 52 cases on the West Coast;[6] these infections would most likely be associated with *D. nihonkaiense* given the preference for that species to parasitize Pacific salmon. Fish from the Great Lakes region also have been implicated, although cases of diphyllobothriasis have been less frequently reported from this focus in recent years.[2] Because "fresh" fish are shipped nationally and internationally, the risk associated with consuming certain fish dishes (such as sushi, ceviche, lightly pickled fish, smoked fish, and gefilte fish) is widespread and human infections may be associated with non-native species of *Diphyllobothrium.*[7–9] *Diphyllobothrium* spp. can be introduced into new regions as a result of aquaculture; one example is the possible introduction of *D. latum* to lakes in South America by means of plerocercoid infection in food fish species.[10]

Clinical Manifestations

Few pathologic changes are observed in the intestinal mucosa of animals with diphyllobothriasis and most infected people are asymptomatic. In a study in eastern Finland, 37% of the 295 tapeworm carriers had symptoms (versus 8% of 832 controls) that included diarrhea, fatigue, change in appetite, and paresthesias; younger persons were less likely to have symptoms.[1] Abdominal pain, nausea, and diarrhea occurred in 2 of 4 cases of diphyllobothriasis in a U.S. outbreak associated with salmon sushi.[11] Parts of the strobila can be passed in stool or vomitus, but proglottids are not very motile and do not spontaneously exit the anus, as can proglottids of the beef tapeworm *Taenia saginata.* Intestinal obstruction can occur when multiple worms are present. Megaloblastic anemia resulting from vitamin B_{12} deficiency is said to occur in up to 2% of *D. latum*-infected Scandinavian adults; pallor, fatigue, hypotrophic glossitis, decreased vibration sense, paresthesia, and central scotoma have been described as clinical features in such patients.

Laboratory Findings and Diagnosis

Mild eosinophilia of 5% to 15% can occur. Intestinal diphyllobothriasis is diagnosed by finding typical eggs in feces ≥5 weeks after ingestion of infected fish. Egg discharge is periodic in intestinal diphyllobothriasis, so the diagnosis can be missed by examining a single stool sample. Eggs are light yellow, operculated, and ovoid, with dimensions ranging from 40 to 80 μm. The microscopist may confuse *Diphyllobothrium* eggs with other operculated eggs produced by flukes of the several genera including *Clonorchis, Fasciola, Nanophyetus,* and *Paragonimus.* The proglottids are of a fleshy consistency and ivory in color (sometimes with central darkening); they are wider (15 mm) than they are long (4 mm). The appearance of these "broad" proglottids is suggestive of the diagnosis of diphyllobothriasis, but a species diagnosis is difficult, even when the proglottids and scolex are recovered and submitted to experts for examination. Although megaloblastic anemia is rare, up to 50% of tapeworm carriers in Finland have reduced serum vitamin B_{12} levels.[12]

Treatment

For intestinal infections, single-dose therapy with praziquantel (5 to 10 mg/kg) is highly efficacious (85% to 95% cure rate); purgatives are not necessary. Niclosamide also is effective as a single dose, but it is no longer available in the U.S. Stool examinations to evaluate for cure may be performed 6 or more weeks after therapy. Cobalamin injections and oral folic acid are indicated in patients with clinical or laboratory evidence of vitamin B_{12} deficiency.

Prevention

Preventing *Diphyllobothrium* infection in humans depends on altering eating habits because regulations for proper disposal of human feces alone will have no impact on contamination of water supplies with eggs from animal sources. Cooking fish to an internal temperature of at least 63°C is recommended. Freezing at −35°C or below and storing at −20°C for 24 hours kills plerocercoids and renders the meat safe for consumption. Canned fish is safe but smoked fish is only safe if the fish was frozen appropriately prior to smoking in order to kill any parasites.[13] Although diphyllobothriasis is not transmitted from person to person, more than one family member can be infected by sharing common meals and having similar eating habits.

DIPYLIDIUM CANINUM

Description of the Pathogen

Dipylidium caninum (the "dog tapeworm" or "double-pored" tapeworm) is a common intestinal cestode of domestic dogs and cats that can infect children who ingest fleas. The head (scolex) of the adult worm has four suckers and is armed with up to seven rows of hooklets. The 15- to 70-cm tapeworm chain (strobila) consists of about 150 proglottids. The proglottids, which are highly motile, are passed whole in feces and easily observed in stool; they later disintegrate in soil to release their eggs. The eggs develop into cysticercoid larvae only if they are consumed by the larval stage fleas. The life cycle is completed when an infected flea is ingested by a dog or cat during its grooming activities.[14]

Epidemiology

Young children can become infected if they swallow fleas while playing with their pets or when crawling in flea-infested areas. From 1973 to 1977, a period when the Centers for Disease Control and Prevention (CDC) was the only source of the drug niclosamide in the U.S., about 8 cases were reported per year.[15]

Clinical Manifestations

Parents usually find proglottids as multiple, motile white objects resembling rice or seeds (often described as cucumber, melon, or pumpkin seeds) in stool or diapers or on the perineum[16] (Figure 279-1A). The child usually is asymptomatic, although anogenital pruritus, rash, irritability, diarrhea, and abdominal pain have been described. Older children can complain of spontaneously passing proglottids per anus. A history of dog or cat pets, fleas, and flea bites are important clues to the diagnosis.

Laboratory Findings and Diagnosis

The differential diagnosis includes enterobiasis (pinworm) and intestinal myiasis (fly larvae). Parents should be advised to place

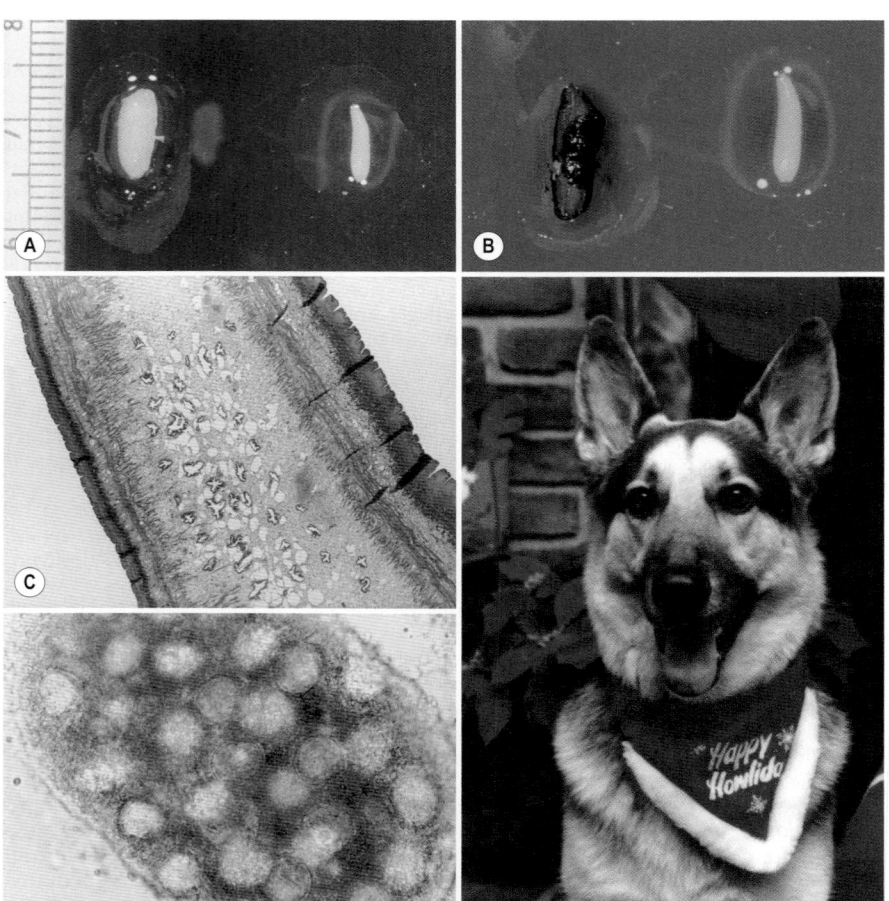

Figure 279-1. A 20-month-old girl was seen in consultation because of "moving rice" in the stool on the diaper. **(A)** A grain of rice from the hospital cafeteria is seen on the left, and the patient's "rice" on the right. **(B)** A drop of iodine shows the typical carbohydrate blackening of rice on the left. Note the 7 mm vase-shape of patient's "rice" on the right. **(C)** Histologic section of "rice" shows typical structure of *Dipylidium caninum*.
(D) Typical egg packet of *Dipylidium caninum* is seen from patient's stool specimen. The veterinarian of the family dog **(E)** did not confirm that his patient had parasites or fleas. (Courtesy of Joel E. Mortensen, PhD, and Sarah S. Long, MD, St. Christopher's Hospital for Children, Philadelphia, PA.)

the proglottids in rubbing alcohol to preserve their differential characteristics for diagnosis. Grossly, a gravid *D. caninum* proglottid measures 3 to 4 mm wide and 10 to 12 mm long, is narrowed at both ends, and has two lateral indentations (pores) at its longitudinal midpoint (Figure 279-1B). Stool examinations usually are negative because few eggs are released from proglottids into the fecal stream. However, characteristic egg packets (a loose membrane usually containing 8 to 63 eggs and measuring 120 to 200 μm in length) can be identified in stool or on perianal adhesive tape ("paddle") preparations (Figure 279-1D).[14,16]

Treatment

Single-dose therapy with praziquantel (5 to 10 mg/kg) is the recommended therapy. Praziquantel is not approved for treatment of children <4 years of age but has been used successfully to treat cases of *D. caninum* infection in children as young as 6 months.[16,17,18] Niclosamide is effective but is not available in the U.S. No purge or follow-up stool examination is indicated, but appearance of proglottids after therapy is indication for retreatment. The infection is self-limiting in the human host and typically clears spontaneously by 6 weeks.

Prevention

Periodic deworming of pets controls this and other canine and feline helminthic infections of pediatric concern (including *Toxocara* species and hookworm). Flea control also is important. Examination of asymptomatic family members rarely is indicated.

HYMENOLEPIS NANA AND *HYMENOLEPIS DIMINUTA*

Description of the Pathogen

Human hymenolepiasis is caused by either *Hymenolepis nana* (the *dwarf tapeworm*) or, rarely, *Hymenolepis diminuta* (the *rodent tapeworm*). The complex life cycles of these cestodes consist of adult (tapeworm) stages in the small bowel of humans and rodents, and larval (cysticercoid) tissue stages in insects. Notably, the cysticercoid stages of *H. nana* also can invade and develop in the human intestine; as a result, *H. nana* is capable of completing its entire life cycle in the human host and, through autoinfection, increase its numbers without having to pass through the insect host. Animal studies demonstrate that T-lymphocyte-mediated immunity is important in preventing hyperinfection by these parasites.[19,20]

H. nana usually is acquired by ingestion of eggs, the hexacanth embryos of which invade the villi of the small intestine. Within 4 to 6 days the embryo develops into a cysticercoid larva that re-enters the lumen, evaginates to become the head (scolex) of the tapeworm, and attaches to the mucosal wall. Morphologically, the scolex has four suckers and numerous hooklets. A body (strobila) measuring 0.5 to 4.5 cm in length and 1 mm in width develops behind the scolex in about 2 weeks. The strobila consists of proglottid segments that periodically break off and rapidly degenerate to release their eggs into the fecal stream. Unlike all other tapeworms that infect humans, *H. nana* eggs are infectious immediately when passed. In addition to being a risk to others, infected people may reingest their own eggs via fecal–hand–mouth transfer (external autoinfection), or alternatively, eggs may hatch in the intestine, reinvade, and develop into new worms (internal autoinfection). A variety of insects that consume feces support development of *H. nana* cysticercoids in their body cavities. Ingestion of these insects by humans or rodents is another route of infection.

The *H. diminuta* tapeworm is much larger than *H. nana* and measures 10 to 60 cm in length and 2 to 4 mm in width. Completion of the life cycle of *H. diminuta* is dependent on development of the cysticercoid stage in the body cavities of insects that ingest eggs they find in rodent feces; autoinfection does not occur. Most commonly minute flour, grain, or dung beetles, fleas, and cockroaches serve as intermediate hosts. Rodents and rarely humans acquire the intestinal stage by consuming uncooked corn, flour, cereal, grains, and dried fruit contaminated with infected insects.

Epidemiology

H. nana is the most common cestode infecting children, with a prevalence ranging from 0.1% to 50% and the highest rates occurring in school-aged children in hot, arid areas of the developing world.[19] Changes in hygienic habits and immunity make *H. nana* infections less common in adults. *H. nana* infections usually are transmitted through fecal–oral contact. In 1987, diagnostic laboratories in the U.S. found *H. nana* eggs in 0.4% of 216,000 stool specimens;[21] however, infection rates in orphanages and institutions were reported to be as much as 10 times higher.[22] Undefined host factors are important. In a 22-month longitudinal study in Pakistan, one-third of children with similar exposure risks were never infected, one-third were infected intermittently, and one-third were always infected.[23] *H. diminuta* infections tend to occur in conditions in which rodents and insects have access to grain stores.

Clinical Manifestations

The intensity of infection, or the worm burden, is the major determinant of symptomatology. Patients whose egg density in stool is greater than 15,000/g invariably have abdominal cramps, diarrhea, and irritability.[24] In light infections, patients are asymptomatic. Based on uncontrolled studies, some authors have suggested that *H. nana* toxins can cause seizures or conjunctivitis. *H. diminuta* infections usually are asymptomatic.[19]

Laboratory Findings and Diagnosis

Mild to moderate eosinophilia is an inconsistent finding, and serologic tests are not available. The diagnosis most often is made by finding characteristic eggs in stool. The *H. nana* egg is round, 30 to 50 μm in diameter and has a double-layered shell that encloses characteristic filaments arising from bipolar thickenings. The enclosed embryo contains 6 hooklets. *H. diminuta* eggs are larger (60 to 85 μm in diameter) and have no polar filaments. Fecal concentration techniques that examine larger amounts of stool are preferred to direct fecal smears. *H. nana* eggs can disintegrate if the specimen is not examined promptly or preserved in formalin. Three stool examinations performed on alternate days are necessary to exclude a suspected infection. The proglottids disintegrate rapidly during their intestinal transit and usually are not observed in feces.

Treatment

A single dose of praziquantel (25 mg/kg) cures 95% to 100% of *H. nana* and *H. diminuta* infections and is the preferred treatment.[19,25] Niclosamide (not available in the U.S.) is not effective as a single dose but must be given daily for 1 week.[15] Repeat stool examinations are recommended 4 weeks after therapy to document cure.

Special Considerations

Family members of patients infected with *H. nana*, particularly siblings, should have stools examined. Simultaneous chemotherapy in institutions and family members may be indicated in some circumstances. Up to 11% of Cambodian refugee children have been reported to have *H. nana* infections.[26] Few examples of *H. nana* dissemination in immunosuppressed humans have been reported, but HIV-infected people who live in *H. nana*-endemic areas have been reported with disseminated disease.[19,27,28]

Prevention

Transmission of *H. nana* can be controlled by measures that decrease fecal–oral contact, particularly hand hygiene after defecation and diaper changing. Hand hygiene after handling pet rodents is advised. Infected food handlers should be treated and cure verified by repeat stool examinations. Rodent and insect control are important, and corn, grain, flour, cereal, and dried fruit stores should be sealed.

280 *Taenia solium, Taenia asiatica,* and *Taenia saginata* (Taeniasis and Cysticercosis)

Michael Cappello, Peter M. Schantz, and A. Clinton White, Jr

Clinical syndromes associated with infection with *Taenia* species tapeworms include intestinal disease caused by adult parasites (taeniasis), as well as single or multiorgan inflammatory conditions attributable to tissue containing larval stages (cysticercosis and coenurosis).[1–3] Distinguishing morphologic features of adult tapeworms include an anterior scolex, followed by a series of segments (proglottids) that extend distally as the worm grows (Figure 280-1). Like most cestodes, *Taenia saginata, T. asiatica,* and *T. solium* require an intermediate host in order to complete their life cycle and infect humans, who are the definitive hosts. In contrast, humans are accidental intermediate hosts for *T. multiceps* and *T. serialis,* the agents of coenurosis (see Chapter 282, *Taenia (Multiceps) multiceps* and *Taenia serialis* (Coenurosis)) and the tissue form or cysticercus of *T. solium* (cysticercosis).

TAENIASIS

Epidemiology and Life Cycle

Taeniasis refers to intestinal infection with the human tapeworms *T. saginata, T. asiatica,* or *T. solium* (class Cestoidea in the phylum Platyhelminthes).[1] The beef tapeworm, *T. saginata,* is endemic in Africa, eastern Europe, Latin America, the Middle East and much of Asia. The prevalence in endemic areas where cattle raising is common, e.g., Africa, can exceed 90%.[4] The pork tapeworm, *T. solium,* also has a worldwide geographic distribution, occurring in rural communities where raising pigs is a common practice.[5–8] Highly endemic areas include Central and South America, Mexico, sub-Saharan Africa, India, and Southeast Asia. The recently identified tapeworm *Taenia asiatica,* which is closely related to *T. saginata,* also is endemic throughout much of Asia.[9–12] Although the clinical presentation and adult worm morphology are very similar to *T. saginata,* the intermediate host of *T. asiatica,* like *T. solium,* is the pig. Although local transmission of *T. solium* has been described in the United States, the majority of these cases involve infection with the larval stages (cysticercosis) and not intestinal taeniasis.[13–15]

Infection with *T. saginata* is acquired by eating undercooked beef that contains cysticerci, which are larval forms of the parasite (Figure 280-2). Upon entering the small intestine, larvae excyst and attach to the mucosal surface using four suckers on the anterior scolex (see Figure 280-1). As it matures, the adult tapeworm extends distally by forming new proglottids, a process referred to as strobilization. These segments pass through the large intestine and are either excreted in the feces or actively exit the host via independent motility. Adult *T. saginata* tapeworms, which can grow to a length of 10 m, can survive within the intestine of an infected individual for up to 25 years, shedding 6 to 10 proglottids daily, each of which contains up to 80,000 eggs. The incubation period from the time of infection to the passage of *T. saginata* segments is approximately 10 weeks. When eggs or proglottids are ingested by the intermediate bovine host, emerging embryos invade the intestinal mucosa and disseminate via the bloodstream to subcutaneous tissues, where they form cysticerci. The life cycle resumes when the definitive human host ingests undercooked beef containing larval cysts. Importantly, unlike *T. solium,* ingested *T. saginata* eggs will not form cysticerci in humans.

Intestinal infection with *T. solium* and *T. asiatica* follows ingestion of undercooked pork containing cysticerci (Figure 280-2). After degradation of the cyst wall, the scolex attaches to the duodenal mucosa and develops into an adult in 6 to 8 weeks. Pigs, the coprophagic intermediate hosts, ingest eggs contained in human waste. The eggs hatch in the stomach and release embryos that penetrate the pig's intestinal wall, and larval stages migrate via the bloodstream to muscle, subcutaneous tissues, or other organs. Humans complete the *T. solium* and *T. asiatica* life cycles by eating pork meat (*T. solium*) or viscera (*T. asiatica*) containing viable cysticerci.

Clinical Manifestations

Most individuals with *T. saginata* or *T. asiatica* infection are asymptomatic, unless they become aware of tapeworm segments passing

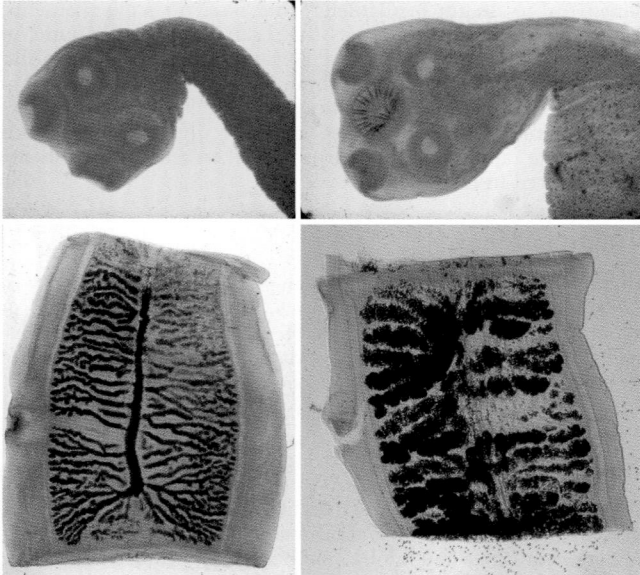

Figure 280-1. Scolices (top) and proglottids (bottom) from the tapeworms *Taenia saginata* (left) and *T. solium* (right). The proglottids are excreted in the feces of infected people. (From U.S. Centers for Disease Control http://dpd.cdc.gov/dpdx/HTML/Image_Library.htm)

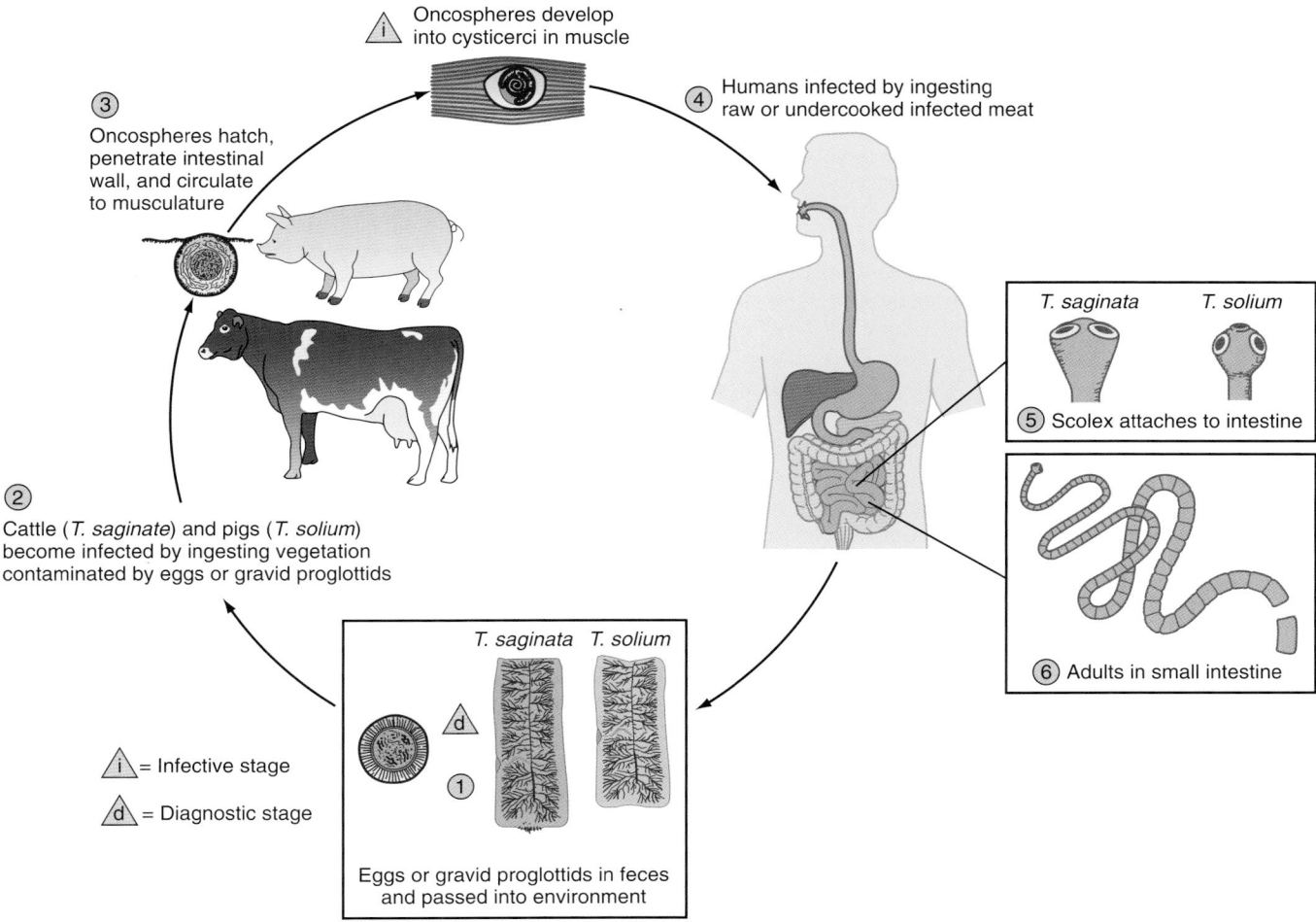

Figure 280-2. Life cycles of *Taenia solium* and *T. saginata.* (Redrawn from the United States Centers for Disease Control and Prevention; http://www.dpd.cdc.gov/dpdx/HTML/ImageLibrary/Taeniasis_il.htm.)

in feces.[4,16] The proglottids often are actively motile and individuals may notice them moving. Mild intermittent gastrointestinal symptoms, such as nausea and epigastric pain, have been reported, as have vomiting, diarrhea, and intestinal obstruction. Migration of proglottids down the thigh can be associated with pruritus.[4] Rarely, proglottid segments are vomited or migrate aberrantly, ultimately leading to appendicitis, cholecystitis, or even colonic perforation.[17–19]

People harboring intestinal *T. solium* frequently are asymptomatic, becoming aware of tapeworm infection only upon fecal passage of proglottids. The *T. solium* proglottid segments are less motile than those of *T. saginata,* so that migration onto the perianal skin is not noted commonly. Anal pruritus and urticaria have been described with heavy infections, sometimes associated with serum eosinophilia. Intestinal symptoms include nausea, abdominal pain, change in appetite, and diarrhea. However, frequent coinfection with other intestinal pathogens makes it difficult to ascribe these symptoms exclusively to taeniasis.

Laboratory Findings and Diagnosis

A definitive diagnosis of intestinal taeniasis requires identification of proglottids or ova excreted from an infected individual. Proglottid specimens should be placed in water or saline prior to analysis.[20] In order to distinguish *T. saginata*/*T. asiatica* from *T. solium,* proglottids can be pressed gently between glass slides and injected with India ink through the lateral pore in order to visualize the uterine branches under light microscopy (see Figure 280-1). *T. saginata* has ≥15 primary uterine branches on each side of the

central core, while *T. solium* usually has <13 per side. Unlike *T. saginata and T. asiatica,* the scolex of *T. solium* possesses two rows of rostellar hooks, which it uses along with four suckers to attach to the mucosa of the small intestine (see Figure 280-1). Because patients infected with adult *T. solium* are at additional risk for cysticercosis secondary to autoinfection, attempts should be made to discriminate between *T. saginata*/*T. asiatica* and *T. solium* infection.[21,22] *Taenia* eggs, which rarely are present in fecal samples, cannot be distinguished based on morphology when viewed by light microscopy. Laboratory tests may reveal mild peripheral blood eosinophilia.

Coproantigen detection of *Taenia*-specific antigens by fecal enzyme immunoassay (EIA) is more sensitive than standard microscopy for detecting infection.[1,23–26] Immunodiagnostic and PCR-based tests can detect *Taenia* antigens or DNA in feces, as well as distinguish between the major species.[26–33] Thus far these assays have been utilized primarily in research settings, and their role in the routine diagnosis of tapeworm infections has not been established. Serodiagnostic testing for *Taenia* infection is used primarily for diagnosing cysticercosis, particularly involving the central nervous system (CNS) (see below). Serologic tests that are specific for the *T. solium* tapeworm carriers also have been developed, but are not available widely.[3,34,35]

Treatment

Anthelmintic drug therapy is recommended for all children found to harbor an intestinal tapeworm. Praziquantel, administered orally in a single dose (5 to 10 mg/kg), is the drug of choice for taeniasis.[36,37] In children with *T. solium* infection, even modest doses of praziquantel occasionally can trigger the destruction of occult CNS cysts, particularly those in the brain parenchyma, perhaps leading to seizures.[38] Albendazole, although effective for treating cysticercosis (see below), is not recommended routinely for the treatment of intestinal tapeworm infection.[39] Niclosamide (currently not marketed in the U.S.) and nitazoxanide can be used as alternatives.[40,41] Effective treatment can be associated with passage of intact or disintegrating proglottids for days. However, purgatives can hasten the process and help identify passage of the scolex (as a test of cure). If the scolex is not identified, a second stool examination should be performed approximately 3 months following anthelmintic therapy, allowing time for regeneration of proglottids from the scolex. Because reinfection is common in endemic areas, repeated courses of therapy may be necessary for long-term control.

Prevention and Control

Thorough cooking of meat is a key measure for the prevention of infection with *Taenia*. In general, transmission of taeniasis can be reduced by improving sanitation and husbandry practices, along with strict inspection of pork or beef prior to sale or consumption.[2,5,42] Unfortunately, in many resource-poor countries, these practices are not feasible economically. Public health measures such as sanitary disposal of human feces and restriction of cattle and pigs from land contaminated by human feces may also prevent transmission. Although freezing of meat at $-20\,^{\circ}$C kills cysticerci, this often is not practical in endemic areas. There is currently no available vaccine for human *T. saginata* infection, although protection of calves from challenge infection has been achieved following immunization with an oncospheral adhesion protein.[43]

Mass chemotherapy programs targeting communities where *T. solium* is highly endemic may reduce transmission from humans to pigs, thereby interrupting the natural life cycle of *T. solium*.[6,44] One intervention study demonstrated that the prevalence of human taeniasis was reduced from 3.5% to 1% within 10 months following treatment, while the seroprevalence of *T. solium* infection in pigs was concomitantly reduced from 55% to 7%.[45] Such strategies will likely have long-term benefit only if education succeeds in reducing the behaviors that encourage the proliferation and transmission of the parasite within high-risk communities. Vaccination of pigs using recombinant *T. solium* proteins also has potential to limit the burden of disease in the porcine host, thus reducing the prevalence of taeniasis (and cysticercosis) in humans.[6,46-49]

CYSTICERCOSIS

Cysticercosis refers to infection of tissues or organs caused by larval stage (cysticercus) of *T. solium*. Neurocysticercosis, or infection of the CNS, is recognized as a significant cause of neurologic disease in developing countries, and is also an emerging disease in the U.S.[13,15,50-58]

Epidemiology and Pathogenesis

The availability of brain imaging studies, especially computed tomography (CT) scans, has led to an increased appreciation of the significance of neurocysticercosis as a common cause of neurologic disease. Studies from Latin America have reported that up to half of patients with adult-onset seizures demonstrated evidence of neurocysticercosis based on results of imaging studies.[59-63] Subsequent population based surveys in Latin America and sub-Saharan Africa have documented CT abnormalities consistent with neurocysticercosis in up to 70% of individuals from rural communities with seizures.[52,64-68] Among patients with focal seizures in India, CT scans demonstrated abnormalities consistent with neurocysticercosis in 40%, including lesions diagnosed as active cysticercosis, typical calcifications, or single enhancing CT lesions (granulomas).[69,70] Similar data were noted for children with seizures and in patients from northern India.[71] Significantly, although single-enhancing CT lesions in this group were frequently attributed to other causes, excisional biopsies demonstrated histopathologic evidence of cysticercosis in most. Neurocysticercosis is also becoming increasingly recognized as a major public health problem throughout Asia.[51,72-75] Worldwide, it has been estimated that neurocysticercosis is responsible for nearly 30% of the burden of epilepsy in endemic areas.[76]

Human cysticercosis follows ingestion of eggs excreted by a tapeworm-infected person, presumably by fecal–oral contamination. Thus it is essential to recognize that neurocysticercosis is not acquired directly from eating pork, as illustrated by cases that have occurred in an Orthodox Jewish community and vegetarians, and even a case of CNS disease in an infant.[72,77,78] However, it is also worth noting that tapeworm carriers can infect themselves via fecal–oral contamination, and thus both stages of the parasite (cysticercus and adult tapeworm) can be found in a single individual. Following ingestion, the eggs hatch and release oncospheres that invade the circulatory system and disseminate to somatic tissues, where they mature into cysticerci. Those that arrest in skeletal and cardiac muscle, subcutaneous tissue, and lung can be from granulomas, which over time calcify. However, the majority of disease attributable to cysticercosis results from invasion of the CNS.

Following tissue invasion, cysticerci reach their final size within a few weeks. Symptoms of neurologic disease, however, usually develop several years after infection.[13,79] Although the parasites secrete a variety of immunomodulatory compounds that can suppress the host inflammatory response, over time, cysticerci eventually trigger a host inflammatory response mediated by a variety of cytokines.[80-88] Degradation of the parasite cyst occurs in stages. During the colloid stage, the cyst wall degenerates, with invasion by inflammatory cells. The cysticercus eventually fibroses and the cavity collapses (*granular-nodular stage*). Finally the granulomatous cyst can calcify (*calcified stage*). It may be possible to detect remnants of the cysticercus (e.g., hooklets) in the calcified lesion.

Clinical Manifestations

A number of factors influence the clinical features of neurocysticercosis in children, with potential impact on management (Figure 280-3).[89-93] Neurocysticercosis typically is separated into parenchymal and extraparenchymal disease based on whether or not there is involvement outside of the brain tissues.[14,94,95] Extraparenchymal locations include the subarachnoid space, ventricles, spinal column, and the eye. It is not uncommon for a single patient to have parenchymal and extraparenchymal infection. Most children with parenchymal neurocysticercosis present with seizures caused by single-enhancing parenchymal cysts, while severe or fatal cases of neurocysticercosis often are associated with extraparenchymal disease.[93,96,97] Patients with parenchymal lesions, particularly those with single enhancing lesions, have a favorable prognosis with medical therapy. By contrast, subarachnoid and ventricular cysts often cause increased intracranial pressure and hydrocephalus, which can be fatal without surgical intervention.

In addition to location, management of neurocysticercosis also requires distinction between viable or degenerating parasites (sometimes called *active disease*) and residua of prior infection (termed *inactive disease*).[98-100] This distinction often is based on the results of neuroimaging studies. Inactive disease implies that the cysts are not viable, and that symptoms occur in response to residual scarring or antigen deposition from prior infection. Imaging studies can reveal calcifications or chronic hydrocephalus but no parasites. Thus, treatment is focused on symptoms. By contrast, viable cysticerci and degenerating parasites demonstrate cystic lesions on imaging studies and often respond to antiparasitic drugs.

Parenchymal Neurocysticercosis

Seizures are the main clinical manifestation of parenchymal neurocysticercosis.[89,90,92,101-103] Seizures usually are focal with

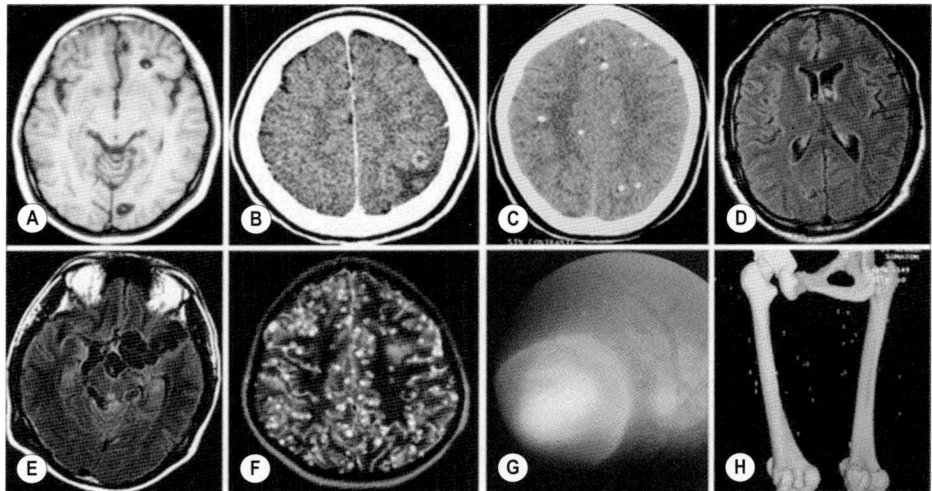

Figure 280-3. Diverse presentations of neurocysticercosis. Multiple viable cysts (vesicular stage; **A);** single enhancing lesion (degenerating cysts; **B);** multiple intraparenchymal calcifications **(C);** intraventricular cyst **(D);** basal subarachnoid cysticercosis (extraparenchymal neurocysticercosis; **E);** cysticercotic encephalitis (extraparenchymal neurocysticercosis; **F);** ocular cysticercosis **(G);** and muscle cysticercosis **(H).** (From Garcia HH, Del Brutto OH. Neurocysticercosis: updated concepts about an old disease. Lancet Neurol 2005;4:653–661.)

secondary generalization, but can be described as generalized or focal.[52,55,65,103-108] Electroencephalogram (EEG) in patients with active disease can reveal focal abnormalities, particularly in those with a single inflamed lesion.[106,109] The majority of patients who present with seizures due to neurocysticercosis have evidence of host inflammation, including edema or contrast enhancement by neuroimaging studies. In contrast, cysts without inflammatory changes are thought to cause few symptoms.[107,108] Thus, the majority of symptomatic infections are likely mediated by host inflammatory responses. Seizures usually can be controlled during treatment with anti-epileptic drugs and often resolve after normalization of imaging studies as the inflammation subsides.[110] Relapse, however, is common, particularly in patients who develop residual calcifications.[104,111]

One uncommon form of parenchymal disease is cysticercal encephalitis, which is characterized by large numbers of inflamed cysts with diffuse cerebral edema, increased intracranial pressure, seizures, and altered mental status. Cysticercal encephalitis occurs more commonly in children than adults, and often is complicated by increased intracranial pressure and diffuse cerebral edema.[111,112]

The hallmark characteristic of inactive parenchymal neurocysticercosis is the presence of calcifications, which typically are solid and measure 2 to 10 mm in diameter.[100,113-116] Children with inactive lesions often present with seizures and infrequently have focal abnormalities on EEG. In some patients, magnetic resonance imaging (MRI) shows that the calcifications are associated with enhancement and edema, which suggests inflammation mediated by release of parasite antigens.

Extraparenchymal Neurocysticercosis

Patients with ventricular neurocysticercosis most often present with symptoms or signs of increased intracranial pressure, including nausea/vomiting, dizziness, vision changes, or altered mental status.[97,112,117-119] The onset of symptoms can be abrupt (due to acute obstruction), intermittent, or gradual. Approximately 10% to 20% of patients with symptomatic neurocysticercosis have evidence of ventricular cysts, which can cause hydrocephalus by obstructing the flow of cerebrospinal fluid (CSF).[120] Cysticerci can develop in any ventricle, and symptoms occur most often when cysts are still viable.[121,122] Computed tomography may show only evidence of obstructive hydrocephalus or distortion of the involved ventricle, while the sensitivity of MRI may be greater for detecting intraventricular cysts.[122,123]

Patients with cysticerci in the gyri of the cerebral convexities (subarachnoid neurocysticercosis) have similar imaging findings and clinical presentation to those with active parenchymal disease. However, these cysts can be larger and not respond as well to chemotherapy. Giant cysticerci, which can grow to several centimeters, can develop within cranial fissures.[123-125] These cysts may

cause a significant mass effect, and often are accompanied by cysticerci in the parenchyma or basilar cisterns. Cysticercosis of the basilar cisterns can be associated with communicating hydrocephalus or arachnoiditis, which can appear on neuroimaging studies as focal or diffuse meningeal enhancement or vasculitis.[100,126,127] Basilar cysticercosis carries a poor prognosis.

Spinal disease occurs rarely in patients with neurocysticercosis, with most cases involving cysticerci in the subarachnoid space.[13,93,97,128-130] Initially, spinal subarachnoid cysticerci are free-floating and can move between levels. When the cysticerci degenerate, they eventually become fixed at one level. The accompanying inflammation can cause mass effect with obstruction of flow demonstrable by myelography. Clinical manifestations include radicular paresthesias or pain, which can progress to myelopathy with bowel or bladder incontinence and paraparesis. Cysticerci rarely are intramedullary, causing cord compression from mass effect or accompanying inflammation.

The most common presentation of ocular cysticercosis is ptosis caused by involvement of extraocular muscles.[131-135] Involvement of the eye usually is subretinal, but can be intravitreal or subconjunctival, and patients can present with altered vision.[136,137] Intraocular disease usually requires surgical removal of cysts.

Mixed Forms of Cysticercosis

Clinical cases, especially those involving dissemination with large numbers of cysticerci, often include >1 of the above forms.[138-145] The pathogenesis and presentation can reflect each location. For example, patients who present with seizures usually have parenchymal cysticerci. However, some also have cysticerci in the basilar cisterns that can progress to hydrocephalus.

Associated Clinical Syndromes

Cysticerci also can be present in skin, muscle, soft tissues, or organs besides the brain, and can be evident as calcifications.[138,139,141-143,145,146] Cysticerci of the subcutaneous tissues may appear as painless cystic lesions that are similar to sebaceous cysts.

Headaches are common among patients with neurocysticercosis, and can occur with parenchymal, ventricular, or cisternal disease.[38,50,93,136,137] Headaches can be hemicranial or bilateral, and are difficult to differentiate from migraine or tension headache. In some cases, headache is an initial symptom of raised intracranial pressure, while the association of parenchymal lesions with migraine-like headaches suggests vascular involvement. Neurocognitive deficits and learning disabilities have been described with cysticercosis.[147-149] There also appears to be an association of cysticercosis with depression and even psychotic episodes.[150-152] By contrast, acute alterations of mental status can reflect ongoing seizures or hydrocephalus. In our experience, altered mental status that does not resolve after a reasonable postictal period usually results from hydrocephalus.

Diagnosis

The most common finding on brain imaging studies in patients with neurocysticercosis is ≥1 parenchymal cystic lesions (see Figure 280-3).[13,79] Parenchymal cysticerci typically measure 4 to 20 mm in diameter and localize to the cerebral cortex, while those that arise within fissures can be as large as 10 cm.[122,153] The fluid within viable cysticerci is isodense with CSF, and the scolex may be visible as a 1 to 3 mm nodule located on the cyst wall.[114,154] In contrast, inflamed cysts appear as ring-enhancing lesions, often with surrounding edema, and the cyst fluid can have increased density. Eventually, cysticerci can evolve into focal areas of enhancement or granulomas. Calcifications within the parenchyma also are a common radiographic finding, and in the absence of an alternative diagnosis (e.g., tuberculosis) should be considered as highly suggestive of neurocysticercosis. MRI may reveal edema and enhancement surrounding calcified lesions, as well as a residual scolex.[121,155] Cysticerci within the ventricles may not be directly visualized by CT, although their presence may be suggested by hydrocephalus. Although CT is more sensitive than MRI at detecting calcifications,[121,122,155,156] MRI provides superior resolution for cysticerci located in the ventricles and subarachnoid space.[157,158]

Issues with sensitivity and specificity have limited the usefulness of serologic assays in the diagnosis of cysticercosis.[35,59,158-164] However, the enzyme-linked immunotransfer blot (EITB), which utilizes a semipurified mixture of *T. solium* membrane antigens, is highly specific, although its sensitivity is limited in patients with single or calcified lesions on brain imaging studies.[160] The test is available through the U.S. Centers for Disease Control and Prevention (www.dpd.cdc.gov/dpdx/HTML/DiagnosticProcedures.htm) as well as commercially. The EITB test also can be performed on CSF, although predictive value is superior with serum.[3,165-167] All of the diagnostic antigens in the EITB test have been cloned and EIAs using the recombinant proteins are in development.[168-173] Assays designed to detect circulating parasite antigens in serum, urine, or CSF have been developed, although the presence of circulating *T. solium* antigens does not necessarily predict risk of clinical sequelae from infection.[35,162,174,175]

Del Brutto and others have proposed specific criteria for the diagnosis of neurocysticercosis combining information from the history (including risk of exposure) with results of neuroimaging studies and serologic tests.[176] A definite diagnosis requires the presence of 1 absolute criterion *or* 2 major criteria plus 2 minor or epidemiologic criteria. Patients with 1 major criterion plus a history of exposure and 2 other criteria, or 3 minor criteria plus exposure are considered probable cases.

In order to meet the **absolute** diagnostic criteria for neurocysticercosis, the parasite must be directly visualized using various modalities, including histology following biopsy of a lesion, fundoscopic examination (in the case of ocular disease), or by identification of the scolex within a cystic lesion using CT or MRI. The **major** diagnostic criteria include results of neuroimaging studies that are highly suggestive of neurocysticercosis (e.g., cystic lesions, single or multiple enhancing ring-like or nodular lesions, and typical parenchymal calcifications). The lesions of neurocysticercosis typically are <20 mm in diameter and rarely cause midline shift.[177] Other **major** criteria include resolution of single or multiple cystic lesions spontaneously or following anticysticercal therapy or satisfaction of clinical criteria for a single enhancing cysticercal granuloma (see below).

Minor criteria include radiographic evidence of lesions that are consistent with, but not pathognomonic for neurocysticercosis (e.g., basilar meningitis, hydrocephalus, or filling defects in the spinal subarachnoid space in the absence of cysticerci). Additional **minor** criteria are symptoms suggestive of neurocysticercosis (including seizures or hydrocephalus), a positive serologic result using a test other than the EITB, and the presence of cysticerci outside the nervous system (e.g., muscle calcifications or

subcutaneous nodules). Risk factors for exposure and infection include residence or prolonged stay in an endemic area and contact with a tapeworm carrier.

Rajshekhar and colleagues developed similar clinical and radiologic criteria for cysticercal granulomas among patients who presented with seizures and single enhancing lesions.[177,178] The combination of a single, round, enhancing lesion <20 mm in diameter and without midline shift, in patients with no signs of increased intracranial pressure, focal neurologic deficits, or evidence of systemic disease, was highly suggestive of neurocysticercosis. These criteria were prospectively studied in 400 patients in India with resulting high sensitivity and specificity. Of note, the differential diagnosis of ring or nodular enhancing lesions also includes tuberculoma, brain abscess, and malignancy.

Treatment and Prognosis

The management and prognosis of neurocysticercosis requires careful consideration of a number of factors, including the stage of the disease (active vs. inactive) as well as the number and location (parenchymal vs. extraparenchymal) (Table 280-1).[13,93,104,106,107,129,179] Poor outcomes, including most fatalities, result from failure to provide effective therapy for complications, such as raised intracranial pressure or seizures. Symptomatic therapy is therefore a key element in the management of neurocysticercosis, and should include anti-epileptic medications for patients with seizures, surgery for patients with hydrocephalus, and corticosteroids for patients with diffuse cerebral edema. In patients with seizures from neurocysticercosis, control of the seizures is the first priority and usually can be accomplished with a established drugs such as phenytoin, phenobarbital, or carbamazepime.[108] Recurrent seizures usually are associated with subtherapeutic anti-epileptic drug levels, most often associated with poor medication adherence.[108,110] Studies suggest that many patients can be tapered off seizure medications after ≥1 year of symptom-free maintenance therapy, providing there is radiographic resolution of the lesion.[103,106-108,180,181] However, the rate of seizures after withdrawal of medications can be as high as 40% in some populations.[120,127,182-185] The presence of residual inflamed or calcified lesions is associated with continued seizure risk and may be an indication to continue anti-epileptic drugs indefinitely.

The use of corticosteroids to control host inflammation is an essential component of therapy for certain forms of neurocysticercosis, including cysticercal encephalitis, subarachnoid neurocysticercosis, and spinal intramedullary cysticercosis. Although data on optimal dose or duration of corticosteroid therapy are lacking, doses of 1 mg/kg/day of prednisone or 0.5 mg/kg/day of dexamethasone are used for severe disease. For individuals with parenchymal lesions, co-administration of corticosteroids with antiparasitic drugs may reduce the potentially harmful host inflammatory reaction to parasite antigens. One randomized trial suggested that treatment with a short course of prednisone (1 mg/kg/day for 10 days) led to a marked reduction in seizures and more rapid resolution in patients with single enhancing lesions.[179,186,187] In patients with obstructive hydrocephalus caused by neurocysticercosis, corticosteroids in conjunction with antiparasitic drug treatment may decrease the rate of ventriculoperitoneal shunt failure.[95]

The role of antiparasitic drugs in the treatment of neurocysticercosis has been controversial.[130,178,188] Early uncontrolled trials in Latin America suggested that antiparasitic drugs were associated with an improved prognosis, while studies in the U.S. demonstrated that many single enhancing lesions resolved without antiparasitic therapy.[186-188] In fact, the first randomized, controlled trials of antiparasitic therapy in the management of neurocysticercosis were not published until the 1990s, and only recently has a consensus on optimal management begun to emerge.[95,96,104,108,191,192]

Praziquantel was the first antiparasitic drug reported effective in the treatment of neurocysticercosis.[193,194] Praziquantel is well absorbed after oral administration, but has extensive first-pass metabolism that is enhanced by anti-epileptic drugs and

TABLE 280-1. Treatment Guidelines for Neurocysticercosis (Modified from Garcia HH, Del Brutto OH. Neurocysticercosis: updated concepts about an old disease. Lancet Neurol 2005;4:653–661)

Parenchymal Neurocysticercosis

VESICULAR CYSTS	
Single	Albendazole 15 mg/kg/day (maximum dose 800 mg) in 2 equally divided doses[a] for 8 days, with simultaneous use of corticosteroids (see text for details)
	Praziquantel 75 mg/kg in 3 equally divided doses is an alternative to albendazole
Moderate infections	Albendazole 15 mg/kg/day in 2 equally divided doses[a] for 8 days, with simultaneous use of corticosteroid
Heavy infections (100 or more cysts)	Albendazole 15 mg/kg/day in 2 equally divided doses[a] for 8 days with high doses of corticosteroid
DEGENERATING (COLLOIDAL) CYSTS	
Single lesions	Albendazole 15 mg/kg/day in 2 equally divided doses[a] for 8 days, with simultaneous use of corticosteroid; or no antiparasitic treatment
Moderate infections	Albendazole 15 mg/kg/day in 2 equally divided doses[a] for 8 days with simultaneous use of corticosteroid
Heavy infections (encephalitis)	High doses of corticosteroid; antiparasitic treatment not indicated
CALCIFICATIONS	
Single or multiple	No antiparasitic treatment
EXTRAPARENCHYMAL NEUROCYSTICERCOSIS	
SUBARACHNOID NEUROCYSTICERCOSIS	
Giant cyst (usually in Sylvian fissure)	Albendazole 15 mg/kg/day in 2 equally divided doses[a] for ≥30 days, with high doses of corticosteroid; or surgical excision
Basal subarachnoid (racemose)	Albendazole 15 mg/kg/day in 2 equally divided doses[a] for ≥30 days, with high doses of corticosteroid
Treatment failure	Albendazole 15 mg/kg/day in 2 equally divided doses[a] for ≥30 days, albendazole 30 mg/kg/day for 15 days, or praziquantel 50–100 mg/kg/day for 30 days, or albendazole 15 mg/kg/day plus praziquantel 50 mg/kg/day for 15 days; either of these plus high dose corticosteroid
Ventricular cysts	Endoscopic or surgical resection; alternatively ventricular shunt plus albendazole 15 mg/kg/day in 2 equally divided doses[a] for ≥30 days, with high doses of corticosteroid or methotrexate
Hydrocephalus	No antiparasitic treatment; ventricular shunt
OTHER FORMS OF NEUROCYSTICERCOSIS	
Spinal cysts	Surgical resection, albendazole with corticosteroid may be used
Ocular cysts	Surgical resection

[a]*Maximum albendazole dose is 800 mg/day (i.e., 400 mg twice a day).*

corticosteroids. Co-administration of cimetidine increases blood levels of praziquantel, but effects of the increased drug levels have not been defined.[123,195–198] Single day regimens of oral praziquantel administered in 3 doses (25 mg/kg/dose) 2 hours apart (with cimetidine) have similar efficacy to longer courses of therapy in patients with parenchymal cysticerci.[198–200] By contrast, higher doses or prolonged duration have been associated with improved efficacy for extraparenchymal diseases.[201] Adverse effects of therapy include worsening neurologic function (e.g., headaches, dizziness, seizures, increased intracranial pressure), presumably due to the host inflammatory response to parasite antigens.[90,95]

Albendazole is a benzimidazole antiparasitic agent with broad-spectrum activity against nematodes, cestodes, and protozoa.[90,95,201,202] The recommended dose of albendazole for the treatment of neurocysticercosis is 15 mg/kg/day in 2 divided doses.[90,92,102,108] Side effects are few, and include mild gastrointestinal discomfort. Higher doses have been used in extraparenchymal infections.[90,95,203] Controlled trials in parenchymal neurocysticercosis suggest no difference in resolution by imaging with treatment for 7 days versus longer courses.[204–207] In fact, a 3-day course of albendazole was associated with more rapid resolution of single parenchymal lesions compared with placebo, although risk of seizure recurrence was not reduced.[208] Praziquantel also has been used in combination with albendazole, and a pharmacokinetic study demonstrated increased levels of the active metabolite of albendazole in subjects receiving combination therapy.[209] However, a study in children with single parenchymal brain lesions did not show statistically significant improvement with combination (albendazole and praziquantel) therapy compared with albendazole alone.[210]

The most common presentation of neurocysticercosis among children includes seizures and a single enhancing lesion on neuroimaging studies. Seizures usually respond to a single anti-epileptic medication. The lesions resolve spontaneously over months to years, but most studies show more rapid radiologic resolution with antiparasitic therapy.[95,96,104,108,178,189,211] Recurrent seizures tend to occur earlier in patients receiving antiparasitic medications, which may facilitate control. Several studies have demonstrated a benefit of corticosteroid therapy in reducing seizures with faster CT resolution of lesions when used in conjunction with anti-epileptic medications.[103,106,107,180]

Children presenting with seizures and multiple cysticerci usually have at least one lesion that is inflamed, but often other cysticerci that also may be viable. Thus, recurrent seizures may be due to sequential degradation of cysticerci. In a placebo-controlled trial, Garcia and colleagues demonstrated a small but statistically significant reduction in generalized seizures in patients treated with albendazole plus corticosteroids compared with placebo.[108] The difference increased after patients were tapered off of anti-seizure medications. Based on these results, most experts now recommend that patients with multiple parenchymal cysticerci should be treated with a course of anthelmintics (albendazole 15 mg/kg/day for 8 days) and a short course of corticosteroids concurrently. In patients with multiple cysticerci who present with diffuse cerebral edema ("cysticercal encephalitis"), antiparasitic therapy is contraindicated because the subsequent inflammatory response may worsen clinical sequelae.[113–115] These patients should be treated with high-dose corticosteroids. In most cases, the cysticerci will resolve spontaneously with anti-inflammatory medications alone.

Antiparasitic drugs are not recommended in children with calcified neurocysticercosis, since no viable parasites are likely to be present. However, because patients with inactive parenchymal lesions often experience recurrent seizures, they should be offered long-term anti-epileptic therapy. Although calcified lesions can exhibit significant ring enhancement and/or edema, it remains to be determined whether treatment with corticosteroids is of benefit in controlling seizures in this circumstance.[113-116]

Increased intracranial pressure may be the result of cerebral edema, which usually can be managed with corticosteroids, or hydrocephalus, which often requires surgery.[129,212] If symptoms are mild or intermittent, elective endoscopic removal of ventricular cysticerci is recommended.[112,213] By contrast, obstructive hydrocephalus caused by active ventricular neurocysticercosis is a medical emergency, and relieving hydrocephalus should be the first priority.[112,120,182,183,185,213,214] Ventricular cysts can be removed using endoscopy, which is the preferred approach.[112,118,212,215-217] For more severe cases of acute hydrocephalus, placement of a ventriculoperitoneal shunt, compared with open craniotomy, is associated with a lower perioperative mortality rate.[218] Patients who receive antiparasitic therapy along with shunting require fewer shunt revisions than those who receive shunts alone, but failure rates remain higher than with endoscopic approaches.[123,125,218,219] Corticosteroids also may reduce the risk of shunt obstruction in the setting of neurocysticercosis.[95,120,123,126,220,221] In some patients, hydrocephalus develops subsequent to infection as a result of chronic inflammation and scarring (e.g., aqueductal stenosis).[95] These patients, who may require placement of a ventriculoperitoneal shunt to relieve chronic hydrocephalus, likely do not benefit from treatment with antiparasitic agents.

Subarachnoid cysticercosis, which can be complicated by significant mass effect, communicating hydrocephalus, cerebral vasculitis, and basilar meningitis, carries a particularly poor prognosis.[112,123,126,220] These patients should receive prolonged courses of anthelmintics (e.g., albendazole 15 mg/kg/day for at least 28 days) along with high doses of corticosteroids (1 mg/kg/day of prednisone or 0.5 mg/kg/day of dexamethasone). Even with this therapy, patients often develop recurrent symptoms, which may respond to repeated courses, prolonged duration, or higher doses of albendazole, or changing to or adding praziquantel. Optimal therapy has not been defined for spinal neurocysticercosis. Intramedullary disease should be treated surgically, due to the risk of paralysis from cord edema. Some cases of spinal subarachnoid cysts may respond to antiparasitic drugs. Surgical removal of ocular cysts generally is recommended, with no clearly defined role for anthelmintic therapy.

Prevention

Cysticercosis remains endemic in areas where pig farming is a common practice, and disease control has remained an elusive goal.[5,51,96,222] Treatment of human tapeworm carriers potentially could eliminate the disease, but the effects of chemotherapy in endemic populations may not result in long-term reduction in risk of neurocysticercosis.[44,223,224] Vaccination of pigs using recombinant *T. solium* antigens, when used in conjunction with anthelmintics, has the potential to reduce transmission to human populations in endemic areas.[47,49] Development of an effective human vaccine against cysticercosis may provide the best potential tool for the eradication of the disease.

281 *Echinococcus* Species (Agents of Cystic, Alveolar, and Polycystic Echinococcosis)

Pedro L. Moro and Peter M. Schantz

ECHINOCOCCUS GRANULOSUS (CYSTIC ECHINOCOCCOSIS)

Description of the Pathogen

Echinococcus granulosus is a cestode whose life cycle involves dogs and other canids, as definitive hosts for the intestinal tapeworm, as well as domestic and wild ungulates as intermediate hosts for the tissue-invading metacestode (larval) stage (Figure 281-1). The metacestode (echinococcal cyst) is a fluid-filled, spherical, unilocular cyst that consists of an inner germinal layer of cells supported by a characteristic acidophilic-staining, acellular, laminated membrane of variable thickness (Figure 281-2).[1] Each cyst is surrounded by a host-produced layer of granulomatous adventitial reaction. Small vesicles called brood capsules bud internally from the germinal layer and produce multiple protoscolices by asexual division. In humans, the slowly growing hydatid cysts can attain a volume of several liters and contain many thousands of protoscolices. With time, internal septations and daughter cysts can form, disrupting the unilocular pattern typical of the young echinococcal cysts.

Epidemiology

Geographically distinct strains of *E. granulosus* exist with different host affinities. Molecular studies using mitochondrial DNA sequences have identified 10 distinct genetic types (G1 to G10) within *E. granulosus*.[2,3] These include two sheep strains (G1, G2), two bovid strains (G3, G5), a horse strain (G4), the camelid strain (G6), a pig strain (G7) and the cervid strain (G8). A ninth genotype (G9) has been described in swine in Poland[2] and a tenth strain (G10) in reindeer in Eurasia. The sheep strain (G1) is the most cosmopolitan form that most commonly is associated with human infections. The other strains appear to be distinct genetically, suggesting that the taxon *E. granulosus* is paraphyletic and may require taxonomic revision.[2,3] The "cervid," or northern sylvatic genotype (G8), is maintained in cycles involving wolves and dogs and moose and reindeer in northern North America and Eurasia. Human infection with this strain is characterized by predominant pulmonary localization, slower and more benign growth, and less frequent occurrence of clinical complications than reported for other forms.[2] The presence of distinct strains of *E. granulosus* has important implications for public health. The shortened maturation time of the adult form of the parasite in the intestine of dogs suggests that the period for administering antiparasitic drugs to infected dogs will have to be shortened in those areas where the G2, G5, and G6 strains occur.[4]

Certain human activities (e.g., widespread rural practice of feeding dogs the viscera of home-butchered sheep) facilitate transmission of the sheep strain and consequently raise the risk that humans will become infected.[5] Dogs infected with *Echinococcus* tapeworms pass eggs in their feces, and humans become infected

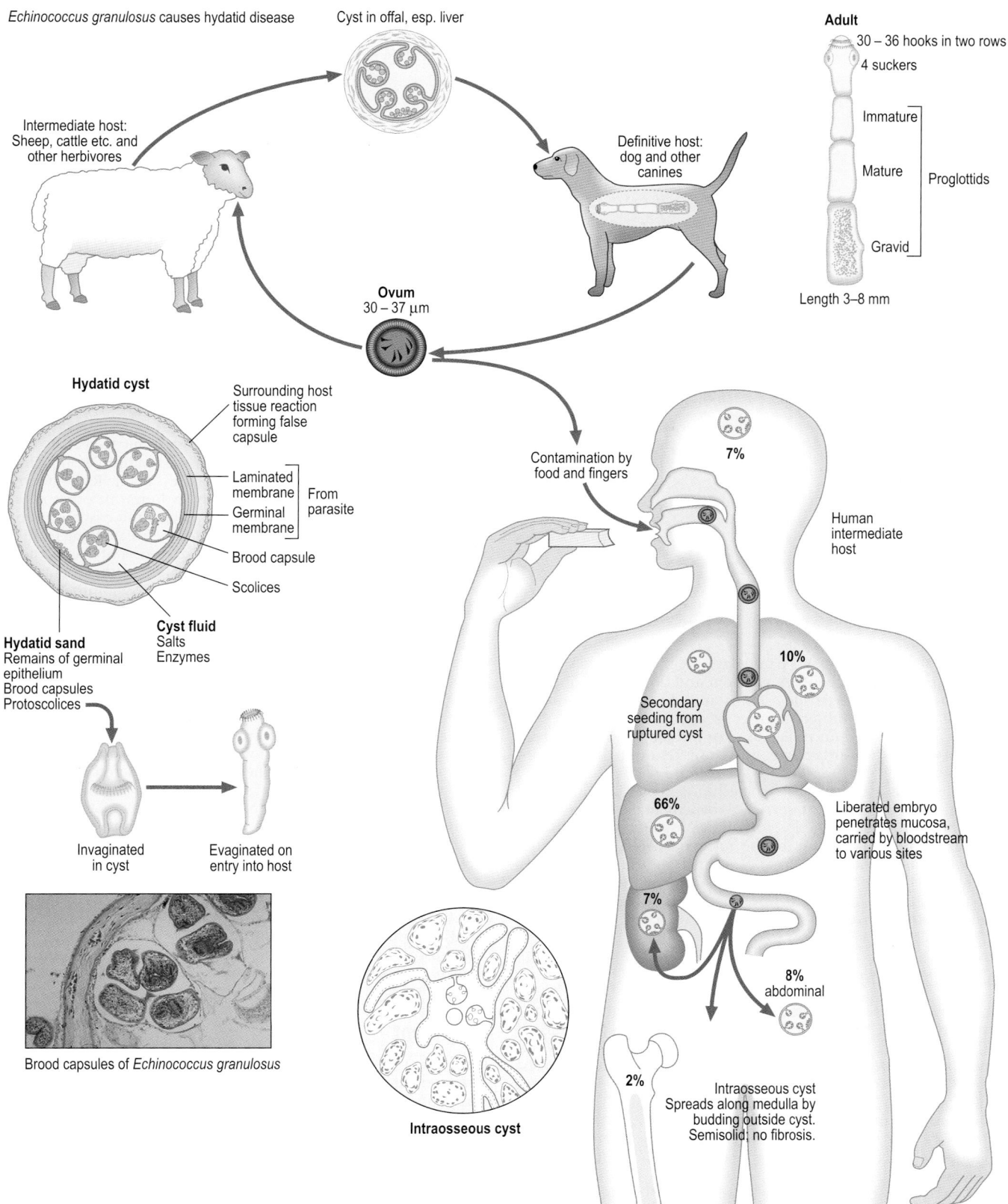

Echinococcus granulosus causes hydatid disease

Cyst in offal, esp. liver

Adult
30 – 36 hooks in two rows
4 suckers

Immature

Mature — Proglottids

Gravid

Length 3–8 mm

Intermediate host:
Sheep, cattle etc. and
other herbivores

Definitive host:
dog and other
canines

Ovum
30 – 37 µm

Hydatid cyst

Surrounding host
tissue reaction
forming false
capsule

Laminated
membrane — From
parasite
Germinal
membrane

Brood capsule

Scolices

Hydatid sand
Remains of germinal
epithelium
Brood capsules
Protoscolices

Cyst fluid
Salts
Enzymes

Invaginated
in cyst

Evaginated on
entry into host

Brood capsules of *Echinococcus granulosus*

Contamination by
food and fingers

7%

Human
intermediate
host

10%

Secondary
seeding from
ruptured cyst

66%

Liberated embryo
penetrates mucosa,
carried by bloodstream
to various sites

7%

8%
abdominal

2%

Intraosseous cyst
Spreads along medulla by
budding outside cyst.
Semisolid; no fibrosis.

Intraosseous cyst

Figure 281-1. Life cycle of *Echinococcus granulosus*. The adult *Echinococcus granulosus* (3 to 6 mm long) resides in the small bowel of the definitive hosts, dogs or other canids. Gravid proglottids release eggs that are passed in the feces. After ingestion by a suitable intermediate host (under natural conditions: sheep, goat, swine, cattle, horses, camel), the egg hatches in the small bowel and releases an oncosphere that penetrates the intestinal wall and migrates through the circulatory system into various organs, especially the liver and lungs. In these organs, the oncosphere develops into a cyst that enlarges gradually, producing protoscolices and daughter cysts that fill the cyst interior. The definitive host becomes infected by ingesting the cyst-containing organs of the infected intermediate host. After ingestion, the protoscolices evaginate, attach to the intestinal mucosa, and develop into adult stages in 32 to 80 days. The same life cycle occurs with *E. multilocularis* (1.2 to 3.7 mm), with the following differences: the definitive hosts are foxes, and to a lesser extent dogs, cats, coyotes, and wolves; the intermediate host are small rodents; and larval growth (in the liver) remains in the proliferative stage indefinitely, resulting in invasion of the surrounding tissues. With *E. vogeli* (up to 5.6 mm long), the definitive hosts are bush dogs and dogs; the intermediate hosts are rodents; and the larval stage (in the liver, lungs, and other organs) develops both externally and internally, resulting in multiple vesicles. *E. oligarthrus* (up to 2.9 mm long) has a life cycle that involves wild felids as definitive hosts and rodents as intermediate hosts. Humans become infected by ingesting eggs, with resulting release of oncospheres in the intestine and the development of cysts in various organs. (Redrawn from data from the Centers for Disease Control and Prevention, http://www.dpd.cdc.gov/dpdx/html/Echinococcosis.htm.)

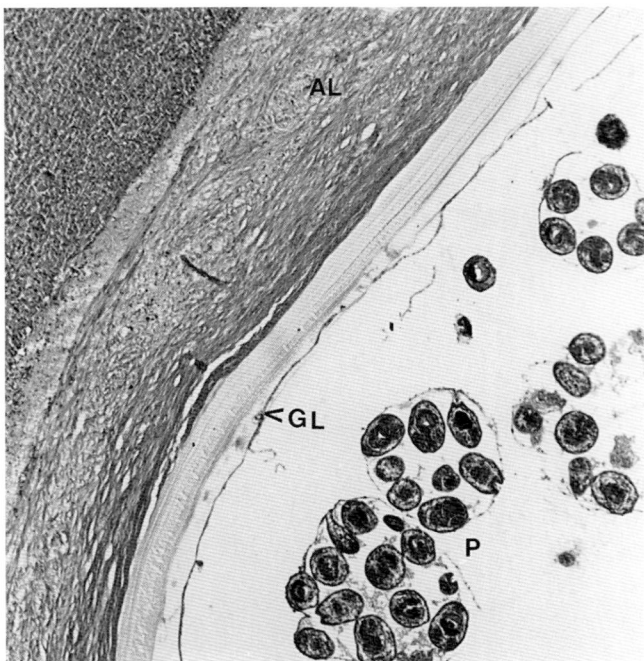

Figure 281-2. Metacestode (hydatid cyst) of *Echinococcus granulosus* showing protoscolices (P) in brood capsules, germinative layer (GL), laminated membrane, and adventitial layer (AL) or ectocyst. (H&E; bar = 100 μm.)

through fecal–oral contact, particularly in the course of playful and intimate contact between children and dogs. Eggs adhere to hairs around an infected dog's anus and also are found on the muzzle and paws. Indirect transfer of eggs, either through contaminated water and uncooked food or through the intermediary of flies and other arthropods, also can result in infection of humans.

The greatest prevalence of cystic echinococcosis in human and animal hosts is found in countries of the temperate zones, including southern South America, the entire Mediterranean littoral, southern and central parts of the former Soviet Union, central Asia, China, Australia, and parts of Africa.[6–8] In the United States, most infections occur in immigrants from countries in which echinococcosis is highly endemic. Sporadic autochthonous transmission is recognized in Alaska, California, Utah, Arizona, and New Mexico.

Clinical Manifestations

After ingestion, *Echinococcus* eggs hatch and release embryos in the small intestine. Penetration through the mucosa leads to bloodstream distribution to the liver and other sites, where development of cysts begins. Most primary infections in humans consist of a single cyst; however, 20% to 40% of infected people have multiple cysts or multiple organ involvement.[9] The liver is the most common site of the echinococcal cyst of the pastoral strains (>65%), followed by lungs (25%); the cyst occurs less frequently in the spleen, kidneys, heart, bone, and central nervous system.

Even though infections can be acquired in childhood, most liver and lung cysts become symptomatic and are diagnosed in adult patients because of the slowly growing nature of the echinococcal cyst. Only 10% to 20% of cases are diagnosed in patients younger than 16 years of age. However, cysts located in the brain or an eye can cause clinical symptoms even when small; thus, most cases of intracerebral echinococcosis are diagnosed in children.

Clinical manifestations of cystic echinococcosis are variable and are determined by the site, size, and condition of the cysts.[9] The rates of growth of cysts are variable, ranging from 1 to 5 cm in diameter per year. The slowly growing echinococcal cyst often is

tolerated well until it causes dysfunction because of its size. Signs and symptoms of hepatic echinococcosis can include hepatic enlargement with or without a palpable mass in the right upper quadrant, right epigastric pain, nausea, and vomiting. If a cyst ruptures, the sudden release of its contents can precipitate allergic reactions ranging from mild to fatal anaphylaxis. In the lungs, ruptured cyst membranes can be evacuated entirely through the bronchi or can be retained to serve as a nidus for bacterial infection. Dissemination of protoscolices can result in multiple secondary echinococcosis disease. Larval growth in bones is atypical; when it occurs, invasion of marrow cavities and spongiosa is common and causes extensive erosion of the bone.

Laboratory Findings and Diagnosis

The presence of a cyst-like mass in a person with a history of exposure to sheepdogs in areas in which *E. granulosus* is endemic supports the diagnosis of cystic echinococcosis. However, echinococcal cysts must be differentiated from benign cysts, cavitary tuberculosis, mycoses, abscesses, and benign or malignant neoplasms. A noninvasive confirmation of the diagnosis usually can be accomplished with the combined use of radiologic imaging and immunodiagnostic techniques (Figure 281-3). Radiography permits detection of echinococcal cysts in lungs; in other sites, however, calcification is necessary for radiographic visualization. Computed tomography (CT), magnetic resonance imaging (MRI), and ultrasonography (US) are useful for diagnosis of deep-seated lesions in all organs and also for determination of the extent and condition of the avascular fluid-filled cysts. Abdominal ultrasonography has emerged as the most widely used imaging technique for echinococcosis because of its widespread availability and usefulness for defining number, site, dimensions, and vitality of cysts.[10] Portable ultrasonography machines have been applied for field surveys with excellent results.[11–13]

Antibody assays are useful to confirm presumptive radiologic diagnoses, although some patients with cystic echinococcosis do not demonstrate a detectable immune response.[14] Hepatic cysts are more likely to elicit an immune response than pulmonary cysts; regardless of location, the sensitivity of serologic tests is related inversely to the degree of sequestration of the echinococcal antigens inside cysts. For example, healthy, intact cysts can elicit minimally detectable response, whereas previously ruptured or leaking cysts are associated with strong responses. Enzyme immunoassay and the indirect hemagglutination test are highly sensitive for initial screening of sera; specific confirmation of reactivity can be obtained by demonstration of echinococcal antigens by immunodiffusion (arc 5) procedures or immunoblot assays (8/12-kd band).[15] Eosinophilia is present in <25% of infected people.

Protoscolices sometimes can be demonstrated in sputum or bronchial washings; identification of hooklets is facilitated by acid-fast stains.

Treatment

Until the 1980s, surgery was the only option for treatment of echinococcal cysts; however, chemotherapy with benzimidazole compounds and, later, treatment with cyst puncture, aspiration, injection of chemicals and re-aspiration were introduced and, increasingly, have supplemented or even replaced surgery as the preferred treatment. The benefits and limitations of current treatment options have been reviewed by the World Health Organization (WHO) Informal Working Group on Echinococcosis.[10,16]

Surgery

Surgical removal of intact hydatid cysts, when possible, remains the treatment with the best potential to remove cysts and lead to an immediate and complete cure. The aim of surgery is total removal of the cyst with avoidance of the adverse consequences of spilling the contents. Pericystectomy is the usual procedure, but simple drainage, capitonnage, marsupialization, and resection of the involved organ can be used, depending on the location and

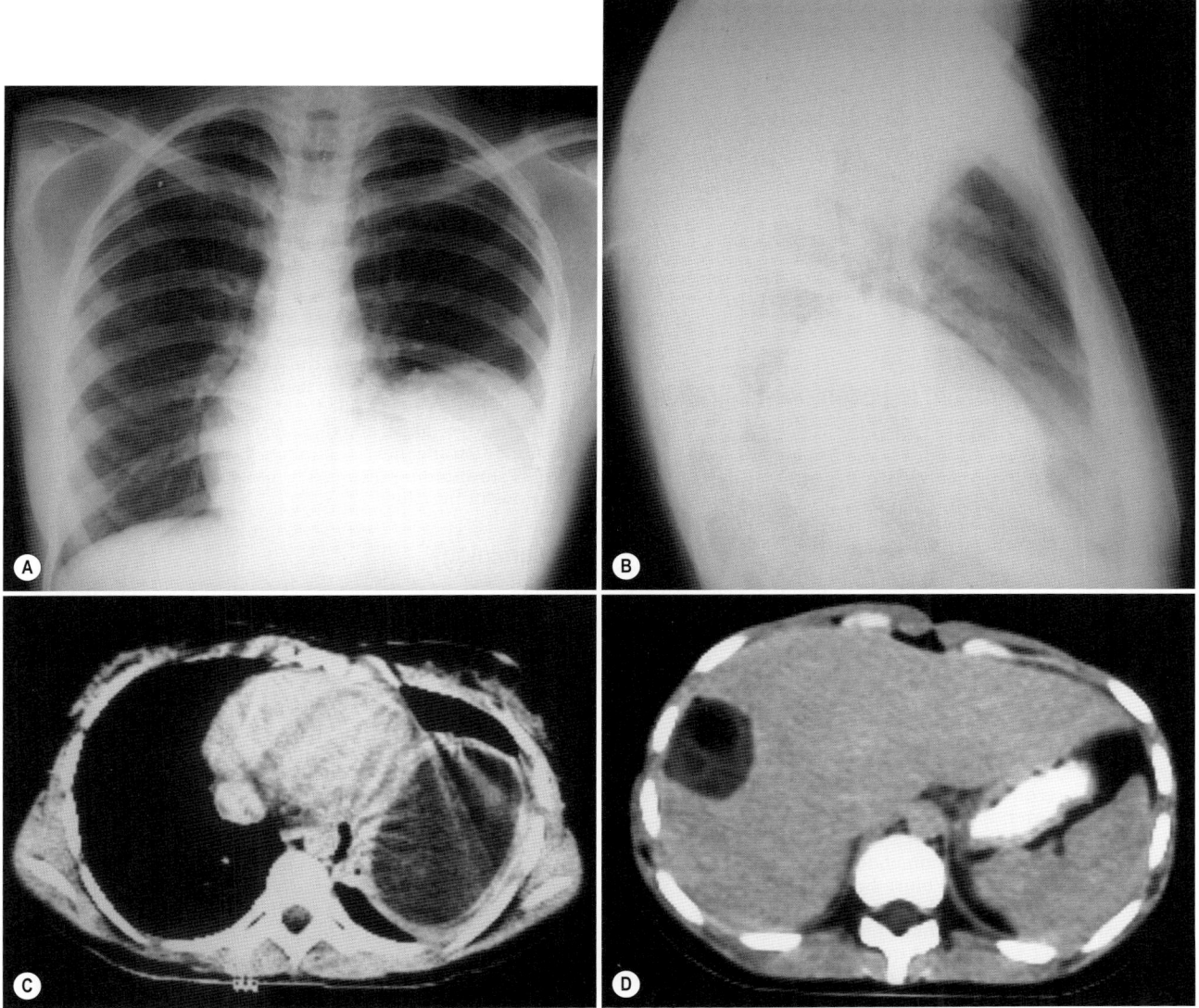

Figure 281-3. Cystic echinococcosis in a 15-year-old girl who came to medical attention in Philadelphia because of cough and pleuritic chest pain and was referred for evaluation for malignancy. This Air Force family had been stationed in Spain and Germany for the preceding 7 years. Plain radiograph frontal **(A)** and lateral **(B)** show a homogeneous left paracardiac mass. Axial computed tomography of the chest **(C)** and abdomen **(D)** without contrast demonstrate large cysts in the lung and liver. Note "daughter" cyst in the liver (D). Serum indirect hemagglutination titer against *Echinococcus* performed at the CDC was 1:1024. (Case courtesy of E.N. Faerber and S.S. Long, St. Christopher's Hospital for Children, Philadelphia, PA.)

condition of the cyst.[17-21] The more radical the intervention, the higher the operative risk but the lower the likelihood of recurrence, and vice versa. Surgery is the preferred treatment when liver cysts are large (>10 cm in diameter), secondarily infected, or located in certain organs (i.e., brain, lung, or kidney).

Surgery is contraindicated in patients who are pregnant, have pre-existing medical conditions that put them at risk, or have multiple cysts that are difficult to access. Surgical risks include those associated with any surgical intervention as well as risks unique to echinococcosis (e.g., anaphylaxis, secondary recurrence). Operative mortality varies from 0.5% to 4% but rises with repeated interventions and when surgery is performed in inadequate facilities.

Chemotherapy

Documentation of experience with chemotherapy using benzimidazole compounds is now extensive, and the medical approach can be recommended for many patients.[7] Approximately one-third of patients treated with benzimidazole drugs are cured (e.g.,

complete and permanent disappearance of cysts) and even higher proportions (30% to 50%) have significant regression of cyst size and alleviation of symptoms.[22-25] However, 20% to 40% of people do not respond favorably. In general, small (<7 mm in diameter), isolated cysts, surrounded by minimal adventitial reaction, respond best, whereas complicated cysts, with multiple compartments or daughter cysts or with thick or calcified surrounding adventitial reactions, are relatively refractory to treatment.

Both albendazole (10 to 15 mg/kg/day) and mebendazole (40 to 50 mg/kg/day) have demonstrated efficacy against cystic echinococcosis; however, the results for albendazole have been superior, probably because of its pharmacokinetic profile, which comparatively favors intestinal absorption and penetration into the cyst.[16,26,27] An intermittent treatment schedule with cycles of 28 days with 14-day periods of rest has been recommended in the past but evidence suggests that continuous treatment may be equally effective.[27] Administration of albendazole with fat-rich meals facilitates absorption and bioavailability. Adverse reactions (neutropenia, liver toxicity, alopecia, and others), reversible upon cessation of treatment, have been noted in a few patients.

Examinations for adverse reactions (aminotransferases and blood count) should be performed regularly, every 2 weeks during the first 3 months and then monthly for one year. Contraindications to chemotherapy include pregnancy, chronic hepatic diseases, and bone marrow depression. Evidence from human case series and experimental animal studies suggest the combination of praziquantel and albendazole may be superior to use of albendazole alone in treatment of hydatid disease.[28,29] Studies in animals suggest nitazoxanide is not effective against cystic echinococcosis.[30]

The combination of praziquantel and albendazole has been used successfully in treatment of hydatid disease.[26-28] Praziquantel used at 50 mg/kg in different regimens (once daily, once weekly or once every 2 weeks) in combination with albendazole has produced very effective and rapid results compared with albendazole therapy alone.[28]

Percutaneous Aspiration, Injection, Re-aspiration

A third option for treatment of hydatid cysts in the liver and some other locations consists of (1) percutaneous puncture using sonographic guidance, (2) aspiration of substantial amounts of the liquid contents, (3) injection of a protoscolicidal agent (e.g., 95% ethanol or hypertonic saline) for at least 15 minutes, and (4) re-aspiration (PAIR).[31-33] PAIR is indicated for patients who cannot undergo surgery and for people who refuse surgery who have single or multiple cysts in the liver, abdominal cavity, spleen, kidney, and bones. PAIR is contraindicated for inaccessible or superficially located liver cysts and for inactive or calcified cystic lesions.

To avoid sclerosing cholangitis, PAIR must not be performed in patients whose cysts have biliary communication; the presence of the latter can be determined by testing the cyst fluid for presence of bilirubin or by intraoperative cholangiogram or endoscopic retrograde cholangiopancreatography. Complications of the procedure include secondary infection of the cavity, acute allergic reactions, and recurrence; however, these have been rare. Application of PAIR to pulmonary cysts has been associated with frequent complications and is not recommended.

The physician using PAIR must be prepared to treat a life-threatening allergic reaction. The possibility of secondary echinococcosis resulting from accidental spillage during this procedure can be minimized by concurrent treatment with benzimidazoles; combined treatment (PAIR with albendazole) may yield better results than either chemotherapy or PAIR alone.[31] The recommended treatment course is 1 month of albendazole after the PAIR procedure. Favorable results have been reported from >2000 PAIR interventions. A meta-analysis comparing the clinical outcomes for 769 patients with hepatic cystic echinococcosis treated with PAIR plus albendazole or mebendazole with 952 era-matched historical control subjects undergoing surgical intervention found greater clinical and parasitologic efficacy, lower rates of morbidity, mortality and disease recurrence, and shorter hospital stays than with surgical treatment.[33]

Monitoring Results of Treatment

The occult nature of the hydatid cyst confounds post-treatment evaluation. Objective response to treatment is best assessed with repeated evaluation of cyst size and consistency at 3-month intervals with US, CT, or MRI. Since the time to recurrence is extremely variable, such monitoring should be continued for at least 3 years. Change in titer of serum antibody values is not reliable in itself to define the outcome of chemotherapy or PAIR.

Prevention

In areas endemic for cystic echinococcosis, personal preventive measures include careful hygiene, strict dietary regulation of pet dogs to preclude ingestion of sheep offal, and avoidance of dogs not so regulated. Periodic prophylactic treatment of pet dogs potentially exposed to E. granulosus sometimes can be necessary.

Control measures include health education, regulation of livestock slaughtering, control of dogs, and periodic mass treatments of dogs with praziquantel (5 mg/kg) to reduce the prevalence of E. granulosus below levels favorable for continued transmission.[5,34] Development of effective vaccines for the metacestode stages of E. granulosus in livestock provides new options for limiting transmission among animal hosts.[35]

ECHINOCOCCUS MULTILOCULARIS (ALVEOLAR ECHINOCOCCOSIS)

Pathogen

Alveolar echinococcosis results from infection by the metacestode (larval) form of *Echinococcus multilocularis*. In rodents, the natural intermediate hosts, the larval mass proliferates rapidly by exogenous budding of germinative tissue and produces an alveolar-like pattern of microvesicles filled with protoscolices.[1] In humans, the larval mass resembles a malignancy in appearance and behavior, because it proliferates indefinitely by exogenous budding and invades surrounding tissues. Protoscolices are observed rarely in infections of humans.

Epidemiology

The life cycle of *E. multilocularis* involves foxes and their rodent prey in ecosystems generally separate from humans.[36] However, there is ecologic overlap with humans, because fox and coyote populations have encroached increasingly upon suburban and urban areas of many regions, and domestic dogs or cats can become infected when they eat infected wild rodents.[36] Alveolar echinococcosis has been reported in parts of central Europe; much of Russia, the central Asian republics, and western China; the northwestern portion of Canada; and western Alaska. Recent surveys in central Europe have extended the known distribution of *E. multilocularis* from 4 countries at the end of the 1980s to 11 countries in 1999, although the annual incidence of disease in humans remains low.[37] There is evidence that parasites are spreading from endemic to previously non-endemic areas in North America and Hokkaido (North Island), Japan, due principally to movement or relocation of foxes.[36] The prevalence and geographic spread in animal hosts appears to be rising in central North America. Hunters, trappers, and persons who work with fox fur are often exposed to alveolar hydatid disease. Hyperendemic foci have been described in some Eskimo villages of the North American tundra and in western China.[38,39] The infection of humans by the larval *E. multilocularis* often is the result of association with dogs and perhaps cats that have eaten infected rodents. Villages within the zone of tundra may constitute hyperendemic foci because of the interaction between dogs and wild rodents that live as commensals in and around dwellings. In central Europe, rodents inhabiting cultivated fields and gardens become infected by ingesting embryophores expelled by foxes and, in turn, may be a source of infection for dogs and cats. A recent case-control study demonstrated a higher risk of alveolar hydatidosis among people who owned dogs that killed game, dogs that roamed outdoors unattended, and farmers and people who owned cats.[40] In rural regions of central North America, the cycle involves foxes and rodents of the genera *Peromyscus* and *Microtus*. Keeping uncontrolled dogs and cats in these regions may be hazardous.

Clinical Manifestations

The liver is the primary location of the metacestode of *E. multilocularis* in humans as well as in natural intermediate hosts. Local extension of the lesion and metastases to lungs and brain may follow.[9] In chronic alveolar echinococcosis infections, the lesion consists of a central necrotic cavity filled with a white amorphous material that is covered with a thin peripheral layer of dense fibrous tissue.[36] Focal areas of calcification exist, as does extensive infiltration by proliferating vesicles. The initial symptoms of

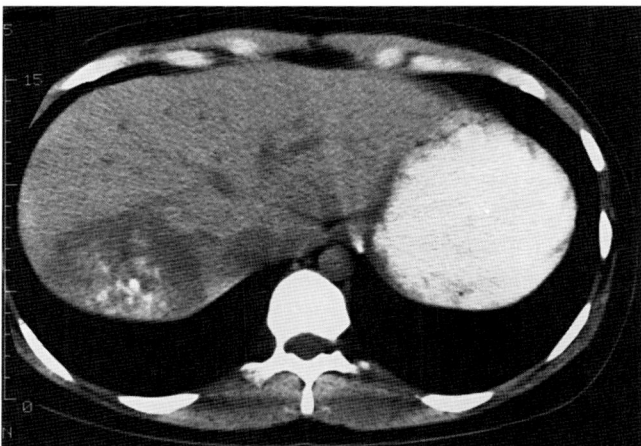

Figure 281-4. Abdominal computed tomography of patient with *Echinococcus multilocularis* lesion in right lobe of the liver. Note irregular low-density zones alternating with scattered areas of calcification. (Courtesy of Joseph F. Wilson, MD)

alveolar hydatid disease usually are vague. Mild upper quadrant and epigastric pain with hepatomegaly may progress to obstructive jaundice. Patients eventually succumb to hepatic failure, invasion of contiguous structures, or, less frequently, metastases to the brain.[38] The mortality in progressive, clinically manifest cases may be 50% to 75%.[38] However, instances of spontaneous death of the cyst during its early stage of development have been reported in people with asymptomatic infection.[41]

Laboratory Findings and Diagnosis

Alveolar echinococcosis typically becomes symptomatic in people of advanced age and closely mimics hepatic carcinoma or cirrhosis. Plain radiographs show hepatomegaly and characteristic scattered areas of radiolucency outlined by calcific rings 2 to 4 mm in diameter. The usual CT image of *E. multilocularis* infection is that of indistinct solid tumors with central necrotic areas and perinecrotic, plaquelike calcifications (Figure 281-4).[41] Results of serologic tests usually are positive at high titers; purified *E. multilocularis* antigens are highly specific and permit serologic discrimination between infections with *E. multilocularis* and *E. granulosus.*[42,43] Needle biopsy of the liver can confirm the diagnosis if larval elements are demonstrated. Exploratory laparotomy often is performed for diagnosis as well as for determining the size and extent of invasion.

Treatment

Surgical resection of the entire larval mass, usually by excision of the entire affected lobe of the liver, is the preferred treatment;

when involvement is extensive, wedge resections of the lesion may be attempted.[36] Because alveolar echinococcosis often is not diagnosed until disease is advanced, the lesion often is inoperable. Long-term treatment with mebendazole (50 mg/kg/day) or albendazole (15 mg/kg/day) inhibits growth of larval *E. multilocularis,* reduces metastasis, and enhances both the quality and length of survival; prolonged therapy eventually can be larvicidal in some patients.[16,44,45] Liver transplantation has been employed successfully in otherwise terminal cases.[46] In a Swiss study, therapy for nonresectable alveolar echinococcosis with mebendazole and albendazole resulted in an increased 10-year survival rate of approximately 80% (versus 29% in untreated historical controls) and a 16- to 20-year survival rate of approximately 70% (versus 0% in historical controls).[36]

Prevention

Eliminating *E. multilocularis* from its wild animal hosts is impractical; therefore, contact with dogs and foxes in areas where the infection is endemic should be avoided. Preventing infection in humans depends on education to improve hygiene and sanitation.[5] Infection in dogs and cats prone to eating infected rodents can be prevented by monthly treatments with praziquantel.

ECHINOCOCCUS VOGELI (POLYCYSTIC ECHINOCOCCOSIS)

A polycystic form of echinococcosis is caused by *Echinococcus vogeli,* the life cycle of which involves the bush dog and possibly other wild canids; domestic dogs also are susceptible. Pacas, agoutis, and spiny rats are the principal intermediate hosts. *E. vogeli* is indigenous to the humid tropical forests in central and northern South America.[2,5] In endemic areas, hunting dogs are often fed the raw viscera of pacas; dogs thus infected then can expose humans. Polycystic echinococcosis has been recognized in humans in Panama, Ecuador, Colombia, Venezuela, and Brazil.[47]

The characteristics of polycystic echinococcosis are intermediate between those of the cystic and alveolar forms.[47] The relatively large cysts are filled with liquid and contain brood capsules with numerous protoscolices. The primary localization is the liver, but cysts may spread to contiguous sites. Techniques useful for diagnosis of cystic or alveolar hydatid disease are also of value in polycystic hydatid disease. Because *E. vogeli* shares antigens with the other *Echinococcus* spp., most available immunodiagnostic tests do not permit species diagnosis. However, the hydatid cysts of *E. vogeli* differ from cysts of other species in the dimensions of the hooks of the protoscolices.

Because lesions in polycystic echinococcosis are so extensive, surgical resection is always difficult and usually incomplete.[47,48] A combination of surgery with albendazole therapy is most likely to be successful. The principles of management for cystic and alveolar echinococcoses also apply to polycystic echinococcosis.

Key Points. Diagnosis and Management of Echinococcal Infection

BIOLOGY	EPIDEMIOLOGY
• Life cycle of *Echinococcus* species involve carnivores (e.g., canids), as definitive hosts and herbivores (e.g., domestic and wild ungulates) as intermediate hosts • The adult stage is small, ranging from 2 to 12 mm in length with 3 to 6 segments, and localized in the lower duodenum and jejunum of the final host • Larval or metacestode stages can develop in any organ (typically the liver) depending on the species of *Echinococcus* as well as species of intermediate host • Humans are incidental intermediate hosts	• Greatest prevalence of cystic echinococcosis found in temperate zones in South America, the entire Mediterranean littoral, southern and central parts of the former Soviet Union, central Asia, China, Australia, and parts of Africa, where dogs often are fed hydatid-infected viscera from home-slaughtered sheep • Alveolar echinococcosis occurs in parts of central Europe; Russia, the Central Asian republics, and western China; the northwestern portion of Canada; and western Alaska and appear to be spreading from endemic to previously non-endemic areas

---

Key Points. Diagnosis and Management of Echinococcal Infection—cont'd

in North America and Hokkaido, Japan, due principally to the movement or relocation of foxes
- Polycystic echinococcosis occurs in humid tropical forests of central and northern South America

CLINICAL FEATURES
- Most echinococcal cysts are asymptomatic
- The liver is the most common site of the echinococcal cyst (>65%), followed by the lungs (25%); cysts occur less frequently in the spleen, kidneys, heart, bone, and central nervous system
- Clinical manifestations are variable and are determined by the site, size, and condition of the cysts
- Dissemination of protoscolices can result in multiple secondary sites of echinococcosis

DIAGNOSIS
- Chest roentgenography permits detection of echinococcal cysts in the lungs

- CT, MRI, and ultrasonography (US) are useful for detecting lesions in the liver and other organs
- Serologic tests are useful to confirm presumptive imaging diagnosis; however, a substantial proportion of patients with cystic echinococcosis may not develop a detectable immune response.

TREATMENT OPTIONS
- Surgery remains the treatment of choice for cysts that are large (>10 cm diameter), secondarily infected, or located in certain organs (e.g., heart, brain)
- Continuous treatment with albendazole (10 to 15 mg/kg/day) or mebendazole (40 to 50 mg/kg/day) is effective
- Percutaneous puncture using US guidance, aspiration of substantial amounts of the liquid contents, injection of a protoscolicidal agent and re-aspiration (PAIR) is an option for treatment of hydatid cysts in the liver and some other locations
- Liver transplantation has been employed successfully in otherwise terminal cases of alveolar echinococcosis

---

282 *Taenia (Multiceps) multiceps* and *Taenia serialis* (Coenurosis)

Michael Cappello, Peter M. Schantz, and A. Clinton White, Jr

COENUROSIS

Human infection with larval forms of the animal tapeworms *Taenia multiceps* (also referred to as *Multiceps multiceps*) or *Taenia serialis* is termed *coenurosis*.[1-8] The coenurus is a fluid-filled cyst that measures from a few millimeters to 2 cm or more in diameter; the wall is a thin, delicate membrane to which multiple invaginated scolices (protoscolices) are attached in rows or clusters. These zoonotic infections occur primarily in tropical and subtropical regions.

Epidemiology and Life Cycle

Fewer than 150 cases of coenurosis in humans have been reported, although potential exposure is common, given the widespread prevalence in dogs and other canids. The majority of cases of coenurosis occur in Africa, although the disease has also been reported in the United Kingdom, France, North America, and the Middle East.[7,9] Most cases from tropical Africa involve subcutaneous sites, while reported cases from South Africa and other temperate regions, including the United States, have a higher frequency of intracranial localization.[10-13] In North America, at least 6 cases of human autochthonous infection have been documented; 3 cases involved the central nervous system, and the others involved intramuscular or subcutaneous localization.[10]

Adult *T. multiceps* and *T. serialis* tapeworms can be recovered from the small intestines of definitive hosts, which include dogs, wolves, foxes, and coyotes.[14,15] Gravid proglottids excreted in feces release eggs that are ingested by an intermediate host. The larval stages of *T. multiceps* are found in various herbivores, such as sheep, goats, or horses, whereas *T. serialis* larvae most often are found in rabbits and squirrels. The oncospheres eventually disseminate to and encyst within various tissues, typically the brain and spinal cord. The inner membrane of the cyst, or bladder, is

composed of multiple protoscolices with additional small protoscolices or metacestodes contained within.

Clinical Manifestations

Human coenurosis occurs when an individual inadvertently ingests eggs or proglottids contained in feces of an infected animal, usually a dog. Human disease frequently involves the central nervous system (CNS), where it causes a cystic lesion that may enlarge.[3,7,8,11-13] Intracerebral cysts can cause seizures or other localizing signs and symptoms and can be confused with neurocysticercosis and echinococcosis. Intraparenchymal lesions of the spinal cord also are reported, and can be associated with meningitis, arteritis, arachnoiditis, ependymitis, and ocular involvement.[12] Subcutaneous and intramuscular cysts are reported most commonly in Africa and involve the intercostal area, axillae, or anterior abdominal wall.[3,14,15] Allergic symptoms, such as recurrent urticaria, fever, and night sweats, also have been reported.

Laboratory Findings and Diagnosis

A presumptive diagnosis of coenurosis most often is based on results of imaging studies, including MRI, CT, or ultrasound.[5,7] The cerebrospinal fluid often is under elevated pressure and may show lymphocytic pleocytosis, as well as reduced glucose and elevated protein concentrations. A definitive diagnosis requires surgical excision and histopathologic identification of the parasite.[7,16] Fine-needle aspiration of a cyst also may yield a diagnosis.[12,17] Coenurus larvae are easily distinguished morphologically from cysticerci and hydatid cysts on the basis of the numbers and characteristics of their protoscolices (Figure 282-1). When protoscolices are absent or not identifiable, coenurid cysts can be distinguished from echinococcal cysts because of their lack of the characteristic acellular, laminated membrane that is typical of the latter.

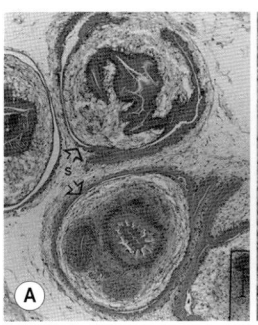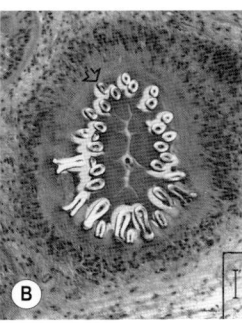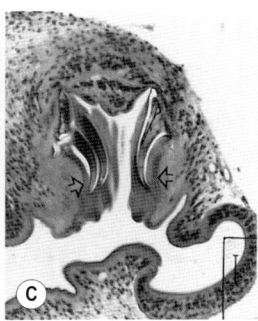

Figure 282-1. (A) Photomicrograph of section of the coenurus. Note two typically formed protoscolices (S, arrows) in late stages of development, with suckers and fully formed rostellum evident (H&E; bar = 100 μm). **(B)** Photomicrograph of transverse section through the rostellum of a fully developed protocolex. Note the typical distribution of approximately 30 rostellar hooks (arrow) in two rows (H&E; bar = 25 μm). **(C)** Photomicrograph of longitudinal section through rostellum. Note structure of the blades in typically formed rostellar hooks (arrows); the guards and handles have not developed (H&E; bar = 25 μm). (From Huss BT, Miller MA, Corwin RM, et al. Fatal cerebral coenurosis in a cat. J Am Vet Med Assoc 1994;205:69.)

However, racemose (acephalic) cysticerci often cannot be differentiated from coenuri because the thin cyst membranes of the two cysts are similar.[2] PCR-based restriction fragment length polymorphism (PCR-RFLP) has been used experimentally to differentiate various species of taeniid cestodes, including *T. multiceps* and *T. serialis*.[10,18] This technique may prove useful for diagnostic and epidemiologic purposes, since at present there is no reliable serologic test for coenurosis.

Treatment

Surgical intervention has been the mainstay of therapy. Excision is indicated in most symptomatic cases involving the CNS, and may be successful in people with small intraparenchymal or single intraventricular cysts. Although treatment of coenurosis often is initiated using anthelmintic drugs, usually praziquantel and albendazole,[7,12] efficacy has not been evaluated in controlled trials.

Prevention

When infection of humans is traced to domesticated dogs and ungulates, transmission can be controlled by strict management of animal slaughter, periodic treatment of dogs, and health education. Transmission from wild animal hosts is more difficult to prevent, and measures are limited to careful avoidance of potentially infected carnivores and adequate hygiene. A recombinant protein vaccine against *T. multiceps* has shown significant protection against infection when administered to sheep in an endemic area.[19,20]

283 Intestinal Trematodes

LeAnne M. Fox

Over 70 species of zoonotic, hermaphroditic intestinal flukes can parasitize the human intestine.[1-4] Most human infections are asymptomatic, but heavy infections are more likely to result in clinical disease. Morphologically, the adult flukes are flat and leaf-shaped, ranging in length from a few millimeters to several centimeters. They attach to the intestinal mucosa by means of oral and ventral suckers, and release eggs having a characteristic operculum at one end of the shell. When deposited into fresh water, the operculum opens to release a miracidia, which finds and penetrates an appropriate snail host, in which further replication occurs. Eventually the infected snail releases thousands of cercariae into water that encyst (as metacercariae) either on aquatic plants, or on or in a second intermediate host (fish, mollusks, crustaceans, and amphibians). Metacercariae, when ingested by humans and other definitive hosts, develop into adult flukes. Some of the more common intestinal trematodes are *Fasciolopsis buski*, *Heterophyes heterophyes*, *Metagonimus yokogawai*, and the echinostomes (Table 283-1). However, *Metorchis conunctus*, *Nanophyetus salmincola*, *Gastrodiscoides hominis*, *Centrocestus formosanus*, *Haplorchis* species, and others infect humans.[1-5] All intestinal trematodes can be treated easily with praziquantel orally.

FASCIOLOPSIASIS

Description. Fasciolopsiasis is a small bowel infection caused by the largest of the intestinal trematodes, *Fasciolopsis buski*, which can measure up to 7.5 by 2.5 cm. Eggs passed in feces hatch and miracidiae infect planorbid snails. Cercariae that emerge encyst on freshwater vegetation (bamboo shoots, water chestnuts, water caltrop, water lilies, hyacinths, and morning glory), and remain infectious for up to 1 year.[6] After ingestion the metacercariae develop into mature flukes in 3 months.[1,2]

Epidemiology. *F. buski* is found throughout the Far East and Southeast Asia, including southern China, Taiwan, Bangladesh, India, Indonesia, Thailand, Malaysia, Sumatra, Kampuchea, Vietnam, Laos, and Myanmar.[1,2] Pigs are important reservoirs of the infection, although dogs and rabbits also can be infected.[1,2] Children, who tend to eat plants, have the highest prevalence rates.

Pathology and symptoms. Most infections are asymptomatic. Ulcers or abscesses develop at the site of attachment to the intestinal mucosa in the duodenum and jejunum and infected individuals may complain of epigastric pain indistinguishable from peptic ulcer disease. Eosinophilia is common. Children can come to medical attention because of systemic allergic manifestations attributed to absorption of parasite metabolites.[1] In heavy infections, an edematous condition resulting from protein-losing enteropathy has been reported. Large numbers of flukes in the intestine may cause ileus or intermittent obstruction.

Diagnosis. Diagnosis is made by identification of large (135 × 80 μm) operculated eggs in stool. Eggs can be confused with those of *Fasciola hepatica*, *Fasciola gigantica*, and the echinostomes, which are similar morphologically. Stool concentration techniques, which allow examination of a gram or more of stool, enhance detection of light infections.

TABLE 283-1. Parasitic Trematodes (Other Than Schistosomes) of Humans

Fluke	Common Name of Disease	Species	Intermediate Host Primary	Intermediate Host Secondary	Location of Adults	Distribution
Intestinal	Fasciolopsiasis	*Fasciolopsis buski*	Snails	Aquatic plants	Small intestine	SE Asia, primarily S. China
	Heterophyiasis	*Heterophyes heterophyes*	Snails	Fish	Small intestine	Middle East
	Metagonimiasis	*Metagonimus yokogawai*	Snails	Fish	Small intestine	Far East
	Echinostomiasis	*Euparyphium ilocanum*	Snails	Fish, amphibians, crustaceans, mollusks	Small intestine	Far East
Liver	Clonorchiasis	*Clonorchis sinensis*	Snails	Fish	Bile ducts	China, SE Asia
	Fascioliasis	*Fasciola hepatica, F. gigantica*	Snails	Watercress	Bile ducts	Worldwide, including British Isles, S. France, Cuba, Algeria
	Opisthorchiasis	*Opisthorchis viverrini, O. felineus*	Snails	Fish	Bile ducts	*O. viverrini* SE Asia; *O. felineus* E Europe and former Soviet Union
Lung	Paragonimiasis	*Paragonimus westermani* (predominate species)	Snails	Crabs	Lungs	Far East, S Asia, Philippines, W Africa, Americas

Principal sources of infection include uncooked plants, water, or poorly cooked, salted, or pickled fish or crustaceans.

Treatment. The drug of choice for both children and adults is praziquantel, 75 mg/kg in one day divided into 3 doses.[5] It is important to note that confusion of fasciolopsiasis eggs with eggs from fascioliasis (a liver fluke infection) will result in ineffective treatment for the latter, which is resistant to praziquantel treatment.

Prevention. In endemic areas, freshwater plants should be cooked before being eaten. Better control of the infection can be achieved by prohibition of night soil use as fertilizer and proper disposal of human and pig excreta.[1,2]

HETEROPHYIASIS AND METAGONIMIASIS

Description. Infection by the intestinal flukes *Heterophyes heterophyes* and *Metagonimus yokogawai* occur in different geographic areas but clinically and pathologically are similar. The importance of these flukes is being increasingly recognized.[7] The adults are small (1.4 × 0.6 mm) and inhabit the small intestine and release eggs that pass in the feces. Miracidiae from eggs infect snails, which release cercariae that encyst (as metacercariae) on the scales and occasionally in muscles of freshwater fish. The fins, tail, and gills are infected most highly. The life cycle is completed when the definitive hosts (including humans) become infected by ingesting raw, or undercooked fish. Incompletely salted or pickled fish also are infectious.[8] The metacercariae are released from the cysts and develop into adults in about 7 days.[1,2]

Epidemiology. Human heterophyiasis is common in Egypt, Iran, Tunisia, Turkey, and Sudan.[1,2] Besides humans, the parasite occurs in dogs, cats, foxes, and a number of other fish-eating mammals. Metagonimiasis occurs in the Far East and Siberia (Taiwan, China, the Philippines, Korea, Indonesia, Japan, and Russia). Adult *M. yokogawai* reside in humans, dogs, cats, pigs, and some other fish-eating birds such as pelicans. Humans are infected from eating undercooked freshwater fish, including salmon and trout. Infection rates can reach 65% in children in places where these fish traditionally are eaten raw.

Pathology and symptoms. Most people are asymptomatic but when large numbers of flukes are present, the clinical picture is one of intermittent diarrhea with mucus, abdominal tenderness, and discomfort. Occasionally, the flukes penetrate the intestinal wall and form granulomas in the peritoneal cavity. Rarely eggs can gain access to the lymphatics and then the bloodstream, embolizing to cause granulomatous lesions in brain, heart, lungs, spleen, and liver, where they can incite serious disease.[2]

Diagnosis. Eosinophilia is common. The diagnosis is based on the finding of characteristic small (30 × 15 μm) operculated eggs in feces or tissues. Stool concentration techniques, which allow examination of a gram or more of stool, enhance detection of light infections. *Heterophyes* and *Metagonimus* eggs are indistinguishable from eggs of the liver flukes *Clonorchis* and *Opisthorchis*.[1,8] All of these flukes are sensitive to praziquantel treatment, so an error in diagnosis does not jeopardize successful treatment.

Treatment. Treatment consists of praziquantel, 75 mg/kg in one day divided into 3 doses.[5]

Prevention. Fish should be carefully cleaned and scaled, and cooked well. Health education should discourage the ingestion of raw, undercooked, or improperly pickled or salted fish.

ECHINOSTOME INFECTIONS

Description. The name "echinostome" refers to the characteristic spines surrounding the oral and ventral suckers of the adult flukes.[1-2] At least 15 species of echinostomes have been observed in humans.[2] The life cycle is similar to that of other intestinal trematodes. Besides humans, reservoir hosts are dogs, cats, rats, and birds.[9] Infection is acquired in humans from ingestion of metacercariae on raw or undercooked fish, mollusks, crustaceans, and amphibians.

Epidemiology. Human infections are found in Korea, Indonesia, the Philippines, Malaysia, Thailand, China, and Taiwan.[1,2]

Pathology and symptoms. Symptoms related to inflammation at the attachment site of adult flukes include abdominal pain, diarrhea, and anorexia. Symptom severity is considered related to infection intensity.

Diagnosis. Diagnosis is made by identification of large (135 × 80 μm) operculated eggs in stool that are difficult to distinguish from eggs of *Fasciola hepatica*, *Fasciola gigantica*, and *Fasciolopsis buski*. Stool concentration techniques, which allow examination of a gram or more of stool, enhance detection of light infections.

Treatment. Praziquantel, 40 mg/kg/day in a single dose is curative. Albendazole 400 mg twice daily for 3 days also is effective. Confusion of echinostome eggs with eggs from fascioliasis (liver fluke infection) will result in ineffective treatment for the latter, which is resistant to praziquantel treatment.

Prevention. In endemic areas, raw or insufficiently cooked snails, fish, frogs, tadpoles, mollusks, and aquatic animals should not be eaten.[10]

284 *Clonorchis, Opisthorchis, Fasciola,* and *Paragonimus* Species

Jeffrey L. Jones

Liver and lung trematodes are hermaphroditic, zoonotic flukes that use snails as intermediate hosts (see Table 283-1). Snails are infected by eggs in feces passed into the environment by humans and other mammals. The snails in turn release cercariae that encyst in a second intermediate host that includes fish, crustaceans, and amphibians, or on water plants. When these are ingested, humans and other definitive hosts become infected. *Clonorchis, Opisthorchis,* and *Fasciola* species invade the biliary tree whereas *Paragonimus* species most often invade the lung. *Clonorchis* and *Opisthorchis* are among the most common causes of biliary fluke infection (an estimated 35 million people and 11.2 million people, respectively). An estimated 10 million people are infected with *Fasciola* species and sporadic infections are caused by *Dicrocoelium dendriticum* and *Eurytrema pancreaticum.*[1-3]

CLONORCHIASIS AND OPISTHORCHIASIS

Description of Pathogens

The adult *Clonorchis* worms are flat, elongated flukes, measuring up to 25 mm long and 5 mm wide. Adult *Opisthorchis* are smaller and measure up to 12 mm long and 3 mm wide. The flukes inhabit the biliary tract, where they produce eggs that are passed into feces. Snails ingest these eggs, become infected, and release thousands of cercariae into water. The cercariae encyst (as metacercariae) in tissues of susceptible fish and shrimp. Over 100 species of freshwater fish and several species of freshwater shrimp are susceptible to infection. When infected raw or undercooked fish (or shrimp) are ingested, the larvae excyst in the duodenum and migrate via the ampulla of Vater to the bile ducts, where they mature to adults in 4 weeks.[3-5] The adult flukes can live as long as 30 years.

Epidemiology

Infections occur where it is customary to eat raw fish dishes. Adult males are most affected in some areas, although in parts of China children will catch and eat small fish and become heavily infected. *Clonorchis sinensis* infects an estimated 15 million people in China. The infection also occurs in Korea, Taiwan, Vietnam, and Japan (rarely).[1,2] Infections in Hong Kong probably are a result of imported fish. Pigs, cats, and dogs are reservoir hosts of *C. sinensis.* *O. viverrini* is endemic in Thailand, Cambodia, and Laos and has reservoirs in dogs, whereas *O. felineus* is found particularly in eastern Europe and Siberia and is most common in cats. An estimated 10 million people are infected with *O. viverrini,* and 1.2 million with *O. felineus.*[2,3] Outbreaks of *O. felineus* infection associated with ingestion of freshwater lake fish have been reported from Italy.[6]

Clinical Manifestations

Adult flukes can be found in bile ducts, the pancreatic duct, and gallbladder. Infection produces inflammatory and hyperplastic changes in the epithelium of bile ducts, with sludging of bile. Eggs and flukes can serve as a nidus for formation of stones. The gallbladder and liver commonly become enlarged, but liver function generally is preserved; portal cirrhosis can occur in chronic infection.[1,3,7,8]

Most infections are asymptomatic or produce only epigastric discomfort. The majority of infections are discovered incidentally on routine screening examination of stool. In endemic areas symptoms often start in the third decade of life.[3] Complications include pyogenic cholangitis, obstructive jaundice, gallstones, pancreatitis, and cholangiocarcinoma.

Laboratory Findings and Diagnosis

An acute syndrome of fever and eosinophilia can occur approximately 2 to 4 weeks after ingestion of infected fish or shrimp.[3] In chronic disease, serum hepatic transaminase levels usually remain normal, but direct and indirect bilirubin and alkaline phosphatase values may be elevated. Definitive diagnosis is made through identification of eggs in stool or in duodenal aspirates, or identification of adult worms during surgery. To improve the chance of finding eggs, multiple examinations using a stool concentration technique may be necessary. *Clonorchis* and *Opisthorchis* eggs are small, approximately 30 by 15 μm, and yellowish brown, with an operculum that rests on a distinctive rim, and often are indistinguishable from each other.[9] Serologic tests are being developed but generally are not available outside of endemic areas. Stool PCR tests also are under investigation.[10] Cholangiography, ultrasonography (US), computed tomography (CT) or magnetic resonance imaging (MRI) demonstrate hepatobiliary dilatation, sludging, stones, and neoplasia. Adult flukes sometimes can be seen as shadows or filling defects in endoscopic retrograde cholangiography.[11] M-mode ultrasonography can show mobile worms in gallbladder ducts.[12]

Treatment

Treatment consists of praziquantel, 25 mg/kg given three times per day for 2 consecutive days.[13,14] Praziquantel is a U.S. Food and Drug Administration (FDA) pregnancy category B medication (animal studies have revealed no evidence of harm to the fetus; however, there are no adequate studies in pregnant women). Side effects include malaise, headache, dizziness, abdominal discomfort (sometimes with nausea), elevated temperature, and urticaria (uncommon); these usually are mild, time-limited, and do not require intervention. Alternative therapy for *C. sinensis* infection is albendazole, 10 mg/kg per day for 7 days. Biliary changes usually are reversible in children but damage from long-standing infection in adults is slow to resolve, and may not resolve. Secondary pyogenic cholangitis is treated with appropriate antimicrobial therapy.

Special Considerations

An increased incidence of cholangiocarcinoma is associated with both *Clonorchis* and *Opisthorchis* infections.[15] Pathologically, tumors are adenocarcinomas originating from the hyperplastic epithelial lining of bile ducts.[1,3,16] *Opisthorchis*-endemic areas may have 15-fold excessive risk of cholangiocarcinoma; *N*-nitrosamines in food may be an important cofactor in inducing the neoplasia.

Prevention

Thoroughly cooking freshwater fish (and shrimp) (63°C; 145°F) prevents infection; freezing (−20°C; −4°F) for 7 days also prevents infection. Travelers should be advised to avoid eating raw fresh-water fish (and shrimp). The practice of using night soil to enrich fish ponds should be discouraged. Repeated mass treatment of populations with praziquantel every 6 to 12 months has been used for clonorchiasis control in China.[17]

FASCIOLIASIS

Description of Pathogens

Fascioliasis is a widespread disease of sheep, goats, and cattle caused by the liver fluke *Fasciola hepatica* and, less commonly, by *F. gigantica*. Humans become infected by eating uncooked, infested aquatic vegetation (classically, watercress). *F. hepatica and F. gigantica* are believed to be resistant to praziquantel.

These large (*Fasciola hepatica:* up to 30 mm by 13 mm; *F. gigantica:* up to 75 mm) flat, leaf-shaped adult flukes inhabit the bile ducts, gallbladder, and occasionally ectopic sites.[2,18] Eggs passed in feces hatch into miracidia and penetrate snails. Cercariae emerge after 4 to 7 weeks and encyst (appearing as small white dots) on watercress or other aquatic plants. Herbivorous mammals (including sheep, goats, cattle, llamas, camels, pigs, deer, and rabbits) become infected by grazing, or indirectly by drinking the surrounding water contaminated with metacercariae.[16,18,19] The metacercariae release larvae that are more invasive in their migration compared with *Clonorchis* and *Opisthorchis* larvae. *Fasciola* larvae penetrate the duodenal wall, invade the peritoneal cavity, and then invade the liver where they cause eosinophilic tracks 1 to 4 mm in diameter and focal necrotic abscesses as they move through the parenchyma. When they reach the bile ducts, they mature into adults and begin to produce eggs 3 to 4 months after infection.[18,19] Adult flukes live up to 10 years.

Epidemiology

Human infection occurs worldwide and is most common among rural people who tend sheep and eat uncooked water vegetables, particularly watercress. Estimates of infection range from 2.4 to 17 million people in Asia, Africa, Europe (including western Europe and the United Kingdom), and the Americas.[2] School-aged shepherds often have parasite burdens of 5000 eggs per gram of feces in Bolivia.[19] Cases have been reported from the U.S.; however, most cases are imported.[20,21] Animals also suffer considerable morbidity from these infections (known as "liver rot").[2]

Clinical Manifestations

The tissue-invasive nature of *Fasciola* larvae can result in an acute or subacute clinical syndrome lasting for many weeks, characterized by fever, eosinophilia, and epigastric or right upper-quadrant abdominal pain, rarely accompanied with ascites or right pleural effusion. Serum hepatic transaminase levels, direct and indirect bilirubin, and alkaline phosphatase values can be elevated. When acute symptoms occur, generally they begin within 6 to 12 weeks after ingestion of metacercariae. After the adult parasites enter the bile ducts, systemic symptoms and laboratory abnormalities abate, and the infection can become asymptomatic. In heavy infections patients can have clinical manifestations similar to clonorchiasis or opisthorchiasis, with jaundice, cholangitis, or gallstones, but cholangiocarcinoma has not been associated with fascioliasis.[1-3,16] An unusual form of fascioliasis can occur after ingestion of raw *Fasciola*-infected liver, when flukes surviving mastication attach to the posterior pharynx, thereby causing hemorrhagic nasopharyngitis and dysphagia, known as *halzoun* in Lebanon and *marrara* in Sudan.[3]

Laboratory Findings and Diagnosis

Acute hepatitis accompanied by eosinophilia and a history of travel or ingestion of watercress is suggestive of facioliasis. Assays for antibody, available at some specialty laboratories, can be helpful in making the diagnosis of acute fascioliasis. Antibody tests are helpful when acute symptoms occur because it takes 1 to 2 months after symptoms develop for eggs to become detectable in the stool. Antibody test sensitivities of >90% have been reported but specificities may not be optimal due to cross-reaction with other helminths.[22] Research on serologic tests for liver flukes is ongoing to develop better antigens and improve sensitivity and specificity.[2] In addition, work also is being done on development of sensitive and specific coproantigen tests.[23] Diagnosis of chronic infections is made through identification in stool of large (130–150 μm long by 60–90 μm wide) eggs with poorly defined opercula.[24] These eggs are confused easily with eggs of the intestinal trematode *Fasciolopsis buski*. Examination of multiple stool specimens using concentration techniques should be undertaken since egg output usually is low. Chronic hepatobiliary tract involvement can be assessed with US, cholangiography, CT, and MRI. US can be negative in acute disease; high-definition CT or MRI can be useful in demonstrating the tracks of migrating larvae in the liver or filling defects in the gallbladder.[16,25] "Spurious fascioliasis" occurs when *Fasciola* eggs are found in uninfected people who recently have ingested (cooked or uncooked) liver from infected animals.

Treatment

Praziquantel is not an effective treatment for fascioliasis, and unfortunately, unlike treatment for other trematode infections, treatment of these cases can be a challenge. Triclabendazole is effective in a single dose of 10 mg/kg for 1 or 2 days, but the human preparation is in short supply and is not FDA approved for general use in the U.S.[13,14] If available, a second course of triclabendazole treatment can be given if parasitologic cure is not achieved after the first course.[26] Bithionol requires a long treatment course of 30 to 50 mg/kg orally (given on alternate days) for 10 to 15 doses, and often causes considerable gastrointestinal tract side effects. Bithionol can be obtained from the Centers for Disease Control and Prevention (CDC) Drug Service (Atlanta, GA 30333; telephone: 404-639-3670). Nitazoxanide most recently has produced cure rates of 60% in adults, 40% in children,[27] with some reported higher cure rates;[19,28] artesunate also has been shown to have some activity.[29] Both artesunate and artemether were effective against *F. hepatica* in animal models.[30] A short course of corticosteroids may be indicated for acute disease.

Special Considerations

Complications of fascioliasis include acute hemorrhage from the biliary tract that can manifest as hematemesis or melena, or aberrant larval migration that can result in ectopic abscesses or nodules in skin, intestine, lung, heart, and brain.

Prevention

Travelers should be advised not to eat uncooked watercress or other aquatic plants. Washing these vegetables in water, vinegar, or lemon juice does not remove the metacercariae. Aquatic vegetable cultivation should be protected from fecal contamination. Where economically feasible, mollusks can be eliminated by drainage of land or use of chemical molluscicides. Oropharyngeal fascioliasis (*halzoun/marrara*) can be prevented by eating well-cooked liver.

PARAGONIMIASIS

Description of Pathogens

Human paragonimiasis is acquired through ingestion of the organism in raw or undercooked crabs or crayfish, and is usually a lung infection. After ingestion, metacercariae excyst in the small intestine and release larvae which penetrate the duodenal wall and enter the peritoneal cavity. Larvae migrate for approximately 1 week, then penetrate the diaphragm, enter the pleural cavity, and migrate directly through lung tissue to reach the bronchi. There they form cystic cavities and develop into adult worms in 5 to 6 weeks.[3] The adult parasites are reddish brown and ovoid, measuring 7.5 to 12 mm by 4 to 6 mm.[3,31] Adult worms induce an inflammatory response in the lungs, generating a fibrous cyst that contains a purulent, bloody effusion and eggs released by the flukes that are passed into the environment via expectoration, or may be swallowed and passed with feces. When deposited in fresh water, eggs hatch to release miracidiae, which then invade specific snail hosts. Thousands of cercariae later are released from the infected snail, which encyst (as metacercariae) in the gills, muscles, legs, and viscera of freshwater crustaceans (crabs or crayfish).

Epidemiology

Eight or nine species (depending on the classification scheme) of *Paragonimus* cause the majority of human infections; the most important is *P. westermani,* which occurs primarily in the Far East (China, the Philippines, Japan, Vietnam, South Korea, Taiwan, and Thailand).[3,32,33] *P. africanus* is an important human pathogen in Africa, as is *P. mexicanus* in Central and South America. Various mammals may be infected, including domestic cats and dogs.[1] Although rare, human paragonimiasis from *P. kellicotti* has been acquired in the U.S., with multiple cases from the midwest.[33,34] Several cases have been associated with ingestion of uncooked crawfish during float trips in Missouri.[34] Specialty dishes and seasonings in which shellfish are consumed raw or prepared in vinegar, brine, or wine without cooking play a key role in transmission of paragonimiasis. Raw crabs or crayfish also are used in traditional medicine practices in Korea, Japan, and some parts of Africa.[3,16]

Clinical Manifestations

An acute syndrome characterized by cough, abdominal pain, malaise, low-grade fever, and eosinophilia can occur 2 to15 days after infection and resolve without treatment. Light infections can be asymptomatic. The clinical picture of chronic paragonimiasis resembles chronic bronchitis or tuberculosis. Patients may complain of cough productive of tenacious coffee-colored or blood-tinged sputum, dyspnea, or pleuritic chest pain (Figure 284-1). Chest radiographs can be negative or show diffuse infiltrates, pleural effusion (often containing a large number of eosinophils), pneumothorax, calcifications, nodules, or cysts.[35]

The infection can be complicated by hemoptysis or secondary pyogenic pulmonary infection. Central nervous system (CNS) involvement occurs in up to 25% of hospitalized patients and can manifest as meningitis and space-occupying lesions. CNS symptoms include headaches, seizures, motor or sensory deficits, and visual disturbances. Skull radiographs can show clusters of calcified cysts (resembling soap bubbles). CT and MRI show aggregated ring-enhancing lesions with edema in the surrounding area. Other extrapulmonary manifestations include migratory skin lesions that resemble cutaneous larva migrans (especially in infections with *P. skrjabini* but can occur with other species). *Paragonimus* flukes also can invade liver, spleen, intestinal wall, peritoneum, and abdominal lymph nodes.

Laboratory Findings and Diagnosis

Peripheral blood eosinophilia is common and can be intense, especially during the early larval migration stages. Many patients have a spectrum of abnormalities on chest radiographs: lobar infiltrates, coin lesions, cavities, calcified nodules, hilar enlargement, pleural thickening and effusions.[3] Ring-shaped opacities of contiguous cavities giving the characteristic appearance of a bunch of grapes are highly suggestive of pulmonary paragonimiasis. Similar "grape bunch" CT findings, characteristically in the temporal and occipital lobes, can be seen in CNS infections.

Eggs are yellowish brown, 80 to 120 μm long by 45 to 70 μm wide, thick-shelled, with an obvious operculum, and their

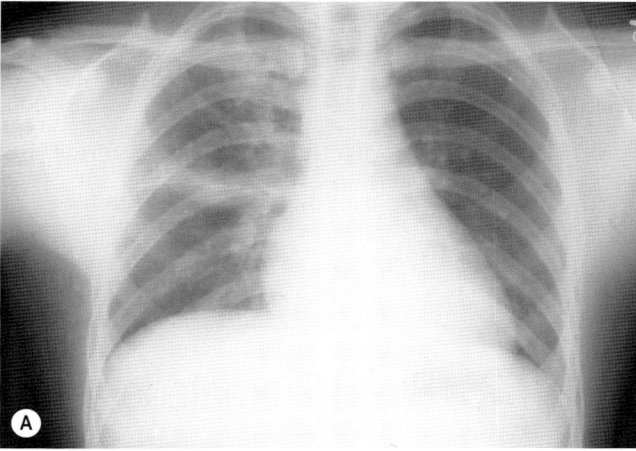

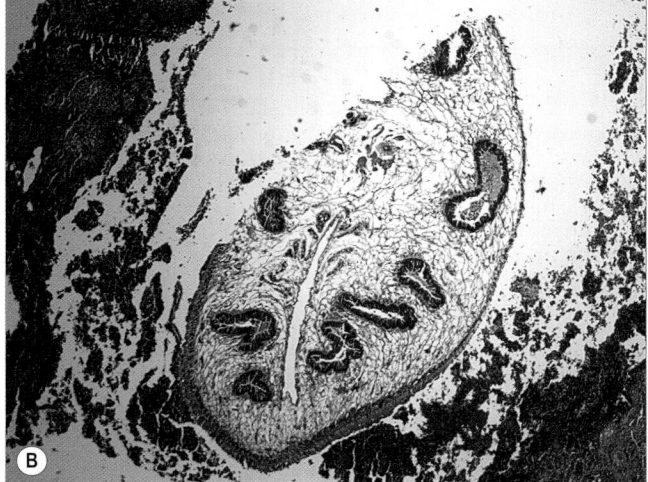

Figure 284-1. A 17-year-old male who had recently emigrated from Laos came to medical attention because of hemoptysis, after a 1-year history of cough, chest pain, and dyspnea on exertion (in Laos). Purified protein derivative was negative; peripheral blood eosinophil count was 3000/mm³. Chest radiograph **(A)** showed right upper-lobe complex cystic disease. Resected lung **(B)** revealed multiple cavitary granulomatous lesions with necrosis and predominant eosinophilic inflammatory response. The gastrointestinal tract of *Paragonimus westermani* was also seen (20×). (Courtesy of D.V. Schidlow, J. Pascasio, and S.S. Long, St. Christopher's Hospital for Children, Philadelphia, PA.)

presence in sputum or stool is diagnostic.[36] Acid-fast staining destroys *Paragonimus* eggs, so the diagnosis cannot be made on sputa prepared with acid-fast stain for tuberculosis testing. Stool examination or gastric aspirates are useful in children. Multiple stools on different days should be examined using a stool concentration technique. Specific and sensitive antibody tests based on *P. westermani* antigens are available through the CDC (telephone: 404-718-4100)[37] and various specialty laboratories. Serologic tests can be useful for early infections (prior to maturation of flukes) or for ectopic infections where eggs are not passed in the stool.

Treatment

Praziquantel, 25 mg/kg given 3 times per day for 2 consecutive days,[13,14] is curative. For cerebral disease, a short course of corticosteroids should be given with the praziquantel to reduce the inflammatory response around dying flukes. Bithionol is an alternative drug. See "Clonorchiasis and Opisthorciasis" for additional information about praziquantel and "Fascioliasis" for additional information about bithionol.

Special Considerations

Ectopic lesions from aberrant migration of flukes can involve any organ, including abdominal viscera, the heart, and the mediastinum. The most clinically recognizable ectopic lesions arise from cerebral paragonimiasis, which, in highly endemic countries, more commonly affects children.[3,33] Children can have eosinophilic meningoencephalitis, seizures, or signs of space-occupying lesions. Many patients with CNS disease also have pulmonary infections. *P. skrjabini* often produces skin nodules, subcutaneous abscesses, or a type of creeping eruption known as "trematode larva migrans."

Prevention

Metacercariae are killed if crabs and crayfish are cooked for at least 5 minutes at 55°C (131°F). Travelers should be advised to avoid traditional meals containing raw or undercooked freshwater crustaceans.

285 Blood Trematodes (Schistosomiasis)

Frank O. Richards, Jr

Schistosomiasis (also known as "Bilharzia" and "snail fever") is a chronic parasitic infection caused by trematodes that reside in the circulatory system. Over 190 million people worldwide are infected with schistosomiasis, and suffer both overt disease as well as subtle hindrance to their day-to-day activities. Infected children have impaired growth and development. Infection occurs from exposure to fresh water into which snails, the intermediate host of the parasite, have liberated cercariae that can penetrate skin. Three main species of schistosomes parasitize humans: *Schistosoma mansoni*, *S. japonicum*, and *S. haematobium*. Gastrointestinal and hepatic disease is caused by infection with either *S. mansoni* or *S. japonicum*, whereas urogenital tract disease results from *S. haematobium*. The other schistosome species more rarely infect humans. *S. intercalatum* is found in Cameroon and the Democratic Republic of Congo, and *S. mekongi* is found primarily in the Mekong River basin. Both of these species inhabit vessels of the large intestine and liver but cause a milder disease than *S. mansoni* and *S. japonicum*. *S. matthei* and *S. bovis* are found primarily in animals but occasionally infect humans.[1]

BIOLOGY

The complicated life cycle alternates between parasitic forms in the snail intermediate host and human definitive host, and free-living forms in water, the cercariae and the miracidia (Figure 285-1). The cercariae are released from infected snails and penetrate intact human skin where they then transform into schistosomulae that travel via the venous system to the lungs, where they reside for approximately 1 week. They then enter the arterial system, reach the liver where they attain sexual maturity in 4 to 6 weeks, and then descend against the blood flow of the portal venous system to the venules of the intestine *(S. mansoni* or *S. japonicum)* or bladder *(S. haematobium)*.

Males and females (schistosomes differ from other trematodes in that they are not hermaphroditic) mate and the females begin to deposit eggs. Eggs must pass through tissue to reach the lumen of the intestine or bladder and then on to the environment in feces or urine. About one-half of the eggs are retained in intestinal or vesicular tissues, where they cause granulomatous inflammation and fibrosis. In the case of the intestinal *Schistosoma* species, eggs also can be swept by the portal blood system back to the liver where they can cause similar pathologic changes. Eggs that exit the body and reach fresh water hatch and release miracidia that infect certain genera of snails. *S. mansoni* infects snails of the *Biomphalaria* species, *S. haematobium* infects *Bulinus* species, and *S. japonicum* infects *Oncomelania* snails. In the receptive snail, a single miracidium will form sporocysts from which thousands of cercariae are released into the water over a period of 6 to 12 months.[1]

EPIDEMIOLOGY

Schistosomiasis is transmitted in 76 countries in tropical and subtropical areas, but 85% of infected people reside in Africa, where *S. mansoni* and *S. haematobium* occur and often are coendemic.[1-3] *S. mansoni* was transplanted with the slave trade to South America (especially Brazil, Venezuela, and Suriname) and several islands in the Caribbean (Antigua, Dominican Republic, Guadeloupe, Martinique, Montserrat, Puerto Rico and Saint Lucia).[3] *S. haematobium* also occurs in a few countries of the Middle East. *S. japonicum* is endemic in China, the Philippines, and Indonesia.[1-3]

People most heavily infected are responsible for the majority of environmental contamination with parasite eggs. Cross-sectional studies of *S. haematobium* and *S. mansoni* show that the highest prevalence of infection occurs in school-aged children 10 to 14

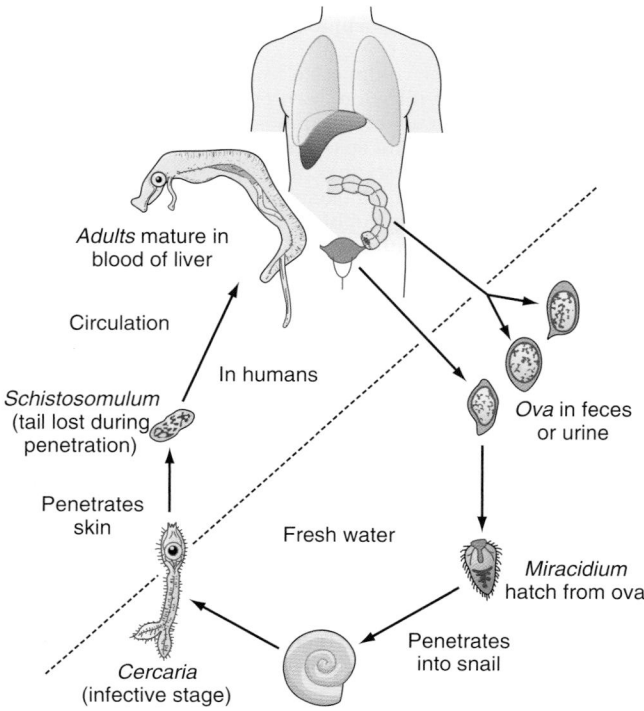

Figure 285-1. Life cycle of *Schistosoma* and occurrence of schistosomiasis.

years of age with rates decreasing (particularly in *S. haematobium*) in adulthood. Infants have been known to be infected from being bathed in irrigation canals or in lake or river water.[4,5] Males are infected twice as often as females, and certain occupations (particularly fishing and farming) are important risk factors. Highly variable community prevalence patterns and disease focality point to complex interactions with both the environment and practices of human waste disposal, water contact, and acquired immunity. Hydraulic dams and irrigation projects often increase snail habitats and the risk of transmission.

Expatriates, missionaries, diplomats, Peace Corps volunteers and other long-term residents of endemic areas are at particular risk. However, tourists also can become infected, particularly those who take part in adventure or ecotourism.[3]

PATHOGENESIS

The host immune response to the variety of stage-specific antigens during schistosomal infection results in the major clinical and pathologic manifestations of schistosomiasis.[1,2] Cercarial penetration of skin can give rise to a local hypersensitivity reaction and macular, papular, or vesicular dermatitis, usually within 72 hours of exposure. Adult worm maturation and sudden exposure to antigens with the onset of egg laying by young female worms can result in an acute illness resembling serum sickness. Chronic organ damage and dysfunction are related to the number of eggs in tissues, which in turn is related to the number of egg-laying female worms; people with a heavy worm load and the heaviest tissue egg load are at greatest risk of disease. Worm burden in humans grows only through repeated exposure to water containing cercariae. Humans acquire some immunity to reinfection but the components of the immune response that are responsible remain incompletely defined.[1]

The developing miracidia within the eggs secrete antigenic materials through microscopic pores in the shell that induce a host granulomatous response with macrophages, lymphocytes, giant cells, and eosinophils. Over time granulomas decrease in size and are replaced by fibrosis. Fibrosis along the portal vein triads of the liver ("periportal fibrosis," "claypipe stem fibrosis") in intestinal schistosomiasis can be complicated by portal hypertension. Liver function remains intact unless there is concurrent insult, such as alcoholic or viral hepatitis. As portal hypertension advances and collateral blood flow channels increase, there can be shunting of eggs to the lungs that can result in pulmonary hypertension and cor pulmonale. In urogenital (*S. haematobium*) schistosomiasis, the bladder shows raised yellow mucosal patches ("sandy patches") and bleeding areas, especially near the trigone. Calcification and fibrosis of the bladder and ureter can result in obstructive uropathy and hydronephrosis. Urogenital schistosomiasis can be complicated by pyelonephritis, calculi, and squamous cell carcinoma.

Other organs less commonly involved include skin, lungs, seminal vesicles, vulva, vagina, cervix, and central nervous system. *S haematobium* is associated with hematospermia (associated with seminal vesicle involvement) in males and cervical ulcerative lesions in females; both can enhance transmission of human immunodeficiency virus (HIV) infection.[6] *S. haematobium* also is associated with human papallomavirus (HPV) infection[7] and infertility.[8]

CLINICAL FEATURES

Acute Schistosomiasis

An acute febrile illness resembling serum sickness can occur 4 to 7 weeks after the initial infection, concurrent with maturation of female worms and the first egg release. This syndrome has been named Katayama fever, after a village in Japan where the entity was first described in association with *S. japonicum* infections. Common signs and symptoms are chills, cough, abdominal pain, diarrhea, nausea, vomiting, headache, rash (often urticarial), lymphadenopathy, and mild hepatosplenomegaly. In contrast to chronic schistosomiasis, peripheral eosinophilia is prominent in acute schistosomiasis.[1]

Intestinal and Hepatosplenic Disease

Patients with intestinal schistosomiasis (*S. mansoni, S. japonicum, S. intercalatum,* and *S. mekongi*) can be asymptomatic, or can have crampy abdominal pain, diarrhea, bloody stools, or colonic polyposis. Physical examination commonly reveals an enlarged, nontender liver, and an enlarged spleen. End-stage disease consists of portal hypertension, ascites, and portosystemic varices with an absence of jaundice. Although esophageal varices can result in severe bleeding, patients often survive these episodes because their blood coagulation function remains intact.

Urogenital Tract Disease

S. haematobium infections can cause microscopic or gross (often terminal) hematuria. In some endemic areas where transmission is intense, hematuria is so common in boys that it is considered a normal passage to manhood, locally described as male menstruation.[9] Other complaints can include dysuria and urinary frequency. Patients with obstructive uropathy or chronic or recurrent pyelonephritis can present with hypertension or end-stage renal disease. Adults can present with a suprapubic mass or urinary obstruction from squamous cell carcinoma of the bladder.

Growth and Development

Children, even with modest and low intensity of infection, may have depressed growth and learning ability.[9-12] Schistosomiasis causes anemia; physical findings in heavily infected children can include pallor and exercise intolerance.[12]

DIAGNOSIS

The history should focus on whether the person has been in an area endemic for schistosomiasis and has swum or bathed in open and likely contaminated freshwater lakes and streams. Ocean beaches and swimming pools are not sources of infection. Depending on the stage of illness, the physical examination can show rash, fever, and hepatosplenomegaly. Eosinophilia characterizes acute schistosomiasis. Hematuria can be present in persons infected with *S. haematobium*. A diagnosis is made by identifying distinctive eggs by microscopy of stool or urine specimens (Figure 285-2). *S. mansoni* eggs are oval (measuring 60×150 µm) with a distinctive lateral spine, *S. haematobium* and *S. intercalatum* are a similar size and shape but with a large terminal spine, whereas *S. japonicum* and *S. mekongi* eggs are smaller (100 µm) and round.[1] In living mature eggs the contained miracidia can be seen. A stool

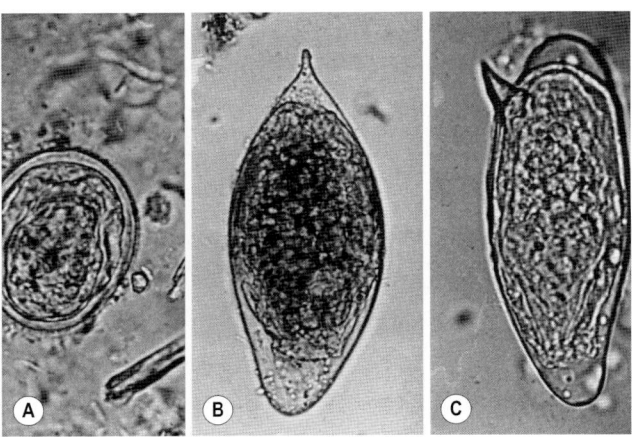

Figure 285-2. Ova in stool or urine of **(A)** *Schistosoma japonicum,* **(B)** *S. haematobium,* and **(C)** *S. mansoni.*

concentration technique (1-g fecal sample) or a Kato preparation (20- or 50-mg fecal sample) optimizes microscopic diagnosis. Rectal biopsy with histologic examination for presence of viable ova may be necessary if repeated stool examinations are negative. The sediment of at least 10 mL of urine should be examined for *S. haematobium* eggs. Sensitivity of urine examination is enhanced by collection of a midday, terminal urine specimen.

Microscopic examination can be negative in patients with acute schistosomiasis or light-intensity infections, and in these people serologic testing is most useful. Antibody detection is useful for screening of ecotourists, missionaries, and Peace Corps volunteers who have had considerable freshwater exposure in endemic areas. A number of specialty laboratories offer a variety of tests; species-specific antibody assays are available through the Centers for Disease Control and Prevention (Atlanta, GA 30333; telephone: 404-639-3311).[3] Travelers with positive antibody results are treated presumptively with praziquantel, but such serology cannot be used reliably to monitor the success of treatment.[13] Interpretation of antibody test results is more difficult in patients who originate from endemic areas, and presumptive treatment in these people based on serologic results alone is controversial. A new commercialized test for detection of antigen in serum and urine appears to be useful for *S. mansoni* diagnosis.[14]

Ultrasonography (US) is most useful for diagnosis and staging of chronic schistosomiasis.[1,15] In intestinal schistosomiasis, characteristic US can demonstrate hepatic findings and the degree of portal hypertension and splenomegaly. In urinary schistosomiasis, US can show bladder wall thickness, dilatation of the ureter and renal pelvis and bladder calculi. Abdominal imaging can show bladder calcification in *S. haematobium* infections.

MANAGEMENT

Praziquantel is the drug of choice for therapy[16] (see Chapter 296, Appendix 296-1). For *S. mansoni* and *S. haematobium* infection, 40 mg/kg in 1 or 2 divided doses orally for 1 day is recommended. For *S. japonicum* infection, 60 mg/kg in 3 divided doses for 1 day is recommended. Side effects of praziquantel are minimal (abdominal pain is most common in treatment of intestinal schistosomiasis). Praziquantel results in parasitologic cure in approximately 80% of cases, but in people who are not cured, egg burden is reduced by 95% to 99%. Oxamniquine is an alternative drug for *S. mansoni*, used primarily in South America. Both drugs periodically are used in school-based or community-based mass treatment programs to reduce the egg burdens of infected people.[17] Treatment in children and young adults promptly results in reversal of much of the disease, cessation of hematuria in urinary schistosomiasis, and regression of hepatosplenomegaly in intestinal disease. Reversal of chronic fibrotic organ damage is uncommon and prognosis is guarded in people with portal hypertension, esophageal varices, cor pulmonale, and hydronephrosis.

Prophylaxis with praziquantel shortly after water exposure is not effective since developing schistosomulae are relatively resistant. However, artemisinins (antimalarial drugs) appear useful against developing stages and may find future use as prophylaxis after skin exposure to infected water sources.[1,18]

Esophageal variceal bleeding initially can be managed conservatively since patients have normal hepatic function. If immediate interventions are needed, balloon tamponade and endoscopic sclerotherapy have been used. Selective distal splenorenal shunts may offer the best survival among options for the surgical management of portal hypertension.[1]

SPECIAL CONSIDERATIONS

Central nervous system schistosomiasis results from aberrant migration of adult worms to the venules draining the brain or spinal cord. Deposition of eggs around these sensitive tissues, and the ensuing granulomatous inflammation, gives rise to serious manifestations that include seizures, headache, and transverse myelitis. Previously unexposed people (i.e., immunologically naive) may be at greater risk for aberrant migration of schistosomes. Use of corticosteroids and/or extended courses of praziquantel in these patients is controversial.

Cercarial dermatitis, also known as "swimmer's itch," is a pruritic macular, papular, or vesicular rash that occurs as a consequence of cercariae penetration of skin. Cercarial dermatitis can occur from exposure to animal (usually avian) schistosomes, often in countries nonendemic for human schistosomiasis, and after exposure to sea, as well as fresh, water. The cercariae die in the skin and the rash responds to symptomatic treatment and topical corticosteroids.

PREVENTION

People planning travel to regions where schistosomiasis may be endemic can consult the CDC's traveler health website for further information on endemic countries.[19] Travelers should avoid entering open fresh water in those areas.

Strategies for controlling schistosomiasis include mass chemotherapy, health education and behavioral modification, improved sewage/sanitation, and control of snails through environmental engineering or use of molluscicides. Large-scale control programs using one or more of these strategies have had varying degrees of success in several countries. Schistosomiasis was eliminated completely from Japan by environmental engineering and improved sanitation. Despite prolonged use of mass praziquantel treatment in a number of country settings, there has been no broadly documented case of emergence of drug resistance,[20] although clinical praziquantel tolerance in travelers requiring 3 days of therapy has been reported.[21] Active research for a vaccine is ongoing and some vaccine candidates are in early human trials.[1]

Key Points. Characteristic Features of Schistosomiasis

MICROBIOLOGY

- Caused by trematodes that reside in the venules of the intestinal tract (*Schistosoma mansoni* and *S. japonicum*) or surrounding the bladder (*S. haematobium*). The female worms lay eggs that exit the body in feces or urine
- If deposited in fresh water, miracidia emerge from eggs and infect specific snails. Cercariae later released from infected snails penetrate intact human skin and establish the infection, completing the life cycle
- Eggs in retained tissue cause granulomatous inflammation that damage host tissues; patients with a heavy worm load are at greatest risk of disease

EPIDEMIOLOGY

- Over 190 million people worldwide are infected, in 76 countries in tropical and subtropical areas, but 85% of infected people reside in Africa, where *S. mansoni* and *S. haematobium* are the most common species and often are co-endemic
- Schistosomiasis occurs in areas with poor sanitation where infected people deposit feces or urine containing eggs directly into fresh water containing the appropriate snails. Other people are later infected or reinfected when these same water bodies are used for swimming, bathing, washing clothes/utensils, and agricultural purposes

Key Points. Characteristic Features of Schistosomiasis—cont'd

CLINICAL FEATURES

- An acute febrile illness resembling serum sickness can occur 4 to 7 weeks after initial infection, concurrent with maturation of female worms and the first egg release ("Katayama fever")
- *S. mansoni* and *S. japonicum* can cause crampy abdominal pain, and an enlarged liver or spleen. End-stage disease can include portal hypertension, ascites, and portosystemic varices
- *S. haematobium* infections can cause microscopic or gross hematuria, dysuria, and urinary frequency. End-stage disease can include genital lesions, obstructive uropathy, and squamous cell carcinoma of the bladder
- Even with light worm burdens, children may have depressed growth and learning ability and anemia

- Dermatitis can occur within 72 hours of exposure to infected water as cercariae penetrate skin. Cercarial dermatitis, also known as "swimmer's itch", also can be due to animal (usually avian) schistosomes, occurring in countries nonendemic for human schistosomiasis and after exposure to sea, as well as fresh, water

DIAGNOSIS

- Detection of eggs in stool or urine. Serologic testing

TREATMENT

- Praziquantel

SECTION A: The Clinician and the Laboratory

286 Laboratory Diagnosis of Infection Due to Bacteria, Fungi, Parasites, and Rickettsiae

John C. Christenson and E. Kent Korgenski

BACTERIA

Collection and Processing of Clinical Specimens

Proper collection and handling of clinical specimens are very important aspects of laboratory medicine. No degree of laboratory expertise can correct the error of inappropriately collected and transported specimens.[1] Common problems include insufficient quantity, contamination, lack of proper transport media, and delay in transport to the laboratory. Dry swabs are commonly sent but are rarely adequate for survival and isolation of bacteria.

Transport media are designed to prevent drying, maintain a balanced physiochemical environment, and prevent oxidation and enzymatic destruction of the pathogen; they provide minimal nutrients. Some transport media contain antimicrobial agents that suppress normal or contaminating flora to enhance the isolation of a specific pathogen or pathogens.

In general, specimens for bacterial culture should not be stored for longer than 24 hours before processing. When specimens cannot be immediately transported to the laboratory, appropriate alternatives are available. Urine is refrigerated at 2°C to 8°C for up to 24 hours. Inoculated blood culture bottles can be held at room temperature for up to 4 hours. Specimens for isolation of *Neisseria gonorrhoeae* should be inoculated on specific media such as modified Thayer–Martin or NYC agar, preferably transported in a self-contained CO_2-generating transport system as soon as possible to the laboratory, and immediately incubated at 35°C in 5% to 10% CO_2. Cerebrospinal fluid (CSF) is held and transported rapidly at room temperature or at 35°C to 37°C and never refrigerated. A dry swab is preferred for detection of *Streptococcus pyogenes* antigen from pharyngeal specimens. Table 286-1 summarizes the specimen collection and transport media commonly used, as well as the specific usefulness of the media. Recommended methods for collection and transport and media for routine microbial isolation are shown in Table 286-2.

Three types of culture media are used: enriched, selective, and differential. Enriched media support the growth of fastidious bacteria. Examples include chocolate agar, sheep blood agar, and thioglycolate broth. Selective media permit the selective growth of certain groups of bacteria while suppressing others. Differential media assist in distinguishing among similar groups of bacteria. Tables 286-3 and 286-4 provide a summary of media used for bacterial isolation.

Specimen-Specific Isolation Methods

Blood

Specimen collection. Many advances have been made to maximize the recovery of bacteria from blood and to minimize contamination during collection. Venipuncture sites are disinfected with chlorhexidine gluconate 2% with 70% isopropyl alcohol or

10% povidone-iodine (allowing either to dry for at least 1 minute, with no wiping).[2] Chlorhexidine should not be used in infants <2 months. Povidone-iodine is preferred in this age group.[3] The rubber stopper of the blood culture bottle or tube is disinfected using 70% isopropyl or ethyl alcohol.

The proportion of blood to broth is important. A ratio of blood to broth >1:5 is desirable.[4,5] Inadequate volume of specimen is the most important cause of a low yield of blood culture. Most broth culture systems contain an anticoagulant, sodium polyanetholesulfonate (SPS), 0.025% to 0.05%, which inhibits phagocytosis and the bactericidal activity of serum, inactivates complement, and neutralizes lysozymes and aminoglycosides. SPS can inhibit the growth of organisms such as *Neisseria* spp., *Streptobacillus moniliformis*, and *Francisella tularensis*. An appropriate ratio of blood to broth volume dilutes SPS, thereby decreasing the natural inhibitory factors, and also dilutes antimicrobial agents if they were present in the patient's bloodstream. Many older "conventional" blood culture systems were suboptimal for pediatric use because the 5- to 10-mL recommended blood volume is inappropriate for infants. Bacteremia in children usually is quantitatively higher than in adults; 1 to 5 mL may be an adequate sample from children, whereas 20 to 30 mL is required from adults.[5] Table 286-5 shows recommended blood volumes according to body weight.

TABLE 286-1. Collection Methods and Transport Media

Method	Use
COMMONLY USED SWABS	
Calcium alginate	Toxic to *Neisseria gonorrhoeae*, herpes simplex virus, ureaplasmas; useful for collection of chlamydiae
Cotton	Residual fatty acids inhibit bacteria and chlamydiae
Dacron	Useful for viruses, culture for *Streptococcus pyogenes*
TRANSPORT SYSTEMS FOR AEROBIC/FACULTATIVE ORGANISMS	
Culturette	Rayon-tipped swab prevents drying, maintains pH
PATHOGEN-SPECIFIC SYSTEMS	
Anaerobic bacteria	Anaswab system, Port-A-Cul vial or swab, Bio Bag environmental system, BD anaerobic specimen collector; aspirate of specimen with expression into vial is always preferred
Neisseria gonorrhoeae	Jemec, Gono–Pak agar systems; contain CO_2-generating tablet ($NaHCO_3$-citric acid tablet); inoculated agar placed in bag and incubated for 18–24 hours before transport

TABLE 286-2. Transport System(s) and Media Inoculated Routinely According to Source of Specimen

Specimen	Transport System	Routine Media
Blood	Blood culture vial(s); if *Neisseria meningitidis*, no SPS	See text
Cerebrospinal fluid	Sterile screw-cap tube	BAP, CHOC (CO$_2$), THIO
Brain abscess	Anaerobic transport medium	BAP, CHOC (CO$_2$), EMB/MAC, BAP-ANA, THIO, MS
Feces	Sterile screw-cap container	BAP, EMB/MAC, CAMPY, HEK, selenite/GN broth, CIN, MAC-S
Rectal swab	Swab transport system	BAP, EMB/MAC, CAMPY, HEK, selenite/GN broth, CIN, MAC-S
Gastric lavage, duodenal aspirate	Sterile screw-cap container	BAP, EMB/MAC, PEA, BAP-ANA, THIO, MS
Biopsied tissue	Sterile screw-cap container with preservative-free 0.85% NaCl	BAP, EMB/MAC, PEA, BAP-ANA, THIO, MS; for lung tissue: no PEA, add CHOC (CO$_2$)
Conjunctival swab	Prepare smears, directly inoculate media	BAP, CHOC (CO$_2$), EMB/MAC, THIO, MS
Genital, anal swab	Swab transport, GC transport system	BAP, EMB/MAC, THIO, CNA, MTM, NYC
Sputum, BAL fluid	Sputum trap, sterile screw-cap container	No anaerobic cultures; BAP, CHOC (CO$_2$), EMB/MAC, MS
Lung aspirate, transtracheal aspirate	Anaerobic transport system or sterile screw-cap container	BAP, CHOC (CO$_2$), EMB/MAC, MS, BAP-ANA, THIO
Throat, nasal, nasopharyngeal swab	Swab transport system	Throat: BAP, SXT-BAP; CHOC (CO$_2$), EMB/MAC, MS
Tympanocentesis fluid, sinus aspirate	Sterile screw-cap tube or anaerobic transport system	BAP, CHOC (CO$_2$), EMB/MAC, MS, BAP-ANA, THIO
Pleural, peritoneal ascites fluid	Sterile screw-cap container or blood culture broth bottle; anaerobic transport system	BAP, CHOC (CO$_2$), EMB/MAC, MS, BAP-ANA, THIO
Urine	Sterile screw-cap container	BAP, EMB/MAC, PEA/CNA
Wound; superficial, deep	Sterile screw-cap container plus anaerobic transport system	BAP, EMB/MAC, PEA, MS; for deep biopsies, add BAP ANA; THIO

BAL, bronchoalveolar lavage; BAP, blood-agar plate; BAP-ANA, blood agar incubated anaerobically; CAMPY, Campylobacter blood agar; CHOC, enriched chocolate agar; CIN, cefsulodin-irgasan-novobiocin agar; CNA, colistin–nalidixic acid; EMB, eosin–methylene blue; GC, gonococcal; GN, gram-negative; HEK, Hektoen enteric agar; MAC, MacConkey medium; MAC-S, MacConkey-sorbitol agar; MS, mannitol salt agar; MTM, modified Thayer–Martin medium; NYC, New York City agar; PEA, phenylethyl alcohol; SPS, sodium polyanetholesulfonate; SXT agar, blood agar with trimethoprim-sulfamethoxazole; THIO, thioglycolate broth.

Although a single sampling may be sufficient for many patients with bacteremia, multiple samples are appropriate in certain circumstances (e.g., in suspected endocarditis, where two to three samples are desirable). The total volume of blood is probably more important in this circumstance than the number of samples. At least two sets of cultures are helpful in children with indwelling intravascular catheters. Bottles should not be inoculated with more than the manufacturer's recommended amount.

Once blood is inoculated into a broth bottle, rapid incubation is essential. Delays in insertion of bottles into automated continuously-monitored blood culture systems results in a delay in detecting the presence of bacteremia.[6]

Media. Advances in blood culture systems have increased yield, reduced the time of recovery, and diminished technologist time. In addition, some systems were developed to maximize recovery of fastidious organisms. Some of these systems are lysis centrifugation-direct plating (Isolator, Wampole), VersaTREK Microbial Detection (Trek Diagnostic Systems), BacT/Alert (BioMérieux), and BACTEC (Becton Dickinson). For the latter three systems, several broth formulas are available, depending on the type of suspected pathogen. No single system is optimal for all microorganisms.

The lysis centrifugation-direct plating system consists of a sterile tube of two different sizes (1.5, 10 mL) that contains saponin and SPS, which lyse red and white blood cells in the blood specimen and inactivate complement and immunoglobulins. Hemoglobin binds to SPS and prevents inhibition of bacteria.[7] The larger tubes are centrifuged at 300 *g* for 30 minutes in a fixed-angle rotor. With the use of an Isostat press, the lysate is removed and inoculated directly onto agar medium, which is incubated and examined daily for growth. Media can be selected to maximize the recovery of suspected pathogens.[8–10] In addition, isolation of certain fungi

is enhanced. As little as 1 mL of blood is required, and direct plating allows quantification of bacteria.[11] Excess contamination can occur with this system. Careful handling and inoculation of agar under laminar flow decreases the likelihood.

Compared with conventional systems, BACTEC has demonstrated increased recovery of organisms and decreased time to detection, particularly for *Mycobacterium*. BACTEC 9240 is a continuous monitoring, "noninvasive" blood culture system that uses internal fluorescent CO$_2$ sensors to detect the metabolic activity of bacteria. BACTEC Plus Aerobic/F, Plus Anaerobic/F, and Peds Plus/F bottles contain resins that may decrease the effect of antibiotics. By utilizing a differential time-to-positivity between a positive culture result from an intravascular catheter site and a peripheral venipuncture site, this system may assist clinicians in identifying an intravascular catheter-related infection.[11]

BacT/Alert and VersaTREK systems are two additional continuous monitoring blood culture systems that have been demonstrated to be useful in the detection of bacteremia and fungemia, with a higher yield of recovery and a reduction in time to detection.

Incubation. Older "conventional" broth bottles were incubated for 7 days. Bottles were inspected for macroscopic growth daily and subcultured blindly. Acridine orange staining was performed after 18 to 24 hours' incubation. With newer systems, bottles are incubated at 35°C usually for 5 days.

Most pediatric pathogens are isolated within 72 hours of incubation. With the newer blood culture systems, most bacterial pathogens are detected within 48 hours.[12–15] Incubation for more than 5 days usually is not warranted except in certain situations (e.g., suspected fungi, *Bartonella henselae*, *Corynebacterium*, *Actinomyces*).

Special pathogens and situations. If brucellosis is suspected, the automated blood culture is held for a minimum of 7 but no more

TABLE 286-3. Commonly Used Culture Media

Medium	Type of Medium	Indicator or Inhibitor	Comments
Sheep blood agar, 5%	N	None	Growth of most medically significant bacteria; allows determination of hemolysis
Horse blood agar, 3–5%	S, N	None	Incubated at 5% CO_2; enhances isolation of *Haemophilus*
MacConkey agar	S, D	Bile salts, crystal violet, lactose, neutral red	Selective agar for Enterobacteriaceae, some other gram-negative rods; differentiates lactose-fermenting and nonlactose-fermenting organisms
MacConkey-sorbitol agar	S, D	MacConkey, sorbitol	Detects *Escherichia coli* O157:H7
Phenylethyl alcohol agar	S	Phenylethyl alcohol	Inhibits gram-negative bacteria; supports gram-positive bacteria
Colistin–nalidixic acid agar	S	Colistin, nalidixic acid, blood agar	Supports gram-positive bacteria; inhibits gram-negative organisms
Mannitol salt agar	S, D	NaCl, mannitol, phenol red	Selects for staphylococci
Selective enterococcal agar	S, D	Oxgall, esculin, sodium azide	Selects for enterococci
Hektoen enteric agar	S, D	Bile salts, ferric ammonium citrate, sodium thiosulfate, lactose, sucrose, salicin, bromthymol blue, fuchsin	Enhances isolation of Enterobacteriaceae, *Shigella*, and *Salmonella* spp.; H_2S production; differentiates lactose-fermenting and nonlactose-fermenting bacteria
Deoxycholate-citrate agar	S, D	Deoxycholate, sodium citrate, ferric citrate, lactose, neutral red	Selects for *Salmonella* and some *Shigella* spp.
Selenite broth	S	Selenium salts	Enrichment for *Salmonella;* inhibits normal flora
Campylobacter agar	S	Amphotericin B, cephalothin, trimethoprim, vancomycin, polymyxin B	Isolation of *Campylobacter* spp.; inhibits normal flora
Chocolate agar	N	None	Enhances growth of bacteria that replicate on blood agar, plus *Haemophilus* spp., *Neisseria gonorrhoeae*, *N. meningitidis*
Thayer–Martin modified agar	S	Vancomycin, colistin, nystatin, trimethoprim	Selects for *N. gonorrhoeae, N. meningitidis;* inhibits normal flora
New York City agar	S	Vancomycin, colistin, amphotericin B, trimethoprim	Same as Thayer–Martin modified agar
Anaerobic blood agar	N	None	Growth of all anaerobic bacteria; should contain yeast extract, vitamin K, and hemin
Salmonella-Shigella agar	S, D	Bile salts, brilliant green, ferric citrate, sodium citrate, sodium thiosulfate, lactose, neutral red	Selects for *Salmonella*, some *Shigella;* inhibits normal flora
Legionella medium	S	Vancomycin, colistin, anisomycin	Selects for *Legionella*
Bordet–Gengou agar, Regan–Lowe medium, Stainer-Scholte medium	S	Cephalexin	Selects for *Bordetella* spp.
Löwenstein–Jensen agar	S	None	Selects for *Mycobacterium* spp.
BC-selective agar	S	Phenol red, ticarcillin, polymyxin B	Selects for *Burkholderia* cepacia
Eosin–methylene blue agar	S, D	Eosin–methylene blue	Selects for gram-negative enteric bacilli
Haemophilus test medium	N	Mueller–Hinton agar, hematin, NAD, yeast extract	Test medium for *Haemophilus*
Haemophilus test broth	N	Mueller–Hinton agar, hematin, NAD, yeast extract	Test medium for *Haemophilus*

BC, Burkholderia cepacia; D, differential; N, enriched nutrient; NAD, nicotinamide adenine dinucleotide; S, selective.

than 10 days. Subculture to a blood agar, chocolate agar, or brucella agar plate and incubation in 5% to 10% CO_2 at 37°C for at least 72 hours usually is adequate. For the isolation of cell wall-deficient bacteria, hypertonic medium (containing 10% sucrose or mannitol) is required. BACTEC NR-8A and BacT/Alert also could be used. Nutritionally deficient organisms such as *Abiotrophia* species should be suspected when organisms are evident on Gram stain but fail to grow when subcultured. Broth can be subcultured onto a blood-agar plate streaked with *Staphylococcus aureus,* or media can be supplemented with 0.001% pyridoxal hydrochloride and 0.05% to 0.1% L-cysteine. A pyridoxal-impregnated disk also can be used. Plates are usually incubated overnight at 35°C to 37°C in 5% to

10% CO_2. Although rare causes of bacteremia and endocarditis, the AACEK (formerly HACEK) group of microorganisms, *Aggregatibacter* (formerly *Haemophilus*) *aphrophilus, Aggregatibacter* (formerly *Actinobacillus*) *actinomycetemcomitans, Cardiobacterium hominis, Eikenella corrodens, Kingella kingae,* grow within the routine incubation period for automated blood culture systems.[16]

Special manipulation is required for isolation of *Bartonella* and should only be performed by laboratories familiar with culture and identification of the organism. The Isolator system is used, with subsequent inoculation onto media enriched with fresh blood (5% rabbit blood), and incubated in CO_2 at 35°C to 37°C for 15 days.

TABLE 286-4. Specific Media Used for Isolation of Common Microorganisms

Microorganism	Media
Staphylococci	Mannitol salt (O_2), PEA, blood agar, CNA (CO_2)
Streptococci	PEA, CNA, blood agar (CO_2)
Enterobacteriaceae	EMB, MAC (O_2), blood agar (O_2)
Escherichia coli O157:H7	MAC-sorbitol (O_2)
Burkholderia cepacia	BCSA (at 32°C), MAC
Neisseria gonorrhoeae	MTM, NYC agar (CO_2), CHOC agar
Haemophilus spp.	CHOC agar, horse blood agar (CO_2)
Salmonella, Shigella spp.	Hektoen agar, SS agar, selenite broth, XLD, MAC
Campylobacter spp.	CAMP-BAP (42°C, 5% O_2, 10% CO_2)
Bordetella spp.	Bordet–Gengou agar, Regan–Lowe (CO_2) medium, Stainer-Scholte medium
Yersinia spp.	Yersinia selective agar, CIN agar (25°C, O_2)
Enterococci	PEA, CNA, blood agar (CO_2), bile esculin (CO_2)
Francisella tularensis	CHOC or MTM (O_2)
Mycobacterium spp.	Middlebrook 7H10, LJ, BACTEC 13A (blood), BACTEC 460 (using Isolator)
Legionella spp.	BCYE (35°C, O_2), BAP (CO_2)
Brucella spp.	Brucella blood agar, MTM, CHOC agar
Anaerobic bacteria	Chopped meat–glucose, TSA, PEA, Brucella blood agar, BAP-ANA, laked blood with kanamycin, vancomycin
Vibrio spp.	TCBS (35–37°C)
Neisseria, Moraxella spp.	CHOC (CO_2), BAP
Aeromonas spp.	BAP-AMP, MAC
Clostridium difficile	CCFA (anaerobic)
Actinomyces, Nocardia spp.	BHI agar, TSA, BAP-ANA (14 days)
Streptococcus pyogenes	SXT agar (CO_2)
Leptospira spp.	Bovine serum albumin–Tween 80
Yersinia pestis	TSA, BAP, BHI agar, CHOC (O_2)
Bacteroides spp.	TSA, BBE, laked blood with kanamycin, vancomycin
Fungi	Isolator (blood), biphasic BHI broth, IMA, SAB

BAP, blood-agar plate; BAP-AMP, blood agar with ampicillin (10 µg/mL); BAP-ANA, blood agar incubated anaerobically; BBE, Bacteroides bile-esculin agar; BCSA, Burkholderia cepacia-selective agar; BCYE, buffered charcoal-yeast extract; BHI, brain–heart infusion; CAMP-BAP, Campylobacter blood-agar plate; CCFA, cycloserinecefoxitin-fructose–egg yolk agar; CHOC, enriched chocolate agar; CIN agar, cefsulodin-irgasan-novobiocin medium; CNA, colistin–nalidixic acid agar; EMB, eosin–methylene blue; IMA, inhibitory mold agar (with gentamicin and chloramphenicol); LJ, Löwenstein–Jensen medium; MAC, MacConkey medium; MTM, modified Thayer–Martin medium; NYC, New York City agar; OFPBL, oxidative-fermentative base–polymyxin B–bacitracin-lactose medium; PEA, phenylethyl alcohol; SAB, Sabouraud dextrose agar; SS agar, Salmonella-Shigella agar; SXT, blood agar with trimethoprim-sulfamethoxazole; TCBS, thiosulfate-citrate–bile salts–sucrose agar; TSA, trypticase soy agar; XLD, xylose-lysine-deoxycholate agar.

TABLE 286-5. Recommended Blood Volumes for Culture for Pediatric-Age Patients[a,b,c]

Patient Weight (kg)	Blood Volume to Collect (mL)	Media Type and Inoculation Volume (mL)	
		BD BACTEC Peds Plus/F	BD BACTEC Lytic/10 Anaerobic/F
<1.5	1	0.5	0.5
1.5–3.9	2	1	1
4–7.9	4	2	2
8–13.9	6	3	3
14–18.9	10	5	5
		BD BACTEC Plus Aerobic/F	BD BACTEC Plus Anaerobic/F
19–25.9	16	8	8
>26	20	10	10

[a]These are the recommended volumes necessary for the optimal isolation of bacterial pathogens.

[b]If unable to obtain sufficient blood for both bottles, inject available blood into aerobic bottle (Peds Plus/F or Plus Aerobic/F).

[c]Plus Aerobic/F and Plus Anaerobic/F are the recommended media for larger children, adolescents and adults.

A combination of systems or potential use of alternative systems according to the anticipated pathogen or pathogens is optimal.

Recent studies have demonstrated the ability of 16S rRNA polymerase chain reaction (PCR) to detect bacteremia within hours of collecting a blood specimen.[17] A multiplex blood PCR can detect the presence of gram-positive and gram-negative bacteria, and fungi in febrile neutropenic patients.[18] PCR was capable of diagnosing and serotyping pneumococcal bacteremic community-acquired pneumonia in children.[19] In persons with S. aureus bacteremia, PCR identified those patients with methicillin-susceptible S. aureus, permitting reduction in vancomycin use, hospital stays, and costs.[20]

Urine

Although clean-voided midstream urine is an acceptable specimen for culture in older children and adults, this technique is difficult in young children. Collection of urine by a bag fixed to the perineum is a poor substitute. In this population, catheterized specimens or specimens collected by suprapubic aspiration are preferred. Because the distal part of the urethra normally is colonized, quantitative culture is required. A known volume of urine (0.01 to 0.001 mL) is inoculated by means of a calibrated loop or pipette onto agar media to permit quantification of isolated colonies. Detection of 10^4 colony-forming units (CFU)/mL of a single bacterial isolate from a clean-voided midstream urine specimen (10^2 CFU/mL from a specimen obtained by catheter) correlates with probable true urinary tract infection. Any bacterial growth from urine obtained by suprapubic aspiration is considered clinically relevant. A prolonged time in ambient temperature from collection to inoculation (2 hours) is associated with a false-positive quantitative culture. Isolation of multiple organisms with low colony counts usually indicates contamination, except in special circumstances such as an inability to concentrate or retain urine and obstructive uropathy.

Gram stain or acridine orange stain of unspun urine in which at least 2 bacteria of the same type per high-power field are demonstrated indicates significant bacteriuria (i.e., 10^5 CFU/mL).

Cerebrospinal Fluid

Specimen collection and processing. CSF must be transported to the laboratory without delay because fluid is hypotonic and bacteria and cells can lyse (thereby affecting the cell count and contributing to falsely abnormal biochemical analysis) or utilize glucose and thus lower measured levels. At room temperature, cell counts decrease approximately 32% by 1 hour and 50% by 2 hours after collection.[21] Neutrophils are affected more than lymphocytes. Refrigeration can render fastidious bacteria nonviable. If delay is expected, samples are stored at room temperature or incubated at 35°C to 37°C to maximize isolation. The first tube collected is sent for microbiologic processing to minimize potential contamination.

Routinely, CSF should be inoculated onto sheep blood agar, enriched chocolate agar, and enriched broth (thioglycolate) and incubated for 4 days at 37°C in 5% to 10% CO_2. If Gram stain is positive but culture demonstrates no growth at 72 hours, the culture is held for an additional 4 days. The minimal volume acceptable for culture of fungi and *Mycobacterium* is 2 mL; 10 to 15 mL is preferred.

Centrifugation by cytospinning (2000 rpm; 350 *g*) to maximize pellet formation of bacteria and cellular elements produces a yield on direct examination of CSF by Gram stain superior to that of unconcentrated samples. Leukocyte morphology is preserved and examination of large numbers of cells improves the validity of the differential cell count. In one study, smears were positive for bacteria in 78% of samples when cytospinning was performed compared with 56% for unconcentrated samples.[22]

Gram stain demonstrates organisms in 75% to 90% of untreated patients with meningitis. Patients with *Streptococcus pneumoniae* and *Haemophilus influenzae* infection are more likely to have a positive Gram stain (90% and 86%, respectively) than are those with *Neisseria meningitidis* (75%).[23] The yield of Gram stain correlates with the density of bacteria in CSF; 97% of infections with $>10^5$ CFU/mL of bacteria and only 25% with $<10^3$ CFU/mL.[24] The yield of Gram stain decreases in patients receiving antimicrobial therapy, even orally.

Acridine orange, or 3,6-*bis*(dimethylamino)acridine staining is a more sensitive technique than Gram stain for detecting bacteria, especially in patients who have received antimicrobial therapy.[25,26]

PCR appears to be an ideal tool for the diagnosis of bacterial meningitis, especially in patients who have received antibiotics.[27,28] Multiple studies have demonstrated its clinical usefulness, with sensitivities similar to routine culture technology but with a shorter turnaround time.[29,30] In one study, 16S rRNA PCR had an overall sensitivity of 93%; with a specificity of 98%.[31]

Bacterial antigen detection usually is not useful in the diagnosis and management of meningitis. Value, if any, appears to be limited to patients whose Gram stain, CSF culture, and blood culture are negative; pretreated patients; and when lumbar puncture is postponed because of the severity of illness.[23,32]

Respiratory Tract

Specimen collection. Tables 286-1 and 286-2 highlight proper collection of respiratory tract specimens for bacterial isolation. Throat swab for the detection of *Streptococcus pyogenes* (GAS) is the most common respiratory tract specimen sent for culture; proper collection of the sample (by swabbing of the tonsillar surface, posterior pharyngeal wall, and opposite tonsillar surface while avoiding the tongue and saliva) affects the yield of the culture.

Rapid tests for GAS. Routine culture on agar requires 24 to 48 hours for results and could delay therapy for some patients. Rapid detection assays for streptococcal antigen can yield results in 10 to 70 minutes. The specificity of various tests is 62% to 100%, but the sensitivity is lower.[33] Although initial studies performed in microbiology laboratories demonstrated high sensitivity, performance in other settings shows variable results. Results are influenced by the skill, experience, and expertise of the person obtaining the throat swab and performing the assay. In a community office-based study, the sensitivity of the office culture for GAS was found to be higher than the rapid antigen-detection test (81% versus 70%). Both tests have specificities greater than 97%.[34] Tests utilizing optical immunoassay have consistently demonstrated sensitivities and specificities higher than other assays.

A reflex culture should be used for individuals with a negative rapid antigen test. Since specificities are high, positive antigen tests do not need to be confirmed by culture.[35,36] Although sensitivity increases with severity of illness, the sensitivity of the assay may not be high enough to avoid performance of a culture.[37] The isolation of GAS on agar permits antimicrobial susceptibility testing for macrolide resistance.

Technology utilizing DNA probes and PCR has demonstrated very high specificity and good sensitivity. Unfortunately, the tests are difficult to perform and are not suitable as point-of-care tests.[38,39]

Antigen detection assays have been used to detect the presence of GAS at extrapharyngeal sites such as in pyogenic arthritis, cellulitis, and parapneumonic effusions. One kit demonstrates high sensitivity and specificity for detecting antigen at skin sites.[40] An enzyme immunoassay (EIA) showed high sensitivity when testing synovial fluid, soft-tissue aspirate, and pleural fluid. No false-positive results were reported.[41]

Special specimens. Tympanocentesis plus sinus aspiration for culture is extremely useful in special situations (e.g., immunocompromised patients, patients with intracranial complications, and those who fail to respond to antimicrobial therapy). Data are conflicting regarding the validity of culture of the nasopharynx in predicting the pathogens of sinusitis and otitis media. Routine use is not indicated.

Collection of sputum from children with lower respiratory tract infections is technically difficult. Aspiration of deep pharyngeal/tracheal secretions (with a Leuken trap) is used by some. In older children, sputum is a valuable specimen. The presence of ≥10 squamous epithelial cells per low-power field is highly suggestive of an oropharyngeal site of collection. Conversely, the presence of >25 white blood cells per low-power field denotes an adequate specimen. Organism isolation at quantities $≥10^4$ CFU/mL is predictive of the pathogen of infection, as proved by biopsy.[42–44] Gram stain should be used to aid in the interpretation of isolates from culture.

Transtracheal aspiration is technically difficult in children and is seldom performed. Bronchoscopy and especially a quantitative bronchoalveolar lavage specimen or protected brush is useful in the diagnosis of *Pneumocystis jirovecii* and mycobacterial, fungal, and bacterial infection.

Burkholderia cepacia. Isolation of *B. cepacia* from the sputum of patients with cystic fibrosis requires the use of selective media. *B. cepacia*-selective agar (BCSA) or oxidative-fermentative base-polymyxin B-bacitracin-lactose (OFPBL) medium have been used.[45,46] It appears that BCSA may be superior to OFPBL.[46]

Bordetella species. Currently available diagnostic tests for *Bordetella* have variable sensitivity, depending on the case definition, level of immunization, adequacy of collection and transport, and diagnostic method.[47] When properly performed, culture is superior to direct immunofluorescence assay on nasopharyngeal secretions. Cultures are more likely to be positive during the first 2 weeks of illness.[48] Serologic tests by EIA (*B. pertussis*-specific immunoglobulin G) are sensitive but difficult to interpret and usually require acute and convalescent sera. PCR assays may provide higher sensitivity with a quicker turnaround.[49–53] In addition, in persons with symptoms for ≥2 weeks, PCR demonstrates a higher sensitivity than culture or DFA.[48,54,55] A combination of culture, serology, and PCR provides a greater sensitivity when performed on previously immunized individuals with cough illness.[47,50] In many diagnostic clinical microbiology laboratories, PCR is the test of choice, and fluorescent staining and culture are no longer being performed. Standardization of PCR assay and false-positive results are problematic. CDC recommendations for primers and test conditions are available at http://www.cdc.gov/pertussi/clinical/diagnostic-testing/index.html.

Synovial and Peritoneal Fluid

Inoculation of synovial fluid and peritoneal fluid into blood culture bottles results in a higher recovery rate of bacteria than inoculation of conventional agar or broth.[56,57] In one study,

Kingella kingae, a cause of septic arthritis, was detected exclusively in specimens inoculated into BACTEC bottles.[58] In another study, BacT/Alert demonstrated high sensitivity.[59]

In patients with spontaneous bacterial peritonitis, inoculation of peritoneal fluid into BACTEC bottles more than doubled the recovery of gram-negative bacteria.[60] Although none of the fluids inoculated into conventional media yielded streptococci and enterococci, 33% of those inoculated into BACTEC bottles grew these organisms. Similar findings have been demonstrated in patients with peritonitis complicating continuous ambulatory peritoneal dialysis.[61,62]

Special Pathogens

Clostridium difficile

Laboratory diagnosis of *C. difficile* remains a challenge and many different testing algorithms can be found. Most algorithms utilize one or more of the following test methods: glutamate dehydrogenase (GDH) antigen, toxin A/B EIA, cytotoxin neutralization, toxigenic culture, or toxin PCR.[63] Laboratories with the capability to perform toxin-detecting PCR or toxigenic culture can use these methods alone as a testing algorithm.[64,65] However, toxigenic culture is complex to perform and results take 2 to 7 days. PCR detection of the toxin B gene (*tcdB*) has been found to have the highest sensitivity and negative predictive value, with the quickest turnaround.[64,66,67] GDH antigen assays are excellent screening tests for *C. difficile* with a high sensitivity and negative predictive value and results usually are available in <24 hours. However, a positive result must be confirmed with a different method for detection of toxin-producing strains. Although many laboratories are utilizing toxin A/B EIA assays alone, there are many published reports indicating that this test alone is not appropriate for toxigenic *C. difficile* detection. Testing should be performed on watery, loose, or unformed specimens only. Neonates frequently can be colonized with toxin-producing strains of *C. difficile* without symptoms; testing is discouraged.

Antimicrobial Susceptibility Testing

A microorganism is considered to be susceptible to an antimicrobial agent if in vitro growth is inhibited at a concentration a fourth to an eighth that achievable in the patient's blood, given a usual dose of the agent. In vitro resistance is highly predictable of clinical failure but in vitro susceptibility does not ensure clinical efficacy. Clinical isolates warrant testing if susceptibility cannot be reliably predicted a priori. The test results of certain antimicrobial agents are reported routinely, whereas other results are reported selectively to gain information about individual and community susceptibility patterns, as well as to control inappropriate use of certain agents, limit cost, and inhibit the emergence of resistant bacteria.

Standard Media and Test Conditions

A variety of methods (e.g., minimum inhibitory concentration (MIC), disk diffusion, and commercial systems, each with advantages and limitations) and media have been developed for susceptibility testing, and standards have been set for interpretation of results. Methods and interpretation are pathogen- and source-specific. Mueller–Hinton (MH) medium is recommended for testing non-fastidious bacteria, including Enterobacteriaceae, *Pseudomonas aeruginosa,* and other non-Enterobacteriaceae, staphylococci, and enterococci. MH medium has good batch-to-batch reproducibility, is low in trimethoprim-sulfamethoxazole (TMP-SMX) and tetracycline inhibitors, and shows a good growth pattern; a large body of data and experience with its use also exist. Cation supplements of calcium and magnesium are necessary when testing certain organisms (*P. aeruginosa*) because the concentration affects the reliability of testing aminoglycosides, tetracycline, and colistin (i.e., excessive levels can cause smaller zones of inhibition; low levels increase the size of such zones).

TABLE 286-6. Special Media/Conditions for Dilution Antimicrobial Susceptibility Testing of Common Bacterial Pathogens

Organism	Medium	Incubation Time[a] (hours)
Haemophilus spp.	HTM[a]	20–24
Listeria monocytogenes	CAMHB with 2–5% LHB	20–24
Staphylococcus aureus for oxacillin testing	CAMHB + 2% NaCl	16–20; 24 for oxacillin and vancomycin
Streptococci	CAMHB with 2–5% LHB	20–24
Enterococci	CAMHB	16–20; 24 for vancomycin
Enterobacteriaceae	CAMHB	16–20
Pseudomonas aeruginosa and other non-Enterobacteriaceae	CAMHB	16–20

CAMHB, cation-adjusted Mueller–Hinton broth; HTM, Haemophilus *test medium;* LHB, lysed horse blood; MHB, Mueller–Hinton broth.

[a]The incubation environment is ambient air, except for streptococci and Haemophilus (Kirby–Bauer), for which CO_2 is also appropriate.

Cation-adjusted (20 to 25 mg/L calcium, 10 to 12.5 mg/L magnesium) MH broth is generally used for microdilution testing. A standardized concentration of organisms is $3–5 \times 10^5$ CFU/mL. Testing of β-lactam agents requires a strictly standardized inoculum (5×10^5 CFU/mL for MIC and 10^8 CFU/mL for disk diffusion testing); an increased inoculum falsely increases the MIC.[68]

MH medium supplemented with 5% sheep blood is recommended for testing non-enterococcal streptococci and *S. pneumoniae. N. gonorrhoeae* should be tested on GC agar base with 1% defined growth supplement and incubated in 5% CO_2 for 20 to 24 hours. *Haemophilus* test medium incubated at 35°C in 5% CO_2 is used for *Haemophilus;* it provides optical clarity, stability, and reproducibility and permits testing of susceptibility to TMP-SMX. Media containing thymidine analogues such as blood or chocolate agar can interfere with the results of TMP-SMX testing. Blood-supplemented MH medium also can antagonize TMP-SMX.

Table 286-6 provides a summary of recommended media for susceptibility testing. Generally, microdilution tests are incubated for 16 to 20 hours at 35°C in ambient air. Tables 286-7, 286-8, and 286-9 provide a summary of MIC interpretative standards for commonly encountered pathogens.

Susceptibility Test Methods

Disk diffusion, or Kirby–Bauer test, is a standardized technique for testing rapidly growing pathogens.[69] Briefly, a standardized inoculum (direct suspension of colonies to yield a standardized inoculum is acceptable) is swabbed onto the surface of MH agar (150 mm). Reproducibility depends on the log growth phase of organisms, therefore fresh subcultures are used. Filter paper disks impregnated with a standardized concentration of an antimicrobial agent are placed on the surface, and the size of the zone of inhibition around the disk is measured after overnight incubation (specific incubation time ranges are outlined in the Clinical Laboratory Standards Institute (CLSI) documents).

The broth microdilution assay is used commonly to determine MICs for antimicrobial agents.[70] MIC trays can be custom-made in the laboratory or purchased commercially. This system allows a quantitative measurement of in vitro activity. Usually, five to eight concentrations representing therapeutically achievable ranges are tested against each organism, or one to three concentrations are used to determine activity at the breakpoint MIC. The latter allows only qualitative assessment of susceptibility; the exact MIC is not known. One must be careful to interpret these

TABLE 286-7. Minimal Inhibitory Concentration (μg/mL) Interpretative Standards for Commonly Used Antimicrobial Agents[a]

Antimicrobial Agent	Susceptible	Intermediate	Resistant
Ampicillin			
Enterobacteriaceae	≤8	16	≥32
Enterococci	≤8	–	≥16
Nafcillin			
Staphylococci	≤2	–	≥4
Oxacillin			
Staphylococcus aureus	≤2	–	≥4
Staphylococcus, coagulase-negative	<0.25	–	>0.5
Extended-spectrum penicillins			
Pseudomonas spp.	≤64	–	≥128
Other gram-negative bacilli	≤16	32–64	≥128
Cefazolin			
Enterobacteriaceae	≤1	2	≥4
Cefotaxime			
Enterobacteriaceae	≤1	2	≥4
Ceftazidime			
Pseudomonas aeruginosa	≤8	16	≥32
Ceftriaxone			
Enterobacteriaceae	≤1	2	≥4
Cefepime			
Enterobacteriaceae	≤8	16	≥32
Cefuroxime oral	≤8	16	≥32
Imipenem			
Enterobacteriaceae	≤4	8	≥16
Vancomycin			
Staphylococcus aureus	≤2	4–8	≥16
Coagulase-negative staphylococci	≤4	8–6	≥32
Enterococci	≤4	8–16	≥32
Amikacin			
Pseudomonas aeruginosa	≤16	32	≥64
Gentamicin			
Enterobacteriaceae	≤4	8	≥16
Enterococci (high-level synergy)	≤500	–	≥500
Other non-Enterobacteriaceae	≤4	8	≥16
Tobramycin			
Enterobacteriaceae	≤4	8	≥16
Erythromycin			
Staphylococci	<0.5	1–4	≥8
Streptococcus pneumoniae	≤0.25	0.5	≥1
Ciprofloxacin			
Enterobacteriaceae	≤1	2	≥4
Clindamycin			
Staphylococci	≤0.5	1–2	≥4
Streptococcus pneumoniae	≤0.25	0.5	≥1
Trimethoprim-sulfamethoxazole	≤2/38	–	≥4/76
Streptococcus pneumoniae	≤0.5/9.5	1/19–2/38	≥4/76

[a]*For organisms other than* Haemophilus *spp.,* Neisseria *spp., and* Streptococcus pneumoniae.

Modified from Performance Standards for Antimicrobial Susceptibility Testing: Twenty-Second Informational Supplement, M100–S202. Clinical and Laboratory Standards Institute, 2012.

somewhat arbitrary standards in the context of the organism, the likely site of infection, the concentration of the organism at the site, and the host's immunocompetence.

Automated instruments can provide results in 2 to 18 hours. Four automated systems commonly used in the United States are the BioMérieux VITEK 2, the Dade MicroScan WalkAway, the BD Phoenix, and the Trek Diagnostic Sensititre. VITEK 2 provides susceptibility and identification as early as 2 hours after inoculation. Plastic reagent cards contain small wells or microcuvettes that allow the simultaneous testing for many different antimicrobial agents. Growth is detected by means of a densitometer. It uses turbidimetrically-determined kinetic measurements of growth to

TABLE 286-8. Minimal Inhibitory Concentration (µg/mL) Interpretative Standards for Commonly Used Antimicrobial Agents for *Haemophilus* Species

Antimicrobial Agent	Susceptible	Intermediate	Resistant
Ampicillin	≤1	2	≥4
Amoxicillin–clavulanic acid	≤4/2	–	≥8/4
Cefixime	≤1	–	–
Cefotaxime	≤2	–	–
Ceftriaxone	≤2	–	–
Cefprozil	≤8	16	≥32
Cefuroxime	≤4	8	≥16
Clarithromycin	≤8	16	≥32
Trimethoprim-sulfamethoxazole	≤0.5/9.5	1/19–2/38	≥4/76

Modified from Performance Standards for Antimicrobial Susceptibility Testing: Twenty-Second Informational Supplement, M100-S202. Clinical and Laboratory Standards Institute, 2012.

TABLE 286-9. Minimal Inhibitory Concentration (MIC: µg/mL) Interpretative Standards for Commonly Used Antimicrobial Agents for *Streptococcus pneumoniae*

Antimicrobial Agent	Susceptible	Intermediate	Resistant
Cefotaxime			
Meningitis	≤0.5	1	≥2
Non-meningitis	<1	2	>4
Cefriaxone			
Meningitis	≤0.5	1	≥2
Non-meningitis	<1	2	>4
Chloramphenicol	≤4	–	≥8
Clarithromycin	≤0.25	0.5	≥1
Clindamycin	≤0.25	0.5	≥1
Penicillin			
Meningitis	≤0.06	0.12–1	≥2
Non-meningitis	≤2	4	≥8
Rifampin	≤1	2	≥4
Trimethoprim-sulfamethoxazole	≤0.5/9.5	1/19–2/38	≥4/76
Vancomycin	≤1	–	–

compute MIC values by regression analysis. MicroScan WalkAway uses substrates that release fluorophores after interaction with bacterial enzymes, a process resulting in increased fluorescence. A major disadvantage is that some bacteria fail to release fluorophores after growth.[71] To solve this problem, MicroScan has incorporated rapid, turbidimetric readers for their panels. Depending on the organism, results are available between 4.5 and 18 hours of incubation. BD Phoenix can accommodate up to 100 simultaneous tests. An indicator is added to the broth of each isolate, and redox indicator measures bacterial growth. Reliable results can be available after approximately 10 hours of incubation.[72] Sensititre is customizable with a choice of completely automated, semi-automated, or manual equipment. The Sensititre ARIS 2X system has a 64-plate capacity and can perform a combination of 192 MIC, breakpoint, or identification tests on a single instrument.

Advantages of automated systems are that they can be connected to the laboratory computer system, provide rapid test results, allow intralaboratory and interlaboratory standardization, are less labor-intensive, and have the potential of artificial intelligence for data review. Disadvantages are noteworthy. Systems may be too restrictive for some laboratories. Panels and cards are formatted by the manufacturer with predetermined antimicrobial agents and concentrations that may not be discerning enough for many clinical situations. Custom-made panels and cards are costly. Systems are not appropriate for all organisms; unacceptable results (usually falsely susceptible test results) can occur for bacteria such as *P. aeruginosa, S. pneumoniae,* enterococci, *Stenotrophomonas maltophilia,* and coagulase-negative staphylococci.[71] The initial capital investment may be prohibitive for some facilities, and a backup system is always needed in case of system failure.[73,74] Data coming through the computer interface needs to be verified for accuracy. Quality control is still dependent on the use of American Tissue Culture Collection organisms.

The E-test (AB Biodisk) is a method that integrates disk diffusion and agar dilution to determine the MIC and provides accurate, reproducible quantitative results. It also allows a simple methodology for testing of anaerobes[75] and fastidious bacteria.[76–78] Briefly, an impervious inert strip carries a marked, continuous concentration gradient of a predefined antibiotic consisting of over 15 2-fold dilutions. After incubation on seeded agar, the MIC is read at the edge of the zone of inhibition as it intersects the strip. Agreement among disk diffusion, agar dilution, and broth microdilution approaches 95%.[79] E-test is especially useful for testing the susceptibility of *S. pneumoniae* to penicillin. Compared with microdilution, it classified all resistant and intermediately resistant strains appropriately.[80] The best results are obtained when the agar is incubated in CO_2.[81–83]

Pathogen- and Mechanism-Specific Testing

Staphylococcus aureus. Testing of staphylococci for methicillin (oxacillin) resistance is best achieved by detection of the *mecA* gene by PCR or its product, penicillin-binding protein (PBP) 2a by latex agglutination (LA).[84] Both tests demonstrate 100% correlation.[85] PCR for *mecA* gene can detect methicillin-resistant *Staphylococcus aureus* (MRSA) rapidly and directly from positive blood culture bottles with high sensitivity and specificity.[86] For smaller laboratories, a Kirby–Bauer test using a cefoxitin disk is a simple and inexpensive method for detecting methicillin resistance. Disk diffusion is still useful in testing staphylococcal isolates. Testing can be performed for TMP-SMX and other antimicrobial agents commonly used for treatment of MRSA that may not be available on automated system panels. Detection of inducible macrolide-lincosamide-streptogramin B resistance in MRSA isolates (D-test) is easily performed using disk diffusion.[87] Disk diffusion is not reliable for detection of vancomycin resistance in staphylococci and MIC testing should be performed. Any *S. aureus* isolate with a vancomycin MIC ≥8 µg/mL should be sent to a reference laboratory.

S. pneumoniae. *S. pneumoniae* isolated from a sterile body site (blood, bone, CSF) or other significant specimen (pleural or mastoid fluid) should be tested directly for MICs. Testing for penicillin, cefotaxime or ceftriaxone, meropenem, and vancomycin should be done routinely on these isolates. An oxacillin disk (1-µg disk on MH blood agar) can be used as a screening test for β-lactam resistance of *S. pneumoniae* in laboratories that cannot perform MIC testing. Penicillin and appropriate β-lactam MIC tests need to be performed on any isolate with a zone diameter of ≤19 mm to determine if the isolate is indeed resistant. CLSI have different interpretative criteria for meningitis and non-meningitis pneumococcal strains for penicillin, cefotaxime, and ceftriaxone, in addition to different criteria for oral penicillin (Table 286-9). Only meningitis interpretations are reported for CSF isolates but all interpretations are reported for isolates from other sources.

Extended-spectrum β-lactamase and carbapenemase. In 2010, CLSI changed their recommendations for testing cephems in Enterobacteriaceae. Previous guidelines recommended specific screening and confirmatory tests for detection of extended-spectrum β-lactamases (ESBLs) produced by certain strains of *Klebsiella* species, *Escherichia coli,* and *Proteus mirabilis* which have been responsible for treatment failures with extended-spectrum cephalosporins. ESBLs also have been detected in isolates of *Salmonella,*

P. aeruginosa, Enterobacter, and *Citrobacter* but are difficult to differentiate from chromosomal *ampC* β-lactamases that are normally found in these isolates. The new CLSI guidelines lower the interpretative standards for cephems, which allow a laboratory to report individual drug results without having to perform the supplemental ESBL screening and confirmatory tests. Unfortunately, many of the commercial systems do not test MIC ranges low enough to use these new standards. For these laboratories, isolates can be detected by testing ESBL-specific screening drugs and then confirming testing using cefotaxime and ceftazidime with and without a β-lactamase inhibitor (clavulanic acid).[88] ESBL-producing isolates are resistant to all penicillins, all cephalosporins, and aztreonam.

Detection of carbapenemase production in Enterobacteriaceae is challenging. The most common is the *K. pneumoniae* carbapenemase (KPC). Laboratories using disk diffusion should screen using an ertapenem or meropenem disk while those using MIC methods can screen using any carbapenem. Screen-positive isolates may indicate carbapenemase production and should be confirmed using a modified Hodge test (MHT).[89] However, false detection of carbapenemase production has been observed with this assay.[90] Clinical efficacy has not been determined for isolates that are MHT-positive but test susceptible for any carbapenem. In these cases, laboratories should report only the MIC value without an interpretation and comment that the isolate is a carbapenemase-producer and treatment of infections caused by these organisms with a carbapenem, despite in vitro susceptibility, is unknown.

β-Lactamase. β-Lactamase production is the most frequent mechanism of resistance with *Haemophilus* species; ampicillin resistance mediated by an alteration in protein binding is relatively uncommon and requires MIC or disk diffusion testing for detection.

Routine testing of *N. gonorrhoeae* isolates is limited to detection of β-lactamase. Any other testing should be referred to a specialized laboratory.[91]

Three methods for detection of β-lactamase are available: the cephalosporin (nitrocefin) method is the most reliable. After inoculation onto a filter paper impregnated with nitrocefin, a color change to red denotes β-lactamase hydrolysis of amide bonds. This method detects most β-lactamases from important isolates such as *Haemophilus, N. gonorrhoeae, Moraxella, Enterococcus faecalis,* and *Bacteroides.* Other assays fail to detect all β-lactamases, and their specificity can be inferior to that of nitrocefin assay.[92-94]

Enterococci. Testing of enterococci for high-level resistance to gentamicin and streptomycin is useful to predict synergistic bacterial killing in combination with a β-lactam or vancomycin. Gentamicin- and streptomycin-containing agar or MIC wells (500 μg gentamicin, 2000 μg streptomycin) are used to detect resistance to high levels of gentamicin or streptomycin. If high-level resistance to gentamicin is noted, resistance to other aminoglycosides is predictable. High-level resistance to streptomycin is specific only to this agent. Incubation for a full 24 hours is necessary (48 hours for streptomycin).

Many susceptibility methods have problems in detecting low-level vancomycin resistance among enterococci. An accurate method for vancomycin screening in enterococci is using an agar dilution plate with brain–heart infusion (BHI) agar with vancomycin 6 μg/mL (vancomycin agar screen plate).[95] Vancomycin agar screen plate can be highly sensitive and specific. However, disk diffusion testing with incubation for at least 24 hours and even broth susceptibility test systems such as VITEK 2 are comparable in their capability to detect resistance.[96] Newer molecular tests such as LC *vanA/van B* detection assay (LC assay, Roche Diagnostics) and the GeneOhm vanR assay (BD Diagnostics-GeneOhm) are capable of detecting glycopeptide resistance genes (especially *vanA* genes) among enterococcal isolates.[84]

Fastitious bacteria. In spite of the standardization of susceptibility testing by CLSI and other professional organizations for common pathogens, there are many organisms that can cause serious infections in which test methods still are not standardized and interpretative guidelines are not available. Among these are *Corynebacterium* spp., *Bacillus* spp., *Listeria monocytogenes, Erysip-* *elothrix rhusiopathiae,* miscellaneous gram-positive cocci like *Leuconostoc* and *Pediococcus; Aeromonas* spp., *Campylobacter* spp., *Pasteurella* spp., the AACEK group of gram-negative bacilli, and others.[97] CLSI document M45-A addresses in vitro susceptibility methods and interpretative criteria for these organisms. Susceptibility testing of anaerobic bacteria requires special qualifications.[98] Testing is indicated for failure of the usual therapeutic regimens or the presence of severe infection when long-term therapy is anticipated (such as for brain abscesses). Agar dilution testing is the referenced standard for determination of MICs. *Brucella* blood agar supports the growth of all anaerobic bacteria. Agar dilution assays are tedious and are not performed in many laboratories. E-test methodology is used more widely.[75] The agar disk diffusion and broth disk elution methods are not recommended because of poor correlation with the agar dilution method. Nitrocefin testing predicts only resistance to ampicillin and penicillin.

Testing of fastidious bacteria should be limited to a few specialized laboratories. Broth microdilution can be used for testing of *Nocardia,* but such testing is not standardized at this time. For mycobacteria, an agar dilution test has been standard for testing. A standardized concentration of test organism is inoculated onto agar (i.e., Middlebrook 7H10) containing the antimicrobial agent to be tested. After incubation for up to 3 weeks (35°C, CO_2), susceptibility is determined by comparing growth on the antibiotic-containing medium with that on antibiotic-free medium.

Mycobacteria. The BACTEC 460TB radiometric system has provided a major advance in the susceptibility testing of slow-growing *Mycobacterium* species. BACTEC 12B or Middlebrook 7H12 broth containing an antimicrobial agent is inoculated with the test organism and incubated for 5 days at 37°C. The growth index is compared with that of a control bottle containing no antimicrobial agent.[99] Automated nonradiometric systems such as BACTEC MGIT 960, and VersaTREK appear to be as reliable as older methods.[100-103]

Antigen Detection Assays

Bacterial antigen detection assays were developed for the rapid diagnosis of bacterial infection. Unfortunately, these tests have poor sensitivity and specificity, and use is not recommended generally.[104,105] A urinary antigen detection assay (EIA) for *Legionella pneumophila* serogroup 1 has been shown to be sensitive and highly specific.[106] Most recently, an immunochromatographic assay has become available. The sensitivity of the assay is higher than that of the EIA test, and results are available within 15 minutes.[107]

Recent studies have resurrected interest in the use of antigen detection assays for the diagnosis of blood culture-negative pneumococcal pneumonia. The sensitivity of this serotype-specific tube latex agglutination assay on urine was 57% for serogroups included in the assay, with a specificity of 98%.[108] The urine pneumococcal rapid immunochromatographic antigen assay (Binax NOW, Binax) has demonstrated a high sensitivity in patients with pneumococcal bacteremia (95%), lobar pneumonia (76%), and bacteremic pneumonia (88%).[109] In children with parapneumonic effusions, the sensitivity and specificity of the assay was 88% and 71%, respectively.[110] Recently, the assay demonstrated a lower sensitivity, but high specificity (96%). In adults with community-acquired pneumonia, a positive test permits optimization of antimicrobial therapy.[111] Unfortunately, false-positive test results were observed in 15% of febrile children with no identifiable pneumococcal infection,[112] probably secondary to nasopharyngeal colonization. Recently, real-time PCR performed on culture-negative parapneumonic fluid samples has substantially increased confirmation of *S. pneumoniae* infection.[113]

FUNGI

Collection and Processing of Clinical Specimens

Specimens submitted for fungal culture are inoculated onto primary isolation media as soon as possible to ensure a high yield of recovery.[1] If a delay is anticipated, the specimen can be stored in the refrigerator at 4°C. Blood and CSF are stored at room temperature or 30°C and dermatologic specimens such as nail scrapings or hair clippings at 15°C to 30°C; respiratory specimens should be processed fresh. Lysis centrifugation-direct plating is the preferred method for recovery of fungi from blood.[1,114] Although this is true for molds, the automated blood culture systems can detect the growth of most *Candida* isolates. It is important to add a small amount of 0.85% saline to a tissue specimen to prevent desiccation. Specimens can then be stored at 4°C for up to 8 hours. Bone marrow should be submitted in a 1.5-mL Isolator tube.

Nails, hair, skin scrapings, fluids, exudates, and biopsy samples for direct microscopic examination can be prepared with 15% potassium hydroxide (with warming of the sample to accelerate the dissolution process). Most samples also can be examined by fluorescent microscopy with 0.1% Calcofluor white, a substance that binds to the chitin and cellulose of cell walls and causes bright fluorescence. Giemsa and Wright stains of blood or bone marrow specimens can reveal intracellular yeast forms such as *Histoplasma capsulatum*. Cryptococcal antigen testing of CSF has replaced India ink staining.

Isolation and Identification

Culture

No single medium is appropriate for all specimens. Sabouraud dextrose and potato flake agar are frequently-used fungal media. The glucose concentration usually is limited to 2.5%; higher concentrations can inhibit some fungi such as *Blastomyces dermatitidis.* To minimize the growth of saprophytes, antimicrobial agents such as gentamicin, chloramphenicol, and cycloheximide, are added to media. Inhibitory mold agar (IMA) is one such medium; it demonstrates higher and more rapid yield.

Agar plates usually are taped and only opened in biologic safety cabinets. Media in tubes provide maximal safety and prevent dehydration and contamination. For fluid specimens, large volumes (>2.0 mL) should be obtained and concentrated through centrifugation at 1500 to 2000 *g* for at least 10 minutes. Tissues are minced and homogenized. Mycosel medium (BBL), which consists of Sabouraud dextrose and cycloheximide, is recommended for isolation of dimorphic fungi. BHI agar containing gentamicin and chloramphenicol in addition to 10% sheep blood is recommended for isolation of *Cryptococcus neoformans* from potentially contaminated fluids such as sputum. Blood obtained in Isolator tubes should be inoculated onto chocolate agar, BHI, and IMA.

After isolation, fungi frequently are identified by the morphologic characteristics of spores and structures. Lactophenol cotton blue mounts are used commonly. The germ tube test, in which yeast is incubated for 2 to 3 hours at 35°C in fresh fetal calf serum, identifies *Candida albicans* by outgrowth of a tube (not all *C. albicans* are germ tube-positive, however). To detect dimorphism, the organism is incubated at 25°C and 37°C to detect the presence of mold or yeast forms, spherules, or endospores, respectively.

Commercial systems can be used to identify many yeasts by assimilation of carbohydrates for growth. A commonly used system is API Analytab 20C yeast identification system. This system is easy to use but does not include rhamnose and urea (the former being necessary for the identification of *C. lusitaniae*). Other frequently used systems are BBL Minitek, BioMérieux VITEK 2, MicroScan, and BD Phoenix.

Antigen Detection

An antigen detection latex agglutination test for *C. neoformans* is available commercially and has been a highly useful clinical tool. However, laboratory personnel should be aware that disinfectants and soaps used to clean ring slides can cause false-positive test results.[115]

Immunoassays performed on urine (and also CSF and blood) can detect *Histoplasma capsulatum* and *Blastomyces dermatitidis* antigens. These tests are particularly useful in the diagnosis of young infants and immunocompromised hosts with disseminated disease.[116-118] Antigenemia and antigenuria also can be detected in acute pulmonary histoplasmosis; but are detected infrequently in individuals with chronic pulmonary disease.[119] Caution in interpreting results is merited since cross-reactivity between fungi occurs. However, at times this may be used as a convenient diagnostic tool. In the southwestern U.S., a positive *Histoplasma* antigen test can aid in the diagnosis of coccidioidomycosis.[120] The diagnosis of pulmonary histoplasmosis and blastomycosis can be made by the detection of antigen in bronchoalveolar lavage fluid. In one study, the overall sensitivity and specificity was 92% and 98.2%, respectively.[121]

Circulating *Aspergillus* galactomannan antigen can be detected in blood specimens from patients with suspected invasive aspergillosis. Frequent screening with this assay may lead to an earlier diagnosis in many immunocompromised individuals.[122,123] Interpretation of positive test results requires careful consideration in patients receiving antibiotic therapy containing β-lactamase inhibitors such as piperacillin-tazobactam, since false-positive results occur.[124] In addition, clinicians should be cautious in interpreting negative results since antifungal therapy appears to decrease test sensitivity.[125]

Bronchoalveolar lavage galactomannan testing has led to the diagnosis of invasive pulmonary aspergillosis in solid-organ transplant recipients and patients with hematologic diseases.[117,126] However, false-positive results are not uncommon in lung transplant recipients.[117] False-positive galactomannan assays have been reported in patients with histoplasmosis.[127]

Antifungal Susceptibility Testing

The emergence of resistance in clinically relevant fungi and yeasts and the availability of new antifungal agents have resulted in the need for standardized methods for antifungal susceptibility testing and interpretation of results. Advances in standardization and guidelines for interpretation permit testing of some yeasts but MIC testing of molds should be performed in reference laboratories. Yeast susceptibility can be performed using either disk diffusion (*Candida* species only, see CLSI document M44-A2)[128] or broth dilution (see CLSI document M27-A3).[69] Unique problems are a slow growth rate, as well as dimorphism. The endpoint MIC for amphotericin B is easily defined, but endpoints for azoles are difficult to determine because of their unique partial inhibition of fungi. Use of the test medium RPMI 1640 with L-glutamine shows the best reproducibility for broth dilution methods. The technical aspects of testing must be carefully controlled to permit reproducibility and to avoid inaccuracies.

CLSI documents have been developed as a reference standard using a consensus process to facilitate agreement between testing methods and measurements. Few data exist that enable correlation of test results with clinical outcomes so caution must be used in interpretation of results.[69,128,129]

Newer antifungal agents such as the echinocandins and voriconazole increase the options for more effective treatment of infections such as aspergillosis. Combinations of these agents may be desirable in some patients since synergy can be present.[130] Susceptibility and interactions are not always predictable. Due to potential inter- and intralaboratory reproducibility problems, testing of filamentous fungi and for effects of combination therapy should be limited to specialized laboratories.[131]

PARASITES

Examination of Feces

Collection and Preservation

Proper collection plus handling of stool specimens is critical for the detection of parasites. Stool should be collected in a clean, wide-mouthed container with a tightly fitting lid. Unpreserved stool specimens are considered potentially infectious and must be handled with care. Stool samples are rejected if they contain mineral oil, bismuth, or barium, which may interfere with accurate examination. The specimen should not be contaminated with urine, or water from the toilet. If transportation to the laboratory is not prompt, the specimen is stored in the refrigerator. Dry samples are not acceptable. A minimum of 3 samples over a period of 7 to 10 days generally is required for accurate testing. For the diagnosis of amebiasis and giardiasis, at least 6 specimens may be required before negative clinical interpretation is appropriate. In one study, only 72% of parasites were detected with a single specimen. Another 28% were identified with 2 additional specimens.[132] In areas of high parasite prevalence (20%), a comprehensive evaluation of a single specimen may have enough sensitivity to be appropriate clinically.

Liquid stool should be examined or preserved within 30 minutes of collection, soft or semi-formed stool within 1 hour, and formed stool on the same day. Two commonly used preservatives are polyvinyl alcohol (PVA) and formalin. PVA provides a good permanent smear and preserves the integrity of trophozoites and cysts. PVA should be handled with care; the substance is poisonous. Formalin is a useful preservative in general and formalin specimens can use a concentration procedure to increase parasite detection, especially cyst and helminth ova (note: trophozoites do not survive the concentration method). Formalin is superior for helminth ova, *Giardia*, and *Cystisospora belli*.

Examination

Stools are examined grossly for consistency, the presence of mucus and blood, and the presence of adult worms or proglottids. Trophic amebas and flagellates are more commonly encountered in liquid and soft specimens; these organisms disintegrate rapidly at room temperature. Trophozoites and cyst forms are more commonly observed in semi-formed stools, and cysts are seen in formed stools.

A direct wet mount smear can be prepared with 0.85% saline or D'Antoni or Lugol iodine. The specimen is scanned at ×10 and then at ×40 magnification. Since wet mount requires fresh stool, it is done infrequently.

Concentration of feces is important when small amounts of organisms are expected. Concentration is designed to facilitate the recovery of protozoan cysts, coccidian oocysts, and helminth eggs and larvae. Either the flotation or the sedimentation (formalin-ethyl acetate) method can be used. Flotation provides a cleaner sample than sedimentation; the higher density of zinc sulfate pushes the protozoan cysts to the surface after centrifugation. The cysts are recovered for examination from the supernatant. Helminth eggs are better recovered with the sedimentation method. Following sedimentation, an iodine stain is performed.

A permanent stain smear is prepared for the identification of intestinal parasites using a PVA-preserved specimen. Wheatly–Gomori tissue trichrome and iron-hematoxylin stains are preferred.

Special Pathogens

Permanent stain with trichrome or iron-hematoxylin allows definition of morphology and provides a slide for reference. *Cryptosporidium* species usually are not seen with the latter stain; they require the use of stain for acid-fast bacilli such as the modified Kinyoun or Ziehl–Neelsen stain. Such stains also can be used to detect *Cystisospora belli* and *Cyclospora* species. If the sediment is mucoid, potassium hydroxide should be added.

Monoclonal antibody assays or direct fluorescent antibody stains for *Giardia* and *Cryptosporidium* are useful when the density of parasites is expected to be low. In specialized laboratories, fecal culture methods or coprocultures (Baerman technique) can be used to recover parasites. These techniques are useful in low-density infestation with hookworms, *Strongyloides*, and *Trichostrongylus*.

A simple way of obtaining larvae and adult worms of *Enterobius vermicularis* for examination is the cellulose tape method. Tape reversed on a tongue depressor is pressed against the anus in the early morning. The tape is then placed over a slide and examined under light microscopy.

Stool antigen detection assays using polyspecific polyclonal antibody are nonspecific and less sensitive in transported/stored samples with fixatives. *Giardia* antigen GSA 65, which is specific to *G. lamblia* and stable in the gastrointestinal tract and in fixatives, is a potentially useful antigen. Detection with a *Giardia* antigen detection method (Prospec T/Giardia, Alexon) is apparently sensitive and specific when testing symptomatic and asymptomatic individuals; the technique has a sensitivity of 96% versus 74% for stool examination for eggs and parasites.[133] Other immunoassays also detect *Cryptosporidium* antigens.[134] These assays have good sensitivity and specificity, are easy to perform, have quick turnarounds, and are reproducible.[135] A multiplex PCR assay has been developed for the detection of *Entamoeba histolytica*, *G. intestinalis*, and *Cryptosporidium* spp.[136]

Trichomonas vaginalis can be observed on direct saline wet mounts from vaginal secretions or first-voided urine (or both) or from other fluids such as respiratory tract secretions from neonates.

Detection of Gastric-Duodenal Pathogens

Helicobacter pylori. Multiple tests are available for the diagnosis of *H. pylori*. Histologic examination of tissue stained with Warthin–Starry silver and hematoxylin and eosin stains is still considered one of the gold standards.[137] In patients with suspected treatment failure, for whom antimicrobial susceptibility testing is desirable, isolation of the organism should be attempted. For culture, commercially available *Brucella* agar plates with 5% horse blood or BHI supplemented with 7% horse blood are the preferred media. Biopsy samples can be tested for the presence of *H. pylori* by testing for urease. The ^{13}C-labeled urea breath test and serology have been advocated as noninvasive methods of diagnosing *H. pylori* disease in children because neither test requires endoscopy. The breath test requires some degree of cooperation for 60 minutes. This assay is highly sensitive and specific.[138-140] An antigen assay performed on stool now has replaced the urea breath test at many institutions.[141] Detection of specific antibodies may not differentiate between acute or past infection, and detection of specific IgM antibody is not sufficiently sensitive to be useful.[142] Although PCR may be a promising diagnostic tool for *H. pylori* infection, the rapid urease testing and histologic examination provide reliable reproducible results. PCR allows for the detection of *H. pylori* and is a culture-independent test for clarithromycin resistance.[143] Rapid office-based technologies have been developed that may obviate the need for invasive procedures for tissue or use of ^{13}C-labeled urea breath test.[144]

Parasites and protozoa. Duodenal contents can be examined for parasites and protozoa by means of the Enterotest capsule. A silicone rubber capsule that contains a spool of string attached to a weight is swallowed; the capsule dissolves, and by peristalsis, the string moves into the small intestine. The string provides an attachment site for duodenal mucus and *Strongyloides* larvae, *Giardia* trophozoites, cryptosporidia, and *Cystisospora* oocysts. No food is allowed during the test, which takes approximately 4 hours. Yellow staining of the string indicates bile. Duodenal aspiration provides an alternative specimen, but the string test is less invasive.

Tissue Specimens

Tissue obtained by biopsy is the preferred specimen for certain severe parasitic infections such as toxoplasmosis. Impression smears, squash preparations, and scrapings from skin and nails are commonly submitted specimens. These specimens are stained and examined microscopically. Giemsa stain of the lung, small intestine, skin, or brain can reveal organisms such as *P. jiroveci*, *Toxoplasma gondii*, *Leishmania*, *Naegleria*, or *Entamoeba*. Other stains such as trichrome and methenamine silver enhance the visualization of parasites. Immunospecific stains such as the TYSGM-9 stain for *E. histolytica* have been developed to improve the sensitivity and specificity of direct microscopy. Modified acid-fast staining of the small intestine allows visualization of *Cryptosporidium parvum*, *C. belli*, and *Cyclospora species*.

Blood Smears

Thin- and thick-film smears stained with Giemsa or Wright stain are still reliable and efficient ways of diagnosing bloodstream parasitic infections caused by *Plasmodium*, *Babesia*, *Trypanosoma*, and *Leishmania*. *Borrelia* and *Yersinia pestis* also can be visualized with these stains. Parasites are observed more easily in the thinner portion of the film. Thick film should be examined for 5 to 10 minutes (about 100 fields) and thin film for 15 to 20 minutes (300 fields). A single blood sample is not sufficient to exclude a diagnosis of these parasitic diseases. Blood samples should be submitted every 6 to 12 hours. Anticoagulated blood (with EDTA) is acceptable only if the sample is <1 hour old. Buffy coat preparations can be stained to visualize the amastigotes of *Leishmania* within monocytes. Finger-stick blood is preferred when examining blood for *Plasmodium*. But times are changing. In a recent study, a rapid diagnostic test for malaria, NOW Malaria Test (Binax), was superior in detecting *P. falciparum* (sensitivity 100%) than a single set of blood smears.[145] Newer diagnostic tests (PCR, loop-mediated isothermal amplification) are becoming more available worldwide.[146] They are valuable in areas in which microscopy is unavailable; and where the availability of antimalarial agents is limited. In some instances, persons testing negative would not require treatment.[147]

RICKETTSIAE

Rickettsial organisms are difficult and hazardous to isolate and also difficult to visualize with light microscopy. Immunofluorescent stain of biopsy samples is useful. Most diagnoses are based on clinical features and confirmed with serologic tests.[148] The most commonly used tests are the indirect fluorescent assay and the microimmunofluorescent test. Additional assays also have been developed. A latex agglutination test can detect IgM and IgG antibody against specific rickettsial antigens. Cross-reactions occur among rickettsial species. False-positive results with indirect fluorescent assays have been reported in users of illicit parenteral drugs. The Weil–Felix assay is rarely used because of its lack of sensitivity and specificity.

IMMUNOSEROLOGY

Documentation of a specific immune response to a pathogenic microorganism provides proof of infection. Nonspecific indicators of infection, such as elevated C-reactive protein, Venereal Disease Research Laboratories (VDRL) antigen, and cytokine levels also assist in the diagnosis and management of serious infections. Methods used for the measurement of antibodies include hemagglutination, EIA, latex agglutination, complement fixation, immunofluorescence, and neutralization assays. Certain methods may be better for certain infections.

The VDRL and rapid plasma reagin are the current screening tests for syphilis, as well as measures of the activity of infection. Observation of spirochetes in body fluids by dark-field examination (or by the direct fluorescent antibody test) or positive specific treponemal antibody tests such as the fluorescent treponemal antibody absorption test confirm infection.[149] The use of new specific treponemal antigens permit a more precise screening of individuals for syphilis. However, the test may have poor positive predictive value in low-risk populations, and cannot distinguish active from treated disease; positive assays must be confirmed with non-treponemal assays.[150]

The immune response to specific pathogenic fungi can assist in diagnosis, as determined by immunodiffusion or completion fixation assays for *Aspergillus*, *Blastomyces*, *Histoplasma*, and *Coccidioides*. However, false-negative test results occur, especially early in the disease or in immunosuppressed hosts.[151]

Febrile agglutinin tests have limited clinical utility in developed countries and should not be used.[152]

NEWER TECHNOLOGIES

Molecular biology has influenced the way in which infectious diseases are diagnosed.[30] DNA and RNA amplification by PCR has become an important resource in the diagnosis of infections. PCR has been shown to be more sensitive than in situ hybridization. PCR has been useful for identifying slowly growing organisms such as *Mycobacterium tuberculosis* and *Borrelia burgdorferi*; and *Rickettsia*, viruses, potential agents of bioterrorism; viruses such as Epstein–Barr virus, human metapneumovirus, and multiple parasites. Quantitative PCRs have revolutionized the way we determine disease activity and response to therapy. It is becoming apparent that we can screen a single specimen for multiple organisms, such as respiratory secretions for respiratory pathogens.[153]

Molecular fingerprinting has become a useful resource in the investigation of nosocomial infections and has fostered the field of molecular epidemiology.[154]

The use of microarrays for the detection of microbial pathogens may revolutionize clinical microbiology in the near future. These arrays have been able to detect and differentiate between viral and bacterial pathogens.[155]

287 Laboratory Diagnosis of Infection Due to Viruses, *Chlamydia*, *Chlamydophila*, and *Mycoplasma*

Tony Mazzulli

VIRUSES

The availability of rapid and reliable viral diagnostic tests, particularly nucleic acid amplification tests (NAATs), facilitates decision-making in the prevention and treatment of viral infections and the practice of effective infection control measures. With specific antiviral therapy now available for many clinically relevant viruses, a correct viral diagnosis is important and also limits further diagnostic testing and unnecessary antibiotic therapy.[1,2]

Two major approaches to diagnosis of viral infection are virologic (detection of virus) and serologic (detection of antibody, antigen, or both). The virologic approach includes: (1) isolation of infectious virus in cell culture; (2) detection of viral antigen by immunologic methods such as fluorescent antibody (FA) testing or enzyme immunoassay (EIA); (3) identification of viral particles by electron microscopy (EM); and (4) detection of viral nucleic acid by direct hybridization or NAATs such as polymerase chain reaction (PCR) which may be qualitative or quantitative.

Cytologic examination of tissues and cells can identify viral effects, prompting further investigation. Occasionally, cytologic changes can be sufficiently specific to suggest a particular agent (e.g., cytomegalovirus (CMV)).[3] The serologic approach to the diagnosis of viral infections includes a demonstration of: (1) immunoglobulin (Ig) G antibodies indicating recent, current, or past infection as well as immunity following recovery or vaccination; (2) a significant rise in virus-specific IgG antibody suggestive of acute or recent infection; (3) virus-specific antigens (e.g., hepatitis B surface antigen (HBsAg)); or (4) virus-specific IgM antibody in late acute- or early recovery-phase sera. As the immune response matures following a viral infection, low-avidity IgG antibodies are replaced with high-avidity antibodies. EIAs capable of measuring the avidity of IgG antibodies to specific viruses have been used to distinguish primary from secondary antibody responses to vaccination or natural infection.[4,5]

In the clinical setting, laboratory tests for the detection of virus infection can be divided into three specific categories: those used to (1) make a specific viral diagnosis; (2) measure viral activity in patients known to be infected (e.g., viral load testing for HIV); and (3) screen for infection (e.g., pretransplant or blood donation).

Specimen Collection and Transport

For the detection of most viruses, it is important to obtain specimens soon after the onset of clinical symptoms (preferably within the first 3 to 4 days) when viral shedding is maximal. Optimal specimens vary depending on the site(s) of disease. In general, tissues, aspirates, and body fluids are superior to swabs. However, in many circumstances, swabs may be the only specimen available. Body sites or lesions that can be sampled easily with a swab include the pharynx or nasopharynx, conjunctiva, urethra, cervix, vagina, and vesicles or ulcers on the skin or mucous membranes. Many types of swabs are available for specimen collection, including plastic, wooden, or those with a flexible wire shaft and a tip made of cotton, Dacron, calcium alginate, or polyurethane.[6] However, certain swabs may not be suitable for detection of some viruses. Swabs with a wooden shaft can contain toxic products that inactivate herpes simplex virus (HSV). Cotton-tipped swabs can contain fatty acids that can interfere with the survival of *Chlamydia* species, but are suitable for the collection of specimens from the vagina, cervix, or urethra for the detection of *Mycoplasma*. Calcium alginate-tipped swabs can be toxic for lipid-enveloped viruses such as herpesviruses and some cell cultures, but are useful for the collection of specimens for *Chlamydia*. Although swabs placed in viral transport media (VTM) can be used for NAATs, many commercial assays for detection of viruses and *Chlamydia* by antigen detection or molecular techniques provide their own swab and transport media, which should be used.

Swabs and tissues for detection of viruses should be placed into VTM to prevent drying, maintain viral viability during transport, and prevent the overgrowth of contaminating organisms.[6] A number of commercially prepared VTMs are available.[7] Swabs collected for bacterial isolation that are placed in bacterial transport medium are unacceptable for detection of viruses.[6] Conversely, VTM contains antimicrobial agents that inhibit most bacteria and fungi. Specimens such as blood, bone marrow, cerebrospinal fluid (CSF), urine, and other body fluids should be placed in clean sterile containers without VTM.

For detection of most respiratory viruses, nasopharyngeal (NP) aspirate or wash, sputum, or bronchoalveolar lavage (BAL) specimen provides a better yield for detection of viruses than NP, nasal, or throat swabs.[7] Multiple samples may be required to maximize yield. Freshly passed stool is superior to a rectal swab for detection of gastrointestinal viruses.[6]

Specific viruses can be found in different blood cells, the plasma/serum, or both (e.g., HIV in lymphocytes and macrophages; CMV in neutrophils and, to a lesser extent, mononuclear cells; enteroviruses in plasma and white blood cells (WBCs)).[8,9] Blood should be collected into Vacutainer tubes containing an anticoagulant such as ethylenediaminetetraacetic acid (EDTA). Recovery rates are higher with EDTA than with heparin.[10] Heparin

can inactivate herpesviruses and can inhibit some NAATs;[11,12] this may be less of a concern for real-time PCR and may be related to the type of heparin (sodium versus lithium) used.[13,14]

For tissue specimens or when the lability of particular viruses (e.g., respiratory syncytial virus (RSV) or varicella-zoster virus (VZV)) is a concern, commercially available VTM containing albumin or serum as a stabilizer should be used.

Most viruses are stable for 2 to 3 days at 4°C (refrigerator or wet ice temperature).[6] Freezing at −20°C (ordinary freezer temperature) destroys or reduces the infectivity of most viruses and can alter the ability to detect viral antigen using some commercially available kits. Beyond 2 to 3 days, specimens should be stored in an ultra-low-temperature freezer (−70°C) and transported on dry ice. For some NAATs (e.g., detection of hepatitis C virus (HCV) RNA in serum/plasma), it is recommended that the serum/plasma be separated within 4 to 6 hours of collection and processed within 72 hours (if kept at 2°C to 8°C) or frozen at −70°C until tested.[7]

For serologic detection of viral antibodies or antigen, blood can be transported at room temperature. If a delay is anticipated, the specimen should be kept refrigerated at 2°C to 8°C. Serum/plasma should be separated as soon as possible after specimen collection. If an extended period will elapse before testing, the serum/plasma sample should be frozen at −20°C or lower. Repeated freeze/thaw cycles should be avoided. For viruses for which an IgM assay is available (e.g., hepatitis A virus (HAV)), an acute-phase specimen can be sufficient for diagnosis. Otherwise, an acute-phase specimen collected within a few days of illness onset followed by a convalescent-phase specimen collected 2 to 4 weeks later should be obtained.

Virus Detection Methods

Virus Isolation

Monolayer cell culture techniques are used in most laboratories for virus isolation. However, many clinically relevant viruses, such as parvovirus, human papillomavirus (HPV), hepatitis viruses, Epstein–Barr virus (EBV), rotaviruses, noroviruses and others, are not cultivatable in the routine diagnostic laboratory; laboratory diagnosis is based on other methods. Although it is possible to cultivate HIV using suspension cultures of lymphocytes, special containment facilities are required; alternative methods are used for routine diagnosis. The major viruses detected by isolation in monolayer cell culture include HSV-1 and HSV-2, CMV, VZV, RSV, influenza A and B viruses, parainfluenza viruses, respiratory adenoviruses, a number of enteroviruses (coxsackievirus, echovirus, poliovirus), and measles virus. Because not all cultivatable viruses replicate in a single cell line, several different cell lines are used for primary isolation. Examples are isolation diploid cell lines (e.g., human foreskin or lung fibroblasts for herpesviruses), primary cell lines such as primary rhesus monkey kidney cells for respiratory viruses and enteroviruses, and heteroploid or continuous human epithelial cell line such as Hep-2 cells for RSV. The types of cell lines used in the diagnostic laboratory are determined by the specimen type, season, epidemiologic data, and clinical information provided. Many viruses cause morphologic changes, i.e., cytopathic effect (CPE), in the cell monolayer. Some viruses cause CPE within 2 days (e.g., HSV), others within a week (e.g., enteroviruses), and others after several weeks (e.g., CMV). For viruses that do not cause typical CPE, detection can be based on the adsorption of red cells to the surface of virus-infected cells in culture (e.g., influenza and parainfluenza viruses) or by the use of interference assays (e.g., rubella virus). Presumptive identification of a particular virus or virus group in cell culture is based on the cell type, the characteristic time of onset, and the appearance of CPE, and is facilitated if the laboratory personnel are informed of the source of the specimen and the suspected clinical diagnosis.

Confirmation of the virus isolated requires immunologic methods such as fluorescein- or peroxidase-conjugated virus-specific monoclonal and polyclonal antibodies. Antibodies to HSV, CMV, VZV, RSV, influenza A and B virus, parainfluenza virus,

TABLE 287-1. Detection Rates[a] of Virus Detection Methods for Selected Viruses

Virus	Shell Vial Culture + Stain		Conventional Tube Culture		Antigen Detection	IFA/DFA	PCR
	Days in Culture	% Detected	Days in Culture	% Detected	% Detected	% Detected	% Detected
HSV	1	66–97	2	40–48	47–89	95	100
CMV	1	68	7	50	100 (Disease); 60–70 (Infection)	N/A	82–100
CMV	2	96					
VZV	2	70–90	5	50	N/A[b]	77–97.5	84–100
Adenovirus (respiratory)	2	97	4	50	N/A	22–67	N/A
Influenza	2	60–100	4	50	39–100	40–90	95.8
RSV	2	95	6	98.2	70–100	80–90	98.6

CMV, cytomegalovirus; CPE, cytopathic effect; DFA, direct immunofluorescence; HSV, herpes simplex virus; IFA, indirect immunofluorescence; PCR, polymerase chain reaction; RSV, respiratory syncytial virus; VZV, varicella-zoster virus.

[a]*Detection rates will vary depending on the specimen type, stage of disease, length of incubation, cell line used for culture and shell vial, and definition of a true positive.*

[b]*N/A, not applicable or data sets include too few isolates for calculation.*

Data from references: 42, 56, 57–60, 65, 76–78, 82–84, 90, 109–114, 137–143, 146, 147, 149–160.

adenovirus, measles virus, and enterovirus antigens are available readily.

Centrifugation of specimens (also referred to as shell vial culture or spin-amplified culture) onto cell monolayers on coverslips placed in the bottom of small vials or in wells, followed by incubation and staining for viral antigen using monoclonal antibody after 1 to 3 days, substantially reduces the time required to detect and confirm the presence of many viruses. For slowly growing viruses such as CMV, the use of monoclonal antibody against nonstructural proteins produced early in the replication cycle (i.e., immediate early antigen or early antigen) allows detection of virus days to weeks before CPE can be observed by traditional cell culture techniques. Because of its speed, the shell vial method has replaced conventional cultures in many laboratories (Table 287-1) and is used routinely for the detection of CMV, HSV, VZV, respiratory viruses, and the enteroviruses.

Two techniques for isolation of some viruses have been developed with comparable sensitivity to standard culture and shell vial methods.[15-17] The use of genetically engineered cell lines such as the ELVIS (enzyme-linked virus-inducible system) was introduced first for the isolation of HSV. A baby hamster kidney cell line has been transformed using an HSV-inducible promoter (UL39 gene) and an *E. coli* β-galactosidase gene. The addition of a substrate for the β-galactosidase enzyme results in formation of a color reaction in the HSV-infected cells. This technique has been adapted for performing rapid HSV antiviral susceptibility testing. Mixing multiple cell types in a single shell vial culture can provide rapid detection of respiratory viruses (R-Mix), HSV, CMV and VZV (H and V Mix), and enteroviruses (E-Mix).

Antigen Detection

Antigen detection tests can be performed directly on a variety of specimen types and are highly specific and rapid.[7] Viable virus is not required for detection. Because virus antigen is cell-associated, collection of an adequate number of infected cells is important. A number of commercial kits (EIA, latex agglutination, FA) are available for the detection of: (1) rotavirus and enteric adenovirus in stool specimens; (2) RSV, influenza A and B viruses, parainfluenza viruses, and adenoviruses in respiratory tract specimens; (3) HBsAg and HIV p24 antigen in serum; (4) HSV and VZV in vesicle/ulcer swab specimens; and (5) CMV in BAL and blood specimens. The FA technique has been used for the detection of rabies virus in brain tissue, mumps virus in throat and urine sediment, and measles virus in conjunctival cells. The detection of CMV pp65

antigen in neutrophils is used commonly in the diagnosis and management of immunocompromised patients with new or reactivated CMV infection.[18]

Electron Microscopy

A variety of specimen types (if collected and processed properly) are suitable for EM.[19,20] An experienced microscopist can identify a viral pathogen morphologically within 10 minutes of arrival of a specimen in the laboratory. Unlike antigen detection and NAATs, which are limited in ability to detect viruses with different antigenic determinants or nucleic acid sequences, respectively, because of the high specificity of reagents used, EM detection is based on morphologic characteristics and can be used broadly to detect members of different virus families as well as potential novel agents.[19]

EM continues to be used for the detection of gastrointestinal pathogens such as rotavirus, enteric adenoviruses, norovirus, and others as well as non-enteric viruses.[21-25] Disadvantages of EM include the large number of virus particles (approximately 1×10^6 per mL of specimen) required for detection, limited throughput, expense, and lack of availability and expertise in many centers.[25]

Nucleic Acid Detection

Molecular hybridization techniques using probes directed at a unique, conserved portion of a viral genome are highly specific and bind only to complementary DNA or RNA sequences.[26] Probes are particularly useful for detecting and typing viruses for which reliable culture methods are not available. Molecular probes are available as commercial kits for the detection of HPV,[27] HIV,[28] HSV,[29] CMV,[30] hepatitis B virus (HBV),[31] and HCV.[32] For some viruses, the concentration of viral genomes in direct patient specimens may be too low to permit detection with adequate sensitivity (e.g., commercially available probes for HSV and CMV detect only 70% to 90% of specimens positive by isolation).[29,30]

The increased sensitivity of NAATs has revolutionized testing in the clinical virology laboratory.[20,33-35] Three approaches have been taken: (1) *target amplification* such as PCR, strand displacement amplification (SDA), nucleic acid sequence-based amplification (NASBA), and transcription-mediated amplification (TMA) systems; (2) *probe amplification*, including Q-beta replicase and ligase chain reaction (LCR); and (3) *signal amplification*, such as branched-chain DNA (bDNA) assay and hybrid capture assay.[20,36-38] Several commercial and in-house ("home-brew") assays have been developed. Quantification of viral genome in plasma or serum can be used to determine prognosis, select patients for antiviral therapy, and monitor response to treatment in a variety of patient populations.[34] Multiplex assays capable of detecting a number of viruses in a single amplification reaction have been developed, e.g., for herpesviruses, enteric, bloodborne, and respiratory viruses.[39-42] The development of automated real-time PCR using fluorescence techniques and continuous detection of amplified product has shortened detection times significantly relative to conventional PCR assays.[43] Because these assays use a closed system (i.e., amplification and detection occur in a single tube that need not be opened once the reaction is completed), they also are less prone to contamination. NAAT has been applied to genotyping of viruses (e.g., HIV, HBV, and HCV) as well as for the detection of mutations that confer resistance to antiviral agents.[34]

Choice of Virus Detection Method

Choosing optimal test(s) depends on the virus being sought, the clinical setting, specimen type, availability of kits, reagents and equipment, experience of laboratory personnel, and cost. Antigen detection methods offer the following advantages: (1) noncritical specimen collection and transport conditions; (2) ability to detect viruses that cannot be cultivated easily; (3) no need for cell culture equipment and highly trained personnel; (4) superior sensitivity compared with culture for certain viruses; and (5) rapid turnaround time (usually within hours). Disadvantages include: (1) lack of available test kits for many clinically important viruses; (2) inferior sensitivity compared with isolation for many cultivatable viruses; and (3) inferior specificity due to nonspecific/cross-reactions particularly with the use of polyclonal antibodies.

Culture is preferred when results are available quickly with the shell vial centrifugation and staining methods (e.g., HSV, CMV, and VZV). Advantages of isolation include: (1) ability to recover a broad range of viruses; (2) availability of the infectious agent for further characterization; (3) 100% specificity; and (4) superior sensitivity compared with antigen detection for some viruses. Disadvantages include: (1) requirement for specialized equipment, supplies, and trained personnel; (2) longer turnaround time; (3) the lability of certain viruses under suboptimal collection and transport conditions; and (4) the inability to culture many clinically relevant viruses.

The use of NAATs is rapidly replacing older viral diagnostic methods due to their rapid turnaround time, superior sensitivity, and the ability to quantify virus density. A number of relatively simple home-brew and commercially available NAATs (including analyte-specific and for research use only) are available for a wide variety of viruses.[34,35]

Serologic Methods

Serologic methods can be used to diagnose a current or recent acute infection, to determine specific susceptibility or immunity, and for epidemiologic and surveillance purposes. Interpretation of serologic results is virus-specific (e.g., the presence of HIV antibodies indicates current infection, whereas the presence of IgG anti-rubella indicates immunity as a result of immunization or recovery from natural infection). Serologic diagnosis of acute infection is more useful when the incubation period is prolonged (e.g., 3 to 6 weeks) and antibody is present in serum concomitantly with signs of illness (e.g., EBV and CMV mononucleosis). Figure 287-1 shows a typical antibody response for an acute, moderate-incubation (several days to 2 weeks) viral illness such as measles. At the onset of rash or other manifestations, antibody is undetectable or is present at low titer. Within 10 to 14 days, appreciable titers of antibody are present. For short-incubation virus infections (e.g., respiratory viruses), a rise in antibody usually does not occur until the late recovery phase or during convalescence and has no value for acute diagnosis. With the use of older serologic methods such as hemagglutination inhibition (HAI) and complement fixation (CF) that detect IgG antibody, a >4-fold rise in titer based on serial dilution endpoints between acute and

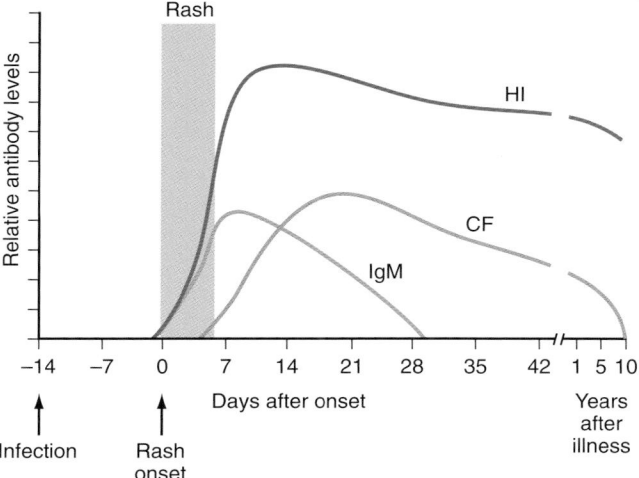

Figure 287-1. Antibody responses during acute measles. HI, hemagglutination inhibition antibody; CF, complement fixation antibody.

convalescent sera tested in parallel confirms a diagnosis. A 4-fold fall in titer also is presumptive evidence of a recent infection whereas unchanging low titers indicate past infection and immunity. The presence of antibody in high titer in a single serum specimen during convalescence usually does not permit a definitive diagnosis. Acute seroconversion also can be used to diagnose an acute or recent infection.

EIA kits and, to a lesser extent, latex agglutination and FA kits have replaced other antibody tests in many laboratories. EIA/ELISA results usually are measured in optical density (OD) units and results reported in international units (IU) or index values. Interpretation of OD units varies with the EIA/ELISA kit used and the virus antibodies being detected. One must refer to the specific kit manufacturer for the criteria defining a significant difference in antibody levels between acute and convalescent sera.

The presence of virus-specific IgM antibody in serum obtained 1 to 2 weeks after the onset of illness permits a diagnosis of acute/recent infection for many viruses. Typically, IgM antibody disappears from serum within a few months after the acute illness, but can persist for an extended time in some individuals and for some viruses.[44] False-positive IgM results can occur through: (1) cross-reactivity (e.g., among herpesviruses or due to polyclonal stimulation secondary to EBV infection);[45] (2) the presence of rheumatoid factor (IgM antibody that binds to the Fc portion of IgG);[46] and (3) inherent testing difficulties.[47] Misinterpretation of IgM antibodies as indicative of an acute/recent infection can occur as a result of: (1) persistence of IgM antibody for several months after the acute illness (e.g., EBV, West Nile virus);[48] or (2) reactivation of latent or chronic viruses (e.g., HSV, HBV).

False-negative IgM tests can result from: (1) an absent, low, or delayed IgM response, especially in immunologically immature hosts (e.g., during infancy, congenital CMV or HIV infection) or in immunosuppressed patients (e.g., patients with AIDS);[48,49] or (2) presence of high-titer IgG antibody (precluding binding of IgM).[20] Many commercially available kits contain reagents to adsorb IgG from the test serum or use a background substraction step, thus reducing the possibility of interference.[50,51]

When using IgG antibody tests to determine susceptibility or immunity to a particular virus, the sensitivity of the method is important. Generally, complement fixation (CF) antibody titers quantitatively are lower than hemagglutination inhibition (HAI) titers and can disappear after several years. Therefore, CF should not be used for determining susceptibility or immunity.

The major advantages of serologic diagnosis of acute viral infection include noncritical specimen handling and wide availability. Disadvantages include: (1) requirement for acute and convalescent sera for IgG antibody tests; (2) false-positive and false-negative IgM antibody results; and (3) delay of 2 to 3 weeks before a diagnosis can be confirmed with short-incubation infections. Because of the many confounding factors (e.g., passive transfer of antibodies from mother to infant, receipt of immunoglobulin, immunocompromised) serologic results always should be interpreted within the context of the clinical situation. Whenever possible, serologic diagnosis should be confirmed with the use of viral isolation or direct detection of virus antigens or nucleic acids.

Depending on the serologic assay, either serum and/or plasma can be used. The use of other specimen types has not been well validated for most viruses. Some exceptions include the use of saliva for the detection of HIV antibodies and CSF in patients with viral central nervous system (CNS) disease.[52,53]

Optimal Tests for Specific Viruses

Table 287-2 lists the medically important viruses, major attributable diseases, optimal diagnostic specimen(s), available tests, and average time to a positive test result. For many tests, the time to obtain a result may be a function of the test itself (e.g., culture), the logistics of laboratory testing schedules, or the need to refer a sample to a reference lab. The preferred test provides the most rapid result with acceptable sensitivity (>90%) and specificity (>95%). Serologic tests remain the mainstay for diagnosis of certain virus infections such as the hepatitis viruses. The preferred diagnostic test or tests can vary, depending on the patient population being tested (e.g., immunocompromised hosts).

In the results summarized herein for individual viruses, assessment of sensitivity and specificity of different tests may be based on a variety of parameters and not simply comparison to culture alone.

Herpes Simplex Virus

For diagnosis of suspected mucocutaneous lesions due to HSV, an aspirate or swab (Dacron, rayon, or cotton on aluminum shafts but not calcium alginate or swabs on wood shafts) of the vesicular fluid or ulcer base placed in VTM is recommended. Other potentially useful samples include blood in EDTA for PCR when viremia is suspected (e.g., neonates), CSF in a sterile container when HSV meningitis or encephalitis is suspected, conjunctival swab or corneal scrapings in VTM in suspected cases of herpes keratitis, and tissue biopsy in VTM or frozen (e.g., disseminated HSV in neonates or immunocompromised patients). In infants, duodenal aspirates may also be collected.

The yield on culture varies depending on the tissue culture cell type used in the laboratory,[54] the stage of the clinical infection (greater during vesicular stage than crusted stage),[55] and the type of specimen (including transportation time and conditions). CPE in a sensitive cell line detects 50% of positives in 24 hours, 80% in 48 hours, and 95% in 72 hours.[56] The shell vial method permits detection of HSV with 66% to 99% sensitivity and 100% specificity by 16 to 24 hours.[54,57] ELVIS has sensitivity similar to both standard and shell vial culture.[15] The use of type-specific monoclonal antibodies distinguishes HSV-1 from HSV-2 in culture.

Direct antigen detection tests for HSV have variable sensitivity (47% to 95%) and specificity (85% to 100%).[58,59] None is sufficiently sensitive to reliably detect asymptomatic shedding.[60] Assays using monoclonal antibodies can distinguish HSV-1 from HSV-2.

In CNS HSV infection, the yield of CSF culture is <5% compared with biopsy-proven cases.[61] HSV PCR performed on CSF (sensitivity of 96% and specificity of 99%)[62] is the diagnostic test of choice for HSV encephalitis and meningitis.[61] PCR is positive at least through the first 6 to 7 days of illness, even in patients receiving acyclovir therapy.[61,63] Conversely, because negative results have been obtained in up to 25% of CSF samples from infants and children, HSV PCR alone cannot exclude HSV encephalitis.[64] HSV PCR also is useful with other clinical specimen types,[65] and can distinguish between HSV-1 and HSV-2. The role of quantitative HSV PCR remains unclear, with conflicting results for amount of HSV in CSF and prognostic value.[66,67] However, successful antiviral therapy is associated with a decline in HSV viral load in CSF.[61]

HSV-specific IgG and IgM antibody is detectable in serum 10 to 20 days after the onset of primary infection. IgG antibodies indicate past or current infection, but not necessarily active disease. The presence of HSV IgG antibody in organ transplant recipients is used as a risk factor for recurrences and has prompted the prophylactic use of acyclovir.[68] Because of fluctuations in HSV IgG antibody titers, serologic tests should not be used to diagnose recurrent HSV infections. IgM antibody is not a reliable indicator of primary infection because reactivation can cause a rise in IgM levels.[68]

Older HSV antibody tests used crude antigen mixtures and could not reliably distinguish between HSV-1 and HSV-2 IgG antibodies. However, commercially available EIA, Western blot (WB), and immunoblot tests based on glycoprotein G antigen now reliably distinguish type-specific HSV antibodies.[69] The use of HSV-2 type-specific assays has provided important information about the insensitivity of clinical history and the epidemiology of genital HSV infection.[70] Recommendations have been proposed for the appropriate use of HSV-2 serologic tests.[71] No IgM test is commercially available that can distinguish HSV-1 and HSV-2 infection.

Guidelines for standardization of in vitro susceptibility testing of HSV have been published.[72] Resistance to acyclovir and other drugs has emerged as a clinical problem in immunocompromised patients receiving prolonged courses of continuous or intermittent suppressive therapy.[73,74] PCR, together with sequence analysis of the DNA polymerase and thymidine kinase genes, can be used to detect mutations conferring drug resistance and have significantly reduced the time for results.[75] However, this approach is limited by the fact that one can only interpret the presence of mutations that have been associated with HSV antiviral resistance. The significance of new or novel mutations requires confirmation.

Cytomegalovirus

CMV can be detected in a variety of clinical specimens by isolation, antigen detection, DNA probes, or NAATs.[18,76-79] It often is difficult to distinguish between asymptomatic shedding (from urine, cervical secretions, semen, saliva, and respiratory tract secretions) and active CMV disease. Isolation of CMV from tissues is good evidence of active infection. The preferred specimen(s) and test(s) for detection and diagnosis of CMV depends on the clinical syndrome and immune function of the patient (see Chapter 206, Cytomegalovirus).[18,80,81]

The shell vial method significantly shortens the detection time for CMV compared with conventional culture. To enhance detection of CMV in various clinical specimens, multiple shell vials should be inoculated (2 for urine, tissue, and BAL and 3 for blood specimens) with staining at 24 hours and 48 hours, and (for blood specimens) observed for CPE for 10 days.[82,83]

Isolation of CMV from urine obtained during the first 3 weeks of life is diagnostic of congenital infection.[80] In all other situations, it is impossible to distinguish CMV viruria related to primary infection, reactivation or reinfection disease, or asymptomatic shedding. Interpretation of the presence of CMV in respiratory tract specimens also is confounded by asymptomatic respiratory tract shedding. In immunosuppressed patients with suspected CMV, testing of a BAL specimen may be useful. Compared with culture of lung biopsy specimens obtained from patients with CMV pneumonia, the sensitivity of isolation from BAL fluid is 70% to 95% and the specificity 50% to 100%.[84,85] Demonstration of CMV antigen in cells from BAL specimens by direct fluorescent antibody (DFA) staining may be more specific for CMV infection, but sensitivity is reduced.[84] Histologic examination of cells obtained by BAL for the presence of characteristic CMV intranuclear inclusions with an "owl's eye" appearance suggests a diagnosis of CMV pneumonia.

Detection of CMV in peripheral WBCs by culture techniques may be useful in the diagnosis of active CMV disease or as a predictor of future CMV pneumonia in transplant recipients and other immunocompromised patients.[86,87] However, the lack of sensitivity of culturing CMV from WBCs has led to the development of the CMV antigenemia assay (an immunocytochemical assay that detects the 65-kd lower-matrix phosphoprotein (pp65)

TABLE 287-2. Optimal Specimen, Preferred Test, and Performance in Confirmation of Specific Infections

Agent/Type or Site of Infection or Host	Major Diseases	Optimal Specimens	Available Tests[a]	Average Time to Positive Results[b]
ADENOVIRUS				
Respiratory	Pharyngitis, pneumonia, undifferentiated febrile illness	NP aspirate/wash, NP swab, throat swab, BAL, lung tissue	Culture[c]	6 days
			PCR	1–2 days
			Antigen detection/FA	2 hours
		Serum	IgG antibody[d]	1–5 days
Eye	Conjunctivitis	Conjunctival swab or scraping	Culture[c]	7 days
			Antigen detection	2 hours
		Serum	IgG antibody[c]	1–5 days
Intestinal (types 40/41)	Gastroenteritis	Stool	Antigen detection	2 hours
			EM	2 hours
Urinary bladder (immunocompromised host)	Hemorrhagic cystitis	Urine	Culture	6 days
			PCR[c]	1–2 days
			EM	2 hours
ARBOVIRUSES				
SLE, California, WEE, EEE, WNV	Fever, meningoencephalitis	Serum, CSF	IgG and IgM antibody[d]	1–5 days
Colorado tick fever	Fever, malaise, neutropenia	Serum	IgG antibody	7 days
Dengue	Febrile illness +/– rash, hemorrhagic fever	Serum	IgG and IgM antibody[c]	1–5 days
			PCR	1–2 days
CHLAMYDIA/CHLAMYDOPHILA				
Chlamydia trachomatis				
Genital	Urethritis, proctitis, cervicitis, salpingitis, pelvic inflammatory disease	Urethral, cervical swab, first-void urine, self-collected vulvovaginal swab, rectal mucosal swab	NAAT[c]	2–6 hours
			Antigen detection	4 hours
			DNA probe	4 hours
			Culture	48–72 hours
Neonatal	Conjunctivitis, pneumonitis	Eye swab, NP aspirate/wash	NAAT[c]	2–6 hours
			Antigen detection	4 hours
			Culture	48–72 hours
Sexual abuse, rape	Vaginitis, urethritis, proctitis	Cervical, urethral, rectal mucosal swab	Culture[e]	48–72 hours
Chlamydophila pneumoniae (TWAR)	Pneumonia, pharyngitis, bronchitis	NP aspirate/swab, throat swab/wash	Culture[c]	4 days
			Antigen detection	4 hours
		Serum	IgG and IgM antibody	1–5 days
Chlamydophila psittaci	Pneumonia	NP aspirate/wash, throat swab/wash	Antigen detection	4 hours
			Culture	2 days
		Serum	IgG antibody[d]	1–5 days
CYTOMEGALOVIRUS				
Congenital	Hepatosplenomegaly, thrombocytopenia, microcephaly, hearing loss, chorioretinitis	Urine, throat swab, EDTA blood, serum, amniotic fluid	Shell vial culture with antigen stain[c]	2 days
			Culture	3–4 weeks
			NAAT[f]	2–5 hours
			IgG and IgM antibody[c]	1–2 days
Postnatal infection	Heterophile-negative infectious mononucleosis	Throat swab, urine, EDTA blood	Shell vial culture with antigen stain[c]	2 days
			Culture	3–4 weeks
		Serum	IgG and IgM antibody[d]	1–2 days
Immunosuppressed patients	Pneumonitis, colitis, retinitis	EDTA blood	Antigenemia assay[c]	4–6 hours
			NAAT[c,f]	2–5 hours
		Bronchoalveolar lavage, rectal swab, vitreous fluid, tissue biopsy	Shell vial culture with antigen stain[c]	2 days
			Culture	3–4 weeks
			NAAT[c,f]	2–5 hours
Pretransplant screening/ immune status	Past infection (donor and recipient)	Serum	IgG antibody	1–2 days

Continued

TABLE 287-2. Optimal Specimen, Preferred Test, and Performance in Confirmation of Specific Infections—cont'd

Agent/Type or Site of Infection or Host	Major Diseases	Optimal Specimens	Available Tests[a]	Average Time to Positive Results[b]
ENTEROVIRUSES				
Coxsackie A and B viruses, echovirus, poliovirus	Aseptic meningitis, fever and rash, herpangina, hand, foot, and mouth disease, myocarditis and pericarditis, paralytic disease	CSF, throat swab, stool, rectal swab, EDTA blood, pericardial fluid, myocardium	Culture	4–7 days
			PCR[c,f]	6 hours
		Serum	Neutralizing[d,g] antibody panel (coxsackie B virus, echovirus and poliovirus)	5 days
EPSTEIN–BARR VIRUS				
Healthy individual	Mononucleosis syndrome	Serum	Slide agglutination test (monospot)[c]	1–3 days
			EBV-specific IgG and IgM antibody[d]	1–3 days
Immunocompromised	Posttransplant lymphoproliferative disease (PTLD)	Serum, plasma, whole blood, leukocytes	PCR (quantitative)[f]	2–5 hours
GASTROINTESTINAL VIRUSES				
Rotaviruses, caliciviridae (norovius and sapovirus), enteric adenoviruses, astroviruses	Gastroenteritis	Stool	EM[c] (rotavirus and enteric adenovirus)[c]	2 hours
			PCR[f]	6 hours
GENITAL *MYCOPLASMA*				
Ureaplasma urealyticum	Urethritis, cervicitis	Urethral, cervical swab; semen	Culture[c]	2 days
Mycoplasma hominis	Pneumonitis, meningitis in neonates	Tracheal aspirate, CSF in neonates	Culture[c]	2 days
HEPATITIS VIRUSES				
Hepatitis A	Acute	Serum	IgM antibody	1–2 days
	Immunity	Serum	Total (IgG and IgM) antibody or IgG antibody	1–2 days
Hepatitis B	Acute	Serum	HBsAg, anti-HBc IgM	1–2 days
	Chronic	Serum	HBsAg, anti-HBc total antibody	1–2 days
		Serum/plasma	NAAT for HBV DNA (quantitative)[f]	1 week
	Immunity	Serum	HBsAb	1–2 days
Hepatitis C	Acute	Serum	Anti-HCV EIA screen	1–2 days
			Anti-HCV RIBA supplementary	5 days
	Chronic	Serum/plasma	NAAT for HCV RNA (quantitative/qualitative)[f]	1 week
Hepatitis D (only occurs in patients with HBV coinfection/ superinfection)	Acute	Serum	HDV Ag, anti-HDV IgM	1–8 days
	Chronic	Serum	HDV Ag, anti-HDV total	1–8 days
Hepatitis E	Acute	Serum	IgG and IgM antibody	1–8 days
HERPES SIMPLEX VIRUS				
Skin, mucous membranes	Oral, genital, cutaneous ulcers or vesicles, herpetic whitlow	Aspirate of vesicle fluid, swab of vesicle fluid or base of ulcer in VTM	Shell vial culture with antigen stain[c,h]	16–24 hours
			Antigen detection (FA)	2 hours
			NAAT[f]	2–5 hours
Past infection	Recurrent genital symptoms but culture negative	Serum	IgG (group- or type-specific) antibody[d]	1–2 days
Neonatal infection	Disseminated disease; hepatitis; pneumonitis; encephalitis; skin, eye, mouth ulcers or vesicles	Swab of lesion(s), EDTA blood, CSF, conjunctiva/nose/mouth swab, rectal swab	Shell vial culture with antigen stain[c,h]	16–24 hours
			Antigen detection (FA)	2 hours
			PCR	2–5 hours
		Serum	IgG and IgM antibody[d]	1–2 days

Continued

TABLE 287-2. Optimal Specimen, Preferred Test, and Performance in Confirmation of Specific Infections—cont'd

Agent/Type or Site of Infection or Host	Major Diseases	Optimal Specimens	Available Tests[a]	Average Time to Positive Results[b]
Ocular herpes	Conjunctivitis, keratitis	Conjunctival or corneal swab or scraping in VTM	Shell vial culture with antigen stain[c,h]	16–24 hours
			Antigen detection (FA)	2 hours
			PCR	2–5 hours
Brain/Meninges	Encephalitis,[i] meningitis	CSF, brain biopsy[j]	PCR[c,f]	2–5 hours
			Antigen/antibody in CSF	2 hours
			Shell vial culture with antigen stain[h]	16–24 hours
		Serum	IgG and IgM antibody[d]	1–2 days
HUMAN HERPESVIRUS 6				
Primary infection	Roseola (exanthem subitum)	Serum	IgG and IgM antibody[d]	1–3 days
Immunocompromised	Transplant recipients, AIDS	EDTA blood for PBMC	PCR[f]	1–2 weeks
HUMAN IMMUNODEFICIENCY VIRUS				
Suspected HIV infection in adult or older child	Symptomatic or asymptomatic	Serum	Screening HIV EIA[c]	1–2 days
			Confirmatory Western blot or IFA	1–3 days
			HIV p24 antigen, NAAT[i]	2–4 days
Newborn	Suspected vertical or perinatal transmission	Serum	Screening HIV EIA	1–2 days
			Confirmatory Western blot or IFA	1–3 days
		EDTA blood	Virus culture	2–3 weeks
			NAAT[c,f,i]	1 week
OTHER VIRUSES				
Human metapneumovirus	Upper respiratory illness, bronchiolitis, pneumonia, croup	NP aspirate/wash, nasal/throat swab, BAL	PCR (including multiplex assays for respiratory viruses)[f]	1 day
Human papillomaviruses	Cervical dysplasia	Cervical swab	RNA probe, hybrid capture, PCR	1–4 days
Influenza viruses	"Flu" syndrome, pneumonia	NP aspirate/wash/swab, throat swab/wash, BAL	PCR (including multiplex assays for respiratory viruses)[c,f]	1 day
			Antigen detection for influenza A and B	30 minutes–2 hours
			Culture[b]	7–9 days
Measles virus	Measles	NP aspirate/wash	Culture[c]	5 days
		Throat swab	Antigen detection[c]	2 hours
		Serum	IgG and IgM antibody[d]	1–2 days
Mumps virus	Parotitis, aseptic meningitis, meningoencephalitis	Urine, throat swab, saliva, CSF, blood	Culture	8 days
		Serum	IgG and IgM antibody[d]	1–2 days
Parainfluenza viruses	Croup, pneumonitis, bronchiolitis	NP aspirate/wash	Culture[c]	4–7 days
			Antigen detection using FA	2 hours
Parvovirus B19	Erythema infectiosum	Blood, serum, bone marrow, amniotic fluid cells, placental tissue, cord	IgG and IgM antibody[d]	2 days
	Aplastic crisis, congenital, hydrops fetalis		PCR	2 days
Polyomavirus (JC and BK)	JC virus – progressive multifocal leukoencephalopathy (PML)	CSF	PCR	1 week
	BK virus – polyomavirus-associated nephropathy (PVAN)	Urine	PCR (quantitative)	1 week
Rabies virus	Encephalomyelitis	Postmortem CNS tissue, Antemorem nuchal biopsy	Direct antigen detection (DFA, IHC, DRIT)[c]	24 to 72 hours / 2 weeks
	Immune status post-vaccination	Serum, CSF		2 weeks
		Saliva (antemortem)	IgG and IgM antibody[d] (IFA)	24 to 72 hours
		Serum, CSF		2 weeks
			Culture	
			RT-PCR	

Continued

TABLE 287-2. Optimal Specimen, Preferred Test, and Performance in Confirmation of Specific Infections—cont'd

Agent/Type or Site of Infection or Host	Major Diseases	Optimal Specimens	Available Tests[a]	Average Time to Positive Results[b]
Respiratory syncytial virus	Bronchiolitis, pneumonia, croup	NP aspirate/wash/swab, throat swab/wash, BAL	Antigen detection[c]	15 minutes–4 hours
			Shell vial with antigen staining	16–48 hours
			Culture	3–7 days
		Serum	PCR (including multiplex assays for respiratory viruses)	1 day
Rhinovirus	Common cold	NP aspirate/wash	Culture	7 days
Rubella	Acquired or congenital rubella	Serum	IgG and IgM antibody[d]	1–2 days
		Throat swab	Culture	5–7 days
VARICELLA-ZOSTER VIRUS				
Skin, disseminated	Chickenpox, herpes zoster, occasional CNS complications	Vesicle fluid, scraping of base of vesicle in VTM, CSF	Antigen detection[c]	2 hours
			Culture	3–7 days
			PCR[c,f]	1 day
		Serum	IgG and IgM antibody[d]	1–2 days
Immune status	Past infection or vaccination	Serum	IgG antibody	1–2 days
MYCOPLASMA PNEUMONIAE	Pneumonia, pharyngitis, Stevens–Johnson syndrome, meningoencephalitis	Throat swab	Culture	3 weeks
		CSF	PCR[f]	4–6 days
		Serum	IgG and IgM antibody[c]	1–5 days

Ag, antigen; AIDS, acquired immunodeficiency syndrome; BAL, bronchoalveolar lavage; CNS, central nervous system; CSF, cerebrospinal fluid; EBV, Epstein–Barr virus; EDTA, ethylenediaminetetraacetic acid; EEE, eastern equine encephalomyelitis; EIA, enzyme immunoassay; EM, electron microscopy; FA, fluorescence antigen detection; HAV, hepatitis A virus; HBc, hepatitis B core; HBsAg, hepatitis B surface antigen; HBV, hepatitis B virus; HCV, hepatitis C virus; HDV, hepatitis D virus; HIV, human immunodeficiency virus; HSV, herpes simplex virus; IFA, indirect fluorescence assay; IgG, immunoglobulin G; NAAT, nucleic acid amplification test (may include: LCR, ligase chain reaction; NASBA, nucleic acid sequence-based amplification; NP, nasopharyngeal; PCR, polymerase chain reaction); PBMCs, peripheral blood mononuclear cells; RIBA, recombinant immunoblot assay; SLE, St. Louis encephalitis; WEE, western equine encephalomyelitis; WNV, West Nile virus.

[a]Available tests may vary by laboratory. Samples may need to be sent to a reference lab for some tests. Not all tests need to be performed in all patients.

[b]The average time to a positive result may be as much a function of the test itself (e.g., culture) as it is the frequency with which the test is performed in the laboratory.

[c]Preferred test on the basis of sensitivity, specificity, and short time to a positive test result.

[d]Acute and convalescent (2 to 4 weeks after the onset of illness) serologic testing is recommended for most viruses. IgM antibody testing is available for CMV, EBV, HAV, HSV, measles, mumps, parvovirus B19, rubella, and varicella-zoster virus.

[e]In cases of sexual abuse or rape, culture is recommended because of concern about false-positive results with nonculture methods.

[f]PCR test times to a positive result vary.

[g]In the echovirus neutralizing antibody panel, four to five of the most prevalent recent serotypes are chosen for the panel.

[h]Serotyping of the isolate as HSV-1 or HSV-2 is available.

[i]Detection of proviral DNA after PCR amplification may be the preferred test in young infants, in adults with mononucleosis syndrome before seroconversion, and in adults with an indeterminate Western blot.

of CMV directly in neutrophils) and a variety of NAATs using WBCs, plasma, serum, or whole blood.[18,88–90] These assays are most widely used in immunocompromised patients and to a lesser extent in infants with congenital CMV infection. Some assays are quantitative or semiquantitative, and several studies support a relationship between the level of CMV in blood and the likelihood of active or emerging CMV disease.[91–94] These assays are used in pre-emptive treatment strategies, as well as for monitoring response to anti-CMV therapy. However, because of variability among commercial as well as in-house quantitative CMV assays, the exact level of CMV DNA or antigenemia that should be used to initiate pre-emptive therapy is not well established. Potential problems with these assays include inhibition of PCR when heparin is used as the anticoagulant,[12] false-negative findings with the CMV antigenemia assay when processing of blood samples is delayed beyond 4 to 6 hours,[95] cost, the need for technical expertise, and labor intensity (e.g., CMV antigenemia). Neither assay has been shown to be clearly superior.

For the diagnosis of CMV mononucleosis in otherwise healthy people, testing for CMV-specific IgM is the preferred test. However, IgM antibodies can be detected in both primary and reactivated CMV infections and can persist for months. False-positive CMV

IgM results can occur in patients with acute EBV infection, as well as in patients with high levels of rheumatoid factor in the presence of CMV-specific IgG.[96] In immunologically immature hosts or in immunosuppressed patients, the CMV IgM response during acute infection can be delayed or absent. Because IgM antibodies do not cross the placenta, their detection in a newborn is diagnostic of congenital infection. However, production of IgM antibodies by the newborn may be delayed or absent in up to 30% of cases and thus a negative result does not exclude congenital infection.[80]

The major use of CMV IgG serology is to determine susceptibility to infection in healthcare or childcare workers[97] and to identify the CMV status of blood and organ/tissue donors and recipients.[98] In pregnant women, CMV-specific IgG avidity assays may be of value.[81] The presence of low-avidity IgG anti-CMV may be a better predictor of recent infection than IgM alone, thus increasing the likelihood of CMV transmission to the fetus. However, substantial variability in performance of different CMV avidity assays precludes clear guidance on use and interpretation.[99] Additional testing such as PCR or virus isolation from amniotic fluid may be required to confirm infection of the fetus.

Standardization of in vitro CMV antiviral susceptibility testing has not been established despite utility in immunocompromised patients in whom resistance correlates with clinical failures.[100] Phenotypic assays are limited by lengthy turnaround time and expertise required for performance. Genotypic assays can detect mutations in the CMV UL97 phosphotransferase gene and the UL 54 DNA polymerase gene conferring antiviral resistance but are not available widely.

Epstein–Barr Virus

In patients with suspected EBV mononucleosis (IM), heterophile antibody remains the serologic test of choice.[101] These IgM antibodies can be detected easily and rapidly using a simple spot agglutination assay (often referred to as a "monospot") or immunochromatographic assays.[102]

Heterophile antibodies develop in approximately 80% to 85% of adolescents and adults with EBV (IM)[101] within 2 to 3 weeks after the onset of illness. Responses can be delayed in some individuals; repeat testing may be required. The heterophile test can be negative in 70% to 80% of EBV infections in children <4 years of age.[102] Heterophile antibodies usually disappear within a few months but can persist for >1 year after acute illness in 20% to 70% of patients[48] and persistence should not be interpreted as recurrent or chronic IM. Cases of heterophile-negative IM in school-aged children are due to CMV in 70% and EBV (proven by EBV-specific serology) in 16%.[103]

EBV serology is indicated when the diagnosis of EBV infection is strongly suspected but the heterophile test is negative.[104] The immunofluorescence antibody (IFA) test is considered the "gold standard" although EIA and immunoblot assays can be used.[101] IFA tests have more uniform performance characteristics, whereas EIAs can vary because of the wide variety of antigen preparations used in different kits. The most useful diagnostic test is IgM anti-EBV viral capsid antigen (VCA), which appears within 1 to 2 weeks after the onset of symptoms, disappears within months, and is 91% to 98% sensitive and 99% specific.[48,101,104] False-positive results can occur due to the presence of rheumatoid factor, other herpesvirus infections, and antinuclear factors in EIA test systems. False-negative results can occur if samples are collected late in the course of the illness. IgG anti-VC is elevated during symptoms of illness and can persist for life, and thus is less useful for the diagnosis of acute infection but remains the most reliable marker of EBV seropositivity. IgG anti-early antigen (EA) rises early, whereas IgG anti-EBNA (Epstein–Barr nuclear antigen) appears late (generally after 6 weeks) and persists for life. Several months after recovering from IM, an individual is expected to have IgG antibodies to VCA and EBNA, but low or absent VCA IgM antibodies as well as low or absent antibodies to EA[101] (see Figure 208-3).

Direct tests for EBV, such as cultivation in cord blood leukocytes, direct detection by immunofluorescence staining, or detection of DNA,[105,106] are performed in some laboratories. EBV can be isolated from oropharyngeal washings or circulating lymphocytes of 80% to 90% of patients with IM. PCR detection of EBV DNA in the CSF of patients with HIV infection is strongly associated with primary CNS lymphoma.[106] Following organ and marrow transplantation, the use of quantitative EBV PCR using blood specimens may help predict the development of posttransplant lymphoproliferative disease.[107] Relative merit of testing whole blood, leukocytes, plasma, or serum is unclear. Elevated levels of EBV DNA in peripheral blood may be an indication to decrease immunosuppressive therapy or to consider therapies such as CD20+ monoclonal antibodies or EBV-specific cytotoxic T lymphocytes.[107]

Rarely, EBV infection is associated with an acute fulminant disease (e.g., X-linked lymphoproliferative syndrome and virus-associated hemophagocytic syndrome).[108] Persistent high-titer EBV antibodies, except against EBNA, are characteristic but may be absent. The diagnosis depends on detection of virus or its genome.

Varicella-Zoster Virus

The diagnosis of chickenpox or herpes zoster (shingles) usually can be made clinically. In selected circumstances, isolation of virus

from vesicular fluid, demonstration of viral antigen in cells scraped from the base of lesions using FA staining, and detection of VZV DNA by PCR in vesicular fluid, skin scrapings, respiratory secretions, blood, or CSF[109–114] may be useful. Skin lesions <4 days old are more likely to yield virus than older ones. Because VZV is extremely labile, transport of samples to the laboratory should occur within 12 hours of collection. Direct detection of VZV antigens by FA of smears from lesions is more sensitive than culture and is the preferred method for diagnosis of VZV skin lesions.[113] Vigorous swabbing to retrieve cellular material from the base of the vesicular lesion optimizes the yield. Vesicular fluid, although good for culture, is inadequate for FA testing.

PCR for detection of VZV DNA compared with culture or FA has advantages of increased sensitivity, in scrapings of older lesions, and ability to distinguish vaccine- versus wild-type VZV. PCR analysis of CSF can confirm the etiology of CNS syndromes that can occur as a complication of varicella or zoster, with or without cutaneous lesions. Detection of VZV DNA in CSF by PCR along with detection of VZV antibody in CSF are recommended to confirm VZV CNS infection.[115] Multiplex PCR assays capable of detecting VZV as well as other herpesviruses have been evaluated and may simplify the diagnosis in patients with overlapping clinical syndromes (e.g., vesicular rash).[33]

IgG anti-VZV is used primarily to assess susceptibility to infection, to determine the need for vaccination or risk of disease in exposed individuals, and to determine the duration of protection post-vaccination.[116,117] During acute VZV infection, VZV antibodies appear within a few days after the onset of rash and peak 2 to 3 weeks later. A >4-fold rise in IgG antibody between serum collected 10 to 14 days apart or the detection of VZV-specific IgM antibodies in a single sample supports a diagnosis of acute infection. However, serologic diagnosis can be confounded by heterotypic HSV antibody increases that can occur in up to one-third of patients with primary HSV infection who have experienced a previous VZV infection.[118] Fluorescent antibody against membrane antigen (FAMA) is considered the gold standard for detection of VZV antibodies.[117] Detection of neutralizing antibodies to VZV in healthy individuals by FAMA or latex agglutination correlates with protection in up to 96% of persons.[119] Occasionally, VZV infection has been reported to occur in patients with low levels of VZV antibodies detected by these assays.[120] EIA assays may have lower sensitivity when compared with FAMA and latex agglutination assays particularly in detecting antibodies post-vaccination.[117] Newer glycoprotein (gp) EIAs appear to have improved sensitivity over older ones.

Human Herpesvirus Types 6, 7, and 8

Primary infection with human herpesvirus 6 (HHV-6) occurs in most children before the age of 2 to 3 years and routine lab testing usually is not performed. Detectable antibodies in primary infection generally appear 3 to 8 days following onset of fever. The following serologic criteria are considered diagnostic of primary HHV-6 infection: (1) antibody seroconversion between acute- and convalescent-phase serum/plasma specimens collected 2 to 4 weeks apart; (2) detection of HHV-6-specific low-avidity IgG antibodies; (3) positive serum IgM in the absence of IgG antibodies; and (4) >4-fold rise in IgG antibody by IFA or anticomplementary immunofluorescence assays.[121] Current commercial assays for IgG anti-HHV-6 do not distinguish between variants A and B and can cross-react with HHV-7 and CMV.[122,123] Antibody avidity testing can be used to differentiate primary HHV-6 from HHV-7 infections. IgM anti-HHV-6 alone is not a reliable indicator of acute or recent infection because IgM also can be found during reactivation or reinfection and approximately 5% of adults have detectable IgM anti-HHV-6 at any time.[121] IgM may not be detectable in some culture-positive children.[122,124] During acute primary HHV-6 infection, virus can be recovered from cultures of peripheral blood mononuclear cells (PBMCs) in 100% of infants, but not after recovery,[125] whereas HHV-6 DNA can be detected by PCR during both acute illness and after recovery.[123,126] Monoclonal antibodies are available for direct detection of HHV-6 antigen and have been used to confirm cell culture CPE and for immunohistochemical staining of tissues.

In immunosuppressed patients, HHV-6 infection can be associated with significant morbidity and mortality.[127,128] Proof of HHV-6 causation is difficult because specific antibodies can be absent and demonstration of viral DNA in PBMCs can represent latent infection. Although PCR detection of HHV-6 DNA in serum/plasma has low sensitivity, it may be a better marker for active infection. PCR was negative in the serum or plasma of 57 healthy adults, but positive in 94% of 17 patients with exanthem subitum, 23% of 13 bone marrow transplant recipients, and 22% of 18 HIV-infected patients.[129,130]

Serologic tests for HHV-7 are not available widely. Some degree of cross-reaction between HHV-6 and HHV-7 antibodies occurs due to cross-reactive epitopes on the viruses.[122] Responses can be distinguished by antibody avidity testing.[122] A significant rise in HHV-7 antibodies with stable or absent antibodies to HHV-6 may indicate active infection with HHV-7. HHV-7 has been isolated from the saliva of 75% of healthy adults[131] as well as from ill individuals, questioning the value of such testing. HHV-7 has been isolated only rarely from PBMCs of healthy asymptomatic individuals compared with those with active infections, suggesting that PBMC cultures may have diagnostic value.[132] Specific primers for PCR amplification of HHV-7 have been developed that do not amplify the DNA from any other human herpesviruses and have been included in a multiplex assay.[133,134]

Testing for HHV-8 is only available in research settings. PCR has been used for detection of HHV-8 DNA in PBMCs and tissues.[135] The use of plasma/serum for HHV-8 PCR has no value for identifying active infections.[121] Serologic assays can detect IgG- but not IgM-anti HHV-8. Useful for seroprevalence studies, the role of serologic tests in diagnosing and managing HHV-8 infections has not been established.[136]

Respiratory Syncytial Virus

NP wash or aspirate is superior to swab sampling for detection of RSV infection. Bronchoalveolar lavage (BAL) and endotracheal tube (ETT) aspirates also are acceptable. Specimens for culture or FA testing should be transported on wet ice or refrigerated as soon after collection as possible as there is substantial loss of cell culture infectivity at room temperature. Samples for antigen detection can be transported at room temperature. Culture for RSV requires a mean of 3 to 7 days. Shell vial culture appears to have a slightly greater sensitivity than standard culture.[137] Culture has the advantage of detecting other respiratory viruses that are recovered from 5% to 10% of specimens submitted for diagnosis of RSV infection. The use of mixed fresh cells has proven to be a rapid and sensitive method for detection of RSV. The sensitivity of antigen detection techniques such as EIA microtiter plate kits, membrane filter EIA, and DFA range from 84% to 96%, with specificity of 92% to 96%.[42,138–140] The membrane filter EIA offers the advantage of providing a result within 15 to 20 minutes.[138,139,141] Some assays can detect multiple respiratory viruses simultaneously.[142] In general, rapid antigen detection tests for RSV have a relatively lower sensitivity in adults than children, which likely reflects the decreased amount and duration of shedding of RSV in respiratory secretions of adults.

The use of serologic tests for the diagnosis of acute RSV infection has little clinical value. In primary RSV infection, detectable IgM antibodies appear approximately 5 to 9 days after onset of symptoms and persist for several weeks. The antibody response may be poor or absent in very young infants, older individuals with repeat infections, and immunocompromised patients.[143] RSV antibody detection may be useful for epidemiologic purposes and for evaluating responses to candidate RSV vaccines.[144] NAATs improve the detection of RSV in respiratory tract specimens and have been used to distinguish between RSV subgroups A and B during community and institutional outbreaks.[145] Multiplex PCR assays capable of detecting several respiratory viruses in the same test have been evaluated.[138,146]

Influenza Viruses

Clinical samples for the detection and isolation of influenza viruses should be collected within 3 days of symptom onset when virus shedding is maximal. Transport to the laboratory should be as prompt as possible and specimens can be stored at 4° C if processing will be delayed beyond 3 to 4 days. Standard tube culture for isolation of influenza viruses requires 3 to 5 days. Shell vial shortens the time for detection to 48 hours but may not be as sensitive as standard culture.[147] Serotyping of influenza A and B viruses isolated in culture can be achieved by inhibition of hemagglutination using serotype-specific antiserum.

Several rapid antigen detection kits, including point-of-care tests, are available for the detection of influenza A only, influenza A and B together (without distinguishing between them), and influenza A or B.[148–150] Evaluations of rapid tests for the detection of seasonal influenza virus as well as the pandemic 2009 H1N1 virus indicate relatively poor sensitivity but high specificity.[147,149,150] These tests have not been evaluated fully for the detection of avian influenza A/H5N1. When good-quality respiratory specimens with well-preserved epithelial cells are used, DFA staining using monoclonal antibodies has a sensitivity of 80% to 90% and specificity of >90%.[151–153] NP aspirates are superior to NP swabs and throat swabs for the detection of influenza A in healthy volunteers.[154,155] A number of different PCR assays including multiplex respiratory virus assays have been evaluated in several studies and show a substantially increased sensitivity compared with other methods, including culture.[42,156–158] Multiplex assays capable of detecting influenza A (including pandemic 2009 H1N1) and B, antiviral resistance mutations (particularly the H275Y substitution conferring resistance to oseltamivir), and multiple other respiratory viruses are available.[156–160]

Other Respiratory Viruses

Numerous other viruses including human parainfluenza viruses types 1, 2, 3, and 4, adenoviruses (subtypes A to E), rhinoviruses, human coronaviruses 229E, OC43, severe acute respiratory syndrome (SARS) coronavirus, and human metapneumovirus (hMPV) can infect the respiratory tract and cause clinical signs and symptoms indistinguishable from influenza and RSV. Laboratory diagnosis may be important for epidemiologic purposes, for implementation of appropriate infection control measures, and for reducing empiric use of antibiotics. Culture for parainfluenza viruses and adenoviruses requires approximately 4 to 6 days for a positive result. Most laboratories do not routinely attempt isolation of rhinoviruses. No routine culture methods are available for isolation of coronaviruses or hMPV. DFA staining is available for parainfluenza viruses and for adenoviruses.[161] Interpretation of the causal role of adenovirus is confounded by latency and reactivation. No antigen detection test is available for rhinoviruses, hMPV, or coronaviruses. Serology is of no value for the diagnosis of acute infection with these viruses. Several of the previously discussed multiplex molecular assays for the detection of respiratory viruses can detect many of these other respiratory viruses.[160]

Hepatitis Viruses

Routine diagnosis for all hepatitis viruses is based on serology. Serum or plasma can be used for most assays and should be separated from blood within 24 hours of collection. The diagnosis of acute HAV is made by demonstration of IgM anti-HAV.[162] Immunity to HAV following natural infection or immunization is determined by measuring hepatitis A IgG or total (IgG and IgM) anti-HAV.[162] Currently, there is no role for reverse transcription (RT)-PCR measurement of HAV RNA for routine diagnosis. In acute and chronic HBV infection both HBsAg and anti-hepatitis B core antibody (HBcAb) usually are present.[163] IgM anti-HBc generally is present in acute HBV infection and occasionally during a flare of inflammation in chronic carriers. Thus, IgM anti-HBc does not always distinguish acute from chronic infection. By definition, a person with persistently positive HBsAg for >6 months is considered chronically infected. Isolated anti-HBc positivity can occur during: (1) acute infection between the loss of detectable HBsAg and emergence of detectable HBsAb ("core window"); (2) late chronic infection when HBsAg levels have fallen below detectable levels; (3) coinfection with HCV or HIV that suppress HBsAg production; (4) infection with a mutant HBV; or (5) a false-positive result. The role of quantitative HBsAg assays is being evaluated for monitoring patients with chronic hepatitis B infection. The presence of HBV e antigen (HBeAg) and the absence of anti-HBe are markers of greater infectivity and correlate with increased risk of progression to chronic hepatitis, cirrhosis, and hepatocellular carcinoma.[163] The presence of anti-HBe is an indicator of likely recovery. The presence of HBsAb at a level >10 IU/mL is considered to protective against acute infection. HBsAb levels can decline below 10 IU/mL after 10 to 12 years in a substantial number of vaccine responders. These individuals remain protected from acute infection likely as a result of immune memory.[164] The presence of HBsAb alone reflects prior immunization whereas the presence of HBsAb together with HBcAb reflects recovery from previous natural infection.[163]

For diagnosis of HCV infection, second- and third-generation EIA and supplementary recombinant immunoblot assay (RIBA) using recombinant structural proteins are available widely.[165,166] Seroconversion occurs by 8 to 12 weeks following acute infection, with sensitivity of 94% to 100% (except in immunosuppressed individuals) and specificity of >97% after the supplementary RIBA test.[32] HCV antibody (anti-HCV) frequently is negative at the onset of jaundice. The presence of HCV antibodies indicates current infection in most patients. No assay is available currently for the detection of IgM anti-HCV. The utility of measuring HCV antigen in serum or plasma has not been established.

Molecular assays for the detection and quantification of HBV and HCV viral nucleic acid in serum are useful for determining prognosis, selecting candidates for therapy, and monitoring response to therapy.[165,167,168] A lower baseline concentration indicates a better prognosis and a greater likelihood of response to treatment. Patients responding to antiviral treatment demonstrate a significant drop in HBV DNA or HCV RNA, whereas nonresponders do not. Molecular assays also are available for HBV and HCV genotyping and antiviral resistance testing.[169] HCV genotyping is useful for epidemiologic purposes and to identify patients most likely to respond to therapy. The role of HBV genotyping is less well established. NAATs that detect HCV RNA in serum 1 to 3 weeks after exposure are being used as part of blood and organ/tissue donor screening and in patients with indeterminate HCV antibody results when the RIBA is inconclusive.

In most clinical situations, testing for hepatitis A, B, and C can be grouped into one of three categories: (1) *acute hepatitis;* (2) *chronic hepatitis;* and (3) *immune status/previous exposure.* For suspected *acute hepatitis,* initial testing for IgM anti-HAV, HBsAg, and anti-HCV should be performed. If all 3 are negative, IgM anti-HBc should be tested. Repeat testing for anti-HCV is recommended in 3 to 4 weeks. In situations where *chronic hepatitis* is suspected, testing should include HBsAg and anti-HCV. Some also may test for anti-HBc. Patients being screened for *immunity* and/or *previous infection* should have the following tests: (1) total or IgG anti-HAV; (2) HBsAb or HBcAb or both (depending on whether previous infection is suspected); and (3) anti-HCV (which is a marker of previous infection and not immunity).

Serologic tests are available for both hepatitis D (delta agent) (HDV) and hepatitis E viruses (HEV) but none have been approved by the Food and Drug Administration (FDA).[170] Because infection with HDV occurs solely in conjunction with HBV infection, testing for anti-HDV only should be performed in patients acutely or chronically infected with HBV. During coinfection with HBV and HDV, anti-HDV disappears within months following recovery from acute infection. However, in HDV superinfection of a HBV chronically infected patient, anti-HDV generally persists indefinitely as infection becomes chronic in most cases. Measurement of HDV RNA by RT-PCR remains a research test. Both IgG and IgM anti-HEV can be measured using research or commercial assays.[171] Due to the use of different antigens, assays show significant

variability in sensitivity and specificity.[172] IgG anti-HEV is positive in most patients 1 to 4 weeks after the onset of disease and becomes undetectable by 3 months. IgG anti-HEV typically declines after infection. In areas where HEV is not endemic, RT-PCR may prove useful as a confirmatory test.

Gastroenteritis Viruses

Stool samples placed in a clean sterile container without VTM or preservative for the detection of enteric viruses should be collected within the first 48 hours of illness. Rectal swabs may not contain sufficient virus for EM detection. Stool specimens are stable at 4°C for up to 1 week. Although freezing at −70°C can permit prolonged storage, EM detection is reduced by repeated freezing and thawing that destroys the morphology of viral structures. None of the enteric viruses can be cultivated readily in conventional cell culture systems, but all can be detected by EM. Commercial EIA, latex agglutination and membrane-based tests with >95% sensitivity and specificity are available for detection of rotaviruses, noroviruses, enteric adenoviruses, and astroviruses.[19,20,173] PCR-based assays for these viruses are becoming available in many state health departments.[41,174] PCR-based assays are now the method of choice for diagnosing enteric viruses, particularly rotaviruses and caliciviruses. There is no role for serologic testing for enteric viruses except during outbreak investigations.

Enteroviruses

Enteroviruses generally are stable and survive in the environment for weeks; rapid transport of clinical specimens to the laboratory is not critical. Enterovirus viability decreases slowly over days to weeks at room temperature and is preserved for decades at −70°C. Appropriate specimens include CSF, serum or whole blood, pericardial fluid, tissue biopsies (e.g., myocardium), urine, stool, and rectal, nasal and throat swabs. Although many enteroviruses can be grown in cell culture, some serotypes (e.g., coxsackievirus A groups 1, 19, and 22) fail to grow in standard cell culture. Isolation of enterovirus requires 4 to 7 days.[175] Virus can be isolated more frequently from stool (80% to 85%) and throat swabs (50% to 60%) than from CSF (40% to 60%) and serum or peripheral leukocytes (40% to 50%). Due to the lack of a common antigen among enteroviruses, immunoassays for direct detection are not available. EM is not useful for diagnosis because of the low numbers of viruses in most clinical samples.

RT-PCR has been used to test CSF, cardiac tissue, pericardial fluid as well as serum and has significantly improved the speed of detection of enteroviruses, with reported sensitivity of 81% to 100% and specificity of 92% to 100%.[176,177] In comparison, culture has a sensitivity of only 40% to 60%.[175] Detection in urine samples is poor, probably due to nonspecific inhibitors of PCR.[178] In respiratory specimens, cross-amplification of some rhinoviruses can occur.

Clinically, the detection of enteroviruses must be interpreted cautiously. Asymptomatic shedding of wild enterovirus from the gastrointestinal tract can occur for weeks or months. Additionally, oral polio vaccine virus can be shed in stool and, less commonly, in the throat of young vaccinated children. Detection of virus in CSF, the genitourinary tract, tissue, or blood is proof of a causative role.

Measuring antibody titers for enteroviruses is of limited diagnostic value. A separate neutralization assay must be performed for each enterovirus subtype.

Measles, Mumps, and Rubella (MMR)

The laboratory diagnosis of MMR viruses can be made by virus isolation, detection of antigen, the use of RT-PCR, or serologic testing. Suitable samples for isolation or detection of viral antigen include whole blood (particularly PBMCs for the isolation of measles), serum, throat and NP secretions, urine and, under appropriate clinical circumstances, CSF, brain and skin biopsies. As these are labile viruses, rapid transport to the laboratory is important. Specimens are best kept at 4°C prior to processing, but may be frozen at −70°C if a delay >48 hours is anticipated. Isolation of virus from blood is greatest 3 to 5 days before rash onset and declines rapidly within 2 to 3 days thereafter. Conjunctival and NP samples for isolation of measles virus can be collected 2 to 4 days before and up to 4 days after the onset of rash. Throat swabs for rubella virus isolation usually are positive (~90%) if collected on the day of rash onset but rapidly become negative within 4 days. Mumps virus can be isolated from saliva 9 days before and up to 8 days after the onset of parotitis. These viruses can be cultivated in conventional cell lines, but isolation requires 7 to 10 days for measles and mumps virus and >3 weeks for rubella virus.[179,180] The shell vial method for measles virus has a sensitivity of 78% at 1 to 2 days and 100% at 5 days. Sensitivity of DFA staining of NP swab specimens for measles virus antigen is 100% compared with culture, but only 67% for throat swabs and 85% for urine specimens. Shell vial culture for detection of mumps virus has comparable sensitivity and specificity to traditional culture.

Molecular diagnosis using virus-specific RT-PCR has been used for detection of all of these viruses and can be used for genotyping to help differentiate wild-type from vaccine-virus strains.[181,182]

Timing of serum specimen collection is critical as many patients do not have IgM antibody at the time of rash onset. For suspected measles virus infection, serum can be collected within 7 to 10 days of rash onset. For rubella virus infection, >90% of patients will have IgM positivity ≥5 days after rash onset. Although the traditional MMR serologic test is HAI for IgG antibody, a number of IFA and EIA IgG and IgM kits are available commercially.[183] With the declining prevalence of these viral diseases, the positive predictive value of IgM tests can be low. The presence of rheumatoid factor can lead to a false-positive IgM result and re-exposure in a previously vaccinated individual or individual with a history of natural infection can result in a secondary IgG or IgM response. Mumps IgM antibody can persist for months after acute illness.[184] Patients with IM,[185] parvovirus B19 infection,[186] measles virus, and CMV infection can have cross-reacting IgM anti-rubella. Similarly infection with parvovirus B19 and rubella virus can result in cross-reacting IgM anti-measles. In pregnant women, IgM anti-rubella should be confirmed with a second IgM assay or detection of a significant rise in IgG antibodies.[187] Avidity assays for IgG antibodies to measles and rubella viruses are available. Measurement of virus-specific IgG antibodies can be used to determine immune status. For mumps virus, cross-reactions with other paramyxoviruses can occur. For rubella virus, an IgG level of >10 IU/mL is thought to represent immunity in most cases.[179]

Human Immunodeficiency Virus

The major diagnostic tests for HIV are serologic (EIA, IFA, and WB for HIV antibody, EIA for p24 antigen), culture, and NAATs for the detection of HIV-1 RNA in plasma or proviral DNA in whole blood or PBMCs. Culture for HIV is no longer used for routine diagnosis.[188] NAATs can be used for the diagnosis of HIV-1 infection in neonates with excellent sensitivity and specificity.[189] Screening tests for HIV-1 RNA have become part of routine blood and organ/tissue donor screening programs since 2002,[190] and also can be used for measuring HIV-1 in other specimen types including CSF, cervical secretions, seminal plasma/semen and serum. The use of NAATs in populations who are not known to be HIV-seropositive has yielded false-positive results.[191] The major use of quantitative HIV-1 viral load assays is for monitoring a patient's response to antiretroviral therapy.[28,192] Because of the intra-assay and biologic variability in HIV-1 RNA levels, a >3-fold change is considered clinically relevant. Different molecular assays also can produce significant differences in HIV-1 viral load and thus baseline values should be repeated when the laboratory testing is changed from one assay to another.[192] Some assays yield lower levels in the same patient if serum is used instead of plasma or if blood is collected in acid-citrate-dextrose anticoagulant rather than EDTA. Currently available commercial assays vary in

specimen volume requirement (range from 50 µL to 2 mL), lower limit of detection, dynamic range, and time to result.[192] Regardless of assay format, plasma must be separated from the blood cells within 6 hours of collection. None of these assays is approved for use in individuals infected with HIV-2 or HIV-1 group O. Other molecular assays are available for HIV-1 genotyping for the detection of antiretroviral resistance mutations.[193] Resistance testing is recommended prior to initiating therapy and when treatment failure occurs. Phenotypic assays can also be performed for this purpose.

The mainstay of diagnosis for HIV remains HIV-specific serology using screening EIAs or, less commonly, particle agglutination assays followed by confirmatory testing using WB or other assay.[190] Both serum and plasma are acceptable specimens. Testing systems for dried blood spots, urine, and saliva also are available. Early EIA had sensitivity and specificity exceeding 95% in the diagnosis of HIV infection in high-risk groups. However, in low-risk groups such as blood donors, 90% of positive results were false due, most commonly, to cross-reacting antibodies against human leukocyte antigens in the cell lysate used in antigen preparation.[190] False-negative results occurred due to antigenic heterogeneity among HIV strains, particularly group O.[194] Recent EIA kits use more purified viral antigens from cell lysates, recombinant viral proteins, and synthetic peptide antigens and can detect group O. These assays have increased sensitivity and specificity and fewer indeterminate results.[190] Most currently available assays detect IgG and IgM anti-HIV-1 and anti-HIV-2 in the same assay.[195] Fourth-generation screening tests can detect both HIV-1/HIV-2 antibodies and p24 antigen at the same time while reducing the seroconversion window period to approximately 16 days.[190] Detuned (also known as "sensitive/less sensitive") EIAs capable of measuring the affinity of HIV antibodies have been used to distinguish recent from past/distant HIV infection and to estimate incidence rates.[196]

WB remains the principal confirmatory test for HIV serology, despite the fact that its sensitivity in seroconversion panels is inferior to third- and fourth-generation screening tests. Separate WB tests must be used to confirm HIV-1 and HIV-2. WB measures the antibody response to 9 HIV-1 proteins (p) or glycoproteins (gp): gp160, gp120, p66, p55, p51, gp41, p31, p24, and p17 but is prone to give a high rate of indeterminate results due to detection of cross-reacting antibodies and nonspecific reactions.[190] The Centers for Disease Control and Prevention (CDC) criterion for confirmation of HIV-1 infection is presence of antibody to any two of the following: p24, gp41, or gp120/160.[197] No antibody response to HIV-1 proteins represents a negative test, whereas the presence of some, but not all, antibodies required for a positive interpretation is an indeterminate result; repeat testing over the next 6 months is recommended, and if WB results remain indeterminate persons are considered not to be infected.[197] In low-risk populations, persons with a positive screening EIA test result and indeterminate WB are rarely, if ever, infected with HIV on follow-up serologic testing.[198,199]

The IFA test can detect both IgG and IgM anti-HIV-1, is quite sensitive and specific, and can be used as an alternative to WB as a confirmatory test.[190] The line immunoassay (LIA) can be used for confirmation of HIV-1 (including group O) and HIV-2 in a single test. Rapid point-of-care tests for both screening and confirmation requiring minimal or no laboratory equipment have been developed that can yield a result in <30 minutes with comparable sensitivity and specificity to third-generation EIA-based tests and other confirmatory assays.[200]

Different laboratory diagnostic strategies are needed for the most common situations in which HIV infection is considered: (1) an *adult or older child who is suspected of having HIV infection;* (2) an *infant with suspected vertically-acquired HIV infection;* and (3) an individual in whom acute infection or seroconversion may develop because of *exposure to an HIV-infected person.*

An *adult or older child who has been infected* with HIV for weeks to months is expected to be antibody positive. The standard approach in this situation is to perform: (1) screening EIA, with a repeat EIA (in duplicate) if the test is positive; and (2) a

TABLE 287-3. Sensitivity (%) of Diagnostic Tests for HIV in Infants According to Age

Method	Age				
	1 week	2–4 weeks	1–2 months	3–6 months	>6 months
Culture	30–50	50	70–90	>95	>95
PCR	30–50	50	70–90	>95	>95
p24	1–25	20–50	30–60	30–50	20–40
IgA	<10	10–30	20–50	50–80	70–90

HIV, human immunodeficiency virus; IgA, immunoglobulin A; PCR, polymerase chain reaction.

Adapted from Report of a Consensus Workshop, Siena, Italy. Early diagnosis of HIV infection in infants. J Acquir Immune Defic Syndr 1992;5:1169–1178.

confirmatory WB test if the repeat EIA is positive.[190] If the results of serologic testing are indeterminate, additional tests for p24 antigen, HIV DNA or RNA, or culture of PBMCs can be performed.[190] In the setting of high risk and clinical features of infection, p24 antigen test has specificity of 99%.[190] The sensitivity of the antigen test varies according to clinical disease status: 4% in asymptomatically infected people, 56% in patients with AIDS-related complex, and 76% in patients with AIDS.[201]

Confirmation of vertical transmission of HIV using EIA or WB is confounded by the presence of maternal antibodies for up to 18 months of age.[189] In a symptomatic infant >4 to 6 months of age, detection of p24 antigen, or HIV genome and culture of the virus from PBMCs are reliable, definitive tests.[202–204] The sensitivities of culture, NAAT, p24 antigen, and IgA anti-HIV-testing for the early diagnosis of HIV infection in young infants are shown in Table 287-3 and discussed further in Chapter 111, Diagnosis and Clinical Manifestation of HIV Infection.[189,202–208] Although culture is considered the "gold standard" for pediatric HIV infection, NAAT for viral DNA or RNA is more sensitive.

In an individual with *known HIV exposure*, antibody to the virus usually can be detected within 2 to 8 weeks after infection. Based on third-generation screening assays, HIV antibodies are detectable in 50% of infected individuals within 3 weeks after infection and in most of the remaining patients within 2 months.[190,209] Virtually all infected, immunocompetent individuals are seropositive 6 months after exposure.[209] A mononucleosis-like syndrome develops in some individuals 2 to 4 weeks after infection; p24 antigen can appear transiently during this period.[209]

Arboviruses

For the majority of arbovirus infections laboratory testing generally is not performed. For arboviruses causing CNS disease only a brief, low level of viremia occurs which clears before the patient seeks medical attention.[210] Thus blood specimen for virus isolation and NAAT rarely yield positive results unless collected prior to the neuroinvasive phase of illness. For some arboviruses, including dengue, yellow fever, sandfly fever, Venezuelan encephalitis, and Colorado tick fever, a relatively high level of viremia occurs that can persist for days or weeks making virus isolation or NAAT from blood specimens possible (in reference laboratories). Virus isolation of neurotropic viruses from brain tissue and CSF occasionally is successful during the acute phase of infection; NAAT is more sensitive in these cases.[211]

For most arbovirus infections, the diagnosis is established by IgG seroconversion or detection of specific IgM antibodies, or both.[210,212] Collection of paired acute (collected during the first week of illness) and convalescent (collected 2 to 3 weeks later) sera is recommended. A single sample may be sufficient for diagnosis if a specific IgM test is available (e.g., eastern equine encephalomyelitis, western equine encephalomyelitis, California (La Crosse) virus, St. Louis encephalitis (SLE), West Nile virus, dengue virus). However, in some cases (e.g., West Nile virus), virus-specific IgM can be detected in serum for ≥2 years following infection. For CNS disease, both serum and CSF specimens should be tested. The sensitivity of some of these tests approaches 100% by the 10th day of illness.[213] Traditional assays such as CF and HAI tests largely have been replaced by FA and EIAs.[210] Serologic cross-reactions can occur among antigenically related viruses (e.g., SLE, West Nile virus, Japanese encephalitis, dengue, Powassan, and other flaviviruses). The neutralization test remains the most specific test for serologic diagnosis of arbovirus infections. Neutralizing antibodies are also felt to be the best indicator of protective immunity.

Parvovirus B19

Parvovirus cannot be cultivated in routine cell culture and thus serology (rising IgG titers or presence of IgM antibody) is the mainstay of diagnosis.[214] IgM antibodies are detectable in serum approximately 10 to 12 days after infection, when the rash or joint symptoms begin, and can persist for several months. The sensitivity of IgM anti-parvovirus exceeds 90% in the first month after the onset of symptoms. IgG antibodies appear within several days after IgM and generally persist for years. Current IgG assays have a sensitivity of >90%; IgG indicates past infection. Re-exposure to parvovirus leads to a rise in IgG antibody levels. IgG avidity assays can help distinguish primary from secondary infections.[215] Immunocompromised individuals may not produce antibody; diagnosis can be made by NAAT detection of viral DNA in serum or other specimen types. Parvovirus-associated aplastic crisis, chronic infection, and congenital infection can be diagnosed by PCR analysis of serum.[214–216] PCR also can be used to detect parvovirus B19 DNA in bone marrow aspirates, cord blood samples, amniotic fluid cells, and biopsy specimens of the placenta and fetal tissues in cases of fetal hydrops. However, parvovirus DNA may be detectable in serum for months after acute infection and for years in other tissues.[217] Thus the diagnosis of acute or chronic parvovirus infection may require both serology and quantitative PCR.

Other Viruses

The recommended specimens and lab tests for other viruses are listed in Table 287-2. For the majority of these viruses, testing is performed in highly specialized research or reference laboratories.

Congenital and Perinatal Viral Infections

The major viruses infecting fetuses and newborn infants include CMV, VZV, HSV, rubella, parvovirus B19, HBV, HCV, HEV, enteroviruses, and HIV.[218] Negative maternal and neonatal serology for any of these viruses generally excludes fetal infection.[218] Detection of virus (via culture, antigen detection, or NAAT) may be required before a correct diagnosis can be made. Cord blood can yield false-positive and false-negative results and should not be relied upon for diagnosis.[218]

Congenital CMV infection is best diagnosed by isolating CMV from the urine of neonates within the first 3 weeks of life. Beyond 3 weeks of age, isolation of CMV from urine cannot distinguish congenital from perinatal or postnatal infection. IgM anti-CMV in a newborn is positive in only 50% to 70% of congenitally infected neonates and the test can yield false-positive results.[219]

Congenital VZV infection can be diagnosed by serology. Perinatal or postnatal infection with VZV, as well as with HSV and enteroviruses, usually can be diagnosed by conventional antigen detection or culture techniques, although NAAT testing is preferred for enteroviruses. Serologic diagnosis of neonatal HSV infections is inappropriate because response may not be detectable for 2 or 3 weeks after infection.[220] Demonstration of rubella IgM in a neonate with features consistent with congenital rubella confirms the diagnosis; virus isolation can require 3 to 4 weeks.[218,220,221]

Parvovirus infection during pregnancy can be diagnosed in the mother by serology; detection of IgM or rising IgG antibody level is diagnostic, whereas a stable IgG titer reflects past infection. In neonates, positive parvovirus B19 antibody at 8 to 12 months suggests infection.[218] Parvovirus B19 infection of a fetus with hydrops can be confirmed using NAAT for viral DNA in fetal blood, amniotic fluid cells, or both.[215,221]

CHLAMYDIA AND CHLAMYDOPHILA

Chlamydia trachomatis, Chlamydophila pneumoniae, and *C. psittaci* cause disease in humans. Psittacosis, rare in children, is confirmed serologically.

Chlamydia trachomatis

Specimen Collection and Transport

Because *C. trachomatis* is an intracellular pathogen, optimal specimens for diagnosis are mucosal epithelial cells rather than purulent material. Preferred specimen types vary for testing methods and age groups tested. The following specimens are acceptable for culture: in postpubertal women, a swab or Cytobrush specimen collected from the cervical os; for prepubertal girls, a vaginal swab; for adult males, a urethral swab inserted 3 to 4 cm and rotated; and for boys, a swab of the urethral meatus (if discharge is present).[222] Infants with suspected chlamydial conjunctivitis should have the purulent discharge removed, followed by swabbing or scraping of the palpebral conjunctiva. The yield of culture is related directly to the quality of the specimen and the transport and storage conditions before testing.[223-225] Urine specimens should not be used for culture because of poor sensitivity.

For culture, Dacron-, cotton- or rayon-tip swabs on an aluminum or plastic shaft are recommended. Swabs with wooden shafts and those with a calcium alginate tip may inhibit growth.[226] In females, pooling of urethral and cervical swab specimens increases culture sensitivity by approximately 20%.[223] Swabs should be placed immediately into chlamydial transport media (containing sucrose phosphate or sucrose phosphate glutamate supplemented with bovine serum and antimicrobial agents) at 2°C to 8°C and transported to the laboratory within 24 hours. Some culture transport media also are acceptable for use with NAAT. Freezing at −70°C can result in a 20% loss of viability. Freezing at −20°C should be avoided.

Collection of endocervical and urethral swab specimens for EIA, DFA, hybridization tests or NAAT generally is similar to that for culture and should follow the instructions of the manufacturer. For EIA and DFA testing, swab specimens do not require refrigeration. Swab specimens for NAAT are stable at room temperature for up to 10 days. Urine, vaginal, rectal, NP, or female urethral specimens should not be tested using EIA, DFA, and hybridization tests due to poor sensitivity.[227]

Acceptable specimens for NAATs include endocervical, vaginal, and urethral swabs as well as urine from adolescents and adults.[223]

NAATs are not approved for use with specimens collected from extragenital sites. NAAT for any specimen type from children has not been approved. First-void urine (10 to 50 mL) collected into a clean sterile container from men and women and self-collected vulvovaginal swab specimens are acceptable for use with NAATs.[228-233] Urine specimens for NAAT are stable for up to 24 hours at room temperature, after which they may be refrigerated for up to 4 days or stored at −20°C or lower for up to 2 months before processing.

Laboratory Test Methods

Tests for *C. trachomatis* can be grouped into four broad categories: *serology, culture, direct detection,* and *molecular diagnosis.*

Serologic tests for *C. trachomatis* genital tract infections are not useful for diagnosis in individual patients.[226] Antibodies to *C. trachomatis* persist for life. In infants, detection of IgM anti-*C. trachomatis* using the microimmunofluorescence (MIF) test is the diagnostic test of choice for chlamydial pneumonia.[223] Maternal IgG antibodies can persist in infants for 6 to 9 months.[226] The MIF test is the most sensitive serologic test and is the only one that detects species- and serovar-specific responses.[223] EIAs for the detection of IgM antibodies in infants have variable performance compared with the MIF test.[226] EIAs detect antibodies to the genus-specific antigen, or lipopolysaccharide (LPS) of chlamydial elementary or reticulate bodies and are not specific for *C. trachomatis*. Interpretation of a single IgG antibody test result is difficult because 50% to 70% of people can have antibodies to *C. pneumoniae*.[234,235] CF tests have been used widely for the diagnosis of psittacosis and lymphogranuloma venereum, but have no value in diagnosing genital tract or neonatal chlamydial infections.

Cell culture has specificity approaching 100%; however it is relatively insensitive compared with NAATs, requires cell culture facilities, and has slow turnaround time (3 to 7 days).[223,226] Barring evaluation using other testing methods, the CDC continues to recommend culture for urethral specimens from women and asymptomatic men, NP specimens from infants, rectal specimens from all patients, and vaginal specimens from prepubertal girls.[222] The shell vial culture method has improved the sensitivity and shortened the detection time (48 to 72 hours) of *C. trachomatis* inclusions.[226]

Diagnosis most often is accomplished by *direct detection* of antigens (EIA or DFA assays) or nucleic acid (hybridization assays), or by cytologic examination for the presence of intracellular inclusions. EIAs use monoclonal or polyclonal antibodies to detect chlamydial LPS and are suited for processing large numbers of specimens; sensitivity generally is less than culture and NAATs. A positive EIA usually requires validation by a second nonculture method, especially in low-prevalence populations.[227] Point-of-care EIAs can provide a result in <30 minutes but their performance is poor and evidence regarding their impact on clinical outcomes is lacking.[236-238] DFA assays using monoclonal antibodies directed against the major outer-membrane protein (MOMP) permit direct visualization of the cellular material obtained (as an assessment of the quality of the specimen) and both elementary bodies and intracellular inclusions can be detected within 30 minutes. However, DFA testing requires a skilled laboratory microscopist, and large numbers of specimens cannot be processed expediently.[239-241] DFA has been used for conjunctival and respiratory specimens from infants. Nucleic acid probes are similar in sensitivity to other antigen detection methods and are relatively specific. However, DNA probe tests (without previous amplification) require special transport media, thus precluding the use of another test on the same specimen to confirm a positive result. DNA probe tests have a sensitivity for male genital secretions inferior to that of other methods. Cytologic examination of direct smears for the presence of intracellular inclusions is useful for detection of chlamydial conjunctivitis in neonates, but not for diagnosing conjunctivitis or genital infection in adolescents.[223]

Three FDA-approved *molecular diagnostic tests* are available for the simultaneous detection of *C. trachomatis* and *Neisseria gonorrhoeae* based on PCR, TMA, and SDA.[226] All have excellent sensitivity and specificity and can be performed in 2 to 5 hours. However, they do not all perform equally well with all specimen types.[242] In 2006, a genetic variant of *C. trachomatis* was identified in Sweden that was undetectable by PCR.[243] Although remaining localized, dissemination to other areas could render the current PCR test useless, highlighting the potential vulnerability of these tests to mutations within the target regions of the organism.

Comparison of Methods

Culture previously was considered the gold standard because of its 100% specificity and excellent sensitivity when optimal techniques are used.[223] However, for genital specimens, its sensitivity is approximately 70% to 80% compared with NAATs, which have become the preferred tests for diagnosis of genital tract infections.[226] For cervical swab specimens, EIA and DFA are less sensitive than hybridization tests and NAATs, whereas NAATs provide the best specificity and positive predictive value. Rapid EIA tests have relatively poor sensitivity using urethral swabs from males and cervical swabs from females and their accuracy for other specimen types has not been well evaluated.[237,238] Testing of first-void urine in men and women by any of the 3 NAATs has a median specificity of >97% and excellent sensitivity resulting in a high positive predictive value.[231]

In infants with conjunctivitis or pneumonitis, testing of conjunctival and NP specimens by culture, DFA, or EIA produces acceptable results. In a study of children ≤13 years of age, SDA and TMA had a sensitivity of 100% for urine specimens and 85% for vaginal swabs.[244] In the same study, the sensitivity of vaginal swab cultures for *C. trachomatis* was only 39%. In cases of suspected rape or sexual abuse, recent studies and guidelines support the use of FDA-approved NAATs when culture is not available; a positive result is confirmed using a different NAAT.[222,245]

Chlamydophila pneumoniae

Accurate laboratory confirmation of acute infection with *C. pneumoniae* is difficult and is most often based on serology.[246,247] The MIF test appears to be the most reliable serologic test, and the following criteria for a positive test have been used: (1) >4-fold rise in titer; (2) IgM titer >1 : 16; or (3) IgG titer >1 : 512. IgG titers between 1 : 16 and 1 : 512 are considered evidence of previous, but not necessarily recent, infection.[235] However, the limitations of the MIF test are lack of standardization and availability of high-quality reagents, and inability to distinguish past from persistent infection.[248] Comparison of EIAs (using species-specific assays) to MIF have shown good sensitivity and specificity in children with respiratory tract diseases and control children.[249] Because some EIAs detect antibodies to LPS, these tests detect antibodies to all *Chlamydia* species. Due to the poor sensitivity, CF tests should not be used for diagnosis.[235,250]

Isolation of *C. pneumoniae* is difficult. The stability of *C. pneumoniae* in clinical specimens has not been well studied, although one study reported that 70% of organisms remain viable after 24 hours at 4°C.[226,251] Throat swabs, sputum, NP, BAL, and other respiratory tract specimens placed in transport media have been used with variable success. Detection of the organism in respiratory secretions does not prove causality because asymptomatic infections occur in children and persistent shedding can occur for months after acute disease in adults.[252,253] Additional problems of culture include: small numbers of organisms present in respiratory secretions, poor recovery unless special transport media and optimal transport and storage conditions are used, and limited availability.

Molecular diagnosis with noncommercial conventional and real-time PCR tests has been evaluated.[254,255] Sensitivities appear to be as good as culture, but specificity is difficult to determine given the lack of a gold standard for comparison.

MYCOPLASMA

Mycoplasma pneumoniae

Rapid and accurate diagnosis of *M. pneumoniae* infection is problematic due to the lack of well-standardized tests.[256] Culture is the most widely accepted method for testing respiratory tract secretions, but availability is limited, specialized broth and agar media are required, and yield is relatively low.[257] For optimal isolation, specimens (BAL, tracheobronchial secretions, sputum, NP aspirates/swabs, tissues, blood, CSF, joint fluid) should be inoculated into appropriate media (e.g., SP4) at the bedside. Most media are acceptable for both isolation and PCR assay. Specimens should be refrigerated if not processed within 24 hours. Because *M. pneumoniae* is relatively slow-growing, cultures should be maintained for 4 weeks before being reported as negative. Shedding of *M. pneumoniae* can persist for several weeks after the onset of illness (particularly in children), confounding the interpretation of a positive culture result.

Direct antigen testing (EIA, DFA, immunoblotting) for respiratory tract secretions such as sputum and NP aspirates perform well in research settings (sensitivity of 90%), but are not available widely.[258,259] Cross-reactivity with other commensal mycoplasmas can occur. Persistent shedding and detection of antigen in asymptomatic individuals confound interpretation of positive results. At present, these tests are not used routinely in the clinical setting.

Conventional and real-time PCR tests for detection of *M. pneumoniae* in respiratory secretions have been widely evaluated.[257-263] PCR tests consistently are more sensitive than culture and antigen detection. Despite relatively high sensitivity, most studies suggest that PCR cannot be used alone to make a diagnosis of acute/recent infection; results must be used in conjunction with other results such as serology.[257,263,264] When performed on CSF, PCR can be useful for the diagnosis of *M. pneumoniae*-associated meningoencephalitis.[265]

CF assay using a chloroform-methanol glycolipid extract of organisms is the best validated test and has often been used as the reference method for serologic diagnosis. Measurement of IgG, IgM, and IgA anti-*M. pneumoniae* can be performed with commercially available EIA, FA, and latex agglutination kits, which are more sensitive and specific than CF and have replaced CF in many diagnostic laboratories.[256,266,267] Usefulness is limited by the fact that many children can be IgM-negative at the time of presentation, and time to seroconversion can be 2 to 4 weeks.[268] In children, adolescents, and young adults, a single positive IgM result can be considered diagnostic, although false-positive test results occur. The combination of serologic results together with culture and/or PCR may provide the most reliable approach to the diagnosis.[257,262,263]

Cold agglutinin antibody titers are simple to perform and widely available. Because only 50% to 75% of those infected with *M. pneumoniae* develop cold agglutinin antibodies and the test lacks sensitivity/specificity, it should not be used for the serologic diagnosis of *M. pneumoniae* infections.[269,270]

Genital Mycoplasmas

The major means for laboratory diagnosis of *U. urealyticum* and *M. hominis* infections is culture of the organism using specialized broth and agar media. Organisms grow rapidly and cultures are positive within 2 to 5 days. PCR (including multiplex assays) has been used to detect *U. urealyticum* and *M. hominis* in clinical specimens.[271-273] *M. genitalium* grows slowly; cultures may not be positive for ≥6 days. PCR-based assays are the mainstay for diagnosis,[271,274] but none is available commercially. Serologic tests for genital mycoplasmas have not been standardized, and none is available commercially. Serologic testing (using EIA, WB, IFA) has little utility except as an epidemiologic tool.[275] *M. genitalium* cross-reacts strongly with *M. pneumoniae*. Patients with invasive *M. hominis* infection almost always have seroconversion or a significant rise in antibody titer.

288 Laboratory Manifestations of Infectious Diseases

Sarah S. Long

ACUTE-PHASE RESPONSE

Inflammatory stimuli of any sort, including infection, trauma, or ischemia, cause marginalization, extravasation, and activation of neutrophils and monocytes with release of multiple proinflammatory cytokines, including interleukin (IL)-1β, IL-6, IL-8, and tumor necrosis factor (TNF-α). These mediators stimulate production of a variety of proteins referred to as acute-phase reactants in macrophages, monocytes, and reticuloendothelial organs. The host–pathogen, damage–response framework conceptualizes consequences of such events, which can be caused primarily by the pathogen or the host, and can be beneficial or detrimental to the host.[1] (See Chapter 10, Fever and the Inflammatory Response, Chapter 11, The Systemic Inflammatory Response Syndrome (SIRS), Sepsis, and Septic Shock.) Expected metabolic changes in the acute-phase response and changes in soluble defense molecules, trace elements, and inflammatory cells are listed in Box 288-1. Over 100 "biomarkers" have been investigated in infection, which have been correlated with magnitude, type, ascent, descent, and duration of acute-phase response. Although measurement provides a guide to the intensity of inflammation or the extent of

BOX 288-1. Expected Manifestations of the Acute-Phase Response

BRAIN

Increased release of corticotropin, endorphin, prolactin, neuropeptides, and neurotransmitters
Increased production of thyroid-stimulating hormone, vasopressin, insulin, and glucagon
Decreased production of insulin-like growth factor I
Fever, diminished appetite, and somnolence

BLOOD CELLS

Neutrophilia, increased neutrophil activation, and redistribution
Thrombocytosis
Reticulocytopenia, eosinopenia
Activation of B lymphocytes (antibody production) and T lymphocytes (lymphokine production)
Redistribution lymphopenia
Anemia of chronic disease

TISSUE

Collagen proliferation by fibroblasts
Demineralization of bone
Proteolysis and amino acid release from muscle

LIVER/OTHER SITES

Increased synthesis/release of complement components and expression of receptors, fibronectin, fibrinogen, mannose-binding protein, lipopolysaccharide-binding protein, hepeidin, ferritin, glycoproteins, C-reactive protein, α1-antitrypsin, α2-macroglobulin, lipids and lipoproteins, and ceruloplasmin
Increased synthesis of serum amyloid A, haptoglobin, and immunoglobulins
Decreased free and total serum iron, zinc, and retinol
Decreased synthesis of albumin, prealbumin and transferrin and cytochromes
Decreased gluconeogenesis

tissue damage, no single marker has exquisite sensitivity, specificity or predictive values as a stand-alone test to exclude need to initiate therapy when serious infection is suspected, or to conclude when therapy can be discontinued in proven infection. Studies suggest superiority of use of combinations of biomarkers in clinical decision rules, but complexity makes this difficult to implement in practice.[2,3] Multiple biomarker panels based on genome-wide expression profiling are under active investigation. If promising, such analyses will require prospective trials of clinical utility and impact on quality of care.[4,5]

ERYTHROCYTE SEDIMENTATION RATE

Physiology and Measurement

Erythrocyte sedimentation rate (ESR) in plasma depends on red blood cell (RBC) mass, volume, and shape; RBC–RBC forces; and the protein constitution of plasma. Electrostatic forces normally cause RBCs to repel each other and inhibit their aggregation. An increased amount of plasma fibrinogen or globulins coat the RBCs, foster their aggregation, and hasten settling, consequently elevating the ESR. Large-molecular-weight, needle-shaped fibrinogen has the greatest effect, followed by β-globulins and distantly by α2-globulins, γ-globulins, and albumin.

The Westergren method of measuring ESR is the most familiar and also the most discriminating at high and low values. It measures the vertical fall of the top of the blood cell column of thoroughly mixed, anticoagulated venous blood over a 1-hour period. For accuracy, care must be taken to anticoagulate and mix the blood adequately and perform the test within 2 hours at room temperature while avoiding any vibration or tilting of the tube. Normal values are age- and sex-dependent (androgens lower the ESR): ≤10 to 20 mm/hour for children 1 month to 12 years old, ≤15 mm/hour for males >12 years, and ≤20 mm/hour for females >12 years. After puberty, the normal top value rises 0.85 mm/hour for every 5-year increase in age. Obese children have higher mean ESRs than lean children (20 versus 10 mm/hour at 9 to 10 years of age).[6]

Elevated Sedimentation Rate

The ESR is elevated in most bacterial, mycobacterial, and fungal infections and is normal or mildly elevated in uncomplicated viral, rickettsial, and ehrlichial infections. An elevated ESR (>20 or 30 mm/hour, depending on the study) has poor discriminating power as a single test (i.e., sensitivity and specificity not exceeding 50%) to predict bacterial infection in children with nonspecific, febrile illnesses of short duration.[7,8] The mean ESR during most viral upper respiratory tract infections is approximately 20 mm/hour (with 90% of values <30 mm/hour), with noteworthy exceptions such as during adenovirus infections in which mean ESR can be 40 mm/hour.[8,9] Normal or mildly elevated ESR is predictive of the eventual diagnosis of a nonserious or viral disease in >90% of cases of fever of unknown origin;[10,11] ESR >50 mm/hour in such patients is an impetus for more extensive evaluation.[11,12]

Usefulness of the ESR in children with osteoarticular conditions has been studied.[13] Several studies of children with bacterial arthritis have documented ESRs >30 mm/hour in 80% to 90% of cases (mean ESR of approximately 65 mm/hour).[14-18] Prospective validation of Kocher criteria for distinguishing pyogenic arthritis of the hip (fever ≥38.5°C, inability to bear weight, ESR ≥40 mm/

BOX 288-2. Effects of Conditions Other than Infectious Diseases on the Erythrocyte Sedimentation Rate (ESR)

INCREASE IN ESR

Noninflammatory or unclear mechanism

Anemias with normal red blood cell shape
Elevated nonfibrinogen proteins: M proteins, macroglobulins, red blood cell agglutinins
Immune globulin intravenous (IGIV)
Heparin therapy, heparin in sample (sodium citrate and ethylenediaminetetraacetic acid do not affect ESR)
Oral contraceptive agents
Obesity
Multiple myeloma
Renal cell carcinoma
Glomerulonephritis
Pregnancy
Hypothyroidism
Hypercholesterolemia
Chronic renal failure
Diabetes and nephropathy
Technical factors (e.g., tilting test tube just 3° from vertical can accelerate up to 30 mm/hour)

Inflammatory or presumed inflammatory mechanism

Hodgkin disease
Lymphoproliferative disorders
Other malignancies
Paraneoplastic syndromes
Collagen vascular disease
Rheumatic and other poststreptococcal syndromes
Myocardial infarction
Postpericardiotomy syndrome

Lymphocytic thyroiditis
Kawasaki disease
Serum sickness
Burn injury
Accidental and surgical trauma
Inflammatory bowel disease
Sinus histiocytosis with massive lymphadenopathy (Rosai–Dorfman disease)
Histiocytic necrotizing lymphadenitis (Kikuchi–Fujimoto disease)
Neutrophilic dermatosis (Sweet syndrome)
Benign hyperplastic lymphadenopathy (Castleman disease)

DECREASE IN ESR

Morphologic abnormalities of red blood cells (e.g., sickle cells, spherocytes, anisocytes, poikilocytes)
Diffuse intravascular coagulation (e.g., associated with infection, hemophagocytic lymphohistiocytosis, macrophage activation syndrome)
Polycythemia
Leukemoid reaction
Dysfibrinoginemia, afibrinogenemia
Extreme elevation of serum bile salt concentration
Congestive heart failure
Valproic acid
Glucocorticoids
Low-molecular-weight dextran
Asparaginase
Cachexia
Technical factors (e.g., sample >2 hours old, nonroom-temperature sample after refrigeration)

---

hour, and blood WBC >12,000 cells/mm³) from toxic synovitis showed area under the receiver operating characteristic (ROC) curve of 0.86.[16] In a recent retrospective case series in a primary referral hospital, positivity of all 4 Koch criteria plus C-reactive protein (CRP) ≥2 mg/dL had predictive value of only 60% for bacterial arthritis.[17] In children with pyogenic arthritis at any site, ESR frequently rises on days 2 to 4 of effective therapy,[14] and ESR >30 mm/hour persists in at least 50% of cases at the conclusion of successful therapy.[14,15] The peak ESR in acute osteomyelitis generally is lower than in bacterial arthritis (mean of approximately 45 mm/hour), with expectations of a gradual fall and normal values at an appropriate conclusion of therapy.[19] In subacute or chronic osteomyelitis, the ESR usually is mildly elevated (25 to 40 mm/hour), but can be normal.

An elevated ESR characteristically occurs in multiple noninfectious inflammatory conditions, as well as in noninflammatory states that affect RBC stearic properties or plasma volume, fibrinogen, globulins, or protein concentrations (Box 288-2). Conversely, during infectious diseases, a number of conditions can result in a "falsely" low ESR.[20] The ESR usually exceeds 30 mm/hour during febrile episodes in children with the PFAPA (periodic fever, aphthous stomatitis, pharyngitis, adenitis) syndrome and autoinflammatory periodic fever symptoms.[21] An ESR <50 mm/hour does not exclude Kawasaki disease but makes the diagnosis unlikely.[22] Discordance between CRP and ESR, i.e., low ESR and high CRP, has been noted in Kawasaki disease[23] and in inflammatory bowel disease.[24] ESR can rise after immune globulin intravenous therapy for Kawasaki disease.[25]

BOX 288-3. Infections and Other Conditions Associated with Erythrocyte Sedimentation Rate >100 mm/hour

INFECTIONS

Miliary tuberculosis
Lymphadenitis or visceral infection caused by *Bartonella henselae*
Soft-tissue or serosal infections caused by *Streptococcus pyogenes* or *Streptococcus pneumoniae*
Pyelonephritis
Bacterial arthritis
Soft-tissue infections of the head and neck
Pelvic inflammatory disease
Ruptured appendicitis
Infective endocarditis

OTHER CONDITIONS

Autoimmune diseases
Autoinflammatory disorders

Kawasaki disease
Postinfectious and rheumatic disorders
Erythema nodosum
Sarcoidosis
Malignant lymphoma
Acute leukemia
Neuroblastoma
Other malignancies, especially metastatic carcinoma
Renal disease and nephrotic syndrome
Multiple myeloma
Visceral inflammatory pseudotumor
Sweet syndrome
Hyper-IgD syndrome
Drug hypersensitivity

Extreme Elevation of the Sedimentation Rate

Box 288-3 shows infectious and noninfectious conditions that should be considered especially when the ESR exceeds 100 mm/hour. Extreme elevation of the ESR is characteristic of certain noninfectious conditions. In children (unlike adults), however, infection still is a likely cause, accounting for 56% of cases in one study of 156 children;[26] miliary tuberculosis is notable among infectious diseases.[10] Collagen vascular, renal and macrophage disorders, and neoplastic disease rise among differential diagnoses. An extreme elevation of the ESR at the diagnosis of bacterial infection does not in itself indicate complicated disease or a guarded prognosis.

Low Erythrocyte Sedimentation Rate

Causes of a low ESR are shown in Box 288-2. In children with infectious diseases, an abnormally low ESR (e.g., <4 mm/hour) is most frequently a sign of disseminated intravascular coagulopathy and reflects low plasma fibrinogen concentrations; elevated fibrinolytic markers (e.g., D-dimer) are expected. Administration of glucocorticoids and possibly high-dose (but not low-dose) salicylates and L-asparaginase lower the sedimentation rate,[27] as does performance of peritoneal dialysis or hemodialysis.[28] The ESR is not valueless in children with sickle-cell disease; in one study, 72% of hospitalized children with an ESR >20 mm/hour had clinical infection (and 38% had vaso-occlusive crisis) compared with 23% with an ESR of ≤20 mm/hour, 74% of whom had vaso-occlusive crisis.[29,30]

C-REACTIVE PROTEIN

Physiology and Measurement

IL-6 released by activated granulocytes stimulates the liver to produce CRP, which was so named because of precipitation with C-polysaccharide of the pneumococcal cell wall. CRP level increases within 4 to 6 hours of an inflammatory stimulus, doubles every 8 hours, peaks at levels 100 to 1000 times normal within 1 to 3 days, and then because of short half-life (4 to 8 hours) falls rapidly once the triggering stimulus ceases. Functional properties of CRP include its ability to activate complement through the classic pathway, modulate the function of phagocytic cells, and augment cell-mediated cytotoxicity.[31,32] Nephelometric assays are the most widely used techniques for measuring CRP; value <1 mg/dL (10 mg/L) is considered normal. Normal range is variable by test used. Modest chronic elevations (>0.3 mg/dL) using high-sensitivity CRP tests have been used as a marker of increased risk of atherosclerosis.[33]

Compared with the ESR, CRP rises more rapidly, peaks earlier, and returns to normal levels more quickly when the stimulus abates. Factors that affect ESR, such as anemia, polycythemia, protein levels, and RBC shape, do not affect CRP levels. Any tissue injury, however, such as trauma, burn injury, ischemia, or infarction, can elicit production of CRP. Because CRP is degraded rapidly, serial determinations can provide additional information on progression of an insult or the effect of therapy.[18]

Clinical Usefulness

In general, CRP levels are elevated substantially (15 to 35 mg/dL) in bacterial infections with a tissue site of infection and only modestly (<2 to 4 mg/dL) in most acute viral infections; a value >10 mg/dL is more likely to be associated with bacterial infection, although infections due to certain viruses (e.g., adenovirus, cytomegalovirus, influenza, measles, and mumps) can cause CRP levels >10 mg/dL.[34] As noted in reviews and systematic reviews published on accuracy of elevated CRP to predict serious bacterial infection (SBI) in neonates and infants with fever without clinical focus of infection, limitations of studies have been variable cutoff values used and low incidence of SBI.[35-38] Pooled estimates in studies with cutoff values of 1 to 7 mg/dL showed sensitivity for BSI of 63% to 95% and specificity 40% to 91%;[36] and 6 studies, 3 of which used

cutoff value of 4 mg/dL, showed sensitivity of 77% and specificity of 79%.[37] In neonates, sensitivity for culture-proven early-onset sepsis was only 39%.[38] Additionally, "elevated" CRP can occur in neonates in the first 48 hours of life (up to 1 mg/dL),[38] in the 48 hours after injections of multiple vaccines (>1 mg/dL),[39] and 1 to 2 days following major surgery (median peak 2 mg/dL).[40] CRP appears to be less sensitive than IL-8 or procalcitonin for detecting SBI in oncologic patients with fever and neutropenia.[41]

CRP level has better predictive value for distinguishing bacterial infection when a tissue focus of infection is identified. A meta-analysis of 8 studies including 1230 children with pneumonia showed positive predictive value (PPV) of CRP >4 mg/dL for bacterial pneumonia of 64%.[42] In one study CRP ≥2 mg/dL distinguished patients with bacterial meningitis despite negative Gram stain (sensitivity 96%, specificity 93%, negative predictive value 99%).[43] In another study, CRP level >2 mg/dL was a strong independent risk factor for pyogenic arthritis (odds ratio 14.5, 95% CI, 3.2 to 64.9) rather than toxic synovitis.[44]

Discordantly high CRP levels compared with other biomarkers of acute-phase response (especially WBC and ESR) have been noted, such as in Kawasaki disease,[23] focal bacterial infections (in one study 26% of cases had WBC count <15,000/mm³ and CRP ≥8 mg/dL),[45] Crohn disease,[46] neoplasms of the liver and reticuloendothelial system (such as lymphoma), Castleman disease, allograft rejection, and graft-versus-host disease.[34,47]

Sequential measurement of CRP is valuable as an assessment of therapeutic control of focal infections, including wound infections following spinal surgery[48] and infective endocarditis,[49] and as a clue to ineffective therapy or complicated infection such as undrained abscess and tissue necrosis.[19,34,35] Serial CRP levels that increase or fail to decrease after 48 hours of therapy suggest treatment failure, a complication, or a noninfectious diagnosis.[35] In neonates, serial serum samples (the first taken at >8 hours of life and subsequent sample(s) separated by ≥24 hours) that continue to show normal CRP levels have negative predictive value (NPV) of >99% for proven early-onset SBI; findings can be used along with negative blood cultures to discontinue empiric antibiotic therapy begun for nonspecific clinical findings and for at-risk infants without clinical abnormalities.[38] Use of point of normalization of CRP in neonates and children with documented infection as the point to halt antibiotic therapy has not been studied adequately.

PROCALCITONIN

Physiology and Measurement

Procalcitonin (PCT) is the prohormone of calcitonin, which known biologic activities are to lower serum calcium concentration by inhibition of bone resorption and to signal bacterial invasion. In animal models, induction of bacterial infection or administration of endotoxin results in synthesis of PCT by virtually all tissues and organs, which is detectable in serum within 4 hours, and peaks at 12 to 48 hours.[50] Relative to other acute-phase reactants, PCT is not increased in response to viral infections.[50]

Normative values of PCT by age and differences in tests and cutoff points in clinical studies confound interpretation of results. Based on highly sensitive research assays, normal PCT level in uninfected adults is 0.033 to 0.003 ng/mL.[50] During the first 48 hours of life in healthy neonates the upper limit of 95% CI increases from 0.7 ng/mL at birth, to 20 ng/mL at 24 hours, declining to 2 ng/mL at 48 hours of age.[38] The first commercially available PCT assay (LUMI test) had a lower limit of sensitivity of 0.5 ng/mL; this cutoff was used for many studies and may be insensitive to detect bacterial infection. The second-generation FDA-approved PCT assay (a time-resolved-cryptate-emission (TRACE), immunoassay) has a functional lower limit of sensitivity of 0.05 ng/mL.[50]

Clinical Studies

Serum PCT levels rise and fall more rapidly than CRP levels during onset and control of bacterial infections and appear to have modestly increased sensitivity, specificity, predictive values, and ROC curve. Usefulness may be offset partially by limitations of determining cutpoints and lower specificity in some populations of interest.[38,50] In a prospective observational study of infants ≤90 days of age with fever without focus of infection, median PCT level was 0.53 ng/mL for infants with SBI, 0.29 ng/mL for infants with recent immunizations without SBI, and 0.17 ng/mL for infants with neither.[51,52] The proposed PCT cutpoint of 0.12 ng/mL showed sensitivity of 96%, specificity of 23% and NPV of 96%. An editorialist questioned disparate PCT levels found at age < and >28 days and for bacterial pathogens, questioning at least generalizability of results.[53] Using cutpoints of 0.5 mg/mL, PCT compared with other biomarkers appeared to have superior ROC performance for SBI in infants <36 months of age with fever for <8 hours,[54] and predictive values for discriminating bacterial infection in febrile neutropenic children with cancer,[55] diarrhea-associated hemolytic-uremic syndrome,[56] bacterial causes of acute hepatic disease,[57] septicemia versus systemic inflammatory response syndrome,[58] bacterial versus aseptic meningitis,[59] bacterial pneumonia,[60] severe Crohn disease (cutoff 0.14 ng/mL),[61] and DMSA-scan-positive urinary tract infection.[62] In one study, PCT discriminated bacterial infection in febrile adults with systemic autoimmune diseases[63] but did not in another study of patients with systemic lupus erythematosus.[64] A multicenter noninferiority randomized trial of use of a PCT algorithm as a decision rule to initiate and stop antibiotics for community-acquired pneumonia in adults (antibiotics discouraged if PCT <0.25 ng/mL and encouraged if PCT >0.5 ng/mL) showed that application of the rule led to similar clinical outcome and reduced antibiotic exposure and adverse events.[65] Letters to the editor questioned superiority compared with pragmatism of CRP measurement,[66] and noted that PCT usefulness was limited primarily to discontinuing antibiotics which likely would have been done without PCT testing.[67] In a study of similar strategy of using PCT cutpoint of 0.5 ng/mL to limit empiric therapy in children <36 months of age with fever without focus, application of the rule would have resulted in a 24% increase in antibiotic use in patients without subsequent diagnosis of SBI.[68]

OTHER ACUTE-PHASE PROTEINS AND CYTOKINES

Because acute-phase proteins are produced in response to proinflammatory cytokines, direct measurement of serum cytokines (e.g., IL-1β, IL-6, IL-8, soluble IL-2 receptor and TNF-α) seems promising. While clinical applications for detection of early points of infection are encouraging (e.g., sensitivity and ROC analyses), cytokine responses are short-lived events and no one mediator is likely to have broad application clinically.[38,40,41]

Ferritin is a highly conserved ubiquitous intracellular protein, control of which depends on multiple genes, regulatory messenger RNA structures, signaling pathways, and protein catalysts. Ferritin tightly controls iron and oxygen chemistry. Expression is upregulated by proinflammatory cytokines; expression also is regulated by thyroid hormone, insulin, insulin growth factors, hypoxia–ischemia, and hyperoxia (nitric oxide). Immunologic activities include binding to T lymphocytes, suppression of delayed-type hypersensitivity and B-lymphocyte antibody production, and regulation of granulomonocytopoiesis. Normal serum ferritin concentrations in adult males is <400 μg/L (<400 ng/mL) and in females <150 μg/L.

Serum ferritin levels are markers of iron deficiency (low) and iron intoxication or overload states (high). Levels also are elevated in inflammation, infection, and hypoxia–ischemia. Clinical interest has escalated because of usefulness as a criteria (serum level >500 μg/L) for hemophagocytic lymphohistiocystosis and macrophage activation syndrome,[69] in which peak levels frequently exceed 10,000 μg/L.[69,70] Moderately elevated ferritin levels (>500 and even >1000 μg/L) also occur in severe sepsis,[71] dengue hemorrhagic fever, lymphoma, systemic lupus erythematosus, and other autoimmune and autoinflammatory conditions.[72,73]

HEMOGLOBIN

Erythrocytosis (polycythemia) secondary to increased erythropoietin production in response to arterial hypoxemia can provide a clue to cryptogenic bronchiectasis. Hemoconcentration (probably primarily a result of plasma leakage; defined as hematocrit level >44% in adult males and >40% in females) also is characteristic of severe or toxic infections such as Hantavirus pulmonary syndrome,[74] dengue hemorrhagic fever,[75] clostridial toxic shock,[76] necrotizing pancreatitis,[77] and generally portends a poor outcome. Methemoglobinemia is well described in young infants with diarrheal disease or urinary tract infection possibly due at least partially to absorption of nitrites produced by enteric organisms.[78]

Anemia in Chronic Infection

The anemia of chronic disease likely is driven by cytokines and reticuloendothelial cells that induce pathologic changes in iron homeostasis, impaired erythropoiesis, blunted erythropoietin response, and decrease in RBC lifespan.[79] Anemia is mildly to moderately severe and is associated with reticulocytopenia. Erythrocyte mean corpuscular hemoglobin and volume are normal, or can be reduced in severe cases. Serum ferritin value frequently is increased. An iron-deficient type of erythropoiesis (low serum iron and increased erythrocyte protoporphyrin concentrations) results despite normal or increased iron stores.

The anemia of chronic disease is expected in clinical tuberculosis, subacute infective endocarditis, human immunodeficiency virus (HIV) infection, hepatitis C, malaria, and chronic osteomyelitis. The severity of the anemia correlates with the degree and duration of the underlying infection. Successful treatment of the infection is the only effective therapy. Noninfectious inflammatory conditions such as autoimmune disorders, malignant solid tumors, and autoinflammatory diseases, such as inflammatory bowel disease, typically are associated with anemia of chronic disease, and in some cases anemia responds to the administration of recombinant erythropoietin. Anemia can be a clue to the diagnosis of Crohn disease in children without overt abdominal symptomatology who are being evaluated for fever of unknown origin. RBC indices also can reflect true iron-deficiency anemia from gastrointestinal blood loss in these patients. Hookworm infestation is another cause of occult blood loss and iron-deficiency anemia.

Anemia in Acute Infection

Mild, readily reversible, normocytic anemia (hemoglobin 9 to 11 mg/dL) is not uncommon in minor bacterial and viral infections and is characterized by mild hemolysis and diminished RBC production (similar to the anemia of chronic infection, but with reversal of the relative importance of mechanisms). A profoundly decreased total and free serum iron concentration (e.g., transferrin saturation <10%) is an acute response to infection or inflammation; measurement during acute infection is inappropriate and frequently leads to incorrect conclusions and therapy.

Approximately 50% of children with serious acute bacterial infections (meningitis, pneumonia, arthritis) have anemia (hemoglobin <11 g/dL) at the time of hospitalization. Moderate to severe acute hemolysis can occur in exotoxin-mediated syndromes secondary to *Staphylococcus aureus* and *Streptococcus pyogenes,* or in septicemia caused by endotoxin-producing enteric bacteria or *Neisseria meningitidis*. Hemolysis occurs with disseminated intravascular coagulopathy associated with severe infection caused by a variety of bacteria, rickettsiae, fungi, viruses, and protozoa; expected associated findings are burred red blood cells, elevated serum lactate dehydrogenase and unconjugated bilirubin, and reduced haptoglobin level. Severe acute hemolysis and thrombosis leading to hemolytic-uremic syndrome is an increasingly reported complication of pneumococcal infection in children, especially complicated pneumonia.[80,81] *Mycoplasma pneumoniae,* Epstein–Barr virus (EBV), and cytomegalovirus (CMV) can produce an immune-mediated hemolytic anemia, and *Vibrio cholerae* can elicit a nonimmune acute hemolytic anemia. *Plasmodium falciparum* malaria and clostridial septicemia classically are associated with marked intravascular hemolysis and profound anemia. Severe and sometimes fatal hemolysis, which probably is immune-mediated, has been associated with initiation of ceftriaxone therapy in several children with a variety of underlying conditions who were previously exposed to ceftriaxone.[82]

Transient erythroblastopenia is an acute-phase response to many infections and usually is of no or minor consequence in previously healthy children. Occasionally erythroblastopenia can be severe and can be associated with autoantibodies against erythroid progenitors or possibly erythropoietin. Viruses causing protracted infections (e.g., EBV, CMV) in immunocompetent and especially in immunosuppressed or immunodeficient children, as well as those with HIV, can result in varying degrees of anemia. Acute human parvovirus B19 infection consistently causes transient reticulocytopenia with little consequence, except in individuals with shortened RBC survival in whom aplastic crisis occurs, in intrauterine life when interrupted erythropoiesis can cause hydrops fetalis, or in immunosuppressed individuals in whom protracted infection leads to significant anemia or pancytopenia.[83] Hepatitis viruses frequently cause suppressed bone marrow during acute infection and rarely can result in permanent aplastic anemia. Hemophagocytic syndromes leading to pancytopenia can be triggered by many infections, especially those caused by herpesviruses and RBC and other intracellular pathogens, such as *Babesia*, parvovirus B19, *Brucella*, *Salmonella*, and *Histoplasma*[84] (see Chapter 12, Hemophagocytic Lymphohistiocytosis and Macrophage Activation Syndrome). In boys with X-linked lymphoproliferative disorder, EBV infection is associated with hepatitis and aplastic anemia, with high mortality.

LEUKOCYTES

Circulating leukocytes are produced by the bone marrow in response to specific growth factors, and normal ranges vary with age[85] (Table 288-1). Leukocytosis is an increase in the total white blood cell (WBC) count above the 95% confidence limits of the mean for age (i.e., approximately >11,000/mm^3 for adults, >13,000 to 15,000/mm^3 for children 4 to 16 years of age, and >20,000/mm^3 for infants 1 to 4 weeks of age). Leukocytosis is less meaningful clinically than are terms that describe the predominant type of leukocyte that is increased.

Neutrophilia

Neutrophils exist in three major anatomic spaces, moving unidirectionally from bone marrow, to peripheral blood, to extravascular spaces. Peripheral blood neutrophils are divided equally between the circulating pool and the marginated pool (where they are attached to or roll along the walls of capillaries or postcapillary venules). The number of neutrophils at each site can be regulated

independently and influenced by various colony-stimulating factors (granulocyte and granulocyte/macrophage CSF, G-CSF and GM-CSF). In an acute inflammatory response, neutrophils are released from the marrow granulocyte reserve (containing 10 to 15 times as many neutrophils as normally are present in circulating blood) into the bloodstream and migrate by margination and diapedesis to extravascular foci of tissue injury. In the bone marrow, CSFs act on progenitor cells to increase mitosis and expand the storage pool. Segmented neutrophils are released preferentially, but as release accelerates, less mature bands and a few metamyelocytes also can be released and produce a "shift to the left." Neutrophilia can occur from movement of neutrophil pools in response to a variety of noninfectious stimuli as well. Endogenous or administered glucocorticoids and epinephrine cause demargination of neutrophils in the bloodstream, and glucocorticoids increase the half-life of neutrophils.[27,86] Immature forms are not expected. Tissue damage or necrosis such as from accidental or surgical trauma, fracture, burn injury, hypoxia, stress, lactic acidosis and ketoacidosis, acute hemolysis or hemorrhage, and systemic autoimmune and inflammatory conditions can induce complex acute-phase responses, mitotic activation in marrow, and redistribution of neutrophils causing neutrophilia, sometimes with a modest release of bands.

Bacterial and fungal cell wall products, exotoxins, and endotoxins are potent stimuli of the acute inflammatory response of neutrophils. Progressive elevation of the WBC count above 15,000/mm^3 with a neutrophil predominance heightens suspicion of bacterial infection but discrimination between viral and bacterial respiratory tract infection is not precise.[9] In one study of 121 children with pneumonia, the mean WBC count was 18,000/mm^3 for *Streptococcus pneumoniae*, 17,000/mm^3 for adenovirus, and 9000/mm^3 for *M. pneumoniae* etiologies.[86] In a retrospective case-control study of 69 children 2 to 24 months of age evaluated in an emergency department for a febrile illness, rate of SBI was only 25% in those with WBC >25,000/mm.[87] Absolute neutrophil count rather than total WBC count, and duration of fever are better predictors of SBI in febrile infants.[88,89]

Serious bacterial infections do not always induce leukocytosis; exotoxin- and endotoxin-producing organisms such as *Staphylococcus aureus*, *Haemophilus influenzae* type b, and *Salmonella* infections are most noteworthy. In one study, only 50% of the children hospitalized with proven bacterial infection had a WBC count >15,000/mm.[3,86] In a prospective observational study performed in 856 neonates >35 weeks of gestation who had been exposed to suspected chorioamnionitis, single or serial neutrophil values did not assist in the diagnosis of early-onset infection.[90]

Extreme Elevations of Neutrophils and Leukemoid Reaction

Any cell type can be involved in a leukemoid reaction, so named because of the simulation of findings in leukemia. A myeloid

TABLE 288-1. Approximate Normal Leukocyte Counts in Children[a]

Age	Total Leukocytes Mean	Total Leukocytes Range	Neutrophils Mean	Neutrophils Range	Neutrophils %	Lymphocytes Mean	Lymphocytes Range	Lymphocytes %	Monocytes Mean	Monocytes %	Eosinophils Mean	Eosinophils %
≤24 hours	20.0	9–35	13.0	5–25	65	5.6	2–11	28	1.1	5	0.5	2
1–4 weeks	11.4	5–20	4.5	1.3–9	40	5.5	2–16	49	1.0	8	0.4	3
1–24 months	11.2	6–17	3.7	1.5–8.5	33	6.7	3–10	59	0.6	5	0.3	3
2–6 years	9.2	5–15	3.9	1.5–8	42	4.6	2–9	50	0.5	5	0.3	3
6–18 years	8.2	4–13	4.4	1.6–8	53	3.2	1.5–6	39	0.4	5	0.2	3
≥21 years	7.4	4–11	4.4	1.8–8	59	2.5	1–5	34	0.3	4	0.2	3

[a]*Numbers of leukocytes are thousands/mm^3; ranges are estimates of 95% confidence limits.*

Modified from McMillan JA, Feigin RD, DeAngelis CD, et al. (eds) Oski's Pediatrics, 4th ed. Philadelphia, Lippincott Williams & Wilkins, 2006, p 2628.

leukemoid reaction is defined as a peripheral WBC count >50,000/mm³ or a differential cell count with >5% immature myeloid cells capable of division (myeloblasts, promyelocytes, and myelocytes). The former type is more frequently encountered in children with infectious diseases. Viral infections do not cause myeloid leukemoid reaction. Box 288-4 lists causes of myeloid leukemoid reaction. Severe bacterial infections are associated most frequently. Disseminated fungal infection can cause mild to profound neutrophilia (e.g., with thrombocytopenia in neonates with candidemia and eosinophilia in disseminated cryptococcosis) or neutropenia (e.g., with thrombocytopenia in disseminated histoplasmosis). Shigellosis, particularly *Shigella dysenteriae,* is associated with leukemoid reaction more frequently in children younger than 4 years and characteristically has predominantly immature neutrophils, but lymphocyte counts can be elevated as well. Leukemoid reactions due to *Clostridium difficile* colitis occur in patients with acquired immunodeficiency syndrome (AIDS) and with toxin-hyperproducing strains and severe disease,[91] as well as due to *C. sordellii* in patients with myonecrosis and septicemia.[92] Malignancies, especially carcinomas, can express certain CSF genes that stimulate neutrophilia inappropriately and sometimes cause paraneoplastic syndrome. Myelogenous leukemia, which is most frequently associated with a leukemoid reaction, usually is distinguished by a disproportionately high number of blast forms in comparison with bands and metamyelocytes, as well as the presence of anemia, thrombocytopenia, eosinophilia, and basophilia.

Young infants with trisomy 21 can have a leukemoid reaction, which usually is transient but can evolve to a leukemic state.[92] Prenatal administration of betamethasone can cause neonatal leukemoid reaction.

Neutropenia

Neutropenia is defined as a peripheral blood neutrophil count below the 95% confidence limit for age (see Table 288-1), usually an absolute count <1500/mm³ in children older than 1 month.[85] Undue susceptibility to infection because of neutropenia correlates best with an absolute neutrophil count <500/mm³. Neutropenia related to infectious diseases can be caused by the infectious agent itself, infection-triggered hemophagocytosis, postinfectious immune mechanisms, or marrow suppression related to antibiotics or other drugs.[93] During severe infection margination and diapedesis of neutrophils into tissues are increased at the expense of circulating cells; peripheral blood neutropenia can occur and typically is associated with bands and metamyelocytes equal to or outnumbering mature neutrophils; cells are vacuolated, with toxic granulations and Döhle bodies. Bone marrow findings can be confusing, with myeloid hyperplasia and "maturation arrest" at the promyelocyte stage. Neutropenia is a poor prognostic sign in rapidly progressive pyogenic infections; in neonates, peripheral blood neutropenia in association with marrow depletion portends death.

Pseudomonas septicemia in previously healthy children, frequently associated with excessive exposure to water (whirlpool, bathing, wet toweling for antipyresis), can cause profound neutropenia with an extreme shift to the left,[94] occasionally with a myeloid leukemoid reaction simulating promyelocytic leukemia.[95] These findings initially can cause confusion because *Pseudomonas* septicemia also complicates congenital and acquired neutropenic states. Toxin-producing bacteria, such as *Staphylococcus aureus, Streptococcus pyogenes,* and enteric gram-negative bacilli (*Escherichia coli, Salmonella, Brucella, Shigella*) have a propensity to cause a disproportionate left shift, frequently with immature neutrophils exceeding mature cells, and a low to normal total neutrophil count; such findings do not indicate a poor prognosis or even bacteremia. Neutropenia or neutrophilia can occur with disseminated tuberculosis and histoplasmosis, and with Rocky Mountain spotted fever (RMSF); in RMSF, when WBC count is <10,000/mm³, bands frequently exceed mature forms.[96] Leukopenia occurs in 60% to 74% of cases of ehrlichiosis and 50% of cases of anaplasmosis with a reduction in mononuclear and polymorphonuclear cells; organisms can be visualized in leukocytes.[97,98]

Mild neutropenia frequently accompanies systemic viral infections. Neutropenia and thrombocytopenia can be a clue to subclinical CMV infection in organ transplant recipients[99], to symptomatic primary infection with HIV, or AIDS.[100] In a report from Israel, a substantial number of children with bacterial and viral infections had aggregated leukocytes that led to false reading of leukopenia by automated cell analyzers.[101]

Left Shift of Neutrophils, Immature Neutrophils

The usefulness of the total WBC count and the ratio of immature to total neutrophils in neonates younger than 7 days to predict bacterial infection has been reported extensively and scored, with disparate results. In a large study, a band neutrophil-to-total neutrophil ratio ≥0.2 had sensitivity and negative predictive values for bacterial infection exceeding 95%.[38] Adenovirus,[102] influenza A,[103] disseminated herpes simplex,[104] and other viral infections can be associated with increased absolute band count simulating bacterial sepsis.[104] In viral infections and in malaria when immature neutrophils are seen in peripheral blood, the total absolute neutrophil count is <10,000/mm³ in almost 90%.[104]

Lymphocytes and Lymphocytosis

Although T and B lymphocytes replicate in multiple anatomic sites (including the lymph nodes, spleen, and bone marrow) and are

---

BOX 288-5. Causes of Abnormal Lymphocyte Counts in Children

LYMPHOCYTOSIS

Infectious

Bordetella pertussis, Epstein–Barr virus, cytomegalovirus, hepatitis viruses, other common viruses, *Toxoplasma*, chronic controlled bacterial infections (e.g., *Treponema, Brucella, Mycobacterium*), recovery from bacterial infections, *Rickettsia*

Noninfectious

Lymphocytic leukemias, thyrotoxicosis

LYMPHOPENIA

Infectious

Acute and chronic viral infection (including human immunodeficiency virus), acute bacterial infection, widespread granulomatous infection (e.g., untreated *Mycobacterium, Cryptococcus, Histoplasma*), malaria

Noninfectious

Protein-calorie malnutrition, radiation or immunosuppressive therapy, monoclonal antibody and anticytokine therapy, congenital immunodeficiency, untreated Hodgkin lymphoma, trauma, stress, glucocorticoids; antibody-mediated destruction, protein-losing enteropathy, chronic right heart failure, lymphangiectasias, thoracic duct interruption

---

capable of leaving and re-entering a given compartment, lymphocytes in peripheral blood are tightly regulated, with T lymphocytes predominating and numbers predictable by age (see Table 288-1). Mean counts decrease with age after a peak of 7300/mm³ (61% of leukocytes) at 6 months of age. Lymphocytosis is present when the count exceeds the 95% confidence limits for age; by definition, a lymphocytic leukemoid reaction requires the presence of immature forms in peripheral blood. Causes of lymphocytosis are shown in Box 288-5.

Bordetella pertussis is the only acute bacterial infection associated typically with lymphocytosis. Lymphocytosis is due to pertussis toxin blocking the normal migration of lymphocytes out of the bloodstream, and the degree is predictive of the severity of illness and fatal outcome (mean leukocyte count in fatal versus nonfatal cases in young infants, 94,000 versus 18,000/mm³).[105,106] Chronic bacterial and granulomatous infections can cause a sustained, modest lymphocytosis.

Although many viral infections cause mild transient lymphocytosis, mononucleosis syndromes related to EBV or CMV, as well as Kikuchi syndrome (of uncertain etiology), induce a sustained lymphocytosis. The atypical lymphocytes in viral infections reflect active proliferation of T lymphocytes; these lymphocytes are large and have a distinctive morphology. Profound atypical lymphocytosis (>50% of lymphocytes) occurs with EBV infection almost exclusively. More modest atypical lymphocytosis can occur with infection due to CMV (including post-perfusion syndrome), HIV (acute), hepatitis A or B, adenovirus, and *Toxoplasma gondii* (congenital and acute), as well as leukemia and lymphoma. Mild atypical lymphocytosis (usually <10%) occurs with drug reactions, serum sickness, infections due to other viruses (rubella, rubeola, human herpesvirus 6, herpes simplex, varicella zoster) and certain bacteria (*M. tuberculosis, Treponema pallidum, Salmonella*). Atypical lymphocytosis is described with malaria, and is a consistent finding in babesiosis (usually <10%) despite normal or mildly depressed peripheral leukocyte count.[107] Multiple infectious, hematologic, and immunologic causes of neutropenia, as well as Addison disease, lead to a relative lymphocytosis without absolute lymphocytosis.

Lymphopenia

Lymphopenia, defined as a peripheral blood lymphocyte count <1500/mm³ (or <2000 in children younger than 6 years), has multiple etiologies, e.g., decreased production, increased loss or destruction, alteration in compartmentalization. Protein-calorie malnutrition is the most common cause of reduced-production lymphopenia worldwide. Viruses (e.g., HIV, rubeola, polioviruses, varicella) can infect lymphocytes and cause destruction, transiently decreased production, or trafficking from the blood compartment. Autoimmune disorders and widespread granulomatous infection, especially tuberculosis, cause lymphopenia, probably by decreased production and redistribution.[10] Acute bacterial infection and infection with *Rickettsia* and *Ehrlichia* cause lymphopenia as part of redistribution during the acute-phase response.

Monocytes and Monocytosis

Absolute deficiency of the highly conserved monocyte-macrophage probably is incompatible with life. Monocytes present antigens to lymphocytes, mediate cellular cytotoxicity, and regulate immune and hematopoietic responses by producing interleukins, interferon, TNF-α, and G-CSF. Stromal cells (e.g., fibroblasts and endothelial cells) produce GM-CSF during inflammation and M-CSF constitutively, which in turn stimulate growth and differentiation of mononuclear phagocytes. These phagocytes are especially effective in killing obligate intracellular parasites such as fungi, viruses, rickettsia, protozoa, and certain bacteria, and participate substantially in all types of granulomatous inflammation. Monocytosis is defined as a peripheral blood monocyte count >800/mm³ in children or >500/mm³ in adults. A monocytic leukemoid reaction is defined as a monocyte count >30% of a WBC count that is >30,000/mm³.

Monocytosis has varied etiologies (Box 288-6). Monocytosis usually precedes recovery from neutropenia, and mild

---

BOX 288-6. Causes of Monocytosis in Children

INFECTIOUS CAUSES

Recovery from acute infections
Bacterial endocarditis
Protozoal infections
Fungal infections
Salmonella enteric fever
Varicella and zoster
Cytomegalovirus
Mycobacterium tuberculosis
Brucella species
Listeria monocytogenes
Treponema pallidum
Rickettsia rickettsiae

NONINFECTIOUS CAUSES

Hodgkin disease and non-Hodgkin lymphoma
Preleukemia
Myelomonocytic and myelogenous leukemia
Myeloproliferative disorders
Carcinomas
Collagen vascular disorders
Sarcoidosis
Inflammatory bowel disease
Cirrhosis
Drug reaction
Congenital and acquired neutropenia
Major depression
Recovery from marrow suppression
Postsplenectomy status

---

monocytosis is common in recovery from acute bacterial and viral illnesses. Monocytosis (average of 15% of the leukocyte count) is a hallmark of symptomatic congenital syphilis,[108] a frequent finding in miliary tuberculosis and congenital toxoplasmosis, and a variable finding in listeriosis (where neutrophilia is more common except in neonates) and malaria. Small premature infants can have monocytosis in the range of 2000 to 7000 cells/mm³ as a reflection of an immature physiologic response to a variety of drugs or infusions of blood and albumin.[109] Several hematologic malignancies and chronic inflammatory states also are associated with peripheral blood monocytosis. In malignant histiocytosis, abnormal mononuclear phagocytes can be seen in the peripheral blood, along with neutropenia or neutrophilia.

Eosinophils and Eosinophilia

Eosinophils are produced from progenitor cells in the bone marrow, largely under the influence of IL-5, IL-3, and GM-CSF. IL-5 promotes proliferation, maturation and survival of eosinophils and facilitates chemotaxis into tissues.[110,111] Increased levels of IL-5 are found in individuals with parasitic infections and other hypereosinophilic syndromes. In parasitic infection, eosinophils exert antibody-dependent (IgG- or IgE-assisted) cellular cytotoxicity and may play a role in the afferent upregulating arm of the immune response through antigen presentation and cytokine secretion. In addition, eosinophils play an immune-modulating role of potentially toxic mast cell degranulation in hypersensitivity reactions.

Eosinophils are predominantly tissue-based cells that spend only 1 to 2 days of their approximate 4-week lifespan in peripheral blood; the tissue-to-blood ratio is at least 100:1. Mature eosinophils are found most prominently in the skin and epithelial lining of the respiratory and gastrointestinal tracts. Inflammatory fluids and tissue exudates (e.g., lung and pleural fluid, cerebrospinal fluid) can be predominantly eosinophilic, are always pathologic, and have unique differential diagnoses. The normal mean peripheral blood eosinophil count in the first week of life is 500/mm³ and falls during the first 6 years to the adult mean of 200/mm³ (normally 2% to 3% of WBCs). Eosinopenia results from adrenocortical hyperfunction and administration of corticosteroids and is part of the acute-phase response. Eosinophilia (>500 cells/mm³) can be classified etiologically as primary (hematologic malignancies and mastocytosis), secondary (allergy, adrenal insufficiency, medications, autoimmune conditions and infections), or idiopathic.[112] Hypereosinophilic syndrome (HES) is defined as AES >1500/mm³ for >6 months leading to end-organ damage from infiltration of the heart, lungs, skin, or nerve tissue. Most cases of HES are idiopathic; a subset have defined molecular bases and specific anti-IL-5 treatment.[113-117]

Table 288-2 delineates infectious and noninfectious conditions associated with mild, moderate, and extreme eosinophilia. Mild eosinophilia (up to 1500 cells/mm³) is common and occurs in the recovery phase of bacterial or viral illness, in response to drugs (usually in the absence of hypersensitivity symptoms), or as a manifestation of any type of atopic disease. Parasites are the most common cause of eosinophilia worldwide, and can induce extreme eosinophilia (>5000 cells/mm³) or eosinophilic leukemoid reaction (>30% eosinophils with a WBC count >30,000/mm³). With the exception of helminthic infections, secondary causes of eosinophilia rarely cause an absolute eosinophil count >1500 cells/mm³.[118] The degree of peripheral eosinophilia in parasitosis usually is proportional to the extent of tissue invasion and is a dynamic process related to the life cycle of the parasite.[118,119] Eosinophilia can occur in the pulmonary migratory phase that precedes gastrointestinal localization by weeks to months, such as with *Ascaris lumbricoides* and *Trichuris trichiura*; in the sustained, highly inflammatory tissue phase, such as with *Trichinella spiralis*, *Toxocara canis*, and *T. cati*; in the sustained, low-grade inflammatory state, such as with *Schistosoma*, *Strongyloides*, *Necator*, and filariae; during episodic tissue movement, such as with *Loa loa*,

Dracunculus, and *Gnathostoma*; or after disruption of cysts or parasitic death, such as with *Echinococcus* and *Taenia solium* (cysticercosis).[119] *Strongyloides* hyperinfection syndrome usually is not associated with eosinophilia. *Enterobius vermicularis* (pinworms) can cause eosinophilia <1000/mm³. Protozoal infections (e.g., giardiasis, malaria, amebiasis, cryptosporidiosis) are not characteristically associated with eosinophilia even though some degree of tissue invasion can occur. *Isospora belli* may be an exception.[120] Adrenal insufficiency, especially due to infection with *Histoplasma*, *Cryptococcus*, cytomegalovirus, or *Mycobacterium*, and to opportunistic infection in compromised hosts, also causes infection-associated eosinophilia.

The life cycle of the parasite, as well as geography, dietary habits, and host factors, must be considered when deciding between performing serologic or microscopic studies in evaluating children with eosinophilia. The prevalence of parasitic infections in new immigrants with eosinophilia ranges from 70% to 95%, compared with 14% to 40% in travelers.[118-122] Exposure greatly affects the likelihood of a parasitic cause of eosinophilia. Travelers who make short visits to urban areas and who adhere to protective dietary measures have low risk. High-risk history includes ingestion of carnivores *(Trichinella)*; raw vegetables, unpeeled fruits or unpurified water (helminths); seafood in Southwest Asia (gastrointestinal, liver, and lung parasites); swimming in fresh water in endemic areas *(Schistosoma)*.[118] Physical examination and identification of organ system(s) involved guide specific diagnostic evaluations. Asymptomatic eosinophilia is neither a highly sensitive nor specific marker for parasitic disease.[119,122] The Centers for Disease Control and Prevention has published domestic guidelines for post-arrival screening for African and Southwest Asian refugees, including measurement for eosinophilia (>400 cells/mm³) and stool examinations for ova and parasites.[123] The differential diagnosis of asymptomatic eosinophila with negative stool evaluations is limited. Recommendations include serologic testing for *Strongyloides* and *Schistosoma* species when AEC exceeds 400 cells/mm³; in a pediatric refugee study, positive predictive value of AEC >400 cells/mm³ for confirming either pathogen was only 58% and negative predictive value was only 75%.[122] From their experience authors conclude that for immigrants who lack documentation of pre-departure treatment, serologic testing should be performed on all African immigrants for both pathogens and on Southeast Asian and Middle Eastern persons for *Strongyloides*.

Fungal infections usually do not elicit eosinophilia, with noteworthy exceptions. *Cryptococcus neoformans* can induce intense eosinophilia in the rare case of the previously healthy young child with disseminated disease. Pulmonary infiltrate with eosinophilia (PIE) syndromes are a group of heterogeneous disorders characterized by eosinophilic infiltration of the lung parenchyma. Eosinophilia in the peripheral blood and systemic symptoms typically but not invariably are present. Parasite-induced PIE is most common in children.[124] Wiskott–Aldrich syndrome, combined immunodeficiency, hyper-IgE syndrome,[125] graft-versus-host disease,[126] and renal and hepatic allograft organ rejection[127] are associated with eosinophilia, as are malignancies (lymphomas, leukemia) and preleukemic states.[128] Eosinophilia can occur in the early stage of HIV infection and in EBV-related lymphoma in AIDS.[129] Organ-specific eosinophilic inflammatory diseases such as eosinophilic gastrointestinal disorders, granuloma of bone, and meningoencephalitis (related to ventricular shunt material, shunt malfunction, vancomycin instillation, bacterial or parasitic infection) do not characteristically cause peripheral blood eosinophilia, but mild elevations can occur, especially in young children.[130-134] In prematurely born neonates, eosinophilia (count >1000/mm³) has been associated with an anabolic state (as well as L-tryptophan exposure), but septicemia also can induce eosinophilia rather than neutrophilia.[135,136] Other causes of eosinophilia are shown in Table 288-2.[137-140] Drug reaction with eosinophilia and systemic symptoms (DRESS) is a newly classified serious multisystem disorder of unknown pathogenesis associated predominantly with aromatic anticonvulsants and sulfonamides.[140]

TABLE 288-2. Causes of Eosinophilia in Children

Conditions	Elevation of Peripheral Blood Eosinophil Count		
	Mild (500–1500 Cells/mm³)	Moderate (1500–5000 Cells/mm³)	Extreme (>5000 Cells/mm³)
COMMON INFECTIOUS CAUSES			
Recovery from bacterial, viral infection	+++	+	
Ascaris lumbricoides (migratory)[a]	++	++	++
Toxocara canis, Toxocara cati[a]		+++	++
Trichinella spiralis[a]		+++	++
LESS COMMON INFECTIOUS CAUSES			
Strongyloides stercoralis[a]	+++ (established)	++ (acute)	+ (acute)
Trichuris trichiura[a]	++		
Ancyclostoma species[a]	+	+	
Filarial worms (tropical eosinophilia)	++ (established)	++ (episodic or treatment)	+++ (episodic or treatment)
Hymenolepis nana[a]	+		
Necator americanus (migrating)[a]	+++	+	
Baylisascaris procyonis[a] (raccoon ascarid)	+	++	
Schistosoma species	++ (established)	++ (acute or treatment)	+ (acute or treatment)
Liver and lung flukes (especially *Paragonimus*)	+ (established)	+++ (acute)	+ (acute)
Echinococcus species	+++ (disruption of cyst)		
Taenia species[a]	+	+++ (treatment of neurocysticercosis)	
Sarcoptis scabiei	++	+	
Isospora belli	++	+	
Histoplasma capsulatum (disseminated)	+		
Cryptococcus neoformans (disseminated)		+	+
Pneumocystis jirovecii pneumonia	++		
Allergic bronchopulmonary aspergillosis	++	++	
Löffler pneumonia (also nonparasitic)	++	+	
Coccidioides immitis	+++ (acute)	+	+++ (progressive) +++ (disseminated)
Epstein–Barr virus mononucleosis	+	+	
Epstein–Barr virus-related lymphoma in human immunodeficiency	+	+	
Human immunodeficiency virus	++	+	
Bartonella henselae lymphadenitis	++	+	
Chlamydia trachomatis pneumonia	++	+	
Streptococcal syndromes (scarlet fever, urticaria, chorea)	+	+	
Mycobacterium tuberculosis (controlled)	+	+	
NONINFECTIOUS CAUSES			
Atopic conditions	+++	+	
Lymphoma, especially Hodgkin (nodular sclerosis and mixed cellularity types)		++	+
Carcinomas		++	+
Leukemia, especially eosinophilic			+++
Preleukemia (myelogenous or lymphocytic)		+	+
Hypereosinophilia syndrome (some genetic)		++	+++
Collagen vascular diseases		++	+
Allergic angiitis (Churg–Strauss)		++	+++
Inflammatory bowel disease	++	+	
Pernicious anemia	++	+	
Addison disease, hypopituitarism	+++	+	

Continued

TABLE 288-2. Causes of Eosinophilia in Children—cont'd

	Elevation of Peripheral Blood Eosinophil Count		
Conditions	Mild (500–1500 Cells/mm³)	Moderate (1500–5000 Cells/mm³)	Extreme (>5000 Cells/mm³)
Chronic pancreatitis	++	+ (exacerbation)	
Cellular immunodeficiencies	+++	++	
Hyperimmunoglobulin E syndromes	+	+++	++
Graft-versus-host disease	++	+	
Organ transplant rejection	+++	+	
Serum sickness, erythema multiforme	+++	++	
Drug hypersensitivity	+++	++	
Premature neonates	++	++	
After abdominal irradiation	++	+	
Chronic peritoneal dialysis	++	+	
Dressler (post-pericardiotomy) syndrome	++	+	
Cholesterol embolus	+	+	
Eosinophilia–myopathy syndrome (L-tryptophan)		++₂	+++
Fasciitis–panniculitis syndromes (Shulman disease)	+	+	
DRESS syndrome	+++	+	

+++, frequently seen in infection or condition; ++, not infrequently seen; +, occasionally seen or cases reported.

ᵃEosinophilia-inducing parasitic infections that can be acquired in the United States.

Basophils

Basophils and mast cells share functional similarities and are involved in immediate hypersensitivity reactions as well as chronic inflammatory or immunologic responses. Basophils secrete cytokines such as IL-4 and histamine, which may play a role in the ongoing allergic response.[141,142] Mast cells are released as precursors from the bone marrow and are found and mature in connective tissue, not circulating in blood. Basophils differentiate and mature in the bone marrow during a 7-day period, have a lifespan of days, circulate in blood, and are not normally found in connective tissue. Basophilia is said to occur when the peripheral blood basophil count exceeds 150/mm³. Infection with parasites often is associated with increased levels of IgE, peripheral basophilia, or the infiltration of basophils and mast cells at sites of infection. Basophilia is highly associated with malignant myeloproliferative disorders and can be seen with Hodgkin disease, hemolytic anemias, hypothyroidism, pregnancy, and nephrotic syndrome and with the use of estrogen and antithyroid medications. Infection, hyperthyroidism, adrenocorticosteroid administration, and chemotherapy or radiation therapy lower the basophil count. Mast cell disease and urticaria pigmentosa are associated with increased basophil counts in tissue and bone marrow, but not usually in peripheral blood.

PLATELETS

Physiology and Measurement

The process of megakaryopoiesis and platelet production is complex, with regulation at multiple steps.[143] Megakaryocytes derive from the hematopoietic stem cell through successive lineage commitment steps, with maturation and eventual shedding of platelets into the sinusoids within the bone marrow. Transcription factors, inflammatory cytokine and hematopoietic cytokine (thrombopoietin) signaling regulate the processes; acquired and inherited disorders have been identified and can result in thrombocytopenia or thrombocytosis.[143] Platelets circulate for 7 to 10 days; approximately one-third are located in the spleen and two-thirds in

the circulation. The normal platelet count range is approximately 80,000 to 450,000 in the first week of life and 150,000 to 400,000/mm³ thereafter. Spuriously high or low platelet counts can be reported when automated instruments are used.[144]

Mature platelets are disk-shaped cells 2 to 4 μm in diameter. In general, platelets tend to be larger in conditions with increased marrow production (acute-phase response) or peripheral destruction (e.g., immune-mediated or mechanical/consumption) and normal to small in size when production defects are present. The spleen is the site of destruction in the presence of platelet antibodies or as a result of sequestration. In hypersplenism, the weight of the spleen correlates directly with the degree of thrombocytopenia regardless of the cause. In thrombocytopenic states, large platelet size is not a completely reliable discriminator of increased destruction because some underproduction states (e.g., Wiskott–Aldrich syndrome) are associated with qualitative abnormalities as well. Exercise or the administration of epinephrine causes immediate thrombocytosis as a result of the redistribution of mature platelets (lasting for minutes to hours), as does splenectomy (lasting indefinitely).

Thrombocytosis

Thrombocytosis is defined as >500,000 platelets/mm³ and usually is a secondary or reactive event related to underlying conditions.[144,145] Primary causes of thrombocytosis (polycythemia vera and essential thrombocythemia, clonal myeloproliferative disorders) are unusual in childhood.[145] Causes of thrombocytosis and extreme thrombocytosis are listed in Table 288-3. Infection (25% to 35% of cases) and rebound after infection (15% of cases) are most common, followed by hematologic causes (25% to 35%). Production of GM-CSF due to any inflammatory response can induce thrombocytosis. The degree of thrombocytosis in bacterial infections is inversely related to age younger than 5 years, the duration of the infection before treatment, and the presence of a tissue site of infection or abscess (e.g., complicated pneumonia, osteomyelitis, pyogenic arthritis, meningitis).[145-148] Thrombocytosis is the hallmark of the second week of Kawasaki disease. Extreme thrombocytosis in pertussis reflects severity of the disease.[105,106]

TABLE 288-3. Causes of Reactive Thrombocytosis in Children

Conditions	Thrombocytosis (500,000–1,000,000 Platelets/mm³)	Extreme Thrombocytosis (>1,000,000 Platelets/mm³)
INFECTIOUS		
Common uncomplicated bacterial infections	+++	+
Bacterial infections with abscess	++	+++
Pertussis	++	+
Chronic bacterial infection (*Mycobacterium, Brucella*)	++	+
Human immunodeficiency virus	+	+
Chronic hepatitis	++	
Disseminated fungal infection	++	
HEMATOLOGIC		
Recovery from infection	++	+
Recovery from cancer chemotherapy	++	
Hemolytic anemia	++	+
Hemorrhage or significant thrombosis	++	+
Iron, vitamin E and B₁₂ deficiency (and treatment)	++	++
Splenectomy or functional asplenia	+++	++
Neuroblastoma, lymphoma	++	+
Histiocytosis	+	
INFLAMMATORY		
Kawasaki disease	+++	++
Burns, surgery, fractures, other trauma or tissue ischemia	+++	+
Collagen vascular disease	+++	+
Postinfectious, postpericardiotomy syndromes	+++	+
Inflammatory bowel disease	++	+
Graft-versus-host disease	++	+
Sarcoidosis	++	
MISCELLANEOUS		
Respiratory acidosis	++	+
Metabolic acidosis, dehydration	++	+
Nephrotic syndrome	+++	++
Chronic renal failure	++	+
Congenital adrenal hyperplasia	+++	+
Antibiotics (especially β-lactams)	+++	
Vinca alkaloids	+++	+
Cocaine exposure (neonate)	+	
Corticosteroid agents	++	
Epinephrine	++	

+++, *frequently seen in infection or condition; ++, not infrequently seen; +, occasionally seen or cases reported.*

Thrombocytosis is unusual in viral infections, except for necrotizing infection and HIV,[149] and in recovery from thrombocytopenia. Multiple drugs, including antibiotics, induce thrombocytosis.

Thrombocytopenia

Thrombocytopenia is defined as <80,000 platelets/mm³ in the first week of life and <150,000 thereafter. Thrombocytopenia can result from several mechanisms and causes[150] (Box 288-7). Infections commonly can downregulate platelet production as part of general hematopoiesis. Immune-mediated destruction during acute, chronic, or congenital infection can occur in several viral infections (such as CMV, EBV, HIV,[151] rubella, and hepatitis B and C[152]) and subacute bacterial infections (such as endocarditis, leptospirosis, and syphilis). Idiopathic thrombocytopenic purpura results from immune-mediated destruction, usually follows nonserious viral infections, and is characterized by profound thrombocytopenia and mucocutaneous bleeding in an otherwise healthy-appearing child.[153] Acute severe infections, viral or bacterial, can cause disseminated intravascular coagulopathy and profound thrombocytopenia on a nonimmunologic basis. Acute infections by *Rickettsia, Ehrlichia* and *Anaplasma,* and *Plasmodium* have a propensity to cause thrombocytopenia without overwhelming infection, and certain bacterial toxins (such as the endotoxins of enteric bacilli and the exotoxins of *S. aureus* and *S. pyogenes*) can cause thrombocytopenia without bacteremia. The Shiga-like toxin of certain *Escherichia coli* and neuraminidase of *S. pneumoniae* are associated with microangiopathic thrombosis and thrombocytopenia in hemolytic-uremic syndrome. The transient mild thrombocytopenia (platelet count of 80,000 to 150,000) that occurs commonly during systemic viral illness is speculated to have marrow-suppressive and peripheral destructive components.

METABOLIC ABNORMALITIES

Many infections result in some degree of associated hepatic dysfunction. Intrahepatic cholestasis secondary to hepatocellular dysfunction is the usual abnormality in systemic bacterial, toxin-mediated, viral, and rickettsial diseases. Serum alanine aminotransferase (ALT) and aspartate aminotransferase (AST) levels are elevated more than 1.5 times normal in >75% of individuals with ehrlichiosis, anaplasmosis,[97] and RMSF[96] and in approximately one-half with staphylococcal toxic shock or streptococcal septicemia or toxin-mediated disease. AST exceeds ALT when hemolysis or rhabdomyolysis occurs. Serum hepatic enzymes are mildly elevated in EBV mononucleosis (almost universally) and CMV mononucleosis (frequently); characteristically, bilirubin (direct greater than the indirect fraction) is disproportionately elevated to the transaminases, with increases to 10 mg/dL or higher in some EBV infections. In acute hepatocellular infections, as with hepatitis viruses, serum levels of the transaminases frequently exceed 1000 mg/dL, with only mildly elevated bilirubin. Neonates with disseminated herpes simplex virus, adenovirus, or enterovirus infection can have severe hepatocellular dysfunction. In a study of 85 episodes of bloodstream infection (BSI) in neonates, 46% of cases due to gram-negative bacilli but only 13% due to coagulase-negative staphylococci were associated with elevated ALT/AST levels.[154] Some bacterial infections (e.g., tuberculosis, brucellosis, syphilis, cat-scratch disease) cause granulomatous space-occupying lesions in the liver resulting in cholestasis and bacterial cholecystitis can cause obstruction. Serum transaminases are mildly elevated in over 50% of children with Kawasaki disease. Hypoglycemia due to impaired gluconeogenesis can be associated with a severe hepatic insult or septicemia. Hyperglycemia sometimes is a clue to candidemia in prematurely born infants.[155]

Hyponatremia is a complication of dehydration and diarrheal loss in childhood infections or a complication of vomiting in pyloric stenosis. Hyponatremia without apparent gastrointestinal fluid loss is a clue to increased vascular permeability and is associated in such situations with decreased albumin and intravascular volume. Hyponatremia is an early and almost universal finding (present in 90% of cases) in RMSF, is present in >50% of individuals with toxic shock syndromes, and is a common finding in nephrotic syndrome and cirrhosis. Edema despite decreased intravascular volume is a hallmark of these conditions. Hyponatremia in individuals with normal hydration and intravascular volume can be associated with inappropriate secretion of antidiuretic hormone as a result of central nervous system or pulmonary infection, or associated with infant botulism.[156] Serum potassium levels rise predictably with hemolysis or with thrombocytosis.[157]

NONSPECIFIC ANTIBODIES

A variety of nonspecific antibodies are produced in response to infectious, neoantigenic, and inflammatory stimuli. Beginning as serendipitous or enigmatic laboratory findings, some tests have become extremely useful in the diagnosis or management of infectious diseases, even though the antigen used does not contain any part of the infectious agent (Table 288-4). Measurement of nonspecific antibodies also can lead to confusion and misdiagnosis.

TABLE 288-4. Nonspecific Antibodies Associated with Infections and Other Conditions

Antibody	Infection/Condition	Antigen/Test	Antibody Class/Timing	Comments
Heterophile antibody	Epstein–Barr virus	Horse or sheep RBC; agglutination (after guinea-pig kidney adsorption step)	IgM Peak at 2–3 weeks of illness; fall by 3 months, negative by 6 months	Positive in Epstein–Barr virus-associated mononucleosis in 90% of adolescents; <50% children <4 years old False positive ≤10% (usually low titer) with multiple bacterial, viral (including human immunodeficiency virus) infections, and autoimmune disease
Cold agglutinin	*Mycoplasma pneumoniae*	Human type O RBC (I antigen); agglutination at 4°C	IgM Peak at 2–3 weeks of illness; positive for months	Titer >1:64 is >90% associated with *Mycoplasma pneumoniae* Titer correlates with severity of pneumonia Titers <1:64 found with respiratory tract viral infections, Epstein–Barr virus, cytomegalovirus, bacterial pneumonia, malaria, lymphoma, hypersensitivity syndromes

Continued

TABLE 288-4. Nonspecific Antibodies Associated with Infections and Other Conditions—cont'd

Antibody	Infection/Condition	Antigen/Test	Antibody Class/Timing	Comments
Reagin antibody	*Treponema pallidum*	Cardiolipin; multiple test methods (e.g., rapid plasma reagin, Venereal Disease Research Laboratory)	IgG/IgM Positive 1–2 weeks after onset of chancre (slightly later than specific antibody); correlates with activity of infection/adequacy of therapy	False-positive test (i.e., negative specific treponemal antibodies) is rarely >1:4; found with *Mycoplasma pneumoniae*, malaria, bacterial and viral infections; after vaccination; illicit drug use and autoimmune diseases
Rheumatoid factor	Autoimmune disorders	Fc fragment of human IgG; latex agglutination, enzyme immunoassays	IgM Titer correlates with activity of infectious disease, not necessarily autoimmune disease	Multiple autoimmune disorders (positive in only 25% with juvenile idiopathic arthritis); can be positive in chronic infections (e.g., endocarditis, and hepatitis) and in neonate against maternal IgG
Antinuclear antibody	Autoimmune disorders	Nuclear and cytoplasmic antigens using Hep-2 cells; indirect immunofluorescence antibody test followed by specific antigen testing	IgG/IgM	Multiple autoimmune disorders; positive in >90% with systemic lupus erythematosus Titer 1:20 in up to 10% of healthy children Titers 1:40 commonly and high titers occasionally with bacterial, viral, toxin-mediated diseases (for up to 8 weeks) Also associated with drug hypersensitivity, malignancy

IgM, immunoglobulin M; RBC, red blood cells.

---

289 Principles of Anti-Infective Therapy

John S. Bradley and Sarah S. Long

When a child develops signs and symptoms consistent with a bacterial infection, the clinician must first decide if the child's illness is caused by an infection or other inflammatory process. For the child who may benefit from antimicrobial therapy, the clinician must select an agent that is the safest and most effective at curing the infection. Inappropriate antibiotic therapy given to a child with a viral infection exposes the child needlessly to the toxicities inherent in the antibiotic, adds to the selective pressure driving antibiotic resistance in bacteria, creates unnecessary costs to the medical system, and may divert the focus of attention from the most appropriate evaluation and therapy for the child's infection.

The selection of optimal antibiotic therapy for presumed bacterial infection is based on the balance of benefits and risks of specific therapy for each child.

SELECTING OPTIMAL ANTIMICROBIAL THERAPY

A number of questions must be addressed sequentially in order to choose optimal empiric and definitive antimicrobial therapy. They revolve around identifying potential or presumed pathogens and considering the relative merits of antimicrobial agents for specific pathogens and circumstances (Box 289-1). The clinician should follow the steps outlined below.

Step 1: Predict the Infecting Organism

The first step in predicting the pathogen is to define the patient's site(s) of infection or the organ systems involved. Bacteria are often tropic for certain tissues; certain species have a proclivity for causing certain infections. Examples are *Neisseria meningitidis*, group B streptococcus, and *Streptococcus pneumoniae* for meningitis; *S. pneumoniae*, *Haemophilus influenzae*, and *Moraxella catarrhalis* for acute otitis media; and *Staphylococcus aureus* and *Streptococcus pyogenes* for cellulitis, osteomyelitis, and pyogenic arthritis.

Step 2: Consider Host Defense Mechanisms

Is the host healthy, with intact immunity and normal integumental barriers to infection? If so, the causative pathogens often are predictable. If the child has an underlying condition such as a defect in granulocyte number or function, nonpathogenic bacteria from both the host and the environment can cause infection. For an immune-competent child with trauma to skin or mucous membranes, a recent surgical procedure, or an indwelling medical device, a variety of relatively nonpathogenic commensals also can be causative pathogens, mandating therapy that provides activity against a much broader range of organisms.

Step 3: Consider the Age of the Child

Infectious agents causing specific target organ infections in immunocompetent hosts often are predictable, based on the age of the child and exposures to pathogens specific to each age group. For example, group B streptococci and *Escherichia coli* are causes of meningitis almost exclusively during the first 90 days of life. Developmental maturation of the immune system as infants approach the third year of life provides improved recognition for polysaccharide-encapsulated pathogens such as *Streptococcus pneumoniae* or *H. influenzae* type b. Group childcare exposures in young infants have been linked to the carriage of and infection by

1. What is the clinical syndrome/site of infection? Pathogens are predictable by site.
2. Does the child have normal defense mechanisms (in which case causative agents are predictable) or are they impaired by underlying conditions, trauma, surgery, or a medical device (in which case causative agents are less reliably predictable)?
3. What is the child's age? Pathogens are predictable by age.
4. What clinical specimen(s) should be obtained to guide empirical definitive therapy?
5. Which antimicrobial agents have activity against the pathogens considered, and what is the current range of susceptibilities for each antibiotic against these pathogens in the practitioner's hospital or clinic?
6. What special pharmacokinetic and pharmacodynamic properties of a therapeutic agent are important regarding the site of the infection and the host?
7. For any given infection site, what percent of children require effective antimicrobial therapy with agents first selected for treatment? Bacterial meningitis requires 100%, whereas 75% may be acceptable for impetigo.
8. What empiric therapy and what definitive therapy would be optimal? Agents with a broad spectrum of activity may be appropriate for empiric therapy, whereas those with a narrow spectrum of activity are preferred for definitive therapy.
9. What special considerations exist regarding drug allergy, drug interaction, route of administration, cost, alteration of flora, or selective pressure in an environment?

antibiotic-resistant strains of *S. pneumoniae* in unimmunized children and may require an increased dosage of amoxicillin in order to achieve the same level of treatment success as that achieved for a child not in group childcare. School-related exposure to *S. pyogenes* is associated with increased age-specific attack rates of streptococcal pharyngitis, which is low in young infants. Similarly, adolescent exposure to sexually transmitted pathogens such as *Neisseria gonorrhoeae* increases the potential etiologies of pyogenic arthritis in that age group.

Step 4: Perform Diagnostic Tests

Every effort should be made to prove the etiology of the infection and to obtain an isolate for susceptibility testing. The Gram stain is a useful rapid test because it provides clues to the pathogen (e.g., swab in neonatal conjunctivitis), pathogenesis (e.g., aspirate in polymicrobial lung abscess), or interpretation of culture results (e.g., tracheal secretions in pneumonia). Although Gram stain result of a tissue sample may lead to the inclusion of additional empiric therapy, it should not necessarily lead to exclusion of antibiotics customarily used in the empiric treatment of that infection. In meningitis, the finding of gram-negative diplococci visualized on Gram stain of cerebrospinal fluid (CSF), suggesting *N. meningitidis*, should not exclude empiric therapy to cover *H. influenzae* type b, or of *S. pneumoniae*. An error in processing or interpreting the Gram stain must not lead to ineffective therapy of bacterial meningitis. Similarly, a Gram stain that demonstrates gram-positive cocci in clusters from endotracheal secretions in a neutropenic child with pneumonia should lead to the addition of agents active against staphylococci, but not to the elimination of agents active against *Pseudomonas aeruginosa*.

Nucleic acid detection is being used more frequently in clinical laboratories for the diagnosis of bacterial, mycobacterial, viral, fungal, and parasitic infection. These techniques do not require the isolation of viable organisms, and can be applied to a variety of tissue specimens. Advantages of improved sensitivity are obvious, but current methods often lack the ability to provide data on antimicrobial susceptibility.

Step 5: Consider Antibiotic Susceptibilities of Suspected Pathogens

Bacteria can have multiple different mechanisms of resistance against a single antibiotic or against multiple types of antibiotics. The most common resistance mechanisms include keeping the antibiotic out of the organism (cell wall permeability changes or efflux pumps), inactivating antibiotics by enzymatic degradation, and altering the antibiotic's target binding site. Bacteria can express resistance continuously (constitutively), or only on exposure to an antibiotic (inducible resistance). With such vast biologic variability in resistance mechanisms and efficient transmission of resistance genes between organisms, it is understandable that a single organism such as *E. coli* can manifest different patterns of antibiotic resistance in different populations within the same region, between regions of a country, and between countries of the world. *E. coli* isolated from urine from a child who was previously healthy and unexposed to antibiotics is likely to demonstrate a very different resistance pattern compared with *E. coli* isolated from a child with relapsed leukemia who has had a prolonged hospitalization in an Oncology Unit in a tertiary care pediatric hospital. The resistance patterns of *E. coli* from cities in the United States differ from those in Buenos Aires and Hong Kong due to local differences in antibiotic pressure and the types of transmissible resistance factors present in each location. Regardless of which population is under study, the range of local susceptibilities to many different antibiotics can always be determined. The hospital antibiogram is a widely available tool that allows the clinician to assess the current local resistance pattern for each pathogen to each antibiotic. These antibiograms are updated annually, as the resistance patterns can change substantially within a 12-month period. The probability that the antibiotic selected for empiric therapy will be effective against the presumed pathogen is directly related to the proportion of susceptible pathogens infecting patients in that location.

Step 6: Consider Pharmacokinetic/ Pharmacodynamic Properties of Drugs

The route of administration, the absorption, tissue distribution, and drug elimination characteristics are all critical pieces of information to guide the selection of both drug and drug dosage in antimicrobial therapy. Eradication of pathogens causing infection requires the appropriate antibiotic exposure at the infected tissue site. For many agents, published data describe the average concentrations and variability of concentrations achieved at specific tissue sites over time. Unfortunately, for many older antibiotics this important information often is unavailable.

To understand best how effective an antibiotic will be in achieving a microbiologic cure using otitis media and amoxicillin treatment as an example, information is required on the range of concentrations achievable in the middle-ear fluid (MEF) following administration of a specific dosage of amoxicillin, as well as the characteristics of amoxicillin elimination from this body site over time. These data provide a measure of exposure of bacteria to amoxicillin in the MEF. Based on the amoxicillin exposure required to achieve an MEF concentration above the minimum inhibitory concentration (MIC) for at least 30% to 40% of each dosing interval, the proportion of children given that specific dosage who would likely respond to treatment is predictable. For different classes of antibiotics, different types of drug exposure may be required for bacterial eradication.[1]

In the treatment of meningitis, adequate antibiotic concentrations in the CSF are critical for cure. The concentration of aminoglycoside antibiotics in the CSF following intravenous infusion is likely to be inadequate to treat meningitis caused by gram-negative pathogens, despite the fact that CSF concentrations are roughly 20% of those achievable in serum. In contrast, the high serum concentration of penicillin after a large dose leads to a bactericidal CSF concentration against pneumococcus if the pathogen is susceptible, even though the CSF concentration of penicillin is only about 5% of that achievable in serum. Within the range of predictable tissue penetration of antimicrobial agents, there is considerable variability among children receiving the same dose of drug. For example, antibiotic concentrations in the middle-ear space can be inadequate in a small but predictable percentage of children all of whom are given the same mg/kg dosage orally. However, unlike acute otitis media, the clinician cannot risk inadequate dosing for even one child with meningitis. The inherent variability among children of serum and site-of-infection tissue concentrations of antibiotics is relevant to other infections, such as pyogenic arthritis, pyomyositis, cellulitis, and pneumonia. Clearly, a single mg/kg dosage of an antibiotic may not be appropriate and effective in all children with the same pathogen causing infection at different tissue sites as the tissue concentration of that antibiotic can differ substantially between sites.

The absorption, distribution, and elimination of drugs are variable in children by age-related developmental changes.[2,3] The volume of distribution of antibiotics varies profoundly during the first few years of life, being greater in the neonate than in the infant. Drug elimination based on organ function generally increases during the first several weeks of life, peaks in infancy, and approaches adult values during adolescence. Many antibiotics require different dosages during these stages of life in order to achieve optimal antibiotic exposure to maximize efficacy and minimize toxicity.

The pharmacodynamic properties of an antibiotic describe how exposure of the antibiotic to the pathogen leads to a bacteriostatic or bactericidal effect and are important in designing an antibiotic dosing regimen (Table 289-1). Aminoglycosides kill bacteria in a concentration-dependent fashion. Therefore, it is desirable to achieve the highest concentration possible at the site of infection in order to achieve the most rapid killing of bacteria. The maximum safe tissue concentration is dictated by the serum aminoglycoside concentration above which renal toxicity occur. For other antibiotic classes, such as the penicillins, achieving

TABLE 289-1. Pharmacodynamic Antibacterial Effect of Antimicrobial Agents by Primary Bacterial Target and by Antibiotic Class

Primary Target[a]	Antibacterial Class	Pharmacodynamics[b]	Intracellular Activity[c]

Cell wall	β-Lactams
	  Penicillins
	  Cephalosporins
	  Monobactams
	  Carbapenems
	Glycopeptides
	  Vancomycin
	  Teicoplanin[d]
		Bactericidal
		Time-dependent
		PAE only against gram-positive organisms
		Carbapenems PAE against gram-positive and gram-negative organisms
			Generally not effective

Cell membrane	Lipopeptides
	  Daptomycin
	Polymyxins
	  Polymyxin B
	  Colistin
		Bactericidal
		Concentration-dependent
		Long PAE (daptomycin)
		PAE (polymyxins)
			Not known

Ribosome	Macrolides, azalides	Bacteriostatic or -cidal Time- and concentration-dependent Long PAE	Yes
	Tetracyclines, glycylcyclines	Bacteriostatic Time-dependent Long PAE	Yes
	Lincosamides (clindamycin)	Bactericidal or -static Time-dependent PAE	Yes
	Aminoglycosides	Bactericidal Concentration-dependent PAE	Generally not effective
	Oxazolidinones	Bacteriostatic (except against *Streptococcus pneumoniae*) Time-dependent PAE	Generally not effective
	Rifamycins	Bactericidal Long PAE	Yes
	Fluoroquinolones	Bactericidal Concentration-dependent Long PAE	Yes
	Streptogramins	Bactericidal (except against *Enterococcus faecium*) Concentration-dependent PAE	Yes
Nucleic acid	Metronidazole	Bactericidal Concentration-dependent PAE	Yes
	Sulfamethoxazole-trimethoprim	Bactericidal Concentration-dependent	Yes

PAE, postantibiotic effect, or the observation of delay in regrowth of organisms following removal of antibiotic from the media.

[a]*The primary antibiotic target within the bacterial pathogen.*

[b]*The type of pharmacodynamic relationship that best describes antibiotic-mediated inhibitory or bactericidal activity.*

[c]*The ability to treat intracellular pathogens, based on the penetration of antibiotic into the host cell by passive diffusion or by active uptake.*

[d]*Not marketed in the United States.*

tissue concentration above the MIC for that pathogen for 30% to 40% of the dosing interval is associated with microbiologic and clinical cure. For the penicillins, a higher concentration of the antibiotic at the infected tissue site, above a certain critical concentration, is not associated with more rapid sterilization of tissues or better clinical outcome.

The postantibiotic effect also is considered in dosing and varies by antibiotic (see Table 289-1). For the aminoglycosides, the postantibiotic effect is profound, i.e., an extended period of time lapses after the antibiotic concentration drops below the MIC before regrowth occurs. On the other hand, other antibiotics (e.g., most macrolides) inhibit growth only until the concentration drops below the MIC. Differences probably reflect molecular mechanisms of antibiotic activity at the target site (e.g., ribosome or cell wall), the avidity of antibiotic binding to the target site, the rate of elimination of the antibiotic from the target site, and whether the damage to the target site structure is reversible or irreversible.

Although growth of a population of organisms generally can be inhibited at a certain antibiotic concentration (the MIC), as defined by standard laboratory techniques, antibiotic concentrations that lead to less frequent emergence of resistance often can be determined using unique assay conditions with higher inocula than those employed in standard clinical assays. For some bacteria, resistance begins with a spontaneous nucleic acid mutation leading to an amino acid change that results in less avid binding of the antibiotic to the target site. This single-step mutation may lead only to a slightly higher MIC. The antibiotic concentration required to inhibit the single-step mutant, however, may not be achievable in infected tissues when a standard antibiotic dosage is used. Second-step mutations may then occur during ongoing exposure to an antibiotic, leading to more profound changes in the MIC, rendering the organisms fully resistant even at the highest attainable antibiotic tissue concentrations. Often it is possible to identify the concentration of antibiotic required to prevent the selection of viable single-step mutants, the mutant prevention concentration (MPC); the MPC often is 2- or 3-fold higher than the MIC.[4,5] If the higher dosage required for the MPC can be prescribed without undue toxicity, the risk of selecting antibiotic-resistant strains that can subsequently infect that child or his/her contacts may be reduced.

Step 7: Consider Target Attainment

In treating any child, the practitioner must assess the seriousness of the infection and the risk of injury or death if the antibiotic is not effective. For infections that are not life-threatening, and cause minimal morbidity (e.g., impetigo), achieving a cure rate of 70% to 80% with a safe and inexpensive antibiotic often is acceptable, especially if the use of an alternative agent to achieve a 98% success rate for that infection carries an excessive risk of toxicity or high cost. For other infections that cause a degree of suffering or risk of organ damage (e.g., pyelonephritis or acute otitis media), a cure rate of 80% to 90% often is desirable. For serious, life-threatening infections (e.g., bacterial meningitis or septicemia in a neutropenic child), an expected cure rate of 100% must be achieved.[1] No formal list of "approved" cure rates, or "target attainment" rates exists. Accepted target attainment rates may differ between infections and hosts as assessed by physicians, families, and societies. Consideration of target attainment rates can help clarify decision-making regarding relative merits, risks, and costs of antimicrobial management.

Step 8: Consider Empiric and Definitive Therapeutic Decisions Separately

For suspected serious infections, antibiotics with appropriately broad antibacterial activity at the highest tolerated dosage are selected for empiric therapy. Adequate empiric therapy is associated with decreased mortality and shorter hospital stays compared with inadequate empiric therapy for seriously ill adults.[6-8] For the

seriously ill child, knowledge of the local resistance patterns for suspected pathogens should lead to selection of antibiotics with a likely achievable cure rate of >95%. Less critically ill children may not require broad-spectrum agents as empiric therapy, particularly if culture results are anticipated to provide information within 48 to 72 hours on the most appropriate antimicrobial therapy, and the risks of delayed appropriate therapy are acceptable to the clinician and the family.

Combination empiric therapy frequently is given when high cure rates are desirable to ensure adequate antimicrobial activity against all potential pathogens. A combination of vancomycin plus a third-generation cephalosporin is used for empiric treatment of community-acquired meningitis since use of a third-generation cephalosporin may provide optimal therapy for *Streptococcus pneumoniae* with decreased susceptibility to β-lactam agents. Empiric therapy for meningitis in the first 2 months of life consists of ampicillin plus a third-generation cephalosporin because the possible pathogens include *Listeria monocytogenes*, group B streptococcus, and *Escherichia coli*. Long-established combination therapies may be used for febrile neutropenic patients to ensure activity against *Pseudomonas aeruginosa*, enteric gram-negative bacilli, and *Staphylococcus aureus*.[9] Once the pathogen is identified, a narrow-spectrum agent frequently can provide the same degree (or higher degree) of bacterial eradication and clinical efficacy with decreased toxicity, decreased selective pressure, and decreased cost. For example, initial therapy with a carbapenem agent for ventilator-associated pneumonia can be narrowed to cefotaxime if the pathogen isolated is a susceptible *Klebsiella* species rather than *Pseudomonas aeruginosa*. A postoperative wound infection treated with vancomycin and cefotaxime can be narrowed to ampicillin if a susceptible *E. coli*, rather than methicillin-resistant *Staphylococcus aureus* (MRSA) or *Enterobacter* species, is isolated. For a patient with catheter-associated septicemia treated with vancomycin and gentamicin from whom ampicillin-susceptible *Enterococcus* is isolated, ampicillin has superior bacterial activity (and less toxicity) than vancomycin. For an outpatient with a cutaneous abscess presumed to be caused by *S. aureus*, empiric clindamycin can be replaced with an oral first-generation cephalosporin or β-lactamase-stable penicillin if the organism is methicillin-susceptible.

Definitive, convalescent outpatient therapy of serious infections initially treated in the hospital is reasonable if the risks of complications of the infection are negligible, the parents and child can adhere to well-defined management plans and can return to hospital quickly for any infection- or therapy-related problem. Situations exist in which either convalescent oral therapy or convalescent parenteral therapy is preferred. High-dose oral β-lactam therapy for bone and joint infections is one of the best evaluated step-down therapies for invasive infection.[10] Parenteral antibiotics, such as ceftriaxone, that can be administered once daily are advantageous for outpatient therapy despite the fact that agents with a narrowor spectrum of activity (or more potent activity) may be available, as they require more frequent closing that may not be available in a home environment.[11]

Step 9: Special Considerations

Considerations of drug allergy impact antimicrobial selection. The degree and type of drug reaction should be ascertained. The history of a morbilliform rash in a child 4 days after commencing amoxicillin therapy does not carry the same risk of a serious drug reaction as the history of hives and airway obstruction following the first dose of amoxicillin. Cost considerations have become a greater issue as health insurers and governmental agencies develop antibiotic formularies that contain "approved," less costly antibiotics with a narrow spectrum of activity. Antibiotic resistance of the suspected pathogen provides guidance for the selection of a particular agent. As antibiotic resistance in a community increases and failures with older, less active agents increase, formularies must be reassessed. An acceptable risk of failure needs to be determined by the treating physicians as well as by medical advisors to government and insurers who determine formularies in order to allow families to achieve acceptable cure rates and continue to have confidence in their healthcare providers.

ANTIMICROBIAL SUSCEPTIBILITY TESTING AND INTERPRETATION

The primary purpose of performing antimicrobial susceptibility testing on clinical isolates is to guide therapeutic decisions for individual children, and amass collective data to inform decisions when a pathogen is not isolated. Susceptibility testing is performed routinely for the vast majority of clinical isolates in order to make decisions for individual children, with a few notable exceptions, such as for *Streptococcus pyogenes* in which susceptibility to penicillin is predictable. A comparison of the antibiograms from sequentially isolated organisms from a child can provide guidance for interpretation of the clinical relevance of two or more isolates (e.g., coagulase-negative staphylococci as a true pathogen vs. contaminant). Company antibiograms from the same bacteria isolated from several children on a hospital ward may provide insight into possible healthcare-associated infections.

Interpretation of Susceptibility Test Results

An assortment of routine susceptibility test methods can be performed, including the disk diffusion (Bauer–Kirby) test, an antibiotic strip gradient-diffusion method (E-test), agar dilution with a mechanized inoculator, broth macrodilution or microdilution, and the short-incubation automated instrument method.[12] Results usually are provided as a measure of the inhibition of growth of a defined inoculum of organisms following incubation in the presence of defined concentrations of an antibiotic. The MIC value provides an operational definition of a strain's intrinsic antibiotic susceptibility, generally reflecting the additive effects of multiple mechanisms of resistance, if present. Standardizing these susceptibility techniques and interpretation largely has been the task of the Food and Drug Administration (FDA) and the Clinical and Laboratory Standards Institute (CLSI), a nonprofit organization comprised of participants from the pharmaceutical industry, the testing device manufacturers, the Centers for Disease Control and Prevention, the FDA, and academic institutions. Interpretation of the clinical relevance and directing clinical applications of MIC values are required beyond simple reporting of an MIC value.[13] Misunderstanding that absolute values of the MICs can be compared across antibiotics can lead to errors in antibiotic management. Examples of misinterpretation could be that ampicillin and gentamicin MICs of 4 µg/mL for *E. coli* denote equivalence, or that the vancomycin MIC of 1 µg/mL and the ampicillin MIC of 2 µg/mL for *Enterococcus* denote the superiority of vancomycin. The variables inherent in disk susceptibility testing were discussed in the landmark report by Ericsson and Sherris,[14] which formed the basis for the categorical interpretations recommended by Bauer and colleagues[15] and subsequently the FDA and the CLSI.[16]

The interpretation of the susceptibility test results is provided by the laboratory report as "S" (susceptible), "I" (intermediate), or "R" (resistant). A report of "S" suggests that treatment with standard FDA-approved dosages could be expected to lead to clinical success if tissue concentration of drug at the infected site is similar to the serum concentration. A report of "I" suggests that some clinical failures can be expected at standard dosages due to decreased susceptibility of the pathogen to that antibiotic. A report of "R" suggests that a microbiologic cure is unlikely as the pathogen is not inhibited by the antibiotic at achievable tissue concentrations. Interpretation is most valid when the distribution of MIC values across several hundred clinical isolates indicate a widely spaced, distinctly bimodal distribution of susceptible and resistant strains, such as *Staphylococcus aureus* for penicillin and *Escherichia coli* for ampicillin. The MIC value at which an organism changes from susceptible to nonsusceptible is called the breakpoint.[13] The uniformity of reporting a single interpretation (S, I, or R) of a

breakpoint for all infections caused by a pathogen frequently is too simplistic and can be misleading, such as demonstrated by selecting a breakpoint when assessing the continuum of MIC values of penicillin for *Streptococcus pneumoniae* or MIC values of aminoglycosides for *P. aeruginosa*. The interpretation by clinicians of the clinical significance of MICs should be based on: (1) the susceptibility values in a large population of isolates (range and mode of distribution, such as unimodal, bimodal, skewed); (2) the clinical pharmacology of the drug (protein binding, volume of distribution, tissue concentrations); and (3) clinical and microbiologic efficacy derived from prospective animal models and human clinical investigations.

At the time an antibiotic is first approved for use by the FDA, MIC interpretative breakpoints are assigned to the antibiotic for various pathogens (sometimes at specific tissue sites). As organisms develop new mechanisms for resistance following widespread use, the interpretation of the susceptibility results (the breakpoints) for a particular organism and a particular antibiotic can change. For example, when ceftriaxone was first approved for use in children, *S. pneumoniae* was considered susceptible if the MIC value was ≤8 µg/mL. Pneumococci then expressed a novel mechanism of resistance, alterations in the penicillin-binding sites on the various cell-wall-synthesizing transpeptidase enzymes. Beginning in 1990, microbiologic failures in the treatment of meningitis occurred in children infected by organisms with ceftriaxone MIC of 2 µg/mL. The breakpoints were subsequently changed so that only organisms with MIC ≤0.5 µg/mL were considered susceptible. However, with the knowledge that ceftriaxone concentrations in tissues other than the CSF are higher, prospective data were collected that documented clinical and microbiologic success of ceftriaxone for infections outside of the central nervous system (CNS) in which the MIC for *Streptococcus pneumoniae* was 2 µg/mL. Therefore, two breakpoints for ceftriaxone now are used: a lower breakpoint of ≤0.5 µg/mL, considered "S" for CNS infections, and a higher breakpoint of ≤1 µg/mL, considered "S" for infections outside of the CNS.

To further add to the confusion regarding multiple breakpoints assigned to a particular antimicrobial agent/pathogen pair, but in recognition that intravenously administered penicillin achieves far higher concentrations in serum and tissues than orally administered drug, two new breakpoints for penicillin/*Streptococcus pneumoniae* also have been accepted: a lower breakpoint of ≤0.06 µg/mL, considered "S" for oral drug administration; and a higher breakpoint of ≤2 µg/mL, considered "S" for intravenous drug administration.[17]

The process of regular review of breakpoints for important pathogens against commonly used older, generic antibiotics is not well standardized. When the MIC value leads to an "S" interpretation in the laboratory report, the clinician should not assume that an antibiotic will be effective for all infections at all tissue sites. Furthermore, since "S" indicates bacterial *inhibition* in the test system, the clinician cannot assume that the antibiotic is bactericidal, which may be required for certain infections.

SITE OF INFECTION

As a rule, only free, nonprotein-bound drug is active in eradicating bacteria. For β-lactam agents, excessive concentrations of antibiotic present at the site of infection are not more efficacious in bacterial eradication, as this class of agents displays time-dependent killing. On the other hand, higher concentrations at the site of infection may enhance killing for aminoglycosides and other concentration-dependent drugs. Additionally, subinhibitory concentrations are not always ineffective; morphology and microbial adherence properties can be altered after exposure to subinhibitory concentrations of some antibiotics, with phagocytosis and intracellular killing subsequently enhanced by neutrophils.

Extracellular Infections

Most bacterial infections occur in interstitial tissue fluid.[18] For such infections, serum concentrations of antibiotics generally predict responses adequately. Antibiotics leave the vascular compartment and enter the extracellular fluid (ECF) via passive diffusion. When the ratio of the surface area of vascular tissue to the site or volume of infection (SAV/V) is high (e.g., in cellulitis, pneumonia, pyelonephritis), antibiotic concentrations at that site are predicted by principles of passive diffusion. This is not the case when the volume of infection exceeds the surface area of the vasculature (e.g., abscess, fibrin clot, or cardiac vegetation). Passive diffusion principles alone also cannot be used to predict the ECF concentration of certain antibiotics at sites with active transport (e.g., urine or bile) or with a barrier to capillary permeability (e.g., into the ocular aqueous humor and CSF). The ability of antibiotics to pass through membranes by nonionic diffusion is related to lipid solubility. Lipid-soluble agents such as rifampin, chloramphenicol, trimethoprim, and isoniazid penetrate membranes and cross the blood–brain barrier better than the more highly ionized aminoglycosides. For meningitis, relatively large dosages of third-generation cephalosporins, penicillin G, ampicillin, or vancomycin are required in order to achieve adequate concentrations in the CSF. Additionally, active transport out of the ECF, including the CSF, also can result in reduced concentrations in CSF of certain antibiotics such as β-lactam agents.

Table 292-1 delineates the distribution characteristics of the major classes of antibiotics. Clinical evidence has indicated the inferiority of antibiotics used for the treatment of infection at sequestered tissue sites where penetration is poor (e.g., brain, eye, bone), and logical preference exists for the use of antibiotics known to accumulate at the site of infection (e.g., urine, bile). The vegetations of endocarditis, devitalized tissue, and bones are areas in which the penetration of most agents may be poor; high-dose and prolonged parenteral therapy usually is required, and surgical debridement may be necessary. The pharmacology of the drug can offer particular advantages. Agents eliminated by glomerular filtration, renal tubular secretion, or both accumulate in urine. Fluoroquinolones, a few β-lactam agents (such as ampicillin, ceftriaxone, and especially cefoperazone), and doxycycline are actively transported into bile, whereas first-generation cephalosporins and aminoglycosides diffuse passively. Clindamycin and the fluoroquinolones achieve excellent concentration in bone, although for infected bone with vascular necrosis, penetration of any antibiotic can be compromised.

Only free drug is considered capable of antibiotic activity.[19] Although only free drug passes through capillary walls and fibrin clots, intercompartmental and pathogen end-target dynamic changes in binding, reversibility of protein binding, and complex interactions at the tissue site probably account for the complexities in prediction of clinical efficacy as a result of the degree of protein binding. Only free drug is considered capable of antibiotic activity.[19] In general, the plasma protein binding of aminoglycosides and fluoroquinolones is low, whereas binding is low to very high for β-lactam agents.

Multiple factors at the site of infection also can alter antimicrobial activity. Examples include the presence of purulent material, which results in a tissue environment with low pH. This leads to a decrease in the cationic aminoglycoside molecule charge that results in decreased binding and decreased antibacterial activity at the site of infection. Pathogens such as *Bacteroides* and *Prevotella* produce β-lactamase and can hydrolyze β-lactam agents.[20] A wound hematoma can lower the SAV/V; hemoglobin can bind penicillins and tetracyclines.[21] Low oxygen tension in abscesses or ischemic tissue impairs active transport of aminoglycosides into bacterial cells. While an acid pH in tissue or urine impairs the activity of aminoglycosides, nitrofurantoin, and methenamine, an alkaline pH enhances the activity of aminoglycosides and clindamycin. A high-bacterial-density infection such as streptococcal necrotizing fasciitis can be associated with slowed growth of bacteria with downregulation of cell wall transpeptidases that are the targets for β-lactam agents, making the organisms less susceptible to β-lactam antibacterial activity.[22] The presence of a foreign body protects some organisms from host bactericidal action through biofilms and inhibition of neutrophil phagocytosis, but probably also protects the pathogens by other less well-defined mechanisms.

Intracellular Infections

The unique properties of antimicrobial agents must be considered when the site of infection is intracellular because many antibiotics do not penetrate into human cells (see Table 289-1). Beta-lactam antibiotics, for example, are confined almost exclusively to plasma water and the interstitial fluid space. Such localization explains some discrepancies between apparent in vitro activity and therapeutic ineffectiveness. Intracellular pathogens include *Listeria monocytogenes, Salmonella, Brucella, Legionella, Mycobacterium, Rickettsia,* and *Toxoplasma,* as well as persisting infections with *Staphylococcus aureus* and *E. coli.* Antibiotics that enter cells do so by a variety of mechanisms, such as diffusion of relatively small lipid-soluble agents across a concentration gradient, pinocytosis of water-soluble agents, and carrier-mediated transport.[23] Cellular accumulation of drug does not necessarily translate into efficacy against intracellular organisms; efficacy depends on whether the microbe and the drug are at the same intracellular site, how avidly the drug is bound to intracellular proteins and to the pathogen target site, and the molecular charge of the antibiotic at its intracellular location.

Clindamycin, macrolides, and azalides are tropic for lysosomes, where they become protonated and concentrated.[24,25] Fluoroquinolones have a large volume of distribution and a high tissue-to-serum ratio, and low-affinity intracellular binding; much of the fluoroquinolone body load thus is present intracellularly. For azithromycin, an even more dramatic intracellular location of antibiotic has been documented within phagocytic cells.[25] The pharmacokinetic properties and intracellular accrual of azithromycin are responsible for successful therapy for intracellular pathogens and for shortened courses with respect to the number of days of antibiotic dosing required (including single dose therapy) of therapy;[26] at the same time, it is noteworthy that azithromycin concentrations in serum, CSF, and the aqueous humor of the eye are almost negligible.[27]

DOSING, ROUTE, AND DURATION OF THERAPY

Optimal dosing of an antimicrobial agent depends on relationships between the time-course of concentration at the site of infection, the characteristics of antimicrobial activity, and adverse effects.

In clinical practice, the route of administration of antibiotics often is based on additional practical considerations. Parenteral administration is required if an agent is absorbed poorly from the gastrointestinal tract, if a condition precludes administration or absorption of a usually well-absorbed drug, if an unusually high tissue concentration of drug is required, or if adherence to an oral regimen for treatment of a significant infection cannot be ensured. Otherwise, substitution of oral for parental agents frequently is possible, even for serious diseases (e.g., pneumonia, osteomyelitis, pyogenic arthritis, orbital cellulitis) during convalescent therapy.

Oral therapy can replace parenteral therapy when highly absorbed and bioavailable agents are used to treat highly susceptible pathogens (e.g., trimethoprim-sulfamethoxazole for *Pneumocystis* pneumonia) and when the tissue concentrations of drugs at relevant sites are uniquely favorable (e.g., clindamycin or fluoroquinolone in bone). With a less favorable profile, parenteral therapy is given for the entire duration of therapy (at home or in the hospital). Abundant evidence for the effectiveness of many approaches is available when patient screening, selection of medical conditions, and follow-up are performed diligently.[11,28,29] Advocacy for the best route of treatment of a child's infection is a paramount consideration with the risk of failure of therapy and the impact of the outcome taken into account.

The appropriate duration of antibiotic therapy has been determined more by experience and by "standard" treatment courses used for FDA antimicrobial drug approval, rather than by prospective, well-controlled studies for most infections in children. Many factors are considered in the decision regarding the duration of therapy, including the intrinsic pathogenicity of the

TABLE 289-2. Duration of Systemic Antibiotic Therapy for Certain Bacterial Infections

Infection	Duration of Therapy	Comments/Duration within Range
Complicated appendicitis[69]	4–7 days	Longer if control of source/infection is not adequate
Cellulitis/impetigo	10 days	Few data
Orbital cellulitis	10 days or longer	Depending on the pathogen (*Haemophilus influenzae, Streptococcus pneumoniae* – shorter) and predisposition (chronic sinusitis in adolescent – longer)
Pharyngitis (streptococcal)[70]	5–10 days	Oral agents that have been evaluated for standard course treatment have not all been evaluated for shorter courses.
Acute otitis media[26,71]	10 days	1-, 3-, and 5-day courses may be adequate in certain cases (older age, rapid response, otoscopic improvement) with certain antibiotics (azithromycin, and certain oral beta-lactams agents)
Acute sinusitis[72]	14–21 days	At least 1 week after resolution of symptoms
Acute mastoiditis	14 days or longer	Generally at least 1 week afebrile
Uncomplicated pneumonia[73]	10 days	Few data; generally at least 5 days afebrile
Complicated pneumonia (necrotizing or with lung abscess, empyema)[74]	14–21 days or longer	Depending on the clinical response, drainage, pathogen (*Staphylococcus aureus, Streptococcus pyogenes* – longer; *Haemophilus influenzae*, anaerobes – shorter); generally at least 1 week afebrile after drainage ceases)
Purulent pericarditis	10–14 days or longer	Depending on the pathogen (*Staphylococcus aureus*, enteric bacilli – longer; *Neisseria meningitidis* – shorter); generally at least 7–10 days afebrile
Endocarditis (native valve)[41]		
Penicillin-susceptible viridans streptococcus or *Streptococcus bovis*	Penicillin, 28 days; *or* Penicillin *plus* Gentamicin, 14 days;[a] *or* Vancomycin, 28 days	
Penicillin-nonsusceptible viridans streptococcus or *Streptococcus bovis*	Pencillin, 28 days *plus* Gentamicin, 14 days;[a] *or* Vancomycin, 28 days	
Enterococcus species (moderately susceptible to ampicillin)[b]	Penicillin, *or* ampicillin, 4–6 weeks; *or* Vancomycin, *plus* Gentamicin, 4–6 weeks[a]	Depending on the duration of symptoms (<3 months – shorter; >3 months – longer)
Methicillin-susceptible *Staphylococcus aureus*[c]	Nafcillin or vancomycin, 4–6 weeks *plus* Optional gentamicin, 3–5 days[a]	
Methicillin-resistant *Staphylococcus aureus*[c]	Vancomycin, 4–6 weeks	Additional therapy with aminoglycoside or rifampin also is given frequently
HACEK microorganisms	Ceftriaxone, 28 days *or* Ampicillin plus gentamicin, 28 days[a]	
Meningitis[74]		
Group B streptococcus	14 days or longer	Gentamicin also is given frequently for 72 hours and until CSF is proved sterile; if isolate is penicillin-tolerant, gentamicin is continued
Listeria monocytogenes	14 days or longer	Gentamicin also is given usually for 72 hours and until CSF is proved sterile
Enteric gram-negative bacilli	21 days or longer	At least 21 days and 14 days after CSF is proved sterile, whichever is longer; longer depending on the presence of infarction, abscess
Streptococcus pneumoniae	10–14 days	A least 7–10 days after CSF is proved sterile; the duration of therapy for meningitis due to pneumococci that are penicillin-nonsusceptible is not known
Haemophilus influenzae	10 days	
Neisseria meningitidis	5–7 days	
Brain abscess	21–28 days or longer	Depending on the pathogen (gram-negative bacilli – longer), drainage (at least 10–14 days after drainage), and diminution on imaging study
Pyelonephritis	10–14 days	
Cystitis[75]	7–10 days	

Continued

TABLE 289-2. Duration of Systemic Antibiotic Therapy for Certain Bacterial Infections—cont'd

Infection	Duration of Therapy	Comments/Duration within Range
Acute pyogenic arthritis[76]	14–21 days or longer	Depending on the course, prompt and adequate drainage, pathogen (*Staphylococcus aureus* – longer), and site (hip or shoulder – longer); generally at least 7–10 days afebrile and after last drainage; therapy for 3–5 days has been adequate for gonococcal arthritis in adults
Acute osteomyelitis[76]	21–42 days or longer	Depending on the course, drainage, and pathogen (*Staphylococcus aureus*, enteric bacilli – longer); generally at least 10–14 days afebrile and until the sedimentation rate is almost normal
Bacteremia without tissue focus	5–7 days or longer	Depending on the underlying condition, persistence of positive blood culture, and pathogen (*Staphylococcus aureus*, enteric bacilli – longer); at least 3–5 days afebrile

CSF, cerebrospinal fluid; HACEK, Aggregatibacter (Haemophilus) aphrophilus, Aggregatibacter (Actinobacillus) actinomycetemcomitans, Cardiobacterium hominis, Eikenella corrodens, Kingella kingae.

aThe gentamicin dose is 3 mg/kg ideal body weight per day.

bSimilar therapy is given for penicillin-resistant viridans Streptococcus (minimal inhibitory concentration, >0.5 µg/mL), for nutritionally variant viridans Streptococcus, and for prosthetic valve endocarditis caused by viridans Streptococcus or Streptococcus bovis.

cIn the presence of a prosthetic valve or other material, nafcillin or vancomycin is given for ≥6 weeks.

microbe, susceptibility to the agent used, the site of infection and penetration of the antibiotic, the use of synergistic combination therapy, the replication rate of the pathogen, the presence of a foreign body, and host factors that impair bactericidal capacity. In many situations, the severity of infection in all children is not uniform (e.g., pyelonephritis, soft-tissue abscess), leading to differences in the time-course of the child's response to antibiotic therapy. In children with pneumonia, treatment can be given parenterally until a clinical (and presumed microbiologic) response has occurred, then oral convalescent "step down" therapy can be provided for a defined time to achieve the desired total duration of therapy. With all infections, a recommendation for duration of therapy is based on the best available information for that child's infection. Longer treatment courses may be more appropriate for more resistant organisms, for more severe infections associated with abscess formation especially if abscesses cannot be drained adequately, or for immunocompromised hosts. Delayed eradication of pathogens from the site of infection can occur in all of these situations. The family should always be cautioned at the end of the treatment course to be alert for the signs and symptoms of relapse. Table 289-2 presents examples of the duration of treatment based on scientific information (when available), consensus, or experience.

ANTIMICROBIAL COMBINATIONS

Prevention of Emergence of Resistance

Antibiotics sometimes are used in combination in an attempt to create synergy, or to prevent or delay the emergence of drug-resistant subpopulations of the pathogen. In most circumstances, clinical data are insufficient to prove these effects.[30,31] *Mycobacterium tuberculosis* provides the best clinically documented example. With a spontaneous resistance mutation frequency of approximately 10^{-8}, the initial use of two or more agents to which the organism is susceptible substantially reduces the probability that resistant organisms will emerge.[32] Treatment of *Pseudomonas* infection with a β-lactam, fluoroquinolone, or aminoglycoside antibiotic alone is associated with the emergence of resistant strains; two-drug combination therapies may reduce the incidence of resistance to either component antibiotic. However, each antibiotic must provide the necessary exposure to pathogens in the infected tissues to ensure eradication of susceptible organisms. Inadequate dosing or poor tissue penetration of one antibiotic in a combination may lead to the selection of organisms resistant to that agent, despite the use of "dual therapy."

Rifampin is one antibiotic that is never used alone for the treatment of infection because of the rapid, frequent development of resistance. Combining rifampin with vancomycin for coagulase-

negative staphylococcal prosthetic valve endocarditis or ventriculoperitoneal shunt infection, or with a semisynthetic penicillin for *S. aureus* infections, may reduce the emergence of resistance while taking advantage of the unique tissue penetrations and target site properties of rifampin.

Inhibition of β-Lactamases

With certain fixed-combination drugs containing a primary β-lactam agent, the site of action of the second drug in the combination is not the vital microbial target binding site but rather a product of the microbe rendering resistance to the primary antimicrobial agent. Antistaphylococcal penicillins such as methicillin and nafcillin are degraded by staphylococcal β-lactamases. β-Lactamase-inhibiting agents such as clavulanic acid, sulbactam, and tazobactam display a specific affinity for and a degree of irreversible binding to the various bacterial β-lactamase enzymes, thereby protecting the companion β-lactam antibiotic from hydrolysis and allowing its access to the target penicillin-binding proteins.[1,33] Amoxicillin-clavulanate is especially useful in children when the potential causative pathogens are susceptible to amoxicillin except for the presence of β-lactamases produced by the pathogen (*Moraxella catarrhalis*, *Haemophilus influenzae*, *Staphylococcus aureus*, and *Bacteroides fragilis*). Piperacillin-tazobactam is a useful agent that extends the spectrum of activity of piperacillin to include additional gram-negative bacilli and methicillin-susceptible staphylococci; it does not, however, add to the activity of piperacillin alone against *Pseudomonas* as tazobactam does not effectively inhibit many of the β-lactamases produced by *P. aeruginosa*.

Synergy

Target Site Synergy

Combinations of antimicrobial agents can have a variety of effects on the target sites of an organism in vitro. The combination can be: (1) *synergistic*, when the combined effect of the drugs is significantly greater than the independent effects when the drugs are tested separately; (2) *antagonistic*, when the combined effect is significantly less than the drugs' independent effects when tested separately; (3) *additive*, when the combined effect is the sum of the separate effects of the drugs tested; or (4) *indifferent*, when the combined effect is simply the effect of the more active drug alone. The clinical applications of these definitions are controversial. Synergy test results depend on the intrinsic activities of each antibiotic on an organism, the test system used, and whether the binding sites are similar or dissimilar.[34–37] Despite the paucity of clinical validation of in vitro results, there is good reason to believe that for certain infections, synergy has clinical relevance.[38] The notion remains appealing because the outcomes of certain severe clinical infections are dependent on rapid bacterial killing, which may be better when combination therapy rather than monotherapy is used. Theoretically, for all infections, enhanced eradication of pathogens could permit a possible shortened course of therapy. Although it is not practical to perform clinical studies of all combinations, concepts regarding classes of drugs and microbes have evolved to guide therapeutic choices. In one retrospective study of severe methicillin-resistant *S. aureus* infections, 50% of children received 3 or 4 agents simultaneously.[39] With the combination of multiple agents, antagonism also can occur, with outcomes that may be worse than using only one or two agents.

Inhibition of Multiple Interrelated Targets

A classic example of synergy of targeted activity at consecutive metabolic steps is represented by the combination of a sulfonamide with a dihydrofolate reductase inhibitor such as trimethoprim. The resulting inhibition of consecutive steps in the folic acid pathway results in a significantly reduced MIC and can also enhance the drug's bactericidal capacity. Streptogramin antibiotics (quinupristin-dalfopristin) include two biochemically distinct bacteriostatic compounds produced by *Streptomyces* that produce bactericidal activity when used in combination. The binding of the type A streptogramin at the acyl-amino tRNA acceptor site on the ribosome both prevents the binding of tRNA and also causes a conformational change in the ribosome, which enhances the binding of the type B streptogramin, which then causes steric hindrance to the extrusion of newly formed polypeptide chains from within the ribosome.

Combination of Cell Wall-Active Agents with Ribosomal-Active Agents

Some instances of antibiotic resistance (e.g., to aminoglycosides) can be due to a permeability barrier that precludes the drug reaching the intracellular target site. Agents that act on the cell wall (e.g., β-lactam agents, vancomycin) should enhance the entry of an aminoglycoside; unless the drug is rendered ineffective by aminoglycoside-modifying enzymes or resistance occurs at the ribosomal level, a combination could be expected to be synergistic. Such bactericidal synergy is demonstrable for viridans streptococci, group B streptococci, enterococci, staphylococci, *Listeria* and *Corynebacterium* species, *P. aeruginosa*, and Enterobacteriaceae. Generally for *Enterococcus*, streptomycin, gentamicin, and tobramycin are predictably synergistic with cell wall-active agents if the enterococcal strain is susceptible to aminoglycosides at 2000 µg/mL; laboratories provide standardized testing at this single-drug concentration.

For gram-negative bacilli, exposure to aminoglycosides can enhance the permeability of the outer cell envelope to β-lactam antibiotics due to aminoglycoside-mediated production of altered, nonfunctional proteins that are incorporated into the cell wall.

The superior clinical efficacy of combination over single-drug therapy has been documented in only limited clinical settings. For the treatment of enterococcal endocarditis, penicillin alone, which provides only bacteriostatic activity against enterococci, results in an unacceptable relapse rate. The addition of an aminoglycoside such as streptomycin or gentamicin results in clinical cure rates comparable with the rates attained in the treatment of endocarditis caused by penicillin-susceptible streptococci.[40] Although similar clinical benefit is demonstrable in the animal model of endocarditis caused by penicillin-tolerant or relatively penicillin-resistant viridans streptococci (MIC of 1 µg/mL), no advantage is shown against fully susceptible strains; nonetheless, combination therapy for 2 weeks in patients with susceptible strains results in success rates comparable with those achieved when penicillin is administered alone for 4 weeks.[40] The combination of nafcillin plus gentamicin is synergistic in vitro against methicillin-susceptible strains of *Staphylococcus aureus*; both retrospective data,

and prospective, comparative trials of nafcillin plus gentamicin versus nafcillin alone in adults with endocarditis, as recently reviewed, failed to show any long-term outcome benefit of combination therapy.[41] Similarly, tolerance to the bactericidal effect of β-lactam agents among streptococci and staphylococci can be overcome in vitro by drug combinations, but superior clinical efficacy in human infections has not been proved. Combinations of ticarcillin or piperacillin with gentamicin, tobramycin, or amikacin exhibit in vitro synergy against many strains of *P. aeruginosa*. One prospective, randomized clinical trial of bacteremic cancer patients confirmed better survival with carbenicillin plus gentamicin versus carbenicillin alone;[42] another prospective, but uncontrolled study of 200 patients with *Pseudomonas* bacteremia documented increased survival in patients receiving combinations, regardless of whether synergy was demonstrable in vitro.[43]

Confirmatory clinical evidence of the superiority of combination therapy for bacteremia caused by other gram-negative bacilli has been limited to neutropenic patients; such evidence documents the critical importance of susceptibility to the β-lactam component.[38,42,44,45] With the advent of more potent, highly bactericidal agents such as the third-generation cephalosporins and carbapenems, the benefit of addition of an aminoglycoside may be difficult to demonstrate except under the most challenging clinical conditions of sequestered pathogens and an absent host response at the site of infection. Prospective, controlled studies under these conditions are not likely to be performed. A recent retrospective analysis of over 4500 bacteremic adults in intensive care units treated early with combination therapy documented decreased mortality and hospital stay compared with those given monotherapy, for both gram-negative and gram-positive pathogens.[46]

Published data exist on the effect of in vitro combination testing for antimicrobial agents approved during the past few decades, against common pathogens. Data on even older drugs also may exist, particularly for currently isolated pathogens that can be multidrug resistant. For example, clindamycin and gentamicin in vitro has been reported to show synergy against some strains of viridans streptococci and antagonism against others.[47] Some studies have shown synergy of trimethoprim-sulfamethoxazole plus amikacin against Enterobacteriaceae for organisms that are susceptible to both drugs.[48] Ciprofloxacin plus an aminoglycoside or various β-lactam agents is infrequently synergistic against Enterobacteriaceae, but can be synergistic occasionally (with aminoglycosides) or frequently (with imipenem) against strains of *P. aeruginosa*;[49] antagonism is rare. When daptomycin was tested in combination with rifampin or gentamicin against methicillin-resistant *S. aureus* (MRSA), additive or indifferent effects usually were observed, without synergy or antagonism. Daptomycin in combination with β-lactam agents showed unexpected synergy in vitro against MRSA. The clinical relevance of these findings requires human clinical investigation.[50] Rifampin has synergistic bactericidal activity with vancomycin against coagulase-negative staphylococci,[51] and with ampicillin against *Listeria*.[52] The unique tissue penetration properties of rifampin make it useful not only in postexposure prophylaxis to prevent or eliminate microbial colonization but in combination therapy for infections related to medical devices.

Antagonism

Despite the paucity of documented reports of the clinical significance of antagonism between antimicrobial agents, multiple examples are demonstrable in vitro; thus, caution is needed in their use, especially in infections in hosts with impaired defenses. Combinations of a bacteriostatic agent with a β-lactam antibiotic can antagonize the bactericidal activity of the β-lactam antibiotic. Combinations of chloramphenicol or tetracycline plus aminoglycosides also are antagonistic for gram-negative bacilli. In addition, chloramphenicol antagonizes the bactericidal effect of ciprofloxacin against *Staphylococcus aureus*, *Escherichia coli*, and *P. aeruginosa*. A combination of agents that bind to similar locations within the ribosome (e.g., clindamycin, erythromycin, spiramycin, chloramphenicol, streptogramins) either complement each other and enhance activity, or compete with each other and antagonize activity.[53]

JUDICIOUS USE OF ANTIBIOTICS

Antimicrobial agents are the principal therapeutic tool for pediatric infectious disease specialists and are among the leading interventions in all of pediatrics. Overuse of this tool is increasingly threatening its effectiveness. Young children have the highest rate of consumption of the approximately 110 million courses of antibiotics prescribed each year in the United States.[54,55] In addition to the many appropriate indications for such drugs, 17 million courses were given to individuals with the common cold.[55] The spread of antimicrobial resistance has led to ongoing concern about such unnecessary use among physicians and increasingly among patients or parents.[56]

Common pathogens such as *Streptococcus pneumoniae* and *Staphylococcus aureus* typically remain treatable, but resistance in these organisms complicates therapy, raises cost, and increases the likelihood of treatment failure. Hospital-associated pathogens such as *Enterobacter, Klebsiella, Acinetobacter, Pseudomonas,* or *Enterococcus* may not be treatable with available agents.[57]

Microbial resistance is driven by antimicrobial exposure. Many studies have linked recent exposure to antimicrobial agents to an increased risk for carrying or being infected with resistant pneumococci.[58,59] During a course of prophylactic antibiotics to prevent acute otitis media, the proportion of children carrying resistant strains of pneumococci, *Haemophilus influenzae,* and *Moraxella*

catarrhalis increased, with a return to baseline levels only after the selective pressure of the antimicrobial regimen was removed.[60] Avoiding such selective pressure that drives resistance by reducing antimicrobial exposure is the focus of a variety of public health strategies to control resistance.

A set of principles for judicious antimicrobial use in children with upper respiratory tract infections summarizing scientific evidence for curtailing such use has been published as a guide to appropriate antibiotic use.[61] Evidence is accumulating that promotion of the judicious use of antimicrobial agents has reduced excess prescribing. Programs for judicious use have been studied in private practice, managed care organizations, emergency departments, and community clinics.[62] Successful reductions in prescribing have been documented when groups in active intervention programs that include both physicians and patients have been compared with groups receiving no intervention other than information. Most importantly, decreased antibiotic use has not led to increased complications.[62,63] Nationwide trends now describe decreased prescribing antibiotics for upper respiratory tract conditions in the U.S.[64,65] More limited but convincing evidence exists that the decrease in prescribing antibiotics is leading to slowing of the spread of resistant bacteria.[56,66–68]

Guidelines for "Antibiotic Stewardship" from the Infectious Diseases Society of America outline strategies to promote appropriate antibiotic selection and duration of therapy and evaluate the potential impact on the development of antibiotic resistance.[56] Unfortunately, there are no prospective, high quality investigations specifically in children that document the impact of improved practices on a decrease in colonization or infection due to resistant organisms.[68]

---

290 Mechanisms and Detection of Antimicrobial Resistance

Melissa B. Miller and Peter H. Gilligan

Microorganisms have survived for millions of years because of their ability to adapt to hostile environments. Over the past 60 years, bacteria that cause human infections have been exposed to ever-increasing antimicrobial pressure, due to appropriate and inappropriate use of these agents. It is estimated that 1,360,800 kg (3 million lb) of antimicrobials are consumed annually in the United States by humans.[1,2] Estimates for animal use are 10-fold higher.[2] The economic benefits in agricultural use versus risk of transfer of resistance to humans are debated.[3,4]

Despite intensive campaigns aimed at reducing inappropriate use of antimicrobial agents, it is estimated that half of children in the industrialized world receive an antimicrobial agent annually and that three-quarters of children 1 to 2 years of age receive these agents.[5,6,7] Even with reduced use, existing levels of antimicrobial resistance are not likely to return to levels prior to the antimicrobial abuse.[8]

Antimicrobial resistance exacts a high economic and human cost. Drug-resistant organisms frequently do not respond to therapy, resulting in hospitalization, surgical interventions, increasing utilization of diagnostic services, and mortality.[9–11] Gram-negative bacilli (GNB) that produce novel β-lactamases with activity against many or, in some cases, all classes of β-lactams are emerging at an alarming rate and spreading globally. These include VIM (**V**erona-**i**ntegron-encoded **m**etallo-β-lactamase), NDM (**N**ew **D**elhi **m**etallo-β-lactamase), and KPC (***K**lebsiella **p**neumoniae **c**arbapenemase).[12–15] It is likely to be years before novel effective antibiotics will become available therapeutically.[12] The specter of extensively drug-resistant (XDR) or totally drug-resistant

(TDR) *Mycobacterium tuberculosis* is of global concern, especially in locales with high rates of HIV infection.[16–19]

GENETICS OF ANTIMICROBIAL RESISTANCE

Intrinsic Resistance

Antimicrobial resistance can be attributed to *intrinsic cellular properties, intrinsic mutations, acquisition of resistance genes,* or *intragenic recombination* resulting in mosaic genes[20] (Table 290-1). Intrinsic resistance can be due to inherent properties of microorganisms, such as cellular membranes, that render them resistant (e.g., gram-negative species to vancomycin). Additionally, intrinsic resistance is mediated by the mutation of chromosomal genes. Although acquired resistance mechanisms are more common, many infections are caused by one or few species, making interspecies gene acquisition difficult in vivo. In these circumstances (as postulated for both *Pseudomonas aeruginosa* in the setting of cystic fibrosis (CF) and *M. tuberculosis*), the organism's primary antibiotic defense mechanism is intrinsic mutations.[21,22] Mutations that contribute to intrinsic antimicrobial resistance include variation in the antimicrobial target site (e.g., quinolones, aminoglycosides), changes in regulatory genes or promoter sequences (e.g., increase in efflux pump or inactivating enzyme expression, decrease in porin expression), and indirect mutations that affect the organism's mutation rate.[21]

Although bacteria have a low mutation rate ($\sim$10^{-8} per base pair) in order to preserve DNA integrity and function, mutations

TABLE 290-1. Common Antibacterial Drug Resistance Mechanisms

Drug Class	Resistance Mechanism	Frequency	Examples
Aminoglycosides	Enzymatic inactivation	Common	Phosphotransferases, acetyltransferases, nucleotidyltransferases in Enterobacteriaceae and *Enterococcus* spp.
	Efflux pump	Uncommon	MexX-MexY efflux pump in Enterobacteriaceae
	Altered binding site	Rare	Streptomycin-resistant *Mycobacterium tuberculosis*
	Altered uptake	Common	Streptococci and all anaerobic bacteria
β-Lactams	Enzymatic inactivation		*Staphylococcus aureus, Haemophilus influenzae,* Enterobacteriaceae
	Ambler class A β-lactamase	Common	ESBL producers: *Escherichia coli, Klebsiella pneumoniae, Proteus mirabilis*
	Ambler class B β-lactamase	Uncommon	Carbapenemase plasmid encoded in *Acinetobacter baumannii, Pseudomonas aeruginosa,* and selected Enterobacteriaceae: chromosomally encoded in *Stenotrophomonas maltophilia*
	Ambler class C β-lactamase	Common	AmpC chromosomal β-lactamase in *Enterobacter* spp.
	Ambler class D β-lactamase	Uncommon	Plasmid encoded in *Pseudomonas aeruginosa* and selected Enterobacteriaceae
	Altered penicillin-binding proteins	Common	Oxacillin-resistant *Staphylococcus aureus* and penicillin-resistant *Streptococcus pneumoniae*
	Efflux pump	Uncommon	MexAB-OprM pump in *Pseudomonas aeruginosa*
	Altered uptake	Uncommon	Loss of OprF and OprD in *Pseudomonas aeruginosa*
Chloramphenicol	Enzymatic inactivation	Common	Chloramphenicol acetyltransferase in a variety of bacteria
	Efflux pump	Uncommon	*Salmonella* Typhimurium DT 104
	Altered uptake	Uncommon	Lack of OmpF protein in *Salmonella* Typhi
Colistin	Altered binding	Uncommon	Altered lipopolysaccharide in *Pseudomonas aeruginosa*
Isoniazid	Altered binding	Common	Mutation of *KatG* in *Mycobacterium tuberculosis*
	Overexpression of target	Uncommon	Overexpression of *inhA* in *Mycobacterium tuberculosis*
Linezolid	Altered binding	Rare	Mutations in 23s rRNA in *Enterococcus* spp.
Macrolides and related compounds	Efflux	Common	Macrolide resistance in streptococci
	Altered binding	Common	Methylation of 23S rRNA conferring resistance to macrolides, streptogramins, and lincosamides in *Staphylococcus* and *Streptococcus* spp.
Metronidazole	Inactivating enzyme	Uncommon	Nitroimidazole reductase in *Bacteroides* spp.
Quinolones	Altered binding	Common	Mutations in *gyr* confers resistance in gram-negative organisms; mutations in *par* confers resistance in gram-positive organisms
	Efflux	Uncommon	Seen in a variety of gram-negative and gram-positive organisms
	Protective protein	Rare	Protein expressed by *Klebsiella pneumoniae* that binds fluoroquinolones, preventing binding to target
Rifampin	Altered binding	Common	Mutations in *rpoB* gene in *Staphylococcus aureus, Mycobacterium tuberculosis,* and *Neisseria meningitidis*
Tetracyclines	Efflux pump	Common	Gram-positive and gram-negative organisms
	Protective proteins	Uncommon	Gram-positive and gram-negative organisms
Trimethoprim-sulfamethoxazole	Overproduction of target	Common	Overproduction of DHFR in a variety of bacteria
	Altered binding	Common	Mutated *dhfr* gene in *Streptococcus pneumoniae*
	Bypass targeted pathway	Uncommon	Thymidine-dependent *Staphylococcus aureus*
Vancomycin	Altered binding	Common	*vanA* and *vanB* in *Enterococcus*
	Overproduction of target	Uncommon	Vancomycin-intermediate *Staphylococcus aureus* (VISA)

DHFR, dihydrofolate reductase; ESBL, extended-spectrum β-lactamase; Opr, outer-protein membrane.

naturally occur that permit evolution toward fitness. Deleterious mutations also can occur, leading to loss of fitness.[23] Induction of a higher mutation rate (i.e., a mutator phenotype) can be beneficial to the organism particularly when the organism is under selective pressure, such as environmental or antibiotic stress. Increased mutation rates are associated with mutations in DNA mismatch repair genes, primarily *mutS, mutL,* and *mutH*.[24,25] Quinolone and aminoglycoside antibiotics have been reported to induce a hypermutable state, leading to antimicrobial resistance.[26,27] The hypermutator state is inducible or transient, allowing for the survival and expansion of the resistant bacterial population; its clinical importance requires further research.[21,28]

Often antimicrobial resistance, and especially multidrug resistance, is due to a combination of resistance determinants (e.g.,

carbapenem resistance due to expression of a β-lactamase plus loss of porin expression). Additionally, resistance mechanisms can be categorized as either intrinsic or acquired resistance depending on the organism. For example, efflux mechanisms are important causes of both single drug and multidrug resistance in a variety of organisms.[29] In general, multidrug resistance conferred by efflux is chromosomally encoded and results from mutations in regulatory genes (intrinsic resistance) while single drug efflux pumps are encoded by mobile genetic elements (acquired resistance).

Acquired Resistance

Acquired resistance occurs via horizontal transfer of resistance genes among organisms by conjugation, transformation, and/or phage-dependent transduction; in some cases, these genes become a stable part of the recipient chromosome.[30] There are two types of mobile genetic elements: those that move between cells and those that move within a cell.[31] However, elements that move only intracellularly (e.g., gene cassettes, resistance transposons, integrons) can "hitch a ride" on intercellular mobile elements such as plasmids and conjugative transposons.

Plasmids are circular, double-stranded extrachromosomal DNA (~4 to 400 kb) that self-replicate. A bacterium can contain multiple compatible plasmids or multiple copies of the same plasmid. Plasmid-based resistance genes can be propagated either by clonal spread of the organism or by horizontal transfer via conjugation, as is the case with R plasmids.[30–32] Resistance genes encoding inactivating enzymes for β-lactam agents (including extended-spectrum β-lactamases (ESBLs) and carbapenemases), macrolides, aminoglycosides, and chloramphenicol; efflux genes for macrolides and tetracyclines; and altered targets for sulfonamides have been found on plasmids.[33–38]

It is not uncommon for plasmid-mediated resistance genes to be located on mobile genetic elements; however, these elements can relocate (either by transposition or site-specific integration) to plasmids or chromosomes, resulting in the intra- and interspecies spread of antimicrobial resistance. These elements are not self-replicating and are maintained by the replication of the plasmid or chromosome on which they reside. Molecular characterization reveals that these elements are derived from a combination of phage, plasmids, and transposons.[39]

Transposons (~2 to 20 kb) contain insertion sequences and a single gene or few linked genes often encoding antimicrobial resistance. In addition, transposons are flanked by inverted sequence repeats and encode for a transposase enzyme required for transposition. Conjugative transposons exist that move directly from one bacterium to another and have been found to mediate the transfer of resistance in gram-positive bacteria. Among the best-studied conjugative transposons are Tn*916* in *Enterococcus faecalis* encoding tetracycline resistance and Tn*1549* in enterococci encoding vancomycin resistance.[40] Nonconjugative transposons (e.g., resistance transposons) generally are transferred from cell to cell via plasmids, and include Tn*1546* implicated in the transfer of vancomycin resistance from *Enterococcus* to *S. aureus*.[41]

Integrons include an integrase, mobile gene cassettes, and an integration site for the gene cassettes to allow for site-specific recombination into plasmids or the bacterial chromosome.[42] Integrons themselves are not mobile but facilitate capture of resistance gene cassettes, which subsequently insert into the chromosome. Integrons encoding antimicrobial resistance determinants have been found in a number of species in the Enterobacteriaceae family, as well as *P. aeruginosa* and *Acinetobacter* species, and have been associated with resistance to β-lactams (including ESBLs), aminoglycosides, chloramphenicol, trimethoprim, and disinfectants.[31,42,43] Integrons can contain multiple gene cassettes and therefore often encode for multidrug resistance. Gene cassettes consist of a coding sequence, usually without promoter sequences, followed by an integrase-specific recombination site, and can either exist in a nonfunctional circularized form or are expressed as part of an integron or transposon.[43] Over 100 gene cassettes have been described.[44]

Mosaicism

Intragenic recombination between a sensitive locus on the host bacterial chromosome and related genes from other bacterial species can result in mosaic genes and antimicrobial resistance.[20] This recombination-dependent mechanism occurs primarily by direct uptake of naked DNA and is therefore limited to organisms that are naturally transformable. Some mosaic alleles, or polymorphisms, are lost or are present only in low numbers due to decreased bacterial fitness. However, if a mosaic allele expresses a phenotype that is favored by antibiotic-selective pressure, the mosaic likely will survive and establish a new resistant population.[20] Examples of successful mosaicism are the penicillin-binding proteins (PBPs) in *Streptococcus pneumoniae* and the pathogenic

Neisseria species, and sulfonamide-resistant dihydropteroate synthase in *N. meningitidis*.[20,45–48]

MECHANISMS OF RESISTANCE

There are at least six basic mechanisms by which bacteria can develop resistance to antimicrobial agents and multiple mechanisms can act concurrently:[49]

1. Enzymatic inactivation
2. Alteration of the antimicrobial binding site
3. Active efflux
4. Alterations in membrane permeability to prevent antimicrobial entry
5. Alterations in enzymatic pathways so that the targeted enzyme is no longer essential for organism survival
6. Overproduction of antimicrobial targets.

In addition, slow rates of growth as seen in small colony variants or in organisms growing in biofilms also can contribute to resistance in vivo that is not detected readily in vitro using standard susceptibility test methods.[50,51]

Aminoglycosides

Antimicrobial resistance in aminoglycosides can be either intrinsic or acquired. Intrinsic resistance is primarily due to inability of these molecules to accumulate in the cytoplasm where they must bind to the 30S ribosome (composed of 16S rRNA and variety of proteins) to have antibacterial effect. This interferes with binding of tRNA to rRNA during translation resulting in inhibition of protein synthesis.[52,53] Aminoglycosides are actively transported into the bacterial cell by a three-step, energy-dependent process.[54] The energy necessary for this process is generated during aerobic respiration. Bacteria, when growing anaerobically, are not able to generate sufficient energy to "drive" this highly charged molecule into the cell.[54] As a result, all anaerobic organisms and those that depend on anaerobic metabolism (such as enterococci) are resistant to aminoglycosides.[52]

Clinically significant, acquired aminoglycoside resistance primarily is due to acquisition of extrachromosomal elements that encode enzymes that chemically modify aminoglycosides to render them unable to bind to the ribosomal target.[42] Three major classes of enzymes inactivate aminoglycosides, and are classified by the specific reaction catalyzed: (1) phosphotransferases (APH) that phosphorylate specific aminoglycoside hydroxyl groups; (2) acetyltransferases (AAC) that modify aminoglycosides via acetylation of selected amino groups; and (3) nucleotidyltransferase (ANT) that adenylates the aminoglycoside by adding AMP to selected hydroxyl groups. More than 100 different enzymes, including 7 classes of APH, 4 classes of AAC, and 5 classes of ANT, have been described.[55] Resistance in clinical isolates is dependent on the specific inactivating enzyme produced by the organism. For example, *P. aeruginosa* can harbor two different types of AAC(6′): one type inactivates tobramycin and amikacin whereas the other inactivates tobramycin and gentamicin.[56] Each enzyme type has variants that can degrade each of the clinically relevant aminoglycosides. However, certain enzyme types predominate. Because of its modified chemical structure, amikacin is not inactivated by as many of these enzymes, resulting in a broader spectrum of activity against gram-negative bacilli compared with gentamicin and tobramycin.[53] One of the predominant aminoglycoside-modifying enzymes among GNB in the U.S. is ANT(2″)I, which confers resistance to both tobramycin and gentamicin but not to amikacin.[55,57]

Aminoglycoside resistance is important among gram-positive organisms (GPOs) as well. In staphylococci, a unique bifunctional enzyme AAC(6′)-I-(APH 2″) produces modification in all three of the most commonly used aminoglycosides (tobramycin, gentamicin, and amikacin), resulting in resistance.[55] Although enterococci are intrinsically resistant to aminoglycosides because of impermeability, treatment with cell wall-active agents such as ampicillin or vancomycin can reverse this resistance, and in combination with an aminoglycoside, can result in synergistic killing.[55]

Resistance due to impermeability is referred as "low-level" resistance (gentamicin minimum inhibitory concentrations (MICs) 16 to 64 µg/mL).[58] High-level resistance also occurs (gentamicin MIC >500 µg/mL), especially among vancomycin-resistant *E. faecium* strains.[58] *E. faecium* strains have a chromosomally encoded AAC (6″)-I that confers resistance to tobramycin but not to gentamicin or streptomycin.[49] Gentamicin resistance in enterococci is due to enzymatic inactivation – primarily the AAC(6′)-I-APH(2″) enzyme.[58] Strains producing this enzyme can be susceptible to high levels of streptomycin.

Aminoglycoside resistance due to efflux of aminoglycosides occurs but is much less common than enzymatic modification.[56] This efflux pump is a three-component membrane structure consisting of the proteins MexX-MexY and an outer-membrane protein (Opr).[29] Both OprM and OprG act as pores in the outer membrane for these efflux pumps.[59,60]

Alteration of the antimicrobial binding site as a mechanism of acquired resistance is observed infrequently, and typically is due to mutation. Since there are multiple genes encoding ribosomes in most bacteria, the likelihood of having the same random mutational event occurring at the same loci in multiple genes is highly unlikely.[53] The lone exception is in *M. tuberculosis*. Because there is only a single ribosomal gene copy, ribosomal mutations can confer resistance to streptomycin.[52]

A second means of alteration of the aminoglycoside binding site has been recognized in a strain of *K. pneumoniae* that possesses a plasmid that encodes a 16S rRNA methyltransferase.[59] Modification of the 16S rRNA results in high-level resistance to gentamicin, tobramycin, and amikacin. Methyltransferase has significant sequence homology with enzymes from aminoglycoside-producing organisms, suggesting that it evolved naturally for self defense.[59] Ribosomal methylase has been found in transposons within plasmids, making horizontal transfer of this resistance gene likely.[61] The 16S rRNA methyltransferase has been detected among Enterobacteriaceae, *Acinetobacter*, and *Pseudomonas*.[62-64]

β-Lactams

Resistance to β-lactam agents is due primarily to production of β-lactamases or alteration in PBPs. In gram-negative organisms, β-lactamase production is the more important resistance mechanism, whereas alteration in PBPs plays a central role in gram-positive organisms, including *S. aureus*, *S. pneumoniae*, and *Enterococcus* spp. Organisms can harbor genes simultaneously that encode both resistance mechanisms, as is seen in methicillin-resistant *S. aureus* (MRSA).[49] Organisms can express >1 β-lactamase gene as well as multiple β-lactam resistance mechanisms concurrently, including β-lactamases, β-lactam efflux, and loss of outer-membrane protein porins (important in the periplasmic drug accumulation in gram-negative organisms (GNOs)).[49]

Classification Systems for β-Lactamases

β-Lactamases are enzymes that degrade the β-lactam ring. They can be encoded chromosomally or on extrachromosomal elements. In GPOs, they are excreted into the extracellular space, whereas in GNOs they are found in the periplasmic space. There are two major classification schemes for β-lactamases, the Ambler and the Bush–Jacoby–Medeiros systems.[33,61] The Ambler system classifies the enzyme into four different groups, A, B, C, D, based on the enzyme structure, whereas the Bush–Jacoby–Medeiros system is based on their substrate profile, i.e., which class of β-lactams is degraded and to what degree activity is inhibited by the β-lactamase inhibitor clavulanic acid.[33,61] In this scheme, organisms are grouped 1 to 4 with subclassification designated by letter, i.e., group 2b. Ambler type A, C, and D β-lactamases are classified as serine β-lactamases because they have serine at the enzyme's active site. Ambler type B enzyme (Bush–Jacoby–Medeiros group 3) is classified as a metalloenzyme because of the requirement for divalent cations, typically Zn^{2+}, at the active site.[33,61] Currently >850 β-lactamses are recognized (http://www.lahey.org/Studies/).[65]

Clinical Relevance of β-Lactam Resistance

The most common type A β-lactamases are TEM and SHV (Bush–Jacoby–Medeiros group 2b).[33] These β-lactamases degrade penicillin G, ampicillin, antipseudomonal penicillins, and first-generation cephalosporins. Clavulanic acid has excellent inhibitory activity against these enzymes and organisms producing these enzymes remain susceptible to aztreonam and third-generation cephalosporins.[65] Over 180 TEM-type enzymes and 130 different SHVs have been identified.[65] TEM frequently is found in *Escherichia coli*, *Haemophilus influenzae*, and *N. gonorrhoeae*, whereas SHV is found in a variety of Enterobacteriaceae and *Pseudomonoas aeruginosa*.[65] Mutations in the region of the active site of these enzymes can expand their spectra to hydrolyze aztreonam and third-generation cephalosporins such as cefotaxime and ceftazidime. Clavulanic acid continues to inhibit these enzymes and these organisms are still susceptible to cephamycins (cefoxitin) and carbapenems (imipenem).[65] Bacteria that are able to express this genotype are described as producing ESBLs.[65] Genes encoding ESBLs frequently are found on large plasmids, which also can encode resistance to other agents such as aminoglycosides and fluoroquinolones.[66] SHV and TEM-type ESBLs are observed most frequently in *E. coli*, *Proteus mirabilis*, and *K. pneumoniae*,[67] and bloodstream infections due to these organisms are associated with significantly increased morbidity and mortality.[68] The number of isolates that harbor ESBLs has increased dramatically over the last 5 years. It is not unusual for as many as 10% to20% of *E. coli* isolates to be both ESBL-producing and MDR.[69]

Another important class A ESBL is CTX-M, so designated because of preferential hydrolytic activity against cefotaxime compared with ceftazidime.[69] Over 90 different types of CTX-M have been identified,[70] and CTX-M has been disseminated on plasmids to many different Enterobacteriaceae, particularly to *Salmonella* strains originating in South America.[69] As with the TEM and SHV enzymes, organisms expressing CTX-M are resistant to all classes of penicillin, aztreonam, and first-, second-, and third-generation cephalosporins. Isolates expressing CTX-M remain susceptible to cephamycins and carbapenems, and like other type A ESBLs, this enzyme is inhibited by clavulanic acid and tazobactam.

The KPC enzymes are an emerging class A ESBL. ESBLs initially were associated most closely with *K. pneumoniae*; however, plasmids encoding KPC now are found in many Enterobacteriaceae. KPCs are an unusual class A ESBL because they can degrade carbapenems such as imipenem in addition to penicillins, aztreonam, and cephalosporins.[71] KPC-producing strains also typically are resistant to aminoglycosides and fluoroquinolones, leaving few therapeutic options.[71] KPC-type β-lactamases are inhibited by clavulanic acid and tazobactam, but isolates expressing KPC can be resistant to β-lactamase inhibitor/β-lactam combinations due to other resistance mechanisms encoded by the KPC-containing plasmid.[71]

The Ambler class B β-lactamases (Bush–Jacoby–Medeiros group 3) are enzymes that require divalent cations, typically Zn^{2+}, to hydrolyze the β-lactam ring.[72] All class B β-lactamases degrade imipenem and are inhibited by chelating agents such as ethylenediaminetetraacetic acid (EDTA) but not by clavulanic acid. The class B enzymes can be chromosomally encoded, as is seen with *Stenotrophomonas maltophilia*, or can be transferred by plasmids or transposons. The most commonly encountered transferable metallo-β-lactamases are IMP and VIM.[72] Metallo-β-lactamase-producing isolates also frequently are resistant to fluoroquinolones and aminoglycosides.[72] IMP is found most commonly in *P. aeruginosa* and *Acinetobacter baumanii* but also can be found in selected Enterobacteriaceae, particularly *Serratia marcescens*.[61] VIM is primarily found in *P. aeruginosa*, but has been reported in Enterobacteriaceae.[72] Aztreonam alone among the β-lactams may demonstrate activity against isolates expressing VIM or IMP.[73] The emergence of the new New Delhi metallo-β-lactamase (NDM) is of significant concern.[13,15] NDM-producing strains are resistant to all antibiotics except tigecycline and colisitin.[15] First seen in the United Kingdom in 2008, NDMs are now the most common carbapenemase-producing organisms recovered clinically in the

U.K.[15] Further, NDMs now have been found in the U.S.,[13] having been brought by patients who received health care in India. There is great concern about NDM spread in the industrialized world.

The Ambler class C β-lactamase (Bush–Jacoby–Medeiros group 1) is referred to as AmpC. AmpC can be chromosomally or plasmid encoded. Chromosomally encoded AmpC β-lactamases typically are inducible and result in low-level resistance to ampicillin, cefazolin, and cefoxitin.[74] Chromosomal AmpC typically is found in *Enterobacter* and *Serratia*.[74] Induction by cephamycin or carbapenems can result in high-level resistance to penicillin and first-, second-, and third-generation cephalosporins. AmpC is not inhibited by clavulanic acid.[65] Plasmid-encoded AmpC was first reported in *K. pneumoniae*. Plasmids carrying AmpC often carry resistance genes for a variety of antibiotics including aminoglycosides, fluoroquinolones, trimethoprim, and tetracylines.[74] Such organisms have constitutive AmpC production and as a result typically are resistant to penicillins including those used in combination with β-lactamase inhibitors, and first-, second- and third-generation cephalosporins.[74] Some, but not all, also are resistant to monobactams. Carbapenems are not degraded by AmpC and remain the best therapeutic option although isolates with mutation in outer-membrane porins can be resistant.[74] The clinical frequency of carbapenem-resistant, AmpC-producing organisms remains unclear.

The prototypic Ambler class D β-lactamase is the OXA family, so designated because of higher rate of hydrolysis of oxacillin compared with benzylpenicillin.[75] A number of OXA enzymes exhibit carbapenemase activity, although this may not confer resistance in vitro.[75] OXA enzymes are resistant to β-lactamase inhibitors.[76] Plasmid-encoded ESBL OXA enzymes have been found in *P. aeruginosa*.[77] However, the most clinically important OXA-carbapenemase-producing organism are *Acinetobacter*.[78] In *Acinetobacter*, OXA-carbapenemases can be encoded chromosomally or on plasmids. Such *Acinetobacter* are resistant to penicillins (including in combination with β-lactamase inhibitors), first-, second-, and third-generation cephalosporins, cefepime, and carbapenems. These isolates also are resistant to aminoglycosides and fluoroquinolones.[78] OXA-carbapenemase-producing *Acinetobacter* has spread globally over the past decade causing nosocomial outbreaks in numerous facilities.[78]

The most clinically relevant β-lactamase among GPOs is Ambler class A penicillinase produced by *S. aureus*, rendering resistance to β-lactams. Semisynthetic penicillins such as methicillin, oxacillin, nafcillin, and others were developed that were poorly hydrolyzed by the *S. aureus* penicillinase, thus maintaining clinical activity. Resistance soon developed in *S. aureus* to penicillinase-stable penicillins due to alteration at the specific penicillin binding protein (PBP) 2 target site. This modified PBP, designated PBP2a, has low affinity for all β-lactam antimicrobial agents.[79] PBP2a is encoded by the *mecA* gene, which when expressed confers resistance to all β-lactam agents.[79] Strains that contain *mecA* are designated as MRSA. Healthcare-associated MRSA (HA-MRSA) arose and frequently were resistant to other agents, including aminoglycosides, macrolides, and fluoroquinolones.[79,80] In the late 1990s, community-associated MRSA (CA-MRSA) appeared, differing from HA-MRSA. CA-MRSA strains, although resistant to β-lactams and containing *mecA*, frequently remain susceptible to other classes of antibiotics.[81] CA-MRSA strains typically carry the gene for Panton–Valentine leukocidin (which is associated with predilection for skin and soft-tissue infections, transmissibility, and virulence), a gene found infrequently in HA-MRSA.[82] CA-MRSA also has a *mecA* encoding region called the staphylococcal chromosomal cassette (SCC) *mec* type IVa, which is much smaller than the SCC most commonly encountered in HA-MRSA and does not contain genes for resistance to other agents.[82] CA-MRSA emerged globally in children, especially associated with soft-tissue infections; in one survey three-quarters of children with CA-S. *aureus* infection had MRSA.[83] The CA-MRSA genotype now has become a nosocomial pathogen in children[80] and virulence properties of CA-MRSA have arisen in MSSA.

With the redefining in 2008 of penicillin resistance for *S. pneumoniae* for non-meningeal isolates from a penicillin MIC ≥2 µg/mL to ≥8 µg/mL, and for meningeal isolates to penicillin MIC ≥0.12 µg/mL, restatement of the epidemiology of drug resistance among pneumococci is necessary.[84] Most isolates with penicillin MIC 2 to 4 µg/mL generally are susceptible to third-generation cephalosporins but frequently are resistant to other classes of antimicrobial agents, including macrolides, sulfonamides, and tetracycline.[85] Isolates with penicillin MIC ≥8.0 µg/mL frequently are resistant to third-generation cephalosporins.[86] Penicillin resistance is due to alterations in PBP2x, 2b, and 1a, resulting in reduced binding of β-lactams coupled with increased production of branched-structure muropeptides.[87,88] Resistance is believed to be encoded by mosaic PBP genes that were transferred to *S. pneumoniae* from commensal respiratory tract streptococci via transformation and recombination.[46]

Penicillins are the drug of choice for treating enterococcal infections[79] but resistance to cell wall-active agents, β-lactams, and vancomycin is common, especially among isolates of *E. faecium*.[79] Intrinsically resistant to cephalosporins and aminoglycosides, enterococci have acquired resistance to both ampicillin and vancomycin.[89] β-Lactamase does not play a role in ampicillin resistance of *E. faecium*.[90] Alteration in PBP5 may be responsible for low-level ampicillin resistance but assigning it a role in high-level resistance has proven problematic.[90]

β-Lactam resistance among *Haemophilus influenzae* can be due to β-lactamases (common) or modification in PBP3 (less common).[91–93] Infrequently, strains are identified that produce β-lactamase and also have altered PBP3.[93] Strains are resistant to ampicillin–β-lactamase inhibitor agents.[92,93] β-Lactamases of *H. influenzae* are Ambler type A and the encoding genes are on plasmids.[93] A recent survey of 6642 *H. influenzae* isolates collected globally identified 25% producing β-lactamase and 1% with altered PBP.[91] However, certain "hot-spots" (e.g., Japan and Spain) have higher rates of resistance due to PBPs.[92,94]

Both efflux mechanisms and alteration in permeability can play a role in β-lactam resistance, particularly among *P. aeruginosa* and *Acinetobacter*.[78,95] Resistance in *P. aeruginosa* to multiple drug classes (including selected β-lactams) can be attributed to the interplay of efflux pumps (most prominently the MexAB-OprM pump) with reduced or loss of expression of porins, OprF (β-lactams), and OprD (imipenem).[96,97] Carbapenem resistance in selected *P. aeruginosa* clinical isolates is due to the interplay of increased expression of efflux systems, decreased expression of the porin protein (OprD), and increased production of AmpC, which is a chromosomally encoded, inducible enzyme.[98] A similar interplay of multiple mechanisms has been observed in MDR-*Acinetobacter*.[76,78]

Chloramphenicol

Chloramphenicol inhibits protein synthesis by binding to the 50S ribosomal subunit and inhibiting peptide chain elongation.[99] The major chloramphenicol resistance mechanism is the acquisition of a chloramphenicol acetyltransferase (CAT). Acetylation prevents drug from binding to its target. Two biochemically distinct types of CAT molecules are designated A and B. The catA gene, which can be found on transposons and plasmids, is the more common and is found in a variety of organisms, including *S. aureus*, *Enterococcus*, *H. influenzae*, and *Salmonella* Typhi. The type B enzyme is produced by GNB such as *P. aeruginosa*, *Vibrio cholerae*, and *S.* Typhimurium.[99]

Genes specific for chloramphenicol efflux also occur among GNBs and have been found on gene clusters in *Salmonella* spp. that encode multiple resistance mechanisms, including β-lactamases and aminoglycoside-inactivating enzymes. Less commonly, bacteria such as *S.* Typhi that lack specific outer-membrane proteins such as OmpF also can be resistant to chloramphenicol.[99]

Colistin

Although it can be nephrotoxic, colistin use is re-emerging due to the increasing number of multidrug-resistant (MDR) gram-negative bacilli. Colistin has been used intravenously, or by aerosol in the case of *P. aeruginosa* exacerbations in CF.[100] However, colistin resistance also has been described,[101] and a number of bacteria are intrinsically resistant to colistin, including all GPOs, all anaerobic bacteria, and select GNB, including *Burkholderia cepacia*, *Proteus*, *Providencia*, and *Serratia* spp.

Colistin (a positively charge peptide) electrostatically interacts with the negatively charged lipid A component of lipopolysaccharide (LPS) in the outer membrane of GNOs. The drug also causes damage to the cytoplasmic membrane, resulting in permeability changes, leakage of cellular material, and ultimately cell lysis and death.[100]

Although reported, development of colistin resistance is uncommon, and transmission of resistance by extrachromosomal elements has not been described. Although the exact mechanism of resistance is uncertain, it is likely due to LPS modifications that decrease the negative charge of LPS and, therefore, lower drug binding affinity. The two-component regulatory systems PmrA-PmrB and PhoP-PhoQ appear to be important in the development of colistin resistance. PmrA-PmrB is essential for colistin resistance and regulates loci responsible for lipid A changes.[101] A number of mutations in *pmrA* or *pmrB* have been identified in colistin-resistant *Salmonella enterica* with apparent minimal fitness costs,[102] although significant fitness costs have been hypothesized for colistin-resistant *A. baumanni*.[103] Although the PmrA-PmrB system is regulated by PhoP-PhoQ, the latter two-component system does not appear to be essential for colistin resistance. However, PhoP-PhoQ upregulates the outer-membrane protein OprH, which is believed to contribute to colistin resistance by occupying membrane magnesium sites thereby reducing colistin binding sites.[101] Additionally, mutations in any of the first three genes of the lipid A biosynthesis pathway (*lpxA*, *lpxC*, and *lpxD*) confer colistin resistance in *A. baumannii*.[104] Colistin heteroresistant strains of *A. baumannii* that would not be detected by routine susceptibility testing are an increasing concern[105] but clinical significance remains to be determined.

Daptomycin

Daptomycin is an acidic cyclic lipopeptide antibiotic that acts in a calcium-dependent manner to disrupt the cell membrane potential and therefore its permeability. The exact mechanism of bacterial killing is unclear, but daptomycin appears to insert into phosphatidylglycerol rich membrane at the cell division septum.[106] Daptomycin also may act on a sensor kinase (YycG) localized at the cell septum leading to rapid cell death without lysis by interfering with the YycF-YycG two-component signal transduction cascade.[106] The *S. aureus* isolates with increased daptomycin MICs display enhanced cell membrane fluidity, increased net positive surface charge, and reduced daptomycin surface binding.[107] Stepwise mutations in several genes (including *mprF*, *yycG*, *rpoB*, and *rpoC*) have been associated with decreased susceptibility to daptomycin likely through effects on the cell wall or membrane.[106,108] Combined mutations, more than single mutations, are associated with higher MICs. Although most vancomycin-intermediate *S. aureus* and all vancomycin-resistant *S. aureus* strains maintain daptomycin susceptibility, there is a correlation between thickness of the *S. aureus* cell wall and nonsusceptibility to daptomycin (see vancomycin discussion below).[109] Most clinical failures of daptomycin involve infections associated with high bacterial load and/or subtherapeutic drug dosing.[110]

Isoniazid

Isoniazid (INH) inhibits a specific enzyme, InhA, in the synthetic pathway of mycolic acid, a key component of the cell wall of *M. tuberculosis*. In order to be active, INH must first be modified to its active form, a hydrazine derivative, by catalase produced by the organism.[111] Mutation in the catalase gene, *katG*, or genetic inactivation of the gene prevents formation of the hydrazine derivative, resulting in INH resistance. Multiple mutations or stop mutations are associated with higher levels of resistance.[112-114] In recent surveys of INH-resistant *M. tuberculosis* isolates, between 65% and

80% were resistant due to modification of the catalase gene.[115,116] A second resistance mechanism, a specific mutation in the *inhA* regulatory region which causes overexpression of *inhA* resulting in low-level INH resistance, was found in <10% to 25% of resistant isolates.[113,114] A recent study suggests that INH resistance can occur in isolates without *katG* or *inhA* genes; INH resistance would not be detected by current molecular detection methods.[113]

Linezolid

Linezolid is the only oxazolidinone approved by the Food and Drug Administration (FDA) for clinical use. Although linezolid inhibits protein synthesis, its unique mechanism of action is due to binding of 50S subunit near the interface with the 30S subunit, thus preventing the formation of the tRNA^{fMet}-70S ribosome-mRNA ternary complex. Even with increasing use, linezolid resistance is relatively uncommon. Recent worldwide surveillance data indicate the incidence of linezolid-resistant enterococci and coagulase-negative staphylococci is 0.5%, with no linezolid resistance among *S. aureus* isolates tested.[115]

The primary mechanism of resistance is specific nucleotide substitutions in the 23S rRNA, although mutations also have been described in ribosomal proteins L3 and L4.[115] Chromosomal mutations usually occur after prolonged linezolid exposure,[116] but have been described in linezolid-naive patients.[117-120] There is a clear association between the number of 23S rRNAs that are mutated and MIC values[121,122] and possibly the number of mutated 23S rRNAs and length of linezolid exposure.[123] Linezolid resistance also can be due to acquisition of the plasmid-encoded *cfr* gene that encodes a 23S rRNA methyltransferase, which alters the target site and confers resistance to other antibiotics.[124] Nosocomial outbreaks of linezolid-resistant *S. aureus* carrying the *cfr* gene have been described.[125,126] Transferable linezolid resistance has not been described for enterococci.

Macrolides and Related Compounds

Macrolides and related compounds act on the 50S ribosomal subunit by binding the peptidyltransferase region and stimulate the premature dissociation of peptidyl-tRNA from ribosomes. These antibiotics are bacteriostatic since they inhibit protein synthesis and include macrolides, lincosamides, streptogramins, and ketolides. Resistance occurs by alteration of target, active efflux, and antibiotic inactivation.[127] Macrolide resistance can occur as resistance to the 14- and 15-membered macrolides (erythromycin, clarithromycin, azithromycin) but not to 16-membered macrolides (spiramycin, josamycin), lincosamides (clindamycin), or streptogramin B (M phenotype); or resistance to all of the above (MLS$_B$ phenotype). M-type resistance generally confers low-level resistance among streptococci (MICs 1 to 32 µg/mL), whereas MLS$_B$ resistance commonly confers high-level resistance (MICs >256 µg/mL).

MLS$_B$ resistance is due to the methylation of the 23S rRNA, which blocks the ribosomal binding site (RBS) for macrolides, lincosamides, and streptogramin B. The methylase is encoded by *erm* (erythromycin ribosome methylase) genes and dimethylates adenine at position 2058, which prevents access to the target either directly or by conformational change.[127] The MLS$_B$ phenotype can be constitutively or inducibly synthesized (MLS$_B$-C or MLS$_B$-I). For MLS$_B$-I strains, *erm* mRNA is inactive in the absence of an inducing macrolide such as erythromycin. Through studies in *S. aureus*, the mechanism of inducibility has been shown to be stem-loop secondary structures in the 5′ *erm* mRNA regulatory region that sequester the RBS.[128] In the presence of low concentrations of erythromycin (the inducer), ribosomes stall in the *erm* regulatory region, resulting in the dissociation of stem-loop structures, which subsequently permits unmasking of the RBS, translation of the *erm* methylase, and the resistant phenotype. There are numerous reports of failed clindamycin therapy for MLS$_B$-I infections, with postulated microbial conversion from the MLS$_B$-I to the MLS$_B$-C phenotype.[128,129] Target alteration by mutations in L4 or L22 ribosomal proteins of the 50S subunit also have been described. These mutations may impair passive transport through the nascent peptide exit tunnel of the ribosome and distort the erythromycin binding site.[130] In *Mycoplasma pneumoniae* and *N. gonorrhoeae*, macrolide resistance is due to mutations in the 23S rRNA gene.[131,132]

M-type resistance is primarily associated with an active efflux system driven by proton motive force.[133] Chromosomally located macrolide efflux (*mef*) genes have been found in a number of bacterial genera, including *Streptococcus, Enterococcus, Staphylococcus, Granulicatella, Gemella, Neisseria,* and *Bacteroides* species,[134] and plasmid-encoded efflux genes (*msrA*) have also been identified in *Staphylococcus* species.[57] In pneumococci, *mef* gene is located on a transposon that can be transferred horizontally.[135,136] Highly resistant *S. pneumoniae* isolates that harbor both *erm* and *mef* resistance mechanisms are reported increasingly.[137]

Macrolide resistance due to drug inactivation rarely is found in clinical isolates and is found more commonly in macrolide-producing organisms as a survival mechanism.[138] *S. aureus* reportedly produces a phosphotransferase that inactivates macrolides but not lincosamides and is encoded by the *mphC* gene.[139] Nucleotidyltransferases encoded by *lnuA/linA* and *lnuB/linB* have been found in staphylococci and enterococci, resulting in inactivation of lincosamides, but not macrolides; low incidence precludes understanding of clinical significance.[139] Antibiotics with activity against MLS$_B$-resistant organisms include the bactericidal streptogramins (i.e., quinupristin-dalfopristin) and the bacteriostatic ketolides (i.e., telithromycin). Quinupristin-dalfopristin, a combination of two streptogramin factors A and B, act synergistically because of dual ribosomal action. Although *erm*-dependent methylation affects the streptogramin B component, synergy is still observed when both A and B components are present.[140] Ketolides are derived from clarithromycin, but are designed to overcome macrolide resistance. The ketolides have activity against MLS$_B$-resistant organisms likely due to >10-fold ribosomal binding affinity; they also do not act as inducers of MLS$_B$ resistance and are not grossly affected by macrolide efflux.[141] Although relatively low numbers of telithromycin-resistant strains have been reported to date,[137] decreased susceptibility to telithromycin has been described among *S. pneumoniae* with mutations in the *erm* mRNA regulatory region, as well as mutations in L4 and L22 ribosomal proteins.[141] Efflux-positive telithromycin-resistant pneumococci have been described as well as efflux-positive *Streptococcus pyogenes* that show decreased telithromycin susceptibility.[142]

Metronidazole

Metronidazole has bactericidal activity against a broad spectrum of anaerobic bacteria and selected protozoans. Metronidazole is a prodrug that is reduced in the cytoplasm by a nitroreductase enzyme; resulting toxic intermediates disrupt nucleic acid structure.[143] It is particularly useful in treating mixed anaerobic infections in which *Bacteroides* or *Prevotella* spp. predominate, and is a widely used therapy for *Clostridium difficile* infection.[143,144] In a recent U.S. survey of *Bacteroides*, metronidazole resistance was found in <1% of isolates.[145]

Metronidazole resistance mechanisms have been best described in *Bacteroides* spp. Resistance is due to the activity of the enzyme nitroimidazole reductase, which catalyzes the conversion of 4- or 5-nitroimidazole to 4- or 5-aminoimidazole. The enzymatic modification prevents the formation of toxic drug intermediates, the active form of metronidazole.[146] This enzyme is encoded on the *nim* gene, has 7 variants described, and can be encoded chromosomally or on plasmids.[147] This gene has been found in *Bacteroides, Helicobacter,* and *Prevotella.*[148,149]

Clinical resistance to metronidazole among *C. difficile* and *H. pylori* is well documented although demonstration in vitro and understanding of the mechanism has proven difficult.[150,151] Emerging data suggest that efflux pumps also may play a role in metronidazole resistance among *Helicobacter.*[150] Heteroresistance to metronidazole has been described in one study in approximately 6% of *C. difficile* isolates directly isolated from clinical specimens.[150] This phenotype, however, is unstable. The mechanism of metronidazole resistance/clinical failure for *C. difficile* currently is unknown. *C. difficile* does not harbor *nim.*[150,152]

Quinolones

Ciprofloxacin reportedly is the most consumed antibacterial agent worldwide,[153,154] and also has widespread use in animals. Multiple resistance mechanisms exist: mutations in target enzymes, changes in intracellular drug concentrations via altered entry and efflux, modification of the drug by bacterial enzymes, and inhibition protection of target enzymes. Quinolones and subsequent derivatives such as the fluoroquinolones act by binding to enzymes that are essential for bacterial replication, transcription, recombination, and DNA repair – DNA gyrase and topoisomerase IV.[155] These enzymes make double-stranded DNA (dsDNA) breaks in the chromosome and introduce negative DNA supercoils to allow subsequent activities such as replication. Quinolones trap and release this dsDNA break intermediately, resulting in activation of the stress (SOS) response and ultimately cell death.

Gyrase and topoisomerase IV comprise two pairs of subunits (A and B). The primary quinolone target appears to be gyrase A (*gyrA*) in GNOs and topoisomerase IV subunit A (*parC*) in GPOs.[154] The most common mutations are in quinolone resistance determining region (QRDR) of *gyrA*. The QRDR of *gyrA* spans amino acids 51 to 106 (*E. coli* numbering) near the catalytic DNA-binding residue Tyr122 of the enzyme; mutational hot spots occur at Ser83 and Asp87.[155] A first-step *gyrA* mutation results in high-level resistance to naladixic acid, but not to fluoroquinolones. When a second mutation occurs either in *gyrA*, or in another quinolone target such as *parC*, high-level resistance to the fluoroquinolones occurs. The same phenomenon has been demonstrated in GPOs, with the first-step mutation generally occurring in *parC*.

Once the primary mutation occurs in either *gyrA* or *parC* (and, more rarely, the B subunit genes, *gyrB* or *parE*), additional mechanisms of resistance can contribute to high-level fluoroquinolone resistance other than secondary mutations in gyrase/topoisomerase IV genes. These include altered permeability and/or efflux. Altered permeability in the absence of other mutations causes low-level resistance and contributes to quinolone resistance in GNOs,[156] and is mediated by decreased expression of outer-membrane porins and/or alterations in the LPS composition that decreases drug entry into cells.[154] Nonspecific adenosine triphosphate-dependent efflux systems also have been described in a number of GNB and GPOs, including *E. coli, P. aeruginosa, S. maltophilia, A. baumannii, S. pneumoniae, S. aureus,* and mycobacteria.[56,154,155] Due to their nonspecific nature, many of the efflux pumps require overexpression to result in the quinolone-resistant phenotype.

All of the above quinolone resistance mechanisms are chromosomally encoded, indicating that quinolone resistance is spread by clonal expansion. Although gyrase and topoisomerase gene mutations are the main mechanisms of quinolone resistance, multiple resistance mechanisms encoded on plasmids can contribute.[157] The Qnr determinant is located on a plasmid-encoded integron, being first described in *K. pneumoniae* and subsequently in *E. coli* and *Enterobacter cloacae.*[155,158–160] The Qnr protein binds and protects DNA gyrase and topoisomerase IV from inhibition by ciprofloxacin.[159] Like first-step *gyrA* mutations, Qnr only causes low-level resistance in the absence of other resistance mechanisms. Commonly, *qnr*-containing plasmids also encode for an AmpC or ESBL.[161,162]

Additional plasmid-encoded genes have been found that also can contribute to quinolone resistance, albeit minor to date.[163] These include a plasmid-encoded aminoglycoside acetyltransferase (AAC(6′)-Ib-cr) that can modify both ciprofloxacin and norfloxacin but not other fluoroquinolones, and efflux pumps (OqxAB and QepA) that appear to be fairly specific for the quinolones.

Rifampin

Rifampin targets the β-subunit of bacterial DNA-dependent RNA polymerase encoded by the gene *rpoB*. Point mutations in *rpoB* can result in amino acid substitutions, decreased binding and resistance.[164] Mutations in *rpoB* have been detected in a variety of bacteria, notably in *S. aureus*,[165] *N. meningitidis*,[166] and *M. tuberculosis*.[167] Because point mutations can result in high-level resistance, rifampin is rarely used alone in order to prevent emergence of resistance. Rifampin resistance does not always persist, suggesting that resistance mutations may adversely affect bacterial fitness.[166] Other mechanisms of resistance to rifampin including rifampin modifying enzymes and efflux pumps are found in environmental GPOs such as *Nocardia* and *Mycobacterium* and GNBs such as *S. maltophilia* and *B. cenocepacia*. Clinical significance of these mechanisms compared with *rpoB* mutations is minor.[168]

Tetracyclines

Tetracyclines have been in use since the 1950s for the broad-spectrum treatment of infections due to gram-negative and gram-positive organisms, including intracellular pathogens such as *Chlamydia, Rickettsia,* and *Mycoplasma*. Widespread use of tetracyclines since the 1950s as therapeutic agents in adults, as a growth promoter in both animals and plants, and as long-term subtherapeutic treatment of noninfectious conditions, has led to substantial resistance.[169] Tetracycline resistance mechanisms have been identified in >75 bacterial genera.[170,171] Doxycycline, minocycline, and a minocycline-derived glycylcycline, tigecycline, are used most frequently.[172] Tigecycline has the same mode of action as other tetracyclines, but is active in the presence of tetracycline resistance genes due to steric hindrance introduced by an additional side chain.[173]

Tetracyclines are bacteriostatic, reversibly inhibiting protein synthesis by binding to the 30S ribosome and preventing elongation by inhibiting tRNA association. Relatively infrequent intrinsic mechanisms of resistance include mutations in outer-membrane porins or LPS that alter cell wall permeability and mutations in the 16S rRNA.[170] Additionally, mutations, such as those that result in upregulation, can allow existing efflux pumps to export tetracyclines (including tigecycline).[172,174,175]

Resistance is most commonly due to the acquisition of genes that encode tetracycline-specific efflux pumps and ribosomal protection proteins. These genes often are located on mobile elements, including plasmids, transposons, and integrons.[169] Of the 40 different tetracycline resistance genes (*tet* and *otr*) described, 26 encode efflux pumps, 11 encode ribosomal protection proteins, and 3 encode tetracycline inactivating enzymes.[171,176] In addition, there are 4 mosaic genes encode ribosomal protection proteins that confer tetracycline resistance. The majority of the efflux genes are found only in GNOs, but two (*tetK* and *tetL*) are found primarily in GPOs. All of these genes except *tetB* confer resistance to tetracycline and doxycycline; *tetB*-containing isolates also are resistant to minocycline, but not to tigecycline. However, in vitro mutations in *tetA* and *tetB* have been produced that result in tigecycline resistance.[177] The genes that encode ribosomal protection proteins confer resistance to tetracycline, doxycycline, and minocycline, TetO and TetM being the most widely distributed determinants. Bearing sequence similarity to translation elongation factors, ribosomal protection proteins appear to be ribosome-binding guanosine triphosphatases that dislodge tetracycline from the ribosome.[171,176,178] The ribosomal protection proteins are found in a variety of bacteria, including GPOs, nonenteric GNOs, and anaerobic bacteria, and often are linked to other resistance genes, such as *erm*.[169,176] Little is known regarding the action or clinical relevance of tetracycline-inactivating enzymes, which appear to be NADPH-requiring oxidoreductases,[179,180] or the roles of reduced antibiotic permeability and target modification in tetracycline resistance.

Trimethoprim-Sulfamethoxazole (TMP-SMX)

Although no longer recommended for treatment of otitis media,[181,182] TMP-SMX has broad use, such as for treatment of skin and soft-tissue infection due to CA-MRSA.[183]

TMP-SMX acts by inhibiting two steps in bacterial folic acid synthesis. Sulfamethoxazole inhibits dihydropteroate synthetase, blocking the formation of dihydrofolate, while trimethoprim inhibits dihydrofolate reductase (DHFR), blocking the formation of tetrahydrofolate. Intrinsic resistance is recognized in *Bacteroides, Neisseria,* and *Clostridium* species due to poor TMP binding to DHFR molecules.[184] TMP resistance can be due to overproduction of DHFR due to mutation in the promoter region controlling its synthesis or to mutations in the *dhfr* gene that result in decreased binding.[184] Resistance to SMX is due to alteration in its target, dihydropteroate synthetase, via point mutation or acquisition of extrachromosomal elements.[184] In *S. pneumoniae,* mutation in the *dhfr* gene resulting in reduced TMP binding plays a central role in TMP-SMX resistance; resistance can be transferred to other strains of pneumococci by transformation.[185]

In patients with cystic fibrosis who have received long-term TMP-SMX treatment for chronic *S. aureus* infection, *S. aureus* become resistant by bypassing the synthetic pathway inhibited by TMP-SMX, becoming auxotrophs for thymidine, a major end-product of this synthetic pathway.[186] Phenotypically, colonies of these thymidine-dependent *S. aureus* strains appear aberrant on sheep blood agar, with a fried-egg appearance and a colony size much smaller than the wild-type strains. So-called "small colony variants (SCV)," although not as fit as wild-type strains, can persist long term in CF patients.[51] SCV-*S. aureus* when occurring in osteomyelitis in children have been found to be refractory to antimicrobial therapy requiring long-term therapy.[187] It is now recognized that mutation in thymidylate synthase encoded by *thyA* is responsible for thymidine dependency.[188] This enzyme catalyzes the conversion of dUMP to dTMP in the thymidine pathway essential for DNA synthesis. Interestingly SCV-*S. aureus* have been shown to be hypermutators. SCV-*S. aureus* is a model for other SCV organisms found in CF patients including SCV-*P. aeruginosa, S. maltophilia,* and *B. cepacia* complex.[189]

Vancomycin

Increased use of vancomycin in the 1980s as oral therapy for *Clostridium difficile* colitis, treatment for MRSA infections, and the increase in glycopeptide use in animal husbandry has been associated with increasing resistance among GPOs.[190-192] Since vancomycin acts by binding an essential substrate for cell wall biosynthesis, it is perhaps not surprising that high-level resistant organisms that were fit enough to survive took some time.

The in vitro activity of vancomycin is considered bacteriostatic or slowly bactericidal owing to its mode of action on the cell wall of GPOs. Vancomycin binds to the D-Ala-D-Ala C-terminus of peptidoglycan precursors, blocking their addition to the growing peptidoglycan chain and preventing the subsequent transglycosylation and transpeptidation steps of cell wall biosynthesis. Since vancomycin must penetrate the peptidoglycan to reach its target, and there are many D-Ala-D-Ala residues in the cell wall, vancomycin is a relatively inefficient drug at obtaining high concentrations around its real targets since drug molecules also become bound by false targets in the peptidoglycan;[193] this phenomenon contributes to slow bactericidal activity. Mechanisms of vancomycin resistance identified to date are: decreased permeability due to cell wall changes; increased intermediate products that are bound; and altered target site.[194]

Enterococci have developed two separate, yet similar, mechanisms of vancomycin resistance. The *van* genes encode the resistance phenotype. Several *van* genes have been described and are characterized by MIC values of vancomycin and teicoplanin, transferability, genetic location in the bacterial host (chromosome versus transposon/plasmid), inducible or constitutive expression, and the modified target produced.[41] High-level resistance (MIC ≥64 µg/mL), generally found in *E. faecium* and *E. faecalis,* generally is conferred by *vanA, vanB,* or *vanD; vanA* and *vanB* display inducible vancomycin resistance whereas *vanD*-mediated resistance is constitutive. The *vanA*-containing organisms are by far the most common in both Europe and the U.S. The *vanA* and *vanB* operons can be located on transposons (i.e., Tn*1546* and Tn*916*-like), which are transferable via plasmids or can be found on large, mobile chromosomal elements.[41,89,195] The transferability of *vanA* and *vanB* genes is the basis for infection control measures to monitor and prevent the spread of vancomycin-resistant enterococci (VRE). Enterococci containing *vanD* appear to carry the gene on the chromosome, and it is thought that this gene is not transferable.[196] The genes *vanA/B/D* encode ligase enzymes that change the acyl-D-Ala-D-Ala C-terminus of lipid II peptidoglycan precursors to acyl-D-Ala-D-Lac (lactate). This altered ligation results in the alteration of the binding site of vancomycin and, thus, ~1000-fold lower affinity for its target.[197] The enzymes needed for this substitution are a D-lactate dehydrogenase (*vanH*), a D-Ala-D-Ala dipeptidase (*vanX*), and a D-Ala-D-Lac ligase (*vanA/B/D*); these enzymes are co-regulated in an operon by a two-component sensor kinase/response regulator pair (*vanS/vanR*).[198] This two-component regulation in response to environmental stimuli and mutations is responsible for the inducible and constitutive vancomycin-resistant phenotypes that are observed among *vanA/B/D*-containing species.[199,200]

Low-level resistance (MIC 2 to 32 µg/mL), found in *Enterococcus gallinarum*, *E. casseliflavus*, and *E. flavescens*, is encoded by the *vanC* genes (*vanC1*, *vanC2*, *vanC3*, respectively). The substitution of acyl-D-Ala-D-Ala with acyl-D-Ala-D-Ser results in an approximately 6-fold lower affinity of vancomycin for its peptidoglycan precursor target.[201] *E. gallinarum* demonstrates constitutive low-level vancomycin resistance, whereas *E. casseliflavus* and *E. flavescens* show inducible low-level resistance (requires 3 to 4 hours in the presence of vancomycin before phenotype is expressed). The two-component regulatory genes for the *vanC*-containing organisms show high homology to the *vanS/R* system of *vanA*-containing species. Unlike *vanA/B*, *vanC* genes are encoded chromosomally and are nontransferable. Therefore, *vanC*-containing species are not considered "true" VRE for infection control purposes. The *vanE* and *vanG* genes are transferable, are found in *E. faecalis* at low frequency, result in acyl-D-Ala-D-Ser peptidoglycan precursors, and confer low-level vancomycin resistance.

Vancomycin resistance can occur in *S. aureus*, including vancomycin-resistant *S. aureus* (VRSA; MIC ≥16 µg/mL) and vancomycin-intermediate *S. aureus* (VISA; MIC 4 to 8 µg/mL). First isolated in 2002, 11 cases of VRSA have been confirmed in the U.S., with 8 isolates from Michigan.[202-204] All VRSA strains tested carry the *vanA* ligase gene, likely originating from a coinfecting/colonizing VRE.[49] Experimentally, *vanA* can be transferred from VRE to *S. aureus*, *Streptococcus sanguinis*, *Lactococcus lactis*, *S. pyogenes*, and *Listeria monocytogenes* via conjugation,[205,206] and case reports indicate that *vanA* also has been transferred to the lactococci, *Cellulosimicrobium* (formerly *Oerskovia*) and *Arcanobacterium* species.[207,208] Risk factors of patients with VRSA infections include older age, compromised blood flow to lower limbs, chronic ulcers, a history of vancomycin therapy, and concomitant or previous isolation of MRSA and/or VRE.[209,210] To date, no VRSA have been found in children. VRSA strains have high MIC values and are detectable readily by routine antimicrobial susceptibility testing; VISA strains have lower MICs, are heterogeneous, and are more difficult to detect.

The mechanism of resistance for VISA strains appears to be a thickened cell wall; VISA isolates do not carry *van* genes.[49] VISA isolates typically have multiple metabolic mutations,[193,211] but the only strict correlation with the VISA phenotype is a thickened cell wall, as shown by electron microscopy.[212] This thickened cell wall, which acts to sequester or "clog" vancomycin in the peptidoglycan, is postulated to reduce susceptibility.[193,213] Some populations of *S. aureus* contain daughter cells that show increased vancomycin MICs of 1 to 4 µg/mL; this is referred to as heterogeneous VISA (hVISA). Although still "susceptible," hVISA subpopulations can proliferate and become the dominant clone under the selective pressure of vancomycin use.[213] Stepwise mutations in certain loci (i.e., the two-component systems GraR-GraS and VraR-VraS) can lead to an hVISA phenotype and then to a true VISA phenotype.[211] Although concerning, the clinical significance of the hVISA phenotype is uncertain.

Certain GPOs are intrinsically resistant to vancomycin, including *Erysipelothrix*, *Leuconostoc*, *Pediococcus*, and *Lactobacillus*.[214] Although these organisms' peptidoglycan precursors end in D-Ala-D-Lac, there is no cross-hybridization between their genomes and the *van* genes from the enterococci, nor polymerase chain reaction (PCR) amplification using multiple primer sets to enterococcal *van* genes.[215,216] *Leuconostoc* D-Ala-D-Lac ligases appear to have evolved independently from the enterococcal *vanA/B/D* ligases, perhaps due to the abundance of lactate in the environment for these organisms.[216] The mechanism of vancomycin resistance in *Erysipelothrix* is unknown.

DETECTION OF ANTIMICROBIAL RESISTANCE

Antimicrobial resistance can be detected using techniques that rely on either phenotypic characteristics of an organism or assessment for genes encoding specific types of resistance. Phenotypic antimicrobial susceptibility testing better predicts resistance, i.e., identifying antimicrobial agents that will be ineffective, than therapeutic effectiveness (susceptibility).[217] Besides intrinsic antibacterial activity, therapeutic effectiveness depends on multiple factors, such as the site of infection, penetration of the agent, and local environmental conditions such as pH and oxygen tension; the mode of growth of the organism (planktonic versus biofilm); pharmacokinetics of the agent and the dosing regimen being used; the immune status of the patient; and adherence to the antimicrobial regimen.[217]

Establishment of Breakpoints

The breakpoints used to determine the susceptibility of a specific organism are based on four types of data, and are assigned by the Clinical and Laboratory Standards Institute (CLSI).[217] First, MICs for bacterial isolates with no known resistance mechanisms are tested to determine the level of activity of a drug against a particular group of organisms. Second, MICs are determined for organisms that are likely to be resistant based on the presence of specific resistance mechanisms in order to find a bimodal distribution pattern in which the specific drug is highly active against the "susceptible" organisms (with low MICs) and poor activity against the "resistant" organisms (with high MICs). Some antimicrobial agents lack a clear bimodal distribution (e.g., polymyxins); newly developed drugs may not have a testable resistant population to characterize (e.g., linezolid). Third, the pharmacokinetics-pharmacodynamics (PK-PD) of the particular drug in serum and occasionally other body compartments such as the central nervous system or urinary tract are considered. Fourth, performance of the drug in clinical trials is considered. Once breakpoints are established and all the regulatory requirements are met, susceptibility can be tested clinically. Susceptibility testing should not be performed when susceptibility (penicillin for *Streptococcus pyogenes*) or resistance (vancomycin for Enterobacteriaceae) is predictable. Susceptibility also should not be performed when in vitro activity is known not to correlate with therapeutic efficacy (cephalosporins for *Listeria monocytogenes*).[218]

Methods of Susceptibility Testing

The reference method or "gold standard" for phenotypic susceptibility testing is MIC determinations. Depending on the organism, testing can be done by either broth microdilution or agar dilution.[218] Automated commercial test systems, such as Vitek (bioMérieux, Hazelwood, MO), Phoenix (BD Bioscience, Sparks, MD), and MicroScan (Dade-Behring, Sacramento, CA), which employ modification of these methods, are used widely. These systems are fast, mechanically reliable, highly reproducible, offer significant cost efficiencies (including interfacing with clinical information systems), and combine susceptibility testing and organism identification in one system. Automated susceptibility testing, however, is not as accurate as reference methods, particularly for detecting inducible resistance and other emerging resistance.[219] Software changes are introduced to address problems but

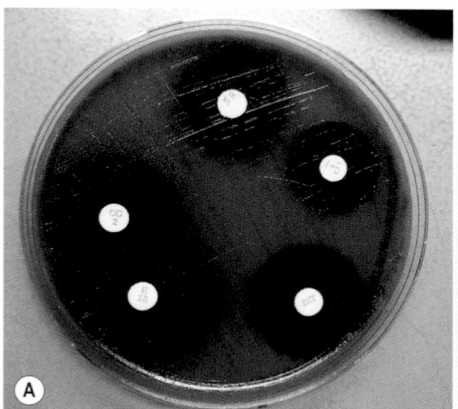
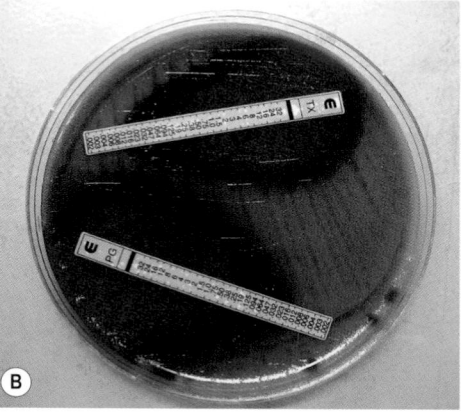

Figure 290-1. Routine susceptibility testing of *Streptococcus pneumoniae*. **(A)** Kirby–Bauer disk diffusion. Disks, counterclockwise from top: vancomycin, levofloxacin, trimethoprim/sulfamethoxazole, erythromycin, and clindamycin. **(B)** Minimum inhibitory concentration (MIC) determination by E-test. TX, ceftriaxone; PG, penicillin. This isolate was susceptible to all antimicrobial agents tested, with ceftriaxone and penicillin MICs of 0.064 µg/mL.

organisms evolve to develop resistance faster than changes can be developed and validated. Perpetually, systems may be a step behind. For example, in mid 2010, CLSI lowered carbapenem susceptibility breakpoints for meropenem and imipenem 4-fold (from ≤4 µg/mL to ≤1 µg/mL) because some carbapenemase-producing Enterobacteriaceae have carbapenem MICs as low as 0.125 µg/mL.[220] But because the automated susceptibility systems are diagnostic devices regulated by the FDA, susceptibility test system manufacturers must perform a complex validation process before breakpoints can be changed on their systems, thus causing conundrums for both laboratorians and clinicians.

In addition to microdilution methods, used by approximately 80% of laboratories in the U.S., disk diffusion susceptibility is used by approximately 15% of laboratories.[219] Disk diffusion testing relies on the use of disks impregnated with specific concentration for each drug. Antimicrobial containing disks are applied to a lawn of bacteria inoculated on a standard medium and, after 16 to 24 hours' incubation, zones of inhibition are measured (Figure 290-1A). Zones of inhibition correlate reasonably well with specific MIC values. Breakpoints for susceptible, intermediate, or resistant have been previously determined for each antibiotic disk based on zone size. Disk diffusion consistently is more accurate than automated commercial systems compared with reference methods,[219] is more flexible for choosing drugs for testing, and may better detect emerging resistance problems.[219] Disadvantages of disk diffusion testing are its labor-intensiveness, less reproducibility because of manual measurement of inhibition zones, lack of breakpoints for all clinically relevant bacteria, and proneness to clerical errors because of manual entry of results into clinical information systems.

Etest (AB Biodisk, Solna, Sweden) is performed in a manner similar to disk diffusion but instead of a disk being placed on a lawn of bacteria, a plastic strip impregnated with a gradient of a specific antimicrobial agent is tested.[221] After appropriate incubation, the MIC is read where the elliptical zone of inhibition of growth meets the strip. Although not as highly standardized as disk diffusion, Etests are particularly useful and accurate compared with reference MIC methods for determining antimicrobial susceptibility for organisms that are fastidious or have a narrow range between drug concentrations considered as susceptible and resistant. For example, determining MICs of penicillin and ceftriaxone for *S. pneumoniae* is best performed by Etest[222] (Figure 290-1B).

Screening for High-Level Aminoglycoside Resistance

All enterococci demonstrate low-level resistance to aminoglycosides but can acquire high-level resistance primarily via production of aminoglycoside-modifying enzymes.[58] Unlike strains with low-level intrinsic resistance, strains with high-level aminoglycoside resistance do not show synergistic inhibition by cell

wall-active agents.[58] Standard susceptibility testing cannot differentiate intrinsic low-level resistance from acquired high-level (gentamicin MICs of >500 µg/mL) resistance. Disks containing high concentrations of gentamicin and streptomycin are highly accurate in detecting high-level resistance compared with reference MIC methods. High level gentamicin resistance of *Enterococcus* also predicts high-level resistance to tobramycin and amikacin.

Molecular Methodologies

Molecular detection is quickly becoming the gold standard in clinical microbiology, particularly in cases where a specific pathogen and/or resistance gene is sought. The molecular detection of clinically relevant resistance can be accomplished using probe hybridization, nucleic acid amplification technologies (NAAT) such as PCR, and DNA sequencing.

Probe detection occurs by hybridization, or annealing, of a labeled probe to a target sequence. The target sequence is released from organisms during lysis, which is followed by hybridization in either a liquid or solid phase. The probe acts to capture the target sequence of interest from a milieu of sequences. The use of solid-phase hybridization on nitrocellulose (i.e., line probe assays) allows for the detection of multiple sequences or polymorphisms from a single preparation. The most commonly used NAAT is PCR and real-time PCR. Real-time PCR (rt-PCR) uses sequence-specific primers and probes to detect gene(s) of interest. Incorporation of the probe detection in the same reaction vessel as the amplification process allows for less contamination, faster turnaround time, and greater sensitivity and specificity compared with traditional NAAT detection platforms. The use of fluorescent probes in rt-PCR allows for the detection of resistance related to acquired genes as well as to intrinsic gene polymorphisms. (See Espy et al.[223] for technology and role of rt-PCR in clinical microbiology).

DNA sequencing can be used to detect resistance mechanisms that rely on intrinsic gene mutations and demonstrate a strict genotype/phenotype correlation. Sequencing and subsequent mutation analysis has long been applied to the detection of antiviral resistance in HIV and, more recently, cytomegalovirus. The use of sequencing for the detection of antimicrobial resistance in bacteria is still largely reserved for research and public health applications. Sequence-based resistance detection in *M. tuberculosis*, for example, detects mutations for rifampin and isoniazid resistance with 97% and 91% sensitivity, respectively, and for ethambutol, pyrazinamide, fluoroquinolone, and kanamycin/capreomycin/amikacin resistance with varying sensitivities.[224]

The interpretation of molecular detection of antimicrobial resistance results can be complicated when: (1) the resistance mechanism is multifactorial; (2) there is an uncertain cause-and-effect, genotype–phenotypic resistance relationship clinically; (3) the infection is polyclonal; or (4) there is synergy among multiple resistance phenotypes. Use should be limited to organisms and

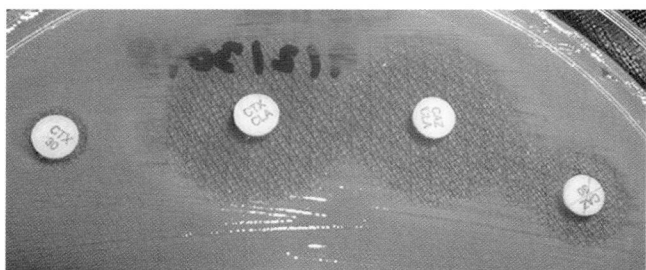

Figure 290-2. Disk diffusion testing for extended spectrum β-lactamase (ESBL) production in *Klebsiella*. Disks, left to right: CTX (cefotaxime), CTX/CLA (cefotaxime + clavulanic acid), CAZ/CLA (ceftazidime + clavulanic acid), CAZ (ceftazidime). Inhibition zones are measured, and an increase of 5 mm in the clavulanic acid-containing disk relative to the corresponding cephalosporin alone indicates production of an ESBL. This isolate produces an ESBL.

infections in which the results can be interpreted with confidence for clinical treatment and/or infection control practices.

SPECIAL CONSIDERATIONS

Detection of ESBL

All *E. coli*, *K. pneumoniae*, *K. oxytoca*, and *Proteus mirabilis* should be screened for the presence of ESBLs if they demonstrate resistance or reduced susceptibility to extended-spectrum cephalosporins. In 2010, CLSI proposed lower cephalosporin breakpoints.[220] Implementation of these lower breakpoints precludes the need for confirmatory testing as ESBL-producing organisms will be interpreted as resistant. However, most automated susceptibility testing systems cannot accommodate these lower breakpoints as the concentration of drug tested is not low enough for some of the cephalosporins. Confirmatory testing is warranted if the revised breakpoints cannot be implemented.

Both phenotypic and molecular methods can be used to detect ESBLs.[67,218] A widely used, highly accurate phenotypic method employs combination disks containing clavulanic acid with either ceftazidime or cefotaxime, versus the cephalosporins alone. If the zone size of inhibition around the combination disk is ≥5 mm around the cephalosporin alone, the isolate is considered to be an ESBL-producer (Figure 290-2).[67,218] Other phenotypic approaches include Etests and MIC tests that detect ≥3-fold lowering by clavulanic acid of MIC of the extended-spectrum cephalosporin. Most automated susceptibility testing systems also include a screen for ESBL production, with acceptable sensitivity and specificity. Using PCR detection of resistance genes as the gold standard, multiple phenotypic methods may be needed to reach optimal sensitivity and specificity.[225] Chromogenic agars can identify possible ESBL-producing isolates for further confirmation, with reported sensitivities of 95% to 97% and specificities of 94% to 95% when testing non-AmpC-producing organisms.[226,227] Because of the wide range of genes encoding ESBLs, molecular approaches are limited to research settings, although multiplex rt-PCR and microarray technologies offer promise for accurate ESBL detection.[228]

Detection of Carbapenem Resistance

Carbapenemase production in Enterobacteriaceae is signaled by decreased susceptibility, although not necessarily resistance, to carbapenems (e.g., MIC ≥2 μg/mL). For Enterobacteriaceae with MIC ≥2 μg/mL of ertapenem, imipenem, or meropenem, confirmatory testing for carbapenemase production should be performed by the modified Hodge test (MHT).[218,229] In the MHT, ertapenem and meropenem disks are placed on a lawn of a susceptible control strain of *E. coli*. A loopful of test organism (one with increased carbapenem MIC) is inoculated in a straight line out from the edge of the disk (Figure 290-3). After incubation,

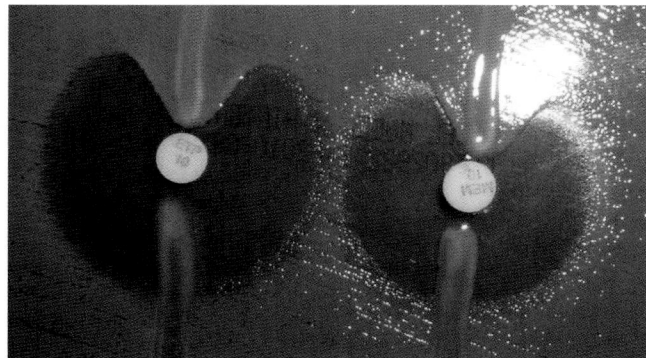

Figure 290-3. Modified Hodge test for the detection of carbapenemase-producing Enterobacteriaceae. A lawn of *Escherichia coli* ATCC 25922 is spread on Mueller–Hinton agar and two disks (10 μg ertapenem and a 10 μg meropenem) are placed in the center of the plate a minimum of 30 mm apart. Test organisms are struck away from the disk with each streak being a minimum of 25 mm. The test organism struck at the top permits growth enhancement of the sensitive *E. coli* strain, indicating production of carbapenemase. No growth enhancement is seen with the test organism struck at the bottom, indicating no production of carbapenemase.

enhanced growth of the control *E. coli* strain at the intersection of the test streak and the carbapenem zone of inhibition indicates carbapenemase production by the test organism. When carbapenemase is detected, resistance is reported for all carbapenems regardless of MICs. Chromogenic agars have been developed for the detection of carbapenem-resistant Enterobacteriaceae. Compared with PCR, sensitivity and specificity of CHROMagar KPC were 100% and 98%, respectively;[230] positive predictive and negative predictive values were calculated as 100% and 99%, respectively.[231] Chromogenic agars may be most beneficial for rectal surveillance cultures. CLSI carbapenem breakpoints also were lowered in mid-2010.[218] If the new, lower breakpoints can be implemented, confirmatory MHT is no longer required unless needed for epidemiologic studies.

Detection of Methicillin/Oxacillin Resistance

Several approaches can be used to detect β-lactam resistance due to altered PBPs in *S. aureus*. The "gold standard" for detection is PCR to detect the *mecA* gene or latex agglutination to detect its gene product, PBP2a. For routine susceptibility testing cefoxitin disk testing is preferred over oxacillin disk testing because clarity of cefoxitin zone of inhibition is superior,[232] but either oxacillin or cefoxitin can be used for MIC testing.[218] The use of agar that contains 6 μg/mL of oxacillin supplemented with 4% NaCl also is utilized for oxacillin resistance screening. All phenotypic methods compare favorably with molecular techniques.[233]

Both molecular and screening culture techniques have been developed for the detection of MRSA carriage. Several selective and differential chromogenic agars commercially available offer MRSA-positive results in 24 to 48 hours directly from clinical specimens and have performance characteristics similar to PCR.[234] Reportedly, broth enrichment prior to chromogenic agar culture improves the sensitivity of culture,[235] but also increases the time to result. Since MRSA colonization often is associated with low bacterial counts, broth enrichment and/or molecular methods may provide the best sensitivity.[235]

Conventional and rt-PCR can detect *mecA* in bacterial isolates and directly on patient specimens. However, direct specimen testing has limitations, often including a lower positive predictive value than culture-based assays.[236–239] Currently, there are three FDA-cleared rt-PCR assays for the detection of MRSA for infection control purposes directly from nasal swabs. (Carriage of CA-MRSA only at sites other than the nose is a limitation.) In addition, there are three FDA-cleared molecular tests available for the detection and differentiation of MRSA and MSSA from positive blood cultures and one from skin and soft-tissue infections.[240] NAAT detection of MRSA has equivalent sensitivity to culture-based methods, but has the advantage of offering a faster turnaround time, which may significantly decrease hospital costs.[223]

Detection of Vancomycin Resistance

Molecular and phenotypic methods are available to detect vancomycin resistance in *Enterococcus* spp. and *S. aureus*. Routine susceptibility testing and isolate screening using brain–heart infusion agar containing 6 µg/mL of vancomycin are the reference methods for detecting vancomycin resistance in *Enterococcus* spp.[218] However, intrinsically resistant enterococci (i.e., due to *vanC*) should be excluded for infection control purposes. Etest and microbroth dilution MICs can be used for detection of VISA and VRSA, but disk diffusion should not be used as it cannot differentiate high-level from low-level resistance accurately and can miss VISA.[211,218]

There is one FDA-cleared assay for the detection of VRE rectal colonization for infection control purposes (Xpert *vanA* Test, Cepheid, Sunnyvale, CA), and numerous homebrew assays are described.[223] It is debated whether these assays should detect both *vanA* and *vanB;* preference largely is dependent on geographic prevalence of resistance determinants. Although both determinants are transferable, detection of *vanB* has a low positive predictive value due to the presence of the gene among anaerobic bacteria, such as *Clostridium* species.[241,242] Thus, *vanB*-positive molecular results should be confirmed by culture. It is controversial whether the assay should detect an *Enterococcus*-specific gene. Since *vanA* rarely is found in non-enterococcal species, many assays do not incorporate an *Enterococcus*-specific target. Two main advantages to molecular detection of VRE are that: (1) amplification technology reportedly increases VRE detection to up to 120%, permitting better infection control; and (2) intrinsically resistant enterococci are excluded, thus mitigating unnecessary contact precautions and cost.[223,243]

Detection of Inducible Clindamycin Resistance

ML$_B$-I organisms appear resistant to erythromycin, but will appear to be susceptible to clindamycin by routine disk diffusion and MIC testing. The D-test detects inducible resistance to clindamycin in the presence of erythromycin. Erythromycin and clindamycin disks are placed in close proximity to each other (15 to 26 mm for staphylococci and 12 mm for streptococci) on agar seeded with the clinical isolate.[218] If inducible resistance is present, there will be a flattening of the clindamycin zone closest to erythromycin, appearing as a "D" (Figure 290-4). Some automated susceptibility testing

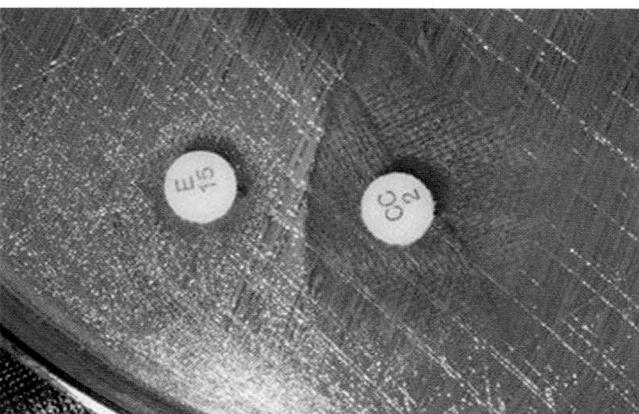

Figure 290-4. D-test for the detection of inducible clindamycin resistance (MLS$_B$-I) in *Staphylococcus aureus*. Disk "CC 2" on the right contains 2 µg of clindamycin; disk "E 15" on the left contains 15 µg of erythromycin. Disks are placed 15 to 26 mm apart, and a flattening of the clindamycin zone proximal to the erythromycin disk is observed, indicating inducible resistance to clindamycin.

systems can screen for inducible clindamycin resistance by comparing susceptibility result from a well containing only clindamycin with that from a well containing both clindamycin and erythromycin. The VITEK2 screen showed 93% sensitivity and 100% specificity compared with the D-test.[244] The CLSI recommends that laboratories screen for inducible clindamycin resistance on all β-hemolytic streptococci and staphylococci.[218] Although the clinical relevance of the detection of inducible resistance in the setting of a patient not receiving erythromycin is debatable in theory, in practice there have been a number of reports of failed clindamycin therapy for infection due to an MLS$_B$-I organism.[129]

Detection of Isoniazid and Rifampin Resistance among *Mycobacterium tuberculosis*

The emergence of multidrug resistant- (MDR-) *M. tuberculosis* (resistant to both rifampin and isoniazid with or without resistance to other first-line drug) and extensively drug resistant (XDR-) *M. tuberculosis* (resistant to both first- and second-line drugs, specifically fluoroquinolones, and one of the injectable agents, capreomycin, amikacin, or kanamycin) has resulted in rethinking the manner in which susceptibility testing is performed.[16–19] The reference method, agar proportion, which technically is similar to agar dilution, is slow and highly labor-intensive. In most clinical laboratories, agar testing has been superseded by automated broth susceptibility testing, which is faster, more convenient, and similar in accuracy.[245] Although faster, automated broth methods still require days to weeks to complete.

Because of the recognition of the high mortality associated with XDR-tuberculosis,[246] the World Health Organization recommends that the Xpert MTB/RIF test (Cepheid, Sunnyvale, CA) be used globally in the fight to reduce the spread of MDR- and XDR-TB (http://www.who.int/tb/en/). Using an automated system, MTB/RIF can detect *M. tuberculosis* and determine strain susceptibility to rifampin directly from clinical specimens in <2 hours.[17] The system detected 99% of TB smear- and culture-positive patients and 90% of smear-negative, culture-positive patients when multiple specimens were tested. Rifampin is a relatively good screening test for the detection of MDR-TB because mutation for isoniazid resistance is found in >95% of rifampin-resistant isolates.[17] This system was found to identify 98% of MDR-TB cases correctly.[17]

Two commercially available assays use a combination of NAAT and a probe-based line blot for the detection of resistance in *M. tuberculosis*. The INNO-LiPA Rif.TB kit (Innogenetics, Ghent, Belgium) detects rifampin resistance using a combination of 5 sensitive probes and 4 resistant probes detecting *rpoB* mutations.[247,248] The Genotype MTBDRpl assays (Hain Lifescience, Nehren, Germany) detects both rifampin and isoniazid resistance by detecting 7 *rpoB* mutations, 2 common *katG* mutations, and 4 *inhA* mutations.[249,250] Sensitivity is greater for the detection of rifampin resistance (>95%) than for isoniazid (~85%), probably due to the wider array of mutations that can confer resistance in isoniazid.[251] A newer generation of the Genotype assay MTBDRsl has been developed for the detection of resistance to ethambutol and second-line drugs.[249,252,253] Performance of this test, with only modest numbers of isolates tested, appears to be reasonably good for the detection of fluoroquinolone, aminoglycoside, and capreomycin resistance (sensitivity and specificity between 75% and 100%) but less sensitive(~60%) for detecting ethambutol resistance.[252,253] Agar proportion susceptibility testing is still the gold standard due to incomplete data on all mutations and/or target genes associated with phenotypic resistance.[249–253] However, if molecular detection is used as an initial assay, resistant isolates can be detected weeks earlier, with significant impact on clinical care.

Susceptibility Testing of *Pseudomonas aeruginosa* Isolates from Patients with Cystic Fibrosis

Susceptibility testing of *P. aeruginosa* from chronically infected CF patients presents a special challenge due to the unique nature of strains, multidrug resistance, a unique mucoid phenotype, and possible growth under anaerobic conditions distal to mucus plugs.[254] Automated systems have inferior accuracy in assessing antimicrobial resistance of mucoid *P. aeruginosa*. Because of the comparatively slow growth of these mucoid organisms, very major errors can occur with automated susceptibility testing systems in which the organism is reported as susceptible when in fact it is resistant to a drug by reference methods. Both Etests and disk diffusion methods compare more favorably with reference methods.[254]

Reference MIC and disk diffusion methods can determine accurately *P. aeruginosa* resistance to several or all classes of antimicrobial agents, with the possible exception of colistin. Agar-based methods for detection of colistin resistance may not be reliable because this large, highly charged molecule diffuses poorly in an agar matrix; microbroth test determinations should be used.[255] Additionally, standard tobramycin breakpoints, which are based on achievable serum concentrations of drug, classify isolates as resistant that in fact have MICs below that achievable by aerosolized tobramycin (lower airway level ≥100 µg/mL). MIC determinations or Etests can be used to determine higher relevant MICs. In one study, 20% of isolates with MICs suggesting intermediate susceptibility or resistance at the serum-achievable level would be susceptible at the aerosol-achievable level; 5% of isolates were resistant to tobramycin at aerosol-achievable levels.[256]

Other alternative strategies for *P. aeruginosa* susceptibility testing include checkerboard synergy testing and testing for multiple combined bactericidal activity.[257] In a randomized trial, clinical outcome for patients whose therapy was based on multiple combination bactericidal antibiotic testing was no better than for those whose therapy was based on standard susceptibility methods.[258] Despite these data, some laboratories continue to perform testing for pan-resistant *P. aeruginosa* and *Burkholderia cepacia* complex because clinicians believe that it provides a rationale basis for 3- and 4-drug combinations. The U.S. Cystic Fibrosis Foundation no longer provides free reference laboratory checkerboard synergy susceptibility testing.

Finally, the mode of growth used in susceptibility testing of *P. aeruginosa* has been studied.[259] When *P. aeruginosa* is grown adherent to biofilms (sessile bacteria), β-lactam antibiotics are much less active than against organisms growing as single cells (planktonically). Aminoglycosides and ciprofloxacin showed similar activity against organisms growing planktonically or in biofilms. Surprisingly, macrolides, usually not thought to be active against *P. aeruginosa*, have activity against biofilm-grown organisms but not planktonic ones.[259] Susceptibility testing of biofilm-grown organisms is complex and questions of clinical utility are unsettled.[258]

291 Pharmacokinetic–Pharmacodynamic Basis of Optimal Antibiotic Therapy

Michael N. Neely and Michael D. Reed

As clinicians continuously strive to practice evidence-based medicine, the use of antibiotics can be frustratingly empiric. Ethical concerns, multiple confounding variables, and unclear endpoints hamper clinical infectious disease research. Empiricism is clearly evident in most recommendations for antibiotic dosing and duration of therapy, especially in children, because only a fraction of published pharmacokinetic (PK) and pharmacodynamic (PD) data are collected from this group of patients. Although pediatric data are more plentiful and better defined for antibiotics than for other drug classes used in children, much more work needs to be done. The lack of specific and sound dosing and safety data for drugs used in children that encompass the pediatric age spectrum continue to hamper the ability to determine an optimal dose regimen rapidly. "Off-label" use of medications in children unfortunately, and necessarily, remains common practice.[1–3]

In response to this lack of pediatric data, the United States Food and Drug Administration (FDA) has been granted additional authority through the Best Pharmaceuticals for Children Act (2002, 2007) and the Pediatric Research Equity Act (2003, 2007), which, respectively, can extend patent exclusivity for 6 months for subsequent research focused towards a pediatric indication, and can mandate that any drug with potential use in children must have data on pediatric dosing unless granted a specific waiver by the FDA. With a growing awareness of the important physiologic differences in children across the age spectrum and their many important influences on drug dosing, knowledge of an antibiotic's PK and PD properties is necessary to determine optimal dosing. This chapter reviews basic PK principles and provides a framework for the clinician to apply these principles at the bedside.

BASIC CONCEPTS OF CLINICAL PHARMACOKINETICS

Pharmacokinetics describes the time course of drug movement in the body; an understanding of a drug's PK profile is essential to the design of an optimal dosage regimen. However, focusing on a drug's PK profile alone provides the clinician with limited information about optimal drug dosing or, more importantly, clinical efficacy. PK principles are of clinical relevance only when they are integrated with the drug's *pharmacodynamic* properties, i.e., the effects of the drug in the patient.

With the exception of intravenous (IV) drug administration, a drug must be absorbed into the systemic circulation from its site of administration. Some drugs may be administered as a prodrug requiring in vivo metabolism to liberate the active moiety. Once absorbed, the drug is distributed within the body to accessible sites that are specific to the individual drug or drug class based on inherent physicochemical characteristics (e.g., lipid solubility, molecular weight, etc.). Factors such as age and disease can influence this distribution. Simultaneous with the processes of absorption and distribution, many drugs undergo metabolism prior to excretion from the body. A drug's disposition profile can be artificially separated into semidiscrete periods of drug absorption, distribution, metabolism, and excretion (Figure 291-1) to permit more accurate quantification. Knowledge of this information allows the clinician to predict drug concentrations and systemic exposures for the active drug that can be achieved at any time over a specified dosing interval after any dose of a given drug. With this information, an optimal drug dose and dosing interval can be determined for any patient with a regimen that accounts for underlying pathophysiology and major organ function.

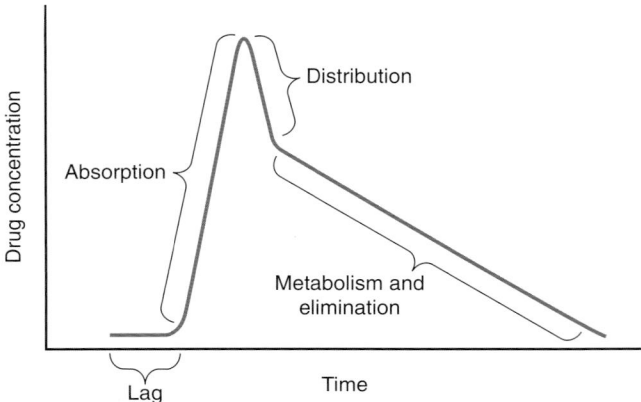

Figure 291-1. Overall biologic fluid (e.g., serum) drug concentration–time curve after extravascular drug administration. Each important process of drug disposition is indicated. Although these processes are compartmentalized graphically in the figure, in reality they occur simultaneously (see text for details).

The PK property *bioavailability* estimates the amount of a drug dose administered extravascularly (e.g., orally, intramuscularly) that is absorbed into the systemic circulation. Bioavailability is calculated as the area under the plasma drug concentration–time curve (AUC) achieved after extravascular drug administration divided by the AUC achieved after IV administration (e.g., AUC_{oral}/AUC_{IV}). Thus, to achieve the same systemic exposure with a drug administered orally as achieved with IV dosing, one simply divides the IV dose by the drug's bioavailability (obtained from the literature) to determine the equivalent oral dose. Lower bioavailability is not necessarily a negative attribute unless the dose required is so large that the patient tolerates it poorly. However, for orally administered antibiotics, poor bioavailability can be a major limitation because unabsorbed drug remaining in the intestinal tract can affect indigenous flora adversely, often leading to intestinal complaints and diarrhea (e.g., ampicillin versus amoxicillin). Conversely, this property sometimes is advantageous therapeutically, as is the case for orally administered vancomycin to treat *Clostridium difficile*-associated colitis or nystatin for mucosal candidiasis.

Bioavailability depends on the solubility and permeability of the drug. Highly soluble and permeable drugs have excellent bioavailability, while the converse results in poor bioavailability. Drugs with opposing solubility and permeability have unpredictable and variable bioavailability, even within the same patient from dose to dose, due to variations in gastrointestinal pH, motility, and food content. Drugs can exhibit complex absorption patterns with delayed or multiple peaks arising from timed-release formulations, enterohepatic recycling, site-specific absorption within the gastrointestinal tract, or variations in gastric emptying and intestinal transit times. A drug's *peak plasma concentration* is the characteristic most affected by changes in the rate and extent of absorption, and reduced peaks theoretically can compromise the efficacy of concentration-dependent antibiotics (discussed later).

Once absorbed into the systemic circulation, the distribution of a drug depends on specific characteristics inherent to the drug molecule. Small, nonprotein-bound, nonionized lipid-soluble molecules usually are distributed widely (e.g., voriconazole), whereas larger, less lipid-soluble (i.e., polar) or highly protein-bound drugs traverse cell membranes poorly, which restricts movement (e.g., aminoglycosides, vancomycin, echinocandins). The PK measurement that attempts to describe this process is the *volume of distribution* (V_d). V_d is a proportionality constant that relates the amount of drug in the body to its plasma concentration. V_d can be conceptualized roughly for an intravenous drug by the following simplified formula: $V_d = dose/C_p$, where C_p is the peak plasma drug concentration. V_d does not correspond to any true anatomic distribution or compartment, although the magnitude of V_d provides clues about a drug's physiologic distribution. For example, for a drug with a very small V_d (i.e., 0.2 L/kg), a larger

proportion of the drug is confined to extracellular fluid (composed of intravascular and interstitial fluid) whereas the distribution of a drug with a large V_d can involve extensive tissue binding, intracellular distribution, or both. Knowing a drug's V_d (expressed in liters per kilogram of body weight) allows the clinician to estimate the dose necessary to achieve any desired plasma drug concentration. For example, the loading dose for a drug can be calculated from the following formula: loading dose = desired plasma drug concentration (mg/L) × V_d (L/kg) × patient body weight (kg). The age-specific V_d for the drug to be prescribed can be obtained from the literature or calculated for the individual patient, as outlined earlier. As inferred from the loading dose calculation, the first (or loading) dose of any drug is independent of an individual's organ function or extent of underlying disease, such as renal failure. A patient's first drug dose is dependent only on the V_d of the specific drug; all subsequent dosing is dependent on the patient's ability to clear (eliminate/metabolize) the drug.

The PK property *clearance* (CL) estimates the volume of solvent (e.g., plasma, serum, or blood) from which all drug is removed per unit time. CL, therefore, is expressed in units of volume per time. Body CL is a composite estimate reflecting all mechanisms of drug CL, including renal, hepatic, and other forms of CL (e.g., lung), and is calculated with the following formulas: CL = 0.693 × $V_d/T_{1/2}$, where $T_{1/2}$ is the drug's elimination half-life, or CL = drug dose × F/AUC, where F is bioavailability. Knowledge of a drug's CL is necessary to determine accurately the need for and proper timing of subsequent doses to maintain any desired drug concentration or degree of systemic exposure. Changes in organ function responsible for drug removal from the body are reflected by changes in a drug's overall CL rate. Although clinically the $T_{1/2}$ often is used at the bedside as a measure of drug CL and to determine subsequent drug dosing, this value merely reflects the time required for a given drug concentration in any biologic fluid to decrease by 50%. Fortunately for many drugs, because V_d usually is constant, $T_{1/2}$ mirrors body CL, thereby permitting bedside application. $T_{1/2}$ can be estimated simply from the measured fall in plasma drug concentration after an individual dose; to calculate the $T_{1/2}$, a preferred method involves the following formula that highlights the dependence of a drug's $T_{1/2}$ on V_d and CL: $T_{1/2}$ = 0.693 × V_d/CL. Although an extremely useful bedside application of PK, the accuracy of the $T_{1/2}$ as a reflection of drug CL diminishes in situations of changing V_d, renal or liver function. For example, a drug's V_d can be altered during extracorporeal membrane oxygenation (ECMO) or severe liver disease with marked ascites.

The PK principles just outlined for V_d, CL, and $T_{1/2}$ assume that the drug follows *first-order* or *linear PK characteristics*. "First-order" means that a constant *fraction* of drug is cleared per unit time; that is, regardless of the initial concentration, the time to clear *x*% is the same. However, for certain drugs, such as voriconazole,[4,5] the CL mechanisms can be saturated at clinically relevant concentrations, and thus their disposition is best described by using *zero-order methodology* or a combination of first-order elimination at lower concentrations and a gradual transition to zero-order elimination at higher concentrations (i.e., *Michaelis–Menten* kinetics). "Zero-order" means that a constant *amount* of drug is cleared per unit time; that is, the higher the initial concentration, the longer it will take to clear *x*%. Fortunately, the vast majority of drugs used clinically follow first-order PK, which is simpler to apply at the bedside. The recognition that a drug's disposition characteristics are first-order allows the clinician to use simple proportions with relative accuracy to define patient-specific drug doses. For example, if a patient's plasma drug steady-state concentration is half that desired (at any time point) and the drug follows first-order PK, the dose can simply be doubled to achieve the desired concentration. In contrast, for a drug with zero-order characteristics, doubling the dose can result in much higher increase in the plasma concentration.

Unfortunately, the clinician encounters many patients who deviate from the proposed PK characteristics found in the literature, especially in pediatrics. A far more sophisticated, powerful, and nuanced approach to dosage individualization is the application of population pharmacokinetic modeling techniques coupled with Bayesian feedback, using specifically designed computer software tools.[6] While these methods have the disadvantage of requiring specialized software, training, and knowledge, there are numerous advantages, including more accurate and rapid attainment of target drug concentrations without the need for steady-state conditions (including patients with unstable pharmacokinetic behavior),[7–11] improved clinical outcomes,[12–15] and reduced costs.[12,16–19] Furthermore, population-based PK data often are more reflective of drug disposition behavior of patients with disease of varying severity. A complete review of this topic is beyond the scope of this chapter, but interested readers are urged to contact experts in the field and consider these approaches when desiring to optimize individual therapy.

DRUG DISPOSITION IN SPECIFIC PATIENT POPULATIONS

Neonates: The Ontogenic Basis of Drug Disposition

Predictably altered pharmacokinetics occur in certain patient populations and PK can influence both the magnitude and the frequency of antibiotic doses. Populations include neonates, patients with organ failure who are undergoing dialysis or ECMO, children with cystic fibrosis (CF), and victims of burns or septic shock.

As children mature physically, they also mature physiologically. This principle has important and clinically relevant implications on both drug PK and PD characteristics.[20–23] Factors that influence drug absorption from the gastrointestinal (GI) tract include the surface area available for absorption, pH, gastric emptying time, exocrine pancreatic function, size of the bile acid pool, and bacterial colonization (Table 291-1). All these functions are variably altered in neonates, particularly those born prematurely, and in young infants relative to older children and adults. Changes in the amount and distribution of body water in neonates, as well as differences in quantitative and qualitative protein-binding characteristics, also are present and affect drug distribution. These ontogenic differences in body water composition (i.e., increased V_d for water-soluble drugs) are reflected by the increased individual doses, on a milligram of drug per kilogram of body weight basis, prescribed for young infants and children in comparison with older children and adults (see Chapters 94 to 96). Although far from fully characterized, both the oxidative and conjugative

hepatic metabolic enzyme systems are immature at birth and reach adult levels of activity at various times throughout early childhood. Renal function and elimination also mature as a function of gestational and postnatal age, with glomerular filtration reaching adult levels in infants of 34 weeks' gestation by about 3 to 5 months of age. Tubular secretion matures more slowly and reaches adult levels by about 8 to 9 months of age (see Table 291-1).

As a result of these physiologic differences (see Table 291-1), infants <44 weeks' postconceptional/postmenstrual age generally have larger V_d and decreased antibiotic CL, which translates clinically to lower peaks, lower overall plasma drug concentrations, and longer $T_{1/2}$ than observed in older infants and children. Furthermore, they may be more susceptible to drug–drug interactions at all levels, which are likely to be significant for other drugs as well as for antibiotics (see the section on The Basis for Drug–Drug Interactions, below).

The physiologic differences of young infants influence not only drug PK but also PD characteristics, which necessarily incorporate the mechanism of drug action. Developmental changes in receptor function are not as relevant to antibiotics because the receptor targets are on the infecting organism. However, host receptors can be involved in therapeutic antibiotic mechanisms (e.g., human kinases that phosphorylate acyclovir) or adverse antibiotic mechanisms. Despite lower CL and prolonged $T_{1/2}$ relative to older children and adults, aminoglycosides cause less nephrotoxicity in neonates.[24] This tolerance is thought to arise from differences in renal disposition characteristics, although the exact mechanism is unknown.

In summary, neonates are physiologically distinct and manifest altered antibiotic PK characteristics. The clinician must be aware of these differences so that recommended antibiotic dosing strategies can be evaluated critically and appropriate prescribing decisions made to assure therapeutic success. In the absence of neonatal dosing recommendations, knowledge of the altered PK patterns will make empiric dosing more rational when extrapolated from dosing recommendations for older children or adults.

Patients with Organ Failure and Principles of Dialyzable Drugs

The major routes of drug elimination are by the kidneys into urine and by the liver into bile. For the vast majority of drugs only minor amounts are eliminated into other body fluids. Alterations in drug disposition result from failure of either of these organs of elimination or failure of the cardiopulmonary system, which perfuses these organs with the oxygenated blood essential for proper function. Patients with cardiopulmonary failure can experience alterations in both V_d as a result of increased total body water and CL as a result of hepatic or renal dysfunction. Knowledge of the PK properties of individual drugs is crucial to understanding the magnitude of such effects. Drugs with a small V_d are more affected because they tend to be distributed to extracellular fluid. The route of metabolism and elimination determines the impact of hepatic or renal dysfunction.

Extracorporeal Membrane Oxygenation (ECMO)

Patients suffering the extremes of organ failure may be maintained by ECMO, which influences drug disposition in several ways. ECMO circuitry can add up to 500 mL of volume to the patient, in which case V_d is increased; children weighing <20 kg are likely to experience a corresponding lower peak concentrations and a longer $T_{1/2}$. Further, drugs can bind to the oxygenation membrane, thereby potentially increasing both V_d and CL.[25] Binding is increased with increasingly lipophilic drugs. CL can be reduced as a consequence of altered perfusion of the liver and kidneys.

Speculations notwithstanding, alterations in the PK characteristics of antibiotics during ECMO have been characterized for gentamicin and vancomycin.[26,27] Although the V_d of aminoglycosides is variably increased, the $T_{1/2}$ can be doubled. Neither drug

TABLE 291-1. Physiologic Changes in Children That Affect the Pharmacokinetic Characteristics of Drugs[20–23]

Parameter	Neonates	Approximate Age Approaching Adult Level
ABSORPTION		
Gastric pH	↑	3 months
Gastric emptying	↓	6–8 months
Pancreatic function	↓	9 months
DISTRIBUTION		
Body water	↑[a]	Adolescence
Protein binding	↓	12 months
METABOLISM		
Hepatic drug-metabolizing	↓	Adolescence
ELIMINATION		
Renal function	↓	Glomerular filtration: 3–5 months
		Tubular secretion: 8–9 months

[a]The distribution of body water depends on age: the total body water (TBW) of neonates is about 75% of body weight, with about 50% intracellular (IC) and 50% extracellular (EC). A gradual decrease in TBW and a shift to IC distribution occur until adult values of 50% to 60% TBW, 33% EC, and 66% IC are reached at puberty.

significantly binds to the oxygenation membrane, as predicted by low liphophilicity. The implication for dosing is that aminoglycosides should be administered every 18 to 24 h initially (or less frequently in those with renal failure) to infants undergoing ECMO (with monitoring of serum drug concentrations), although no efficacy studies are available to support this recommendation. For vancomycin, V_d and $T_{1/2}$ are increased, and CL decreased, resulting in a suggested initial dose of 20 mg/kg IV every 18 to 24 h for infants with a serum creatinine value <1.5 mg/dL. For infants with a higher serum creatinine concentration, the dosing interval must be extended. In all cases, serum vancomycin concentrations should be monitored.

Increased ECMO-associated cefotaxime V_d has been documented, but the percentage of the dosing interval above organism minimal inhibitory concentration (MIC) after standard doses while on ECMO is not significantly different from the same doses off ECMO, leading to no required dosing changes.[28] There are some reports of lowered plasma voriconazole concentrations requiring higher doses in patients on ECMO, which is consistent with its high lipophilicity; therapeutic drug monitoring is recommended.[29,30] Caspofungin, which is less lipophilic, had reportedly lowered[31] and unaltered[30] concentrations in a total of three patients receiving ECMO, resulting in no clear recommendation. Oseltamivir pharmacokinetics do not appear to be changed significantly.[32]

For other antimicrobial agents for which plasma drug concentrations are unavailable, the clinician can only estimate dosing modifications based upon the expected changes described above. In general, V_d and $T_{1/2}$ are the same or are increased. Lipophilic drugs are more affected than hydrophilic drugs. However, to complicate the setting further, patients undergoing ECMO usually have multiorgan failure, with renal failure being the most problematic for determining many antibiotic regimens.

Dialysis

For patients with acute or chronic renal failure who require dialysis, several options can be used for extracorporeal therapy, including intermittent or continuous hemodialysis (HD), hemofiltration (HF), and peritoneal dialysis. HD and HF can be combined. HD removes an antibiotic by diffusion across the dialysis membrane into the dialysate according to the drug's concentration gradient. The amount of blood flow past the dialysis membrane and the composition and flow of dialysate influence the amount of drug removed. HF (without HD) removes antibiotics in the ultrafiltrate, which is a hydrostatically generated flow of water containing the dissolved drug. There is no drug concentration gradient. Peritoneal dialysis, in general, removes most antibiotics minimally. The volume of peritoneal dialysis fluid is generally small (0.05 to 0.2 L/kg) in comparison with the V_d of antibiotics (0.2 to >100 L/kg), so only a very small percentage of the total drug in the body is distributed to the peritoneal dialysis fluid unless the antibiotic has a similarly small V_d. Furthermore, the intraperitoneal concentration of antibiotics is proportional to the concentration of free, nonprotein-bound drug. The protein content of typical dialysate fluid is zero, so highly protein-bound antibiotics are poorly distributed to the peritoneal fluid. Increasing the amount of peritoneal dialysate or the frequency of exchange increases the amount of drug extracted, but a cumulative amount extracted of <25% during a dosing interval usually is insignificant. In contrast, antibiotics administered into the peritoneal dialysate can reach therapeutic plasma concentrations if they can cross the peritoneal membrane, passage through which is enhanced in the presence of inflammation. Since the potential extra-abdominal volume for an antibiotic to diffuse into is much larger than the intra-abdominal volume, with equal concentrations across the peritoneal membrane at equilibrium, the amount of drug in the body is greater than in the peritoneal dialysate.

All these modalities partially restore the ability of the body to eliminate an antibiotic that would normally be cleared by the kidneys. Although there are several thorough reviews on the use of antimicrobial agents in these patients, it must be emphasized

TABLE 291-2. Factors That Increase the Likelihood of Antibiotic Removal by Dialysis

Factors Intrinsic to the Antibiotic	Factors Intrinsic to the Mode of Dialysis
Smaller Vd (<1 L/kd)	CVVHDF[a] > CVVH > CVVHD[a] > IHD >> PD
Smaller molecular mass (<2 kd)	Frequent dialysis
Reduced protein binding (<2 kd)	High flow rate of blood and/or dialysate
Neutral charge	Filter capacity and selectivity
Normally eliminated by kidneys (>30%)	Dialysate composition

CVVH, continuous venovenous hemofiltration; CVVHD, continuous venovenous hemodialysis; CVVHDF, continuous venovenous hemodiafiltration; IHD, intermittent hemodialysis; PD, peritoneal dialysis; Vd, volume of distribution.

[a]The differences in drug clearance between the continuous modes of hemodialysis and/or hemofiltration are less significant for small molecules, which includes most hydrophilic antibiotics that are likely to be cleared by these modes. Among these, the largest are teicoplanin (1.9 kd), colistimethate, aka colistin (1.8 kd) and vancomycin (1.5 kd).

that none of the guidelines has pediatric dosing, and all of them strongly convey the same message: antimicrobial concentrations are highly dependent on factors intrinsic to the mode of dialysis itself and the drug's PK properties (Table 291-2). This variability could have significant clinical implications.[33] While the clinician can apply principles outlined here to an individual patient to generate a qualitative assessment of the need for dose adjustment, confirmatory measurement of drug concentrations is crucial when possible.

Drugs with a small V_d (<1.0 L/kg) that are primarily confined to the extracellular compartment are available for filtration across the dialysis membrane. The pore size of HD membranes is approximately 0.5 kd, whereas HF membranes are usually about 50 kd. Most antibiotics are <1 kd. Passage across a membrane is inversely proportional to the square root of the molecular mass. Drug–protein complexes are too large to pass through the pores of intact dialysis membranes, so highly protein-bound antibiotics (>80%) pass through the membrane poorly. Further, the membranes carry a net negative charge; highly polar molecules do not cross the membrane efficiently. Antibiotics that are eliminated mainly by a functioning kidney are more likely to be eliminated by dialysis, and a simplistic "rule of thumb" predicts some removal of drugs that are eliminated in the urine >30% unchanged in patients with normal renal function. However, the fraction of an antibiotic normally cleared by active tubular secretion is not compensated for by dialysis, and this should be considered in any patient manifesting unexplained signs or symptoms of drug toxicity.

Antibiotic dose adjustment in the absence of measurable drug concentrations in blood, dialysate, or ultrafiltrate is a crude estimate, at best. Unfortunately, most pharmacology references consulted to determine dose recommendations use complicated formulas that require information the clinician often does not possess. Therefore, a more intuitive approach is typical, and the clinician first should consider the relevance of potential drug accumulation by monitoring the patient closely for desired and undesired drug effect(s). Fortunately, most antibiotics have a very high therapeutic index, i.e., the ratio of therapeutic-to-toxic doses. "Safe" drugs generally can be allowed to accumulate moderately without risk of serious or irreversible toxicity or both. In contrast, more rigorous dose adjustments should be applied for antibiotics that can be associated with toxicity, e.g., the aminoglycosides, as, in general, patients with renal failure, especially if uremic, are more prone to adverse effects from all drugs. Regardless of the dosing scheme selected, the clinician must monitor patients closely for specific evidence of toxicity related to the drug in question as well as expected clinical response(s). On the other hand, unaccounted-for extracorporeal elimination has major importance when subtherapeutic drug concentrations lead to clinical failure. This can occur when a drug is dosed based on a patient's intrinsic renal function without accounting for dialysis-mediated drug clearance. Therefore, for most antibiotics, it is more important to avoid underdosing. Appendix 291-1 lists suggested adjustments for selected antibiotics in response to renal failure with or without dialysis.

Cystic Fibrosis

Cystic fibrosis (CF) is the most common potentially lethal genetic disorder in white people and remains a therapeutic challenge for pediatric and adult practitioners. The disease is characterized by an elevated sweat chloride concentration, pancreatic exocrine insufficiency, thick tenacious mucous secretions, and chronic obstructive pulmonary disease.[34,35] A hallmark of CF is chronic microbial colonization of the lung with resultant repeated acute pulmonary infections or exacerbations.[36] Most CF morbidity and mortality is due to the pulmonary component of this disease, and treatment (e.g., antibiotics, ibuprofen) focuses on decreasing the inflammation that is responsible for the progressive, irreversible deterioration in lung function[37] (see Chapter 108, Infectious

Complications in Special Hosts). However, optimal antibiotic therapy in CF patients is complicated by differences in the disposition of many drugs.[38,39] Unfortunately, the lack of adequate control groups in many studies precludes definitive conclusions regarding CF-induced alterations in drug PK.[36] Nevertheless, these data do provide consensus findings that CF patients exhibit a larger V_d and enhanced body CL in comparison with non-CF patients for many antibiotics, including aminoglycoside and β-lactam agents.[38,39] The reasons for these differences are unknown. CF-induced differences in drug V_d may merely reflect the difference in body composition in CF patients, specifically, their limited adipose tissue. When the V_d for various drugs is expressed as a function of lean body mass rather than body weight characterized by kilograms, differences in drug V_d diminish. Because drug dosing in pediatrics usually is based on the patient's body weight in kilograms, the real differences in the body composition of CF patients necessitate higher individual milligram-per-kilogram drug dosing to achieve systemic drug exposure similar to that of non-CF patients.

Drug elimination also appears to be enhanced in CF patients.[38,39] Despite well-characterized CF-induced hepatic dysfunction, particularly in CF patients older than 15 years, the CL of many drugs

TABLE 291-3. Pharmacokinetic Alterations of Specific Antibiotics with Suggested Dosing Strategies in Patients with Septic Shock or Extensive Burns

Antibiotic	Pharmacokinetic Change	Suggested Dose Adjustment
Aminoglycosides (gentamicin, tobramycin, amikacin)	Generally increased CL and V_d	1. Administer twice the standard multiple-daily dose[a] 2. Measure drug concentration at end of infusion and 4 h after end of infusion 3. If 4-hour concentration is <2 µg/mL (gentamicin, tobramycin) or <5 µg/mL (amikacin), administer another dose; otherwise, estimate V_d and $T_{1/2}$ and administer second dose when trough concentration expected to be at target. 4. Continue dose and schedule from step 3. **Dosing based on traditional peaks and troughs:**[a] 1. Administer high end of standard dose 2. Obtain serum concentrations 15 minutes, 1 hour, and 3 hours after end of infusion 3. Calculate individual V_d and $T_{1/2}$ 4. Adjust dose based on pharmacokinetic calculations 5. Confirm therapeutic trough and peak 3–5 doses later
Glycopeptides (vancomycin, teicoplanin)	Generally increased CL; fair correlation with CLCr. V_d is not affected	1. Measure CLCr as soon as possible (after initial 48 hours postburn) 2. Administer highest end of standard dose based on shortest dosing interval 3. Measure peak concentration at end of infusion. 4. Time the measurement of trough level on CLCr, if available;[b] if unavailable, measure trough before next dose is due after standard short interval 5. Adjust dose/interval based on serum troughs[c]
β-Lactams (cefepime ceftazidime, ticarcillin-clavulanate, piperacillin-tazobactam)	V_d is substantially increased; total CL generally is correlated with CLCr. $T_{1/2}$ is variably increased, but initial serum concentrations are less than normal	1. Measure CLCr as soon as possible (after initial 48 hours postburn) 2. Consider 50% increase over highest usual dose 3. Dosing interval depends on CLCr. If above normal, choose moderate interval; if below normal, choose long interval
Carbapenems/monopenems (imipenem, meropenem, aztreonam)	CL correlates well with CLCr; no change in V_d	1. Measure CLCr as soon as possible (after initial 48 hours postburn) 2. Use high end of standard dose 3. Dosing interval depends on CLCr. If above normal, choose short interval; if below normal, choose long interva

CL, clearance; CLCr, creatine clearance; $T_{1/2}$, drug's elimination half-life; V_d, volume of distribution.

[a]Once-daily dosing of aminoglycosides has been shown to result in extended periods of sub-therapeutic plasma concentrations in excess of those seen in non-burned patients, potentially compromising efficacy, and standard multiple-daily dosing carries a significant risk of subtherapeutic peaks. Therefore, higher dose multiple daily dosing is preferred initially.[46]

[b]The standard dose of vancomycin in children with the shortest interval is 15 mg/kg every 6 hours. If CLCr is 100% of normal for age/weight/sex, measure trough 5 hours after the end of infusion (1 × normal dosing interval). If CLCr is 50% of normal, measure trough 11 hours after the end of infusion (2 × normal dosing interval). If CLCr is 200% of normal, measure trough 2 hours after the end of infusion (0.5 × normal dosing interval).

[c]Based on the pharmacokinetic/pharmacodynamic characteristics of vancomycin, continuous infusion may be an alternative for patients with rapid clearance to avoid excessively large or frequent doses. Clinical data are limited, and the best targeted serum concentration is not clear, but is likely at least 8 × MIC, with the understanding that particular caution or alternate therapies should be considered if sustained vancomycin concentrations >20 ug/mL are considered necessary.[303]

Adapted from reviews,[301,302] except where noted.

that undergo liver metabolism is increased in CF patients. Emerging data are revealing that the function of phase I mixed-function oxidases is selectively affected; the functional capacity of the cytochrome P450 (CYP) system isoforms 1A2 and 2C8 appear to be enhanced, whereas CYP2C9 and 3A4 are unaffected. With phase II reactions, the activity of glucuronyl transferase, *N*-acetyltransferase, and sulfotransferase may be increased. Moreover, the renal CL of many drugs is increased in patients with CF.[40] The mechanism for the increase in renal CL also is unknown but does not appear to be related to any disease-associated effect on the activity of the primary renal efflux transporter, P glycoprotein.[41] Nevertheless based on this information, it is necessary to increase the amount and possibly the frequency of individual doses to compensate for the larger V_d and CL, as tolerated by the patient. Regardless of the dosing strategy used, close clinical monitoring for antimicrobial efficacy and safety is necessary to ensure optimal safe drug therapy.

Additionally, in patients with CF, the amount and composition of sputum, as well as bacterial density, have been shown to reduce the bioactivity of many antibiotics (i.e., inoculum effect).[39,42–44] These pathophysiologic variables must be considered when devising antibiotic regimens, including increasing systemic doses and attempting topical application via aerosol antibiotic administration.[45]

Septic Shock or Burns

Children who are in septic shock or are severely burned can suffer dramatic physiologic changes.[46,47] One can assume that any child with hemodynamic changes requiring significant fluid resuscitation and/or pharmacologic pressor support will be neither physiologically nor pharmacokinetically normal. The timing of physiologic changes is somewhat more characteristic for burns than for septic shock, as the former insult is of defined duration. The first phase in the 48 h after a severe burn is characterized by an acute decrease in glomerular filtration as a result of hypovolemia and shock, with a rapid shift of intravascular fluid to the interstitial spaces. After 48 h, with adequate resuscitation, the second phase is characterized by increased cardiac output, increased glomerular filtration (although not tubular secretion), hypoalbuminemia with reduced drug protein binding, and edema. Unfortunately, burned patients frequently sustain hypovolemic renal injury, which can antagonize the postburn increased glomerular filtration. Additionally, the function of hepatic CYP450 enzymes appears to be depressed in burned patients. These factors and others have an important impact on drug disposition and require dose adjustments.

Similar changes can be observed with septic shock, with early increases in the volume of distribution of hydrophilic drugs associated with increased capillary leak and fluid resuscitation, as well as organ blood flow associated with a hyperdynamic cardiac output. Subsequent infection- and immune-mediated tissue damage then can compromise organ function, including drug metabolism and elimination. The temporal variability of the pathophysiologic changes associated with septic shock and burns makes the PK of antibiotics quite unpredictable. Nonetheless, some studies have revealed class-dependent patterns that can make antibiotic dosing more rational. Table 291-3 indicates the PK changes observed for various commonly used antibiotics and provides suggested dosing strategies. Ongoing awareness of the patient's physiologic status and further monitoring of serum antibiotic concentrations or secondary markers such as creatinine CL and albumin are required to ensure that the most effective dosing regimens are maintained.

THE BASIS FOR DRUG–DRUG INTERACTIONS

Pharmacokinetic Interactions

A drug–drug interaction can exist at any phase of the PK profile (see Figure 291-1) – absorption, distribution, metabolism, or elimination. Frequently, these interactions are predictable

qualitatively, if not always quantitatively. For example, knowing that clarithromycin inhibits the same hepatic enzyme responsible for metabolizing cyclosporine leads one to predict that clarithromycin is likely to raise the cyclosporine serum concentration and that a lower dose of the latter may be required. However, actual quantitative adjustment of the cyclosporine dose must be based on measurement of the serum concentration or close patient monitoring (or both) for defined endpoints of efficacy and side effects.

The first step is awareness of the possibility of a drug–drug interaction and knowledge of the PK properties of the respective drugs. The second step is assessment of the clinical relevance of a potential interaction. Clinical importance occurs when the amount of free (active) drug in the body is significantly altered such that therapeutic efficacy is compromised or toxicity is increased. An assessment of possible specific influences on each aspect of a drug's disposition profile is outlined in the following sections.

Absorption

The absorption of orally administered drugs can be altered by numerous factors:

1. Alterations in GI motility by pharmacologic or nonpharmacologic means. Intestinal motility can be influenced by the administration of gastrokinetic medications (e.g., metoclopramide) or decreased by drugs with anticholinergic or opiate properties.
2. The presence of food in the GI tract. Food can affect the absorption of many antibiotics. For example, itraconazole tablets are better absorbed in the presence of fatty food, whereas itraconazole solution is better absorbed in the fasting state.
3. Alterations in gastric pH. Drugs that are highly charged cross membranes poorly, including the GI mucosal surface. In the normally acidic environment of the stomach, drugs that are weak acids are nonpolar; weak bases are charged. As the pH increases with the use of antacids, H_2-blocking agents, and proton pump inhibitors, weak acids become more polar and are thus absorbed less, while weak bases become less polar and are absorbed more readily. For example, increased gastric and proximal duodenal pH reduces the absorption of cefpodoxime,[48] itraconazole capsules but not solution,[49] oral ampicillin (product literature), and the antiretroviral drugs atazanavir and indinavir.[50] In contrast, absorption of the antiretroviral drug raltegravir is enhanced by concomitant omeprazole.[51] These examples notwithstanding, since most drug absorption occurs in the small intestine, gastric pH generally plays a minor role in overall bioavailability of orally administered drugs.
4. Binding substances. Fluoroquinolones and tetracyclines are poorly absorbed in the presence of cationic ions such as bismuth, calcium, aluminum, and magnesium ions found in vitamin supplements and antacids; concomitant use of these medications should be avoided. Such complex interactions can be avoided by separating antibiotic administration by a minimum of 2 to 4 hours.

Distribution

Drug interactions influencing distribution can occur as a result of interactions that affect drug displacement from plasma proteins, most notably serum albumin, or are due to drug transporters. Drug–drug protein displacement interactions represent drug interactions of common clinical concern but of rare clinical significance, specifically, displacement of one drug or substance (e.g., bilirubin) by another drug or substance from its binding site or sites (e.g., albumin) leading to an increased concentration of free drug. The resultant increased free drug concentration undergoes distribution and clearance and also is available for enhanced PD effect. However, *all* the following criteria must be fulfilled before such an interaction becomes problematic:

TABLE 291-4. Antibiotics Classified According to their Possible Ability to Displace Bilirubin from Albumin in Cord Blood Serum in Vitro

High[a]	Intermediate	Low	No Data[b]
Cefoperazone	Ampicillin	Aminoglycosides	Acyclovir
Ceftriaxone	Cefonicid	Amoxicillin	Amantadine
Dicloxacillin	Cefoxitin	Aztreonam	Amphotericin B[c]
Sulfamethoxazole	Cephalexin	Cefamandole	Cidofovir
Sulfisoxazole	Erythromycin	Cefazolin	Clindamycin
	Imipenem	Cefotaxime	Fluconazole
	Nafcillin	Ceftazidime	Ganciclovir
	Vancomycin	Cefuroxime	Meropenem
		Ciprofloxacin	Metronidazole
		Penicillin G	Neuraminidase inhibitors
		Piperacillin	Protease inhibitors[c]
		Ticarcillin	Reverse transcriptase inhibitors

[a]Avoid in neonates unless no alternative is available.

[b]Although specific data regarding the ability of these antimicrobials to displace bilirubin are lacking, they appear to be safe in this regard based on clinical experience and/or a low degree of protein binding.

[c]Infants receiving amphotericin B or the protease inhibitors indinavir and atazanavir can have elevated total serum bilirubin, but not because of displacement from albumin.

1. The antibiotic must be highly protein bound (>80%).
2. The drug must have a small V_d (<1 L/kg). A larger V_d means that the bulk of the drug is extravascular and is not affected by changes in serum protein binding.
3. The drug must have a long $T_{1/2}$. As drug is displaced from serum protein, it not only becomes biologically active but also becomes available for distribution to extravascular sites, metabolism, and excretion. For drugs with a short $T_{1/2}$, any displaced excess free drug is redistributed quickly, inactivated, or eliminated from the body, promptly reaching a new equilibrium (within 3 to 5 half-lives). A lower amount of total drug (and thus a larger apparent V_d) characterizes this new equilibrium, and although the free fraction is higher, the absolute concentration of free active drug is the *same* as before. This disposition occurs with all displaced drugs, but the $T_{1/2}$ of the displaced free drug is the most significant factor because it determines the time for the displaced free drug to re-equilibrate. The longer the free drug $T_{1/2}$, the greater the amount of time that elevated active drug concentrations are available to augment the therapeutic or toxic effects (or both). The implication of a decreased total serum concentration but the same free concentration is that highly protein-bound drugs with therapeutic levels based on the total serum concentrations (e.g., voriconazole) can appear falsely subtherapeutic because the active free drug concentration is not being measured.
4. The antibiotic must have a low therapeutic index; that is, significant toxicity occurs at a serum concentration only slightly above therapeutic concentrations.

Although several antibiotics meet some of the criteria just outlined, none meets all of them. Therefore, concern about toxicity caused by the displacement of antibiotics from serum proteins appears to be unwarranted.

The converse question is whether highly protein-bound antibiotics can displace potentially harmful substances that are bound to serum proteins. The area of biggest concern in pediatrics is displacement of albumin-bound bilirubin and subsequent kernicterus in a neonate. The most commonly implicated drugs are the sulfa antibiotics and ceftriaxone. The pathophysiology of kernicterus is incompletely understood but is more complex than simple displacement of albumin-bound bilirubin. The only antibiotic that has actually been associated with kernicterus is IV sulfisoxazole.[52] Nonetheless, because the development of kernicterus involves the transfer of bilirubin from serum and tissue albumin to brain parenchyma in neonates,[53] especially premature infants, it seems prudent to avoid the use of antibiotics that do or could potentially displace bilirubin unless no other choice is available. Commonly used antimicrobial agents and their ability to displace bilirubin are listed in Table 291-4.[54-56]

Metabolism

Many drug–drug interactions occur at the level of drug CL, particularly for drugs that undergo metabolism. The CYP450 enzyme system is responsible for the metabolism of many drugs, including antibiotics. These enzymes can be inhibited, induced, and/or saturated by substrate. For antibiotics that are primarily metabolized by one P450 isoform, the potential exists for significant changes in serum concentration as CL is either increased or decreased because of changes in enzyme activity. The highest concentration of these enzymes is in the liver, but the intestinal mucosa also contains CYP450 enzymes and is the site of numerous drug–drug interactions that affect bioavailability. To predict a clinically significant drug–drug interaction, therefore, similar questions are asked regarding whether the antibiotic is primarily metabolized by one CYP450 isoform or has alternative or parallel metabolic pathways and whether a change in serum concentration would have significance. Specifically, if lowered, could the antibiotic concentration–time course ratio fall short of the optimal PK-PD-predicted concentration–time course ratio? If raised, could toxicity occur?

Table 291-5 lists antimicrobial agents that modulate specific CYP450 isoforms that predispose a patient to potential drug–drug interactions when coadministered with drugs metabolized via similar pathways. Knowledge of which isoform is primarily responsible for a drug's metabolism provides the clinician with the insight at least to question the possibility of a metabolically based drug–drug interaction. For specific drug–drug interactions, refer to individual agents in Chapter 292, Antimicrobial Agents.

Elimination

The primary mechanisms of antibiotic elimination from the body involve elimination via bile, feces, urine, or combinations of these mechanisms. Drugs that are eliminated in the bile are subject to enterohepatic recirculation. Amoxicillin can lower the effectiveness of oral contraceptives by altering the GI flora, reducing enterohepatic recirculation of the contraceptive, and enhancing elimination. Agents eliminated in urine can be filtered at the glomerular level and secreted at the tubular level. Fortunately, few drugs cause unwanted alterations at these sites. However, any agent that can reduce glomerular filtration (e.g., amphotericin B, cisplatin) can decrease the CL of the concurrently administered and filtered antibiotic, potentially necessitating dose adjustment.

TABLE 291-5. Antibiotic–Cytochrome P450 Interactions

Isoenzyme	Substrate	Inhibitor	Inducer
1A2[304]	Efavirenz	Fluoroquinolones (esp. ciprofloxacin) Isoniazid	Nafcillin Ritonavir
2B6[305]	Artemisinin Efavirenz Nevirapine		Artemisinin Efavirenz Rifampin Ritonavir
2C8[306]	Amodiaquine Chloroquine Dapsone	Ketoconazole Trimethoprim	Rifampin
2C9[307]	Etravirine[308]	Chloramphenicol Fluconazole Isoniazid Sulfamethoxazole Trimethoprim Voriconazole	Rifampin Ritonavir
2C19[309]	Etravirine[308] Nelfinavir Proguanil Voriconazole	Chloramphenicol Ketoconazole Probenecid	Artemisinin Rifampin Ritonavir
2D6		Ritonavir[310]	Rifampin
2E1[311]		Isoniazid	Isoniazid
3A4,5,7[312]	Azoles Chloroquine Dapsone Efavirenz Etravirine[308] HIV protease inhibitors Macrolides Mefloquine Primaquine Rifampin Trimethoprim	Azoles Ciprofloxacin HIV protease inhibitors Macrolides Norfloxacin	Efavirenz HIV protease inhibitors Nafcillin Nevirapine Rifampin

TABLE 291-6. Examples of Pharmacodynamic Interactions

Efficacy	Toxicity
INCREASED Numerous examples exist: synergistic activity of β-lactam plus aminoglycoside against enterococci; β-lactam plus β-lactamase inhibitor for extended gram-negative and anaerobic coverage; trimethoprim plus sulfamethoxazole; quinupristin plus dalfopristin	**INCREASED** Two potentially nephrotoxic antibiotics such as vancomycin plus an aminoglycoside can increase the likelihood of renal injury
DECREASED The antiretroviral drugs zidovudine and stavudine are antagonistic when coadministered, likely due to an interaction at the level of intracellular, molecular targets	**DECREASED** Probenecid mitigates nephrotoxicity of cidofovir[313]

quantitatively. Thus, changes in the balance of cellular efflux or uptake in the intestine can decrease or increase bioavailability, while changes in tissues can affect V_d and drug CL. Antimicrobial agents that are substrates for the P-GP efflux transporter include select protease inhibitors, erythromycin, and the antifungal drugs ketoconazole and itraconazole. Substrates for OATs include the penicillins and select cephalosporins. Probenecid inhibition of OATP activity is still used as a part of the amoxicillin-probenecid drug combination for treatment of uncomplicated *N. gonorrhoeae* (amoxicillin-susceptible) infection.

PHARMACODYNAMIC INTERACTIONS

PD interactions can affect efficacy or toxicity, and drugs can interact to diminish or augment either effect. As discussed in Chapter 289, Principles of Anti-infective Therapy, these interactions can be synergistic, additive, indifferent, or antagonistic. Because PD interactions arise from relationships between a drug's mechanism(s) of action, the clinician must be aware of these mechanisms. The appropriate question is whether the mechanisms of action of a patient's medications are likely to be related in any way. Table 291-6 outlines some frequent examples of each type of PD-based interaction.

INTEGRATION OF PHARMACOKINETIC AND PHARMACODYNAMIC PRINCIPLES FOR OPTIMAL ANTIBIOTIC DOSING REGIMENS

Identification and definition of optimal doses and dosing intervals for antimicrobial agents have eluded clinicians and investigators for decades. This problem can be attributed to the difficulty and delay in measuring outcomes, specifically, clinical improvement, microbiologic eradication, or survival. This difficulty in quantifying the effect of antibiotics is in contrast to other classes of drugs used in clinical medicine, such as antihypertensive drugs, for example. Substantial research to date has described the PK properties for most antimicrobial drugs used in pediatric practice. The challenge remains to determine objective PD markers or endpoints that reflect optimal dosing to achieve the desired therapeutic response.[60]

Antibacterial Agents

Antibacterial agents influence the life cycle of organisms in various ways. To alter bacterial growth, antibiotics must bind to a cellular target[61] (Figure 291-2). Binding of the drug to its target results in alteration of the normal function of the bacterium, leading to either inhibition of growth or cell death. In addition to the ability of an antimicrobial agent to reach its target site of action (i.e., the receptor), the drug also must possess sufficient affinity for its receptor and it must achieve a sufficient concentration to affect

A notable example that has been used therapeutically is probenecid, a drug that inhibits the tubular secretion of organic acids by antagonizing the efflux effects of select OATs (see Transporters, below). Probenecid can be coadministered with penicillin to reduce the extent of the antibiotic's tubular secretion and promote its accumulation in the body. Nevertheless, the lack of adequate guidelines for pediatric dosing of probenecid, the unpredictability of the drug–drug interaction, and the exact amount of drug accumulation and the potential that probenecid also can interfere with in vivo antibiotic distribution (antagonism by probenecid of the organic acid transport used by selected β-lactams into target tissue) preclude the common use of probenecid for this use in children or adults.

Transporters

Transporters important to cellular homeostasis influence the bioavailability, distribution, and elimination of many drugs.[57–59] Examples of such transporters are P glycoprotein (P-GP) and the organic anion transport polypeptides (OATP)/organic cation transporters (OCT), which often are associated with drug efflux out of the cell or facilitation of intracellular drug uptake. Transporters are found in many organs and tissues including the intestinal tract, placenta, blood–brain barrier, liver, and kidney and are also subject to induction and inhibition.[58,59] Drugs can serve as substrates, inhibitors, inducers, or any combination of the three, resulting in complex interactions that can be difficult to predict

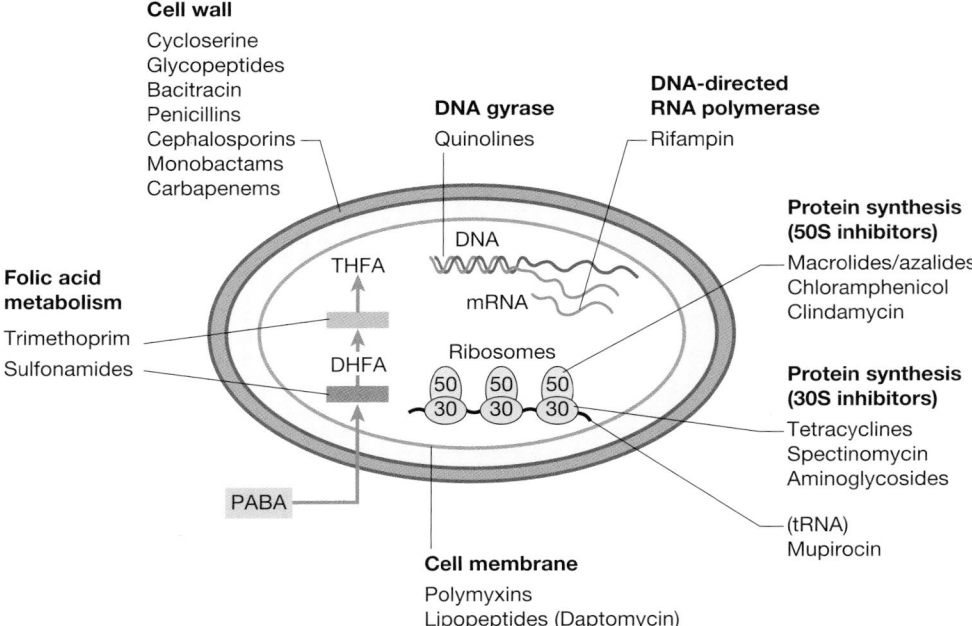

Figure 291-2. Sites of action for major antibacterial drugs. DHFA, dihydrofolic acid; PABA, *para*-aminobenzoic acid; THFA, tetrahydrofolic acid. (Adapted from Neu HC. The crisis in antibiotic resistance. Science 1992;257:1064–1073.)

bacterial function. These pharmacologic characteristics are the primary determinants of antimicrobial activity.

Unfortunately, we are unable to directly quantify these characteristics clinically. As such, surrogate markers have been developed in an attempt to reflect these crucial cellular interactions. For antibacterial agents, in vitro tests such as the minimal inhibitory concentration (MIC) and the minimal bactericidal concentration (MBC) are used as indirect measures to predict in vivo activity.[60,62,63] However, these markers do not provide sufficient information on the temporal pattern of exposure of an organism to antimicrobial agents or the antimicrobial concentration that must be achieved relative to the MIC/MBC to ensure a sufficient therapeutic response.

Consideration of the laboratory procedures involved in the determination of MICs and MBCs raises additional questions regarding the overall usefulness of these in vitro tests as primary indicators of clinical antimicrobial activity. First, measurements of MIC and MBC are obtained in bacterial growth media that are devoid of protein, which can have implications for agents that are highly bound to plasma proteins (e.g., >70% bound). Thus, antibiotic concentrations used to determine MICs or MBCs represent 100% free active drug. Similar concentrations of free drug at the anatomic site of infection may not be achievable clinically because of extensive protein binding, drug molecular weight, and degree of ionization at pathophysiologic pH. Second, measuring MICs and MBCs usually involves maintaining a constant concentration of free drug for a standard period (generally 18 h). Such a constant concentration simulates a continuous infusion of antibiotic whereas clinically, antibiotics usually are administered intermittently, which results in peaks and troughs rather than constant concentrations. Third, MICs or MBCs are measured on a standard inoculum of bacteria that may or may not reflect the actual density of bacteria present at the site of infection. Finally, the laboratory procedures used to determine the MIC and MBC do not account for the antimicrobial activity of various host defenses, including immunoglobulins and macrophages.

Intuitively, it is important to select an antibiotic with demonstrated activity against the pathogen, and in vitro susceptibility testing is especially valuable in identifying antimicrobial agents that will be ineffective in eradicating the pathogen. On the other hand, a pathogen can appear susceptible to a particular agent from in vitro testing (i.e., low MIC), yet information is lacking on the ability of the agent to achieve the necessary concentrations for a sufficient period at the site of infection to eradicate the pathogen. The immense importance of integrating such data with therapeutic outcome is exemplified by the PK–PD correlates in the successful treatment of bacterial meningitis.[64] The time course of the drug must be integrated with the concentration at the receptor site to reflect the in vivo antibiotic–bacteria interaction adequately.[62]

As a result of the differences in the mechanisms by which antibiotics kill bacteria and the position of safely achievable concentrations on the concentration–response curve, specific PK–PD properties can be correlated with efficacy (Table 291-7). The first pattern of activity is for drugs with concentrations near the upper, flat portion of the concentration–response curve, and which have minimal post-antibiotic effect, i.e., ongoing killing after serum concentrations have dropped below the MIC. The activity of these drugs depends on the duration of time that the antibiotic concentration exceeds the MIC (T >MIC).[65] Examples of T >MIC are shown in Figures 291-3 and 291-4. For these antibiotics, saturation of the bacterial killing rate is observed at certain multiples of the MIC, usually two to four times, and antibiotic concentrations exceeding this level generally do not achieve any greater killing rate. Clearly, the duration that the antibiotic concentration exceeds the MIC of the pathogen is influenced by several factors, including the dosing interval, the pathogen, and the site of infection. Drugs that demonstrate this type of PK–PD relationship are referred to as *time-dependent*. Some refer to this class as concentration-independent antibiotics, but this term is not preferred because all antibiotics require a minimal concentration for efficacy. Examples of drugs that exhibit time-dependent killing include all of the β-lactams (see Table 291-7).

In contrast, a second pattern of bacterial killing has been characterized for drugs that have concentrations in the steeper portion of the concentration–response curve, and that have some degree of post-antibiotic effect.[66,67] The bactericidal ability of agents in this group depends on the *peak concentration to MIC (peak/MIC)* within the dosing interval. In other words, the higher the antibiotic peak concentration, the greater the bacterial kill. Agents that demonstrate this type of PK–PD interface are referred to as *concentration-dependent* antibiotics and include aminoglycosides and fluoroquinolones.

A third class of drugs also have a post-antibiotic effect, but lie near the upper portion of the concentration–response curve, such

TABLE 291-7. Classification of Selected Antibacterial Agents Based on Their Pattern of Antimicrobial Activity

Pattern	Drug	Target
Peak/MIC Concentration-dependent killing, prolonged post-antibiotic effects	Aminoglycosides	10
	Daptomycin[314]	100 (*S. aureus*) 36 (*S. pneumoniae*) 0.25 (*E. faecium*)
	Fluoroquinolones	10
	Metronidazole	?
Time >MIC Time-dependent killing, minimal post-antibiotic effects	Carbapenems, aztreonam	>20–40%
	Cephalosporins	>20–40%
	Penicillins	>40–60%
AUC/MIC Time-dependent killing, moderate to prolonged persistent antibiotic effects	Azithromycin	25 (in vitro, immediate release)[315] 5 (clinical, extended release)[316]
	Clindamycin	?
	Telithromycin	3[317]
	Linezolid	80 (or trough >1 × MIC)[318]
	Macrolides	30[319,320]
	Quinupristin/dalfopristin	?
	Telavancin	?
	Tetracyclines	10
	Tigecycline	18 (gram-positive organism)[321] 7 (gram-negative organism)[322]
	Vancomycin	400 (trough ~8 × MIC)[303]

AUC, area under the curve; MIC, minimal inhibitory concentration.

Data are from references 323,324 unless otherwise noted.

that it is simply the *area under the plasma (serum) drug concentration–time curve (AUC) to MIC (AUC/MIC)* ratio that best describes activity. These are also called time-dependent drugs, but the post-antibiotic effect makes the choice of dose interval less critical than the time-dependent drugs with little to no post-antibiotic effect. Examples include vancomycin and azithromycin.

The clinical challenge relative to the PK–PD properties of *T* >MIC and peak/MIC or AUC/MIC is determining the target range for each that correlates with bacteriologic response. These are summarized in Table 291-7.

The Clinical Utility of Correlates of Antibiotic Pharmacokinetic–Pharmacodynamic Characteristics

The superior ability to predict bacteriologic cure by using integrated PK–PD characteristics rather than MIC or MBC information solely (see Table 291-7) helps standardize antimicrobial dosing in clinical trials and assists in guiding antimicrobial therapy for individual patients.[62,65,66] Furthermore, providing adequate amounts

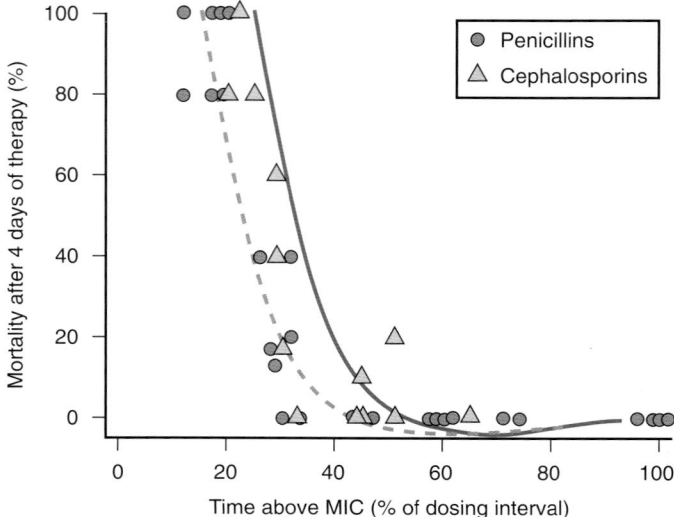

Figure 291-3. Efficacy of β-lactam antibiotics against *Streptococcus pneumoniae* in animal models. MIC, minimal inhibitory concentration. (Adapted from Craig WA. Pharmacokinetic/pharmacodynamic parameters: rationale for antibacterial dosing of mice and men. Clin Infect Dis 1998;26:1–10.)

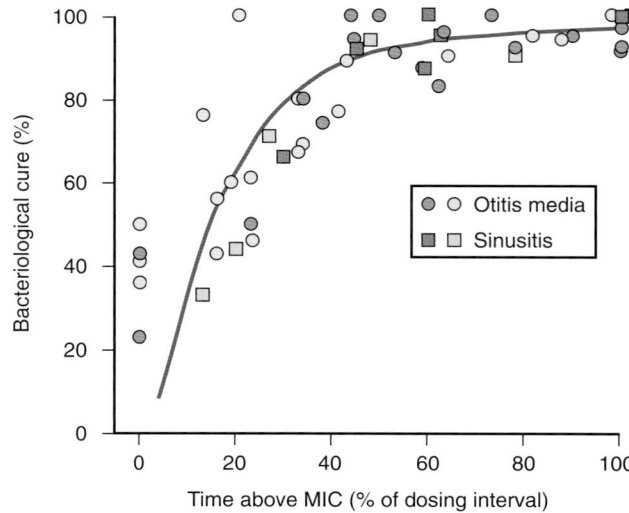

Figure 291-4. The relationship between time of antibiotic serum concentration above the minimal inhibitory concentration for 90% of organisms (MIC90) and bacteriologic cure in *Streptococcus pneumoniae* (dark symbols) and *Haemophilus influenzae* (light symbols) otitis media and sinusitis. (Adapted from Craig WA, Andes D. Pharmacokinetics and pharmacodynamics of antibiotics in otitis media. Pediatr Infect Dis J 1996;15:255–259.)

of antibiotic for sufficient periods via optimal dosing based on PK–PD properties also can decrease the rate and extent of bacterial resistance. One example of the application of PK–PD principles to antibiotic dosing is the current wide acceptance of once-daily aminoglycoside dosing for the treatment of systemic infections. An appreciation of the PK–PD characteristics of aminoglycosides, combined with a better understanding of their safety profiles, led to a once-daily dosing of aminoglycosides that can take advantage of the concentration-dependent killing characteristics of this class of antibiotics.[68]

In patients with a poor clinical response, an understanding of a particular drug's PK–PD characteristics allows the clinician rationally to assess the potential contribution of suboptimal dosing and to develop an effective, alternative regimen. In their assessment of published data, Craig and Andes demonstrated that the $T > $MIC for β-lactam antibiotics predicted bacteriologic efficacy with accuracy similar to that of the ratio of middle-ear fluid concentration to MIC.[69] Moreover, when the $T > $MIC exceeded 40% to 50% of the dosing interval, bacteriologic and clinical cure was achieved in 80% to 85% of the patients studied. Although most of the *Streptococcus pneumoniae* isolates in these studies were susceptible to penicillin, the same principles apply in an era of increasing resistance. For example, conventional amoxicillin dosing (13.3 mg/kg per dose three times daily) would be expected to exceed the target $T > $MIC for penicillin-susceptible and penicillin-intermediate *S. pneumoniae*, whereas higher doses (45 to 50 mg/kg per dose twice daily) often are required to achieve the target $T > $MIC for resistant isolates. Note that it is not the increased dose of amoxicillin per se that correlates with increased efficacy but the longer $T > $MIC afforded by higher initial concentrations. As an extension of this work, much attention has been paid recently to modeling improved efficacy of prolonged infusion of β-lactam agents against resistant gram-negative organisms,[70] although to our knowledge clinical benefit has yet to be demonstrated prospectively.

An awareness of PK–PD characteristics also permits more sophisticated interpretation of the breakpoints for in vitro susceptibility. Frequently, clinical laboratories do not report actual MICs for drugs against cultured pathogens but assign descriptive categories of "susceptible," "intermediate," or "resistant" to the organism based on defined guidelines for interpreting MICs. In general, these guidelines are derived from the likelihood of bacteriologic success relative to the MIC of the infecting organism and the projected achievable *serum* concentration of antibiotic. A major exception is the breakpoint reporting for *S. pneumoniae*, which is based on projected achievable concentrations, i.e., with oral dosing for simple infections and intravenous dosing for meningitis versus non-meningitis infections. Thus, if the infection is in an anatomic location other than that for which the breakpoints were derived, the breakpoints may be less relevant.

OTHER ANTIMICROBIAL AGENTS

Maximizing desirable PD outcomes while minimizing undesirable adverse effects necessarily requires the ability to quantify such endpoints. Furthermore, an objective index variable must be identified to which therapy can be linked to achieve the therapeutic goals. Although our knowledge of PK–PD relationships for other antimicrobial agents (e.g., antifungal, antiviral, antimycobacterial) is not yet as advanced as for antibacterial agents, some progress has been made.

Antifungal MICs are determined most reliably for yeasts (e.g., *Candida* and *Cryptococcus*). The value of MICs lies in the assignment of susceptibility breakpoints – drug concentrations above which the isolate is considered resistant and below which it is considered susceptible. These breakpoints allow clinicians to choose appropriate antimicrobial therapy.

The Clinical Laboratory Standards Institute (CLSI) and the European Committee on Antimicrobial Susceptibility Testing (EUCAST) have established breakpoints for azoles, echinocandins, and flucytosine against *Candida* spp. Although there is some reliability similar to MIC breakpoints for bacterial infections,[71] controversy still surrounds the exact thresholds for susceptibility.[72,73] Breakpoints for filamentous fungal infections, such as *Aspergillus*, still do not exist, and will be very difficult to generate

TABLE 291-8. Proposed Pharmacokinetic–Pharmacodynamic (PK–PD) Relationships for Antifungal Drugs

Drug	PK–PD Relationship	Notes
Amphotericin B	Peak/MIC?	Single, large daily doses are more effective than smaller, frequent doses; the dosage is limited by toxicity to a maximum of 1.5 mg/kg per day
Lipid amphotericin B (AmBisome, Abelcet, Amphotec)	Peak/MIC?	As above, but the pharmacokinetics of the three preparations are different and more studies are required to determine whether PD differences also exist. Lower toxicity in general permits a higher dosing of 5 mg/kg per day, and tolerability up to 15 mg/kg per day (Ambisome[325]) and 10 mg/kg per day (Abelcet[326]) has been reported, but added efficacy at the higher doses has not been demonstrated and may result in increased nephrotoxicity[327]
Fluconazole	AUC/MIC	Optimal dosing is 3–6 mg/kg per day IV/PO for susceptible isolates, 6–12 mg/kg per day for dose-dependent isolates. Doses >12 mg/kg offer unproven additional benefit and increase the risk of toxicity. A dose/MIC ratio of >50 or AUC/MIC ratio of >25 have been suggested as targets[328]
Itraconazole	AUC/MIC	Target trough concentrations of >0.5 µg/mL are recommended[329]
Posaconazole	AUC/MIC	Concentrations demonstrate a great deal of inter-patient variability; in two pivotal Phase III studies analyzed by the FDA, a plasma concentration of >0.35 µg/mL 3–5 h after dosing on day 2, was predictive of a concentration of >0.7 µg/mL at the same time on day 7, which was associated with *prevention* of invasive fungal infections.[329] Another study reported best *treatment* outcomes with average concentrations of >1.25 µg/mL.[330] In practice such concentrations are difficult to achieve in children[331]
Voriconazole	AUC/MIC	Target trough concentrations of >1.0 mg/mL have been associated with survival benefit in children[4]
Flucytosine	T>MIC	In vitro data suggest that peak efficacy occurs at a serum concentration–MIC ratio of 4 : 1. No data exist on the most effective duration of serum concentration above the MIC. If toxicity is problematic (typically with peak >100 µg/mL), smaller, more frequent doses or even continuous infusion may be more effective, but human data are lacking
Echinocandins (caspofungin, micafungin, anidulafungin, aminocandin)	AUC/MIC	Clinical data are lacking, but in vitro and animal models suggest for *Candida* species, a free drug AUC/MIC ratio of 5–20 (high end for *C. albicans*) may be adequate,[332] while for *Aspergillus* species, the target is a free C_{max}/MEC ratio of about 10[333]

MIC, minimal inhibitory concentration; MEC, minimum effective concentration which, is the minimum amount of drug to cause transition to a compact rounded hyphal form; C_{max}, maximum concentration.

now that combination therapy is widely employed for *Aspergillus* and other filamentous fungal infections.[74] We are only in the early stages of understanding optimal PK-based dosing of antifungal drugs. Table 291-8 shows the hypothesized relationships and dosing implications.[75]

PK–PD dosing for antiviral drugs, as shown in Table 291-9, has been most applied to therapy for human immunodeficiency virus

(HIV) infection. The concept of MIC determination translates as the inhibitory concentration, or IC_{xx}, where "xx" is the percentage reduction of viral concentration in vitro, and typically is expressed as IC_{50}. Numerous studies have demonstrated a dose–response relationship for both protease inhibitors and non-nucleoside reverse transcriptase inhibitors and have identified threshold trough serum concentrations, or AUC, above which efficacy is

TABLE 291-9. Pharmacokinetic–Pharmacodynamic Targets for Antiretroviral and Antiviral Drugs Based on Clinical Data

Antiretroviral Drugs				
Drug	Minimum (Naive)	Minimum (Experienced)	Maximum	Notes
NRTI				
Didanosine	*AUC 600 µg·h/L*[295]	ND	ND	Not in DHHS Guidelines
Lamivudine	400 ng/mL[14]	ND	ND	Not in DHHS Guidelines
Tenofovir	AUC 3.8 µg·h/mL[334]	ND	ND	Not in DHHS Guidelines
Zidovudine	*430 ng/mL*[335]	ND	ND	Not in DHHS Guidelines
NNRTI				
Efavirenz	*1000 ng/mL*[336] *AUC 50 µg·h/mL*[336]	ND	4000 ng/mL[337,338]	Good agreement between children and adults
Nevirapine	3000 or >4300[339] ng/mL	ND	ND	The higher target has been associated with reduced emergence of resistance mutations
PI				
Amprenavir	400 ng/mL	1600 ng/mL[340] gIQ 300 ng/mL/mutation	4000 ng/mL[341]	A free-drug gIQ target of 80 ng/mL/mutation has been reported[342]
Atazanavir	150 ng/mL *600 ng/mL*[343] *AUC 45 µg·h/mL*[343]	pIQ 1 gIQ 100 ng/mL/ mutation	ND	A target gIQ of 200 ng/mL/mutation has been reported in more recent studies;[344,345] C_{trough} >850 ng/mL has been associated with increased odds of hyperbilirubinemia,[346] but this generally is not treatment limiting
Darunavir	ND	pIQ 60[347] gIQ 1400[347] or 1800 ng/mL/mutation vIQ 800 ng/mL/unit fold change[348]	ND	
Indinavir	*100 ng/mL*[295] *AUC 15 µg·h/mL*[296]	ND	C_{trough}: 500 ng/mL[349] C_{max}: 10000 ng/mL[350]	
Lopinavir	1000 ng/mL	nIQ 1[351] pIQ 15, 25[352] gIQ 900 ng/mL/mutation	22,000 ng/mL[353]	For nIQ target, significant benefit only occurred when baseline regimen contained at least 70% PI activity (see footnote) Maximum reported concentration in one study with little toxicity[353]
Nelfinavir	*800 ng/mL*[354]	ND	12000 ng/mL[355]	
Saquinavir	100–250 ng/mL	nIQ 1[351] pIQ 1 gIQ 40 ng/mL/mutation	6000 ng/mL[350]	For nIQ target, significant benefit only occurred when baseline regimen contained at least 70% PI activity (see footnote)
Tipranavir	ND	20500 ng/mL pIQ 76 gIQ 4700 ng/mL/mutation vIQ 6000 ng/mL/unit fold change[356]	ND	In a head-to-head comparison, vIQ had the best PPV and LHR+[356] The gIQ target is consistent with pediatric data[357]
Entry inhibitor				
Maraviroc	ND	50 ng/mL	ND	

Non-antiretroviral Agents		
Drug	Target	Notes
Ganciclovir	AUC 35–50 µg·h/mL	For prevention of CMV infection

Concentration targets are from Department of Health and Human Services (DHHS) pediatric treatment guidelines[358] (which have been adopted from adult guidelines[359]), except where indicated. Inhibitory quotient targets are from adult recommendation by la Porte et al.,[360] unless indicated. Recommendations from studies specifically conducted in children are italicized. Targets, particularly maxima, should be viewed as approximate and taken in the context of the patient response. Several antiretroviral agents, particularly the NRTIs, have conflicting data where no association was found and these are discussed in the text.

NRTI, nucleoside reverse transcriptase inhibiting agent; NNRTI, non-nucleoside reverse transcriptase inhibiting agent; PI, protease inhibiting agent; ND = no data; gIQ = genotypic inhibitory quotient, the ratio of the drug concentration to the number of drug-specific mutations; pIQ = phenotypic inhibitory quotient, the ratio of drug concentration and viral 50% inhibitory concentration; nIQ = normalized inhibitory quotient, the pIQ normalized to a reference pIQ; C_{max}, maximum concentration; C_{trough}, trough concentration.

improved (as measured by the reduction in viral load and increased CD4+ T-lymphocyte count). Studies also have demonstrated the safety and feasibility of antiretroviral therapeutic regimens tailored for specific patients to maintain serum drug concentrations within a predetermined range, although efficacy studies are yet to come.

For non-HIV viral infections, some data suggest that the acyclovir effect is time-dependent and that if the serum drug concentration remains above the IC_{50} of herpes simplex virus or varicella-zoster virus for at least 12 h a day, clinical efficacy is maximized. Ganciclovir has been reported to have near-maximal efficacy to prevent cytomegalovirus infection when a target AUC of 35 to 50 μg/mL per hour is reached, with a concomitant 10% to 20% and 30% to 50% probability of developing neutropenia and leukopenia, respectively.[76]

CONCLUSIONS

As our knowledge of PK–PD relationships expands, drug dosing increasingly will be based on achieving PK–PD targets in individual patients rather than the traditional population-based recommendations of dosing ranges. Therefore, studies of new antimicrobial agents must include an assessment of PK–PD relationships. The ongoing challenge in pediatrics is to assure that the

determination of these important surrogate markers/endpoints incorporate the important changes that occur with increasing age. Box 291-1 synthesizes the information presented in this chapter into questions that a thorough clinician should consider at the bedside of every patient to whom antibiotics are to be administered. Finally, Box 291-2 provides a listing of useful websites.

Acknowledgment

This work was supported in part by NIAID K23 AI076106-01 (MN).

APPENDIX 291-1. Usual Dosing, Therapeutic Targets, and Suggestions for Maintenance Dosing of Selected Antimicrobial Agents in Individuals with Impaired Renal Function[a]

Drug (Route)	Usual Dosing: Maintenance (Daily Max.)	Adjustment of Usual Dosing for Renal Failure: GFR (mL/min/1.73 m²)[b]			Adjustment for Dialysis[c]
		>60–90	30–60	<30	
AMINOGLYCOSIDES[d]					
Amikacin (IM, IV)[79,83–88]	5–7 mg/kg q8h	60–90% q12h	30–70% q12–18h	20–30% q24–48h	H: 66% after H P: 15–20 mg/L IP C: As for CrCl 30–60
Gentamicin (IM, IV)[85,89–92]	2.5 mg/kg q8h	60–90% q8h	30–70% q12h	20–30% q24–48h	H: 66% after H P: 3–4 mg/L IP C: As for CrCl 30–60
Streptomycin (IM, IV)[85,93–95]	20–40 mg/kg q24h (2 g/day)	Usual dosing	100% q24–72h	100% q72–96h	H: 50% after H P: 20–40 mg/L IP C: As for CrCl 30–60
Tobramycin (IV)[85,96–98]	2.5 mg/kg q8h	60–90% q8h	30–70% q12h	20–30% q24–48h	H: 66% after H P: 3–4 mg/L IP C: As for CrCl 30–60

Continued

APPENDIX 291-1. Usual Dosing, Therapeutic Targets, and Suggestions for Maintenance Dosing of Selected Antimicrobial Agents in Individuals with Impaired Renal Function—cont'd

Drug (Route)	Usual Dosing: Maintenance (Daily Max.)	Adjustment of Usual Dosing for Renal Failure: GFR (mL/min/1.73 m²)[b]			Adjustment for Dialysis[c]
		>60–90	30–60	<30	
Cephalosporins[e]					
Cefaclor (PO)[99]	10–15 mg/kg q8h (4 g/day)	Usual dosing	Usual dosing	50% q8h	H: 50–75% q8h P: No significant clearance C: Usual dosing
Cefadroxil (PO)[100]	15 mg/kg q12h (4 g/day)	Usual dosing	100% q24h	100% q48h	H: 100% q48h P: No significant clearance C: As for CrCl 30–60
Cefazolin (IV)[101-104]	20–35 mg/kg q8h (12 g/day)	Usual dosing	100% q12h	100% q24h	H: 100% q24h P: 15 mg/kg IP q24h C: As for CrCl 30–60
Cefdinir (PO)[105,106]	14 mg/kg q24h (600 mg/day)	Usual dosing	Usual dosing	50% q24h	H: 50% q48h P: No significant clearance C: As for CrCl 30–60
Cefepime (IV)[101,107-109]	50 mg/kg q8–12h (6 g/day)	100% q12h	100% q16–24h	100% q24–48h	H: 50% q24h P: 15 mg/kg IP q24h C: As for CrCl >60–90
Cefixime (PO)[110]	8 mg/kg q24h (400 mg/day)	Usual dosing	75% q24h	50% q24h	H: 75% q24h P: No significant clearance C: As for CrCl 30–60
Cefotaxime[f] (IV)[111,112]	50–75 mg/kg q6–8h (12 g/day)	Usual dosing	Usual dosing	50% q6–8h	H: 50% q6-8h P: 500 mg IP q24h C: As for CrCl 30–60
Cefoxitin (IV)[113,114]	20–40 mg/kg q6h (12 g/day)	100% q8h	100% q8–12h	100% q24–48h	H: 100% q24–48h P: No significant clearance C: As for CrCl 30–60
Cefpodoxime (PO)[115-117]	5 mg/kg q12h (800 mg/day)	Usual dosing	Usual dosing	50% q12h	H: 50% q12h P: No significant clearance C: As for CrCl 30–60
Cefprozil (PO)[118]	15 mg/kg q12h (1 g/day)	Usual dosing	Usual dosing	100% q24h	H: 100% q24h P: Significant clearance unlikely C: Likely as for CrCl 30–60
Ceftaroline[g] (IV)	>12 years: 8 mg/kg q12h (1.2 g/day)	Usual dosing	50–75% q12h	50% q12h	H: 50% q12h P: No significant clearance C: As for CrCl 30–60
Ceftazidime (IV)[104,119-122]	50 mg/kg q8h (6 g/day)	Usual dosing	100% q12h	100% q24h	H: 100% q24h P: 50% IV q24h OR- 125 mg/L continuous IP -OR- 15–20 mg/kg q24h IP C: 50–75% q12h
Ceftriaxone (IV, IM)[123-126]	50–75 mg/kg/day divided q12–24h (4 g/day)	Usual dosing	Usual dosing	Usual dosing	H: Usual dosing P: 50 mg/kg IP q24h C: Usual dosing
Cefuroxime sodium (IV)[120]	35–80 mg/kg q8h (9 g/day)	Usual dosing	100% q8–12h	100% q24h	H: 100% q24h P: 15 mg/kg IP q24h C: As for CrCl 30–60
Cefuroxime axetil (PO)[120,127]	15 mg/kg q12h (1 g/day)	Usual dosing	100% q12h	100% q24h	H: 100% q24h P: No significant clearance C: As for CrCl 30–60
Cephalexin[h] (PO)[128]	25 mg/kg q6h (4 g/day)	Usual dosing	Usual dosing	50% q6h	H: 50% q6h P: No significant clearance C: Usual dosing
Penicillins					
Amoxicillin (PO)	40–90 mg/kg/day divided q8–12h (3 g/day)	Usual dosing	Usual dosing	100% q12–24h	H: 100% q24h P: Significant clearance unlikely C: Usual dosing
Ampicillin ± sulbactam (IV, IM)[129,130]	50 mg/kg q6h (14 g/day – amp) (8 g/day – amp/sul)	Usual dosing	100% q8h	100% q12h	H: 100% q24h P: 100% q12h IP C: Usual dosing

Continued

APPENDIX 291-1. Usual Dosing, Therapeutic Targets, and Suggestions for Maintenance Dosing of Selected Antimicrobial Agents in Individuals with Impaired Renal Function—cont'd

Drug (Route)	Usual Dosing: Maintenance (Daily Max.)	Adjustment of Usual Dosing for Renal Failure: GFR (mL/min/1.73 m²)[b]			Adjustment for Dialysis[c]
		>60–90	30–60	<30	
Dicloxacillin (PO)	6.25 mg/kg q6h (4 g/day)	Usual dosing	Usual dosing	Usual dosing	H/P: No significant clearance C: Usual dosing
Nafcillin[j] (IV)[131]	25–50 mg/kg q6h (12 g/day)	Usual dosing	Usual dosing	Usual dosing	H/P: No significant clearance C: Usual dosing
Penicillin G (IV)	150–300 kU/kg/day divided q4–6h (80 MU/day)	Usual dosing	50% q4–5h	50% q8h	H: 50% q8h P: No significant clearance C: 50% q4–5h
Penicillin VK (PO)	25–50 mg/kg/day divided q6–8h (7.2 g/day)	Usual dosing	50% q4–5h	50% q8h	H: 50% q8h P: No significant clearance C: 50% q4–5h
Piperacillin ± tazobactam (IV)[132–136]	2–9 months: 80 mg/kg q8h >9 months: 100 mg/kg q8h >40 kg: 3.375 g q6h (18 g/day)	Usual dosing	66% q6–8h	66% q8h	H: 66% q12h + 20% after H P: No significant clearance and IP tazobactam not well absorbed C: As for CrCl 30–60
Ticarcillin ± clavulanate (IV)[137,138]	50 mg/kg q4–6h (24 g/day)	66% q4–6h	66% q8h	66% q8–12h	H: 66% q12h + 100% after H P: 100% q12h IV C: As for CrCl 30–60
MONOBACTAM					
Aztreonam (IV)[139–141]	30–40 mg/kg q8h (8 g/day)	Usual dosing	50–75% q8h	25% q8h	H: 25% q8h + 12.5% after H P: 100% q8h IP or 25% q8h IV C: As for CrCl 30–60
CARBAPENEMS					
Doripenem[j] (IV)[143]	3 months to 2 years: 10 mg/kg q8h ≥2 years: 15 mg/kg q8h (1.5 g/day)	Usual dosing	50–75% q8h	50–75% q12h	H: Likely similar to other carbapenems P: Significant clearance unlikely C: As for CrCl 30–60
Ertapenem (IV)[144–146]	<13 years: 15 mg/kg q12h ≥13 years: 1 g q24h (1 g/day)	Usual dosing	Usual dosing	50% q12h	H: 50% q12h + 15% after H if H <6h after last dose P: Significant clearance unlikely C: Likely as for CrCl 30–60
Imipenem[k] (IV)[147–156]	15–25 mg/kg q6h (4 g/day)	Usual dosing	50% q8h	50% q12h	H: 50% q12h + 25% after H if H <6 h after last dose P: No significant clearance C: As for CrCl 30–60
Meropenem (IV)[157–166]	20–40 mg/kg q8h (6 g/day)	Usual dosing	100% q12h	50% q12–24h	H: 50% q24h –OR- 100% q48h P: No significant clearance C: As for CrCl 30–60
FLUOROQUINOLONES					
Ciprofloxacin (IV, PO)[167–170]	10–20 mg/kg q12h (1.5 g/day)	Usual dosing	50% q12h	50% q18h	H: No significant clearance P: No significant clearance C: As for CrCl 30–60
Levofloxacin[171–179] (IV, PO)	<50 kg: 8 mg/kg q12h ≥50 kg: 500–750 mg q24h (750 mg/day)	Usual dosing	50% q24h	50% q48h	H: No significant clearance P: No significant clearance C: As for CrCl 30–60
Moxifloxacin[j] (IV, PO)[182,183]	8–10 mg/kg q24h (400 mg/day)	Usual dosing	Usual dosing	Usual dosing	H: No significant clearance P: No significant clearance C: Significant clearance unlikely
MACROLIDES + LINCOSAMIDES					
Azithromycin (IV, PO)[184]	5–12 mg/kg q24h (2 g/day)	Usual dosing	Usual dosing	Usual dosing	H/P/C: Usual dosing
Clarithromycin (PO)	7.5 mg/kg q12h (1 g/day)	Usual dosing	Usual dosing	50% q12h	H/P/C: Significant clearance Unlikely
Clindamycin (IM, IV)[185]	20–40 mg/kg divided q6–8h (4.8 g/day)	Usual dosing	Usual dosing	Usual dosing	H/P/C: Usual dosing
Clindamycin (PO)	10–30 mg/kg divided q6–8h (2.7 g/day)	Usual dosing	Usual dosing	Usual dosing	H/P/C: Usual dosing

Continued

APPENDIX 291-1. Usual Dosing, Therapeutic Targets, and Suggestions for Maintenance Dosing of Selected Antimicrobial Agents in Individuals with Impaired Renal Function—cont'd

Drug (Route)	Usual Dosing: Maintenance (Daily Max.)	Adjustment of Usual Dosing for Renal Failure: GFR (mL/min/1.73 m²)[b]			Adjustment for Dialysis[c]
		>60–90	30–60	<30	
Erythromycin[m] (IV, PO)[186]	10 mg/kg q6h (4 g/day)	Usual dosing	Usual dosing	Usual dosing	H/P/C: Usual dosing
Telithromycin (PO)	No data (800 mg/day)	Usual dosing	Usual dosing	Usual dosing	H: 66% q24h P: Significant clearance unlikely C: Usual dosing
TETRACYCLINES					
Doxycycline[n] (IV, PO)[187]	2.2 mg/kg q12h (200 mg/day)	Usual dosing	Usual dosing	Usual dosing	H/P/C: No significant clearance
Tigecycline[o] (IV)	No data (100 mg/day)	Usual dosing	Usual dosing	Usual dosing	H/P/C: No significant clearance
OTHER ANTIBACTERIAL AGENTS					
Chloramphenicol (IV)[190,191]	12.5–25 mg/kg q6h (4 g/day)	Usual dosing	Usual dosing	Usual dosing	H: Usual dosing P/C: No significant clearance
Daptomycin[p] (IV)[196–199]	4–6 mg/kg q24h (6 mg/kg/day)	Usual dosing	Usual dosing	100% q48h	H: 100% q48h P: 100% q48h OR 7 mg/kg IP q24h C: 8 mg/kg IV q48h
Linezolid (IV, PO)[200–204]	10 mg/kg q8h (1.2 g/day)	Usual dosing	Usual dosing	Usual dosing	H: Usual dosing P: Significant clearance unlikely C: Usual dosing
Metronidazole[q] (IV, PO)[205–207]	11.6–16.6 mg/kg q8h (4 g/day)	Usual dosing	Usual dosing	75% q6h	H: Usual dosing P: No significant clearance C: Usual dosing
Nitrofurantoin (PO)	1–2 mg/kg q6h (400 mg/day)	Usual dosing	Avoid	Avoid	H/P/C: avoid
Quinupristin-dalfopristin[r] (IV)[208,209]	7.5 mg/kg q8h (22.5 mg/kg/day)	Usual dosing	Usual dosing	Usual dosing	H/P/C: No significant clearance
Trimethoprim-sulfamethoxazole (IV, PO)[210–212]	4–6 mg/kg q12h *Pneumocystis:* 5 mg/kg q6–8h (20 mg/kg/day)	Usual dosing Usual dosing	Usual dosing 100% q8h	100% q12–24h 100% q12–24h	H: 100% q24h P: No significant clearance C: As for CrCl 30–60
Vancomycin[s] (IV)[139,213–217]	15 mg/kg q6h (2 g/day)	q12–24h	10 mg/kg q24–96h	10 mg/kg q4–10 days	H: 10 mg/kg after H P: 50–100% IP q24h C: As for CrCl 30–60
ANTITUBERCULOUS AGENTS					
Ethambutol (PO)[218–220]	15–25 mg/kg q24h (2.5 g/day)	Usual dosing	Usual dosing	100% q48h	H: 100% q48h P: No significant clearance C: Likely usual dosing
Ethionamide (PO)[221]	15–20 mg/kg q24h (1 g/day)	Usual dosing	Usual dosing	50% q24h	H: 50% q24h P: No significant clearance C: Likely usual dosing
Isoniazid (IV, PO)[219,222–224]	10–20 mg/kg q24h (300 mg/day)	Usual dosing	Usual dosing	Usual dosing	H/P/C: Usual dosing
Para-aminosalicylic acid (PO)[93,221]	100–150 mg/kg q12h (10 g/day)	Usual dosing	Usual dosing	Usual dosing	H/P/C: Usual dosing
Pyrazinamide[t] (PO)[93,219,222,225,226]	15–30 mg/kg q24h (2 g/day)	Usual dosing	Usual dosing	100% q48–72h	H: As for CrCl < 10 P: As for CrCl < 10 C: No data
Rifampin (IV, PO)[93,219,222]	10–20 mg/kg q12h (600 mg/day)	Usual dosing	Usual dosing	Usual dosing	H/P/C: No significant clearance
ANTIFUNGAL AGENTS					
Polyenes					
Amphotericin B (IV)	0.5–1.5 mg/kg q24h (1.5 mg/kg/day)	Usual dosing	Usual dosing	100% q24–48h	H/P/C: No significant clearance
AmBisome (liposomal amphotericin B) (IV)	3–5 mg/kg q24h (7.5 mg/kg/day)	Usual dosing	Usual dosing	100% q24–48h	H/P/C: No significant clearance

Continued

APPENDIX 291-1. Usual Dosing, Therapeutic Targets, and Suggestions for Maintenance Dosing of Selected Antimicrobial Agents in Individuals with Impaired Renal Function—cont'd

Drug (Route)	Usual Dosing: Maintenance (Daily Max.)	Adjustment of Usual Dosing for Renal Failure: GFR (mL/min/1.73 m²)[b]			Adjustment for Dialysis[c]
		>60–90	30–60	<30	
Abelcet, Amphotec (lipid amphotericin B) (IV)	5 mg/kg q24h *(5 mg/kg/day)*	Usual dosing	Usual dosing	100% q24–48h	H/P/C: No significant clearance
Azoles					
Fluconazole (IV,PO)[227–232]	3–12 mg/kg q24h *(400 mg/day)*	Usual dosing	50% q24h	50% q48h	H: 100% after H P: As for CrCl <30 C: As for CrCl 30–60
Itraconazole[u] (IV, PO)[233,234]	2.5 mg/kg q12h *(200 mg/day)*	Usual dosing	Usual dosing	Usual dosing	H/P/C: No significant clearance
Posaconazole[v] (PO)[235]	200 mg q8h *(800 mg/day)*	Usual dosing	Usual dosing	Usual dosing	H/P/C: No significant clearance
Voriconazole[u,xxi] (IV, PO)[236–239]	7 mg/kg q12h *(800 mg/day)*	Usual dosing	Usual dosing	Usual dosing	H/P/C: No significant clearance
Echinocandins					
Anidulafungin[ww] (IV)	1.5 mg/kg q24h *(100 mg/day)*	Usual dosing	Usual dosing	Usual dosing	H/P/C: No significant clearance
Caspofungin (IV)	50 mg/m² q24h *(50 mg/day)*	Usual dosing	Usual dosing	Usual dosing	H/P/C: No significant clearance
Micafungin[x] (IV)	1–4 mg/kg q24h *(150 mg/day)*	Usual dosing	Usual dosing	Usual dosing	H/P/C: No significant clearance
Other antifungal agents					
Flucytosine[y] (IV,PO)[243,244]	12.5–37.5 mg/kg q6h *(150 mg/kg/day)*	100% q12h	100% q18h	100% q24h	H: 100% after H P: No significant clearance C: As for CrCl 30–60
Griseofulvin ultramicrosize (PO)	1.5 mg/kg q24h *(750 mg/day)*	Usual dosing	Usual dosing	Usual dosing	H/P/C: No significant clearance
Terbinafine[z] (PO)	<25 kg: 125 mg q24h 25–35 kg: 125 mg q24h >35 kg: 250 mg q24h *(250 mg/day)*	Usual dosing	Usual dosing	Usual dosing	H/P/C: Significant clearance unlikely
ANTIVIRAL AGENTS					
Anti-herpesviruses					
Acyclovir[aa] (IV, PO)[247–252]	10–20 mg/kg q8h (IV) *(60 mg/kg/day IV)* 20 mg/kg q6h (PO) *(4.8 g/day PO)*	100% q8h 100% q6h	100% q12h 100% q6h	50–100% q24h 100% q8–12h	H: 50% q24h P: 50% q24h C: 100% q24h
Cidofovir[bb] (IV)	No established pediatric dose or frequency	Usual dosing	Contraindicated, but consider 40–60%	Contraindicated, but consider 10–30%	H: Consider 100% 2 h before HD P: Consider 10% C: No data
Foscarnet (IV)[258–260]	Induction: 40–90 mg/kg q12h Maintenance: 90–120 mg/kg q24h *(180 mg/kg/day)*	50–75% q12h 50–75% q24h	50–75% q24h 50–75% q48h	Avoid Avoid	H: 50% after H P: 75% q48–72h C: No data
Ganciclovir[cc] (IV)[261–265]	Induction: 5 mg/kg q12h Maintenance: 5 mg/kg q24h *(10 mg/kg/day)*	50–100% q12h 50–100% q24h	50% q24h 25% q24h	25% q24h 12.5% q24h	H: 25% after H P: No significant clearance C: 100% q48h
Valacyclovir (PO)[266]	20 mg/kg q8–12h *(3 g/day)*	Usual dose	Usual dose	50–100% q24h	H/P/C: As for acyclovir
Valganciclovir (PO)	Induction: 7 mg × BSA × CrCl q12h Maintenance: 7 mg × BSA × CrCl q24h *(1.8 g/day)*	Usual dosing Usual dosing	Usual dosing Usual dosing	Usual dosing Usual dosing	H/P/C: No data, but likely as for ganciclovir

Continued

APPENDIX 291-1. Usual Dosing, Therapeutic Targets, and Suggestions for Maintenance Dosing of Selected Antimicrobial Agents in Individuals with Impaired Renal Function—cont'd

Drug (Route)	Usual Dosing: Maintenance (Daily Max.)	Adjustment of Usual Dosing for Renal Failure: GFR (mL/min/1.73 m²)[b]			Adjustment for Dialysis[c]
		>60–90	30–60	<30	
Anti-influenza agents					
Amantadine[dd] (PO)[267,268]	2.2–4.4 mg/kg q12h (200 mg/day)	Usual dosing	100% q24h	100% q48h	H/P: 100% once weekly C: No data
Oseltamivir (PO)[269-271]	2 mg/kg q12h (150 mg/day)	Usual dosing	100% q24h	50% q24h	H: 0.5 mg/kg after H P: 50% once weekly C: As for CrCl 30–60
Peramivir[ee] (IV)	All doses are mg/kg q24h: 0–30 days: 6 31–90 days: 8 91–180 days: 10 181 days to 5 years: 12 6–17 years: 10 (600 mg/day)	Usual dosing	25% q24h	16% q24h	H: 2.5% q24h P/C: No data
Rimantidine[ff] (PO)	1–9 years: 5 mg/kg q24h (150 mg/day) ≥10 years: 100 mg q12h (200 mg/day)	Usual dosing Usual dosing	Usual dosing Usual dosing	75% q24h 75% q12h	H: No significant clearance P/C: Significant clearance unlikely
Zanamivir (Inhaled)	10 mg q12h	Usual dosing	Usual dosing	Usual dosing	H/P/C: No significant systemic absorption from inhalation
ANTIRETROVIRAL AGENTS					
Nucleoside reverse transcriptase inhibitors					
Abacavir (PO)[272]	8 mg/kg q12h (600 mg/day)	Usual dosing	Usual dosing	Usual dosing	H: No significant clearance P/C: Significant clearance unlikely
Didanosine (PO)[273,274]	>8 months: 100 mg/m² q12h (400 mg/day) EC formulation: 20–<25 kg: 200 mg q24h 25–<60 kg: 250 mg q24h >60 kg: 400 mg q24h (400 mg/day)	Usual dosing Usual dosing Usual dosing Usual dosing	100% q24h 50% q24h 50% q24h 50% q24h	50% q24h Avoid Avoid 50% q24h	H: 37.5% q24h P: 37.5% q24h C: No data
Emtricitabine (PO)	0–3 months: 3 mg/kg q24h >3 months: 6 mg/kg q24h (240 mg/day)	Usual dosing (capsule) Usual dosing (solution)	100% q48h (capsule) 50% q24h (solution)	100% q72h (capsule) 33% q24h (solution)	H: 100% q96h (capsule) 25% q24h (solution) P/C: No data, likely some clearance
Lamivudine (PO)[275-277]	4 mg/kg q12h (300 mg/day)	Usual dosing	100% q24h	16–66% q24h	H: No significant clearance P: No significant clearance C: As for CrCl 30–60
Stavudine (PO)[278]	<30 kg: 1 mg/kg q12h 30–60 kg: 30 mg q12h >60 kg: 40 mg q12h (80 mg/day)	Usual dosing	50% q12h	50% q24h	H: 50% q24h P: Likely as for CrCl <30 C: Likely as for CrCl 30–60
Tenofovir (PO)[279]	>35 kg: 300 mg q24h (300 mg/day)	Usual dosing	100% q48h	100% q72–96h	H: 100% once weekly P: Significant clearance unlikely C: No data
Zidovudine (IV,PO)[280-284]	Treatment: 240 mg/m² q12h Prevention: 2 mg/kg q6h (PO) 1.5 mg/kg q6h (IV) (600 mg/day)	Usual dosing	Usual dosing	Usual dosing	H: 50% q8h P: 50% q8h C: Likely usual dosing
Non-nucleoside reverse transcriptase inhibitors					
Efavirenz (PO)[285-287]	200 mg + 50 mg/5 kg over 15 kg q24h (600 mg/day)	Usual dosing	Usual dosing	Usual dosing	H/P/C: No significant clearance
Etravirine (PO)[288]	100 mg + 25 mg/5 kg over 20 kg q12h (400 mg/day)	Usual dosing	Usual dosing	Usual dosing	H/P/C: No significant clearance

Continued

APPENDIX 291-1. Usual Dosing, Therapeutic Targets, and Suggestions for Maintenance Dosing of Selected Antimicrobial Agents in Individuals with Impaired Renal Function—cont'd

Drug (Route)	Usual Dosing: Maintenance (Daily Max.)	Adjustment of Usual Dosing for Renal Failure: GFR (mL/min/1.73 m²)[b]			Adjustment for Dialysis[c]
		>60–90	30–60	<30	
Nevirapine (PO)[289–291]	150 mg/m² q12h (400 mg/day)	Usual dosing	Usual dosing	Usual dosing	H: Usual dosing after H P: Usual dosing C: Likely usual dosing
Protease inhibitors					
Atazanavir (PO)[292]	100 + 50 mg/10 kg over 15 kg q24h (800 mg/day)	Usual dosing	Usual dosing	Usual dosing	H/P/C: No significant clearance
Darunavir (PO)[288]	20–30 kg: 375 mg q12h ≥30–40 kg: 450 mg q12h ≥40 kg: 600 mg q12h (1.2 g/day)	Usual dosing	Usual dosing	Usual dosing	H/P/C: No significant clearance
Fosamprenavir (PO)	30 mg/kg q12h (2.8 g/day) OR 18 mg/kg + 3 mg/kg ritonavir q12h (1400 mg/day)	Usual dosing	Usual dosing	Usual dosing	H/P/C: No significant clearance
Indinavir[99] (PO)	500 mg/m² q8h (2.4 g/day)	Usual dosing	Usual dosing	Usual dosing	H/P/C: No significant clearance
Lopinavir (PO)[286]	230 mg/m² q12h (800 mg/day)	Usual dosing	Usual dosing	Usual dosing	H/P/C: No significant clearance
Nelfinavir (PO)[291,300]	45–55 mg/kg q12h (2.5 g/day)	Usual dosing	Usual dosing	Usual dosing	H/P/C: No significant clearance
Ritonavir (PO)[290]	400 mg/m² q12h (600 mg/day)	Usual dosing	Usual dosing	Usual dosing	H/P/C: No significant clearance
Saquinavir (PO)	No established pediatric dose (2 g/day)	Usual dosing	Usual dosing	Usual dosing	H/P/C: No significant clearance
Tipranavir (PO)	14 mg/kg q12h (1 g/day)	Usual dosing	Usual dosing	Usual dosing	H/P/C: No significant clearance
Other antiretrovirals					
Maraviroc (PO)	No established pediatric dose (1.2 g/day)	Likely usual dosing	Likely usual dosing	Likely usual dosing	H/P/C: Significant clearance unlikely
Raltegravir (PO)[288]	No established pediatric dose (800 mg/day)	Likely usual dosing	Likely usual dosing	Likely usual dosing	H/P/C: Significant clearance unlikely
Anti-hepati					
Adefovir (PO)	>12 years: 10 mg q24h (10 mg/day)	Usual dosing	100% q48h	100% q72h	H: 100% weekly P/C: No data
Entecavir (PO)	>16 years: 0.5–1 mg q24h (1 mg/day)	Usual dosing	100% q48h	100% q72h	H: 100% weekly
Ribavirin (PO)	7.5 mg/kg q12h (15 mg/kg/day)	Usual dosing	Avoid	Avoid	H/P/C: Avoid

BSA, body surface area; C, continuous renal replacement; CrCl, creatinine clearance (calculated or measured); ESRD, end-stage renal disease; H, intermittent hemodialysis; HIV, human immunodeficiency virus; IM, intramuscular; IP, intraperitoneal; IV, intravenous; kU, thousand units; MU, million units; P, continuous peritoneal dialysis; PO, orally.

[a]*Package inserts and several review articles[77–81] on antibiotic dosing in renal failure and the various modes of dialysis were consulted for each drug. Recommendations are a synthesis of these sources and the pharmacokinetic characteristics of each drug; where available, supplemental references are included. Data are based primarily on studies in adults as there are very few pediatric studies reported in any literature source. Usual doses are for children with normal renal function beyond the neonatal period and for maintenance of systemic drug levels after an initial loading dose (which is typically standard in patients with impaired renal function). Doses herein may differ from those recommended by manufacturers (see package inserts) and in many cases are not approved for children.*

[b]*The preferred method for estimating GFR in children is the revised Schwartz formula: GFR (ml/min/1.73 m²) = 0.413 × height (cm)/plasma creatinine (mg/dL).[82] This formula is most accurate in the GFR range of 15–75 ml/min/1.73 m², and values outside this range should be reported only as less than or below these limits.*

Continued

APPENDIX 291-1. Usual Dosing, Therapeutic Targets, and Suggestions for Maintenance Dosing of Selected Antimicrobial Agents in Individuals with Impaired Renal Function—cont'd

*c*These dose projections are only guidelines and based on standard intermittent hemodialysis three times weekly, continuous peritoneal ambulatory dialysis with 3–4 daily exchanges, and continuous renal replacement with ultrafiltration rates approximately 1L/h. The advent of high-flux or extended intermittent hemodialysis, earlier use of continuous renal replacement in critically ill patients who have residual renal function, and the myriad of settings possible for all forms of ultrafiltration/ dialysis make the possibility of clinically significant under- or over-dosing very real indeed. Measurement of serum drug concentrations must be used when feasible. "No significant clearance" means that the drug should be dosed according to the recommendation for a given degree of renal failure, without regard to dialysis schedule. For intermittent hemodialysis, unless there is "no significant clearance," dialysis should always be timed to give the scheduled dose at the end of the dialysis session. If this is not possible, clinicians must use their best judgment about administering a supplemental dose after dialysis, depending on when the next regular dose is due and the relative risks of drug toxicity versus subtherapeutic concentrations. Peritoneal dialysis, as discussed in the text, removes most drugs poorly from blood; therefore, unless indicated, oral or intravenous drugs should be administered according to the underlying renal function. However, many drugs can achieve therapeutic serum concentrations when administered intraperitoneally; hence, recommendations for this route are included.

*d*Serum drug concentrations should be monitored. Concurrent administration with penicillins may result in subtherapeutic gentamicin or tobramycin. Peritoneal absorption increases with inflammation. Doses for once daily aminoglycoside regimens in patients with normal renal function generally should not be used in those with compromised renal function; hence they are not reported here.

*e*Peritoneal absorption of cephalosporins is generally good.

*f*Active metabolite of cefotaxime also accumulates in ESRD. The dose should be further reduced for hepatic and renal failure.

*g*Usual dose of ceftaroline is if >12 years; not approved <18 years of age.

*h*To treat urinary tract infection in ESRD with cephalexin, the dose should be the usual dose.

*i*Drugs with renal and hepatic excretion like nafcillin require little change unless both mechanisms are impaired.

*j*Doripenem is not approved <18 years of age. Doses in children are under study.[142]

*k*Imipenem neurotoxicity can occur, especially in ESRD.

*l*Moxifloxacin is not approved <18 years of age. Dose recommendation is based on allometric scaling from adult dose and a case report.[180] There is also a case report of 13 mg/kg q24h used in an infant.[181]

*m*Ototoxicity from erythromycin can occur with prolonged high doses in ESRD.

*n*Doxycycline is the preferred member of the tetracycline class for use in individuals with impaired renal function.

*o*Tigecycline is not approved in children. There are two case reports of use in children at doses of 1 mg/kg q12h[188] or 2 mg/kg q8h.[189]

*p*Daptomycin is not approved for use in children. There are reports of dosing and pharmacokinetics in children at the same dose as for adults (4–6 mg/kg q24h), although the exposure may be lower in the pediatric patients relative to the adults.[192–194] There is even a report of intraventricular daptomycin in a toddler at a dose of 2.5 mg in 5 mL normal saline, administered via ventriculostomy tubing every 24 hours, which was locked for 30 minutes after administration and then reopened.[189] Of note, one study found that daptomycin failure was independently associated with severe renal failure, raising the question of whether the recommended dosing for these patients is suboptimal.[195]

*q*Dosage adjustment of metronidazole is necessary because the metabolite accumulates in ESRD, although this is cleared by hemodialysis and continuous renal replacement.

*r*Microbiologically active metabolites of quinupristin-dalfopristin can accumulate in renal failure, and be cleared by dialysis.

*s*Serum vancomycin concentrations should be monitored.

*t*Serum pyrazinamide concentrations are the best guide.

*u*β-Cyclodextrin, the vehicle for the oral liquid and intravenous itraconazole and voriconazole preparations, is cleared by the kidneys and accumulates with significant renal failure after intravenous administration; oral dosing is therefore preferred in patients with CrCl<50. Absorption of liquid itraconazole is superior to the capsules; thus liquid itraconazole is preferred for oral therapy.

*v*Posaconazole dosing in children has not been established.

*w*Anidulafungin is not approved in children, but 1.5 mg/kg/day results in similar exposures to adults who receive 100 mg/day.[240]

*x*Micafungin is not approved in children, but doses of 1–4 mg/kg/day (the higher doses in younger children) appear to replicate adult exposures from 50–150 mg/day. There appear to be few safety concerns associated with mild overdosing of micafungin or the other echinocandins.[241,242]

*y*Serum flucytosine concentrations should be monitored; bone marrow suppression is more common in azotemic individuals.

*z*Terbinafine is not approved in children. The usual dosing in the table has been shown to reproduce adult exposures from 250 mg/day.[245,246]

*aa*Acyclovir impairs urate secretion and can cause gout; uric acid levels should be monitored.

*bb*There is no established pediatric dose for cidofovir. Dosing ranging from 5 mg/kg weekly (induction) followed by 3–5 mg/kg weekly to biweekly (maintenance), to 1 mg/kg thrice weekly, to 0.25–1 mg/kg every other week have been used for adenovirus, cytomegalovirus, and polyoma viral infections in children.[253–256] Although the package insert states that the drug is contraindicated in renal failure, the reported dosing guidelines were developed with the intent to change the label.[257]

*cc*The maintenance ganciclovir dose is half the induction dose; bone marrow suppression is more common in azotemic individuals.

*dd*Amantadine neurotoxicity is more common in ESRD.

*ee*Peramivir is not licensed by the FDA for use in humans. It is available through an emergency use protocol through the FDA (http://www.fda.gov/Drugs/ DevelopmentApprovalProcess/HowDrugsareDevelopedandApproved/ApprovalApplications/InvestigationalNewDrugINDApplication/ucm090039.htm) or enrollment in a clinical trial.

*ff*These doses are for prophylaxis only. Rimantidine is not indicated for influenza treatment in patients <16 years of age.

*gg*Indinavir is not approved in children. Doses shown to approximate adult exposures include 50 mg/kg, 500 mg/m² and 600 mg/m², all every 8 hours.[293–299]

292 Antimicrobial Agents

John S. Bradley and Jason B. Sauberan

Antimicrobial agents are essential in the therapy of bacterial infections. The approach to antimicrobial therapy is outlined in Chapter 289 (Principles of Anti-Infective Therapy), providing the clinician with an overview of the selection of agents based on the characteristics of infected children with respect to their pathogens and antibiotic susceptibilities, sites of infection, drug absorption, distribution and elimination, comorbidities, and a consideration of the benefits versus the risks of antimicrobial therapy. In this chapter, the agents themselves are discussed, providing a background on mechanism of action, spectrum of antibacterial activity, antibiotic resistance, and current clinical use. A more detailed discussion for specific infections is found in each chapter describing that infection. An in-depth discussion of antibiotic resistance and the ways to detect resistance is presented in Chapter 291. Pharmacokinetic-pharmacodynamic basis of optimal antibiotic therapy is discussed in Chapter 292. Table 292-1 provides a summary of the pharmacokinetics, tissue distribution, metabolism, and excretion of commonly used antimicrobial agents within each of the antibiotic classes. Table 292-2 provides the spectrum of activity of each antibiotic. Appendices 292-1 and 292-2 provide dosages of antibiotics.

Text continued on page 1465.

TABLE 292-1. Pharmacokinetics, Tissue Distribution, Metabolism, and Excretion of Antimicrobial Agents

Agent	Oral Bioavailability	Protein Binding	Body Distribution and CSF Penetration	Metabolism	Excretion	$t_{1/2}$[a] (Elimination)
AMINOGLYCOSIDES						
Gentamicin, amikacin, kanamycin, tobramycin	Poorly absorbed	<25%	Primarily to extracellular fluids and vascularized tissues, fetus, ascitic, synovial, and amniotic fluid; minimally into CSF	None	Renal	Neonates <1 week, 5–14 hours (varies inversely with birthweight) Neonates >1 week and infants, 3–5 hours Children/adults, ~2 hours
Streptomycin	Poorly absorbed	35%	Same as gentamicin	10–30% at unknown site	Renal	Neonates, 4–10 hours Adults, 2–3 hours
β-LACTAMS						
Penicillin G	Erratic, 15–80% Not available in oral formulation	60–65%	Penetrates most tissues, fetus, and amniotic fluid; poorly into CSF[b]	Hepatic <30%	Renal	Neonates, 1–3 hours varies inversely with (postnatal age) Infants/children, 0.5–1.2 hours
Penicillin V	60%	80%	Penetrates most tissues; poorly into CSF, not used to treat meningitis	Same as penicillin G with additional gut inactivation (metabolized) of 35–70% of an oral dose	Same as penicillin G	Adults, 0.5 hour
PENICILLINASE-RESISTANT PENICILLINS						
Dicloxacillin	35–76% Give on empty stomach	98%	Penetrates most tissues, fetus, and amniotic fluid; poorly into CSF	Hepatic 10%	Renal	Adults, 30–40 minutes
Oxacillin	No oral form available	94%	Penetrates most tissues, fetus, and amniotic fluid; poorly into CSF[b]	Hepatic ~50%	Renal	Neonates and infants, 1–2 hours Adults, 30–60 minutes
Nafcillin	Not administered orally	90%	Penetrates most tissues, fetus, and amniotic fluid; poorly into CSF[b]	Hepatic 60%	Biliary (with enterohepatic recirculation); renal 10–30%	Neonates, 2.2–5.5 hours Infants, 1–2 hours Children and adults, 30–90 minutes

Continued

TABLE 292-1. Pharmacokinetics, Tissue Distribution, Metabolism, and Excretion of Antimicrobial Agents—cont'd

Agent	Oral Bioavailability	Protein Binding	Body Distribution and CSF Penetration	Metabolism	Excretion	$t_{1/2}$[a] (Elimination)
AMINOPENICILLINS						
Amoxicillin	85%	20%	Penetrates most tissues, fetus, and amniotic fluid; poorly into CSF[b]	Hepatic 10%	Renal	Neonates, 3.7 hours Children, 1–2 hours Adults, 1–1.5 hours
Clavulanate (amoxicillin pharmacokinetics not affected by clavulanate)	Well absorbed	25%	Penetrates most tissues, fetus, and amniotic fluid; poorly into CSF	Hepatic extensive	Renal 25–40%	Adults, 1 hour
Ampicillin	50%	22% 10% in neonates	Penetrates most tissues, fetus, and amniotic fluid; poorly into CSF[b]	Hepatic 10%	Renal	Neonates, <1 week, 3–6 hours Neonates, >1 week, 2–4 hours Children, 1–2 hours Adults, 1–1.5 hours
Sulbactam	Not administered orally	38%	Penetrates most tissues, fetus, and amniotic fluid; poorly into CSF[b]	Hepatic 10%	Renal	Adults 1–1.5 hours
EXTENDED-SPECTRUM PENICILLINS						
Carbenicillin (as indanyl sodium)	30–40%	50%	Penetrates most tissues, fetus, and amniotic fluid; poorly into CSF[b]	Hepatic minimal	Renal	Neonates, ~3 hours Children/adults, ~1 hour
Ticarcillin	Not administered orally	45%	Penetrates most tissues, fetus, and amniotic fluid; poorly into CSF[b]	Hepatic 10%	Renal	Neonates <1 week, 4–5 hours Neonates >1 week, ~2 hours Infants/children, ~1 hour
Piperacillin	Not administered orally	15–20%	Penetrates most tissues, fetus, and amniotic fluid; poorly into CSF[b]	Hepatic minimal	Renal; biliary <20%	Neonates, 2–3 hours Infants/children, 0.5–1 hour Adults, 0.5 hour (increases to 1–1.5 hours for high dose due to saturation of hepatobiliary excretion (dose-dependent $t_{1/2}$))
Tazobactam (piperacillin kinetics are unaffected by tazobactam)	Not administered orally	20–23%	Penetrates most tissues, fetus, and amniotic fluid; poorly into CSF[b]	Hepatic minimal	Renal	Infants, 1.6 hours Children/adults, 45 minutes–1 hour
CEPHALOSPORINS **FIRST-GENERATION**						
Cefadroxil	Well absorbed	20%	Penetrates most tissues, fetus, and amniotic fluid; minimally into CSF	None	Renal (slower excretion rate than cephalexin)	Adult, 1–2 hours
Cefazolin	Not administered orally	80%	Penetrates most tissues, fetus, and amniotic fluid; minimally into CSF	None	Renal	Neonates, 3–5 hours Adult, 1.5–2.5 hours
Cephalexin	Well absorbed; ↓ with food	6%	Penetrates most tissues, fetus, and amniotic fluid; minimally into CSF	None	Renal; some biliary	Neonates, 5 hours Infants, 2.5 hours Children/adults, 1 hour
Cephradine	Well absorbed; ↓ with food	10%	Penetrates most tissues, fetus, and amniotic fluid; minimally into CSF	None	Renal; some biliary	Children/adults, ~1 hour

Continued

TABLE 292-1. Pharmacokinetics, Tissue Distribution, Metabolism, and Excretion of Antimicrobial Agents—cont'd

Agent	Oral Bioavailability	Protein Binding	Body Distribution and CSF Penetration	Metabolism	Excretion	t$_{1/2}$[a] (Elimination)
SECOND-GENERATION						
Cefaclor	Well absorbed	25%	Penetrates most tissues; unknown fetal, amniotic, and CSF distribution	Unknown	Renal (nonrenal: elimination at unknown site in renal failure)	Adults, 0.5–1 hour
Cefprozil	95%	36%	Penetrates middle-ear fluids and tonsillar, adenoidal, skin, and soft tissues well; unknown fetal, amniotic and CSF distribution	Unknown	Renal; nonrenal 30%	Infants/children, 1.5–2 hours Adults, 1–1.5 hours
Cefuroxime	37% (as axetil); ↑ to 52% when given with food	50%	Penetrates most tissues, fetus, and amniotic fluid; minimally into CSF	None	Renal	Neonates, 3–6 hours Infants/children, 1.5–2 hours Adults, 1.2 hours
Cefoxitin	Not administered orally	75%	Penetrates most tissues, fetus, and amniotic fluid; minimally into CSF[a]	Hepatic minimal	Renal	Neonates, 1.4 hours Infants/children/adults, ~45 minutes
Loracarbef	90% but can with food	25%	Penetrates most tissues, unknown fetal, amniotic and CSF distribution	None	Renal	Children/adults, ~1 hour
THIRD-GENERATION						
Cefdinir	16–21% cap; 25% suspension	60–70%	Penetrates most tissues; unknown fetal, amniotic and CSF distribution	None	Renal	Adults, 1.7 hours
Cefixime	40–50%	65–70%	Not well studied	Unknown	Renal, biliary	Adults, 3–4 hours
Cefoperazone	Not administered orally	90%	Penetrates most tissues, fetus, and amniotic fluid; minimally into CSF[a]	Hepatic <20%	Biliary, renal 20–30%	Neonates, 6–10 hours (varies inversely with postnatal age) Infants/children, 2.2–2.3 hours Adults, ~2 hours
Cefotaxime	Not administered orally	35–40%	Penetrates most tissues, fetus, and amniotic fluid; adequately into CSF[b]	Hepatic	Renal	Neonates, 2–6 hours (varies inversely with gestational and postnatal age) Infants/children, 1–1.5 hours Older children/adults, 45 minutes–1 hour
Cefpodoxime	50%	20–30%	Penetrates most tissues, unknown fetal, amniotic, and CSF distribution	None	Renal	Adults, 2–3 hours
Ceftazidime	Not administered orally	<10%	Penetrates most tissues, fetus, and amniotic fluid; adequately into CSF[b]	None	Renal	Neonates, 4–7 hours (varies inversely with gestational age) Adults, 1.4–2 hours
Ceftibuten	>90%	65–77%	Penetrates most tissues, unknown fetal, amniotic, and CSF distribution	Hepatic minimal	Renal	Children/adults, 1.5–2.5 hours
Ceftizoxime	Not administered orally	31%	Penetrates most tissues, fetus, and amniotic fluid; minimally into CSF[b]	None	Renal	Neonates, 2–4 hours Adults, 1–2 hours

Continued

TABLE 292-1. Pharmacokinetics, Tissue Distribution, Metabolism, and Excretion of Antimicrobial Agents—cont'd

Agent	Oral Bioavailability	Protein Binding	Body Distribution and CSF Penetration	Metabolism	Excretion	$t_{1/2}$[a] (Elimination)
Ceftriaxone	Not administered orally	95%	Penetrates most tissues, fetus, and amniotic fluid; adequately into CSF[b]	None	Renal; biliary	Neonates, 9–19 hours Children, 4–7 hours Adults, 6–9 hours
FOURTH-GENERATION						
Cefepime	Not administered orally	20%	Penetrates most tissues, fetus, and amniotic fluid; adequately into CSF[b]	Hepatic minimal	Renal	Neonates, 3–7 hours Children/adults, ~2 hours
OTHER β-LACTAMS, MONOBACTAMS						
Aztreonam	Not administered orally	50–70%	Penetrates most tissues, fetus, and amniotic fluid; minimally into CSF[b]	Minimal hydrolysis at unknown site	Renal; biliary minor	Neonates <1 week, 6–10 hours (varies inversely with birthweight) Neonates >1 week, ~3 hours Children/adults, 1.5–2 hours
CARBAPENEMS						
Meropenem	Not administered orally	Minimal	Penetrates most tissues, fetus, and amniotic fluid; adequately into CSF[b]	Renal, serum, hepatic 20–25%	Renal; biliary minor	Neonates, 2–3 hours Infants, 1.5 hours Adults, 1 hour
Imipenem (I) + cilastatin (C)	Not administered orally	20% (I) 40% (C)	Penetrates most tissues, fetus, and amniotic fluid; adequately into CSF[b] but relatively contraindicated for meningitis	Renal, serum, hepatic 20–25%	Renal; biliary minor	Neonates, 1.5–2.5 hours (cilastatin 3–8 hours) Infants/children, 1–1.4 hours Adults, ~1 hour
Ertapenem	Not administered orally	95%	Penetrates interstitial fluids; unknown fetal, amniotic, and CSF distribution	Renal 20%, hepatic minor	Renal; biliary minor	Infants/children, 2.5 hours Adolescents/adults, 4 hours
CHLORAMPHENICOL SUCCINATE (INJECTION)	PO forms (base and palmitate salt) not available	~50%	Widely distributed including fetal, amniotic, and CSF	Hepatic	Renal (as succinate salt and glucuronide metabolite) biliary minimal	Highly variable; see text
FLUOROQUINOLONES AND QUINOLONES						
Ciprofloxacin	60–80%; >90% in adolescents with CF	20–40%	Penetrates most tissues, fetus, amniotic fluid; minimally into CSF[b]	Hepatic <20%	Renal, feces	Neonates/infants/children/ adults, ~3–5 hours
Gatifloxacin	96%	20%	Penetrates most tissues including CSF; fetal, amniotic unknown	Minimal	Renal	Infants/children, 4–7 hours Adults, 7–8 hours
Levofloxacin	99%	24–38%	Penetrates most tissues, fetus, amniotic fluid, CSF	Minimal	Renal	Infants/children, 4–7 hours Adults, 6–8 hours
Norfloxacin	30–40%	10–15%	Penetrates GU and GI, fetus and amniotic fluid; CSF unknown	Hepatic extensive	Renal, biliary	Adults, 3–4 hours
Nalidixic acid	>90%	90–95%	Not widely distributed; penetrates renal tissue well; crosses placenta	Hepatic, renal	Renal (85% as inactive form)	Adults, 1.5 hours

Continued

TABLE 292-1. Pharmacokinetics, Tissue Distribution, Metabolism, and Excretion of Antimicrobial Agents—cont'd

Agent	Oral Bioavailability	Protein Binding	Body Distribution and CSF Penetration	Metabolism	Excretion	$t_{1/2}$[a] (Elimination)
KETOLIDES						
Telithromycin	57%	60–70%	Widely distributed; fetal, amniotic fluid and CSF unknown	Hepatic	Renal, biliary	Adults, 9–10 hours
LINCOSAMIDES						
Clindamycin	90%	94%	Penetrates most tissues, fetus, amniotic fluid; minimally into uninflamed CSF, but adequately into inflamed CSF or brain abscess	Hepatic	Biliary; renal minor	Neonates, 3.6–8.7 hours (inversely related to gestational age and birthweight) Infants/children/adults, ~2–3.5 hours
LIPOPEPTIDES						
Daptomycin	Not administered orally	~90%	Limited distribution; fetal, amniotic, and CSF penetration unknown	Renal	Renal	Adults, 7–10 hours
MACROLIDES AND AZALIDES						
Azithromycin	37%	20–50%	Widely distributed including fetus, amniotic fluid; minimally into CSF[b]	Hepatic	Biliary; renal, minimal	Infants/children, >50 hours Adults, 35–40 hours
Clarithromycin	50–55%	60–70%	Penetrates most tissues, fetus; CSF penetration unknown	Hepatic	Renal 40–50% (as drug and active metabolite)	Infants/children/adults, 3–7 hours (dose-dependent)
Erythromycin	Poor, 25–65% depending on salt and form	80–90%	Penetrates most tissues, fetus, amniotic fluid; minimally into CSF[b]	Hepatic	Biliary, renal minimal	Adult, 1–2 hours (estolate 3–8 hours)
METRONIDAZOLE	100%	<20%	Widely distributed, including fetus, amniotic fluid, CSF	Hepatic	Renal (60–80% with 10–20% as unchanged drug); biliary minor	Neonates, 22.5 to 109 hours (varies inversely with gestational age) Children/adults, 6–14 hours
NITROFURANTOIN	Well absorbed	90%	Mainly urinary tract, prostate, and placenta	Tissues	Renal, biliary	Adults, 20 minutes
OXAZOLIDINONES						
Linezolid	100%	31%	Penetrates most tissues, including CSF; fetus, amniotic fluid unknown	Hepatic	Renal	Neonates, 1.5–10 hours (varies inversely with gestational age) Infants/children, 2–3 hours Adults, 3–6 hours
POLYMYXINS						
Colistimethate (injection)	Not administered orally	Minimal	Penetrates most tissues, fetus and amniotic fluid; minimal to pleural or joint cavities or to CSF	Tissue minor and slow	Renal	Children, 2–3 hours Adults, 1.5–3 hours
RIFAMYCINS						
Rifampin	90–95%	60–90%	Widely distributed including fetus, amniotic fluid; minimally into CSF[b]	Hepatic	Biliary, renal	Infants/children/adults, ~2–4 hours

Continued

TABLE 292-1. Pharmacokinetics, Tissue Distribution, Metabolism, and Excretion of Antimicrobial Agents—cont'd

Agent	Oral Bioavailability	Protein Binding	Body Distribution and CSF Penetration	Metabolism	Excretion	$t_{1/2}$[a] (Elimination)
Rifaximin	Poorly absorbed	N/A	Minimal systemic distribution due to poor oral bioavailability, but high intraluminal GI concentrations	Hepatic minimal	Feces absorption	Minimal systemic
STREPTOGRAMINS						
Quinupristin-dalfopristin	Not administered orally	55–78% (Q) 11–26% (D)	Penetrates most tissues; minimally into CSF; fetus, amniotic fluid unknown	Hepatic, conversion to several active metabolites	Biliary; renal ~15%	Adults, 0.85 hours (Q) 0.75 hours (D) 2.5–3.5 hours (Q + m) ~1 hour (D + m): m = metabolites
SULFONAMIDES AND TRIMETHOPRIM						
Sulfadiazine	100%	20%	Widely distributed, including fetus, amniotic fluid, CSF	Hepatic wide individual variation	Renal (free and conjugated forms)	Adults, 7–17 hours
Sulfamethoxazole	100%	65%	Widely distributed, including fetus, amniotic fluid, CSF	Hepatic wide individual variation	Renal (free and conjugated forms)	Adults, 9–12 hours
Sulfisoxazole	100%	85%	Widely distributed, including fetus, amniotic fluid, CSF	Hepatic wide individual variation	Renal (free and conjugated forms)	Adults, 5–8 hours
Trimethoprim	100%	~45%	Widely distributed, including fetus, amniotic fluid, CSF	Hepatic <20%	Renal	Infants/children, 3–5.5 hours Adults, 8–10 hours
TETRACYCLINES AND GLYCYLCYCLINES						
Doxycycline	90–100%	82%	Widely distributed including fetus, amniotic fluid; minimally into CSF[b]	Hepatic	Renal, biliary	Adults, ~20 hours
Minocycline	90–100%	76%	Widely distributed including fetus, amniotic fluid; minimally into CSF[b]	Hepatic minimal	Biliary, renal	Adults, 11–22 hours
Tetracycline (T), Demeclocycine (D)	75–80%; decreases significantly with food	65% (T) 41–91% (D)	Widely distributed including fetus, amniotic fluid; minimally into CSF[b]	Hepatic minimal	Renal, biliary	Adults, 7–10 hours (T) Adults, 10–17 hours (D)
Tigecycline	Not administered orally	70–90%	Widely distributed; fetal, amniotic fluid and CSF unknown	Hepatic 5–20%	Biliary, renal	Adults, 40 hours
GLYCOPEPTIDES						
Vancomycin	Negligible	30%	Penetrates most tissues, fetus, amniotic fluid; adequately but erratically into CSF[b]	None	Renal; biliary minimal	Neonates, 4–11 hours (varies inversely with gestational age) Infants, 2–4 hours Children, 2–2.5 hours Adults, 4–6 hours

CF, cystic fibrosis; CSF, cerebrospinal fluid; GI, gastrointestinal; GU, genitourinary; IV, intravenous; PO, orally.

[a]Agents with both minimal metabolism and urinary excretion will have a prolonged $t_{1/2}$ in a patient with renal impairment.

[b]Concentration of drug in CSF significantly increased with inflamed meninges.

I. Cell Wall-Active Agents			I. Cell Wall-Active Agents		
A. Antibiotic Class: Transpeptidase Inhibitors			A. Antibiotic Class: Transpeptidase Inhibitors		
	β-Lactam Antibiotics	Spectrum of Activity[a]		β-Lactam Antibiotics	Spectrum of Activity[a]
PENICILLINS				Ampicillin/ sulbactam	Adds activity to ampicillin:
Natural penicillins	Penicillin G	**Gram-positive**			*Staphylococcus aureus* (except MRSA)
	Penicillin V	Streptococci			*Escherichia coli*, β-lactamase-producing strains
	Benzathine penicillin G	Groups A, B, C, G, F			*Klebsiella* species
	Procaine penicillin G	Viridans group streptococci			*Proteus mirabilis*
	Benzathine/ procaine penicillin G combinations	*Streptococcus pneumoniae*			*Proteus vulgaris*
		Enterococcus faecalis[b]			*Providencia rettgeri*
		Enterococcus faecium[b]			*Providencia stuartii*
		Actinomyces			*Morganella morganii*
		Bacillus anthracis			**Anaerobes**
		Listeria monocytogenes			As above for penicillins, but now includes:
		Gram-negative			*Bacteroides* and *Prevotella* species (β-lactamase-producing strains)
		Eikenella corrodens	Extended-spectrum penicillins	Carbenicillin	**Gram-positive**
		Neisseria meningitidis		Ticarcillin	Streptococci (as above for penicillins)
		Neisseria gonorrhoeae		Piperacillin	**Gram-negative**
		Pasteurella multocida			*Escherichia coli*
		Borrelia burgdorferi			*Haemophilus influenzae*
		Spirillum minus			*Proteus mirabilis*
		Streptobacillus moniliformis			*Proteus vulgaris*
		Treponema pallidum			*Morganella morganii*
		Leptospira species			*Pseudomonas aeruginosa*
		Anaerobes			*Providencia rettgeri*
		Bacteroides and *Prevotella* species (non-β-lactamase-producing strains)			*Enterobacter* species
		Fusobacterium species			**Anaerobes**
		Veillonella species			*Bacteroides* and *Prevotella* species (non-β-lactamase-producing strains)
		Clostridium species			*Fusobacterium* species
		Eubacterium species			*Veillonella* species
		Peptococcus species			*Clostridium* species
		Peptostreptococcus species			*Eubacterium* species
		Propionibacterium species			*Peptococcus* species
Penicillinase-stable penicillins	Methicillin	**Gram-positive**			*Peptostreptococcus* species
	Oxacillin	Streptococci (as above for penicillins)		Ticarcillin/ clavulanate	Adds β-lactamase-producing strains of:
	Nafcillin	*Staphylococcus aureus* (except MRSA)		Piperacillin/ tazobactam	*Staphylococcus aureus* (except MRSA)
	Cloxacillin				*Escherichia coli*
	Dicloxacillin				*Haemophilus influenzae*
Aminopenicillins	Ampicillin	**Gram-positive**			*Klebsiella* species
	Amoxicillin	Streptococci (as above for penicillins)			*Serratia marcescens*
		Enterococcus faecalis[b]			*Citrobacter* species
		Enterococcus faecium[b]			*Enterobacter* species
		Listeria monocytogenes			**Anaerobes**
		Gram-negative			*Bacteroides* and *Prevotella* species (including β-lactamase-producing strains)
		Escherichia coli			*Fusobacterium* species
		Haemophilus influenzae			*Veillonella* species
		Neisseria meningitidis			*Clostridium* species
		Anaerobes			*Eubacterium* species
		For ampicillin: as above for penicillins			*Peptococcus* species
	Amoxicillin/ clavulanate	Adds activity to amoxicillin:			*Peptostreptococcus* species
		Staphylococcus aureus (except MRSA)			
		Haemophilus influenzae, β-lactamase-producing strains			
		Anaerobes			
		As above for penicillins, but now includes:			
		Bacteroides and *Prevotella* species, β-lactamase-producing strains			

Continued

TABLE 292-2. Spectrum of Activity of Antimicrobial Agents by Microbial Site of Activity and Antimicrobial Drug Class—cont'd

I. Cell Wall-Active Agents			I. Cell Wall-Active Agents		
A. Antibiotic Class: Transpeptidase Inhibitors			**A. Antibiotic Class: Transpeptidase Inhibitors**		
	β-Lactam Antibiotics	Spectrum of Activity[a]		β-Lactam Antibiotics	Spectrum of Activity[a]
CEPHALOSPORINS					*Proteus mirabilis*
First-generation	Cephalothin	**Gram-positive**			*Proteus vulgaris*
	Cephapirin	Streptococci			*Providencia rettgeri*
	Cefazolin	Groups A, B, C, G, F			*Providencia stuartii*
	Cephalexin	Viridans group streptococci			*Serratia marcescens*
	Cephradine	*Streptococcus pneumoniae*			For ceftazidime and cefoperazone:
	Cefadroxil	*Staphylococcus aureus* (except MRSA)			*Pseudomonas aeruginosa*
		Gram-negative			**Anaerobes**
		Escherichia coli			*Bacteroides* and *Prevotella* species (non-β-lactamase-producing strains)
		Proteus mirabilis			*Fusobacterium* species
Second-generation	Cefamandole	**Gram-positive**			*Eubacterium* species
	Cefuroxime	Streptococci			*Peptococcus* species
	Cefonicid	Groups A, B, C, G, F	Fourth-generation	Cefepime	**Gram-positive**
	Ceforanide	Viridans group streptococci			Streptococci
	Cefaclor	*Streptococcus pneumoniae*			Groups A, B, C, G, F
	Cefoxitin	*Staphylococcus aureus* (except MRSA)			Viridans group streptococci
	Cefotetan	**Gram-negative**			*Streptococcus pneumoniae*
		Escherichia coli			*Staphylococcus aureus* (except MRSA)
		Haemophilus influenzae (including β-lactamase-producing strains)			**Gram-negative**
		Klebsiella species			As above for third-generation cephalosporins, but including *Pseudomonas aeruginosa*)
		Moraxella catarrhalis			**Anaerobes**
		Neisseria gonorrhoeae			*Bacteroides* and *Prevotella* species (non-β-lactamase-producing strains)
		Neisseria meningitidis			*Fusobacterium* species
		Proteus mirabilis			*Veillonella* species
		Providencia rettgeri			*Eubacterium* species
		Salmonella species			*Peptococcus* species
		Shigella species	Fifth-generation	Ceftaroline	As above for third-generation cephalosporins, but also includes MRSA strains of *Staphylococcus aureus*
		Anaerobes			
		Bacteroides and *Prevotella* species (non-β-lactamase-producing strains, except for cefoxitin and, to a lesser extent, cefotetan)	CARBAPENEMS	Imipenem (with cilastatin)	**Gram-positive**
		Fusobacterium species		Meropenem	Streptococci
		Veillonella species		Ertapenem	Groups A, B, C, D, G, F
		Eubacterium species		Doripenem	Viridans group streptococci
		Peptococcus species			*Streptococcus pneumoniae*
		Peptostreptococcus species			*Enterococcus faecalis*
Third-generation	Cefotaxime	**Gram-positive**			*Staphylococcus aureus* (except MRSA)
	Ceftriaxone	Streptococci			**Gram-negative**
	Ceftazidime	Groups A, B, C, G, F			*Acinetobacter* species
	Cefoperazone	Viridans group streptococci			*Citrobacter* species
	Ceftizoxime	*Streptococcus pneumoniae*			*Enterobacter* species
	Cefixime	*Staphylococcus aureus* (except MRSA)			*Escherichia coli* (including ESBL-producing strains)
	Cefpodoxime	**Gram-negative**			*Gardnerella vaginalis*
	Ceftibuten	*Citrobacter* species			*Haemophilus influenzae*
	Cefdinir	*Enterobacter* species			*Klebsiella* species (including ESBL-producing strains)
		Escherichia coli			*Morganella morganii*
		Haemophilus influenzae (including β-lactamase-producing strains)			*Proteus vulgaris*
		Klebsiella species			*Providencia rettgeri*
		Morganella morganii			*Pseudomonas aeruginosa* (except ertapenem)
		Neisseria gonorrhoeae (including β-lactamase-producing strains)			*Serratia* species
		Neisseria meningitidis			

Continued

TABLE 292-2. Spectrum of Activity of Antimicrobial Agents by Microbial Site of Activity and Antimicrobial Drug Class—cont'd

I. Cell Wall-Active Agents

A. Antibiotic Class: Transpeptidase Inhibitors

	β-Lactam Antibiotics	Spectrum of Activity[a]
CARBAPENEMS (cont'd)		**Anaerobes**
		Bifidobacterium species
		Clostridium species
		Eubacterium species
		Peptococcus species
		Peptostreptococcus species
		Propionibacterium species
		Bacteroides and *Prevotella* species (including β-lactamase-producing strains)
		Fusobacterium species
MONOBACTANS	Aztreonam	**Gram-negative**
		Citrobacter species
		Enterobacter species
		Escherichia coli
		Haemophilus influenzae (including β-lactamase-producing strains)
		Klebsiella species
		Proteus mirabilis
		Pseudomonas aeruginosa
		Serratia species

B. Antibiotic Class: Transglycosylase Inhibitors

		Spectrum of Activity[a]
GLYCOPEPTIDES	Vancomycin Teicoplanin (not available in the United States)	**Gram-positive**
		Streptococci
		Groups A, B, C, G, F
		Viridans group streptococci
		Streptococcus pneumoniae
		Enterococcus faecalis[b]
		Enterococcus faecium[b]
		Staphylococcus aureus (including MRSA, but not vancomycin-intermediate or vancomycin-resistant strains)
		Staphylococcus epidermidis
		Actinomyces species
		Lactobacillus species
		Listeria monocytogenes
		Anaerobes
		Clostridium difficile

II. Cell Membrane Active Agents

A. Antibiotic Class: Lipopeptides

		Spectrum of Activity[a]
	Daptomycin	*Staphylococcus aureus* (including methicillin-resistant and vancomycin-resistant strains)
		Enterococcus faecalis (vancomycin-susceptible and -resistant strains)
		Enterococcus faecium (vancomycin-susceptible and -resistant strains)
		Streptococci
		Groups A, B
		Viridans group streptococci

B. Antibiotic Class: Polymyxins

	Colistin	*Enterobacter aerogenes*
		Escherichia coli
		Klebsiella pneumoniae
		Pseudomonas aeruginosa
		Actinobacter species
		Citrobacter species

II. Cell Membrane Active Agents

B. Antibiotic Class: Polymyxins

		Haemophilus species
		Salmonella species
		Shigella species

III. Ribosome-Active Agents

A. Antibiotic Class: Macrolides

MACROLIDES	Erythromycin	**Gram-positive**
		Corynebacterium diphtheriae
		Corynebacterium minutissimum
		Listeria monocytogenes
		Staphylococcus aureus
		Streptococcus pneumoniae
		Streptococcus pyogenes
		Gram-negative
		Bordetella pertussis
		Legionella pneumophila
		Neisseria gonorrhoeae
		Other pathogens
		Chlamydia trachomatis
		Entamoeba histolytica
		Mycoplasma pneumoniae
		Treponema pallidum
		Ureaplasma urealyticum
	Clarithromycin	**Gram-positive**
		Staphylococcus aureus
		Streptococcus pneumoniae
		Streptococcus pyogenes
		Gram-negative
		Haemophilus influenzae
		Moraxella catarrhalis
		Helicobacter pylori
		Other pathogens
		Mycoplasma pneumoniae
		Chlamydophila pneumoniae
		Mycobacterium avium complex
AZALIDES	Azithromycin	**Gram-positive**
		Staphylococcus aureus
		Streptococci
		Groups A, B C, F, G
		Viridans group streptococci
		Streptococcus pneumoniae
		Bordetella pertussis
		Gram-negative
		Haemophilus influenzae
		Haemophilus ducreyi
		Moraxella catarrhalis
		Neisseria gonorrhoeae
		Other pathogens
		Chlamydophila pneumoniae
		Chlamydia trachomatis
		Legionella pneumophila
		Mycoplasma hominis
		Mycoplasma pneumoniae
		Ureaplasma urealyticum
KETOLIDES	Telithromycin	**Gram-positive**
		Staphylococcus aureus
		Streptococci
		Groups A, C and G
		Viridans group streptococci
		Gram-negative
		Haemophilus influenzae
		Moraxella catarrhalis
		Other pathogens
		Bordetella pertussis
		Mycoplasma pneumoniae
		Legionella pneumophila
		Chlamydophila pneumoniae

TABLE 292-2. Spectrum of Activity of Antimicrobial Agents by Microbial Site of Activity and Antimicrobial Drug Class—cont'd

III. Ribosome-Active Agents				III. Ribosome-Active Agents			
B. Antibiotic Class: Tetracyclines				**C. Antibiotic Class: Lincosamides**			
TETRACYCLINES	Tetracycline Minocycline Doxycycline	**Gram-positive** *Actinomyces* species **Gram-negative** *Vibrio cholerae* *Brucella* species *Campylobacter* species *Francisella tularensis* *Listeria monocytogenes* *Yersinia pestis* *Neisseria meningitidis* *Neisseria gonorrhoeae* **Other pathogens** *Borrelia recurrentis* *Chlamydophila psittaci* *Chlamydia trachomatis* *Mycoplasma pneumoniae* *Ureaplasma* *Treponema pallidum* *Entamoeba* species				**Anaerobes** *Bacteroides fragilis* *Prevotella melaninogenica* *Fusobacterium* species *Peptococcus* species *Peptostreptococcus* species *Actinomyces* species *Clostridium perfringens* *Propionibacterium* species	
				D. Antibiotic Class: Aminoglycosides			

GLYCYLCYCLINES	Tigecycline	**Gram-positive**
		Streptococci
		  Groups A, B
		    Viridans group streptococci
		    Streptococcus pneumoniae
		Enterococcus faecalis
		Enterococcus faecium
		Staphylococcus aureus
		Listeria monocytogenes
		Clostridium perfringens
		Peptostreptococcus species
		Gram-negative
		Acinetobacter baumannii
		Aeromonas hydrophila
		Citrobacter freundii
		Citrobacter koseri
		Enterobacter cloacae
		Enterobacter aerogenes
		Escherichia coli
		Klebsiella oxytoca
		Klebsiella pneumoniae
		Pasteurella multocida
		Serratia marcescens
		Stenotrophomonas maltophilia
		Bacteroides species
		Other pathogens
		Chlamydia trachomatis
		Mycoplasma pneumoniae
		Ureaplasma
		Mycobacterium abscessus
		Mycobacterium chelonae
		Mycobacterium fortuitum
				AMINOGLYCOSIDES	Streptomycin	**Gram-negative**
						Brucella species
						Francisella species
						Mycobacterium tuberculosis	

					Gentamicin Netilmicin Tobramycin Amikacin	**Gram-positive** *Staphylococcus aureus* **Gram-negative** *Escherichia coli* *Klebsiella* species *Enterobacter* species *Serratia* species *Citrobacter* species *Morganella morganii* *Acinetobacter* species *Providencia* species *Proteus mirabilis* *Proteus vulgaris* *Pseudomonas aeruginosa*	
					Paromomycin	*Entamoeba histolytica* *Dientamoeba fragilis* *Cryptosporidium* species	
				E. Antibiotic Class: Oxazolidinones			

				OXAZOLIDINONES	Linezolid	**Gram-positive**
						Streptococci
						  Groups A, B
						    Viridans group streptococci
						    Streptococcus pneumoniae
						Staphylococcus aureus
						Enterococcus faecium
						Enterococcus faecalis	

				F. Antibiotic Class: Streptogramins			
				STREPTOGRAMINS	Quinupristin/ dalfopristin	**Gram-positive** Streptococci Groups A, B *Staphylococcus aureus* *Enterococcus faecium*	
				IV. Nucleic Acid-Active Antibiotics			
				A. Antibiotic Class: Rifamycins			
C. Antibiotic Class: Lincosamides				RIFAMYCINS	Rifampin	**Gram-positive** *Staphylococcus aureus* **Gram-negative** *Neisseria meningitidis* *Haemophilus influenzae* **Other** *Mycobacterium tuberculosis* *Mycobacterium avium* complex	

LINCOSAMIDES	Clindamycin	**Gram-positive**
		Streptococci
		  Groups A, B
		    Streptococcus pneumoniae
		Staphylococcus aureus					

Continued

TABLE 292-2. Spectrum of Activity of Antimicrobial Agents by Microbial Site of Activity and Antimicrobial Drug Class—cont'd

IV. Nucleic Acid-Active Antibiotics

A. Antibiotic Class: Rifamycins

	Rifabutin	*Mycobacterium tuberculosis*
	Rifapentine	*Mycobacterium avium* complex
	Rifaximin	Susceptible at concentrations achieved within the gastrointestinal lumen:
		Campylobacter
		Escherichia coli
		Salmonella species
		Shigella species
		Vibrio species
		Yersinia species

B. Antibiotic Class: Quinolones

QUINOLONES — Nalidixic acid

Gram-negative
Escherichia coli
Enterobacter species
Morganella morganii
Proteus mirabilis
Proteus vulgaris
Providencia rettgeri

FLUOROQUINOLONES — Ciprofloxacin

Gram-positive
Streptococcus pyogenes
Streptococcus pneumoniae
Staphylococcus aureus
Enterococcus faecalis
Bacillus anthracis
Gram-negative
Aeromonas species
Acinetobacter species
Escherichia coli
Klebsiella pneumoniae
Enterobacter cloacae
Citrobacter diversus
Citrobacter freundii
Campylobacter jejuni
Proteus mirabilis
Proteus vulgaris
Providencia rettgeri
Providencia stuartii
Serratia marcescens
Pseudomonas aeruginosa
Morganella morganii
Salmonella species
Shigella species
Haemophilus influenzae
Haemophilus parainfluenzae
Moraxella catarrhalis
Neisseria gonorrhoeae[b]
Pasteurella multocida
Vibrio species
Yersinia enterocolitica
Other pathogens
Legionella pneumophila

IV. Nucleic Acid-Active Antibiotics

B. Antibiotic Class: Quinolones

Levofloxacin
Gemifloxacin
Moxifloxacin

Gram-positive
Streptococci
  Group A
    Viridans group streptococci
    Streptococcus pneumoniae
Enterococcus faecalis
Staphylococcus aureus
Actinomyces species
Bacillus anthracis
Listeria monocytogenes
Gram-negative
Acinetobacter species
Escherichia coli
Enterobacter species
Klebsiella species
Proteus species
Providencia species
Serratia marcescens
Citrobacter species
Morganella morganii
Pseudomonas aeruginosa
Haemophilus influenzae
Moraxella catarrhalis
Anaerobes
Clostridium perfringens
Other pathogens
Legionella pneumophila
Mycoplasma pneumoniae
Chlamydophila pneumoniae

C. Antibiotic Class: Nitroimadazoles

NITROIMADAZOLES — Metronidazole

Anaerobes
Clostridium species
Eubacterium species
Peptococcus species
Peptostreptococcus species
Bacteroides fragilis
Fusobacterium species

D. Antibiotic Class: Sulfonamides

SULFONAMIDES — Sulfisoxazole / Sulfamethoxazole

SULFA IN COMBINATION WITH ANOTHER ANTIMICROBIAL AGENT — Sulfamethoxazole plus trimethoprim

Gram-positive
Streptococcus pneumoniae[b]
Gram-negative
Escherichia coli
Klebsiella species
Enterobacter species
Morganella morganii
Proteus mirabilis
Proteus vulgaris
Shigella species
Haemophilus influenze
Other pathogens
Pneumocystis jirovecii

Sulfadiazine plus pyramethamine — *Toxoplasma gondii* / *Plasmodium* species

ESBL, extended-spectrum β-lactamases; MRSA, methicillin-resistant Staphylococcus aureus.

[a]A majority of strains of the listed bacteria are susceptible; however, some organisms within the group may be less susceptible or resistant to one or more agents listed. Susceptibility pattern for each pathogen and antibiotic may be available to physicians through local health care institutions.

[b]Important exceptions exist.

CELL WALL-ACTIVE AGENTS

The synthesis of the bacterial cell wall is remarkably complicated and still is not understood fully.[1-3] Several steps are involved in cell wall creation, from the synthesis of precursors within the bacterial cytoplasm to the intricate construction of a lattice-like structure around the organism that maintains cell shape and osmotic integrity. Gram-negative cell walls consist of inner (plasma) and outer membranes, and are more complicated than those of gram-positive organisms that contain a single membrane. Many steps in cell wall synthesis have been exploited as targets of currently available antimicrobial agents and others provide potential targets for ongoing anti-infective research (Figure 292-1). Our understanding of mechanisms of cell death following interruption of cell wall synthesis has increased to include both direct mechanisms from cell wall damage, as well as initiation of metabolic pathways for programmed cell death.[3]

The saccharide precursors of cell walls, N-acetylmuramic acid (MurNAc), and N-acetylglucosamine (GlcNAc) are modified enzymatically by a series of steps, with MurNAc acquiring a side chain consisting of five peptides, incorporating D-alanine, D-alanine as the terminal two amino acids in this chain. This MurNAc-pentapeptide is subsequently attached to a GlcNAc saccharide unit, completing the disaccharide pentapeptide building block required for cell wall peptidoglycan formation (see Figure 292-1). Agents that inhibit these initial steps have been identified in a research setting and many are currently under investigation as clinically important targets.[4,5] The disaccharide pentapeptide building block subsequently is transferred through the cell membrane to undergo further modification ultimately to create the peptidoglycan structure either outside the cell membrane (in gram-positive organisms), or between the inner plasma membrane and outer membrane within the cell wall (in gram-negative organisms). Linking of the disaccharide pentapeptide building blocks occurs by transglycosylation, and creates repeating disaccharide subunits (Glc NAc-MurNAc-pentapeptide) to produce long glycan chains.[6] Vancomycin and related glycopeptide antibiotics inhibit this step in cell wall synthesis by binding to the terminal D-ala, D-ala of the pentapeptide attached to MurNAc, and interfering sterically with the enzymatic function of the transglycosylase.[7]

The mature glycan chains containing the repeating disaccharide units are subsequently linked by connecting the pentapeptides located on the MurNAc units from adjacent glycan chains. In this transpeptidation step, a stable bridge is created between glycan chains to form the two-dimensional peptidoglycan structure.[6] The β-lactam class of antibiotics inhibits the transpeptidase function by binding covalently to the active serine site of the enzyme responsible for linking the two pentapeptide arms from MurNAc units on adjacent glycan strands.[8] The structure of enzymes that are responsible for transglycosylation and transpeptidation varies somewhat between bacteria. Fortunately, the active sites of these enzymes tend to be quite conserved. An organism often contains several transpeptidases, each responsible for a different cell wall function, including repair, elongation, septation, and cell wall thickening, among others. Some of these enzymes contain both transglycosylation and transpeptidation functions. Historically, these enzymes were identified by penicillin attachment to them, and are also known as penicillin-binding proteins, or PBPs.

β-Lactam Antibiotics

The β-lactam antibiotics all share the capacity to inhibit the transpeptidase cross-linking of peptidoglycan in the final steps of

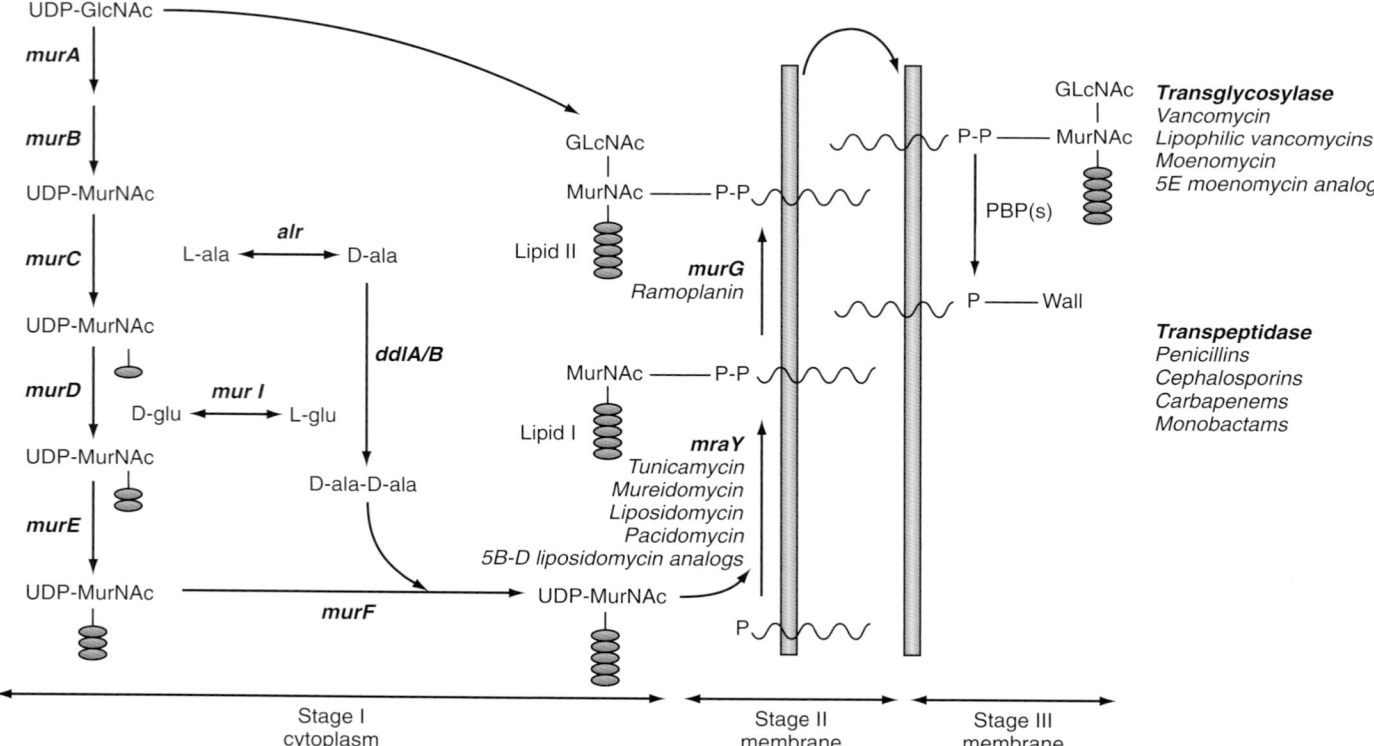

UDP, uridine diphosphate; MurNAc, N-Acetylmuramic acid; GLcNAc, N-Acetylglucosamine; PBP(s), penicillin binding proteins (transpeptidase); L-ala, L-alanine; D-ala, D-alanine.

Figure 292-1. The peptidoglycan synthesis pathway in cell wall formation. (Redrawn with modification from Wong VK, Pompliano DL Peptidoglycan biosynthesis: unexploited targets within a familiar pathway. In: Rosen BP, Mobashery S (eds) Resolving the Antibiotic Paradox. New York, Kluwer Academic/Plenum Publishers, 1998, pp 197–217.)

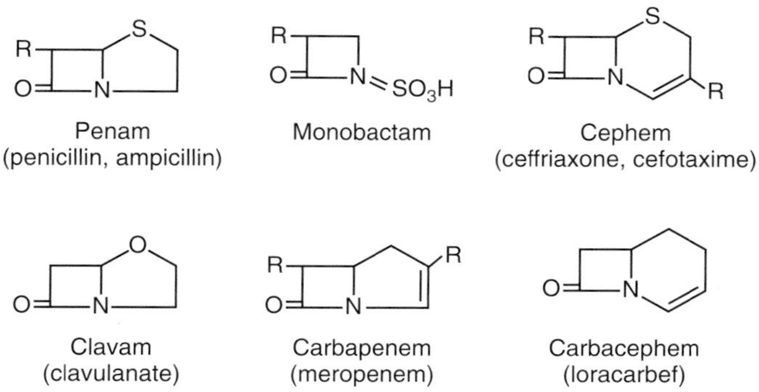

Figure 292-2. β-Lactam antibiotic structures.

formation of the cell wall. Whereas the β-lactam structure itself is consistent across all antibiotics in this class, the ring to which the lactam moiety is fused is variable, with relatively small differences in the composition of the ring allowing for variable activity against the PBPs of both gram-positive and gram-negative bacteria (Figure 292-2). The addition of chemical "chains" to the ring structures enhances activity against certain organisms, but simultaneously can decrease activity against others. Differences in the charges of the antibiotic molecule affect the ability of the compound to reach and to bind to its target, particularly for gram-negative pathogens.

In general, the β-lactam antibiotics are bactericidal with the concentrations required for killing being very close to those required for inhibition of growth. The maximal bactericidal effect occurs on rapidly growing bacteria; in stationary phase, this class of antibiotics has substantially less impact on the viability of organisms.[9]

Resistance to β-Lactam Antibiotics

Probably just as ancient as the natural antibiotics are natural mechanisms of resistance to them (Figure 292-3). Resistance to the β-lactam antibiotics occurs primarily in four ways: (1) enzymatic hydrolysis of the β-lactam ring by bacterial β-lactamases, rendering the antibiotic harmless; (2) alterations in the structure of the transpeptidase, so that binding of the antibiotic to the active serine site of the transpeptidase does not occur; (3) efflux pumps that, in gram-negative organisms, quickly and efficiently remove the antibiotics from the periplasmic space before they can bind to the transpeptidases; and (4) alterations in the gram-negative outer membrane proteins that prevent the antibiotic from entering the periplasmic space. Each of these resistance mechanisms is variably effective and can lead either to profound resistance or merely to slightly increased resistance that has no clinical impact. Unfortunately, some pathogens combine several resistance mechanisms, each creating incremental increases in β-lactam resistance, ultimately leading to the development of an organism that is no longer susceptible to these antibiotics.

Chemical modifications of the β-lactam ring and associated drug structure can enhance the intrinsic activity of a drug against bacterial pathogens. Modifications that alter ionic charges on the molecule can allow the new agent (e.g., ampicillin) to enter the gram-negative bacterial periplasmic space, in contrast to an older agent (e.g., penicillin G) that could not. Side chains can create enhanced stability of the antibiotic against one or more of the hundreds of β-lactamases that have been identified, or can enhance binding to bactericidal targets within the organism.[4] Unfortunately, new, more active and broader-spectrum β-lactamases are reported with disturbing regularity.[10] Although many different efflux pump systems exist, changes in the structure and charge of the antibiotic can decrease the affinity of the antibiotic for the pump, while hopefully not decreasing its affinity for the target transpeptidase.

Penicillins

The penicillins are the most commonly used antibiotics in pediatrics, and can be divided broadly into four different groups: (1) natural penicillins; (2) penicillinase-stable penicillins; (3) aminopenicillins; and (4) extended-spectrum penicillins.

Natural Penicillins

Natural penicillins are the natural products of *Penicillium chrysogenum*. It is likely that both penicillins and penicillin-resistance mechanisms evolved millions of years ago as result of competition for survival between single-cell organisms.[11] Fleming's observations in the 1920s led to the identification of penicillin, and the discovery of the mechanism by which *Penicillium* killed other bacteria, paving the way for the modern era of antibacterial therapy. The basic structure of penicillin, 6-aminopenicillanic acid, is characteristic of the lactam ring fused to a larger ring structure to create a penam nucleus that is the basic structure of all penicillins (see Figure 292-2). Of the natural penicillins, only penicillin G (crystalline penicillin G, benzyl penicillin G) and penicillin V (phenoxymethyl-penicillin) currently are available commercially. Penicillin G is available in both oral and parenteral formulations. For intramuscular injection, penicillin G is also available in repository forms of the drug. Procaine penicillin G and benzathine penicillin G both have much longer serum elimination half-lives as a result of prolonged absorption from the muscle injection site, compared with crystalline penicillin G. However, the peak serum concentrations of the repository forms of penicillin G are considerably lower than those achieved with intravenous administration of crystalline penicillin G. Therefore, the only situations in which the repository forms of penicillin are effective are those in which the targeted organisms are exquisitely susceptible to penicillin, in tissues with good perfusion. Intramuscular procaine penicillin has a half-life of approximately 12 hours and achieves peak serum concentrations of about 2 μg/mL, compared with a half-life of 30 to 50 minutes for crystalline penicillin G, and achieved peak serum concentrations of approximately 20 μg/mL. Benzathine penicillin G yields even lower serum concentrations (only about 1.5 μg/mL), but can remain above 0.2 μg/mL for 3 weeks or longer. Combinations of procaine and benzathine penicillin, either in equal amounts or as a 3:1 (benzathine:procaine) mixture, also are available. As these repository forms of penicillin are used infrequently, extreme caution must be taken never to administer them intravenously, which can be lethal.

In clinical practice, although active against a wide range of bacteria (see Table 292-2), the natural penicillins are used most widely for treatment and prevention of infections caused by streptococci. Pharyngitis, lower respiratory tract infection, skin and skin structure infections, and bloodstream infection (BSI) caused by group A streptococcus (*Streptococcus pyogenes*) are effectively treated with penicillin. The in vitro susceptibility of these organisms has remained unchanged over the past several decades,[12] although the efficacy in the treatment of streptococcal pharyngitis in more recent studies is less than expected, for reasons that are not well understood.[13] Intramuscular injections of benzathine penicillin every 3 to 4 weeks are effective in the prevention of rheumatic fever due to the prolonged tonsillar tissue concentrations of penicillin G.

Empiric penicillin therapy of infections suspected to be caused by *Streptococcus pneumoniae* has not been appropriate during the past decade as a result of widespread decreased susceptibility of pneumococci to penicillin. By mutation, stable alterations in the structure of several pneumococcal PBPs yield penicillin-nonsusceptible organisms, treatment of which requires use of higher dosages of penicillins or agents from other antibiotic classes. However, if culture results document susceptibility, penicillin still represents highly effective therapy.

Most anaerobes, with the exception of β-lactamase-producing strains of *Bacteroides* sp. and *Prevotella* sp. are highly susceptible to penicillin G. However, due to the common presence of *Bacteroides fragilis* among the anaerobes present in intra-abdominal infections

GRAM-POSITIVE BACTERIAL CELL WALL

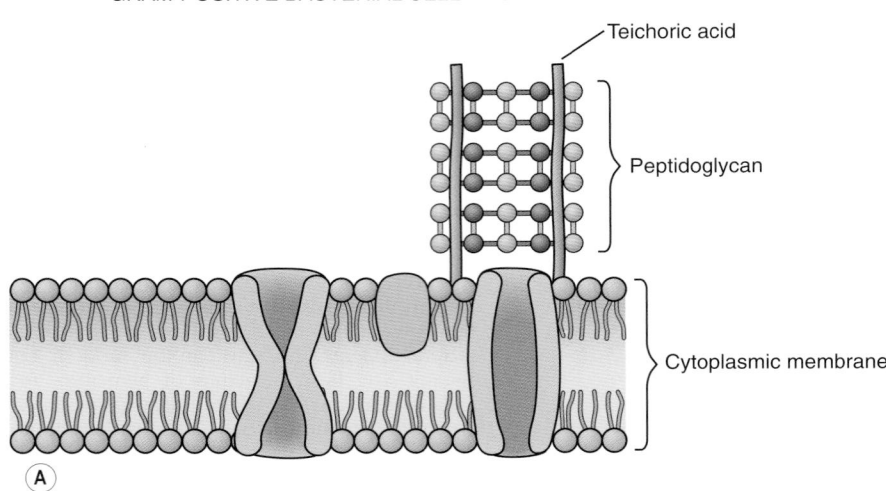

GRAM-NEGATIVE BACTERIAL CELL WALL

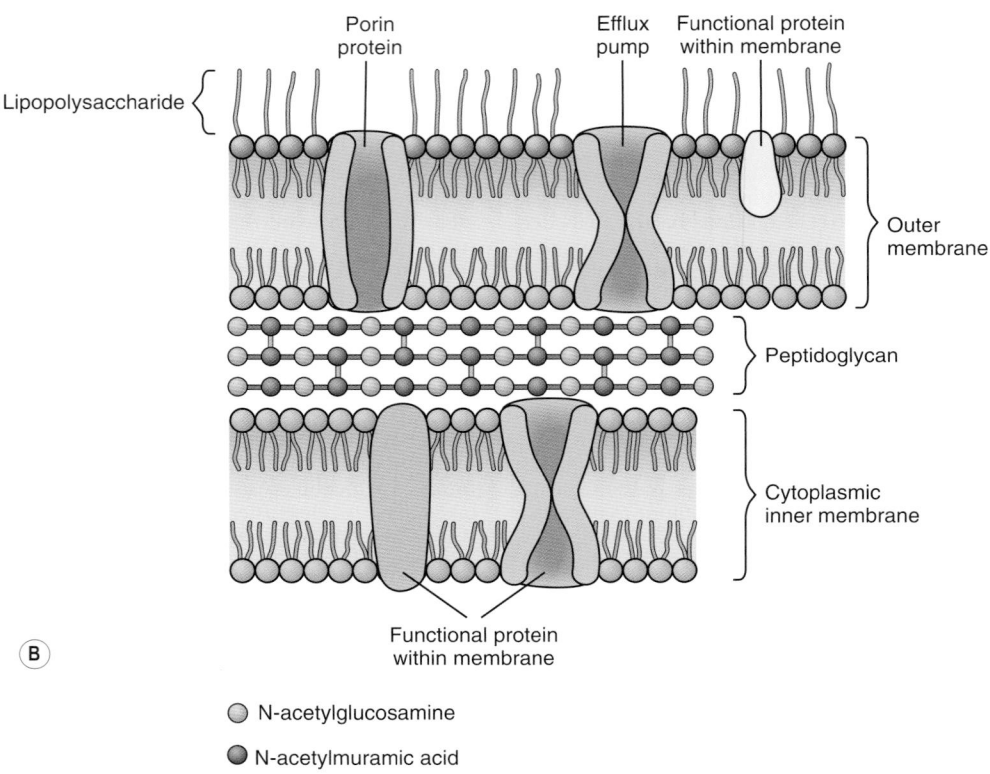

○ N-acetylglucosamine

● N-acetylmuramic acid

Figure 292-3. Structure of bacterial cell walls of gram-positive and gram-negative bacteria.

and *Prevotella melaninogenica* among the organisms causing sinus-related and deep head and neck space infections, including brain abscesses, agents active against β-lactamase-producing anaerobes are preferred to treat infections at these sites.

Penicillin G continues to play a role in the treatment of infections caused by other α- and β-hemolytic streptococci, most of which remain susceptible. For life-threatening infections such as bacterial endocarditis, susceptibility testing should be performed to ensure that the organisms do not exhibit penicillin tolerance, which may decrease treatment success using single drug therapy at standard dosages.

Penicillin G is effective therapy of less common infections, including diphtheria, naturally occurring anthrax, actinomycosis, leptospirosis, and syphilis.

Penicillinase-Resistant Penicillins

This class of semisynthetic penicillins was created to meet the challenge of the development of penicillin-resistant *Staphylococcus aureus*. The bulky side chains prevent the staphylococcal β-lactamases from binding to and hydrolyzing the lactam ring of the molecule. However, these antibiotics are resistant only to staphylococcal penicillinases, and not to the β-lactamases of gram-negative organisms, to which they remain vulnerable. These antibiotics are not active against methicillin-resistant strains of *S. aureus* (MRSA) due to the presence of a transpeptidase (PBP 2a) which had not been capable of being bound and inactivated by any β-lactam antibiotic until the advent of ceftaroline (approved by the Food and Drug Administration (FDA) in 2010).

In clinical practice, these antibiotics are used to treat infections caused by susceptible strains of *S. aureus*. They are available in both parenteral and oral formulations. With the emergence of community-associated (CA)-MRSA, their long-standing role in the empiric therapy of presumed staphylococcal infections is now compromised. For susceptible strains of *S. aureus*, however, they remain among the safest and most effective therapeutic agents available.

Aminopenicillins

This class of semisynthetic penicillins (as represented by ampicillin and amoxicillin) contains an amino substitution in the phenyl acetamido side chain of the penam nucleus, providing a polar charge on the molecule that allows activity against gram-negative pathogens, including *Escherichia coli* and *Haemophilus influenzae* (see Table 292-2). However, aminopenicillins are not stable to staphylococcal penicillinases, or to the hundreds of different β-lactamases provided by gram-negative pathogens. Their activity against other gram-positive organisms, such as group A and group B streptococci still is excellent, and activity against most enterococci is equivalent to or better than penicillin G.

As a means of enhancing the activity of the aminopenicillins against β-lactamase-producing pathogens, the concurrent use of a second agent that binds irreversibly to a pathogen's β-lactamase has led to a useful group of drugs. These concurrently used agents, called β-lactamase inhibitors, have little antibiotic activity on their own as they have been selected for avid binding characteristics to specific β-lactamases, rather than to PBPs. However, just as diversity exists in the affinity of binding of penicillin to the target PBPs of various pathogens, diversity also exists in the binding affinity of each β-lactamase inhibitor to the β-lactamases of different organisms. Currently, clavulanate is paired with amoxicillin in an oral formulation in the United States (and a parenteral formulation in other parts of the world), and ampicillin is paired with sulbactam in a parenteral preparation (see Table 292-2).

The clinical uses of ampicillin and amoxicillin are extensive. The enhanced activity against *E. coli* and other gram-negative enteric bacilli compared with penicillin G permits ampicillin and amoxicillin to be used for the treatment of some urinary tract infections (UTIs) and gastrointestinal infections. The excellent activity against β-lactamase-negative strains of *Haemophilus influenzae* allows ampicillin and amoxicillin to be used in the treatment of upper and lower respiratory tract infections. Ampicillin is one of the most bactericidal agents (when used together with gentamicin) for susceptible strains of *Enterococcus*. Unfortunately, the development of resistance in *E. coli*, *Shigella*, *Salmonella*, and *H. influenzae* has limited the usefulness of aminopenicillins against these pathogens.

However, the addition of clavulanate to amoxicillin allows activity against β-lactamase-producing strains of *H. influenzae* and *Moraxella catarrhalis* as well as *S. aureus*. This combination increases the clinical usefulness of amoxicillin in the treatment of community-associated upper and lower respiratory tract infections (e.g., acute otitis media, sinusitis, and pneumonia), in addition to skin and skin structure infections. The addition of sulbactam to ampicillin allows activity against an array of β-lactamase-producing organisms, including staphylococci, many enteric gram-negative bacilli, and *Bacteroides fragilis*. This allows for the treatment of skin and skin structure infections as well as some intra-abdominal infections, not possible with ampicillin alone.

Extended-Spectrum Penicillins

These semisynthetic penicillins are designed to increase activity against gram-negative pathogens, including *Klebsiella*, *Enterobacter*, and, for some agents, *Pseudomonas* (see Table 292-2). The two major classes are the carboxypenicillins, represented by ticarcillin and carbenicillin, and the acylureidopenicillins, represented by piperacillin. Although the spectrum of activity of these antibiotics has been enhanced beyond the aminopenicillins, they remain susceptible to hydrolysis by many β-lactamases, including those of staphylococcus. Similar to the aminopenicillins, activity of these drugs has been enhanced by pairing them with β-lactamase inhibitors, such as ticarcillin-clavulanate and piperacillin-tazobactam.

The clinical uses of these antibiotics reflect their broad activity against gram-negative enteric bacilli and *Pseudomonas aeruginosa*. While originally available as a single-antibiotic agent, ticarcillin now is only available in combination with clavulanate, while piperacillin still is available and may be used as a single agent for therapy for a variety of gram-negative infections. However, an enhanced antibacterial spectrum when paired with a β-lactamase inhibitor increases the activity against many organisms, including *S. aureus*, *B. fragilis*, *P. melaninogenica*, and many gram-negative enteric bacilli (*E. coli* and *Klebsiella* sp.) (see Table 292-2). This allows for successful therapy for skin and skin structure infections, intra-abdominal infections, and, gram-positive and gram-negative hospital-associated infections, such as wound infections, UTIs, and pneumonia. The extended-spectrum penicillins also retain good activity against ampicillin-susceptible strains of *Enterococcus*.

Cephalosporins

Cephalosporins, like the penicillins, are β-lactam antibiotics found in nature. Cephalosporin C, the precursor molecule for antibiotics used in humans, was originally isolated from *Cephalosporium acremonium*. Successive modifications of the cephem ring structure have resulted in "generations" of cephalosporin antibiotics. There is no official scientific designation of generations; rather, the description of enhanced activity of the second generation over the first was created as a marketing tool.[14] However, the ability to distinguish the relative activity of the large number of cephalosporin antibiotics by generation is quite useful (see Table 292-2).

In general, the first-generation cephalosporins (represented by cefazolin intramuscularly (IM)/intravenously (IV) and cephalexin orally (PO)) are active against gram-positive pathogens, group A streptococcus, and penicillinase-producing *S. aureus* (methicillin-susceptible strains) (MSSA), which has led to their use for skin and skin structure infections and surgical prophylaxis, as well as for invasive infections caused by these organisms. Although they are better tolerated than the penicillinase-stable penicillins (e.g., methicillin), they are somewhat less active in vitro against *S. aureus*, and may not be as effective in the treatment of serious infections such as endocarditis. Cephalosporins uniformly lack activity against all enterococci.

The cephalosporins are active against many strains of *Escherichia coli*, allowing treatment of urinary tract and intestinal infections. However, increasing resistance to first-generation cephalosporins during the past few decades has limited the usefulness of these agents in the treatment of both community-associated and hospital-associated infections.

The second-generation cephalosporins have enhanced activity against gram-negative pathogens as well as demonstrating enhanced stability against β-lactamases compared with first-generation agents (see Table 292-2). This increases the spectrum of activity of these agents to include many enteric gram-negative bacilli, and β-lactamase-positive strains of *Haemophilus influenzae*. The activity of second-generation agents against staphylococci is decreased, although not sufficiently to lead to clinical failures in treatment of mild to moderate staphylococcal infections. This broad spectrum of activity allows for single-drug therapy of staphylococcal, streptococcal, and *Haemophilus influenzae* infections in children. However, due to poor penetration of the first- and second-generation cephalosporins into cerebrospinal fluid (CSF), use is limited for the treatment of invasive BSIs caused by *S. pneumoniae* and *H. influenzae*. Within the second generation of agents, all of which share the cephem ring structure (see Figure 292-2), are both true cephalosporins and the cephamycins. The cephamycins were originally isolated from *Streptomyces* sp., and contain an additional side chain that enhances stability to β-lactamases, providing these agents (cefoxitin and cefotetan) with improved activity against β-lactamase-containing strains of *B. fragilis*. Given reasonable activity against gram-positive organisms (except enterococci), gram-negative enteric bacilli, and anaerobes, these antibiotics are effective in the treatment of intra-abdominal infections.

Oral second-generation agents were used widely for the treatment of upper and lower respiratory tract infections in children. However, with increasing β-lactam resistance in *S. pneumoniae* caused by changes in the PBP structures of these pathogens, treatment failures of pneumococcal infections using the oral second-generation cephalosporins occur more commonly than previously.

The third-generation cephalosporins have further enhanced gram-negative activity, which extends to *P. aeruginosa* for ceftazidime, but at the expense of a further decrease in activity against staphylococci. They lack activity against enterococci. Enhanced activity against enteric gram-negative bacilli has led to successful therapy of UTIs and many nosocomial infections. Therapy of infections caused by *Enterobacter*, *Serratia*, and *Citrobacter* species, which have the ability to produce chromosomally mediated (inducible) β-lactamases, may fail. Failure is likely to be due to the selection of organisms at the site of infection, which based on alterations in β-lactamase gene regulation, constitutively hyperproduce these enzymes, conferring resistance to third-generation agents.[15] The third-generation cephalosporins are, in general, also hydrolyzed by the extended-spectrum β-lactamases (ESBLs) produced most commonly by *E. coli* and *Klebsiella* sp.[10,16] The activity of the third-generation agents is superb against virtually all strains of *H. influenzae*. These agents, in general, achieve CSF concentrations that are effective for treatment of bacterial meningitis caused by all three major pediatric pathogens: *H. influenzae*, *S. pneumoniae*, and *Neisseria meningitidis*. Of note, certain penicillin-resistant strains of *S. pneumoniae* have decreased susceptibility to these cephalosporins and have been associated with clinical and microbiologic failure at tissue sites with decreased antibiotic penetration, such as the central nervous system (CNS).[17,18] However, the most active of the third-generation cephalosporins against *S. pneumoniae*, ceftriaxone and cefotaxime, have not been associated with treatment failure of respiratory tract infections caused by penicillin-resistant strains when appropriate dosing regimens are used. None of the third-generation agents should be considered optimal for the treatment of infections caused by MSSA as other cephalosporins and penicillinase-stable penicillins are more active against this pathogen.

Of the third-generation agents, ceftriaxone has a prolonged serum half-life compared with the other agents, allowing for its once-daily use for treatment of exquisitely susceptible organisms. The infrequent dosing and the ability to use either intramuscular or intravenous routes of administration have allowed for outpatient therapy of serious, invasive infections at a point when the child's clinical condition is stable.[19]

The fourth-generation cephalosporin, cefepime, maintains activity against *P. aeruginosa*, displays enhanced stability to the ampC chromosomal β-lactamases of *Enterobacter*, *Serratia*, and *Citrobacter* species, while retaining significant (but not optimal) activity against *S. aureus* (see Table 292-2).[20] This broad activity allows for empiric therapy of neutropenic children with fever, and allows for treatment of a wide variety of nosocomial gram-negative infections.[20-24] However, lack of activity against β-lactamase-positive strains of *B. fragilis* and against *Enterococcus* limits the ability to treat intra-abdominal infections with cefepime alone.

The fifth generation of cephalosporins, represented currently by only one available product, ceftaroline, combines the gram-negative and gram-positive activity of the third- and fourth-generation cephalosporins with in vitro and clinically demonstrable activity against CA-MRSA. These agents have been designed to bind to and inactivate PBP2a, which confers resistance of MRSA to all other currently available β-lactam agents.[25] However, ceftaroline is not active against *Pseudomonas*, and is not stable to ESBLs.

Carbapenems

Carbapenems, also naturally occurring, were initially isolated from a species of *Streptomyces*, with the β-lactam moiety contained within a carbapenem nucleus (see Figure 292-2). Carbapenems demonstrate the broadest spectrum of activity of all of the β-lactam antibiotics and currently include imipenem, meropenem, doripenem, and ertapenem.[26] Carbapenems are active against both gram-positive pathogens, including MSSA but not MRSA and streptococci (with moderate activity against ampicillin-susceptible enterococci) and gram-negative pathogens, including *P. aeruginosa* for imipenem and meropenem, with enhanced stability against both the chromosomal ampC β-lactamases of *Enterobacter*, *Serratia*, and *Citrobacter* species and the ESBLs of *E. coli* and *Klebsiella* (see Table 292-2). They are highly active against anaerobic organisms, including β-lactamase-producing strains of *Bacteroides* and *Prevotella*. Of these agents, the antibacterial spectrum of activity of imipenem, meropenem, and doripenem is similar, whereas ertapenem matches the activity of the other carbapenems against enteric bacilli, but is not as potent against *P. aeruginosa*. Imipenem is paired with cilastatin, a renal dehydropeptidase inhibitor that inhibits the destruction of imipenem by renal tubular enzymes providing both an increase in the serum half-life of imipenem and a decrease in the renal toxicity of the compound. Imipenem use was associated with unexpected seizures in an open, noncomparative clinical trial in children with meningitis,[27] probably attributable to competitive inhibition of the inhibitory CNS neural pathways. Therefore, meropenem, which does not produce clinically detectable CNS side effects, is the preferred carbapenem agent for treatment of CNS infections, including meningitis, brain abscess, epidural abscess, and subdural empyema. Ertapenem has the most prolonged serum half-life of the carbapenems, and requires only once-daily dosing in older children (≥13 years of age) and once- or twice-a-day dosing in younger children. Carbapenems are used primarily for nosocomial infections or infections in immunocompromised hosts when exceptionally broad spectrum of activity is essential. Data support clinical and microbiologic efficacy in pneumonia, UTIs, wound infections, bone and joint infections, and skin and skin structure infections.[28] Imipenem and meropenem have been used as single-drug empiric therapy of fever and neutropenia in immunocompromised children.[21] Carbapenems provide good, but not optimal, activity against *S. aureus*. They provide the best activity of all β-lactam agents against pathogens harboring either chromosomally mediated ampC β-lactamases or ESBLs. Recent emergence of carbapenemase-producing *Klebsiella* and other gram-negative pathogens may limit the usefulness of these broad-spectrum agents in the near future.[29] Use of such broad-spectrum agents must be weighed against the risk of promoting resistance and profoundly altering normal flora.

Monobactams

This unique β-lactam structure is a naturally occurring antibiotic isolated from *Chromobacterium* sp.; it is not fused to an adjacent ring, in contrast to penicillins, cephalosporins, and carbapenems. Aztreonam, the only available agent in this class, has been modified chemically with side chains,[30] and demonstrates gram-negative activity comparable with the third-generation cephalosporins but without significant gram-positive or anaerobic activity. Clinical use in pediatrics is limited primarily to treatment of community-acquired infections in which enteric gram-negative organisms are suspected or proven pathogens and aminoglycosides are not adequate or appropriate therapy. Aztreonam was recently FDA-approved as an inhalational antibiotic for children with cystic fibrosis who are 7 years of age and older, for the treatment of *P. aeruginosa* lower respiratory tract infection, with doses given three times daily for 28 days.

Glycopeptide Antibiotics

Glycopeptides interfere with cell wall formation in the steps that create the glycan chains prior to cross-linking the chains in the formation of peptidoglycan (see Figure 292-1). These antibiotics have a large, complex structure that consists of multiple peptides linked together into three rings, with various side-chain substitutions, including large saccharide moieties attached to the central polycyclic structure. Strong hydrogen bonds occur between a glycopeptide antibiotic and the terminal D-alanine, D-alanine dipeptide of the pentapeptide side chains of the MurNAc subunits of the glycan chain. Once bound, the glycopeptides sterically prevent the transglycosylation steps required for lengthening the glycan chain.[5] Glycopeptide antibiotics are primarily active against gram-positive organisms, in which the cell wall construction occurs outside the cell membrane (see Figure 292-3). Little activity is demonstrated against gram-negative organisms, as the large structure does not cross the gram-negative outer membrane easily, preventing contact with enzymes responsible for transglycosylation in the periplasmic space. Recent documented resistance in gram-positive pathogens to vancomycin has led to intense investigation of derivatives of vancomycin and teicoplanin, another parenteral glycopeptide antibiotic that has been available outside the U.S. for several years.

Vancomycin

Vancomycin is a natural product, originally isolated from *Streptomyces* sp. in 1956. Vancomycin is the only glycopeptide currently available in the U.S. Originally developed to treat staphylococcal infections, vancomycin was rarely used following the availability of the penicillinase-stable penicillins, which were tolerated better. However, since the first appearance of healthcare-associated (HA)-MRSA four decades ago, vancomycin has played a continuing role in the treatment of nosocomial *S. aureus* infections. Recently, with the increasing prevalence of CA-MRSA, vancomycin is now routinely used in the empiric therapy of serious suspected staphylococcal infections.[31,32] Concern for decreased bactericidal activity and clinical efficacy of vancomycin compared with the penicillinase-stable penicillins for treatment of MSSA, as well as greater toxicity, make vancomycin non-preferred therapy for infections caused by MSSA.

Resistance to vancomycin has developed in several ways. In *Enterococcus* sp., *vanA*-mediated resistance, the most common resistance seen in clinical isolates, leads to complete resistance to vancomycin. A transmissible set of 7 genes, which encode a series of biologic functions that allows *Enterococcus* to sense the presence of vancomycin, to cleave the D-alanine, D-alanine dipeptide from the pentapeptide chain, and to substitute D-alanine, D-lactate at the terminus of the pentapeptide, results in a 1000-fold decrease in binding of vancomycin.[33,34] The new pentapeptide appears to be as viable a precursor for peptidoglycan formation as the original pentapeptide. The *vanA* resistance mechanism has now been detected in *S. aureus* infecting adult patients, creating vancomycin-resistant *S. aureus* (VRSA). A more common resistance mechanism of *S. aureus* to vancomycin, producing a heterogeneous population of intermediately susceptible strains or hVISA, is proliferation of the D-alanine, D-alanine glycan structures, creating a disorganized, thickened cell wall, leading to increases in the binding and trapping of vancomycin to nonfunctional dipeptides.[35–38] Under vancomycin pressure, these strains, which are present in every large population of staphylococci, are selected. However, as these strains are not fully resistant to vancomycin, retrospective data suggest that higher dosages of vancomycin (if tolerated by the patient) can remain effective therapy for hVISA.[39,40]

Three new glycopeptide antibiotics, dalbavancin, telavancin, and oritavancin, have demonstrated clinical efficacy in small clinical trials, but none is yet approved for use.[41] Modifications of the glycopeptide to enhance binding to targets, to increase stability of antibiotic binding by creating glycopeptide dimers, and to anchor the glycopeptide to the cell membrane have all been successful strategies for enhancing the activity of this class of agents. Although these newer agents have shown increased in vitro activity against *S. aureus* compared with vancomycin, prospective, controlled clinical data to document improved outcomes in adults are not available, and no data exist currently for children.

Clinical uses of vancomycin include therapy for gram-positive infections in children who are penicillin-allergic, therapy of infections caused by *S. pneumoniae* that are resistant to penicillin,[42] and therapy of infections caused by MRSA. Treatment of *Clostridium difficile* infections with orally administered vancomycin is highly effective, but is not first-line therapy because of the emergence of vancomycin-resistant enterococci (VRE) following oral vancomycin therapy. In selected cases of metronidazole failure, vancomycin represents effective alternative therapy.[43]

A common reaction can occur with the rapid infusion of vancomycin, the red-man or red-neck syndrome, characterized by flushing and hypotension. This reaction is histamine-mediated and not immunoglobulin E-mediated and is distinct from anaphylaxis. The risk of this reaction varies directly with the rapidity of the vancomycin infusion; therefore, each dose of vancomycin usually is infused over 1 hour. For children who develop red-man syndrome, prolonging the infusion time or pretreating with an antihistamine may permit continuation of therapy with vancomycin.

Cell Membrane Active Antibiotics

Daptomycin

Daptomycin, a natural product derived from *Streptomyces* sp., is a novel lipopeptide antibiotic that is rapidly bactericidal based on effects on the gram-positive cell membrane. Daptomycin has a unique structure that consists of 13 amino acids, including a cyclic peptide containing 9 amino acids, attached to a lipophilic fatty acid tail that inserts into the cell membrane. The mechanism of action of daptomycin is not well understood, but it appears that depolarization of the membrane occurs as the antibiotic polymerizes within the bacterial cell membrane, producing channels in the membrane that result in leakage of cell contents, inhibition of protein, DNA and RNA synthesis, and cell death. Based on in vitro assays, daptomycin is one of the most rapidly bactericidal antibiotics against *S. aureus* and is active against a wide variety of gram-positive organisms, including MSSA, MRSA, VRSA, streptococci, and enterococci (including VRE) (see Table 292-2).[44]

Clinical use of daptomycin has focused on MRSA infections that are unresponsive to vancomycin. Efficacy has been demonstrated in adults for skin and skin structure infections, and for BSI. Surprisingly, daptomycin is not effective for the treatment of pneumonia, based on clinical trials in which response rates were not equivalent to comparator agents. Daptomycin is inactivated by surfactant, yielding relatively low concentrations in bronchial-alveolar epithelial lining fluid and lung parenchyma.[45] Limited pharmacokinetic and clinical data have been reported in children.[46–48] The prolonged half-life in adults of 8 to 9 hours allows for once-daily dosing.

In the first human clinical trials five decades ago, daptomycin was associated with a high incidence of myalgias and muscle weakness accompanied by elevations in serum creatine kinase. This adverse effect appears to depend on the frequency of dosing, with less adverse effect noted with a decreased frequency of dosing. While toxicity was prohibitive when daptomycin was administered every 6 to 8 hours, the drug demonstrated no greater toxicity than comparator agents when administered to adults in a dose of 4 mg/kg once daily.[37] As the approved dosage of daptomycin was increased to 6 mg/kg daily in adults for the treatment of BSI and endocarditis, no significant muscle toxicity was noted.[49]

Colistin

Colistin is a polymyxin antibiotic that is a natural product isolated from *Bacillus polymyxa*, and consists of 10 linked amino acids, with 6 forming a peptide ring structure attached to a fatty-acid side chain. Colistin is also known as polymyxin E, structurally similar to polymyxin B, which is used extensively as a topical agent. The polymyxin antibiotics were first discovered in 1947, with the first clinical use of colistin in the U.S. in 1959.[50] Colistin is available in the U.S. as a sodium methanesulfonate salt, known as colistimethate. The dosage is calculated as the colistin base, at 2.5 to

5.0 mg/kg per day given in 2 to 4 divided doses. Colistimethate is hydrolyzed to colistin, but the rate and extent of hydrolysis and the contributions of biologic activity of the parent compound and products of metabolism are not well known. The mechanism of bactericidal activity against the cytoplasmic membrane is based on cationic detergent activity, binding to lipopolysaccharides in the outer cell membrane, displacing calcium and magnesium and disrupting the lipid component of the cell membrane. Permeability changes subsequently occur in the membrane, disrupting the osmotic gradient of the cell and impacting cellular metabolism and nucleic acid synthesis.[51]

Colistin has been used as both intravenous and inhalational treatment for multidrug resistant gram-negative pathogens in children with cystic fibrosis (CF),[52] and more recently, in non-CF patients with gram-negative pneumonia.[53] For treatment of gram-negative CNS infections, colistin has been injected intrathecally.[54,55] Only limited, retrospective clinical data are available to guide therapy with this agent.[54,55]

Colistin has significant toxicity, primarily renal and neurologic. Renal side effects include decreased urine output with elevated blood urea nitrogen and serum creatinine, proteinuria, hematuria, and acute tubular necrosis. Because colistin is eliminated by renal excretion, it is imperative to assess renal function closely during therapy, decreasing the dosage if any degree of renal insufficiency is noted. Drug accumulation and additional renal toxicity occur if dosing is not altered when renal insufficiency first occurs. Renal toxicity usually is reversible if detected early. Neuromuscular side effects had been noted in adults and children treated with colistin in case series reported up to 50 years ago, most often manifest as oral and perioral paresthesias, weakness, lethargy, confusion, ataxia, and respiratory muscle paralysis. However, more recent experience with colistin, particularly in children, has not described this neuromuscular toxicity.[54,55] Colistin also crosses the placenta and has been shown to be teratogenic in certain laboratory animals following drug exposures in pregnant animals.

Due to the toxicity, clinical use of parenteral colistimethate is limited to therapy of infections caused by multidrug-resistant gram-negative pathogens for which no other option is available. Other clinical uses include inhaled therapy in ventilated patients with nosocomial multidrug-resistant gram-negative pulmonary infections[56] and aerosolized colistimethate in children with CF as adjunctive antimicrobial therapy.[57,58]

RIBOSOME-ACTIVE ANTIBIOTICS

The bacterial ribosome, highly conserved over millions of years, has long been a target of antibiotics. As our ability to understand the function of the ribosome has increased, and with recent advances in our ability to visualize ribosomal structures with crystallography, our knowledge of the mechanism of activity of both older and newer agents and our ability to design more effective antibiotics has improved substantially. The ribosome contains a 30S and a 50S subunit, each comprising rRNA and ribosomal proteins. Several sites have been documented to be antibiotic targets on each of the subunits and at the junction of the subunits. Targets include: the entry site of mRNA, the initial recognition and binding site of tRNAs, the site of attachment of the tRNA-peptide chain where peptide bonds are formed (the peptidyl transferase center), and the exit channel of the growing polypeptide.[59-61] The critical chemical and structural relationships between the ribosomal rRNA and the peptidyl transferase center, which promote the chemical reactions to create a new peptide, as well as movement of mRNA and the newly formed peptide through the ribosome, provide opportunities for interference in bacterial protein synthesis.

Macrolides

The currently available macrolides consist of the erythromycins, azithromycin, and clarithromycin. All share structural similarities with either a 14-member lactone ring (erythromycin, clarithromycin) or a 15-member ring (azithromycin). All bind to at least one site in common within the peptide exit tunnel of the ribosome: domain V of the 23S RNA within the 50S subunit. To achieve activity in most bacteria, binding to a specific adenine residue of the rRNA, A2058, within this channel prevents the orderly movement of protein out of the ribosome.[62]

Clarithromycin is similar structurally to erythromycin, with only the addition of a single methyl group to the erythromycin ring, primarily conferring improved stability to gastric acid. While erythromycin, clarithromycin, and azithromycin contain a cladinose carbohydrate attached to the lactone ring, a new class of ketolides, represented by telithromycin, substitutes a ketone in this position while adding highly charged side chains to the C11 and C12 positions. These changes improve the binding characteristics to both the peptide tunnel binding site within domain V, and create an additional unique binding site at adjacent domain II within the ribosome, improving activity against many macrolide-resistant gram-positive organisms. Azithromycin is structurally similar to erythromycin, but contains a 15-member ring with the addition of a nitrogen atom within the ring itself, structurally changing the drug from a macrolide to an azalide, but containing the same side chain-attached carbohydrate moieties as erythromycin. This change improves gram-negative activity as well as increasing gastric acid stability. The degradation products of azithromycin provide far less stimulation of gastric motility, improving the tolerability of azithromycin over erythromycin.

In general, the macrolides are inhibitory, not bactericidal, to bacteria and therefore are not used for the treatment of serious and life-threatening infections when other bactericidal agents can be used. The various macrolide agents have different binding affinities for their ribosomal targets in different organisms. Binding generally is reversible, with a prolonged rate of dissociation off the ribosome potentially adding to a more prolonged antibiotic effect seen with some macrolides (see Table 290-1).[63]

The macrolides are most active against gram-positive cocci and bacilli, and, to a lesser extent, gram-negative bacilli (see Table 292-2). Some of these agents also are active against spirochetes and certain mycobacteria. Pathogens that lack a formal cell wall (e.g., *Mycoplasma* and *Ureaplasma*) and are not susceptible to β-lactam antibiotics often remain susceptible to macrolides.

All of the macrolides achieve high antibiotic concentrations within phagocytic cells. These concentrations often are much higher than those measured in serum, providing access of these antibiotics to infected tissue spaces by means of neutrophils and establishing a higher tissue concentration than antibiotics that enter primarily by diffusion alone. However, presence in the intracellular location leads to less free drug available to expose extracellular pathogens. Macrolides are particularly effective therapy against susceptible intracellular pathogens.

In general, macrolides are well tolerated. Clarithromycin and azithromycin are better tolerated than erythromycin, which has problematic gastrointestinal side effects in some children. With the exception of azithromycin, this class of antibiotics is metabolized by hepatic cytochrome P450 system, and drug–antibiotic interactions should be considered as they may increase or decrease the macrolide and concurrent drug concentrations.[64] Azithromycin has demonstrated minimal drug–drug interactions, and may represent the preferred macrolide in certain situations, particularly for immunocompromised children receiving multiple medications concurrently.

Resistance to the macrolides occurs when molecular changes occur at the critical ribosomal attachment site, most commonly a mono- or dimethylation of the A2058 adenine binding site. A rapidly increasing number of recognized methyltransferase enzymes have now been reported. Most of these are encoded by gram-positive organisms, are most often inducible, but may be constitutively produced and lead to high-level resistance to erythromycin, clarithromycin, and azithromycin.[65] Less frequent alterations at this site also impact binding, with either substitution of guanine for adenine or structural changes in the L4 ribosomal protein.[66] Efflux pumps represent another common mechanism of resistance in gram-positive pathogens, including pneumococcus, group A streptococcus, and *S. aureus.* The most common pumps are active against all the macrolides – erythromycin, clarithromycin, and azithromycin.[65,67]

Erythromycin

Erythromycin, a natural product isolated from *Saccharopolyspora erythraea* (formerly *Streptomyces*) in 1949, was first approved for clinical use in 1952. Erythromycin is degraded by gastric acid, and has long been associated with stimulation of motilin receptors in the stomach and possibly in the colon, leading to adverse gastrointestinal side effects, including cramping and diarrhea.[68,69] Many preparations have attempted to bypass exposure of erythromycin to gastric acid, thereby avoiding products of macrolide hydrolysis. These preparations include enteric coating of orally administered tablets, delayed-release formulations, polymer coating of beads, and various formulations of salts and esters.[70] The lactobionate salt used for intravenous administration of erythromycin can cause phlebitis at the site of injection.

Erythromycin is used for the treatment of group A streptococcal infections in children who are penicillin-allergic. Erythromycin is an alternative treatment for both streptococcal pharyngitis and streptococcal or staphylococcal impetigo. The usefulness of erythromycin for respiratory tract infections caused by *S. pneumoniae* has been greatly diminished by the development of widespread resistance to the macrolides.[42] Macrolide therapy of upper respiratory tract infections (otitis media and sinusitis) or lower respiratory tract infections (pneumonia) potentially caused by *S. pneumoniae* has a relatively high likelihood of failure, particularly in younger children who are at highest risk of infections caused by antibiotic-resistant strains. For upper respiratory tract infections, erythromycin has inadequate activity against *H. influenzae*, and must be paired with another agent such as a sulfonamide for empiric therapy. Macrolides are effective therapy for pneumonia caused by *Mycoplasma pneumoniae*, *Chlamydophila pneumoniae*, or *Legionella pneumophila*.

Erythromycin and azithromycin are the preferred antibiotics for treatment of *Campylobacter* gastroenteritis. Erythromycin also remains the most appropriate therapy for diphtheria (*Corynebacterium diphtheriae*). Erythromycin, clarithromycin, or azithromycin is recommended for treatment or prophylaxis of pertussis (*Bordetella pertussis*).[71] Azithromycin is preferred for treatment or prophylaxis for pertussis in neonates, based on concerns for the development of pyloric stenosis.[71] Efficacy of erythromycin also has been demonstrated in infections caused by *Chlamydophila pneumoniae* and *Chlamydia trachomatis*, including neonatal conjunctivitis and pneumonia, as well as urogenital infections during pregnancy. Erythromycin is active in vitro against *Ureaplasma urealyticum*, but its role in the treatment of neonatal infections associated with this organism is not well defined.[72]

Clarithromycin

With the improved activity demonstrated against *H. influenzae* and improved tolerability compared with erythromycin, treatment of respiratory tract infections is the most common clinical use for clarithromycin. FDA-approved indications include pharyngitis/tonsillitis, acute otitis media, acute maxillary sinusitis, and community-acquired pneumonia caused by susceptible strains of *S. pneumoniae*, *H. influenzae*, *M. catarrhalis*, *M. pneumoniae*, *C. pneumoniae*, and *L. pneumophila*. For *S. pneumoniae*, strains that are resistant to erythromycin from either methyltransferase or efflux mechanisms also are resistant to clarithromycin. The activity of clarithromycin against *H. influenzae* is only moderate, but in noninferiority-designed clinical trials of clarithromycin for the treatment of respiratory tract infections, the microbiologic and clinical efficacy was not significantly less than that of other approved agents.

Clarithromycin is one of the most effective macrolides for treatment and prevention of disseminated mycobacterial infections due to *Mycobacterium avium* complex (MAC) in human immunodeficiency virus (HIV)-infected persons. Although not well studied in immunocompetent children, clarithromycin may play a role in

the treatment of cervical adenitis and pneumonia caused by MAC (or other nontuberculous mycobacteria proved to be susceptible in vitro), in conjunction with other antibiotics and/or surgery.[73]

Clarithromycin plays a role in the treatment of *Helicobacter pylori* infections in combination with amoxicillin and lansoprazole, or omeprazole, or in combination with ranitidine.[74,75] Clarithromycin has demonstrated efficacy similar to erythromycin in pertussis infections in small clinical trials, and is considered as one of three first-line drugs. Although approved for treatment of skin and skin structure infections, clarithromycin is not often used for this indication as other more cost-effective or more active agents are available in the treatment of infections caused by *S. aureus*. Similarly, other β-lactam and macrolide antibiotics are preferred for the treatment of streptococcal pharyngitis.

Azithromycin

Azithromycin has among the highest intracellular concentrations of the macrolides and provides the most prolonged tissue concentrations at the site of infection, allowing the antibiotic to be administered for very short courses for respiratory tract infections without compromising prolonged tissue site activity. Erythromycin-resistant strains of *S. pneumoniae* also are resistant to azithromycin. Group A streptococcus has variable resistance to macrolides. Activity against *H. influenzae* is moderate, with in vitro activity increased compared with erythromycin, but decreased compared with clarithromycin. However, the relatively small differences in susceptibility may be offset by higher concentrations of antibiotic if there is an intracellular site of infection. Azithromycin also is active against the pathogens causing atypical pneumonia (see Table 292-2).

Azithromycin is far better tolerated than erythromycin, can be given once daily, and is available in both oral and intravenous formulations. Based on noninferiority-designed clinical trials, azithromycin is approved for treatment of streptococcal pharyngitis, acute otitis media, sinusitis, and community-acquired pneumonia in children. Because of prolonged tissue concentrations, particularly using larger azithromycin dosages, 5-day, 3-day, and 1-day treatment courses, all providing a total treatment dosage of 30 mg/kg, have been shown to be comparable for clinical and microbiologic outcomes with 10-day treatment courses of comparator β-lactam antibiotics in acute, uncomplicated otitis media. However, as the dose increases, the gastrointestinal tolerability of the antibiotic decreases, with vomiting and diarrhea occurring in about 10% of children receiving 30 mg/kg as a single dose.[76] Although clinical data on single-dose treatment courses for otitis media are available, data exist only for treatment courses of 3 and 5 days for sinusitis, and for 5 days for treatment of community-acquired pneumonia and streptococcal pharyngitis. The dosage for treatment of streptococcal pharyngitis is 12 mg/kg per day once daily for 5 days, which is larger than that for otitis and provides a total dosage of 60 mg/kg.

Azithromycin has the widest use in children for the treatment of upper and lower respiratory tract infections.[77] However, other uses have been documented in clinical trials, although FDA approval for many of these infections has not been requested. Treatment of pertussis has been shown to be effective in small trials.[78] Azithromycin is the recommended macrolide for prophylaxis or treatment of infants under 1 month of age and is considered equal to erythromycin and clarithromycin in older individuals.[71]

Azithromycin also is used in the treatment of sexually transmitted infections, including *Chlamydia trachomatis*-caused infections (urethritis, cervicitis, and lymphogranuloma venereum), chancroid, granuloma inguinale, and gonorrhea.[79]

Similar to clarithromycin, azithromycin has been shown to play a role in the prophylaxis and therapy of MAC infections in HIV-infected children.[80] Azithromycin also may have a role in therapy of cutaneous and lymph node infection caused by these pathogens in healthy children.

Azithromycin has enhanced activity compared with the other macrolides against many gastrointestinal pathogens, including *E. coli*, *Salmonella*, *Shigella*, and *Campylobacter*.[81] In vitro activity demonstrated against *Salmonella* is particularly advantageous given the intracellular location of this pathogen.[82] With widespread resistance among gastrointestinal pathogens to β-lactam antibiotics, fluoroquinolones, and trimethoprim-sulfamethoxazole in certain parts of the world, the utility of empiric azithromycin therapy for traveler's diarrhea has increased.[83]

Azithromycin is the only antibiotic that has been prospectively evaluated for the treatment of cat-scratch lymphadenitis.[84] However, the clinical response to treatment of lymph node disease is not dramatic, and azithromycin has not been evaluated prospectively for the treatment in other tissue sites of infection, such as liver, bone, or CNS.

Tetracyclines

The tetracyclines were derived as natural products from *Streptomyces* spp., with discovery in the 1940s and subsequent availability of two agents by 1948, chlortetracycline and oxytetracycline.[85] Tetracyclines bind reversibly to the ribosome at the aminoacyl acceptor site (A site) where the amino acid-charged tRNA binds to the ribosome immediately adjacent to the site on the ribosome holding the mRNA strand.

The aminoacyl tRNA binds to the A site together with an elongation factor (EF-Tu) and guanosine triphosphate (GTP), which supplies the energy required to drive protein synthesis. The protein synthesis step includes the chemical reaction to attach the amino acid to the growing peptide chain, together with changes in the conformation of the ribosome that are associated with movement of the protein chain and the mRNA through the ribosome, followed by the subsequent release of the "empty" tRNA.[86] It appears that the flat, four-ring structure characteristic of the tetracyclines binds to at least two locations within the ribosome. Binding at the classically recognized A site appears to prevent movement of the tRNA/mRNA/EF-Tu complex into the "P site" (peptidyl site) by steric hindrance, which prevents elongation of the growing peptide. Binding to a second site in the 30S ribosome may stabilize the ribosome in an inappropriate conformation at the crucial site of recognition of the aminoacyl tRNA's anticodon with the corresponding codon within the mRNA, thereby preventing placement of the correct amino acid in the elongating chain.[87] Inhibition of peptide formation by tetracyclines occurs after the binding of the tRNA to the complex and after expenditure of GTP-mediated energy, presenting the bacteria with an energy cost in addition to blocking the synthesis of a new protein.

The tetracyclines are effective against many gram-positive and gram-negative bacteria as well as against cell wall-deficient pathogens (*Mycoplasma, Rickettsia*) and certain single-cell parasites (see Table 292-2). Eukaryotic cells have elongation factors different than bacteria, and are therefore not susceptible to the protein synthesis inhibition activity of this class of antibiotics. The tetracyclines enter the gram-negative cell wall through outer membrane porin proteins and are sufficiently lipophilic to allow passage through the cytoplasmic membrane of both gram-negative and gram-positive bacteria. The tetracyclines are, in general, bacteriostatic.

Resistance to tetracyclines occurred quickly following their availability for clinical use, primarily based on efflux pumps and, to a lesser extent, on the presence of ribosomal protection proteins and tetracycline-inactivating enzymes. Of concern, the number of resistance genes and the number of bacterial species that contain them continues to increase.[85,88] These resistance mechanisms are present on plasmids, conjugative transposons, and integrons, allowing free exchange of resistance determinants between a wide range of bacteria. Over 200 different efflux pumps have been characterized, most of which are active against tetracycline, some of which also are active against minocycline, and fewer of which also are active against the most recently available tetracycline, tigecycline. The ribosomal protection proteins have sequence homologies with bacterial elongation factors present in the tRNA/mRNA/EF-Tu complex. It is believed that, as these protection proteins themselves bind to the ribosome, changes in the conformation at the tetracycline binding site occur, preventing the binding of tetracycline but not interfering with protein synthesis.

Resistance at the second 30S ribosomal binding site also has been described, due to base substitutions in the rRNA of the 30S unit.

Advances in the design of the structure of the early tetracyclines led to doxycycline (in 1967) and minocycline (in 1972), both of which provide a greater spectrum of activity and improved solubility, creating improvements in both oral and parenteral preparations (see Table 292-2). Doxycycline and minocycline can be taken with food (with the exceptions noted below). In most cases, doxycycline and minocycline demonstrate increased activity against gram-positive organisms, and decreased activity against gram-negative organisms compared with tetracycline. Activity against *Enterococcus faecium*, but not *E. faecalis*, is achieved with newer agents. Minocycline, however, demonstrates improved activity against gram-negative organisms, including *H. influenzae*, *M. catarrhalis*, *E. coli*, and *Klebsiella* spp. compared with tetracycline, but only fair activity against *Salmonella* and *Shigella* spp. and *Pseudomonas aeruginosa*. Tigecycline, a derivative of minocycline, increases the spectrum of activity against many enteric gram-negative bacilli and anaerobes, including *B. fragilis*, but still lacks a high degree of activity against *P. aeruginosa* (see Table 292-2). Historically, clinical use in pediatrics has been limited by the binding of tetracyclines to teeth and bones in growing children. Permanent staining of the teeth (not affecting the structural integrity of the tooth) and enamel hypoplasia occurs with any tetracycline antibiotic, with the degree of staining directly proportional to the number of tetracycline courses prescribed. A single course of therapy is not associated with clinically detectable changes.[89-91] Stable calcium complexes also can develop in bone, and reversible decreases in long-bone growth rates in juvenile animals have been observed. The clinical impact of these observations for children is not well defined but has been a cause for concern, limiting the use of tetracyclines to children 8 years of age and older.[92] In addition, the tetracyclines cross the placenta to expose the fetus; skeletal embryopathy in experimental animals has been noted. The oral tetracyclines cannot be taken with dairy products due to the insoluble chelation complexes that form with calcium; similar complexes form with magnesium and iron ions. When ingested with foods containing these ions, absorption from the gastrointestinal tract is blocked.

In adults and older children, the tetracyclines have been used for the treatment of mild to moderate respiratory tract infections, skin and skin structure infections (most commonly acne), and sexually transmitted infections. Some agents in this class demonstrate activity against strains of CA-MRSA,[93] penicillin-resistant pneumococci, and VRE, and have been used in the treatment of these infections. However, few prospective, comparative data are available to assess the efficacy of tetracyclines against these pathogens, with the exception of recent studies on tigecycline (see below).

Tetracyclines are first-line therapy for infections caused by *Rickettsia, Ehrlichia,* and *Anaplasma* spp. (most notably Rocky Mountain spotted fever), tularemia (oral therapy for less severe infections), brucellosis (with rifampin), cholera, *Chlamydia* genital infections, and Lyme disease (*Borrelia burgdorferi*) in older children.

Tigecycline

Tigecycline is a chemically modified minocycline, with the addition of a *t*-butylglycylamido side chain to the C9 carbon of the "D" tetracycline ring.[94] Tigecycline is not affected by the majority of efflux pumps and ribosomal protection proteins that decrease the activity of other tetracyclines. Tigecycline has a higher binding affinity to the ribosomal binding site than the previous tetracyclines[85] and has a broader spectrum of activity than any other tetracycline agent (see Table 292-2). In rat models, bone discoloration was documented, suggesting that tigecycline forms calcium complexes in bone similar to other tetracyclines.

In adults, tigecycline is approved for treatment of complicated skin and skin structure infections and complicated intra-abdominal infections given its activity against enteric gram-negative bacilli and anaerobes, including *B. fragilis.* Tigecycline retains activity against the agents of atypical pneumonia that is equivalent to, or better than, earlier tetracyclines.

The ultimate clinical role of tigecycline has yet to be defined in the treatment of nosocomial infections caused by multidrug-resistant gram-negative and gram-positive organisms that remain susceptible to tigecycline. For children, the risks of bone toxicity and tooth staining need to be balanced with the benefits of therapy, particularly for drug-resistant pathogens. For situations in which no alternatives exist, the tetracyclines represent effective therapy.

Lincosamides

The lincosamides are naturally occurring compounds derived from *Streptomyces* spp. Clindamycin, approved in 1966, is the only lincosamide available in the U.S. and is a semisynthetic derivative of lincomycin. The lincosamide antibiotics bind to the 50S subunit at a site which overlaps both the A and P sites on the ribosome, preventing the docking of charged tRNAs and their movement through the peptidyl transferase center, thus inhibiting the formation of protein. The P-site attachment of clindamycin occurs at the same ribosomal-RNA structural bases as the macrolide binding sites (A2058, A2059), explaining the competitive inhibition between binding of the two classes of antibiotics for the ribosome, as well the resistance that occurs to both antibiotics by altering a single base.[95] The lincosamides generally are considered bacteriostatic, although bactericidal activity can be demonstrated against certain organisms at antibiotic concentrations 2 to 4 times the minimum inhibitory concentration (MIC).[96]

Resistance to the lincosamides occurs primarily in bacteria that constitutively produce the methyltransferase that mono- or dimethylates the A2058 adenine present at the outlet of the ribosomal peptidyl transferase center. This inducible enzyme most often is activated only in the presence of the appropriate substrate, usually a macrolide. In contrast, the lincosamides appear to be poor inducers of the methylase enzyme. Therefore, organisms that have inducible resistance may remain susceptible to clindamycin, even following exposure to the antibiotic. However, genetically altered strains that have lost gene regulation and constitutively produce methylase occur at a rate of approximately one in 10^7 S. *aureus;* selection of constitutive mutants can occur during therapy with subsequent treatment failure.[67,97] This situation is most likely to occur in serious, deep, high-density bacterial infections, but not with mild to moderate skin infections or cutaneous and soft-tissue abscesses that can be incised and drained. The commonly encountered efflux pumps that are active against the macrolides are not active against clindamycin.

High intracellular concentrations of clindamycin in phagocytic cells are believed to be beneficial in certain clinical infections.[98] However, no prospectively collected data have confirmed the benefit in clinical or microbiologic cure of infection either as a result of improved intracellular killing of organisms such as staphylococci, or improved delivery of clindamycin to the site of infection through phagocytic cell migration.

Clinical use of clindamycin has changed substantially over the past decade. Commonly used for its activity against anaerobes in the treatment of intra-abdominal infections such as appendicitis, clindamycin resistance of *Bacteroides fragilis* has increased and clindamycin no longer is recommended as the anaerobic agent of choice.[99,100] Clindamycin continues to have a good spectrum of activity for use in deep head and neck space infections, dental abscesses, and aspiration pneumonia (with or without empyema). Less common uses continue for treatment of gram-positive cocci, such as failures of penicillin in group A streptococcal pharyngitis, and for treatment of *S. aureus* infections due to susceptible organisms.

In the early 1990s, the emergence of penicillin- and macrolide-resistant *S. pneumoniae* causing upper and lower respiratory tract infections promoted the use of clindamycin in the treatment of mild to moderate respiratory tract infections in children. Although no formal, randomized prospective comparative studies were performed in acute otitis media, sinusitis, and pneumonia,

clindamycin has been recommended for treatment of infection due to penicillin-resistant pneumococci.[101]

Since the mid-1990s, with the dramatic emergence of CA-MRSA, the use of clindamycin for skin and skin structure infections and bone and joint infections has increased substantially. Although most published data on the efficacy of clindamycin in the treatment of MRSA are retrospective, clindamycin appears to be effective for these pathogens.[102,103] While some regions of the U.S. in which MRSA is prevalent have documented decreasing resistance to clindamycin due to spread in the community of certain clindamycin-susceptible clones,[83] other areas may experience increasing clindamycin resistance, particularly with methylase-harboring organisms that confer resistance to both clindamycin and macrolides. Susceptibility of MRSA and MSSA should be assessed locally to determine empiric therapy for serious infections.[104,105]

The ability of clindamycin to target ribosomal protein production has led to use in the treatment of toxin-mediated infections caused by *S. aureus* (toxic shock syndrome) and *S. pyogenes* (toxic shock-like illness), either alone or in combination with a cell wall-active antibiotic agent. In vitro data and retrospectively analyzed human data suggest some benefit of combined therapy.[106]

The principal adverse event associated with clindamycin is a direct function of its activity against normal anaerobic gastrointestinal flora – diarrhea.[85] *Clostridium difficile*-mediated pseudomembranous colitis is a potential complication of virtually any broad-spectrum antibiotic, including clindamycin.[107] Accurate, prospectively collected data on the incidence of *C. difficile* enterocolitis are not available for clindamycin-treated children, but increasing reports of enterocolitis have not occurred with the increased use of clindamycin for pneumococcal and staphylococcal infections.

Aminoglycosides

The aminoglycoside/aminocyclitol class of antibiotics is derived from *Streptomyces* spp. and *Micromonospora* spp. In general, these antibiotics contain a 2-deoxystreptamine ring attached to two or three additional moieties, most often amino sugars, all connected together by glycosidic linkages. Medicinal chemists have created substitutions at up to 10 different positions on the three rings or associated amino groups that have led to the creation of several semisynthetic aminoglycoside antibiotics. However, given the nephrotoxicity and ototoxicity inherent to aminoglycosides, little recent activity has occurred in the development of newer agents for community infections. All aminoglycosides currently available in the U.S. are generic formulations, with gentamicin, tobramycin, and amikacin representing those most often used in children.

All of the aminoglycoside antibiotics share a common binding region within the 30S ribosome, which is located at the peptidyl transferase center where charged tRNAs are first recognized and attach to the A site. With aminoglycoside binding close to the A site, conformational changes occur at the ribosomal tRNA docking site that creates enhanced affinity for tRNA binding, facilitating incorrect binding of noncognate tRNAs that do not match the corresponding codon on the mRNA. With attachment of incorrect tRNAs, misreading occurs and amino acid sequences in the resulting peptide are incorrect, leading to the creation of nonfunctional proteins. With binding of the aminoglycoside, proofreading for the accuracy of the attached tRNA also is compromised, as subsequent conformational changes that should occur in the 30S unit to allow for exact recognition of the attached tRNA cannot take place.[86,108–110] The structures of two of the larger aminoglycosides, streptomycin and spectinomycin, allow for additional binding sites within the 30S ribosome. Streptomycin attaches at four different domains within the 30S rRNA, as well as having a unique attachment to one of the ribosomal proteins. Spectinomycin, a larger structure with fused rings, appears to bind at the A site in a unique manner which also blocks the movement of the aminoacyl tRNA/peptidyl tRNA/EF-Tu complex from the A site to the P site during the peptidyl transferase reaction. With the production of abnormal proteins that may be incorporated into cellular structures such as the cell membrane, increased permeability of the membrane occurs. With increased permeability, the aminoglycosides demonstrate enhanced entry into the cells, allowing further saturation of aminoglycoside binding sites on the ribosome, thus preventing the formation of new, functional ribosomes, which ultimately results in cell death. The aminoglycosides are bactericidal, and show concentration-dependent killing of bacteria (Table 289-1).

Resistance to aminoglycosides occurs primarily with the acquisition of a variety of aminoglycoside-modifying enzymes, many of which are carried on plasmids and transposons for efficient spread between bacteria. The most common are acetyltransferases, adenyltransferases, and phosphotransferases.[109] Many different efflux pump systems also play a major role in aminoglycoside resistance, particularly in gram-negative bacilli.[109] Ribosomal RNA methylase genes from *Actinomyces* that confer resistance to aminoglycosides recently have been identified in clinical isolates of enteric gram-negative bacilli and *Pseudomonas aeruginosa*.[111] Although this mechanism of resistance currently is uncommon, these genes now have the potential to spread quickly within clinical settings.

The clinical use of aminoglycosides occurs primarily for the treatment of gram-negative facultative bacillary infections – from the premature neonate through the adolescent.[112-114] Aminoglycosides are strongly polar, with high solubility in water but poor solubility in lipids resulting in poor penetration into the CNS, vitreous, bronchial secretions, and saliva. Aminoglycosides are concentrated in the proximal renal tubules and excreted in urine and achieve urinary tract concentrations up to 100 times the serum concentration. Due to the toxicity of the aminoglycosides at serum concentrations that are only 5- to 10-fold above the bacterial MICs, they are not usually used as the sole agents for treatment of serious infections. The aminoglycosides frequently are paired with a β-lactam antibiotic to create synergistic antibacterial activity and potentially to retard the emergence of antibiotic resistance, although the clinical impact of combination therapy has not been well demonstrated beyond the immunocompromised host.[115] Empiric and definitive therapy of early- and late-onset neonatal septicemia with gentamicin-containing combinations for enteric gram-negative infections is still considered appropriate three decades following the first recommendations in this age group, although well-controlled, prospective, comparative studies generally have not been performed.[112,113,116] Therapy of nosocomial infections with aminoglycoside-containing regimens is still acceptable in institutions in which nosocomial gram-negative pathogens remain susceptible.[117]

In gram-positive infections, the aminoglycosides add enhanced bacterial killing to cell wall-active agents, particularly in the treatment of serious infections.[118] Enterococcal infections are treated with ampicillin or vancomycin in combination with gentamicin in order to achieve bactericidal activity. The combination of penicillin plus gentamicin, or nafcillin plus gentamicin, are considered by some experts to be the most effective therapy for infective endocarditis caused by susceptible strains of viridans streptococci and *S. aureus*, respectively, especially for initial therapy.[119] However, controversy exists over the role of aminoglycosides in combination therapy, as clinical benefits have not been documented to be substantial, while renal toxicity is not uncommon.[120]

Empiric therapy of nosocomial infections and infections in immunocompromised hosts has included combination regimens containing aminoglycosides to enhance the spectrum of β-lactam agents, to provide potential synergy, and to minimize the emergence of resistant pathogens.[21] Aminoglycosides are also used in combination with other agents in the treatment of intra-abdominal infections. However, the cationic charges on the aminoglycoside molecule change as the pH changes in infected tissues, with the acidic environment of an abscess decreasing the ability of these antibiotics to enter bacterial cells (as documented by MICs that can be higher than those safely achievable in serum).[121] In addition, the active transport of aminoglycosides through the inner cell membrane into the cytoplasm of the bacteria requires an oxygen-dependent transport system not present in anaerobes, explaining the lack of activity of this class of agent in the treatment of anaerobic infections.

Given the high level of activity against certain gram-negative pathogens and lack of current prospective treatment trials using newer agents, the aminoglycosides still represent preferred therapy for tularemia and plague.

Streptomycin remains highly active against most strains of *Mycobacterium tuberculosis* requiring parenteral therapy, which leads to use in treatment of multidrug-resistant tuberculosis. Streptomycin may be particularly useful in the treatment of serious, life-threatening tuberculosis, including tuberculous meningitis. Although originally approved for use in 1952 and previously important for the treatment of infections caused by *Brucella* and *Francisella* spp., streptomycin has been replaced by gentamicin because of concerns for streptomycin-induced vestibular, auditory, and renal toxicity.

Paromomycin is an oral, nonabsorbable aminoglycoside. This agent is effective in the treatment of intestinal protozoal infections, including amebiasis and cryptosporidiosis.

Inhaled aminoglycosides, most commonly tobramycin, are used clinically to treat cystic fibrosis. Achieving high enough antibiotic concentrations in respiratory tract secretions and at the bronchial mucosa to be effective against *P. aeruginosa* is not usually possible with parenterally administered aminoglycosides, but high concentrations can be achieved with inhaled tobramycin, without concern for nephro- or ototoxicity.[122] The use of aerosolized aminoglycosides in patients with pneumonia caused by other multidrug-resistant gram-negative pathogens has not been prospectively investigated in controlled studies, but case series in adults suggest their potential role.[123]

Nephrotoxicity of aminoglycosides is dose-dependent and primarily is tubular. Monitoring renal function or aminoglycoside serum concentrations during therapy permits early detection of decreased renal function attributable to the aminoglycoside. Aminoglycoside ototoxicity can be either cochlear (with hearing loss) or vestibular (with vertigo), and correlates with increasing serum trough concentration as a function of overall drug exposure, rather than the peak serum concentration.[124]

Providing children with a single daily dose of aminoglycosides to decrease nephrotoxicity while maintaining or increasing efficacy has not been widely accepted due to the lack of well-controlled studies in children. However, limited data that exist in children, taken together with convincing data in adults, suggest that once-daily dosing could become routine for children, except possibly for certain severe infections, such as meningitis or persistent BSI.[125,126]

While streptomycin was the first aminoglycoside available for use, the toxicity and rapid development of resistance in bacteria limited its long-term viability. Kanamycin was approved for use in 1957 but was replaced by the less nephrotoxic gentamicin in 1963 as a more broadly active antibiotic against resistant gram-negative pathogens. Tobramycin was approved in 1968 and provided a small but predictable increase in in vitro activity against *P. aeruginosa* with a concomitant small but clinically insignificant decrease in activity against enteric gram-negative bacilli, allowing its use as the anti-pseudomonal aminoglycoside of choice. Amikacin, a semisynthetic derivative of kanamycin, was approved in 1972, and offered enhanced activity against many gentamicin- and tobramycin-resistant pathogens, in addition to providing serum antibiotic concentrations approximately 3- to 4-fold greater than those achievable with gentamicin or tobramycin. Amikacin also is useful in the treatment of infections caused by some strains of nontuberculous mycobacteria.

Streptogramins A and B

The streptogramins are two of a series of naturally occurring antibiotics isolated from *Streptomyces pristinaespiralis*. Two antibiotics have been modified from the naturally occurring pristinomycins I and IIA to create the semisynthetic antibiotics quinupristin (streptogramin B) and dalfopristin (streptogramin A), respectively. These two antibiotics are present in the FDA-approved combination Synercid in a 70:30 ratio.[127] Quinupristin and dalfopristin have completely different chemical structures, each with a distinct but overlapping binding region within the P site of the peptidyl transferase center in the ribosome. Binding of dalfopristin to this region produces a conformational change that significantly increases the affinity of binding of quinupristin, in part explaining the synergy observed when the combination is used. Dalfopristin inhibits protein synthesis by interfering with substrate attachment to both A and P sites of the 50S subunit, while quinupristin blocks peptide bond synthesis during elongation by causing incorrect positioning of the peptidyl tRNA at the P site.[128] Once elongation has been initiated, quinupristin triggers the premature release of the elongating peptide chain. Quinupristin binds to the peptidyl transferase site at a similar location as the macrolides and lincosamides; methylation of the A2058 adenine at this important binding site prevents binding of quinupristin as well as the macrolides and clindamycin, and creates the macrolide-lincosamide-streptogramin (MLS) resistance phenotype.

Unfortunately, many mechanisms of bacterial resistance limit the clinical utility of quinupristin/dalfopristin, with resistance developing in some patients soon after starting therapy. Alterations of target binding sites, efflux removal of antibiotics from cytoplasm, and enzymatic alteration of the antibiotic structure all have been reported.[65,129] Although each of the streptogramins independently produces inhibitory effects on protein synthesis, the combination is bactericidal for a number of gram-positive pathogens, including *S. aureus*.

The agents have been available in Europe for several years as topical therapy, but with the development and spread of enterococci that are resistant to vancomycin, β-lactams, and aminoglycosides, an urgent need for quinupristin/dalfopristin was well documented. Clinical use is largely limited to serious infections caused by vancomycin-resistant strains of *Enterococcus faecium* (VRE). The combination is not active against the more common enterococcal pathogen, *Enterococcus faecalis*. Although quinupristin/dalfopristin also is FDA-approved for treatment of skin and skin structure infections caused by *S. aureus*, there are better evaluated and tolerated agents for therapy in children.

Quinupristin/dalfopristin significantly inhibits cytochrome P450 CYP3A function and may impact serum concentrations of concomitant drugs which are eliminated by this pathway. Phlebitis was a major side effect in quinupristin/dalfopristin-treated patients, occurring in almost half of adults receiving therapy. This combination agent has not been systematically studied for children under 16 years of age.

Oxazolidinones

Linezolid is the first antibiotic in the oxazolidinone class to be approved and used in children. This class of antibiotics is unique in that members are not natural products, but were discovered as one of a number of compounds created as potential monoamine oxidase-inhibiting agents.[130] However, some of these compounds also demonstrated antibacterial activity, although initially, many were associated with significant toxicity. Subsequent chemical modifications led to the development of linezolid, which demonstrated a reasonable balance between antimicrobial activity, clinical efficacy, and acceptable clinical toxicity. The oxazolidinones have a unique mechanism of action on the ribosome, distinct from all other classes of antimicrobial agents. The antibiotic binds to an area close to the ribosomal peptidyl transferase center and inhibits the initiation of protein synthesis by preventing the formation of the initiation complex of fMet-tRNA/elongation factors/mRNA/GTP at the peptidyl transferase center. The movement of the complex from the ribosome's "A site" of tRNA attachment to the peptidyl "P site" is blocked and coupling of amino acids and lengthening of the peptide chain cannot occur.[131]

Linezolid demonstrates bactericidal activity against *S. pneumoniae*, but bacteriostatic activity against *S. aureus* and *Enterococcus* species. However, limited studies comparing vancomycin, a bactericidal agent (with limitations in activity in infected lung), with linezolid in the treatment of nosocomial pneumonia caused by MRSA suggest equivalent clinical outcomes.[132,133] Activity of linezolid is primarily limited to gram-positive bacteria, due to the presence of an efflux pump (AcrAB) present in many gram-negative organisms. Linezolid is not active against *Mycoplasma* or *Ureaplasma*.[134]

Resistance to linezolid has been described and consists of structural changes at the linezolid binding site that prevent attachment.[65,135] These relatively infrequent changes, which tend to occur more frequently with more prolonged therapy, are primarily single-base changes in the rRNA occurring around the peptidyl transferase site. Transferable resistance to the oxazolidinones through conjugative transposons has been documented.[65]

Linezolid has been studied clinically for nosocomial and community-acquired pneumonia, and for complicated and uncomplicated skin and skin structure infections.[136,137] The clinical and microbiologic response rates for each of these tissue-specific infections in children were equivalent to comparator agents, usually vancomycin. The in vitro activity and clinical efficacy of linezolid in the treatment of infections caused by penicillin- and macrolide-resistant pneumococci, VRE, MRSA, and VRSA support a role for linezolid when other, better-studied agents are not available or are not tolerated. The most common current clinical use of linezolid in children is for the treatment of MRSA-associated skin or respiratory tract infections.[138] Little data other than case reports are available for the use of linezolid in treatment of bone and joint infections[139] and CNS infections.[140]

Data on pharmacokinetics for both parenterally and orally administered linezolid are available in children, including premature neonates.[141] Linezolid is virtually 100% absorbed by the oral route, allowing equivalent mg/kg dosing for both intravenous and oral formulations. Linezolid is not metabolized by the cytochrome P450 system, and does not induce this enzyme or compete with other drugs in P450-mediated metabolism. Some concerns have been raised regarding hematologic toxicity, including neutropenia and thrombocytopenia, which was found to be dependent on dose and duration of therapy.[130] However, prospective, comparative data in the pediatric FDA registration studies failed to demonstrate a significant difference in toxicity compared with other agents. Also of concern in the early pediatric clinical trials of linezolid was the possibility of hypertension due to effects of the antibiotic's mild monoamine oxidase (MAO) inhibitor activity. However, no MAO inhibitor side effects were noted in any phase I to III pediatric trial, permitting children to remain on usual diets while receiving treatment.[142]

NUCLEIC ACID-ACTIVE ANTIBIOTICS

RNA Polymerase

Rifamycins

The rifamycins, rifampin (also called rifampicin), rifabutin, rifapentine, and the oral nonabsorbed rifaximin, are all semisynthetic derivatives of natural products of *Streptomyces* spp. The intracellular target for the rifamycins is DNA-dependent RNA polymerase and has been well defined on a molecular level.[143] During the creation of an RNA strand from the bacterial DNA strand, the polymerase requires functional channels within the enzyme for both the DNA template strand and complementary strand, as well as for the elongating RNA strand. As the RNA bases dock sequentially at the active site within the polymerase, the newly created RNA strand moves forward, one base at a time. The rifamycins bind in the channel occupied by the newly created RNA strand, approximately 2 to 3 bases downstream from the active site, blocking the RNA strand from moving out of the polymerase and terminating the further elongation of that RNA segment as it also uncouples the RNA strand from the active site.[143,144] Although the actual active site of the polymerase is highly conserved between bacterial species, there is some diversity between bacteria around the active site with respect to the RNA polymerase structure. This diversity alters the binding affinity for rifampin across bacterial and mycobacterial species and provides one basis for the variable susceptibility to this class of agents. Rifampin demonstrates bactericidal activity against susceptible organisms.

Given the large size of the rifamycin molecule, multiple binding sites within the polymerase, and the restricted target binding pocket in the polymerase, it is not surprising that many different single amino acid substitutions from mutational events within the polymerase will lead to decreased rifamycin binding and stable resistance with little impact on the viability of the organism. In *S. aureus*, at least 18 genotypes resistant to rifampin have been characterized, some of which contain multiple base substitutions.[145] Each of these mutations is likely to affect either the binding affinity or the access of rifampin to the binding pocket to a different degree. Most mutations causing rifampin resistance also produce resistance to rifabutin and rifapentine.[146]

The rifamycins have a remarkably broad spectrum of activity that includes *Staphylococcus* spp., *S. pyogenes*, *Neisseria* spp., *H. influenzae*, *Campylobacter jejuni*, *H. pylori*, *C. trachomatis*, both tuberculous and nontuberculous *Mycobacterium* spp., *Aspergillus* spp., *Naegleria fowleri*, and *Toxoplasma gondii* (see Table 292-2). Rifabutin has increased in vitro activity against *M. tuberculosis* compared with rifampin, but has not been documented to result in improved microbiologic outcomes in treated patients.[147] Rifabutin also has increased activity against MAC compared with rifampin, most likely due to binding to additional sites within the polymerase.[143,148,149] Rifapentine has both increased in vitro activity against *M. tuberculosis* in addition to an extended serum elimination half-life (16 hours) compared with rifampin (2 to 3 hours).

Rifamycins achieve high intracellular concentrations, between 5- and 20-fold greater than extracellular concentrations.[148] This likely explains the effectiveness of this class in the therapy for mycobacterial infections, in which pathogens are sequestered intracellularly.

Of the rifamycins, rifampin is the agent most commonly used in pediatrics. Rifabutin and rifapentine were developed for treatment of mycobacterial infections, and neither is currently FDA-approved for use in children. Rifampin is used in children as part of combination therapy for tuberculosis. Rifampin also can be used in combination therapy for treatment of nontuberculous mycobacterial infections such as adenitis, cellulitis, or pneumonia. For treatment of bacterial infections, rapid emergence of resistance in virtually every pathogen dictates a need for combination antibiotic therapy. Combination therapy may allow for eradication of rifampin-resistant strains before they become clinically important. Rifampin has been used in combination therapy of *Bartonella henselae* infections (cat-scratch disease), multidrug-resistant *S. aureus* infections (particularly MRSA), and multidrug-resistant pneumococcal infections, including meningitis.[150] Although not well studied in prospective comparative clinical trials, the excellent tissue penetration of rifampin may provide improved clinical outcomes compared with β-lactam antibiotic therapy alone in deep bone and joint infections and in foreign-body or device infections associated with intravascular catheters or implanted devices. As single-drug therapy, rifampin is only used for the eradication of colonization of *N. meningitidis* and in the prophylaxis when indicated for *N. meningitidis* and *H. influenzae* type b.

Rifabutin has documented efficacy in both prophylaxis and therapy of MAC (in combination with other agents) in HIV-infected adults, but clarithromycin and azithromycin are recommended as preferred therapy for HIV-infected children.[80] Only limited data are available in children with MAC infections.[73,151,152] The extended half-life of rifapentine provides a rationale for once-weekly therapy, although the failure rate in those with more serious tuberculosis, and the bacteriologic relapse rate was slightly higher in those treated with rifapentine compared with rifampin.[147,153] Rifapentine has not been evaluated in children.

Rifaximin is an oral agent that is not absorbed from the gastrointestinal tract and produces high intraluminal antibiotic concentrations with little systemic toxicity. Microbiologic activity has been demonstrated in vitro at achievable intraluminal antibiotic concentrations against *E. coli*, *Salmonella*, *Shigella*, *Vibrio*, *Yersinia*, and *Campylobacter* species. Although the susceptibility of these enteric pathogens is about 32 to 64 µg/mL, a concentration not achievable in tissues, the concentrations achieved in the gastrointestinal tract are as high as 8000 µg/mL, providing an antibiotic

exposure that is well above that required for an antibacterial effect.[154] Although this antibiotic is currently only approved for traveler's diarrhea in adults,[155] an oral nonabsorbable, broad-spectrum agent for other gastrointestinal pathogens could have considerable value for children.

The most common clinical side effect of treatment with rifampin is nausea, which appears to decrease as the treatment course progresses. The most common adverse effect of treatment is hepatotoxicity, as assessed by elevation of hepatic transaminase levels; however, most children receiving rifampin for tuberculosis therapy also receive other hepatotoxic agents, preventing an accurate assessment of the role of rifampin as a single agent causing liver injury.[156] Children receiving multiple hepatotoxic agents should be assessed at regular intervals for evidence of hepatic injury.

The drug–drug interaction profile of the rifamycins frequently complicates clinical management. The P450 CYP3A system is activated by the rifamycins. If the child is receiving other drug(s) metabolized by this system, decreased, potentially ineffective serum concentrations of that drug may be present. In addition, if the concurrent drug represents a competitive substrate for P450 metabolism, increased and potentially toxic serum concentrations of that drug may result from decreased metabolism.[148] The potency of CYP3A induction is greatest with rifampin and least with rifabutin. Rifabutin is also a CYP3A substrate itself, resulting in higher rifabutin serum concentrations when given concomitantly with CYP3A inhibitors.

DNA-Dependent DNA Polymerase

Quinolones and Fluoroquinolones

The quinolones are a diverse group of antibiotics that target DNA synthesis and are active against a wide range of bacteria, *Mycoplasma*, *Chlamydia*, and *Chlamydophila* spp., and, for some agents, mycobacteria.[157,158] The first of the quinolone antibiotics was discovered during the commercial preparation of the antimalarial agent chloroquine, and was subsequently modified for antibacterial use in humans.[157] The first approved quinolone agent, nalidixic acid, has a limited gram-negative spectrum of activity and a poor pharmacokinetic profile for treatment of invasive infections. With chemical modifications to the basic quinolone (and the closely related naphthyridone) ring structure, the spectrum of activity and pharmacokinetics have been greatly enhanced, allowing for once-daily dosing for infections in many different tissue sites. The 6-fluoroquinolones (beginning with norfloxacin and ciprofloxacin) demonstrated a significant improvement in antibacterial activity, and virtually all subsequently approved compounds are fluoroquinolones.

The quinolones all interfere with DNA synthesis by interfering with two closely related type II topoisomerase enzymes involved in DNA synthesis: DNA gyrase and topoisomerase IV.[158,159] Each of these enzymes comprised 4 subunits: DNA gyrase contains 2 subunits of GyrA and 2 of GyrB, whereas topoisomerase IV consists of 2 subunits of ParC and 2 of ParE (in *Staphylococcus aureus*, these topoisomerase IV subunits are termed GrlA and GrlB). The DNA gyrase is responsible for uncoiling DNA ahead of the replication fork to allow for DNA strand replication by DNA polymerase, or for the creation of RNA strands by RNA polymerase. In the process of uncoiling and coiling, strands of DNA are cut and then religated by these enzymes in order to maintain a stable double-helix structure. The topoisomerase IV appears to be primarily responsible for stabilizing the newly created strands of DNA as they separate from template strands following replication. The quinolones bind to these enzymes at specific nucleic acid strand attachment sites, producing conformational changes in the DNA gyrase/DNA or topoisomerase IV/DNA complexes and stabilizing them, thus "freezing" the complex. This leads to an inability to translocate the entire DNA replication complex along the DNA strand, halting the process of nucleic acid replication. Binding of the fluoroquinolones leads to single- and double-strand DNA breaks without religation, and the subsequent release of DNA fragments into the cell, which leads to cell death in ways that are not well understood. The

DNA gyrase/DNA replication complex may also be involved in altering the formation and stability of DNA loops involved in the transcription process, representing another mechanism by which fluoroquinolones impact cell function.

Although quinolones can bind to some extent to both of these enzymes, structural characteristics of each quinolone create unique binding characteristics to each of these two enzymes for every drug in this class. The differences in binding to DNA gyrase and topoisomerase IV lead to differences in the susceptibility of organisms to the various quinolones as well as differences in the development of resistance. In general, the quinolones preferentially bind to DNA gyrase in gram-negative bacteria, and to topoisomerase IV in gram-positive bacteria, although some of the newer quinolones bind to both enzymes equally well. Binding to DNA gyrase, occurring before the replication fork of DNA synthesis, produces a more rapid effect on the formation of DNA, whereas binding to the topoisomerase IV after strand duplication has occurred creates a less immediate effect on cell death. However, as both enzymes function to nick and religate strands of DNA during the coiling/uncoiling process, the quinolone effects after binding to either, or both enzymes, can lead to cell death. These agents display bactericidal activity against bacterial pathogens, with dose-dependent pharmacodynamic activity best described by the ratio of AUC:MIC (the ratio of the area under the serum concentration versus time curve to the MIC of the antibiotic for that organism).[160]

As with many antibiotics, resistance can develop in many different ways, and resistance from multiple different mechanisms can be additive. The most common resistance occurs from alterations in the amino acids present at certain critical and virtually identical sites on the two enzymes, DNA gyrase, and topoisomerase IV, that prevent avid binding of the quinolone. Single gene mutations leading to these amino acid changes are primarily found in the quinolone resistance-determining regions of *gyrA* and *parC*.[161] Additional but less common mutations have been detected in *gyrB* and *parE*. For *E. coli,* accumulating additional amino acid changes leads to increasing resistance. The first-step mutation in *E. coli* most often occurs in the *gyrA* subunit of DNA gyrase, leading to a mild-to-moderate increase in the MIC, depending on the quinolone being assessed. A second-step mutation, usually in *parC*, generally leads to resistance that cannot be overcome at achievable tissue concentrations. For *S. pneumoniae* and *S. aureus,* the first-step mutation most often occurs in the *parC* (or *GrlA*) subunit of topoisomerase IV.[161,162] Depending on both drug and bacteria, mutations in one of the subunit sites can lead to substantial increases in resistance for a particular drug, but for drugs that bind to both gyrase and topoisomerase IV sites, a mutation at one site does not effectively raise the MIC to a level that usually leads to treatment failure. When two or more mutations occur that affect binding to both enzymes, clinical failures become more common.

Efflux pumps also are effective mechanisms to prevent quinolone binding intracellularly to the gyrase and topoisomerase targets. Efflux pumps affect intracellular concentrations of different quinolones to differing degrees.[162] In addition, newly described mutations in aminoglycoside acetyltransferases confer the ability to acetylate ciprofloxacin, decreasing its activity against *E. coli* 2- to 4-fold, with the modified enzyme still retaining activity against the aminoglycosides. This mechanism of resistance is transferable to other bacteria, in contrast to the *gyrA* or *parC* mutations which only spread horizontally from patient to patient. It is not known how problematic these strains will become.[163]

Safety issues for children have been a concern for this entire class of agents. Although nalidixic acid was approved for children by the FDA in 1963, more extensive animal toxicology studies were available for the agents that followed. Preclinical juvenile animal toxicity data for ciprofloxacin in the late 1970s suggested the potential for damage to joints in young children. Therefore, no routine pediatric drug development was undertaken for this compound or any other fluoroquinolone until the need for potential use of these agents for children was demonstrated to the FDA in 1997.[164] No quinolone-associated arthropathy has yet been documented clearly in children for agents available in the U.S. although a suggestion of transient arthralgia exists from an FDA

safety database of ciprofloxacin.[165] Long-term toxicity studies currently are in progress, but are not of sufficient size to be able to detect or define rates of rare adverse effects on joints or tendons. It is encouraging, nonetheless, that lack of reported toxicity from current published data and from data presented to the FDA suggests that joint toxicity is not a common problem in children, if it exists at all.[166]

Nalidixic Acid, Norfloxacin

Nalidixic acid was approved in 1963 for use in children down to 3 months of age for the treatment of UTI. Norfloxacin, used for treatment of UTIs in children in other areas of the world, is not FDA-approved for children in the U.S. With the FDA approval of ciprofloxacin for children with UTIs in 2004, ciprofloxacin is the preferred quinolone agent for these infections when a fluoroquinolone is needed for gram-negative pathogens, based on the quality of prospectively collected data regarding both safety and efficacy in children.

Ciprofloxacin

Ciprofloxacin was one of the first of the 6-fluoroquinolones to be FDA-approved for adults, but large clinical trial investigations in children did not begin until the late 1990s, with the exception of studies in children with cystic fibrosis. Ciprofloxacin was recently studied for complicated UTI, and was the first 6-fluoroquinolone to be approved for use in pediatrics. Although all of the fluoroquinolones have a bitter taste, a tolerable suspension formulation of ciprofloxacin is available for children. Current usage of the fluoroquinolones is limited, based on concerns of cartilage toxicity. The antimicrobial activity of ciprofloxacin is provided in Table 292-2, and includes most of the enteric gram-negative bacilli as well as *P. aeruginosa.* Activity against the gram-positive pathogens and anaerobic pathogens generally is only fair.

Current clinical use of ciprofloxacin centers on gram-negative infections for which no other oral antibiotic agent is available.[165,167] In this setting, ciprofloxacin and other fluoroquinolones represent effective therapy in which the risk/benefit assessment favors treatment with an oral quinolone agent rather than parenteral therapy with a nonquinolone agent. These infections may be located in virtually any tissue site except the CNS. Examples of infections, many of which are hospital-associated, include complicated UTI, bone or joint infection (including those caused by *P. aeruginosa*), soft-tissue infection, and lower respiratory tract infection. Many of these children have comorbid conditions that have created a need for previous courses of antibiotics and therefore the selection of multidrug-resistant pathogens. Because these infections are uncommon, no prospective, randomized, controlled clinical trials of use of ciprofloxacin in children are available. In addition, some reluctance may exist on the part of the pharmaceutical industry to perform these studies due to potential toxicity. In addition to complicated UTI, FDA approval has also been given for the treatment of inhalational anthrax in children.

Fluoroquinolones achieve effective concentrations in the gastrointestinal tract and have an advantage over β-lactam antibiotics in that they also achieve high intracellular antibiotic concentrations, particularly effective in the treatment of *Salmonella* infections. Ciprofloxacin has been studied in children for shigellosis and salmonellosis, and provides equivalent or superior rates of eradication compared with standard agents.[168,169]

With the high bioavailability of orally administered fluoroquinolones and activity against most gram-negative pathogens for immunocompromised children, selective use of these agents (with or without additional oral therapy for gram-positive pathogens) in low-risk children with fever and neutropenia is a promising area of clinical investigation.[170]

Levofloxacin

Levofloxacin was the first available agent in a series of newer fluoroquinolone agents with enhanced activity against gram-positive pathogens, including *S. pneumoniae* and *S. aureus*. Levofloxacin has been clinically effective in treatment of upper and lower respiratory tract infections in adults,[171] with successfully completed clinical trials in children in both acute otitis media and community-acquired pneumonia. No safety issues of significant concern were raised in adult or pediatric clinical programs. No joint-related toxicity was noted in children, with a sufficiently large number of subjects prospectively studied to detect a 1% adverse event rate. The most acknowledged clinical need for levofloxacin in children is for the treatment of unresponsive or recurrent otitis media due to pneumococci resistant to β-lactam and macrolide agents.[172] Use for therapy of serious infections is appropriate in situations for which no other class of active parenteral agent exists, or use as oral therapy of infections in situations for which only nonquinolone parenteral therapies exist.[165] Levofloxacin also is approved for treatment of inhalational anthrax in children.

Moxifloxacin, Gemifloxacin

New generations of fluoroquinolones demonstrate increased activity against *S. pneumoniae* compared with earlier fluoroquinolones.[173] None of these newer agents have been studied adequately or approved for use in children.

Nitroimidazoles

Metronidazole

Metronidazole is a synthetic nitroimidazole antibiotic with a poorly defined mechanism of action despite decades of extensive use. Originally introduced for the treatment of *Trichomonas* infections (hence the original trade name, Flagyl), use in pediatrics has been most extensive for treatment of anaerobic infections, despite the fact that the antibiotic has never been approved by the FDA for use in children for these indications. Metronidazole is taken into cells by passive diffusion and the nitro side chain on the imidazole ring is reduced intracellularly by the pyruvate-ferredoxin reductase complex into a toxic nitro radical that reacts with DNA, leading to DNA strand breaks, helix destabilization, and ultimately cell death in both dividing and nondividing cells.[150,151] Metronidazole demonstrates concentration-dependent bactericidal activity. One of the major metabolites, a hydroxy derivative, retains significant antibiotic activity. Metronidazole is active against anaerobic bacteria and certain protozoa, including *Trichomonas*, *Entamoeba*, and *Giardia* (see Table 292-2).

In addition to direct bactericidal activity, metronidazole also appears to have direct effects on decreasing neutrophil generation of hydrogen peroxide and hydroxyl radicals, which may lead to decreased inflammation at the site of infection. Some evidence suggests that metronidazole may also inhibit lymphocyte transformation and granuloma formation.[152] The clinical relevance of these observations is not known.

Although resistance to metronidazole is uncommon, a number of bacteria, including some strains of *B. fragilis*, contain *nim* genes which code for an inactivating enzyme that may exist on both plasmids and within chromosomes. This enzyme effectively reduces the nitro group on metronidazole into a stable and inactive amine.[174-176]

Metronidazole is available in intravenous, oral tablet and capsule formulations, and topical formulations. Although metronidazole has a very bitter taste and is not well tolerated when pulverized and placed in suspension, the absorption from the gastrointestinal tract is excellent, with >90% bioavailability. Although rectal administration yields approximately 70% to 80% bioavailability, this route of administration has never gained widespread acceptance for children. Metronidazole provides excellent therapeutic concentrations in a wide range of tissue sites, including CSF, in which concentrations are very close to those achieved in serum.[177-179] Although the serum elimination half-life is approximately 8 hours, early studies performed in adults for FDA approval used 6-hour dosing regimens, which remains the current FDA dosing recommendation in the package label. The observed

half-life with oral administration appears to be longer than that found for IV administration, for unknown reasons. For most clinical situations, based on the pharmacodynamics of antibiotic exposure, dosing every 8 hours should be adequate. One of the metabolites of metronidazole that displays significant antibacterial activity has a more extended half-life, averaging 11 to 13 hours, providing another rationale for less frequent dosing.

Clinical use in pediatrics primarily is for the treatment of anaerobic infections.[174,180] Given the excellent tissue penetration characteristics of metronidazole, activity against all susceptible anaerobes is achievable in most tissue sites. However, data from randomized, prospective clinical trials may not be available for many sites of infection. As most infections involving anaerobes also involve facultative or aerobic organisms, additional antibiotics are necessary.

Metronidazole is bactericidal for *Bacteroides* spp. and has been used extensively in the treatment of intra-abdominal infections, including complicated appendicitis, penetrating injury to the bowel, and colitis.[99] These infections often involve multiple susceptible anaerobic species, including *B. fragilis*. Other mixed aerobic/anaerobic infections include deep head and neck space infections (e.g., parapharyngeal abscesses, Ludwig angina) and necrotizing fasciitis/cellulitis (e.g., necrotizing synergistic fasciitis, Fournier gangrene, and omphalitis). *Clostridia* spp. also are susceptible to metronidazole, and can be effectively treated when causing deep-tissue infections. Some penicillin-susceptible anaerobic gram-positive cocci, however, are not susceptible to metronidazole.

Metronidazole, in combination with other antibiotics and proton pump inhibitors, is part of a treatment regimen for *H. pylori*-mediated ulcer disease.[181] In addition, some benefit from metronidazole in the treatment of Crohn disease may occur;[182] antibiotic and anti-inflammatory properties of the agent both may play a role.

Given the excellent penetration into CSF and bactericidal capacity, metronidazole treatment of anaerobic organisms causing meningitis or ventriculitis (traumatic, postsurgical, or nosocomial), or treatment of anaerobic brain abscesses is effective.[178] Prospective, comparative data to document efficacy for these indications are not available.

Metronidazole also can be used for female genital tract infections, including bacterial vaginosis, and as part of antimicrobial therapy of pelvic inflammatory disease.

One of the most common pediatric uses for metronidazole is in the treatment of *Clostridium difficile* enterocolitis.[43] Following the documented increases in vancomycin resistance of gastrointestinal tract flora with the use of oral vancomycin in adults for *C. difficile* colitis, metronidazole became the drug of choice in therapy for children as well as adults. Although clinical response rates comparing oral metronidazole therapy with oral vancomycin therapy for *C. difficile* infection have been equivalent in the past, currently there is concern regarding the efficacy of metronidazole in the treatment of *C. difficile* infection.[183]

Entamoeba histolytica trophozoites (but not cysts) are susceptible to metronidazole, allowing therapy for both intestinal and extraintestinal amebiasis, including amebic liver abscess.[184] Metronidazole is one of the drugs of choice for treatment of *Giardia* intestinal infections and is an alternative treatment for *Dientamoeba* infections.[184] For sexually active adolescent females and males, metronidazole still remains effective therapy for *Trichomonas* infections.[185]

Sulfonamides (Single Agents or in Combination with Trimethoprim or Pyrimethamine)

Sulfisoxazole, Sulfamethoxazole, Sulfadiazine

The sulfonamide class was one of the first available antibiotics for human use, with striking clinical responses documented in 1937 in the treatment of erysipelas by sulfanilamide and its prodrug.[186,187] Unfortunately, due to widespread resistance in common bacterial pathogens after decades of extensive use, sulfonamides now are focused in a few areas of remaining effectiveness. However, for pathogens that remain susceptible to sulfonamides, either used alone or since 1968 when used in combination with trimethoprim, these agents have a long history of efficacy with reasonable safety. Sulfonamides now are used almost exclusively in combination with trimethoprim for the treatment or prophylaxis of bacterial infections.[188] Sulfadiazine currently is used in combination with pyrimethamine for the treatment of toxoplasmosis.

The sulfonamides are bacteriostatic by means of competitive inhibition of *para*-aminobenzoic acid, utilized by dihydropteroate synthase in the synthesis of dihydrofolic acid, a precursor of purine bases in the formation of nucleic acid. Bacteria that are required to synthesize folic acid are susceptible to this class of compounds.

Sulfa agents are well absorbed from the gastrointestinal tract and are, in general, metabolized by the liver and excreted by the kidney. Both sulfisoxazole and sulfamethoxazole are highly protein-bound (70% to 80%). Due to sulfonamide binding to albumin, bilirubin may be displaced from its albumin binding sites, causing kernicterus in ill, acidotic neonates with hyperbilirubinemia as a result of subsequent bilirubin binding to CNS tissue. However, no cases of kernicterus have been documented in full-term, well-appearing infants. Despite FDA labeling cautions against the use of this class of agents in infants under 2 months of age, they are safe in nonacidotic term infants as early as the second week of life, as physiologic neonatal jaundice is resolving.

Sulfonamides are responsible for one of the most serious drug-related adverse events, an intense immune-mediated separation of skin at the dermal-epidermal junction. This immune reaction also can result in separation of the respiratory and gastrointestinal tract mucosa from supporting connective tissue. Variously called Stevens–Johnson syndrome, toxic epidermal necrolysis, or erythema multiforme major, the spectrum of reactions varies from a cutaneous erythematous, blistering rash to severe, extensive, life-threatening sloughing of skin and mucosa of the respiratory and gastrointestinal tract.[189,190] At the first sign of a skin reaction in a child receiving sulfa therapy, the child should be evaluated, the sulfonamide discontinued, and careful observation begun.

Trimethoprim plus Sulfamethoxazole (TMP-SMX)

Trimethoprim, available as a single agent but used far more commonly in children in combination with sulfamethoxazole, acts at the metabolic step following that inhibited by sulfonamides in the synthesis of purine bases.[188] TMP-SMX prevents the formation of tetrahydrofolic acid from dihydrofolic acid by binding to and reversibly inhibiting dihydrofolate reductase. The combination of sulfamethoxazole and trimethoprim blocks two consecutive steps in the synthesis of thymidine, providing both synergistic activity against most pathogens, and decreasing the risk of development of resistance to either the sulfa agent or the trimethoprim. Trimethoprim displays bactericidal activity against bacteria, as does the combination.

Current clinical uses of TMP-SMX are limited in the treatment of UTI due to increasing resistance of *E. coli*, but TMP-SMX therapy is effective in regions where susceptibility remains substantial. For children with urinary tract anomalies and significant reflux, TMP-SMX prophylaxis has been documented to decrease the number of recurrent UTIs.[191]

In the treatment of respiratory tract infections, the rate of pneumococcal resistance to sulfa in most areas of the U.S. is greater than 40%, precluding it as first-line therapy of acute otitis media, sinusitis, or community-acquired pneumonia. Despite in vitro susceptibility of *S. pyogenes*, TMP-SMX is not recommended for treatment of streptococcal pharyngitis since host immune response to streptococci is not prevented reliably (which is required in order to prevent the development of acute rheumatic fever).

TMP-SMX has been used increasingly for the treatment of CA-MRSA skin and skin structure infections although prospective, controlled studies were never performed for skin and skin structure infections at the time of original antibiotic approval, or since the emergence of CA-MRSA. In vitro susceptibility of CA-MRSA to TMP-SMX is almost universal; data on comparable efficacy with

clindamycin are limited and conflicting depending on lesions and outcomes studied.[192,193]

TMP-SMX is used for certain hospital-associated infections caused by multidrug-resistant (MDR) enteric gram-negative bacilli such as *Enterobacter* and *Klebsiella* species and *Stenotrophomonas maltophilia* (which often remains susceptible). TMP-SMX is generally bactericidal, although not consistently for high-density inocula of gram-negative bacilli. TMP-SMX is considered safer than most other options (e.g., colistin, fluoroquinolones) in the treatment of MDR gram-negative infections, and may provide an adequate therapy for infections in most tissue sites, including meningitis, in situations for which no other well-evaluated therapy options exist.

Gastrointestinal infections caused by *Salmonella* and *Shigella* spp. and enteropathogenic strains of *E. coli* often were treated successfully with TMP-SMX in the past; however, the value of TMP-SMX has decreased as resistance in these gastrointestinal pathogens has increased.[83,155] The intracellular activity of TMP-SMX has been particularly advantageous in the treatment of susceptible strains of *Salmonella. Yersinia enterocolitica* and *Vibrio cholera* often are susceptible to TMP-SMX. Susceptibility of enteric bacterial pathogens should be assessed before TMP-SMX is selected for therapy in serious infections. For parasitic infections of the gastrointestinal tract caused by *Cyclospora* sp. and *Cystoisospora* (formerly *Isospora*), TMP-SMX remains the treatment of choice.[194]

TMP-SMX remains effective therapy for brucellosis, nocardiosis (with exceptions), and some infections caused by the nontuberculous mycobacteria. Prophylaxis and treatment of *Pneumocystis* pneumonia in immunocompromised children remains highly effective.

Sulfadiazine plus Pyrimethamine

The combination of sulfadiazine and pyrimethamine is active against a number of protozoa, including *Toxoplasma* and *Plasmodium*. Clinical use in children is primarily limited to congenital toxoplasmosis, with treatment starting as soon as physiologic jaundice has resolved, and to older children who have documented toxoplasmosis associated with immune deficiencies (primarily HIV-related).

Miscellaneous

Nitrofurantoin

Nitrofurantoin is a unique antibiotic, characterized by a hydantoin ring with a nitro-substituted furanyl side chain that is metabolized within the bacteria to produce reactive compounds that are bactericidal. The mechanism of antibacterial activity is not well understood, but presumably occurs by altering ribosomal proteins and other important intracellular structures. Both gram-positive bacteria (including staphylococci and streptococci) and gram-negative bacteria (*E. coli*, *Klebsiella*, and *Citrobacter* spp.) are susceptible. Mechanisms of resistance have not been well defined, but no cross-resistance occurs with other antibiotic classes. Recent data from the U.S. on susceptibility of pediatric uropathogens document that, overall, resistance to nitrofurantoin across all pathogens and pediatric age groups is approximately 5% to 10%.[195]

Nitrofurantoin was originally FDA-approved in 1953 for the treatment of uncomplicated UTIs. Nitrofurantoin is well absorbed orally and is rapidly cleared from the serum, producing subtherapeutic concentrations in serum, but bactericidal concentrations in urine. Currently available formulations include a rapidly absorbed monohydrate salt, a monohydrate salt in slow-release matrix, and crystalline nitrofurantoin that is also more slowly absorbed. Dosages should be decreased in children with any degree of renal insufficiency.

In clinical practice, nitrofurantoin has been used primarily for prophylaxis of UTI, although few prospective comparative data are available on which to base recommendations.[196–199] Serious pulmonary toxicities, both acute and chronic, were reported in the decade following availability of nitrofurantoin.[166,167] Acute lung injury, felt to be immune-mediated, and chronic fibrosis have been reported in adults during long-term therapy. The rate and severity of these multiple pulmonary toxicities have not been evaluated prospectively in children. However, no reports of pulmonary toxicity in young children receiving nitrofurantoin prophylaxis for UTI have been published in the past two decades, despite continued use. In addition to pulmonary toxicity, hemolysis secondary to glucose-6-phosphate dehydrogenase deficiency has also been documented.

Methenamine

Methenamine hippurate is used exclusively for the prevention of UTI. Initially available in 1967 and FDA-approved for patients ≥12 years of age, methenamine is a salt that ultimately exerts an antibacterial effect in the urine as it becomes converted into formaldehyde. This effect occurs when the urine pH is below 5.5. Formaldehyde has nonspecific bactericidal activity on both gram-positive and gram-negative bacteria. However, as the generation of formaldehyde is dependent on an acidic urinary pH, methenamine may not be active in situations in which a more alkaline pH is created by diet, or by urea-splitting bacteria in the urine, such as *Proteus* and *Pseudomonas*. A recent review of previously published data on clinical trials of methenamine prophylaxis, some of which were published as early as 1975, suggested efficacy for short-term use (<1 week), in adults with normal urinary tract anatomy.[200] Data collected in children in Finland from 1960 to 1974 suggest a benefit that is equivalent to, or superior to sulfa and nitrofurantoin, although failures were not uncommon.[201] The clinical use of methenamine in children is not well defined currently due to lack of high quality data on the safety and efficacy in children, and particularly for long-term prophylaxis.

APPENDIX 292-1. Dosage of Antibacterial Drugs for Infants, Older Children, and Adolescents

Drug Generic (Trade)	Route	Dosage (per kg/day)[a]	Comments
AMINOGLYCOSIDES[b]			Dosage adjusted according to serum concentration(s).
Amikacin (Amikin)	IV, IM	15–22.5 mg divided into 3 doses	
Gentamicin (Garamycin)	IV, IM	3–7.5 mg divided into 3 doses	8–10 mg for cystic fibrosis
	Intraventricular	1–2 mg per dose (adult 3 mg)	
Kanamycin (Kantrex)	IV, IM	15–30 mg divided into 3 doses (adult maximum 1.5 g/day)	
Neomycin (numerous)	PO	100 mg divided into 4 doses (adult, 4–8 g/day)	Minimally absorbed from GI tract
Streptomycin	IM, IV	20–30 mg divided into 2 doses (adult 1–2 g/day)	
Tobramycin (Nebcin)	IV, IM	3–7.5 mg divided into 3 doses	8–10 mg for cystic fibrosis
β-LACTAM AGENTS[c]			
MONOLACTAMS			
Aztreonam (Azactam)	IV, IM	90–120 mg divided into 4 doses (adult 3–6 g/day, maximum 8 g/day)	
CARBAPENEMS[c]			
Doripenem (Doribax)	IV	Adults 1500 mg per day in 3 doses	
Ertapenem (Invanz)	IV, IM	30 mg divided into 2 doses, maximum 1 g/day (children ≥12 years and adults, 1 g/day once daily)	
Imipenem-cilastatin (Primaxin)	IV, IM	60–100 mg divided into 4 doses (adult 1–2 g/day)	Seizures at high doses; not used for meningitis
Meropenem (Merrem)	IV	60 mg divided into 3 doses (adult 3–6 g/day)	120 mg for meningitis
CEPHALOSPORINS[c]			Methicillin-resistant staphylococci are resistant to all currently available cephalosporins, except ceftaroline
Cefaclor (Ceclor)	PO	20–40 mg divided into 2 or 3 doses (adult 1–1.5 g/day, maximum 4 g/day)	
Cefadroxil (Duricef, Ultracef)	PO	30 mg divided into 2 doses (adult 1–2 g/day, maximum 4 g/day)	
Cefazolin (Kefzol, Ancef)	IV, IM	50–100 mg divided into 3 doses (adult 1.5–6 g/day, maximum 12 g/day)	
Cefdinir (Omnicef)	PO	14 mg once daily, maximum 600 mg/day	
Cefditoren (Spectracef)	PO	400–800 mg (not per kg) divided into 2 doses	
Cefepime (Maxipime)	IV, IM	100–150 mg divided into 2–3 doses (adult 2–6 g/day, maximum 6 g/day)	
Cefixime (Suprax)	PO	8 mg divided into 1 or 2 doses (adult 400 mg/day)	Poor antistaphylococcal activity Single-dose gonorrhea treatment 400 mg ×1 in children ≥45 kg
Cefotaxime (Claforan)	IV, IM	50–180 mg divided into 3 or 4 doses (adult 3–6 g/day, maximum 12 g/day)	200–300 mg divided into 4 doses for meningitis
Cefotetan (Cefotan)	IV, IM	60–100 mg divided into 2 doses (adult 2–4 g/day, maximum 6 g/day)	
Cefoxitin (Mefoxin)	IV, IM	80–160 mg divided into 4 doses (adult 4–6 g/day, maximum 12 g/day)	

Continued

APPENDIX 292-1. Dosage of Antibacterial Drugs for Infants, Older Children, and Adolescents—cont'd

Drug Generic (Trade)	Route	Dosage (per kg/day)[a]	Comments
Cefpodoxime proxetil (Vantin)	PO	10 mg divided into 2 doses (adult 200–400 mg/day, maximum 800 mg/day)	
Cefprozil (Cefzil)	PO	15–30 mg divided into 2 doses (adult 0.5–1 g/day, maximum 1 g/day)	
Ceftazidime (Fortaz, Tazicef, Tazidime)	IV, IM	100–150 mg divided into 3 doses (adult 3–6 g/day, maximum 6 g/day)	200–300 mg for serious *Pseudomonas* infection
Ceftibuten (Cedax)	PO	9 mg once daily (adult 400 mg/day)	
Ceftizoxime (Cefizox)	IV, IM	150–200 mg divided into 3 doses (adult 3–6 g/day, maximum 12 g/day)	
Ceftriaxone (Rocephin)	IV, IM	50–100 mg divided into 1 or 2 doses (adult 1–2 g/day, maximum 4 g/day)	100 mg for meningitis and penicillin-resistant pneumococcal pneumonia
Cefuroxime (Zinacef)	IV, IM	75–150 mg divided into 3 doses (adult 2.25–4.5 g/day)	Should not be used for meningitis
Cefuroxime axetil (Ceftin)	PO	20–30 mg divided into 2 doses, maximum 1 g/day	
Cephalexin (Keflex)	PO	25–50 mg divided into 3 or 4 doses (adult 1–4 g/day)	100 mg for oral step-down therapy to replace parenteral therapy
PENICILLINS[c]			
PENICILLIN G and V			
Penicillin G, crystalline K or Na	IV, IM	100,000–300,000 units divided into 4–6 doses (adult 8–24 million units/day)	
Penicillin G, procaine	IM	25,000–50,000 units divided into 1–2 doses (adult 600,000–1.2 million units/day, maximum 4.8 million units/day)	
Penicillin G, benzathine (Bicillin LA)	IM	50,000 units/kg once for neonates/infants <27 kg (60 lb) 300,000–600,000 units (not per kg) once ≥27 kg (60 lb) 900,000 units (not per kg) once (adult 1.2–2.4 million units once)	
Penicillin G benzathine/ procaine (Bicillin CR)	IM	<14 kg (30 lb) 600,000 units (not per kg) once 14–27 kg (30–60 lb) 900,000–1,200,000 units (not per kg) once ≥27 kg (60 lb) 2,400,000 units (not per kg) once	
Penicillin V K (numerous)	PO	25–50 mg divided into 3 or 4 doses (adult 0.5–2 g/day)	Optimal administration on empty stomach
PENICILLINASE-RESISTANT PENICILLINS			Methicillin-resistant staphylococci are resistant to all penicillins
Oxacillin (Bactocill)	IV, IM	100–200 mg divided into 4–6 doses (adult 4–6 g/day, maximum 12 g/day)	
Nafcillin (Unipen, Nafcil)	IV, IM	100–200 mg divided into 4–6 doses (adult 4–6 g/day, maximum 12 g/day)	
Dicloxacillin (Dynapen, Pathocil)	PO	12.5–25 mg divided into 4 doses (adult 0.5–2 g/day, maximum 4 g/day)	100 mg for oral step-down therapy to replace parenteral therapy
AMINOPENICILLINS			
Amoxicillin (Amoxil)	PO	25–50 mg divided into 3 doses (adult 0.75–3 g/day)	90 mg in 2 doses for AOM 80–100 mg in 3 doses for oral step-down therapy to replace parenteral therapy
Amoxicillin-clavulanate (Augmentin)	PO	14:1 formulation: 90 mg amoxicillin component divided into 2 doses 7:1 formulation: 25–45 mg amoxicillin component divided into 2 doses 4:1 formulation: 20–40 mg amoxicillin component divided into 3 doses	
Ampicillin	IV, IM	100–200 mg divided into 4 doses (adult 4–12 g/day)	200–400 mg divided into 4 doses for meningitis
Ampicillin-sulbactam (Unasyn)	IV	100–200 mg ampicillin component divided into 4 doses (adult 4–8 g day)	
Ampicillin/ampicillin trihydrate (Principen)	PO	50–100 mg divided into 4 doses (adult 2–4 g/day)	
BROAD-SPECTRUM PENICILLINS			
Piperacillin (Pipracil)	IV, IM	200–400 divided into 3–6 doses (adult 6–18 g/day, maximum 24 g/day)	

Continued

APPENDIX 292-1. Dosage of Antibacterial Drugs for Infants, Older Children, and Adolescents—cont'd

Drug Generic (Trade)	Route	Dosage (per kg/day)[a]	Comments
Piperacillin-tazobactam (Zosyn)	IV	240–300 mg piperacillin component divided into 3–4 doses (adult 9–16 g piperacillin/day)	
Ticarcillin-clavulanate (Timentin)	IV	200–300 mg ticarcillin component divided into 4–6 doses (adult 12–18 g ticarcillin/day, maximum 24 g/day)	300–600 mg divided into 4 doses for cystic fibrosis
Chloramphenicol (Chloromycetin) sodium-succinate	IV	50–100 mg divided into 4 doses (adult 2–4 g/day)	Dosage adjusted according to serum concentration(s)
FLUOROQUINOLONES			Arthropathy is a potential fluoroquinolone-class side effect in children
Norfloxacin (Noroxin)	PO	9–14 mg divided into 2 doses (adult 400–800 mg/day, maximum 1.2 g/day)	
Ciprofloxacin (Cipro)	PO	20–40 mg divided into 2 doses, maximum 2 g/day	
	IV	20–30 mg divided into 2–3 doses, maximum 1.2 g/day	
Levofloxacin (Levaquin)	PO, IV	20 mg divided into 2 doses (children <5 years); 10 mg once-daily (children ≥5 years) (adult 500–750 mg/day)	
LINCOSAMIDES Clindamycin (Cleocin)	IM, IV	20–40 mg divided into 3 doses (adult 900 mg–2.7 g/day, maximum 4.8 g/day)	
	PO	10–30 mg divided into 3–4 doses (adult 600 mg–1.8 g/day, maximum 2.7 mg/day)	30–40 mg for AOM and CA-MRSA infection
LIPOPEPTIDES Daptomycin (Cubicin)	IV	4–6 mg once daily for children ≥12 years; 7 mg once daily for 6–12 years; 8–10 mg once daily for 2–6 years (adult 4–6 mg/kg once daily)	
MACROLIDES/AZALIDES Erythromycin (numerous)	PO	50 mg divided into 2–4 doses (adult 1–2 g/day, maximum 4 g/day)	Available as base, stearate, ethyl succinate preparations, and as erythromycin-sulfisoxazole
	IV	20 mg divided into 4 doses (adult 1–2 g/day, maximum 4 g/day)	Administer over at least 60 min to potentially prevent cardiac arrhythmias
Clarithromycin (Biaxin)	PO	15 mg divided into 2 doses (adult 0.5–1 g/day)	
Azithromycin (Zithromax)	PO, IV	All doses once daily: AOM: 10 mg × 3 days; *or* 30 mg × 1 day; *or* 10 mg × 1 day, then 5 mg × 4 days Pharyngitis: 12 mg × 5 days Sinusitis: 10 mg × 3 days; *or* 10 mg ×1 days, then 5 mg × 4 days Pneumonia: 10 mg × 1 day, then 5 mg × 4 days; *or* 60 mg × 1 day of Zmax susp if >6 months of age Shigellosis: 12 mg × 1 day, then 6 mg × 4 days	
MISCELLANEOUS Methenamine mandelate (Mandelamine)	PO	50–75 mg divided into 2–4 doses (adult 2–4 g/day)	For UTI prophylaxis
Nitrofurantoin (Furadantin)	PO	5–7 mg divided into 4 doses (adult 200–400 mg/day, maximum 7 mg/kg per day)	1–2 mg once-daily for UTI prophylaxis
NITROIMIDAZOLES Metronidazole (Flagyl)	PO	30–50 mg divided into 3 doses (adult 0.75–2.25 g/day)	
	IV	22.5–40 mg divided into 3 doses (adult 1–2 g/day, maximum 4 g/day)	
OXAZOLIDINONES Linezolid (Zyvox)	PO, IV	For children <12 years of age: 30 mg in 3 doses For adolescents ≥12 years and adults: 1200 mg per day (not per kg) in 2 doses	Myelosuppression increases with duration of therapy over 10 days
POLYMYXINS Colistin (as Colistimethate, Coly-Mycin M)	IV, IM	5–7 mg colistin base, divided into 3 doses	Reserved for multidrug-resistant gram-negative pathogens because of neuro- and nephrotoxicity
Quinupristin-dalfopristin (Synercid)	IV	15–22.5 mg divided into 2–3 doses (adult dose same)	

Continued

APPENDIX 292-1. Dosage of Antibacterial Drugs for Infants, Older Children, and Adolescents—cont'd

Drug Generic (Trade)	Route	Dosage (per kg/day)[a]	Comments
RIFAMYCINS			
Rifampin (Rifadin)	PO, IV	10–20 mg divided into 1–2 doses (adult 600 mg/day)	
Rifaximin (Xifaxan)	PO	≥12 years of age:600 mg/day (not per kg) divided into 3 doses	
SULFONAMIDES			
Sulfadiazine	PO	120–150 mg divided into 4 doses (adult 4–6 g/day)	
Sulfisoxazole (Gantrisin)	PO	120–150 mg divided into 4 doses (adult 2–4 g/day)	10–20 mg in 2 doses for UTI prophylaxis
Trimethoprim-sulfamethoxazole (TMP-SMX) (Bactrim, Septra)	IV, PO	8–12 mg TMP divided into 2 doses (adult 160–320 mg TMP/day, maximum 15 mg TMP/kg per day)	20 mg TMP divided into 4 doses for *Pneumocystis* pneumonia (PCP) 2 mg TMP once daily for UTI prophylaxis 5 mg TMP divided into 2 doses for 3 consecutive days per week for PCP prophylaxis
TETRACYCLINES			Tetracycline-class antibiotics stain unerupted teeth; use in children <8 years of age if benefits exceed risks
Tetracycline (numerous)	PO	25–50 mg divided into 4 doses (adult 1–2 g/day)	
Minocycline (Minocin)	PO, IV	4 mg divided into 2 doses (adult 200 mg/day PO, 200–400 mg/day IV)	
Doxycycline (numerous)	PO, IV	2–4 mg divided into 1–2 doses (adult 100–200 mg/day)	
Tigecycline (Tygacil)	IV	2 mg divided into 2 doses (adult 100 mg/day)	
VANCOMYCIN (VANCOCIN)	IV	40 mg divided into 3–4 doses (adult 1–2 g/day)	Dosage adjusted according to serum concentration(s) Consider dose of 60 mg/kg per day for meningitis, and for invasive CA-MRSA
	PO	40 mg divided into 4 doses (adult, 500 mg divided into 4 doses)	Not absorbed from GI tract
	Intraventricular	1–2 mg daily	

AOM, acute otitis media; GI, gastrointestinal; IV, intravenous; IM, intramuscular; PO, orally; UTI, urinary tract infection.

[a]*Doses for children are listed as the number of dosing units (e.g. mg, µg, etc.) per kilogram per day along with an absolute maximum dose if known. The corresponding parenthetic adult doses are the common adult dose range (not per kg per day, unless specified) followed by the adult maximum dose, if known.*

[b]*Once daily IV aminoglycoside dosing (amikacin 15–20 mg/kg; gentamicin/tobramycin 4.5–7.5 mg/kg) may provide equal efficacy with reduced toxicity and can be used as an alternative to multiple daily dosing.[202]*

[c]*In patients with a history of immediate hypersensitivity (anaphylaxis) to penicillin, other penicillins, cephalosporins, or carbapenems should not be used.*

Data for Appendix 293–1 from references 126, 203–208.

APPENDIX 292-2. Table of Antibiotic Dosages for Neonates

Drug	Route	Dosage (mg/kg per dose) and Frequency of Administration[a]			
		Body weight ≤2 kg		Body weight >2 kg	
		≤7 days old	8–28 days old[b]	≤7 days old	8–28 days old
AMINOGLYCOSIDES[c,d]					
Amikacin	IV, IM	15 every 48 h	15 every 24–48 h	15 every 24 h	15 every 12–24 h
Gentamicin	IV, IM	5 every 48 h	4–5 every 24–48 h	4 every 24 h	4 every 12–24 h
Tobramycin	IV, IM	5 every 48 h	4–5 every 24–48 h	4 every 24 h	4 every 12–24 h
CARBAPENEMS					
Imipenem/cilastatin	IV	25 every 12 h	25 every 12 h	25 every 12 h	25 every 8 h
Meropenem[e]	IV	20 every 12 h	20 every 8 h	20 every 8 h	20 every 8 h
for meningitis		40 every 12 h	40 every 8 h	40 every 8 h	40 every 8 h
CEPHALOSPORINS					
Cefepime[e]	IV, IM	30 every 12 h	30 every 12 h	30 every 12 h	30 every 12 h
Cefotaxime	IV, IM	50 every 12 h	50 every 8–12 h	50 every 12 h	50 every 8 h
for meningitis	IV	50 every 12 h	50 every 8 h	50 every 8 h	50 every 6 h
Cefazolin	IV, IM	25 every 12 h	25 every 12 h	25 every 12 h	25 every 8 h

Continued

APPENDIX 292-2. Table of Antibiotic Dosages for Neonates—cont'd

| | | Dosage (mg/kg per dose) and Frequency of Administration[a] | | | |
| | | Body weight ≤2 kg | | Body weight >2 kg | |
Drug	Route	≤7 days old	8–28 days old[b]	≤7 days old	8–28 days old
Ceftazidime	IV, IM	50 every 12 h	50 every 8–12 h	50 every 12 h	50 every 8 h
Ceftriaxone[f]	IV, IM	50 every 24 h	50 every 24 h	50 every 24 h	50 every 24 h
Cefuroxime	IV, IM	50 every 12 h	50 every 8–12 h	50 every 12 h	50 every 8 h
PENICILLINS					
Ampicillin	IV, IM	50 every 12 h[g]	50 every 8 h	50 every 8 h	50 every 6 h
for meningitis	IV	100 every 12 h	100 every 8 h	100 every 8 h	75 every 6 h
Nafcillin, Oxacillin	IV, IM	25 every 12 h	25 every 8 h	25 every 8 h	25 every 6 h
for meningitis	IV	50 every 12 h	50 every 8 h	50 every 8 h	50 every 6 h
Penicillin G crystalline[h]	IV, IM	50,000 units every 12 h	50,000 units every 8 h	50,000 units every 12 h	50,000 units every 8 h
for meningitis	IV	100,000 units every 12 h	100,000 units every 8 h	100,000 units every 8 h	100, 000 units every 6 h
Penicillin G procaine	IM only	50,000 units every 24 h	50,000 units every 24 h	50,000 units every 24 h	50,000 units every 24 h
Piperacillin-Tazobactam	IV	100 every 12 h	100 every 8 h	100 every 12 h	100 every 8 h
Ticarcillin-Clavulanate	IV	75 every 12 h	75 every 8 h	75 every 12 h	75 every 8 h
OTHER AGENTS					
Azithromycin	PO, IV	10 every 24 h	10 every 24 h	10 every 24 h	10 every 24 h
Aztreonam[e]	IV, IM	30 every 12 h	30 every 8–12 h	30 every 8 h	30 every 6 h
Clindamycin	IV, IM, PO	5 every 12 h	5 every 8 h	5 every 8 h	5 every 6 h
Erythromycin	PO, IV	10 every 12 h	10 every 8 h	10 every 12 h	10 every 8 h
Linezolid	IV	10 every 12 h	10 every 8 h	10 every 8 h	10 every 8 h
Metronidazole	IV	7.5 every 24–48 h[i]	15 every 24 h	15 every 24 h	15 every 12 h
Vancomycin	IV	See comment[j]			

IV. intravenous; IM, intramuscular; PO, oral.

[a]*In milligrams (mg) unless otherwise specified. Dosages may need to be adjusted in neonates with severe renal or hepatic impairment.*

[b]*May use the longer dosing interval (if given) in extremely low-birthweight (less than 1000 g) neonates until 2 weeks of life.*

[c]*Dosages for aminoglycosides may differ from those recommended by the manufacturer and approved by the FDA.*

[d]*Optimal, individualized dosage should be based on determination of serum concentrations.*

[e]*50 mg/kg/dose may be required for Pseudomonas infections.*

[f]*Neonates should not receive ceftriaxone intravenously if they are also receiving, or are expected to receive, intravenous calcium in any form, including parenteral nutrition. See Pediatrics 2009;123;e609. Cefotaxime is the preferred 3rd generation cephalosporin in neonates.*

[g]*100 mg/kg/dose every 12 hours is also acceptable for empiric therapy of early onset sepsis.*

[h]*Dosage applies to treatment of congenital syphilis and empiric therapy of early onset sepsis. Some experts recommend 200–300,000 units/kg/day for other invasive infections.*

[i]*May begin therapy with a 15 mg/kg loading dose, then use the longer dosing interval for extremely low-birthweight (less than 1000 g) neonates.*

[j]*Dosing algorithm based on serum creatinine; if <0.7 then 15 mg/kg every 12 h, if 0.7–0.9 then 20 mg/kg every 24 h, if 1–1.2 then 15 mg/kg every 24 h, if 1.3–1.6 then 10 mg/kg every 24h, if >1.6 then 15 mg/kg every 48h. Add 0.2 to serum creatinine when using algorithm in neonates ≤28 weeks gestational age.*

Reproduced from Bradley JS and Nelson JD, ed. Antiinfective therapy for newborns. In: Nelson's Pocketbook of Pediatric Antimicrobial Therapy, 19th ed. Elk Grove Village, IL American Academy of Pediatrics; 2012.

293 Antifungal Agents

William J. Steinbach and Christopher C. Dvorak

Fungal pathogens generally can be divided into superficial infections that can affect children with normal immune systems, and invasive infections that tend to occur primarily in children who are immunocompromised due to a genetic defect, a hematopoietic cell or solid-organ transplantation, or following one of the potent chemotherapeutic regimens used for childhood malignancies. Fortunately, there has been a recent surge in the development of antifungal therapies, and several new studies have expanded our knowledge on how to optimize the utility of new agents. However, because of the paucity of pediatric data, many recommendations for the use of systemic antifungal drugs in children are derived from experience in adults, which is problematic in light of the pharmacokinetic differences between small children and adults. This chapter provides a brief review of topical antifungal therapy and an overview of the current state of systemic antifungal therapy. The preferred treatment for each pathogen is covered in pathogen-specific chapters.

ANTIFUNGAL AGENTS FOR TREATMENT OF SUPERFICIAL INFECTIONS

Among the therapeutic options available for treatment of fungal infections of the hair, skin, and nails, few have been tested in children, and fewer are approved for use in children younger than 13 years. Furthermore, extrapolating data from adults treated for dermatomycoses to infants and children may not be justified. For example, *Trichophyton tonsurans*, although uncommon in adults, is the most common cause of tinea capitis and tinea corporis in children.

The use of topical agents should be confined to infections of the epidermis, hair, and nails. The choice of treating superficial fungal infections with a topical or a systemic agent depends on the fungal pathogen, the site of infection, and the extent of the lesion. For example, systemic antifungal therapy almost always is used for ringworm of the scalp, nails, palms, or soles; creams or solutions are preferred for fissured or intertriginous areas.

Over-the-Counter Preparations

Undecylenic acid is an unsaturated fatty acid antifungal agent available as an ointment, powder, or liquid. Its therapeutic efficacy was first recognized in the 1940s in treating superficial fungal diseases affecting military troops. However, it has little efficacy compared with newer agents. Tolnaftate has similar activity against dermatophytes, with cure rates of 60% to 90%, but tinea pedis, tinea cruris, and tinea corporis resolve spontaneously in 20% to 30% of cases.[1] Tinea capitis and tinea unguinum frequently are resistant, probably because of poor penetration of tolnaftate into involved areas. The advantages of these compounds are that they are safe, inexpensive, and rarely cause local irritation.

Topical Polyenes

Nystatin is a polyene antifungal agent named after New York State. It binds to ergosterol in the fungal cell membrane and causes changes in cell permeability and, eventually, cell lysis. Nystatin is useful for the treatment of oral, mucosal, and cutaneous infections caused by *Candida* species. Nystatin is available as a suspension, powder, cream, or ointment (100,000 U/mL or U/g, respectively); a pastille (200,000 U) to be dissolved in the mouth; an oral tablet (500,000 U); and a vaginal tablet (100,000 U). Oral forms are administered four or more times daily and are well tolerated, since there is no significant systemic absorption, although large oral doses of the suspension can cause nausea. Nystatin is not effective against the dermatophytes.

Azoles

The azole class (divided into imidazoles and triazoles based on chemical structure) inhibit ergosterol synthesis in the fungal cell membrane. Clotrimazole is an imidazole with broad-spectrum activity against *Candida* species and the dermatophytes *T. tonsurans*, *Trichophyton rubrum*, *Trichophyton mentagrophytes*, *Epidermophyton floccosum*, and *Microsporum canis* (Table 293-1). Clotrimazole also is effective against *Malassezia furfur*, the cause of tinea versicolor. Clotrimazole is one of the few topical antifungal agents studied in children. The 1% cream, lotion, and solution are available over the counter for the treatment of tinea pedis, tinea cruris, and tinea corporis. High concentrations of clotrimazole are achieved topically, but systemic absorption is negligible. Topical application generally is well tolerated but can cause local irritation or urticaria. Clotrimazole also is available with 0.05% betamethasone and appears to foster more rapid healing in adults. However, this combination cream is not recommended for use in children because of the potential for systemic absorption of the corticosteroid.

Miconazole is an imidazole available over the counter as a 2% cream. Its spectrum of activity is identical to that of clotrimazole, and in clinical trials it has demonstrated equivalent efficacy. Its efficacy in the treatment of superficial *Candida* infections is better than that of nystatin, and it has the advantage of once-a-day application. Local side effects, such as those seen with clotrimazole, can occur, and miconazole should be used sparingly in intertriginous areas to avoid maceration of the skin.

Ketoconazole is an imidazole available as a 2% cream. Ketoconazole is effective therapy for dermatomycoses caused by *Candida* species, *T. rubrum*, *T. mentagrophytes*, *E. floccosum*, and *M. furfur*. Although it has in vitro activity against *T. tonsurans* and *Microsporum*, the clinical relevance of these data to efficacy is not known. Ketoconazole applied topically is not absorbed systemically; but it can cause local irritation.

Econazole is an imidazole nearly identical in structure to miconazole. Its activity and adverse reactions are similar. Published studies demonstrate cure rates for dermatomycoses similar to those of other topical imidazoles, but comparative studies have not been performed, and econazole has no clear advantage over other topical azoles.

Newer topical azoles include oxiconazole and terconazole. Oxiconazole is an imidazole that is approved for the treatment of tinea pedis, tinea cruris, tinea corporis, and tinea versicolor. Terconazole is an imidazole formulated only for vaginal use in the treatment of *Candida* vaginitis.

TABLE 293-1. Categories and Activities of Antifungal Agents against Dermatomycoses

Agent	Category	Trade Name	Activity Against			
			Candida Species	*Trichophyton tonsurans*	Other Dermatophytes	*Malassezia furfur*
Nystatin	Topical polyene	Mycostatin	+	−	−	−
Clotrimazole	Imidazole	Lotrimin	+	+	+	+
Miconazole	Imidazole	Desenex	+	+	+	+
Ketoconazole	Imidazole	Nizoral	+	?	+	+
Terbinafine	Allylamine	Lamisil	−	?	+	−
Oxiconazole	Imidazole	Oxistat	+	+	+	+
Naftifine	Allylamine	Naftin	−	?	+	−
Butenafine	Benzylamine	Mentax	−	+	+	−
Griseofulvin	*Penicillium* derivative	Fulvicin	−	+	+	−

+, activity; −, no activity; ?, variable activity.

Griseofulvin

Griseofulvin is U.S. Food and Drug Administration (FDA) approved for tinea capitis (daily for 6 to 8 weeks), a condition almost uniformly resistant to treatment with topical agents and therefore requiring oral antifungal therapy. Studies in children have demonstrated the superiority of griseofulvin over ketoconazole for the treatment of tinea capitis.[2] The exact mechanism of action is not known, but griseofulvin is deposited in keratin precursor cells and becomes bound to newly formed keratin, thereby preventing fungal invasion. Griseofulvin is only fungistatic against *Trichophyton*, *E. floccosum*, and *Microsporum*, and is not active against *Candida* or *M. furfur*. Absorption of griseofulvin from the gastrointestinal tract varies considerably but is increased by decreasing the size of the crystals and administering the drug with a meal high in fat content. Historically the usual dose of griseofulvin for children was 10 to 15 mg/kg/day, but due to increasing resistance many experts now recommend 20 to 25 mg/kg/day.

Griseofulvin has a long-standing history of safety and efficacy, and comes as an oral suspension. Because it is metabolized in the liver, adjustment in dosage is not necessary in patients with renal impairment. Side effects are infrequent but include hypersensitivity rash, urticaria, nausea, vomiting, diarrhea, headache, fatigue, proteinuria, and leukopenia. Elevated levels of serum hepatic enzymes can occur. Griseofulvin can decrease the effects of oral anticoagulant and contraceptive agents. Its antifungal effect can be decreased by the concurrent administration of phenobarbital.

Squalene Epoxidase Inhibitors

The allylamine terbinafine acts by inhibiting squalene epoxidase, an enzyme in the pathway leading to the synthesis of ergosterol in the fungal cell membrane. Terbinafine is available as both a topical preparation and an oral tablet. Topical terbinafine is at least as effective as other topical antifungal agents. Its main advantage is that 1-week treatment with 1% terbinafine cream applied twice daily is superior to 4-week treatment with 1% clotrimazole cream.[3] The oral tablet has high absorportion (>70%) and a long half-life (approximately 36 hours), penetrates keratinized tissues, and maintains concentrations higher in skin/nails than serum for one week after stopping treatment. Unlike griseofulvin, no liquid formulation is available.[4] Both griseofulvin and terbinafine are active against the common dermatophytes and have proven efficacy in the treatment of dermatomycoses in adults. In a meta-analysis comparing terbinafine with griseofulvin for the treatment of tinea capitis, all analyses favored terbinafine (OR 0.65 to 0.86). This suggests that 2 to 4 weeks of terbinafine therapy is at least as effective as 6 to 8 weeks of griseofulvin for *Trichophyton* tinea capitis, with no differences in tolerability or adverse effects and an overall cost saving with the 4-week therapy.[5] In contrast, some studies suggest that griseofulvin may be the preferred agent over terbinafine against tinea capitis due to *Microsporum* species.[6] However, terbinafine dosing is very important. Based on dose modeling in other studies and one clinical trial, there was a clear effect with higher doses (7 to 12.5 mg/kg/day) of terbinafine resulting in greater mycologic cure even against the more recalcitrant *M. canis*.[7]

Butenafine is a benzylamine with a mechanism of action similar to that of the allylamine class of antifungal agents. Butenafine is indicated for the topical treatment of tinea pedis, tinea corporis, and tinea cruris.

ANTIFUNGAL AGENTS FOR TREATMENT OF INVASIVE INFECTIONS

The armamentarium of antifungal choices for invasive fungal infections has increased substantially in recent years (Tables 293-2 and 293-3). While choices once were limited and often ineffective, clinicians must now consider many factors before deciding on therapy, including the organism and its epidemiology, antifungal

TABLE 293-2. Spectrum of Activity of Selected Systemic Antifungal Agents

Antifungal	Important Clinical Uses
Amphotericin B	*Blastomyces dermatitidis, Coccidioides immitis, Cryptococcus neoformans, Histoplasma capsulatum, Paracoccidioides brasiliensis, Sporothrix schenckii*, most *Candida* species, *Aspergillus*, Mucormycosis (formerly Zygomycetes) (**not** *A. terreus, Candida lusitaniae, Scedosporium, Fusarium, Trichosporon*)
5-Fluorocytosine	Only in combination therapy for *Candida, C. neoformans*, dematiaceous molds
Fluconazole	Most *Candida, C. neoformans, B. dermatitidis, H. capsulatum, C. immitis, P. brasiliensis* (**not** *C. krusei, C. glabrata, Aspergillus* species)
Itraconazole	*Candida, Aspergillus, B. dermatitidis, H. capsulatum, C. immitis, P. brasiliensis*
Voriconazole	*Candida, Aspergillus, Fusarium, B. dermatitidis, H. capsulatum, C. immitis, Malassezia* species, *Scedosporium*, dematiaceous molds (**not** Mucormycosis; **caution** *C. glabrata*)
Posaconazole	Mucormycosis, *Candida, Aspergillus, Fusarium, B. dermatitidis, H. capsulatum, C. immitis, Malassezia* species, *Scedosporium*, dematiaceous molds
Caspofungin	*Candida, Aspergillus* (**not** *C. neoformans, Fusarium*, Mucormycosis)
Micafungin	*Candida, Aspergillus* (**not** *C. neoformans, Fusarium*, Mucormycosis)
Anidulafungin	*Candida, Aspergillus* (**not** *C. neoformans, Fusarium*, Mucormycosis)

resistance patterns, and prior antifungal therapy. Currently licensed systemic antifungal agents include amphotericin B and its lipid derivatives; 5-fluorocytosine; the triazoles, including fluconazole, itraconazole, voriconazole, and posaconazole; and the echinocandins, including caspofungin, micafungin, and anidulafungin.

Polyenes

Amphotericin B

Mechanism of action. The oldest antifungal class is the polyene macrolides – amphotericin B and nystatin. Since its initial approval for use in 1958, amphotericin B deoxycholate remained for years the "gold standard" for the therapy of many invasive fungal infections, as well as the comparative agent for newer antifungal agents. Amphotericin B binds to ergosterol, the major sterol found in fungal cytoplasmic membranes, creating transmembrane channels resulting in an increased permeability to monovalent cations. Fungicidal activity is believed to be caused by leakage of essential nutrients from the fungal cell. Fungicidal activity appears lost against some fungi, such as *Aspergillus terreus*, where amphotericin B is an ineffective option.[8]

Pharmacology and toxicities. The fungicidal activity of amphotericin B is concentration-dependent, increasing directly with the amount of drug attained at the site of infection. Amphotericin B also has a prolonged post-antifungal effect, allowing antifungal activity to persist even after the concentration of drug falls below the minimum inhibitory concentration (MIC) needed to kill the fungus. These pharmacodynamic characteristics suggest that a single daily dose of amphotericin B will be effective.[9] Although there is a relationship between total dose administered and tissue concentrations,[10] there is no conclusive clinical evidence that doses higher than 1 mg/kg/day of amphotericin B deoxycholate

TABLE 293-3. Preferred Pediatric Dosing of Approved Systemic Antifungal Agents

Drug Class	Antifungal Drug	Preferred Adult Dosing	Preferred Pediatric Dosing	Pediatric Dosing Comments
Polyene	Amphotericin B deoxycholate (Fungizone)	1–1.5 mg/kg/day	1–1.5 mg/kg/day	Children generally tolerate higher doses than adults
	Amphotericin B Lipid Complex (ABLC; Abelcet)	5 mg/kg/day	5 mg/kg/day	
	Liposomal Amphotericin B (L-AmB; AmBisome)	5 mg/kg/day	5 mg/kg/day	
Pyrimidine analogue	5-Fluorocytosine (Ancoban)	150 mg/kg/day divided q6h	150 mg/kg/day divided q6h	Use caution with large oral volume for neonates
Triazole	Fluconazole (Diflucan)	100–800 mg/day; 3–6 mg/kg/day	6–12 mg/kg/day	Dose higher in children due to shorter half-life; neonates require further special dosing
	Itraconazole (Sporanox)	200–400 mg/day	2.5–5 mg/kg/dose bid	Dosing bid preferred in children
	Voriconazole (VFend)	Load: 6 mg/kg/dose bid × 1 day Maintenance: 3–4 mg/kg/dose bid	Load: 9 mg/kg/dose bid × 1 day Maintenance: 8 mg/kg/dose bid	Linear pharmacokinetics in children Pediatric dosing can be increased more easily than in adult patients due to linear pharmacokinetics versus non-linear in adult patients
	Posaconazole (Noxafil)	400 mg bid	200 mg qid or 400 mg bid q6–12h	Exact pediatric dosing unknown; appears that dose should be divided more frequently in children
Echinocandin	Caspofungin (Cancidas)	Load: 70 mg qd × 1 day Maintenance: 50 mg qd	Load: 70 mg/m² qd × 1 day Maintenance: 50 mg/m² qd	Dosing for hepatic insufficiency in children is 35 mg/m² qd, similar to the adult decrease to 35 mg qd
	Micafungin (Mycamine)	50–150 mg/day	2–10 mg/kg per day	Very dependent on age of child as neonates require far more drug than pediatric patients
	Anidulafungin (Eraxis)	Load: 200mg qd × 1 day Maintenance: 100mg qd	Load: 3 mg/kg/qd × 1 day Maintenance: 1.5 mg/kg/qd	

q6h = once every 6 hours; qd = once daily; bid = twice daily.

ABLC is recommended officially at 5mg/kg/day, ABCD at 3–5 mg/kg/day, and L-AmB at 1–5 mg/kg/day. Most clinical data have been obtained with the use of these preparations at 5 mg/kg/day and most clinicians use and prefer this higher dosing.

are necessary for successful therapy.[11] Cerebrospinal fluid (CSF) concentrations are only 2% to 4% of serum concentrations,[12] so this agent is a poor choice as monotherapy for the treatment of meningitis. Amphotericin B is eliminated primarily via the kidneys, although dose adjustments generally are not needed with renal impairment. Amphotericin B has few direct drug interactions, although nephrotoxic medications can cause additive toxic effects.

In addition to fungal ergosterol, amphotericin B binds to cholesterol in human cell membranes, likely accounting for its toxicity.[13] Lipid formulations of amphotericin B generally are better tolerated, with less infusion-related toxicities (such as fever, chills, or headache), than the conventional deoxycholate preparation, perhaps because the lipid stabilizes the drug in a self-associated state so that drug cannot interact with the cholesterol of human cellular membranes.[14,15] The reduced nephrotoxicity of lipid formulations also may result from their preferential binding to serum high-density lipoproteins. High-density lipoprotein-bound amphotericin B appears to be released to the kidney more slowly, or to a lesser degree, than conventional amphotericin B that is bound to low density lipoproteins.[16]

Several lipid-associated formulations of amphotericin B offer the advantage of an increased daily dose of the parent drug, better delivery to the primary reticuloendothelial organs (lungs, liver, spleen),[17,18] and reduced toxicity. The FDA approved amphotericin B lipid complex (ABLC; Abelcet, Enzon Corporation, Bridgewater, NJ) in December 1995 and liposomal amphotericin B (L-AmB; AmBisome, Astellas Pharma US, Deerfield, IL) in August 1997.[19] It is postulated that activated monocytes/macrophages take up drug-laden lipid formulations and transport them to the site of infection where phospholipases release free drug.[19,20] A multicenter maximum tolerated dose study of liposomal amphotericin B in adult patients using doses from 7.5 to 15 mg/kg/day found

a nonlinear plasma pharmacokinetic profile with a maximal concentration at 10 mg/kg/day and no demonstrable dose-limiting nephrotoxicity or infusion-related toxicity.[21] A more recent randomized clinical trial comparing liposomal amphotericin B at a standard dose of 3 mg/kg/day versus a higher dose of 10 mg/kg/day failed to show any improvement in efficacy and yielded more nephrotoxicity with the higher dose.[22]

Amphotericin B nephrotoxicity generally is less severe in infants and children than adults, likely due to the more rapid clearance of the drug in children. Reports of reduced nephrotoxicity with a lipid formulation in adults also have been observed in children[23,24] and neonates.[25] A pharmacokinetic study of liposomal amphotericin B conducted in 39 children observed no dose-related trends in adverse events and a maximally-tolerated dose of 10 mg/kg/day (Gilead Sciences, data on file). These results are similar to those in studies conducted in adults.[21] A 56-center prospective study evaluated the safety and efficacy of L-amphotericin B administered to 260 adults, 242 children (<15 years), and 43 infants <2 months of age.[26] In general, the infants and children tolerated the largest doses of liposomal amphotericin B administered for the longest period of time (median of 16 days),[26] dispelling historical notions that children were unable to tolerate such a potentially toxic antifungal agent.

Amphotericin B is available as an intravenous preparation and does not have an active oral formulation. While there are anecdotal reports of using intravenous amphotericin B in numerous instillation or irrigation methods (including intrathecal, intrapleural, or intra-articular instillation or bladder irrigation), there are no controlled data to support these uses of amphotericin B. Often the drug will prove irritating to the surrounding tissue, potentially creating more side effects than clinical benefit. Inhaled amphotericin B has been used successfully as prophylaxis in lung transplant recipients, but has not been shown to be effective as adjunctive therapy in a broader patient population.

Clinical experience and pediatric data. The optimal duration of amphotericin B therapy is unknown but likely is dependent on underlying disease, extent of fungal infection, resolution of neutropenia, degree of immunosuppression, and graft function following transplantation. There is no specific total cumulative dose of amphotericin B recommended currently, rather a standard approach is to initiate therapy with 1 mg/kg/day, reducing the dose if toxicity develops.[27] While mortality was slightly lower in patients treated with liposomal AmB compared with conventional AmB in one study with a small number of patients,[28] there are no convincing data indicating that any of the amphotericin B lipid formulation are more clinically effective than conventional amphotericin B.[17,19,29–31] A study of 56 infants with candidiasis, including 52 preterm infants, showed no differences in mortality or time to resolution of candidemia between neonates receiving conventional amphotericin B (n=34), liposomal amphotericin B (n=6), or amphotericin B colloidal dispersion (n=16).[32] Therefore, the decision to prescribe a lipid formulation of amphotericin B should be based on the potential of reducing nephrotoxicity or infusion-related toxicity rather than anticipated therapeutic benefit.

In noncomparative studies, ABLC has been found to be an effective antifungal agent in children. In an open-label pediatric trial, complete or partial therapeutic response was observed in 70% (38/54) of patients, including 56% (14/25) of those with aspergillosis and 81% (22/27) of those with candidiasis.[24] A retrospective study of 46 children treated with ABLC reported an overall response rate of 83% (38/46), including 78% (18/23) against aspergillosis and 89% (17/19) against candidiasis.[33]

There are few published data on the use of lipid formulations of amphotericin B in neonates. One study that included 40 preterm neonates (mean birthweight 1090 grams, mean gestational age 28.4 weeks) noted that liposomal amphotericin B was associated with clinical resolution in over 70% of patients with candidiasis;[34] other uncontrolled studies have confirmed high response rates. For example, in three other studies, 83% to 100% of neonates with candidiasis cleared their infections.[35]

Pyrimidine Analogues

5-Fluorocytosine

Mechanism of action. 5-Fluorocytosine (5-FC; Ancoban, ICN Pharmaceuticals, Costa Mesa, CA) is a fluorinated analogue of cytosine which has antimycotic activity resulting from the rapid conversion of 5-FC into 5-fluorouracil (5-FU) within susceptible fungal cells.[36,37] 5-FU inhibits fungal protein synthesis following incorporation into fungal RNA in place of uridylic acid or through inhibition of thymidylate synthetase, thus inhibiting fungal DNA synthesis.[37] 5-FC has little inherent activity against molds[38] and most reports detail clinical failure with monotherapy against yeast infections.[39] Antifungal resistance develops quickly to 5-FC monotherapy, so the drug should be used only in combination with other agents. 5-FC is thought to enhance the antifungal activity of amphotericin B, especially in anatomic sites where amphotericin B penetration is poor, such as CSF, heart valves, and the ocular vitreous.[40] One explanation for the synergy detected with amphotericin B plus 5-FC is that the membrane-permeabilizing effects of low concentrations of amphotericin B facilitate penetration of 5-FC into the cell interior.[41]

Pharmacology and toxicities. 5-FC is well-absorbed after oral administration.[37] 5-FC distributes widely, attaining therapeutic concentrations in most body sites such as the CSF, vitreous and peritoneal fluids, and into inflamed joints because it is small and highly water soluble and not bound by serum proteins to a great extent.[37] It is often technically difficult to treat neonates with 5-FC because of the large volume necessitated by using the oral formulation and the lack of an intravenous formulation available in the U.S. 5-FC is no longer recommended for treatment of neonatal candidiasis.

5-FC toxicity appears to be due to its conversion to 5-FU, with reports of 5-FU concentrations being in the range found after chemotherapeutic doses.[42] 5-FC can exacerbate myelosuppression in patients with neutropenia and trough serum concentrations of ≥100 µg/mL are associated with bone marrow aplasia. Therefore, 5-FC serum concentrations should be monitored closely and levels maintained at approximately 40 to 80 µg/mL. In a review of a multicenter trial of 194 patients who received amphotericin B plus 5-FC for cryptococcal meningitis, hematologic toxicity appeared in the first 2 weeks of therapy in 56% of patients, and in the first 4 weeks of therapy in 87%.[43] Neonates have slower clearance of 5-FC and can be dosed every 12 to 24 hours, but older children and adults require every 6 hour dosing. Clearance is via the kidneys, and the interval between doses should be prolonged in the setting of renal dysfunction.

Clinical experience and pediatric data. A pivotal trial showed that the combination of amphotericin B plus 5-FC was more effective than amphotericin B alone in the treatment of cryptococcal meningitis.[44] A subsequent multicenter study of 194 patients with cryptococcal meningitis concluded that 4 weeks of amphotericin B plus 5-FC was adequate for immunocompetent patients without neurologic complications such as hydrocephalus. However, among immunocompromised patients 6 weeks of combination therapy resulted in fewer relapses.[45] Amphotericin B in combination with 5-FC currently is recommended as initial therapy for cryptococcal meningitis.[46] These two agents also are suggested for use in patients with candidal meningitis.[47] While there are many historic reports of 5-FC combined with amphotericin B to penetrate difficult sites of infection such as the joints, eyes, or brain, this use for 5-FC has diminished with the advent of newer antifungal agents with an improved pharmacodynamic profile.

There are limited data regarding the use of 5-FC in children. One review of 17 cases of candidal meningitis (including 11 patients under 12 months of age) noted improvement in 15 patients treated with amphotericin B and 5-FC.[48]

Azoles

The azole antifungal agents are heterocyclic synthetic compounds that inhibit the fungal cytochrome $P450_{14DM}$ (also known as lanosterol 14α-demethylase), which catalyzes a late step in ergosterol biosynthesis. The drugs bind through a nitrogen group in their 5-membered azole ring to the heme group in the target protein and block demethylation of the C14 of lanosterol, leading to substitution of methylated sterols in the membrane and depletion of ergosterol. The result is an accumulation of precursors with abnormalities in fungal membrane permeability, membrane-bound enzyme activity, and coordination of chitin synthesis.[49,50]

The azoles are subdivided into imidazoles and triazoles on the basis of the number of nitrogens in the azole ring,[51] with the structural differences resulting in different binding affinities of the azole pharmacophore for the cytochrome P450 (CYP) enzyme system. With the exception of ketoconazole, the imidazoles are limited to superficial mycoses and none, including ketoconazole, have activity against molds such as *Aspergillus*.

Fluconazole

Pharmacology and toxicities. Fluconazole (Diflucan, Pfizer Inc., New York, NY) is a triazole that was approved by the FDA for therapy of cryptococcosis and *Candida* infections in 1990. Fluconazole's activity is concentration-independent; effect does not increase once the maximal fungistatic concentration is attained.[52] Fluconazole is available as either an oral or intravenous form, and oral fluconazole is approximately 90% bioavailable. Unchanged drug is predominantly cleared by the kidneys; metabolism accounts for only a minor proportion of fluconazole clearance.[53] Through interaction with the CYP enzyme system, fluconazole can increase blood levels of various medications, including cyclosporine and tacrolimus, albeit to a lesser degree than seen with mold-active triazoles. Fluconazole passes into tissues and fluids rapidly, probably due to its relatively low lipophilicity and limited binding to plasma proteins. Drug concentrations in CSF and vitreous fluid are approximately 80% of those found in blood.[54] Concentrations of fluconazole are 10- to 20-fold higher in the urine than blood and therefore fluconazole is particularly appropriate for the therapy of fungal urinary tract infections.

The pharmacokinetics of fluconazole differ between adults and children. A review of five separate fluconazole pharmacokinetic studies that included 101 infants and children ranging in age from 2 weeks to 16 years[53] demonstrated that fluconazole clearance is more rapid in children than in adults. The mean plasma half-life was approximately 20 hours in children, compared with 30 hours in adults. Therefore, to achieve comparable drug exposure, the daily fluconazole dose needs to be approximately doubled for children over 3 months of age to 6 to 12 mg/kg/day.

The volume of distribution of fluconazole is greater and more variable in neonates than in infants and children. However, there is also a slow elimination of fluconazole, with a mean half-life of 88.6 hours at birth, decreasing to approximately 55 hours by 2 weeks of age. Therefore, neonates should be treated with a higher dose of fluconazole to compensate for increased volume of distribution, but the frequency of dosing needs to be decreased due to slow elimination. The pharmacologic consequence of such a long half-life is that patients require at least 8 days to reach steady-state.[55] A subsequent population pharmacokinetic study of young infants showed that clearance doubled from birth to 28 days of age and stressed the importance of dosing in the very smallest infants.[56]

Side effects of fluconazole are uncommon. In one study of 24 immunocompromised children, elevated serum hepatic transaminases were observed in only 2 cases.[57] Another review of 562 children confirmed that pediatric results mirror the excellent safety profile seen in adults. The most common side effects were gastrointestinal upset (7.7%) (vomiting, diarrhea, nausea), or a skin rash (1.2%).[58]

Clinical experience and pediatric data. In one clinical trial of 206 non-neutropenic adults with invasive candidiasis, the rate of successful therapy with 0.5 to 0.6 mg/kg/day of amphotericin B (79%) was similar to that of 400 mg/day of fluconazole (70%).[59] Another multicenter trial of 219 mostly non-neutropenic adults with invasive candidiasis found that those treated with a combination of fluconazole and amphotericin B (n=112) showed no difference in time to blood sterilization compared with those treated with fluconazole alone (n=107).[60] Although a secondary analysis suggested that combination therapy was superior in efficacy to fluconazole alone, the difference in favorable outcome was small (69% vs. 56%; P=0.043). A definitive conclusion regarding the benefit of this combination therapy to treat candidiasis remains unproven.

Clinical and mycologic response was observed in 97% of 40 neonates and infants with candidiasis treated with fluconazole. These children either had been nonresponsive or intolerant to standard antifungal therapy.[61] In another report, 80% of 40 neonates with invasive candidiasis were treated successfully with fluconazole. Although 3 of these patients relapsed, they ultimately were cured with an increased dose of fluconazole (10 mg/kg/day).[62] Finally, a prospective randomized study that compared fluconazole with amphotericin B in 24 infants with candidemia, noted a slight survival benefit among those treated with fluconazole (67%) compared with amphotericin B (55%).[63]

Fluconazole also has been evaluated for antifungal prophylaxis. Randomized, placebo-controlled clinical trials have demonstrated that the prophylactic use of fluconazole following allogeneic bone marrow transplantation results in lower rates of candidal infection and graft-versus-host disease (GvHD).[64] Studies conducted in adult stem cell transplant recipients have observed that 200 mg/day of prophylactic fluconazole is as effective as 400 mg/day.[65,66] One concern with this patient population continues to be the lack of activity of fluconazole against *Aspergillus* species. A prospective, placebo-controlled, randomized, double-blind evaluation of prophylactic fluconazole has been conducted in 100 low birthweight (<1000 grams) infants. Six weeks of fluconazole therapy resulted in a statistically significant reduction in the incidence of fungal

colonization (22% vs. 60%) as well as a decrease in the development of invasive fungal infection (0% vs. 20%).[67] Neonatal fluconazole prophylaxis currently is thought to be effective only at centers with a higher incidence of candidiasis.

Itraconazole

Pharmacology and toxicities. Itraconazole (Sporanox, Janssen Pharmaceuticals, Titusville, NJ) is fungicidal and has been available for clinical use since 1990.[68] Limitations of itraconazole include: erratic oral absorption in high risk patients, and frequent drug interactions.

Itraconazole has a high volume of distribution and accumulates in tissues.[50] Drug is not absorbed reliably from the gastrointestinal tract and has high protein binding.[9] H_2-receptor antagonists may result in decreased drug absorption, whereas acidic beverages such as colas or cranberry juice may enhance absorption.[69] Administration of the capsular formulation with food increases absorption, but the oral suspension is better absorbed on an empty stomach.[12] Elimination of itraconazole is hepatic primarily; there is no need for dosage adjustment in the presence of impairment of renal function.[50]

Serum concentrations of itraconazole are much lower in children than in adults after administration of the oral solution. This is especially true in children less than 5 years of age.[70] Therefore, children usually need twice daily dosing, whereas single daily dosing is appropriate for adults. However, due to the importance of effectively monitoring itraconazole concentrations, and the erratic absorption of the capsular formulation, clinicians should use itraconazole in children with caution.

Itraconazole can be difficult to tolerate, with nausea and vomiting occurring in about 10% of subjects and elevated serum hepatic transaminases in 5%.[71] Rare cases of cardiomyopathy have been reported in adults but no cases have been described in children. Itraconazole is a potent inhibitor of the CYP3A4 enzyme and therefore can result in important drug interactions. Prior or concurrent use of rifampin, phenytoin, carbamazepime, and phenobarbital should be avoided, and concomitant use with cyclophosphamide should be discouraged.[72] Any drug handled by this cytochrome pathway with normally low bioavailability, extensive first-pass metabolism, or a narrow therapeutic window – such as cyclosporine or tacrolimus – may be especially vulnerable.[73]

Clinical experience and pediatric data. Itraconazole has roles in the therapy of numerous fungal infections, including therapy for coccidioidomycosis,[74] histoplasmosis,[75] and others. A multi-center open-label study was performed in 31 patients with invasive pulmonary aspergillosis who received 14 days of itraconazole intravenously followed by 12 weeks of capsules orally. The intravenous form was well tolerated and target therapeutic concentrations were obtained within 2 days in 91% of patients and in all patients within one week of intravenous treatment. These levels also were maintained after changing to oral therapy and a complete or partial response was seen in 48% (15/31) of patients.[76]

Itraconazole currently is more appealing as a prophylactic rather than a therapeutic agent and may be superior to fluconazole for this purpose. In one large randomized controlled trial conducted in 445 patients with hematologic malignancy, itraconazole oral solution prevented more fungal infections than fluconazole suspension. Specifically, 6 proven fungal infections, including 4 fatal cases, occurred among the fluconazole recipients compared with one nonfatal case of candidiasis among the itraconazole recipients.[77] Additionally, while there were no cases of invasive aspergillosis among the patients receiving itraconazole, 4 cases of aspergillosis were diagnosed among those receiving fluconazole. However, itraconazole and fluconazole prophylaxis had similar prophylactic efficacy in a trial conducted in liver transplant recipients.[78] Itraconazole also has been shown to be an effective prophylactic agent in patients infected with HIV. A double-blind, placebo-controlled trial conducted in 63 patients with HIV infection in Thailand demonstrated a reduction in fungal infections from 16.7% in the placebo recipients to 1.6% in those taking itraconazole.[79]

There are no pivotal studies of itraconazole prophylaxis in children, and the few children enrolled in the larger prophylaxis studies were not analyzed separately. A phase I study in 26 HIV-infected children did show the cyclodextrin itraconazole solution was well-tolerated and efficacious against oropharyngeal candidiasis, including responses in all patients with fluconazole-resistant isolates.[80]

Voriconazole

Voriconazole (VFend, Pfizer Inc., New York, NY) is a second generation triazole and a synthetic derivative of fluconazole. Voriconazole combines the broad spectrum of antifungal activity of itraconazole with the increased bioavailability of fluconazole. It is fungicidal against *Aspergillus* and fungistatic against *Candida* species.[68,81–83]

Pharmacology and toxicities. Children require higher doses of voriconazole than adults to attain similar serum concentrations over time because the drug exhibits nonlinear pharmacokinetics in adults but exhibits linearity in children. This linearity was based on initial pharmacokinetic analyses of children from 2 to 11 years old where it appears that a higher pediatric dosage was needed to approximate bioequivalence to an adult dosage of 4 mg/kg given every 12 hours.[84] Therefore, using voriconazole at recommended doses for adults may lead to clinical failures in children less than 12 years of age.

A subsequent pharmacokinetic study was performed to evaluate doses of 4 to 8 mg/kg/dose and determined that a loading dose of 7 mg/kg/dose, followed by a maintenance dose remaining at 7 mg/kg/dose, was more acceptable.[85] Importantly, this analysis also uncovered a greatly decreased pediatric oral bioavailability (44%). A later study found that dosing at 8 mg/kg/dose was likely preferable, and confirmed a lower pediatric bioavailability (65%).[86] Due to the inherent linear pharmacokinetics in children, even using this "higher" dose in children affords room for further escalation in the setting of clinical nonresponsiveness. It is our practice often to escalate the maintenance dose slowly to 8 to 10 mg/kg/dose for serious infections while closely monitoring for toxicity.

Although available in a parenteral formulation, voriconazole has nearly complete oral absorption followed by extensive metabolism by the liver. As a result of a genetic polymorphism from a point mutation in the gene encoding CYP2C19, some individuals are poor metabolizers and some are extensive metabolizers.[87] About 5% to 7% of white people and 20% of non-Indian Asians have a deficiency in expressing this enzyme. As a result, voriconazole levels are as much as 4-fold greater in these subjects than in those homozygous subjects who metabolize the drug more extensively.[88] Voriconazole has excellent central nervous system penetrance (as seen by its side effects) and offers a proven option for treatment of cerebral fungal infection.[89] Monitoring voriconazole levels appears important both to gauge adequacy of treatment (most experts suggest a serum trough level of at least 1 μg/mL to overcome the MIC of the infecting organism), as well as to avoid potential toxicities.

Voriconazole's main side effects include reversible dose-dependent visual disturbances (increased brightness, blurred vision)[90] in as many as one-third of treated patients; elevated serum hepatic transaminases with increasing doses;[91,92] and occasional skin reactions, likely due to photosensitization.[49,81,93] Similar to the other triazoles, drug interactions also can be problematic due to inhibition of the CYP enzyme system. For instance, concomitant use with sirolimus is contraindicated as concentrations of the immunosuppressant can be increased 2- to 10-fold.[94] Intravenous voriconazole is solubilized in sulfobutyl ether β-cyclodextrin (SBECD) and because elimination of cyclodextrin is dependent on glomerular filtration the vehicle can accumulate in patients with significant impaired renal function, but clinical significance has yet to be determined fully.[95]

Clinical experience and pediatric data. Voriconazole is statistically superior for the therapy of aspergillosis compared with amphotericin B deoxycholate. In a prospective clinical trial of 392 patients with invasive aspergillosis, over 50% of those initially treated with voriconazole compared with only about 30% of those treated with conventional amphotericin B had complete or partial responses. Improved survival also was observed among those initially treated with voriconazole.[96] Similar positive experience with voriconazole was noted in an open-label multicenter study of 116 patients with invasive aspergillosis treated with voriconazole as either primary (60 patients) or salvage therapy (56 patients).[97] Additional analyses also have shown the significant benefit of early administration of voriconazole over amphotericin B.[98] These data have led clinicians to conclude that voriconazole is the preferred agent for treatment of invasive aspergillosis.

Despite its fungistatic activity, voriconazole also is effective in the treatment of *Candida* infections. In a multicenter evaluation of the therapy of esophageal candidiasis in 391 immunocompromised patients, voriconazole was successful in 98% and fluconazole in 95%.[99] In another study of 422 patients with invasive candidiasis, approximately 40% of patients were successfully treated with voriconazole. This rate of success was virtually identical to that of amphotericin B therapy, followed by oral fluconazole.[100] Voriconazole also has been evaluated in the management of febrile neutropenic patients. In one large study of over 800 episodes of fever and neutropenia, voriconazole was slightly inferior to L-amphotericin B. Voriconazole was effective in 26% of 415 subjects and L-amphotericin B was effective in 30% of 422. However, there were more breakthrough infections in the L-amphotericin B recipients, including 13 cases of invasive aspergillosis versus only 4 cases in the voriconazole recipients.[101]

The largest pediatric report of voriconazole is an open-label, compassionate-use evaluation of the drug in 58 children with proven or probable invasive fungal infection refractory to or intolerant of conventional antifungal therapy.[102] Voriconazole was administered as a loading dose of 6 mg/kg every 12 hours on the first day of therapy, followed by 4 mg/kg every 12 hours on subsequent days. When possible, the conversion to oral therapy was made with a dose of 100 or 200 mg twice a day for patients weighing <40 kg and ≥40 kg, respectively. Almost three-quarters of the patients had invasive aspergillosis. The most common treatment-related adverse reactions were elevations of serum hepatic transaminase or bilirubin in 13.8%, rash in 13.8%, abnormal vision (photophobia or blurred vision) in 5.1%, and photosensitivity reactions in 5.1% of patients. Only three patients discontinued voriconazole due to toxicity. Despite dosage lower than recommended currently, complete or partial response was observed in 43% of children with aspergillosis, 50% with candidemia, and 63% with scedosporiosis.

Voriconazole has not been tested formally in neonates. Due to the reports of visual adverse events in adults and pediatric patients there is concern over the unknown interactions with the developing retina and there are no planned clinical trials in neonates.

Posaconazole

Pharmacology and toxicities. Posaconazole (Noxafil, Merck & Co, Whitehouse Station, NJ) is a second-generation triazole that became available in the U.S. in 2006. It is closely related to itraconazole, fungicidal in vitro against *Aspergillus*, and has a half-life of at least 24 hours in humans.[49,103] Posaconazole has dose-proportional pharmacokinetics up to 800 mg/day with bioavailability greatest when administered in divided doses, and has a large apparent volume of distribution with slow elimination, suggesting an extensive distribution into tissues.[104] Chronic renal impairment has no effect on the pharmacokinetics of posaconazole.[105] Posaconazole has lower central nervous system (CNS) penetrance than voriconazole; however, there are well-documented cases of clinical success for treatment of CNS fungal infection.[106] Posaconazole currently is available as an oral formulation, but an intravenous prodrug also is under development. Posaconazole was found to be effective and well tolerated in a multicenter study in patients refractory to other antifungal agents.[107]

One retrospective study analyzed the pharmacokinetic profile of posaconazole for 12 pediatric patients (<18 years old) with resistant or refractory invasive fungal infections. These patients received a maintenance dose of 800 mg/day of posaconazole oral suspension given in two or three divided daily doses, compared with adult patients (18 to 64 years old) who received a maintenance dose of 800 mg/day. The overall success rate and adverse event profile were similar for pediatric and adult patients.[108] These preliminary data suggested that posaconazole pharmacokinetics are similar in adults and the children examined in this study, but a complete pediatric pharmacokinetic study is underway.

Clinical experience and pediatric data. Posaconazole showed a survival benefit over historic controls in treating invasive aspergillosis as salvage antifungal therapy,[109] but has not been examined as primary therapy. Anecdotal experience has suggested that the newer triazoles, posaconazole and voriconazole, are both effective anti-*Aspergillus* agents, but no comparative trials exist. Due to voriconazole's lack of activity against Zygomycetes infections, there is excitement due to posaconazole's in vitro activity as well as clinical efficacy as a salvage therapy against these emerging infections.[110]

Posaconazole has been best studied as antifungal prophylaxis, including a large trial in patients with acute myelogenous leukemia or myelodysplastic syndrome, which demonstrated less invasive fungal infections (2%) with posaconazole versus either fluconazole or itraconazole (8%). Survival also was significantly longer in patients who received posaconazole.[111] Similarly, in patients with active graft-versus-host disease, posaconazole was similar to fluconazole in preventing invasive fungal infections, but superior to fluconazole in preventing invasive aspergillosis as well as reducing death due to invasive fungal infections.[112]

Experience with posaconazole in children is very limited. An open-label study of 8 patients with chronic granulomatous disease and invasive mold infection treated with posaconazole salvage therapy included 7 pediatric patients. All patients had received itraconazole prophylaxis and had prior antifungal therapy with either voriconazole, caspofungin, or a lipid formulation of amphotericin B.[113] There was a complete response with posaconazole in 7 of 8 patients, including 6 of 7 pediatric patients. Posaconazole will have an important role in antifungal management in the future, but devoted pediatric clinical studies have yet to be performed.

Echinocandins

For years, development of new systemic antifungals focused on chemically modifying existing classes. An entirely new class of antifungals, the echinocandins, interferes with cell wall biosynthesis by noncompetitive inhibition of 1,3-β-D-glucan synthase, an enzyme present in fungi, but absent in mammalian cells.[49,103] This enzyme produces 1,3-β-D-glucan, which forms a fibril of three helically-entwined linear polysaccharides and provides essential structural integrity to the fungal cell wall.[114,115]

Echinocandins are fungicidal against *Candida* but fungistatic against *Aspergillus* as they inhibit hyphal tip and branch point growth, converting the mycelium to small clumps of cells, but the older septated cells with little glucan synthesis are not killed.[116] These agents are not metabolized through the CYP enzyme system but through a presumed *O*-methyltransferase, lessening some of the drug interactions and side effects seen with the azoles. Due to the water insolubility of the molecules, the echinocandins are only available in a parenteral formulation and have relatively poor CNS penetrance.

Caspofungin

Pharmacology and toxicities. Caspofungin (Cancidas, Merck & Co., Whitehouse Station, NJ) is a fungicidal semisynthetic derivative of the natural product pneumocandin B_0. Caspofungin has linear pharmacokinetics,[117] is excreted primarily by the liver, has a beta-phase half-life of 9 to 10 hours,[118] and is well tolerated.[119-122]

It is not metabolized by the CYP isoenzyme system[123] and at present there is no known maximal tolerated dose and no toxicity-defined maximal length of therapy. Elevations of caspofungin plasma concentrations are observed in patients with mild hepatic insufficiency and a dose reduction in adults from 50 mg to 35 mg daily following the standard 70 mg loading dose is recommended in this setting.[91]

A pharmacokinetic study conducted in children evaluated 39 patients between the ages of 2 and 17 years. Data were analyzed on the basis of both weight (1 mg/kg/day) and body surface area (50 or 70 mg/m^2/day).[124] Compared with plasma concentrations attained in adults treated with 50 mg/day, the weight-based approach resulted in suboptimal plasma concentrations, whereas the 50 mg/m^2/day dose yielded similar plasma concentrations in children. Caspofungin's half-life is approximately one-third less in children than in adults. Based on this initial study, subsequent dosing in children has been proposed to include a loading dose of 70 mg/m^2 followed by daily maintenance dosing of 50 mg/m^2.

Since 1,3-β-glucan is a selective target present only in fungal cell walls and not in mammalian cells, caspofungin has few adverse effects.[114] The drug has no apparent myelotoxicity or nephrotoxicity.[125] Plasma concentrations of tacrolimus are reduced by about 20% when co-administered with caspofungin, but tacrolimus does not alter the pharmacokinetics of caspofungin.[126] Cyclosporine increases the concentration of caspofungin by about 35%, but plasma concentrations of cyclosporine are not altered by co-administration of caspofungin.[127] A retrospective analysis of compassionate-use caspofungin in 25 immunocompromised children, most of whom also received other antifungal agents, noted that only 3 (12%) had a possible drug-related adverse event, which included hypokalemia and elevated serum bilirubin or hepatic transaminases.[128] Another study of 65 immunocompromised children revealed that caspofungin was not discontinued in any patients due to adverse events, and clinical adverse events were mild to moderate and observed in 23 patients (43%). Mean aspartate aminotransferase and alanine aminotransferase values were slightly (P<0.05) higher at end of therapy, but creatinine, bilirubin, and alkaline phosphatase levels were not different from baseline.[129]

Clinical experience and pediatric data. In the pivotal clinical study that led to FDA approval, 56 adults with acute invasive aspergillosis received caspofungin as "salvage" therapy after failing primary therapy for more than a week or developing significant nephrotoxicity. More than 40% of the patients had a favorable response to therapy.[130] A follow-up report found 45% (37/83) had a complete or partial response, including 50% (32/64) with pulmonary aspergillosis and 23% (3/13) with disseminated infection.[131]

A study of therapy comparing caspofungin with conventional amphotericin B in 224 adults with invasive candidiasis found that the response to caspofungin (81%) was slightly better than response to amphotericin B (65%).[132] Caspofungin was as effective as amphotericin B against all the major species of *Candida*. Mortality was similar in both groups, and the proportion of patients with drug-related adverse events was substantially higher in the amphotericin B group. More recently, caspofungin (n=556) was compared with liposomal amphotericin B (n=539) in febrile neutropenic patients; overall success was virtually identical (~33%).[133]

A multicenter retrospective survey in Germany analyzed 53 immunocompromised pediatric patients considered to require caspofungin therapy[129] for refractory infection (n=35), intolerance of standard agents (n=7), or as the best perceived therapeutic option (n=11). In 13 evaluable patients with proven infection, complete responses (4/13), partial responses (6/13), or stabilization (2/13) were observed. The majority (11/13) of patients on empiric therapy completed without breakthrough fungal infection. Overall survival was 72% at end of therapy and 64% (44 evaluable patients) at 3 months post-end of therapy.[129]

A multicenter, open-label comparative study evaluating the safety, tolerability, and efficacy of caspofungin in children with documented *Candida* or *Aspergillus* infections found similarly high rates of success as seen in adult patients. The drug also appears to be well tolerated in children.[134] There have been limited reports of caspofungin use in neonates with invasive candidiasis. In one report, caspofungin was added to either amphotericin B, fluconazole, or 5-FC in 13 infants with a median birthweight of 800 grams whose candidemia persisted despite conventional antifungal therapy. After addition of caspofungin, blood sterilization occurred in a mean of 3 days.[135] Caspofungin has been studied in 18 children <3 months of age and a dose of 25 mg/m²/day appeared to be similar to adults receiving a maintenance dose of 50 mg/day.[136] However, large scale neonatal trials with caspofungin have not been done.

Micafungin

Pharmacology and toxicities. Micafungin (Mycamine, Astellas PharmaUS, Inc., Deerfield, IL) is an echinocandin lipopeptide compound[49,137,138] with a half-life of approximately 12 hours. As with other echinocandins, it is fungicidal against *Candida* and fungistatic against *Aspergillus*.[139] The highest drug concentrations of this agent are detected in the lung, followed by the liver, spleen, and kidney. Micafungin was undetectable in the CSF, with low levels detected in the brain tissue, choroidal layer, and vitreous fluid, but not the aqueous fluid of the eye.[117]

One open-label study assessed the safety and pharmacokinetics of micafungin in young infants with suspected *Candida* infection and found that micafungin dosages of 7 and 10 mg/kg/day are well tolerated and provide exposure levels that have been shown in animal models to be adequate for CNS coverage.[140] This compares with a dose of 15 mg/kg, which has been shown to be equivalent in premature infants.[141]

A phase I pediatric (2 to 17 years old) study in patients with fever and neutropenia found that doses up to 4 mg/kg/day were well tolerated with no side effects. A total of 78 children (mean age 7.1 years) received at least one dose of micafungin with no signs of nephrotoxicity or hepatotoxicity. The micafungin pharmacokinetics were dose proportional over the range tested and mean half-life values were relatively constant on days 1 and 4.[142] Dosing in children under the age of 8 years old appears to yield a 1.3 to 1.5 times greater clearance of micafungin, resulting in the likely need for an increased dose in this age cohort. In general, the terminal half-life of micafungin does not change appreciably in pediatric versus adult patients, and the volume of distribution is only slightly higher in children.[143] These early pharmacokinetic studies, and a recent population pharmacokinetic analysis,[144] show that a relatively high weight-based dose is required, especially in smaller infants and neonates.

Clinical experience and pediatric data. A study of micafungin in combination with a second antifungal agent in pediatric and adult bone marrow transplant recipients with invasive aspergillosis revealed an overall complete or partial response of 39% in adult patients and 38% in pediatric (n=16) patients.[145] Other studies have demonstrated the efficacy of micafungin in the primary therapy of esophageal candidiasis,[146] and as rescue therapy in those failing to respond to first-line antifungal agents.[147] In an open-label noncomparative study of new or refractory candidemia including 15% (18/119) pediatric patients, the overall complete or partial response was 85% (86/101) in adults but only 72% (13/18) in pediatric patients,[148] possibly due to inadequate dosing in children.

A study comparing prophylaxis in 882 stem cell transplant recipients found that micafungin (80%) was more effective than fluconazole (74%) for preventing yeast and mold infections.[149] This study included 84 patients <16 years and found the success in those patients was 69% (27/39) in the micafungin arm and 53% (24/45) in the fluconazole arm. These values are both worse than the results for patients aged 16 to 64 years, where micafungin was 81% effective and fluconazole was 76% effective.

A pediatric substudy as part of a double-blind, randomized, multinational trial comparing micafungin (2 mg/kg) with liposomal amphotericin B (3 mg/kg) as first-line treatment of invasive

candidiasis found similar efficacy.[150] At present there are no large-scale clinical trial reports of micafungin in neonates, but a large phase III trial comparing micafungin with amphotericin B for neonatal candidiasis is underway currently.

Anidulafungin

Pharmacology and toxicities. Anidulafungin (Eraxis, Pfizer Inc., New York, NY) has linear pharmacokinetics,[103] with the longest half-life of all the echinocandins (approximately 18 hours).[119,151] Its in vitro activity is similar to that of the other echinocandins.[152] Neither end-stage renal impairment nor dialysis substantially alters the pharmacokinetics of anidulafungin.[153] Tissue concentrations after multiple dosing were highest in lung and liver, followed by spleen and kidney, with measurable concentrations in the brain tissue similar to the other echinocandins. The pharmacokinetics showed approximately 6-fold lower mean peak concentrations in plasma, and 2-fold lower area under the curve values compared to values with similar doses of caspofungin and micafungin.

Clinical experience and pediatric data. Adult dosage of anidulafungin is 50 mg/day for esophageal candidiasis and 100 mg/day for invasive mycoses. A phase I/II dose escalation study of anidulafungin involving 5 centers enrolled children with persistent neutropenia who were at risk for invasive fungal infection and data were determined in 12 patients (0.75 mg/kg/day) and 7 patients (1.5 mg/kg/day) following the first and fifth dose of anidulafungin. No drug-related serious adverse events were observed; one patient had fever and one patient had rash/facial erythema that resolved with slowing the infusion rate. Anidulafungin in pediatric patients was well tolerated and can be dosed based on body weight. Pediatric patients receiving 0.75 mg/kg/day or 1.5 mg/kg/day have pharmacokinetics similar to adults receiving 50 or 100 mg/day, respectively.[154] This important fact separates anidulafungin from caspofungin, which necessitated a higher dosing based on body-surface area.

A study of 601 patients with esophageal candidiasis compared anidulafungin with oral fluconazole and found endoscopic success exceeding 95%.[155] A subsequent study found superiority of anidulafungin over fluconazole for candidemia, solidifying the role of the echinocandins in treating invasive candidiasis.[156]

SUMMARY

For over 40 years, there has been limited progress in the treatment of invasive fungal infections and the field of pediatric antifungal therapy has been largely ignored. Although conventional amphotericin B deoxycholate was the drug of choice for many invasive fungal infections for years, newer, safer, and more effective agents have largely relegated it to antiquity. Lipid formulations of amphotericin B have reduced the toxicity of conventional amphotericin B and these agents still have a role in the management of several specific diseases, such as zygomycosis. The newer triazoles – voriconazole and posaconazole – have expanded our options for therapy against mold infections such as invasive aspergillosis. The echinocandins offer a new class of antifungal therapy where for the first time there is no cross-reactivity with a human substrate, leading to very minimal toxicities.

There are now numerous nuances to choosing the correct antifungal, including the fungistatic versus fungicidal activity of certain antifungal classes against the various genera or even species of fungal pathogens. One of the most important aspects for successful management of pediatric invasive fungal infections is the development of a solid understanding of the differences in the pharmacokinetics of the drug in children and adults, which results in more optimal dosing. Unfortunately, there have been very few antifungal studies conducted in children. Consequently, most information for the pediatrician has been extrapolated from adult data. Through the efforts of dedicated clinicians and collaboration, pediatric indications and dosing strategies will eventually be discovered that will directly benefit pediatric patients.

Topical Antimicrobial Agents

Jane M. Gould and Gail L. Rodgers

Topical antimicrobial therapy dates back to ancient times, when a wide variety of substances such as grease, lint oil, wine, and metallic salts were applied to wounds. Since then, topical antibiotics have been developed. They are most frequently used to treat infections affecting the skin and mucous membranes. Agents include topical preparations of parenterally administered antibiotics, as well as antibiotics and antiseptics not given by any other route because of their toxicity. As a general principle, agents used topically should not be those relied upon for systemic use as resistance develops rapidly. Precise recommendations for use of topical agents are limited by the difficulty of in vitro assays, establishment of breakpoints for susceptibility, effect of the vehicle on delivery, and lack of clinical efficacy trials. Antifungal and antiviral agents are described in Chapter 295, Antiviral Agents, and Chapter 296, Antiparasitic Agents.

OPHTHALMIC THERAPY

Antibiotics administered topically are used for the prophylaxis and treatment of many ophthalmologic pathogens. Topical agents are used for the prophylaxis of neonatal conjunctivitis, perioperative infections, and ophthalmologic trauma such as corneal abrasions, foreign bodies, and ruptured globes. They are used for the treatment of blepharitis, chronic dacryocystitis, conjunctivitis, corneal ulcers, and endophthalmitis. Selection of an antimicrobial agent should be based on its activity against the most likely pathogenic organisms and lack of adverse effects (Table 294-1).[1-14] Different routes of administration (topical, subconjunctival, retrobulbar, and intravitreal) can be used, depending on the site of infection. Formulations are available as ointments or solutions (Table 294-2). To optimize antibiotic delivery, devices impregnated with antibiotics, such as the collagen shield, have been developed. These devices act as reservoirs that prolong contact of the antibiotic with the ocular surface so that sustained antibiotic concentrations are delivered to the affected area.[15]

Blepharitis

Blepharitis is commonly caused by *Staphylococcus aureus*, and treatment consists of the topical application of an antistaphylococcal agent in ointment form to the eyelids.

Dacryocystitis

Acute dacryocystitis and dacryoadenitis are commonly caused by *S. aureus* and should be treated systemically. Chronic dacryocystitis is not usually infectious, but infection can occur secondary to stasis and obstruction of the lacrimal duct. Treatment consists of relief of the obstruction by irrigation of the lacrimal outflow tract. The use of a topical antibiotic is controversial.[6]

Conjunctivitis

Acute conjunctivitis in children is bacterial in >50% of cases;[16] nontypable *Haemophilus influenzae* and *Streptococcus pneumoniae* are the most common causative agents. Although conjunctivitis is usually self-limited, treatment with topical antibiotics has been shown to shorten the duration of clinical illness.[17] Treatment consists of a topical agent active against major pathogens in solution form (sulfacetamide, erythromycin, azithromycin, gentamicin, gatifloxacin, ofloxacin, or besifloxacin). Topical preparations of aminoglycosides and fluoroquinolones have been shown to be equally efficacious (84% to 90%) in the treatment of acute conjunctivitis,[18] but in view of the high spontaneous cure rate, these topical preparations should be reserved for serious infections when gram-negative bacilli are causative, especially *Pseudomonas aeruginosa*. It is important to keep in mind, however, that drops are washed out rapidly in a crying child. In infants, ointments may be preferable for ease of application, but the resultant visual blurring can be discomforting to older children. When otitis media accompanies conjunctivitis, as is frequently the case with nontypable *H. influenzae*, treatment should consist of the administration of an appropriate antibiotic orally; concomitant topical therapy is not necessary. Such is also the case for chlamydial conjunctivitis, which is treated systemically to eradicate nasopharyngeal colonization; topical therapy is not necessary.

Neonatal Conjunctivitis

Antibiotic prophylaxis has greatly reduced the incidence of ophthalmia neonatorum in the United States. The use of topical silver nitrate reduced the incidence of gonococcal ophthalmia neonatorum from 10% to 0.3%.[19] It does not prevent chlamydial conjunctivitis, which is presently the most common cause of neonatal conjunctivitis.[20] One percent silver nitrate causes chemical conjunctivitis in 10% of patients;[21] 0.5% erythromycin ointment or 1% tetracycline may be the preferred prophylactic agent.[22-24] Each is ineffective for the prevention of chlamydial infection. A 2.5% povidone-iodine solution was shown in a study in Kenya to be effective in preventing ophthalmia neonatorum; it demonstrated efficacy against *Neisseria gonorrhoeae* similar to that of erythromycin or silver nitrate and was superior to these drugs against *Chlamydia trachomatis*; the incidence of the latter was reduced to 5.5% (as compared with 7.4% for erythromycin and 10.5% for silver nitrate).[12,25]

Keratitis

Bacterial infections of corneal ulceration are rare in children and most commonly follow corneal abrasion, a scratch, or a foreign-body injury. The usual bacterial etiologies include *S. aureus*, coagulase-negative staphylococci (CoNS), *S. pneumoniae*, *Moraxella catarrhalis*, and gram-negative bacilli, especially *P. aeruginosa*.[26] Adequate evaluation and treatment are essential to prevent permanent corneal injury. For existing infection, Gram stain and culture of the ulcer surface are essential to determine the causative organism, direct antimicrobial therapy, and distinguish bacterial keratitis from herpetic and fungal keratitis. Treatment consists of the frequent administration of antimicrobial agents topically by subconjunctival instillation.

The achievable concentration of antibiotic in corneal stroma after topical application is limited because the corneal epithelium is a barrier to drug transport. The damaged cornea allows greater penetration of antibiotics into the cornea, and lipophilic antibiotics such as chloramphenicol achieve higher concentrations. "Fortified drops" are solutions prepared extemporaneously to contain higher concentrations of antibiotics than available commercially or antibiotics not commercially available for ophthalmic application; they are frequently used for the treatment of bacterial corneal ulcers and endophthalmitis.[6,13] Some commonly used "fortified drops" are listed in Table 294-2.

Subconjunctival injection bypasses the corneal epithelial barrier and provides high concentrations of agents in the cornea. Unfortunately, levels fall rapidly, so readministration is required.

TABLE 294-1. Commercially Available Topical Ophthalmic Antimicrobial Agents

	Concentration	Mechanism of Action	Spectrum of Activity		Chlamydia	Anaerobes	Adverse Effects
			Gram-Positive Organisms	Gram-Negative Organisms[a]			
SINGLE AGENTS							
Azithromycin (Azasite)	Solution, 1%	Inhibits protein synthesis	+++	++	+	+	Skin and eye irritation, altered taste
Bacitracin (generic)	Ointment, 500 U/g	Inhibits early steps in peptidoglycan biosynthesis, thus inhibiting cell wall synthesis; also changes membrane permeability	+++ (group B streptococci, usually R)	+ (Enterobacteriaceae and Pseudomonas spp. R)	ND	++	Hypersensitivity skin reactions
Besifloxacin (Besivance)	Solution, 0.6%	Inhibits DNA gyrase and topoisomerase IV	+++	+++	+++	+	Hyper sensitivity reaction
Chloramphenicol (generic)	Ointment, 1% Solution, 0.5%	Inhibits protein synthesis	++ (Staphylococcus aureus R)	+++ (Pseudomonas spp. R)	++	++	Absorbed into blood; can cause aplastic anemia[3]
Ciprofloxacin (Ciloxan)	Ointment, solution, 0.3%	Inhibits DNA gyrase	++	+++	+++	–	Local burning and discomfort; reversible crystalline corneal deposits[4]
Erythromycin (generic)	Ointment, 0.5%	Inhibits protein synthesis	+++	+/– (Enterobacteriaceae and Pseudomonas spp. R)	++	+	
Gatifloxacin (Zymar)	Solution, 0.3%	Inhibits DNA gyrase and topoisomerase IV	+++	++	+++	+	
Gentamicin (generic)	Ointment, 0.3% Solution, 0.3%	Inhibits protein synthesis	–	+++	ND	–	Eyelid and facial dermatitis in 10%; keratitis with chronic use[4]
Levofloxacin (Quixen)	Solution, 0.5%	Inhibits DNA gyrase and topoisomerase IV	+++	++	+++	–	
Moxifloxacin (Vigamox)	Solution, 0.5%	Inhibits DNA gyrase and topoisomerase IV	+++	++	+++	–	
Norfloxacin (Chibroxin)	Solution, 0.3%	Inhibits DNA gyrase	++	+++	++	–	Local burning and discomfort; reversible crystalline corneal deposits[4]
Ofloxacin (Ocuflox)	Solution, 0.3%	Inhibits DNA gyrase	++	++	++	–	Local burning and discomfort
Povidone-iodine	Solution, 2.5%	Unknown	+++	+++	++	++	Discolors conjunctiva temporarily
Silver nitrate	Solution, 1%	Inhibits DNA replication; modifies cell membrane and disrupts superficial cells[11]	+	++	–	ND	Chemical conjunctivitis in 10%
Sulfacetamide (generic)	Ointment, 10% Solution, 10%, 15%, 30%	Inhibits folic acid synthesis	++	++ (Pseudomonas spp. R)	++	–	Painful; absorption can cause Stevens–Johnson syndrome[5]
Sulfisoxazole diolamine (Gantrisin)	Ointment, 4% Solution, 4%	Inhibits folic acid synthesis	++	++ (Pseudomonas spp. R)	++	–	Same as sulfacetamide
Tetracycline (Achromycin)	Solution, 1%	Inhibits protein synthesis	+	++ (Pseudomonas spp. R)	++	+	Photosensitivity

Continued

TABLE 294-1. Commercially Available Topical Ophthalmic Antimicrobial Agents—cont'd

	Concentration	Mechanism of Action	Spectrum of Activity		Chlamydia	Anaerobes	Adverse Effects
			Gram-Positive Organisms	Gram-Negative Organisms[a]			
Tobramycin (generic)	Ointment, 0.3% Solution, 0.3%	Inhibits protein	−	+++	+	−	Eyelid/facial dermatitis in 10%; keratitis with chronic use[4]
COMBINATION PREPARATIONS							
Neomycin + Polymyxin B/ bacitracin + Polymyxin B + Polymyxin B/ gramicidin	Various concentrations	Inhibits protein synthesis	+	++ (Pseudomonas spp. R)	ND	−	Allergic reaction manifested as follicular conjunctivitis
Polymyxin B + Bacitracin + Neomycin + Neomycin/ bacitracin + Neomycin/ gramicidin + Oxytetracycline + Trimethoprim	Various concentrations	Attaches to cell membrane, with disruption of osmotic properties leading to cell death	−	+++ (Neisseria gonorrhoeae R, Proteus spp. R)	ND	+ (Bacillus fragilis R)	Adverse effects of components
Trimethoprim + Polymyxin B	Various concentrations	Inhibits dihydrofolic acid reductase	++	++ (Pseudomonas spp. and Neissseria gonorrhoeae R)	ND	−	Adverse effects of components
Gramicidin + Polymyxin B/ neomycin	Various concentrations	Uncouples oxidative phosphorylation	++	−	ND	−	Adverse effects of components

+++, excellent activity and spectrum; ++, good activity and spectrum; +, fair activity and spectrum; −, no activity; ND, no or limited data; R, resistant.

[a]Gram-negative organisms include Haemophilus spp., Neisseria spp., Enterobacteriaceae, and Pseudomonas spp., unless otherwise indicated.

Data from references 1–14.

2006 Physician's Desk Reference, 60th ed. Thomson PDR, Montvale, NJ.

TABLE 294-2. Commonly Used Fortified Drops

Antibiotic	Concentration
Amikacin	6.7 mg/mL
Bacitracin	9600 U/mL
Carbenicillin	6.2 mg/mL
Cefazolin	33 mg/mL
Gentamicin	14 mg/mL
Neomycin	33 mg/mL
Oxacillin	66 mg/mL
Penicillin G	333,000 U/mL
Pipercillin	12.5 mg/mL
Ticarcillin	6.3 mg/mL
Tobramycin	5 mg/mL
Vancomycin	31 mg/mL

Adapted from Baum JL. Antibiotic use in ophthalmology. In: Tasman W, Jaeger EA (eds) Duane's Clinical Ophthalmology. Philadelphia, Lippincott-Raven, 1989, pp 1–20.

Collagen shields impregnated with antibiotics are an alternative to subconjunctival injection because they deliver therapeutic levels of antibiotic to the cornea in a less invasive way.[15] Collagen shields have also been demonstrated to promote epithelial healing after surgical procedures involving the anterior segment.[27,28] Frequent topical use of fortified drops may produce a more sustained concentration, and such application is easier to implement. The average drop volume far exceeds the capacity of the inferior cul-de-sac of the eye; spillage or drainage into the lacrimal sac is rapid.[6] Drug draining through the lacrimal system is absorbed systemically and may be of sufficient amount in patients with hepatic or renal insufficiency to cause toxicity. To avoid lacrimal sac drainage and systemic absorption, the puncta in the medial canthal area can be occluded by digital pressure for 15 to 20 seconds after administration of an eyedrop.[4] Systemic antibiotics have little role in the treatment of bacterial corneal ulcers because concentrations achieved in the cornea are inferior to those attained by topical or subconjunctival administration.

Endophthalmitis

Infectious endophthalmitis is a virulent, sight-threatening infection of intraocular tissue. Prompt diagnosis and therapy are essential. Risk factors for endophthalmitis include ocular trauma or surgery, periocular infection, and systemic infection.[29,30] Common bacterial pathogens include S. aureus, CoNS, streptococci, and gram-negative bacilli. When endophthalmitis is suspected, aspiration of vitreous humor for culture is essential to determine the pathogen or pathogens and to guide antimicrobial therapy. The corneal epithelium, retinal capillaries, and pigmented retinal epithelium provide mechanical barriers to antimicrobial penetration into the vitreous humor. In addition, the flow of aqueous humor anteriorly impairs the movement of drugs to the vitreous humor. Thus, administration of antibiotics by the topical, subconjunctival, or systemic route may not achieve an adequate intravitreal concentration (Table 294-3). The optimal route of administration

TABLE 294-3. Concentrations of Antimicrobial Agents in Human Eyes after Systemic Administration

Antibiotic	Dosage	Vitreous Humor (Uninflamed Eye) (μg/mL)
Cefazolin	2 g IV	0.33–4.6
Cefotaxime	1 g IM	<0.2
Chloramphenicol	3 g PO	5–15
Ciprofloxacin	200 mg IV × 3	0.16–0.44
	750 mg PO	
Gentamicin	1.6 mg/kg IM	<0.2
Imipenem	1 g IV	1.4–3.6[a]
Oxacillin	2 g IV	<0.25–4.5

IM, intramuscular; IV, intravenous; PO, orally.

[a]A concentration of 13 μg/mL was achieved in one patient with an inflamed eye.

Adapted from Barza M. Antibacterial agents in treatment of ocular infections. Infect Dis Clin North Am 1989;3:533.

TABLE 294-4. Suggested Doses of Antibiotics for Subconjunctival and Intravitreal Administration[a]

Antibiotic	Dose Subconjunctival (mg)	Dose Intravitreal (μg)	Interval (hours)
Amikacin[b]	25	400	24–48
Ampicillin	50–150	500–5000	48
Aztreonam	100		
Bacitracin[c]	5000–10,000 U		
Carbenicillin	100	250–2000	16–24
Cefazolin	100	2000–2500	24
Ceftazidime	200	2000–2200	72
Ceftriaxone	100	3000	48–72
Cefuroxime	100	250	
Chloramphenicol	50–100	2000	24
Clindamycin	15–150	1000	24
Erythromycin	100	500	24
Gentamicin	10–40[d]	100–400	72–96
Kanamycin	30	400	72
Neomycin	125–500		
Oxacillin		500	24
Penicillin G	0.5–1 million U	600 U	24
Polymyxin B[c]	100,000 U		
Ticarcillin	100–150		
Tetracycline	2.5–5		
Tobramycin	10–40	100–400	72–96
Vancomycin[c]	25	1000–2000	72

[a]Doses are for adults; guidelines for intravitreal injections have not been established in neonates or infants.

[b]Less toxic to the retina than gentamicin or tobramycin when given intravitreally.

[c]May cause tissue necrosis/sloughing when administered subconjunctivally.

[d]In children <40 kg, the dose should not exceed half of a single IV dose.

Data from Baum JL. Antibiotic use in ophthalmology. In: Tasman W, Jaeger EA (eds) Duane's Clinical Ophthalmology. Philadelphia, Lippincott-Raven, 1989, pp 1–20; and Gigliotti F, Hendley JO, Morgan J, et al. Efficacy of topical antibiotic therapy in acute conjunctivitis in children. J Pediatr 1984;104:623.

is intravitreal instillation (see Chapter 86, Endophthalmitis). Many parenterally administered antibiotics have been used for intravitreal injection (Table 294-4). Disadvantages of intravitreal administration are possible damage to the retina and intraocular structures, as well as the need for anesthesia for injection. Adjuvant therapy consists of subconjunctivally and parenterally administered antibiotics, vitrectomy, and corticosteroids (systemically, intraocularly, or by both routes).[13]

For treatment of endogenous fungal endophthalmitis, systemically administered antifungal agents have variable penetration into the posterior segment of the eye. Therapeutic concentrations of fluconazole and voriconazole usually can be achieved, but not amphotericin B, posaconazole or the echinocandins.[31] Intravitreal injection of amphotericin B (5 to 10 μg) or voriconazole (100 μg) usually is used for sight-threatening involvement to achieve high local antifungal activity as rapidly as possible.

OTIC THERAPY

Topical antibiotic therapy is used in the treatment of otitis externa and chronic suppurative otitis media (CSOM) and as prophylaxis for surgery. Controlled studies documenting efficacy or assessing safety are generally lacking.

Otitis Externa

Otitis externa describes an inflammatory condition of the auricle, ear canal, or outer surface of the tympanic membrane.[32] Infectious etiologies include bacteria (most commonly S. aureus, P. aeruginosa, and anaerobic bacteria), fungi, and mycobacteria. Therapy for otitis externa consists of cleansing of the canal, elimination of pathogens, reduction of the accompanying inflammation and edema, symptomatic relief, restoration of the oil and water content of the skin, and elimination or control of predisposing factors.[32] The most commonly used topical antibiotics are listed in Table 294-5. Commercial preparations for the treatment of external otitis are combinations of broad-spectrum antibiotics, often with anti-inflammatory agents (Table 294-6). Topical preparations of ciprofloxacin (with hydrocortisone) and ofloxacin have been shown to be efficacious in the treatment of otitis externa,[37-40] thus leading to Food and Drug Administration (FDA) approval in patients 1 year and older. Topical antibacterial therapy for otitis externa should be used in conjunction with aural toilet because prolonged use of topical agents alone may induce fungal overgrowth.

Chronic Suppurative Otitis Media

CSOM is defined as otorrhea through a nonintact tympanic membrane that lasts more than 6 weeks and is unresponsive to medical management.[41] This condition is usually a complication of acute otitis media with chronic mastoiditis. The pathogens, however, are different in this condition, with P. aeruginosa, S. aureus, and anaerobic bacteria most commonly implicated. Therapy requires systemic antimicrobial agents in conjunction with aural toilet. A Cochrane Review of 24 randomized treatment trials of patients with perforated tympanic membranes and persistent otorrhea revealed that treatment of CSOM with aural toilet and topical antibiotics especially the fluoroquinolones is effective in eradicating bacteria from the middle ear and resolving otorrhea.[42]

A study in 44 children with tympanostomy tubes for CSOM who received topical otic therapy did not demonstrate excessive hearing loss, as measured by a change in bone conduction thresholds.[43] Despite the lack of extensive safety data, topical otic agents (see Table 294-5) have been used extensively, alone or in combination with systemic therapy, with apparent success and without

TABLE 294-5. Topical Otic Antimicrobial Agents

| Agent | Concentration | Mechanism | Spectrum of Activity | | Adverse Effects |
			Gram-Positive Organisms	Gram-Negative Organisms[a]	
Acetic acid	36% solution	Unknown	ND	*Pseudomonas aeruginosa*[33,34]	
Boric acid	2.75–5% solution	Unknown	ND; yeasts > bacteria[35]	ND	Marked systemic absorption can lead to shock and death
Ciprofloxacin (Cipro HC Otic)	Ciprofloxacin, 2 mg/mL Hydrocortisone, 10 mg/mL	Interferes with DNA gyrase	++	+++ *Pseudomonas aeruginosa*	Pruritus rarely
Colistin (polymyxin E)	3 mg/mL	Same as polymyxin	–	++ (*Pseudomonas* spp. R)	Renal toxicity; neurotoxicity if absorbed
Modified Burow solution (water, aluminum, and sodium acetate)		Unknown	ND	ND	
Neomycin	3.3–3.5 mg/mL	Inhibits protein synthesis	+	++ (*Pseudomonas* spp. R)	
Ofloxacin (Floxin)	0.3% solution	Interferes with DNA gyrase	++	+++	Taste perversion, pruritus, site irritation; dizziness, earache, and vertigo in ~1% of patients studied
Polymyxin B	10,000 U/mL	Attaches to cell membrane, with disruption of osmotic properties leading to cell death	–	+++	Renal toxicity if absorbed

+++, excellent activity and spectrum; ++, good activity and spectrum; +, fair activity and spectrum; –, no activity; ND, no or limited data; R, resistant.

[a]Gram-negative organisms include Haemophilus spp., Neisseria spp., Enterobacteriaceae, and Pseudomonas spp., or as otherwise indicated.

Data from references 7, 10, 33–36.

adverse effects attributed solely to their use. Cortisporin is used most commonly. Topical aminoglycosides also are used frequently because of their antipseudomonal activity. No otic preparations of aminoglycosides are commercially available; thus ophthalmic preparations are frequently substituted. Topical ofloxacin is

FDA-approved for the treatment of CSOM in individuals 12 years and older and for acute otitis media in children 1 year and older with tympanostomy tubes because of its microbiologic profile and favorable performance in clinical trials.[44,45] Combined medical therapy and surgical debridement are frequently necessary. Failure

TABLE 294-6. Commercially Available Topical Otic Preparations

Trade Name	Composition	Trade Name	Composition
Cipro HC Otic	Ciprofloxacin, 2 mg/mL Hydrocortisone, 10 mg/mL	Otic Tridesilon solution	Acetic acid, 2% Desonide, 0.5% (nonfluorinated corticosteroid)
Ciprodex	Ciprofloxacin, 3 mg/mL Dexamethasone, 1 mg/mL	Pedotic suspension	Neomycin sulfate, 3.5 mg/mL Polymyxin B sulfate, 10,000 U/mL Hydrocortisone, 10 mg/mL
Coly-Mycin S Otic	Colistin sulfate, 3 mg/mL Neomycin sulfate, 3.3 mg/mL Thonzonium bromide, 0.5 mg/mL Hydrocortisone acetate, 10 mg/mL		
		Star-Otic ear solution	Acetic acid, 2% Burow solution (aluminum acetate) Boric acid
Cortisporin (solution, suspension)	Neomycin, 3.5 mg/mL Polymyxin B, 10,000 U/mL Hydrocortisone, 10 mg/mL	Tobra Dex	Tobramycin, 0.3% Dexamethasone, 0.1%
Floxin	Ofloxacin, 0.3%	VōSol HC Otic	Acetic acid, 2% Hydrocortisone, 10 mg/mL
LazerSporin-C solution	Neomycin sulfate, 3.5 mg/mL Polymyxin B, 10,000 U/mL Hydrocortisone, 10 mg/mL	VōSol Otic	Acetic acid, 2%
Otic Domeboro solution	Acetic acid, 2% Modified Burow solution (water, aluminum acetate, and sodium acetate)		

of management or the presence of cholesteatoma is an indication for surgical intervention.

Prophylaxis after Tympanostomy Tube Placement

Topical otic therapy has been used as prophylaxis for otorrhea after tympanostomy tube placement. Studies performed to determine whether this strategy is efficacious have had conflicting results. The use of Cortisporin in one study[46] and a solution of polymyxin B, neomycin, sulfonamide, and hydrocortisone in another[47] proved to be efficacious, whereas the use of topical gentamicin after tympanostomy tube placement had no significant effect on subsequent otorrhea.[48]

THERAPY FOR SKIN INFECTIONS

Topical antibiotics are used for the prophylaxis and treatment of a wide variety of skin infections (Table 294-7). Topical

TABLE 294-7. Topical Antibiotics for Use on Skin

Agent (Trade Name)	Mechanism of Action	Spectrum of Activity				Adverse Effects
		Gram-Positive Organisms	Gram-Negative Organisms[a]	Anaerobes	Yeast	
Bacitracin[b] 400, 500 U/g (generic)	Inhibits early steps in peptidoglycan biosynthesis, inhibits cell wall synthesis; changes membrane permeability	+++ (group B streptococci R)	+ (Enterobacteriaceae R, *Pseudomonas* spp. R)	++	–	Hypersensitivity skin reactions
Clindamycin, 10 mg/mL (Cleocin)	Inhibits protein synthesis	+++	–	+++	–	Pseudomembranous colitis has been reported with topical use
Erythromycin, 2%, 3% (many preparations)	Inhibits protein synthesis	+++	++	–	–	
Fusidic acid, 2% (Fucidin)	Inhibits protein synthesis	+++	+ (Enterobacteriaceae R, *Pseudomonas* spp. R)	++	–	Resistance develops during therapy; not available in the United States
Gentamicin, 0.1%	Inhibits protein synthesis	+	+++	–	–	
Meclocycline, 1% (Meclan)	Inhibits protein synthesis	+	++ (*Pseudomonas* spp. R)		+	
Metronidazole, 0.75% (MetroGel)	Interacts with bacterial DNA; precise mechanism unknown	–	–	+++ (*Propionibacterium acnes* R)	–	
Mupirocin, 2% (Bactroban)	Inhibits protein synthesis by acting on bacterial isoleucyl transfer RNA synthetase	+++	+/–	–	–	Application to open wound can cause pain
Neomycin, 3.5 mg/g[b] (many)	Inhibits protein synthesis	+	++ (*Pseudomonas* spp. R)	–	–	Hypersensitivity reactions (rash) – uncommon
Polymyxin B[b]	Attaches to cell membrane, with disruption of osmotic properties leading to cell death	–	+++ (*Proteus* spp. R, *Serratia* spp. R)	+ (*Bacteroides fragilis* R)	+/– (in high concentrations)	Hypersensitivity reaction; renal toxicity if absorbed
Retapamulin 1% ointment (Altabax, Altargo)	Inhibits protein synthesis (novel site of action on 50S ribosomal subunit)	+++	–	+	–	Rare allergic contact dermatitis; localized irritation (pruritus)
Sulfacetamide, 10% (Novacet, Sulfacet-R)	Inhibits folic acid synthesis	++	++ (*Pseudomonas* spp. R)	–	–	Absorption can causes Stevens–Johnson syndrome
Tetracycline, 2.2 mg/mL (Topicycline)	Inhibits protein synthesis	+	++ (*Pseudomonas* spp. R)	+		Photosensitivity

+++, excellent activity and spectrum; ++, good activity and spectrum; +, fair activity and spectrum; –, no activity; R, resistant.

[a]Gram-negative organisms include Haemophilus spp., Neisseria spp., Enterobacteriaceae, and Pseudomonas spp., unless otherwise specified.

[b]Many commercial preparations combine bacitracin, neomycin, and polymyxin B.

Data from references 8, 10, 49–57.

TABLE 294-8. Antiseptics Used on Skin

| Agent (Trade Name) | Spectrum of Activity[a] | | | | Adverse Effects |
	Gram-Positive Organisms	Gram-Negative Organisms[b]	Anaerobes	Yeast	
Acid electrolytic water (AEW)	S	S			
Benzalkonium chloride (Lanax, Zephiran, many brands)	S	S[c]		S	Nosocomial gram-negative bacilli and yeast infections from open contaminated solutions
Benzethonium chloride (many brands)	S	S		S	
Benzoyl peroxide (many brands)	S				Irritation and dryness
Chlorhexidine gluconate, solutions 2% and 4% (Hibiclens)	S	S		S	Possible CNS toxicity if broad application to neonate
Clioquinol (Vioform)	S				
Hexachlorophene (pHisoHex)	S				CNS toxicity if broad application to neonate
Phenol (Castellani Paint, Anbesol, Campho-Phenique)	S	S		S	Hyperbilirubinemia in neonates; ? carcinogenic potential
Povidone-iodine (Betadine)	S	S	S	S	Excessive area of application can cause thyroid dysfunction
Triple dye (brilliant green, proflavine hemisulfate, gentian violet)	S				Can be deleterious to wound healing
Triclosan	S				Limited against gram-negative bacilli; may lead to Pseudomonas aeruginosa overgrowth

[a]S, susceptible; blanks indicate resistance or insufficient data.

[b]Gram-negative organisms include Haemophilus spp., Neisseria spp., Enterobacteriaceae, and Pseudomonas spp.

[c]Pseudomonas is frequently resistant.

Data from references 57, 62–68.

antimicrobial agents often are used at intravascular catheter sites to prevent infection. The most common conditions for which the use of topical therapy has been found to be efficacious are acne, impetigo, and burns.

Acne

Minor acne can be treated with topical antibiotics, keratolytics, and drying agents. Antibiotics active against *Propionibacterium acnes* are frequently used as adjunctive therapy. Topical erythromycin and clindamycin have been shown to decrease *P. acnes* colonization and to lessen the percentage of free fatty acids in surface lipids.[53] For more severe acne, systemic antibiotics (erythromycin, clindamycin, or tetracycline) and retinoids (topical and systemic) are added to the therapeutic regimen.

Impetigo

Impetigo is caused by *Streptococcus pyogenes* alone or in combination with *S. aureus*.[58,59] Topical therapy is sufficient for minor localized infection in a well child. Mupirocin has exquisite activity against these organisms and is the topical agent of choice for impetigo.[60] Retapamulin 1% ointment, FDA approved in 2007 for the treatment of impetigo secondary to *S. pyogenes* or methicillin-susceptible *S. aureus*, is a 1% semisynthetic pleuromutilin compound with in vitro activity against most gram-positive bacteria and anaerobes. Pleuromutilin may be active against some mupirocin-resistant *S. aureus* strains.[61] Systemic antibiotic therapy is required for a febrile or ill-appearing child (because of the possibility of bacteremia or toxin-mediated manifestations) or if there are multiple or deep lesions. When choosing antibiotic therapy, healthcare practitioners should bear in mind the increasing incidence of community-associated methicillin-resistant *S. aureus* (CA-MRSA) skin infections.

Prophylaxis and Treatment of Wounds

Although topical antibacterial agents are used commonly for the prophylaxis of minor cuts and abrasions, no study has demonstrated that their use prevents infection. In addition to topical antibiotics, antiseptic agents are used for cleansing and treating wounds. Antiseptic agents comprise a wide variety of substances that are applied to living tissues to inhibit or kill microorganisms. The mechanism of action of most agents is not clearly understood. Because methods of testing are not well standardized and it is difficult to make comparisons of antimicrobial activity between compounds, no quantification of the antimicrobial activity of antiseptic agents has been made. Table 294-8 lists antiseptics commonly used for the treatment of skin infections.

Topical agents such as mupirocin have been used intranasally in an attempt to eliminate colonization with *S. aureus*. Mupirocin is especially advantageous because of efficacy against MRSA. Unfortunately, increasing use has been associated with the emergence of mupirocin resistance and failure to eradicate CA-MRSA.[66]

THERAPY FOR BURNS

Infections are a leading cause of death in burn victims who are successfully resuscitated. The burn wound is often the source of infection in these patients. Aggressive, early surgical debridement and wound closure in combination with routine use of topical antimicrobial agents have contributed immensely to prevention and control of burn wound sepsis. Burn wound infection is defined as bacterial invasion into the underlying viable tissue and usually correlates with more than 10^5 colony-forming units per gram of tissue. Topical antimicrobial agents do not sterilize the wound, but decrease the number of colonizing bacteria and the risk of deeper bacterial invasion into underlying viable tissue.

BOX 294-1. Characteristics of an Ideal Topical Antimicrobial Agent

GENERAL

Painless on application
Nonallergenic
No systemic absorption
Long lasting
Ease of use
Inexpensive

PERTINENT TO BURN WOUNDS

Penetrates burn wounds to a sufficient depth
Prevents desiccation
Does not impair the ability to examine wounds
Controls bacterial proliferation
Does not promote bacterial resistance
Does not inhibit re-epithelization
Does not injure viable cells

BOX 294-2. Parenteral Agents Used Topically in the Care of Burns

ANTIBACTERIAL AGENTS	ANTIFUNGAL AGENTS
Amikacin	Amphotericin B
Cefoperazone	Fluconazole
Ciprofloxacin	Ketoconazole
Clavulanate potassium	Nystatin
Imipenem	
Kanamycin	
Norfloxacin	
Piperacillin	
Ticarcillin	
Tobramycin	
Vancomycin	

Thus, their major role is one of prophylaxis. For established burn wound sepsis, topical therapy is used in conjunction with aggressive surgical debridement and parenteral antibiotic therapy. Many topical agents are used, all differing in their antimicrobial spectrum of activity and side effects, but none is ideal. The characteristics of an ideal agent are listed in Box 294-1.

The most commonly used agents are shown in Table 294-9. The agent used most widely has been silver sulfadiazine because of its broad antibacterial spectrum and relatively minor side effects. Other nonconventional topical agents such as acetic acid, formalin, and honey are used occasionally.[33,34,92-96] To some extent, all topical antimicrobial agents inhibit the rate of wound epithelialization, but on balance, their prophylactic efficacy against burn wound infection merits use.[97,98] Although susceptibility testing can be performed by several methods (most commonly the Nathan agar well diffusion assay), such methods are poorly standardized for topical antimicrobial testing and results have varied widely.[70,71,99-103] In vitro results do not always correlate with clinical efficacy; thus, susceptibility testing is rarely used in clinical practice. Selection of agents is based on known or expected colonizing organisms and their presumed susceptibilities, timing of injury, knowledge of organisms indigenous to the burn unit, and possible adverse reactions of agents. In addition to the commonly used antimicrobial agents, preparations of systemically administered antibiotics are occasionally used topically when an infection is due to a resistant organism or when cultured autografts are used because many routine preparations can be toxic to keratinocytes. Several of the parenteral agents used topically are listed in Box 294-2.

The toxicity of antibiotics on cultured skin and skin substitutes varies extensively, and the choice of agents should be based on the manufacturer's guidelines and the antimicrobial susceptibility of the organisms isolated. Solutions of topical antimicrobial agents and parenteral antibiotics have been used via subeschar clysis (administration by needles under the eschar) for the treatment of burn wound infection, although this practice has been replaced to a great extent by early surgical intervention.

TABLE 294-9. Topical Antimicrobial Agents Used in the Treatment of Burns

Agent (Trade Name)	Mechanism of Action	Antimicrobial Activity					Adverse Effects
		Gram-Positive Organisms	Gram-Negative Organisms[a]	Anaerobes	Yeast		
Acetic acid	Unknown	ND	*Pseudomonas aeruginosa*	ND	ND		
Bacitracin, 400, 500 U/g (generic)	Inhibits early steps in peptidoglycan biosynthesis resulting in inhibition of cell wall synthesis; also changes cell membrane permeability	+++ (group B streptococci R)	+	++	−		Allergic reaction (rare)
Cerium nitrate, 2.2%	Unknown	+++	+++	ND	+++		Methemoglobinemia (rare); ? inactivates silver sulfadiazine
Chlorhexidine	Unknown	+++	+++	ND	+		Possible central nervous system toxicity if broad application
Fusidic acid, 2% (Fucidin)	Inhibits protein synthesis	+++	+ (Enterobacteriaceae, *Pseudomonas* spp. R)	++	−		Resistance develops during therapy; not available in the United States

Continued

TABLE 294-9. Topical Antimicrobial Agents Used in the Treatment of Burns—cont'd

Agent (Trade Name)	Mechanism of Action	Antimicrobial Activity				Adverse Effects
		Gram-Positive Organisms	Gram-Negative Organisms[a]	Anaerobes	Yeast	
Gentamicin, 0.1% (Garamycin)	Inhibits protein synthesis	+ (synergy for *Staphylococcus aureus* and *Enterococcus* spp.)	+++	–	–	High rate of systemic absorption with neuro/ototoxicities; resistance develops during therapy with possible cross-resistance to silver sulfadiazine
Mafenide acetate, 11.1% cream, 5% solution (Sulfamylon)	Unknown	+	+++	+++	+	Allergic reaction in 10%; painful on application; electrolyte disturbances; metabolic acidosis
Mupirocin, 2% (Bactroban)	Inhibits protein synthesis by irreversibly binding to bacterial isoleucyl transfer RNA synthesis	+++	+/– (*Pseudomonas* spp. R)	+/–	–	Some MRSA-resistant
Neomycin, 3.5 mg/g	Inhibits protein synthesis	+	++ (*Pseudomonas* spp. R)	–	–	Allergic reaction in 6–8%; renal toxicity; neuromuscular blockade
Nitrofurazone, 0.2% cream, solution (Furacin)	Inhibits several bacterial enzymes involved in carbohydrate metabolism	+++	+++	++	–	Contact dermatitis in 1%; fatal hypersensitivity (rare); fungal overgrowth; mild pain on application secondary to vehicle
Polymyxin B, 5000, 10,000 U/g	Attaches to cell membrane, with disruption of osmotic properties leading to cell death	–	+++ (*Proteus* spp. R; *Serratia* spp. R)	+/– (*Bacillus fragilis* R)	+/– (in high concentrations)	Allergic reaction (rare)
Povidone-iodine, 5% cream, 10% ointment (Betadine)	Unknown	+++	+++	++	++	Allergic reaction in 20%; inactivated by wound exudate; absorption of iodine leads to thyroid dysfunction; short antibacterial effect requires frequent reapplication
Silver nitrate, 0.5% solution	Silver ion inhibits DNA replication; modifies cell membrane	+	++	+	+	No penetration of burn eschar; causes a decrease in serum osmolality, sodium, potassium, chloride, and calcium; methemoglobinemia (rare); staining
Silver sulfadiazine, 1% cream (Silvadene, Thermazene)	Silver ion inhibits DNA replication; modifies cell membrane	++	+++	++	++	Allergic reaction in 5%; transient, reversible leukopenia in 5–15% (probably due to margination); moderate penetration into burn eschar; causes "pseudoeschar", a proteinaceous exudate confused with purulence; resistance of gram-negative bacilli (especially *Pseudomonas* spp.) develops; serum hyperosmolality secondary to propylene glycol in cream base

+++, excellent activity and spectrum; ++, good activity and spectrum; +, fair activity and spectrum; –, no activity; MRSA, methicillin-resistant Staphylococcus aureus; ND, no or limited data; R, resistant.

[a]Gram-negative organisms include Haemophilus spp., Neisseria spp., Enterobacteriaceae, and Pseudomonas spp., unless otherwise specified.

Data from references 33, 34, 69–91.

295 Antiviral Agents

David W. Kimberlin

The first antiviral compound to be licensed by the United States Food and Drug Administration (FDA) was idoxuridine for the topical treatment of herpes simplex virus (HSV) keratitis, in 1963. This was followed shortly by licensure of amantadine in 1966, as the first systemic antiviral compound, for the treatment of influenza A infection. During the 1970s, only vidarabine (1976) received licensure for the systemic treatment of HSV central nervous system (CNS) infections. The licensure of acyclovir in 1982 opened the field of clinical antiviral drug intervention and heralded the era of rapid development of new drugs.

In addition to antiretroviral drugs for the treatment of the human immunodeficiency virus (HIV), three additional non-HIV antiviral drugs were licensed in the 1980s: trifluridine (1980), ribavirin (1985), and interferon (1986). Ten non-HIV antiviral drugs were licensed in the 1990s: foscarnet (1991), rimantadine (1993), ganciclovir (1994), famciclovir (1994), valacyclovir (1995), topical penciclovir (1996), cidofovir (1996), palivizumab (1998), zanamivir (1999), and oseltamivir (1999). Additionally, lamivudine, which was approved originally as an HIV medication, was licensed for the treatment of chronic hepatitis B virus (HBV) infection in 1998. Fewer new antiviral agents were brought to market in the first decade of the 21st century, and all except valganciclovir were for the treatment of hepatitis B: valganciclovir (2001), tenofovir disoproxil fumarate (2001), adefovir dipivoxil (2002), pegylated interferon (2003), entecavir (2005), and telbivudine (2006). These antiviral agents have demonstrated efficacy in the treatment of infections caused by HSV, cytomegalovirus (CMV), varicella-zoster virus (VZV), HIV, respiratory syncytial

virus (RSV), influenza A and B, hepatitis B and C, human papillomavirus (HPV), and Lassa virus.[1] Major sites of action of antiviral agents are presented in Table 295-1. Mechanisms of antiviral resistance are presented in Table 295-2.

Non-HIV antiviral agents and interferons that are licensed currently by the FDA are the primary focus of this chapter. Monoclonal and polyclonal antibody preparations, also utilized in the treatment and prevention of viral infections, are addressed in pathogen-specific chapters and in Chapter 5, Passive Immunization.

SPECIFIC ANTIVIRAL AGENTS

Nucleoside and Nucleotide Analogues

Acyclovir (Acycloguanosine, Zovirax, ACV) and Valacyclovir (Valtrex)

Chemistry, mechanism of action, spectrum, and resistance. Acyclovir is a deoxyguanosine analogue with an acyclic side chain that lacks the 3′-hydoxyl group of natural nucleosides.[2] Following preferential uptake by infected cells, acyclovir is monophosphorylated by virus-encoded thymidine kinase. Subsequent diphosphorylation and triphosphorylation are catalyzed by host cell enzymes, resulting in acyclovir triphosphate concentrations that are 40 to 100 times higher in HSV-infected cells than in noninfected cells.[3] Acyclovir triphosphate prevents viral DNA

TABLE 295-1. Major Sites of Action of Antiviral Agents

Major Site of Action	Antiviral Agent	Indicated for Management of Infections Caused by
Viral entry, adsorption, penetration, or uncoating	Amantadine	Influenza A
	Rimantadine	Influenza A
Transcription or replication of viral genome	Acyclovir/valacyclovir	HSV, VZV
	Adefovir dipivoxil	HBV
	Cidofovir	CMV, HSV, HPV
	Entecavir	HBV
	Famciclovir/penciclovir	HSV, VZV
	Foscarnet	HSV, VZV, CMV
	Ganciclovir/valganciclovir	CMV
	Lamivudine	HBV, HIV
	Ribavirin	RSV, HCV, Lassa virus
	Telbivudine	HBV
	Tenofovir	HBV, HIV
	Trifluridine	HSV
	Vidarabine	HSV, VZV
Viral protein synthesis	Interferon	HPV, HBV, HCV
Viral assembly, release, or deaggregation	Interferon	RNA tumor viruses
	Oseltamivir	Influenza A and B
	Zanamivir	Influenza A and B

CMV, cytomegalovirus; HBV, hepatitis B virus; HCV, hepatitis C virus; HIV, human immunodeficiency virus; HPV, human papillomavirus; HSV, herpes simplex virus; RSV, respiratory syncytial virus; VZV, varicella-zoster virus.

TABLE 295-2. Mechanisms of Antiviral Resistance

Antiviral	Virus(es)	Mechanism of Resistance	Clinical Correlates of Resistance	Alternative Antiviral Agent(s)
Acyclovir Valacyclovir	HSV, VZV	Usually due to mutations in thymidine kinase gene resulting in absent or altered thymidine kinase; rarely due to mutation in DNA polymerase gene	Persistent or progressive infection due to resistant strains isolated from patients with severely compromised immunity (e.g., bone marrow transplant recipients and those with AIDS); isolates of HSV from healthy individuals described in those receiving long-term suppressive therapy	Foscarnet
Amantadine Rimantadine	Influenza A	Mutation in RNA sequence encoding for M2 protein transmembrane domain	Usually recovered from drug recipients within 2 days of starting therapy, and their infected household contacts; clinical relevance undefined	Oseltamivir Zanamivir
Cidofovir	CMV, HSV	Mutation in DNA polymerase gene	Only rare clinical isolates have been reported	Foscarnet
Famciclovir Penciclovir	HSV, VZV	Usually due to mutations in thymidine kinase gene resulting in absent or altered thymidine kinase; also can be due to mutation in DNA polymerase gene	Persistent or progressive infection due to resistant strains isolated from patients with severely compromised immunity (e.g., bone marrow transplant recipients and those with AIDS); isolates of HSV from healthy individuals described in those receiving long-term suppressive therapy	Foscarnet Acyclovir
Foscarnet	HSV, VZV, CMV	Mutations in viral DNA polymerase gene	Only rare clinical isolates have been reported	Acyclovir Cidofovir
Ganciclovir Valganciclovir	CMV	Decreased intracellular phosphorylation due to mutations in the CMV UL97 gene with decreased expression of CMV phosphotransferase enzymes or mutation in viral DNA polymerase gene	Responsible for severe, rapidly progressive infection in patients with severely compromised immunity (e.g., bone marrow transplant recipients and those with AIDS)	Foscarnet Cidofovir
Lamivudine	HBV	Mutation in HBV polymerase gene	Reappearance of HBV DNA in serum after its initial disappearance, although most patients continue to have lower serum HBV DNA and ALT levels compared with pretreatment levels	Adefovir Entecavir

AIDS, acquired immunodeficiency syndrome; ALT, alanine transferase; CMV, cytomegalovirus; HBV, hepatitis B virus; HSV, herpes simplex virus; VZV, varicella-zoster virus.

synthesis by inhibiting the viral DNA polymerase. In vitro, acyclovir triphosphate competes with deoxyguanosine triphosphate as a substrate for viral DNA polymerase. Because acyclovir triphosphate lacks the 3′-hydroxyl group required for elongation of the DNA chain, the growing chain of DNA is terminated. In the presence of the deoxynucleoside triphosphate complementary to the next template position, the viral DNA polymerase is functionally inactivated.[4] In addition, acyclovir triphosphate is a much better substrate for the viral polymerase than for cellular DNA polymerase, resulting in little incorporation of acyclovir into cellular DNA. The higher concentration of the active triphosphate metabolite in infected cells plus the affinity for viral polymerases result in the very low toxicity of acyclovir in noninfected host cells.

Acyclovir is most active in vitro against HSV, with activity against VZV being about 10-fold less but still substantial. Although Epstein–Barr virus (EBV) has only minimal thymidine kinase activity, EBV DNA polymerase is susceptible to inhibition by acyclovir triphosphate. Therefore, EBV is moderately susceptible to acyclovir in vitro. Activity against CMV is limited because CMV does not encode for thymidine kinase, and CMV DNA polymerase is poorly inhibited by acyclovir triphosphate. In vitro susceptibility of viruses to acyclovir depends on a number of factors, including cell line, viral inoculum, incubation conditions, and the specific assay system used. Currently, no standardized method of susceptibility testing is universally accepted, and therefore wide disparities in specific inhibitory concentrations of antiviral agents are reported. Given the limitations of susceptibility testing and variations in reporting, the relative activity of an antiviral agent is more meaningful than is the absolute inhibitory concentration. The relative activities of drugs used in the treatment of herpesvirus infections are summarized in Table 295-3.

Resistance of HSV to acyclovir has long been recognized. However, it has only become an important clinical problem during the past two decades. In some referral centers, 5% to 14% of HSV isolates from immunocompromised patients are resistant to acyclovir.[5] Viral resistance to acyclovir can result from mutations in either the viral TK gene or the viral DNA polymerase gene. Although these acyclovir-resistant isolates exhibit diminished virulence in animal models, among HIV-infected patients they can cause severe, progressive, debilitating mucosal disease and, rarely, visceral dissemination.[6,7] Acyclovir-resistant strains of HSV also have been recovered from patients receiving cancer chemotherapy, bone marrow and solid organ transplant recipients, children with congenital immunodeficiency syndromes, and neonates.[8,9] Although it is uncommon, genital herpes caused by acyclovir-resistant isolates has also been reported in immunocompetent hosts, who usually have received chronic acyclovir therapy.[10]

Acyclovir-resistant strains of VZV have also been reported. Resistance is due to mechanisms the same as those described for HSV isolates. Most acyclovir-resistant VZV strains have been isolated from HIV-infected children and adults who have profound depletion of CD4 cells ($\leq 100/mm^3$) and previously have received acyclovir therapy for prolonged periods of time.[11] Changes in the susceptibility of VZV isolates to acyclovir can develop after only 4 to 12 weeks.[8]

Foscarnet is the drug of choice for both HSV and VZV infections caused by acyclovir-resistant strains.[8]

Valacyclovir is the L-valyl ester of acyclovir that is rapidly converted to acyclovir after oral administration by first-pass metabolism in the liver.[12] Its mechanism of action, antiviral spectrum, and resistance are the same as those of its parent drug, acyclovir.

TABLE 295-3. Relative In Vitro Activity of Nucleoside Analogues against Herpesviruses

Virus	Acyclovir	Penciclovir	Vidarabine	Foscarnet	Ganciclovir
HSV-1	+++	++	++	++	+++
HSV-2	+++	++	++	++	+++
VZV	+++	+++	++	++	++
CMV	±	±	±	++	++
EBV	+	–	–	+	++

CMV, cytomegalovirus; EBV, Epstein–Barr virus; HSV, herpes simplex virus; VZV, varicella-zoster virus; +++, high degree of activity; ++, moderate degree of activity; +, minimal degree of activity; ±, minimal to no activity; –, no useful activity.

Pharmacokinetics. Acyclovir is available as a topical formulation, as oral formulations (capsules, tablets, and suspension), and as a sterile powder for intravenous infusion. The topical formulation licensed in the United States is an ointment, whereas a cream is available in Europe. Although these topical products are not absorbed systemically, a substantial concentration of the drug reaches the basal epidermis in cutaneous infections. Only 15% to 30% of the oral formulations of acyclovir is absorbed; peak concentrations of approximately 0.5 μg/mL are attained 1.5 to 2.5 hours after a 200 mg dose.[2,13] Higher doses result in higher serum concentrations, and food does not appear to alter the extent of absorption substantially. Steady-state concentrations of acyclovir after intravenous doses of 2.5 to 15 mg/kg range from 6.7 to 20.6 μg/mL. The disposition of acyclovir is not affected by the duration or frequency of dosing.

Systemically administered acyclovir is distributed widely, attaining high concentrations in the kidneys, lung, liver, heart, and skin vesicles; concentrations attained in the cerebrospinal fluid (CSF) are approximately 50% of those in the plasma.[2] Acyclovir readily crosses the placenta and also accumulates in breast milk. Protein binding ranges from 9% to 33% and is independent of plasma drug concentration. Less than 20% of acyclovir is metabolized to a biologically inactive metabolite; more than 60% of administered drug is excreted intact in the urine. The half-life of acyclovir is 2 to 3 hours in older children and adults and 2.5 to 5 hours in neonates with normal creatinine clearance (CrCl).[2] Elimination of acyclovir is prolonged in patients with renal dysfunction, with a half-life of approximately 20 hours in persons with end-stage renal disease.[14] Dosage modifications are necessary for those with CrCl <50 mL/min per 1.73 m² (for dosing guidelines for various degrees of renal dysfunction, see Table 295-4). Acyclovir is readily hemodialyzable. The mean plasma half-life in patients during hemodialysis is about 5 hours, requiring that patients receive an additional dose of acyclovir after each dialysis (Table 295-5).[15] The half-life of acyclovir is 13 to 18 hours during continuous ambulatory peritoneal dialysis (CAPD), and no supplemental dose is necessary after adjustment of the dosing interval.

After oral administration of valacyclovir, rapid and complete conversion to acyclovir occurs with first-pass intestinal and hepatic metabolism. The bioavailability of valacyclovir in adults exceeds 50%, which is three to five times greater than that of acyclovir.[16] Peak serum concentrations, attained about 1.5 hours after a dose has been given, are proportional to the amount of drug administered; they range from 0.8 to 8.5 μg/mL for doses of 100 to 2000 mg.[17] The area under the drug concentration time curve approximates that seen after intravenous acyclovir. All other pharmacokinetic characteristics are similar to those of acyclovir. Valacyclovir oral suspension has been studied in children 1 month to 12 years of age.[18] Bioavailability was estimated to be 45% to 51% in all age groups except those 3 months through 5 months of age, in whom the bioavailability is lower at 22%. Approximate dose proportionality in C_{max} and AUC was seen across the 10 mg/kg to 25 mg/kg dose range (i.e., dose normalized differences generally within ≤~30%) with the exception of children 2 years through 5 years of age, for whom a near doubling in C_{max} and AUC was noted with only a modest increase in dose from 20 to 25 mg/kg.[18]

Toxicity and drug interactions. Acyclovir consistently has demonstrated a favorable safety profile. The topical formulation can cause transient burning, especially when applied to ulcerated mucosal lesions. Oral acyclovir sometimes is associated with mild gastrointestinal upset, rash, and headache, but even long-term administration usually is well tolerated. Intravenous acyclovir is also well tolerated unless it extravasates at the injection site or is given too rapidly or to a dehydrated patient. Because of its alkalinity (pH 9 to 11), extravasation of drug can cause severe inflammation, phlebitis, and sometimes a vesicular eruption leading to cutaneous necrosis. Reversible nephrotoxicity occurs if acyclovir is given by rapid intravenous infusion or to patients who are poorly hydrated or who have pre-existing renal compromise. Obstructive nephropathy results from the formation of acyclovir crystals that precipitate in renal tubules. Other reported side effects of intravenous acyclovir include rash, sweating, nausea, headache, hematuria, and hypotension. The use of high doses of intravenous acyclovir (60 mg/kg per day) for the treatment of neonatal disease has been associated with neutropenia in some patients.[19]

The most serious side effect of acyclovir is neurotoxicity.[20] When this occurs, lethargy, confusion, hallucinations, tremors, myoclonus, seizures, extrapyramidal signs, and changes in state of consciousness develop within the first few days of starting therapy. Neurotoxicity usually occurs in subjects with compromised renal function who attain high serum concentrations of the drug.[21] Other risk factors may include concurrent administration of interferon or intrathecal methotrexate. Neurotoxic manifestations usually resolve spontaneously within several days after the discontinuation of acyclovir; hemodialysis may be useful in severe cases associated with high serum concentrations of the drug.

TABLE 295-4. Dosage Adjustment of Acyclovir in Individuals with Renal Dysfunction

Creatinine Clearance (mL/min per 1.73 m²)	Suggested Modifications of Standard Intravenous Dose	Suggested Modification of Standard Oral Dose
>50	No modification necessary	No modification necessary
25–50	Maintain unit dose, but increase the dosing interval by 50%	No modification necessary
10–25	Maintain unit dose, but double the dosing interval	Maintain unit dose, but double the dosing interval
0–10	Reduce dose by 50%, *and* double the dosing interval	Maintain unit dose, but triple the dosing interval

Data from Wagstaff et al.[2] and Laskin et al.[14]

TABLE 295-5. Dosage Adjustments Necessary for Antiviral Agents in Individuals with Renal Dysfunction[a]

	Creatinine Clearance Necessitating Dose Adjustment (mL/min per 1.73 m^2)	Need for Supplementary Dose Following Hemodialysis
Acyclovir	<50	Yes
Adefovir	<50	No[b]
Amantadine	<80	No
Entecavir	<50	No[b]
Famciclovir (for VZV)	<60	Yes
Famciclovir (for HSV)	<40	Yes
Foscarnet	<100	Yes
Ganciclovir	<80	Yes
Lamivudine	<50	Unknown
Oseltamivir	<30	Unknown
Ribavirin	–	No
Rimantadine	–	No

HSV, herpes simplex virus; VZV, varicella-zoster virus.

[a]Cidofovir dosing must be adjusted for renal dysfunction but is based on changes in creatinine from baseline. See section on cidofovir in this chapter for details.

[b]Administer recommended dose at the appropriate interval following hemodialysis.

Although acyclovir is mutagenic at high concentrations in some in vitro assays, it is not teratogenic in various animal models. Although acyclovir is not recommended for use in pregnant women, limited data suggest that such use is not associated with congenital defects or other adverse gestational outcomes.[22] The finding of neutropenia in infants given acyclovir orally to suppress HSV reactivation after neonatal infection is not well explained.

A limited number of adverse drug interactions have been reported with acyclovir use. Subjects being treated with both zidovudine and acyclovir can develop severe somnolence and lethargy. The likelihood of renal toxicity is increased when acyclovir is administered with nephrotoxic drugs, such as cyclosporine and amphotericin B. Concomitant administration of probenecid decreases renal clearance of acyclovir and prolongs its half-life; conversely, acyclovir can decrease the clearance of drugs, such as methotrexate, that are eliminated by active renal secretion.

The profiles of adverse effects and potential drug interactions observed with valacyclovir therapy are the same as those observed with acyclovir treatment. Neurotoxicity has not been reported in humans to date, although it has been observed in animal models.[12] Manifestations resembling thrombotic microangiopathy have been described in patients with advanced HIV disease receiving very high doses of valacyclovir, but the multitude of other medications being administered to such patients makes the establishment of a causal relationship between valacyclovir use and the manifestations difficult.[23]

Clinical uses and dosage. Acyclovir is effective for the treatment of infections caused by HSV and VZV in immunocompetent and immunocompromised hosts.[24] Table 295-6 outlines the infections for which acyclovir is effective, the recommended dosage, and the magnitude of anticipated benefits. Unless otherwise stated in the table, the anticipated benefits of acyclovir therapy are based on the results of randomized controlled trials.

Therapy clearly is indicated for life-threatening infections and for disease associated with severe morbidity and death, such as HSV encephalitis, neonatal HSV infections, and VZV infections in compromised hosts.[19,25-30] Acyclovir therapy also is indicated for mucocutaneous HSV infections in immunocompromised hosts and for disseminated HSV and VZV infections in otherwise normal hosts, including pregnant women.[31-33] Acyclovir is effective for the treatment of primary genital HSV infections,[34-37] reducing the median duration of viral shedding, pain, and length of time to complete healing.[38] Intravenous and oral acyclovir therapies are almost equally efficacious, with topical treatment providing less

benefit. Neither intravenous nor oral treatment with acyclovir for primary or recurrent genital HSV disease reduces the frequency of recurrences.[39-41] Acyclovir probably reduces the ocular morbidity of zoster ophthalmicus.[42] The advantages of treating previously healthy individuals with herpes labialis,[43,44] recurrent genital herpes,[37,39,45] varicella,[46-49] and herpes zoster[50,51] are less dramatic, and the treatment of patients with these conditions should be individualized.

In general, the favorable effects of therapy are more probable among those who begin acyclovir earlier, rather than later, after the onset of infection. For example, previously healthy persons with primary varicella may benefit only if acyclovir is begun within 24 hours of appearance of the first cutaneous lesions.[46-48] Benefit, however, can be observed in the treatment of severe, life-threatening infections caused by HSV and VZV, even if acyclovir is commenced several days after the onset of infection, provided that irreversible damage has not occurred.

Possible indications for prophylactic acyclovir therapy are summarized in Table 295-7. Prophylactic acyclovir is almost exclusively used for the suppression of HSV infections; its efficacy for CMV infections is inferior to that of ganciclovir.[52] The most frequent indication for long-term prophylactic therapy is in patients with frequently recurrent genital infections,[37] in whom daily administration of acyclovir reduces the frequency of recurrences by at least 75%. Acyclovir has been shown to maintain a high degree of efficacy and little toxicity even after more than 5 years of continuous suppressive therapy.[53] The use of prophylactic acyclovir therapy in pregnant women has been explored in several small studies,[54-56] but the numbers of patients evaluated to date are insufficient to prove definitively its safety or efficacy in this population. Brief courses of acyclovir can be given to HSV-1-infected individuals to suppress reactivation of HSV that predictably follows certain stimuli, such as exposure to ultraviolet radiation[57] or facial surgery.[58] Longer courses can be given to those with frequently recurrent oral HSV infections,[53,58-60] and to people after ocular HSV disease to prevent recurrence.[61] Prophylactic acyclovir also has proved to be a useful strategy for postponing the inevitable reactivation of HSV infection after severe immunosuppression of HSV-infected patients.[58] Anecdotal data suggest that prophylactic acyclovir can reduce the frequency of attacks of erythema multiforme temporally related to HSV.[62]

Data published in 2011 describe the benefit of oral acyclovir suppressive therapy following parenteral acyclovir therapy for acute neonatal HSV disease.[63] The NIAID Collaborative Antiviral

TABLE 295-6. Potential Indications for Acyclovir Use

Infection	Dosage	Anticipated Benefits	Factors Favoring Beneficial Effect of Therapy	Strength of Indication
Initial genital HSV	15 mg/kg per day IV in 3 divided doses for 5–7 days *or* 40–80 mg/kg per day (maximum 1000 mg/day) PO in 3–4 divided doses for 5–10 days[a]	4–12-day reduction in duration of viral shedding, 3–12-day reduction in time to healing, and 1–10-day reduction in duration of pain; therapy is not associated with reduced frequency of subsequent recurrences[34-36]	Intravenous, rather than oral, therapy; therapy for primary, rather than less severe first episode, nonprimary infections	++
Recurrent genital HSV	1000 mg/day in 5 divided doses for 5 days *or* 1600 mg/day in 2 divided doses for 5 days *or* 2400 mg/day in 3 divided *or* doses for 2 days[a]	1–2-day reduction in duration of viral shedding and time to healing; no difference in duration of pain or frequency of subsequent recurrences[39,45,346]	Initiation during prodromal phase of infection	±
Primary HSV labialis	2400 mg/m² per day PO in 4 divided doses for 10 days	6-day reduction in the duration of viral shedding and 2–4-day reduction in the duration of drooling, gum swelling, and healing of oral and cutaneous lesions[44]	Initiation within 4 days of onset of signs of infection	++
Recurrent HSV labialis	1000 mg/day PO in 5 divided doses for 5 days	0.5–2-day reduction in the duration of pain and time to healing[43]	Initiation during prodromal or erythema stage	±
Mucocutaneous HSV in compromised hosts	30 mg/kg per day IV in 3 divided doses for 7–14 days	60–80% reduction in the duration of viral shedding, 30–60% reduction in healing time and the duration of pain[33]	Recovery of immune function	+++
Viscerally disseminated HSV in pregnant women and transplant recipients	30 mg/kg per day IV in 3 divided doses for 7–14 days	Improved likelihood of recovery based on anecdotal reports, rather than controlled trials[31,32]		+++
HSV encephalitis	30–45 mg/kg per day IV in 3 divided doses for 14–21 days	Reduced mortality and improved long-term neurologic outcome[25]	High (>6) Glasgow Coma Score at time of initiation of therapy; young age (<30 years)	++++
Neonatal HSV	60 mg/kg per day IV in 3 divided doses for 14 (SEM) to 21 (CNS, disseminated) days	Reduced mortality and improved long-term neurologic outcome[19,27]	Infection limited to the skin, eye, and mucosal membranes; absence of seizures at initiation of therapy for CNS infection	++++
Primary varicella in normal children, adolescents, and adults	80 mg/kg per day (maximum 3200 mg/day) PO in 4 divided doses for 5 days	1–3-day reduction in new lesion formation and fever; reduced maximum number of lesions[46-48]	Initiation of therapy within 24 hours of onset of infection; older subjects and secondary cases in household benefit more than younger subjects and those with community-acquired infections	+/++
Disseminated varicella in previously healthy subjects	30 mg/kg per day IV in 3 divided doses for 7–10 days	Improved likelihood of recovery based on anecdotal reports, rather than controlled trials[347]		+++
Zoster in normal hosts	80 mg/kg per day (maximum 4000 mg/day) PO in 5 divided doses for 5–7 days	Reduced time to healing of skin lesions, duration of acute pain, and duration of viral shedding[50,51]	Initiation of therapy within 24–48 hours of onset of infection	+
Zoster ophthalmicus in normal hosts	80 mg/kg per day (maximum 4000 mg/day) PO in 5 divided doses for 5–7 days	Reduced incidence of keratitis and anterior uveitis[42]		++
Primary varicella in compromised hosts	30 mg/kg per day IV in 3 divided doses for 7–10 days	Reduced incidence of cutaneous and visceral dissemination; reduced duration of lesion formation and time to healing[27,28]	Initiation of therapy within 24–48 hours of onset of infection and mild degree of immunologic dysfunction	++++
Zoster in compromised hosts	30 mg/kg per day IV in 3 divided doses for 7–10 days	Reduced risk of cutaneous dissemination and visceral complications[26,30]	Initiation of therapy within 24–48 hours of onset of infection and mild degree of immunologic dysfunction	++++

CNS, central nervous system; HSV, herpes simplex virus; IV, intravenous; PO, orally; ±, benefit is limited, therefore therapy usually not indicated; +, benefit is consistent but limited, costs of therapy should be weighed against small amount of anticipated benefit and decision to treat individualized; ++, therapeutic benefit usually favors treatment; +++, therapy indicated, although supporting data not definitive; ++++, therapy is clearly indicated and is based on the results of controlled clinical trials.

[a]*Topical acyclovir is not recommended, since its effects on duration of viral shedding, pain, and lesions are much less than those of systemic therapy in patients with primary infections.*

TABLE 295-7. Potential Indications for Prophylactic Antiviral Therapy

Antiviral Agent	Clinical Indication	Expected Effect	Dosage
Acyclovir	Frequently recurrent genital HSV	70–90% reduction in frequency of clinical episodes of infection;[53,58,59] frequency of asymptomatic shedding also reduced, but not eliminated[348]	Start with 1000 mg/day in divided doses and slowly reduce to minimum effective dose; attempt withdrawal after 6–12 months; if symptoms recur, restart therapy
	Frequently recurrent HSV labialis	53% reduction in number of clinical recurrences[60]	400 mg bid for 4 months
	Skiers with histories of sun-induced recurrences of HSV labialis	73% reduction in risk of recurrence[57]	400 mg bid for 1 week
	Suppressive therapy following treatment of acute neonatal HSV disease	30% reduction in cutaneous recurrence (all disease categories); improved neurodevelopmental outcomes (CNS category)[63]	300 mg/m²/dose tid for 6 months; monitor absolute neutrophil counts at 2 and 4 weeks, then monthly during therapy
	Reactivations of HSV associated with serious systemic complications, such as erythema multiforme, aseptic meningitis, and eczema herpeticum	Reduction in the frequency of serious complications associated with HSV infection	Use is supported by theoretical benefit and anecdotal reports, rather than controlled trials;[58,62] dosage is empirical
	Dermabrasion of facial skin or surgery involving the trigeminal ganglion in patients previously infected with HSV-1	Reduction in the frequency of postoperative outbreaks of herpes labialis[58,62]	Use is supported by theoretical benefit and anecdotal reports, rather than controlled trials; dosage is empirical
	HSV-seropositive persons undergoing bone marrow or solid-organ transplantation or induction chemotherapy for hematologic malignancy	50–60% decrease in the number of herpetic recurrences during the time of drug administration[58]	500–750 mg/m² per day begun prior to transplantation or induction chemotherapy and continued for about 6 weeks thereafter; intravenous therapy initially and oral therapy when tolerated
	CMV-seropositive persons undergoing bone marrow or solid-organ transplantation	As much as 50% reduction in the frequency of CMV infection and disease in CMV-seropositive recipients[349] and, to a lesser extent, in recipients at risk for primary infection;[350] however, ganciclovir is drug of choice[57]	1500 mg/m² per day begun prior to transplantation and continued for 1–3 months thereafter; intravenous therapy initially, and oral therapy when tolerated
Ganciclovir	CMV-seropositive solid-organ transplant recipients	Reduction in frequency of CMV disease	10 mg/kg per day in 2 divided doses, started several days before transplantation and continued for 2–3 weeks after transplantation; 5 mg/kg per day in single dose thereafter
	CMV-seropositive renal or liver transplant recipients beginning OKT3 suppressive therapy	Reduction in frequency of CMV disease	10 mg/kg per day in 2 divided doses for 2–3 weeks after OKT3 initiated
	Bone marrow transplant recipients with positive CMV surveillance culture (see text)	Reduction in frequency of CMV disease	10 mg/kg per day in 2 divided doses for 2–3 weeks after transplantation; 5 mg/kg per day in single dose thereafter

CMV, cytomegalovirus; HSV, herpes simplex virus.

Study Group conducted an evaluation of 6 months of oral acyclovir suppression following neonatal herpes. Subjects with neonatal HSV CNS disease who were randomized immediately at the conclusion of intravenous therapy to oral acyclovir for suppression had more favorable neurodevelopmental outcomes at 12 months of age compared with subjects in whom antiviral suppression was delayed until cutaneous recurrences were noted. Additionally, suppressive oral acyclovir therapy delayed the development of cutaneous recurrences in all categories of neonatal HSV disease.[63]

The indications for valacyclovir therapy are the same as those for acyclovir.[37,64–66] Adult treatment doses are as follows: (1) 1 g orally (PO) tid for 7 days for herpes zoster in patients older than 50 years of age; (2) 1 g PO bid for 10 days for first-episode genital herpes; (3) 500 mg PO bid for 3 days for episodic treatment of recurrent genital HSV disease; (4) 1 g PO once daily for suppression of recurrent genital HSV; and (5) 2 g PO bid for 1 day for recurrent herpes labialis (≥12 years of age). Efficacy of valacyclovir has been demonstrated in the short-term treatment of recurrent herpes labialis (2 g PO bid for 1 day)[67] and in the suppression of recurrent herpes labialis (500 mg given once daily).[68] In children, valacyclovir dosing is 20 mg/kg per dose (dose not to exceed 1 g) administered either tid (for VZV) or bid (for HSV).[18] In the U.S.,

valacyclovir is licensed for the treatment of pediatric patients with orolabial HSV recurrences (12 years of age and older) and chickenpox (2 years through 17 years of age). Although comparative data from controlled studies are limited, valacyclovir may be advantageous in treating infections caused by viruses that are relatively less sensitive to acyclovir than is HSV (e.g., VZV and CMV).

Adefovir dipivoxil (Hepsera)

Chemistry, mechanism of action, spectrum, and resistance. Adefovir dipivoxil is the oral prodrug of adefovir, which is an acyclic nucleotide analogue of deoxyadenosine-5′-monophosphate (dAMP).[69,70] Conversion of the prodrug to the active adefovir diphosphate is accomplished by cellular adenylate kinase. Adefovir diphosphate then acts as a competitive inhibitor of deoxyadenosine triphosphate for viral DNA polymerase, resulting in DNA chain termination following its incorporation in HBV DNA.[69,70] In addition to HBV, adefovir diphosphate competitively inhibits deoxyadenosine triphosphate as a substrate for HIV-1 reverse transcriptase, resulting in chain termination following its incorporation in HIV DNA.[71–73] In vitro, adefovir has an additive effect when combined with lamivudine, entecavir, or telbivudine.[74]

Resistance to adefovir is a limiting factor with prolonged use. The N236T mutation and the A181V mutation in the HBV polymerase both confer in vitro and in vivo antiviral resistance to adefovir diphosphate.[75] Rates of resistance to adefovir at 1, 2, 4, and 5 years are 0%, 3%, 18%, and 29%, respectively.[76] HBV strains with the A181V mutation also are resistant to lamivudine.

Pharmacokinetics. Adefovir dipivoxil is absorbed rapidly following oral administration. Following a single oral dose, the bioavailability is ~59%.[77] Food does not substantially impact absorption of adefovir dipivoxil, so the drug may be administered without regard to meals.[77] Half-life at steady state is ~7 hours. Following absorption, adefovir dipivoxil is cleaved to adefovir by extracellular esterases.[77] Adefovir then is phosphorylated to the active moiety adefovir diphosphate by cellular adenylate kinase. The intracellular half-life of adefovir diphosphate is estimated to be 16 to 18 hours.[72] Adefovir is excreted renally as unchanged drug by tubular secretion and glomerular filtration. Dosing in patients with baseline creatinine clearance values <50 mL/min requires adjustment in the dosing interval.[77] The dose of adefovir dipivoxil does not need to be adjusted in patients with hepatic impairment.

Toxicity and drug interactions. Adefovir dipivoxil generally is well tolerated over prolonged periods of administration.[76,78] In randomized, controlled trials, diarrhea, headache, and abdominal pain occurred slightly more frequently in adefovir-treated patients compared with placebo-treated patients.[79,80] Long-term administration may result in nephrotoxicity, but the risk in patients with adequate renal function is low.[76,81] In vitro, adefovir does not inhibit cytochrome P450. No clinically relevant drug interactions have been reported in clinical trials.[77]

Clinical uses and recommended doses. Adefovir has been studied in children with HBV infection, and is approved for use in those 12 years of age and older. It is the preferred oral treatment option for children ages 12 through 15 years, after which they can be treated with entecavir.[82] In HBeAg-positive children from 2 through 17 years of age with alanine transferase (ALT0 values at least 1.5 times the upper limit of normal), adefovir therapy resulted in favorable virologic and hepatic results (e.g., achievement of undetectable HSV DNA and normal ALT) in 12- through 17-year-olds but not in 2- through 11-year-olds.[83] In this trial of 173 children, no adverse effects associated with adefovir were identified,[83] and the drug was well tolerated in all age groups. In adult patients with a greater number of approved anti-HBV treatment options, adefovir dipivoxil is not as effective as other antiviral agents, and is no longer favored for the treatment of chronic HBV infection. In adults, adefovir dipivoxil therapy is associated with a 12% rate of HBeAg seroconversion, 21% rate of undetectable serum HBV DNA, and 53% rate of histologic improvement in HBeAg-positive patients after 1 year of therapy.[80] Once seroconversion occurs, it is sustained in 91% of patients.[84,85] In adults, persistence of high levels of HBV DNA after 48 weeks of adefovir therapy predicts the emergence of resistance.[76]

The optimal duration of adefovir treatment in children is not known. In the pivotal pediatric study,[83] children were treated for 48 weeks. For those who did not seroconvert during this time, continued treatment for up to 2 years was provided. Results from this extended therapy have not been reported yet. Children with HBeAg-positive chronic HBV infection should continue on treatment for at least 6 months after seroconversion.[82] Monitoring for several months following cessation of therapy is recommended since posttreatment flares have been reported in adults.[77,86] The recommended dose of adefovir dipivoxil in chronic hepatitis B patients for patients ≥12 years of age with adequate renal function is 10 mg, once daily, taken orally, without regard to food.

Cidofovir (HPMPC, Vistide)

Chemistry, mechanism of action, spectrum, and resistance. Cidofovir, or (5)-1-(3-hydroxy-2-(phosphonylmethoxy)-propyl)cytosine, is a novel acyclic phosphonate nucleotide analogue. Cidofovir has a mechanism of action that is similar to that of the nucleoside analogues, such as acyclovir and ganciclovir. In its native form, however, cidofovir already has a single phosphate group attached. As such, viral enzymes are not required for the initial phosphorylation of the drug. Cellular kinases sequentially attach two additional phosphate groups, converting cidofovir to its most active form. This active compound then serves as a competitive inhibitor of DNA polymerase.[87] Although cidofovir is taken up by both virus-infected and noninfected cells, the active form of the drug exhibits a 25- to 50-fold greater affinity for the viral DNA polymerase, compared with the cellular DNA polymerase, thereby selectively inhibiting viral replication.[87,88] Incorporation into the growing viral DNA chain results in reductions in the rate of viral DNA synthesis.

Cidofovir has demonstrable activity against HSV and CMV. Owing to its unique phosphorylation requirements for activation, the drug usually maintains activity against acyclovir- and foscarnet-resistant HSV isolates, as well as ganciclovir- and foscarnet-resistant CMV mutants. Cidofovir exhibits marked activity against CMV, with inhibitory concentrations of 0.1 µg/mL for susceptible clinical isolates.[89] Although cidofovir is less potent in vitro against HSV than is acyclovir, its favorable pharmacokinetic profile increases its anti-HSV activity. Cidofovir also has demonstrated in vitro activity against VZV, EBV, human herpesvirus 6, human herpesvirus 8, polyomaviruses, orthopoxviruses, adenovirus, BK virus, and HPV.

Only a small number of cidofovir-resistant CMV isolates have been described, and an appreciation of the full spectrum of antiviral resistance to this compound currently is lacking. Some cidofovir-resistant CMV isolates also are resistant to ganciclovir because of mutations within the DNA polymerase gene but remain sensitive to foscarnet.[90-92]

Pharmacokinetics. After intravenous administration of cidofovir, the plasma half-life is 2.6 hours, although cidofovir persists in cells for prolonged periods.[93] In addition, active intracellular metabolites of cidofovir have long half-lives of 17 to 48 hours.[88] Such prolonged intracellular activity allows for an intermittent dosing schedule that is attractive compared with that for ganciclovir or foscarnet. Ninety percent of the drug is excreted in the urine, primarily by renal tubular secretion.[94,95]

Toxicity and drug interactions. Nephrotoxicity is the principal adverse event associated with systemic administration of cidofovir.[94,95] Cidofovir concentrates in renal cells in amounts 100 times greater than in other tissues, producing severe nephrotoxicity involving the proximal convoluted tubule when concomitant hydration and administration of probenecid are not employed.[96] Renal toxicity manifests as proteinuria and glycosuria.[97] To decrease the potential for nephrotoxicity, aggressive intravenous prehydration and coadministration of probenecid are required with each cidofovir dose. Within 48 hours prior to delivery of each dose of cidofovir, serum creatinine and urine protein concentrations must be determined, with adjustment in dose as indicated. Cidofovir should not be administered concomitantly with other nephrotoxic agents. Cidofovir is contraindicated in patients with a serum creatinine >1.5 mg/dL, a calculated CrCl of ≤55 mL/min, or a urine protein of ≥100 mg/dL (equivalent to ≥2+ proteinuria). The maintenance dose of cidofovir must be reduced from 5 mg/kg to 3 mg/kg for an increase in serum creatinine of 0.3 to 0.4 mg/dL above baseline. Cidofovir therapy must be discontinued if serum creatinine increases ≥0.5 mg/dL above baseline.

In animal studies, cidofovir has been shown to be carcinogenic and teratogenic, and to cause hypospermia.

Owing to poor oral bioavailability (2% to 26%),[98] cidofovir can be administered only intravenously or topically. Intravitreal administration has been associated with ocular hypotony.

Clinical uses and recommended doses. Cidofovir has been evaluated for the treatment of CMV retinitis in patients with acquired immunodeficiency syndrome (AIDS);[99,100] therapy delays retinal disease progression.[99,100] In one study, patients who had failed or were intolerant of traditional therapy (ganciclovir or foscarnet) were treated with a 2-week induction course of cidofovir (5 mg/kg administered weekly) followed by randomization to maintenance with either a dose of 5 mg/kg or 3 mg/kg every other week.[99] At the higher maintenance dose of cidofovir, disease progression was delayed for 115 days, compared with 49 days in the lower-dose cohort. Cidofovir also has been used successfully in the management of disease caused by acyclovir-resistant HSV isolates.[96]

The safety and efficacy of cidofovir in children have not been studied. The use of cidofovir in children with AIDS warrants caution because of the risk of long-term carcinogenicity and reproductive toxicity.

Intralesional injection of cidofovir has been reported in several small, uncontrolled studies in patients with laryngeal papillomatosis caused by HPV infection.[101,102] Some patients have experienced dramatic improvement, although the anecdotal nature of the trials prevents definitive conclusions regarding efficacy.[103] Recent uncontrolled studies have reported less impressive therapeutic responses to cidofovir therapy,[104–106] raising further questions about cidofovir's efficacy and safety in laryngeal papillomatosis. Case reports and small case series suggest that cidofovir may be beneficial in the management of adenovirus infections[107–109] and BK virus infections[110,111] in immunocompromised patients.

The recommended induction dose of cidofovir for patients with CMV disease with a serum creatinine of ≤1.5 mg/dL, a calculated CrCl >55 mL/min, and a urine protein <100 mg/dL (equivalent to <2+ proteinuria) is 5 mg/kg administered once per week for 2 consecutive weeks. The recommended maintenance dose of cidofovir is 5 mg/kg administered once every 2 weeks. The drug should be administered with probenecid, and hydration should be assured.

Entecavir (Baraclude)

Chemistry, mechanism of action, spectrum, and resistance. Entecavir is a guanosine nucleoside analogue, which, following phosphorylation to the active triphosphate form, exhibits potent activity against HBV polymerase.[112–114] Entecavir triphosphate inhibits HBV polymerase base priming, reverse transcription of the negative strand from the pregenomic messenger RNA, and synthesis of positive-strand HBV DNA. It is approximately 30-fold more potent than lamivudine in vitro.[112] Entecavir triphosphate is a weak inhibitor of cellular DNA polymerases, and does not demonstrate activity against HIV-1 replication.[115,116]

Both in vitro and in vivo data suggest that emergence of resistance to entecavir is rare in nucleoside-naive patients.[117–122] However, approximately 7% of lamivudine-refractory patients with HBV infection develop entecavir resistance-associated substitutions at rtI169, rtT184, rtS202, and/or rtM250 when pre-existing lamivudine resistance mutations reL180M and/or rtM204V/I are present.[123] Additional mutations within the HBV viral polymerase are required for entecavir resistance to develop.[118,119,121] Five-year entecavir-resistance rates are 1.2% in nucleoside-naive and 51% in lamivudine-refractory patients[117,124] Entecavir is active against adefovir-resistant mutants,[112] and since additional mutations are required to develop resistance to entecavir the drug also remains active against lamivudine-resistant mutants.[117,125] Emergence of entecavir resistance mutations is usually associated with virologic rebound during therapy.[119]

Pharmacokinetics. Entecavir peak plasma concentrations occur between 0.5 and 1.5 hours following oral administration in adults. Steady state is achieved following 6 to 10 days of once-daily administration, with approximately 2-fold accumulation. At steady state, C_{max} is 4.2 ng/mL and C_{trough} is 0.3 ng/mL. Due to decreases of approximately 20% in area under the curve (AUC) when administered with food, entecavir should only be given at least 2 hours before or after a meal. The intracellular half-life of entecavir triphosphate is 15 hours. Approximately two-thirds to three-quarters of drug is excreted unchanged in the urine.

Pharmacokinetic studies of entecavir have not been conducted in children younger than 16 years of age.

Toxicity and drug interactions. Coadministration of entecavir in vitro with several HIV nucleoside reverse transcriptase inhibitors (NRTIs) had no negative impact on entecavir's anti-HBV activity. Conversely, entecavir did not have a detrimental effect on the activity of the NRTIs' anti-HIV activity. Entecavir is not a substrate, inhibitor, or inducer of the cytochrome P450 enzyme system. As such, entecavir pharmacokinetics are unlikely to be affected by drugs that affect or are metabolized by the cytochrome (CY) P450 system. Steady-state pharmacokinetics of entecavir are not altered when the drug is coadministered with lamivudine, adefovir dipivoxil, and tenofovir disoproxil fumarate.

As with other therapies for chronic HBV infections, severe acute exacerbations of hepatitis B have been reported in patients who have discontinued entecavir therapy. Therefore, hepatic function should be closely monitored with both clinical and laboratory follow-up for at least several months in patients who discontinue HBV therapy.

Clinical uses and recommended dosage. Entecavir is indicated for the treatment of chronic HBV infection in adults with evidence of active viral replication and either evidence of persistent elevations in serum aminotransferases or histologically active liver disease. Entecavir is superior to lamivudine in the treatment of chronic HBV infection,[126] and is the most potent anti-HBV agent available.[127,128] When entecavir (0.5 mg once daily) was compared with lamivudine (100 mg once daily) for 52 weeks in nucleoside-naive patients with compensated liver disease, more patients receiving entecavir experienced improvement in histologic Knodell necro-inflammatory scores in both hepatitis B e antigen (HBeAg)-positive (72% versus 62%, P<0.05) and HBeAg-negative (70% versus 61%, P<0.05) patients. Similarly, more patients developed normal serum ALT concentrations during therapy with entecavir compared with lamivudine (68% versus 60% for HBeAg-positive patients, P<0.05; 78% versus 71% for HBeAg-negative patients, P<0.05). Also, more patients cleared viremia on entecavir compared with lamivudine (67% versus 36% for HBeAg-positive patients, P<0.05; 90% versus 72% for HBeAg-negative patients, P<0.05).[129–131] Responses endure through the second year of therapy.[132]

Among patients with lamivudine-refractory chronic HBV infection, changing to entecavir (1 mg once daily) was superior to continuing lamivudine (100 mg once daily).[133] More patients receiving entecavir experienced improvement in histologic Knodell necro-inflammatory scores (55% versus 28%, P<0.01), in Ishak fibrosis score (34% versus 16%, P<0.01), normalization of ALT concentration (61% versus 15%, P<0.0001), and clearance of viremia (19% versus 1%, P<0.0001).[124,129]

Entecavir also is superior to adefovir dipivoxil in nucleoside-naive, HBeAg-positive patients.[134] At 12 weeks, mean change in serum HBV DNA concentration was −6.23 log10 copies/mL in the entecavir group, versus −4.42 log10 copies/mL in the adefovir dipivoxil group. After 96 weeks of treatment, 97% of entecavir-treated patients had achieved ALT normalization, compared with 85% of adefovir-treated patients (95% CI, 5.4 to 28.6).[134]

The recommended dose of entecavir for chronic HBV infection in nucleoside-naive adults and adolescents ≥16 years of age is 0.5 mg once daily. In HBV-infected persons ≥16 years of age who have a history of HBV viremia while receiving lamivudine or who have a known lamivudine resistance mutation, the entecavir dose should be increased to 1.0 mg once daily. The optimal duration of therapy with entecavir is not known. A phase IIB pharmacokinetic and efficacy trial of entecavir in children 2 years of age and older is nearing completion, and a phase III trial in this age group already has started.[82]

Hemodialysis removes approximately 13% of the entecavir dose over 4 hours, whereas CAPD removes approximately 0.3% of the dose over 7 days. In patients with renal impairment, the apparent oral clearance of entecavir decreases as CrCl decreases. Dosage adjustment is recommended for patients with CrCl <50 mL/min, including patients on hemodialysis or CAPD. Dosage is 0.25 mg once daily for CrCl 30 to <50 mL/min, 0.15 mg once daily for CrCl 10 to <30 mL/min, and 0.05 mg once daily for CrCl <10 mL/min or CAPD. A dose should be administered after hemodialysis. These doses are doubled for individuals refractory to lamivudine.

Famciclovir (Famvir) and Topical Penciclovir (Denavir)

Chemistry, mechanism of action, spectrum, and resistance. Famciclovir is the inactive diacetyl ester prodrug of penciclovir, an acyclic nucleoside analogue with a spectrum of activity against herpesviruses similar to that of acyclovir. Its activation by viral and host cell enzymes and its mechanism of action are also akin to that of acyclovir, except that it is neither an obligate DNA chain terminator nor an inactivator of the DNA polymerase. However, laboratory studies suggest that penciclovir triphosphate retards the rate of subsequent nucleotide incorporation. Penciclovir is approximately 100-fold less potent than acyclovir in inhibiting herpesvirus DNA polymerase activity. However, it remains an effective antiviral agent because of high intracellular concentrations and long half-life. Because penciclovir, like acyclovir, must be activated by the viral-encoded TK enzyme, TK-deficient viral strains are resistant to both acyclovir and penciclovir. Penciclovir persists in high intracellular concentrations much longer than acyclovir; its antiviral effect is more sustained, and the drug can be administered less frequently than acyclovir.

Pharmacokinetics. After oral administration of famciclovir, the bioavailability of penciclovir is about 70%. Food delays absorption but does not affect the final plasma drug concentration. Peak concentrations of drug after intravenous administration of 10 mg/kg are approximately 6-fold higher than those attained after oral doses of 250 mg. Drug half-life is 2.5 hours; almost 75% of administered drug is recovered unchanged in the urine, and dose reduction is recommended for those with compromised renal function. A 12-hour dosing interval is recommended for those with CrCl between 30 and 50 mL/min per 1.73 m^2, and a 24-hour interval for those with CrCl <30 mL/min per 1.73 m^2.[135] Measurable penciclovir concentrations are not detectable in plasma or urine after topical administration of penciclovir cream. Famciclovir pharmacokinetics have been assessed in a single-dose pediatric study of infants 1 to 12 months of age who were given famciclovir sprinkles orally.[136] Infants under 6 months of age had substantially lower systemic exposure compared with 6- to 12-month-olds.

Toxicity and drug interactions. Famciclovir is as well tolerated as acyclovir. Complaints of nausea, diarrhea, and headache occurred in clinical trials, but at frequencies similar to those reported by placebo recipients.[137] No clinically significant drug interactions have been reported to date, although concentrations of famciclovir among volunteers increase by about 20% in patients receiving concomitant cimetidine or theophylline administration.[138]

Clinical uses and recommended dosage. The efficacy of famciclovir in the treatment of uncomplicated herpes zoster was studied in a placebo-controlled, double-blind trial of 419 immunocompetent adults.[139] Treatment was begun within 72 hours of the appearance of lesions, and therapy was continued for 7 days. Famciclovir therapy decreased the median time to full crusting by 2 days. The effects of famciclovir were greater when therapy was initiated within 48 hours of the onset of rash; effects also were more pronounced in patients 50 years of age or older. There were no overall differences in the duration of pain before healing of rash between the famciclovir-treated and the placebo groups. In addition, there was no difference in the incidence of postherpetic neuralgia between the treatment groups. Among patients who developed postherpetic neuralgia, however, the median duration of symptoms was shorter in patients treated with famciclovir than in those given placebo (63 days and 119 days, respectively).

A double-blind, controlled trial in 545 immunocompetent adults with uncomplicated herpes zoster treated within 72 hours of the appearance of lesions compared three doses of famciclovir with acyclovir at a dose of 800 mg 5 times per day. Times to full lesion crusting and times to loss of acute pain were comparable for all groups, and there were no statistically significant differences in the times to resolution of postherpetic neuralgia between famciclovir- and acyclovir-treated groups.

Placebo-controlled studies of famciclovir for the episodic treatment of genital HSV[140] and for suppression of genital HSV

TABLE 295-8. Famciclovir: Indications and Dosages

Infection	Dosage	Duration
Zoster	500 mg tid	7 days
Recurrent genital HSV, immunocompetent host (episodic therapy)	1000 mg bid	1 day
Recurrent genital HSV, immunocompetent host (suppressive therapy)	250 mg bid	Up to 1 year
Recurrent genital HSV, immunocompromised host (episodic therapy in compromised hosts)	500 mg bid	7 days
Recurrent orolabial HSV, immunocompromised host (episodic therapy)	500 mg bid	7 days
Recurrent orolabial HSV, immunocompetent host (episodic therapy)	1500 mg	Administer as a single dose

HSV, herpes simplex virus.

recurrences[141,142] also have been performed. Famciclovir was well tolerated and efficacious in these investigations.[37]

Famciclovir was approved by the FDA for the treatment of herpes zoster in 1994, and subsequently was approved for the treatment and suppression of genital HSV disease. The indications for and recommended dosages of famciclovir are presented in Table 295-8. Dosing in infants and young children has been studied.[136] Dosing recommendations in children 6 months to 12 years of age are based on pharmacokinetic modeling, and have not been studied adequately to warrant dosing recommendations in this age group.

Topical penciclovir for the treatment of recurrent herpes labialis reduces the time to healing and the duration of pain by about half a day.[143,144] Application of medicine should begin as early as possible, preferably during the prodromal phase, and should be continued every 2 hours during waking hours for 4 days.

Ganciclovir (DHPG, Cytovene, GCV) and Valganciclovir (Valcyte, VGCV)

Chemistry, mechanism of action, spectrum, and resistance. Ganciclovir is a nucleoside analogue that differs from acyclovir by having an extra hydroxymethyl group on the acyclic side chain.[145] Ganciclovir's greatest in vitro activity is against CMV (see Table 295-3), although it is also as active as acyclovir against HSV-1 and HSV-2 and almost as active against VZV. As with acyclovir and penciclovir, the first step in ganciclovir phosphorylation is carried out by a virus-encoded enzyme, and the final steps by cellular enzymes. Because CMV lacks the gene for thymidine kinase, the enzyme that catalyzes the initial phosphorylation of ganciclovir in CMV-infected cells is the phosphotransferase encoded by the *UL97* gene.[146,147] Intracellular ganciclovir triphosphate concentrations are at least 10-fold higher in CMV-infected cells than in noninfected cells,[148] and intracellular ganciclovir triphosphate has a half-life of more than 24 hours. Ganciclovir triphosphate serves as a competitive inhibitor of herpesviral DNA polymerases, although it also has some activity against cellular DNA polymerases. This potential for incorporation into host cellular DNA accounts for ganciclovir's significant toxicity. Incorporation of ganciclovir triphosphate into the growing viral DNA chain results in slowing and subsequent cessation of DNA chain elongation.[149]

Valganciclovir was approved by the FDA in 2001. Because valganciclovir is well absorbed after oral administration, it may represent a favorable alternative to intravenously administered ganciclovir for the treatment and suppression of CMV infections in immunocompromised hosts. Valganciclovir is an L-valine ester prodrug of ganciclovir and has the same mechanism of action and antiviral spectrum as ganciclovir.[150]

Ganciclovir resistance among CMV isolates is conferred by mutations in either the *UL97* gene or the CMV DNA polymerase gene. Of these two mechanisms of antiviral resistance, ganciclovir-resistant CMV isolates with mutations in the *UL97* open reading frame are the predominant phenotype.[90] Specific mutations within the *UL97* region can be detected rapidly in plasma and serum by direct sequencing of polymerase chain reaction amplified CMV DNA.[151] Resistant strains of CMV should be suspected when progressive disease and continued recovery of virus occur despite ganciclovir therapy. In one study, 8% of 72 patients with AIDS had progressive infection associated with isolation of ganciclovir-resistant strains of CMV after 3 months of continuous ganciclovir therapy.[152] Resistance may be more likely to occur in patients treated with oral ganciclovir than in those treated with intravenous ganciclovir, possibly owing to the selective pressure applied by the lower concentrations of drug achieved with oral administration.[153] By contrast, CMV isolates from solid-organ transplant recipients who have been exposed to ganciclovir appear less likely to develop resistance to the drug.[154] Foscarnet may be useful in the treatment of CMV infections caused by ganciclovir-resistant isolates.[155] Occasionally, strains of HSV that are resistant to acyclovir because of TK deficiency also are much less susceptible to ganciclovir.[156] Ganciclovir-resistant isolates of HSV due to mutations in DNA polymerase have been demonstrated in the laboratory but have not yet become a clinical problem.

The mechanisms of resistance to ganciclovir and valganciclovir are the same.[150] Since selective pressure resulting from exposure to lower concentrations of drug appears to increase the likelihood of resistance developing among CMV isolates,[153] it is believed that the higher serum and tissue concentrations of ganciclovir achieved with administration of valganciclovir will produce less emergence of resistance compared with oral ganciclovir. Small studies have indicated that rates of resistance among valganciclovir recipients are similar to those of intravenous ganciclovir recipients[157] and are less than those of patients taking oral ganciclovir.[158]

Pharmacokinetics. Peak serum concentrations of ganciclovir attained after 5 mg/kg administered intravenously range from 8 to 11 μg/mL.[145] Concentrations sufficient to inhibit susceptible strains of CMV are attained in aqueous humor, subretinal fluid, CSF, and brain tissue. Most of an administered dose of ganciclovir is eliminated unchanged in the urine; the elimination half-life is 2 to 3 hours.[13] Dose reduction, roughly proportional to the degree of reduction in CrCl, is necessary in persons with impaired renal function (see Table 295-5).[151,159] For CrCl 50 to <80 mL/min per 1.73 m², half of the usual dose should be given every 12 hours. This same dose should be given every 24 hours for CrCl 25 to <50 mL/min per 1.73 m², and 25% of the usual dose should be given every 24 hours for CrCl <25 mL/min per 1.73 m². Because ganciclovir is removed efficiently by hemodialysis, a supplemental dose is recommended after dialysis.[159]

The pharmacokinetics of ganciclovir in the neonatal population are similar to those of adults.[160] After intravenous administration of 6 mg/kg ganciclovir, peak concentrations of 7.0 μg/mL are achieved. The mean elimination half-life is 2.4 hours. In addition, pharmacokinetics in this population of oral valganciclovir have been compared with parenteral ganciclovir.[161] Intravenous ganciclovir clearance nearly doubled and AUC_{12} was reduced by almost one-half over the first 6 weeks of life. In comparison, only a marginal decrease in AUC_{12} was noted following administration of valganciclovir oral solution, possibly because bioavailability increased by 32% over the same time period.

Oral bioavailability of ganciclovir is poor, with <10% of the drug being absorbed following oral administration.[162] Despite this, an oral dose of 1000 mg ganciclovir produces a peak plasma concentration of 1 μg/mL, a level that is above the inhibitory concentration of most CMV clinical isolates. Intravitreal drug concentration achieved during intravenous induction therapy averages 1 μg/mL, whereas subretinal concentration is comparable

with plasma.[163,164] Concentration of ganciclovir in the CNS ranges from 24% to 70% of those in the plasma, with brain concentration approximately 38% of plasma level.[165]

Valganciclovir is rapidly converted to ganciclovir, with a mean plasma half-life of about 30 minutes.[166] The absolute bioavailability of valganciclovir exceeds 60% and is enhanced by about 30% with concomitant administration of food.[167] Oral valganciclovir produces exposures of ganciclovir exceeding those attained with oral ganciclovir, and similar to those reported after standard intravenous administration of ganciclovir.[168] Patients with impaired renal function require dosage reduction roughly proportional to their reduction in CrCl.[150]

Toxicity and drug interactions. The most important toxic effect of ganciclovir is myelosuppression. Dose-related neutropenia, defined as a >50% decrease in absolute neutrophil count from baseline or <1000/mm³, is the most consistent hematologic disturbance.[145] The incidence of neutropenia during a 2-week course is about 40%. It is dose-limiting in about 15% of courses, and is reversible on cessation of drug.[145] The likelihood of neutropenia occurring following oral administration of ganciclovir is lower, with 14% to 24% of patients developing an absolute neutrophil count of <1000/mm³.[169] Hematopoietic growth factors may be useful in preventing or counteracting neutropenia.[170] Thrombocytopenia (<50,000 platelets/mm³) occurs in approximately 20% of treated patients. Anemia occurs in only about 2% of ganciclovir recipients.

Approximately 5% of ganciclovir recipients experience some combination of headache, confusion, altered mental status, hallucinations, nightmares, anxiety, ataxia, tremors, and seizures. About 2% of recipients develop fever, rash, and abnormal levels of serum hepatic enzymes. Intraocular injection of ganciclovir can cause transient increases in intraocular pressure with associated intense pain and amaurosis lasting up to 30 minutes.[171]

In preclinical test systems, ganciclovir is mutagenic, carcinogenic, and teratogenic. Additionally, it causes irreversible reproductive toxicity in animals.[172]

The most common side effects associated with valganciclovir therapy include diarrhea (41%), nausea (30%), neutropenia (27%), anemia (26%), and headache (22%).[150] Long-term (up to 5 years) treatment with valganciclovir is well tolerated in patients with AIDS, and the type and incidence of adverse events experienced long-term appear to be similar to those observed at 1 year.[173]

Clinical uses and recommended dosage. Ganciclovir is indicated for the treatment and prevention of life- and sight-threatening CMV infections occurring in immunosuppressed patients.[145] It is approved in the U.S. for the treatment and suppression of retinitis caused by CMV in immunocompromised patients and for the prevention of CMV disease in transplant recipients, but it is frequently used for a number of other serious CMV infections. In almost 90% of patients with CMV retinitis, there is improvement or stabilization of the ocular disease and then clearing of the condition, or a more than 100-fold reduction in viral titers, from urine, blood, and throat after 1 to 2 weeks of ganciclovir therapy.[170] Relapse of retinitis is virtually inevitable in patients with AIDS; thus, ganciclovir should be continued long-term for CMV suppression after induction therapy. Patients in whom ganciclovir therapy has failed may benefit from treatment with a combination of foscarnet and ganciclovir.[174] Patients with AIDS who have CNS disease caused by CMV also have been treated successfully with a combination of ganciclovir and foscarnet.[175] As many as 25% of ganciclovir recipients develop resistance within 9 months of the initiation of therapy.[176,177]

Patients with AIDS and recipients of solid-organ transplants who have gastrointestinal disease attributed to CMV appear to benefit from ganciclovir therapy.[178,179] Ganciclovir monotherapy does not appear to benefit bone marrow transplant recipients with CMV gastrointestinal infections.[180]

Limited and uncontrolled data suggest that ganciclovir therapy may be useful in patients with AIDS and CMV pneumonia.[145] By contrast, bone marrow transplant recipients with CMV pneumonia fail to respond to ganciclovir therapy alone[181] but may benefit from therapy with intravenous CMV hyperimmunoglobulin and ganciclovir given together.[182,183]

Ganciclovir has been evaluated in the treatment of neonates congenitally infected with CMV. In a phase III randomized controlled trial, ganciclovir therapy (6 mg/kg per dose administered every 12 hours intravenously for 6 weeks) protected infants from hearing deterioration beyond 1 year of life,[184] and may improve neurologic outcomes.[185] Transient positive effects on growth also were seen, as was a decreased time to resolution of serum hepatic transaminase elevation. Approximately two-thirds of treated patients, however, developed neutropenia, with half of these requiring dose modification. A phase I/II pharmacokinetic and pharmacodynamic study of oral valganciclovir has established that a 16 mg/kg dose of oral valganciclovir produces similar systemic exposure to a 6 mg/kg dose of intravenous ganciclovir.[161] With these data, a study of 6 weeks versus 6 months of oral valganciclovir for the treatment of symptomatic congenital CMV disease is being conducted, and analysis of the impact of longer-term treatment on hearing and developmental outcomes is expected in 2013.

Ganciclovir is useful for prevention of CMV infections in high-risk immunocompromised subjects, including bone marrow and solid organ transplant recipients (see Table 295-7). Strategies that have been used to reduce the frequency of posttransplantation disease include routine administration of ganciclovir to all transplant recipients at risk and pre-emptive administration to those who have a positive culture for CMV after transplantation. Pre-emptive therapy has been demonstrated to reduce CMV disease effectively in recipients of liver,[186] lung,[187] heart,[188] and bone marrow transplants.[189–191] CMV-seropositive recipients of heart, lung, or liver transplants who receive routine prophylaxis with ganciclovir for 1 month also have significant reductions in post-transplant CMV infection and disease.[33,192–195] Pre-emptive administration of ganciclovir improves survival in bone marrow transplant recipients,[196,197] whereas routine initiation of prophylactic ganciclovir prior to bone marrow transplantation in patients who are CMV-seropositive does not have an impact on survival.[197,198] Ultimately, however, the best strategy has not been determined for preventing primary CMV infections in CMV-seronegative solid-organ transplant recipients who receive an organ from a CMV-seropositive donor.

The usual therapeutic and prophylactic dose of ganciclovir is 10 mg/kg per day IV divided every 12 hours for 2 to 3 weeks. For continued suppressive therapy to prevent relapse of infection (e.g., in patients with AIDS) or long-term prophylaxis, either of the following may be used: (1) 5 mg/kg as a single daily dose each day of the week; or (2) 6 mg/kg administered as a single dose 5 days a week. Prophylactic oral ganciclovir (1000 mg tid) significantly reduces the risk of CMV disease in persons with advanced AIDS.[199]

Indications for valganciclovir are similar to those for ganciclovir. However, based on limited controlled trials published to date, valganciclovir currently is approved only for the induction and maintenance therapy for CMV retinitis.[200] The recommended dose of valganciclovir for induction therapy is 900 mg twice daily for 2 weeks. The recommended dose for maintenance therapy is 900 mg once daily. Orally administered valganciclovir appears to be as effective as intravenous ganciclovir for induction treatment and is convenient and effective for the long-term management of CMV retinitis in patients with AIDS.

The greater systemic exposure to ganciclovir delivered by valganciclovir when used prophylactically is safe and is associated with delayed development of viremia in solid-organ transplant recipients, compared with oral ganciclovir.[201–203] Valganciclovir also is effective as pre-emptive therapy[204–206] and as treatment for CMV disease[207] in solid-organ transplant recipients.

Lamivudine (Epivir, 3TC)

Chemistry, mechanism of action, spectrum, and resistance. Lamivudine is a nucleoside analogue that is phosphorylated to lamivudine triphosphate by cellular kinases. Lamivudine inhibits the reverse transcriptase of both HBV and HIV, and is indicated for the treatment of HIV and chronic HBV infection.

Lamivudine-resistant HBV mutants occur in up to one-third of subjects by the end of 1 year of therapy, and in up to two-thirds by the end of 4 years of drug exposure.[208] The most common mutation affects the tyrosine-methionine-aspartate-aspartate (YMDD) motif in the catalytic domain of the HBV polymerase, resulting in a change from methionine to valine (M522V) or isoleucine (M522I).

Pharmacokinetics. Lamivudine at a dose of 4 mg/kg administered twice daily produces an AUC_{12} of 5.16 mg • h/L and half-life of 1.76 hours. This half-life in children is less than the half-life in adults (3.5 hours).[209]

Toxicity and drug interactions. Adverse reactions include pancreatitis, paresthesia, peripheral neuropathy, neutropenia, anemia, rashes, nausea, vomiting, and hair loss.

Clinical uses and recommended dosage. In the treatment of chronic HBV infection, lamivudine decreases serum HBV DNA by 3 to 4 log copies per mL in most patients. Among patients who are HBeAg-positive, approximately 20% achieve HBeAg seroconversion and undetectable serum HBV DNA at the end of 1 year of lamivudine therapy.[208,210,211] Slightly more than half of patients experience improvement in histologic liver abnormalities. Similar findings have been seen in children.[212] Lamivudine resistance usually is manifest as breakthrough infection defined as reappearance of HBV DNA in serum after its initial disappearance,[213] and occurs in approximately two-thirds of patients within 3 years of therapy.[214] Most patients continue to have lower serum HBV DNA and serum ALT levels compared with pretreatment values, perhaps due to decreased fitness of the lamivudine-resistant mutants. Upon cessation of lamivudine therapy, most patients experience an increase in serum HBV DNA concentrations.[215]

Lamivudine is indicated for the treatment of HIV and chronic HBV infection. Of note, Epivir-HBV tablets and oral solution contain a lower dose of lamivudine than do Epivir tablets and oral solution used for HIV infection. Therefore, the formulation and dosage of lamivudine in Epivir-HBV are not appropriate for patients dually infected with HIV and HBV; rapid emergence of HIV resistance is likely to result because of the subtherapeutic dose for HIV. The recommended oral dose of lamivudine in adult HBV-infected patients is 100 mg once daily. For HBV-infected children 2 through 17 years of age, the dose is 3 mg/kg (maximum dose 100 mg) administered once daily.

Ribavirin (Virazole; Rebetron Combination Therapy)

Chemistry, mechanism of action, spectrum, and resistance. Ribavirin is a synthetic nucleoside analogue developed in 1972 that most closely resembles guanosine in structure.[216] Ribavirin is absorbed rapidly across cell membranes and is enzymatically converted by host cell enzymes into its 5′-phosphate derivatives and the deribosylated base.[217] These metabolites interfere with the capping and elongation of messenger RNA. Ribavirin also appears to reduce guanine nucleosides via feedback inhibition.[218] Although more potent against RNA viruses, ribavirin is active in vitro against a wide range of both RNA and DNA viruses, including myxoviruses, paramyxoviruses, arenaviruses, bunyaviruses, herpesviruses, adenoviruses, poxviruses, and retroviruses.[219,220] It is approved in the U.S. for the treatment of RSV infections and, in combination with interferon, for hepatitis C virus infections. Viral resistance to ribavirin has not been observed, although Sindbis virus mutants with diminished susceptibility to ribavirin have been reported.[221]

Pharmacokinetics. Ribavirin can be administered orally, intravenously, or by aerosol. Only the aerosolized formulation of drug (Virazole) and the oral formulation (in combination in interferon-α (Rebetol) or peginterferon α-2a (Copegus)) are approved for use in the U.S. About 40% of orally administered ribavirin is absorbed; following doses ranging from 600 to 2400 mg, peak plasma concentrations range from 1.3 to 3.2 μg/mL.[222] Peak concentrations after intravenous therapy are approximately 10-fold greater. Ribavirin and its metabolites concentrate in red blood cells. The levels in CSF are approximately 70% of the plasma concentration of the drug.[223] About one-quarter to one-third of systemically administered ribavirin is recovered unchanged in urine, and an additional 6% to 30% is excreted as metabolites. The terminal half-life of ribavirin is 18 to 36 hours, but some drug persists in red blood cells for several weeks after administration.[222]

Toxicity and drug interactions. Ribavirin administered by the oral and intravenous routes causes dose-related, reversible anemia.[222] At low doses of the drug, anemia is due to extravascular hemolysis, whereas at high doses anemia is due to bone marrow suppression. Increases in serum bilirubin, iron, and uric acid also occur with systemic ribavirin therapy.

Clinical uses and recommended dosage. Systemic ribavirin has demonstrated efficacy in the management of life-threatening infections caused by Lassa fever and hemorrhagic fever with renal syndrome.[224,225] Orally and intravenously administered ribavirin substantially reduce the mortality and morbidity directly attributable to each of these infections, and oral ribavirin has been recommended for prophylaxis against Lassa fever in exposed contacts.[226] Clinical benefit also has been observed in the treatment of Argentine and Bolivian hemorrhagic fever[227] and laboratory-acquired Sabia virus infection.[228]

Telbivudine (Tyzeka)

Chemistry, mechanism of action, spectrum, and resistance. Telbivudine is the unmodified L-enantiomer of the naturally occurring nucleoside D-thymidine.[229,230] Host cell kinases phophorylate telbivudine to telbivudine-5′-triphosphate, which then is incorporated into HBV DNA resulting in viral DNA chain termination.[230,231] Telbivudine preferentially inhibits HBV second strand (DNA-dependent) DNA synthesis.[232] In comparison, lamivudine preferentially inhibits first strand (RNA-dependent) DNA synthesis.[232] Telbivudine is active only against hepadnaviruses.[230,231] Coadministration of telbivudine with lamivudine does not produce additive or synergistic effects.[233]

In vitro, telbivudine-5′-triphosphate has no inhibitory effect on host cell DNA polymerases α, β, or γ at concentrations up to 100 μmol/L.[229,231] In contrast, the mean 50% effective concentration (EC_{50}) inhibiting HBV DNA polymerase is 0.12 to 0.24 μmol/L,[231] illustrating the specificity and potency of the drug for HBV replication. At concentrations up to 10 μmol/L, telbivudine has minimal toxic effect on host cell mitochondria and does not increase lactic acid production.[229,231]

The key determinant of telbivudine resistance is the *M204I* mutation in the YMDD motif.[231] The principal mutations conferring in vivo lamivudine resistance do not produce cross-resistance to telbivudine,[234] but cross-resistance can be induced in vitro.[235] Telbivudine is active or has slightly reduced activity in vitro against adefovir-resistant HBV strains.[234]

Pharmacokinetics. Telbivudine is abdorbed rapidly after oral administration. Absorption is not influenced by food.[236] The half-life of telbivudine is ~40 hours. Approximately 40% of the dose is excreted as the unchanged active substance by the kidneys, likely via renal filtration.[231] Systemic exposure to telbivudine is increased in patients with impaired renal function, and in patients with moderate to severe renal impairment (creatinine clearance <50 mL/min) or end-stage renal disease requiring dialysis, the dosing interval requires adjustment.[237] Dosage adjustment is not required for patients with impaired hepatic function.

Toxicity and drug interactions. No dose-related or dose-limiting toxicities have been identified in healthy volunteers or patients with chronic hepatitis B infection.[238,239] Elevated serum creatine kinase (CK) concentrations are the most frequent adverse event related to telbivudine. Cases of myopathy during telbivudine therapy have been described, but they did not correlate with the magnitude or timing of CK elevations.[231,240] Nevertheless, treatment should be discontinued if persistent, unexplained muscle-related symptoms occur.[231,240] Patients receiving telbivudine along with other drugs associated with myopathy, such as cyclosporine or HMG-CoA reductase inhibitors, should be monitored closely

for signs and symptoms of myopathy.[231] There are no clinically significant interactions between telbivudine and adefovir, tenofovir, and lamivudine.[241] The drug does not induce or inhibit CYP450. Coadministration of telbivudine with drugs that affect renal function (e.g., aminoglycosides, amphotericin B) may impact plasma concentrations of either drug.[231]

Clinical uses and recommended doses. Telbivudine is licensed for use in adolescents and adults (≥16 years of age). It has not been studied in children with HBV infection. In HBeAg-seropositive and -seronegative adults, telbivudine is superior to lamivudine after 1 and 2 years of therapy.[242,243] The rate of HBeAg seroconversion was 22%, and viral suppression (<300 copies/mL) was achieved in 60% of HBeAg-positive patients after 1 year of therapy.[233] Telbivudine also has better early viral suppression compared to adefovir at week 24 in HBeAg-positive patients regardless of whether the patients were treated initially with telbivudine or switched from adefovir to telbivudine.[244] The early virological suppression resulted in better rates of HBeAg seroconversion, serum ALT normalization, and viral suppression.[245]

Tenofovir Disoproxil Fumarate (Viread)

Chemistry, mechanism of action, spectrum, and resistance. Tenofovir disoproxil fumarate is a nucleoside phosphonate diester analogue of deoxyadenosine 5′-monophosphate and a prodrug of tenofovir.[246,247] Following absorption from the gastrointestinal tract, the prodrug is hydrolyzed to tenofovir, which then is taken up in target cells and phosphorylated to the active drug tenofovir diphosphate. Tenofovir diphosphate is a competitive inhibitor of the nucleotide deoxyadenosine 5′-triphosphate for incorporation by HBV polymerase into viral DNA, and inhibits HBV DNA replication by leading to chain termination.[246,248] In addition to HBV, tenofovir diphosphate competitively inhibits deoxyadenosine triphosphate as a substrate for HIV-1 reverse transcriptase, resulting in chain termination following its incorporation in HIV DNA.

Tenofovir diphosphate selectively inhibits viral DNA polymerase, and has only weak inhibition of human cellular DNA polymerase α, β, and γ.[248] The active compound is a potent inhibitor of HBV DNA polymerase, with an inhibition constant (K_i) of 0.18 μmol/L.[249] At in vitro concentrations of ≤300 μmol/L, tenofovir diphosphate does not inhibit synthesis of mitochondrial DNA or result in lactic acid production.[246]

Resistance to tenofovir can be generated in HBV in vitro, but antiviral resistance does not appear to be a clinical problem resulting in virologic breakthrough in vivo. In clinical studies, no HBV mutations associated with resistance to tenofovir disoproxil fumarate have been identified, even after 96 weeks of treatment and in both immunocompetent and HIV-infected patients.[246,250-254] Cross-resistance between tenofovir and adefovir has been demonstrated from in vivo isolates,[249] but not for telbivudine or lamivudine.[255]

Pharmacokinetics. Following oral administration, tenofovir disoproxil fumarate is rapidly absorbed and converted to tenofovir. Oral bioavailability is ~25% in fasting individuals or after a light meal, and is ~39% after a high-fat meal.[246,247,256] The half-life of tenofovir is approximately 17 hours.[246] The intracellular half-life of tenofovir diphosphate is estimated to be 95 hours.[249] Approximately 70% to 80% of the tenofovir dose is excreted unchanged in the urine up to 72 hours after administration.[246,247] In patients with moderate to severe renal impairment (creatinine clearance <50 mL/min), the dosing interval requires adjustment. Dosage adjustment is not required for patients with impaired hepatic function.[246,247]

Toxicity and drug interactions. Tenofovir disoproxil fumarate is generally well tolerated for extended periods of time.[246,250] Mild adverse reactions to therapy include headache, nasopharyngitis, and gastrointestinal upset. Neither tenofovir disoproxil fumarate nor tenofovir is metabolized by CYP450 enzymes. While decreased metabolism of CYP1A substrates has been observed,[247] drug interactions mediated via CYP450 enzymes are minimal with tenofovir. Coadministration of tenofovir disoproxil fumarate with nephrotoxic drugs or compounds that compete for active tubular secretion can result in increased serum concentrations of tenofovir. Tenofovir disoproxil fumarate should not be administered with adefovir dipivoxil.[247] Renal function should be closely monitored if tenofovir disoproxil fumarate is coadministered with tacrolimus.[246] No drug interactions were noted with coadministration with telbivudine,[257] and use with entecavir has not been evaluated.[246,247]

Clinical uses and recommended doses. While tenofovir is licensed for use in children 12 years of age and older with HIV infection, it is not approved for use in the treatment of HBV in children. There is no recommended dose in children with HBV infection. In adults, tenofovir is more potent than adefovir in achieving viral suppression (76% vs. 13% with <400 copies/mL), histologic improvement (67% vs. 12%), and higher rates of HBsAg loss (3.2% vs. 0%) at 48 weeks in HBeAg-seropositive patients with chronic hepatitis B infection.[250] Eighty-nine percent of patients maintained serum HBV DNA <400 copies/mL when continued on tenofovir disoproxil fumarate for 72 weeks. Seventy-eight percent of patients who did not achieve complete viral suppression did so after 24 weeks of tenofovir therapy.[258] Similar results have been observed in other studies.[257] The recommended adult dose is 300 mg orally once daily without regard to food.

Trifluridine (TFT, Trifluorothymidine, Viroptic)

Trifluridine is a pyrimidine nucleoside active in vitro against HSV-1 and HSV-2 (including acyclovir-resistant strains), CMV, and certain adenoviruses.[259] DNA polymerase activity and viral DNA synthesis are inhibited after phosphorylation to trifluridine triphosphate. Selection of trifluridine-resistant HSV strains with altered TK substrate specificity can be accomplished in the laboratory. Trifluridine is approved only for topical use in the management of primary keratoconjunctivitis and recurrent keratitis caused by HSV. Trifluridine is more active than idoxuridine in HSV ocular infections[260] and is the treatment of choice for the topical treatment of HSV keratitis. Adverse effects include local discomfort, irritation, edema, and, less commonly, hypersensitivity reactions as well as superficial punctate or epithelial keratopathy. It is supplied as a 1% ophthalmic solution, one drop to be instilled in each eye, up to nine times a day.

Vidarabine (ARA-A, Adenine Arabinoside, Vira-A Ophthalmic Ointment)

Licensed for use in the U.S. in 1977 as a systemic treatment for life-threatening HSV and VZV infections, intravenous vidarabine has not been available in the U.S. since 1992 due to the more favorable toxicity profile of intravenous acyclovir. However, a topical preparation remains on the market for the treatment of HSV keratitis.

Vidarabine is phosphorylated by cellular enzymes to the active triphosphate form. Thus, unlike acyclovir, conversion of vidarabine to its active intracellular derivative does not require viral enzymes at any step of the triphosphorylation process; this lack of specificity accounts for at least some of its toxicity. Vidarabine triphosphate then acts as a competitive inhibitor of viral and, to a lesser extent, cellular DNA polymerase. It functions as a chain terminator after incorporation into the growing chain of both viral and cellular DNA.[261] Vidarabine triphosphate also inhibits ribonucleoside reductase, RNA polyadenylation, and S-adenosylhomocysteine hydrolase (SAHH), an enzyme involved in transmethylation reactions. Inhibition of SAHH and the resulting inhibition of adenosine deaminase may contribute to vidarabine's antiviral and toxic effects.[262,263]

Resistance to vidarabine is conferred by mutations in the viral DNA polymerase gene. The degree of maximal resistance to vidarabine in polymerase mutants is 4-fold, much lower than the 100-fold resistance to acyclovir that can result from similar mutations. Acyclovir-resistant clinical HSV isolates virtually always retain in vitro susceptibility to vidarabine.[264]

Although trifluridine is the antiviral agent of choice for the topical treatment of HSV keratitis, vidarabine is a suitable alternative in patients in whom trifluridine cannot be used.[265-267] Topical vidarabine is superior to idoxuridine in the treatment of HSV ocular infections.[260]

Tricyclic Amines

Amantadine (Symmetrel) and Rimantadine (Flumadine)

Chemistry, mechanism of action, spectrum, and resistance. Amantadine (1-adamantanamine hydrochloride) and rimantadine (α-methyl-1-adamantanemethylamine hydrochloride) are symmetric tricyclic amines with cagelike structures that are closely related structurally to one another. Amantadine was the first antiviral agent to be licensed for systemic use in the U.S. The activity of amantadine and rimantadine is limited to influenza A viruses. Rimantadine is 4- to 10-fold more active than amantadine.[268] The target of the inhibitory action for both amantadine and rimantadine is the influenza A virus M2 protein. Resistance to amantadine and rimantadine results from a point mutation in the RNA sequence encoding for the M2 protein transmembrane domain.[269] Resistance typically appears in the treated subject and his or her close contacts within 2 to 3 days of the initiation of therapy; as many as one-third of treated adults and children shed resistant strains of influenza by the fifth day of treatment.[270]

Pharmacokinetics. Amantadine is well absorbed after oral administration, with >90% of an orally administered dose being excreted unchanged in the urine.[271] Rimantadine is also well absorbed. In contrast with amantadine, however, rimantadine is metabolized extensively, with <15% of the drug being excreted unchanged in the urine.[272] Food does not appear to interfere with the absorption of either drug.

Toxicity and drug interactions. Generally, rimantadine is tolerated better than amantadine; the types of adverse reactions associated with both drugs are qualitatively similar but less frequent with rimantadine. The most common minor complaints associated with the administration of both drugs are dose-related gastrointestinal and CNS disturbances.

Clinical uses and dosage. Until the 2005–2006 influenza season, amantadine and rimantadine were useful in the prevention and treatment of infections caused by influenza A.[273] However, extremely high rates of resistance emerged rapidly in 2005, and at the current time neither amantadine nor rimantadine is recommended for treatment or prophylaxis of influenza.

Inorganic Pyrophosphate Analogues

Foscarnet (PFA, Foscavir)

Chemistry, mechanism of action, spectrum, and resistance. Foscarnet is an inorganic pyrophosphate analogue that inhibits all known human herpesviruses, including most ganciclovir-resistant CMV isolates and acyclovir-resistant HSV and VZV strains (see Table 295-3).[274] Foscarnet also is active against HIV. This antiviral agent directly inhibits DNA polymerase by blocking the pyrophosphate binding site and preventing cleavage of pyrophosphate from deoxynucleotide triphosphates.[275] Foscarnet is a noncompetitive inhibitor of viral DNA polymerases or HIV reverse transcriptase and is not incorporated into the growing viral DNA chain. It is approximately 100-fold more active against viral enzymes than against host cellular enzymes.[275] Resistance occurs as a result of DNA polymerase mutations; strains of CMV, HSV, and VZV with 3-fold to 5-fold reduced sensitivity to foscarnet have been reported.[276,277] These isolates may respond to therapy with acyclovir[276] or cidofovir.[277]

Pharmacokinetics. Foscarnet is absorbed poorly after oral administration, with a bioavailability of only about 20%.[274] This limits foscarnet's delivery to the intravenous route. Maximum serum concentration attained after a dose of 60 mg/kg is approximately 500 μmol/L. Data regarding tissue distribution are limited, but CSF concentrations are about two-thirds of those in serum.[278]

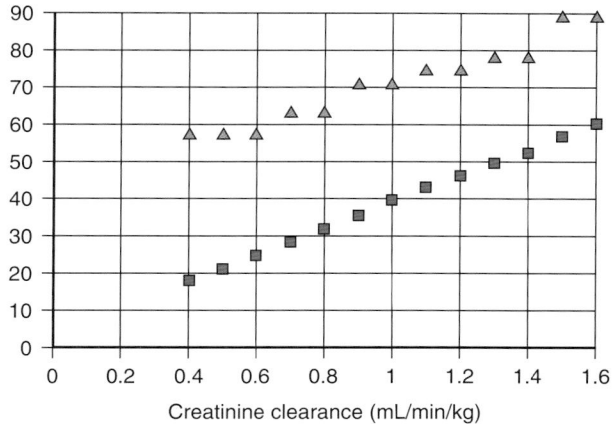

Figure 295-1. Recommended dosage of foscarnet in patients with varying degrees of renal impairment. Triangles indicate maintenance dose (mg/kg per day); squares indicate induction dose (mg/kg per 8 h). (Adapted from MacGregor RR, Graziani AL, Weiss R, et al. Successful foscarnet therapy for cytomegalovirus retinitis in an AIDS patient undergoing hemodialysis: rationale for empiric dosing and plasma level monitoring. J Infect Dis 1991;164:785–787, with permission.)

Eighty percent of an administered dose of foscarnet is eliminated unchanged in the urine; the half-life is 48 hours, and dosage adjustments are necessary even in the presence of minimal degrees of renal dysfunction (see Table 295-5). The degree of dose reduction is proportional to the degree of reduction in CrCl; when CrCl is 50% of normal, the dose should be reduced by about 50% (Figure 295-1). Hemodialysis efficiently eliminates foscarnet, and therefore an extra dose of drug is recommended after a 3-hour dialysis run.[279] There are no pharmacokinetic data for foscarnet in neonates.

Toxicity and drug interactions. The most common and serious adverse effects of foscarnet therapy are nephrotoxicity and metabolic derangements. Azotemia, proteinuria, acute tubular necrosis, crystalluria, and interstitial nephritis can occur,[280] and serum creatinine concentrations increase, usually during the second week of therapy, in as many as 50% of patients. In most affected patients, renal function returns to normal within 2 to 4 weeks after stopping therapy. Risk factors for developing renal dysfunction include pre-existing renal disease, concurrent use of other nephrotoxic drugs, dehydration, rapid injection of large doses, and continuous intravenous infusion of drug.[281] Electrolyte disturbances, including symptomatic hypocalcemia and hypercalcemia and hypophosphatemia and hyperphosphatemia, can be caused by foscarnet therapy. Hypocalcemia is due to direct chelation of ionized calcium by the drug, and patients can have symptoms such as paresthesias, tetany, seizures, and arrhythmias.[282] Metabolic disturbances can be minimized if foscarnet is administered by slow infusion, with rates not exceeding 1 mg/kg per minute. Common CNS symptoms associated with foscarnet therapy are headache, tremor, irritability, seizures, and hallucinations. Fever, nausea, vomiting, abnormal serum hepatic enzymes, anemia, granulocytopenia, and genital ulcerations also have been reported. The genital ulcerations appear to be associated with high urinary concentrations of drug.[283] Concomitant use of amphotericin B, cyclosporine, gentamicin, and other nephrotoxic drugs increases the likelihood of renal dysfunction associated with foscarnet therapy. Hypocalcemia is more common with coadministration of pentamidine, and anemia and neutropenia are more common when patients are treated with both foscarnet and zidovudine.

Clinical uses and recommended dosage. The most important indication for foscarnet is for therapy for sight-threatening chorioretinitis caused by CMV in patients with AIDS.[274] Several controlled trials have demonstrated that foscarnet is as effective as ganciclovir in managing this infection and may offer a survival advantage because of its inherent activity against HIV.[280] In refractory cases of chorioretinitis, foscarnet and ganciclovir therapy have been given in combination.[174] Foscarnet is also effective in the treatment of CMV infections caused by ganciclovir-resistant strains of CMV.[284] Limited data in patients with AIDS suggest that foscarnet may be of benefit when administered to those with gastrointestinal and pulmonary infections caused by CMV.[155,216] The usual dosage regimen of foscarnet for CMV infection is 180 mg/kg per day in three divided doses for 14 to 21 days, followed by a daily maintenance dose of 90 to 120 mg/kg. About 90% of patients have stabilization of their retinitis, and the time to progression of infection is prolonged to about 3 months.[285]

Infections caused by acyclovir-resistant strains of HSV and VZV also have been successfully controlled with foscarnet.[286,287] The dosage of foscarnet used for these infections is 120 mg/kg per day in 3 divided doses. In patients with AIDS, foscarnet therapy should be initiated within 7 to 10 days of suspicion of infection caused by acyclovir-resistant HSV or VZV.[288] Therapy should be continued until lesions have resolved.

Interferons and Pegylated Interferons

Chemistry, mechanism of action, spectrum, and resistance. Interferons are a family of nonspecific regulatory proteins associated with a variety of antiviral, antiproliferative, and immunomodulating activities.[289,290] There are two major types of interferons. Type 1 (α and β) interferons are secreted by all nucleated cells after viral infection; interferon-α is predominantly produced by virus-infected leukocytes, and interferon-β by fibroblasts. There are about 20 subtypes of interferon-α that share a high degree of amino acid sequence homology but have different antiviral and biologic effects on human cells in vitro.[291] Type II (γ, or immune) interferon is the product of antigen- or mitogen-stimulated lymphocytes. In addition to being produced by different cells, the major types of interferon are immunologically distinct and have unique biologic effects and physicochemical properties.[290] Interferons are active against a broad range of viruses; in general, RNA viruses are more susceptible than DNA viruses.

Interferons do not have direct antiviral activity, but rather exert antiviral effects by inducing production of more than two dozen effector proteins in exposed cells. Antiviral effects are mediated by inhibition of viral penetration or uncoating, synthesis or methylation of mRNA, viral protein translation, or viral assembly and release.[292] The main inhibitory effect for specific viruses differs among virus families, and individual viruses can be inhibited at more than one step. Antiviral activity also can be facilitated by the complex interactions between interferons and other components of the immune system, resulting in modification of host response to infection.[290]

Pharmacokinetics. Interferons are administered by intramuscular or subcutaneous routes, or by direct injection into viral lesions. Absorption of interferon-α is more than 80% complete after intramuscular or subcutaneous injection; plasma levels peak at 4 to 8 hours.[293] Plasma half-life is approximately 2 to 4 hours, but the antiviral state peaks at 24 hours and then slowly decreases to baseline over about 6 days.[294] Negligible plasma levels of interferon-β are detected after intramuscular or subcutaneous injection, and concentrations of interferon-γ are variable. After parenteral administration, only low concentrations of interferon are detectable in body tissues and fluid, including the CSF.[293] Interferon is eliminated by inactivation in various body fluids and metabolism in a number of organs, including the kidneys, liver, heart, skeletal muscle, and lungs. Negligible amounts are excreted in the urine.

Toxicity and drug interactions. Interferons cause immediate and late-onset adverse effects that are dose related.[295] With interferon doses at and above 1 to 2 million IU, most persons develop an influenza-like illness, with fever, chills, headache, myalgia, arthralgia, and gastrointestinal disturbances. These symptoms typically appear during the first week of therapy and remit with continued therapy. They rarely necessitate discontinuing therapy or modifying dosage.

Major therapy-limiting toxicities of systemically administered interferon are neuropsychiatric complications and bone marrow suppression.[296] About 10% to 20% of interferon recipients develop neuropsychiatric problems, with greatest frequency in elderly people; those with pre-existing CNS injuries, insults, or psychosis; and those with cirrhosis. Symptoms usually develop 2 to 3 months after the initiation of therapy and include somnolence, confusion, behavioral disturbances, depression, neurasthenia with profound fatigue, anorexia, weight loss, and occasionally seizures and coma. Neutropenia and thrombocytopenia are the most common signs of bone marrow suppression; they occur most frequently in patients with pre-existing portal hypertension.[297] Most persons have a 40% decline in absolute neutrophil count within the first week of therapy; therefore, therapy should be avoided in those with a neutrophil count <1500/mm^3 before therapy. The dose of interferon should be reduced by 50% if the neutrophil count drops to <1000/mm^3, and therapy should be discontinued if there is no increase in the count within 1 to 2 weeks. A 20% decline in platelet count also usually occurs in interferon recipients. The fall usually occurs within the first day or days of therapy. Interferon should be avoided in persons with pretreatment platelet counts <80,000/mm^3. The dosage should be reduced by 50% in those whose counts drop to <50,000/mm^3 during treatment, and the drug should be discontinued if there is no increase in the count within 1 to 2 weeks.

Less common side effects of interferon include exacerbation or development of autoimmune disorders (e.g., hypothyroidism and hyperthyroidism); renal dysfunction (e.g., proteinuria, interstitial nephritis, renal insufficiency, and acute rejection and nephrotic syndrome in renal transplant recipients); cardiac dysfunction (e.g., hypotension, arrhythmias, cardiomyopathy); diabetes; pulmonary infiltrates; hepatic dysfunction (elevated transaminases and triglyceride concentrations); alopecia; and impaired hormone levels and fertility among women.[296-298] Intralesional injection of interferon can be associated with development of influenza-like illness, leukopenia, and local pain, tenderness, and erythema.

Pegylated interferon has fewer side effects and is better tolerated overall than the nonpegylated interferons.

Interferon interferes with the function of the hepatic CYP450 enzymes and, as a result, significantly increases the half-lives and concentrations of drugs metabolized by these enzymes, such as theophylline. Interferon also increases the hematopoietic toxicity of myelotoxic drugs, such as zidovudine.

Clinical uses and recommended dosage. Interferon has been evaluated in the management of a wide variety of infections, and is currently approved for the following: (1) the treatment of chronic hepatitis caused by HBV and HCV, as well as papillomavirus-induced anogenital disease (interferon-α); (2) the treatment of multiple sclerosis (interferon-β); and (3) reduction of the frequency and severity of infections associated with chronic granulomatous disease (interferon-γ). The use of interferon for the treatment of other viral infections has been limited by dose-limiting side effects, a relative lack of potency, and the availability of less toxic, more active agents.

The use of interferon-α for the treatment of chronic hepatitis B and C infections is supported by a large number of controlled clinical trials.[299,300] A total of 30% to 40% of patients with chronic hepatitis B infection have biochemical and histologic improvement in response to parenteral administration of interferon-α; improvement is associated with a prompt decline of HBV DNA and polymerase activity.[299] Sustained inhibition of viral replication occurs in 30% to 40% of individuals with chronic infection, and 10% to 20% actually lose hepatitis B surface antigen.[301] The response to therapy often is associated with an elevation in serum transaminase levels and a hepatitis-like illness, thought to be related to the immune clearance of infected hepatocytes. Interferon does not appear to be of benefit in the management of acute hepatitis B or hepatitis delta (D) infection, although it may, at least transiently, benefit about 50% of patients with chronic hepatitis D infection.[302] Interferon therapy also seems to benefit some patients with hepatitis B-associated nephrotic syndrome and glomerulonephritis.[303,304]

Pegylated interferon α-2a recently has been approved for the treatment of chronic HBV infection.[305] Pegylated interferon α-2a monotherapy in HBeAg-positive patients with chronic hepatitis B results in loss of HBeAg in 35% of patients after 1 year. Combination therapy with lamivudine provided no additional benefit.[306]

Interferon-α results in normalized serum hepatic transaminase levels and histologic improvement in about 45% of individuals with chronic hepatitis C infection.[301,307] The response usually is associated with the loss of detectable serum hepatitis C virus RNA.[308] Unfortunately, 1 to 2 months after treatment is stopped, relapse occurs in approximately 50%; most patients who relapse respond to retreatment. Sustained responders tend to have lower pretreatment viral titers than those of nonresponders or those who relapse.[309] In an attempt to enhance therapeutic efficacy, oral ribavirin is used in combination with interferon-α (Rebetron) and peginterferon α-2a (Copegus), with improved outcomes. Forty-one percent of interferon-naive patients treated with interferon-α and oral ribavirin for 48 weeks had a sustained virologic response, compared with 16% of patients treated with interferon monotherapy.[310,311] Hepatitis C genotypes 2 and 3 are much more likely to respond to therapy than is genotype 1. Fifty percent of patients who relapsed after a previous course of interferon monotherapy had a sustained virologic response after 24 weeks of combination therapy.[312]

Interferon-α is indicated for the treatment of recalcitrant anogenital warts (condylomata acuminata) caused by papillomaviruses.[313] Both intralesional injection and systemic administration of interferon have been shown to produce some regression of warts. Intralesional injection is associated with complete clearing of injected warts in as many as 60% of treated individuals, but noninjected warts do not regress.[313,314] Systemic therapy may be indicated for those with extensive or refractory disease, but among these patients toxicity often limits utility. Systemic interferon-α also has been shown to have variable efficacy in the management of recurrent respiratory papillomatosis. Clinical relapse occurs in approximately one-third of patients who demonstrate an initial response to therapy.[315]

The dosage of systemic interferon-α varies with the indication for treatment. The highest doses, 10 million IU/1.73 m^2 given 3 times a week for 16 weeks, are needed for the treatment of chronic hepatitis B infections; children have been treated with 2 to 6 MU/m^2 at a similar interval.[316] Chronic hepatitis C infections are usually treated with 3 million IU given 3 times a week for 16 to 24 weeks. The dosage of pegylated interferon α-2a for monotherapy of chronic HBV or HCV infection is 180 µg once weekly for 48 weeks by subcutaneous injection. This dose also is used in combination with ribavirin for the treatment of chronic HCV infection. The usual dose of interferon used for intralesional therapy of HPV is 1 million IU injected into up to five warts 3 times a week for 3 weeks.

Neuraminidase Inhibitors

Oseltamivir Phosphate (Tamiflu)

Chemistry, mechanism of action, spectrum, and resistance. Oseltamivir is one of two licensed medications that specifically target the neuraminidase protein common to influenza A and B viruses. Oseltamivir is an ethyl ester prodrug that, following hydrolysis by hepatic esterases, is converted to the active compound, oseltamivir carboxylate. The prodrug masks the polarity of the active compound, allowing for enhanced oral bioavailability. The mechanism of action for this class of compounds is the specific inhibition of the influenza neuraminidase, with subsequent interference with the deaggregation and release of the viral progeny. The influenza neuraminidase enzyme is highly conserved, being common to type A H1N1, type A H2N2, type A H3N2, type A H5N1, and type B influenza viruses. Therefore, oseltamivir has activity against both influenza A and B viruses. Antiviral activity in vitro is dependent on the assay utilized and the viral strain evaluated.

In human challenge studies, only 3% of posttreatment isolates were resistant to oseltamivir. However, a phase IV study from Japan identified neuraminidase mutations conferring resistance to neuraminidase inhibitors in 18% of treated children.[317]

Pharmacokinetics. Oseltamivir has good oral bioavailability; at least 75% of orally administered drug reaches the systemic circulation in the form of oseltamivir carboxylate. The C_{max} and the AUC for the active compound following a multiple 75 mg bid oral dosing regimen are 348 ng/mL and 2719 ng • h/mL, respectively. Coadministration with food has no significant effect on the peak plasma concentration. Neither oseltamivir nor oseltamivir carboxylate is metabolized by CYP450 isoforms. Protein binding of oseltamivir carboxylate is only 3%, whereas the protein binding of the prodrug is 42%.

The half-life of oseltamivir after oral administration is 1 to 3 hours, whereas the half-life of oseltamivir carboxylate is 6 to 10 hours.[318] The primary route of elimination of oseltamivir is by conversion to the active drug, with more than 90% of the prodrug being metabolized to oseltamivir carboxylate. Oseltamivir carboxylate is not further metabolized, and it is entirely eliminated by renal excretion through glomerular filtration and anionic tubular secretion. Serum concentrations of oseltamivir carboxylate increase in the presence of declining renal function, and dose adjustment is recommended for patients with a CrCl below 30 mL/min. Administration of oseltamivir to patients with renal failure (CrCl <10 mL/min) has not been evaluated.

Toxicity and drug interactions. The most common adverse effect reported with oseltamivir use is nausea, with or without vomiting. In controlled clinical trials, approximately 10% of patients reported nausea without vomiting, and an additional 10% experienced vomiting. The nausea and vomiting episodes generally were mild to moderate and usually occurred on the first 2 days of oseltamivir administration. Fewer than 1% of study subjects discontinued participation in the clinical trials prematurely because of nausea and/or vomiting. Food may help to alleviate these gastrointestinal side effects in some patients.[319] Insomnia and vertigo also were reported more frequently among oseltamivir recipients than those receiving placebo.

No drug interactions have been described to date for oseltamivir or oseltamivir carboxylate. Neither the prodrug nor the active metabolite is metabolized by CYP450 isoforms. No dose adjustments are required when oseltamivir is coadministered with probenecid.

Clinical uses and recommended doses. Oseltamivir is licensed for the treatment and prophylaxis of influenza infection in patients 1 year of age and older. During 2009–2010, the FDA issued temporary emergency use authorization for treatment and prevention of 2009 H1N1 influenza in infants as young as 3 months of age. The efficacy of oseltamivir for the treatment of influenza has been established in two large phase III studies, one conducted at 60 centers throughout the U.S.,[320] and the other conducted at 63 centers in Europe, Canada, and China.[321] A total of 1355 patients were enrolled into these two trials, of whom 849 (63%) were subsequently confirmed to be infected with influenza. The vast majority (95%) of patients were infected with influenza A. Patients had to be enrolled within 36 hours of the onset of symptoms. The duration of illness among oseltamivir recipients was reduced by approximately 1.3 days compared with placebo recipients in both studies.[320,321] Among patients treated within 24 hours of the onset of symptoms, illness duration was reduced by almost 2 days.[321] Oseltamivir recipients compared with patients receiving placebo also had a more rapid return to normal health and activity.[320] No serious drug-related adverse events were noted. The proportions of oseltamivir recipients who experienced nausea were 17% and 12% for the U.S. and international studies, respectively. The frequency of physician-diagnosed secondary complications leading to antibiotic prescriptions also was reduced among oseltamivir recipients.[322] Similar results were observed in a randomized double-blind, placebo-controlled study conducted in children with influenza infection.[323]

Compared with placebo, administration of oseltamivir for 6 weeks during the peak of the influenza season significantly reduced the risk of contracting influenza.[324] The protective efficacy for the prevention of culture-proven influenza approached 90%,[324,325] which is comparable with that achievable with amantadine and rimantadine for influenza A.

The recommended oral dose of oseltamivir for the treatment of influenza in adults and adolescents 13 years and older is 75 mg bid for 5 days. For children 1 through 12 years of age, dose is based upon weight: (1) ≤15 kg (≤33 lb), 30 mg bid; (2) >15 kg to 23 kg (>33 lb to 51 lb), 45 mg bid; (3) >23 kg to 40 kg (>51 lb to 88 lb), 60 mg bid; and (4) >40 kg (>88 lb), 75 mg bid. Duration of treatment is 5 days. Data from the NIAID Collaborative Antiviral Study Group before and during the 2009 H1N1 pandemic determined that the appropriate dose of oseltamivir in infants from birth through 11 months of age is 3 mg/kg per dose given twice daily.[326] This same group assessed dosing in premature neonates, and estimated that 1 mg/kg per dose is the appropriate amount to administer in this at-risk group.[327] If possible, treatment should begin within 2 days of the onset of symptoms of influenza. Oseltamivir may be taken with or without food; when taken with food, tolerability may be enhanced in some patients.

The recommended oral dose of oseltamivir for the prophylaxis of influenza in adults and adolescents 13 years and older is 75 mg once daily for at least 7 days. Therapy should begin within 2 days of close contact with an infected person. Safety and efficacy have been demonstrated for up to 6 weeks.[324]

No dose adjustment is necessary for patients with CrCl >30 mL/min. In patients with CrCl <30 mL/min, it is recommended that the dose of oseltamivir be reduced to 75 mg once daily for 5 days. Caution is advised when one administers oseltamivir to patients with CrCl <10 mL/min, because the use of the compound has not been evaluated in this population. At present, oseltamivir is licensed by the FDA for use only in adults for the treatment of influenza A and B infections.

Zanamivir (Relenza)

Chemistry, mechanism of action, spectrum, and resistance. Zanamivir also interferes with the function of the influenza neuraminidase enzyme, with subsequent interference with the deaggregation and release of the viral progeny. Zanamivir has poor oral bioavailability and therefore is administered by oral inhalation. Although the amount of zanamivir that is delivered to the respiratory tract during inhalation depends on patient factors, such as inspiratory flow, the supplied delivery device delivers 4 mg of zanamivir when tested in vitro under conditions that approximate inhalation pressures achievable in vivo. Antiviral activity in vitro is dependent on the assay utilized and the viral strain evaluated.

Antiviral resistance can be induced in vitro by performing passage of the virus in the presence of increasing concentrations of zanamivir.[328,329] Decreased susceptibility to zanamivir was associated with mutations resulting in amino acid changes in the viral neuraminidase and/or hemagglutinin. Resistance has also been documented in clinical specimens isolated from a zanamivir recipient. After 2 weeks of therapy with zanamivir, an immunocompromised patient infected with influenza B shed a resistant isolate that was shown to have mutations in both the viral hemagglutinin and the viral neuraminidase.[330] The neuraminidase mutation resulted in a 1000-fold reduction in enzyme activity. Cross-resistance between zanamivir and oseltamivir has been demonstrated as well in resistant isolates generated in vitro. Accurate estimation of the risk of emergence of oseltamivir resistance in the clinical setting will be determined only by careful phase IV monitoring postlicensure.

Pharmacokinetics. More than 75% of an orally inhaled dose of zanamivir is deposited in the oropharynx, most of which is swallowed. Approximately 13% of the dose distributes to the airways and lungs, and the remainder is retained in the delivery device.[331] Inhaled zanamivir provides local concentrations in respiratory tract mucosa that greatly exceed inhibitory concentrations for influenza A and B viruses;[331,332] median zanamivir concentrations exceed 1000 ng/mL in sputum 6 hours after inhalation and remain detectable for 24 hours.[333] Between 4% and 17% of an inhaled dose of zanamivir is absorbed systemically. No metabolites of zanamivir have been identified, and all absorbed drug is excreted unchanged in the urine. Although serum zanamivir concentrations increase with decreasing CrCl, no adjustment in dosing is necessary in cases of renal insufficiency. Unabsorbed drug is excreted in the feces.

Toxicity and drug interactions. Zanamivir is well tolerated.[334] The most serious adverse event associated with its use is respiratory distress. Decline in pulmonary function and bronchospasm have been reported in some patients receiving zanamivir.[335,336] Many, but not all, of these patients had underlying airways disease, such as asthma or chronic obstructive pulmonary disease. Although influenza itself can cause such deteriorations, zanamivir is generally not recommended for the treatment of patients with underlying airways disease because of the risk of adverse events and the lack of demonstrated efficacy in this population. Zanamivir should be discontinued in any patient who develops bronchospasm or a decline in respiratory function.

No drug interactions with zanamivir have been reported.[337] Zanamivir does not affect CYP450 isoenzymes in human liver microsomes.

Clinical uses and recommended doses. The efficacy of zanamivir in the management of influenza A and B virus infections has been demonstrated in three placebo-controlled studies.[338-340] A total of 1588 patients were enrolled in these three investigations, of whom 1167 (73%) were infected with influenza. Patients received zanamivir, 10 mg inhaled bid, versus placebo inhaled bid. The zanamivir-treated patients improved 1.0 to 2.5 days faster than did the placebo recipients. Combined analysis of these trials indicated that zanamivir reduces the duration of symptoms by approximately 1.5 days.[336] Similar findings have been demonstrated in influenza-infected children.[341] Efficacy has been documented for both influenza A and influenza B.[342] Zanamivir therapy also reduces the frequency of antibiotic prescriptions for lower respiratory complications by 40%, although it does not reduce prescriptions for presumed upper respiratory tract complications.[343]

Inhaled zanamivir, 10 mg once daily administered for 4 weeks as seasonal prophylaxis, reduces the likelihood of laboratory-confirmed influenza infection (with or without symptoms) by 31%, influenza disease by 67%, and influenza disease with fever by 84%.[344] A study of zanamivir administered once daily to healthy household contacts of influenza-infected index subjects demonstrated a 79% reduction in influenza illness.[345]

Zanamivir is indicated for the treatment of uncomplicated illness due to influenza A and B virus of no more than 2 days' duration. The recommended dose of zanamivir for the treatment of influenza in adults and children aged 7 years and older is two inhalations of 5 mg each administered bid for 5 days. Two doses should be taken on the first day of treatment whenever possible, provided that there is at least 2 hours between doses. On subsequent days, the doses should be approximately 12 hours apart. Patients scheduled to use an inhaled bronchodilator at the same time as zanamivir should use their bronchodilator before taking zamanivir.

No dose adjustments are indicated in patients with impaired renal function.

296 Antiparasitic Agents

Craig M. Wilson

This chapter provides an overview of antiparasitic therapy organized broadly into: (1) agents active against luminal protozoans; (2) agents active against the kinetoplastid protozoans; (3) agents active against the malarial parasites; (4) antibacterial agents with antiprotozoan activity; and (5) anthelmintics. These divisions are somewhat arbitrary, because some drugs are pertinent to more than one category. Appendix 296-1 is a reproduction with permission of the *Drugs for Parasitic Infections*, 2010 edition, published by The Medical Letter, Inc., and is organized by organism.[1] Currently recommended dosing indications for individual drugs are given in the table and can vary by organism. Most of the drugs and their particular indications in specific disease states, as well as recommendations for treatment and prophylaxis are discussed more extensively in pathogen-specific chapters. A few drugs that are not available in the United States but are used extensively in other countries are discussed.

The tables in the Medical Letter provide recommendations that are likely to be consistent in many cases with those of the American Academy of Pediatrics (AAP) Committee on Infectious Diseases, as given in the disease-specific chapters. However, because the Medical Letter recommendations are developed independently, these recommendations occasionally may differ from recommendations of the AAP. Accordingly, both should be consulted. The AAP appreciate the consideration of the Medical Letter in allowing this information to be printed. These recommendations periodically (usually every other year) are updated and, thus, are likely to be superseded by new ones before the next edition of this publication is printed.

Commercial production and distribution of several widely used antiparasitic agents have ceased in the U.S. over the past several years, because of commercial nonprofitability for their manufacturers in the domestic market.[2] These agents include niclosamide, quinacrine, diloxanide furoate, and furazolidone. Specialized compounding pharmacies may import bulk powder of all of these compounds previously approved by the U.S. Food and Drug Administration (FDA). Expert Compounding Pharmacy and Medical Center Pharmacy have well-established reputations within the tropical disease community. A listing of compounding pharmacies is available at www.pccarx.com. Diethylcarbamazine (DEC), melarsoprol, nifurtimox, sodium stibogluconate, suramin, dehydroemetine, and bithionol now are only available through the Centers for Disease Control and Prevention (CDC). Telephone numbers for the above-mentioned companies and the CDC are given in Appendix 296-1. Intravenous quinidine for treatment of severe malaria is no longer stocked routinely by most hospitals because it has fallen into disuse as a cardiac agent.

There are multiple other informative resources about antiparasitic therapy, including a more detailed discussion of pharmacokinetics and adverse reactions.[3] *Martindale: The Complete Drug Reference* contains comprehensive information on antiparasitic drugs available worldwide, including brand names.[4] For particular recommendations regarding malaria prophylaxis and advice for physicians on case management, the telephone numbers are given in Chapter 271, *Plasmodium* Species (Malaria).

TREATMENT OF LUMINAL PROTOZOA

Therapy for luminal protozoa has changed little in the past decade. However, some advances have been made in management of luminal protozoa that increasingly are being recognized as pathogens, initially in patients with the acquired immunodeficiency syndrome (AIDS) and then in other community settings, such as in group childcare. In addition, tinidazole and nitazoxanide have been approved for use.

Metronidazole and Tinidazole

Metronidazole and tinidazole are synthetic nitroimidazoles with selective activity against organisms that utilize anaerobic metabolism. Metronidazole has been shown to be efficacious for the following protozoan infections: *Entamoeba histolytica,*[5] *E. polecki,*[6] *Giardia intestinalis,*[7] *Trichomonas vaginalis,*[8] *Blastocystis hominis,*[9] and *Balantidium coli.*[10] The approval of tinidazole was based on studies done predominantly in the 1970s and 1980s prior to its use in European countries. Tinidazole is approved for use against giardiasis and amebiasis in adults and children >3 years of age and for trichomoniasis in adults.[11] For amebiasis, these drugs are active against the trophozoite stage of the parasite life cycle and can be used to treat the luminal and tissue phases of the infection, including liver abscesses. Patients with invasive colonic disease or liver abscess also are treated with iodoquinol or other luminally active amebicides to eliminate residual cyst forms of the parasite. Metronidazole and tinidazole are the only effective therapy available in the U.S. for trichomoniasis, with cure rates approaching 95% with single-dose regimens of both drugs.[12] Tinidazole has in vitro activity against metronidazole-resistant strains of *T vaginalis.*[13] Both drugs are effective against giardiasis.[14] Generally, tinidazole is as effective as metronidazole for most clinical indications and is modestly better tolerated. Tinidazole is used as a single-dose regimen for giardiasis and trichomoniasis and the recommended course for amebiasis is shorter. Despite this, a course of tinidazole is considerably more expensive than generic metronidazole for all indications.[11] Tinidazole is not available in suspension but can be formulated by crushing the tablets. Ornidazole is another nitroimidazole with a similar pharmacokinetic profile to tinidazole and also with extensive clinical experience in non-U.S. settings.[15]

Both metronidazole and tinidazole generally are well tolerated, with tinidazole being modestly more favorable compared with metronidazole at the high single-dose regimens or at the higher doses used for amebiasis. Side effects of both drugs include nausea, vomiting, epigastric discomfort, anorexia, and a metallic or bitter taste. Seizures and peripheral neuropathy have been reported uncommonly with both drugs. Patients taking either drug should avoid alcohol (including that found commonly in suspensions of children's medicines) because of the disulfiram-like effects.

Furazolidone

Furazolidone is a nitrofuran derivative most commonly used in treatment of giardiasis in children because of its availability in a liquid preparation, although it is no longer commercially available in the U.S. This agent has been used for a variety of bacterial pathogens of the intestine, including *Vibrio cholerae.* The gastrointestinal tract side effects of nausea and vomiting are the most common complaints associated with furazolidone therapy. Allergic reactions, including pulmonary infiltration, hypotension, urticaria, fever, and vesicular rash, occur occasionally. Other potential complications of furazolidone therapy are a disulfiram-like reaction with concurrent use of alcohol-containing medications, hemolytic anemia either in infants <1 month of age or in patients with glucose-6-phosphate dehydrogenase (G6PD) deficiency, and reactions due to the drug's monoamine oxidase inhibitor activity.

Nitazoxanide

Nitazoxanide is an antiparasitic agent with specific indications for treatment of cryptosporidiosis and giardiasis in children.[16] Nitazoxanide is a nitrothiazolyl-salicylamide derivative, whose activity appears to be at the level of electron transfer of anaerobic metabolism.[17] Cure rates in small, randomized trials were comparable with standard agents for giardiasis.[18] Treatment trials using nitazoxanide for cryptosporidiosis have shown greater efficacy compared with placebo in nonimmunocompromised hosts but no effect in immunocompromised children.[19–21] Nitazoxanide has been shown in limited trials with limited follow-up to have some activity against *Ascaris, Trichuris,* and *Hymenolepis* and amebiasis but is not regarded at this time as being either a first-line or alternative therapy for these infections.[22–24] Nitazoxanide generally is well tolerated with side-effect profiles comparable with placebo in multiple studies. Rarely yellow sclera are noted which clear with discontinuation of the drug.

Iodoquinol

Iodoquinol, or diiodohydroxyquin, is a halogenated oxyquinoline; it is a luminally active agent with efficacy for *E. histolytica, Dientamoeba fragilis, Blastocystis hominis,* and *Balantidium coli.*[25] For *E. histolytica,* iodoquinol is used to treat patients with asymptomatic shedding of cysts or as adjunctive therapy for patients being treated with other agents for invasive disease. Gastrointestinal tract complaints, including nausea, cramps, and diarrhea, are the most common problems associated with iodoquinol therapy. Other side effects occasionally associated with its use are rash, acne, anal pruritus, and slight enlargement of the thyroid gland.

Diloxanide Furoate

A dichloroacetamide derivative of an acetanilide, diloxanide furoate has amebicidal activity at low concentrations. It is a luminally active agent with activity against *E. histolytica* and *E. polecki.* Diloxanide furoate has no activity against the extraluminal forms of *E. histolytica.* Its only common side effect is flatulence; nausea, vomiting, and diarrhea are occasional side effects. The drug is well tolerated and inexpensive; however, it is not readily available in most countries and may be available through a compounding pharmacy listed in Appendix 296-1.

Paromomycin

Paromomycin, an aminoglycoside, is poorly absorbed from the gastrointestinal tract but is active as a luminal agent for *E. histolytica, D. fragilis,* and *G. intestinalis.* Paromomycin also has activity against human tapeworms but not against the extraluminal forms of *E. histolytica.* The use of paromomycin for giardiasis is limited but may be indicated for treatment of giardiasis during pregnancy. Paromomycin also has been used to treat cryptosporidiosis in a limited number of people and, when combined with azithromycin, appears to impact malabsorption and diarrhea in patients with AIDS.[26,27] The frequent side effects of paromomycin with oral use are gastrointestinal tract disturbances, which are self-limited.

TREATMENT OF KINETOPLASTIDAE INFECTIONS

Treatment of infections with either *Trypanosoma* or *Leishmania* spp. generally is difficult because of drug toxicity, the refractory nature of the organisms to available therapies, and the need for prolonged therapy. The first-line drugs for these infections are available from the CDC.

Suramin

Suramin sodium is a nonmetallic compound developed in the 1920s on the basis of structural similarities to trypanocidal dyestuffs. Suramin is active against the hemolymphatic stages of

African trypanosomes (*Trypanosoma brucei rhodesiense* and *T. b. gambiense*) and also has been used prophylactically for workers in areas where *T. b. gambiense* is highly endemic. Suramin is available from the CDC and only in a parenteral formulation. The side effects of suramin are protean and can be life-threatening. Frequently encountered side effects include vomiting and acute hypersensitivity-like reactions (pruritus, urticaria, paresthesias, hyperesthesia of hands and feet, and photophobia) and, later, neurologic, ocular, renal, and hepatic toxicities. Arsenic-based compounds or eflornithine are recommended for central nervous system (CNS) trypanosomiasis. Suramin also is one of the only compounds active against the adult stages of onchocerciasis, but toxicity limits its overall usefulness.

Melarsoprol

Melarsoprol, a trivalent antimonial compound, is used exclusively for treatment of CNS trypanosomiasis caused by *T. b. rhodesiense*. It is only available from the CDC and in a parenteral formulation. Severe side effects are common and include fever, vomiting, a delayed drug-induced reactive encephalopathy (which is potentially fatal), myocardial damage, albuminuria, hypertension, colic, Herxheimer-type reaction, and peripheral neuropathy. Multiple other toxic effects include gastrointestinal tract complaints, hypersensitivity reactions, renal and hepatic dysfunction, and a severe hemolytic anemia in G6PD-deficient patients. Eflornithine has become the drug of choice for CNS trypanosomiasis caused by *T. b. gambiense*.

Eflornithine

Eflornithine, or difluoromethylornithine (DFMO), is an irreversible inhibitor of the enzyme ornithine decarboxylase and is active preferentially against many protozoan parasites. Eflornithine is a drug of choice, alone or in combination to treat people with African sleeping sickness caused by *T. b. gambiense*, including people with advanced CNS disease.[28–30] Eflornithine has limited side effects compared with other available agents, but its use in endemic areas is limited by its cost and labor intensive administration. East African sleeping sickness caused by *T. b. rhodesiense* is less responsive to this therapy. Eflornithine causes mild reversible bone marrow toxicity, which is manifest as anemia, leukopenia, and, occasionally, thrombocytopenia; diarrhea; seizures; and occasional transient hearing loss. Eflornithine is available from the World Health Organization (WHO).

Nifurtimox

Nifurtimox is a nitrofuran with activity against both African and American (*T. cruzi*, Chagas disease) trypanosomiasis. It is the agent most commonly used for treatment of acute infections with *T cruzi*, for which it is about 80% effective.[31] The efficacy of nifurtimox for the chronic forms of Chagas disease appears to be more geographically variable, with better results in Chile, Venezuela, Argentina, and southern Brazil than in central Brazil.

Therapy with nifurtimox generally is prolonged, and another agent commonly is substituted because of toxicity. Toxic effects of nifurtimox usually are reversible. They include gastrointestinal tract symptoms (anorexia, vomiting), weight loss, memory loss, sleep disorders, weakness, and nervous system disorders (tremor, paresthesias, polyneuritis, and, rarely, convulsions). Other rare complications are fever, pulmonary infiltrates, and pleural effusion. Children generally tolerate therapy better than adults.

Sodium Stibogluconate

Sodium stibogluconate, a synthetic pentavalent antimonial agent, is the drug of choice for treatment of leishmaniasis in the U.S.[32,33] Meglumine antimonate is a related compound used more extensively in francophone countries and in Central and South America.[34] These compounds probably are as active against leishmaniasis as the trivalent antimonial agents but generally are better

tolerated. Side effects of sodium stibogluconate include gastrointestinal tract complaints (nausea, diarrhea), musculoskeletal complaints (muscle and joint pain), fatigue, serum transaminase elevations, T-wave inversion or flattening, pancreatitis, and, rarely, myocardial, renal, and hepatic damage.

Pentamidine

A diamidine, pentamidine is effective as a second-line agent for visceral or cutaneous leishmaniasis and also for the hemolymphatic stages of African trypanosomiasis.[35] Pentamidine is used most commonly in the U.S. as a second-line agent for treatment or prophylaxis of *Pneumocystis* pneumonia (PCP).[36]

Pentamidine is available in a parenteral preparation or for aerosolization therapy for PCP. A high incidence of side effects is associated with the parenteral administration of pentamidine. These include hypoglycemia, hyperglycemia, pain at the injection site, hypotension, gastrointestinal tract disturbances, including vomiting, reversible nephrotoxicity, serum transaminase elevations, electrolyte disturbances, and bone marrow toxicities. Less common toxicities are anaphylaxis, acute pancreatitis, hyperkalemia, and cardiotoxicity Pentamidine should not be used concurrently with didanosine, foscarnet, nephrotoxic drugs, or erythromycin, because it can potentiate these agents' toxicities. There are few systemic side effects with the aerosolized therapy, although bronchospasm is common, as is difficulty delivering this therapy effectively to younger children.

Parenteral pentamidine for therapy and aerosolized pentamidine for prophylaxis of PCP usually are reserved for patients who cannot tolerate or (rarely) whose disease does not respond to trimethoprim-sulfamethoxazole (TMP-SMX) therapy.

Amphotericin B

Amphotericin B has been shown to be useful as an alternative therapy for treatment of various forms of leishmaniasis, especially mucocutaneous disease. This agent generally is reserved for use when antimonial therapy has failed. The overall use of amphotericin B for leishmaniasis is limited by toxicity of the drug and the need for prolonged intravenous therapy. Lipid micelle formulations of amphotericin B are useful because they are less toxic.[37,38] The FDA has approved the liposomal preparation of amphotericin B for treatment of visceral leishmaniasis.[39] Amphotericin B also has been used in a limited number of cases to treat primary meningoencephalitis due to free-living amebas.[40] Other second-line therapies not commonly used in the U.S. for trypanosomiasis (benznidazole) and leishmaniasis (meglumine and miltefosine) are noted in Appendix 296-1.

ANTIMALARIAL THERAPY

Therapy and prophylaxis for malaria are becoming more complex because of the spread of drug resistance, initially with *Plasmodium falciparum* but now also with *P. vivax*. The *qinghaosu* derivatives or artemisinin-based compounds are being used extensively worldwide as antimalarial agents, with good results in areas where multidrug-resistant parasites are a problem.[41–43] Artemether/lumefantrine is now available in the U.S. for treatment of *P. vivax* acquired in areas where chlororquine resistance has been reported. Reports of resistance to artemisinin-based compounds are beginning to emerge.[44]

Chloroquine

Chloroquine, a 4-amino-quinoline, has been the backbone of antimalarial therapy and prophylaxis for >50 years. The incessant spread of resistance to chloroquine by *P. falciparum* is leading to a resurgence of malaria in most endemic areas. Extensive reports of chloroquine treatment failures with *P. vivax* have been reported from Papua New Guinea and Indonesia along with sporadic reports from Brazil, Myanmar, India, Guyana, and Colombia.[45,46] However, most cases of malaria due to *P. vivax*, *P. malariae*, or *P.*

ovale remain responsive to chloroquine. Like most antimalarial agents, chloroquine is active against the erythrocytic stages of the parasite; other agents are necessary for the radical cure of *P. vivax* and *P. ovale* infections. Chloroquine has been used as adjunctive therapy with dehydroemetine for invasive amebiasis unresponsive to initial therapy as well as for therapy of connective tissue autoimmune diseases unresponsive to other agents.

Chloroquine is well tolerated by most people, even for long-term therapy. The side effects include mild gastrointestinal tract complaints (which are usually alleviated if the drug is taken with meals), occasional headaches, blurred vision, dizziness, fatigue, confusion, depigmentation of hair, skin eruptions, corneal opacity, weight loss, and myalgias. Intense pruritus, a common complaint among black Africans taking the drug, usually is relieved with antihistamines. Chloroquine is contraindicated in patients with psoriasis, retinal disease, or porphyria.

The preparations of chloroquine available in the U.S. are bitter-tasting tablets; hydroxychloroquine is better tolerated in children. Suspensions of chloroquine are available widely elsewhere for pediatric use and are much better tolerated. The use of intravenous chloroquine for patients unable to take chloroquine orally largely has been supplanted by use of intravenous quinidine in the U.S.

Quinine

Quinine, a cinchona alkaloid, was the first commercially available antimalarial agent; its use was supplanted when chloroquine became available. Well known for its antimalarial effects, quinine also is effective when used in combination with clindamycin for treatment of babesiosis. The use of this agent has grown with the spread of chloroquine resistance, and now there are increasing reports of clinical resistance to quinine in multiple geographic regions.

Oral quinine sulfate, in combination with pyrimethamine-sulfadoxine, tetracycline, or clindamycin, is the recommended therapy for *P. falciparum* malaria (falciparum malaria) acquired in areas of chloroquine resistance. For patients unable to take oral medication, intravenous quinidine gluconate is the drug of choice because of its safety compared with intravenous quinine hydrochloride.[47]

Quinine commonly causes a group of side effects known collectively as *cinchonism*, which in the mild form consists of tinnitus, impaired vision, headache, nausea, and abdominal pain and, in its more severe form, of cardiovascular, gastrointestinal, and dermal manifestations. Blood glucose levels must be monitored carefully in any patient receiving quinine, because hypoglycemia occurs commonly, particularly in the setting of high parasitemia. An idiosyncratic hypersensitivity reaction to quinine also can occur, most commonly manifesting as extensive skin flushing with an intense, generalized pruritus; this is a contraindication to further use of the drug.

Quinidine

Quinidine, the dextrostereoisomer of quinine, is the drug of choice when parenteral antimalarial therapy is required.[47] Quinidine gluconate is as potent an antimalarial agent as quinine and generally is available. (See Appendix 296-1 if availability is a problem.) The potential side effects, similar to those seen with quinine, include cinchonism, idiosyncratic hypersensitivity reactions, and risk of hypoglycemia in the setting of high parasitemia. The usual precautions associated with use of quinine, such as careful cardiac monitoring, should always be followed. Patients requiring quinidine should be changed to oral therapy, whether chloroquine, quinine, or other antimalarial drugs, as soon as tolerated.

Mefloquine

A 4-quinolinemethanol analogue of quinine, mefloquine is most commonly used for prophylaxis of malaria in areas of chloroquine-resistant malaria.[48] When used for treatment, mefloquine generally is effective when administered as a single dose.[49] Clinical resistance to mefloquine has emerged rapidly in areas where the drug is widely available, particularly in border areas of Thailand with Myanmar and Cambodia. Most resistant isolates also are resistant to halofantrine.

Nausea and vomiting have been problematic in children taking mefloquine. Other reported side effects include headache, insomnia, abnormal dreams, visual disturbances, depression, anxiety disorder, and dizziness. Rare serious adverse reactions include acute reversible severe neuropsychiatric reaction, seizures, and cardiac conduction abnormalities. Mefloquine is safe to use in pregnancy, although data on use in the first trimester are limited. Mefloquine is contraindicated in people with active depression, a recent history of depression, generalized anxiety disorder, psychosis, schizophrenia, other major psychiatric disorders, or seizures (but not including typical febrile seizures). It should be used with caution in people with psychiatric disturbances or a previous history of depression. Generally, mefloquine should not be prescribed for anyone taking other cardioactive medications.

Halofantrine

Halofantrine is a 9-phenanthrenemethanol that was developed nearly in parallel with mefloquine and is available outside the U.S.[50] Halofantrine has been approved by the FDA for treatment of malaria; however, it is not marketed in the U.S. It is used both prophylactically and for treatment in areas of chloroquine-resistant malaria. Resistance is emerging rapidly in areas of widespread use of halofantrine, and there is evidence of cross-resistance with mefloquine.

Halofantrine generally is well tolerated, but it must be taken with a fatty meal to ensure consistent absorption. Occasional side effects of halofantrine are prolongation of the QT and PR interval, diarrhea, abdominal pain, and pruritus. Halofantrine must be used with caution in patients with cardiovascular problems.

Primaquine

An 8-aminoquinoline, primaquine is the only drug available for treating the latent hepatic life cycle forms of *P. vivax* and *P. ovale*. Thus, primaquine is recommended for the radical cure of these infections once chloroquine treatment has been initiated for the erythrocytic stages of infection.

Primaquine generally is well tolerated except in people with G6PD deficiency, in whom it can lead to brisk hemolysis. Patients should be screened for G6PD deficiency before primaquine therapy. Patients with the Mediterranean or Caucasian type of G6PD deficiency should not be treated with primaquine; those with the milder type seen in African American populations can be treated with the dosage given here. Other occasional side effects are neutropenia, gastrointestinal tract disturbance, and methemoglobinemia. Relapses of *P. vivax* after primaquine therapy have responded to retreatment with chloroquine and either higher doses or more prolonged courses of primaquine.[51] Primaquine also has been used with clindamycin in a limited number of patients with AIDS who have PCP and in whom other therapies have failed.[52]

Atovaquone

Atovaquone, a hydroxynaphthoquinone, is a ubiquinone analogue that has been studied most extensively as an antimalarial agent. Atovaquone has been released in the U.S. for treatment of PCP[53] and toxoplasmosis.[54] Atovaquone is approved by the FDA in fixed-dose combination with proguanil (Malarone in both adult and pediatric dosages) for both treatment and prophylaxis of *P. falciparum* infections. Atovaquone was combined with proguanil because of rapid development of resistance in vitro and in early clinical trials when atovaquone was used alone for malaria. Multiple studies have documented efficacy of the combination for both treatment and prophylaxis of *P. falciparum* malaria,[55] and there is a growing experience in treatment of infections with *P.*

vivax. The combination of atovaquone with azithromycin has been shown to be an effective therapy for babesiosis with a better side effect profile than clindamycin and quinine.[56]

For PCP, studies have indicated that atovaquone is slightly less efficacious but is tolerated moderately better than either TMP-SMX or pentamidine.[57] There are no efficacy data in children; however, pharmacokinetic data are similar to those in adults. The most common side effects are fever, nausea, diarrhea, and rashes. Unlike most of the currently used therapies, atovaquone has been shown to be active against the tissue cyst stages of *Toxoplasma gondii* in animal models. Atovaquone has been used alone or in combination with pyrimethamine for treatment of CNS toxoplasmosis in AIDS patients.[58]

ANTIBACTERIAL AGENTS WITH ANTIPROTOZOAN ACTIVITY

Tetracycline and Doxycycline

Agents with antiprotozoan activity increasingly have been used as antimalarial compounds, mainly in areas where drug-resistant malaria is a problem. When used for treatment, these compounds should always be given in combination with more rapidly acting drugs such as quinine, because generally they are slowly malariacidal. Tetracycline has been used more extensively for treatment of acute malaria, and doxycycline more commonly for prophylaxis. The drugs generally are well tolerated except for common gastrointestinal tract complaints.

Photosensitivity and secondary *Candida* vaginitis are concerns with more prolonged prophylactic use of tetracycline and doxycycline. Use of this class of compounds is restricted in pregnancy and generally in children younger than 8 years because of potential toxicity. Tetracycline also is efficacious for treatment of balantidiasis and can be used as adjunctive therapy with metronidazole to treat amebiasis.

Clindamycin

Clindamycin is a macrolide antibiotic, which, when used as an antiprotozoan agent, always is combined with other therapies for treatment of falciparum malaria, toxoplasmosis, and babesiosis. Clindamycin plus quinine is one of the alternative regimens useful for treatment of malaria during pregnancy and in people from areas with chloroquine resistance.[59] Clindamycin plus pyrimethamine is effective as an alternative for treatment of *Toxoplasma* encephalitis in patients infected with human immunodeficiency virus (HIV) who cannot tolerate sulfadiazine.[60] Clindamycin with quinine (or quinidine) is a recommended therapy for babesiosis,[61] although atovaquone with azithromycin has better side effect profile.[56] Clindamycin has been used in combination with primaquine for treatment of PCP in a limited number of patients.[52]

Generally, clindamycin is well tolerated in children who have a less apparent risk for development of pseudomembranous colitis as a complication of therapy.

Spiramycin

Spiramycin is a macrolide antibiotic used more extensively in Europe for treatment of toxoplasmosis in pregnancy. Spiramycin has been used in the U.S. for treatment of congenital toxoplasmosis in patients who are intolerant of other therapies. Spiramycin has been used to treat cryptosporidiosis in HIV-infected patients, but its efficacy is questionable.[62] The drug generally is well tolerated and is available in the U.S. from the FDA (telephone: 301-443-4280). Occasional side effects are gastrointestinal tract disturbances.

Folate Metabolism Inhibitors

Many antiprotozoan compounds have been developed that take advantage of reliance of a parasite on the synthesis or scavenging of folate precursors. These compounds include the dihydrofolate reductase (DHFR) inhibitors, which preferentially inhibit the parasite enzyme, and also sulfonamides, which act as para-aminobenzoic acid analogues and either inhibit, or act as suicide substrates in the folate biosynthetic pathways. These two classes of compounds are often formulated in combinations for various indications. DHFR inhibitors used for antiparasitic therapy include pyrimethamine, trimethoprim, proguanil, and trimetrexate. The sulfonamides have varying pharmacokinetic properties, which are taken advantage of in the formulations used for treatment of parasitic infections.

Pyrimethamine with sulfadiazine is the treatment of choice for toxoplasmosis in most clinical settings. A limiting factor in HIV-infected patients who require prolonged therapy for toxoplasmosis is the high incidence of side effects, mainly attributed to the sulfonamide component. Pyrimethamine has been used with clindamycin in this clinical setting to circumvent these problems.[60] Supplementation with folinic acid often is recommended with prolonged use of pyrimethamine, to lessen the bone marrow-suppressive effects of this drug and to prevent folic acid deficiency.

TMP-SMX, commonly formulated in a 1:5 ratio, is the treatment and prophylaxis of choice for PCP in both HIV-infected patients and patients receiving immunosuppressive therapy.[63] The only limitation of this regimen is the high incidence (up to 65%) of untoward reactions in HIV-infected patients.[64] Trimethoprim with dapsone has been shown to be efficacious for PCP prophylaxis, although toxicity still remains a problem. TMP-SMX is the recommended therapy for any patient with *Cystoisospora belli* infection, although relapse in patients with AIDS is common.[65] TMP-SMX also has been shown to have efficacy for *Cyclospora cayetanensis* infections in HIV-infected patients.[66,67] TMP-SMX has been used for treatment of toxoplasmosis, but pyrimethamine-sulfadiazine should be considered the treatment of choice. TMP-SMX also has been used for prophylaxis against *T. gondii* in patients with AIDS who test positive for antibodies to *T. gondii* and thus have a 25% to 50% risk for toxoplasmic encephalitis. This combination also has been used to treat malaria in areas where drug resistance is not a major problem, although it is not a recommended therapy.

Proguanil, the prototype of the DHFR inhibitors, is not available in the U.S. but is available overseas. Proguanil has been approved by the FDA to be used in a fixed-dose combination with atovaquone (see earlier) for both treatment and prophylaxis of infections with *P. falciparum*. Trimetrexate is a lipid-soluble, potent DHFR inhibitor with the lowest therapeutic index in this group of compounds. It is available in the U.S. for treatment of PCP and also has been used for treatment of toxoplasmosis.[68] Generally, trimetrexate is used in combination with folinic acid (20 mg/m² per dose 4 times daily) to prevent bone marrow toxicity. Toxicity is a problem with the combinations of DHFR inhibitors and sulfonamides, particularly in patients with AIDS. Most of these untoward reactions are attributed to the sulfonamide components of the combination. The common side effects of sulfonamides are rashes, fever, bone marrow suppression, gastrointestinal tract complaints, and hepatotoxicity. More severe but less common reactions include toxic epidermal necrolysis, Stevens–Johnson syndrome, erythema multiforme, and serum sickness. The toxicity most commonly associated with the DHFR inhibitors is bone marrow suppression, which usually can be alleviated by folinic acid supplementation. Proguanil also is associated with oral ulcerations, hair loss, scaling of palms and soles, and urticaria. Trimetrexate occasionally causes rash, peripheral neuropathy, and a rise in serum aminotransferase values.

TREATMENT OF HELMINTHIC INFECTIONS

Therapy of helminthic infection often is confusing to the clinician for the following reasons: (1) a large number of available compounds have overlapping activity; (2) for mostly commercial reasons, these compounds are variably available in different countries; and (3) the spectrum of activity for the individual drugs often does not parallel the common biologic classification of helminths into nematodes, trematodes, and cestodes. If all drugs were available universally, the use of just three highly efficacious and safe drugs – praziquantel, albendazole, and ivermectin – would cover essentially all human helminthic infections.[69] These three drugs and all anthelmintics marketed in the U.S. are described here. Because some drugs have broad activity, the grouping of drugs according to their most common indications is overly simplistic but provides a general framework.

INTESTINAL NEMATODES

Mebendazole

Mebendazole, a synthetic benzimidazole, is the agent used most widely in the U.S. for treatment of intestinal helminthiasis, including ascariasis, hookworm infection, trichuriasis, trichostrongyliasis, and enterobiasis. Regimens of mebendazole consisting of a single high dose generally yield lower cure rates compared with regimens of single-dose albendazole. Treatment of capillariasis, infection with a nematode that is rare outside a circumscribed area of the Philippines, requires administration of mebendazole orally for 20 days, but albendazole generally is preferred for this indication. High-dose mebendazole often is used as a secondary agent in the treatment of trichinellosis; systemic corticosteroids must be used concomitantly. Because neither DEC nor ivermectin is effective against *Mansonella perstans* infection, mebendazole is thought to be the optimal treatment.[70] Mebendazole has been used in the past to treat *Angiostrongylus cantonensis*, *Gnathostoma spinigerum*, and echinococcal disease. Due to the poor tissue penetration of mebendazole and the current availability of albendazole in all countries, mebendazole should no longer be used for these indications.

Mebendazole binds irreversibly to colchicine-sensitive sites on tubulin, blocking microtubule assembly. Glucose uptake by the organism is thus inhibited without an effect on serum glucose levels in humans. Because of poor gastrointestinal tract absorption (<10%), side effects from the usual low-dose regimens are restricted to abdominal pain and diarrhea, mostly in people with heavy worm burdens, in whom an *Ascaris* worm occasionally migrates to the nose or mouth. With high-dose regimens, monitoring for bone marrow suppression (leukopenia, agranulocytosis) and hepatic transaminase elevation is required.

Mebendazole tablets can be chewed, swallowed whole, or crushed with food. Test of cure should not be performed for at least 1 week after therapy. Lack of data in children <2 years of age has precluded specific U.S. labeling for or establishment of dosage in this age group though the label leaves the physician some discretion in electing to treat children <2 years of age. A recent review has led the WHO to recommend use of mebendazole, if otherwise indicated, in children as young as 1 year of age.[71] There are no data on the agent's excretion in human milk, but little is excreted in animal milk; caution is indicated but breastfeeding women can be treated if necessary. Pediatric dosage is identical to adult dosage. Mebendazole is teratogenic in rats and generally has been avoided during pregnancy. Data now suggest no increase in major congenital defects, so mebendazole can be recommended for use in the second and third trimesters if absolutely necessary.[72]

Albendazole

Albendazole is a synthetic nitroimidazole with a broad spectrum of antinematodal activity similar to that of mebendazole but also with anticestodal and some antiprotozoal action. The advantage of albendazole over mebendazole is its activity in a single oral dose of 400 mg (200 mg for children <2 years of age) against ascariasis, hookworm infection, enterobiasis, trichostrongylosis, and, to a slightly lesser extent, trichuriasis. Because intestinal helminthiasis is typically multiparasitic, albendazole is an almost ideal agent.[73,74] It has good activity in multiple doses against both cutaneous larva migrans and strongyloidiasis, but single-dose therapy with ivermectin is more effective for these two helminthic

infections.[75,76] Successful treatment of visceral larva migrans has been reported.[77] Efficacy against the microfilarial stage of *Wuchereria bancrofti*, *Brugia malayi*, and *Loa loa* is well documented, although DEC remains the drug of choice for treatment of individual patients with these filarial infections.[78-80] DEC and albendazole in combination has superior activity against adult *W. bancrofti* compared with either drug alone.[81] Reports with limited numbers of patients have documented the activity of albendazole in giardiasis,[82] microsporidiosis,[83] clonorchiasis, trichinellosis, and capillariasis, but its role in treatment of these infections has yet to be defined. The benefit of any existing chemotherapy for gnathostomiasis or angiostrongyliasis is doubtful, but albendazole is thought to be the most active benzimidazole.[84]

Prolonged high-dose regimens of albendazole constitute the most effective medical treatment of larval cestode disease caused by *Echinococcus granulosus*, *E. multilocularis*, and *E. vogelii*.[85] Some studies suggest that an initial trial of medical therapy can obviate surgical intervention in relatively uncomplicated disease.[86] Dosage is not defined in children <6 years of age. Treatment is individualized to response and normally is required for a minimum of several months. Concentration in cyst fluid is approximately 25% of plasma concentration. Earlier recommendations and FDA labeling of cycles of 28 days of therapy followed by 14 days of rest before the next cycle of therapy are now thought to be unnecessary. Albendazole should be started several days before any surgical intervention to minimize the effect of intraoperative spillage of cyst contents.

The necessity for anticestodal chemotherapy in neurocysticercosis is controversial.[87-90] In comparative nonblinded trials, albendazole appeared to have slightly higher activity than praziquantel. Cerebrospinal fluid levels of albendazole are approximately 40% plasma levels. Either 8 or 28 days of therapy has been used, with cycles repeated according to clinical judgment. Corticosteroids, which increase plasma levels of albendazole up to 50%, usually are administered concomitantly. Albendazole has activity in multiple doses against adult *Taenia* spp., but its use is discouraged for this indication.

The mode of action of albendazole is identical to that already described for mebendazole. Intake with a fatty meal is necessary to attain tissue levels required to treat extraluminal helminths. Detectable levels are achieved in serum, cerebrospinal fluid, cyst fluid, and bile with a serum half-life of 8 to 15 hours depending on the dose. Rapid extensive hepatic biotransformation to the active metabolite, albendazole sulfoxide, occurs, but the major route of excretion is not clear. Side effects of low-dose albendazole therapy are minimal, consisting of diarrhea, abdominal pain, migration of *Ascaris* through the mouth or nose, and rare hypersensitivity. With high-dose therapy, elevations of hepatic transaminases, dizziness, neutropenia, and alopecia are most common.[91] Serum hepatic enzyme levels and blood count should be monitored every 2 weeks during high-dose therapy. No problems specific to children have been documented and considerations in using albendazole <2 years of age for soil-transmitted helminthiasis are identical to those for mebendazole (see above). However, significant embryotoxic potential precludes the use of albendazole in pregnancy. Albendazole is manufactured as a suspension as well as tablets that can be crushed with food, chewed, or taken whole.

Pyrantel Pamoate

Pyrantel pamoate, a broad-spectrum anthelmintic drug, is only available as an over-the-counter oral suspension in the U.S. This drug has been supplanted by the benzimidazoles, except for its continued popularity for the treatment of enterobiasis. A single-dose regimen is sufficient for ascariasis and trichostrongylosis, but three such doses on consecutive days are required for hookworm infection. Pyrantel pamoate is ineffective for trichuriasis.

The agent is nonvermicidal but causes depolarizing neuromuscular blockade of helminth musculature. Paralyzed worms are expelled with intestinal peristalsis. Because of poor absorption from the gastrointestinal tract, side effects are restricted to infrequent occurrence of abdominal pain, diarrhea, dizziness, insomnia, rash, and headache. Pyrantel pamoate should be used with caution in people with hepatic dysfunction. Although no specific data exist on its use in children younger than 2 years of age, no age-related problems have been documented. Few data exist on use in pregnancy, and pyrantel pamoate is nonembryotoxic in animals. If absolutely necessary, it can be used in pregnancy after the first trimester. Pyrantel pamoate should not be administered concurrently with piperazine.

SYSTEMIC NEMATODES

Diethylcarbamazine (DEC)

DEC is a piperazine derivative used primarily in treatment of selected human filarial infections. Because of frequent unacceptable side effects in persons infected with *Onchocerca volvulus*, DEC should not be used for microfilaricidal treatment of this parasite; ivermectin is the drug of choice. DEC is ineffective for treatment of *Mansonella* spp. and should not be used to treat visceral larva migrans.

For lymphatic filariasis (*W. bancrofti, Brugia malayi*, and *B. timori*) and loiasis, relatively low-dose microfilaricidal regimens are often used in the developing world as part of mass treatment campaigns. In the treatment of the individual patient, however, the aim is macrofilaricidal activity, with use of multiple aggressive courses of therapy.[92] Dosage regimens are not well established in children, but infection is rare in children <2 years of age. Use of weekly DEC for prophylaxis of loiasis is effective.[93]

DEC, which should be taken after a meal, is absorbed readily, is distributed into all body compartments, and undergoes renal excretion with a serum half-life of 8 hours. The mechanism of action is not documented clearly. Side effects, which often correlate with microfilarial load, most commonly include nausea, dizziness, headache, visual disturbances, and fever. Transient microscopic hematuria is common.[94] The gastrointestinal tract side effects are dose-related, and some patients cannot tolerate the 9 mg/kg per day dose. In lymphatic filariasis, the death of adult worms often results in lymphadenopathy or lymphangitis, frequently in the genital region. Encephalopathy can occur after treatment for loiasis in people with high microfilarial counts.[95]

Ivermectin

Ivermectin, a semisynthetic lactone originally developed in the 1970s for veterinary use, is the most potent anthelmintic ever developed. Receptor-mediated hyperpolarization of cells after an influx of negatively charged ions occurs through a novel glutamate-sensitive chloride channel present in nematodes. The drug is well absorbed when taken orally, and excretion is almost entirely in the feces, with a serum half-life of 12 hours.

Originally developed for human use in onchocerciasis, ivermectin is now the treatment of choice for *O. volvulus* in a single microfilaricidal dose. Ivermectin is also microfilaricidal for *W. bancrofti, B. malayi*, and *L. loa*; it was also microfilaricidal in a single patient with *Mansonella ozzardi*.

At doses studied to date, ivermectin apparently is not macrofilaricidal. Determination of the true macrofilaricidal potential awaits further studies of the range of dosages of this remarkably nontoxic compound.[96,97] Until then, DEC, which has macrofilaricidal activity, remains the drug of choice for *W. bancrofti, B. malayi*, and *L. loa*. Ivermectin is inactive against *M. perstans*.

Ivermectin, as a single dose or as two doses 1 day apart, is the drug of choice for uncomplicated strongyloidiasis.[98] Its efficacy rate far exceeds that of any other available drug, and only mild adverse reactions have been documented. Thiabendazole, previously the drug of choice, is no longer available. Dosing of oral ivermectin in disseminated strongyloidiasis is not well studied[99] and subcutaneous administration of veterinary preparations has been reported in life-threatening cases.[100] A single dose of ivermectin is curative in up to 100% of cases of cutaneous larval migrans and similarly will supersede older therapies for this indication.[101,102] Single-dose ivermectin is equal in efficacy to other

available agents for treatment of ascariasis, enterobiasis, and trichuriasis but is poorly active against hookworm.

Ivermectin itself is nontoxic. All adverse effects are due to reactions to the release of endosymbiotic bacteria from dying parasites.[103] This so-called Mazzotti-type reaction can occur in onchocerciasis and filariasis and consists of fever, pruritus, urticaria, headache, myalgia, joint and bone pain, and tender lymphadenopathy.[104] In general, severity of the reaction is proportionate to microfilarial load and rapidity of death of microfilariae. Thus, reactions are less marked in *B. malayi* infection, in which microfilarial clearance occurs over days rather than hours. In lymphatic filariasis and loiasis, severity of adverse effects with ivermectin is equivalent to those found with DEC. Ivermectin should not be used in patients who have loiasis with more than 5000 microfilariae per mL of blood, and all patients with microfilaremic loiasis require premedication with corticosteroids. Adverse outcomes have not been observed in women accidentally treated while pregnant; use in pregnancy is not recommended.

TREMATODES AND CESTODES

Praziquantel

Praziquantel, which is almost universally available, is the drug of choice for all fluke infections except for *Fasciola hepatica* (sheep liver fluke), and for all cestode infections.[105] It is effective for all species and clinical manifestations of schistosomiasis, including CNS disease, in a single dose.[106] For liver and intestinal flukes including *Clonorchis sinensis* (Chinese liver fluke), *Opisthorchis viverrini* (liver fluke), *Fasciolopsis buski* (intestinal fluke), *Heterophyes heterophyes* (intestinal fluke), *Paragonimus westermani* (lung fluke), and *Metagonimus yokogawai* (intestinal fluke), multidose therapy is required.

A single dose of praziquantel is an effective treatment for adult stages of the tapeworms *Taenia saginata* (beef), *T. solium* (pork), and *Diphyllobothrium latum* (fish). Although it is more expensive and is absorbed systemically, single-dose praziquantel offers the advantage over niclosamide of not requiring purging and of theoretical guarding against cysticercosis. Because praziquantel is effective against intraluminal cysticerci, a single dose is required for *Hymenolepis nana*, in contrast to a 7-day course of niclosamide.

The necessity for anticestodal chemotherapy in neurocysticercosis due to *T. solium* is controversial (see above). In comparative nonblinded trials, albendazole appears to have slightly higher activity than praziquantel and is the current drug of choice. The often-practiced concomitant administration of dexamethasone can reduce serum levels of praziquantel by as much as 50%.

Praziquantel is a heterocyclic prazinoisoquinoline derivative, the precise mechanism of action of which is unknown. The agent is rapidly taken up by helminths, with resultant loss of intracellular calcium causing blebbing and bursting of the tegument. Exposure of worm antigens in this way may allow the host immune system to play a role in final parasite death. Oral absorption is rapid, with extensive first-pass metabolism by the liver. High levels (10% to 25% of serum levels) are achieved in cerebrospinal fluid, bile, feces, and human milk. Serum half-life is 1 to 1.5 hours with rapid renal excretion. Plasma concentrations can be higher in patients with hepatic compromise. Side effects, including lassitude, malaise, headache, and dizziness, are common but are mild and transient. More uncommonly, sedation, fever, pruritus, rash, sweating, and severe abdominal discomfort occur. No specific data on the use of praziquantel in children <4 years of age are available, but no age-specific problems have been reported. Nursing mothers must stop breastfeeding during and for 72 hours after completion of treatment. Tablets must be swallowed whole.

Niclosamide

Niclosamide is a highly effective single-dose treatment for adult stages of *T. saginata, T. solium*, and *D. latum* tapeworm infections.[107]

Its production has been discontinued in the U.S. This agent kills the scolex and proximal segments of the cestodes on contact by uncoupling oxidative phosphorylation. Because niclosamide causes degeneration of proglottids, a laxative purge 1 to 2 hours after treatment is recommended to reduce the theoretical risk of cysticercosis from release of eggs. Treatment can be repeated in a few days if it is not effective. Mild nausea and abdominal pain are the only reported side effects of this negligibly absorbed compound.

Other Anthelmintic Drugs

Because *F. hepatica* infection may not respond to praziquantel, a single dose of triclabendazole is now regarded by the World Health Organization as the drug of choice for this disorder.[108–110] Efforts to register triclabendazole are ongoing in many endemic countries, and in the U.S., the drug can be obtained on a "compassionate-release" basis from the manufacturer.

An older drug for *F. hepatica*, bithionol, can be obtained from the CDC. Bithionol is also an alternative drug for the treatment of *P. westermani* (lung fluke). Side effects include photosensitivity reactions, urticaria, and gastrointestinal complaints (vomiting, diarrhea, abdominal pain). Production of bithionol ceased >30 years ago, but apparently, current stocks retain potency.

Oxamniquine and metrifonate are effective, well-tolerated antischistosomal drugs most frequently used in the developing world. Piperazine citrate, piperazine adipate, and piperazine hexahydrate are inexpensive and quite effective treatments for ascariasis or enterobiasis, but because of potential toxicity and the need for prolonged treatment, they should not be used when other agents are available.[111] Pyrvinium pamoate, used in some places for enterobiasis, is no longer available commercially in the U.S.

Drugs for
Parasitic Infections

With increasing travel, immigration, use of immunosuppressive drugs and the spread of AIDS, physicians anywhere may see infections caused by parasites. The table below lists first-choice and alternative drugs for most parasitic infections. The table on page 12 summarizes the known prenatal risks of antiparasitic drugs. The brand names and manufacturers of the drugs are listed on page 14.

Infection		Drug	Adult dosage	Pediatric dosage
ACANTHAMOEBA keratitis				
Drug of choice:		See footnote 1		
AMEBIASIS *(Entamoeba histolytica)*				
asymptomatic				
Drug of choice:		Iodoquinol[2]	650 mg PO tid x 20d	30-40 mg/kg/d (max. 2g) PO in 3 doses x 20d
	OR	Paromomycin[3]	25-35 mg/kg/d PO in 3 doses x 7d	25-35 mg/kg/d PO in 3 doses x 7d
	OR	Diloxanide furoate[4]*	500 mg PO tid x 10d	20 mg/kg/d PO in 3 doses x 10d
mild to moderate intestinal disease				
Drug of choice:[5]		Metronidazole	500-750 mg PO tid x 7-10d	35-50 mg/kg/d PO in 3 doses x 7-10d
	OR	Tinidazole[6]	2 g once PO daily x 3d	≥3yrs: 50 mg/kg/d (max. 2g) PO in 1 dose x 3d
		either followed by		
		Iodoquinol[2]	650 mg PO tid x 20d	30-40 mg/kg/d (max. 2g) PO in 3 doses x 20d
	OR	Paromomycin[3]*	25-35 mg/kg/d PO in 3 doses x 7d	25-35 mg/kg/d PO in 3 doses x 7d
severe intestinal and extraintestinal disease				
Drug of choice:		Metronidazole	750 mg PO tid x 7-10d	35-50 mg/kg/d PO in 3 doses x 7-10d
	OR	Tinidazole[6]	2 g once PO daily x 5d	≥3yrs: 50 mg/kg/d (max. 2g) PO in 1 dose x 5d
		either followed by		
		Iodoquinol[2]	650 mg PO tid x 20d	30-40 mg/kg/d (max. 2g) PO in 3 doses x 20d
	OR	Paromomycin[3]*	25-35 mg/kg/d PO in 3 doses x 7d	25-35 mg/kg/d PO in 3 doses x 7d
AMEBIC MENINGOENCEPHALITIS, primary and granulomatous				
Naegleria fowleri				
Drug of choice:		Amphotericin B[7,8]	1.5 mg/kg/d IV in 2 doses x 3d, then 1 mg/kg/d x 6d plus 1.5 mg/d intrathecally x 2d, then 1 mg/d every other day x 8d	1.5 mg/kg/d IV in 2 doses x 3d, then 1 mg/kg/d x 6d plus 1.5 mg/d intrathecally x 2d, then 1 mg/d every other day x 8d
Acanthamoeba spp.				
Drug of choice:		See footnote 9		

* Availability problems. See table on page 16.
1. Keratitis is typically associated with contact lens use (FR Carvalho et al, Cornea 2009; 28:516). Topical 0.02% chlorhexidine and polyhexamethylene biguanide (PHMB, 0.02%), either alone or in combination, have been used successfully in a large number of patients. Treatment with either chlorhexidine or PHMB is often combined with propamidine isethionate *(Brolene)* or hexamidine *(Desmodine)*. None of these drugs is commercially available or approved for use in the US, but they can be obtained from compounding pharmacies (see footnote 4). Leiter's Park Avenue Pharmacy, San Jose, CA (800-292-6773; www.leiterrx.com) is a compounding pharmacy that specializes in ophthalmic drugs. Propamidine is available over the counter in the UK and Australia. Hexamidine is available in France. The combination of chlorhexidine, natamycin (pimaricin) and debridement also has been successful (K Kitagawa et al, Jpn J Ophthalmol 2003; 47:616), as has 0.1% sodium diclofenac (AL Agahan et al, Ann Acad Med Singapore 2009; 38: 175) in a small series of 3 patients. Debridement is most useful during the stage of corneal epithelial infection; keratoplasty in medically unresponsive keratitis was successful in 31 patients (AS Kitzmann et al, Ophthalmology 2009; 116: 864). Most cysts are resistant to neomycin; its use is no longer recommended. Azole antifungal drugs (ketoconazole, itraconazole) have been used as oral or topical adjuncts. Use of corticosteroids is controversial. Prolonged therapy (≥6 months) may be necessary (JK Dart et al, Am J Ophthalmol 2009; 148:487).
2. Iodoquinol should be taken after meals.
3. Paromomycin should be taken with a meal.
4. Not available commercially. It may be obtained through compounding pharmacies such as Expert Compounding Pharmacy, 6744 Balboa Blvd, Lake Balboa, CA 91406 (800-247-9767) or Medical Center Pharmacy, New Haven, CT (203-688-7064). Other compounding pharmacies may be found through the National Association of Compounding Pharmacies (800-687-7850) or the Professional Compounding Centers of America (800-331-2498, www.pccarx.com).
5. Nitazoxanide may be effective against a variety of protozoan and helminth infections (DA Bobak, Curr Infect Dis Rep 2006; 8:91; E Diaz et al, Am J Trop Med Hyg 2003; 68:384). It is effective against mild to moderate amebiasis, 500 mg bid x 3d (JF Rossignol et al, Trans R Soc Trop Med Hyg 2007; 101:1025; AE Escobedo et al, Arch Dis Child 2009; 94:478). It is FDA-approved only for treatment of diarrhea caused by *Giardia* or *Cryptosporidium* (Med Lett Drugs Ther 2003; 45:29). Nitazoxanide is available in 500-mg tablets and an oral suspension; it should be taken with food.
6. A nitroimidazole similar to metronidazole, tinidazole appears to be as effective as metronidazole and better tolerated (Med Lett Drugs Ther 2004; 46:70). It should be taken with food to minimize GI adverse effects. For children and patients unable to take tablets, a pharmacist can crush the tablets and mix them with cherry syrup *(Humco,* and others). The syrup suspension is good for 7 days at room temperature and must be shaken before use (HB Fung and TL Doan, Clin Ther 2005; 27:1859). Ornidazole, a similar drug, is also used outside the US.
7. Not FDA-approved for this indication.

e1

Appendix 296-1. Drugs for parasitic infections. (Reprinted with permission from Drugs for Parasitic Infections. Treatment Guidelines from The Medical Letter 2010;8(Suppl):e1–e20.)

Infection	Drug	Adult dosage	Pediatric dosage
AMEBIC MENINGOENCEPHALITIS (continued)			
Balamuthia mandrillaris			
Drug of choice:	See footnote 10		
Sappinia diploidea			
Drug of choice:	See footnote 11		
ANCYLOSTOMA caninum (Eosinophilic enterocolitis)			
Drug of choice:	Albendazole[7,12]	400 mg PO once	400 mg PO once
OR	Mebendazole	100 mg PO bid x 3d	100 mg PO bid x 3d
OR	Endoscopic removal		
Ancylostoma duodenale, see HOOKWORM			
ANGIOSTRONGYLIASIS (*Angiostrongylus cantonensis, Angiostrongylus costaricensis*)			
Drug of choice:	See footnote 13		
ANISAKIASIS (*Anisakis* spp.)			
Treatment of choice:[14]	Surgical or endoscopic removal		
ASCARIASIS (*Ascaris lumbricoides,* roundworm)			
Drug of choice:[5]	Albendazole[7,12]	400 mg PO once	400 mg PO once
OR	Mebendazole	100 mg bid PO x 3d or 500 mg once	100 mg PO bid x 3d or 500 mg once
OR	Ivermectin[7,15]	150-200 mcg/kg PO once	150-200 mcg/kg PO once
BABESIOSIS			
Drug of choice:[16]	Atovaquone[7,17]	750 mg PO bid x 7-10d	40 mg/kg/d PO in 2 doses x 7-10d
	plus azithromycin[7]	500-1000 mg PO on d1, then 250-1000 mg PO on d2-10	10 mg/kg (max 500 mg/dose) PO on d 1, then 5 mg/kg/d (max 250 mg dose) PO on d 2-10
OR	Clindamycin[7,18]	300-600 mg IV qid or 600 mg PO tid x 7-10d	20-40 mg/kg/d PO in 3 doses x 7-10d
	plus quinine[7,19]	650 mg PO tid x 7-10d	30 mg/kg/d PO in 3 doses x 7-10d
Balamuthia mandrillaris, see AMEBIC MENINGOENCEPHALITIS, PRIMARY			
BALANTIDIASIS (*Balantidium coli*)			
Drug of choice:	Tetracycline[7,20]	500 mg PO qid x 10d	40 mg/kg/d (max. 2 g) PO in 4 doses x 10d
Alternative:	Metronidazole[7]	500-750 mg PO tid x 5d	35-50 mg/kg/d PO in 3 doses x 5d
OR	Iodoquinol[2,7]	650 mg PO tid x 20d	30-40 mg/kg/d (max 2 g) PO in 3 doses x 20d

* Availability problems. See table on page 16.

8. A *Naegleria fowleri* infection was treated successfully in a 9-year old girl with combination of amphotericin B and miconazole (both drugs given intravenously and intrathecally) plus oral rifampin (JS Seidel et al NEJM 1982; 306:346). While amphotericin B and miconazole appear to have a synergistic effect, Medical Letter consultants believe the rifampin probably had no additional effect (GS Visvesvara et al, FEMS Immunol Med Microbiol 2007; 50:1). Parenteral miconazole is no longer available in the US. Azithromycin (changed to clarithromycin during therapy because of toxicity concerns and for better CNS penetration) has been used in multidrug combination regimens to treat *Balamuthia* infection. *In vitro*, azithromycin is more active than clarithromycin against *Naegleria*, so may be a better choice combined with amphotericin B for treatment of *Naegleria* (TR Deetz et al, Clin Infect Dis 2003; 37:1304; FL Schuster and GS Visvesvara, Drug Resistance Updates 2004; 7:41). Combinations of amphotericin B, ornidazole and rifampin (R Jain et al, Neurol India 2002; 50:470), amphotericin B, fluconazole (IV and PO) and rifampin (J Vargas-Zepeda et al, Arch Med Research 2005;36:83) and amphotericin B, chloramphicol and rifampacin have also been used (R Rai et al, Indian Pediatr 2008; 45:1004). Case reports of other successful therapy have been published (FL Schuster and GS Visvesvara, Int J Parasitiol 2004; 34:1001).
9. Several patients with granulomatous amebic encephalitis (GAE) have been successfully treated with combinations of pentamidine, sulfadiazine, flucytosine, and either fluconazole or itraconazole (GS Visvesvara et al, FEMS Immunol Med Microbiol 2007; 50:1). GAE in an AIDS patient was treated successfully with sulfadiazine, pyrimethamine and fluconazole combined with surgical resection of the CNS lesion (M Seijo Martinez et al, J Clin Microbiol 2000; 38:3892). Chronic *Acanthamoeba* meningitis was successfully treated in 2 children with a combination of oral trimethoprim/sulfamethoxazole, rifampin and ketoconazole (T Singhal et al, Pediatr Infect Dis J 2001; 20:623). Disseminated cutaneous infection in an immunocompromised patient was treated successfully with IV pentamidine, topical chlorhexidine and 2% ketoconazole cream, followed by PO itraconazole (CA Slater et al, N Engl J Med 1994; 331:85) and with voriconazole and amphotericin B lipid complex (R Walia et al, Transplant Infect Dis 2007; 9:51). Other reports of successful therapy have been described (FL Schuster and GS Visvesvara, Drug Resistance Updates 2004; 7:41; AC Aichelburg et al, Emerg Infect Dis 2008; 14:1743). Susceptibility testing of *Acanthamoeba* isolates has shown differences in drug sensitivity between species and even among strains of a single species; antimicrobial susceptibility testing is advisable (FL Schuster and GS Visvesvara, Int J Parasitiol 2004; 34:1001).
10. *B. mandrillaris* is a free-living ameba that causes subacute to fatal granulomatous amebic encephalitis (GAE) and cutaneous disease (MMWR 2008; 57:768; FL Schuster et al, Clin Infect Dis 2009; 48:879). Three cases of *Balamuthia* encephalitis have been successfully treated with pentamidine, flucytosine, fluconazole and sulfadiazine plus either azithromycin or clarithromycin combined with surgical resection of the CNS lesion; in two cases flucytosine was given as well. Clarithromycin may have less toxicity and better penetration into CSF than azithromycin (TR Deetz et al, Clin Infect Dis 2003; 37:1304; S Jung et al, Arch Pathol Lab Med 2004; 128:466).
11. A free-living ameba that may rarely be pathogenic to humans (GS Visvesvara et al, FEMS Immunol Med Microbiol 2007; 50:1; F Marciano-Cabral, J Infect Dis 2009; 199: 1104). *S. diploidea* has been successfully treated with azithromycin, pentamidine, itraconazole and flucytosine combined with surgical resection of the CNS lesion (BB Gelman et al, J Neuropathol Exp Neurol 2003; 62:990).
12. Albendazole must be taken with food; a fatty meal increases oral bioavailability.
13. *A. cantonensis* causes predominantly neurotropic disease (QP Wang et al, Lancet Infect Dis 2008; 8:621). *A. costaricensis* causes gastrointestinal disease. Most patients infected with either species have a self-limited course and recover completely. Analgesics, corticosteroids and periodic removal of CSF can relieve symptoms from increased intracranial pressure (L Ramirez-Avila et al, Clin Infect Dis 2009; 48:322). Treatment of *A. cantonensis* is controversial and varies across endemic areas. No antihelminthic drug is proven to be effective and some patients have worsened with therapy. Mebendazole or albendazole each with or without a corticosteroid appear to shorten the course of infection (K Sawanyawisuth and K Sawanyawisuth, Trans R Soc Trop Med Hyg 2008; 102:990; V Chotmongkol et al. Am J Trop Med Hyg 2009; 81:443).
14. Gastric anisakiasis can usually be diagnosed and treated by endoscopic removal of the worm. Enteric anisakiasis is more difficult to diagnose; it can be managed without worm removal as the worms eventually die. Surgery may be needed in the event of intestinal obstruction or peritonitis (A Repiso Ortega et al, Gastroenterol Hepatol 2003; 26:341; K Nakaji, Intern Med 2009; 48:573). Successful treatment of anisakiasis with albendazole 400 mg PO bid x 3-5d has been reported, but diagnosis was presumptive (DA Moore et al, Lancet 2002; 360:54; E Pacios et al, Clin Infect Dis 2005; 41:1825).
15. Safety of ivermectin in young children (<15 kg) and pregnant women remains to be established. Ivermectin should be taken on an empty stomach with water (NM Fox, Curr Opin Infect Dis 2006; 19:588).
16. E Vannier et al, Infect Dis Clin North Am 2008; 22:469; GP Wormser et al, Clin Infect Dis 2006; 43:1089. *B. microti* is most common in the US. Most disease in Europe is attributed to *B. divergens* and is generally more severe. Several cases caused by various *B. divergens*-like agents have also been documented in the US (BL Herwaldt et al, Emerg Infect Dis 2004; 10:622). Exchange transfusion has been used in combination with drug treatment in severely ill patients and those with high (>10%) parasitemia. In non-immunosuppressed patients infected with *B. microti* who were not severely ill, combination therapy with atovaquone and azithromycin was as effective as clindamycin and quinine and better tolerated (PJ Krause et al, N Engl J Med 2000; 343:1454). Immunosuppressed patients and those with asplenia should be treated a minimum of 6 weeks and at least 2 weeks past the last positive smear. Resistance to azithromycin-atovaquone treatment has been reported in immunocompromised patients (GP Wormser et al. Clin Infect Dis 2010; 50:381). Some patients may be co-infected with the etiologic agents of Lyme disease and human granulocytic anaplasmosis.
17. Atovaquone is available in an oral suspension that should be taken with a meal to increase absorption.
18. Oral clindamycin should be taken with a full glass of water to minimize esophageal ulceration.

e2

Infection	Drug	Adult dosage	Pediatric dosage
BAYLISASCARIASIS (*Baylisascaris procyonis*)			
Drug of choice:	See footnote 21		
***BLASTOCYSTIS* spp.** infection			
Drug of choice:	See footnote 22		
CAPILLARIASIS (*Capillaria philippinensis*)			
Drug of choice:	Mebendazole[7]	200 mg PO bid x 20d	200 mg PO bid x 20d
Alternative:	Albendazole[7,12]	400 mg PO daily x 10d	400 mg PO daily x 10d
Chagas' disease, see TRYPANOSOMIASIS			
Clonorchis sinensis, see FLUKE infection			
CRYPTOSPORIDIOSIS (*Cryptosporidium*) Non-HIV infected			
Drug of choice:	Nitazoxanide[5]	500 mg PO bid x 3d	1-3yrs: 100 mg PO bid x 3d 4-11yrs: 200 mg PO bid x 3d >12yrs: 500 mg PO bid x 3d
HIV infected			
Drug of choice:	See footnote 23		
CUTANEOUS LARVA MIGRANS (creeping eruption, dog and cat hookworm)			
Drug of choice:[24]	Albendazole[7,12]	400 mg PO daily x 3d	400 mg PO daily x 3d
OR	Ivermectin[7,15]	200 mcg/kg PO daily x 1-2d	200 mcg/kg PO daily x 1-2d
CYCLOSPORIASIS (*Cyclospora cayetanensis*)			
Drug of choice:[25]	Trimethoprim/ sulfamethoxazole[7]	TMP 160 mg/SMX 800 mg (1 DS tab) PO bid x 7-10d	TMP 10 mg/kg/SMX 50 mg/kg/d PO in 2 doses x 7-10d
Alternative:	Ciprofloxacin[7]	500 mg PO bid x 7d	—
CYSTICERCOSIS, see TAPEWORM infection			
CYSTOISOSPORIASIS (*Cystoisospora belli,* formerly known as *Isospora*)			
Drug of choice:[26]	Trimethoprim- sulfamethoxazole[7]	TMP 160 mg/SMX 800 mg (1 DS tab) PO bid x 10d	TMP 10 mg/kg/d/SMX 50 mg/kg/d PO in 2 doses x 10d
***DIENTAMOEBA fragilis* infection**[27]			
Drug of choice:[28]	Iodoquinol[2,7]	650 mg PO tid x 20d	30-40 mg/kg/d (max. 2g) PO in 3 doses x 20d
OR	Paromomycin[3,7*]	25-35 mg/kg/d PO in 3 doses x 7d	25-35 mg/kg/d PO in 3 doses x 7d
OR	Metronidazole[7]	500-750 mg PO tid x 10d	35-50 mg/kg/d PO in 3 doses x 10d
Diphyllobothrium latum, see TAPEWORM infection			
DRACUNCULUS medinensis (guinea worm) infection			
Drug of choice:	See footnote 29		
Echinococcus, see TAPEWORM infection			
Entamoeba histolytica, see AMEBIASIS			
ENTEROBIUS vermicularis (pinworm) infection			
Drug of choice:[30]	Albendazole[7,12]	400 mg PO once; repeat in 2wks	400 mg PO once; repeat in 2wks
OR	Mebendazole	100 mg PO once; repeat in 2wks	100 mg PO once; repeat in 2wks
OR	Pyrantel pamoate[31*]	11 mg/kg base PO once (max. 1 g); repeat in 2wks	11 mg/kg base PO once (max. 1 g); repeat in 2wks
Fasciola hepatica, see FLUKE infection			
FILARIASIS[32, 33]			
Wuchereria bancrofti, Brugia malayi, Brugia timori			
Drug of choice:[34]	Diethylcarbamazine*	6 mg/kg/d PO in 3 doses x 12d[35,36]	6 mg/kg/d PO in 3 doses x 12d[35,36]
Loa loa			
Drug of choice:[37]	Diethylcarbamazine*	9 mg/kg/d PO in 3 doses x 12d[35,36]	9 mg/kg/d PO in 3 doses x 12d[35,36]

*   Availability problems. See table on page 16.

19. Quinine should be taken with or after a meal to decrease gastrointestinal adverse effects.

20. Use of tetracyclines is contraindicated in pregnancy and in children <8 years old. Tetracycline should be taken 1 hour before or 2 hours after meals and/or dairy products.

21. No drug has been demonstrated to be effective. Albendazole 25 mg/kg/d PO x 20d started as soon as possible (up to 3d after possible infection) might prevent clinical disease and is recommended for children with known exposure (ingestion of raccoon stool or contaminated soil) (WJ Murray and KR Kazacos, Clin Infect Dis 2004; 39:1484). Mebendazole, levamisole or ivermectin could be tried if albendazole is not available. Steroid therapy may be helpful, especially in eye and CNS infections (PJ Gavin et al, Clin Microbiol Rev 2005; 18:703). Ocular baylisascariasis has been treated successfully using laser photocoagulation therapy to destroy the intraretinal larvae (CA Garcia et al, Eye (Lond) 2004; 18:624).

22. Blastocystis has been reclassified as a fungus. Clinical significance of these organisms is controversial; metronidazole 750 mg PO tid x 10d, iodoquinol 650 mg PO tid x 20d or trimethoprim/sulfamethoxazole 1 DS tab PO bid x 7d have been reported to be effective (KS Tan, Clin Microbiol Rev 2008; 21:639). Metronidazole resistance may be common in some areas (J Yakoob et al, Br J Biomed Sci 2004; 61:75). Nitazoxanide has been effective in clearing organisms and improving symptoms (E Diaz et al, Am J Trop Med Hyg 2003; 68:384; JF Rossignol, Clin Gastroenterol Hepatol 2005; 3:987).

23. No drug has proven efficacy against cryptosporidiosis in advanced AIDS (I Abubakar et al, Cochrane Database Syst Rev 2007; 1:CD004932). Potent antiretroviral therapy (ART) is the mainstay of treatment. Nitazoxanide, paromomycin, or a combination of paromomycin and azithromycin may be tried to decrease diarrhea and recalcitrant malabsorption of antimicrobial drugs, which can occur with chronic cryptosporidiosis (B Pantenburg et al, Expert Rev Anti Infect Ther 2009; 7:385).

24. J Heukelbach and H Feldmeier, Lancet Infect Dis 2008; 8:302.

25. CA Warren, Curr Infect Dis Rep 2009; 11:108. In one study of HIV-infected patients with *Cyclospora* infection, ciprofloxacin treatment led to resolution in 87% of patients compared to 100% with TMP/SMX (RI Verdier et al, Ann Intern Med 2000; 132:885). HIV-infected patients may need higher dosage and long-term maintenance. Nitazoxanide (see also footnote 5) has also been used in a few patients (SM Zimmer et al, Clin Infect Dis 2007; 44:466; E Diaz et al, Am J Trop Med Hyg 2003; 68:384).

26. *Isospora belli* has been renamed and included the *Cystoisospora* genus. Usually a self-limited illness in immunocompetent patients. Immunosuppressed patients may need higher doses and longer duration (TMP/SMX qid for up to 3 to 4 weeks (Morbid Mortal Wkly Rep 2009; 58 RR4:1). They may require secondary prophylaxis (TMP/SMX DS tiw). In sulfa-allergic patients, pyrimethamine 50-75 mg daily in divided doses (plus leucovorin 10-25 mg/d) has been effective.

27. DJ Stark et al, Trends Parasitol 2006; 22:92; O Vandenberg et al, Pediatr Infect Dis J 2007; 26:88.

28. In one study, single-dose ornidazole, a nitroimidazole similar to metronidazole that is available in Europe, was effective and better tolerated than 5 days of metronidazole (O Kurt, Clin Microbiol Infect 2008; 14:601).

29. No drug is curative against *Dracunculus*. A program for monitoring local sources of drinking water to eliminate transmission has dramatically decreased the number of cases worldwide. The treatment of choice is slow extraction of worm combined with wound care and pain management (Morbid Mortal Wkly Rep 2009; 58:1123).

30. Since family members are usually infected, treatment of the entire household is recommended; retreatment after 14-21d may be needed.

31. Pyrantel pamoate suspension can be mixed with milk or fruit juice.

e3

Infection	Drug	Adult dosage	Pediatric dosage
FILARIASIS (continued)[32,33]			
Mansonella ozzardi			
Drug of choice:	See footnote 38		
Mansonella perstans			
Drug of choice[39]	Albendazole[7,12]	400 mg PO bid x 10d	400 mg PO bid x 10d
OR	Mebendazole[7]	100 mg PO bid x 30d	100 mg PO bid x 30d
Mansonella streptocerca			
Drug of choice:[40]	Diethylcarba-mazine*	6 mg/kg/d PO in 3 doses x 12d[36]	6 mg/kg/d PO in 3 doses x 12d[36]
OR	Ivermectin[7,15]	150 mcg/kg PO once	150 mcg/kg PO once
Tropical Pulmonary Eosinophilia (TPE)[41]			
Drug of choice:	Diethylcarba-mazine*	6 mg/kg/d in 3 doses x 12-21d[36]	6 mg/kg/d in 3 doses x 12-21d[36]
Onchocerca volvulus (River blindness)			
Drug of choice:	Ivermectin[15,42]	150 mcg/kg PO once, repeated every 6-12mos until asymptomatic	150 mcg/kg PO once, repeated every 6-12mos until asymptomatic
FLUKE, hermaphroditic, infection			
Clonorchis sinensis (Chinese liver fluke)[43]			
Drug of choice:	Praziquantel[44]	75 mg/kg/d PO in 3 doses x 2d	75 mg/kg/d PO in 3 doses x 2d
OR	Albendazole[7,12]	10 mg/kg/d PO x 7d	10 mg/kg/d PO x 7d
Fasciola hepatica (sheep liver fluke)[43]			
Drug of choice:[45]	Triclabendazole*	10 mg/kg PO once or twice	10 mg/kg PO once or twice
Alternative:	Bithionol*	30-50 mg/kg on alternate days x 10-15 doses	30-50 mg/kg on alternate days x 10-15 doses
OR	Nitazoxanide[5,7]	500 mg PO bid x 7d	1-3yrs: 100 mg PO bid x 7d 4-11yrs: 200 mg PO bid x 7d >12yrs: 500 mg PO bid x 7d
Fasciolopsis buski, Heterophyes heterophyes, Metagonimus yokogawai (intestinal flukes)			
Drug of choice:	Praziquantel[7,44]	75 mg/kg/d PO in 3 doses x 1d	75 mg/kg/d PO in 3 doses x 1d
Metorchis conjunctus (North American liver fluke)			
Drug of choice:	Praziquantel[7,44]	75 mg/kg/d PO in 3 doses x 1d	75 mg/kg/d PO in 3 doses x 1d
Nanophyetus salmincola			
Drug of choice:	Praziquantel[7,44]	60 mg/kg/d PO in 3 doses x 1d	60 mg/kg/d PO in 3 doses x 1d
Opisthorchis viverrini (Southeast Asian liver fluke)[43]			
Drug of choice:	Praziquantel[44]	75 mg/kg/d PO in 3 doses x 2d	75 mg/kg/d PO in 3 doses x 2d
Paragonimiasis (*P. westermani, P. miyazaki, P. skrjabini, P. hueitungensis, P. heterotrema, P. utcerobilaterus, P. Africanus, P. Mexicanus, P. Kellicotti,*) (lung fluke)			
Drug of choice:	Praziquantel[7,44]	75 mg/kg/d PO in 3 doses x 2d	75 mg/kg/d PO in 3 doses x 2d
Alternative:	Triclabendazole[46]*	10 mg/kg PO once or twice	10 mg/kg PO once or twice
	Bithionol*	30-50 mg/kg on alternate days x 10-15 doses	30-50 mg/kg on alternate days x 10-15 doses

* Availability problems. See table on page 16.

32. Antihistamines or corticosteroids may be required to decrease allergic reactions to components of disintegrating microfilariae that result from treatment, especially in infection caused by *Loa loa*.

33. Endosymbiotic *Wolbachia* bacteria, which are present in most human filariae except *Loa loa*, are essential to filarial growth, development, embryogenesis and survival and represent an additional target for therapy. Doxycycline 100 or 200 mg/d PO x 6-8wks in lymphatic filariasis, onchocerciasis, and *Mansonella perstans* has resulted in substantial loss of *Wolbachia* and decrease in both micro- and macrofilariae (MJ Bockarie et al, Expert Rev Anti Infect Ther 2009; 7:595; A Hoerauf Curr Opin Infect Dis 2008; 21:673; YI Coulibaly et al, N Engl J Med 2009; 361:1448). Use of tetracyclines is contraindicated in pregnancy and in children <8 yrs old.

34. Most symptoms are caused by adult worm. A single-dose combination of albendazole (400 mg PO) with either ivermectin (200 mcg/kg PO) or diethylcarbamazine (6 mg/kg PO) is effective for reduction or suppression of *W. bancrofti* microfilaria; none of these drug combinations kills all the adult worms (D Addiss et al, Cochrane Database Syst Rev 2004; CD003753).

35. For patients with microfilaria in the blood, Medical Letter consultants start with a lower dosage and scale up: d1: 50 mg; d2: 50 mg tid; d3: 100 mg tid; d4-14: 6 mg/kg/d in 3 doses (for *Loa Loa* d4-14: 9 mg/kg/d in 3 doses). Multi-dose regimens have been shown to provide more rapid reduction in microfilaria than single-dose diethylcarbamazine, but microfilaria levels are similar 6-12 months after treatment (LD Andrade et al, Trans R Soc Trop Med Hyg 1995; 89:319; PE Simonsen et al, Am J Trop Med Hyg 1995; 53:267). A single dose of 6 mg/kg is used in endemic areas for mass treatment, but there are no studies directly comparing the efficacy of the single-dose regimen to a 12-day course. It should be used cautiously in geographic regions where *O. volvulus* coexists with other filariae. One review concluded that the 12-day regimen did not have a higher macrofilaricidal effect than single dose (A Hoerauf, Curr Opin Infect Dis 2008; 21: 673; J Figueredo-Silva et al, Trans R Soc Trop Med Hyg 1996; 90:192; J Noroes et al, Trans R Soc Trop Med Hyg 1997; 91:78).

36. Diethylcarbamazine should not be used for treatment of *Onchocerca volvulus* due to the risk of increased ocular side effects (including blindness) associated with rapid killing of the worms. It should be used cautiously in geographic regions where *O. volvulus* coexists with other filariae. Diethylcarbamazine is contraindicated during pregnancy. See also footnote 42.

37. In heavy infections with *Loa loa*, rapid killing of microfilariae can provoke encephalopathy. Apheresis has been reported to be effective in lowering microfilarial counts in patients heavily infected with *Loa loa* (EA Ottesen, Infect Dis Clin North Am 1993; 7:619). Albendazole may be useful for treatment of loiasis when diethylcarbamazine is ineffective or cannot be used, but repeated courses may be necessary (AD Klion et al, Clin Infect Dis 1999; 29:680; TE Tabi et al, Am J Trop Med Hyg 2004; 71:211). Ivermectin has also been used to reduce microfilaremia, but albendazole is preferred because of its slower onset of action and lower risk of precipitating encephalopathy (AD Klion et al, J Infect Dis 1993; 168:202; M Kombila et al, Am J Trop Med Hyg 1998; 58:458). Diethylcarbamazine, 300 mg PO once/wk, has been recommended for prevention of loiasis (TB Nutman et al, N Engl J Med 1988; 319:752).

38. Diethylcarbamazine has no effect. A single dose of ivermectin 200 mcg/kg PO reduces microfilaria densities and provides both short- and long-term reductions in *M. ozzardi* microfilaremia (AA Gonzalez et al, W Indian Med J 1999; 48:231).

39. One small study compared single-dose ivermectin to albendazole alone or the two together although the combination reduced microfilaremia 1 and 3 months post treatment, the effect was not significant at 6 and 12 months (SM Asio et al, Ann Trop Med Parasitol 2009; 103:31).

40. Diethylcarbamazine is potentially curative due to activity against both adult worms and microfilariae. Ivermectin is active only against microfilariae.

41. VK Vijayan, Curr Opin Pulm Med 2007; 13:428. Relapses occur and can be treated with a repeated course of diethylcarbamazine.

42. Diethylcarbamazine should not be used for treatment of this disease because rapid killing of the worms can lead to blindness. Periodic treatment with ivermectin (every 3-12 months), 150 mcg/kg PO, can prevent blindness due to ocular onchocerciasis (DN Udall, Clin Infect Dis 2007; 44:53). Skin reactions after ivermectin treatment are often reported in persons with high microfilarial skin densities. Ivermectin has been inadvertently given to pregnant women during mass treatment pro-

e4

Appendix 296-1, cont'd.

Infection		Drug	Adult dosage	Pediatric dosage
GIARDIASIS (*Giardia duodenalis*)				
Drug of choice:		Metronidazole[7]	250 mg PO tid x 5-7d	15 mg/kg/d PO in 3 doses x 5-7d
	OR	Tinidazole[6]	2 g PO once	≥3yrs: 50 mg/kg PO once (max. 2 g)
	OR	Nitazoxanide[5]	500 mg PO bid x 3d	1-3yrs: 100 mg PO bid x 3d
				4-11yrs: 200 mg PO bid x 3d
				>12yrs: 500 mg PO bid x 3d
Alternative:[47]		Paromomycin[3,7,48]*	25-35 mg/kg/d PO in 3 doses x 5-10d	25-35 mg/kg/d PO in 3 doses x 5-10d
	OR	Furazolidone*	100 mg PO qid x 7-10d	6 mg/kg/d PO in 4 doses x 7-10d
	OR	Quinacrine[4,49]*	100 mg PO tid x 5d	6 mg/kg/d PO in 3 doses x 5d (max 300 mg/d)
GNATHOSTOMIASIS (*Gnathostoma spinigerum*) [50]				
Treatment of choice:		Albendazole[7,12]	400 mg PO bid x 21d	400 mg PO bid x 21d
	OR	Ivermectin[7,15]	200 mcg/kg/d PO x 2d	200 mcg/kg/d PO x 2d
		either		
	±	Surgical removal		
GONGYLONEMIASIS (*Gongylonema* sp.) [51]				
Treatment of choice:		Surgical removal		
	OR	Albendazole[7,12]	400 mg/d PO x 3d	400 mg/d PO x 3d
HOOKWORM infection (*Ancylostoma duodenale, Necator americanus*)				
Drug of choice:		Albendazole[7,12]	400 mg PO once	400 mg PO once
	OR	Mebendazole	100 mg PO bid x 3d or 500 mg once	100 mg PO bid x 3d or 500 mg once
	OR	Pyrantel pamoate[7,31]*	11 mg/kg (max. 1g) PO daily x 3d	11 mg/kg (max. 1g) PO daily x 3d
Hydatid cyst, see TAPEWORM infection				
Hymenolepis nana, see TAPEWORM infection				
Isospora belli, see *Cystoisospora*				
LEISHMANIASIS				
Visceral[52,53]				
Drug of choice:		Liposomal amphotericin B[54]	3 mg/kg/d IV d 1-5, 14 and 21[55]	3 mg/kg/d IV d 1-5, 14 and 21[55]
	OR	Sodium stibo-gluconate*	20 mg Sb/kg/d IV or IM x 28d	20 mg Sb/kg/d IV or IM x 28d
	OR	Meglumine antimonate*	20 mg Sb/kg/d IV or IM x 28d	20 mg Sb/kg/d IV or IM x 28d
	OR	Miltefosine[56,57]*	2.5 mg/kg/d PO (max 150 mg/d) x 28d	2.5 mg/kg/d PO (max 150 mg/d) x 28d
Alternative:	OR	Amphotericin B[7]	1 mg/kg IV daily x 15-20d or every second day for up to 8 wks (total usually 15-20 mg/kg)	1 mg/kg IV daily x 15-20d or every second day for up to 8 wks (total usually 15-20 mg/kg)
	OR	Paromomycin[3,7,58]* sulfate	15 mg/kg/d IM x 21d	15 mg/kg/d IM x 21d

* Availability problems. See table on page 16.

grams; the rates of congenital abnormalities were similar in treated and untreated women. Because of the high risk of blindness from onchocerciasis, the use of ivermectin after the first trimester is considered acceptable according to the WHO. Addition of 6-8 weeks of doxycycline to ivermectin is increasingly common. Doxycycline (100 mg/day PO for 6 weeks), followed by a single 150 mcg/kg PO dose of ivermectin, resulted in up to 19 months of amicrofilaridermia and 100% elimination of *Wolbachia* species (A Hoeraut et al, Lancet 2001; 357:1415).

43. LA Marcos, Curr Opin Infect Dis 2008; 21:523.

44. Praziquantel should be taken with liquids during a meal.

45. Unlike infections with other flukes, *Fasciola hepatica* infections may not respond to praziquantel. Triclabendazole (*Egaten* - Novartis) appears to be safe and effective, but data are limited (J Keiser et al, Expert Opin Investig Drugs 2005; 14:1513). It is available from Victoria Pharmacy, Zurich, Switzerland (www.pharmaworld.com; 011-4143-344-60-60) and should be given with food for better absorption. Nitazoxanide also appears to have efficacy in treating fascioliasis in adults and in children (L Favennec et al, Aliment Pharmacol Ther 2003; 17:265; JF Rossignol et al, Trans R Soc Trop Med Hyg 1998; 92:103; SM Kabil et al, Curr Ther Res 2000; 61:339).

46. J Keiser et al, Expert Opin Investig Drugs 2005; 14:1513. See footnote 45 for availability.

47. Additional option: albendazole (400 mg/d PO x 5d in adults and 10 mg/kg PO x 5d in children) (K Yereli et al, Clin Microbiol Infect 2004; 10:527; O Karabay et al, World J Gastroenterol 2004; 10:1215). Refractory disease: standard doses of metronidazole plus quinacrine x 3wks (TE Nash et al, Clin Infect Dis 2001; 33:22). In one study, nitazoxanide was used successfully in high doses (1.5 g PO bid x 30d) to treat a case of *Giardia* resistant to metronidazole and albendazole (P Abboud et al, Clin Infect Dis 2001; 32:1792).

48. Poorly absorbed; may be useful for treatment of giardiasis in pregnancy.

49. Quinacrine should be taken with liquids after a meal. It is not available in the US but can be compounded by Gallipot Pharmacy (www.gallipot.com; 800-423-6967).

50. All patients should be treated with medication whether surgery is attempted or not. JS Herman and PL Chiodini, Clin Microbiol Rev 2009; 22:484; L Ramirez-Avila et al, Clin Infect Dis 2009; 48:322.

51. S Pasuralertsakul et al, Am Trop Med Parasitol 2008; 102:455; G Molavi et al, J Helminth 2006; 80:425.

52. To maximize effectiveness and minimize toxicity, the choice of drug, dosage and duration of therapy should be individualized based on the region of disease acquisition, likely infecting species, and host factors such as immune status (BL Herwaldt, Lancet 1999; 354:1191). Some of the listed drugs and regimens are effective only against certain *Leishmania* species/strains and only in certain areas of the world (J Arevalo et al, J Infect Dis 2007; 195:1846). Medical Letter consultants recommend consultation with physicians experienced in management of this disease.

53. Visceral infection is most commonly due to the Old World species *L. donovani* (kala-azar) and *L. infantum* (referred to as *L. chagasi* in the New World).

54. Liposomal amphotericin B (*AmBisome*) is the only lipid formulation of amphotericin B FDA-approved for treatment of visceral leishmania, largely based on clinical trials in patients infected with *L. infantum* (A Meyerhoff, Clin Infect Dis 1999; 28:42). In one open-label study one 10 mg/kg dose of liposomal amphotericin B was as effective as 15 infusions of amphotericin B (1 mg/kg/d) on alternate days (S Sundar et al, N Engl J Med 2010; 362:504). It is the drug of choice for visceral leishmania in pregnancy. Two other amphotericin B lipid formulations, amphotericin B lipid complex (*Abelcet*) and amphotericin B cholesteryl sulfate (*Amphotec*) have been used, but are considered investigational for this condition and may not be as effective (C Bern et al, Clin Infect Dis 2006; 43:917).

55. The FDA-approved dosage regimen for immunocompromised patients (e.g., HIV infected) is 4 mg/kg/d IV on days 1-5, 10, 17, 24, 31 and 38. The relapse rate is high; maintenance therapy (secondary prevention) may be indicated, but there is no consensus as to dosage or duration.

56. Miltefosine (*Impavido*) is manufactured in 10- or 50-mg capsules by Paladin (Montreal, Canada) and is not available in the US. The drug is contraindicated in pregnancy; a negative pregnancy test before drug initiation and effective contraception during and for 2 months after treatment is recommended (HW Murray et al, Lancet 2005; 366:1561).

57. Miltefosine is effective for both antimony-sensitive and -resistant *L. donovani* (Indian).

Appendix 296-1, cont'd.

Infection		Drug	Adult dosage	Pediatric dosage
LEISHMANIASIS (continued)				
Cutaneous[52,59]				
Drugs of choice:		Sodium stibo-gluconate*	20 mg Sb/kg/d IV or IM x 20d	20 mg Sb/kg/d IV or IM x 20d
	OR	Meglumine antimonate*	20 mg Sb/kg/d IV or IM x 20d	20 mg Sb/kg/d IV or IM x 20d
	OR	Miltefosine[56,60]*	2.5 mg/kg/d PO (max 150 mg/d) x 28d	2.5 mg/kg/d PO (max 150 mg/d) x 28d
Alternative:[61]		Paromomycin[3,7,58]*	Topically 2x/d x 10-20d	Topically 2x/d x 10-20d
	OR	Pentamidine[7]	2-3 mg/kg IV or IM daily or every second day x 4-7 doses[62]	2-3 mg/kg IV or IM daily or every second day x 4-7 doses[62]
Mucosal[52,63]				
Drug of choice:		Sodium stibo-gluconate*	20 mg Sb/kg/d IV or IM x 28d	20 mg Sb/kg/d IV or IM x 28d
	OR	Meglumine antimonate*	20 mg Sb/kg/d IV or IM x 28d	20 mg Sb/kg/d IV or IM x 28d
	OR	Amphotericin B[7]	0.5-1 mg/kg IV daily or every second day for up to 8wks	0.5-1 mg/kg IV daily or every second day for up to 8wks
	OR	Miltefosine[56,64]*	2.5 mg/kg/d PO (max 150 mg/d) x 28d	2.5 mg/kg/d PO (max 150 mg/d) x 28d
LICE infestation (*Pediculus humanus, P. capitis, Phthirus pubis*)[65]				
Drug of choice:		Pyrethrins with piperonyl butoxide[66]	Topically, 2 x at least 7d apart	Topically, 2 x at least 7d apart
	OR	1% Permethrin[66]	Topically, 2 x at least 7d apart	Topically, 2 x at least 7d apart
	OR	5% Benzyl alcohol lotion[67]	Topically, 2 x at least 7d apart	Topically, 2 x at least 7d apart
	OR	0.5% Malathion[68]	Topically, 2 x at least 7d apart	Topically, 2 x at least 7d apart
Alternative:		Ivermectin[7,15,69]	200 or 400 mcg/kg PO	≥15kg: 200 or 400 mcg/kg PO
Loa loa, see FILARIASIS				
MALARIA, Treatment of (*Plasmodium falciparum,*[70] *P. vivax,*[71] *P. ovale, P. malariae*[72] and *P. knowlesi*[73])				
ORAL (Uncomplicated or mild infection)[74]				
P. falciparum or unidentified species[75] acquired in areas of chloroquine-resistant *P. falciparum*[70]				
Drug of choice:		Atovaquone/proguanil[76]	4 adult tabs PO once/d or 2 adult tabs PO bid[77] x 3d	<5kg: not indicated 5-8kg: 2 peds tabs PO once/d x 3d 9-10kg: 3 peds tabs PO once/d x 3d 11-20kg: 1 adult tab PO once/d x 3d 21-30kg: 2 adult tabs PO once/d x 3d 31-40kg: 3 adult tabs PO once/d x 3d >40kg: 4 adult tabs PO once/d x 3d[77]
	OR	Artemether/lumefantrine[78,79]	6 doses over 3d (4 tabs/dose at 0, 8, 24, 36, 48 and 60 hours)	6 doses over 3d at same intervals as adults; 5-15kg: 1 tab/dose ≥15-25kg: 2 tabs/dose ≥25-35kg: 3 tabs/dose ≥35kg: 4 tabs/dose

* Availability problems. See table on page 16.

58. Paromomycin IM has been effective against *Leishmania* in India; it has not yet been tested in South America or the Mediterranean and there are insufficient data to support its use in pregnancy (S Sundar et al, N Engl J Med 2007; 356:2571; S Sundar and J Chakravarty, Expert Opin Investig Drugs 2008; 17:787). One study in India used a 14-day course of paromomycin (S Sundar et al, Clin Infect Dis 2009; 49:914). Topical paromomycin should be used only in geographic regions where cutaneous leishmaniasis species have low potential for mucosal spread. A formulation of 15% paromomycin/12% methylbenzethonium chloride (*Leshcutan*) in soft white paraffin for topical use has been reported to be partially effective against cutaneous leishmaniasis due to *L. major* in Israel and *L. mexicana* and *L. (V.) braziliensis* in Guatemala, where mucosal spread is very rare (BA Arana et al, Am J Trop Med Hyg 2001; 65:466; DH Kim et al, PLoS Negl Trop Dis 2009; 3:e381). The methylbenzethonium is irritating to the skin; lesions may worsen before they improve.

59. Cutaneous infection is most commonly due to the Old World species *L. major* and *L. tropica* and the New World species *L. mexicana, L. (Vianna) braziliensis, L. (V.) panamensis* and others.

60. In a placebo-controlled trial in patients ≥12 years old, miltefosine was effective for treatment of cutaneous leishmaniasis due to *L.(V.) panamensis* in Colombia, but not *L.(V.) braziliensis* or *L. mexicana* in Guatemala (J Soto et al, Clin Infect Dis 2004; 38:1266). For forms of disease that require long periods of treatment, such as diffuse cutaneous leishmaniasis and post kala-azar dermal leishmaniasis, miltefosine might be a useful treatment (JJ Berman, Expert Opin Drug Metab Toxicol 2008; 4:1209).

61. Although azole drugs (fluconazole, ketoconazole, itraconazole) have been used to treat cutaneous disease, they are not reliably effective and have very limited if any efficacy against mucosal disease (JA Blum and CS Hatz, J Travel Med 2009; 16:123). For treatment of *L. major* cutaneous lesions, a study in Saudi Arabia found that oral fluconazole, 200 mg once/d x 6wks appeared to modestly accelerate the healing process (AA Alrajhi et al, N Engl J Med 2002; 346:891). Thermotherapy may be an option for some cases of cutaneous *L. tropica* infection (R Reithinger et al, Clin Infect Dis 2005; 40:1148). A device that generates focused and controlled heating of the skin is being marketed (*ThermoMed* – ThermoSurgery Technologies Inc., Phoenix, AZ, 602-264-7300; www.thermo-surgery.com). In one small study after 12 months of followup localized thermal heat was as effective as 10 doses of sodium stibogluconate with less toxicity (NE Aronson et al, PLOS Negl Trop Dis 2010; 4:e628).

62. At this dosage pentamidine has been effective in Colombia predominantly against *L. (V.) panamensis* (J Soto-Mancipe et al, Clin Infect Dis 1993; 16:417; J Soto et al, Am J Trop Med Hyg 1994; 50:107). Activity against other species is not well established.

63. Mucosal infection (espundia) is most commonly due to New World species *L. (V.) braziliensis, L. (V.) panamensis,* or *L. (V.) guyanensis.*

64. Miltefosine has been effective for mucosal leishmania due to *L.(V.) braziliensis* in Bolivia (J Soto et al, Clin Infect Dis 2007; 44:350; J Soto et al, Am J Trop Med Hyg 2009; 81:387).

65. Pediculocides should not be used for infestations of the eyelashes. Such infestations are treated with petrolatum ointment applied 2-4x/d x 8-10d. Oral TMP/SMX has also been used (TL Meinking and D Taplin, Curr Probl Dermatol 1996; 24:157). For pubic lice, treat with 5% permethrin or ivermectin as for scabies (see page 10). TMP/SMX has also been effective when used together with permethrin for head lice (RB Hipolito et al, Pediatrics 2001; 107:E30).

66. Permethrin and pyrethrin are pediculocidal; retreatment in 7-10d is needed to eradicate the infestation. Some lice are resistant to pyrethrins and permethrin (TL Meinking et al, Arch Dermatol 2002; 138:220). Medical Letter consultants prefer pyrethrin products with a benzyl alcohol vehicle.

e6

Appendix 296-1, cont'd.

Infection	Drug	Adult dosage	Pediatric dosage
MALARIA, Treatment of (continued)			
ORAL (continued)			
P. falciparum (continued)			
OR	Quinine sulfate	650 mg PO q8h x 3 **or** 7d[80]	30 mg/kg/d PO in 3 doses x 3 **or** 7d[80]
	plus		
	doxycycline[7,20,81]	100 mg PO bid x 7d	4 mg/kg/d PO in 2 doses x 7d
	or plus		
	tetracycline[7,20]	250 mg PO qid x 7d	25 mg/kg/d PO in 4 doses x 7d
	or plus		
	clindamycin[7,18,82]	20 mg/kg/d PO in 3 doses x 7d[83]	20 mg/kg/d PO in 3 doses x 7d[83]
Alternative:	Mefloquine[84,85]	750 mg PO followed 12 hrs later by 500 mg	15 mg/kg PO followed 12 hrs later by 10 mg/kg
OR	Artesunate[78]*	4 mg/kg/d PO x 3d	4 mg/kg/d PO x 3d
	plus see footnote 86		
P. vivax acquired in areas of chloroquine-resistant *P. vivax*[71]			
Drug of choice:	Artemether/ lumefantrine[78,79]	6 doses over 3d (4 tabs/dose at 0, 8, 24, 36, 48 and 60 hours)	6 doses over 3d at same intervals as adults; 5-15kg: 1 tab/dose ≥15-25kg: 2 tabs/dose ≥25-35kg: 3 tabs/dose ≥35kg: 4 tabs/dose
OR	Atovaquone/ proguanil[76]	4 adult tabs PO once/d or 2 adult tabs bid[77] x 3d	<5kg: not indicated 5-8kg: 2 peds tabs PO once/d x 3d 9-10kg: 3 peds tabs PO once/d x 3d 11-20kg: 1 adult tab PO once/d x 3d 21-30kg: 2 adult tabs PO once/d x 3d 31-40kg: 3 adult tabs PO once/d x 3d >40kg: 4 adult tabs PO once/d x 3d[77]
OR	Quinine sulfate	650 mg PO q8h x 3-7d[80]	30 mg/kg/d PO in 3 doses x 3-7d[80]
	plus		
	doxycycline[7,20,81]	100 mg PO bid x 7d	4 mg/kg/d PO in 2 doses x 7d
ALL PLUS	primaquine phosphate[75,87]	30 mg base/d PO x 14d	0.5 mg/kg/d PO x 14d
Alternative:	Mefloquine[84]	750 mg PO followed 12 hrs later by 500 mg	15 mg/kg PO followed 12 hrs later by 10 mg/kg
	Chloroquine phosphate[88,89]	25 mg base/kg PO in 3 doses over 48 hrs	25 mg base/kg PO in 3 doses over 48 hrs
	plus		
	doxycycline[7,20,81]	100 mg PO bid x 7d	4 mg/kg/d PO in 2 doses x 7d
ALL PLUS	primaquine phosphate[75,87]	30 mg base/d PO x 14d	0.5 mg/kg/d PO x 14d
All *Plasmodium* species except chloroquine-resistant *P. falciparum*[70] and chloroquine-resistant *P. vivax*[71]			
Drug of choice:[75]	Chloroquine phosphate[88]	1 g (600 mg base) PO, then 500 mg (300 mg base) 6 hrs later, then 500mg (300 mg base) at 24 and 48 hrs	10 mg base/kg (max. 600 mg base) PO, then 5 mg base/kg 6 hrs later, then 5 mg base/kg at 24 and 48 hrs

* Availability problems. See table on page 16.

67. FDA-approved to treat head lice in 2009, benzyl alcohol prevents lice from closing their respiratory spiracles and the lotion vehicle then obstructs their airway causing them to asphyxiate. It is not ovicidal. Two applications at least 7d apart are generally necessary to kill all lice and nits. Resistance, which is a problem with other drugs, is unlikely to develop (Med Lett Drugs Ther 2009; 51:57).

68. Malathion is both ovicidal and pediculocidal; 2 applications at least 7d apart are generally necessary to kill all lice and nits.

69. Ivermectin is pediculocidal, but not ovicidal; more than one dose is generally necessary to eradicate the infestation (KN Jones and JC English 3rd, Clin Infect Dis 2003; 36:1355). The number of doses and interval between doses has not been established. In one study for treatment of head lice, 2 doses of ivermectin (400 mcg/kg) 7 days apart was more effective than treatment with topical malathion (O Chosidow et al, N Engl J Med 2010; 362:896). In one study for treatment of body lice, 3 doses of ivermectin (12 mg each) administered at 7d intervals were effective (C Fouault et al, J Infect Dis 2006; 193:474).

70. Chloroquine-resistant *P. falciparum* occurs in all malarious areas except Central America (including Panama north and west of the Canal Zone), Mexico, Haiti, the Dominican Republic, Paraguay, northern Argentina, North and South Korea, Georgia, Armenia, most of rural China and some countries in the Middle East (chloroquine resistance has been reported in Yemen, Saudi Arabia and Iran). For treatment of multiple-drug-resistant *P. falciparum* in Southeast Asia, especially Thailand, where mefloquine resistance is frequent, atovaquone/proguanil, quinine plus either doxycycline or clindamycin, or artemether/lumefantrine may be used.

71. *P. vivax* with decreased susceptibility to chloroquine is a significant problem in Papua-New Guinea and Indonesia. There are also reports of resistance from Myanmar, Vietnam, Korea, India, the Solomon Islands, Vanuatu, Indonesia, Guyana, Brazil, Colombia and Peru (JK Baird, Clin Microbiol Rev 2009; 22:508).

72. Chloroquine-resistant *P. malariae* has been reported from Sumatra (JD Maguire et al, Lancet 2002; 360:58).

73. Human infection with the simian species, *P. knowlesi* has been reported in Malaysia where it was initially misdiagnosed as *P. malariae*. Additional cases have been reported from Thailand, Myanmar, Singapore, the Thai-Burma border, and the Philippines (J Cox-Singh et al, Clin Infect Dis 2008; 46:165; MMWR 2009; 58:229). Treatment with the usual antimalarials, such as chloroquine and atovaquone/proguanil appear to be effective.

74. Uncomplicated or mild malaria may be treated with oral drugs. Severe malaria (e.g. impaired consciousness, parasitemia >5%, shock, etc.) should be treated with parenteral drugs (KS Griffin et al, JAMA 2007; 297:2264).

75. Primaquine is given as part of primary treatment to prevent relapse after infection with *P. vivax* or *P. ovale*. Some experts also prescribe primaquine phosphate 30 mg base/d (0.6 mg base/kg/d for children) for 14d after departure from areas where these species are endemic (Presumptive Anti-Relapse Therapy [PART], "terminal prophylaxis"). Since this is not always effective as prophylaxis (E Schwartz et al, N Engl J Med 2003; 349:1510), others prefer to rely on surveillance to detect cases when they occur, particularly when exposure was limited or doubtful. See also footnote 87.

76. Atovaquone/proguanil is available as a fixed-dose combination tablet: adult tablets (*Malarone*; atovaquone 250 mg/proguanil 100 mg) and pediatric tablets (*Malarone Pediatric*; atovaquone 62.5 mg/proguanil 25 mg). To enhance absorption and reduce nausea and vomiting, it should be taken with food or a milky drink. Safety in pregnancy is unknown; in a few small studies; outcomes were normal in women treated with the combination in the 2nd and 3rd trimester (AK Boggild et al, Am J Trop Med Hyg 2007; 76:208). The drug should not be given to patients with severe renal impairment (creatinine clearance <30mL/min). There have been isolated case reports of resistance in *P. falciparum* in Africa, but Medical Letter consultants do not believe there is a high risk for acquisition of *Malarone*-resistant disease (E Schwartz et al, Clin Infect Dis 2003; 37:450; A Farnert et al, BMJ 2003; 326:628; S Kuhn et al, Am J Trop Med Hyg 2005; 72:407; CT Happi et al, Malaria Journal 2006; 5:82).

e7

Appendix 296-1, cont'd.

Infection	Drug	Adult dosage	Pediatric dosage
PARENTERAL (severe infection)[74]			
All Plasmodium species (Chloroquine-sensitive and resistant)			
Drug of choice:[75,90]	Quinidine gluconate[91]	10 mg/kg IV loading dose (max. 600 mg) in normal saline over 1-2 hrs, followed by continuous infusion of 0.02 mg/kg/min until PO therapy can be started	10 mg/kg IV loading dose (max. 600 mg) in normal saline over 1-2 hrs, followed by continuous infusion of 0.02 mg/kg/min until PO therapy can be started
OR	Quinine dihydro-chloride[91]*	20 mg/kg IV loading dose in 5% dextrose over 4 hrs, followed by 10 mg/kg over 2-4 hrs q8h (max. 1800 mg/d) until PO therapy can be started	20 mg/kg IV loading dose in 5% dextrose over 4 hrs, followed by 10 mg/kg over 2-4 hrs q8h (max. 1800 mg/d) until PO therapy can be started
OR	Artesunate[78]*	2.4 mg/kg/dose IV x 3d at 0, 12, 24, 48 and 72 hrs	2.4 mg/kg/dose IV x 3d at 0, 12, 24, 48 and 72 hrs
	plus see footnote 86		
MALARIA, Prevention of[92]			
All Plasmodium species in chloroquine-resistant areas[70-73]			
Drug of choice:[75]	Atovaquone/ proguanil[76]	1 adult tab/d[93]	5-8kg: ½ peds tab/d[76,93] 9-10kg: ¾ peds tab/d[76,93] 11-20kg: 1 peds tab/d[76,93] 21-30kg: 2 peds tabs/d[76,93] 31-40kg: 3 peds tabs/d[76,93] >40kg: 1 adult tab/d[76,93]
OR	Doxycycline[20,81]	100 mg PO daily[94]	2 mg/kg/d PO, up to 100 mg/d[94]
OR	Mefloquine[85,95]	250 mg PO once/wk[96]	≤ 9kg: 5 mg/kg salt once/wk[96] 9-19kg: ¼ tab once/wk[96] >19-30kg: ½ tab once/wk[96] >31-45kg: ¾ tab once/wk[96] >45kg: 1 tab once/wk[96]
Alternative:[97]	Primaquine[7,87] phosphate	30 mg base PO daily[98]	0.5 mg/kg base PO daily[98]
All Plasmodium species in chloroquine-sensitive areas[70-73]			
Drug of choice:[75,99]	Chloroquine phosphate[88,100]	500 mg (300 mg base) PO once/wk[101]	5 mg/kg base PO once/wk, up to adult dose of 300 mg base[101]

* Availability problems. See table on page 16.

77. Although approved for once-daily dosing, Medical Letter consultants usually divide the dose in two to decrease nausea and vomiting.

78. The artemisinin-derivatives, artemether and artesunate, are both frequently used globally in combination regimens to treat malaria. Both are available in oral, parenteral and rectal formulations, but manufacturing standards are not consistent (HA Karunajeewa et al, JAMA 2007; 297:2381; EA Ashley and NJ White, Curr Opin Infect Dis 2005; 18:531). Oral artesunate is not available in the US; the IV formulation is available through the CDC Malaria branch (M-F, 8am-4:30pm ET, 770-488-7788, or after hours, 770-488-7100) under an IND for patients with severe disease who do not have timely access, cannot tolerate, or fail to respond to IV quinidine (Med Lett Drugs Ther 2008; 50:37). To avoid development of resistance, monotherapy should be avoided (PE Duffy and CH Sibley, Lancet 2005; 366:1908). Reduced susceptibility to artesunate characterized by slow parasitic clearance has been reported in Cambodia (WO Rogers et al, Malaria J 2009; 8:10; AM Dundorp et al, N Engl J Med 2009; 361:455). Based on the few studies available, artemisin have been relatively safe during pregnancy (I Adam et al, Am Trop Med Parisito 2009; 103; 205), but some experts would not prescribe them in the 1st trimester (RL Clark, Reprod Toxicol 2009; 28:285).

79. Artemether/lumefantrine is available as a fixed-dose combination tablet (*Coartem* in the US and in countries with endemic malaria, *Riamet* in Europe and countries without endemic malaria); each tablet contains artemeter 20 mg and lumefantrine 120 mg. It is FDA-approved for treatment of uncomplicated malaria and should not be used for severe infection or for prophylaxis. It is contraindicated during the 1st trimester of pregnancy; safety during the 2nd and 3rd trimester is not known. The tablets should be taken with fatty food (tablets may be crushed and mixed with 1-2 tsp water, and taken with milk). Artemether/lumefantrine should not be used in patients with cardiac arrhythmias, bradycardia, severe cardiac disease or QT prolongation. Concomitant use of drugs that prolong the QT interval or are metabolized by CYP2D6 is contraindicated (Med Lett Drugs Ther 2009; 51:75).

80. Available in the US in a 324-mg capsule; 2 capsules suffice for adult dosage. In Southeast Asia, relative resistance to quinine has increased and treatment should be continued for 7d. Quinine should be taken with or after meals to decrease gastrointestinal adverse effects. It is generally considered safe in pregnancy.

81. Doxycycline should be taken with adequate water to avoid esophageal irritation. It can be taken with food to minimize gastrointestinal adverse effects.

82. For use in pregnancy and in children <8 yrs.

83. B Lell and PG Kremsner, Antimicrob Agents Chemother 2002; 46:2315; M Ramharter et al, Clin Infect Dis 2005; 40:1777.

84. At this dosage, adverse effects include nausea, vomiting, diarrhea and dizziness. Disturbed sense of balance, toxic psychosis and seizures can also occur. Mefloquine should not be used for treatment of malaria in pregnancy unless there is not another treatment option (F Nosten et al, Curr Drug Saf 2006; 1:1). It should be avoided for treatment of malaria in persons with active depression or with a history of psychosis or seizures and should be used with caution in persons with any psychiatric illness. Mefloquine should not be used in patients with conduction abnormalities; it can be given to patients taking β-blockers if they do not have an underlying arrhythmia. Mefloquine should not be given together with quinine or quinidine, and caution is required in using quinine or quinidine to treat patients with malaria who have taken mefloquine for prophylaxis. Mefloquine should not be taken on an empty stomach; it should be taken with at least 8 oz of water.

85. *P. falciparum* with resistance to mefloquine is a significant problem in the malarious areas of Thailand and in areas of Myanmar and Cambodia that border on Thailand. It has also been reported on the borders between Myanmar and China, Laos and Myanmar, and in Southern Vietnam. In the US, a 250-mg tablet of mefloquine contains 228 mg mefloquine base. Outside the US, each 275-mg tablet contains 250 mg base.

86. Adults treated with artesunate should also receive oral treatment doses of either atovaquone/proguanil, doxycycline, clindamycin or mefloquine; children should take either atovaquone/proguanil, clindamycin or mefloquine (F Nosten et al, Lancet 2000; 356:297; M van Vugt, Clin Infect Dis 2002; 35:1498; F Smithuis et al, Trans R Soc Trop Med Hyg 2004; 98:182). If artesunate is given IV, oral medication should be started when the patient is able to tolerate it (SEAQUAMAT group, Lancet 2005; 366:717).

87. Primaquine phosphate can cause hemolytic anemia, especially in patients whose red cells are deficient in G-6-PD. This deficiency is most common in African, Asian and Mediterranean peoples. Patients should be screened for G-6-PD deficiency before treatment. Primaquine should not be used during pregnancy. It should be taken with food to minimize nausea and abdominal pain. Primaquine-tolerant *P. vivax* can be found globally. Relapses of primaquine-resistant strains may be retreated with 30 mg (base) x 28d.

88. Chloroquine should be taken with food to decrease gastrointestinal adverse effects. If chloroquine phosphate is not available, hydroxychloroquine sulfate is as effective; 400 mg of hydroxychloroquine sulfate is equivalent to 500 mg of chloroquine phosphate.

89. Chloroquine combined with primaquine was effective in 85% of patients with *P. vivax* resistant to chloroquine and could be a reasonable choice in areas where other alternatives are not available (JK Baird et al, J Infect Dis 1995; 171:1678).

90. Exchange transfusion is controversial, but has been helpful for some patients with high-density (>10%) parasitemia, altered mental status, pulmonary edema or renal complications (PJ Van Genderen et al, Transfusion 2009; Nov 20 epub).

91. Continuous EKG, blood pressure and glucose monitoring are recommended. Quinine IV is not available in the US. Quinidine may have greater antimalarial activity than quinine. The loading dose should be decreased or omitted in patients who have received quinine or mefloquine. If more than 48 hours of parenteral treat-

e8

Infection	Drug	Adult dosage	Pediatric dosage
MALARIA, Prevention of relapses: _P. vivax_ and _P. ovale_[75]			
Drug of choice:	Primaquine phosphate[87]	30 mg base/d PO x 14d	0.5 mg base/kg/d PO x 14d
MALARIA, Self-Presumptive Treatment[102]			
Drug of Choice:	Atovaquone/ proguanil[7,76]	4 adult tabs once/d or 2 adult tabs bid x 3d[77]	<5kg: not indicated 5-8kg: 2 peds tabs once/d x 3 9-10kg: 3 peds tabs once/d x 3 11-20kg: 1 adult tab once/d x 3 21-30kg: 2 adult tabs once/d x 3 31-40kg: 3 adult tabs once/d x 3 >40kg: 4 adult tabs once/d x 3d[77]
OR	Artemether/ lumefantrine[7,78,79]	6 doses over 3d (4 tabs/dose at 0, 8, 24, 36, 48 and 60 hours)	6 doses over 3d at same intervals as adults; 5-15kg: 1 tab/dose 15-25kg: 2 tabs/dose 25-35kg: 3 tabs/dose >35kg: 4 tabs/dose
OR	Quinine sulfate **plus**	650 mg PO q8h x 3 or 7d[70]	30 mg/kg/d PO in 3 doses x 3 or 7d[70]
	doxycycline[7,20,81]	100 mg PO bid x 7d	4 mg/kg/d PO in 2 doses x 7d
OR	Artesunate[78]* **plus** see footnote 86	4 mg/kg/d PO x 3d	4 mg/kg/d PO x 3d
MICROSPORIDIOSIS			
Ocular (_Encephalitozoon hellem, E. cuniculi, Vittaforma [Nosema] corneae_)			
Drug of choice:	Fumagillin[103]* **plus**		
	albendazole[7,12]	400 mg PO bid	15 mg/kg/d in 2 doses (max 400 mg/dose)
Intestinal (_E. bieneusi, E. [Septata] intestinalis_) _E. bieneusi_			
Drug of choice: _E. intestinalis_	Fumagillin[104]*	20 mg PO tid x 14d	
Drug of choice:	Albendazole[7,12]	400 mg PO bid x 21d	15 mg/kg/d in 2 doses (max 400 mg/dose)
Disseminated (_E. hellem, E. cuniculi, E. intestinalis, Pleistophora sp., Trachipleistophora sp._ and _Anncaliia [Brachiola] vesicularum_)			
Drug of choice:[105]	Albendazole[7,12]	400 mg PO bid	15 mg/kg/d in 2 doses (max 400 mg/dose)
Mites, see SCABIES			
MONILIFORMIS _moniliformis_ infection			
Drug of choice:	Pyrantel pamoate[7,31]*	11 mg/kg PO once, repeat twice, 2wks apart	11 mg/kg PO once, repeat twice, 2wks apart

* Availability problems. See table on page 16.

ment is required, the quinine or quinidine dose should be reduced by 30-50%. Intrarectal quinine has been tried for the treatment of cerebral malaria in children (J Achan et al, Clin Infect Dis 2007; 45:1446).

92. No drug guarantees protection against malaria. Travelers should be advised to seek medical attention if fever develops after they return. Insect repellents, insecticide-impregnated bed nets and proper clothing are important adjuncts for malaria prophylaxis (Treat Guidel Med Lett 2009; 7:83). Malaria in pregnancy is particularly serious for both mother and fetus; prophylaxis is indicated if exposure cannot be avoided.

93. Beginning 1-2 d before travel and continuing for the duration of stay and for 1wk after leaving malarious zone. In one study of malaria prophylaxis, atovaquone/proguanil was better tolerated than mefloquine in nonimmune travelers (D Overbosch et al, Clin Infect Dis 2001; 33:1015). The protective efficacy of _Malarone_ against _P. vivax_ is variable ranging from 84% in Indonesian New Guinea (J Ling et al, Clin Infect Dis 2002; 35:825) to 100% in Colombia (J Soto et al, Am J Trop Med Hyg 2006; 75:430). Some Medical Letter consultants prefer alternate drugs if traveling to areas where _P. vivax_ predominates.

94. Beginning 1-2 d before travel and continuing for the duration of stay and for 4wks after leaving malarious zone. Doxycycline can cause gastrointestinal disturbances, vaginal moniliasis and photosensitivity reactions.

95. Mefloquine has not been approved for use during pregnancy. However, it has been reported to be safe for prophylactic use during the second and third trimester of pregnancy and possibly during early pregnancy as well (CDC Health Information for International Travel, 2010, page 141). Not recommended for use in travelers with active depression or with a history of psychosis or seizures and should be used with caution in persons with psychiatric illness. Mefloquine should not be used in patients with conduction abnormalities; it can be given to patients taking β-blockers if they do not have an underlying arrhythmia.

96. Beginning 1-2 wks before travel and continuing weekly for the duration of stay and for 4wks after leaving malarious zone. Most adverse events occur within 3 doses. Some Medical Letter consultants favor starting mefloquine 3 weeks prior to travel and monitoring the patient for adverse events, this allows time to change to an alternative regimen if mefloquine is not tolerated. Mefloquine should not be taken on an empty stomach; it should be taken with at least 8 oz of water. For pediatric doses <½ tablet, it is advisable to have a pharmacist crush the tablet, estimate doses by weighing, and package them in gelatin capsules. There is no data for use in children <5 kg, but based on dosages in other weight groups, a dose of 5 mg/kg can be used.

97. The combination of weekly chloroquine (300 mg base) and daily proguanil (200 mg) is recommended by the World Health Organization (www.WHO.int) for use in selected areas; this combination is no longer recommended by the CDC. Proguanil (_Paludrine_ – AstraZeneca, United Kingdom) is not available alone in the US but is widely available in Canada and Europe. Prophylaxis is recommended during exposure and for 4 weeks afterwards. Proguanil has been used in pregnancy without evidence of toxicity (PA Phillips-Howard and D Wood, Drug Saf 1996; 14:131).

98. Studies have shown that daily primaquine beginning 1d before departure and continued until 3-7 d after leaving the malarious area provides effective prophylaxis against chloroquine-resistant _P. falciparum_ (DR Hill et al, Am J Trop Med Hyg 2006; 75:402). Nausea and abdominal pain can be diminished by taking with food.

99. Alternatives for patients who are unable to take chloroquine include atovaquone/proguanil, mefloquine, doxycycline or primaquine dosed as for chloroquine-resistant areas.

100. Has been used extensively and safely for prophylaxis in pregnancy.

101. Beginning 1-2wks before travel and continuing weekly for the duration of stay and for 4 wks after leaving malarious zone.

102. A traveler can be given a course of medication for presumptive self-treatment of febrile illness. The drug given for self-treatment should be different from that used for prophylaxis. This approach should be used only in very rare circumstances when a traveler would not be able to get medical care promptly.

103. CM Chan et al, Ophthalmology 2003; 110:1420. Ocular lesions due to _E. hellem_ in HIV-infected patients have responded to fumagillin eyedrops prepared from _Fumidil-B_ (bicyclohexyl ammonium fumagillin) used to control a microsporidial disease of honey bees (MJ Garvey et al, Ann Pharmacother 1995; 29:872), available from Leiter's Park Avenue Pharmacy (see footnote 1). For lesions due to _V. corneae_, topical therapy is generally not effective and keratoplasty may be required (RM Davis et al, Ophthalmology 1990; 97:953).

104. Oral fumagillin (_Flisint_ – Sanofi-Aventis, France) has been effective in treating _E. bieneusi_ in patients with HIV or solid organ transplants (J-M Molina et al, N Engl J Med 2002; 346:1963; F Lanternier et al, Transpl Infect Dis 2009; 11:83), but has been associated with thrombocytopenia and neutropenia. Potent anti

Appendix 296-1, cont'd.

Infection		Drug	Adult dosage	Pediatric dosage
Naegleria species, see AMEBIC MENINGOENCEPHALITIS, PRIMARY				
Necator americanus, see HOOKWORM infection				
OESOPHAGOSTOMUM bifurcum				
Drug of choice:		See footnote 106		
Onchocerca volvulus, see FILARIASIS				
Opisthorchis viverrini, see FLUKE infection				
Paragonimus westermani, see FLUKE infection				
Pediculus capitis, humanus, Phthirus pubis, see LICE				
Pinworm, see ENTEROBIUS				
PNEUMOCYSTIS JIROVECII (formerly *carinii*) pneumonia (PCP)[107]				
Moderate to severe disease[108]				
Drug of choice:		Trimethoprim/ sulfamethoxazole	TMP 15-20 mg/kg/d SMX 75-100 mg/kg/d PO or IV in 3 or 4 doses (change to PO after clinical improvement) x 21d	TMP 15-20 mg/kg/d SMX 75-100 mg/kg/d PO or IV in 3 or 4 doses (change to PO after clinical improvement) x 21d
Alternative:		Pentamidine	3-4 mg/kg IV daily x 21d	3-4 mg/kg IV daily x 21d
	OR	Primaquine[7,87]	30 mg base PO daily x 21d	0.3 mg/kg base PO (max. 30 mg) daily x 21d
		plus		
		clindamycin[7,18]	600-900 mg IV tid or qid x 21d, or 300-450 mg PO tid or qid x 21d (change to PO after clinical improvement)	15-25 mg/kg IV tid or qid (max 600 mg/dose) x 21 d, or 10 mg/kg PO tid or qid (max 300-450 mg/dose)x 21d (change to PO after clinical improvement)
Mild to moderate disease				
Drug of Choice:		Trimethoprim/ sulfamethoxazole	2 DS tablets (160 mg/800 mg) PO tid x 21d	TMP 15-20 mg/kg/SMX 75-100 mg/kg/d PO in 3 or 4 doses x 21d
Alternative:		Dapsone[7]	100 mg PO daily x 21d	2 mg/kg/d (max. 100 mg) PO x 21d
		plus		
		Trimethoprim[7]	15 mg/kg/d PO in 3 doses	15 mg/kg/d PO in 3 doses
	OR	Primaquine[7,87]	30 mg base PO daily x 21d	0.3 mg/kg base PO daily (max. 30 mg) x 21d
		plus		
		clindamycin[7,18]	300-450 mg PO tid or qid x 21 d	10 mg/kg PO tid or qid (max 300-450 mg/dose) x 21d
	OR	Atovaquone[17]	750 mg PO bid x 21d	1-3 mos: 30 mg/kg/d PO x 21d 4-24 mos: 45 mg/kg/d PO x 21d >24 mos: 30 mg/kg/d PO x 21d
Primary and secondary prophylaxis[109]				
Drug of Choice:		Trimethoprim/ sulfamethoxazole	1 tab (SS or DS) daily or 1 DS tab PO 3d/wk	TMP 150 mg/SMX 750 mg/m^2/d PO in 2 doses 3d/wk
Alternative:		Dapsone[7]	50 mg PO bid or 100 mg PO daily	≥ 1 mos: 2 mg/kg/d (max. 100 mg) PO or 4 mg/kg (max. 200 mg) PO each wk
	OR	Dapsone[7] **plus** pyrimeth-amine[110]	50 mg PO daily or 200 mg PO each wk 50 mg PO daily or 75 mg PO each wk	
	OR	Atovaquone[7,17]	1500 mg/d PO in 1 or 2 doses	1-3mos: 30 mg/kg/d PO 4-24mos: 45 mg/kg/d PO >24mos: 30 mg/kg/d PO
	OR	Pentamidine	300 mg aerosol inhaled monthly via *Respirgard II* nebulizer	≥5yrs: 300 mg inhaled monthly via *Respirgard II* nebulizer
River Blindness, see FILARIASIS				
Roundworm, see ASCARIASIS				
Sappinia diploidea, See AMEBIC MENINGOENCEPHALITIS, PRIMARY				
SARCOCYSTIS spp. (intestinal and muscular), see footnote 111				
SCABIES (*Sarcoptes scabiei*)[112]				
Drug of choice:		5% Permethrin	Topically, 2x at least 7 d apart	Topically, 2x at least 7 d apart
Alternative:[113]		Ivermectin[7,15]	200 mcg/kg PO 2x at least 7 d apart[114]	200 mcg/kg PO, 2x at least 7 d apart[114]
		10% Crotamiton	Topically overnight on days 1, 2, 3, 8	Topically overnight on days 1, 2, 3, 8

* Availability problems. See table on page 16.
  retroviral therapy (ART) may lead to microbiologic and clinical response in HIV-infected patients with microsporidial diarrhea. Octreotide (*Sandostatin*) has provided symptomatic relief in some patients with large-volume diarrhea.
105. J-M Molina et al, J Infect Dis 1995; 171:245. There is no established treatment for *Pleistophora*. For disseminated disease due to *Trachipleistophora* or *Anncaliia*, itraconazole 400 mg PO once/d plus albendazole may also be tried (CM Coyle et al, N Engl J Med 2004; 351:42).
106. Albendazole or pyrantel pamoate may be effective (JB Ziem et al, Ann Trop Med Parasitol 2004; 98:385).
107. Pneumocystis has been reclassified as a fungus.

e10

Appendix 296-1, cont'd.

Infection	Drug	Adult dosage	Pediatric dosage
SCHISTOSOMIASIS *(Bilharziasis)*			
S. haematobium			
Drug of choice:	Praziquantel[44,115]	40 mg/kg/d PO in 1 or 2 doses x 1d	40 mg/kg/d PO in 2 doses x 1d
S. intercalatum[116]			
Drug of Choice:	Praziquantel[44,115]	40 mg/kg/d PO in 1 or 2 doses x 1d	40 mg/kg/d PO x 1d
S. japonicum			
Drug of choice:	Praziquantel[44,115]	60 mg/kg/d PO in 2 or 3 doses x 1d	60 mg/kg/d PO in 3 doses x 1d
S. mansoni			
Drug of choice:	Praziquantel[44,115]	40 mg/kg/d PO in 1 or 2 doses x 1d	40 mg/kg/d PO in 2 doses x 1d
Alternative:	Oxamniquine[117]*	15 mg/kg PO once[118]	20 mg/kg/d PO in 2 doses x 1d[118]
S. mekongi			
Drug of choice:	Praziquantel[44,115]	60 mg/kg/d PO in 2 or 3 doses x 1d	60 mg/kg/d PO in 3 doses x 1d
Sleeping sickness, see TRYPANOSOMIASIS			
STRONGYLOIDIASIS *(Strongyloides stercoralis)*			
Drug of choice:[119]	Ivermectin[15]	200 mcg/kg/d PO x 2d	200 mcg/kg/d PO x 2d
Alternative:	Albendazole[7,12]	400 mg PO bid x 7d	400 mg PO bid x 7d
TAPEWORM infection			
— **Adult** (intestinal stage)			
Diphyllobothrium latum (fish), ***Taenia saginata*** (beef), ***Taenia solium*** (pork), ***Dipylidium caninum*** (dog)			
Drug of choice:	Praziquantel[7,44]	5-10 mg/kg PO once	5-10 mg/kg PO once
Alternative:	Niclosamide[120]*	2 g PO once	50 mg/kg PO once
Hymenolepis nana (dwarf tapeworm)			
Drug of choice:	Praziquantel[7,44]	25 mg/kg PO once	25 mg/kg PO once
Alternative:[121]	Niclosamide[120]*	2 g PO daily x 7 d	11-34 kg: 1 g PO on d 1 then 500 mg/d PO x 6 days > 34 kg: 1.5 g PO on d 1 then 1 g/d PO x 6 days
— **Larval** (tissue stage)			
Echinococcus granulosus (hydatid cyst)			
Drug of choice:[122]	Albendazole[12]	400 mg PO bid x 1-6mos	15 mg/kg/d (max. 800 mg) PO in 2 doses x 1-6mos
Echinococcus multilocularis			
Treatment of choice:	See footnote 123		
Taenia solium (Cysticercosis)			
Treatment of choice:	See footnote 124		
Alternative:	Albendazole[12]	400 mg PO bid x 8-30d; can be repeated as necessary	15 mg/kg/d (max. 800 mg) PO in 2 doses x 8-30d; can be repeated as necessary
	OR Praziquantel[7,44]	100 mg/kg/d PO in 3 doses x 1 day then 50 mg/kg/d in 3 doses x 29 days	100 mg/kg/d PO in 3 doses x 1 day then 50 mg/kg/d in 3 doses x 29 days

*   Availability problems. See table on page 16.

108. In severe disease with room air $PO_2 \leq 70$ mmHg or Aa gradient ≥ 35 mmHg, prednisone or its IV equivalent should also be used. For adults: d 1-5: 40 mg PO bid; d 6-10: 40 mg PO daily; d 11-21: 20 mg PO daily. For children: d 1-5: 2 mg/kg/d PO in 2 doses; d 6-10: 1 mg/kg/d PO in 2 doses; d 11-21: 0.5 mg/kg/d PO daily (JE Kaplan et al, Morbid Mortal Wkly Rep 2009; 58(RR04):1; Morbid Mortal Wkly Rep 2009; 58(RR11):1).

109. Primary/secondary prophylaxis in patients with HIV can be discontinued after CD4 count increases to >200 x 10^6/L for >3mos.

110. Plus leucovorin 25 mg with each dose of pyrimethamine. Pyrimethamine should be taken with food to minimize gastrointestinal adverse effects.

111. Sarcocystis in humans is acquired by ingesting sporocysts in infected meat, infections characterized by nausea, abdominal pain and diarrhea. Muscular infections are usually mild or subclinical (R Fayer, Clin Microbiol Rev 2004; 17:894). Albendazole was reported to be efficacious (MK Arness et al, Am J Trop Med Hyg 1999; 61:548).

112. TL Meinking et al, Infestations in LA Schachner and RA Hansen, eds. *Pediatric Dermatology*. 3rd ed. St Louis: Mosby; 2003, page 1291.

113. Lindane (γ-benzene hexachloride) should be reserved for treatment of patients who fail to respond to other drugs. The FDA has recommended it not be used for immunocompromised patients, young children, the elderly, pregnant and breast-feeding women, and patients weighing <50 kg.

114. BJ Currie and JS McCarthy, N Engl J Med 2010; 362:717. A second ivermectin dose taken 2 weeks later increased the cure rate to 95%, which is equivalent to that of 5% permethrin (V Usha et al, J Am Acad Dermatol 2000; 42:236). Ivermectin, either alone or in combination with a topical scabicide, is the drug of choice for crusted scabies in immunocompromised patients (P del Giudice, Curr Opin Infect Dis 2004; 15:123).

115. MJ Doenhoff et al, Curr Opin Infect Dis 2008; 21:659.

116. Geographically restricted to Central Western Africa and the island of São Tomé. Usually a disease of the lower GI tract; there are also case reports of complications including central nervous system, liver and cardiopulmonary involvement (A Murinello et al, GE - J Port Gastrenterol 2006; 13:97).

117. Oxamniquine, which is not available in the US, is generally not as effective as praziquantel. It has been useful, however, in some areas in which praziquantel is less effective (ML Ferrari et al, Bull World Health Organ 2003; 81:190; A Harder, Parasitol Res 2002; 88:395). Oxamniquine is contraindicated in pregnancy. It should be taken after food.

118. In East Africa, the dose should be increased to 30 mg/kg PO, and in Egypt and South Africa to 30 mg/kg/d PO x 2d. Some experts recommend 40-60 mg/kg PO over 2-3d in all of Africa (KC Shekhar, Drugs 1991; 42:379).

119. In immunocompromised patients or disseminated disease, it may be necessary to prolong or repeat therapy, or to use other agents. Veterinary parenteral and enema formulations of ivermectin have been used in severely ill patients with hyperinfection who were unable to take or reliably absorb oral medications (FM Marty et al, Clin Infect Dis 2005; 41:e5; P Lichtenberger et al, Transpl Infect Dis 2009; 11:137). In disseminated strongyloidiasis, combination therapy with albendazole and ivermectin has been suggested (M Seqarra, Ann Pharmacother 2007; 41:1992).

120. Niclosamide must be thoroughly chewed or crushed and swallowed with a small amount of water.

121. Nitazoxanide may be an alternative (JJ Ortiz et al, Trans R Soc Trop Med Hyg 2002; 96:193; JC Chero et al, Trans R Soc Trop Med Hyg 2007; 101:203; E Diaz et al, Am J Trop Med Hyg 2003; 68:384).

122. Patients may benefit from surgical resection or percutaneous drainage of cysts. Praziquantel is useful preoperatively or in case of spillage of cyst contents during surgery. Percutaneous aspiration-injection-reaspiration (PAIR) with ultrasound guidance plus albendazole therapy has been effective for management of hepatic hydatid cyst disease (P Moro and PM Schantz, Int J Infect Dis 2009; 13:125.).

123. Surgical excision is the only reliable means of cure. Reports have suggested that in nonresectable cases use of albendazole (400 mg bid) can stabilize and sometimes cure infection (P Moro and PM Schantz, Int J Infect Dis 2009; 13:125).

124. Advances in neuroimaging using CT and MRI have facilitated the ability to make an accurate diagnosis (AC White Jr, J Infect Dis 2009; 199:1261). Initial therapy for patients with inflamed parenchymal cysticercosis should focus on symptomatic treatment with anti-seizure medication (S Sinha and BS Sharma, J Clin Neurosci 2009; 16:867). Patients with live parenchymal cysts who have seizures should be treated with albendazole together with steroids and an anti-seizure

e11

Infection	Drug	Adult dosage	Pediatric dosage
Toxocariasis, see VISCERAL LARVA MIGRANS			
TOXOPLASMOSIS *(Toxoplasma gondii)*			
CNS disease[125]			
Drug of choice:	Pyrimethamine[126]	200 mg PO x 1 then 50-75 mg/d PO x 3-6 wks	2 mg/kg/d PO x 2d, then 1 mg/kg/d (max. 25 mg/d) x 3-6 wks
	plus		
	sulfadiazine[127]	1-1.5 g PO qid x 3-6 wks	100-200 mg/kg/d PO x 3-6 wks
OR	**plus**		
	clindamycin[7,128]	1.8-2.4 g/d IV or PO in 3 or 4 doses	5-7.5 mg/kg/d IV or PO in 3 or 4 doses (max 600 mg/dose)
OR	**plus**		
	atovaquone[7,17,128]	1500 mg PO bid	1500 mg PO bid
Alternative:	Trimethoprim/ sulfamethox-azole[7]	15-20 mg/kg/SMX 75-100 mg/kg/d PO or IV in 3 or 4 doses	15-20 mg/kg/SMX 75-100 mg/kg/d PO or IV in 3 or 4 doses
Primary infection in pregnancy			
Treatment of choice:	See footnote 129		
TRICHINELLOSIS *(Trichinella spiralis)*			
Drug of choice:[130]	Steroids for severe symptoms, e.g.	prednisone 30-60 mg PO daily x10-15 d	
	plus		
	Albendazole[7,12]	400 mg PO bid x 8-14d	400 mg PO bid x 8-14d
Alternative:	Mebendazole[7]	200-400 mg PO tid x 3d, then 400-500 mg tid x 10d	200-400 mg PO tid x 3d, then 400-500 mg tid x 10d
TRICHOMONIASIS *(Trichomonas vaginalis)*			
Drug of choice:[131]	Metronidazole	2 g PO once	15 mg/kg/d PO in 3 doses x 7d
OR	Tinidazole[6]	2 g PO once	50 mg/kg once (max. 2 g)
TRICHOSTRONGYLUS infection			
Drug of choice:	Pyrantel pamoate[7,31*]	11 mg/kg base PO once (max. 1 g)	11 mg/kg PO once (max. 1 g)
Alternative:	Mebendazole[7]	100 mg PO bid x 3d	100 mg PO bid x 3d
OR	Albendazole[7,12]	400 mg PO once	400 mg PO once
TRICHURIASIS *(Trichuris trichiura,* whipworm)			
Drug of choice:	Albendazole[7,12]	400 mg PO x 3d	400 mg PO x 3d
Alternative:	Mebendazole	100 mg PO bid x 3d	100 mg PO bid x 3d
OR	Ivermectin[7,15]	200 mcg/kg/d PO x 3d	200 mcg/kg/d PO x 3d
TRYPANOSOMIASIS			
T. cruzi (American trypanosomiasis, Chagas' disease)[132]			
Drug of choice:	Nifurtimox*	8-10 mg/kg/d PO in 3-4 doses x 90-120d	1-10yrs: 15-20 mg/kg/d PO in 4 doses x 90-120d 11-16yrs: 12.5-15 mg/kg/d PO in 4 doses x 90-120d
OR	Benznidazole[133*]	5-7 mg/kg/d PO in 2 doses x 60-90d	≤12yrs: 10 mg/kg/d PO in 2 doses x 60-90d >12 yrs: 5-7 mg/kg/d PO in 2 doses x 60-90d
T. brucei gambiense (West African trypanosomiasis, sleeping sickness)[134]			
Hemolymphatic stage			
Drug of choice:[135]	Pentamidine[7]	4 mg/kg/d IM x 7d	4 mg/kg/d IM x 7d
Alternative:	Suramin*	100-200 mg (test dose) IV, then 1 g IV on days 1,3,7,14 and 21	20 mg/kg on d 1,3,7,14 and 21
Late disease with CNS involvement			
Drug of Choice:[136]	Eflornithine[137*]	400 mg/kg/d IV in 4 doses x 14d	400 mg/kg/d IV in 4 doses x 14d
OR	Eflornithine[137*]	400 mg/kg IV in 2 doses x 7d	
	plus		
	Nitfurtimox	15 mg/kg/d PO in 3 doses x 10d	
OR	Melarsoprol[138]	2.2 mg/kg/d IV x 10d	2.2 mg/kg/d IV x 10d

* Availability problems. See table on page 16.
medication (HH Garcia et al, N Engl J Med 2004; 350:249). Patients with subarachnoid cysts or giant cysts in the fissures should be treated for at least 30d (JV Proaño et al, N Engl J Med 2001; 345:879). Surgical intervention (especially neuroendoscopic removal) or CSF diversion followed by albendazole and steroids is indicated for obstructive hydocephalus. Arachnoiditis, vasculitis or cerebral edema is treated with albendazole or praziquantel plus prednisone (60 mg/d) or dexamethasone (4-6 mg/d). Any cysticercocidal drug may cause irreparable damage when used to treat ocular or spinal cysts, even when corticosteroids are used. An ophthalmic exam should always precede treatment to rule out intraocular cysts.
125. Treatment is followed by chronic suppression with lower dosage regimens of the same drugs. For primary prophylaxis in HIV patients with CD4 <100 x 10[6] cells/L, either trimethoprim-sulfamethoxazole, pyrimethamine with dapsone, or atovaquone with or without pyrimethamine can be used. Primary or secondary prophylaxis may be discontinued when the CD4 count increases to >200 x 10[6] cells/L for >3mos (MMWR Morb Mortal Wkly Rep 2009; 58 [RR4]:1). In ocular toxoplasmosis with macular involvement, corticosteroids are recommended in addition to antiparasitic therapy (JG Montoya and O Liesenfeld, Lancet 2004; 363:1965).
126. Plus leucovorin 10-25 mg with each dose of pyrimethamine. Pyrimethamine should be taken with food to minimize gastrointestinal adverse effects.
127. Sulfadiazine should be taken on an empty stomach with adequate water.
128. Clindamycin has been used in combination with pyrimethamine to treat CNS toxoplasmosis in HIV infected patients who developed sulfonamide sensitivity while on sulfadiazine (G Beraud et al, Am J Trop Med Hygiene 2009; 80:583). Atovaquone has also been used to treat sulfonamide-intolerant patients (K Chirgwin et al, Clin Infect Dis 2002; 34:1243).
129. Women who develop toxoplasmosis during the first trimester of pregnancy should be treated with spiramycin (3-4 g/d). After the first trimester, if there is no documented transmission to the fetus, spiramycin can be continued until term. Spiramycin is not currently available in the US but can be obtained at no cost

e12

Appendix 296-1, cont'd.

Infection	Drug	Adult dosage	Pediatric dosage
TRYPANOSOMIASIS (continued)			
T. b. rhodesiense (East African trypanosomiasis, sleeping sickness)[134]			
Hemolymphatic stage			
Drug of choice:	Suramin*	100-200 mg (test dose) IV, then 1 g IV on days 1,3,7,14 and 21	20 mg/kg IV on d 1,3,7,14 and 21
Late disease with CNS involvement			
Drug of choice:	Melarsoprol[138]	2-3.6 mg/kg/d IV x 3d; after 7d 3.6 mg/kg/d x 3d; repeat again after 7d	2-3.6 mg/kg/d IV x 3d; after 7d 3.6 mg/kg/d x 3d; repeat again after 7d
VISCERAL LARVA MIGRANS[139] *(Toxocariasis)*			
Drug of choice:	Albendazole[7,12]	400 mg PO bid x 5d	400 mg PO bid x 5d
OR	Mebendazole[7]	100-200 mg PO bid x 5d	100-200 mg PO bid x 5d
Whipworm, see TRICHURIASIS			
Wuchereria bancrofti, see FILARIASIS			

*   Availability problems. See table on page 16.
    from Palo Alto Medical Foundation Toxoplasma Serology Laboratory (PAMF-TSL, 650-853-4828), US National Collaborative Treatment Trials Study (773-834-4152), or the FDA (301-796-1600). If transmission has occurred *in utero*, therapy with pyrimethamine and sulfadiazine should be started. Pyrimethamine is a potential teratogen and should be used only after the first trimester (JG Montoya and JS Remington, Clin Infect Dis 2008; 47:554). Congenitally infected new borns should be treated with pyrimethamine every 2 or 3 days and a sulfonamide daily for about one year (JS Remington and G Desmonts in JS Remington and JO Klein, eds, *Infectious Disease of the Fetus and Newborn Infant*, 6th ed, Philadelphia:Saunders, 2006, page 1038).
130.   B Gottstein et al. Clin Microbiol Rev 2009; 22:127.
131.   Sexual partners should be treated simultaneously with same dosage. If treatment failure occurs and reinfection is excluded, treat with metronidazole 500 mg PO bid x7d, or tinidazole 2 g PO once (MMWR Morb Mortal Wkly Rep 2006; 55 [RR11]:1).
132.   Treatment of chronic or indeterminate Chagas' disease with benznidazole has been associated with reduced progression and increased negative seroconversion (C Bern et al, JAMA 2007; 298:2171; JA Perez-Molina et al, J Antimicrob Chemother 2009; 64:1139).
133.   Benznidazole should be taken with meals to minimize gastrointestinal adverse effects. It is contraindicated during pregnancy.
134.   PG Kennedy, Ann Neurol 2008; 64:116.
135.   Pentamidine and suramin have equal efficacy, but pentamidine is better tolerated.
136.   In one study eflornithine for 7 days combined with nifurtimox x 10 d was more effective and less toxic than eflornithine x 14 d (G Priotto et al, Lancet 2009; 374:56).
137.   Eflornithine is highly effective in *T.b. gambiense*, but not in *T.b. rhodesiense* infections. In one study of treatment of CNS disease due to *T.b. gambiense*, there were fewer serious complications with eflornithine than with melarsoprol (PG Kennedy, Ann Neurol 2008; 64:116). Eflornithine is available in limited supply only from the WHO. It is contraindicated during pregnancy.
138.   E Schmid et al, J Infect Dis 2005; 191:1922. Corticosteroids have been used to prevent arsenical encephalopathy (J Pepin et al, Trans R Soc Trop Med Hyg 1995; 89:92). Up to 20% of patients with *T.b.gambiense* fail to respond to melarsoprol (MP Barrett, Lancet 1999; 353:1113). In one study, a combination of low-dose melarsoprol (1.2 mg/kg/d IV) and nifurtimox (7.5 mg/kg PO bid) x 10 d was more effective than standard-dose melarsoprol alone (S Bisser et al, J Infect Dis 2007; 195:322).
139.   Optimum duration of therapy is not known; some Medical Letter consultants would treat x 20 d. For severe symptoms or eye involvement, corticosteroids can be used in addition (D Despommier, Clin Microbiol Rev 2003; 16:265).

e13

Appendix 296-1, cont'd.

PRINCIPAL ADVERSE EFFECTS OF
ANTIPARASITIC DRUGS

Adverse effects of antiparasitic drugs vary with dosage, duration of administration, concomitant therapy, renal and hepatic function, immune competence, and the age of the patient. The principal adverse effects of antiparasitic agents are listed in the following table. The designation of adverse effects as "frequent," "occasional" or "rare" is based on published reports and on the experience of Medical Letter consultants. Information about adverse interactions between drugs, including probable mechanisms and recommendations for clinical management, are available in the Medical Letter Adverse Drug Interactions Program.

ALBENDAZOLE (*Albenza*)
  Occasional: abdominal pain; reversible alopecia; increased serum transaminases
  Rare: leukopenia; rash; renal toxicity

AMPHOTERICIN B DEOXYCHOLATE (*Fungizone*, and others)
  Frequent: renal damage; hypokalemia; thrombophlebitis at site of peripheral vein infusion; anorexia; headache; nausea; weight loss; bone marrow suppression with reversible decline in hematocrit; chills, fever, vomiting during infusion, possibly with delirium, hypotension or hypertension, wheezing, and hypoxemia, especially in cardiac or pulmonary diease
  Occasional: hypomagnesemia; normocytic, normochromic anemia
  Rare: hemorrhagic gastroenteritis; blood dyscrasias; rash; blurred vision; peripheral neuropathy; convulsions; anaphylaxis; arrhythmias; acute liver failure; reversible nephrogenic diabetes insipidus; hearing loss; acute pulmonary edema; spinal cord damage with intrathecal use

AMPHOTERICIN B LIPID FORMULATIONS (*AmBisone, Abelcet, Amphotec*)
  Similar to amphotericin B but generally better tolerated. Nephrotoxicity is less common and less severe with the lipid-based formulations. Acute infusion reactions are worse with *Amphotec*, less with *Abelcet* and least with *AmBisome*. Liver toxicity has been reported.

ARTEMETHER (*Artenam*)
  Occasional: neurological toxicity; possible increase in length of coma; increased convulsions; prolongation of QTc interval

ARTEMETHER/LUMEFANTRINE (*Coatem, Riamet*)
  Frequent: abdominal pain; anorexia; headache; dizziness; diarrhea; vomiting; nausea; palpitations; arthralgia; myalgia; asthenia; fatigue; pruritus; rash; sleep disorder; cough
  Occasional: somnolence; involuntary muscle contractions; paresthesia; hypoesthesia; abnormal gait; ataxia
  Rare: Hypersensitivity

ARTESUNATE
  Occasional: ataxia; slurred speech; neurological toxicity; possible increase in length of coma; increased convulsions; prolongation of QTc interval

ATOVAQUONE (*Mepron, Malarone* [with *proguanil*])
  Frequent: rash; nausea
  Occasional: diarrhea; increased amino-transferases; cholestasis

AZITHROMYCIN (*Zithromax*, and others)
  Occasional: nausea; diarrhea; abdominal pain; headache; dizziness; vaginitis
  Rare: angioedema; cholestatic jaundice; photosensitivity; reversible dose-related hearing loss

BENZNIDAZOLE (*Rochagan*)
  Frequent: allergic rash; dose-dependent polyneuropathy; GI disturbance; psychic disturbances

BENZYL ALCOHOL (*Ulesfia Lotion*)
  Frequent: eye irritation; contact dermatitis

BITHIONOL (*Bitin*)
  Frequent: photosensitivity reactions; vomiting; diarrhea; abdominal pain; urticaria
  Rare: leukopenia; toxic hepatitis

CHLOROQUINE HCL and **CHLOROQUINE PHOSPHATE** (*Aralen*, and others)
  Occasional: pruritus; vomiting; headache; confusion; depigmentation of hair; skin eruptions; corneal opacity; weight loss; partial alopecia; extraocular muscle palsies; exacerbation of psoriasis, eczema, and other exfoliative dermatoses; myalgias; photophobia
  Rare: irreversible retinal injury (especially when total dosage exceeds 100 grams); discoloration of nails and mucus membranes; nerve-type deafness; peripheral neuropathy and myopathy; heart block; blood dyscrasias; hematemesis

CLARITHROMYCIN (*Biaxin*, and others)
  Occasional: nausea; diarrhea; abdominal pain; abnormal taste; headache; dizziness
  Rare: reversible dose-related hearing loss; pseudomembranous colitis; pancreatitis; torsades de pointes

CLINDAMYCIN (*Cleocin*, and others)
  Frequent: diarrhea; allergic reactions
  Occasional: pseudomembranous colitis, sometimes severe, can occur even with topical use
  Rare: blood dyscrasias; esophageal ulceration; hepatotoxicity; arrhythmia due to QTc prolongation

CROTAMITON (*Eurax*)
  Occasional: rash

DAPSONE
  Frequent: rash; transient headache; GI irritation; anorexia; infectious mononucleosis-like syndrome
  Occasional: cyanosis due to methemoglobinemia and sulfhemoglobinemia; other blood dyscrasias, including hemolytic anemia; nephrotic syndrome; liver damage; peripheral neuropathy; hypersensitivity reactions; increased risk of lepra reactions; insomnia; irritability; uncoordinated speech; agitation; acute psychosis
  Rare: renal papillary necrosis; severe hypoalbuminemia; epidermal necrolysis; optic atrophy; agranulocytosis; neonatal hyperbilirubinemia after use in pregnancy

e14

Appendix 296-1, cont'd.

DIETHYLCARBAMAZINE CITRATE (*Hetrazan*)
Frequent: allergic or febrile reactions, which may be severe, in patients with microfilaria in the blood or the skin; GI disturbance
Rare: encephalopathy

DILOXANIDE FUROATE (*Furamide*)
Frequent: flatulence
Occasional: nausea; vomiting; diarrhea
Rare: diplopia; dizziness; urticaria; pruritus

EFLORNITHINE (Difluoromethylornithine, DFMO, *Ornidyl*)
Frequent: anemia; leukopenia
Occasional: diarrhea; thrombocytopenia; seizures
Rare: hearing loss

FLUCONAZOLE (*Diflucan*, and others)
Occasional: nausea; vomiting; diarrhea; abdominal pain; headache; rash; increased aminotransferases
Rare: severe hepatic toxicity; exfoliative dermatitis; anaphylaxis; Stevens-Johnson syndrome; toxic epidermal necrolysis; hair loss

FLUCYTOSINE (*Ancobon*)
Frequent: blood dyscrasias, including pancytopenia and fatal agranulocytosis; GI disturbance, including severe diarrhea and ulcerative colitis; rash; hepatic dysfunction
Occasional: confusion; hallucinations
Rare: anaphylaxis

FURAZOLIDONE (*Furoxone*)
Frequent: nausea; vomiting
Occasional: allergic reactions, including pulmonary infiltration; hypotension; urticaria; fever; vesicular rash; hypoglycemia; headache
Rare: hemolytic anemia in G-6-PD deficiency and neonates; disulfiram-like reaction with alcohol; MAO-inhibitor interactions; polyneuritis

IODOQUINOL (*Yodoxin*, and others)
Occasional: rash; acne; slight enlargement of the thyroid gland; nausea; diarrhea; cramps; anal pruritus
Rare: optic neuritis, atrophy and loss of vision; peripheral neuropathy after prolonged use in high dosage (for months); iodine sensitivity

ITRACONAZOLE (*Sporanox*, and others)
Occasional: nausea; epigastric pain; headache; dizziness; edema; hypokalemia; rash; hepatic toxicity
Rare: congestive heart failure

IVERMECTIN (*Stromectol*)
Occasional: Mazzotti-type reaction seen in onchocerciasis, including fever; pruritus; tender lymph nodes; headache; and joint and bone pain
Rare: hypotension

KETOCONAZOLE (*Nizoral*, and others)
Frequent: nausea; vomiting
Occasional: decreased testosterone synthesis; gynecomastia; oligospermia and impotence in men; abdomina pain; rash; hepatitis; pruritus; dizziness; constipation; diarrhea; fever and chills; photophobia; headache
Rare: fatal hepatic necrosis; liver injury with jaundice; transient elevated transaminase; severe epigastric burning and pain; may interfere with adrenal function; anaphylaxis

MALATHION (*Ovide*)
Occasional: local irritation

MEBENDAZOLE (*Vermox*)
Occasional: diarrhea; abdominal pain
Rare: leukopenia; agranulocytosis; hypospermia

MEFLOQUINE (*Lariam*)
Frequent: vertigo; lightheadedness; nausea; other GI disturbances; nightmares; visual disturbances; headache; insomnia
Occasional: confusion
Rare: psychosis; hypotension; convulsions; coma; paresthesias

MEGLUMINE ANTIMONIATE (*Glucantime*)
— Similar to sodium stibogluconate

MELARSOPROL (*Mel B*)
Frequent: myocardial damage; albuminuria; hypertension; colic; Herxheimer-type reaction; encephalopathy; vomiting; peripheral neuropathy
Rare: shock

METRONIDAZOLE (*Flagyl*, and others)
Frequent: nausea; headache; anorexia; metallic taste
Occasional: vomiting; diarrhea; insomnia; weakness; dry mouth; stomatitis; vertigo; tinnitus; paresthesias; rash; dark urine; urethral burning; disulfiram-like reaction with alcohol; candidiasis
Rare: pseudomembranous colitis; leukopenia; pancreatitis; seizures; peripheral neuropathy; encephalopathy; cerebellar syndrome with ataxia, dysarthria and MRI abnormalities

MICONAZOLE (*Monistat i.v.*)
Occasional: phlebitis; thrombocytosis; chills; intense, persistent pruritus; rash; vomiting; hyperlipidemia; dizziness; blurred vision; local burning and irritation with topical use
Rare: anemia; thrombocytopenia; hyponatremia; renal insufficiency; anaphylaxis; cardiac and respiratory arrest with initial dose

MILTEFOSINE (*Impavido*)
Frequent: nausea; vomiting; diarrhea; motion sickness; increased creatinine

NICLOSAMIDE (*Niclocide*)
Occasional: nausea; abdominal pain

e15

Appendix 296-1, cont'd.

NITAZOXANIDE (*Alinia*)
Occasional: GI disturbance; headache
Rare: yellow discoloration of sclera; allergic reactions; increased creatinine; dizziness; flatulence; malaise; salivary gland enlargement; discolored urine; anemia; leukoytosis

ORNIDAZOLE (*Tiberal*)
Occasional: dizziness; headache; GI disturbance
Rare: reversible peripheral neuropathy

OXAMNIQUINE (*Vansil*)
Occasional: headache; fever; dizziness; somnolence and insomnia; nausea; diarrhea; rash; increased aminotransferases; ECG changes; EEG changes; orange-red discoloration of urine
Rare: seizures; neuropsychiatric disturbances

PAROMOMYCIN (aminosidine; *Humatin*)
Frequent: GI disturbance with oral use
Rare: eighth-nerve damage (mainly auditory) and renal damage when aminosidine is given IV; vertigo; pancreatitis

PENTAMIDINE ISETHIONATE (*Pentam 300, NebuPent*, and others)
Frequent: hypotension; hypoglycemia often followed by diabetes mellitus; vomiting; blood dyscrasias; renal damage; pain at injection site; GI disturbance
Occasional: may aggravate diabetes; shock; hypocalcemia; liver damage; cardiotoxicity; delirium; rash
Rare: Herxheimer-type reaction; anaphylaxis; acute pancreatitis; hyperkalemia

PERMETHRIN (*Nix,* and others)
Occasional: burning; stinging; numbness; increased pruritus; pain; edema; erythema; rash

PRAZIQUANTEL (*Biltricide*)
Frequent: abdominal pain; diarrhea; malaise; headache; dizziness
Occasional: sedation; fever; sweating; nausea; eosinophilia
Rare: pruritus; rash; edema; hiccups

PRIMAQUINE PHOSPHATE
Frequent: hemolytic anemia in G-6-PD deficiency
Occasional: neutropenia; GI disturbance; methemoglobinemia
Rare: CNS symptoms; hypertension; arrhythmias

PROGUANIL (*Paludrine; Malarone* [with atovaquone])
Occasional: oral ulceration; hair loss; scaling of palms and soles; urticaria
Rare: hematuria (with large doses); vomiting; abdominal pain; diarrhea (with large doses); thrombocytopenia

PYRANTEL PAMOATE (*Antiminth*, and others)
Occasional: GI disturbance; headache; dizziness; rash; fever

PYRETHRINS with PIPERONYL BUTOXIDE (*A-200,* and others)
Occasional: allergic reactions

PYRIMETHAMINE (*Daraprim*)
Occasional: blood dyscrasias; folic acid deficiency
Rare: rash; vomiting; convulsions; shock; possibly pulmonary eosinophilia; fatal cutaneous reactions with pyrimethamine-sulfadoxine (*Fansidar*)

QUINACRINE
Frequent: disulfiram-like reaction with alcohol; nausea and vomiting; colors skin and urine yellow
Occasional: headache; dizziness
Rare: rash; fever; psychosis; extensive exfoliative dermatitis in patients with psoriasis

QUININE DIHYDROCHLORIDE and QUININE SULFATE
Frequent: cinchonism (tinnitus, headache, nausea, abdominal pain, visual disturbance)
Occasional: deafness; hemolytic anemia; other blood dyscrasias; photosensitivity reactions; hypoglycemia; arrhythmias; hypotension; fever
Rare: blindness; sudden death if injected too rapidly; hypersensitivity reaction with TTP-HUS

SODIUM STIBOGLUCONATE (*Pentostam*)
Frequent: myalgia and arthralgia (typically, large joint, may or may not br symmetric); malaise, fatigue and weakness; headache; anorexia; nausea; increased aminotransferases; increased amylase and lipase; T-wave flattening or inversion
Occasional: abdominal pain; liver damage; bradycardia; leukopenia; thrombocytopenia; rash; vomiting
Rare: diarrhea; pruritus; myocardial damage; hemolytic anemia; renal damage; shock; sudden death

SPIRAMYCIN (*Rovamycine*)
Occasional: GI disturbance
Rare: allergic reactions

SULFONAMIDES
Frequent: allergic reactions (rash, photosensitivity, drug fever)
Occasional: kernicterus in newborn; renal damage; liver damage; Stevens-Johnson syndrome (particularly with long-acting sulfonamides); hemolytic anemia; other blood dyscrasias; vasculitis
Rare: transient acute myopia; pseudomembranous colitis; reversible infertility in men with sulfasalazine; CNS toxicity with trimethoprim-sulfamethoxazole in patients with AIDS

SURAMIN SODIUM
Frequent: vomiting; pruritus; urticaria; paresthesias; hyperesthesia of hands and feet; peripheral neuropathy; photophobia
Occasional: kidney damage; blood dyscrasias; shock; optic atrophy

TETRACYCLINES
(doxycycline – *Vibramycin*, and others; tetracycline hydrochloride – *Sumycin*, and others)
Frequent: GI disturbance; bone lesions and staining and deformity of teeth in children up to 8 years old, and in the newborn when given to pregnant women after the fourth month of pregnancy

e16

Appendix 296-1, cont'd.

Occasional: malabsorption; enterocolitis; photosensitivity reactions; increased azotemia with renal insufficiency (except doxycycline, but exacerbation of renal failure with doxycycline has been reported); hepatic injury; parenteral doses may cause serious liver damage, especially in pregnant women and patients with renal disease receiving 1 gram or more daily; esophageal ulcerations; cutaneous and mucosal hyperpigmentation

Rare: allergic reactions, including serum sickness and anaphylaxis; pseudomembranous colitis; blood dyscrasias; drug-induced lupus; autoimmune hepatitis; increased intracranial pressure; fixed-drug eruptions; transient acute myopia; blurred vision; diplopia; papilledema; photoonycholysis and onycholysis; aggravation of myasthenic symptoms with IV injection, reversed with calcium; possibly transient neuropathy; hemolytic anemia

TINIDAZOLE (*Tindamax*)
    Occasional: metallic taste; GI symptoms; rash
    Rare: weakness

TRIMETHOPRIM (*Proloprim*, and others)
    Frequent: nausea and vomiting with high doses
    Occasional: megaloblastic anemia; thrombocytopenia; neutropenia; rash; fixed drug eruption
    Rare: pancytopenia; hyperkalemia

TRIMETHOPRIM/SULFAMETHOXAZOLE (*Bactrim, Septra*, and others)
    Frequent: rash; fever; nausea and vomiting
    Occasional: hemolysis in G-6-PD deficiency; acute megaloblastic anemia; granulocytopenia; thrombocytopenia; pseudomembranous colitis; kernicterus in newborn; hyperkalemia
    Rare: agranulocytosis; aplastic anemia; hepatotoxicity; Stevens-Johnson syndrome; aseptic meningitis; fever; confusion; depression; hallucinations; deterioration in renal disease; intrahepatic cholestasis; methemoglobinemia; pancreatitis; ataxia; CNS toxicity in patients with AIDS; renal tubular acidosis; hyperkalemia

e17

Appendix 296-1, cont'd.

SAFETY OF ANTIPARASITIC DRUGS IN PREGNANCY

Drug	Toxicity in Pregnancy	Recommendations	FDA
Albendazole (*Albenza*)	Teratogenic and embryotoxic in animals	Caution*	C
Amphotericin B (*Fungizone*, and others)	None known	Caution*	B
Amphotericin B liposomal (*AmBisome*)	None known	Caution*	B
Artemether/lumefantrine (*Coartem, Riamet*)[1]	Unknown	Contraindicated during 1st trimester; caution 2nd and 3rd trimesters*	C
Artesunate[2]	Embryocidal and teratogenic in rats	Contraindicated during 1st trimester; caution 2nd and 3rd trimesters*	N/A
Atovaquone (*Mepron*)	Maternal and fetal toxicity in animals	Caution*	C
Atovaquone/proguanil (*Malarone*)[3]	Maternal and fetal toxicity in animals	Caution*	C
Azithromycin (*Zithromax*, and others)	None known	Probably safe	B
Benznidazole (*Rochagan*)	Unknown	Contraindicated	N/A
Benzyl alcohol lotion (*Ulesfia Lotion*)	Unknown	Probably safe	B
Chloroquine (*Aralen*, and others)	None known with doses recommended for malaria prophylaxis	Probably safe in low doses	C
Clarithromycin (*Biaxin*, and others)	Teratogenic in animals	Contraindicated	C
Clindamycin (*Cleocin*, and others)[4]	None known	Caution*	B
Crotamiton (*Eurax*)	Unknown	Caution*	C
Dapsone	None known; carcinogenic in rats and mice; hemolytic reactions in neonates	Caution*, especially at term	C
Diethylcarbamazine (DEC; *Hetrazan*)	Not known; abortifacient in one study in rabbits	Contraindicated	N/A
Diloxanide (*Furamide*)	Safety not established	Caution*	N/A
Doxycycline (*Vibramycin*, and others)	Tooth discoloration and dysplasia inhibition of bone growth in fetus; hepatic toxicity and azotemia with IV use in pregnant patients with decreased renal function or with overdosage	Contraindicated	D
Eflornithine (*Ornidyl*)	Embryocidal in animals	Contraindicated	C
Fluconazole (*Diflucan*, and others)	Teratogenic	Contraindicated for high dose; caution* for single dose	C
Flucytosine (*Ancoban*)	Teratogenic in rats	Contraindicated	C
Furazolidone (*Furoxone*)	None known; carcinogenic in rodents; hemolysis with G-6-PD deficiency in newborn	Caution*; contraindicated at term	N/A
Hydroxychloroquine (*Plaquenil*)	None known with doses recommended for malaria prophylaxis	Probably safe in low doses	C
Itraconazole (*Sporanox*, and others)	Teratogenic and embryotoxic in rats	Caution*	C
Iodoquinol (*Yodoxin*, and others)	Unknown	Caution*	C
Ivermectin (*Stromectol*)[5]	Teratogenic in animals	Contraindicated	C
Ketoconazole (*Nizoral*, and others)	Teratogenic and embryotoxic in rats	Contraindicated; topical probably safe	C
Lindane	Absorbed from the skin; potential CNS toxicity in fetus	Contraindicated	C
Malathion, topical	None known	Probably safe	B
Mebendazole (*Vermox*)	Teratogenic and embryotoxic in rats	Caution*	C
Mefloquine[6]	Teratogenic in animals	Caution*	C
Meglumine (*Glucantine*)	Not known	Caution*	N/A
Metronidazole (*Flagyl*, and others)	None known – carcinogenic in rats and mice	Caution*	B
Miconazole (*Monistat i.v.*)	None known	Caution*	C

e18

Appendix 296-1, cont'd.

Miltefosine (*Impavido*)	Teratogenic in rats and induces abortions inanimals	Contraindicated; effective contraception must be used for 2 months after the last dose	N/A
Niclosamide (*Niclocide*)	Not absorbed; no known toxicity in fetus	Probably safe	B
Nitazoxanide (*Alinia*)	None known	Probably safe	B
Oxamniquine (*Vansil*)	Embryocidal in animals	Contraindicated	N/A
Paromomycin	Poorly absorbed; toxicity in fetus unknown	Oral capsules probably safe	C
Pentamidine (*Pentam 300, NebuPent,* and others)	Safety not established	Caution*	C
Permethrin (*Nix,* and others)	Poorly absorbed; no known toxicity in fetus	Probably safe	B
Praziquantel (*Biltricide*)	None known	Caution	B
Primaquine	Hemolysis in G-6-PD deficiency	Contraindicated	C
Pyrantel pamoate (*Antiminth,* and others)	Absorbed in small amounts; no known toxicity in fetus	Probably safe	C
Pyrethrins and piperonyl butoxide (*A-200,* and others)	Poorly absorbed; no known toxicity in fetus	Probably safe	C
Pyrimethamine (*Daraprim*)[7]	Teratogenic in animals	Caution*; contraindicated during 1st trimester	C
Quinacrine (*Atabrine*)	Safety not established	Caution*	N/A
Quinidine	Large doses can cause abortion	Probably safe	C
Quinine (*Qualaquin*)	Large doses can cause abortion; auditory nerve hypoplasia, deafness in fetus; visual changes, limb anomalies, visceral defects also reported	Caution*	C
Sodium stibogluconate (*Pentostam*)	Not known	Caution*	N/A
Spiramycin (*Rovamycine*)[7]	None known	Probably safe	N/A
Sulfonamides	Teratogenic in some animal studies;hemolysis in newborn with G-6-PD deficiency; increased risk of kernicterus in newborn	Caution*; contraindicated at term	C
Suramin sodium (*Germanin*)	Teratogenic in mice	Caution*	N/A
Tetracycline (*Sumycin,* and others)	Tooth discoloration and dysplasia, inhibition of bone growth in fetus; hepatic toxicity and azotemia with IV use in pregnant patients with decreased renal function or with overdosage	Contraindicated	D
Tinidazole (*Tindamax*)	Increased fetal mortality in rats	Caution*	C
Trimethoprim	Folate antagonism; teratogenic in rats	Caution*	C
Trimethoprim-sulfamethoxazole (*Bactrim,* and others)	Same as sulfonamides and trimethoprim	Caution*; contraindicated at term	C

N/A= FDA pregnancy category not available

*Use only for strong clinical indication in absence of suitable alternative.
1. See also footnotes 78 and 79 on page 8.
2. See also footnote 78 on page 8.
3. See also footnote 76 on page 7.
4. See also footnote 82 on page 8.
5. See also footnote 42 on page 4.
6. See also footnotes 84 and 95 on pages 8 and 9.
7. See also footnote 129 on page 12.

e19

Appendix 296-1, cont'd.

MANUFACTURERS OF DRUGS USED TO TREAT PARASITIC INFECTIONS

A-200 (Hogil) – pyrethrins and piperonyl butoxide
albendazole – *Albenza* (GlaxoSmithKline)
Albenza (GlaxoSmithKline) – albendazole
Alinia (Romark) – nitazoxanide
AmBisome (Gilead) – amphotericin B, liposomal
amphotericin B – *Fungizone* (Apothecon), others
amphotericin B, liposomal – *AmBisome* (Gilead)
Ancobon (Valeant) – flucytosine
§ *Antiminth* (Pfizer) – pyrantel pamoate
• *Aralen* (sanofi-aventis) – chloroquine HCl and chloroquine phosphate
§ artemether – *Artenam* (Arenco, Belgium)
artemether/lumefantrine – *Coartem, Riamet* (Novartis)
§ *Artenam* (Arenco, Belgium) – artemether
• † artesunate – (Guilin No. 1 Factory, People's Republic of China)
atovaquone – *Mepron* (GlaxoSmithKline)
atovaquone/proguanil – *Malarone* (GlaxoSmithKline)
azithromycin – *Zithromax* (Pfizer), others
• *Bactrim* (AR Scientific) – TMP/Sulfa
Benzyl alcohol lotion – *Ulesfia* (Sciele)
§ benznidazole – *Rochagan* (Brazil)
• *Biaxin* (Abbott) – clarithromycin
Biltricide (Bayer) – praziquantel
† bithionol – *Bitin* (Tanabe, Japan)
† *Bitin* (Tanabe, Japan) – bithionol
§ *Brolene* (Aventis, Canada) – propamidine isethionate
chloroquine HCl and chloroquine phosphate – *Aralen* (sanofi-aventis), others
• clarithromycin – *Biaxin* (Abbott), others
• *Cleocin* (Pfizer) – clindamycin
clindamycin – *Cleocin* (Pfizer), others
Coartem (Novartis) – artemether/lumefantrine
crotamiton – *Eurax* (Ranbaxy)
dapsone – (Jacobus)
§ *Daraprim* (GlaxoSmithKline) – pyrimethamine USP
† diethylcarbamazine citrate (DEC) – *Hetrazan*
• *Diflucan* (Pfizer) – fluconazole
§ diloxanide furoate – *Furamide*
doxycycline – *Vibramycin* (Pfizer), others
§ eflornithine (Difluoromethylornithine, DFMO) – *Ornidyl* (Aventis)
§ *Egaten* (Novartis) – triclabendazole
Elimite (Allergan) – permethrin
Eurax (Ranbaxy) – crotamiton
• *Flagyl* (Pfizer) – metronidazole
§ *Flisint* (Sanofi-Aventis, France) – fumagillin
fluconazole – *Diflucan* (Pfizer), others
flucytosine – *Ancobon* (Valeant)
§ fumagillin – *Flisint* (Sanofi-Aventis, France)
• *Fungizone* (Apothecon) – amphotericin
§ *Furamide* – diloxanide furoate
§ furazolidone – *Furoxone* (Roberts)
§ *Furoxone* (Roberts) – furazolidone
† *Germanin* (Bayer, Germany) – suramin sodium
§ *Glucantime* (Aventis, France) – meglumine antimonate
† *Hetrazan* – diethylcarbamazine citrate (DEC)
§ *Impavido* (Paladin, Montreal, Canada) – miltefosine
iodoquinol – *Yodoxin* (Glenwood), others
itraconazole – *Sporanox* (Ortho-McNeil-Janssen), others
ivermectin – *Stromectol* (Merck)
ketoconazole – *Nizoral* (Janssen), others
† *Lampit* (Bayer, Germany) – nifurtimox
§ *Leshcutan* (Teva, Israel) – topical paromomycin
lumefantrine/artemether – *Coartem, Riamet* (Novartis)
Malarone (GlaxoSmithKline) – atovaquone/proguanil
malathion – *Ovide* (Taro)
mebendazole
mefloquine
§ meglumine antimonate – *Glucantime* (Aventis, France)

† melarsoprol – *Mel-B*
† *Mel-B* – melarsoprol
Mepron (GlaxoSmithKline) – atovaquone
metronidazole – *Flagyl* (Pfizer), others
§ miconazole – *Monistat i.v.*
§ miltefosine – *Impavido* (Paladin, Montreal, Canada)
§ *Monistat i.v.* – miconazole
NebuPent (Fujisawa) – pentamidine isethionate
Neutrexin (US Bioscience) – trimetrexate
§ niclosamide – *Yomesan* (Bayer, Germany)
† nifurtimox – *Lampit* (Bayer, Germany)
nitazoxanide – *Alinia* (Romark)
• *Nizoral* (Janssen) – ketoconazole
Nix (GlaxoSmithKline) – permethrin
§ ornidazole – *Tiberal* (Roche, France)
Ornidyl (Aventis) – eflornithine (Difluoromethylornithine, DFMO)
Ovide (Taro) – malathion
§ oxamniquine – *Vansil* (Pfizer)
§ *Paludrine* (AstraZeneca, United Kingdom) – proguanil
§ paromomycin – Oral generics; *Leshcutan* (Teva, Israel; (topical formulation not available in US)
Pentam 300 (Fujisawa) – pentamidine isethionate
pentamidine isethionate – *Pentam 300* (Fujisawa), *NebuPent* (Fujisawa)
† *Pentostam* (GlaxoSmithKline, United Kingdom) – sodium stibogluconate
permethrin – *Nix* (GlaxoSmithKline), *Elimite* (Allergan)
praziquantel – *Biltricide* (Bayer)
primaquine phosphate USP
§ proguanil – *Paludrine* (AstraZeneca, United Kingdom)
proguanil/atovaquone – *Malarone* (GlaxoSmithKline)
§ propamidine isethionate – *Brolene* (Aventis, Canada)
§ pyrantel pamoate – *Antiminth* (Pfizer)
pyrethrins and piperonyl butoxide – *A-200* (Hogil), others
§ pyrimethamine USP – *Daraprim* (GlaxoSmithKline)
Qualaquin – quinine sulfate (AR Scientific)
quinidine gluconate
§ quinine dihydrochloride
quinine sulfate – *Qualaquin* (AR Scientific)
Riamet (Novartis) – artemether/lumefantrine
• *Rifadin* (sanofi-aventis) – rifampin
rifampin – *Rifadin* (sanofi-aventis), others
§ *Rochagan* (Brazil) – benznidazole
* *Rovamycine* (Aventis) – spiramycin
† sodium stibogluconate – *Pentostam* (GlaxoSmithKline, United Kingdom)
* spiramycin – *Rovamycine* (Aventis)
• *Sporanox* (Ortho-McNeil-Janssen) – itraconazole
Stromectol (Merck) – ivermectin
sulfadiazine
† suramin sodium – *Germanin* (Bayer, Germany)
§ *Tiberal* (Roche, France) – ornidazole
Tindamax (Mission) – tinidazole
tinidazole – *Tindamax* (Mission)
TMP/Sulfa – *Bactrim* (AR Scientific), others
§ triclabendazole – *Egaten* (Novartis)
trimetrexate – *Neutrexin* (US Bioscience)
Ulesfia – benzyl alcohol
§ *Vansil* (Pfizer) – oxamniquine
• *Vibramycin* (Pfizer) – doxycycline
§ *Yodoxin* (Glenwood) – iodoquinol
§ *Yomesan* (Bayer, Germany) – niclosamide
• *Zithromax* (Pfizer) – azithromycin

---

§ Not available in the US; may be available through a compounding pharmacy (see footnote 4).
† Available from the CDC Drug Service, Centers for Disease Control and Prevention, Atlanta, Georgia 30333; 404-639-3670 (evenings, weekends, or holidays: 770-488-7100).
• Also available generically.

e20

Subject Index

Note

Cross-reference terms in italics are general cross-references, or refer to subentry terms within the main entry (the main entry is not repeated to save space).

Page numbers suffixed by 'b', 'f', and 't', refer to boxes, figures and tables respectively.

This index is alphabetized in word-by-word order.

Abbreviations

CGD – chronic granulomatous disease
CLABSIs – central line associated bloodstream infections
CMV – cytomegalovirus
CVC – central venous catheter
EBV – Epstein–Barr virus
GAS – group A streptococci
GBS – group B streptococci
HAIs – healthcare-associated infections
HAV – hepatitis A virus
HBV – hepatitis B virus
HCV – hepatitis C virus
HLH – hemophagocytic lymphohistiocytosis
HSCT – hematopoietic stem cell transplantation
HSV – herpes simplex virus
IGIV – immune globulin intravenous
MIC – minimum inhibitory concentration
PFAPA – periodic fever with aphthous stomatitis, pharyngitis and adenitis syndrome
RSV – respiratory syncytial virus
VZV – varicella zoster virus

A

AACEK organisms, 257, 835–836, 939
  Aggregatibacter actinomycetemcomitans, 939
  blood cultures, 1374–1375
  Cardiobacterium hominis, 940
  Eikenella corrodens, 835–836
  endocarditis due to, 257, 260–261, 1418t–1419t
    complications, 264
    management, 263–264
  Kingella kingae, 921
AAP Red Book Report of the Committee on Infectious Diseases (COID), 68
Abacavir, 664, 665t
  dosage, 1445t–1452t
Abdominal abscess, 423–427
  anaerobic gram-negative bacilli, 984

see also Intra-abdominal abscess; Retroperitoneal abscess; Visceral abscesses
Abdominal distention
  necrotizing enterocolitis, 389
  peritonitis, 417
  visceral leishmaniasis, 1287
Abdominal examination, in acute abdominal pain, 172
Abdominal infections
  appendiceal *see* Appendicitis
  hepatitis *see* Hepatitis
  peritonitis *see* Peritonitis
  trauma-related, 512t, 514–515
  see also Intra-abdominal infections
Abdominal lymph nodes, 155–156, 156f
  biopsy, 157
Abdominal lymphadenopathy, 155–157
  causes, 155
    infectious, 155–156
    noninfectious, 155, 157
  differential diagnosis, 155–157
  epidemiology, 155–157
  evaluation, 156b
Abdominal mass, acute pancreatitis, 410
Abdominal migraine, 176
Abdominal pain
  acute, 171–174
    associated symptoms, 171
    character and severity, 171–172
    differential diagnosis, 421b
    history, 171
    location of pain, 171
    physical examination, 172
    radiation sites, 171
  acute pancreatitis, 410
  Angiostrongylus costaricensis causing, 1338
  appendicitis, 171–172, 420
  Ascaris lumbricoides infections, 1328
  biliary colic, 171
  Blastocystis hominis associated, 1268
  bowel obstruction, 171
  Campylobacter jejuni infections, 174, 876
  causes, 172–174
  cholecystitis and cholelithiasis, 173, 413
  chronic (CAP) or recurrent (RAP), 174–176
    associated conditions, 175
    causes, 176t
    diagnostic criteria, 174–175
    diagnostic guidelines, 175
    expanded diagnosis, 176t
    management, 176
    nonorganic causes, 175, 175t–176t
    nonorganic *vs.* organic causes, 175t
    organic causes, 175–176, 175t–176t
  Clostridium difficile infections, 174, 978
  Cyclospora causing, 1283

Cystoisospora belli causing, 1283–1284
  diagnosis and management, 176
  Dientamoeba fragilis infection, 1279
  Diphyllobothrium infection, 1347
  Entamoeba histolytica infection, 1275–1276, 1275t
  enteric infections, 174
  Enterobius vermicularis, 174
  epigastric, 171
  Epstein–Barr virus (EBV) causing, 174
  Escherichia coli O157:H7, 174
  familial Mediterranean fever, 124–125
  functional (FAP), 174–175
    management, 176
  gallbladder disease, 173
  gastroenteritis, 171
  granulomatous hepatitis, 409
  Helicobacter pylori, 908, 912
  Henoch–Schönlein purpura (HSP), 173–174
  hookworm infections, 1329
  hypogastric, 171
  intra-abdominal abscess, 424
  intussusception, 174
  liver abscess, 425
  mesenteric adenitis, 172–173
  pancreatitis, 171, 173, 176, 410
  pelvic inflammatory disease, 173
  peritonitis, 171–172, 417
  pneumonia, 173
  postprandial, 174
  pyelonephritis, 173
  referred, 171–173
  renal/ureteral colic, 171
  Rocky Mountain Spotted Fever, 533
  Salmonella, 174
  Shigella, 174
  Streptococcus pyogenes, 174
  Trichinella spiralis infections, 1341
  volvulus, 174
  Yersinia infections, 174
Abdominal radiography
  appendicitis, 421
  necrotizing enterocolitis, 389–390, 389f
Abdominal surgery, infection chemoprophylaxis, 73
Abdominal symptom complexes, 171–176
  acute pain *see* Abdominal pain
Abdominal trauma, 513t, 514–515
  blunt *vs* penetrating, 514
  management, 513t, 514
  pathogens and infection prophylaxis, 512t, 514
Abelcet, 1443t, 1445t–1452t
Abiotrophia, 716–719
  antimicrobial resistance, 718
  blood cultures, 1374–1375

endocarditis due to, 258, 717
  complications, 264
Abiotrophia defectiva, endocarditis treatment, 263
Abortion
  Borrelia infections, 957–958
  Leptospira infections, 951–952
  septic, 981
  spontaneous
    Listeria monocytogenes infection, 764
    rubella virus infection, 1115
    Ureaplasma urealyticum infection, 1000–1001, 1115
    viral infections associated, 546–547
Abscess, 456–459
  abdominal *see* Abdominal abscess; Intra-abdominal abscess
  Aggregatibacter actinomycetemcomitans, 939–940
  amebic liver *see* Amebic liver abscess
  anaerobic infections causing, 962
  Aspergillus, 319
  Bacteroides fragilis, 962
  Bezold, 223, 225
  breast *see* Breast abscess
  Brodie, 469
  Brucella causing, 863
  cerebral *see* Brain abscess
  Citilli, 223
  coagulase-negative staphylococci causing, 693
  cutaneous/subcutaneous
    Aggregatibacter actinomycetemcomitans, 939–940
    etiology, 456b
    predisposing factors, 455b
  definition, 456
  dental *see* Dental abscess
  drainage, 146
  Eikenella infection, 836
  endocardial, 264
  epidural *see* Epidural abscess
  etiology, 423–424
  extracerebral *see* Epidural abscess; Septic venous thrombosis; Subdural empyema
  fingerstick site, 836–837
  frontal lobe *see* Frontal lobe abscess
  Fusobacterium causing, 986
  hepatic *see* Liver, abscess
  iliopsoas *see* Iliopsoas abscess
  intra-abdominal *see* Intra-abdominal abscess
  lateral pharyngeal, 207–208
  lung *see* Lung, abscess
  lymph nodes, 681
  management, 424, 426–427
  metastatic, in Lemierre disease, 210
  muscle *see* Muscle, abscess
  Mycobacterium tuberculosis, 778
  myocardial, 595–596
  nasolacrimal duct, 681
  neck *see* Neck, abscess
  Nocardia causing, 794
  obturator internus, 680
  orbital, 510
  pancreatic, 426
  Paragonimus skrjabini causing, 1368

parapharyngeal *see* Parapharyngeal abscess
paraspinal, 778
paraspinal, *Mycobacterium tuberculosis*, 778
parietal lobe, 322–323, 322b
perianal, 458
periapical, 191
periappendiceal, 768
perinephric (perirenal), 344, 425
periodontal *see* Periodontal abscess
perirectal, 458
peritonsillar *see* Peritonsillar abscess
psoas muscle *see* Psoas muscle abscess
renal (intrarenal and perinephric) *see* Renal abscess
retroperitoneal *see* Retroperitoneal abscess
retropharyngeal *see* Retropharyngeal abscess
scalp *see* Scalp, abscess
splenic, 426
Staphylococcus aureus see *Staphylococcus aureus*
stellate, lymphogranuloma venereum, 129
subdural *see* Subdural abscess
subperiosteal *see* Subperiosteal abscess
sweat gland, 457–458
temporal lobe *see* Temporal lobe abscess
tubo-ovarian, 364
valve ring, 595
visceral *see* Visceral abscesses
Absidiaceae, 1212–1213
Absolute lymphocyte count (ALC), SCID, 629
Absolute risk reduction (ARR), 2t, 5
Absorption, of drugs, 1433, 1434f, 1438
  age *vs.*, 1435, 1435t
Abuse, child *see* Sexual abuse
AC/HS test (differential agglutination), *Toxoplasma gondii*, 1313
Acanthamoeba, 1295–1297
  characteristics, 1295t
  clinical manifestations, 1296
  culture, 1296–1297
  cutaneous infections, 1296
    treatment, 1297
  description and taxonomy, 1295–1296
  diagnosis, 1296–1297
  encephalitis due to, 303–304, 307
  epidemiology, 1296
  granulomatous amebic encephalitis, 1294, 1295t, 1296
    diagnosis, 1296–1297
    epidemiology, 1296
    treatment, 1297
  keratitis, 497, 1296, 1297f
    prevention, 1297
    treatment, 498, 1297
  laboratory testing, 308t–311t
  mortality, 1296
  Naegleria fowleri infections *vs.*, 1294–1295, 1295t
  prevention, 1297
  trophozoites, 1296–1297, 1296f
Acanthamoeba astronyxis, 1296
Acanthamoeba castellanii, 1296

Acanthamoeba culbertsoni, 1296
Acanthamoeba griffini, 1296
Acanthamoeba hatchetti, 1296
Acanthamoeba lugdunensis, 1296
Acanthamoeba palestinensis, 1296
Acanthamoeba polyphagia, 1296
Acanthamoeba quina, 1296
Acanthamoeba rhysodes, 1296
ACE inhibitors, in myocarditis, 267–268
Acetaminophen, antipyretic action, 92
Acetic acid
  burns treatment, 1500t–1501t
  ear infection treatment, 1497t
Acholeplasma laidlawii, 998t
Acholeplasma oculi, 998t
Achromobacter, 832–833
Achromobacter denitrificans, 832
Achromobacter piechaudii, 832
Achromobacter xylosoxidans, 832
  in cystic fibrosis, 639
Acid electrolytic water (AEW), skin antiseptic, 1499t
Acid-fast bacilli (AFB), 673, 771–772
  see also Mycobacterium
Acidosis
  lactic, antiretroviral drugs causing, 672
  metabolic *see* Metabolic acidosis
  respiratory, tachypnea in, 168–169
Acidovorax, 833
Acinetobacter, 828–830
  antimicrobial susceptibility/resistance, 829
  bloodstream infections, 829
  clinical features, 829
  meningitis, 829
  microbiology and epidemiology, 828–829
  nosocomial infections, 829
  septicemia, 829
  treatment, 829–830
Acinetobacter anitratus, 828
Acinetobacter baumannii, 828
  antimicrobial resistance, healthcare-associated infections, 14t
  antimicrobial susceptibility/resistance, 829
Acinetobacter calcoaceticus, 828–829
Acinetobacter calcoaceticus-Acinetobacter baumannii complex, 828
Acinetobacter haemolyticus, 828
Acinetobacter johnsonii, 828
Acinetobacter junii, 828
Acinetobacter lwoffii, 828
Acinetobacter radioresistens, 828
ACIP *see* Advisory Committee on Immunization Practices
Acne vulgaris
  Malassezia folliculitis *vs.*, 1217
  treatment, 1499
Aconoidasida, 1261
Acquired immunodeficiency syndrome (AIDS) *see* Human immunodeficiency virus (HIV)/AIDS
3,6-*bis*(dimethylamino) Acridine, 1374, 1376–1377
Acridine orange, 1374, 1376–1377
Act A, *Listeria monocytogenes* protein, 763–764

Actinobacillus, 939
  animal bites, 521–522
Actinobacillus actinomycetemcomitans see
  Aggregatibacter actinomycetemcomitans
Actinobacillus hominis, 939
Actinobacillus israelii, 939
Actinobacillus lignieresii, 939
Actinobacillus ureae, 939
Actinomyces, 990–992
  abdominal actinomycosis, 991
  antibiotic susceptibility, 966t, 991
  cervicofacial actinomycosis, 991
  classification, 959t
  clinical manifestations, 991
  culture media, 1376t
  diagnosis/detection, 963–964, 991
  gastrointestinal actinomycosis, 990–991
  isolation and identification, 991
  mandibular osteomyelitis, 196
  meningitis, 281–282
  microbiology, 990
  mycetoma, 1250
  neck infection, management, 146
  Nocardia vs., 990
  osteomyelitis, 476f
  pathogenesis of infections, 990–991
  pelvic actinomycosis, 991
  pulmonary actinomycosis, 990–991
  soft tissue abscess, 962
  synergistic infections, 991
  thoracic actinomycosis, 991, 992f
  treatment of infections, 991
Actinomyces gerencseriae, 990
Actinomyces israelii, 962, 990
  unilateral cervical lymphadenitis due to,
    141
Actinomyces meyeri, 990
Actinomyces naeslundii, 990
Actinomyces odontolyticus, 990
Actinomyces viscosus, 990
Actinomycetes, cell wall and Gram staining,
    673
Actinomycosis *see Actinomyces*
Action potentials, muscle, *Clostridium
    botulinum* infection, 974
Activated protein C (aPC)
  in meningococcal septicemia treatment,
    737
  in sepsis, 101t–102t
Activation-induced cytidine deaminase
    (AID) deficiency, 610t, 613, 632
  characteristics, 602t
Active immunization *see* Immunization
Active surveillance, 1, 16
Active surveillance cultures, 16
Acute chest syndrome, 251
  sickle-cell disease, 634
Acute disseminated encephalomyelitis
    (ADEM), 178–179, 304, 314–317
  clinical features, 317
  diagnosis, 317
  differential diagnosis, 317
  etiology, 314t
  imaging, 307f
  incidence, 316–317
  MRI, 317, 317f
  postinfectious, differential diagnosis, 325
  recurrent, 317

Acute flaccid paralysis (AFP), 1176
Acute focal bacterial nephritis (AFBN),
    343–345
Acute inflammatory demyelinating
    polyneuropathy (AIDP) *see* Guillain–
    Barré syndrome
Acute lymphoblastic leukemia (ALL)
  eosinophilic meningitis, 333
  mediastinal masses, 154
Acute lymphocytic leukemia (ALL), varicella
    vaccine use, 62
Acute motor axonal neuropathy (AMAN),
    Campylobacter jejuni infections, 877
Acute necrotizing ulcerative gingivitis
    (ANUG), 193t, 194
Acute otitis media (AOM) *see* Otitis media
Acute-phase proteins, 1400
  in Kawasaki disease, 113
  negative, 94
  positive, 94
  synthesis, 94
  see also C-reactive protein (CRP)
Acute-phase response, 94, 1400
  magnitude, extent of inflammation, 94
  manifestations, 1400b
  mineral changes, 94
  see also C-reactive protein (CRP)
Acute respiratory distress syndrome (ARDS)
  Plasmodium infection, 1299, 1303
  in sepsis, 98
Acute retinal necrosis (ARN), VZV
    infections, 502
Acute rheumatic fever (ARF) *see Streptococcus
    pyogenes* (group A streptococcus)
Acute suppurative sialadenitis, 195
Acyclovir, 1502–1507
  adverse effects, 1504–1505
  chemistry, 1502–1503
  clinical uses, 1505–1507, 1506t
  dosage, 1445t–1452t, 1505–1507,
    1506t
    in renal dysfunction, 1445t–1452t,
      1504, 1504t–1505t
  drug interactions, 1504–1505
  EBV infection, 1062
  HSV infections, 1033, 1033t
    compromised hosts, 1034
    congenital/perinatal infections, 1034
    conjunctivitis, 489
    genital herpes, 1033–1034
    gingivostomatitis, 192, 204
    guidelines for use, 1033t
    long-term use, 1034–1035
    neonatal, 548
    orolabial herpes, 1033
    prophylactic use, 1033, 1035
    role, types of infections, 1033t
    stomatitis, 192
    topical, 1033
  HSV-related meningitis, 296
  mechanism of action, 1041, 1502–1503,
    1502t
  metabolism, 1041
  neonatal infections, 538, 548
  pharmacokinetics, 1504
  prophylactic, 70t–71t, 71, 1505, 1507t
    HSV infections, 71
    neonatal HSV prevention, 71

resistance to, 1502–1503, 1503t
  HSV, 1034
spectrum of activity, 1502–1503, 1504t
viral keratitis, 497
VZV infection prevention, 1042
VZV infection treatment, 1040–1041,
    1040b
  dosages and optimal use, 1041
  healthy children/adolescents, 1041
  herpes zoster, 1041
  immunocompromised children, 1041
  intravenous, 1041
  neonatal, 548
  oral, 1041
  resistance, 1041
  varicella, 1040b, 1041
VZV postexposure prophylaxis, 39
Adamantanes
  influenza treatment, 1154
  influenza virus resistance, 1155
  see also Amantadine; Rimantadine
Adaptive immune response *see* Immune
    response
ADCC *see* Antibody-dependent cell-
    mediated cytotoxicity (ADCC)
Adefovir, HBV infection treatment,
    1083–1084
Adefovir dipivoxil, 1502t, 1507–1508
Adenitis *see* Lymphadenitis/
    lymphadenopathy
Adeno-associated virus-2, preterm birth and,
    546
Adenoidectomy, 231
  sinusitis, 231
Adenoids, anatomy, 127
Adenopathy *see* Lymphadenitis/
    lymphadenopathy
Adenosine deaminase (ADA), 627
  deficiency, 627, 628t, 629
    diagnosis, 629
    management, 629
  enzyme replacement, 629
Adenoviridae, 1016t, 1067
  infections, 1017t
Adenoviruses, 378, 1067–1070
  acute bilateral cervical lymphadenitis,
    138
  acute respiratory disease due to, 138,
    1069
  in AIDS, 1070
  antigens, detection, 1070
  Bordetella pertussis infections *vs.*, 869
  bronchiolitis due to, 231
  bronchiolitis obliterans due to, 250,
    1069
  cardiac infections, 1069
  cell culture, 1070
  clinical manifestations, 1068–1070,
    1068t, 1071b
  conjunctivitis due to, 108–110, 491
    treatment, 493
  cystitis due to, 339, 1069
  cytopathic effects, 1070
  diagnosis/detection, 113, 1070, 1071b
    detection rates, 1386t
    optimal tests, 1389t–1392t
  disseminated disease, 1068
  DNA, detection, 1070

encephalitis due to, 1069
enteric, 378, 1068t, 1069
   clinical features, 380t
   description, 379f
   diagnosis, 1386, 1389t–1392t, 1395
   diarrhea, 26t
   epidemiology, 380, 380t
   group childcare and, 25t
   transmission, 380
epidemic keratoconjunctivitis due to,
   1068–1069, 1068t
epidemiology, 197f, 1067–1068, 1071b,
   1131f
fetal/neonatal infections, 1070
   nosocomial, 551
gastrointestinal infections, 1068t, 1069
   clinical features, 380t
   healthcare-associated infections, 584
   see also Adenoviruses, enteric
generalized lymphadenopathy due to,
   132
genitourinary infections, 1068t, 1069
group childcare and, 25t
HSCT recipients, 564
immunization against, 1070
immunocompromised hosts, 1068t,
   1069–1070
keratitis due to, 496
laboratory testing, 308t–311t
myocarditis due to, 265–266
neurologic infections, 1069
neutrophilia due to, 1404
nosocomial infections, 551, 1068
obliterative bronchiolitis due to, 250,
   1069
ocular infections, 491, 1068t, 1069
persistence on hands, 1068
pharyngitis due to, 201
pharyngoconjunctival fever, 138, 1068t,
   1069
pneumonia due to, 238
   persistent pneumonia, 246
prevention of infections, 1070
respiratory, 1068t, 1069
   diagnosis/detection, 1385
   group childcare and, 25t
serotype 7, 1069
skin lesions due to, 112
subgroups/serotypes, 1067–1068
   diseases associated, 1068–1069, 1068t
   identification, 1070
transmission, 1067–1068
transplant recipients, 559, 564
treatment of infections, 1070, 1071b
urethritis due to, 353
virology, 1071b
Adenylate kinase 2 (AK2) gene, 628t
Adhesins, Klebsiella, 800
Adhesion molecules, 85, 85f
Aditus ad antrum, 222–223, 223f
Adjuvants, 45
   sites of vaccine administration, 46
Adolescents
   anaerobic infections, 963t
   back pain, 187
   Bordetella pertussis infections, 866, 866f
   cervical lymphadenitis, 138, 144
   cervicitis and ectropion, 361–362, 362t

chronic fatigue syndrome, 1011–1013,
   1015
dysuria in females, 354
HIV infection, 672
   clinical features, 657
   HIV replication, 648–649
   natural history, 643
   opportunistic infections, 657
   postexposure prophylaxis, 648
   prevention, 648, 648b
   testing, 648
   transmission, 648, 657
immunization, 54
   catch-up schedule, 49f
   meningococcal, 65
   MMR and MMRV, 59
   schedule, 49f
   Tdap, 56, 758, 872
   varicella, 62
inclusion conjunctivitis, 494
juvenile periodontitis, 191
Mycoplasma hominis infections, 998,
   998t
Mycoplasma pneumoniae infections, 993
myopericarditis due to enteroviruses,
   1177
ocular larva migrans, 1336
pelvic inflammatory disease, 353
   see also Pelvic inflammatory disease
   (PID)
peritonsillar abscess (quinsy), 206
pneumonia, 169–170, 170t, 236–239
   persistent pneumonia, 246
pyogenic arthritis, 478
SARS-CoV infection, 1119
urethritis, 354
urinary tract infections, 340
varicella complications, 1038
   treatment, 1041
vulvitis, 361
Adoption, international see Refugee and
   internationally adopted children
Adrenal failure, in septic shock, 100
Adrenal insufficiency, chronic fatigue
   syndrome pathogenesis, 1008–1010
α-adrenergic agonists, RSV infection, 1133
β-adrenergic agonists see β-adrenergic agents
   (under beta)
Adult infectious diseases
   group childcare infections and, 31
   in healthcare personnel see Healthcare
     personnel
Adult seborrheic eczema (ASE), Malassezia,
   1217
Adult T-cell leukemia/lymphoma (ATLL),
   1165
Adverse effects of drugs
   see individual drugs
Advisory Committee on Immunization
   Practices (ACIP), 27
   hepatitis A virus recommendations, 1184
   licensure of vaccines, 47
   PCV7 recommendations, 726
   structure and role, 47
Aedes mosquito, 81
   Chikungunya virus transmission,
     1097–1098
   dengue virus transmission, 1100

   Ross River virus transmission, 1098
   yellow fever transmission, 1099
Aerobic bacteria, strict aerobes, 959t
Aerococcus
   antibiotic susceptibility, 730
   biochemical differentiation, 729t
Aerococcus viridans, 729–730
Aeromonas, 830–831
   antimicrobial susceptibility/resistance,
     831
   clinical manifestations, 830–831
   culture media, 1376t
   gastroenteritis due to, 830
   laboratory findings/diagnosis, 376, 831
   septicemia due to, 831
   skin and soft-tissue infections, 830–831
   treatment of infections, 831
   virulence factors and enterotoxins,
     830
Aeromonas caviae, 830
Aeromonas hydrophila, 830
   inflammatory enteritis due to, 383
   skin and soft-tissue infections, 830–831
   skin infections after trauma, 514
Aeromonas sobria, 830
Aerophobia, rabies, 1147
Aerosol transmission
   classification (obligate, preferential,
     opportunistic), 12–13
   common cold viruses, 197
   healthcare-associated infections, 12–13
   small-particle and large-particle, 197
Afelimomab, 101t–102t
Affective disorders
   chronic fatigue syndrome and, 1012
   see also Depression
Aflatoxin, 1203
African Programme for Onchocerciasis
   Control (APOC), 1345
African sleeping sickness see Trypanosoma
   (Trypanozoon) brucei
African tickbite fever, 935–937
   see also Rickettsiosis
African trypanosomiasis see Trypanosoma
   (Trypanozoon) brucei
Agammaglobulinemia
   autosomal, 610–611, 610t
   characteristics, 602t
   X-linked see X-linked
     agammaglobulinemia
Agar, for culture see Culture media
Agar dilution testing, antimicrobial
   susceptibility testing, 1381
Age
   antimicrobial agent selection and,
     1412–1413
   cervical lymphadenitis etiology, 135t,
     136
   cystic fibrosis, infections in, 639t
   immune response to immunization and,
     46
   neonatal antibiotic dosage, 1483t–1484t
   normal rectal temperatures, 117, 117f
   in pharmacokinetics, 1414, 1434–1435,
     1435t
   sepsis incidence and estimates, 97t
   solid-organ transplant infections, 551
   see also specific infections

Agglutination test
  Leptospira, 951
  see also Latex agglutination (LA)
Agglutinin tests, 1384
Aggregatibacter, 907–908, 938
  brain abscess, 320
  differential characteristics of species, 906t
  microbiology, 938
  species, 907–908, 938
Aggregatibacter (Actinobacillus) actinomycetemcomitans, 939–940
  early-onset periodontitis, 191
  endocarditis, 257, 939
  isolation, 940
  treatment, 940
Aggregatibacter (Haemophilus) aphrophilus, 907–908
Aggregatibacter (Haemophilus) parainfluenzae see Haemophilus parainfluenzae
Aggregatibacter (Haemophilus) segnis, 907–908
AID (activation-induced cytidine deaminase), deficiency, 610t, 613, 632
  characteristics, 602t
AIDS *see* Human immunodeficiency virus (HIV)/AIDS
Air crescent sign, *Aspergillus* infections, 1207
Air trapping, viral pneumonia, 238
Airborne infections
  healthcare-associated infections, 12–13
  Mycobacterium tuberculosis, 772
Airborne Precautions, 18
Airflow
  infant lung, 233
  resistance, RSV infection, 1132
Airway
  compression
    cough in, 167t
    persistent pneumonia, 247
  congenital abnormalities, persistent pneumonia, 247
  extrathoracic, narrowing in inspiration, 165
  hyperreactive, cough in, 167t
  intrathoracic, narrowing in expiration, 165
  reactive
    chest pain, 189
    cough in, 167t
Airway infections
  lower *see* Lower respiratory tract infections (LRTIs)
  middle *see* Supraglottic infections
  upper *see* Upper respiratory tract infections (URTIs)
Airway management
  acute epiglottitis (supraglottitis), 210–211
  bacterial tracheitis, 212
  laryngotracheitis, 211
Airway obstruction
  laryngotracheitis, 211
  lower tract, in bronchiolitis, 233
  necrotizing pneumonia and lung abscess, 243
  upper *see* Upper airway obstruction

Ajellomyces capsulatus, 1194
Ajellomyces dermatitidis, 1194, 1234
Alagille syndrome, 402–403
Alanine aminotransferase (ALT), 1411
  CMV infection, 1046–1047
  HAV infection, 1183, 1183f
  HBV infection, 1080
  HCV infection, 1107–1108, 1110
  HIV infection, 655
Alastrim (variola minor), 1021, 1022t
Albendazole
  adverse reactions, 1355, 1359–1360, 1523
  contraindications, 1359–1360
  mechanism of action, 1523
  treatment of
    Angiostrongylus infections, 1338
    Ascaris lumbricoides infections, 1328
    Clonorchis and *Opisthorchis* infections, 1365
    cutaneous larva migrans, 1339
    Echinococcus granulosus infections, 1359–1360
    Echinococcus multilocularis infections, 1361
    echinostomiasis, 1364
    Enterobius vermicularis infections, 1332
    Giardia intestinalis (giardiasis) infections, 1281t, 1282
    Gnathostoma spinigerum infections, 1338
    hookworm infections, 1330
    intestinal nematode infections, 1326–1327
    Loa loa infections, 1346
    lymphatic filariasis, 1344
    Mansonella perstans infections, 1346
    nematodes, 1523
    Sarcocystis infections, 1308
    Strongyloides infections, 1334
    Taenia infections, 1351–1352
    Taenia solium neurocysticercosis, 1355, 1355t
    Toxocara infections, 1337
    Trichinella spiralis infection, 1341
    Trichuris trichiura infections, 1331
Albumin, nasal secretions, elevated levels in colds, 197–198
Albuterol
  Bordetella pertussis infection, 878
  bronchiolitis management, 234
Alcaligenaceae, 832
Alcaligenes, 832–833
Alcaligenes faecalis, 832
Alcohol-based hand gels, common cold prevention, 199
Alexithymia, 1012
Alkaline phosphatase
  elevated, *Cryptosporidium* infections, 1270
  hepatitis A virus infection, 1183
Allergic bronchopulmonary aspergillosis (ABPA), 1205, 1408t–1409t
Allergic reactions
  to animals/pets, 529
  in common variable immunodeficiency, 612

to drugs
    antimicrobial agent selection and, 1415–1416
    penicillins, 218, 219t
  hydatid cyst rupture, 1358
  to immunization
    DTaP, 56
    rotavirus vaccine, 66
    rubeola virus (measles) vaccine, 1143
  see also Anaphylaxis
  recurrent sinusitis, 230
  to *Taenia serialis* (coenurosis), 1362
  see also Hypersensitivity reactions
Allergic rhinitis, 164
  common colds *vs.*, 198
  diagnosis, 164t, 198
  differential diagnosis, 164t
  epidemiology, 164
  features, and treatment, 164t
  mucopurulent rhinorrhea, 164–165
Allylamines, 1486
  see also individual agents
Alopecia, tinea capitis, 1246f, 1247
Alopecia areata, 1247
Alphaherpesvirinae, 1026, 1026t, 1035
Alphaviruses, 1097–1099
  diagnosis, 1098–1099
  prevention, 1099
ALPS syndrome, 603t–604t
Alternaria, 1211–1212
Alveolar-capillary block, 777
Alveolar echinococcosis *see Echinococcus multilocularis* (alveolar echinococcosis)
Alveolar macrophage, 238
  Mycobacterium tuberculosis infections, 772
Alveoli, rupture, 239
Amanita, 397t, 399
Amanita muscaria, 397t
Amanita pantherina, 397t
Amantadine, 1514
  adverse effects, 1514
  clinical uses, 1514
  dosage, 1514
    in renal dysfunction, 1445t–1452t, 1505t
  drug interactions, 1514
  influenza treatment, 1154
  prophylactic, 70t–71t, 72, 1507t, 1514
  resistance to, 1155, 1158, 1503t, 1514
Amastigotes
  Leishmania, 1285–1288, 1286f
  Trypanosoma (Schizotrypanum) cruzi, 1322, 1324f
Amatoxin, 397t
AmBisome, dosage, 1445t–1452t, 1487t
  pharmacokinetic-pharmacodynamic relationships, 1443t
Ambler classification system, 1424
Ameba, free-living, 1293
  avoidance/control, 1295
  laboratory testing, 308t–311t
  see also Acanthamoeba; Naegleria fowleri
Amebapore, 1274
Amebiasis *see Entamoeba histolytica*

Amebic colitis (intestinal amebiasis),
1273–1275, 1275f, 1275t
diagnosis, 1277
treatment, 1277, 1277b
Amebic liver abscess (ALA), 425, 1273–
1274, 1276, 1276t
diagnosis, 1276–1277, 1276f
treatment, 1277, 1277b
Amebic meningoencephalitis, 1520
Ameboma, 1276
American Academy of Pediatrics (AAP)
acute otitis media treatment, 217–218,
218t–219t, 725
hepatitis A vaccine recommendations,
1184, 1185t
influenza vaccine recommendation, 1156
mumps vaccine recommendations, 1129
Neisseria meningitidis vaccines, 734
PCV7 recommendations, 726
rubella vaccination, 1117
tuberculin skin test recommendations,
773b
tuberculosis treatment recommendations,
784
American Association of Blood Banks, 581
American Heart Association (AHA)
endocarditis
prophylaxis, recommendations, 75,
75b
surgical intervention, guidelines, 264,
264t
viridans streptococcal, treatment, 718,
719t
Kawasaki disease, 1003–1006
American Public Health Association, Red
Book: Report of the Committee on
Infectious Diseases, 68
American Red Cross Blood Services,
580–581
American Thoracic Society
nontuberculous mycobacterial infection
diagnosis, 790
tuberculosis treatment recommendations,
784
American trypanosomiasis see Trypanosoma
(Schizotrypanum) cruzi
American Veterinary Medical Association
(AVMA), 529, 531
Amikacin
dosage, 1445t–1452t, 1480t–1484t
dose adjustment
burned patients, 1437t
renal failure, 1445t–1452t
pharmacology, 1453t–1458t
spectrum of activity, 1459t–1463t, 1474
treatment of
eye infections, 1494t–1496t
Francisella tularensis infections,
898–899
Klebsiella infections, 802
Nocardia infections, 795
Proteus, Providencia, Morganella
infections, 812
tuberculosis, 780t
Amine (whiff) test, 770
Aminoglycosides, 1473–1474
cell wall-active agents with, 1420
clinical uses, 1474

combination therapy, 1415, 1420,
1423–1424
antagonism, 1420–1421
concentration-dependent killing, 1441,
1442t
distribution, 1417
dosage, 1445t–1452t, 1480t–1483t
dose adjustment in burned patients,
1437t
enzymes modifying, Pseudomonas
aeruginosa, 845
inhaled, 1474
mechanism of action, 1473–1474
pharmacodynamic properties, 1414–
1415, 1414t
pharmacology, 1453t–1458t
postantibiotic effect, 1414t, 1415
resistance, 1421–1424, 1422t, 1474
Enterococcus, 714–715
screening for, 1430
viridans group streptococci, 718
spectrum of activity, 1459t–1463t, 1474
structure, 1473
toxicity, 1474
treatment of
endocarditis, 263, 718
infections after burns, 520, 1437t
infections in neutropenia in cancer,
570
nosocomial neonatal infections, 552
Proteus, Providencia, Morganella
infections, 812
Pseudomonas aeruginosa infections,
846
Staphylococcus aureus infection, 688
Ureaplasma urealyticum infections,
1001
viridans group streptococci infections,
718
urinary tract infection, 341
Aminopenicillins, 1453t–1458t, 1467,
1480t–1483t
clinical uses, 1467
dosage, 1480t–1483t
pharmacology, 1453t–1458t
spectrum of activity, 1459t–1463t,
1467
para-Aminosalicylic acid see Para-
aminosalicylic acid (PAS)
Aminotransferases see Alanine
aminotransferase (ALT); Aspartate
transaminase (AST)
Amnionitis, Mycoplasma hominis infections,
998
Amniotic fluid, Toxoplasma gondii infection
diagnosis, 1313
Amniotic membrane rupture, Mycoplasma
hominis infections, 998
Amoxicillin
allergy to, 1415–1416
chemoprophylactic use, 74t
clinical uses, 1467
dosage, 1445t–1452t, 1480t–1483t
pharmacology, 1453t–1458t
spectrum of activity, 1459t–1463t
treatment of
acute bacterial sinusitis, 229–230,
229t

acute otitis media, 216t, 217–218,
218t, 220, 725
Bacillus anthracis infections, 753
fever without localizing signs, 116
GAS pharyngitis treatment, 203–204
Haemophilus infections, 908
Helicobacter pylori treatment, 914
pneumococcal pneumonia, 726
pneumonia, 240, 726
Amoxicillin-clavulanate
bite wound infection prevention, 73
dosage, 1480t–1483t
mechanism of action, 1467
spectrum of activity, 1459t–1463t, 1467
treatment of
acute otitis media, 218, 218t, 725
bite wound infection, 526
Nocardia infections, 795
Amoxicillin-potassium clavulanate, acute
bacterial sinusitis, 230
AmpC β-lactamase see β-Lactamase (under
lactamase); B-lactamase (under
lactamase)
Amphibians, Salmonella transmission, 528
Amphotec, dosage, 1445t–1452t
pharmacokinetic-pharmacodynamic
relationships, 1443t
Amphotericin B, 1486–1488
adverse effects, 1243, 1486–1488
dosage, 1445t–1452t, 1486–1487,
1487t
pharmacokinetic-pharmacodynamic
relationships, 1443t
infections in phagocytic disorders,
622–623
lipid-preparations
Blastomyces dermatitidis
(blastomycosis), 1237, 1238t
in cancer, 578
Candida infections, 1200
dosage, 1445t–1452t
mucormycosis, 1214
pharmacokinetic-pharmacodynamic
relationships, 1443t
liposomal
Aspergillus infections, 1208–1209
Blastomyces dermatitidis
(blastomycosis), 1237–1238,
1238t
dosage, 1445t–1452t, 1487t
Histoplasma capsulatum
(histoplasmosis), 1229
neutropenia associated with cancer,
571
pharmacokinetic-pharmacodynamic
relationships, 1443t
sporotrichosis, 1220
mechanism of action, 1486
minimum inhibitory concentration
(MIC), 1382
pharmacology, 1486–1488
resistance
Fusarium, 1210
Scedosporium apiospermum, 1210
spectrum of activity, 1486t
toxicity, 1243, 1486–1488
nephrotoxicity, 1487
treatment of

Aspergillus infections, 576–577, 1208–1209
Blastomyces dermatitidis (blastomycosis), 1237, 1238t
Coccidioides immitis (coccidioidomycosis), 1243–1244
Coccidioides immitis meningitis, 1243–1244
cryptococcal meningitis, 1222–1223
eumycotic mycetoma, 1252
fungal endocarditis, 263
fungal endophthalmitis, 505
fungal pericarditis, 271
hepatic candidiasis, 578
Histoplasma capsulatum (histoplasmosis), 1228t, 1229
infections in HSCT recipients, 565
leishmaniasis, 1520
mucocutaneous leishmaniasis, 1290
mucormycosis, 1214
Naegleria fowleri (naegleriasis), 1295
neonatal infections, 538
neutropenia associated with cancer, 571
Sporothrix schenckii (sporotrichosis), 1220
visceral leishmaniasis, 1289–1290, 1290t
trial data, 1488
Amphotericin B deoxycholate
Aspergillus infections, 1208
Blastomyces dermatitidis (blastomycosis), 1237, 1238t
Candida infections, 1201, 1201t
Cryptococcus infections, 1222
mucormycosis, 1214
phaeohyphomycosis, 1212
visceral leishmaniasis, 1290, 1290t
Ampicillin
adverse effects, 277
chemoprophylactic use, 70t–71t
Streptococcus agalactiae (group B streptococcus), 711
clinical uses, 1467
dosage, 1445t–1452t, 1480t–1483t
MICs, 1379t
pharmacology, 1453t–1458t
resistance, 275–276
Haemophilus influenzae, 904
spectrum of activity, 1459t–1463t
treatment of
endocarditis, 263t, 1418t–1419t
Enterococcus infections, 715
eye infections, 1496t
Haemophilus infections, 908
Haemophilus influenzae, 907
infants with fever without localizing signs, 116
Kingella kingae, 921
Listeria monocytogenes infections, 766
meningitis, 276–277
neonatal infections, 538, 542–543, 552
nosocomial neonatal infections, 552
rash in EBV infection and, 1061
Salmonella infections, 818, 818t
Shigella infections, 822, 822t
urinary tract infection, 340–341

Ampicillin/ampicillin trihydrate, 1480t–1483t
Ampicillin–sulbactam
clinical uses, 1467
dosage, 1480t–1483t
spectrum of activity, 1459t–1463t, 1467
treatment of
orbital infections, 512
preseptal cellulitis due to sinusitis, 510
Amplified fragment length polymorphism (AFLP) analysis
bacterial identification, 674
Malassezia, 1216
Amprenavir, 1444t–1452t
Amyloidosis, in TRAPS, 126
Anaerobic bacteria, 135t, 958–966
acute bacterial sinusitis due to, 229
antibiotic resistance mechanisms, 965
antibiotic susceptibility, 965–966, 966t
antibiotic susceptibility testing, 964–965, 1381
problems, 964–965
bite wound infections due to, 521
burn wound infections due to, 517–519
cellulitis due to *see* Anaerobic cellulitis
cervical lymphadenitis due to, 135
acute unilateral, 139t, 140
management, 147t
classification, 958–959, 959t
clinical clues to and approach, 962, 963t
clinically important genera, 959, 959t
cocci, 988–990
gram-negative, 960t, 988
gram-positive *see* Anaerobic gram-positive cocci
culture media, 1376t
facultative, 959t
establishment of normal flora, 959
genera and species, 959t
gram-negative bacilli *see* Anaerobic gram-negative bacilli (AGNB)
gram-negative cocci, 960t, 988
gram-positive bacilli, 960t
non-spore-forming *see* Anaerobic gram-positive nonsporulating bacilli
gram-positive cocci *see* Anaerobic gram-positive cocci
host susceptibility factors, 961
intra-abdominal infections, pathogenesis, 962
β-lactamase production, 961, 965
microbiologic methods for detection, 962–965
direct examination, 963–964
primary isolation and media for, 964, 964t
specimen collection, 962–963, 964t
transport of samples, 963, 964t
mortality, 965
necrotizing enterocolitis due to, 390
necrotizing pneumonia and lung abscess due to, 243, 243t
neonatal infections, 539, 539t
neutropenia associated with cancer, 567

normal flora, 958–961
establishment, 959–960
see also Flora
orthopedic device infections, 598
osteomyelitis due to, 475–476
oxygen-reducing potential, 959
oxygen sensitivity, 959
pathogenesis of infections, 961–962
synergistic, 962
pelvic inflammatory disease due to, 364
pericarditis due to, 269
renal abscess due to, 344
septicemia, pathogenesis, 962
specimen collection/processing, transport media, 1373t
spore-forming, 959t
strict anaerobes, 959t
subcutaneous abscess due to, 456
supraglottic infections due to, 205–206
T lymphocyte-mediated response, 961
treatment of infections, 965–966
antibiotics, 965–966, 966t
choice of antibiotics, 966t
combination therapy, 966
principles, 965
toxin neutralization, 965
virulence factors, 962
see also individual genera
Anaerobic bacteria agar, 1375t
Anaerobic cellulitis, 461
clostridial, 466t
nonclostridial, 461, 466t
Anaerobic gram-negative bacilli (AGNB), 960t, 982–985
bacteremia, 984
clinical manifestations, 983–984
female genital tract infections, 984
genera included, 982
intra-abdominal infections, 984
osteomyelitis and pyogenic arthritis, 984
pathophysiology, 983
pleuropulmonary infections, 983–984
prevention of infections, 985
skin/soft tissue infections, 984
treatment of infections, 985
see also Bacteroides; Prevotella
Anaerobic gram-negative cocci, 960t
Anaerobic gram-positive cocci, 959t–960t, 988–990
clinical manifestations, 989
mixed infections, 989–990
pathophysiology, 988–989
Peptococcus, anaerobic cellulitis, 461
predisposing conditions, 988–989
synergistic infections, 988–989
treatment of infections, 989–990
see also Peptostreptococcus
Anaerobic gram-positive nonsporulating bacilli, 959t, 990–992
see also Actinomyces; Propionibacterium
Anaerobic protozoa, *Trichomonas vaginalis*, 1318
Anakinra
in CAPS, 126–127
in TRAPS, 126
Anal discharge, 347
Anal discharge/proctitis/proctocolitis/ enteritis syndrome, 346t, 347

Anal intercourse, 347
Anal pruritus
    Enterobius vermicularis, 1332
    Taenia solium, 1351
Analytic epidemiology, 1–7
    case-control studies, 3t, 4
    cohort studies, 3, 3t
    cross-sectional studies, 3–4
    ecological (trend) studies, 2
    observational studies, 2
    study design, 2–4
Anamorphs, 1194
Anaphylatoxins, 94, 616
Anaphylaxis
    immune globulin intravenous (IGIV)
        causing, 42–43
    urticaria with, 447
    vaccine precaution/contraindication, 56,
        59
        influenza vaccine, 64
        MMR, 60
    see also Allergic reactions
Anaplasma, 893–896
    clinical features of infection, 894–895,
        894t
    diagnosis of infections, 895–896,
        896b
    differential diagnosis, 895
    epidemiology, 894
    fever of unknown origin due to,
        119t–120t
    generalized lymphadenopathy due to,
        132
    immune evasion by, 893
    infections, 108
    laboratory findings, 895
    laboratory testing, 308t–311t
    microbiology, 894
    neutropenia in, 1405
    pathogenesis of infections, 893–894
    prevention, 896
    thrombocytopenia due to, 1410–1411
    treatment of infections, 896, 896b
Anaplasma phagocytophilum, 893
    Babesia infection with, 1261–1263
    Borrelia burgdorferi coinfection, 894
    cross-reactivity with *E. chaffeensis*, 535
    detection, 895–896
    human granulocytic anaplasmosis
        clinical manifestations, 894
        epidemiology, 532t
        laboratory findings and diagnosis,
            533t–534t
    laboratory testing, 308t–311t
    morulae, 893
    in pregnancy, 896
    transmission, by ticks, 533
Anaplasmataceae, 673, 893
Ancylostoma, eosinophilia, 1408t–1409t
Ancylostoma braziliense, 1338–1339
    cutaneous larva migrans, 1338–1339
Ancylostoma caninum, 1329, 1338, 1338f
    clinical features, 1327b, 1330, 1338
    cutaneous larva migrans, 1338, 1338f
    neuroretinitis, 502
Ancylostoma ceylanicum, 1326, 1329–1330
    clinical manifestations, 1327b
    epidemiology, 1329

Ancylostoma duodenale, 1326, 1329–1330
    clinical manifestations, 1327b, 1329
    epidemiology, 1329
    infection route, 1326
    neonatal infection, 1327t
    see also Hookworms
Anelloviridae, 1016t
    infections, 1017t
Anemia
    in acute infections, 1403–1404
    aplastic, chloramphenicol associated,
        928–929
    Babesia causing, 1263
    in *Brucella* infections, 863
    in chronic infections, 1403
    hemolytic *see* Hemolytic anemia
    in HIV infection, 656, 671
        management, 671
    in hookworm infections, 1329, 1403
    in inflammatory response, 94
    iron deficiency *see* Iron deficiency
        anemia
    in *Leptospira* infections, 951
    megaloblastic, *Diphyllobothrium* infection,
        1347
    in *Neisseria meningitidis* infections, 736,
        1403–1404
    normocytic, in acute infections, 1403
    parvovirus B19 infection causing, 41
    in *Plasmodium* infections, 1299–1300
    in *Trichuris trichiura* infections, 1331
    in visceral leishmaniasis, 1287
Anergy
    cell, 92
    to fungal antigens, 1243
Aneurysms
    coronary artery *see* Coronary artery
        aneurysm
    Trypanosoma cruzi infections, 1324
Angina, Ludwig, 194
Angioedema, 447
    erythematous, *Loa loa* causing,
        1345–1346
Angiostrongylus, 1337–1338
    description and life cycle, 1337
    encephalitis, 304
    eosinophilic meningoencephalitis, 1337
    meningitis, 283t
Angiostrongylus cantonensis, 1337
    clinical features, 1337
    CNS migration, 330
    eosinophilic meningitis, 330–333, 331t
        diagnosis, 333
        management, 333
        symptoms and diagnosis, 330–333
    geographic distribution, 330
    intermediate host, 330
    life cycle, 330
    optic neuritis, 316
Angiostrongylus costaricensis, 1337
    clinical features, 1338
Angiotensin-converting enzyme (ACE)
    inhibitors, in myocarditis, 267–268
Anidulafungin, 1492
    clinical uses, 1492
    dosage, 1487t, 1492
    pharmacology, 1492
    spectrum of activity, 1486t

    treatment of *Candida* infections, 1201,
        1201t
Animal(s)
    allergies associated, 529
    antibiotics in feeds, 392
    Babesia infections, 1262–1263
    Balantidium coli infections, 1266–1267
    bites *see* Bites
    Blastocystis hominis infections, 1268
    Coxiella burnetii transmission, 891
    Echinococcus granulosus, 1356
    Echinococcus multilocularis, 1360
    exotic, 526–531
        see also Pet(s), nontraditional
    Helicobacter infections/colonization, 916
    infections associated
        group childcare setting, 25, 30–31
        see also Zoonotic infections
    injuries from, 529
        prevention, 530
    Leishmania reservoir, 1286
    models, cytokine role in antibacterial
        defense, 100
    Mycoplasma infections, 999
    nontyphoidal *Salmonella*, 815, 815t
    pets *see* Pet(s)
    plasma, immunoglobulin products
        prepared from, 42
    in public settings, 529b
        diseases associated, 528–529
        recommendations and guidelines,
            530b, 531
        reportable diseases from, 529–530
    rabies, 1145–1146, 1146f
    recommendations and guidelines, 531
    Sarcocystis infections, 1306
    Toxoplasma gondii transmission, 1309,
        1309f
    Trichinella spiralis infections, 1339
    wildlife, endemic rabies, 1145–1146,
        1146t
    wounds by, care in rabies prevention,
        1148–1149, 1148t
    see also Cat(s); Dog(s); Pig(s); Wildlife;
        Zoonotic infections
Anisakis, 1339
Anncaliia, 1292t
Anogenital warts, HPV associated,
    1072–1073
    treatment, 1074, 1074b
Anopheles mosquito
    malaria transmission, 80
    O'nyong Nyong virus transmission,
        1098
    Plasmodium transmission, 1298–1299,
        1298f, 1304–1306
Anorectal bleeding, 347
Anorectal discharge, sexually transmitted
    infections, 347
Anorectal infections, *Neisseria gonorrhoeae*,
    744
Antagonism, combination antimicrobial
    therapy, 1419–1421
Anterior chamber of eye, Stevens–Johnson
    syndrome, 110–111
Anterior fossa, anomalies, recurrent
    meningitis, 287b
Anterior triangle, neck, 136

Anthelmintics
  intestinal nematode infections,
    1326–1327
    see also Benzimidazoles
  resistance, in hookworms, 1330
  Taenia infections, 1351–1352
    neurocysticercosis, 1354–1356, 1355t
  see also individual drugs
Anthrax see Bacillus anthracis
Anti-C-polysaccharide antibodies, 722
Anti-DNAse B (ADB), Streptococcus pyogenes,
    699
Anti-HIV agents see under Human
    immunodeficiency virus (HIV)/AIDS
Anti-inflammatory agents
  in cystic fibrosis, 641
  see also Non-steroidal anti-inflammatory
    drugs (NSAIDs)
Anti-inflammatory mediators, imbalance
    with inflammatory mediators, 98
Anti-inflammatory pathways, 94–95
Anti-inflammatory therapy, acute rheumatic
    fever (ARF), 705, 705t
Antibacterial therapy see Antibiotics
Antibiotic-associated colitis see
    Antimicrobial-associated colitis (AAC)
Antibiotic-associated diarrhea see Diarrhea
Antibiotic cleansers, topical, folliculitis, 430
Antibiotics, 1453–1484
  acute cervical lymphadenitis treatment,
    146, 147t
  administration routes, 1417–1419
  allergy consideration, 1415–1416
  in animal feeds, 392
  aseptic meningitis induced by, 295–296
  bacterial targets, 1414t, 1441f
  bactericidal vs. bacteriostatic, 262–263
  broad-spectrum
    acute bacterial sinusitis, 230
    children with fever without localizing
      signs, 116
    costs and risks associated, 115–116
    infants with fever without localizing
      signs, 115–116
    in pneumonia, 240
  cell membrane active, 1414t, 1459t–
    1463t, 1469–1470
  cell wall-active agents, 1414t, 1464–1470
    ribosomal-active agents with, 1420
    transglycosylase inhibitors, 1459t–
      1463t, 1464f
    transpeptidase inhibitors, 1459t–
      1463t, 1464f
  Clostridium difficile associated, 978, 979b
    see also Antimicrobial-associated
      colitis (AAC)
  combination therapy, 1415, 1419–1421
  contraindications, in common cold, 199
  dialysis and, 1435, 1436t
  diarrhea due to see Diarrhea
  distribution, 1414, 1414t, 1417
  dosage see Dosage
  duration of therapy, 1417–1419,
    1418t–1419t
  empiric therapy, 1415
    abdominal trauma-related infections,
      514
    endocarditis treatment, 262–263

fever without localizing signs,
    115–116
  Pseudomonas aeruginosa infections,
    845
  Shigella infections, 822
  endocarditis treatment, 262–264,
    262t–263t
  extracellular infections, 1416–1417
  intracellular infections, 1417
  intracellular penetration, for Legionella,
    924–925, 925t
  intravenous, chronic mastoiditis
    management, 227
  judicious use of, 1421
  localized lymphadenitis management,
    159b, 160
  normal flora affected by, 961
  nucleic acid-active, 1414t, 1459t–1463t,
    1475–1480
    DNA-dependent DNA polymerase,
      1476–1478
    RNA polymerase, 1475–1476
  otic, otitis externa management, 221
  overuse, 1421
  parenteral
    Pasteurella multocida infections, 838
    urinary tract infections, 341
  peritonsillar abscess, 206
  pharmacokinetics/pharmacodynamics
    as basis of optimal therapy,
      1433–1452
    burns patients, 520
    dose determination and, 1445b
    properties, 1413–1415, 1414t
  pharmacology, 1453t–1458t
  prophylaxis
    acute rheumatic fever, 704, 705t
    appendicitis, 422
    in asplenia, 637
    bite wounds, 525
    Borrelia burgdorferi (Lyme disease),
      956
    burn patients, 521
    coagulase-negative staphylococcal
      infections, 694
    endocarditis prevention, 76
    fever in HIV infection, 660
    infections in neutropenia in cancer,
      573
    infections in phagocyte disorders,
      624, 624t
    intrapartum see Intrapartum
      antibiotic prophylaxis
    intravascular catheter infections, 594
    material intrapartum, 542
    Mycoplasma pneumoniae infections,
      997
    Neisseria meningitidis infection, 739,
      739t
    Pasteurella multocida infections, 838
    recurrent meningitis, 292
    recurrent otitis media, 219
    Rocky Mountain spotted fever
      (Rickettsia rickettsii), 929
    Shigella infections, 823
    in sickle-cell disease, 636
    Streptococcus pneumoniae infections,
      728

in surgery, 72–73
  surgical site infections, 586–587
  tickborne infections, 535
  trauma-related infection prevention,
    512t, 513
  Yersinia pestis infections, 827
  see also Chemoprophylaxis
  resistance to, 1413, 1415–1416
    urinary tract infections, 75
    see also Antimicrobial drug resistance
  ribosome-active, 1414t, 1459t–1463t,
    1470–1475
    cell wall-active agents with, 1420
  selection of, 1412–1416, 1413b
  sepsis, 99, 99t
  site of infection vs., 1412, 1416–1417
  spectrum of activity, 1459t–1463t
  structures, 1465f
  subconjunctival, 505–506
  surrogate markers, 1441
  susceptibility testing see Susceptibility
    testing
  synergistic, in coagulase-negative
    staphylococcal infections, 694
  target attainment, 1415
  time-dependent, 1441, 1442f, 1442t
  topical see Topical antimicrobial agents
  use in childcare centers, 31
Antibodies, 609
  actions, 45–46
  active production of, 89
  agglutinating, to Brucella, 863
  antigen binding, 609
  bactericidal, role in Neisseria meningitidis
    infections, 731
  deficiency, 89, 609–615, 611f
    characteristics, 602t
    detection, 608t
    diagnosis, 609
    as meningitis risk factor, 273t
    specific, normal Ig levels, 610t,
      614–615, 614t
    transcobalamin II deficiency with,
      602t
    see also Agammaglobulinemia;
      Hypogammaglobulinemia;
      Immunodeficiency;
      Immunoglobulin(s), deficiencies
  formation, 45–46, 611f
    active production, 89
    induced by vaccines, 46
  function, 609
  heterophile, EBV infection, 1061–1062,
    1393, 1411t–1412t
  immaturity of antibody responsiveness,
    615
  Leishmania (leishmaniasis), 1286, 1289
  levels from birth to 6 months, 87
  maternal, 615
    measurement, 548
    transplacental transfer, 87, 544–545
  mechanism of action, 45–46
  monoclonal see Monoclonal antibodies
  neutralizing
    in acquired rubella infection,
      1112–1113, 1113f
    to EBV, 1062–1063
    to HHV-6, 1053

to rabies virus, 1145
to rubeola virus, 1137–1138, 1141
nonspecific, 1411, 1411t–1412t
passively-acquired, 87–89
Plasmodium infections, 1300
production/formation, 87
response during infections, 1387f
to RSV, 1130–1132
specific, deficiency (SAD), 610t, 614–615, 614t
specificity, 87
structure, 609
virus isolation/identification, 1384–1386, 1387f
antibody response over time, 1387f
see also Immunoglobulin(s); *specific pathogens*
Antibody-dependent cell-mediated cytotoxicity (ADCC), 87
HIV infection, 649–650
HSV infections, 1027
influenza virus infections, 1151
Anticholinergic poisoning, infant botulism *vs.*, 974t
Anticoagulants
endocarditis management, 264
Lemierre disease treatment, 210
prosthetic valve infections, 595
sepsis management, 101t–102t, 102
septic venous thrombosis management, 328
Anticytokine therapy, 100, 101t–102t
Antidiarrheal agents, *Cryptosporidium* infections, 1270–1271
Antiemetics, foodborne/waterborne disease, 398
Antiendotoxin therapy
in meningococcal disease, 737
in sepsis, 100, 101t–102t
statin therapy, 101t–102t
Antifungal agents, 1484–1492
dosage, 1443–1444, 1445t–1452t
pharmacokinetic-pharmacodynamic relationships, 1443t
empiric, infections in neutropenia in cancer, 571–572
in HIV agents, 662
infections in phagocytic disorders, 622–623
neonatal infections, nosocomial, 552
prophylactic, infections in neutropenia in cancer, 573
susceptibility testing, 1382
systemic, 1486–1492
topical, 1485–1486
treatment of
Aspergillus infections, 1208–1209
Blastomyces dermatitidis (blastomycosis), 1237–1238, 1238t
Coccidioides immitis (coccidioidomycosis), 1243, 1245
recommendations, 1243–1244
eumycotic mycetoma, 1252
focal CNS infections, 329, 329t
Histoplasma capsulatum (histoplasmosis), 1228–1229, 1228t

infections in neutropenia in cancer, 571–572
invasive *Candida* infections, 1200–1201
Malassezia infections, 1217–1218
mucormycosis, 1214–1215
oral candidiasis, 192–194
otitis externa, 221
Pseudallescheria boydii infections, 1253
superficial *Candida* infections, 1200
vulvovaginitis, 360
see also individual fungal infections
Antigen(s)
polysaccharide, response failure, 612
presentation, 45, 92
processing, 45
thymus (T)-dependent, 632–633
thymus (T)-independent
development of response to, 89
NEMO mutation with immunodeficiency, 632–633
see also specific pathogens
Antigen detection tests
bacterial, 1381
cerebrospinal fluid (CSF), 1377
Candida, 1200
Chlamydia trachomatis, 1398
Cryptococcus neoformans, 1222
Legionella pneumophila, 924, 1381
Mycoplasma pneumoniae, 1399
rapid *see* Rapid antigen detection tests (RADTs)
Streptococcus pneumoniae, 1381
viruses, 1386, 1386t
calicivirus, 381
causing bronchiolitis, 233–234
CMV, 1386
HSV, 1386t, 1388
influenza viruses, 1394
RSV, 1394
VZV, 1040, 1386, 1393
Antigen-presenting cells (APCs), 92, 627
dendritic cells as, 85–86
Antigen–antibody complexes *see* Immune complexes
Antigenic drift
influenza viruses, 1150
RSV, 1130
Antigenic shift
influenza viruses, 1150, 1158
rubeola virus, 1137
Antigenic variation, RSV, 1130
Antiheart antibodies, 266
Antihistamines
treatment of, common colds, 198
urticaria treatment, 447
Antimalarial therapy, 1520–1522
Antimicrobial agents, 1412–1421, 1518–1526
antiprotozoan activity, 1522
bacterial infections *see* Antibiotics
fungal infections *see* Antifungal agents
parasitic infections *see* Antiparasitic agents
prophylactic, 68
duration limited, 69
in transplant recipients, 560–561

selection, pharmacodynamic principles, 216–217, 216t
selection pressure, 12
sepsis, 99, 99t
topical *see* Topical antimicrobial agents
virus infections *see* Antiviral agents
Antimicrobial-associated colitis (AAC), 382
presentation, 382
see also Clostridium difficile
Antimicrobial drug resistance, 1421–1433
acquired, 1422–1423
acute bacterial meningitis treatment, 275–276
antibiotics, 1421–1433
antimalarial agents, 1520–1522
antiviral agents, 1503t
in childcare centers, 31
combination therapy, 1419
cost of, 1421
detection, 1429–1431
see also Susceptibility testing
genetics, 1421–1423
healthcare-associated infections, 13–14, 14t
intragenic recombination (mosaicism), 1423
intrinsic, 1421–1422
mechanisms, 1413, 1422t, 1423–1429
aminoglycosides, 1422t, 1423–1424, 1474
antiviral agents, 1503t
acyclovir, 1502–1503, 1503t
adefovir dipivoxil, 1508
amantadine, 1503t, 1514
cidofovir, 1503t, 1508
famciclovir, 1503t, 1510
foscarnet, 1503t, 1514
ganciclovir, 1503t, 1510–1511
lamivudine, 1503t, 1512
oseltamivir, 1517
penciclovir, 1503t, 1510
rimantadine, 1503t, 1514
tenofovir, 1513
valacyclovir, 1503t
valganciclovir, 1503t, 1511
vidarabine, 1514
zanamivir, 1517
chloramphenicol, 1422t, 1425
colistin, 1422t, 1425–1426
daptomycin, 1426
isoniazid, 1422t, 1426
β-lactams, 1422t, 1424–1425, 1465
lincosamides (clindamycin), 1473
linezolid, 1422t, 1426, 1475
macrolides, 1422t, 1426–1427
metronidazole, 1422t, 1427, 1478
nitrofurantoin, 1479
quinolones, 1422t, 1427, 1477
quinupristin-dalfopristin, 1475
rifampin, 1422t, 1427–1428, 1476
streptogramins, 1475
tetracyclines, 1422t, 1428, 1472
trimethoprim/sulfamethoxazole, 1422t, 1428
vancomycin, 1422t, 1428–1429, 1469
nasopharyngeal colonization with otopathogens, 217
in *Plasmodium*, 1520

susceptibility testing and see
 Susceptibility testing
see also individual drugs and pathogens
Antimicrobial peptides, in innate immune
 system, 83–84
Antimicrobial proteins (AMPs), 569
Antimicrobial susceptibility, testing *see*
 Susceptibility testing
Antimotility agents
 avoidance
  in hemolytic uremic syndrome, 799
  in shigellosis, 822
 Escherichia coli infections, 798
 see also Antiperistaltic agents
Antimycobacterial therapy *see*
 Antituberculosis agents
Antinuclear antibodies, 1411t–1412t
Antiparasitic agents, 1518–1526
 discontinued production, 1518
 manufacturers, 1518
 treatment of
  eosinophilic meningitis, 333
  fluke infection, 1524–1525
  helminthic infections, 1522–1523
  intestinal nematodes, 1523–1524
  Kinetoplastidae infections,
   1519–1520
  luminal protozoa, 1519
  malaria, 1520–1522
  tapeworm infection, 1524–1525
 see also individual drugs
Antiperistaltic agents
 contraindications, *Clostridium difficile*
  infections, 585
 foodborne/waterborne disease, 398
 gastrointestinal tract infection, 377
 inflammatory enteritis, 387
 see also Antimotility agents
Antiplatelet antibodies, EBV infection, 1062
Antipseudomonal agents, 845
Antipyretic therapy, 91–92
 drugs included, 92
 sepsis management, 99
Antiretroviral therapy, 664–667
 after sexual abuse, 371–372
 HAART *see* Highly active antiretroviral
  therapy (HAART)
 selection of drugs, 667
 side effects, 664, 666
 see also Human immunodeficiency virus
  (HIV)/AIDS
Antistaphylococcal agents, 686–688
 orthopedic device infections, 599
Antistreptococcal antibody titers
 acute rheumatic fever, 704
 GAS pharyngitis diagnosis, 203
Antistreptolysin O (ASO), 699
 groups C and G streptococci, 720
Antithrombin, sepsis management,
 101t–102t
α_1-Antitrypsin deficiency
 acute hepatitis, 403
 chronic hepatitis, 407
Antituberculosis agents, 780t, 781–782
 in cervical lymphadenitis, 146
 chronic meningitis treatment, 286
 dosage, 780t, 1445t–1452t
 follow-up after, 785

rifamycins, 1475–1476
streptomycin, 1474
tuberculous osteomyelitis, 475
tuberculous pericarditis, 271
see also Mycobacterium tuberculosis,
 treatment; *individual drugs*
Antitussives, 198
Antiviral agents, 1502–1518
 bronchiolitis management, 235
 dosage, 1445t–1452t
 history, 1502
 inorganic pyrophosphate analogues as,
  1514–1516
 mechanisms of action, 1502t
 in myocarditis, 268
 neuraminidase inhibitors as, 1516–1518
 nucleoside/nucleotide analogues as,
  1502–1514, 1504t
 pharmacology, 1444–1445, 1444t
 prophylactic therapy, 1507t
 resistance to, 1503t
  see also Antimicrobial drug resistance
 tricyclic amines as, 1514
 see also Antiretroviral therapy; *individual*
  agents
Antrum (mastoid), 222
Anxiety, chronic/recurrent abdominal pain
 due to, 175
Aortic dissection, chest pain, 190t
Aortic valve, endocarditis, 258f
Aortic valve disease, in acute rheumatic
 fever, 703
APECED, 603t–604t, 630t, 631
 Candida infection, 631
 genetic and clinical features, 630t
Apheresis, extracorporeal, 101t–102t
Aphthous stomatitis, 193t
Aphthous ulcers, HIV infection, 662
API Analytab 20C yeast identification
 system, 1382
Apicomplexa, 1255
Aplastic crisis, transient, parvovirus B19
 causing, 1088f, 1089, 1089t, 1091
Apnea
 Bordetella pertussis infection, 868f
 in bronchiolitis, 233
 RSV-related, 233, 1132–1133
APOBEC 3 family of proteins, 1167
Apophysomyces, 1212–1213
Apophysomyces elegans, 1214
Apoptosis, host cells, by *Entamoeba*
 histolytica, 1274
Appendectomy, 422
 interval, 422
 laparoscopic *vs.* open, 422
 postoperative antibiotics, 422
Appendiceal obstruction, abdominal pain
 migration, 171
Appendiceal rupture, 172, 420
Appendicitis, 172, 420–423
 abdominal pain, 171–172
 Actinomyces infection, 991
 acute
  differential diagnosis, 421b
  pelvic inflammatory disease *vs.*,
   365
 Angiostrongylus costaricensis mimicking,
  1338

Balantidium coli infections mimicking,
 1267
clinical manifestations, 420–421, 420t
complicated, 422–423
diagnosis, 420–421
Enterobius vermicularis and, 1332
epidemiology, 420
etiology, 420
imaging, 421
in infants, 172
laboratory studies, 421
left-sided, 172
mesenteric adenitis with/*vs.*, 172–173
mumps orchitis *vs.*, 368–369
pathogenesis, 420
patient position, 172
perforated
 anaerobic gram-negative bacilli
  infections, 984
 intra-abdominal abscess, 422–423
 management, 422
 rate, 420
retrocecal, 351
scoring system (MANTRELS), 421,
 421t
sequence of events, 172, 172b
treatment, 422–423
Appetite, loss, acute abdominal pain with,
 171
"Apple-core" lesions, *Entamoeba histolytica*
 infection, 1276
Aqueous humor, infection *see*
 Endophthalmitis
D-Arabinitol, *Candida* metabolite detection,
 1200
D-Arabinitol/L-arabinitol ratio (DA/LA
 ratio), *Candida* metabolite detection,
 1200
Arachidonic acid, 100
 fever induction mechanism, 91, 91f
 metabolic products, 100
 in sepsis, 100, 101t–102t
Arachidonic acid inhibitor therapy, in sepsis,
 100, 101t–102t
Arachnoid cyst, 291f
Arboviruses
 arthritis due to, 481
 aseptic meningitis due to, 293–295,
  297
 chronic fatigue syndrome pathogenesis,
  1008t–1009t
 diagnosis/detection, 296, 1397
  optimal tests, 1389t–1392t
 encephalitis due to, 302–304
 laboratory testing, 308t–311t
 pathogenesis, 294–295
 transmission, 294–295
Arcanobacterium haemolyticum, 750–751
 coinfections, 751
 pharyngitis due to, 199, 201, 203, 750
 septicemia due to, 751
Arcanobacterium pyogenes, 959t
Archeozoa, 1254–1255, 1254b–1255b,
 1255t
 evolutionary transition, 1255
Arcobacter, 874t
Arenaviridae, 1016t, 1159
 infections, 1017t

Arenaviruses, 1159–1164
  aseptic meningitis due to, 294
  clinical manifestations, 1161–1162
  epidemiology and transmission, 1159, 1160t
  laboratory findings and diagnosis, 1162–1163, 1162t
  New World, 1159–1161, 1160t
  Old World, 1159, 1160t
  pathobiology, 1160–1161
  prevention of infections, 1163–1164
  treatment of infections, 1163
Argentine hemorrhagic fever, 1160t, 1161, 1163–1164
Arginine, metabolism, *Mycoplasma hominis*, 999
Arithmetic mean, 5
Artemether
  Fasciola infections, 1366
  Schistosoma (schistosomiasis) prophylaxis, 1370
Artemether-lumefantrine, *Plasmodium* infections, 1301t–1303t, 1303–1304, 1520
Artemis deficiency, 628t
Artemisinin, *Plasmodium* infections, 1520
Arteriovenous fistula infection, *Rothia dentocariosa*, 768
Artesunate, *Fasciola* infections, 1366
Arthralgia
  mumps virus infection, 1127
  Streptobacillus moniliformis (rat-bite fever), 938–939
  see also Joint, pain
Arthritis, 477–483
  in acute rheumatic fever, 704t
  Aspergillus, 482
  bacterial *see* Arthritis, pyogenic
  Blastomyces dermatitidis, 482
  Borrelia burgdorferi (Lyme disease), 481, 533, 955
  Candida, 482
  Coccidioides immitis (coccidioidomycosis), 482, 1242
  Cryptococcus neoformans, 482
  epidemiology and etiology, 477
  fungal infections, 482
  in Henoch–Schönlein purpura, 173–174
  Histoplasma capsulatum, 482
  infectious *see* Arthritis, pyogenic
  limb pain, 184
  Mycoplasma, 481–482
  Mycoplasma pneumoniae infections, 481–482, 994t, 995
  neonatal, 480
  noninfectious inflammatory, 184
    causes, 184–186
  poststreptococcal reactive (PSRA), 706
  pyogenic (bacterial), 184, 185t, 477–480
    anaerobic gram-negative bacilli, 984
    anaerobic gram-positive cocci, 989
    Bartonella henselae, 477
    bite wound complication, 526
    Brucella causing, 477, 863
    burns patients, 519
    clinical features, 477–478
    Corynebacterium diphtheriae, 756
    diagnosis, 478, 478t

disseminated gonococcal infection, 744
    ESR elevation, 1400–1401
    in group childcare, 27
    Haemophilus influenzae type b (Hib), 477, 902
    hip, 184, 479
      iliopsoas abscess *vs.*, 426
    joints involved, 477–478, 478t
    Kingella kingae, 27, 477, 920
    in Lemierre disease, 209f, 210
    Moraxella, 840
    Neisseria gonorrhoeae, 744
    Neisseria meningitidis, 477
    neonatal, 541
    Pantoea causing, 805
    pathogenesis, 477
    prognosis and sequelae, 480
    Pseudomonas aeruginosa, 477
    sickle-cell disease, 635
    Staphylococcus aureus, 184, 477, 680
    Streptococcus agalactiae (group B streptococcus), 709
    Streptococcus pneumoniae, 477
    Streptococcus pyogenes, 477
    transient synovitis *vs.*, 486
    treatment, 478–480, 479t, 1418t–1419t
  reactive, 184–185, 185t, 482–483
    after foodborne disease, 399
    after *Neisseria meningitidis* infections, 738
    Campylobacter infections, 877
    definition, 482
    etiology, 482b, 483
    Haemophilus influenzae type b (Hib), 902
    polyarticular, 483
    Salmonella gastroenteritis, 816
    Shigella infections, 821
    Streptococcus pyogenes, 483
    Yersinia enterocolitica, 824
    Yersinia pseudotuberculosis, 825
    see also Reiter syndrome
  rheumatoid *see* Rheumatoid arthritis
  rubella vaccination association, 60
  Scedosporium, 482
  septic *see* Arthritis, pyogenic (bacterial)
  Sporothrix schenckii (sporotrichosis), 1219
  tuberculous (*Mycobacterium tuberculosis*), 482
  varicella complication, 1038
  viral, 481
Arthritis–dermatitis syndrome (disseminated gonococcal infection), 349, 744
Arthroconidia, *Coccidioides*, 1239–1240, 1239f
Arthropathy
  acquired rubella complication, 1116
  limb pain, 185t
Arthroscopy, pyogenic arthritis, 479
Arthus-type hypersensitivity
  diphtheria toxoid and, 759
  Mantoux tuberculin skin test, 779
Aryepiglottic folds, edema, 210f
Ascariasis *see* *Ascaris lumbricoides*
Ascaris lumbricoides, 1255, 1256t, 1327–1329

acute pancreatitis due to, 411
  biliary obstruction due to, 412
  chronic infections, 1327–1328
  clinical manifestations, 1327–1328, 1327b
  differential diagnosis, 1328
  eggs, 1327, 1327f
    number, 1256
  eosinophilia due to, 1407, 1408t–1409t
  eosinophilic meningitis due to, 331t
  epidemiology, 1327
  infection route, 1326–1327
  intestinal obstruction due to, 1327–1328, 1328f
  laboratory findings and diagnosis, 1326, 1327f, 1328
  life cycle, 1327
  neonatal infection, 1327, 1327t
  prevention of infections, 1328–1329
  treatment of infection, 1328
Ascites, 638
  liver disease associated, 638
  peritonitis association, 638
  specimen collection/transport, 1374t
Ascitic fluid, composition, 638
Aspartate transaminase (AST), 1411
  elevated
    Ehrlichia and *Anaplasma* causing, 895
    Rickettsia felis infections, 933
    in varicella, 1038
    hepatitis A virus infection, 1183
    HIV infection, 655
Aspergilloma, pulmonary, 1205
Aspergillosis
  allergic bronchopulmonary, 1205, 1408t–1409t
  chronic pulmonary, 1205
Aspergillus, 1203–1209, 1209b
  aflatoxin, 1203
  allergic bronchopulmonary aspergillosis, 1205, 1408t–1409t
  antigens, 1207
  arthritis due to, 482
  aspergilloma due to, 1205
  brain abscess due to, 319, 1204–1205, 1205f
  burn wound infections due to, 518
  cerebral infection, 1204–1205, 1205f
  chronic aspergillosis, 1205
  chronic necrotizing pulmonary aspergillosis, 1205
  clinical manifestations, 1203–1205, 1209b
  CNS infections due to, 1204–1205, 1205f
  in cancer, 579
  colonization process, 1203
  conidia, 1203, 1205
  description and structure, 1203
  diagnosis, 1206–1208, 1209b
    bronchoalveolar lavage, 1207
    culture, 1206
    galactomannan antigen testing, 1207–1208, 1382
    (1,3)-β-D-glucan, 1208
    polymerase chain reaction, 1208
    radiology, 1207
    serologic testing, 1207

disseminated disease, 1204–1205
endocarditis due to, 260t
   management, 263
epidemiology, 1205–1206, 1209b
fungemia, 1206
galactomannan antigen, 563, 1207–
   1208, 1382
(1,3)-β-D-glucan, 1208
growth, 1203
hemorrhage due to, 1207, 1209
host defense mechanisms, 1203
hyphae, 1203–1206
immunocompromised hosts, 1203
infections in heart transplant recipients,
   558
infections in HSCT recipient, 563, 563f
invasive disease
   liver transplant recipients, 557
   treatment, 576
keratitis due to, 496–497
meningitis due to, 282–284, 284t
mortality, 1205–1206, 1209
necrotizing otitis externa, 222
neutropenia associated with cancer, 567,
   571
osteomyelitis due to, 475
otitis externa, 221
pathogenesis of infection, 563
in phagocytic disorders, 620t, 622f
pneumonia due to, 246, 251, 575–576
   diagnosis, 254–255
   transplant-associated, 254
prognosis, 1209
pulmonary infection, 1203–1204, 1204f
   in cancer, 575–576
reproduction (sexual/asexual), 1203
risk factors for infection, 1206
semi-invasive aspergillosis, 1205
sinusitis due to, 577, 1204, 1204f
skin infections, 1205
   in cancer, 574
treatment of infections, 1208–1209,
   1209b
   combination, 1208–1209
   surgical, 1209
whole-genome sequencing, 1203
Aspergillus flavus, 1203
neutropenia associated with cancer, 567,
   571
Aspergillus fumigatus, 1203
allergic bronchopulmonary aspergillosis,
   1205
colonization process, 1203
in cystic fibrosis, 639
necrotizing otitis externa, 222
neutropenia associated with cancer, 567,
   571
virulence, 1203
Aspergillus nidulans, 1203
pulmonary and invasive disease, 1204
Aspergillus niger, 1203
otitis externa due to, 221
Aspergillus terreus, 1203, 1486
adventitious sporulation, 1206
Aspiration
foreign body *see* Foreign body
lung abscess pathogenesis, 243–244
pneumonia pathogenesis, 243–244, 581

Aspiration pneumonia, 243–244, 581
Aspirin
antipyretic action, 92
avoidance, in dengue fever, 1100
Kawasaki disease treatment, 41, 1002,
   1006
low-dose, Kawasaki disease, 1006
Asplenia, 636–637
Babesia infections, 1263, 1265
Capnocytophaga canimorsus infections, 881
congenital, 636
functional, 636–637
infection chemoprophylaxis, 73–74, 74t,
   637
   travelers, 83
infection prevention, 637
infection risk, 73–74
infections associated, 636
isolated congenital, 637
meningitis associated, 273t
pathogenesis of infections, 636–637
Streptococcus pneumoniae infections, 636,
   723
treatment of infections, 637
vaccination in, 74, 83, 637
   meningococcal conjugate vaccine, 65
Association for Professionals in Infection
   Control and Epidemiology (APIC),
   19–20
Association measures and risk, 2t, 5
Asteroid bodies, 162
Sporothrix schenckii, 1219
Asthma
allergic bronchopulmonary aspergillosis,
   1205
bronchiolitis linked to, 235
cough in, 166–167
diagnosis, 252
exacerbations, 199
   Chlamydophila (Chlamydia)
     pneumoniae, 882
   human metapneumovirus (hMPV),
     1137
   Mycoplasma pneumoniae infection, 994
   prevention by influenza vaccination,
     1156–1157
human parainfluenza viruses (HPIVs)
   and, 1123
pneumonia linked to, 239, 248–251,
   249f
   persistent/recurrent pneumonia,
     248–251
RSV infection and, 1133
Asthma-like condition, visceral larva
   migrans, 1336
Astrakhan spotted fever, 923t
Astroviridae, 1016t, 1190
infections, 1017t
Astroviruses, 378, 1190–1191
clinical manifestations, 1191
description and structure, 378, 379f,
   1190, 1190f
diagnosis/detection, 381, 1191, 1395
   optimal tests, 1389t–1392t
epidemiology, 379–380, 380t, 1190–1191
gastroenteritis due to, 378, 1190–1191
   clinical features, 380t
   diarrhea, 26t

healthcare-associated infections, 584
infections in group childcare, 25t
prevention, 1191
serotypes, 378, 1190
shedding, 380
transmission, 380, 1191
treatment, 1191
Ataxia, 180
causes, 180
cerebellar, 316
chronic, 180
differential diagnosis, 180, 180t
history and physical examination, 180
Ataxia telangiectasia, 603t–604t, 629–631,
   630t
genetic and clinical features, 629–631,
   630t
immunizations in, 52t–53t
Atazanavir, 665t, 1444t–1452t
Atelectasis, 234f
in bronchiolitis, 233, 234f
in infant botulism, 976
persistent pneumonia and, 246–247
Atherosclerotic heart disease, *Chlamydophila*
   (Chlamydia) pneumoniae and, 882
Athlete's foot (tinea pedis), 1247–1248
ATM gene, 629–631
Atopic dermatitis, 83
tinea capitis *vs.*, 1247
Atopobium vaginae, bacterial vaginosis, 358
Atopy, respiratory syncytial virus infection
   and, 1133
Atovaquone
Babesia (babesiosis), 1265
Plasmodium (malaria), 1521–1522
Pneumocystis jirovecii infection, 1232t,
   1233
Toxoplasma gondii infections, 1314–1315,
   1316t, 1317
Atovaquone-proguanil
adverse effects, 1304
Plasmodium infections, 1301t–1303t,
   1303–1304
prophylaxis, 80–81, 1304, 1305t
Attack rates (AR), 1
Attapulgite, diarrhea, 377t
Attributable risk, 5
Aural lavage, otitis externa management,
   221
Aural toilet, chronic mastoiditis
   management, 227
Auralgan, in acute otitis media, 218
Auscultation, musculoskeletal pain, 183
Australia antigen *see* Hepatitis B virus
   (HBV), HBsAg (surface antigen)
Autism, MMR vaccine and, 51
Autoantibodies, in EBV infection, 1062
Autoimmune disorders
acute hepatitis, 403
chronic active hepatitis, HAV, 1183
chronic hepatitis, 406
fever of unknown origin due to, 124
generalized lymphadenopathy, 134
Autoimmune lymphoproliferative syndrome
   (ALPS), 603t–604t
Autoimmune polyendocrinopathy–
   candidiasis–ectodermal dysplasia *see*
   APECED

Autoimmune regulator (AIRE) gene, 630t, 631
Autoimmunity
    acute rheumatic fever pathogenesis, 703
    in PANDAS, 706
Autoinflammatory disorders, generalized lymphadenopathy, 134
Autoinflammatory syndrome, 124
    see also Hereditary periodic fever syndromes
Autolysin, from coagulase-negative staphylococci, 690–691
Autonomic dysfunction
    congenital varicella, 1038
    infant botulism, 973
Autonomic pathway, in fever, 91
Autosensitization, 453–454, 454b
Autosomal agammaglobulinemia, 611, 611t
Autosomal SCID, 603t–604t
Avian influenza (H5N1 strain), 82, 1158
    clinical features and management, 1158
    diagnosis, 1394
    inflammatory response and TLR4, 92–93
    myocarditis due to, 265–266
    pneumonia due to, 236–237
    transmission, 1158
    travelers and, 82
Avian pneumovirus, 1134
Avoidant behavior, chronic fatigue syndrome, 1012
Axillary lymph nodes, palpable in normal children, 158
Axillary lymphadenopathy, 158t, 159–160
    Bartonella henselae infection, 858f–859f
Axonal loss, rabies, 1145
Azalides
    distribution, 1417
    dosage, 1480t–1483t
    pharmacodynamic properties, 1414t
    pharmacology, 1453t–1458t
    spectrum of activity, 1459t–1463t
Azathioprine, in myocarditis, 268
Azidothymidine (AZT) see Zidovudine
Azithromycin, 1471–1472
    chemoprophylactic use, 70t–71t, 71–72
        meningococcal meningitis, 279
    clinical uses, 1471
    in cystic fibrosis, 640
    distribution, 1417
    dosage, 1445t–1452t, 1480t–1483t
    pelvic inflammatory disease, 357
    pharmacology, 1453t–1458t, 1471
    spectrum of activity, 1459t–1463t, 1471
    structure, 1470
    treatment of, 860
        acute bacterial cystitis, 356
        acute bacterial sinusitis, 229t
        acute otitis media, 216–217
        Babesia (babesiosis), 1265
        Bartonella henselae infections, 860
        bite wound infections, 521–522, 526
        Bordetella pertussis infections, 871
        Campylobacter infections, 877–878
        Chlamydia conjunctivitis, 488
        Chlamydia trachomatis infections, 888t
        Chlamydophila pneumoniae, 883
        Haemophilus ducreyi (chancroid), 907
        Klebsiella granulomatis infection, 803

Legionella infections, 924, 925t
Mycoplasma genitalium, 356
Mycoplasma pneumoniae infections, 996–997
Naegleria fowleri (naegleriasis), 1295
Neisseria gonorrhoeae infections, 746–747
nontuberculous mycobacterial infection, 792
Rhodococcus equi infections, 769
Rickettsia infections, 938
Shigella infections, 822, 822t
travelers' diarrhea, 82
Ureaplasma urealyticum infections, 1002
urethritis, 356
vulvovaginitis, 358
Azole antifungal agents, 1194
    Blastomyces dermatitidis (blastomycosis), 1237–1238, 1238t
    Histoplasma capsulatum (histoplasmosis), 1228t, 1229
    infections in HSCT recipients, 565
    infections in neutropenia in cancer, 571
    as topical antifungal agents, 1485, 1485t
    treatment of systemic infections, 1488–1491
    see also Fluconazole; Itraconazole; Ketoconazole; Miconazole
AZT see Zidovudine (AZT)
Aztreonam
    clinical use, 1468
    in cystic fibrosis, 640
    dosage, 1480t–1483t
    dose adjustment in burned patients, 1437t
    eye infection treatment, 1496t
    pharmacology, 1453t–1458t
    spectrum of activity, 1459t–1463t, 1468

B

B cells see B lymphocytes
B-lymphocyte linker protein (BLNK), 611
B lymphocytes, 87, 92
    activation, 89, 609
        by EBV, 1059, 1062–1063
        visceral leishmaniasis, 1287
    antibody synthesis, 609
    CD19+, deficiency, 610
    chronic fatigue syndrome, 1010t
    in common variable immunoglobulin deficiency, 612
    defective, hyper-IgM syndrome, 631–632
    deficiency, 612
        immunizations in, 52t–53t
        pneumonia, 252–253, 253t
        SCID see Severe combined immunodeficiency (SCID)
    development, 87, 88f, 89, 609
    EBV infection, 1060
    fetal, 89
    function, 89
    hemophagocytic lymphohistiocytosis, 106
    in HIV infection, 649b, 658
    Ig isotype expression, 609

immortalization and activation, by EBV, 1059–1060, 1062–1063
    in immune response, 45
    lymphoblastoid transformation, 1062
    memory, EBV persistence, 1060
    posttransplant lymphoproliferative disease (PTLD), 1063
    signaling, 89
        via CD40, 612–613
    surface markers, 87
    T cell interaction, 626–627
    X-linked lymphoproliferative syndrome, 1064
B virus see Herpes B virus (herpes simiae)
BabA, Helicobacter pylori expressing, 908–909
Babesia (babesiosis), 1261–1265, 1265b
    Borrelia burgdorferi infection with, 1261–1263
    clinical manifestations, 1263, 1263t
    description, 1261–1262, 1265b
    diagnosis, 1384
    epidemiology, 532t, 1262–1263, 1262f, 1265b
    hemolysis and anemia due to, 1263
    immunocompromised hosts, 1261, 1263, 1265
    laboratory findings and diagnosis, 533t–534t, 1263–1265, 1264f, 1264t, 1265b
    Plasmodium infections vs., 1264t
    prevention of infection, 1265
    treatment, 535
    treatment of infections, 1265, 1265b, 1521–1522
    vectors, 532t
Babesia divergens, 1261–1263, 1265
Babesia duncani, 1261, 1263
Babesia microti, 1261
    in asplenia, 636
    clinical manifestations, 1263, 1263t
    epidemiology, 1262–1263
    immunocompromised hosts, 1265
    laboratory findings and diagnosis, 1263, 1263t–1264t
Babesia MO1, 1261
Babesia venatorum, 1261, 1263
Babesia WA1, 1261
Babesiidae, 1261
BabyBIG, 975
Bacillary angiomatosis see Bartonella henselae; Bartonella quintana
Bacillary dysentery see Shigella dysenteriae type 1
Bacillary peliosis see Bartonella henselae; Bartonella quintana
Bacille Calmette-Guérin (BCG) vaccine see Calmette-Guérin bacillus (BCG) vaccine
Bacilli, 673
    anaerobic gram-negative see Anaerobic gram-negative bacilli (AGNB)
    anaerobic gram-positive nonsporulating, 990–992
    see also Actinomyces
    gram-negative see Gram-negative bacilli
    gram-positive see Gram-positive bacilli
Bacillus, 751–754

Bacillus alvei, 754
Bacillus anthracis (anthrax), 752–753
  as biological weapon, 751–753
    diagnosis, isolation and treatment, 753
  cutaneous anthrax, 432, 433f, 751–752
    cowpox *vs.*, 1024
    management, 753
    Rickettsia akari (rickettsialpox) infection *vs.*, 934
  eyelid cellulitis due to, 509
  gastrointestinal disease, 752
  inhalational anthrax, 752–753
  pharyngeal anthrax, 752
  postexposure prophylaxis, 753
  septicemia and meningitis due to, 752
  vaccines, 753
Bacillus brevis, 754
Bacillus cereus, 753–754
  endophthalmitis due to, 503–504, 754
  food poisoning, 393–395, 394t, 398t, 753
    "emetic syndrome", 395
  group childcare and, 25
  ophthalmitis due to, 754
  toxins, 375, 393–394, 394t, 753
Bacillus circulans, 754
Bacillus coagulans, 754
Bacillus fusiformis, 194
Bacillus laterosporus, 754
Bacillus licheniformis, 754
Bacillus macerans, 754
Bacillus pumilus, 754
Bacillus sphaericus, 754
Bacillus subtilis, 754
Bacillus thuringiensis, 754
Bacitracin
  resistance, groups C and G streptococci, 720
  treatment of
    burns, 1500t–1501t
    Clostridium difficile infections, 979b
    eye infections, 1494t–1496t
    skin infections, 1498t
    staphylococcal blepharitis, 493–494
Bacitracin disk test, GAS pharyngitis diagnosis, 203
Bacitracin-polymyxin, acute conjunctivitis treatment, 492–493
Back pain, 187–188, 187b, 188t
  causes, 187b
    infectious, 187–188, 187b
    noninfectious, 184b, 188
  diskitis, 484
BacT/Alert system, 1374
BACTEC system, 1374, 1381
Bacteremia
  anaerobic gram-negative bacilli (AGNB), 984
  Bacillus cereus infections, 754
  Bartonella henselae, 857
  Borrelia infections, 957
  Brevundimonas vesicularis, 833
  burns patients, 519
  Campylobacter, 874t, 876
  cancer patients, 574
  Candida, 553
  Capnocytophaga, 880

catheter-related
  in cancer, 574
  Staphylococcus epidermidis causing, 563, 692
  causes in very young infants, 114t
  Clostridium perfringens, 980t
  coagulase-negative staphylococci, 553–554
  Corynebacterium, 760t–761t
  Corynebacterium jeikeium, 762
  detection, quantitation, 1373–1374
  endocarditis pathogenesis, 258, 260
  Enterobacter, 805
  Enterobacteriaceae, 554
  Gardnerella vaginalis, 769
  Haemophilus influenzae, 902–903
  Helicobacter infections, 918
  indwelling central venous catheter causing, 257
  Kingella kingae, 921
  Listeria monocytogenes, 763, 765
  meningitis pathogenesis, 273
  Mycobacterium tuberculosis, 776
  neonatal, 541
  neutropenia in cancer, 567
  "occult", 723
  occult pneumococcal, 115
  persistent
    causes, 259–260
    neonatal, 554
  in pneumonia, 235–236
  prosthetic valve infections, 595
  rate associated with various procedures, 258t
  rate for various procedures, 258
  rates, after various procedures, 258t
  rates in children with fever, 114–115
  renal abscess complication, 344
  risk in children with fever, 115
  Staphylococcus aureus, 554
  Streptococcus agalactiae (group B streptococcus), 708, 710t
  Streptococcus pneumoniae, 4f, 115, 721, 723
  treatment, 1418t–1419t
  viridans group streptococci, 717–718
  see also Bloodstream infections (BSIs); Septicemia
Bacteria
  adherence, biofilm formation, 690–691, 690f
  attachment, urinary tract, 339
  cell wall, 673f
    structure, 673, 1466f
    synthesis, 1464, 1464f
    synthesis inhibitors, 1441f, 1459t–1463t, 1464, 1464f
  cell wall-deficient, blood cultures, 1374–1375
  classification, 673–675
  colonization by *see* Colonization; *individual bacteria*
  fastidious, antimicrobial susceptibility testing, 1381
  genome, 674
  genome sequencing, 675
  identification
    by molecular techniques, 674–675

    by phenotypic characteristics, 673–674
  nonspore-forming, 690
    see also Staphylococcus (staphylococci)
  normal flora *see* Flora, normal
  obligate intracellular, 673
  outer membrane, 673
  phylogenetic tree, 674f
  ribosomes, 1470
  species, 673
  synergism, 460
  translocation, burn wounds, 518
Bacterial infections
  elevated C-reactive protein (CRP), 1402
  fever of unknown origin, 119t–120t
  group childcare and, 25t, 28
  invasive, group childcare setting, 28
  laboratory diagnosis *see* Laboratory diagnosis
  lymphadenopathy *see* Lymphadenitis/ lymphadenopathy
  necrotizing enterocolitis pathogenesis, 388
  neonatal *see* Neonatal infections
  in neutropenia associated with cancer, 567, 569t
  neutrophil response, 1404
  viral infections differentiation, ocular features, 108–110
  see also individual infections
Bacterial overgrowth, 391
  burns and, 518
  diagnosis and treatment, 391
  toxigenic *Clostridium difficile*, 382
Bacterial vaginosis (BV), 358
  cervicitis and, 361
  clinical features, 354, 359t
  complications, 361
  diagnosis, 355f, 359–360, 359t
  etiology/causative agents, 358
  Gardnerella vaginalis, 769
  HIV and, 359, 361
  outcome and complications, 361
  pelvic inflammatory disease, 361, 364
  recurrence, treatment, 358
  risk factors, 358
  treatment, 360
Bactericidal/permeability-increasing protein (BPI), 85
  recombinant (rBPI₂₁), 101t–102t
    in meningococcal disease, 737
Bacteriocins, *Streptococcus pyogenes* (group A streptococcus), 698
Bacteriophage
  lysogenic, *Corynebacterium diphtheriae*, 754
  role in *Streptococcus pyogenes*, 698
Bacteriuria
  covert/asymptomatic, 342
  pathogenesis, 339
  risk factors, 339–340
Bacteroidaceae, 959
  classification, 959t
Bacteroides, 982–985
  anaerobic cellulitis due to, 461
  antimicrobial resistance
    metronidazole, 1422t, 1427
    trimethoprim/sulfamethoxazole, 1428

bacterial vaginosis due to, 358
Clostridium botulinum inhibition, 971
CNS infections, 983
culture media, 1376t
diagnosis/detection, 963–964
female genital tract infections, 984
head and neck infections, 983
intra-abdominal infections, 984
necrotizing fasciitis due to, 459–460
neutropenia associated with cancer, 567
normal flora, 959
osteomyelitis due to, 984
pathophysiology, 983
peritonsillar abscess, 205–206
pleuropulmonary infections, 983–984
prevention of infections, 985
pyogenic arthritis due to, 984
secondary peritonitis due to, 416–417
skin/soft tissue infections, 984
subcutaneous abscess due to, 456
treatment of infections, 985
virulence factors, 983
Bacteroides corrodens (Bacteroides ureolyticus), 835
Bacteroides distasonis, 982
Bacteroides forsythus, 982
Bacteroides fragilis, 962
abscess due to, 962
antibiotic susceptibility, 966t
appendicitis due to, 420
endotoxin, 962
normal flora, 959
oxygen sensitivity, 959
surgical site infection, prevention, 587
T lymphocyte-mediated response, 961
Bacteroides fragilis group, 982
penicillin resistance, 982
Bacteroides gracilis, 982
Bacteroides melaninogenicus, 959
Bacteroides melaninogenicus group, 982
Bacteroides ovatus, 982
Bacteroides thetaiotaomicron, 982
Bacteroides ureolyticus (Bacteroides corrodens), 835, 982
Bacteroides vulgatus, 982
Bactibilia, 412
Baerman technique, 1383
BAFF receptor deficiency, characteristics, 602t
Bairnsdale ulcer, 788
Baker cyst, in Lyme disease, 954f, 955
Balamuthia mandrillaris, 1294
encephalitis due to, 303–304, 307, 307f
laboratory testing, 308t–311t
Balance disturbances, after acute bacterial meningitis, 278
Balanitis, *Gardnerella vaginalis*, 769–770
Balanoposthitis, *Candida*, 351–352
Balantidium coli (balantidiasis), 1266–1268
clinical manifestations, 1267, 1267f
description and structure, 1266, 1267f
diagnosis/detection, 385t, 1267
life cycle, 1266, 1266f
prevention of infection, 1268
treatment, 1267–1268
water contamination, 384
Ballooning degeneration, HSV infection, 1027

Bare lymphocyte syndrome, 603t–604t
Barmah Forest virus, 1098
arthritis, 481
Bartonella, 856–861, 940
blood cultures, 1375
clinical manifestations, 857–859, 858f–859f
epidemiology, 857
laboratory findings/diagnosis, 857
microbiology, 857
species, 940
treatment of infections, 860
Bartonella bacilliformis, 856, 940
epidemiology, 857
generalized lymphadenopathy, 130, 131t–132t
optic neuritis, 316
Oroya fever, 130
Bartonella henselae, 856–861
abdominal computed tomography in, 858f–859f
abdominal lymphadenopathy due to, 156
after cat bites, 523
antimicrobial susceptibility, 860
arthritis due to, 477
axillary lymphadenopathy due to, 159–160, 858f–859f
bacillary angiomatosis, 857–858, 860
bacillary peliosis, 857–860
bacteremia, 857
cat-scratch disease, 140–141, 857, 858f–859f
abdominal lymphadenopathy, 156
adenitis, 159f
adenitis, diagnosis, 160
clinical manifestations, 119t–120t, 857–859
complications, 860
diagnosis, 859–860
eosinophilia, 1408t–1409t
generalized lymphadenopathy, 130, 131t–132t
management, 146, 147t
prevention, 860–861
systemic, 857
treatment, 860
unilateral cervical lymphadenitis, 139t, 140–141
cervical lymphadenitis due to, 135t
management, 146, 147t
subacute unilateral, 139t, 140–141
chronic fatigue syndrome pathogenesis, 1008t–1009t
clinical manifestations, 119t–120t, 857–859
complications and sequelae, 860
detection, 860
encephalopathy due to, 179–180, 303, 313, 860
endocarditis due to, 260t
epidemiology, 857
erythema nodosum due to, 858f–859f
fever of unknown origin due to, 119t–120t
granulomatous conjunctivitis, 159f, 858f–859f

histologic specimen of neck mass due to, 858f–859f
histology of infections, 860
iliac/femoral lymphadenitis due to, 160
inguinal adenopathy without genital ulcers, 351, 352t
laboratory findings/diagnosis, 160–161, 857
laboratory testing, 308t–311t
lymphadenitis due to, 130
localized, 159
lymphadenopathy due to, 156, 159, 858f–859f
facial/anterior cervical, 159f
generalized, 130, 131t–132t
preauricular, 159, 159f, 858f–859f
management, 160
mediastinal lymphadenopathy, 153
osteomyelitis due to, 469
outbreaks and seasonality, 857
papular lesions due to, 858f–859f
Parinaud oculoglandular syndrome due to, 129, 138, 138b, 140–141, 159, 857
organisms associated, 138b, 140–141, 159
preauricular node involvement, 159
prevention of infection, 860–861
prognosis, 860
superficial necrotizing mass in neck due to, 858f–859f
Bartonella quintana, 856
bacillary angiomatosis, 857–858, 860
bacillary peliosis, 857–860
endocarditis due to, 260t
epidemiology, 857
genome size, 674
laboratory findings/diagnosis, 859–860
treatment of infections, 860
Bartonellaceae, 940
Bartonellosis *see Bartonella bacilliformis*
Basal cell(s), HPV infection, 1071
Basal ganglia, calcification, in HIV infection, 654f
Basement membrane, skin, 438
Basidiobolus, 1212–1213
Basilar artery migraine, 180, 180t
Basilar skull fracture, pathogens and infection prophylaxis, 512t, 515
Basophilia, 1409
Basophils, 619, 1409
Bat bites, rabies and, 303f
Bath toys, contaminated, 13
Bauer–Kirby test, 1416
Baylisascaris procyonis, 1335–1337
antibodies and enzyme immunoassay, 1336
CNS migration, 332
encephalitis, 304, 307, 307f
eosinophilia due to, 1408t–1409t
eosinophilic meningitis due to, 330, 331t, 332–333, 1336
management, 333
epidemiology, 1336
laboratory testing, 308t–311t
larvae, 1336, 1336f
meningitis due to, 280t, 283t

ocular larva migrans due to, 1335–1336
retinitis due to, 502
BC-selective agar, 1375t
BCG vaccine *see* Calmette-Guérin bacillus (BCG) vaccine
Beau lines, 1003
Beck triad, 270
Bednets
    Leishmania control, 1290
    Plasmodium infection prevention, 1304–1306
Behavior, recurrent abdominal pain associated, 175
Behavioral problems, after acute bacterial meningitis, 278–279
Behçet syndrome
    clinical features, 108, 111
    oral mucosal features, 193t
    uveitis, 110–111
Bejel (*Treponema pallidum* subsp. *endemicum*), 941
Bell palsy, 315–316
    see also Facial nerve palsy
Benign paroxysmal vertigo, 180t
Benzalkonium chloride, skin antiseptic, 1499t
Benzathine penicillin G *see* Penicillin G, benzathine
Benzethonium chloride, skin antiseptic, 1499t
Benzimidazoles
    Angiostrongylus infections, 1338
    Ascaris lumbricoides infections, 1328
    Enterobius vermicularis infections, 1332
    hookworm infections, 1330
    hydatid cysts (*Echinococcus granulosus*), 1359–1360
    intestinal nematode infections, 1326–1327
    Toxocara infections, 1337
    Trichuris trichiura infections, 1331
    see also Albendazole; Mebendazole; Thiabendazole
Benznidazole
    side effects, 1325
    Trypanosoma cruzi infections, 1325
Benzoyl peroxide, skin antiseptic, 1499t
Benzyl alcohol, pediculosis treatment, 1258–1259
Benzyl benzoate, scabies treatment, 1260
Benzylpenicillin sodium *see* Penicillin G
Bergeyella, 834
Bergeyella zoohelcum (*Weeksella zoohelcum*), 832
    animal bites, 521
Beryllium exposure, generalized lymphadenopathy, 135
β-adrenergic agents
    bronchiolitis management, 234
    RSV infection, 1133
Beta-lactam antibiotics *see* β-Lactam antibiotics (*under lactam*)
Betaherpesvirinae, 1026t, 1044, 1052, 1057
Bethesda system, 1071–1072, 1072t
Bezold abscess, 223, 225
Bias, 4, 9
    affecting validity of study, 4
    diagnostic, 4

estimation of exposure, 5
impact, 4–5
minimization, 9
potential sources, 4
selection for case-control studies, 5
sources, 5b
types, 4
Bifidobacterium, 991–992
    chronic otitis media, 991–992
    classification, 959t
    normal flora, 959
Bifidobacterium bifidum, infant formula supplemented with, 961
Bifidobacterium breve, nosocomial infection prevention, 555
Bifidobacterium infantis, in probiotic, necrotizing enterocolitis reduction, 961
Bile, 412
    culture, 413
    stagnant, superinfection, 412
Bile acid metabolism disorders, 404
Bile ducts
    Fasciola infections, 1366
    inflammation *see* Cholangitis
Bilharzia *see Schistosoma* (schistosomiasis)
Biliary atresia, 402–403, 413–414
    Kasai procedure, 412–413
Biliary colic, site and radiation of pain, 171
Biliary drainage
    impairment, 412
    surgical, 413
Biliary dyskinesia, acute abdominal pain, 173
Biliary obstruction, 412
Biliary sepsis, 413
Biliary stones, 412
    sickle-cell disease, 414
Biliary tract disease
    Cryptosporidium infections, 1270
    intra-abdominal abscess, 424
Bilirubin
    CMV infection, 1046–1047
    displacement by antibiotics, 1439, 1439t
    intra-abdominal abscess, 424
Bilophila wadsworthia, 962
Bioavailability, antibiotics, 1434
    oral, 1453t–1458t
Biofilm, 191, 690, 690f
    Candida, 1200, 1202
    device-related infections, 588
    formation by coagulase-negative staphylococci, 690, 690f
    bacterial adherence, 690
    intravascular catheter placement duration and, 590
    otitis media with effusion, 220
    Pseudomonas aeruginosa, 639, 843
    ventilator-associated pneumonia, 581–582
Biopsy
    abdominal lymph nodes, 157
    brain *see* Brain biopsy
    cervical lymph nodes *see* Cervical lymph nodes
    duodenal, *Giardia intestinalis*, 1282
    endomyocardial, 267
    gastric, *Helicobacter pylori*, 913–914

intestinal, 386
liver, HCV infection, 1110
lung *see* Lung, biopsy
lymph nodes *see* Lymph nodes, biopsy
mediastinal, 151
pericardial, tuberculosis, 776
rectal, *Schistosoma* infections, 1369–1370
renal, poststreptococcal acute glomerulonephritis, 705
skin *see* Skin, biopsy
small bowel, *Cyclospora* or *Cystoisospora*, 1284
supraclavicular lymph nodes, 151
tissue specimen collection/transport, bacterial infections, 1374t, 1383–1384
Bioterrorism, biological agents used, 751–752
Bunyaviridae, 1102
Biotin-dependent multiple carboxylase deficiency, 603t–604t
Bioweapons
    exposure management in pregnant healthcare worker, 22t–23t
    see also Bioterrorism
Bipolaris, 1211–1212
Birds
    avian influenza, 1158
    see also Avian influenza (H5N1 strain)
    Campylobacter transmission, 875
    Toxocara egg dispersal, 1337
Birth history, recurrent infections, 606–607
Birthweight
    categories, central line associated bloodstream infections (CLABSIs), 12t
    necrotizing enterocolitis association, 388
    Streptococcus agalactiae (group B streptococcus) infections and, 708
    see also Low-birthweight infants; Very low birthweight infants
Bismuth subsalicylate
    diarrhea treatment, 377t
    inflammatory enteritis treatment, 387
Bites, infections after, 521–526
    bat bites, 523
    cat bites, 521, 522t
        clinical features, 523f
        epidemiology, 523
        infections transmitted by, 523
        Pasteurella multocida infections, 521
        pathogenesis, 523
        pathogens causing infections, 521, 523
        rabies prevention, 1148
    causative agents, 514, 521–523, 522t, 529
    chemoprophylaxis, 73, 525–526
        indications, 525b
    clinical features and differential diagnosis, 523–524
    complications, 526
    dog bites, 521, 527
        anatomic sites, 523
        Capnocytophaga canimorsus infection, 881
        epidemiology, 522
        fatalities, 523

management, 525
Pasteurella canis infections, 521
pathogenesis, 523
pathogens causing infections, 521, 522t, 523
prevention, 526
rabies, 525
rabies prevention, 1148
Eikenella corrodens infections, 521, 523, 836
epidemiology, 521–523
fatalities, 523
hepatitis B virus transmission, 29
history and physical examination, 524b
HIV transmission, 29
horse bites, 521–522
human bites, 521
   anaerobic gram-negative bacilli infections, 984
   clinical features, 523–524
   epidemiology, 523
   infections transmitted by, 522t, 523
   infectious agents, 521, 522t
   postexposure prophylaxis, 525
incidence/prevalence, 521, 529
infection rates by site, 523t
insect *see* Insect bites
laboratory findings and diagnosis, 524
management, 513t, 524–526
   empiric, 525b, 526
   immediate postexposure, 524–526
   postexposure prophylaxis, 525–526, 525b
   presumptive therapy, 524–526
   wound closure, 524–525
   wound debridement, 524
Pasteurella multocida infections, 521, 523, 836, 837f
   prevention and management, 838
pathogenesis, 523
pathogens causing infections, 514, 521–523, 522t, 529
pig, bites, 521–522
precautions for travelers, 76
prevention, 526
prognosis and sequelae, 526
puncture wounds, 523–524
rat bites, 521–523
   Spirillum minus infections, 958
risk of infections, 513t
self-inflicted bites, 523
septicemia after, 523
simian, 521–522
sites, 523–524, 523t
snake bites, 521–522
wound infections, 521, 523
Bithionol, 1525
Fasciola infections, 1366
Paragonimus infections, 1367
BK virus (BKV), 1075–1076
chronic fatigue syndrome pathogenesis, 1008t–1009t
cystitis due to, 339
diagnosis, 1076
disseminated disease, 1075–1076
epidemiology, 1075
hemorrhagic cystitis in HSCT recipients, 1076

nephritis in HSCT recipients, 1076
nephritis in renal transplant patients, 1076
primary infection, 1075
reactivation, 1076
transmission, 1075
treatment of infections, 1076
viruria, 1076
Black Death *see Yersinia pestis* (plague)
Black fever *see Leishmania* (leishmaniasis), visceral
Black piedra, 1250
Blackflies (*Simulium*), 1344
Blackwater fever, 1299–1300
Bladder
calcification, *Schistosoma* infections, 1369–1370
paralysis, poliovirus causing, 1170
Schistosoma infections, 1369
Blastocystis hominis, 1268–1269
diagnosis, 1268–1269, 1269f
treatment and prevention, 1269
Blastomyces dermatitidis (blastomycosis), 1194, 1234–1238
antigens, cross-reactivity, 1237
antigenuria, 1237
arthritis due to, 482
clinical manifestations, 1234f, 1235–1236
CNS infections, 1234, 1236–1238, 1238t
culture, 1236–1237
cutaneous infection, 1234f, 1236, 1236f, 1236t
description and structure, 1234, 1234f
encephalitis, 303
epidemiology, 1235, 1235f
extrapulmonary infection, 1234, 1236, 1236t
genitourinary tract infections, 1234, 1236t
in HIV infection, 1238
immune response to, 1234
immunosuppressed hosts, 1236, 1238, 1238t
laboratory findings and diagnosis, 1236–1237, 1382
laboratory testing, 308t–311t
meningitis, 280t, 282–283, 283t–284t
mortality, 1237–1238
osseous infections, 1236, 1236f, 1236t
pathogenesis, 1234–1235
persistent pneumonia due to, 246
pneumonia due to *see* Pneumonia
in pregnancy, 1238, 1238t
prevention, 1238
pulmonary infection, 1234–1236, 1234f
   acute, 1234f–1235f, 1235
   chronic, 1235
   treatment, 1237–1238, 1238t
transmission, 1235
treatment of infections, 1237–1238
   recommendations, 1237–1238, 1238t
vaccine development, 1238
virulence, 1234
WI-1 (BAD1) protein, 1234
Blepharitis, 493, 1493
angular, 494
anterior and posterior types, 493

staphylococcal, 493–494
ulcerative, 494
Blindness
infective keratitis causing, 494
ocular larva migrans, 1336
Onchocerca volvulus causing, 1344–1345
trachoma causing, 494
Blisters *see* Bullae; Vesicles
BLNK deficiency, 602t
Blood
donation *see* Blood transfusions
specimen collection, 1373–1374
   see also Blood cultures
viral infection specimens, 1385
Blood agar cultures, pharyngitis, 202
Blood counts
persistent/recurrent pneumonia, 251
in refugee and internationally adopted children, 36
see also White blood cell (WBC) count
Blood cultures
acute bacterial meningitis diagnosis, 275
Aspergillus, 1206
bacterial infections, 1373–1376
   blood to broth ratio, 1373–1374
   "conventional" systems, 1373–1374
   incubation time, 1374
   media for, 1374, 1374t
   specific pathogens, 1374–1376
   specimen collection/processing, 1373–1374
   specimen transport, 1374t
   volume of specimen, 1373–1374, 1376t
Candida infections, 1200
CLABSI, 590–591
   blood volume, 591
   positive predictive value (PPV), 590–591
   sensitivity, 591
   timing of cultures, 591
coagulase-negative staphylococci, 692
computer-assisted automatic, 542
contaminants, coagulase-negative staphylococci, 692
CVC-associated bloodstream infection, 590–591
diskitis, 483, 483t
endocarditis, 257, 260–261, 260t
endophthalmitis, 504–505
Fusarium, 1210
infections in neutropenia with cancer, 570
Malassezia, 1217
Mycoplasma hominis, 999
necrotizing enterocolitis, 390
Neisseria meningitidis, 736
neonatal infections, 537
neonatal nosocomial infection, 549–550
neonatal septicemia diagnosis, 542
Nocardia, 794
pneumococcal infections, 723
prosthetic valves/patches infections, 595
pyogenic arthritis, 478
quantitative, coagulase-negative staphylococci detection, 692
Salmonella, 817
septic thrombophlebitis, 265

Staphylococcus aureus, 684
Streptococcus agalactiae (group B
    streptococcus), 709
Trypanosoma cruzi infections, 1325
vertebral osteomyelitis, 474
Yersinia pestis, 827
Blood dyscrasias, petechiae and, 443
Blood flow, turbulent, endocarditis
    pathogenesis, 258
Blood flukes *see* Schistosoma
Blood groups
    O blood group
        cholera severity and, 850
        norovirus infection susceptibility,
            1187
    P antigen, 1088
    P1 blood group, urinary tract infection
        association, 339
    urinary tract infection association, 339
Blood pressure, sepsis, 99
Blood products
    contamination rate, 580
    infections associated, 580–581
        clinical manifestations, 581
        epidemiology and pathogenesis,
            580–581
        etiology, 580–581, 581t
        management, 581
        prevention, 581
    see also Blood transfusions
Blood smears/films, 1384
    detection of
        Babesia, 1263–1265, 1264f
        Plasmodium, 1300, 1384
        Trypanosoma (*Trypanozoon*) *brucei*,
            1320f, 1321–1322, 1384
        Trypanosoma cruzi, 1325
        Wuchereria bancrofti, 1343, 1343f
Blood-to-broth ratio, 591
Blood transfusions
    Babesia divergens infections, 1265
    CMV infection *see* Cytomegalovirus
        (CMV)
    contamination rate, 580
    donation contraindication, 581
    donor screening, 580–581
    exchange, *Plasmodium* infections, 1303
    HBV transmission, 1078
    HCV transmission, 1107–1108
    HIV transmission, 642–643
    infections associated, 580–581
        clinical manifestations, 581
        epidemiology and pathogenesis,
            580–581
        etiology, 580–581, 581t
        management, 581
        prevention, 581
        skin contamination causing, 581
    leukocytes, 623
    mortality and complications, 581
    parvovirus B19 transmission, 1089
    Trypanosoma cruzi transmission,
        1322–1325
    vCJD transmission link, 337
    West Nile virus transmission, 1101
    see also Blood products; Bloodborne viral
        pathogens
Blood trematodes *see* Schistosoma

Bloodborne viral pathogens
    group childcare setting, 29
    hepatitis A virus, 1180
    HTLV-1 and HTLV-2, 1165
    see also Blood transfusions; Hepatitis B
        virus (HBV); Hepatitis C virus (HCV);
        Human immunodeficiency virus
        (HIV)/AIDS
Blood–brain barrier, 91, 1416–1417
    disruption, bacterial meningitis, 95
    meningitis pathogenesis, 273
Bloodstream infections (BSIs)
    Campylobacter upsaliensis, 880
    Candida, 1196, 1198
    catheter-related *see* Central line
        associated bloodstream infections
        (CLABSIs); Central venous catheter
        (CVC)-related infections; Intravascular
        catheters
    causative agents, 581t
    costs and mortality, 97
    cystic fibrosis, 640
    device-associated, 580
    healthcare-associated, 580–581
    in HIV infection, 659
    HSCT recipients, 565
    laboratory-confirmed (LCBI), late-onset
        neonatal, 551
    late-onset in neonates *see* Neonatal
        infections, late-onset sepsis
    liver transplant recipients, 557
    neonatal *see* Neonatal infections,
        late-onset sepsis
    recurrent, anatomic/physiologic
        abnormalities predisposing, 600t
    in sickle cell disease, 634
    transient, 98
    urinary tract infection complication,
        344
        neonatal, 550
    see also Bacteremia; *individual pathogens*
Bocavirus *see* Human bocavirus (HBoV)
Body louse *see* Pediculus humanus humanus
    (body louse) infestation
Body piercings, infections after, 513t, 514
Body temperature *see* Temperature
Boils *see* Furuncle (boil)
Bolivian hemorrhagic fever, 1160t, 1164
Bone
    abnormalities in congenital syphilis,
        943–944
    damage in eumycotic mycetoma, 1251,
        1251f
    destruction, sickle-cell disease, 635
    diseases, limb pain, 186
    health, HIV infection treatment and, 671
    pain
        causes, 186
        at night, 186
    sclerosis, 470
    tumors
        bone pain, 186
        neutropenia and infections, 568
Bone infections, 469–477
    Blastomyces dermatitidis (blastomycosis),
        1236, 1236f, 1236t
    Candida, 1199–1200
    Cryptococcus, 1222

Echinococcus granulosus, 1358
Mycobacterium tuberculosis, 778, 784
neonatal, 541, 541t
nontuberculous mycobacteria, 788–789
Pseudomonas aeruginosa, 843t
recurrent, anatomic/physiologic
    abnormalities predisposing, 600t
sickle-cell disease, 635–636, 635f
see also Osteoarticular infections;
    Osteomyelitis
Bone marrow
    aspiration, visceral leishmaniasis
        diagnosis, 1287
    chronic failure, parvovirus B19 and,
        1088f, 1089
    Leishmania infiltration, 1287
    suppression, interferon treatment in
        HCV infection, 1111
Bone marrow transplantation
    adenovirus infections, 1069
    Corynebacterium jeikeium infections, 762
    indication for IGIV, 40–41, 40t
    neutropenia in cancer, 572
    posttransplant lymphoproliferative
        disease (PTLD), 1063
    VZV infection prevention, 1041–1042
Bone mineral density (BMD), decreased, in
    HIV infection, 671
Bone–joint devices, in cancer, neutropenia
    and infections, 568
Bony ankylosis, diskitis complication, 485
Boostrix, 55t
Bordet-Gengou agar, 1375t
Bordetella, 867
    agglutinogens (fimbrial proteins), 867
    culture media, 1376t, 1377
    specimen collection, 1377
Bordetella bronchiseptica
    antimicrobial susceptibility, 871
    etiology, 865
    microbiology, 867
Bordetella hinzii, 865
Bordetella holmesii, 865, 871
Bordetella parapertussis
    antimicrobial susceptibility, 871
    etiology, 865
    microbiology, 867
Bordetella pertussis (pertussis), 856–861
    acute bronchitis due to, 213
    adolescent infections, 866, 866f
    agglutinogens (fimbrial proteins), 867
    antigens in vaccines, 55t
    antimicrobial susceptibility, 871
    bronchiolitis due to, 231
    chemoprophylaxis, 70t–71t, 72
    clinical manifestations, 868–869, 868f
        cadence of symptoms, 868–869
        spectrum of symptoms, 868f, 869
    complications, 870
    control measure, 872
    culture and culture media, 869
    deaths due to, 870
    differential diagnosis, 869–870
    epidemiology, 865–867, 866f
        incidence and group childcare, 27
    etiology, 865–867
    filamentous hemagglutinin (FHA), 867
    group childcare and, 25t, 27

household/contacts, care, 872
hyperimmune serum, 872
immunity to, 867, 867t
laboratory findings/diagnosis, 869–870
leukocytosis due to, 869, 1406
lymphocytosis due to, 1406
management, 870–872
    supportive care, 870–871
    therapeutic agents, 871–872, 871t
microbiology, 867
outcome, 870
pathophysiology, 867–868
pertactin, 868
pertussis
    assessment of severity, 871t
    case definition, 869
    clinical features, 868–869
    complications and outcome, 870
    control, 871t
    cough in, 167–168, 167t, 865, 868
    differential diagnosis, 869–870
    epidemiology, 865–867, 866f
    etiology, 865
    laboratory diagnosis, 869–870
    leukocytosis, 869t
    morbidity reduced by vaccine, 48t
    postexposure prophylaxis, 872
    stages, 868f, 870f
pertussis immune globulin intravenous,
    872
pertussis toxin (PT), 867t
    antibody to, 867
    structure, 868
pneumonia due to, 168t, 169, 236, 238,
    865
    clinical features, 168t
    management, 240
postexposure prophylaxis (PEP), 872
prevention of infections, 872–873
rapid diagnostic testing, 869–870
respiratory tract epithelial damage due
    to, 250
severity assessment, 871t
silent reinfection, 867
tracheal cytotoxin (TCT), 867
transmission, 867
    by healthcare personnel, 869–870
vaccination/immunization, 55–56,
    865–867
    contraindications, diphtheria vaccine,
        759
    indications for Tdap, 56
    measurement of response, 46
    schedule, recommended, 55–56
    see also Diphtheria, tetanus, and
        pertussis (DTP) vaccination/
        vaccines
vaccines
    acellular (DTaP), 47, 49f
    adverse events and IoM findings,
        50t
    interchangeability, 48–50
    Tdap, 865
        see also Diphtheria, tetanus, and
            pertussis (DTP) vaccination/
            vaccines
virulence and pathogenesis, 867–868,
    867t

Boric acid
    Candida vulvovaginitis, 360
    ear infection treatment, 1497t
Borna disease virus, chronic fatigue
    syndrome pathogenesis, 1008t–1009t
Bornaviridae, 1016t
    infections, 1017t
Bornholm disease (epidemic pleurodynia),
    1176
Borrelia, 673, 952–958
    antigenic structure changes, 957
    microbiology, 957
    relapsing fever, 957–958
        causes, 957t
        clinical manifestations, 957–958
        epidemiology, 957–958
        laboratory findings and diagnosis,
            533t–534t, 958, 1384
        louse-borne see Borrelia recurrentis
        in pregnancy, 957–958
        relapsing phase, 957–958
        tickborne, 532t–534t, 957
        transmission, 957
        treatment and prevention, 958
    transmission
        by lice, 957
        by ticks, 532–533, 957
Borrelia afzelli, 952
Borrelia burgdorferi (Lyme disease),
    952–956
    Anaplasma phagocytophilum coinfection,
        894
    anterior uveitis due to, 499, 499t
    antibodies to (IgM and IgG), 955–956,
        1411t–1412t
    arthritis due to, 481, 533, 955
    aseptic meningitis due to, 294–295,
        954–955
    asymptomatic infection, 952–954
    Babesia infection with, 1261–1263
    Baker cyst, 954f, 955
    chronic fatigue syndrome pathogenesis,
        1008t–1009t
    chronic infections, 952
    chronic myositis due to, 464
    clinical manifestations, 281, 533,
        953–955, 953b, 954f
    congenital disease, 956
    cross-reactivity with other species, 535
    diagnosis/detection, 281, 955
    early disseminated disease, 952, 953b,
        954–955
    early localized disease, 953–954, 953b
    ecology, 952–953
    encephalitis due to, 303
    eosinophilia due to, 1408t–1409t
    epidemiology, 281, 532t, 952–953,
        953f
    facial nerve palsy, 315
    generalized lymphadenopathy due to,
        130, 131t–132t
    immunity to, 952
    isolation, 952, 955
    laboratory findings and diagnosis, 281,
        533t–534t, 955
    laboratory testing, 308t–311t
    late disease, 953b, 955, 956b
    long-term sequelae, 957–958

meningitis due to, 275t, 280t, 281, 283t,
    295
    diagnosis, 281
microbiology, 952
myocarditis due to, 266
outcomes, 956
outer-surface proteins (OspA, OspB,
    OspC), 952, 956
pathogenesis, 281, 952
persistence, 952
in pregnancy, 956
prevention, 535–536, 956
prophylactic antibiotics, 535–536
pyogenic arthritis due to, 184
routine testing not recommended, 956
strains, 952
transmission, 953, 957
    risk factors for, 953
    by ticks, 533, 957
treatment, 481, 955–956, 956b
    "failures", 956
vaccine (OspA), 956
vectors, 532t
Borrelia duttonii, 957t
Borrelia garinii, 952
Borrelia hermsii, 957t
Borrelia lonestari, 533
Borrelia mazzottii, 957t
Borrelia parkeri, 957t
Borrelia persica, 957t
Borrelia recurrentis, 957, 957t
    tickborne relapsing fever, 121
Borrelia vincenti, 194
Botanical oils, pediculosis treatment, 1259
Botulism see Clostridium botulinum
Botulism immune globulin intravenous
    (BIG-IGIV), 42
    indications and dose, 42
Boutonneuse fever, 935–938
    see also Rickettsiosis
Bovine papular stomatitis virus, 1020t, 1024
    clinical features, 1024
    infection, 1024
Bovine spongiform encephalopathy (BSE),
    334–335
Bowel
    gangrenous, 390
    obstruction see Intestinal obstruction
Brachyspira, 673
Bradykinin, in nasal secretions in colds,
    197–198
Bradyzoites
    Sarcocystis, 1306, 1307f
    Toxoplasma gondii, 1309, 1311
Brain
    CMV infection damage, 1045,
        1047–1048
    midline shift, Taenia solium
        neurocysticercosis, 1354
    in Toxoplasma gondii infection, 1311–1312
    see also Entries beginning cerebral
Brain abscess
    amebic, 319, 1276
    anaerobic gram-negative bacilli, 983
    anaerobic gram-positive cocci, 989
    Aspergillus, 319, 1204–1205, 1205f
    Bacillus cereus, 754
    burns patients, 519

Candida, 319
Citrobacter, 806–807, 807f
clinical features, 322–323, 323t, 683
 headache, 177–178, 177t
 by site, 322b
complications and prognosis, 329–330
CT, 325, 326f
differential diagnosis, 323t, 324–325
Eikenella corrodens, 718f
Entamoeba histolytica, 319, 1276
epidemiology, 321
etiology, 319–321, 320t
 organisms by site, 321t
 uncommon pathogens, 320t
fungal, 319, 329
imaging, 325
laboratory findings and diagnosis, 325
Listeria monocytogenes, 319, 765
management, 327–329, 683,
 1418t–1419t
 corticosteroids, 683
 drainage, 812
 empirical antibiotics, 328–329, 329t
 indications for antibiotics, 327–328
mortality, 329–330, 683
MRI, 325
Mycobacterium tuberculosis, 320
Nocardia, 329
nuchal rigidity, 177–178
pathogenesis, 321–322
 contiguous spread, 322
 hematogenous spread, 320–321
predisposing factors, 321–322, 321b
Proteus, Providencia, Morganella, 812
Salmonella, 817
specimen collection/transport, 1374t
Staphylococcus aureus, 320, 683
stereotactic aspiration, 328
Streptococcus intermedius, 718f
Toxoplasma gondii, 319, 1312
Ureaplasma urealyticum, 1001
viridans group streptococci, 718
Brain biopsy
 CJD diagnosis, 336
 encephalitis diagnosis, 308–312
 subacute sclerosing panencephalitis
  diagnosis, 1142–1143
Brain cysts
 Enterobacter causing, 805
 Taenia serialis (coenurosis), 1362
Brain tumor
 altered mental status, 179t
 ataxia, 180
 headache in, 177–178, 177t
 tuberculoma *vs.*, 778
Brainstem encephalitis (rhombencephalitis)
 enteroviruses causing, 1176
 Listeria monocytogenes, 765
Brainstem glioma, ataxia in, 180
Branched-chain DNA (bDNA) assay, virus
 detection, 1386–1387
Branchial cleft cysts, 138–139, 142t
Branchial cleft sinuses, 138–139, 142t
Brazilian hemorrhagic fever, 1160t
Brazilian purpuric fever (BPF), 491
Breast, enlargement, breast abscess and, 457
Breast abscess, 457
 cellulitis after, 457

coagulase-negative staphylococci causing,
 693
Staphylococcus aureus, 457, 678
Breast milk, gastrointestinal tract infection
 management, 377
Breastfeeding/breastmilk
 avoidance, HIV transmission prevention,
  647
 immunizations, yellow fever vaccine
  contraindicated, 68
 infant botulism risk, 972
 infection protection/prevention
  astrovirus infections, 1191
  gastrointestinal infection prevention,
   377
  recurrent acute otitis media
   prevention, 722
  rotavirus infection protection, 1097
  Vibrio cholerae protection, 850
  viral gastroenteritis prevention, 381
 normal flora establishment, 959
 nosocomial neonatal infection
  prevention, 555
 pathogen transmission by
  Ancylostoma, 1330
  CMV, 1046, 1048
  Ebola virus, 1159
  HBV, 1078, 1085
  HCV, 1106, 1111
  HHV-7, 1057–1058
  HIV, 545, 642, 646–648
  Strongyloides, 1330, 1333
  viral infections, 545, 546t
 response to vaccination and, 51–52
 rotavirus infection management,
  1096–1097
 tuberculosis treatment, 784
 viral gastroenteritis management, 381
Breath
 malodorous, acute bacterial sinusitis,
  228
 odor, putrid, 962
Breath sounds, 169
 diminished, 169
 tubular, 169
Breath test
 ¹³C-labeled urea *see* Urea breath test
  (UBT)
 hydrogen, 391
 necrotizing enterocolitis, 389–390
Breathing
 bronchial, in pneumonia, 238
 rate *see* Respiratory rate
Brevundimonas, 833
Brevundimonas diminuta, 833
Brevundimonas vesicularis, 833
Bright disease (poststreptococcal acute
 glomerulonephritis) *see under*
 *Streptococcus pyogenes (group A
 streptococcus)*
Brill–Zinsser disease *see Rickettsia prowazekii*
Brodie abscess, 469
Bronchi
 obstruction
  persistent pneumonia, 246–247
  pulmonary tuberculosis, 774
 tracheal, 247
Bronchial breathing, in pneumonia, 238

Bronchiectasis
 in ciliary dysfunction, 638
 in cystic fibrosis, 640f
 mediastinal lymphadenopathy in, 153
 persistent pneumonia with, 246
Bronchiolitis, 231–235
 acute, 233
 adenoviruses, 231
 Bordetella pertussis (pertussis), 231
 clinical features, 233
 complications, 233, 235
 in congenital heart disease, 233
 cough in, 167t
 course, 233
 definition, 231
 diagnosis, 233–234
 differential diagnosis, 233
 epidemics, 231
 epidemiology, 231–233, 232f
 etiologic agents, 231, 232t
 hospitalization rates, 231–233
 hospitalization risk, 233
 human metapneumovirus (hMPV), 231,
  1123
 human parainfluenza viruses, 231, 232f,
  1121, 1123, 1123f
 imaging, 233, 234f
 influenza viruses, 231
 management, 234–235
 mortality, 231
 Mycoplasma pneumoniae, 231
 obliterative, adenoviruses causing,
  1069
 pathogenesis and pathology, 233
 prevention, 235
 prognosis, 235
 respiratory syncytial virus (RSV), 231,
  1130, 1132–1133
 risk factors, 231
Bronchiolitis obliterans, 227, 250
Bronchiolitis obliterans organizing
 pneumonia, 250
Bronchitis
 acute, 213
  bacterial infection, 213
  clinical features and management,
   213
  etiology, 213
 bacterial, protracted, 168
 in ciliary dysfunction, 638
Bronchoalveolar lavage (BAL)
 Aspergillus infections, 1207
 CMV pneumonia, 254
 in persistent pneumonia, 248, 252
 Pneumocystis jirovecii (carinii) detection,
  1231, 1231t
 pneumonia in HIV infection, 660–661
 pneumonia in SCID, 629
 specimen collection/transport, 1374t
 ventilator-associated pneumonia, 582
Bronchodilators
 bronchiolitis management, 234
 in ciliary dysfunction, 638
 human metapneumovirus (hMPV)
  infection, 1136–1137
Bronchogenic cysts, persistent pneumonia,
 247
Bronchomediastinal lymphatic trunk, 149

Bronchopleural fistula, 242
  tuberculosis, 775–776
Bronchopneumonia, 238
  influenza viruses causing, 1153
  see also Pneumonia
Bronchopulmonary lymph nodes, 148–149
Bronchoscopy
  bacterial tracheitis, 213f
  CMV pneumonia, 254
  indications, 962
  in persistent pneumonia, 248, 252
  pneumonia diagnosis, 252
  pneumonia in immunocompromised,
    254–255
  specimen collection/transport, 1377
Bronchus-associated lymphoid tissue
    (BALT), 254
Brood capsules, Echinococcus granulosus,
    1356, 1358f
Broth microdilution assay, 1378–1379
Brucella (brucellosis), 861–864
  clinical manifestations, 119t–120t, 862t,
    863
  culture media, 1376t
  endocarditis due to, 863
  epidemiology and transmission,
    862–863
  fever of unknown origin due to,
    119t–120t
  fever pattern, 863
  hepatic granulomas due to, 863
  immune response to, 861–862
  infection routes, 862t
  joint infections, 477
  laboratory findings/diagnosis, 863–864
    blood cultures, 1374–1375
  laboratory testing, 308t–311t
  meningitis due to, 280t, 281, 863
  microbiology and pathogenesis, 861–862
  noncaseating granuloma due to,
    129–130
  organs involved, 863
  pathogenesis, 861–862
  in pregnancy, 862, 864
  prevention and vaccines, 864
  species and hosts, 861, 861t
  transmission route, 862t
  treatment and outcome, 864, 864t
  virulence factors, 861
Brucella abortus
  biovars and host, 861t
  clinical manifestations, 863
  cross-reaction with Yersinia enterocolitica,
    824
  pneumonia due to, 237t
  transmission route, 862t
Brucella abortus strain, 863, 865
Brucella canis
  biovars and host, 861t
  diagnosis, 863–864
Brucella melitensis
  biovars and host, 861t
  clinical manifestations, 863
  endocarditis due to, 260t
  epidemiology, 862–863
  strain Rev-1, 864
  transmission route, 862t
Brucella neotomae, biovars and host, 861t

Brucella ovis, 861t
Brucella suis
  biovars and host, 861t
  clinical manifestations, 863
  transmission route, 862t
Brucellosis see Brucella
Brudzinski sign, 274, 295, 1175
Brugia malayi, 1342–1344
  characteristics, 1342t
  epidemiology, 1342
  treatment of infections, 1344
  see also Wuchereria bancrofti
Brugia timori, 1342
  characteristics, 1342t
  epidemiology, 1342
  see also Wuchereria bancrofti
Bruises see Ecchymoses (bruises)
Bruton agammaglobulinemia, 611
Bruton agammaglobulinemia tyrosine
    kinase (BTK), 611
BSI see Bloodstream infections
Bubo(es)
  chancroid, 351
  Yersinia pestis, 140, 826
Bubonic plague, 826
  see also Yersinia pestis
Buccal mucosa
  bacteria colonizing, 190
  infections, 191–194, 193t
Buccal ulceration, 111
Budesonide
  acute sinusitis management, 230
  nebulized, laryngotracheitis therapy, 211
Bull-neck appearance, 138–140, 201–202
  diphtheria, 755–757
  Ludwig angina, 194
Bullae, 427t, 438–441
  etiology, 438–440
  hemorrhagic, 111
  mucocutaneous syndromes, 111
  size, 438–439
Bullous impetigo, 428, 428f, 440, 678
Bull's eye lesions, 578
Bunyaviridae, 1016t, 1102–1104
  clinical manifestations, 1103–1104, 1104t
  epidemiology, 1102–1103, 1103t
  infections, 1017t
  laboratory findings and diagnosis, 1104
  prevention, 1104
  treatment, 1104
Burkholderia, 846–848
  patient-to-patient transmission, 24
Burkholderia cenocepacia
  in cystic fibrosis, 639
  infection in lung transplant recipient,
    558
Burkholderia cepacia, 248–249, 846–848
  antibiotic resistance, 848, 1425–1426,
    1433
  cable (Cbl) pilus, 847
  in chronic granulomatous disease, 622f,
    846–847, 847t
  culture media, 1376t, 1377
  in cystic fibrosis, 248–249, 639–640,
    847, 847t
  epidemiology, 847
  infection in lung transplant recipient,
    558

persistence in disinfectants, 846–847
in phagocytic disorders, 620t, 624
Pseudomonas aeruginosa coinfection, 848
pulmonary infections, 248–249, 251,
    848
specimen collection, 1377
subspecies (genomovars), 846–847, 847t
treatment of infections, 848
virulence and pathogenesis, 847
Burkholderia cepacia complex, 846–848
  clinical manifestations, 847t, 848
Burkholderia gladioli, 846, 847t, 848
Burkholderia mallei, 846, 847t, 848
Burkholderia pseudomallei, 846
  clinical manifestations, 847t, 848
  septicemia, 848
  treatment of infections, 848
Burkitt lymphoma, 133, 1064
  oral EBV infections, 192t
Burns, 516–521
  care, 520
  child survival and burn extent, 516
  first-/second-/third-degree, 516
  full-thickness, 516–517
  infections after (not wound), 516–521
    bacteremia, 519
    catheter-related, 516, 519
    CNS infections, 519
    diagnosis, 516–517
    incidence, 516
    intra-abdominal, 519
    management of outpatients, 520–521
    prevention, 521
    Pseudomonas aeruginosa, 518, 844t
    respiratory tract, 519
    risk factors, 516
    treatment, 520
    urinary tract, 519
    viral, 519–520
    see also Burns, wound infections
  mortality, 516
  partial-thickness, 516–517
    care, 520
  pharmacokinetics, 1437t, 1438
  total body surface area (TBSA) and
    outcome, 516
  treatment, 520, 1499–1500, 1500b,
    1500t–1501t
    debridement, 519–520
    dressings, 520–521, 520t
    outpatients, 520–521
    systemic antimicrobials, 520
    topical antimicrobials, 520, 520t
  wound infections, 517–519
    anaerobic, 517–519
    biopsy findings, 517, 517b
    blood supply affecting, 517
    characteristics, 517b
    colonization by pathogens, 517–518
    debridement, 519–520
    definition, 517
    diagnosis, 517, 517b
    early infections, 518
    etiology, 518
    factors influencing (wound/host
      factors), 517–518, 518t
    fungal, 518
    group A streptococcal, 517–518

immune system dysfunction, 518, 518t
later infections, 518
local/systemic signs, 517b
management, 519–520
organism number effect, 518
outpatient management, 520–521
prevention, 521
prophylactic antibiotics, 521
Pseudomonas aeruginosa, 518, 844t
Staphylococcus aureus, 518
temporary membranes for, 520
tetanus, 518
wound septicemia, 517–518
Burow solution
ear infections, 1497t
tinea pedis, 1248–1249
Bursitis, *Staphylococcus aureus*, 678–679
Buruli ulcer, 788
Bush yaws, 1289
Bush–Jacoby–Medeiros classification system, 1424
Butenafine, treatment of superficial infections, 1485t, 1486

C

C-reactive protein (CRP), 94, 1402
acute bacterial meningitis, 274
acute rheumatic fever, 704
clinical usefulness, 1402
focal suppurative CNS infections, 325
function, 94
increased levels, 1402
causes, 1402
pelvic inflammatory disease, 348
infections after burns, 517
Kawasaki disease, 113, 1005
neonatal infections, 537
nosocomial, 552
neonatal septicemia diagnosis, 541t, 542
osteomyelitis, 470
physiology and measurement, 1402
pyogenic arthritis, 478
sequential determinations, 1402
staphylococcal osteomyelitis, 679
transient synovitis, 486
C1 component, 615
C1 deficiency, 604t–605t
C1 esterase inhibitor deficiency, 617
C1q component, 615
deficiency, 617
C1r component, 615
deficiency, 617
C1s component, 615
deficiency, 617
C2, 615
deficiency, 604t–605t, 618
C3, 615–616
activation, 616, 618
decreased in *Mycoplasma pneumoniae* infections, 995
deficiency, 604t–605t, 617–618
C3(H₂O), 616
C3-convertase, 616
"priming" and "amplification", 616
C3a, 94, 616
C3b, 616

C4, 615–616
deficiency, 604t–605t, 618
recurrent meningitis associated, 288
C5, 616–617
deficiency, 604t–605t, 618
recurrent meningitis associated, 288
C5a, 94, 616
deficiency, 86
role, 86
C5a peptidase, *Streptococcus pyogenes*, 702
C5b, 616, 618
C6, 616
deficiency, 604t–605t, 618
recurrent meningitis association, 288
C7 deficiency, 604t–605t, 618
recurrent meningitis association, 288
C8, 618
deficiency, 604t–605t, 618–619
recurrent meningitis association, 288
C9 deficiency, 604t–605t, 618
CA-MRSA *see Staphylococcus aureus*, community-associated methicillin-resistant (CA-MRSA)
CA-UTI *see* Catheter-associated urinary tract infection (CA-UTI)
Calabar swellings, 1345–1346
Calcification
intracerebral, congenital toxoplasmosis, 1312, 1314
neurocysticercosis (*Taenia solium*), 1352–1354, 1353f, 1355t
Calcium, *Entamoeba histolytica* infection effect, 1274
Calcium alginate swabs, 1373t
Calcium channel deficiency, characteristics, 603t–604t
Calcofluor white, 1382
Caliciviridae, 1016t, 1187
infections, 1017t
Caliciviruses, 378, 1187–1189
antigen detection, 381
clinical manifestations, 1189
description and structure, 378, 1187, 1187f
diagnosis/detection, 381, 1389t–1392t
diarrhea due to, 26t
epidemiology, 1188–1189, 1188f–1189f
gastroenteritis due to, 26t, 378
laboratory findings and diagnosis, 1189
prevention, 1189
treatment, 1189
see also Norovirus(es)
California encephalitis virus, diagnosis/detection, 1389t–1392t, 1397
California serogroup viruses, 1103
Calmette-Guérin bacillus (BCG) vaccine, 67, 785–786
adverse events, 67
axillary lymphadenopathy due to, 159–160
clinical efficacy trials, 786
complications, 786
contraindications, 786
effect on *Mycobacterium tuberculosis* incidence, 772
evaluation problems, 785–786
false-positive reactions to tuberculin, 779–780

in HIV infection, 669
immune response to, 785–786
indications, 80
neonates, 779–780
recommendations for, 67, 786
for refugee and internationally adopted children, 34–35
schedule/dose for travelers, 79t, 80
unilateral cervical lymphadenitis due to, 141
Calymmatobacterium granulomatis see Klebsiella (Calymmatobacterium) granulomatis
Campylobacter, 873, 878–880, 878b
bloodstream infections, 876
clinical manifestations, 876–877
cytotoxins, 875
description and microbiology, 873–874
diagnosis/detection, 385t, 877
stool cultures, 376
epidemiology, 874–875
flagella, 873–875
foodborne infections, 394, 394t
genome, 873–874
growth and culture, 874
culture media, 1376t
immunity, 876
inflammatory enteritis due to, 387
intestinal epithelial cell invasion, 875
location of and diseases due to, 878t
mode of transmission, 875
pathogenesis of infections, 875–876
phylogenetic trees, 878–879
prognosis of infections, 878
reservoirs and diseases due to, 874t
species, 874, 874t
number, 878
treatment of infections, 877–878
virulence factor, 875
Campylobacter agar, 1375t
Campylobacter coli, 873–878, 874t
bloodstream infection, 876
description and microbiology, 874–875
epidemiology, 874–875
Campylobacter concisus, 874t, 880
diarrhea, 880
Campylobacter curvus, 874t, 880
Campylobacter fetus, 874, 874t, 878t
antimicrobial susceptibility, 879
bloodstream infection, 876, 879
clinical manifestations, 879
enteric fever due to, 879
infections in pregnancy, 879
management of infections, 879
microbiology and epidemiology, 879
mortality due to, 879
pathogenesis and pathology, 879
perinatal infections, 877, 879
virulence factor, 879
Campylobacter fetus subsp. *fetus*, 874t, 879
microbiology, 879
Campylobacter fetus subsp. *venerealis*, 879
Campylobacter gracilis, 878t
Campylobacter helveticus, 878t
Campylobacter hyointestinalis, 874t, 878t, 880
Campylobacter jejuni, 873–878
abdominal pain due to, 174, 876
adhesins, 875

antibodies to, 876
bloodstream infections, 876
clinical manifestations, 876–877
colonization and adherence, 875
cytotoxins, 875
description and microbiology, 873–874
diagnosis, 877
diarrhea due to, 874
group childcare and, 25
number of organisms needed, 875
types, 876
enteric infections, 875–876
epidemiology, 874–875
extraintestinal infections, 875–877
fecal shedding, 876
foodborne infections, 394, 394t
group childcare setting, 25, 25t, 30–31
Guillain-Barré syndrome and, 877
immunity to, 876
immunoreactive complications, 877
incubation period, 875
infections, 876
inflammatory enteritis due to, 383, 383t
mesenteric lymphadenitis due to, 876
milkborne, 874–875
mortality due to, 874–875
nonmotile variants, 875
pathogenesis of infections, 875–876
pathology, 875
perinatal infections, 877
phylogenetic tree, 878, 878t
prognosis of infections, 878
recurrent infections, 876
reservoir for, 383
travelers' diarrhea due to, 373
treatment of infections, 877–878
Trichuris trichiura synergy, 1327
vaccine development, 81
in X-linked agammaglobulinemia, 610
Campylobacter jejuni subsp. *doylei*, 874t, 876
Campylobacter jejuni subsp. *jejuni*, 874t, 876
Campylobacter lari, 874, 874t, 880
microbiology and infections, 880
Campylobacter mucosalis, 878t
Campylobacter pyloridis see *Helicobacter pylori*
Campylobacter rectus, 874t
Campylobacter showae, 878t
Campylobacter sputorum, 874t
Campylobacter upsaliensis, 874t, 876, 879–880
bloodstream infections, 880
diarrhea due to, 879–880
epidemiology and clinical manifestations, 879–880
microbiology, 879
phylogenetic tree, 878, 878t
septicemia due to, 880
Campylobacteraceae, 873–874, 874t
classification, 959t
Campylobacteriosis see *Campylobacter*
Cancer
human polyomaviruses and, 1077
infections in, 567–579
adenovirus infections, 1070
Aspergillus infections, 1204f, 1206
catheter-related and soft-tissue, 573–574

CNS, 579
cystitis, 579
diagnosis and management, 573–579
ear and sinus, 577
gastrointestinal, 577
intra-abdominal infections, 578
mucormycosis, 1213–1214
mucositis and esophagitis, 577–578
osteoarticular, 579
pulmonary, 575–577, 575t
sites and types, 574t
skin, 574–575
see also Neutropenia, fever in
lymphadenopathy see Lymphadenitis/
lymphadenopathy
neutropenia in see Neutropenia
varicella complications, 1039
see also Chemotherapy
Candida, 1196–1202, 1202b
abscess due to, 1198, 1198f–1199f
antifungal resistance, 360, 664
in APECED, 631
arthritis due to, 482
biofilm formation, 1200, 1202
bloodstream infections, 1196, 1198
bone/joint infections, 1199–1200
brain abscess due to, 319
burn wound infections, 518
candidemia see Candidemia
chronic disseminated candidiasis, 1199, 1199f
in cancer, 578
chronic meningitis, 282–283
treatment, 578
chronic fatigue syndrome pathogenesis, 1008t–1009t
chronic mucocutaneous candidiasis, 1197
characteristics, 603t–604t
CLABSIs in neonates, 553
clinical manifestations, 1196–1200, 1202b
CNS candidiasis, 1198, 1198f
colonization, risk factors increasing, 1201
congenital cutaneous candidiasis, 1197–1198, 1197f
diagnosis/detection, 1200, 1202b
antigens, 1200
blood culture, 1200
DNA polymerase chain reaction, 1200
metabolites, 1200
routine tests, 1200
serology, 1200
diskitis due to, 483
endocarditis due to, 1199
complications, 264
epidemiology, 1196, 1202b
esophageal candidiasis, in HIV infection, 659, 662
esophagitis in cancer due to, 578
genital dermatosis, 351–352
healthcare-associated infections, 14
hepatosplenic candidiasis, 1199, 1199f
in cancer, 578
in HIV infection, 659, 661–662
prevention, 664

infections in heart transplant recipients, 558
infections in HSCT recipient, 563
infections in liver transplant recipients, 557
infections in premature infants *see under* Premature infants
infections in renal transplant recipients, 557
inflammatory enteritis due to, 384–385
intravascular catheter-related infection, 589–590, 593
invasion, risk factors increasing, 1201–1202
invasive fungal dermatitis, 1198, 1198f
invasive infections, 1195–1196, 1198–1200
definition, 1198
pathogenesis and risk factors, 1201–1202
prophylaxis, 1202
signs and symptoms, 1198
treatment, 1200–1201, 1201t
joint infections, 477
meningitis due to, 282–284, 284t, 286
meningoencephalitis due to, 1198, 1198f
mucosal (buccal) infection, 192–194, 193t
neonatal infections, 539
nosocomial, 549t, 550
nosocomial, prevention, 555
nosocomial, treatment, 552
persistent, 554
neutropenia associated with cancer, 567
optic complications, 1199
oral infection, 192–194, 193t
in cancer, 577–578
in HIV infection, 659, 662
management, 192–194
prevention in HIV infection, 664
osteomyelitis due to, 475
neonatal, 541
otitis externa due to, 221
in phagocytic disorders, 620t, 625
pneumonia in cancer due to, 575
prevention, in transplant recipients, 561
pseudomembranous infection, 192–194, 193t
renal/urinary tract infections, 1198–1199, 1199f
risk factors, 14
skin infections, in cancer, 574
species, 1196
superficial and mucosal infections, 1196–1198
chronic mucocutaneous candidiasis, 1197
diaper dermatitis, 1197, 1198f, 1200
esophagitis, 1197
neonatal presentations, 1197–1198, 1197f–1198f
oropharyngeal candidiasis (thrush), 1196–1197, 1197f
treatment, 1200
vulvovaginitis, 1197, 1200
treatment of infections, 360, 1200–1201, 1201t, 1202b
urinary catheter-related infection, 599

vertical transmission, 1201
vulvovaginitis due to, 356–359
  treatment, 358, 360
see also Candida albicans
Candida albicans, 1196
  arthritis due to, 482
  bloodstream infections, 503
  breakpoints against, 1443, 1443t
  CLABSIs in neonates, 553
  detection method, 1382
  endophthalmitis due to, 503
  genital dermatosis due to, 351
  infections in HSCT recipient, 563
  keratitis due to, 496–497
  monoclonal antibody development, 44
  mucocutaneous candidiasis, innate
    immunity, 83
  nail infections, 1249
  neutropenia associated with cancer, 567
  oral cavity colonization, 192–194
  paronychia due to, 432
  skin colonization, 429–430
  urinary tract infection, 342
  vaginitis, 358–359
    clinical features, 359, 359t
    diagnosis and laboratory findings,
      359t, 360
    treatment, 359t, 360
  vernix extracts action against, 83
  vulvovaginitis due to, 356–359
    clinical features, 359, 359t
    diagnosis, 359t, 360
    HIV and, 361
    recurrent, 358–360
    risk factors, 358–359
    treatment, 359t, 360
    uncomplicated vs complicated,
      358–359
  see also Candida
Candida dubliniensis, 1196
Candida glabrata, 1196
  genital dermatosis due to, 351
  urinary tract infection, 342
  vaginitis due to, 358–359
    diagnosis, 360
    treatment, 360
Candida guilliermondi, 1196
Candida intermedia, 1196
Candida kefyr, 1196
Candida krusei, 1196
Candida lusitaniae, 1196
Candida parapsilosis, 1196
  neutropenia associated with cancer,
    571–572
Candida pseudotropicalis, 1196
Candida stellatoidea, 1196
Candida tropicalis, 1196
  infections in HSCT recipient, 563
Candidemia, 1196, 1198
  extremely-low-birthweight neonates, 538
  intravascular catheter-related infection,
    593
  persistence and biofilm role, 1202
Canine heartworm disease, 1346
Cannibalism, 334
Cannula, indwelling, infections in
  transplant recipients, 556
Capillary hemangiomas, 143

Capillary invasion, purpura pathogenesis,
  441
Capillary leakage, peritonitis
  pathophysiology, 415
Capnocytophaga, 880–881
  bacteremia, 880
  canine (DF-2) group, 881
  clinical manifestations and treatment,
    880–881
  human (DF-1) group, 880–881
  microbiology and epidemiology,
    880–881
  species, 880
Capnocytophaga canimorsus, 881
  animal bite wounds, 521, 523
  in asplenia, 636
  dog-bite wounds, 881
Capnocytophaga cynodegmi, 881
Capnocytophaga gingivalis, 880
Capnocytophaga granulosa, 880
Capnocytophaga haemolytica, 880
Capnocytophaga sputigena, 880
Capreomycin, tuberculosis treatment, 782
CAPS see Cryopyrin-associated periodic
  syndromes (CAPS)
Capsule, Staphylococcus aureus, 676
Carbacephem, structure, 1465f
Carbapenem(s), 1468
  clinical uses, 1468
  dosage, 1445t–1452t, 1480t–1483t
  dose adjustment
    burned patients, 1437t
    renal failure, 1445t–1452t
  pharmacodynamic properties, 1414t
  pharmacology, 1453t–1458t
  resistance, 1422, 1424–1425
    detection, 1431, 1431f
    Enterococcus, 714–715
  spectrum of activity, 1459t–1463t,
    1468
  structure, 1465f, 1468
  treatment of
    Pseudomonas aeruginosa infections,
      846
    sepsis, 99
    Serratia infections, 813
Carbapenemases, Serratia marcescens, 813
Carbaryl, pediculosis treatment, 1259
Carbenicillin
  dosage, 1480t–1483t
  eye infection treatment, 1494t–1496t
  pharmacology, 1453t–1458t
  spectrum of activity, 1459t–1463t
Carbohydrate metabolism disorders
  acute hepatitis, 403–404
  chronic hepatitis, 407
Carbohydrates, utilization, in inflammatory
  response, 94
Carbuncle, 431–432
Carcinogenesis, 1164
CARD-9 protein, 83
Card agglutination test for trypanosomiasis
  (CATT), 1321–1322
Cardiac abnormalities
  in congenital rubella, 1115
  infection chemoprophylaxis, 75–76, 75b
  in Leptospira infections, 951
  persistent/recurrent pneumonia in, 251

quinidine use in Plasmodium infections,
  1303
  in Trypanosoma cruzi infections,
    1324–1325
  see also Cardiovascular abnormalities
Cardiac arrhythmias, Corynebacterium
  diphtheriae causing, 756
Cardiac disease
  adenoviruses causing, 1068t, 1069
  in HIV infection, 655–656, 670
  Mycobacterium tuberculosis causing, 776
  in Mycoplasma pneumoniae infections,
    994t
  persistent pneumonia, 251
Cardiac features, EBV infection, 1061
Cardiac infections, 256–265
  see also Endocarditis; Myocarditis;
    Pericarditis
Cardiac insufficiency, viral infections in
  fetus/neonate, 547
Cardiac muscle disease, enterovirus
  infections, 1176–1177
Cardiac surgery
  infection chemoprophylaxis, 72–73
  mediastinitis after, 587
Cardiac tamponade
  clinical features, 270
  pathogenesis, 269
Cardiobacterium hominis, 940
  endocarditis due to, 257, 940
Cardiomyopathy
  chronic dilated, enterovirus infections,
    1177
  Corynebacterium diphtheriae causing, 756
  in HIV infection, 655–656
    management, 670
  idiopathic dilated, 265–266
Cardiovascular abnormalities
  chronic fatigue syndrome etiology, 1008
  in HIV infection, 655–656, 670
  Trypanosoma cruzi infections, 1324–1325,
    1324f
  see also Cardiac abnormalities
Cardiovascular infections, Staphylococcus
  aureus, 681–683
Cardiovascular shock, in meningococcal
  disease, 737
Carditis
  in acute rheumatic fever, 703, 704t
  Borrelia burgdorferi (Lyme disease), 954
  rheumatic, 703
Caries, dental see Dental caries
Caroli disease, 403
Carrión disease, 940
  see also Bartonella bacilliformis
Cartilage hair hypoplasia (CHH) syndrome,
  627, 628t
  diagnosis, 629
Case ascertainment, bias in, 5
Case-control efficacy studies, 7
Case-control studies, 3t, 4
  advantages, 3t, 4
  bias in selection, 5
  disadvantages, 3t, 4
  outbreak investigations, 7
  vaccine efficacy, 7
Case-crossover analysis, 6–7
Case definition, 1

Case series analysis, 6–7
Caseating necrosis, 134, 151–153
　tuberculosis, 151–153
Caspase (host), activation, by *Entamoeba*
　　histolytica, 1274
Caspase 1, 126
Caspofungin, 1491–1492
　adverse effects, 1491
　clinical trials, 1491–1492
　dosage, 1445t–1452t, 1487t, 1491
　pharmacology, 1491
　spectrum of activity, 1486t
　treatment of
　　Aspergillus infections, 576, 1208–1209
　　Candida infections, 1201, 1201t
　　Coccidioides immitis
　　　(coccidioidomycosis), 1245
　　fever in neutropenia (in cancer),
　　　571–572
　　fungal endocarditis, 263
　　fungal infections in cancer, 576
　　hepatic candidiasis, 578
Castleman disease, 134
　generalized lymphadenopathy, 131t–
　　132t, 134
　HHV-8 association, 155
　mediastinal lymphadenopathy, 155
　multicentric, 134
　neck masses, 142t
Cat(s), infections related to
　bites *see* Bites, infections after
　cat-scratch disease *see Bartonella henselae*
　reservoir for *Bartonella henselae*, 857
　scratches, *Pasteurella multocida* infections,
　　837
　tapeworm (*Dipylidium caninum*),
　　1348–1349, 1348f
　Toxocara infection transmission, 1335,
　　1337
　Toxoplasma gondii, 1309, 1309f
　　prevention, 1317, 1317t
　see also Pet(s)
Cat fleas, 931–932
Cat-scratch disease *see Bartonella henselae*
Cathelicidins, 83
Catheter(s)
　antibiotic-impregnated, coagulase-
　　negative staphylococcal infection
　　prevention, 694
　central venous *see* Central line associated
　　bloodstream infections (CLABSIs);
　　Central venous catheter (CVC)-related
　　infections
　intravascular *see* Intravascular catheters
　peripheral intravascular, changing,
　　infection risk, 11–12
　peritoneal *see* Peritoneal catheters
　subdural, infections, 596
　urethral, nosocomial infection of
　　neonates, 550
　urinary
　　antiseptic-impregnated, 599
　　infections, 599
　ventriculostomy, infections, 596–597
　see also Device-related infections
Catheter-associated urinary tract infection
　　(CA-UTI), 342, 599
　pathogens, 580t

Catheter hubs, 594
Catheter-related bloodstream infections,
　　589
　burns patients, 516, 519
　in cancer, 573–574
　clinical features, 591t
　coagulase-negative staphylococcal
　　infection, 692, 694
　late-onset sepsis in neonates, 549
　neonatal, 538
　　urinary catheters, 550
　prevention, coagulase-negative
　　staphylococcal infection, 694
　see also Central line associated
　　bloodstream infections (CLABSIs)
Catheter-related infections, peritonitis *see*
　　Peritonitis
Caulobacteraceae, 832
Causal inference, 4–5
　single hypothesis *vs.* multiple, 9
CAUTI (catheter-associated UTI) *see*
　　Catheter-associated urinary tract
　　infection (CA-UTI)
Cavernous hemangioma, parotid masses,
　　143
Cavernous sinus thrombosis
　septic, 323t, 324
　staphylococcal orbital infection
　　complication, 679
CCR5, 1166
CD3- zeta-associated protein (ZAP-70)
　　kinase, 627
CD4⁺ molecule, HIV receptor, 1166
CD4 receptor, HIV binding, 666
CD4⁺ T cells *see* T lymphocytes, CD4⁺
　　(helper)
CD8 deficiency, characteristics, 603t–604t
CD8⁺ T cells *see* T lymphocytes, CD8⁺
CD14
　endotoxin interaction, 102–103
　monoclonal antibodies against, 103
CD19 deficiency, characteristics, 602t
CD20, 87, 89, 1063
CD21, 87, 89, 616
　EBV receptor, 1060
CD22, 89
CD25
　hemophagocytic lymphohistiocytosis,
　　107
　macrophage activation syndrome, 107
CD34⁺ cells, 85–86
CD35, 616
CD40, 87, 90, 626–627
　CD40L interaction, 631
　deficiency, 610t, 612–613
　　autosomal recessive hyper-IgM
　　　syndrome, 630t, 631–632
　EBV protein mimicking, 1059
　impaired signalling, 632–633
CD40 ligand (CD40L), 626–627
　CD40 interaction, 631
　deficiency, 609–610, 610t, 612–613, 630t,
　　632
　mutations, 612–613
　Pneumocystis jirovecii (carinii) pneumonia
　　and, 1230–1231
　role, 632–633
CD45, 627

CD45 tyrosine phosphatase, 627
CD45RA⁺ cells, 90
CD46, 491
　HHV-6 receptor, 1053
CD80, 92
CD86, 92
CD127, 627
CD132, 627
　deficiency, 628t
CD150, 633
CD154, 626–627, 630t
CDC *see* Centers for Disease Control and
　　Prevention
Cecitis, neutropenic, in cancer, 578
Cedecea, 808
Cefaclor
　dosage, 1445t–1452t, 1480t–1483t
　pharmacology, 1453t–1458t
　spectrum of activity, 1459t–1463t
Cefadroxil
　dosage, 1445t–1452t, 1480t–1483t
　pharmacology, 1453t–1458t
　spectrum of activity, 1459t–1463t
Cefamandole, spectrum of activity,
　　1459t–1463t
Cefazolin
　clinical uses, 1467
　dosage, 1445t–1452t, 1480t–1483t
　pharmacology, 1453t–1458t
　spectrum of activity, 1459t–1463t,
　　1467
　Streptococcus agalactiae (group B
　　streptococcus) prevention, 711
　surgical site infection prevention, 587
　treatment of
　　anaerobic gram-negative bacilli
　　　infections, 985
　　bacterial keratitis, 497–498
　　dacryocystitis, 509
　　endocarditis, 263t
　　endophthalmitis, 505
　　eye infections, 1494t–1496t
　　Staphylococcus aureus infections, 686
Cefdinir
　acute bacterial sinusitis treatment, 229t
　dosage, 1480t–1483t
　pharmacology, 1453t–1458t
　spectrum of activity, 1459t–1463t
Cefepime
　acute bacterial meningitis treatment,
　　277
　clinical uses, 1468
　dosage, 1445t–1452t, 1480t–1483t
　dose adjustment
　　burned patients, 1437t
　　renal failure, 1445t–1452t
　mortality, in neutropenia associated with
　　cancer, 571
　pharmacology, 1453t–1458t
　spectrum of activity, 1459t–1463t, 1468
Cefixime
　chemoprophylactic use, 70t–71t
　dosage, 1445t–1452t, 1480t–1483t
　pharmacology, 1453t–1458t
　spectrum of activity, 1459t–1463t
　treatment of
　　acute otitis media, 219t
　　Escherichia coli infections, 798

Neisseria gonorrhoeae infections, 747
  Shigella infections, 387, 822t
  urinary tract infections, 341
Cefonicid
  infection prophylaxis after trauma, 73
  spectrum of activity, 1459t–1463t
Cefoperazone
  dosage, 1480t–1483t
  pharmacology, 1453t–1458t
  spectrum of activity, 1459t–1463t
Ceforanide, spectrum of activity,
    1459t–1463t
Cefotaxime
  dosage, 1445t–1452t, 1480t–1483t
  pharmacology, 1453t–1458t
  spectrum of activity, 1459t–1463t,
    1468
  structure, 1465f
  treatment of
    acute bacterial meningitis, 275–276,
      543, 725
    acute bacterial meningitis in
      neonates, 543
    acute bacterial sinusitis, 230
    eye infections, 1496t
    fever without localizing signs, 116
    H. influenzae biogroup *aegyptius*, 907
    Haemophilus influenzae, 904–905
    Leptospira infections, 951
    Neisseria gonorrhoeae infections, 746
    neonatal infections, 538, 542
    Salmonella infections, 818t
    Streptococcus pneumoniae infections,
      724–725
Cefotetan
  clinical uses, 1467–1468
  spectrum of activity, 1459t–1463t,
    1467–1468
Cefoxitin
  clinical uses, 1467–1468
  dosage, 1445t–1452t, 1480t–1483t
  Neisseria gonorrhoeae infection treatment,
    747
  pharmacology, 1453t–1458t
  spectrum of activity, 1459t–1463t,
    1467–1468
  surgical site infection prevention, 587
Cefpodoxime
  dosage, 1445t–1452t, 1480t–1483t
  Neisseria gonorrhoeae infections, 747
  pharmacology, 1453t–1458t
  spectrum of activity, 1459t–1463t
Cefpodoxime proxetil, acute bacterial
    sinusitis, 229t
Cefprozil
  dosage, 1445t–1452t, 1480t–1483t
  pharmacology, 1453t–1458t
  treatment of
    acute bacterial sinusitis, 229t, 230
    acute otitis media, 218, 219t
Ceftazidime, 227
  dosage, 1445t–1452t, 1480t–1483t
  dose adjustment
    burned patients, 1437t
    renal failure, 1445t–1452t
  pharmacology, 1453t–1458t
  spectrum of activity, 1459t–1463t,
    1468

treatment of
  acute mastoiditis, 225–226
  eye infections, 1496t
  infections in HSCT recipients, 565
Ceftibuten
  dosage, 1480t–1483t
  pharmacology, 1453t–1458t
  spectrum of activity, 1459t–1463t
Ceftizoxime
  dosage, 1480t–1483t
  Neisseria gonorrhoeae infection treatment,
    747
  pharmacology, 1453t–1458t
  spectrum of activity, 1459t–1463t
Ceftobiprole, spectrum of activity,
    1459t–1463t
Ceftriaxone
  adverse effects, 277
  chemoprophylactic use, 70t–71t, 72
  dosage, 1445t–1452t, 1480t–1483t
  fatal hemolysis due to, 1403–1404
  Neisseria meningitidis infection
    prophylaxis, 69, 739
  pharmacology, 1453t–1458t, 1468
  spectrum of activity, 1459t–1463t,
    1468
  structure, 1465f
  susceptibility testing, 1416
  treatment of
    acute bacterial meningitis, 275–277,
      725
    acute bacterial sinusitis, 230
    acute otitis media, 217–218
    brain abscess and subdural empyema,
      328–329
    endocarditis, 262t–263t, 1418t–1419t
    epididymitis, 367
    eye infections, 1496t
    fever without localizing signs, 116
    Haemophilus ducreyi, 907
    Haemophilus influenzae, 904–905
    Haemophilus influenzae biogroup
      aegyptius, 907
    Neisseria gonorrhoeae infections, 489,
      745
    ophthalmia neonatorum, 489
    Salmonella infections, 818, 818t
    Shigella infections, 822, 822t
    Streptococcus pneumoniae infections,
      724–725
    vulvovaginitis, 358
Cefuroxime
  dosage, 1445t–1452t, 1480t–1483t
  pharmacology, 1453t–1458t
  spectrum of activity, 1459t–1463t
  treatment of
    acute bacterial sinusitis, 229t,
      230
    acute otitis media, 218, 219t
    Borrelia burgdorferi (Lyme disease),
      955–956
    eye infections, 1496t
    preseptal cellulitis due to sinusitis,
      510
Celiac disease
  abdominal pain, 176
  chronic hepatitis, 407
Cell adhesion molecules, 85, 85f

Cell culture
  Chlamydia trachomatis see *Chlamydia
    trachomatis*
  for specific viruses, 1386t
    HSV, 351, 1388
  virus isolation, 1385–1387, 1386t
Cell-mediated immunity, 45–46, 89–90,
    626–627
  acquired rubella infection, 1113
  Blastomyces dermatitidis, 1235
  CMV infections, 1045
  deficiency/defects, 626–633
    pathogens associated, 569t
    persistent/recurrent pneumonia,
      251
    pneumonia, 238, 253, 253t
  disorders, 626
  functions, 626–627
  HHV-6 infections, 1053
  Histoplasma capsulatum, 1224
  HSV infections, 1027
  human parainfluenza virus infections,
    1121
  Leishmania (leishmaniasis), 1286,
    1288–1289
  in respiratory tract, 238
  see also T lymphocytes
Cell wall
  Staphylococcus aureus, 676
  Streptococcus pyogenes, 698
  see also Bacteria, cell wall
Cellulitis, 434–435
  Aeromonas causing, 830–831
  anaerobic see Anaerobic cellulitis
  breast abscess causing, 457
  buccal (*H. influenzae*), 902–903, 903f
  Capnocytophaga canimorsus causing, 881
  Clostridium causing, 461, 980t
  etiology, 434–435
  eyelid, *Bacillus anthracis* causing, 509
  facial, 434–435, 902–903, 903f
  Haemophilus influenzae type b (Hib)
    causing, 434–435, 902–903, 903f
  limb pain, 187
  necrotizing, *Streptococcus pyogenes* (group
    A streptococcus), 701f
  orbital (postseptal) see Orbit, cellulitis
  Pasteurella multocida causing, 837f
  pathogens causing, 144t
  perianal, in cancer, 578–579
  periorbital see Periorbital cellulitis
  preseptal see Preseptal cellulitis
  secondary infections in varicella, 1037
  Staphylococcus aureus causing, 434–435,
    678–679
  Streptococcus causing, 434–435
  Streptococcus pneumoniae causing,
    434–435, 510
  Streptococcus pyogenes (group A
    streptococcus), 434–435, 701f
  trauma causing, 514
  treatment, 1418t–1419t
  Trichophyton causing, 509
Cellulose tape method, 1383
Cellulosimicrobium (*Oerskovia*), 771
Cellulosimicrobium funkei (*Oerskovia
    xanthineolytica*), 771
CEM-15, 1167

Centers for Disease Control and Prevention (CDC), 69
  antiparasitic agent availability, 1518
  chronic fatigue syndrome definition, 1007, 1013t
  Clostridium botulinum management, 399
  congenital syphilis case definition and evaluation, 945
  diphtheria antitoxin source, 757
  hand hygiene guidelines, neonatal nosocomial infection prevention, 554
  Healthcare Infection Control Practice Advisory Committee, 13
  influenza vaccine recommendation, 1156
  information sources on vaccines, 68
  Listeria monocytogenes infection rates, 763
  Malaria Hotline, 1303–1304
  Plasmodium infection prophylaxis, 1304
  PulseNet, 763
  recommendations on surveillance, 16
  sexually transmitted disease treatment, 803
  smallpox clinical features, 1021–1022, 1022t
  surveillance for vaccine-preventable diseases, 55
  tuberculin skin test recommendations, 773b
Centers for Disease Control and Prevention (CDC) enteric group, 804
Centers for Disease Control and Prevention (CDC) group JK *see Corynebacterium jeikeium*
Centers for Disease Control and Prevention (CDC) group M1 *see Kingella kingae*
Central line associated bloodstream infections (CLABSIs), 10–12, 265, 553
  in cancer, 573–574
    pathogens, 573–574
    risk, antibiotics due to, 573–574
  clinical features and diagnosis, 590–592, 591t
  complications, 593
  definition, 590
  infection rates
    by birthweight category, 12t
    by ICU type, 11t
  late-onset sepsis in neonates, 549
  management and outcome, 592–593, 592t
  mortality, 593
  neonatal, 549, 553
    Candida, 553
    clinical features, 551
    coagulase-negative staphylococci, 553
    Enterobacteriaceae, 554
    management, 549–550, 553–554
    persistent infections, 554
    polymicrobial, 554
    prevention, 554–555
    S. aureus, 554
    with CVC removal, 554
    without CVC removal, 554
  pathogens, 580t, 589
  prevention, 593–594, 594b
  removal, neonates, 554

risk factors
    catheter, 589–590
    host actors, 590
  sepsis, causes, 97–98
  terminology, 589
  see also Central venous catheter (CVC)-related infections; Intravascular catheters
Central nervous system (CNS)
  anomalies, recurrent meningitis, 287, 289
  bacterial invasion, 273
  Bordetella pertussis infection complications, 870
  defects, congenital rubella with, 1115–1116
  in HIV infection, 653–654, 653t, 654f
  trauma, hypotonia, 181t
Central nervous system (CNS) devices
  infections, 596–597, 597b
    clinical features and diagnosis, 597
    management and outcome, 597
    prevention, 597
  malfunction, infections, 597
Central nervous system (CNS) features
  hemophagocytic lymphohistiocytosis, 105–106
  lymphocytic choriomeningitis virus infection, 1162, 1162f
  Plasmodium infection, 1299
Central nervous system (CNS) infections, 272–279
  adenoviruses, 1068t, 1069
  anaerobic cocci, 989
  anaerobic gram-negative bacilli (AGNB), 983–984
  Aspergillus, 1204–1205, 1205f
  Blastomyces dermatitidis (blastomycosis), 1234, 1236–1238, 1238t
  Brucella, 863
  in burns patients, 519
  in cancer, 579
  Candida, 1198, 1198f
  CMV, 1045–1047, 1047t
  EBV, 1061
  enteroviruses, 1175–1176, 1179
  Escherichia coli, 797
  focal suppurative infections, 319–330
    bacterial, 319–321
    clinical features, 322–324, 323t
    complications and prognosis, 329–330
    differential diagnosis, 323t, 324–325
    epidemiology, 321
    etiology, 319–321, 320t
    etiology by site, 321t
    fungal, 319
    imaging, 325–327, 326f
    laboratory tests and diagnosis, 325–327
    management, 327–329, 329t
    risk factors, 319
    see also Brain abscess; Subdural empyema
  HHV-6 (roseola), 1054–1056
  in HIV infection, 653–654, 653t, 654f, 661
  HSV, 1030, 1034

Listeria monocytogenes see Listeria monocytogenes
  mucormycosis, 1214
  mumps virus, 1126–1127
  Mycoplasma pneumoniae, 994t, 995
  neonatal, viral, 547
  Pseudomonas aeruginosa, 844t, 846
  Schistosoma (schistosomiasis), 1370
  in sickle-cell disease, 634–635
  slow infections *see* Prion diseases
  Staphylococcus aureus, 683–684
Central venous catheter (CVC), 589
  antimicrobial coatings, 594
  classification/types, 589
  insertion, infection prevention, 593
Central venous catheter (CVC)-related infections, 589
  antibiotic-impregnated, 588–589, 594
  in cancer, neutropenia and infections, 568
  clinical features, 590–592, 591t
  coagulase-negative staphylococcal infections, 691–692
  complications, 593
  diagnosis, 590–592
  endocarditis, 257
  hematopoietic stem cell transplant recipients, 562–563
  invasive *Candida* infections, 1202
    treatment, 1200
  management and outcome, 592–593, 592t
  mortality, 593
  neonatal, 547, 592–593
    signs, 551
  nontuberculous mycobacterial infections, 786–787, 792
  osteomyelitis treatment, 472
  pathogens, 589, 589b
  prevention, 588–589, 593–594, 594b
  removal, 592–593
  risk reduction, 588–589
  sepsis, 97–98
  Staphylococcus aureus infections, 684
  Staphylococcus epidermidis infections, 691–692
  systemic *Malassezia* infections, 1216–1218
  thrombin sheath formation, *Candida* role, 1202
  thrombosis, 593
    detection, 593
  see also Central line associated bloodstream infections (CLABSIs); Intravascular catheters
Centrifugation, specimens in viral infections, 1386
Cephalexin
  dosage, 1445t–1452t, 1480t–1483t
  pharmacology, 1453t–1458t
  spectrum of activity, 1459t–1463t
Cephalosporin(s), 1467–1468
  antipseudomonal, 846
  bite wound infection, 526
  clinical uses, 1467
  dosage, 1480t–1483t
    in renal failure, 1445t–1452t
  fifth-generation, 1459t–1463t, 1468

first-generation, 1453t–1463t, 1467
    GAS pharyngitis treatment, 204, 204t
    Staphylococcus aureus infections, 686
fourth-generation, 1453t–1463t, 1468
peritonitis prevention, 419
pharmacodynamics, 1414t
pharmacology, 1453t–1458t
resistance
    Enterococcus, 714–715
    Neisseria gonorrhoea infections, 743
second-generation, 1453t–1463t,
    1467–1468
    abdominal trauma-related infections,
      514
spectrum of activity, 1459t–1463t,
    1467–1468
third-generation, 1453t–1463t, 1468
    Actinobacillus actinomycetemcomitans
      infections, 940
    acute bacterial meningitis treatment,
      276–277
    after abdominal trauma, 514
    exposure, impact on infection rate, 12
    Haemophilus influenzae infections, 904
    infants with fever without localizing
      signs, 116
    infections in neutropenia in cancer,
      571
    meningococcal meningitis, 736–737
    urinary tract infection, 341
treatment of, 1467–1468
    bacteremic periorbital cellulitis, 510
    bacterial keratitis, 497–498
    chronic mastoiditis, 227
    GAS pharyngitis, 204, 921
    Neisseria gonorrhoeae infections, 745
    nosocomial neonatal infections, 552
    urinary tract infection, 341
Cephalosporin (nitrocefin) method, 1381
Cephalosporinase, *Bacillus anthracis*,
    752–753
Cephalothin, spectrum of activity,
    1459t–1463t
Cephamycins, 1467–1468
Cephapirin, spectrum of activity,
    1459t–1463t
Cephradine
    dosage, 1480t–1483t
    pharmacology, 1453t–1458t
    spectrum of activity, 1459t–1463t
Cercariae, 1256, 1365
    Fasciola, 1366
    intestinal trematodes, 1363
Cerebellar abscess
    etiology, 320
    see also Brain abscess
Cerebellar ataxia
    acute, 316
    in kuru and CJD, 334
    in varicella, 1037–1038
Cerebellar disease, site, ataxia and, 180
Cerebellar dysfunction, ataxia due to, 180
Cerebellar herniation, meningitis, 273
Cerebellitis, 316, 316f
    acute, 180t, 316
    etiology, 314t, 316
    management, 316
    postinfectious, 180t

Cerebral abscess *see* Brain abscess
Cerebral aspergillosis, 1204–1205, 1205f
Cerebral cortex, vacuolation, 335f, 336
Cerebral edema
    encephalitis complication, 312–313
    Plasmodium infections, 1303
Cerebral herniation, lumbar puncture
    before, 178
Cerebral infarction, *Mycobacterium*
    tuberculosis infection, 777
Cerebral mucormycosis, 1214
Cerebral paragonimiasis, 1367–1368
Cerebritis, 325
Cerebrospinal fluid (CSF)
    analysis/features in
      Acanthamoeba infection, 1295t,
        1296–1297
      Borrelia infections, 958
      Coccidioides immitis
        (coccidioidomycosis), 1242–1244
      congenital syphilis, 943–944
      cryptococcal meningitis, 1222
      Ehrlichia and *Anaplasma* infections,
        895–896
      encephalitis, 308, 312
      focal suppurating CNS infections,
        325
      in Guillain–Barré syndrome, 319
      hemophagocytic lymphohistiocytosis,
        105–107
      herpes simplex encephalitis,
        1030–1031
      HHV-6 infection, 1055
      latent syphilis, 942
      Leptospira infections, 951
      meningitis diagnosis *see below*
      Mycoplasma hominis infections,
        998–999
      Mycoplasma pneumoniae infections,
        993
      Naegleria fowleri, 1294–1295, 1295t
      neonatal meningitis, 542
      neonatal nosocomial infection
        diagnosis, 551–552
      rabies, 1147
      recurrent meningitis, 290–291
      subacute sclerosing panencephalitis,
        1142–1143
      Taenia solium neurocysticercosis,
        1354
      Toxoplasma gondii infection, 1314
      Trypanosoma (Trypanozoon) brucei
        infection, 1321–1322
      Trypanosoma cruzi infections, 1325
      tuberculous meningitis, 777–778
      Ureaplasma urealyticum, 1001
      VZV infections, 1040
    antimicrobial agent penetration,
      1416–1417, 1453t–1458t
    bacterial antigen detection, 1377
    in bacterial meningitis pathogenesis,
      273
    culture, 1377
      head trauma and, 515
      Neisseria meningitidis, 736
      neonatal infection diagnosis, 542
    eosinophilia, 285, 332–333
      see also Eosinophilia

eosinophilic pleocytosis, 332–333
glucose
    meningitis diagnosis, 274
    Naegleria fowleri, 1294–1295
Haemophilus influenzae capsular
    polysaccharide, 904
Haemophilus influenzae detection,
    903–904
leak
    clinical features, 290
    diagnosis, 291
    head trauma and, 515
    management, 292
    meningitis associated, 273, 273t
    recurrent meningitis, 287–290
leukocytes
    chronic meningitis, 280, 285t
    congenital syphilis, 943–944
    herpes simplex encephalitis,
      1030–1031
    mumps virus infection, 1127
lumbar drainage, *Cryptococcus* meningitis,
    1223
lymphocytic pleocytosis, 280, 285
in meningitis diagnosis, 274
    acute bacterial meningitis, 274–275,
      275t, 277
    Borrelia, 281
    chronic meningitis, 279, 285–286,
      286t
    Cryptococcal infections, 282
    Histoplasma infections, 282
    syphilis, 281
    tuberculous, 280
meningococcal antigen in, 736
neutrophilic pleocytosis, 285, 325
otorrhea, 287, 291
    management, 292
    recurrent meningitis, 287, 290
PCR
    acute bacterial meningitis diagnosis,
      274
    HSV infections, 1388
pleocytosis, 325
    aseptic meningitis, 296
    in CJD, 338
    encephalitis, 312
    enterovirus infections, 1175–1176
    eosinophilic meningitis, 332
    mumps virus infection, 1127
    VZV infections, 1040
    in X-linked agammaglobulinemia,
      610–611
protein
    aseptic meningitis, 296
    in CJD, 338
    encephalitis, 312
    meningitis diagnosis, 274
pseudocyst, 416
red blood cells, HSV encephalitis,
    1030
rhinorrhea, 287, 291
    management, 292
    recurrent meningitis, 287, 290
specimen collection/transport, 1373,
    1374t, 1376–1377
    refrigeration, 1376–1377
treponemes in, 942

Cerebrospinal fluid (CSF) fistula
  diagnosis, 291
  recurrent meningitis risk, 287, 288f
  repair, 292
Cerebrospinal fluid (CSF) shunt, infections
  management, 693
  meningitis associated, 683
  Staphylococcus aureus infections, 683–684
  Staphylococcus epidermidis causing, 693
  see also Ventriculoperitoneal shunt
Cerebrovascular accident
  infant botulism *vs.*, 974t
  in sickle-cell disease, 635
Cerium nitrate, burns treatment,
  1500t–1501t
Cerumen, 220–221
Cervical cancer, HPV association *see* Human
  papillomavirus (HPV)
Cervical cytology, 1071–1074, 1072t
Cervical ectopy, 363, 363f
Cervical lymph nodes, 136–137
  anterior cervical, infections/pathogens,
    145t
  biopsy, 145–146
    contraindications, 145–146
    guidelines, 144, 146b
    staining, 145–146
  characteristics, 144t
    by pathogen and mode of onset,
      144t–145t
  deep, 136–137, 136f–137f, 136t
    infections/pathogens, 145t
    inferior, 136t, 137, 148–149
    superior, 136–137, 136t
  deep lateral (spinal accessory) chain, 136
  groups and area drained, 136t
  infections by specific nodes, 145t
  lymphatic flow, 136–138
  palpable in normal children, 158
  "posterior", 136
    infections/pathogens, 145t
  superficial, 136, 136f, 136t
  superficial anterior, 136
  surgical excision, 146
  see also Lymph nodes
Cervical lymphadenitis, 135–147, 146b
  acute, 144t
    causes, 136
  acute bacterial, management, 147t
  acute bilateral, 144
    causes, 138–139
    diagnosis, 144
  acute unilateral, 138
    causes, 139–140, 139t
    diagnosis, 143
  age-specific causes, 135t, 136
  asymptomatic, diagnosis, 144
  characteristics, by pathogen and mode of
    onset, 144t–145t
  chronic, 144t
  complications, 147
  definition, 135
  diagnosis, 143–146
  epidemiology, 135–136
  Haemophilus aphrophilus causing,
    907–908
  infectious causes, 138–141
  lymph nodes involved, 136–137

  management, 146, 147t, 791
    abscess drainage, 146
    surgical and long-term, 146
  needle aspiration, 144–145
  nonspecific lymphoid hyperplasia, 135
  nontuberculous mycobacteria causing,
    789, 791
  subacute, 144t
  subacute/chronic unilateral, 140–141
  suppurative, 144t
  see also Cervical lymphadenopathy
Cervical lymphadenopathy, 135
  in acute bacterial sinusitis, 228
  acute epiglottitis, 210
  Bartonella henselae infection, 159f
  complications, 147
  diagnostic approach, 143–146
  diseases and organisms causing,
    131t–132t
  epidemiology, 135–136
  infectious etiology, 135–136, 138–141
    age-specific, 135t
  inherited immunodeficiency syndromes,
    134
  Kawasaki disease, 1003
  management, 146
    bacterial infections, 147t
    drainage, 146
  noninfectious causes, 135, 141–142,
    142t
  nonspecific reactive hyperplasia, 135
  reactive, 135
  see also Cervical lymphadenitis; Neck,
    masses
Cervicitis, 361–363
  bacterial vaginitis and, 361
  clinical features, 362
  coinfection with vulvovaginitis, 359
  complications, 363
  diagnosis, 362
  epidemiology, 361–362
  etiology, 361–362
  gonococcal, 744
  mucopurulent, 362
    Chlamydia trachomatis, 889
  treatment, 362, 362t
Cervicofacial syndrome, *Nocardia* causing,
  794
Cervix
  cytology, 1071–1074, 1072t
  screening, in HIV infection, 672
  in *Trichomonas vaginalis* infections, 1318
  ulcerative lesions, *Schistosoma* infections,
    1369
Cesarean section, elective, HIV transmission
  prevention, 645–646
Cestodes, 1256, 1256t, 1347–1350,
  1362–1363
  infections in refugee and internationally
    adopted children, 35–36, 35t
  pseudophyllidean, 1347
  see also Tapeworms; *individual cestodes*;
    individual cestodes (listed page 1228)
CH50 assay, 291
Chagas disease *see Trypanosoma*
  (Schizotrypanum) cruzi
Chalazion, 508
  blepharitis complication, 493

Chancre
  differential diagnosis, 1321
  Treponema pallidum (primary syphilis),
    348, 942
  Trypanosoma, 1320
Chancroid *see Haemophilus ducreyi*
Charcot–Leyden crystals, 1328, 1331
  phaeohyphomycosis, 1211
CHARGE syndrome, 627–629, 628t
Chédiak–Higashi syndrome, 104, 104t,
  604t–605t, 620, 626
  characteristics, 619t
  clinical features, 621t, 626
  complications of infections, 620t
  generalized lymphadenopathy, 134
  infection management, 626
  infection prevention, 624
  infections associated, 620t, 626
Chemokines, 84, 90
  CC and CXC types, 1166
  encoded by NFκB-regulated gene, 94
  HHV-6 infection, 1053
  in inflammatory response, 94
  receptors, HIV coreceptors, 1166
Chemoprophylaxis, 68–76
  antiviral agents, 1507t
  benefits, 69
  in burns, 1499–1500, 1500t–1501t
  in children predisposed to infections,
    73–76, 74t
  definition, 68
  general, 68–69
  general principles/criteria, 69
  in healthy children, specific pathogens,
    69–72, 70t–71t
  pneumonia in immunocompromised
    patients, 256
  recommendations for, 68
  sexually transmitted infections, 72
  in special situations, 73–76
  specific *vs* general type, 68–69
  for surgical procedures, 72–73
  for trauma, 73
  tympanostomy tube placement, 1498
  see also individual drugs and infections
Chemotactic factors, released by *Blastomyces
  dermatitidis*, 1235
Chemotaxis, 85, 85f
  defects, 85
Chemotherapy
  effect on immune response, 569
  effect on normal flora, 569
  HLH treatment, 107
  intravascular catheter-related infections,
    590
  mucositis, 577–578
  neutropenia
    bacterial infections, 568
    see also Neutropenia, fever in
  pneumonia associated, 253
  see also Cancer, infections in
CHER trial, 666
Chest CT, fever of unknown origin, 117–118
Chest pain, 188–190
  cardiac causes, 189
  causes, 189b, 190t
  miscellaneous causes, 189–190
  musculoskeletal causes, 188–189

pleural, in pneumonia, 242
pleuritic, *Paragonimus* infections, 1367
precordial, pericarditis, 269–270
pulmonary causes, 189
Chest radiographs
    Aspergillus infections, 1205, 1207
    Blastomyces dermatitidis (blastomycosis), 1235f, 1236
    bronchiolitis, 233, 234f
    Coccidioides immitis (coccidioidomycosis), 1241f, 1242
    cystic fibrosis, 640f
    diskitis diagnosis, 484
    Histoplasma capsulatum (histoplasmosis), 1225f, 1226, 1227f
    infections in neutropenia with cancer, 570
    Mycobacterium tuberculosis, 151f–152f, 774f–776f, 785
        refugee and internationally adopted children, 34
    Mycoplasma pneumoniae infections, 996, 996f
    necrotizing pneumonia, 244, 244f
    Paragonimus infections, 1367, 1367f
    pericarditis, 270
    pleural effusions, 242, 242f, 244f
    Pneumocystis jirovecii (carinii) pneumonia, 1231, 1231f
    pneumonia, 239f
        in immunocompromised patients, 254, 256t
Chest wall lesions, *Aggregatibacter actinomycetemcomitans*, 939–940
Cheyne–Stokes respiration, 171
CHH syndrome *see* Cartilage hair hypoplasia (CHH) syndrome
Chikungunya virus, 1097–1098
    arthritis, 481
    maternal infection and transmission to neonate, 546
    transmission, 546
ChILD, 251
Child abuse, sexual *see* Sexual abuse
Childcare
    arrangements, 10–13
        number of facilities, 24
    group *see* Group childcare, infections associated
Children
    cervical lymphadenopathy diagnosis, 144
    group care *see* Group childcare, infections associated
    immunization, catch-up schedule, 49f
    immunization schedule, 49f
    see also specific topics
Chilomastix mesnili, 1279
Chinese paralytic syndrome, 877
Chlamydia
    chronic fatigue syndrome pathogenesis, 1008t–1009t
    detection methods, specimens, 1385
    endocarditis due to, 260t
    pneumonia, clinical features, 167–168, 167t
Chlamydia pneumoniae see Chlamydophila (Chlamydia) pneumoniae

Chlamydia psittaci see Chlamydophila (Chlamydia) psittaci
Chlamydia trachomatis, 883–889
    antibodies to, 488, 1398
    Bordetella pertussis infections *vs.*, 886
    cell culture methods, 887, 1398
        as gold standard test, 354
        in urethritis, 354–355
    chemoprophylaxis, 70t–71t
    classification, 884
    clinical manifestations, 885–887
    complications and sequelae, 889
    conjunctivitis due to, 885–886, 885f
        inclusion, 159, 885–886, 885f
        inclusion, in adolescents, 494
        Neisseria gonorrhoeae vs., 488t, 884
        neonatal *see Chlamydia trachomatis, ophthalmia neonatorum*
        treatment, 888
    contract tracing and treatment, 888
    cough due to, 167–168, 167t
    cytoplasmic inclusions, 884, 887–888
    diagnosis/detection, 240, 385t, 488, 1398–1399
        antigen detection, 1398
        cell culture, 1398
        comparison of methods, 1399
        DNA probes, 1398
        methods, 1398–1399
        nucleic acid amplification, 354–355, 362, 364–365, 370, 488, 887
        optimal tests, 1389t–1392t
        PCR, 1399
        in pelvic inflammatory disease, 364–365
        rapid "point-of-care" tests, 1398
        serologic tests, 1398
        specimen collection for nonculture tests, 1398
        specimen collection/transport, 1398
        in suspected child abuse, 353–355, 362, 364–365
        in urethritis, 354–355
        in vulvovaginitis, 357
        see also Laboratory diagnosis (below)
    elementary body (EB), 884, 884f
        detection, 1398
    endocervicitis due to, 361–362
    endometritis due to, 886
    eosinophilia due to, 1408t–1409t
    epidemiology, 353, 363–364, 884–885, 885t
    epididymitis due to, 367, 889
    Fitz-Hugh–Curtis syndrome (acute perihepatitis), 886
    genital discharge/dysuria syndrome, 346
    genital infections, diagnosis, 1389t–1392t
    genital ulcers with lymphadenopathy, 348–349, 350t
    immune evasion, 884
    immune response to, 884
    incubation period, 884, 886
    infection route, 884
    infertility due to, 886, 886f, 889
    intracellular inclusions, detection, 1398
    laboratory diagnosis, 887–888
        cell culture, 887

direct fluorescent antibody assays (DFAs), 887
    nonculture tests, 887–888
    nucleic acid amplification, 354–355, 362, 488, 887
    specimens, 351t, 887
    see also Diagnosis/detection (above)
    leukocyte esterase (LE) urine test, 887
    life cycle and replication, 884, 884f
    lymphogranuloma venereum (LGV) due to, 129, 349, 887
        clinical features, 350t, 887
        epidemiology, 347
        genital ulcers/lymphadenopathy, 348
        serovars associated, 884, 887
        treatment, 350t, 889
    major outer membrane protein (MOMP), 883
    microbiology, 883
    natural course of infections, 884, 886
    Neisseria gonorrhoeae coinfection, 745, 747
    neonatal infections
        diagnosis, 1389t–1392t
        ocular *see Chlamydia trachomatis, ophthalmia neonatorum*
    oculogenital disease, 886
        serovars associated, 884
        treatment, 888–889
    ophthalmia neonatorum, 487–488, 488t, 885
        diagnosis, 488
        pneumonia after, 488
        preauricular lymphadenopathy, 159
        prevention, 490
        treatment, 488
    outer membrane, 883
    pathogenesis, 884
    pelvic inflammatory disease due to, 173, 346t, 348, 363–364, 366, 886, 889
    perinatal infections, 885
        prevention, 889
        treatment, 888
    persistence, 885
    pneumonia *see* Pneumonia
    pregnancy and, 886–887
        PCR, 886–887
    prevention, 70t–71t, 889
    proctitis and proctocolitis due to, 886–887
    prostatitis due to, 369
    reinfection, 887
    Reiter syndrome due to, 886, 889
    reticulate body (RB), 884, 884f
    salpingitis due to, 886
    screening for, 887, 889
        pelvic inflammatory disease prevention, 366
    serological tests, 887–888
    serovars, 884
    serovars L1, L2, L3, genital ulcers with lymphadenopathy, 348–349
    sexual abuse, 370–371
    sexual transmission, diagnosis, 1389t–1392t
    sexually transmitted infection, 346–347
        anal discharge/proctitis syndrome, 347

discharge/dysuria syndrome, 346
pelvic inflammatory disease, 346t, 348
screening, 346
scrotal pain, 346t, 348–349
urethritis, 353
trachoma due to, 494, 887
oculoglandular syndrome in, 159
pannus formation and scarring, 887
prevention and WHO's SAFE program, 889
serovars associated, 884
treatment, 494, 889
transmission routes, 884
treatment of infections, 888–889, 888t
empiric treatment, 72
urethritis due to, 347, 353, 355, 886
diagnosis, 354
follow-up, 355–356
management, 355–356
vaccines, 889
vaginitis due to, 886
vulvovaginitis due to, 356–357
management, 358
Chlamydiaceae, 673
Chlamydophila, 881
laboratory diagnosis, 1398–1399
Chlamydophila (Chlamydia) pneumoniae, 881–883
acute bronchitis due to, 213
acute infections, epidemiology, 881–882
acute otitis media due to, 882
acute sinusitis due to, 882
antibiotic susceptibility, 883
antibodies to (IgM and IgG), 882–883, 1399
atherosclerotic heart disease and, 882
biovar TWAR, 881, 1389t–1392t
biovars, 883
classification, 881
clinical manifestations, 882, 882t
colonization, 881–882
complications, 883
cough due to, 865
diagnosis/detection, 240, 1399
optimal tests, 1389t–1392t
diseases associated, 882, 882t
elementary body and reticulate body, 881
epidemics, 882
epidemiology, 881–882
genome, 881
growth and culture, 883
laboratory diagnosis, 882–883
microbiology, 881
persistent infections, 883
pharyngitis due to, 199
pneumonia due to, 169–170, 236–237, 239–240, 239f, 882
replication, 881
shedding, 882
in sickle-cell disease, 634
staining with monoclonal antibodies, 883
transmission, 882
group childcare and, 27
treatment of infections, 883

Chlamydophila (Chlamydia) psittaci, 889–891
antibiotic susceptibility, 891
clinical manifestations, 890, 890b, 890f
diagnosis, 890–891, 1398
optimal tests, 1389t–1392t
epidemiology, 890, 890f
microbiology, 889–890, 890f
outbreaks, 890
pneumonia due to, 237, 237t, 890
persistent pneumonia, 245–246
transmission, 890
treatment, 891
Chloramphenicol, 1425
adverse effects, 277, 928–929
distribution, 1416–1417
dosage, 1445t–1452t, 1480t–1483t
mechanism of action, 1425
pharmacology, 1453t–1458t
resistance to, 275–276, 1422t, 1425
Salmonella Typhi, 816
treatment of
acute bacterial meningitis, 277
Bartonella bacilliformis, 940
Ehrlichia and *Anaplasma* infections, 896
eye infections, 1494t–1496t
meningococcal meningitis, 736
Rickettsia akari (rickettsialpox) infection, 934
Rickettsia felis infections, 933
Rickettsia infections, 938
Rickettsia prowazekii, 931
Rickettsia typhi (murine typhus), 932
Rocky Mountain spotted fever (*Rickettsia rickettsii*), 928–929
Salmonella infections, 818, 818t
Yersinia pestis infection, 827
Chlorhexidine
for central venous catheter insertion, CLABSI prevention, 593
skin antiseptic, 1499t
Staphylococcus aureus infection prevention, 689
treatment of burns, 1500t–1501t
Chlorhexidine gluconate (CHG), 555
Chloroquine
adverse effects, 1304
Plasmodium infections, 1301t–1303t, 1303–1304
failure rates, 1304
prophylaxis, 80–81, 1304, 1305t, 1520–1521
prophylaxis in pregnancy, 1306
resistance, *Plasmodium*, 1303–1304
Chocolate agar, 1375t
Cholangiocarcinoma, *Clonorchis* and *Opisthorchis* infections, 1365
Cholangitis, 412–414
ascending, liver transplant recipients, 557
chronic, 413
clinical/laboratory features, 413
diagnosis, 413
etiology, 412–413
microsporidia association, 1291–1292
pathogenesis, 412

sclerosing, 403
Cryptosporidium infections, 1270
Echinococcus granulosus cysts, 1360
treatment, 413
Cholecystitis, 412–414
acalculous, 412
in *Leptospira* infections, 950–951
acute
acute abdominal pain, 173
burns patients, 519
clinical/laboratory features, 413
diagnosis, 413
etiology, 412–413
pathogenesis, 412
treatment, 413
Cholecystography, 413
Choledochal cysts, 403
Cholelithiasis, acute abdominal pain, 173
Cholera see *Vibrio cholerae*
Cholestasis, intrahepatic, 1411
Cholestyramine, *Clostridium difficile* infections, 979
Chorea
in acute rheumatic fever, 703–704, 704t
Sydenham, 703–704
Chorioamnionitis
Capnocytophaga causing, 880
Chlamydia trachomatis causing, 886–887
early-onset neonatal GBS infections after, 708, 711
Ureaplasma urealyticum causing, 1000–1001
Chorioretinal lesions, *Candida*, 1199
Chorioretinal scar, 500f
Chorioretinitis, 499–503
Acanthamoeba, 1296
in chronic meningitis, 284t
CMV, transplant recipients, 558
toxoplasmic see *Toxoplasma gondii* (toxoplasmosis)
Treponema pallidum, 499
viral infections in neonates, 547–548
West Nile virus associated, 502, 1101
see also Retinitis
Choroid plexitis, 273, 295
Choroiditis
focal, 502–503
multifocal, 502–503
Chromista, 1268
Chromobacterium, 835–839
microbiology and epidemiology, 835–836
Chromobacterium violaceum, 835–836
clinical manifestations, 836–837
treatment of infections, 838–839
Chromosome 22, deletions (22q11.2 deletion syndrome), 631
Chronic disseminated candidiasis, 1199, 1199f
Chronic fatigue syndrome (CFS), 1007–1015
case definition (CDC), 1007, 1013t
case series, 1013t
chronic active EBV infection *vs.*, 1065
clinical manifestations, 1012–1013, 1012t
symptoms, 1012, 1012t
diagnosis/evaluation, 1013–1014
acknowledgment of condition, 1013–1015

alternative diagnosis, 1013b
psychological, 1014
tests, 1014b
when to suspect, 1013b
epidemiology, 1007–1008
etiology/pathogenesis, 1008–1012
cardiovascular physiology, 1008
connective tissue disease, 1008
genomics, 1011
hypothalamic-pituitary-adrenal axis,
1008–1010
immune dysfunction, 1008, 1010,
1010t, 1012
infectious agents, 1008, 1008t–1009t
Mycoplasma infections associated,
999
neurobiology and sleep, 1010–1011
psychology, 1011–1012, 1011t
viral, 1007–1008, 1008t–1009t, 1013
follow-up, 1015
management, 1013
activity, 1015
medical, 1014
psychological, 1014–1015
reassurance, 1015
outcome and natural history, 1013
pathogenic models, 1012
risk factors, 1013
subgroups, 1007
Chronic granulomatous disease (CGD), 85,
604t–605t, 619, 624–626
Burkholderia cepacia infections, 622f,
846–847, 847t
characteristics, 619t
Chromobacterium violaceum infections,
837
clinical features, 621t, 624
complications of infections, 620t,
621f–622f, 623
diagnosis/screening, 624
fungal infections, management, 622–624
fungal pneumonia, 622f, 624
gastrointestinal granulomatosis, 623f
generalized lymphadenopathy, 134
hepatic abscess, 624, 625f
imaging, 622f–623f, 625f
immunizations in, 52t–53t
infection management, 623
infections associated, 85, 251, 253, 620t
clinical manifestations, 624
invasive *Aspergillus* infection
galactomannan antigen test,
1207–1208
invasive pulmonary aspergillosis,
1203–1204, 1204f
invasive *Candida* infections, 1202
mediastinal lymphadenopathy, 155
osteomyelitis, 624
pathologic findings, 620, 621f
phagocytes action and defect, 624
pneumonia, 622f, 624
persistent/recurrent, 251, 253
prevention, 256
prevention, 624
prognosis and sequelae, 623–624
RSV infection, 1133
Serratia infections, 813
unilateral cervical lymphadenitis, 140

Chronic interstitial or diffuse lung diseases
of children (ChILD), 251
Chronic lymphocytic leukemia (CLL),
indication for IGIV, 40, 40t
Chronic mucocutaneous candidiasis, 1197
Chronic pulmonary aspergillosis, 1205
Chronic recurrent multifocal osteomyelitis
(CRMO), 186
Chronic suppurative otitis media (CSOM)
see Otitis media
Chryseobacterium, 832, 834
animal bites, 521–522
Chryseobacterium indologenes, 832
bloodstream infections, 834
*Chryseobacterium meningosepticum see
Elizabethkingia meningoseptica*
Chryseomonas luteola (Pseudomonas luteola),
841, 841t
Chrysops, 1345
Chylocele, filarial, 1343
Chyluria, *Wuchereria bancrofti* causing, 1343,
1344t
CIAS1 gene, 126
Cidofovir, 1508–1509
adverse effects, 1508
chemistry, 1508
clinical uses, 1508–1509
dosage, 1508–1509
mechanism of action, 1508
pharmacokinetics, 1508
resistance to, 1503t, 1508
spectrum of activity, 1508
treatment of
adenovirus infections, 1070
BC virus treatment, 1076
JC virus treatment, 1076–1077
smallpox, 1022–1023
zoonotic poxvirus infections, 1024
Ciguatera fish poisoning, 393, 396t, 397
management, 399
Cilastatin *see* Imipenem-cilastatin
Cilia, respiratory tract, 83–84
Ciliary dysfunction, 638
Ciliary dyskinesia, primary, 638
persistent/recurrent pneumonia,
250–251
Ciliary function, in paranasal sinuses, 227
Ciliophora, 1255
Cimetidine
PFAPA treatment, 123
Taenia solium neurocysticercosis,
1354–1355
CINCA syndrome, 126
Cinchonism, 1521
Ciprofloxacin, 1477
chemoprophylactic use, 70t–71t
Neisseria meningitidis infection, 69,
279, 739
clinical uses, 1477
dosage, 1445t–1452t, 1480t–1483t
pharmacology, 1453t–1458t, 1477
resistance to, 1427, 1477
spectrum of activity, 1459t–1463t
treatment of
Bacillus anthracis infections, 752–753
ear infections, 1496, 1497t
eye infections, 1494t–1496t
fever in neutropenia (in cancer), 572

Francisella tularensis infections,
898–899
Haemophilus ducreyi (chancroid), 907
infections in cystic fibrosis, 640
Klebsiella granulomatis infection, 803
Legionella infections, 925t
Mycoplasma hominis infections, 999
osteomyelitis, 472
Shigella infections, 387
travelers' diarrhea, 82
tuberculosis, 780t
Vibrio cholerae infection, 853
Circling disease of sheep, 765
Circulatory collapse, in *Leptospira* infections,
951
Circulatory congestion, in poststreptococcal
acute glomerulonephritis, 705–706
Circumcision, urinary tract infection
reduction, 339–340
Cirrhosis
HBV infection, 1079–1080
HCV infection, 1108, 1110
Indian childhood, 404
portal, *Clonorchis* and *Opisthorchis*
infections, 1365
Citilli abscess, 223
Citrobacter, 806–807
clinical manifestations, 806–807
epidemiology and pathogenesis, 806
meningitis due to, 806–807
plasmids and antibiotic resistance, 807
septicemia due to, 806–807
species and microbiology, 806
treatment of infections, 807
urinary tract infection, 807
Citrobacter amalonaticus, 806
Citrobacter braakii, 806
Citrobacter freundii, 806
antibiotic resistance, 807
outbreak, 806
Citrobacter koseri, 806
Citrobacter rodentium, 806
Citrobacter youngae, 806
CLABSI *see* Central line associated
bloodstream infections (CLABSIs)
Cladophialophora, 1211–1212
Cladosporium, chronic meningitis, 284t
Clarithromycin, 1471
chemoprophylactic use, 70t–71t, 72
dosage, 1445t–1452t, 1480t–1483t
pharmacology, 1453t–1458t
resistance, *Helicobacter pylori*, 914
spectrum of activity, 1459t–1463t,
1471
structure, 1470
treatment of, 1471
acute bacterial sinusitis, 229t
*Chlamydophila (Chlamydia)
pneumoniae* infections, 883
Helicobacter pylori treatment, 914
Legionella infections, 925t
Mycoplasma pneumoniae infections,
997
nontuberculous mycobacterial
infection, 792
Clavulanate
pharmacology, 1453t–1458t
structure, 1465f

Cleaning
   definition, 21
   prevention of HAIs, 13
Clearance, drug, 1434
Clindamycin
   adverse effects, 686, 1473
   chemoprophylactic use, 74t
   clinical uses, 1473
   Clostridium difficile infection associated
      with, 978
   distribution, 1417
   dosage, 1445t–1452t, 1480t–1483t
   mechanism of action, 686, 1473
   pharmacodynamic properties, 1414t
   pharmacology, 1453t–1458t
   resistance, 1426–1427, 1473
      community-associated MRSA
         (CA-MRSA), 686
      detection of, 1432, 1432f
      Staphylococcus aureus, 686
   spectrum of activity, 1459t–1463t
   treatment of
      acute mastoiditis, 225–226
      acute otitis media, 218
      acute pyogenic lymphadenitis, 160
      anaerobic gram-positive coccal
         infections, 989
      Babesia (babesiosis), 1265
      bacterial vaginosis, 360
      Clostridium perfringens, 982
      community-associated methicillin-
         resistant (CA-MRSA), 468
      dacryoadenitis, 508
      eye infections, 1496t
      Gardnerella vaginalis, 770
      GAS carrier management, 203–204
      group A streptococcal infections, 702
      infections in phagocyte disorders,
         624t
      lung abscess, 244
      necrotizing fasciitis, 514
      osteomyelitis, 472
      Plasmodium infections, 1300–1304,
         1301t–1303t
      Pneumocystis jirovecii (carinii)
         pneumonia, 1232t, 1233
      protozoan infections, 1522
      pyomyositis, 468
      skin infections, 1498t
      Staphylococcus aureus infections, 686
      Toxoplasma gondii infections,
         1314–1316, 1316t
Clinical Immunization Safety Assessment
   centers, 51
Clinical Laboratory Standards Institute
   (CLSI)
   acute otitis media treatment, 216t, 217
   antimicrobial susceptibility definitions,
      of *Streptococcus pneumoniae*, 724, 724t
   antimicrobial susceptibility testing, 1378,
      1381
   ESBL-producing *Enterobacter*, 805
   ESBL-producing *Klebsiella*, 801
Clinical Pulmonary Infection Score (CPIS),
   ventilator-associated pneumonia,
   582
Clioquinol, skin antiseptic, 1499t
Clitocybe, 397t

Clonorchis sinensis, 1365–1366
   acute pancreatitis, 411
   biliary obstruction, 412
Clostridium, 979–982
   antibiotic susceptibility, 966t
   appendicitis due to, 420
   cellulitis due to, 461, 980t, 982
   classification, 959t
   clinical manifestations, 980–981, 980t
   description and microbiology, 979
   diagnosis of infections, 981
   diseases associated, 980t
   food poisoning due to, 980, 982
      prevention/treatment, 982
   histotoxic infections, 980–981, 980t
      prevention/treatment, 982
   myonecrosis due to, 461
   necrotizing fasciitis due to, 463
   subcutaneous tissue infections, 460
   trimethoprim/sulfamethoxazole
      resistance, 1428
Clostridium baratii, 971
   toxin type F, 971
Clostridium bifermentans, 980
Clostridium botulinum (botulism), 970–977
   adult intestinal toxemia botulism,
      970–971
   antitoxin, 42, 971
   botulism immune globulin intravenous
      (BIG-IV), 975
   clinical manifestations, 973, 973t
   description and microbiology, 971
   diagnosis, 397, 974
      neurologic tests, 974
   differential diagnosis, 973–974, 974t
   epidemiology, 971–972
      environmental exposures, 971–972
      geographic distribution, 971–972,
         972f
   equine antitoxin, 975
   etiology and sources, 971
   foodborne botulism, 373, 394–395, 399,
      970–971, 976–977
      diagnosis, 397
   history and physical examination, 973
   hospital course of botulism, 974–975
   host susceptibility, 972
   iatrogenic botulism, 970–971
   immunity to, 972
   infant botulism, 970–971
      clinical features, 973t
      complications, 975, 975t
      diagnosis, 974
      epidemiology, 971
      fluid and electrolyte disorders, 975
      honey and corn syrup associated,
         971–972, 976
      hypotonia, 181t
      management, 975–976
      pathophysiology, 971, 972f
      progression, 973–975
      respiratory dysfunction, 974–976
      risk factors, 971–972
      sudden infant death syndrome, 973
      susceptibility, normal flora effect,
         961
   inhalational botulism, 970–971
   isolation and identification, 974

   management, 399, 975–976
      antimicrobial therapy, 975
      antitoxin therapy, 975
      nutrition, 976
      respiratory support, 975–976
   neurotoxins, 375, 971
      identification, 974
      mechanism of action, 971
      mouse bioassay, 974
      potency, 971
      type A, 971–972
      type B, 971
   outcome and prevention, 976
   spores, 971
      sources, 971
   susceptibility, normal flora effect,
      960–961
   transmission control, 976
   wound botulism, 970–971, 977
Clostridium butyricum, 959, 971
Clostridium difficile, 583–584, 977–979
   antibiotic resistance, 382
      fluoroquinolone resistance, 978
      metronidazole resistance, 1427
   antibiotics associated, 978, 979b
      clindamycin, 978
   in cancer, 578
   clinical manifestations, 584, 978
      acute abdominal pain, 174, 978
      diarrhea, 26t, 374, 584, 978, 979b
      diarrhea in cancer, 578
   colitis, 382
      diagnosis, 386
      in HIV infection, 382
      pathogenesis, 384
      susceptibility, normal flora effect,
         961
      see also Pseudomembranous colitis
   colonization, 977–978
      rates, 374
   culture media, 1376t
   cytokines released by, 384
   cytotoxin A, 384
   description and microbiology, 977
   diagnosis/detection, 584, 1378
      stool cultures, 376
   differential diagnosis, 978
   enterocolitis due to
      clindamycin and, 1473
      treatment, metronidazole, 1478
   epidemiology, 583–584, 977–978
   group childcare and, 25t
   in HIV infection, 662
   HSCT recipients, 563–564
   inflammatory enteritis, 383t
   intestinal flora, 960
   isolation and detection, 978
   neutropenia associated with cancer,
      567
   outcome, 585
   pathogenesis of infections, 382, 384,
      584, 962, 977
   pathology, 977
   prevention of infections, 585, 979
   profound neutrophilia due to,
      1404–1405
   relapses, 585
      treatment, 979, 979b

risk factors for, 978
spores, 977
   sporicidal cleaning agents, 979
toxigenic, overgrowth, 382
toxins, 584, 978
   detection, 1378
   neutralization, 1378
   toxin A, 584, 978
   toxin B, 584, 978
   types and actions, 384
transmission, 584–585, 979
treatment of infections, 578, 585, 966t,
   978–979, 979b
Clostridium histolyticum, 980
Clostridium novyi, 980
Clostridium perfringens
   abdominal pain due to, 981
   anaerobic cellulitis, 461
   antibiotic susceptibility, 966t
   bacteremia, 980t
   clinical manifestations, 980t, 981
   diagnosis of infections, 981
   food poisoning due to, 393–394, 394t,
      398t, 980, 982
      clinical features, 981
      differential diagnosis, 981
      treatment, 982
   gas gangrene due to, 980–981
      clinical features, 981
      diagnosis, 981
      treatment, 982
   histotoxic infections, 980–981
      clinical features, 980–981, 980t
   intestinal flora, 960
   pathogenesis of infections, 962
   prevention of infections, 982
   spores, 980–981
Clostridium perfringens type C, 393–394
Clostridium ramosum, 960, 981
Clostridium septicum, 962, 980
   anaerobic cellulitis due to, 461
   gas gangrene due to, 463
   neutropenia associated with cancer, 567,
      571
   septicemia due to, 980t, 981
      in cancer, 578
Clostridium sordellii, infections, 980
Clostridium tetani (tetanus), 966–970
   antitoxin level target, 969–970
   bite wound infection prevention, 525
   burn wound infections, 518
   elimination goal, 47
   exotoxins, 967
   immune globulin intravenous (IGIV),
      968–969, 969t
      infection prevention after trauma,
         512–513
   microbiology, 967
   myocarditis due to, 266
   pathogenesis, 967
   spores, 967
   tetanus
      antimicrobial drugs, 969, 969t
      causes, 967
      cephalic, 968
      clinical manifestations, 967–968
      complications, 969t
      diagnosis, 968

differential diagnosis, 968
epidemiology, 966–967
generalized, 967–968
localized, 968
morbidity reduced by vaccine, 48t
neonatal, 968
ophthalmoplegic, 968
prevalence reduced by vaccines, 47
prevention, 56, 969–970, 970t
time of injury to symptoms, 967
treatment and outcome, 968–969,
   969t
tetanus and diphtheria toxoids (Td), 45
   in pregnancy, 51–52
   shortage, 54
   see also Diphtheria, tetanus, and
      pertussis (DTP) vaccination/
      vaccines
tetanus antitoxin (TAT), 968–969, 969t
tetanus immune globulin (TIG), 37t,
   968–970
   burn wound infection prevention,
      518
   indications and dose, 39, 969t
tetanus prophylaxis, 969–970, 970t
   wound management, 56
tetanus toxoid, 39, 55, 759
   antigen content (US vaccines), 872,
      873t
   in vaccines, 55, 55t
      see also Diphtheria, tetanus, and
         pertussis (DTP) vaccination/
         vaccines
vaccination, 55–56, 525
   burn wound infection prevention,
      518
   infection prevention after trauma,
      512–513
   in pregnancy, 51–52
   see also Diphtheria, tetanus, and
      pertussis (DTP) vaccination/
      vaccines
Clostridium welchii see Clostridium perfringens
Clotrimazole, treatment of superficial
   infections, 1485, 1485t
Cloxacillin, spectrum of activity,
   1459t–1463t
Clue cells, 355f, 359–360
Clutton joints, 944
CMV *see* Cytomegalovirus (CMV)
CNS *see* Central nervous system (CNS)
Co-bedding, infection risk associated, 12
Co-trimoxazole *see*
   Trimethoprim-sulfamethoxazole
Coagulase, *Staphylococcus aureus*, 676
Coagulase-negative staphylococci *see*
   Staphylococcus (staphylococci)
Coagulation, activation, in sepsis, 98
Coagulopathy
   consumptive, *Plasmodium* infections,
      1299–1300
   Neisseria meningitidis infections, 736
Cobalamin, *Diphyllobothrium*
   (diphyllobothriasis), 1348
Cocci, 673
   anaerobic gram-negative, 960t
   anaerobic gram-positive *see* Anaerobic
      gram-positive cocci

gram-negative *see* Gram-negative cocci
gram-positive *see* Gram-positive cocci
Coccidian-like bodies, 1283
Coccidioides immitis (coccidioidomycosis),
   153, 1239–1245, 1245b
   antibodies, 1242–1243
   antigens and processing of, 1239–1240,
      1243
   arthritis due to, 482, 1242
   chronic pulmonary complications, 1241,
      1241f
   clinical manifestations, 1241–1242
   description and structure, 1239,
      1239f–1240f, 1245b
   diagnosis, 1242–1243, 1245b
      direct examination and culture,
         1242–1243
      serologic tests, 1243
      skin tests, 1243
   disseminated infection
      generalized lymphadenopathy, 130,
         131t–132t
      risk factors, 1242
   encephalitis, 303
   eosinophilia due to, 1408t–1409t
   eosinophilic meningitis due to, 331t,
      332
   epidemiology, 1240–1241, 1240f, 1245b
   extrapulmonary infections, 1242
      treatment recommendation, 1244
   in HIV infection, 1244–1245
   immune response to, 1239–1240
   immunity, 1239–1240
   incubation period, 1241
   laboratory testing, 308t–311t
   life cycle, 1239, 1239f
   mediastinal lymphadenitis due to,
      153–154
   meningitis due to, 280t, 282, 283t–284t,
      1242–1243
      diagnosis, 282
      eosinophilic meningitis, 331t, 332
      treatment, 1243–1245
   neonatal infection, 1242, 1245
   neutropenia associated with cancer, 567,
      571
   osteomyelitis due to, 1242
   pathogenesis, 1239
   persistent pneumonia due to, 246
   pneumonia due to, 237, 237t
   pneumonitis in cancer due to, 575
   poor prognosis, factors for, 1242b
   in pregnancy, 1242–1245
   prevention of infection, 1245
   primary pulmonary infection, 1241
      treatment recommendation,
         1243–1244
   recrudescence, 1244
   relapse and treatment failure, 1244
   risk factors for infection, 1239–1240,
      1242, 1244
   skin infections, 1242, 1242f
   solid-organ transplant recipients, 560
   spherules, 1239, 1239f–1240f,
      1242–1243
   treatment of infection, 1243, 1245b
      recommendations, 1243–1244
      surgical management, 1245

unilateral cervical lymphadenitis, 140
virulence, 1239
Coccidioides posadasii, 1239–1245, 1245b
epidemiology, 1239
microbiology, 1239
pathogenesis, 1239
see also Coccidioides immitis
(coccidioidomycosis)
Coccidioidomycosis *see Coccidioides immitis*;
Coccidioides posadasii
Coccobacilli, 674
gram-negative, 856–861, 939–941
Cochlear dysplasia, 288f
Cochlear implantation, 292
Streptococcus pneumoniae infections, 722
Coenurosis (*Taenia serialis*), 1362–1363,
1363f
Coenurus, 1362–1363, 1363f
Cognitive behavioral therapy (CBT), chronic
fatigue syndrome therapy, 1014–1015
Cognitive complications, *Entamoeba*
histolytica infections, 1276
Cognitive deficits, *Taenia solium*
neurocysticercosis, 1353–1354
Cohort studies, 3, 3t
disadvantages, 3, 3t
outbreak investigations, 7
prospective and retrospective, 3
vaccine efficacy, 7
COID (Committee on Infectious Diseases),
47
"Coin lesions", pulmonary dirofilariasis,
1346
Cokermyces, 1212–1213
Colchicine, familial Mediterranean fever,
125
Cold-agglutinating antibodies, 1411t–1412t
Mycoplasma pneumoniae, 995
Cold agglutinin test
Mycoplasma pneumoniae, 1399
pneumonia etiology determination,
240
Cold enrichment, *Listeria monocytogenes*
growth, 762
Cold shock, 98
Cold sores, 192
Colds *see* Common colds
Coliforms, in normal flora, 961
Colistimethate
dosage, 1480t–1483t
pharmacology, 1453t–1458t, 1469–1470
Colistin, 1469–1470
adverse effects, 1470
clinical uses, 1470
mechanism of action, 1426
pharmacodynamics, 1414t
resistance to, 1422t, 1425–1426, 1433
spectrum of activity, 1459t–1463t
treatment of ear infections, 1497t
Colistin–nalidixic acid agar, 1375t
Colitis
acute fulminant (necrotizing), 1275–
1276, 1275f
amebic *see* Amebic colitis (intestinal
amebiasis)
antimicrobial-associated, 382
see also Clostridium difficile
chronic, *Trichuris trichiura* causing, 1331

neutropenic, 390
pseudomembranous *see*
Pseudomembranous colitis
Shigella causing, 821
Trichuris, 1331
ulcerative, *Entamoeba histolytica* infection
vs., 1275
Colonic inflammation *see* Enteritis
Colonization
burns wound infections, 517–518
female genital tract, *Lactobacillus*, 769
gastric mucosa, *Helicobacter pylori*, 908
micro-organisms
Achromobacter xylosoxidans, 639
Aspergillus, 1203
Campylobacter jejuni, 875
Candida, 1201
Candida albicans, 192–194
Clostridium difficile, 374, 977–978
coagulase-negative staphylococci
(CONS), 690, 959
Entamoeba dispar, 1275
Entamoeba histolytica, 1274
Enterococcus, 713
Giardia intestinalis (giardiasis), 1279
gram-negative bacteria, 427
gram-positive bacteria, 427
Haemophilus influenzae, 273
Malassezia, 1216
Mycoplasma hominis, 998
Neisseria meningitidis, 273, 731,
733–734
Serratia, 813
Staphylococcus aureus see Staphylococcus
aureus
Staphylococcus epidermidis, 690
Streptococcus agalactiae (group B
streptococcus), 708
Streptococcus pneumoniae see
Streptococcus pneumoniae
Streptococcus pyogenes (group A
streptococcus), 698
Ureaplasma urealyticum, 1000–1001
Veillonella, 190
mucous membranes, 192–194, 690
nasopharynx, 273
neonates, 536
oral cavity, 190
respiratory tract, 83–84, 273
Haemophilus influenzae, 900–901,
904
tooth, 190–191
urinary tract, 339
vaginal, 1000–1001
see also Flora, normal; *specific organisms*
Colonoscopy, *Entamoeba histolytica*, 1277
Colony-stimulating factors (CSFs)
recombinant human, in neutropenia
with fever, 572
see also Granulocyte colony-stimulating
factor (G-CSF); Granulocyte-
macrophage colony-stimulating factor
(GM-CSF)
Colorado tick virus
epidemiology and vectors, 532
laboratory findings and diagnosis,
533t–534t
Colposcopy, 1073–1074

Coltivirus (Colorado tick fever), 1092–1094
antibodies to, 296, 1093
antigens, 1093
clinical/laboratory findings, 295–296,
1093, 1093b
diagnosis, 1093–1094, 1093b
optimal tests, 1389t–1392t
epidemiology, 1092–1093, 1092b, 1092f
Rocky Mountain spotted fever *vs.*, 1093
tick vector and vertebrate hosts, 1092
treatment and prevention, 1094
Coma
acute bacterial meningitis, 273–274
Naegleria fowleri infection, 1294
Plasmodium infection, 1299
rabies, 1147
Comamonadaceae, 832
Comamonas, 833
Comamonas acidovorans (Delftia acidovorans),
833
Comamonas testosteroni, 833
Combination therapy, 1419–1421
antagonism, 1419–1421
β-lactamase inhibition, 1419
cell wall-active agents with ribosome-
active agents, 1420
empiric treatment, 1415
resistance prevention, 1419
synergy, 1419–1420
see also individual drugs/drug combinations
Commensal bacteria *see* Flora, normal
Committee on Infectious Diseases (COID),
licensure of vaccines, 47
Common bile duct
stenosis, *Cryptosporidium* infections, 1270
stones, 412
Common colds, 196–199
clinical approach, 198
clinical features, 198, 198t
complications, 199
definition, 196
differential diagnosis, 198
epidemiology, 197, 197f
etiology, 196–197
coronaviruses, 1119
rhinoviruses, 1186–1187
ginseng in prevention of, 1120
immunity to viruses, 196, 197t
management, 198–199
mucopurulent rhinorrhea in, 163
pathogenesis, 197–198
prevention and hygiene, 199
recent advances, 199
susceptibility/risk factors, 196
vaccines, 199
virus transmission, 197
Common gamma chain (γc) gene, 627, 628t
Common variable immunoglobulin
deficiency (CVID), 40, 609, 612, 612t
characteristics, 602t, 610t, 612t
genetic basis, 612
infections associated, 612, 612t
Community-associated (CA)-MRSA *see under*
Staphylococcus aureus
Community-associated pneumonia (CAP),
235–237
Mycoplasma pneumoniae infections, 993
see also Pneumonia

"Compensatory anti-inflammatory response", 100
Complement, 86
    activation, 86, 94
        alternative pathway, 86, 616, 616f
        classical pathway, 86, 615–616, 616f
        control, 617
        lectin pathway, 616
        in sickle cell disease, 634
        in trauma, 512
    biochemistry and biology, 615–617, 616f
    CH50 assay, 291, 619
    components, 86
        see also individual components (e.g. C3)
    deficiency, 86, 604t–605t, 615–619
        detection, 608t
        diagnosis, 291, 619
        frequency, 288
        genetically determined, 617–618, 617t
        Haemophilus influenzae infections, 617–618
        immunizations in, 52t–53t, 619
        incidence of meningococcal disease, 288
        individual components, 604t–605t
        infection prevention, 292
        infections associated, 617
        management, 292, 619
        meningitis associated, 272–273, 273t
        Neisseria gonorrhoeae infection, 744
        Neisseria meningitidis infections, 617–618, 732
        neonatal, 618
        nephrotic syndrome, 618
        persistent/recurrent pneumonia, 251
        recurrent meningitis associated, 288–289
        secondary, 618–619
        sickle-cell disease, 619
        vaccines in, meningococcal conjugate vaccine, 65
        see also individual complement components
    Entamoeba histolytica infection, 1275
    levels in infants, 86
    MBL pathway, 86
    receptors, 616
    role in Haemophilus influenzae infections, 901
    role in host defense, 615, 617
    terminal component(s), 616
    terminal component deficiency, 604t–605t
        Neisseria meningitidis infections, 732
        recurrent meningitis and, 288
        vaccines in, 733
    timing of protective effects, 617
    see also individual components
Complement fixation test
    Blastomyces dermatitidis, 1237
    Chlamydophila (Chlamydia) psittaci, 882–883
    Coccidioides immitis (coccidioidomycosis), 1243
    Histoplasma capsulatum (histoplasmosis), 1227, 1227t
    Mycoplasma pneumoniae, 994–995, 1399
    in viral infections, 1387, 1387f

Complement-fixing (CF) antibodies, acquired rubella infection, 1112–1113, 1113f
Computed tomography (CT)
    abdominal lymphadenopathy, 157
    Acanthamoeba infection, 1296–1297
    acute bacterial sinusitis, 228–229
    acute mastoiditis, 224–225, 224f–225f
    amebic liver abscess, 1276f
    Aspergillus infections, 1204f, 1207
    Candida infections, 1199f
    cochlear dysplasia, 288f
    contrast-enhanced, retropharyngeal abscess, 208f
    cystic fibrosis, 640f
    cysticercosis (Taenia solium), 1352, 1354
    diskitis diagnosis, 484
    Echinococcus granulosus, 1358, 1359f
    Echinococcus multilocularis, 1361, 1361f
    encephalitis diagnosis, 308
    focal suppurative CNS infections, 325–327, 326f–327f
    intra-abdominal abscess, 424f
    lung abscess, 244, 244f
    mediastinal masses, 150–151, 154f
        pulmonary histoplasmosis, 153f
    meningococcal infections, 736
    Mycoplasma pneumoniae infections, 996f
    in necrotizing otitis externa, 222
    necrotizing pneumonia, 244, 244f
    parapneumonic effusion, 242
    pericarditis, 270
    in persistent pneumonia, 248
    pneumonia, in immunocompromised patients, 254
    postoperative mediastinitis, 587
    pyogenic arthritis, 478
    pyomyositis, 468
    recurrent meningitis, 291
    recurrent pneumonia, 248, 248f
    renal abscess, 344, 344f
    retropharyngeal abscess, 208f
    Toxoplasma gondii infection, 1314
Computed tomography (CT)-stereotactic methods, focal suppurative CNS infection management, 327
Concentration-dependent antibiotics, 1441, 1442t
Condyloma, HPV associated, 1072–1073
    treatment, 1074, 1074b
Condyloma acuminatum, 352
Confidence intervals, 2t, 5, 7
Confounding variables, 6, 6f, 9
    control of, 6–7
    impact, 6f
Congenital anomalies
    Borrelia burgdorferi (Lyme disease), 956
    healthcare-associated infection risk, 10
    recurrent meningitis associated, 287–288, 287b
    rubella virus infection, 1115
    see also specific congenital infections
Congenital cutaneous candidiasis, 1197–1198, 1197f
Congenital cystadenomatoid malformation (CCAM), 247, 248f
Congenital cysts, neck masses, 142–143, 142t

Congenital heart disease
    bronchiolitis risk, 233
    cyanotic
        brain abscess and, 321
        focal suppurative CNS infections, 321
    endocarditis associated, 257–258, 257t
Congenital hepatic fibrosis, 403
Congenital infections see Fetal infections; Neonatal infections; individual infections
Congenital rubella see Rubella virus
Congenital sinuses, neck masses, 142–143
Congenital syndromes, generalized lymphadenopathy, 131t–132t, 133
Congenital vascular rings, cough in, 167t
Congestive heart failure (CHF), cough in, 167t
Conidia, 1209
    Aspergillus, 1203, 1205
Conidiobolus, 1212–1213
Conidiogenesis, 1194
Conidiophores, 1194
Conjunctiva
    cicatrization, 494
    discharge, 490
    Kawasaki disease, 490, 1003, 1004f, 1005–1006
    in mucocutaneous syndromes, 108–111, 109t–110t
    nontypable Haemophilus influenzae infections, 903
    scrapings, 488
    ulcers, Francisella tularensis causing, 898
Conjunctival hyperemia, 490
Conjunctival swabs, specimen collection/transport, 1374t
Conjunctivitis, 490–494
    acute, 490–492
        bacterial causes, 110, 490–491
        clinical features, 491t
        diagnosis, 492
        Haemophilus influenzae biogroup aegyptius, 906
        treatment, 492–493
        viral causes, 491–492
    acute follicular, 491, 492t
    acute hemorrhagic
        adenoviruses causing, 1068t
        enteroviruses causing, 1174t, 1177
    adenoviral, 108–110, 491
        treatment, 493
    Chlamydia trachomatis see under Chlamydia trachomatis
    chlamydial neonatal inclusion, preauricular lymphadenopathy, 159
    chronic, 493–494
        chlamydial, 494
        viral, 494
    differential diagnosis, 490
    etiology, 490–492, 508
    gonococcal, 743–744
    granulomatous, Bartonella henselae, 159f
    HSV, 491–492
        treatment, 493
    inclusion, 494
        of adolescents, 494

chlamydial neonatal, preauricular
lymphadenopathy, 159
see also Chlamydia trachomatis
infants/children, 490–494
Listeria monocytogenes, 764–765
Loa loa causing, 1345–1346
Neisseria gonorrhoeae, 747
neonatal *see* Neonatal infections;
Ophthalmia neonatorum
neonatal nosocomial, 550
Pseudomonas aeruginosa, 541
Psychrobacter immobilis, 941
purulent, *Staphylococcus aureus*, 679
rubeola virus (measles), 492t, 1140
Staphylococcus aureus, 489
Streptococcus pneumoniae, 723
treatment, 1493
Conjunctivitis-otitis syndrome, 492–493
diagnosis and treatment, 492
Connective tissue disease, chronic fatigue
syndrome etiology, 1008
Consciousness loss
in acute bacterial meningitis, 273–274
see also Coma
Consolidated Standards of Reporting Trials
(CONSORT), 9
Constipation, 174
Cyclospora causing, 1283–1284
Contact dermatitis, 439f
Contact lens
Acanthamoeba keratitis, 497, 1296–1297
see also Acanthamoeba
infective keratitis due to, 495
storage and solutions for, infection
prevention, 1297
Contact Precautions, 18
Contact route of transmission, healthcare-
associated infections, 12
Contagious pustular dermatitis (orf), 1024
Continuous ambulatory peritoneal dialysis
(CAPD), 417, 418f
infection prevention, 419
peritonitis, 414–416
training, 419
Contraceptives, oral, pelvic inflammatory
disease and, 363
Contracoecum, 1339
Control of Communicable Diseases in Man,
68
Controls, for outbreak investigation studies,
7
Convalescent outpatient therapy, antibiotics,
1415
Conversion disorder, weakness in, weakness
due to, differential diagnosis,
181t–182t
Convulsions *see* Seizures
Cooling *see* Fever, management
Coombs test, in visceral leishmaniasis, 1287
Copepods, 1347
Copper, increased serum levels in acute-
phase response, 94
Coprinus atramentarius, 397t
Coproantigen, *Taenia* detection, 1351
Cornea
burn wound infections, 519
exposure, infective keratitis due to, 495
infections, 494–495

in gonococcal conjunctivitis,
488–489
microsporidial, 1291
inflammation *see* Keratitis
opacification, 495
perforation, in gonococcal conjunctivitis,
488–489
scarring, 498
scrapings, 497
transplants, 498
trauma, 495
ulceration
Acanthamoeba keratitis, 1296
burns, 519
Chlamydia trachomatis, 885
Coronary artery abnormalities, Kawasaki
disease, 1003, 1004f, 1005t, 1006
Coronary artery aneurysm
chest pain, 189
Kawasaki disease, 1003, 1004f, 1006
Coronary artery atherosclerosis, CMV
infection in transplant recipients,
1048
Coronaviridae, 1016t, 1117
infections, 1017t
Coronaviruses *see* Human coronaviruses
(HCoV)
Coronin 1A deficiency, 627
Corpus callosum, absent, fever in,
119t–120t
Corticosteroids
acute pancreatitis due to, 411
antipyretic action, 92
as *Aspergillus* infection risk factor,
1206
candidiasis risk with, 1202
contraindications
Corynebacterium diphtheriae infections,
757
Kawasaki disease, 113, 1006
cortisol replacement in sepsis, 100
lymphocytolytic effects, 1228
macrophage suppression, 1206
in management of
Acanthamoeba infections, 1297
acute bacterial meningitis, 278
acute epiglottitis, 211
acute rheumatic fever, 704
allergic bronchopulmonary
aspergillosis, 1205
brain abscess, 328
brain abscess due to *Staphylococcus*
aureus, 684
bronchiolitis, 234
chronic granulomatous disease
(CGD), 623
chronic meningitis, 286
EBV infection, 1062
enterovirus infections, 1177
hemophagocytic lymphohistiocytosis,
107
Histoplasma capsulatum infections,
1228, 1228t
human metapneumovirus (hMPV)
infection, 1136–1137
laryngotracheitis (croup), 211
Loa loa infections, 1345–1346
meningococcal meningitis, 737

Mycobacterium tuberculosis infections,
785
nephrotic syndrome, 637
otitis externa, 221
periodic fever syndrome, 122
Pneumocystis jirovecii (carinii)
infections, 1233
RSV infections, 1133
Salmonella Typhi infection, 818
sepsis/septic shock, 100–102
Taenia solium neurocysticercosis,
1354–1356, 1355t
Trichinella spiralis infection, 1341
urticaria, 447
see also Dexamethasone
Cortisol, reduced levels, chronic fatigue
syndrome pathogenesis, 1010
Corynebacterium, 759–762
CNS device infection, 597
device-related infections, 588
identification and characteristics,
759–762, 760t–761t
pitted keratolysis due to, 430
pneumonia, 760t–761t
prosthetic device infections, 759–762
skin flora, 427
treatment and features of infections,
760t–761t
Corynebacterium accolens, 762
Corynebacterium afermentans, 760t–761t, 762
Corynebacterium amycolatum, 760t–761t, 762
Corynebacterium aquaticum, 760t–761t
Corynebacterium argentoratense, 762
Corynebacterium auris, 762
Corynebacterium bovis, 760t–761t
Corynebacterium coyleae, 760t–761t
Corynebacterium diphtheriae, 164, 754–759
acute bilateral cervical lymphadenitis
due to, 139
antimicrobial resistance, 757
antimicrobial susceptibility, 757
antitoxin, 433
Arcanobacterium haemolyticum similarity,
750–751
bullneck diphtheria, 755–757
carriers, 758
chemoprophylaxis, 70t–71t
clinical manifestations, 755–757
cutaneous diphtheria, 432–433,
755–757
outbreaks, 755–756
Seattle outbreak, 756
secondary bacterial infections,
432–433
differential diagnosis, 756
diphtheria antitoxin (DAT), 42, 757–758
administration and dosage, 757
serum sickness due to, 757
sources, 757
diphtheria toxin, 433, 754–755
genes, 754–755
diphtheria toxoid, 55
antigen content (US vaccines), 872,
873t
indications, 758
limit of flocculation (Lf) content, 758
DTap *see under* Diphtheria, tetanus, and
pertussis (DTP) vaccination/vaccines

elimination goal, 47
endocarditis, 756
epidemiology of infections, 755
etiology, 754–755
faucial diphtheria, 756f
growth conditions, 754, 757
laboratory diagnosis, 757
laryngeal diphtheria, 211, 755–756
management, 757–758
    antimicrobial, 757
    asymptomatic carriers, 758
    asymptomatic case contacts, 758
    exposed persons, 758
microbiology, 754
morbidity reduced by vaccine, 48t
mortality due to, 755, 757
myocarditis due to, 266, 268
nontoxigenic strains, 754–755
notification cessation, 55
outbreaks, 754–755
pathogenesis of infection, 755
pharyngeal diphtheria, 201–202,
    755–757
pharyngitis due to, 199, 201–202
phenotypes, 754
prevalence, 55
    reduced by vaccines, 47
prevention of infection, 758–759
prognosis, 757
respiratory tract diphtheria, 755–756
    pseudomembrane, 754–756
    sporadic, 755
risk factors for infection, 755
Russian outbreak, 755
septicemia due to, 756
Tdap see under Diphtheria, tetanus, and
    pertussis (DTP) vaccination/vaccines
toxic myocardiopathy due to, 756
toxic neuropathy due to, 756–757
toxigenic strains, 754–755
transmission, 755, 758
vaccines/vaccination, 758
    in pregnancy, 51–52
    preparations, 758
    requirements, 755
    schedules, 758–759
    underimmunization, 755
    see also Diphtheria, tetanus, and
        pertussis (DTP) vaccination/
        vaccines
virulence factors, 755
Corynebacterium equi, 768–769
Corynebacterium glucuronolyticum, 762
Corynebacterium jeikeium, 760t–761t, 762
    prosthetic device infections, 762
Corynebacterium kutscheri, 760t–761t, 762
Corynebacterium macginleyi, 760t–761t, 762
Corynebacterium minutissimum, 760t–761t,
    762
    erythrasma, 430
Corynebacterium ovis, 760t–761t
Corynebacterium pilosum, 760t–761t
Corynebacterium propinquum, 762
Corynebacterium pseudodiphtheriticum,
    760t–761t
Corynebacterium pseudotuberculosis, 760t–761t
Corynebacterium striatum, 760t–761t, 762
Corynebacterium ulcerans, 760t–761t

Corynebacterium urealyticum, 760t–761t
Corynebacterium vaginale see Gardnerella
    vaginalis
Corynebacterium xerosis, 760t–761t, 762
Coryneform bacteria see Corynebacterium
    diphtheriae
Cost considerations
    antimicrobial agent selection, 1415–
        1416
    antimicrobial drug resistance, 1421
    broad-spectrum antibiotics, 115–116
    enteric infections in group childcare, 31
    varicella vaccines, 1044
Cost-effectiveness, 8
Cost–benefit analysis, 8–9
Costimulatory molecules, 92
Costochondritis, 189
    chest pain, 190t
Cost–utility analysis, 8
Cough, 166–168, 167t
    acute bacterial sinusitis, 228
    acute bronchitis, 213
    Aspergillus infections, 1203
    Bordetella pertussis (pertussis), 167–168,
        167t, 865, 868
    bronchiolitis, 233
    Brucella causing, 863
    characteristics, 166
    Chlamydophila pneumoniae causing, 890
    chronic, 166–167
        after Chlamydia trachomatis
            pneumonia, 239
    dry, 166–167
    EBV infection, 1061
    empiric transmission-based precautions,
        20t
    etiology, 166–168
    hookworm infections, 1329
    in infants, CRADLE mnemonic, 167
    infectious causes, 166–168, 167t
    influenza, 1152
    laryngotracheitis (croup), 211
    Legionella, 923
    Mycoplasma pneumoniae infections, 994
    nature (characteristics) and diseases
        causing, 167t
    nocturnal, 248–251
    non-typable Haemophilus influenzae
        causing, 900
    noninfectious causes, 166–167, 167t
    Paragonimus infections, 1367
    pathologic, 166
    pertussis, 865, 868
    pneumonia, 167–169, 238–239
    productive, 166
    protracted, causes, Bordetella pertussis,
        865
    psychogenic, 167t
    pulmonary Mycobacterium tuberculosis
        infection, 774
    respiratory syncytial virus (RSV)
        infections, 1132–1133
    rubeola virus (measles), 1140
    SARS, 1119
    types, defined, 166
    wet, 166–167
    whooping see Bordetella pertussis
        (pertussis)

Cough etiquette, standard precautions, 17,
    18t
Cough reflex, 238, 248
    loss, 248–251
Cough suppressants, in common colds, 198
Council for State and Territorial
    Epidemiologists (CSTE), mumps
    definition, 1127
Cow(s), diseases related to, Sarcocystis
    infections, 1306
Cowdry inclusion bodies, 1141–1142
Cowpox virus, 1020t, 1024
    clinical features, 1024
Cow's milk protein allergy, 251, 445
Coxiella burnetii (Q fever), 891–893
    acute Q fever, 892
    antibodies to, 892
    antigenic phases of lipopolysaccharide,
        891
    asymptomatic infection, 892
    as Category B bioterrorism agent, 891
    chronic Q fever, 892
    clinical manifestations, 119t–120t, 892
    detection, in endocarditis, 260–261
    endocarditis due to, 260t
    epidemiology, 891, 891f
    fever of unknown origin due to,
        119t–120t
    laboratory findings and diagnosis, 892
    laboratory testing, 308t–311t
    microbiology, 891
    pneumonia due to, 237t, 238–239, 892
        persistent pneumonia, 246
    prevention, 893
    special considerations, 892–893
    transmission, 891
    treatment of infections, 892
    vaccines, 893
Coxiellaceae, 891
Coxsackievirus(es)
    myocarditis, 265–266
    oral infections, 192t
Coxsackievirus A, 1172–1180
    clinical manifestations, 1174t, 1175f
    diagnosis, optimal tests, 1389t–1392t
    in immunodeficiency children, 1179
    serotypes, 1172, 1172t–1173t
    see also Enterovirus(es)
Coxsackievirus A7, clinical manifestations,
    1176
Coxsackievirus A9, 1173t, 1176–1177
Coxsackievirus A16, hand, foot and mouth
    disease, 1174–1175, 1175f
Coxsackievirus A24
    acute hemorrhagic conjunctivitis, 1177
    conjunctivitis, 492, 492t
Coxsackievirus-adenovirus receptor (CAR),
    266
Coxsackievirus B, 1172–1180
    aseptic meningitis due to, 295,
        1174–1175
    cardiac muscle disease, 1176
    clinical manifestations, 1174, 1174t
    diagnosis, optimal tests, 1389t–1392t
    epidemiology, 1173–1174
    hepatitis due to, 1178–1179
    in immunodeficiency children, 1179
    juvenile dermatomyositis and, 464–465

myocarditis due to, 1178
myopericarditis due to, 1176
neonatal infections, 1178
serotypes, 1172, 1172t–1173t
see also Enterovirus(es)
Coxsackievirus B1, juvenile dermatomyositis and, 464–465
Coxsackievirus B2, 1173t, 1175–1176
Coxsackievirus B5, 1173t, 1175, 1177–1178
aseptic meningitis, 295
Coxsackievirus B6, 1173–1174, 1176
Crab louse *see Phthirus pubis* (crab louse) infestation
Crackles (breath sounds)
coarse, 169
fine, 169
in pneumonia, 238
CRADLE mnemonic, 167
Cranial nerve abnormalities
Campylobacter jejuni infection, 877
facial, *Borrelia burgdorferi* (Lyme disease), 954–955
headache with, 177
herpes zoster, 1039
infant botulism, 973
Mycobacterium tuberculosis infection, 777
poliovirus causing, 1170
Cranial nerve palsies, 315–316
Angiostrongylus cantonensis causing, 1337
sixth, in acute bacterial meningitis, 274
Cranial neuropathy
Borrelia burgdorferi (Lyme disease), 954–955
in chronic meningitis, 284t
Corynebacterium diphtheriae, 756–757
Craniotomy, 328
Creatinine clearance, burns infection treatment and, 520
Credé method, 599
Creeping eruption, 1338f, 1339
Paragonimus skrjabini causing, 1368
Cremasteric reflex, 367
Creutzfeldt–Jakob disease (CJD), 333–334
diagnosis, 338
familial, 337–338
genetics, 337–338, 337f
iatrogenic transmission, 334
dura mater grafts, 334
human pituitary hormones and, 334
other sources, 334–335
laboratory findings and MRI, 335–336, 335f, 338
origin of name, 333–334
pathology, 336f
prevention, 338
sporadic, 333–334, 337
diagnosis, 338
EEG, 338
epidemiology, 334, 336t, 337
neuropathology, 336f, 337–338
variant CJD *vs.*, 335–336
treatment, 338
variant (vCJD), 335–337
clinical features, 335–336
diagnosis, 336
epidemiology, 335
latent/asymptomatic, 337
management, 338

MRI, 335–336, 335f
pathology, 335–336, 336f
sporadic CJD *vs.*, 335–336
transfusions linked to, 337
Cribriform fracture, acute bacterial meningitis after, 272–273
Crimean–Congo hemorrhagic fever
clinical manifestations, 1104, 1104t
epidemiology, 532t, 1103, 1103t
laboratory findings and diagnosis, 533t–534t
prevention, 536
treatment, 1104
vectors, 532t
Critical care, principles, 99
Critical equipment, 21
Critical evaluation, medical literature, 9, 9b
Critical review, of medical literature, 9, 9b
Crohn disease
anemia, 1403
rubeola virus (measles) vaccine association, 1143
Cronobacter (*Enterobacter sakazakii*), 804–806
neonatal meningitis, 805
nomenclature and microbiology, 804
treatment, 805
Cross-sectional studies, 3–4, 3t
Crotamiton
pediculosis treatment, 1259
scabies treatment, 1261
Croup *see* Laryngotracheitis (croup)
"Crumbling-bone disease", 635
Cryopyrin, 126
Cryopyrin-associated periodic syndromes (CAPS), 122t, 126–127
cardinal clinical features, 126
course, treatment and outcome, 126–127
epidemiology and etiology, 126
Cryptococcus, 1220–1223, 1223b
bone infections, 1222
clinical manifestations, 1221–1222, 1223b
CNS cryptococcosis, 1222–1223
description and structure, 1220, 1223b
diagnosis, 1222, 1223b
epidemiology, 1221, 1223b
in hyper-IgM syndromes, 613
in immunocompromised hosts, 1220–1221, 1223
infections in heart transplant recipients, 555
invasive cryptococcosis, 1195–1196
meningitis *see under Cryptococcus neoformans*
neutropenia associated with cancer, 567
ocular infections, 1222
pneumonitis, in cancer, 575
prevention of infections, 1223
pulmonary cryptococcosis, 1221–1222
refractory infections, 1223
skin lesions, 1222
species and serotypes, 1220, 1221t
treatment of infections, 1222–1223, 1223b
Cryptococcus gattii
characteristics, 1220, 1221t
diagnostic testing for, 1222
epidemiology, 1221

Cryptococcus neoformans
antigen, in CSF, 282, 286, 1222
antigen detection, 1222
arthritis due to, 482
capsule and acapsular strains, 1220–1221
characteristics, 1220, 1221t
clinical features, 282
in CSF, 1222
culture and growth, 1222
diagnostic testing for, 1222, 1382
eosinophilia, 1407, 1408t–1409t
epidemiology, 282, 1221
focal CNS infections, 319
in HIV infection, 661
immune response, 1220–1221
meningitis due to, 282, 284t, 1221–1222
diagnosis, 282, 1222
eosinophilic, 331t, 332
treatment, 1222–1223
monoclonal antibody development, 44
pathogenesis, 282
pneumonitis, in cancer, 575
pulmonary infection, 1221
serotypes A and D, 1221t, 1222
treatment of infections, 1222
virulence, 1220–1221
Cryptococcus neoformans var. *gattii*, 1220
Cryptococcus neoformans var. *grubii*, 1220
Cryptococcus neoformans var. *neoformans*, 1220
Cryptosporidium, 1269–1271, 1271b
in AIDS/HIV infection, 662
clinical manifestations, 1270, 1271b
description and life cycle, 1270–1271
diagnosis/detection, 385t, 1270, 1270f, 1271b, 1383–1384
epidemiology, 1269–1270, 1271b
in HIV infections, 1270–1271
in hyper-IgM syndrome, 613, 631–632
inflammatory enteritis, 387
laboratory findings, 1383–1384
neutropenia associated with cancer, 568
oocysts and oocyst shedding, 1269–1271
outbreaks, 377
in childcare centers, 1271
prevention of infection, 1271
transmission, 1269, 1271
treatment of infections, 1270–1271, 1271b, 1519
water contamination, 384, 1269
Cryptosporidium hominis, 1269
Cryptosporidium parvum, 1269
acute pancreatitis, 411
in childcare setting, 25t, 26, 30–31
diarrhea due to, 26t
genome, 1255
refugee and internationally adopted children, 35–36
waterborne disease, 396
"CSF-oma", 596–597
Ctenocephalides felis (cat flea), 931–932
CTX-M enzyme, in drug resistance, 1424
Culex mosquito, 81
Japanese encephalitis virus transmission, 1100
Ross River virus transmission, 1098
West Nile virus transmission, 1101

Cullen sign, 173
Culture
    adenoviruses, 1070
    bile, 413
    blood *see* Blood cultures
    in endocarditis *see* Endocarditis
    intravascular catheter infection diagnosis, 591
    nasopharyngeal, 240
    peritoneal fluid, 390
    sputum, 640
    stool *see* Stool culture
    throat, pharyngitis, 202–203
    tube culture, HSV, 1386t
    urine *see* Urine, culture
    see also individual micro-organisms
Culture media, 1373
    Actinomyces, 1376t
    antibiotic susceptibility testing, 1378, 1378t
    for bacterial infections, 1375t
        anaerobic bacteria, 964t, 1375t–1376t
        by species, 1376t
        by specimen type, 1374t
    commonly used types, 1375t
    differential, 1373, 1375t
    enriched, 1373, 1375t
    for fungi, 1376t, 1382
    selective, 1373, 1375t
    for specific organisms, 1376t
    transport media *see* Transport media
Cumulative hazard, 3
Cumulative hazard curves, 3, 4f
Cumulative incidence, 1
Cunninghamella, 1212–1213
"Currant jelly stool", 174
Cushing triad, 171
Cutaneous amebiasis, 1276
Cutaneous infections *see* Skin infections
Cutaneous larva migrans (CLM), *Ancylostoma braziliense* causing, 1338–1339
CVID *see* Common variable immunoglobulin deficiency (CVID)
CXCR4 (LESTR; fusin), 1166
CXCR4 chemokine receptor, 666
Cyanobacteria-like bodies, 1283
Cyanosis, in pneumonia, 240
Cyanotic congenital heart disease, brain abscess and, 321
Cyclic hematopoiesis, 604t–605t
    see also Cyclic neutropenia
Cyclic neutropenia, 122t, 123–124, 604t–605t
    cardinal clinical features, 123–124
    characteristics, 604t–605t
    course, treatment and outcome, 124
    diagnosis, 124
    differential diagnosis, 122t
    epidemiology and etiology, 123
    mutations, 123
Cyclic neutropenia and agranulocytosis, oral mucosal features, 193t
Cyclitis, Fuch heterochromic, 501
Cyclooxygenase (COX)
    increased expression in fever, 91, 91f
    inhibitors, 92

Cycloserine, tuberculosis treatment, 780t, 782
Cyclospora (cyclosporiasis), 1283–1284
    clinical manifestations, 1283–1284
    description, 1283
    epidemiology, 1283
    foodborne, 397–398
    laboratory findings and diagnosis, 1284, 1284f, 1383
    prevention, 1284
    refugee and internationally adopted children, 35–36
    treatment, 1284
Cyclospora cayetanensis
    description, 1283
    epidemiology, 1283
    foodborne, 398
    gastrointestinal symptoms, 394t
    laboratory findings and diagnosis, 1284, 1284f
Cyclosporine/cyclosporine A (CSA)
    HLH treatment, 107
    in myocarditis, 268
Cyst(s)
    arachnoid, 291f
    Balantidium coli, 1266–1267, 1266f–1267f
    brain *see* Brain cysts
    branchial cleft, 142t, 143
    bronchogenic, 247
    choledochal, 403
    congenital, neck masses, 142–143, 142t
    dermal, 289f
    dermoid *see* Dermoid cysts
    echinococcal *see* Echinococcus granulosus (cystic echinococcosis)
    Endolimax nana, 1271–1272, 1272f
    Entamoeba, 1278
    Entamoeba histolytica, 1273f–1274f, 1274
    epidermoid *see* Epidermoid cysts
    Giardia intestinalis, 1279–1282
    hydatid *see* Echinococcus granulosus (cystic echinococcosis)
    lung, 247
    mediastinal, 149
    midline, 142t, 143
    muscle, *Taenia serialis* (coenurosis), 1362
    Naegleria fowleri, 1293–1295, 1293f, 1295t
    parasitic, resistance to chlorination, 384
    resistance and survival, *Entamoeba histolytica*, 1274
    Taenia solium neurocysticercosis, 1352, 1353f, 1354
    thyroglossal duct, 142t
    Toxoplasma gondii, 1309–1310
    ventricular, *Taenia solium*, 1352–1353, 1353f, 1355t
Cystic cystadenomatoid malformation (CCAM), 247
Cystic echinococcosis *see* Echinococcus granulosus
Cystic fibrosis, 83–84, 638–641
    Achromobacter xylosoxidans colonization, 639
    acute hepatitis, 403
    allergic bronchopulmonary aspergillosis, 1205

bacterial pathogens transmitted to, 24
bloodstream infection, 640
Burkholderia cepacia infections, 639–641, 847, 847t, 1433
Burkholderia infections, 639, 846, 847t
chronic hepatitis, 407
clinical features, 248–249, 1437
cough, 166–167, 167t
diagnosis, 248–249, 403
epidemiology of infections, 639
gene therapy, 641
immunizations in, 641
infections in
    age-related, 639t
    antibiotic selection issues, 641
    clinical features, 639
    epidemiology, 639
    etiology, 639–640, 639t
    laboratory findings/imaging, 640, 640f
    management, 640–641
    pathogenesis, 639
    pre-emptive therapy, 640
    prevention, 641
    recent advances for, 641
    in transplant recipients, 555
influenza virus infections, 1153
inheritance, 248–249
mutations, 248–249
nontuberculous mycobacterial infection, 786–787, 790
    diagnostic criteria, 790
    differential diagnosis, 790
pharmacokinetics, 1437–1438
Pseudomonas aeruginosa infections, 639, 843–844, 844t, 846, 1425–1426, 1432–1433
    management, 640
    prevention, 640–641
recurrent pneumonia, 248–249
respiratory infections, 248–249, 639
sinusitis, 638–639
Staphylococcus aureus infections, 639, 1428
Stenotrophomonas maltophilia, 639
treatment, inhaled aminoglycosides, 1474
Cystic fibrosis transmembrane regulator (CFTR), 638
cDNA, administration, 641
Cystic hygroma, 142t, 143, 143f
Cysticercoids, *Hymenolepis nana*, 1349
Cysticercosis, 1256, 1256t, 1350, 1352–1356, 1355t
    chronic myositis, 464
    meningitis, 283, 283t
    see also Taenia solium; Tapeworms
Cysticercus, meningitis, 280t
Cystisospora, in AIDS/HIV infection, 662
Cystitis
    acute bacterial
        treatment, 356
        urethritis and vulvovaginitis *vs.*, 354, 354t
    acute hemorrhagic, 341, 1069
    adenoviruses causing, 339, 1069
    in cancer, 579
    hemorrhagic

BK virus, 1076
  in cancer, 579
  in HSCT recipients, 563, 1076
  in solid-organ transplant recipients, 559
  treatment, 1418t–1419t
  urinary catheter-related infection, 599
Cystoisospora (cystisosporiasis), 1283–1284
  clinical manifestations, 1283–1284
  description, 1283
  epidemiology, 1283
  laboratory diagnosis, 1284, 1284f, 1383
Cystoisospora belli, 1283–1284
  eosinophilia, 1408t–1409t
  laboratory findings, 1284, 1284f
Cystoscopy, elective, endocarditis prevention, 76
Cytochrome P-450 (CYP)
  activation by rifamycin, 1476
  burned patients, 1438
  cystic fibrosis, 1437–1438
  in drug-drug interactions, 1439, 1440t
  inhibition by itraconazole, 1489
"Cytokine storm"
  chronic active EBV infection, 1065
  hemophagocytic lymphohistiocytosis pathogenesis, 105
Cytokines, 85f, 90
  acute-phase response, 1400
  aerobic vaginitis and, 361
  anti-inflammatory, 94–95, 100
    antibacterial defense impaired by, 100
  antibacterial defense mechanism, 100
  anticytokine therapy, in sepsis, 100
  chronic fatigue syndrome, 1010t
  common cold pathogenesis, 197–198
  dermatophytic ("id") reactions, 453–454
  elevated, in HLH, 105
  encoded by NFκB-regulated gene, 94
  erythema multiforme pathogenesis, 448
  functions and types, 100
  HHV-6 infection, 1053
  in immune response to vaccines, 45
  induced by *Shigella*, 820
  monocyte deactivation reversal, 100
  in *Neisseria meningitidis* infections, 731, 737
  produced by T cells, 90
  proinflammatory, 92, 94, 100
    elevated in HLH, 105
    host defense role, 100
    inhibition, 100
    stimulated by *Pseudomonas aeruginosa*, 842–843
  pyogenic arthritis pathogenesis, 477
  pyrogenic, 91–92
    inhibitors, 92
  release, *Clostridium difficile*, 384
  in sepsis, 98, 100
  therapeutic, 624
  upregulation, Kawasaki disease, 1003
Cytolysis, by *Entamoeba histolytica*, mechanism, 1274
Cytomegalovirus (CMV), 1044–1051, 1052b
  acquired infection (healthy hosts), 1046–1047
    diagnosis/detection, 1049

acute bilateral cervical lymphadenitis due to, 138
in AIDS/HIV infection *see* Human immunodeficiency virus (HIV)/AIDS
antibodies to, 1049
antigenemia, 1049, 1388–1392
antiviral drug resistance, 1051
cell types infected by, 1044
chemokines, 1044
chorioretinitis, transplant recipients, 558
chronic fatigue syndrome pathogenesis, 1008t–1009t
chronic hepatitis due to, 406
chronic meningitis, 283
clinical manifestations, 1044, 1046–1049
  acquired infection in healthy hosts, 1046–1047
  in AIDS, 1048–1049
  complications, 1047
  congenital infection, 1045–1048, 1047t
    premature newborns, 1048
    transplant recipients, 1048
congenital infection, 545, 547t
  anomalies, 1045–1048
  asymptomatic, 1047
  clinical features, 537t, 1045–1048, 1047t
  CNS features, 1045–1047, 1047t
  diagnosis, 538t, 1049, 1388, 1389t–1392t, 1398
  epidemiology, 1046
  fetal development impaired, 1045
  hearing loss, 548, 1045–1049
  imaging, 1047
  laboratory features, 1047, 1047t
  pathogenesis, 1045–1046
  pathology, 1045
  prevention, 1051
  sequelae, 1045–1047, 1045t, 1047t
  transmission, 1045
  treatment, 1050
cytopathology, 1044, 1049
cytoplasmic inclusions, 1044
description and structure, 1044
diagnosis/detection, 385t, 1044, 1049, 1388–1393
  antigen detection, 1386
  antigenemia assay, 1049
  blood samples, 1385
  congenital infection, 1049
  culture, 1388
  detection rates, 1386t
  DNA probes, 1386, 1388
  IgM and IgG, 1388
  immunocompromised patients, 1049
  lack of standardization, 1049
  optimal tests, 1389t–1392t
  in peripheral white blood cells, 1388–1392
  serologic tests, 1049, 1049b
  shell vial method, 1386, 1388
  specimens, 1388
  transplant recipients, 558
dissemination, 1044

DNA, 1044
  detection, 1049
  probes, 1386, 1388
  quantitation, 1049
in drug-induced immunodeficiency, 253–254
drug resistance, 1051, 1503t
encephalitis, 314, 1047
epidemiology, 1044, 1046
  age-related prevalence, 1046
  congenital infection, 1046
exposure management in pregnant healthcare worker, 22t–23t
ganciclovir resistance, 1050
generalized lymphadenopathy due to, 130–132, 131t–132t
genome, 1044
glycoprotein B (gB), 1045
group childcare and, 25t, 28–29
  in adults attending/care providers, 31
hepatic enzyme elevation, 1046–1047, 1411
in HIV infection/AIDS, 659
  clinical features, 1048–1049
  treatment, 1050
HSCT recipients, 562, 564, 1048–1051
  management, 566
  prevention, 566
hyperimmune globulin, transplant recipient treatment, 558
immune evasion, 1044
immune globulin (CMVIG), 1050–1051
  CMV infection prophylaxis in transplant recipients, 561
immune globulin intravenous (CMV-IGIV), 37t, 41–42
  indications and dosage, 41–42
immune response, 1045
immunity, maternal and lack of, 1045
immunocompromised patients, 1511–1512
  clinical features, 1048–1049
  diagnosis/detection, 1049, 1389t–1392t, 1392
  treatment, 1050–1051
infection process, 1044
infections after burns, 519
inflammatory enteritis due to, 386–387
intranuclear inclusions, 1388
laboratory findings, 1049
laboratory testing, 308t–311t
mononucleosis syndrome due to, 1046
  diagnosis, 1392
  outcome and complications, 1047
neonatal infection, 545, 1045
  premature newborns, 1048
neutropenia in, 1405
nosocomial infections
  epidemiology, 1046
  management in pregnant healthcare worker, 22t–23t
  prevention, 1051
occupational infection, 1046
oral infections, 192t
outcome, 1047
passive immunization, 1045
pathogenesis of infections, 1044–1046
  congenital infection, 1045–1046

pericarditis due to, 268–269
persistence, 1044, 1047
pneumonia due to, 168t, 236–237
  in cancer, 577
  diagnosis, 254
  HSCT recipients, 564, 566
  in immunocompromised, 236, 253–254
  prediction, 1388–1392
  risk factors, 577
  treatment, 577
pneumonitis due to, in transplant recipients, 1048
post-transfusion, 1046
postnatal infections
  community-acquired, 546
  diagnosis, 1389t–1392t
in pregnancy, 1045–1046
  prevention, 22t–23t, 1051
in premature neonates, 1048
pretransplant screening, 1389t–1392t
prevention of infections, 1044, 1051
  CDC recommendations, 1051b
  chemoprophylaxis, 1507t, 1511–1512
  maternal/congenital infections, 1051
  nosocomial infections, 1051
  passive immunization, 1050–1051
  transplant recipients, 561, 1050–1051
proteins, synthesis, 1044
replication, 1044
retinitis due to, 501, 501f, 1047–1048, 1050
shedding, 1044–1046, 1048, 1388
spontaneous abortion/stillbirth, 546–547
structure, 1044
tegument protein pp65, 1049
tissue culture, 1049
tissue tropism, 1044
transfusion-acquired, 1046, 1048
  infants, 544–545
  premature newborns, 1048
  prevention, 1051
transmission, 1046, 1051
  assisted reproductive technology, 1051
  breastmilk, 545, 1046, 1048
  intrapartum, 545
  saliva, 1046
  sexual, 1046
  sources of maternal infection, 545–546
  vertical, 536, 1045–1046
in transplant associated pneumonia, 254
transplant recipients, 558, 1045–1046, 1048
  bone marrow transplants, 1046
  breakthrough disease, 1050
  chorioretinitis, 558
  clinical features, 558, 1048
  coinfections, 1048
  detection, 558, 1049
  disseminated infection, 558
  donor positive/recipient negative (D⁺/R⁻), 1048, 1050–1051
  gastrointestinal disease, 1048
  hematopoietic stem cell transplant, 1048

HSCT see Cytomegalovirus (CMV), HSCT recipients
immunization (CMV gB) before, 1051
  pneumonitis, 1048
  prevention, 561, 1048, 1050–1051
  solid-organ transplants, 558, 1048
  source of infection, 1048
  treatment, 558, 1050–1051
treatment of infections, 1049–1051, 1052b, 1504t, 1508–1509, 1511–1512, 1515
  congenital infection, 1050
  immunocompromised patients, 1050–1051
  transplant recipients, 1050–1051
UL97 and UL54 genes, mutations, 1051
vaccines, 1051
  glycoprotein B (gB), 1045, 1051
  recombinant subunit, 1051
  Towne strain live-attenuated, 1051
viremia, 1044
virology, 1044
Cytopathic effects, 1385
  adenoviruses, 1070
  enteroviruses, 1179
  herpes simplex virus, 1031–1033
  human herpesvirus 7 (HHV-7), 1057
  human metapneumovirus (hMPV), 1134, 1136
  human parainfluenza viruses, 1121
  mumps virus, 1125, 1127–1128
  rubella virus, 1112
Cytopenia
  detection, 608t
  immune-mediated, IGIV use, 41
Cytospinning, CSF, 1377
Cytotoxic chemotherapy see Chemotherapy
Cytotoxic/cytolytic T lymphocytes (CTL), 46, 89, 626–627
  CMV-specific, 1045
  EBV-specific, 1060–1061
    X-linked lymphoproliferative syndrome, 1064
  hepatitis B virus spread, 1078
  HIV infection, 648–649
  influenza virus infection, 1151
  NK cells compared, 86t
  pathogens killed by, 89–90
  Pneumocystis jirovecii (carinii) infection, 1230
  see also T lymphocytes, CD8⁺
Cytotoxicity
  antibody-dependent cell-mediated see Antibody-dependent cell-mediated cytotoxicity (ADCC)
  perforin-mediated, defective, 104–105
Cytotrophoblasts, CMV infection, 1045

D

D test (disk diffusion), 686
D4T see Stavudine (d4T)
Dacryoadenitis, 508, 508f
Dacryocystitis, 508–509, 509f, 1493
Dactylitis
  blistering distal, 432
  sickle-cell disease, 635

Dade MicroScan WalkAway system, 1379–1380
Dalbavancin, 1469
  coagulase-negative staphylococcal infections, 694
Dalfopristin (streptogramin A)
  mechanism of action, 1474–1475
  see also Streptogramins
Damage-associated molecular patterns (DAMPs), 92–93
Dandruff, Malassezia, 1217
Dane particle, 1077
Dapsone
  chemoprophylactic use, 70t–71t
  Pneumocystis jirovecii (carinii) pneumonia, 1233, 1233t
  Toxoplasma gondii infection, 1314–1315, 1316t, 1317
Daptacel, 55t
Daptomycin, 1469
  adverse effects, 1469
  clinical uses, 1469
  dosage, 1480t–1483t
  mechanism of action, 687–688, 1426, 1469
  pharmacodynamic properties, 1414t
  pharmacology, 1453t–1458t
  resistance, 1426
  spectrum of activity, 1459t–1463t, 1469
  structure, 1469
  treatment of
    Ca-MRSA infections, 472
    coagulase-negative staphylococcal infections, 694
    Enterococcus infections, 715
    infections in neutropenia with cancer, 571
    Leuconostoc infection, 730
    Staphylococcus aureus infections, 687–688
Darkfield microscopy, 673
  Treponema pallidum, 945
Darunavir, 665t
De Quervain thyroiditis, 143
Deafness see Hearing loss
DEBONEL, 935–938
Deconditioning, fatigue of see Fatigue
Decongestants, in common colds, 198
Decubitus ulcers, anaerobic gram-positive cocci causing, 989
Deerfly (Chrysops), 1345
Deerpox virus, 1020t
DEET
  Plasmodium infection prevention, 81, 81b, 1304–1306
  precautions for use, 81b
  Rickettsia infection prevention, 938
  Rickettsia parkeri infection prevention, 935
  Rocky Mountain spotted fever (Rickettsia rickettsii) prevention, 929
  tick repellent, 535
Defensins, 83
  α-defensins, 83
  β-defensins, 83
Deferoxamine, as mucormycosis risk factor, 1213

Dehydration
infant botulism vs., 974t
management, 376
see also Oral rehydration therapy (ORT)
orolabial HSV infection, 1028
Shigella infection causing, 821
Vibrio cholerae infection causing, 851
management, 852–853, 852b
viral gastroenteritis causing, 381
Delayed-type hypersensitivity
cutaneous leishmaniasis, 1288
Mantoux tuberculin skin test, 779
rubeola virus infection (measles), 1138
Toxocara infections, 1335–1336
Delftia, 833
Delftia acidovorans (Comamonas acidovorans), 833
Delirium, recrudescent typhus (*Rickettsia prowazekii*), 931
Delta antigen (HDAg), 1086–1087
Delta hepatitis *see* Hepatitis D virus (HDV, delta agent)
Delta sign, 326
Delta viruses, 1016t–1017t
see also Hepatitis D virus (HDV, delta agent)
Demeclocycline, pharmacology, 1453t–1458t
Demyelinating disorders, HHV-6 role, 1057
Demyelination, hemophagocytic lymphohistiocytosis, 105
Dendritic cells, 85–86, 134, 627
antigen presentation, 86
congenital CMV infection, 1045
development, 85–86
function, 86
in histiocytosis, 134
in HIV infection, 649b, 1167
myeloid, 627
plasmacytoid, 627
Dengue fever, 1100
in returning travelers, 83
Dengue hemorrhagic fever (DHF), 1100
Dengue shock syndrome (DSS), 1100
Dengue viruses, 1100
maternal infection, 546
serotypes, 1100
transmission, 546
to neonate, 546
Dental abscess
anaerobic infections after, 140
management, 138
Dental caries, 191
Rothia dentocariosa role, 768
Dental infections, 190–191
anaerobic gram-negative bacilli, 983
anaerobic gram-positive cocci, 989
viridans group streptococci, 717
see also Odontogenic infection
Dental plaque, 191
Dental procedures
endocarditis pathogenesis, 258
endocarditis prevention, 75, 75b
Dental trauma, endocarditis associated, 717
Deoxycholate-citrate agar, 1375t
Deoxyribonuclease, recombinant human, 641

Depression
chronic fatigue syndrome and, 1012
in HCV infection treatment, 1111
mefloquine contraindication, 1304, 1305t
Taenia solium neurocysticercosis, 1353–1354
Dermacentor andersoni
appearance, 1092f
coltivirus (Colorado tick fever) transmission, 1092
geographical distribution, 1092, 1092f
Dermal cyst, 289f
Dermal sinus tract, 289f
meningitis associated, 273t
recurrent meningitis, 287–289, 289f
Dermatitis
atopic *see* Atopic dermatitis
cercarial ("swimmer's itch"), 1370
contact, 439f
contagious pustular (orf) *see* Orf virus
diaper (*Candida*), 1197, 1198f, 1200
disseminated gonococcal infection, 744
hookworm infections, 1329
inflammatory, otitis externa, 221
invasive fungal, 1198, 1198f
molluscum, 1025
pruritic, *Onchocerca volvulus* (onchocerciasis), 1345
Schistosoma (schistosomiasis), 1369–1370
seborrheic *see* Seborrheic dermatitis
Dermatologic infections *see* Skin infections
Dermatolymphangioadenitis, acute, *Wuchereria bancrofti* causing, 1343, 1344t
Dermatomyositis
clinical features, 186
juvenile *see* Juvenile dermatomyositis
muscle pain, 186
Dermatophytes, 1246–1250
genital dermatosis due to, 352
transmission, 1246
treatment of infections, 1485t
Dermatophytic ("id") reactions, 453–454, 454b, 1246–1247
Dermoid cysts, 142t, 143, 290f
CSF leak, 290f
recurrent meningitis associated, 287–289
subarachnoid space connection, 290f
Dermonecrosis, leukocidins role, 676
Descriptive epidemiology *see* Epidemiology
Desquamation
Kawasaki disease, 112–113
staphylococcal exfoliative toxin syndrome, 112–113
Developmental delays
congenital rubella, 1115–1116
metabolic diseases causing acute hepatitis, 403
Device-related infections, 10–12, 580, 588–599
bloodstream infections, 580
"bundles" for risk reduction, 588–589
in cancer, neutropenia and, 568, 568t
CNS devices, 596–597, 597b
determinants and risk factors, 588b
devices involved, 588

intravascular catheters *see* Central line associated bloodstream infections (CLABSIs); Central venous catheter (CVC)-related infections; Intravascular catheters
orthopedic devices, 598–599
pacemakers and ventricular assist devices, 596
pathogens, 588–589, 588b
peritoneal catheters, 597–598
prosthetic valves/patches and vascular grafts, 594–596, 595b–596b
risk factors, 588, 588b
risk reduction measures, 588–589
sources and rates, 10–12
urinary catheters, 599
Deworming programs
Ascaris lumbricoides, 1328–1329
pets, *Dipylidium caninum* prevention, 1349
Dexamethasone
in acute bacterial meningitis, 278, 725–726
Haemophilus influenzae, 904
adverse effects, 725–726
bronchiolitis management, 234
laryngotracheitis therapy, 211
very low birthweight infants, 555
see also Corticosteroids
DF-2 bacillus *see* Capnocytophaga canimorsus
Diabetes insipidus, fever of unknown origin due to, 119t–120t
Diabetes mellitus
Coccidioides immitis (coccidioidomycosis) in, 1241
insulin-dependent
in congenital rubella, 1115
enterovirus role in etiology, 1177–1178
as mucormycosis risk factor, 1213
necrotizing otitis externa, 221
subcutaneous tissue infection pathogenesis, 460
Diagnosis/diagnostic testing *see* Laboratory diagnosis; *individual pathogens*
Dialysis
antibiotic dose adjustment, 1445t–1452t
pharmacokinetics, 1436–1437, 1436t
see also Hemodialysis; Peritoneal dialysis
Dialyzers, sterilization and reuse protocols, 596
Diaper dermatitis, 1197, 1198f, 1200
Diapers
advice to travelers, 76
infections associated, group childcare, 26
Diaphragm, splinting, 172
Diaphragmatic hernia, congenital, persistent pneumonia, 247f
Diaphragmatic irritation
abdominal pain in pneumonia, 173
acute pain, 171
Diarrhea
acute infectious
in childcare, 26, 374
Giardia intestinalis (giardiasis), 1281–1282
adenoviruses, 1069
Aeromonas causing, 830–831

in AIDS/HIV infection, 386–387,
  661–662
antimicrobial-associated, 374
  healthcare-associated, 584–585
  HSCT recipients, 563–564
  see also Clostridium difficile
Bacillus cereus infections causing, 753
Balantidium coli causing, 1267
bloody, 375
  differential diagnosis, 1275
  Entamoeba histolytica infection, 1275
  foodborne disease, 398
  hemolytic uremic syndrome,
    798–799
  Salmonella Typhi, 817
  Shigella, 821
  Yersinia enterocolitica, 824
Campylobacter jejuni causing *see*
  Campylobacter jejuni
Campylobacter upsaliensis causing,
  879–880
chronic
  Cystoisospora and *Cyclospora* causing,
    1283–1284
  Giardia intestinalis (giardiasis),
    1281–1282
  microsporidia causing, 1291–1292
Clostridium difficile associated *see*
  Clostridium difficile
Clostridium perfringens causing, 397
Cryptosporidium causing, 1269–1270
Cyclospora causing, 1283–1284
Cystoisospora belli causing, 1283–1284
Dientamoeba fragilis causing, 1279
Diphyllobothrium causing, 1347
electrolyte imbalances in, 1411
empiric transmission-based precautions,
  20t
enteroviruses causing, 1177
Escherichia coli causing, 797–798
etiology, 24–27, 26t
  assessment, 373f
  inoculum required, 372t
foodborne, 373
  Staphylococcus aureus food poisoning,
    394t
foodborne diseases causing, 393, 394t
Giardia intestinalis (giardiasis) causing,
  1279–1281, 1281t
group childcare and, 24–27, 26t, 374
  transmission and risk factors, 374
Helicobacter infections causing, 911,
  918
Helicobacter pylori causing, 912
in hospitals, 374–375
HSCT recipients, 563–564
immunosuppressed children, 374
inflammatory, 375
  Campylobacter jejuni, 876
Listeria monocytogenes causing, 765–766
microsporidia causing, 1291–1292
noninflammatory, 375
norovirus infections, 1187, 1188t, 1189
osmotic, rotavirus causing, 380
pathogen transmission and attack rates,
  24–25
pathogenesis, 375
pathogens causing, 24–27, 26t

persistent, 375
  bacterial overgrowth, 391
person-to-person transmission, 372, 372t
Plesiomonas shigelloides causing, 810
rotavirus causing, 380, 1094–1095
Salmonella causing, 816
  group childcare infections and, 25
secretory
  Campylobacter jejuni, 873–874
  rotavirus causing, 380, 584
Shigella causing, 26t, 821
short-gut syndrome, 391
Staphylococcus aureus food poisoning,
  394t
Strongyloides causing, 1333
Strongyloides fuelleborni causing, 1333
travelers', 81–82, 373–374
  Aeromonas, 830
  causative agents, 81
  chemoprophylaxis, 81–82
  Cryptosporidium, 1269
  Cystoisospora belli, 1283
  etiology and risk factors, 373–374
  preventive measures, 81–82, 82b, 374
  risk, 81
  treatment, 82
Trichinella spiralis causing, 1341
Trichuris trichiura causing, 1331
viral gastroenteritis causing, 380
watery, 375
  Aeromonas causing, 830
  astroviruses causing, 1191
  Campylobacter jejuni, 873–874
  clinical features (in cholera), 851t
  Clostridium difficile, 584
  Cryptosporidium causing, 1270
  differential diagnosis, 822
  Escherichia coli causing, 797–798
  Plesiomonas shigelloides, 810
  Shigella causing, 821
  Vibrio cholerae infection, 851
see also Gastroenteritis
Diarrheal illness, epidemic curve, 8f
Diazepam, *Clostridium tetani* infections, 969
Dibromopropamidine, *Acanthamoeba*
  keratitis, 1297
Dicloxacillin
  dacryoadenitis, 508
  dosage, 1445t–1452t, 1480t–1483t
  infections in phagocyte disorders, 624t
  pharmacology, 1453t–1458t
  spectrum of activity, 1459t–1463t
Dicrocoelium dendriticum, 1365
Dictyostelium discoideum, 1273–1274
Didanosine (ddI), 664, 665t
  dosage, 1445t–1452t
Dientamoeba fragilis, 1279
  diagnosis and treatment, 1279
  Enterobius vermicularis association, 1279
N, N-Diethyl-meta-toluamide see DEET
Diethylcarbamazine (DEC)
  adverse reactions, 1343, 1345–1346,
    1524
  Loa loa infections, 1346
  lymphatic filariasis, 1342t, 1343
  Mansonella ozzardi, 1346
  Mansonella perstans, 1346
  Mansonella streptocerca, 1346

Onchocerca volvulus detection by Mazzotti
  reaction, 1345
  systemic nematode infections, 1524
Diethyltoluamide *see* DEET
Difenoxin, diarrhea, 377t
DiGeorge syndrome, 627, 630t, 631
  characteristics, 603t–604t
  clinical features, 630t, 631
  Giardia intestinalis (giardiasis), 1281
  immunizations in, 52t–53t
  pneumonia, 251, 253
  SCID associated, 626–627, 630t
Digoxin
  metabolism, 961
  in myocarditis, 267–268
Dihydrofolate reductase (DHFR) inhibitors,
  1479, 1522
Diloxanide furoate, protozoan infection
  treatment, 1519
  Entamoeba histolytica (amebiasis), 1277,
    1519
3,6-*bis*(Dimethylamino) acridine, 1374,
  1376–1377
Dimeticones, pediculosis treatment, 1259
Dimorphic fungi
  Blastomyces dermatitidis, 1234
  Coccidioides, 1239, 1239f
  detection, 1382
  Histoplasma capsulatum, 1224
Dinoflagellates, poisoning due to, 396t
Dipetalogaster maximus, 1322, 1323f
Diphenoxylate hydrochloride
  diarrhea, 377t
  inflammatory enteritis, 387
Diphtheria *see Corynebacterium diphtheriae*
Diphtheria, tetanus, and pertussis (DTP)
  vaccination/vaccines, 55–56,
    872–873, 873t
  adverse events and IoM findings, 50t, 56
  adverse reactions, 873
  cocoon strategy, 872–873
  contraindications/precautions, 56
    adolescents to 18 years, 56
  diphtheria–tetanus (dT) vaccine,
    758–759
  DTaP, 55–56, 758, 873
    composition, types and indications,
      55, 55t
    dosages, 55t
    reasons for deferral, 56
    recommendations for children over 7
      years, 55–56, 55t, 757
    recommendations for children under
      7 years, 51, 55t, 758, 872
    schedule, 49f, 55–56
    tetanus prevention, 970t
    for travelers, 77–78, 78t
  group childcare and, 30t
  indications, 55
  schedule, 49f, 55–56, 758–759
    by age, 758
    pertussis contraindication, 759
  Tdap, 55t, 56, 758, 872
    decennial booster, 872
    indications, 758
    licensure, 873
    pregnant healthcare personnels,
      22–24

recommendations for adolescents, 56, 758–759
special situations (for single dose), 56
trauma-related infection prevention, 512–513
whole-cell DTP, 55
adverse reactions, 55
see also Bordetella pertussis; Clostridium tetani; Corynebacterium diphtheriae
Diphtheria antitoxin see under Corynebacterium diphtheriae
Diphtheria toxoid see under Corynebacterium diphtheriae
Diphtheria–tetanus (dT) vaccine, 758–759
"Diphtheroids" see Corynebacterium diphtheriae
Diphyllobothrium (diphyllobothriasis), 1347–1348
clinical manifestations, 1347
description, 1347
eggs and egg discharge, 1347
epidemiology, 1347
laboratory findings and diagnosis, 1347
larvae (sparganum), 1347
life cycle and stages, 1347
prevention, 1348
treatment of infections, 1348
Diphyllobothrium cordatum, 1347
Diphyllobothrium dalliae, 1347
Diphyllobothrium dendriticum, 1347
Diphyllobothrium lanceolatum, 1347
Diphyllobothrium latum, 1347
Diphyllobothrium nihonkaiense, 1347
Diphyllobothrium pacificum, 1347
Diphyllobothrium ursi, 1347
Dipylidium caninum, 1348–1349, 1348f
Direct fluorescent antibody (DFA)
Bordetella pertussis, 869–870
Chlamydia trachomatis, 887, 1398
Giardia intestinalis, 1281–1282
Legionella, 924
Rickettsia akari (rickettsialpox) infection, 934
for specific viruses, 1386t
adenoviruses, 1070
measles virus, 1395–1396
RSV, 233–234, 1394
Treponema pallidum test (DFA-TP), 945
Directly observed therapy (DOTS), tuberculosis, 784–785
follow-up, 785
latent Mycobacterium tuberculosis infection treatment, 783
Dirofilaria (dirofilariasis), 1346
pulmonary, 1346
subcutaneous, 1346
Dirofilaria immitis, 1342t, 1346
Dirofilaria repens, 1342t, 1346
Dirofilaria tenuis, 1342t, 1346
Disability-adjusted life years (DALYs)
Campylobacter jejuni infections, 874–875
parasitic infection burden, 1254–1255
Disaccharidase deficiency, Giardia intestinalis (giardiasis), 1280
Discharge/dysuria syndrome, 346–347, 346t
clinical features, 346–347
Discharge/proctitis/proctocolitis/enteritis syndrome, 346t, 347

Disclosure, HIV infection, 670
Disease control, 7–9
public health policy and, 7–9
see also Infection prevention and control (IPC)
Disease outcome, confounding variable and risk relationship, 6f
Disease prevention see Infection prevention and control (IPC)
Diseases of possible infectious origin see Chronic fatigue syndrome; Kawasaki disease (KD)
Disinfectants
norovirus infection prevention, 1189
resistance to, 18
Disinfection, 21
deficiencies, 21
definition, 21
Disk diffusion D testing, 686, 1378, 1430, 1430f–1431f
Diskitis, 483–485
back pain due to, 187, 188t
Candida, 483
clinical features, 484, 484t
definition, 483
diagnosis, 483t, 484–485
differential diagnosis, 484
epidemiology and etiology, 483
Kingella kingae, 483
management and outcome, 485
Mycobacterium, 483
pathogenesis and pathology, 483–484
Staphylococcus aureus, 483, 680
Streptococcus epidermidis, 483
Streptococcus pneumoniae, 483
vertebral osteomyelitis vs., 474, 483, 680
Disseminated intravascular coagulation (DIC), 94, 1402–1404
Distribution, drug, 1433, 1434f, 1438–1439
age vs., 1435, 1435t
antimicrobial agents, 1453t–1458t
volume of, 1434
see also individual drugs
DNA-DNA hybridization, bacterial identification by, 674
DNA probe assay
bacterial vaginosis diagnosis, 360
Chlamydia trachomatis, 1398
cytomegalovirus (CMV), 1386, 1388
Gardnerella vaginalis, 360
resistance detection, 1430
Trichomonas vaginalis, 360
viruses, 1386–1387
DNA sequencing
resistance detection, 1430
see also Genome
DNA viruses, 1018f
Dobrava virus, 1103–1104, 1103t–1104t
Dog(s), infections related to, 527
bites see Bites, infections after
Echinococcus granulosus, 1356, 1357f
Echinococcus multilocularis, 1360
Echinococcus vogeli, 1361
Leishmania reservoir, 1286, 1290
rabies, 1146–1147
Strongyloides (strongyloidiasis), 1332
Taenia serialis, 1362–1363

tapeworms (Dipylidium caninum), 1348–1349, 1348f
Toxocara infection transmission, 1335, 1337
Trypanosoma (Schizotrypanum) cruzi reservoir, 1324
Döhle bodies, 1405
Domoic acid, poisoning, 396t
Donovan bodies, 803
Donovanosis see Klebsiella (Calymmatobacterium) granulomatis (donovanosis)
Dopamine, septic shock management, 99
Doppler flow imaging, endocarditis, 261
Dorsal root ganglion, latent VZV infection, 1035–1036
Dosage
antifungal agents, 1443–1444, 1443t
antimicrobial agents, 1417–1419, 1480t–1483t
burned patients, 1437t, 1438
neonates, 1483t–1484t
optimal regimens, 1440–1443
pharmacokinetic/pharmacodynamic issues for consideration, 1445b
renal dysfunction, 1435–1437, 1445t–1452t
antiretroviral agents, 1445t–1452t
antiviral agents, 1445t–1452t
see also specific agents and diseases
Dose–response relationship, 9
Double hockey stick sign, 335f
Double sickening, 228
Downey cells, 1061
Doxycycline
adverse effects, 1304
chemoprophylactic use, 70t–71t
dosage, 1445t–1452t, 1480t–1483t
life-threatening reaction to, 938
pharmacology, 1453t–1458t
in prion diseases, 338
prophylaxis
Lyme disease, 535–536
malaria, 80–81, 1522
Plasmodium, 1304, 1305t
protozoan infections, 1522
Yersinia pestis infection, 827
resistance to, 1428
spectrum of activity, 1459t–1463t, 1472
staining of teeth by, 892
treatment of, 935
acute bacterial cystitis, 356
Babesia (babesiosis), 1265
Bacillus anthracis infections, 752–753
Borrelia burgdorferi (Lyme disease), 955
Borrelia infections, 958
Brucella infections, 864, 864t
Chlamydia trachomatis infections, 888t
Coxiella burnetii infections, 892
Ehrlichia and Anaplasma infections, 896
epididymitis, 367
Leptospira infections, 951
Mansonella perstans infections, 1346
murine typhus (Rickettsia typhi), 932
Mycoplasma pneumoniae infections, 997

Neisseria gonorrhoeae infections, 746–747
Onchocerca volvulus infection, 1345
Plasmodium infections, 1300–1304, 1301t–1303t
in pneumonia, 240
Rickettsia akari (rickettsialpox) infection, 934
Rickettsia felis infections, 933
Rickettsia prowazekii infections, 931
Rocky Mountain spotted fever (*Rickettsia rickettsii*), 928
Staphylococcus aureus infection, 687
tickborne infections, 535
Ureaplasma urealyticum infections, 1001
urethritis, 356
Vibrio cholerae infection, 853
vulvovaginitis, 358
Dracunculus, eosinophilia, 1407
DRESS syndrome, 133–134
Dressler syndrome, 270
Droplet Precautions, 18
Droplet transmission, healthcare-associated infections, 12
Drug absorption *see* Absorption, of drugs
Drug abuse, intravenous
Bacillus cereus infections, 754
Corynebacterium diphtheriae infections, 756
eosinophilic meningitis, 333
HCV transmission, 1105–1107
HIV transmission, 642–643, 648
viral infections in neonates *vs.*, 548
wound botulism, 977
Drug distribution *see* Distribution, drug
Drug hypersensitivity reactions, 108
Drug-induced disorders
acute pancreatitis, 411
aseptic meningitis, 295–296
chronic hepatitis, 407
eosinophilic meningitis, 333
generalized lymphadenopathy, 133–134
granulomatous hepatitis, 409
hypersensitivity, 133–134
fever of unknown origin due to, 119t–120t
maculopapular rashes, 436
recurrent meningitis, 289
stomatitis, 193t
urticaria, 445
Drug resistance *see* Antimicrobial drug resistance
Drug–drug interactions, 1438–1440, 1440t
see also under individual drugs
Dry eyes, infective keratitis due to, 495
DTaP vaccine *see* Diphtheria, tetanus, and pertussis (DTP) vaccination/vaccines
Dual energy X-ray absorptiometry (DXA), in HIV infection, 671
"Duck hunter's itch", 1338
Duffy blood group antigen, 1298
Duke schema, endocarditis diagnostic criteria, 261b, 262
Duodenal aspirate, specimen collection/transport, 1374t, 1383
Duodenal biopsy, *Giardia intestinalis*, 1282

Duodenal injury, retroperitoneal abscess after, 426
Duodenal ulcer *see* Peptic ulcer
Dura mater grafts, CJD and, 334
Dural venous sinuses, septic thrombosis *see* Septic venous thrombosis
Duration of therapy, antibiotics, 1417–1419, 1418t–1419t
Dysautonomia, fever of unknown origin due to, 119t–120t
Dysentery, 375
acute, 382
amebic, 384, 1275–1276, 1275t
bacillary *see Shigella dysenteriae* type 1
Trichuris, 1331
Dyslipidemia, after HAART in HIV infection, 670
Dyspnea
Aspergillus infections, 1203
in bacterial tracheitis, 212
SARS, 1119
Dysuria
discharge/dysuria syndrome, 346–347
epididymitis, 367
external/internal, 354
female, 353–354
urethritis, 354, 354t
urinary tract infection, 340

E

E-cadherin, internalin interaction, 763–764
E-test, 965, 1380–1381, 1416, 1430, 1430f
Ear, 253t
cartilage, burn wound infections, 519
congenital abnormalities, recurrent meningitis with, 287–289
infections
in cancer, 577
treatment, 1496–1498, 1497t
see also Middle ear; Otitis externa; Otitis media
Ear drops, 1496–1498, 1497t
Earache, mumps virus infection, 1126
Earthworms, *Toxocara* eggs distribution, 1337
Eastern Association for the Surgery of Trauma (EAST), 515
Eastern equine encephalitis virus (EEEV), 1098
diagnosis/detection, 1397
optimal tests, 1389t–1392t
encephalitis due to, 302–303, 313
Ebola virus, 1159, 1160t
epidemiology, 1159, 1160t
treatment and prevention of infections, 1163–1164
see also Filoviruses
Ecchymoses (bruises)
etiology, 443–444
pathogenesis, 443
Echinacea, in common colds, 198, 1187
Echinocandins, 1491–1492
Aspergillus infection treatment, 1208–1209
Candida infection treatment, 1201
Cryptococcus infections, 1223

neutropenia associated with cancer, 571–572
Echinococcosis
alveolar *see Echinococcus multilocularis*
cystic *see Echinococcus granulosus*
hepatic, 1358
polycystic, 1357f, 1361
Echinococcus, 1356–1361, 1361b–1362b
eosinophilia, 1407, 1408t–1409t
Echinococcus granulosus (cystic echinococcosis), 1356–1360
biliary obstruction, 412
"cervid" type, 1356
clinical manifestations, 1358
description, 1356, 1358f
eosinophilic meningitis, 331t
epidemiology, 1356–1358
genetic types and strains, 1356
hydatid cysts, 1356, 1358f
diagnosis, 1358, 1359f
liver, 1358, 1359f
lung, 1358, 1359f
percutaneous aspiration, 1360
rupture, 1358
surgical removal, 1358–1359
laboratory findings and diagnosis, 1358, 1359f
life cycle, 1356, 1357f
prevention, 1360
treatment, 1358
chemotherapy, 1359–1360
monitoring results, 1360
percutaneous aspiration, injection, respiration (PAIR), 1358, 1360
surgery, 1358–1359
Echinococcus multilocularis (alveolar echinococcosis), 1360–1361
clinical manifestations, 1360–1361
description of pathogen, 1360
epidemiology, 1360
laboratory findings and diagnosis, 1361, 1361f
prevention, 1361
treatment, 1361
Echinococcus vogeli (polycystic echinococcosis), 1357f, 1361
Echinostome infections, 1364
Echocardiography
acute rheumatic fever, 704
endocarditis, 261–262
Kawasaki disease, 1005
M-mode, pericarditis, 270
myocarditis, 267
pericarditis, 270
transesophageal *see* Transesophageal echocardiography (TEE)
two-dimensional, pericarditis, 270
Echovirus(es), 1172–1180
aseptic meningitis due to, 1175
clinical manifestations, 1174, 1174t
diagnosis, optimal tests, 1389t–1392t
diarrhea due to, 1177
group childcare setting, 28
in adults attending/care providers, 28
in immunodeficiency children, 1179
myositis due to, 1176
neonatal infections, 1178
reclassification, 297–302

serotypes, 1172–1174, 1172t–1173t
see also Enterovirus(es)
Echovirus 6 infection, 1173t, 1177
Echovirus 11, neonatal hepatitis, 1178–1179
"Ecological fallacy", 2
Econazole, superficial infection treatment, 1485
Economic analysis, disease prevention, 8–9
Economic impact, of group childcare illness, 31
Ecthyma, 434
Ecthyma contagiosum, 1024
Ecthyma gangrenosum, 434, 434f
  Aeromonas causing, 830–831
  Pseudomonas aeruginosa, 550, 844f, 844t
  Stenotrophomonas maltophilia, 849
Ectocervicitis, 361
Ectocervix, inflammation *see* Cervicitis
Ectodermal dysplasia, 632–633
  hypohidrotic, 602t
Ectoocervix, infections, 361
Ectoparasites, 1257–1261
  lice *see* Pediculosis
  scabies *see* Sarcoptes scabiei (scabies)
Ectopic pregnancy
  pelvic inflammatory disease complication, 366
  pelvic inflammatory disease *vs.*, 365t
Ectopy, cervical, 353, 363, 363f
Ectropion, 361
Eczema *see* Dermatitis
Eczema vaccinatum, 1023–1024, 1023f
Edema, 1411
  aryepiglottic folds, 210f
  cerebral *see* Cerebral edema
  inflammatory, sinusitis causing, 510
  mucosal, *Trichuris trichiura* causing, 1331
  periorbital, *Trichinella spiralis* infections, 1341
  pulmonary *see* Pulmonary edema
Education, infection prevention in childcare centers, 31–32
Edwardsiella, 808
Edwardsiella tarda, 808
  bloodstream infections, 808
  meningitis, 808
Efavirenz, 664–666, 665t, 1444t–1452t
Effect modifiers, 6
  control of, 6–7
  impact, 6f
Eflornithine, *Trypanosoma brucei* infection, 1322t, 1520
Ehrlichia, 893–896
  chronic fatigue syndrome pathogenesis, 1008t–1009t
  clinical manifestations, 108, 894–895, 894t
  diagnosis of infections, 895–896, 896b
  differential diagnosis, 108, 895
  epidemiology, 894, 894t
  fever of unknown origin due to, 119t–120t
  laboratory findings, 895
  lymphopenia due to, 1406
  microbiology, 894
  morulae, 893
  neutropenia due to, 1405
  opportunistic infections, 895

  pathogenesis, 893–894
  prevention, 896
  thrombocytopenia due to, 1410–1411
  treatment of infections, 896, 896b
Ehrlichia chaffeensis, 893–896
  cross-reactivity with *Anaplasma phagocytophila*, 535
  generalized lymphadenopathy, 131t–132t
  human monocytic ehrlichiosis epidemiology, 532t
  laboratory findings and diagnosis, 533t–534t
  laboratory testing, 308t–311t
Ehrlichia ewingii, 894, 896
  epidemiology and vectors, 532t
  laboratory findings and diagnosis, 533t–534t
  laboratory testing, 308t–311t
Ehrlichia phagocytophilum see Anaplasma phagocytophilum
Ehrlichia sennetsu
  generalized lymphadenopathy, 131t–132t, 132
  see also Sennetsu fever
Ehrlichiosis *see* Ehrlichia
Eikenella, 835–839
  clinical manifestations, 836–837
  microbiology and epidemiology, 835–836
Eikenella corrodens, 835–836
  bite and fist fight infections, 836
  brain abscess due to, 718f
  clinical manifestations, 836, 837f
  endocarditis due to, 257
  growth and culture, 835–836
  human bites, 521, 523, 526
  paronychia due to, 432
  puncture wound infections, 515
  skin infection after trauma, 514
  treatment of infections, 838–839
  virulence factors and pilus proteins, 836
Ekiri syndrome, 821
Elastase, neutrophil, in cyclic neutropenia, 123
Electrocardiography (ECG)
  myocarditis, 267
  pericarditis, 270
  PR interval prolongation
    in acute rheumatic fever, 704
    Corynebacterium diphtheriae causing, 756
  QRS complex, quinidine use in *Plasmodium* infections, 1303
  Trichinella spiralis infections, 1341
Electroencephalography (EEG)
  in altered mental status, 178–179
  encephalitis diagnosis, 308
  HSV encephalitis, 1030–1031
  rabies, 1147
  sporadic CJD, 338
  subacute sclerosing panencephalitis, 1142–1143
Electrolytes
  composition of oral rehydration solution, 851t
  diarrheal stools in cholera, 851t

  imbalance
    Plasmodium infections, 1300
    Vibrio cholerae infection, 851–852
Electromyography (EMG), *Clostridium botulinum*, 974
Electron microscopy, viruses, 1386
Elek test, 754–755
Elementary body (EB)
  Chlamydia trachomatis, 884, 884f
  Chlamydophila (Chlamydia) pneumoniae, 881
Elephantiasis, *Wuchereria bancrofti* causing, 1343–1344, 1344t
Elimination, antimicrobial agents, 1434–1435, 1434f, 1439–1440, 1453t–1458t
  age *vs.*, 1435, 1435t
Elizabethkingia meningoseptica, 832, 834
  antibiotic resistance, 834
  neonatal meningitis, 834
  nosocomial infections, 834
  treatment, 834
Emboli
  endocarditis complication, 264
  endocarditis pathogenesis, 259
  septic
    brain abscess due to, 321
    endocarditis complication, 264
Embryopathy, varicella in pregnancy, 1038
Emerging infectious diseases
  nosocomial neonatal infections, 551
  travelers, 82
Emesis *see* Vomiting
Emotions, recurrent abdominal pain associated, 175
Empedobacter, 834
Empedobacter brevis (Flavobacterium breve), 832
Emphysema, obstructive, pulmonary tuberculosis, 774–775
Empiric (Syndromic) Precautions, 18
Empiric therapy, antibiotics *see* Antibiotics
Empyema
  complicated, 241
  pleural, 241–243
    trauma-associated, 516
    Streptococcus pneumoniae, 723
  subdural *see* Subdural empyema
Empyema necessitans, 242
Emtricitabine, 665t
  dosage, 1445t–1452t
  HBV infection treatment, 1083
Enanthems, enterovirus infections, 1174–1175, 1174t, 1175f
Encephalitis, 297–314
  Acanthamoeba, 1296
  acute, rubeola virus (measles), 1141
  acute disseminated *see* Acute disseminated encephalomyelitis (ADEM)
  adenoviruses, 1069
  altered mental status, 179t
  amebas (free-living) causing, 303–304, 307
  anaerobic gram-negative bacilli, 983
  arboviruses, 302–304
  bacterial causes, 178, 303
  Bartonella henselae, 303, 313

Borrelia burgdorferi (Lyme disease), 303
brainstem *see* Brainstem encephalitis
  (rhombencephalitis)
clinical approach, 312b
clinical features, 297, 304–308,
  305t–306t
complications and prognosis, 313
conditions mimicking, 302b
cytomegalovirus (CMV), 314, 1047
definition, 297
differential diagnosis, 302b, 304–308,
  312t
Eastern equine encephalitis virus,
  302–303
enteroviruses causing, 297, 302, 1174t,
  1176
  brainstem encephalitis, 1176
epidemiology, 297–304, 298t–302t
Epstein–Barr virus (EBV), 302, 313
etiologic agents, 297–304, 298t–302t
  new pathogens, 297
  viral/bacterial, 178, 297–303
fungi causing, 303, 314
granulomatous amebic *see*
  Granulomatous amebic encephalitis
  (GAE)
HHV-6 causing, 1055
histology, 304
HSV causing *see* Herpes simplex virus
  (HSV), encephalitis
human parechoviruses, 297–302
immunocompromised hosts, 314
infant botulism *vs.*, 974t
infectious, 297–304
influenza-associated, 303–304, 1153
Japanese encephalitis virus, 303
  see also Japanese encephalitis virus
  (JEV)
La Crosse virus (LACV), 303, 1103–1104,
  1104t
laboratory findings, 305t–306t, 312
laboratory tests (organism-specific),
  308t–311t
LCMV causing, 303
Listeria monocytogenes, 313, 765
management, 312–313
  future directions, 313
measles complication, 303, 1141
  subacute, 1143
MMR vaccine associated, 60
Mycoplasma, 304, 307
Mycoplasma pneumoniae, 994t, 995
neonatal, 312t, 313
NMDAR, 179–180, 304, 307–308, 313
paraneoplastic limbic, 178–179
parasites causing, 303–304
pathogenesis, 304
Plasmodium falciparum, 304
postinfectious, epidemiology, 304
Powassan virus, 303
prevention, 313
primary amebic *see* Primary amebic
  meningoencephalitis (PAM)
rabies vaccine-associated autoimmune,
  1147
rabies virus (rabies), 303, 1145–1146
Rift Valley fever, 1104
Rocky Mountain spotted fever, 303

rubella, 1116
rubeola virus (measles), 1141
St Louis encephalitis virus causing,
  302–303
Taenia solium, 1353–1354, 1353f, 1355t
Toxoplasma, 304
toxoplasmic *see Toxoplasma gondii*
varicella (VZV), 1037–1039
viruses causing, 178, 297–303
West Nile virus, 303, 1101, 1170
yellow fever vaccine associated, 79
Encephalitozoon cuniculi, 1291, 1292t
Encephalitozoon hellem, 1292t
Encephalitozoon intestinalis, 1292, 1292t
Encephalocele, recurrent meningitis and,
  288–289
Encephalomyelitis, acute disseminated *see*
  Acute disseminated encephalomyelitis
  (ADEM)
Encephalopathy
  acute necrotizing (ANE), 306–307, 306b
  bovine spongiform (BSE), 334–335
  cat-scratch (*Bartonella henselae*),
    179–180, 860
  HHV-6 causing, 1055
  HSCT recipients, 564, 565b
  influenza complication, 1153
  metabolic, *Plasmodium* infection, 1299
  progressive HIV, 652b, 653, 653t
  RSV infection, 1132–1133
  toxic *see* Toxic encephalopathy
Endocardial abscess, 264
Endocardial fibroelastosis (EFE), 1127
Endocardial thrombosis, in *Trypanosoma
  cruzi* infections, 1324
Endocardial vegetations, 256–257, 259,
  259f, 261f
  indications for surgical intervention,
    264t
Endocarditis, infective, 256–265
  Abiotrophia, 258, 717
  acute, 259
  in acute rheumatic fever, 703
  Aggregatibacter actinomycetemcomitans,
    257, 939
  Aggregatibacter parainfluenzae, 257
  aortic valve, *Kurthia bessonii* causing, 771
  Bacillus cereus, 754
  bacteremia associated, 258, 260
  blood cultures, 260
    negative results, 257, 260–263, 260t
  brain abscess in, 321, 329
  Brucella, 863, 864t
  burns patients, 519
  Candida, 1199
  Cardiobacterium hominis, 940
  catheter-associated, 257–258, 592
  Cellulosimicrobium (*Oerskovia*), 771
  clinical features, 259–260, 259t, 681,
    692
    signs, 259t
    symptoms, 259, 259t
  coagulase-negative staphylococci
    (CONS), 257
  complications, 260, 264
  congenital heart disease and, 257, 257t
  Corynebacterium, 760t–761t
  Corynebacterium diphtheriae, 756

Coxiella burnetii causing, 260–261, 892
culture-negative, 257, 717
definition, 256–257
dental trauma associated, 75, 717
diagnosis, 260–262, 692–693
  adjuvant, culture-negative
    endocarditis, 260t
  diagnostic imaging, 261–262
  microbiologic evaluation, 260–261
diagnostic criteria, 262
  Duke Schema, 261b, 262, 681
differential diagnosis, 259–260
  myocarditis *vs.*, 266–267
Enterococcus, 714
  treatment, 262t, 263, 1418t–1419t
Enterococcus faecalis, 713, 715
epidemiology, 257, 257t
Erysipelothrix rhusiopathiae, 767
etiologic agents, 257, 257t
fever of unknown origin due to,
  119t–120t
fungi causing, 257
  management, 263–264
gonococcal, 744
Granulicatella, 717
Haemophilus parainfluenzae, 908
histopathology, 259f
imaging (diagnostic), 261–262
Kingella kingae, 257, 920–921
laboratory findings, 260–262, 260t
  culture-negative, 260t
Lactobacillus, 770
left-sided, 259, 263
Listeria monocytogenes, 765
management, 262–264, 681,
  1418t–1419t
  anticoagulants, 264
  coagulase-negative staphylococcal
    infections, 694
  definitive antibiotic therapy, 262t,
    263–264
  doses of antimicrobials, 263t
  duration of therapy, 263–264
  empiric antibiotics, 262–263
  oral antibiotics, 264
  by organism, 262t
  outpatient, 264
  surgical, 264, 264t
methicillin-resistant *Staphylococcus aureus*,
  1418t–1419t
mortality, 257, 265
  in neonates, 692–693
neonatal, 257, 549, 692–693
pathogenesis, 258–259, 717
  native valve, 258, 681, 692
  pacemaker-/ventricular assist devices,
    258–259
  postoperative, 258
  prosthetic valve, 681, 692
pathology, 258f–259f, 259
physical examination, 259
postoperative, 257–258
prevention, 74t, 75–76, 75b, 261–262,
  265
  chemoprophylaxis, 74t, 75, 268
  chemoprophylaxis recommendations
    of AHA, 75, 75b
  dental care/procedures, 75, 75b

gastrointestinal tract procedures, 76
genitourinary tract procedures, 76
prosthetic valve/patch use, 596
respiratory tract procedures, 76
viridans streptococci causing, 719
prognosis, 264–265
prognostic factors, 265
prosthetic valves, 595, 681, 692
Pseudomonas aeruginosa, 843t
right-sided, 258–259
risk factors, 257, 264
Rothia dentocariosa, 768
Staphylococcus, 257
Staphylococcus aureus, 257–258, 263,
   592–593, 681, 683, 686
Staphylococcus epidermidis, 692–693
Staphylococcus lugdunensis, 692
Streptococcus, 257
Streptococcus bovis, 1418t–1419t
Streptococcus pneumoniae, 257, 263
Streptococcus viridans, 1418t–1419t
subacute, 259
viridans group streptococci, 257, 717
   treatment recommendations, 718,
      719t
"Endocarditis-like" intravascular infections,
   265
Endocervicitis, 361–363
clinical features, 362
complications, 363
differential diagnosis, 362
etiology and epidemiology, 361–362
laboratory findings and diagnosis, 362
management, 362, 362t
prevention, 363
Endocervix
infections, 361
inflammation *see* Cervicitis
Endogenous pyrogens, 91
Endolimax nana, 1271–1272, 1272f
Endomyocardial biopsy, 267
Endophthalmitis, 503–506, 504f
Bacillus cereus infections, 754
bleb-related, 503
in chronic meningitis, 284t
clinical manifestations, 504
coagulase-negative staphylococci causing,
   693
diagnosis, 504–505
endogenous, 503
epidemiology and host factors, 503–504
etiologic agents, 503
exogenous, 503
management, 505, 505t, 1495–1496
outcome, 505
pathophysiology, 504
postoperative, 503, 505
posttraumatic, 503–504, 506
prevention, 506
Staphylococcus aureus, 679
Endoscopy, endocarditis prevention, 76
Endospores, *Coccidioides immitis*
   (coccidioidomycosis), 1239,
   1239f–1240f
Endothelial cells
dysregulation/damage in sepsis, 102
   therapy targeted at, 101t–102t, 102
meningitis pathology, 273

stimulation in inflammatory response,
   94
Treponema pallidum adherence, 941–942
Endotoxin (lipopolysaccharide), 100, 673
actions, 100
antibodies against, 101t–102t
antiendotoxin therapies, 100
CD14 interaction, 102–103
as exogenous pyrogen, 91
in inflammation, 100
as pathogen-associated molecular pattern
   (PAMP), 92–93
Pseudomonas aeruginosa, 842t, 843
release, *Neisseria meningitidis* infections,
   731
removal therapy, 101t–102t
statin therapy effect on, 101t–102t
toxicity, TNF-α role, 100
Endotracheal intubation
in infant botulism, 975
in meningococcal disease, 737
in ventilator-associated pneumonia,
   581–582
Enfuvirtide, 665t, 666, 1445t–1452t
Entamoeba, 1273, 1278
Entamoeba chattoni, 1278
Entamoeba coli, 1271, 1272f, 1279
Entamoeba dispar, 1273, 1278
description and infections, 1274–1275
Entamoeba histolytica vs., 1276–1277
epidemiology, 1274
Entamoeba gingivalis, 1278
Entamoeba histolytica vs., 1278
Entamoeba hartmanni, 1271, 1272f,
   1278–1279
Entamoeba histolytica (amebiasis), 1273–
   1277, 1277b–1278b
amebic meningoencephalitis, treatment,
   1520
clinical manifestations, 1275–1276,
   1277b–1278b
   acute fulminant (necrotizing) colitis,
      1275–1276, 1275f
   amebic colitis (intestinal amebiasis),
      1273–1275, 1275f, 1275t
   ameboma, 1276
   brain abscess, 319, 1276
   colonic ulcers, 1274
   extraintestinal, 1276
   growth and cognitive complications,
      1276
   liver abscess, 1273–1274, 1276,
      1276f, 1276t
   noninvasive intestinal infection, 1275
   signs/symptoms, 1275t–1276t
colonization, 1274
cytolysis mechanism, 1274
description and life cycle, 1273–1274,
   1273f–1274f, 1277b–1278b
diagnosis/detection, 385t
differential diagnosis, 1275–1276
   Entamoeba gingivalis vs., 1278
differentiation from nonpathogenic
   Entamoeba, 1277
dissemination, 383
epidemiology, 1274, 1277b–1278b
Gal/GalNAc lectin, 1274
genome, 1255

immunity (innate and acquired), 1275
inflammatory enteritis, 383t, 384
laboratory findings and diagnosis, 1274f,
   1276–1277, 1276f, 1277b–1278b
   biopsy specimen, 1383–1384
   specimen collection, 1382–1383
mortality, 1274–1276
pathogenesis of infection, 1274
prevention, 1277
proteinase, 1275
surgery indications, 1275–1276
treatment of infections, 1277, 1277b,
   1519
trophozoites, 384
water contamination, 384
Entamoeba invadens, 1278
Entamoeba moshkovskii, 1273–1274, 1276,
   1278
Entamoeba polecki, 1271, 1272f, 1278
Entecavir, 1509
HBV infection treatment, 1083–1084
Enteric fever
Campylobacter fetus, 879
generalized lymphadenopathy, 130,
   131t–132t
Salmonella see Salmonella Typhi
Enteric gram-negative bacilli, meningitis,
   1418t–1419t
Enteric infections
acute abdominal pain, 174
generalized lymphadenopathy, 130,
   131t–132t
group childcare and, 24–27, 25t, 30–31
   costs and economic impact, 31
HSCT recipients, 563–564
refugee and internationally adopted
   children, 35–36
see also Gastroenteritis; Gastrointestinal
   tract infections
Enteric pathogens
diagnosis/detection, 384–386, 385t
effect of normal flora on, 961
focal suppurative CNS infections, 319
group childcare and, 24–27, 25t
transmission and epidemiology, 373
treatment, 376–377, 377t
see also individual organisms
Enteric viruses, group childcare infections
   and, 25
Enteritis
in AIDS/HIV infection, 661–662
Campylobacter jejuni, 875–876
eosinophilic, *Ancylostoma caninum*
   causing, 1329
inflammatory, 382–387
   acute, 382t
   causes, 383–384, 383t
   chronic, 382, 382t
   complications, 383t
   definition, 382
   diagnosis of pathogen, 385t
   diagnostic evaluation, 384–386, 385t
   differential diagnosis, 382t
   epidemiology, 384
   etiology confirmatory tests, 385–386,
      385t
   immunocompromised host,
      386–387, 386b

management, 387
noninfectious causes, 382
pathogenesis, 383t, 384
risk factors, 384, 384t
tuberculous, 778
see also Diarrhea; Gastroenteritis
Enteritis necroticans (pigbel), 981
Enterobacter, 804–806
ampC β-lactamase, 805
antimicrobial resistance, healthcare-associated infections, 14t
appendicitis due to, 420
bacteremia due to, 805
clinical manifestations, 804–805
epidemiology, 804
extended-spectrum β-lactamase, 805
folliculitis due to, 431
fracture-associated infection, 515
meningitis due to, 806
microbiology and pathogenesis, 804
necrotizing soft-tissue infection, 459–460
nosocomial infections and risk factors, 804
nosocomial infections of neonates, 551
plasmids, 805
species, 804
"stably depressed mutants", 805
treatment, 805–806
Enterobacter aerogenes, 804
prostatitis due to, 369
Enterobacter agglomerans, 804
Yersinia pestis vs., 827
Enterobacter cloacae, 804
Enterobacter sakazakii see Cronobacter
Enterobacteriaceae
antimicrobial susceptibility testing, 1378, 1378t
CLABSI in neonates, 554
culture media, 1376t
less commonly encountered genera, 808–810
meningitis due to, treatment, 276t
surgical site infection, prevention, 587
see also Escherichia coli; Klebsiella; Proteus mirabilis
Enterobius vermicularis, 1326, 1331–1332
acute abdominal pain due to, 174
appendix infection, 1332, 1332f
clinical manifestations, 1327b, 1332
Dientamoeba fragilis association, 1279
eggs, 1327f, 1331–1332
eosinophilia due to, 1407
epidemiology, 1331–1332
infection route, 1326, 1331–1332
laboratory findings and diagnosis, 1327f, 1332, 1383
life cycle, 1332
prevention, 1332
treatment of infections, 1332
urinary tract infections, 339
vulvovaginitis due to, 357
Enterococcal agar, selective, 1375t
Enterococcus, 696b, 696t, 712–716
antimicrobial resistance, 713–714, 1381, 1423
aminoglycosides, 1430
carbapenems, 714–715

healthcare-associated infections, 14t
high- and low-level, 714–715
intrinsic *vs.* acquired, 714, 714b
linezolid, 1426
mechanisms, 714
vancomycin, 1429, 1432, 1469
antimicrobial susceptibility testing, 1378t, 1381
in asplenia, 636
biochemical differentiation, 729t
bloodstream infections, 713
classification, 712, 713t
clinical manifestations, 713–714
colonization by, 713
culture media, 1376t
detection/differentiation, 713
endocarditis, 714
treatment, 262t, 263, 1418t–1419t
epidemiology, 713
Esp virulence factor, 713
growth characteristics, 713t
infection after abdominal trauma, 514
infections in older children, 714
intra-abdominal abscess due to, 714
meningitis due to, 277, 714
microbiology, 713
neonatal infections, 538, 551t, 713–714
normal flora, 959
nosocomial infections of neonates, 549t, 551
prevention of infections, 715–716
risk factors for infections by, 714
treatment of infections, 714–715, 714t
strategies, 715
urinary catheter-related infection, 599
urinary tract infections, 341, 714
vanA and *vanB* genes, 715
vancomycin-resistant *see* Vancomycin-resistant enterococci (VRE)
virulence factors, 713
Enterococcus faecalis, 713
antibiotic resistance, 1423, 1428–1429
carbapenems, 714–715
antibiotic sensitivity, 714, 714t
biochemical/growth characteristics, 713t
catheter-associated BSI, 715
clinical manifestations, 713
cytolysin, 713
endocarditis due to, 713, 715
epidemiology and transmission, 713
neonatal infections, 713
septicemia due to, 713
strain V583, genome, 713
treatment of infections, 714–715, 714t
quinupristin-dalfopristin, 715
Enterococcus faecium, 713
antibiotic resistance, 1423–1425, 1428–1429
carbapenems, 714–715
antibiotic sensitivity, 714, 714t
biochemical/growth characteristics, 713t
infections in neutropenia in cancer, 567
Enterocolitis
Clostridium difficile, 1473, 1478
necrotizing *see* Necrotizing enterocolitis (NEC)
neutropenic, 981
Salmonella, 814

Enterocytozoon bieneusi, 1292, 1292t
Enterohepatic disease, *Helicobacter* causing, 918
Enteropathogens *see* Enteric pathogens
Enterotest capsule, 1383
Enterotoxin, staphylococcal, 676, 684
Enterovirus(es), 1167–1168, 1172–1180
acute bilateral cervical lymphadenitis due to, 138
acute pancreatitis due to, 411, 1177
antibodies, 1173–1174, 1179, 1395
aseptic meningitis due to, 293–296, 1174–1176
treatment, 296
cell culture, 1179, 1395
chest pain due to, 189, 1176
chronic fatigue syndrome pathogenesis, 1008t–1009t
chronic meningitis due to, 283
classification, 1172, 1172t–1173t
clinical manifestations, 1174–1178, 1174t, 1175f
CNS infections, 1175–1176, 1179
congenital infection, clinical features, 537t
cytopathic effects, 1179
diabetes mellitus and, 1177–1178
diagnosis/detection, 293, 296, 1179, 1395
optimal tests, 1389t–1392t
RT-PCR, 1395
specimen collection/transport, 1395
encephalitis due to, 297, 1174t, 1176
brainstem encephalitis, 1176
neonates, 313
epidemiology, 546, 1173–1174, 1173t
erythematous macules/papules due to, 436
exanthems/enanthems due to, 1174–1175, 1175f
fever and prodrome, 1174
generalized lymphadenopathy due to, 132
hand–foot–mouth disease, 1174–1175, 1175f
oral features, 192t
oral mucosal infection, 192t
pharyngitis, 201
skin lesions, 112
herpangina, oral features, 192t
immune response to, 1173
in immunodeficiency, 1179
incubation period, 1174
isolation methods, 1395
laboratory findings, 1179
laboratory testing, 308t–311t
meningoencephalitis, in X-linked agammaglobulinemia, 610–611
mucocutaneous findings, fever and prodrome, 108
myocarditis due to, 265–266, 547, 1176, 1178
neonatal infections, 546–547, 1178–1179
nosocomial, 551
newer types, 1174t
nosocomial postnatal infections, 1178
passive immunity to, 1173

pathogenesis, 1172–1173
pericarditis due to, 268–270, 1176
pharyngitis due to, 201
in pregnancy, 1178
prevention of infection, 1180
replication, 294
replication site, 1172–1173
seasonal infections, neonates, 546
serotypes, 293, 1172, 1172t–1173t
shedding, 1172–1174
skin lesions due to, 112, 1174–1175,
    1175f
spectrum of illness, 1174t
tissue culture, 293, 296
transmission, 294, 546, 1174
    prevention, 297
treatment of infections, 296, 1179–1180
vesiculobullous rash due to, 438–439
viremia, 1173
wild, shedding, 1395
see also Coxsackievirus A; Coxsackievirus
    B; Echovirus(es)
Enterovirus 70, 1173–1174, 1179
    acute hemorrhagic conjunctivitis, 1175f,
        1177
    conjunctivitis, 492, 492t
Enterovirus 71, 1177
    clinical manifestations, 1177
    encephalitis, 297, 304
Environmental control
    prevention of HAIs, 13
    standard precautions, 18t
    transmission-based precaution, 19t
Environmental service personnel, education,
    healthcare-associated infections, 18
Environmental sources, Legionella infections,
    922–923
Enzyme immunoassay (EIA)
    alphavirus diagnosis, 1099
    astrovirus, 381
    Baylisascaris procyonis, 1336
    Blastomyces dermatitidis, 1237
    Bordetella pertussis, 870
    Borrelia burgdorferi, 955
    Burkholderia pseudomallei, 848
    Chlamydia trachomatis, 887, 1398
    Clostridium difficile, 978, 1378
    CMV infection, 1049
    coltivirus (Colorado tick fever), 1093
    Cryptosporidium, 1270
    Echinococcus granulosus cysts, 1358
    Entamoeba histolytica, 1276–1277
    Epstein–Barr virus (EBV), 1393
    eumycotic mycetoma agents, 1251
    flavivirus infections, 1102
    galactomannan antigen testing, 1207
    Giardia intestinalis, 1281–1282
    HCV infections, 1109–1110, 1395
    Helicobacter pylori, 913
    Histoplasma capsulatum, 1227–1228,
        1227t
    HIV testing, 651, 1396
    HSV, 1388
    Legionella pneumophila, 924
    meningitis etiologic agents, 274
    MMR, 1396
    mumps virus, 1128
    Mycoplasma pneumoniae, 995

Rickettsia prowazekii, 931
Rickettsia rickettsii, 928
rotavirus infections, 1096
RSV, 1394
Streptococcus pyogenes (group A
    streptococcus), 1377
Taenia, 1351, 1354
Toxocara, 1336–1337
Treponema pallidum, 944
Trichinella spiralis, 1341
Trypanosoma cruzi, 1325
viral gastroenteritis diagnosis, 381
viral infection diagnosis, 1384–1385,
    1387
VZV, 1040, 1393
Enzyme-immunotransfer blot (EITB), Taenia
    solium neurocysticercosis, 1354
Enzyme-linked virus-inducible system
    (ELVIS), 1386
Eosin–methylene blue agar, 1375t
Eosinophil(s), 619, 1407
    in CSF, in chronic meningitis, 285, 285t
    life span, 1407
    normal counts, 1404t, 1407
    recruitment, Ascaris lumbricoides
        infections, 1327–1328
    tissue-to-blood ratio, 1407
Eosinophilia, 1407
    causes, 1407, 1408t–1409t
        non-infectious, 1408t–1409t
    Clonorchis and Opisthorchis infections,
        1365
    CSF, 285, 332–333
        chronic meningitis, 285
        eosinophilic meningitis, 332
    Diphyllobothrium infections, 1347
    Enterobius vermicularis infections, 1332
    Fasciola infections, 1366
    Fasciolopsis buski (fasciolopsiasis), 1363
    Heterophyes and Metagonimus infections,
        1364
    hookworm infections, 1330
    Paragonimus infections, 1367
    parasitic infections, 1407, 1408t–1409t
    refugee and internationally adopted
        children, 36
    Schistosoma infections, 1369–1370
    Strongyloides infections, 1333
    Toxocara infections, 1335–1337
    Trichinella spiralis infections, 1341
    tropical pulmonary see Tropical
        pulmonary eosinophilia (TPE)
Eosinophilic deposit, Splenore–Hoeppli
    reaction, 1251
Eosinophilic inclusions, rabies-specific, 1145
Eosinophilic meningitis, 330–333
    Angiostrongylus cantonensis, 330–333,
        331t
    Ascaris lumbricoides, 331t
    Baylisascaris procyonis, 330, 331t,
        332–333, 1336
    clinical features, 330–332
    definition, 330
    diagnosis, 332–333
    Gnathostoma spinigerum, 331t, 332, 1338
    infectious causes, 330–333, 331t
        bacteria, 331t, 332
        helminths, 330–332

    parasites, 330–332, 331t
    viruses and fungi, 331t, 332
    management, 333
    noninfectious causes, 331t, 332–333
Epi-Info, sample size calculation, 6
Epidemic curve, 7, 8f
    examples, 8f
Epidemic keratoconjunctivitis, 492t
    adenoviruses, 1068–1069, 1068t
    preauricular lymphadenopathy in, 159
Epidemic pleurodynia, 1176
Epidemic typhus see Rickettsia prowazekii
Epidemiologic studies, hypothesis testing, 3
"Epidemiologically important organisms",
    13
Epidemiology, 1–9
    analytic see Analytic epidemiology
    calculation of parameters, 2t
    causal inference and impact of bias, 4–5
    critical review of literature, 9, 9b
    definitions and formulae, 1, 2t
    describing illness by person, place or
        time, 2
    descriptive, 1–2
        case definition, 1
        illness by person, place and time, 2
        sensitivity, specificity and predictive
            value, 1
        surveillance, 1
    group childcare and, 24–30
    principles, 1–9
Epidermodysplasia verruciformis
    HPV causing, 1073
    malignant transformation, 1073
Epidermoid cysts, 142t, 143
    recurrent meningitis associated,
        287–288, 290
Epidermophyton, 1246
Epidermophyton floccosum
    genital dermatosis due to, 352
    tinea corporis due to, 1248
    tinea cruris due to, 1248
    tinea pedis due to, 1247
    tinea unguium due to, 1249
Epididymitis, 346t, 367–368, 368t
    Brucella, 863
    clinical features and differential
        diagnosis, 367, 368t
    etiology and epidemiology, 367, 367t
    laboratory findings and diagnosis, 367,
        368t
    management and complications,
        367–368
    pathogenesis, 367
    scrotal pain, 348–349
    sexually transmitted, 367
    tuberculous, 779
    urethritis complication, 356
Epididymo-orchitis, 368–369
Epidural abscess, 187–188
    clinical features, 323t
    cranial
        clinical features, 323, 323t
        complications and prognosis, 330
        CT and MRI, 326, 327f
        differential diagnosis, 325
        drainage and therapy, 328
        epidemiology, 321

etiology, 320–321, 320t
pathogenesis, 322
etiology, 320t
posterior fossa, 321
spinal, 320–321
back pain due to, 187–188, 188t
clinical features, 323, 684
complications and prognosis, 330
differential diagnosis, 325, 684
epidemiology, 321
etiology, 320t
laboratory findings and diagnosis, 325
management, 328, 684
MRI, 327
pathogenesis, 322
Staphylococcus aureus, 684
Epigastric pain, *Clonorchis* and *Opisthorchis* infections, 1365
Epiglottitis
acute, 210–211
clinical features, 206t, 210
complications and prognosis, 211
differential diagnosis, 210
epidemiology and pathogenesis, 210
etiology, 210
management, 210–211
radiography, 210, 210f
Haemophilus influenzae type b (Hib), 210, 901, 902f
Haemophilus paraphrophilus, 907–908
necrotizing, 210
stridor and, 165
"thumbprint" sign, 210, 210f
see also Supraglottitis
Epimastigotes, *Trypanosoma (Schizotrypanum) cruzi*, 1322
Epinephrine
nebulised
acute epiglottitis (supraglottitis), 210–211
bronchiolitis management, 234
laryngotracheitis (croup), 211
racemic, laryngotracheitis (croup), 211
thrombocytosis due to, 1409
Epithelial cells, influenza virus infection, 1151
Epitrochlear lymphadenopathy, 158t, 160
Epstein–Barr virus (EBV), 1059–1065
abdominal lymphadenopathy due to, 156–157
acquired HLH associated, 104–105, 1064, 1064b
management, 107
acute abdominal pain due to, 174
acute bilateral cervical lymphadenitis due to, 138
biopsy avoidance, 145–146
acute fulminant disease, diagnosis, 1393
acute pancreatitis due to, 411
in AIDS, 1063–1064
leiomyosarcoma, 1064
lymphocytic interstitial pneumonitis, 1063–1064
non-Hodgkin lymphoma, 1064
oral "hairy" leukoplakia, 1064
anti-early antigen (EA) antibodies, 1393

antibodies, 1061–1062, 1393
anti-early antigen (EA), 1393
chronic active EBV infection, 1065
detection, 1061–1062
to EB nuclear antigen (EBNA), 1393
heterophile, 1061–1062, 1393, 1411t–1412t
neutralizing, 1062–1063
time course, 1062, 1062f
antigens, 1059
antibodies to, 1061
detection, 1062
arthritis due to, 481
autoantibodies, 1062
B lymphocytes, immortalization and activation, 1059–1060
burns patients, 519–520
chronic active infections (CAEBVI), 1064–1065
chronic fatigue syndrome *vs.*, 1065
clinical features, 1065
NK-cell form, 1065
T-cell form, 1065
chronic fatigue syndrome pathogenesis, 1007–1008, 1008t–1009t, 1013
chronic fatigue syndrome *vs.*, 1065
chronic hepatitis due to, 406
congenital, 1065
description and structure, 1059
diagnosis/detection, 1062, 1393
antibodies, 1061–1062
direct tests, 1393
heterophile antibodies, 1061–1062, 1393, 1411t–1412t
IgM, 1061–1062, 1393
optimal tests, 1389t–1392t
PCR, 559, 1062, 1393
serologic, 1061–1062, 1062t
virus detection, 1062
DNA, 1059
detection, 1062, 1393
lymphocytic interstitial pneumonitis, 1063–1064
in posttransplant lymphoproliferative disease, 1063
early antigens (EAs), 1059, 1065
antibodies to, 1393
EBNA-1 (nuclear antigen-1), 1059
antibodies to, 1062
encephalitis due to, 302, 313
epidemiology, 1059–1060, 1059f
fever due to, 1061
fever of unknown origin due to, 119t–120t
generalized lymphadenopathy due to, 130, 131t–132t, 154, 1061
genome (DNA), 1059
hemoptysis in, 171
hepatic enzyme elevation, 1061, 1411
HSCT recipients and, 562
hypercytokinemia after, 105
hypogammaglobulinemia after, 633
immune response, 1060–1063
immunosuppressed hosts, 559, 1062–1065
in AIDS, 1063–1064
pathogenesis and clinical features, 1062–1065

PTLD *see* Posttransplant lymphoproliferative disease (PTLD)
X-linked lymphoproliferative syndrome, 1064–1065
incubation period, 1061
infectious mononucleosis, 1059, 1061–1062
anterior uveitis, 499t
clinical features, 1060f, 1061
eosinophilia, 1408t–1409t
laboratory findings/diagnosis, 1061
mortality, 1061
oral infections, 192t
treatment, 1062
keratitis due to, 496
laboratory testing, 308t–311t
latency, 1059, 1062
latent membrane protein-1 (LMP-1), 1059
life cycle, 1059
lymphadenopathy due to, 130, 131t–132t, 1061
lymphocyte appearance, 201, 202f, 1060–1061
lymphocytic interstitial pneumonitis, 253
lymphocytosis, 1061, 1406
lymphoma due to, 1062–1064, 1393
lymphoproliferative syndromes due to, 156
mediastinal lymphadenopathy due to, 154, 1061
myocarditis due to, 265–266
oral hairy leukoplakia, 192t
oral infections, 192t
pathogenesis, 1060–1061, 1060f
in immunosuppressed children, 1062–1065
persistence, 1059–1060, 1062–1063
pharyngitis due to, 199, 201, 201f–202f, 1061
pneumonia due to, 253, 1061
posttransplant, 559
pneumonia, 253–254
in pregnancy, 1065
primary CNS lymphoma and, 1393
primary infection, 1060–1061
proteins, 1059
receptor on B cells (CD21), 1060
relapse, 559
replication, 1059
chronic active EBV infection, 1065
RNA (EBER) probe, 559
serological findings, 1061–1062, 1062t
shedding, 1060
small RNAs (EBERs), 1062
transient synovitis due to, 485–486
transmission, 1060
transplant recipients, 253–254, 559
see also Posttransplant lymphoproliferative disease (PTLD)
treatment, 1504t
tropism for T lymphocytes, 105
viral capsid antigen (VCA), 1059, 1065
antibodies to, 1062
IgM, 1393

virology, 1059
X-linked lymphoproliferative disease, 627, 633
Equipment
soiled, standard precautions, 18t
Spaulding classification, 21
sterilization, 21
Equivalence, 6
"Erasive edema", 139
Erb palsy, 541
Ertapenem
dosage, 1480t–1483t
pharmacology, 1453t–1458t, 1468
spectrum of activity, 1459t–1463t, 1468
Erwinia, 804
Erysipelas, 434
Erysipeloid, 435, 767
Erysipelothrix, vancomycin resistance, 1429
Erysipelothrix rhusiopathiae, 767–768
bloodstream infections, 768
clinical manifestations, 767–768
diagnosis, 768
epidemiology, 767
microbiology, 767
treatment, 768
Erythema
Kawasaki disease, 1003, 1004f
toxic, 441
Erythema arthriticum epidemicum, 938
Erythema infectiosum *see* Parvovirus B19
Erythema marginatum, in acute rheumatic fever, 704
Erythema migrans, 953–955, 954f, 956b
in chronic meningitis, 284–285
differential diagnosis, 955
pathogenesis, 952
treatment, 956b
see also Borrelia burgdorferi
Erythema multiforme, 448–449
bullous, 111
clinical features and diagnosis, 448–449
etiology, 445b, 448
HSV infections of oral cavity, 192t
management, 449
pathogenesis and pathology, 448
recurrent, 448
HSV causing, 1030
Erythema multiforme major *see* Stevens–Johnson syndrome (SJS)
Erythema multiforme minor, 445
Erythema nodosum, 453
Bartonella henselae infection, 858f–859f
in chronic meningitis, 284–285, 284t
Coccidioides immitis (coccidioidomycosis), 1241
cutaneous tuberculosis, 779
Histoplasma capsulatum, 1225–1226
infectious causes, 452b, 453
pneumonia with, 246
Yersinia enterocolitica infections, 824
Erythrasma, 430
Corynebacterium minutissimum, 760t–761t
Erythroblastopenia, transient, 1404
Erythrocyte(s)
cold storage, blood transfusions, 580, 581t
erythrocyte sedimentation rate and, 1400
"knobs" on, in malaria, 1299

parasitization
Babesia, 1261, 1264f, 1264t
Bartonella bacilliformis, 940
Plasmodium, 1298
pitted/pocked, 636
Erythrocyte sedimentation rate (ESR), 1400–1402
acute rheumatic fever, 704
basis for, 94
Coccidioides immitis (coccidioidomycosis), 1242
decreased, 1401b, 1402
causes, 1401b
diskitis, 484
elevated, 1400–1401
causes, 1400–1401, 1401b
extreme, 1401b, 1402
pelvic inflammatory disease, 348
"falsely" low, 1401
focal suppurative CNS infections, 325
Kawasaki disease, 1003, 1005, 1401
neonatal septicemia diagnosis, 541t
normal values, 1400
osteomyelitis, 470, 679
physiology and measurement, 1400
pyogenic arthritis, 478
staphylococcal osteomyelitis, 679
transient synovitis, 486
Westergren measurement method, 1400
Erythrocytosis, 1403
Erythroderma
indurative, 112
toxic shock syndrome, 112
Erythroid progenitor cells, parvovirus B19 infection, 1088
Erythromycin, 1471
adverse effects, 1471
chemoprophylactic use, 70t–71t, 72, 74t
clinical uses, 1471
dosage, 1445t–1452t, 1480t–1483t
pharmacology, 1453t–1458t
resistance
Bordetella pertussis, 871, 871t
Corynebacterium diphtheriae, 757
spectrum of activity, 1459t–1463t, 1471
structure, 1470
topical, *Chlamydia* conjunctivitis, 488
treatment of, 1471
acute conjunctivitis, 492–493
acute rheumatic fever, 704–705
Bartonella bacilliformis, 940
Bordetella pertussis (pertussis), 871
Campylobacter jejuni, 877–878
Chlamydia trachomatis, 888t
Chlamydophila pneumoniae, 883
Corynebacterium diphtheriae infections, 757–758
eye infections, 1494t–1496t
GAS pharyngitis, 204t
Haemophilus ducreyi (chancroid), 907
impetigo, 429
Legionella infections, 924, 925t
Mycoplasma pneumoniae infections, 997
skin infections, 1498t
staphylococcal blepharitis, 493–494
trachoma, 494

Ureaplasma urealyticum infections, 1001
vulvovaginitis, 358
Erythromycin estolate, *Chlamydia* conjunctivitis, 488
Erythropoietin, increased levels, 1403
Erythrovirus genus, 1088
ESBLs *see* Extended-spectrum beta-lactamase(s) (ESBLs)
Eschar, 517
Escherichia coli, 796–799
antibiotic resistance, 31, 1416
amoxicillin, 341
healthcare-associated infections, 14t
antigens, 339
appendicitis due to, 420
bundle-forming pilus (BFP), 796
clinical manifestations, 797–798
CNS infections, 797
colonization factor antigens (CFAs), 796
diagnosis/detection, 798
stool cultures, 376
diarrheagenic, 796–797, 796t
prevention, 799
disseminated infections, 797
enteroaggregative (EAEC), 383, 796t, 797–798, 798t
diagnosis/detection, 385t
pathogenesis, 797
enterohemorrhagic (EHEC), 383, 796t, 798t, 799
"attaching and effacing" lesion, 797f
pathogenesis, 796
serotypes, 798
see also Escherichia coli O157:H7
enteroinvasive (EIEC), 383, 796t, 797–798, 798t, 820
pathogenesis, 796
enteropathogenic (EPEC), 383, 796t, 797–798, 798t
pathogenesis, 796
enterotoxigenic (ETEC), 383, 796t, 797–799, 798t
diagnosis, 397
pathogenesis, 796
vaccine development, 81
epidemiology, 797
fimbriae
aggregative adherence, 797
P fimbriae, 339, 796
S fimbriae, 797
folliculitis due to, 431
heat-labile (LT) and heat-stable (ST) toxins, 397, 796
hemolytic uremic syndrome, 796, 798–799
management, 799
see also Hemolytic uremic syndrome (HUS)
in HIV infection, 661–662
infections in HSCT recipient, 563
inflammatory enteritis due to, 383, 383t
K1 antigen, 797, 799
meningitis due to, 277, 797–798
necrotizing fasciitis due to, 459–460
necrotizing soft-tissue infection, 459–460

neonatal infections, 538–539, 797
orchitis due to, 369
osteomyelitis, vertebral, 474
P-fimbriae, 339, 796
P-pili, 339
pathogenesis, 796–797, 796t
pathotypes, 797
peritonitis due to, 415
in phagocytic disorders, 620t
phagocytosis in neonates, 85
pneumonia due to, 236
prevention of infections, 799
prostatitis due to, 369
scalp abscess due to, 458–459
screening tests for, 801
septicemia due to, 797
neonatal, 538–539
shiga-like toxin (STx), 796, 798
antibiotic contraindication, 387
Shiga toxin-producing (STEC)
diagnosis, 397
foodborne disease, 397, 398t
public settings, diseases associated,
528–529
travelers' diarrhea, 373
treatment of infections, 798
in sepsis, 99
urinary catheter-related infection, 599
urinary tract infections, 339, 796
uropathogenic (UPEC), 796
vaccines, 799
virulence factors, 339, 375
virulence markers, 339
xanthogranulomatous pyelonephritis,
344
Escherichia coli O111:K58, diarrhea, 26t
Escherichia coli O114:NM, diarrhea, 26t
Escherichia coli O157:H7, 798
acute abdominal pain due to, 174
animals in public settings associated,
528–529
antibiotic therapy effect, 377
Citrobacter braakii cross-reaction, 806
culture media, 1376t
diagnosis, 385, 385t
diarrhea due to, 26t
group childcare and, 25, 25t
hand hygiene inadequacy causing,
30–31
hemolytic-uremic syndrome due to *see*
Hemolytic uremic syndrome (HUS)
outbreaks, 25, 528–529
thrombocytopenia due to, 1410–1411
Esculin, 713
Esophageal variceal bleeding, 1369–1370
Esophagitis
in cancer, 577–578
Candida causing, 578, 1197
in HIV infection, 662
Esophagography, barium, 662
Esophagus, HSV infections, 1030
Estrogen, vaginal pH and flora, 358
Ethambutol
adverse reactions, 781–782, 785
dosage, 1445t–1452t
nontuberculous mycobacterial infection,
791
tuberculosis treatment, 780t, 781–782

Ethionamide
dosage, 1445t–1452t
tuberculosis treatment, 780t, 782
Ethmoid sinuses, in preseptal cellulitis due
to sinusitis, 510
Ethnic factors
Chlamydia trachomatis infections, 885
Helicobacter pylori prevalence, 909
invasive pneumococcal disease, 722
Kawasaki disease, 1002
urinary tract infection (UTI), 339
Ethylenediaminetetraacetic acid (EDTA),
1385
Etoposide
HLH treatment, 107
infection-associated hemophagocytic
syndrome, 1065
Etravirine, 665t
Eubacterium, 959, 991–992
classification, 959t
Eubacterium lentum, 961
Eucalyptus oil, tick repellent, 535
Eumycotic mycetoma, 1250–1253, 1254b
agents causing, 1250–1251, 1250b,
1254b
anatomic alterations due to, 1251f, 1252,
1252t
antibodies, 1251
clinical manifestations, 1251–1252,
1251f, 1252t, 1254b
definition, 1250, 1254b
epidemiology, 1251, 1254b
laboratory findings and diagnosis, 1251f,
1252, 1254b
pathogenesis, 1251
prevention, 1253
treatment, 1252–1253, 1254b
virulence and immunity, 1251
see also Pseudallescheria boydii
European tickborne encephalitis virus,
epidemiology and vectors, 532t
Eurytrema pancreaticum, 1365
Eustachian tube
anatomy, 222, 223f
dysfunction, 214
acute otitis media complication,
222–223
Ewingella americana, 808–809
Exanthem(s)
in encephalitis, 305t–306t
enterovirus infections, 1174–1175, 1174t,
1175f
evolution and resolution, 111
in mucocutaneous syndromes, 109t–110t,
111–112
Rickettsia akari (rickettsialpox) infection,
934
varicella lesions, 1037, 1037f
viral infection, 112
maculopapular rashes, 436, 437t
see also Rash(es)
Exanthem subitum *see* Human herpesvirus 6
(HHV-6), roseola
Exanthematous syndromes, generalized
lymphadenopathy, 130, 131t–132t
Excretion, antimicrobial agents *see*
Elimination, antimicrobial agents
Exercise intolerance, pericarditis, 269

Exogenous pyrogens, 91
Exophiala, 1211–1212
Exophiala werneckii, 1249–1250
Exophilia jeanselmei, 1250
Expectorants, in common cold, 198
Experimental studies, 2–3
Exposure, 9
accidental, 17–18
Exposure control plan, 17–18
Exposures of concern, control, 17
Extended-spectrum beta-lactamase(s)
(ESBLs), 1422t, 1424
detection, 1380–1381, 1431, 1431f
hydrolysis of third-generation
cephalosporins, 1468
Extended-spectrum beta-lactamase (ESBL)-
producing organisms
antimicrobial therapy in sepsis, 99
Enterobacter, 805
Klebsiella, 800–801
Pseudomonas aeruginosa, 845
Serratia marcescens, 813
Extended-spectrum penicillins, 1459t–
1463t, 1467
clinical uses, 1467
MICs, 1379t
pharmacology, 1453t–1458t, 1467
spectrum of activity, 1459t–1463t, 1467
Extensive limb swelling (ELS), DTaP
association, 873
External validity, 9
Extracerebral abscess *see* Epidural abscess;
Septic venous thrombosis; Subdural
empyema
Extracorporeal membrane oxygenation
(ECMO), pharmacokinetics,
1435–1436
Extreme sports, risks and advice, 76
Extremely low birthweight infants (ELBW)
Candida infection, 1196
prevention, 1202
candidemia, 538
neonatal infections, 538
neonatal sepsis, 538
nosocomial infections, 549
prevention, 555
Exudates, pleural effusion, 241
Eyach virus, 1094
Eye
anatomy, 506, 507f
black, 506
in chronic meningitis, 284t, 285
disease *see* Ocular disease
dry, infective keratitis due to, 495
infections *see* Ocular infections
pain
infective keratitis, 495
mucocutaneous syndromes, 110–111
red
allergic disorders, 110
anterior uveitis, 498
endophthalmitis, 504
swollen, 506, 506f, 510
tumors, 506
*see also Entries beginning ocular; specific
anatomical regions of eye*
Eye drops, 1493, 1494t–1496t
fortified, 1493, 1495t

Eyelids
  cellulitis, 509
  in HHV-6 infection (roseola), 1054
  staphylococcal infection, 493
  swelling, 506
    bacteremic periorbital cellulitis,
      509–510
    preseptal cellulitis due to sinusitis,
      510
    upper outer aspect, 508

F

Face
  bites to, 523–524
  cellulitis, 434–435
    H. influenzae, 902–903, 903f
  osteomyelitis, 476
  tenderness in acute bacterial sinusitis,
    228
Face shield, transmission-based precaution,
  19t
Facial lymph nodes, 136t
Facial lymphadenopathy, *Bartonella henselae*
  infection, 159f
Facial nerve palsy, 315–316
  Borrelia burgdorferi (Lyme disease),
    954–955
  etiology, 314t, 315
  incidence, 315
  in necrotizing otitis externa, 221–222
  pathogenesis, 315
  treatment, 315–316
  see also Facial palsy/paralysis
Facial pain, unilateral, epidural abscess,
  323
Facial palsy/paralysis
  acute mastoiditis complication, 225
  acute otitis media complication, 220
  see also Facial nerve palsy
Factitious fever, fever of unknown origin,
  119t–120t
Factor V, for *Haemophilus influenzae* growth,
  899
Factor X, for *Haemophilus influenzae* growth,
  899
Factor B, 616, 618
Factor D, deficiency, 604t–605t, 618–619
Factor G,(1,3)-β-D-glucan detection, 1208
Factor H, 86
  deficiency, 618
Factor I, 618
  deficiency, 618–619
Failure to thrive
  pulmonary tuberculosis, 775
  SCID, 627–628
Fallopian tubes
  pelvic inflammatory disease
    pathogenesis, 364
  tuberculosis, 779
Fallot, tetralogy
  brain abscess, 321
  endocarditis pathogenesis, 257
Famciclovir, 1503t, 1510, 1510t
  VZV infections, 1041
Familial cold autoinflammatory syndrome
  (FCAS), 126
Familial cold urticaria, 126

Familial hemophagocytic
  lymphohistiocytosis *see*
  Hemophagocytic lymphohistiocytosis
  (HLH)
Familial hemophagocytic
  lymphohistiocytosis (HLH),
  604t–605t
Familial hemophagocytic reticulosis *see*
  Hemophagocytic lymphohistiocytosis
  (HLH)
Familial Mediterranean fever (FMF), 122t,
  124–125
  cardinal clinical features, 124–125
  course, treatment and outcome, 125
  epidemiology and etiology, 124
  mutations, 124
Family history, recurrent infections, 606
Far-eastern tickborne encephalitis virus,
  epidemiology and vectors, 532t
Farber disease, generalized
  lymphadenopathy, 135
Farm animals, infections associated, 528
Fascia
  deep and superficial, 454
  diseases, limb pain, 187
Fasciitis
  Clostridium, 980t
  necrotizing *see* Necrotizing fasciitis
Fasciola gigantica, 1366
Fasciola hepatica (fascioliasis), 1365–1366
  eosinophilic meningitis, 331t
  oropharyngeal fascioliasis, 1366
Fasciolopsis buski (fasciolopsiasis),
  1363–1364
Fastidious pathogens, endocarditis due to,
  257
Fatal familial insomnia (FFI), 338
Fatigue, 1007–1008, 1012
  of deconditioning, 121
    clinical features, 121b
    definition, 121
    management, 121b
  HCV infection, 1107–1108
  persistent, 1007–1008, 1013
    see also Chronic fatigue syndrome
      (CFS)
  postinfectious, syndrome (PIFS), 1008,
    1010t
Fatty acids, volatile, 960
Favus (tinea favosa), 1249
Febrile agglutinin tests, 1384
Feces *see* Stool
Femoral adenitis, 160
Femoral lymph nodes, enlarged, 158t,
  160
  visceral leishmaniasis, 1287
Femur, osteomyelitis, neonates, 541
Ferrets, bites, 529
Ferriprotoporphyrin IX, *Plasmodium*,
  1298–1299
Ferritin, 1403
  serum, elevated, in HLH, 105
Fetal infections, 536
  adenovirus infections, 1070
  CMV, 1045
  HSV, 1031
  parvovirus B19, 1089–1091
  Pasteurella multocida, 837

  rubella *see* Rubella virus, congenital
    rubella
  Toxoplasma gondii see Toxoplasma gondii,
    congenital
  Toxoplasma gondii diagnosis, 1313–
    1314
  viral, 544–548
    diagnosis, 1397–1398
    pathogenesis, 544–545
  see also individual congenital infections
Fetal monitoring, source of healthcare-
  associated infection, 10
Fetor oris, in gingivitis, 191
Fetus
  gestation age, viral infections, 544
  IgA and IgG levels, 87, 89
  immune system immaturity, 544
  loss, parvovirus B19, 1089–1090
  susceptibility to rubella virus, 1113
  see also Pregnancy
Fever, 91–95, 117–127
  acute bacterial meningitis, 278, 278b
  acute bacterial sinusitis, 228
  aseptic meningitis, 295
  Aspergillus infections, 1203
  bacteremic periorbital cellulitis, 509
  beneficial effects, 91–92
  brain abscess, 323
  Brucella causing, 863
  in cancer, 570
    see also Neutropenia, fever in
  clinical features, 91
  CMV infection, 1046
  Coccidioides immitis (coccidioidomycosis),
    1241–1242, 1244
  Cystoisospora belli causing, 1283–1284
  definition, 91
  early-onset/late-onset neonatal sepsis,
    540
  EBV infection, 1061
  Entamoeba histolytica infection, 1275–
    1277, 1275t
  enterovirus infections, 1174
  factitious, 119t–120t
  fatigue of deconditioning with, 121,
    121b
  gastrointestinal infections, 375
  granulocytopenic, 567–573
    see also Neutropenia
  HHV-6 infection (roseola), 1054–
    1055
  high/persistent, infections associated,
    108
  HIV infection, 659–660, 659b
    antibiotic prophylaxis, 660
    antibiotic treatment, 660
    clinical approach to, 659–660
    hospitalizations, 659
  hyperthermia *vs.*, 91
  induction mechanism, 91, 91f
  infants and small children, 91
  infections due to burns, 516–517
  infectious encephalitis, 304
  influenza, 1152
  intra-abdominal abscess, 424
  intravascular catheter-related infections,
    590
  low-grade or falsely perceived, 121

management
  antipyretic therapy, 91–92
  cooling, 91–92
measurement, 91
mucocutaneous symptom complexes,
  108
mucocutaneous syndromes, 108
Neisseria meningitidis infections, 734
in neutropenia *see* Neutropenia
pancreatitis, 173
pathogenesis, 91
patterns, 117, 117b
periodic, 117, 117b, 121–122
  clockwork cycle, 121–124
  definition, 121–122
  hereditary syndromes *see* Hereditary
    periodic fever syndromes
  syndromes, differentiating features,
    122t
peritonitis, 417
physical examination, 118b
Plasmodium infections, 1299
pneumonia, 238, 254
prolonged, 117b, 121
  bacterial meningitis, 278, 278b
  HIV infection, 659
prolonged insignificant/resolved, 121
pulmonary *Mycobacterium tuberculosis*
  infection, 774
rabies, 1147
recurrent, 117b, 121
relapsing infections causing, 121
Rickettsia akari (rickettsialpox) infection,
  934
Rickettsia prowazekii (epidemic typhus),
  930–931
Rickettsia rickettsii (Rocky Mountain
  spotted fever), 926
Rickettsia typhi (murine typhus), 932
rubeola virus (measles), 1140
Salmonella Typhi infection, 817
in sepsis, 99
Streptobacillus moniliformis (rat-bite fever),
  938–939
subdural empyema, 323
transfusion-associated infection, 581
Trichinella spiralis infections, 1341
Trypanosoma (Trypanozoon) brucei
  infection, 1320
Trypanosoma cruzi infections, 1324
of unknown origin (FUO), 117–119,
  117b
  causes, frequency, 117–118, 118t
  clinical approach, 660
  definition and criteria for, 117–118
  diagnostic clues, 118
  duration, 117–118
  ESR elevation, 1400
  in HIV infection, 659b, 660
  infectious causes, 118–119, 118t–120t
  investigations, 118, 118b
  noninfectious causes, 118–119, 119b,
    119t–120t
varicella, 1037
viral nasopharyngitis, 163
viral upper respiratory tract infections,
  228
visceral leishmaniasis, 1287

without localizing signs, 114–117
  children older than 3 months,
    115–116
  children younger than 3 months,
    114–116, 114t
  diagnosis, 114–115
  epidemiology, 114–115
  etiologic agents, 114, 114t
  laboratory findings, 115
  management, 115–117
  outcome, 116
Yersinia pestis infection (bubonic plague),
  826
Fever syndromes, 118
Fibrinogen
  effect on ESR, 1400
  in hemophagocytic lymphohistiocytosis,
    105
  low levels, decreased ESR, 1402
  synthesis, by *Enterococcus faecalis*, 713
Fibrinogen-binding protein, from coagulase-
  negative staphylococci, 690f
Fibromyalgia syndrome, 186
  diagnostic criteria, 186
  Mycoplasma infections associated, 999
Fibronectin
  neonatal septicemia diagnosis, 541t
  ventilator-associated pneumonia,
    581–582
Fibrosis
  "claypipe stem", 1369
  periportal, 1369
  Schistosoma (schistosomiasis), 1369
Fibrous dysplasia, *Actinomyces* infections,
  991
Ficolins, 616
"Fifth disease" *see* Parvovirus B19, erythema
  infectiosum
"Filarial dance sign", 1342–1343
Filarial infections (filariasis), 1342–1346
  characteristics of pathogens, 1342t
  chronic sequelae, 1342
  eosinophilia, 1408t–1409t
  generalized lymphadenopathy, 131t–
    132t, 132
  IgG, 1342
  Loa loa see Loa loa (loiasis)
  lymphatic, 1342–1344
    clinical manifestations, 1342–1343
    epidemiology, 1342
    laboratory findings and diagnosis,
      1343, 1344t
    in pregnancy and infants, 1344
    prevention, 1344
    treatment, 1343–1344, 1344t
    see also Brugia malayi; Brugia timori;
      Wuchereria bancrofti
  Mansonella species, 1342t, 1346
  Onchocerca volvulus see Onchocerca
    volvulus (onchocerciasis)
  treatment, 1523–1524
  see also individual species
Filoviridae, 1016t, 1159
  infections, 1017t
Filoviruses, 1159–1164
  clinical manifestations, 1161–1162
  epidemiology and transmission, 1159,
    1160t

laboratory findings and diagnosis,
  1162–1163, 1162t
pathobiology, 1160–1161
prevention of infections, 1163–1164
treatment of infections, 1163
Fimbriae
  Escherichia coli see Escherichia coli
  Klebsiella, 800
  Streptococcus pyogenes, 698
Finegoldia, 988
Fish
  cooking, *Diphyllobothrium* prevention,
    1348
  Diphyllobothrium transmission, 1347
  Heterophyes transmission, 1364
  infections associated, 528
  poisoning, 396t, 397
  raw, visceral larva migrans after
    consuming, 1339
Fitz-Hugh–Curtis syndrome (acute
  perihepatitis), 747
  Chlamydia trachomatis, 886
  peritonitis complication, 416
Flagella
  Campylobacter, 873–875
  Helicobacter, 918
  Pseudomonas aeruginosa, 842t, 843
Flank pain, renal abscess, 344
Flatworms *see* Platyhelminthes (flatworms)
Flavimonas oryzihabitans (Pseudomonas
  oryzihabitans), 841, 841t
Flaviviridae, 1016t, 1105
  arthritis, 481b
  infections, 1017t
Flaviviruses, 1099–1102
  diagnosis, 1102
  encephalitic, 1099–1102
  miscellaneous, 1102
  prevention of infection, 1102
  see also Dengue viruses; Yellow fever
    virus
Flavobacteriaceae, 832
Flavobacterium see Chryseobacterium
  indologenes
Flavobacterium breve (Empedobacter brevis),
  832
Flea bites, 529
Flea-borne disease
  Dipylidium caninum transmission,
    1348
  endemic typhus *see Rickettsia typhi*
  Yersinia pestis (plague), 826
Flea control
  murine typhus (*Rickettsia typhi*)
    prevention, 932
  Yersinia pestis infection prevention, 827
Flebogamma, 38t
Flora, normal
  anaerobes, 958–961
    by body site, 960t
    Clostridium, 979–980
    cocci, 988–989
    genera and species, 959t
    see also Anaerobic bacteria
  antibiotics effect on, 961
  cancer and, 569
  establishment and composition,
    959–960

gastrointestinal
  Actinomyces, 990–991
  effect of antibiotics, 961
  Enterobacter, 804
  establishment, 960
  Fusobacterium, 985
  Proteus, Providencia and *Morganella,*
    811
genitourinary tract, 960t
  Fusobacterium, 985
gingival crevices, 959
mouth, *Lactobacillus,* 770
nasopharyngeal, 163, 961
  effect of antibiotics, 961
neonates, 536
oral cavity, 190
  Actinobacillus actinomycetemcomitans,
    938–939
  Actinomyces, 990–991
  Bacteroides, 982–983
  Capnocytophaga, 880
  Eikenella corrodens, 835–836
  establishment of flora, 959
  Fusobacterium, 985
  Prevotella, 982–983
oropharynx
  effect of antibiotics, 961
  establishment of flora, 961
resistance to antimicrobial peptides,
    84
respiratory tract, 960t
  Eikenella corrodens, 835–836
  Haemophilus influenzae, 273
  Moraxella, 840
  Pasteurella, 836
role, 960–961
skin, 427, 517
  blood transfusion-related infections,
    581
  CNS device contamination, 596
  intravascular catheter infection risk,
    590
  Malassezia, 1216
source of healthcare-associated infection,
    10
staphylococci, 690
vaginal, 358
  establishment, 959–960
  hydrogen peroxide formation, 960
  see also Colonization
Flow cytometry
  Cyclospora, 1284
  in hemophagocytic lymphohistiocytosis,
    107
Fluconazole, 1488–1489
  adverse effects, 1489
  breakpoint for, 1443t
  clinical trials, 1489
  dosage, 1445t–1452t, 1487t, 1489
    pharmacokinetic-pharmacodynamic
      relationships, 1443t
  pharmacology, 1202, 1488–1489
  prophylactic
    Candida infection prophylaxis, 1196,
      1201–1202
    HSCT recipients, 566
    nosocomial neonatal infection
      prevention, 555

very high-risk low-birthweight infants,
    14
  resistance, *Candida,* 1196, 1201
  spectrum of activity, 1486t
  treatment of
    Acanthamoeba infections, 1297
    bacterial vaginosis, 360
    Blastomyces dermatitidis
      (blastomycosis), 1237–1238,
      1238t
    Candida infection, 1201, 1201t
    Candida vulvovaginitis, 360
    Coccidioides immitis
      (coccidioidomycosis), 1243–1244
    Cryptococcus neoformans, 1222–1223
    endocarditis, 263
    fever in neutropenia (in cancer), 571,
      573
    Histoplasma capsulatum
      (histoplasmosis), 1228t, 1229
    Malassezia infections, 1218
    Naegleria fowleri (naegleriasis), 1295
    neonatal infections, 538
    pityriasis versicolor, 1249
    Sporothrix schenckii (sporotrichosis),
      1219–1220
    tinea capitis, 1247
Flucytosine (5-fluorocytosine), 1488
  adverse effects, 1222, 1488
  breakpoint for, 1443t
  clinical uses, 1488
  dosage, 1445t–1452t
    pharmacokinetic-pharmacodynamic
      relationships, 1443t
  mechanism of action, 1488
  pharmacology, 1488
  resistance, *Cryptococcus* infections, 1222
  spectrum of activity, 1486t
  treatment of
    Acanthamoeba infections, 1297
    Candida infections, 1201
    cryptococcal meningitis, 1222–1223
    Cryptococcus infections, 1222
  trial data, 1488
Fluid restriction, in acute bacterial
    meningitis, 278
Fluid resuscitation
  sepsis, 99
  Shigella infections, 822
  Vibrio cholerae infection, 852–853, 852b
  see also Oral rehydration therapy (ORT)
Fluid therapy
  acute bacterial meningitis, 278
  pneumonia, 240
  see also Oral rehydration therapy (ORT)
Flukes
  blood *see Schistosoma*
  intestinal, 1363–1364
  liver and lung, 1365–1368
    eosinophilia, 1408t–1409t
  treatment of infections, 1524–1525
Fluorescent antibody against membrane
    antigen (FAMA), VZV diagnosis, 1393
Fluorescent antibody methods
  EBV, 1393
  RSV, 1394
  viral infection diagnosis, 1384–1386
  VZV, 1393

see also Direct fluorescent antibody
    (DFA); Indirect immunofluorescence
    antibody (IFA) assay
Fluorescent immunohistology, rabies, 1147
Fluorescent treponemal antibody-absorbed
    test (FTA-ABS), 944–945
  syphilitic meningitis diagnosis, 281
Fluorocytosine *see* Flucytosine
    (5-fluorocytosine)
Fluorodeoxyglucose positron emission
    tomography (FDG-PET), fever of
    unknown origin (FUO), 118
Fluoroquinolones, 1476–1477
  dosage, 1480t–1483t
  mechanism of action, 1476–1477
  pharmacology, 1453t–1458t
  prophylactic
    infections in neutropenia in cancer,
      573
    meningococcal disease, 69
  resistance to, 1477
    Clostridium difficile, 382, 978
    Klebsiella, 802
    Mycobacterium tuberculosis, 785
    Mycoplasma hominis, 999
    Neisseria gonorrhoea, 743, 743f
    Proteus mirabilis, 812
    Salmonella Choleraesuis, 816
    Salmonella Typhi, 816
  spectrum of activity, 1459t–1463t
  treatment of
    acute bacterial meningitis, 277
    bacterial keratitis, 497–498
    bite wound infections, 521–522, 526
    Campylobacter jejuni infections,
      877–878
    endophthalmitis, 505
    Escherichia coli infections, 798
    infections in cystic fibrosis, 640–641
    infections in sickle cell disease, 635
    Mycoplasma pneumoniae infections,
      996–997
    necrotizing otitis externa, 222
    Neisseria gonorrhoeae infections, 743
    otitis externa, 221–222
    travelers' diarrhea, 82
    urinary tract infection, 341
  see also Quinolones
Focal epithelial hyperplasia (Heck disease),
    192t
Focal intestinal perforation (FIP), 550
Folate deficiency, *Strongyloides* causing,
    1333
Folate metabolism inhibitors, 1428, 1479
  protozoan infection treatment, 1522
Folinic acid *see* Leucovorin (folinic acid)
Folliculitis, 430–431
  Enterobacter, 431
  Escherichia coli, 431
  HIV, 431
  hot-tub, 431
  Klebsiella, 431
  Malassezia, 1216–1218
    acne vulgaris *vs.,* 1217
  Malassezia furfur, 431
  Pseudomonas aeruginosa, 431, 843–844,
    843t
  Staphylococcus aureus, 431

Fontanelle, bulging
  acute bacterial meningitis, 274, 540
  aseptic meningitis, 295
  HHV-6 infection (roseola), 1054–1055
  subdural empyema, 323
Food(s)
  foodborne disease management,
    398–399
  gastrointestinal tract infections due to,
    393–396
  Helicobacter pylori infection treatment,
    914–915
  precautions for travelers, 76, 81
  raw, prevention of infections, 399
Food and Drug Administration (FDA),
    vaccine licensing, 47
Food handlers, norovirus infection
    prevention, 1189
Food vacuole, *Plasmodium*, 1298–1299
Foodborne disease and food poisoning,
    373, 392–400
  Bacillus cereus, 393–395, 394t, 398t, 753
  botulism *see Clostridium botulinum*,
    foodborne botulism
  Campylobacter, 394, 394t, 875
  Campylobacter jejuni, 394, 394t
  characteristics and causes, 394t
  chemicals causing, 396t
  Citrobacter, 807
  clinical syndromes, 393
  Clostridium perfringens causing *see*
    Clostridium perfringens
  complications, 399
  Cyclospora (cyclosporiasis), 397–398,
    1283
  Cyclospora cayetanensis, 398t
  diagnosis, 393–398
    epidemiologic clues, 393–396, 398t
    laboratory diagnosis, 397–398, 398t
  diarrhea, 373–374
    see also Diarrhea
  epidemiology, 392, 395t
  Escherichia coli, 797, 799
    Shiga toxin-producing, 398t
  fish and shellfish causing, 396t, 397
  Giardia intestinalis (giardiasis), 1280
  group childcare and, 25
  groups C and G streptococci causing,
    720
  hepatitis A virus infection, 1180
  infectious causes, 393–395
  inflammatory enteritis, 384, 384t
  listeriosis *see Listeria monocytogenes*
  management, 373, 398–399
  microbial agents/toxins causing,
    393–395, 394t
  mushrooms causing, 396, 397t
  noroviruses, 393–394, 394t
  outbreaks
    definition, 373
    epidemiology, 395t
    number, 392
  pathogenesis, 393
  prevention, 377, 399
    regulatory/industry role, 399
  reporting, 373
  Salmonella, 393–394, 394t, 397, 398t,
    817

Shigella, 394, 394t, 397, 398t, 820–821
Staphylococcus aureus, 394t, 395, 398t,
    676, 680–681
Vibrio cholerae, 395
Vibrio cholerae non-O1, 398t
Vibrio cholerae O1, 398t
Vibrio parahaemolyticus, 395, 398t
viral gastroenteritis, 380
websites on, 399
Yersinia enterocolitica, 393–394, 394t,
    396, 398t, 823–824
Foodborne Surveillance Network (FoodNet),
    Salmonella (nontyphoidal) infections,
    815
Foot
  nontuberculous mycobacterial infections,
    788–789
  puncture wounds, 515
    infection risk and management, 512t
    osteochondritis, 476
Foreign body
  aspiration, persistent pneumonia due to,
    246–247
  infections associated, 588–589
  nasal, 164
    see also Rhinitis, foreign body-related
  rhinitis, 164t
Forkhead box N1 deficiency, 627
  characteristics, 603t–604t
Formalin, stool sample preservation, 1383
Fosamprenavir, 665t, 1445t–1452t
Foscarnet, 1514–1515
  adverse effects, 1515
  chemistry, 1514
  clinical uses, 1515
  dosage, 1445t–1452t, 1515
    in renal impairment, 1514–1515,
    1515f
  drug interactions, 1515
  mechanism of action, 1514
  resistance to, 1503t, 1514
  spectrum of activity, 1504t, 1514
  treatment of
    CMV infection, 1050
    VZV infection, 1041
Fractures, 515
  infection risk and management, 512t
  open
    classification, 515
    infection rate, 515
    pathogens and infection prophylaxis,
    512t, 515
Francisella tularensis (*Pasteurella tularensis*)
    (tularemia), 897–899, 899b
  acute unilateral cervical lymphadenitis,
    140
    management, 147t
  antibodies to, 898
  bites associated, 529
  clinical manifestations, 897–898, 897t
  culture and growth, 898
    culture media, 1376t
  description and microbiology, 897
  diagnosis, 160, 533t–534t, 898
  epidemiology, 532t, 897
  fever of unknown origin due to,
    119t–120t
  glandular disease, 897–898

immunity to, 897
inguinal adenopathy without genital
    ulcers, 351, 352t
laboratory findings, 533t–534t, 898
lymphadenitis due to, 130, 131t–132t
lymphadenopathy due to, 897–898
occipital lymph node involvement, 159
oculoglandular, 140, 898
oropharyngeal, 898
pathogenesis and immunity, 897
pharyngitis due to, 199
pneumonia due to, 237t, 898
prevention of infections, 899
subspecies, 897
subspecies B, 897, 899
transmission, 897
    by ticks, 532
treatment of infections, 898–899
typhoidal, 898
ulceroglandular tularemia, 140, 140f,
    897–898
    clinical features, 533
vaccine, 899
vectors, 532t
Fremitus
  increased, 169
  tactile, musculoskeletal pain with, 183
Frequency matching, 6–7
Frontal lobe abscess
  clinical features, 322–323, 322b
  complications, 329–330
  etiology, 320
FSME-IMMUN vaccine, 535
FTA-ABS *see* Fluorescent treponemal
    antibody-absorbed test (FTA-ABS)
Fuch heterochromic cyclitis, 501
Fungal infections, 1195t
  arthritis, 482
  classification, 1195–1196, 1195t
  clinical manifestations, 1195–1196
  CNS device infection, 597
  disseminated, profound neutrophilia,
    1404–1405
  endocarditis due to, 257
    management, 263
  eosinophilia, 1407
  eosinophilic meningitis, 331t, 332
  fever of unknown origin, 119t–120t
  healthcare-associated infections, 14
  HSCT recipients, 563
  inflammatory enteritis, 387
  inoculation/contamination, 1195–1196,
    1195t
  intravascular catheter-related infections,
    589, 591
  liver transplant recipients, 557
  lung transplant recipients, 558
  neutropenia associated with cancer, 567,
    569t
  neutrophil response, 1404
  opportunistic, 1195–1196, 1195t
  osteomyelitis, 475
  otitis externa due to, 221
  pneumonia due to, 253
    transplant-associated, 254
  predisposing factors, 1195t
  primary systemic, 1195–1196, 1195t
  pulmonary infections, in cancer, 575

recurrent, 606
renal transplant recipients, 557
SCID, 628
sinus infections, in cancer, 577
skin infections, in cancer, 574
treatment see Antifungal agents
see also individual fungi
Fungemia, endocarditis pathogenesis, 258, 260
Fungi, 1194–1196, 1250–1253
 classification, 1194–1196
 cross-reactivity, diagnosis/detection, 1382
 culture media, 1194–1195, 1376t
 description and structure, 1194–1195
 diagnosis/detection, 1381–1382
 dimorphic, 1194
 growth, 1194
 host interactions, 1195, 1195t
 immune response, 1384
 isolation and identification, 1382
 laboratory testing, 308t–311t
 lymphangitis due to, 161
 molds see Molds
 saprophytic, Toxocara larvicidal activity, 1337
 specimen collection/processing, 1194–1195, 1381–1382
 susceptibility testing, 1382
 yeasts, 1194
Fungi imperfecti, 1250
Funguria, 342
Fungus balls, 342
Furazolidone, 1519
 adverse effects, 1519
 treatment of
  Giardia intestinalis (giardiasis), 1281t, 1282
  protozoan infections, 1519
Furuncle (boil), 431–432
 recurrent, 431
 Staphylococcus aureus, 431, 432f, 678
Furunculosis, recurrent, 678
Fusarium, 1210–1211
 amphotericin B resistance, 1210
 burn wound infections, 518
 clinical manifestations, 1210, 1210f
 in cystic fibrosis, 639
 disseminated fusariosis, 1210
 keratitis due to, 496–497
 macroconidia, 1211f
 neutropenia associated with cancer, 567
 pulmonary infections, in cancer, 575–576
 skin infections, in cancer, 574
Fusarium falciforme, 1250
Fusarium solani, keratitis, 496–497
Fusidic acid
 burns treatment, 1500t–1501t
 skin infection treatment, 1498t
Fusiform bacteria, 674
Fusion inhibitors (FI), 666
Fusobacterium, 164, 985–988
 abscesses due to, 986
 antibiotic susceptibility, 966t
 classification, 959t
 clinical manifestations, 986–988
 diagnosis/detection, 963–964

endotoxin, 962
head and neck infections, 986–988
 β-lactamase, 986, 988
 Lemierre syndrome associated, 138, 265
 management of infections, 988
 normal flora, 985
 pathogenesis of infections, 985–986
 postanginal sepsis due to, 985
 pulmonary infections, 986
 treatment of infections, 985
 wound infections, 987–988
Fusobacterium gonidiaformans, 985
Fusobacterium mortiferum, 985
Fusobacterium naviforme, 985
Fusobacterium necrophorum, 962, 986, 986t
 antibiotic resistance, 208
 antibiotics for, 208
 clinical manifestations, 986–987
 Lemierre disease, 194–195, 208, 265
 lung abscesses due to, 243
 pharyngitis, 199, 202
Fusobacterium nucleatum, 962, 985
 clinical manifestations, 986–987
Fusobacterium varium, 985

G

G + C content, bacterial identification by, 674
Gait, antalgic, 185
Galactomannan, 1207
Galactomannan antigen, 248, 254–255
 Aspergillus, 563, 1382
 testing, Aspergillus, 1207–1208
Galerina, 397t
Gallbladder
 disease/infections, acute abdominal pain, 173
 inflammation see Cholecystitis
 transient hydrops, 113
Gallium scan
 myocarditis, 261
 necrotizing otitis externa, 222
 osteomyelitis, 472
Gallstones, 412
 sickle-cell disease, 414
Gambierdiscus toxicus, 396t
Gametocytes, Plasmodium, 1298, 1298f, 1300, 1303
Gammaherpesvirinae, 1026t, 1059, 1066
Ganciclovir, 1444t, 1445, 1510–1512
 adenovirus infection treatment, 1070
 adverse effects, 1511
 chemistry, 1510
 clinical uses, 1511–1512
 CMV infection prophylaxis
  in AIDS, 1050
  transplant recipients, 561
 CMV infection treatment
  congenital, 1050
  HIV/AIDS patients, 1050
  resistance, 1051
  retinitis, 501
  transplant recipients, 558, 1050–1051
 dosage, 1445t–1452t, 1511–1512
 EBV infection treatment, 1062
 mechanism of action, 1051, 1510–1511
 pharmacokinetics, 1511

prophylactic, 1507t, 1512
 resistance to, 1503t, 1511
 spectrum of activity, 1504t, 1510–1511
 VZV infection treatment, 1041
Ganglion cells, in Trypanosoma cruzi infections, 1324
Gangrene
 bacterial synergistic, 459–460, 466t
  clinical features, 461
  Staphylococcus aureus, 461
 digital, Kawasaki disease, 112, 112f
 gas see Gas gangrene
 hemolytic streptococcal see Necrotizing fasciitis
 hospital see Necrotizing fasciitis
 skin, meningococcal disease, 735, 737
 Yersinia pestis infection (bubonic plague), 826
Gangrenous stomatitis (noma), 193t
Gardnerella vaginalis, 769–770
 bacterial vaginosis due to, 358
  diagnosis, 359–360
 clinical manifestations, 769–770
 diagnosis, 770
 DNA probe assay, 360
 microbiology, 769
 pathogenesis, 769
 treatment, 770
 vulvovaginitis due to, 356–357, 360
Garré sclerosing osteomyelitis, 196
GAS (group A streptococcus) see Streptococcus pyogenes
Gas gangrene, 460–461, 980t
 clinical features, 466t, 981
 clostridial antitoxin for, 965
 etiology, 466t, 513t, 514
  see also Clostridium perfringens
 trauma association, 513t, 514
 treatment, 468, 982
Gastric acidity
 as barrier to infection, 815
 reduced, invasive Candida infections associated, 1201
Gastric aspirates, acid-fast smears, congenital tuberculosis, 779
Gastric biopsy, Helicobacter pylori detection, 913
Gastric cancer, Helicobacter pylori causing, 912
Gastric lavage, specimen collection/ transport, 1374t
Gastric mucosal inflammation, Helicobacter pylori infection, 908
Gastric ulcer see Peptic ulcer
Gastritis, Helicobacter pylori see Helicobacter pylori
Gastroduodenal pathogens, detection, 1383
Gastroduodenal ulcer disease
 Helicobacter pylori, 912
 Helicobacter species associated, 911, 918
 see also Peptic ulcer
Gastroenteritis
 abdominal pain, 171–172
 Aeromonas causing, 830
 astroviruses causing, 1190–1191
 Citrobacter causing, 807
 Edwardsiella tarda causing, 808

enteroviruses causing, 1177
etiology, 372t
healthcare-associated, 583–584
  risk factors, 584
Helicobacter causing, 918
in HIV infection, 661–662
household attack rates, 26
Listeria monocytogenes causing, 765–766
norovirus causing, 398t, 1187–1189, 1190b
Plesiomonas shigelloides causing, 810
rotavirus causing, 66, 1094–1095
Salmonella causing, 816, 818
Trichinella spiralis infections, 1341
Vibrio parahaemolyticus causing, 856
Vibrio vulnificus causing, 856
viral, 377–381, 584–585
  clinical features, 380–381, 380t
  complications, 381
  diagnosis, 381
  endemic/epidemic, 378
  epidemiology, 378–380, 380t
  etiology, 378
  foods associated, 380
  pathogenesis, 380
  prevention, 381
  treatment, 381
  see also Adenoviruses, enteric;
    Astroviruses; Caliciviruses;
    Rotaviruses
  see also Diarrhea; Enteric infections;
    Enteritis; Gastrointestinal tract
    infections
Gastroenterology, infection rates associated, 10
Gastroesophageal reflux
  cough in, 167t
  persistent/recurrent pneumonia, 250
  recurrent abdominal pain due to, 175
Gastroesophageal reflux disease (GERD),
  Helicobacter pylori, 912
Gastrointestinal bleeding
  hookworm infections causing, 1329
  Trichuris trichiura causing, 1331
Gastrointestinal disease
  chest pain due to, 189
  functional, 174
Gastrointestinal granulomatosis, in CGD,
  622f–623f, 623
Gastrointestinal infections *see*
    Gastroenteritis; Gastrointestinal tract
    infections
Gastrointestinal pathogens
  healthcare-associated infections, 584
  viruses, 584
Gastrointestinal perforation *see* Intestinal
    perforation
Gastrointestinal symptoms
  Ehrlichia infections, 894
  HIV infection, 655
  hookworm infections, 1329–1330
  influenza, 1152
  Kawasaki disease, 1005t
  murine typhus (*Rickettsia typhi*), 932
  Plasmodium infections, 1299
  Sarcocystis infections, 1307
  Strongyloides infections, 1333

Trypanosoma cruzi infections, 1324–1325
  see also Abdominal pain; Diarrhea; *Other
    symptoms*
Gastrointestinal tract
  drug absorption, 1434–1435, 1435t,
    1438
  features in tickborne infections, 533
  host defense systems in, 83–84
    Entamoeba histolytica infection
      prevention, 1275
    mucins, 1275
    multisystem organ dysfunction, in sepsis,
      100
  normal flora *see* Flora, normal
  procedures, endocarditis prevention,
    76
Gastrointestinal tract infections
  adenoviruses, 1068t, 1069
  in cancer, 577
  clinical features, 375
    extraintestinal, 375, 375t
  diagnosis, 375–376
  diagnostic approach, 372–377
  epidemiology, 372–373
  etiology, assessment, 373–375, 373f
  healthcare-associated *see* Healthcare-
    associated infection (HAI)
  history-taking, 375
  immunosuppressed children, 374
  mucormycosis, 1214
  nematode, treatment, 1523–1524
  pathogenesis, 375
  prevention, 377
  protozoan, treatment, 1519
  stool examination, 375–376
  transmission of enteric pathogens, 372
  treatment, 376–377
    antimicrobial therapy, 377
    antiperistaltic agents, 376t, 377
    dietary intake/refeeding, 376
    fluid and electrolytes, 376, 376t
    see also Diarrhea; Enteric infections;
      Foodborne disease and food
      poisoning; Gastroenteritis; *individual
      pathogens*
Gastrointestinal viruses, diagnosis/detection,
  1395
  optimal tests, 1389t–1392t
  specimens, 1385
Gastrospirillum hominis see Helicobacter
  heilmannii
Gatifloxacin
  pharmacology, 1453t–1458t
  spectrum of activity, 1459t–1463t
  treatment of
    eye infection, 1494t–1495t
    Mycoplasma hominis infections, 999
    Mycoplasma pneumoniae infections,
      996–997
Gaucher disease, 135
GB virus C *see* Hepatitis GB virus C
  (HGBV-C)
GBS *see* Guillain–Barré syndrome
GBS (group B streptococcus) *see* Streptococcus
  agalactiae
GBV agents, 1193–1194
Gelatin, allergy, mumps vaccine caution,
  1129

Gemella, 729–730
  antibiotic susceptibility, 730
  biochemical differentiation, 729t
Gemifloxacin, 1478
Gene(s)
  candidate, familial HLH, 103, 104t
  sequencing of 16s rRNA, 674–675
Gene cassettes, acquired drug resistance,
  1423
Gene therapy, cystic fibrosis, 641
General paresis (tertiary syphilis), 942–943
Genetic testing, immunodeficiency
  disorders, 608
Genetics
  antimicrobial drug resistance, 1421–1423
  Creutzfeldt–Jakob disease (CJD),
    337–338, 337f
  familial HLH, 103, 104t
  Staphylococcus aureus (CA-MRSA),
    462–464
  Streptococcus pyogenes infection
    predisposition, 703
Genital dermatosis, 351–352
  Candida, 351–352
Genital discharge *see* Urethral discharge;
  Vaginal discharge
Genital discharge/dysuria syndrome,
  346–347, 346t
Genital herpes *see* Herpes simplex virus
  (HSV), genital herpes
Genital tract infections *see* Genitourinary
  tract infections
Genital ulcer(s), 346t
  Calymmatobacterium granulomatis, 348
  chancroid *see* Haemophilus ducreyi
  Treponema pallidum subsp. *pallidum*, 348,
    350t
  with lymphadenopathy, 347–348
    see also Genital ulcer disease (GUD)
  without lymphadenopathy, 351
Genital ulcer disease (GUD), 347–351
  lymphadenopathy with, 347–351
    clinical features, 348, 350–351, 350t
    differential diagnosis, 350–351, 352t
    etiology and epidemiology, 349–350
    laboratory diagnosis, 350t–351t, 351
    management, 350t, 351
  see also Genital ulcer(s)
Genital ulcer/lymphadenopathy syndrome,
  346t, 347–348
  see also Genital ulcer disease (GUD)
Genital warts, 349, 352, 352f
  HPV associated, 1072–1073
    treatment, 1074, 1074b
  sexual abuse and, 371
Genitourinary surgery, infection
  chemoprophylaxis, 73
Genitourinary tract
  anomalies, urinary tract infection risk
    factor, 340
  normal flora *see* Flora, normal
  procedures, endocarditis prevention, 76
  symptoms, Kawasaki disease, 1005t
Genitourinary tract infections, 342
  adenoviruses, 1068t, 1069
  Blastomyces dermatitidis (blastomycosis),
    1234, 1236t
  Brucella, 863

cervicitis see Cervicitis
female
    anaerobic gram-negative bacilli, 984
    anaerobic gram-positive cocci, 989
genital dermatosis, 351–352
genital ulcers see Genital ulcer(s)
Mycoplasma hominis, 998–999
sexual abuse and see Sexual abuse
tuberculosis, 778–779
urethritis see Urethritis
vulvovaginitis see Vulvovaginitis
see also Sexually transmitted infections;
    Urinary tract infection (UTI)
Genome
bacterial, 674
    sequencing, 676–677
see also specific microorganisms
Genomics, chronic fatigue syndrome
    etiology, 1010–1011
Gentamicin
chemoprophylactic use, 74t
dosage, 1445t–1452t, 1480t–1484t
dose adjustment
    burned patients, 1437t
    renal failure, 1445t–1452t
MICs, 1379t
pharmacology, 1453t–1458t
spectrum of activity, 1459t–1463t,
    1474
treatment of
    Brucella infections, 864t
    burns, 1500t–1501t
    endocarditis, 263, 263t, 1418t–
        1419t
    endophthalmitis, 505
    eye infections, 1494t–1496t
    Francisella tularensis infections,
        898–899
    infants with fever without localizing
        signs, 116
    infections in phagocyte disorders,
        624t
    Listeria monocytogenes infections,
        766
    meningitis, 1418t–1419t
    neonatal infections, 538, 542
    skin infections, 1498t
    Staphylococcus aureus infection, 688
    urinary tract infections, 341
    Yersinia pestis infection, 827
Geometric mean, 5
Germ tube test, 1382
Germicides, HCV inactivation, 1105
Gerstmann–Sträussler–Scheinker (GSS)
    syndrome, 338
Gianotti–Crosti syndrome (papular
    acrodermatitis), 453, 453b
    generalized lymphadenopathy, 135
Giant cell(s)
    formation, viral pneumonia, 238
    VZV infections, 1040
Giant cell myocarditis, 266
Giant cell pneumonia, rubeola virus
    (measles), 1143
Giant lymph node hyperplasia see
    Castleman disease
Giardia duodenalis see Giardia intestinalis
    (giardiasis)

Giardia intestinalis (giardiasis), 1279–1282,
    1283b
antibodies to, 1280
    detection, 1282
antigens, 1279
    detection, 1281–1282, 1383
asymptomatic carriage, 1281–1282
clinical manifestations, 1281, 1281t,
    1283b
colonization, 1279
cysts, 1279–1282
description, 1255, 1279–1280, 1280f,
    1283b
diagnosis/detection, 1281–1282, 1283b,
    1383
    Chilomastix mesnili vs., 1279
    specimen collection, 1382–1383
diarrhea due to, 26, 26t
epidemiology, 1280, 1280f, 1283b
group childcare and, 25t, 26, 30–31,
    1280
in HIV infection, 661–662
incubation period, 1279
pathogenesis, 1279–1280
prevention, 1282
proctocolitis, 347
recurrence, 1282
refugee and internationally adopted
    children, 35
transmission and high-risk groups, 1280
treatment of infections, 1281t, 1282,
    1283b, 1519
    combinations, 1282
in X-linked agammaglobulinemia, 610
Giardia lamblia see Giardia intestinalis
    (giardiasis)
Giardia muris, 1280
Giardin, 1279
Giemsa stain, 1194–1195, 1383–1384
Gingiva
    cystic lesions, 193t
    inflammation (periodontitis), 191
    ulceration, 111
Gingivitis, 191, 193t
    acute necrotizing ulcerative, 193t, 194,
        983
    anaerobic gram-negative bacilli, 983
    in cancer, 577–578
    in cyclic neutropenia, 123–124
    in immunodeficiency, 194
    necrotizing, 194
Gingivostomatitis
    HSV, 191–192, 192t
        in childcare settings, 30
        treatment, 192, 204
    see also Stomatitis
Ginseng, common cold prevention, 1120
Glanders see Burkholderia mallei
Glasgow Coma Scale, 179
Glaucoma
    congenital rubella with, 1115
    surgery, postoperative endophthalmitis
        after, 503
Global Alliance for Vaccines and
    Immunization (GAVI), 44, 68
Globe, penetration, endophthalmitis after,
    503–504
Globoside, 1088

Glomerulonephritis
    in endocarditis, 260
    mumps virus infection, 1127
    Mycoplasma pneumoniae-associated, 995
    Plasmodium infection, 1299–1300
    postinfectious
        groups C and G streptococci causing,
            720
        see also Streptococcus pyogenes (group A
            streptococcus)
        poststreptococcal acute (PSAGN) see
            under Streptococcus pyogenes (group A
            streptococcus)
Glossina, Trypanosoma (Trypanozoon) brucei
    transmission, 1319–1320
Glossina palpalis, 1320
Glossina tachinoides, 1320
Glossitis, 193t
Glossopharyngeal nerve, compression,
    cough, 167t
Gloves
    standard precautions, 18t
    transmission-based precaution, 19t
"Gloves-and-socks" syndrome, 443
(1,3)-β-D-Glucan
    Aspergillus detection, 1208
    Candida detection, 1200
β-D-Glucan, Pneumocystis jiroveciii marker,
    254–255
Glucocorticoids see Corticosteroids
Gluconeogenesis, in inflammatory response,
    94
Glucose, blood, in sepsis management, 100
Glucose-6-phosphate dehydrogenase,
    deficiency, Plasmodium infections and,
    1299–1300, 1304
Glucose dysmetabolism, 1523
γ-Glutamyl transpeptidase, elevated,
    Cryptosporidium infections, 1270
Gluten-sensitive enteropathy see Celiac
    disease
Glycerol, oral, in bacterial meningitis, 278
Glycopeptides
    dose adjustment in burned patients,
        1437t
    mechanism of action, 1468–1469
    pharmacodynamic properties, 1414t
    pharmacology, 1453t–1458t
    spectrum of activity, 1459t–1463t,
        1468–1469
    structure, 1468–1469
    see also Teicoplanin; Vancomycin
Glycylcyclines
    pharmacodynamic properties, 1414t
    pharmacology, 1453t–1458t
    spectrum of activity, 1459t–1463t
Gnathostoma spinigerum (gnathostomiasis),
    1338
    encephalitis, 304
    eosinophilia due to, 1407
    eosinophilic meningitis, 331t, 332–333
Goggles, transmission-based precaution, 19t
Gomori methenamine silver (GMS) stain,
    1194–1195, 1252
Gonococcal ophthalmia neonatorum see
    Neisseria gonorrhoeae
Gonococcus see Neisseria gonorrhoeae
Gonorrhea see Neisseria gonorrhoeae

Gordona aurantiaca see Tsukamurella
Gower sign, 484
Gown(s)
  standard precautions, 18t
  transmission-based precaution, 19t
Gradenigo sign, 324
Gradenigo syndrome, acute mastoiditis
    complication, 225, 225f
Graft-*versus*-host disease (GvHD), 562
  as *Aspergillus* infection risk factor, 1206
  chronic, HSCT recipients, 565
  pulmonary mucormycosis in, 1213
  in SCID, 628–629
Gram-negative bacilli
  anaerobic, 960t
  combination therapy antagonism,
    1420–1421
  conjunctivitis due to, 491
  endocarditis due to, 257
    management, 263
  endophthalmitis due to, 503
  enteric, neonatal septicemia, 539t
  Enterobacteriaceae *see* Enterobacteriaceae
  healthcare-associated infection, 13–14
  intravascular catheter-related infections,
    589, 593
  nonenteric, less common genera,
    832–835
  normal flora, 960t
  nosocomial infections of neonates, 549t,
    551t
  renal abscess, 344
  ventilator-associated pneumonia, 582
Gram-negative bacteria, 673
  cell wall, 673, 673f, 1464
    structure, 673f, 1466f
  focal suppurative CNS infections, 319
  folliculitis due to, 431
  infections in neutropenia in cancer, 567
  meningitis due to, 277
  otitis externa due to, 221
  subdural empyema due to, 320
Gram-negative cocci, 730–741, 748–750
  anaerobic, 960t
  normal flora, 960t
  see also Neisseria
Gram-negative coccobacilli, 856–861,
    939–941
Gram-negative diplococcus, *Neisseria
    gonorrhoeae*, 741–742, 744–745
Gram-positive bacilli, 750–751, 767–771,
    792–795
  Bacillus see Bacillus
  Corynebacterium see Corynebacterium
  endospore-forming, anaerobic, 959t
  Listeria see Listeria monocytogenes
  non-spore-forming, anaerobic, 959t
  normal flora, 960t
Gram-positive bacteria, 673
  cell wall, 673, 673f, 1464
    structure, 673f, 1466f
  infections in neutropenia, 567
  neonatal nosocomial infections, 550
    late-onset, 549t, 551
  toxic shock syndrome due to *see* Toxic
    shock syndrome (TSS)
Gram-positive cocci, 729–730
  anaerobic, 959t

catalase-negative, 696b, 729–730
  biochemical differentiation, 729t
  see also Enterococcus; Streptococcus
    (streptococci); Streptococcus
    pneumoniae
  coagulase-negative *see* Staphylococcus
    (staphylococci), coagulase-negative
  coagulase-positive *see* Staphylococcus
    aureus
  normal flora, 960t
Gram-positive diplococci, pneumococcal
    infections, 723
Gram stain, 1413
  CSF samples, 1377
  fungi, 1194–1195
  urethritis diagnosis, 354
  Yersinia pestis infection, 826–827
Gramicidin, eye infection treatment,
    1494t–1495t
Granules (sclerotia), mycetoma, 1250, 1253
Granulicatella, 716–719
  antimicrobial resistance, 718
  endocarditis, 717
    treatment, 263
Granulocyte colony-stimulating factor
    (G-CSF), 84, 94
  adverse effects, 124
  cyclic neutropenia management, 124
  HIV infection management, 658
  infections in neutropenia in cancer, 572
  in inflammatory response, 94
  nosocomial neonatal infection
    treatment, 544, 552–553
  recombinant human, 544, 658
Granulocyte-macrophage colony-stimulating
    factor (GM-CSF), 84, 1406–1407,
    1409–1410
  infections in neutropenia in cancer, 572
  neonatal infection diagnosis, 544
  nosocomial neonatal infection
    treatment, 552–553
Granulocytic anaplasmosis *see* Anaplasma
    phagocytophilum
Granulocytopenia
  fever with (in cancer) *see* Neutropenia,
    fever in
  HIV infection, 660
  see also Neutropenia
Granuloma
  caseating, 129
  Coccidioides immitis (coccidioidomycosis),
    1241
  cutaneous leishmaniasis, 1288
  eosinophilic
    Angiostrongylus infections, 1338
    Anisakis infections, 1339
  fish-handlers', 161–162
  foreign-body, persistent pneumonia, 247
  formation, 129
  hyperplastic, ameboma, 1276
  noncaseating, 129–130
  pericardial, 269
  swimming-pool, 161–162
  tinea corporis form, 1248
Granuloma annulare, 1248
Granuloma inguinale *see* Klebsiella
    (*Calymmatobacterium*) *granulomatis*
    (donovanosis)

Granulomatosis
  gastrointestinal, in CGD, 623f
  Wegener, 155
Granulomatosis infantiseptica, 764
Granulomatous amebic encephalitis (GAE)
  Acanthamoeba causing, 1294, 1295t,
    1296–1297
  clinical features, 1294, 1295t, 1296
  diagnosis, 1296–1297
  epidemiology, 1296
  treatment, 1297
Granulomatous conjunctivitis, *Bartonella
    henselae* infection, 858f–859f
Granulomatous disease
  caseating, in tuberculous pneumonia,
    238
  lung disease, 149
Granulomatous hepatitis, 407–409
  clinical manifestations, 408–409
  diagnosis, 409, 409f
  infectious causes, 408–409, 408t
  management and outcome, 409
  noninfectious causes, 408t, 409
  pathogenesis and pathology, 407–408
Granulomatous infections,
    lymphadenopathy, 129
Granulomatous reaction
  cutaneous leishmaniasis, 1288–1289
  Schistosoma (schistosomiasis), 1369
Granzymes, 87
Graves' disease, mediastinal
    lymphadenopathy, 155
Gray-baby syndrome, 277
  chloramphenicol causing, 928–929
Grey Turner sign, 173
Griesinger sign, 324
Griscelli syndrome, 104, 104t, 604t–605t
Griseofulvin
  dosage, 1445t–1452t
  treatment of
    eumycotic mycetoma, 1252
    superficial infections, 1485t, 1486
    tinea capitis, 1247
    tinea unguium, 1249
Ground itch, 1329
Group A coxsackievirus *see* Coxsackievirus A
Group A streptococcus (GAS) *see*
    Streptococcus pyogenes
Group B coxsackievirus *see* Coxsackievirus B
Group B streptococcal cellulitis–adenitis
    syndrome, 139–140
Group B streptococcus (GBS) *see*
    Streptococcus agalactiae
Group C streptococci *see* Streptococcus
    (streptococci), group C
Group childcare, arrangements, 24
  closure, influenza pandemics, 28
  number of facilities, 24
  types of facilities, 24
Group childcare, infections associated,
    24–32
  adult infections, 31
  age of children and, 24
  animal contact association, 25
  animals, infections associated, 30–31
  antibiotic use and resistance, 31
  Cryptosporidium, 1271
  economic impact, 31

Enterobius vermicularis, 1331
epidemiology and etiology, 24–30
  bloodborne viral pathogens, 29
  cytomegalovirus infections, 28–29
  echovirus infections, 28
  enteric infections, 24–27, 25t–26t, 30–31, 374, 1280
  hepatitis A virus infection, 401–402
  invasive bacterial infections, 28
  MRSA infections, 30
  multiple organ infections, 25t
  parvovirus B19, 28–29
  respiratory tract infections, 25t, 27–28
  RSV infections, 232–233
  skin infections, 25t, 29–30
  Giardia intestinalis (giardiasis), 1280
prevention, 31–32, 377
  hand hygiene, 27, 32
  policies and guidelines, 32
types of childcare, 24
vaccine-preventable diseases, 30, 30t
Group childcare settings, 24
Group D streptococci, 712, 713t
  see also Enterococcus
Group G streptococci *see* Streptococcus (streptococci), group G
Group sequential method, 6
"Growing pains", 186
Growth, in HIV infection, 669–670
Growth hormone deficiency, X-linked agammaglobulinemia with, 602t
Growth retardation
  Ascaris lumbricoides infections, 1327
  Entamoeba histolytica infections, 1276
  Helicobacter pylori infections, 913
  hookworm infections, 1329–1330
  Schistosoma infections, 1369
Grunting, 169
  in acute bacterial meningitis, 273
Guaifenesin, in common colds, 198
Guanarito virus (Venezuelan hemorrhagic fever), 1159, 1160t
Guillain–Barré syndrome, 319
  Campylobacter association, 877
  Campylobacter jejuni association, 877
  clinical features, 319
  Corynebacterium diphtheriae infection *vs.*, 757
  enterovirus infections, 1176
  etiology, 315t, 319
  immune globulin intravenous (IGIV) use, 41
  infant botulism *vs.*, 974t
  influenza vaccine associated, 64–65
  investigations, 319
  MCV4 vaccine association, 740
  Miller–Fisher variant, 316
  MRI, 318f
  oral poliovirus vaccine associated, 50–51
  poliomyelitis *vs.*, 1170
  prognosis, 319
  rabies *vs.*, 1147
  vaccine association, 50t
  weakness due to, differential diagnosis, 181t–182t
West Nile virus associated, 1101

Gulf War syndrome, *Mycoplasma* infections associated, 999
Gum(s)
  bleeding, in gingivitis, 191
  infections/inflammation *see* Gingivitis
Gummas, syphilis, 941–943
Guthrie card blood spots, 627–628
Gyrase, *Salmonella*, 817
Gyromitra, 397t, 399

H

H_1 receptor, 447
H_2 receptor, 447
H_2 receptor blockers
  invasive *Candida* infections associated, 1201
  nosocomial neonatal infection prevention, 555
HA-1A monoclonal antibody
  to lipid A, 101t–102t
  in meningococcal disease, 737
Habitus *see* Patient position
HACEK organisms, 257, 835–836, 939
  see also AACEK organisms
Haemogogus mosquitoes, yellow fever transmission, 1099
Haemophilus, 906–908
  antibiotic resistance, 1379t, 1381
  antimicrobial susceptibility testing, 1378, 1378t, 1380t
  culture medium/broth, 1375t–1376t
  description of genus, 906
  differential characteristics, 906t
  oral and pharyngeal species, 907–908
  urethritis, 353
  urinary tract infections due to, 339
  see also Aggregatibacter
Haemophilus aegyptius see *Haemophilus influenzae* biogroup *aegyptius*
Haemophilus aphrophilus, 907–908
Haemophilus ducreyi (chancroid), 907
  clinical features, 907
  diagnosis, 907
  differential characteristics, 906t
  epidemiology, 348, 350
  genital ulcers with lymphadenopathy, 348–349
  features and treatment, 350t
  laboratory diagnosis and specimens, 351t
  lymphadenopathy, 907
  microbiology, 906
  pathogenesis, 907
  transmission, 907
  treatment of infections, 907
Haemophilus influenzae, 899–905
  acute bacterial sinusitis, 229, 229t
  after head trauma, 515
  antibiotic resistance, 31, 904, 1379t
  antibodies to, 901
  antimicrobial susceptibility, 215–218, 216t, 904
  bacteremia due to, 900–901
  bacteremic periorbital cellulitis due to, 510
  bacterial tracheitis due to, 212
  biotypes, 899–900, 900t
  capsule composition, 900, 900t

chemoprophylaxis, 905
classification, 899, 906
clinical manifestations, 901–903
colonization of respiratory tract, 900–901, 904
conjunctivitis due to, 490
in cystic fibrosis, 639
diagnosis, 903–904, 905b
epidemiology, 900, 905b
genome, 899
group childcare and, 27
growth requirements, 899
historical aspects, 899–900
immunity, 901
infections in complement deficiency, 617–618
keratitis due to, 496
laboratory findings, CSF specimens, 1377
lipopolysaccharide, 900
microbiology, 899–900, 905b, 906
morbidity reduced by vaccine, 48t
neonatal otitis media, 540
non-typable (NTHi), 900
  acute otitis media, 214–215, 214f, 217, 901, 903–904
  antibiotic resistance mechanism, 218
  antibiotic susceptibility, 218
  clinical manifestations, 903
  conjunctivitis-otitis syndrome, 492, 508
  endophthalmitis, 503
  immunity, 901
  lactamase producing, 214
  meningitis, 272–273, 903
  neonatal infections, 903
  as otopathogen, 214
  pneumonia due to, 237
  recurrent meningitis, 287
  recurrent otitis media prevention, 219
  sinusitis, 229, 900, 903
  vaccine, 905
non-type b strains, 900
nonencapsulated, 899–900
ophthalmia neonatorum due to, 489
pathogenesis of infections, 900–901
peritonitis due to, 416
peritonsillar/retropharyngeal abscess, 205–206
persistent/progressive pneumonia due to, 245–246
pneumonia, in cancer, 575
prevention, 904–905
protection from, HBD2 and LL-37 role, 83–84
protein D (GlpQ), 900
  vaccine, 905
recurrent meningitis due to, 287, 289
subdural empyema due to, 320
transmission, 900
treatment of infections, 904, 904t, 905b
type b see *Haemophilus influenzae* type b (Hib)
vaccines
  containing diphtheria toxoid (PRP-D), 759
  PRP (polysaccharide (polyribosylribitol phosphate)), 56–58, 904–905

see also *Haemophilus influenzae* type b (Hib) vaccines
viral nasopharyngitis and, 163
see also *Haemophilus influenzae* type b (Hib)
Haemophilus influenzae biogroup *aegyptius*, 906–907
Brazilian purpuric fever, 906
Brazilian purpuric fever strains, 906
classification/nomenclature, 906
conjunctivitis, 906
Koch–Weeks bacillus, 906
treatment, 907
Haemophilus influenzae type b (Hib), 901–903
antibiotic resistance, 904
meningitis treatment and, 275–276
antibodies, 901
in asplenia, 636
capsular polysaccharide secretion/detection, 904
cellulitis due to, 434–435, 902–903, 903f
chemoprophylaxis, 69, 70t–71t, 905
indication, 69
clinical manifestations, 901–903
colonization by, 273, 900–901
diagnosis, 903–904, 905b
elimination goal, 47
epidemiology, 56, 900, 905b
epididymitis due to, 367
epiglottitis due to, 210, 901, 902f
fever without localizing features, 114–115
group childcare and, 25t, 28
immune response to, 901
invasive disease, 900
meningitis due to, 272, 900–901
clinical features, 901
CSF features, 274
dexamethasone in, 278
diagnosis, 903–904
incidence, 272f
treatment, 275, 276t, 904, 1418t–1419t
nasopharynx colonization, 273
osteoarticular infection, 902
osteomyelitis due to, 469, 472, 902–903
pericarditis due to, 269, 271
pneumonia due to, 237, 900, 902
prevention of infections, 904–905
pyogenic arthritis due to, 477
risk factors, 900
sepsis due to, 98
in sickle-cell disease, 634
treatment of infections, 472, 904, 904t, 905b
in X-linked agammaglobulinemia, 610
Haemophilus influenzae type b (Hib) vaccines, 56–58, 904–905, 904t
10-valent, protein D, 905
adverse events, IoM findings, 50t
background and initial licensing, 56–58
benefits in childcare setting, 28
components and combinations, 56–58
conjugate, 904–905, 904t
use/coverage, 47
contraindications/precautions, 58

effect on Hib pneumonia, 241
group childcare and, 30t
HbOC, 904t
in HIV infection, 663
indications, 905
meningitis prevalence reduction, 272, 279
occult bacteremia reduction by, 115
polyribosylribitol phosphate (PRP), 904–905
PRP-OMP, 58, 904–905, 904t
PRP-T, 58, 904–905, 904t
recommendations for immunization, 58
reduced incidence of acute epiglottitis, 210
schedule, 49f
special patient groups, 58
for travelers, 77–78, 78t
Haemophilus parainfluenzae, 907–908
endocarditis due to, 257, 907–908
meningitis due to, 907–908
Haemophilus paraphrophilus, 907–908
Haemophilus segnis, 907–908
Haemophilus vaginalis see *Gardnerella vaginalis*
Hafnia, 809
Hafnia alvei, 809
HAI see Healthcare-associated infection
Hair, fractured, 1247
Halazone, water treatment, *Giardia* prevention, 1282
Halo device use, brain abscess after, 322
Halo sign
invasive pulmonary aspergillosis, 1204
pulmonary mucormycosis, 1213
Halofantrine, *Plasmodium* infections, 1521
Halomonas venusta, animal bites, 521–522
Halzoun, 1366
Hamsters, infections associated, 528
Hand(s)
bites to, 523
exposure of concern, management, 17
infection transmission route, 12
Hand, foot and mouth disease see Enterovirus(es)
Hand hygiene
adenovirus infection prevention, 1068
CDC guidelines, neonatal nosocomial infection prevention, 554
Clostridium difficile transmission prevention, 585
common cold prevention, 199
Giardia intestinalis (giardiasis) prevention, 1282
group childcare centers, 30–32
Hymenolepis nana infection prevention, 1350
inadequate, zoonotic infections in group childcare, 30–31
influenza transmission prevention, 28
pneumonia prevention, 241
pregnant healthcare workers, 13, 17
recommendations, group childcare, 31
Salmonella infection prevention, 818
standard precautions, 18t
transmission-based precaution, 19t
see also Handwashing
Hand sanitizer, alcohol-based, infection prevention, in group childcare, 32

Handwashing
acute respiratory tract infection prevention, 27
Clostridium difficile prevention, 979
CMV infection prevention, 1046, 1051
coagulase-negative staphylococcal infection prevention, 694
inadequate, infections from petting zoos, 529
infection prevention
in group childcare, 28, 32
in travelers, 81
necrotizing enterocolitis prevention, 390
see also Hand hygiene
Hantaan virus, 1103–1104, 1103t–1104t
Hantavirus(es), 1102–1103, 1103t
hantavirus pulmonary syndrome, 1102–1104, 1103t–1104t
hemorrhagic fever with renal syndrome, 1103–1104, 1103t–1104t
nephropathia epidemica, 1103–1104
pneumonia due to, 237t
Hantavirus pulmonary syndrome (HPS), 1102–1104, 1103t–1104t
"Happy wheezers", 233
HAV see Hepatitis A virus
Haverhill fever, 938
Hazard curves, cumulative, 3, 4f
Hazard ratio, 3, 3t, 5
HCap18/LL-37 (cathelicidin), 83
Head
lymphatic system, 136–138, 136f, 136t
trauma, 513t, 515
acute bacterial meningitis risk, 272–273, 273t
brain abscess after, 322
recurrent meningitis after, 287–288
Head and neck
infections
anaerobic gram-negative bacilli (AGNB), 983
Eikenella corrodens, 836
Fusobacterium, 986–988
Staphylococcus aureus, 680–681
lymphoid system, 136–138, 136f, 136t
surgery
infection after, anaerobic gram-negative bacilli, 983
infection chemoprophylaxis, 72
tumors, 142
see also Neck
Head louse (lice) see *Pediculus humanus capitis* (head louse) infestation
Headache, 177–178
Angiostrongylus cantonensis causing, 1337
aseptic meningitis, 295
brain abscess, 323
causes, 177t
chronic, 177
differential diagnosis, 171
Ehrlichia and *Anaplasma* causing, 894–895
eosinophilic meningitis, 330–332
epidemic typhus (*Rickettsia prowazekii*), 930–931
evaluation, 178
history, 177
intracranial disease, 177

Naegleria fowleri infection, 1294
persisting focalization, 177
physical examination, 177–178
prevalence, 171
Rickettsia akari (rickettsialpox) infection, 934
Rocky Mountain spotted fever (*Rickettsia rickettsii*), 926–927
Taenia solium neurocysticercosis, 1353–1354
tension headache, 177t
therapy, 178
Trypanosoma (Trypanozoon) brucei infection, 1320–1321
Trypanosoma cruzi infections, 1324
Health Information for International Travel, 68
Healthcare-associated infection (HAI), 579–588
  adult infection comparison, 579
  antimicrobial resistance, 13–14, 14t
  blood transfusion-associated *see* Blood transfusions
  bloodstream *see* Bloodstream infections (BSIs)
  catheters *see* Catheter-related bloodstream infections; Central line associated bloodstream infections (CLABSIs); Intravascular catheters
  definitions, 10, 16, 579
  epidemiology, 579, 580t
  fungal UTI, 342
  gastrointestinal infections, 583–585
    clinical features and diagnosis, 584
    epidemiology and pathogenesis, 583–584
    management, outcome, control, 585
    risk factors, 584
    viruses, 584–585
    see also Clostridium difficile; Rotaviruses
  host (intrinsic) factors affecting, 10
  isolation precautions *see* Isolation precautions
  neonatal *see* Neonatal infections, nosocomial
  occupational health and, 21–24
  pathogens, 13–14, 14t, 580t
  pneumonia, 581–582
    prevention, 583b
    see also Ventilator-associated pneumonia
  postoperative mediastinitis, 587–588
    see also Mediastinitis, postoperative
  postoperative sternal osteomyelitis, 587–588
    see also Osteomyelitis
  prevention and control, 9–24
    administrative factors, 15
    ambulatory settings, 24
    bundled practices (best practices), 14–15
    disinfection, sterilization and waste removal, 21
    environmental measures, 18
    IPC guidelines, 14
    IPC team, 15–16
    isolation precautions *see* Isolation precautions

microbiology laboratory role, 16
occupational health, 21–24
pets and, 19–21
pharmacy role, 16–17
resources for recommendations, 15
single-patient rooms, 13
surveillance, 16–17
visitation policies, 19–21
see also Infection prevention and control (IPC); Surveillance
rates, 10, 579, 580t
respiratory tract infections, 581–583
  clinical features and diagnosis, 582
  epidemiology and pathogenesis, 581–582
  management and outcome, 583
  pneumonia *see Above*
  prevention, 583
  viral, 582
  see also Ventilator-associated pneumonia (VAP)
respiratory tract viruses, 13
risk factors, 10–13, 579
  extrinsic factors, 10–12
  host (intrinsic) factors, 10
role in patient safety, 9
sources of extrinsic causes, 10–12
  antimicrobial selection pressure, 12
  devices, 10–12
  practices, 12
surgical site infections *see* Surgical site infections
surveillance, 16–17
  CDC recommendations, 15–16
  data sources, 15–16
susceptibility, 10
transmission, 12–13
  environmental surfaces and, 13
  by healthcare personnel, 12–13
  infants and young children, 13
  modes, 12–13
  multi-bed *vs* single-patient rooms, 13
  pathogens, 13
  preschool children, 13
  routes, 12–13
  see also Healthcare personnel
  see also Device-related infections; Nosocomial infections
Healthcare facility waste, definition, 21
Healthcare Infection Control Practices Advisory Committee (HICPAC), 583
Healthcare personnel
  advice on nontraditional pets, 530–531
  BCG vaccine recommendation, 786
  with children, infection preventive procedures, 21–22
  Coccidioides immitis (coccidioidomycosis) avoidance, 1243
  exposure control plan, 17–18
  guidance on isolation precautions, 17
  HCV screening, 1108–1109
  HCV transmission to/from, 1107
  HIV prophylaxis, 71
  immunization of, 21–24
  implementation of standard precautions, 17
  infected, infection transmission by, 21–22

infection prevention and control team, 15–16
infection preventive procedures, 21–22
infection risk increased, 21
infection transmission by, 12–13
  bacterial and fungal, 20t
  hand contamination, 13, 17
  to own children, 21–22
  viral, 20t, 22–24, 22t–23t
infection transmission to, 21–24
influenza vaccine coverage, 21
occupational health and, 21–24
  special concerns, 21–24
precautions, anthrax prevention, 753
pregnant, 22–24
  exposure management (specific infections), 22t–23t
  guidelines for infection prevention, 14–15
  influenza vaccination, 22–24
  pathogens of concern, 22–24
  Tdap immunization, 22–24
protection against viral hemorrhagic fever, 1163
rubeola virus infection (measles) immunity, 1144
screening for immune status, 21
screening for TB, 21
Standard Precautions implementation, 17, 18t
VZV exposure, 21–22
see also Healthcare-associated infection (HAI)
Healthy People 202, objectives, 47
Hearing loss
  after acute bacterial meningitis, 278, 725–726
  conductive, otitis media with effusion, 220
  congenital CMV, 548, 1045–1049
  congenital rubella, 548, 1115
  sensorineural, recurrent meningitis, 287–288, 292
Heart
  abnormalities *see* Cardiac abnormalities
  disease *see* Cardiac disease
  failure
    endocarditis complication, 264
    management, 267–268
    myocarditis, 268
  rate
    abnormal, nosocomial neonatal infections, 551
    in sepsis, 99
  Sarcocystis in muscle, 1307–1308
  sounds, muffled
    musculoskeletal pain with, 183
    pericarditis, 270
  transplantation, infections after, 558
  Trypanosoma cruzi infections, 1324, 1324f
Heart valves
  damage, endocarditis complication, 264
  endocarditis pathogenesis, 258
Heart–lung transplantation, infections, 558
Heartworm disease, canine, 1346
Heat
  injuries *see* Burns
  loss, 91

Heat-labile toxin (LT), *Escherichia coli*, 397, 796

Heat-stable toxin (ST), *Escherichia coli*, 796

Heavy chains, immunoglobulin, 609
   deficiency, characteristics, 602t
   deletions, 610t, 613

Heavy-metal poisoning, 395, 399

Heck disease (focal epithelial hyperplasia), 192t

Hedgehogs
   hives from, 529
   infections associated, 528

Hektoen enteric agar, 1375t

Helicobacter, 916–919
   clinical manifestations, 917–918
   diagnosis, 918
   enterohepatic species, 909–912, 916, 916t
   epidemiology, 916–917
   flagellae, 918
   growth and culture, 918
   hepatobiliary species, 916
   immunity and immune evasion, 916–917
   infections due to, 908
   inflammatory bowel disease and, 916–917
   liver disease, 918
   MALT lymphomas and, 916
   non-pylori species, 916–919
      animals infected, 917
   species, 908, 916t
   taxonomic classification, 916
   transmission routes, 916
   treatment of infections, 918–919

Helicobacter bilis, 910, 916, 916t

Helicobacter bizzozeronii, 916

Helicobacter canadensis, 908, 916t

Helicobacter canis, 911, 916

Helicobacter cholecystus, 916

Helicobacter cinaedi, 916–917, 916t
   clinical features of infection, 918

Helicobacter felis, 916

Helicobacter fennelliae, 911, 916t, 917
   clinical features of infection, 918

Helicobacter flexispirataxon 5, 916t

Helicobacter heilmannii, 908, 910, 916t, 917
   clinical features of infection, 917–918
   diagnosis, 918
   gastritis, 911, 917
   gastroduodenal disease, 917–918
   Helicobacter pylori vs., 918
   MALTomas, 918
   treatment of infections, 918–919

Helicobacter hepaticus, 916

Helicobacter mainz, 916t

Helicobacter muridarum, 916

Helicobacter pametensis, 916

Helicobacter pullorum, 910–911, 916, 916t

Helicobacter pylori, 908–916
   abdominal pain due to, 908, 912
   adherence, 908–909
   antibiotic resistance, 914
   antibodies to, 913
   asymptomatic infections, 911–912
   BabA, role in pathogenesis, 908–910
   blood groups and, 908–910
   *cag*A pathogenicity island, 908–911
   *cag*A⁺ variants, 910–911

carcinogenesis mechanism, 910

clinical manifestations, 908, 911–913
   extraintestinal disease, 912–913
   intestinal disease, 911–912

colonization of gastric mucosa, 908, 910, 916–917

description and microbiology, 908–909

diagnosis, 913–914, 1383
   antibodies, 914
   biopsy as gold standard, 913–914
   guidelines, 913
   string test, 913–914
   testing indications, 913
   tests, 913, 1383
   urea breath test, 913–914

diarrhea disease due to, 912

discovery, 908

enzymes, 908

epidemiology, 909–910
   declining seroprevalence, 909, 909f

follow-up, 914

fucosyltransferase gene, 908–909

gastric cancer due to, 912

gastric mucosal inflammation due to, 910–911

gastritis due to, 911–912

gastroduodenal ulcer disease due to, 175–176, 912

gastroesophageal reflux disease due to, 912

genetic diversity, 911

genome, 908

genotyping, 910f, 911

growth retardation, 913

idiopathic thrombocytopenic purpura and, 913

iron deficiency anemia and, 912–913

isolates from families, 909

MALToma development, 908, 910–912

natural history of infections, 911f, 912

non-pathogenic strains, 911

pathogenesis, 908, 910–911, 911f

reinfection/recurrent infections, 909

screening, 913

short stature and growth retardation, 913

strains, 916

transmission routes, 909–910

transport medium for, 913–914

treatment of infections, 914–915, 915b, 915f, 1471, 1478
   algorithm, 915f
   first line, 914, 915b
   guidelines, 914
   novel therapy, 914–915

type IV secretion system (TFSS), 908–909

urease, 908, 910
   binding to MHC class II, 911
   detection, 913–914

vacuolating cytotoxin (VacA), 908–910

virulence, 908, 911

Helicobacter rappini, 911, 916

Helicobacter salomonis, 916

Helicobacter westmeadii, 916, 916t

Helminths, 1254–1256
   endoparasitic, 1254–1255
   eosinophilia due to, 1407
   refugee and internationally adopted children, 35, 35t

soil-transmitted *see* Nematodes (roundworms), intestinal

treatment of infections, 1522–1523

see also specific helminths

Helper T cells *see* T lymphocytes, CD4⁺ (helper)

Hemagglutination inhibition (HAI), in viral infections, 1387, 1387f
   acquired rubella infection, 1112–1113, 1113f, 1116
   measles, mumps and rubella, 1396
   mumps virus, 1127–1128

Hemagglutinin (HA)
   antibodies, 1149, 1150f
   influenza viruses, 1149, 1150f

Hemangioma-like nodules, *Bartonella bacilliformis*, 940

Hematologic abnormalities
   HIV infection, 656
   viral infections in neonates *vs.*, 548

Hematologic disease, *Mycoplasma pneumoniae* infections, 994t

Hematopoiesis, cyclic, 604t–605t

Hematopoietic stem cell(s) (HSC), 85–87
   T cell development, 90

Hematopoietic stem cell transplantation (HSCT), 562–566
   active immunizations, 566, 566t
   adenovirus infections, 564, 1069
   Aspergillus infections, 563
      cerebral, 1204–1205
      cutaneous, 1205
      diagnosis, 1206–1207
      epidemiology and mortality, 1205–1206
      risk factors, 1206
   BK virus infection, 1076
   bloodstream infections (BSIs), 565
   clinical syndromes and differential diagnosis, 563–565
   CMV infection, 562, 564, 1048
      diagnosis, 1049
      prevention, 566, 1048
      treatment, 566, 1050–1051
   Coccidioides immitis (coccidioidomycosis), 1244–1245
   conditioning regimen, 562
   CVC-related bloodstream infections, 562–563
   early period (before engraftment), 563–564
   EBV infection, 1063
   encephalopathy, 564, 565b
   enteric infections, 563–564
   epidemiology of infections, 562–563
   etiology of infections, 562
      temporal association, 562f
   fungal infections, 563
   in hemophagocytic lymphohistiocytosis, 107
   hemorrhagic cystitis, 563, 564b
      BK virus causing, 1076
   hepatitis, 565, 565b
   HSV infection, 562–563, 566
   infection predisposing factors, 562, 562b
   laboratory findings and diagnosis, 565
   late posttransplant period, 565
   management, 565–566

middle posttransplant period, 564
nephritis, BK virus causing, 1076
passive immunization, 566
Pneumocystis jirovecii pneumonia, 562, 564
pneumonitis, 564, 564b
posttransplant lymphoproliferative disease, 1063
  see also Posttransplant lymphoproliferative disease (PTLD)
presumptive therapy, 565–566
pretransplant evaluation, 563t
prevention, 566
pulmonary mucormycosis, 1213
septicemia, coagulase-negative staphylococci causing, 691–692
toxoplasmosis, 564
viral infections, 563–564
VZV infection, 562, 565
Hematospermia, *Schistosoma* infections, 1369
Hematoxylin–eosin stain, 1383
Hematuria
  gross, poststreptococcal acute glomerulonephritis, 705–706
  mumps virus infection, 1127
  Schistosoma haematobium causing, 1369–1370
Hemoconcentration, 1403
Hemodialysis
  antibiotic dose adjustment, 1445t–1452t
  infection risk, 637
  intravascular catheter-related infection risk, 590
  pharmacokinetics, 1436–1437, 1436t
Hemodialysis grafts, infections, 595–596
Hemofiltration, pharmacokinetics, 1436–1437, 1436t
Hemoglobin, 1403–1404
  abnormalities
    anemia *see* Anemia
    erythrocytosis, 1403
    see also Hemoglobinopathies
  sickle cell, 633–634
Hemoglobinopathies
  sickle *see* Sickle-cell disease
  transient aplastic crisis in, parvovirus B19 and, 1089, 1089t, 1091
Hemolysis
  Babesia causing, 1263
  causes, 1403–1404
  fatal, causes, 1403–1404
  Plasmodium infections, 1299–1300
Hemolytic anemia, 1403–1404
  Bartonella bacilliformis causing, 940
  Salmonella bloodstream infection with, 817
Hemolytic streptococcal gangrene *see* Necrotizing fasciitis
Hemolytic uremic syndrome (HUS), 86, 798–799
  clinical features, 798–799
  Clostridium septicum septicemia with, 980
  Shigella infection complication, 821
  subgroups, 798
  treatment, 798–799
  see also Escherichia coli O157:H7

Hemophagocytic lymphohistiocytosis (HLH), 103–107, 604t–605t, 1064, 1064b
  acquired (AHL), 104, 104t
    fever of unknown origin due to, 119t–120t
  classification, 103, 104t
  clinical features, 103, 105, 105t
    CNS manifestations, 105
    systemic manifestations, 105
  diagnosis/diagnostic criteria, 106–107, 106b
  differential diagnosis, 107
  etiology and incidence, 103–104
    primary HLH, 103–104
    secondary LHL, 104
  familial (FHL), 103, 104t, 1064–1065, 1064b
    diagnosis, 106
    fever of unknown origin due to, 119t–120t
    FHL1-FHL5 subtypes, 103, 104t
    incidence, 103
    X-linked, 104
  in fetus and neonate, 105
  genetics, 103, 104t, 107
  immunology, 106
  infections associated, 104–105, 104t, 1064b, 1065
  investigations, 106
  management, 107
  laboratory/pathologic findings, 105–106, 106t
  lymphoid malignancies associated, 104
  natural history, 107
  pathogenesis, 104–105
  pathology, 106
  primary/secondary forms, 103–104
  prognosis, 107
  radiologic features, 105
  treatment, 107
    hematopoietic stem cell transplantation, 107
    immunosuppression and chemotherapy, 107
  X-linked familial, 104
Hemophagocytic syndrome
  Burkholderia cepacia infection causing, 848
  infection-associated, 134, 1065
  in SCID, 628
Hemophagocytosis, 87, 103
  X-linked lymphoproliferative disease, 633
Hemophilia
  HCV infection, 1107–1108
  HIV transmission, 642–643
Hemoptysis, 170–171
  Aspergillus infections, 1203, 1209
  causes, 170–171, 171t
  definition, 170–171
  mechanisms, 170–171
Hemorrhage
  Aspergillus infections, 1207, 1209
  Ebola and Marburg viruses causing, 1160t
  Lassa virus infection causing, 1161, 1161f
  pulmonary *see* Pulmonary hemorrhage

scleral, *Bordetella pertussis* infection, 870f
varicella in malignancy causing, 1039
Hemorrhagic fever
  Argentine, 1160t, 1161, 1163–1164
  Bolivian, 1160t, 1164
  Brazilian, 1160t
  Crimean–Congo *see* Crimean–Congo hemorrhagic fever
  dengue, 1100
  hemorrhagic fever with renal syndrome, 1103–1104, 1103t–1104t
  Omsk, 1102
  Venezuelan, 1160t, 1161–1162
  see also Viral hemorrhagic fevers
Hemorrhagic fever with renal syndrome, 1103–1104, 1103t–1104t
Hemosiderosis, pulmonary hemorrhage with, 251
Hemostatic tissue factor (TF), 94
Hemothorax, 516
Henderson-Patterson bodies, 451
Henoch–Schönlein purpura (HSP)
  abdominal pain, 172–174
  distinguishing features, 173–174
  parvovirus B19 infection, 1089
  patient position and pain, 172
  purpura in, 173–174
HEPA-filtered rooms, 563
Hepacivirus genus, 1105
Hepadnaviridae, 1016t, 1077
  arthritis, 481b
  infections, 1017t
  see also Hepatitis B virus (HBV); Hepatitis D virus (HDV, delta agent)
Heparin, CMV assays and, 1388–1392
Hepatic abscess *see* Liver, abscess
Hepatic carcinoma, *Helicobacter* associated, 916
Hepatic cirrhosis *see* Cirrhosis
Hepatic disease *see* Liver disease
Hepatic enzymes
  elevated, 1411
  hepatitis A virus infection, 1183, 1183f
  see also individual enzymes
Hepatic fibrosis *see under* Liver
Hepatic function, in HIV infection treatment, 670
Hepatic necrosis, fulminant, adenoviruses causing, 1069
Hepatic transaminase, CMV infection, 1046–1047
Hepatitis
  acute, 400–404
    acute abdominal pain, 174
    age of onset, 401t
    age-specific evaluation, 402t
    anatomic causes, 402–403
    approach to evaluation, 400, 401b, 402t
    autoimmune causes, 403
    disseminated infections, 400
    Fasciola infections, 1366
    hepatitis viruses causing, 401–402
    infectious causes, 400–402, 401t
    metabolic causes, 403–404
    toxins causing, 404
  autoimmune chronic active, hepatitis A virus, 1183

cholestatic, hepatitis A virus, 1183
chronic, 404–407
    approach to evaluation, 404–405,
        405b
    autoimmune causes, 406
    causes, 405–407
    causes by age, 405t
    idiopathic and anatomic causes, 407
    infections after burns, 519–520
    nonalcoholic fatty liver disease, 406
    toxins/drugs causing, 407
chronic active, 1183
cryptogenic, 407
EBV infection causing, 1061
enteroviral, 1178–1179, 1178f
granulomatous see Granulomatous
    hepatitis
HIV infection, 655
    differential diagnosis, 655b
HSCT recipients, 565, 565b
neonatal, 407
non-A, non-B, transfusion-associated see
    Hepatitis C virus (HCV)
non-A-E, 1193–1194
relapsing, hepatitis A virus (HAV), 1183
transient anicteric, in measles, 1140
varicella causing, 1038
viral, jaundice associated, 349
see also specific hepatitis viruses
Hepatitis A virus (HAV), 1180–1185, 1185b
    acute hepatitis, 401–402, 1180, 1183
    anicteric, generalized lymphadenopathy,
        131t–132t, 132
    anti-HAV IgM, 1183, 1183f, 1394–1395
        screening, 33
    antibodies, 1183, 1183f, 1394–1395
    classification, 1167–1168
    clinical manifestations, 1182–1183,
        1185b
        atypical, 1183
    description and structure, 1180, 1185b
    diagnosis/detection, 1183, 1183f, 1185b,
        1394–1395
        optimal tests, 1389t–1392t
        PCR, 1180, 1183
        serologic tests, 1183, 1183f
    epidemic curve, 8f
    epidemiology, 62, 1180–1182, 1185b
        age-specific, 1181–1182, 1181f
        geographic distribution, 1180, 1181f
        US incidence, 62, 1181–1182,
            1181f–1182f
        vaccine effect on, 1181–1182,
            1181f–1182f
    foodborne, 1180
    fulminant, 1183
    group childcare and, 25t, 26–27, 1182
        in adults attending/care providers, 31
        costs and economic impact, 31
    immune response to, 1180
    infection risk and asymptomatic
        infection likelihood, 1180
    laboratory findings, 1183, 1183f
    nosocomial infection, 1182
    pathogenesis, 1180
    postexposure prophylaxis, 38
        dosages by age group, 38
        immune globulin, 1184

    in pregnant healthcare worker,
        22t–23t
    prevention of infection, 26–27,
        1184–1185, 1185b
    refugee and internationally adopted
        children, 33
    relapsing hepatitis, 1183
    replication, 1168, 1180
    transmission, 26–27, 401–402, 1180
    travelers, 1180–1182
    treatment of infections, 1183, 1185b
    vaccine, 26–27, 62–64, 1184–1185
        adverse reactions, 1184
        combined with hepatitis B, 78,
            78t–79t
        contraindications/precautions, 64
        dose and administration routes, 1184
        duration of protection, 1184
        efficacy/effectiveness, 1184
        group childcare and, 26–27, 30t
        inactivated, 1184
        indications, 1184–1185, 1185t
        postexposure, 1184
        pre-exposure, 1184, 1185t
        recommendations for, 64, 1184–1185,
            1185t
        schedule, 49f, 64
        for travelers, 78, 78t
    viremia, 1180
Hepatitis B virus (HBV), 1077–1087
    acute hepatitis, 401–402, 1078
        clinical features, 1080
        extrahepatic manifestations, 1080
        incidence in US, 1079, 1079f
        outcome, 1080, 1081f
        resolution, 1078, 1081–1082, 1082f,
            1082t
        resolved, 1081
        risk factors, 1078–1079
        serology, 1081, 1082f, 1082t
        treatment, 1083
    acute pancreatitis, 411
    anicteric, generalized lymphadenopathy,
        132
    antibodies, 1394–1395
    antiviral drug resistance, 1503t
    arthritis due to, 481
    carriers
        neonatal infections, 545
        pregnant, hepatitis B immune
            globulin use, 38–39
    chronic fatigue syndrome pathogenesis,
        1008t–1009t
    chronic hepatitis, 405–406, 1078
        clinical features, 1080
        extrahepatic manifestations, 1080
        management, 1084
        monitoring, 1082–1083
        natural history and outcome,
            1080–1081, 1081f
        prevalence, 1079–1080, 1079f
        recovery phase, 1081
        screening, 1081
        serology, 1082, 1082f, 1082t
        treatment, 1083–1084
    clinical manifestations, 1080
        age influence, 1080–1081, 1081f
        extrahepatic, 1080

    congenital, 545
    contacts, management, 1084
    core antigen (HBcAg), 1077
        IgM, 1078, 1081, 1082f, 1082t
    description and structure, 1077–1078
    diagnosis/detection, 1394–1395
        optimal tests, 1389t–1392t
        in refugee and internationally
            adopted children, 33–34, 33t
        serologic testing, 32–33, 33t,
            1081–1082, 1082t
    DNA, 1078, 1080–1081
        detection, 1395
        integration into host DNA, 1078
    DNA polymerase, 1077
        YMDD mutations, 1083
    elimination goal, 47
    elimination strategy, 58
    epidemiology, 1078–1080
        global prevalence, 58, 1079f, 1080
        impact of HBV vaccine, 1079, 1084
        incidence in US, 1079, 1079f
        low/intermediate/high endemicity
            areas, 1079f, 1080
        prevalence in resource-poor countries,
            32
    exposure management in pregnant
        healthcare worker, 22t–23t
    fulminant infection, 1080
    genome, 1077, 1077f
    genotypes, 1077–1078, 1078t
        influence on infection, 1081
    Gianotti–Crosti syndrome (papular
        acrodermatitis) due to, 453
    group childcare and, 25t, 29
    HBe antigen, 1077–1078, 1081, 1082f,
        1083
        –negative chronic hepatitis B, 1080
        –positive, 1078, 1080–1081
        –positive, treatment, 1083–1084
        antibodies, 1078, 1081–1082, 1082f,
            1394–1395
        clearance, 1080–1081
        clearance, treatment effect, 1083
        influence on infection, 1080–1081
        seroconversion, 1080–1081
    HBsAg (surface antigen), 1077–1078,
        1080
        antibodies, 1078, 1394–1395
        antibody detection, 1386, 1395
        clearance, 1081
        detection/testing, 1081–1082, 1082f,
            1082t, 1084
        persistence, 1080, 1082
        prevalence, 1079f, 1080
        screening, 33
        vaccine formed from, 58, 1084
    HBsAg (surface antigen) carrier state,
        1087
        in childcare setting, 29
        pregnant, hepatitis B immune
            globulin indication, 39
    HBV-HDV coinfection, 1086–1087
    hepatocellular carcinoma risk, 1078,
        1080–1081
        screening for, 1081–1083
    HIV coinfection, 643, 655, 670
    immune active phase of infection, 1080

immune globulin (HBIG), 37t, 38–39, 1085
immune inactive phase of infection, 1080
immune tolerant phase of infection, 1080
incubation period, 1080
maternal infection sources, 545–546
monitoring for disease progression, 1082–1083
in neonates, 401–402
pathogenesis, 1078
perinatal infection
    prevention by vaccines, 1084–1085
    serology, 1082
in pregnancy, 1081, 1084–1085
prevention and control, 1084–1086
reactivation phase of infection, 1080
refugee and internationally adopted children, 33–34
replication via RNA intermediate, 1077
resolution of infection, 1078, 1081–1082, 1082f, 1082t
risk factors, 1078–1079
screening, 1081
subtypes, 1077–1078, 1078t
transmission, 401–402, 1078
    by bites, 29, 525
    blood products, 580–581
    blood transfusions, 1078
    breast milk, 545
    in childcare setting, 29
    global prevalence and, 1080
    horizontal, 1078
    in utero, 545, 1078
    intrapartum, 545
    perinatal, 545, 1078, 1081
    sexual, 1078
treatment of infection, 1083–1084, 1508–1509, 1512–1514
    antiviral drugs, 1083–1084
    interferon-based, 1083
vaccination, 1084b
    measurement of response, 46
    pre-/postvaccination testing, 1085
    preterm infants, 1085
    recommendations, 58–59
    schedule, 49f, 58, 1084
    strategies, 1084, 1084b
vaccines, 58–59, 1084
    adverse events and IoM findings, 50t
    in childcare setting, 29
    combination, 1084
    combined with hepatitis A, 78, 78t–79t
    components, 58
    contraindications/precautions, 59, 1085
    dosage/administration route, 58, 1085
    efficacy, 1085
    group childcare and, 30t
    HDV infection prevention, 1087
    hyper-accelerated schedule, 78
    immunogenicity, 1085
    long-term protection, 1085–1086, 1086t
    response in premature infants, 51

response to, 58–59
safety, 1085
for travelers, 78, 78t
types licensed, 58t
Hepatitis C virus (HCV), 1105–1111, 1112b
    acute hepatitis, 402, 1107, 1110
        treatment, 1110–1111
    after burns, 519–520
    anti-HCV immune globulin, 1105
    antibodies, 1395
    arthritis due to, 481
    breastfeeding and, 1106, 1111
    chronic fatigue syndrome pathogenesis, 1008t–1009t
    chronic hepatitis, 406, 1107–1108, 1107f
        management, 1110
        treatment, 1111
    chronic liver disease, 1108
    clinical manifestations, 1107–1108, 1112b
    congenital, 545
    counseling messages for, 1108b, 1109, 1111
    culture, 1105
    description and structure, 1105
    diagnosis/detection, 1108–1110, 1112b, 1394–1395
        anti-HCV tests, 1109–1110
        of antibodies, 43
        nucleic acid detection, 1386, 1395
        nucleic acid testing, 1110
        optimal tests, 1389t–1392t
        recommendations, 1106b
        refugee and internationally adopted children, 33t, 34
        serologic assays, 33t, 34, 43, 1109–1110
        testing algorithm, 1109f
        virus genotyping, 1110
    epidemiology, 1105–1107, 1112b
    evaluation of liver damage, 1110
    exposure management in pregnant healthcare worker, 22t–23t
    fulminant, 1107
    genome, 1105
    genotypes, 1105
    granulomatous hepatitis, 408
    group childcare and, 25t, 29
    HIV coinfection, 670, 1107–1108
        maternal, 1106
    HSCT recipients, 565
    immune response, 1105
    inactivation methods, 1105
    injection drug use, 1105
    laboratory testing, 308t–311t
    management of infection, 1110
    maternal infection sources, 545–546
    myocarditis due to, 265–266
    natural history, 1107–1108, 1107f
    neonatal infections, 545
    oral features, 192t
    pathogenesis, 1105
    perinatal infections, 402
    persistent infection, 1107–1108
    prevalence and incidence, 1105
    prevention, 1111
    refugee and internationally adopted children, 34
    resolution, 1107–1108

RNA, 1105
    detection, 1395
    maternal blood, 1106
    mutations and quasispecies, 1105
    testing, 1105–1106, 1109–1110
    viremia in infants, 545
screening, 1108–1109
serum aminotransferase levels, 1107–1108, 1110
transmission, 402, 1105
    bite wounds, 525
    blood/blood products, 1107–1108
    blood products, 580–581
    breast milk, 545
    healthcare settings, 1107
    household contacts, 1107
    by immune globulin intravenous (IGIV), 43
    perinatal, 1105–1106
    by plasma donors, 43
    sexual, 1107
    through injection drug use, 1106–1107
    vertical, 545
treatment of infection, 1110–1111, 1112b, 1512, 1516
    future treatments, 1111
vaccine, 1111
viremia, 1106, 1108–1109
Hepatitis D virus (HDV, delta agent), 1086–1087
    acute hepatitis, 402
    antibodies, 1087
    chronic hepatitis, 405–406
    clinical manifestations, 1087
    diagnosis/detection, 1087, 1395
        optimal tests, 1389t–1392t
    epidemiology, 1087
    HBV-HDV coinfection, 1086–1087
    HDV superinfection, 1086–1087
    laboratory findings, 1087
    pathogenesis, 1086–1087
    prevention, 1087
    structure, 1086–1087, 1086f
    transmission, 1087
    treatment, 1087
Hepatitis E virus (HEV), 1191–1194
    acute hepatitis, 402
    antibodies, 1191, 1192f, 1193, 1193t, 1395
    clinical manifestations, 1192–1193
    description and structure, 1191–1192
    diagnosis/detection, 1193, 1193t, 1395
        optimal tests, 1389t–1392t
    epidemiology, 1192, 1192f
    fulminant, 1192–1193
    immune response, 1191, 1192f
    outbreaks, 1192–1193, 1192f
    in pregnancy, 1193
    prevention, 1193
    transmission, 1192
    treatment, 1193
    vaccine, 1193
Hepatitis G virus (HGV), 402, 1193–1194
    see also Hepatitis GB virus C (HGBV-C)
Hepatitis GB virus C (HGBV-C)
    chronic fatigue syndrome pathogenesis, 1008t–1009t

neonatal infection, 545
RNA, maternal, infant infections, 545
Hepatitis viruses
acute hepatitis due to, 401–402
arthritis due to, 481
see also individual viruses
Hepatobiliary disease
Ascaris lumbricoides infections, 1328
Fasciola infections, 1366
Hepatobiliary gas, 389f
Hepatocellular carcinoma (hepatoma)
HBV causing *see* Hepatitis B virus (HBV)
HCV infection, 1108, 1110
Helicobacter causing, 918
Hepatocytes, HCV infection, 1105
Hepatoma *see* Hepatocellular carcinoma (hepatoma)
Hepatomegaly
in chronic meningitis, 284t, 285
in congenital syphilis, 943
EBV infection, 1061
in murine typhus (*Rickettsia typhi*), 932
Hepatosplenic disease
Candida causing, 1199, 1199f
Schistosoma causing, 1368–1369
Hepatosplenomegaly
autoinflammatory/autoimmune
disorders, 134
diseases and organisms causing,
131t–132t
Francisella tularensis infection, 898
Histoplasma capsulatum infection, 1226,
1226f
Hodgkin and non-Hodgkin lymphoma,
133
Hepatotoxicity, isoniazid, 781, 785
Hepatotoxins, 404
Hepeviridae, 1016t, 1191
infections, 1017t
Hepevirus, 1191
Herbert pits, 494
Hereditary periodic fever syndromes, 124
clinical features and pathogenesis, 124
mutations, 124
Herpangina, 1174, 1174t
oral mucosal features, 192t
pharyngitis, 201
Herpes B virus (herpes simiae)
infection prevention after bites, 525–526
primates associated, 528
Herpes gladiatorum, 1029
Herpes labialis, 192t, 1033, 1506t–1507t,
1507, 1510
prevention, 1033
Herpes simiae *see* Herpes B virus (herpes
simiae)
Herpes simplex encephalitis *see under*
Herpes simplex virus (HSV)
Herpes simplex virus (HSV), 87, 1026–1035
acute bilateral cervical lymphadenitis,
138
acyclovir resistance, 1034
after burns, 519
anterior uveitis due to, 499t
antibodies, 1027–1028, 1033, 1388
IgG, 1033, 1388
antiviral drug resistance, 1503, 1503t
aseptic meningitis due to, 294–297

attachment to cell receptors, 1026
Bell (facial nerve) palsy, 315
capsid, 1026
cerebral infections, diagnosis,
1389t–1392t
characteristics, 1026
chronic fatigue syndrome pathogenesis,
1008t–1009t
clinical syndromes, 1028–1031
see also specific clinical features below
CNS infections, 1030–1031
treatment, 1034
see also Herpes simplex virus (HSV),
encephalitis
congenital infection, 547t, 1031
clinical features, 537t
diagnosis, 538t
conjunctivitis due to, 491–492, 492f,
492t
treatment, 493
see also Herpes simplex virus (HSV),
keratoconjunctivitis due to
CSF culture, 296
culture, 351, 1031, 1388
cutaneous infections, 1029–1030, 1029f
in cancer, 574
perinatal, 1031
treatment, 1034
cytopathic effects, 1031–1033
diagnosis/detection, 385t, 1033, 1388
antigen detection, 1386, 1388
in cervicitis, 362
culture, 351, 351t, 1031, 1388
detection rates, 1386t
IgG and IgM, 1033, 1388
optimal tests, 1389t–1392t
PCR, 1033, 1388
sample collection/transport, 1033,
1388
shell vial method, 1386, 1388
*see also Laboratory diagnosis and
specimens (below)*
disseminated/generalized infections,
1027, 1031, 1505, 1506t
neonatal, 537
encephalitis, 302, 304, 1030, 1030f,
1506t
brain biopsy and diagnosis, 1388
clinical features, 302
complications, 313
diagnosis, 308
epidemiology, 302
management, 179–180, 312
mortality, 1034
neonatal, 313
pathogenesis, 304
treatment, 1034, 1506t
epidemiology, 349–350, 1027–1028
sexual practices affecting, 353
erythema multiforme, 448, 1030
exposure management in pregnant
healthcare worker, 22t–23t
gene products, 1026
genital herpes, 346t, 347–348,
1028–1029
clinical features, 348
epidemiology, 1028
first episode, 348

nonprimary first episode infection,
1028–1029
primary infection, 1029
recurrent, 1028–1029, 1033–1034
recurrent episode, 348
treatment, 1033–1034
genital infection, 1505, 1506t–1507t,
1510, 1510t
genital ulcer disease with inguinal
lymphadenopathy, 347–350
features and treatment, 350t
recurrence, 350
genome, 1026–1027
gingivostomatitis, 191–192, 192t
clinical features, 191
complications, 192
HSCT recipients, 563
treatment, 192
glycoproteins, 351, 1026
group childcare and, 25t
gingivostomatitis, 30
in *Haemophilus ducreyi* (chancroid)
infection, 907
in HIV infection, 659
HIV interaction, 350–351
HSCT recipients, 562–563, 566
HSV-1, 1026
cross-reaction with HSV-2, 1033
cutaneous infection, 1029
encephalitis, 1030
genital herpes, 346t, 347–348,
1028
genital ulcer disease, 350, 350t
immunity to, 1027
keratoconjunctivitis, 1029
laboratory diagnosis, 351, 351t
laboratory testing, 308t–311t
oral infections, 192t
orolabial infections, 1028, 1028f
pharyngeal infections, 349, 1028
recurrent infection, 1027
sexual abuse, 371
urethritis, 353
HSV-2, 1026
cross-reaction with HSV-1, 1033
cutaneous infection, 1029
encephalitis, 1030f
epidemiology, 1028
genital herpes, 346t, 347–348,
1028–1029
genital shedding, 1029
genital ulcer disease, 350, 350t
laboratory diagnosis, 351, 351t
laboratory testing, 308t–311t
monoclonal antibodies, 1033
neonatal exposure, 1027
neonatal infection prevention, 71
pharyngeal infections, 349
recurrent infection, 1027
retinitis, 502
sexual abuse, 371
shedding, 348
transmission, 1028
urethritis, 353
identification, 1031–1033
immediate early/early and late proteins,
1026
immunity to, 87, 1027

immunocompromised hosts, 1031, 1034, 1505, 1506t
in vitro susceptibility testing, 1388
infection process and replication, 1026
infection route, 1027
infective keratitis due to, 495, 495f
innate immune response against, 87
intrauterine/perinatal infections, 1031
   diagnosis, 1397
   management, 1034
   prevention, 1034
keratoconjunctivitis due to, 495
   treatment, 1034
   see also Herpes simplex virus (HSV), conjunctivitis due to
labialis see Herpes labialis
laboratory diagnosis and specimens, 351t, 1031–1033
   rapid diagnosis, 1033
   serology, 1033
   specimen collection, 1033
latency, 1026–1027
latency-associated transcripts (LATs), 1027
maternal infection, diagnosis, 71
Mollaret meningitis associated, 290–291
monoclonal antibodies, 1033
mucocutaneous infection, 1505, 1506t
mucocutaneous lesions, 1032f
mucous membrane infections, 1027
   diagnosis, 1389t–1392t
neonatal infections, 545t, 546–547, 1027, 1032f, 1506t
   characteristics, 1031, 1031t
   chemoprophylaxis, 71
   diagnosis, 1389t–1392t
   epidemiology, 1027
   management, 1034
   skin, eyes and mouth (SEM) infection, 1031
neutropenia associated with cancer, 568
ophthalmia neonatorum due to, 489
orolabial infection, 194, 1028
   in cancer, 577–578
   HIV infection, 662
   pharyngitis with, 199, 201
   primary, 1028, 1028f
   reactivation, 1028
   treatment, 1033, 1033t
   see also Herpes labialis
pathophysiology, 1027
pharyngeal infections, 349, 1028
pneumonia, 236
   in cancer, 577
   in immunocompromised, 253
   in immunodeficiency, 253–254
polypeptides, 1026
prevention of infections, 1034–1035
   chemoprophylaxis, 70t–71t, 71, 1505, 1507t
   prophylactic acyclovir, 1033, 1035
primary infections, 348
reactivation, 192, 1027–1028
   burns patients, 519
   gingivostomatitis, 192
   prevention, 1035
   stimuli precipitating, 1028–1029
   vesiculobullous rash, 439f

recurrence of infection, 1027
recurrent intraoral, 192t
relapse, prevention, 1035
retinitis due to, 501
scalp abscess vs., 459
sexual abuse, 371
sexually transmitted infection
   anal discharge/proctitis syndrome, 347
   discharge/dysuria syndrome, 346
shedding, 348, 351, 1027, 1029
   prevention, 1034–1035
skin infections see Herpes simplex virus (HSV), cutaneous infections
spontaneous abortion/stillbirth, 546–547
spread, 1027
stomatitis due to, 191–192, 192t
structure, 1026
transmission, 1027–1028
   intrapartum, 544–545
   prevention, 1034
   sources of maternal infection, 545–546
treatment of infection, 1033–1034, 1033t, 1505–1507, 1506t
   see also Acyclovir
ulcerative blepharitis due to, 494
urethritis due to, 353
vaccines, candidate, 1034
vertical transmission prevention, 1034
vesiculobullous rash due to, 438–439, 439f
viremia, 1028, 1030
whitlow due to, 432, 524, 1029, 1029f
Herpes zoster see Varicella zoster virus (VZV)
Herpes zoster keratouveitis, 497
Herpes zoster ophthalmicus, 496
Herpesviridae, 1016t, 1025, 1066–1067
   arthritis due to, 481b
   chronic fatigue syndrome pathogenesis, 1008t–1009t
   common features of family, 1025, 1026b
   genome, 1025, 1026b
   infections, 1017t
   latency and persistence, 1025, 1026b
   subfamilies, 1025, 1026t
   see also individual viruses
Herpesvirus 1, cercopithecine see Herpes B virus (herpes simiae)
Herpesvirus 6 (HHV-6) see Human herpesvirus 6 (HHV-6)
Herpetic whitlow, 432, 524, 1029, 1029f
Heterophyes heterophyes (heterophyiasis), 1364
Hexachlorophene, skin antiseptic, 1499t
Hexaplex, 233–234
Hib see Haemophilus influenzae type b (Hib)
Hickman-Broviac-type catheters, in cancer, neutropenia and infections, 568
Hidradenitis suppurativa, 159–160, 431
   axillary lymphadenopathy due to, 159–160
HIDS see Hyperimmunoglobulinemia D with periodic fever syndrome (HIDS)
Highly active antiretroviral therapy (HAART), 664, 667–669
   bone health and, 671

cardiovascular health after, 670
clinical/laboratory monitoring, 667–669
Cryptosporidium infection improvement, 1271
drug selection for initial regimen, 667
effect on Cryptococcus infections, 1221, 1223
effect on Histoplasma capsulatum infections, 1226, 1229
growth after, 669
hematologic abnormalities and, 671–672
hepatic function after, 670
HIV infection prognosis, 658
immune reconstitution syndrome after, 658
malignancies and, 672
neurologic function and, 670
Pneumocystis jirovecii (carinii) pneumonia prevention, 663, 1233
in pregnancy, 643–644
pulmonary abnormalities and, 671
renal health and, 670–671
successful, effects, 667–669
see also individual drugs
Hilar lymph nodes, 148
Hilar lymphadenopathy, 148–155
   bilateral, lymphomas, 149
   diagnostic approach, 155
   EBV infection, 1061
   Mycoplasma pneumoniae infections, 996
   nontuberculous mycobacterial infection, 790
   pneumonia, 239
   pulmonary Mycobacterium tuberculosis infection, 151, 774, 774f, 783–784
Hilar masses, diagnosis by CT, 150–151
Hip
   pain
      diskitis, 484
      infectious causes, 184
      structural abnormalities causing, 185
   pyogenic arthritis, 184, 478–479
      transient synovitis vs., 486
   septic arthritis, 426
   transient synovitis, ESR elevation, 1400–1401
Histamine, 447
Histamine fish poisoning (scombroid), 393, 396t, 397
Histatins, 84
L-Histidine decarboxylase, 812
Histiocytes, sinus, 134
Histiocytic necrotizing lymphadenitis (Kikuchi disease), 134
   cervical lymphadenopathy, 141–142
   clinical features, 141–142
   etiology, 141–142
   fever of unknown origin, 119t–120t
   generalized lymphadenopathy, 134
   lymphocytosis, 1406
   neck masses, 142t
Histiocytic system, 134
Histiocytosis, 134
   generalized lymphadenopathy, 134
   sinus see Sinus histiocytosis with massive lymphadenopathy (Rosai–Dorfman disease)
Histo spots, 502

Histoplasma capsulatum (histoplasmosis),
    1194, 1224–1229, 1229b
    antigen, 1226–1229
    arthritis due to, 482
    clinical manifestations, 153–154, 282,
        1225–1226, 1225b, 1229b
        immunocompetent host, 1225–1226
        immunocompromised host, 153,
          1226
    culture, 1227, 1227t
    description and structure, 1224, 1224f,
        1229b
    detection/diagnostic methods, 155, 1382
    differential diagnosis, 1228
    disseminated infections, 1224, 1226–
        1228, 1228t
        acute, generalized lymphadenopathy,
          130, 131t–132t
    encephalitis, 303
    eosinophilia, 1408t–1409t
    epidemiology, 282, 1225, 1225b, 1225f,
        1229b
    in HIV infections, 1225–1226, 1226b,
        1228t, 1229
    immunity to, 1224
    immunocompromised hosts, 1224,
        1226–1228, 1227t
        treatment, 1229
    inflammatory enteritis due to, 386
    laboratory findings and diagnosis,
        1226–1228, 1227t, 1229b
    laboratory testing, 308t–311t
    mediastinal granuloma due to, 152f, 153
    mediastinal lymphadenitis due to, 149,
        152f–153f, 153–154
        isolated, differential diagnosis, 153
    mediastinitis due to, 1225–1226, 1228t
    meningitis due to, 280t, 282, 283t–284t,
        1226, 1228t
        diagnosis, 282
    neutropenia associated with cancer, 567
    neutropenia in, 1405
    ocular infection, 1229
    oral mucosal features, 193t
    pathogenesis, 282, 1224
    persistent pneumonia due to, 246
    pneumonia due to, 237, 237t
    pneumonitis, in cancer, 575
    prevention, 1229
    progressive disseminated histoplasmosis
        of infancy, 1226, 1226f
    pulmonary infection, 153–154
        symptomatic, 1228
    recurrent, 1228
    reinfection, 1224
    retinitis due to, 502
    risk factors for, 1225, 1225b
    self-limited infections, 1226–1228
    severe, risk factors for, 1226, 1226b
    transplacental infection, 1229
    treatment of infections, 153, 1228–1229,
        1228t, 1229b
        indications, 1228
Histoplasma capsulatum var. *capsulatum*, 1224
Histoplasmosis *see Histoplasma capsulatum*
HIV *see* Human immunodeficiency virus
    (HIV)/AIDS
HIV encephalopathy, 652b, 653, 653t

HIV entry inhibitors, 665t, 666
HIV Paediatric Prognostic Markers
    Collaborative Study (HPPMCS), 656
Hives
    animals associated, 529
    see also Urticaria
HLA-B27, *Yersinia enterocolitica* infections
    and, 824
Hodgkin lymphoma (HL), 133
    clinical features, 133, 154
    eosinophilic meningitis, 333
    epidemiology, 133
    generalized lymphadenopathy, 133
    lymph nodes involved, 133
    mediastinal masses, 154, 154f
    mixed-cell
        CT scans, 154f
        mediastinal lymphadenopathy, 154f
    neck masses, 135, 142
Homoserine lactone derivatives, 843
Homosexual males *see* Men who have sex
    with men (MSM)
Hookworms, 1329–1330
    attachment to intestinal mucosa, 1329,
        1329f
    clinical manifestations, 1329–1330
    diagnosis, 1326, 1327f
    dog *see Ancylostoma caninum*
    eggs, 1327f, 1329
    epidemiology, 1329
    iron deficiency anemia, 1329, 1403
    laboratory findings and diagnosis, 1330
    larvae, 1329
    life cycle, 1329
    mode of transmission, 1256t
    neonatal infections, 1327t, 1330
    oral cavity, 1256
    in pregnancy, 1329–1330
    prevention, 1330
    reinfections, 1330
    treatment of infection, 1330
    vaccines, 1330
    see also Ancylostoma ceylanicum;
        Ancylostoma duodenale; Necator
        americanus
Hordeolum, 508, 679
Horse blood agar, 1375t
Hortae werneckii, 1249–1250
Hospital-acquired infections *see* Healthcare-
    associated infection (HAI)
Hospital-associated pneumonia (HAP) *see*
    Pneumonia, healthcare-associated
Hospital gangrene *see* Necrotizing fasciitis
Hospital-onset infections *see* Healthcare-
    associated infection (HAI)
Hospitalization
    fever in HIV infection, 659
    fever without localizing signs without,
        116
    gastroenteritis, 372–373
    human metapneumovirus (hMPV), 1134,
        1136
    human parainfluenza virus infections,
        1121–1123, 1122t
    indications, pneumonia, 240
    infections associated *see* Healthcare-
        associated infection (HAI)
    influenza, 1149, 1151–1153, 1152t

Pasteurella multocida infections, 838
Plasmodium infections, 1300–1303
    rates, bronchiolitis, 231–233
    rotavirus infections, 1094
    RSV infections, 232–233, 1130–1131,
        1133
Host defense mechanisms
    adaptive immune response *see* Immune
        response
    anatomic abnormalities altering, 600,
        600t
    antimicrobial agent selection and, 1412
    complement role, 617
    defects/deficient
        recurrent pneumonia, 251–252
        see also Complement, deficiency;
          Immunodeficiency
    gastrointestinal system, 83–84
    innate immune response *see* Innate
        immune response
    lung, 238
    lymphoid system, 127
    skin and mucosal barriers, 83–84, 517
    trauma adversely affecting, 512
    urinary tract, 339
Host factors, susceptibility to healthcare-
    associated infections, 10, 590
Howell–Jolly bodies, 636
HSCT *see* Hematopoietic stem cell
    transplantation (HSCT)
HSV *see* Herpes simplex virus (HSV)
HTLV-1-associated myelopathy/tropical
    spastic paraparesis (HAM/TSP),
    1165
Human β-defensin 2 (HBD2), 83–84
Human B-lymphotropic herpesvirus *see*
    Human herpesvirus 6 (HHV-6)
Human bocavirus (HBoV), 1087
    common cold and, 196–197
Human CMV *see* Cytomegalovirus (CMV)
Human coronaviruses (HCoV), 1117–1120,
    1120b
    clinical manifestations, 1119, 1120b
    common cold due to, 196, 197f, 1119
    description and structure, 1117, 1118f
    diagnosis/detection, 1119–1120, 1120b,
        1394
    epidemiology, 197, 197f, 1118–1119,
        1120b
    gastroenteritis, 378
    HCoV 229E, 1118–1120, 1118t
        clinical manifestations, 1119
        incubation period, 1119
        pathogenesis and immunity, 1119
    HCoV HKU1, 1118–1120, 1118t
    HCoV NL63 (NH63), 1118–1120, 1118t
        laryngotracheitis (croup), 211
    HCoV OC43, 1118–1120, 1118t
    immune response, 1119
    neonatal infections, nosocomial, 551
    novel viruses, 1118
    pathogenesis, 1119
    prevention of infections, 1120
    SARS-CoV, 82, 1118f, 1118t
        antibodies, 1119
        clinical features, 1119
        diagnosis, 1119–1120
        epidemiology, 1118

gastroenteritis, 378
pathogenesis and immunity, 1119
pneumonia due to, 236–237
in pregnancy, 1119
prevention, 1120
transmission, 12–13, 1118–1119
treatment, 1120
strains, 1118, 1118t
transmission, 197, 1118–1119
treatment of infections, 1120, 1120b
Human enterovirus C, 1015–1018
Human enteroviruses (HEVs)
classification, 1172, 1172t–1173t
pathogenesis, 1172–1173
see also Enterovirus(es)
Human granulocytic anaplasmosis *see*
Anaplasma phagocytophilum
Human growth hormone, CJD and, 334
Human herpesvirus 6 (HHV-6), 439,
1052–1059
acute bilateral cervical lymphadenitis,
138
antibodies, 1053, 1056, 1393–1394
HHV-7 antibodies cross-reacting,
1057
maternal, 1053
antibody conversion, 1393–1394
binding/infection, 1053
cells infected., 1052–1053, 1057
chromosomally integrated virus
(CI-HHV-6), 1054
chronic fatigue syndrome pathogenesis,
1008t–1009t
congenital infections, 1054
demyelinating disease and, 1057
description and structure, 1052–1053
diagnosis/detection, 1055–1056, 1058t,
1393–1394
optimal tests, 1389t–1392t
serologic, 1056, 1058t
DNA, detection, 1055–1056, 1058t
DNA genome, 1052–1054
effect on immune system, 1053
epidemiology, 1053, 1053f
HHV-6A, 1052
HHV-6B, 1052
congenital infections, 1054
HHV-7 differentiation, 1393–1394
HHV-7 relationship, 1057
HIV coinfection, 1057
immune evasion, 1053
immune response to, 1053
immunosuppressed patients, 1394
immunosuppressive effect of, 1053,
1055f
incubation period, 1054
laboratory testing, 308t–311t
latency, 1054
multiple sclerosis association, 1057
neurotropism, 1057
persistence, 1053
pneumonia due to, 253–254
primary infection, 1054
reactivation, 1053, 1057
immunocompromised hosts, 1057
roseola
acute bilateral cervical lymphadenitis,
138

clinical features, 1054–1056,
1054f–1055f
CNS features, 1054–1056
complications in special populations,
1057
course, 1054, 1055f
diagnosis, 1055–1056
treatment, 1057
shedding, 1053–1054
simian immunodeficiency disease and,
1057
subgroups/variants, 1052
T cell infection, 1052–1053, 1057
transmission, 1053–1054
congenital infections, 1054
postnatal, 1053–1054
postnatal infections, 1053–1054
transplacental, 1054
vertical, 1054
transplant-related, 1054, 1057
treatment, resistance, 1057
viremia, 1056
virology, 1052–1057
Human herpesvirus 7 (HHV-7), 1057–1059
acute bilateral cervical lymphadenitis,
138
antibodies, 1057, 1393–1394
HHV-6 antibodies cross-reacting,
1057
cellular tropism, 1057–1058
chronic fatigue syndrome pathogenesis,
1008t–1009t
clinical manifestations, 1058, 1058t
cytopathic effect, 1057
description and structure, 1057
diagnosis/detection, 1058, 1058t,
1393–1394
epidemiology, 1057–1058
HHV-6 differentiation, 1393–1394
HHV-6 relationship, 1057
immunocompromised patients, 1058
immunosuppressive effect, 1057–1058
latent infection, 1057
persistent infection, 1057
pityriasis rosea and, 1058
in pregnancy, 1057–1058
reactivation, 1058
transmission, 1057–1058
transplant patients, 1058
treatment of infections, 1058–1059
Human herpesvirus 8 (HHV-8), 1066–1067
acute bilateral cervical lymphadenitis,
138–139
Castleman disease associated, 155
cell culture, 1066
cells infected, 1066
chronic fatigue syndrome pathogenesis,
1008t–1009t
clinical manifestations, 1066–1067,
1066f
description and structure, 1066
diagnosis/detection, 1067
PCR, 1067, 1394
DNA, 1066
epidemiology, 1066
IgG antibodies, 1394
Kaposi sarcoma due to, 138–139,
1066–1067

AIDS-associated, 1067
clinical features, 1066–1067, 1066f
endemic, 1066–1067
epidemic form, 1067
treatment, 1067
variants, 1066–1067
multicentric Castleman disease, 134
oral infections, 192t
transmission
nonsexual, 1066
sexual, 1066
treatment of infections, 1067
Human immunodeficiency virus (HIV)/
AIDS, 641–657, 661, 1166–1167
abdominal lymphadenopathy due to,
157
Acanthamoeba infections, 1296–1297
acute inflammatory syndrome, 650
acute pancreatitis due to, 411
adenovirus infections in, 1070
adolescents, 648, 657
clinical manifestations, 657
routine care, 672
AIDS-defining criteria, 386, 643, 653,
656–659
infections, 658t
pulmonary tuberculosis, 773
antibodies, 1396
detection, 651–652, 651t, 1387, 1396
in HIV-associated encephalopathy,
653
transplacental acquisition, 650–651
antiretroviral prophylaxis, 71, 643
adverse events, 645
breastfeeding infants, 647–648
combination regimens, 644
effectiveness, 645
guidelines in pregnancy, 644
initiation in pregnancy, 644
during labour, 644
maternal HAART in pregnancy,
643–644
mechanism of action, 644
postnatal, 644–645
in pregnancy, 643–644, 643b
regimens for perinatal transmission
prevention, 644–645
timing, 645
WHO guidelines, 645
zidovudine, 647
zidovudine with lamivudine, 644
antiretroviral therapy, 664–672
clinical/laboratory monitoring,
667–669, 667t–668t
drug selection, 667
effect on hematological function,
656, 671–672
effect on HIV encephalopathy, 654
effect on immune function, 650
failure, 667t–668t, 669
hematologic abnormalities and,
671–672
immune reconstitution after, 650,
669
indications, 666–667, 666t
mechanism of action, 665f
prognosis after, 656
pulmonary conditions and, 671

resistance, 644
specific organ systems affected *see under Management (below)*
WHO recommendations, 666t
see also Highly active antiretroviral therapy (HAART); *specific drugs*
bacterial vaginosis and, 359, 361
Blastocystis hominis infections, 1268
Blastomyces dermatitidis (blastomycosis), 1238
bloodstream infections (BSIs), 659
in body fluids, 642–643
breastfeeding safety issue, 545
candidiasis and, 659, 662
prevention, 664
cardiomyopathy in, 655–656, 670
CDC classification, 643
cerebral toxoplasmosis, 661
chronic meningitis, 283
chronic myositis, 463t, 464
chronic phase, 650
classification of infection, 651t, 652b
infants, 651t
clinical manifestations, 643, 653
adolescents, 657
bones/bone density, 671
cardiovascular, 655–656, 670
clinical categories, 652b
delayed presentation, 666
dermatologic, 656
early signs/symptoms, vertical infection, 653
fever *see* Fever
gastrointestinal, 655
hematologic, 656, 671–672
hepatic function, 670
infancy, 656
late signs/symptoms, 656
malignancies, 655, 672
management of *see Management (below)*
metabolic, management, 669–670
neurologic features, 653–654, 653t, 654f, 670
organ system specific, 653–656
pulmonary features, 654–655, 654f, 671
renal, 656, 670–671
Clostridium difficile colitis, 382, 662
CMV infection, 659, 1048–1049
retinitis, 501
treatment, 1050, 1508–1509, 1511, 1515
CNS infections, 661
CNS mass lesions, 661
Coccidioides immitis (coccidioidomycosis), 1244–1245
congenital infection, diagnosis, 538t
congenital syndrome, 653
Cryptococcus infections, 661, 1221
treatment and prevention, 1223
Cryptococcus neoformans infection, 282
Cryptosporidium infections, 662, 1270–1271
culture, 651t, 1396
Cyclospora infection, 1283–1284
Cystoisospora belli infection, 1283–1284
delayed puberty, 669–670

diagnosis/detection, 650–653, 1396–1397
after *Haemophilus ducreyi* infections, 907
antibodies, 651–652, 651t, 1387, 1396
assays, 651–653, 651t
blood samples, 1385
confirmatory antibody tests, 651–652
enzyme immunoassays, 651
immunofluorescence assays, 651–652
in infants, 651
non-breastfed infants, 653
nucleic acid detection, 652–653
in older children, 651t, 652–653, 1396–1397
optimal tests, 1389t–1392t
p24 antigen, 651t, 652–653
PCR, 651t, 652–653, 1167
rapid tests, 651
RNA levels, 650–651, 653, 1167
screening tests, 651
sensitivity of tests, 1397, 1397t
vertical transmission confirmation, 1397
Western blot, 651, 651t
diagnostic test sensitivity by age, 1397, 1397t
diarrhea in, 374, 386–387, 661–662
disclosure, 670
early infection process, 1166–1167
EBV infections, 1063–1064
encephalopathy in, 652b, 653–654, 653t
Entamoeba gingivalis infection, 1278
Entamoeba histolytica infection, 1274
eosinophilia, 1407, 1408t–1409t
epidemiology, 641–648
perinatally acquired, 642
prevalence in children, 642
in women of childbearing age, 642
Escherichia coli infection, 661–662
esophagitis in, 662
exposure management in pregnant healthcare worker, 22t–23t
fever of unknown origin due to, 119t–120t
folliculitis in, 431
generalized lymphadenopathy, 131t–132t, 132
Castleman's disease and, 134
genes, 1166
genetic variability, 653
genome, 1166
detection, 1397
Giardia infection, 661–662
gp41 protein, 666
gp120, 1166
group childcare and, 25t, 29
growth in, 669–670
in *Haemophilus ducreyi* (chancroid) infection, after accidental exposures, 907
HBV coinfection, 643, 655, 670
HCV coinfection, 670, 1107–1108
maternal, 1106
Helicobacter infections, 918
hepatitis in, 655, 655b
HHV-6 infection as cofactor, 1057

HHV-8 coinfection, 1067
Histoplasma capsulatum infections, 1225–1226, 1226b, 1228t, 1229
HIV-1, 650, 1166–1167, 1166t
diagnosis, 1396–1397
HIV-2 comparison, 1166t
refugee and internationally adopted children, 34
testing, refugee and internationally adopted children, 33t, 34
HIV-2, 1166t, 1167
diagnosis, 1396–1397
testing, refugee and internationally adopted children, 33t, 34
HPV infection, 1072–1074
HPV-related neoplasia, 1073
HSV infections in, 659, 662
HSV interactions, 350–351
HTLV-1 coinfection, 1165
human parainfluenza virus infections, 1124
hypergammaglobulinemia of, 653
persistent/recurrent pneumonia, 251
hyperimmunoglobulinemia, 653
immune consequences, 648, 650, 658
antiretroviral therapy effect, 650
see also T lymphocytes
immune reconstitution after therapy, 650
immune reconstitution inflammatory syndrome (IRIS), 650, 658, 662–663, 669
immune response, 653, 658, 669
immunizations in, 52, 62, 669
BCG, 669
influenza, 663
meningococcal conjugate vaccine, 65
MMR vaccine and, 1117
MMRV, 663
passive, 663
pneumococcal, schedule, 663
response to, 669
routine, 662–663, 669
immunopathogenesis, 648–650
indication for IGIV, 40, 40t
infants, ADCC defect, 87
infection prophylaxis, 662–664, 669
bacterial infections, 40
fungal infections, 664
IGIV, 40, 40t, 663
Mycobacterium avium complex, 663–664
pneumococcal vaccine, 663
Pneumocystis jirovecii (carinii) pneumonia, 663, 669
viral infections, 663
infectious complications, 657–664
bacterial, 659
clinical approach, 659–662
CNS infections, 661
diarrhea, 661–662
epidemiology and etiology, 658–659, 658t
fever, 659–660, 659b
fungal, 659
incidence (by infection), 658t
pathogenesis, 657–658
pneumonia, 660–661
pre-post-HAART, 658–659, 658t

prognosis, 664
see also Fever; Pneumonia
influenza virus infection, 1156
intravascular catheter-related infections, 590
isolation precautions and, 17
JC virus infection, 661, 662f
Kaposi sarcoma, 655, 672
Klebsiella granulomatis infections, 803
laboratory abnormalities, early, 653
laboratory testing, 308t–311t, 667–669
    of antiretroviral therapy, 308t–311t, 667–669
Leishmania co-infection, 1287
life-cycle, 665f, 1166
Listeria monocytogenes infections, 764
lymphadenopathy, 132
lymphomas, 655
Malassezia folliculitis, 1217
management, 664–672
    bone health and antiretroviral drugs, 671
    cardiovascular health and, 670
    clinical/laboratory monitoring, 667–669, 667t–668t
    comorbid infections, 667, 672
    dosage, 1445t–1452t
    hematologic abnormalities and, 671–672
    hepatic function and, 670
    infection prevention *see Above*
    international settings, 672
    lactic acidosis, 672
    lamivudine, 1512
    malignancies and, 672
    mitochondrial dysfunction, 672
    neurologic function, 670
    nutrition, 669–670
    pharmacokinetic-pharmacodynamic targets, 1444–1445, 1444t
    pulmonary abnormalities and, 671
    renal health and, 670–671
    reproductive health, 672
    routine monitoring, 667–669, 667t–668t
    transition to adult care, 672
    see also Human immunodeficiency virus (HIV)/AIDS, antiretroviral therapy
meningitis in, 283, 661
microsporidial infections, 1291–1292
molluscum contagiosum and, 352, 1025
mortality, 656–657, 666
mother-to-child transmission, 545, 642, 667
    intrapartum period, 645–646
    prevention *see Perinatal infection prevention (below)*
    risk factors and predictors, 642
    timing, 643
Mycobacterium avium-intracellulare, 658, 790–791
Mycobacterium tuberculosis infection *see Mycobacterium tuberculosis*
Mycoplasma infections and, 999
myocarditis in, 265–266, 655–656, 668
natural history, 643
neonatal infection, 545

neurologic features, 653–654, 653t, 654f, 670
neurologic function, 670
Nocardia infections and relapses, 795
non-Hodgkin lymphoma (NHL), 655
non-perinatally acquired, 657
opportunistic infections, 657, 669
    see also Infectious complications (above)
oral infections, 662
p24 antigen, 651t
    detection tests, 652–653, 1396–1397
passive immunization, 663
perinatal infection
    breastfeeding avoidance, 647
    early signs/symptoms, 653
    natural history, 643
    treatment, 548
perinatal infection prevention, 71, 643–648
    antiretroviral therapy, 643b, 644–645
    in breastfeeding infants, 646–648
    cesarean section, 645–646
    interventions, 643–648
    mechanism of action, 644
    mother-to-child transmission prevention (PMTCT), 667
    prophylaxis in labour, 644
    recommendations, 643b
    see also Antiretroviral prophylaxis (above); Human immunodeficiency virus (HIV)/AIDS, antiretroviral prophylaxis
perinatally acquired, 10
periodontitis, gingivitis and mucositis, 194
Pneumocystis jirovecii pneumonia *see Pneumocystis jirovecii (carinii)*, pneumonia
pneumonia *see Pneumocystis jirovecii (carinii)*; Pneumonia
postexposure prophylaxis (PEP)
    adolescents, 648
    indications, 371
    infants, 644
    sexual abuse and, 371–372
preterm infants, 87
prevention
    adolescents, 648, 648b
    antiretroviral drugs *see Above*
    perinatal infection *see Above*
    postexposure *see Above*
prognosis, 656, 664
progression, 643
    variations, 643
progressive multifocal leukoencephalopathy, 661, 662f
progressive necrotizing retinitis, 502
proteins, 1166
Pseudomonas aeruginosa infections, 844t
receptor and coreceptors, 1166
recurrent otitis media in, 219
replication, 648–650
    site, 648–649
reverse transcriptase, 664, 1166
Rhodococcus (Corynebacterium) equi infections, 769
risk factors, 642
RNA levels, 650–651, 653

rubeola virus infection (measles), 1143–1144
Salmonella gastroenteritis in, 816
screening, 1396
seroconversion syndrome, 132
sexual abuse and, 371–372
    postexposure prophylaxis, 371–372
sexually transmitted infections with, 648, 672
Shigella infections in, 821
SIV relationship and genomic analyses, 1166
spontaneous abortion/stillbirth, 546–547
Streptococcus pneumoniae infections with, 659, 722, 728
subtype B, diagnosis, 653
subtype C, diagnosis, 653
syphilis associated *see Treponema pallidum* subsp. *pallidum*
testing, 651
    adolescents, 648
time to AIDS, perinatal infections, 643
Toxoplasma gondii infections, 661, 1311–1312, 1314, 1317
    prevention, 669
transfusion/hemophilia-associated, 642–643
transmission, 642–643, 642t
    adolescents, 648, 657
    bite wounds, 521–522, 525
    blood products, 580–581
    breast milk, 545, 642, 646–648
    childcare setting, 29
    drug abuse, 642–643, 648
    genital ulcer disease role, 350
    healthcare setting, 642–643
    hemophilia-associated, 642–643
    heterosexual, 648
    HIV-2, 1167
    intrapartum, 545, 645–646
    intrauterine, 545, 642
    mother-to-child *see Mother-to-child transmission (above)*
    perinatal *see Perinatal transmission (above)*
    postnatal, 642–643, 645
    sexual, 648, 657
    transfusions, 642–643
    vertical, 371, 642, 1167
Trichomonas vaginalis infection and, 361
Trypanosoma cruzi infections in, 1325
tuberculosis, 671
tumors in, 655
Vibrio cholerae infections, 661–662
Vibrio cholerae vaccine and, 854
viral loads, 643–644
    HAART effect, 667–669
    measurement, 1396
viremia, 648–650
    antiretroviral drug effect, 667–669
    "set point", 648–650
vitamin D deficiency, 670
VZV infection, 1036
wasting syndrome, 652b, 655
Human metapneumovirus (hMPV), 1130, 1134–1137, 1137b
    acute otitis media due to, 1136

age of infection, 1136, 1136b
asthma exacerbation, 1137
bronchiolitis due to, 231, 1123
clinical manifestations, 1136, 1136b–
    1137b, 1136t
description and virology, 1134–1135,
    1134f–1135f, 1135t
diagnosis/detection, 1136, 1137b, 1394
epidemiological pattern, 1131f
epidemiology, 1135–1136, 1137b
F and G protein, 1134
genogroups, 1134–1135
group childcare and, 25t
hospitalizations, 1134, 1136
immune response to, 1135
immunity to, 1134–1135
in immunocompromised hosts,
    1136–1137
laboratory testing, 308t–311t
lower respiratory tract infections, 1136
pathogenesis, 1135
pathology, 1135
pneumonia due to, 236–237
prevention of infection, 1137
recombinant, 1137
reinfection, 1134–1135
replication, 1135
RNA genome, 1134, 1135f, 1135t
subgroups A and B, 1134–1135
transmission, 1136
treatment of infection, 1136–1137, 1137b
upper respiratory tract infections, 1134,
    1136
Human monkeypox, 527
Human papillomavirus (HPV), 66,
    1071–1074, 1075b
anogenital cancers, 1072–1073
anogenital tract infections, 1072, 1074
anogenital warts, 1072–1073
    treatment, 1074, 1074b
antibodies, 1072
antigens, 1071
cervical cancer, 1071–1072
    in HIV-infected women, 1073–1074
    prevention, 1074, 1074b
    screening and management,
        1071–1074, 1072t
clinical manifestations, 1072–1073
condyloma acuminatum, 352
    oral features, 192t
cutaneous warts due to, 1072–1074
description and structure, 1071–1072,
    1075b
diagnosis/detection, 1073, 1075b
    nucleic acid amplification,
        1386–1387
    optimal tests, 1389t–1392t
    sexual abuse detection, 371
DNA genome, 1071
E6 and E7 proteins, 1071
    in cervical cancer, 1071–1072
epidemiology, 1072–1073, 1075b
epidermodysplasia verruciformis due to,
    1073
epitheliotropic, 1071
focal epithelial hyperplasia (Heck
    disease), 192t
genital warts due to, 349, 352

groups and types, 66, 1072
HPV-1, 1072
HPV-2, 1072
HPV-6, 1072–1073
HPV-11, 1072–1073
HPV-16, 66, 371, 1072
HPV-18, 66, 371, 1072
immune response, 1072
immunocompromised hosts, 1072–1074
laryngeal papilloma due to, 349
oral infections and cancers, 192t, 1073
pathogenesis, 1071–1072
persistent infections, 1072
prevention of infections, 1074, 1074b
recurrent respiratory papillomatosis,
    juvenile, 1072–1073
screening, 1073, 1075b
sexual abuse, 371
sexually transmitted infection, 349
    dermatologic syndromes, 349
squamous cell papilloma, oral features,
    192t
subtypes, sexual abuse and, 371
transmission, 1072
treatment of infections, 1073–1074,
    1074b–1075b, 1509
vaccines, 66–67, 1072, 1074
    bivalent, 67, 1074, 1074b
    contraindications/precautions, 66–67.
    group childcare settings, 30t
    indications, 66
    quadrivalent, 66–67, 1074, 1074b
    recommendations for, 66–67
    schedule, 49f
    for travelers, 79
verruca vulgaris, oral features, 192t
vulvovaginitis due to, 356–357
Human parainfluenza viruses (HPIVs),
    1121–1124, 1124b
antibodies, 1121, 1123–1124
aseptic meningitis due to, 294
asthma and, 1123
bronchiolitis due to, 231, 232f, 1121,
    1123, 1123f
cell culture, 1123–1124
clinical manifestations, 1122–1123,
    1123f, 1124b
colds, 196, 197f
common cold due to, 196
croup (laryngotracheobronchitis), 211,
    1121–1123, 1123f
cytopathic effects, 1121
description and structure, 1121, 1124b
diagnosis/detection, 1123–1124, 1124b,
    1394
    optimal tests, 1389t–1392t
epidemiology, 197, 197f, 1122, 1122f,
    1122t, 1124b, 1131f
group childcare and, 25t
health impact and costs, 1122
in HIV infection, 1124
hospitalization due to, 1121–1123, 1122t
HPIV-1, 1122t
    bronchiolitis, 232f
    clinical manifestations, 1122–1123
    epidemiology, 1122, 1122f, 1122t
    immune response, 1121
    vaccine, 1124

HPIV-2, 1122t
    bronchiolitis, 232f
    clinical manifestations, 1122–1123
    epidemiology, 1122, 1122f, 1122t
    immune response, 1121
    vaccine, 1124
HPIV-3, 1122t
    bronchiolitis, 232f
    clinical manifestations, 1122–1123
    epidemiology, 1122, 1122f, 1122t
    immune response, 1121
    immunocompromised hosts, 1124
HPIV-4, 1122t, 1123–1124
    epidemiology, 1122, 1122f, 1122t
    immune response, 1121
    immunocompromised hosts, 1124
lower respiratory tract infections, 1121,
    1123f
neonatal infections, 1123
neurotropic, 1123
otitis media, 1123, 1123f
pathogenesis, 1121
pneumonia due to, 236–237, 1121,
    1123–1124, 1123f
    treatment, 1124
prevention of infections, 1124
recombinant chimeric bovine/human,
    vaccine to hMPV, 1137
reinfections, 1121
RNA genome, 1121
seasonal outbreaks, 232, 232f, 1122
serotypes and subgroups/genotypes,
    1121
transmission, 1122
in transplant recipients, 559–560
treatment of infections, 1124, 1124b
upper respiratory tract infections, 1121,
    1123, 1123f
vaccines, 1124
Human parechovirus(es), 293, 1172, 1177
aseptic meningitis due to, 293
encephalitis, 297–302
    neonates, 313
neonatal infections, 1178
    CNS infection, 1179
    hepatitis, 1178–1179
serotypes, 1172, 1177
Human parechovirus 1 (HPEV-1),
    pneumonia due to, 236–237
Human parechovirus 3 (HPEV-3), aseptic
    meningitis due to, 293, 295
Human parvovirus B19 see Parvovirus B19
Human parvoviruses see Parvovirus B19
Human pituitary hormones, CJD and, 334
Human polyomaviruses, 1075–1077
cancer and, 1077
description, 1075
epidemiology, 1075
KI polyomavirus, 1075, 1077
Merkel cell polyomavirus (MCV), 1075,
    1077
pathogenesis, 1075
permissive and nonpermissive hosts,
    1075
trichodysplasia spinulosa-associated
    polyomavirus (TSV), 1075, 1077
WU polyomavirus, 1075, 1077
see also BK virus; JC virus

Human T-lymphocyte lymphotropic viruses
(HTLV), 1165
clinical manifestations, 1165
epidemiology, 1165
HIV coinfection, 1165
HTLV-1, 1165
Strongyloides stercoralis infections and,
1332–1333
transmission by blood products,
580–581
transmission in breast milk, 545
HTLV-2, 1165
HTLV-3, 1165
HTLV-4, 1165
transmission, 1165
Humidification of air, laryngotracheitis,
211
Humoral immune response, 609
developmental milestones, 89t
in HIV infection, 658
HSV infections, 1027
to vaccines, 45
see also Antibodies; B lymphocytes;
Immune response, adaptive;
Immunoglobulin
Hutchinson teeth, 944
Hyalohyphomycosis, 1209–1212, 1212b
clinical manifestations, 1210, 1210f,
1212b
diagnosis, 1210, 1211f, 1212b
epidemiology, 1210, 1212b
microbiology, 1210–1211, 1212b
therapy and prevention, 1210–1211,
1212b
Hyalomma (ticks), vectors for *Rickettsia
prowazekii*, 930
Hybrid study designs, 3
Hydatid cysts *see Echinococcus granulosus*
(cystic echinococcosis)
Hydrocele, filarial, 1342–1344, 1344t
Hydrocephalus
acute, after acute bacterial meningitis,
278
communicating, *Mycobacterium
tuberculosis* infection, 777
congenital toxoplasmosis, 1311–1312,
1314
obstructive
Coccidioides immitis meningitis, 1244
in meningitis, 273
Taenia solium neurocysticercosis,
1353–1354, 1356
Hydrocortisone, septic shock management,
100–102
Hydrogen breath test, 391
Hydrogen peroxide, 85
formation, by vaginal flora, 960
Mycoplasma pneumoniae infections, 993
Hydrogenosomes, *Trichomonas vaginalis*,
1317–1318
Hydronephrosis, suppurative
(pyonephrosis), 343
Hydrophobia, rabies, 1147
Hydrops fetalis
nonimmune, in hemophagocytic
lymphohistiocytosis, 105
parvovirus B19, 546–547, 1089–1091,
1089t

Hydroxychloroquine
Coxiella burnetii infections, 892
Plasmodium infections, 1301t–1303t,
1304
prophylaxis, 1301t–1303t, 1304
Hygiene
enterovirus infection prevention, 1180
hands *see* Hand hygiene
poor, *Helicobacter pylori* prevalence, 909
rotavirus infection prevention, 1097
Staphylococcus aureus infection
prevention, 689
Vibrio cholerae infection prevention,
853–854
Hymenolepis diminuta, 1349–1350
clinical manifestations, 1349
description, 1349
epidemiology, 1349
laboratory findings and diagnosis, 1349
treatment, 1349
Hymenolepis nana, 1349–1350
clinical manifestations, 1349
description, 1349
eosinophilia, 1408t–1409t
epidemiology, 1349
laboratory findings and diagnosis, 1349
prevention, 1350
treatment, 1349
Hyper-IgE/recurrent infection syndrome
(Job syndrome), 140, 604t–605t, 625
characteristics, 619t
clinical features, 621t, 625
infection prevention, 624
infections associated, 620t, 625
infectious complications, 620t
invasive *Aspergillus* infection, 1207–1208
as multisystem disease, 620t, 625
Hyper-IgE syndrome
autosomal dominant, 630t, 631
characteristics, 603t–604t
Hyper-IgM syndrome, 610t, 612–613, 613t,
630t, 631–632
AID and UNG deficiencies, 613
autosomal recessive, 632
characteristics, 602t
genetic and clinical features, 630t,
631–632
genetic basis, 612–613
indication for IGIV, 40
Pneumocystis jirovecii (carinii) infections,
1230–1231
X-linked, 631–632
Hyperbaric oxygen (HBO)
anaerobic gram-negative bacilli, 985
anaerobic infections, 965
Clostridium perfringens gas gangrene, 982
mucormycosis, 1214
Hyperbilirubinemia, 670
Hypercalcemia, in *Histoplasma capsulatum*
infections, 1225–1226
Hyperemia, conjunctival, 490
Hypereosinophilia, *Loa loa* infections, 1346
Hypereosinophilic syndrome
definition, 1407
eosinophilic meningitis, 333
idiopathic, 1408t–1409t
Hyperesthesia, streptococcal soft-tissue
infection causing, 112

Hypergammaglobulinemia
of HIV infection, 251, 658
in *Toxocara* infections, 1336–1337
Hyperglycemia, 1411
invasive *Candida* infections associated,
1201
reactive, in inflammatory response, 94
Vibrio cholerae infection, 851–852
Hyperimmune serum, *Bordetella pertussis*
infection, 872
Hyperimmunization, *Clostridium tetani*
prevention, 970
Hyperimmunoglobulin M syndrome *see*
Hyper-IgM syndrome
Hyperimmunoglobulinemia, in HIV
infection, 653
Hyperimmunoglobulinemia D with periodic
fever syndrome (HIDS), 122t, 125
cardinal clinical features, 125
course, treatment and outcome, 125
epidemiology and etiology, 125
mutations, 125
Hyperkalemia, 1520
Hypermetabolic state, in inflammatory
response, 94
Hypersalivation, rabies, 1147
Hypersensitivity reactions
drug-induced lymph node hyperplasia,
133–134
to immune globulin intravenous (IGIV),
42–43
to mumps virus vaccine, 1129
in *Mycobacterium tuberculosis* infection,
776
to *Schistosoma* (schistosomiasis), 1369
see also Allergic reactions
Hypersplenism, 1409
Hypertension, poststreptococcal acute
glomerulonephritis, 705
Hyperthermia, fever *vs.*, 91
Hyperthyroidism, generalized
lymphadenopathy, 135
Hyphae, 1194
Hypnozoite, *Plasmodium*, 1298, 1298f,
1304
Hypochlorhydria, gastric cancer in
Helicobacter pylori infections, 912
Hypofibrinogenemia, in hemophagocytic
lymphohistiocytosis, 105
Hypogammaglobulinemia
in EBV infection, 633, 1062
indication for IGIV, 40
measles infection in, 1138
Mycoplasma pneumoniae infection in,
995
Neisseria meningitidis infections in,
731–732
nephrotic syndrome with, infections,
637
transient, of infancy, 610t, 615, 615t
Hypoglycemia, 1411
early-onset/late-onset neonatal sepsis,
540
Plasmodium infections, 1299–1303
Shigella infection causing, 821
Vibrio cholerae infection, 851–852
Hypokalemia, *Vibrio cholerae* infection,
851–852

Hyponatremia, 1411
  infant botulism and, 974t
  Rocky Mountain spotted fever (*Rickettsia rickettsii*), 928
  Shigella infection causing, 821
Hypopigmentation, varicella lesions, 1037
Hypoproteinemia, 506
Hypopyon, 504, 504f
Hypotension
  infections after burns, 517
  orthostatic, chronic fatigue syndrome pathogenesis, 1008
  septic shock, 97
Hypothalamic-pituitary-adrenal (HPA) axis, chronic fatigue syndrome pathogenesis, 1008–1010
Hypothalamic set-point, changes in/after fever, 91
Hypothermia
  early-onset/late-onset neonatal sepsis, 540
  infections after burns, 517
Hypothyroidism, infant botulism *vs.*, 974t
Hypotonia, 180–182, 181t
  therapy, 182
Hypovolemia, *Vibrio cholerae* infection, 851
Hypoxemia
  in bronchiolitis, 233
  in pneumonia, 240
  tachypnea in, 168–169
Hypoxia, poliovirus causing, 1170
Hyrtl fissure, 288–289

I

Ibuprofen
  sepsis, 101t–102t
  transient synovitis, 486–487
IC14 (monoclonal antibody to CD14), 103
ICAM-1, 1186
ICAMs, 85
ICOS deficiency, characteristics, 602t
"Id" (dermatophytic) reactions, 453–454, 454b, 1246–1247
Idiopathic hypereosinophilic syndrome, 1408t–1409t
Idiopathic hypertrophic pyloric stenosis (IHPS), 72
Idiopathic thrombocytopenic purpura (ITP), 1410–1411
  Helicobacter pylori infections, 913
  indication for IGIV, 40–41, 40t
  parvovirus B19, 1089
IFN-γ release assays (IGRA), *Mycobacterium*, non-tuberculosis, 788
IGIV *see* Intravenous immune globulin (IGIV)
Ikaros transcription factor, 85–86
IL-1R-associated kinase (IRAK), 84
Ileitis
  hookworm causing, 1330
  terminal, 130
  Trichuris trichiura causing, 1331
  Yersinia enterocolitica causing, 824
  see also Enteritis
Ileocolitis, eosinophilic, *Enterobius vermicularis*, 1332

Iliac adenitis, 160
  suppurative, 158t, 160
Iliac lymph nodes, enlarged, 158t, 160
Iliopsoas abscess, 680
  etiology, 423–424
  Staphylococcus aureus, 680
Imaging
  acute bacterial sinusitis, 228–229
  myocarditis, 267
  responsible, and radiation risks, 345
  see also Computed tomography (CT); Magnetic resonance imaging (MRI); Radiography
Imidazole, *Malassezia* infections, 1217–1218
Imipenem
  adverse effects, 1468
  clinical uses, 1468
  dosage, 1445t–1452t
  dose adjustment in burned patients, 1437t
  eye infection treatment, 1496t
  Nocardia infection treatment, 795
  spectrum of activity, 1468
Imipenem-cilastatin
  acute bacterial meningitis treatment, 277
  dosage, 1480t–1483t
  pharmacology, 1453t–1458t, 1468
  spectrum of activity, 1459t–1463t
Immediate-type hypersensitivity
  basophils and mast cells, 1409
  Toxocara infections, 1335–1336
Immigrants to USA, 32
  immunizations, 52
  travel advice for visiting home countries, 76
  see also Refugee and internationally adopted children
Immobile children, persistent pneumonia, 247
Immortalization, 1059
Immortalization assay, EBV, 1062
Immotile cilia syndrome, 83–84, 638
Immune complexes
  complement activation, 615
  deposition, *Neisseria meningitidis* infections, 737
  poststreptococcal acute glomerulonephritis, 705–706
  urticaria pathogenesis, 445–446
Immune deficiencies *see* Immunodeficiency
Immune evasion
  Anaplasma, 893
  Chlamydia trachomatis, 884
  CMV, 1044
  Ehrlichia and *Anaplasma*, 893
  Haemophilus influenzae, 900
  Helicobacter, 916–917
  HHV-6, 1053
  Listeria monocytogenes, 763–764
  Neisseria gonorrhoeae, 742
  Staphylococcus epidermidis, 691
  Streptococcus pneumoniae, 722
  Streptococcus pyogenes, 698
  Treponema pallidum subsp. *pallidum*, 941
Immune globulin/immunoglobulin (human Ig), 38
  active immunization after, 77
  adenovirus infections, 1070

administration routes, 37t
adverse reactions, 42–43, 42b
  mechanism, 42–43
  transmission of viruses/prions, 43
available products, 38t
background to, 37
bronchiolitis management, 235
Cryptosporidium infections, 1270
diphtheria management, 757
future prospects, 44
hepatitis A prophylaxis, 38
hepatitis A virus infection management, 1184
hepatitis E virus infection prevention, 1193
indications, 37
interference with active immunization, 43
intramuscular administration, 37–39, 37t
  HBV, 38–39
  rabies, 39
  tetanus, 39
  VZV, 39
intravenous (IGIV) *see* Intravenous immune globulin (IGIV)
intravenous administration, 37, 37t
measles prophylaxis, 38
mumps virus, 1129
myocarditis treatment, 268
origin of use in passive immunization, 37
pneumonia in immunocompromised patients, 256
polyclonal, human metapneumovirus (hMPV) infections, 1136–1137
preparation method, 37–38, 1184
  to prevent prion transmission, 43
  to prevent virus transmission, 43
product shortages, 43
products, names and abbreviations, 38t
RSV prevention, 235
rubella prophylaxis, 38
rubeola virus (measles) prevention, 1144
specific types, 38–39
  for intravenous use, 41–42
VZV infection prevention, 1041–1042
  see also individual immune globulins (e.g. hepatitis B immune globulin)
Immune-mediated cytopenia, IGIV use, 41
Immune-modulating agents *see* Immunomodulation
Immune reconstitution, after antiretroviral therapy in HIV infection, 650
Immune reconstitution inflammatory syndrome (IRIS), 669
  ART effect in *Cryptococcus* infections, 1223
  in HIV infection, 650, 658, 662–663
  infections associated, 658
  Mycobacterium avium complex role, 791
  Mycobacterium tuberculosis, 774
Immune response, 83–90
  to active immunization *see* Immunization (active)
  adaptive, 87–90, 92, 93f
    effector cells, 87

innate response interaction, 95
see also Antibodies; B lymphocytes; T lymphocytes
cell-mediated *see* Cell-mediated immunity
chemotherapy effect, 569
developmental milestones, 89t
hemophagocytic lymphohistiocytosis, 104–105, 107
HHV-6 effects on, 1053
humoral *see* Humoral immune response
immediate, 92
immunity induced by vaccination, 45–46
to infections
see individual infections
innate *see* Innate immune response
interrelationships and future, 90
maternal, 544–545
pathogen interrelationships, 90
primary, 45
to vaccines, 45
see also Immune system
Immune serum globulin (ISG), enteroviral meningitis treatment, 296–297
Immune system, 83–90
abnormalities
chronic fatigue syndrome pathogenesis, 1008, 1010, 1010t, 1012
persistent/recurrent pneumonia, 249t, 251
recurrent meningitis associated, 288–289
see also Immunodeficiency
development, 83–90
defects, 609
milestones, 89t
invasive *Candida* infections and, 1201
see also Immune response
Immune thrombocytopenic purpura (ITP)
see Idiopathic thrombocytopenic purpura (ITP)
Immunization, 37–68
active *see* Immunization (active)(*below*)
in complement deficiency, 52t–53t, 619
definition, 44
passive *see* Passive immunization
post-transplant, 561
see also specific agents/pathogens
Immunization (active), 44–68
administration routes, effect on response, 46
adverse events *see* Vaccine(s), adverse events/reactions
after immune globulin, for travelers, 77
in asplenia, 74
audits, 54
benefits, 44, 47
morbidity reduction, 48t
boosters, rationale/mechanism, 609
contraindications, in immunodeficiencies, 52t–53t, 629
cost–benefits, 44
coverage (USA), 47, 48t
strategies for improving, 54
cystic fibrosis, 641
definition, 44

disease reduction by, 47, 48t
group childcare settings, diseases prevented, 29, 30t
schedule/doses, 30t
HCST recipients, 566, 566t
in HIV infection *see* Human immunodeficiency virus (HIV)/AIDS
immigrants, 52
immune globulin use interfering with, 43
immune response to, 45–46
determinants of, 46
host factors, 46
measurement (test types), 46
immunocompromised people, 52
in immunodeficiency (primary/secondary), 52, 52t–53t
infections in neutropenia in cancer, 572–573
information sources on vaccines, 68
international adoptees, 52
intradermal administration, 46
intramuscular administration, 46
in Kawasaki disease, 1006
mass, polio, 44
mucosal administration, 46
in pregnancy, 51–52
premature infants, 51
programs
issues relating to, 54–55
principles, 47–55
records, 52
refugee and internationally adopted children, 36–37, 37t, 52
responsibility for, 52
routine vaccines, 29, 48, 55–67
see also individual vaccines
schedules, 48, 49f
catch-up schedule, 49f
for travelers, 77–79, 78t–79t
sites of vaccine administration, 46
special situations, 51–52
standards/practice guidelines, 54
status evaluation, refugee and internationally adopted children, 36, 37t
travelers, 52, 76–77
advice/information source, 52, 77b
vaccine spacing, 48
see also individual vaccines
Immunoassays, group A streptococci, 1377
Immunoblot test *see* Western blot
Immunochromatographic assay, *Legionella pneumophila*, 924
Immunochromatographic capillary flow assay, *Trichomonas vaginalis*, 360
Immunocompromised hosts, 1069
adenovirus infections, 1068t, 1069–1070
animal bite infections, 523
Arcanobacterium haemolyticum infections, 751
Aspergillus infections, 1203
babesiosis, 1261, 1263, 1265
Bacillus infections, 750
bacterial infections in neutropenia, 567, 569t
Balantidium coli infections, 1267

Bartonella infections, 859
Blastomyces dermatitidis (blastomycosis), 1236, 1238, 1238t
chemoprophylaxis, 74–75
Coxiella burnetii causing, 892
Cryptococcus infections, 1220–1221
Cryptosporidium infections, 1270
Cyclospora infections, 1283–1284
diarrhea, 374
in AIDS, 386–387
encephalitis, 314
herpes zoster, 1039–1040
HHV-6 reactivation, 1057
HHV-7 infection, 1058
HHV-8 infection, 1067
Histoplasma capsulatum (histoplasmosis), 1224, 1226–1228, 1227t
treatment, 1229
HPV infection, 1072–1074
HSV infection, 1031, 1034
human metapneumovirus (hMPV) infections, 1136–1137
human parainfluenza virus infections, 1124
immunization in, 52
MMR contraindication, 60
inflammatory enteritis, 386–387, 386b
influenza virus infections, 1155–1156
Lactobacillus infections, 770
Legionella pneumonia, 923
nontuberculous mycobacterial infections, 790
Pneumocystis jirovecii (carinii), 1230
pneumonia *see* Pneumonia
Pseudallescheria boydii infections, 1253
Pseudomonas aeruginosa infection treatment, 845
Pseudomonas infections, 841
RSV infection, 1132–1133
rubeola virus (measles), 1143
Salmonella infection, 815
subcutaneous tissue infections, 460
Toxoplasma gondii infection *see Toxoplasma gondii*
travelers, 82–83
VZV infection, 1039–1040
see also Human immunodeficiency virus (HIV)/AIDS; Immunodeficiency; Neutropenia
Immunodeficiency, 600–609
antibody deficiency *see* Antibodies, deficiency
burn wound infections, 518, 518t
common variable *see* Common variable immunoglobulin deficiency (CVID)
drug-induced, 253–254
enteroviral infections, 1179
Giardia intestinalis (giardiasis), 1280
healthcare-associated infection risk, 10
HSCT recipients, 562
HSV infections, 1506t
immunization in, 52, 52t–53t
immunoglobulin deficiency *see* Immunoglobulin(s)
infections/pathogens, 600–609
inherited, generalized lymphadenopathy, 133b, 134
Listeria monocytogenes infections, 764

lymphocyte abnormalities *see* B
   lymphocytes; T lymphocytes
lymphoproliferative disorders associated,
   133b
mucosal, respiratory tract infections, 254
mucositis, 194
mumps vaccine not recommended, 1129
Mycoplasma pneumoniae infection, 994
"normal but unlucky child" *vs.*, 600,
   600b, 607
pathogens in, 569t
periodontitis, and gingivitis, 194
pneumonia *see* Pneumonia, in
   immunocompromised patients
primary, 600–601, 601b, 611f
   approach to patient, 609–610
   cell-mediated *see* Cell-mediated
      immunity
   characteristics, 601b
   chemoprophylaxis, 75
   classification, 609
   frequency, 600–601, 601t
   generalized lymphadenopathy, 133
   genetic testing, 608
   identification, 600–601
   immunizations, 52, 52t–53t
   immunoglobulins, disorders, 602t,
      610t
   indication for IGIV, 40, 40t
   innate immunity disorders,
      604t–605t
   intravenous IgG, 40
   recurrent infections *see* Recurrent
      infections
   screening tests, 608t
   specific testing, 607b, 608, 608t
   T lymphocyte disorders, 603t–604t
   vaccine-associated paralytic polio risk,
      50, 61
secondary
   generalized lymphadenopathy, 133
   immunizations, 52, 52t–53t
   indication for IGIV, 40, 40t
sentinel pathogens, 606t
sepsis in, 98
severe combined *see* Severe combined
   immunodeficiency (SCID)
Streptococcus pneumoniae infections, 722
structural abnormalities with,
   pneumonia due to, 254
subcutaneous tissue infections, 460
suspected, evaluation, 600–609
   abnormalities associated, 600, 600t
   conditions predisposing to, 600–601,
      601t
   "normal but unlucky child", 600,
      600b, 608
   pathogens, 606
   see also Recurrent infections
travelers, infection prevention, 82–83
varicella, 1039
VZV infections, 1036, 1039, 1506t
see also Immunoglobulin(s), deficiencies;
   *individual immunodeficiency syndromes
   (e.g. immunoglobulin A (IgA),
   deficiency)*
Immunodiffusion complement fixation
   (IDCF) test, *Coccidioides immitis*, 1243

Immunodiffusion precipitin test
   Blastomyces dermatitidis, 1237
   Coccidioides immitis, 1243
   Histoplasma capsulatum, 1227
Immunofluorescence staining/assays
   anaerobic infections, 963–964
   direct *see* Direct fluorescent antibody
      (DFA)
   HIV, 651–652
   human parainfluenza viruses, 1123–1124
   indirect *see* Indirect immunofluorescence
      antibody (IFA) assay
   mumps virus, 1128
   rabies, 1147
   VZV detection, 1040
Immunoglobulin(s)
   chronic fatigue syndrome, 1010t
   deficiencies, 610–611, 610t, 611f
      all isotypes, 610–611, 610t
      approach to patient, 609–610
      isotype deficiency, 612–613, 614t
      persistent/recurrent pneumonia, 251
      see also Antibodies, deficiency;
         Immunodeficiency; *specific
         immunoglobulins*
   heavy-chain deletion, 610t, 613
   products
      from animal plasma, 42
      from human plasma *see* Immune
         globulin/immunoglobulin
         (human Ig)
   structure, 609
   "switch recombination", 609, 612–613
Immunoglobulin A (IgA)
   antibodies to, 43
   in common variable immunoglobulin
      deficiency, 612
   deficiency, 610t, 614
      brain abscess and, 322
      characteristics, 602t, 614t
      IgG₂ deficiency with, 610t, 614, 614t
      recurrent acute parotitis, 195
      recurrent otitis media, 218–219
      urinary tract infection risk factor, 340
   elevated
      in HIDS, 125
      Wiskott–Aldrich syndrome, 633
   Entamoeba histolytica infection, 1275
   functions, in respiratory tract, 238, 254
   Giardia intestinalis (giardiasis), 1280
   infusion-related reactions to immune
      globulins, 43
   Kawasaki disease, 1003
   mucosal immunization inducing, 46
   Mycoplasma pneumoniae, 1399
   poliomyelitis virus infection, 1171
   RSV infections, 1132
   rubella virus, 1116
   secretory
      deficiency, 614
      deficiency, *Giardia intestinalis*
         (giardiasis), 1281
      enterovirus infections, 1173
      in fetus, 89
   Shigella infections, 815
   Toxoplasma gondii, 1312, 1314
Immunoglobulin A (IgA) 1 protease, 731
   Haemophilus influenzae, 900

Immunoglobulin D (IgD), elevated *see*
   Hyperimmunoglobulinemia D with
   periodic fever syndrome (HIDS)
Immunoglobulin E (IgE)
   elevated, in Wiskott–Aldrich syndrome,
      633
   human parainfluenza viruses, 1121
   Toxoplasma gondii, 1312
   urticaria pathogenesis, 445–446
Immunoglobulin G (IgG)
   autoantibodies, urticaria pathogenesis,
      445–446
   Borrelia burgdorferi, 955
   Chlamydia trachomatis, 1398
   CMV, 1049, 1392
   common variable immunoglobulin
      deficiency, 612
   in cord blood, 87
   deficiency
      brain abscess and, 322
      characteristics, 602t
      with IgA deficiency, 610t
      urinary tract infection risk factor, 340
      variable IgM levels, 612–613
   Entamoeba histolytica, 1275, 1277
   to filarial worms, 1342–1343
   formed after immunization, 46
   Giardia intestinalis (giardiasis), 1280
   hepatitis A virus (HAV), 1183, 1183f,
      1395
   hepatitis E virus (HEV), 1191, 1192f,
      1193, 1193t, 1395
   HHV-6, 1053, 1393–1394
   HHV-8, 1394
   HSV, 1033, 1388
   hyperimmune, burn wound infection
      prevention, 521
   IgG₂, phagocyte binding defect, *Neisseria
      meningitidis* infection, 732
   IgG₂ deficiency
      with IgA deficiency, 610t, 614, 614t
      recurrent meningitis and, 288
   IgG₃, deficiency, recurrent meningitis
      and, 288
   levels in infants and fetus, 87, 89, 89t
   maternal, 628
   maturational delay, 615
   measles, mumps and rubella, 1396
   mumps virus, 1126–1128
   Mycoplasma pneumoniae infections, 1399
   parvovirus B19, 1088, 1091, 1397
   placental transfer, 87
      role against group B streptococci, 87
   rubella virus infection, 1113, 1113f, 1116
   subclasses, 87
      deficiencies, characteristics, 602t, 610t,
         613–614
      functions, 613
      IgA deficiency with, 610t, 614–615,
         614t
      normal levels, 613
      quantifying, 609
   Toxoplasma gondii, 1312–1313
   transient hypogammaglobulinemia of
      infancy, 610t, 615, 615t
   Trypanosoma cruzi infections, 1325
   viral infection diagnosis, 1384–1385
      neonatal, 548

virus-specific, 1384–1385, 1387
VZV infection, 1040, 1393
Immunoglobulin M (IgM)
    AID and UNG deficiencies, 613
    alphaviruses, 1099
    arboviruses, 1397
    autoantibodies, *Mycoplasma pneumoniae*, 995
    Borrelia burgdorferi, 955
    Chlamydia trachomatis, 1398
    CMV, 1049, 1392
    Coccidioides immitis (coccidioidomycosis), 1243
    coltivirus (Colorado tick fever), 1093
    complement C1 activation, 615
    deficiency, characteristics, 602t
    development, 89
    E5, monoclonal antibody to endotoxin, 101t–102t
    EBV, 1393
    flavivirus infections, 1102
    formed after immunization, 46
    Giardia intestinalis (giardiasis), 1280
    hepatitis A virus (HAV), 1183, 1183f, 1395
    hepatitis B virus (HBV), 1078, 1081, 1082f, 1082t
    hepatitis E virus (HEV), 1191, 1192f, 1193, 1193t, 1395
    HHV-6, 1053, 1393–1394
    HSV, 1033, 1388
    Kawasaki disease, 1003
    Listeria monocytogenes opsonization, 764
    measles, mumps and rubella, 1396
    mumps virus, 1126–1128
    Mycoplasma pneumoniae infections, 995, 1399
    no placental transfer, 87
    nonspecific antibodies, 1411t–1412t
    parvovirus B19, 1088, 1091, 1397
    production, spleen role, 636–637
    response during viral infections, 1387f
    rubella virus, 1113, 1113f, 1116
    rubeola virus, 1141
    Toxoplasma gondii, 1312–1314
    Treponema pallidum subsp. *pallidum*, 945
    Trypanosoma (Trypanozoon) brucei infection, 1320, 1322
    viral infection diagnosis, 1384–1385
        neonatal, 548
    virus-specific, 1384–1385, 1387
        false-negatives/positives, 1387
    VZV infection, 1040, 1393
    in Wiskott–Aldrich syndrome, 633
Immunohistochemical diagnosis
    Rickettsia, 938
    Rickettsia prowazekii, 931
    Rickettsia rickettsii, 928
Immunologic memory, 87
Immunologic tolerance, 90
Immunomodulation, 40–41
    by IGIV, 40, 40t
    in myocarditis, 268
    see also Immune globulin/immunoglobulin (human Ig)
Immunoparalysis, in sepsis, 100
Immunosuppressed patients *see* Immunocompromised hosts

Immunosuppression
    in burns patients, infections after, 518, 518t
    hematopoietic stem cell transplantation, 562
    HHV-6 causing, 1053, 1055f
    HHV-7 causing, 1057–1058
    HLH treatment, 107
    in myocarditis, 268
    posttransplant lymphoproliferative disease (PTLD) after, 1063
    response to vaccines and, 46
    transplant recipients, infection risk factors, 556, 556b
Immunotherapy, adoptive, infections in HSCT recipients, 566
Impetigo, 427–429
    bullous, 428, 428f, 440, 678
    group childcare and, 25t, 29
    nonbullous, 428
    secondary infections in varicella, 1037
    Staphylococcus aureus, 428, 440, 678–679
    Streptococcus pyogenes (group A streptococcus), 428, 702
    treatment, 1418t–1419t, 1499
In situ hybridization, EBV detection, 1062
Inappropriate antidiuretic hormone secretion *see* Syndrome of inappropriate antidiuretic hormone secretion (SIADH)
Inborn errors of metabolism
    infectious encephalitis *vs.*, 302b
    viral infections in neonates *vs.*, 548
Incidence, 1–2
Incidence density, 1
Inclusion(s)
    eosinophilic, rabies-specific, 1145
    intranuclear, CMV, 1388
    "owl's eye", 1044
    viral, viral pneumonia, 238
Inclusion bodies, cytoplasmic
    cytomegalovirus (CMV), 1044
    human metapneumovirus (hMPV) infections, 1135
    Kawasaki disease, 1003
Inclusion conjunctivitis *see* Conjunctivitis, inclusion
Indinavir, 665t, 1444t–1452t
Indirect-cohort method, 7
Indirect hemagglutination antibody assay
    Burkholderia pseudomallei, 848
    Echinococcus granulosus, 1358
    Entamoeba histolytica, 1277
    Trypanosoma cruzi, 1325
Indirect immunofluorescence antibody (IFA) assay
    Anaplasma and *Ehrlichia* infections, 895–896
    Babesia (babesiosis), 1263–1265
    Coxiella burnetii, 892
    Cryptosporidium, 1270
    HIV, 1396
    Legionella, 924
    Rickettsia prowazekii, 931
    Rickettsia rickettsii, 928
    for specific viruses, 1386t
    Trypanosoma cruzi infections, 1325
Indium-111 scanning, osteomyelitis, 472

Indwelling vascular catheters *see* Intravascular catheters
Infant(s)
    airflow in lung, 233
    appendicitis, 172
    Bordetella pertussis infection, 865–866, 866f, 869
        treatment, 871
    botulism *see* *Clostridium botulinum*, infant botulism
    bronchiolitis, 231, 233
    cervical lymphadenopathy diagnosis, 143
    CNS infections, *Treponema pallidum*, 281
    complement component levels, 86
    enterovirus infections, 1173
    fever without localizing signs, 114–115, 114t
    HIV, classification of infection, 651t
    hypotonia, causes, 181t
    IgG and IgA levels, 87, 89, 89t
    immunization schedule, 49f
        DtaP, 55
        MMR, 59
        poliovirus vaccine, 61
        rotavirus vaccine, 66
    influenza vaccination, 1156
    Kawasaki disease course, 112f, 113
    mucopurulent rhinorrhea, 163
    myocarditis, 266
    osteomyelitis, 469
    passively-acquired antibodies, 87
    pneumonia, 168t, 169, 236–238, 236t
    progressive disseminated histoplasmosis, 1226, 1226f
    pulmonary tuberculosis, 775
    pyogenic arthritis, 184
    RSV bronchiolitis, 231, 233
    urinary tract infections, 340–341
    see also Neonate(s); Perinatal infections; Premature infants
Infant formulae, *Salmonella* infections and, 394
Infantile hypertrophic pyloric stenosis, after *Chlamydia trachomatis* infection treatment, 888
Infantile maxillary osteomyelitis, 196
Infantile periarteritis nodosa *see* Kawasaki disease (KD)
Infantile seborrheic eczema (ISE), *Malassezia*, 1217
Infection-associated hemophagocytic syndrome (IAHS), 134, 1064–1065
Infection prevention and control (IPC), 9–24, 37–44, 76–83
    active immunization *see* Immunization (active)
    bundled practices (best practices), 14–15
    chemoprophylaxis *see* Chemoprophylaxis
    Committee, 15
    definition, 10
    economic analysis, 8–9
    goals, 14
    group childcare centers, 31–32
    guidelines, 14–15
    healthcare-associated infections *see* Healthcare-associated infection (HAI)
    immune response *see* Immune response
    impact and economic analysis, 8–9

passive immunization *see* Passive immunization
program, 15
recommendations, resources for, 15
in refugee and internationally adopted children, 36–37
team, 15–16
Infection preventionists (IPs), 15–16
ratio (number to beds), 15–16
responsibilities, 15–16
Infection route, 83–84
Infectious mononucleosis
causes, non-EBV, 1061
CMV *see under* Cytomegalovirus (CMV)
diagnosis, 1393
EBV *see* Epstein–Barr virus (EBV)
X-linked lymphoproliferative disease, 633
see also Mononucleosis syndromes
Infectious mononucleosis-like syndrome, adenoviruses, 1068t, 1069
Infectious waste, definition, 21
Infective endocarditis *see* Endocarditis
Infertility, pelvic inflammatory disease complication, 366
Infestations, skin *see* Skin infections
Inflammasome, 45, 126
Inflammation-mediated syndromes, 97–103
see also Sepsis; Systemic inflammatory response syndrome (SIRS)
Inflammatory bowel disease
clinical features, 119t–120t
fever of unknown origin due to, 119, 119t–120t
Helicobacter associated, 916–917
oral mucosal features, 193t
recurrent abdominal pain due to, 175
Salmonella gastroenteritis in, 816
Inflammatory edema, sinusitis causing, 510
Inflammatory enteritis *see* Enteritis
Inflammatory mediators
anti-inflammatory mediators imbalance with, 98
infections after burns, 517
overproduction, 94–95
rhinovirus infection, 1186
see also Cytokines
Inflammatory response, 92–95
abnormal acute, 620
absent, phagocytic cell disorders, 621
in cutaneous leishmaniasis, 1288
endotoxin action, 100
in *Enterobius vermicularis* infections, 1332
in eumycotic mycetoma, 1251, 1251f
functions and role, 92
immediate and later stages, 92, 95
in Kawasaki disease, 1003
model, 92–93
neutrophils in, 1404
to peritoneum, 415
regulation, 92, 94–95
suppression *see* Immunosuppression
in *Toxocara* infections, 1335–1336
in *Trypanosoma (Trypanozoon) brucei* infection, 1320
in *Trypanosoma cruzi* infections, 1324
Infliximab, in TRAPS, 126
Influenza bacillus see Haemophilus influenzae

Influenza H5N1 *see* Avian influenza (H5N1 strain)
Influenza virus(es), 1149–1159, 1158b–1159b
acute otitis media due to, 1153, 1153t
anterior uveitis due to, 499t
antibodies, 1150–1152
antigenic changes, 64
antigenic shift/drift, 1150, 1158
antivirals, resistance, 1155
bronchiolitis due to, 231
burden of, and mortality, 13
chemoprophylaxis, 72, 1157
clinical manifestations, 1152–1153, 1153t
complications, 1153
croup syndrome *vs.*, 1153
culture, 1154
description and structure, 1149–1151, 1150f, 1158b–1159b
diagnosis/detection, 1153–1154, 1154t, 1158b–1159b, 1394
antigen detection, 1394
detection rates, 1386t
optimal tests, 1389t–1392t
PCR, 1394
sample collection and transport, 1394
tube culture, 1394
encephalitis associated, 303–304
epidemics, 1150–1151
seasonal, 1151
epidemiological pattern, 1131f
epidemiology, 197f, 1151–1152, 1158b–1159b
genetic reassortment, 1150, 1158
genome, 1150
glycoproteins, 1149
group childcare and, 25t, 28
H1N1, 64, 1149–1151, 1155
2009 pandemic, 1150–1153, 1150f, 1155
pandemic, group childcare center closure, 28
Spanish flu pandemic, 1151
transmission route, 12–13
travelers and, 82
H2N2, 1150–1151
Asian flu pandemic, 1150–1151
H3N2, 64, 1150–1152, 1155
Hong Kong flu pandemic, 1150–1151
H5N1 *see* Avian influenza (H5N1 strain)
healthcare-associated, 582
in HIV infection, 1156
immunity, 1151
immunocompromised hosts, 1155–1156
impact on children, 1151–1152, 1152t
infant infections, 1152
infection rates, young children in childcare, 28
influenza A *see* Influenza virus(es), type A
influenza B *see* Influenza virus(es), type B
laboratory findings, 1153
laboratory testing, 308t–311t
laryngotracheitis (croup) due to, 211–212
lips in, 111
mortality and morbidity due to, 1151–1152, 1155–1156

muscle pain due to, 186
natural hosts, 1150
nomenclature, 1150, 1150b
pandemics, 64, 1150–1151, 1158
2009 influenza A (H1N1) pandemic, 1150–1153, 1150f, 1155
H2N2 Asian flu pandemic, 1150–1151
H3N2 Hong Kong flu pandemic, 1150–1151
preparedness, 1158
pathogenesis, 1151
pneumonia due to, 236–237, 1153, 1153t
postexposure prophylaxis, 1157
pregnant healthcare workers, 22t–23t
in pregnancy, 1156
prevalence, 64
prevention of infection, 1156–1157, 1517
rashes, 112
shedding, 1151
transmission, 12, 1151
group childcare and, 28
interspecies, 1157–1158
prevention, visitation policies, 19
in transplant recipients, 559–560
treatment of infections, 241t, 1154–1155, 1158b–1159b
antiviral agents, 1517
in pneumonia, 241
type A, 1149
acute otitis media, 214
birds as reservoir, 1150, 1158
chemoprophylaxis, 70t–71t, 72
H1N1 *see Above*
H3N2 *see Above*
H5N1 *see* Avian influenza (H5N1 strain)
prevention, 1156–1157
prophylaxis/treatment, 1507t, 1514
treatment, 1154–1155
type B, 1149
chemoprophylaxis, 72
treatment of infections, 1154–1155
type C, 1149
vaccination, 64–65
asthma exacerbation prevention, 1156–1157
CDC recommendations, 1156
childcare settings, 28, 30t, 1156
of close contact of young children, 1156
contraindication/precautions, 64–65, 1156
coverage of healthcare personnel, 21
cystic fibrosis families, 641
efficacy and otitis media prevention, 28, 1156
healthcare personnel, 21–24
HSCT recipients, 566
in pregnancy, 22–24, 51–52, 1157
recommendations for, 64, 1156
schedule, 49f
in sickle-cell disease, 636
universal, in childhood, 1156
vaccines, 64–65, 1156
efficacy, 64, 1156–1157
high-risk children and, 64
in HIV infection, 663

intranasal, 28
live-attenuated (LAIV), 64–65, 1157
schedule, 64
shortage, 54
for travelers, 78
trivalent inactivated (TIV), 64,
1156–1157
zoonotic influenza, 1157–1158
see also Avian influenza (H5N1 strain)
Infusion-related reactions, to immune
globulin intravenous (IGIV), 42–43,
42b
Inguinal lymph nodes
enlarged, visceral leishmaniasis, 1287
palpable in normal children, 158
see also Lymphadenitis/
lymphadenopathy, inguinal
Inhalation injuries, 519
Inhibitory mold agar (IMA), 1382
Injection practices
safe, 18t
unsafe
HBV transmission, 1078
HCV transmission, 1105–1107
Injuries *see* Trauma
Innate immune response, 45, 83–87, 92,
93f, 102–103
activation, in sepsis, 98
adaptive response interaction, 95
antimicrobial peptides, 83–84
antimicrobial products, 83–84
cells and functions, 85f
chemotaxis, 85
complement activation, 86, 615–617
deficiency
infection rates associated, 10
pneumonia, 253
dendritic cells, 85–86
detrimental effects, 98
disorders, 604t–605t
induction, Toll-like receptor role,
102–103
natural killer cells, 86–87
pathogen receptors, 84
phagocytes role, 85
receptors, 92–94
skin and mucosal barriers, 83–84
Toll-like receptors, 84, 102–103
VZV infection, 1036
*see also individual components (e.g. natural
killer cells)*
Inner-ear malformation, recurrent
meningitis, 287–289, 292
Inocybe, 397t
Inoue–Melnick virus, chronic fatigue
syndrome pathogenesis, 1008t–1009t
InPouch culture system, 354–355, 360
InPouch TV culture system, 1318–1319
Insect bites, protection against, 81
Insect repellents, 81
Borrelia burgdorferi infection prevention,
956
Insecticides, 81
Trypanosoma brucei infection prevention,
1322
Trypanosoma cruzi infection prevention,
1326
Insomnia, fatal syndromes, 338

Institute for Child Health and Human
Development (NICHD) Neonatal
Research Network, 538–539
Institute of Medicine (IOM)
immunization safety review, 50–51,
51b
vaccine adverse events and, 50–51, 50t
Integrase inhibitors, 665t, 666
Integrins, 85
Integrons, acquired drug resistance, 1423
Intensive care units (ICUs)
Candida infections, 1196, 1201–1202
central line associated bloodstream
infections, 10–12
by ICU type, 11t
infection rates, 10
ventilator-associated pneumonia
management, 583
see also Neonatal intensive care units
(NICUs)
Intent-to-treat analysis, 9
Interferon(s), 1515–1516
adverse effects, 1515–1516
chemistry, 1515
clinical uses, 1516
dosage, 1516
drug interactions, 1515–1516
mechanism of action, 1515
pegylated, 1515–1516
chronic HCV infection, 1111
HBV infection treatment, 1083
pharmacokinetics, 1515
production, by human parainfluenza
viruses, 1121
resistance, 1515
spectrum of activity, 1515
West Nile virus infection, 1101
yellow fever treatment, 1099
Interferon-α, 1515–1516
chronic HCV infection, 1111
adverse effects, 1111
human coronavirus infection prevention,
1120
influenza A virus infection, 1151
myocarditis treatment, 268
rhinovirus infections, 1187
VZV infection, 1036
Interferon alfa-2a, 1516
HBV infection treatment, 1083
HDV infection treatment, 1087
Interferon-β, 1515–1516
innate immune system, 84
myocarditis treatment, 268
Interferon-γ, 1515–1516
burn wound infection prevention, 521
Coccidioides immitis infection treatment,
1245
elevated in hemophagocytic
lymphohistiocytosis, 106
in immune response to vaccines, 45
infections in phagocyte disorders, 624
production by Th1 cells, 89–90, 92
receptor, 632
receptor deficiency, 604t–605t, 630t,
632
diagnosis, 632
partial, 632
RSV infection, 1133

release
hemophagocytic lymphohistiocytosis,
105
tuberculosis diagnosis, 780
Interferon-γ release assay (IGRA), 660–661
in HIV infection, 660–661
Mycobacterium tuberculosis, 34
tuberculous pneumonia diagnosis, 240
Interim analyses, 6
Interleukin(s)
chronic fatigue syndrome, 1010t
in immune response to vaccines, 45
infections after burns, 517
Interleukin-1 (IL-1), 94–95
inflammatory response, 94
neutralization by IL-1ra, 100
proinflammatory cytokine, 100
pyrogenic cytokine, 92
recombinant (IL-1ra), 100, 101t–102t
in sepsis, 100
Interleukin-1 (IL-1) receptor, inhibitor *see*
Anakinra
Interleukin-1 (IL-1) receptor-associated
kinase (IRAK), 84
Interleukin-2 (IL-2), receptor, deficiency,
603t–604t
Interleukin-4 (IL-4)
anti-inflammatory cytokine, 94–95
Th2 differentiation, 92
Interleukin-5 (IL-5), eosinophil production,
1407
Interleukin-6 (IL-6)
Afelimomab effect, 101t–102t
elevated in hemophagocytic
lymphohistiocytosis, 106
inflammatory response, 94
influenza A virus infection, 1151
neonatal septicemia diagnosis, 541t,
542
pyrogenic cytokine, 92
Interleukin-7 (IL-7)
receptor, 627, 628t, 632
in SCID, 628t
Interleukin-8 (IL-8)
chemoattractant for neutrophils,
197–198
influenza A virus infection, 1151
neonatal septicemia diagnosis, 541t
Interleukin-10 (IL-10)
anti-inflammatory cytokine, 94–95, 100
elevated in hemophagocytic
lymphohistiocytosis, 106
functions, 100
Interleukin-12 (IL-12)
deficiency, 604t–605t, 630t, 632
receptor deficiency, 604t–605t, 630t, 632
in sepsis, 100
structure and function, 632
Th1 cell differentiation, 92
Interleukin-13 (IL-13), 83
Interleukin-15 (IL-15), 86–87
Interleukin-23 (IL-23), 627
Interleukin-27 (IL-27), 627
Internal jugular vein, anaerobic
thrombophlebitis, 194–195, 208
see also Lemierre disease
Internalin, *Listeria monocytogenes* virulence
factor, 763–764

International Committee on Taxonomy of
    Viruses (ICTV), 1015
International Travel and Health, 77b
Internationally adopted children *see* Refugee
    and internationally adopted children
Interpretation of studies, 9
Interquartile range, 5
Intervertebral disk
    composition, 484
    inflammation *see* Diskitis
Intervertebral disk spaces
    aspiration and culture, 484–485
    blood supply, 483–484
Intestinal amebiasis *see* Amebic colitis
    (intestinal amebiasis)
Intestinal biopsy, inflammatory enteritis,
    386
Intestinal flukes, 1256
Intestinal nematodes *see* Nematodes
    (roundworms)
Intestinal obstruction
    Ascaris lumbricoides, 1327–1328, 1328f
    Diphyllobothrium infection, 1347
    vomiting and abdominal pain, 171
Intestinal pathogens, refugee and
    internationally adopted children,
    35–36, 35t
Intestinal perforation
    necrotizing enterocolitis, 388, 390
    neonatal (nosocomial), 550
    Salmonella Typhi infection, 818
Intestinal schistosomiasis, 1368–1369
Intestinal stricture, *Entamoeba histolytica*
    infection, 1276
Intestinal transplantation, infections after,
    557–558
Intestinal trematodes, 1363–1364
Intimin, 796
Intra-abdominal abscess, 423–424
    anaerobic infections, 962
    clinical manifestations, 423–424
    Enterococcus, 714
    etiology, 423–424, 423t, 962
    management, 424
    pathogenesis, 423
    percutaneous drainage, 424, 425f
    perforated appendix leading to, 422
    postoperative, 424f
    viridans group streptococci, 718
Intra-abdominal infections
    anaerobic gram-positive cocci causing,
        989
    burns patients, 519
    in cancer, 578
    see also individual infections
Intracellular adhesion molecules (ICAMs),
    85
Intracellular pathogens
    Coxiella burnetii, 891
    Francisella tularensis, 897
    Legionella, 922
    Leishmania, 1285
    Rhodococcus equi, 768
    Rickettsia rickettsii, 926
    see also Macrophage
Intracellular signaling, Toll-like receptors, 94
Intracerebral calcification, congenital
    toxoplasmosis, 1312, 1314

Intracranial abscess, acute sinusitis
    complication, 230
Intracranial calcifications, LCMV infection,
    1162f
Intracranial disease, headache, 171, 177
Intracranial pressure, increased, 172
    ataxia in, 180
    CNS cryptococcosis, 1222–1223
    management, in acute bacterial
        meningitis, 278
    meningococcal disease, 737
    Naegleria fowleri infection, 1294
    Taenia solium neurocysticercosis, 1354,
        1356
Intracranial septic thrombosis *see* Septic
    thrombophlebitis, intracranial
Intragenic recombination, drug resistance,
    1423
Intralipid, neonatal septicemia due to
    Staphylococcus epidermidis, 692
Intramedullary tumors, back pain due to,
    188
Intranuclear inclusions, CMV, 1388
Intrapartum antibiotic prophylaxis (IAP),
    542, 544
    Streptococcus agalactiae (group B
        streptococcus) infections, 710, 711t,
        712f
Intrapulmonary lymph nodes, 148–149
Intrarenal abscess, 343–344
Intrasinal pressure (paranasal sinuses), 227
Intrauterine contraceptive device
    Actinomyces infections associated,
        990–991
    pelvic inflammatory disease and, 353
Intrauterine infections, *Ureaplasma
    urealyticum*, 1000–1001
Intravascular catheters
    antibiotic-impregnated, 588–589, 594,
        694
    antibiotic prophylaxis, 588–589, 594
    bloodstream infections, 590
    care of, infection prevention, 593–594
    CVC *see* Central venous catheter
        (CVC)-related infections
    dressings for, 594
    exit site infections, 590, 591t
        management, 592
    indwelling, *Staphylococcus aureus*
        infections, 684
    infections, 589–594
        Candida, 589–590, 593
        catheter-related risk factors, 588–590,
            588b
        clinical features and diagnosis,
            590–592, 591t
        coagulase-negative staphylococci, 589,
            592, 691–692, 694
        complications, 593
        cultures for diagnosis, 590–591
        duration of placement, 590
        epidemiology, 589
        fungi, 589, 591
        gram-negative bacilli, 589, 593
        host risk factors, 590
        management and outcome, 592–593,
            592t
        mortality, 593

nontuberculous mycobacteria, 593
        pathogenesis, 589
        pathogens, 588b, 589
        prevention, 593–594, 594b
        relapse, 592–593
        risk factors, 590b
        routes of infection, 589–590, 589b
        Staphylococcus aureus, 589, 592–593
        types, 590, 591t
    infusates, infection risk factor, 590
    needleless connection systems, 594
    outpatient management, 594
    peripheral *see* Peripheral intravascular
        catheters
    placement
        duration, infection risk, 590
        site, infection risk factor, 589
    pocket infections, 590, 591t, 592
    removal, 592–593
    subcutaneously implanted, 594
    tunnel infections, 589, 591t
    see also Catheter-related bloodstream
        infections; Central line associated
        bloodstream infections (CLABSIs)
Intravascular infections, "endocarditis-like",
    265
Intravenous fluids, contamination, infection
    risk, 590
Intravenous immune globulin (IGIV),
    37–41, 295–296
    administration, 37, 37t
    adverse reactions, 37, 42–43, 42b
    anti-inflammatory actions/mechanisms,
        40
    future prospects, 44
    high-dose use, 42–43
    immunomodulation by, 40–41, 40t
    indications, 40–41, 40t
        acute disseminated encephalomyelitis,
            317
        antibody deficiencies, 40, 40t,
            609–610
        burns infections prevention, 521
        Clostridium tetani infections, 968–969,
            969t
        enteroviral meningitis, 296–297
        enterovirus infections, 1173, 1177,
            1179–1180
        group A streptococcal infections,
            702
        Guillain–Barré syndrome, 314
        in HIV infection, 663
        HSCT recipients, 566
        hyper-IgM syndrome, 613, 631–632
        immune deficiencies, 40, 40t,
            609–610
        infection prevention in HIV infection,
            663
        Kawasaki disease, 40t, 41, 114, 1002,
            1005–1006
        necrotizing fasciitis, 468t
        NEMO immunodeficiency, 633
        neonatal septicemia, 544
        nosocomial neonatal infection
            prevention, 552–553
        parvovirus B19 infection, 1091
        in SCID, 629
        sepsis, 100

Streptococcus pneumoniae infections, 725
toxic shock syndrome, 468, 685
X-linked agammaglobulinemia, 611
interference with active immunization, 43
lot-to-lot consistency, 39–40
minimum number of antibodies, 39–40
off-label use, 41, 44
pertussis (PIG-IGIV), 872
physiologic properties, 39–40
preparation, 39, 43
product shortages, 43
specific immune globulins, 41–42
transmission of viruses/prions by, 43
see also Immune globulin/
immunoglobulin (human Ig)
Intraventricular shunts, in cancer, infections, 579
Intravitreal injection, 505t, 506
Intussusception
acute abdominal pain, 174
altered mental status in, 179
patient position and abdominal pain, 172
rotavirus infection causing, 1095
rotavirus vaccine association, 66, 1096–1097
Involucrum, 469
Iodamoeba butschlii, 1271, 1272f, 1279
Iodoquinol, protozoan infection treatment, 1519
Entamoeba histolytica (amebiasis), 1277, 1519
IPEX syndrome, 603t–604t
IRAK-4 deficiency, 604t–605t
pneumonia, 253
Iritis, after *Neisseria meningitidis* infections, 738
Iron
acquisition, *Staphylococcus aureus* cell wall, 676
in acute-phase response, 94
decreased serum levels, 94, 1403
overload
infections associated, 637–638
Yersinia enterocolitica infections in, 824
Yersinia pseudotuberculosis infections in, 825
requirement for bacterial growth, 637
scavenging, *Listeria monocytogenes*, 763–764
supplementation, hookworm infections, 1330
Iron deficiency anemia, 1403
Helicobacter pylori, 912–913
hookworm infections, 1329, 1403
Iron-dextran, 637–638
Irritable bowel-like syndrome, *Strongyloides* causing, 1333
Irritable bowel syndrome (IBS)
amebic colitis *vs.*, 1275
Campylobacter jejuni infection, 877
Ischemic limb, after *Neisseria meningitidis* infection, 738

Isolation precautions, 17–18
categories based on transmission routes, 18, 19t
Corynebacterium diphtheriae infections, 757
guidelines, 17
rubella virus infection, 1117
rubeola virus infection (measles), 1144
standard precautions *see* Standard precautions
transmission-based precautions, 18, 19t–20t
Isoniazid, 781, 1426
distribution, 1416–1417
dosage, 780t, 1445t–1452t
hepatotoxicity, 781, 785
mechanism of action, 1426
resistance to, 1422t, 1426
detection, 1430, 1432
tuberculosis prophylaxis, 71
tuberculosis treatment, 780t, 781, 783
breastfeeding and in pregnancy, 784
infants in contagious household, 784
latent infection, 782–783
resistance mechanisms, 785
Isospora belli see Cystoisospora belli
Isosporiasis *see Cystoisospora* (cystisosporiasis)
Itk deficiency, characteristics, 603t–604t
Itraconazole, 1489–1490
adverse effects, 1489
breakpoint for, 1443t
clinical uses, 1489–1490
dosage, 1445t–1452t, 1487t, 1489
pharmacokinetic-pharmacodynamic relationships, 1443t
pharmacology, 1489
spectrum of activity, 1486t
treatment of
Blastomyces dermatitidis (blastomycosis), 1237, 1238t
Coccidioides immitis (coccidioidomycosis), 1243–1244
Cryptococcus infections, 1222–1223
Histoplasma capsulatum (histoplasmosis), 1228t, 1229
hyalohyphomycosis, 1210–1211
infections in phagocyte disorders, 624
lymphocutaneous sporotrichosis, 162
Malassezia infections, 1217–1218
phaeohyphomycosis, 1212
Sporothrix schenckii (sporotrichosis), 1220
tinea capitis, 1247
trial data, 1489–1490
Ivemark syndrome, 636
Ivermectin
adverse effects, 1524
treatment of
cutaneous larva migrans, 1339
Loa loa infections, 1346
nematode infections, 1524
Onchocerca volvulus infection, 1345
pediculosis, 1259
scabies, 1260–1261
Strongyloides infections, 1334
Trichuris trichiura infections, 1331
Wuchereria bancrofti infections, 1344

Ixodes, diseases transmitted by, 894
Babesia (babesiosis) transmission, 1261–1263
Borrelia burgdorferi infection transmission, 952–953, 957

J

JAK-3 kinase, 627
deficiency, 628t
Janeway lesions, 259
Janus kinase-3 *see* JAK-3 kinase
Japan, Kawasaki disease, 1002–1003
Japanese encephalitis virus (JEV), 67, 1100–1101
aseptic meningitis due to, 294
clinical features and treatment, 1100–1101
encephalitis, 303
epidemiology, 80
prevention, 1102
transmission, 80, 1100
vaccine, 67, 80, 1101
indications, 67
JE-VAX and JE-VC types, 67, 80
schedule/dosing for travelers, 79t, 80
for travelers, 80
Jarisch–Herxheimer reaction
Borrelia infections, 955, 958
Leptospira infections, 951
symptoms and treatment, 955
Treponema pallidum subsp. *pallidum* infections, 947
Jaundice
Cryptosporidium infections, 1270
hepatitis A virus and, 1182–1183
in pancreatitis, 173
viral hepatitis and, 349
Jaw
Actinomyces infections, 991
osteomyelitis, 196
JC polyomavirus, laboratory testing, 308t–311t
JC virus (JCV), 1075–1077
chronic fatigue syndrome pathogenesis, 1008t–1009t
encephalitis, 314
in HIV infection, 661
progressive multifocal leukoencephalopathy, 631–632, 661, 662f, 1076–1077
transmission, 1075
Job syndrome *see* Hyper-IgE/recurrent infection syndrome
Jock itch (tinea cruris), 1248–1249
Joint
disease, limb pain, 184–186, 185t
hypermobility, chronic fatigue syndrome pathogenesis, 1008
infections
Candida, 1199–1200
Mycobacterium tuberculosis, 778, 784
neonatal, 541, 541t
sickle-cell disease, 635, 635f
see also Arthritis; Diskitis; Osteoarticular infections; Transient synovitis

pain
  diseases with, 184–186, 185t
  pyogenic arthritis, 477
  see also Arthralgia
prosthetic, infections, 598–599
Jones criteria, acute rheumatic fever (ARF), 703–704, 703b
Jugulo-omohyoid lymph nodes, 137
Junin virus (Argentine hemorrhagic fever), 1159, 1160t
Juvenile dermatomyositis, 464
  chronic myositis, 464
  etiology, 464–465
Juvenile idiopathic arthritis (JIA), 184–185
  arthritis in acute rheumatic fever *vs.*, 704, 704t
  fever of unknown origin, 119t–120t
  generalized lymphadenopathy, 134
  granulomatous hepatitis and, 409
  limb pain, 184–185, 185t
  macrophage activation syndrome association, 107
  oligoarthritis/polyarthritis, 184–185
  systemic, 184–185
  uveitis, 110–111
Juvenile recurrent respiratory papillomatosis, HPV causing, 1072–1073

K

K1 antigen, *Escherichia coli*, 797, 799
Kala-azar *see Leishmania*, visceral; *Leishmania* (leishmaniasis), visceral
Kanamycin, 1474
  dosage, 1480t–1483t
  eye infection treatment, 1496t
  pharmacology, 1453t–1458t
  tuberculosis treatment, 782
Kangaroo care (co-bedding), infection risk associated, 12
Kaplan criteria, 381
Kaplan–Meier survival curves, 3, 4f
Kaposi sarcoma
  HHV-8 causing *see* Human herpesvirus 8 (HHV-8)
  in HIV infection, 655, 672
K light-chain deficiency, 610t, 613
Kartagener syndrome, 638
Kartagener triad, 247–248
Kasai procedure, 412–413
Katayama fever, 131t–132t, 132, 1369
  see also Schistosoma (schistosomiasis)
Kato preparation, *Schistosoma* infections, 1369–1370
Kawasaki disease (KD), 1002–1007
  acute-phase proteins, 113, 1005, 1005t
  cardinal feature, 113, 1003
  Chlamydophila (Chlamydia) pneumoniae and, 882
  clinical features, 109t–110t, 113, 1003–1005, 1003b, 1004f, 1005t, 1007b
    anterior uveitis, 499, 499t
    chest pain, 189
    conjunctival, 1003, 1004f, 1005–1006
    desquamation, 112–113, 1003, 1004f
    exanthem, 111–113, 1004f

extremity changes, 112, 112f, 1003, 1004f
generalized lymphadenopathy, 141–142
hair and nail changes, 112–113, 1003, 1004f
hypotension, 108
lips in, 111
musculoskeletal pain, 183
ocular features, 108–111, 113, 1003, 1004f, 1005–1006
oral mucosal, 193t
oropharynx, 111
prodrome and fever, 108, 113, 1003
rash and lesions, 112, 1003, 1004f
uveitis, 110–111
coronary artery abnormalities, 1003, 1004f, 1005t, 1006
corticosteroid contraindication, 113, 1006
cytoplasmic inclusion bodies, 1003
diagnosis, 109t–110t, 113–114, 1003b, 1005–1006, 1007b
  group A streptococcal disease *vs.*, 1005
  measles *vs.*, 1005
epidemiology, 1002–1003
ESR elevation, 1003, 1005, 1401
ethnic factors, 1002
etiology, 1002–1003
fever of unknown origin due to, 119, 119t–120t
historical background, 1002
immune response, 1003
incomplete, 1003–1005
laboratory features, 109t–110t, 1005–1006, 1005t
meningitis, 295
pathology, 1003
progression in infants, 112f, 113, 1006
refractory, 1003
thrombocytosis, 113, 1005, 1409–1410
treatment, 109t–110t, 114, 1002, 1006
  aspirin, 41, 1006
  corticosteroids, 1006
  IGIV, 1006
  IGIV indications, 40t, 41, 43, 114
Yersinia pseudotuberculosis infection relationship, 825
Kawasaki disease-like disease, adenovirus infections, 1069
Kayser-Fleischer ring, 407
Kerandel sign, 1320
Keratinocytes, 438
Keratitis, infective, 494–498
  Acanthamoeba see Acanthamoeba
  Aspergillus, 496–497
  bacterial, 496–498
  Candida albicans, 496–497
  causes, 495–497
  chronic staphylococcal, 493–494
  clinical features, 495
  complications, 498
  dendritic, 496f
  diagnosis, 497
  disciform, 496f
  etiological agents, 495–497, 1493

fungal, 496–498
Fusarium, 496–497
Haemophilus influenzae, 496
herpes zoster, 1039f
herpetic, 495, 495f
HSV infection, 489, 495
interstitial, 497
marginal, 497
Moraxella catarrhalis, 496
pathogenesis, 494–495
Pseudomonas aeruginosa, 496
risk factors, 495b
trauma causing, 495
treatment, 497–498, 1493–1495, 1495t
ulcerative, 496
viral, 495–497
Keratoconjunctivitis
  epidemic *see* Epidemic keratoconjunctivitis
  HSV infection, 489, 495, 1029, 1034
Keratolysis, pitted, 430
Kerion, 1246, 1246f
Kernicterus, displacement of bilirubin by antibiotics, 1439, 1439t
Kernig sign, 274, 295, 734–735, 1175
Ketoconazole
  Blastomyces dermatitidis (blastomycosis), 1237–1238
  Coccidioides immitis (coccidioidomycosis), 1243–1244
  eumycotic mycetoma, 1252
  Malassezia infections, 1217
  Sporothrix schenckii (sporotrichosis), 1219–1220
  superficial infection treatment, 1485, 1485t
Ketoconazole shampoo, *Malassezia* infections, 1217
Ketolides
  dosage, 1480t–1483t
  pharmacology, 1453t–1458t
  spectrum of activity, 1459t–1463t
KI polyomavirus, 1075, 1077
Kidney
  acute inflammatory changes, 345
  focal infections, sites, 343f
  see also Entries beginning renal
Kikuchi disease (Kikuchi–Fujimoto disease) *see* Histiocytic necrotizing lymphadenitis (Kikuchi disease)
Kimura disease, cervical lymphadenopathy, 142, 142t
KINDLIN3 gene, 626
Kinetoplast, *Leishmania*, 1286f
Kinetoplastida, treatment of infections, 1519–1520
Kingella, 919–921
Kingella denitrificans, 919
Kingella kingae
  bacteremia and septicemia, 921
  carriage, 919–920, 920f
  child-to-child transmission, 27
  clinical manifestations, 920–921, 922b
  culture detection, 921
  diagnosis, 921, 922b
  diskitis due to, 187, 483
  endocarditis due to, 257, 920–921

epidemiology and transmission, 919–920, 920f, 922b
group childcare and, 25t, 27
immunity to, 919
invasive infections, 920, 920f
lower respiratory tract infections, 921
meningitis, 921
microbiology, 919, 919f, 922b
nucleic acid amplification, 921
ocular infections, 921
osteoarticular infections, 920–921
osteomyelitis due to, 27, 469, 920
pathogenesis and virulence, 919
prognosis, 922b
pyogenic arthritis due to, 477
soft-tissue infections, 921
treatment of infections, 472, 921, 922b
Kingella oralis, 919
Kingella potus, 919
Kinins, nasal secretions, in colds, 197–198
Kirby–Bauer test, 1378
Klebsiella, 799–802
AmpC β-lactamases, 802
appendicitis and, 420
clinical manifestations, 800
extended-spectrum β-lactamases (ESBLs), 800–801
folliculitis due to, 431
infections in HSCT recipient, 563
in iron overload state, 637–638
meningitis due to, 277
microbiology and epidemiology, 799–800
mortality due to, 800
neonatal infections, 800
orchitis due to, 369
prostatitis due to, 369
screening tests, 801
treatment of infections, 800–802
urinary tract infections, 800
virulence factors, 800
Klebsiella (Calymmatobacterium) granulomatis (donovanosis), 799, 802–803
chemoprophylaxis, 70t–71t
clinical features, 803, 803f
differential diagnosis, 803
epidemiology, 348, 350, 802
genital ulcers, 348
genital ulcers with lymphadenopathy, 348–350, 350t
in HIV infection, 803
laboratory diagnosis, 351t, 803
in pregnancy, treatment, 803
transmission, 802
treatment and prevention, 803
Klebsiella oxytoca, 799
antibiotic susceptibility, 800–801
screening tests for, 801
Klebsiella pneumoniae
antibiotic susceptibility, 800–801
antimicrobial resistance, 13–14
aminoglycosides, 1424
cephalosporins, 14t
healthcare-associated infections, 14t
carrier rates, 800
endophthalmitis due to, 503–504
polysaccharide vaccines, 802
subspecies, 799

Klebsiella pneumoniae subsp. *pneumoniae*, 800
Klippel–Feil syndrome, recurrent meningitis, 289
Kluyvera, 809
Knee
pain
causes, 186
osteomyelitis, 183f
structural abnormalities causing, 185
pyogenic arthritis, 477–478
Koch–Weeks bacillus *see Haemophilus influenzae* biogroup *aegyptius*
Koebner phenomenon, 453
Koplik spots, 1140
Koserella trabulsii (Yokenella regensburgei), 810
Kostmann disease, 604t–605t
KPC enzymes, in drug resistance, 1424
Kurthia, 771
Kurthia bessonii, 771
Kuru
clinical features, 334
etiology, 334
pathogenesis, 334
Kussmaul breathing, 172
Kussmaul sign, 270
Kyasanur Forest disease virus, 1102

L

L-selectin, 85
La Crosse virus (LACV), 1103, 1103t
aseptic meningitis due to, 294
encephalitis due to, 303, 313, 1103–1104, 1104t
Laboratory diagnosis, 1373–1399
bacterial infections, 1373–1381
antibiotic susceptibility *see* Susceptibility testing
antigen detection assays, 1381
see also Antigen detection tests
blood/blood cultures *see* Blood cultures
CSF specimens, 1376–1377
peritoneal fluid specimens, 1377–1378
respiratory tract specimens, 1377
specific pathogens, 1378
specimen collection and processing, 1373
specimen-specific isolation methods, 1373–1378
synovial fluid specimens, 1377–1378
transport media, 1373, 1373t
urine cultures, 1376
Chlamydia trachomatis, 1398–1399
Chlamydophila species, 1398–1399
fungi, 1381–1382
antigen detection, 1382
culture, 1382
specimen collection/processing, 1381–1382
susceptibility testing, 1382
gastro-duodenal pathogens, 1383
genital ulcer with lymphadenopathy syndrome, 351, 351t
parasites, 1382–1384
rickettsiae, 1384
urethritis, 354–355

viruses, 1384–1398
antigen detection *see* Antigen detection tests
choice of method, 1387
congenital/perinatal infections, 1389t–1392t, 1397–1398
cross-reactions, 1387
culture, 1385–1387, 1386t
cytological, 1384–1385
detection methods, 1385–1388, 1386t
electron microscopy, 1386
isolation of viruses, 1385–1386
not cultivatable types, 1385, 1387
nucleic acid detection, 1386–1387, 1386t
optimal tests for specific viruses, 1388–1398, 1389t–1392t
sample sites, 1385
serologic approach, 1384–1385, 1386t, 1387–1388, 1387f
specimen collection/transport, 1385
specimen storage/temperatures, 1385
timing of specimen collection, 1385
virologic approach, 1384–1388
see also Cell culture; Shell vial method
see also individual pathogens/diseases, and tests
Laboratory manifestations of infections, 1400–1411
acute-phase response *see* Acute-phase response
C-reactive protein *see* C-reactive protein (CRP)
ESR *see* Erythrocyte sedimentation rate (ESR)
ferritin, 1403
hemoglobin, 1403–1404
see also Anemia
leukocytes, 1404–1409
see also individual cell types
metabolic abnormalities, 1411
nonspecific antibodies, 1411, 1411t–1412t
procalcitonin *see* Procalcitonin (PCT)
Labyrinthitis, acute otitis media complication, 220
Lacerations, animal bites, 523
Lacrimal sac
compression (digital), 493
infections (dacryocystitis), 508–509, 509f
LaCrosse virus (LACV) *see* La Crosse virus (LACV)
β-Lactam antibiotics, 1464–1465
alternatives, in acute otitis media, 218
β-lactamase inhibitor with, *Staphylococcus aureus* infections, 686
combination therapy, 1419–1421
dosage, 1480t–1483t
in burned patients, 1437t
pharmacodynamics, 1414t, 1465
pharmacology, 1453t–1458t
resistance, 1419
Bacillus cereus, 754
Enterococcus, 714–715
mechanisms, 1422t, 1424–1425, 1465

Rhodococcus equi, 769
Staphylococcus aureus, 676
Streptococcus pneumoniae, 724–725, 724t
ribosomal-active agents with, 1420
spectrum of activity, 1459t–1463t
structure, 1465f
time-dependent killing, 1441, 1442f, 1442t
treatment of
acute bacterial meningitis ., 276–277
acute otitis media, 216–218
endocarditis, 263
infections in neutropenia in cancer, 570
osteomyelitis, 472
Staphylococcus aureus infections, 686
see also Cephalosporin(s); Penicillin(s); *specific antibiotics*
β-Lactamase
Aeromonas, 831
AmpC
Citrobacter, 807
Enterobacter, 805
Klebsiella, 802
Morganella morganii, 812
Pseudomonas aeruginosa, 845
Serratia marcescens, 813
anaerobic gram-negative bacilli, 983, 985
Bacteroides, 983, 985
BRO-1 and BRO-2, *Moraxella catarrhalis*, 841
Burkholderia cepacia, 848
Bush group 1/class C *see* β-Lactamase, AmpC
classification systems, 1424
detection methods, 1381
in drug resistance, 1422t, 1424–1425
extended-spectrum *see* Extended-spectrum beta-lactamase (ESBL)-producing organisms
Fusobacterium, 986, 988
inhibition of, 1419
Kingella kingae, 921
Klebsiella, 800–801
Pasteurella multocida, 838
plasmid-mediated, 801–802, 845
production, by anaerobes, 961, 965
production at site of infection, 1417
Pseudomonas aeruginosa, 845
Staphylococcus aureus, 1425
TEM-type, *Pseudomonas aeruginosa*, 845
Lactation *see* Breastfeeding/breastmilk
Lactic acidosis, antiretroviral drugs causing, 672
Lactobacillus, 770, 991–992
classification, 959t
Clostridium botulinum inhibition, 971
Clostridium difficile infection treatment, 585
endocarditis due to, 770
female genital tract colonization, 769
vancomycin resistance, 1429
Lactobacillus acidophilus, 770
in probiotic, necrotizing enterocolitis reduction, 961

Lactobacillus casei, 770
Helicobacter pylori infection treatment, 914–915
nosocomial infection prevention, 555
Lactobacillus catenaforme, 770
Lactobacillus fermentum, 770
Lactobacillus jensenii, 770
Lactobacillus plantarum, 770
Lactobacillus rhamnosus, 770
Lactobacillus rhamnosus GG, 770
Lactobacillus salivarius, 770
Lactococcus, 729–730
biochemical differentiation, 729t
Lactoferrin, 84, 385
deficiency, 626
fecal, inflammatory enteritis, 385
Lactophenol cotton blue, 1382
Lagovirus, 1187
Lamina lucida, 438
Lamivudine (3TC), 664, 665t, 1512
adverse effects, 1512
chemistry, 1512
clinical uses, 1512
dosage, 1445t–1452t, 1512
mechanism of action, 1512
pharmacokinetics, 1512
resistance to, 1503t, 1512
treatment of
HBV infection, 1083
HIV infection, 1512
zidovudine with, HIV prophylaxis, 644, 647
Langerhans cells, 85–86
distribution, 86
in histiocytosis, 134
Language delay, otitis media with effusion, 220
Lantibiotics, formation, by *Staphylococcus epidermidis*, 691
Laparoscopy, pelvic inflammatory disease, 364
Larva currens (racing larva), 1333
Larva migrans
cutaneous, 1338–1339
ocular *see* Ocular larva migrans (OLM)
visceral *see* Visceral larva migrans (VLM)
Laryngeal diphtheria, 211
Laryngeal papilloma, 349
Laryngitis
acute, 212
Candida albicans, 1196–1197, 1197f
Laryngomalacia, 165
Laryngotracheitis (croup), 165, 211–212
clinical features, 167t, 206t, 211
complications, prognosis, 212
differential diagnosis, 211
epidemiology and etiology, 211
human parainfluenza viruses, 1121–1123, 1123f
infectious *see* Laryngotracheitis, viral
influenza *vs.*, 1153
management, 211–212
noninfectious causes, recurrent, 211
pathogenesis, 211
RSV causing, 1132
spasmodic, 211
viral, 211–212
causes and stridor in, 165–166, 211

clinical features and diagnosis, 166t
cough in, 167t, 211
Laryngotracheobronchitis *see* Laryngotracheitis (croup)
Lassa virus infection, 1159–1161, 1160t
clinical manifestations, 1161–1162, 1161f
treatment, 1163, 1513
Lateral pharyngeal abscess, 207–208
see also Parapharyngeal abscess
Lateral pharyngeal space, 137–138, 137f, 207
Lateral sinus septic thrombosis, 322, 323t, 324
Latex agglutination (LA), 203
Cryptococcus neoformans, 1382
meningitis etiologic agents, 274
rickettsiae, 1384
Staphylococcus antibiotic susceptibility testing, 1380–1381
VZV detection, 1040
Laundry, standard precautions, 18t
LCMV *see* Lymphocytic choriomeningitis virus (LCMV)
Lead, blood levels, in refugee and internationally adopted children, 36
Learned helplessness, chronic fatigue syndrome, 1012
Leclercia, 809
Lectin pathway, complement activation, 616
Lectins
C-type, 84
mannose-binding *see* Mannose-binding lectins (MBLs)
neonatal immunodeficiency, infections, 540
Left ventricular assist devices (LVAD), infections, 596
Leg pain, transient synovitis, 486
Legg–Calvé–Perthes (LCP) disease, 185
Legionella, 922–925
antigens, detection, 924
antimicrobial susceptibility, 924, 925t
clinical manifestations, 923–924, 925b
copathogens, 923
cross-reactions with other pathogens, 924
culture and growth, 924
culture media, 1375t–1376t
epidemiology, 922–923, 925b
extrapulmonary infection, 923–924
incubation period, 923
laboratory diagnosis, 924, 925b
bacterial detection, 924
serology, 924
microbiology, 922
nosocomial infections, 923
pathogenesis, 922–923
pneumonia due to *see* Pneumonia
Pontiac fever, 923
prevention, 925
pulmonary nodules and pleural effusion, 923
seroconversion, 924
subclinical infection, 923
transmission, 922–923
treatment of infections, 923t, 924–925
urine antigen testing, 924
virulence, 922

Legionella longbeachae, 922–923
Legionella micdadei, 922
Legionella pneumophila, 922–925
  antigen detection assays, 924, 1381
  clinical features of infection, 923–924
  diagnosis, 924
  endocarditis due to, 260t
  generalized lymphadenopathy, 130,
    131t–132t
  genome size, 674
  infection of macrophages, 922
  pneumonia due to, 237, 237t
    in cancer, 575
    see also Legionella
  serogroups, 922
  TLR-5 role in susceptibility to, 84
  see also Entries under Legionella
Legionellaceae, 922
Legionnaire disease, 922
  due to *Legionella longbeachae*, 922–923
  due to *Legionella pneumophila see*
    Legionella pneumophila
Leiomyoma, in HIV infection, 655
Leiomyosarcoma
  EBV association, 1064
  in HIV infection, 655
Leishmania (leishmaniasis), 1285–1290,
  1291b
  amastigotes, 1285–1288, 1286f
  antibodies, 1286, 1289
  classification, 1286
  clinical manifestations, 1286, 1291b
  cutaneous disease, 1285–1286, 1288f
    New World *see Below*
    Old World *see Below*
  description and life cycle, 1285–1286,
    1285f–1286f, 1291b
  diagnosis/detection, 1287–1289, 1291b
    biopsy specimen, 1383–1384
    blood smears, 1384
  diffuse cutaneous disease, 1288–1289
  epidemiology, 1286
  HIV co-infection, 1287
  immune response, 1286, 1288–1289
  leishmaniasis recidivans, 1288–1289
    treatment, 1290
  lymphangitis due to, 161
  mucocutaneous disease, 1286, 1289
    treatment, 1290, 1520
  New World, 1285
  New World cutaneous, 1289
    clinical features, 1289
    diagnosis, 1289
    epidemiology, 1289
    lymphangitis due to, 161–162, 161t
    pathology and pathogenesis, 1289
    prevention, 162
    treatment, 162, 1290
  Old World, 1285
  Old World cutaneous disease,
    1288–1289
    clinical features, 1288, 1288f
    diagnosis, 1288–1289
    epidemiology, 1288
    incubation period, 1288
    pathogenesis, 1288
    treatment, 1290
  prevention and control, 162, 1290

  promastigotes, 1285–1288
  resistance to pentavalent antimony, 1289
  subgenus *Leishmania*, 1285–1286
  subgenus *Viannia*, 1285–1286, 1289
  treatment, 1520
  visceral (kala-azar), 1286–1287
    clinical manifestations, 1287
    cultures, 1287
    diagnosis, 1287
    epidemiology, 1286–1287
    generalized lymphadenopathy,
      119t–120t, 132
    in HIV infection, 1287
    mortality, 1286–1287
    pathology and pathogenesis, 1287
    post-kala-azar dermal leishmaniasis,
      1287–1288
    relapses, 1287
    species causing, 1286
    sporadic, 1286
    treatment, 1289–1290, 1290t
Leishmania aethiopica, 1286, 1288
Leishmania amazonensis, 1286, 1289–1290
Leishmania braziliensis (L. (Viannia)
  braziliensis), 1286, 1289–1290
  lymphangitis due to, 161–162, 161t
Leishmania chagasi (L. d. chagasi), 1289
Leishmania donovani (L. d. donovani), 1286
Leishmania donovani complex, 1286
Leishmania guyanensis, 1289–1290
Leishmania infantum, 1286, 1289
Leishmania major, 1286, 1288
Leishmania mexicana (Leishmania (L.)
  mexicana), 1286, 1289
  lymphangitis due to, 161–162, 161t
Leishmania panamensis, 1289–1290
Leishmania peruviana, 1289
Leishmania skin test, Old World cutaneous
  leishmaniasis, 1288–1289
Leishmania tropica, 1286, 1288
  viscerotropic infection, 1288
Lemierre disease, 194–195, 202, 208–210,
  243, 321, 962
  clinical features, 206t, 208–210, 209f,
    265
  complications and prognosis, 210
  CT scans, 209f
  differential diagnosis, 209–210
  epidemiology and pathogenesis,
    208–209
  etiology, 194–195, 208, 265
  management, 210
Lemierre syndrome, 138
Leminorella, 809
Leprosy *see Mycobacterium leprae* (leprosy)
Leptosphaeria senegalensis, 1250
Leptospira (leptospirosis), 108, 673, 949–
  952
  anicteric leptospirosis, 950–951, 950f
  clinical features, 119t–120t, 950–951
  congenital leptospirosis, 951–952
  culture and growth, 951
    culture media, 1376t
  epidemiology, 949–950
  fever of unknown origin due to,
    119t–120t
  generalized lymphadenopathy, 130,
    131t–132t

  icteric leptospirosis (Weil syndrome),
    950–951, 950f
  "immune" phase, 950
  incubation period, 950
  infection route, 950
  laboratory findings and diagnosis, 951
  laboratory testing, 308t–311t
  meningitis due to, 280t, 281–282, 283t,
    295
  pathogenesis of infections, 949
  pneumonia due to, 237t
  precautions for travelers, 76
  in pregnancy, 952
  prevention, 952
  "septicemic" phase, 950
  serologic tests, 951
  transmission by animal bites, 521–522
  treatment of infections, 951
Leptospira biflexa, 949
Leptospira interrogans, 949–950
  Weil syndrome, 950–951, 950f
Leptospira interrogans serovar
  icterohaemorrhagiae, 949–950
Leptospira interrogans serovar *pomona*,
  941–942
Leptospirosis *see Leptospira*
Leuconostoc, 729
  antibiotic resistance, 730
    vancomycin, 1429
  biochemical differentiation, 729t
  bloodstream infections, 729
  pneumonia and meningitis, 729
  therapy of infections, 730
Leuconostoc mesenteroides, 729
Leuconostoc paramesenteroides, 729
Leucovorin (folinic acid)
  Pneumocystis jirovecii (carinii) pneumonia,
    1232t, 1233
  Toxoplasma gondii infections, 1315–1316,
    1315t–1316t
Leukemia
  acute lymphoblastic, 578
  acute lymphocytic, varicella vaccine use,
    62
  chronic lymphocytic, 40, 40t
  congenital, 548
  infections in
    Aspergillus infections, 1204f, 1206
    mucormycosis, 1213–1214
  large granular lymphocytic, HTLV-2
    causing, 1165
  myelogenous, 1404–1405
  Oka-Merck varicella vaccine in, 1043
Leukemoid reaction, 1404–1405
  eosinophilic, 1407
  Kawasaki disease, 113
  monocytic, 1406
  myeloid, 1404–1405, 1405b
γ-Leukocidin, 676
Leukocidins, *Staphylococcus aureus*, 676
Leukocyte adhesion, 94
Leukocyte adhesion deficiency/defects,
  603t–604t, 616, 620, 625–626
  adhesion molecule expression defects, 85
  characteristics, 619t
  clinical features, 621t, 625–626
  complications of infections, 620t
  immunizations in, 52t–53t

infections associated, 620t, 625–626
types I, II and III, 625–626
Leukocyte esterase (LE), 340
    pyuria diagnosis, 354
    urethritis diagnosis, 353–354
    urinary tract infections, 340
Leukocyte transfusions, 623
Leukocytes *see* White blood cell(s) (WBC)
Leukocytosis, 1404
    Bordetella pertussis infection, 869
    Borrelia infections, 958
    left shift, cholecystitis and cholangitis, 413
    Leptospira infections, 951
    see also White blood cell (WBC) count
Leukomalacia, periventricular, 710
Leukopenia
    adenoviral infections, 113
    coltivirus (Colorado tick fever) infection, 1093
    Ehrlichia and *Anaplasma* infections, 895
    HIV infection, 656
    Rickettsia akari (rickettsialpox) infection, 934
Leukoplakia, oral "hairy", EBV association, 1064
Leukorrhea, 358
Levofloxacin, 1477–1478
    dosage, 1480t–1483t
    pharmacology, 1453t–1458t
    prophylactic, infections in neutropenia in cancer, 573
    spectrum of activity, 1459t–1463t, 1477–1478
    treatment of, 925t
        bacterial keratitis, 497–498
        eye infection treatment, 1494t–1495t
        Helicobacter pylori infections, 914
        Legionella, 924
        Mycoplasma hominis infections, 999
        Mycoplasma pneumoniae infections, 996–997
        tuberculosis, 780t, 782
Lewis X antigen, 85
Libman–Sachs vegetations, 259–260
Lice
    body, vectors for *Rickettsia prowazekii*, 930
    pubic *see Phthirus pubis* (crab louse) infestation
Lice infestation *see* Pediculosis
Lichenification of skin, 352
Light-chain deficiency, 610t, 613, 614t
Light chains, immunoglobulin, 609
Limb anomalies, congenital varicella, 1038
Limb compartment syndromes, after *Neisseria meningitidis* infection, 738
Limb pain, 184–187
    causes, 184b
    diseases involving bone, 186
    diseases involving joints, 184–186
    infectious causes, 184, 186
    in meningococcal septicemia, 735
    muscle diseases causing, 186
    noninfectious causes, 184–186
    soft tissue/fascia diseases causing, 187
    transient synovitis, 486

Limb paralysis, poliovirus causing, 1170
Limp
    causes, 184b
    diskitis, 484
    pyogenic arthritis, 477
    sickle-cell disease, 635
Lincosamides, 1473
    dosage, 1480t–1483t
    resistance, *Streptococcus pyogenes* (group A streptococcus), 204
    see also Clindamycin
Lindane
    pediculosis treatment, 1259
    scabies treatment, 1261
Linezolid, 1426, 1475
    adverse reactions, 687, 1475
    clinical use, 1475
    dosage, 1445t–1452t, 1483t–1484t
    formulations and costs, 687
    mechanism of action, 687, 1426
    pharmacology, 1453t–1458t, 1475
    resistance to, 687, 1422t, 1426, 1475
    spectrum of activity, 1459t–1463t, 1475
    treatment of
        acute bacterial meningitis, 277
        acute pyogenic lymphadenitis, 160
        Ca-MRSA infections, 472
        coagulase-negative staphylococcal infections, 694
        endocarditis, 264
        Enterococcus infections, 637, 715
        Mycoplasma pneumoniae infections, 996–997
        Nocardia infections, 795
        Staphylococcus aureus infections, 687
Lip(s)
    Kawasaki disease (KD), 111, 1003, 1005–1006
    mucocutaneous syndromes, 109t–110t, 111
    rubeola virus (measles), 111
    Stevens–Johnson syndrome, 111, 111f
Lipid(s), utilization, in inflammatory response, 94
Lipid A, monoclonal antibodies to (HA-1A), 101t–102t
Lipid amphotericin B *see* Amphotericin B
Lipid-rich infusions, systemic *Malassezia* infections, 1216–1217
    management, 1218
Lipid storage diseases
    acute hepatitis, 404
    generalized lymphadenopathy, 135
Liponyssoides sanguineus (house mite), 933–934
Lipopeptides
    dosage, 1480t–1483t
    pharmacodynamic properties, 1414t
    pharmacology, 1453t–1458t
    spectrum of activity, 1459t–1463t
Lipopolysaccharide (LPS) *see* Endotoxin (lipopolysaccharide)
Lipopolysaccharide binding protein (LBP), 103
Liposomal amphotericin B *see* Amphotericin B, liposomal
Lipoteichoic acid, *Streptococcus pyogenes*, 698

Listeria
    in interferon-γ receptor deficiency, 632
    species, 763
Listeria grayi, 763
Listeria innocua, 763
Listeria ivanovii, 763
Listeria monocytogenes, 762–766
    antimicrobial susceptibility testing, 1378t
    ataxia due to, 180
    bacteremia due to, 763, 765
    brain abscess due to, 319, 765
    brainstem encephalitis (rhombencephalitis), 765
    clinical manifestations, 764–767
    CNS infection, 763, 765
    coinfections, 763
    conjunctivitis due to, 764–765
    diagnosis, 766–767, 766b
    encephalitis due to, 313
    endocarditis due to, 765
    epidemiology, 763, 763f, 767
    febrile gastroenteritis, 765–766
    food contamination by, 763
    foodborne, 394, 398t, 765–766
        epidemiology and outbreaks, 763, 765–766
        prevention, 766b
    growth conditions, 762
    immune evasion, 763–764
    immunity to, 764
    infection in pregnancy, 763–764
    in iron overload state, 637–638
    iron scavenging, 763–764
    laboratory misidentification, 762–763
    laboratory testing, 308t–311t
    localized infections, 765
    macrophage invasion and spread via, 763–764, 764f
    meningitis due to, 272–273, 277, 765–766, 765t
        neonatal, treatment, 543
        treatment, 1418t–1419t
    microbiology, 762–763
    neonatal infections (early-/late-onset), 764–765
    pathogenesis of infections, 763–764
    perinatal infections, 764
    pneumonia due to, 236
    prevention, 764, 766, 766b
    proliferation in placenta, 763–764
    resistance to, in HIV infection, 764
    serotypes, 763
    transmission, 763
    treatment of infections, 329, 766–767
    urinary tract infection, 341
    virulence factors, 763–764
Listeria seeligeri, 763
Listeria welshimeri, 763
Listeriolysin, 763–764
Listeriolysin O, antibodies, 766
Listeriosis *see Listeria monocytogenes*
Literature, critical evaluation, 9, 9b
Liver
    abscess, 425
        amebic *see* Amebic liver abscess
        Ascaris lumbricoides infections, 1328

chronic granulomatous disease, 624, 625f
clinical manifestations, 425
liver transplant recipients, 557
post-transplant, 557
pyogenic, 425
Staphylococcus aureus, 680
treatment, 426
bacterial clearance role, 638
biopsy, HCV infection, 1110
carcinoma *see* Hepatocellular carcinoma
in chronic meningitis, 284t, 285
cirrhosis *see* Cirrhosis
drug metabolism in, 1439, 1440t
dysfunction, in *Mycoplasma pneumoniae* infections, 994t
Echinococcus multilocularis infections, 1360–1361, 1361f
failure, *Bacillus cereus* infections, 753
fibrosis
congenital, 403
HCV infection, 1108, 1110
function, in HIV infection treatment, 670
granulomas due to *Brucella* (brucellosis), 863
HSV infection, 1031
hydatid cysts (*Echinococcus granulosus*), 1358, 1359f
metabolic abnormalities, 1411
necrosis, fulminant, adenoviruses causing, 1069
transplantation
adenovirus infections, 1069–1070
in *Amanita* poisoning, 399
for chronic hepatitis D, 1087
CMV infection, 1048
Echinococcus multilocularis infections, 1361
for hepatitis A virus infection, 1183
infections after, 557
orthotopic, 414
polysplenia syndrome, 636
trauma, abscess after, 425
trematode infections, 1365
tumors, 404
visceral leishmaniasis, 1287
Liver disease
ascites associated, 638
chronic, HCV causing *see* Hepatitis C virus (HCV)
viral infections in neonates *vs.*, 548
"Liver rot", 1366
LL-37 (cathelicidin), 83–84
Loa loa (loiasis), 1345–1346
characteristics, 1342t
eosinophilia, 1407
Onchocerca volvulus (onchocerciasis) with, 1346
refugee and internationally adopted children, 35
Lockjaw (trismus) *see* Trismus
Löeffler pneumonia
Ascaris lumbricoides causing, 1327–1328
eosinophilia, 1408t–1409t
Loperamide
diarrhea, 377t
inflammatory enteritis, 387
travelers' diarrhea, 82

Lopinavir, 665t, 1444t
Loracarbef
dosage, 1480t–1483t
pharmacology, 1453t–1458t
structure, 1465f
Louping ill virus, 1102
Louseborne diseases
epidemic typhus *see Rickettsia prowazekii*
relapsing fever (*Borrelia recurrentis*), 957–958
Low-birthweight infants
HBV immunization, 1085
systemic *Malassezia* infections, 1216–1217
Löwenstein-Jensen agar, 1375t
Lower respiratory tract, spontaneous hemorrhage, 246–247
Lower respiratory tract infections (LRTIs), 231–235
acute, neutrophilia, 1404
adenovirus, 1068t, 1069
bronchiolitis *see* Bronchiolitis
human coronaviruses causing, 1119–1120
human metapneumovirus, 1136
human parainfluenza viruses, 1121, 1123f
influenza, 1153
Kingella kingae, 921
pneumonia *see* Pneumonia
Staphylococcus aureus, 681
tachypnea in, 169
see also Entries beginning lung; Pneumonia
Ludwig angina, 138, 194
Lumbar puncture
contraindications, 178, 274–275, 325, 736
Acanthamoeba infection, 1296–1297
encephalitis diagnosis, 308
herniation after, 178
in meningitis, 274
after treatment, 725–726
brain imaging prior to, 178
Neisseria meningitidis meningitis, 736
neonatal infection diagnosis, 542
spinal epidural abscess, 684
Streptococcus agalactiae (group B streptococcus) infections, 709
"Lumpy jaw", 991
Lung
abscess, 243–245
anaerobic, 243, 243t
anaerobic gram-negative bacilli, 983
clinical features, 244
diagnosis, 244, 244f
differential diagnosis, 244
etiologic agents, 243, 243t
management, 244
mediastinal lymphadenopathy, 153
Pasteurella multocida, 838
pathogenesis, 243–244
percutaneous drainage, 244
prognosis and complications, 245
Staphylococcus aureus, 681
treatment, 965
aspirate, specimen collection/transport, 1374t
bilateral dense infiltrates in pneumonia, 239

biopsy
in persistent/recurrent pneumonia, 252
Pneumocystis jirovecii (carinii) detection, 1231, 1231t
pneumonia diagnosis, 254–255
pneumonia in SCID, 629
in chronic meningitis, 284t, 285
congenital abnormalities, persistent pneumonia, 247
congenital cysts, persistent pneumonia, 247
congenital overinflation, persistent pneumonia, 247
consolidation, tuberculosis, 774f
cysts, congenital, persistent pneumonia, 247
defense mechanisms, 238
dense focal/multifocal infiltrates, causes, 248, 249t
diffuse interstitial infiltrates, 256t
in cancer, 576–577, 577f
causes, 249t, 251
focal consolidative infiltrates, 254–255, 256t
hemorrhage *see* Pulmonary hemorrhage
hydatid cysts (*Echinococcus granulosus*), 1358, 1359f
hyperinflation, respiratory syncytial virus infection, 1132
infections *see* Pulmonary infections
inflammation *see* Pneumonia
lobar consolidation, pneumococcal pneumonia, 723
localized infiltrates, in cancer, 575–576
lymphatic drainage, 148–149, 148f, 148t
nodular and micronodular infiltrates, 254–255, 256t
parenchymal necrosis, 243–244
parenchymal volume loss *see* Atelectasis
reticulonodular infiltrates, 251
right middle lobe pneumonia, 247
transplant recipients
adenovirus infections, 1069–1070
in cystic fibrosis, 641
human metapneumovirus infections, 1135
infections, 558
nontuberculous mycobacterial infections, 790
RSV infection, 1133
trematode infections, 1365
tuberculosis *see Mycobacterium tuberculosis*, pulmonary
unilateral hyperlucent, 250
see also Entries beginning pulmonary; Pneumonia
Lung disease
chronic, of prematurity, 1001
chronic pyogenic, brain abscess and, 322
granulomatous, 149
in HIV infection, 654–655, 654f, 654t
persistent/recurrent pneumonia, 251
see also Pulmonary infections
Lutzomyia, Leishmania transmission, 1285, 1289
Lyme disease *see Borrelia burgdorferi* (Lyme disease)

Lymph, 127
  flow in abdomen, 156f
  flow in head and neck, 136–138
  flow in lungs and pleura, 149
  see also Lymphatic drainage
Lymph nodes, 127, 127t
  abdominal, 155–156, 156f
  abscess, Staphylococcus aureus, 681
  acute pyogenic infections, 129
  aspirates, Trypanosoma brucei detection,
    1322
  axillary, 159–160
  biopsy, 145–146, 160
    guidelines, 144, 146b
  cervical see Cervical lymph nodes
  enlarged see Lymphadenitis/
    lymphadenopathy
  femoral, 158t, 160, 1287
  fixation, 158
  fluctuation, 158
  in head and neck, 136–138, 136f
  infection etiology, clinical clues, 159b
  inflammation see Lymphadenitis/
    lymphadenopathy
  inguinal see Inguinal lymph nodes
  invasion by neutrophils, 158
  location, 127, 128t
  mediastinal see Mediastinal lymph nodes
  microbes in, lymphadenopathy
    pathogenesis, 129
  in neonates, 128
  nonspecific hyperplasia, 128, 160–161
  palpable, frequency in healthy children,
    128, 128t, 158
  palpation, 128
  primary neoplasms, 128
    see also Histiocytosis; Lymphoma
  regional, disease, 157–158
  size increase
    antigen exposure causing, 128, 158
    see also Lymphadenitis/
      lymphadenopathy
  Sporothrix schenckii (sporotrichosis)
    infection, 1219
  visceral leishmaniasis, 1287
  see also specific lymph nodes
Lymphadenitis/lymphadenopathy, 135, 155,
  157–161
  abdominal see Abdominal
    lymphadenopathy
  acute, 155
  acute pyogenic, pathogenesis, 129
  axillary, 158t, 159–160
  bacterial infection causing, 128t, 129
    characteristics, 128t
  Bartonella henselae causing, 857
  bilateral, 128
  cervical see Cervical lymphadenitis;
    Cervical lymphadenopathy
  characteristics, 128–129, 128t
    node size, 128
    by pathogen and mode of onset, 144t
  chronic, 155
  Corynebacterium species, 760t–761t
  definitions, 135, 155
  development in infections, 129
  differential diagnosis, 158–160
  drug-induced hyperplasia, 133–134

EBV infection, 1061
epitrochlear region, 128, 158t, 160
etiology, clinical clues, 159b
femoral, 158t, 160
Francisella tularensis infection, 897–898
generalized, 128–129, 144t
  autoinflammatory and autoimmune
    disorders, 134
  definition, 128–129
  EBV infection, 1061
  evaluation method, 129b
  histiocytic necrotizing lymphadenitis,
    134
  histiocytosis, 134
  infection-associated hemophagocytic
    syndrome, 134
  infectious causes, 128t, 129–133,
    131t–132t
  inherited immunodeficiency, 134
  lipid storage diseases, 135
  lymphomas, 133
  lymphoproliferative diseases, 133
  malignant causes, 128t, 133–135
  metastatic neoplasms, 134
  miscellaneous disorders, 135
  multicentric Castleman disease, 134
  noninfectious causes, 133–135, 133b
  occipital node involvement, 136
  papular acrodermatitis, 135
  reactive hyperplasia, 135
  Rosai–Dorfman disease, 134
  sarcoidosis, 135
genital ulcer with see Genital ulcer
  disease (GUD)
granulomatous, 134
Haemophilus ducreyi (chancroid), 907
hilar see Hilar lymphadenopathy
histiocytic necrotizing, 134
histopathology, 129
HIV infection, 653
iliac, 158t, 160
inflammatory, 128
inguinal, 128
  differential diagnosis, 352t
  genital ulcers with see Genital ulcer
    disease (GUD)
  management, 351
  without genital ulcers, 351
localized, 157–162, 158t
  acute, 158
  acute, causes, 158
  acute, treatment, 160
  clinical features, 158
  diagnosis, 160–161
  differential diagnosis, 158–160
  etiologic agents, 158, 158t
  history, 158
  investigations, 160–161
  management, 160–161, 160b
  pathogenesis, 158
  subacute, causes, 158
in lymphoma, 128
massive, inhalational anthrax, 752
mediastinal see Mediastinal
  lymphadenopathy/lymphadenitis
mesenteric infectious see Mesenteric
  lymphadenopathy
monkeypox virus infection, 1024

musculoskeletal pain with, 183
necrotizing, 680f
nontuberculous mycobacteria causing see
  Mycobacterium, non-tuberculosis
in normal children, 128, 158
occipital, 158t, 159
paratracheal, 151f
pathogenesis, 129, 129b, 158
popliteal, 160
preauricular, 132, 136, 158t, 159, 159f,
  898
pulmonary Mycobacterium tuberculosis
  infection, 774, 774f
purulence, 129
pyogenic, 129
regional, 128–129
  occipital node involvement, 136
rubella virus infection, 1114
suppurative, chronic granulomatous
  disease, 624
supraclavicular, 148–149, 151
Toxoplasma gondii infections, 1311, 1314
tracheobronchial, 151f
Treponema pallidum subsp. pallidum, 942
Trypanosoma (Trypanozoon) brucei
  infection, 1320
Trypanosoma cruzi infection, 1324–1325
tuberculous, 141, 777, 790
unilateral, 128
viral infections causing, 158
  characteristics, 128t, 129
Wuchereria bancrofti causing, 1342–1343,
  1343f
Yersinia pestis infection (bubonic plague),
  826
Lymphangiomas, 143
Lymphangiomatosis, skull, recurrent
  meningitis associated, 287–288
Lymphangitis, 161–162
  acute bacterial, 160, 161t
    differential diagnosis, 161
  acute filarial, 1343, 1344t
  clinical features, 161
  definition, 161
  differential diagnosis, 161–162
  etiologic agents, 161, 161t
  groups C and G streptococci causing,
    720
  Nocardia causing, 794
  nodular, 161–162, 161t, 162f, 449
    chronic, 162
    differential diagnosis, 161–162
    etiology, 161–162, 161t
  therapy, 162
Lymphangitis-associated rickettsiosis,
  935–938
  see also Rickettsiosis
Lymphatic drainage
  of abdomen, 156f
  of head and neck, 136–138, 136f
  of lungs and pleura, 148–149, 148f,
    148t
  peritonitis pathophysiology, 415
Lymphatic filariasis see Filarial infections
  (filariasis)
Lymphatic system see Lymphoid system
Lymphatic vessels, 127
  Wuchereria bancrofti infections, 1342

Lymphedema, filarial, 1342–1344, 1344t
Lymphoblastoid transformation, in EBV
    infection, 1062
Lymphocutaneous sporotrichosis,
    1219–1220
Lymphocutaneous syndrome, 129
    etiologic agents, 161, 161t
    Nocardia brasiliensis causing, 141
    organisms causing, 138b
    see also Lymphangitis, nodular
Lymphocytes, 1405–1406
    absolute count (ALC), SCID, 629
    atypical, EBV infection, 1060–1061
    in CSF, in chronic meningitis, 285, 285t
    cytolysis, by *Entamoeba histolytica*, 1274
    deficiency/depressed number
        HHV-6 infection, 1053
        HHV-7 infection, 1058
        pneumonia in, 253
    lymphatic circulation, 127
    migration, 127
    normal counts, 90, 1404t
    see also B lymphocytes; T lymphocytes
Lymphocytic choriomeningitis virus
    (LCMV), 1159, 1160t, 1162
    aseptic meningitis due to, 293–295, 297
    chronic meningitis, 283
    clinical manifestations, 1162, 1162f
    congenital infection, 546, 547t
    encephalitis, 303
    eosinophilic meningitis, 331t
    hamsters associated, 528
    laboratory testing, 308t–311t
    transmission, 294
    treatment of infections, 1163
Lymphocytic interstitial pneumonitis (LIP)
    see Lymphoid interstitial pneumonitis
    (LIP)
Lymphocytosis, 1405–1406
    acute infectious, 1406
    atypical, 1406
    causes, 1406b
    CMV infection, 1046–1047
Lymphogranuloma venereum *see* Chlamydia
    trachomatis
Lymphoid hyperplasia, AID and UNG
    deficiency, 613
Lymphoid hyperplasia syndromes, 133b
Lymphoid interstitial pneumonitis (LIP),
    251, 253, 1063–1064
    clinical course, 655
    clinical features, 654
    in HIV infection, 653–655, 654f, 660,
        661f, 671
        management, 671
    imaging, 654f, 660, 660f
    Pneumocystis jirovecii pneumonia *vs.*, 654t
    presumptive diagnosis, 654–655
Lymphoid nodules, 127, 127t
Lymphoid system, 127–135
    abdominal, 156f
    anatomy and function, 127
    developmental changes, 133–134
    head and neck, 136–138, 136f
    thoracic, 148–149, 148f
Lymphoid tissue
    anatomy and function, 127, 127t
    atrophy, 128

bronchus-associated (BALT), 254
    development, 128
Lymphoma
    bilateral hilar adenopathy, 149
    Burkitt, 1064
    CNS
        EBV association, 1393
        in HIV infection, 655
    EBV infection associated, 1064, 1393
    enlarged lymph nodes, 128
    Hodgkin *see* Hodgkin lymphoma (HL)
    lymph node biopsy, 145–146
    mediastinal masses, 154
    non-Hodgkin *see* Non-Hodgkin
        lymphoma (NHL)
    prevalence, 133
Lymphopenia, 1406, 1406b
Lymphopoiesis, 87
Lymphoproliferative disorders, 133
    Castleman disease *see* Castleman disease
    Cryptococcus infections, 1221
    EBV causing, 157
    generalized lymphadenopathy, 133
    immunodeficiency associated, 133b
Lymphoreticular malignancies
    fever of unknown origin due to,
        119t–120t
    see also Leukemia; Lymphoma
Lysis centrifugation-direct plating system,
    1374
Lysosomal trafficking regulator gene (LYST),
    626
Lysosomes, 85
Lysozyme, 84
Lyssavirus, 1145

M

M cells, *Shigella* pathogenesis, 820
MAC *see* Mycobacterium avium-intracellulare
MAC-1, 86
MacConkey agar, 1375t
MacConkey-sorbitol agar, 1375t
Machupo virus (Bolivian hemorrhagic
    fever), 1159, 1160t
Macrolide antibiotics, 1426–1427,
    1470–1472
    dosage, 1445t–1452t, 1480t–1483t
    mechanism of action, 1426–1427
    metabolism, 1470
    pharmacodynamic properties, 1414t
    pharmacology, 1453t–1458t, 1470
    resistance, 1426–1427, 1470–1471
        GAS pharyngitis, 204
        Mycobacterium, non-tuberculosis, 791
        Streptococcus pneumoniae, 724–725,
            724t
    spectrum of activity, 1459t–1463t, 1470
    structure, 1470
    treatment of
        acute otitis media, 725
        Mycoplasma pneumoniae infections,
            997
        pneumococcal pneumonia, 726
        pneumonia, 240, 726
        tickborne infections, 535
Macrophage, 84, 619
    accumulation, histiocytosis, 134

activation
    in *Toxoplasma gondii* infection, 1311
    by *Treponema pallidum* subsp.
        pallidum, 941
acute-phase proteins from, 1400
alveolar, 238, 772
Aspergillus infections, 1203, 1206
Blastomyces dermatitidis phagocytosis,
    1234
development, 84
dysfunction, *Aspergillus* infections, 1206
enterovirus infections, 1173
excess activation
    in hemophagocytic
        lymphohistiocytosis, 103
    in macrophage activation syndrome,
        107
Histoplasma capsulatum, 1224
HIV infection, 649b, 1166
    in CNS, 653–654
in infection-associated hemophagocytic
    syndrome, 1065
Legionella multiplication in, 922
Leishmania amastigotes in, 1285–1288,
    1286f
Listeria monocytogenes invasion/spread,
    763–764, 764f
mucormycosis, 1213
Mycobacterium tuberculosis infections, 772
phagocytosis, *Shigella* infection
    pathogenesis, 820
suppression by corticosteroids, 1206
Trichomonas vaginalis infections, 1318
see also Monocytes
Macrophage activation syndrome (MAS),
    103, 107, 1065
Macrophage colony-stimulating factor
    (M-CSF), 84
Macrophage mannose receptor (MMR), 84
Macula
    detachment, 500–501
    scarring, CMV infection, 500–501
    in *Toxoplasma gondii* infection, 1312
Maculae cerulae, 1257, 1257f
"Maculatum agent", 934
Maculatum infection, 934–935
Macules, 427t, 436
    blanching, Rocky Mountain spotted fever
        (*Rickettsia rickettsii*), 926–927
    erythematous, 435–436
    secondary syphilis, 942
Madura foot *see* Mycetoma
Madurella grisea, 1250
Madurella mycetomatis, 1250
    clinical manifestations, 1251f
    treatment, 1252
Maduromycosis *see* Mycetoma
Mafenide acetate, burn wound infections,
    520, 520t, 1500t–1501t
Magnesium sulfate, neutrophil motility
    reduction, 85
Magnetic resonance angiography (MRA),
    327
Magnetic resonance
    cholangiopancreatography (MRCP),
    413
Magnetic resonance cisternography,
    recurrent meningitis, 291

Magnetic resonance imaging (MRI), 270
  acute disseminated encephalomyelitis, 317, 317f
  acute mastoiditis, 225
  Aspergillus infections, 1205f, 1207
  diskitis diagnosis, 484
  encephalitis diagnosis, 307f, 308
  focal suppurative CNS infections, 327, 327f
  gadolinium-enhanced
    brain abscess due to *Staphylococcus aureus*, 683
    osteomyelitis, 472
    postoperative mediastinitis, 587
  Guillain–Barré syndrome, 318f
  mediastinal masses, 150–151
  in musculoskeletal pain, 183–184
  myocarditis, 267
  necrotizing fasciitis, 467f
  necrotizing otitis externa, 222
  osteomyelitis, 472, 679
  pyogenic arthritis, 478
  pyomyositis, 468
  recurrent meningitis, 291
  sporadic CJD, 338
  staphylococcal osteomyelitis diagnosis, 679
  subacute sclerosing panencephalitis, 1142–1143, 1142f
  Taenia solium neurocysticercosis, 1353–1354
  transient synovitis, 486
  transverse myelitis, 318f
  variant CJD, 335–336
Magnetic resonance imaging (MRI)-stereotactic methods, focal suppurative CNS infection management, 327
Magnitude of effect, 5–6
Majocchi granuloma, 1248
Major histocompatibility complex (MHC)
  antigen presentation with, 45–46, 89–90, 627
  class I, 89
  class II, 89
    deficiency, 628t
  CMV infection, 1044
  Helicobacter pylori urease binding, 911
  polymorphism, vaccine response and, 46
Malabsorption
  Ascaris lumbricoides infections, 1328
  Giardia intestinalis (giardiasis), 1280–1281
  hookworm infections, 1329–1330
  Strongyloides causing, 1333
  viral gastroenteritis, 381
Malaria *see* Plasmodium
Malarone *see* Atovaquone-proguanil
Malassezia, 1215–1218, 1218b
  clinical manifestations, 1216–1217, 1218b
  culture, 1217
  description and structure, 1215–1216, 1218b
  diagnosis, 1217, 1218b
  epidemiology, 1216, 1218b
  folliculitis, 1216–1218
  fungemia, 1217–1218

nosocomial outbreaks, 1216
  pityriasis versicolor, 1216–1217
  seborrheic eczema/dermatitis, 1216–1218
  septicemia due to, 1217
  skin colonization, 1216
  species, 1215–1216
  superficial infections, 1216–1218, 1218b
  systemic infections, 1217–1218, 1218b
  transmission, 1216
  treatment of infections, 1217–1218, 1218b
Malassezia caprae, 1215–1216
Malassezia dermatis, 1215–1216
Malassezia equina, 1215–1216
Malassezia furfur, 1215–1216
  folliculitis, 431
Malassezia globosa, 1215–1217
Malassezia japonica, 1215–1216
Malassezia nana, 1215–1216
Malassezia obtusa, 1215–1216
Malassezia pachydermatis, 1215–1216
Malassezia restricta, 1215–1217
Malassezia slooffiae, 1215–1217
Malassezia sympodialis, 1215–1217
Malassezia yamatoensis, 1215–1216
Malasseziales, 1215
Malathion, pediculosis treatment, 1259
Malignancies *see* Cancer
"Malignant pustule" *see* Bacillus anthracis (anthrax), cutaneous anthrax
Malnutrition/malnourishment
  Ascaris lumbricoides infections, 1328
  Balantidium coli infections, 1267
  shigellosis complications, 821
MALToma
  development, *Helicobacter pylori* infections, 908, 910–912
  Helicobacter heilmannii, 918
  Helicobacter species associated, 916
Mandibular osteomyelitis, 196
Mannheimia, 835
Mannitol, in acute bacterial meningitis, 278
Mannitol salt agar, 1375t
Mannose-binding lectins (MBLs), 84
  complement activation, 616
  deficiency, 604t–605t, 618
  MBL pathway of complement activation, 86
  normal levels, 618
Mannose-binding lectins (MBLs) associated serine proteases (MASPs), 616
Mansonella ozzardi, 1342t, 1346
Mansonella perstans, 1342t, 1346
Mansonella streptocerca, 1342t, 1346
Mantel–Haentzel odds ratio, 7
Mantoux intradermal tuberculin skin test, 779–780
  in abdominal lymphadenopathy, 157
  for communities with high TB rates, 779–780
  false-positive reactions, 779
  in HIV infection, 660–661
  interpretation and induration diameters, 773b, 779–780
  in localized lymphadenopathy, 160
  nonreactive, reasons, 779, 780b
  in persistent pneumonia, 247–248
  in pleural effusion, 243

recommendations, 773b
  refugee and internationally adopted children, 33t, 34
  screening children for risk factors, 780
  technique, 779
  tuberculous pneumonia diagnosis, 240
Maraviroc, 665t, 666
Marburg virus, 1159, 1160t
  see also Filoviruses
Marenostrin, 124
Marfan disease, chest pain due to, 189–190
Marine mammals, ascarids of, 1339
Marrara, 1366
Mask
  standard precautions, 18t
  transmission-based precaution, 19t
  use, recommendations, 17
MASP-2 deficiency, 604t–605t
Mast cells, 1409
Mastoid (mastoid air cells)
  anatomy, 222, 223f
  clouding, 224–225, 224f–225f
  coalescence, 224–225, 224f
  development, 222
  necrotizing otitis externa, 222, 222f
Mastoid infections, anaerobic gram-negative bacilli, 983
Mastoidectomy, 225
Mastoiditis, 222–227
  acute, 222–226
    clinical features, 223–224
    complications, 223b, 225, 225f
    diagnosis, 224–225, 224b
    incidence, 222
    management, 225–226
    microbiology, 224, 224t
    pathogenesis, 222–223
    treatment, 1418t–1419t
  acute coalescent, 222–223
  acute otitis media complication, 215–216, 220, 222–223, 223f
  in cancer, 577
  chronic, 226–227
    anaerobic gram-negative bacilli, 983
    anaerobic gram-positive cocci, 989
    bacteriology, 226
    diagnosis, 226, 226b
    management, 226–227
    pathogenesis, 226
    see also Otitis media, chronic suppurative (CSOM)
  masked, 224
  pathogens causing, 220
  Proteus mirabilis, 812
  subacute, 224
Maternal infections, source of healthcare-associated infection, 10
Mathematical modeling, 7
Matrix-assisted laser desorption ionization of flight mass spectrometry (MALDI-TOF), bacterial identification, 675
Maxillary osteomyelitis, infantile, 196
Maxillary sinuses, 231f
  aspiration, 229
Mayaro virus, 1098
  arthritis, 481
Mazzotti reaction, 1345

MCV4 (tetravalent meningococcal conjugate vaccine) *see under Neisseria meningitidis*
MDR tuberculosis, 785
  see also Mycobacterium tuberculosis
Mean (arithmetic), 5
Measles *see* Rubeola virus (measles)
Measles, mumps, and rubella (MMR) vaccine, 59–60, 1117, 1143
  adverse events, 60
    IoM findings, 50t, 60
  autism controversy/concerns, 51
  childcare settings, 30t
  contraindications, 60, 1117
    after IGIV, 43
    pregnancy, 51–52
  in HIV infection, 52
  mumps prevention, 195, 1128
  precautions, 60
  recommendations for immunization, 59–60
  schedule, 49f, 59
    single dose or two doses, 59
    timing recommendations, 59
    for travelers, 78, 78t
  timing, after immune globulins, 43, 48
Measles, mumps, rubella and varicella (MMRV) vaccine, 59, 62, 1043, 1117, 1143
  contraindications/precautions, 60
  in HIV infection, 663
  recommendations for, 62
Measles virus *see* Rubeola virus (measles)
Meat
  inspection, *Trichinella spiralis* infection prevention, 1341
  Sarcocystis infection prevention, 1308
  Taenia infection prevention, 1352
  Toxoplasma gondii infection from, 1310
    prevention, 1317, 1317t
  Trichinella spiralis infections from, 1339, 1341
Mebendazole
  adverse effects, 1523
  mechanism of action, 1523
  treatment of
    Angiostrongylus infections, 1338
    Ascaris lumbricoides infections, 1328
    Echinococcus granulosus infections, 1359–1360
    Echinococcus multilocularis infections, 1361
    Enterobius vermicularis infections, 1332
    hookworm infections, 1330
    Mansonella perstans infections, 1346
    nematode infections, 1523
    Toxocara infections, 1337
    Trichinella spiralis infection, 1341
    Trichuris trichiura infections, 1331
Meclocycline, skin infection treatment, 1498t
Meconium, gram-staining, 764
Medawar, Sir Peter, 90
Media *see* Culture media
Median, 5
Mediastinal compression, persistent pneumonia, 247

Mediastinal cysts, 149
Mediastinal granuloma, histoplasmosis, 152f, 153
Mediastinal lymph nodes
  abscess, 150t
  anterior, 148
  calcified, 149, 150t, 151
    tuberculosis, 151
  middle, 148
  posterior, 148
  size, 149
Mediastinal lymphadenopathy/lymphadenitis, 128–130, 131t–132t, 133, 148–155
  asymptomatic, 149–150
  biopsy, 151
    conditions not requiring, 149
  characteristics, 149
  clinical features, 149–150, 149t
    of compression, 149t
  diagnosis, 150–151
  diagnostic approach, 155
  diseases and organisms causing, 131t–132t
  epidemiology, 149
  infectious causes, 150t, 151–154
    bacterial, 150t, 151–153
    fungal, 150t, 153–154
    histoplasmosis, 149, 152f–153f, 153–154, 1228
    viral, 150t, 154
  lymphomas, 133, 154, 154f
  noninfectious causes, 150t, 154–155
Mediastinal masses, 148
  anterior, 155
  benign tumors, 149
  clinical features, 149–150, 149t
  diagnosis, 150–151
  epidemiology, 149
  malignant *vs* nonmalignant, 149
  noninfectious causes, frequencies, 149t
  tumors causing, 154
  see also Mediastinal lymphadenopathy/lymphadenitis
Mediastinal widening, 149–150
Mediastinitis
  heart transplant recipients, 558
  Histoplasma capsulatum (histoplasmosis), 1225–1226, 1228t
  postoperative, 587–588
    clinical features and diagnosis, 587
    coagulase-negative staphylococci causing, 693
    epidemiology and pathogenesis, 587
    management and outcome, 587–588
    prevention, 588
    risk factors, 587
Mediastinum, 148
  anatomy, 148
  anterior/posterior, 148
  lymphatic drainage, 148–149, 148f
  middle, 148
  widened, inhalational anthrax, 752
Medical devices, 588
  in cancer, neutropenia and infections, 568, 568t
  Cellulosimicrobium infections, 771

  infections associated *see* Device-related infections
  reprocessing and sterilization, 21
  Tsukamurella infections, 770–771
  use, and indications, 588–589
  see also Device-related infections; Prosthetic device infections
Medical history, recurrent infections, 606
Medical literature, evaluation, 9, 9b
Medical waste, definition, 21
Mediterranean spotted fever, 935–938
  see also Rickettsiosis
Mefloquine
  adverse effects, 1304
  contraindications, 1304
  Plasmodium infections, 1301t–1303t, 1303–1304
    prophylaxis, 80–81, 1304, 1305t, 1521
    prophylaxis in pregnancy, 1306
MEFV gene, 124
Megakaryocytes, 1409
Meglumine antimoniate
  cutaneous leishmaniasis, 1290
  visceral leishmaniasis, 1290, 1290t
Melanin, production by
  Blastomyces dermatitidis, 1234
  Cryptococcus, 1220–1221
Melarsoprol, *Trypanosoma* (*Trypanozoon*) *brucei* infection, 1322t, 1520
Meleney synergistic gangrene, 466t
Meleney ulcer, 461
Melioidosis *see Burkholderia pseudomallei*
Membrane attack complex, 617
Membrane cofactor protein (MCP; CD46), 86
Membranes, rupture, early-onset neonatal infection risk factor, 539–540, 540t
Men who have sex with men (MSM)
  Blastocystis hominis infections, 1268
  Entamoeba histolytica infection, 1274
  HBV transmission, 1078
  HHV-8 infection, 1066
  HPV infection, 1072–1074
  Neisseria gonorrhoeae infection, 742, 744
  syphilis transmission, 942
Meningeal irritation, 279
Meningeal syphilis, 942–943
Meningismus, 325
  Angiostrongylus cantonensis causing, 1337
Meningitis
  Acinetobacter, 829
  Actinomyces, 281–282
  acute bacterial, 272–279
    adjunctive measures, 278
    antimicrobial resistance and, 275–276
    blood–brain barrier disruption, 95
    brain abscess development, 322
    clinical features, 273–274
    conditions associated, 272–273, 273t
    contacts, management, 279
    CSF findings, 274–275, 275t, 277
    differential diagnosis, 274
    dosages of antibiotics, 275
    empiric antibiotics, 275
    epidemiology, 272–273, 272f
    etiologic agents, 272–273

GBS, 708, 709t–710t
head trauma before, 272–273
laboratory findings/diagnosis, 274–275, 275t, 1377
life-threatening complications, 277–278, 322
management, 275–277, 276t, 710t
monitoring of therapy, 277
mortality, 278
neurosurgery before, 272–273
pathogenesis, 273
pathology, 273
patterns, presentation forms, 274
patterns of features, 274
prevention, 279
prognosis and sequelae, 278–279, 278b
supportive care, 277–278
therapy duration, 277
unusual organisms causing, 277
anaerobic gram-negative bacilli, 983
Angiostrongylus, 280t, 283t
antibiotic concentrations in CSF, 1413–1414
arboviruses causing, 294–297
arenaviruses causing, 294
aseptic/viral, 292–297
clinical features, 292–293, 295
complications, 296–297
definition, 292
diagnostic methods, 296
differential diagnosis, 295–296
etiology and epidemiology, 293–294, 293b, 293f
high-dose IGIV associated, 42–43
laboratory findings and diagnosis, 296
in *Leptospira* infections, 950–951
noninfectious causes, 293b
pathogenesis and pathology, 294–295
prevention, 297
prognosis and sequelae, 296–297
recurrent, 287b, 289
seasonal incidence, 293f
terminology, 292
treatment, 296
see also specific viruses (above/below under 'meningitis')
Aspergillus, 282–284, 284t
Bacillus anthracis, 752
Bacillus cereus, 754
Baylisascaris, 280t, 283t
Blastomyces dermatitidis, 280t, 282–283, 283t–284t, 286
Borrelia burgdorferi, 275t, 280t, 281, 283t, 294–295, 954–955
Brucella, 280t, 281, 283t, 863, 864t
in cancer, 579
Candida, 282–284, 284t, 286
causes in very young infants, 114t
Cellulosimicrobium, 771
cerebrospinal fluid analysis, 1413
chronic, 279–286
characteristics of etiologic agents, 279–283
clinical features, 283f, 284t
CSF analysis, 280, 285–286, 285t
definition, 279

diagnosis, 283–286, 283t, 286t
diagnostic algorithm, 283f
epidemiology, 279
etiology, 279, 280t
evaluation, 283–286
fungal, 282–283
history-taking, 283–284
imaging, 285
noninfectious causes, 280b
parameningeal infections manifesting as, 280b
parasites causing, 283
physical examination, 284–285
predisposing conditions, 284t
therapy, 286
viral, 283
Citrobacter, 806–807
Coccidioides immitis, 280t, 282, 283t–284t, 1242–1243
newer drugs, 1245
treatment, 1243–1245
Corynebacterium species, 760t–761t
Cronobacter (*Enterobacter sakazakii*), 805
cryptococcal, 1221–1222
diagnosis, 282, 1222
in HIV infection, 661
treatment, 1222–1223
Cryptococcus neoformans, 282, 284t
in cysticercosis, 280t, 283, 283t
drug-induced, 295–296
Edwardsiella tarda, 808
Elizabethkingia meningoseptica, 834
empiric transmission-based precautions, 20t
enteric gram-negative bacilli, 1418t–1419t
Enterobacter, 805–806
Enterobacteriaceae causing, 276t
Enterococcus, 277, 714
enteroviruses causing, 293–296, 1174–1176
treatment, 296
eosinophilic *see* Eosinophilic meningitis
Escherichia coli, 277, 797
recurrent meningitis, 287
fungal, 275t
gram-negative bacteria causing, 277, 1418t–1419t
group B streptococci causing, 287
Haemophilus influenzae see Haemophilus influenzae
Haemophilus influenzae type b (Hib) *see Haemophilus influenzae* type b (Hib)
Haemophilus parainfluenzae, 907–908
head trauma and, 515
headache in, 177t, 178
herpesviruses causing, 294–297
Histoplasma capsulatum, 280t, 282, 283t–284t, 1226, 1228t
in HIV infection, 283, 661
human parainfluenza viruses causing, 294
infant botulism *vs.*, 974t
intracranial pressure elevation, 178
investigations, 178
Kingella kingae, 921
Klebsiella, 277, 802
late-onset neonatal, 549–550

in leptospirosis, 280t, 283t
Leuconostoc, 729
Listeria monocytogenes, 272–273, 277, 765–766, 765t, 1418t–1419t
treatment, 276t
lumbar puncture *see* Lumbar puncture
in Lyme disease *see* Meningitis, *Borrelia burgdorferi*
lymphocytic choriomeningitis virus (LCMV), 293–295, 297
management, 1418t–1419t
antibiotics before diagnosis, 274
meningococcal *see Neisseria meningitidis*, meningitis
Mollaret *see* Mollaret meningitis
mumps vaccine-associated, 1129
mumps virus, 294–297, 1127
Mycobacterium tuberculosis see Mycobacterium tuberculosis
Mycoplasma hominis, 281–282
Mycoplasma pneumoniae, 295, 994t, 995
Neisseria gonorrhoea, 744
Neisseria meningitidis see Neisseria meningitidis
neonates *see* Neonatal infections
Nocardia, 280t, 281–282, 284t, 794–795
non-typable *Haemophilus influenzae see Haemophilus influenzae*
nuchal rigidity, 177–178
Paracoccidioides, 280t
paramyxoviruses causing, 294
parechoviruses causing, 293, 295
Pasteurella multocida, 837
pneumococcal *see Streptococcus pneumoniae*, meningitis
posttraumatic, 287–289
Proteus, 287
Proteus mirabilis, 812
Pseudomonas, 277
Pseudomonas aeruginosa, treatment, 276t
Psychrobacter immobilis, 840, 941
recurrent, 287–292
anatomic/physiologic abnormalities predisposing, 600t
aseptic, 287, 287b, 289
clinical features, 290
diagnosis, 290–291
drug-induced, 289
epidemiology, 287–288
etiologic agents, 287
Haemophilus influenzae causing, 287
immunologic defects, 288–289
lymphocytic, 290
parameningeal foci, 288b
pathogenesis, 288–290
prophylaxis, 292
trauma and congenital defects, 287–289
treatment, 291–292
recurrent benign lymphocytic (RBLM), 295
risk in children over 3 months with fever, 115
risk in occult bacteremia, 115
risk in young infants with fever, 114–115
Salmonella, 272–273
Serratia marcescens, 813–814
in sickle-cell disease, 634–635

Sporothrix, 280t, 283t
Sporothrix schenckii infection, 1219
Staphylococcus aureus, 277, 683
  recurrent meningitis, 287
Staphylococcus epidermidis, 693
Streptococcus agalactiae, treatment, 276t,
  1418t–1419t
Streptococcus pneumoniae see *Streptococcus*
  pneumoniae
symptoms, 42–43
syphilitic see *Treponema pallidum* subsp.
  pallidum
Taenia, 283
Toxoplasma gondii, 283, 284t
trauma preceding, 515
tuberculous see under *Mycobacterium*
  tuberculosis
Ureaplasma urealyticum, 281–282, 295
viral, 290, 292–297
  CSF findings, 275t
  see also Meningitis, aseptic/viral
viridans group streptococci, 718
West Nile virus infection, 294–295, 297
Yersinia pestis, 826
"Meningitis belt" travel, 80
Meningococcal disease see *Neisseria*
  meningitidis
Meningococcus see *Neisseria meningitidis*
Meningoencephalitic syndrome, epidemic
  typhus (*Rickettsia prowazekii*),
  930–931
Meningoencephalitis, 297
  amebic, 1520
  aseptic meningitis progressing to,
    296–297
  Candida, 1198, 1198f
  chronic, enteroviral, 1179
  enteroviral, in X-linked
    agammaglobulinemia, 610–611
  eosinophilic, 332
    Angiostrongylus causing, 1337
    see also Eosinophilic meningitis
  headache in, 177t
  Mycoplasma hominis infections, 998–999
  Paragonimus infections, 1368
  primary amebic (PEM), 1293–1295
  rotavirus causing, 1095
  Trypanosoma (Trypanozoon) brucei
    infection, 1320–1321
  Trypanosoma cruzi infection, 1324
  varicella, 1037–1038
  see also Encephalitis
Meningomyelocele, meningitis associated,
  273t
Mental status
  altered, 178–180
    causes, 178, 178t
    differential diagnosis of causes, 179t
    evaluation, 179
    history and physical examination,
      179
    Taenia solium neurocysticercosis,
      1353–1354
    therapy, 179–180
  in brain abscess, 323
  in vCJD, 335–336
Meperidine hydrochloride, acute pancreatitis
  treatment, 411

Mercury, exposure from vaccines
  (thimerosal), 45
Merkel cell carcinoma (MCC), 1077
Merkel cell polyomavirus (MCV), 1075,
  1077
Merogony, 1291
Meropenem
  clinical uses, 1468
  dosage, 1445t–1452t, 1480t–1484t
  dose adjustment
    burned patients, 1437t
    renal failure, 1445t–1452t
  pharmacology, 1453t–1458t
  spectrum of activity, 1459t–1463t, 1468
  structure, 1465f
  treatment of
    Acinetobacter infections, 829–830
    acute bacterial meningitis, 277
    Enterobacter meningitis, 806
    Nocardia infections, 795
    perianal cellulitis in cancer, 578–579
Merozoites
  Plasmodium, 1298–1299, 1298f
  Sarcocystis, 1306, 1307f
Mesenteric arteritis, *Angiostrongylus* causing,
  1337
Mesenteric lymph nodes, 156
Mesenteric lymphadenitis (adenitis), 130,
  155, 172–173
  appendicitis with or vs., 172–173
  clinical features and treatment, 172–173
  definition, 155
  infectious, 129, 156
    evaluation, 156b
  tuberculous, 778
  Yersinia enterocolitica, 824
  Yersinia pseudotuberculosis causing, 825
Mesenteric lymphadenopathy, 129,
  156–157
  diagnostic tests, 157
    biopsy, 157
    clinical and laboratory tests, 157
    imaging, 157
  EBV infection, 1061
  evaluation, 156b
  infectious cause, 156
  in intussusception, 174
  noninfectious cause, 157
  therapy, 157
Mesenteric lymphadenopathy syndromes,
  131t–132t
Metabolic abnormalities, 1411
Metabolic acidosis, 168–169
  antiretroviral drugs causing, 672
  necrotizing enterocolitis, 390
Metabolic changes, in acute-phase response,
  1400
Metabolic disorders
  acute hepatitis, 403–404
  chronic hepatitis, 406–407
  genetic, infant botulism vs., 974t
Metabolism, antimicrobial agents, 1434f,
  1435, 1435t, 1439, 1440t,
  1453t–1458t
  burned patients, 1438
  cystic fibrosis, 1437–1438
Metacercariae
  Clonorchis and *Opisthorchis*, 1365

Fasciola, 1366
Heterophyes and *Metagonimus*, 1364
  intestinal trematodes, 1363
Metacestodes, *Echinococcus granulosus*, 1356,
  1358f
Metagonimus yokogawai (metagonimiasis),
  1364
Metal metabolism, disorders, acute
  hepatitis, 404
Metalloproteinase, *Coccidioides immitis*
  (coccidioidomycosis), 1239
Metamyelocytes, 1404
Metapneumovirus see Human
  metapneumovirus (hMPV)
Metastatic tumors, generalized
  lymphadenopathy, 134
Methemoglobinemia, 1403
Methenamine, 1480, 1480t–1483t
Methenamine silver, 1383–1384
Methicillin
  resistance, 1425
    detection, 1431–1432
    resistance, *Staphylococcus epidermidis*, 694
    spectrum of activity, 1459t–1463t
Methicillin-resistant *Staphylococcus aureus*
  (MRSA) see *Staphylococcus aureus*
Methicillin-sensitive *Staphylococcus aureus*
  (MSSA) see *Staphylococcus aureus*
N-Methyl-D-aspartate receptor (NMDAR)
  antibodies, 178–179
  encephalitis, 179–180, 304, 307–308,
    313
Methylbenzethonium, cutaneous
  leishmaniasis, 1290
Methylene blue, 399
Methylobacteriaceae, 832–833
Methylobacterium, 834
Methylobacterium mesophilica, 834
Methylprednisolone see Corticosteroids
Metrifonate, 1525
Metronidazole, 514, 1427, 1478
  adverse effects, 1519
  clinical uses, 1427, 1478
  dosage, 1445t–1452t, 1480t–1484t
  formulations, 1282
  mechanism of action, 1427, 1478
  pharmacodynamic properties, 1414t
  pharmacology, 1453t–1458t, 1478
  resistance, 1478
    Helicobacter pylori, 914
    mechanisms, 1427
  spectrum of activity, 1459t–1463t, 1478
  treatment of
    abdominal trauma-related infections,
      514
    anaerobic gram-positive coccal
      infections, 989
    bacterial vaginosis, 360
    Balantidium coli infection, 1267–1268
    Blastocystis hominis infections, 1269
    Clostridium difficile infections, 585,
      978–979, 979b
    Clostridium tetani infections, 969t
    Entamoeba histolytica (amebiasis),
      1277, 1277b
    Gardnerella vaginalis, 770
    Giardia intestinalis (giardiasis), 1281t,
      1282

Helicobacter pylori infection, 915b
protozoan infections, 1519
skin infections, 1498t
Trichomonas vaginalis infection, 355–356, 360–361, 1319
Mevalonate kinase (MVK), 125
deficiency *see*
Hyperimmunoglobulinemia D with periodic fever syndrome (HIDS)
Micafungin, 1492
clinical trials, 1492
dosage, 1445t–1452t, 1487t, 1492
pharmacology, 1492
prophylactic, HSCT recipients, 566
spectrum of activity, 1486t, 1492
treatment of
Aspergillus infections, 1208–1209
Candida infections, 1200–1201, 1201t
fever in neutropenia (in cancer), 571–572
Mice
B-lymphocyte-deficient (MuMT), 1230–1231
lymphocytic choriomeningitis virus transmission, 1159
mites, *Rickettsia akari* transmission, 933–934
see also Rodents
Miconazole
Candida infection prophylaxis, 1202
superficial infection treatment, 1485, 1485t
Microagglutination assay, *Francisella tularensis*, 898
Microarray analysis, *Shigella* infections, 822
Microbial surface components recognizing adhesive matrix molecules (MSCRAMMs), 258, 676
Microbiology laboratory, surveillance role for HAIs, 16
Microcephaly, congenital rubella, 1115–1116
Micrococcaceae, 690
coagulase-negative, 694–695
see also Staphylococcus (staphylococci)
Micrococcus, 694–695
Micrococcus luteus, 694–695
Micrococcus mucilaginosus (Stomatococcus mucilaginosus), 695
Microconidia, *Histoplasma capsulatum*, 1224
Microdilution methods, susceptibility testing, 1429–1430
Microfilaremia, 1342
peripheral, 1343
Microfilariae, 1342–1343, 1343f
circulation periodicity, 1343
Microhemagglutination test for *T. pallidum* (MHA-TP), 944
Microimmunofluorescence (MIF) test
Chlamydia trachomatis, 1398
Chlamydophila pneumoniae, 1399
Chlamydophila psittaci, 882–883
Microscopic agglutination test, *Leptospira*, 951
Microscopy
darkfield, 673
Treponema pallidum detection, 945
hepatitis A virus (HAV), 1183
Leptospira infections diagnosis, 951

Microsporidia, 1291–1292
clinical diseases, 1291–1292, 1292t
description and structure, 1291, 1292f
epidemiology of microsporidial disease, 1291
HIV infection with, 1291–1292
prevention of infection, 1292
treatment of infection, 1292
Microsporidium (microsporidiosis), 1292t
Microsporum, 1246
Microsporum audouinii, tinea capitis, 1246–1247
Microsporum canis
tinea capitis, 1246–1247
tinea corporis, 1248
Middle airway infections *see* Supraglottic infections
Middle ear
anatomy, 222, 223f
brain abscess pathogenesis, 322
chronic infections, 319
in common cold, 198
infections, anaerobic gram-negative bacilli, 983
pathogens, 540
Middle-ear disease, ataxia in, 180
Middle-ear effusion
acute otitis media with, 216
AAP guidelines for treatment, 218
in masked mastoiditis, 224
Midges, *Mansonella* transmission, 1346
Midline sinuses/cysts, 142t, 143
Migraine, 177t
abdominal, 176
Military recruits
anthrax prevention, 753
Mycoplasma pneumoniae, 993
Neisseria meningitidis, 733–734
Milk
raw, infections associated, 394
source of healthcare-associated infection, 10
Milkborne pathogens
Campylobacter fetus, 879
Campylobacter jejuni, 874–875
Milker's nodules/pseudocowpox, 1024
Miller Fisher syndrome, *Campylobacter jejuni* infection, 877
Millisievert, 345
Miltefosine
cutaneous leishmaniasis, 1290
side effects, 1290
visceral leishmaniasis, 1290, 1290t
Mineral oil, contamination, *Listeria monocytogenes*, 763
Minerals, changes in acute-phase response, 94
Minimal bactericidal concentration (MBC), *Streptococcus agalactiae* (group B streptococcus) infections, 710
Minimum inhibitory concentration (MIC)
antibiotics, 1413–1416, 1440–1442
acute bacterial meningitis treatment, 275
antifungal agents, 1443
antiviral agents, 1444–1445
breakpoints for *Nocardia*, 794
broth microdilution assay, 1378–1379

Streptococcus agalactiae (group B streptococcus) infections, 709
for susceptible/intermediate/resistant organisms, 1379t
Minocycline
dosage, 1480t–1483t
pharmacology, 1453t–1458t
resistance to, 1428
spectrum of activity, 1459t–1463t, 1472
ventricular drain impregnated, eosinophilic meningitis and, 332–333
Miracidia, 1256
Schistosoma, 1368–1369, 1368f
Miscarriage *see* Abortion, spontaneous
Mites, 531
Mitochondrial abnormalities, antiretrovirals causing, 672
Mitochondrial fatty acid oxidation disorders, 404
Mitral valve disease, acute rheumatic fever, 703
Mitral valve prolapse, endocarditis associated, 258f, 259, 261f
MMR *see* Measles, mumps, and rubella (MMR) vaccine
MMRV *see* Measles, mumps, rubella and varicella (MMRV) vaccine
Mobiluncus, 990
bacterial vaginosis, 358
Mode, 5
Moellerella, 809
Molds, 1194, 1209, 1212–1213
spore-bearing, 1194
Molecular fingerprinting, 1384
Molecular methodologies, drug resistance detection, 1430–1431
Molecular mimicry concept
acute rheumatic fever pathogenesis, 703
enteroviruses and diabetes mellitus, 1178
in Kawasaki disease, 1003
Molecular probes, viruses, 1386–1387
Mollaret meningitis, 289–290
diagnosis and clinical features, 289–291
etiology, 290
management, 292
prevention, 292
Molluscicides, 1370
Molluscipoxvirus, 1020t
see also Molluscum contagiosum
Molluscum bodies, 451
Molluscum contagiosum, 349, 352, 450–453, 1020t, 1024–1025
autoinoculation, 1024–1025
clinical features, 451, 452f, 1025
conjunctivitis, 494
diagnosis and treatment, 1025, 1025b
epidemiology, 1024–1025
etiology, 352, 450–451
group childcare and, 30
oral features, 192t
refugee and internationally adopted children, 36
Molluscum dermatitis, 1025
Mondini dysplasia, 287–289
CMV infection, 1045

Monkey(s)
bites, 521–522
infections associated, 528
Monkeypox, 527
laboratory findings/diagnosis, 1024
treatment, 1024
Monkeypox virus, 1020t, 1024
clinical features, 1024
Monobactams, 1468
clinical use, 1468
dosage, 1480t–1483t
pharmacodynamic properties, 1414t
spectrum of activity, 1459t–1463t, 1468
structure, 1465f
Monoclonal antibodies, 42
to *Candida albicans*, 44
to *Cryptococcus neoformans*, 44
development and uses, 42
to herpes simplex virus (HSV), 1033
humanized murine, 44
indications for use, 44
infection prevention by, 44
licensed for use, 44
to Lipid A, 101t–102t
parasite detection by, 1383
product development, 42
to *Staphylococcus aureus*, 44
to tumor necrosis factor-α (TNF-α), 101t–102t
virus isolation/identification, 1386
see also Palivizumab
Monocytes, 84, 619, 1406–1407
activation, in trauma, 512
acute-phase proteins from, 1400
in HIV infection, 649b
normal counts, 1404t
role/function, 1406
see also Macrophage
Monocytic ehrlichiosis *see Ehrlichia chaffeensis*
Monocytosis
causes, 1406b
definition, 1406
Mononuclear cells
chronic fatigue syndrome, 1010t
see also Macrophage; Monocytes
Mononucleosis syndromes
abdominal lymphadenopathy, 156
CMV causing, 1046
EBV causing *see* Epstein–Barr virus (EBV)
generalized lymphadenopathy, 130–132, 131t–132t
see also Infectious mononucleosis
Monopenems, 1437t
Montenegro test (leishmania skin test), 1288–1289
Moraxella, 839–841
culture media, 1376t
Moraxella canis, 840
Moraxella catarrhalis, 839
acute bacterial sinusitis due to, 229, 229t
acute otitis media due to, 214–215, 214f, 839–840
antimicrobial susceptibility, 216t
testing, 1378t
bacterial tracheitis due to, 212
bloodstream infections, 840

clinical manifestations, 840
epidemiology, 839–840
keratitis due to, 496
microbiology, pathogenesis, 839–840
as otopathogen, 214
treatment of infections, 840–841
Moraxella kingii see Kingella kingae
Moraxella lacunata, 840
Moraxella-like organisms, 839
Moraxella lincolnii, 840
Moraxella nonliquefaciens, 840
Moraxella osloensis, 840
Moraxellaceae, 828
Morbidity and Mortality Weekly Report, 68
Morbillivirus, 1137
Morganella, 811–812
clinical manifestations, 812
microbiology and epidemiology, 811
treatment, 812
Morganella morganii, 811
AmpC β-lactamase, 812
cross-reaction with *Yersinia enterocolitica*, 824
neonatal infections, 812
treatment of infections, 812
Mosaicism, drug resistance, 1423
Mosquito-borne diseases, 81
malaria *see Plasmodium* (malaria)
see also individual mosquito species
Mosquitoes, species, 81
Motor disturbances, in subacute sclerosing panencephalitis, 1142–1143
Motor neuron disease, enteroviruses causing, 1174–1175
Motor paralysis, acute *see* Botulism; Poliovirus
Motor vehicle accidents, 515–516
travelers, 76
Moulds *see* Molds
Mouse *see* Mice
Mouse bioassays, *Clostridium botulinum* neurotoxins, 974
Mouth, infections *see* Oral cavity
Mouth ulcers *see* Oral ulceration
Moxifloxacin, 1478
bacterial keratitis, 497–498
eye infection treatment, 1494t–1495t
Mycoplasma hominis infections, 999
Mycoplasma pneumoniae infections, 996–997
Nocardia infections, 795
MRSA *see Staphylococcus aureus*
MSCRAMMS (microbial surface components that recognise adhesive matrix molecules), 258, 676
MSSA *see Staphylococcus aureus*
Muckle–Wells syndrome (MWS), 126
Mucociliary clearance/transport
reduced in cystic fibrosis, 639
respiratory tract, 238
therapy for improving, 641
Mucocutaneous symptom complexes, 108–114
"best" diagnosis, 108
conjunctiva, 108–111, 109t–110t
diagnosis, 108, 109t–110t, 113–114
differential diagnosis, 109t–110t
distinguishing characteristics, 108–113

exanthems, 109t–110t, 111–112
evolution and resolution, 112–113
extremity changes, 112, 112f
fever and prodrome, 108, 113
infection differentiation, 109t–110t
lesions, 112, 112f
lips, 109t–110t, 111
oropharynx, 109t–110t, 111
secondary syphilis, 942
treatment, 109t–110t, 113–114
see also Kawasaki disease; *Staphylococcus aureus*, exfoliative toxin syndrome; Stevens–Johnson syndrome; Toxic shock syndrome (TSS)
Mucopurulent rhinorrhea *see* Rhinorrhea, mucopurulent
Mucor, 1212–1213
neutropenia associated with cancer, 567
Mucorales, 1212–1213
necrotizing soft-tissue infection, 459
Mucormycosis (zygomycosis), 1212–1214, 1215b
clinical manifestations, 1213–1214, 1215b
cutaneous, 1214
diagnosis, 1214, 1215b
disseminated, 1214
epidemiology, 1213, 1215b
focal CNS infections, 1214
gastrointestinal, 1214
microbiology, 1212–1213, 1215b
nosocomial, 1213
prevention, 1214
pulmonary, 1213
rhinocerebral, 1213
sinus infections, 1204
treatment, 1214, 1215b
Mucosal barrier to pathogens, 83–84
Mucosal edema, *Trichuris trichiura* causing, 1331
Mucosal infections, oral, 191–194, 192t–193t
Mucositis
in cancer, 577–578
chemotherapy associated, 568
in immunodeficiency, 194
of rectal mucosa, in cancer, 578–579
Stevens–Johnson syndrome *vs.*, 111
see also Stomatitis
Mucous membranes
colonization, by coagulase-negative staphylococci, 690
infections, 349–352
involvement in infections *see* Mucocutaneous symptom complexes
lesions, HSV infection, 1027
Mucus, antimicrobial properties, 83–84
Mueller–Hinton medium, 1378
cation-adjusted, 1378
Multi-organ failure, systemic inflammatory response syndrome, 98
Multiceps multiceps, 1362–1363, 1363f
Multicollinearity, 7
Multidrug resistance (MDR)
Mycobacterium tuberculosis, 783, 785
Salmonella, 816–817
Streptococcus pneumoniae, 725
Yersinia pestis, 827

Multidrug resistant organisms (MDROs), healthcare-associated infections, 13–14

Multilocus enzyme electrophoresis (MEE), bacterial identification, 674

Multilocus sequence typing (MLST), bacterial identification, 675, 677

Multiorgan dysfunction syndrome, sepsis/septic shock leading to, management, 100

Multiple sclerosis, HHV-6 association, 1057

Multivariable model, 7, 9

Mumps virus, 1125–1129
  acute pancreatitis due to, 411
  anterior uveitis due to, 499t
  antibodies to, 296, 1126–1127, 1396
  arthritis due to, 1127
  aseptic meningitis due to, 294, 296–297
  clinical manifestations, 1126–1127, 1126f
  CNS infection, 1126–1127
  complications, 1127
  control measures, 1129
  cytopathic effects, 1125, 1127–1128
  description and structure, 1125
  diagnosis/detection, 296, 1127–1128, 1395–1396
    IgM antibodies, 195
    optimal tests, 1389t–1392t
  differential diagnosis, 195
  elimination goal, 47
  epidemiology, 1125–1126, 1125f
    incidence, 58–59
    outbreak in 2006 (USA), 294
  genome, 1125
  growth in cell lines, 1125
  immune globulin, 1129
  immune response, 1126
  incubation period, 1126
  keratitis due to, 496
  laboratory testing, 308t–311t
  meningitis due to, 294–297, 1127
  morbidity reduced by vaccine, 48t
  oral features, 192t
  orchitis due to, 368–369, 1126–1127
  pancreatitis due to, 1127
  parotitis due to, 195, 294–295, 411, 1125–1127, 1126f
  pathogenesis, 1126
  in pregnancy, 1127
  prevention of infections, 1128–1129
  prodrome, 195
  proteins, 1125
  renal features, 1127
  replication site, 1126
  treatment, 1128–1129
  vaccination
    efficacy, 1128
    recommendations, 1128, 1128b
  vaccine, 59, 195, 1128
    adverse events, 60, 1129
    adverse events and IoM findings, 50t
    antibody development, 1128
    contraindications, 1129
    hypersensitivity, 1129
    live-attenuated Jeryl Lynn strain, 1128
    pregnancy and, 1129
    response to, 59

  see also Measles, mumps; Measles, mumps, and rubella (MMR) vaccine
vaccine-associated meningitis, 1129

Munc13-4 protein, in familial HLH, 104–105, 104t

Munc18-2 protein, in familial HLH, 104–105

Munchausen syndrome by proxy, 119t–120t

Mupirocin
  intranasal, Staphylococcus aureus infection prevention, 689
  peritonitis prevention, 419
  treatment of
    burns, 1500t–1501t
    impetigo, 429
    neonatal pustulosis, 543
    peritoneal catheter-associated infection, 598
    skin infections, 1498t

Murray Valley encephalitis virus, 1102

Muscle
  abscess
    back pain due to, 188
    staphylococcal, 465
    see also Psoas muscle abscess; Pyomyositis
  biopsy, Trichinella spiralis diagnosis, 1341
  cysts, Taenia serialis (coenurosis), 1362
  disease, limb pain in, 186
  disintegration, in pyomyositis, 465
  pain, 186
    poliovirus causing, 1170
    see also Musculoskeletal pain
  strength, 180
  tenderness, Trichinella spiralis infections, 1341
  tone, 180
  weakness, 180–182
    proximal, Corynebacterium diphtheriae, 757
    see also Weakness

Muscle enzymes, Trichinella spiralis infection diagnosis, 1341

Muscle infections, 186
  enterovirus, 1176–1177
  Sarcocystis, 1307–1308, 1308f
  Trichinella spiralis, 1340
  types and causes, 463t
  see also Myositis; Pyomyositis

Musculoskeletal infections, endocarditis prevention, 76

Musculoskeletal pain, 182
  acute and chronic, 183
  back pain, 187–188, 187b, 188t
  history, 183
  laboratory evaluation and imaging, 183–184
  limb pain, 184–187
  physical examination, 183
  see also Muscle, pain

Musculoskeletal symptom complexes, 182–190
  back pain, 187–188, 187b, 188t
  chest pain, 188–190
  history, 183
  in Kawasaki disease, 1005t

  laboratory evaluation and imaging, 183–184
  limb pain, 184–187
  physical examination, 183
  see also Back pain; Chest pain; Limb pain

Mushroom poisoning, 373, 396, 397t
  management, 399

Mutant prevention concentration (MPC), antibiotics, 1415

Myalgia see Muscle, pain

Myalgic encephalomyelitis (ME) see Chronic fatigue syndrome (CFS)

Myasthenia gravis
  hypotonia, 181t
  infant botulism vs., 974t
  Tensilon test, 974

Mycelia, 1194

"Mycelia sterilia", 1211–1212

Mycetoma, 794, 1195–1196, 1250
  actinomycotic, 1250
  eumycotic see Eumycotic mycetoma
  granules (sclerotia), 1250, 1253

Mycobacterial infections, non-tuberculous see Mycobacterium, non-tuberculosis

Mycobacterium, 771–772
  antimicrobial susceptibility testing, 1381
  cell wall, 673
  culture media, 1376t
  diagnosis/detection, 385t
  diskitis, 483
  diversity, 771–772
  in interferon-γ receptor deficiency, 632
  skin infections, 449

Mycobacterium, non-tuberculosis, 786–792
  antibiotic resistance, 791
  antibiotic susceptibility, 788
  bone infections, 788–789
  cervical lymphadenitis, 135t, 789, 789f
    differential diagnosis, 790
    management, 146, 147t, 791
    subacute/chronic unilateral, 139t, 140, 141f
    surgical excision, 146, 791
  clinical manifestations, 787t, 788–791
  culture and growth requirements, 787
  cutaneous/skeletal infections, 787t, 788–789, 791
  diagnosis/detection, 786–788
  disseminated infections, 787t, 790–792
  epidemiology, 786
  false-positive reactions to tuberculin, 779
  fever of unknown origin due to, 119t–120t
  intravascular catheter-related infections, 593
  lymphadenitis/lymphadenopathy, 787t, 789–791
    M. tuberculosis vs., 777
    treatment, 791
  mediastinal lymphadenopathy, 153
  in NEMO mutation with immunodeficiency, 632–633
  otitis media, 790
  pathogenesis, 786–787
  pneumonia due to, 253t
  prophylaxis in AIDS, 792
  pulmonary infections, 787t, 790
    treatment, 791–792

species, 786
staining methods, 787
treatment of infections, 791–792
virulence factors, 787
Mycobacterium abscessus, 786
clinical manifestations, 787t, 788–790
treatment, 791–792
Mycobacterium africanum, 771–772
Mycobacterium avium, 786
Mycobacterium avium complex, 786
abdominal lymphadenopathy due to, 157
in AIDS, 658, 791
prevention, 663–664
cervical lymphadenitis, 135t
clinical manifestations, 787t, 789–791, 789f
inflammatory enteritis, 387
prophylaxis in AIDS, 792
Mycobacterium avium-intracellulare, in HIV infection, 658, 1476
Mycobacterium bovis, 771–772
abdominal lymphadenopathy due to, 156–157
chronic mastoiditis, 226
chronic suppurative otitis media, 226
peritonitis due to, 415–416
refugee and internationally adopted children, 35f
scrofula due to, 777
Mycobacterium chelonae, 786
clinical manifestations, 787t, 788–790
lymphangitis due to, 161–162, 161t
necrotizing soft-tissue infection, 459–460
treatment, 791
Mycobacterium fortuitum, 786
clinical manifestations, 787t, 788–789
erm gene, 791
treatment, 791
Mycobacterium gastri, abdominal lymphadenopathy due to, 156–157
Mycobacterium goodii, 786–787, 789
Mycobacterium haemophilum
clinical manifestations, 787t, 790
lymphadenitis, 789
Mycobacterium intracellulare, 786
Mycobacterium kansasii, 786
clinical manifestations, 787t, 789–790
necrotizing soft-tissue infection, 459–460
treatment, 791–792
Mycobacterium leprae (leprosy)
anterior uveitis, 499t
chemoprophylaxis, 70t–71t
Mycobacterium malmoense, 786
Mycobacterium marinum, 786
clinical manifestations, 787t, 788
detection, 162
lymphangitis due to, 161–162, 161t, 162f
management, 162
rodents associated, 528
skin infections after trauma, 514
Mycobacterium mucogenicum, 786
Mycobacterium scrofulaceum, 789
Mycobacterium simiae, 786
Mycobacterium smegmatis, 632

Mycobacterium tuberculosis, 771–786
abdominal lymphadenopathy due to, 156–157
abdominal tuberculosis, 156–157, 778
adenitis, nontuberculous mycobacterial *vs.*, 140
anterior uveitis due to, 499, 499t
arthritis due to, 482
aspergilloma development, 1205
bacteremia due to, 776
brain abscess due to, 320
breastfeeding and, treatment in, 784
cardiac disease due to, 776
caseous necrosis due to, 775–777, 775f
cervical lymphadenitis due to, 136, 141f, 777
bilateral, 141
diagnosis and management, 144–146
superficial nodes, 141
unilateral, 139t, 140–141
chemoprophylaxis, 71
chest radiography, 151f–152f, 239, 774f–776f
choroiditis due to, 503
chronic inflammatory enteritis, 382
chronic mastoiditis, 226
chronic suppurative otitis media, 226
clinical manifestations, 774–779
extrathoracic, 776–779
intrathoracic, 774–776
CNS disease, 777–778
congenital disease, 779
treatment, 784
contagiousness, markers of, 772
control failure, 786
control measures, 786
see also Calmette-Guérin bacillus (BCG) vaccine
culture, 780t, 781
sputum induction technique, 781
cutaneous tuberculosis, 449
diagnosis/detection, 779–781
DNA methods, 780t, 781
IFN-γ release test, 34, 780
PCR, 781
in pleural fluid, 240
refugee and internationally adopted children, 33t, 34
serological testing, 781
tuberculin skin test *see* Mantoux intradermal tuberculin skin test
dissemination, 772, 776, 784
drug resistance, 785, 1419
detection, 1432
factors contributing to, 785
isoniazid, 1422t, 1426, 1432
mechanisms, 785
multiple resistance, 783, 785
mutations, 783
prevalence, 785
rifampin, 1427–1428, 1432
selection for, bacterial density, 783
streptomycin, 1424
treatment, 785
eosinophilia, 1408t–1409t
eosinophilic meningitis, 331t, 332
epidemiology, 34, 772
childhood infections, 772, 773f

estimated total risk, 772
ethnicity, age and sex influences, 772
prevalence in refugee and internationally adopted children, 34
prevalence in USA, 34
epididymitis due to, 367
exposure management in pregnant healthcare worker, 22t–23t
extrathoracic, 776–779
therapy, 784
fever of unknown origin due to, 119t–120t
gastrointestinal disease due to, 778
gene sequences for detection, 781
generalized lymphadenopathy, 130, 131t–132t
genitourinary disease, 778
granuloma due to, 776
granulomatous hepatitis due to, 408
group childcare and, 25t, 27, 30–31
growth conditions, 781
in HIV infection, 658, 660, 671
epidemiology, 773
latent infection, treatment, 783
therapy, 784
treatment, 661
immigrant populations, 246, 772
immunity to and immune response, 772
effect on clinical features, 772
ineffective, 772
immunocompromised children, 773–774
inguinal adenopathy without genital ulcers, 351, 352t
insertion sequence IS6110, 781
intraparenchymal lymphangitis due to, 151–153
laboratory diagnosis, 780–781, 780t
laboratory testing, 308t–311t
latent (LTBI), 782–783
refugee and internationally adopted children, 34
treatment, 782–783
lymph nodes involved, 151, 777
lymphadenitis, 140–141, 777
cervical *see Above*
mediastinal, unilateral, 151–153
nontuberculous mycobacteria *vs.*, 777, 790
regional, 151–153
lymphatic disease, 777
lymphohematogenous disease, 776–777
maternal, treatment of infants, 784
mediastinal lymphadenitis, unilateral, 151–153
mediastinal lymphadenopathy, 151–153, 151f–152f
meningitis due to, 279–280, 284t, 295, 777
clinical features, 280, 777
CSF findings, 275t, 280, 777–778
CT, 778f
diagnosis, 280, 777–778
epidemiology, 279
laboratory findings/tests, 280
lymphocytic pleocytosis in CSF, 280
pathogenesis, 279–280

stages (I-III), 777
treatment, 777, 784
tuberculoma during therapy of, 778
miliary tuberculosis, 776–777, 784
diagnosis and prognosis, 777
elevated ESR, 1402
viral infections in neonates *vs.*, 548
mortality, 772
neonatal, in contagious household, treatment, 784
noninfectious, 772
osteoarticular disease due to, 778, 784
osteomyelitis due to, 475
outbreaks, 772–773
drug-resistant, factors leading to, 785
group childcare and, 27
pericarditis due to, 268–270, 776
peritonitis due to, 415–416, 777–778
persistent pneumonia due to, 246–247
placental infection, 779
pleural disease due to, 776
pleurisy, 772
pneumonia due to, 237, 240, 253t, 775f
features, 170t
transplant-associated, 254
in pregnancy, treatment, 785
preseptal cellulitis, 509
prevention by BCG vaccine, 67
see also Calmette-Guérin bacillus (BCG) vaccine
psoas muscle abscess due to, 188
pulmonary tuberculosis, 151–153, 774–776
as AIDS defining condition, 773
calcified caseous lesion, 775–776, 775f
clinical features, 774–776, 774f–775f
mortality, 775–776
primary complex, 774
progressive primary, 772
reactivation, 776, 776f
segmental lesions, 774, 774f
short-course chemotherapy, 783
silent, 774
treatment, 783
visceral leishmaniasis complication, 1287
reactivated tuberculosis
chest radiograph, 152f
pulmonary disease, 776, 776f
treatment, 783
reactivation, 772
refugee and internationally adopted children, 34–35
treatment of tuberculosis, 34
regional cutaneous, 159–160
renal disease due to, 778–779
resurgence of, 772
risk factors for, 772–773
screening children, 780
screening, of healthcare personnel, 21
scrofuloderma, 159–160
scrotal pain syndrome due to, 348–349
skeletal disease, 482, 778
skin disease, 779
strains, distinguishing, 781
transmission, 12–13, 772, 779
kangaroo care and, 12

in transplant recipients, 560
treatment of tuberculosis, 781–785
adjunctive, 785
anticipatory guidance with, 785
antituberculous agents, 780t, 781–782
congenital disease, 784
current recommendations, isoniazid-sensitive, 784
dosages of drugs, 780t, 1445t–1452t
extrathoracic disease, 784
factors for success, 783
follow-up after/during, 785
in HIV infection, 784
latent infection (LTBI), 782–783
monitoring for adverse reactions, 785
multiple drug regimens, 781, 783–784
neonates in contagious household, 784
in pregnancy and lactation, 785
principles, 783
pulmonary disease, 783
refugee and internationally adopted children, 34
rifamycins, 1476
streptomycin, 1474
see also Directly observed therapy (DOTS)
tuberculin skin test *see* Mantoux intradermal tuberculin skin test
urinary tract infections due to, 339
vaccine *see* Calmette-Guérin bacillus (BCG) vaccine
vertebral osteomyelitis due to, 187, 778
Mycobacterium tuberculosis complex, 771–772
Mycobacterium ulcerans, 786
clinical manifestations, 787t, 788
treatment, 791
Mycobacterium xenopi, 786
Mycolactone, 787
Mycoplasma, 673, 998–999
bacterial vaginosis, 358
Bordetella pertussis infections *vs.*, 865
cell wall absent, 993
chronic fatigue syndrome pathogenesis, 1008t–1009t
in cystic fibrosis, 639
diagnosis/detection, 1399
specimens, 1385
genital, diagnosis, 1389t–1392t
HIV infections and, 999
"T-strain", 1000
see also Ureaplasma
tracheobronchitis, cough in, 167t
transient synovitis, 485–486
in X-linked agammaglobulinemia, 610
Mycoplasma amphoriforme, 998t
Mycoplasma buccale, 998t
Mycoplasma faucium, 998t
Mycoplasma fermentans, 998t, 999
Mycoplasma genitalium, 998t, 999
diagnosis, in cervicitis, 362
discharge/dysuria syndrome due to, 346
endocervicitis due to, 361–362
management, 362
genital discharge/dysuria syndrome, 346–347

nongonococcal urethritis, 999
pelvic inflammatory disease due to, 364
scrotal pain syndrome due to, 348–349
urethritis, 353, 356
Mycoplasma hominis, 998–999, 998t
antibiotic susceptibility, 999
arthritis due to, 481–482
aseptic meningitis due to, 295
bacterial vaginosis due to, 358
clinical manifestations, 998–999, 998t
colonization and rates of, 998
diagnosis, optimal tests, 1389t–1392t
genital discharge/dysuria syndrome, 346
genitourinary tract infections, 998
isolation and identification, 998–999
Mycoplasma lipophilum, 998t
Mycoplasma orale, 998t
Mycoplasma penetrans, 998t, 999
Mycoplasma pneumoniae, 993–997, 998t
acute bilateral cervical lymphadenitis due to, 139
acute bronchitis due to, 213
altered mental status and, 178
antibiotic susceptibility/resistance, 996–997
antibodies to, 1399
cold-agglutinating, 995, 1411t–1412t
testing for, 240, 995
arthritis due to, 481–482
aseptic meningitis due to, 295
bronchiolitis due to, 231
clinical course, 994f
clinical manifestations, 993–995
cough due to, 167–168, 994
culture, 240, 995, 1399
description and microbiology, 993
diagnosis/detection, 240, 995–996, 1399
optimal tests, 1389t–1392t
encephalitis, 304, 307
endocarditis due to, 260t
epidemic infections, 993
epidemiology, 993
extrapulmonary disease, 994–995, 994t
generalized lymphadenopathy, 130, 131t–132t
laboratory findings, 995–996
laboratory testing, 308t–311t
mediastinal lymphadenopathy due to, 153
neutrophilia due to, 1404
parapneumonic effusion, 241–242
pathogenesis of infection, 993
pharyngitis due to, 199
pneumonia due to, 169–170, 236–237, 239–240, 246, 993–994
features, 170t
in immunocompromised, diagnosis, 254
necrotizing pneumonia, 243
persistent pneumonia, 245–246
respiratory tract disease, 993–994
respiratory tract epithelial damage due to, 250
in sickle-cell disease, 634
size, 993
skin lesions due to, 112
treatment of infections, 996–997
viral infections with, 993–994

Mycoplasma salivarium, 481–482, 998t
Mycoplasma spermatophilum, 998t
Mycoplasmataceae, 673, 999
Mycosel medium, 1382
Mycosis fungoides, HTLV-2 causing, 1165
Mycotoxins, *Fusarium*, 1210
MyD88 deficiency
    characteristics, 604t–605t
    pneumonia, 253
Myelitis, acute transverse *see* Transverse
    myelitis, acute
Myeloid differentiation factor 88 (MyD88),
    84
Myeloperoxidase (MPO) deficiency,
    603t–604t, 625
    characteristics, 619t, 625
    clinical features, 621t
    immunizations in, 52t–53t
    infections associated, 620t, 625
    infectious complications, 620t
Myiasis, 76
Myocardial abscess, 596
Myocardial infarction
    chest pain, 189, 190t
    differential diagnosis
        myocarditis *vs.*, 266–267
        pericarditis *vs.*, 270
Myocardial ischemia, 189
    drug abuse causing, 270
Myocardiopathy *see* Cardiomyopathy
Myocarditis, 265–268
    active and borderline types, 266
    in acute rheumatic fever, 703
    adenovirus infections, 1069
    bacterial, 266
    clinical features, 266
    complications and prognosis, 268
    Corynebacterium diphtheriae causing,
        756–757
    cough in, 167t
    Dallas criteria, 266
    definition, 265
    differential diagnosis, 266–267
    diphtheritic, 266, 268
    enteroviral, 1176
        neonatal, 547, 1178
    epidemiology, 266
    etiology, 265–266
        noninfectious, 267b
    giant-cell, 266
    in HIV infection, 655–656
    idiopathic, 266–267
    influenza complication, 1153
    Kawasaki disease, 1003
    laboratory findings and diagnosis, 267
        specific organisms, 267
    lymphocytic, 266–267
    management, 267–268
    mortality, 266, 268
    mumps virus, 1127
    Naegleria fowleri infection, 1294
    neonatal, enteroviruses causing, 547,
        1178
    parasites causing, 266
    pathogenesis, 266
    pathology, 266
    prevention, 268
    toxin-mediated, 266

Trichinella spiralis infections, 1341
Trypanosoma cruzi infection, 1324–1325
    viral, 265–266, 547
    viral prodrome, 266
Myocarditis Treatment Trial, 268
Myocardium, in *Trypanosoma cruzi*
    infections, 1324
Myonecrosis
    clostridial, 463
    Clostridium, 461, 463, 466t
Myopathy, hypotonia, 181t
Myopericarditis, enterovirus infections,
    1176–1177
Myositis, 186, 462–465
    acute, causes, 463t
    bacterial, 462–464
        causes, 186
    chronic, causes, 463t
    chronic inflammatory, 464–465
    enterovirus infections, 1176
    fungal, 464
    influenza complication, 1153
    necrotizing group A streptococcal,
        465
    parasitic, 464
        causes, 186
    viral, 464
        causes, 186
Myringitis, bullous, *Mycoplasma pneumoniae*
    infections, 993–994
Myroides, 834
Myroides odoratimimus, 834
Myroides odoratus, 834

N

NADPH oxidase enzyme complex, in
    phagocytosis, 85
Naegleria australiensis, 1293
Naegleria fowleri (naegleriasis), 1293–1295
    Acanthamoeba infections *vs.*, 1294–1295,
        1295t
    characteristics, 1295t
    clinical manifestations, 1294
    description and life cycle, 1293,
        1293f–1294f, 1295t
    diagnosis, 1294–1295, 1383–1384
    epidemiology, 1294
    laboratory testing, 308t–311t
    prevention, 1295
    primary amebic meningoencephalitis,
        303–304, 307, 1293–1295
    treatment, 1295
    trophozoites, 1293–1295, 1293f–1294f,
        1295t
Naegleria italica, 1293
Nafcillin
    dosage, 1445t–1452t, 1480t–1484t
    MICs, 1379t
    pharmacology, 1453t–1458t
    spectrum of activity, 1459t–1463t
    treatment of
        dacryocystitis, 509
        endocarditis, 263t, 1418t–1419t
        necrotizing fasciitis, 514
        neonatal infections, 543
Nagayama spots, HHV-6 infection (roseola),
    1054

Nail bed, deformities, Kawasaki disease,
    112–113
Nail dystrophy, differential diagnosis, 1249
Nail fold infections, 432
Nail infections, tinea unguium, 1249
Nails, artificial, 13
Nairovirus, 1102, 1103t
Nalidixic acid, 1477
    dosage, 1480t–1483t
    pharmacology, 1453t–1458t
    resistance, *Salmonella*, 817
    spectrum of activity, 1459t–1463t
NALP family of receptors, 45
Nanocrystalline silver dressings, 520t
Nanofiltration, for IGIV preparation, 43
Nasal congestion
    acute bacterial sinusitis, 228
    common colds, 198
        management, 198–199
    rhinocerebral mucormycosis, 1213
    subacute/chronic sinusitis, 228
    viral upper respiratory tract infections,
        228
Nasal discharge
    acute bacterial sinusitis, 227–228
    bronchiolitis, 233
    characteristics, 164t
    common colds, 197–198
    non-typable *Haemophilus influenzae*
        causing, 903
    purulent *see* Rhinorrhea, mucopurulent
    subacute/chronic sinusitis, 228
    unilateral, 163
    viral nasopharyngitis, 163
    viral upper respiratory tract infections,
        228
    see also Nasal secretions
Nasal flaring, in pneumonia, 238
Nasal lavage, mucopurulent rhinorrhea, 164
Nasal mucosa, 227
    in acute bacterial sinusitis, 228
    in common cold, 1180–1181
Nasal pain, rhinocerebral mucormycosis,
    1213
"Nasal salute", 198
Nasal secretions, 227
    characteristics in colds, 197–198
    screening for pathogens by monoclonal
        antibodies, 233–234
    see also Nasal discharge
Nasal swabs, specimen collection/transport,
    1374t
Nasoenteric feeding, in infant botulism, 976
Nasolacrimal duct
    abscess, *Staphylococcus aureus*, 681
    obstruction, 493
Nasopharyngeal carcinoma, oral features,
    192t
Nasopharyngeal culture, 240
Nasopharyngeal secretions, collection,
    1123–1124
Nasopharyngeal swabs, specimen collection/
    transport, 1374t
Nasopharyngitis
    hemorrhagic, *Fasciola* infections, 1366
    streptococcal, 164t
        mucopurulent rhinorrhea in, 163
    viral, 163, 164t

Nasopharynx
  anatomy, 127
  bacterial colonization
    Haemophilus influenzae type b (Hib), 273
    meningitis pathogenesis, 273
  carcinoma, neck masses, 142, 142t
  normal flora, 163
  radiograph, retropharyngeal abscess, 207, 208f
National Association of State and Public Health Veterinarians (NASPHV), 529, 531
National Childhood Vaccine Injury Act (NCVIA), 47, 50, 50t
National Committee for Clinical Laboratory Standards (NCCLS) *see* Clinical Laboratory Standards Institute (CLSI)
National Health and Nutrition Examination Survey (NHANES), HCV prevalence, 1105
National Healthcare Safety Network (NHSN), 9, 549, 579, 580t, 585–586
  antimicrobial resistance, trends, 14t
  central line associated bloodstream infections, 10–12
National Institute for Child Health and Development (NICHD), Neonatal Research Network, 549, 555
National Nosocomial Infection Surveillance (NNIS) system, 9, 374, 579, 580t
  Acinetobacter infections, 829
  Enterobacter infections, 805, 805t
  late-onset sepsis in neonates, 549
  Proteus mirabilis infections, 811
  Serratia marcescens infections, 813
  ventilator-associated pneumonia, 250–251
  see also National Healthcare Safety Network (NHSN)
National Notifiable Disease Surveillance System, vaccine-preventable diseases, 62–64
National Vaccine Advisory Committee, standards for child/adolescent immunization, 54
National Vaccine Injury Compensation Program (NVICP), 54
Natriuretic peptide, B-type, in endocarditis, 260
Natural killer (NK) cells, 46, 86–87, 627
  activity levels, 87
  chronic fatigue syndrome, 1010t
  cytolytic T cell comparison, 86t
  defects, 87
  deficiency, 629–633, 630t
    SCID *see* Severe combined immunodeficiency (SCID)
  development, 86–87, 88f
  disorders, 626, 629–633, 630t
  EBV infection, 1060–1063
  HIV infection, 649b
  low/reduced, in HLH, 104–107
  macrophage activation syndrome, 107
  mechanism of action, 87
  NEMO-deficient, 633
  in X-linked lymphoproliferative disease, 633

Natural penicillins *see* Penicillin(s)
Nausea
  acute abdominal pain with, 171
  foodborne diseases, 393, 394t
Necator americanus, 1326, 1329–1330
  clinical manifestations, 1327b
  eosinophilia, 1407, 1408t–1409t
  infection route, 1326
  see also Hookworms
Neck
  abscess
    drainage, 146
    Staphylococcus aureus causing, 139, 139f, 146
  deep infections, 137–138
    anaerobic gram-negative bacilli, 983
  fascia, 136–138
  infections, 135–147
  lymphatic system, 136–138, 136f, 136t
  masses
    epidemiology, 135–136
    malignant tumors, 135
    noninfectious causes, 142t
    nonspecific lymphoid hyperplasia, 135
    not involving lymph nodes, 142–143, 142t
    persistent, causes, 135
    in posterior triangle, 142
    tumors, 142
    see also Cervical lymphadenopathy
  stiffness
    in acute bacterial meningitis, 273–274
    see also Nuchal rigidity
    see also Cervical lymphadenitis; Head and neck
Necrosis, 456
Necrotizing cellulitis *see* Anaerobic cellulitis; Cellulitis
Necrotizing enterocolitis (NEC), 382, 388–391
  modified Bell staging, 389–390, 390t
  in neonates, 388–391
    clinical manifestations, 389–390, 389b
    management, 390
    nosocomial, 550
    pathology and pathogenesis, 388–389, 388t
    risk factors, 388b, 388t
  prevention, 391
    probiotics role, 961
  secondary peritonitis, 419
  Staphylococcus epidermidis, 691–692
Necrotizing fasciitis, 465–466
  Bacteroides, 459–460
  causes, 187, 463t, 514
  chest wall, 189
  clinical features, 466
  diagnosis, 462, 468
  epidemiology, 465
  Escherichia coli, 459–460
  limb pain, 187
  predisposing conditions, 465
  Serratia marcescens, 813
  Staphylococcus aureus, 680

Streptococcus pyogenes (group A streptococcus), 460, 467f, 700–702
  trauma, 514
    risk and management, 513t
  treatment, 468, 514
  type 1, 466, 466t
  type 2, 466, 466t
  type 3, 466
  varicella complication, 1037f
  Vibrio causing, 856
Necrotizing group A streptococcal myositis, 463f, 465
  treatment, 468
Necrotizing pneumonia *see* Pneumonia, necrotizing parenchymal
Necrotizing soft-tissue infections, 466t
  classification, 454–455
  etiology, 459–460, 460b
  polymicrobial, 459–460
  suprafascial, 461
  see also Anaerobic cellulitis; Gas gangrene; Necrotizing fasciitis
Needle(s), infected, sharing of, *Leishmania* transmission, 1286
Needle aspiration
  cervical lymph nodes, 144–145
  in localized lymphadenopathy, 160
Needlestick injuries
  HCV transmission, 1107
  HIV transmission, 642–643
Negative predictive value (NPV), 2f, 2t
Negri bodies, 1145, 1147
Neisseria, 730
  clinical manifestations, 749–750
  commensal species, 748–750
    antibiotic resistance transfer, 750
    prevention, 750
  culture media, 1376t
  epidemiology, 749
  microbiology and laboratory diagnosis, 748–749, 749t
  trimethoprim/sulfamethoxazole resistance, 1428
Neisseria bacilliformis, 749–750
Neisseria canis, animal bites, 521
Neisseria cinerea, 749, 749t
  ophthalmia neonatorum, 489
Neisseria elongata, 749, 749t
  clinical manifestations, 749
Neisseria elongata subsp. *nitroreducens*, 839
Neisseria flavescens, 749, 749t
Neisseria gonorrhoeae, 741–748
  antibiotic resistance, 743, 743f
    fluoroquinolone resistance, 357
    transfer by commensal *Neisseria*, 750
  antibodies to, 741–742
  antimicrobial susceptibility testing, 1381
  biochemical characteristics, 730, 745
  capillary invasion, 441
  chemoprophylaxis, 70t–71t, 72
  Chlamydia trachomatis coinfection, 745, 747
  clinical manifestations, 743–744
  commensal *Neisseria* species *vs.*, 748–749, 749t
  conjunctivitis due to, 491, 743–744, 747
  culture media, 1376t, 1378
  culture techniques, 745, 1373

diagnosis/detection, 355f, 489, 744–745, 748
  in cervicitis, 362
  confirmatory identification, 744
  gram stain evaluation, 744–745
  NAATs, 354–355, 362, 364–365, 370
  nonculture tests, 745
  in pelvic inflammatory disease, 364–365
  serology, 745
  specimen collection/transport media, 1373t
  in urethritis, 354–355
  in vulvovaginitis, 357
disseminated infection (DGI), 349, 744
  arthritis/dermatitis syndrome, 349
  treatment, 747
endocarditis due to, 744
endocervicitis due to, 361–362
  management, 362
epidemiology, 353, 742, 742f, 748
  age/sex-specific rates, 742, 742f
  prevalence, 741–742
epididymitis, 367
expedited partner therapy, 748
genital discharge/dysuria syndrome, 346
immune evasion, 742
immunity to, 741–742
meningitis due to, 744
notifiable disease, 746
oculogenital infection, 744
  treatment, 747
ophthalmia neonatorum, 487–489, 487t, 743
  chemoprophylaxis, 70t–71t
  clinical features, 488–489
  diagnosis and differential diagnosis, 488t, 489
  epidemiology, 488
  prevention, 490, 747–748
  treatment, 489, 746
partner therapy, 748
pathogenesis of infection, 741–742
pelvic inflammatory disease, 173, 353, 363–364
  management, 357
penicillinase-producing strains, 743
perinatal infections, 743–744
  treatment, 746
peritonitis due to, 416
pharyngeal infections, 349, 744, 746–747
pharyngitis due to, 199–200
prevention of infection, 747–748
pyogenic arthritis due to, 184, 744
scalp abscesses due to, 744
screening, 748
sexual abuse, 370–371
as sexually transmitted infection, 346–347
  anal discharge/proctitis syndrome, 347
  discharge/dysuria syndrome, 346
  pelvic inflammatory disease, 346t, 348
  screening, 346
  scrotal pain, 346t, 348–349
systemic infections, 744

transmission, 741–742, 744
  likelihood and risk factors, 742
treatment of infections, 743, 745–748, 746t
urethritis due to, 353, 355f, 744, 747
  clinical features, 353, 354t
  diagnosis, 354–355
  follow-up, 355–356
  management, 355–356
vaccines, 748
vulvovaginitis due to, 356–357
  management, 358
Neisseria lactamica
  carriage, 732, 749
  clinical manifestations, 750
  "natural" immunity to *N. meningitidis*, 749
Neisseria meningitidis, 730–741
  after head trauma, 515
  antibiotic resistance, 736–737, 739
    meningitis treatment and, 276
    rifampin, 1427–1428
    transfer by commensal *Neisseria*, 750
  in asplenia, 636
  asymptomatic carriers, 733–734
  biochemical characteristics, 730
  capillary invasion, 441
  capsular polysaccharide, 730–731
    vaccine development, 65
  carriage, 732–734, 749
    transmission prevention, 739
  cell envelope and surface structures, 730, 730f
  chemoprophylaxis, 69, 70t–71t, 279
  clinical manifestations, 734–736, 735f, 741
  colonization, 273, 731, 733–734
  commensal *Neisseria* species *vs.*, 748–749, 749t
  conjunctivitis due to, 491
  contacts, management, 738–739, 738b
  cytokines role in infections, 731, 737
  diagnosis/laboratory findings, 736, 741
    CSF specimens, 1377
  differential diagnosis, 734
    Rocky Mountain spotted fever (*Rickettsia rickettsii*), 929
  ecchymoses due to, 443–444
  endophthalmitis due to, 503
  endotoxin release in infections, 731
  epidemic disease, 732
  epidemiology, 732–734, 741
    age-specific incidence, 731, 732f
    incidence, in complement deficiency, 289
    prevalence, 65
  factors predisposing to, 733, 733b
  fever of unknown origin due to, 119t–120t
  fever without localizing features, 114–115
  genome, 731
  group childcare and, 25t, 28
  growth requirements, 736
  hemolysis and anemia due to, 1403–1404
  hyperinvasive lineages, 733
  IgA1 protease, 731

  immunity to, 731–732, 749
    natural, 732
  in immunodeficiency, 731, 733
  infections in complement deficiency, 617–618
  meningitis due to, 272, 1418t–1419t
    clinical features, 734–735
    CSF features, 274
    duration of therapy, 737
    lumbar puncture, 736
    prognosis/mortality, 737–738
    recurrent meningitis, 287, 289–291
    serogroups B and C, 272
    treatment, 276–279, 276t, 736–737, 1418t–1419t
  meningococcemia
    benign or unsuspected, 734
    chronic, 735–736
    fulminant, 734
    prognosis/mortality, 737
  metabolic and hematologic abnormalities, 736
  microbiology, 730–731
  in military recruits, 733–734
  mortality due to, 737–738
  nasopharyngeal colonization, 273
  nontypable, carriage, 732
  outbreaks, 734
    risk factors, 734b
  outcome of infections, 737–738
  outer membrane proteins (OMPs), 730f, 731–732
    Por A and Por B, 731–732, 740
  pathogenesis of infections, 731
  petechiae due to, 444
  phagocytosis and killing mechanism, 732
  phase variation of surface structures, 731
  pneumonia due to, 735
  postinfectious inflammatory syndromes, 738
  prevention of infections, 738–740
    chemoprophylaxis, 69, 70t–71t, 279
    management of contacts, 738–739, 738b
    mass prophylaxis, 739
  prognosis, 737–738
  purpura due to, 444
  pyogenic arthritis due to, 477
  recurrent infections, 606
  risk factors for, 733, 733b–734b
  sepsis due to, 98
  septicemia due to, 443–444, 735
    clinical features and mortality, 735
  serogroup A, 80, 732
    vaccine development, 740
    vaccines, 739–740
  serogroup B, 80, 732
    carriage, 734
    meningitis, 272
    outbreaks, 734
    outcome of infections, 738, 738t
    polysaccharide vaccine, 740
    vaccines, 80, 740
  serogroup C, 732
    disease reduction by vaccine, 740
    meningitis, 272
    outbreaks, 734

outcome of infections, 738, 738t
vaccines, 279, 734, 740
   MCV4 (tetravalent meningococcal
      conjugate vaccine) *see Neisseria
      meningitidis* vaccines
serogroup W135, 80, 732
   vaccines, 740
serogroup Y, vaccines, 740
serogroups, 80, 730
serum bactericidal activity to, 731, 732f
severity of disease, factors influencing,
   733
in sickle-cell disease, 634
susceptibility to infection by, 731, 732f
   factors influencing, 733
transmission, 733–734
treatment of infections, 736–737, 741
   cardiovascular resuscitation, 733
   emergency, 737
urethritis due to, 353
virulence, 731
Neisseria meningitidis vaccines, 65, 739–741
A/C/Y/W-135, 78, 79t, 80, 272, 739
   adverse reactions, 739
   recurrent meningitis prevention, 292
after splenectomy, 515
candidate proteins, 731
conjugated, 79t
   advantages and efficacy, 740
   adverse reactions, 740
   in asplenia, 637
   HSCT recipients, 566
conjugated group C, 740
contraindications/precautions, 65
development, 65, 740
group childcare settings, 30t
in HIV infected patients, 65
MCV4 (tetravalent meningococcal
   conjugate vaccine), 65, 78, 79t, 80,
   740
   administration, Tdap with and
      timing, 56
   adverse reaction, 65, 740
   contraindications, 65
   doses, 65
   in immune deficiency and asplenia,
      65
   immune response to, 65
   meningitis epidemiology, 272
   meningitis prevention, 279
   recommendations, 65
   recurrent meningitis prevention, 292
   UK vaccine licensed, 65
   US MCVs licensed, 65
meningitis prevention, 279, 740
OMP vaccines, for group B, 65
polysaccharide (MPS), 65, 739–740
   contraindications, 65
   serogroup B, 65
   for travelers, 78
in pregnancy, 65
recommendations for, 65, 734, 739b
response to, 65
schedule/dosing, 49f
   for travelers, 79t
serogroup A, 739–740
serogroup B, 80, 740
serogroup C, 279, 734, 740

serogroup W135, 740
serogroup Y, 740
for travelers, 78, 79t, 80
Neisseria mucosa, 749–750, 749t
Neisseria perflava, 749
Neisseria polysaccharea, 749t, 750
Neisseria sicca, 749t, 750
Neisseria subflava, 749t, 750
Neisseria weaveri, 748–750, 749t
   animal bites, 521
Neisseriaceae, 835
Nelfinavir, 665t, 1444t–1452t
Nematoda, 1254–1255
   classification, 1254b, 1256, 1256t
   see also specific nematodes
Nematodes (roundworms), 1254–1255,
   1326–1334, 1342–1346
   blood and tissue (filarial worms),
      1342–1346
   see also Filarial infections
   genome projects, 1256
   intestinal, 1326–1334, 1334b
      chronic infections, 1326
      clinical features, 1327b
      diagnosis, 1326, 1327f, 1334b
      epidemiology, 1326, 1334b
      high intensity infections, 1326
      importance and species, 1326
      infection routes, 1326
      neonatal syndromes, 1327t
      reinfections and treatment failures,
         1326–1327
      treatment, 1326–1327, 1334b
      *see also Ancylostoma ceylanicum;
         Ancylostoma duodenale; Ascaris
         lumbricoides; Enterobius vermicularis;
         Necator americanus; Strongyloides
         stercoralis; Trichuris trichiura*
   prevalence, 1255
   in refugee and internationally adopted
      children, 35, 35t
   size/length, 1256
   tissue, 1334–1341
      see also Ocular larva migrans (OLM);
         Visceral larva migrans
   transmission modes, 1256t
   treatment of infections, 1523–1524
NEMO mutation with immunodeficiency,
   630t, 632–633
NEMO protein, 632–633
Neomycin
   allergy, mumps vaccine caution, 1129
   dosage, 1480t–1483t
   treatment of
      burns, 1500t–1501t
      ear infections, 1497t
      eye infections, 1494t–1496t
      otitis externa, 221
      skin infections, 1498t
Neonatal infections, 536–538, 547
   adenovirus, 1068t, 1070
   arthritis due to, 480
   aseptic meningitis, 295
   bacterial, 537–544
      clinical manifestations, 540–541,
         540t
      definitive therapy, 543
      diagnosis, 541–542, 541t

empiric therapy, 542–543, 543t
epidemiology and mortality, 539
etiologic agents, 538–539, 539t
management, 542–543, 543t
pathogenesis, 539–540
prevention, 544
recent advances, 544
BCG vaccination, 779–780
bloodstream infections
   persistent, management, 554
   Streptococcus bovis, 718
   viridans group streptococci, 717
   see also Neonatal infections, late-onset
      sepsis
bone and joint infections, 541, 541t
   treatment, 543t
brain abscess, 321, 329
breast abscess, 457
Candida, 1197–1198, 1197f–1198f
   osteomyelitis, 541
cardiac insufficiency, 547
Citrobacter, 806–807
clinical approach, 536–538
clinical manifestations, 537, 537t,
   540–541, 540t–541t
Clostridium difficile infections, 977–978
CMV, 544–546, 1045
   clinical features, 1047–1048
CNS infections, viral, 547
Coccidioides immitis (coccidioidomycosis),
   1242, 1245
community acquired, 546
congenital rubella, 1115, 1115t
conjunctivitis, 541
   nosocomial, 550
   prevention, 1493
   see also Chlamydia trachomatis;
      Ophthalmia neonatorum
CVC-related *see* Central venous catheter
   (CVC)-related infections
deafness, 548
early-onset, 536
early-onset sepsis, 538–539
   causative agents, 538, 539t
   clinical manifestations, 540
   late-onset *vs.*, 539t
   management, 543t
   maternal risk factors, 539–540, 540t
   treatment, 542
   see also Streptococcus agalactiae (group
      B streptococcus)
elevated C-reactive protein (CRP), 1402
Elizabethkingia meningoseptica, 834
encephalitis, 312t, 313
endocarditis, 257, 692–693
Enterobacter, 805
enteroviruses, 1178–1179
epidemiology, 536
erysipelas, 434
Escherichia coli, 797
etiology, 536
gastrointestinal infections, treatment,
   543t
group B streptococcal *see Streptococcus
   agalactiae* (group B streptococcus)
healthcare-associated *see* Neonatal
   infections, nosocomial
hepatitis, 407

hepatitis B virus (HBV), 401–402
hookworm infections, 1327t, 1330
HSV *see* Herpes simplex virus (HSV)
human parainfluenza viruses, 1123
influenza, 1152
intestinal nematodes, 1327t
Klebsiella, 800
laboratory evaluation, 541–542, 541t
laboratory findings and diagnosis, 537
late-late-onset sepsis, 536, 539
late-onset sepsis, 536, 538–539
    causative agents, 539t, 550–551, 551t
    clinical manifestations, 540
    CVCs causing *see* Central venous
        catheter (CVC)-related infections
    definition, 549
    emerging pathogens, 551
    epidemiology, 549
    treatment, 542–543
Legionella pneumonia, 923
Listeria monocytogenes, 764–765
management, 538
meningitis, 537–538, 540, 543
    aseptic meningitis, 295
    complications, 543–544
    definitive therapy, 543
    diagnosis, 542, 544
    late-onset, nosocomial, 549–550
    Listeria monocytogenes, 765
    management, 542–543, 543t
    Staphylococcus epidermidis causing, 693
Morganella morganii, 812
Mycoplasma hominis infections, 998–999,
    998t
necrotizing enterocolitis, 388–391, 692
neutropenia and septicemia, 84
neutrophil count, 84
non-typable *Haemophilus influenzae*, 903
nosocomial, 537, 546, 548–555
    adjunctive therapy, 552–553
    anatomic sites, 549–550, 549t, 552t
    causes, 549–550, 549t
    clinical manifestations, 551
    conjunctivitis, 550
    CVC *see* Central venous catheter
        (CVC)-related infections
    emerging infections, 551
    empiric therapy, 552, 552t
    epidemiology, 549–550, 549t
    intestinal perforation and peritonitis,
        550
    laboratory diagnosis, 551–552
    persistent bloodstream infections,
        554
    prevention, 554–555
    treatment, 552–553
    treatment duration, 552, 552t
    viral, 546, 549t, 551–552
    see also Central line associated
        bloodstream infections (CLABSIs)
ocular abnormalities, 547–548
ocular infections, 547–548, 547t
    see also Conjunctivitis
osteomyelitis *see* Osteomyelitis
otitis media, 540–541
Pasteurella multocida, 837
pathogenesis, 539–540
peritonitis, 416–417

pneumonia *see* Pneumonia, in neonates
    and young infants
postnatal infections, 546
pulmonary disease, 547
pyogenic arthritis, 541, 541t
response to killed vaccines, 46
risk of serious bacterial infection with
    fever, 114–115
sepsis, 98, 537
septicemia, 537
    clinical manifestations, 540
    Escherichia coli, 538–539
    IGIV for, 544
    management, 542–543, 543t
    pathogenesis, 540
    prevention, 544
    screening tests, 541–542, 541t
    Staphylococcus epidermidis, 692
Serratia marcescens, 813
Shigella, 821–822
skin and soft-tissue, 541
Streptococcus agalactiae see Streptococcus
    agalactiae (group B streptococcus)
Strongyloides, 1327t, 1332–1333
susceptibility, 536
tetanus, 968
timing of infections, 536
Toxoplasma gondii infection diagnosis,
    1314
transmission, 536
    periods for various infections, 536t
Trichomonas vaginalis infections, 1318
Ureaplasma urealyticum, 1000–1001
urinary tract infections, nosocomial, 550
varicella, 1038–1039
ventilator-associated pneumonia (VAP),
    549t, 550
very-late-onset sepsis, 539
viral infections, 544–548
    chronic viremia, 545
    clinical approach, 548
    clinical manifestations, 546–548
    congenital infection syndrome, 547,
        547t
    diagnosis, 1397–1398
    differential diagnosis, 548
    epidemiology, 545–546, 545t
    horizontal transmission route, 546
    intrapartum and via breastmilk, 545,
        546t
    laboratory diagnosis, 548, 552
    maternal infection sources, 545–546
    nosocomial, 546, 549t, 551
    pathogenesis, 544–545
    prevention, 548
    transmission, 544–545
    transmission routes, 545t–546t
    treatment, 548
    vertical transmission, 545, 545t
    virus types, 544–545
    see also Infant(s); Perinatal infections;
        Premature infants; *individual*
        congenital infections
Neonatal intensive care units (NICUs), 539,
    548
    Candida infections, 1196, 1201–1202
    control, 552
    emerging infections, 551

    infection rates, 10, 550, 579
    late-onset sepsis
        epidemiology, 549, 551t
        etiology, 550–551, 551t
    prevention of infections, 554–555
    single-patient rooms, 13
    sites and causes of infections, 549–550,
        549t
    urinary tract infections, 550
    ventilator-associated pneumonia,
        582–583
    viral infections, 551
Neonatal-onset multisystemic inflammatory
    disease syndrome (NOMID), 126
Neonatal sialadenitis, 195
Neonate(s), 536
    antibiotic dosages, 1483t–1484t
    antibiotic resistance, 543
    colonization by microflora, 536
    complement deficiency, 618
    drug disposition, 1435
    immune response, 544–545
    lymph nodes (healthy infants), 128
    morbidity, delivery type in HIV infection,
        646
    passively-acquired antibodies, 87
    pharmacokinetics, 1435, 1435t
    T lymphocytes, 90, 90t
    see also Neonatal infections
Neotestudina rosatii, 1250–1251
Nephelometric assay, C-reactive protein
    (CRP), 1402
Nephritis
    acute focal bacterial, 343–345
    in Henoch–Schönlein purpura, 173–174
    HSCT recipients, BK virus causing, 1076
    interstitial, in *Leptospira* infections,
        950–951
    renal transplant patients, BK virus
        causing, 1076
    varicella complication, 1038
Nephronia, lobar, focal bacterial nephritis
    and, 343–345
Nephropathia epidemica, 1103–1104
Nephropathy, HIV infection in, 656
Nephrotic syndrome
    in complement deficiency, 618
    in congenital syphilis, 943–944
    HIV infection in, 656
    infections in, 637
    peritonitis and, 415
    Plasmodium infection, 1299–1300
    varicella complication, 1038
Nephrotoxicity
    trimethoprim-sulfamethoxazole,
        794–795
    see also Renal dysfunction/failure
Netilmicin, spectrum of activity,
    1459t–1463t
Neuraminidase (NA), influenza viruses,
    1149, 1150f
Neuraminidase inhibitors, 1516–1518
    adverse effects, 1155
    chemoprophylactic use, 72
    influenza prevention, 1157
    influenza treatment, 1154–1155
Neurobiology, chronic fatigue syndrome
    pathogenesis, 1010–1012

Neuroblastoma
  ataxia in, 180, 180t
  neck masses, 142, 142t
  viral infections in neonate *vs.*, 548
Neurocysticercosis *see Taenia solium*
Neurogenic tumors, mediastinal, 149
Neurologic dysfunction
  foodborne diseases, 399
  persistent/recurrent pneumonia due to, 250
Neurologic examination
  in altered mental status, 179
  in chronic meningitis, 285
  in headache, 177
  musculoskeletal pain with, 183
Neurologic infections, adenoviruses, 1069
Neurologic sequelae (of)
  acute bacterial meningitis, 278, 278b
  Bartonella henselae infections, 860
  Corynebacterium diphtheriae infections, 756–757
  Neisseria meningitidis infections, 738
  Trypanosoma cruzi infections, 1325
  varicella, 1037–1038
Neurologic symptom complexes, 176–182
  altered mental status, 178–180
  ataxia, 180
  headache, 177–178
  hypotonia and weakness, 180–182, 181t–182t
  see also Each of the above symptoms
Neurologic symptoms
  hemophagocytic lymphohistiocytosis, 105
  Kawasaki disease, 1005t
  Shigella infections, 821
  Trypanosoma cruzi infections, 1325
Neurologic syndromes, para-/postinfectious
  see Postinfectious neurologic syndromes
Neuronal cell adhesion molecule (NCAM), 1145
Neuronal specific enolase (NSE), 338
Neuropathies
  cranial *see* Cranial neuropathy
  peripheral, 181t
  toxic, *Corynebacterium diphtheriae* causing, 756–757
Neuroretinitis
  Bartonella henselae infection complication, 860
  diffuse unilateral subacute, 502
Neurosurgery
  acute bacterial meningitis risk, 272–273
  brain abscess after, 322
  focal suppurative CNS infection management, 328
  infection chemoprophylaxis, 72
  recurrent meningitis risk, 287
Neurosyphilis *see Treponema pallidum* subsp. *pallidum*
Neurotoxic shellfish poisoning, 396t, 397
Neurotrichinellosis, 1341
Neurotropism, *Nocardia*, 794
Neutropenia, 568–569, 1405
  Aspergillus infections, 1203–1204, 1206–1207
  in cancer, 568–569

causes, 1406
in cell-mediated immunity, infections, 569t
congenital, 604t–605t
cyclic *see* Cyclic neutropenia
definition, 570, 1405
fever in (in cancer), 567–573
  active immunization, 572–573
  anatomic disruptions/devices causing, 568, 568t
  antibiotic resistance, 570
  antifungal treatment, 571–572
  bacterial infections, 567, 569t
  clinical approach to diagnosis in, 570
  empiric antifungal therapy, 571–572
  empiric regimens, 570–571
  epidemiology, 568
  etiologic agents, 567
  fungal infections, 567, 569t, 577
  intravascular catheter-related infections, 574, 577
  management, 570–572, 576t
  monotherapy, 570–571
  parasitic infections, 568
  passive immunization, 573
  pathogenesis and etiology, 568–569
  presumptive therapy, 570–572
  prevention, 572–573
  prognosis and sequelae, 572
  prophylactic antimicrobials, 573
  pulmonary infections, 575
  risk stratification, 572
  sites of infection, 574t
  surveillance programmes, 570
  therapy duration/modification, 571
  viral infections, 568
  see also Cancer
in HIV infection, 656, 658, 672
  management, 672
in hyper-IgM syndrome, 631–632
as mucormycosis risk factor, 1213
mucositis associated, 568
neonatal, 84
neutrophil count, 1405
pathogens associated, 568t–569t
pneumonia, 253, 253t
Pseudomonas aeruginosa infections, 844t
sepsis in, 98
X-linked congenital, 604t–605t
Neutropenic enterocolitis, 981
Neutrophil(s), 84, 619, 1404
  in acute inflammatory response, 1404
  adhesion and extravasation, 94
  apoptosis, 123
  Aspergillus infections, 1203–1204, 1206
  Blastomyces dermatitidis infections, 1235
  chemotaxis, 85, 85f, 197–198
  circulating pool, 1404
  common cold pathogenesis, 197–198
  count, neonatal, 84
  Cryptococcus neoformans infections, 1220–1221
  in CSF
    chronic meningitis, 285, 285t
    meningitis diagnosis, 274
    pleocytosis, 285, 325
  in cyclic neutropenia, 123–124

defective, 89
  invasive *Candida* infections, 1201–1202
  pneumonia, 253–254, 253t
deficiency, 604t–605t
  see also Neutropenia
degranulation, 94
  abnormal, 626
elastase, mutations, 123
granules, 626
in HIV infection, 649b, 658
immature, 1405
infiltration, pneumonia, 238
killing of, by *Shigella*, 820
left shift, 1404–1405
marginated pool, 1404
mucopurulent cervicitis, 362
mucormycosis, 1213
normal count, 1404t
peripheral blood, 1404
recruitment, *Ascaris lumbricoides* infections, 1327–1328
response to
  Neisseria gonorrhoeae, 741–742
  Trichomonas vaginalis, 1318
role
  Candida infections, 1202
  in oral cavity, 192–194
segmented, 1404
Neutrophil deficiency syndrome, 604t–605t
Neutrophilia, 1404
  adenoviruses, 1404
  causes, 1404
  extreme elevations, 1404–1405
  Leptospira infections, 951
Nevirapine, 664–666, 665t, 1444t–1452t
  short-course zidovudine with, HIV prophylaxis, breastfeeding infants, 647–648
New Castle disease, 492t
New York City agar, 1375t
Nezelof syndrome, 603t–604t
NFκB, 632–633
  activation, 632–633
    by TLRs, 94
  inhibitors, 632–633
NFκB essential modulator (NEMO) protein, 632–633
  NEMO mutation with immunodeficiency, 630t, 632–633
Niclosamide
  Diphyllobothrium (diphyllobothriasis), 1348
  Dipylidium caninum infections, 1349
  Hymenolepis infections, 1349
  Taenia infections, 1351–1352
  tapeworm infection treatment, 1524–1525
NICUs *see* Neonatal intensive care units
Niemann–Pick disease, 135
Nifurtimox, 1520
  side effects, 1325, 1520
  Trypanosoma brucei infection, 1322t, 1520
  Trypanosoma cruzi infections, 1325, 1520
Nikolsky sign, 111, 438
  staphylococcal scalded-skin syndrome, 684–685

Nitazoxanide
  Ascaris lumbricoides infections, 1328
  Cryptosporidium infections, 1270
  Fasciola infections, 1366
  Giardia intestinalis (giardiasis), 1281t,
    1282
  hookworm infections, 1330
  protozoan infections, 1519
  Trichuris trichiura infections, 1331
Nitric oxide
  increased production, in sepsis, 102
  mechanism of action, 102
  RSV infection, 1133
  in sepsis, 102
  synthesis, 102
Nitrite reaction, urinary tract infections,
    340
Nitroblue tetrazolium test, 624
Nitrocefin test, 838, 965, 1381
Nitrofurantoin, 1479–1480
  adverse reactions, 1479–1480
  chemoprophylactic use, 74t, 75
  clinical uses, 1479–1480
  dosage, 1445t–1452t, 1480t–1483t
  mechanism of action, 1479
  pharmacology, 1453t–1458t, 1479
  resistance, 1479
    Proteus mirabilis, 812
  structure, 1479
  treatment of
    Enterococcus infections, 715
    urinary tract infection, 341
Nitrofurazone, burn wound infections,
    520t
Nitroimidazoles, 1478
  bacterial vaginosis treatment, 360
  protozoan infections treatment, 1519
  spectrum of activity, 1459t–1463t
  see also Metronidazole; Tinidazole
Nitzchia pungens, 396t
NK cells *see* Natural killer (NK) cells
NMDAR antibodies, 178–179
NMDAR encephalitis, 179–180, 304,
    307–308, 313
NNT (number needed to treat), 2t, 5, 8
Nocardia, 792–795
  Actinomyces vs., 990
  antibiotic resistance, 795
  antibiotic susceptibility and MIC
    breakpoints, 794
  antimicrobial susceptibility testing,
    1381
  brain abscess, treatment, 329
  clinical manifestations, 794
  culture and growth, 792–794
    culture media, 1376t
  diagnosis, 794
  epidemiology, 793
  "granules"/"grains", 794
  groups and classification, 792, 793t
  identification, 792–793
  immune response to, 793–794
  laboratory findings, 794
  meningitis due to, 280t, 281–282, 284t,
    794–795
  microbiology, 792–793
  microscopy and staining, 792–793,
    793f

  pathogenesis, 793–794
  in phagocytic disorders, 620t
  prognosis of infections, 795
  pulmonary disease due to, 793–794
  relapses in AIDS, 795
  skin disease due to, 793–794
  treatment of infections, 794–795
Nocardia abscessus, 792, 793t
Nocardia asteroides, 794
Nocardia asteroides complex, 792, 793t
Nocardia brasiliensis, 792, 793t, 794–795
  detection, 162
  lymphangitis due to, 161–162, 161t
    management, 162
  preseptal cellulitis, 509
  unilateral cervical lymphadenitis due to,
    140–141
Nocardia brevicatina, 792
Nocardia cyriaciageorgia, 792, 793t, 794
Nocardia farcinica, 792–794, 793t
  treatment of infections, 795
Nocardia nova, 792, 793t, 795
Nocardia otitidiscaviarum, 792, 793t, 794
  treatment of infections, 795
Nocardia pseudobrasiliensis, 792, 793t
Nocardia transvalensis, 792, 793t
Nocardiaceae, 792–793
Nocardiosis *see* Nocardia
NOD-like receptors (NLRs), 45, 93–94
Nodular lymphangitis *see* Lymphangitis,
    nodular
Nodules, 427t, 449–454
  Acanthamoeba infection, 1296
  cutaneous leishmaniasis, 1288–1289
  erythema nodosum, 449–454
  infectious causes, 450t
  milker's, 1024
  noninfectious causes, 451t
  Onchocerca volvulus (onchocerciasis),
    1344–1345, 1344f
  pulmonary, in cancer, 575–576
  sterile, 452t
  subcutaneous *see* Subcutaneous nodules
Noma (gangrenous stomatitis), 193t
Non-A, non-B hepatitis (NANBH) *see*
    Hepatitis C virus (HCV)
Non-A-through-E (non-A-E) hepatitis,
    1193–1194
Non-absorbable oral agents, *Candida*
    infection prevention, 1202
Non-Hodgkin lymphoma (NHL), 133
  clinical features, 133
  EBV association in AIDS, 1064
  generalized lymphadenopathy, 133
  in HIV infection, 655
  lymph nodes involved, 142
  mediastinal masses, 154
  neck masses, 135, 142
  prevalence, 133
  prognosis, 154
  subtypes, 133
Non-nucleoside reverse transcriptase
    inhibitors (non-NRTIs), 664–666,
    665t
  cross-resistance, 664–666
  in HIV encephalopathy, 654
  hypersensitivity to, 666
  initial HAART regimen, 667

  side effects, 666, 670
  specificity against HIV-1, 664–666
Non-steroidal anti-inflammatory drugs
    (NSAIDs)
  aseptic meningitis caused by, 295–296
  fever management, 92
  transient synovitis, 486–487
Nonalcoholic fatty liver disease (NAFLD),
    406
Nonalcoholic steatohepatitis (NASH), 406
Noncritical equipment, 21
Noninferiority, 6
Nonspecific vaginosis *see* Bacterial vaginosis
    (BV)
Nonsuppurative ossifying periostitis (Garré
    sclerosing osteomyelitis), 196
Nonsystematic error, 4
Nontuberculous mycobacteria (NTM) *see*
    Mycobacterium, non-*tuberculosis*
Norfloxacin, 1477
  dosage, 1480t–1483t
  eye infections treatment, 1494t–1495t
  pharmacology, 1453t–1458t
"Normal but unlucky child", 600, 600b
Normal counts/values
  eosinophils, 1404t, 1407
  ESR, 1400
  leukocyte counts, 1404, 1404t
  monocytes, 1404t
  neutrophils, 1404t
  platelets, 1409
  T cells, 90
Normal flora *see* Flora, normal
Norovirus(es), 378, 1187–1189
  antibodies, 1187
  characteristics, 1188t
  clinical manifestations, 1189, 1190b
  diagnosis, 397, 1189, 1190b
  diagnostic criteria, 397
  epidemiology, 379, 380t, 1188,
    1188f–1189f, 1190b
  foodborne disease due to, 393–394,
    394t
  gastroenteritis due to, 378, 398t,
    1187–1189, 1190b
    clinical features, 380t
    diagnosis, 397
    prevention, 381
  genogroups, 378, 1187
  group childcare and, 25t
  healthcare-associated infections,
    583–584
  outbreaks in institutions, 380
  pathogenesis and immune response,
    1187
  prevention, 1189
  receptors for, 1187
  shedding, 380
  structure, 1187, 1187f
  transmission, 380, 1188–1189, 1188f,
    1188t
  treatment, 1189, 1190b
  vaccines, 381
  see also Caliciviruses
Norwalk-like viruses, 378, 1188t
Norwalk virus, 1187, 1188t
  gastroenteritis, 378
Nose, anatomy, 231f

Nose-blowing
  bacterial contamination of paranasal
    sinuses, 198, 227
  virus spread, 198
Nosocomial infections, 10, 579
  definition, 10
  diarrhea, 374
  human metapneumovirus (hMPV), 1136
  Legionella, 923
  neonatal *see* Neonatal infections,
    nosocomial
  pneumonia *see* Pneumonia,
    healthcare-associated
  RSV, 1131
  Stenotrophomonas maltophilia, 849
  susceptibility, after sepsis, 100
  transplant recipients, 556
  see also Healthcare-associated infection
    (HAI)
Notification
  foodborne disease, 373
  Vibrio cholerae infections, 854
NSAIDs *see* Non-steroidal anti-inflammatory
    drugs (NSAIDs)
NTM *see* Mycobacterium, non-*tuberculosis*
Nuchal rigidity, 177–178
  aseptic meningitis, 295
  Borrelia infections, 957
  Listeria monocytogenes brainstem
    encephalitis, 765
  neonatal meningitis, 540
Nuclear imaging, in myocarditis, 267
Nucleic acid amplification
  Chlamydia trachomatis, 488, 1398
  CMV, 1388–1392
  Kingella kingae, 921
  Neisseria gonorrhoeae detection, 745
  parvovirus B19, 1397
  RSV, 1394
  techniques, 1386–1387
  virus detection, 1384, 1386–1387
  see also Polymerase chain reaction (PCR)
Nucleic acid amplification tests (NAATs)
  Chlamydia trachomatis, 354–355, 362,
    364–365, 370, 887
  Neisseria gonorrhoeae, 354–355, 362,
    364–365, 370
  resistance detection, 1430
  Trichomonas vaginalis, 354–355
  urethritis diagnosis, 354–355
  virus meningitis diagnosis, 296
  see also Polymerase chain reaction (PCR)
Nucleic acid detection tests, HIV, 652–653
Nucleic acid hybridization
  EBV detection, 1062
  Neisseria gonorrhoeae detection, 745
Nucleoside/nucleotide analogues, as
    antiviral agents, 1502–1514, 1504t
Nucleoside reverse transcriptase inhibitors
    (NRTIs), 664
  drugs included, 664, 665t
  initial HAART regimen, 667
  mechanism of action, 664
  side effects, 664, 670
Nucleotide reverse transcriptase inhibitors
    (NtRTI), 664
  drugs included, 664, 665t
  side effects, 664

Null hypothesis, 6
Number needed to treat (NNT), 2t, 5, 8
Nurseries
  neonatal infections from, 546
  see also Group childcare, arrangements
Nutrition
  HIV infection management, 669–670
  infection prevention after trauma, 513
  in pneumonia, 240
Nutritionally variant streptococci (NVS) *see*
    Streptococcus (streptococci),
    nutritionally variant (NVS)
Nystatin
  Candida infection prophylaxis, 1202
  oropharyngeal candidiasis prevention,
    561
  superficial fungal infection treatment,
    1485, 1485t

O

Observational studies, 5
Obsessive-compulsive symptoms, in
    PANDAS, 706
Obstetric procedures, HCV transmission
    and, 1106
Obturator internus abscess, *Staphylococcus
    aureus*, 680
Occipital lymph nodes, 136, 136t, 159
  pathogens infecting, 145t
Occipital lymphadenopathy, 158t, 159
Occupational health, 21–24
  CMV infections, 1046
  Helicobacter pylori transmission, 909–910
  see also Healthcare personnel
Occupational Safety and Health
    Administration (OSHA), isolation
    precautions, 17
Ochrobactrum, 834
Ocular abnormalities, viral infections in
    neonates, 547–548, 547t
Ocular cysticercosis, 1353–1354, 1353f,
    1355t
Ocular discharge, *Chlamydia trachomatis*, 885
Ocular disease
  in *Mycoplasma pneumoniae* infections,
    994t
  in *Onchocerca volvulus* infections, 1345
Ocular features
  congenital rubella, 1115
  mucocutaneous syndromes, 108–111
Ocular infections
  Candida, 1199
  conjunctivitis *see* Conjunctivitis
  Cryptococcus, 1222
  enterovirus infections, 1175f, 1177
  Histoplasma capsulatum, 1229
  Kingella kingae, 921
  Pseudomonas aeruginosa, 843t, 846
  Serratia marcescens, 813
  Shigella, 821
  Staphylococcus aureus, 679
  treatment, 1493–1496, 1494t–1496t
    zoster ophthalmicus, 1506t
  viral, neonatal, 547–548, 547t
Ocular larva migrans (OLM), 502
  diagnosis, 1337
  Gnathostoma spinigerum causing, 1338

Toxocara and *Baylisascaris* causing,
    1335–1337
  treatment, 1337
Ocular motor nerve palsies, 316
Oculoglandular syndrome, 129
  of Parinaud *see under Bartonella henselae*
  in trachoma, 159
Oculoglandular tularemia, 140
Oculomotor neuropathy, etiology, 314t
Odds ratio (OR), 2t, 4–5
Odontogenic infection, 190–191
  anaerobic gram-negative bacilli, 983
  complications, 194–195
  fever of unknown origin due to,
    119t–120t
  see also Dental infections; Periodontal
    abscess
Odynophagia
  acute epiglottitis, 210
  peritonsillar abscess (quinsy), 206
Oerskovia (*Cellulosimicrobium*), 771
Oerskovia xanthineolytica (*Cellulosimicrobium
    funkei*), 771
Ofloxacin
  Neisseria meningitidis infection
    prophylaxis, 739
  treatment of
    Chlamydia trachomatis infections, 888t
    ear infections, 1496, 1497t
    eye infections, 1494t–1495t
    Mycoplasma pneumoniae infections,
      996–997
Ofloxacin otic solution, chronic mastoiditis
    management, 227
OFPBL medium, 1375t
OKT3, aseptic meningitis caused by,
    295–296
Oligella, 834–835
Oligella ureolytica, 832, 834–835
Oligella urethralis, 834–835
Oligoarthritis, juvenile idiopathic, limb
    pain, 184–185, 185t
Oliguria, in poststreptococcal acute
    glomerulonephritis, 705–706
Omenn syndrome, 628–629, 628t
  diagnosis, 629
Omeprazole, *Helicobacter pylori* treatment,
    914
Ommaya reservoirs, infections related to,
    568
Omphalitis, coagulase-negative
    staphylococci causing, 693
Omsk hemorrhagic fever virus, 1102
Onchocerca volvulus (onchocerciasis),
    1344–1345
  characteristics, 1342t
  clinical manifestations, 1344f, 1345
  conjunctivitis due to, 490
  epidemiology, 1345
  laboratory findings and diagnosis, 1345
  loiasis with, 1346
  prevention, 1345
  transmission, 490
  treatment, 1345
Onchocercoma, 1344f, 1345
Oncogenes, 1164
Oncogenic transformation, 1164
Oncology, infection rates associated, 10

Online Mendelian Inheritance in Man (OMIM), 602t–605t, 608
Onychomycosis (tinea unguium), 1249
O'nyong-nyong virus, 1098
  arthritis, 481
Oocysts
  Cryptosporidium, 1269–1271
  Cyclospora, 1283–1284, 1284f
  Cystoisospora belli, 1283–1284, 1284f
  Plasmodium, 1298f, 1299
  Sarcocystis, 1306, 1307f–1308f
  Toxoplasma gondii, 1309, 1309f, 1311
Ookinete, *Plasmodium*, 1298f, 1299
Operative wounds *see* Surgical wounds
Ophthalmia neonatorum, 487–490, 541
  chemoprophylaxis, 70t–71t
  Chlamydia trachomatis see Chlamydia trachomatis
  differential diagnosis, 489
  etiology, 488–490
    prevalence of pathogens, 487t
  gonococcal *see Neisseria gonorrhoeae*
  hospital-associated, 487
  HSV, 489
  miscellaneous bacterial causes, 489–490
  pathogenesis, 487
  prophylaxis, 490
  treatment, 1493
Ophthalmic infections *see* Ocular infections
Ophthalmitis, posttraumatic, *Bacillus cereus* infections, 754
Ophthalmoscopy, indirect, viral infections in neonates, 547–548
Opisthorchis felineus, 1365
Opisthorchis viverrini, 1365
Opium, tincture of, diarrhea, 377t
Opportunistic infections
  Acinetobacter, 828
  in CMV infections in transplant recipients, 1048
  Enterobacter, 804
  fungal, 1195–1196, 1195t
    Malassezia, 1215
  in HIV infection *see* Human immunodeficiency virus (HIV)/AIDS
  Klebsiella, 800
  Pantoea, 804
  pneumonia due to, 253–254, 253t
  Pseudomonas aeruginosa, 842
  solid-organ transplant recipients, 560
  Stomatococcus mucilaginosus, 695
  visceral leishmaniasis as, 1287
  see also individual infections and diseases
Opsoclonus–ataxia, 180
Opsonins, 85
Opsonization, 45–46
  Mycoplasma pneumoniae, 993
Opsonophagocytosis, of serogroup B meningococci, 732
Optic neuritis, 316
  Bartonella henselae infection complication, 860
  clinical features, 316
  epidemiology, 316
  etiology, 314t, 316
  treatment, 316
OR (odds ratio), 2t, 4–5

Oral cavity
  flora, 190
  infections, 190–196
    bacterial, 193t
    enterovirus, 1174–1175, 1175f
    fungal, 193t
    in HIV infection, 662
    HPV, 1073
    viral, 192t
  mucosal infections, 191–194, 192t–193t
  odontogenic infections *see* Odontogenic infection
  salivary gland infections, 195–196
  viral infections, 192t
Oral contraceptives, pelvic inflammatory disease and, 363
Oral hygiene, in phagocyte disorders, 624
Oral polio vaccine *see* Poliovirus vaccine, oral
Oral rehydration therapy (ORT), 82, 376, 376t
  astrovirus infections, 1191
  composition, 376t, 851t
  foodborne/waterborne disease, 398
  formulation, 82t
  glucose-electrolyte solutions, 376, 376t
  rice-based, 852–853
  rotavirus infection, 1096
  Shigella infections, 822
  Vibrio cholerae infection, 852–853, 852b
  viral gastroenteritis, 381
  WHO recommended solutions, 852–853
Oral ulceration
  aphthous, in HIV infection, 662
  recurrent, 193t
  see also Stomatitis
Orbit
  abscess, 510
  cellulitis, 110, 507, 679
    causes, 507b
    treatment, 1418t–1419t
  pseudotumor, 506
  valveless venous system, 506, 507f
Orbital infections, 510–512, 511f
  acute sinusitis complication, 230
  differential diagnosis, 506
  pathogenesis, 506–507
Orbital septum, 507f
Orchitis, 368–369, 368t
  bacterial, 367, 368t
  Brucella, 863
  EBV infection, 1061
  enteroviruses causing, 1177
  Escherichia coli, 369
  Klebsiella, 369
  mumps virus, 368–369, 368t, 1126–1127
  Pseudomonas aeruginosa, 369
  Toxoplasma gondii (toxoplasmosis), 369
  tuberculous, 779
Orf virus, 1020t, 1024
  clinical features, 1024
Organ failure, pharmacokinetics, 1435
Organ perfusion impairment, after *Neisseria meningitidis* infection, 738
Organomegaly, hemophagocytic lymphohistiocytosis, 105

Orientia tsutsugamushi, scrub typhus, generalized lymphadenopathy, 131t–132t, 132
Oritavancin, 1469
Ornidazole, 1519
Ornithodoros ticks, 957
Ornithosis *see Chlamydophila (Chlamydia) psittaci*
Oropharynx
  candidiasis (thrush), 1196–1197, 1197f
  fascioliasis, 1366
  in mucocutaneous syndromes, 109t–110t, 111
  secretions, aspiration pneumonia, 581
  tularemia, 898
Oroya fever, 940
  generalized lymphadenopathy, 130, 131t–132t
  see also Bartonella bacilliformis
Orthokeratology, 495
Orthomyxoviridae, 1016t, 1149–1159
  infections, 1017t
Orthopedic devices, infections, 598–599
Orthopedic surgery, infection chemoprophylaxis, 73
Orthopoxvirus, 1020t, 1024
  epidemiology, 1024
Orthostatic intolerance, chronic fatigue syndrome pathogenesis, 1008
Oseltamivir, 1516–1517
  chemoprophylactic use, 72
  dosage, 1445t–1452t, 1517
  influenza prevention, 1157, 1517
  influenza treatment, 241t, 1154–1155, 1517
  pneumonia treatment, 241t
Osgood–Schlatter disease, 186
Osler nodes, 259
Osteoarticular infections
  anaerobic cocci, 988
  Brucella, 863–864
  in cancer, 579
  causes in very young infants, 114t
  Kingella kingae, 920–921
    abortive infections, 920
  see also Bone infections; Joint, infections
Osteochondritis
  congenital syphilis, 943, 943f
  puncture wounds leading to, 515
    of foot, 476
Osteochondritis dissecans, 186
Osteomyelitis, 186, 469–477
  Actinomyces, 196, 476f, 991
  acute hematogenous, 469–472
    pathogenesis, 469–472
  anaerobic bacterial, 475–476
  anaerobic gram-negative bacilli, 984
  anaerobic gram-positive cocci, 989
  Aspergillus, 475
  Bacillus cereus, 754
  Bacteroides, 469, 984
  Bartonella henselae, 469
  bite wound complication, 526
  Blastomyces dermatitidis, 1236, 1236f
  Candida, 475, 541
  cervical spine, *Pasteurella multocida*, 837
  chest pain due to, 190t

chronic, 476–477
in chronic granulomatous disease, 624
chronic recurrent multifocal (CRMO),
186, 476
clinical features, 470, 541, 541t
coagulase-negative staphylococci causing,
693
Coccidioides immitis (coccidioidomycosis),
1242
Coxiella burnetii causing, 892
diagnosis, 470, 679
differential diagnosis, 470, 472
Eikenella infection, 836
epidemiology, 469
Escherichia coli, 474
etiology, 469–470
facial, 476
fungal, 475
Gardnerella vaginalis, 769–770
Garré, 196
Haemophilus influenzae type b (Hib), 469,
472, 902–903
hematogenous, 679–680
infantile maxillary, 196
of jaw, 196
Kingella kingae causing, 469, 920
in group childcare, 27
limb pain, 183f, 186
mandibular, 196
neonatal, 472–474, 474f, 474t, 541,
541t, 549
clinical features, 541, 541t
nonhematogenous, 476
nontuberculous mycobacteria causing,
789
patellar, 183f
pelvic, 186, 474–475
fever of unknown origin due to,
119t–120t
Prevotella, 984
Pseudomonas aeruginosa, 845
pyogenic arthritis complication, 477–478
ribs, sternum, 188–189
Salmonella, 475
secondary to soft-tissue infection,
679–680
in sickle-cell disease, 475, 475b,
635–636, 635f
simple acute, 679
sites, 470f
skull base, 221
see also Otitis externa, necrotizing
*Staphylococcus aureus see Staphylococcus
aureus*
sternal postoperative, 587–588
clinical features and diagnosis, 587
epidemiology and pathogenesis, 587
management and outcome, 587–588
prevention, 588
Streptococcus agalactiae (group B
streptococcus), 709
Streptococcus pneumoniae, 469
Streptococcus pyogenes, 469
treatment, 472–473, 679, 1418t–1419t
antibiotic choice, 472–473, 473t
tuberculous, 475
vertebral, 474
back pain due to, 187, 188t

chronic granulomatous disease, 624
diskitis *vs.*, 474, 483, 680
fever of unknown origin due to,
119t–120t
Mycobacterium tuberculosis, 187, 778
see also Bone infections
Osteonecrosis, in HIV infection, 671
Osteopenia, 470
Osteoporosis, in HIV infection, 671
Osteosarcoma, neutropenia and infections,
568
Ostiomeatal complex
endoscopic sinus surgery, 231
in sinusitis, 231, 231f
Otalgia, in necrotizing otitis externa, 221
Otalgia, in mastoiditis, 223
Otic fistula, meningitis associated, 273t
Otitis-conjunctivitis syndrome, 215
Otitis externa, 220–222
acute, 220–221
in cancer, 577
chronic, 221
clinical features, 221
epidemiology, 220–221
etiologic agents, 221
malignant *see* Otitis externa, necrotizing
management, 221
mild/moderate, 221
necrotizing, 221–222, 577
clinical features, 221–222
complications, 222
epidemiology, 221–222
etiology, 222
imaging, 222, 222f
management, 222
prognosis, 222
prevention, 221
Pseudomonas aeruginosa, 221, 843t, 845
severe, 221
treatment, 1496, 1497t
Otitis media, 213–220
acute (AOM), 214–220
AAP guidelines for treatment,
217–218, 218t–219t, 725
antimicrobial resistance, 216t
antimicrobial selection, 216–217,
216t
antimicrobial susceptibility, 214–215,
724t, 725
bacterial and viral coinfection, 214,
214f, 219
chemoprophylaxis, 219
*Chlamydophila (Chlamydia)
pneumoniae*, 882
clinical/microbiologic outcomes, 216t
complications, 215–216, 220,
222–223, 223f, 839–840
epidemiology, 213, 214f, 215
group childcare and, 27
guidelines for drug selection, 216–217
Haemophilus influenzae, 214f, 215,
903–904
human metapneumovirus (hMPV),
1134, 1136
influenza vaccines effect, 1156
influenza viruses causing, 1153, 1153t
microbiology, 214–215, 214f, 214t,
224, 229

Moraxella catarrhalis, 214f, 215, 840
natural history, 215–216, 216t, 220
neonatal, 540–541
pathogenesis, 214, 214f
in penicillin allergy, 218, 219t
presumptive pathogens, 217, 217f
Pseudomonas aeruginosa, 220
recurrent, evaluation, 218–219
relapse and recurrence, 217–218
respiratory tract viruses, 214
risk factors, 215
rubeola virus causing, 1141
spontaneous resolution, 216
Staphylococcus aureus, 215, 220,
680–681
Staphylococcus epidermidis, 215
Streptococcus agalactiae (group B
streptococcus), 215
*Streptococcus pneumoniae see
Streptococcus pneumoniae*
Streptococcus pyogenes (group A
streptococcus), 214f, 215
treatment, 27, 215, 725, 1418t–
1419t
treatment failure, 222–223, 225f
treatment failure rates, 216–218
viral, 214t
"watchful waiting", 216, 218
bacterial, as common cold complication,
198
in burns patients, 519
in cancer, 577
chronic suppurative (CSOM), 220, 226
anaerobic gram-negative bacilli,
983
bacteriology, 226, 226t
Bifidobacterium causing, 991–992
diagnosis, 226, 226b
otitis externa with, 226
pathogenesis, 226
Proteus, Providencia and *Morganella*
causing, 812
Pseudomonas aeruginosa, 226–227,
843t
treatment, 226–227, 1496–1498,
1497t
conjunctivitis with *see* Conjunctivitis-
otitis syndrome
Corynebacterium species, 760t–761t
with effusion (OME), 215–216, 220
comorbid conditions, 220b
human parainfluenza virus infection
complication, 1123, 1123f
neonatal, 540–541
nontuberculous mycobacteria causing,
790
recurrent
chemoprophylaxis, 74t, 75, 219
ciliary dysfunction syndromes, 638
evaluation, 218–219
prevention, 219–220
vaccination, 219–220, 219t
RSV infection, 1131, 1133
Otitis-prone child, 215
Otopathogens, bacterial, 214
antibiotic sensitivity/resistance, 217–218
nasopharyngeal colonization,
217–218

colonization and recurrent otitis media, 219–220
treatment selection, 216–217
Otorrhea, 215–216, 291
chronic, after acute otitis media, 215–216
chronic mastoiditis and CSOM, 226
CSF see Cerebrospinal fluid (CSF)
in mastoiditis, 223
in meningitis, 287, 290–291
in necrotizing otitis externa, 221
Ototoxicity, aminoglycosides, 1474
Outbreaks
identification, 7
investigations, 7
Outcome variables, 9
Outpatient therapy, convalescent, antibiotics, 1415
"Owl's eye" inclusions, 1044
Oxacillin
dosage, 1480t–1484t
MICs, 1379t
pharmacology, 1453t–1458t
resistance, 1425
detection, 1431–1432
spectrum of activity, 1459t–1463t
susceptibility testing, 1380–1381
treatment of
endocarditis, 262t–263t
eye infections, 1494t–1496t
infections in phagocyte disorders, 624t
Oxamniquine, 1525
Schistosoma (schistosomiasis), 1370
Oxantel, Trichuris trichiura infections, 1331
Oxazolidinones, 1475
mechanism of action, 1475
pharmacodynamic properties, 1414t
pharmacology, 1453t–1458t
spectrum of activity, 1459t–1463t
Oxazolines, enterovirus infection treatment, 1180
Oxiconazole, superficial infection treatment, 1485, 1485t
Oxygen
arterial tension (PaO$_2$), Pneumocystis jirovecii (carinii) infection, 1230, 1233
saturation assessment, in pneumonia, 240
supplemental, laryngotracheitis (croup), 211–212
Oxygen-reducing potential, anaerobes, 959
Oxygen therapy
bronchiolitis, 234
hyperbaric see Hyperbaric oxygen (HBO)
laryngotracheitis therapy, 211–212
in RSV infection, 1132–1133
Oxytetracycline, Mycoplasma pneumoniae infections, 997
Oysters, Vibrio infections associated, 856
Ozena, 799

P

P-selectin, Anaplasma phagocytophilum binding to, 893

P value, 2f, 5
p24 antigen see under Human immunodeficiency virus (HIV)/AIDS
p53, inactivation by HPV, 1071
p75 neurotrophin receptor (p75NTR), 1145
Pacemakers
endocarditis pathogenesis, 258–259
infections associated, 596
Paecilomyces, 1210–1211
Pain
abdominal see Abdominal pain
back see Back pain
chest see Chest pain
epigastric, Clonorchis and Opisthorchis infections, 1365
facial, unilateral, 323
limb see Limb pain
musculoskeletal see Musculoskeletal pain
nasal, rhinocerebral mucormycosis, 1213
pelvic see Pelvic pain
phrenic, 173
scrotal see Scrotal pain
vertebral, site and radiation, 171
see also individual causes of pain
Palatal petechiae, 111
Palifermin, 194
Palivizumab, 42
bronchiolitis prevention, 235
RSV infection prevention, 42, 241, 1133–1134
Palpation, abdomen, in acute abdominal pain, 172
Pancreatic abscess, 426
Pancreatic injury, 410
Pancreatitis
acute, 410–411
burns patients, 519
clinical course, 411
clinical features, 173, 410
diagnosis, 410
differential diagnosis, 410–411
fever in, 173
mumps virus, 411
pathogenesis, 410
treatment, 411
acute abdominal pain, 171, 173
chronic, abdominal pain, 176
Cryptosporidium infections, 1270
enteroviruses causing, 1177
hemorrhagic, 173
hereditary, 411
mumps virus infection, 411, 1127
in Mycoplasma pneumoniae infections, 994t
necrotizing, 411
traumatic, 411
vomiting in, 171
Pancytopenia, 1404
PANDAS, 73, 706
Panencephalitis, late-onset progressive, congenital rubella, 1115–1116
Paneth cells, α-defensin release, 84
Panophthalmitis, Clostridium perfringens, 981
Pantoea, 804–806
Pantoea agglomerans, 804
Pantoea dispersa, 804
Panton–Valentine leukocidin, 676

Panton–Valentine leukocidin-producing Staphylococcus aureus see Staphylococcus aureus
Papanicolaou (Pap) smears
HPV infections, 1071–1073
HSV identification, 1033
Trichomonas vaginalis diagnosis, 360
Papilledema
in acute bacterial meningitis, 273–274
headache with, 171
Papillomaviridae, 1016t
infections, 1017t
see also Human papillomavirus (HPV)
Papoviridae, 1075
Papular acrodermatitis see Gianotti–Crosti syndrome (papular acrodermatitis)
Papular-purpuric gloves and socks syndrome (PPGSS), 1089
Papules, 427t, 436, 449–454
in cutaneous anthrax, 751–752
in cutaneous leishmaniasis, 1288–1289
erythematous, 435–436
etiology and pathogenesis, 436
in Gianotti-Crosti syndrome, 453
infectious causes, 450–451, 450t
in Klebsiella (Calymmatobacterium) granulomatis infection, 803
in molluscum contagiosum, 450–453
Mycobacterium causing, 449
noninfectious causes, 451t
in primary syphilis, 942
in Rickettsia akari infection, 934
sterile, 452t
Papulonecrotic tuberculids, 779
Papulovesicular acro-located syndrome, 453
Para-aminosalicylic acid (PAS)
dosage, 1445t–1452t
tuberculosis treatment, 782
Parabasal cells, HPV infection, 1071
Paracoccidioides
generalized lymphadenopathy, 130, 131t–132t
mediastinal lymphadenopathy, 154
meningitis, 280t
Paracoccidioides brasiliensis, inflammatory enteritis, 384–385
Paracoccidioidomycosis see Paracoccidioides
Paragonimus (paragonimiasis), 1366–1368, 1367f
cerebral paragonimiasis, 1367–1368
Paragonimus africanus, 1367
Paragonimus kellicotti, 1367
Paragonimus mexicanus, 1367
Paragonimus skrjabini, 1367–1368
Paragonimus westermani, 1367, 1367f
eosinophilic meningitis, 331t
Parainfectious neurologic syndromes, 314–319
Parainfluenza viruses see Human parainfluenza viruses (HPIVs)
Paralysis
bladder, poliovirus causing, 1170
facial see Facial palsy/paralysis
flaccid, West Nile virus, 1101
foodborne botulism, 399
foodborne disease, 399
poliomyelitis, 1170
rabies, 1147

soft palate, *Corynebacterium diphtheriae*, 756–757
tetanospasmin causing, 967
vocal cord, 165
Paralytic disorders, acute *see* Botulism; Poliovirus
Paralytic shellfish poisoning (PSP), 373, 396t, 399
management, 399
Parameningeal infections
manifesting as chronic meningitis, 280b
recurrent meningitis associated, 288b
Paramyxoviridae, 1016t, 1121–1124, 1137–1144
arthritis due to, 481b
infections, 1017t
see also Human metapneumovirus (hMPV); Human parainfluenza viruses (HPIVs); Mumps virus; Respiratory syncytial virus (RSV); Rubeola virus (measles)
Paramyxoviruses, aseptic meningitis due to, 294
Paranasal sinuses
air–fluid level, 228–229, 231f
anatomy, 227, 231f, 506–507, 507f
aspiration in sinusitis, 229–231
bacterial contamination during nose-blowing, 198, 227
brain abscess pathogenesis, 322
in cancer, 577
in common colds, 198
drainage and sinusitis pathogenesis, 227
endoscopic surgery, 231
fracture through, recurrent meningitis, 288
infections, in cancer, 577
maxillary, 231f
Aspergillus infection, 1204, 1204f
normal physiology, 227
phaeohyphomycosis, 1211
pressure, 227
rhinocerebral mucormycosis, 1213
secretion retention, 227
tumors, 577
see also Sinusitis
Paraneoplastic limbic encephalitis, 178–179
Paraneoplastic syndrome, ataxia in, 180
Paraneoplastic vasculitis, 108
Parapharyngeal abscess, 207–208
clinical features, 206t, 207
diagnosis, 207
etiology, epidemiology and pathogenesis, 207
lateral, 207–208
management, prognosis, 208
Parapharyngeal space, 207
Parapneumonic effusion, 241–243
clinical features and radiology, 242, 242f
complicated (CPPE), 241
diagnosis and laboratory findings, 242–243
etiologic agents, 241–242
management, 243
Mycoplasma pneumoniae infection, 994
necrotizing pneumonia complication, 244

pathogenesis and pathology, 242
prognosis, 243
uncomplicated (UPPE), 241
Parapoxvirus, 1020t, 1024
epidemiology, 1024
molluscum contagiosum, 352
Parasites
Archeozoa, 1254–1255, 1254b–1255b, 1255t
classification, 1254–1256
evolutionary transition, 1255
helminths *see* Helminths
laboratory diagnosis, 1382–1384
laboratory testing, 308t–311t
protozoa *see* Protozoa
specimen collection and processing, 1382–1383
see also individual parasites
Parasitic animalia *see* Nematodes (roundworms); Platyhelminthes (flatworms)
Parasitic infections
burden, disability adjusted life years (DALYs), 1254–1255
eosinophilia, 1407, 1408t–1409t
fever of unknown origin, 119t–120t
group childcare and, 25t
intestinal, refugee and internationally adopted children, 35–36
as neglected diseases, 1254–1255
neutropenia associated with cancer, 568
precautions for travelers, 76
Parasitology, 1254
Paraspinal abscess, *Mycobacterium tuberculosis*, 778
Paratracheal lymph nodes, 148–149
tuberculosis, 151–153
Paratracheal lymphadenopathy, 151f
Paravaccinia virus, 1020t
Parechoviruses *see* Human parechovirus(es)
Parenteral nutrition, infection risk, 590
Parents, responsibility over immunizations, 52
Paresthesia, *Angiostrongylus cantonensis* causing, 1337
Parietal lobe abscess, clinical features, 322–323, 322b
Parinaud oculoglandular syndrome *see under Bartonella henselae*
Paromomycin, 1474
spectrum of activity, 1459t–1463t
treatment of
cutaneous leishmaniasis, 1290
Entamoeba histolytica (amebiasis), 1277
Giardia intestinalis (giardiasis), 1281t, 1282
protozoan infections, 1519
visceral leishmaniasis, 1290, 1290t
Paronychia, 432
Paronychial infections, 524
Parotid gland
acute suppurative sialadenitis, 195
calculi, 143
enlargement, 136, 143, 194–195
infections, 195
masses, 143

swelling, mumps virus infection, 1126, 1126f
tumors, 142t, 143
Parotid lymph nodes, 136t
Parotitis, 195–196
acute, enteroviruses causing, 1177
differential diagnosis, 1126f, 1127
granulomatous, 196
juvenile recurrent, 195–196
mumps virus infection, 294–295, 411, 1125–1127, 1126f
mycobacterial and fungal, 195
neonatal, 195
recurrent acute, 195
suppurative, 195
viral, 195
Paroxysmal lateralizing epileptiform discharges (PLEDs), 1030
Parrot fever *see Chlamydophila (Chlamydia) psittaci*
Parv4/5 viruses, 1087
Parvoviridae, 1016t
infections, 1017t
Parvovirus(es), 1087–1091
adeno-associated virus, 1087
arthritis due to, 481b
human bocavirus, 1087
Parv4/5, 1087
see also Parvovirus B19
Parvovirus B19, 1087–1091
acute bilateral cervical lymphadenitis due to, 139
antibodies, 1088, 1091, 1397
arthritis due to, 481
cardiac insufficiency in neonate, 547
chronic bone marrow failure, 1088f, 1089
chronic fatigue syndrome pathogenesis, 1008t–1009t
clinical manifestations, 1089–1091, 1089t, 1090b–1091b
congenital infection, 41, 544–545
clinical features, 537t
diagnosis, 538t, 1398
culture, 1091
diagnosis/detection, 1091, 1091b, 1397
optimal tests, 1389t–1392t
PCR, 1088, 1091
DNA, 1088, 1091, 1397
epidemiology, 1088–1089, 1091b
erythema infectiosum due to, 436, 1088f, 1089, 1089t, 1090f, 1091b
exposure management in pregnant healthcare worker, 22t–23t
generalized lymphadenopathy, 130, 131t–132t
group childcare and, 25t, 28–29
in adults attending/care providers, 31
hydrops fetalis due to, 546–547, 1089–1091, 1089t
immune globulin intravenous (IGIV) use, 41
laboratory testing, 308t–311t
papular-purpuric gloves and socks syndrome (PPGSS), 1089
pathogenesis, 1088, 1088f, 1091b
petechiae due to, 443

polyarthropathy syndrome due to, 1089, 1089t
  in pregnancy, 28–29, 1089–1091
  pure red cell aplasia due to, 1089, 1089t, 1091
  rash due to, 436
  receptor (globoside), 1088
  in sickle-cell disease, 636
  spontaneous abortion/stillbirth, 546–547
  structure and replication, 1088
  transient aplastic crisis, 1088f, 1089, 1089t, 1091
  transient reticulocytopenia, 1404
  transient synovitis, 485–486
  transmission, 1088–1089, 1091
  treatment and prevention, 1091, 1091b
  viremia, 1088, 1091
Passive immunization, 37–44
  antibodies acquired by neonates, 87
  background to, 37
  definition, 44
  in HIV infection, 663
  HSCT recipients, 566
  indications, 37
  infections in neutropenia in cancer, 572–573
  Streptococcus pneumoniae, 728
  see also Immune globulin/immunoglobulin (human Ig)
Passive surveillance, 1
Pasteurella, 835–839
  bite wound infections, 521–522, 526
  classification changes, 835
  clinical manifestations, 837
  growth and culture, 836
  lymphangitis due to, 161
  microbiology and epidemiology, 835–836
  treatment of infections, 838–839
  virulence factors, 836
Pasteurella aerogenes, 835, 837
Pasteurella bettyae, 835, 837
Pasteurella caballi, 521–522
Pasteurella canis, 835, 837
  bite wound infections, 521, 523
  lymphangitis due to, 161
Pasteurella dagmatis, 835, 837
Pasteurella gallinarum, 835
Pasteurella hemolytica, 835
Pasteurella multocida, 835
  acute unilateral cervical lymphadenitis, 140
    management, 147t
  animal bite infections, 521, 523, 836
  brain abscess, 837
  growth and culture, 836
  human bite wound infections, 523
  lymphangitis due to, 161, 161t
  meningitis due to, 837
  pneumonia due to, 837
  preseptal cellulitis due to, 509
  skin infection after trauma, 514
  treatment of infections, 838–839
Pasteurella pneumotropica, 835, 837
Pasteurella stomatis, 835, 837
Pasteurella tularensis see Francisella tularensis (Pasteurella tularensis) (tularemia)

Pasteurellaceae, 835, 906
Pastia lines, 201
Pastia sign, 112
Patches (skin), 427t
Patellofemoral pain syndrome, 186
Pathogen-associated molecular pattern (PAMP), 84, 92–93, 93f, 102
Pathogen-associated molecular patterns (PAMPs), 45
Pathogen receptors, 84
Pathogenicity island
  Burkholderia cepacia, 847
  cytotoxin-associated gene (cag) see Helicobacter pylori
  Enterococcus virulence factors, 713
Pathogens
  group childcare infections, 24–30, 25t
  receptors for, 84
  recognition by innate immune system, 84
  see also individual micro-organisms
Patient placement
  standard precautions, 18t
  transmission-based precaution, 19t
Patient position
  in acute abdominal pain, 172
  tripod, in acute epiglottitis, 210
Pattern recognition receptors (PRRs), 45, 92–93, 102
Paul–Bunnell heterophil test, 1061–1062
PCP see Pneumocystis jirovecii (carinii), pneumonia
PCR see Polymerase chain reaction (PCR)
PCV7 see Streptococcus pneumoniae, pneumococcal conjugate vaccine, 7 valent (PCV7)
Peak plasma concentration, of drugs, 1434
Pediarix, 58t
Pediatric autoimmune neuropsychiatric disorders associated with streptococcus (PANDAS), 73, 706
Pediculosis, 1257–1259, 1259b
  clinical manifestations, 1257, 1257f–1258f
  diagnosis, 1257
  epidemiology, 1257, 1259b
  group childcare and, 25t
  microbiology, 1257, 1259b
  pathogenesis, 1257
  prevention, 1259
  refugee and internationally adopted children, 36
  treatment, 1258–1259, 1258t, 1259b
    alternative agents, 1259
    second-line treatments, 1259
    toxic effects of pesticides, 1259
    treatment of choice, 1258–1259
  virulence, 1257
  see also Phthirus pubis (crab louse) infestation
Pediculus humanus capitis (head louse) infestation, 1257, 1257f
  clinical manifestations, 1257
  diagnosis, 1257, 1257f–1258f
  epidemiology, 1257
  group childcare settings and, 30
  not involved in epidemic typhus, 931
  pathogenesis, 1257

prevention, 1259
  treatment, 1258–1259, 1258t
Pediculus humanus corporis, louse-borne relapsing fever transmission, 930, 957
Pediculus humanus humanus (body louse) infestation, 1257, 1257f
  clinical manifestations, 1257, 1257f
  epidemiology, 1257
  treatment, 1258–1259, 1258t
  vectors for Rickettsia prowazekii, 930
Pediococcus, 729
  biochemical differentiation, 729t
  vancomycin resistance, 1429
Pediococcus acidilactici, 729
Pediococcus pentosaceus, 729
Pegylated interferon see Interferon(s), pegylated
Pegylated interferons, 1515–1516
Pelvic inflammatory disease (PID), 346t, 363–366
  abdominal pain, 173
  adolescents, 353
  bacterial vaginosis and, 361, 364
  cervicitis and, 361–363
  Chlamydia trachomatis, 346t, 348, 363–364, 885t, 886
  clinical manifestations, 173, 348, 364, 364b
  complications and sequelae, 366
  diagnosis, 364
  diagnostic criteria, 174b, 364b
  differential diagnosis, 365b, 365t
  endocervicitis complication, 363
  epidemiology, 353, 363
  etiology/infections associated, 173, 363–364
    mono-microbial/polymicrobial phases, 364
  laboratory findings and diagnosis, 364–365, 365t
  management, 365–366, 366b
  morbidity, 353
  Mycoplasma genitalium causing, 999
  Neisseria gonorrhoeae causing, 346t, 348, 363–364, 747
  pain, 173, 364
  pathogenesis and pathology, 364
  prevention, 366
  recurrence, 365
  risk factors, 363–364
  sexually transmitted infection causing, 346t, 348
  silent, 363–364
  urethritis complication, 356
Pelvic pain
  chronic, prostatitis, 369
  pelvic inflammatory disease, 364
  sexually transmitted infection, 346t, 348–349
Pelvis, osteomyelitis, 186, 474–475
  fever of unknown origin due to, 119t–120t
Pemphigus syphiliticus, 943
Penciclovir
  resistance to, 1503t
  spectrum of activity, 1504t
  topical, 1510
Pendred syndrome, 289

Penicillin(s), 1465–1467
  allergy, acute otitis media treatment, 218, 219t
  aminopenicillins see Aminopenicillins
  cephalosporins vs, GAS pharyngitis, 204
  dosage, 1480t–1483t
    GAS pharyngitis treatment, 204
    in renal failure, 1445t–1452t
  extended-spectrum see Extended-spectrum penicillins
  natural, 1459t–1463t, 1465–1466
    clinical uses, 1465
    pharmacokinetics, 1465
    spectrum of activity, 1459t–1463t, 1465
  penicillinase-resistant see Penicillinase-resistant penicillin
  pharmacodynamics, 1414t
  pharmacology, 1453t–1458t
  prophylaxis
    meningococcal disease, 69
    in sickle-cell disease, 636
    Streptococcus pneumoniae infections, 728
  resistance, 204, 941
    Bacteroides fragilis group, 982
    Enterococcus, 714–715
    Leuconostoc, 730
    in meningitis, 275–276
    Neisseria meningitidis, 736–737
    Staphylococcus aureus, 676–677
    Staphylococcus epidermidis, 693–694
    Streptococcus pneumoniae, 724–725, 724t, 1425
    viridans group streptococci, 718
  spectrum of activity, 1459t–1463t
  structure, 1465f
  treatment of, 940
    Actinobacillus actinomycetemcomitans infections, 940
    Actinomyces infection, 991
    acute bacterial meningitis, 725
    acute pyogenic lymphadenitis, 162
    Arcanobacterium haemolyticum infections, 751
    chronic mastoiditis, 227
    Corynebacterium diphtheriae infections, 757–758
    endocarditis, 718, 719t, 1418t–1419t
    Erysipelothrix rhusiopathiae infections, 768
    GAS pharyngitis, 203–204, 204t
    groups C and G streptococcal infections, 721
    Pasteurella multocida infections, 838
    Rothia dentocariosa infections, 768
    Staphylococcus aureus infections, 686
    Streptobacillus moniliformis (rat-bite fever), 939
    Streptococcus agalactiae (group B streptococcus) infections, 709
    Streptococcus bovis infection, 719
    viridans group streptococcal infections, 718–719, 719t
  types, 1465
Penicillin, benzathine (bicillin)
  in acute rheumatic fever (ARF), 704, 705t
  allergy, Treponema pallidum infections, 947
  chemoprophylactic use, 70t–71t, 73
  GAS carrier management, 205
  GAS pharyngitis treatment, 203–204, 204t
  nonvenereal Treponema infections, 949
  Treponema pallidum subsp. pallidum (syphilis), 945–946, 947t
    congenital, 946–947
  see also Penicillin G, benzathine
Penicillin-binding proteins (PBPs), 1463
  β-lactamase resistance, 1422t, 1424–1425, 1431
  PBP 2, in meningococcal infections, 736–737
  viridans group streptococci, 718
Penicillin G
  chemoprophylactic use, 70t–71t, 74t
  clinical uses, 1465
  dosage, 1445t–1452t, 1480t–1484t
  pharmacology, 1453t–1458t, 1465
  spectrum of activity, 1459t–1463t, 1465
  Streptococcus agalactiae (group B streptococcus) prevention, 711
  treatment of
    acute bacterial meningitis, 276–277
    anaerobic gram-positive coccal infections, 989
    Clostridium perfringens gas gangrene, 982
    Clostridium tetani infections, 969t
    endocarditis, 262t–263t, 263
    eye infections, 1494t–1495t
    group A streptococcal infections, 702
    Leptospira infections, 951
    meningococcal meningitis, 276, 736
    necrotizing fasciitis, 514
    neonatal meningitis, 543
    in pneumococcal pneumonia, 726
    Treponema pallidum subsp. pallidum (syphilis), 946–947, 947t
  see also Procaine penicillin G
Penicillin G, benzathine
  dosage, 1483t–1484t
  pharmacology, 1465
  spectrum of activity, 1459t–1463t
  see also Penicillin, benzathine (bicillin)
Penicillin V, 1465
  chemoprophylactic use, 73–74, 74t
  dosage, 1480t–1483t
  pharmacology, 1453t–1458t
  spectrum of activity, 1459t–1463t
  Streptococcus pyogenes infection treatment, 162
Penicillinase-resistant penicillin, 1453t–1458t, 1466–1467, 1480t–1483t
  clinical uses, 1467
  dosage, 1480t–1483t
  pharmacology, 1453t–1458t
Penicillium, 1210–1211
Penicillium chrysogenum, 1465
Penile ulcers, Klebsiella (Calymmatobacterium) granulomatis, 803f
Pentamidine, 1520
  treatment of
    Babesia infections, 1265
    leishmaniasis, 1520
    Pneumocystis jirovecii pneumonia, 1520
    Trypanosoma brucei infection, 1322, 1322t, 1520
Pentamidine isethionate
  adverse reactions, 1232
  Pneumocystis jirovecii (carinii) infections, 1232, 1232t
Pentavalent antimony
  cutaneous leishmaniasis, 1290
  Leishmania resistance, 1289
  side effects, 1290
  visceral leishmaniasis, 1290, 1290t
Pentosan polysulfate (PPS), in prion diseases, 338
Pentoxifylline, in sepsis, 101t–102t
Peptic ulcer
  Helicobacter pylori infection, 175–176
  recurrent abdominal pain due to, 175–176
  see also Gastroduodenal ulcer disease
Peptidoglycan, 673, 676, 698
Peptococcus, anaerobic cellulitis, 461
Peptostreptococcus, 962, 988
  anaerobic cellulitis due to, 461
  antibiotic susceptibility, 966t
  appendicitis due to, 420
  peritonsillar abscess, 205–206
  viral nasopharyngitis due to, 163
Percussion, abdomen, in acute abdominal pain, 172
Percutaneous aspiration, injection, respiration (PAIR), hydatid cysts, 1358, 1360
Perforin, 87, 104–105
  defect, infection-associated hemophagocytic syndrome, 1065
  deficiency, in familial HLH, 104–105, 104t
  release, 104–105
Perianal abscess, 458
Perianal cellulitis, in cancer, 578–579
Perianal dermatitis, 429
Perianal infections, Enterobius vermicularis, 1331–1332
Perianal pruritus see Anal pruritus
Periapical abscess, 191
Periappendiceal abscess, Rothia dentocariosa role, 768
Pericardial effusion
  chest pain with, 189
  management, 271
  noninfectious causes, 270
Pericardial fluid, 269
  examination in pericarditis, 270
  in Histoplasma capsulatum infections, 1225–1226
  removal/drainage, 271
Pericardial friction rub, 270, 776
  enteroviruses causing, 1177
Pericardial inflammation see Pericarditis
Pericardiectomy, 271
Pericardiocentesis, 271
Pericarditis, 268–271
  acute, tuberculosis, 775–776
  in acute rheumatic fever, 703
  adenovirus infections, 1069
  bacterial, 269

chest pain, 189, 190t
clinical features, 269–270
complications, 271
constrictive, 268–269
Corynebacterium species, 760t–761t
definition, 268
differential diagnosis, 270
    myocarditis *vs.*, 266–267
enteroviruses causing, 268–270
epidemiology, 269
etiology, 268–269
    noninfectious, 268
fungal, 269
    management, 271
Haemophilus influenzae type b, 269, 271
laboratory finding and diagnosis,
    270–271
management, 271, 271t
mortality, 271
Mycobacterium tuberculosis, 268–269, 776
pathogenesis, 269
purulent, 268–269
    causes, 269, 269t
    cough in, 167t
    Haemophilus influenzae type b (Hib),
        902
    management, 271t
    treatment, 1418t–1419t
recurrence, 271
serofibrinous, 776
Staphylococcus aureus, 269, 271t, 683
tuberculous, 268–270
viral, 268–270
Pericardium
    anatomy, 269
    biopsy, tuberculosis, 776
    granulomas, 269
Pericoronitis, 191
Pericystectomy, hydatid cysts (*Echinococcus
    granulosus*), 1358–1359
Perihepatitis, acute (Fitz-Hugh–Curtis
    syndrome), 747
Perinatal care, sources of healthcare-
    associated infections, 13–14
Perinatal infections
    Campylobacter, 877, 879
    Campylobacter fetus, 879
    Chlamydia trachomatis, 885
    epidemiology, 536
    HSV, 1031, 1034
    Listeria monocytogenes, 764
    viral, epidemiology, 545, 545t
    see also Infant(s); Neonatal infections
Perinephric (perirenal) abscess, 344, 425
Periocular cellulitis, 509
Periodic fever syndromes
    differentiating features, 122t
    see also Fever, periodic
Periodic fever with aphthous stomatitis,
    pharyngitis and adenitis (PFAPA)
    syndrome, 108, 121–124
    cervical lymphadenopathy in, 141
    clinical features, 122, 122t–123t
    diagnosis, 122
    differential diagnosis, 122t
    epidemiology, 122, 123t
    ESR elevation, 1401
    etiology, 122

first description of, 122
mutations, 124
oral mucosal features, 193t
outcome/resolution, 123
treatment, 123
Periodontal abscess
    anaerobic gram-positive cocci causing,
        989
    anaerobic infections after, 140
    management, 138
Periodontal bacteria, 191
Periodontal infections, 191
Periodontitis, 191
    anaerobic gram-negative bacilli, 983
    in cyclic neutropenia, 123–124
    early-onset, 191
    in immunodeficiency, 194
    juvenile, 191
Periodontium, 191
Periorbital cellulitis, 110, 507, 679
    bacteremic, 509–510
    see also Preseptal cellulitis
Periorbital edema
    Bordetella pertussis infection, 870f
    Trichinella spiralis infections, 1341
Periorbital infections, 506–512
    differential diagnosis, 506
    pathogenesis, 506–507
Periostitis
    Actinomyces, 991
    congenital syphilis, 943
Periostitis ossificans (Garré sclerosing
    osteomyelitis), 196
Peripheral blood mononuclear cells
    (PBMCs), culture, HHV-6 diagnosis,
    1393–1394
Peripheral intravascular catheters
    in cancer, neutropenia and infections,
        568
    changing, infection risk, 11–12
Peripheral neuropathy, hypotonia, 181t
Peripherally inserted central catheters
    (PICCs), 589–590
    in cancer, neutropenia and infections,
        568
Periporitis (sweat gland abscess), 457–458
Periporitis staphylogenes, 457–458
Perirectal abscess, 458
Perirenal (perinephric) abscess, 425
Peritoneal catheters
    infections, 597–598
    removal, 598
Peritoneal dialysis
    antibiotic dose adjustment, 1445t–1452t
    continuous ambulatory *see* Continuous
        ambulatory peritoneal dialysis
        (CAPD)
    infection risk, 637
    infections associated, 597–598
    pharmacokinetics, 1436–1437, 1436t
Peritoneal fluid
    culture, necrotizing enterocolitis, 390
    specimen collection/analysis, 1377–1378
Peritonitis, 414–419
    abdominal pain, 171–172, 417
    abdominal trauma association, 514
    ascites association, 638
    Bacteroides, 416–417

in burns patients, 519
in cancer, 578
catheter-related, 415–416, 415t–416t
    management, 417–419, 418t
    prevention, 419
    Staphylococcus epidermidis causing, 693
Cellulosimicrobium, 771
clinical features, 417
coagulase-negative staphylococci, 693
complications and prognosis, 419
    CNS device infection, 597
in continuous ambulatory peritoneal
    dialysis, 414–417, 418f
diagnosis, 417
epidemiology, 414–415
Escherichia coli, 415
etiology, 415–417, 416t
fecal, 419
fungal, 416–418
Haemophilus influenzae, 416
infectious, 414
management, 417–419, 418f
mortality, 419
Mycobacterium bovis, 415–416
Mycobacterium tuberculosis, 415–416,
    777–778
Neisseria gonorrhoeae, 416
neonatal, 416–417
    nosocomial, 550
neonatal idiopathic primary, 415
in nephrotic syndrome, 415
pathophysiology, 415, 415t
peritoneal dialysis catheter-associated,
    598
    Staphylococcus epidermidis causing, 693
prevention, 419
primary (spontaneous) bacterial, 415,
    415t–416t, 417–419
    ascites, 638
    in cancer, 578
    etiology, 415–416
    management, 417–419, 638
Pseudomonas, 416
relapsing, 418–419
Rothia dentocariosa, 768
secondary bacterial, 414, 415t–416t,
    416–417
    management, 419
Staphylococcus aureus, 416
Staphylococcus epidermidis, 693
Streptococcus pneumoniae, 415
    ascites, 638
Peritonsillar abscess, 138, 165, 205–207
    clinical features, 206, 206t
    diagnosis, 206
    epidemiology, pathogenesis, 206
    etiology, 205–206
    Fusobacterium, 986–987
    treatment and complications, 206–207
Permethrin
    chemoprophylactic use, 70t–71t
    insecticide, 81
    treatment of
        pediculosis, 1259
        scabies, 1260
Person, place or time, describing illness by,
    2
Personal protective equipment (PPE), 17

Pertussis *see Bordetella pertussis*
Pertussis-like illness, adenoviruses, 1068t, 1069
Pet(s), 526–531
    bites *see* Bites, infections after
    categories, 527
    exotic, 527
    exposure to/households with, 526–527
    infections related to, 526–531
        from nontraditional pets, 527
        prevention, 530–531
    injuries from, 529
        prevention, 530–531
    nontraditional, 527, 527t
        fish, 528
        healthcare professional/veterinarian input, 530–531
        injuries from, 529
        nonhuman primates, 528
        other sources of infection, 528
        recommendations and guidelines, 531
        reportable diseases from, 529–530
        reptiles, 528
        risks associated, 527
        rodents, 528
        zoonoses associated, 527–528
        see also Zoonotic infections
    prevention of HAIs and, 19–21
    traditional, 527
    see also Cat(s), infections related to; Dog(s), infections related to; Zoonotic infections
Pet foods, contaminated, infections from, 528
Pet treats, contaminated, infections from, 528
Petechiae
    EBV infection, 1061
    etiology, 441–444
    palatal, 443
    pathogenesis, 442
    Rocky Mountain spotted fever (*Rickettsia rickettsii*), 926–927
Petechial hemorrhages, *Trichinella spiralis* infections, 1341
Peyer patches, 129
    hypertrophy, 174
PFAPA *see* Periodic fever with aphthous stomatitis, pharyngitis and adenitis (PFAPA) syndrome
Phaeohyphomycosis, 1209–1212, 1212b
    clinical manifestations, 1211, 1212b
    diagnosis, 1211–1212, 1212b
    epidemiology, 1211, 1212b
    microbiology, 1211–1212, 1212b
    neutropenia associated with cancer, 567
    treatment and prevention, 1212, 1212b
Phagocytic cells, 84–85, 619
    adherence, 617t
    chemotaxis, 617t
    cord blood, bacterial killing by, 85
    defects/dysfunction, infections, 85, 619–626
        characteristics, 619t
        clinical approach, 621
        clinical manifestations, 620, 621t
        complications, 620t, 623

detection, 608t
identification of infection site/agent, 620t, 621
identification of infectious agent, 621
immunizations in, 52t–53t
infection etiology, 620–621, 620t
infectious complications, 620t
management, 621–623
pathology, 620
patterns of illness, 621t
persistent/recurrent pneumonia, 251
prevention of infections, 624, 624t
prognosis and sequelae, 623–624
prophylactic antibiotics, 624t
recent advances, 624
RSV infection, 1133
specific treatment, 622–623
surgical prophylaxis, 624t
tissue involvement/debridement, 621–622
development, 84
disorders, 604t–605t, 619–626, 620t
function, 85, 85f
in histiocytosis, 134
in HIV infection, 658
in lymph nodes, 127
microbicidal activity, 617t
mononuclear, 619
polymorphonuclear, 619
see also Phagocytosis; *individual cell types*
Phagocytosis, 45–46, 85
    Coccidioides immitis (coccidioidomycosis), 1239
    defective, 85
        Coccidioides immitis infection in, 1239
    of *Neisseria meningitidis*, 732
    process, 85
    toxic products produced, 85
    see also Phagocytic cells
Pharmacodynamics, 1433
    antibiotic selection and, 1413–1415, 1414t
    drug interactions, 1440, 1440t
    pharmacokinetics and
        antifungal dosage, 1443–1444, 1443t
        optimal antibiotic dosage, 1440–1443
Pharmacokinetics
    antibiotic selection and, 1413–1415
    as basis of optimal antibiotic therapy, 1433–1452
    burned patients, 1437t, 1438
    in cystic fibrosis, 1437–1438
    definition, 1433
    dialysis, 1436–1437, 1436t
    distribution in, 1435t
    drug absorption *see* Absorption, of drugs
    drug distribution *see* Distribution, drug
    drug elimination *see* Elimination, antimicrobial agents
    drug metabolism *see* Metabolism, antimicrobial agents
    drug–drug interactions, 1438–1440, 1440t
    in kidney failure, 1435
    neonates, 1435, 1435t
    in organ failure, 1435

pharmacodynamics and *see under* Pharmacodynamics
    principles, 1433–1435, 1434f
    in septic shock, 1437t, 1438
Pharmacology, antimicrobial agents, 1453t–1458t
Pharmacy, role in surveillance of HAIs, 16–17
Pharyngeal diphtheria, 201–202
Pharyngeal erythema, HHV-6 infection (roseola), 1054
Pharyngeal infections, *Neisseria gonorrhoeae*, 744
Pharyngitis, 199–205
    adenoviruses causing, 201
    Arcanobacterium haemolyticum, 199, 201, 203, 750–751
    bacterial, 199–202, 200t
    chlamydial, 200t
    Chlamydophila (Chlamydia) pneumoniae, 199
    clinical features, 200–202, 200b
        group A streptococci *vs.* viral, 200b
    Corynebacterium, 760t–761t
    Corynebacterium diphtheriae, 199, 201–202
    diagnosis, 202–203
        follow-up testing, 203
        guidelines, 202
        rapid antigen detection tests, 200, 203
        throat cultures, 202–203
    EBV infection, 199, 201, 201f–202f, 1061
    enteroviruses, 201
    epidemiology, 200
    etiology, 199, 200t
    Fusobacterium, 986–987
    Fusobacterium necrophorum, 202
    GAS (group A streptococci), 199–200, 200b, 201f, 203, 698–699, 700f
        acute glomerulonephritis after, 705
        acute rheumatic fever after, 702, 704
        antimicrobial agents, 203–204
        antimicrobial dosing and duration, 204
        apparent bacteriologic failure, 205
        carrier management, 204–205
        carrier state, 204–205
        clinical features, 200–201, 200b
        complications, 205
        diagnosis, 202–203
        monitoring of therapy, 205
        outcome, 204–205
        recurrences, 204–205
        repeated episodes, 205
        treatment, 203–204, 204t, 1418t–1419t
        treatment failure, 204–205
        treatment failure (true *vs.* apparent), 205
        viral disease *vs.*, 200b, 201–202
    gonococcal, 199–200
    group A streptococci *see Above*
    group C streptococci, 199–200, 204, 720
    group G streptococci, 199–200, 204, 720
    HSV causing, 199, 201, 1028
    influenza virus infection, 1153
    Lassa virus infection, 1161

Mycoplasma pneumoniae, 199
mycoplasmal, 200t
Neisseria gonorrhoeae, 199–200
nonexudative, streptococcal infection, 113
Streptococcus pyogenes see Pharyngitis, GAS (group A streptococci)
treatment, 203–204, 1418t–1419t
viral, 199, 200b, 200t, 201
Yersinia enterocolitica, 199
Pharyngoconjunctival fever, 201
acute bilateral cervical lymphadenitis, 138
acute follicular conjunctivitis, 492t
adenoviruses, 491, 1068t, 1069
generalized lymphadenopathy, 132
preauricular lymphadenopathy, 159
Phase variation of surface structures, *Neisseria meningitidis*, 731
Phenobarbital, in Sydenham chorea, 704
Phenol, skin antiseptic, 1499t
Phenosafranin stain, 1284
Phenoxymethylpenicillin *see* Penicillin V
Phenylephrine, in common colds, 198
Phenylethyl alcohol agar, 1375t
Pheohyphomycoses *see* Phaeohyphomycosis
Pheromones, antibiotic resistance in *Enterococcus* and, 714
Phlebitis
catheter-related complication, 593
suppurative, *Staphylococcus aureus*, 683
Phlebotomus, Leishmania transmission, 1285–1286, 1288
Phlebovirus, 1102, 1103t
Phocanema, 1339
Phoenix System, 1379–1380
Phospholipase, *Gardnerella vaginalis*, 769
Phospholipase A$_2$, 84
fever induction mechanism, 91, 91f
Photophobia
acute bacterial meningitis, 273–274
aseptic meningitis, 295
mucocutaneous syndromes, 110–111
Photorhabdus, 809
Phrenic nerve, compression, cough, 167t
Phrenic pain, 173
Phthirus pubis (crab louse) infestation, 1257, 1258f
clinical manifestations, 1257
diagnosis, 1257, 1258f
transmission, 349, 352, 1257
treatment, 1258–1259, 1258t
see also Pediculosis
Physical activity, chronic fatigue syndrome therapy, 1015
Physicians' Desk Reference (PDR), 68
Pian bois, 1289
see also Leishmania (leishmaniasis), New World
Pica, history of, *Toxocara* infections, 1334, 1336–1337
Picaridin
insect repellent, 81
Plasmodium infection prevention, 1304–1306
tick repellent, 535
Picobirnavirus, gastroenteritis, 378
Picornaviridae, 1016t, 1167–1168, 1180

arthritis due to, 481b
classification, 1167, 1168t
conjunctivitis due to, 492
description and structure, 1168, 1168b
infections, 1017t
serotypes, 1167–1168
Piedra, 1250
Piedraia hortae, 1249–1250
Pig(s), diseases related to
Balantidium coli infections, 1266–1267
Entamoeba polecki, 1278
Fasciolopsis buski infection, 1363
hepatitis E virus transmission, 1192
influenza viruses, 1150–1151, 1158
Sarcocystis infections, 1306
tapeworms (*Taenia solium*), 1350, 1351f, 1352, 1356
Trichinella spiralis, 1339, 1341
Pigbel, 981
Pigmentation of skin, postinflammatory changes, 438
Pili, *Streptococcus agalactiae* (group B streptococcus), 707
Pinna, in mastoiditis, 223
Pinta (*Treponema carateum*), 941, 949
Pintids, 949
Pinworm *see Enterobius vermicularis*
Piperacillin
eye infection treatment, 1494t–1495t
pharmacology, 1453t–1458t
spectrum of activity, 1459t–1463t
Piperacillin-tazobactam
clinical uses, 1467
dosage, 1445t–1452t, 1483t–1484t
dose adjustment
burned patients, 1437t
renal failure, 1445t–1452t
spectrum of activity, 1459t–1463t, 1467
treatment of
acute mastoiditis, 227
Klebsiella infections, 802
Piperazine, 1525
Ascaris lumbricoides infections, 1328
Piperonal, as head louse repellent, 1259
Piperonyl butoxide, pediculosis treatment, 1259
Piroplasmidora, 1261
Pituitary hormones, human, CJD from, 334
Pityriasis rosea, HHV-7 association, 1058
Pityriasis versicolor, 1249, 1249b
clinical manifestations, 1216–1217, 1249, 1249b, 1249f
diagnosis, 1217, 1249, 1249b
epidemiology, 1216, 1249b
treatment, 1217, 1249, 1249b
see also Malassezia
Pizotifen, treatment of, abdominal migraine, 176
Placenta
CMV infection/transmission, 1045
susceptibility to rubella virus, 1113
syphilis transmission, 943
Placental membranes, premature rupture *see* Premature rupture of membranes
Plague *see Yersinia pestis*
Plants, freshwater, *Fasciolopsis buski* infection due to, 1363–1364

Plaque-reduction neutralization test (PRNT), flavivirus infections, 1102
Plaques (skin lesion), 427t, 436
Plasma cells, 87
hyperplasia, 1063
Plasma-derived blood products, HCV transmission, 1107
Plasmapheresis
endotoxin removal, 101t–102t
in *Loa loa* infections, 1346
Plasmids
antimicrobial resistance, 801–802, 845, 1423
Citrobacter, 807
Enterobacter, 805
Yersinia pestis (plague), 823
Plasminogen activator inhibitor (PAI), in sepsis, 101t–102t
Plasmodium (malaria), 80, 1298–1306, 1306b
"algid" malaria, 1299–1300
cerebral malaria, 1299–1300, 1303
clinical manifestations, 83, 119t–120t, 1299–1300, 1306b
complications, 1299, 1303, 1306
description of pathogen, 1298–1299
deterioration despite therapy, 1303
diagnosis, 1300, 1306b
blood smears, 1300, 1384
epidemiology, 1299, 1306b
prevalence, 80
fever of unknown origin due to, 119t–120t
hyperparasitemia, 1299
incubation period, 1298
laboratory findings, 1300
Babesia (babesiosis) *vs.*, 1264t
life cycle, 1298, 1298f
mortality, 80, 1299–1300
nonimmune persons, clinical features in, 1299
post-travel, 83
in pregnancy, 1306
prophylaxis, 80, 1304–1306, 1305t, 1520–1522
capsules for children, 1306
chemoprophylaxis, 80–81, 1304–1306, 1305t
in pregnancy, 1306
protective measures, 81, 1304–1306
screening, refugee and internationally adopted children, 36
severe malaria
management, 1300–1303, 1300b, 1301t–1303t
manifestations, 1300b
see also Plasmodium falciparum (malaria)
thrombocytopenia in, 1410–1411
tolerance to infections, 1299
travelers, 1298–1300
prophylaxis, 1304–1306, 1305t
treatment, 1300–1304, 1301t–1303t, 1306b, 1520–1522
uncomplicated malaria, management, 1301t–1303t, 1303–1304, 1306b
Plasmodium falciparum (malaria), 1298
clinical manifestations, 1299

diagnosis, 1300
encephalitis, 304
epidemiology, 1299
genome, 1255
life cycle, 1298, 1298f
mortality, 1254–1255, 1299
prophylaxis, 1304, 1305t, 1306
treatment, 1300–1303, 1301t–1303t, 1520–1522
see also Plasmodium (malaria)
Plasmodium malariae, 1298–1299
life cycle, 1298, 1298f
treatment, 1301t–1303t, 1520–1521
see also Plasmodium (malaria)
Plasmodium ovale, 1298
life cycle, 1298, 1298f
treatment, 1301t–1303t, 1304, 1520–1521
see also Plasmodium (malaria)
Plasmodium vivax, 1298
laboratory findings, 1300
life cycle, 1298–1299, 1298f
treatment, 1301t–1303t, 1304, 1520–1522
see also Plasmodium (malaria)
Plastic surgery, cutaneous leishmaniasis, 1290
Platelet(s), 1409–1411
count, neonatal septicemia diagnosis, 541t
destruction, thrombocytopenia, 1410–1411
endothelial cell activation, 94
in hemophagocytic lymphohistiocytosis, 105
normal count, 1409
physiology and measurement, 1409
transfusions
Bacillus cereus infection after, 754
infections associated, 580, 581t
see also Thrombocytopenia
Platelet activating factor (PAF), necrotizing enterocolitis pathogenesis, 391
Platelet activating factor (PAF) acetylhydrolase (PAF-AH), 101t–102t
Platyhelminthes (flatworms), 1254–1256
classification, 1254, 1254b, 1256, 1256t
transmission modes, 1256t
see also Cestodes; Trematodes
Pleconaril
enteroviral infection treatment, 1179–1180
enteroviral meningitis treatment, 296
rhinovirus infection treatment, 1187
Pleocytosis, hemophagocytic lymphohistiocytosis, 106–107
Plesiomonas shigelloides, 810–811
clinical features, 810
cytotoxin, 810
description, 810
diagnosis, 811
epidemiology, 810
gastroenteritis, 810
pathogenesis, 810
treatment, 811
Pleura, lymphatic drainage, 148–149, 148f, 148t

Pleural disease, Mycobacterium tuberculosis infection, 776
Pleural effusion, 241–243
biochemical characteristics, 241t
Burkholderia cepacia infection causing, 848
clinical features and radiology, 242, 242f
diagnosis and laboratory findings, 242–243
Entamoeba histolytica infection, 1276
infectious agents, 241–242
management, 243
Mycoplasma pneumoniae infections, 996
noninfectious causes, 242t
pathogenesis and pathology, 242
in pneumonia, 239
prognosis and mortality, 243
Staphylococcus aureus causing, 681
transudate vs. exudate, 241, 241t
Pleural empyema see Empyema
Pleural fluid, 242
analysis, 241
fibrinopurulent, 242
in Mycobacterium tuberculosis infection, 776
pH (acidic), 242
pneumonia diagnosis, 254–255
purulent, 242
specimen collection/transport, 1374t
Pleural space, 242
Pleurisy, tuberculous, 772
Pleurodynia
chest pain, 190t
cough in, 167t
enterovirus infections, 1176
Pleuropulmonary infections
amebiasis, 1276
anaerobic gram-positive cocci causing, 989
Eikenella corrodens, 836
Pneumatoceles, 239
Staphylococcus aureus causing, 681, 682f
Pneumatosis cystoides intestinalis, 981
Pneumatosis intestinalis, 389f
Pneumococcal pneumonia see Streptococcus pneumoniae
Pneumococcal vaccines see Streptococcus pneumoniae
Pneumococcus see Streptococcus pneumoniae
Pneumocystis carinii
nomenclature, 1230
see also Pneumocystis jirovecii (carinii)
Pneumocystis jirovecii (carinii), 1230–1233
in AIDS/HIV infection, 1230–1231
pneumonia see Below
prevention, 40, 663, 669, 1233, 1233t
breakthrough infections, 1233
chemoprophylaxis, 1233, 1233t
clinical manifestations, 1230
culture not yet achieved, 1230
description and structure, 1230
eosinophilia, 1408t–1409t
epidemiology, 1230
immune response to, 1230
immunocompromised hosts, 1230
laboratory findings and diagnosis, 1230–1232, 1377

diagnostic testing for, 248
staining methods, 1231–1232, 1231f
mediastinal disease due to, 149
mediastinal lymphadenopathy due to, 154
neutropenia associated with cancer, 567
nomenclature, 1230
pneumonia (PCP), 237, 237t, 246, 248, 253–254, 663, 1230
in cancer, 576–577, 577f
clinical features, 654, 1230, 1231f
diagnosis, 254–255
diagnostic evaluation, 660–661
endemic infantile form, 1230
epidemiology, 1230
HIV infection, 653–654, 657–659, 660f, 671
HSCT recipients, 562, 564
in hyper-IgM syndromes, 613
imaging, in HIV infection, 660f
indications for prophylaxis, 663
laboratory findings/diagnosis, 1230–1232
lymphoid interstitial pneumonitis (LIP) vs., 654t
neutropenia associated with cancer, 567, 573
persistent, 246
prevention, 566, 1233, 1233t
prevention in HIV infection, 40, 663, 669, 1233, 1233t
prevention in neutropenia in cancer, 573
prognosis, 664
recurrences, in cancer, 576–577
risk factors, 1230–1231, 1233
in SCID, 627–628
solid-organ transplant recipients, 556, 560
TMP-SMX for, 663
treatment, 255, 576–577, 1232–1233, 1232t, 1520
in young infants, 169
prevention of infections, 1233, 1233t
prognosis affected by inflammation, 1230
specimen collection, 1231, 1377
transmission, 1230
treatment of infections, 1232–1233, 1232t
presumptive diagnosis, 1232
PneumoCystis pneumonia see Pneumocystis jirovecii (carinii), pneumonia (PCP)
Pneumolysin, 721
Pneumonia
acute, 235–245
definition, 235
etiology and epidemiology, 235–236
incidence, 235
acute abdominal pain in, 173
adenoviruses causing, 238, 246, 1069
adolescents, 236–237, 246
"afebrile", 169
Aspergillus causing, 246, 575–576
aspiration of bacteria causing, 236, 238
aspiration of secretions, 581
bacterial, 236–238, 723
clinical features, 238–239

diagnosis, 240
in immunodeficiency, 253, 253t
pathologic patterns, 238
Blastomyces dermatitidis, 237t, 246, 1234f, 1235, 1237
persistent pneumonia, 246
Bordetella pertussis see *Bordetella pertussis* (pertussis)
as bronchiolitis complication, 233
bronchiolitis obliterans organizing, 250
Brucella abortus, 237t
in burns patients, 519
in cancer, 575, 577
Candida, 575
chemical, 239
chest pain due to, 189, 190t
Chlamydia trachomatis, 168t, 236, 238, 240–241, 886
conjunctivitis complication, 488
cough, 167–168, 167t
in infancy, 886
Chlamydophila pneumoniae causing, 236–237, 239–240, 882
Chlamydophila psittaci causing, 237, 237t, 246, 890
Chromobacterium violaceum, 837
in chronic granulomatous disease, 622f, 624
classification, neonatal nosocomial infections, 550
clinical course, 238
clinical features, 168t, 169, 238–239
bacterial pneumonia, 238–239
infants (less than 3 months), 168t, 169, 238
older infants/children/adolescents, 169–170, 170t, 238–239
viral pneumonia, 238
CMV infection see Cytomegalovirus (CMV)
coagulase-negative staphylococci, 693
Coccidioides immitis causing, 237, 246
community-acquired, 235–237
Chlamydophila pneumoniae causing, 882
etiology, 236–237, 236t
management, 169
normal resolution, 245
persistent, 245
community-acquired necrotizing, 681, 683f
complications, 241, 245–246, 248
consolidative, 239f, 254–255, 256t
Corynebacterium species, 760t–761t
cough in, 167–169, 167t, 238
Coxiella burnetii causing, 237, 237t, 239, 246, 892
definition, 235
diagnosis, 239
of bacteria, 240
of specific etiologic agents, 240
of viruses, 239–240
differential diagnosis, 169–170, 239
EBV causing, 253, 1061
epidemiology, 235–236, 681
Escherichia coli, 236
etiologic agents, 235–236
by age, 236t

bacteria, 236–237, 236t, 240, 723
diagnosis of specific agents, 240
infants, children and adolescents, 236–237, 236t
neonates and young infants, 236, 236t
occasional pathogens, 237, 237t, 240
viruses, 236–237, 240
Francisella tularensis, 237t, 898
fungal, 246, 624
in immunodeficiency, 253, 253t
generalized lymphadenopathy in, 130, 131t–132t
giant cell, rubeola virus (measles), 1143
gonococcal, ophthalmia neonatorum complication, 489
groups C and G streptococci causing, 720
Haemophilus influenzae, 900, 902
Haemophilus influenzae type b (Hib), 237, 245–246, 900, 902
healthcare-associated, 250–251, 581–582
causative agents, 580t
coagulase-negative staphylococci causing, 693
prevention, 583b
Serratia marcescens, 813
trauma associated, 515–516
treatment, 583
Histoplasma capsulatum causing, 237, 237t, 246
in HIV infection/AIDS, 253, 660–661
bacterial pathogens, 660
diagnostic evaluation, 660–661, 660f
empiric antibiotics, 661
imaging, 660, 660f–661f
persistent, 251
hospital-associated, 235
hospitalization indications, 240
HSV infection see Herpes simplex virus (HSV)
human coronaviruses (HCoV), 236–237
human herpesvirus 6 (HHV-6), 253–254
human immunodeficiency virus (HIV)/ AIDS, 660–661
see also *Pneumocystis jirovecii (carinii)*
human metapneumovirus (hMPV), 236–237
human paraechovirus 1 (HPEV-1), 236–237
human parainfluenza viruses, 236–237, 1121, 1123–1124, 1123f
treatment, 1124
in immunocompromised patients, 239, 252–256
bacterial and fungal, 253
clinical diagnosis, 254–255, 255f
epidemiology, 252–254
etiologic agents, 253–254, 253t
immunodeficiency, 253
management and therapy, 255–256
nosocomial acquisition, 254
pathogenesis and pathology, 254
prevention, 256
radiography, 254–255, 256t
transplant recipients, 253–254
viral, 253–254
incidence, 235

infants see Pneumonia, in neonates and young infants
influenza viruses causing, 236–237, 1153, 1153t
interstitial, EBV infection, 1061
investigations, 168t
laboratory findings, 239
laboratory tests, 239
Legionella, 237, 237t, 922–923, 923t
in cancer, 575
Leptospira (leptospirosis), 237t
Leuconostoc causing, 729
Listeria monocytogenes causing, 236
lobar, 238
Löeffler
Ascaris lumbricoides causing, 1327–1328
eosinophilia, 1408t–1409t
lung transplant recipients, 558
lymphocytic interstitial, 251, 253
management, 240, 1418t–1419t
antimicrobial, 240–241
antiviral agents, 240–241, 241t
mortality, 241
Mycobacterium tuberculosis causing see *Mycobacterium tuberculosis*
Mycoplasma, 236
Mycoplasma pneumoniae causing see *Mycoplasma pneumoniae*, pneumonia
necrotizing parenchymal, 238, 243–245, 681, 683f, 983
clinical features, 244
diagnosis, 244, 244f
endocarditis complication, 264
etiologic agents, 243–245, 243t
management, 244
pathogenesis, 243–244
pneumococcal, 243
prognosis and complications, 245
Neisseria gonorrhoeae, 489
Neisseria meningitidis, 735
in neonates and young infants, 236, 236t, 547
causes and differential diagnosis, 169
differential diagnosis, 169
enteroviruses, 1179
etiology, 169, 236, 236t
nodular, 254–255, 256t
nosocomial see Pneumonia, healthcare-associated
Pasteurella multocida, 837
pathogenesis and pathology, 238
bacterial pneumonia, 238
viral pneumonia, 238
persistent, 245–252
definition, 245
differential diagnosis, 245
persistent/progressive at one site, 245–248, 245t
congenital abnormalities, 247
diagnostic approach, 247–248
extrinsic obstructing lesions causing, 247
host-related causes, 246
intraluminal obstructing lesions causing, 246–247
pathogen-related causes, 245–246

persistent/recurrent not confined to one
site, 248–252
dense focal or multifocal infiltrates,
248, 249t
diagnostic approach, 251–252
diffuse interstitial infiltrates, 249t,
251
immunological abnormalities, 249t,
251
most common causes, 249t, 252,
252t
respiratory tract anomalies, 248–251,
249t
respiratory tract disorders, 248–251
phaeohyphomycosis, 1211
Pneumocystis jirovecii (carinii) causing see
Pneumocystis jirovecii (carinii)
prevention, 241
Prevotella melaninogenica causing,
245–246
primary atypical, Mycoplasma pneumoniae
causing, 993–994
prognosis and sequelae, 241
Pseudomonas aeruginosa, 248–250, 582,
846
Pseudomonas pseudomallei, 237t
radiography, 239, 239f
rapidly progressive, Staphylococcus aureus,
681, 682f
recurrent, 245–252, 245t
anatomic/physiologic abnormalities
predisposing, 600t
bacterial, 239
CT, 248, 248f
definition, 245
diagnosis, 248
differential diagnosis, 248
most common causes, 252
not confined to one site, 248–252
see also Pneumonia, persistent/
recurrent
recurrent right middle lobe, 247
respiratory tract viruses, 168t, 236–237,
253
rhinoviruses, 236–237
Rhodococcus (Corynebacterium) equi, 769
Rothia dentocariosa, 768
RSV causing, 168t, 236–237, 241,
1131–1133
in SCID, 629
severity assessment, 238
in sickle-cell disease, 634–635
Sporothrix schenckii (sporotrichosis)
infection, 1219
Staphylococcus aureus causing, 245–246,
253, 681, 682f
Streptococcus pneumoniae, 237, 245–246,
253, 723
tuberculous, 237–239, 775f
diagnosis, 240
see also Mycobacterium tuberculosis
Ureaplasma, 236, 238
Ureaplasma urealyticum, 169
varicella, 1038–1039
varicella-zoster virus (VZV), 253–254,
1038–1039
ventilator-associated see Ventilator-
associated pneumonia (VAP)

"verminous", Ascaris lumbricoides causing,
1327–1328
viral, 236–238, 245–246
bacterial superinfection rate, 240–241
clinical features, 238
diagnosis, 239–240
in immunodeficiency, 253–254, 253t
neonatal, 547
visceral leishmaniasis complication,
1287
"walking", 994
Yersinia pestis, 826
see also Bronchopneumonia
Pneumonitis
anaerobic gram-negative bacilli infection,
983
chemical, 581
CMV infection
stem cell transplant recipients, 1048
transplant recipients, 1048
Corynebacterium species, 760t–761t
hookworm, 1329
HSCT recipients, 564, 564b
lymphocytic interstitial, 251, 253,
1063–1064
necrotizing, Mycoplasma pneumoniae
infection, 994
primary viral, rubeola virus (measles),
1143
Pneumoperitoneum, necrotizing
enterocolitis, 389–390
Pneumovirinae, 1130
Point estimate, 5
Point source exposure, 7
Poison oak, 439f
Poisoning
fish and shellfish, 396t, 397
food see Foodborne disease
heavy-metal, 395, 399
Poliomyelitis-like illness, enterovirus
infections, 1176
Poliomyelitis virus see Poliovirus
Poliovirus, 1168–1172
antibodies, 1169–1170
IgA, 1171
clinical manifestations, 1170
CNS entry, 294
CNS infection, 1168, 1170
description and structure, 1168–1169
diagnosis, 1170
optimal tests, 1389t–1392t
diseases mimicking, 1170
endemic (countries), 61
epidemiology, 1169–1170, 1169f
prevalence in US, 61, 1169
eradication, 44, 47, 1169–1170
immune response to, 1169
morbidity reduced by vaccine, 48t
paralytic polio, 1170
infant botulism vs., 974t
weakness due to, differential
diagnosis, 181t–182t
pathogenesis, 1168–1169, 1168t
in pregnancy, 1170
prevention, 1170–1171
replication site, 1168, 1168t
RNA and proteins, 1168
shedding of virus, 1168, 1170

spinal poliomyelitis, 1170
transmission, 1168, 1169f
treatment of infections, 1170
type 3 poliovirus, 1171
vaccine-associated paralytic poliomyelitis
(VAPP), 50, 61, 1170–1171
case number, 1169f, 1171
frequency and risk, 61
in X-linked agammaglobulinemia,
610–611
vaccine/vaccination see Poliovirus vaccine
Poliovirus vaccine, 61
combined schedule (eIPV then OPV),
1171–1172
efficacy, 1170–1171
enhanced-potency (eIPV), 1171
group childcare settings, 30t
inactivated (IPV), 61, 1170
adverse events and IoM findings,
50t
contraindications/precautions, 48
enhanced, 61
HSCT recipients, 566
immunocompromised travelers,
82–83
oral vaccine vs., 1170–1172
outbreaks associated, 1171
schedule, 49f, 1171–1172
for travelers, 78, 78t, 1171–1172
oral (OPV), 61, 1170
adverse events, 50–51, 61
adverse events and IoM findings, 50t
contraindications/precautions, 61,
1171–1172
failure, 1170–1171
immunocompromised travelers,
82–83
monovalent (mOPV), 1171
for travelers, 78, 78t
recommendations for, 61, 1171
vaccination
campaigns, 44
measurement of response, 46
in pregnancy, 1171–1172
schedule in US, 1171–1172
Polyarthritis, 480–481
epidemic, 481
juvenile idiopathic, limb pain, 184–185,
185t
migratory
in acute rheumatic fever, 703–704
disseminated gonococcal infection,
744
Streptobacillus moniliformis (rat-bite fever),
938–939
Polyarthropathy syndrome, parvovirus B19
causing, 1089, 1089t
Polycystic echinococcosis (Echinococcus
vogeli), 1357f, 1361
Polycythemia, 1403
Polyenes
systemic, 1486–1488, 1486t
topical, 1485, 1485t
Polymerase chain reaction (PCR), 1384
cervical lymphadenitis etiology, 135–136
CSF specimens, 1377
acute bacterial meningitis diagnosis,
274

disease/pathogen detection, 354–355
  adenoviruses, 1070
  Anaplasma and *Ehrlichia* infections, 896
  Aspergillus, 1208
  Babesia (babesiosis), 1263–1265, 1264t
  bacterial identification, 674
  BK virus, 1076
  Bordetella pertussis, 869–870
  Burkholderia pseudomallei, 848
  Candida, 1200
  Chlamydia trachomatis, 353, 1399
  Chlamydophila pneumoniae, 883, 1399
  chronic meningitis diagnosis, 286
  Clostridium botulinum, 974
  CMV infection, 1049
  coltivirus (Colorado tick fever), 1093
  Coxiella burnetii, 892
  cutaneous leishmaniasis, 1288
  Cyclospora, 1284
  EBV, 1062, 1393
  Ehrlichia and *Anaplasma*, 896
  encephalitis diagnosis, 308
  endocarditis diagnosis, 260–261
  Entamoeba histolytica, 1277
  enteroviruses, 1179
  Giardia intestinalis, 1281–1282
  Helicobacter pylori, 914, 1383
  hepatitis A virus (HAV), 1180, 1183
  hepatitis viruses, 402
  HHV-6, 1394
  HHV-7, 1394
  HHV-8, 1067, 1394
  HIV, 651t, 652–653, 1167
  HSV, 1033, 1388
  human parainfluenza viruses, 1123–1124
  infections in HSCT recipients, 565
  influenza viruses, 1154, 1394
  Legionella, 924
  Malassezia, 1216–1217
  microsporidia, 1292
  Mycobacterium tuberculosis, 781
  Mycoplasma genitalium, 999
  Mycoplasma hominis, 998–999
  Mycoplasma pneumoniae, 993–995, 1399
  Neisseria meningitidis, 736
  parvovirus B19, 1088, 1091, 1397
  Plasmodium infections, 1300
  Rickettsia akari (rickettsialpox) infection, 934
  Rickettsia felis, 933
  Rickettsia prowazekii, 931
  Rickettsia rickettsii, 928
  RSV, 1394
  for specific viruses, 1386t
  Streptobacillus moniliformis (rat-bite fever), 939
  Taenia, 1351
  Taenia multiceps, 1362–1363
  Taenia serialis (coenurosis), 1362–1363
  Toxoplasma gondii infection, 1313–1314
  Trichinella spiralis diagnosis, 1341
  Trichomonas vaginalis, 1318–1319

  Trypanosoma brucei infection, 1322
  Trypanosoma cruzi infections, 1325
  Ureaplasma urealyticum, 1000
  variola (smallpox) virus, 1021–1022
  virus detection, 1386–1387, 1386t
  visceral leishmaniasis, 1287
  VZV, 1040, 1393
  Wuchereria bancrofti, 1343
drug resistance detection, 1430
group A streptococcal pharyngitis, 203
meningitis etiologic agents, 274
multiplex assays
  influenza viruses, 1394
  RSV, 1394
myocarditis etiologic agents, 265–267
neonatal infection diagnosis, 544
pericarditis etiologic agents, 270
pneumonia diagnosis, 240
prenatal screening of *Toxoplasma gondii*, 1313
quantitative, 1384
real-time (RT-PCR), CMV infection, 1049
see also Reverse transcription PCR (RT-PCR)
Polymorphonuclear cells (PMNs) *see* Neutrophil(s)
Polymorphonuclear phagocytes *see* Basophils; Eosinophil(s); Neutrophil(s); Phagocytic cells
Polymyxin B, treatment of
  burns, 1500t–1501t
  ear infections, 1497t
  eye infections, 1494t–1496t
  skin infections, 1498t
Polymyxin B–neosporin-hydrocortisone, otitis externa, 221
Polymyxins
  dosage, 1480t–1483t
  pharmacodynamics, 1414t
  pharmacology, 1453t–1458t
  spectrum of activity, 1459t–1463t
  see also Colistin
Polyneuropathy, symmetric, *Corynebacterium diphtheriae*, 756–757
Polyomaviridae, 1016t, 1075
  infections, 1017t
Polyomaviruses
  SV40, 1075
  see also Human polyomaviruses
Polyribosylribitol phosphate (PRP) vaccine *see Haemophilus influenzae*
Polysaccharide antigen, in CSF, meningitis diagnosis, 274
Polysplenia, 636
Polythetic, definition, 1015
Polyvinyl alcohol (PVA), 1383
Pontiac fever, *Legionella*, 923
  see also Legionella
Popliteal lymph nodes, enlarged, 160
Population attributable fraction, 2t, 5–6
Populations in statistical analysis, 5
Porcine circovirus, 66
Porphyromonas
  antibiotic susceptibility, 966t
  classification, 959t
  treatment of infections, 985
Porphyromonas asaccharolytica, 982
Porphyromonas gingivalis, 84

Port-a-Cul specimen collector, 963
Portal hypertension, *Schistosoma* infections, 1369–1370
Portoenterostomy (Kasai procedure), 412–413
Posaconazole, 1490–1491
  dosage, 1487t, 1491
  pediatric data, 1491
  pharmacology, 1490–1491
  spectrum of activity, 1486t
  treatment of
    Aspergillus infections, 1208
    Blastomyces dermatitidis (blastomycosis), 1237
    Coccidioides immitis (coccidioidomycosis), 1245
    Cryptococcus infections, 1222–1223
    Cryptococcus neoformans, 1222–1223
    eumycotic mycetoma, 1252
    hyalohyphomycosis, 1210–1211
    mucormycosis, 1214
    phaeohyphomycosis, 1212
    Pseudallescheria boydii infections, 1253
Positive predictive value (PPV), 2f, 2t
Post-kala-azar dermal leishmaniasis, 1287–1288
Post-partum fever, *Mycoplasma hominis* infections, 998–999
Postanginal sepsis, *Fusobacterium*, 985
Postantibiotic effect, 1414t, 1415, 1440–1442, 1442t
Postauricular (mastoid) lymph nodes, 136t
  pathogens infecting, 145t
Postauricular lymphadenopathy, otitis externa, 221
Postcardiotomy syndrome, 271
Postinfectious encephalitis *see* Encephalitis
Postinfectious fatigue syndrome (PIFS), 1008, 1012
Postinfectious neurologic syndromes, 314–319
  ADEM *see* Acute disseminated encephalomyelitis (ADEM)
  cerebellitis, 316
  cranial nerve palsies, 315–316
  etiologies, 314t
  Guillain–Barré syndrome *see* Guillain–Barré syndrome
  transverse myelitis *see* Transverse myelitis, acute
Postinfectious syndromes, foodborne infections, 399
Postinflammatory pigmentary changes, 438
Postmarketing surveillance, of vaccines, 47
Postnatal infections, 546
Postoperative mediastinitis *see* Mediastinitis
Postpericardiotomy syndrome, 270
Postpolio syndrome, 1170
  chronic fatigue syndrome *vs.*, 1010–1011
  clinical features, 1010–1011
Poststreptococcal acute glomerulonephritis (PSAGN) *see under Streptococcus pyogenes* (group A streptococcus)
Poststreptococcal reactive arthritis (PSRA), 706
Posttransplant lymphoproliferative disease (PTLD), 559, 1063
  asymptomatic, management, 1063

diagnosis, 559, 1063
histology, 1063
occult, diagnosis, 559
prevention, 559, 1063
risk factors and causes, 1063
secondary therapy, 1063
treatment, 559, 1063
Postviral fatigue syndrome *see* Chronic
fatigue syndrome (CFS)
Potassium, serum level elevation, 1411
Potassium hydroxide
fungi specimens, 1194–1195, 1246–1247
in vaginitis diagnosis, 360
in vulvovaginitis diagnosis, 357
Pott disease, 778
Pott puffy tumor, 324, 324f
Poultry, *Salmonella* infection from, 528
Povidone-iodine
ophthalmia neonatorum prevention, 490
skin antiseptic, 1499t
treatment of
acute conjunctivitis, 493
burns, 1500t–1501t
eye infections, 1494t–1495t
POW virus, aseptic meningitis due to, 294
Powassan virus, 1102
encephalitis, 303
epidemiology and vectors, 532t
laboratory findings and diagnosis,
533t–534t
Poxviridae, 1016t, 1020–1025, 1020t
description, 1020
genome, 1020
infections, 1017t, 1020t
replications, 1020
Poxviruses, 1020
zoonotic, 1024
clinical features, 1024
epidemiology, 1024
laboratory findings/diagnosis, 1024
prevention, 1024
treatment, 1024
PPV23 *see Streptococcus pneumoniae*
Praziquantel
adverse effects, 1354–1355, 1370, 1524
mass treatment, schistosomiasis
prevention, 1370
resistance, *Schistosoma*, concerns, 1370
treatment of
Clonorchis and *Opisthorchis* infections,
1365
Diphyllobothrium (diphyllobothriasis),
1348
Dipylidium caninum infections, 1349
Echinococcus granulosus infections,
1359–1360
echinostomiasis, 1364
Fasciolopsis buski infection, 1364
fluke infection, 1524
Heterophyes and *Metagonimus*
infections, 1364
Hymenolepis infections, 1349
Paragonimus infections, 1367
Schistosoma (schistosomiasis), 1370
Taenia infections, 1351–1352
Taenia solium neurocysticercosis,
1354–1355, 1355t
tapeworm infection, 1524

Preauricular lymph nodes, 136, 136t, 159
pathogens infecting, 145t, 159
Preauricular lymphadenitis, 132, 136, 138
Preauricular lymphadenopathy, 132, 136,
138, 158t, 159, 898
Bartonella henselae infection, 159f,
858f–859f
otitis externa, 221
Prebiotics, *Helicobacter pylori* infection
treatment, 915
Precautions against infection *see* Infection
prevention and control (IPC)
Precipitated sulfur, scabies treatment, 1260
Predictive value, 1
positive and negative, 2t
Pregnancy
Anaplasma phagocytophilum, 896
bacterial vaginosis, 361
Blastomyces dermatitidis (blastomycosis),
1238, 1238t
Borrelia burgdorferi (Lyme disease), 956
Borrelia infections, 957–958
Brucella infections, 862, 864, 864t
Campylobacter fetus infections, 879
Chlamydia trachomatis, 886–887
screening, 889
chronic viral infections, 544–545
Clostridium tetani (tetanus), 51–52
CMV infection, 1045–1046
prevention, 1051
Coccidioides immitis (coccidioidomycosis),
1242–1245
Coxiella burnetii infections, 892–893
EBV infection, 1065
ectopic *see* Ectopic pregnancy
enterovirus infections, 1178
gonorrhea during, 747
HAART during, 644
healthcare workers *see under* Healthcare
personnel
hepatitis B virus (HBV) infection, 1081,
1084–1085
hepatitis E virus infection, 1193
HHV-7 transmission, 1057–1058
HIV/AIDS epidemiology, 642
see also Human immunodeficiency
virus (HIV)/AIDS
HIV infection prophylaxis *see under*
Human immunodeficiency virus
(HIV)/AIDS
hookworm infections, 1329–1330
human granulocytic anaplasmosis, 896
immunization in, 51–52
HPV vaccine not recommended,
66–67
meningococcal vaccines, 65
MMR contraindication, 60
mumps virus vaccine, 1129
poliovirus vaccine, 1171–1172
response to vaccines, 46
Tdap, 56
varicella vaccine after, 62
yellow fever vaccine contraindicated,
68
influenza virus infection, 1156
innate immune response during, 83
Klebsiella (*Calymmatobacterium*)
granulomatis, 803

Leptospira infections, 952
Listeria monocytogenes infections,
763–764
lymphatic filariasis, 1344
mumps virus, 1127
Mycobacterium tuberculosis treatment, 785
parvovirus B19 infection, 28–29,
1089–1091
Plasmodium infections, 1306
poliomyelitis virus, 1170
risk factors for early-onset neonatal
infections, 539–540, 540t
Rocky Mountain spotted fever (*Rickettsia
rickettsii*), 928–929
rubella virus infection, 1113
rubeola virus (measles), 1143
SARS-CoV infection, 1119
stillbirth due to *Chlamydia trachomatis*,
886–887
Streptococcus agalactiae (group B
streptococcus), 710
syphilis, 942, 945
treatment, 947t
tetracycline contraindication, 929
Toxoplasma gondii see Toxoplasma gondii
Trichomonas vaginalis infections, 361,
1318
outcome, 1319
Trypanosoma (*Schizotrypanum*) *cruzi*,
1325
tuberculosis treatment, 785
Ureaplasma urealyticum infections, 1000
varicella complications, 1038–1039
Vibrio cholerae infection, 851–853
Prehn sign, 348–349, 367
Premature infants
bacterial vaginosis outcome, 361
bronchiolitis, 233
Candida infections, 1196–1197
invasive, 1198, 1201
treatment, 1201
CMV infection, 1048
early-onset neonatal septicemia, 538,
539t
pathogenesis, 540
eosinophilia, 1407
HIV infection, 87
IgG levels, 87, 89t
immune globulin intravenous (IGIV)
use, 39, 41
immunization, 51–52
HBV vaccination, 1085
response to, 87
rotavirus vaccine, 66
infective keratitis, 495
monocytosis, 1406–1407
necrotizing enterocolitis, 388
nosocomial infection prevention, 555
ophthalmia neonatorum, 487
otitis media, 540–541
prolonged vitamin E use, 548
rhinovirus infection, 1187
RSV infections, 1131
septicemia risk, 540
Trichomonas vaginalis infections in
pregnancy and, 1319
Ureaplasma urealyticum infections,
1000–1001

viral infections, 546
  see also Neonatal infections; Neonate(s)
Premature rupture of membranes, 487
  GBS septicemia and, 539–540
Prenatal screening, *Toxoplasma gondii*,
    1311–1313
Preschool children, transmission of
    respiratory tract infections, 13
Preseptal cellulitis, 507, 679
  after trauma, 509, 509f
  causes, 507b
  inflammatory edema of sinusitis causing,
    510
  see also Periorbital cellulitis
Preseptal infections, 507–510
Preservatives, for vaccines, 45
Preterm infants *see* Premature infants
Prevalence, 1–2
Prevented fraction (PF), 8
Prevention and control of infections *see*
    Infection prevention and control
    (IPC)
Prevertebral space, 137–138, 137f
Prevotella, 982–985
  antibiotic susceptibility, 966t
  classification, 959t
  CNS infections, 983
  female genital tract infections, 984
  head and neck infections, 983
  intra-abdominal infections, 984
  nonpigmented, 982
  osteomyelitis due to, 984
  pathophysiology, 983
  peritonsillar abscess, 205–206
  pigmented, 982
  pleuropulmonary infections, 983–984
  prevention of infections, 985
  pyogenic arthritis due to, 984
  skin/soft tissue infections, 984
  treatment of infections, 985
Prevotella bivia, 960, 982
Prevotella disiens, 960, 982
Prevotella intermedia, 982
Prevotella melaninogenica, 962, 983
  endotoxin, 962
  gingival crevices flora, 959
  persistent/progressive pneumonia,
    245–246
  viral nasopharyngitis, 163
Prevotella oralis, 982
Prevotella oris, 982
Primaquine
  Plasmodium infection prophylaxis, 80–81,
    1304, 1305t, 1521
  Plasmodium infection treatment,
    1301t–1303t, 1304
  Pneumocystis jirovecii (carinii) pneumonia,
    1232t, 1233
Primary amebic meningoencephalitis
    (PAM), 1293–1295, 1520
Primary biliary cirrhosis (PBC), 406
Primary ciliary dyskinesia, 250–251, 638
Primary sclerosing cholangitis (PSC), 406
Primates, nonhuman, infections associated,
    528
"Prion", 333
Prion diseases, 333–338
  acquired

clinical features, 334–337
  see also Creutzfeldt–Jakob disease
    (CJD)
  diagnosis, 338
  diseases included, 333
  epidemiology and transmission, 334
  etiology, 333–334
  genetic/familial, 337–338
  laboratory findings, 338
  management, 338
  neuropathology, 336f
  prevention, and disinfection, 338
  transmission by IGIV, 43
  see also Creutzfeldt–Jakob disease (CJD)
Prion protein (PrP), 333–334
  cellular (PrP^C), 334
  characteristics, 334
  scrapie-type (PrP^{Sc}), 334, 336
  structure and conformation, 334
PRNP gene, 334, 337f
  mutations, 334, 337f
    acquired prion disease, 334, 337
    genetic prion diseases, 337–338
  structure, 337f
Probe hybridization, resistance detection,
    1430
Probiotics
  Clostridium difficile infections and, 585
  Helicobacter pylori infection treatment,
    914–915
  necrotizing enterocolitis reduction, 961
  nosocomial infection prevention, 555
  viral gastroenteritis management, 381
Procaine penicillin G
  congenital syphilis, 946–947
  dosage, 1483t–1484t
  pharmacology, 1465
  spectrum of activity, 1459t–1463t
Procalcitonin (PCT), 1402–1403
  clinical studies, 1402–1403
  elevated, causes, 1402
  neonatal infections, nosocomial, 552
  neonatal septicemia diagnosis, 541t,
    542
  physiology and measurement, 1402
Proctitis
  in anal discharge/proctitis syndrome,
    346t, 347
  Chlamydia trachomatis, 886–887
  diagnosis of pathogen, 385t
  etiology, 382t
  sexually transmitted infections, 347
  ulcerative, 382
Proctocolitis, sexually transmitted infections,
    347
Proctosigmoidoscopy, 376
Prodigiosin, 813
Product (for geometric mean), 5
Proglottids, 1256
  Diphyllobothrium, 1347
  Dipylidium caninum, 1348
  Hymenolepis, 1349
  Taenia, 1350–1351, 1350f
  Taenia multiceps, 1362
  Taenia serialis, 1362
PROGRAMS trial, 544
Progressive disseminated histoplasmosis of
    infancy, 1226, 1226f

Progressive multifocal leukoencephalopathy
    (PML), 1076–1077
  in hyper-IgM syndrome, 631–632
  JC virus causing, 631–632
Proguanil, 1521–1522
  Ty21a vaccine contraindication, 79
Promastigotes, *Leishmania*, 1285–1288
Propamidine isethionate, *Acanthamoeba*
    keratitis, 1297
Properdin, 618
  deficiency, 604t–605t, 617–619
    Neisseria meningitidis infections, 733
    recurrent meningitis associated, 288
Prophylaxis, definition, 68
Propionibacterium, 962
  classification, 959t
  clinical manifestations, 990
  free fatty acids produced, 960
  microbiology, 990
  skin flora, 427
Propionibacterium acnes, 991
  CNS device infection, 597
  endophthalmitis due to, 503
  skin colonization, 959–960
Propionibacterium propionica, 990
Propionibacterium propionicum, diagnosis/
    detection, 963–964
Proptosis, orbital infections, 510
Prostaglandin E$_2$ (PGE$_2$), fever induction
    mechanism, 91, 91f
  fever management, 92
Prostate, in prostatitis, 369
Prostatic massage, 369
Prostatic secretions, 369
Prostatitic localization 4-cup urine
    collection test, 369
Prostatitis, 369
  clinical features and differential
    diagnosis, 369
  complications, 369
  etiology, pathogenesis, epidemiology,
    369
  laboratory findings and diagnosis, 369
  management, 369
  nonbacterial (inflammatory), 369
  urethritis complication, 356
Prosthetic device infections, 594–596,
    595b
  Corynebacterium, 759–762
Prosthetic joints, infections, 598–599
Prosthetic valves/patches, infections
    associated, 594–596, 595b–596b
  clinical features and diagnosis, 595,
    595b
  complications, 595
  epidemiology and pathogenesis,
    594–595
  infection routes, 595b
  management and outcome, 595
  prevention, 595–596, 596b
Proteae, 811
  indole-positive members, 812
Protease inhibitors, 665t, 666
  in HIV encephalopathy, 654
  mechanism of action, 666
  toxicity and adverse effects, 666, 670
Protected specimen brushing (PSB),
    ventilator-associated pneumonia, 582

Protein(s)
  metabolism, disorders, acute hepatitis, 404
  utilization, in inflammatory response, 94
Protein A, *Staphylococcus aureus*, 676
Protein C, reduced in meningococcal infections, 736–737
Protein–calorie malnutrition, 1406
Proteinuria
  mumps virus infection, 1127
  persistent, HIV infection, 656
Proteus, 811–812
  clinical manifestations, 811–812
  microbiology and epidemiology, 811
  OX19 antigen, cross-reactivity with *R. prowazekii*, 931
  recurrent meningitis due to, 287
  treatment of infections, 812
  urinary tract infections, 811–812
  xanthogranulomatous pyelonephritis, 344
Proteus mirabilis, 811–812
  axillary lymphadenopathy due to, 159–160
  chronic otitis media, 812
  clinical manifestations, 811–812
  meningitis due to, 812
  screening tests for, 801
  treatment of infections, 812
Proteus penneri, 811
Proteus vulgaris, 811
Proton pump inhibitor
  Helicobacter pylori treatment, 914
  invasive *Candida* infections associated, 1201
Protozoa, 1261–1265, 1319–1326
  classification, 1254–1255, 1254b–1255b
  endoparasitic, 1254–1255
  eosinophilia in infections, 1407
  genomes, 1255
  laboratory diagnosis, gastro-duodenal parasites, 1383
  in refugee and internationally adopted children, 35–36, 35t
  transmission modes, 1255t
  treatment
    with antibacterial agents, 1522
    kinetoplastidae infections, 1519–1520
    luminal infection, 1519
  see also specific protozoa
Providencia, 811–812
  clinical manifestations, 812
  microbiology and epidemiology, 811
  treatment, 812
Providencia alcalifaciens, 812
Providencia rettgeri, 811
Providencia rustigianii, 811
Providencia stuartii, 811
Prozone effect, 944
PRP (polysaccharide (polyribosylribitol phosphate)) vaccine *see Haemophilus influenzae*, vaccines
Pruritic papular eruption (PPE), in HIV infection, 656
Pruritus
  anal, *Taenia solium*, 1351
  Malassezia folliculitis, 1217
  perianal, *Enterobius vermicularis*, 1332

pityriasis versicolor, 1216–1217
vulvovaginal, *Candida*, 351–352
PRV *see* Rotaviruses, vaccines
Pseudallescheria boydii, 1210–1211, 1250, 1253
  clinical manifestations, 1253
  diagnosis, 1253
  epidemiology, 1253
  microbiology, 1253
  mycetoma, 1253
  treatment, 1253
Pseudallescheria minutispora, 1250
Pseudo-TORCH syndrome, 548
Pseudoappendicitis *see* Mesenteric lymphadenitis (adenitis)
Pseudocowpox (milker's nodules), 1024
Pseudohyphae, 1194
Pseudomembrane
  in diphtheria, 754–756
  in Lemierre syndrome, 209
Pseudomembranous colitis, 584
  in cancer, 578
  clinical features, 584
  Clostridium difficile associated, 978, 979b
  neutropenia associated with cancer, 567
  see also Clostridium difficile
Pseudomonadaceae, 832–833
Pseudomonas, 841
  antibiotic resistance, 1419
  appendicitis due to, 420
  blood product contamination, 581
  Burkholderia relationship, 846
  closely related genera, 841, 841b
  fracture-associated infection, 515
  otitis externa due to, 221
  peritonitis due to, 416
  septicemia due to, neutropenia in, 1405
  Stenotrophomonas maltophilia
    reclassification from, 849
  in X-linked agammaglobulinemia, 610
Pseudomonas aeruginosa, 841–846
  acute mastoiditis due to, 224
  acute otitis media due to, 220
  alginate exopolysaccharide, 639
  animal bites, 521–523
  antimicrobial resistance, 842, 844–845
    aminoglycoside-modifying enzymes, 845
    β-lactams and lactamases, 640–641, 845, 1424–1425
    healthcare-associated infections, 14t
    mechanisms, 844–845
    permeability factors and efflux pumps, 844–845
    trends and surveillance, 844
  antimicrobial susceptibility testing, 1378, 1378t, 1380, 1416
    cystic fibrosis, 1432–1433
  biofilm, 639, 843
  bloodstream infections, 845
  Burkholderia cepacia coinfection, 848
  burn wound infections, 518
  capillary invasion, 441
  chronic mastoiditis due to, 226–227
  chronic suppurative otitis media, 843t
  clinical manifestations, 843–845, 843t
    special hosts, 844t
  CNS infections, 846

community-acquired infections, 843t
in cystic fibrosis, 639, 843–844, 844t, 846
  management, 640
  prevention, 641
  respiratory infections, 248–249, 842, 846
device-related infections, 589
ear infections in cancer, 577
ecthyma gangrenosum due to, 844f, 844t
  neonatal, 550
epidemiology, 843–845, 843t–844t
ExoU, ExoT and ExoS, 842–843, 842t
flagella and Toll-like receptor interactions, 842t, 843
fluorescent siderophores, 842
focal suppurative CNS infections, 319
folliculitis due to, 431, 843–844, 843t
genome and gene expression, 842–844
in HIV infections, 844t
in HSCT recipients, 563
keratitis due to, 496
late-onset sepsis etiology, 550–551, 551t
meningitis, treatment, 276t
mexAB operon, 844–845
microbiology, 842
muc mutants, 843
necrotizing otitis externa, 222
neonatal conjunctivitis, 541
neutropenia in, 1405
nosocomial infections, 843t
ocular infections, 843t, 846
ophthalmia neonatorum, 489–490
orchitis due to, 369
osteochondritis of foot, 476
osteomyelitis due to, 845
otitis externa due to, 220–221, 843t, 845
patient-to-patient transmission, 24
in phagocytic disorders, 620t
pneumonia, 248–250, 253, 582, 846
prevention of infections, 846
prostatitis due to, 369
pulmonary infections, 845
  in cystic fibrosis, 248–249, 842, 846
puncture wound infections, 515
pyogenic arthritis due to, 477
quorum sensing, 843–845
receptors for, 639
renal infections, 845–846
sepsis, 98
septicemia, 435f, 844f, 844t
skin infections, 845f
  after trauma, 514
  in cancer, 574, 574f
transmission, by contaminated toys, 13
treatment of infections, 845–846
  immunocompromised patients, 845
  uncomplicated infections, 845
urinary tract infections, 843t
vaccine, 846
  adverse reactions, 521
  burn wound infection prevention, 521
ventilator-associated pneumonia due to, 250
virulence factors and pathogenesis, 842–843, 842t
Pseudomonas fluorescens, 841, 841t

Pseudomonas luteola (Chryseomonas luteola), 835, 841, 841t
Pseudomonas monteilii, 841t
Pseudomonas oryzihabitans (Flavimonas oryzihabitans), 835, 841, 841t
Pseudomonas paucimobilis (Sphingomonas paucimobilis), 835, 841
Pseudomonas pseudomallei, 237t
Pseudomonas putida, 841, 841t
    septicemia, 841
Pseudomonas stutzeri, 841, 841t
Pseudomonas veronii, 841t
Pseudoparalysis, 541
    pyogenic arthritis, 477, 541
Pseudoparalysis of Parrot, 943
Pseudotumor, inflammatory, fever of unknown origin due to, 119t–120t
Pseudotumor cerebri, headache in, 177t
Psilocybe, 397t
Psilocybin, 397t
Psittacosis *see Chlamydophila (Chlamydia) psittaci*
Psoas muscle abscess, 464
    back pain due to, 188, 188t
    etiology and clinical features, 426
Psoas sign, 188
Psoriasin, 83
Psoriasis, 83
    tinea capitis *vs.*, 1247
Psorophora mosquito, Venezuelan equine encephalitis virus (VEEV) transmission, 1098
Psychiatric features
    congenital rubella, 1115–1116
    Trypanosoma (Trypanozoon) brucei infection, 1320–1321
    see also Depression
Psychological interventions, chronic fatigue syndrome, 1014–1015
Psychological problems, chronic fatigue syndrome pathogenesis, 1011–1012, 1011t
Psychrobacter, 839–841
    clinical features, 840
    treatment, 840–841
Psychrobacter immobilis, 840, 941
    conjunctivitis, 941
    meningitis, 840, 941
Psychrobacter phenylpyruvicus, 840
    treatment of infections, 840–841
PU.1 transcription factor, 85–86
Puberty, delayed, HIV infection, 669–670
Pubic lice *see Phthirus pubis* (crab louse) infestation
Public health
    principles, 1–9
    surveillance for unusual infections, 17
Public health policy, 7–9
    impact/economic analysis of disease prevention, 8–9
    outbreak investigations, 7
Pulmonary arteriovenous malformations, 322
Pulmonary artery catheterization, infections, 592
Pulmonary contusions, management, 512
Pulmonary cysts, congenital, 247
Pulmonary disease, neonatal, 547

Pulmonary edema
    enterovirus 71 causing, 1177
    hantavirus pulmonary syndrome, 1103
Pulmonary embolus, chest pain, 189, 190t
Pulmonary features, EBV infection, 1061
Pulmonary hemorrhage
    Bacillus cereus infections, 753
    in hemosiderosis, 251
    spontaneous, 246–247
Pulmonary hypertension, *Bordetella pertussis* infection complication, 870
Pulmonary infections
    Aspergillus, 1203–1204, 1204f
    Blastomyces dermatitidis see Blastomyces dermatitidis (blastomycosis)
    Burkholderia cepacia, 848
    in cancer, 575–577, 575t
        treatment, 576t
    Cryptococcus, 1221–1222
    generalized lymphadenopathy, 130, 131t–132t
    mucormycosis, 1213
    Pseudomonas aeruginosa, 846
    Sporothrix schenckii (sporotrichosis), 1219–1220
    Tsukamurella, 770–771
    see also Lung; Respiratory tract infections; *specific infections*
Pulmonary infiltrate with eosinophilia (PIE) syndromes, 1407
Pulmonary lymphoid hyperplasia, in HIV infection, 654–655, 654f, 660, 661f
    see also Lymphoid interstitial pneumonitis (LIP)
Pulmonary microhemorrhage, *Ascaris lumbricoides* causing, 1327–1328
Pulmonary nodules, in cancer, 575–576
Pulmonary sequestrations, persistent pneumonia, 247
Pulmonary sling, cough, 167t
Pulpitis, 191
Pulse oximetry, in pneumonia, 240
Pulsed-field gel electrophoresis (PFGE), bacterial identification, 674
PulseNet, 763
Pulsus paradoxicus, 189, 270
Pulvinar sign, 335–336, 335f
Puncture wound(s)
    infections, 512t, 515
    osteochondritis, of foot, 476
Pupils (eye)
    in headache assessment, 171
    infant botulism, 973
Pure red cell aplasia, parvovirus B19 and, 1089, 1089t, 1091
Purgatives, *Taenia* infection treatment, 1351–1352
Purified protein derivative (PPD), tuberculosis diagnosis, 779
    transplant recipients, 560
    see also Mantoux intradermal tuberculin skin test
Purine nucleoside phosphorylase, deficiency, 603t–604t, 628t, 629
Purpura, 441–444
    etiology, 441–444, 443b
    Henoch–Schönlein *see* Henoch–Schönlein purpura (HSP)

    palpable, 444
        etiology, 443b, 444
        pathogenesis, 444
Purpura fulminans, 444
    pneumococcal, 734
    varicella complication, 1038
Pustules, 427t
    smallpox, 1021
Puumala virus, 1103–1104, 1103t–1104t
Pyelonephritis
    acute abdominal pain, 173
    anatomy and, 343f
    clinical features, 340
    complications, 343
    Corynebacterium minutissimum, 760t–761t
    focal, 343–344
    recurrent, 342
    treatment, 1418t–1419t
    xanthogranulomatous, 344, 811–812
Pyochelin, *Pseudomonas aeruginosa* producing, 842, 842t
Pyoderma, *Streptococcus pyogenes* (group A streptococcus), 705–706
Pyoderma gangrenosum, in cancer, 574, 574f
Pyogenic arthritis *see* Arthritis, pyogenic
Pyogenic neck infections *see* Cervical lymphadenitis
Pyogranuloma, in chronic granulomatous disease, 621f
Pyomyositis, 186, 465
    burn wound complications, 519
    chest wall, 189
    clinical features, 465
    diagnosis, 468
    epidemiology, 465
    etiology, 465, 514
    group A streptococcus, 463f, 465
    necrotizing group A streptococcal, 463f, 465, 468
    pathogenesis, 465
    Staphylococcus aureus, 465, 466f, 680
    trauma causing, 513t, 514
    treatment, 468
    "tropical" (staphylococcal), 465
Pyonephrosis (suppurative hydronephrosis), 343
Pyopneumothorax, tuberculosis, 775–776
Pyoverdin, *Pseudomonas aeruginosa* producing, 842, 842t
PYR reaction
    enterococci, 713
    groups C and G streptococci, 720
Pyrantel pamoate
    piperazine interaction, 1328
    treatment of
        Ascaris lumbricoides infections, 1328
        Enterobius vermicularis infections, 1332
        hookworm infections, 1330
        nematodes, 1523–1524
        Trichuris trichiura infections, 1331
Pyrazinamide
    adverse reactions, 781
    dosage, 1445t–1452t
    tuberculosis treatment, 780t, 781, 783
Pyrenochaeta, 1250–1251
Pyrethrins, pediculosis treatment, 1259

Pyrethroid, tick repellent, 535
Pyrexia *see* Fever
Pyrexia of unknown origin (PUO) *see* Fever, of unknown origin (FUO)
Pyridine hydrochloride, 399
Pyrimethamine, *Toxoplasma gondii* infection treatment, 1315–1316, 1315t–1316t
Pyrimidine analogs, systemic fungal infections, 1487t, 1488
Pyrin protein, 124
Pyrogens, endogenous/exogenous, 91
Pyrvinium pamoate, 1525
Pyuria, 340
    sterile, 346–347
        urinary catheter-related infection, 599

Q

Q fever *see Coxiella burnetii* (Q fever)
QALYS, 8
Qinghaosu, *Plasmodium* infections, 1520
Quality-adjusted life-years (QALYs), 8
Quasispecies
    HCV, 1105
    retroviruses, 1164
Query (Q) fever *see Coxiella burnetii*
Quinacrine
    Giardia intestinalis (giardiasis), 1281t, 1282
    in prion diseases, 338
Quinidine
    intravenous, *Plasmodium* infections, 1303
    monitoring use and adverse effects, 1303
    Plasmodium infections, 1301t–1303t, 1303, 1521
Quinine
    Babesia (babesiosis), 1265
    Plasmodium infections, 1299–1300, 1301t–1303t, 1303–1304, 1521
Quinolones, 1427, 1476–1477
    chronic suppurative otitis media, 227
    distribution, 1417
    dosage, 1480t–1483t
    mechanism of action, 1427, 1476–1477
    pharmacodynamic properties, 1414t
    pharmacology, 1453t–1458t
    resistance, 1419, 1477
        mechanisms, 1421–1422, 1422t, 1427
        Salmonella Paratyphi A, 816
    safety issues, 1477
    spectrum of activity, 1459t–1463t, 1476
    see also Fluoroquinolones
Quinsy *see* Peritonsillar abscess
Quinupristin (streptogramin B), mechanism of action, 1474–1475
Quinupristin-dalfopristin
    adverse effect, 1475
    clinical use, 1475
    dosage, 1445t–1452t, 1480t–1483t
    mechanism of action, 687
    pharmacology, 1453t–1458t
    resistance to, 1475
    spectrum of activity, 1459t–1463t
    treatment of
        Enterococcus infections, 715
        Staphylococcus aureus infection, 687

Ureaplasma urealyticum infections, 1001
Quorum sensing, *Pseudomonas aeruginosa*, 843–845

R

Rabbit Infectivity Testing (RIT), 943–945
Rabbits, *Francisella tularensis* infections, 897
Rabies virus (rabies), 529, 1145–1149, 1149b
    in animals, 1145–1146, 1146f, 1146t
        "furious" and "dumb" phases, 1146
    antibodies, 1145
    bites
        animal bites, 523
        bat bites and, 303f
        management, 80
    clinical manifestations, 1146–1147, 1149b
    description and virology, 1145, 1145f, 1149b
    diagnosis, 1147, 1149b
    distribution, 80
    encephalitis due to, 302–303, 1145–1146
    endemic rabies in wildlife, 1145–1146, 1146t
    epidemiology, 1145–1146, 1146f, 1149b
    "furious" form, 1147
    human rabies immune globulin (HRIG), 1148
    immune globulin (RIG), 37t, 39, 80, 1148
        indications and dose, 39
    incubation period, 1145–1147
    laboratory testing, 308t–311t
    mortality from, 1147
    neurological features, 1147
    "paralytic" form, 1147
    paralytic *vs* furious forms, 306
    pathogenesis of infections, 1145
    postexposure prophylaxis (PEP), 529, 1147t–1148t, 1148–1149
        bite wounds, 525
    pre-exposure prophylaxis, 1147t, 1148
    prevention of infection, 529, 1147–1149, 1149b
        in animals, 1148
    replication, 1145
    transmission, 1146
        animal contact in childcare, 31
        human-to-human, 1148–1149
    treatment of infection, 1147, 1149b
    vaccine, 80, 1147–1148
        encephalitis associated, 1147
        human diploid cell vaccine (HDCV), 80, 1147–1148
        pre-exposure, 80
        primary chick embryo cell vaccine (PCECV), 80, 1147–1148
        purified duck embryo vaccine (PDEV), 1147–1148
        rhesus lung cell vaccine (RVA), 1147–1148
        schedule/dosing for travelers, 79t, 80, 1147–1148, 1147t
        for travelers, 80

Vero cell vaccine (PVRV), 1147–1148
    for wild animals, 529
virulence and immunity, 1145
wildlife reservoirs, control, 529
Rac2, 85
Raccoon
    dangers/infections associated, 333
    parasites, *Baylisascaris procyonis*, 332, 1336
Radiation
    background, 345
    exposures by examination, 345, 345t
    responsible imaging, 345
    risks, 345
        minimization, 345
Radiation-induced stomatitis, 193t
Radiculoneuritis, *Borrelia burgdorferi* (Lyme disease), 954–955
Radiography
    abdominal *see* Abdominal radiography
    in acute bacterial sinusitis, 228–229
    chest *see* Chest radiographs
    diskitis diagnosis, 484, 485f
    Echinococcus granulosus cysts, 1358, 1359f
    in musculoskeletal pain, 183–184
    necrotizing enterocolitis (NEC), 389–390, 389f
    osteomyelitis, 470
    peritonitis, 417
    pyogenic arthritis, 478
    transient synovitis, 486
Radioimmunoassay (RIA), *Legionella pneumophila*, 924
Radiology, *Aspergillus* infections, 1207
Radionuclide cisternography, recurrent meningitis, 291
Radionuclide scan
    bone, osteomyelitis, 470–472, 471t
    epididymitis, 367
RAG-1 and RAG-2 proteins, 627–629, 628t
    deficiency, 627, 628t
Rahnella aquatilis, 809
Ralstonia, 841
Ralstonia pickettii, 841
Ralstonia respiraculi, 841
Raltegravir, 665t, 666
Ramsay Hunt syndrome, 221, 315
Random misclassification, 4
Randomized controlled trials (RCT)
    design and reporting, 9
    vaccine efficacy, 7
Range, 5
Ranitidine bismuth citrate, *Helicobacter pylori* treatment, 914
RANTES, 90
Raoultella, 799–802
    clinical manifestations, 800
    microbiology and epidemiology, 799–800
    treatment of infections, 800–802
Raoultella planticola, 800
Rape
    Chlamydia trachomatis, 1389t–1392t
    see also Sexual abuse
Rapid antigen detection tests (RADTs)
    GAS pharyngitis, 200, 203, 1377
        GAS pharyngitis *vs.* GAS carriers, 203

monitoring of treatment, 205
specificity and sensitivity, 203
methods, 203
Streptococcus agalactiae (group B streptococcus), 709
Streptococcus pneumoniae, 724
Rapid Diagnostic Tests (RDTs), *Plasmodium* infections, 1300
Rapid fluorescent focus inhibition test (RFFIT), rabies, 1147
Rapid plasma reagin (RPR) test, 944, 1384
Rapid urease test, *Helicobacter pylori* detection, 913
Rash(es)
    acute bacterial meningitis, 274
    adenoviral infections, 112
    Arcanobacterium haemolyticum causing, 751
    Borrelia infections, 957
    coltivirus (Colorado tick fever), 1093
    congenital syphilis, 943
    EBV infection, 1061
        ampicillin association, 1061
    Ehrlichia causing, 894
    empiric transmission-based precautions, 20t
    enterovirus infections, 1174–1175, 1174t, 1175f
    epidemic typhus (*Rickettsia prowazekii*), 930–931
    erythema migrans *see* Erythema migrans
    herpes zoster, 1039
    HHV-6 infection (roseola), 1054, 1055f
    HHV-8 association, 1066f, 1067
    in HIV infection, 656
    Kawasaki disease, 111, 1003, 1004f
    Leptospira infections, 950–951
    in Lyme disease, 953–954
    maculopapular, 436
        acute bacterial meningitis, 274
        etiology, 437t
    measles, 112
    morbilliform, 436
    murine typhus (*Rickettsia typhi*), 932
    petechial, *Neisseria meningitidis* infections, 734–735, 735f
    Rickettsia infections, 932, 934–935
    Rickettsia parkeri infection, 934
    Rocky Mountain spotted fever (*Rickettsia rickettsii*), 926–927, 928f
    rubella virus infection, 1114
    rubelliform, 112, 436
    rubeola virus (measles), 1140, 1140f
    scarlatiniform, 436
        Arcanobacterium haemolyticum causing, 751
    Spirillum minus infections, 958
    Streptobacillus moniliformis (rat-bite fever), 938–939
    Strongyloides infection, 1333
    toxic shock syndrome, 685
    trimethoprim-sulfamethoxazole causing, 1232
    varicella, 1037, 1037f
    varicella vaccine-related, 1043
    vesiculobullous, 438–441
        differential diagnosis, 441

viral infections, 112
    see also Exanthem(s)
Rat(s) *see* Rodents
Rat bite fever *see Streptobacillus moniliformis*
Rat bites *see* Bites, rat
Reactive arthritis *see* Arthritis, reactive
Reagin antibody, 1411t–1412t
Recombinant immunoblot assay (RIBA)
    HCV, 1109–1110
    hepatitis C virus, 1395
Recombinase-activating gene (RAG), 87, 90
Recombination, intragenic, drug resistance, 1423
Rectal biopsy, *Schistosoma* infections, 1369–1370
Rectal examination, in acute abdominal pain, 172
Rectal swabs
    gastrointestinal virus detection, 1395
    specimen collection/transport, 1374t
    Vibrio cholerae infection, 852
Recurrent infections, 601
    common variable immunodeficiency, 612
    evaluation, 606–608
        birth history, 606–607
        family history, 606
        genetic testing, 608
        history-taking, 600, 606
        medical history, 606
        physical examination, 607, 607b
        screening laboratory tests, 607, 608t
        social history, 607
        specialized testing, 607–608, 608t
        systems review, 607
    management, 608–609
    pathogens, 606
    predisposing anatomic/physiologic abnormalities, 600, 600t
    predisposing conditions, 600–601, 601b
        frequencies, 601t
    sentinel pathogens for specific conditions, 606t
    X-linked agammaglobulinemia, 610
    see also Immunodeficiency; *individual infections*
Recurrent respiratory papillomatosis, HPV causing, 1072–1073
Recurrent vulvovaginal candidiasis (RVVC), 358–360
Red blood cells (RBCs) *see* Erythrocyte(s)
Red Book: Report of the Committee on Infectious Diseases (COID), 68
Red-man (red-neck) syndrome, 688, 1469
Reduviidae, 1322
Refeeding
    gastrointestinal tract infection management, 377
    in inflammatory enteritis, 387
Refugee and internationally adopted children, 32–37
    evaluation guidelines, 33–36
        Chagas disease, 36
        enteric infections, 35–36
        hepatitis A, 33
        hepatitis B, 33–34
        hepatitis C, 34
        HIV-1 and HIV-2, 34

intestinal pathogens, 35–36
less common infections, 36
other testing, 36
recommended tests, 33t
skin infections, 36
syphilis, 36
tuberculosis, 34–35
upper respiratory tract infections, 36
immunizations, 36–37, 52
numbers and countries of origin, 32
prevention of infections, 36–37
screening before immigration to US, 32–36
serologic testing for immunization status, 36–37, 37t
Regan-Lowe medium, 1375t
Rehydration
    in inflammatory enteritis, 387
    intravenous, viral gastroenteritis, 381
    oral see Oral rehydration therapy (ORT)
    see also Fluid resuscitation
Reiter syndrome, 482–483
    Chlamydia trachomatis, 886, 889
    urethritis complication, 356
Relapsing fever *see Borrelia*
Relative risk, 2t, 3–5
Relative risk/risk ratio (RR), 2t–3t
RelB transcription factor, 85–86
Renal abnormalities
    EBV infection, 1061
    varicella complication, 1038
Renal abscess, 343–345, 425
    epidemiology and pathogenesis, 344
    etiology, 344
    intrarenal, 343–344
    laboratory and imaging studies, 344, 344f, 345t
    management, 344
    risk factors (conditions), 343b
Renal biopsy, in poststreptococcal acute glomerulonephritis, 705
Renal calculi, xanthogranulomatous pyelonephritis, 344
Renal colic, site and radiation of pain, 171
Renal damage, risk factors, 339–340
Renal disease
    end-stage, 637
    in HIV infection, 656
        management, 670–671
    infections in, 637
    in *Plasmodium* infection, 1299
Renal dysfunction/failure
    acute, IGIV causing, 42–43
    amantadine dosage, 1445t–1452t, 1505t
    aminoglycoside-induced, 1474
    amphotericin-induced, 1487
    antimicrobial dosage, 1435–1437, 1445t–1452t
    antiviral agent dosage, 1505t
    cidofovir-induced, 1508
    foscarnet dosage, 1505t, 1514–1515, 1515f
    foscarnet-induced, 1515
    hemolytic uremic syndrome complication, 798–799
    Leptospira infections, 951
    pharmacokinetics, 1435, 1436t

Yersinia pseudotuberculosis, 825
see also Pyelonephritis
Renal infections
    Candida, 1198–1199, 1199f
    Nocardia causing, 794
    Pseudomonas aeruginosa, 845–846
    see also Pyelonephritis
Renal transplantation
    adenovirus infections, 1070
    meningitis associated, 273t
    nephritis, BK virus causing, 1076
    septicemia and infections after, 557
    VZV infections after, 559
Renal tuberculosis, 778–779
Reoviridae, 1016t, 1092, 1094
    infections, 1017t
Reporting of disease *see* Notification
Reproductive health, HIV infection and, 672
Reptiles
    bites, 529
    infection transmission, 528
    Salmonella transmission, 528
Research hypotheses, 9
Resource-poor countries
    children adopted from *see* Refugee and internationally adopted children
    hepatitis B and delta hepatitis prevalence, 32
Respiratory acidosis, tachypnea in, 168–169
Respiratory arrest, infant botulism, 975
Respiratory burst, defective, 620, 624
Respiratory distress
    in bronchiolitis, 233
    in *Plasmodium* infection, 1299, 1303
    in SARS, 1119
    signs, 172
Respiratory failure, in bronchiolitis, 233
Respiratory hygiene, standard precautions, 17, 18t
Respiratory mucosa, 227
Respiratory rate, 165
    in abdominal pain, 172
    in bronchiolitis, 233
    raised *see* Tachypnea
Respiratory sounds, adventitial, 169
Respiratory syncytial virus (RSV), 196, 1130–1134
    antibodies to, 233–235, 1130–1132, 1394
    apnea due to, 233, 1132–1133
    A and B strains, 232, 1130
    bronchiolitis, 231, 1130, 1132–1133
    clinical manifestations, 1132–1133, 1132b
    co-pathogenicity with other infections, 1131
    common cold due to, 196–197, 197f
    cough due to, 1132
    culture, 233–234, 1133
    in cystic fibrosis, 639
    description and virology, 1130
    diagnosis/detection, 233–234, 1133, 1394
        detection rates, 1386t
        optimal tests, 1389t–1392t
        rapid testing, 1131, 1133
    epidemics, 1130–1131

epidemiology, 197f, 231–232, 232f, 1130–1131
    seasonal pattern, 1130, 1131f
F (fusion) protein, 235
    antibodies to, 233
glycoproteins F and G, 1130
group childcare and, 25t
health-care associated infections, 583
    epidemiology and pathogenesis, 581–582
    treatment, 583
hospitalization due to, 232–233, 1130–1131, 1133
in HSCT recipients, 564
IgG to, effect on bronchiolitis, 233
immune globulin, 235, 1133–1134
immune response, 1132
immunity to, 1130
immunocompromised hosts, 1132–1133
immunotherapy, 583
infections in cancer, 577
laboratory testing, 308t–311t
laryngotracheitis (croup) due to, 211, 1132
monoclonal antibodies to, 42, 233–234, 241, 582–583, 1133–1134
    see also Palivizumab
mortality, 1130–1131, 1133
nasal discharge due to, 163
neonatal infections, 547
    nosocomial, 551
neurological complications, 1132–1133
nucleocapsid and genome, 1130
outbreaks, timing, 231–232, 232f, 1130, 1131f
pathogenesis of infection, 1132
pathology, 1132
pneumonia due to, 235–236, 240–241, 1131–1133
    clinical features, 168t
    prevention, 241
prevention of infections, 1133–1134
reinfection, 1131
risk factors, 232–233, 1131, 1131b, 1133
serotypes and antigenic subgroups, 1130
severe infection in infants/children, risk factors, 1131, 1131b, 1133
shedding, 1131
skin lesions due to, 112
spread from upper to lower airway, 233, 1132
transmission, 13, 582, 1131
    kangaroo care and, 12
    via outpatient clinic, 24
    in transplant recipients, 559–560
treatment of infections, 1133, 1502t, 1512
vaccine, 1134
    candidates, 235
    DNA vaccine development, 235
    formalin-inactivated and enhanced disease, 1132
Respiratory tract
    colonization, *Haemophilus influenzae*, 273, 900–901, 904
    congenital abnormalities, persistent pneumonia, 247
    defense mechanisms, 83–84, 238, 254

epithelial damage due to viruses/bacteria, 250
hemophagocytic lymphohistiocytosis, 105
procedures, endocarditis prevention, 76
specimen collection, 1123–1124, 1377
    Aspergillus culture, 1206
    see also Airway; Lung
Respiratory tract disorders, persistent and recurrent pneumonia with, 248–251
Respiratory tract infections
    Brucella, 863
    burns patients, 519
    chemoprophylaxis, 71–72
    cystic fibrosis, 639
    empiric transmission-based precautions, 20t
    group childcare and, 25t, 27–28
    healthcare-associated *see* Healthcare-associated infection (HAI)
    lower tract *see* Lower respiratory tract infections (LRTIs)
    non-typable *Haemophilus influenzae*, 903
    Pseudallescheria boydii, 1253
    Pseudomonas aeruginosa, 842, 843t, 846
    severe acute syndrome *see under* Human coronaviruses (HCoV)
    sickle-cell disease, 634
    upper tract *see* Upper respiratory tract infections (URTIs)
    viral, healthcare-associated, 582
        clinical features and diagnosis, 582
        management and outcome, 583
    viridans group streptococci, 718
    see also Pulmonary infections; *individual anatomical structures; individual infections*
Respiratory tract symptom complexes, 162–171
    cough, 166–168, 167t
    hemoptysis, 170–171
    mucopurulent rhinorrhea, 162–165, 164t
    stridor, 165–166, 165t
    tachypnea, 168–169
    see also Each of the above symptoms
Respiratory tract symptoms (in)
    Cryptosporidium infections, 1270
    HIV infection, 654–655, 654f, 654t
        management, 671
    Kawasaki disease, 1005t
    rubeola virus (measles), 1141
Respiratory tract viruses
    acute bacterial sinusitis after, 229
    acute otitis media due to, 214
    cell culture, 1394
    chronic fatigue syndrome pathogenesis, 1008t–1009t
    diagnosis/detection, 1394
        shell vial method, 1386
        specimens, 1385
    epidemiology, seasonality, 231–232
    healthcare-associated infections, 13
    infection, fever and prodrome, 108
    infections in cancer, 575
    neonatal infections, 547
    pneumonia due to, 168t, 236–237, 246

see also Upper respiratory tract infections (URTIs)
Restriction fragment length polymorphism (RFLP)
  Mycobacterium tuberculosis diagnosis, 781
  Taenia multiceps, 1362–1363
  Taenia serialis, 1362–1363
Resuscitation equipment, standard precautions, 18t
Retapamulin, impetigo, 678
Reticular dysgenesis, 603t–604t, 628t
Reticulate body (RB)
  Chlamydia trachomatis, 884, 884f
  Chlamydophila pneumoniae, 881
  Chlamydophila (Chlamydia) psittaci, 890f
Reticulocytopenia, 1403
  parvovirus B19 infection, 1088–1089, 1088f
  transient, 1404
Retina
  acute necrosis, HSV infection, 1031
  ocular larva migrans, 1335–1336, 1336f
Retinal neovascularization, congenital rubella with, 1115
Retinitis, 499–503
  causes, 499–503, 499t
  CMV, 501, 501f, 1047–1048, 1050
  HSV, 501
  progressive necrotizing, in AIDS, 502
  Rift Valley fever, 1104
  rubella virus causing, 500–501, 500f
  VZV, 501–502
  see also Chorioretinitis
Retinoblastoma, *Toxocara* infection misdiagnosis, 1335–1336
Retinochoroiditis *see* Chorioretinitis
Retinopathy, "salt-and-pepper", in congenital rubella, 500–501, 500f, 1115
Retinopathy of prematurity, *Candida* infections, 1199
Retroperitoneal abscess, 424, 426–427
  clinical features, 426
  etiology, 423t, 426–427
  fever of unknown origin due to, 119t–120t
  management, 426–427
Retroperitoneal blood, management, 512
Retroperitoneal lymphadenopathy, 155–157
  causes, 155
  diagnosis and therapy, 157
  differential diagnosis, 155–157
  epidemiology, 155–157
Retropharyngeal abscess, 165, 207
  clinical features, 166t, 206t, 207
  complications and prognosis, 207
  diagnosis, 166t, 207
  differential diagnosis, 207
  epidemiology and pathogenesis, 207
  etiology, 207
  management, 207
  parapharyngeal abscess relationship, 207
  radiography and CT, 207, 208f
Retropharyngeal space, 137–138, 137f, 207
  infection, 138
Retroviridae, 1016t, 1164
  arthritis due to, 481b
  infections, 1017t

Retroviruses
  chronic fatigue syndrome pathogenesis, 1008t–1009t
  delta-retroviruses, 1165
  endogenous, 1164
  exogenous, 1164
  genomic diversity and reasons, 1164
  proviral DNA integration, 1164–1165
  quasispecies, 1164
  RNA and genes, 1164
  structure, 1164
  see also Human immunodeficiency virus (HIV)/AIDS; Human T-lymphocyte lymphotropic viruses (HTLV)
Reverse genetics, human metapneumovirus (hMPV) infection prevention, 1137
Reverse transcriptase, HIV, 664, 1166
Reverse transcription PCR (RT-PCR)
  alphavirus, 1099
  astrovirus, 381
  calicivirus, 381
  enteroviruses, 1395
  HCV, 1110
  hepatitis viruses, 1395
  human coronaviruses, 1119
  human metapneumovirus (hMPV), 1134
  human parainfluenza viruses, 1123–1124
  measles and rubella viruses, 1396
  rabies, 1147
  rhinoviruses, 1186–1187
  rotavirus, 381, 1096
  RSV, 1133
  see also Polymerase chain reaction (PCR)
Reye-like syndrome, *Shigella* infection causing, 821
Reye syndrome
  altered mental status, 179, 179t
  aspirin association, 92
  influenza complication, 1153
  influenza vaccine and, 64–65
  varicella with, 1038
RFXANK, 627
RFXAP, 627
Rhabdomyolysis, 186
  Bacillus cereus infections, 753
  transient acute myositis, 464
Rhabdomyosarcoma, neck masses, 142, 142t
Rhabdoviridae, 1016t, 1145–1149
  infections, 1017t
Rheumatic fever, acute *see Streptococcus pyogenes* (group A streptococcus)
Rheumatic heart disease, 703
  acute rheumatic fever *see under Streptococcus pyogenes*
  epidemiology, 702
Rheumatoid arthritis
  migratory polyarthritis in acute rheumatic fever *vs.*, 703
  rubella association, 1116
Rheumatoid factor, 1411t–1412t
Rheumatologic diseases, axillary lymphadenopathy due to, 159–160
Rhinitis
  allergic *see* Allergic rhinitis
  atrophic, 799
  in congenital syphilis, 943–944
  foreign body-related, 164t

  differential diagnosis, 164t
  mucopurulent rhinorrhea, 164
  recurrent mucopurulent, 638
  serosanguineous erosive (in diphtheria), 755–756
  vasomotor, 198
    common colds *vs.*, 198
  see also Nasopharyngitis
Rhinocerebral mucormycosis, 577, 1213
Rhinorrhea
  in common colds, 198
  CSF *see* Cerebrospinal fluid (CSF)
  mucopurulent, 162–165
    acute, 163–164, 163t
    acute sporadic, 163
    causes, 163–164, 163t
    chronic and/or recurrent, 163, 163t
    description and epidemiology, 162–163
    duration, 163–165
    management, 163–165
    onset, 163
  Mycoplasma pneumoniae infections, 993–994
  in pneumonia, 238
Rhinoscleroma, 799
Rhinoscopy, causes of nasal discharge, 164t
Rhinoviruses, 1167–1168, 1186–1187
  clinical manifestations, 1186, 1186f
  common colds due to, 196–197, 1186
  description, 1186
  diagnosis, 1186–1187, 1394
    optimal tests, 1389t–1392t
  epidemiology, 197, 1186
  group childcare and, 25t
  laboratory findings, 1186–1187
  pathogenesis/infection process, 1186
  pneumonia due to, 236–237
  prevention of infection, 1187
  transmission, 197, 1186
  treatment of infection, 1187
Rhipicehalus sanguineus (brown dog tick)
  vector for *Rickettsia akari*, 929
  vector for *Rickettsia rickettsii*, 926
Rhizobiaceae, 833
Rhizobium radiobacter, 833–834
Rhizomucor, 1212–1213
Rhizopoda, 1255
Rhizopus, 1212–1214
Rhizopus oryzae, 1213
Rho proteins, 384
Rhodococcus (Corynebacterium) equi, 768–769
Rhombencephalitis *see* Brainstem encephalitis (rhombencephalitis)
Rhonchi, 169
Ribavirin, 1512–1513
  adverse effects, 1111, 1513
  chemistry, 1512
  clinical uses, 1513
  dosage, 1445t–1452t, 1513
  mechanism of action, 1512
  pharmacokinetics, 1512–1513
  spectrum of activity, 1512
  treatment of
    adenovirus infections, 1070
    bronchiolitis, 235
    chronic HCV infection, 1111

Crimean-Congo hemorrhagic fever, 1104
hemorrhagic fever with renal syndrome, 1104
human coronavirus infections, 1120
human metapneumovirus (hMPV) infection, 1136–1137
human parainfluenza virus infections, 1124
RSV infection, 583, 1133
rubeola virus infection (measles), 1141
viral hemorrhagic fever, 1163
West Nile virus infection, 1101
Ribosomes
bacterial, 1470
RNA see 16s rRNA
Ribs, osteomyelitis, 188–189
"Rice-water stools", 851
Rickettsia, laboratory testing, 308t–311t
Rickettsia
aseptic meningitis due to, 294
chronic fatigue syndrome pathogenesis, 1008t–1009t
clinical manifestations, 937
diagnosis, 938, 1384
fever of unknown origin, 119t–120t
generalized lymphadenopathy, 131t–132t, 132
laboratory testing, 308t–311t
lymphopenia in, 1406
prevention, 938
in returning travelers, 83
spotted fever group, 935–937
Rickettsia prowazekii vs., 930
thrombocytopenia due to, 1410–1411
transmission, by ticks, 532–533
treatment of infections, 938
vasculitis due to, 444
Rickettsia aeschlimanii, 936t–937t
Rickettsia africae, 935–937, 936t–937t
Rickettsia akari, 933–934, 936t–937t
clinical manifestations, 934
description, 933
epidemiology, 933–934
laboratory findings and diagnosis, 934
prevention, 934
treatment, 934
Rickettsia australis, 936t–937t
Rickettsia conorii, 936t–937t
Mediterranean spotted fever, 935–937
epidemiology, 532t
laboratory findings and diagnosis, 533t–534t
Rickettsia conorii subsp. caspia, 935–937, 936t–937t
Rickettsia conorii subsp. conorii, 935–937, 936t–937t
Rickettsia conorii subsp. Israelensis, 935–937, 936t–937t
Rickettsia felis, 932–933, 936t–937t
antibodies to, 933
clinical manifestations, 933
description, 932
epidemiology, 932–933
laboratory findings and diagnosis, 933
prevention, 933
treatment, 933

Rickettsia heilongjiangensis, 936t–937t
Rickettsia honei, 936t–937t
Rickettsia japonica, 936t–937t
Rickettsia-like endosymbiotic bacteria see Wolbachia
Rickettsia marmionii, 936t–937t
Rickettsia massiliae, 935–937, 936t–937t
Rickettsia parkeri, 934–935, 936t–937t
clinical manifestations, 934
description, 934
epidemiology, 934
laboratory findings and diagnosis, 934–935
prevention, 935
treatment, 935
Rickettsia prowazekii, 930–938
bioterrorism agent, 930
clinical manifestations, 930–931
description and microbiology, 930
epidemic typhus, 930–931
clinical features, 930–931
complications, 930–931
diagnosis, 931
epidemiology, 930
treatment, 931
epidemiology, 930
humans as reservoir for, 930
immune response, 930
laboratory findings and diagnosis, 931
prevention and control, 931
relapse (Brill-Zinsser disease), 930
clinical features, 931
prevention, 931
treatment, 931
Rickettsia raoultii, 936t–937t
Rickettsia rickettsii, 926–929, 936t–937t
antibiotic resistance, 929
antibodies to, 926
description and microbiology, 926
eosinophilic meningitis, 331t
epidemiology, 926, 926f–927f
hyponatremia, 1411
neutropenia in, 1405
pathogenesis of infections, 926
rickettsial outer membrane protein (rompA), 926
Rocky Mountain spotted fever, 108, 926–929
clinical features, 108, 533, 926–927
coltivirus (Colorado tick fever) vs., 1093
complications and sequelae, 929
differential diagnosis, 929
encephalitis, 303–304
epidemiology, 532t, 923–924, 926f–927f
laboratory findings and diagnosis, 533t–534t, 928
mortality, 927–928
natural course, 929
prevention and control, 929
tick bites, 533
treatment of infections, 928–929
vectors, 532t
strains, 926
Rickettsia sibirica, 936t–937t
Rickettsia sibirica subsp. mongolotimonae, 936t–937t

Rickettsia slovaca, 936t–937t
Rickettsia species 364D, 935
clinical manifestations, 935
description, 935
epidemiology, 935
treatment, 935
Rickettsia typhi, 931–932
clinical manifestations, 932
description, 931
epidemiology, 931–932
laboratory findings and diagnosis, 932
murine typhus due to, 931–932
prevention, 932
treatment, 932
Rickettsiaceae, 673
Rickettsiales, 893
Rickettsialpox (Rickettsia akari), 933–934
Rickettsiosis, 935–938
clinical manifestations, 937
description of pathogens, 923t, 935–937
diagnosis, 938
differential diagnosis, 936t–937t
epidemiology, 935–937
lymphangitis-associated, 935–937
prevention, 938
rifampin-resistant, 935–937
spotted fever, 935–938, 936t–937t
travel-associated, 935–937
treatment, 938
Rifabutin
clinical use, 1476
mechanism of action, 1475
spectrum of activity, 1459t–1463t, 1476
treatment of
nontuberculous mycobacterial infection, 792
tuberculosis, 783–784
Rifampin, 1427–1428, 1475–1476
adverse reactions, 781, 785, 1476
chemoprophylactic use, 70t–71t
Haemophilus influenzae infection, 905
Haemophilus influenzae type b (Hib), 69
Hib infection, 69
Neisseria meningitidis infection, 69, 278, 739
clinical use, 1476
combination therapy, 1419–1420
synergistic activity, 1420
distribution, 1416–1417
dosage, 1445t–1452t, 1480t–1484t
drug interactions, 69
excretion, 69
mechanism of action, 688, 1459
pharmacology, 1453t–1458t, 1476
resistance to, 1419, 1422t, 1427–1428, 1476
detection, 1430, 1432
Rickettisa species, 938
safety, 69
spectrum of activity, 1459t–1463t, 1476
treatment of
acute bacterial meningitis, 276–277
bacteremic periorbital cellulitis, 510
Brucella infections, 864, 864t, 871
Ca-MRSA infections, 472
coagulase-negative staphylococcal infections, 694

Elizabethkingia meningoseptica
    infections, 834
Haemophilus influenzae biogroup
    aegyptius, 907
Legionella, 924
Listeria monocytogenes infection, 766
Naegleria fowleri (naegleriasis), 1295
nontuberculous mycobacterial
    infection, 791–792
Staphylococcus aureus infection, 688
Streptococcus agalactiae (group B
    streptococcus) infections, 710
tuberculosis treatment, 780t, 781, 783
    drug resistance mechanism, 785
    latent infection treatment, 783
ventricular drain impregnated,
    eosinophilic meningitis associated,
    332–333
Rifamycins, 1475–1476
    clinical uses, 1476
    dosage, 1480t–1483t
    mechanism of action, 1475
    pharmacodynamic properties, 1414t
    pharmacology, 1453t–1458t, 1476
    resistance to, 1476
    spectrum of activity, 1459t–1463t, 1476
Rifapentine
    clinical use, 1476
    mechanism of action, 1475
    spectrum of activity, 1459t–1463t,
        1476
Rifaximin
    dosage, 1480t–1483t
    mechanism of action, 1475
    pharmacology, 1453t–1458t, 1476
    spectrum of activity, 1459t–1463t,
        1476
    for travelers' diarrhea, 82
Rift Valley fever
    clinical manifestations, 1104, 1104t
    epidemiology, 1103, 1103t
    treatment, 1104
Right bundle branch, damage in
    Trypanosoma cruzi infections, 1324
Right middle lobe syndrome, 247
Rimantadine, 1514
    adverse effects, 1514
    chemoprophylactic use, 70t–71t, 72
    clinical uses, 1514
    influenza treatment, 1154
    pharmacokinetics, 1514
    prophylactic, 1507t, 1514
    resistance to, 1503t
        influenza virus, 1155
Ringer lactate, *Vibrio cholerae* infection, 853
Rings, trophozoite (*Plasmodium*),
    1298–1299
Ringworm (tinea corporis), 1248, 1248b
    group childcare and, 25t
Risk
    difference, 5
    excess, 5
    measures, 2t
    relative/risk ratio in statistical analysis,
        2t–3t, 3–5
Risk ratio (RR), 2t, 3–5
Risus sardonicus, 967
Ritonavir, 665t, 666, 1445t–1452t

Rituximab
    EBV infections after transplants, 559
    in HIV infection, 656
    posttransplant lymphoproliferative
        disease therapy, 1063
River blindness *see Onchocerca volvulus*
    (onchocerciasis)
RNA viruses
    negative-sense RNA, 1019f
    positive-sense mRNA, 1018f
    see also individual viruses
Rocky Mountain spotted fever *see Rickettsia
    rickettsii*
Rocky Mountain wood tick *see Dermacentor
    andersoni*
Rodents
    Angiostrongylus transmission, 1337
    arenavirus infection transmission, 1159
    bites, infections after, 521–523
    control
        arenavirus infection prevention, 1164
        murine typhus (*Rickettsia typhi*)
            prevention, 932
    hantavirus transmission, 1102–1103
    infections from, 528
    Leishmania reservoir, 1286, 1290
    Leptospira transmission, 949–950
    Rickettsia akari transmission, 933–934
    Streptobacillus moniliformis transmission,
        938
Romaña sign, 1324, 1324f
Romberg test, 180
Rosai–Dorfman disease *see* Sinus
    histiocytosis with massive
    lymphadenopathy
Rose spots, 817
Roseola *see* Human herpesvirus 6 (HHV-6)
Roseolovirus genus, 1052, 1057
Roseomonas, 834
Roseomonas gilardi, 834
Ross River virus (RRV), 1098
    epidemic polyarthritis, 481
Rotaviruses, 378, 1094–1097
    antibodies, 381
    clinical manifestations, 66, 584, 1095
    description and structure, 378, 379f,
        1094, 1094f
    diagnosis/detection, 381, 584, 1095–
        1096, 1395
        optimal tests, 1389t–1392t
    diarrhea due to, 25–26, 26t, 380,
        583–584, 1094–1095
        epidemiology, 378–379, 380t
        hospitalizations, 372–373
    epidemiology, 66, 380t, 1095, 1095f
    gastroenteritis due to, 378, 1094–1095
        clinical features, 380t
        extraintestinal complications, 381
        mortality, 66
        prevention, 381
    genome (dsRNA), 378, 1094
    group A, 378, 1094
        G and P types, 1094
    group B and group C, 378, 1094
    group childcare and, 25t, 26
    healthcare-associated infections, 13,
        583–584
    laboratory findings, 1095–1096

laboratory testing, 308t–311t
    mortality, 1094–1095, 1095f
    neonatal infections, nosocomial, 551
    prevention of infections, 1096–1097
    proteins, 378
        VP6, 1094
    serotypes, 1094
    shedding, 380
    structure, 378
    transmission, 26, 1095
        prevention, 26
    treatment of infections, 585, 1096
    vaccines, 26, 56, 377, 381, 1096
        adverse events, 66, 1096–1097
        contraindications/precautions, 66
        future vaccines, 1097
        group childcare settings, 30t
        impact, 1096, 1097f
        live-attenuated tetravalent, 66
        monovalent (oral)(RV1), 66, 1096
        pentavalent reassortant (PRV)(RV5),
            66, 1096
        recommendations for, 66
        safety, 1096–1097
        schedule, 49f
        tetravalent rhesus (RRV), 47
        tetravalent rhesus (RRV), adverse
            events, 47
        for travelers, 79
Roth spots, 259
Rothia dentocariosa, 768
Roundworms *see* Nematodes
Roux-en-Y loop, 414
RRNA, 674–675, 697
16s rRNA
    bacterial identification, 674–675, 674f
        streptococci, 697, 697t
    genes, 674–675
    Nocardia identification, 794
    nonenteric gram-negative bacilli, 832
    streptococci, 697, 697t
    viridans group streptococci, 716–717
RSV *see* Respiratory syncytial virus (RSV)
Rubella virus, 1112–1117
    acquired rubella, 1112
        clinical features, 1114–1115
        complications, 1116
        differential diagnosis, 1116
        epidemiology, 1113–1114, 1114f
        immune response, 1112–1113, 1113f
        laboratory findings and diagnosis,
            1116
        pathogenesis/transmission, 1112
    acute bilateral cervical lymphadenitis
        due to, 139
    antibodies, 1112–1113, 1116, 1396
    arthritis due to, 481, 1116
    chronic fatigue syndrome pathogenesis,
        1008t–1009t
    clinical manifestations, 1114–1116
    congenital rubella, 536, 547t, 1112
        clinical features, 537t, 1115–1116,
            1115f, 1115t
        deafness, 548
        diagnosis, 538t, 1116, 1116t, 1398
        epidemiology, 1114, 1114f
        immune response, 1113, 1113f
        incidence, 58–59

long-term sequelae, 1116
morbidity reduced by vaccine, 48t
pathogenesis, 1113
retinopathy, 500–501, 500f
conjunctivitis due to, 492t
description and structure, 1112–1113
diagnosis/detection, 402, 1116, 1395–1396
optimal tests, 1389t–1392t
sample collection/transport, 1395–1396
elimination goal, 47
encephalitis due to, 1116
epidemiology, 1113–1114, 1114f
exposure management in pregnant healthcare worker, 22t–23t
immune globulin, 1117
immune response, 1112–1113, 1113f
inactivation methods, 1112
incubation period, 1114
laboratory findings, 1116
laboratory testing, 308t–311t
oral features, 192t
in pregnancy, 1113
prevention, 1117
active immunity, 1117
isolation procedures, 1117
passive immunity, 1117
public health measures, 1117
proteins, 1112
reinfection, 1114–1115
retinitis due to, 500–501, 500f
rheumatoid arthritis and, 1116
RNA genome, 1112
transmission, 1112
breast milk, 545
fetal, 536
treatment of infections, 1116
vaccination, 1112–1114, 1114f
adults, 60
adverse events, 60, 1117
adverse events and IoM findings, 50t, 60
contraindications, 1117
generalized lymphadenopathy, 130, 131t–132t
measurement of response, 46
strategies, 1114
US programs, 1114
vaccines, 59
fetal infection, 60
MMR see Measles, mumps, and rubella (MMR) vaccine
RA 27/3 live-attenuated, 59, 1112–1113, 1117
recommendations, 60
response to, 59
see also Measles, mumps, and rubella (MMR) vaccine
Rubeola virus (measles), 1137–1144, 1144b
acute otitis media, 1141
anterior uveitis due to, 499t
antibodies to, 1137–1138, 1141, 1396
maternal, effect on vaccination, 1143
aseptic meningitis due to, 294
bronchiolitis due to, 231
cell-associated viremia, 1138

chronic fatigue syndrome pathogenesis, 1008t–1009t
clinical manifestations, 1140, 1144b
atypical measles, 1140
modified measles, 1140
typical measles, 1140, 1140f
complications, 1141–1143
conjunctivitis due to, 492t, 1140
description and virology, 1137–1138
diagnosis/detection, 1141, 1144b, 1395–1396
optimal tests, 1389t–1392t
differential diagnosis, 1141
Kawasaki disease vs., 1005
elimination goal, 47
encephalitis after, 303, 1141, 1143
see also Subacute sclerosing panencephalitis (SSPE)
epidemics, 1137–1139
epidemiology, 1138–1140, 1138f–1139f, 1144b
prevalence, 59
generalized lymphadenopathy, 130, 131t–132t
healthcare-associated infections, 13
hemorrhagic (black) measles, 1140
in HIV infection, 1143–1144
immune globulin, 38, 1144
modified measles after, 1140
vaccine deferment after, 1144
immune response, 1138, 1141–1142
immunity to, 1137–1138
transplacental, 1140
in immunocompromised hosts, 1143
incubation period, 1140
institution-associated measles, 1144
isolation procedures, 1144
keratitis due to, 496
laboratory findings, 1141
laboratory testing, 308t–311t
lipid envelope and inactivation, 1138
lips in, 111
mediastinal lymphadenopathy due to, 154
Moraten strain, 1143
morbidity reduced by vaccine, 48t, 1139
mortality, 78, 1138–1139, 1141, 1143
nonpreventable cases, 1139
oral features, 192t
oral mucosal features, 192t, 1140
pathogenesis of infection, 1138
pathology, 1138
in pregnancy, 1143
prevention, 1143–1144, 1144b
active immunity, 1143–1144
passive immunity, 38, 1144
public health measures and outbreak control, 1144
public health measures and outbreak control, 1144
replication, 1138
resurgence of measles, 1139
RNA genome, 1137
structural proteins, 1137–1138
susceptibility to and risk factors, 1139–1140
transient anicteric hepatitis in, 1140
transmission, 1138

treatment of infection, 1141, 1144b
vaccination/immunization, 1143–1144
adverse events, 46, 60, 1143
adverse events and IoM findings, 50t
allergic reactions, 1143
contraindications, 1143
Crohn disease association, 1143
deferment after immune globulin, 1144
effect of maternal antibody, 1143
formalin-inactivated, 46
IGIV effect, 38, 1144
immunity induced by, 1143
measurement of response, 46
recommendations, 1143–1144
reduced measles incidence, 1139
timing, 46
vaccine, 59, 1139, 1143–1144
development, 59
high-titre, 1143–1144
inactivated, 46, 1139
live-attenuated, 1138–1139, 1143
sensitization to wild virus, 46
for travelers, 78, 78t
two-dose program, 1143–1144
see also Measles, mumps, rubella and varicella (MMRV) vaccine
Rubivirus genus, 1112
Rubulavirus genus, 1125

S

Sabia virus (Brazilian hemorrhagic fever), 1160t
Saccharomyces boulardii, Clostridium difficile infection treatment, 585
Saccharomyces cerevisiae, allergy to, hepatitis B vaccine risk, 59
Saddle nose, congenital syphilis, 944
Safety, for travelers see Travelers, protection of
S(ain)t Louis encephalitis virus see St Louis encephalitis virus
Saksenaea, 1212–1213
Salbutamol, bronchiolitis management, 234
Salicylates, acute rheumatic fever response, 704
Saline
nebulized hypertonic, 641
nose drops, mucopurulent rhinorrhea, 164
Saliva, HIV transmission, 642–643
Salivary gland infections, 195–196
Salivary gland masses, 143
Salmon River virus, 1094
Salmonella, 814–818
antimicrobial resistance, 816–817
in asplenia, 636
asymptomatic infection, 817
bloodstream infection, 816–817
brain abscess due to, 817
clinical manifestations, 119t–120t, 816–817
acute abdominal pain, 174
cross-reaction with Yersinia enterocolitica, 824
culture media, 1376t
description, 814

diagnosis/detection, 385t, 817
diarrhea, 816
  group childcare infections and, 25
differential diagnosis, 818
enteric fever, generalized
    lymphadenopathy, 130
epidemiology, 815–816
epididymitis due to, 367
excretion, 816–817
experimental infection, normal flora
    effect, 961
extraintestinal focal infections, 817
factors predisposing to, 815t, 816
fever of unknown origin due to,
    119t–120t
foodborne infections, 393–394, 394t,
    398t, 817
gastroenteritis due to, 816, 818
generalized lymphadenopathy due to,
    130, 131t–132t
genome, 814–815
genome sequencing, 814–815
group childcare and, 25, 25t
healthcare-associated infections, 816
in HIV infection, 662
host defences against, 815
inflammatory enteritis due to, 384
in interferon-γ receptor deficiency, 632
in iron overload state, 638
meningitis due to, 272–273
microbiology, 814
multidrug-resistant (MDR), 816
nomenclature, 814, 814t
nontyphoidal, 814–818
    epidemiology, 815–816
    foodborne disease, 393–394
    inflammatory enteritis, 383, 383t
    reservoir, 815
    serotypes, 815, 815t
number ingested for disease, 816
osteomyelitis, in sickle-cell disease, 475
pathogenesis, 814–815
pathology, 814
poultry transmitting, 528
prevention of infections, 818, 819t
prognosis, 818
pyogenic arthritis, 477
reduced HBD1 and LL-37 expression, 84
sepsis due to, 98
septicemia due to, 817
serotypes, 814
    animal-associated, 815, 815t
sickle-cell disease, 634–635
transmission from reptiles, 528
transmission prevention, 531
travelers' diarrhea due to, 373
treatment of infections, 818
typhoid see Salmonella Typhi
typhoid fever (non S. Typhi), 817
in X-linked agammaglobulinemia, 610
Salmonella Choleraesuis, 635, 816
Salmonella Dublin, 814–815
Salmonella enterica, 814
Salmonella enteritica serotype Typhimurium
    see Salmonella Typhimurium
Salmonella Enteritidis
    bloodstream infection, 816–817
    definitive phage type 104 (DT104), 816

Salmonella heidelberg, 635
Salmonella Paratyphi A, 814
    antimicrobial resistance, 816
    clinical features, 817
    epidemiology, 816
Salmonella serotype Tilene, rodents
    associated, 528
Salmonella Typhi, 814
    antimicrobial resistance, 816
    epidemiology, 816
    genome, 814–815
    prognosis and recurrence, 818
    typhoid fever
        clinical features, 817
        differential diagnosis, 818
        fever, 817
        generalized lymphadenopathy, 130,
            131t–132t
        prevention, 818, 819t
        treatment, 818
    vaccine, 67, 79, 377, 818, 819t
        adverse effects, 67
        immunocompromised travelers,
            82–83
        schedule/dosing for travelers, 79t
        for travelers, 79
        Ty21a, 67, 79, 818, 819t
        Vi conjugate, 818, 819t
        Vi vaccine, 67, 79
    Vi antigen, 67
Salmonella Typhimurium
    bloodstream infection, 816–817
    in childcare setting, 30–31
    genome, 814–815
Salmonellosis see Salmonella
Salpingitis, acute, Neisseria gonorrhoeae
    causing, 747
Samples, in statistical analysis, 6
    size, 6, 9
San Joaquin valley fever see Coccidioides
    immitis (coccidioidomycosis)
Sandflies, Leishmania transmission,
    1285–1286, 1285f, 1288–1289
Sandifer syndrome, persistent/recurrent
    pneumonia, 250
Santorini, fissures, 221
Sapovirus(es), 378, 1187–1189
    characteristics, 1188t
    clinical manifestations, 1189
    epidemiology, 379, 380t, 1189
    gastroenteritis, 378, 380t
        sporadic, 379
    genogroups, 1187
    pathogenesis and immune response,
        1187
Sapporo-like viruses, 378, 1188t
Sapporo virus, 1188t
Saprophytes, 1194
    culture media, 1382
    Histoplasma capsulatum, 1224
    skin, 517
Saquinavir, 665t, 1444t–1452t
Sarcina, 674
Sarcocystis, 1306–1308
    description and structure, 1306, 1308f
    diagnosis, 1308, 1308f
    life cycle, 1306, 1307f
Sarcocystis hominis, 1306

Sarcocystis suihominis, 1306
Sarcoidosis
    cervical lymphadenopathy, 141
    clinical features, 119t–120t
    eosinophilic meningitis, 333
    fever of unknown origin due to,
        119t–120t
    generalized lymphadenopathy, 135
    mediastinal lymphadenopathy, 155
Sarcoptes scabiei (scabies), 1259–1261,
        1261b
    chemoprophylaxis, 70t–71t
    clinical manifestations, 1260, 1260f
    crusted scabies, 1259–1260
        treatment, 1261
    diagnosis, 1260, 1260f
    eosinophilia, 1408t–1409t
    epidemiology, 1259–1260, 1261b
    group childcare and, 25t, 29
    microbiology, 1259, 1261b
    Norwegian (crusted), in cancer, 575
    pathogenesis, 1259
    prevention, 1261
    refugee and internationally adopted
        children, 36
    sexual transmission, 349
    transmission, 352
    treatment, 1258t, 1260–1261, 1261b
        crusted scabies, 1261
        first-line treatments, 1260–1261
        second-line treatments, 1261
    virulence, 1259
SARS-CoV see Human coronaviruses
    (HCoV), SARS-CoV
Satellite virus, HDV as, 1086–1087
Saturated potassium iodide solution
    (SSKI)
    adverse effects, 1219–1220
    Sporothrix schenckii (sporotrichosis),
        1219–1220
Scabies see Sarcoptes scabiei (scabies)
Scald injuries, 516
Scalded skin syndrome, staphylococcal
    (SSSS), 676, 684–685
    clinical features, 440
Scalp
    abscess, 458–459
        coagulase-negative staphylococci
            causing, 693
        Escherichia coli, 458–459
        etiology, 458–459
        Neisseria gonorrhoea, 744
    animal bites, 523–524
    infections
        tinea capitis see Tinea capitis
        tinea favosa (favus), 1249
Scarlatina/scarlet fever see Streptococcus
    pyogenes
Scars, varicella lesions, 1037
Scedosporium, arthritis, 482
Scedosporium apiospermum, 1210, 1253
    amphotericin B resistance, 1210
    microbiology, 1253
Scedosporium aurantiacum, 1250
Scedosporium prolificans, 1211–1212
Scheuermann's kyphosis, back pain due to,
    188
Schick test, 758

Schistosoma (schistosomiasis), 1368–1371, 1370b–1371b
  acute, 1369
  cercarial dermatitis due to, 1370
  clinical features, 1369, 1370b–1371b
  CNS schistosomiasis, 1370
  description and life cycle, 1368, 1368f, 1370b–1371b
  diagnosis/detection, 385t, 1369–1370, 1369f, 1370b–1371b
  drug resistance concerns, 1370
  effect on growth and development, 1369
  eosinophilia due to, 1407, 1408t–1409t
  epidemiology, 1368–1369, 1370b–1371b
  generalized lymphadenopathy, 131t–132t, 132
  hepatosplenic disease, 1368–1369
  intestinal schistosomiasis, 1368–1369
  pathogenesis and immune response, 1369
  precautions for travelers, 76
  prevention, 1370
  refugee and internationally adopted children, 35–36
  treatment, 1370, 1370b–1371b
  urinary schistosomiasis, 1368–1369
Schistosoma bovis, 1368
Schistosoma haematobium, 1368–1369
  epidemiology, 1256, 1368
  ova, 1369–1370, 1369f
  pathogenesis, 1369
  urinary schistosomiasis, 1369
Schistosoma intercalatum, 1368–1370
Schistosoma japonicum, 1368
  clinical manifestations, 1369
  eosinophilic meningitis, 331t
  epidemiology, 1368
  ova, 1369–1370, 1369f
Schistosoma mansoni, 1368
  clinical manifestations, 1369
  epidemiology, 1256, 1368
  ova, 1369–1370, 1369f
Schistosoma matthei, 1368
Schistosoma mekongi, 1368–1370
Schistosomiasis *see Schistosoma* (schistosomiasis)
Schistosomulae, 1368
Schizogony, 1291, 1298
  exo-erythrocytic, 1298
Schizont, *Plasmodium*, 1298f, 1299
Schizonticides, 1304
School absenteeism, chronic fatigue syndrome, 1012, 1015
Scleral hemorrhage, *Bordetella pertussis* infection, 870, 870f
Scleritis, after *Neisseria meningitidis* infections, 738
Scolices, *Taenia*, 1350f
Scombroid poisoning, 812
Scrapie, 334–335
Screening
  abdominal pain causes, 176
  post-travel, 83
  refugee and internationally adopted children, 32–36
  tests in recurrent/persistent pneumonia, 252
  see also individual infections

Scrofula, 777
Scrofuloderma, 779
Scrotal pain, 346t
  chronic, prostatitis, 369
  epididymitis, 367
  sexually transmitted infection causing, 346t, 348–349
Scrub typhus, 131t–132t, 132, 935–938
  see also Rickettsiosis
"Scrum-pox", 1029
Seadornavirus, 1094
Seafood
  raw, ingestion, eosinophilic meningitis, 330, 332
  see also Fish; Shellfish-borne disease
Seal finger, 521–522, 999
Sealpox virus, 1020t
Seborrheic dermatitis
  in HIV infection, 656
  Malassezia, 1216–1218
  tinea capitis *vs.*, 1247
Secondary granule deficiency, 603t–604t, 619t
Seizures
  acute bacterial meningitis, 273–274, 278
  aseptic meningitis, 295
  brain abscess complication, 329–330
  CNS device infections, 597
  cysticercosis (*Taenia solium*), 1352–1353
    recurrent, 1355
    treatment, 1354–1355
  HHV-6 infection (roseola), 1055
  infant botulism, 975
  neonatal meningitis, 540
  Plasmodium infections, 1299
  RSV infection, 1132–1133
  Shigella infections, 821
  subacute sclerosing panencephalitis, 1142–1143
  Toxocara canis infection, 1336
Selectins, 85, 94
Selective IgA deficiency *see* Immunoglobulin A (IgA), deficiency
Selenite broth, 1375t
Selenium sulfide
  Malassezia infections, 1217
  tinea capitis, 1247
Semicritical equipment, 21
Sendai virus, 1193–1194
Sennetsu fever, generalized lymphadenopathy, 131t–132t, 132
Sensitivity, 1, 2t
Sensitivity analysis, 8–9
Sensory ganglia, HSV infection, 1027
Sepsis, 97–103
  biologic markers, 99
  clinical features, 98–99
  controlled phase III trials, 103
  cytokine levels, 100
  definition, 97, 98b
  etiology, 97–98
  incidence and estimates by age, 97t
  laboratory findings, 99
  management, 99–103, 101t–102t
    anticoagulants, 102
    anticytokine therapy, 100
    antiendotoxin therapy, 100

  antimicrobial therapy, 99, 99t
  arachidonic acid inhibition, 100
  corticosteroids, 100–102
  endothelial-targeted therapy, 102
  future prospects, 103
  IVIG, 100
  supportive care, 99–100
  morbidity and mortality, 97, 97t
  neonatal, 537
  neonatal syndrome, 547
  pathophysiology, 98
    arachidonic acid metabolites, 100
    cytokines, 100
    endotoxin actions, 100
    risk factors, 98
  severe
    definition, 98b, 685
    Staphylococcus aureus causing, 685–686
  see also Septicemia
Septic arthritis *see* Arthritis, pyogenic (bacterial)
Septic shock, 97–103
  Burkholderia pseudomallei, 848
  definition, 97, 98b
  management, 99–103
    glucocorticoids, 100–102
    see also Sepsis, management
  Pasteurella multocida infections, 837
  pharmacokinetics, 1437t, 1438
Septic thrombophlebitis, 265
  diagnosis, 265
  intracranial
    clinical features, 323–324, 323t
    CT and MRI, 326
    differential diagnosis, 325
    epidemiology, 321
    etiology, 321
    management, 328
  management and complications, 265
  risk factors and pathogenesis, 265
  Staphylococcus aureus, 683
  symptoms, 265
  see also Septic venous thrombosis
Septic venous thrombosis
  clinical features, 323–324, 323t
  complications and prognosis, 330
  CT and MRI, 326, 327f
  differential diagnosis, 325
  etiology, 321
  management, 328
  in necrotizing otitis externa, 222
  pathogenesis, 322
  see also Septic thrombophlebitis
Septicemia, infections causing
  Acinetobacter, 829
  Aeromonas, 831
  anaerobic infections, 962
  animal bites leading to, 523
  Arcanobacterium haemolyticum, 751
  in asplenia, 636
  Bacillus anthracis, 752
  Bacillus cereus infections, 754
  Burkholderia pseudomallei, 848
  burn wound, 517–518
  Campylobacter upsaliensis, 880
  Citrobacter, 806–807
  Clostridium septicum, 980t, 981

coagulase-negative staphylococci, 691–692
Corynebacterium diphtheriae, 756
early-onset, in neonates, 537
Edwardsiella tarda, 808
Enterococcus faecalis, 713
Erysipelothrix rhusiopathiae, 768
Escherichia coli, 797
groups C and G streptococci, 720
Helicobacter associated, 916
infant botulism *vs.*, 974t
Kingella kingae, 921
Malassezia, 1217
meningococcal *see Neisseria meningitidis*
neonatal *see* Neonatal infections, septicemia
neutropenia in neonates, 84
in polysplenia, 636
postpartum/postabortion, *Gardnerella vaginalis*, 769
Pseudomonas aeruginosa, 435f, 844f, 844t
Pseudomonas putida, 841
puerperal, 981
recurrent, *Salmonella*, 817
renal transplant recipients, 557
secondary infections in varicella, 1037
Serratia marcescens, 813
sickle-cell disease, 635
in stem cell transplant recipients, 691–692
Vibrio vulnificus, 855–856
viridans group streptococci, 717–718
Yersinia pestis, 826
Yersinia pseudotuberculosis, 825
see also Bacteremia; Sepsis
Sequestra, 469
Serologic tests, 1384
adenoviruses, 1070
Aspergillus, 1207
Bartonella henselae, 859–860
Blastomyces dermatitidis, 1237
Bordetella pertussis, 870
Borrelia burgdorferi, 955
pitfalls and problems, 955
Candida infections, 1200
Chlamydia trachomatis, 887–888, 1398
Chlamydophila pneumoniae, 882–883
CMV infection, 1049, 1049b
Coccidioides immitis (coccidioidomycosis), 1243
Coxiella burnetii, 892
Echinococcus multilocularis, 1361
Entamoeba histolytica, 1277
Enterobius vermicularis, 1332
enteroviruses, 1179
Francisella tularensis, 898
HCV, 1109–1110
hepatitis A virus, 1183, 1183f
HHV-6, 1393–1394
HHV-7, 1393–1394
HIV, 1388
HSV, 1033, 1396
human parainfluenza viruses, 1123–1124
influenza viruses, 1154
Leptospira, 951
measles, mumps and rubella, 1396
Mycobacterium tuberculosis, 781
Mycoplasma pneumoniae, 995

Neisseria gonorrhoeae detection, 745
in persistent pneumonia, 248
Plasmodium, 1300
Rickettsia, 938
Rickettsia prowazekii, 931
Rickettsia typhi, 932
Schistosoma, 1370
Strongyloides, 1333
Toxocara, 1336–1337
Toxoplasma gondii, 1312–1314
Treponema pallidum subsp. *pallidum* (syphilis), 944
Trypanosoma (Trypanozoon) brucei infection, 1321–1322
Trypanosoma cruzi infection, 1325
visceral leishmaniasis diagnosis, 1287
VZV, 1393
Yersinia pestis, 826–827
Serratia, 813–814
clinical features, 813
microbiology and epidemiology, 813
prostatitis due to, 369
treatment of infections, 813–814
Serratia ficaria, 813
Serratia fonticola, 813
Serratia liquefaciens, 813
Serratia marcescens, 813
clinical features, 813
β-lactamases, 813
meningitis, 813–814
microbiology and epidemiology, 813
neonatal infections, 813
in phagocytic disorders, 620t
septicemia, 813
treatment of infections, 813–814
urinary tract infection (UTI), 813
Serratia odorifera, 813
Serratia plymuthica, 813
Serratia rubidaea, 813
Serum amyloid A, neonatal septicemia diagnosis, 541t
Serum opacity factor (SOF), *Streptococcus pyogenes* (group A streptococcus), 698
Serum sickness
acute schistosomiasis resembling, 1369
diphtheria antitoxin associated, 757
Severe acute respiratory syndrome (SARS) *see* Human coronaviruses (HCoV)
Severe acute respiratory syndrome-coronavirus *see* Human coronaviruses (HCoV), SARS-CoV
Severe combined immunodeficiency (SCID), 627–629
autosomal, 603t–604t
bacterial infections, 628
characteristic infections, 627–629
definition, 627
diagnosis, 629
forms, clinical features, 627, 628t
fungal infections, 628
gene defects and inheritance, 627, 628t
GvHD, 628–629
immunization contraindication, 629
rotavirus vaccine, 66
indication for IGIV, 40
Pneumocystis jirovecii (carinii) infection, 627–628, 1230, 1233
pneumonia, 629

"radiosensitive", 603t–604t
T lymphocytes, 627
treatment, 629
viral infections, 627–628
X-linked, 603t–604t, 627, 629
Sewage, contamination of water, *Cryptosporidium*, 1269–1270
Sexual abuse, infections associated, 370–372
Chlamydia trachomatis, 370–371, 370f, 1389t–1392t, 1399
culture of pathogens, 357
diagnosis of abuse, 353–356
evaluation, 370, 370f
herpes simplex virus (HSV), 371
HIV, 371–372
human papillomavirus (HPV), 371
Neisseria gonorrhoeae, 370–371, 370f, 744
Treponema pallidum subsp. *pallidum* infections, 371, 945
Trichomonas vaginalis, 1318
vulvovaginitis, 356–357
Sexual activity, urinary tract infection risk factor, 340
Sexual transmission of pathogens *see individual pathogens*
Sexually transmitted infections (STIs), 345–349
asymptomatic, 346
chemoprophylaxis, 72
Chlamydia trachomatis, 885t, 886
see also Chlamydia trachomatis
concurrent infections, 351
endocervicitis etiology, 362
epidemiology, 345–346
epididymitis associated, 346t, 348–349, 367
gonorrhea *see Neisseria gonorrhoeae*
Haemophilus ducreyi (chancroid), 907
HCV, 1107
HIV co-infection, 672
HIV transmission, 648, 657
Neisseria gonorrhoeae see Neisseria gonorrhoeae
office and laboratory tests, 347t
pelvic inflammatory disease and, 353
sexual abuse and *see* Sexual abuse
symptomatic infections/syndromes, 346–349, 346t
anal discharge/proctitis syndrome, 346t, 347
dermatologic syndromes, 346t, 349
discharge/dysuria syndrome, 346–347, 346t
genital ulcer/lymphadenopathy syndrome, 346t, 347–351
jaundice associated with viral hepatitis, 349
pelvic pain syndrome, 346t, 348–349
pharyngeal infections, 346t, 349
scrotal pain syndrome, 346t, 348–349
see also Genital ulcer disease (GUD)
treatment, CDC/WHO guidelines, 803
Treponema pallidum see Treponema pallidum subsp. *pallidum* (syphilis)
Trichomonas vaginalis, 1318
urethritis, 353–356
see also individual pathogens

SH2 domain protein 1A/*SAP* gene, 633
SH2D1A (SH2 domain protein 1A) gene
    mutations, 633
Sheep blood agar, 1375t
    CSF inoculation, 1377
Shell vial method, 233–234, 1386, 1386t
    Chlamydia trachomatis, 1398
    CMV, 1386, 1388
    HSV, 1386, 1388
    RSV, 1394
    for specific viruses, 1386t
Shellfish-borne disease, 395
    neurotoxic poisoning, 396t, 397
    Paragonimus infections, 1367–1368
    paralytic, 373, 396t
    Vibrio cholerae, 395
Shewanella, 835
Shewanella algae, 835
Shewanella putrefaciens, 835
Shewanellaceae, 833
Shiga-like toxin (STx), *Escherichia coli*, 796
Shiga toxin, 820
Shigella, 819–823
    acute abdominal pain due to, 174
    antimicrobial resistance, 822
    bloodstream infection, 821
    chromosomal virulence genes, 820
    clinical manifestations, 821–822
    complications of infections, 821–822
    culture media, 1376t
    description and microbiology, 819
    diagnosis/detection, 385t, 822
    diarrhea due to, 26t, 373
    dysentery *see Shigella dysenteriae* type 1
    epidemiology, 820–821
    experimental infection, normal flora
        effect, 961
    extraintestinal infections, 821
    foodborne infections, 394, 394t, 397,
        398t
    group childcare outbreaks, 24–26, 25t
    immune response to, 815
    inflammatory enteritis, 383–384
    ipaABCD (plasmid antigens), 820
    laboratory findings, 822
    musculoskeletal symptoms, 821
    neonatal infections, 821–822
    neurologic symptoms, 821
    pathogenesis, 820
    pathology, 820
    plasmid virulence genes, 820
    prevention, 822–823
    reduced HBD1 and LL-37 expression, 84
    serogroups, 819
    surgical complications, 821
    travelers' diarrhea due to, 373
    treatment of infections, 822, 822t
    uncomplicated shigellosis, 821
    vaccine development, 81, 823
    vulvovaginitis due to, 357, 821
Shigella dysenteriae type 1
    bacillary dysentery due to, epidemiology,
        821
    bloodstream infection, 821
    hemolytic uremic syndrome, 798
    prevalence, 821
    profound neutrophilia due to,
        1404–1405

Shiga toxin, 820
    treatment, 387
Shigella flexneri
    bloodstream infection, 821
    prevalence, 821
    Reye-like syndrome, 821
    treatment, 822
Shigella sonnei
    antibiotic resistance, 31
    group childcare outbreaks, 25–26
    inflammatory enteritis, 383–384, 383t
    prevalence, 821
    Reye-like syndrome, 821
    treatment, 822
Shingles *see* Varicella zoster virus (VZV),
    herpes zoster
Shock
    endotoxic, *Yersinia pestis* infection
        (bubonic plague), 826
    septic *see* Septic shock
    warm *vs* cold, 97
Shock syndrome, bacterial
    staphylococcal *see* Toxic shock syndrome
        (TSS)
    streptococcal *see Streptococcus pyogenes*
Short-gut syndrome, 391, 729
Short-limbed dwarfism/cartilage-hair
    dysplasia, 603t–604t
Short stature, *Helicobacter pylori* infections,
    913
Shunting procedures, persistent pneumonia,
    247
SHV enzymes, in drug resistance, 1424
Sialadenitis
    acute suppurative, 195
    neonatal, 195
    recurrent acute, 195
Sialectasia, recurrent, 143
Sialic acid, 85, 797
Sialyl-Lewis X, 85, 626
Siberian tickborne encephalitis virus,
    epidemiology and vectors, 532t
Siblings, visiting, infections from, 19
Sickle-cell disease, 632–641
    bone and joint infections, 635–636,
        635f
    bone pain, 186
    clinical manifestations, 634
    CNS infections, 634–635
    complement deficiency, 619
    epidemiology of infections, 634
    erythrocyte sedimentation rate, 1402
    gallstones, 414
    infection etiology, 634
    influenza vaccine, 636
    intra-abdominal abscess in, 424
    management and presumptive therapy,
        635–636
    meningitis, 634–635
    mortality, 633–634
    Mycoplasma pneumoniae infection, 634
    osteomyelitis, 475, 475b
    parvovirus B19 infection, 636
    pathogenesis/pathology, 634
    persistent/recurrent pneumonia, 251
    pneumococcal conjugate vaccine, 636
    pneumococcal polysaccharide vaccine,
        636

    pneumonia, 634–635
    prevention of infections, 636
    pulmonary infections, 634–635
    Salmonella infection, 634–635
    septicemia, 635
    Streptococcus pneumoniae infections,
        634–636, 722
    transient aplastic crisis, 636
    vaso-occlusive disease (stroke), 634–635
Siderophores, 763–764
    fluorescent, *Pseudomonas aeruginosa*
        producing, 842, 842t
    Klebsiella, 800
Sigma factor, σ^B, 676
Sigmoidoscopy, *Clostridium difficile*
    infections, 978
Signal transduction system, *Staphylococcus
    aureus*, 676
Signaling pathways, Toll-like receptors
    (TLRs), 84, 102–103
Silver nitrate
    burns, treatment, 1500t–1501t
    eye infection treatment, 1494t–1495t
    gonococcal ophthalmia neonatorum
        prevention, 490, 747–748
Silver sulfadiazine, burn wound infections,
    520, 520t, 1500t–1501t
Simian immunodeficiency virus (SIV),
    1166
    HHV-6 cofactor, 1057
Simian T-lymphotropic viruses (STLV),
    1165
Simian vacuolated polyomavirus (SV40),
    1075
Simulium (blackflies), 1344
Sindbis virus, 1098
    arthritis, 481
Single-patient room, HAI prevention
    strategies, 13
Sinus(es), paranasal *see* Paranasal sinuses
Sinus histiocytes, 134
Sinus histiocytosis with massive
    lymphadenopathy (Rosai–Dorfman
    disease), 134, 142t
    cervical lymphadenopathy in, 141
Sinus ostia, obstruction, 227
    predisposing factors, 227, 227t
Sinusitis, 227–231
    acute bacterial (ABS), 163–165, 227
        biphasic, 228
        *Chlamydophila (Chlamydia)
            pneumoniae*, 882
        clinical features, 164t, 228, 228b
        common cold complication, 199
        common colds *vs.*, 198
        complications, 230, 230b
        diagnosis, 164t
        diagnostic methods, 228–229
        differential diagnosis, 164t
        Haemophilus influenzae, 900, 903
        management, 164t, 229–230, 229t,
            1418t–1419t
        microbiology, 229, 229t
        outcome of treatment, 230–231
        persistence of symptoms, 228
        prevalence, 227
        severity, symptoms, 228
        sinus aspiration, 229

surgical management, 230–231
treatment failure, 237t
viral infections preceding, 227–228, 228f
worsening of symptoms, 228
anaerobic gram-negative bacilli, 983
aspergillosis *vs.* zygomycosis, 1204
Aspergillus, 1204, 1204f
in burns patients, 519
in cancer, 577
chronic, 228, 230
anaerobic gram-positive cocci, 989
bacteriology, 229t
management, 230
clinical features, 228
viral infections, 228
cough in, 167t
in cystic fibrosis, 638–639
diagnostic methods, 228–229
frontal, 324f
fungal, 577
headache in, 177t, 178, 228
inflammatory edema, preseptal cellulitis
due to, 510
management, 229–230
microbiology, 229
Moraxella catarrhalis, 840
mucopurulent rhinorrhea in, 163
pathogenesis, 227
phaeohyphomycosis, 1211
recurrent, 230
Staphylococcus aureus, 680–681
subacute, 228, 229t
viral infections
pathogens, 229
recurrent sinusitis, 230
time course, 228f
SIRS *see* Systemic inflammatory response
syndrome
"Sixth exanthematous disease of childhood"
see Human herpesvirus 6 (HHV-6)
Sjögren syndrome, viral parotitis *vs.*, 195
Skin
antiseptics for, 1499, 1499t
intravascular catheter infection
prevention, 593
barrier to infections, 83–84, 512
biopsy
burn wound infections, 517, 517b
Onchocerca volvulus infections, 1345
in chronic meningitis, 284–285, 284t
colonization, *Malassezia*, 1216
darkening, visceral leishmaniasis, 1287
defense mechanism *vs.* pathogen
virulence, 427
epithelial colonization by pathogens,
427
HIV transmission, 642–643
host defense, 517
lesions
in familial Mediterranean fever,
124–125
in HIDS, 125
in TRAPS, 126
types, 427t
normal flora, 427
blood transfusion-associated infection
due to, 581

scrapings
Malassezia, 1217
Sporothrix schenckii, 1219
sexually transmitted infection
syndromes, 346t, 349, 351–352
snips, *Onchocerca volvulus* infections,
1345
structure, 427, 438, 438f
trauma, pathogens and infection
prophylaxis, 513–514
infection risk and management, 513t
Skin disease, in HIV infection, 656
Skin infections, 349–352
Aeromonas, 830–831
anaerobic gram-negative bacilli, 984
anaerobic gram-positive cocci causing,
989
Aspergillus, 574, 1205
Bacillus cereus, 754
Blastomyces dermatitidis (blastomycosis),
1234f, 1236, 1236f, 1236t
in cancer, 574–575
Clostridium causing, 980t
Coccidioides immitis (coccidioidomycosis),
1242, 1242f
Cryptococcus, 1222
diphtheria *see* *Corynebacterium diphtheriae*
empiric transmission-based precautions,
20t
endocarditis prevention, 76
Erysipelothrix rhusiopathiae, 767
fungal *see* Dermatophytes
Fusarium, 1210, 1210f
group childcare and, 25t, 29–30
groups C and G streptococci causing,
720
HSV, 1029–1030, 1029f, 1034
Leishmania *see* *Leishmania* (leishmaniasis)
Malassezia, 1216–1218, 1218b
mucormycosis, 1214
Mycobacterium tuberculosis, 779
Mycoplasma pneumoniae, 994t
neonatal, 541
nosocomial, 550
nontuberculous mycobacteria, 787t,
788–789
primary, 427, 454–455
prophylaxis/treatment, 1498–1499,
1498t–1499t
duration, 1418t–1419t
in refugee and internationally adopted
children, 36
rodents associated, 528
secondary, 454–455
Sporothrix schenckii (sporotrichosis),
1219–1220
superficial, 427–430, 428t
bacterial, 427–435
Yersinia enterocolitica, 824
see also Soft-tissue infections; *individual
infections*
Skull
congenital defects, recurrent meningitis
risk, 287–288
fracture, 515
antibiotic prophylaxis, 292, 512t, 515
pathogens, 512t, 515
recurrent meningitis, 288

lymphangiomatosis, recurrent meningitis
associated, 287–288
SLAM receptor, 633
"Slapped cheek disease" *see* Parvovirus B19,
erythema infectiosum
Sleep, chronic fatigue syndrome
pathogenesis, 1010–1011
Sleep disorders, in *Trypanosoma brucei*
infection, 1321
Sleeping sickness *see* *Trypanosoma
(Trypanozoon) brucei*
"Slim disease", 655
Slime, 691
formation by *Staphylococcus epidermidis*,
691
Slipped capital femoral epiphysis (SCFE),
185–186
Slow infections of CNS *see* Prion diseases
Slow viral infections, 333
Small bowel
biopsy, *Cyclospora* or *Cystoisospora*, 1284
obstruction, vomiting and abdominal
pain, 171
Small round structured virus (SRSV), 1188t
Smallpox *see* Variola virus (smallpox)
Smoke inhalation, 516
Smoking, response to vaccines and, 46
"Snail fever" *see* *Schistosoma*
(schistosomiasis)
Snails
control, *Schistosoma* infection prevention,
1370
liver/lung trematode transmission,
1365
Schistosoma development, 1368
Social history, recurrent infections, 607
Sodium polyanetholesulfonate (SPS),
1373–1374
Sodium stibogluconate, leishmaniasis
treatment, 1520
visceral leishmaniasis, 1290, 1290t
Sodium sulfacetamide, conjunctivitis
treatment, 492–493
Soduka (spirillary rat-bite fever), 938, 958
Soft palate, paralysis, *Corynebacterium
diphtheriae*, 756–757
Soft tissue abscesses *see* Abscess
Soft tissue diseases
limb pain, 187
Streptococcus pyogenes causing, 700f–701f
Soft-tissue infections
Aeromonas, 830–831
anaerobic gram-negative bacilli, 984
anaerobic gram-positive cocci causing,
989
in cancer, 573–574
Clostridium causing, 980t
Corynebacterium species, 760t–761t
definition/description, 454–455
groups C and G streptococci causing,
720
Kingella kingae, 921
necrotizing *see* Necrotizing soft-tissue
infections
neonatal, 541
nontuberculous mycobacteria, 787t,
788–789
Pseudomonas aeruginosa, 843t

recurrent, anatomic/physiologic abnormalities predisposing, 600t
Streptococcus pneumoniae, 723
subcutaneous, 454–462
see also Skin infections
Soft-tissue necrosis, bite wound complication, 526
Soft-tissue sarcoma, neck masses, 142
Soft-tissue trauma, infections, 513–514
Soil-transmitted helminths see Nematodes (roundworms), intestinal
Solid-organ transplant recipients, infections, 555–561
   bacterial and fungal, 556–558, 560
   CMV see Cytomegalovirus (CMV)
   from donors, 560, 561t
   EBV infection, 559, 1063
   management, 560–561
   opportunistic infections, 560
   Pneumocystis jirovecii pneumonia, 560
   postoperative/posttransplant, 557
   predisposing factors, 555–556, 556b
      intraoperative, 556, 556b
      posttransplant factors, 556, 556b
      pretransplant, 555–556, 556b
   pretransplant evaluation, 560, 561t
   prevention, 560–561
   screening tests, 560, 561t
   timing (early to late period), 556–557, 557t
   Toxoplasma gondii infections, 560, 1311, 1314, 1317
   tuberculosis, 560
   viral infections, 556–560
      community-associated, 559–560
   see also individual organ transplants
Solvent-detergent treatment, use in intravenous IG preparation, 43
Somnolence, Trypanosoma brucei infection, 1321
Sore throat
   GAS pharyngitis, 200–201
   prevalence, 203
   respiratory tract diphtheria, 755–756
   severe, peritonsillar abscess (quinsy), 206
   subacute/chronic sinusitis, 228
Southern tick-associated rash illness (STARI), 532t, 533
   laboratory findings and diagnosis, 533t–534t
Space-occupying lesions, altered mental status, 179t
SPACEY group, 961
Spaulding classification, equipment, 21
Species, virus, 1015
Specific granule deficiency, 626
   characteristics, 619t
   clinical features, 621t
   infections associated, 620t
   infectious complications, 620t
Specificity, 1, 2t
Specimen collection/processing, fungi, 1194–1195
Specimens see Laboratory diagnosis
Spectinomycin
   mechanism of action, 1473–1474
   Neisseria gonorrhoeae infections, 747

Spherules, Coccidioides, 1239, 1239f–1240f, 1242–1243
Sphingobacteriaceae, 833
Sphingobacterium, 835
Sphingobacterium multivorum, 835
Sphingobacterium spritivorum, 835
Sphingomonadaceae, 833
Sphingomonas, 835
Sphingomonas paucimobilis (Pseudomonas paucimobilis), 835, 841
Sphingomyelinase, 676
Spin-amplified culture, 1386
   see also Shell vial method
Spinal cord tumor
   back pain due to, 188
   weakness due to, differential diagnosis, 181t–182t
Spinal disease, neurocysticercosis (Taenia solium), 1353, 1355t
Spinal epidural abscess see Epidural abscess
Spinal muscular atrophy, hypotonia, 181t
Spine
   abscess, epidural see Epidural abscess, spinal
   defects, recurrent meningitis association, 287b
   immobilization, diskitis, 485
   see also Vertebrae
Spiral organisms see Treponema
Spiramycin
   protozoan infection treatment, 1522
   Toxoplasma gondii infections, 1310–1311, 1313, 1315, 1315t
Spirilla, definition, 673
Spirillum, 673
Spirillum minor
   axillary lymphadenopathy due to, 159–160
   lymphangitis due to, 161, 161t
   treatment, 162
Spirillum minus, 938, 958
   clinical features, 958
   treatment of infections, 958
Spirochetes, 673, 941
   generalized lymphadenopathy, 130, 131t–132t
   see also Borrelia; Leptospira; Treponema pallidum
Spirometry, persistent/recurrent pneumonia, 252
Spleen
   abscess, 426
   anatomy and function, 127, 127t
   aspiration, visceral leishmaniasis diagnosis, 1287
   platelet destruction, 1409
   roles, 634, 636–637
   rupture
      EBV infection, 1061
      infections after, 514–515
   sickle-cell disease, 634
   smears, visceral leishmaniasis diagnosis, 1287
   visceral leishmaniasis, 1287
Splenectomy
   in HIV infection, 656
   immunization before, 637
   infection prevention, 515, 637

infections after, 514–515, 636
   pathogens and infection prophylaxis, 512t, 515
   splenic abscess treatment, 426
   see also Asplenia
Splenomegaly
   EBV infection, 1061
   murine typhus (Rickettsia typhi), 932
Spondylodiskitis, Kingella kingae, 920
Spondylolisthesis, back pain due to, 188
Spondylosis, back pain due to, 188
Sporangiophores, 1212–1213
Sporangiospores, 1212–1213
Sporangium, 1212–1213
Spores
   Clostridium botulinum, 971
   Clostridium difficile, 977
   Clostridium tetani, 967
   microsporidia, 1291, 1292f
Sporogony, 1291
Sporothrix, meningitis, 280t, 282–283, 283t, 286t
Sporothrix schenckii (sporotrichosis), 1218–1220, 1220b
   arthritis due to, 482, 1219
   clinical manifestations, 1219, 1220b
   cutaneous disease, 1219–1220
   diagnosis, 162, 1219, 1220b
   epidemiology, 1219, 1220b
   "fixed" infections, 1219–1220
   lymphangitis due to, 161–162, 161t, 162f
   lymphocutaneous, 1219–1220
   meningitis, 1219
   microbiology, 1218, 1220b
   in Peru, 1219
   pneumonia due to, 1219
   prevention of infections, 1220
   pulmonary disease, 1219–1220
   replication, 1219
   treatment of infections, 162, 1219–1220, 1220b
Sporotrichosis see Sporothrix schenckii (sporotrichosis)
Sporozoites
   Plasmodium, 1298–1299, 1298f
   Pneumocystis jirovecii (carinii), 1230
   Sarcocystis, 1306, 1307f
   Toxoplasma gondii, 1309, 1311
Sporulation, adventitious, 1206
Spot map, 7
Spotted fevers, 935–938
   see also Rickettsia; Rickettsiosis
Sputum
   contamination, non-typable Haemophilus influenzae detection, 903
   culture, cystic fibrosis, 640
   examination, Paragonimus infections, 1367
   induction technique, 1231
      tuberculosis diagnosis, 781
   Pneumocystis jirovecii (carinii) detection, 1231, 1231t
   pneumonia etiology determination, 240
   specimen collection/transport, 1374t, 1377
Squalene epoxidase inhibitors, 1486
ST-246, smallpox therapy, 1022–1023

St Louis encephalitis virus, 1102
aseptic meningitis due to, 294
diagnosis/detection, 1397
optimal tests, 1389t–1392t
encephalitis due to, 302–303
neuroinvasive disease (SLEND), 294
St Vitus dance (Sydenham chorea), 703–704
Stainer-Scholte medium, 1375t
Standard deviation, 2t, 5
Standard error, 2t, 5
Standard precautions
isolation precautions, 17–18
implementation, 17
indications for use, 17
recent additions, 17
recommendations for applying, 18t
see also Isolation precautions
Staphylococcal lid disease, 497, 497f
Staphylococcal toxic shock *see* Toxic shock
syndrome (TSS)
Staphylococcus (staphylococci)
antimicrobial susceptibility testing,
1380–1381
characteristics, 696t
coagulase-negative (CONS), 689–695
abscesses, 693
antimicrobial resistance, 693
AtlE, 690–691
biofilm formation, 690–691, 690f
bloodstream infections, 691–692
central venous catheter infections,
684
CLABSIs in cancer, 573
CLABSIs in neonates, 553
clinical manifestations, 691–693
CNS device infection, 597
colonization by, 690, 959
CSF shunt infection and meningitis,
693
device-related infections, 588, 597
dominant strains, 691
endocarditis due to, 257, 262t
epidemiology, 691
intravascular catheter-related
infections, 591–592, 691–692
late-onset sepsis etiology, 549t,
550–551, 551t
management, 592
neonatal focal intestinal perforation,
692
neonatal septicemia, 538–539, 692
in neonates (CVC-related infections),
553
nosocomial infections of neonates,
549t, 550
orthopedic device infections, 598
osteomyelitis, 469
pathogenesis of infections, 690–691
peritonitis due to, 416, 693
persistent bacteremia, 553–554
pneumonia, 693
polysaccharide capsular adhesin
(PS/A), 690–691
postoperative mediastinitis due to,
587
prevention of infections, 694
prosthetic valve infections, 594–595
SSP-1 and SSP-2 proteins, 690–691

treatment of infections, 552, 592,
693–694
typing and identification, 691
urinary tract infections, 693
see also Staphylococcus epidermidis
coagulase-positive *see Staphylococcus
aureus*
culture media, 1376t
endocarditis due to, 257
flora (normal), 690
growth conditions, 690
linezolid resistance, 1426
Staphylococcus albus, 690
Staphylococcus aureus, 675–689
abscess due to, 678
in head and neck, 681
muscular and visceral, 680
acute bacterial sinusitis due to, 229, 229t
acute mastoiditis due to, 224
acute otitis media due to, 215, 220
agr locus, 676
animal bites, 521–522
anticlumping factor A antibody effect,
690
antimicrobial resistance, 14t, 676–677,
1380–1381
erythromycin, 677–678, 686
β-lactam resistance, 1424–1425
linezolid, 1426
macrolides, 1426–1427
mechanisms, 676, 686
penicillin, 676–677, 1466–1467
rifampin, 1427–1428
trimethoprim/sulfamethoxazole, 1428
vancomycin *see Staphylococcus aureus*,
vancomycin-resistant
antimicrobial susceptibility testing,
1378t, 1380–1381, 1416
β-lactamase-producing, 676–677, 1424
bacterial synergistic gangrene, 461
bacterial tracheitis due to, 165, 212, 213f
bactericidal agents, 686–687
bacteriostatic agents, 687
blepharitis due to, 493
blistering distal dactylitis due to, 432
blood cultures, 1374–1375
bloodstream infection, 676–677,
680–681, 684
brain abscess due to, 320, 683
breast abscess due to, 457, 678
bullous impetigo due to, 428
burn wound infections, 518
bursitis due to, 678–679
CA-MRSA *see Community-associated
(below)*
candidate vaccines, 689
capsular polysaccharide types, 676
capsule, 676
cardiovascular infections, 681–683
catheter-related peritonitis, 416
cell wall, 676
cellulitis due to, 434–435, 678
orbital (postseptal), 679
preseptal (periorbital), 679
cervical lymphadenitis due to, 135, 135t,
144
acute unilateral, 139, 139t
management, 138, 147t

as sole cause, controversy, 139
suppurative submandibular, 139
in Chédiak–Higashi syndrome, 626
chromosome cassette *mec* (SCC*mec*),
677
in chronic granulomatous disease, 251
chronic sinusitis due to, 680–681
chronic suppurative otitis media due to,
226
CLABSI in neonates, 554
clinical manifestations, 678–686
CNS infections, 683–684
in cancer, 579
coagulase, 676
colonization by, 677
eradication, 689
community-associated infections,
677–678
empiric therapy, 688, 688f
epidemiology, 677–678
community-associated methicillin-
resistant (CA-MRSA), 677–678, 686
acute lymphadenitis treatment, 160
acute otitis media, 215, 220
acute unilateral cervical
lymphadenitis, 139
cervical lymphadenitis, 135
clindamycin resistance rates, 686
clinical features, 462
complicated parapneumonic effusion,
241–242
emergence, 13–14
endocarditis due to, 257
epidemiology, 465
genetics, 462–464
in group childcare, 30
HA-MRSA *vs.*, 677–678
healthcare-associated infection and,
13–14
in healthcare personnel, transmission,
24
infections in neutropenia in cancer,
567
macrolide-lincosamide-streptogramin
resistance, 567
management, 514
needle aspiration in localized
lymphadenopathy, 160
neonatal infections, 538–539
nosocomial neonatal infections, 550
osteomyelitis, 470
pneumonia due to, 237, 240
skin and soft-tissue infections, 468t
treatment, 468, 468t, 472, 687–688
wound cellulitis, 514
conjunctivitis due to, 491, 679
in cystic fibrosis, 639
dacryocystitis due to, 508–509
device-related infections, 589, 684
diskitis due to, 187, 483, 680
empyema or pleural effusion due to,
241–242, 681
endocarditis due to, 258, 592–593, 681,
683, 686
complications, 264
management, 262t, 263
"endocarditis-like" intravascular
infections, 265

endophthalmitis due to, 679
enterotoxin, 676, 684
enterotoxin A, 676
epidemiology, 677–678
epidural abscess (spinal and cranial), 320–321
exfoliative toxin syndrome
    clinical features, 109t–110t, 113
    desquamation, 112–113
    diagnosis, 109t–110t
    fever and prodrome, 108
    laboratory features, 109t–110t
    skin lesions, 112, 112f
    treatment, 109t–110t
exfoliative toxins (ETA, ETB), 676, 684–685
exit-site infections, 684
exotoxins, 676, 678
eyelid infection, 497, 497f
folliculitis due to, 430
food poisoning, 394t, 395, 398t, 676, 680–681
fracture-associated infection, 515
furuncle due to, 431, 432f, 678
genetic basis, 676–677
genome, 676
glycopeptide-intermediately susceptible (GISA), 678
    endocarditis, management, 263
head and neck infections, 680–681
healthcare-associated infections, 677
heart transplant recipients, 558
heart–lung transplant recipients, 558
hemodialysis graft infections, 595–596
hemolysins, 676
hemolysis and anemia due to, 1403–1404
hordeolum (style) due to, 508, 679
hospital-acquired infections, 684
    empiric therapy, 688–689
hyper-IgE–AD syndrome, 631
iliopsoas abscess due to, 680
impetigo due to, 678
infections in HSCT recipient, 563
influenza complication, 1153
intravascular catheter-related infections, 592
    management, 592–593
invasive infections, 679–680
keratitis due to, 496
liver abscess due to, 680
localized lymphadenitis due to, 158
lower respiratory tract infections, 681
lung abscesses due to, 243, 681
lymphangitis due to, 161
macrolide-lincosamide-streptogramin B (MLS$_B$) phenotype, 686
mecA gene, 677, 1380–1381
meningitis due to, 277, 683
    in cancer, 579
    recurrent, 287, 290–291
methicillin-resistant (MRSA), 677, 1424–1425
    acute pyogenic lymphadenitis, therapy, 160
    antimicrobial therapy, in sepsis, 99
    brain abscess, 320
    burn wound infections, 518

colonization, antibiotics associated, 30
detection of, 1431
endocarditis due to, 257, 264–265, 1418t–1419t
    epidemiology, 677
    eradication of colonization, 689
    group childcare setting, 30–31
    hospital-acquired, management, 687
    hospital-acquired vs. CA-MRSA, 677–678
    impetigo treatment, 429
    infections in neutropenia in cancer, 567
    nosocomial infections of neonates, 550
    persistent/progressive pneumonia, 245–246
    pneumonia in HIV infection, 661
    purulent pericarditis, 271
    pyogenic arthritis, 477
    skin infections after trauma, 514
    surgical prophylaxis, 72
    testing for, 1380–1381
    treatment, 160, 686–687
        clindamycin, 1473
        linezolid, 1475
        rifampin, 1476
methicillin-sensitive (MSSA), 677
    endocarditis, 1418t–1419t
    hospital-acquired, 677
    nasal carriage and impetigo, 429
    neonatal CVC-related infection, 550
    osteomyelitis treatment, 472
    pyogenic arthritis, 477
    pyomyositis, 465
    treatment, 687
microbiology, 675–677
monoclonal antibody development, 44
muscle infections, 186
muscular abscess due to, 680
nasal carriage, 598, 677
neck abscess due to, 139, 139f, 146
necrotizing fasciitis due to, 680
necrotizing otitis externa due to, 222
necrotizing pneumonia due to, 243
neonatal infections, 538–539
    central venous catheter-related, 554, 592–593
    persistent bacteremia, 554
neonatal otitis media, 540
nonbullous impetigo due to, 428
nosocomial infections of neonates, 549, 549t
    late-onset sepsis, 551t
obturator internus abscess due to, 680
ocular infections, 679
ophthalmia neonatorum due to, 489
orthopedic device infections, 598
osteochondritis of foot due to, 476
osteomyelitis due to, 469, 679–680
    neonatal, 474
    in sickle-cell disease, 475
    vertebral, 187, 474
otitis externa due to, 221
otitis media due to, 680–681
Panton–Valentine leukocidin-producing, 678

necrotizing fasciitis, 462–464
osteomyelitis, 470
pneumonia, 171
paronychia due to, 432
pathogenesis of infections, 675–677
pathogenicity, 675–677, 675f
    regulation, 676–677
pericarditis due to, 269, 683
peritonitis due to, 416
peritonsillar/retropharyngeal abscess, 205–206
in phagocytic disorders, 620t, 626
pneumonia due to, 253, 681, 682f
postoperative mediastinitis due to, 587
prevention of infections, 689
    infection control, 689
    vaccines, 689
prosthetic valve infections due to, 594–595
psoas muscle abscess due to, 188
pyogenic arthritis due to, 184, 477, 680
pyomyositis due to, 466f, 680
renal abscess due to, 344
retropharyngeal abscess due to, 208f
scalded skin syndrome, 676, 684–685
secondary infection in varicella, 1037
sepsis due to, 98–99
septic intracranial thrombophlebitis, 321
septic thrombophlebitis, 683
severe sepsis syndrome, 685–686
in sickle-cell disease, 634
signal transduction system, 676
sinusitis due to, 229, 680–681
skin and soft-tissue infections, 678–679
    after trauma, 514
    in atopic dermatitis, 83
    neonatal (nosocomial), 550
skin defence mechanism against, 427
skin resistance to, 427
spinal epidural abscess due to, 684
Staphylococcus epidermidis vs., 690
subcutaneous abscess due to, 456
subdural empyema due to, 320
superantigens, 467
suppurative parotitis due to, 195
suppurative phlebitis due to, 683
surface proteins, 675f, 676
surgical site infections, 585, 587
sweat gland abscess (periporitis), 457–458
toxic shock syndrome (TSS), 108, 676, 685
    in bacterial tracheitis, 213
    case definition, 685b
    clinical features, 109t–110t, 113, 685
    diagnosis, 109t–110t
    etiology and pathogenesis, 685
    IGIV use, 41
    laboratory features, 109t–110t
    lips in, 111
    management, 109t–110t, 113, 685
    ocular features, 108–110
    oral mucosal features, 193t
    prodrome and fever, 108
    risk factors, 685
    skin lesions, 112
    streptococcal TSS vs., 108, 111t

toxic shock syndrome (TSS) toxin-1 (TSST-1), 676, 685
toxin-mediated diseases, 676, 684–686
toxins, 375, 676
   CA-MRSA *vs.*HA-MRSA, 678
tracheitis due to, 681
treatment of infections, 592–593, 686–688
   antistaphylococcal, 686–688
   empiric, 688
unencapsulated type 336 isolates, 676
upper respiratory tract infections, 680–681
urinary tract infections, 339
vaccines, 689
   candidate, 689
vancomycin-intermediate (VISA), 678, 687–689
vancomycin-resistant (VRSA), 678, 687–689, 1429, 1432, 1469
ventilator-associated pneumonia due to, 250
vertebral osteomyelitis, 187, 474
vesiculobullous rash due to, 438–439
virulence factors, 467, 675f, 676
visceral abscess due to, 680
wound infections, 678–679
in X-linked agammaglobulinemia, 610
Staphylococcus epidermidis, 689–695
accumulation-associated protein (AAP), 691
acute otitis media due to, 215
adhesion and adhesion proteins, 691
antimicrobial resistance, 693
   vancomycin, 693
biofilm formation, 690–691, 690f
bloodstream infections, 690–692
   nosocomial, prevention, 691
   recurrent, 692
catheter-related bacteremia, 692
   HSCT recipient, 563
clinical manifestations, 690–693
colonization, 690
conjunctivitis due to, 491
CSF shunts, 693
dacryocystitis due to, 508–509
diagnosis/detection, 690
   quantitative blood cultures, 692
diskitis due to, 483
endocarditis associated, 692–693
   management, 263
endophthalmitis due to, 503
epidemiology, 691
growth conditions, 690
immune evasion, 691
intravascular catheter-related infections, 691–692
keratitis due to, 496
lantibiotic formation, 691
meningitis due to, 693
microbiology, 690
necrotizing enterocolitis, 691–692
neonatal focal intestinal perforation, 692
neonatal meningitis due to, 693
neonatal septicemia due to, 692
pathogenesis of infections, 690–691, 690f

peritoneal dialysis catheter-associated peritonitis, 693
polysaccharide intercellular adhesion (PIA), 691
prevention of infections, 694
slime formation, 691
Staphylococcus aureus vs., 690
treatment of infections, 693–694
unilateral cervical lymphadenitis due to, 140
urinary tract infections, 693
see also Staphylococcus (staphylococci), coagulase-negative
Staphylococcus haemolyticus, 690, 693
   urinary tract infections, 693
Staphylococcus intermedius, animal bites, 521
Staphylococcus lugdunensis, 690, 692
   endocarditis, 692
Staphylococcus salivarius (Stomatococcus mucilaginosus), 695
Staphylococcus saprophyticus, 690–691
   pathogenesis of infections and Ssp, 691
   urinary tract infections, 693
Staphylococcus schleiferi, 690
Staphylothrombin, 676
STAT3 mutations, 630t, 631
STAT5b deficiency, characteristics, 603t–604t
Statins, as antiendotoxin therapy in sepsis, 101t–102t
Statistical analysis, 5
   population/sample characteristics, 5
   sample size, 6
Statistical inference, 6–7
Statistical significance, 5–6
   interpretation, pitfalls, 5–6
Statistical tests, types, 6t
Stavudine (d4T), 664, 665t
   dosage, 1445t–1452t
"Stealth" virus, chronic fatigue syndrome pathogenesis, 1008t–1009t
Stem cells
   CMV persistence, 1044
   transplant recipients *see* Hematopoietic stem cell transplantation (HSCT)
Stenotrophomonas maltophilia, 849
   bloodstream infections, 849
   clinical features and treatment, 849
   in cystic fibrosis, 639, 849
   epidemiology and risk factors, 849, 849b
   persistence in disinfectants, 849
   pneumonia due to, 253
   respiratory infection in cystic fibrosis, 248–249
   virulence factors, 849
Sterilization, 21
   deficiencies, 21
   definition, 21
Sternocleidomastoid muscle, 136–137
   branchial cleft cysts/sinuses, 143
Sternocleidomastoid tumor, 142t
Sternum, osteomyelitis, 188–189
   postoperative *see* Osteomyelitis
Stevens–Johnson syndrome (SJS), 108, 440, 1479
   clinical features, 108, 109t–110t, 113
      anterior segment features, 110–111
      fever and prodrome, 108, 113
      lesions, 111

      lips, 111, 111f
      ocular features, 110–111
      oral mucosal features, 193t
      treatment, 109t–110t, 113
      urethritis, 353
   corticosteroid controversy, 113
   diagnosis/laboratory features, 109t–110t
   management, 113
   mucositis *vs.*, 111
   trimethoprim-sulfamethoxazole causing, 1232
Stibogluconate, visceral leishmaniasis, 1290, 1290t
Stillbirth, viral infections associated, 546–547
Stings, insect *see* Insect bites
Stomach, herniation, in CGD, 622f
Stomatitis
   aphthous (recurrent oral ulcers), 193t
   drug-induced, 193t
   gangrenous, 193t
   HSV, 191–192
   radiation-induced, 193t
   see also Gingivostomatitis
Stomatococcus, 695
Stomatococcus mucilaginosus, 695
Stool(s)
   blood in, 375–376
      Clostridium difficile infection, 978
      necrotizing enterocolitis, 389
   Clostridium difficile toxin detection, 978
   collection and preservation, 1382–1383
   leukocytes
      Entamoeba histolytica infection, 1275
      inflammatory enteritis, 385
   mucus, leukocyte assay, 385
   specimen collection/transport, 376, 1374t
Stool culture, 376
   bacillary dysentery, 822
   Yersinia enterocolitica, 824
Stool examination, 1382–1383
   antigen detection assays, 1383
   antigen test for *Helicobacter pylori*, 913
   concentration technique, 1383
      Clonorchis and *Opisthorchis* infections, 1365
      Schistosoma infections, 1369–1370
   detection of
      Ascaris, 1328
      Balantidium coli, 1267, 1267f
      Blastocystis, 1268–1269, 1269f
      Cryptosporidium, 1270
      Cyclospora, 1284
      Cystoisospora, 1284
      Dientamoeba fragilis, 1279
      Diphyllobothrium, 1347
      Dipylidium caninum, 1348–1349
      Endolimax nana, 1272
      Entamoeba histolytica, 1274f, 1277
      Fasciola, 1366
      Fasciolopsis buski, 1363
      Giardia intestinalis, 1281–1282
      Heterophyes and *Metagonimus*, 1364
      hookworms, 1330
      Hymenolepis nana, 1349
      Paragonimus, 1367
      Schistosoma, 1369–1370

specific pathogens, 1383–1384
Strongyloides, 1333, 1333f
Trichuris trichiura, 1331
direct wet mount smear, 1383
in eosinophilic meningitis, 333
gastrointestinal infections/diarrhea, 375–376
inflammatory enteritis, 385–386, 385t
permanent stain smear, 1383
process, 1383
refugee and internationally adopted children, 33t, 35–36
rotaviruses, 1095–1096
specific pathogens, 1383–1384
Stratified analyses, 7
Stratum corneum, 427, 438
Stratum-specific estimates, 7
Strawberry tongue, 111
Kawasaki disease, 1003, 1005–1006
streptococcal *see Streptococcus pyogenes* (group A streptococcus)
Streptobacillus moniliformis, 938–939
animal bite infections, 523
clinical findings, 938–939
description and microbiology, 938
diagnosis, 939
epidemiology, 938
erythema arthriticum epidemicum, 938
Haverhill fever, 938
microbiology, 938
prevention, 939
Soduka (spirillary rat-bite fever), 938, 958
treatment, 939
Streptococcus (streptococci)
α-hemolytic, 696, 696t
infections in neutropenia in cancer, 567
unilateral cervical lymphadenitis due to, 140
antimicrobial susceptibility testing, 1378t
beta-hemolytic, 696–697, 696t, 719–720
group A *see Streptococcus pyogenes* (group A streptococcus)
biochemical differentiation, 729t
classification, 695–697
colonial morphology, 696–697
culture media, 1376t
eosinophilia due to, 1408t–1409t
group A *see Streptococcus pyogenes* (group A streptococcus)
group B *see Streptococcus agalactiae* (group B streptococcus)
group C, 719–721
antimicrobial resistance, 720
biochemical characteristics, 720t
clinical manifestations, 720–721
differentiation from other streptococci, 720t
epidemiology, 720
microbiology, 720
pharyngitis, 199–201, 720
speciation, 720
treatment of infections, 721
virulence, 720
group D, 712, 713t
see also Enterococcus

group G, 719–721
antimicrobial resistance, 720
bacitracin-resistance, 200
clinical manifestations, 720–721
differentiation from other streptococci, 720t
epidemiology, 720
erysipelas, 434
microbiology, 720
pharyngitis, 199–200, 720
speciation, 720
treatment of infections, 721
virulence, 720
Lancefield Groups, 696–697, 696t
microaerophilic, 988
nonhemolytic, 696, 696t
nutritionally variant (NVS), 717
see also Abiotrophia; Gemella; Granulicatella
oral, endocarditis pathogenesis, 257–258
penicillin resistance, endocarditis treatment, 262t, 263
penicillin susceptibility, endocarditis treatment, 262t, 263
in phagocytic disorders, 620t
phylogenetic relationship, 697f
16s rRNA sequencing, 697, 697t
soft-tissue infection, skin lesions, 112
toxic shock-like syndrome *see under Streptococcus pyogenes*
viridans group *see* Viridans group streptococci
Streptococcus agalactiae (group B streptococcus), 696t, 707–712
acute otitis media due to, 215
in asplenia, 636
bacteremia due to, 708, 710t
blistering distal dactylitis due to, 432
capsular polysaccharide mimicking Lewis X, 85
carriage in pregnancy, screening, 710
cervical lymphadenitis due to, 135t, 144
acute unilateral, 139–140, 139t
management, 147t
chemoprophylaxis, 70t–71t, 71
clinical manifestations, 708–709
colonization by, 708
culture-based screening, 711, 712f
dacryocystitis due to, 508–509
early-onset neonatal infections, 536, 538–539, 708
clinical features, 708, 709t
late-onset infections *vs.*, 708t
pathogenesis, 707t, 708
prevention, 710, 712f
epidemiology, 708
laboratory findings and diagnosis, 709
late, late-onset infection, 538–539, 708t, 709
late-onset infections, 538–539, 551t, 708–709, 708t
clinical features, 708–709
meningitis due to, 708–709, 709t, 1418t–1419t
treatment, 276t, 710t
mortality due to, 710
neonatal infections, 536, 551t
osteomyelitis due to, 709

pathogenesis of infection, 707
pili, 707
pneumonia due to, 236
pneumonia in young infants, 236
prevention, 710–712, 712f
guidelines, 711
prognosis, 710
protein C, 707
pyogenic arthritis due to, 709
recurrent infections, 710
screening, 711, 712f
sensitivity to penicillin, 709
septicemia due to, 710t
serotypes, 707, 707t
transplacental IgG role against, 87
treatment of infections, 543, 709–710, 710t
type III strains, 707
vaccines, 711–712
virulence and virulence factors, 707
Streptococcus anginosus, 716, 718
focal suppurative CNS infections, 319
group C and G streptococci *vs.*, 720t
lung abscesses due to, 243
Streptococcus anginosus group, 719–720
Streptococcus bovis, 696t, 712, 716–719
biochemical/growth characteristics, 713t, 716t
biotypes, 717
endocarditis due to, 1418t–1419t
neonatal BSI, 718
septicemia due to, 718
treatment of infections, 719
Streptococcus canis, 696t, 720
Streptococcus constellatus, focal suppurative CNS infections, 319
Streptococcus dysgalactiae, 720
Streptococcus dysgalactiae subsp. *equisimilis*, 696t
Streptococcus equinus, 712
Streptococcus equisimilis, 720
Streptococcus intermedius, 718f
focal suppurative CNS infections, 319
Streptococcus milleri group, 319
Streptococcus mitis, 717
endocarditis, 257
infections in neutropenia in cancer, 567
septicemia due to, 717
Streptococcus mutans, 190–191, 718
endocarditis, 257
Streptococcus pneumoniae, 696–697, 696t, 721–728
acute bacterial sinusitis, 229, 229t
acute mastoiditis due to, 224
acute otitis media due to, 214–215, 214f–215f
AAP guidelines for treatment, 725
antibiotic resistance likelihood after, 217–218, 218f
incidence, 723
penicillin sensitivity, 217, 218f
prevention, vaccine role, 726
prognosis, 726
serotypes causing, 721
treatment, 725
after head trauma, 515
age-specific infections, 722, 722f

antibiotic resistance, 31, 215, 724–725, 724t
  childcare settings, 28
  likelihood after otitis media treatment, 217, 218f
  macrolides, 724–725, 724t
  mechanisms, 724–725, 724t
  meningitis treatment and, 275–276
  MLS$_a$ phenotype (macrolide resistance), 724–725
  multidrug resistance, 217, 725
  occurrence, and antibiotic types, 217t
  penicillin see Streptococcus pneumoniae, penicillin-resistant
  quinolones, 724t
  surveillance, 725
  telithromycin, 1427
  testing, 1380, 1380t
  trimethoprim, 724t
  trimethoprim/sulfamethoxazole, 1428
antibiotic susceptibility, 216t–217t, 217–218, 724–725, 724t–725t
  in meningitis, 276t
  NCCLS definitions, 724, 724t
  reduced, risk factors, 217
antimicrobial susceptibility testing, 724, 1380, 1380t, 1416
  interpretation, 276
in asplenia, 636
autolysis by, 274, 721
bacteremia due to, 4f, 723
  serotypes causing, 721
bacterial tracheitis due to, 212
C-polysaccharide and antibodies to, 722
cellulitis due to, 434–435, 510
clinical manifestations, 723
colonization, 217–218, 721–722
  group childcare settings, 28
  nasopharyngeal see Below
conjunctivitis due to, 490, 508, 723
dacryocystitis due to, 508–509
diskitis due to, 187, 483
empyema due to, 723
endocarditis due to, 257, 263
epidemiology, 722, 722f
epididymitis due to, 367
fever without localizing features, 114–115
focal suppurative CNS infections, 319–321, 328–329
group childcare and, 25t, 28
heart transplant recipients, 558
in HIV infection, 659, 722, 728
immune evasion by, 722
immunity to, 722
in immunodeficiency, 722
influenza complication, 1153
invasive disease
  decline due to vaccines, 726–728, 727f, 727t
  epidemiology, 722
keratitis due to, 496f
laboratory findings and diagnosis, 723–724
  antigen detection assays, 1381
  CSF specimens, 1377
meningitis due to, 272
  in cancer, 579

CSF features, 274
  dexamethasone in, 278
  diagnosis, 274, 724
  recurrent, 287, 289–291, 722
  sequelae, 726
  serotypes causing, 721
  in sickle-cell disease, 634–635
  treatment, 272, 275–277, 276t, 725–726, 1418t–1419t
microbiology, 721
mortality, 726
nasopharyngeal colonization, 217–218, 273, 722
necrotizing pneumonia due to, 243
neonatal infections, 538–539
neonatal otitis media, 540
neutrophilia due to, 1404
non-vaccine serotypes (NV-Sp), 215
  acute otitis media, 215
  recurrent otitis media prevention, 217–218
ophthalmia neonatorum due to, 489
osteomyelitis due to, 469
as otopathogen, 214–215
pathogenesis of infections, 721–722
penicillin-resistant, 230, 275–276, 724–725, 724t, 1425
  classification, 230
  management of acute sinusitis, 229–230, 229t
  persistent/progressive pneumonia, 245–246
  testing, 1380
peritonitis due to, 415
pleural effusion due to, 241–242
pneumococcal conjugate vaccine, 60–61
  after abdominal trauma and splenectomy, 515
  contraindications/precautions, 61
  recommendations for use, 61
pneumococcal conjugate vaccine, 7 valent (PCV7), 60, 215, 721, 726
  acute mastoiditis incidence, 224
  acute otitis media decline, 215, 229
  acute otitis media microbiology change, 214–215
  acute otitis media prevention, 726
  antibiotic resistance after, 217
  in asplenia, 637
  composition and development, 60, 726
  development, 726
  effect on invasive disease, 722, 726
  effect on pneumonia complications, 241
  efficacy, 726
  indications, 727t
  meningitis prevention, 279
  PCV$_{CRM}$ and PCV$_{OMP}$, 219
  pneumococcal disease reduction by, 48
  pneumonia prevention, 726
  pneumonia prevention in HIV infection, 663
  pneumonia reduced by use, 169
  postlicensure surveillance, 727
  recommendations for use, 61, 723t, 726

recurrent otitis media prevention, 219–220, 219t
  schedule in HIV infection, 663
  serotypes included, 726
  shift in Streptococcus pneumoniae serotypes, 215, 215f
  shortage in US, 54
  in sickle-cell disease, 636
  sinusitis decline, 229
  for travelers, 78, 78t
  universal immunization, 726
pneumococcal conjugate vaccine, 9 valent (PCV9), meningitis prevention, 279
pneumococcal conjugate vaccine, 13 valent (PCV13), 60–61, 727–728
  recurrent meningitis prevention, 292
pneumococcal polysaccharide vaccine (PPSV23), 60–61
  after abdominal trauma and splenectomy, 515
  composition and development, 60
  contraindications/precautions, 61
  in HIV infection, 663
  meningitis reduction with, 272, 279
  recommendations for use, 61
  response to and efficacy, 60
  vaccine efficacy, 7, 219t
pneumococcal polysaccharide vaccine (PPV23), 726
  background to use and efficacy, 726
  in cystic fibrosis, 641
  recurrent meningitis prevention, 292
  in sickle-cell disease, 636
pneumococcal surface protein A (Psp A), 721
pneumonia due to, 169–170, 237, 240, 723
  in cancer, 575
  in immunocompromised, 253
  necrotizing, 243
  PCV7 vaccine role, 726
  prodrome and clinical features, 723
  sickle-cell disease, 634
  treatment, 726
polysaccharide capsule, 721, 724
prevalence, 60
prevention of infections, 726–728
  chemoprophylaxis, 728
  in contacts, 728
  passive immunoprophylaxis, 728
  vaccines see Below
prognosis of infections, 726
purpura fulminans due to, 734
pyogenic arthritis due to, 477
recurrent infections, 722
in renal disease, 637
sepsis due to, 98
serotype 19A, meningitis, 272
serotypes, 215, 721
  antibiotic resistance, 275–276
  meningitis due to, 272
shift in serotypes with use of PCV7, 215, 215f
sickle-cell disease, 634–636
soft-tissue infections, 723
subdural empyema due to, 328–329
survival plots, 4f

tolerance to antibiotics, 276
transmission, 722
treatment of infections, 724–726
  antimicrobial, 725–726, 725t
  MICs, 1380t
  in sickle-cell disease, 635
unilateral cervical lymphadenitis due to,
  140
V-Sp, 215
vaccines, 30, 726–728
  after splenectomy, 515
  decline of invasive disease, 726–727,
    727f, 727t
  development, 726
  group childcare settings, 30t
  historical perspective, 726
  routine childhood immunization
    schedule, 28
  schedule, 49f
  see also individual vaccines listed above
viral nasopharyngitis, 163
viridans group streptococci vs., 716
virulence, 721–722
in X-linked agammaglobulinemia, 610
Streptococcus pyogenes (group A
  streptococcus), 200–201, 696t,
  698–706
acute abdominal pain due to, 174
acute glomerulonephritis (PSAGN),
  705–706
  clinical features, 705, 705b
  epidemiology, 705
  laboratory findings, 705–706
  pathogenesis, 705
  pathology, 705
  treatment and prevention, 706
acute mastoiditis due to, 224
acute otitis media due to, 214–215, 214f
acute pharyngitis due to, 699–700, 700f
acute rheumatic fever (ARF), 698,
  702–705
  anti-inflammatory therapy, 705, 705t
  carditis, 703
  cause of heart disease, 703
  chorea, 703–704
  clinical features, 703
  diagnostic criteria (Jones), 703–704,
    703b
  differential diagnosis, 704, 704t
  epidemiology, 702–703
  erythema marginatum, 704
  GAS pharyngitis complication, 702,
    704
  genetics, 703
  host factors contributing to, 702
  infection chemoprophylaxis, 73, 74t
  limb pain, 185, 185t
  major manifestations, 703–704
  migratory polyarthritis, 703–704
  minor manifestations, 704
  mortality, 702
  pathogenesis, 703
  prevention, 704–705, 705t
  prognosis, 703, 705
  recurrent, 704–705
  subcutaneous nodules, 704
  treatment, 704
animal bites, 521–522

antibody titers, 203
antigens, rapid testing, 1377
antimicrobial resistance
  lincosamide, 204
  macrolides, 204
  telithromycin, 1427
bacterial tracheitis due to, 165
bacteriocins, 698
blistering distal dactylitis due to, 432
burn wound infections, 517–518
carrier state and eradication, 212
carriers vs. pharyngitis, diagnosis, 203
cell structure, 698
cell wall, 698
cellulitis due to, 434–435
cervical lymphadenitis due to, 135, 135t,
  144
  abscess drainage, 146
  acute unilateral, 139, 139t
  management, 138, 147t
characteristics, 698
chemoprophylaxis, 73
clinical manifestations, 700–701, 700f
colonization, 698, 960
complications of infections, 702
culture media, 1376t
emm gene, 698
epidemiology, 698–700
erysipelas due to, 434
femoral adenitis due to, 160
group C and G streptococci vs., 720t
group childcare and, 25t, 27
  in adults attending/care providers, 31
head trauma, 515
hemolysis and anemia due to,
  1403–1404
human bites, 521
hyaluronic acid capsule, 460–461
immune evasion mechanisms, 698
immunologic response to, 699
impetigo due to, 428, 702
impetigo strains, 428
infection sequelae, 73
invasive infections, 699
Kawasaki disease vs., 1005
laboratory findings and diagnosis, 701,
  1377
  specimen collection/processing, 1373,
    1377
localized lymphadenitis, 158
lymphangitis due to, 161, 161t
  management, 162
M protein, 467, 698, 702–703, 705
  antibodies to, 699
  "C-repeat", 702
  immunity elicited by, 702
microbiology, 698
morbidity and mortality due to, 698
mucoid strains, 703
muscle infections, 186
necrotizing cellulitis due to, 701f
necrotizing fasciitis due to, 460,
  462–463, 467f, 700–702
necrotizing pneumonia due to, 243
necrotizing soft-tissue infection,
  455–456, 460–461
neonatal infections, 699
nephritogenic strains, 429

nonbullous impetigo due to, 428
osteomyelitis due to, 469
otitis externa due to, 221
as otopathogen, 214
PANDAS, 706
paronychia due to, 432
pathogenesis of infections, 699
perianal dermatitis due to, 429
peritonsillar/retropharyngeal abscess due
  to, 205–206
phagocytosis in neonates, 85
pharyngitis see Pharyngitis
pleural effusion due to, 241–242
pneumonia due to, 237
poststreptococcal reactive arthritis, 73,
  706
prevention of infections, 73, 702
pyoderma due to, 705–706
pyogenic arthritis due to, 477
pyomyositis due to, 463f, 465, 468
pyrogenic exotoxin (erythrogenic
  toxin)-producing, 201
pyrogenic exotoxins (SPEs), 698–699
reactive arthritis due to, 483
recurrent infection, acute rheumatic fever
  after, 704
rheumatic fever see Above
scarlet fever/scarlatina due to
  clinical features, 109t–110t, 201
  diagnosis/laboratory features,
    109t–110t
  generalized lymphadenopathy, 130,
    131t–132t
  oral mucosal features, 193t
  pharyngitis, 199–201
  rash, 441
  skin lesions, 112
  treatment, 109t–110t
secondary infection in varicella, 1037
serotypes and typing, 698, 703
serum opacity factor (SOF), 698
skin defence mechanism against, 427
skin infection after trauma, 514
strawberry tongue, 111, 193t
streptococcal nasopharyngitis, 163, 164t
superantigens, 467, 698
suppurative infections, 699–702
supraglottic infection, 205–206
T antigen, 698
toxic shock-like syndrome (STSS), 108,
  702
  clinical features, 109t–110t, 113
  diagnosis, 109t–110t
  laboratory features, 109t–110t
  management, 113
  in necrotizing fasciitis, 461
  staphylococcal toxic shock vs., 108,
    111t
  susceptibility to, 698
  treatment, 109t–110t
transient synovitis, 485–486
transmission, 699, 702
treatment of infections, 162, 701–702
urticaria due to, 445
vaccines, 702
varicella as risk factor, 699–700, 701f
vesiculobullous rash due to, 438–439
virulence, 699

virulence factors, 460–461, 467
vulvovaginitis, 357–358
Streptococcus pyogenes-like organisms *see*
Streptococcus (streptococci), group C;
Streptococcus (streptococci), group G
Streptococcus salivarius, 190
endocarditis, 257
Streptococcus sanguis
endocarditis, 257
infections in neutropenia in cancer,
567
Streptococcus thermophilus, 961
Streptococcus viridans see Viridans group
streptococci
Streptogramins, 1474–1475
clinical use, 1475
combination therapy, 1420–1421
mechanisms of action, 1474–1475
pharmacodynamic properties, 1414t
pharmacology, 1453t–1458t
resistance to, 1475
spectrum of activity, 1459t–1463t
structures, 1474–1475
Streptokinase, *Streptococcus pyogenes*, 699
Streptolysin O, 698–699
Streptolysin S, 698
groups C and G streptococci, 720
Streptomycin
dosage, 1445t–1452t, 1480t–1483t
mechanism of action, 1473–1474
pharmacology, 1453t–1458t
spectrum of activity, 1459t–1463t, 1474
treatment of
endocarditis, 263t
Francisella tularensis infections,
898–899
tuberculosis, 780t, 781, 783
Yersinia pestis infection, 827
Stridor, 165–166, 165t, 251
acute, 165t
acute infectious, clinical features,
165–166
in bacterial tracheitis, 212
characteristics, 165
definition, 165
etiology, 165, 165t
clues to, 165
expiratory/inspiratory, 165
laryngotracheitis, 211
persistent, 165t
"String test", *Helicobacter pylori*, 913–914
Strobila *see* Proglottids
Stroke
in sickle-cell disease, 635
see also Cerebrovascular accident
Strongyloides (strongyloidiasis), 1332–1334
bacterial infections with, 1334
clinical manifestations, 1327b, 1333
description and life cycle, 1332, 1333f
disseminated infection, 1333–1334
eosinophilia, 1407
epidemiology, 1332–1333
hyperinfection, 1332–1333
infection route, 1326, 1332
internal autoinfection, 1332–1333
laboratory findings and diagnosis, 1326,
1333, 1383
mortality, 1334

neonatal infection, 1327t, 1332–1333
prevention, 1334, 1524
treatment, 1334, 1524
Strongyloides fuelleborni, 1326, 1332–1334
infantile infection, 1333
neonatal infection, 1327t, 1332
Strongyloides procyonis, 1338
Strongyloides stercoralis, 1326, 1332–1334,
1333f
clinical manifestations, 1327b
eosinophilia, 1407, 1408t–1409t
neonatal infection, 1327t
refugee and internationally adopted
children, 35–36
size and virulence, 1256
see also Strongyloides
Strychnine poisoning, 968
Study on Efficacy of Nosocomial Infection
Control (SENIC), 15–16, 579
Style (hordeolum), 679
Subacute sclerosing panencephalitis (SSPE),
78, 303, 1141–1143, 1142f
CJD *vs*, 338
MMR vaccine associated, 60
Subarachnoid exudate, purulent, 273
Subarachnoid neurocysticercosis, 1353,
1353f, 1355t, 1356
Subcarinal lymph nodes, 148–149
enlarged, pulmonary tuberculosis,
774–775
Subcutaneous compartment, 454
Subcutaneous nodules
in acute rheumatic fever, 704
in eumycotic mycetoma, 1251–1252
in nodular lymphangitis, 161
Subcutaneous tissue infections, 454–462
etiology, 459–460
human, 984
noninfectious diseases *vs.*, 456b
pathogenesis, 460–461
predisposing factors, 455b
tertiary, 454–455
see also Abscess; Necrotizing soft-tissue
infections
Subdural abscess, spinal
clinical features, 323
epidemiology, 321
management, 328
MRI, 327
outcome, 330
Subdural empyema, 325–326
anaerobic gram-positive cocci, 989
clinical features, 323, 323t
complications and prognosis, 330
CT and MRI, 325–326, 326f
differential diagnosis, 325
epidemiology, 321
etiology, 320, 320t
laboratory findings and diagnosis, 325
management, 328–329
pathogenesis, 322
Subglottic polyps, bacterial tracheitis
complication, 213
Subglottic stenosis
bacterial tracheitis complication, 213
congenital, 165
Submandibular lymph nodes, 136t
Submandibular space, infection, 138

Submaxillary lymph nodes, 136–137, 136t
infections/pathogens, 145t
pathogens infecting, 145t
Submaxillary triangle, abscess, 191
Submental lymph nodes, 136, 136t
Subperiosteal abscess
acute sinusitis complication, 230
of long bones, 265
in mastoiditis, 223
Sudden death, in myocarditis, 266
Sudden infant death syndrome (SIDS)
Bordetella pertussis association, 869
Clostridium botulinum associated, 973
human parainfluenza virus infections,
1123
myocarditis involvement, 266
Sulbactam
Acinetobacter infections, 829–830
pharmacology, 1453t–1458t
Sulfacetamide, treatment of
eye infections, 1494t–1495t
skin infections, 1498t
Sulfadiazine, 1478–1479
dosage, 1480t–1483t
Neisseria meningitidis infection
prophylaxis, 739
pharmacology, 1453t–1458t
Toxoplasma gondii infections, 1315–1316,
1315t–1316t
Sulfadiazine-pyrimethamine, 1479
protozoan infection treatment, 1522
spectrum of activity, 1459t–1463t
Sulfamethoxazole (SMX), 1478–1479
Cystoisospora (cystisosporiasis), 1284
pharmacology, 1453t–1458t
spectrum of activity, 1459t–1463t
see also Trimethoprim-sulfamethoxazole
(TMP-SMX)
Sulfamethoxazole/trimethoprim *see*
Trimethoprim-sulfamethoxazole
(TMP-SMX)
Sulfisoxazole
chemoprophylactic use, 74t
dosage, 1480t–1483t
pharmacology, 1453t–1458t
spectrum of activity, 1459t–1463t
treatment of
acute otitis media, 218
eye infection, 1494t–1495t
Sulfonamides, 1478–1479
chemoprophylactic use, 70t–71t
dosage, 1480t–1483t
Ehrlichia and *Anaplasma* infections,
delayed diagnosis, 896
mechanism of action, 1479
pharmacology, 1453t–1458t, 1479
reaction to, 1479
resistance to, 1478–1479
spectrum of activity, 1459t–1463t
Sulfur, scabies treatment, 1260
Sulfur granules, 162, 991, 992f
Sun exposure, precautions for travelers, 76
Sun screens, 76
Sunblock, precaution for travelers, 76
Superantigen toxins, IGIV use against, 41
Superantigens, 467
inhibition, necrotizing fasciitis treatment,
468

Kawasaki disease, 1003
  Staphylococcus aureus, 467
  Streptococcus pyogenes, 467, 698
Superior sagittal sinus, septic thrombosis, 323t, 326, 330
Superior vena cava
  obstruction, 149–150, 149t
  petechiae around, 443
Superior vena cava syndrome, 265
Superoxide, 85
  in HIV infection, 658
  Mycoplasma pneumoniae infections, 993
Supportive care, for sepsis, 99–100
Suppurative jugular thrombophlebitis *see* Lemierre disease
Suppurative thrombophlebitis *see* Septic thrombophlebitis
Supraclavicular lymph nodes, 137
  biopsy, 151
  pathogens infecting, 145t
Supraclavicular lymphadenopathy, 148–149
Supraglottic infections, 205–213
  acute bronchitis, 213
  acute epiglottitis, 210–211
  acute laryngitis, 212
  bacterial tracheitis, 212–213
  conditions included, 205
  definitions, infections included, 205
  laryngotracheitis, 211–212
  Lemierre disease *see* Lemierre disease
  parapharyngeal abscess, 207–208
  peritonsillar abscess, 205–207
  retropharyngeal abscess, 207
  see also Each of the above infections
Supraglottitis, 210–211
  clinical features and diagnosis, 165, 166t
  stridor, 165
Suramin sodium, *Trypanosoma (Trypanozoon) brucei* infection, 1322, 1322t, 1519–1520
Surfactant-associated proteins, 84
Surfactant protein A (SP-A), 84
Surfactant protein D (SP-D), 84
Surgery
  anaerobic infection treatment, 965
  Aspergillus infection treatment, 1209
  Blastomyces dermatitidis (blastomycosis), 1238
  chemoprophylaxis for, 72–73
    in phagocyte disorders, 624t
    recommendations, 72–73
  Coccidioides immitis infection treatment, 1245
  Echinococcus granulosus (cystic echinococcosis), 1358–1359
  Echinococcus multilocularis (alveolar echinococcosis), 1361
  Echinococcus vogeli (polycystic echinococcosis), 1361
  eumycotic mycetoma, 1252–1253
  infection risk, 72
    principles, 72
  necrotizing enterocolitis, 390
  in prosthetic valve/patch infections, 594–595
  see also specific types of surgery (e.g. cardiac surgery)

Surgical drainage
  parapharyngeal abscess, 208
  peritonsillar abscess, 206
  retropharyngeal abscess, 207
Surgical site infections, 585–587
  classification, 585–586
  clinical features and diagnosis, 585–586
  deep incisional, 586
  definition, 10
  epidemiology and pathogenesis, 585, 585t
  management and outcome, 586
  organ or space infection, 586
  prevalence by site/operation, 585t–586t
  prevention, 586–587
  risk factors, 585
Surgical wounds, 585–587
  classification and risk of infection, 69t
  infection chemoprophylaxis, 72–73
    principles, 72
    surgical procedures/surgery types, 72–73
  Pseudomonas aeruginosa infections, 843t
Surveillance, 1
  active, 1, 16
  data sources for, 16b
  HAIs *see* Healthcare-associated infection (HAI)
  healthcare-associated infections, 16–17
  methods, 16
  microbiology laboratory role, 16
  passive, 1
  pharmacy role, 16–17
  prospective, 16
  sources of data for, 16b
  unusual infections, 17
  vaccine-preventable diseases, 55
Surveillance and Control of Pathogens of Epidemiologic Importance (SCOPE), 800
Survey of Income and Program Participation (SIPP), 24
Susceptibility testing, 1373–1381, 1416
  of bacteria
    anaerobic bacteria, 1381
    antibiotics, 1416
    automated systems, 1379–1380
    breakpoint establishment, 1429
    definition/description, 1378
    fastidious bacteria, 1381
    interpretation of results, 1416
    media and test conditions, 1378, 1378t
    media recommended (for specific pathogens), 1378t
    methods, 1429–1430, 1430f
    minimum inhibitory concentrations (MICs), 1379t, 1413–1416, 1429–1430, 1430f
    pathogen- and mechanism-specific, 1380–1381
    purpose of, 1413
    quality control, 1380
    resistance detection, 1429–1431
    standardization, 1378, 1381
    test methods, 1378–1380
    see also individual pathogens

  of fungi, to antifungals, 1382
  of viruses, HSV, 1386
Susceptibility to infection, 83–90
Suturing, bite wounds, 524–525
SV40, 1075
Swabs
  for bacterial infection detection, 1373t
  viral infection diagnosis, 1385
Sweat gland abscess (periporitis), 457–458
Sweet syndrome, 453
Swimmer's ear, *Pseudomonas aeruginosa*, 220–221, 843t
  treatment of infections, normal host, 845
Swimmer's itch, 1370
Swimming
  Giardia intestinalis (giardiasis) prevention, 1282
  Naegleria fowleri infections, 1294–1295
  nontuberculous mycobacterial infections from, 788
  otitis externa association, 220–221
  Schistosoma infections, 1369–1370
  subcutaneously implanted vascular catheters, 594
  Toxocara infection, 1337
Swimming pool
  chlorine recommendations, *Naegleria fowleri* prevention, 1295
  pharyngoconjunctival fever and, 491
  water contamination
    Acanthamoeba, 1296
    Cryptosporidium, 1269–1270
    Naegleria fowleri, 1294
Swollen belly syndrome, 1327t, 1332
Swyer-James syndrome (unilateral hyperlucent lung), 250
Sydenham chorea, 703–704
Sympathetic effusion, sinusitis causing, 510
Symptom complexes
  see individual symptoms/complexes
Syncephalastrum, 1212–1213
Syncytial cytopathic effect, RSV, 1133
Syndrome of inappropriate antidiuretic hormone secretion (SIADH), 240
  encephalitis complication, 312–313
  Mycobacterium tuberculosis infection, 777
  varicella in cancer causing, 1039
Syndromic Precautions, 18
Synercid *see* Quinupristin-dalfopristin
Synergism
  cell wall-active agents with ribosomal active agents, 1420
  combination antimicrobial therapy, 1419–1420
Synovial fluid
  examination
    in musculoskeletal pain, 183
    transient synovitis, 486
  Mycoplasma pneumoniae infection, 995
  pyogenic arthritis, 478
  specimen collection/analysis, 1377–1378
Synovial infections, *Mycobacterium avium* complex, 789
Synovitis, transient *see* Transient synovitis
Syntaxin 11 (STX11), defective, in familial HLH, 104t

Syphilis
  endemic, 941, 948–949
  venereal *see Treponema pallidum* subsp.
    pallidum
Systematic error, 4
Systemic inflammatory response syndrome
    (SIRS), 94, 97–103, 512
  biologic markers, 99
  clinical features, 99
  cytokine levels, 100
  definition, 97, 98b
  etiology, 97–98
  laboratory findings, 99
  management, 99–103, 101t–102t
    anticoagulants, 102
    anticytokine therapy, 100
    antimicrobial therapy, 99, 99t
    arachidonic acid inhibition, 100
    corticosteroids, 100–102
    endothelial-targeted therapy, 102
    future prospects, 103
    immunoparalysis, 100
    intravenous immunoglobulin therapy,
      100
    nitric oxide balance, 102
    supportive care, 99–100
  pathophysiology, 98
  see also Sepsis; Septic shock
Systemic lupus erythematosus (SLE)
  arthritis in acute rheumatic fever *vs.*, 704
  diagnostic criteria, 184–185
  fever of unknown origin due to,
    119t–120t
  Libman–Sachs vegetations, 259–260
  limb pain, 184–185, 185t

T

T-cell receptor (TCR), 89–90, 626–627
  gene recombination, 90
T cells *see* T lymphocytes
T lymphocytes, 87, 89–90, 92, 626–627
  in 22q11.2 deletion syndrome, 630t, 631
  αβ, 90, 626–627, 631
  abnormal counts, 1405–1406
  activation, deregulated in HLH, 104–105
  anaerobic infections, 961
  antigen presentation to, 45, 89
  apoptosis, prevention in HLH, 107
  B cell interactions, 626–627
  CD4+ (helper), 45, 90, 92, 626–627
    counts, *M. avium* Complex
      prophylaxis, 663–664
    counts in HIV infection, 658
    Cryptococcus neoformans infections,
      1220–1221, 1223
    cytokines released, 92
    decline in HIV infection, 649–650,
      656
    deficiency, 627–628
    deficiency, *Giardia intestinalis*
      (giardiasis), 1281
    downregulation of CD4 expression by
      HHV-7, 1058
    function, 626–627
    HHV-7 latency, 1057
    HIV infection, 658, 1166–1167
    HIV replication, 648–649

HTLV-1 infection, 1165
  intestinal *vs.* peripheral, in HIV
    infection, 650
  in *Leishmania* infections, 1286
  low counts in *Pneumocystis jirovecii*
    infection, 1230
  restoration after antiretrovirals in
    HIV, 650
  in SCID, 627–629
  Th1 and Th2 types, 45, 90, 92
  Th1 cells, 626–627
  Th1 cells, *Coccidioides immitis*
    infection, 1239–1240
  Toxoplasma gondii infection, 1311
CD8+, 46, 90, 626–627
  decreased, Kawasaki disease, 1003
  HIV replication and, 648–649
  reduced in HLH, 104–106
  Toxoplasma gondii infection, 1311
  see also Cytotoxic/cytolytic T
    lymphocytes (CTL)
chronic fatigue syndrome, 1010t
chronic hepatitis B, 1078
CMV infection, 1045
cytokines produced, 90, 626–627, 772
cytolytic *see* Cytotoxic/cytolytic T
  lymphocytes
decreased function, 90
deficiency, 90, 603t–604t, 627
  detection, 608t
  Giardia intestinalis (giardiasis), 1281
  immunizations in, 52t–53t
  pneumonia, 251, 253t
  rubeola virus infection (measles),
    1143
  SCID *see* Severe combined
    immunodeficiency (SCID)
depletion
  HHV-6 immune evasion method,
    1053
  HHV-7 immune evasion method,
    1058
development, 88f, 90
disorders, 626
  non-SCID, 629–633, 630t
  SCID, 627
    see also Severe combined
      immunodeficiency (SCID)
EBV infection, 1062–1063
EBV tropism, 105
enterovirus infections, 1173
functions, 89, 626–627
γδ, 90, 626–627
HHV-6 infection of, 1052–1053, 1057
Histoplasma capsulatum infections, 1224
in HIV infection, 649b, 650
  see also T lymphocytes, CD4+
maturation, 90
memory, 90
  congenital CMV infection, 1045
  VZV infection, 1036
MHC restriction, 45–46, 627
Mycobacterium tuberculosis infections, 772
naive, 90, 92
in neonate, 90, 544
  vs adult, 90t
normal counts, 90
pathogens killed by, 89–90

proliferation, 90
receptors *see* T-cell receptor (TCR)
regulation, defective in HLH, 104–105
regulatory, 90
response to vaccines, 45–46
role in *Neisseria meningitidis* infections,
  732
RSV infection, 1132
signaling pathway defect in X-linked
  lymphoproliferative syndrome, 1064
Th17 cells, 626–628
  HIV infection, 650
  VZV infection, 1035–1036
X-linked lymphoproliferative syndrome,
  1064
T-tau, in CJD, 338
Tabes dorsalis, 942–943
Tachycardia
  Corynebacterium diphtheriae causing, 756
  definition, 98
  orthostatic, chronic fatigue syndrome
    pathogenesis, 1008
  in sepsis, 99
  in systemic inflammatory response
    syndrome, 98
Tachypnea, 168–169
  in acute abdominal pain, 172
  causes, 168–169
  in cystic fibrosis, 639
  in pneumonia, 169, 238
  in sepsis, 99
  stridor associated, 165
Tachyzoites, *Toxoplasma gondii*, 1309, 1311,
  1313
Taenia
  eosinophilia, 1408t–1409t
  meningitis, 283
Taenia asiatica, 1350
  life cycle, 1350, 1351f
  taeniasis, 1350–1352
    clinical manifestations, 1350–1351
    epidemiology, 1350
    laboratory findings and diagnosis,
      1351
Taenia (Multiceps) multiceps, 1362–1363,
  1363f
Taenia saginata, 1350, 1350f
  life cycle, 1350, 1351f
  T. solium vs., 1350f, 1351
  taeniasis, 1350–1352
    clinical manifestations, 1350–1351
    epidemiology, 1350
    laboratory findings and diagnosis,
      1350f, 1351
Taenia serialis (coenurosis), 1350, 1362–
  1363, 1363f
Taenia solium, 1350–1356
  autoinfection, 1350
  chronic myositis, 463t, 464
  cysticercosis, 1256, 1256t, 1350,
    1352–1356
    associated syndromes, 1353–1354
    calcifications, 1352–1354, 1353f,
      1355t
    clinical manifestations, 1352–1354
    eggs and autoinfection, 1352
    encephalitis, 1353–1354, 1353f,
      1355t

epidemiology, 1352
mixed forms, 1353
muscle, 1353f
pathogenesis, 1352
prevention, 1356
treatment and prognosis, 1354–1356,
1355t
vaccine, 1356
eosinophilia, 1407
eosinophilic meningitis, 331t
epidemiology and life cycle, 1350,
1351f
neurocysticercosis, 319, 1352–1354
diagnosis, 1353f, 1354
extraparenchymal, 1352–1353,
1355t
ocular, 1353–1354, 1353f, 1355t
parenchymal, 1352–1353, 1355t
spinal, 1353, 1355t
subarachnoid, 1353, 1353f, 1355t,
1356
treatment and prognosis, 1354–1356,
1355t
ventricular, 1353–1354, 1355t
T. saginata vs., 1350f, 1351
taeniasis, 1350–1352
clinical manifestations, 1350–1351
laboratory findings and diagnosis,
1351
prevention and control, 1352
treatment, 1351–1352
Tamm–Horsfall protein, 339
Tampons, toxic shock syndrome, 685
Tanapox, 1024
Tanapox virus, 1020t, 1024
Tapeworms (cestodes)
beef see Taenia saginata
dog (double-pored) (Dipylidium
caninum), 1348–1349, 1348f
dwarf see Hymenolepis nana
fish (broad), 1347
larval forms see Taenia (Multiceps)
multiceps; Taenia serialis (coenurosis)
pork see Taenia solium
rodent, 1349
treatment of infections, 1524–1525
Target attainment, antibiotic selection and,
1415
Target lesions, 111
Tattoos, infections after, 513t, 514
Tatumella, 809
Tau, in CJD, 338
Tazobactam, pharmacology, 1453t–1458t
3TC see Lamivudine
Tdap see under Diphtheria, tetanus, and
pertussis (DTP) vaccination/vaccines
Tears, reduced secretory rate, 487
Technetium 99 methylene phosphonate,
staphylococcal osteomyelitis
diagnosis, 679
Technetium-labeled bone scanning, 470,
471f, 471t
Technetium phosphate radionuclide scans,
pyogenic arthritis, 478
Teicoplanin, 1459t–1463t, 1468–1469
dose adjustment in burned patients,
1437t
pharmacodynamic properties, 1414t

Telavancin, 1469
treatment of, Staphylococcus aureus
infection, 688
Telbivudine, 1513
HBV infection treatment, 1083
Teleomorphic fungal stages, 1194
Telithromycin
dosage, 1480t–1483t
pharmacology, 1453t–1458t
spectrum of activity, 1459t–1463t
structure, 1470
Ureaplasma urealyticum infections,
1001
TEM enzymes, in drug resistance, 1424
Temperature (body)
aural, 91
axillary, 91
diurnal variations, 91
measurement methods, 91
normal variations, 91
oral, 91
raised see Fever
rectal, 91
normal by age/gender, 117, 117f
Temporal bone, anomalies
CMV infection, 1045
recurrent meningitis, 287b, 292
Temporal lobe abscess, 320
complications, 329–330
Tendon reflexes, deep, loss in spinal cord
tumors, 188
Tenesmus, 347
Tenofovir, 664, 665t, 1513–1514
dosage, 1445t–1452t, 1514
HBV infection treatment, 1083
Tenosynovitis, disseminated gonococcal
infection, 349
Tensilon test, 974
Teratogenicity
lymphocytic choriomeningitis virus,
1162
ribavirin, 1111
Terbinafine
dosage, 1445t–1452t
Sporothrix schenckii (sporotrichosis),
1219–1220
superficial infection treatment, 1485t,
1486
tinea capitis, 1247
Terconazole, 1485
Terminal fragment length polymorphism
(tFLP), Malassezia, 1216
Terranova, 1339
Terrorism, biological see Bioterrorism
Testis
inflammation see Orchitis
torsion, 368t
Tetanolysin, 967
Tetanospasmin, 967
duration of effect, 968
mechanism of action, 967
paralysis due to, 967
Tetanus toxin see Tetanospasmin
Tetanus toxoid see Clostridium tetani
Tetanus–diphtheria–acellular pertussis
(Tdap) vaccine see under Diphtheria,
tetanus, and pertussis (DTP)
vaccination/vaccines

Tetracycline(s), 1428, 1472–1473
chemoprophylactic use, 70t–71t
clinical uses, 1472
contraindication, pregnancy, 929
dosage, 1480t–1483t
mechanism of action, 687, 1428, 1472
pharmacodynamic properties, 1414t
pharmacology, 1453t–1458t
resistance to, 1422t, 1428, 1472
spectrum of activity, 1428, 1459t–1463t,
1472
staining of teeth by, 928
treatment of
Balantidium coli infection, 1267–1268
Bartonella bacilliformis, 940
bite wound infections, 521–522, 526
Borrelia infections, 958
Brucella infections, 864t
Chlamydophila (Chlamydia) psittaci,
891
Clostridium tetani infections, 969t
eye infections, 1494t–1496t
murine typhus (Rickettsia typhi), 932
Plasmodium infections, 1300–1304,
1301t–1303t, 1522
protozoan infections, 1522
Rickettsia prowazekii, 931
Rocky Mountain spotted fever
(Rickettsia rickettsii), 928
skin infections, 1498t
skin wound infections, 514
Staphylococcus aureus infections, 687
trachoma, 494
Treponema pallidum subsp. pallidum
(syphilis), 947
Textiles, standard precautions, 18t
Thayer-Martin modified agar, 1375t
Thermoregulation, fever, 91
Thermoregulatory neurons, 91
Thiabendazole
cutaneous larva migrans, 1339
Strongyloides infections, 1334
Toxocara infections, 1337
Thimerosal, 45, 51
Thioctic acid, 399
Thoracic surgery, infection
chemoprophylaxis, 72
Thoracic trauma, 513t, 515–516
pathogens and infection prophylaxis,
512t–513t, 516
Thoracoscopic surgery, video-assisted
(VATS), 243
Thoracostomy, pneumonia after, 516
Thoracotomy, infection prophylaxis, 516
Throat cultures, pharyngitis, 202–203
Throat swabs, specimen collection/transport,
1374t, 1377
Thrombi, formation, endocarditis
pathogenesis, 259
Thrombin, generation, in sepsis, 98
Thrombocytopenia, 1410–1411
Babesia infections, 1263, 1264f
Candida infections, 1200
causes, 1410–1411, 1411b
EBV infection, 1061
Ehrlichia and Anaplasma infections, 895
hemophagocytic lymphohistiocytosis,
106–107

HIV infection, 656, 672
MMR vaccine associated, 60
mucocutaneous syndromes with, 113
neutropenia with, 1405
Plasmodium infections, 1299–1300
Rickettsia felis infections, 933
varicella complication, 1038
Wiskott–Aldrich syndrome, 633
Thrombocytopenic purpura
acquired rubella, 1115–1116
congenital rubella, 1115
see also Idiopathic thrombocytopenic
purpura (ITP)
Thrombocytosis, 1409–1410
causes, 1409–1410, 1410t
epinephrine causing, 1409
Kawasaki disease, 113, 1003, 1409–1410
Thrombophlebitis
acute bacterial lymphangitis *vs.*, 161
septic *see* Septic thrombophlebitis
superficial, 265
suppurative
after burns, 519
catheter-related complication, 593
suppurative jugular *see* Lemierre disease
Thrombosis
burn wound infections, 517
central venous catheter-related, 592–593
innate immune response causing, 98
Thrush *see* Candida
"Thumb sign", acute epiglottitis, 210, 210f
Thymoma, with immunodeficiency, 602t
Thymus
anatomy and function, 127, 127t
destruction in HIV infection, 658
developmental changes, 128
weight in children *vs.* adults, 128
Thyroglossal duct cyst, 142t
Thyroid disorders, in congenital rubella,
1115
Thyroid gland
cancer, neck masses, 142t, 143
infections and pathogens causing, 143
masses, 143
Thyroid tissue, embryology, 143
Thyroiditis, subacute (de Quervain), 143
Thyrotropin-receptor autoantibodies, 155
TIBOLA/DEBONEL, 935–938
see also Rickettsiosis
Tic disorders, in PANDAS, 706
Ticarcillin
dosage, 1483t–1484t
eye infection treatment, 1494t–1496t
pharmacology, 1453t–1458t
spectrum of activity, 1459t–1463t
Ticarcillin-clavulanate
clinical uses, 1467
dosage, 1445t–1452t, 1483t–1484t
dose adjustment
burned patients, 1437t
renal failure, 1445t–1452t
spectrum of activity, 1459t–1463t,
1467
Tick(s), 531
ataxia associated, 180
attachment sites, 535
bites, occipital lymphadenopathy, 159
control, 535–536, 1094

Borrelia burgdorferi (Lyme disease),
956
Rickettsia parkeri infection, 935
Rocky Mountain spotted fever
(*Rickettsia rickettsii*) prevention,
929
distribution, 532t
endemic areas, precautions, 535
hard and soft types, 531
life cycle, 532
lifespan, 531
removal, 535
repellents and avoidance, 535
vectors for coltivirus (Colorado tick
fever), 1092
as vectors for pathogens, 532t, 533–535
Tick paralysis, weakness in, 531–532
differential diagnosis, 181t–182t
Tick repellents *see* DEET
Tickbite fever, African, 935–938
see also Rickettsiosis
Tickborne diseases
Babesia (babesiosis), 1261–1263, 1265
Borrelia burgdorferi infection, 952–953
Ehrlichia and *Anaplasma*, 893
Francisella tularensis, 895, 897
granulomatous hepatitis due to, 408
relapsing fever (*Borrelia*), 957–958
Rickettsia parkeri infection, 934–935
Rocky Mountain spotted fever (*Rickettsia
rickettsii*), 922–923, 926
Tickborne encephalitis
epidemiology and vectors, 532t
laboratory findings and diagnosis,
533t–534t
vaccines, 535
Tickborne encephalitis virus (TBEV),
1101–1102
aseptic meningitis, 293–295
vaccine, 80, 535
Tickborne infections, 531–536, 532t
clinical features and diagnosis, 533–535,
533t–534t
diagnosis, 533t–534t, 535
epidemiology, 531–532
factors influencing, 531–532
laboratory findings, 533t–534t
pathogenesis, 532–533
pathogens transmitted, 532
types, vectors and distribution, 532t
prevention, 535–536
control of host reservoirs, 535
prognosis and sequelae, 535
treatment, 535
vaccines, 535
see also specific infections
Tickborne relapsing fever, *Borrelia recurrentis*
see Borrelia recurrentis
Tickborne spotted fever, 83
Tietze syndrome, 189
Tigecycline, 1428, 1472–1473
clinical uses, 1472–1473
dosage, 1480t–1483t
pharmacology, 1453t–1458t
resistance to, 1428
spectrum of activity, 1459t–1463t,
1472–1473
structure, 1472

treatment of
Ca-MRSA infections, 472
Enterococcus infections, 715
Staphylococcus aureus infection, 687
Tight junctions, 83
Time-dependent antibiotics, 1441, 1442f,
1442t
Time-to-event analyses, 3, 5
Tine versicolor *see* Pityriasis versicolor
"Tinea", definition, 1246
Tinea capitis, 1246–1247, 1247b
clinical manifestations, 1246–1247,
1246f
differential diagnosis, 1247
epidemiology, 1246, 1247b
microbiology, 1246, 1247b
treatment, 1247, 1247b
Tinea corporis *see* Ringworm (tinea
corporis)
Tinea cruris (jock itch), 1248–1249
Tinea favosa (favus), 1249
Tinea gladiatorum, 1248
Tinea nigra, 1249–1250
Tinea pedis (athlete's foot), 1247–1248
Tinea unguium (onychomycosis), 1249
Tinidazole, treatment of
Giardia intestinalis (giardiasis), 1281t,
1282
protozoan infection, 1519
Trichomonas vaginalis, 360, 1319
Tipranavir, 665t, 1444t–1452t
Tissue culture, CMV infection, 1049
Tissue factor pathway inhibitor (TFPI),
101t–102t
Tissue flukes, 1256
Tissue necrosis, 456
Tissue nematodes *see* Nematodes
(roundworms)
Tissue plasminogen activator (tPA),
101t–102t
TMP-SMX *see* Trimethoprim-
sulfamethoxazole (TMP-SMX)
TNF-α *see* Tumor necrosis factor-α (TNF-α)
Tobramycin, 1474
in cystic fibrosis, 640
dosage, 1445t–1452t, 1480t–1484t
dose adjustment
burned patients, 1437t
renal failure, 1445t–1452t
eye infection treatment, 1494t–1496t
inhaled, 1474
pharmacology, 1453t–1458t
spectrum of activity, 1459t–1463t, 1474
Togaviridae, 1016t, 1097, 1112
arthritis, 481b
infections, 1017t
Toll-like receptors (TLRs), 45, 84, 92–93,
93f, 93t, 102–103, 569
activation, 95
NEMO role, 632–633
cells expressing, 93–94
chemotherapy effect on immune
response, 569
engagement and activation, 94
functions, 84, 92–93, 93f
intracellular signaling pathways, 84, 94,
102–103
microbial ligands, 93t

NEMO role, NEMO immunodeficiency, 632–633
NFκB activation, and effects, 94
pathogen evasion and, 93–94
polymorphism, 84
Pseudomonas aeruginosa flagella interactions, 842t, 843
recognition of microbial products, 84
signaling, 102–103
TLR 2, TLR5, TLR9, 102–103
TLR 3, TLR7, TLR9, 94
TLR 3 deficiency, characteristics, 604t–605t
TLR 4, 92–93, 102–103
urinary tract, 339
Toll receptors, 84
Tolnaftate, superficial fungal infections, 1485
Tongue
infections, 193t
in mucocutaneous syndromes, 111
strawberry *see* Strawberry tongue
Tonsillar lymph nodes, pathogens infecting, 145t
Tonsillar membrane, respiratory tract diphtheria, 755–756
Tonsillectomy
peritonsillar abscess, 206
in PFAPA, 123
in recurrent GAS pharyngitis, 205
Tonsillitis
adenoviruses causing, 1069
chronic, anaerobic gram-negative bacilli, 983
Tonsils, faucial (palatine)
anatomy, 127
lymphatic drainage, 136
prominent, in children, 128
Tooth
colonization, 190–191
demineralization, 191
infections *see* Dental infections
Toothpick puncture injury, 515
Topical antifungal agents, 1485–1486
Topical antimicrobial agents, 1493–1501
characteristics of ideal agents, 1500b
treatment of
burns, 520, 520t, 1499–1500, 1500b, 1500t–1501t
ear infections, 1496–1498, 1497t
eye infections, 1493–1496, 1494t–1496t
skin infections, 1498–1499, 1498t–1499t
Topoisomerase IV, *Salmonella*, 817
TORCH screen, 402, 548
Torovirus, gastroenteritis, 378
Torticollis, 129
Total body surface area (TBSA), 516
Total parenteral nutrition, infection risk, 590
Total serum hemolytic complement (CH$_{50}$) assay, 619
Tourniquet test, dengue fever, 1100
Toxic encephalopathy
encephalitis *vs.*, 302b
Proteus causing, 811–812
Shigella causing, 821

Toxic epidermal necrolysis (TEN), 1479
Toxic erythema, 441
Toxic ingestions
altered mental status, 179, 179t
ataxia in, 180t
Toxic shock syndrome (TSS), 108
necrotizing fasciitis with, 514
staphylococcal *see Staphylococcus aureus*
streptococcal *see Streptococcus pyogenes*
streptococcal group C and G causing, 720
syndromes comparison, 108, 109t–111t
Toxins
acute hepatitis due to, 404
chronic hepatitis due to, 407
foodborne, 392–396
granulomatous hepatitis due to, 409
rashes due to, 441
see also individual micro-organisms
Toxocara (toxocariasis), 1335–1337
clinical features, 1335–1336
"covert", 1335
diagnosis, 1336–1337
eggs, 1335–1336, 1335f
larvae, 1335–1336, 1336f
larvicidal activity against, 1337
life cycle and description, 1335–1336, 1335f–1336f
medical ecology, 1337
ocular larva migrans, 1335–1337, 1336f
treatment and prevention, 1337
visceral larva migrans, 1335–1337
Toxocara canis, 1335–1337
clinical features, 1335–1336
diagnosis, 1336–1337
eosinophilia due to, 1407, 1408t–1409t
fever of unknown origin due to, 119t–120t
larvae, 1336f
life cycle and description, 1335, 1335f, 1337
ocular infections, 502
retinitis due to, 502
Toxocara cati, 1335–1337
diagnosis, 1336–1337
eosinophilia due to, 1407, 1408t–1409t
fever of unknown origin due to, 119t–120t
life cycle and description, 1335, 1335f, 1337
Toxoids, 44–45
Toxoplasma gondii (toxoplasmosis), 1308–1317
acute infection, 1308, 1311
diagnosis, 1312
prevention, 1317
risk factors, 1310
antibodies, 1311–1312, 1314
asymptomatic infection, 1308, 1311
bradyzoites, 1309, 1311
brain abscess due to, 319, 1312
cerebral infection, in HIV infection, 661
cervical lymphadenitis due to, 135t
unilateral, 139t, 140
unilateral, biopsy avoidance, 145–146
chorioretinitis due to, 499–500, 500f
clinical features, 1311–1312, 1312f

diagnosis, 1313–1314
epidemiology, 1312
examination for, 1311
prevention of relapses, 1317
prognosis, 1311–1312
treatment, 1315t
chronic fatigue syndrome pathogenesis, 1008t–1009t
chronic infection, 1308
diagnosis, 1312
in immunocompetent children, 1312
reactivation in immunocompromised patients, 1308, 1311–1312
chronic myositis due to, 464
clinical manifestations, 1311–1312
chronic infection in immunocompetent children, 1312
congenital toxoplasmosis, 1311–1312, 1312f
primary infection in immunocompetent hosts, 1311
reactivation of chronic infections in immunocompromised patients, 1312
CNS infection, 304
congenital toxoplasmosis, 536
chorioretinitis, 1311–1312, 1312f
clinical features, 537t, 1311–1312, 1312f
CT, 1314
diagnosis, 538t
diagnosis in neonates, 1314
epidemiology, 1309–1310
generalized lymphadenopathy, 131t–132t, 133
in utero treatment, prognosis, 1315–1316
incidence, 1311
neonatal evaluation, 1312
pathogenesis, 1311
prenatal diagnosis by PCR, 1313
prognosis (after treatment), 1316
retinitis, 499t
sequelae, 1312
signs before diagnosis/treatment, 1311–1312
transmission prevention, 1310–1311, 1313, 1315, 1315t
treatment, 1315t, 1316
description of pathogen, 1309
diagnosis, 1312–1314
AC/HS test (differential agglutination), 1313
acute and chronic infection, 1312
biopsy specimen, 1383–1384
chorioretinitis, 1313–1314
immunocompetent children, 1314
immunocompromised children, 1314
in neonates, 1314
in pregnancy, 1313–1314
Sarcocystis vs., 1308
serologic tests, 1312–1314
toxoplasmosis, 1313
encephalitis due to, 304, 1311–1312
diagnosis, 1313–1314
prophylaxis, 1317
eosinophilic meningitis due to, 331t
epidemiology, 1310–1311

fetal infection *see Toxoplasma gondii* (toxoplasmosis), congenital toxoplasmosis
genome, 1309
in HIV/AIDS, 661, 1311–1312, 1314, 1317
   prevention, 669
HSCT recipients, 564
immune response, 1311
immunocompromised hosts
   clinical manifestations, 1310, 1312
   diagnosis, 1314
   immune response, 1311
   prophylaxis against activation of latent infection, 1317
   treatment, 1316, 1316t
laboratory testing, 308t–311t
life cycle, 1309, 1309f
lymph nodes in, 129
lymphadenopathy due to, 1311, 1314
   generalized lymphadenopathy, 131t–132t, 132, 1311
meningitis due to, 283, 284t, 331t
neonatal infection, clinical manifestations, 537t
neutropenia associated with cancer, 568
ocular toxoplasmosis, 499–500
oocysts, 1309, 1309f, 1311
orchitis due to, 369
pathogenesis, 1311
in pregnancy, 1310
   clinical manifestations, 1311
   diagnosis, 1313–1314
   transmission prevention, 1310–1311, 1313, 1315, 1315t
   transmission rates, 1310–1311, 1310f
   treatment, 1315–1316, 1315t, 1316f
prevention of infection, 1317
   primary infection, 1317, 1317t
   reactivation of latent infection, 1317
primary infection, clinical manifestations, 1311
prognosis
   acute infection in immunocompetent children, 1311
   congenital infection, 1311–1312
   congenital infection, after treatment, 1316
   immunocompromised patients, 1311–1312
proteins, 1314
reactivation of infection, 1308, 1311–1312
   clinical manifestations, 1312
   prevention, 1317
retinitis due to, 499–500, 500f
   see also Chorioretinitis (above)
screening, 1311–1313
solid-organ transplant recipients, 560
sporozoites, 1309, 1311
tachyzoites, 1309, 1311, 1313
transmission to fetus in utero, 536, 1310
   incidence, 1311
   prevention, 1310–1311, 1313, 1315, 1315t
   rates and gestation age, 1310–1311, 1310f

treatment of infection, 1314–1316, 1315t, 1521–1522
   immunocompetent children, 1316, 1316t
   immunocompromised children, 1316, 1316t
   neonates, 1315t, 1316
   in pregnancy, 1315–1316, 1315t, 1316f
Toxoplasmosis *see Toxoplasma gondii*
Trabulsiella, 810
Tracheal aspiration, pneumonia diagnosis, 240
Tracheal bronchus, 247
Tracheal lymph nodes, 148–149
Tracheal secretions, aspiration, rigid, 212
Tracheitis, bacterial, 165, 212–213
   clinical features, 166t, 206t, 212
   complications and prognosis, 213
   diagnosis, 166t, 212
   management, 212
   pathophysiology and etiology, 212
   radiography, 212, 213f
   Staphylococcus aureus, 681
   stridor, 165, 212
Tracheobronchial lymph nodes, 148–149
   pulmonary *Mycobacterium tuberculosis* infection, 151
   tuberculosis, 151–153
Tracheobronchial lymphadenopathy, 151f
Tracheobronchial tree, congenital cystic anomalies, pneumonia, 247
Tracheobronchitis
   burns patients, 519
   mycoplasmal, cough in, 167t
   necrotizing/exudative, HSV infection, 1030
   viral, stridor, 165
   see also Laryngotracheitis (croup)
Tracheoesophageal anomalies, persistent/recurrent pneumonia, 250
Tracheoesophageal fistula, H-type, persistent/recurrent pneumonia, 250
Tracheoesophagitis, cough in, 167t
Tracheostomy, infant botulism, 975–976
Trachipleistophora, 1292t
Trachoma *see Chlamydia trachomatis*, trachoma
Transcobalamin II deficiency, antibiotic deficiency with, 602t
Transcription-mediated amplification (TMA), *Trichomonas vaginalis* (trichomoniasis) diagnosis, 354–355
Transesophageal echocardiography (TEE)
   endocarditis, 261
   pericarditis, 270
β_2-Transferrin, in CSF, recurrent meningitis, 291
Transforming growth factor-β (TGF-β), anti-inflammatory cytokine, 94–95
Transfusion-transmitted viruses (TTVs), 1193–1194
Transfusions, infections transmitted by *see* Blood transfusions
Transient hypogammaglobulinemia of infancy, 610t, 615, 615t
Transient synovitis, 184, 185t, 485–487
   clinical manifestations, 486

diagnosis, 486
differential diagnosis, 486
etiology and epidemiology, 485–486
of hip, ESR elevation, 1400–1401
treatment and prognosis, 486–487
Transmissible spongiform encephalopathies (TSEs), 333–338
   see also Creutzfeldt–Jakob disease (CJD); Prion diseases
Transmission-based precautions, 18, 19t–20t
   clinical syndromes warranting, 20t
Transmission of infections, 12–13
   group childcare and, 24
      see also Group childcare, infections associated
   healthcare-associated infection *see* Healthcare-associated infection (HAI)
   horizontal, 12
   modes, 12–13
   see also individual infections
Transplant recipients, infections, 555–561
   adenoviruses, 1068t, 1069–1070
   Aspergillus infections, 1205–1206
   CMV infection *see* Cytomegalovirus (CMV)
   Coccidioides immitis (coccidioidomycosis), 1244–1245
   EBV infection, 559, 1063
   HHV-6 infection, 1054, 1057
   HHV-7 infection, 1058
   immunization after, 561
   Nocardia infections, 794
   organisms causing pneumonia, 253–254
   pulmonary histoplasmosis, 153
   Toxoplasma gondii infections, 1308, 1310–1311, 1314, 1317
   varicella, 1039
   see also Hematopoietic stem cell transplantation (HSCT); Solid-organ transplant recipients; *individual organs*
Transport, transmission-based precaution, 19t
Transport media
   bacteria, 1373, 1373t–1374t
   viral (VTM), 1385
Transporters, drug, 1440
Transposons, acquired drug resistance, 1423
Transtracheal aspiration, specimen collection/transport, 1377
Transudates, 241
Transverse myelitis, acute, 317
   diagnosis, 317
   enterovirus infections, 1176
   epidemiology, 317
   etiology, 314t, 317
   MRI, 318f
   treatment, 317
   varicella with, 1039
   weakness due to, differential diagnosis, 181t–182t
TRAPS, 122, 122t
Trauma
   adverse effects on host defense, 512
   from animals, 529
   bites *see* Bites, infections after
   chronic fatigue syndrome pathogenesis, 1012

epidemiology, 512
infections due to, 512–516
  antibiotic prophylaxis, 512t, 513
  chemoprophylaxis, 73
  incidence, 512
  management, 512–513
  pathogenesis, 512, 512t
  risk factors, 512
  travelers, 76
Travel medicine kit, 76, 77b
Travel-related illness, 83
  in immunocompromised people, 82
Travelers
  eosinophilia, 1407
  hepatitis A virus infection, 1180–1182
  posttravel screening, 83
  return after, infections, 83
Travelers, protection of, 76–83
  diarrhea *see* Diarrhea, travelers'
  education on food/drink safety, 374
  emerging infectious diseases, 82
  Escherichia coli infection prevention, 799
  Fasciola infection prevention, 1366
  general advice for, 76, 854b
  hepatitis A postexposure prophylaxis, 38
  immunization, 52, 76–77
    acceleration of routine schedules, 77, 78t
    co-administration of vaccines, 77
    MMR, 60
    poliovirus vaccine, 1171–1172
    required and recommended vaccines, 77, 79–80, 79t
    routine vaccines, 77–79
    schedule and dosing, 77–79, 78t–79t
    vaccines available, 67–68
  immunocompromised, 82–83
  information sources, 77b
  malaria prophylaxis, 80–81
  Plasmodium infection *see* *Plasmodium* (malaria)
  preparation for travel, 76–80
  pretravel evaluation, 76
  Schistosoma infection prevention, 1370
  Vibrio cholerae infection prevention, 854, 854b
  Wuchereria bancrofti prevention, 1344
Trematode larva migrans, *Paragonimus skrjabini* causing, 1368
Trematodes, 1363–1364, 1368–1371
  infections, refugee and internationally adopted children, 35
  see also Flukes
Trench fever, louse-borne *see* *Bartonella quintana*
Trench mouth (acute necrotizing ulcerative gingivitis (ANUG)), 194, 983
Treponema, 673, 941, 948–949
  diseases caused, 941
    evolution/development, 941
  meningitis due to, 294–295
  nonvenereal infections, 941
    treatment, 949
  serologic tests, 941
  structure/characteristics, 941
Treponema carateum (pinta), 941, 949
Treponema pallidum particle agglutination test (TPPA), 944

Treponema pallidum subsp. *endemicum* (endemic syphilis/bejel), 941, 948–949
Treponema pallidum subsp. *pallidum* (syphilis), 941–948
  acquired syphilis, 942–943, 945
  acquisition route, 942
  anterior uveitis due to, 499, 499t
  antibodies, 941
  cardiovascular syphilis, 941–943
  chemoprophylaxis, 70t–71t
  chorioretinitis due to, 499
  clinical manifestations, 942–944, 948b
  congenital syphilis, 133, 942–944, 943f
    assessment and management, 946f
    case definitions (CDC), 945
    clinical features, 537t
    diagnosis, 538t
    early-onset disease, 943–944
    evaluation, 945, 946f
    generalized lymphadenopathy, 131t–132t
    laboratory evaluation/diagnosis, 945
    late-onset disease, 944
    meningitis, 280–281
    nasal discharge, 164
    prenatal treatment, 946
    presumed *vs* confirmed case, 945
    treatment, 946–947, 947t
  description and microbiology, 941–942
  diagnosis/detection, 385t, 941, 944–945, 948b
    antibody tests, 944–945
    false-negative and false-positive, 944
    IgM tests, 945–947, 948b
    nontreponemal tests, 944–945
    organism tests, 945
    in refugee and internationally adopted children, 33t, 36
    serologic tests, 33t, 36
    specimens, 351t
    treponemal tests, 944–945
  DNA sequence, 941
  endothelial cell adherence, 941–942
  eosinophilic meningitis, 331t, 332
  epidemiology, 348, 350, 941–942, 948b
  exposure management in pregnant healthcare worker, 22t–23t
  follow-up, 947
  general paresis due to, 942–943
  generalized lymphadenopathy due to, 130, 131t–132t, 942
  genital ulcers with lymphadenopathy, 348–349
    epidemiology, 350
    features and treatment, 350t
  gummas due to, 941–943
  historical aspects, 941
  in HIV infection, 942–943, 945–947
    treatment, 947t
  immune evasion, 941
  immune response to, 941
  incubation period, 942
  laboratory evaluation, 945
  laboratory testing, 308t–311t
  latent syphilis, 942
    follow-up, 947
    treatment, 942–943

lipoproteins and antigens, 941
macrolide resistance, 947
meningeal, 942–943
meningitis, 280–281, 942
  clinical features, 281
  diagnosis and laboratory findings, 281
  epidemiology, 280–281
  pathogenesis, 280–281
microbiology, 941–942
neurosyphilis, 942–944
  treatment, 947t
oral mucosal features, 193t
outer membrane proteins (TROMP), 941
pathogenesis, 941–942
pharyngeal infections, 349
in pregnancy, 942–943
  adverse outcomes, 944–945
  screening, 945
  seroreactive, 945
  treatment, 942–943, 946
prevention, 947
primary disease, 941–942
Reagin antibody, 1411t–1412t
refugee and immigrant children, 945
refugee and internationally adopted children, 36
screening, 944–945
secondary syphilis, 941–942
  epitrochlear lymphadenopathy, 160
  lesions, 349
seroreversion, 944
sexual abuse, 371
structure, 941
syphilis, genital ulcers/lymphadenopathy, 348
tabes dorsalis, 942–943
tertiary disease, 941–943
  "benign", 943
transmission
  sexual, 942
  vertical, 942–943
treatment, 945–947, 947t, 948b
  failures, 945–946
Treponema pallidum subsp. *pertenue*, 941, 948
yaws, 941
  clinical features, 948
  diagnosis, 948
  latent, 948
  treatment, 949
Treponemataceae, 941–958
  genera included, 673
Triatoma infestans, 1322–1323
Triatomine bugs, 1322, 1323f
Trichinella britovi, 1339
Trichinella murrelli, 1339
Trichinella nativa, 1339, 1341
Trichinella nelsoni, 1339
Trichinella paupae, 1339
Trichinella pseudospiralis, 1339
Trichinella spiralis (trichinellosis), 1339–1341
  chronic myositis, 463t, 464
  clinical manifestations, 1341
  diagnosis, 1341
  eosinophilia, 1407, 1408t–1409t
  eosinophilic meningitis, 331t
  epidemiology, 1339

larvae, 1339, 1340f
life cycle, 1339–1340, 1340f
misdiagnosis reasons, 1341
muscle cell infections, 1340
nurse cell-larva complex, 1339–1341, 1340f
prevention, 1341
treatment, 1341
Trichoderma, 1210–1211
Trichodysplasia spinulosa (TS), 1077
Trichodysplasia spinulosa-associated polyomavirus (TSV), 1075, 1077
Trichomonas vaginalis (trichomoniasis), 1317–1319
cervicitis, diagnosis, 362
clinical manifestations, 1318
culture, 354–355, 360
description and structure, 1317–1318, 1318f
diagnosis, 353, 355, 360
DNA probes, 360
transcription-mediated amplification, 354–355
in vulvovaginitis, 357, 359
differential diagnosis, 1318
discharge/dysuria syndrome, 346
epidemiology, 353, 359, 1318
fishy odor, 359–360
genital discharge/dysuria syndrome, 346
HIV infection and, 359, 361
immune response to, 1318
laboratory diagnosis, 1318–1319, 1383
in neonates, 1318
in pregnancy, 361, 1318
outcome, 1319
prevention, 1319
sexually transmitted infection, 346
transmission, 1318
treatment of infections, 1319, 1519
resistance and failures, 1319
urethritis, 353
diagnosis, 353–355
in males, 1318
management, 355–356
vaginitis, 359, 1318
diagnosis, 360
management, 360–361
vulvovaginitis, 356–357, 359
clinical features, 359t
diagnosis, 357, 359, 359t
treatment, 359t, 360–361
wet-mount technique, 1318–1319
Trichophyton, 1246
preseptal cellulitis, 509
Trichophyton mentagrophytes
genital dermatosis, 352
tinea capitis, 1246
tinea corporis, 1248
tinea cruris, 1248
tinea pedis, 1247
tinea unguium, 1249
treatment, 1485
Trichophyton rubrum
genital dermatosis, 352
tinea corporis, 1248
tinea cruris, 1248
tinea pedis, 1247

tinea unguium, 1249
treatment, 1485
Trichophyton schoenleinii, tinea favosa, 1249
Trichophyton tonsurans
tinea capitis, 1246–1247, 1246f
tinea corporis, 1248
treatment, 1485, 1485t
Trichophyton violaceum, tinea capitis, 1246
Trichosporon, neutropenia associated with cancer, 567
Trichosporon beigelii, 1250
Trichostrongylus, 1383
Trichotillomania, 1247
Trichrome stain, 1383–1384
Giardia intestinalis (giardiasis), 1281–1282
Trichuris trichiura, 1326, 1330–1331
Campylobacter jejuni synergy, 1331
clinical manifestations, 1327b, 1331
description, 1330, 1330f–1331f
diagnosis, 1326, 1327f, 1331
eggs, 1327f, 1330–1331
eosinophilia, 1407, 1408t–1409t
epidemiology, 1330–1331
infection route, 1326, 1330
prevention, 1331
treatment, 1331
Triclabendazole, 1525
Fasciola infections, 1366
Triclosan, skin antiseptic, 1499t
Tricyclic amines, as antiviral agents, 1514
Trifluorothymidine, viral keratitis, 497
Trifluridine, 1514
adenovirus infections, 1070
HSV infections, conjunctivitis, 489
Trigger points, 186
TRIM-5α, 1167
Trimethoprim
mechanism of action, 1479
pharmacology, 1416–1417, 1453t–1458t
treatment of
Cystoisospora (cystisosporiasis), 1284
eye infections, 1494t–1495t
Pneumocystis jirovecii (carinii) pneumonia, 1232t
Trimethoprim-sulfamethoxazole (TMP-SMX), 1479
adverse reactions, 687, 1232
chemoprophylactic use, 70t–71t, 74t, 75
cholangitis prevention, 413
Listeria monocytogenes prevention, 764
Pneumocystis jirovecii (carinii), 1233, 1233t
clinical uses, 1428, 1479
dosage, 1445t–1452t, 1480t–1483t
mechanism of action, 687, 1428, 1479
nephrotoxicity, 794–795
pharmacodynamic properties, 1414t
resistance, 1422t, 1428
Proteus mirabilis, 812
Shigella, 822
spectrum of activity, 1459t–1463t
susceptibility testing, 1378
treatment of, 624, 624t
acute otitis media, 216–217
Aeromonas infections, 831
Babesia divergens infections, 1265

bite wound infections, 526
Blastocystis hominis infections, 1269
Brucella infections, 871, 871t
cholecystitis and cholangitis, 414
Cystoisospora (cystisosporiasis), 1284
dacryoadenitis, 508
infections in CGD, 624
infections in phagocyte disorders, 624t
Klebsiella granulomatis infection, 803
Listeria monocytogenes infections, 766
Nocardia brain abscess, 329
Nocardia infections, 794–795
pediculosis, 1259
Pneumocystis jirovecii (carinii), 663, 1232, 1232t
Pneumocystis jirovecii (carinii) in cancer, 576–577
pneumonia in immunocompromised patients, 255
Proteus mirabilis, 812
protozoan infections, 1522
Rocky Mountain spotted fever, 535
Salmonella infections, 818, 818t
Shigella infections, 822t
Staphylococcus aureus infections, 687
tickborne infections, 535
Toxoplasma gondii infection, 1316, 1316t
urinary tract infections, 341
Yersinia pestis infection prevention, 827
Trimetrexate, *Pneumocystis jirovecii (carinii)* infections, 1232t, 1233
Triple dye, skin antiseptic, 1499t
Tripod position, in acute epiglottitis, 210
Trismus
Clostridium tetani causing, 967
in peritonsillar abscess, 165
Troisier sign, 137
Tropheryma whipplei
endocarditis due to, 260t
meningitis, 281–282
Trophozoites
Acanthamoeba, 1296–1297, 1296f
Babesia, 1261
Balantidium coli, 1266–1267, 1266f–1267f
Dientamoeba fragilis, 1279
Endolimax nana, 1271–1272, 1272f
Entamoeba histolytica, 383, 1273–1274, 1273f–1274f
Giardia intestinalis, 1279–1282, 1280f
Naegleria fowleri, 1293–1295, 1293f–1294f, 1295t
Plasmodium, 1298–1300, 1298f
Pneumocystis jirovecii (carinii), 1230
stool examination, 1383
Tropical pulmonary eosinophilia (TPE), 1343
diagnosis, 1344t
treatment, 1342t, 1344
Troponin I
in endocarditis, 260
in myocarditis, 267
pericarditis, 270
Troponin T, in myocarditis, 267

Trypanosoma, 1319–1326
  classification, 1319
  detection in blood smears, 1384
  Salivaria, 1319
  Stercoraria, 1319
Trypanosoma (Trypanozoon) brucei, 1319–
    1322, 1326b
  antibodies to, 1322
  chronic stage, 1320–1321
  classification, 1319–1320
  clinical course, 1320–1321
  CNS disease, 1320, 1322
  description and life cycle, 1320, 1320f
  diagnosis, 1321–1322
  differential diagnosis, 1321
  epidemiology, 1320
  generalized lymphadenopathy, 131t–
    132t, 132, 1320
  genome, 1255
  lymphadenopathy, 1320
  pathogenesis and pathology, 1320
  prevention, 1322
  prognosis, 1322
  transmission, 1320
  treatment, 1322, 1322t, 1519–1520
  Trypanosoma cruzi vs., 1326b
  trypomastigotes, 1320
Trypanosoma (Trypanozoon) brucei gambiense,
    1319–1322
Trypanosoma (Trypanozoon) brucei rhodesiense,
    1319–1322
Trypanosoma (Schizotrypanum) cruzi, 1319,
    1322–1326, 1326b
  acute phase, 1324
  amastigotes, 1322, 1324f
  asymptomatic, 1324
  cardiac abnormalities, 1324–1325, 1324f
  chronic phase, 1324
  clinical manifestations, 1324–1325,
    1324f
  congenital infection, 1325
  description and life cycle, 1322, 1323f
  diagnosis, 1325
  epidemiology, 1322–1324
  epimastigotes, 1322
  generalized lymphadenopathy, 131t–
    132t, 132
  genome, 1255
  immune response, 1324
  intrauterine infection, 1325
  myocarditis due to, 266
  pathogenesis and pathology, 1324, 1324f
  in pregnancy, 1325
  prevention, 1326
  prognosis, 1325
  refugee and internationally adopted
    children, 36
  transmission, 1322–1323
    by blood transfusions, 1322–1323,
      1325
    congenital, 1325
  treatment, 1325–1326, 1520
  Trypanosoma brucei vs., 1326b
  trypomastigotes, 1322, 1323f
Trypanosomatidae, 1320
Trypanosomiasis
  African *see Trypanosoma (Trypanozoon)
    brucei*

American *see Trypanosoma
    (Schizotrypanum) cruzi*
Trypanozoon, 1319–1320
Trypomastigotes
  Trypanosoma (Trypanozoon) brucei, 1320
  Trypanosoma (Schizotrypanum) cruzi, 1322,
    1323f
Tsetse flies
  Trypanosoma (Trypanozoon) brucei
    transmission, 1319–1320
  see also Glossina
TSST-1 *see under Staphylococcus aureus*
Tsukamurella, 770
  Tsukamurella paurometabola, 770
  Tsukamurella pulmonis, 770
  Tsukamurella strandjordae, 770
TT virus, infant infections, 545
Tuberculid reactions, 454
Tuberculin skin test *see* Mantoux
    intradermal tuberculin skin test
Tuberculin units (TU), 779
  see also Mantoux intradermal tuberculin
    skin test
Tuberculoma, 778
  during tuberculous meningitis therapy,
    778
Tuberculosis *see Mycobacterium tuberculosis*
Tubo-ovarian abscess, 364
Tularemia *see Francisella tularensis
    (Pasteurella tularensis)* (tularemia)
Tumbu fly, 76
Tumefaction, 1252
Tumor fever *see* Neutropenia, fever in
Tumor necrosis factor-α (TNF-α), 100
  antagonists, *Histoplasma capsulatum*
    infections, 1226
  elevated levels
    HIV encephalopathy, 653–654
    in HLH, 105
    Histoplasma capsulatum infections, 1224
  inflammatory response, 94
  influenza A virus infection, 1151
  microbe binding to Toll-like receptors
    releasing, 84
  monoclonal antibody (Afelimomab),
    101t–102t
  Mycobacterium tuberculosis infections,
    772
  as proinflammatory cytokine, 100
  as pyrogenic cytokine, 92
  receptors, soluble, 94–95, 100
  role in endotoxin toxicity, 100
  in sepsis, 100
  soluble receptor constructs, 101t–102t
Tumor necrosis factor receptor 1 (TNFR1),
    126
Tumor necrosis factor receptor-associated
    periodic syndromes (TRAPS), 122,
    122t, 125–126
  cardinal clinical features, 126
  course, treatment and outcome, 126
  epidemiology and etiology, 125–126
  mutations, 126
Tumor suppressor gene 101 (TSG-101), 1167
Tumor suppressor proteins, inactivation, by
    HPV, 1071
Tumors *see* Cancer; *specific tumors*
Turtles, *Salmonella* transmission, 528

Tympanic membrane
  bulging opaque, in mastoiditis, 223
  examination, chronic mastoiditis
    diagnosis, 226
  perforation
    acute otitis media complication, 220
    chronic mastoiditis in, 226
  temperature measurement, 91
Tympanocentesis
  acute mastoiditis treatment, 225
  specimen collection/transport, 1374t,
    1377
Tympanostomy tube insertion
  chemoprophylaxis, 1498
  otitis media with effusion, 220
  in recurrent otitis media, 219
Type I error, 5
Type II error, 6
Type III secretion system (TTSS)
  Pseudomonas aeruginosa, 842–843, 842t
  Yersinia, 823
Typhlitis, 386, 981
  in cancer, 578
Typhoid fever *see Salmonella* Typhi
Typhus
  epidemic *see Rickettsia prowazekii*
  murine (fleaborne) *see Rickettsia typhi*
  recrudescent *see Rickettsia prowazekii*
  Rickettsia prowazekii (epidemic typhus),
    930–931
Tyrosine kinase (BTK) gene, 611
TYSGM-9 stain, 1383–1384

U

Ulcer(s), 449–454
  aphthous, HIV infection, 662
  Blastomyces dermatitidis (blastomycosis),
    1236, 1236f
  colonic
    Entamoeba dispar, 1278
    Entamoeba histolytica, 1274
  corneal, *Acanthamoeba* keratitis, 1296
  cutaneous, leishmaniasis, 1287–1289,
    1288f
  decubitus, anaerobic gram-positive cocci,
    989
  Francisella tularensis infection, 897–898
  genital *see* Genital ulcer(s)
  infectious causes, 450t
  *Klebsiella (Calymmatobacterium)
    granulomatis* infection, 803
  mouth *see* Oral ulceration
  noninfectious causes, 451t
  penile, donovanosis, 803, 803f
  skin, *Acanthamoeba* infection, 1296
  visceral leishmaniasis, 1287
Ulcerative colitis, *Entamoeba histolytica*
    infection *vs.*, 1275
Ulceroglandular tularemia *see Francisella
    tularensis (Pasteurella tularensis)*
    (tularemia)
Ulesfia (benzyl alcohol), pediculosis
    treatment, 1258–1259
Ultrasonography
  acute pancreatitis, 410
  appendicitis, 421
  cholecystitis and cholangitis, 413

cranial, *Candida* infections, 1198, 1198f
Echinococcus granulosus cysts, 1358
fetal, *Toxoplasma gondii* infections, 1313–1314
intravascular catheter-related infections, 592
Onchocerca volvulus infections, 1345
peritonitis, 417
pyogenic arthritis, 478
renal, *Candida* infections, 1198–1199, 1199f
Schistosoma infections, 1370
transient synovitis, 486
Wuchereria bancrofti, 1343
Umbilical cord care, 606–607
Umbilical infections, neonatal tetanus, 968
UN International Children's Emergency Fund, vitamin A in measles, 1141
UNC93B protein mutation, 604t–605t
Undecylenic acid, superficial fungal infections, 1485
Undulant fever, 863
  see also Brucella
UNG deficiency, 610t, 613, 632
United Nations Children's (Emergency) Fund, oral rehydration therapy, 376
Upper airway obstruction
  causes, 166t
  course and sequelae, 166t
  differential diagnosis, 165t
Upper respiratory tract infections (URTIs), 196–220, 227–231
  adenoviruses, 1068t, 1069
  anaerobic gram-positive cocci, 989
  colds *see* Common colds
  group childcare and, 27, 31
  human coronaviruses causing, 1119–1120
  human metapneumovirus, 1134, 1136
  human parainfluenza viruses, 1121, 1123, 1123f
  influenza, 1153
  judicious antimicrobial use, 1421
  mastoiditis *see* Mastoiditis
  otitis media *see* Otitis media
  pharyngitis, 199
  refugee and internationally adopted children, 36
  respiratory syncytial virus infection, 1133
  sinusitis *see* Sinusitis
  Staphylococcus aureus, 680–681
  supraglottic *see* Supraglottic infections
  viral, 227
    clinical features, 228
    natural history, 228
    recurrent, 230
    see also Sinusitis
  see also Respiratory tract infections; Respiratory tract viruses
Uracil-DNA glycosylase (UNG) deficiency, 610t, 613, 632
Urea breath test (UBT), *Helicobacter pylori* infections, 913–914, 1383
Ureaplasma, 673
  pneumonia due to, 236, 238
  in X-linked agammaglobulinemia, 610
Ureaplasma parvum, 998t, 1000–1001
Ureaplasma urealyticum, 998t, 1000–1002
  arthritis due to, 481–482

aseptic meningitis due to, 295
asymptomatic urethral carriage, 1000
biovars, 353
chronic lung disease of prematurity, 1001
clinical manifestations, 1000–1001
culture and growth, 355
diagnosis/detection, 1001, 1399
  optimal tests, 1389t–1392t
  in urethritis, 355
epidemiology, 353, 1000
genital discharge/dysuria syndrome, 346
genome, 1000
intrauterine and neonatal infections, 1000–1001
  treatment, 1001
laboratory findings, 1001
pneumonia in young infants, 169
preterm deliveries and, 1000
serotypes and biovars, 1000
sexually transmitted infection
  discharge/dysuria syndrome, 346
  scrotal pain syndrome, 348–349
treatment of infections, 1001–1002
urethritis, 353
  diagnosis, 355
  treatment, 356
vaginal colonization, 1000–1001
Urease, rapid test, *Helicobacter pylori* detection, 913
Ureteral colic, site and radiation of pain, 171
Urethral catheterization, nosocomial infection of neonates, 550
Urethral catheters, infections associated, 342
Urethral discharge
  diagnosis of pathogen, 354, 355f
  discharge/dysuria syndrome, 347
  in epididymitis, 367
  HSV infection, 1029
  sexually transmitted infections, 347
  in urethritis, 354, 354t
Urethral strictures, 356
Urethral syndrome, 353–354
Urethritis, 353–363
  clinical manifestations, 354, 354t
  complications, 356
  definition, 353
  diagnostic criteria, 353
  differential diagnosis, 354, 354t
  epidemiology, 353–354
  etiology, 353
    infectious, 353
    noninfectious, 353
  females, 353–355
  gonococcal *see* Neisseria gonorrhoeae
  laboratory findings and diagnosis, 354–355
  males, 353–355
  management, 355–356, 356t
  nongonococcal (NGU), 353
    Chlamydia trachomatis see Chlamydia trachomatis
    clinical features, 354, 354t
    Mycoplasma genitalium, 347, 353, 1000
    Trichomonas vaginalis see Trichomonas vaginalis

Ureaplasma urealyticum causing, 353, 1000
prevention, 356
sexually transmitted pathogens causing, 353–354
Urinalysis
  fever without localizing signs, 116–117
  Plasmodium infections, 1300
  refugee and internationally adopted children, 33t, 36
  urinary tract infections, 340
  see also Urine
Urinary catheterization, clean intermittent, 599
Urinary catheters
  antiseptic-impregnated, 599
  infections, 599
Urinary leukocyte esterase *see* Leukocyte esterase
Urinary schistosomiasis, 1368–1369
Urinary tract
  anomalies, urinary tract infection risk factor, 340
  bacterial colonization, 339
  obstruction, infections associated, 341
Urinary tract infection (UTI), 339–343
  antibiotic-resistant, 75
  asymptomatic, 342
  atypical, 341
  Bacillus cereus, 754
  bacteriologic ecology and drug resistance, 75
  burns patients, 519
  Candida, 342, 1198–1199, 1199f
  catheter-associated, 342
  causes in very young infants, 114t
  Citrobacter, 807
  clinical features, 173, 340
  complications, 342
  Corynebacterium species, 760t–761t
  covert, 342
  diagnostic tests, 340
  differential diagnosis, urethritis *vs*, 354
  Enterobius vermicularis, 1332
  epidemiology, 339–340
  etiologic agents, 339, 341
  fever without localizing signs, 116–117
  follow-up imaging, 342
  Gardnerella vaginalis, 769
  imaging evaluation, 341–342
    acute infection, 341
    image findings, 342
    responsible, and radiation risks, 345
  Klebsiella, 800
  laboratory findings and diagnosis, 340
    basis for diagnosis (CFU/mL), 340
  management, 341
    oral antimicrobials, 341
    parenteral antimicrobials, 341
  nosocomial, 342
    causative agents, 580t
    neonatal, 550
  pathogenesis, 339
  prophylaxis, 341
  Proteus, 811–812
  Pseudomonas aeruginosa, 843t
  recurrence rate, 339

recurrent
  anatomic/physiologic abnormalities
    predisposing, 600t
  chemoprophylaxis, 74t, 75, 341
  with normal GU system, 75
recurrent abdominal pain due to, 175
Serratia marcescens, 813
Staphylococcus saprophyticus, 693
symptoms and abdominal pain, 173
treatment/prophylaxis
  methenamine, 1480
  nitrofurantoin, 1479–1480
  trimethoprim-sulfamethoxazole, 1479
urinary catheter-related infection, 599
urine sample collection, 340
Urine
  analysis *see* Urinalysis
  bacterial antigen detection assays, 1381
  CMV culture, 1388
  culture, 340, 1376
    infections in neutropenia with cancer,
      570
    neonatal infections, 537, 542
    neonatal nosocomial infection,
      549–550
    quantitative, 340
  first-void (FVU), *Chlamydia trachomatis*
    detection sample, 1398–1399
  fishy amine-like odor, 770
  specimen, 340
    for UTI diagnosis, 340
  specimen collection/transport, 340,
    1374t, 1376
    bag specimen, 340
    midstream voided, 340
    suprapubic, 340
  sterile, reflux, 369
  see also Urinalysis
Urogenital infections, *Neisseria gonorrhoeae*,
  744
Urokinase, central venous catheter-related
  thrombosis, 593
Uropathogens, 339–340
  epididymitis due to, 367
  prostatitis due to, 369
Urticaria, 445–449
  acute and chronic types, 445
  anaphylaxis with, 447
  diagnosis and management, 446–447
  differential diagnosis, 448–449
  etiology, 445
    infectious, 445b
    noninfectious, 445b
  papular, 446–447
  pathogenesis, 445–446
  Taenia solium, 1351
Uta, 1289
  see also Leishmania (leishmaniasis), New
    World
Uveitis, 498–503
  anterior, 110–111, 113, 498–499
    causes, 499t
  intermediate, 498
  mucocutaneous syndromes, 110–111
  posterior, 498–503
    see also Chorioretinitis; Retinitis
  Yersinia enterocolitica infections, 824
Uvulitis, 111, 193t

V

Vaccination *see* Immunization (active);
  Vaccine(s)
Vaccine(s), 46
  adjuvants with, 45–46
  administration, 48
  administration routes and responses to,
    46
  adverse events/reactions, 47
    case-crossover analysis, 6–7
    causality, 50–51
    compensation for, 50–51
    monitoring, 47
    reporting system, 51
    surveillance, 55
  antibody-containing product spacing
    with, 48–50
  benefits, 44
  booster doses, 45
  constituents, 45
  content, 44–45
  definition, 44–45
  determinants of response to, 46
  efficacy (VE), 7
    cohort studies, 7
    studies, 7
  financing, 54–55, 54t
  historical aspects, 44
  immunogenicity, 46
  immunologic basis of response, 45–46
  impact, 44
  inactivated, 44–45
    formalin-inactivated, 46
    immune response to, 45–46
    response to and factors affecting, 46
    sensitization to wild virus, 46
    timing, 46
    types, 44–45
    see also Vaccine(s), killed
  infant susceptibility to infections
    prevented by, 10
  information sources, 68
  interchangeability, 48–50
  killed, 44–45, 82–83
    for immunocompromised people,
      52
    response to and factors affecting,
      46
    timing, 46
  licensure and approval, 47, 47f
  live-attenuated, 44–45
    contraindication after IGIV, 43
    contraindications, 46, 52
    immune response to, 45
    interference between, 48
    optimal timing, 45–46
    two or more, 77
  manufacturers, decrease in number, 54
  pneumonia in immunocompromised
    patients, 256
  polysaccharide antigens, 45
  prelicensure clinical trials, 47
  purified antigens in, 45
  recommendations for, development of,
    47, 47f
  routes of administration, 46
  routine, 55–67

safety, 50–51
  monitoring, 51
  studies, 44, 50–51
shortages, 54
simultaneous administration, 48
sites of administration, 46
spacing (timing), 48
storage and handling, 54
types, 45–47
whole organism, 44–45
see also specific vaccines
Vaccine Adverse Event Reporting System
  (VAERS), 51, 55
  pneumococcal conjugate vaccine (PCV7),
    726
Vaccine Injury Compensation Program
  (VICP), 47
Vaccine-preventable diseases, surveillance,
  55
Vaccine Safety Datalink (VSD), 51
Vaccines for Children Program, 54–55, 54t
Vaccinia virus, 1020–1024, 1020t
  accidental inoculation with, 1023–1024,
    1023f
  epidemiology, 1020–1021, 1024
  host range, 1021
  immune globulin (VIG), 42, 1023–1024
  immune globulin intravenous (VIG-
    IGIV), 37t, 42
  smallpox vaccine, 1021, 1023f
    contraindications, 1024
    see also Variola virus
Vacuolation, cerebral cortex, 335f
Vagina
  inflammation *see* Vulvovaginitis
  normal flora *see* Flora, normal
  pH, 358
Vaginal discharge
  bacterial vaginosis, 359
  clinical features, 359
  diagnosis, 357, 357b
  discharge/dysuria syndrome, 346–347
  endocervicitis, 362
  fishy odor, 359–360
  HSV infection, 1029
  Neisseria gonorrhoeae infections, 744
  sexually transmitted infections, 346–347
  Trichomonas vaginalis, 1318
  vulvovaginitis, 357
Vaginal specimens
  swab, specimen collection/transport,
    1374t
  urethritis diagnosis, 355
  vaginitis diagnosis, 360
  vulvovaginitis diagnosis, 357, 357b
Vaginitis
  Enterobius vermicularis, 1332
  nonspecific *see* Bacterial vaginosis (BV)
  pubertal females, 358–361
    clinical features, 359, 359t
    complications, 361
    diagnosis, 359, 359t
    etiology and epidemiology, 358–359
    laboratory findings and diagnosis,
      359–360
    management, 359t, 360–361
  Trichomonas vaginalis, 1318
  see also Vulvovaginitis

Vaginosis, bacterial *see* Bacterial vaginosis (BV)
Vahlkampfiid family, 1293
Valacyclovir, 1502–1507, 1502t
  adverse effects, 1505
  chemistry, 1503
  clinical uses, 1507
  dosage, 1504
  pharmacokinetics, 1504
  prophylactic, HSV infections, 71
  resistance to, 1503t
  treatment of
    EBV infection, 1062
    VZV infections, 1041
Valganciclovir, 1510–1512
  adverse effects, 1511
  chemistry, 1510–1511
  clinical uses, 1512
  CMV infection prophylaxis, transplant recipients, 561, 1050
  CMV infection treatment, transplant recipients, 558
  congenital CMV infection treatment, 1050
  dosage, 1512
  mechanism of action, 1510–1511
  pharmacokinetics, 1511
  resistance to, 1503t, 1511
Validity, 4
  external, 9
Validity of studies, 4
Valley fever, 1241
  see also Coccidioides immitis (coccidioidomycosis)
Valve ring abscess, 595
Vancomycin, 1469
  adverse reactions, 686, 1469
  chemoprophylactic use
    CVC-related infection prevention, 594
    Streptococcus agalactiae (group B streptococcus) prevention, 711
  clinical uses, 1469
  dosage, 1445t–1452t, 1480t–1484t
  dose adjustment in burned patients, 1437t
  exposure, impact on infection rate, 12
  mechanism of action, 1428, 1468–1469
  pharmacodynamics, 1414t
  pharmacology, 1453t–1458t
  resistance, 1422t, 1423, 1428–1429, 1469
    detection of, 1432
    Enterococcus see Vancomycin-resistant enterococci (VRE)
    Erysipelothrix rhusiopathiae infections, 768
    intermediate, *Staphylococcus aureus*, 678, 686, 688–689
    Lactobacillus, 770
    Leuconostoc, 730
    Pediococcus, 730
    Staphylococcus aureus, 678, 687–689, 1429, 1432, 1469
    Staphylococcus epidermidis, 693
  spectrum of activity, 1459t–1463t, 1469
  treatment of, 1469
    acute bacterial meningitis, 276–277, 725

acute mastoiditis, 225
bacteremic periorbital cellulitis, 510
brain abscess and subdural empyema, 328–329
Clostridium difficile infections, 585, 978, 979b
CNS infections, 328–329
coagulase-negative staphylococcal infections, 693–694
Corynebacterium jeikeium infections, 762
CVC-related infection in neonates, 553
dacryoadenitis, 508
Elizabethkingia meningoseptica infections, 834
in end-stage renal disease, 637
endocarditis, 263, 263t, 1418t–1419t
eye infections, 1494t–1496t
infections after burns, 520
infections in neutropenia with cancer, 571
Listeria monocytogenes infection, 766
necrotizing enterocolitis, 390
necrotizing otitis externa, 222
neonatal infections, 538, 543
nosocomial neonatal infections, 552
osteomyelitis, 472
Staphylococcus aureus infections, 684, 686–689
viridans group streptococcal infections, 718–719
Vancomycin-resistant enterococci (VRE), 714–715
  endocarditis, management, 263
  in renal disease, 637
Variance, 2t, 5
Varicella *see* Varicella zoster virus (VZV), varicella
Varicella gangrenosa, 1037
Varicella hepatitis, 1038
Varicella pneumonia, 1038–1039
Varicella zoster virus (VZV), 1035–1044
  acute cerebellar ataxia due to, 316
  acute retinal necrosis due to, 502
  anterior uveitis due to, 499, 499t
  antibodies to, 1036, 1040
    IgG, 1040
    IgM, 1040, 1393
    passive immunization, 1041–1042
  antigen detection, 1040, 1386, 1393
  antiviral drug resistance, 1503, 1503t
    acyclovir-resistant, 1041
  aseptic meningitis due to, 294
  chronic fatigue syndrome pathogenesis, 1008t–1009t
  congenital infection, 547t
    clinical features, 537t
    diagnosis, 538t
    epidemiology, 545
    retinitis, 501–502
    varicella, 1038
  diagnosis/detection, 1040, 1393
    antigen detection, 1040, 1386, 1393
    detection rates, 1386t
    DNA, 1393
    enzyme immunoassays, 1040
    optimal tests, 1389t–1392t

PCR, 1393
    serologic tests, 1393
    shell vial method, 1386
    specimen collection/transport, 1393
  in drug-induced immunodeficiency, 253–254
  epidemiology, 1036
  exposure
    healthcare personnel, 21–22
    management in pregnant healthcare worker, 22t–23t
  generalized lymphadenopathy, 130, 131t–132t
  group childcare and, 25t, 29
  hepatitis due to, 1038
  herpes zoster, 1035–1036, 1039–1040
    anterior uveitis, 499t
    clinical features, 1039, 1039f
    complications, 1039–1040
    epidemiology, 1036
    immunocompromised children, 1039–1040
    keratitis, 1039f
    keratouveitis, 497
    lumbosacral, 1039
    oral infections, 192t
    rash, 440
    retinochoroiditis, 502
    risk after varicella vaccination, 62
    treatment, 1041, 1506t
  herpes zoster ophthalmicus, 502
  HIV coinfection, 1036
  HSCT recipients, 562, 565–566
  immune globulin (VariZIG), 37t, 39, 1041–1042, 1042b
    indication and dose, 39
    infections in neutropenia in cancer, 573
    postexposure prophylaxis, 39
  immune globulin (VZIG), 1041–1042, 1042b
    in HIV infection, 663
    in nephrotic syndrome, 637
    neutropenia in cancer, 573
    posttransplant, 559
  immune response, 1036
  immunity
    assessment, 1040
    persistent, 1036, 1043
  incubation period, 1035–1037
  infection process, 1035–1036
  keratitis due to, 495–496
  labile virus, 1393
  laboratory findings/diagnosis, 1040
  laboratory testing, 308t–311t
  latent infection, 1035–1036
  in neutropenia associated with cancer, 568
  Oka strain, 61–62
  oral infections, 192t
  oral mucosal infections, 192t
  pathogenesis of infection, 1035–1036, 1036f
  perinatal infections, diagnosis, 1397
  pneumonia due to, 236–237, 1038–1039
    in cancer, 577
    in immunocompromised, 253

prevention of infections, 1041–1044
  antivirals, 1042
  healthcare workers, 1041
  passive antibody prophylaxis, 1041–1042, 1042b
  varicella vaccines, 1042–1044, 1043b
pyomyositis due to, 465
Ramsay Hunt syndrome, 315
reactivation, 1036, 1039, 1043–1044
  keratitis, 496
reinfection, 1036
SCID-hu mouse model, 1035–1036
shingles see Varicella zoster virus (VZV), herpes zoster
skin infections, in cancer, 574–575
transmission, 1035–1036, 1036f
  to neonates, 544–545
  prevention, 1041
in transplant recipients, 559
treatment of infections, 1040–1041, 1504t, 1505, 1506t, 1514
  acyclovir see Acyclovir
vaccines, 61–62, 1042–1044, 1043b
  2-dose schedule, 62
  in acute lymphocytic leukemia, 62
  adverse effects, 62, 1043
  breakthrough infections, 61–62, 1043
  catch-up use, 62, 1043
  complications, 29
  contraindication in pregnancy, 51–52
  contraindications/precautions, 62, 559
  costs, 1044
  dosage, 1043
  dose number, 62
  efficacy, 29, 62, 1043
  group childcare settings, 30t
  in HIV infection, 52, 62
  indications, 62
  live-attenuated, 61–62
  live-attenuated Oka-Merck, 1043, 1043b
  MMRV, 1043
  Oka strain, 61–62
  posttransplant, 559
  pregnancy and, 51–52, 62
  recommendations for, 62
  routine use, 1043
  schedule, 49f
  for travelers, 78, 78t
  see also Measles, mumps, rubella and varicella (MMRV) vaccine
varicella (chickenpox), 1035, 1037–1039
  anterior uveitis, 499, 499t
  arthritis, 1038
  bullous, 1037
  in cancer, 574–575
  clinical features, 438f, 440
  complications in adolescents, 1038
  complications in healthy children, 1038–1039
  complications in high-risk children, 1038–1039
  congenital, 1038, 1038b
  differential diagnosis, 1037
  epidemiology, 1036
  group childcare and outbreaks, 29
  healthcare-associated infections, 13

hepatitis, 1038
immunocompromised children, 1039, 1041
in immunodeficiency, 1039
malignancy, 1039
morbidity reduced by vaccine, 48t
neonatal, 1038–1039
in nephrotic syndrome, 637
neurologic, 1037–1038
oral infections, 192t
pneumonia, 1038–1039
in pregnancy, 1038–1039
progressive, in cancer, 1039
Rickettsia akari (rickettsialpox) infection vs., 934
risk factor for Streptococcus pyogenes (GAS), 699–700, 701f
secondary bacterial infections, 1037, 1037f
severity, 1042
smallpox vs, 1023t
treatment, 1040b, 1041
vesiculobullous rash, 438–439, 439f, 1037, 1037f
viremia, 1035–1036
wild-type strains, 1036
zoster see Varicella zoster virus (VZV), herpes zoster
Variola major, 1021, 1022t
Variola minor (alastrim), 1021, 1022t
Variola sine eruptione, 1021
Variola virus (smallpox), 1020–1024, 1020t
  biosafety level for, 1021–1022
  mortality, 1021
  smallpox
    bioterrorism and, 1020
    chickenpox vs, 1023t
    clinical features, 1021, 1022t, 1023f
    differential diagnosis, 1022, 1023b
    epidemiology, 1020–1021
    eradication, 44, 47, 1020
    history, 1020, 1021b
    laboratory findings and diagnosis, 1021–1022
    patient evaluation algorithm, 1021–1022, 1022f
    risk factors, 1021–1022, 1022t
    treatment, 1022–1023
  smallpox vaccination, 1021, 1023–1024
    adverse events, 1023–1024, 1023f
    contraindications, 1024
    first to third generation vaccines, 1023
    history, 1021b, 1023
    licensed vaccine, 1023
    vaccine delivery, 1023
    see also Vaccinia virus
  spread and transmission, 1020, 1020t
VariZIG see Varicella zoster virus (VZV), immune globulin (VariZIG)
Vascular catheters see Intravascular catheters
Vascular grafts, infections associated, 594–596
  clinical features and diagnosis, 595
  management and outcome, 595
  prevention, 595–596
Vascular thrombosis, subcutaneous tissue infection pathogenesis, 460

Vasculitis
  after Neisseria meningitidis infections, 738
  CNS, infectious encephalitis vs., 308
  diffuse, rickettsiae causing, 441
  familial Mediterranean fever, 124–125
  fever of unknown origin due to, 119t–120t
  paraneoplastic, 108
  in TRAPS, 126
  Trypanosoma (Trypanozoon) brucei infection, 1320
Vaso-occlusive crises, 186
  sickle-cell disease, 634
Vaso-occlusive disease, in sickle-cell disease, 635
Vasodilatation, heat loss, 91
Vasomotor rhinitis, 198
Vasomotor tone, in sepsis, 102
VE see Vaccine(s), efficacy (VE)
Vegetations
  in endocarditis, 256–257, 259, 259f
    indications for surgical intervention, 264t
  Libman–Sachs, 259
Veillonella, 190
  buccal mucosal colonization, 190
  diagnosis/detection, 963–964
Veillonella parvula, 989
Veillonellaceae, classification, 959t
Velocardial facial syndrome, 629, 630t, 631
Venereal Disease Research Laboratory (VDRL), 942, 1384
  syphilitic meningitis diagnosis, 281
  Treponema pallidum subsp. pallidum (syphilis), 944
Venezuelan equine encephalitis virus (VEEV), 1098
Venezuelan hemorrhagic fever, 1160t, 1161–1162
Venipuncture, sites, specimen collection, 1373
Venous access devices, in cancer, neutropenia and infections, 568
Venous sinuses, dural, septic thrombosis see Septic venous thrombosis
Ventilator-associated pneumonia (VAP), 250–251, 579, 581–582
  clinical features and diagnosis, 250–251, 582
  management and outcome, 250–251, 583
  neonatal, 549t, 550
    diagnosis, 550
  pathogenesis, 581–582
  pathogens, 580t, 582
  prevention, 250–251, 583, 583b
  risk factors, 250, 582
Ventricular assist devices, infections, 596
  endocarditis pathogenesis, 258–259
Ventricular cysts, Taenia solium, 1352–1353, 1353f, 1355t, 1356
Ventricular drain, eosinophilic meningitis associated, 332–333
Ventricular fibrillation, in Trypanosoma cruzi infections, 1324
Ventricular neurocysticercosis (Taenia solium), 1353–1354, 1355t

Ventricular septal defect, endocarditis pathogenesis, 258, 717
Ventriculitis
  complications, 597
  Corynebacterium species, 760t–761t
  as meningitis risk factor, 272–273
Ventriculoatrial shunts, infections, 597b
Ventriculoperitoneal shunt
  anaerobic gram-negative bacilli, 983
  brain abscess and, 322
  in cancer, neutropenia and infections, 568
  catheter-related peritonitis, 416
  complications, 597
  CSF eosinophilia, 332
  eosinophilic meningitis associated, 332
  infection chemoprophylaxis, 71–72
  infections, 596–597
  as meningitis risk factor, 272–273, 273t
    recurrent meningitis, 289
  Staphylococcus aureus infections, 684
  Taenia solium neurocysticercosis, 1355t, 1356
  see also Cerebrospinal fluid (CSF) shunt
Ventriculopleural shunts, infections, 597, 597b
Ventriculostomy, 693
Venturi effect, 520
Veronate™, 689
Verruca peruana, 940
  see also Bartonella bacilliformis
Verrucosa cutis, 779
Verrucous lesions, *Blastomyces dermatitidis* (blastomycosis), 1236, 1236f
Versajet tool, 520
VersaTREK Microbial Detection system, 1374
Vertebrae
  erosion, 149–150
  osteomyelitis *see* Osteomyelitis, vertebral
  pain, site and radiation, 171
  in tuberculosis, 778
Vertebral bodies
  anomalies, recurrent meningitis, 289
  blood supply, 483–484
  infection, 187
Vertebral body endplates, inflammation *see* Diskitis
Vertigo, benign paroxysmal, 180t
Very low birthweight infants
  Candida infections, 1196–1197, 1199–1201
    prevention, 1202
  dexamethasone, 555
  early-onset sepsis, 538
  healthcare-associated infection risk, 10
  late late-onset sepsis, 539
  late-onset infections, 539, 549
    etiology, 550–551, 551t
    meningitis, 549–550
  necrotizing enterocolitis association, 388
  neonatal sepsis, 538–539
    treatment, 552
  nosocomial infection prevention, 555
  urinary tract infections, 550
  ventilator-associated pneumonia, 549t, 550
  viral infections, 546

Vesicles, 427t, 438–441
  etiology, 438–440
  genital herpes, 348
  herpes zoster, 1039, 1039f
  HSV infection, 1029, 1032f
  size, 438–439
  varicella lesions, 1037, 1037f
Vesico-ulcerative lesions, orolabial HSV infection, 1028, 1028f
Vesicoureteral reflux (VUR), 340
Vesicular lesions, mucocutaneous syndromes, 111
Vesiculobullous diseases, 438–441
  sites, 438f
Vesivirus, 1187
Veterinarians, advice on nontraditional pets, 530–531
Vibrio, 854–856
  culture media, 1376t
Vibrio alginolyticus, 855t
Vibrio carchariae, 855–856
Vibrio cholerae, 849–854
  antimicrobial susceptibility, 852
  carriage, 850
  chromosomes I and II, 850
  classic biotype, 850, 852
  clinical manifestations, 851–852
  description, 850
  El Tor biotype, 850, 852
    pandemic, 850–851
  epidemiology, 850–851
  genome, 850
  in HIV infection, 661–662
  immunity to and immune response, 850
  laboratory findings/diagnosis, 852
    stool cultures, 376
  microbiology, 850
  mortality due to, 850
  natural reservoirs and transmission, 851
  non-O1, 852, 855t
    foodborne disease, 395, 398t
  non-O1, non-O139 strains, 852
    clinical manifestations, 856
    epidemiology, 855
  nontoxigenic strains, 852, 855t
  O antigens, 852
  pandemics and epidemics, 850
  pathogenesis, 850
  in pregnancy, 851–853
  prevention of infection, 853–854
    chemoprophylaxis, 70t–71t
    epidemiological, 854
    hygiene and public health, 853–854
  serogroups, 849
  toxin, 850
  toxin coregulated pilus (TCP), 850
  treatment of infection, 852–853, 853t
  vaccines, 67, 854
    for travelers, 79
  virulence, 850
Vibrio cholerae O1, 849
  endemic foci, 851
  foodborne disease, 394t, 395, 398t
  serotypes and biotypes, 852
Vibrio cholerae O139, 849
Vibrio cholerae O139 Bengal, 851
Vibrio cincinnatiensis, 855–856
Vibrio fluvialis, 855t

Vibrio furnissii, 855–856
Vibrio hollisae, 855t
Vibrio metschnikovii, 855–856
Vibrio mimicus, 855t
Vibrio parahaemolyticus, 855, 855t
  clinical features, 856
  epidemiology, 855
  foodborne disease, 395, 398t
  gastroenteritis, 856
  inflammatory enteritis, 383–384
  laboratory findings/diagnosis, stool cultures, 376
  treatment and prevention, 856
Vibrio vulnificus, 855, 855t
  clinical features, 856
  epidemiology, 855
  gastroenteritis, 855–856
  in iron overload state, 638
  septicemia, 855–856
  skin infections after trauma, 514
  treatment and prevention, 856
  wound infections, 855–856
Vibrionaceae, 850
Vibrios, 673
Vidarabine, 1504t, 1514
  congenital HSV infection, 1034
  viral keratitis treatment, 497
Video-assisted thoracoscopic surgery (VATS), 243
Villous atrophy, *Giardia intestinalis* (giardiasis), 1279
Vimentin, *Streptococcus pyogenes*, 700
Vincent disease (acute necrotizing ulcerative gingivitis (ANUG)), 194, 983
Vinegar solution, otitis externa management, 221
Viral gastroenteritis *see* Gastroenteritis
Viral hemorrhagic fevers, 1159
  arenaviruses, 1160t, 1161–1162, 1161f, 1162t
  clinical manifestations, 1161–1162
  diagnosis, 1162–1163, 1162t
  filoviruses, 1160t, 1161–1162, 1162t
  prevention, 1163–1164
    contact tracing, 1163
    personal protection, 1163
    postexposure prophylaxis, 1164
    precautions for healthcare workers, 1163
    reservoir and vector control, 1164
    vaccines, 1164
  treatment, 1163
  see also Hemorrhagic fever
Viral inclusions, viral pneumonia, 238
Viral infections
  acquired HLH associated, 104
  anemia due to, 1403
  arthritis, 481, 481b
  bacterial infections differentiation, 108
  in burns patients, 519–520
  clinical features, 109t–110t, 112–113
  congenital, 545, 545t
  diagnosis, 109t–110t
  elevated C-reactive protein, 1402
  ESR elevation, 1400
  fever of unknown origin, 119t–120t
  fever without localizing signs, 116–117

generalized lymphadenopathy, 131t–132t, 132–133
group childcare and, 25t
laboratory features, 109t–110t
lymphadenopathy see Lymphadenitis/lymphadenopathy
of muscle, 186
necrotizing enterocolitis pathogenesis, 389
neonatal sepsis, 97–98
neutropenia associated with cancer, 568
neutropenia in, 1405
oral cavity, 192t
postnatal, 546
skin lesions, 112
slow virus infections, 333
solid-organ transplant recipients, 558–560
transient lymphocytosis, 1406
transmission
    fetal/neonatal, 544–545, 545t
    see also Neonatal infections
treatment, 109t–110t
see also individual viral infections
Viral transport media (VTM), 1385
Virchow–Troisier node, 137
Viridans group streptococci, 696–697, 696t, 716–719
abscesses due to, 718
antimicrobial resistance, 718
bacteremia due to, 717–718
biochemical/growth characteristics, 716t
clinical manifestations, 717–718
dental infections, 718
dextran exopolysaccharide, 717
endocarditis due to, 257–258, 717, 1418t–1419t
    management, 263–264
    treatment recommendations, 718, 719t, 1418t–1419t
epidemiology, 717
infections in HSCT recipient, 563
meningitis due to, 718
microbiology, 716
neonatal BSI due to, 717
penicillin-binding proteins (PBPs), 718
prevention of infections, 719
respiratory tract infections, 718
sepsis/septicemia due to, 98, 717–718
speciation and identification, 716–717
Streptococcus pneumoniae vs., 716
treatment of infections, 718–719
virulence properties, 717
see also Streptococcus (streptococci)
Viridans streptococci see Viridans group streptococci
Viruses
amplification (shell vial method), 233–234
classification, 1015–1019
    biologic, 1019
    criteria for, 1016t
    by genomes, 1018f–1019f
    recent changes, 1015
families, 1015, 1016t
    subdivisions, 1015
genome, quantification methods, 1386–1387

inactivation, preparation of IGIV, 43
isolation methods, 1385–1386
laboratory diagnosis see Laboratory diagnosis
neutralization by antibody, 45–46
nomenclature, 1015
orders, 1018
respiratory tract see Respiratory tract viruses
species, 1015
    classification system, 1015–1018
    criteria for, 1015
transmission routes, 1019b
Visceral abscesses, 425–426
etiology, 423t, 425–426
Visceral larva migrans (VLM)
Angiostrongylus causing, 1337–1338
clinical features, 1335–1336
diagnosis, 1336–1337
Gnathostoma spinigerum causing, 1337–1338
marine mammal ascarids causing, 1339
Toxocara and Baylisascaris causing, 1335–1337
see also Toxocara canis
Visceral leishmaniasis see Leishmania (leishmaniasis)
Visitation policies, 19–21
pets and, 19–21
prevention of HAIs and, 19–21
recommendations, 19
Visual loss see Blindness
Vital signs, in headache assessment, 171
Vital signs, in acute abdominal pain, 172
Vitamin, deficiencies, bacterial overgrowth, 391
Vitamin A
bronchiolitis therapy, 235
deficiency, Shigella infection treatment, 822
rubeola virus infection (measles), 1141
Vitamin B_{12} deficiency
Diphyllobothrium infection, 1347–1348
Strongyloides causing, 1333
Vitamin D deficiency, in HIV infection, 670
Vitamin E, intravenous, prolonged use, 548
VITEK2 System, 1379–1380
Vitreal reaction, 500f
Vitrectomy, 505
Vitreous
aspiration, 504–505, 504f
culture, 504–505
injection, endophthalmitis management, 505t, 506
Vocal cord, paralysis, 165
Voges–Proskauer test, 697
Voice, in acute laryngitis, 212
Voiding cystourethrogram (VCUG), urinary tract infection, 341
Volume depletion
Vibrio cholerae infection, 851–853
see also Dehydration
Volume of distribution, drug, 1434
Volvulus, abdominal pain, 174
Vomiting, 375
acute abdominal pain with, 171
Borrelia infections, 958

chronic/recurrent abdominal pain with, 175
foodborne diseases, 393, 394t
gastrointestinal tract infections, 375
    see also Gastroenteritis
norovirus infections, 1189
posttussive (in pertussis), 868–869
rotavirus infections, 1095
sequelae, 399
Staphylococcus aureus food poisoning, 394t
Trichinella spiralis infections, 1341
Vibrio cholerae infection, 851
viral gastroenteritis, 380
Voriconazole, 1490
adverse effects, 1490
breakpoint for, 1443t
clinical trials, 1490
dosage, 1445t–1452t, 1487t, 1490
    pharmacokinetic-pharmacodynamic relationships, 1443t
long-term use, mucormycosis association, 1214
pharmacology, 1490
spectrum of activity, 1486t, 1490
susceptibility testing, 1382
treatment of
    Aspergillus infections, 576–577, 1208
    Blastomyces dermatitidis (blastomycosis), 1237–1238, 1238t
    Candida infections, 1201, 1201t
    Coccidioides immitis (coccidioidomycosis), 1245
    Cryptococcus infections, 1223
    eumycotic mycetoma, 1252
    fever in neutropenia (in cancer), 571
    hyalohyphomycosis, 1210–1211
    phaeohyphomycosis, 1212
    Pseudallescheria boydii infections, 1253
"Vulnerable child" syndrome, 115–116
Vulva, inflammation see Vulvovaginitis
Vulvitis, adolescents, 361
Vulvovaginitis, 356–361
bacterial vaginosis see Bacterial vaginosis (BV)
Candida, 351–352, 356–357, 1197, 1200
Candida albicans, 358–359
Candida glabrata, 358–359
clinical features, 357
diagnosis and laboratory findings, 357, 357b
differential diagnosis, 357
Enterobius vermicularis, 357
etiology and epidemiology, 356–357, 357b
Gardnerella vaginalis, 356–358
management, 358
prepubertal females, 356–358, 357b
prognosis and sequelae, 358
pubertal females, 356–358
recurrences, 358
sexual abuse, 354–355, 362, 364–365
sexually transmitted infections causing, 356–357
Shigella causing, 821
Streptococcus pyogenes, 357–358

Trichomonas vaginalis, 356–357, 359–360
urethritis and cystitis *vs.*, 354t
VZV *see* Varicella zoster virus (VZV)

W

Wakana disease, 1329
Waldeyer ring, 127, 127t, 136
generalized hyperplasia, 129
Warfare, biological *see* Bioterrorism
Warfarin, Kawasaki disease, 1006
Warm shock, 98
Warthin–Starry stain, *Bartonella henselae* infections, 860
Warthin–Starry stain, 160–161, 1383
Warts
cutaneous, HPV associated, 1072–1074
genital *see* Genital warts
Waste disposal, 21
types of waste, 21
Wasting syndrome, HIV, 655
Water
chlorination
Naegleria fowleri prevention, 1295
Salmonella infection prevention, 818
contamination, infections associated
Acanthamoeba, 1296
Balantidium coli, 384
Cryptosporidium, 384, 1269
Cyclospora, 1283
Cystoisospora belli, 1283
Diphyllobothrium, 1347–1348
Entamoeba histolytica, 384
Giardia intestinalis (giardiasis), 1280
inflammatory enteritis, 384t
Legionella, 922–923
Naegleria fowleri, 1294
Sarcocystis, 1308
Shigella transmission, 820–821
Toxocara, 1337
Toxoplasma gondii, 1310, 1317t
Vibrio cholerae, 851
see also Waterborne disease
filtration, *Giardia* prevention, 1282
hot water systems, *Legionella* infections, 922–923
hyperchlorination, 925
infections related to trauma, 513t
precautions for travelers, 76, 81, 1282
prevention of infections, 399
purification, 1282
Giardia intestinalis (giardiasis) prevention, 1282
Water filters, 1282
Water–alcohol bathing, 92
Waterborne disease, 392–400
causes, 395–396, 395t
complications, 399
Cryptosporidium parvum, 396
diagnosis, 393–398
epidemiology, 392–393
Helicobacter pylori infection, 909–910
hepatitis E virus, 1192
inflammatory enteritis, 384, 384t
management, 398–399
outbreak, definition, 373
prevention, 377, 399
see also Water, contamination

Watercress, *Fasciola* infections associated, 1366
Wayson staining, *Yersinia pestis* infection, 826–827
Weakness, 180–182, 181t–182t
causes, 181t–182t
Guillain–Barré syndrome, 319
therapy, 182
see also Muscle, weakness
Websites, useful, 1445b
Weeksella, 834
Weeksella virosa, 832, 834
Weeksella zoohelcum (*Bergeyella zoohelcum*), 832
Wegener granulomatosis, 155
Weight
HIV infection prognosis, 656
loss, interferon treatment in HCV infection, 1111
Weil syndrome, 950–951, 950f
see also Leptospira interrogans
Weil–Felix febrile agglutination test, 1384
Rickettsia prowazekii, 931
"Welts" *see* Urticaria
West Nile virus (WNV), 1101
acute flaccid paralysis, weakness due to, differential diagnosis, 181t–182t
aseptic meningitis, 294, 297
clinical features, 295, 1101
CNS infection, 294
diagnosis/detection, 296, 1397
optimal tests, 1389t–1392t
encephalitis due to, 302–303
poliomyelitis *vs.*, 1170
global distribution, 1101
laboratory testing, 308t–311t
maternal infection, transmission, 546
neuroinvasive disease, 293–294, 297, 302–303, 313
New York City outbreak, 1101
prevention of infections, 1102
retinitis, 502
transmission, 1101
treatment of infections, 1101
vaccines, 1101
Westergren measurement method, ESR, 1400
Western blot
Borrelia burgdorferi, 955
Helicobacter pylori, 914
HIV, 651, 652b
Western equine encephalitis virus (WEEV), 1098
diagnosis/detection, 1389t–1392t, 1397
Wet-mount technique, *Trichomonas vaginalis*, 1318–1319
Wheezes/wheezing (expiratory stridor), 169, 251
in bronchiolitis, 233, 235
common cold complication, 199
definition and causes, 169
in pneumonia, 238
recurrent, bronchiolitis linked to, 235
virus-induced, 233
Whiff test (amine test), 770
WHIM syndrome, characteristics, 602t, 606
Whipworms *see* Trichuris trichiura
White blood cell(s) (WBC), 1404–1409

adhesion and transmigration, 94
Candida infections, 1197–1198, 1200
CMV infection detection, 1049
diskitis, 484
HHV-6 infection, 1055f
neonatal septicemia diagnosis, 541–542, 541t
transfusions, 623
transient synovitis, 486
urethritis diagnosis, 353
VZV infections, 1040
see also specific white cell types
White blood cell (WBC) count
bacillary dysentery, 822
brain abscess, 325
Campylobacter jejuni infections, 876
Chlamydophila (*Chlamydia*) *pneumoniae* infections, 883
CSF, meningitis diagnosis, 274
fever without localizing signs, 115
Mycoplasma pneumoniae infections, 996
normal, 90, 1404, 1404t
in pneumonia, 239
Trichinella spiralis infections, 1341
see also Leukocytosis
White piedra, 1250
Whitlow, 432
herpetic, 524, 1029, 1029f
Whooping cough *see Bordetella pertussis* (pertussis)
Wildlife
endemic rabies, 1145–1146, 1146t
Toxoplasma gondii transmission, 1309, 1309f
Trichinella spiralis infections, 1339, 1341
see also Animal(s)
Wilson disease, 404
Wimberger sign, congenital syphilis, 943, 943f
Winterbottom sign, 1320
Wiskott–Aldrich syndrome, 603t–604t, 630t, 633
diagnosis, 633
genetic and clinical features, 630t, 633
immunizations in, 52t–53t
infections associated, 633
Wiskott–Aldrich syndrome protein (WASP), 633
deficiency, 633
Wolbachia, 1342, 1346
treatment, 1344–1345
Wolman disease, 135
Wood's light, 1217
tinea capitis diagnosis, 1246–1247
tinea pedis diagnosis, 1247–1248
tinea versicolor diagnosis, 1249
Woolsorters' disease (inhalational anthrax), 752–753
World Health Organization (WHO)
antiretroviral prophylaxis guidance, 645
HIV prevalence, 641–642
information on vaccines, 68
oral rehydration therapy, 376
poliovirus eradication strategies, 1169–1170
rubeola virus (measles) vaccine, 1143–1144
SAFE, trachoma prevention strategy, 889

sexually transmitted infection treatment, 803
vitamin A in measles, 1141
Wuchereria bancrofti elimination, 1344
Worms *see* Filarial infections (filariasis); Nematodes (roundworms); *specific worms*
Wound(s)
cellulitis, 514
closure, bite wounds, 524–525
infection risk, 69t
operative, classification, 69t
see also Burns
Wound infections
Bacillus cereus, 754
Clostridium tetani, 967, 969
Edwardsiella tarda, 808
empiric transmission-based precautions, 20t
Fusobacterium, 987–988
human, 984
nontuberculous mycobacterial, 788–789
odor, *Clostridium perfringens* (gas gangrene), 981
Pasteurella multocida infections, 837
prophylaxis/treatment, 1498t–1499t, 1499
Proteus, 811
specimen collection/transport, 1374t
Staphylococcus aureus, 678–679
Vibrio vulnificus, 856
see also Bites, infections after; Burns, wound infections
WU polyomavirus, 1075, 1077
Wuchereria bancrofti, 1342–1344, 1343f
antigens, 1343
characteristics, 1342t
clinical manifestations, 1342–1343, 1343f
diagnosis, 1342–1343
epidemiology, 1342
lymphangitis due to, 161, 161t
prevention, 1344
treatment, 1343–1344

X

X-linked agammaglobulinemia (XLA), 610t
characteristics, 602t, 610t
clinical features, diagnosis and treatment, 610–611
with growth hormone deficiency, 602t
indication for IGIV, 40
infections and etiology, 610–611
mutations, 611
persistent/recurrent pneumonia, 251
X-linked congenital neutropenia, 604t–605t
X-linked disorders, immunodeficiency, 609
X-linked hyper-IgM syndrome, 609–610, 631–632
X-linked lymphoproliferative (XLP) disease/syndrome, 103–104, 104t, 603t–604t, 627, 633, 1064–1065
aproliferative disease, 1064, 1064b
diagnosis, 107
genetic and clinical features, 630t
immune response, 1064
infections associated, 633

pathogenesis, 105
proliferative response, 1064, 1064b
SAP and XIAP defects, 1064
X-linked SCID, 603t–604t, 627, 629
Xanthogranulomatous pyelonephritis, 344
epidemiology, 344
etiology, 344
Xanthoma cells, 344
Xanthomonas, Stenotrophomonas maltophilia reclassification from, 849
Xenodiagnosis, 1325
Trypanosoma cruzi infections, 1325
Xenopsylla cheopis (rat flea), 931
Xenotropic murine leukemia virus (XMRV), chronic fatigue syndrome, 1008, 1008t–1009t
Xylitol, recurrent otitis media prevention, 219

Y

Yaba-like disease virus of monkeys, 1020t
Yatapoxvirus, 1020t, 1024
clinical features, 1024
epidemiology, 1024
treatment, 1024
Yaws *see Treponema pallidum* subsp. *pertenue*
Years of potential life lost (YPLLs), 8
Yeast identification systems, API Analytab 20C, 1382
Yeastlike organisms, 1194
Yeasts, 1194
Yellow fever virus, 1099–1100
epidemiology and transmission, 1099
prevalence of infection, 67
travelers' infected, 67
vaccine, 67–68, 79, 1099–1100
adverse events, 67–68
contraindication in pregnancy, 68
encephalitis syndrome associated, 79
recommendations, 67–68
schedule/dosing for travelers, 79t
for travelers, 79
Yersinia, 823–827
culture media, 1376t
microbiology, 823
toxins, 823
type III secretion system in virulence plasmid, 823
Yersinia enterocolitica, 823–825
acute abdominal pain due to, 174
blood product contamination, 581
bloodstream infection, 824
clinical features, 638
clinical syndromes, 824
cross-reactions, 824
diagnosis/detection, 385t, 824
stool cultures, 376
enterocolitis and diarrhea due to, 824
epidemiology, 823–824
extraintestinal manifestations, 824
fever of unknown origin due to, 119t–120t
foodborne disease, 393–394, 394t, 396, 398t
generalized lymphadenopathy, 130, 131t–132t
inflammatory enteritis, 383, 383t

in iron overload state, 637–638
laboratory findings, 824
lymph nodes in, 129
mediastinal lymphadenopathy, 153
pharyngitis due to, 199
treatment and prevention, 824–825
unilateral cervical lymphadenitis due to, 140
virulence gene and enterotoxin, 823
Yersinia pestis (plague), 823, 826–827
acute unilateral cervical lymphadenitis, 140
antibiotic resistance, 827
bubonic plague, 826
chemoprophylaxis, 70t–71t
clinical manifestations, 826
culture media, 1376t
differential diagnosis, 827
Enterobacter agglomerans vs., 827
inguinal adenopathy without genital ulcers, 351, 352t
laboratory findings/diagnosis, 826–827, 1384
delayed diagnosis, 826
meningitis, 826
plague as biological weapon, 827
diagnosis, isolation and treatment, 827
plague pandemics, 826
plasmids and virulence, 823
pneumonia due to, 826
pneumonic plague, 826
prognosis, 827
rodents transmitting, 528
septicemia due to, 826
treatment of infections, 827
vaccines, 827
Yersinia pseudotuberculosis, 823, 825–826
acute abdominal pain, 174
clinical manifestations, 825
generalized lymphadenopathy, 130, 131t–132t
rodents associated, 528
treatment and prevention, 825
Yersiniosis *see Yersinia enterocolitica*
Yokenella, 810
Yokenella regensburgei, 810

Z

Zalcitabine (ddC), dosage, 1445t–1452t
Zanamivir, 1517–1518
chemoprophylactic use, 72
dosage, 1445t–1452t, 1518
influenza prophylaxis/treatment, 241t, 1154–1155, 1157, 1518
pneumonia treatment, 241t
Zeta-associated protein (ZAP-70) kinase, 627, 628t, 629
deficiency, 628t, 629
Zidovudine (AZT), 664, 665t
dosage, 1445t–1452t
HIV prophylaxis, 71
combination regimens, 644
for infants, 645
lamivudine with, 644, 647
nevirapine with, 647–648
timing, 645

mechanism of action, 664
perinatal HIV transmission prevention, 644
platelet counts after, 656
resistance, 644
Zinc
decreased serum levels in acute-phase response, 94
supplementation, for travelers, 82
Zoo(s), petting, 529, 531
Zoonotic infections
Ancylostoma caninum, 1329–1330
anthrax *see Bacillus anthracis*
Borrelia burgdorferi infections, 952–953
brucellosis *see Brucella*

Cryptosporidium transmission, 1269–1270
emerging diseases, 527
enteric, 393
group childcare setting, 30–31
Leishmania (leishmaniasis), 1286, 1288–1289
Leptospira, 949–950
Listeria monocytogenes, 763
nontraditional pets associated, 527–528
from reptiles, 528
transmission and risk, 528
poxviruses *see* Poxviruses, zoonotic
prevalence, childcare setting, 30–31
Sarcocystis, 1306

Trypanosoma (Schizotrypanum) cruzi infections, 1322
see also Animal(s); Pet(s)
Zoster *see* Varicella zoster virus (VZV), herpes zoster
Zoster sine herpete, 1039
Zygomatic mast cells, 223
Zygomycetes
in iron overload state, 638
meningitis due to, 284t
neonatal skin infections, 550
Zygomycosis *see* Mucormycosis (zygomycosis)
Zygotes, *Plasmodium*, 1298f, 1299